NATIONAL LIBRARY of MEDICINE

# BIBLIOGRAPHY
## OF THE
# HISTORY OF MEDICINE

NUMBER 20

1980-1984

U.S. DEPARTMENT OF HEALTH AND HUMAN SERVICES
Public Health Service
National Institutes of Health

NATIONAL LIBRARY OF MEDICINE
8600 Rockville Pike
Bethesda, Maryland 20894

NIH Publication No. 85-1224

For sale by the Superintendent of Documents, U.S. Government Printing Office
Washington, D.C. 20402

**National Library of Medicine Cataloging in Publication**

ZWZ 40 B582

Bibliography of the history of medicine / National Library of Medicine. -- No. 1 (1965)- . -- Bethesda, Md. : U.S. Dept. of Health, Education, and Welfare, Public Health Service ; Washington, D.C. : For sale by the Supt. of Docs., U.S. G.P.O., 1966-

v.

Annual, each 5th issue being a quinquennial cumulation.

Vols. for 1965-68 issued as Public Health Service publication ; no. 1540; for 1969-77 as DHEW publication ; no. (NIH) 71-297, etc.: for 1978- as NIH publication ; no. 80-315, etc.

ISSN 0067-7280 = Bibliography of the history of medicine.

1. Bibliography of medicine 2. History of Medicine - indexes I. National Library of Medicine (U.S.). II. Series: DHEW publication ; no. (NIH) 71-297, etc. III. Series: NIH publication ; no. 80-315, etc. IV. Series: Public Health Service publication ; no. 1540

# INTRODUCTION

This cumulative volume is the twentieth in a series of bibliographies of the history of medicine. It includes and supersedes the material contained in the last four annual volumes which preceded it. It also incorporates citations to several thousand articles and monographs which have been indexed since Bibliography Number 19 (1983) was published. This volume indexes mainly publications that were issued from 1980 through 1984, but includes in addition scattered citations to literature back to 1964.

The bibliography is prepared from citations added to the file monthly and stored in the National Library of Medicine's computerized data base in the history of medicine, known as HISTLINE. Detailed online searches of this same material, as well as of the entire history data base, may be made from computer terminals at any of over 3,000 medical schools, hospitals, universities, and businesses that have access to NLM's MEDLARS. Further information on making such searches may be obtained from the MEDLARS Management Section, National Library of Medicine, Bethesda, MD 20894.

The *Bibliography of the History of Medicine* focuses on the history of medicine and its related sciences, professions, and institutions. The general history and philosophy of science have been admitted only sparingly. All chronological periods and geographic areas are covered. Journal articles, monographs, and analytical entries for symposia, congresses, and similar composite publications, as well as historical chapters in general monographs, are included.

A substantial proportion of the journal citations in this bibliography have come from the National Library of Medicine's *Index Medicus*. The Library regularly indexes over 2,700 medical and related serials, the titles of which are given in its *List of Journals Indexed in Index Medicus*. The journal title abbreviations are those used in *Index Medicus* or are based upon the same principles. The majority of monographs are from the *Current Catalog*, which lists all monographs and other works received and catalogued in the National Library of Medicine. Further citations have been obtained by regularly reviewing a select group of additional journals in the history of medicine and science and by scanning bibliographies, abstracts, and lists of recent articles from fields such as classics and general history. Persons using the *Bibliography of the History of Medicine* as well as HISTLINE should be aware that most of the citations from these nonmedical periodicals are to journals that are not in the National Library of Medicine collections. The presence of these journals should be verified in SERLINE or in the most recent edition of the *Index of NLM Serial Titles* before they are requested on interlibrary loan.

The bibliography is divided into three main parts: Part I, "Biographies," Part II, "Subjects," and Part III, "Authors." Part I includes citations to works dealing with the medical history of famous nonmedical persons, or with medical aspects of the work of literary figures, composers, artists, etc., as well as those dealing with lives and contributions of physicians, scientists, and others in professions related to health. In Part II, where applicable, the citations under each subject heading are subdivided by chronologic and/or geographic subheadings. The same citation may appear under more than one heading. The subject headings used are based primarily on medical sciences and specialties, diseases, and institutions. In Part III, the citations in Parts I and II are listed alphabetically by author (or by title where there is no author). Cross references are given for co-authors and editors when appropriate.

The Library acknowledges its indebtedness to a number of authors who sent reprints of their publications for inclusion in the bibliography. All authors who wish to insure prompt consideration of articles appearing in journals not indexed in *Index Medicus* are invited to send reprints, including complete citations to the original publications, to the following address:

History of Medicine Division
National Library of Medicine
Bethesda, MD 20894

# CONTENTS

# DISEASES INDEXED IN PART II

Articles dealing with the history of individual diseases (see Contents: Diseases and Injuries) are included in Part II from among the following standard disease terms:

Headache
Hearing Disorders
Heart
Helminthiasis
Hemophilia
Hemorrhage
Hernia
Herpes
Hookworm Infection
Hypersensitivity
Iatrogenic
Infectious
Infectious Mononucleosis
Influenza
Jaundice
Kidney
Laurence-Moon-Biedl Syndrome
Leishmaniasis
Leprosy
Leptospirosis
Leukemia
Liver
Lymphatic
Malaria
Marfan's Syndrome
Measles
Meningitis
Mental Disorders
Mental Retardation

Schistosomiasis
Scrofula
Scurvy
Sex Deviation
Sex Disorders
Shock
Sjogren's Syndrome
Skin
Smallpox
Speech Disorders
Splenic
Spontaneous Combustion
Sweating Sickness
Syphilis
Tetanus
Thymus
Thyroid
Tonsillitis
Toxoplasmosis
Treponemal Infection
Trichinosis
Trypanosomiasis
Tuberculosis
Tularemia
Typhoid
Typhus
Urinary Calculi
Urogenital System
Vascular
Venereal
Vision Disorders
Waterhouse-Friderichsen Syndrome
Whooping Cough
Wound Infection
Wounds and Injuries
Yellow Fever

# PART I. BIOGRAPHIES

## A. COLLECTIVE BIOGRAPHIES

**Abbott D:** The biographical dictionary of scientists: biologists. London and New York, Blond Educational and Bedrick, 1984. 182 p.

**Ackerknecht EH:** From barber-surgeon to modern doctor. **Bull Hist Med** 1984 Winter;58(4):545–53

**Ackerman LV:** H. P. Smith Award lecture. Tumor pathologists I have known. **Am J Clin Pathol** 1982 Apr;77(4):385–90

**Adeloye A:** Nigerian pioneers of modern medicine. Selected writings. Ibadan, Nigeria, Ibadan University Press, 1977. xiv. 299 p.

**Asimov I:** Asimov's biographical encyclopedia of science and technology. The lives and achievements of 1510 great scientists from ancient times to the present chronologically arranged. Second revised edition. Garden City, New York, Doubleday, 1982. xxxv, 941 p.

**Bankhofer H:** Die grossen Naturheiler. Ihr Leben – ihre Lehren. Frankfurt, Ullstein, 1982. 359 p.

**Baumann HU:** Ueber Mehrfachentdeckungen. Eine Darstellung des allgemeinen Problems mit Beispielen aus drei Teilgebieten der theoretischen Medizin. Diss. Münster, 1972. 133 p.

**Birch CA:** Names we remember: 56 eponymous medical biographies. Beckenham, Kent: Ravenswood, 1979. xi, 165 p.

**Breitenecker MT:** [Biographical] Lexikon. In Sournia JC, Martiny M, Poulet J, ed: Illustrierte Geschichte der Medizin. Salzburg, Andreas, 1984. Vol. 9. p. 3201-503.

**Brennan JF:** History and systems of psychology. Englewood Cliffs, Prentice-Hall, 1982. x, 374 p.

**Buess H, Portmann ML:** Berühmte Schweizer Arzte. **Gesnerus** 1980;37(3/4):289–306

**Donáth T:** Nagy anatómusok jubileuma. **Orv Hetil** 1984 Feb 5;125(6):344–6

**Downs RB:** Landmarks in science, Hippocrates to Carson. Littleton, Colo., Libraries Unlimited, 1982. 305 p.

**Eberson F:** Profiles, giants in social medicine. St. Petersburg, Valkyrie Press, 1980. 103 p.

**Eberson F:** Apostles and prophets. Medicine for society's ills. Hicksville, Exposition Press, 1977. xi, 106 p.

**Erickson RP:** Ohrwall, Henning and von Skramlik; the foundations of the four primary positions in taste. **Neurosci Biobehav Rev** 1984 Spring;8(1):105–27

**Falk LA:** Black Abolitionist doctors and healers, 1810–1885. **Bull Hist Med** 1980 Summer;54(2):258–72

**Feldman A, Ford P:** Scientists & inventors. New York, Facts On File, 1979. 336 p.

**Greene EL:** Landmarks of botanical history. Ed., F. N. Egerton, with contributions by R. P. McIntosh and R. McVaugh. 2 vols. Stanford, Stanford University Press, 1983. 1139 p. (Vol. I first published 1909)

**Guerra F:** El medico politico. Estudios biográficos sobre la influencia del médico en la Historia Politica de Hispanoamérica y Filipinas. Madrid, Afrodisio Aguado, 1975. 350 p.

**Howells JG, Osborn ML:** A reference companion to the history of abnormal psychology. Westport, Conn., Greenwood Press, 1984. 2 v. xviii, 1141 p.

**Jasper HH, Sourkes TL:** Nobel laureates in neuroscience: 1904–1981. **Annu Rev Neurosci** 1983;6:1–42

**Jordi González R:** Activitat del col.legi de Farmacèutics de Barcelona durant la Renaixença. **Figueres** 1981 (Separata: Ciència Renaixença Catalana)

**Kean BH, Mott K, Russell AJ:** Tropical medicine and parasitology: classic investigations. 2 v. Ithaca, N. Y., Cornell Univ. Press, 1978. xxiii, 677 p.

**Kemper R:** Zur Syphillis-Erkrankung des Conrad Celtis zum 'Vaticinium' Ulsens und zum sogenannten 'Pestbild' Dürers. **Arch Kulturgesch** 1977;59:99–118

**Killian H:** Meister der Chirurgie und die Chirurgenschulen im gesamten deutschen Sprachraum. 2., neubearbeitete Auflage. Stuttgart, Thieme, 1980. xii, 492 p.

**Kleeberg J, ed:** Eide und Bekenntnisse in der Medizin, eine Anthologie. Basel, München, Karger, 1979. 81 p.

**Kyle RA, Shampo MA:** [Historical aspects of medicine and philately]. **JAMA** 1982 Feb 12;247(6):796 (continued regularly)

**Labuda G, Rodzik I:** Scientists and scholars of Polish origin and Polish men of learning active abroad: their share in the development of science. **Rev Pol Acad Sci (Warsz)** 1980;25(1-2):105–23

**Levin BS:** Women and medicine. Metuchen, N. J., London, Scarecrow, 1980. vii, 257 p.

**Mazzei Uzcátegui M:** Los medicos en la aventura y en la exploracion. **Rev Soc Venez Hist Med** 1972–73;20–21(34–35):161–96

**Murphy RL, Nodyne KR:** The healing science in the Mountain State: some notable medical personalities of West Virginia. **W Va Hist** 1981 Spring–Summer;42(3–4):285–306

**National Institute of General Medical Sciences. Office of Research Reports:** Nobel prize laureates. [Bethesda, Md.], National Institutes of Health, Dept. of Health, Education, and Welfare. [1978]. 24 p.

**Palmer C, Horowitz M, ed:** Shaman woman, mainline lady: women's writings on the drug experience. New York, Morrow, 1982. 285 p.

**Pascal JN:** Bordeu, Bouvart et Rostain: trois médecins face à la tuberculose in 1772 (documents inédits). In J. Proust, ed: Recherches nouvelles sur quelques érivains des lumières (II). Montpellier, Univ. Paul Valéry, 1979. p. 63–71.

**Pelletier PA, ed:** Prominent scientists. An index to collective biographies. New York, Neal-Schuman, 1980. xxviii, 311 p.

**Politzer A:** History of otology. Volume I. From earliest times to the middle of the nineteenth century. An English translation by S. Milstein, C. Portnoff, A. Coleman from the original German edition (Stuttgart, 1907). Phoenix, Columella Press, 1981. xv, 324 p.

**Porter R, ed:** Liber amicorum. Repertorio biografico di storia della medicina e delle scienze naturali. **Kos Liber Amicorum** 1984;1- (continued regularly)

**Postel J, Quétel C, ed:** Nouvelle histoire de la psychiatrie. Toulouse, Privat, 1983. 774 p. Contributions by J. Bancaud, P. Berner, F. Bing.

**Raju TN:** Some famous 'high risk' newborn babies. In Smith GF, Smith PN, Vidyasagar D, ed: Historical review and recent advances in neonatal and perinatal medicine. [Chicago?], Mead Johnson Nutritional Division,

1983. Vol. II. p. 187–9.

**Rosoff L:** Roger Bacon, William of Occam and Lord Houghton: guides for the perplexed physician. **Am J Surg** 1981 Jan;141(1):2–9

**Ryslavy K:** Materialien zur Geschichte der Apotheken und Apotheker im Burgenland. Eisenstadt, Amt der Burgenländischen Landesregierung, Landesarchiv, 1979. 285 p. (Burgenländische Forschungen, Heft/68).

**Sastri R:** Bharata ke pranacarya: Aśivanikumara, Dhanvantari, Susruta, Atreya Punarvasu, Kaśyapa, Kumara Bhartr Jivaka, Caraka, Nagarjuna, Vagbhata sambandhi ayurvedika, aitihasika sahitya evam puratatva ke gambhira adhyayana, Bharatiya sabhyata, aura Samskrti ka gaveshana-purna paricaya. Dilli [Delhi, India], Atmarama, 1976. xvii, 895 p.

**Savodnik I, ed:** The origins of structure in biology. Oceanside, Dabor, 1977. xvi, 154 p.

**Savodnik I, ed:** Concept and explanation in biology. Oceanside, Dabor, 1977. xvii, 240 p.

**Schoenberg DG, Schoenberg BS:** [Eponyms in medical history] **South Med J** 1979 Dec;72(12):1590–1 (continued periodically)

**Schulz-Schaeffer J:** History of cytogenetics. In his: Cytogenetics--plants, animals, humans. New York, Springer, 1980. p. 2–29.

**Shampo MA, Kyle RA:** [Contributions to the history of medical philately]. **JAMA** 1981 Dec 4;246(22):2572 (continued periodically)

**Silló-Seidl G:** Arzte ohne Nobelpreis deren Entdeckungen Millionen Menschen geholfen haben. Genf, Ariston, 1978. 256 p.

**Sladen A:** Landmark perspective: Closed-chest massage, Kouwenhoven, Jude, Knickerbocker. **JAMA** 1984 Jun 15;251(23):3137–40

**Smith SB:** The great mental calculators: the psychology, methods, and lives of calculating prodigies, past and present. New York, Columbia University Press, 1983. xviii, 374 p.

**Smith WD:** Under the influence. A history of nitrous oxide and oxygen anaesthesia. London, Macmillan, 1982. xxviii, 188 p.

**Stafleu FA, Cowan RS:** Taxonomic literature. A selective guide to botanical publications and collections with dates, commentaries and types. Second edition. Utrecht; Bohn, Scheltema and Holkema; The Hague, Junk; Vol. II, 1979, 991 p; Vol. III, 1981, xii, 980 p.

**[The caricature of the teacher]: Indiana Med Hist Q** 1977;3(2):23–37

**Van Buskirk EL:** Fort Wayne College of Medicine. Includes The practice of medicine in the Fort Wayne area written in 1889 by B. S. Woodworth. **Indiana Med Hist Q** 1977;3(2):4–6

**Verheyden CN:** The history of Dupuytren's contracture. In Romm S, ed: Symposium on historical perspectives of plastic surgery. Philadelphia, Saunders, 1983. p. 619–25.

**Walsh J:** New niche for science on reference shelf. **Science** 1981 Jan 16;211(4479):263–4

**Wangensteen OH:** A few renowned European military surgeons. In Ganzinger K, Skopec M, Wyklicky H, ed: Festschrift für Erna Lesky zum 70. Geburtstag. Wien, Brüder Hollinek, 1981. p. 167–84.

**Wells EB:** Scientists' libraries: a handlist of printed sources. **Ann Sci** 1983 Jul;40(4):317–89

**Who was who in American history - science and technology:** (A component of Who's who in American history). Chicago, Marquis, 1976. xiii, 688 p.

**Wiench P, ed:** Die grossen Arzte. Geschichte der Medizin in Lebensbildern. München, Kindler, 1982. 335 p.

**Williams TI, Withers S, ed:** A biographical dictionary of scientists. 3rd ed. London, A. & C. Black, 1982. xiv, 674 p.

**Williams TI, ed, Withers S, ed:** A biographical dictionary of scientists. New York, Wiley, [1974]. 641 p.

**Argentina**

**Semorile A:** Quienes ejercieron la medicina hasta el año 1.800. In Congreso de Historia de la Medicina Argentina [Transactions], 5th, Mendoza, 1983. p. 141–4.

**Austria**

**Hochenegg H:** Tiroler Aerzte und Pharmazeuten als Künstler und Schriftsteller, Forscher und Volksvertreter. **Tirol Heimat** 1976;40:135–62

**Leitner H:** Die jüdischen Arzte in Osterreich und ihr Beitrag zur medizinischen Wissenschaft. In K. Lohrmann, ed: 1000 Jahre Osterreichisches Judentum. Ausstellungskatalog. Eisenstadt, 1982. p. 161–92.

**Denmark**

**Brix J:** Laegevirke i Sønderjylland før 1864. **Dan Medicinhist Arbog** 1980;:9–10

**Laeger i Sønderjylland indtil 1864: Dan Medicinhist Arbog** 1980;:11–65

**France**

**Dillemann G:** Les illustres pharmaciens dont les noms ont été donnés aux amphithéatres de la Faculté de Pharmacie de Paris. **Bull Ordre Natl Pharm** 1979 Apr;221:517–41

**Dulieu L:** La pharmacie à Montpellier de ses origines à nos jours. [Marseilles], Presses Universelles, 1973. 343 p.

**Germany**

**Benedum J, Giese C:** Die Professoren der Medizin in der giessener Gemäldegalerie. Giessen, Schmitz, 1983. 230 p. (Arbeiten zur Geschichte der Medizin in Giessen, Bd. 5)

**Hein WH, Schwarz HD, ed:** Deutsche Apotheker-Biographie. Band II, M–Z. Stuttgart, Wissenschaftliche Verlagsgesellschaft, 1978. p. 393–788. (Veröffentlichungen der Internationalen Gesellschaft für Geschichte der Pharmazie, Neue Folge, Band 46).

**Kohlhauer CE:** Mediziner und Naturwissenschaftler im Fürstentum Ansbach. [Ansbach, s. n., 1964]. 30 p.

**Sommer R:** Zur Geschichte des Medizinal- und Apothekenwesens in einem kleinen souveränen Staat (Schaumburg-Lippe). Diss. Braunschweig, 1979. vi, 295 p. (Veröffentlichungen aus dem Pharmaziegeschichtlichen Seminar der Technischen Universität Braunschweig, 19).

**Great Britain**

**David GR, ed:** The manuscript papers of British scientists, 1600–1940. London, H.M.S.O., 1982. 109 p.

**Whittet TD, White PM:** Some midland apothecaries. **Pharm Hist (London)** 1978 Jul;8(2):6–8

**Hungary**

**Duka Zólyomi N:** Die Leopoldinische Akademie und die ungarländische Medizin und Naturwissenschaft bis zum Ende des 18. Jahrhunderts. **Acta Hist Leopoldina** 1980;13:51–101

**Mester AF:** Six great men in Hungarian otorhinolaryngology. **Am J Otolaryngol** 1982 Jan–Feb;3(1):67–72

**Süle T:** Az Erzsébet Tudományegyetem Orvosi Kara, az önálló Pécsi Orvostudományi Egyetem rövid története és numizmatikai emlékei. **Orvostort Kozl** 1982;28(1–3):227–39

**Zsebök Z:** Famous Hungarian doctors. **New Hung Q** 1982;23(85):131–4

**Netherlands**

**Bosman-Jelgersma HA:** Vijf eeuwen delftse apothekers, een bronnenstudie over de geschiedenis van de farmacie in een hollandse stad. Amsterdam, Ronald Meesters, 1979. xx, 446 p. (Thesis, Amsterdam).

**Hes HS:** Jewish physicians in the Netherlands 1600–1940. Assen, Van Gorcum, 1980. xxi, 206 p.

**Scandinavia**

**Kay E, ed:** Dictionary of Scandinavian biography. Second edition. Cambridge, International Biographical Centre, 1976. xxviii, 497 p.

**Spain**

**Zubiri Vidal F:** Médicos aragoneses ilustres. Zaragoza, Diputación Provincial, Institución 'Fernando El Católico', [1983]. 395 p.

**Sweden**

**Clemedson CJ:** Berömda svenska böcker inom medicin och farmaci. **Nord Medicinhist Arsb** 1980;Suppl 6:35–51

**Strandell B:** Svenska medicinska medaljer. **Nord Medicinhist Arsb** 1980;Supp 6:52–6

**Switzerland**

**Balmer H:** Walliser Naturforscher. **Gesnerus** 1979;36(1/2):35–49

**United States**

**Eberson F:** Early physicians of the West. Forerunners of modern medicine. St. Petersburg, Valkyrie Press, 1979. ix, 140 p.

**Lender ME:** Dictionary of American temperance biography: from temperance reform to alcohol research, the 1600s to the 1980s. Westport, Conn., Greenwood Press, 1984. xiv, 572 p.

**Thomas KB:** Some early Welsh contributors to American medicine: the family of Jones. In J. Cule, ed: Wales and medicine. London, British Society for the History of Medicine, 1975. p. 10–22.

### Before 500 A.D.

**Greece**

**Byl S:** Note sur huit recentiores du livre IV Du régime. **Rev Philol (Paris)** 1978;52:37–49

### 500 A.D.–1450

**France**

**Jacquart D:** Le milieu médical en France du XIIe au XVe siècle: en annexe 2e supplément au 'Dictionnaire' d'Ernest Wickersheimer. Genève, Droz; Paris, Champion, 1981. 487 p. (Centre de recherches d'histoire et de philologie de la IVe section de l'Ecole pratique des hautes études. V, Hautes études médiévales et modernes ; 46)

**Keil G:** Randnotizen zu Danielle Jacquarts Wickersheimer-Supplements. **Sudhoffs Arch** 1982;66(2):172–86

### 1450–1700

**Bosch K:** Zur Vorgeschichte chemiatrischer Pharmakopöepräparate im 16./17. Jahrhundert. Braunschweig, 1980. 223 p. (Veröffentlichungen aus dem Pharmaziegeschichtlichen Seminar der Technischen Universität Braunschweig, 21).

**Yates FA:** The occult philosophy in the Elizabethan age. London, Boston, Routledge & Kegan Paul, 1979. x, 217 p.

**France**

**Dulieu L:** La médecine à Montpellier. Tome II. La Renaissance. Avignon, Presses Universelles, 1979. 481 p.

**Great Britain**

**Kealey EJ:** Medieval medicus. A social history of Anglo-Norman medicine. Baltimore, Johns Hopkins University Press, 1981. x, 211 p.

**Mexico**

**Somolinos d'Ardois G:** Relacion alfabetica de los profesionistas medicos, o en conexion con la medicina, que practicaron en territorio mexicano (1521–1618). México, Sociedad Mexicana de Historia y Filosofía de la Medicina, [1979?]. (Capitulos de historia medica mexicana, III). p. 175–312.

### 1700 to Present

**American Academy of Arts and Sciences, American Philosophical Society:** Survey of sources for the history of biochemistry and molecular biology. **Surv Sources Newsl** 1975–1981;1(1–10):various pagings

**Camp J:** One hundred years of medical murder. London, Bodley Head, 1982. 221 p.

**Carlson PA:** Three contributors to cardiac catheterization. **J Thorac Cardiovasc Surg** 1980 May;79(5):782–8

**Franken FH:** Krankheit und Tod grosser Komponisten. Baden-Baden, New York, Witzstrock, 1979. 280 p.

**Garnham PC:** Some contributions of Scotland to tropical medicine. In Passmore R, ed: Proceedings of the Royal College of Physicians of Edinburgh Tercentenary Congress, 1981. Edinburgh, Royal College of Physicians of Edinburgh, 1982. p. 128–42.

**Hoffman W, Shields J:** Doctors on the new frontier: breaking through the barriers of modern medicine. New York, Macmillan, 1981. xi, 207 p.

**Huard P, Grmek MD:** Coup d'oeil sur les élèves étrangers de Laennec. In: Congrès National des Sociétés Savantes, 97e, Nantes, 1972. Comptes Rendus. Paris, 1976. Section des Sciences, Tome 1. p. 21–35.

**Keel O:** Les conditions de la décomposition 'analytique' de l'organisme: Haller, Hunter, Bichat. **Etud Philos** 1982;:37–62

**Krause RM:** The restless tide. The persistent challenge of the microbial world. Washington, D. C., National Foundation for Infectious Diseases, 1981. 152 p.

**Magner LN:** Women and the scientific idiom: textual episodes from Wollstonecraft, Fuller, Gilman, and Firestone. **Signs** 1978;4(1):61–80

**Mayr E, Provine WB, ed:** The evolutionary synthesis: perspectives on the unification of biology. Cambridge, Mass., and London, England, Harvard University Press, 1980. xi, 487 p. Contributions by M. B. Adams, G. E. Allen, E. Boesiger, R. W. Burkhardt, H. L. Carson, F. B. Churchill, W. Coleman, C. D. Darlington, T. Dobzhansky, E. B. Ford, M. T. Ghiselin, S. J. Gould, V. Hamburger, R. C. Lewontin, C. Limoges, B. Rensch, D. Shapere, G. L. Stebbins, A. Weinstein.

**Nobel lectures in molecular biology, 1933–1975:** New York, Elsevier, 1977. ix, 534 p.

**O'Connell AN, Russo NF, ed:** Models of achievement. Reflections of eminent women in psychology. New York, Columbia University Press, 1983. xiii, 338 p.

**O'Donnell S:** Irish-American scientists. **Eire Irel** 1979;14(2):106–9

**Rattner J, ed:** Wandlungen der Psychoanalyse. Wien, Europaverlag, 1980. 373 p.

**Sapira JD:** Quincke, de Musset, Duroziez, and Hill: some aortic regurgitations. **South Med J** 1981 Apr;74(4):459–67

**Stolorow RD, Atwood GE:** Faces in a cloud: subjectivity in personality theory. New York, Aronson, 1979. 217 p.

**Willier BH, Oppenheimer JM, ed:** Foundations of experimental embryology. 2nd ed., enlarged and with a new introduction, by J. M. Oppenheimer. New York, Hafner, 1974. xx, 277 p. Selections from various authors.

**Americas**

**Plaza Izquierdo F:** Medicos presidentes de America. **Rev Soc Venez Hist Med** 1976;24(38):19–36

**Argentina**

**Martín de Codoni EL:** Apuntes para un estudio de los pioneros de la medicina en Mendoza en el siglo XIX. In Congreso de Historia de la Medicina Argentina [Transactions], 5th, Mendoza, 1983. p. 145–82.

**Pennini de Vega E, Landáburu AJ, Kohn Loncarica AG, et al:** La inmigración médica española en la Argentina. In International Congress of the History of Medicine, 27th, Barcelona, 1980. Actas. Barcelona, Académia de Ciències Mèdiques de Catalunya i Balears, 1981. p. 188–94.

**Australia**

**Leggett CA:** The founders of the College. **Aust NZ J Surg** 1981 Oct;51(5):508–12

**Wilson G:** The pioneering anaesthetists of Australia. **Anaesth Intensive Care** 1979 Nov;7(4):311–21

**Austria**

**Lesky E:** American medicine as viewed by Viennese physicians, 1893–1912. **Bull Hist Med** 1982 Fall;56(3):368–76

**Mitterstiller S:** 100 Jahre Chirurgische Klinik in Innsbruck. **Tirol Heimat** 1970;34:17–38

**Rüden AD von:** Medicina Graecensis. Das medizinisch-chirurgische Studium in Graz (1782–1862). Diss. Technischen Universität München, 1978. 195 p.

**Canada**

**Bonenfant JL:** La pathologie à l'âge des incertitudes. **Union Med Can** 1984 May;113(5):352–4

**Chile**

**Neghme A:** La obra literaria de los médicos chilenos. **Rev Med Chil** 1981 Jun;109(6):557–64; Jul;109(7):683–91

**Neghme A:** Obra literaria de los médicos chilenos. (III, IV). **Rev Med Chil** 1981 Aug-Sep;109(8,9):789–93, 895–900 (continued periodically)

**China**

**Chan H:** [A description of demographic cognition during the Ch'ing Dynasty] (Chi). **Ssu yu Yen** 1973;10(6):425–31

**Czechoslovakia**

**Slavětínský M:** Naši lékaři-archeologové. **Vnitr Lek** 1980 Mar;26(3):415-6

**Denmark**

**Marvitz L, Rasmussen EG:** Tandlaegeskaebner fra perioden 1790-1850. **Dan Medicinhist Arbog** 1983;12:23-36

**France**

**Didier C:** Aperçu sur les médecins et chirurgiens à Colmar au XVIIIe siècle. In Livet G, Schaff G, ed: Médecine et assistance en Alsace, XVIe-XXe siècle. Strasbourg, Istra, 1976. p. 87-111.

**Dillemann G:** Les cumuls d'emplois en 1821. **Rev Hist Pharm (Paris)** 1981 Jun;28(249):109-11

**Fabre A, ed:** Histoire de la médecine aux armées. Tome 2. De la Révolution française au conflit mondial de 1914. Paris, Charles-Lavazelle, 1984. 491 p.

**Fischer JL, Smith J:** French embryology and the 'Mechanics of development' from 1887 to 1910: L. Chabry, Y. Delage & E. Bataillon. **Hist Philos Life Sci** 1984;6(1):25-39

**Paul CB:** Science and immortality. The eloges of the Paris Academy of Sciences (1699-1791). Berkeley, University of California Press, 1980. x, 202 p.

**Germany**

**Abe HR:** Zum Leben und Werk bedeutender Thüringischer Apotheker. **Pharmazie** 1981 Jun;36(6):435-7

**Bach H:** Die Entwicklung der künstlichen Niere aus Hydrodiffusion und Hämodialyse, von J. A. Nollet bis G. Haas. Der Ursprung des ersten Künstlichen inneren Organs. Giessen, Schmitz, 1983. 334 p. (Arbeiten zur Geschichte der Medizin in Giessen, Bd. 7)

**Balde JH:** Dreizehn biographische Skizzen. In Balde JH, Schmiking W, ed: Festschrift zum 86. Deutschen Arztetag in Kassel. Kassel, Arztevereins, 1983. p. 51-86.

**Blodi FC:** Ophthalmology and philately. **Arch Ophthalmol** 1982 Mar;100(3):425,44 (continuing periodically)

**Goerke H, ed:** Berliner Aerzte. 2d ed. Berlin, Berlin Verlag, 1984. 328 p.

**Hinze E:** Feldscherer und Feldmedici in deutschen wie fremden Heeren und Flotten. (Biographisches Lexikon deutscher Militärärzte bis 1870) Band I. Hannover, Im Selbstverlag, 1979. 43 p.

**Hoppe B:** Adolf Windaus, Heinrich Wieland, Richard Kuhn, Leopold Ružička, Alexander Todd und Adolf Bunenandt. Die Erforschung der Vitamine und der Hormone. In: Die Grossen der Weltgeschichte. Zürich, Kindler, 1978. p. 336-81.

**Klaschka F, Rauhut K, ed:** 100 Jahre Dermatologie in Berlin. Beiträge und Aufzeichnungen anlässlich der Festsitzung der Berliner Dermatologischen Gesellschaft am 12. und 13 Februar 1982. Berlin, Grosse Verlag, 1984. 152 p.

**Meinel C:** Die Chemie an der Universität Marburg seit Beginn des 19. Jahrhunderts. Ein Beitrag zu ihrer Entwicklung als Hochschulfach. Marburg, Elwert, 1978. xvi, 669 p. (Academia Marburgensis. Herausgegeben von der Philipps-Universität Marburg, Band 3).

**Müller-Jahncke WD:** Weitere Apothekerbildnisse auf Medaillen und Plaketten des deutschsprachigen Raums. **Beitr Gesch Pharm** 1984;31(24):205-9

**Prentner H:** Geschichte der Urologie in Würzburg. Diss. Würzburg, 1981. 68 p.

**Winau R, Vaubel E:** Chirurgen in Berlin. 100 Porträts. Berlin, New York, Walter de Gruyter, 1983. 106 p.

**Great Britain**

**Abse D, ed:** My medical school. London, Robson, 1978. 211 p.

**Fozzard JA:** Professors of anatomy in the University of Cambridge: the first two hundred and sixty-one years of the Cambridge University Department of Anatomy, 1707-1968. Cambridge, FOSSLIA, 1983. 87 p.

**Kingsley Brown A:** 'Mony a mickle...' **Trans Hunter Soc** 1978-80;37-38:7-33

**McGuckin A:** Nineteenth-century pharmacists of Newcastle. **Pharm Hist (London)** 1971 Jul;2(2):4-6

**Peel J:** The lives of the fellows of the Royal College of Obstetricians and Gynaecologists, 1929-1969. London, Heinemann, 1976. xviii, 390 p.

**Posner E:** Josiah Wedgwood's doctors. **Pharm Hist (London)** 1973 Sep;3(2):2-5

**Ross JP, LeFanu WR, ed:** Lives of the Fellows of the Royal College of Surgeons of England 1965-1973. London, Pitman Medical, 1981. 405 p.

**Scott-Moncrieff R:** The classical period in chemical genetics; recollections of Muriel Wheldale Onslow, Robert and Gertrude Robinson and J. B. S. Haldane. **Notes Rec R Soc Lond** 1981;36(1):125-54

**Shellard EJ:** Some early women research workers in British pharmacy 1886-1912. **Pharm Hist (London)** 1982 Aug;12(2):2-3

**Hungary**

**Huszár G:** Az önéletrajzok, mint fogorvostörténelmünk forrásai. **Orvostort Kozl** 1980;89-91(26 no 1-3):157-74

**India**

**Husain SA:** Physicians of Hyderabad during Nizam II & III. **Bull Indian Inst Hist Med (Hyderabad)** 1980;10(1-4):40-7

**Israel**

**Margalith D:** Physicians, forerunners of modern Israel. Tel-Aviv, Jerusalem Academy of Medicine, 1973. 192, iv, 12 p.

**Italy**

**Pini UA:** Medici e chirurghi parmigiani dell'ottocento. Notizie sulla vita e sulle opere. III. **Minerva Med** 1980 Sep 1;71(31):2245-7 (continued periodically)

**Pini UA:** Medici e chirurghi parmigiani dell'ottocento. Notizie sulla vita e sulle opere. **Minerva Med** 1980 May 12;71(19-20):1393-8, 1461-6

**Japan**

**Lifton RJ, Kato S, Reich MR:** Six lives, six deaths. Portraits from modern Japan. New Haven and London, Yale University Press, 1979. xiii, 305 p.

**Poland**

**Gaertner H:** Ordynatorzy oddziału chirurgicznego Krakowskiego Szpitala Braci Miłosiernych (obecnie im. Edmunda Biernackiego). **Nasza Przeslosc** 1979;(51):179-204

**Skład osobowy władz Polskiego Towarzystwa Historii Medycyny i Farmacji: Arch Hist Med (Warsz)** 1984;47(2):269-85

**Romania**

**Costea V:** Cîteva date din activitatea primilor trei profesori titulari ai clinicii dermato-venerologice: Gh. Demetriade, E. I. Mironescu şi Gh. Nastase (1901-1962). **Rev Med Chir Soc Med Nat Iasi** 1983 Jan-Mar;87(1):149-55

**Spain**

**d'Ors A:** Cuatro precursores de la ciencia española de nuestro tiempo. **Rev Med Univ Navarra** 1980 Dec;24(4):55-60

**Garcia Gonzalez R, Prieto Cantero A:** Licenciados en medicina y cirugia graduados en la Universidad de Valladolid (1871-1936). Vallodolid, Universidad de Valladolid, 1979. 383 p. (Acta Historico-Medica Vallisoletana, Monografias, IX)

**Matilla V:** Cuatro secretarios perpetuos ejemplares de la Real Academia Nacional de Medicina. **An R Acad Nac Med (Madr)** 1981;98(1):31-68

**Switzerland**

**Heller S:** Boerhaaves Schweizer Studenten: ein Beitrag zur Geschichte des Medizinstudiums. Zürich, Juris, 1984. 111 p. (Zürcher Medizingeschichtliche Abhandlungen, Neue Reihe, Nr. 169)

**United States**

**Bowers JZ:** Alpha Omega Alpha program of audiovisual memoirs of leaders in American medicine. **Bull Hist Med** 1973 Jul-Aug;47(4):409-16

**Browne HS:** Newport's revolutionary physicians. **Newport Hist** 1981;54(1):4-34

**Butterworth VE:** The girls in white. Independence, Mo., Herald Publishing House, 1979. 176 p.

**Cobb WM:** The Black American in medicine. **J Natl Med Assoc** 1981

Dec;73 Suppl:1185–244

**Dexter RW:** The impact of evolutionary theories on the Salem group of Agassiz zoologists (Morse, Hyatt, Packard, Putnam). **Essex Inst Hist Collect** 1979;115(3):144–71

**Edgar II:** A history of early Jewish physicians in the State of Michigan. New York, Philosophical Library, 1982. 249 p.

**Elliott CA:** Models of the American scientist: a look at collective biography. **Isis** 1982 Mar;73(266):77–93

**Gault EW, Attwood HD:** Medical men in the early history of the Austin Hospital. Five doctors of widely varying ages and backgrounds were associated with the formative years of the Austin Hospital. **Med J Aust** 1981 Dec 12–26;2(12–13):680–3

**Harvey AM:** Research and discovery in medicine. Contributions from Johns Hopkins. Baltimore and London, Johns Hopkins University Press, 1981. xiii, 322 p. [Collected historical papers reprinted from various journals].

**Hess AJ:** History of medicine in Harrison County, West Virginia. Clarksburg, Harrison County Medical Society, 1978. xxiii, 662 p.

**Holloway L:** Medical obituaries: American physicians, biographical notices in selected medical journals before 1907. New York, Garland, 1982. xiv, 513 p.

**Morantz RM, Pomerleau CS, Fenichel CH, ed:** In her own words: oral histories of women physicians. Westport, Conn., Greenwood, 1982. xiv, 284 p. (Contributions in Medical History, 8).

**Nevins MA:** Bergen County's poet-physicians. **J Med Soc NJ** 1980 Nov;77(12):831–3

**Noble I:** Contemporary women scientists in America. New York, Messner, 1979. 158 p.

**Ono J:** Legacies of Jefferson men to Japanese medicine. **Ann Otol Rhinol Laryngol [Suppl]** 1981 Sep–Oct;90(5 pt 2 Suppl 87):1–10

**Poirier S:** The physician and authority: portraits by four physician-writers. In Jones AH, ed: Images of healers. Albany, State University of New York Press, 1983. p. 21–40.

**The presidents: J Am Dent Assoc** 1979 Oct;99(4):601 (continued periodically)

**Profile:** four academic pioneers who stayed to help the Health Center grow. **J Fla Med Assoc** 1980 Mar;67(3):298–301

**Ryan TA:** Psychology at Cornell after Titchener: Madison Bentley to Robert Macleod, 1928–1948. **J Hist Behav Sci** 1982 Oct;18(4):347–69

**Scannell JG:** Some thoracic surgeons of Boston--before the cardiac balloon went up. **Pharos** 1984 Fall;47(4):26–30

**Stern MB, comp:** A phrenological dictionary of nineteenth-century Americans. Westport, Conn., Greenwood Press, 1982. xx, 430 p.

**Stumpf DA:** The founding of pediatric neurology in America. **Bull NY Acad Med** 1981 Nov;57(9):804–16

**Wilson JL:** American Thoracic Society--five great teachers in the field of tuberculosis. **Am Rev Respir Dis** 1981 May;123(5):571–5

**Wilson LG, ed:** Benjamin Silliman and his circle: Studies on the influence of Benjamin Silliman on science in America. Prepared in honor of Elizabeth H. Thomson. New York, Science History Publications, 1979. x, 227 p. Contributions by S. D Beckham, J. C. Greene, L. I. Kuslan, G. Robinson, M. W. Rossiter.

### USSR

**Beliaev DK:** Vydaiushchiesia sovetskie genetiki: sbornik biograficheskikh ocherkov. Moskva, Nauka, 1980. 147 p.

**Müller-Dietz HE:** Aerzte im Russland des achtzehnten Jahrhunderts. Esslingen/Neckar, Robugen, 1973. 111 p.

### Venezuela

**Salfelder K, Novoa Montero D:** Patologos alemanes en Venezuela 1936–1981. Merida, Universidad de los Andes, 1982. 131 p.

**Vélez Boza F:** Historia de la microscopia en Venezuela. **Rev Soc Venez Hist Med** 1981;30(45–46):125–97

# B. INDIVIDUAL BIOGRAPHIES

## A

**Aaskow, Urban Bruun, 1742-1806**
Winge M: Urban Bruun Aaskow. **Dan Medicinhist Arbog** 1981;:94-127

**Abakeliia, Iosif Konstantinovich, 1883-1938?**
Batiashvili OG: I. K. Abakeliia--osnovopolozhnik ftiziatrii i organizator bor'by s tuberkulezom v Gruzii (k 100-letiiu dnia rozhdeniia). **Probl Tuberk** 1983 Jul;(7):73-4

**Abbe, Robert, d. 1928**
Frileck SP: More on Robert Abbe's contributions to the field of plastic surgery. **Ann Plast Surg** 1979 Oct;3(4):357-60

**Abbott, Albert Clifford, 1897-**
Beamish RE: Dr. Albert Clifford Abbott: a pioneer surgeon of western Canada. **Can Med Assoc J** 1983 Apr 1;128(7):862-4

**Abbott, Anderson Ruffin, 1837-1913**
Robinson HS: Anderson Ruffin Abbott, MD, 1837-1913. **J Natl Med Assoc** 1980 Jul;72(7):713-6

**Abbott, Edward Gilbert, 1825-1855**
Vandam LD, Abbott JA: Edward Gilbert Abbott: enigmatic figure of the ether demonstration. **N Engl J Med** 1984 Oct 11;311(15):991-4

**Abbott, Maude Elizabeth Seymour, 1869-1940**
Smith K: Maude Abbott: pathologist and historian. **Can Med Assoc J** 1982 Oct 15;127(8):774-6
Wiglesworth FW: Maude E. Abbott. **Perspect Pediatr Pathol** 1984 Winter;8(4):291-4

**Abd Al-Malik Ibn Habib al-Sulami al Ilbiri, ca. 790-854**
Alvarez de Morales C, Irueste FG: Medicina creencial y medicina racional en la España arabe del siglo IX: el Mujtasar Fi L-tibb (compendio de medicina) de 'Abd al-Malik Ibn Habib al-Ilbiri (c. 790-854). **Asclepio** 1982;34:283-94

**Abderhalden, Emil, 1877-1950**
Sackmann W: Der Arzt und Biochemiker Emil Abderhalden (1877-1950) und seine Beziehungen zur Tiermedizin. **Schweiz Arch Tierheilkd** 1982 Jan;124(1):1-10
Schmidt V: Emil Abderhalden. Laege, professor, Geheimrat, kolonihavemand, afholdsmand -- og glemt! **Dan Medicinhist Arbog** 1979;116-29

**Abel, John Jacob, 1857-1938**
Becker RA: The John Jacob Abel papers--primary sources for the history of American pharmacology. **Pharm Hist** 1982;24(3):115-6
Parascandola J: John J. Abel and the early development of pharmacology at the Johns Hopkins University. **Bull Hist Med** 1982;56(4):512-27
Parascandola J: John J. Abel and the founding of ASPET. **Pharmacologist** 1984;26(1):37-40

**Abonyi, Jozsef**
Huszár G: Abonyi József, a hazai protetika úttörője. **Fogorv Sz** 1980 Jun;73(6):187-91

**Abrahám, Ambrus, 1893-**
Csillik B: Prof. Dr. Ambrus Abrahám. **Acta Biol Acad Sci Hung** 1983;34(2-3):131-5

**Abraham, Karl, 1877-1925**
Rattner J: Karl Abraham. In J. Rattner, ed: Wandlungen der Psychoanalyse. Wien, Europaverlag, 1980. p. 9-29.

**Abrahams, Adolphe, 1884-**
Hansell P: A backward glance -- 2. **J Audiov Media Med** 1979 Jul;2(3):107-11

**Abrams, Albert, 1863-1924**
Pollack CV: Electronic therapeutics of Albert Abrams, M.D. **Pharm Hist** 1984;26(2):109-13

**Abu Mansur al-Hasan b. Nuh al-Qumri, 10th cent.**
Karmi Ghada: Arabic medicine in the 10th century---a study based on the book Ghina wa Muna by Abu Mansur al-Hasan b. Nuh al-Qumri. In: International Symposium for the History of Arabic Science, 1st, University of Aleppo, 1976. Proceedings. Aleppo, Syria, 1976. Papers in European Languages, Vol. II. p. 326-35.

**Abu Muhammad 'Ali ibn Hazm, 994-1063**
Linage Conde A: Ibn Hazm de Cordoba y la neurosis. **Asclepio** 1981;33:349-77

**Abulcasis, 936?-1013?**
Buniiatov ZM, Kagramanov KM: O 30-m traktate Abu-l-kasima Khalafa Ibn Abbasa Az-Zakhravi. **Vestn Akad Med Nauk SSSR** 1980;9:75-8
Drinnan AJ: Odontophilately (Abul Kasim). **NY State Dent J** 1979 Aug-Sep;45(7):332
Hamarneh SK, Hamarneh NT: The physician-surgeon al-Zahrawi and the natural origins and manufacture of drugs. In A. R. El-Gindy, ed: Proceedings of the Second International Conference on Islamic Medicine. No. IV. Kuwait, Islamic Medicine Organization, 1982. (Bulletin of Islamic Medicine, v. 2). p. 375-82, 401-406.
Nabri IA: El Zahrawi (936-1013 AD), the father of operative surgery. **Ann R Coll Surg Engl** 1983 Mar;65(2):132-4
Wijesinha SS: El Zahrawi (936-1013 AD), the father of operative surgery. **Ann R Coll Surg Engl** 1983 Nov;65(6):423

**Aburel, Eugen Bogdan, 1899-1975**
Curelaru I, Sandu L: Eugen Bogdan Aburel (1899-1975). The pioneer of regional analgesia for pain relief in childbirth. **Anaesthesia** 1982 Jun;37(6):663-9

**Acarí, Santiago de Parcos de, fl. 1593**
Visita de Acarí (1593): **Hist Cult (Peru)** 1973;7:129-209

**Achard, François, d. 1853**
Aurel D: De l'histoire des relations médicales franco-roumaines -- au 120e anniversaire de la mort de François Achard -- l'activité de François Achard en Roumanie. **Soc Fr Hist Art Dent** 1979 Sep-Dec;(5-6):30-3

**Acheson, James Alexander, 1892-1968**
Lowenthal MN: The yaws notebook of Dr. Acheson. **Trans R Soc Trop Med Hyg** 1982;76(5):627-9

**Achillini, Alessandro, 1463-1512**
Matsen HS: Giovanni Garzoni (1419-1505) to Alessandro Achillini (1463-1512): An unpublished letter and defense. In Edward P Mahoney, ed. Philosophy and humanism: Renaissance essays in honor of Paul Oskar Kristeller. New York: Columbia Univ. Press, 1976. p. 518-530.

**Achúcarro, Nicolás, 1880-1918**
Bustamante M: Nicolás Achúcarro: el hombre y su obra. **Arch Neurobiol (Madr)** 1982 Jan-Feb;45(1):55-72

**Acosta, Cristavão, ca. 1525-1594**
Falcao RF: A proposito do quarto centenario de publicão do 'Tratado de las drogas' de Cristóvão da Costa. **Rev Port Farm** 1980;30:234-44

**Acosta, José, 1539-1600**
Gilbert DL: The first documented description of mountain sickness: the Andean or Pariacaca story. **Respir Physiol** 1983 Jun;52(3):327-47

**Acrel, Olof af, 1717-1806**
Ljunggren B: Reflexioner kring en hjärnsvulst hos 'En förnäm herre af 30 år'. **Sydsven Medicinhist Sallsk Arsskr** 1983;:87-102

**Adamkiewicz, Albert Wojciech, 1850-1921**
Sokołowska-Pituchowa J: Two monographs on the spinal cord vascularization. **Folia Morphol (Warsz)** 1980;39(1):1-8

**Adams Family**
Musto DF: Continuity across generations: the Adams Family myth.

In M. Albin, R. J. Devlin, G. Heeger, ed: New directions in psychohistory. The Adelphi papers in honor of Erik H. Erikson. Lexington, Toronto, D. C. Heath, 1980. p. 117–29.

**Adams, Scott, 1909–1982**
Scott Adams: A continuing force in the age of discontinuity: **Bull Am Soc Inf Sci** 1982 Dec;9(2):16–8

**Addams, Jane, 1860–1935**
Agris J: 'Jane Addams'. Medical student, social worker and activist, humanitarian. **J Dermatol Surg Oncol** 1979 Dec;5(12):936
Cavallo D: Sexual politics and social reform: Jane Addams, from childhood to Hull House. In: Albin, Mel, ed. New Directions in Psychohistory: The Adelphi Papers in Honor of Erik H. Erikson. Lexingon, Mass., Health, 1980: 161–82.
Greenstone JD: Dorothea Dix and Jane Addams: from transcendentalism to pragmatism in American social reform. **Soc Serv Rev** 1979;53(4):527–59

**Addenbrooke, John, 1680–1719**
Rook A, Martin L: John Addenbrooke M.D. (1680–1719). **Med Hist** 1982 Apr;26(2):169–78

**Addison, Christopher, 1869–1951**
Morgan KO: Dr. Christopher Addison and social reform. **Soc Soc Hist Med Bull (Lond)** 1981 Dec;29:21–5

**Addison, Thomas, 1795–1860**
Stoffregen MH: Thomas Addison (1793–1860), zum 120. Todestag. **Med Welt** 1981;21:3–4
White IR, MacDonald DM: Thomas Addison, M.D. First dermatologist at Guy's Hospital. **J Am Acad Dermatol** 1982 Mar;6(3):426–30

**Adelphus, Johannes, fl. 1500–1523**
Johannes Adelphus: Ausgewählte Schriften. 3. Band. Das Buch des Lebens. Ed. A. R. Arthur, B. Gotzkowsky. Berlin, New York, De Gruyter, 1980. 413 p.

**Adil Mustafa (Adil-Bey), 1871–1904**
Erk N: Adil Mustafa (Adil-Bey), a pioneer veterinary bacteriologist in Turkey. **Hist Med Vet** 1977;2(4):99–101

**Adler, Alfred, 1870–1937**
Ansbacher HL: Discussion of Alfred Alder's preface to The Diary of Vaslav Nijinsky. **Arch Gen Psychiatry** 1981 Jul;38(7):834–41
Ansbacher HL: 'To love and to work'. Adlerian thoughts on an anecdote about Freud. **Bull Menninger Clin** 1981 Sep;45(5):439–41
Beckh-Widmannstetter HA: Zur Geschichte der Individualpsychologie: Julius Wagner-Jauregg über Alfred Adler. **Unsere Heimat** 1965;36(10–12):182–8
Pinkham JR: The dentist and child-patient encounter: an Adlerian analysis. **ASDC J Dent Child** 1982 Jul–Aug;49(4):266–72
Rattner J: Alfred Adler. New York, Frederick Ungar, 1983. 226 p.
Rodríguez A: Samuel Ramos: influencia de Adler y Jung en su estudio sobre el carácter del Mexicano. **Cuad Hispanoam** 1977;109(326–327):420–30
Schachter M: Alfred Adler (1870–1937), et sa psycho-pédagogie clinique. **Rev Hist Med Heb** 1981 Dec;139(34 no 4):53–6

**Adler, Cyril, 1903–**
Melzer R, Kahn A, Kriel J, ed: Festschrift in honour of Dr. Cyril Adler on the occasion of his 80th birthday.

**Adler, Kurt A., 1905–**
Adler KA: A personal autobiography. **J Individ Psychol** 1981 Nov;37(2):196–204

**Adlung, Alfred, 1875–**
Wankmüller A: Entstehung des 'Grundriss der Geschichte der deutschen Pharmazie' von Adlung und Urdang. **Pharm Ztg** 1980;125:403–6

**Adrian, Edgar Douglas, 1889–1977**
Moruzzi G: In memoriam Lord Adrian (1889–1977). **Rev Physiol Biochem Pharmacol** 1980;87:1–24

**Adrianov, Nikolai Konstantinovich, 1869–1931**
Alekseev GA, Sergeev TS, Galkina ND: N. K. Adrianov--pervyĭ vrach-chuvash. **Sov Zdravookhr** 1981;(11):65–7

**Ady, Endre, 1877–1919**
Huszár G: Ady Endre fogbántalmairól. **Orv Hetil** 1984 Oct 14;125(42):2575–6

**Aelius Aristides, 117–180**
Van der Horst PW: Aelius Aristides and the New Testament. Leiden, E. J. Brill, 1980. ix, 115 p. (Studia ad Corpus Hellenisticum Novi Testamenti. Volumen Sextum.)

**Aepli, Johann Melchior, 1744–1813**
Ort-Wädensweiler L: Johann Melchior Aepli: zur Verbesserung des Medizinalwesens in der Schweiz (1783/88). Zürich, Juris Druck, 1984. 70 p. (Zürcher Medizingeschichtliche Abhandlungen, Neue Reihe, Nr. 167).
Peter CH: Der Briefwechsel zwischen Paulus Usteri und Melchior Aepli. Zürich, Juris Druck, 1983. 161 p. (Zürcher Medizingeschichtliche Abhandlungen, Neue Reihe, Nr. 155).

**Aesculapius, God of Medicine**
Briceño Maaz T: Santuario de Esculapio en Epidauro. **Rev Soc Venez Hist Med** 1972–73;20–21(34–35):51–65
Delbrel R: Asclépios et les secrets d'epidaure. **Atlantis** 1981 Jan–Feb;:173–247
Kerényi K: Der göttliche Arzt. Studien über Asklepios und seine Kultstätten. Darmstadt, Wissenschaftliche Buchgesellschaft, 1975, 3rd ed. xxi, 113 p.
Siefert H: Inkubation, Imagination und Kommunikation im antiken Asklepioskult. In Leuner H, ed: Katathymes Bilderleben. Ergebnisse in Theorie und Praxis. Bern, Stuttgart, Wien, Huber, 1980. p. 324–45.
Vincelet L: Asklépios, dieu grec de la médecine ou simple praticien grec mortel? **Arch Med Normandie** 1978 Oct, Dec;9(8,10):427–9, 543–4

**Aetius, of Amida**
Conti Bizzarro F, et al: Per l'edizione dei libri medicinali di Aezio Amideno. **Koinonia** 1978;2:169–97

**Agassiz, Louis, 1807–1873**
Dexter RW: The impact of evolutionary theories on the Salem group of Agassiz zoologists (Morse, Hyatt, Packard, Putnam). **Essex Inst Hist Collect** 1979;115(3):144–71
Winsor MP: Louis Agassiz and the species question. **Stud Hist Biol** 1979;3:89–138

**Agatha, Saint**
Marí VJ: El martirio de Santa Agatha, un precedente de la mastectomia. Représentacion artistica con especial referencia a una coleccion de tallas. In International Congress of the History of Medicine. 26th, Plovdiv, 1978. Actes du Congress. Sofia, 1981. Volume II. p. 150–7.

**Agathias**
Théodoridès J: Quelle était la maladie décrite par l'historien Agathias (VIe siècle A.D.)? **Hist Sci Med** 1981;15(2):153–8

**Aggrey, James E. Kadwo Kwegyir, 1875–1927**
Gryfe CI: James E. Kadwo Kwegyir Aggrey, D.D., D.O., 1875–1927. **Scalpel Tongs** 1981;25:53–5

**Agnew, David Hayes, 1818–1892**
Schneck JM: S. Weir Mitchell, M.D. (1829 to 1914) and D. Hayes Agnew, M.D. (1818 to 1892). Neuropsychiatrist's poetic tribute to a surgeon. **NY State J Med** 1982 Jul;82(8):1264–8

**Agrippa von Nettesheim, Heinrich Cornelius, 1486–1535**
Müller-Jahncke WD: Agrippa von Nettesheim in Antwerpen. Ein Beitrag zur Geschichte des 'Englischen Schweiss'. In Dilg P, et al., ed: Perspektiven der Pharmaziegeschichte. Graz, Austria, Akademische Druck- u. Verlagsanstalt, 1983. p. 243–68.
Newman W: Thomas Vaughan as an interpreter of Agrippa von Nettesheim. **Ambix** 1982 Nov;29(3):125–40
Starobinski J: D'Agrippa de Nettesheim à Montaigne: l'embarras de médecins devant l'origine de la semence. **Gesnerus** 1983;40(1–2):175–83

**Aguilar, Francisco, fl. ca. 1590**
Gonzalez Iglesias J: Los Borbones y el desarrollo de la odontologia en Espãna. **Bol Inf Dent (Madr)** 1978;Spec no:63–92

**Aguilon, François d', 1566–1617**
Jaeger W: Die Ordnungsprinzipien der Farbsysteme des 17. Jahrhunderts. (Franciscus Aguilonius--Athanasius Kircher--Isaac Newton). **Klin Monatsbl Augenheilkd** 1984 Apr;184(4):321–5

**Ahmad ibn Ibrāhim, called Ibn al-Jazzār, d. ca. 1009**
Catahier S: A l'occasion du millénaire de la mort d'Ibnoul-Jazzar (Algizar). **Hist Sci Med** 1984;18(3):247–53

**Aikenhead, Mary, 1787–1858**
Okamura A: [A long road to the hospice movement--life of Mother Mary Aikenhead] (Jpn). **Kango Kyoiku** 1984 Jan;25(1):38–45;25(2):104–11 (continued periodically)

**Akhutin, Mikhail Nikiforovich, 1898–1948**
Aleksanian IV, Knopov MSh: Akhutinskoe dvizhenie. **Voen Med Zh** 1981;(7):74–5

**Akimovich, V. V., 1912–1968**
Zykin LF, Metlin VN: Nauchnaia deiatel'nost' professora V. V. Akimovicha. **Zh Mikrobiol Epidemiol Immunobiol** 1984 Apr;(4):113–4

**Aladashvili, Aleksandr Stepanovich**
Bakhtadze G: Akademik Aleksandr Stepanovich Aladashvili: zhizn' i deiatel'nost. Tbilisi, Metsniereba, 1980. 147 p.

**Albarran, Joaquin, 1860–1912**
Puigvert A: The young Albarrán in Spain. **Eur Urol** 1981;7(1):57–9
Pytel' AIa: Ioakhim Al'barran i ego rol' v razvitii urologii. **Urol Nefrol (Mosk)** 1981 Nov–Dec;(6):56–61

**Alberca Lorente, Roman, 1903–1967**
Marín Fernández JL: Aspectos bibliometricos de la obra de Roman Alberca Lorente (1903–1967). **Asclepio** 1980;32:229–53

**Albert, Eduard, 1841–1900**
Paul U: Das chirurgische Erbe. Eduard Albert. **Zentralbl Chir** 1982;107(23):1535–7

**Albert III, Duke of Saxony, 1443–1500**
Cadden J: The medieval philosophy and biology of growth: Albertus

Magnus, Thomas Aquinas, Albert of Saxony and Masilius of Inghen on Book I, Chapter V, of Aristotle's 'De generatione et corruptione.' With translated texts of Albertus Magnus and Thomas Aquinas. Ph. D. Diss. Indiana University. Bloomington, 1971. vii, 267 leaves.

**Albert, Joseph, 1825–1886**

Schmutz HK: Rüdingers 'Atlas des peripherischen Nervensystems des menschlichen Körpers' mit Photographien von Joseph Albert; zur Frühgeschichte der medizinischen Photographie. **Gesnerus** 1980;37(1/2):83–90

**Albert, Prince Consort, 1819–1861**

Illustrations from the Wellcome Institute library: The last moments of H. R. H. the Prince Consort. **Med Hist** 1982 Jul;26(3):321–4

**Alberti, Leon Battista, 1404–1472**

Aiken J: Leon Battista Alberti's system of human proportions. **J Warburg Courtauld Inst** 1980;43:68–96

**Albertus Magnus, Saint, Bp. of Ratisbon, 1193?–1280**

Akdogan C: Optics in Albert the Great's De sensu et sensato; an edition, English translation, and analysis. Ph.D. Diss., University of Wisconsin. Madison, 1978. iv, 267 leaves.

Cadden J: The medieval philosophy and biology of growth: Albertus Magnus, Thomas Aquinas, Albert of Saxony and Masilius of Inghen on Book I, Chapter V, of Aristotle's 'De generatione et corruptione.' With translated texts of Albertus Magnus and Thomas Aquinas. Ph. D. Diss. Indiana University. Bloomington, 1971. vii, 267 leaves.

Cadden J: A matter of life and death: water in the natural philosophy of Albertus Magnus. **Hist Philos Life Sci** 1980;2(2):241–52

Caroti S: Problèmes textuels et lexicographiques dans l'oeuvre scientifique d'Albert le Grand. **Ann Ist Mus Stor Sci Fir** 1981;6(1):187–202

Goldstein-Préaud T: Albert le Grand et les questions du XIIIe siècle sur le De animalibus d'Aristote. **Hist Philos Life Sci** 1981;3(1):61–71

Jacquart D, Thomasset C: Albert le Grand et les problèmes de la sexualité. **Hist Philos Life Sci** 1981;3(1):73–93

John Paul II Pope: Discurso de Juan Pablo II a los profesores y estudiantes universitarios en la catedral de Colonia (Aalemania), 15.XI.1980. **Rev Med Univ Navarra** 1981 Jun;25(2):61–4

Schipperges H: Das medizinische Denken bei Albertus Magnus. In: Albertus Magnus, Doctor universalis, 1280/1980; hrsg. von G. Meyer, A. Zimmermann. Mainz, Matthias-Grünewald, 1980. p. 279–94.

Schipperges H: Eine 'summa medicinae' bei Albertus Magnus. **Jahrb Gorres Ges** 1981;:5–24

Weisheipl JA, ed: Albertus Magnus and the sciences: commenmorative essays 1980. Toronto, Pontifical Institute of Mediaeval Studies, 1980. xiv, 657 p.

**Albinus, Bernard Siegfried, 1697–1770**

Hilloowala R: Illustrations from the Wellcome Institute Library: the origin of the Wellcome anatomical waxes Albinus and the Florentine collection at La Specola. **Med Hist** 1984 Oct;28(4):432–7

**Albrant, Meister, fl. 13th cent.**

Bauer B: Studien zum ersten altdeutschen Pferdearzneibuch des anonymen Kopenhagener Ms. Thott Nr. 202. DMV Diss. Hannover, 1980. 99 p.

**Albright, Fuller, 1900–1969**

Gordan GS: Fuller Albright and postmenopausal osteoporosis: a personal appreciation. **Perspect Biol Med** 1981 Summer;24(4):547–60

Howard JE: Fuller Albright: the endocrinologists' clinical endocrinologist. **Perspect Biol Med** 1981 Spring;24(3):374–81

**Alcmaeon, of Crotona, fl. 5th cent. B.C.**

Leikola A: Alkmaion – den vetenskapliga medicinens pionjär. **Nord Medicinhist Arsbok** 1983;:59–63

Mansfeld J: Alcmaeon: 'Physikos' or physician? With some remarks on Calcidius' 'On vision' compared to Galen's Plac. Hipp. Plat. VII. In J. Mansfeld, L. M. de Rijk, eds. Kephalaion: Studies in Greek philosophy and its continuation. Assen, Van Gorcum, 1975. p. 26–38.

**Alcón, Andrés, 1782–1850**

Puerto Sarmiento FJ: Andrés Alcón (1782–1850), farmacéutico, político y profesor de Química. **Bol Soc Esp Hist Farm** 1984 Sep;35(139):143–64

**Alcott, Louisa May, 1832–1888**

Nursing revisited: Louisa May Alcott: **Mass Nurse** 1983 Jun;52(6):13

Van Buren J: Louisa May Alcott: a study in persona and idealization. **Psychohist Rev** 1981;9(4):282–99

**Alder, Albert, 1888–1980**

Späth HU: Der Hämatologe Albert Alder, 1888–1980. Zürich, Juris Druck, 1983. 81 p. (Zürcher Medizingeschichtliche Abhandlungen, Neue Reihe, 164).

**Alderotti, Taddeo, 1223–1295?**

Siraisi NG: Taddeo Alderotti and his pupils. Two generations of Italian medical learning. Princeton, Princeton University Press, 1981. xxiii, 461 p.

**Aldrovandi, Ulisse, 1522–1605**

Olmi G: Osservazione della natura e raffiguarazione in Ulisse Aldrovandi (1522–1605). **Ann Ist Stor Italo-Ger** 1977;3:105–81

Simili A: Spigolature medicine fra gli inediti aldrovandiani. **Archiginnasio (Italy)** 1968–70;63–65(1):361–488

**Alekseev, A. A., 1882–1950**

Zasukhin DN, Alekseev GA: Vydaiushchiĭ protozoolog A. G. Alekseev (1882–1950). **Parazitologiia** 1982 May–Jun;16(3):262–4

**Alekseev, Nikolai Aleksandrovich, 1873–**

Chernobrov IV: Vrach-revoliutsioner N. A. Alekseev. **Sov Zdravookhr** 1983;(11):57–9

**Alessandri, Hernán, 1900–**

Chamorro G: El Dr. Hernán Alessandri y el desarrollo de la medicina interna en el Hospital de Salvador. **Rev Med Chil** 1979 May;107(5):438–40

Neghme A: La medicina chilena esta de duelo. **Rev Med Chil** 1980 May;108(5):399–406

**Aletrino, Arnold, 1858–1916**

Bakker-van der Kooij C: De zoekende zusters. Enige beschouwingen naar aanleiding van de herdruk van de roman 'Zuster Bertha', geschreven door Arnold Aletrino en voor het eerst uitgegeven in 1891. **Tijdschr Ziekenverpl** 1983 Apr 26;36(9):275–8

Hekma G: Homoseksualiteit: van zonde tot geaardheid. **Spiegel Hist** 1980;15(9):484–91

**Alexander, Alexander, 1849–1928**

Parry NA: Pioneers of physical education in the 19th century: Alexander Alexander. [1849–1928]. **Bull Hist Educ Soc** 1978;22:21–38

**Alexander, Eben, Jr., 1913–**

Kelly DL: Eben Alexander, Jr., M.D.: a biographical sketch. **Clin Neurosurg** 1981;28:xiii–xx

**Alexander, Franz Gabriel, 1981–1964**

Lerner EA: Franz Gabriel Alexander. In Dictionary of American Biography, 1961–1965. Suppl. 7, 1981. p. 5–7.

**Alexander, Frederick Matthias, 1869–1955**

Tengwall R. A note on the influence of F. M. Alexander on the development of Gestalt therapy. **J Hist Behav Sci** 1981 Jan;17(1):126–30

**Alexander, Hattie Elizabeth, 1901–1968**

Dubos R: Hattie Elizabeth Alexander. In: Notable American women. The modern period. Cambridge, Mass., Belknap-Harvard Univ. Press, 1980. 4:10–1.

**Alexander, John, 1891–**

Just Viera JO: Mitral valve commissurotomy by John Alexander: repeat surgery 28 years later. **Bol Asoc Med PR** 1981 Feb;73(2):56–8

**Alexander, King of Poland, 1461–1506**

Dudziński W: Choroby i zgon króla Aleksandra Jagiellończyka. **Wiad Lek** 1981 Jul 15;34(14):1227–32

**Alexander, Samuel, 1888–1952**

Alexander SF: Samuel Alexander, M.D., and the Uniform Medical Practice Act. **J Med Soc NJ** 1984 Sep;81(9):759–62

**Alexander the Great, 356–323 B.C.**

Angulo Arvelo LA: Acerca de la probable causa de la muerte de Alejandro el Grande. **Rev Soc Venez Hist Med** 1981;30(45–46):105–10

Coulomb J: La mort d'Alexandre Le Grand. **Hist Sci Med** 1984;18(2):137–45

Hughes JD: The dreams of Alexander the Great. **J Psychohist** 1984 Fall;12(2):168–92

**Alexander, Vojtech, 1857–1916**

Kutarňa A, Sajter V: Subtrakcia a harmonizácia kontrastu röntgenového obrazu v diele prof. MUDr. Vojtecha Alexandra (1857–1916). **Bratisl Lek Listy** 1983 Dec;80(6):717–24

**Alexis, Crown Prince of Russia, 1904–1918**

Willbanks OL, Willbanks SE: Femoral neuropathy due to retroperitoneal bleeding. A red herring in medicine complicates anticoagulant therapy and influences the Russian Communist Revolution (Crown Prince Alexis, Rasputin). **Am J Surg** 1983 Feb;145(2):193–8

**Alfonso XII, King of Spain, 1857–1885**

de Andrés Turrión ML: Medicacíon vegetal para el rey Alfonso XII. **Bol Soc Esp Hist Farm** 1984 Sep;35(139):187–98

**Alhazen, 965–1039**

Lindberg DC, ed: Opticae thesaurus. Alhazeni Arabis libri septem, nuncprimùm editi. Eiusdem liber De Crepusculis et nubium ascensionibus. Item Vitellonis Thuringopoloni libri X. Reprint of the 1572 ed. New York, Johnson Reprint Corp., 1972. xxxiv, 288, 474 p.

Mawas LJ, Mawas E, Weiss JB: Intérêt en strabologie de la plaquette modifiée de Al Hazen. **Bull Soc Belge Ophtalmol** 1981;196:53–65

Omar S: Ibn Al-Haytham's theory of knowledge and its significânce for later science. **Arab Stud Q** 1979;1(1):67–82

**Alibert, Jean Louis Marie, 1766?–1837**

Dahm S: Frühe Krankenbildnisse: Alibert Esquirol Baumgartner. Köln, 1981. (Kölner medizinhistorische Beiträge; Arbeiten der Forschungsstelle des Instituts für Geschichte der Medizin der Universität zu Köln, Band 21).

Everett MA: Jean Louis Alibert. The father of French dermatology. **Int J Dermatol** 1984 Jun;23(5):351–6

Goldwyn RM: Keloid. **Plast Reconstr Surg** 1981 Oct;68(4):640–1

**Alice Maud Mary, Princess of Great Britain, 1843–1878**
Whitfield AG: The kiss of death (Princess Alice). **Ann R Coll Surg Engl** 1979 Sep;61(5):390–2

**Aliev, A. M.**
Fel' II, Truman GL: A. M. Aliev--vydaiushchiĭsia pertiĭnyĭ, gosudarstvennyĭ deiatel', organizator zdravookhraneniia i meditsinskoĭ nauki v Sovetskom Azerbaĭdzhane. **Sov Zdravookhr** 1982;(8):57–9

**Alison, William Pulteney, 1790–1859**
Leys R: Background to the reflex controversy: William Alison and the doctrine of sympathy before Hall. **Stud Hist Biol** 1980;4:1–66

**Alkindus, Jacobus, d. ca. 870**
Habib KM: Pharmacology and materiae medicae in the medical formulary of Al-Kindi. **Hamdard** 1981;24(1–2):92–101

**Allen, William, 1770–1843**
Trease GE: William Allen 1770–1843. **Br J Pharm Pract** 1981;3(4):33–4

**Allende, Salvador, 1908–1973**
Ionov IuV: Sal'vador Al'ende i ego meditsinskaia deiatel'nost'. **Feldsher Akush** 1981;46(2):39–41

**Allison, William David, 1854–1928**
McDonell KM: W. D. Allison: manufacturer of physicians' furniture. **Snakeroot Extr** 1984 Oct;(3):2–3

**Allport, Floyd Henry, 1890–1978**
Gorman M: Pre-war conformity research in social psychology: the approaches of Floyd H. Allport and Muzafer Sherif. **J Hist Behav Sci** 1981 Jan;17(1):3–14
Post DL: Floyd H. Allport and the launching of modern social psychology. **J Hist Behav Sci** 1980 Oct;16(4):369–76

**Allport, Gordon Willard, 1897–1967**
Evans RI: Dialogue with Gordon Allport. New York, Praeger, 1981. xxv, 157 p.
High RP, Woodward WR: William James and Gordon Allport: parallels in their maturing conceptions of self and personality. In R. W. Rieber, K. Salzinger, ed: Psychology: theoretical-historical perspectives. New York, Academic Press, 1980. p. 57–79.

**Almon, William James, 1755–1817**
Kernaghan LK: William James Almon. In Dictionary of Canadian biography, 1801 to 1820. Volume 5, 1983. p. 23–4.

**Alpago, Andrea, d. 1521**
Lucchetta F: La data della morte di Andrea Alpago. **Quad Stor Univ Padova** 1982;15:147–8

**Altenähr, Eberhard, 1940–1981**
Eberhard Altenähr (4. 12. 1940 bis 5. 4. 1981): **Verh Dtsch Ges Pathol** 1981;65:561–70

**Althoff, Friedrich**
Kaiser W, Skrobacki A: Królewieckie listy Jana Mukulicza de Fryderyka Althoffa. **Komun Mazursko Warm** 1975;4(130):455–65

**Alvarado, Lisandro**
Octavio O: Algunos momentos familiares de Don Lisandro Alvarado. **Bol Acad Nac Hist (Caracas)** 1981;64(254):419–23

**Alvares, Manuel, 1545–1612**
David-Peyre Y: Manuel Alvares, ou la synthèse de la littérature médicale sur la préservation contre la peste. **Bull Etud Port Bres** 1965;26:67–87

**Alvarez Chanca, Diego, fl. 1493**
Brotóns Picó J: Un medico en el descubrimiento de America. **Rev Gen Mar** 1980 Jul;199:3–11
Paniagua JA: Tradicion y renovacion en la obra del doctor Chanca. **Asclepio** 1978–79;30–31:365–9

**Amar, Jules, 1879–1935**
Colas des Francs G: L'oeuvre de Jules Amar entre 1914 et 1918. Thèse, Université René-Descartes, Faculté Cochin-Port-Royal. Paris, 1984. 21, 29, 7, 70 p.

**Ames, Blanche Ames, 1878–1969**
Friedell JN: Blanche Ames Ames. In: Notable American women. The modern period. Cambridge, Mass., Belknap-Harvard Univ. Press, 1980. 4:15–6.

**Amesse Family**
Delaney JJ: The doctors Amesse. **Colo Med** 1984 Mar;81(3):77–9

**Amoroso, Emmanuel Ciprian**
Short RV: The scientific contributions of Professor Emmanuel Ciprian Amoroso, CBE, TC, FRS. **J Reprod Fertil [Suppl]** 1982 Nov;31:1–8

**Ampère, André-Marie, 1775–1836**
Mammerickx M: André-Marie Ampère et Claude-Julien Bredin, II. Ampère, Bredin et le magnétisme animal, ou la petite histoire d'une grande découverte. **Hist Med Vet** 1977;2(3):69–75
Mammerickx M: André-Marie Ampère et Claude-Julien Bredin, I. Ampère, Bredin et la philosophie, ou la belle histoire d'une amitié. **Hist Med Vet** 1977;2(1):11–19

**Amstein, Johann Georg, 1819–1892**
Sieber CF: Johann Georg Amstein 'der Jüngere' (1819–1892): ein gelehrter Bündner Arzt und Naturforscher des 19. Jahrhunderts. Zürich, Juris Druck, 1984. 72 p. (Zürcher Medizingeschichtliche Abhandlungen, Neue Rheihe, Nr. 168).

**Andersen, Dorothy Hansine, 1901–1963**
Machol L: Dorothy Hansine Andersen. In: Notable American women. The modern period. Cambridge, Mass., Belknap-Harvard Univ. Press, 1980. 4:18–20.

**Andersen, Hans Christian, 1805–1875**
Greenacre P: Hans Christian Andersen and children. **Psychoanal Study Child** 1983;38:617–35

**Anderson, Charles Henry**
Dummett CO: Health professional emancipators: examples in excellence. **J Natl Med Assoc** 1984 Sep;76(9):925–30

**Anderson, Elda Emma, 1899–1961**
Kathren RL: Elda Emma Anderson. In: Notable American women. The modern period. Cambridge, Mass., Belknap-Harvard Univ. Press, 1980. 4:20–1.

**Anderson, Elizabeth Garrett, 1836–1917**
Wilkinson M: Elizabeth Garrett Anderson and migraine. In Rose FC, Bynum WF, ed: Historical aspects of the neurosciences. New York, Raven, 1982. p. 165–9.

**Anderson, Victor Vance, 1879–1960**
Sulman AM: Victor Vance Anderson. In Dictionary of American Biography, Suppl. 6, 1956–1960. p. 16–17, 1980.

**Anderson, William Wallace**
Woosley AI: Fort Burgwin's hospital. **Palacio** 86(1):3–7, 36–9

**Andrade, Corino**
Guerra M: Corino Andrade na história da medicina Portuguesa. **Acta Med Port** 1983 Apr–May;4(4–5):239–43

**Andral, Gabriel, 1797–1876**
Andral G: Pathological hematology: an essay on the blood in disease. Reprint of the 1844 ed. With a historical introduction by L. A. May. Oceanside, N. Y. Dabor Science Publications, 1977. 129 p.
Huard P, Imbault-Huart MJ: Gabriel Andral (1797–1876). **Rev Hist Sci** 1982;35(2):131–53

**Andreevskii, Stepan Semenovich, 1760–1818**
Palkin BN: S. S. Andreevskiĭ v Astrakhani. **Sov Zdravookhr** 1981;(6):66–8

**Andric, Ivo, 1892–**
Striković J: Analiza jednog samoubistva u delu Ive Andrića 'Na Drini Cuprija'. **Srp Arh Celok Lek** 1979 Sep;107(9):477–82

**Andrus, Edwin Cowles, 1896–**
Gantt WH: E. Cowles Andrus (1896--1978), eighth president of the Pavlovian Society. **Pavlov J Biol Sci** 1979 Jan–Mar;14(1):74–5

**Andrzejewski, Antoni, 1807–1883**
Michalczak W, Lisiewicz J: Antoni Andrzejewski (1807–1883) -- lekarz powiatu kieleckiego. **Przegl Lek** 1980;37(10):717–8

**Anel, Dominique, 1679–1730**
Amalric P: Dominique Anel et les Quinze Vingts de Paris. **Bull Soc Ophtalmol Fr** 1982 Jan;82(1):87–90

**Angel, John Lawrence**
Stewart TD: J. Lawrence Angel. **Am J Phys Anthropol** 1979 Nov;51(4):509–16

**Anger, Hal O., 1920–**
Powell MR: H.O. Anger and his work at the Donner Laboratory. **Semin Nucl Med** 1979 Jul;9(3):164–8

**Angibaud, Charles, fl. 1678–1728**
Burnby J: The mortar of Charles Angibaud. **Pharm Hist (London)** 1979 Apr;9(1):6–8

**Anglada, Joseph, 1775–1833**
Rivet R: Un médecin de Perpignan, professeur à l'Université de Montpellier: Joseph Anglada (1775–1833). In: Congrès National des Sociétés Savantes, 106e, Perpignan, 1981. Comptes Rendus. Paris, Bibliothèque Nationale, 1982. Fasc. IV. p. 111–7.

**Anglade, Jean, 1698–1764**
Bergasse JD: Jean Anglade (1698–1764) et la fondation de l'hôpital rural de Cazouls-les-Béziers au XVIIIe siècle. Bergasse (ed.) Hommage à Jacques Fabre de Morlhon. Albi, O.J.S., 1978. p. 133–47.

**Angle, Edward Hartley, 1855–1930**
Kurashima K: [Angle's orthodontics: a critical review. I. Angle's quest for science, and his classification of malocclusion] (Jpn). **Nippon Kyosei Shika Gakkai Zasshi** 1983 Sep;42(3):379–84

**Angrist, Alfred Alvin, 1902–**
Alfred A. Angrist: **NY State J Med** 1983 May;83(6):809–11, 872–6

**Angus, Samuel, 1784–1840**
Langley HD: Respect for civilian authority: the tragic career of Captain Angus. **Am Neptune** 1980;40(1):23–37

**Annan, Ebenezer, fl. 1836–1843**
Birchall S: A disowned apothecary. **Pharm Hist (London)** 1984 Sep;14(3):8

**Annaratone, Carlo**
Pankhurst R: Le piaghe d'Etiopia. **Kos** 1984 Jul-Aug;1(6):33-50

**Anne Boleyn, Queen, consort of Henry VIII, 1507-1536**
Dewhurst J: The alleged miscarriages of Catherine of Aragon and Anne Boleyn. **Med Hist** 1984 Jan;28(1):49-56

**Anne of Austria, Queen of France, 1601-1666**
Kleinmann R: Facing cancer in the seventeenth century: the last illness of Anne of Austria, 1664-1666. **Adv Thanatol** 1978;4:37-55

**Anokhin, Petr Kusmich, 1898-1974**
Kokina NN: P. K. Anokhin's concept of systems genesis and its subsequent development. **Neurosci Behav Physiol** 1980 Mar-Apr;10(2):142-6
Roslakova NA: Contribution of academician P. K. Anokhin to physiology. **Agressologie** 1982;23(5):165-6

**Anselmino, Otto, 1873-1955**
Friedrich C, Seidlein HJ: Otto Anselmino--Seine Bedeutung für die Entwicklung der Pharmazeutischen Wissenschaft, insbesondere an der Universität Greifswald. **Pharmazie** 1981 Dec;36(12):846-52

**Anthony, Francis, 1550-1623**
Proust J: Francis Anthonie, charlatan elisabéthain. In: Devins et charlatans au temps de la Renaissance. ed. M.T. Jones-Davies. Paris, Université, Centre de Recherches sur la Renaissance, 1979. p. 101-11.

**Antommarchi, Francesco A., 1780-1838**
Dumaitre P: Les planches anatomiques d'Antommarchi. **Clio Med** 1981 Sep;16(1):13-23
Poulet J: Le cas Antommarchi. **Rev Inst Napoleon (Paris)** 1971;(120)131-8

**Anzoux, Louis Thomas Jérome, 1797-1880**
Mulder WJ: De 'Anatomie clastique' van Dr. L. T. J. Anzoux. **Tijdschr Geschied Geneeskd** 1981:4(3):133-43

**Apert, Eugene, 1868-1940**
Steffen C: Eugène Apert (1868-1940). **Am J Dermatopathol** 1984 Jun;6(3):223-4

**Apgar, Virginia, 1909-1974**
Calmes SH: Virginia Apgar: a woman physician's career in a developing specialty. **J Am Med Wom Assoc** 1984 Nov-Dec;39(6):184-8
Waldinger RJ: Virginia Apgar. In: Notable American women. The modern period. Cambridge, Mass., Belknap-Harvard Univ. Press, 1980. 4:27-8.

**Apollonia of Alexandria, Saint**
Deutsch-Kasimir M: Die Heilige Apollonia. **Quintessenz J** 1982 Nov;12(11):1025-6
Eramo S: L'odontoiatria nell'arte. Su un affresco raffigurante S. Apollonia nella Basilica di Santa Maria di Collemaggio a l'Aquila. **Dent Cadmos** 1984 Apr;52(4):135-7
Rocchietta S: Iconografia statuaria e pittorica di Santa Apollonia nel Duomo di Milano. **Minerva Med** 1981 Jan 14;72(1):45-9
Rocchietta S: Due raffigurazioni di santa Apollonia. (sec. XVI e sec. XVIII). **Minerva Med** 1983 Oct 6;74(38):2245-6
Sct Apollonia og dansk odontologi: **Tandlaegebladet** 1984 Jan;88(1):5-8
Tronnberg G: S:ta Apollonia av Alexandra--tandlakarnas skyddshelgon. **Odontol Foren Tidskr** 1980 Dec;44(5):22-8

**Apollonius, of Tyana**
Weisser U, ed: Buch über das Geheimnis der Schöpfung und die Darstellung der Natur (Buch der Ursachen), von Pseudo-Apollonios von Tyana. Aleppo, Institute for the History of Arabic Science, University of Aleppo, 1979. 66 p. (Sources and Studies in the History of Arabic-Islamic Science, Natural Sciences Series 1).

**Appel, Kenneth Ellwaker, 1896-1979**
Blain D: Twentieth century psychiatry--living history in the life of Kenneth E. Appel, M.D., 1896-1979. **Trans Stud Coll Physicians Phila** 1980 Jun;5(2 no 2):144-54

**Appert, Nicolas, 1749-1841**
Laissus J: Les conserves alimentaires: Nicolas Appert (1749-1841) bienfaiteur de l'humanité. In: Congrès National des Sociétés Savantes, 93e, Tours, 1968. Comptes Rendus. Paris, 1971. Section des Sciences, Tome II. p. 137-57.

**Appia, Louis, 1818-1898**
Zanobio B: Je le pansai, Dieu le guérit. Gli aforismi di chirurgia militare di Louis Appia (1818-1898) sulla cura delle ferite d'armi da fuoco. **G Accad Med Torino** 1980;143(Spec No):7-95

**Apuleius Barbarus**
Disertori B, Piazza M: L'epilettologia di Apuleio. **Ann Osp Maria Vittoria Torino** 1977 Jul-Dec;20(7-12):341-53

**Aragáo, Joáo Moniz Barreto de, 1874-1922**
Souza LC: João Moniz Barreto de Aragão-médico militar e pioneiro da veterinária brasileira. **Rev Inst Hist Georgr Bras** 1974;305:51-68

**Aragon, Enrique O., 1880-1942**
Colotla VA, Jurado S: Contributions to the history of psychology: XXXIV. Enrique O. Aragon, a pioneer in Mexican psychology. **Percept Mot Skills** 1983 Dec;57(3 Pt 1):1013-4

**Aragon, Louis, 1897-1982**
Decourt J: Aragon, tendre et fidèle. **Sem Hop Paris** 1983 May 12;59(19):1489-92
Matot JP: Filiation problématique roman familial et secret (à propos de Louis Aragon. **Psychiatr Enfant** 1984;27(2):523-38

**Aranguren, Manuel Bernardino de, 1743-1794**
Elósegui J: Un guipuzcoano benemérito del siglo XVIII, Manuel Bernardino de Aranguren, médico (1743-1794). **Bol Real Soc Vascongada Amigos Pais** 1973;29(1-3):171-91

**Arany, János, 1817-1882**
Szállási A: Arany János tanártársa Lengyel Dániel doktor. **Orv Hetil** 1983 Apr 3;124(14):833-4

**Arbuthnot, John, 1667-1735**
Bruneteau C: John Arbuthnot (1667-1735) et les idées au début XVIIIe siècle. Univ. de Paris III, 1973. 949 p.

**Arcimboldo, Giuseppe, 1527?-1593**
Bresgen C: Homo omnis creatura. Arcimboldo und Paracelsus - eine Gegenüberstellung aus der Sicht des Künstlers. **Salzburger Beitr Paracelsusforsch** 1984;23:36-49

**Arderne, John, fl. 1307-1370**
Classic articles in colonic and rectal surgery: John Arderne 1307-1380 (?). **Dis Colon Rectum** 1982 Nov-Dec;25(8):832-40

**Areilza, Enrique de, 1860-1926**
Victoria Ortiz M: Vida y obra del doctor Areilza. Bilbao, La Gran Enciclopedia Vasca, 1975. 329 p.

**Arejula, Juan Manuel de, 1755-1830**
Carrillo JL, Gago R: Memoria sobre una nueva y metodica clasificacion de los fluidos elasticos permanentes y gaseosos de Juan Manuel de Arejula (1755-1830). Introduccion, transcripcion y notas. Malaga, Universidad de Malaga, 1980. 47 p.

**Arenal, Concepción, 1820-1893**
Fernández Picón L: Concepcion Arenal en la historia de la medicina. Ideas medicas de Concepcion Arenal. **Asclepio** 1980;32:161-70

**Aretaeus of Cappadocia**
Marketos SG, Ballas CN: Bronchial asthma in the medical literature of Greek antiquity. **J Asthma** 1982;19(4):263-9

**Ariès, Philippe, 1914-1984**
Mitchell A: Philippe Ariès and the French way of death. **Fr Hist Stud** 1978;10(4):684-95
Poussou JP: In memoriam: Philippe Aries (1914-1984). **Ann Demogr Hist (Paris)** 1984;:5-6
Spagnoli PG: Philippe Ariès, historian of the family. **J Fam Hist** 1981 Winter;6(4):434-41

**Ariosto, Lodovico, 1474-1533**
Ferroni G: Nota sull' Erbolato. **Rass Lett Ital** 1979;7(1-2):202-14

**Ariss, E. A.**
Barkley S: A nurse who made a difference. **Pulse** 1984 May;20(5):1-2

**Aristotle**
Abdullaev MS: Aristotel'i razvitie predstavlenii o nervnoĭ sisteme. **Arkh Anat Gistol Embriol** 1984 Sep;87(9):97-103
Abdullaev MS: Anatomiia v trudakh Aristotelia. **Arkh Anat Gistol Embriol** 1984 Mar;86(3):95-9
Azeez Pasha M: Biography of the Unani physician Arestu. **Bull Indian Inst Hist Med (Hyderabad)** 1978;8(1-4):26-31
Barnes J: Aristotle's de Motu Animalium. **Classical Rev** 1980;30(2):222-6
Bodson L: Aristotle's statement on the reproduction of sharks. **J Hist Biol** 1983 Fall;16(3):391-407
Boylan M: The digestive and 'circulatory' systems in Aristotle's biology. **J Hist Biol** 1982 Spring;15(1):89-118
Boylan M: Mechanism and teleology in Aristotle's biology. **Apeiron** 1981, reçu 1982;15(2):96-102
Boylan M: The Galenic and Hippocratic challenges to Aristotle's conception theory. **J Hist Biol** 1984 Spring;17(1):83-112
Bugaj R: Koncepcje elementów ognia i powietrza u Arystotelesa i ich rola w procesach spalania i oddychania. **Kwart Hist Nauki Tech** 1980;25(1):89-103
Cadden J: The medieval philosophy and biology of growth: Albertus Magnus, Thomas Aquinas, Albert of Saxony and Masilius of Inghen on Book I, Chapter V, of Aristotle's 'De generatione et corruptione.' With translated texts of Albertus Magnus and Thomas Aquinas. Ph. D. Diss. Indiana University. Bloomington, 1971. vii, 267 leaves.
Cappelletti AJ: El sentido del olfato, segun Aristoteles. **Rev Soc Venez Hist Med** 1978;27(41):9-40
Cappelletti AJ: El sentido del gusto, segun Aristoteles. **Rev Soc Venez Hist Med** 1978;27(41):41-57
Gaukroger S: Aristotle on the function of sense perception. **Stud Hist Philos Sci** 1981 Mar;12(1):75-89
Goldstein-Préaud T: Albert le Grand et les questions du XIIIe siècle sur le De animalibus d'Aristote. **Hist Philos Life Sci** 1981;3(1):61-71
Gracia D: The structure of medical knowledge in Aristotle's philosophy. **Sudhoffs Arch** 1978;62(1):1-36
Kruk R: Aristoteles semitico-latinus. The Arabic version of Aristotle's Parts of animals. Book XI-XIV of the Kitab al-Hayawan. A critical edition with introduction and selected glossary. Amsterdam, Oxford, North-Holland Publishing Co., 1979. 96 [107] p.
Kullmann W: Aristoteles' Grundgedanken zu Aufbau und Funktion der Körpergewebe. **Sudhoffs Arch** 1982;66(3):209-38

Kullmann W: Wesen und Bedeutung der 'Zweckursache' bei Aristoteles. **Ber Wissenschaftsgesch** 1982;5:25–39
Kung J: Aristotle's De motu animalium and the separability of the sciences. **J Hist Philos** 1982;20:65–76
Lefèvre C: Sur l'évolution d'Aristote en psychologie. Louvain, Editions de l'Institut supérieur de philosophie, 1972. ix, 345 p.
Lennox J: Teleology, chance, and Aristotle's theory of spontaneous generation. **J Hist Philos** 1981;19:219–38
Lohr CH: Renaissance Latin Aristotle Commentaries: authors N–Ph. **Renaiss Q** 1979 Winter;32(4):529–80 (continued periodically)
Nussbaum MC, ed: Aristotle's De motu animalium. Text with translation, commentary, and interpretive essays. Princeton, Princeton University Press, 1978. xxiii, 430 p.
Oppenheimer JM: Aristotle as a biologist. **Scientia** 1971;65(106):649–58
Osborne C: Aristotle's De anima 3.2: how do we perceive that we see and hear? **Classical Q** 1983;33:401–11
Ott S: Aristotle among the Basques: the 'cheese analogy' of conception. **Man** 1979;14:699–711
Pack RA ed: Pseudo-Aristotelis Epistola ad Alexandrum der regimine sanitatis a quodam Nicolao versificata. **Arch Hist Doctrinale Litt Moyen Age** 1978;53:307–25
Pitskhelauri GZ: Aristotle's knowledge in the field of natural and medical sciences (on celebrating 2300 years since his death). **Sante Publique (Bucur)** 1980;23(4):375–9
Pratt V: Aristotle and the essence of natural history. **Hist Philos Life Sci** 1982;4(2):203–23
Robert F: Hippocrate, Platon, Aristote et les notions de genre et d'espèce. **Hist Philos Life Sci** 1982;4(2):173–201
Roselli A: Aristotele e il sistema della sensazione. **Physis** 1980;22(2):157–73
Roussel M: Ether et chaleur dans l'embryologie aristotélienne: influences archaïques. In: Mélanges d'études anciennes offerts à Maurice Lebel. St-Jean-Chrysostôme, Québec, 1980. p. 157–60.
Roussel M: Physique et biologie dans la 'Génération des animaux' d'Aristote. **Rev Etud Grec** 1980, reçu 1981:93(440–441):42–71
Schöffler HH: Die Akademie von Gondischapur. Aristoteles auf dem Wege in den Orient. Stuttgart, Freies Geistesleben, 1979. 154 p.
Seidler MJ: The medical paradigm in Aristotelian ethics. **Thomist** 1978;42:400–33
Thomasen AL: 'Historia animalium' contra 'Gynaecia' in der Literatur des Mittelalters. **Clio Med** 1980;15(1/2):5–23
Ushida N: Etude comparative de la psychologie d'Aristote, d'Avicenne et de St. Thomas d'Aquin. Tokyo, Keio Institute of Cultural and Linguistic Studies, 1968. vi, 231 p. (Studies in the humanities and social relations; v. 11.).
Van Praagh R, Van Praagh S: Aristotle's 'triventricular' heart and the relevant early history of the cardiovascular system. **Chest** 1983 Oct;84(4):462–8

**Aristovskiĭ, Viacheslav Mikhaĭlovich, 1882–**
Koroliuk AM: K stoletiiu so dnia rozhdeniia Viacheslava Mikhaĭlovicha Aristovskogo. **Zh Mikrobiol Epidemiol Immunobiol** 1983 Mar;(3):109–12

**Arkövy, József, 1851–1922**
Huszár G: A magyar fogászat feilődése Arkövytól napjainkig. **Orv Hetil** 1982 May 16;123(20):1243–6

**Armengandus Blasii, fl. 1280–1309**
Daems WF: Ermengald Blasius' Tabellen zum 'Antidotarium Nicolai'. **Pharm Acta Helv** 1979;54(4):101–5

**Armengaud, André, 1920–1980**
Biraben JN: André Armengaud, 1920–1980. **Ann Demogr Hist (Paris)** 1980;:7–10

**Armstrong, Fergus, 1887–**
Morris AD: Two Colliery doctors: the brothers Armstrong of Treorchy. In J. Cule, ed: Wales and medicine. London, British Society for the History of Medicine, 1975. p. 208–15.

**Armstrong, John Richard, 1872–1931**
Morris AD: Two Colliery doctors: the brothers Armstrong of Treorchy. In J. Cule, ed: Wales and medicine. London, British Society for the History of Medicine, 1975. p. 208–15.

**Arnald, George, 1763–1841**
Paly D: Portrait of William Norris. Broadside, 1815, with etched portrait (1814) entitled 'William Norris: confined in this manner in Bethlem Hospital'; George Arnald, A.R.A., artist, etcher, and publisher. **Radic Hist Rev** 1979 Spring/Summer;Spec:65

**Arnaldus de Villanova, d. 1313?**
Haven M: La vie et les oeuvres de Maître Arnaud de Villenauve. Genève, Slatkine Reprints, 1972. [192] p.
Hussenot C: Sur un Erbier de Me Arnauld de Villeneuve (manuscrit médiéval). Thèse de doctorat, Université René-Descartes. Paris, 1983. 119 leaves. (U. E. R. des Sciences pharm. et biol. de Paris-Luxembourg, 1982–1983, no U 558).
Paniagua Arellano JA, Arnau de Vilanova: El maravilloso regimiento y orden de vivir (una versión castellana del Regimen sanitatis ad regem Aragonum). **Cuad Aragon Hist Med Cienc (B)** 1980;3:1–106
Rodrigo Lizondo M: La protesta de Valencia de 1318 y otros documentos inéditos referentes a Arnau de Vilanova. **Dynamis** 1981;1:241–73

**Arnold, Harry Loren, 1912–**
Goltz RW: WWII, the 147th General hospital & Harry Arnold. **Hawaii Med J** 1982 Nov;41(11):410

**Arnott, Neil, 1788–1874**
Bayliss RA, Ellis CW: Neil Arnott, F.R.S., reformer, innovator and popularizer of science, 1788–1874. **Notes Rec R Soc Lond** 1981;36(1):103–24

**Arnstein, Margaret Gene, 1904–1972**
Milio N: Margaret Gene Arnstein. In: Notable American women. The modern period. Cambridge, Mass., Belknap-Harvard Univ. Press, 1980. 4:37–8.

**Arrhenius, Svante, 1859–1927**
Rubin LP: Styles in scientific explanations: Paul Ehrlich and Svante Arrhenius on immunochemistry. **J Hist Med Allied Sci** 1980 Oct;35(4):397–425

**Arsenijevic, Milan, 1901–1981**
Mićić R: General prof. dr Milan Arsenijević (24. III 1901 - 10. XI 1981). **Srp Arh Celok Lek** 1982 Sep;110(9):1109–13

**Arsonval, Asène d', 1851–1940**
Borell M: D'Arsonval's calorimeter: measurement of animal heat, 1877. **Med Instrum** 1982 Nov–Dec;16(6):307–8

**Arthurs, Robert, fl. 1886**
Arthurs R: The man who played doctor. **Civ War Times Illus** 1980;19(5):36–8

**Artur, Jacques-François, 1708–1779**
Chaïa J: Sur une correspondance, entre 1739 et 1749, de Duhamel du Monceau avec J.-F. Artur, médecin du roy a Cayenne. In: Congrès National des Sociétés Savantes, 102e, Limoges, 1977. Comptes Rendus. Paris, 1977. Section des Sciences, Fasc. III. p. 21–6.

**Artzybasheff, Boris, 1899–1965**
Astrow A: Anxiety - frustration - repressed hostility. An original drawing, painted in gouache, by Boris Artzybasheff. **J Hist Med Allied Sci** 1980 Oct;35(4):453

**Asaph Ha-Yehoudi, 7th cent.**
Pines S: The oath of Asaph the Physician and Yohanan Ben Zabda: Its relation to the Hippocratic Oath and the Doctrina duarum viarium of the Didaché. **Proc Isr Acad Sci Humanit** 1971–76;5:223–64
Simon I: L'influence hippocratique sur la médecine hébraique, surtout chez Assaph, Isaac Israèli et Maimonide. In La collection hippocratique et son rôle dans l'histoire de la médecine. Colloque de Strasbourg (23–27 octobre 1972) organisé par le Centre de Recherches sur la Grèce Antique, avec le concours des Facultés de Philosophie et des Langues Classiques. Leiden, E. J. Brill, 1975. 275–89.

**Asch, Morris Joseph, 1833–1902**
Romm S: Morris Joseph Asch. **Plast Reconstr Surg** 1983 May;71(5):724–8

**Asche, Justice**
The rights of the child: **Aust Paediatr J** 1982 Mar;18(1):6–12

**Asclepiades Bithynus**
Harig G: Die philosophischen Grundlagen des medizinischen Systems des Asklepiades von Bithynien. **Philologus** 1983;127:43–60
Rawson E: The life and death of Asclepiades of Bithynia. **Classical Q** 1982;32(2):358–70

**Ash, James Earle, 1884–1984**
Stewart HL: Reflections on Colonel James Earle Ash on the occasion of his 100th birthday September 8, 1984. **Lab Invest** 1984 Jan;50(1):1–2

**Ash, John, ca. 1821–1886**
Teece WK: John Ash. In Dictionary of Canadian biography, 1881–1890. 1982;11:32–3.

**Asratian, Ezras Asratovich, 1903–**
Kol'tsova MM: Mekhanizmy integratsii uslovnykh refleksov v trudakh E. A. Asratiana. **Zh Vyssh Nerv Deiat** 1983 Mar–Apr;33(2):216–20
Podachin VP: Cherty nauchnogo tvorchestva. E. A. Asratiana (k 80-letiiu so dnia rozhdeniia). **Usp Fiziol Nauk** 1983 Jul–Sep;14(3):3–13
Pressman IaM: E. A. Asratian i nauchnoe sodruzhestvo neĭrofiziologiov sotsialisticheskikh stran. **Zh Vyssh Nerv Deiat** 1983 Mar–Apr;33(2):211–5
Shingarov GKh: Filosofskie voprosy ucheniia o vyssheĭ nervnoĭ deiatel'nosti v tvorchestve E. A. Asratiana. **Zh Vyssh Nerv Deiat** 1983 Mar–Apr;33(2):204–10
Simonov PV: Polveka neotstupnykh iskaniĭ istiny (k 80-letiiu so dnia rozhdeniia E. A. Asratiana). **Zh Vyssh Nerv Deiat** 1983 Mar–Apr;33(2):197–203
Simonov PV: Podkrepliaiushchaia funktsiia émotsiĭ (k 80-letiiu so dnia rozhdeniia Ezrasa Asratovicha Asratiana). **Fiziol Zh SSSR** 1983 May;69(5):577–86
Simonov PV: Half a century of pursuing the truth. Dedicated to the 80th anniversary of E. A. Asratyan. **Pavlov J Biol Sci** 1983 Apr–Jun;18(2):63–8
Zieliński K: Ezras A. Asratyan. **Acta Neurobiol Exp (Warsz)** 1981;41(6):521–42

**Astaurov, Boris L'vovich, 1904–**
Berg RL: The life and research of Boris L. Astaurov. **Q Rev Biol** 1979 Dec;54(4):397–419

**Astbury, William Thomas, 1898–1961**
Edsall JT: The papers of W.T. Astbury and J.D. Bernal. **Surv Sources Newsl** 1981 Apr;10:2–6
Preston RD: William Thomas Astbury. In Dictionary of national biography, 1961–1970. Suppl. 8, 1981. p. 41–2.
Witkowski JA: W. T. Astbury and Ross G. Harrison: the search for the molecular determination of form in the developing embryo. **Notes Rec R Soc Lond** 1980 Dec;35(2):195–219

**Astruc de Sestiers, fl. early 15th cent.**
Iancu-Agou D: L'inventaire de la bibliothèque et du mobilier d'un médecin juif d'Aix en Provence au milieu du XVe siècle. **Rev Etud Juives** 1975;134(1–2):47–80

**Astruc, Jean, 1684–1766**
Jottras PL: Jean Astruc, médecin humaniste. **Hist Sci Med** 1984;18(3):271–7

**Atkins, Hedley, 1905–**
Atkins H: Memoirs of a surgeon. London, Springwood, 1977. xiv, 265 p.

**Atreya, Maharshi**
Raison A, ed: La Haritasamhita: texte médical sanskrit; avec un index de nomenclature ayurvédique. Pondichéry, Institut français d'indologie, 1974. xlvi, 396 p. (Publications de l'Institut français d'indologie; no. 52).

**Attenhofer, Heinrich Ludwig, 1783–1856**
Scalabrin HR: Heinrich Ludwig Attenhofer, 1783–1856. Arzt und Politiker. Zürich, Juris Druck, 1983. 67 p. (Zürcher Medizingeschichtliche Abhhandlungen, Neue Reihe, Nr. 158).

**Atwater, Wilbur Olin, 1844–1907**
Aronson N: Nutrition as a social problem: a case study of entrepreneurial strategy in science. **Soc Probl** 1982;29(5):474–87

**Aub, Joseph Charles, 1890–**
Harvey AM: Joseph Charles Aub: applying the tools of the basic sciences to clinical investigation. **Am J Med** 1981 Jul;71(1):13–5

**Aubert, Hermann Rudolf, 1826–1892**
Dodt E: Die erste Beschreibung des Knicks in der Dunkeladaptationskurve durch H. Aubert (1865). **Klin Monatsbl Augenheilkd** 1983 Jan;182(1):107–8

**Aubri, Claude, 17th cent.**
Belloni L: Claudius Aubrius a Francesco M. Fiorentini sull'assunzione di latte da parte del feto nell'utero. **Physis** 1977;19(1–4):378–82

**Audibran, Joseph, 1801–1867**
Sugden KC: Dentists in the rare books. Joseph Audibran and incorruptible artificial teeth. **Br Dent J** 1983 Dec 24;155(12):420

**Audouard Family**
Chalbert P: Une lignée d'apothicaires et de pharmaciens languedociens: les Audouard, d'Agde, Béziers et Castres. **Rev Hist Pharm (Paris)** 1980 Sep;27(246):175–88

**Audouard, Maxence, 1776–1856**
Chabbert P: Maxence Audouard (1776–1856). In: Congrès National des Sociétés Savantes, 96e, Toulouse, 1971. Comptes Rendus. Paris, 1974. Histoire des Sciences, Tome 1. p. 83–97.

**Auenbrugger, Leopold, 1722–1809**
Landsberger M: Percussion discovered. **Trans Stud Coll Physicians Phila** 1981 Dec;5(3 no 4):255

**Augiéras Family**
Bonnemain H: Une famille médico-pharmaceutique: les Augiéras-Bernou. **Rev Hist Pharm (Paris)** 1981;28(248):14–20

**Augustus II (the Strong), 1670–1733**
Wunderlich P: Die Anfänge der Staatlichen Waisen-Fürsorge in Sachsen unter August dem Starken (Waldheim 1716). **Kinderarztl Prax** 1984 Nov;52(11):510–20

**Augustus III, King of Poland, 1696–1763**
Dudziński W: Choroba i zgon króla Augusta III Sasa. **Wiad Lek** 1981 Sep 1;34(17):1479–84

**Aurach, Georges, fl. 1470**
Aurach G: Le jardin de richesses. Texte calligraphié et préface par B. Biebel. Neuilly-sur-Seine, Arma Artis, 1978. xix, 83 p.

**Aurelianus, Caelius**
Pujol F: L'odontologie à la fin de l'empire romain: Caelius Aurelianus. **Chir Dent Fr** 1984 May 31;54(252):21–5
Vidal F: Caelius Aurelianus et la douleur dentaire: 'de dolore dentium'. **Inf Dent** 1984 Jul 12–19;66(28–29):2875–88

**Auspitz, Heinrich, 1835–1886**
King DF: Modern textbooks of dermatopathology and acantholysis of Auspitz. **J Am Acad Dermatol** 1984 Aug;11(2 Pt 1):301–3

**Auzoux, Louis Thomas Jérome, 1797–1880**
Net echt!: De anatomische wereld van Dr. Auzoux. [Exhibition, Museum Boerhaave, Leiden.] **Tijdschr Geschied Geneeskd** 1981;4(1):50–2

**Avenzoar, d. ca. 1162**
Giran Irueste F: La medicina practica en la España arabe del siglo XII: El 'Kitab al-Yami fi-l-asriba wa-l-Ma ayin de Abu Marwan abd al-Malik ibn Zuhr (Avenzoar). Edicion, traduccion y comentarios. Resumen of Diss. 209. Granada, 1978. 33 p.
Pena Munoz C, Girón Irueste F: Aspectos ineditos de la obra medica de Avenzoar: el prologo del 'Kitab al-Taysir'. Edicion, traduccion y comentarios. **Misc Estud Arabes Hebraicos** 1977;26(1):103–16

**Averroes, 1126–1198**
Barcia Goyanes JJ: Los arabismos en las ediciones latinas del libro I del Colliget de Averroes. **Med Esp** 1984 Jan–Feb;83:9–29
Gracia D: En torno al averroismo medico latino. **Asclepio** 1978–79;30–31:233–64
Peña Muñoz C, ed: Indice de sustancias medicinales citadas en el Kitab al-Kulliyyat de Averroes. Granada, Universidad de Granada, 1980. 18 [20] p. (Estudios del Departamento de Historia de la Farmacia y Legislacion Farmaceutica, 5).

**Avery, Oswald Theodore, 1877–1955**
Bendiner E: Avery: making sense of a 'stupid tetranucleotide'. **Hosp Pract** 1982 Oct;17(10):195, 199, 202–3 passim

**Avicenna, 980?–1037**
Abdullaev AKh, Sharafiddinov TA: Abu Ali Ibn-Sina (Avitsenna) o lepre. **Vestn Dermatol Venerol** 1981 May;(5):76–9
Ammar S: Introduction à l'étude de la médecine arabo-islamique. **Tunis Med** 1980 Jul–Aug;58(4):544–55, 562–77
Arnaldez R: The theory and practice of science according to Ibn Sina and al-Biruni. **Stud Philos Med** 1977 Mar;1(1):58–69
Aroua A: L'hygiène et la prevention chez Ibn Sina. **Tunis Med** 1980 Jul–Aug;58(4):556–61
Aroua A: Hygiene et prevention médicale chez Ibnou Sina (Avicenne). Alger, S.N.E.D., [1974?]. 106 p.
Arzumetov IuS: Voprosy gepatologii v 'Kanone vrachebnoĭ nauki' Ibn-Sina. **Sov Zdravookhr** 1980;(5):67–9
Arzumetov IuS: Ibn Sina--vrach-éntsiklopedist i nekotorye osnovy ego ucheniia o zdorov'e i bolezni (k 1000-letiiu so dnia rozhdeniia). **Fiziol Zh SSSR** 1980 Sep;66(9):1273–7
Asimov MS, et al: Avicenna. **Unesco Cour** 1980 Oct;33:1–46
Asimov MS, et al: [On the 1000th anniversary of Avicenna] (Rus). **Vopr Istor Estestvozn Tekh** 1980,4:69–76
Asimova MZ, Kuznetsov VK, Piotrovskiĭ SM: Abu Ali Ibn-Sina i znachenie ego nauchnogo naslediia v istorii akusherstva. **Feldsher Akush** 1980;45(5):59–61
Atabaev ShT, Babakhodzhaev NK, Il'inskiĭ II: Gigiencheskie vzgliady Abu Ali ibn-Siny (k 1000-letiiu so dnia rozhdeniia). **Gig Sanit** 1979 Dec;(12):36–40
El avicenismo: **Med Tradic** 1980;3(10):33–6
Bano M, Ali MI: Cosmetics according to Avicenna. **Bull Indian Inst Hist Med (Hyderabad)** 1981;1–4:110–7
Bečka J: Otec lékařu Avicenna v naší vědě a kultuře. Abú Alí ibn Síná (980–1037). **Cas Lek Cesk** 1980 Jan 5;119(1):17–23
Belolapotkova AV: Voprosy stomatologii v 'Kanone vrachebnoĭ nauki' Ibn-Siny. **Stomatologiia (Mosk)** 1980 Nov–Dec;59(6):69–70
Belova LV: Znachenie tvochestva Ibn Sina dlia sovremennoĭ meditsiny. **Med Sestra** 1983 Nov;42(11):46–51
Belova LV, Mirakhmedov UM: Vklad Abu Ali ibn-Sina v dermato-venerologiiu. **Vestn Dermatol Venerol** 1983 Dec;(12):60–4
Belova LV: Vklad Abu Ali ibn-Siny v kosmetologiiu. **Sov Zdravookhr** 1984;(9):53–6
Birtalan G: Avicenna Kánonja és az európai orvostudomány. **Orvostort Kozl** 1980;89–91(26 no 1–3):25–43
Brahmaji Rao U: Avicenna's contribution to the understanding of anatomy and pathology of heart. **Bull Indian Inst Hist Med (Hyderabad)** 1981;1–4:91–4
Brandenburg D: Das Portrait des Ibn Sînâ (Avicenna). **Med Welt** 1983 Jun 10;34(23):682–4
Carreras Panchón A: Sobre el concepto de pestilencia (WABA') en el Canon de Avicena. **Asclepio** 1981;33:265–73
Demirhan A: Ibn Sina's canon and some patterns. **Med Bull Istanbul Med Fac** 1979;12:158–62
Denisenko PP, Nuraliev IuN: Abu Ali Ibn-Sina i farmakologiia; k 1000-letiiu so dnia rozhdeniia Avitsenny. **Farmakol Toksikol** 1980 Nov–Dec;43(6):753–4
Durrany KS, Uddin Siddiqui T: Al-Adwiyat al-Qalbiya. **Stud Hist Med** 1980 Mar;4(1):29–38
Durrany KS: Ibn Sinā's concept of man. **Stud Hist Med** 1982 Sep;6(3):161–94
East-west discord over the prince of scholars [Avicenna]: **New Sci** 1981;91:395
Egri B: Arab triangulum **Orv Hetil** 1981 Jun 28;122(26):1595–600
Egri B: Keleti géniusz. Emlékezés Avicennára, születésének 1000. évfordulóján. **Orv Hetil** 1980 Dec 28;121(52):3207–12
En el milenario de Avicena: **Med Tradic** 1980;2(8):5–9
Estestvennye i preformirovannye fizicheskie faktory vo vrachebnoĭ deiatel'nosti Abu-Ali Ibn-Siny (k 1000-letiiu so dnia rozhdneiia): **Vopr Kurortol Fizioter Lech Fiz Kult** 1981 Jan–Feb;(1):64–6
Gracia D, Vidal JL: Avicena, sobre el corazón. In International Congress of the History of Medicine, 27th, Barcelona, 1980. Actas. Barcelona, Académia de Ciències Médiques de Catalunya i Balears, 1981. p. 711–22.
Gracia D, Vidal JL: Avicena, sobre la definición de la medicina. In

International Congress of the History of Medicine, 27th, Barcelona, 1980. Actas. Barcelona, Académia de Ciències Médiques de Catalunya i Balears, 1981. p. 723-30.
Guerra F: The description of syphilis in Avicenna. In International Congress of the History of Medicine, 27th, Barcelona, 1980. Actas. Barcelona, Académia de Ciències Médiques de Catalunya i Balears, 1981. p. 731-3.
Habibullah CM: Avicenna, a physician and his approach to medicine. **Bull Indian Inst Hist Med (Hyderabad)** 1981;1-4:75-7
Haddad FS, Richter-Bernburg L: A hitherto unknown eighth-century commentary on Avicenna's 'Kulliyyat'. **J Hist Arabic Sci** 1980;4:253-8
Hadžiomeragić M: Prikaz znanja o bolestima jezika prije 1000 godina. **Stomatol Vjesn** 1983;12(3-4):147-51
Hijazi AR: L'anesthésie chez Avicenne et les techniques anesthésiques au XIe siècle. **Ann Fr Anesth Reanim** 1984;3(1):76-8
Iqbal Ali M: Contribution of Avicenna to medicine. **Bull Indian Inst Hist Med (Hyderabad)** 1981;1-4:139-45
Iskandar AZ: Another fragment from the autograph of Ibn Al-Tilmidh's 'Marginal commentary on Ibn Sina's Canon of medicine'. **Bull Sch Orient Afr Stud** 1981;44:253-61
Iskhaki IuB, Kal'shteĭn LI: Rol' Abu Ali Ibn-Siny v razvitii otorinolaringologii. **Vestn Otorinolaringol** 1980 Nov-Dec;(6):81-5
Ismail M, Raheem Rafeeq MA: Anatomy of eye and the mechanism of vision according to Avicenna. **Bull Indian Inst Hist Med (Hyderabad)** 1981;1-4:146-51
Kahle E: Avicenna (Ibn Sina) über Kinderkrankheiten im Kinderregimen seines Qanun. Erlangen, Verlagsbuchhandlung Hannelore Lüling, 1979. 53, [14] p.
Kahle E: Das Ammenregimen des Avicenna (Ibn Sina) in seinem Qanun. Erlangen, Verlagsbuchhandlung Hannelore Lüling, 1980. 45, [13] p.
Kâhya E: Renal calculi and their treatment in Ibn Sina. In International Congress of the History of Medicine, 27th, Barcelona, 1980. Actas. Barcelona, Académia de Ciències Médiques de Catalunya i Balears, 1981. p. 734-8.
Kakhorov GK: Gigienicheskie vzgliady Avitsenny. **Feldsher Akush** 1984 Feb;49(2):52
Katsenovich RA, Mirzaev NL: Kardiologicheskoe nasledie Abu Ali Ibn-Siny (k 1000-letiu so dnia rozhdeniia). **Kardiologiia** 1980 Nov;20(11):120-2
Khadri SK: 'Shaik -al - Rais' Abu Ali Ibn Sina (Avicenna) and his contribution to the science and art of medicine. **Bull Indian Inst Hist Med (Hyderabad)** 1981;1-4:130-8
Khaleefathullah S: Avicenna as a physician and medical writer. **Bull Indian Inst Hist Med (Hyderabad)** 1981;1-4:123-9
Kottek SS, Metzger M, Metzger T: Manuscrits hebraiques décorés ou illustrés du Canon d'Avicenne. In International Congress of the History of Medicine, 27th, Barcelona, 1980. Actas. Barcelona, Académia de Ciències Médiques de Catalunya i Balears, 1981. p. 739-45.
Kucharz E: Avicenna (Abu Ali Ibn Sina) - życie i działalność Lekarska. **Wiad Lek** 1981 Aug 15;34(16):1405-9
Kuz'min MK, Bukharov PL: Ibn-Sina (Avitsenna) i narodnaia meditsina. **Feldsher Akush** 1981;46(3):50-2
Lakshmipathi G: Avicenna on ear, nose and throat diseases. **Bull Indian Inst Hist Med (Hyderabad)** 1981;1-4:79-82
Leibowitz JO: Ibn Sina in Hebrew. **Koroth** 1981;8(1-2):3-8
Ley H: Ibn Sina (Avicenna, 980-1037): Gründe für 1000 Jahre Rückerinnerung. **Dtsch Z Philos** 1980;28(11):1309-23
Mansursov KhKh: Vrachebnoe nasledie Ibn-Siny i sovremennaia klinicheskaia meditsina. **Ter Arkh** 1980;52(11):149-51
Marmura ME: Avicenna on the division of the sciences in the 'Isagoge' of his 'Shifa'. **J Hist Arabic Sci** 1980;4:239-51
Mihic DN: Die erste orotracheale Intubation. **Anaesthesist** 1983 Sep;32(9):450-1
Moshkov VA: Abu Ali Ibn-Sina (Avitsenna) o fizicheskikh uprazhneniiakh i massazhe. **Vopr Kurortol Fizioter Lech Fiz Kult** 1981 Jan-Feb;(1):66-7
Muhammad U: Avicenna as a clinician. **Bull Indian Inst Hist Med (Hyderabad)** 1981;1-4:87-90
Mukhitdinov BN: Eticheskie printsipy Abu Ali Ibn-Siny (Avitsenny) i voprosy sovremennoĭ deontologii (k 1000-letiiu so dnia rozhdeniia). **Vestn Rentgenol Radiol** 1980 May-Jun;(3):80-2
Mukhtarov AM, Bolgarskiĭ IS: Voprosy urologii v trudakh Abu Ali Ibn-Siny. **Urol Nefrol (Mosk)** 1980 Nov-Dec;(6):52-5
Musaev TM: Vzgliady Abu Ali Ibn Siny (Avitsenny) na opukholevye zabolevaniia. **Vopr Onkol** 1980;26(9):72-4
Nuralev IuN: Abu Ali Ibn-Sina i voprosy vrachebnoĭ étiki. **Klin Med (Mosk)** 1980 Oct;58(10):112-4
Nuseibeh S: Avicenna: medicine and scepticism. **Koroth** 1981;8(1-2):9-20
Omirov RIu, Mardanov LM: Nekotorye voprosy khirurgii v trudakh Abu Ali Ibn Siny (k 1000-letiiu so dnia rozhdeniia). **Klin Khir** 1980 Mar;(3):66-8
Petrov BD: Voprosy okhrany zdorov'ia v 'Kanone' Ibn-Siny (k 1000-letiiu so dnia rozhdeniia). **Gig Sanit** 1980 May;(5):22-5
Petrov BD: Diagnostika v sisteme meditsinskikh vzgliadov Ibn Siny. **Klin Med (Mosk)** 1979 Dec;57(12):91-6
Petrov BD: Meditsinskoe nasledie Ibn-Siny. **Sov Zdravookhr** 1980;(9):53-6
Petrov BD: Ibn-Sina--Avitsenna (K 1000-letiiu so dnia rozhdeniia). **Med Sestra** 1980 Aug;39(8):45-51
Petrov BD: Study on the medical heritage of Avicenna (Ibn Sina). In E. Schultheisz, ed: History of physiology. Oxford, Elmsford, New York, Pergamon, 1981. xvi, 208 p. (Advances in Physiological Sciences. Proceedings of the 28th International Congress of Physiological Sciences, Budapest, 1980. Volume 21). p. 49-51.
Petrov BD: Study of Ibn Sina's medical heritage. In International Congress of the History of Medicine, 27th, Barcelona, 1980. Actas. Barcelona, Académia de Ciències Médiques de Catalunya i Balears, 1981. p. 746-9.
Pulatov AM: Abuali Ibn-Sina (Avitsenna) i ego nauchno-meditsinskoe nasledie. **Vrach Delo** 1980 Sep;(9):1-6
Rahman F: Essence and existence in Ibn Sina: the myth and the reality. **Hamdard** 1981;4(1):3-14
Rahman SA: Avicenna on digestion of food. **Bull Indian Inst Hist Med (Hyderabad)** 1981;1-4:59-63
Rahman Baig MA: Avicenna's principles of dietetics. **Bull Indian Inst Hist Med (Hyderabad)** 1981;1-4:95-8
Rama Rao GS: Contribution of Avicenna in therapeutics reflecting on modern medicine. **Bull Indian Inst Hist Med (Hyderabad)** 1981;1-4:118-22
Rasheed BM: Avicenna's influence on European medicine. **Bull Indian Inst Hist Med (Hyderabad)** 1981;1-4:99-102
Richler B: Manuscripts of Avicenna's Kanon in Hebrew translation: a revised and up-to-date list. **Koroth** 1982 Aug;8(3/4):145-68
Said HM: Zuviel Erfolg für Avicenna? **Med Welt** 1981 Sep 25;32(39):62-3
Sankaran JR: Avicenna's thoughts and concepts of the pulse (sphygmology). **Bull Indian Inst Hist Med (Hyderabad)** 1981;1-4:64-74
Schultheisz E: Avicenna és a psychosomatika gyökerei. **Orv Hetil** 1980 Dec 28;121(52):3171-3
Shamansurov SS, Madzhidova AT: Ibn-Sina i bolezni detskogo vozrasta. **Pediatriia** 1980 Jul;(7):70-1
Sharma OA: Avicenna's description of tuberculosis. **Bull Indian Inst Hist Med (Hyderabad)** 1981;1-4:83-6
Shetty PS: A critical analysis of Avicenna's contribution to physiology. **Bull Indian Inst Hist Med (Hyderabad)** 1981;1-4:152-60
Shvabe IuIa: Voprosy travmatologii v trudakh Ibn-Siny (Avitsenny). **Ortop Travmatol Protez** 1979 Sep;(9):68-70
Shvabe IuIa: Lechenie travmaticheskikh povrezhdeniĭ v trudakh Ibn-Siny (Avitsenny) (k 1000-letiiu so dnia rozhdeniia Abu Ali Ibn-Siny). **Feldsher Akush** 1980;45(8):47-8
Smith RD: Avicenna and the Canon of Medicine: a millennial tribute. **West J Med** 1980 Oct;133(4):367-70
Smith RD: Tribute to Avicenna: one thousand years of the art of preserving health. **J Kans Med Soc** 1981;82:359-60, 372
Terzioglu A: Zur Avicenna (Ibn Sina) - Forschung in der Türkei. In International Congress of the History of Medicine, 27th, Barcelona, 1980. Actas. Barcelona, Académia de Ciències Médiques de Catalunya i Balears, 1981. p. 750-5.
Théodoridès J: Ibn Sina et la rage. In International Congress of the History of Medicine, 27th, Barcelona, 1980. Actas. Barcelona, Académia de Ciències Médiques de Catalunya i Balears, 1981. p. 756-60.
Tirmizi SM: Ibn Sina as a scientist. **Stud Hist Med** 1981 Sep;5(3):233-8
Tóth A: Avicenna-kötet a keszthelyi Helikon Könyvtárban. Velencei kiadás, 1564. **Orv Hetil** 1980 Dec 28;121(52):3212-3
Tratner E: 1. Tracheotomy in the Hebrew translation of Ibn-Sina. 2. Intubation mentioned in the Talmud and by Jacob Ben Asher (14th Century). **Koroth** 1983 Aug;8(7-8):333-8
Uddinahmed R: Single drugs mentioned by Avicenna for cardiac ailments in his canon and Kitab-Ul-Adwiyyah Qalbiyyah. **Bull Indian Inst Hist Med (Hyderabad)** 1979;9:46-66
Ushida N: Etude comparative de la psychologie d'Aristote, d'Avicenne et de St. Thomas d'Aquin. Tokyo, Keio Institute of Cultural and Linguistic Studies, 1968. vi, 231 p. (Studies in the humanities and social relations; v. 11.).
Usmanova RA: Fiziologiia pishchevareniia v trudakh Ibn Siny. **Fiziol Zh SSSR** 1980 Sep;66(9):1424-8
Usmanova RA: Ibn Sina o Kostnoĭ i myshechnoĭ sisteme. **Arkh Anat Gistol Embriol** 1980 Sep;79(9):112-4
Vakhidov VV: K 1000-letiiu Avitsenny. **Khirurgiia (Mosk)** 1980 Jul;(7):110-4
Van Riet S, ed: Avicenna Latinus. Liber de philosophia prima sive scientia divina, I-IV. Louvain, Peeters; Leiden, Brill, 1977. 225 p.
Viesca Trevino C: La medicina de Avicena. **Med Tradic** 1980;3(9):45-52
Viesca Treviño C: El avicenismo. **Med Tradic** 1980;3(10):33-6
Wahab Zuhuri MA: Influence on Ibn Sina on Unani medicine in subsequent ages. **Bull Indian Inst Hist Med (Hyderabad)** 1981;1-4:103-9
Weisser U: Beiträge Ibn Sina's zur Kenntnis der weiblichen Genitalien und zur Embryologie. Eine kritische Betrachtung. In International Congress of the History of Medicine, 27th, Barcelona, 1980. Actas. Barcelona, Académia de Ciències Médiques de Catalunya i Balears, 1981. p. 761-5.
Weisser U: Ibn Sina und die Medizin des arabisch-islamischen Mittelalters - Alte und neue Urteile und Vorurteile. **Medizinhist J** 1983;18(4):283-305

Willemot J: Le nez et la gorge dans le poème de la médecine et le premier livre du Canon d'Avicenne. In International Congress of the History of Medicine, 27th, Barcelona, 1980. Actas. Barcelona, Académia de Ciències Médiques de Catalunya i Balears, 1981. p. 766–70.
Zedler BH: The prince of physicians on the nature of man. **Mod Schoolman** 1978;55(2):165–77
14L 1000-letiiu so dnia rozhdenii a Abu Ali Ibn-Siny (980–1037): **Zh Nevropatol Psikhiatr** 1980;80(8):1221–8

**Axhausen, Georg, 1877–**
Taubert E: Das chirurgische Erbe. Das Wirken Georg Axhausens an der Chirurgischen Klinik der Charité--Berlin. **Zentralbl Chir** 1983;108(14):913–7

**Aykroyd, Wallace Ruddell, 1899–1979**
Passmore R. Obituary Notice. Wallace Ruddell Aykroyd, CBE, MD, ScD (30 July 1899–7 February 1979). **Br J Nutr** 1980 Mar;43(2):245–50

**Aziz al-Din**
Chandpuri K: Hakim Aziz al-Din; foreign minister of the Sikh kingdom. **Stud Hist Med** 1979 Sep;3(3):178–80

## B

**Babar, Emperor of Hindostan, 1483–1530**
Beg MH: Zaheeruddin Mohammad Babar. **JPMA** 1981;31(5):114–7

**Babel, Isaac, 1894–1941**
Mendelson G, Mendelson D: Psychological aspects of bronchial asthma in the writings of Isaac Babel. **Isr J Psychiatr Relat Sci** 1981;18(1):31–9

**Babes, Victor, 1854–1926**
Babes V: Opere alese. Vol. I. Bucuresti, Editura Academiei Republicii Socialiste Romania, 1979. 330 p. Biographical contributions by B. Dutescu, N. Marcu, and I. Moraru
Babeş VT: Some less well-known priorities of Victor Babeş. **Virologie** 1979 Jul–Sep;30(3):235–6
Calciu M: La 125 de ani de la naşterea lui V. Babes (1854–1979). contribuţiile lui Victor Babes la edificarea ftiziologiei ştiinţifice. **Rev Ig [Pneumoftiziol]** 1979 Jul–Sep;28(3):187–91
Negru I: Concepţia profesorului Victor Babeş asupra instruirii şi formării agentului sanitar. **Viata Med [Medii Sanit]** 1983 Sep;31(9):211–4
On the 125th anniversary of Victor Babeş birth: **Virologie** 1979 Jul–Sep;30(3):169–70

**Babinski, Joseph François Félix, 1857–1932**
Cohn DF: Joseph Babinski and his reflex (1857–1932). **Koroth** 1982 Aug;8(3/4):191–4
Kenéz J: Joseph Babinski (1857–1932) a francia klinikai neurológia egyik úttörője. **Orv Hetil** 1984 Jan 22;125(4):222–7
Sternbach G: Joseph Babinski: the phenomenon of the toes. **J Emerg Med** 1984;1(3):263–6

**Babits, Mihály, 1883–1941**
Bíró I: Babits Mihály szenvedései. **Orv Hetil** 1983 Nov 27;124(48):2937–9
Gyenes G: Adatok Babits betegségéhez. **Orv Hetil** 1983 Nov 27;124(48):2942–6
Gyenes G: Adatok Babits Mihaly betegségéhez. **Orvostort Kozl** 1981;93–96(27 No 1–4):193–200
Szállási A: Babits betegségei a tracheotomia elött. **Orv Hetil** 1981 Sep 6;122(36):2235–9
Szállási A: Babits betegségei. **Orv Hetil** 1983 Nov 27;124(48):2940–2

**Babmindra, Viktor Petrovich, 1923–**
Viktor Petrovich Babmindra (k 60-letiiu so dnia rozhdeniia): **Arkh Anat Gistol Embriol** 1983 Oct;85(10):102–4

**Bach, Edward, 1886–1936**
Weeks N: The medical discoveries of Edward Bach, physician. New Canaan, Conn., Keats, 1973. 141 p.

**Bacharach, Alfred Louis, 1891–1966**
Pyke M: Alfred Louis Bacharach. In Dictionary of national biography, 1961–1970. Suppl. 8, 1981, p. 59–60.

**Bachelard, Gaston, 1884?–1962**
Yáñez Cortés RJ: La intervención de conceptos psicoanalíticos en el pensamiento epistemológico de Gastón Bachelard. **Acta Psiquiatr Psicol Am Lat** 1979 Jun;25(2):135–41

**Bachmann, Christian Ludwig, 1763–1813**
Isliker B: Christian Ludwig Bachmanns Dissertation 'Uber die Wirkungen der Musik auf den Menschen' (Erlangen 1792). Zürich, Juris Druck, 1982. 76 p. (Zürcher Medizingeschichtliche Abhandlungen, Neue Reihe, Nr. 154).

**Bacon, Francis, 1561–1626**
Bloch H: Francis Bacon (1561–1626), his interest and influence in education, science, and medicine. **NY State J Med** 1981 Jun;81(7):1120–2
Gregory RL: Bacon's last egg?--the Exploratory. **Perception** 1982;11(4):371–5
Klein J: Sir Francis Bacon's 'Valerius Terminus' (1603). **Sudhoffs Arch** 1982;66(1):38–69
Koch CH: Petrus Severinus, Francis Bacon og Naturiagttagelsen. **Dan Medicinhist Arbog** 1979;161–72

**Bacq, Zénon M., 1903–1983**
Lecomte J: Apologie de Zénon Bacq 1903–1983. **Rev Med Liege** 1983 Sep 1;38(17):627–30

**Bacsó, Bálint, 1789–1855**
Varga P: Bacsó Bálint debreceni orvos-gyógyszerész élete és munkássága. **Orvostort Kozl** 1982;28(1–3):155–67

**Badelard, Philippe-Louis-François, 1728–1802**
Bernier J: Philippe-Louis-François Badelard. In Dictionary of Canadian biography, 1801 to 1820. Volume 5, 1983. p. 46–7.

**Badger, John, fl. 1683**
Whittet TD: John Badger, apothecaryite. **Pharm Hist (London)** 1973 May;3(1):2–4

**Badger, Robert, 1829–**
Robinson HS: Robert and Roderick Badger, pioneer Georgia dentists. **Negro Hist Bull** 1961;24(4):77–80

**Badger, Roderick, 1834–1890**
Robinson HS: Robert and Roderick Badger, pioneer Georgia dentists. **Negro Hist Bull** 1961;24(4):77–80

**Badiano, Juan, fl. 16th cent.**
Bárcena A, Barrera A, Ruiz E, et al: Interpretación etnobotánica de la iconografía del Códice de la Cruz-Badiano. **An Soc Mex Hist Cienc Tec** 1979;5:35–48

**Badurski, Andrzej, 1740–1789**
Lejman K: Andrzej Badurski (1740–1789) jako założyciel szpitala akademickiego i inicjator klinicznego nauczania meydycyny. **Przegl Lek** 1981;38(7):567–70

**Baelz, Erwin, 1849–1913**
Matsuki A: [Current findings on the studies of the history of anesthesiology (8) -- Erwin Von Baelz and obstetrical anesthesia] (Jpn). **Masui** 1980 Mar;29(3):287–90
Matsuki A: [Erwin von Baelz as a pioneer in obstetrical anaesthesia in Japan.] (Jpn). **Nihon I-Shigaku Zasshi** 1981;27(1):47–55

**Baer, Karl Ernst von, 1792–1876**
Baer KE von: Reden gehalten in wissenschaftlichen Versammlungen und kleinere Aufsätze vermischten Inhalts. With an introduction by K. B. Sterling. New York, Arno Press, 1978. Three volumes in two. (Reprint. St. Petersburg, 1864/1876/1873).
Mikhaĭlov VP: Nikolaĭ Varnek i Karl Bér. **Arkh Anat Gistol Embriol** 1982 Apr;82(4):86–95

**Baer, William Stevenson, 1872–1931**
Harvey AM: Orthopaedic surgery at Johns Hopkins: a heritage of excellence in clinical practice, training and research. **Johns Hopkins Med J** 1982 Jun;150(6):221–45

**Bagdasar, Dimitrie, 1893–1946**
Niculescu SI: Pe marginea corespondenţei dintre Harvey Cushing şi Dumitru Bagdasar. **Rev Med Interna [Neurol Psihiatr]** 1981 Jul–Sep;26(3):229–33

**Bagley, William Chandler, 1874–1946**
Cole RA, Rudnicky AI: What's new in speech perception? The research and ideas of William Chandler Bagley, 1874–1946. **Psychol Rev** 1983 Jan;90(1):94–101

**Baglivi, Giorgio, 1668?–1707?**
Olagüe G: La 'teoria fibrilar' en la obra de Giorgio Baglivi (1668–1707). Introduccion, traduccion de los capitulos I y II del libro I de su specimen Quatuor librorum de fibra motrice et morbosa (Perusa, 1700), y notas. **Morfol Norm Patol** 1979;3:335–56

**Bagration, P. I.**
Popov MIa: Ranenie i smert' bagrationa. **Vopr Istor** 1975;(3):211–4

**Bailey, Harriet**
Church OM, Buckwalter KC: Harriet Bailey---a psychiatric nurse pioneer. **Perspect Psychiatr Care** 1980 Mar–Apr;18(2):62–6

**Bailey, Jacob Whitman, 1811–1857**
Edgar RK: An annotated bibliography of the American microscopist and diatomist Jacob Whitman Bailey (1811–1857). **Occas Pap Farlow Herb Cryptogam Bot Harv Univ** 1977;11:1–26

**Bailey, Liberty Hyde, 1858–1954**
MacRoberts MH: L. H. Bailey's citations to Gregor Mendel. **J Hered** 1984 Nov–Dec;75(6):500–1

**Bailey, Percival Sylvester, 1892–**
Cain AM, ed: A catalog of the Percival Bailey collection of neurology & psychiatry. Chicago, Library of the Health Sciences, University of Illinois at the Medical Center, Chicago, 1973. viii, 230 p.
Handa H: [Percival Bailey (author's transl)] (Jpn). **No Shinkei Geka** 1981 Mar;9(4):538–41

**Baillie, Matthew, 1761–1823**
Attwood HD: Matthew Baillie--a possible early description of amniotic fluid embolism. **Aust NZ J Obstet Gynaecol** 1979 Aug;19(3):176–7
Crainz F: The editions and translations of Dr. Matthew Baillie's Morbid Anatomy. **Med Hist** 1982 Oct;26(4):443–52

**Bailly, Nicolas, 1817–1907**
Trocme C: L'atélectasie découverte et délaissée: Claude-Auguste Reynaud et Nicolas Bailly. **Hist Sci Med** 1979;13(4):441–50

**Baintner, Ferenc, 1805–1883**
Leblancné Kelemen M: Adalékok a reformkori Nógrád megye egészségügyi helyzetéröl Baintner Ferenc megyei föorvos jelentései alapján. **Orvostort Kozl** 1979;87–88(25 no 1–2):269–75

**Bairati, Angelo, 1901 or 11–**
Bairati A: Ultrastructure of the protoplasm. The 'pioneer' work by A. Bairati and F. E. Lehmann revisited. **J Submicrosc Cytol** 1981 Apr;13(2):117–25

**Baker, Burton Lowell, 1912–1978**
Knigge KM: Burton Lowell Baker 1912–1978. **Am J Anat** 1980 Aug;158(4):391–4

**Baker, Edward, 1818–1902**
Searle CG: A soldier pharmacist. **Pharm Hist (London)** 1974 Jan;4(1):2–3

**Baker, William Morrant, 1839–1896**
Hershman MJ: William Morrant Baker (1839–1896). **Int J Dermatol** 1980 Sep;19(7):409–12

**Bakewell, Robert Hall, 1831–1908**
Wright-St Clair RE: Robert Hall Bakewell, letter writer. **NZ Med J** 1982 Nov 24;95(720):820–2

**Balassa, János, 1814–1868**
Csillag I: Elfelejtett kórházak nyomában. Balassa és Semmelweis a régi zsidó kórházban. **Orv Hetil** 1981 Feb 22;122(8):463–5
Robicsek F, Littmann L: The first reported case of external heart massage (János Balassa). **Clin Cardiol** 1983 Nov;6(11):569, 571
Vas G, Hidvégi J: Balassa érsebészeti munkásságáról. **Orv Hetil** 1983 Mar 20;124(12):709–10

**Baldwin, James Mark, 1861–1934**
Continenza B: L'effetto Baldwin. **Stor Crit Psicol** 1982 Dec;3(2):335–42

**Baldwin, William, 1779–1819**
Ewan J: Five pupils of Benjamin Smith Barton: the men and their minds. **Trans Stud Coll Physicians Phila** 1983 Dec;5(5 no 4):309–20

**Balint, Michael, 1896–**
Dervin D: Michael Balint's contributions to the psychoanalysis of literature. **Psychoanal Rev** 1979–80 Winter;66(4):553–70
Sutherland JD: The British object relations theorists: Balint, Winnicott, Fairbairn, Guntrip. **J Am Psychoanal Assoc** 1980;28(4):829–60

**Balogh, Kálmán, 1853–1888**
Kerekes L: Miért vallott kudarcot Balogh Kálmán, a bakteriológia magyar úttörője? **Orvostort Kozl** 1982;28(1–3):65–85

**Balser, Georg Friedrich Wilhelm, 1780–1846**
Handrack C: Georg Friedrich Wilhelm Balser (1780–1846). Giessen, Schmitz, 1979. 388 p. (Arbeiten zur Geschichte der Medizin in Giessen, 2).

**Baltar Domínguez, Ramón, 1902–1981**
Ramón Baltar Domínguez: **Rev Esp Enferm Apar Dig** 1981 Oct;60(4):413–5

**Balzac, Honoré de, 1799–1850**
Balzac et la médecine de son temps: [Paris], Maison de Balzac, [1976?]. [98] p.
Bonalumi F: Il medico di Balzac e il curato di Ravizza. **Aevum** 1979;53(3):519–32
Mainetti JA: Leyendo con Freud La peau de chagrin de Balzac. **Asclepio** 1982;34:265–81
Rossier A: Une jalousie mortelle (Honoré de Balzac). **Ann Pediatr (Paris)** 1981 Apr;28(4):298–300
Rossier A: L'enfant maudit. **Ann Pediatr (Paris)** 1980 Mar;27(3):195–6

**Bancroft, Jessie Hubbell, 1867–1952**
Remley ML: Jessie Hubbell Bancroft. In: Notable American women. The modern period. Cambridge, Mass., Belknap-Harvard Univ. Press, 1980. 4:46–7.

**Bandeira, Manuel, 1886–1968**
Montenegro TH: A tuberculose na vida e obra de Manuel Bandeira. **Interam Rev Bibliogr** 1969;19(3):278–300

**Bandurska, Halina**
Czapska I, Kamińska A: Whołdzie najlepszym (Halina Bandurska). **Pieleg Polozna** 1983;(5):27, 31

**Bánfihunyadi, János, d. 1646**
Gömöri G: Bejegyzések Bánfihunyadi János oxfordi bibliájában és adalekok Angliai működéséhez. **Magyar Könyvsz** 1978;94(1):93–9

**Bang, Bernhard, 1848–1932**
Bang F: From a visit in America. **Hist Med Vet** 1979;4(2):25–30

**Banks, Joseph, 1743–1820**
Lyte C: Sir Joseph Banks, 18th century explorer, botanist and entrepreneur. London, David & Charles, 1980. 248 p.
Meynell G: Banks papers in the Kent Archives Offices, including notebooks by Joseph Banks and Francis Bauer. **Arch Nat Hist** 1981;10(1):77–88
Smith E: The life of Sir Joseph Banks. New York, Arno Press, 1975. xvi, 348 p.

**Banting, Frederick Grant, 1891–1941**
Bliss M, ed: Banting's, Best's, and Collip's accounts of the discovery of insulin. **Bull Hist Med** 1982;56(4):554–68
Dr. Frederick Banting getting out of town: **Can Med Assoc J** 1984 May 1;130(9):1215–23
Jain KM, Swan KG, Casey KF: Nobel prize winners in surgery. Part 3. (Frederick Grant Banting, Walter Rudolph Hess). **Am Surg** 1982 Jul;48(7):287–90
Katz S: A new, informal glimpse of Dr. Frederick Banting. **Can Med Assoc J** 1983 Dec 1;129(11):1229–32
Krosnick A: The art of Banting. **J Med Soc NJ** 1984 Feb;81(2):138–9
Pitt B: Insulin. **Br Herit** 1981;2(3):28–38
Quinn KF: Banting and his biographers: maker of miracles, makers of myth. **Queens Q** 1982;89(2):243–59
Rafter GW: Banting and Best and the sources of useful knowledge. **Perspect Biol Med** 1983 Winter;26(2):281–6
Shortt SE: Banting, insulin and the question of simultaneous discovery. **Queens Q** 1982;89(2):260–73
Vipond M: A Canadian hero of the 1920s: Dr. Frederick G. Banting. **Can Hist Rev** 1982;63(4):461–86

**Bao Qianguang, fl. 310–363**
Zeng Shixin: Bao Gu, the distinguished woman physician of the Jin Dynasty. **Chung Hua I Shih Tsa Chih** 1981;11:75–7

**Baptista, José María, 1908–**
Palabras pronunciadas por el doctor Mario Mazzei Uzcategui, con motivo de la colocacion del retrato del doctor Josa Maria Baptista, en la sede de la Sociedad Venezolana de Historia de la Medicina, en Caracas. Sesion del 8 de febrero de 1972.: **Rev Soc Venez Hist Med** 1972–73;20–21(34–35):41–9

**Bárány, Robert, 1876–1936**
Diamant H: Robert Bárány och Nobel-priset. **Sydsven Medicinhist Sallsk Arsskr** 1984;21:123–8
Jain KM, Swan KG, Casey KF: Nobel Prize winner in surgery. Part 2. **Am Surg** 1982 May;48(5):191–6
Pappas DG: Barany's History of Vestibular Physiology. Translation and commentary. **Ann Otol Rhinol Laryngol [Suppl]** 1984 Mar–Apr;110:1–16
Torok N: Robert Bárány. **JAMA** 1980 Dec 5;244(22):2520

**Barbeau, Victor, 1896–**
Trépanier P: Victor Barbeau et Albiny Paquette. **Action Natl** 1978;68(4):324–30

**Barber, Marshall Albert, 1868–1953**
Terreros DA, Grantham JJ: Marshall Barber and the origins of micropipette methods. **Am J Physiol** 1982 Mar;242(3):F293–6

**Barbot, Jean, 1655–1713**
Hair PE: A note on Jean Barbot (1655–1713). **Proc Huguenot Soc Lond** 1981;23:295–308

**Barchusen, Johann Conrad, 1666–1723**
Jüttner G: Ein 'Pharmacopoeus spagyricus': Johann Conrad Barkhausen (1666–1723) und die Pharmazie. In Dilg P, et al., ed: Perspektiven der Pharmaziegeschichte. Graz, Austria, Akademische Druck- u. Verlagsanstalt, 1983. p. 147–64.

**Barcroft, Joseph, 1872–1947**
Eskes TK: Classic illustrations: Researches on prenatal life. **Eur J Obstet Gynecol Reprod Biol** 1981 May;11(6):435–6

**Bardadin, Tadeusz**
Waspomnienie pósmiertne o prof. dr med. Tadeuszu Bardadinie.: **Otolaryngol Pol** 1980;34(1):I–VI

**Bardeleben, Karl Heinrich von, 1849–1919**
Linss W: Karl von Bardeleben--der Begründer des 'Anatomischen Anzeigers'. **Anat Anz** 1981;150(1–2):5–10

**Bargmann, Wolfgang, 1906–1978**
Fleischhauer K: In memoriam Wolfgang Bargmann. **Anat Anz** 1979;146(8):209–34

**Barker, Edward John, 1799–1884**
Spurr JW: Edward John Barker. In Dictionary of Canadian biography, 1881–1890. 1982;11:47–9.

**Barlaeus, Caspar, 1584–1648**
Van der Horst K: Inventaire de la correspondance de Caspar Barlaeus (1602–1648). Assen, Van Gorcum, 1978. 214 p.

**Barlow, Thomas, 1845–1945**
Evans PR: Infantile scurvy: the centenary of Barlow's disease. **Br Med J [Clin Res]** 1983 Dec 17;287(6408):1862–3

**Barnardo, Thomas John, 1845–1905**
Montague L: Ambassadors of the king. **Nurs Times** 1983 Dec 14–20;79(50):57–60

**Barnes, Djuna, 1892–1982**
Fuchs M: Dr. Matthew O'Connor: the unhealthy healer of Djuna Barnes's Nightwood. In Jones AH, ed: Images of healers. Albany, State University of New York Press, 1983. p. 125–34.

**Barneveld, Willem van, 1747–1826**
Snelders HA: The Amsterdam pharmacist Willem van Barneveld (1747–1826) and the discovery of photosynthesis (1778). **Janus** 1981;68:1–14

**Barnhill, John Finch, 1865–1943**
Barnhill JF: An epoch of medical education. **Indiana Med Hist Q** 1975;3(1):53–63

**Barnum, Sanford Christie, 1838–1885**
Abrams RA, Drake CW, Segal H: Dr. Sanford C. Barnum and the invention of the rubber dam. **Gen Dent** 1982 Jul–Aug;30(4):320–2

**Barraquer Roviralta, Lluis, 1855–1928**
Barraquer i Bordás L, Gutiérrez Gómez D: En el centenario de la neurología clínica española. **Arch Neurobiol (Madr)** 1982 Mar–Apr;45(2):157–62

**Barreda, Gabino, 1818–1881**
Somolinos-Palencia J: Gabino Barreda, el educador. **Gac Med Mex** 1981 Sep;117(9):377–81

**Barrès, Auguste Maurice, 1862–1923**
Baumont M: Maurice Barrès et les morts de la guerre de 1914–18. **Inf Hist** 1969;31(1):30–5

**Barrett, Michael, 1816–1887**
Craig GM: Michael Barrett. In Dictionary of Canadian biography, 1881–1890. 1982;11:53–4.

**Barrios, Juan de, fl. 1590–1610**
Comas J: Influencia de la farmacopea y terapéutica indígenas de Nueva España en la obra de Juan de Barrios (1607). **An Antropol** 1971;8:125–50

**Barry, James, 1795–1865**
Smith KM: Dr. James Barry: military man--or woman? **Can Med Assoc J** 1982 Apr 1;126(7):854–7

**Barthez, Paul Joseph, 1734–1806**
Di Trocchio F: Paul-Joseph Barthez e l' 'Encyclopédie'. **Physis** 1980;22(3–4):379–92

**Bartholin, Thomas, 1616–1680**
Gysel C: Thomas Bartholinus (1616–1680–1980), zijn nederlandse relaties en de tandheelkunde (II). **Ned Tijdschr Tandheelkd** 1982 Oct;89(10):414–9
Gysel C: Thomas Bartholinus (1616–1680–1980), zijn Zederlandse relaties en de tandheelkunde (I). **Ned Tijdschr Tandheelkd** 1982 Jan;89(1):39–43

**Bartholomaeus Anglicus, fl. 1230–1250**
Bitterling K: Zwei bisher unbeachtete Fragmente der mittelenglischen Uebersetzung von Bartholomaeus Anglicus, 'De rerum proprietatibus'. **Neuphilol Mitt** 1977;78:47–56
Seymour MC, et al, ed: On the properties of things. John Trevisa's translation of Bartholomaeus Anglicus De proprietatibus rerum. A critical text. 2 vols. Oxford, Oxford University Press, 1975. xix, 1397 p.

**Bartholow, Roberts, 1831–1904**
Holmes GL: Roberts Bartholow. In search of anatomic localization. **NY State J Med** 1982 Feb;82(2):238–41
Morgan JP: The first reported case of electrical stimulation of the human brain. **J Hist Med Allied Sci** 1982 Jan;37(1):51–64

**Bartisch, Georg, 1535–1606**
Albert DM: 400th anniversary of Batisch's Der Augendienst. **Arch Ophthalmol** 1983 Dec;101(12):1857
Stefani FH, Riedel K: 400 Jahre Augendienst von George Bartisch (1535–1606). **Klin Monatsbl Augenheilkd** 1984 Jan;184(1):64–5

**Bartlett, Edwin Lewis, 1904–1968**
Naske CM: Bob Bartlett and the Alaska Mental Health Act. **Pac Northwest Q** 1980;71(1):31–9

**Bartlett, Frederick Charles, 1886–1969**
Broadbent DE: Sir Frederic Charles Bartlett. In Dictionary of national biography, 1961–1970. Suppl. 8, 1981. p. 77–9.

**Bartlett, Josiah, 1729–1795**
Mevers FC, ed: The papers of Josiah Bartlett, Hanover, University Press of New England, for the New Hampshire Historical Society, 1979. xxxvii, 477 p.

**Bartók, Béla, 1881–1945**
Böhme G: Medizinische Porträts berühmter Komponisten: Wolfgang Amadeus Mozart, Ludwig van Beethoven, Carl Maria von Weber, Frédéric Chopin, Peter Iljitsch Tschaikowski, Béla Bartók. 2. verbesserte und erweiterte Auflage. Stuttgart, New York, Gustav Fischer Verlag, 1981. xi, 199 p.
Kerner D: Béla Bartóks Tod in New York. Zu seinem 100. Geburtstag am 25. März 1981. **MMW** 1981 Mar 27;123(13):525–9

**Bartolotti, Gian Giacomo, ca. 1470–ca. 1530**
Kapronczay K: Két kevéssé ismert 15. századi orvostörténeti munka. **Orv Hetil** 1983 Jul 10;124(28):1701–5
Schupbach W: Doctor Parma's medicinal macaronic: poem by Bartolotti, pictures by Giorgione and Titian. [Wellcome MS 461]. **J Warburg Courtauld Inst** 1978;41:147–91, 350

**Barton, Benjamin Smith, 1766–1815**
Ewan J: Five pupils of Benjamin Smith Barton: the men and their minds. **Trans Stud Coll Physicians Phila** 1983 Dec;5(5 no 4):309–20

**Barton, Clarissa Harlowe, 1821–1912**
Gilbo PF: Candid 'cranky' Clara Barton gave us the Red Cross. **Smithsonian** 1981;12(2):126–42
Hanron J: Nursing revisited: Clarissa Harlow Barton. **Mass Nurse** 1983 Sep;52(9):9, 27
Stewart S: Sharing more than marble palaces. **DAR Mag** 1981;115(3):188–91

**Barton, Edward Hall, d. 1857?**
Aldrete JA, Marron GM, Wright AJ: The first administration of anesthesia in military surgery: on occasion of the Mexican-American War. **Anesthesiology** 1984 Nov;61(5):585–8
Health in the southern United States: New York, Arno, 1977. Various paginations. Facsimiles of works by David Ramsay (1790 and 1796), Josiah C. Nott (1847), Edward H. Barton (1851), Wickliffe Rose (1910), Joseph Goldberger (1916).

**Barton, William Paul Crillon, 1786–1856**
Patton WK: Deficit spending (Dr. William P.C. Barton). **US Navy Med** 1982 Feb;73(2):16–7

**Bartram, John, 1699–1777**
Berkeley E, Berkeley DS: The life and travels of John Bartram: from Lake Ontario to the River St. John. Tallahassee, University Presses of Florida, 1982. xvi, 376 p.

**Baruch, Simon, 1840–1921**
Moerchel J: Simon Baruch (1840–1921) und die öffentliche Gesundheitspflege in New York. **Medizinhist J** 1982;17(1/2):138–47

**Basch, Samuel von, 1837–1905**
Křížek V: Samuel von Basch. Sto let od vynálezu nekrvavého měření krevního tlaku. **Cas Lek Cesk** 1980 Nov 28;119(48):1322–5

**Bashenin, Viktor Andreevich, 1882–**
Rykushin IuP, Smorodintsev AA, Shliakhtenko LI, et al: Professor V. A. Bashenin--odin iz osnovopolozhnikov otechestvennoĭ épidemiologii. **Zh Mikrobiol Epidemiol Immunobiol** 1983 Apr;(4):112–6

**Basiādes, Erokles**
Stavros T: Erokles basiades o teleytaios iatrophilosophos. **Epeirotike Hestia** 1975;24(279–280):419–32

**Bass, Charles Cassedy, 1875–1975**
Christen AG: Charles C. Bass, M.D.--1875–1975: that cantankerous genius of preventive dentistry. **Bull Hist Dent** 1982 Apr;30(1):8–18

**Bass, Heinrich, 1690–1754**
Tautz P, Hein G: Frühformen orthopädischen Denkens und orthopädischer Methoden in den ersten 120 Jahren der Universität Halle (Saale) (III). Heinrich Bass (1690–1754), genannt, 'Bandagen-Bass'. **Beitr Orthop Traumatol** 1979;26(12):705–12

**Bass, Mary Elizabeth, 1876–1956**
Burns C, Nelson M: Mary Elizabeth Bass. In: Notable American women. The modern period. Cambridge, Mass., Belknap-Harvard Univ. Press, 1980. 4:63–5.

**Bassini, Edoardo, 1844–1924**
Read RD: Marcy's priority in the development of inguinal herniorrphaphy. **Surgery** 1980 Nov;88(5):682–5

**Bastian, Henry Charlton, 1837–1915**
Dixon B: Spontaneous generation. **New Sci** 1981;91:553

**Batawia, Stanisław**
Jaroszewski Z: Działalność profesora Stanisława Batawii na polu alkohologii i walki z alkoholizmem. **Psychiatr Pol** 1979 Sep–Oct;13(5):445–9
Uszkiewiczowa L: Działalność profesora Stanisława Batawii w dziedzinie psychiatrii sądowej. **Psychiatr Pol** 1979 Sep–Oct;13(5):441–3

**Bate, George, 1608–1669**
Bruce-Chwatt LJ: George Bate--Cromwell's devious physician. **J R Coll Physicians Lond** 1983 Apr;17(2):144–6

**Bateman, Harry, 1882–1946**
Kratochvíl L, Lustig M: K historii tzv. Batemanovy funkce. **Cesk Farm** 1984 Jun;33(5):210–2

**Baten'kov, G. S.**
Katsnel'bogen AG: Dekabrist G. S. Baten'kov. **Sov Zdravookhr** 1982;(8):62–7

**Bates, Katharine Lee, 1859–1929**
Schwarz J: Yellow clover: Katharine Lee Bates and Katharine Coman. **Frontiers** 1979;4(1):59–67

**Bateson, Gregory, 1904–**
Delahousse J: Gregory Bateson et les Alcooliques Anonymes. **Soins** 1984 Jan;(421–422):52–3

**Bateson, William, 1861–1926**
Bateson W: Problems of genetics. Reprint of 1913 ed. Historical introduction by G. E. Hutchinson and S. Rachootin. New Haven and London, Yale University Press, 1979. xxii, 258 p.
Cock AG: William Bateson's pilgrimages to Brno. Cesty Williama Batesona do Brna. **Folia Mendeliana** 1980;65(15):243–50
Cock AG: William Bateson's rejection and eventual acceptance of chromosome theory. **Ann Sci** 1983 Jan;40:19–59

**Batllés y Torres de Amat, Mariano, 1798–1865**
Guerra F: La neurosis del exilio en Mariano Batllés, 1827. In

International Congress of the History of Medicine, 27th, Barcelona, 1980. Actas. Barcelona, Acadèmia de Ciències Mèdiques de Catalunya i Balears, 1981. p. 177–80.

**Batthyány, Boldizar, fl. 1572**
Barlay OS: Boldizsár Batthyány und sein Humanisten-Kreis. Die ersten Jahrzehnten der Güssinger Bibliothek. **Magy Konyvsz** 1979;95(3):231–51

**Baudeau, Pierre, 1643–1708**
Biron H: Pierre Baudeau. In Dictionary of Canadian biography, 1701 to 1740. Volume 2, 1969. p. 47–48.

**Baudelaire, Charles Pierre, 1821–1867**
Stäuble-Lipman Wulf, M: De Quincey, Baudelaire, e i 'Paradisi artificiali'. **Nuova Antologia** 1972;514(2054):245–54

**Baudelocque, Jean Louis, 1745?–1810**
Houtzager HL: Jean Louis Baudelocque. **Eur J Obstet Gynecol Reprod Biol** 1982 Aug;13(5):323–4

**Baudens, Jean Baptiste Lucien, 1804–1857**
Courtine JC: L'Armée d'Afrique et l'anesthésie-réanimation: de Baudens (1853) au Corps expéditionnaire française à la Première Armée (1942–1945) et à la guerre d'Algérie. **Hist Sci Med** 1983;17(4):411–17

**Baumé, Antoine, 1728–1804**
Julien P: Les 'Eléments de pharmacie' de Baumé et la contrefaçon. **Rev Hist Pharm (Paris)** 1981 Jun;28(249):103–6

**Baumès, Prosper, 1791–1871**
Prosper Baumès, dermatologist of Lyon 1791–1871 and the Willan-Alibert controversy: **Br J Dermatol** 1981 Dec;105(6):727–31

**Baumgärtner, Karl Heinrich, 1798–1886**
Dahm S: Frühe Krankenbildnisse: Alibert Esquirol Baumgartner. Köln, 1981. (Kölner medizinhistorische Beiträge; Arbeiten der Forschungsstelle des Instituts für Geschichte der Medizin der Universität zu Köln, Band 21).

**Bausner, Bartholomaeus, 1629–1682**
Bugyi B: Bausner Bertalan (1629–1682). **Orv Hetil** 1984 Jul 22;125(30):1831–2

**Baxley, H. Willis**
Jensen JE: A Med-Chi physician's travelog 1860–62 (Dr. H. Willis Baxley). **Md State Med J** 1984 Feb;33(2):90–2

**Bayer, Karl, fl. 1891**
Konjhodžić F, Simunović V: Prve operacije na glavi i mozgu u akufskoj bolnici u Sarajeve. **Med Arh** 1978 Sep–Oct;32(5):325–8

**Bayle, Juan del, fl. 1698**
Gago R, Olagüe G, Carrillo JL: Aportación al estudio del movimiento novator en España: el Laboratorio Químico del Palacio Real (1694) y la obra del boticario aragonés Juan del Bayle (fl. 1698). **Bol Soc Esp Hist Farm** 1981 Jun;32(126):95–107

**Bayne-Jones, Stanhope, 1888–1970**
Harvey AM: Stanhope Bayne-Jones, 1886–1970: the story of a lifetime devoted to country and to medicine. **Johns Hopkins Med J** 1981 Oct;149(4):150–66

**Bean, William Bennett, 1909–**
Bean WB: Personal reflections on clinical investigations. **Annu Rev Nutr** 1982;2:1–20

**Beanes, William, 1749–1828?**
Jensen JE: 166 years ago this month ... William Beanes: the doctor behind 'The Star-Spangled Banner'. **Md State Med J** 1980 Sep;29(9):60–5

**Beaney, James George, 1826–1891**
Gandevia B, Clasen U: James George Beaney: his authorship. **Med J Aust** 1981 Aug 8;2(3):160

**Beard, George Miller, 1839–1883**
Gruman GJ, ed: The 'Fixed period' controversy: prelude to modern ageism. New York, Arno Press, 1979. Various paginations. Reprint of passages by George M. Beard, William Osler, and James Crichton-Browne.
Roth N: Electrotherapy, 19th-century neurasthenia, and the case of Alice James. **Med Instrum** 1981 Mar–Apr;15(2):116

**Beatson, George Thomas, 1848–1933**
Stockwell S: Classics in oncology. George Thomas Beatson, M.D. (1848–1933). **CA** 1983 Mar–Apr;33(2):105–21

**Beaubien, Pierre, 1796–1881**
Bernier J: Pierre Beaubien. In Dictionary of Canadian biography, 1881–1890. 1982;11:57–8.

**Beaumont, William, 1785–1853**
Cohen IB, ed: The career of William Beaumont and the reception of his discovery. New York, Arno Press, 1980. Various pagings. Reprint of G. Miller: William Beaumont's formative years: two early notebooks 1811–1821 (1946); G. Rosen: The reception of William Beaumont's discovery in Europe (1942); G. Rosen: Notes on the reception and influence of William Beaumont's discovery (1943). (Three centuries of Science in America).
Crispell KR: Beaumont and Dunglison: who was Dunglison? **Trans Am Clin Climatol Assoc** 1980;92:194–8
Higgins GA: Problems in clinical trials: lessons from the 'tuck uppers'. **Cancer** 1981;47:2167–71
Myer JS: William Beaumont: a pioneer American physiologist. New ed. of his: Life and letters of Dr. William Beaumont. With historical introductions by E. Brodman and R. E. Shank. Includes reprint of 1833 ed. of Beaumont's Experiments and observations on the gastric juice and the physiology of digestion. St. Louis, Mosby, 1981. xi, 394 p.
Numbers RL, Orr WJ: William Beaumont's reception at home and abroad. **Isis** 1981 Dec;72(264):590–612
Zollinger RM: The legacies of William Beaumont, pioneer investigator. **Pharos** 1983 Winter;46(1):20–3

**Beauperthuy, Louis Daniel, 1807–1871**
Beauperthuy de Benedetti R: Repercusion en la Argentina en 1871 del descubrimiento del vector de la fiebre amarilla realizado por Beauperthuy en Venezuela. **Rev Soc Venez Hist Med** 1980;29(43–44):87–93
Beauperthuy de Benedetti R: Beauperthuy y su microscopio. **Rev Soc Venez Hist Med** 1978;27(41):59–64
Beauperthuy de Benedetti R: Bref commentaire à un travail de Sir William Osler et sa reconnaissance de la théorie scientifique de Beauperthuy sur la fièvre jaune. In: Congrès international d'histoire de la médecine, XXVe, Québec, 1976. Actes. Québec, 1977. p. 487–92.
Beauperthuy de Benedetti R: Informe sobre la publicacion del señor Cesar Rodriguez Exposito. **Rev Soc Venez Hist Med** 1972–73;20–21(34–35):141–50
Beauperthuy de Benedetti R: Resonancia del descurbrimiento del agente transmisor de la fiebre amarilla que hizo Beauperthuy en Venezuela. **Rev Soc Venez Hist Med** 1972–73;20–21(34–35):67–77
Beauperthuy de Benedetti R: Laveran y Beauperthuy. **Acta Med Venez** 1981 Jan–Mar;28(1):47–52
Beauperthuy de Benedetti R: Beauperthuy. La herpetología y Venuzuela. In International Congress of the History of Medicine, 27th, Barcelona, 1980. Actas. Barcelona, Acadèmia de Ciències Mèdiques de Catalunya i Balears, 1981. p. 454–7.
Osuna A: Beuperthuy 'Descubridor'. **Rev Soc Venez Hist Med** 1972–73;20–21(34–35):197–201
Stroppiana L: Correspondencia cientifica de 1858 entre el doctor Beauperthuy de Caracas y el doctor Socrate Cadet de Roma. **Rev Soc Venez Hist Med** 1979;28(42):37–44

**Beccaria, Giovanni Battista, 1715–1781**
Cremona GF: Studi di biologia e medicina nell'opera del fisico piemontese G. B. Beccaria. **Ann Osp Maria Vittoria Torino** 1982 Jul–Dec;25(7–12):259–68

**Béchamp, Pierre Jacques Antoine, 1816–1908**
Decourt P: Les zymases ou ferments solubles de Béchamp à la lumière des connaissances du XXe siècle. **Hist Sci Med** 1984;18(2):147–51
Nonclercq M: Un chapitre ignoré de l'histoire des sciences: l'oeuvre de Béchamp. In: Congrés National des Sociétés Savantes, 103e, Nancy, 1978. Comptes Rendus. Paris, 1978. Section des Sciences, Fasc. V. p. 157–69.
Nonclercq M: Antoine Béchamp 1816–1908: l'homme et le savant originalité et fécondité de son oeuvre. Preface et note documentaire par le Docteur Philippe Decourt. Paris, Maloine, 1982. 249 p.
Nonclercq M: A. Béchamp, un' ingiustizia nella storia delle scienze. **Empedocle** 1983 Sep–Oct;1(1):39–49

**Beck, Henryk, 1896–1946**
Jaworska J: Henryka Becka 'Bunkier 1944 roku'. Wrocław, Zakład Narodowy im. Ossolińskich, 1982. 119 p.

**Beck, Theodric Romeyn, 1791–1855**
Grob GN, ed: The beginnings of American psychiatric thought and practice. Five accounts, 1811–1830. New York, Arno, 1973. Various paginations. Includes Account of the rise and progress of the Asylum . . . near Philadelphia (1814), and works by Theodric Romeyn Beck (1811); Thomas Eddy (1815); George Parkman (1814); and Rufus Wyman (1830).

**Beckett, Samuel, 1906–**
Culik H: Mindful of the body: medical allusions in Beckett's Murphy. **Eire-Irel** 1977 Spring;14:84–101

**Béclaed, Jules**
Sicard A: Un doyen misogyne et un recteur féministe. **Hist Sci Med** 1982;16(1):15–20

**Béclère, Antoine, 1856–1939**
Ratti A: Antoinette Béclère e il Centro per le Relazioni internazionali in Radiologia. **Radiol Med (Torino)** 1982 Nov;68(11):785–7

**Beddoes, Thomas, 1760–1808**
Levere TH: Dr. Thomas Beddoes at Oxford: radical politics in 1788–1793 and the fate of the Regius Chair in Chemistry. **Ambix** 1981 Jul;28(2):61–9
Levere TH: Dr. Thomas Beddoes: the interaction of pneumatic and preventive medicine with chemistry. **Interdiscip Sci Rev** 1982;7:137–47
Levere TH: Dr. Thomas Beddoes (1750–1808): science and medicine in politics and society. **Br J Hist Sci** 1984 Jul;17(56 pt 2):187–204

**Beddome, Henry Septimus, ca. 1830–1881**
Bredin TF: Henry Septimus Beddome. In Dictionary of Canadian

biography, 1881–1890. 1982;11:63–4.

**Bede (the Venerable), 673–735**
Gardner R: Miracles of healing in Anglo-Celtic Northumbria as recorded by the venerable Bede and his contemporaries: a reappraisal in the light of twentieth century experience. **Br Med J [Clin Res]** 1983 Dec 24–31;287(6409):1927–33

**Bednarz, Józef**
Petelski M: Dr Józef Bednarz. **Przegl Lek** 1981;38(1):173–5

**Bedson, Samuel Phillips, 1886–1969**
Downie AW: Sir Samuel Phillips Bedson. In Dictionary of national biography, 1961–1970. Suppl. 8, 1981. p. 86–7.

**Beecher, Catharine Esther, 1800–1878**
Vertinsky P: Sexual equality and the legacy of Catharine Beecher. **J Sport Hist** 1979;6(1):38–49

**Beer, Benjamin Ben Elizah Harofe**
Kottek S: The humble physician, explanation of and notes on a Renaissance medal. **Koroth** 1980 Jun;7(11–12):747–53

**Beer-Hofmann, Richard, 1866–1945**
Berlin JB: Richard Beer-Hofmann and Theodor Reik: a letter in exile. **Psychoanal Rev** 1981–82 Winter;68(4):479–86

**Beers, Clifford Whittingham, 1876–1943**
Dain N: Clifford W. Beers: advocate for the insane. Pittsburgh, Univ. of Pittsburgh Press, 1980. xxix, 392 p.
Griffin JD: The amazing careers of Hincks and Beers. **Can J Psychiatry** 1982 Dec;27(8):668–71

**Beethoven, Ludwig van, 1770–1827**
Aterman K, MacSween HM, Perry PE, et al: Recurrent infections, diarrhea, ascites and phonophobia in a 57-year-old man. **Can Med Assoc J** 1982 Mar 15;126(6):623–8
Böhme G: Medizinische Porträts berühmter Komponisten: Wolfgang Amadeus Mozart, Ludwig van Beethoven, Carl Maria von Weber, Frédéric Chopin, Peter Iljitsch Tschaikowski, Béla Bartók. 2. verbesserte und erweiterte Auflage. Stuttgart, New York, Gustav Fischer Verlag, 1981. xi, 199 p.
Chalat NI: Some psychologic aspects of deafness: Beethoven, Goya, and Oscar Wilde. **Am J Otol** 1980 Apr;1(4):240–6
Czeizel A: Ludwig van Beethoven. **Ther Hung** 1982;30(1):43–7
Reichsman F: Life experiences and creativity of great composers: a psychosomaticist's view. **Psychosom Med** 1981 Aug;43(4):291–300
Wurmser L: Idealization and aggression in Beethoven's creativity. **Am Imago** 1979 Winter;36(4):328–44
Zagarra MJ: Ludwig van Beethoven: hipótesis sobre su sordera. **CERON** 1979 Dec;4(3):7–9

**Behal, Auguste, 1859–1941**
Bouriez J: Lens, trois savants oubliés: Auguste Behal, Amand Valeur, Raymond Delaby. [France], Société de recherches historiques de la région d'Henin-Carvin, [1981] 69 leaves.

**Behr, Georg Heinrich, 1708–1761**
Bachoffner P: Vulgarisation théraputique à travers la 'Materia Medica' de Georges-Henri Behr, médecin strasbourgeois. In Livet G, Schaff G, ed: Médecine et assistance en Alsace, XVIe–XXe siècle. Strasbourg, Istra, 1976. p. 145–53.

**Behring, Emil Adolf von, 1854–1917**
Cooper EL: Prix D'Immunologie Behring-Metschnikoff. **Dev Comp Immunol** 1982 Summer;6(3):389–90
Schadewaldt H: Emil von Behring und die Entwicklung der deutschen Immunologie. **Med Welt** 1979;30(48):1795–801

**Beilhardt, Jacob, 1846–1908**
Fogarty RS, Grant HR: Free love in Ohio: Jacob Beilhardt and the Spirit Fruit Colony. **Ohio Hist** 1980;89(2):206–21

**Bekhterev, Vladimir Mikhaĭlovich, 1857–1927**
Arkhangel'skiĭ GV: K prioritetu opisaniia akademikom V. M. Bekhterevym khoreicheskoĭ paducheĭ. **Zh Nevropatol Psikhiatr** 1981;81(6):929–30
Arkhangel'skiĭ GV: V. M. Bekhterev--vydaiushchiĭsia deiatel' otechestvennoĭ nauki (k 125-letiiu so dnia rozhdeniia). **Klin Med (Mosk)** 1983 Feb;61(2):106–10
Bal'dysh G: Bekhterev v Peterburge-Leningrade. Leningrad, Lenizdat, 1979. 318 p.
Briskman AM: O 'khoreicheskoĭ paducheĭ' Bekhtereva i mioklonus-epilepsii. **Zh Nevropatol Psikhiatr** 1984;84(1):122–5
Kelemen G: 125 éve született V. M. Bekhterev. **Orv Hetil** 1983 Apr 3;124(14):831–3
Kukuev LA: V. M. Bekhterev i znachenie ego trudov dlia sovremennoĭ nevrologii i meditsiny. **Klin Med (Mosk)** 1982 Oct;60(10):118–21
Panchenko PM, Shereshevskiĭ AM: V. M. Bekhterev i neĭrokhirurgiia (k 125-letiiu so dnia rozhdeniia). **Zh Vopr Neirokhir** 1982 Sep–Oct;(5):59–61

**Bekkers, L. A., 1831–**
Serebrennikov AB: Khirurg L. A. Bekkers - uchenik N. I. Pirogova. **Klin Med (Mosk)** 1983 Mar;61(3):113–5

**Beklemishev, Vladimir Nikolaevich, 1890–1962**
Kupriianova ES, Detinova TS, Anufrieva VN, et al: Osnovnye napravleniia rabot V. N. Baklemisheva v oblasti meditsinskoĭ éntomologii i ikh znachenie v épidemiologii i profilaktike transmissivnykh bolezneĭ. **Med Parazitol (Mosk)** 1982 Jan–Feb;51(1):33–9
Shipitsina NK: Vliianie issledovaniĭ V. N. Beklemisheva v oblasti obshcheĭ biologii, parazitologii i épidemiologii transmissivnykh bolezneĭ na razvitie étikh otrasleĭ nauki (k 90-letiiu so dnia rozhdeniia). **Med Parazitol (Mosk)** 1982 Mar–Apr;60(2):86–8
Tamarina NA, Lange AB: Razvitie ideĭ V. N. Beklemisheva v oblasti sravnitel'noĭ parazitologii. **Med Parazitol (Mosk)** 1982 Jan–Feb;51(1):3–9

**Beletskiĭ, P. K., 1871–**
Ionov IuV, Ionov AIu: Fel'dsher P. K. Beletskiĭ--pisatel', publitsist, étnograf, obshchestvennyĭ deiatel'. **Feldsher Akush** 1982;47(1):55–8

**Beliaev, I. V.**
Sivoloh NI: Vklad I.V. Beliaeva v organizatsiiu sanitarnogo dela v Donbasse. **Sov Zdravookhr** 1984;(5):65–7

**Belinskiĭ, Vissarion Grigor'evich, 1811–1848**
Brzheskiĭ VCh, Evdokimov PP: K istorii bolezni V.G. Belinskogo. **Klin Med (Mosk)** 1984 Aug;62(8):150–2

**Bell, Alexander Graham, 1847–1922**
Pappas DG: Alexander Graham Bell: teacher of the deaf. **Am J Otol** 1983 Jan;4(3):263–5

**Bell, Andrew, 1753–1832**
Stephen K: Andrew Bell F.R.S.E. (1753–1832). Edinburgh, University of Edinburgh, 1982. [10 p.] (Scottish Men of Letters).

**Bell, Charles, 1774–1842**
Gallistel CR: Bell, Magendie, and the proposals to restrict the use of animals in neurobehavioral research. **Am Psychol** 1981 Apr;36(4):357–60
Loudon IS: Sir Charles Bell and the anatomy of expression. **Br Med J [Clin Res]** 1982 Dec 18–25;285(6357):1794–6
McHenry LC: L'idea e la mano. **Kos** 1984 Jul–Aug;1(6):79–90

**Bell, Gordon, 1863–1923**
Dudley HA: From Edinburgh, an academic surgeon. **Aust NZ J Surg** 1981 Jun;51(3):247–50

**Bell, John, 1845–1878**
Fishman N: John Bell, MD--teacher to William Osler. **Can Med Assoc J** 1981 Nov 1;125(9):1042, 1044

**Bell, Joseph, 1837–1911**
Mann RJ, Key JD: Joseph Bell, M.D., F.R.C.S.: 'notes on a case of paralysis following diphtheria'. **Pharos** 1982 Spring;45(2):27–9
Massey EW: Joseph Bell, MD, FRCS - Mr. Sherlock Holmes? **South Med J** 1980;73:1635–6

**Belliarminov, Leonid Gorovich, 1859–1930**
Krasnikov PG: L. G. Belliarminov--vydaiushchiĭsia uchenyĭ, obshchestvennyĭ deiatel' i organizator oftal'mologicheskoĭ pomoshchi naseleniiu (k 125-letiiu so dnia rozhdeniia). **Vestn Oftalmol** 1984 Sep–Oct;(5):69–70

**Bellini, Vincenzo, 1801–1835**
Kerner D: Bellinis Tod in Paris. **Orchester** 1976;24:712–6

**Belogolovyĭ, Nikolaĭ Andreevich, 1834–1895**
Arkhangel'skiĭ GA: N. A. Belogolovyĭ--obshchestvennyĭ vrach, zhurnalist (k 150-letiiu so dnia rozhdeniia). **Sov Zdravookhr** 1984;(10):67–70

**Ben-Gurion, David, 1886–1973**
Sherman ED: David Ben-Gurion (1886–1973). **J Am Geriatr Soc** 1983 Aug;31(8):501–5

**Ben Zabda, Yohanan**
Pines S: The oath of Asaph the Physician and Yohanan Ben Zabda: Its relation to the Hippocratic Oath and the Doctrina duarum viarium of the Didaché. **Proc Isr Acad Sci Humanit** 1971–76;5:223–64

**Benavente, Samuel de Lion, 1643–1723**
Kerner S: Samuel de Lion Benavente; chirurgien et lithotomiste (1643–1723). **Rev Hist Med Heb** 1981 Jul;34(2):29–30

**Benckiser, Robert, fl. 1831**
Duchatel F: Insertion vélamenteuse du cordon ombilical et hémorragie de Benckiser. **Hist Sci Med** 1982;16(3):185–92

**Benedetto Greco da Salerno, fl. 1401**
Billanovich MC: I libri di Benedetto Greco da Salerno, studente a Padova in medicina (1401). **Quad Stor Univ Padova** 1974;7:1–15

**Benedict of Nursia, Saint, ca. 480–ca. 544**
Beya y Alonso E: Prescripciones medicas y sanitarias en la Regla de San Benito. **Bol Soc Esp Hist Farm** 1984;35(137):61–7
Daglio P: San Benedetto da Norcia patrono d'Europa, nella medicina e nella storia. **Minerva Med** 1982 Sep 8;73(34):2193–8
Ferrari Sacco A: Benedetto da Norcia e la medicina conventuale in Europa (nel 1500th anniversario della nascita). **Minerva Med** 1981 Mar 10;72(9):585–7

**Benes, Eduard, 1884–1948**
Winters SB: The health of Edvard Beneš: an unpublished letter from 1948. **East Cent Eur** 1977;4:60–6

**Benion, Samuel, 1673–1708**
Howie WB: Samuel Benion--Glasgow University's first Doctor of Medicine. **Scott Med J** 1979 Jan;24(1):76–9

**Benítez, José María, 1790-1855**
O'Neill YV: Jose Maria Benites' informe--alta California's first medical account. In International Congress of the History of Medicine, 27th, Barcelona, 1980. Actas. Barcelona, Académia de Ciències Médiques de Catalunya i Balears, 1981. p. 203-6.
Vélez Boza F: Licenciado Jose Maria Benitez; maestro en artes, médico y botánico. **Rev Soc Venez Hist Med** 1977;25(39):71-92

**Benjamin, Georg, 1895-1942**
Benjamin H: Georg Benjamin: eine Biographie. 2d ed. Leipzig, S. Hirzel, 1982. 363 p.

**Bennet, Jesse, 1769-1842**
Nipe GM: 'Jessee Bennett decided to operate on his wife at once'. **Va Med** 1979 Dec;106(12):884-5

**Bennet, Sara**
Rawlings FH: Two 17th century women apothecaries. **Pharm Hist (London)** 1984 Sep;14(3):7

**Bennett, Alexander Hughes, 1848-1901**
Kirkpatrick DB: The first primary brain-tumor operation. **J Neurosurg** 1984 Nov;61(5):809-13

**Bennett, Arnold, 1867-1931**
Perkin GD: Arnold Bennett and medicine: with particular reference to his description of dressing apraxia. **Br Med J [Clin Res]** 1981 Dec 19;283(6307):1666-8

**Bennett, Francis Oswald, 1898-1976**
Bennett F: A Canterbury tale. The autobiography of Dr. Francis Bennett. Wellington, Oxford University Press, 1980. 249 p.

**Bennett, George Eli, 1885-**
Harvey AM: Orthopaedic surgery at Johns Hopkins: a heritage of excellence in clinical practice, training and research. **Johns Hopkins Med J** 1982 Jun;150(6):221-45

**Bennett, Jesse, 1769-1842**
Grubb JM: The first successful cesarean section and the first oophorectomy in the Americas. **W Va Med J** 1984 Oct;80(10):221-3

**Bennetts, Harold William, 1898-**
Underwood EJ: The contribution of H. W. Bennetts to the solution and control of animal disease problems in Western Australia. **Hist Rec Aust Sci** 1980;5(1):59-67

**Bensley, Robert Russell, 1867-1956**
Garrett CG: Robert Russell Bensley. In Dictionary of American Biography, Suppl. 6, 1956-1960. p. 53-4, 1980.

**Bentham, Jeremy, 1748-1832**
C[one] TE: Jeremy Bentham's list of data needed to understand the growth and development of children (1797). **Pediatrics** 1981;68:447

**Bentley, Arthur Fisher, 1870-1957**
Ward JF: Arthur F. Bentley and the foundations of behavioral science. **J Hist Behav Sci** 1981;17:222-31

**Bentley, Charles Edwin, 1859-1929**
Dummett CO: Charles Edwin Bentley: a genuine emancipator. **Crisis** 1979;86(4):133-5
Dummett CO: Prevention began early: Charles Edwin Bentley, DDS 1859-1929. **J Natl Med Assoc** 1983 Dec;75(12):1235-6
Dummett CO: Health professional emancipators: examples in excellence. **J Natl Med Assoc** 1984 Sep;76(9):925-30

**Bentley, Edwin, 1824-1917**
Cobb WM: Edwin Bentley, MD, 1824-1917: Connecticut Yankee in Washington and Little Rock. **J Natl Med Assoc** 1980;72:1012-4

**Bentom, Clark, ca. 1774-ca. 1820**
Cook CS: Clark Bentom. In Dictionary of Canadian biography, 1801 to 1820. Volume 5, 1983. p. 68-9.

**Benton, Arthur Lester, 1909-**
Distinguished Professional Contribution Award for 1978: (Arthur L. Benton). **Am Psychol** 1979 Jan;34(1):56-64

**Berg, Albert Ashton, 1872-**
Robbins C: The collector's legacy. **MD** 1982 May;26(6):193-6, 201

**Berger, Hans, 1873-1941**
Jung R, Berger W: Fünfzig Jahre EEG. Hans Bergers Entdeckung des Elektrenkephalogramms und seine ersten Befunde 1924--1931. **Arch Psychiatr Nervenkr** 1979 Dec;227(4):279-300
Zani A: Le origini storiche dell'elettroencefalografia. **Stor Crit Psicol** 1981;2(1):119-84

**Bergh, Henry, 1811-1888**
Kaufman M, Kaufman HJ: Henry Bergh, Kit Burns, and the sportsmen of New York. **NY Folkl Q** 1972;28(1):15-29

**Bergman, Hjalmar Frederik Elgerus, 1883-1931**
Bergström CO: Den sjuka människan i Hjalmar Bergmans diktning. **Nord Medicinhist Arsb** 1984;:165-73

**Bergman, Per, 1874-**
Marks LS, Maxwell MH: Tigerstedt and the discovery of renin. An historical note. **Hypertension** 1979 Jul-Aug;1(4):384-8

**Bergmann, Carl, 1814-1865**
Coleman W: Bergmann's rule: animal heat as a biological phenomenon. **Stud Hist Biol** 1979;3:67-88

**Bergmann, Ernst von, 1836-1907**
Linde E: Ernst von Bergmann. Rückblick auf das Leben anlässlich der Einweihung der Sanitätsakademie in München. **MMW** 1981 May 1;123(18):751-2

**Bergmann, Max, 1886-1944**
Miller M: The Max Bergmann papers. **Surv Sources Newsl** 1976Dec;4:7-8

**Bergson, Henri Louis, 1859-1941**
Gunter PA: Bergson and Jung. **J Hist Ideas** 1982 Oct-Dec;43(4):635-52

**Berkeley, George, Bp. of Cloyne, 1685-1753**
Gaustad ES: George Berkeley in America. New Haven, Yale University Press, 1979. xi, 225 p.

**Berman, Mones, 1920-1982**
Rall JE: Mones Berman--the man and his legacy to quantitative biology. **Am J Physiol** 1983 Nov;245(5 Pt 1):R618-9

**Bernal, John Desmond, 1901-1971**
Edsall JT: The papers of W.T. Astbury and J.D. Bernal. **Surv Sources Newsl** 1981 Apr;10:2-6

**Bernard, Camille, 1802-1879**
Pons J, Davoust B, Pons ML: Qui êtes-vous Monsieur Camille Bernard? **Ann Chir Plast Esthet** 1983;28(2):199-200

**Bernard, Claude, 1813-1878**
Albury WR: Going beyond the introduction: Claude Bernard scholarship in the 1970s, an essay review. **Bull Hist Med** 1982 Summer;56(2):271-5
Amalric P: Claude Bernard et l'ophtalmologie. **Bull Soc Ophtalmol Fr** 1979 Nov-Dec;79(11-12):995-7
Bacq ZM: Le centenaire de la mort de Claude Bernard. **Rev Med Liege** 1979 Jun 1;34(11):525-8
Belloni L: Un circolo bernardiano in Italia: la Società delle Scienze Biologiche in Torino. Luigi Vella de la curaroterapia del tetano. **Physis** 1981;23(3):301-10
Bourguignon A: Certains problèmes épistemologiques évoqués par Claude Bernard. In Poirier J, Poirier JL, ed: Médecine et philosophie à la fin du XIXe siècle. Paris, Université de Paris XII - Val de Marne, [1980?]. p. 85-100.
Cappelletti V: Bernard, oltre meccanicismo e vitalismo. **Med Secoli** 1979 Jan-Apr;16(1):5-11
Cappelletti V: Claude Bernard between history and the 'principles' of science. **Riv Biol** 1980 Spring;73(1):21-33
Cimino G: Claude Bernard sulle 'funzioni del cervello'. **Physis** 1980;22(1):85-119
Claude Bernard fut-il un médecin praticien?: Entretiens de Bichat, Faculté de médecine, Pitié-Salpêtrière, Paris, 29 septembre-8 Octobre 1978. [France], Expansion scientifique, 1978 printing. [32] p.
Dillemann G: L'éloge de Magendie par Claude Bernard. **Hist Sci Med** 1983;17(4):345-9
Dreyfus G: Médecine scientifique et art médical. Une controverse à propos de Claude Bernard. **Sem Hop Paris** 1983 May 19;59(20):1569-71
Federspil G: Lo sviluppo delle teorie sulla glicogenesi e il diabete in Claude Bernard e oggi. **Med Secoli** 1979 Jan-Apr;16(1):31-50
Huard P: Claude Bernard et la morphologie. In: Congrès National des Sociétés Savantes, 107e. Brest, 1982. Comptes Rendus, Paris, 1983. Section des Sciences, Fasc. IV. p. 273-9.
Huard P: Claude Bernard et la chirurgie. In: Congrès National des Sociétés Savantes, 107e. Brest, 1982. Comptes Rendus, Paris, 1983. Section des Sciences, Fasc. IV. p. 267-71.
Huard P: Claude Bernard et le système vasculaire. In: Congrès National des Sociétés Savantes, 107e. Brest, 1982. Comptes Rendus, Paris, 1983. Section des Sciences, Fasc. IV. p. 281-6.
Knaus WA: Claude Bernard fut-il l'inventeur de l'indice de gravité? **Presse Med** 1983 Jul 2;12(28):1755-6
La Vergata A: Claude Bernard, 'punti di vista fisiologici', ed economia della natura. **Riv Filos** 1982;73:361-95
Lagoutte J: Claude Bernard, un physiologiste, un philosophe. Lyon, Centre régional de documentation pédagogique, 1978. 40 p.
Medaer R: Classics in neurology. Etching showing Claude Bernard doing an experiment surrounded by his colleagues. **Neurology** 1982 Oct;32(10):1145
Miles A: Reports by Louis Pasteur and Claude Bernard on the organization of scientific teaching and research. **Notes Rec R Soc Lond** 1982 Aug;37(1):101-18
Poggi S: Ricerca della verità e metodo sperimentale in Claude Bernard. **Intersezioni** 1981;1:361-79
Pozo EC del: La medicina como ciencia en Claudio Bernard. Homenaje en el primer centenario de su muerte. **Gac Med Mex** 1979 Jun;115(6):245-56
Premuda L: Claude Bernard e gli indirizzi della fisiologia e della medicina nel secolo XIX. **Minerva Med** 1982 Feb 25;73(7):329-35
Pyke DA: Claude Bernard et l'étiologie du diabète. **Journ Annu Diabetol Hotel Dieu** 1981;:153-61
Robin ED, ed: Claude Bernard and the internal environment: a memorial symposium. New York, Dekker, 1979. xvi, 299 p. Historical contributions by J. Bernard, M. Bertrand, J. S. Fruton, R. H. Unger, J. P. Changeux, A. Cournand, F. Morel, R. Guillemin, H. Rahn, S. S. Cohen.

Sloan AW: Claude Bernard's philosophy of medical science. **S Afr Med J** 1984 May 19;65(20):817–9

Théodoridès J: Claude Bernard et les parasites. (Contribution au centenaire de la mort de Claude Bernard). **Hist Nat** 1979;(14):31–8

Théodoridès J: Claude Bernard et la microbiologie médicale. In: Congrès international d'histoire de la médecine, XXVe, Québec, 1976. Actes. Québec, 1977. p. 1354–60.

Trease GE: Claude Bernard 1813–1878. **Br J Pharm Pract** 1981;3(2):21–2

Weissmann G: The introduction is over. **Arthritis Rheum** 1983 Nov;26(11):1297–302

**Bernard de Gordon, fl. ca. 1283–ca. 1308**

Demaitre LE: Doctor Bernard de Gordon: professor and practitioner. Toronto, Pontifical Institute of Mediaeval Studies, 1980. xii, 236 p.

**Bernard, Jean Jacques, 1888–**

Golliet P, Binet JL: Deux historiens du sang, ou Réponse de Lucien Lévy-Bruhl et de Wifredo Lam à Jean Bernard. **Nouv Rev Fr Hematol** 1983;25(5):337–41

**Bernay, Paul, fl. 1872**

Ness DE: C'est fini. . . .le pouls ne bat plus! Drawn by Paul Bernay, for Le Charivari, in 1872. **J Hist Med Allied Sci** 1980 Jul;35(3):312

**Bernfeld, Siegfried, 1892–1953**

Grubrich-Simitis I: Siegfried Bernfeld: Historiker der Psychoanalyse und Freud-Biograph. **Psyche (Stuttg)** 1981 May;35(5):397–434

**Bernhard, Wilhelm, 1920–1978**

Marbach JU: Wilhelm Bernhard, 1920–1978. **Gesnerus** 1979;36(3–4):303–11

**Bernheim, Hippolyte, 1840–1919**

Barrucand D: Bernheim. Importance historique et actualité de l'Ecole de Nancy. In: Congrès National des Sociétés Savantes, 103e, Nancy, 1978. Comptes Rendus. Paris, 1978. Section des Sciences, Fasc. V. p. 75–86.

Sandor RS, ed: Bernheim's New studies in hypnotism. New York, International Universities Press, 1980. xix, 407 p. Translation of Hypnotisme, suggestion, psychothérapie: Etudes nouvelles, 1891.

Théodoridès J: Hippolyte Bernheim et la pathologie infectieuse. In: Congrès National des Sociétés Savantes, 103e, Nancy, 1978. Comptes Rendus. Paris, 1978. Section des Sciences, Fasc. V. p. 87–94.

Weitzenhoffer AM: What did he (Bernheim) say? A postscript and an addendum. **Int J Clin Exp Hypn** 1980 July;28(3):252–60

**Bernhisel, John Milton, 1799–1881**

Barrett G: Delegate John M. Bernhisel, Salt Lake physician following the Civil War. **Utah Hist Q** 1982;50(4):354–60

**Bernou Family**

Bonnemain H: Une famille médico-pharmaceutique: les Augiéras-Bernou. **Rev Hist Pharm (Paris)** 1981;28(248):14–20

**Bernoulli, Daniel, 1700–1782**

Guess HA: Bernoulli's cost-benefit analysis of smallpox immunization. **N Engl J Med** 1981 Aug 6;305(6):347

**Bernstein, Julius, 1839–1917**

Kaiser W, Völker A: Der Arbeitskreis um den halleschen Physiologen Julius Bernstein (1839–1917) und seine Bedeutung für die klinische Medizin. **Wiss Z Martin Luther Univ (Math)** 1982;31(6):75–100

**Berovich, Petr, 1799–1871**

Kozhokaru I, Maslev S: Novootkriti dokumenti ot i za D–R Petur Beron. **Izv Inst Istor** 1968;20:229–341

**Berruti, Giuseppe, 19th cent.**

Bèttica-Giovannini R: Giuseppe Berruti e l'Ospizio Marino Piemontese per ragazzi scrofolosi poveri con una nota su la fondazione dell'Ospedale Maria Vittoria di Torino (1887). **Ann Osp Maria Vittoria Torino** 1977 Jul–Dec;20(7–12):227–340

**Berryhill, Walter Reece, 1900–1979**

Blythe WB, et al: Walter Reece Berryhill. **NC Med J** 1984 Oct;45(10):615–29

**Bert, Paul, 1833–1886**

Bert P: La pression barométrique. Recherches de physiologie expérimentale. Facsimile of 1878 edition. Biographical introduction by P. Dejour. Paris, Editions du Centre National de la Recherche Scientifique, 1979. viii, 1183 p.

**Bertalanffy, Ludwig von, 1901–1972**

Nierhaus G: Ludwig von Bertalanffy 1901–1972. **Sudhoffs Arch** 1981;65(2):144–72

**Bertele, Georg, 1767–1818**

Oldenburg D: Georg August Bertele (1767–1818) und die Arzneimittellehre der romantischen Naturphilosophie. **Medizinhist J** 1981;16(3):240–56

**Bertenson, Iosef Vasil'evich, 1833–1895**

Lotova EI, Egorysheva IV: Gigienist i obshchestvennyĭ deiatel' I. V. Bertenson (k 150-letiiu so dnia rozhdeniia). **Sov Zdravookhr** 1984;(1):57–60

**Berthelot, Marcellin Pierre Eugène, 1827–1907**

Halleux R: Marcellin Berthelot, historien de l'alchimie. In: Congrès National des Sociétés Savantes, 104e, Bordeaux, 1979. Comptes Rendus. Paris, 1979. Section des Sciences, Fasc. IV. p. 169–80.

**Bertier, Michel, 1695–1740**

Boissonnault CM: Michel Bertier. In Dictionary of Canadian biography, 1701 to 1740. Volume 2, 1969. p. 60.

**Bertillon family**

Dupaquier M: La famille Bertillon et la naissance d'une nouvelle science sociale: la démographie. **Ann Demogr Hist (Paris)** 1983;:293–310

**Bertin, René Joseph Hyacinthe, 1767–1828**

Lellouch A, Rullière R: René Joseph Hyacinthe Bertin (1767–1827). **Hist Sci Med** 1980;14:325–36

**Berzelius, Jöns Jacob, 1779–1848**

Ekström S: Jöns Jacob Berzelius--ett 200-årsminne. **Sven Farm Tidskr** 1979;83:635–51

Gutt RW: Jons Jacob Berzelius (1779–1848) i poczatki chemii fizjologicznej). **Arch Hist Med (Warsz)** 1979;42(1):83–92

Křížek V, Nevoral V: Jöns Jacob Berzelius a české minerální vody. **Fysiatr Reumatol Vestn** 1980 Aug;58(4):238–42

Krook H: Jacob Berzelius privat. **Nord Medicinhist Arsb** 1980;:81–9

Melhado EM: Jacob Berzelius. The emergence of his chemical system. Stockholm, Almqvist & Wiksell International; Madison, University of Wisconsin Press, 1981. 357 p. (Also published as 'Studies and sources published by the Swedish History of Science Society No. 34').

Nevoral V, Křížek V: J. J. Berzelius jako analytik minerálních vod. **Fysiatr Reumatol Vestn** 1980 Aug;58(4):244–7

Obermajer J: Neznámé dopisy Purkyňova tchána K. A. Rudolphiho J. J. Berzeliovi. **Cas Lek Cesk** 1984 Feb 17;123(7):199–203

Trofast J: Jöns Jacob Berzelius och djurkemien. **Sydsven Medicinhist Sallsk Arsskr** 1981;:170–84

**Berzin, Robert Iur'evich, 1887–1950**

Apostolov M: D-r Robert Iur'evich Berzin (1887–1950 g.) i bolnitsata na ruskiia Cherven krust v Sofiia. **Khirurgiia (Sofiia)** 1982;35(2):223–7

**Berzins, Elfrida K., 1904–**

Gregory CJ: Elfrida K. Berzins: world record holder, olympic athlete, concert soloist, author, and pioneer physical educator. **Can J Hist Sport Phys Educ** 1979;10(2):1–14

**Berzsenyi, Daniel, 1776–1836**

Merényi O: Berzsenyi Dániel (1776–1836) betegségei és halála. **Orvostort Kozl** 1979;87–88(25 no 1–2):243–7

**Besant, Annie, 1847–1933**

Chandrasekhar S: 'A dirty, filthy book.' The writings of Charles Knowlton and Annie Besant on reproductive physiology and birth control and an account of the Bradlaugh-Besant trial. With the definitive texts of Fruits of philosophy by Charles Knowlton; The law of population by Annie Besant; Theosophy and the law of population by Annie Besant. Berkeley, University of California Press, 1981. xi, 217 p.

**Best, Charles Herbert, 1899–1978**

Bliss M, ed: Banting's, Best's, and Collip's accounts of the discovery of insulin. **Bull Hist Med** 1982;56(4):554–68

Pitt B: Insulin. **Br Herit** 1981;2(3):28–38

Rafter GW: Banting and Best and the sources of useful knowledge. **Perspect Biol Med** 1983 Winter;26(2):281–6

Sunday ME: Canada's Best. **Harv Med Alumni Bull** 1980 Dec;54(6):10–15

**Betances, Ramón Emeterio, 1830–1898**

Figueroa L: Betances, el irreductible. **Atenea (Puerto Rico)** 1972;9(3–4):29–39

Veray FX: Betances, el médico. **Bol Asoc Med PR** 1983 Mar;75(3):110–3

**Bethlen, Gabor, prince of Transylvania, 1580–1629**

Szilágyi I: Bethlen Gábor betegsége és halála. **Orv Hetil** 1984 May 13;125(20):1205–10

**Bethune, Henry Norman, 1890–1939**

Barootes EW: Dr. Norman Bethune: inspiration for a modern China. **Can Med Assoc J** 1980 May 24;122(10):1176–84

Bethune manuscripts in the Osler Library: **HSTC Bull** 1980;15/16:3

Chi nien Pai Ch'iu-en: in memory of Norman Bethune. Pei-ching, Jen min ch'u pan she, 1979. 285 p.

Shephard DA, Lévesque A, ed: Norman Bethune. His time and his legacy. Ottawa, Canadian Public Health Association, 1982. xii, 253 p.

Stewart R: Bethune. 2nd ed. Hamden, Connecticut, Archon, 1979. 210 p.

Stewart R: The mind of Norman Bethune. Toronto, Fitzhenry and Whiteside, 1977. ix, 150 p.

Summers GV: Norman Bethune, Canadian surgeon: his Chinese connection. **Can J Surg** 1983 Jul;26(4):379–82

Walt AJ: The world's best-known surgeon. **Surgery** 1983 Oct;94(4):582–90

**Beuys, Joseph, 1921–**

Murken AH: Joseph Beuys und die Medizin. Münster, Coppenrath, 1979. 160 p. German and English.

Schellmann B: Kunst und Pathologie: Joseph Beuys--'zeige deine Wunde'. **Pathologe** 1983 Nov;4(6):325–7

**Bevan, Arthur Dean, 1861–1943**
Criado FJ, Wilson TH: Posterior transsphincteric approach for surgery of the rectum: the Bevan operation. **Dis Colon Rectum** 1981;24:145–50

**Beveridge, William, 1879–1963**
Harris J: William Beveridge. A biography. Oxford, Clarendon Press, 1977. 488 p.

**Beverwijck, Johan van, 1594–1647**
Van Lieburg MJ: De dichter-medicus Daniël Jonctys (1611–1654), zijn strijd tegen het bijgeloof en zijn relatie tot Johan van Beverwijck, William Harvey en Daniël Sennert. **Tijdschr Geschied Geneeskd** 1979;2(4):137–67

**Beyle, Marie Henri, 1783–1842**
Rocchietta S: Una ricetta contro la gotta trascritta da Stendhal in italiano. **Minerva Med** 1981 Feb 25;72(6):305

**Bharadvaja**
Rama Rao B: Rasapradipika; a Sanskrit medical work attributed to Bharadvaja. **Bull Indian Inst Hist Med (Hyderabad)** 1975 Jul;5(3):123–8

**Bhatia, Sohan Lal, 1891–1981**
Hameed A: A historian of medicine, Major General (Dr) S. L. Bhatia, passes away. **Stud Hist Med** 1981 Sept;5(3):239–41
Subba Reddy DV: Major General S. L. Bhatia (1891–1982). **Bull Indian Inst Hist Med Hyderabad** 1982;12(1–4):88–91

**Bialet Massé, Juan, 1840–1907**
Aznárez EP: Juan Bialet Massé, ilustre médico catalán emigrado a la Argentina. In International Congress of the History of Medicine, 27th, Barcelona, 1980. Actas. Barcelona, Acadèmia de Ciències Mèdiques de Catalunya i Balears, 1981. p. 165–7.

**Bichat, Marie Francois Xavier, 1771–1802**
Duchesneau F: Vers une théorie analytique de l'organisme (Bichat). **Arch Int Hist Idees** 1982;95:431–76
Heywood C: D. H. Lawrence's 'blood consciousness' and the work of Xavier Bichat and Marshall Hall. **Etud Anglaises** 1979;32:397–413
Keel O: John Hunter et Xavier Bichat: les rapports de leurs travaux en pathologie tissulaire. In International Congress of the History of Medicine, 27th, Barcelona, 1980. Actas. Barcelona, Acadèmia de Ciències Mèdiques de Catalunya i Balears, 1981. p. 535–49.
Pickstone JV: Bureaucracy, liberalism and the body in post-revolutionary France: Bichat's physiology and the Paris school of medicine. **Hist Sci** 1981 Jun;19(44 pt 2):115–42
Sutton G: The physical and chemical path to vitalism: Xavier Bichat's Physiological Researches on Life and Death. **Bull Hist Med** 1984 Spring;58(1):53–71

**Bicker, Lambertus, 1732–1801**
Snelders HA: Lambertus Bicker (1732–1801). An early adherent of Lavoisier in the Netherlands. **Janus** 1980;67(1–2–3):101–23

**Bickerdyke, Mary Ann Ball, 1817–1901**
Robbins P: General Grant's calico colonel. **Am Hist Illus** 1979;14(1):4–7, 43–8

**Bidloo, Govard, 1649–1713**
Dumaitre P: La curieuse destinée des planches anatomiques de Gérard de Lairesse, peintre en Hollande - Lairesse, Bidloo, Cowper. Amsterdam, Rodopi, 1982. xvii, 107 p. (Nieuwe Nederlandse Bijdragen tot de Geschiedenis der Geneeskunde en der Natuurwetenschappen, no. 6).
Lindeboom GA: Cowper's brutale 'plagiaat' van Bidloo's Anatomische Atlas. **Ned Tijdschr Geneeskd** 1982 Oct 9;126(41):1878–82

**Biegański, Władysław, 1857–1917**
Jasińska Z, Komorowska W: Władysław Biegański (1857–1917). Spis prac w układzie chronologicznym. **Ann Univ Mariae Curie Sklodowska [Med]** 1978;33:15–27
Matysiak W: Doktor Władysław Biegański -- żywa karta historii polskiej medycyny. **Ann Univ Mariae Curie Sklodowska [Med]** 1978;33:1–5

**Bielschowsky, Alfred, 1871–**
Hertzberg R: Bielschowsky's sign. Its genesis and other observations by Bielschowsky. **Aust J Ophthalmol** 1982 Nov;10(4):282–4

**Bier, August, 1861–1949**
Riet AV: August Bier en de homoeopathie. Eindhoven, Gema, 1978. 320 p. (Diss. Amsterdam).
Waas G: Die Berufung von August Bier (1861–1949) an die Berliner Universität im Jahre 1907. **Z Arztl Fortbild (Jena)** 1980 Oct 15;74(20):982–7

**Bierkowski, Ludwig Jozef, 1801–1860**
Skrobacki A, Völker A: Ze starań Profesora Ludwika Bierkowskiego o pozyskanie katedry w berlinie w 1847 r. **Arch Hist Med (Warsz)** 1979;42(3):303–8

**Bigelow Family**
Lindskog GE: Three generations of Doctors Bigelow at Harvard. **Conn Med** 1983 Dec;47(12):763–9

**Bigelow, Jacob, 1786–1879**
Ewan J: Five pupils of Benjamin Smith Barton: the men and their minds. **Trans Stud Coll Physicians Phila** 1983 Dec;5(5 no 4):309–20
Wolfe RJ: Jacob Bigelow's American medical botany 1817–1821. An examination of the origin, printing, binding and distribution of America's first color plate book. With special emphasis on the manner of making and printing its colored plates. North Hills, Pennsylvania, and Boston, Bird & Bull Press and Boston Medical Library, 1979. 121 p.

**Biggs, Hermann Michael, 1859–1923**
Models for action: **J Public Health Policy** 1980;1(2):103–9

**Biggs, Noah**
Tigertt WD: Noah Biggs, author, fl. 1651. **J Hist Med Allied Sci** 1983 Oct;38(4):452–5

**Bigsby, John Jeremiah, 1792–1881**
Rasporich AW: John Jeremiah Bigsby. In Dictionary of Canadian biography, 1881–1890. 1982;11:72–3.

**Bilharz, Theodor, 1825–1862**
Althoff A: Wissenschaftlicher Briefwechsel von und mit Theodor Bilharz. Düsseldorf, Triltsch, 1980. 133 p. (Düsseldorfer Arbeiten zur Geschichte der Medizin, 56; also Diss.) **Dusseld Arb Gesch Med Hefte** 1980;56:1–133
Classics in infectious diseases: A contribution to human helminthology: Theodore Bilharz (1825–1862). **Rev Infect Dis** 1982 May–Jun;4(3):727–32
Pytel' AIa: Ob otkrytii Bil'gartsem vozbuditelia urinarnogo shistosomoza. **Urol Nefrol (Mosk)** 1980 May–Jun;(3):67–70

**Bilibin, Aleksandr Fedorovich**
Korotkikh RV: Vklad A. F. Bilibina v razvitie problwm meditsinskoĭ deontologii. **Ter Arkh** 1982;54(10):103–6

**Bilikiewicz, Tadeusz, 1901–1980**
Sulestrowska H: Zasługi prof. dr. Tadeusza Bilikiewicza dla rozwoju psychiatrii dziecięcej w Polsce. **Psychiatr Pol** 1982;16(4):321–8
Tadeusz Bilikiewicz (1901–1980)---historyk medycyny i filozof: **Kwart Hist Nauki Tech** 1981;26(2):435–48

**Billings, John Shaw, 1838–1913**
Bleser C, ed: The Hammonds of Redcliffe. New York, Oxford, Oxford University Press, 1981. xxii, 421 p.
Bonsett CA: Museum notes [John Shaw Billings' birthplace] **J Indiana State Med Assoc** 1981;74:348
Cummings MM: Comments on John Shaw Billings. **J Indiana State Med Assoc** 1981 Oct;74(10):638
Havighurst W: The mind of John Shaw Billings. In his: Men of old Miami, 1809–1873, a book of portraits. New York, Putnams, 1974. p. 189–207.
Keys TE, Key JD: Osler and Billings: their friendship and contributions to librarianship. **Am Coll Physicians Obs** 1981 Aug;1(8):1, 4–5
Miles WD: A history of the National Library of Medicine. The nation's treasury of medical knowledge. Bethesda, National Library of Medicine, 1982. viii, 531 p. (NIH Publication No. 82–1904).
Rózsa G: 70 éve halt meg John Shaw Billings. **Orv Hetil** 1983 Sep 4;124(36):2191–2
Waserman M: An important John Shaw Billings find. **Bull Med Libr Assoc** 1984 Jan;72(1):23–5
Webb WM: There's a doctor in the library. The story of John Shaw Billings, M.D. (1838–1913). **J Indiana State Med Assoc** 1981 Jun;74(6):360–6

**Billroth, Theodor, 1829–1894**
Absolon KB: The surgeon's surgeon. Theodor Billroth 1829–1894. Vol. I. Lawrence, Kansas, Coronado Press, 1979. xxi, 282 p.
Absolon KB: Ein einmaliger Brief - Der zwanzigjährige Billroth beschreibt seine Reise durch Thüringen im Jahre 1849. **Pommern** 1982;4:18–27
Absolon KB: The surgeon's surgeon. Theodor Billroth 1829–1894. Volume II. Lawrence, Kansas, Coronado Press, 1981. 232 p.
Absolon KB: Theodor Billroth and cardiac surgery. **J Thorac Cardiovasc Surg** 1983 Sep;86(3):451–2
Allgöwer M, Tröhler U: Biographical note on Theodor Billroth. **Br J Surg** 1981 Oct;68(10):678–9
Andree C: Theodor Billroth (1829–1894) zum 150. Geburtstag. **Med Welt** 1979 Dec 7;30(49):1857–62
Caldamone AA: Theodor Billroth: the urologist. **Urology** 1981 Sep;18(3):316–24
Casal A: Hace cien años, 1881–1981--Billroth y la primera gastrectomía. **Acta Gastroenterol Latinoam** 1981;11(2):326–8
Genschorek W: Wegbereiter der Chirurgis: Johann Friedrich Dieffenbach, Theodor Billroth. Leipzig, Hirzel, Teubner, 1983. 252 p.
Helmer F: Das chirurgische Erbe. Der Einfluss Theodor Billroths auf die heutige Abdominalchirurgie. **Zentralbl Chir** 1982;107(22):1469–80
Holinka C: Theodor Billroth: the life of a surgeon in the spirit of music. **Mt Sinai J Med (NY)** 1981 Jan–Feb;48(1):21–41
Imanaga H: [Honoring Theodor Billroth by attaining a hundred years since his first success in gastric cancer resection (author's transl)] (Jpn). **Nippon Gan Chiryo Gakkai Shi** 1981 Jun 20;16(3):405–8
Kern E: Das chirurgische Erbe. Theodor Billroth und die Musik. **Zentralbl Chir** 1982;107(21):1408–16
Littmann I: Theodor Billroth (1829–1894). **Orvostort Kozl** 1979;87–88(25 no 1–2):123–39
Majno G, Joris I: Billroth and Penicillium. **Rev Infect Dis** 1979 Sep–Oct;1(5):880–4
Schein CJ, Koch E: Jenny Lind's concert in Göttingen. Billroth's letter

to his mother. **NY State J Med** 1979 Oct;79(11):1786-1891
Schober KL: The quotation about the heart. Comments on Theodor Billroth's attitude towards cardiac surgery. **Thorac Cardiovasc Surg** 1981 Jun;29(3):131-7
Schober KL: Teodor Bil'rot i sovremennaia khirurgiia. **Khirurgiia (Mosk)** 1981 Feb;(2):116-7
Schober KL: Das chirurgische Erbe. Theodor Billroth und die Karzinomchirurgie des Intestinaltraktes. **Zentralbl Chir** 1981;106(10):693-9
Schober KL: Das chirurgische Erbe. Theodor Billroth und seine norddeutsche Heimat. **Zentralbl Chir** 1982;107(20):1317-23
Schreiber HW: Wo steht die Carcinom-Chirurgie des Magens 100 Jahre nach der ersten erfolgreichen Magenresektion durch Theodor Billroth? **Langenbecks Arch Chir** 1982;358:53-5
Shafar J: The Brahms Billroth friendship. **Br Med J** 1981;282:1775
Vara López R: Teodoro Billroth (con motivo del centenario de la primera gastrectomía). **An R Acad Nac Med (Madr)** 1981;98(2):283-310
Weir NF: Theodor Billroth and Johannes Brahms--a thirty year friendship. **Hist Med (Lond)** 1975 Autumn-Winter;6(3-4):8-14
Wolff H: Billroth in Berlin. **Zentralbl Chir** 1982;107(20):1324-6
Wondrák E: Ke 100. výročí velkého výkonu v chirurgii žaludku. **Cas Lek Cesk** 1981 May 28;120(21):646-50
Wyklicky H: Vor hundert Jahren. Billroths erste Pylorusresektion, seine diesbezüglichen Publikationen in der 'Wiener Medizinischen Wochenschrift' und ein Rückblick auf seine Zeit. **Wien Med Wochenschr** 1981 Jan 15;131(1):1-13

**Binet, Alfred, 1857-1911**
Stocking GW: Innovation in the Malinowskian mode: an essay review of long-term field research in social anthropology. **J Hist Behav Sci** 1980 Jul;16(3):281-6

**Bing, R. Abraham, 1752-1841**
Prayer composed during cholera epidemic outbreak 1831 and 1847?: by R. Abraham Bing of Würzburg. **Koroth** 1979 Nov;7(9-10):719-20

**Binswanger, Ludwig, 1881-1966**
Pivnicki D: Paradoxes of psychotherapy. In honor and memory of Ludwig Binswanger. **Confin Psychiatr** 1979;22(4):197-203

**Biourge, Philibert, 1864-1942**
Hennebert GL: Philibert Biourge, microbiologiste et mycologue (1864-1942). Colloque d'histoire des sciences III. Louvain, 1979. p. 61-98.

**Birčák, Ján, 1923-**
Houštěk J: Professor MUDr. Ján Birčák šedesátiletý. **Cesk Pediatr** 1983 Feb;38(2):117-9

**Bircher, Willy, 1898-1970**
Dr. med. Willy Bircher-Schwarzenbach (1898-1970): s. l., s. n., 1970?. 28 p.

**Biriukov, Dmitriĭ Andreevich, 1904-1969**
Bogdanov OV: Vklad D. A. Biriukova v émbriofiziologiiu i dal'neĭshee razvitie ego ideĭ. **Fiziol Zh SSSR** 1984 Sep;70(9):1248-55
Vasilevskiĭ NN: D. A. Biriukov, 1904-1969. Moskva, Meditsina, 1981 95 p.

**al-Biruni, 973?-1048**
Arnaldez R: The theory and practice of science according to Ibn Sina and al-Biruni. **Stud Philos Med** 1977 Mar;1(1):58-69
Hamarneh SK: Al-Biruni, the father of Arabic pharmacy and marine biology as demonstrated in al-Saydanah. In: International Congress held in Pakistan on the occasion of Millenary of Abu Raihan Muhammad ibn Ahmad al-Biruni (973-ca 1051 A.D.) November 26, 1973 thru December 12, 1973. Proceedings. Karachi, Hamdard National Foundation, 1979. p. 479-500.
Hermelink H: Zur Bestimmung von Birunis Todestag. **Sudhoffs Arch** 1977;61(3):298-300

**Bissell, Emily Perkins, 1861-1948**
Agris J: Stamps commemorating medicine: Emily Bissell. **J Dermatol Surg Oncol** 1980;6(9):705
Higgins A: John Janvier Black (1837-1909): an ornament to his profession. **Del Med J** 1982 Apr;54(4):233-7

**Bizzozero, Giulio Cesare, 1846-1901**
Coller BS: Bizzozero and the discovery of the blood platelet. **Lancet** 1984 Apr 7;1(8380):804
Tavassoli M: Selected items from the history of pathology - Giulio Bizzozero (1846-1901). **Am J Pathol** 1980;101(1):50

**Bjerrum, Jannik Petersen, 1851-1920**
Ehlers H: Bjerrum's Clinic. **Surv Ophthalmol** 1981 Sep-Oct;26(1):101-2

**Black, Greene Vardiman, 1836-1915**
Herschfeld JJ: G. V. Black and the search for a better amalgam. **Bull Hist Dent** 1980 Oct;28(2):76-82
Mann WV: G. V. Black revisited. **J Dent Educ** 1981 Jun;45(6):338-9
Pappas CN: The life and times of G. V. Black. Chicago, Quintessence Pub. Co., 1983. 128 p.

**Black, John Janvier, 1837-1909**
Higgins A: John Janvier Black (1837-1909): an ornament to his profession. **Del Med J** 1982 Apr;54(4):233-7

**Black, Joseph, 1728-1799**
Buchanan WW, Brown DH: Joseph Black (1728-1799): Scottish physician and chemist. **Practitioner** 1980 Jun;224(1344):663-6
Perrin CE: A reluctant catalyst: Joseph Black and the Edinburgh reception of Lavoisier's chemistry. **Ambix** 1982 Nov;29(3):141-76

**Blackburn, Luke Pryor, 1816-1887**
Baird ND: Luke Pryor Blackburn: physician, governor, reformer. Lexington, University Press of Kentucky, 1979. viii, 127 p.

**Blackely, Carlos**
Deschamps Chapeaux P: El negro en la economía Habanera del siglo XIX. Flebotomianos y dentistas. **Rev Bibl Nac Jose Marti** 1971;13(1):75-86

**Blacklock, Donald Breadalbane, 1879-**
Crosskey RW, Post RJ: Which cytospecies of the Simulium damnosum complex did Blacklock incriminate in the transmission of Onchocerca volvulus? **Ann Trop Med Parasitol** 1981 Oct;75(5):569-71

**Blackwell, Elizabeth, 1821-1910**
Bendiner E: Past and present: Elizabeth Blackwell: 'heresy with intelligence'. **Hosp Pract** Jun;15(6):1821-1910
Farley F: Two generations of women physicians: the New York Infirmary, 1870-1899. **J Am Med Wom Assoc** 1984 Nov-Dec;39(6):189-91
Fischoff E: Elizabeth Blackwell: first woman M.D. **Pearson Mus Monogr Ser** 1981;4:1-22
Morantz RM: Feminism, professionalism, and germs: the thought of Mary Putnam Jacobi and Elizabeth Blackwell. **Amer Q** 1982;34:459-78
Smith D: A persistent rebel. **Am Hist Illus** 1981;15(9):28-35

**Blackwell Family, 19th cent.**
Horn M: 'Sisters worthy of respect': family dynamics and women's roles in the Blackwell family. **J Fam Hist** 1983 Winter;8(4):367-82

**Blackwood, Thomas**
Franklin WE: Thomas Blackwood, frontier physician. **Mich Hist** 1970;54(4):216-30

**Bláhnik Family**
Hanzlíček Z: První česká lékárna v Chicagu. **Cesk Farm** 1981 May;30(3-4):125-30

**Blainville, Henri Marie Ducrotay de, 1777-1850**
Legée G: Henri Ducrotay de Blainville (1777-1850) et la physiologie. In: Congrès National des Sociétés Savantes, 105e, Caen, 1980. Comptes Rendus, Paris, 1980. Section des Sciences, Fasc. V. p. 49-59.

**Blake, Charles, 1746-1810**
Janson G: Charles Blake. In Dictionary of Canadian biography, 1801 to 1820. Volume 5, 1983. p. 88-9.

**Blake, I. F.**
Davis E: Irene's diary of nursing in World War I. **Australas Nurses J** 1980 Dec;10(1):16-8

**Blake, John Ballard, 1922-**
Stevenson LG: The Blake era at HMD. **Bull Hist Med** 1982;56(4):455-9

**Blake, William, 1757-1827**
Curtis FB: William Blake and eighteenth-century medicine. **Blake Stud** 1979;8:187-99
Lee RV: The generalist: a jaundiced view. **Am J Med** 1983 Dec;75(6):902-5

**Blalock, Alfred, 1899-1964**
Harvey AM: Alfred Blalock. In Dictionary of American biography, 1961-1965. Suppl. 7, 1981. p. 59.
Longmire WP: Two great American surgeons, each with four aces. **Pharos** 1983 Summer;46(3):9-14
McNamara DG: Landmark perspective: the Blalock-Taussig operation and subsequent progress in surgical treatment of cardiovascular diseases. **JAMA** 1984 Apr 27;251(16):2139-41
Ravitch MM: Progress in resection of the chest wall for tumor with reminiscences of Dr. Blalock. **Johns Hopkins Med J** 1982 Aug;151(2):43-53
Scott HW: A tribute to Barney Brooks, Alfred Blalock, and the Vanderbilt Surgical Staff (1925 to 1982). **South Med J** 1982 Dec;75(12):1439-52

**Blanchet, François, 1776-1830**
Bernier J: François Blanchet et le mouvement réformiste en médecine au début du XIXe siècle. **Rev Hist Am Fr** 1980;34(2):223-44

**Blanchet, Joseph-Godric, 1829-1890**
Caissie F: Joseph-Godric Blanchet. In Dictionary of Canadian biography, 1881-1890. 1982;11:85-6.

**Blanchfield, Florence Aby, 1882-1971**
Henry LJ: Florence Aby Blanchfield. In: Notable American women. The modern period. Cambridge, Mass., Belknap-Harvard Univ. Press, 1980. 4:83-5.

**Bland, Theodorick, 1777-1846**
Trice ER: Theodorick Bland, Jr: Virginia physician, cuirassier. **Va Med** 1980 Feb;107(2):88-9

**Blane, Gilbert, 1749-1834**
Leach RD: Sir Gilbert Blane, Bart, MD FRS (1749-1832). **Ann R Coll Surg Engl** 1980 May;62(3):232-9

Wharton M: Sir Gilbert Blane Bt (1749-1834). **Ann R Coll Surg Engl** 1984 Sep;66(5):375-6

**Blankaart, Stephanus, 1650-1702**
Blankaart S: Den Nederlandschen Herbarius. Facsimile of 1698 ed. Edited by D. A. Wittop Koning. Alphen, Stafleu-Brussel. 621 p.
Jarcho S: Blankaart's Dictionary, an index to 17th century medicine. **Bull NY Acad Med** 1982 Sep;58(6):568-77

**Blasco, Manuel, 1899-**
Jordi R: Manuel Blasco, pintor, escritor y bohemio. **Circ Farm** 1981 Mar;12(136):83-8

**Blaser, Robert Henry**
Blaser RH: Paracelsus in Basel. Festschrift für Professor Dr. Robert-Henri Blaser zum 60. Geburtstag. Herausgegeben von der Schweizerischen Paracelsus-Gesellschaft. Biographical introduction by K. Goldammer. Muttenz/Basel, St. Arbogast Verlag, 1979. 210 p. (Reprint of 7 works by Blaser).

**Blasius, Ernst, 1802-1875**
Hauben DJ: Ernst Blasius's contributions to plastic surgery. **Plast Reconstr Surg** 1984 Oct;74(4):561-70
Schober KL: Vor etwa 100 Jahren (8). Amputatio talo-calcanea von Dr. E. Blasius Geh. Medicinalrath und Professor in Halle. **Zentralbl Chir** 1979;104(11):739-41

**Blasius, Gerard, 1626-1682**
Gysel C: Een vulgarisator van de anatomie van het kauwstelsel: Gerard Blasius (1626-1682-1982). **Ned Tijdschr Tandheelkd** 1984 Jun;91(6):153-8

**Blaszkowski, Thomas**
Welsh JS: The trial pharmacist. **Am Pharm** 19(5):16-7, 33, May 79

**Blest, Guillermo Cunningham, 1800-1884**
Costa-Casaretto C: Don Diego Portales y el Dr. Guillermo C. Blest. **Rev Med Chil** 1984 Jun;112(6):625-31
Costa-Casaretto C: Presentacion del Dr. Guillermo C. Blest. **Rev Med Chil** 1983 Apr;111(4):364-7

**Bleuler, Eugen, 1857-1939**
Bleuler M: Eugen Bleuler and schizophrenia. **Br J Psychiatry** 1984 Mar;144:327-8
Hitomi K: [Historical progress and the present interpretation of schizophrenic theory held by Bleuler's school] (Jpn). **Seishin Shinkeigaku Zasshi** 1982;84(10):735-42
Hoenig J: The concept of Schizophrenia. Kraepelin-Bleuler-Schneider. **Br J Psychiatry** 1983 Jun;142:547-56

**Bleuler, Manfred Eugen, 1902-1983**
Jarosz M: Manfred Bleuler i inni o wyst epowaniu prawidłowych stanów psychicznych u chorych na schizofrenię. **Psychiatr Pol** 1981 Jul-Dec;15(4-6):403-9
Rihner F: Professor Dr. Manfred Bleuler zum 80. Geburtstag. Zürich, Woodtli, 1982. 43 p.

**Bleyer, Adrian, 1879-1965?**
Karp LE: Adrien Bleyer: in the right place at the wrong time. **Am J Med Genet** 1981;10(3):209-11

**Bloch, Bruno, 1878-1933**
Sulzberger MB: Three lessons learned in Bloch's clinic. **Am J Dermatopathol** 1980 Winter;2(4):321-5

**Block, Dr., d. 1892**
Schober KL: Das chirurgische Erbe: Tragische Chirurgenschicksale. 1882: Die Tragödie des Dr. Block. **Zentralbl Chir** 1984;109(5):366-73

**Blomefylde, Myles, 1525-1603**
Baker DC, Murphy JL: Myles Blomefylde, Elizabethan physician, alchemist and book collector: a sketch of a life. **Bodleian Libr Rec** 1982 Nov;11(1):35-46

**Blonski, Pavel Petrovich**
Kozulin A: Peter Blonsky and Russian progressivism: the early years. **Stud Sov Thought** 1982;24(1):11-21

**Blood, Peter, 1653-**
Dauber LG: Peter Blood and the Brethren of the Coast. Fictional physicians afield. **NY State J Med** 1982 Jun;82(7):1107-9

**Blos, Peter, 1904-**
Muuss RE: Peter Blos' modern psychoanalytic interpretation of adolescence. **J Adolesc** 1980 sep;3(3):229-52

**Blumenbach, Johann Friedrich, 1752-1840**
Gysel C: Les relations du jeune Blumenbach avec Camper vieillissant. **Hist Sci Med** 1983;17(2):135-9
Lenoir T: Kant, Blumenbach, and vital materialism in German biology. **Isis** 1980 Mar;71(256):77-108

**Blundell, James, 1790-1878**
Sørensen T: James Blundell 27.XII.1790-15.I.1878. Professor i fysiologi og obstetrik ved Guy's Hospital 1823-1834. **Ugeskr Laeger** 1983 Jun 27;145 Spec No:5-49

**Blunt, Katharine, 1876-1954**
Trecker JL: Katharine Blunt. In: Notable American women. The modern period. Cambridge, Mass., Belknap-Harvard Univ. Press, 1980. 4:87-8.

**Blyth, Edward, 1810-1873**
Eiseley L: Darwin and the mysterious Mr. X: new light on the evolutionists. New York and London, Harcourt Brace Jovanovich, 1981. xii, 278 p.

**Boaistuau, Pierre, d. 1566**
Simonin M: Michel de Nostredame, Pierre Boaistuau, Chavigny et la peste aixoise de 1546. **Bibl Hum Renaissance** 1983;45(1):127-30

**Boardman, Mabel Thorp, 1860-1946**
Stewart S: Sharing more than marble palaces. **DAR Mag** 1981;115(3):188-91

**Bobbs, John Stough, 1809-1870**
Bonsett CA: The world's first gall bladder surgeon was a Hoosier. **J Indiana State Med Assoc** 1980 Apr;73(4):201
Carmichael AG, ed: [John S. Bobbs]. **Indiana Med Hist Q** 1982;8(2):3-24
Greenwood RD: 19th century medicine in Indiana. An 1869 clinical report by J. S. Bobbs. **Indiana Med** 1984 Jun;77(6):476

**Bobon, Jean**
Dor J: Jean Bobon et la psychopathologie du langage. **Acta Psychiatr Belg** 1983 May-Jun;83(3):197-206

**Bocage, André, 1892-1953**
Mercier P: André Bocage et la naissance de la tomographie. **Bull Acad Natl Med (Paris)** 1979;3:188-91

**Bochdalka, Vincence Alexandra, 1801-1883**
Wondrák E: Cesky anatom a patolog V. A. Bochdalek--100 let od smrti. **Cas Lek Cesk** 1983 Oct 28;122(43):1334-7

**Boczoń, Tadeusz**
Marczyński A: Dr Tadeusz Boczoń. **Przegl Lek** 1984;41(1):127-31

**Bodington, George, 1799-1882**
Keers RY: Two forgotten pioneers. James Carson and George Bodington. **Thorax** 1980 Jul;35(7):483-9

**Bodio, Luigi, 1840-1920**
Kármán T: A nemzetközi összehasonlító népesedésstatisztika fejlödese a XIX. század utolsó negyedében (Luigi Bodio). **Demografia** 1978;21(4):493-504

**Bodley, Rachel Littler, 1831-1888**
Abram RJ: Documenting our past. Daughters of Aesculapius. **J Am Med Wom Assoc** 1983 May-Jun;38(3):71-2, 82

**Bodoni, Giovanni Battista, 1740-1813**
Rocchietta S: Libri di interesse medico stampati da Giambattista Bodoni (1740-1813). **Minerva Med** 1983 Oct 13;74(39):2327-8

**Boeck, Caesar, 1845-1917**
Epstein WL: 'Multiple benign sarkoid of the skin' by Boeck, December 1899. Commentary: What begot Boeck? **Arch Dermatol** 1982 Oct;118(10):711-22

**Boecler, Jean, 1737-1808**
Jacquel R: Trois Alsaciens et les débuts--modestes--de la médecine sociale en Pologne pendant l'époque des lumières (troisième tiers du XVIIIe siècle). Les médecins strasbourgeois Jacques Reinbold Spielmann (1722-1783) et Jean Boecler (1737-1808) et le savant mulhousien Jean-Henri Lambert (1728-1777). In Livet G, Schaff G, ed: Médecine et assistance en Alsace, XVIe-XXe siècle. Strasbourg, Istra, 1976. p. 155-200.

**Boerhaave, Herman, 1668-1738**
Donnellan WL: Medicine and society in the sixteenth and seventeenth centuries: their influence on the life and work of Herman Boerhaave, 1668-1738. Ph.D. Diss., Northwestern University. Evanston, 1981. vii, 483 p.
Groos KS: Enkele opmerkingen met betrekking tot het graf van Herman Boerhaave in de Pieterskerk te Leiden. **Tijdschr Geschied Geneeskd** 1979;2(4):176-81
Heller S: Boerhaaves Schweizer Studenten: ein Beitrag zur Geschichte des Medizinstudiums. Zürich, Juris, 1984. 111 p. (Zürcher Medizingeschichtliche Abhandlungen, Neue Reihe, Nr. 169)
Houtzager HL: A letter from Herman Boerhaave to Johan Philip Burggraaf jr. **Janus** 1980:67(1-2-3):201-5
Kegel-Brinkgreve E, Luyendijk-Elshout AM, ed: Boerhaave's orations. Leiden, Leiden University Press, 1983. vi, 374 p.
Lindeboom GA, ed: Boerhaave's correspondence. Part 3. Leiden, Brill, 1979. viii, 281 p. (Part 1 was published 1962, and Part 2 in 1964).
Luyendijk-Elshout AM: Samuel Musgrave's attack upon Stahl's and Boerhaave's doctrines in 1763. **Janus** 1980;67(1-2-3):141-56
Luyendijk-Elshout AM: Mechanicisme contra vitalisme de school van Herman Boerhaave en de beginselen van het leven. **Tijdschr Geschied Geneeskd** 1982;5(1):16-26
Maat GJ: Boerhaave en zijn tijdgenoten, en de betekenis van hun lichaamslengte (een fysisch-antropologisch onderzoek van begravenen in de Pieterskerk te Leiden). **Ned Tijdschr Geneeskd** 1982 Apr 17;126(16):705-12
Schmid-Schönbein H: Die Ursprünge der medizinischen Hämorheologie im 18. Jahrhundert: H. Boerhaave, A. v. Haller und G. van Swieten. **Vasa** 1984;Suppl 12:10-31
Scopa JP: Boerhaave on alchemy. **Synthesis** 1979;4(4):24-37
Van der Star P, ed: Fahrenheit's letters to Leibniz and Boerhaave. Amsterdam, Rodopi, 1983. 195 p. (Nieuwe Nederlandse bijdragen

tot de geschiedenis der geneeskunde en der natuurwetenschappen, no. 10).

**Bogdanov, Ivan Luk'ianovich, 1903–**
Ivan Luk'ianovich Bogdanov (k 80-letiiu so dnia rozhdeniia): **Vrach Delo** 1983 Aug;(8):125–6

**Bogdanovskiĭ, Evstafii Ivanovich**
Mirskiĭ MB: Vydaiushchiĭsia russkiĭ khirurg E. I. Bogdanovskiĭ (k 150-letiiu so dnia rozhdeniia). **Vestn Khir** 1984 Mar;132(3):143–5

**Bogisic, Baltazar, 1834–1908**
Grujić V: Nekolike korespondentne veze ismedju Vladana Djordjevića i Valtazara Bogišića. **Srp Ark Celok Lek** 1981 Jan;109(1):161–8

**Bogomolets, Aleksandr Aleksandrovich, 1881–1946**
Ado AD: Razvitie ideĭ A. A. Bogomol'tsa v sovremennoĭ allergologii. **Fiziol Zh** 1981 May–Jun;27(3):354–7
Ado AD: A. A. Bogomolets i sovremennaia allergologiia. **Patol Fiziol Eksp Ter** 1981 Mar–Apr;(2): 70–3
Berezhnaia NM: Uchenie o reaktivnosti A. A. Bogomolets i razvitie sovremennoĭ allergologii. **Fiziol Zh** 1981 May–Jun;27(3):358–68
Berezovskiĭ VA: Ritmy biologicheskikh protsessov kak proiavlenie individual'noĭ reaktivnosti i konstitutsii individa. **Patol Fiziol Eksp Ter** 1981 May–Jun;(3):3–7
Chebotarev DF: Idei A. A. Bogomol'tsa razvitie sovremenno i gerontologii. **Fiziol Zh** 1981 May–Jun;27(3):400–6
Chebotarev DF, Duplenko IuK: Vklad A. A. Bogomol'tsa v razrabotku aktual'nyk problem medikobiologicheskoĭ nauki (k 100-letiiu so dnia rozhdeniia). **Vrach Delo** 1981 May;(5):6–10
Fedorov NA, Movshed BE: Teoriia A. A. Bogomol'tsa o kolloidoklazii v mekhanizme deĭstviia perelivaniia krovi i ee sovremennoe razvitie. **Probl Gematol Pereliv Krovi** 1981 May;26(5):5–13
Il'chevich NV, Spasokukotskiĭ IuA, Alekseeva IN, et al: Razvitie ideĭ A. A. Bogomol'tsa v oblasti ėksperimental'nogo izucheniia i primeneniia v praktike tsitotoksicheskikh syvorotok. **Fiziol Zh** 1981 May–Jun;27(3):339–46
K 100-letiiu so dnia rozhdeniia A. A. Bogomol'tsa: **Klin Med (Mosk)** 1981 Nov;59(11):3–8
K 100-letiiu so dnia rozhdeniia akademika A. A. Bogomol'tsa: **Fiziol Zh** 1981 May–Jun;27(3):291–443
Komissarenko PV: Znachenie issledovaniĭ A. A. Bogomol'tsa v razvitii sovremennoĭ ėndokrinologii. **Fiziol Zh** 1981 May–Jun;27(3):388–93
Komissarenko VP: Idei A. A. Bogomol'tsa v razvitii sovremennoĭ ėndokrinologii. **Patol Fiziol Eksp Ter** 1981 Mar–Apr;(2):82–9
Miagkaia IP: Antiretikuliarnaia tsitotoksicheskaia syvorotka A. A. Bogomol'tsa kak sredstvo patogeneticheskoĭ terapii razlichnykh zabolevaniĭ. **Patol Fiziol Eksp Ter** 1981 Mar–Apr;(2):39–46
Miagkaia IP: Sovremennye predstavleniia o mekhanizme deĭstviia antiretikuliarnoĭ tsitotoksicheskoĭ syvorotki Bogomol'tsa. **Fiziol Zh** 1981 May–Jun;27(3):347–53
Movshev BE: Razvitie ucheniia A. A. Bogomol'tsa o mekhanizme deĭstviia perelivaniia krovi. **Gematol Transfuziol** 1984 Jan;29(1):6–12
Neiman IM: Predvidenie--osnovnaia osobennost' tvorchestva Aleksandra Aleksandrovicha Bogomol'tsa. **Fiziol Zh** 1981 May–Jun;27(3):307–10
Nichik VM: Filosofskie vzgliady A. A. Bogomol'tsa. **Patol Fiziol Eksp Ter** 1981 Mar–Apr;(2):20–30, also in Fiziol Zh 1981 May–Jun;27(3):302–6
Nikitin VN, Perskiĭ EE, Utevskiĭ LA: Molekuliarnye mekhanizmy vozrastnogo razvitiia kollagenovykh struktur i teoriia stareniia A. A. Bogomol'tsa. **Fiziol Zh** 1981 May–Jun;27(3):407–12
Nikitin VN, Perskiĭ EE, Utevskaia LA: Uchenie A. A. Bogomol'tsa o roli soedinitel'noĭ tkani v starenii i sovremennye predstavleniia o mekhanizmakh vozrastnogo razvitiia kollagenovyk struktur. **Patol Fiziol Eksp Ter** 1981 Mar–Apr;(2):30–9
Pinchuk VG: Razvitie ideĭ A. A. Bogomolets v oblasti izucheniia reaktivnosti organizma pri opukholevom protsesse. **Fiziol Zh** 1981 May–Jun;27(3):327–31
Serkov FN: Problemy normal'noĭ fiziologii v issledovaniiakh A. A. Bogomolets. **Fiziol Zh** 1981 May–Jun;27(3):438–43
Terekhov NT: Razvitie idei akademika A. A. Bogomol'tsa v sovremennoĭ transfuziologii. **Fiziol Zh** 1981 May–Jun;27(3):384–7
Uzhanskiĭ IaG: K nauchno-literaturnomu nasledstvu akademika Aleksandra Aleksandrovicha Bogomol'tsa (ob osobennostiakh pis'ma akademika A. A. Bogomol'tsa v nauchnykh trudakh). **Patol Fiziol Eksp Ter** 1981 Mar–Apr;(2):16–20
Uzhanskiĭ IaG: K mekhanizmu stimuliatsii funksiĭ i regeneratsii kletok i tkaneĭ po A. A. Bogomol'tsa. **Fiziol Zh** 1981 May–Jun;27(3):322–6
Zaĭko NN: A. A. Bogomolets kak pedagog. **Patol Fiziol Eksp Ter** 1981 Mar–Apr;(2):9–16
Zaiko NN: A. A. Bogomolets, zhizn i deiatel nost. K 100-letiiu so dnia rozhdeniia. **Fiziol Zh** 1981 May–Jun;27(3):291–301

**Boháč, Antonín, 1882–1950**
Subrtová A: Antonín Bohác--statistik a demograf: život a dílo. **Sb Nar Muzea Praze Rada A Hist** 1977;32(1–3):1–198

**Bohn, Johann, 1640–1718**
Trevisani F: 'Ratio' und 'Experimentum': Johannes Bohn (1640–1718) und die italienische Experimentalphysiologie. **Clio Med** 1983 Mar;17(4):199–206

**Boillaud, Jean Baptiste, 1796–1887**
Borodulin VI: Klinicheskaia shkola Korvizara i ee rol' v razvitii ucheniia o bolezniakh serdtsa (k 100-letiiu so dnia smerti Zhana Batista Buĭo). **Kardiologiia** 1982 Jan;22(1):113–5

**Boisen, Anton Theophilus, 1876–1965**
Asquith GH: Anton T. Boisen and the study of 'living human documents.' **J Presbyt Hist** 1982;60(3):244–65
Powell RC: Anton Theophilus Boisen. In Dictionary of American biography, 1961–1965. Suppl. 7, 1981. p. 63–5.

**Bókay, János, 1858–1937**
Gegesi Kiss P: Bókay János junior a tanítvány szemével. **Orv Hetil** 1983 May 29;124(22):1329–34
Kiss PG: János Bókay junior as seen by a disciple. **Acta Paediatr Hung** 1984;25(1–2):7–10
Miltényi M: Emlékezés ifjú Bókay Jánosra. **Orv Hetil** 1983 May 29;124(22):1327–9
Miltényi M: Professor János Bókay, Jr. **Acta Paediatr Hung** 1984;25(1–2):3–5

**Bolívar, Simón, 1783–1830**
Febres-Cordero F: Datos sobre el estado de salud dentaria del Libertador. **Thorax** 1979;6(1):29–31
Febres-Cordero F: Datos sobre el estado de la salud dentaria del Libertador. Caracas, 1983. [2 p.]
Figueroa Marroquin H: De qué murió Simon Bolivar? **Bol Soc Mex Hist Filos Med** 1981 Dec;5(37):217–47
Figueroa Marroquín H: De que murio Simon Bolivar? **Bol Hist Antig (Bogota)** 1981;68(733):385–419
Laclé A: La falsa ciclotimia de Bolivar. **Rev Soc Bolivar Venez** 1979;36(121):71–3
Mérida F: Semblanzas de Alejandro Prospero Révérend, primicias para calificar su actuacion frente a la ultima enfermedad del Libertador. **Rev Soc Venez Hist Med** 1981;30(47):71–80
Mérida F: Las enfermedades odontologicas y dermatologicas del Libertador. **Rev Soc Venez Hist Med** 1981;30(47):81–7
Mérida MT: Las enfermedades odontológicas y dermatológicas del Liberatador. **Acta Odontol Venez** 1983 May–Aug;21(2):154–61
Reverend AP: La enfermedad y los ultimos momentos de Simon Bolivar, libertador de Colombia y del Peru. **Rev Soc Bolivar Venez** 1980;37(128):57–94
Torres M: La nueva perspectiva psicologica de Bolivar. **Bol Hist Antiq (Bogota)** 1980;67(728):69–85

**Boll, Franz, 1849–1879**
Belloni L: Hermann Helmholtz und Franz Boll. **Medizinhist J** 1982;17(1/2):129–37

**Boltzmann, Ludwig Edward, 1844–1906**
Broda E: Ludwig Boltzmann als evolutionistischer Philosoph. **Ber Wissenschaftsgesch** 1983;6(1–4):103–14

**Bolzano, Bernard, 1781–1848**
Daněk K: Bernard Bolzano v historii medicíny. **Cas Lek Cesk** 1981 Sep 24;120(38)1160–3

**Bonaparte, Marie, 1882–1962**
Buckley NL: Women psychoanalysts and the theory of feminine development: a study of Karen Horney, Helene Deutsch, and Marie Bonaparte. Ph.D. Diss., University of California. Los Angeles, 1982. 178 p.

**Bonavita, Juan María, fl. 1832**
Beauperthuy de Benedetti R: Un cirujano y un medico de Montpellier en el siglo pasado en Caracas. **Rev Soc Venez Hist Med** 1979;28(42):29–30

**Bond, Charles John, 1856–1939**
Walker JB: Charles John Bond of Leicester (1856–1939). **J R Soc Med** 1984 Apr;77(4):316–24

**Bond, Thomas, 1712–1784**
Brock CH: Dr. Thomas Bond of Philadelphia and his 'Worm'. **Trans Stud Coll Physicians Phila** 1981 Sep;5(3 no 3):209–13

**Bonet, Théophile, 1620–1689**
Crellin J: Théophile Bonet (1620–1689). **Am J Pathol** 1980 Jan;98(1):212
Trebbin H: Frühe Pathologie. **MMW** 1980 Feb 8;122(6):209–11

**Bonhoeffer, Karl, 1868–1948**
Propping P: Genetic disorders presenting as 'schizophrenia'. Karl Bonhoeffer's early view of the psychoses in the light of medical genetics. **Hum Genet** 1983;65(1):1–10
Schulze HA: Karl Bonhoeffer, seine Persönlichkeit, sein Werk, seine Wirkung. **Psychiatr Neurol Med Psychol (Leipz)** 1981 Jun;33(6):321–6

**Boniface VIII, Pope, 1235?–1303**
Brown EA: Death and the human body in the later Middle Ages: the legislation of Boniface VIII on the division of the corpse. **Viator** 1981;12:221–70

**Bonilla-Naar, Alfonso, 1916–**
Hernández de Alba G: Una obra postuma cientifica monumental: la bibliografia medica Colombiana (1782–1976). **Bol Cult Bibliogr (Bogota)** 1976;16(7–8):176–9

**Bonnafont, Jean-Pierre, 1805–1891**
Ségal A: Le médecin principal de 1re classe Jean-Pierre Bonnafont (1805–1891); sa place prépondérante dans l'histoire de l'endoscopie aus XIXe siècle. **Hist Sci Med** 1983;17(1):63–70

**Bonnet, Charles, 1720–1793**
Marx J: Charles Bonnet contre les Lumières. 2 v. Oxford, Voltaire Foundation at the Taylor Institution, 1976. 782 p.

**Bonwill, William G. A., 1833–1899**
Herschfeld JJ: W.G.A. Bonwill and the 'anatomical articulator.' **Bull Hist Dent** 1980 Apr;28(1):29–34

**Booker, William, fl. 1682**
Burnby J: Three 17th century London apothecaries; Richard Meynell, Charles Needham, William Booker. **Pharm Hist (London)** 1975 May;5(1):2–3

**Boone, Levi Day, 1808–1882**
Beatty WK: Levi Day Boone--Physician and politician. **Proc Inst Med Chic** 1980 Oct–Dec;33(4):139–41

**Booth, William, 1829–1912**
Matsufuji G: [Phosphor-poisoning in match factories and the Salvation Army General Booth] (Jpn). **Igakushi Kenkyu** 1980;54:1–6

**Bordet, Jules, 1870–1961**
Silverstein AM: History of immunology. Development of the concept of immunologic specificity, I. **Cell Immunol** 1982 Mar 1;67(2):396–409

**Borelli, Giovanni Alfonso, 1608–1679**
Middleton WE: Some unpublished correspondence of Giovanni Alfonso Borelli. **Ann Ist Mus Stor Sci Fir** 1984;9(2):99–132
Sourander P: Drottning Christina och Giovanni Alfonso Borelli till 300–årsminnet av kinesiologins födelse. **Nord Medicinhist Arsb** 1982;:56–65

**Boric, Dusan, 1889–1978**
Djordjević SP: Akademik prof. dr Dušan Borić (1. IX 1889–3. IX 1978). **Srp Arh Celok Lek** 1980 May;108(5):541–53

**Borja de Guzman, Pedro, 1908–**
Swanson BZ: Spain's private dental museum. **Bull Hist Dent** 1984;32(1):27–30

**Bormann, Martin, 1900–1945?**
Sognnaes RF: Hitler and Bormann identifications compared by postmortem craniofacial and dental characteristics. **Am J Forensic Med Pathol** 1980 Jun;1(2):105–15

**Borodin, Aleksandr Porfir'evich, 1833–1887**
Ionov IuV, Ionov AIu: A. P. Borodin - vrach, khimik, pedagog (k 150–letiiu so dnia rozhdeniia). **Sov Zdravookhr** 1984;(1):61–4
Lasky II: Medicine and music. **NY State J Med** 1982 Dec;82(13):1862–4
Liashenko NI: Aleksandr Porfir'evich Borodin (k 150 letiiu so dnia rozhdeniia). **Voen Med Zh** 1983 Nov;(11):66–9
Shul'tsev GP: Aleksandr Porfir'evich Borodin (k 150–letiiu so dnia rozhdeniia). **Klin Med (Mosk)** 1984 Jul;62(7):144–7

**Bory de Saint-Vincent, Jean-Baptiste Marcellin, 1778–1846**
Arvy L: Jean-Baptiste Marcellin Bory de Saint-Vincent (1778–1846) et les 'Animaux Spermatiques'. In: Congrès National des Sociétés Savantes, 104e, Bordeaux, 1979. Comptes Rendus. Paris, 1979. Section des Sciences, Fasc. IV. p. 21–5.

**Borzenkov, Ia A., 1825–1883**
Bliakher LI: Ia. A. Borzenkov-istorik biologii. **Vopr Istor Estestvozn Tekh** 1982;1:36–44

**Bosch, Hieronymus van Aken, known as, d. 1516**
Dixon LS: Alchemical imagery in Bosch's Garden of Delights. Ann Arbor, UMI Research Press, 1981. xxii, 225 p. (Studies in the Fine Arts: Iconography, no. 2).
Kierulf H: L'ergotisme chez Bosch et Grünewald. In International Congress of the History of Medicine, 27th, Barcelona, 1980. Actas. Barcelona, Académia de Ciències Médiques de Catalunya i Balears, 1981. p. 81–90.
Kierulf H: L'ergotisme chez Bosch et Grünewald. **Nouv Presse Med** 1982 Oct 2;11(38):2803–9
Tschassovnikarov D, Markov G: Personologische Untersuchungen über einige Urbilder im Schaffen von Hieronymus Bosch. **Psychiatr Neurol Med Psychol (Leipz)** 1980 Oct;32(10):623–30

**Boseman, Benjamin A., Jr., 1840–1881**
Hine WC: Dr. Benjamin A. Boseman, Jr.: Charleston's black physician-politician. In Rabinowitz HN, ed: Southern Black leaders of the reconstruction era. Urbana, University of Illinois Press, 1982. p. 335–62.

**Boss, Medard, 1903–**
Rattner J: Medard Boss. In J. Rattner, ed: Wandlungen der Psychoanalyse. Wien, Europaverlag, 1980. p. 281–308.

**Bossuet, Jacques Bénigne, Bp. of Meaux, 1627–1704**
Demoulin B: Bossuet et la Mort. In Congrès National des Sociétés Savantes, 102e, Limoges, 1977. Actes. Paris, 1978. Tome I, p. 263–79.

**Bostroem, Eugen Woldemar, 1850–1928**
Krumholz W: Eugen Woldemar Bostroem (1850–1928), Lehrer der Bathologie und Förderer der Medizin in Giessen. Giessen, Schmitz, 1983. 311 p. (Arbeiten zur Geschichte der Medizin in Giessen, Bd. 8)

**Boswell, James, 1740–1795**
Rix KJ: Boswell and his doctors. **Hist Med** 1981;9(1):9–12, 17

**Botey, Ricardo, 1855–1927**
Botey i Puig A: L'obra del Dr. Ricard Botey i Ducoing. In Congrés Internacional d'Historie de la Medicina Catalana, 1st, Barcelona-Montpellier, 1970. Barcelona, Editorial Scientia, 1971. v 4, p. 20–6.
Perello J: The Bordeaux School of ENT in the nineteenth century as seen by a Spanish practitioner, Ricardo Botey. **Rev Laryngol Otol Rhinol (Bord)** 1980 Jan–Feb;101(1–2):15–30

**Botkin, Sergeĭ Petrovich, 1832–1889**
Al'bitskiĭ VIu: K 150–letiiu so dnia rozhdeniia Nikolaia Andreevicha Vinogradova - uchenika S. P. Botkina. **Klin Med (Mosk)** 1982 Sep;60(9):121–3
Anisimov VE: Ucheniki i psoledovateli S. P. Botkina v. Kazani. **Klin Med (Mosk)** 1982 Sep;60(9):113–6
Arkhangel'skiĭ GV: A. I. Gertsen i S. P. Botkin. **Klin Med (Mosk)** 1982 Nov;60(11):118–20
Arkhangel'skiĭ GV: S. P. Botkin i pisateli–revoliutsionery demokraty. **Sov Zdravookhr** 1983;(2):60
Arkhangel'skii GV: S. P. Botkin i otechestvennye deiateli muzykal'noĭ i khudozhestvennoĭ kul'tury. **Klin Med (Mosk)** 1982 May;60(5):112–7
Arkhangel'skiĭ GV: Teoreticheskie vzgliady S. P. Botkina po klinicheskim i obshchepatologicheskim voprosam meditsiny (k 150–letiiu so dnia rozhdeniia). **Klin Med (Mosk)** 1981 Nov;59(11):109–13
Arkhangel'skiĭ GV: S. P. Botkin i M. E. Saltykov–Shchedrin. **Klin Med (Mosk)** 1982 Oct;60(10):114–8
Arkhangel'skiĭ GV: Znachenie S. P. Botkina v razvitii otechestvennoĭ nevrologii. **Klin Med (Mosk)** 1983 Apr;61(4):105–9
Bagdasarian SM: Velikiĭ Russkiĭ klinitsist S. P. Botkin (k 150–letiiu so dnia rozhdeniia). **Klin Med (Mosk)** 1982 Dec;60(12):94–9
Belitskaia EIa: Gigienicheskie i sotsial'no–gigienicheskie vzgliady S. P. Botkina (k 150–letiiu so dnia rozhdeniia). **Gig Sanit** 1982 Jul;(7):34–8
Borisova MA, Bychkovskiĭ AV: Vklad Sergeia Petrovicha Bokina v izuchenie infektsionnykh bolezneĭ (k 150–letiiu so dnia rozhdeniia). **Vrach Delo** 1982 Sep;(9):116–9
Gembitskiĭ EV: S. P. Botkin kak voennyĭ terapevt. **Klin Med (Mosk)** 1982 Sep;60(9):22–7
Georgievskiĭ AS: Vklad S. P. Botkina v razvitie otechestvennoĭ voennoĭ meditsiny. **Sov Zdravookhr** 1983;6:62–6
Grebenev AL: S. P. Botkin o N. I. Pirogove. **Klin Med (Mosk)** 1982 Sep;60(9):108–10
Ianushkevichus ZI: Razvitie ideĭ i rabot S. P. Botkina i ego shkoly v kardiologii i klinicheskoĭ farmakologii. **Vestn Akad Med Nauk SSSR** 1983;(3):14–7
Ivanov NG, Georgievskiĭ AS: Sergeĭ Petrovich Botkin i voenno–meditsinskaia akademiia. **Vestn Akad Med Nauk SSSR** 1983;(3):8–14
Kliachkin LM: Ucheniki S. P. Botkina v. Saratove. **Klin Med (Mosk)** 1982 Sep;60(9):119–21
Komarov FI: S. P. Botkin--vydaiushchiisia deiatel' otechestvennoi meditsiny. **Vestn Akad Med Nauk SSSR** 1983;(3):3–7
Kotel'nikov VP: Znachenie nauchnogo naslediia S. P. Botkina v khirurgii. **Klin Med (Mosk)** 1983 Jul;61(7):140–2
Lisitsyn IuP, Arkhangel'skiĭ GV: S. P. Botkin--nevrolog. **Zh Nevropatol Psikhiatr** 1982;82(10):127–30
Mikirtichan GL: S. P. Botkin i okhrana zdorov'ia deteĭ (k 150–letiiu so dnia rozhdeniia). **Pediatriia** 1982 Oct;(10):62–4
Peleshchuk AP, Koliadenko VG, Zhukovskiĭ LI: Ucheniki S. P. Botkina na Ukraine. **Klin Med (Mosk)** 1982 Sep;60(9):110–3
Petrov BD: Izuchenie nauchnogo naslediia S. P. Botkina. **Sov Zdravookhr** 1983;(2):57–9
Petrov NS: Idei S. P. Botkina v funktsional'noĭ gematologii i ikh dal'neishee razvitie. **Vestn Akad Med Nauk SSSR** 1983;(3):47–51
Petrov NS: Sergeĭ Petrovich Botkin (k 150–letiius so dnia rozhdeniia). **Probl Gematol Pereliv Krovi** 1982 Dec;27(12):49–51
Petrov NS, Georgievskiĭ AS, Antonov VB: Sergeĭ Petrovich Botkin i voennaia meditsina (k 150–letiiu so dnia rozhdeniia). **Voen Med Zh** 1982;(9):64–6
Polenova IV: N. A. Iaroshenko i ucheniki S. P. Botkina. **Klin Med (Mosk)** 1982 Sep;60(9):117–9
Riabov SI, Stavskaia VV: Idei S. P. Botkina v nefrologii. **Klin Med (Mosk)** 1982 Sep;60(9):27–32
Shul'tsev GP: Zhizn' i deiatel'nost' Sergeia Petrovicha Botkina. **Klin Med (Mosk)** 1982 Sep;60(9):12–21
Shul'tsev GP: Perechityvaia 'Klinicheskie Lektsii' S. P. Botkina (k 100–letiu so dnia izdaniia). **Klin Med (Mosk)** 1983 Oct;61(10):132–6
Shul'tsev GP: Khronologiia zhizni i deiatel'nosti Sergeia Petrovicha Botkina (k 150–letiiu so dnia rozhdenia). **Klin Med (Mosk)** 1983 Oct;61(10):142–8
Shurygin DIa: Razvitie ideĭ S. P. Botkina v oblasti épidemiologii. **Klin Med (Mosk)** 1982 Apr;60(4):112–5
Shuvalova EP: Razvitie ideĭ S. P. Botkina v klinike infektsionnykh bolezneĭ. **Vestn Akad Med Nauk SSSR** 1983;(3):35–40
Smirnov EI, Garin NS: Vklad S. P. Botkina v razvitie épidemiologii (k 150–letiiu so dnia rozhdeniia). **Zh Mikrobiol Epidemiol Immunobiol** 1982 May;(5):109–15
Smirnov EI, Garin NS: S. P. Botkin o variabel'nosti klinicheskogo techeniia infektsionnykh bolezneĭ i épidemiologicheskikh aspektakh étoĭ problemy (K 150–letiiu so dnia rozhdeniia). **Vestn Akad Med Nauk SSSR** 1982;(10):3–9

Tareev EM: Sergeĭ Petrovich Botkin i sovremennaia klinika. **Klin Med (Mosk)** 1982 Sep;60(9):4–11
Vzaimootnosheniia A.I. Gertsena i S. P. Botkina: **Klin Med (Mosk)** 1983 Jun;61(6):108–10

**Botteri, Albert, 1879–1955**
Pavišić Z, Dugački V: Značenje znanstvenog, stručnog i nastavnog rada prof. dr. Alberta Botterija za razvoj oftalmologije u Jugoslaviji. **Lijec Vjesn** 1980 Jan;102(1):43–7

**Botticelli, Sandro, 1444 or 45–1510**
Alarcón-Segovia D, Laffón A, Alcocer-Varela J: Probable depiction of juvenile arthritis by Sandro Botticelli. **Arthritis Rheum** 1983 Oct;26(10):1266–8
Dequeker J: Arthritis in the paintings of Sandro Botticelli. **Arthritis Rheum** 1984 Oct;27(10):1196–7
Leden I: Doubts about Sandro Botticelli's depiction of juvenile rheumatoid arthritis. **Arthritis Rheum** 1984 Oct;27(10):1197–8

**Bouchardat, Apollinaire, 1806–1886**
Major V: Live in peace and joy. In: Congrès international d'histoire de la médecine, XXVe, Québec, 1976. Actes. Québec, 1977. p. 944–50.

**Boucher, André, 1903–1980**
Clement A: André Boucher. **Bull Acad Chir Dent (Paris)** 1981–82;27(27):99–102

**Bouestard, Jean-Jacques, 1730–1810**
Stofft H: Bouestard, médecin des épidémies à Morlaix. **Hist Sci Med** 1984;18(3):223–45

**Boule, Marcellin, 1861–1942**
Hammond M: The expulsion of the Neanderthals from human ancestry: Marcellin Boule and the social context of scientific research. **Soc Stud Sci** 1982 Feb;12(1):1–36

**Bourbon Family**
Gonzalez Iglesias J: Los Borbones y el desarrollo de la odontologia en Espāna. **Bol Inf Dent (Madr)** 1978;Spec no:63–92

**Bourdelin, Claude, ca. 1621–1699**
Rendinger C de: Un apothicaire du 'Grand Siècle', Claude Bourdelin (1621–1699), de l'Académie des Sciences, sa vie et les événements de son temps. **Bull Ordre Natl Pharm** 1980 Sep;236:1415–24

**Bourdon, Marguerite, 1642–1706**
Voisine N: Marguerite Bourdon. In Dictionary of Canadian biography, 1701 to 1740. Volume 2, 1969. p. 92–3.

**Bourgelat, Claude, 1712–1779**
Blin PC: Bourgelat, founder of veterinary teaching, 1712–1779. **Comp Immunol Microbiol Infect Dis** 1980;3(1–2):xiii–xvi

**Bourgeois, Jacques, ca. 1620–1701**
Cormier C: Jacques Bourgeois. In Dictionary of Canadian biography, 1701 to 1740. Volume 2, 1969. p. 94.

**Bourguet, Julien, 1877–**
Marchac D: Julien Bourguet. The pioneer in aesthetic surgery of the neck. **Clin Plast Surg** 1983 Jul;10(3):363–5

**Bourrus, Josep, 1865–**
Bourrus R: Le Docteur Bourrus, professeur et médecin à Mont-de-Marsan (1820–1897). **Bull Soc Borda** 1982;107(386):197–200

**Boursier, Louise (Bourgeois), 1563–1636**
Kalisch PA, Scobey M, Kalisch BJ: Louyse Bourgeois and the emergence of modern midwifery. **J Nurse Midwife** 1981 Jul–Aug;26(4):3–17

**Bovie, William T., 1882–1958**
Beatty WK: William T. Bovie, inventor and teacher. **Trans Stud Coll Physicians Phila** 1979 Jun;5(1 no 2):138–44
Beatty WK: William T. Bovie. In Dictionary of American Biography, Suppl. 6, 1956–1960. p. 69–70, 1980.

**Bowden, Edmund, 1801–1847**
Forster FM: David D. Davis' Obstetric Atlas in Tasmania in 1846. Edmund Bowden's gift to Robert Officer. **Aust NZ J Obstet Gynaecol** 1983 May;23(2):88–92

**Bowditch, Henry Pickering, 1840–1911**
Benison S, Barger AC, Wolfe EL: Changing of the guard. **Harv Med Alumni Bull** 1982 Spring;56(2):34–41
Bowditch HP: The life and writings of Henry Pickering Bowditch. 2 vols. New York, Arno Press, 1980. Various paginations.
Fye WB: Why a physiologist?--the case of Henry P. Bowditch. **Bull Hist Med** 1982 Spring;56(1):19–29

**Bowen, John Templeton, 1857–**
Bernhard JD, Elliot AD: A letter from Darier to Bowen on the naming of Bowen's disease. **Arch Dermatol** 1983 Mar;119(3):261–2
King DF: Chronic atypical epithelial proliferation of Bowen. A historical and biographical note. **Am J Dermatopathol** 1984 Feb;6(1):35–8

**Bowen, Thomas Aubrey, 1837–1893**
Lowe RF: T. Aubrey Bowen, oculist, 1837–93. **Aust J Ophthalmol** 1981 May;9(2):155–62
Lowe RF: T. Aubrey Bowen, Oculist, 1837–93: his bequests to English charities. **Br J Ophthalmol** 1982 Oct;66(10):622–4
Lowe RF: T. Aubrey Bowen, oculist, 1837–93. His charitable bequest in Victoria. **Aust NZ J Surg** 1983 Apr;53(2):183–7
Lowe RF: T. Aubrey Bowen and his house at 167 Collins Street East, Melbourne. **Aust NZ J Surg** 1981;51:102–5

**Bowers, Jacob, 1841–1922**
Wells LA: Rural psychiatry on the nineteenth-century frontier: the career of Jacob Bowers. **Perspect Biol Med** 1981 Winter;24(2):270–81

**Bowlby, John Mostyn, 1907–**
Newcombe N, Lerner JC: Britain between the wars: the historical context of Bowlby's theory of attachment. **Psychiatry** 1982 Feb;45(1):1–12

**Box, John, 1863–1934**
Lowe RF: John Box (1863-1934) and William Box (1905–1982). **Aust J Ophthalmol** 1983 Feb;11(1):51–3

**Box, William, 1905–1982**
Lowe RF: John Box (1863–1934) and William Box (1905–1982). **Aust J Ophthalmol** 1983 Feb;11(1):51–3

**Boyd, David R.**
Ellison RC, ed: A pioneer Alabama doctor's ledger. **Ala Hist Q** 1981;43(4):315–32

**Boyd, William, 1885–**
Barrie HJ: Sir William Boyd: a legacy in print. **Can Med Assoc J** 1982 Feb 15;126(4):421,423–4

**Boyden, Edward Allen, 1886–**
Scannell JG: A sidelight of cholecystography. **Pharos** 1983 Summer;46(3):42

**Boyle, Robert, 1627–1691**
Bylebyl JJ: Boyle and Harvey on the valves in the veins. **Bull Hist Med** 1982 Fall;56(3):351–67
Debus AG: Thomas Sherley's philosophical essay (1672): Helmontian mechanism as the basis of a new philosophy. **Ambix** 1980 Jul;27(2):124–35
Steneck NH: Greatrakes the stroker: the interpretations of historians. **ISIS** 1982 Jun;73(267):161–77
Stewart MA: The authenticity of Robert Boyle's anonymous writings on reason. **Bodleian Libr Rec** 1981 Aug;10(5):280–9

**Boylston, Zabdiel, 1680–1766**
Moore FD: Zabdiel Boylston and colonial surgery. American surgery and public health in the early 18th century. **Bull Am Coll Surg** 1983 May;68(5):13–7

**Bradlaugh, Charles, 1833–1891**
Chandrasekhar S: 'A dirty, filthy book.' The writings of Charles Knowlton and Annie Besant on reproductive physiology and birth control and an account of the Bradlaugh-Besant trial. With the definitive texts of Fruits of philosophy by Charles Knowlton; The law of population by Annie Besant; Theosophy and the law of population by Annie Besant. Berkeley, University of California Press, 1981. xi, 217 p.

**Bradshaw, William, 1830–1861**
Thompson FG: Assistant surgeon William Bradshaw, V.C. **Ir Sword** 1981;14(56):237–9

**Bradwardine, Thomas, Abp. of Canterbury, 1290?–1349**
Rowland B: Bishop Bradwardine on the artificial memory. **J Warburg Courtauld Inst** 1978;41:307–12

**Bragg, William Henry, 1862–1942**
Del Regato JA: William Henry Bragg. **Int J Radiat Oncol Biol Phys** 1981 Jan;7(1):83–97

**Brahe, Tycho, 1546–1601**
Greisman HC: Tycho Brahe: astronomer of renaissance Denmark. In Romm S, ed: Symposium on historical perspectives of plastic surgery. Philadelphia, Saunders, 1983. p. 629–33.

**Brahms, Johannes, 1833–1897**
Kern E: Das chirurgische Erbe. Theodor Billroth und die Musik. **Zentralbl Chir** 1982;107(21):1408–16
Kerner D: El último Brahms. **Folia Hum (Barc)** 1981;19:27–34
Shafar J: The Brahms-Billroth friendship. **Br Med J** 1981;282:1775
Weir NF: Theodor Billroth and Johannes Brahms--a thirty year friendship. **Hist Med (Lond)** 1975 Autumn-Winter;6(3–4):8–14

**Braid, James, 1795–1860**
Gravitz MA, Gerton MI: Origins of the term hypnotism prior to Braid. **Am J Clin Hypn** 1984 Oct;27(2):107–10

**Brain, Walter Russell, 1895–1966**
Pickering G: Walter Russell Brain. In Dictionary of national biography, 1961–1970. Suppl. 8, 1981. p. 127–9.

**Bräker, Ulrich, 1735–1798**
Stettler A: Vorläufige medizinhistorische und pathographische Bemerkungen zu Ulrich Bräker. **Gesnerus** 1983;40(1–2):185–92

**Brambilla, Giovanni Alessandro, 1728–1800**
Giovanni Alessandro Brambilla nella cultura medica del Settecento Europeo: Milano, Istituto Editoriale Cisalpino-La Goliardica, 1980. 371 p.
Miniati M: Lo strumentario di G. A. Brambilla. **Kos** 1984 Feb;1(1):74–6

**Bramwell, Byrom, 1847–1931**
Ashworth B: The Bramwells and neurology in Edinburgh. **Scott Med J** 1981 Oct;26(4):364–70

**Bramwell, Edwin, 1873–1955**
Ashworth B: The Bramwells and neurology in Edinburgh. **Scott Med J** 1981 Oct;26(4):364–70

**Brancusi, Constantin, 1876–1957**
Meares R: Body feeling in human relations: the possible examples of Brancusi and Giacometti. **Psychiatry** 1980 May;43(2):160–7

**Brand, Johannes Henricus, 1823–1888**
Retief FP: President J. H. Brand en sy siekte-geskiedenis. **S Afr Med J** 1981 Mar 14;59(11):384–6

**Brand, Paul Wilson, 1914–**
Wilson DC: Ten fingers for God: [the complete biography of Dr. Paul Brand]. Nashville, Nelson Publ, 1983. vii, 275 p.

**Brandt, Josef, 1838–1912**
Spielmann J: Ein siebenbürgischer Pionier der Nephrektomie: Josef Brandt (1838–1912). **Sudhoffs Arch** 1980;64(2):151–62

**Brant, Sebastian, 1458–1521**
Calagan JL: The conjoined twins born near Worms, 1495. **J Hist Med Allied Sci** 1983 Oct;38(4):450–1

**Brascu, Stefan S., 1895–1965**
Sărmăşanu-Cortez ML, Cortez PP: Un distins psihiatru la confluenta dintre muzică şi medicină: dr. Stefan S. Braşcu (1895–1965). **Rev Med Interna [Neurol Psihiatr]** 1980 Apr–Jun;24(2):143–8

**Brass, Arnold, 1854–**
Szyfman L: Les prétendues falsifications d'Ernst Haeckel et son triomphe sur ses diffamateurs. **Bull Biol Fr Belg** 1980;113(4):375–406

**Bratton, James Rufus, 1821–1897**
Leland TM: James Rufus Bratton 1821–1897. **J SC Med Assoc** 1984 Feb;80(2):84

**Brauer, John Charles, 1905–**
Pioneers in pedodontics: influential leaders of the past (John C. Brauer): **Pediatr Dent** 1982 Jun;4(2):143–4

**Brauer, Ludolph, 1865–1951**
Hein J: Ludolph Brauer--Der Wegbereiter der modernen Pneumologie. **Prax Klin Pneumol** 1984 Oct;38(10):471–3

**Bravo, Francisco, fl. ca. 1553**
Somolinos d'Ardois G: Francisco Bravo y su opera medicinalia. **Bol Inst Invest Bibliogr** 1970;4:337–88

**Brdlík, Jiří**
Tichý M, Volná A: Bratislavské roky profesora Brdlíka. **Cesk Zdrav** 1983 Jul;31(6):250–5

**Brdlík, Jiří, 1883–1965**
Houštěk J: Sto let od narození profesora MUDr. Jiřího Brdlíka, DrSc., vedoucí osobnosti československé pediatrie (24. října 1883--6. července 1965). **Cesk Pediatr** 1983 Nov;38(11):680–1

**Breckinridge, Mary, 1881–1965**
Dye NS: Mary Breckinridge, the Frontier Nursing Service and the introduction of nurse-midwifery in the United States. **Bull Hist Med** 1983 Winter;57(4):485–507
Faust DG: Mary Breckinridge. In: Notable American women. The modern period. Cambridge, Mass., Belknap-Harvard Univ. Press, 1980. 4:103–5.
Kiser TS: A story of true devotion (Mary Breckinridge). **Front Nurs Serv Q Bull** 1981 Autumn;57(2):16–8
Matthies K: Mary Breckinridge and the frontier nursing service. **DAR Mag** 1980;114(5):692–4
Pletsch PK: Mary Breckinridge: a pioneer who made her mark. **Am J Nurs** 1981 Dec;81(12):2188–90

**Breda, Achille, 1850–1934**
Pampiglione S: Il contributo di Achille Breda alla conoscenza della leishmaniosi muco-cutanea americana. **Parassitologia** 1979 Dec;21(1–3):35–58

**Bredin, Claude-Julien, 1776–1854**
Mammerickx M: André-Marie Ampère et Claude-Julien Bredin, II. Ampère, Bredin et le magnétisme animal, ou la petite histoire d'une grande découverte. **Hist Med Vet** 1977;2(3):69–75
Mammerickx M: André-Marie Ampère et Claude-Julien Bredin, I. Ampère, Bredin et la philosophie, ou la belle histoire d'une amitié. **Hist Med Vet** 1977;2(1):11–19

**Breese, Frederick, 1866–1945**
Gelbier S: Frederick Breese and London's first school dental clinic. **Br Dent J** 1981 Nov 3;151(9):309–11

**Brenner, Charles, 1913–**
Abend SM: Charles Brenner. An appreciation. **Psychoanal Q** 1984 Jan;53(1):1–12

**Brenner, Friedrich, 1809–1874**
Ober WB: History of the Brenner tumor of the ovary. **Pathol Annu** 1979;14 Pt 2:107–24

**Brenner, József, 1887–1919**
Szentgyörgyvölgyi G: Csáth Géza--Dr. Brenner József (1887–1919). **Orv Hetil** 1984 Sep 30;125(40):2446–8

**Brent, Charles Henry, 1862–1929**
Pargas K: Bishop Charles Henry Brent (1862–1929)--a retrospective. 'That damned opium mess has started again'. **J Addict Res Found** 1979;8(9):7

**Brethel, Alexandre, 1834–1901**
Massa F: Alexandre Brethel, pharmacien et planteur au Carangolo: recherche sur sa correspondence brésilienne (1862–1901). Rennes, Université de Haute-Bretagne, Institut Armoricain de recherches économiques et humaines de Rennes, 1977. v, 462 p.

**Breton, André, 1896–1966**
Robert BP: Profiles de 'La fruite des idées' et surréalisme. **Rev Univ Ottawa** 1977;47(3):345–64
Robert BP: Origines du surréalisme. **Univ Ottawa Q** 1982;52(2):190–205

**Bretonneau, Pierre Fidèle, 1778–1862**
Aron E: Bretonneau et sa légende. **Hist Sci Med** 1980;14(2):187–91

**Breuer, Josef, 1842–1925**
Hollender MH: The case of Anna O.: a reformulation. **Am J Psychiatry** 1980 Jul;137(7):797–800
Knight IF: Freud's 'Project': a theory for Studies on Hysteria. **J Hist Behav Sci** 1984 Oct;20(4):340–58
Pilleri G: Josef Breuer, 1842–1925. Waldau-Bern (Schweiz), Verlag des Hiranatomischen Institutes, 1983. 81 p.
Schneck JM: Sigmund Freud, Josef Breuer, and Freud's self-observations on meralgia paresthetica. **NY State J Med** 1983 Jun;83(7):968–9
Schott HG: Elemente der Selbstanalyse in den 'Studien über Hysterie'. **Gesnerus** 1980;37(3/4):235–56

**Brewster, David, 1781–1868**
Campbell R: Sir David Brewster (1781–1868). Edinburgh, History of Medicine and Science Unit, University of Edinburgh, [1982?] [12] p.

**Bridgeman, Laura Dewey, 1829–1889**
Oppenheim RW: Laura Bridgeman's brain: an early consideration of functional adaptations in neural development. **Dev Psychobiol** 1979 Nov;12(6):533–7

**Briggs, William, ca. 1650–1704**
Amalric P: La naissance de la neuro-ophtalmologie à Montpellier au XVIIme siècle à travers l'oeuvre de Raymond Vieussens et de Guilhem Briggs. **Bull Soc Ophtalmol Fr** 1983 Jan;83(1):83–8

**Brigham, Amariah, 1798–1849**
Grob GN, ed: The beginnings of mental hygiene in America. Three selected essays 1833–1850. New York, Arno, 1973. Various paginations. Includes works by Amariah Brigham (1833); William Sweetser (1850); Samuel B. Woodward (1840).

**Brighenti, Alberto, 1886–**
Bonuzzi L: Alberto Brighenti nella storia della fisiologia. **Acta Med Hist Patav** 1981/82;28:21–8

**Bright, Richard, 1789–1858**
Boss J: Richard Bright's Reports of Medical Cases (1827): a sesquicentennial note. **Bristol Med Chir J** 1978 Jan–Apr;93(345–346):5–6, 18
Bright P: Dr. Richard Bright (1789–1858). London, Bodley Head, 1983. 312 p.
Hakulinen E: Mannen bakom syndromet: Richard Bright. En av de stora inom njurforskningen--hans 'Reports of medical cases' epokgörande. **Lakartidningen** 1984 Apr 25;81(17):1722–3
Kark RM, Moore DT: The life, work, and geological collections of Richard Bright, M.D. (1789–1858); with a note on the collections of other members of the family. **Arch Nat Hist** 1981 Apr;10(1):119–51
Naiken VS: Richard Bright, physician and budding socio-cultural anthropologist. In: Congrès international d'histoire de la médecine, XXVe, Québec, 1976. Actes. Québec, 1977. p. 999–1001.
Peitzman SJ: Bright's disease and Bright's generation--toward exact medicine at Guy's Hospital. **Bull Hist Med** 1981;55(3):307–21

**Brinkhous, Kenneth Merle, 1909–**
Sherry S: A tribute to Kenneth M. Brinkhous, M.D. **Thromb Haemost** 1979 Feb 28;40(1):3–23

**Briquet, Paul, d. 1882**
Dongier M: Briquet and Briquet's syndrome viewed from France. **Can J Psychiatry** 1983 Oct;28(6):422–7
Mai FM, Merskey H: Briquet's concept of hysteria: an historical perspective. **Can J Psychiatry** 1981 Feb;26(1):57–63
Mai FM: Pierre Briquet: 19th century savant with 20th century ideas. **Can J Psychiatry** 1983 Oct;28(6):418–21

**Broca, Pierre Paul, 1824–1880**
Alajouanine T, Signoret JL: Paul Broca et l'aphasie. **Bull Acad Natl Med (Paris)** 1980;164(6):545–51
Bibliographie des travaux de P. Broca consacrés à l'aphasie.: **Rev Neurol (Paris)** 1980;136(10):663–4
Castaigne P: Photographies et tomodensitométrie des deux cerveaux sur lesquels Broca fonda sa conception anatomoclinique de l'"aphémie'. **Bull Acad Natl Med (Paris)** 1979 Oct;163(7):663–7
Castaigne P, Lhermitte F, Signoret JL, et al: Description et étude scannographique du cerveau de Leborgne. La découverte de Broca.

**Rev Neurol (Paris)** 1980;136(10):563-83
Commémoration du centenaire de la mort de Paul Broca: **Chirurgie** 1980;106(10):773-93
D'Aubigné RM: Paul Broca et la chirurgie de l'appareil moteur. **Chirurgie** 1980;106(10):791-3
Dechaume M, Huard P: Paul Broca (1824-1880). Stomatologiste ou la stomatologie du siècle dernier. **Actual Odontostomatol (Paris)** 1980;(132):537-43
Delmas A: Paul Broca et l'anatomie. **Bull Acad Natl Med (Paris)** 1980;164(6):552-6
Delmas A: Paul Broca (1824-1880). Esquisse biographique. Le chirurgien et l'anatomiste. **Cah Anthropol** 1980;1-2:15-45
Denoix P: Paul Broca. L'anatomie pathologique, le cancer, la statistique. **Chirurgie** 1980;106(10).787-90
Galaburda AM: La région de Broca: observations anatomiques faites un siècle après la mort de son découvreur. **Rev Neurol (Paris)** 1980;136(10):609-16
Hamanaka Y: [Jackson's theory of stratification of neurological functions--a controversy involving Broca at a symposium (1868) at Norwich] (Jpn). **No To Shinkei** 1982 Oct;34(10):1018-9
Houdart R: Paul Broca, précurseur des disciplines neurologiques. **Chirurgie** 1980;106(10):783-6
Huard P: Paul Broca anatomiste. **Chirurgie** 1980;106(10):774-6
Huard P, Aaron C, Askienazy S, et al: La mort de Paul Broca (1824-1880). **Bull Acad Natl Med (Paris)** 1980 Oct;164(7):682-5
Huard P, Aaron C, Askienazy S, et al: Le cerveau de Paul Broca (1824-1880). Confrontation anatomo-pathologique et tomo-densitométrique. **J Radiol** 1982 Mar;63(3):175-80
Joynt RJ: The great confrontation: the meeting between Broca and Jackson in 1868. In Rose FC, Bynum WF, ed: Historical aspects of the neurosciences. New York, Raven, 1982. p. 99-102.
Kraetschmer K: Broca's localization theory reconsidered. **Br J Disord Commun** 1980 May;15(1):5-8
Lee DA: Paul Broca and the history of aphasia. **Neurology** 1981 May;31(5):600-2
Lukács D: Pierre Paul Broca, az antropológia és a beszéd agykérgi központjának felfedezöje. **Orv Hetil** 1980 Aug 24;121(34):2081-2
Merle d'Aubigné R: Paul Broca (1824-1880). **Bull Soc Hist Protestantisme Fr** 1980;126(4):509-24
Monod-Broca P: Paul Broca (1824-1880). Le chirurgien, l'homme. **Bull Acad Natl Med (Paris)** 1980;164(6):536-44
Natali J: Paul Broca, chirurgien vasculaire. **Chirurgie** 1980;106(10):777-82
Pineau H: Paul Broca et l'anthropologie. **Bull Acad Natl Med (Paris)** 1980;164(6):557-62
Pineau H: Paul Broca. L'anthropologiste et le biologiste. **Cah Anthropol** 1980;1-2:47-93
Pineau H: Remarque sur la bibliographie des oeuvres de Paul Broca. **Cah Anthropol** 1980;3-4:245-83
Schiller F: Paul Broca, founder of French anthropology, explorer of the brain. Berkeley, University of California Press, 1979. ix, 350 p.
Schiller F: Paul Broca and the history of aphasia. **Neurosci Behav Physiol** 1983 May;33(5):667
Signoret JL, Castaigne P, Lhermitte F, et al: Rediscovery of Leborgne's brain: anatomical description with CT scan. **Brain Lang** 1984 Jul;22(2):303-19
Valette G, et al: Centenaire de la mort de Paul Broca (1824-1880). **Bull Acad Natl Med (Paris)** 1980;164:535-62

**Brock, Frederick W.**
Wittenberg S: Brock's research in stereopsis. **Am J Optom Physiol Opt** 1981 Aug;58(8):663-6, 667-70

**Brodie, Benjamin Collins, 1783-1862**
Russell JR: The three royal doctors of Betchworth. **Practitioner** 1981 Jul;225(1357):1070-1
Wharton M: Sir Benjamin Brodie, Bt. (1783-1862). **Ann R Coll Surg Engl** 1983 Nov;65(6):418-9

**Brodniewicz, Anita Zofia**
Czapska I: Whołdzie najlepszym (Anita Zofia Brodniewicz). **Pieleg Polozna** 1983;(6):28-9

**Bromberg, Walter, 1900-**
Bromberg W: Psychiatry between the wars, 1918-1945. A recollection. Westport, London, Greenwood Press, 1982. xxxii, 184 p. (Contributions in Medical History, No. 10).

**Brongersma, H. R., 1869-1944**
Karthaus PP, Brongersma LD: H. R. G. J. Brongersma en de Nederlandse Vereniging voor Urologie. **Ned Tijdschr Geneeskd** 1983 Sep 3;127(36):1642-3

**Bronner, Augusta Fox, 1881-1866**
Burnham JC: Augusta Fox Bronner. In: Notable American women. The modern period. Cambridge, Mass., Belknap-Harvard Univ. Press, 1980. 4:108-10.

**Brooks, Barney, 1884-**
Scott HW: A tribute to Barney Brooks, Alfred Blalock, and the Vanderbilt Surgical Staff (1925 to 1982). **South Med J** 1982 Dec;75(12):1439-52

**Brooks, William Keith, 1848-1908**
Benson KR: 'William Keith Brooks (1848-1908): primary resource material'. **Mendel Newsl** 1983 Nov;23:7-11
Benson KR: William Keith Brooks (1848-1908): a case study in morphology and the development of American biology. Ph.D. Diss. Oregon State University. Corvallis, 1979. 356 leaves.

**Brouillet, André, 1857-1914**
Signoret JL: Une leçon clinique a la Salpêtrière (1887) par André Brouillet. **Rev Neurol (Paris)** 1983;139(12):687-701

**Brouse, William Henry, 1824-1881**
Swainson D: William Henry Brouse. In Dictionary of Canadian biography, 1881-1890. 1982;11:114.

**Broussais, François Joseph Victor, 1772-1838**
Cid F: Broussais, su concepto de irritación en el cuadro de la locura durante el siglo XIX. **Med Hist (Barc)** 1984;(5):3-7
Wickwar H, Bryan CS: Broussais in Columbia, South Carolina - 1831. **J SC Med Assoc** 1981 Dec;77(12):615-22

**Browicz, Tadeusz, 1847-1928**
Szymańska R, Schmidt-Pospuła M: Z historii badań tadeusza Browicza (1847-1928) i Karola Kupffera (1829--1902) nad komórkami siateczkowo-śródbłonkowymi watroby. **Arch Hist Med (Warsz)** 1979;42(3):331-6

**Brown, Charles Brockden, 1771-1810**
Ferguson RA: Yellow fever and Charles Brockden Brown: the contest of the emerging novelist. **Early Am Lit** 1979-80;14(3):293-305

**Brown, Charles, 1783-1879**
Savitt TL: Patient letters to an early nineteenth century Virginia physician. **J Fla Med Assoc** 1982 Aug;69(8):688-94

**Brown, Isaac Baker, 1812-1873**
Sheehan E: Victorian clitoridectomy: Isaac Baker Brown and his harmless operative procedure. **Med Anthropol Newsl** 1981;12(4):9-15

**Brown, John, 1735-1788**
Daněk K: Incitabilita, stenie a astenie. K 200. výročí Brownových Základu medicíny. **Cas Lek Cesk** 1980 Jul 11;119(27-28):774-6
Henkelmann T: Zur Geschichte des pathophysiologischen Denkens. John Brown (1735-1788) und sein System der Medizin. Berlin, New York, Springer, 1981. 104 p.
Overmier JA: John Brown's Elementa medicinae: an introductory bibliographical essay. **Bull Med Libr Assoc** 1982 Jul;70(3):310-7
Schwanitz HJ: Homöopathie und Brownianismus 1795-1844. Zwei wissenschaftstheoretische Fallstudien aus der praktischen Medizin. Stuttgart Fischer, 1983. 202 p. (Medizin in Geschichte und Kultur, 15).
Trotter WR: John Brown, and the nonspecific component of human sickness. **Perspect Biol Med** 1978 Winter;21(2):258-64

**Brown, Lucius Polk, 1867-1935**
Wolfe MR: Lucius Polk Brown and progressive food and drug control. Tennessee and New York City 1908-1920. Lawrence, Regents Press of Kansas, 1978. 194 p.

**Brown, Rachel, 1898-1980**
Baldwin RS: The fungus fighters: two women scientists and their discovery. Ithaca, Cornell University Press, 1981. 212 p.

**Brown, Robert, 1773-1858**
Edwards PI: Robert Brown (1773-1858) and the natural history of Matthew Flinders' voyage in H.M.S. Investigator, 1801-1805. **J Soc Bibliogr Nat Hist** 1976;7(4):385-407
Hatfield G: Robert Brown A.M., F.R.S.E. (1773-1858). Edinburgh, History of Medicine and Science Unit, University of Edinburgh, [1981?]. [11] p.

**Brown-Séquard, Charles Edouard, 1817-1894**
Gooddy W: Dr. Brown-Sequard in space and time. **Trans Hunter Soc** 1978-80;37-38:153-9
Gooddy W: Charles Edward Brown-Séquard. In Rose FC, Bynum WF, ed: Historical aspects of the neurosciences. New York, Raven, 1982. p. 371-8.
Role A: La vie étrange d'un grand savant: le professeur Brown-Sequard, 1817-1894. Paris, Plon, 1977. 219 p.
Tyler HR, Tyler KL: Charles Edouard Brown-Séquard: professor of physiology and pathology of the nervous system at Harvard Medical School. **Neurology** 1984 Sep;34(9):1231-6

**Brown, Solyman, 1790-1876**
Gardiner JF: Solyman Brown and his epic poem 'Dentologia'. **Bull Hist Dent** 1984;32(1):44-51

**Brown, Thomas**
Olson GD: Dr. David Ramsay and Lt. Colonel Thomas Brown: patriot historian and loyalist critic. **SC Hist Mag** 1976;77:256-67

**Brown, Thomas Graham, 1882-1965**
Evans C: Thomas Graham Brown. In Dictionary of national biography, 1961-1970. Suppl. 8, 1981. p. 151-2.

**Brown, Thomas, 1778-1820**
Robinson DN, ed: Significant contributions to the history of psychology 1750-1920. Series A. Orientations. Volume I: E. Condillac, T. Brown. Washington, D. C., University Publications of America, 1977. Various pagings.

**Brown, William Michael Court, 1918-1968**
Doll R: William Michael Court Brown. In Dictionary of national biography, 1961-1970. Suppl. 8, 1981. p. 152-3.

**Brown, William, 1748–1792**
Scarchuk JM, ed: The first pharmacopoeia published in the Federated States of America, by William Brown, entitled Pharmacopoeia Simpliciorum et Efficiorum in Usum Nosocomii Militaris, published by Styner Cist. 1778. Coventry, Conn., the Author, 1976. xii, 32 p.

**Browne, Charles Albert, 1870–1947**
Liebenau J: Charles Albert Browne (1870–1947). **Surv Sources Newsl** 1977 May;5:10–1

**Browne, Edward, 1644–1708**
Levental Z: Medizinisches in den Schriften Edward Brownes (1642–1708). **Gesnerus** 1982;39(2):215–35

**Browne, Thomas, 1605–1682**
Ardolino F: The saving hand of God: the significance of the emblematic frontispiece of the Religio medici. **Engl Lang Notes** 1977;15:19–23
Dirckx JH: Sir Thomas Browne (1605-1682). A model for medical humanists. **JAMA** 1982 Oct 15;248(15):1845–7
Felts JH: Browne spots. **NC Med J** 1982 Aug;43(8):591
Geis G, Bunn I: Sir Thomas Browne and witchcraft: a cautionary tale for contemporary law and psychiatry. **Int J Law Psychiatry** 1981;4(1–2):1–11
Huntley FL: 'Well Sir Thomas?': oration to commemorate the tercentenary of the death of Sir Thomas Browne. **Br Med J [Clin Res]** 1982 Jul 3;285(6334):43–7
Massey RU: Reflections from the Dean's office. The cheerful physicians. **Conn Med** 1979 Nov;43(11):747
Miller E: The Browne doublet: 'Religio medici' in the history of English prose style. **Bull Res Humanit** 1979;82:213–21
Shaw AB: Sir Thomas Browne: the man and the physician. **Br Med J [Clin Res]** 1982 Jul 3;285(6334):40–2
Webster A: Threefold cord of religion, science, and literature in the character of Sir Thomas Browne. **Br Med J [Clin Res]** 1982 Dec 18–25;285(6357):1801–2

**Brownlee, John, 1868–1927**
Fine PE: John Brownlee and the measurement of infectiousness: an historical study in epidemic theory. **J R Stat Soc** 1979;142:347–62

**Brownrigg, William, 1712–1800**
Beckett JV: An eighteenth-century case history: Carlisle Spedding 1738. **Med Hist** 1982 Jul;26(3):303–6

**Bruce, David, 1855–1931**
Fry J: First David Bruce lecture in the David Bruce tradition. The evolution of general practice in the British Army. **J R Army Med Corps** 1982 Oct;128(3):152–9

**Bruce, James, 1730–1794**
Pankhurst R: The medical activities in eighteenth century Ethiopia of James Bruce the explorer. **Medizinhist J** 1982;17(3):256–76

**Bruce, John Mitchell, 1846–1929**
John Mitchell Bruce (1846–1929): **Practitioner** 1982 Apr;226(1366):800

**Bruce, William, 1835–1920**
Mowat AG: Strathpeffer Spa: Dr. William Bruce and polymyalgia rheumatica. **Ann Rheum Dis** 1981 Oct;40(5):503–6

**Brücke, Ernst Wilhelm von, 1819–1892**
Brücke EW von: Briefe an Emil Du Bois-Reymond. Ed. H. Brücke, W. Hilger, W. Höflechner, W. W. Swoboda. Erster Teil. Graz, Akademische Druck- und Verlagsanstalt, 1978. 308 p. (Publikationen aus dem Archiv der Universität Graz, Band 8/1).

**Brueghel, Jan, the Elder, 1568–1625**
Hoppe B: Darstellung der Alchemie in Gemälden von Jan Brueghel d. A. (1568–1625). **Beitr Gesch Pharm** 1983;31(18/19):144–9

**Brugmans, Sebald Instinus, 1763–1819**
Zambon JV: Brugmans, voorloper van Semmelweis. **Ned Tijdschr Geneeskd** 1983 Jun 11;127(24):1060–4

**Brugsch, Theodor, 1878–1963**
Brugsch T: Arzt seit fünf Jahrzehnten. Berlin, Rütten & Loening, 1978. 390 p.
Luther E: Theodor Brugsch und das ärztliche Ethos. **Wiss Z Martin Luther Univ (Math)** 1980;29(2):91–6

**Brun, Rudolf, 1885–1969**
Aeschlimann J: Rudolf Brun (1885–1969). Leben und Werk des Zürcher Neurologen, Psychoanalytikers and Entomologen. Zürich, Juris, 1980. 70p. (Zürcher medizingeschichtliche Abhandlungen. Neue Reihe, Nr. 144).

**Brunfels, Otto, 1488–1534**
Dilg P: Die 'Reformation der Apotecken' (1536) des Berner Stadtarztes Otto Brunfels. **Gesnerus** 1979;36(3–4):181–205
Plowman T: Brunfelsia in ethnomedicine. **Bot Mus Leafl Harv Univ** 1977;25:289–320

**Brunner, Alfred, 1890–1972**
Tanner-Weder C: Alfred Brunner und die Entwicklung der Thoraxchirurgie. Zürich, Juris, 1980. 37p. (Zürcher Medizingeschichtliche Abhandlungen, Neue Reihe, Nr. 142).

**Brupbacher, Fritz, 1874–1945**
Lang K: Kritiker, Ketzer, Kämpfer: das Leben des Arbeiterarztes Fritz Brupbacher. Zürich, Limmat, 1983. 360 p.

**Brush, Clinton E., 1879–1981**
Kampmeier RH: Practice in Nashville--1905 and succeeding years. **J Tenn Med Assoc** 1983 Jan;76(1):9–15

**Bruteanu, Mircea, 1882–1957**
Sărmăşanu-Cortez ML, Cortez P: Un luptător neobosit pentru progresul psihiatriei româneşti: dr. Mircea Bruteanu (1882--1957). **Rev Med Interna [Neurol Psihiatr]** 1979 Apr–Jun;24(2):137–42

**Bryant, Louise Frances Stevens, 1885–1959**
Reed J: Louise Frances Stevens Bryant. In Dictionary of American Biography, Suppl. 6, 1956–1960. p. 80–2, 1980.

**Buber, Martin, 1878–1965**
Tellenbach H: Martin Bubers Einfluss auf die anthropologische Wende in der Medizin. **Nervenarzt** 1980 May;51(5):302–6
Wachinger L: Buber und Freud. **Stimmen Zeit** 1978;196(11):754–62

**Buccella, Nicola, d. 1610**
Szpilczyński S: Das traditionelle und progressive Gesicht der Medizin in der Renaissance-Epoche im Lichte der Polemik zwischen S. Simonius und N. Buccella nach dem Tode des Königs Stefan Batory. **Organon** 1979;15:229–37

**Buchan, John, 1769–1847**
Rechtman J: L'asepsie et son histoire; le Dr Buchan précède le Dr Semmelweis de plus d'un siècle (1769–1847). **Soc Fr Hist Art Dent** 1979 Sep-Dec;(5–6):15–17

**Buchan, William, 1729–1805**
Rechtman J: Un précurseur génial de la prévention et de la diététique, du bouche à bouche et du massage cardiaque externe de l'asepsie et parrain de J. P. Marat: Le docteur William Buchan (1729–1805). Diss. Paris VII, 1979. 115 p.
Rosenberg CE: Medical text and social context: explaining William Buchans's Domestic Medicine. **Bull Hist Med** 1983;57(1):22–42

**Buchheim, Rudolf, 1820–1879**
Benedum J: Vom Giessener pharmakologischen Institut unter Rudolf Buchheim und Karl Gaehtgens (1867–1898). **Medizinhist J** 1980;15(1/2):103–19

**Buchner, Eduard, 1860–1917**
Sinohara H: [Eduard Buchner (1860–1917): a biographical essay] (Jpn). **Seikagaku** 1981;53(10):1139–60

**Buck, Gurdon, 1807–1877**
Burns SB: Early medical photography in America (1839--1883); IV. Early wet-plate era. **NY State J Med** 1979 Nov;79(12):1931–8

**Bucke, Richard Maurice, 1837–1902**
Mitchinson W: R. M. Bucke: a Victorian asylum superintendent. **Ont Hist** 1981;73(4):239–54
Shortt SE: R. M. Bucke: vital force, evolution and somatic psychiatry, 1862–1902. In International Congress of the History of Medicine, 27th, Barcelona, 1980. Actas. Barcelona, Académia de Ciències Mèdiques de Catalunya i Balears, 1981. p. 149–53.

**Buckley, Wilfred, 1873–1933**
Sheail P: Hampshire man [Wilfred Buckley] and the quest for clean milk. **Hampshire** 1981 Mar;:60–2

**Bucknill, John Charles, 1817–1897**
Langley GE: Sir John Charles Bucknill 1817–1897: our founder. **Br J Psychiatry** 1980;137:105–10

**Budd, William, 1811–1880**
Smith DC: William Budd manuscript at the National Library of Medicine. **J Hist Med Allied Sci** 1980 Jul;35(3):318–19
Smith DC, ed: 'On the causes of fevers' (1839) by William Budd. Baltimore and London, Johns Hopkins University Press, 1984. xi, 164 p. (Henry E. Sigerist Supplements to the Bulletin of the History of Medicine, n.s., no. 9)

**Budden, William Alfred, 1884–1954**
Gatterman MI: W. A. Budden: the transition through proprietary education, 1924–1954. **Chiropr Hist** 1982;2(1):21–5

**Buddha**
Murthy CK: Sculpture of fasting Buddha; artist's knowledge of anatomy in ancient India. **Bull Inst Hist Med (Hyderabad)** 1973 Oct;3(4):186–8
Winder M: Il Buddha della medicina. **Kos** 1984 Apr;1(3):55–74

**Budisavljevic, Julije, 1882–1981**
Djordjević SP: Prof. dr Julije Budisavljević (2. III 1882--5. V 1981). **Srp Arh Celok Lek** 1983 Jun;111(6):861–4
Djordjević SP: Sećanja na rad u vojnom sanitetu Srbije u toku II balkanskog rata 1913. godine. Iz sećanja dr Julija Budisavljevinja i njegovih kolega iz Hirurške klinike u Insbruku. **Srp Arh Celok Lek** 1983 Jun;111(6):853–9

**Buerger, Leo, 1879–1943**
Fagrell B: Först med stort patientmaterial på rökbetingad allergi. **Lakartidningen** 1982 Oct 13;79(41):3669–7

**Buffi da Bertipaglia, Leonardo, fl. 1448**
Pesenti Marañgon T: 'Professores chirurgie', 'medici ciroici' e 'barbitonsores' a Padova nell' età di Leonardo Buffi da Bertipaglia (dopo il 1448). Quad. Stor Univ. Padova, 1978;11:1–38.

**Buffon, Georges Louis Leclerc, 1707–1788**
Eddy JH: Buffon, organic alterations, and man. **Stud Hist Biol** 1984;7:1–45

**Bugát, Pál, 1793–1865**
Batári G: Erik Ingman finn orvos látogatása Pesten Bugát Pálnál 1847-ben. **Orvostort Kozl** 1981;93–96(27 No 1–4):189–92

**Bühler, Charlotte Bertha, 1893–1974**
Allen M: Charlotte Bertha Bühler. In: Notable American women. The modern period. Cambridge, Mass., Belknap–Harvard Univ. Press, 1980. 4:119–21.

**Bühler, Karl, 1879–1963**
Marion P: La psicologia del pensiero dalla polemica di Wundt alla Entwicklungspsychologie di Bühler. **Stor Crit Psicol** 1982 Dec;3(2):249–79
Marion P: La polemica tra Henning e Bühler. **Stor Crit Psicol** 1980;1(2):297–310

**Buĭnovskiĭ, A. A., 1844–**
Alekseev GA, Butsevitskiĭ VS, Galkina ND: Revoliutsionnaia deiatel'nost' vracha A.A. Buĭnovskogo. **Sov Zdravookhr** 1979;(8):54–5

**Bujwid, Odon, 1857–1942**
Kucharz E: Odo Bujwid - the pioneer in microbiology in Poland. In International Congress of the History of Medicine. 26th, Plovdiv, 1978. Actes du Congress. Sofia, 1981. Volume II. p. 128–9.

**Bukhtishu' ibn Jibrail, d. 870**
Hajal F: Psychological treatment of anorexia: a case from the ninth century. **J Hist Med Allied Sci** 1982 Jul;37(3):325–8

**Bukowiecki, Henryk, 1903–**
Pankiewicz H: Prof. dr hab. Henryk Bukowiecki jako historyk farmacji. **Arch Hist Med (Warsz)** 1984;47(3):389–93

**Bularski, Jan**
Sikorski J: Płk dr Jan Bularski. **Przegl Lek** 1981;38(1):175–7

**Bullitt, James Bell, 1874–1964**
Graham JB: James Bell Bullitt, M.D., 1874–1964: a University of North Carolina medical giant. **NC Med J** 1984 Feb;45(2):88–92

**Bumm, Ernst, 1778–1820**
Danilishina EI: Ernst Bumm (k 125-letiiu so dnia rozhdeniia). **Akush Ginekol (Mosk)** 1984 Jan;(1):69–70

**Bumm, Ernst, 1858–1925**
Schneck P: Ernst Bumm (1858–1925) und die Gynäkologie seiner Zeit. Eine bioergographische Skizze anlässlich seines 125. Geburtstages. **Zentralbl Gynakol** 1983;105(10):662–5

**Bunnell, Sterling, 1882–1957**
Sterling Bunnell; 1882–1957: **J Hand Surg** 1982 May;7(3):217–20

**Bunnell, Walls Willard, 1902–**
Paul JR, Bunnell WW: Classics in infectious diseases. The presence of heterophile antibodies in infectious mononucleosis by John R. Paul and W. W. Bunnell. American Journal of the Medical Sciences, 1932.

**Bunsen, Robert Wilhelm Eberhard, 1811–1899**
Trease GE: Robert Wilhelm Eberhard Bunsen (1811–1899). **Br J Pharm Pract** 1981;3(5):38–9

**Burchenal, Elizabeth, 1876?–1959**
Weissman MB: Elizabeth Burchenal. In: Notable American women. The modern period. Cambridge, Mass., Belknap–Harvard Univ. Press, 1980. 4:121–2.

**Burd, Joseph G.**
Burd JG: Forty years on the same job (or orthopedic surgery can be fun). **J Tenn Med Assoc** 1979 Jul;72(7):534–6

**Burdenko, Nikolai Nilovich, 1876–1946**
Bagdasar'ian SM: Vydaiushchiĭsia sovetskiĭ uchenyĭ (k 40-letiiu prisvoeniia zvaniia Geroia Sotsialisticheskogo Truda N. N. Burdenko). **Voen Med Zh** 1983 May;5:64–8

**Burdett-Coutts, Angelina Georgina, 1814–1906**
Sakula A: Baroness Burdett-Coutts' garden party: the International Medical Congress, London, 1881. **Med Hist** 1982 Apr;26(2):183–90

**Burgers, Thomas François, 1834?–1881**
Appelgryn MS: Die siektetoestand en laaste dae van president T. F. Burgers. **Kleio (S Afr)** 1980;12(1–2):18–31

**Burgesser, William Slater, 1853–1927**
Vining JW: Slater Burgesser and his famous spring. **West Ill Reg Stud** 1982;5(2):184–95

**Burggraaf jr., Johannes Philips, 1700–1775**
Houtzager HL: A letter from Herman Boerhaave to Johan Philip Burggraaf jr. **Janus** 1980:67(1–2–3):201–5

**Burgkmair, Hans, the Elder, 1473–ca. 1531**
Cone TE: A rachitic infant painted by Burgkmair 136 years before Dr. Whistler described rickets. **Clin Pediatr (Phila)** 1980 Mar;19(3):194

**Burijan, Richard**
Kostić AD: Osvrt na ličnost prof. dr. Riharda Burijana i na vreme osnivanja medicinskog fakulteta univerziteta u Beogradu. **Srp Arh Celok Lek** 1982 Mar;110(3):387–98

**Burke, Edmund, 1729–1797**
Kaufman P: Burke, Freud, and the Gothic **Stud Burke Time** 1972;13(3):2179–92

**Burke, Thomas, 1886–1945**
Watterson J, ed: Poetic justice; or, an illfated epic by Thomas Burke. **NC Hist Rev** 1978;55(3):339–46

**Burke, William, 1792–1829**
Douglas H: Burke and Hare. **Br Hist Illus** 1978–79;5(5):32–43

**Burlingham, Dorothy, 1891–1979**
In memoriam. Dorothy Burlingham. 1891–1979.: **Psychoanal Study Child** 1980;35:ix–xxii
Jackson DL: Contributions to the history of psychology: XXXV. Dorothy Burlingham. **Psychol Rep** 1984 Jun;54(3):855–63

**Burn, Joshua Harold, 1892–1981**
Bülbring E, Walker JM: Joshua Harold Burn: 6 March 1892–13 July 1981. **Biogr Mem Fellows R Soc** 1984;30:45–89

**Burney, Fanny, 1752–1840**
Kris K: A 70-year follow-up of a childhood learning disability. The case of Fanny Burney. **Psychoanal Study Child** 1983;38:637–52

**Burns, Allan, 1781–1813**
Kligfield P: The early pathophysiolic understanding of angina pectoris (Edward Jenner, Caleb Hillier Parry, Allan Burns). **Am J Cardiol** 1982 Dec;50(6):1433–5

**Burns, Kit**
Kaufman M, Kaufman HJ: Henry Bergh, Kit Burns, and the sportsmen of New York. **NY Folkl Q** 1972;28(1):15–29

**Burns, Louisa, 1870–1958**
Northup GW: Louisa Burns Memorial Lecture: Re--search. **J Am Osteopath Assoc** 1984 Sep;84(1):67–70

**Burns, Robert, 1759–1796**
Buchanan WW, Kean WF: Robert Burn's illness revisited. **Scott Med J** 1982 Jan;27(1):75–88

**Burow, Carl August, 1809–1874**
Goldwyn RM: Carl August Burow. **Plast Reconstr Surg** 1984 Apr;73(4):687–90

**Burrough, William, fl. 1825–1850**
Moes RJ: The elusive Dr. Burrough: Alta California's first physician. **South Calif Q** 1982;64(4):265–80

**Burroughs, Silas Mainville, 1846–1895**
Garner J: Burroughs and Wellcome: American architects of a British empire. **Can Pharm J** 1980 Dec;:417–9

**Burt, Cyril, 1883–1971**
Hearnshaw LS: Cyril Burt, psychologist. Ithaca, Cornell University Press, 1979. xi, 370 p.
Karier C: In praise of great men. **Hist Educ Q** 1980;20(4):473–86
Norton B: Psychologists and class. In C. Webster, ed: Biology, medicine and society 1840–1940. Cambridge, Cambridge University Press, 1981. p. 289–314.
Sutherland G, Sharp S: 'The fust official psychologist in the wurrld': aspects of the professionalization of psychology in early twentieth century Britain. **Hist Sci** 1980 Sep;18(41 pt 3):181–208

**Burton, Robert, 1577–1640**
Brink A: Depression and loss: a theme in Robert Burton's 'Anatomy of melancholy' (1621). **Can J Psychiatry** 1979 Dec;24(8):767–72
Faulkner TC: Computer applications for an edition of Robert Burton's The anatomy of melancholy: a system for scholarly publishing. **Comput Hum** 1981 Nov;15(3):163–82
Heyd M: Robert Burton's sources on enthusiasm and melancholy: from a medical tradition to religious controversy. **Hist Eur Ideas** 1984;5:17–44

**Burton, William, 1609–1657**
Alsop JD: The fatal illness of the antiquary William Burton (1609–57). **Notes Queries** 1979 Oct;26(5):424–5

**Busanny-Caspari, Willi, 1922–1982**
Willi Busanny-Caspari (8. 4. 1922 bis 7. 7. 1982): **Verh Dtsch Ges Pathol** 1983;67:772–3

**Busbecq, Ogier Ghiselin de, 1522–1592**
Bourilkova L, Israel S: Données sur la médecine et l'hygiène dans les terres bulgares d'après la description du voyageur Ogier Ghiselin de Busbecq (1522–1592). In International Congress of the History of Medicine. 26th, Plovdiv, 1978. Actes du Congress. Sofia, 1981. Volume II. p. 62–3.

**Busby, John**
Peacock EG: Early Idaho panhandle doctor reached patients on horseback, boats and rails. **Pac Northwest** 1979;23(1):1–15

**Busch, Wilhelm, 1832–1908**
Bienengräber A: Wilhelm Busch und die Medizin. **Zentralbl Chir** 1980;105(24):1644–52

**Bustillos, José Vicente, 1803–1873**
Presentación de José Vicente Bustillos. Una paradoja?: **Rev Med Chil** 1983 Oct;111(10):1075–84

**Butler, Harry B., d. 1965**
Miller GH: A drill in either hand. **CAL** 1981 Mar;44(9):14-5, 18-9

**Butler, Mary Joseph, Mother, 1901-**
Holland MM, Dean L: Mother Joseph: founder, architect, beggar. **Hosp Prog** 1980 Apr;61(4):70-3

**Buzzi, Francesco, 1751-1805**
Belloni L: Der Beitrag von Francesco Buzzi zur Entdeckung der 'Macula lutea' under 'Fovea centralis' des menschlichen Auges. **Gesnerus** 1983;40(1-2):23-30

**Byron, George Gordon Noël, 1788-1824**
Lundström B: Medicinska aspekter på Lord Byron. **Sydsven Medicinhist Sallsk Arsskr** 1980;:112-23

# C

**Cabanis, Pierre Jean Georges, 1757-1808**
Levin A: Venel, Lavoisier, Fourcroy, Cabanis and the idea of scientific revolution: the French political context and the general patterns of conceptualization of scientific change. **Hist Sci** 1984 Sep;22(57 pt 3):303-20
Mitchell H: The passions according to Adam Smith and Pierre-Jean-Georges-Cabanis. Two sciences of man(1). **Soc Soc Hist Med Bull (Lond)** 1979 Dec;25:20-7
Pigeaud J: Cabanis et les rapports du physique et du moral. **Sci Tech Persp** 1981-82;1:8.1-.13
Staum MS: Cabanis. Enlightenment and medical philosophy in the French Revolution. Princeton, Princeton University Press, 1980. xi, 430 p.

**Cabot, Richard Clarke, 1868-1939**
Burns CR: Richard Cabot and 'The American type' of psychotherapy. In International Congress of the History of Medicine, 27th, Barcelona, 1980. Actas. Barcelona, Acadèmia de Ciències Mèdiques de Catalunya i Balears, 1981. p. 39-41.

**Cabrol, Barthélemy, b. 1529**
Luyendijk-Elshout AM: The introduction of Juan Valverde's and Bartholomy Cabrol's anatomy into Low Countries between 1568-1633. In International Congress of the History of Medicine, 27th, Barcelona, 1980. Actas. Barcelona, Acadèmia de Ciències Mèdiques de Catalunya i Balears, 1981. p. 298-303.

**Cade, John F.**
Schou M: Lithium perspectives. **Neuropsychobiology** 1983;10(1):7-12

**Cade, John Frederick Joseph, d. 1980**
Lithium salts in the treatment of psychotic excitement: John F Cade: **Aust NZ J Psychiatry** 1982 Sep;16(3):129-33

**Cadet de Gassicourt, Charles Louis, 1769-1821**
Flahaut S: Le pharmacien Charles-Louis Cadet de Gassicourt, bâtard de Louis XV, et sa famille. **Rev Hist Pharm (Paris)** 1980 Mar;27(244):53-61

**Cadet, Sócrate, 1808-1879**
Stroppiana L: Correspondencia cientifica de 1858 entre el doctor Beauperthuy de Caracas y el doctor Socrate Cadet de Roma. **Rev Soc Venez Hist Med** 1979;28(42):37-44

**Cadogan, William, 1711-1797**
Wilson AF: The Enlightenment and infant care. **Soc Soc Hist Med Bull (Lond)** 1979 Dec;25:44-7

**Caillié, René-Auguste, 1799-1838**
Logeay R: Le voyage de René Caillé à Tombouctou; ce qu'il lui en a coûté. **Hist Sci Med** 1982;16(4):273-83

**Cairns, Hugh William Bell, 1896-1952**
McEwin R: Florey and Cairns--early work on penicillin. **Med J Aust** 1982 Jan 9;1(1):12-3
Travers R: Florey and Cairns--early work on penicillin. **Med J Aust** 1982 Jul 10;2(1):10-1

**Cairns, Thomas**
Johnson KM, Scribner Cl, McCormick JB: Ecology of ebola virus: a first clue? **J Infect Dis** 1981 May;143(5):749-51

**Caius, John, 1510-1573**
Nutton V: John Caius und Johannes Lange: medizinischer Humanismus zur Zeit Vesals. **NTM** 1984;21(2):81-7

**Calcar, Jan Stephan van, 1499-1546?**
Speransky LS, Bocharov VJ, Goncharov NI: The personages of Jan Stephan van Calcar's frontispiece to Andreas Vesalius' book 'On the Structure of the Human Body'. **Anat Anz** 1983;153(5):465-79

**Calcidius, fl. 400**
Mansfeld J: Alcmaeon: 'Physikos' or physician? With some remarks on Calcidius' 'On vision' compared to Galen's Plac. Hipp. Plat. VII. In J. Mansfeld, L. M. de Rijk, eds. Kephalaion: Studies in Greek philosophy and its continuation. Assen, Van Gorcum, 1975. p. 26-38.

**Caldwell, Charles, 1772-1853**
Erickson P: The anthropology of Charles Caldwell, M.D. **ISIS** 1981 Jun;72(262):252-6

**Calef, John, 1725-1812**
Condon AG: John Caleff. In Dictionary of Canadian biography, 1801 to 1820. Volume 5, 1983. p. 134-5.
Hall CA: Doctors afield: John Calef, M.D. **N Engl J Med** 1981 Oct 29;305(18):1048-51

**Call i Morros, Josep**
Parellada i Feliu D: Comentaris al llibre 'Higiene del alma' del doctor Josep Call i Morros (editat a Barcelona l'any 1888). In Congrés International d'Història de la Medicina Catalana, 2nd, Barcelona, 1975. Llibre d'Actes. Barcelona, Socitra, 1977. p. 263-71.

**Callahan, John Ross, 1853-1918**
Dew WC: John Ross Callahan: a man, a memorial, an award. **Ohio Dent J** 1982 Jul-Aug;56(7-8):46-52

**Calmette, Albert, 1863-1933**
Dodin A: Albert Calmette. Président de la Société de Pathologie Exotique. **Bull Soc Pathol Exot Filiales** 1983 May-Jun;76(3):211-4
Hourlier: 7 juin 1983: Cérémonie d'hommage public à Calmette (Hôpital des Armées de Lorient). **Bull Soc Pathol Exot Filiales** 1983 May-Jun;76(3):312-6
Saenz A, Boisvert H: Correspondance inédite d'Albert Calmette (1863-1933). **Hist Sci Med** 1983;17(4):419-27
Sakula A: BCG: who were Calmette and Guérin? **Thorax** 1983 Nov;38(11):806-12

**Calot, Jean François, 1861-1944**
Rocko JM, Di Gioia JM: Calot's triangle revisited. **Surg Gynecol Obstet** 1981 Sep;153(3):410-4

**Calvin, John, 1509-1564**
Bouwsma WJ: John Calvin's anxiety. **Proc Am Philos Soc** 1984 Sep;128(3):252-6

**Calvo Asensio, Pedro, 1821-1863**
Javier Puerto F: Pedro Calvo Asensio (1821-1863): farmaceutico liberal. **Bol Soc Esp Hist Farm** 1983;34(136):203-28

**Camac, Charles Nicoll Bancker, 1868-1940**
Nation EF, McGovern JP, ed: Student and chief: the Osler-Camac correspondence. Pasadena, Castle Press, 1980. 131 p.

**Cambournac, Francisco, 1903-**
Sessão solene de homenagem ao Prof. Dr. Francisco Cambournac, por ocasião da atribuição do prémio e medalha da Fundação Léon Bernard pela Organização Mundial de Saúde--22 de Junho de 1978: **An Inst Hig Med Trop (Lisb)** 1977-1978;5(1-4):37-53

**Cameron, D. Ewen, 1901-1967**
Goldman DL, Arvanitakis K: D. Ewen Cameron's Day Hospital and the day hospital movement. **Can J Psychiatry** 1981 Aug;26(5):365-8

**Cameron, Gordon Roy, 1899-1966**
Oakley CL: Sir Gordon Roy Cameron. In Dictionary of national biography, 1961-1970. Suppl. 8, 1981. p. 167-9.

**Camões, Luis Vaz de, 1524?-1580**
Collet AJ: Luis Vaz de Camões. **Scalpel Tongs** 1981;25:52
Collet AJ: Luiz Vaz de Camões (1524?-1580). **Scalpel Tongs** 1981;25:44-5

**Campani, Giuseppe, 1635-1715**
Bonelli ML, Helden A van: Divini and Campani: a forgotten chapter in the history of the Academia del Cimento. **Ann Ist Mus Stor Sci Fir** 1981;6(1):3-176

**Campbell, Alfred Walter, 1868-1937**
Eadie MJ: A. W. Campbell: Australia's first neurologist. **Clin Exp Neurol** 1980;17:27-35

**Campbell, C. S.**
Sternbach G: C.S. Campbell: Gamekeeper's thumb. **J Emerg Med** 1984;1(4):345-7

**Campbell, George William, 1810-1882**
Roland CG: George William Campbell. In Dictionary of Canadian biography, 1881-1890. 1982;11:148-9.

**Campbell, John Logan, 1817-1912**
Wright-St Clair RE: The medical qualifications of Sir John Logan Campbell. **NZ Med J** 1983 Mar 23;96(728):212-3

**Campbell Swinton, Alan A., d. 1930**
Ramsey LJ: Some notable early contributors to radiography--Thompson, Jackson and Campbell Swinton. **Radiography** 1980 Dec;46(552):289-97

**Camper, John E., d. 1977**
Cahn JD: A doctor's legacy: Dr. John E. T. Camper and the MeDeSo. **J Natl Med Assoc** 1980 Mar;72(3):283-7

**Camper, Petrus, 1722-1789**
Gysel C: Conférence autour de Camper (1722-1789) et de 'son' angle facial. **Orthod Fr** 1980;51:LIX-XCVII
Gysel C: Les relations du jeune Blumenbach avec Camper vieillissant. **Hist Sci Med** 1983;17(2):135-9
Hellmich S, Hellmich J: Der Zwischenkieferknochen und Goethes Mephistopheles. **Laryngol Rhinol Otol (Stuttg)** 1982 Oct;61(10):552-6
Kobes LW: Quellenstudie zu Petrus Camper und der nach ihm benannten Schädelebene. **Dtsch Zahnarztl Z** 1983;38(3):268-70

**Campo Posada, Arturo, 1909-**
Campo Posada A: Una vida, un médico. Bogota, Colombia, Ediciones Fondo Cultural Cafetero, [1982]. 248 p.

**Camus, Albert, 1913–1960**
Montiel L: La enfermedad como símbolo: la peste en la obra de Albert Camus. **Asclepio** 1983;35:171–6

**Cañas, Ricardo Moreno, 1890–1938**
Low SM: Dr. Moreno Cañas: a symbolic bridge to the demedicalization of healing. **Soc Sci Med** 1982;16(5):527–31

**Candau, Marcolino Gomes, 1911–1983**
Dr. Marcolino Gomes Candau (30.05.1911--23.01.1983): **Rev Bras Malariol Doencas Trop** 1982;34:119–22

**Candolle, Alphonse de, 1806–1893**
Fancher RE: Alphonse de Candolle, Francis Galton, and the early history of the nature-nurture controversy. **J Hist Behav Sci** 1983 Oct;19(4):341-52
Mikulinskij SR, Markova LA, Starostin BA: Alphonse de Candolle (1806–1893). Jena, Fischer, 1980. 224 p. (Biographien bedeutender Biologen, Band 3).

**Cane, Florence, 1882–1952**
Detre KC, Frank T, Kniazzeh CR, et al: Roots of art therapy. Margaret Naumburg (1890–1983) and Florence Cane (1882–1952). A family portrait. **Am J Art Ther** 1983 Jul;22(4):111–23

**Cannon, Claude Clenton**
Mosteller JH: 'Practices dentistry in Fayette, Alabama'. A tardy but sincere tribute to Claude Clenton Cannon. **J Ala Dent Assoc** 1977 Oct;61(4):19–24

**Cannon, Ida Maud, 1877–1960**
Vogel MJ: Ida Maud Canon. In Dictionary of American Biography, Suppl. 6, 1956–1960. p. 97–8, 1980.

**Cannon, Walter Bradford, 1871–1945**
Barger AC: New technology for a new century: Walter B. Cannon and the invisible rays. **AJR** 1981 Jan;136(1):187–95
Benison S, Barger AC, Wolfe EL: Changing of the guard. **Harv Med Alumni Bull** 1982 Spring;56(2):34–41
Cannon B: Walter Bradford Cannon, M. D.: Reflections on the physician, the man, and his contributions. **Gastrointest Radiol** 1982;7(1):1–6
Chang S: In memory of our visiting professor: Walter B. Cannon at Peking. **Physiologist** 1980 Jun;23(3):39–40
Davenport HW: Signs of anxiety, rage, or distress. **Physiologist** 1981 Oct–Nov;24(5):1–5
Miller M: The Walter Bradford Cannon Papers. **Surv Sources Newsl** 1977 May;5:8–9
Schlesinger MC: Snatched from oblivion: a Cambridge memoir. Boston, Little Brown, 1979. 243 p.

**Cantacuzino, Serban, 1640–1688**
Milin M, Popescu A: Sfîrsitul Lui Serban Cantacuzino. **Mag Istor** 1980;14(9):53–8

**Cantémir, Demetris, 1673–1723**
Todericiu D: Prolongements méconnus de la philosophie chimique de Jean-Baptiste Van Helmont (1578–1644) en Europe centrale et orientale. L'éloge à Van Helmont du savant roumain Démètre Cantémir (1701). **Bull Cl Sci Acad R Belg** 1979;65:228–38

**Carbonell y Bravo, Francisco, 1768–1837**
Beya Alonso E: Un comentario sobre los 'Elementos de Farmacia', de Carbonell. **Bol Soc Esp Hist Farm** 1980/81 Dec–Mar;31-32(124–5):315–22
Rof Carballo MC: Biografía y labor docente de Francisco Carbonell y Bravo. Diss. Barcelona, Facultad de Farmacia, Universidad de Barcelona, 1975. 189 p. (Publicaciones del Seminario de Historia de la Farmacia).

**Cardano, Girolamo, 1501–1576**
Fierz M: Girolamo Cardano (1501–1576): Arzt, Naturphilosoph, Mathematiker, Astronom, und Traumdeuter. Basel, Birkhäuser, 1977. 138 p.
Fierz M: Girolamo Cardano, 1501–1576. Physician, natural philosopher, mathematician, astrologer, and interpreter of dreams. Boston, Birkhäuser, 1983. xxii, 202 p.
Müller-Jahncke WD: Kleiner Beitrag zum Prioritätenstreit um die Metoposkopie: Hájek contra Cardano. **Sudhoffs Arch** 1982;66(1):79–84

**Cardenas, Juan de, 1563–1609**
Cardenas J de: Primera parte de los problemas y secretos maravillosos de las Indias. Edicion, estudio preliminar y notas para X. Lozoya. Mexico, Academia Nacional de Medicina, 1980. 320 p.

**Carew, Richard, b. 1555**
Lewis TH: Richard Carew on the treatment of a 'Franticke person' in Medieval Cornwall. **J Hist Med Allied Sci** 1981 Jan;36(1)64–6

**Carli, Christopher, 1811–1887**
Rosenthal R: Dr. Christopher Carli, pioneer physician of Minnesota. **Minn Med** 1982 Dec;65(12):765–8

**Carlier, Francois**
Fernandez D: Francois Carlier, La Prostitution antiphysique (1857). Précédé de La Pederastie (1887) par Ambroise Tardieu. Paris, Le Sycomore, 1981. ix, 250 p.

**Carlos III, King of Spain, 1716–1788**
Puente Veloso S: Aportación de la botánica a la medicina en el reinado de Carlos III. **An R Acad Nac Med (Madr)** 1982;99(3):437–501

**Carlos, Prince of Asturias, 1545–1568**
Floriano AC: En torno a la enfermedad y muerte del príncipe Don Carlos (hijo de Felipe II). In: Homenaje al Profesor Carriazo. Seville, Univ. of Seville, 1973. vol. 2. p. 203–31.

**Carlson, Anton Julius, 1875–1956**
Garrett CG: Anton Julius Carlson. In Dictionary of American Biography, Suppl. 6, 1956–1960. p. 99–100, 1980.

**Carlyle, Thomas, 1795–1881**
Spear JL: Filaments, females, families and social fabric: Carlyle's extension of a biological analogy. In Paradis J, Postlewait T, ed: Victorian science and Victorian values: literary perspectives. New York, New York Academy of Sciences, 1981. p. 69–84.

**Carmichael, Edward Arnold, 1896–**
Merton PA: Neurophysiology on man. **J Neurol Neurosurg Psychiatry** 1981 Oct;44(10):861–70

**Carmichael, John Leslie, 1897–**
Carmichael JL: Medical reminiscences. **Ala Med** 1984 Jun;53(12):16–27; July;54(1):13–5, 17

**Carmona y Valle, Manuel, 1827–1902**
Pérez Gallardo R: El monumento del Dr. Manuel Carmona y Valle. **Bol Soc Mex Hist Filos Med** 1981 Mar;5(34):147–58

**Carnegie, Andrew, 1835?–1919**
Farrah MA: Andrew Carnegie: a psychohistorical sketch. D. A. Diss. Carnegie-Mellon University. Pittsburgh, 1982. ix. 183 p.

**Carnegie, Dale, 1888–1955**
Parker GT: How to win friends and influence people: Dale Carnegie and the problem of sincerity. **Am Q** 1977;29(5):506–18

**Carnot, Marie François Sadi, 1837–1894**
Peset JL: La sociedad enferma: algunas reflexiones sobre la muerte del presidente Carnot (1894). **Asclepio** 1983;35:177–88

**Carnwath, Thomas, 1878–**
Elwood JH: Thomas Carnwath. **Ulster Med J** 1982;51(2):98–109

**Carpenter, Edward, 1844–1929**
Martin RK: Edward Carpenter and the double structure of Maurice. **J Homosex** 1983 Spring–Summer;8(3–4):35–46

**Carr-Saunders, Alexander Morris, 1886–1966**
Brown HP: Sir Alexander Carr-Saunders. In Dictionary of national biography, 1961–1970. Suppl. 8, 1981. p. 175–6.

**Carracido, José Rodríguez, 1856–1928**
Sanchez-Moscoso A: José Rodríguez Carracido. **Bol Soc Esp Hist Farm** 1971 Jun;22(86):54–84

**Carrel, Alexis, 1873–1944**
Bing RJ: Carrel: a personal reminiscence. **JAMA** 1983 Dec 23–30;250(24):3297–8
Chambers RW, Durkin JT, ed: Papers of the Alexis Carrel centennial conference, Georgetown University June 28, 1973. Washington, Georgetown University, 1973. 107 p. Contributions by C. A. Lindbergh, A. Gros, S. Maggio, L. G. Walker, C. A. Hufnagel, T. I. Malinin.
Converse JM: Alexis Carrel: the man, the unknown. **Plast Reconstr Surg** 1981 Oct;68(4):629–39
d'Allaines C: Alexis Carrel (1873–1944), visionnaire de la chirurgie cardio-vasculaire. **Arch Mal Coeur** 1984 Sep;77(9):1074–7
Dr. Alexis Carrel and tissue culture: **JAMA** 1984 Jul 6;252(1):44–5
Edwards WS: Alexis Carrel's contributions to thoracic surgery. **Ann Thorac Surg** 1983 Jan;35(1):111–4
Hardy JD: Landmark perspective. Transplantation of blood vessels, organs, and limbs. **JAMA** 1983 Aug 19;250(7):954–7
Jain KM, Swan KG, Casey KF: Nobel Prize winner in surgery. Part 2. **Am Surg** 1982 May;48(5):191–6
Malinin TI: Surgery and life: the extraordinary career of Alexis Carrel. New York, Harcourt Brace Jovanovich, 1979. xiii, 242 p.
Moseley J: Alexis Carrel, the man unknown. Journey of an idea. **JAMA** 1980 Sep 5;244(10):1119–21
Najafi H: Landmark perspective: Dr. Alexis Carrel and tissue culture. **JAMA** 1983 Aug 26;250(8):1086–9
Rutkow IM: The letters of William Halsted and Alexis Carrel. **Surg Gynecol Obstet** 1980 Nov;151(5):676–88
Schmitt W: Das chirurgische Erbe. Alexis Carrel (1873–1944). **Zentralbl Chir** 1983;108(8):495–503
Windsor HM: Direct blood transfusion. **Med J Aust** 1980 Feb 9;1(3):136
Witkowski JA: Dr. Carrel's immortal cells. **Med Hist** 1980 Apr;24(2):129–42

**Carro, Jean de, 1770–1857**
Subrtová A: Jean de Carro (1770–1857) - příspěvek k biografi. **Cas Nar Muz** 1980;149(1–2):45–61

**Carroll, Lewis, 1832–1898**
Keller EF: Lewis Carroll: a study of mathematical inhibition. **J Am Psychoanal Assoc** 1980;28(1):133–60
Murray TJ: The neurology of Alice in Wonderland. **Can J Neurol Sci** 1982 Nov;9(4):453–7

**Carson, James, 1772-1843**
Keers RY: Two forgotten pioneers. James Carson and George Bodington. **Thorax** 1980 Jul;35(7):483-9

**Carson, Rachel Louise, 1907-1964**
Brooks P: Rachel Louise Carson. In: Notable American women. The modern period. Cambridge, Mass., Belknap-Harvard Univ. Press, 1980. 4:138-41.

**Carswell, John, 1856-1931**
Sclare AB: John Carswell: a pioneer in Scottish psychiatry. **Scott Med J** 1981 Jul;26(3):265-70

**Carswell, Robert, 1793-1857**
Behan PO, Behan WM: Sir Robert Carswell: Scotland's pioneer pathologist. In Rose FC, Bynum WF, ed: Historical aspects of the neurosciences. New York, Raven, 1982. p. 273-92.
Reckert H: Das unbekannte Werk des Pathologen, Robert Carswell (1793-1857). Köln, 1982. 283 p. (Kölner medizinhistorische Beiträge, Band 22)

**Cartegni da Bagnone, Giovanbattista, 1559-1624**
Pagni U: Giovanbattista Cartegni da Bagnone lettore di medicina nello Studio di Pisa. **Arch Stor Prov Parmensi** 1979;31:91-102

**Carter, Robert Brudenell, 1828-1918**
Kane A, Carlson ET: A different drummer: Robert B. Carter and Nineteenth Century hysteria. **Bull NY Acad Med** 1982 Sep;58(6):519-34

**Cartier, Jacques, 1491-1557**
Cadotte M: A propos de la description par Jacques Cartier d'une 'grosse maladie' survenue au cours de son deuxième voyage au Canada. **Union Med Can** 1984 Aug;113(8):651-5

**Carvallo, Temislocles, 1885-1964**
Mazzei Uzcátegui M: Dos figuras medicas venezolanas. **Rev Soc Venez Hist Med** 1969-71;17-19(31-33):163-94

**Casabona, Giuseppe, d. 1595**
Tomasi LT: L'isola dei semplici. **Kos** 1984 Jun;1(5):61-84

**Casal, Gaspar, 1680-1759**
Albarracín A: Gaspar Casal y el concepto moderno de especie morbosa. **Asclepio** 1983;35:189-95

**Casanova, Danielle, 1909-1943**
Fouré J: A French woman dentist who gave her life as a freedom fighter against the Nazis. **Bull Hist Dent** 1984 Oct;32(2):133-4

**Casanova, Giacomo Girolamo, 1725-1798**
Fechner PU, Fechner MU: Tadini, the man who invented the artificial lens. **J Am Intraocul Implant Soc** 1979 Jan;5(1):22-3

**Casimir IV, King of Poland, 1427-1492**
Dudziński W: Smierć króla Kazimierza Jagiellończyka. **Wiad Lek** 1981 Jun 15;34(12):1041-4

**Casona, Alejandro, 1903-1965**
Jiménez Herrero F: La medicina y los médicos en el teatro de Casona. **Bol Inst Estud Asturianos** 1968;22(64-65):319-51

**Casotti, Luigi, 1891-1959**
Bellagarda M, Bellagarda G: L'attività storico-scientifica di Luigi Casotti (1891-1959). **Minerva Med** 1984 Nov 17;75(44):2695-704

**Caspersson, Torbjörn Oskar, 1910-**
Klein G, Klein E: Torbjörn Caspersson: some personal perspectives. **Cytometry** 1984 Jul;5(4):318
Mayall BH: Torbjörn Oskar Caspersson: curriculum vitae and selected publications. **Cytometry** 1984 Jul;5(4):314-7

**Cassel, John C., 1921-1976**
Ibrahim MA, Kaplan BH, Patrick RC, et al: The legacy of John C. Cassel. **Am J Epidemiol** 1980 Jul;112(1):1-7

**Cassiodorus, Flavius Magnus Aurelius, ca. 487-ca. 580**
Petrocchi M: Cassiodore, son temps et la Formula Comitis Archiatrorum. In International Congress of the History of Medicine. 26th, Plovdiv, 1978. Actes du Congress. Sofia, 1981. Volume II. p. 183-7.

**Castelo Branco, Camilo, 1825-1890**
Pina L de, Meneses MO de: Camilo e a historia da medicina. **Arch Hist Med Port** 1968-70;3(1-4):91-116

**Castle, William B., 1897-**
Brecher G: A further note on red cell discoveries. William B. Castle's contribution to the discovery of hemoglobin S. **Blood Cells** 1982;8(2):471-2
Herbert V: Landmark perspective: An 'extrinsic factor' and pernicious anemia. **JAMA** 1984 Jan 27;251(4):522-3

**Castro, Fidel, 1927-**
Richmond JB: A conversation with Fidel Castro about health services. **N Engl J Med** 1984 Apr 12;310(15):994-5

**Castro, Rosalía de, 1837-1885**
Bouza Brey F: Las enfermedades infantiles de Rosalia de Castro y los ritos de medicina magica en Galicia. **Cuad Estud Gallegos** 1967;22(67):183-97

**Catalani, Vincenzo, 1769-1843**
Imerti AD: Vincenzo Catalani, Neapolitan Jacobin, jurist, reformer (1769-1843), with an appendix containing a translation of his work 'A digression on vaccination.' Lawrence, Kansas, Coronado Press, 1976. 155 p.

**Catherine II, the Great, of Russia, 1729-1796**
Alexander JT: Catherine the great and public health. **J Hist Med Allied Sci** 1981 Apr;36(2):185-204
Griffiths J: Doctor Thomas Dimsdale, and smallpox in Russia. The variolation of the Empress Catherine the Great. **Bristol Med Chir J** 1984 Jan;99(369):14-6

**Catherine, of Aragon, queen consort of Henry VIII, 1485-1536**
Dewhurst J: The alleged miscarriages of Catherine of Aragon and Anne Boleyn. **Med Hist** 1984 Jan;28(1):49-56

**Catlin, George, 1796-1872**
Onsager LW: That curious book 'The breath of life' by George Catlin. **Int J Oral Myol** 1980 Oct;6(4):7-10

**Cato, Marcus Porcius, 234-149 B.C.**
Janiszewski J: Veterinärmedizin Catos des Aelteren. **Hist Med Vet** 1979;4(2):42-5

**Cattaneo, Carlo, 1801-1869**
Doise W: Dalla filosofia alla psicologia sociale. Una 'lettura' di Carlo Cattaneo. **Stor Crit Psicol** 1983;4(1):117-29

**Cattell, James McKeen, 1860-1944**
Sokal MM: Science and James McKeen Cattell, 1894 to 1945. **Science** 1980 Jul 4;209(4452):43-52
Sokal MM: James McKeen Cattell and American psychology in the 1920s. In J. Brozĕk, ed: Explorations in the history of psychology in the United States. Lewisburg, Bucknell University Press, 1984. p. 273-323.
Sokal MM, ed: An education in psychology: James McKeen Cattell's journal and letters from Germany and England. 1880-1888. Cambridge, Mass., MIT Press, 1981, xxvii, 372 p.

**Caujole, Paul, 1978-1961**
Gilbrin E: Le docteur Paul Caujole: l'hôpital français d'Oumiah (septembre 1917 - avril 1918). **Hist Sci Med** 1980;14(2):155-64

**Cave, Charles J. B., 1879-1939**
Phillips GO: Barbados' Battle Creek doctor Charles J. B. Cave 1879-1939. **Advent Herit** 1978;5(2):22-33

**Cavell, Edith Louisa, 1865-1915**
Guntrip G: The unknown Edith Cavell. **Nurs Times** 1984 Apr 25-May 1;80(17):63-4
Sadler C: Edith Cavell: from Blakeney Point to Brussels. **Nurs Mirror** 1982 Sep 15;155(11):52-4
Weller B: The spy who nursed me (Edith Cavell). **Nurs Times** 1984 Oct 17-23;80(42):18-9

**Cavina, Cesare, 1888-1935**
Favero GA: Odontoiatria del passato. La stomatologia nelle opere di Cessare Cavina (1888-1935). **Dent Cadmos** 1982 Oct;50(10):83-91

**Cawker, Lenore Harrison**
Palmer VA: Lenore H. Cawker, the animals' friend. **Milw Hist** 1979;2(2):43-8

**Cawthorne, Terence Edward, 1902-1970**
Macbeth R: Sir Terence Edward Cawthorne. In Dictionary of national biography, 1961-1970. Suppl. 8, 1981. p. 179-80.

**Céloron, Marie-Catherine-Françoise, 1744-1809**
Ducharme J: Marie-Catherine-Françoise Céloron. In Dictionary of Canadian biography, 1801 to 1820. Volume 5, 1983. p. 174.

**Celsus, Aulus Cornelius**
Dirckx JH: Dermatologic terms in the De Medicina of Celsus. **Am J Dermatopathol** 1983 Aug;5(4):363-9
Dolzani C: Un 'prelievo' di sangue adombrato in una poesia di Giovanni Pascoli? **Acta Med Hist Patav** 1982-83;29:25-8
Gentile DP: 'Urethrolithotomy': an ingenious approach of the ancients. **J Urol** 1984 Aug;132(2):359-60
Hauben DJ: Aulus (Aurelius) Cornelius Celsus (25 v.u.Z.-50 n.u.Z.) - Vater der plastischen Chirurgie. **Zentralbl Chir** 1984;109(6):441-3
Marmelzat Wl: Medicine in history. Celsus (Ad 25), plastic surgeon: on the repair of defects of the ears, lips, and nose. **J Dermatol Surg Oncol** 1982 Dec;8(12):1012-4
Ollero Granados D: New light Celsus' 'De medicina'. **Sudhoffs Arch** 1978;62(4):359-77
Rubin JP: Celsus' decircumcision operation: medical and historical implications. **Urology** 1980 Jul;16(1):121-4
Villey R: Die Medizin in Rom: Galen. In Sournia JC, Martiny M, Poulet J, ed: Illustrierte Geschichte der Medizin. Salzburg, Andreas, 1980. Vol. 2. p. 411-39.

**Cendala y Gómez, Isabel, fl. 1805**
Bustamente ME: La primera enfermera en la historia de la salud pública, Isabel Cendala y Gómez. **Rev Col Nac Enferm** 1980 Jul, 1981 Feb;27-28(107):7-12

**Cermák, Josef, 1825-1872**
Vencovský E: Mudr. Josef Cermák a jeho zásluhy o vybudování psychiatrické léčebny v Cernovicích. **Cesk Psychiatr** 1984 Jun;80(3):200-3

**Cervantes Saavedra, Miguel de, 1547–1616**
Gracia D: Chirino en el Retablo de las Maravillas. **Asclepio** 1978–79;30–31:265–76
Grinberg L, Rodríguez JF: The influence of Cervantes on the future creator of psychoanalysis. **Int J Psychoanal** 1984;65(Pt 2):155–68

**Cerveňanský, Ján, 1905–**
Cerveňanská N: Ian Chervenianskiĭ––osnovopolozhnik chekhoslovatsko–sovetskikh sviazeĭ v ortopedii. **Ortop Travmatol Protez** 1983 Apr;(4):68–71

**Cesalpino, Andrea, 1524–1603**
Morton AG: Marginalia to Andrea Cesalpino's work on botany. **Arch Nat Hist** 1981 Apr;10(1):31–6

**Cesi, Nicolò, fl. 1391**
Pesce L: Due inventari di libri del medico umanista trevigiano Nicolò Cesi. **Quad Stor Univ Padova** 1978;11:125–7

**Cestoni, Giacinto, 1637–1718**
Testoni G: Una lettera di Cestoni a Vallisneri (1710). **Riv Biol** 1983 Spring;76(1):125–31

**Chabbert, Pierre, 1924–1981**
Théodoridès J: Pierre Chabbert (1924–1981). **Hist Sci Med** 1981;15(4):287–92

**Chadwick, Edwin, 1800–1890**
Budnick LD: The spirit of Chadwick. **NY State J Med** 1983 Dec;83(13):1345–6

**Chadwick, Samuel Taylor, 1809–1873**
Felstein I, Naqvi N: Samuel Taylor Chadwick: 1809–73. **Br Med J [Clin Res]** 1983 Jun 25;286(6383):2031–2

**Chagas, Carlos Ribeiro Justiniano, 1879–1934**
Bergoglio RM: En el centenario del nacimiento de Carlos Chagas. **Rev Fac Cien Med Univ Nac Cordoba** 1981 Jan–Dec;39(1–4):87–9
Lewinsohn R: Carlos Chagas and the discovery of Chagas' disease (American trypanosomiasis). **J R Soc Med** 1981 Jun;74(6):451–5
Neghme A: Semblanza del Dr. Carlos R. Chagas, figura señera de la medicina. **Rev Med Chil** 1979 Sep;107(9):876–8

**Chagovets, Rotislav Vsesolodovich, 1904–1982**
Khalmuradov AG, Rybina AA: Tvorcheskiĭ vklad akademika AN USSR R. V. Chagovtsa v razvitie biokhimii. **Ukr Biokhim Zh** 1984 Sep–Oct;56(5):576–86

**Chain, Ernst Boris, 1906–1979**
Abraham EP: Ernst Chain and Paul Garrod. **J Antimicrob Chemother** 1980 Jul;6(4):423–4
Sheppard J: Illustrations from the Wellcome Institute Library: the Chain papers. **Med Hist** 1983 Oct;27(4):434–5

**Chaliapin, Feodor Ivanovich, 1873–1938**
Evdokimov PP: K istorii bolezni F. I. Shaliapina. **Klin Med (Mosk)** 1983 May;61(5):115–6

**Chałubiński, Tytus, 1820–1889**
Kempa K: Tytus Chałubiński w opiniach współczesnych mu przedstawicieli literatury i sztuki. **Wiad Lek** 1980 Dec;33(23):1931–4

**Champier, Symphorien, 1471 or 2–ca. 1539**
Copenhaver BP: Symphorien Champier and the reception of the occultist tradition in Renaissance France. The Hague, New York, Mouton, 1978. 368 p.

**Chandler, Raymond, 1888–1959**
Skinner RE: Narcotics, barred windows, and murder: the medical practitioner in the writings of Raymond Chandler. **Perspect Biol Med** 1983 Autumn;27(1):127–34

**Chang and Eng, 1811–1874**
Schuknecht HF: The Siamese twins, Eng and Chang: their lives and their hearing losses. **Arch Otolaryngol** 1979 Dec;105(12):737–40

**Chao, Hsüeh-min, fl. 1765**
Unschuld PU: Das Ch'uan-ya und die Praxis chinesischer Landärzte im 18. Jahrhundert. **Sudhoffs Arch** 1978;62(4):378–407

**Chapanis, Alphonse Robert Everysta, 1917–**
Distinguished contribution for applications in psychology award for 1978 (Alphonse Chapanis).: **Am Psychol** 1979 Jan;34(1):48–55

**Chapin, Charles Value, 1856–1941**
Cassedy JH: Charles V. Chapin re-visited: an appreciation. **RI Med J** 1983 Jan;66(1):41–4
Models for action: **J Public Health Policy** 1980;1(2):103–9

**Chaplin, Charles, 1889–1977**
Benson F: Blood tests showing nonpaternity–conclusive or rebuttable evidence? The Chaplin case revisited. **Am J Forensic Med Pathol** 1981 Sep;2(3):221–3

**Chapman, Nathaniel, 1780–1853**
D'Amato NA: Nathaniel Chapman: first president of the American Medical Association. **Va Med** 1984 Nov;111(11):708–10

**Chappuis, Charles, 1822–1897**
Wrotnowska D: Un ami de Pasteur: Charles Chappuis. In: Congrès National des Sociétés Savantes, 99e, Besançon, 1974. Comptes Rendus. Paris, 1976. Section des Sciences, Fasc. V. p. 171–84.

**Charcot, Jean Baptiste, 1867–1936**
Lanchou G, Veron C: Un évadé de la médecine: Jean-Baptiste Charcot (1867–1936). **Hist Sci Med** 1980;14(1):43–50
Sicard A: L'aide des médecins de la Salpêtrière à la première expédition polaire de Jean-Baptiste Charcot. **Hist Sci Med** 1983;17(2):129–33

**Charcot, Jean-Martin, 1825–1893**
Capildeo R: Charcot in the 80s. In Rose FC, Bynum WF, ed: Historical aspects of the neurosciences. New York, Raven, 1982. p. 383–96.
Chertok L: Hypnosis and suggestion in a century of psychotherapy: an epistemological assessment. **J Am Acad Psychoanal** 1984 Apr;12(2):211–32
Chertok L: On the centenary of Charcot: hysteria, suggestibility and hypnosis. **Br J Med Psychol** 1984 Jun;57(Pt 2):111–20
Didi-Huberman G: Invention de l'hystérie: Charcot et l'iconographie photographique de la Salpêtrière. Paris, Macula, 1982. 303 p.
Ekbom K: Mannen bakom syndromen: Jean-Martin Charcot. Under hans inspirerande ledning skapades den klassiska franska neurologin. **Lakartidningen** 1984 Jun 6;81(23):2363–4
Huard P: La gérontologie de J. M. Charcot. **Rev Neurol (Paris)** 1982;138(12):989–95
Leden I: Doubts about Sandro Botticelli's depiction of juvenile rheumatoid arthritis. **Arthritis Rheum** 1984 Oct;27(10):1197–8
Ryckewaert A, Naveau B: Principaux apports de Charcot et de Pierre Marie à la pathologie ostéo–articulaire. **Rev Rhum Mal Osteoartic** 1984 Jul–Sep;51(7–8):405–13
Signoret JL: La création de la chaire de Charcot. **Rev Neurol (Paris)** 1982;138(12):887–92
Telson HW: Une leçon du Docteur Charcot à la Salpêtrière. Lithograph by Eugene Pirodon after a painting (1887) by André Brouillet. **J Hist Med Allied Sci** 1980 Jan;35(1):58

**Chargaff, Erwin, 1905–**
Abir-Am P: From biochemistry to molecular biology: DNA and the acculturated journey of the critic of science Erwin Chargaff. **Hist Philos Life Sci** 1980;2(1):3–60

**Charles I, King of England, 1600–1649**
Carlton C: Towards a psychobiography of Charles I. **J Psychohist** 1984 Spring;11(4):513–31

**Charles II, King of Great Britain, 1630–1685**
Fraser A: King Charles II, 'The Father of His People'. In Passmore R, ed: Proceedings of the Royal College of Physicians of Edinburgh Tercentenary Congress, 1981. Edinburgh, Royal College of Physicians of Edinburgh, 1982. p. 23–43.
Madsen V: Medicine in history. Dryden on the doctors and the death of Charles II. **J Dermatol Surg Oncol** 1981 May;7(5):366–9

**Charles, Jacques Alexandre César, 1746–1823**
Shampo MA, Kyle RA: Jacques–Alexandre–César Charles. **JAMA** 1984 May 18;251(19):2547

**Charles VI, King of France, 1368–1422**
Lesný I: Sílenství francouzského krále Karla VI. **Cas Lek Cesk** 1982 May 14;121(19):597–600

**Charlotte Augusta, of Wales, Consort of Prince Leopold of Saxe-Coburg-Saalfeld, 1796–1817**
Croft C: The confinement and death of Princess Charlotte. **St Thomas Hosp Gaz** 1981;79:46–9

**Charlotte, Consort of Maximilian, Emperor of Mexico, 1840–1927**
Müller C: Historische Reminiszenz: die schizophrene Psychose der Kaiserin von Mexiko. **Fortschr Neurol Psychiatr** 1979 Oct;47(10):550–2

**Charnley, John, 1911–1982**
Husberg K, Räf L: John Charnley efter 30 års arbete med höftledskirurgi: 'intuition och slump hjälpte fram genombrotten men protesens livslängd måste förbättras'. **Lakartidningen** 1982 Jun 9;79(23):2301–3
Nisbet NW, Woodruff M: John Charnley: 29 August 1911–5 August 1982. **Biogr Mem Fellows R Soc** 1984;30:119–37
Poal–Manresa J: Comentarios sobre la evolución de la prótesis de cadera: a propósito de la muerte de Sir John Charnley. **Med Clin (Barc)** 1983 May 7;80(16):715–6

**Charters, Werrett Wallace, Sr., 1875–1952**
Russell JC: Werrett Wallace Charters, Sr. (1875–1952): his life, career and influence upon pharmaceutical education. Ph.D. Diss., Loyola University. Chicago, 1981. vii, 259 leaves.

**Charukovskiĭ, Prokhor Alekseevich, 1790–1842**
Shabunin AV: Prokhor Charukovskiĭ i ego 'Opyt sistemy prakticheskoĭ meditsiny' (k 150–letiiu so dnia vykhoda pervoĭ chasti truda). **Klin Med (Mosk)** 1983 Nov;61(11):145–7

**Charvet, A. P., fl. 1826**
Siegel RK, Hirschman AE: Charvet and the first psychopharmacological studies on opium: a historical note and translation. **J Psychoactive Drugs** 1983 Oct–Dec;15(4):323–9

**Chase, Alvin Wood, 1817–1885**
100 years ago: household medicine and treatment: the gospel according to Dr. Chase: **One One** 1981 May–Jun;3(3):4–5

**Chastenet, Armand-Marie, Marquis de Puségur, fl. 1784**
Conn JH: Nature of magnetic treatment.

J Am Soc Psychosom Dent Med 1982;29(2):44–53

**Chaucer, Geoffrey, 1344–1400**
Benson CD: The astrological medicine of Chaucer's physician and Nicholas of Lynn's Kalendarium. **Am Notes Queries** 1984 Jan–Feb;22(5–6):62–6
Mandel SL: Chaucer's vivid medical word pictures (reflections of yore afflictions). **Int J Dermatol** 1983 Jun;22(5):329–31
Rowland B: Chaucer's idea of the pardoner. **Chaucer Rev** 1979–80;14(2):138–54

**Chaudillon, Antoine, 1643–1707**
Biron H: Antoine Chaudillon. In Dictionary of Canadian biography, 1701 to 1740. Volume 2, 1969. p. 140–1.

**Chauffard, Anatole Marie Emile, 1855–1932**
Binet JL: Histoire de la sphèrocytose congénitale. **Nouv Rev Fr Hematol** 1981 Sep;23(3):177–84

**Chauveau, Jean Baptiste Auguste, 1827–1917**
Espinosa RE, Vlietstra RE, Mann RJ: J. B. A. Chauveau, E. J. Marey, and their resolution of the apex beat controversy through intracardiac pressure recordings. **Mayo Clin Proc** 1983 Mar;58(3):197–202

**Chávez, Ignacio, 1897–1979**
Somolinos-Palencia J, Martínez-Cortés F, Sepúlveda B, et al: Etapas de la educación médica en México. **Gac Med Mex** 1984 Jun;120(6):213–28
Véjar-Lacave C: El maestro Ignacio Chávez, la medicina y los problemas educacionales. **Gac Med Mex** 1980 Jan;116(1):43–6
40 aniversario del Institute Nacional de Cardiología de México: **Arch Inst Cardiol Mex** 1984 Jul–Aug;54(4):411–26

**Chekhov, Anton Pavlovich, 1860–1904**
Bugyi B: Csehov, az orvos. **Orv Hetil** 1980 Nov 16;121(46):2834–7
Guyotjeannin C: Les médicaments de Tchékhov. **Monit Pharm** 1983;37(1557):1248–50
Ionov IuV: A. P. Chekhov i meditsina. **Feldsher Akush** 1980;45(6):51–4
Melzer R: Chekhov's doctors. **Adler Mus Bull** 1981 Oct;7(3):15–9
Szállási A: Csehov és Maugham a Nyugat kedvenc írói. **Orv Hetil** 1980 Jan 27;121(4):226–9

**Chemodanov, Mikhail Mikhailovich, 1856–1908**
Viduta VK: Vrach, revoliutsioner, uchenyĭ M. M. Chemodanov. **Sov Zdravookhr** 1983;(4):58–60

**Cherkinskiĭ, Samuil Naumovich**
Akulov KI, Shlepnina TG: Nauchnoe obosnovanie standartizatsii kachestva pit'evoĭ vody v trudakh prof. S. N. Cherkinskogo. **Gig Sanit** 1982 Aug;(8):50–3

**Chernogubov, A., fl. 1892**
Denko CW: Chernogubov's syndrome: a translation of the first modern case report of the Ehlers-Danlos syndrome. **J Rheumatol** 1978 Fall;5(3):347–52

**Chernomordik, Solomon Isaevich, 1880–1938**
Idel'chik KhI: Vrachi-bol'sheviki S. I. Mitskevich i S. I. Chernomordik u istokov Tsentral'nogo muzeia revoliutsii SSSR (k 60-letiiu muzeia). **Sov Zdravookhr** 1984;(9):56–9

**Chernorutskiĭ, Mikhail Vasil'evich, 1884–1957**
Uspenskaia EP: Mikhail Vasil'evich Chernorutskiĭ (k 100-letiiu so dnia rozhdeniia). **Ter Arkh** 1984;56(7):151–3

**Cheshire, Johnathan Singleton, 1830–1891**
Peyton R: A Webster parish country doctor's record. **North La Hist Assoc J** 1979;10(3):103–10

**Chesterton, Gilbert Keith, 1874–1936**
Schall JV: The rarest of all revolutions: G. K. Chesterton on the relation of human life to Christian doctrine. **Am Benedictine Rev** 1981;32(4):304–27

**Chetyrkin, Roman Sergeevich, 1797–1865**
Shabunin AV: K 150-letiiu izdaniia truda R. S. Chetyrkina 'Opyt voenno-meditsinskoĭ politsii ili pravila k sokhraneniiu zdorov'ia russkikh soldat v sukhoputnoĭ sluzhbe'. **Gig Sanit** 1984 Jun;(6):35–6

**Chevreul, Michel Eugène, 1786–1889**
Kalugai I: Michel-Eugène Chevreul, 1786–1889. **Koroth** 1980 Jun;7(11–12):796–802
Schmitt R: Henri Loewel, chimiste alsacien, élève, collaborateur et ami du savant Angevin Michel-Eugène Chevreul. In: Congrès National des Sociétés Savantes, 93e, Tours, 1968. Comptes Rendus. Paris, 1971. Section des Sciences, Tome II. p. 175–88.

**Chichagov, Leonid Mikhailovich, 1853–1938**
Kvitnitskiĭ-Ryzhov IuN: Iz istorii populiarizatsii meditsinskikh znaniĭ v Rosii. L.M. Chichagov i ego 'Meditsinskie besedy'. **Sov Zdravookhr** 1984;(8):66–70

**Chidley, William, 1860–1916**
Edwards GA, Hall W: The case of William Chidley: a study in psychiatry, morality and lunacy law. **Aust NZ J Psychiatry** 1980 Jun;14(2):133–9
Finnane M: The popular defence of Chidley. **Labour Hist** 1981;41:57–73

**Childs, Richard Spencer, 1882–1978**
Hirschhorn B: Richard Spencer Childs (1882–1978). His role in modernization of medicolegal investigation in America. **Am J Forensic Med Pathol** 1983 Sep;4(3):245–54

**Chilov, Konstantin, 1898–1955**
Petkova M: Naukometrichna kharakteristika na publikuvanoto nauchno tvorchestvo na professor Konstantin Chilov. **Vutr Boles** 1984;23(4):102–8

**Chirac, Pierre, 1650–1732**
Dulieu L: Pierre Chirac et les maladies des équipages des vaisseaux. **Rev Hist Sci (Paris)** 1984 Jan;37(1):65–70

**Chirino, Alonso, d. 1430?**
Gracia D: Chirino en el Retablo de las Maravillas. **Asclepio** 1978–79;30–31:265–76

**Chisolm, Julian John, 1830–1903**
Leland TM: Anesthesiology in the Civil War (Dr. Julian John Chisolm). **J SC Med Assoc** 1981 Nov;77(11):524

**Chivers, Thomas Holley, 1809–1858**
Tucker EL: A new letter by Thomas Holley Chivers. **Ga Hist Q** 1971;55(4):582–8

**Chodounský, Karel, 1843–**
Novák J: Stočtyřicet let od narození prof. MUDr. Karla Chodounského. **Cas Lek Cesk** 1983 May 13;122(19):600–1

**Chodźko, Witold, 1875–1954**
Maćkowiak Z: Uwagi o życiu i działalności Witolda Chodźki (1875–1954). **Przegl Lek** 1980;37(4):437–40

**Cholewa, Leon**
Kieć E, et al: Prof. Dr. Leon Cholewa. **Przegl Lek** 1984;41(7):465–76

**Chomakov, Stoian, 1819–1893**
Zaprianov NI, Kazandzhiev NK: D-r Stoian Chomakov. Sofiia, Meditsina i fizkultura, 1979.

**Chopin, Frédéric Francois, 1810–1849**
Böhme G: Medizinische Porträts berühmter Komponisten: Wolfgang Amadeus Mozart, Ludwig van Beethoven, Carl Maria von Weber, Frédéric Chopin, Peter Iljitsch Tschaikowski, Béla Bartók. 2. verbesserte und erweiterte Auflage. Stuttgart, New York, Gustav Fischer Verlag, 1981. xi, 199 p.
Godlewski G: Chopin génie asexué. **Sem Hop Paris** 1979 Dec 18–25;55(43–44):2051–63
Pačes V: Uvahy o nemoci Fryderyka Chopina. **Vnitr Lek** 1980 Oct;26(10):1027–31
Sielużycki C: Choroby Fryderyka Chopina, ich patogeneza i leczenie. **Arch Hist Med (Warsz)** 1981;44(3/4):237–56

**Chopra, Ram Nath, 1882–**
Ramalingaswami V, Satyavati GV: Sir Ram Nath Chopra. **Indian J Med Res** 1982 Dec;76 Suppl:V–VI

**Chowning, William M.**
Ormsbee RA: A review: 'Studies in Pyroplasmosis hominis ('spotted fever' or 'tick fever' of the Rocky Mountains)' by Louis B. Wilson and William M. Chowning, published in The Journal of Infectious Diseases 1:31–57, 1904. **Rev Infect Dis** 1979 May–Jun;1(3):559–62

**Christie, Agatha, 1891?–1976**
Bardell EB: Dame Agatha's dispensary. **Pharm Hist** 1984;26(1):13–9

**Christoffel, Hans, 1888–1959**
Kaiser W: Leben und Werk des Basler Psychiaters und Psychoanalytikers Hans Christoffel (1888–1959. Zürich, Juris Druck, 1982. 267 p. (Zürcher Medizingeschichtliche Abhandlungen, Neue Reihe, Nr. 152.)

**Christophe, Pierre, 1758–1826**
Brullard P: Pierre Christophe (1758–1826), médecin, soldat et humaniste. In: Congrès National des Sociétés Savantes, 103e, Nancy, 1978. Comptes Rendus. Paris, 1978. Section des Sciences, Fasc. V. p. 43–53.

**Chu, Judy**
Paung PP: [The memoirs of Judy Chu] (Chi). **Hu Li Tsa Chih** 1980 Jul;27(3):63–71

**Chunyu, Yi, ca. 205–ca. 134 B.C.**
He A: [Exploration on the date of birth and death of Chunyu Yi] (Chi). **Chung Hua I Shih Tsa Chih** 1984;14(2):80–4
Lin P: [Textual research on the date of birth and death of Chunyu Yi and his appointment] (Chi). **Chung Hua I Shih Tsa Chih** 1984;14(2):78–9

**Churchill, Randolph, 1849–1895**
Greenblatt RB: The humiliating demise of Lord Randolph Churchill, 1849–1895. **Postgrad Med** 1984 Jan;75(1):129–31, 134

**Cibat, Antonio, 1770–1812**
Riera J: Antonio Cibat y la catedra de fisica experimental de Barcelona (un proyecto de 1807). **Asclepio** 1980;32:383–8

**Cicero, Marcus Tullius**
Richardson WF: Medicine: the art of guessing? **NZ Med J** 1984 Jul 11;97(759):453–5

**Cirillo, Domenico, 1739–1799**
Marbach JU: Domenico Cirillo; ein Lebenslauf, 1739–1799. **Gesnerus** 1980;37(3/4):257–69

**Ciucă, Mihai, 1883–1969**
Alexa I: La 100 ani de la naşterea doctorului Mihai Ciucă (1883–1983).

**Rev Med Chir Soc Med Nat Iasi** 1983 Oct-Dec;87(4):731-6
Franche M: Omagiu Profesorului Mihai Ciucă, la 100 ani de la naştere. Profesorul Mihai Ciucă şi spitalul clinic de boli contagioase 'izolarea' Iaşi. **Rev Med Chir Soc Med Nat Iasi** 1983 Oct-Dec;87(4):726-8
Panaitescu D, Mihalcu F, Neguţ M: Activitatea stiinţifică a prof. Mihai Ciucă. **Rev Iq [Bacteriol]** 1984 Jan-Mar;29(1):80-8
Sefer M, Sefer M: [10 years after the death of Professor Mihai Ciucă (18 July 1883 - 20 Feb. 1969). Mihai Ciucă and the study of bacteriophage, recorded in his working notebooks.] (Rum) **Rev Ig [Bacteriol]** 1979;24:123-6
Ungureanu EM: Contribuţia Academicianului Mihai Ciucă pe plan naţional şi internaţional în domeniul combaterii malariei. **Rev Med Chir Soc Med Nat Iasi** 1983 Oct-Dec;87(4):729-30

**Clagett, Horatio C., 1793-1858**
Mason EM: Some insights into the life of a country doctor. **Md State Med J** 1981 Nov;30(11):20-1

**Clapers, Bernat dez, d. 1311**
Rubio Vela A: Una fundación burguesa en la Valencia medieval: El Hospital de En Clapers (1311). **Dynamis** 1981;1:18-49

**Clark, Duncan, ca. 1759-1808**
Kernaghan LK: Duncan Clark. In Dictionary of Canadian biography, 1801 to 1820. Volume 5, 1983. p. 187-8.

**Clark, Kenneth Bancroft, 1914-**
Distinguished contribution to psychology in the public interest.: **Am Psychol** 1979 Jan;34(1):65-8

**Clark, William Mansfield, 1884-1964**
Edsall JT: William Mansfield Clark papers. **Surv Sources Newsl** 1978 Mar;7:2-5
Edsall JT: The William Mansfield Clark papers: a second installment. **Surv Sources Newsl** 1981;10:1

**Clarke, Hans Thacher, 1887-1972**
Miller M: Hans Thacher Clarke Papers. **Surv Sources Newsl** 1977 May;5:12-3

**Clayton, Robert, 1629-1707**
Cockett FB: The statue of Sir Robert Clayton. **St Thomas Hosp Gaz** 1981;79:52-5

**Cleave, Thomas Latimer, 1906-**
Heaton KW: T. L. Cleave and the fibre story. **J R Nav Med Serv** 1980;66(1):5-10

**Clemenceau, Georges, 1841-1929**
Godlewski G: Le Docteur Clemenceau. **Sem Hop Paris** 1981 Dec 18-25;57(47-48):2057-71
Royer J, Haut J, Amalric P: L'opération de la cataracte de Claude Monet, correspondence inédite du peintre et de G.-Clemenceau au docteur Coutela. **Hist Sci Med** 1984;18(2):109-27

**Clemens, Samuel Langhorne, 1835-1910**
Francke OC: Tandbehandling för 100 år sedan och Mark Twain som patient. **Nord Medicinhist Arsb** 1984;:137-40
Morgan WG: Mark Twain: behaviorist. **J Behav Ther Exp Psychiatry** 1984 Jun;15(2):99
Reed JF: Samuel Clemens and family: the Hartfold connection and Hartford physicians. **Am J Surg** 1981 Apr;141(4):401-10

**Cleveland, Grover, 1837-1908**
Barber D: Secret operation on US president. **Probe (Lond)** 1982 May;23(11):415-6
Brooks JJ, Enterline HT, Aponte GE: The final diagnosis of President Cleveland's lesion. **Trans Stud Coll Physicians Phila** 1980 Mar;(2 no 1):1-25
Cross W, Moses J: 'My God, sir, I think the president is doomed!' [Grover Cleveland's cancer surgery] **Am Hist Illus** 1982 Nov;17:40-5

**Cleyer, Andreas, 1634-1697 or 8**
Kraft ES: Andreas Cleyer. In Balde JH, Schmiking W, ed: Festschrift zum 86. Deutschen Arztetag in Kassel. Kassel, Arztevereins, 1983. p.40.

**Clift, Caroline Amelia, 1801-1873**
Austin F, Jones B: The Clifts and the arts. **Ann R Coll Surg Engl** 1984 Jan;66(1):63-70

**Clift, William Home, 1803-1832**
Austin F: The Letters of William Home Clift, 1803-1832. Dorset, Meldon House, 1983. ix, 115 p.
Austin F, Jones B: The Clifts and the arts. **Ann R Coll Surg Engl** 1984 Jan;66(1):63-70

**Clift, William, 1775-1849**
Austin F, Jones B: William Home Clift: the first assistant Conservator of the Hunterian Museum. **Ann R Coll Surg Engl** 1980 Jul;62(4):299-303
Austin F, Jones B: The Clifts and the arts. **Ann R Coll Surg Engl** 1984 Jan;66(1):63-70

**Clinch, John, 1749-1819**
Jones F: John Clinch. In Dictionary of Canadian biography, 1801 to 1820. Volume 5, 1983. p. 189-190.

**Close, Harold George, 1898-**
Close HG: A genetic Odyssey. **S Afr Med J** 1982 Jun 26;61(26):1010-2

**Clot, Antoine-Barthélemy, 1793-1868**
Ghoneim M: Antoine-Barthelemy Clot créateur de l'école de médecine. **Cah Hist** 1969;11:125-36

**Clough, Arthur Hugh, 1819-1861**
Oliver H: The Shore Smith family library: Arthur Hugh Clough and Florence Nightingale. **Book Collect** 1979;28:521-9

**Clowes, George Henry Alexander, 1877-1958**
Clowes GH: George Henry Alexander Clowes, PhD, DSc, LLD (1877-1958): a man of science for all seasons. **J Surg Oncol** 1981;18(2):197-217

**Clubbe, Charles, 1854-1932**
Jones PG: 'A man and his hospital'. **Aust Paediatr J** 1981 Mar;17(1):5-14

**Clyman, Martin J., 1914-1979**
Cohen MR: A tribute to Martin J. Clyman, M.D., 1914-1979. **J Reprod Med** 1983 Apr;28(4):233-4
Kase NG: Gynecologic endocrinology and infertility. A tribute to Martin J. Clyman, M.D. **J Reprod Med** 1983 Apr;28(4):231-2

**Cmunt, Eduard, 1878-**
Skodáček P: Prof. MUDr Eduard Cmunt, prvý slovanský balneológ v Piešt'anoch. **Fysiatr Reumatol Vestn** 1984 Feb;62(1):44-6

**Coates, Samuel, 1748-1830**
Tomes N: The domesticated madman: changing concepts of insanity at the Pennsylvania Hospital, 1780-1830. **Pa Mag Hist Biogr** 1982;106(2):271-86

**Cobb, David, 1748-1830**
Simpson HN: Doctors afield: David Cobb, M.D. **N Engl J Med** 1980 Dec 25;303(26):1517-9

**Cobb, William Montague, 1904-**
Spady JG: Dr. W. Montague Cobb: anatomist, physician, physical anthropologist, editor emeritus of the Journal of the National Medical Association, and first black president of NAACP. **J Natl Med Assoc** 1984 Jul;76(7):739-44

**Cobbe, Frances Power, 1822-1904**
Bauer C, Ritt L: 'The little health of ladies.' An anatomy of female invalidism in the nineteenth century. **J Am Med Wom Assoc** 1981 Oct;36(10):300-6

**Cobbett, William, 1763-1835**
Davies NE, Davies GH, Sanders ED: William Cobbett, Benjamin Rush, and the death of General Washington. **JAMA** 1983 Feb 18;249(7):912-5

**Coca, Arthur F., 1875-1959**
Chase MW: Irreverent recollections from Cooke and Coca, 1928-1978. **J Allergy Clin Immunol** 1979 Nov;64(5):306-20

**Codman, Ernest Amory, 1869-1940**
Reverby S: Stealing the golden eggs: Ernest Amory Codman and the science and management of medicine. **Bull Hist Med** 1981 Summer;55(2):156-71

**Codorníu y Ferreras, Manuel**
Parrilla Hermida M: La direccion de Sanidad Militar---su primer director. **Asclepio** 1980;32:295-302

**Coeuershof, Christiaen, 1596-1659**
Slenders J: De Anatomische les van Dr. Zacheus de Jager (1640). **Tijdschr Geschied Geneeskd** 1981;4(4):159-67

**Cogan, Thomas, 1545?-1607**
Bowman IA: Thomas Cogan on studying. **Bookman** 1980 Feb;7(2):5-10

**Cogswell, Henry D., 1820-**
Foley GP: A treasury of dentistry. Henry Cogswell. **J Am Coll Dent** 1984 Summer;51(2):20-1

**Cohen, Abraham, of Zante, 1678-1722**
Benayahu M: Rabbi Abraham Hacohen of Zante and the Padua group of doctor-poets. **Hasifrut** 1978;26:108-40

**Cohn, Alfred Einstein, 1879-1957**
Cranefield PF: Alfred Einstein Cohn. In Dictionary of American Biography, Suppl. 6, 1956-1960. p. 117-18, 1980.
Krikler DM: Wolff-Parkinson-White syndrome: long follow up and an Anglo-American historical note. **J Am Coll Cardiol** 1983 Dec;2(6):1216-8

**Cohn, Ferdinand Julius, 1828-1898**
Hoppe B: Die Biologie der Mikroorganismen von F. J. Cohn (1828-1898). **Sudhoffs Arch** 1983;67(2):158-89

**Cohn, Tobias, 1652-1729**
Allan N: Illustrations from the Wellcome Institute Library: a Jewish physician in the seventeenth century. **Med Hist** 1984 Jul;28(3):324-8

**Coindet, Jean-François, 1774-1834**
Rentchnick P: Iode et goitre. A propos du 150e anniversaire de la mort du Dr Jean-François Coindet (12 juillet 1774-11 février 1834). **Med Hyg (Geneve)** 1984 Feb 15;42(1551):465-6, 469-70, 472-4, 477-8

**Colden, Cadwallader, 1688-1776**
Swinton WE: Cadwallader Colden: physician, historian and government official. **Can Med Assoc J** 1981 Mar 15;124(6):805-9

**Cole, Warren Henry, 1899–**
Cole WH: The development of cholecystography. **J Thorac Cardiovasc Surg** 1984 Nov;88(5 Pt 2):827–33

**Colebrook, Leonard, 1883–1967**
Abraham EP: Leonard Colebrook. In Dictionary of national biography, 1961–1970. Suppl. 8, 1981. p. 230–2.
Lowbury EJ: Leonard Colebrook (1883–1967). **Br Med J [Clin Res]** 1983 Dec 24–31;287(6409):1981–3

**Coleridge, Samuel Taylor, 1772–1834**
Corrigan TJ: Biographia Literaria and the language of science. **J Hist Ideas** 1980 Jul–Sep;41(3):399–419
Levere TH: Poetry realized in nature. Samuel Taylor Coleridge and early nineteenth-century science. Cambridge, Cambridge University Press, 1981. xiii, 271 p.

**Coles, Robert Martin, 1929–**
Schnell RL: Contributions to psychohistory: IV. Individual experience in historiography and psychoanalysis: significance of Erik Erikson and Robert Coles. **Psychol Rep** 1980 Apr;46(2):591–612

**Colledge, Thomas Richardson, 1796–1879**
Taylor S: Thomas Richardson Colledge FRCS, 1796–1879. **Ann R Coll Surg Engl** 1982 Jul;64(4):266–7

**Colles, Abraham, 1773–1843**
Strmeň J: Abraham Colles (1773–1843) a ním v roku 1814 popísaná zlomenina radia. **Rozhl Chir** 1984 Oct;63(10):701–4
Zarzycki D, Zarzycka M: Abraham Colles życie i twórczość. **Chir Narzadow Ruchu Ortop Pol** 1980;45(1):103–4

**Collingwood, Edward Foyle, 1900–1970**
Cartwright ML: Sir Edward Foyle Collingwood. In Dictionary of national biography, 1961–1970. Suppl. 8, 1981. p. 232–4.

**Collins, Wilkie, 1824–1889**
Siegel S: Wilkie Collins: Victorian novelist as psychopharmacologist. **J Hist Med Allied Sci** 1983 Apr;38(2):161–75

**Collins, William, 1721–1759**
Wendorf R: 'Poor Collins' reconsidered. **Huntington Libr Q** 1979;42(2):91–116

**Collip, James Bertram, 1892–1965**
Barr ML: James Bertram Collip (1892–1965): a Canadian pioneer in endocrinology. In: Congrès international d'histoire de la médecine, XXVe, Québec, 1976. Actes. Québec, 1977. p. 469–76.
Bliss M, ed: Banting's, Best's, and Collip's accounts of the discovery of insulin. **Bull Hist Med** 1982;56(4):554–68

**Collomb, Henri, 1913–1979**
Zempléni A: Henri Collomb (1913–1979) et l'équipe de Fann. **Soc Sci Med [Med Anthropol]** 1980 May;14(2):85–90

**Colombat, Emile, 1839–1891**
Michel J: Notice historique sur la création de l'orthophonie et de la phonologie par M. Colombat de l'Isère (1828). **J Fr Otorhinolaryngol** 1981 May;30(5):281–3

**Colombo, Realdo, ca. 1515–1559**
Donáth T: Egy évforduló ürügyén. **Orv Hetil** 1984 Sep 30;125(40):2441–4

**Colonna Egidio, 1247?–1316**
Houtzager HL: Giles of Rome. **Eur J Obstet Gynecol Reprod Biol** 1981 Aug;12(2):127–9

**Colston, Joseph, fl. 1664**
Alsop JD: A footnote on the circulation of the blood: Joseph Colston and Harvey's discovery in 1642. **J Hist Med Allied Sci** 1981 Jul;36(3):331–4

**Columbus, Christopher, 1446–1506**
Alegría C: Medicos que estimularon a Cristobal Colón en su actividad precursora al descubrimiento de America. **Rev Soc Venez Hist Med** 1969–71;17–19(31–33):199–203
Allison DJ: Christopher Columbus: first case of Reiter's disease in the Old World? **Lancet** 1980 Dec 13;2(8207):1309
Columbus: was it Reiter's disease?: **Lancet** 1981 Jan 10;1(8211):94–5
Shizusawa K: [Columbus as the 1st known patient with Reiter's disease?] (Jpn). **Kango** 1981 Apr;33(4):83

**Coman, Katharine, 1857–1915**
Schwarz J: Yellow clover: Katharine Lee Bates and Katharine Coman. **Frontiers** 1979;4(1):59–67

**Combes, Justin Louis Emile, 1835–1921**
Godlewski G: Le docteur Combes, pourfendeur de l'Eglise. **Sem Hop Paris** 1982 Dec 23;58(47):2802–13

**Combiescu, Dumitru, 1887–1961**
Sefer M, Sefer M: Evocare: Dumitru Combiescu (6 ianuarie 1887 25 noiembrie 1961)] (Rom). **Rev Ig [Bacteriol]** 1981 Jul–Sep;26(3):199–204

**Comenge y Ferrer, Luis, 1854–1916**
Marí Balcells VJ: Tres historiadores de la medicina española: Villalba, Hernandez Morejon y Comenge, e influencia del primero en la obra de los otros dos. In: Sociedad Española de Historia de la Medicina. V Congreso Nacional. Madrid, 1977. **Asclepio** 1977;29:167–76

**Compain, Pierre-Joseph, 1740–1806**
Janson G: Pierre-Joseph Compain. In Dictionary of Canadian biography, 1801 to 1820. Volume 5, 1983. p. 201–202.

**Compton, Arthur Holly, 1892–**
Del Regato JA: The tracks of the Compton effect. **Med Phys** 1981 Nov–Dec;8(6):761–5

**Comstock, Oliver E.**
Hall D: Ointment of love: Oliver E. Comstock and Tuscon's [sic] tent city. **J Ariz Hist** 19(2):111–30, 1978

**Comte, Auguste, 1798–1857**
Hawkins MJ: Reason and sense perception in Comte's theory of mind. **Hist Eur Ideas** 1984;5:149–63
Poirier JL: La réorganisation des études médicales selon Auguste Comte. In Poirier J, Poirier JL, ed: Médecine et philosophie à la fin du XIXe siècle. Paris, Université de Paris XII - Val de Marne, [1980?]. p. 47–59.
Stanguennec A: Le scalpel contre le microscope: Auguste Comte et la théorie cellulaire. **Sci Tech Perspect** 1981–82;1:11.1–.12

**Condillac, Etienne Bonnôt de, 1714–1780**
Rauch A: Le souci du corps chez Condillac. **Stadion** 1977;3(1):60–89
Robinson DN, ed: Significant contributions to the history of psychology 1750–1920. Series A. Orientations. Volume I: E. Condillac, T. Brown. Washington, D. C., University Publications of America, 1977. Various pagings.
Stratone M: Metoda analizei la E.B. Condillac. **Rev Med Chir Soc Med Nat Iasi** 1979 Jan–Mar;83(1):163–6

**Condorcet, Marie Jean Antoine Nicolas de Coritat, 1743–1794**
Tzonis A: Un 'Mémoire sur les hôpitaux' de Condorcet. **Dix-Huit Siecle** 1977;9:109–14

**Conner, Eugene Hayward, 1921–**
Young DM: Eugene H. Conner, M.D., KMA historian. **J Ky Med Assoc** 1982 Apr;80(4):224–6

**Connor, Bernard, 1666–1698**
Dalitz RH, Stone GC: Doctor Bernard Connor: physician to King Jan III Sobieski and author of the History of Poland (1698). **Oxf Slav Pap** 1981;14:14–35

**Conolly, John, 1794–1866**
Scull A: A brilliant career? John Conolly and Victorian psychiatry. **Victorian Stud** 1984;27:203–35

**Conscience, Hendrik, 1812–1883**
Dieckhöfer K: Der flämische Schriftsteller Hendrik Conscience (1812–1883) und die psychisch Kranken von Geel. **Z Psychosom Med Psychoanal** 1984;30(2):179–90

**Conseil, Ernest Alfred, 1879–**
Gaumer B: Contribution de Ernest Conseil à la naissance de l'épidémiologie en Tunisie. **Arch Inst Pasteur Tunis** 1983 Mar–Sep;60(1–2):49–64

**Consolazio, Carlo Frank, 1913–1976**
Johnson RE: Carlo Frank Consolazio: March 9, 1913--December 23, 1976. **Prog Food Nutr Sci** 1983;7(1–2):1–10

**Constantin, Paul**
Niaussat P, Huard P: Problèmes acoustiques communs à la médecine, à la marine et aux télécommunications, étudiés par le Docteur Paul Constantin. In: Congrès National des Sociétés Savantes, 106e, Perpignan, 1981. Comptes Rendus. Paris, Bibliothèque Nationale, 1982. Fasc. IV. p. 81–9.

**Constantini Family**
Giebel A: Drei Generationen Constantini als Hofapotheker in Rotenburg a. d. Fulda. **Hess Familienkd** 1977;13:445–8

**Conta, Vasile, 1845–1882**
Stratone N: Spaţiul si timpul in concepţia lui Vasile Conta (1845–1882). **Rev Med Chir Soc Med Nat Iasi** 1982 Jul–Sep;86(3):513–5

**Cook, Albert Ruskin, 1870–1951**
Foster WD: The Church Missionary Society and modern medicine in Uganda. The life of Sir Albert Cook, K.C.M.G., 1870–1951. Newhaven, Sussex, [The author], 1978. 234 p.
Ofcansky TP: The life and times of Sir Albert Ruskin Cook. **J Hist Med Allied Sci** 1982 Apr;37(2):225–8

**Cook, James, 1728–1779**
Lloyd C: Cook and scurvy. **Mar Mirror** 1979 Feb;65:23–8
Tilghman RC: Captain James Cook (1728–1779). **Trans Am Clin Climatol Assoc** 1980;92:1–15

**Cooke, Elisha, Jr., 1678–1737**
Kaiser LM: Feriis Festisque Diebus: the salutatory oration of Elisha Cooke, Jr., 7 July 1697. **Harv Libr Bull** 1980 Oct;28(4):380–90

**Cooke, Robert Anderson, 1880–1960**
Chase MW: Irreverent recollections from Cooke and Coca, 1928–1978. **J Allergy Clin Immunol** 1979 Nov;64(5):306–20
Hast A: Robert Anderson Cooke. In Dictionary of American Biography, Suppl. 6, 1956–1960. p. 123–4, 1980.

**Cookworthy, William, 1705–1780**
Selleck AD: William Cookworthy, an 18th century polymath. **Pharm Hist (London)** 1979 Dec;9(3):8–12

**Cooper, Astley Paston, 1768–1841**
McGovern FH: Sir Astley Cooper and his otological papers. **Ann Otol Rhinol Laryngol** 1984 Nov–Dec;93(6 Pt 1):531–3
Ravitch MM: Sir Astley Paston Cooper. **Bull Am Coll Surg** 1977 Feb;62(2):17–20
Wilson TG: Historical vignette. Sir Astley Cooper. **Am J Otol** 1984 Jul;5(5):411–4

**Cooper, Thomas Henry, 1813–1881**
Allen DE: The plagiarisms of Thomas Henry Cooper. **J Soc Bibliogr Nat Hist** 1979 Nov;9(3):275–9

**Cooper, Thomas, 1759–1839**
Cohen SS: Two refugee chemists in the United States, 1794: how we see them. **Proc Am Philos Soc** 1982 Aug;126(4):301–15

**Cope, Freeman Widener, 1930–1982**
Damadian R: In memoriam--Freeman Widener Cope--1930–1982. **Physiol Chem Phys** 1982;14(5):411–4

**Copernicus, Nicolaus, 1473–1543**
Bart C: L'astronome Nicolas Copernic a-t-il été médecin? In: Congrès international d'histoire de la médecine, XXVe, Québec, 1976. Actes. Québec, 1977. p. 477–86.
Miller JM: Copernicus, medicine, and the heliocentric concept. **South Med J** 1983 Sep;76(9):1167–8
Skulimowski M: Mikołaj Kopernik, wybitny predstawiciel medycyny XVI wieku w Polsce. Kraków, Akademia Medyczna, 1978. 84 p.

**Copley, Alfred Lewin, 1910–**
A. L. Copley: curriculum vitae and publications: **Biorheology** 1981;18(3–6):703--23
Perspectives in biorheology: Festschrift for A. L. Copley. **Biorheology** 1981;18(3–6):305–729

**Corachán, Juan Bautista, 1661–1741**
Navarro Brotóns V: Juan Bautista Corachán y la enseñanza universitaria. In: Estudios de historia de Valencia. Valencia, Universidad, Facultad de Derecho. 1978. p. 279–92.

**Coram, Thomas, 1668–1751**
Jones PG: 'A man and his hospital'. **Aust Paediatr J** 1981 Mar;17(1):5–14
McClure RK: Coram's children, the London Foundling Hospital in the eighteenth century. New Haven, Yale University Press, 1981. xiii, 321 p.

**Cori, Gerty Theresa Radnitz, 1896–1957**
Brown BI: Gerty Theresa Radnitz Cori. In Dictionary of American Biography, Suppl. 6, 1956–1960. p. 126–7, 1980.
Parascandola J: Gerty Theresa Radnitz Cori. In: Notable American women. The modern period. Cambridge, Mass., Belknap-Harvard Univ. Press, 1980. 4:165–7.

**Cornarius, Janus, 1500–1558**
Richter W: Janus Cornarius, ein 'philologischer Mediziner' des 16. Jahrhunderts, und seine Beziehungen zur Rostocker Universität. **Wiss Z Univ Rostock** 1978;27(3):181–9

**Cornelio, Tommaso, 1614–1686**
Trevisani F, Moscheo R: Between ancients and moderns: Tommaso Cornelio's medical teaching and an unpublished comment by him on the Galenic Ars parva. **Nouv Repub Lett** 1983;(2):59–73

**Cornelio, Vittorio, b. ca. 1760**
Sugden KC: Dentists in the rare books. 2. Vittorio Cornelio. **Br Dent J** 1983 Oct 22;155(8):278

**Cornelius, Elias, 1758–1823**
Ackerman EB: The activities of a country doctor in New York State: Dr. Elias Cornelius of Somers, 1794–1803. **Hist Reflect** 1982 Spring–Summer;9:181–93

**Corner, George Washington, 1889–1981**
Bell WJ: George W. Corner (1889–1981): historian. **Bull Hist Med** 1982 Spring;56(1):93–8
Corner GW: The seven ages of a medical scientist, an autobiography. Philadelphia, University of Pennsylvania Press, 1981. xi, 411 p.
Oppenheimer JM, Whitfield JB: Biographical Memoirs: George Washington Corner (1889–1981). **Misc Am Philos Soc** 1982?;9 p.

**Corner, Thomas Cromwell, 1865–1938**
Szczepaniak AS: Thomas Cromwell Corner, Baltimore Portrait artist. **Md State Med J** 1980 Apr;29(4):78–9

**Cornfield, Jerome, 1912–1979**
Ederer F: Jerome Cornfield's contributions to the conduct of clinical trials. **Biometrics** 1982 Mar;38 Suppl:25–32
Greenhouse SW: Jerome Cornfield's contributions to epidemiology. **Biometrics** 1982 Mar;38 Suppl:33–45
Jerome Cornfield's publications: contributions to the literature as they appeared from 1941 through 1980: **Biometrics** 1982 Mar;38 Suppl:47–52
Mantel N: Jerome Cornfield and statistical applications to laboratory research: a personal reminiscence. **Biometrics** 1982 Mar;38 Suppl:17–23
Zelen M: The contributions of Jerome Cornfield to the theory of statistics. **Biometrics** 1982 Mar;38 Suppl:11–5

**Correns, Carl Franz Joseph Erich, 1864–1933**
Saha MS: The Carl Correns papers. **Mendel Newsl** 1981 Nov;21:1–6

**Corrigan, Dominic John, 1802–1880**
Connolly DC, Mann RJ: Dominic J. Corrigan (1802–1880) and his description of the pericardial knock. **Mayo Clin Proc** 1980 Dec;55(12):771–3
Counihan HE: Corrigan on pulmonary disease. **J Ir Coll Physicians Surg** 1980 Jul;10(1):38–40
Doyle JS: Corrigan on fever. **J Ir Coll Physicians Surg** 1980 Jul;10(1):44–5
Fielding J: Corrigan on abdominal disease. **J Ir Coll Physicians Surg** 1980 Jul;10(1):41–3
Holland D: Corrigan and The House of Industry Hospital. **J Ir Coll Physicians Surg** 1980 Jul;10(1):24–6
Horgan J: Corrigan on cardiac disease. **J Ir Coll Physicians Surg** 1980 Jul;10(1):27–31
Mills R, O'Brien E: Corrigan bibliography. **J Ir Coll Physicians Surg** 1980 Jul;10(1):50–4
Mills R, O'Brien E: Memorabilia and letters of Dominic Corrigan: catalogue of an exhibition. **J Ir Coll Physicians Surg** 1980 Jul;10(1):55–7
O'Brien E: The Lancet maketh the man? Sir Dominic John Corrigan (1802–80). **Lancet** 1980 Dec 20–27;2(8208–8209):1356–7
O'Brien E: Corrigan's disease. **J Ir Coll Physicians Surg** 1980 Jul;10(1):32–7
O'Brien E: Sir Dominic Corrigan (1802–1880). **J Ir Coll Physicians Surg** 1980 Jul;10(1):11–9
O'Brien ET: The man behind the eponym: Sir Dominic John Corrigan (1802–1880). **N Engl J Med** 1981 Feb 5;304(6):365–6
O'Dwyer WF: Corrigan and the Charitable Infirmary. **J Ir Coll Physicians Surg** 1980 Jul;10(1):21–3

**Cortona, Pietro Berrettini, 1596–1669**
Duhme L: Die Tabulae anatomicae des Pietro Berrettini da Cortona. Köln, Universität zu Köln, 1980. 185 p. (Kölner medizinhistorische Beiträge, 18) (also Diss.).

**Corvisart des Marets, Jean Nicolas, 1755–1821**
Albury WR: Heart of darkness: J. N. Corvisart and the medicalization of life. **Hist Reflect** 1982;9(1–2):17–31.
Borodulin VI: Klinicheskaia shkola Korvizara i ee rol' v razvitii ucheniia o bolezniakh serdtsa (k 100-letiiu so dnia smerti Zhana Batista Buĭo). **Kardiologiia** 1982 Jan;22(1):113–5

**Coschwitz, Georg Daniel, 1679–1729**
Kaiser W: Medizinisches Grundlagenstudium im frühen 18. Jahrhundert. Zur 300. Wiederkehr des Geburtstages von Georg Daniel Coschwitz (1679–1729). **Z Gesamte Inn Med** 1979 Aug 1;34(15):419–28

**Cosmas and Damian, Saints**
Alberti H: Die heiligen Kosmas und Damian auf einer Prozessionsfahne im Deutschen Apotheken-Museum. **Dtsch Apoth Ztg** 1979 Jun 14;119(24):948–50 (also in Pharm Ztg 1979 Jun 14;24:1155–7
Bano-Fleischmann M, Zalai K: Gegenstände der Erinnerung an Kosma und Damian in Ungarn. **Ther Hung** 1981;29(3):152–6
Berle EJ: Legenden om en senantikk bentransplantasjon. **Sydsven Medicinhist Sallsk Arsskr** 1984;21:135–40
David-Danel ML: Un ex-libris non professionnel à l'effigie de saint Côme. **Rev Hist Pharm (Paris)** 1982;29(252):171–2
Dobras W: Cosmas und Damian in oberbayerischen Kirchen. **Pharm Ztg** 1981 Dec 24;126(52–53):2715–6
Fleishmann-Bánó M, Zalai K: St. Cosmas and St. Damian relics in Hungary. **Ther Hung** 1981;29(3):142–6
Julien P: Le point sur les ex-libris professionnels à l'effigie des saints Côme et Damien. **Rev Hist Pharm (Paris)** 1982;29(252):176–8
Julien P: Culte et iconographie des saints médecins Come et Damien dans une province française. In International Congress of the History of Medicine, 27th, Barcelona, 1980. Actas. Barcelona, Académia de Ciències Mèdiques de Catalunya i Balears, 1981. p. 530–4.
Julien P: Une miniature des saints Côme et Damien (fin XVe - début XVIe siècle). **Rev Hist Pharm (Paris)** 1982 Sep;29(254):175–6
Julien P: Deux saints médecins et pharmaciens, Côme et Damien. **Bull Liaison Assoc Amis Mus Pharm Montp** 1982;:(7):13–35
Kahan BD: Cosmas and Damian revisited. **Transplant Proc** 1983 Dec;15(4 Suppl 1–2):2211–6
Manzi L: I santi protettori degli artisti dello studio bolognese... Santi Cosma e Damiano. **Strenna Stor Bolognese** 1977;27:179–93
Rocchietta S: Un 'Christ à la pharmacie' ou 'Les Saints Côme et Damien'? **Rev Hist Pharm (Paris)** 1984 Jun;31(261):131–3
Verellen T: Cosmas and Damian in the New Sacristy [Medici Chapel of San Lorenzo, Florence]. **J Warburg Courtauld Inst** 1979;42:274–7
Vida M: A Kozma- és Damján-tisztelet írásos és tárgyi emlékei Magyarországon. **Orvostort Kozl** 1980;89–91(26 no 1–3):257–65
Vida M: Ursprung und Deutung der Verehrung der Heiligen Kosmas und Damian in Ungarn (11–14. Jahrhundert). **Orvostort Kozl** 1980;89–91(26 no 1–3):45–95
Zuring J: Saint Côme et Saint Damien dans la philatélie. **Rev Hist Pharm (Paris)** 1984 Mar;31(260):69–72

**Cosslett, Vernon Ellis, 1908–**
Barer R: Cosslett's contribution to microscopy (Ellis Cosslett). **J Microsc** 1979 Sep;117(1):5–10
Hirsch PB: Foreword: the Cosslett festschrift (Ellis Cosslett).

**J Microsc** 1979 Sep;117(1):1-4

**Costa Barreto, Manuel Alves de, fl. 1797**
Ribeiro de Araujo A: O ensaio sobre as fracturas do cirurgiao Manuel Alves da Costa Barreto. **Rev Inst Hist Geogr Bras** 1977;317:100-31

**Costa Ben Luca, fl. 870**
Wilcox J: Problems in the Latin manuscript tradition of De differentia spiritus et animae by the physician Costa ben Luca (9/10 cent.). In International Congress of the History of Medicine, 27th, Barcelona, 1980. Actas. Barcelona, Acadèmia de Ciències Mèdiques de Catalunya i Balears, 1981. p. 363-5.

**Coste, Jean François, 1741-1819**
Peumery JJ: La prodigieuse carrière de Jean-François Coste (1741-1819) médicin-chef des armées. **Hist Sci Med** 1980;14(2):177-86

**Cotard, Jules, 1840-1889**
Bourgeois M: Jules Cotard et son syndrome cent ans après. **Ann Med Psychol (Paris)** 1980 Dec;138(10);1165-80

**Cotta, John, 1575?-1650?**
McConchie RW: Additions to OED from John Cotta's Ignorant Practisers of Physicke, 1612. **Notes Queries** 1981 Dec;28(6):490-3

**Cottam, Nephi, 1883-1966**
Cottam C, Smith EM: The roots of cranial manipulation: Nephi Cottam and 'craniopathy'. **Chiropr Hist** 1981;1(1):31-5

**Cotterman, Charles William, 1914-**
Opitz JM: Cotterman and combinatorial genetics. **Am J Med Genet** 1983 Nov;16(3):389-92

**Cotugno, Domenico, 1736-1822**
Belloni L: Il Morgagni tra il Malpighi e il Cotugno. **Gesnerus** 1982;39(2):195-213
Milstein S: Domenico Cotugno. **Am J Otol** 1982 Jul;4(1):95-7

**Cotzias, George C., 1918-1977**
Tang LC: A personal and scientific biography of Dr. George C. Cotzias. **Neurotoxicology (Park Forest Il)** 1984 Spring;5(1):5-12

**Coues, Elliott, 1842-1899**
Cutright PR, Brodhead MJ: Elliott Coues: naturalist and frontier historian. Urbana, University of Illinois Press, 1981. xv, 509 p.

**Councilman, William Thomas, 1854-1933**
Harvey AM: Amebic dysentery gets its name: the story of William Thomas Councilman. **Johns Hopkins Med J** 1980 May;146(5):185-92, 199-201

**Couney, Martin A., 1860 or 70-1950**
Silverman WA: Incubator-baby side shows (Dr. Martin A. Couney). **Pediatrics** 64(2):127-41, Aug 79

**Courville, Cyril Brian, 1900-1968**
Manson Thomas ML, Cooper WC, ed: Catalog of works in the neurological sciences collected by Cyril Brian Courville, M.D., representative of clinical neurology, neuroanatomy and neuropathology, with particular reference to head trauma, and books from historical medicine in the Medical Sciences Library, University of California, Irvine. Irvine, University of California, 1978. 239 p.

**Cousins, Norman, 1912-**
Ruderman FA: A placebo for the doctor. **Commentary** 1980;69(5):54-60

**Coutela, Charles, 1876-1969**
Royer J, Haut J, Amalric P: L'opération de la cataracte de Claude Monet, correspondence inédite du peintre et de G.-Clemenceau au docteur Coutela. **Hist Sci Med** 1984;18(2):109-27

**Cove, John William, 1838-1901**
Campbell BJ: Springhill's first doctor. **NS Hist Q** 1979;9(4):297-312

**Cowper, William, 1731-1800**
Dumaitre P: La curieuse destinée des planches anatomiques de Gérard de Lairesse, peintre en Hollande - Lairesse, Bidloo, Cowper. Amsterdam, Rodopi, 1982. xvii, 107 p. (Nieuwe Nederlandse Bijdragen tot de Geschiedenis der Geneeskunde en der Natuurwetenschappen, no. 6).
Lindeboom GA: Cowper's brutale 'plagiaat' van Bidloo's Anatomische Atlas. **Ned Tijdschr Geneeskd** 1982 Oct 9;126(41):1878-82
Meyer JE, Meyer R: Selbstschilderungen eines Depressiven--Zur Pathobiographie William Cowper's. **Fortschr Neurol Psychiatr** 1984 Apr;52(4):107-12

**Cox, Alfred, 1866-1954**
James T: Dr. Alfred Cox and the South African Medical Association. **S Afr Med J** 1980 Mar 15;57(11):416-21

**Craig, Winchell McKendree, 1892-1960**
Key JD: Winchell McKendree Craig. In Dictionary of American Biography, Suppl. 6, 1956-1960. p. 130-31, 1980.

**Craik, James, 1730-1814**
Adams RR: Dr. James Craik, George Washington's physician and friend. **Record** 1980 May, Sep;1-4,1-3

**Craik, Kenneth James Williams, 1914-1945**
Cordeschi R: Craik e la psicologia meccanicistica. **Stor Crit Psicol** 1984 Jun;5(1):161-75
Gregory RL: Forty years on: Kenneth Craik's The Nature of Explanation (1943). **Perception** 1983;12(3):233-7

**Cranach, Lucas, 1472-1553**
Eberle MW: Lucas Cranach's cupid as honey thief paintings: allegories of syphilis? **Com J Mediev Renaiss Stud** 1979-80;10:21-30

**Crane, Caroline Julia Bartlett, 1858-1938**
Brown AS: Caroline Bartlett Crane and urban reform. **Mich Hist** 1972;56(4):287-301

**Crane, John, 1571-1652**
Martin L: John Crane (1571-1652); the Cambridge apothecary and philanthropist. **Med Hist** 1980;24(4):432-46

**Crapper, Thomas, 1837-1910**
Hinton BT: Thomas Crapper (1837-1910). **Invest Urol** 1980 May;17(6):534-5

**Crawford, Adair, 1748-1795**
Gago R, Carrillo JL: La obra fisiológica de Ignacio María Ruiz de Luzuriaga (1763-1822) y su plagio del cientifico británico Adair Crawford (1748-1795). **Dynamis** 1981;1:87-100

**Crawford, James, 1682-1731**
Doyle WP: James Crawford (1682-1731), M. D. Edinburgh, University of Edinburgh, [1981]. 10 p. (Scottish men of science).

**Crawford, Thomas, 1824-1895**
Eakins WA: Thomas Crawford, regimental medical officer in the Crimea, 1855. **Ulster Med J** 1982;51(1):46-51

**Credé, Carl S. F., 1819-1892**
Fodor F: 100 de ani de la introducerea procedeului profilactic Credé. **Rev Chir [Oftalmol]** 1981 Jul-Sep;25(3):161-3
Newell FW: Centenary of Credé prophylaxis. **Am J Ophthalmol** 1980 Dec;90(6):874-5

**Cree, Edward Hodges, 1814-1901**
Levien M, ed: Naval surgeon. The voyages of Dr. Edward H. Cree, Royal Navy, as related in his private journals, 1837-1856. New York, E. P. Dutton, 1982. 275 p.

**Creus y Manso, Juan, 1828-1897**
Herrera Casado A: Vída y obra del doctor D. Juan Creus y Manso (1828-1897). **An Otorrinolaringol Ibero Am** 1980;7(2):109-32

**Crevier, Joseph Alexandre, 1824-1889**
Lortie L: Joseph-Alexandre Crevier. In Dictionary of Canadian biography, 1881-1890. 1982;11:217-8.

**Crichton, Alexander, 1763-1856**
Tansey EM: The life and works of Sir Alexander Crichton, F.R.S. (1763-1856): a Scottish physician to the Imperial Russian Court. **Notes Rec R Soc Lond** 1984;38(2):241-59

**Crichton Browne, James, 1840-1938**
Gruman GJ, ed: The 'Fixed period' controversy: prelude to modern ageism. New York, Arno Press, 1979. Various paginations. Reprint of passages by George M. Beard, William Osler, and James Crichton-Browne.

**Crichton, Eric Cuthbert, 1888-1962**
Daubenton F: Professor Cuthbert Crichton--the man and his times. **S Afr Med J** 1979 Dec 15;56(25):1064-75
Louw JH: Professor Eric Cuthbert Crichton's contribution to the medical school. **S Afr Med J** 1979 Dec 15;56(25):1075-84
Sharp RG: Tribute to a great teacher. **S Afr Med J** 1979 Dec 15;56(25):1059-64

**Crichton, Michael, 1942-**
Graham PW: A mirror for medicine: Richard Selzer, Michael Crichton, and Walker Percy. **Perspect Biol Med** 1981 Winter;24(2):229-39

**Crick, Francis Harry, 1916-**
Thirty years of DNA--and after: **Nature** 1983 Apr 14;302(5909):557-8

**Crile, George Washington, 1864-1943**
English PC: Shock, physiological surgery, and George Washington Crile. Medical innovation in the Progressive era. Westport, Connecticut, and London, Greenwood, 1980. xi, 271 p. (Contributions in medical history, 5)

**Cristofano di Giulio, Cessini, d. 1642**
Cipolla CM: Cristofano e la peste. Bologna, Il Mulino, 1976. 157 p.

**Critchley, Macdonald, 1900-**
Rose FC, Bynum WF, ed: Historical aspects of the neurosciences. A festschrift for Macdonald Critchley. New York, Raven Press, 1982. xix, 537 p.

**Crohn, Burrill Bernard, 1884-**
Janowitz HD: Crohn and his disease. **Lancet** 1983 Nov 12;2(8359):1140
Kirsner JB: Landmark perspective. Crohn's disease. **JAMA** 1984 Jan 6;251(1):80-1

**Croll, Oswald, ca. 1560-1609**
Klutz M: Die Rezepte in Oswald Crolls Basilica Chymica (1609) und ihre Beziehungen zu Paracelsus. Braunschweig, 1974. 124 p. (Veröffentlichungen aus dem Pharmaziegeschichtlichen Seminar der Technischen Universität Braunschweig, 14).

**Cromwell, Frances Elisabeth, 1875-1950**
Vickers ED: F. Elisabeth Cromwell: Pensacola's pioneer nurse. **J Fla Med Assoc** 1983 Aug;70(8):642-6

**Cromwell, Oliver, 1599–1658**
- Bruce-Chwatt LJ: Medical sense and nonsense in biography. **Br Med J [Clin Res]** 1983 Apr 16;286(6373):1281
- Bruce-Chwatt LJ: George Bate--Cromwell's devious physician. **J R Coll Physicians Lond** 1983 Apr;17(2):144–6
- Bruce-Chwatt LJ: Myth of quartan malaria. **Trans R Soc Trop Med Hyg** 1982;76(1):133–4
- Morris GC: Which Molins treated Cromwell for stone--and did not prescribe for Pepys? **Med Hist** 1982 Oct;26(4):429–35
- Okamura A: [A long road to the hospice movement--life of Mother Mary Aikenhead] (Jpn). **Kango Kyoiku** 1984 Jan;25(1):38–45;25(2):104–11 (continued periodically)

**Crosse, Andrew, 1784–1855**
- Roth N: Bugs and blasphemy: Andrew Crosse and the Acarus electricus. **Med Instrum** 1979 Nov–Dec;13(6):357

**Crowe, Samuel James, 1883–1955**
- Catlin FI: Pulmonary complications of tonsillectomy as originally described by Samuel J. Crowe, M.D. **Laryngoscope** 1981 Jan;91(1):52–61

**Crowell, Edward Payson, 1856–1934**
- Rogers FB: Dr. Edward P. Crowell (1856–1934), Cape Codder, and the Black Slipper. **J Hist Med Allied Sci** 1981 Oct;36(4):493–4

**Crowley, Ralph Manning, 1905–**
- Schimel JL: Ralph M. Crowley: psychoanalytic pioneer. **J Am Acad Psychoanal** 1981 Oct;9(4):489–91

**Cruikshank, George, 1792–1878**
- Carty MA: The examination of a young surgeon. Hand-colored etching by George Cruikshank, from The Scourge, 1811. **J Hist Med Allied Sci** 1981 Apr;36(2):214

**Cruveilhier, Jean, 1791–1874**
- Grebeneva LS: K 150-letiiu opisaniia Kruivel'e prostoĭ khronicheskoĭ iazvy zheludka. **Klin Med (Mosk)** 1981 May;59(5):112–4

**Cruz Jobim, José Martin da**
- Fernandes R: Jose Martins da Cruz Jobim, um fundador da Academia Nacional de Medicina. **Rev Inst Hist Geogr Bras** 1980;327:247–68

**Cruz, Oswaldo Gonçalves, 1872–1917**
- Fraga C: Vida e obra de Osvaldo Cruz. Rio de Janeiro, Livraria José Olympio Editôra em convênio com o Instituto Nacional do Livro, [1972]. 186 p.
- Freitas CA de: A memória de Oswaldo Cruz. **Rev Bras Malariol Doencas Trop** 1978;30:129–33

**Csáth, Géza, 1887–1919**
- Szentgyörgyvölgyi G: Csáth Géza--Dr. Brenner József (1887–1919). **Orv Hetil** 1984 Sep 30;125(40):2446–8

**Csipkés, György Komáromi, 1628–1678**
- Bolyki J: Komáromi Csipkés György: Pestis pestise (1664). **Orvostort Kozl** 1979;86(24 no 4):81–9

**Csokonai, Vitéz Mihály, 1773–1805**
- Ferenczy M: Csokonai Vitéz Mihály egészségügyi tanácsai. **Orv Hetil** 1982 Nov 28;123(48):2973–4

**Csorba, József**
- Frankl J, Bodosi M: Csorba József emlékezete. **Orv Hetil** 1984 Aug 19;125(34):2087–9

**Csörsz, Károly, 1892–1935**
- Czeizel A: A historical evaluation of the doctrine of heredodegeneration. **Orvostort Kozl** 1979;87–88(25 no 1–2):157–79

**Cuefner, Johannes**
- Kostenzer O: Dr. Johannes Cuefner aus Rattenberg (biographische Notizen). **Tirol Heimatbl** 1971;46(1–3):18–20

**Cuénot, Lucien, 1866–1951**
- Buican D: Lucien Cuénot et la redécouverte de la génétique. **Pour Sci** 1981;45:21–9

**Culpeper, Nicholas, 1616–1654**
- Bloch H: Nicholas Culpeper, M.D. (1616 to 1654). Medical maverick in seventeenth-century England. **NY State J Med** 1982 Dec;82(13):1865–7
- Jones DA: Nicholas Culpeper and his Pharmacopoeia. **Pharm Hist (London)** 1980 Aug;10(2):9–10
- Potterton D: Alternative medicine: Culpeper and his cure-alls. **Health Soc Serv J** 1983 Feb 3;93(4832):145–6

**Cummings, Martin Marc, 1920–**
- Davis NE, Huth EJ: Martin M. Cummings and the National Library of Medicine. **Ann Intern Med** 1983 Dec;99(6):860–1
- Premio Abraham Horwitz. Dr. Martin M. Cummings: **Bol Of Sanit Panam** 1984 Jan;96(1):73–8

**Cummins, Harold, 1893–**
- Rife DC, et al: Dr. Harold Cummins and dermatoglyphics. **Birth Defects** 1979;15(6):1–797, passim

**Cumston, Charles Greene, 1868–1928**
- Röthlisberger P: Charles Greene Cumston (1868–1928): Medizinhistoriker in zwei Kontinenten. **Gesnerus** 1984;41(1/2):137–51

**Cupples, George H., 1816–1865**
- Banks CS: Two pioneer physicians of San Antonio. **Friends P. I. Nixon Med Hist Libr** 1973 Oct;2:2–17

**Curie, Marie Skłodowska, 1867–1934**
- Bendiner E: The Curies: pioneers and victims of the atomic era. **Hosp Pract** 1981 Dec;16(12):80, 82–4 passim
- Chrzanowski A: Dar Narodowy dla pani Marii Skłodowska-Curie. **Nowotwory** 1980 Jan–Mar;30(1):93–7
- Hevesy GC de: Marie Curie and her contemporaries. **J Nucl Med** 1984 Jan;25(1):116–31
- Hurwic J: Nieznany list Marii Skłodowskiej-Curie. **Kwart Hist Nauki Tech** 1984;29(3–4):557–8
- Róziewicz J: Zwiazki Marii Skłodowskiej-Curie z nauka rosyjska i radziecka. **Kwart Hist Nauki Tech** 1984;29(3–4):535–55

**Curie, Pierre, 1859–1906**
- Bendiner E: The Curies: pioneers and victims of the atomic era. **Hosp Pract** 1981 Dec;16(12):80, 82–4 passim
- Sztanyik BL: Curie és az orvostudomány. **Orv Hetil** 1981 Apr 19;;122(16):961–4

**Curran, Edward J., 1873–1962**
- Feibel RM: Edward J. Curran and the concept of relative pupillary block. **Surv Ophthalmol** 1981 Jan–Feb;25(4):270–8

**Currey, Richard Owen**
- Corgan JX: Richard Owen Currey, a little known intellectual figure of antebellum Tennessee. **East Tenn Hist Soc Publ** 1978;50:58–70

**Cushing, George Hoppin, 1829–1900**
- The presidents. George Hoppin Cushing, 1871–1872: **J Am Dent Assoc** 1979 Dec;99(6):956

**Cushing, Harvey Williams, 1869–1939**
- Alexander E, Alexander E (3d): German influences on the work of Harvey Cushing, the pioneer of neurosurgery in America. **Neurosurgery** 1981 Nov;9(5):501–5
- Altschule MD: Occasional notes. A near miss: Osler's early description of Cushing's syndrome with, regrettably, no post-mortem examination. **N Engl J Med** 1980 May 15;302(20):1153–5
- Christy NP: Harvey Cushing as clinical investigator and laboratory worker. **Am J Med Sci** 1981 Mar–Apr;281(2):79–96
- Dalessio DJ: Trigeminal neuralgia, Cushing. **JAMA** 1983 Jul 22–29;250(4):529–31
- Fulton JF: History of medicine–Arnold Klebs and Harvey Cushing at the 1st International Neurological Congress at Berne in 1931. **Int J Neurol** 1980;14(1):103–15
- Gillingham FJ: The influence of Harvey Cushing on British and European neurosurgery. **Surg Neurol** 1982 May;17(5):344–9
- Horrax G: Some of Harvey's Cushing's contributions to neurological surgery. **J Neurosurg** 1981 Apr;54(4):436–47
- Kenéz J: Harvey Williams Cushing (1869–1939) und die moderne Hirnchirurgie. **Med Welt** 1980 Sep 5;31(36):1295–7
- Ljunggren B: Cushing och Sven Hedin. **Lakartidningen** 1982 Aug 11;79(32–33):2790–2
- Ljunggren B: The case of General Wood. **J Neurosurg** 1982 Apr;56(4):471–4
- Ljunggren B: Harvey Cushing and Sven Hedin. **Surg Neurol** 1982 Mar;17(3):165–71
- Ljunggren B: Pionjärer inom hjärnkirurgi. **Lakartidningen** 1982 Apr 7;79(14):1377–8
- Moore TJ: Credit for describing Cushing's syndrome. **N Engl J Med** 1983 Sep 22;309(12):735
- Niculescu SI: Pe marginea corespondenţei dintre Harvey Cushing şi Dumitru Bagdasar. **Rev Med Interna [Neurol Psihiatr]** 1981 Jul–Sep;26(3):229–33
- Rosegay H: Cushing's legacy to transsphenoidal surgery. **J Neurosurg** 1981 Apr;54(4):448–54
- Sano K: [Harvey Williams Cushing] (Jpn). **No Shinkei Geka** 1981 Jan;9(1):32–5
- Teichman SL, Aldea PA: Pioneers in pituitary physiology: Harvey Cushing and Nicolas Paulescu. **J Hist Med Allied Sci** 1985 Jan;40(1):68–72
- Thomson EH: Madeline Earle Stanton, disciple: the years 1920 to 1941. **J Hist Med Allied Sci** 1981 Apr,36(2):151–67
- Thomson EH: Harvey Cushing, surgeon, author, artist. New York, Neale Watson Academic Publications, 1981, xvii, 347 p.
- Tilney NL: Harvey Cushing and the surgical research laboratory. **Surg Gynecol Obstet** 1980 Aug;151(2):263–70
- Tilney NL: Cushing, Cutler and the mitral valve. **Surg Gynecol Obstet** 1981 Jan;152(1):91–6
- Tilney NL: Harvey Cushing and the Oxford connection. **Surg Gynecol Obstet** 1982 Jul;155(1):89–94
- Tilney NL: The marrow of the tragedy (Harvey Cushing). **Surg Gynecol Obstet** 1983 Oct;157(4):380–8

**Custer, George Armstrong, 1839–1876**
- Rowe WF: Discussion of 'George Armstrong Custer and the Battle of the Little Bighorn: homicide or mass suicide'. **J Forensic Sci** 1984 Jul;29(3):696–9
- Spencer JD: George Armstrong Custer and the Battle of the Little Bighorn: homicide or mass suicide? **J Forensic Sci** 1983 Jul;28(3):756–61

**Cuthbert, Saint, d. 687**
- Rubin S: St Cuthbert of Lindisfarne: a medical reconstruction. **Trans Archit Archaeol Soc Durham Northumberl** 1978 Sep;4:101–3

**Cutler, Elliott Carr, 1888–1947**
Tilney NL: Cushing, Cutler and the mitral valve. **Surg Gynecol Obstet** 1981 Jan;152(1):91–6

**Cuvier, George, 1769–1832**
Theunissen B: Theorie en praktijk van Cuviers Recherches sur les ossemens fossiles. **Tijdschr Geschied Geneeskd** 1983;6(1):1–17

**Cysat, Renward, 1545–1614**
Brunner-Wildisen B: Medizinisches aus den Schriften des Renward Cysat, 1545–1614. Zürich, Juris, 1980. 75 p. (Zürcher Medizingeschichtliche Abhandlungen, Neue Reihe, Nr. 138).
Daems WF: Renward Cysat und Paracelsus. **Gesnerus** 1982;39(3–4):469–72

**Czermák, Johann Nepomuk, 1828–1873**
Antall J, Kapronczay K: Jan Nepomuk Czermak in Hungary. In E. Schultheisz, ed: History of physiology. Oxford, Elmsford, New York, Pergamon, 1981. xvi, 208 p. (Advances in Physiological Sciences. Proceedings of the 28th International Congress of Physiological Sciences, Budapest, 1980. Volume 21). p. 77–84.

**Czerny, Adalbert, 1863–1941**
Wunderlich P: Zur Geschichte der Universitäts-Kinderklinik in Breslau unter Adalbert Czerny (1863--1941) von 1894--1910. **Arch Hist Med (Warsz)** 1979;42(3):337–43

# D

**DaCosta, Jacob Mendez, 1833–1900**
Wooley CF: Jacob Mendez DaCosta: medical teacher, clinician, and clinical investigator. **Am J Cardiol** 1982 Nov;50(5):1145–8
Wooley CF: From irritable heart to mitral valve prolapse: the Osler connection. **Am J Cardiol** 1984 Mar 1;53(6):870–4

**Dagomari, Paolo, ca. 1281–1365**
Van Egmond W: New light on Paolo dell'Abbaco. **Ann Ist Mus Stor Sci Fir** 1977;2(2):3–21

**Dagonet, Henri**
Esman AH: Henri Dagonet. Pioneer of psychiatric photography. **NY State J Med** 1984 Feb;84(2):79–81

**Dahl, Haldoe Christian, fl. 1800**
Excerpt of a letter from veterinary surgeon Haldoe Dahl: from the Diocese of Trondheim to Professor E. Viborg. **Hist Med Vet** 1977;2(1):4–9

**Dailey, Ulysses Grant, 1885–1961**
Johnston GA: Tribute to a Chicago surgeon: Ulysses Grant Dailey. **IMJ** 1983 Jan;163(1):35–6

**Dain, Harry Guy, 1870–1966**
Stevenson D: Sir Harry Guy Dain. In Dictionary of national biography, 1961–1970. Suppl. 8, 1981. p. 262.

**Dakin, Henry Drysdale, 1880–1952**
Baguenier-Desormeaux L: Henry Drysdale Dakin à Compiègne, en 1915. **Rev Hist Pharm (Paris)** 1981 Jun;28(249):79–88

**Dalcq, Albert, 1893–1973**
Pasteels JJ: Albert Dalcq, 1893–1973. In Florilège des Sciences en Belgique - II. Bruxelles, Académie Royale de Belgique, 1980. p. 625–39.

**Dale, Henry Hallett, 1875–1968**
Feldberg W: Sir Henry Hallett Dale. In Dictionary of national biography, 1961–1970. Suppl. 8, 1981. p. 262–5.

**Daléchamps, Jacques, 1513–1588**
Bono JJ, Schmitt CB: An unknown letter of Jacques Daléchamps to Jean Fernel: local autonomy versus centralized government. **Bull Hist Med** 1979 Spring;53(1):100–27

**Daley, William Allen, 1887–1969**
Stewart AB: Sir William Allen Daley. In Dictionary of national biography, 1961–1970. Suppl. 8, 1981. p. 265–6.

**Dalhana**
Sharma PV: Dalhana's version of the Suśruta Samhita. **Bull Indian Inst Hist Med (Hyderabad)** 1979;9:27–32

**Dalmahoy, Alexander, ca. 1723–1783**
Hopkinson GD: Alexander Dalmahoy: chemist to Her Majesty. **Pharm Hist (London)** 1984 Dec;14(4):8–11

**Dalton, John Call, 1825–1889**
Loew FM: Animal experimentation. **Bull Hist Med** 1982 Spring;56(1):123–6

**Dalton, John, 1766–1844**
Cardwell D, Mottram J: Fresh light on John Dalton. **Notes Rec R Soc Lond** 1984 Sep;39(1):29–40

**Dancer, John Benjamin, 1812–1887**
Nuttali RH: An early microscope by John Benjamin Dancer of Manchester. **Microscope** 1980;28(3/4):93–100

**Dandy, Walter Edward, 1886–1946**
Pinkus RL: Innovation in neurosurgery: Walter Dandy in his day. **Neurosurgery** 1984 May;14(5):623–31
Woodhall B: Walter Dandy, M.D.: personal reminiscences. **Neurosurgery** 1979 Jan;4(1):3–6

**Dann, Georg Edmund, 1898–**
Schneider W: Pharmaziegeschichte und ihre Repräsentanten im 20. Jahrhundert. Zum 80. Geburtstag von Prof. Dr. Georg Edmund Dann. **Pharm Ztg** 1978;123:1265–71

**Danta, Júlio, 1876–1962**
Iria A: Evocação de Júlio Dantas no 1. centenário do seu nascimento: duas raridades bibliográficas do médico militar. **An Acad Port Hist** 1979;25:359–84

**Dapper, Olfert, 1636 or 37–1689**
Faust E: Arabien 1680. Olfert Dappers Arabienbuch und seine Quellen, geprüft an Nachrichten über Kaffee, Sesam und Träumen. Köln, Universität zu Köln, 1977, 256 p. (Kölner medizinhistorische Beiträge, 5; also Diss).

**Dar-mo Sman-ram Blo-bzan-chos-grags**
Dar-mo Sman-ram Blo-bzan-chos-grags: Dar Mo Bka' Brgya Ma. Man nag zab mo kun gyi snin khu bsdus pa dar-mo sman-rams-pa'i gdams nag bka rgya ma. A collection of profound instructions on the methods and rituals of Tibetan healing transmitted by the physician of the 5th Dalia Lama. Reproduced from a print from the Sde-Dge blocks, 2 vols; and from the Ska-' Bum blocks, 2 vols. Leh, Ladakh, T. S Tashigangpa, 1978. n.p. (Smanrtsis Shesrig Spendzog, Vols. 88–91).

**Darier, Jean, 1856–1938**
Bernhard JD, Elliot AD: A letter from Darier to Bowen on the naming of Bowen's disease. **Arch Dermatol** 1983 Mar;119(3):261–2
Civatte J: Jean Darier: a memoir. **Am J Dermatopathol** 1979 Spring;1(1):57–60

**Darling, Samuel Taylor, 1872–1925**
Chaves-Carballo E: Samuel T. Darling: studies on malaria and the Panama Canal. **Bull Hist Med** 1980 Spring;54(1):95–100

**Darlington, William, 1782–1863**
Ewan J: Five pupils of Benjamin Smith Barton: the men and their minds. **Trans Stud Coll Physicians Phila** 1983 Dec;5(5 no 4):309–20
Stuckey RL: Dr. William Darlington's botanical contacts on the western American frontier. **Trans Stud Coll Physicians Phila** 1983 Sep;5(5 No 3):213–43

**Darré, Richard Walther, 1895–1953**
Heinrich WL: Richard Walther Darré und der Hegehofgedanke. Diss. Mainz, 1980. 161 p.

**Darwin, Charles Robert, 1809–1882**
Arquiola E: Darwinism in the Société d'Anthropologie de Paris. **Clio Med** 1980 May;14(2):119–28
Ayala FJ: Darwin y la idea de progreso. **Arbor** 1982;113(441–2):59–75
Beatty J: What's in a word? Coming to terms in the Darwinian revolution. With a comment by D. Hull. In M. Ruse, ed: Nature animated. Historical and philosophical case studies in Greek medicine, nineteenth-century and recent biology, psychiatry, and psychoanalysis. Volume II. Dordrecht, D. Reidel, 1983. p. 79–111.
Beer CG: Darwin, instinct, and ethology. **J Hist Behav Sci** 1983 Jan;19(1):68–80
Beer G: Anxiety and interchange: Daniel Deronda and the implications of Darwin's writing. **J Hist Behav Sci** 1983 Jan;19(1):31–44
Bendall DS, ed: Evolution from molecules to men. Cambridge, Cambridge University Press, 1983. xiii, 594 p.
Bendiner E: The descent of man and the ascent of the Darwins. **Hosp Pract** 1982 Dec;17(12):160, 165, 173–4 passim
Bernstein RE: What was Charles Darwin's illness? **S Afr Med J** 1982 Jun 19;61(25):939
Bernstein RE: Darwin's alter ego: co-originator Alfred Wallace. **Perspect Biol Med** 1984;27(2):234–8
Bernstein RE: Darwin's illness: Chagas' disease resurgens. **J R Soc Med** 1984 Jul;77(7):608–9
Browne J: Darwin's botanical arithmetic and the 'principle of divergence,' 1854–1858. **J Hist Biol** 1980 Spring;13(1):53–89
Browne J: Essay review: new developments in Darwins studies? **J Hist Biol** 1982 Summer;15(2):275–80
Bynum WF: Darwin and the doctors: evolution, diathesis, and germs in 19th-century Britain. **Gesnerus** 1983;40(1–2):43–53
Castagnino HE, Thompson AC: Sufrió Darwin la enfermedad de Chagas? **Medicina (B Aires)** 1981;41(2):263–4
Charles Darwin, 1809–1882; Anton Dohrn, 1840–1909: Correspondence. Napoli, Macchiaroli, 1982. 118 p.
Colp R: Charles Darwin's coffin, and its maker. **J Hist Med Allied Sci** 1980 Jan;35(1):59–74
Colp R: 'I was born a naturalist': Charles Darwin's 1838 notes about himself. **J Hist Med Allied Sci** 1980 Jan;35(1):8–39
Colp R: Charles Darwin, Dr. Edward Lane, and the 'Singular Trial' of Robinson v. Robinson and Lane. **J Hist Med Allied Sci** 1981 Apr;36(2):205–13
Colp R: Charles Darwin's reprobation of nature. 'Clumsy, wasteful, blundering low and horribly cruel.' **NY State J Med** 1981 Jun;81(7):1116–9
Colp R: The Darwin exhibition at the Cambridge University Library. **Bull NY Acad Med** 1983 Jun;59(5):526–8
Colp R: [Charles Darwin: Essay-Review] **Trans Stud Coll Physicians Phila** 1983 Dec;5(5 no 4):353–75

Conry Y: Organisme et organisation: de Darwin à la génétique des populations. In Actes du Colloques R.A. Fisher.... Paris, 5–6 déc. 1979. p. 291–330. **Rev Synth (Paris)** 1981;102(103–104)
Continenza B: Darwin e la psicologia. **Stor Crit Psicol** 1981;2(1):99–105
Cornell JF: Analogy and technology in Darwin's vision of nature. **J Hist Biol** 1984 Fall;17(3):303–44
Crook DP: Darwinism – the political implications. **Hist Eur Ideas** 1981;5:99–139
Darwin CR: The descent of man, and selection in relation to sex. 2 vols in 1. Reprint of 1871 ed, with historical introduction by J. T. Bonner and R. M. May. Princeton, Princeton University Press, 1981. xli, 475, x, p.
Diamond P: The natural theologians and Darwin: a case of divergent evolution in the history of ideas. **Aust J Polit Hist** 1980;26(2):204–11
Di Gregorio MA: Order or process of nature: Huxley's and Darwin's different approaches to natural sciences. **Hist Philos Life Sci** 1981;3(2):217–41
Egozcue J: Darwin y el origen del hombre. **Arbor** 1982;113(441–2):77–86
Egri B: Mecsnyikov a cambridge-i Darwin-emlékünnepségekröl. **Orv Hetil** 1982 Nov 14;123(46):2858–60
Eiseley L: Darwin and the mysterious Mr. X: new light on the evolutionists. New York and London, Harcourt Brace Jovanovich, 1981. xii, 278 p.
Evans LT: Darwin's use of the analogy between artificial and natural selection. **J Hist Biol** 1984 Spring;17(1):113–40
Freeman D: The evolutionary theories of Charles Darwin and Herbert Spencer. **Curr Anthropol** 1974;15(3):211–21
Freeman RB: The works of Charles Darwin: an annotated bibliographical handlist. 2d. ed. Folkestone, England, Dawson, 1977. 235 p.
George W: Darwin. Glasgow, Fontana Paperbacks, 1982. 160 p.
Gould SJ: Darwinism and the expansion of evolutionary theory. **Science** 1982 Apr 23;216(4544):380–7
Groeben C, ed: Guida alla Mostra allestita nella Sala degli Affreschi della Stazione Zoologica nella Villa Comunale (6 luglio – 30 settembre 1982) su Charles Darwin e la Stazione Zoologica di Napoli.
Gruber HE: Darwin on man: a psychological study of scientific creativity. 2d. ed. Chicago, University of Chicago Press, 1981. xxvii, 310 p.
Gruber HE: Darwin on psychology and its relation to evolutionary thought. In R. W. Rieber, K. Salzinger, ed: Psychology: theoretical-historical perspectives. New York, Academic Press, 1980. p. 145–74.
Gruber HE: History and creative work: from the most ordinary to the most exalted. **J Hist Behav Sci** 1983 Jan;19(1):4–14
Gruber HE, Keegan RT, ed: Charles Darwin and the human sciences. Special issue. **J Hist Behav Sci** 1983 Jan;19(1):3–113
Gruber HE: Cognitive psychology, scientific creativity, and the case study method. In M. D. Grmek, R. S. Cohen, G. Cimino, ed: On scientific discovery. The Erice Lectures 1977. Dordrecht, D. Reidel, 1981. p. 295–322. (Boston Studies in the Philosophy of Science, v. 34).
Gruber HE: The evolving systems approach to creative scientific work: Charles Darwin's early thought. In T. Nickles, ed: Scientific discovery: case studies. Dordrecht, D. Reidel, 1980. (Boston Studies in the Philosophy of Science, v. 60). p. 113–30.
Hamrum CL, ed: Darwin's legacy. Nobel Conference XVIII, Gustavus Adolphus College. St. Peter, Minnesota, held October 5–6, 1982. San Francisco, Harper & Row, 1983. 125 p. Contributions by S. J. Gould, I. Stone, R. E. Leakey, P. B. Medawar, E. O. Wilson, J. Pelikan.
Haugen LK: Darwin, evolusjonen og medisinen. **Tidsskr Nor Laegeforen** 1982 Dec 10;102(34–36):1835–8
Herbert S, ed: The red notebook of Charles Darwin. Ithaca and London, Cornell University Press and British Museum (Natural History), 1980. 164 p.
Howard J: Darwin. New York, Hill and Wang, 1982. viii, 101 p.
James PJ: 'A theory by which to work': Mr. Darwin reminisces. **Hist Philos Life Sci** 1982;4(2):255–70
K 100-letiiu so dnia smerti Charlza Darvina: **Arkh Anat Gistol Embriol** 1982 Nov;83(11):5–6
Keegan RT, Gruber HE: Love, death, and continuity in Darwin's thinking. **J Hist Behav Sci** 1983 Jan;19(1):15–30
Kirsop W: W. R. Greg and Charles Darwin in Edinburgh and after: an antipodean gloss. **Trans Camb Bibliogr Soc** 1979;7(3):376–90
Kleiner SA: Problem solving and discovery in the growth of Darwin's theories of evolution. **Synthese** 1981;47(1):119–62
Kohn D: Theories to work by: rejected theories, reproduction, and Darwin's path to natural selection. **Stud Hist Biol** 1980;4:67–70
Kohn D, Stauffer RC, Smith S: New light on The foundations of the origin of species: A reconstruction of the archival record. **J Hist Biol** 1982 Fall;15(3):419–42
Kottler MJ: Darwin, Wallace, and the origin of sexual dimorphism. **Proc Am Philos Soc** 1980 Jun;124(3):203–26
Lewin R: Darwin died at a most propitious time. **Science** 1982 Aug 20;217(4561):717–8
Manier E: Darwin's language and logic. **Stud Hist Philos Sci** 1980;11:305–23
Márquez-Monter H: Conmemoración del centenario de la muerte de Charles R. Darwin. **Gac Med Mex** 1983 May;119(5):212–8
Martucci V: Il discusso fascino di una ipotesi: la pangenesi di Darwin e gli studiosi italiani (1868–1888). **Hist Philos Life Sci** 1981;3(2):243–57
Maynard-Smith J: The century since Darwin. **Nature** 1982 Apr 15;296(5858):599–601
Meagher LR: The influence of Darwinian theory upon biological research of the late nineteenth century. Ph.D. Diss., Duke University. Durham, 1979. xii, 329 leaves.
Novák VJ: Zakladatel moderní biologie. Sto let od smrti Ch. R. Darwina. **Cas Lek Cesk** 1982 Apr 16;121(15):449–50
Obál F: Emlékezés Charles Robert Darwin-ra (1809–1882) halála centenáriuma alkalmából. **Orv Hetil** 1982 Nov 14;123(46):2857–8
Oldroyd DR: Darwinian impacts. An introduction to the Darwinian revolution. Atlantic Highlands, N. J., Humanities Press, 1980. xiv, 399 p.
Ospovat D: God and natural selection: the Darwinian idea of design. **J Hist Biol** 1980 Fall;13(2):169–94
Ospovat D: The development of Darwin's theory: natural history, natural theology, and natural selection, 1838–1859. Cambridge, New York, Cambridge University Press, 1981. xii, 301 p.
Porter R: The descent of genius: Charles Darwin's brilliant career. **Hist Today** 1982 Jul;32:16–22
Rabasa SL: Dificultades del neo-darwinismo a los 100 años de la muerte de Darwin (19-IV-1882). **Medicina (B Aires)** 1982;42(2):213–6
Rheinberger HJ, McLaughlin P: Darwin's experimental natural history. **J Hist Biol** 1984 Fall;17(3):345–68
Rhodes FH: Gradualism, punctuated equilibrium and the Origin of Species. **Nature** 1983 Sep 22–28;305(5932):269–72
Richards RJ: Instinct and intelligence in British natural theology: some contributions to Darwin's theory of the evolution of behavior. **J Hist Biol** 1981 Fall;14(2):193–230
Richards RJ: Why Darwin delayed, or interesting problems and models in the history of science. **J Hist Behav Sci** 1983 Jan;19(1):45–53
Ruffié J. Darwin, cent ans après. **Biomed Pharmacother** 1982;36(3):170–3
Ruse M: Charles Darwin and group selection. **Ann Sci** 1980;37(6):615–30
Ruse M: Charles Darwin and the Beagle. **Wilson Q** 1982;6(1):164–75
Ruse M: Darwin's theory: an exercise in science. **New Sci** 1981;90:828–30
Ruse M: Ought philosophers consider scientific discovery? A Darwinian case-study. In T. Nickles, ed: Scientific discovery: case studies. Dordrecht, D. Reidel, 1980. (Boston Studies in the Philosophy of Science, v. 60). p. 131–49.
Schweber SS: Darwin and the political economists: divergence of character. **J Hist Biol** 1980 Fall;13(2):195–289
Secord JA: Nature's fancy: Charles Darwin and the breeding of pigeons. **Isis** 1981;72:163–86
Sheets-Pyenson S: Darwin's data: his reading of natural history journals, 1837–1842. **J Hist Biol** 1981 Fall;14(2):231–48
Shepherd JA: Lawson Tait – disciple of Charles Darwin. **Br Med J [Clin Res]** 1982 May;284(6326):1386–7
Sulloway FJ: Geographic isolation in Darwin's thinking: the vicissitudes of a crucial idea. **Stud Hist Biol** 1979;3:23–65
Sulloway FJ: Darwin's conversion: the Beagle voyage and its aftermath. **J Hist Biol** 1982 Fall;15(3):325–96
Sulloway FJ: Further remarks on Darwin's spelling habits and the dating of Beagle voyage manuscripts. **J Hist Biol** 1983 Fall;16(3):361–90
Swinton WE: Charles Darwin as an 'invalid recluse'. **Can Med Assoc J** 1982 Nov 15;127(10):1042–5
Templado J: Darwin: ayer y hoy. **Arbor** 1982;113(441–2):7–20
Tobach E: The relationship between Preyer's concept of psychogenesis and his views of Darwin's theory of evolution. **Z Psychol** 1983;191(4):388–95
Van der Peet R: Florence Nightingale en haar visie op verplegen in relatie tot het leven en werk van Charles Darwin. **Tijdschr Ziekenverpl** 1983 Aug 23;36(17):530–6
Vidal F, Buscaglia M, Vonèche JJ: Darwinism and developmental psychology. **J Hist Behav Sci** 1983 Jan;19(1):81–94

**Darwin, Erasmus, 1731–1802**
Bendiner E: The descent of man and the ascent of the Darwins. **Hosp Pract** 1982 Dec;17(12):160, 165, 173–4 passim
Cohen B: Erasmus Darwin's observations on rotation and vertigo. **Hum Neurobiol** 1984;3(3):121–8
Colp R: Dr. Erasmus Darwin consults with another physician. **Radic Hist Rev** 1979 Spring/Summer;Spec:66–71
King-Hele D, ed: The letters of Erasmus Darwin. Cambridge, Cambridge University Press, 1981. xxxii, 363 p.

**d'Attenhoven, Gerald, d. 1413**
De Backer C: Gérard d'Attenhoven, apothicaire liégois de la fin du XIVe siècle. **Rev Hist Pharm (Paris)** 1982 Jun;29(253):107–8

**Daubenton, Louis Jean Marie, 1716–1799**
Gysel C: Daubenton (1716–1800) et ses recherches sur le trou occipital. **Orthod Fr** 1979;50:377–92

**Daubrawa, Ferdinand**
Hošek E: Dr. phil. PhMr. Ferdinand Daubrawa, světlý zjev mezi lékárníky Moravského venkova v 19. století. **Cesk Farm** 1979 Jun;28(5):223–4

**Daudet, Alphonse, 1840-1897**
Godonnèche J: La Doulou: auto-observation d'Alphonse Daudet. **Hist Sci Med** 1981;15(4):321-5

**Daumier, Honoré, 1808-1879**
Handelsman A: Le médecin hydropathe---color lithograph by Honoré Daumier. **J Hist Med Allied Sci** 1981 Jan;36(1)63
Julien P: Le Dr. Véron et Daumier, ou le fabricant de pâté pectorale en proie à la caricature. In: Congrès international d'histoire de la médecine, XXVe, Québec, 1976. Actes. Québec, 1977. p. 807-21.
Moskow BS: The dental cartoons of Honoré Daumier (1808-1879). **J Am Dent Assoc** 1981 Jan;102(1):82-6
Rocchietta S: Caricature di Daumier correlate alla medicina in una mostra commemorativa. **Minerva Med** 1981 May 7;72(18):1157-8

**Davaine, Casimir-Joseph, 1812-1882**
Théodoridès J: Un centenaire oublié: Casimir-Joseph Davaine (1812-1882). **Hist Sci Med** 1982;16(4):263-6

**DaVega, Columbus, 1830-1882**
Leland TM: DaVega's Floating Hospital. **J SC Med Assoc** 1984 Nov;80(11):581

**Davenport, Horace Willard, 1912-**
Davenport HW: Carbonic anhydrase, or, the strange case of the disappearing scientist. **Physiologist** 1980 Apr;23(2):11-5

**David, Jacques Louis, 1748-1825**
Dotz W: Jean Paul Marat. His life, cutaneous disease, death, and depiction by Jacques Louis David. **Am J Dermatopathol** 1979 Fall;1(3):247-50

**Davidenkov, Sergeĭ Nikolaevich, 1880-**
Bochkov NP: Vklad s. n. Davidenkova v razrabotku probelmy nasledstvennykh nervynkh i psikhicheskikh zabolevaniĭ. **Zh Nevropatol Psikhiatr** 1982;82(3):1-4
Davidenkova EF: Zanchenie nauchnogo naslediia S. N. Davidenkova v razvitii klinicheskoĭ genetiki (k 100-letiiu so dnai rozhdeniia). **Klin Med (Mosk)** 1981;59(4):112-6
Dogel' LV, Shalagina TL: S. N. Davidenkov v Leningradskom gosudarstvennom institute usovershenstvovaniia vracheĭ. **Zh Nevropatol Psikhiatr** 1982;82(3):107-9

**Davidoff, Leo Max, 1898-1975**
Jacobson HG: A revisit with Leo M. Davidoff, M.D.--a titan of his time: some personal notes (1898-1975). **Neurosurgery** 1983 Nov;13(5):601-6

**Davidson, Maurice, 1883-1967**
Scadding JG: Maurice Davidson 1883-1967--progress in respiratory medicine since his time. **Postgrad Med J** 1984 Mar;60(701):178-82

**Daviel, Jacques, 1693-1762**
Figarella J: Jacques Daviel, chirurgien marseillais. **Marseille** 1978;113:42-56
Figarella J: Jacques Daviel à Marseille. **Hist Sci Med** 1979;13(4):347-62

**Davila, Carol, 1828-1884**
Cotrău M: Procesful cottorului Carol Davila (Iaşi, 1872). **Rev Med Chir Soc Med Nat Iasi** 1980 Apr-Jun;84(2):325-6

**Davis, Adelle, 1904-1974**
Young JH: Adelle Davis. In: Notable American women. The modern period. Cambridge, Mass., Belknap-Harvard Univ. Press, 1980. 4:179-80.

**Davis, David Daniel, 1777-1841**
Forster FM: David D. Davis' Obstetric Atlas in Tasmania in 1846. Edmund Bowden's gift to Robert Officer. **Aust NZ J Obstet Gynaecol** 1983 May;23(2):88-92

**Davis, Egerton Yorrick, ca.1850-ca.1920**
Graner JL: An introduction to the writings of Egerton Yorrick Davis. **IMJ** 1983 Jul;164(1):47-8
Robb-Smith AH: Egerton Y. Davis, M.D., and placentophagy. **Bull NY Acad Med** 1980 Mar;56(2):258-60
Tigertt WD: An annotated life of Egerton Yorrick Davis, M.D., an intimate of Sir William Osler. **J Hist Med Allied Sci** 1983 Jul;38(3):259-97

**Davis, Frances Elliot, 1882?-1965**
Elmore JA: Frances Elliott Davis. In: Notable American women. The modern period. Cambridge, Mass., Belknap-Harvard Univ. Press, 1980. 4:180-2.

**Davis, John Staige, 1872-1946**
Sargent LA, Morgan RF, Davis WB: John Staige Davis: pioneer American plastic surgeon. In Romm S, ed: Symposium on historical perspectives of plastic surgery. Philadelphia, Saunders, 1983. p. 653-6.

**Davis, Loyal Edward, 1896-1982**
Beahrs OH: Surgery of the head and neck--1896-1982. **Surg Gynecol Obstet** 1983 Aug;157(2):180-4
Davis RA: A surgeon at war. **Surg Gynecol Obstet** 1983 Aug;157(2):147-59
Laufman H: Loyal Davis and the young surgeon. **Surg Gynecol Obstet** 1983 Aug;157(2):123-8
Longmire WP: Loyal Davis' personal qualities and their influence on American surgery. **Surg Gynecol Obstet** 1983 Aug;157(2):114-7
Method HL: Doctor Loyal Davis--the editor. **Surg Gynecol Obstet** 1983 Aug;157(2):144-6
Perret GE: Doctor Loyal Davis--the neurosurgeon. **Surg Gynecol Obstet** 1983 Aug;157(2):140-3
Starzl TE: Loyal Davis, surgery of the liver and transplantation of the kidney. **Surg Gynecol Obstet** 1983 Aug;157(2):160-3
Stephenson GW: Loyal Davis, M.D., Fellow of the American College of Surgeons. **Surg Gynecol Obstet** 1983 Aug;157(2):118-22
Wetzel N: Loyal Davis; Allen Kanavel; surgery, gynecology and obstetrics, and the development of neurosurgery. **Surg Gynecol Obstet** 1983 Aug;157(2):135-9
Zollinger RM: Overview biography--Doctor Loyal Davis. **Surg Gynecol Obstet** 1983 Aug;157(2):111-3

**Davis, Mary Ellen, 1840-1924**
Doona ME: The cause is just: Mary E. P. Davis. **Mass Nurse** 1982 Jul;51(7):4-6

**Davis, Nathan Smith, 1817-1904**
Beatty WK: Nathan Smith Davis: observer, motivator, and doer. **Proc Inst Med Chic** 1980 Jul-Sep;33(3):88-90

**Davison, William, 1781-1858**
Pharmacist -cum-printer: **Pharm Hist (London)** 1971 Dec;2(3):5-6

**Davy, Humphry, 1778-1829**
Forgan S, ed: Science and the sons of genius: studies on Humphry Davy. London, Science Reviews, 1980. xii, 247 p. Contributions by M. Neve, T. H. Levere, J. Z. Fullmer, M. Crosland, J. H. Brooke, R. Siegfried, D. Knight, E. B. Smith.
Hartley H: Humphry Davy. London, Nelson, 1966. viii, 160 p.
Levere TH: Humphry Davy and the idea of glory. **Trans R Soc Can** 1980;18:247-61

**Davydovskiĭ, Ippolit Vasil'evich, 1887-**
Chekareva GA: I. V. Davydovskiĭ, 1887-1968. Moskva, Meditsina, 1980. 79 p.

**Dawson, Anne, d. 1769**
Agnew LR: An 18th century amputation (Lady Anne Dawson). **Lancet** 1983 Nov 5;2(8358):1074-5

**Dawson, William, 1820-1899**
Cornell JF: From creation to evolution: Sir William Dawson and The idea of design in the nineteenth century. **J Hist Biol** 1983 Spring;16(1):137-70

**Dax, Gustave, 1815-1893**
Critchley M: Dax's law. **Int J Neurol** 1978;11(4):404-11

**Dax, Marc, 1770-1837**
Critchley M: Dax's law. **Int J Neurol** 1978;11(4):404-11

**Day, Paul Louis, 1899-1980**
Totter JR, Darby WJ: Paul Louis Day (1899-1980). A biographical sketch. **J Nutr** 1984 Feb;114(2):241-6

**Dayan, Moshe, 1915-**
Falk A: Moshe Dyan: the infantile roots of political action. **J Psychohist** 1983 Fall;11(2):271-88

**Dazille, Jean Barthélemy, 1733-1812**
Reusch C: Die medizinische Versorgung auf den französischen Westindischen Inseln im 18. Jhd. im Spiegel des Werkes von J.B. Dazille 'Les Maladies des Nègres, leurs causes, leur traitement, et les moyens de les prévenir.' Diss., Universität Düsseldorf. Düsseldorf, 1982. 117 p.

**Dean-Throckmorton, Jeannette, 1883-1963**
Schroeder MJ: Manuscript collections: The Jeannette Dean-Throckmorton papers. **Ann Iowa** 1979;44(7):551-4

**Dearborn, Henry, 1751-1829**
Agris J: 'Henry Dearborn'. Physician, soldier, civil servant, diplomat. **J Dermatol Surg Oncol** 1979 Sep;9(5):677

**Dearborn, J. G., fl. 1886**
Morer G: Naissance d'un vocable. **Hist Sci Med** 1984;18(2):165-71

**Dearin, John Joseph, ca. 1818-1890**
Hiller JK: John Joseph Dearin. In Dictionary of Canadian biography, 1881-1890. 1982;11:239-40.

**Debaisieux, Paul, 1886-1978**
Demal J: Paul Debaisieux, 1886-1978. In Florilège des Sciences en Belgique - II. Bruxelles, Académie Royale de Belgique, 1980. p. 617-23.

**DeBakey, Michael Ellis, 1908-**
A tribute: Michael E. DeBakey, M.D. **Compr Ther** 1984 Feb;10(2):3-5

**De Bap, Jean-César, 1718-1785**
Théodoridès J: L'abbé de Bap, curé de Sommières, et son prétendu remède antirabique. **Rev Hist Pharm (Paris)** 1979 Dec;26(243):269-79

**DeBeer, Gavin Rylands, 1899-1972**
Gershenowitz H: Gavin De Beer and the Neo-Lamarckians. **Indian J Hist Sci** 1978, reçu 1982;13(1):23-7

**Debray, Charles, 1907-1979**
Roux M: Eloge de Charles Debray, 1907-1979. **Bull Acad Natl Med (Paris)** 1979 Dec;163(9):897-906

**Debré, Robert, 1882–1978**
Bernard J: Robert Debré: l'humanisme et les académies. **Bull Acad Natl Med (Paris)** 1982 Dec;166(9):1281–4
Debré M: Robert Debré, réformateur. **Bull Acad Natl Med (Paris)** 1982 Dec;166(9):1295–303
Mande R: Robert Debré et la pédiatrie sociale. **Bull Acad Natl Med (Paris)** 1982 Dec;166(9):1275–9
Marie J: Robert Debré (1882–1978): l'homme, le médecin, le professeur. **Bull Acad Natl Med (Paris)** 1982 Dec;166(9):1257–64
Mercier P: L'oeuvre scientifique de Robert Debré. **Bull Acad Natl Med (Paris)** 1982 Dec;166(9):1285–94
Popescu V: Centenar Robert Debré. **Rev Pediatr Obstet Ginecol [Pediatr]** 1983 Apr–Jun;32(2):97–100
Thieffry S: La vie quotidienne avec Robert Debré, pionnier de la pédiatrie; le médecin d'enfants, le chef de service, le chef d'école. **Bull Acad Natl Med (Paris)** 1982 Dec;166(9):1265–77

**Déclat, Gilbert, 1827–1896**
Wrotnowska D: Lettres inédites de Gilbert Déclat à Louis Pasteur. **Hist Sci Med** 1982;16(2):115–23

**Dee, Arthur, 1579–1651**
Appleby JH: Dr. Arthur Dee: merchant and litigant. **Slav East Eur Rev** 1979;57(1):32–55

**Defoe, Daniel, 1660–1731**
Cone TE: Daniel Defoe on the deplorable effect of the great London plague of 1665 on women with child. **Pediatrics** 1981;67:221

**Dega, Wiktor, 1897?–**
Dega W: Zapiski do autobiografii moja droga zyciowa do wiedzy i zawodu. **Kwart Hist Nauki Tech** 1984;29(2):259–322
Marciniak W: Zagadnienia wrodzonego zwichni ęcia biodra w pracach prof. dr Wiktora Degi – z okazji 85 rocznicy urodzin. **Chir Narzadow Ruchu Ortop Pol** 1982;47(3):219–23

**De Gama Pinto, M. R., 1853–1945**
Blodi FC: Ophthalmology and philately: I. Ophthalmologist on stamps--M.R. de Gama Pinto (1853–1945). **Arch Ophthalmol** 1980 Jan;98(1):143

**Deigendesch, Johannes**
Hepding L: Das Rossarzneibuch des Scharfrichters Johannes Deigendesch von 1716. **DTW** 1983 Apr 6;90(4):147–50

**Déjerine, Joseph Jules, 1849–1917**
Valla JP: L'oeuvre psychothérapeutique de Déjerine. **Inf Psychiatr** 1978 Feb;54(2):171–8

**De la Quadra Family**
Figuerola JE, Figuerola I: La cuenta de medicinas administradas a la hija del Marques de la Quadra. **Bol Soc Esp Hist Farm** 1980 Mar–Jun;3(121–2)

**Delaby, Raymond, 1891–1958**
Bouriez J: Lens, trois savants oubliés: Auguste Behal, Amand Valeur, Raymond Delaby. [France], Société de recherches historiques de la région d'Henin-Carvin, [1981] 69 leaves.

**Delachaux, Armand, 1911–**
Hommage au professeur Armand Delachaux à l'occasion de son 70e anniversaire: **Soz Praventivmed** 1982 May;27(2–3):59–67

**Delage, Yves, 1854–1920**
Fischer JL: Yves Delage (1854–1920): l'epigenèse néo-lamarckienne contre la prédétermination weismannienne. **Rev Synth (Paris)** 1979;100(95–6):443–61

**Delagenière, Henry, 1858–1930**
Monod-Broca P: Henry Delagenière, 1858–1930. **Chirurgie** 1982;108(1):17–25

**Delano, Jane Arminda, 1862–1919**
Thompson ME: Sixty years of progress: nursing and the times in U. S. A. – and Vermont, 1919. An overview of nursing's accomplishment in World War I – under its chief – Jane A. Delano. **Vt Regist Nurse** 1979 Jul;:6–8

**Delany, Martin Robinson, 1812–1885**
Cameron S, Falk LA: Some black medical history: Dr. Martin R. Delany's Canadian years as medical practitioner and abolitionist (1856–1864). In: Congrès international d'histoire de la médecine, XXVe, Québec, 1976. Actes. Québec, 1977. p. 537–45.
Cash P: Pride, prejudice and politics. **Harv Med Alumni Bull** 1980 Dec;54(6):20–5
Kass AM, Kass EH: Doctors afield. Martin Delany, Thomas Hodgkin, and the Black Nationalist movement. **N Engl J Med** 1981 Sep 17;305(12):682–4
Kass AM: Dr Thomas Hodgkin, Dr Martin Delany, and the 'Return to Africa'. **Med Hist** 1983 Oct;27(4):373–93

**Delaunay, Paul, 1878–1958**
Fossard J: Un inédit d'un fondateur de la Société française d'histoire de la médecine, le docteur Paul Delaunay. **Hist Sci Med** 1981;15(4):305–6

**Delbrück, Max, 1906–1981**
Edgar RS: Max Delbrück. **Annu Rev Genet** 1982;16:501–5
Stent GS: Max Delbrück, 1906–1981. **Genetics** 1982 May;101(1):1–16

**Delgado, Honorio**
Saavedra A: Honorio Delgado y la psiquiatría Peruana. **Rev Neuropsiquiatr** 1980 Jun;43(2):67–86

**Delgado y Amestoy, Claudio, 1843–1916**
Martínez-Fortún y Foyo O: Dr. Claudio Delgado y su aportación al estudio de la fiebre amarilla. La Habana [Consejo Científico, Ministerio de la Salud Pública] 1967. 130 p.

**Delioux de Savignac, Joseph François, 1812–1876**
Niaussat PM: Delioux de Savignac et le traitement des dysenteries. In: Congrès National des Sociétés Savantes, 107e. Brest, 1982. Comptes Rendus, Paris, 1983. Section des Sciences, Fasc. IV. p. 299–309.

**Delius, Frederick, 1862–1934**
Wainapel SF: Frederick Delius: medical assessment. **NY State J Med** 1980 Nov;80(12):1886–7

**Delmedigo, Joseph Solomon, 1591–1655**
David M: Critical edition of Hippocrates' Aphorisms, translated into Hebrew by J. S. Delmedigo (1591–1655), sections VI–VIII (cont. and end). **Koroth** 1980 Jun;7(11–12):764–94
David M: Critical edition of Hippocrates' Aphorisms translated into Hebrew by J.S. Delmedigo (1591–1655), sections IV, V. **Koroth** 1979 Nov;7(9–10):680–709

**Delpech, Jacques Matthieu, 1777–1832**
Huard P: Jacques Delpech (1777–1832). In: Congrès National des Sociétés Savantes, 96e, Toulouse, 1971. Comptes Rendus. Paris, 1974. Histoire des Sciences, Tome 1. p. 99–105.
Peltier LF: The 'back school' of Delpech in Montpellier. **Clin Orthop** 1983 Oct;179:4–9

**Del Pozo, Efrén C., 1907–1979**
Guzmán-Flores C: El Doctor Efrén C. Del Pozo, Fisiólogo y Maestro. **Bol Estud Med Biol** 1980 Jul–Oct;31(3–4):116–26
Lozoya X: La herbolaria medicinal en Mexico y el Doctor Del Pozo. **Bol Soc Mex Hist Filos Med** 1980 Mar;3(30):11–6

**Del Río-Hortega, Pío, 1882–1945**
Ortiz Picón JM: Pío del Río Hortega. Un estudio biográfico. **Arch Neurobiol (Madr)** 1983 May–Jun;46(3):209–26

**Demich, V. F., 1858–1930**
Kvitnitskiĭ-Ryzhov IN: Vydaiushchiĭsia issledovatel' otechestvennoĭ narodnoĭ meditsiny V. F. Demich (1858–1930). **Sov Zdravookhr** 1982;7:70–4

**Democritus, ca. 460–ca. 370 B.C.**
López Férez JA: Algunos datos sobre la influencia de la teoria embriologica de Democrito en el corpus hippocraticum. Gemelos y abortos. **Asclepio** 1981;33:379–90
López Férez JA: Ideas embriologicas de Democrito. **Asclepio** 1982;34:317–26
López Férez JA: El falso Demócrito y los escritos medicos pseudodemocritos. **An Hist Antigua Mediev** 1977–80;20:175–87

**De Morogan, Campbell, 1811–1876**
Rosser EM: Campbell De Morgan and his spots. **Ann R Coll Surg Engl** 1983 Jul;65(4):266–8

**De Morti, Mark**
Tomashevich GV, ed: Some of the incidents in the life of Mark De Mortie. **Afro-Am NY Life Hist** 1979;3(1):61–71

**Demosthenes, 385?–322 B.C.**
Wooten CW: Unnoticed medical language in Demosthenes. **Hermes** 1979;107:157–60

**Dénéchaud, Jacques, 1728–1810**
Desjardins E: Jacques Dénéchaud. In Dictionary of Canadian biography, 1801 to 1820. Volume 5, 1983. p. 248–9.

**Denigès, Georges, 1859–1951**
Casaux-Bussière M: Georges Denigès (1859-1951). Essai biographique. Thèse, Bordeaux II, 1981. 374 leaves.

**Denis, Jean Baptiste, 1640?–1704**
Farr AD: The first human blood transfusion. **Med Hist** 1980 Apr;24(2):143–62

**Dentz, S. N., Jr., 1817–1872**
Wolff JD: Over chloroform-narcose en een Nederlandse pionier (S.N. Dentz Jr.). **Ned Tijdschr Geneeskd** 1981 Oct 17;125(42):1719–22

**DePauw, Cornelius**
Michel D: Corps sauvages, corps étranges. **Dix-Huit Siecle** 1977;9:27–38

**Déplanche, Emile, 1824–1875**
McKee ME, McKee HS: E. Vieillard et E. Deplanche, deux grands botanistes collecteurs en Nouvelle-Calédonie. **Hist Nat** 1980–81;17–18:49–68

**De Quervain, Johann Friedrich, 1868–1940**
De Quervain's stenosing tenovaginitis: Fritz de Quervain, 1868–1940: **Orthop Nurs** 1982 Sep–Oct;1(5):24–5

**De Quincey, Thomas, 1785–1859**
Schiller F: Thomas de Quincey's lifelong addiction. **Perspect Biol Med** 1976 Autumn;20(1):131–41
Stäuble-Lipman Wulf, M: De Quincey, Baudelaire, e i 'Paradisi

artificiali'. **Nuova Antologia** 1972;514(2054):245-54

**De Ribera, J., 1588-1656**
Sullivan EJ: Art in dermatopathology. Jusepe de Ribera. An interpreter of the skin through art. **Am J Dermatopathol** 1979 Summer;1(2):159-62

**Descartes, René, 1596-1650**
Ahlström CG, Ekström P, Persson O: Cartesius' kranium. **Sydsven Medicinhist Sallsk Arsskr** 1983;:23-50
Arbini R: Did Descartes have a philosophical theory of sense perception? **J Hist Philos** 1983;21:317-37
Blom JJ, ed: Descartes, his moral philosophy and psychology. Hassocks, Sussex, Harvester Press, 1978. xxi, 288 p.
Carter RB: Descartes' medical philosophy. The organic solution to the mind-body problem. Baltimore, London, Johns Hopkins University Press, 1983. xi, 301 p.
Carter RB: Gilbert and Descartes: the science of conserving the compound body. **Z Allg Wissenschaftstheorie** 1982;13(2):224-33
Farina P: Il corpuscolarismo di Henricus Regius: materialismo e medicina in un cartesiano olandese del Seicento. In: Ricerche sull'atomismo del Seicento. Florence: La Nuova Italia, 1977. p. 119-78.
Gysel C: Cartesianisme en tandheelkunde bij Henricus Regius (1598--1679--1979). **Rev Belge Med Dent** 1979;34(2):213-22
Gysel C: Odontologie et cartesianisme naissant (1637--1650). **Rev Belge Med Dent** 1979;34(2):223-30
Gysel C: Odontoiatria e cartesianesimo nascente (1637-1650). **Dent Cadmos** 1980 Mar;48(3):53-5
Gysel C: Les implications cartésiennes de la nosologie bucco-dentaire de Pierre Fauchard (1678-1761-1978). **Rev Belge Med Dent** 1979;34(3):313-20
Gysel C: Jan Swammerdam (1637-1680-1980), zijn Cartesianisme en de fysiologie van het kauwstelsel (II). **Ned Tijdschr Tandheelkd** 1981 Jul-Aug;88(7-8):274-7
Gysel C: Jan Swammerdam (1637-1680-1980), zijn Cartesianism en de fysiologie van het kauwstelsel (I). **Ned Tijdschr Tandheelkd** 1981 Jun;88(6):238-41
Gysel C: Jan Swammerdam (1637- 1680- 1980), zijn Cartesianisme en de fysiologie van het kauwstelsel (SLOT). **Ned Tijdschr Tandheelkd** 1981 Nov;88(11):414-6
Legrenzi P, Sonino M: Fisica ingenua a teoria cartesiana degli urti. **Stor Crit Psicol** 1984;5(2):213-28
Limbrick E: Franciscus Sanchez 'Scepticus': un médecin philosophe précurseur de Descartes (1550-1623). **Renaiss Reformation** 1982;18:264-72
Lindeboom GA: Descartes and medicine. Amsterdam, Rodopi, 1979. 134 p. (Nieuwe Nederlandse Bijdragen tot de Geschiedenis der Geneeskunde, No. 1).
Locke D: Mind, matter, and the 'Meditations'. **Mind** 1981;90:343-66
Perret L: René Descartes--drottning Kristinas Cartesius--filosof, matematiker och medicinsk läromästare. **Nord Medicinhist Arsb** 1981;:52-8
Pflug G: Descartes und das mechanistische Menschenbild. **Medizinhist J** 1982;17(1/2):3-19
Reed ES: Descartes' corporeal ideas hypothesis and the origin of scientific psychology. **Rev Metaphys** 1982;35:731-52
Stone MH: Modern concepts of emotion as prefigured in Descartes' 'Passions of the Soul'. **J Am Acad Psychoanal** 1980;8:473-95
Sutton GV: A science for a polite society: Cartesian natural philosophy in Paris during the reigns of Louis XIII and XIV. Ph.D. Diss., Princeton University. Princeton, 1982. xi, 481 leaves.
Tomaselli S: The first person: Descartes, Locke and mind-body dualism. **Hist Sci** 1984;22(pt 2):185-205
Trevisani F: Un corrispondente di Cartesio: alcune note su Lazare Meyssonnier (1611/12-1673), medico e astrologo lionese e sulla sua Belle Magie (1669). **Hist Philos Life Sci** 1979;1(2):285-308
Vetter T: Louis de la Forge (1632-1667?) angevin et fidèle adepte de la physiologie cartésienne. In: Congrès National des Sociétés Savantes, 93e, Tours, 1968. Comptes Rendus. Paris, 1971. Section des Sciences, Tome II. p. 31-50.
Weckowicz TE, Liebel-Weckowicz H: Typologies of the theory of behaviorism since Descartes. **Sudhoffs Arch** 1982;66(2):129-51
Wilson C: Sensation and explanation: the problem of consciousness in Descartes. **Nat Syst** 1982;4:151-65
Yolton JW: Perceptual cognition with Descartes. **Stud Cartesiana** 1981;2:63-83

**Deschiens, Robert, 1893-**
Lamy LH: Sur un point particulier de la contribution de Robert Deschiens à la connaissance des amibes. **Bull Soc Pathol Exot Filiales** 1978;71 Spec No:502-8
Séance du 11 octobre 1978: Séance solennelle à la mémoire du Professeur Robert Deschiens (Professeur et Chef de Service honoraire à l'Institut Pasteur, Membre de l'Académie Nationale de Médecine, Secrétaire Général de la Société de Pathologie Exotique). **Bull Soc Pathol Exot Filiales** 1978;71 Spec No:499-511

**De Schweinitz, Georg Edmund, 1858-1938**
McDonald PR: Evolution of cataract surgery since the deSchweinitz era. **Ophthalmic Surg** 1979 May;10(5):44-52

**Desfontaines, René, 1750?-1833**
Laissus J: La succession de Le Monnier au Jardin du Roi: Antoine-Laurent de Jussieu et René Louiche-Desfontaines. In: Congrès National des Sociétés Savantes, 91e, Rennes, 1966. Comptes Rendus. Paris, 1967. Section des Sciences, Tome 1. p. 137-52.
Laissus Y: Lettres inédites de René Desfontaines à Louis-Guillaume le Monnier, conservées à la Bibliothèque centrale du Muséum national d'histoire naturelle. In: Congrès National des Sociétés Savantes, 91e, Rennes, 1966. Comptes Rendus. Paris, 1967. Section des Sciences, Tome 1. p. 153-69.

**Desgenettes, René Nicolas Dufriche, 1762-1837**
Egeblad K: Militaerkirurgen Dominique Jean Larrey: Om pesten i felttoget til Aegypten og Syrien 1798-1801. **Dan Medicinhist Arbog** 1979;132-59

**Despars, Jacques, 1380-1458**
Jacquart D: Le regard d'un médecin sur son temps: Jacques Despars (1380?-1458). **Bibl Ec Chartres** 1980;138:35-86

**Destot, Etienne Auguste Joseph, 1864-1918**
Arnulf G: A propos de la naissance de la radiologie en France. L'oeuvre d'Etienne Destot à Lyon. **Bull Acad Natl Med (Paris)** 1981 Oct;165(7):955-9

**De Théis, Constance Marie, 1767-1845**
Huard P, Théodoridès J: Jean-Baptiste Pipelet (1759-1823), Constance de Théis (1767-1845), Josef de Salm-Dyck (1773-1861) ou le chirurgien, la poétesse et le botaniste. In: Congrès National des Sociétés Savantes, 93e, Tours, 1968. Comptes Rendus. Paris, 1971. Section des Sciences, Tome II. p. 127-36.

**De Trey, Emil, 1846-1898**
Odontoiatria del passato: La storia di De Trey. **Dent Cadmos** 1983 Mar;51(3):75-81

**Deutsch, Felix, 1884-1964**
Roazen P: A note on the Vienna Psychoanalytic Society: Felix Deutsch's letters, 1923 and 1935. **J Hist Behav Sci** 1984 Oct;20(4):359-62

**Deutsch, Helene, 1884-1982**
Buckley NL: Women psychoanalysts and the theory of feminine development: a study of Karen Horney, Helene Deutsch, and Marie Bonaparte. Ph.D. Diss., University of California. Los Angeles, 1982. 178 p.
Roazen P: Two cases of induced insanity. Helene Deutsch, Cambridge, Mass. **Int J Psychoanal** 1981;62(pt 2):139-50
Roazen P: Anorexia nervosa: Helene Deutsch, M.D. **Bull Menninger Clin** 1981 Nov;45(6):499-501
Roazen P: A note on the Vienna Psychoanalytic Society: Felix Deutsch's letters, 1923 and 1935. **J Hist Behav Sci** 1984 Oct;20(4):359-62
Roazen P: The menopause. By Helene Deutsch. **Int J Psychoanal** 1984;65(Pt 1):55-62

**Deventer, Hendrik van, 1651-1724**
Benedek-Jaszmann LJ: Hendrik van Deventer (1651-1724); the silversmith who became the co-founder of modern obstetrics. **Orvostort Kozl** 1980;89-91(26 no 1-3):241-9

**Devoto, Luigi, 1864-1936**
Malamani A: Medicina ottocentesca e medicina del lavoro: l'opera scientifico-sociale di Luigi Devoto a Pavia. **G Ital Med Lav** 1983 Jan;5(1):1-16

**Dezeimeris, Jean-Eugène, 1799-1852**
Dumaître P: Jean Dezeimeris, médecin et historien (1799-1852). In: Congrès National des Sociétés Savantes, 104e, Bordeaux, 1979. Comptes Rendus. Paris, 1979. Section des Sciences, Fasc. IV. p. 69-80.

**Dhur, Lorenz, b. ca.1515**
Kuchowicz Z, Ojrzyński J: Czy twardowski był niemcem? **Przegl Hist** 1978;69(2):309-15

**Diad'kovskiĭ, Iustin Evdokimovich, 1784-1841**
Belitskaia EI: Systema morborum (klassifikatsiia bolezneĭ) I. I. Diad'kovskogo (k 150-letiiu opublikovaniia). **Sov Zdravookhr** 1983;5:63-6
Katsnel'bogen AG: Delo o rassmotrenii lektsiĭ I. E. Diad'kovskogo. **Klin Med (Mosk)** 1981;59(4):116-8

**Diamond, Hugh Welch, 1809-1886**
Burrows A, Schumacher I: Doktor Diamonds Bildnisse von Geisteskranken. Transl. of Doctor Diamond's portraits of the insane. Frankfurt am Main, Syndikat, 1979. 159 p.

**Diamond, Louis Klein, 1902-**
Pochedly C: Dr. James A. Wolff. I. Early progress in treatment of Rh hemolytic disease. **Am J Pediatr Hematol Oncol** 1984 Fall;6(3):319-23

**Diaz del Castillo, Bernal, ca. 1498-ca. 1568**
Ehlers AP. Medizinisches und Pharmazeutisches in Bernal Diaz del Castillos, 'Historia verdadera de la conquista de la Nueva-España,' Madrid, 1632. Diss. Düsseldorf, 1980. 118 p.

**Díaz, Eloísa, 1866-1950**
Costa-Casaretto C: Dra. Eloísa Díaz. Centenario del ingreso de la mujer chilena al estudio de las profesiones universitarias. **Rev Med Chil** 1981 Apr;109(4):355-66

**Díaz Rodríguez, Manuel, 1871–1927**
Bonadies A: Manuel Diaz Rodriguez: maestro del estilismo y medico. **Rev Soc Venez Hist Med** 1969–71;17–19(31–33):109–15

**Dibner, Bern**
Holden C: Bern Dibner: science bibliophile. **Science** 1980 May 30;208(4447):1012–4

**Dick, Elisha, 1762?–1825**
Schneck JM: Elisha Dick, Benjamin Rush, and George Washington. **JAMA** 1983 Jul 8;250(2):164

**Dick, Gladys Rowena Henry, 1881–1963**
Rubin LP: Gladys Rowena Henry Dick. In: Notable American women. The modern period. Cambridge, Mass., Belknap-Harvard Univ. Press, 1980. 4:191–2.

**Dickens, Charles, 1812–1870**
Bernard CA: Dickens and Victorian dream theory. In Paradis J, Postlewait T, ed: Victorian science and Victorian values: literary perspectives. New York, New York Academy of Sciences, 1981. p. 197–216.
Charles DC, Charles LA: Charles Dickens' old people. **Int J Aging Hum Dev** 1979–80;10(3):231–7
Dauber LG: Dickens and doctors; physicians in fiction of Charles Dickens. **NY State J Med** 1981 Sep;81(10):1522–6
Jacoby E: Der Aufstieg ins Bürgertum und sein Preis. Charles Dickens als Beispiel. **Psyche (Stuttg)** 1982 Jul;36(7):609–29
Johnson JP: Herbert Hoover and David Copperfield: a tale of two childhoods. **J Psychohist** 1980 Spring;7(4):467–75
Smithers DW: Dicken's doctors. Oxford, New York, Pergamon, 1979. xiii, 111 p.
Stetz MD: Charles Dickens and 'The Sanatorium': an unpublished letter and manuscript. **Dickensian** 1980;76(390)22–30
Tucker WS: Osler and sleep apnea. **Arch Intern Med** 1984 May;144(5):1085

**Dickinson, Emily, 1830–1886**
Burbick J: Emily Dickinson and the revenge of the nerves. **Womens Stud** 1980;7(1–2):95–109
Wand M, Sewall RB: 'Eyes be blind, heart be still': a new perspective on Emily Dickinson's eye problem. **N Engl Q** 1979;52(3):400–6

**Dickson, David James, 1780–1850**
Lattimore MI: Sir David James Hamilton Dickson, MD (1780–1850). **J R Nav Med Serv** 1981;67(2):92–100

**Dickson, Earle Ensign, 1892–1961**
Sweeney JK: Earle Ensign Dickson. In Dictionary of American biography, 1961–1965. Suppl. 7, 1981. p. 182–3.

**Dickson, John Robinson, 1819–1882**
Angus MS: John Robinson Dickson. In Dictionary of Canadian biography, 1881–1890. 1982;11:263–4.

**Diderot, Denis, 1713–1784**
Buffat M: Diderot, le corps le la machine. **Rev Sci Hum** 1982–3;186–7:185–97
Gregory RL: French without fears: Denis Diderot. **Perception** 1983;12(5):509–12
Mayer J: Quand Diderot corrige Diderot: l'élaboration des Eléments de physiologie. In J. Proust, ed: Recherches nouvelles sur quelques écrivains des lumières (II). Montpellier, Univ. Paul Valéry, 1979. p. 73–129.

**Dieck, Wilhelm, 1867–1935**
Hoffmann-Axthelm W: Wilhelm Dieck--Lehrer, Forscher und Standespolitiker. **Quintessenz** 1984 Feb;35(2):365–9

**Dieffenbach, Johann Friedrich, 1792–1847**
Genschorek W: Wegbereiter der Chirurgis: Johann Friedrich Dieffenbach, Theodor Billroth. Leipzig, Hirzel, Teubner, 1983. 252 p.

**Diehl, Harold Sheely, 1891–1973**
Garfinkel L: A tribute to Harold S. Diehl (1891-1973) - changing patterns of smoking and disease. **CA** 1981;31:114–9

**Dièreville, fl. 1699–1711**
Rousseau J: Dièreville. In Dictionary of Canadian biography, 1701 to 1740. Volume 2, 1969. p. 188–9.

**Dietl, Jósef, 1804–1878**
Berezowski S: Joseph Dietl, a great Polish physician of the 19th century. In International Congress of the History of Medicine. 26th, Plovdiv, 1978. Actes du Congress. Sofia, 1981. Volume II. p. 64–5.
Kucharz E: The life and achievements of Joseph Dietl. **Clio Med** 1981 Sep;16(1):25–35
Skulimowski M, Sliwinski S: Joseph Dietl's contributions to European medicine development. In International Congress of the History of Medicine. 26th, Plovdiv, 1978. Actes du Congress. Sofia, 1981. Volume II. p. 96–7.
Stevenson LG: Joseph Dietl, William Osler and the definition of therapeutic nihilism. In Ganzinger K, Skopec M, Wyklicky H, ed: Festschrift für Erna Lesky zum 70. Geburtstag. Wien, Brüder Hollinek, 1981. p. 149–52.

**Dieulafoy, Georges, 1839–1911**
Huard P, Imbault-Huart MJ: Le professeur Georges Dieulafoy (1839-1911). In: Congrès National des Sociétés Savantes, 96e, Toulouse, 1971. Comptes Rendus. Paris, 1974. Histoire des Sciences, Tome 1. p. 201–5.

**Diller, Hans, 1905–1977**
Lichtenthaeler C: [A tribute to Hans Diller.] **Hermes** 1979;109:270–86

**Dimsdale, Thomas, 1712–1800**
Griffiths J: Doctor Thomas Dimsdale, and smallpox in Russia. The variolation of the Empress Catherine the Great. **Bristol Med Chir J** 1984 Jan;99(369):14–6

**Dionis, Pierre, 1643–1718**
Rullière R: Les morts subites à la Cour de Louis XIV de 1690 à 1709, d'après Pierre Dionis. **Hist Sci Med** 1984;18(1):19–24

**Dionne quintuplets**
Kalisch BJ, Kalisch PA: The Dionne quintuplets legacy: establishing the 'good doctor and his loyal nurse' image in American culture. **Nurs Health Care** 1984 May;5(5):242–51

**Dioscorides, Pedanius, of Anazarbos**
Hein WH: Ein arabisches Apothekeninterieur vom Jahre 1222. **Pharm Ztg** 1979 Jan 4;124(1):3–4
Riddle JM: Pseudo-Dioscorides' Ex herbis femininis and early medieval medical botany. **J Hist Biol** 1981 Spring;14(1):43–81
Riddle JM: Dioscorides. In Cranz FE, Kristeller PO, ed: Catalogus translationum et commentariorum: mediaeval and Renaissance Latin translations and commentaries. Annotated lists and guides. Vol. IV. Washington, D.C., Catholic University of America Press, 1980. p. 1–143.

**Diósszilágyi, Samuel, 1882–**
Somló G: Megemlékezés Diósszilágyi Sámuelröl Makón. **Orv Hetil** 1983 Jul 10;124(28):1705–6
Szállási A: Diósszilágyi Sámuel, az írók orvosa és az orvosok írója. **Orv Hetil** 1981 Jun 14;122(24):1467–72

**Disney, Walter E., 1901–1966**
Knudson KG: Walt Disney, dentistry and the armed forces during World War II. **Bull Hist Dent** 1984 Oct;32(2):112–7

**Disraeli, Benjamin, 1804–1881**
Whitfield AG: Disraeli's doctors. **J R Coll Physicians Lond** 1980 Jul;14(3):202–4

**Diterikhs, Mikhail Konstantinovich, 1874–**
Galin LL: Shina Diterikhsa. **Feldsher Akush** 1983 Nov;48(11):46–8

**Divini, Eustachio, 1610–1685**
Bonelli ML, Helden A van: Divini and Campani: a forgotten chapter in the history of the Academia del Cimento. **Ann Ist Mus Stor Sci Fir** 1981;6(1):3–176

**Dix, Dorothea Lynde, 1802–1887**
Greenstone JD: Dorothea Dix and Jane Addams: from transcendentalism to pragmatism in American social reform. **Soc Serv Rev** 1979;53(4):527–59

**Diya Muhammad Masud Rashid Zangi Umar Ghaznavi**
Muhammad Abad al-Wahab Zahuri: A medical treatise of the time of King Muhammad Tughlaq. **Stud Hist Med** 3(3):173–77, Sep 79

**Dizy, Marguerite, 1663–ca. 1730**
Vachon A: Marguerite Dizy. In Dictionary of Canadian biography, 1701 to 1740. Volume 2, 1969. p. 189–90.

**Djahiz, 776–868**
Bel-Haj Mahmoud N: La psychologie des animaux chez les arabes, notamment à travers le kitab al-hayawan de Djahiz. Paris, Klincksieck, 1977. xxiii, 231 p. (Etudes arabes et islamiques, Série 3; Etudes et documents, 8).

**Długosz, Jan**
Dobrzyniecki Z: 'Dzieje Polskie' Jana Długosza jako źródło do dziejów medycyny w Polsce w XIV i XV w. **Arch Hist Med (Warsz)** 1981;44(3/4):265–76

**Dobbs, Harriet, 1808–1887**
Angus MS: Harriet (Cartwright) Dobbs. In Dictionary of Canadian biography, 1881–1890. 1982;11:265–6.

**Döblin, Alfred, 1878–1957**
Neumann H: Leben, wissenschaftliche Studien, Krankheiten und Tod Alfred Döblins. St. Michael [Austria], Bläschke, 1982. 110 p.

**Dobroslavin, Aleksei Petrovich, 1842–1889**
Vavilin PA: Rol' A. P. Dobroslavina v stanovlenii otechestvennoĭ gigienicheskoĭ nauki (k 90-letiiu so dnia smerti). **Gig Sanit** 1980 Mar;(3):45–7
Vavilin PA: Gigienicheskie prognozy v trudakh A. P. Dobroslavina. **Gig Sanit** 1980 May;(5):25–9
Vavilin PA: A. P. Dobroslavin--ego obshchestvennaia i prakticheskaia deiatel'nost' (k 140-letiiu so dnia rozdeniia). **Gig Sanit** 1982 Sep;(9):53–6

**Dobzhansky, Theodosius Grigorievich, 1900–1975**
Fuller MB: Theodosius Dobzhansky Papers. **Mendel Newsl** 1980 Jun;(18):1–8
Lewontin RC, Moore JA, Provine WB, et al: Dobzhansky's genetics of natural populations, I–XLIII. New York, Columbia University Press, 1981. xiv, 942 p. Includes Provine WB: Origins of the Genetics of natural populations series, p. 1–76.

**Dock, George, 1860–1951**
Bean WB: George Dock: excerpts from the 34th Dock lecture. **South Med J** 1979 Mar;72(3):348–50

**Dock, Lavinia Lloyd, 1858–1956**
James JW: Lavinia Lloyd Dock. In: Notable American women. The modern period. Cambridge, Mass., Belknap-Harvard Univ. Press, 1980. 4:195–8.
Trolander JA: Lavinia Lloyd Dock. In Dictionary of American Biography, Suppl. 6, 1956–1960. p. 166–8, 1980.

**Dodds, Edward Charles, 1899–1973**
Sporn MB: Edward Charles Dodds: diethylstilbestrol. **Cancer Res** 1983 Sep;43(9):preceding 3981

**Dodoens, Rembert, 1517–1585**
Dodoens R: Histoire des plantes. Traduction française, suivie du Petit recueil, auquel est contenue la description d'aucunes gommes et liqueurs etc., par Charles de l'Escluse (1557). Fac-similé avec introduction, commentaires et la concordance avec la terminologie scientifique moderne, par J.-E. Opsomer. Bruxelles, Centre National d'Histoire des Sciences, 1978. 78, 584 p. (Publications du Centre National d'Histoire des Sciences, V).

**Dogel, Valentin Aleksandrovich, 1882–**
Smirnova KV: O razvitii ėkologicheskoĭ parazitologii v Kazakhstane. **Parazitologiia** 1982 Jan–Feb;16(1):85–7

**Dogiel, Valentin Aleksandrovich, 1882–1955**
Gusev AV: Commemorating the 100th birthday of Valentin Aleksandrovich Dogiel (1882–1955). **J Parasitol** 1982 Dec;68(6):1188–9

**Dohrn, Anton, 1840–1909**
Charles Darwin, 1809–1882; Anton Dohrn, 1840–1909: Correspondence. Napoli, Macchiaroli, 1982. 118 p.
Sloan JB: The founding of the Naples Table Association for promoting scientific research by women, 1897. **Signs** 1978;4(1):208–16

**Dolliner, Jan, 1808–**
Berezowski S: Jan Dolliner--chirurg bocheński (przyczynek do historii zdobywania doktoratów chirurgii w Uniwersytecie Jagiellońskim). **Pol Tyg Lek** 1979 Aug 27;34(35):1403–5

**Domashiavichius, A. I.**
Liepa A: Ikh imena nosiat meditsinskie uchilischcha. **Med Sestra** 1980 Sep;37(9):54–6

**D'Ombrain, Arthur, d. 1963**
Hertzberg R: Three great ophthalmologists (E. C. Temple-Smith, Norman Gregg, Arthur D'Ombrain). **Med J Aust** 1979 Dec 15;2(12):649–50

**Dominik, Małgorzata, 1941–1979**
Drozdowski P, Fortuna D, Nieniewska M, et al: Dr med. Małgorzata Dominik (1941–1979). **Psychiatr Pol** 1980 Sep–Oct;14(5):549–54

**Donáth, Gyula**
Szállási A: Donath Gyula és a Klinikai Füzetek. **Orv Hetil** 1984 Apr 15;125(16):960–3

**Donne, John, 1573–1631**
Hawkins A: Two pathographies: a study in illness and literature. **J Med Philos** 1984 Aug;9(3):231–52
Nelson TG: Death, dung, the devil, and worldly delights: a metaphysical conceit in Harington, Donne, and Herbert. **Stud Philol** 1979 Summer;76(3):272–87

**Donovan, John Charles, d. 1976**
Wilbush J: Climacteric symptom formation: Donovan's contribution. **Maturitas** 1981 Aug;3(2):99–105

**Dooley, Thomas Anthony, 1927–1961**
Blantz TE: Thomas Anthony Dooley. In Dictionary of American biography, 1961–1965. Suppl. 7, 1981. p. 190–1.

**Doolin, William, 1887–1962**
Lyons JB: Letters to an editor. The William Doolin Memorial Lecture. **Ir Med J** 1980 Sep;73(9):323–30
Walsh J: Who was William Doolin? **Ir Med J** 1983 Oct;76(10):436–7

**Doolittle, Hilda, 1886–1961**
DuPlessis RB, Friedman SS: 'Woman is perfect': H. D.'s debate with Freud. **Feminist Stud** 1981;7(3):407–30

**Dordevic, Vladan, 1844–1930**
Dragić M: Dr. Vladan Djordjević i zakon o zaštiti narodnog zdravlja u Srbiji iz 1881. godine. **Srp Arh Celok Lek** 1982 Jun;110(6):791–8
Grujić V: Nekolike korespondentne veze ismedju Vladana Djordjevića i Valtazara Bogišića. **Srp Ark Celok Lek** 1981 Jan;109(1):161–8
Krajinović S: Povodom stogodišnjice jednog izveštaja dr Vladana Djordjevića objavljenog y 'Srpskom Arhivu' 1883. godine. **Srp Arh Celok Lek** 1983 Jul;111(7):1005–8

**Dorn, Harold Fred, 1906–1963**
Henson PM: Harold Fred Dorn. In Dictionary of American biography, 1961–1965. Suppl. 7, 1981. p. 191–3.

**Doroshevskiĭ, Nikolai Antonovich, 1857–1910**
Popushoĭ EP, Ioksa VA: N. A. Doroshevskiĭ – peredovoĭ vrach, uchastnik revoliutsionne-demokraticheskogo dvizheniia. **Sov Zdravookhr** 1982;(11):55–7

**Dorsey, John Morris, 1900–1978**
Dorsey JM: University Professor John M. Dorsey. Detroit, Wayne State University Press, 1980. 282 p.

**Dorvault, François Laurent Marie, 1815–1879**
Boussel P: Dorvault, sa vie et son oeuvre. Honfleur [France], Editions de la porte verte, 1979. 301 p.
Cotereau Y: L'"Officine' de Dorvault. **Rev Hist Pharm (Paris)** 1980 Jun;27(245):95–107
Folch Jou G: L'influence de Dorvault en Espagne. **Rev Hist Pharm (Paris)** 1980 Jun;27(245):109–18
Hossard J: Une rencontre inattendue: Flaubert et Dorvault. **Rev Hist Pharm (Paris)** 1980 Jun;27(245):119–22
Julien P: Remarque sur l'édition 1936 de 'l'Officine' de Dorvault. **Rev Hist Pharm (Paris)** 1982 Mar;29(252):37–8
Mory B: Dorvault et la 'Pharmacie centrale de France.' **Rev Hist Pharm (Paris)** 1980 Jun;27(245):79–90

**Dosios, Anastase Andrei Periclis, 1900–1974**
Cortez P, Sărmăşeanu-Cortez ML: Un psihiatru în căutarea propriului său destin. Dr. Anastse Andrei Periclis Dosis (1900–1974). **Rev Med Interna [Neurol Psihiatr]** 1980 Jul–Sep;25(3):231–7

**Dostoevskii, Fedor Mikhaĭlovich, 1821–1881**
Brunclík J: Freud o dostojevském – či naopak. **Cas Lek Cesk** 1982 Aug 13;121(32):1015–6
Gastaut H: New comments on the epilepsy of Fyodor Dostoevsky. **Epilepsia** 1984 Aug;25(4):408–11
Miksanek T: Dostoevsky's The Idiot and psychic disorders in epilepsy. **Perspect Biol Med** 1982 Winter;25(2):231–7
Retamal P: Consideraciones psicopatológicas sobre el diagnóstico de la enfermedad de Fedor Dostoyevski. **Actas Luso Esp Neurol Psiquiatr** 1983 May–Jun;11(3):231–4
Rice JL: Dostoevsky's medical history: diagnosis and dialectic. **Russ Rev** 1983;42(2):131–61
Skvortsov VI, Skvortsova AI: F. M. Dostoevskiĭ i meditsina. **Klin Med (Mosk)** 1982 Feb;60(2):112–6
Voskuil PH: The epilepsy of Fyodor Mikhailovitch Dostoevsky (1821–1881). **Epilepsia** 1983 Dec;24(6):658–67

**Doué, Pierre-Alphonse, 1832–1895**
Servat A, Servat C: Pierre-Alphonse Doué, médecin de marine, médecin major de 'l'Aigle' à l'inauguration du canal de Suez. **Med Armees** 1981;9:453–68

**Doughty, Charles Montagu, 1843–1926**
James T: Medicine in Arabia Deserta. **Adler Mus Bull** 1981;7(2):13–6

**Douglas, Claude Gordon, 1882–1963**
Cunningham DJ: Claude Gordon Douglas. In Dictionary of national biography, 1961–1970. Suppl. 8, 1981. p. 303–4.

**Douglas, George Mellis, 1809?–1864**
Swinton WE: George Mellis Douglas: typhus and tragedy. **Can Med Assoc J** 1981 Dec 1;125(11):1284–6

**Douglas, James, 1675–1742**
Brock CH: James Douglas (1675–1742), botanist. **J Soc Bibliogr Nat Hist** 1979 Apr;9(2):137–45

**Douglas, James, 1800–1886**
Leblond S: James Douglas. In Dictionary of Canadian biography, 1881–1890. 1982;11:271–2.
Leblond S: Le Dr James Douglas, de Québec, remonté le Nil en 1860–61. **Cah Dix** 1979;42:101–23

**Douglass, William, ca. 1691–1752**
C[one] TE: William Douglass on the first reported cases of scarlet fever in New England, 1736. **Pediatrics** 1981;68:230

**Doull, James Angus, 1889–1963**
Brandt AM: James Angus Doull. In Dictionary of American biography, 1961–1965. Suppl. 7, 1981. p. 194–5.

**Doulton, Henry, d. 1897**
Haugh MC: The Doulton story (Henry Doulton). **Nurs Times** 1979 Jul 19;75(29):1207–8

**Dover, Thomas, 1662–1742**
Monk BE: Thomas Dover, physician and pirate. **J R Coll Physicians Lond** 1982 Jan;16(1):60–1

**Dow, Margaret Cornelius**
Ingells DT: Miss Cora Dow. **Cinci Hist Soc Bull** 1982;40(3):151–66

**Down, John Langdon Haydon, 1828–1896**
Gustavson KH: Mannen bakom syndromet: John Down. Banade väg för den kliniska kromosomforskningen. **Lakartidningen** 1984 May 30;81(22):2261–3

**Doyen, Eugene Louis, 1859–1916**
Brahma B, Singh M: The man behind the name: Eugene Louis Doyen 1859–1916. **NATNEWS** 1981 Dec;18(12):14

**Doyle, Arthur Conan, 1859–1930**
Aronson ME: Sherlock Holmes, father of forensic pathology. **Trans Stud Coll Physicians Phila** 1978 Jul;45(5):258–61
Beerman H: Sherlock Holmes and medical history. **Trans Stud Coll Physicians Phila** 1978 Jul;45(5):243–8
Dirckx JH: Doctor Watson's brothers. **Pharos** 1981 Summer;44(3):24–7
Foster R: United States place names and Sherlock Holmes.

**Trans Stud Coll Physicians Phila** 1978 Jul;45(5):249-51
Gabriel A: Sir Arthur Conan Doyle: to see and to be seen. **Bull Menninger Clin** 1982 Nov;46(6):530-8
Ginzburg C: Morelli, Freud and Sherlock Holmes: clues and scientific method. **Hist Workshop J** 1980;9:5-36
Hart ED: Conan Doyle as rheumatologist. **Ann Rheum Dis** 1982 Aug;41(4):437-8
Key JD, Rodin AE: William Osler and Arthur Conan Doyle versus the antivivisectionists: some lessons from history for today. **Mayo Clin Proc** 1984 Mar;59(3):189-96
Kittle CF: Sir Arthur Conan Doyle--physician and detective. **Proc Inst Med Chic** 1981 Jan-Mar;34(1):7-11
Lasky II: A most benevolent Victorian (Sir Arthur Conan Doyle). **Md State Med J** 1982 Dec;31(12):22-4
Miller WH: The habit of Sherlock Holmes. **Trans Stud Coll Physicians Phila** 1978 Jul;45(5):252-7
Rodin AE: Autoexperimentation with a drug by Arthur Conan Doyle. **J Hist Med Allied Sci** 1980 Oct;35(4):426-30
Rodin AE, Key JD: Arthur Conan Doyle's thesis on tabes dorsalis. **JAMA** 1982 Feb 5;247(5):646-50
Rodin AE, Key JD: Assessment and significance of Arthur Conan Doyle's medical writings. **South Med J** 1982 Nov;75(11):1392-9
Sugar O: Doyle on tabes dorsalis. **JAMA** 1982 May 21;247(19):2659-60

**Dragendorff, Johann Georg Noël, 1836-1898**
Jack DB: Dastardly deeds at Dorpat. **Pharm Hist (London)** 1984 Sep;14(3):9-12
Kokoska U: Johann Georg Noël Dragendorff (20.4.1836 - 7.4.1898): Sein Beitrag zur Gerichtsmedizin, Pharmakologie und Pharmazie an der Universität Dorpat. Diss. Berlin, 1983. 234 p.

**Dragstedt, Lester Reynold, 1893-**
Landor JH: Lester Reynold Dragstedt--physiologist-surgeon. **Gastroenterology** 1981 Apr;80(4):846-53
Mysh VG: L. R. Dragstedt (vklad v uchenie o patogeneze i lechenii iazvennoi bolezni). **Khirurgiia (Mosk)** 1983 Jul;7:140-1
Woodward ER: Dr. Dragstedt's first vagotomy. **World J Surg** 1983 Jul;7(4):554

**Drake, Daniel, 1785-1852**
Snively WD: Daniel Drake: the Ohio Valley's man for all season. **Indiana Med Hist Q** 1976;2(4):61-4

**Drake, John Poad, 1794?-1883**
Bensley EH: John Poad Drake (1794-1883), the first artist to portray the Hospital. **Montreal Gen Hosp News** 1981;19(1):8-9

**Drane, Robert, 1833-1914**
Burnby JG: Robert Drane: no ordinary pharmacist. **Pharm Hist (London)** 1984 Dec;14(4):3-6

**Dreiser, Theodore, 1871-1945**
Spangler GM: Suicide and social criticism: Durkheim, Dreiser, Wharton, and London. **Am Q** 1979;31(4):496-516

**Dreuschuch, Frantisek, 1855-1938**
Vilček E: O prvom röntgenológovi z Moravy. **Cesk Radiol** 1980 Mar;34(2):138-43

**Drew, Charles Richard, 1904-1950**
Agris J: Stamps commemorating medicine. 'Dr. Charles R. Drew'. **J Dermatol Surg Oncol** 1982 Feb;8(2):96
Chakravorty RC: Charles Richard Drew (1904-1950). **Scalpel Tongs** 1981;25:69-70
Drew GR: The Dr. Charles R. Drew stamp. **J Afro-Am Hist Geneol Soc** 1981;2(4):139-42
Lichello R: Pioneer in blood plasma; Dr. Charles Richard Drew. New York, Messner, [1968]. 190 p.
Yancey AG: US postage stamp issued in honor of Charles R. Drew, MD, MDSc. **J Natl Med Assoc** 1982 Jun;74(6):561-5

**Driesch, Hans Adolf Eduard, 1867-1941**
Mocek R: Wilhelm Roux--Hans Driesch. Zur Geschichte der Entwicklungsphysiologie der Tiere ['Entwicklungsmechanik']. Jena, Fischer, 1974. 229 p. (Biographien bedeutender Biologen, Band 1).

**Drinker, Cecil Kent, 1887-1956**
Beatty W: Cecil Kent Drinker. In Dictionary of American Biography, Suppl. 6, 1956-1960. p. 174-5, 1980.

**Drost-Hülshoff, Annette Elizabeth, Freiin von, 1797-1848**
Meyer-Schwickerath G: Das Annette von Droste-Hülshoff-Syndrom. **Klin Monatsbl Augenheilkd** 1984 Jun;184(6):574-7

**Drummond, Adam, 1679-1758**
Drummond CG: Adam Drummond of Megginch, surgeon-apothecary. **Pharm Hist (London)** 1971 Dec;2(3):3-5

**Dryden, John, 1631-1700**
Madsen V: Medicine in history. Dryden on the doctors and the death of Charles II. **J Dermatol Surg Oncol** 1981 May;7(5):366-9
Ormsby-Lennon H: Radical physicians and conservative poets in Restoration England: Dryden among the doctors. **Stud Eighteenth Cent Cult** 1978;7:389-411

**Du Bois-Reymond, Emil Heinrich, 1818-1896**
Brücke EW von: Briefe an Emil Du Bois-Reymond. Ed. H. Brücke, W. Hilger, W. Höflechner, W. W. Swoboda. Erster Teil. Graz, Akademische Druck- und Verlagsanstalt, 1978. 308 p. (Publikationen aus dem Archiv der Universität Graz, Band 8/1).
Cranefield PF, ed: Two great scientists of the nineteenth century. Correspondence of Emil Du Bois-Reymond and Carl Ludwig. Collected by Estelle Du Bois-Reymond. Foreword, notes, and indexes by Paul Diepgen. Translation of 1927 German ed. Baltimore, London, Johns Hopkins Univ. Press, 1982. xix, 183 p.
Mann G: Geschichte als Wissenschaft und Wissenschaftsgeschichte bei Du Bois-Reymond. **Hist Z** 1980;231:75-100
Mann G, ed: Naturwissen und Erkenntnis im 19. Jahrhundert: Emil Du Bois-Reymond. Hildesheim, Gerstenberg, 1981. 243 p. Contributions by K. E. Rothschuh, H. Hensel, R. Malter, C. von Campenhausen, B. Lohff, H. Lübbe, D. von Engelhardt, W. F. Gutmann, K. Bonink, C. Andree

**Du Gardin, Louis, fl. 1617**
Gysel C: Odontoiatria del passato. L'odontostomatologia nel contesto delle 'vere e solide fondamenta della medicine', definite da Louis Du Gardin, Professore all'Università di Douai, sotto il regno di Alberto ed Isabella. **Dent Cadmos** 1983 Apr;51(4):91-5 contd
Gysel C: L'odonto-stomatologie d'après les 'vrais et solides fondements de la médecine', établis par Louis du Gardin, professeur à l'université de Douai, sous le règne d'Albert et d'Isabelle. **Rev Belge Med Dent** 1982 Jul;37(4):164-71
Gysel G: Odontoiatria del passato. L'odontostomatologia nel contesto delle 'vere e solide fondamenta della medicina', definite da Louis Du Gardin, Professore all'Università di Douai, sotto il regno di Alberto ed Isabella. II. **Dent Cadmos** 1983 May;51(5):107-9, 112

**Du Vigneaud, Vincent, 1901-1978**
Bing FC: Vincent du Vigneaud (1901-1978): a biographical sketch. **J Nutr** 1982 Aug;112(8):1463-73

**Dubb, Per, 1750-1834**
Höök O: Pehr Dubb -- en medicinsk storman inom västsvensk sjukvård på 1700-talet. **Lakartidningen** 1979 Dec 19;76(51):4710-3

**Dubois de Chemant, Nicolas, 1753-1824**
Herschfeld JJ: Nicholas Dubois de Chemant and the invention of mineral teeth. **Bull Hist Dent** 1982 Apr;30(1):40-3
Sugden KC: Nicolas Dubois de Chemant and the disputed invention of mineral teeth. **Br Dent J** 1983 Sep 24;155(6):202

**Dubois, J. A., 1765-1848**
Sastry VV: Health habits of South Indians as recorded by Abbe J. A. Dubois. **Bull Indian Inst Hist Med (Hyderabad)** 1980;10(1-4):84-9

**Dubois, Paul, 1848-1918**
Ducommun C: Paul Dubois (1848-1918). Sa place dans l'histoire de la psychothérapie. **Gesnerus** 1984;41(1/2):61-99

**DuBois, W. E. B., 1868-1963**
Taylor CM: W. E. B. Dubois's challenge to scientific racism. **J Black Stud** 1981;11(4):449-60

**Duckworth, Dyce, 1840-1928**
Russell JR: The three royal doctors of Betchworth. **Practitioner** 1981 Jul;225(1357):1070-1

**Dudith, András, Bp. of Pécs, 1533-1589**
Glesinger L: Der Humanist Andreas Dudith im Kreise der Antiparacelsisten. Wien, 1967. (Salzburger Beiträge zur Paracelsusforschung, 7). p. 3-12.

**Dudits, Andor, 1866-1944**
Monsées Y: 'Klinisches Ambulatorium' von Andor Dudits, 1890. **Medizinhist J** 1981;16(4):454-8

**Duff, William, 1732-1815**
Duff W: An essay on original genius and its various modes of exertion in philosophy and the fine arts, particularly in poetry (1767). Facsimile. Ed. by J. L. Mahoney. Delmar, New York, Scholars' Facsimiles and Reprints, 1978. ix, 296 p.

**Dugay, Jacques, ca. 1647-1727**
Douville R: Jacques Dugay. In Dictionary of Canadian biography, 1701 to 1740. Volume 2, 1969. p. 202-3.

**Duhamel du Monceau, Henri Louis, 1700-1781?**
Chaïa J: Sur une correspondance, entre 1739 et 1749, de Duhamel du Monceau avec J.-F. Artur, médecin du roy a Cayenne. In: Congrès National des Sociétés Savantes, 102e, Limoges, 1977. Comptes Rendus. Paris, 1977. Section des Sciences, Fasc. III. p. 21-6.
Portal C, Rideau M, Viel C: Quelques aspects de l'oeuvre de Duhamel de Monceau dans le domaine des sciences naturelles et des sciences physiques. In: Congrès National des Sociétés Savantes, 107e. Brest, 1982. Comptes Rendus, Paris, 1982. Section des Sciences, Fasc. IV. p. 341-50.

**Duhamel, Georges, 1884-1966**
Szállá A: Arthur Schnitzler és Georges Duhamel a Nyugatban. **Orv Hetil** 1982 Sep 5;123(36):2246-50
Vieuville P: Duhamel et la médecine. **Hist Sci Med** 1980;14(1):71-6

**Duhring, Louis Adolphus, 1845-1913**
Zivković K: Sečanje na prof. Dr. Luisa A. Djuringa (23. XII 1854 - 8. V 1913). **Srp Arh Celok Lek** 1982 Apr;110(4):523-4

**Duka, Tivadar, 1825-1908**
Vida M: Tivadar Duka (1825-1908). **Orvostort Kozl** 1979;86(24 no 4):9-23

**Duke, William Waddel, 1882–1946**
Brinkhous KM: W. W. Duke and his bleeding time test. A commentary on platelet function. **JAMA** 1983 Sep 2;250(9):1210–14

**Dumarest, Frédéric, 1862–1951**
Roda JJ: Histoire de la fondation du premier sanatorium populaire français. Ses origines et ses vingt-cinq premières années d'existence (Sanatorium Mangini Hauteville). Thèse. Lyon I, 1976. 85 p.

**Dumas, Alexandre, 1802–1870**
Hernández EI: Sindrome de enclaustramiento. **Medicina (B Aires)** 1983;43(1):117–8

**Dumas, Jean-Baptiste, 1800–1884**
Castellani C: Una rilettura ottocentesca di Spallanzani: la nouvelle théorie de la génération di Prévost e Dumas (1824). **Hist Philos Life Sci** 1979;1(2):215–59
Castellani C: Fra preformismo e epigenesi: le teorie di Prevost e Dumas. **Hist Philos Life Sci** 1980;2(2):253–68

**Dummer, Ethel Sturges, 1866–1954**
Mennel RM: Ethel Sturges Dummer. In: Notable American women. The modern period. Cambridge, Mass., Belknap-Harvard Univ. Press, 1980. 4:208–10.

**Dumont, Fritz Ludwig, 1854–1932**
Lewerenz-Steinsiepe M: Fritz Ludwig Dumont: ein moderner Anaesthesist. **Anaesthesist** 1982 Jun;31(6):302–5

**Dumont, Henri Joseph, 1824–1878**
Rivero de la Calle M, Collado Lopez O: Reporte sobre las primeras mediciones craneometricas de tipo comparativo realizadas en Cuba. [H. J. Dumont.]. **Cienc Habana Ser 9** 1976;6:3–27

**Dunant, Jean Henri, 1828–1910**
Morgenstern S: Henri Dunant and the Red Cross. **Bull NY Acad Med** 1979 Nov;55(10):949–56
Morgenstern S: Henri Dunant and the Red Cross. **Bull NY Acad Med** 1981 May;57(4):311–26

**Dunash ben Tamin, 10th cent.**
Vajda G: La structure du corps humain d'après le commentaire de Dunash ben Tamin sur le 'Livre de la Création'. **J Semit Stud** 1978;23(1):88–94

**Dunbar, Helen Flanders, 1902–1959**
Powell RC: (Helen) Flanders Dunbar. In Dictionary of American Biography, Suppl. 6, 1956–1960. p. 180–1, 1980.
Stokes GA: Helen Flanders Dunbar. In: Notable American women. The modern period. Cambridge, Mass., Belknap-Harvard Univ. Press, 1980. 4:210–2.

**Duncan, Andrew, 1744–1828**
Rosner LM: Andrew Duncan M.D., F.R.S.E. (1744–1828). Edinburgh, History of Medicine and Science Unit, University of Edinburgh, [1981?]. [12] p.

**Duncan, James Matthews, 1826–1890**
Drury MI: Diabetes in pregnancy--Matthews Duncan revisited. **Ir J Med Sci** 1984 Apr;153(4):144–51

**Duncan, William Henry, 1805–1863**
Chave SP: Duncan of Liverpool--and some lessons for today. **Community Med** 1984 Feb;6(1):61–71

**Dunglison, Robley, 1798–1869**
Crispell KR: Beaumont and Dunglison: who was Dunglison? **Trans Am Clin Climatol Assoc** 1980;92:194–8

**Dunham, Ethel Collins, 1883–1969**
Schmidt WM: Ethel Collins Dunham. In: Notable American women. The modern period. Cambridge, Mass., Belknap-Harvard Univ. Press, 1980. 4:212–3.

**Dunn, Charles Wesley, 1885–1959**
Janssen WF: FDLI's unforgettable character: Charles Wesley Dunn. **Food Drug Cosmet Law J** 1982 Oct;37(4):446–56

**Dupuytren, Guillaume, 1777–1835**
Arvy L, Rivet R: Dupuytren (1777–1835) face à l'énigme qu'était la fièvre jaune en 1826. In: Congrès National des Sociétés Savantes, 102e, Limoges, 1977. Comptes Rendus. Paris, 1977. Section des Sciences, Fasc. III. p. 27–32.
Bloch H: Guillaume Dupuytren, M.D. (1777–1835). Surgeon of Hôtel Dieu and his American students. **NY State J Med** 1981 Feb;81(2):259–60
Gutmann RA: Une lettre de Marjolin sur ses rapports avec Dupuytren. **Hist Sci Med** 1981;15(2):123–7
Hauben DJ: Das chirurgische Erbe. Guillaume Dupuytren (1777–1835). **Zentralbl Chir** 1984;109(11):765–6
Lugnegård H: Mannen bakom dupuytrens kontraktur: 'vilddjuret vid Seine' - sin tids mest namnkunnige kirurg. **Lakartidningen** 1983 Dec 28;80(52):5068–9

**Duran, R. Simon ben Zemah, 1361–1444**
Leibowitz JO: R. Simon ben Zemah Duran (1361–1444) and his conception of metabolism in Magen Avot. **Koroth** 1979 Nov;7(9–10):CLXIX–XXIX(626–33)

**Durant, Sálvano Velasco, 1833–1905**
Mazzei Uzcátegui M: Dos figuras medicas venezolanas. **Rev Soc Venez Hist Med** 1969–71;17–19(31–33):163–94

**Durante, Francesco, 1844–1934**
Guidetti B: Francesco Durante. June 29, 1844 to October 2, 1934. **Surg Neurol** 1983 Jul;20(1):1–3

**Dürer, Albrecht, 1471–1528**
Dotz W: Albrecht Dürer. Depictions of facies as expressions of personality. **Am J Dermatopathol** 1981 Spring;3(1):59–65

**Durham, James, fl. 1802**
Plummer BL: Document: letters of James Durham to Benjamin Rush. **J Negro Hist** 1980;65(3):261–9
Wynes CE: Dr. James Durham, mysterious eighteenth-century black physician: man or myth? **Pa Mag Hist Biogr** 1979;103(3):325–33

**Düring, Ernst Eduard Kamille von, 1858–1944**
Winkelmann O: Zur Erinnerung an Ernst von Düring-Pascha (1858–1944). In: First International Congress on the History of Turkish-Islamic Science and Technology, ITU 14–18 September 1981. Proceedings Vol. IV, p. 32–44.

**Durkheim, Emile, 1858–1917**
Spangler GM: Suicide and social criticism: Durkheim, Dreiser, Wharton, and London. **Am Q** 1979;31(4):496–516

**Durocher, Marie Josephine, 1809–1894**
Lobo FB: Duas pioneiras-Madame Dubocher, Rita Lobato. **Rev Inst Hist Geogr Bras** 1980;(328):53–6

**Dussaus, Marie-Angélique, 1737–1809**
Séguin G: Marie-Angélique Dussaus. In Dictionary of Canadian biography, 1801 to 1820. Volume 5, 1983. p. 293.

**Dutrochet, René Joachim Henri, 1776–1847**
Schiller J: Henri Dutrochet et la terminologie scientifique. In: Congrès National des Sociétés Savantes, 97e, Nantes, 1972. Comptes Rendus. Paris, 1976. Section des Sciences, Tome 1. p. 83–9.
Schiller N: Henri Dutrochet contributions biographiques et iconographiques. In: Congrès National des Sociétés Savantes, 97e, Nantes, 1972. Comptes Rendus. Paris, 1976. Section des Sciences, Tome 1. p. 71–82.

**Duverney, Guichard Joseph, 1648–1730**
Peltier LF: Joseph Guichard Duverney (1648–1730). Champion of applied comparative anatomy. **Clin Orthop** 1984 Jul–Aug;(187):308–11

**Dvorzhak, Milan, 1929–**
Cech S: Milan Dvorzhak (k 50-letiiu so dnia rozhdeniia). **Arkh Anat Gistol Embriol** 1980 Jul;79(7):121–5

**Dyer, Charles Volney, 1808–1878**
Beatty WK: Charles Volney Dyer: physician, promoter, and abolitionist. **Proc Inst Med Chic** 1982 Apr–Jun;35(2):45–8

**Dzhanelidze, Iustin Iulianovich, 1883–1950**
Gvozdev MP, Petrov VA: Iustin Iulianovich Dzhanelidze (K 100-letiiu so dnia rozhdeniia). **Voen Med Zh** 1983 Aug;(8):72–4
Ternovoĭ KS, Shalimov AA: Vydaiushchiĭsia sovetskiĭ khirurg I. I. Dzhanelidze (k 100-letiiu so dnia rozhdeniia). **Klin Khir** 1983 Jul;(8):76–9
Uglov FG, Afanas'eva AV: Iustin Iulianovich Dzhanelidze (k 100-letiiu so dnia rozhdeniia). **Vestn Khir** 1983 Aug;131(8):131–4

## E

**Earle, Sylvester Zobieski, 1822–1888**
McGahan EW: Sylvester Zobieski Earle. In Dictionary of Canadian biography, 1881–1890. 1982;11:295–6.

**Easlick, Kenneth Alexander, 1893–1979**
Pike JS, Ireland RL: Pioneers in pedodontics. Kenneth Alexander Easlick, 1893–1979. **Pediatr Dent** 1982 Sep;4(3):268–9

**Eastman, Joseph, 1842–1902**
MacDougall JD: Joseph Eastman, M.D., LL.D; citizen, soldier, surgeon and medical educator. **Indiana Med Hist Q** 1974;1(2):26–30

**Ebbinghaus, Hermann, 1850–1909**
Klix F: Hermann Ebbinghaus---Ursprünge und Anfang psychologischer Forschungen an der Berliner Universität. In Eckardt G, ed: Zur Geschichte der Psychologie. Berlin, VEB Deutscher Verlag der Wissenschaften, 1979. p. 85–109.

**Eckstein, Ferenc, 1769–1833**
Csillag I: Eckstein Ferenc és a hadisebészet a Napóleon elleni háborúban. **Orv Hetil** 1984 Feb 19;125(8):467–70

**Economo, Constantin von, 1876–1931**
Wyklicky H: Economo als Psychiater. **Osterr Arzteztg** 1982;37(8):533

**Eddy, Mary Baker, 1821–1910**
Johnson RA: On the psychology of the aging woman. Mary Baker Eddy as a religious leader. **J Geriatr Psychiatry** 1979;12(1):27–35
Kenyon FE: Mary Baker Eddy, founder of Christian Science; the sublime hysteric. **Hist Med (Lond)** 1975 Autumn-Winter;6(3-4):29–46
Silberger J: On the psychology of the aging woman. Mourning and transformation: how Mary Baker Eddy found in middle age a way of making a new life for herself. **J Geriatr Psychiatry** 1979;12(1):9–25

**Eddy, Thomas, 1758–1827**
Grob GN, ed: The beginnings of American psychiatric thought and

practice. Five accounts, 1811–1830. New York, Arno, 1973. Various paginations. Includes Account of the rise and progress of the Asylum . . . near Philadelphia (1814), and works by Theodric Romeyn Beck (1811); Thomas Eddy (1815); George Parkman (1814); and Rufus Wyman (1830).

**Edelfelt, Albert, 1854–1905**
Sourander P: Edelfelts berömda pasteurporträtt – originalet och repliken. **Nord Medicinhist Arsbok** 1983;:149–54

**Edward, Derrick Graham, 1910–1978**
Freundt EA: Derrick Graham ffarington Edward: a pioneer in mycoplasmology. **Rev Infect Dis** 1982 May–Jun;(4 Suppl):S3–7

**Edward VII, King of Great Britain, 1841–1910**
Williams GR: A history of appendicitis. With anecdotes illustrating its importance. **Ann Surg** 1983 May;197(5):495–506

**Edwardes, David, fl. 16th cent.**
Rook A, Newbold M: David Edwardes: his activities at Cambridge. **Med Hist** 1975 Oct;19(4):389–92

**Edwards, Charles Cornell, 1923–**
Elliott J: Orthopedist is pioneer in prosthetic design. **JAMA** 1976 Oct 26;242(17):1831–3, 1837

**Edwards, Jonathan, 1703–1758**
Blight JG: Jonathan Edwards's theory of the mind: its applications and implications. In J. Brozěk, ed: Explorations in the history of psychology in the United States. Lewisburg, Bucknell University Press, 1984. p. 61–120.
Erdt T: Jonathan Edwards: art and the sense of heart. Amherst, University of Massachusetts Press, 1980. xiv, 123 p.
Hoopes J: Jonathan Edwards's religious psychology. **J Am Hist** 1983;69(4):849–65
Williams DR: Horses, pigeons, and the therapy of conversion: a psychological reading of Jonathan Edwards's theology. **Harv Theol Rev** 1981;74(4):337–52

**Eeden, Frederik van, 1860–1932**
Bulhof IN: From psychotherapy to psychoanalysis: Frederik van Eeden and Albert Willem van Renterghem. **J Hist Behav Sci** 1981;17:209–21

**Ehlers, Ernst Heinrich, 1835–1925**
Hawkins H: Transatlantic discipleship: two American biologists and their German mentor. **Isis** 1980 Jun;71(257):197–210

**Ehrenberg, Christian Gottfried, 1795–1876**
Siesser WG: Christian Gottfried Ehrenberg: Founder of micropaleontology. **Centaurus** 1981;25(3):166–88

**Ehrenfels, Christian von, 1859–1932**
Oppitz R: Freiherr von Ehrenfels (1859–1932) und die Entwicklung des 'Neuen Menschen' zu Beginn des 20. Jahrhunderts. Diss. Mainz, 1980. 256 p.

**Ehrlich, Paul, 1854–1915**
Bäumler E: Paul Ehrlich, Forscher für das Leben. Frankfurt, Societäts-Verlag, 1979. 370 p.
Bendiner E: Ehrlich: immunologist, chemotherapist, prophet. **Hum Dev** 1980 Nov;15(11):129, 133, 138–9 passim
Borek F: Eighty years of Ehrlich's side-chain theory. **J Immunol Methods** 1980;33(4):393
Costa-Casaretto C: Por que se les otorgo el Premio Nobel de medicina y fisiologia a Ehrlich y a Metchnikoff en 1908? **Rev Med Chil** 1980;108:775–6
Gergely J: Ehrlich 'varázslövedéke' a megvalósulás útján (gyógyszerek irányított célbajuttatása specifikus ellenanyagokkal). **Orv Hetil** 1982 Sep 19;123(38):2331–6
Kallós P: Immunity and concomitant immunity in infectious diseases. Introduction. **Prog Allergy** 1982;31:IX–XV
Kleeberg J: Uber Ehrlichs Benzaldehyd-Reaktion (auf Urobilinogen) nach 80 Jahren. **Z Gastroenterol** 1982 Aug;20(8):424–8
Parascandola J: The theoretical basis of Paul Ehrlich's chemotherapy. **J Hist Med Allied Sci** 1981 Jan;36(1)19–43
Rubin LP: Styles in scientific explanations: Paul Ehrlich and Svante Arrhenius on immunochemistry. **J Hist Med Allied Sci** 1980 Oct;35(4):397–425
Schneck P: Die Briefe Paul Ehrlichs an den Moskauer Mikrobiologen Georgij Norbertovič Gabričevskij. **NTM** 1982;19(2):81–7
Siefert G, Stöckl T: Die Entdeckung der Mastzellen durch den Freiburger Medizinstudenten Paul Ehrlich. **Medizinhist J** 1983;18(3):227–37
Silverstein AM: History of immunology. Development of the concept of immunologic specificity, I. **Cell Immunol** 1982 Mar 1;67(2):396–409
Thorburn AL: Paul Ehrlich: pioneer of chemotherapy and cure by arsenic (1854–1915). **Br J Vener Dis** 1983 Dec;59(6):404–5
Ward PS: The American reception of Salvarsan. **J Hist Med Allied Sci** 1981 Jan;36(1)44–62

**Ehrmann, Albert, 1821–1871**
Steimle R: Albert Ehrmann (1821–1871). **Hist Sci Med** 1984;18(3):208–14

**Ehrmann, Martin, fl. 1836–1866**
Santavý F: Prof. Dr. chem. PhMr. Martin Ehrmann a jeho pusobení na medicínskochirurgickém učilišti v Olomouci v letech 1836––1866. **Cesk Farm** 1979 Jun;28(5):221–2

**Eichhorst, Hermann, 1849–1921**
Fasol E: Der Internist Hermann Eichhorst, 1849–1921. Zürich, Juris Druck, 1983. 98 P. (Zürcher Medizingeschichtliche Abhandlungen, Neue Reihe, Nr. 159).

**Einthoven, Willem, 1860–1927**
Lamas GA, Koller LR, Antman EM, et al: Electrocardiogram by Einthoven 63 years earlier. **Am J Cardiol** 1984 Nov 1;54(8):1163–5

**Eiselsberg, Anton von, 1860–1939**
Rutkow IM: The letters of William Halsted and Anton von Eiselsberg: a very special friendship. **Arch Surg** 1980 Aug;115(8):993–1001

**Eisenbarth, Johann Andreas, 1663–1727**
Pies E: Ich bin der Doktor Eisenbarth. Arzt der Landstrasse. Eine Bildbiographie über das Leben und Wirken des volkstümlichen und berümten Chirurgen Johann Andreas Eisenbarth (1663–1727). Genf, Ariston, 1977. 306 p.
Rocchietta S: Vita avventurosa di Johann Andreas Eisenbarth (1663–1727), chirurgo e medico girovago. **Minerva Med** 1981 Jan 28;72(3):173–4

**Eisenhower, Dwight David, 1890–1969**
Pillsbury DM: General Eisenhower's 'melanoma'. **J Am Acad Dermatol** 1981 May;4(5):631–2

**Eisler, Robert, 1882–1949**
Greisman HC: Social structure, psychoanalysis, and collective aggression. **Hist Eur Ideas** 1981;2(1):35–48

**Ekman, Olof Jacob, 1764–1839**
Peltier LF: The classic: congenital osteomalacia. Olaus Jacob Ekman. **Clin Orthop** 1981 Sep;159:3–5

**Elanski, A. N., 1894–1964**
Kuzin M, Antipenko E: Zhizn' otdannaia nauke. **Voen Istor Zh** 1969;11(12):47–50

**Elfinger, Anton, 1821–1864**
Poch-Kalous M, Till R: Cajetan. Ein Wiener Mediziner und Karikaturist um die Mitte des 19. Jahrhunderts. **Wien Geschichtsbl** 1967;22(3):220–4
Skopec M: Anton Elfinger (1821–1864)––a forgotten medical illustrator. **Int J Dermatol** 1983 May;22(4):256–9

**Elguero, Jose Ramón, fl. 1862**
Costa-Casaretto C: Ideario psiquiátrico del médico de la Casa de Locos de Santiago en 1862. **Rev Med Chil** 1980 Jun;108(6):559–67

**Elin, Vladimir Leont'evich, 1883–1962**
Vasil'ev KG, Vasil'ev KK: Vrach-revoliutsioner V. L. Elin. **Sov Zdravookhr** 1983;(8):57–8

**Eliot, Charles William, 1834–1926**
Eliot's farewell address, May 1, 1909: **Harv Med Alumni Bull** 1982 Spring;56(2):14–6

**Eliot, George, 1819–1880**
Beer G: Anxiety and interchange: Daniel Deronda and the implications of Darwin's writing. **J Hist Behav Sci** 1983 Jan;19(1):31–44
Shuttleworth SA: The language of science and psychology in George Eliot's Daniel Deronda. In Paradis J, Postlewait T, ed: Victorian science and Victorian values: literary perspectives. New York, New York Academy of Sciences, 1981. p. 269–98.

**Elischer, Gyula, 1846–1909**
Hrabovszky Z: [Gyula Elischer: as seen by one of his students] (Hun). **Orv Hetil** 1980;121:2831–4
Szállási A: Id. Elischer Gyula élete––a mügyüjtés apológiája. **Orv Hetil** 1984 Oct 14;125(42):2567–9

**Eliseev, Aleksandr Vasil'evich, 1858–1895**
Buianov MI: Vrach-puteshestvennik A. V. Eliseev. **Klin Med (Mosk)** 1982;60(8):113–4
Veselov EI, Belevitin AB: A. V. Eliseev––vrach, puteshestvennik, uchenyĭ (k 125-letiiu so dnia rozhdeniia). **Voen Med Zh** 1984 Sep;(9):68–9

**Elizabeth, of Hungary, Saint, 1207–1231**
Hofmann B: Kranker und Krankheit um 1500. Die Darstellung des Kranken im Zusammenhang mit den spätgotischen Bildnissen der Heiligen Elisabeth. Herzogenrath, Verlag Murken-Altrogge, 1983. 226 p. (Studien zur Medizin-, Kunst- und Literaturgeschichte, Bd. 3).
Van der May-de Leur AP: Moderne pelgrimage: Sint Elisabeth-expositie Marburg 1981. **Tijdschr Ziekenverpl** 1982 Feb 2;35(3):83–6

**Elkin, Daniel Collier, 1893–1958**
Kinnaird DW: Kentucky's Doctors Elkin contributions to growth of Emory's medical school. **J Ky Med Assoc** 1984 Jun;82(6):291–3

**Elkin, William Simpson, 1858–**
Kinnaird DW: Kentucky's Doctors Elkin contributions to growth of Emory's medical school. **J Ky Med Assoc** 1984 Jun;82(6):291–3

**Elkind, Mortimer Murray, 1922–**
Elkind MM: Radiobiology in radiotherapy: a personal history. **Int J Radiat Oncol Biol Phys** 1984 Jul;10(7):1143–8

**Elliotson, John, 1791–1868**
Miller J: A Gower Street scandal. The Samuel Gee lecture 1982.

**J R Coll Physicians Lond** 1983 Oct;17(4):181–5, 188–91

**Elliott, Thomas Renton, 1877–1961**
Himsworth H: Thomas Renton Elliott. In Dictionary of national biography, 1961–1970. Suppl. 8, 1981. p. 329–30.

**Ellis, Arthur William Mickle, 1883–1966**
Wilson C: Sir Arthur William Mickle Ellis. In Dictionary of national biography, 1961–1970. Suppl. 8, 1981. p. 330–2.

**Ellis, Calvin, 1826–1883**
Wolfe EL: Calvin Ellis, the forgotten dean. **Harv Med Alumni Bull** 1982 Spring;56(2):27–31

**Ellis, Havelock, 1859–1939**
Bowman IA: 'My life'; an important Ellis manuscript. **Bookman** 1981 Apr;8(4):3–7
Brome V: Havelock Ellis, philospher of sex: a biography. London, Boston, Routledge & Kegan Paul, 1979. xiv, 271 p.
Cott NF: Passionlessness: an interpretation of Victorian sexual ideology, 1790–1850. **Signs** 1978;4(2):219–36
Grosskurth P: Havelock Ellis: biography. New York, Knopf, 1980. xvi, 492 p.

**Elman, Robert, 1897–1956**
Olch PD: Robert Elman. In Dictionary of American Biography, Suppl. 6, 1956–1960. p. 189–90, 1980.

**Elmhirst, William, 1721–1773**
Sigsworth EM, Swan P: An eighteenth-century surgeon and apothecary: William Elmhirst (1721–1773). **Med Hist** 1982 Apr;26(2):191–8
Sigsworth EM: William Elmhirst 1721–1773: surgeon-apothecary--and medical frontiersman. **Pharm Hist (London)** 1984 Sep;14(3):6–7

**Eloesser, Leo, 1881?–1976**
Shumacker HB: An American surgeon's contribution to Chinese health care. **Am J Surg** 1981 Mar;141(3):311–6
Shumacker HB: Leo Eloesser, M.D.: eulogy for a free spirit. New York, Philosophical Library, 1982. 483 p.

**Elpat'evskiĭ, Sergeĭ Iakovievich, 1854–1933**
Galaĭ IuG: Novye dokumenty o vrache-pisatele S. Ia. Elpat'evskom. **Sov Zdravookhr** 1983;(9):59–62
Skachilov VA: S. Ia. Elpat'evskiĭ v Ufimskoĭ ssylke. **Sov Zdravookhr** 1980;(8):56–9

**Elsaesser, Armin Emil, 1875–1952**
Aellen HP: Dr. Med. Armin Emil Elsaesser (1875–1952), Schueler von Theodor Kocher: sein Werden und Wirken in der Schweiz und in den Vereinigten Staaten von Amerika. Bern, [s.n.], 1982. x, 187 p.

**Elschnig, Anton, 1863–1939**
Libicky H: A personal sketch of Professor Anton Elschnig. **Surv Ophthalmol** 1982 Mar–Apr;26(5):266–8

**Elsheimer, Adam, 1578–1610**
Schupbach WM: Elsheimer il malinconico. **Kos** 1984 Jun;1(5):85–100

**Elsner, John, 1844–1922**
Hornbein M: Dr. John Elsner, a Colorado pioneer. **West States Jew Hist Q** 1981;13(4):291–302

**Elvehjem, Conrad Arnold, 1901–1962**
Ihde AJ: Conrad Arnold Elvehjem. In Dictionary of American biography, 1961–1965. Suppl. 7, 1981. p. 223–4.

**Elyot, Thomas, 1490?–1546**
Payne LM: A trap for the unwary. **J R Coll Physicians Lond** 1981;15:168

**Emerson, Haven, 1874–1957**
Duffy J: Haven Emerson. In Dictionary of American Biography, Suppl. 6, 1956–1960. p. 192–3, 1980.

**Emerson, Louville Eugene, 1873–1939**
Taylor E: Louville Eugene Emerson: psychotherapy, Harvard, and the early Boston scene. **Harv Med Alumni Bull** 1982 Spring;56(2):42–8

**Emery-Coderre, Joseph, 1813–1888**
Desjardins E: Joseph Emery-Coderre. In Dictionary of Canadian biography, 1881–1890. 1982;11:302–3.

**Emmens, Stephen H., ca. 1845–**
Kauffman GB: The mystery of Stephen H. Emmens: successful alchemist or ingenious swindler?. **Ambix** 1983 Jul;30(2):65–88

**Emmeram, Saint, d. ca. 660**
Röhrer-Ertl O: Bemerkungen zur Identifikation des Hl. Emmeram aus St. Emmeram in Regensburg. Ein methodenkritischer Vergleich. **Anthropol Anz** 1981 Sep;39(3):173–88

**Enault de Barbaucannes, Philippe, 1651–ca. 1708**
MacBeath G: Philippe Enault de Barbaucannes. In Dictionary of Canadian biography, 1701 to 1740. Volume 2, 1969. p. 217.

**Encarnación Valencia, José de la**
Deschamps Chapeaux P: El negro en la economía Habanera del siglo XIX. Flebotomianos y dentistas. **Rev Bibl Nac Jose Marti** 1971;13(1):75–86

**Enders, John Franklin, 1897–**
Bendiner E: Enders, Weller, and Robbins: the trio that 'fished in troubled waters'. **Hosp Pract** 1982 Jan;17(1):163, 169, 174–5 passim

**Eng, Helga Kristine, 1875–**
Svebak S: Helga Eng: a Norwegian precursor to Darrow and Lacey. **Psychophysiology** 1983 Sep;20(5):600–1

**Engel, George Libman, 1913–**
Ader R, Schmale AH: George Libman Engel: on the occasion of his retirement. **Psychosom Med** 1980;42(1 Suppl):79–101

**Engel, Rudolph, 1904–**
Halberg F, Halberg E: Circadian rhythms in the mammalian central nervous system, blood pressure and parasites - hobbies of Rudolf Engel. **Int J Chronobiol** 1979;7(1):1–16

**Engelin, Jakob, ca. 1365–1420**
Bergmann H: Neufunde zum Pesttraktat Jakob Engelins von Ulm. **Sudhoffs Arch** 1978;62(3):282–93

**Engelmann, George Julius, 1847–1903**
Dieckmann I: Untersuchungen des menschlichen Endometriums durch Hanns Kundrat (1845–1893) und George Julius Engelmann (1847–1903). Diss. Erlangen-Nürnberg, 1980. 73 p.

**Engels, Friedrich, 1820–1895**
Löhr HG: Ein Vierteljahrhundert gemeinsamen Weges von Karl Marx und Friedrich Engels mit ihrem treuen Freund und Kampfgefährten Carl Schorlemmer. **Pharmazie** 1983 Nov;38(11):768–72
Löther I, Löther R: Engels' 'Ludwig Feuerbach und der Ausgang der klassischen deutschen Philosophie', die Grundrichtungen des philosophischen Denkens und die Medizin. **Med Ges** 1979;(5):79–91
Löther R, ed: Philosophische Schriften von Marx, Engels und Lenin und ihre Bedeutung für die Medizin heute. Jena, Fischer, 1979. 127 p. Contributions by U. Körner, I. Löther, P. W. Ruff, R. Stach, G. Straass.

**Enghoff, Henrik, 1894–**
Nunn JB, Holmdahl MH: Henrik Enghoff and the volumen inefficax. **Ups J Med Sci** 1979;84(2):105–8

**Enríquez Jorge, Enrique, fl. 1594**
Sanchez-Moscoso Hermida A: Distinción entre alimento y medicamento en un texto médico del siglo XVI. **Bol Soc Esp Hist Farm** 1980 Oct;31(123):151–90

**Entz, Béla, 1877–1959**
Frankl J: Entz Béla professzor tudomanyos müködése. **Orvostort Kozl** 1979;86(24 no 4):107–11
Lambrecht M: Entz Béla, a klinikai pathológia egyik hazai úttöröje. **Orv Hetil** 1984 Oct 28;125(44):2694–5

**Eppinger, Hans, 1879–1946**
Spiro HM: Eppinger of Vienna: scientist and villain? **J Clin Gastroenterol** 1984 Dec;6(6):493–7

**Erasistratus, fl. ca. 250 B.C.**
Kudlien F: A new testimony for Erasistratus? **Clio Med** 1981 Apr;15(3–4):137–42
Smith WD: Erasistratus's dietetic medicine. **Bull Hist Med** 1982 Fall;56(3):398–409

**Erasmus, Desiderius, d. 1536**
Benedek TG: The gout of Desiderius Erasmus and Willibald Pirckheimer: medical autobiography and its literary reflections. **Bull Hist Med** 1983 Winter;57(4):526–44
Sheerin DJ: A Carolingian cure recovered: Erasmus' citation of Hucbald of St. Amand's Ecloga de caluis. **Bibl Hum Renaissance** 1980 Jan;42(1):167–71
Veltheer W: Erasmus, in de grond niet so slecht. **Spiegel Hist** 1982;17(4):190–6

**Erb, Wilhelm Heinrich, 1840–1921**
Thom A: Zur disziplinären Genese der Neurologie im ausgehenden 19. Jahrhundert--aus den Briefen Wilhelm Erbs an Adolf Strümpell. **Z Gesamte Inn Med** 1982 Jun 1;37(11):340–6

**Erichsen, Johann Gottfried, 1712–1768**
Erichsen SW: Dronning Caroline Mathildes reiseapotek og litt om Stadsfysikus Johan Gotfried Erichsen. **Aust Agder Arv** 1977–78;:55–69

**Erickson, Milton Hyland, 1901–1980**
Hammond DC: Myths about Erickson and Ericksonian hypnosis. **Am J Clin Hypn** 1984 Apr;26(4):236–45
Rosen S: The psychotherapeutic and hypnotherapeutic approaches of Milton H. Erickson, M.D. **Am J Psychoanal** 1984 Summer;44(2):133–45

**Erikson, Erik Homburger, 1902–**
Albin M, Devlin RJ, Heeger G, ed: New directions in psychohistory. The Adelphi papers in honor of Erik H. Erikson. Lexington, Toronto, D. C. Heath, 1980. xx, 217 p. Includes contributions by E. S. Wolf, M. F. Shore, G. M. Platt, H. Feinstein, S. H. Rudolph, L. I. Rudolph.
Evans RI: Dialogue with Erik Erikson. New York, London, Harper & Row, 1967. xvi, 142 p.
Kushner HI: Americanization of the ego. **Can Rev Am Stud** 1979;10(1):95–101
Roazen P: Erik H. Erikson's America: the political implications of ego psychology. **J Hist Behav Sci** 1980 Oct;16(4):333–41
Schnell RL: Contributions to psychohistory: IV. Individual experience in historiography and psychoanalysis: significance of Erik Erikson and Robert Coles. **Psychol Rep** 1980 Apr;46(2):591–612

Weinstein F: On the social function of intellectuals: a consideration of Erik H. Erikson's contribution to psychoanalysis and psychohistory. In M. Albin, R. J. Devlin, G. Heeger, ed: New directions in psychohistory. The Adelphi papers in honor of Erik H. Erikson. Lexington, Toronto, D. C. Heath, 1980. p. 3–19.
Zahn WM: Erik H. Erikson. In J. Rattner, ed: Wandlungen der Psychoanalyse. Wien, Europaverlag, 1980. p. 187–210.
Zimmerman J: Transcendent psychology: Erik H. Erikson, Erich Fromm, Karen Horney, Abraham H. Maslow, and Harry Stack Sullivan and the quest for a healthy humanity. Ph.D. Diss., Northwestern University. Evanston, 1982. vi, 498 p.

**Erisman, Friedrich Huldreich, 1842–1915**
Dogle NV: Issledovaniia F. F. Erismana v Moskovskoĭ gubernii i sovremennost'. **Gig Tr Prof Zabol** 1983 Jul;(7):38–41

**Erlanger, Joseph, 1874–1965**
Ludmerer KM: Joseph Erlanger. In Dictionary of American biography, 1961–1965. Suppl. 7, 1981. p. 225–7.

**Ermengem, Emile P. van, 1851–1932**
Gunn RA: Botulism: from van Ermengem to the present. A comment. **Rev Infect Dis** 1979 Jul–Aug;1(4):720–1

**Erni, Hans, 1909–**
Rogers BO: Hans Erni: humanistic and aesthetic artist. **Aesthetic Plast Surg** 1983;7(1):51–67

**Erskine, Robert, 1677–1718**
Appleby JH: Robert Erskine--Scottish pioneer of Russian natural history. **Arch Nat Hist** 1982 Apr;10(3):377–98

**Erskine, Robert, 1735–1780**
Appleby JH, Cunningham A: Robert Erskine and Archibald Pitcairne: two Scottish physicians' outstanding libraries. **Bibliotheck** 1982;11:3–16

**Erspamer, Vittorio, 1909–**
Mutt V: An appreciation of the work of Vittorio Erspamer. **Peptides (Fayetteville)** 1981;2(Suppl 2):3–6

**Ertl, Johann von, 1881–**
Ertl JW von: Die Versorgung von Amputationsstümpfen durch Osteo-Myoplastik nach v. Ertl. **Z Plast Chir** 1981 Sep;5(3):184–9

**Erxleben, Dorthea Christiana, 1715–1762**
Erxleben DC: Gründliche Untersuchung der Ursachen, die das weibliche Geschlecht vom Studieren abhalten. Reprint of the Berlin, 1742, ed., mit einem Nachwort von G. Rechenberg. Hildesheim, New York, Olms, 1977. [68], 250 p.

**Escherich, Theodor, 1857–1911**
Morowitz HJ: How E. coli got its name. **Hosp Pract** 1982 Dec;17(12):58–9

**Esdaile, James, 1808–1859**
Newman JL: Acupuncture, anaesthesia, and all that. **NZ Med J** 1982 Jan 13;95(699):22

**Eshmun, God of Sidon**
Levin S: Eshmun, healing of God of Sidon. **Adler Mus Bull** 1983 Nov;Spec issue:39–42

**Eskuchen, Karl, 1885–1955**
Loebe FM: Karl Eskuchen--ein fast vergessener Pionier der Liquorforschung. **Psychiatr Neurol Med Psychol (Leipz)** 1983 Sep;35(9):561–5

**Esmarch, Friedrich von, 1823–1908**
Romm S: Johann Friedrich August von Esmarch. **Plast Reconstr Surg** 1983 Feb;71(2):271–3
Schmauss AK: Das chirurgische Erbe. Johann Friedrich August von Esmarch--Leben und Werk (9. 1. 1823–23. 2. 1908). **Zentralbl Chir** 1983;108(24):1577–83

**Espinosa de los Reyes, Isidro, 1887–1951**
Espinosa de los Reyes V: El doctor Isidro Espinosa de los Reyes y los inicios de la atención materno-infantil en México. **Gac Med Mex** 1981 Feb;117(2):81–7

**Esquirol, Jean Etienne Dominique, 1772–1840**
Dahm S: Frühe Krankenbildnisse: Alibert Esquirol Baumgartner. Köln, 1981. (Kölner medizinhistorische Beiträge; Arbeiten der Forschungsstelle des Instituts für Geschichte der Medizin der Universität zu Köln, Band 21).
Gourevitch M: Esquirol et la medicalisation de la psychiatrie: théorie médicale et pratique clinique. In International Congress of the History of Medicine, 27th, Barcelona, 1980. Actas. Barcelona, Académia de Ciències Médiques de Catalunya i Balears, 1981. p. 74–7.
Ledermann F: La psychiatrie française et les médicaments: Pomme, Pinel, Esquirol, Morel. **Rev Hist Pharm (Paris)** 1982 Sep;29(254):189–206
Legée G: Evolution de l'étude clinique, sociale et juridique de l'aliénation mentale, sous l'impulsion de Jean-Etienne-Dominique Esquirol (1772–1840), médecin aliéniste d'origine Toulousaine. In: Congrès National des Sociétés Savantes, 96e, Toulouse, 1971. Comptes Rendus. Paris, 1974. Histoire des Sciences, Tome 1. p. 63–81.

**Esteyneffer, Juan de, 1664–1716**
Esteyneffer J de: Florilegio medicinal. Edicion, estudio preliminar, notas, glosario e indice analitico by M. del Carmen Anzures y Bolaños. México, Academía Nacional de Medicina, 1978. 2 v. xxiii, 973 p.
Kay MA: The Florilegio Medicinal: source of Southwest ethnomedicine. **Ethnohistory** 1977;24(3):251–9

**Estrada, Dr., fl. 1584**
Torre E: Las 'Conclusiones' del doctor Estrada de Madrid, contra los 'Avisos particulares' del doctor Hidalgo de Aguero, sevillano. **Asclepio** 1978–79;30–31:389–401

**Estrada, José, fl. 1821**
Moses RJ: Smallpox immunization in Alta California: a story based on José Estrada's 1821 postscript. **South Calif Q** 1979;61(2):123–43

**Euclid**
Theisen WR: 'Liber de visu': the Greco-Latin translation of Euclid's 'Optics'. **Mediaev Stud** 1979;41:44–105

**Euler, Leonhard, 1707–1783**
Kunze G: Die Anfänge einer biomathematisch - biophysikalischen Denkweise in der Physiologie im Spiegel einiger Arbeiten Leonhard Eulers (1707–1783). Diss., Johannes-Gutenberg-Universität. Mainz, 1981. 182 p.

**Euler, Ulf Svante von, 1905–1983**
Ottoson D: Ulf von Euler. Tre milstolpar inom medicinen: substans P, prostaglandin och noradrenalin. **Lakartidningen** 1983 Apr 13;80(15):1579–82

**Eulner, Hans-Heinz, 1925–1980**
Winkelmann H, Mildner S: Schriftenverzeichnis Hans-Heinz Eulner (19. 4. 1925 - 17. 10. 1980). **Medizinhist J** 1982;17(1/2):148–55

**Eustachi, Bartolomeo, d. 1574**
Belloni L: Bartolomeo Eustachi, anatomico del cinquecento, al lume di recenti ricerche. **Arch Int Hist Sci (Paris)** 1979 Jun–Dec;29(104):5–10
Belloni L: Ancora sul manoscritto 'De dissensionibus, et controversis anatomicis' di Bartolomeo Eustachi. **Physis** 1981;23(4):581–7
Eden AR, Opland J: Bartolommeo Eustachio's De Auditus Organis and the unique murder plot in Shakespeare's Hamlet. **N Engl J Med** 1982 Jul 22;307(4):259–61
Herschfeld JJ: Bartholomeus Eustachius--the first great dental anatomist. **Bull Hist Dent** 1982 Oct;30(2):123–8
Karlan MS: An anatomic plate from Bartolomeo Eustachi. **J Hist Med Allied Sci** 1980 Jul;35(3):316–18
Roberts KB: Eustachius and his anatomical plates. **Newsl Can Soc Hist** 1979 Apr;:9–13

**Evans, Alice, 1881–1975**
O'Hern EM: Alice Catherine Evans. In: Notable American women. The modern period. Cambridge, Mass., Belknap-Harvard Univ. Press, 1980. 4:219–21.

**Evans, Amos Alexander, 1785–1848**
Cushman P: Amos Evans, M.D.; surgeon on U.S.S. Constitution in War of 1812. **NY State J Med** 1980 Oct;80(11):1753–6

**Evans, Charles Arthur Lovatt, 1884–1968**
Smyth DH: Sir Charles Arthur Lovatt Evans. In Dictionary of national biography, 1961–1970. Suppl. 8, 1981. p. 334–6.

**Evans, Griffith, 1835–1935**
Cule J: Griffith Evans (1835–1935) and his trypanosome. **Vet Hist** 1979–80;1(3):94–101
Durrant GR: Griffith Evans--a pioneer in tropical medicine. **Br Army Rev** 1980;65:66–8
Ware J, Hunt H: The several lives of a Victorian vet. London, Bachman and Turner, 1979. 213 p.

**Evans, Herbert McLean, 1882–1971**
Grumbach MM: Herbert McLean Evans, revolutionary in modern endocrinology: a tale of great expectations. **J Clin Endocrinol Metab** 1982 Dec;55(6):1240–7
Raacke ID: Herbert Mclean Evans (1882–1971). A biographical sketch. **J Nutr** 1983 May;113(5):929–43

**Evans, Horace, 1903–1963**
Wilson C: Horace Evans. In Dictionary of national biography, 1961–1970. Suppl. 8, 1981. p. 336–7.

**Evans, Thomas Wiltberger, 1823–1897**
Besombes A: Odonto-stomatologie et diplomatie de l'Impératrice Eugénie à Clemenceau. **Hist Sci Med** 1983;17(1):13–22
Carr MW: Thomas W. Evans: his life and influence on the development of dentistry as a learned profession. **J Am Coll Dent** 1979 Apr;46(2):87–100
Carson G: The dentist and the empress. The adventures of Dr. Tom Evans in gas-lit Paris. Boston, Houghton Mifflin, 1983. xiii, 222 p.

**Evans, Warren Felt, 1817–1889**
Teahan JF: Warren Felt Evans and mental healing: romantic idealism and practical mysticism in nineteenth-century America. **Church Hist** 1979 Mar;48(1):63–80

**Evdokimov, Aleksandr Ivanovich, 1883–**
Osnovipolozhnik sovetskoĭ stomatologii (k 100-letiiu so dnia rozhdeniia

Aleksandra Ivanovicha Evdokimova): **Stomatologiia (Mosk)** 1984 Jan–Feb;63(1):4–6
Troianskiĭ GN, Krechmer MI: A. I. Evdokimov--odin iz osnovopolozhnikov sovetskoĭ stomatologii. **Sov Zdravookhr** 1984;(10):60–4

**Evrat, Louis-Antoine, 1797–1876**
Biéder J: Un aliéniste du XIXe siècle: Louis-Antoine Evrat (1797–1876). **Ann Med Psychol (Paris)** 1983 Jan;141(1):122–33

**Ey, Henri, 1900–1977**
Bernard H: L'histoire de la psychiatrie selon Ey (sa forme et son sens, le mythe). **Rev Int Hist Psychiatr** 1983;1(1):59–77
Nica-Udangiu S: Henri Ey (1900–1977). **Rev Med Interna [Neurol Psihiatr]** 1984 Apr–Jun;29(2):151–6

**Eyck, Jan van, ca. 1390–1440**
Dequeker JV: Polymyalgia rheumatica with temporal arteritis, as painted by Jan van Eyck in 1436. **Can Med Assoc J** 1981 Jun 15;124(12):1597–8

**Ezekiel (prophet)**
Bron B: Zur Psychopathologie und Verkündigung des Propheten Ezechiel. Zum Phänomen der prophetischen Ekstase. **Schweiz Arch Neurol Neurochir Psychiatr** 1981;128(1):21–31

# F

**Faber, Tamás, fl. 1710–1719**
Frankl J: Faber Tamás dr., Somogy els ó megyei orvosa. **Orv Hetil** 1983 Feb 20;124(8):466–7

**Fabi, Mauritius, 1738–1801**
Zalai K: 'Systema Artis Pharmaceuticae'. La première dissertation à la Faculté Hongroise de médecine, présentée par Maritius Fabi. **Beitr Gesch Pharm** 1983;31(20):25–7

**Fábián, Daniel**
Szállási A: Fábián Dániel és József Attila. **Orv Hetil** 1983 Feb 20;124(8):464–6

**Fabricius, Hieronymus, ab Aquapendente, ca. 1533–1619**
Huizink L: Die Abhandlung über das Sehen von Hieronymus Fabricius ab Aquapendente (1537–1619): Ubersetzung von 'De actione oculorum' mit Kommentar. Zürich, Juris Druck, 1984. 58 p. (Zürcher Medizingeschichtliche Abhandlungen, Neue Reihe, Nr. 166).
Pariente L: Le De venarum ostiolis de Jerome Fabrice d'Acquapendente: sa place dans l'histoire de la découverte de la circulation du sang. Paris, Louis Pariente, 1981. 2 volumes.
Scarano GB: Le malattie della bocca e dei denti nell'opera di Girolamo Fabrizio d'Acquapendente. **Med Secoli** 1982 Jan–Apr;19(1):101–23

**Fabricius von Hilden, Wilhelm, 1560–1634**
Schärli AF: Kinder mit Missbildungen in der Renaissance (nach den Aufzeichnungen von Fabricius Hildanus, 1560–1634). **Z Kinderchir** 1984 Oct;39(5):296–301
Schneider-Hiltbrunner V: Wilhelm Fabry von Hilden 1560–1634. Verzeichnis der Werke und des Briefwechsels. Bern, Hans Huber, 1976. 172 p. (Berner Beiträge zur Geschichte der Medizin und der Naturwissenschaften, 8).

**Fafard, Théogène, 1855–1890**
Painchaud R: Théogène Fafard. In Dictionary of Canadian biography, 1881–1890. 1982;11:306–7.

**Faget, Jean-Charles, 1818–**
Tomlinson WK, Perret JJ: Jean-Charles Faget and the yellow fever controversy in New Orleans. In: Congrès international d'histoire de la médecine, XXVe, Québec, 1976. Actes. Québec, 1977. p. 1361–73.

**Fahrenheit, Gabriel Daniel, 1686–1736**
Van der Star P, ed: Fahrenheit's letters to Leibniz and Boerhaave. Amsterdam, Rodopi, 1983. 195 p. (Nieuwe Nederlandse bijdragen tot de geschiedenis der geneeskunde en der natuurwetenschappen, no. 10).

**Fairbairn, William Ronald Dodds, 1889–1964**
Sutherland JD: The British object relations theorists: Balint, Winnicott, Fairbairn, Guntrip. **J Am Psychoanal Assoc** 1980;28(4):829–60

**Fairley, Neil Hamilton, 1891–1966**
Boyd J: Sir Neil Hamilton Fairley. In Dictionary of national biography, 1961–1970. Suppl. 8, 1981. p. 344–6.

**Fajardo, Francisco de Paula, d. 1906**
Rezende de Castro Monteiro A: 'Hypnotisme'. Analyse de la thèse présentée à la Faculté de Médecine de Rio de Janeiro par Francisco de Paula Fajardo Junior, en vue d'obtenir le grade de docteur en médecine - Rio de Janeiro, 1888. In: Congrès international d'histoire de la médecine, XXVe, Québec, 1976. Actes. Québec, 1977. p. 980–91.

**Falkberget, Johan Petter, 1879–1967**
Kierulf H: Farsottenes rolle i dikteren Johan Falkbergets trilogi 'Christianus Sextus' (1720 årene). **Nord Medicinhist Arsb** 1980;Suppl 6:82–9

**Fallot, Arthur, 1850–1911**
Bjarke B: Mannen bakom syndromet: Arthur Fallot. En medicinens 'doldis'--fransmannen vars namn alla känner men få vet någonting om. **Lakartidningen** 1984 Oct 24;81(43):3934–5

**Falret, Jean Pierre, 1794–1870**
Sedler MJ: Falret's discovery: the origin of the concept of bipolar affective illness. Translated by M. J. Sedler and Eric C. Dessain. **Am J Psychiatry** 1983 Sep;140(9):1127–33

**Fankuchen, Isidor, 1905–1964**
Pnina Abir-Am: The I. Fankuchen papers: their relevance to the historian of molecular biology. **Surv Sources Newsl** 1981 Apr;10:6–9

**Fanon, Frantz, 1925–1961**
Bulhan HA: Frantz Fanon: the revolutionary psychiatrist. **Race Cl** 1980 Winter;21:251–72
Butts HF: Frantz Fanon's contribution to psychiatry: the psychology of racism and colonialism. **J Natl Med Assoc** 1979 Oct;71(10):1015–8

**Fantus, Bernard, 1874–1940**
Myhre BA: Landmark perspective: the significance of Dr. Fantus' report. **JAMA** 1984 Feb 3;251(5):650–2

**Farabeuf, Louis Hubert, 1841–1910**
Guarner V: El pequeño farabeuf, aquel gigante de mi vida estudiantil. **Bol Soc Mex Hist Filos Med** 1982 Mar;6(38):15–22
Guarner V: Louis-Hubert Farabeuf (1841–1910). **Gac Med Mex** 1982 Dec;118(12):505–8

**Farini, Juan Angel, 1901–**
Quiroga M: Juan Angel Farini, medico. **Bol Acad Nac Hist (Argentina)** 1967;40:348–53

**Farkas, Géza, 1872–1934**
Néhány F: Farkas Géza professzorról a tanítványai. **Orv Hetil** 1984 Nov 11;125(46):2817
Szállási A: Farkas Géza-akinek élete volt a fömüve. **Orv Hetil** 1984 Sep 16;125(38):2324–7

**Farmer, Joseph John, 1854–1930**
Forsythe-Jauch WE: L Cpl Joseph John Farmer, VC, AHC. Centenary of the battle of Majuba 1881. **J R Army Med Corps** 1981 Jun;127(2):100–2

**Farquhar, Walter, 1738–1819**
Whitfield AG: Physician to the Prince of Wales. **J R Coll Physicians Lond** 1983 Oct;17(4):231–4

**Farr, Archer, fl. 1865**
Jackson WA: Farr's Patent Ampulla. **Pharm Hist (London)** 1977 Dec;7(3):2–3

**Farr, William, 1807–1883**
C[one] TE: A plea to give weakly children a fair chance, by William Farr (1865). **Pediatrics** 1981;68:49
Carpenter M: William Farr: a pioneer of public health. **Nurs Times** 1983 Jun 15–21;79(24):9–11
Eyler JM: The conceptual origins of William Farr's epidemiology: numerical methods and social thought in the 1830s. In Lilienfeld AM, ed: Times, plaes, and persons. Baltimore, London, Johns Hopkins Univ. Press, 1980. (Sigerist suppl. to the Bull Hist Med, n.s., no 4) p. 1–21.
Richards T: Farr sighted. **Br Med J [Clin Res]** 1983 May 28;286(6379):1736–7

**Farrell Family**
Bogard MO: Peoria's pioneer druggists, the Farrells, and Farrell's Arabian liniment. **Pharm Hist** 1982;24(3):99–105

**Fastlicht, Samuel, 1902–1983**
Sanfilippo J: The life and accomplishments of Dr. Samuel Fastlicht. **Bull Hist Dent** 1983 Oct;31(2):87–92
Sanfilippo J: Bibliografía histórico-odontológica del Dr. Samuel Fastlicht. **Bol Soc Mex Hist Filos Med** 1984 Jun;7(47):317–24
Sanfilippo J: Semblanza del doctor Samuel Fastlicht. **Bol Soc Mex Hist Filos Med** 1984 Jun;7(47):309–15

**Fatio, Johannes, 1649–1691**
Rickham PP: Johannes Fatio: Sein Leben, sein Werk und sein schreckliches Ende. **Z Kinderchir** 1984 Oct;39(5):289–95
Rintelen F: Der Basler Chirurg und Rebell Johannes Fatio 1649–1691. **Gesnerus** 1983;40(1–2):149–58

**Fauchard, Pierre, 1678–1761**
Angot JL: Pierre Fauchard (1677?–1761). Expert pour les dents, et maître chirurgien de Saint-Côme de Paris. **Clio Med** 1983 Mar;17(4):207–21
Besombes A: La triste fin de Pierre-Nicolas Gaulard (1713–1740) 'élève-associé de Fauchard'. **Hist Sci Med** 1980;14(2):213–20
Gysel C: Les implications cartésiennes de la nosologie bucco-dentaire de Pierre Fauchard (1678–1761–1978). **Rev Belge Med Dent** 1979;34(3):313–20
Gysel C: Il dentista Fauchard. **Dent Cadmos** 1980 Jan;48(1):61–3. Feb;48(2):49–52
'Le chirurgien-dentiste' di Pierre Fauchard, I and II: **Dent Cadmos** 1980 May;48(5):57–60, (6):53–7
Marmasse A: Soins de canaux de Fauchard à aujourd'hui. **Actual Odontostomatol (Paris)** 1980;34(129):37–49
Premuda L: Significativi ritorni: Pierre Fauchard (1690–1761). **G Stomatol Ortognatodonzia** 1982 Apr–Jun;1(1):5–9
Tanzer G: Aus der Geschichte der Zahnheilkunde. Pierre Fauchard. **Zahnarzt** 1983 Nov;27(11):713–7

**Faulkner, William, 1897–1962**
Liles DM: William Faulkner's Absalom, Absalom!: an exegesis of the homoerotic configurations in the novel. **J Homosex** 1983 Spring–Summer;8(3–4):99–111

**Fautrart, Thomas, fl. 1670**
Burnby J: The Thomas Fautrart pill tile. **Pharm Hist (London)** 1977 Dec;7(3):6

**Fawcett, Benjamin, ca. 1817–1890**
Forster FM: Benjamin Fawcett, a 19th century Australian quack-doctor. In: International Congress of the History of Medicine, 26th, Plovdiv (Bulgaria), 1978. Actes du Congres, Vol. 1. Sofia, 1980. p. 111–2.
Forster FM: B. Fawcett, a nineteenth-century Australian quack doctor. **J R Aust Hist Soc** 1981;67(3):272–82

**Fay, Cyrus, 1778–1839**
Cohen RA: Cyrus Fay, a pioneer in forceps design. **Bull Hist Dent** 1983 Apr;31(1):32–3

**Fayyad bin Hakim Wahhaj**
Abdul Hai Farooqi: Dafi al-Amrad; an important medical manuscript. **Stud Hist Med** 3(3):199–203, Sep 79

**Featherstone, Henry Walter**
Helliwell PJ: Henry Walter Featherstone, first President of the Association of Anesthetists of Great Britain and Ireland (1932–34). **Anaesthesia** 1982 Apr;37(4):394–7

**Fébres-Cordero, Focion, 1910–**
Fébres-Cordero F: Hoja de servicios (1929–1979). Datos biográficos, actividades, labor intelectual y algunos juicios y comentarios sobre la obra realizada. Caracas, Publicaciones del Consejo de Profesores Universitarios Jubilados, 1979. 256 p.

**Fechner, Gustav Theodor, 1801–1887**
Adler HE: Vicissitudes of Fechnerian psychophysics in America. In R. W. Rieber, K. Salzinger, ed. Psychology: theoretical-historical perspectives. New York, Academic Press, 1980. p. 11–23.
Eckhardt G, ed: Zur Geschichte der Psychologie. Berlin, VEB Deutscher Verlag der Wissenschaften, 1979. 128p. Mit Beiträgen von H. Hiebsch, F. Klix, W. Schreier, und L. Sprung.
Marshall ME: Biographical genre and biographical archetype: five studies of Gustav Theodor Fechner. **Stor Crit Psicol** 1980;1(2):197–233
Schreier W: Ueber historische Wurzeln von Fechners Psychophysik. In Eckardt G, ed: Zur Geschichte der Psychologie. Berlin, VEB Deutscher Verlag der Wissenschaften, 1979. p. 61–71.

**Fedorov, Nikolay Aleksandrovich, 1904–**
Koziner VB, Iarochkin VS: Razvitie problemy krovezamenitelei v trudakh akademika N. A. Fedorova i ego shkoly. **Gematol Transfuziol** 1984 Jan;29(1):12–6

**Fehling, Hermann Johannes Karl, 1847–1925**
Blönningen J: Die Osteomalazie als Indikation für eine bilaterale Oophorektomie im späten 19. und frühen 20. Jahrhundert. Ergebnisse und Erklärungsversuche. Diss. Erlangen-Nürnberg, 1980. 113 p.
Wankmüller A: Anfänge des Chemie- und Pharmaziestudiums in Stuttgart unter Professor Hermann Fehling. **Dtsch Apoth Ztg** 1982 Sep 9;122(36):1805–6

**Feldberg, Wilhelm Siegmund, 1900–**
Bacq ZM: Les expériences de W. Feldberg en l'année 1932. **Bull Mem Acad R Med Belg** 1982;137 Suppl:9–30

**Feldman, William Hugh, 1892–**
Comroe JH: Pay dirt: the story of streptomycin. Part II. Feldman and Hinshaw; Lehmann. **Am Rev Respir Dis** 1978 May;117(5):957–68

**Felix, Iacob, 1832–**
Anastasatu C: Aportul lui Iacob Felix la combaterea tuberculozei în ţara noastră (cu acasia aniversarii a 150 de ani de la naştere). **Rev Ig [Pneumoftiziol]** 1983 Oct–Dec;32(4):379–80

**Felixmüller, Conrad, 1897–1977**
Schulze W: Conrad Felixmüller 1897 - 1977—ein Maler der Tierärzte. **Hist Med Vet** 1977;2(2):51–5

**Felke, Emanuel, 1856–1926**
Rothschuh KE: Aus der Geschichte der Naturheilbewegung (VII). Die Heilkräfte von Licht, Luft und Erde. Arnold Rikli, Adolf Just und Pastor Felke. **ZFA (Stuttgart)** 1983 Jun 10;59(16):933–40

**Felsenfeld, Oscar**
Felsenfeld O: Selected bibliography O. Felsenfeld. **Acta Trop (Basel)** 1979 Jun;36(2):193–8

**Felty, Augustus Roi, 1895–**
Hedfors E: Mannen bakom syndromet: Augustus Roi Felty. Fann ovanlig symtomkonstellation: artrit, splenomegali, leukopeni. **Lakartidningen** 1983 Sep 14;80(37):3281

**Feltz, Victor Thimothé, 1835–1893**
Wrotnowska D: Pasteur et Victor Feltz de Nancy. Correspondance inédite. In: Congrès National des Sociétés Savantes, 103e, Nancy, 1978. Comptes Rendus. Paris, 1978. Section des Sciences, Fasc. V. p. 131–44.

**Fencl, Zdeněk, 1922–1981**
Dr. Zdeněk Fencl 1922–1981: **Folia Microbiol (Praha)** 1982;27(5):285–94

**Fenn, Wallace Osgood, 1893–1971**
Dustan A, ed: In memoriam Wallace O. Fenn 1893–1971. [S.l., s.n.] 1979? [127] p.

**Fenton, Joseph, fl. 1623–1634**
Alsop JD: The fatal illness of the antiquary William Burton (1609–57). **Notes Queries** 1979 Oct;26(5):424–5

**Ferenczi, Sándor, 1873–1933**
Cremerius J: 'Die Sprache der Zärtlichkeit und der Leidenschaft'. Reflexionen zu Sándor Ferenczis Wiesbadener Vortrag von 1932. **Psyche (Stuttg)** 1983 Nov;37(11):988–1015
Hárdi I: Ferenczi Sándor jelentösége a mai orvostudomány számára. **Orv Hetil** 1983 Aug 21;124(34):2067–70
Harmat P, Hebenstreit G: Freud, Ferenczi und die Psychoanalyse in Ungarn. **Wien Med Wochenschr** 1982 Feb 15;132(3):63–6
Harmat P, Hebenstreit G: Sándor Ferenczis theoretisches Werk. **Wien Med Wochenschr** 1984 Jan 31;134(2):49–53
Szállási A: Freud, Ferenczi és a Nyugat. **Orv Hetil** 1980 May 18;121(20):1207–8
Walter H: Sándor Ferenczi. In J. Rattner, ed: Wandlungen der Psychoanalyse. Wien, Europaverlag, 1980. p. 53–86.

**Ferguson, John Creery, 1802–1865**
Pinkerton JH: John Creery Ferguson 1802–1865: Physician and fetologist. **Ulster Med J** 1981;50(1):10–20
Pinkerton JH: John Creery Ferguson. Friend of William Stokes and pioneer of auscultation of the fetal heart in the British Isles. **Br J Obstet Gynaecol** 1980 Apr;87(4):257–60

**Fergusson, William, 1773–1846**
Bennett JP: Sir William Fergusson and the Indian Rhinoplasty. **Ann R Coll Surg Engl** 1984 Nov;66(6):444–8

**Fermi, Enrico, 1901–1954**
Regato JA del: Enrico Fermi. **Int J Radiat Oncol Biol Phys** 1982 Aug;8(8):1393–416

**Fernel, Jean François, 1506 or 7–1558**
Bono JJ, Schmitt CB: An unknown letter of Jacques Daléchamps to Jean Fernel: local autonomy versus centralized government. **Bull Hist Med** 1979 Spring;53(1):100–27

**Ferran y Clua, Jaime, 1852–1929**
Bornside GH: Jaime Ferran and preventive inoculation against cholera. **Bull Hist Med** 1981 Winter;55(4):516–32
Bornside GH: Waldemar Haffkine's cholera vaccines and the Ferran–Haffkine priority dispute. **J Hist Med Allied Sci** 1982 Oct;37(4):399–422
Wrotnowska D: Pasteur et Ferran y Clua, correspondance inédite. In International Congress of the History of Medicine, 27th, Barcelona, 1980. Actas. Barcelona, Acadèmia de Ciències Mèdiques de Catalunya i Balears, 1981. p. 699–707.

**Ferrari, Antonio de, Galateo, 1444–1517**
Tateo F: L'esperienza scientifica di A. de Ferrariis Galateo: Osservazioni sul De podagra. In S. Bertelli, G. Ramakus, ed: Essays presented to Myron P. Gilmore. Vol. 1. Florence, La Nuova Italia, 1978.

**Ferrata, Adolfo, 1880–1946**
Baserga A, Zavagli G: Ferrata's stem cells: an historical review on hemocytoblasts and hemohistioblasts. **Blood Cells** 1981;7(3):537–45

**Ferreira, Luiz Gomes, fl. 1735–1745**
Costa Filho M: O Erário mineral de Luiz Gomes Ferreira. **Rev Inst Hist Geogr Bras** 1957;235:331–40

**Ferriar, John, 1764–1815**
Pickstone JV: Ferriar's fever and Kay's cholera: disease and social structure in Cottonopolis. **Soc Soc Hist Med Bull (Lond)** 1980;27:19–22
Pickstone JV: Ferriar's fever to Kay's cholera: disease and social structure in cottonopolis. **Hist Sci** 1984 Dec;22(58 pt 4):401–19

**Ferrier, Auger, 1513–1585**
Martinez Conesa JA: Sobre 'De somniis' de Augerius Ferrerius. **Helmantica** 1975;26:341–55

**Feuchtersleben, Ernst von, 1806–1849**
Laor N: Szasz, Feuchtersleben, and the history of psychiatry. **Psychiatry** 1982;45(4):316–24
Laor N: The myth of mental illness: the Feuchtersleben version. **Gesnerus** 1984;41(1/2):3–32
Rissmann W: Ernst Freiherr von Feuchtersleben (1806–1849). Sein Beitrag zur medizinischen Anthropologie und Psychopathologie. Freiburg im Breisgau, Schulz, 1980. 243 p. (Freiburger Forschungen zur Medizingeschichte, Neue Folge, Band 12).

**Feuerbach, Ludwig Andreas, 1804–1872**
Löther I, Löther R: Engels' 'Ludwig Feuerbach und der Ausgang der klassischen deutschen Philosophie', die Grundrichtungen des philosophischen Denkens und die Medizin. **Med Ges** 1979;(5):79–91

**Feydeau, Georges Léon Jules Marie, 1862–1921**
Cremerius J: Die ödipal verkleidete präödipale Liebe oder Feydeaus professionelles Missverständnis. **Psyche (Stuttg)** 1981;35:253–67

**Fezl-e-Ali-Shifa-ee Khan**
Hussain SA: Ilajul Atfal: a treatise on pediatrics by Fezl-e-Ali-Shifa-ee Khan. **Bull Indian Inst Hist Med Hyderabad** 1982;12(1-4):45-50

**Fibiger, Johannes Andreas Grib, 1867-1928**
Clemmesen J: Johannes Fibiger. Copenhagen, Munksgaard, 1978. 13 p.

**Ficino, Marsilio, 1433-1499**
Ficino M: The book of life. A translation by Charles Boer of Liber de Vita (or De Vita Triplici). Irving, Texas, Spring Publications, 1980. xix, 217 p.
Johannes Adelphus: Ausgewählte Schriften. 3. Band. Das Buch des Lebens. Ed. A. R. Arthur, B. Gotzkowsky. Berlin, New York, De Gruyter, 1980. 413 p.

**Field, Edward, 1782?-1840**
Langley HD: Edward Field: a pioneer practitioner of the old Navy. **Conn Med** 1982 Nov;46(11):667-72

**Fielding, George Hunsley, 1801-1871**
Read MB: A 19th-century weatherman, Dr. George Henry [sic] Fielding of Grove House, Tonbridge. **Cantium** 1972;3,4(4):99-100

**Figueredo y Diaz, Félix, 1828-1892**
Expósito CR: Dr. Félix Figueredo y Diaz (Un hombre del 68 y de la Protesta de Baraguá). Habana, Organismos, 1973. 417 p. (Cuadernos de Historia de la Salud Pública, 55).
Figueredo Díaz F: La guerra de Cuba en 1878 (La protesta de Baragua). Habana, Organismos, 1973. 338 p. (Cuadernos de Historia de la Salud Pública, 56).

**Fikentscher, Richard, 1903-**
Richter K: Die II. Frauenklinik der Universität München und Richard Fikentscher. **MMW** 1983 Sep 23;125(38):827-30

**Filatov, Antonin Nikolaevich, 1902-1974**
Bogomolova LG, Andrianova LG, Selivanov EA: Zaslugi A. N. Filatova v razvitie problemy sozdaniia lechebnykh preparatov krovi i krovezameniteleĭ. **Vestn Khir** 1982 Oct;129(10):9-13
Fedorova ZD: Osnovnye napravleniia rabot A. N. Filatova po probleme svertyvaniia krovi. **Vestn Khir** 1982 Oct;129(10):13-6
Golovin GV, Depp ME, Dutkevich IG: Vydaiushchiĭsia sovetskiĭ khirurg i transfuziolog (k 80-letiiu so dnia rozhdeniia A. N. Filatova). **Vestn Khir** 1982 Oct;129(10):3-8
Kovalev MM, Suslov VS: Antonin Nikolaevich Filatov, ego rol' v razvitii sovremennoĭ khirurgii. **Klin Khir** 1983 Mar;(3):58-60
Zinevich VP: Razvitie ideĭ A. N. Filatova po probleme parenteral'nogo pitaniia v khirurgii. **Vestn Khir** 1982 Oct;129(10):16-20

**Filelfo, Francesco, 1398-1481**
Kraye J: Francesco Filelfo on emotions, virtues and vices: a re-examination of his sources. **Bibl Hum Renaissance** 1981;43(1):129-40

**Filipchenko, IuA, 1882-1930**
Golda DM: Iu. A. Filipchenko--osnovopolozhnik otechestvennoĭ genetiki (1882-1930 gg.). **Tsitol Genet** 1982;16(1):73 passim

**Filliozat, Jean, 1906-1982**
Mazars G: Jean Filliozat (1906-1982). **Watermark** 1983 Jan;12:3-7
Subba Reddy DV: Prof. Jean Filliozat (1906-1981). **Bull Indian Inst Hist Med Hyderabad** 1982;12(1-4):85-8

**Finfrock, John H., 1836-1893**
Palmieri A, Humberson C: Medical incidents in the life of Dr. John H. Finfrock. **Ann Wyo** 1981;53(2):64-9

**Finkelnburg, D. C., fl. 1870**
Duffy RJ, Liles BZ: A translation of Finkelnburg's (1870) lecture on aphasia as 'asymbolia' with commentary. **J Speech Hear Disord** 1979 May;144(2):156-68

**Finlay, Carlos Juan, 1833-1915**
Belozerov VN: 150-letie so dnia rozhdeniia Karlosa Kh. Finleia. **Parazitologiia** 1983 Nov-Dec;17(6):498-9
Centenario del descubrimiento del agente trasmisor de la fiebre amarilla: **Rev Cubana Med Trop** 1981 Jan-Apr;33(1):3-7
Echemendia V: Zum 100. Jahrestag der Entdeckung des Vektors des Gelbfiebers durch den kubanischen Gelehrten Carlos J. Finlay. **Z Gesamte Hyg** 1983 Jan;29(1):35-6
Finlay Seiglie A: Datos interesantes y anecdóticos sobre el sabio cubano Carlos J. Finlay, descubridor del agente trasmisor de la fiebre amarilla. **Rev Cubana Med Trop** 1981 Jan-Apr;33(1):8-12
Guerra FS, Flores GK: Carlos J. Finlay y Barrés (1833-1915). **Trans R Soc Trop Med Hyg** 1983;77(6):850
López Sánchez J: Karlos KH. Finlai i teoriia peredachi infektsii. **Vopr Istor Estestvozn Tekh** 1981;(4):29-34
Lopez Sanchez J: Carlos J. Finlay and the conception of contagion. **Indian J Hist Sci** 1981;16(2):156-68

**Finot, André, 1884-1980**
Pecker A: André Finot (24 mars 1884 - 3 janvier 1980). **Hist Sci Med** 1980;14(1):23-7

**Finsen, Niels Ryberg, 1860-1904**
Kock W: Nordens första medicinska Nobelpris. **Nord Medicinhist Arsb** 1982;:110-21

**Fischelis, Robert P., 1891-1981**
Cowen DL: Robert P. Fischelis 1891-1981. **NJ J Pharm** 1982 Feb;55(2):12-4

**Fischer, Albert, 1891-1956**
Rasmussen L: En forstander og hans assistent. **Dan Medicinhist Arbog** 1981;:130-40

**Fischer, Carl, d. 1893**
Gluckman LK: Dr. Carl Fischer MD and the history of homeopathy in Auckland in the 19th century. **NZ Med J** 1979 Jul 25;90(640):66-9
Gluckman LK: Dr. Carl Frank Fischer M.D.: an early Auckland physician, botanist and viticulturalist. **J Auckl Waikato Hist Soc** 1980;(37):18-20

**Fischer, Johann Nepomuk, 1777-1847**
Kadlecová V: Počátky oční kliniky v Praze, její první profesor J. N. Fischer a jeho asistenti. **Cesk Oftalmol** 1983 May;39(3):202-14
Kadlecová V: Počátky oční kliniky v Praze, Jej í první profesor J.N. Fischer a jeho asistenti. III. První profesor pražské oční kliniky J.N. Fischer: jeho život; Fischer - učitel, operatér, člověk. **Cesk Oftalmol** 1983 Jul;39(4):268-80

**Fishbein, Morris, 1889-1976**
Bean WB: Occasional notes. My sampler of editors: a Fishbein, a Fox, and a Garland. **N Engl J Med** 1980 Jul 24;303(4):229-33

**Fisher, C. Miller, 1913-**
Ojemann RG: Biography of C. Miller Fisher, M.D. **Clin Neurosurg** 1983;31:xiii-xxviii

**Fisher, George Jackson, 1825-1893**
Burns SB: Early medical photography in America (1839--1883); IV. Early wet-plate era. **NY State J Med** 1979 Nov;79(12):1931-8

**Fisher, Ronald Aylmer, 1890-1962**
Box JF: R. A. Fisher: the life of a scientist. New York, Wiley, 1978. xii, 512 p.
Norton B: Fisher and the neo-Darwinian synthesis. In Forbes EG, ed: Human implications of scientific advance. Edinburgh, Edinburgh University Press, 1978. p. 481-94.
Norton B: La situation intellectuelle au moment des débuts de Fisher en génétique des populations. In Actes du Colloque R.A. Fisher.... Paris, 5-6 déc. 1979. p. 231-50. **Rev Synth (Paris)** 1981;102(103-104)
Race RR, Sanger R: Fisher's contribution to Rh. **Vox Sang** 1982;43(6):354-6
Van Loghem JJ: Classic illustration (Sir Ronald Fisher). **Eur J Obstet Gynecol Reprod Biol** 1983 Oct;16(2):147-8
Yates F: Sir Ronald Aylmer Fisher. In Dictionary of national biography, 1961-1970. Suppl. 8, 1981. p. 361-2.

**Fisher, Russell Sylvester, 1916-**
Petty CS: The medical examiner and medical education (Russell S. Fisher). **Hum Pathol** 1980 Mar;11(2):101-3

**Fiske, John, 1842-1901**
Lester JF: John Fiske's philosophy of science: the union of science and religion through the principle of evolution. Ph.D. Diss., Oregon State University, Corvallis, 1979. 275 leaves.

**Fitz, Reginal Heber, 1843-1913**
Morer G: Naissance d'un vocable. **Hist Sci Med** 1984;18(2):165-71

**Fitzgerald, Alice Louise Florence, 1875-1962**
Weigold ME: Alice Louise Florence Fitzgerald. In Dictionary of American biography, 1961-1965. Suppl. 7, 1981. p. 247-8.

**Fitzpatrick, Thomas Bernard, 1919-**
Curriculum vitae: Thomas Bernard Fitzpatrick. **J Invest Dermatol** 1983 Jun;80 Suppl:6s-11s
Parrish JA: Festschrift: Thomas B. Fitzpatrick--a powerful difference. **J Invest Dermatol** 1983 Jun;80 Suppl:3s-5s

**Flaubert, Achille Cléophas, 1784-1846**
Sagaert LLC: Un grand chirurgien français: le docteur Achille-Cléophas Flaubert. **Hist Sci Med** 1980;14:449-52

**Flaubert, Gustave, 1821-1880**
Baudry FD: Adolescent love and self-analysis as contributors to Flaubert's creativity. **Psychoanal Study Child** 1980;35:377-416
Bugyi B: G. Flaubert (1821-1880) és az orvosok. **Orv Hetil** 1980 Jun 1;121(22):1339-40
Gastaut H, Gastaut Y: La maladie de Gustave Flaubert. **Rev Neurol (Paris)** 1982;138(6-7):467-92
Gastaut H, Gastaut Y, Broughton R: Gustave Flaubert's illness: a case report in evidence against the erroneous notion of psychogenic epilepsy. **Epilepsia** 1984 Oct;25(5):622-37
Godlewski G: Flaubert l'inassouvi. **Sem Hop Paris** 1980 Dec 18-25;56(47-68):2051-62
Hossard J: Une rencontre inattendue: Flaubert et Dorvault. **Rev Hist Pharm (Paris)** 1980 Jun;27(245):119-22
Hossard J, ed: Flaubert et la médecine. [Catalog of an exhibition July 5-27, 1980.] Rouen, Musée Flaubert, Hôtel Dieu de Rouen, 1980. n. p.
Lemaire JF: Gustave Flaubert, médecin passif. **Nouv Rev Deux Mondes** 1981;9:580-92
Mitzman A: The unstrung Orpheus: Flaubert's youth and the psycho-social origins of art for art's sake. **Psychohist Rev** 6(1):27-42, Summer 77

Mitzman A: Sartres Flaubert. **Psyche (Stuttg)** 1981 Mar;35(3):268-98
Romay Garcia Arias L: La medicina en la obra literaria de Gustave Flaubert. **Galicia Clin** 1978;50:604, 671, 759
Vigliani F, Vigliani MC: La strefopodia nella fantasia e nell'arte di Gustave Flaubert. **Chir Organi Mov** 1980 Jul-Aug;66(4):533-43

**Flechsig, Paul Emil, 1847-1929**
Meyer A: Paul Flechsig's system of myelogenetic cortical localization in the light of recent research in neuroanatomy and neurophysiology part II. **Can J Neurol Sci** 1981 May;8(2):95-104
Meyer A: Paul Flechsig's system of myelogenetic cortical localization in the light of recent research in neuroanatomy and neurophysiology. Part I. **Can J Neurol Sci** 1981 Feb;8(1):1-6

**Fleck, Ludwik, 1896-1961**
Kielanowski T: My meetings with Ludwik Fleck in Lublin during the years 1945-1950. **Kwart Hist Nauki Tech** 1983;28(3-4):583-7
Porus VN: Ludwick Flecks's epistemological conception and contemporary discussion on the nature and dynamics of scientific knowledge. **Kwart Hist Nauki Tech** 1983;28(3-4):545-60
Schnelle T: Ludwik Fleck - a classical scholar of the sociology of science and of epistemology. **Kwart Hist Nauki Tech** 1983;28(3-4):525-43
Tsouyopoulos N: Auf der Suche nach einer adäquaten Methode für die Geschichte und Theorie der Medizin. Auseinandersetzung mit Ludwik Flecks 'Entstehung und Entwicklung einer wissenschaftlichen Tatsache'. **Medizinhist J** 1982;17(1/2):20-36
Weissmann G: In quest of Fleck: science from the holocaust. **Hosp Pract** 1980 Oct;15(10):48-9, 52, 54-5 passim

**Fleming, Alexander, 1881-1955**
Abraham EP: Fleming's discovery. **Rev Infect Dis** 1980 Jan-Feb;2(1):129-140
Chain E: A short history of the penicillin discovery from Fleming's early observations in 1929 to the present time. In J. Parascandola, ed: The history of antibiotics. Madison, American Institute of the History of Pharmacy, 1980. p. 15-29.
Fleming y la penicilina: **Rev Col Nac Enferm** 1979 Aug-Dec;26(105):16-8
Hankiss J: A tudományos teljesítmény értékelése. Fleming felfedezése tükrében. **Orv Hetil** 1980 Jan 13;121(2):95-8
Hare R: The scientific activities of Alexander Fleming, other than the discovery of penicillin. **Med Hist** 1983 Oct;27(4):347-72
Jones G: Alexander Fleming. **New Sci** 1981;91:349-51
Kempler K: Tervszerü kutatás, vagy véletlen? Gondolatok Fleming születésének centenáriumán. **Orv Hetil** 1981 Nov 29;122(48):2967-9
Macfarlane RG: Alexander Fleming: the man and the myth. London, Chatto & Windus, The Hogarth Press, 1984. xiv, 304 p.
Milders JW: Taking a look at the invisible. **Hindustan Antibiot Bull** 1982 Aug-Nov;24(3-4):93-6
Rihner F: Sir Alexander Fleming - zum 25. Todestag. **Med Welt** 1980;31:1564-5
Starzycki Z: W 40 rocznice wprowadzenia penicyliny do leczenia kiły i rzeżaczki. **Przegl Lek** 1984;41(6):453-7
Tovarova II, Shamin AN: Istoriia penitsillinov (k 100-letiiu so dnia rozhdeniia Aleksandra Eleminga). **Vopr Istor Estestvozn Tekh** 1981;3:65-75
Voyatzakis E, et al: [The research work of Sir Alexander Fleming] (Gre). **Mater Med Greca** 1981;9:367-76
Zikeev PD: Aleksandr Fleming (k 100-letiiu so dnia rozhdeniia). **Klin Med (Mosk)** 1983 Feb;61(2):110-2

**Fleming, William, 1728-1795**
Shields RT: He helped shape Virginia: Dr. Wiliam Fleming, 1728-1795. **Va Med** 1982 Jul;109(7):441-5

**Flemming, Walther, 1843-1905**
Breathnach CS: Biographical sketches No. 18--Flemming. **Ir Med J** 1982 Jun;75(6):177

**Fletcher, Horace, 1849-1919**
Whorton JC: 'Physiologic optimism': Horace Fletcher and hygienic ideology in progressive America. **Bull Hist Med** 1981 Spring;55(1):59-87

**Fletcher, William Baldwin, 1837-1907**
Cone TE: On dressing the American newborn infant a century ago. **Pediatrics** 1981;67:268

**Fleurimont, Sieur de, fl. 1682**
Gysel C: Un tricentenaire: la prophylaxie dentaire du Sieur de Fleurimont (1682-1982) (I). **Med Hyg (Geneve)** 1983 Jul 15;41(1525):2549-50; Jul 30;41(1526):2622-3

**Flexner, Abraham, 1866-1959**
Cangi EC: Abraham Flexner's philanthrophy: the full-time system in the department of surgery at the University of Cincinnati College of Medicine, 1910-1930. **Bull Hist Med** 1982 Summer;56(2):160-74
Donatucci CF: In anticipation of Flexner. **Trans Stud Coll Physicians Phila** 1978 Jul;45(5):280-9
Fox DM: Abraham Flexner's unpublished report: foundations and medical education, 1909-1928. **Bull Hist Med** 1980 Winter;54(4):475-96
Harris MR: Abraham Flexner. In Dictionary of American Biography, Suppl. 6, 1956-1960. p. 207-9, 1980.
King LS: Medicine in the USA: historical vignettes. XX. The Flexner report of 1910. **JAMA** 1984 Feb 24;251(8):1079-86
Lemann N: Let the nurses do it. **Wash Mon** 1979;11(2):29-36
Lovell RR: The university medical presence in hospitals seventy years after Flexner and a look ahead. **Aust NZ J Med** 1983 Apr;13(2):187-94
Medical school reformer: **MD** 1978 Jul;22(7):133-8

**Flexner, Simon, 1863-1946**
Hatcher J: Simon Flexner. **Gaz Inst Med Lab Sci** 1981;25:317-8
Miller M: The Simon Flexner papers. **Surv Sources Newsl** 1979 Apr;9:2-4

**Fliedner, Theodor, 1800-1864**
Sticker DA: [Theodor Fliedner and nursing] (Jpn). **Sogo Kango** 1980;15(4):146-55

**Fliess, Wilhelm, 1858-1928**
Schott H: Freuds Selbstanalyse (Freud und Fliess). In International Congress of the History of Medicine, 27th, Barcelona, 1980. Actas. Barcelona, Académia de Ciències Médiques de Catalunya i Balears, 1981. p. 145-8.
Wentges RT: Wilhelm Fliess en de nasale reflexneurose. **Ned Tijdschr Geneeskd** 1981 Feb 14;125(7):278-84

**Florén Lozano, Luis, 1913-**
Hernández de Alba G: Una obra postuma cientifica monumental: la bibliografia medica Colombiana (1782-1976). **Bol Cult Bibliogr (Bogota)** 1976;16(7-8):176-9

**Flores y Troncoso, Francisco de Asis, 1855-1931**
Flores y Troncoso FA: Historia de la medicina en México desde la época de los indios hasta la presente. Facsimile of 1886 ed. plus new indices. 4 vols. México, Instituto Mexicano del Seguro Social, 1982. Various pagings. Historical and biographical chapters by V. M. Ruiz Naufal, A. G. Medrano, C. Viesca, G. A. Beltrán, J. S. Palencia, J. S. Riquer, B. F. Hernández.

**Florey, Howard Walter, 1898-1968**
McEwin R: Florey and Cairns--early work on penicillin. **Med J Aust** 1982 Jan 9;1(1):12-3
Macfarlane RG: Howard Florey; the making of a great scientist. Oxford and New York, Oxford University Press, 1979. xvi, 396 p.
Macfarlane RG: Howard Walter Florey. In Dictionary of national biography, 1961-1970. Suppl. 8, 1981. p. 370-4.
Travers R: Florey and Cairns--early work on penicillin. **Med J Aust** 1982 Jul 10;2(1):10-1

**Florkin, Marcel, 1900-1979**
Bacq ZM: Marcel Florkin. Harvard et Californie 1929-1930. **Rev Med Liege** 1983 Apr 1;38(7):257-60
Bacq ZM: Marcel Florkin, 1900-1979. In Florilège des Sciences en Belgique - II. Bruxelles, Académie Royale de Belgique, 1980. p. 675-78.
Brachet J: Marcel Florkin. **Bull Cl Sci Acad R Belg** 1980;5(66):188-94
Edsall JT: Marcel Florkin, August 15, 1900--May 3, 1979. **Isis** 1980 Jun;71(257):286-8
Fruton JS: Marcel Florkin, 1900-1979, historian of biochemistry. **Hist Philos Life Sci** 1980;2(1):167-71
Huard P: Marcel Florkin (1900-1979). **Clio Med** 1980 May;14(2):93-5
In memoriam Professor Dr. Marcel Florkin (1900-1979): **Clio Med** 1980 May;14(2):89-90
Schoffeniels E: In memoriam Marcel Florkin (Liège, 15 août 1900-3 mai 1979). Les chênes qu'on abat. **Rev Med Liege** 1979 Jun 1;34(11):481-7
Schoffeniels E: Marcel Florkin et les aspects moleculaires de la biologie. **Bull Mem Acad R Med Belg** 1979 Nov 24;134(10):604-16
Schoffeniels E: Marcel Florkin: founding father of comparative biochemistry. **Comp Biochem Physiol** 1980;67B:353-8
Théodoridès J: Marcel Florkin (1900-1979). **Rev Hist Sci (Paris)** 1980 Jan;33(1):75-6
Théodoridès J: Marcel Florkin (1900-1979). **Hist Sci Med** 1980;14(2):145-50

**Florschütz, Vatroslav, 1876-1967**
Marinović I: 'Balkanski okvir' (ram) ili 'Balkanska metoda' i njegov tvorac. **Srp Arh Celok Lek** 1984 Jan;112(1):127-36

**Flourens, Marie Jean Pierre, 1794-1867**
Legée G: P. Flourens (1794-1867) et la psychiatrie de son temps. In: Congrès National des Sociétés Savantes, 103e, Nancy, 1978. Comptes Rendus. Paris, 1978. Section des Sciences, Fasc. V. p. 113-23.
Légée G: A. Vulpien (1826-1887), physiologiste élève de P. Flourens (1794-1867). In: Congrès international d'histoire de la médecine, XXVe, Québec, 1976. Actes. Québec, 1977. p. 873-80.
Legée G: L'activité parisienne d'un physiologiste languedocien Marie-Jean-Pierre Flourens (1794-1867). In: Congrès National des Sociétés Savantes, 96e, Toulouse, 1971. Comptes Rendus. Paris, 1974. Histoire des Sciences, Tome 1. p. 107-22.
Legée G: Les concepts de localisation et de coordination dans la neurophysiologie de Maire-Jean-Pierre Flourens (1794-1867). In: Congrès National des Sociétés Savantes, 96e, Toulouse, 1971. Comptes Rendus. Paris, 1974. Histoire des Sciences, Tome 1. p. 123-51.
Legée G: Physiologie et phrenologie au temps du physiologiste Pierre Flourens (1794-1867). In International Congress of the History of Medicine, 27th, Barcelona, 1980. Actas. Barcelona, Académia de

Ciències Médiques de Catalunya i Balears, 1981. p. 91-7.
Legée G: Lettres inédites des Félix Archimède Pouchet (1800-1872) au physiologiste Pierre Flourens (1794-1867). In International Congress of the History of Medicine. 26th, Plovdiv, 1978. Actes du Congress. Sofia, 1981. Volume II. p. 130-8.
Legée G: Les relations épistolaires de P. Flourens et de ses collègues de l'Institut de France. In: Congrès National des Sociétés Savantes, 106e, Perpignan, 1981. Comptes Rendus. Paris, Bibliothèque Nationale, 1982. Fasc. IV. p. 171-85.
Legee G: P. Flourens, historien des sciences: valeur de son histoire de la découverte de la circulation du sang. In: Congrès National des Sociétés Savantes, 107e. Brest, 1982. Comptes Rendus, Paris, 1983. Section des Sciences, Fasc. IV. p. 313-31.
Legée G: Influence du vitalisme montpelliérain sur la neurophysiologie de Pierre Flourens. **Hist Nat** 1982;21:13-45

**Flournoy, Théodore, 1854-1920**
Witzig JS: Theodore Flournoy-a friend indeed. **J Anal Psychol** 1982 Apr;27(2):131-48

**Floyer, John, 1649-1734**
Sakula A: Sir John Floyer's A Treatise of the Asthma (1698). **Thorax** 1984 Apr;39(4):248-54
Viniaker H: L'asthme et son environnement selon Sir John Floyer (1649-1734). **Hist Sci Med** 1984;18(1):77-82

**Fludd, Robert, 1574-1637**
Godwin J: Robert Fludd: hermetic philosopher and surveyor of two worlds. London, Thames and Hudson, 1979. 96 p. An annotated collection of plates from Fludds's works.

**Flynn, John, 1880-1951**
Daley EA: The Royal Flying Doctor Service of Australia. **Victorian Hist Mag** 1970;41(3-4):375-95

**Fodor, József, 1843-1901**
Kapronczay K: Markusovszky Lajos utolsó levele Fodor Józsefhez. **Orvostort Kozl** 1980;89-91(26 no 1-3):269-71
Kapronczay K: Markusovszky Lajos utolsó levele Fodor Józsefhez. **Orv Hetil** 1982 Dec 26;123(52):3213-4

**Fogarty, John Edward, 1913-1967**
Bair B: 'The full light of the dawn': Congressman John Fogarty and the historical cycle of community mental health policy in Rhode Island. **RI Hist** 1982;41(4):127-38

**Foix, Charles, 1882-1927**
Pretresco A: Dos conmemoraciones. **Rev Neuropsiquiatr** 1980 Jun;43(2):115-23

**Fokker, Abraham Peter, 1840-1906**
de Knecht-van Eekelen A: Abraham Pieter Fokker (1840-1906) en de serumtherapie bij difterie. **Tijdschr Geschied Geneeskd Natuurwet Wiskd Tech** 1984;7(4):161-71

**Földi, János, 1755-1801**
Nagy S: Szépirodalom--orvostörténelem. **Orv Hetil** 1980 Sep 28;121(39):2421

**Folin, Otto, 1867-1934**
Meites S: Otto Folin's decade in Minnesota, 1882-1892: a brief review. **Clin Chem** 1982 Oct;28(10):2173-7
Meites S: The first call for clinical chemists in the United States. **Clin Chem** 1983 Oct;29(10):1852-3

**Folks, Homer, 1867-1963**
Trattner WI: Homer Folks. In Dictionary of American biography, 1961-1965. Suppl. 7, 1981. p. 250-2.

**Folley, Sydney John, 1906-1970**
Parkes AS: Sydney John Folley. In Dictionary of national biography, 1961-1970. Suppl. 8, 1981. p. 375-6.

**Folsom, James Elisha, 1908-**
Morris JT: Clinical notes on His Excellency James Elisha 'Big Jim' Folsom--Governor of Alabama (1947-1951 and 1955-1959). **J Med Assoc State Ala** 1982 Jan;51(7):36, 39-41, 46

**Fonck, Francisco, 1830-1912**
Costa-Casaretto C: Chile en dueda con el Doctor Francisco Fonck. **Rev Med Chil** 1981 Nov;109(11):1119-25

**Fontana, Felice, 1730-1805**
Disertori B, Piazza M: Felice Fontana precursore delle moderne neuroscienze. **Ann Osp Maria Vittoria Torino** 1981 Jan-Jun;24(1-6)178-209
Knoefel PK: Felice Fontana on Poisons. **Clio Med** 1980;15(1/2):35-65
Knoefel PK: Felice Fontana: light thrown on his character by the case of the 'spazzino' Guidetti. **Med Secoli** 1981 May-Aug;18(2):229-42

**Fontana, Giovanni, ca. 1395-ca. 1455**
Clagett M: The life and works of Giovanni Fontana. **Ann Ist Mus Stor Sci Fir** 1976;1(1):5-28

**Fontane, Theodor, 1819-1898**
Faber-Castell, K von: Arzt, Krankheit und Tod im erzählerischen Werk Theodor Fontanes. Zürich, Juris Druck, 1983. 97 p. (Zürcher Medizingeschichtliche Abhandlungen, Neue Reihe, Nr. 157).

**Fonzi, Giuseppangelo Lucinto, 1768-1840**
Tanzer G: Aus der Geschichte der Zahnheilkunde. Giuseppangelo Fonzi, 13.7.1768-31.8.1840. **Zahnarzt** 1983 Dec;27(12):765-9

**Foote, Edward Bliss, 1829-1906**
Cirillo VJ: Edward Bliss Foote: pioneer American advocate of birth control. **Bull Hist Med** 1973 Sep-Oct;47(5):471-9

**Foote, Frank William, 1911-**
Hutter RV: Classics in Oncology. Lobular carcinoma in situ by Foote and Stewart. **CA** 1982 Jul-Aug;32(4):232-7

**Forberger, Georg, ca. 1543-ca. 1604**
Zaunick R: Der sächsische Paracelsist Georg Forberger. Wiesbaden, Steiner, 1977. xii, 110 p. (Kosmosophie, IV).

**Fordyce, George, 1736-1802**
Heinecke H: Die Kontrolle im Tierversuch--eine historische Studie über Tierversuche von G. F. Fordyce. **Z Versuchstierkd** 1983;25(4):223-6

**Forel, Auguste Henri, 1848-1931**
Müller C: Historische Vignette. August Forel und der Nationalsozialismus. **Nervenarzt** 1984 Sep;55(9):504-5
Vader JP: August Forel defends the persecuted Persian Baha'is, 1925-27. **Gesnerus** 1984;41(1/2):53-60
Walser HH: Ist das Wohl des Landesherrn in Wein zu trinken? Carl und Gerhart Hauptmann bei August Forel in Zürich. **Gesnerus** 1981;38:207-14

**Forestier, Antoine, 1646-1717**
Boissonnault CM: Antoine Forestier. In Dictionary of Canadian biography, 1701 to 1740. Volume 2, 1969. p. 226.

**Forestier, Thomas, fl. 1485**
Walton MT: Stinking air, corrupt water, and the English Sweat: a footnote to the quality of life in fifteenth-century London. **J Hist Med Allied Sci** 1981 Jan;36(1):67-8
Walton MT: Thomas Forestier and the 'False Lechys' of London. **J Hist Med Allied Sci** 1982 Jan;37(1):71-3

**Forlanini, Carlo, 1847-1918**
Berti Bock G, Vial F, Heymans G, et al: Considerazioni critiche sull'opera di Carlo Forlanini (1847-1918). **Minerva Med** 1980 Jun 30;71(26):1879-83
Sakula A: Carlo Forlanini, inventor of artificial pneumothorax for treatment of pulmonary tuberculosis. **Thorax** 1983 May;38(5):326-32

**Formey, Johann Ludwig F., 1766-1823**
Hiller I: Ludwig Formeys 'Versuch einer medicinischen Topographie von Berlin' und kommunale Umweltproblematik im 18. Jahrhundert. **Z Exp Chir** 1982 Jul;28(7):474-6

**Forssell, Gösta, 1876-1950**
Nicou G, Kock W, ed: Från Gösta Forssells och den Svenska röntgenologiens ungdomstid. Södertälje, Sweden, Fingraf Tryckeri, 1984. 84 p. (Nordisk Medicinhistorisk Arsbok, Supplementum X, 1984)

**Forssmann, Werner, 1904-1979**
Jain KM, Swan KG, Casey KF: Nobel prize winners in surgery. **Am Surg** 1982 Oct;48(10):495-500
Steckelberg JM, et al: Werner Forssmann (1904-1979) and his unusual success story. **Conn Med** 1981;45(2):110-2

**Forster, Georg, 1754-1794**
Kaiser W: Johann Reinhold Forster (1729-1798) und Johann Georg Forster (1754-1794) in Halle. Zur 250. Wiederkehr des Geburtstages von Johann Reinhold Forster. **Z Gesamte Inn Med** 1979 Jul 15;34(14):373-81

**Forster, Johann Reinhold, 1729-1798**
Kaiser W: Johann Reinhold Forster (1729-1798) und Johann Georg Forster (1754-1794) in Halle. Zur 250. Wiederkehr des Geburtstages von Johann Reinhold Forster. **Z Gesamte Inn Med** 1979 Jul 15;34(14):373-81
Kaiser W, Völker A: Johann Reinhold Forster (1729-1798) als Ordinarius in Halle. **Wiss Z Martin Luther Univ (Math)** 1981;30(2):61-79

**Fortas, Abe, 1910-1982**
Rioch MJ: In memoriam: Abe Fortas. **Psychiatry** 1983;46(1):83-6

**Fortin, Pierre-Etienne, 1823-1888**
Bilas I: Pierre-Etienne Fortin. In Dictionary of Canadian biography, 1881-1890. 1982;11:320-1.

**Foster, Abigail Kelley, 1810-1887**
Bernard J: Authority, autonomy, and radical commitment: Stephen and Abby Kelley Foster. **Proc Am Antiq Soc** 1980:90(2):347-86

**Foster, Stephen Symonds, 1809-1881**
Bernard J: Authority, autonomy, and radical commitment: Stephen and Abby Kelley Foster. **Proc Am Antiq Soc** 1980:90(2):347-86

**Fothergill, John, 1712-1780**
Fothergill J: Observations on the recovery of a man dead in appearance by distending the lungs with air. Facsimile of London 1745 edition, with biographical note by K. G. Huston. Van Nuys, California, Hoffman, 1980. 13 p.
Lysaght A: A letter from Sydney Parkinson in Batavia to Dr. John Fothergill. **Notes Rec R Soc Lond** 1981;36(1):79-81

**Foucault, Michel Jean Pierre, 1925–**
Forrester J: Michel Foucault and the history of psychoanalysis. **Hist Sci** 1980 Dec;18(42 pt 4):286–303
Midelfort HC: Madness and civilization in early modern Europe: a reappraisal of Michel Foucault. In Malament, Barbara C., ed. After the Reformation: Essays in honor of J. H. Hexter, Philadelphia; U. of Pennsylvania Press, 1980. p. 247–65.
Russ, J: Histoire de la folie [de] Michel Foucault: analyse critique. Paris, Hatier, 1979. 79 p.
Sedgwick P: Michel Foucault: the anti-history of psychiatry. **Psychol Med** 1981 May;11(2):235–48

**Foucher, Emile, 1823–1867**
Peltier LF: The classic. Separations of the epiphyses. By Jean Timothée Emile Foucher. 1867. **Clin Orthop** 1984 Sep;(188):3–9

**Fougerat, André Jacques**
Joblin J: Monseigneur André Jacques Fougerat; ecclesiastical advisor of CICIAMS (1952–1982). **Nouv Com Int Cathol Infirm Assist Med Soc** 1983;(3):1–8

**Fouquet, Marie (de Maupeon), 1590–1681**
Rocchietta S: Le edizioni italiane del ricettario di Madame Fouquet. **Minerva Med** 1981 Jan 21;72(2):111–2

**Fourcroy, Antoine François de, 1755–1809**
Kursanova TA: A. F. Fourcroy and zoochemistry in France at the beginning of the XIXth century. **Istor Biol Issled** 1983;9:176–86
Levin A: Venel, Lavoisier, Fourcroy, Cabanis and the idea of scientific revolution: the French political context and the general patterns of conceptualization of scientific change. **Hist Sci** 1984 Sep;22(57 pt 3):303–20

**Fournier de Lempdes, J.-F., 1783–1861**
Sarazin M: Le docteur Fournier de Lempdes (1783–1861). **Bull Hist Sci Auvergne** 1984;92(680):37–47

**Fournier, Jean Alfred, 1832–1914**
Kampmeier RH: Syphilis and marriage by Alfred Fournier. **Sex Transm Dis** 1981 Jan–Mar;8(1):29–32
Studnitsin AA, Rukavishnikova VM: K 150-letiiu Zhana Al'freda Furn'e. **Vestn Dermatol Venerol** 1982 Apr;(4):75–7

**Fowler, Russell Story, 1874–1959**
Saffron MH: Russell Story Fowler. In Dictionary of American Biography, Suppl. 6, 1956–1960. p. 214–15, 1980.

**Fox, Charles James, 1830–1896**
Illustrations from the Wellcome Institute Library: John Monro MD and Charles James Fox: etching by Thomas Rowlandson. **Med Hist** 1983 Jan;27(1):80–3

**Fox, Joseph, d. 1816**
Herschfeld JJ: Joseph Fox - pioneer dental investigator and author of The Natural History of the Human Teeth. **Bull Hist Dent** 1983 Oct;31(2):101–7

**Fox, Theodor, 1899–**
Bean WB: Occasional notes. My sampler of editors: a Fishbein, a Fox, and a Garland. **N Engl J Med** 1980 Jul 24;303(4):229–33

**Foy, Maximilien-Sebastien, 1775–1825**
Théodoridès J: La médecine et les sciences dans les 'Notes journalières du général Foy'. **Hist Sci Med** 1980;14:305–15

**Fracastoro, Girolamo, 1483–1553**
Chakravorty RC: Girolamo Fracastoro, a man of the Renaissance. **Hist Med (Lond)** 1975 Autumn–Winter;6(3–4):65–7
Graziani R: Fracastoro's 'syphilis' and Priapus. **Clio Med** 1981 Dec;16(2/3):93–9
Heidel G: Zur wahrscheinlich ältesten deutschen Ubersetzung des Syphilisgedichtes von Girolamo Fracastoro. **Dermatol Monatsschr** 1983;169(2):130–5
Peruzzi E: Un trattato inedito di farmacologia di Gerolamo Fracastoro. **Rinascimento** 1978;18:183–228
Rodriguez-Castellon JA: Selected items from the history of pathology - Girolamo Fracastoro (1478–1553). **Am J Pathol** 1980;101(1):62

**Fragonard, Jean Honoré, 1732–1806**
Ellenberger M: Fragonard, l'anatomiste. **Pour Sci** 1982;53:98–108

**Fragoso, Juan, d. 1597**
Carreras Panchon A: La obra de Juan de Villarreal y otros estudios historico-medicos. Salamanca, Ediciones Universidad de Salamanca, 1978. 69 p. (Cuadernos de Historia de la Medicina Española, Mongrafias, XXXIII).

**Fraiberg, Selma, 1918–**
Selective bibliography of Selma Fraiberg (1945–1982): **Psychoanal Q** 1982;51(4):636–41

**France, Anatole, 1844–1924**
Rocchietta S: Alchimia e medicina nel romanzo 'La rosticceria della regina Pedoca' di Anatole France. **Minerva Med** 1980 Oct 31;71(42):3091–2

**Francesco, d'Assisi, Saint, 1182–1226**
Touati FO: François d'Assise et la diffusion d'un modèle thérapeutique a XIIIe siècle. **Hist Sci Med** 1982;16(3):175–84

**Francis of Assisi, Saint, 1182–1226**
Casanovas J: La enfermedad ocular de Francisco de Asís. **Klin Oczna** 1980 May;82(5):243–4

**Francke, Donald Eugene, 1910–**
McLeod DC, Whitney HA: The legacy of Donald E. Francke: DICP--a fifteen-year commitment to clinical pharmacy. **Drug Intell Clin Pharm** 1981 Dec;15(12):990–1

**Franco, Francisco, 1892–1975**
Plaza Izquierdo F: Enfermedad final de Francisco Franco, a proposito de los que mueren en el poder. **Rev Soc Venez Hist Med** 1980;29(43–44):95–124

**Franco, Pierre, ca. 1505–ca. 1579**
Ayer E, Montandon D: Pierre Franco (1506–1580) and the treatment of a cheek ulcer. **Chir Plast** 1980;5(4):289–93

**Frank, Anne, 1929–1945**
Dalsimer K: Female adolescent development. A study of the Diary of Anne Frank. **Psychoanal Study Child** 1982;37:487–522

**Frank, Jerome, 1889–1957**
Chase A: Jerome Frank and American psychoanalytic jurisprudence. **Int J Law Psychiatry** 1979;2(1):29–54

**Frank, Johann Peter, 1745–1821**
Breyer H: Johann Peter Frank. 'Fürst unter den Arzten Europas.' Leipzig, S. Hirzel, 1983. 184 p.
Ganzinger K: Johann Peter Frank und die Apothekerordnung für die österreichische Lombardei. In Ganzinger K, Skopec M, Wyklicky H, ed: Festschrift für Erna Lesky zum 70. Geburtstag. Wien, Brüder Hollinek, 1981. p. 39–47.
Ganzinger K: Johann Peter Frank und die Apothekerordnung für die österreichische Lombardei. **Osterr Apoth Ztg** 1981;35:410–4
Odontoiatria del passato: Dei campanelli de Loreto. **Dent Cadmos** 1981 Jul;49(7):59–60
Vasil'ev KG, Vasil'ev KK: Rol' I. P. Franka a razvitii vysshego meditsinskogo obrazovaniia v Rossii. **Sov Zdravookhr** 1980;(10):62–5

**Fränkel, Albert, 1864–1938**
Szállási A: 100 éve ismert a Pneumococcus pathogén természete. **Orv Hetil** 1984 Dec 9;125(50):3059–62

**Fränkel, Moritz Ottomar, 1814–1902**
Kaiser W: Moritz O. Fränkel (1814–1902) als Mitarbeiter der 'Allgemeinen Zeitschrift für Psychiatrie'. **Wiss Z Martin Luther Univ (Math)** 1983;32(2):89–94

**Frankenthal, Käte, 1889–1976**
Der dreifache Fluch: Jüdin, Intellektuelle, Sozialistin: Lebenserinnerungen einer Arztin in Deutschland und im Exil: Frankfurt/Main, New York, Campus Verlag, 1981. 320 p.

**Frankl, Viktor Emil, 1905–**
Baruk H: Viktor Frankl et la psychanalyse. **Ann Med Psychol (Paris)** 1982 Apr;140(4):438–42
Doering D: Die Logotherapie Viktor Emil Frankls. Köln, 1981, 272 p. (Kölner medizinhistorische Beiträge; Arbeiten der Forschungsstelle des Instituts für Geschichte der Medizin der Universität zu Köln, Band 19).

**Frankland, Edward, 1825–1899**
Hamlin C: Edward Frankland's early career as London's official water analyst, 1865–1876: the context of 'previous sewage contamination'. **Bull Hist Med** 1982 Spring;56(1):56–76

**Franklin, Benjamin, 1706–1790**
Lemay JA, Rousseau GS: The Renaissance man in the eighteenth century. Papers read at a Clark Library seminar, 9 October 1976. Los Angeles, William Andrews Clark Memorial Library, UCLA, 1978. xi, 139 p.

**Frantz, Virginia Kneeland, 1896–1967**
Brandt AM: Virginia Kneeland Frantz. In: Notable American women. The modern period. Cambridge, Mass., Belknap–Harvard Univ. Press, 1980. 4:247–8.

**Franz Family**
Merwe DW van der: Bochum-Blauberg: die ontstaan, stigting en ontwikkeling van die Helene Franz-Hospital, 1895–1935. **Kleio (S Afr)** 1978;10(1–2):2–20

**Fraser, Francis Richard, 1885–1964**
Krikler DM: Wolff-Parkinson-White syndrome: long follow-up and an Anglo-American historical note. **J Am Coll Cardiol** 1983 Dec;2(6):1216–8
McMichael J: Sir Francis Richard Fraser. In Dictionary of national biography, 1961–1970. Suppl. 8, 1981. p. 393–4.

**Fraser, John, 1885–1947**
Woodruff M: The master surgeon. **J R Coll Surg Edinb** 1981 Sep;26(5):257–63

**Frazer, Alastair Campbell, 1909–1969**
Young FG: Alastair Campbell Frazer. In Dictionary of national biography, 1961–1970. Suppl. 8, 1981. p. 397–8.

**Frederic II, King of Prussia, 1712–1786**
Schachter M: La personnalité de Frédéric II Le Grand, Roi de Prusse (1712–1786). Essai de psychologie adlérienne. **Hist Sci Med** 1984;18(2):181–7

**Frederick II, Emperor of Germany, 1194–1250**
Mallach HJ: Gibt es Ansätze zur Gerichtlichen Medizin in Friedrichs II. von Hohenstaufen Konstitutionen von Melfi? **Beitr Gerichtl Med** 1982;40:463–72

**Frederick II, King of Denmark, 1534–1588**
Karker A: Kong Frederik 2.s dod. **Jyske Saml** 1964;6(3):252–81

**Frederick III, Emperor of Germany, 1831–1888**
Chalat NI: Sir Morell Mackenzie revisited. **Laryngoscope** 1984 Oct;94(10):1307–10
Lee M: The 99 day Emperor, a misdiagnosis of historical importance. **Rostrum** 1981;(100):1–3
Lin JI: Virchow's pathological reports on Frederick III's cancer. **N Engl J Med** 1984 Nov 8;311(19):1261–4
Wyk AJ: Medisyne uit Suid-Afrika vir die Keiser. **Historia (S Afr)** 1979;24(1):63–5

**Frederick of Olomouc**
Wondrák E: Olomoucký Mistr Fridrich--zapomenutý lékař králuv a císařuv. **Cas Lek Cesk** 1984 May 4;123(18):551–2

**Fredericq, Leon, 1851–1935**
Florkin M, Théodoridès J: Henri de Lacaze-Duthiers et Léon Fredericq: correspondance (1876–1900). **Arch Int Physiol Biochim** 1982 Jul;90(2):Suppl 1–94
Florkin M: L'Ecole Liégeoise de Physiologie et son Maître Léon Fredericq (1851–1935), pionnier de la zoologie chimique. Liège, Vaillant-Carmanne, 1979. 211 p. (Publication des Archives Internationales de Physiologie et de Biochimie, Médecine et Médicins au Pays de Liège, IV).
Lecomte J, Schoffeniels E: L'oeuvre de Léon Frédéricq et son école (1853–1934) à travers les Archives de Biologie (1880–1904). **Arch Biol (Liege)** 1980;91(2):267–70

**Fredrik I, King of Sweden, 1676–1751**
Modig M: Kungliga hus--och reseapotek. **Livrustkammaren** 1980;15(1):1–16

**Freeman, Leonard, 1860–1935**
Delaney JJ: Leonard Freeman. **Colo Med** 1983 Aug;80(8):219–20

**Freixas i Freixas, Joan, 1860–1933**
Cornudella J: L'obra mèdica del Dr. Joan Freixas i Freixas. In Congrés Internacional d'Historie de la Medicina Catalana, 1st, Barcelona-Montpellier, 1970. Llibr d'Actes. Barcelona, Editorial Scientia, 1971. v 4, p. 362–5.

**French, Dexter, 1918–1981**
Pazur JH: Dexter French 1918–1981. **Adv Carbohydr Chem Biochem** 1984;42:1–13

**Frenkel-Brunswik, Else, 1908–1958**
Smith MB: Else Frenkel-Brunswik. In: Notable American women. The modern period. Cambridge, Mass., Belknap-Harvard Univ. Press, 1980. 4:250–2.

**Frenkel', Zakhariĭ Grigor'evich, 1869–1970**
Alekseeva LP: Z. G. Frenkel'. Moskva, Meditsina, 1971. 126 p.

**Freud, Anna, 1895–1982**
Edgcumbe R: Anna Freud--child analyst. **Int J Psychoanal** 1983;64 (Pt 4):427–33
Ekstein R: As I remember her: Anna Freud, 1895–1982. **Adolesc Psychiatry** 1983;11:5–8
Freeman T: Anna Freud--psychiatrist. **Int J Psychoanal** 1983;64 (Pt 4):441–4
Goldstein J: Anna Freud in law. **Psychoanal Study Child** 1984;39:3–13
Hellman I: Work in the Hampstead war nurseries. **Int J Psychoanal** 1983;64 (Pt 4):435–9
Kennedy H: Anna Freud, 1895–1982. **Psychoanal Q** 1983 Oct;52(4):501–6
Kris AO: The analyst's conceptual freedom in the method of free association. **Int J Psychoanal** 1983;64 (Pt 4):407–11
Lebovici S: L'oeuvre D'Anna Freud (1895–1982). **Psychiatr Enfant** 1984;27(1):5–34
Limentani A: Anna Freud's contribution to the work of the International Psychoanalytical Association. **Int J Psychoanal** 1983;64 (Pt 4):375–7
Lipton MA: A letter from Anna Freud. **Am J Psychiatry** 1983 Dec;140(12):1583–4
Neubauer PB: Anna Freud's legacy. **Psychoanal Q** 1983 Oct;52(4):507–13
Paediatrics and psychoanalysis--Miss Anna Freud: **Arch Dis Child** 1983 Jun;58(6):472–3
Peters UH: Anna Freud. Ein Leben für das Kind. München, Kindler, 1979. 309 p.
Rangell L: The Anna Freud experience. **Psychoanal Study Child** 1984;39:29–43
Roth JK: Verleihung des Ehrendoktors der Johann-Wolfgang-Goethe-Universität an Anna Freud. **Psyche (Stuttg)** 1982 Oct;36(10):951–3
Sandler J, Sandler AM: The 'second censorship', the 'three box model' and some technical implications. **Int J Psychoanal** 1983;64 (Pt 4):413–25
Sandler J: Discussions with Anna Freud on The Ego and the Mechanisms of Defence: The Ego and the Id at Puberty. **Int J Psychoanal** 1983;64 (Pt 4):401–6
Solnit AJ: Anna Freud 1895–1982. **Am J Psychiatry** 1983 Dec;140(12):1632–3
Solnit AJ: Anna Freud. December 3, 1895–October 9, 1982. **J Am Acad Child Psychiatry** 1984 Mar;23(2):233–6
Solnit AJ, Newman LM: Anna Freud: the child expert. **Psychoanal Study Child** 1984;39:45–63
Solnit AJ: Anna Freud's contributions to child and applied analysis. **Int J Psychoanal** 1983;64 (Pt 4):379–90
Strotzka H: Laudatio auf Anna Freud. **Wien Klin Wochenschr** 1983 Jan 21;95(2):35–7
Vikár G: Emlékezés Anna Freudra. **Orv Hetil** 1983 Nov 13;124(46):2819–20
Wallerstein RS: Anna Freud: radical innovator and staunch conservative. **Psychoanal Study Child** 1984;39:65–80
Yorke C: Anna Freud, CBE (1895–1982). **J Child Psychol Psychiatry** 1983 Jul;24(3):333–8
Yorke C: Anna Freud and the psychoanalytic study and treatment of adults. **Int J Psychoanal** 1983;64 (Pt 4):391–400

**Freud, Sigmund, 1856–1939**
Aaron PG, Clouse RG: Freud's psychohistory of Leonardo de Vinci: A matter of being right or left. **J Interdiscip Hist** 1982;13(1):1–16
Aberbach D: Freud's Jewish problem. **Commentary** 1980;69(6):35–9
Accardo PJ: Freud on diplegia. Commentary and translation. **Am J Dis Child** 1982 May;136(5):452–6
Albarello B, Collorio C: Analisi dei collegamenti tra l'opera freudiana e il positivismo ottocentesco. **Acta Med Hist Patav** 1982–83;29:9–18
Albarello B: Il concetto di regressione in Freud. **Minerva Psichiatr** 1984 Jan-Mar;25(1):23–36
Alexander LB: Social work's Freudian deluge: myth or reality? **Soc Serv Rev** 1972;46(4):517–38
Ansbacher HL: 'To love and to work'. Adlerian thoughts on an anecdote about Freud. **Bull Menninger Clin** 1981 Sep;45(5):439–41
Antal G: Freud in Hungary. An interview with Imre Hermann, the psychoanalyst. **New Hung Q** 1982;23(85):88–95
Bakan D: Freud e la tradizione mistica ebraica: psicoanalisi e cabala. **Comunita** 1976;39(176):206–44
Baruk H: Moïse, Freud et le veau d'or. **Rev Hist Med Heb** 1984 Jul;37(2):19–23
Bay E: Sigmund Freud's contribution to the early history of aphasiology. In Rose FC, Bynum WF, ed: Historical aspects of the neurosciences. New York, Raven, 1982. p. 103–7.
Beierlein C: Zum Leben und Schaffen von Sigmund Freud (1856–1939) im Umfeld seiner Zeit. **Wiss Z Martin Luther Univ (Math)** 1984;33(2):101–12
Berliner AK: Psychoanalysis and society. The social thought of Sigmund Freud. Washington, D.C., University Press of America, 1983. x, 205 p.
Bernays EL: Uncle Sigi. **J Hist Med Allied Sci** 1980 Apr;35(2):216–23
Bernfeld S: Freuds früheste Theorien und die Helmholtz-Schule (1944). **Psyche (Stuttg)** 1981 May;35(5):435–55
Bettelheim B: Reflections: Freud and the Soul [as perceived in America]. **New Yorker** 1982;68(2):52–93
Bocock R: Freud and modern society. An outline and analysis of Freud's sociology. New York, Holmes & Meier, 1978. xv, 200 p.
Bocock R: Sigmund Freud. Chichester, Horwood; London; New York, Tavistock, 1983. 145 p.
Bori PC: Materiale storico-religioso nella biblioteca di Sigmund Freud: alcuni rilievi sul catalogo. **Ann Ist Stor Italo-Ger** 1975;1:281–9
Brun D: Les sources infantiles de la théorie chez Freud. Une scène d'enfance dans l'après-coup. **Rev Fr Psychanal** 1982;46(3):583–99
Brunclík J: Freud o dostojevském – či naopak. **Cas Lek Cesk** 1982 Aug 13;121(32):1015–6
Burnham JC, McGuire W: Jelliffe: American psychoanalyst and physician & his correspondence with Sigmund Freud and C. G. Jung. Chicago, University of Chicago Press, 1983. xx, 324 p. With contributions by A. R. D'Amore and J. E. Sauer.
Caire JB: A holographic model of a psychosomatic pattern: Freud's specimen dream re-interpreted. **Psychother Psychosom** 1981;36(2):132–42
Camus CH: La psychoanalyse, avènement d'une connaissance originale (Sigmund Freud). **Soins Psychiatr** 1980 Dec;(6):3–8
Carotenuto A: A secret symmetry: Sabina Spielrein between Jung and Freud. New York, Pantheon Books, 1982. xix, 250 p.
Carter KC: Germ theory, hysteria, and Freud's early work in psychopathology. **Med Hist** 1980 Jul;24(3):259–74
Castorina JA, Lerner BD: Comentarios sobre la investigación clínica en Freud y Piaget. **Acta Psiquiatr Psicol Am Lat** 1983 Jun;29(2):85–95
Chabot CB: Freud on Schreber. Psychoanalytic theory and the critical act. Amherst, University of Massachusetts Press, 1982. 171 p.
Chertok L: Hypnosis and suggestion in a century of psychotherapy: an epistemological assessment. **J Am Acad Psychoanal** 1984 Apr;12(2):211–32
Chessick RD: Freud teaches psychotherapy. Indianapolis, Cambridge, Hackett, 1980. viii, 342 p.
Clark RW: Freud: the man the cause. New York, Random House, 1980. 652 p.
Clark RW: Sigmund Freud's sortie to America. **Am Heritage** 1980;3(3):34–43
Covert C: A view of the press in the twenties. **Journalism Hist** 1975;2(3):66–7, 92–6
Cremerius J: Freuds Sterben--Die Identität von Denken, Leben und

Sterben. **Psychother Psychosom Med Psychol** 1983 Sep;33(5):163–6
Dacquino G: Psicoanalisi e ipnosi nella dottrina e nella pratica clinica. **Minerva Med** 1982 Nov 24;73(45):3207–12
Decker HS: Freud and Dora: constraints on medical progress. **J Soc Hist** 1981;14(3):445–64
Decker HS: The choice of a name: 'Dora' and Freud's relationship with Breuer. **J Am Psychoanal Assoc** 1982;30(1):113–36
Delion P: Freud, l'hystérique et la psychanalyse. **Soins Psychiatr** 1983 Jan;(27):7–10
Diamond S: Sigmund Freud, his Jewishness, and scientific method: the seen and the unseen as evidence. **J Hist Ideas** 1982 Oct–Dec;43(4):613–34
Dilman I: Freud and human nature. Oxford, Basil Blackwell, 1983. 207 p.
DuPlessis RB, Friedman SS: 'Woman is perfect': H. D.'s debate with Freud. **Feminist Stud** 1981;7(3):407–30
Eissler KR: Freud und Wagner–Jauregg vor der Kommission zur Erhebung militärischer Pflichtverletzungen. Wien, Löcker, 1979. 333 p.
Eissler KR: K. R. Eissler on errors regarding Freud. **Int J Psychoanal** 1981;62(3):371–2
Eissler KR: Victor Tausk's suicide. New York, International Universities Press, 1983. 322 p.
Eng E: Locke's Tabula Rasa and Freud's 'Mystic writing pad.' **J Hist Ideas** 1980 Jan–Mar;41(1):133–40
Engelman E: Berggasse 19, Sigmund Freud's home and offices, Vienna, 1938: the photographs of Edmund Engelman. Chicago, University of Chicago Press, 1981. 153 p.
Erdheim M: Freuds Grössenphantasien, sein Konzept des Unbewussten und die Wiener Décadence. **Psyche (Stuttg)** 1981 Oct;35(10):857–74;Nov;35(11):1006–33
Fisher S, Greenberg RP, ed: The scientific evaluation of Freud's theories and therapy; a book of readings. New York, Basic Books, 1978. xv, 446 p. (Reprinted articles of various authors).
Freeman L, Strean HS: Freud and women. New York, Frederick Ungar, 1981. xiii, 238 p.
Frey–Rohn L: Von Freud zu Jung. Eine vergleichende Studie zur Psychologie des Unbewussten. (2. überarbeitete Ausgabe) Zürich, Daimon Verlag, 1980?. 456 p.
Fullinwider SP: Sigmund Freud, John Hughlings Jackson, and speech. **J Hist Ideas** 1983 Jan–Mar;44(1):151–8
Galati D: Lacan: un ritorno a Freud? **Stor Crit Psicol** 1980;1(1):79–91
Gautier J: Freud a menti. Périgny–sur–Yerres, Mandres–les–Roses, Edition de 'La vie claire, 1977. vii, 566 p.
Gershenowitz H: The influence of Lamarckism on the development of Freud's psychoanalytic theory. **Indian J Hist Sci** 1979 Nov;14(2):105–13
Gichlhorn R: Eine Episode aus S. Freuds Mittelschulzeit. **Unsere Heimat** 1965;36(1–3):18–24
Gilman SL: Freud and the prostitute: male stereotypes of female sexuality in fin–de–siècle Vienna. **J Am Acad Psychoanal** 1981 Jul;9(3):337–60
Ginzburg C: Morelli, Freud and Sherlock Holmes: clues and scientific method. **Hist Workshop J** 1980;9:5–36
Glenn J: 'The open–air closet'. **Am J Psychoanal** 1980 Summer;40(2):165–8
Glymour C: The theory of your dreams. In R.S. Cohen, L. Laudan, ed: Physics, philosophy and psychoanalysis. Dordrecht, D. Reidel, 1983. p. 57–71.
Gmelin OF: Anti–Freud: von der Psychoanalyse zur Medienwissenschaft. Mit einem Beitrag von Helene Saussure. Frankfurt am Main, Haag and Herchen, 1979. 175 p.
Goering JD: Sigmund Freud, Carl Jung and religion. **Mennon Q Rev** 1982;56(1):47–56
Goldstein RL: Sigmund Freud: forensic psychiatrist. **Bull Am Acad Psychiatry Law** 1983;11(3):273–7
Golub S: Coping with cancer: Freud's experiences. **Psychoanal Rev** 1981 Summer;68(2):191–200
Gravitz MA, Gerton MI: Freud and hypnosis: report of post–rejection use. **J Hist Behav Sci** 1981 Jan;17(1):68–74
Gravitz MA, Gerton MI: Polgar as Freud's hypnotist? contrary evidence. **Am J Clin Hypn** 1982 Apr;24(4):272–6
Grinberg L, Rodríguez JF: The influence of Cervantes on the future creator of psychoanalysis. **Int J Psychoanal** 1984;65(Pt 2):155–68
Grinstein A: Sigmund Freud's dreams. New York, International Universities Press, 1980. 486 p.
Grubrich–Simitis I: Siegfried Bernfeld: Historiker der Psychoanalyse und Freud–Biograph. **Psyche (Stuttg)** 1981 May;35(5):397–434
Gutmann A: Freud versus feminism. **Dissent** 1979;26(2):204–12
Harmat P, Hebenstreit G: Freud, Ferenczi und die Psychoanalyse in Ungarn. **Wien Med Wochenschr** 1982 Feb 15;132(3):63–6
Herren R: Freud und die Kriminologie: Einführung in die psychoanalytische Kriminologie. Stuttgart, Enke, 1973. x, 281 p.
Hoffman LE: War, revolution, and psychoanalysis: Freudian thought begins to grapple with social reality. **J Hist Behav Sci** 1981;17:251–69
Hogenson GB: Jung's struggle with Freud. Notre Dame, London, University of Notre Dame Press, 1983. xi, 180 p.
Holland NN: Freud, physics, and literature. **J Am Acad Psychoanal** 1984 Jul;12(3):301–20
Hurst LC: Freud and the great neurosis: discussion paper. **J R Soc Med** 1983 Jan;76(1):57–61
Jaffe NC: A second opinion on delusions and dreams. A reading of Freud's interpretation of Jensen. In Jones AH, ed: Images of healers. Albany, State University of New York Press, 1983. p. 101–7.
Jarrick A: Freud och historien. **Scandia** 1982;48(1):107–48
Kanzer M, Glenn J, ed., et al: Freud and his patients. New York and London, Aronson, 1980. 452 p.
Kanzer M, Glenn J, ed: Freud and his self–analysis. New York and London, Aronson, 1979. x, 308 p. (Downstate Psychoanalytic Institute, Twenty–Fifth Anniversary Series, Vol. I). Includes reprinted papers by various authors.
Kanzer M: Freud, Theodor Lipps, and 'scientific psychology'. **Psychoanal Q** 1981;50(3):393–410
Kardiner A: My analysis with Freud. New York, Norton, 1977. 123 p.
Kästle O: Zwei wiederentdeckte Rezensionen Sigmund Freuds von 1895. Wissenschaftlicher Kontext und biographischer Hintergrund. **Psyche (Stuttg)** 1983 Sep;37(9):805–27
Kätzel S: Individuum contra Gesellschaft? Ein Beitrag zur Kritik der Gesellschaftsauffassung von Sigmund Freud. **Wiss Z Karl Marx Univ Math Natur Wiss Reihe** 1973;22(5):467–82
Katzenstein A, Thom A: Die historische Leistung und die Grenzen des Werkes von Sigmund Freud (1856–1939). **Psychiatr Neurol Med Psychol (Leipz)** 1982 Feb;34(2):68–78
Kaufman P: Burke, Freud, and the Gothic **Stud Burke Time** 1972;13(3):2179–92
Kern S: The prehistory of Freud's dream theory: Freud's masterpiece anticipated. **Hist Med (Lond)** 1975 Autumn–Winter;6(3–4):83–92
Kern SR: Freud and the emergence of child psychology. [New York, s. n.], 1973. 3, vii, 415 leaves.
Kirsch J: Jung's transference on Freud: its Jewish element. **Am Imago** 1984;41:63–84
Klein DB: Jewish origins of the psychoanalytic movement. New York, Praeger, 1981. xvi, 198 p.
Knight IF: Freud's 'Project': a theory for Studies on Hysteria. **J Hist Behav Sci** 1984 Oct;20(4):340–58
Knoepfmacher H: Sigmund Freud in high school. **Am Imago** 1979 Fall;36(3):287–300
Køppe S: The psychology of the neuron: Freud, Cajal and Golgi. **Scand J Psychol** 1983;24(1):1–12
Kottayarikil C: Sigmund Freud on religion and morality: a challenge to Christianity. Innsbruck, Resch, 1977. xx, 399 p.
Kovel J: Marx and Freud. In M. Albin, R. J. Devlin, G. Heeger, ed: New directions in psychohistory. The Adelphi papers in honor of Erik H. Erikson. Lexington, Toronto, D. C. Heath, 1980. p. 21–6.
Krüll M: Freud und sein Vater. München, Beck, 1979. 344 p.
Lebzeltern G: Eine interessante Fehlleistung S. Freuds. **Z Klin Psychol Psychother** 1980;28(1):14–20
Lebzeltern G: Ein vielsagender Irrtum S. Freuds. **Z Klin Psychol Psychother** 1982;30(1):25–30
Lebzeltern G: S. Freud und das Kokain. **Wien Klin Wochenschr** 1983 Nov 11;95(21):765–9
Lipton SD: An addendum to 'The advantages of Freud's technique, as shown in his analysis of the Rat Man'. **Int J Psychoanal** 1979;60(pt2):215–6
Lomax EM, Kagan J, Rosenkrantz BG: Science and patterns of child care. San Francisco, W. H. Freeman, 1978. xiv, 247 p.
Luce EA: The ordeal of Sigmund Freud. In Romm S, ed: Symposium on historical perspectives of plastic surgery. Philadelphia, Saunders, 1983. p. 715–6.
McCarthy T: Freud and the problem of sexuality. **J Hist Behav Sci** 1981;17:332–9
McGuinness BF: Freud e Wittgenstein. **Ann Sc Norm Super Pisa** 1979;9(1):409–24
McLaren A: Contraception and its discontents: Sigmund Freud and birth control. **J Soc Hist** 1979;12(4):513–29
Macmillan MB: Freud and Lindner on pleasure sucking. **Stor Crit Psicol** 1980;1(1):111–43
Mahony P: Freud as a writer. New York, International Universities Press, 1982. xv, 227 p.
Mainetti JA: Leyendo con Freud La peau de chagrin de Balzac. **Asclepio** 1982;34:265–81
May R: Freud and the phallic defense. **Psychiatry** 1979;42(2):147–56
Meisel P, ed: Freud: a collection of critical essays. Englewood Cliffs, New Jersey, Prentice–Hall, 1981. 240 p. Reprinted works by literary figures.
Menaker E: Otto Rank: a rediscovered legacy. New York, Columbia University Press, 1982. xvii, 166 p.
Merani AL: Freud y el Talmud: seguido de crítica de los fundamentos de la psicopatología. México, Grijalbo, 1974. 159 p.
Meynell GG: Freud translated: an historical and bibliographical note. **J R Soc Med** 1981 Apr;74(4):306–9
Miller J: Interpretations of Freud's Jewishness, 1924–1974. **J Hist Behav Sci** 1981;17:357–74
Milner M: Freud et l'interprétation de la littérature. Paris, Société d'édition d'enseignement supérieur, 1980. 328 p.
Montiel L: Freud y el psicoanálisis en dos conferencias de Thomas Mann. In International Congress of the History of Medicine, 27th, Barcelona, 1980. Actas. Barcelona, Académia de Ciències Mèdiques de Catalunya i Balears, 1981. p. 111–5.
Mora Merida JA: Freud: De la libido al eros. La coherencia del

discurso freudiano. Malaga, Universidad de Malaga, 1979. 284 p.
Muldworf B: Freud. Paris, Les Editeurs français réunis, 1976. 349 p.
Musatti C: Freud e l'ebraismo. **Belfagor** 1980;35(6):687–96
Obermeit W: Die Wirklichkeit des Fiktiven. Literatur und Psychoanalyse. **Psyche (Stuttg)** 1981 Mar;35(3):193–208
Obholzer K: The Wolf-man. Conversations with Freud's patient--sixty years later. New York, Continuum, 1982. 250 p.
Oring E: The jokes of Sigmund Freud: a study in humor and Jewish identity. Philadelphia, University of Pennsylvania Press, 1984. xiii, 151 p.
Pagel G: Narziss und Prometheus: die Theorie der Phantasie bei Freud und Gehlen. Würzburg, Königshausen & Neumann, 1984. 195 p. (Studien zur Anthropologie, Band 8).
Pansera MT: Per un'antropologia filosofica freudiana: il valore della negazione. **Physis** 1982;24(1):76–108
Parson T: The articulation of the personality and the social-action system: Sigmund Freud and Max Weber. In M. Albin, R. J. Devlin, G. Heeger, ed: New directions in psychohistory. The Adelphi papers in honor of Erik H. Erikson. Lexington, Toronto, D. C. Heath, 1980. p. 27–35.
Paskaukas RA: Sigmund Freud and Arthur Schopenhauer reexamined. In International Congress of the History of Medicine, 27th, Barcelona, 1980. Actas. Barcelona, Acadèmia de Ciències Mèdiques de Catalunya i Balears, 1981. p. 125–9.
Peck W, Diethelm O: Review of the Freud library. In International Congress of the History of Medicine, 27th, Barcelona, 1980. Actas. Barcelona, Acadèmia de Ciències Mèdiques de Catalunya i Balears, 1981. p. 130–3.
Pletsch C: Freud's case studies. **Partisan Rev** 1982;49(1):101–18
Ramas M: Freud's Dora, Dora's hysteria: the negation of a woman's rebellion. **Feminist Stud** 1980;6(3):472–510
Rausky F: Le discours freudien sur l'antisémitisme.
Rice JL: Russian stereotypes in the Freud-Jung correspondence. **Slavic Rev** 1982 Spring;41(1):19–34
Roazen P: Freud and America. **Soc Res (NY)** 1972;39(4):720–32
Roazen P: Paul Roazen on errors regarding Freud. **Int J Psychoanal** 1982;63(pt 2):260–1
Romm S, Luce EA: Hans Pichler: oral surgeon to Sigmund Freud. **Oral Surg** 1984 Jan;57(1):31–2
Romm S: The oral cancer of Sigmund Freud. In Romm S, ed: Symposium on historical perspectives of plastic surgery. Philadelphia, Saunders, 1983. p. 709–14.
Roustang F: Dire mastery. Discipleship from Freud to Lacan. Translated by Ned Lukacher. Baltimore, London, Johns Hopkins University Press, 1982. (Translation of: Un destin si funeste).
Rubinstein BB: Freud's early theories of hysteria. In R.S. Cohen, L. Laudan, ed: Physics, philosophy and psychoanalysis. Dordrecht, D. Reidel, 1983. p. 169–90.
Ruse M: Medicine as social science: the case of Freud on homosexuality. **J Med Philos** 1981 Nov;6(4):361–86
Rychlak JF: Freud's confrontation with the telic mind. **J Hist Behav Sci** 1981;17:176–83
Scheidhauer M: Un problème épineux entre Freud et Jung: le rêve. **Rev Hist Philos Relig** 1981;61(4):413–25
Schneck JM: Sigmund Freud, Josef Breuer, and Freud's self-observations on meralgia paresthetica. **NY State J Med** 1983 Jun;83(7):968–9
Schöpf A: Sigmund Freud. München, Beck, 1982. 244 p.
Schorske CF: Freud: the psycho-archeology of civilizations. **Mass Hist Soc Proc** 1980;92:52–67
Schott H: Traum und Geschichte. Zur Freudschen Geschichtsauffassung im Kontext der Traumdeutung. **Sudhoffs Arch** 1980;64(3):298–312
Schott H: Freuds Selbstanalyse (Freud und Fliess). In International Congress of the History of Medicine, 27th, Barcelona, 1980. Actas. Barcelona, Acadèmia de Ciències Mèdiques de Catalunya i Balears, 1981. p. 145–8.
Schott HG: Elemente der Selbstanalyse in den 'Studien über Hysterie'. **Gesnerus** 1980;37(3/4):235–56
Schwaber P: Scientific art: the interpretation of dreams. **Colby Libr Q** 1977;13(1):5–18
Schwaber P: Freud and the twenties. **Mass Rev** 1981;22(1):133–51
Sebald H: Freud: instinctivist or behaviorist? The mirages of American sociology. **J Hist Sociol** 1982;4(2):64–89
Seidler E, Kindt H, Schaub N: Jaspers und Freud. **Sudhoffs Arch** 1978;62(1):37–63
Sherman MH, ed: Psychoanalysis and old Vienna: Freud, Reik, Schnitzler, Kraus. New York, Human Sciences Press, 1978. 192 p.
Siefert H: Sigmund Freud, Georg Groddeck und die psychosomatische Medizin. **Prax Psychother Psychosom** 1979;24:63–78
Sirkin M, Fleming M: Freud's 'Project' and its relationship to psychoanalytic theory. **J Hist Behav Sci** 1982 Jul;18(3):230–41
Sirota M: On the Freud-Jung correspondence. **Mod Stud** 1977;2(3):45–8
Slochower H: The permanence of our Freudian heritage. **Mod Stud** 1977;2(3):13–18
Sparvieri F: Teorie freudiane e psicologia aeronautica. **Riv Med Aeronaut Spaz** 1980 Jan-Jun;43(1–2):81–103
Stannard DE: Shrinking history. On Freud and the failure of psychohistory. New York, Oxford University Press, 1980. xx, 187 p.
Steele RS, Swinney SV: Freud and Jung: conflicts of interpretation. London, Boston, Routledge and Kegan Paul, 1982. x, 390 p.
Steiner H: Freud against himself. **Perspect Biol Med** 1977 Summer;20(4):510–27
Sulloway FJ: Freud, biologist of the mind: beyond the psychoanalytic legend. New York, Basic Books, 1979. xxvi, 612 p.
Sulloway FJ: Freud as psychobiologist: a study in scientific revolution and revolutionary ideology. Ph.D. Diss. Harvard University. Cambridge, Mass., 1979.
Szállási A: Freud, Ferenczi és a Nyugat. **Orv Hetil** 1980 May 18;121(20):1207–8
Székács I: Freud és pszichoanalízis természettudományos alapjai. **Orv Hetil** 1982 Dec 12;123(50):3091–9
Tedeschi G: Jung-Freud: un dilemma inattuale. Roma, Astrolabio, 1979. 88 p.
Thomas DM: Freud and the 'White Hotel'. **Br Med J [Clin Res]** 1983 Dec 24–31;287(6409):1957–60
Thornton EM: Freud and cocaine: the Freudian fallacy. London, Blond & Briggs, 1983. 340 p.
Ventura P: Freud e la giuridicità della coesistenza. Per un ritorno filosofico alla psicologia del profondo. Vol. I. La psicoanalisi individuale. Milano, Giuffrè, 1979. xvi, 420 p.
Wachinger L: Buber und Freud. **Stimmen Zeit** 1978;196(11):754–62
Wallace ER: A commentary on the Freud-Jung letters. **Psychoanal Rev** 1980 Spring;67(1):112–37
Wallace ER: The primal parricide. **Bull Hist Med** 1980 Summer;54(2):153–65
Wallace ER: Freud and anthropology. A history and reappraisal. New York, International Universities Press, 1983. xi, 306 p. (Psychological Issues, Monograph 55).
Weinstein MA, Weinstein D: Freud's encounter with religion: a study in bad faith. **Thought** 1981;56:463–76
Woodman RG: Freud and Jung: the parting of the ways. **Queens Q** 1978;85(1):93–108
Zaretsky E: Evolutionary biology and psychoanalysis: a review essay on Frank J. Sulloway's Freud: biologist of the mind. **Psychohist Rev** 1981;10(2):109–22

**Frey, Heinrich, 1822–1890**
Jonecko A: Uwagi o podręczniku histochemii Freya z roku 1870 na tle osiągnięć histochemicznych połowy XIX wieku. **Wiad Lek** 1979 Dec 15;32(24):1811–4

**Frick, George, 1793–1870**
Snyder C: A look at George Frick's Treatise on diseases of the eye. In: Congrès international d'histoire de la médecine, XXVe, Québec, 1976. Actes. Québec, 1977. p. 1289–1300.

**Fricke, Johann Karl Georg, 1790–1841**
Rodegra H: Johann Carl Georg Fricke (1790–1841): Wegbereiter einer klinischen Chirurgie in Deutschland. Herzogenrath, Murken-Altrogge, 1983. 203 p. (Studien zur Geschichte des Krankenhauswesens, 20)

**Friedenwald Family**
Pelner L: The distinguished doctors Friedenwald. **Koroth** 1981;8(1–2):45–50

**Friedenwald, Jonas Stein, 1897–**
Alpern M: Presentation of the Procter Medal for Research in vision and Ophthalmology to Gerald Westheimer. **Invest Ophthalmol Vis Sci** 1979 Sep;18(9):883–92
Patz A: Jonas S. Friedenwald, man of science. **Invest Ophthalmol Vis Sci** 1980 Oct;19(10):1139–49

**Friedman, Israel, 1906–1980**
Mascia AV: In memoriam Israel Friedman (1906–1980). **J Asthma** 1982;19(1):59–60

**Friedmann, Richard**
Vencovský E: Ceskoslovenský psychiatr spolupracovníkem profesora dr. Alberta Schweitzera v Lambarène. **Cesk Psychiatr** 1984 Apr;80(2):125–8

**Fries, Jakob Friedrich, 1773–1843**
Leary DE: The psychology of Jakob Friedrich Fries (1773–1843): its context, nature, and historical significance. **Stor Crit Psicol** 1982 Dec;3(2):217–48

**Fritzsche, Christian Friedrich, 1851–1938**
Stoffel G: Christian Friedrich Fritzsche, 1851–1938. Erster Glarner Spitalarzt und Beschreiber der Akromealie. Zürich, Juris Druck, 1983. 66 p. (Zürcher Medizingeschichtliche Abhandlungen, Neue Reihe, Nr. 161).

**Froelicher, Hans, Jr.**
Stakem KA: Hans Froelicher, Jr.: civic educator. **Md Hist Mag** 1982;77(2):193–201

**Fromm, Erich, 1900–**
Campillo-Sainz C, et al: Homenaje al Doctor Erich Fromm. **Gac Med Mex** 1980;116:431–45
Homenaje al Doctor Erich Fromm: **Gac Med Mex** 1980 Oct;116(10):431–45
Zimmerman J: Transcendent psychology: Erik H. Erikson, Erich Fromm, Karen Horney, Abraham H. Maslow, and Harry Stack Sullivan and the quest for a healthy humanity. Ph.D. Diss., Northwestern University. Evanston, 1982. vi, 498 p.

**Fromm-Reichmann, Frieda, 1889-1957**
Bruch H: Personal reminiscences of Frieda Fromm-Reichmann. **Psychiatry** 1982;45(2):98-104
Cohen RA: Notes on the life and work of Frieda Fromm-Reichmann. **Psychiatry** 1982;45(2):90-8
Crowley RM: Frieda Fromm-Reichmann: recollections of a student. **Psychiatry** 1982;45(2):105-7
Frieda Fromm-Reichmann: A seminar in the history of psychiatry. **Psychiatry** 1982 May;45(2):89-136
Frieda Fromm-Reichmann discusses the 'Rose garden' case: **Psychiatry** 1982 May;45(2):128-36
Frommknecht M: Frieda Fromm-Reichmann. In J. Rattner, ed: Wandlungen der Psychoanalyse. Wien, Europaverlag, 1980. p. 115 39.
Gunst VK: Memoirs-Professional and personal: a decade with Frieda Fromm-Reichmann. **Psychiatry** 1982;45(2):107-15
Hoff SG: Frieda Fromm-Reichmann. In Dictionary of American Biography, Suppl. 6, 1956-1960. p. 219-20, 1980.
Powell RC, Hoff SG: Frieda Fromm-Reichmann. In: Notable American women. The modern period. Cambridge, Mass., Belknap-Harvard Univ. Press, 1980. 4:252-5.
Stanton AH: Frieda Fromm-Reichmann, MD: her impact on American psychiatry. **Psychiatry** 1982;45(2):121-7

**Fronczak, Francis Eustace, 1874-1955**
Jones MJ: The Francis E. Fronczak Collection. **Niagara Frontier** 1978;25(4):96-9

**Froriep, Robert Friedrich, 1804-1861**
Froriep R: Aspects of tongue (1828). Original Latin text edited and translated by C. Garton, J. D. Gerencser, A. J. Drinnan. Buffalo, Dept. of Classics, State University of N. Y., 1982. xix, 109, 108a p. (Arethusa Monographs IX).

**Frost, Wade Hampton, 1880-1938**
Lilienfeld AM: Wade Hampton Frost: contributions to epidemiology and public health. **Am J Epidemiol** 1983 Apr;117(4):379-83

**Frugoni, Carlo Innocenzo, 1692-1768**
Pini UA: I medici parmigiani nelle poesie di Carlo Innocenzo Frugoni. **Minerva Med** 1980 Apr 7;71(14):1059-61
Pini UA: I medici parmigiani nelle poesie del Frugoni. Il medico dormiglione. **Minerva Med** 1980 Sep 22;71(35):2515

**Fryer, Douglas Henry, 1891-1960**
Smith HC: Douglas Henry Fryer. In Dictionary of American Biography, Suppl. 6, 1956-1960. p. 222, 1980.

**Fuchs, Ernst, 1851-1930**
Streiff B: Ernst Fuchs (1851-1930)--Gedächtnisvorlesung Wien 31. 5. 1984. **Klin Monatsbl Augenheilkd** 1984 Nov;185(5):316-20

**Fuchs, Leonhart, 1501-1566**
Bernus A von, ed: Alt-Kräuterbüchlein. Nach dem 'New-Kreüterbüchlein' des Leonhart Fuchs. Mit einem Nachwort von E. Mittler. Frankfurt am Main, Insel, 1980. 153 p.
Guédès M: Une variante de la page de titre du De historia stirpium de L. Fuchs (1542). **J Soc Bibliogr Nat Hist** 1974;7(1):81-5

**Fugger, Octavianus Secundus, 1549-1600**
Zimmermann A: Pharmazeutisches aus dem Nachlassinventar des Octavianus Secundus Fugger (1549-1600). **Beitr Gesch Pharm** 1981;31(12):89-91

**Fuller, Margaret, 1810-1850**
Stern MB: Margaret Fuller and the phrenologist-publishers. **Stud Am Renaiss** 1980;229:37

**Fully, Georges, 1926-1973**
Stewart TD: A tribute to the French forensic anthropologist Georges Fully (1926-1973). **J Forensic Sci** 1979 Oct;24(4):916-24

**Fulton, John Farquhar, 1899-1960**
Thomson EH: John Farquhar Fulton. In Dictionary of American Biography, Suppl. 6, 1956-1960. p. 222-4, 1980.
Thomson EH: Madeline Earle Stanton, disciple: the years 1920 to 1941. **J Hist Med Allied Sci** 1981 Apr,36(2):151-67

**Fulton, John, 1837-1887**
Roland CG: John Fulton, In Dictionary of Canadian biography, 1881-1890. 1982;11:328-9.

**Furmaga, Stefan, 1924-1983**
Gundłach JL: Prof. Dr Stefan Furmaga (1924-1983). Wspomnienie pośmiertne. **Wiad Parazytol** 1984;30(3):385-91

**Furness, Richard, 1791-1857**
Riddington Young J: Medicus Magus. **J Hist Med Allied Sci** 1980 Jan;35(1):40-57

**Fusco, Silvain, 1903-1940**
Simeoni CE, Mouren MC, Aulas JJ: Psychose et créativité. Réflexions à propos d'un peintre autiste: Sykvain Fusco. **Confin Psychiatr** 1980;23(3):151-63

**Fusek Family**
Pabis-Braunstein M: Aptekarstwo w Bieczu. Dzieje rodziny Fusków. **Arch Hist Med (Warsz)** 1984;47(2):191-206

**Fuszek, Rudolf, 1882-1941**
Kálmán G: Libéria egykori magyar minisztere Fuszek Rudolf dr.

# G

**Gaaz, Fedor Petrovich, 1780-1853**
Arkhangel'skiĭ GV: Moskovskiĭ vrach-gumanist Fedor Petrovich Gaaz (1780-1853) i ego znachenie v razvitii otechestvennoĭ meditsiny. **Klin Med (Mosk)** 1981 Feb;59(2):118-20
Fokina EN: Fedor Petrovich Gaaz i ego issledovaniia po izucheniiu lechebnykh mineral'nykh istochnikov Kavkaza. **Vopr Kurortol Fizioter Lech Fiz Kult** 1980 Sep-Oct;(5):65-6
Kotel'nikov VP: F. P. Gaaz (k 200-letiiu so dnia roxhdeniia). **Klin Med (Mosk)** 1982 Jul;60(7):115-7

**Gabričevskij, Georgij Norbertovič, 1860-1907**
Schneck P: Die Briefe Paul Ehrlichs an den Moskauer Mikrobiologen Georgij Norbertovič Gabričevskij. **NTM** 1982;19(2):81-7

**Gachet, Paul Fernand, 1828-1909**
Southgate MT: Vincent van Gogh, portrait of Dr. Gachet. **JAMA** 1981 Feb 20;245(7):657, 688

**Gadadhara, 7th and 8th cent.**
Pandey AN, Rama Rao B, Raghunathan K: Gadadhara. **Bull Indian Inst Hist Med (Hyderabad)** 1975 Oct;5(4):193-7

**Gaddum, John Henry, 1900-1965**
Feldberg W: Sir John Henry Gaddum. In Dictionary of national biography, 1961-1970. Suppl. 8, 1981. p. 412-3.

**Gaehtgens, Carl, fl. 1881-1898**
Benedum J: Vom Giessener pharmakologischen Institut unter Rudolf Buchheim und Karl Gaehtgens (1867-1898). **Medizinhist J** 1980;15(1/2):103-19

**Gaines, Walter Lee, 1881-1950**
Dreifuss JJ: W. L. Gaines, précurseur du concept de réflexe neuroendocrine. **Gesnerus** 1981;38(3/4):331-8

**Gairdner, Douglas**
Dobbs R, Robinson R, MacCarthy D, et al: Douglas Gairdner, editor of the Archives 1964-79. **Arch Dis Child** 1979 Nov;54(11):813, 815-21

**Gajdusek, Daniel Carleton, 1923-**
Farquhar J, Gajdusek DC, ed: Kuru: Early letters and field notes from the collection of D. Carleton Gajdusek. New York, Raven Press, 1981. xxviii, 338 p.

**Galbraith, James Garber, 1914-**
James Garber Galbraith, M.D.: **Clin Neurosurg** 1982;29:xiii-xix

**Galen**
Anastassiou A: Zur hippokratischen Schrift De locis in homine und zum Hippokratesglossar des Galen. **Rheinisches Mus Philol** 1982;125:193-201
Azeez Pasha M: Jalinoos [Galen] the famous physician of Yunan (Greece). **Bull Indian Inst Hist Med (Hyderabad)** 1975 Oct;5(4):211-24
Barcia Goyanes JJ: Las correcciones de Vesalio a la anatomia de Galeno. **Med Esp** 1980;79:1-16
Boylan M: The Galenic and Hippocratic challenges to Aristotle's conception theory. **J Hist Biol** 1984 Spring;17(1):83-112
Cheng Zhifan: [Galen's thought, physiology and anatomy as taught by him] (Chi). **Chin J Med Hist** 1980;10:92-5
De Lacy PH: Galen's concept of continuity. **Greek Roman Byz Stud (Cambridge, Mass.)** 1979;20:355-69
Durling R: Corrigenda and addenda to Diels' Galenica: II. codices miscellanei. **Traditio** 1981;37:373-81
Durling RJ: Lexicographical notes on Galen's pharmacological writings. **Glotta** 1979;57(3-4):218-24
Durling RJ: Lexicographical notes on Galen's writings (part II). **Glotta** 1980;58(3-4):260-5
Durling RJ: Lexicographical notes on Galen's writings. **Glotta** 1981;59:108-16
Eastwood BS: Cosmology and physiology in Galenic visual theory: Hunayn Ibn Ishaq. **Trans Stud Coll Physicians Phila** 1980 Dec;5(2 no 4):276-83
Fehlmann HR: Ceratum Galeni. Zur Geschichte von Unguentum leniens. In Dilg P, et al., ed: Perspektiven der Pharmaziegeschichte. Graz, Austria, Akademische Druck- u. Verlagsanstalt, 1983. p. 65-77.
French RK, Lloyd GE: Greek fragments of the lost books of Galen's Anatomical procedures. **Sudhoffs Arch** 1978;62(3):235-49
Galen: On the doctrines of Hippocrates and Plato. Edition, translation and commentary by P De Lacy. Second Part: Books VI-IX. Berlin, Akademie Verlag, 1980. p. 361-609. (Corpus Medicorum Graecorum, V, 4, 1, 2).
García-Ballester L: Studies on Hippocrates and Galen in modern Spain. **Trans Stud Coll Physicians Phila** 1979 Sep;5(1 No 3):215-29
García Ballester L: Experiencia y especulación en el diagnóstico galénico. **Dynamis** 1981;1:203-23
Goss CM, Chodkowski EG: 'On Bones for Beginners' by Galen of Pergamon: a translation with commentary. **Am J Anat** 1984 Jan;169(1):59-74
Hajal F: Galen's ethical psychotherapy: its influence on a medieval Near Eastern physician. **J Hist Med Allied Sci** 1983 Jul;38(3):320-33
Harig G, Kollesch J: Galen und Hippokrates. In La collection hippocratique et son rôle dans l'histoire de la médecine. Colloque

de Strasbourg (23–27 octobre 1972) organisé par le Centre de Recherches sur la Grèce Antique, avec le concours des Facultés de Philosophie et des Langues Classiques. Leiden, E. J. Brill, 1975. p. 257–74.
Jouanna J: Une forme étymologique retrouvée: omelesis dans le Glossaire hippocratique de Galien et dans le traité hippocratique des Maladies II c, 31. **Rev Philol (Paris)** 1979;53:260–63
Klein-Franke F: The Arabic version of Galen's Periethon. **Jerus Stud Arabic Islam** 1979;1:125–50
Kollesch J: Galen als Vertreter der zweiten Sophistik. **Orvostort Kozl** 1981;93–96(27 No 1–4):47–54
McVaugh MR: The authorship of the Galenic compendium de interioribus, 'Quoniam diversitas...'. **Dynamis** 1981;1:225–9
Mansfeld J: Alcmaeon: 'Physikos' or physician? With some remarks on Calcidius' 'On vision' compared to Galen's Plac. Hipp. Plat. VII. In J. Mansfeld, L. M. de Rijk, eds. Kephalaion: Studies in Greek philosophy and its continuation. Assen, Van Gorcum, 1975. p. 26–38.
Marinone N: Galeno, De victu attenuante, 79 e 98. **Riv Filol Istruz Classica** 1976;104:328–36
Marketos SG, Ballas CN: Bronchial asthma in the medical literature of Greek antiquity. **J Asthma** 1982;19(4):263–9
Maróth M: Apodeiksis und Endeiksis bei Galen. **Orvostort Kozl** 1981;93–96(27 No 1–4):55–62
Moszyński J: Galenus - De victu attenuante. **Arch Hist Med (Warsz)** 1982;45(1–4):61–75
Mugnai Carrara D: Una polemica umanistico-scolastica circa l'interpretazione delle tre dottrine ordinate di Galeno. **Ann Ist Mus Stor Sci Fir** 1983;8(1):31–57
Nickel D: Galens Untersuchungen zur embryonalen Blutbewegung. **Orvostort Kozl** 1981;93–96(27 No 1–4):25–35
Nutton V: Galen's autobiographies. In International Congress of the History of Medicine. 26th, Plovdiv, 1978. Actes du Congress. Sofia, 1981. Volume II. p. 173–5.
Nutton V: Galeno salvato dalle acque. **Kos** 1984 Mar;1(2):33–50
Nutton V: Galen in the eyes of his contemporaries. **Bull Hist Med** 1984 Fall;58(3):315–24
Nutton V, ed: Galen On prognosis. Berlin, Akademie-Verlag, 1979. 262 p. (Corpus Medicorum Graecorum, vol. 5, pt. 8, fasc. 1).
Nutton V, ed: Karl Gottlob Kühn and his edition of the works of Galen. Oxford, Oxford Microform Publications, 1976. 35 p. (First published with the microfiche edition of Kühn's edition of The works of Galen, March 1976).
Oberhelman SM: Galen, On Diagnosis from Dreams. **J Hist Med Allied Sci** 1983 Jan;38(1):36–47
Oide S: Der Einfluss der galenischen Pneumatheorie auf die cusanische Spiritustheorie. Eine Anmerkung zu 'De quaerendo deum'. **Mitt Forschungsbeitr Cusanus Ges** 1978;13:198–207
O'Neill YV: Ossa mandibulae inferioris duo. **Clio Med** 1980 May;14(2):97–104
Palmieri N: Un antico commento a Galeno della scuola medica di Ravenna. **Physis** 1981;23:197–296
Pearcy LT: Galen and Stoic rhetoric. **Greek Roman Byz Stud** 1983;24:259–72
Petersen ES: Galen: the most maligned physician. **Proc Inst Med Chic** 1981;34:12
Scarborough J: The Galenic question. **Sudhoffs Arch** 1981;65(1):1–31
Sider D, McVaugh M: Galen On tremor, palpitation, spasm, and rigor; Galeni De tremore, palpitatione, convulsione, et rigore. **Trans Stud Coll Physicians Phila** 1979 Sep;5(1 No 3):183–210
Smith WD: Galen on Coans versus Cnidians. **Bull Hist Med** 1973 Nov–Dec;47(6):569–85
Trevisani F, Moscheo R: Between ancients and moderns: Tommaso Cornelio's medical teaching and an unpublished comment by him on the Galenic Ars parva. **Nouv Repub Lett** 1983;(2):59–73
Villey R: Die Medizin in Rom: Galen. In Sournia JC, Martiny M, Poulet J, ed: Illustrierte Geschichte der Medizin. Salzburg, Andreas, 1980. Vol. 2. p. 411–39.
Weisser U: Die hippokratische Lehre von den Siebenmonatskindern bei Galen und Tabit ibn Qurra. **Sudhoffs Arch** 1979;63(3):209–38
Winkler L: Galens Schrift 'De Antidotis'. Ein Beitrag zur Geschichte von Antidot und Theriak. Diss. rer. nat. Marburg, 1980. 390 p.

**Gálfalvi Domby, Sámuel, 1729–1807**
Gyárfás A: Gálfalvi Domby Sámuel, Borsod vármegye fõorvosa (1729–1807)]. **Orv Hetil** 1982 Aug 22;123(34):2123–5

**Galifret-Granjon, Nadine**
Schmid-Kitsikis E: Un certain regard sur l'oeuvre de N. Galifret-Granjon. **Psychiatr Enfant** 1984;27(1):35–48

**Galilei, Galileo, 1564–1642**
Barcaro U: Galileo e il mondo biologico. **Physis** 1982;24(3):357–79
DelChicca S, Tedeschi J: L'insonnia di Galileo in una lettera inedita di Francesco Redi. **Arch Stor Ital** 1979;173(4):615–8

**Galka, Jozef**
Klodziński S: Dr Józef Gałka. **Przegl Lek** 1981;38(1):184–7

**Gall, Franz Joseph, 1758–1828**
Fischer W: Franz Joseph Gall und Johann Kaspar Spurzheim--Vorläufer einer biologischen Psychiatrie. **Psychiatr Neurol Med Psychol (Leipz)** 1984 Jul;36(7):433–7
Goscilo H: Lermontov's debt to Lavater and Gall. **Slav East Eur Rev** 1981;59(4):500–15
Holck P: Galls frenologi. **Tidsskr Nor Laegeforen** 1983 Sep 20;103(26):1805–7
Lesky E: Das Portrait: Franz Joseph Gall 1758–1828. **Med Unserer Zeit** 1980;4(2):57–61
Lesky E: Der angeklagte Gall. **Gesnerus** 1981;38(3/4):301–11
Lesky E, ed: Franz Joseph Gall, 1758–1828, Naturforscher und Anthropologe. Wien, Huber, 1979. (Hubers Klassiker der Medizin und der Naturwissenschaften, Band 15) 217 p.
Mann G: Franz Joseph Galls kranioskopische Reise durch Europa (1805–1807). Fundierung und Rechtfertigung neuer Wissenschaft. **Nachrichtenbl Dtsch Ges Gesch Med Naturwiss Tech** 1984;34(3):86–114
Wegner PC: Phrenologische Schnupftabakdosen; ein Beitrag zur Wirkung Franz Joseph Galls bei seiner Ankunft in Paris. **Medizinhist J** 1983;18(1–2):69–99
Wegner PC: Le docteur Gall à Cynthère. **Medizinhist J** 1984;19(3):233–43

**Gallard, Charlotte, 1648–1725**
Bernier H: Charlotte Gallard. In Dictionary of Canadian biography, 1701 to 1740. Volume 2, 1969. p. 235–6.

**Gallaudet, Thomas Hopkins, 1787–1851**
Fernandes JJ: Thomas Hopkins Gallaudet on language and communication: a reassessment. **Am Ann Deaf** 1983 Aug;128(4):467–73

**Galton, Francis, 1822–1911**
Billig M: The origins of race psychology - I. **Patterns Prejudice** 1982;16(3):3–16
Corney G: Sir Francis Galton, 1822–1911. **Acta Genet Med Gemellol (Roma)** 1984;33(1):13–8
Diamond S: Francis Galton and American psychology. In R. W. Rieber, K. Salzinger, ed: Psychology: theoretical-historical perspectives. New York, Academic Press, 1980. p. 43–55.
Fancher RE: Francis Galton's African ethnography and its role in the development of his psychology. **Br J Hist Sci** 1983 Mar;16(12 No. 1):67–79
Fancher RE: Alphonse de Candolle, Francis Galton, and the early history of the nature-nurture controversy. **J Hist Behav Sci** 1983 Oct;19(4):341–52
Merrington M, Golden J, ed: A list of the papers and correspondence of Sir Francis Galton (1822–1911) held in the Manuscripts Room, The Library, University College London. London, Galton Laboratory University College London, 1978. 80 p.

**Gamaleia, Nikolai Fedorovich, 1859–1949**
Bardell D: An 1898 report by Gamaleya for a lytic agent specific for Bacillus anthracis. **J Hist Med Allied Sci** 1982 Apr;37(2):222–5

**Gamble, Clarence James, 1894–1966**
Williams D, Williams G: Every child a wanted child. Clarence James Gamble, M.D., and his work in the birth control movement. Ed. E. P. Flint. Boston, Harvard University Press for Countway Library of Medicine, 1978. xvii, 445 p.

**Gamble, James Lawder, 1883–1959**
Bing FC: James Lawder Gamble (1883–1959). A biographical sketch. **J Nutr** 1981;111:203–7

**Gamelin, Jacques, 1738–1803**
Fossard J: Faut-il rendre à Gamelin l'Ecorché de Bayonne attribué à Géricault? **Hist Sci Med** 1984;18(2):153–8

**Gamgee, John, 1831–1894**
Fisher J: Professor Gamgee and the farmers. **Vet Hist** 1979–80;1(2):47–63

**Gandhi, Mohandas Karamchand, 1869–1948**
Adelman H: Hitler and Gandhi: the will as spirit and as flesh. **Psychoanal Rev** 1980 Winter;67(4):543–61

**Gându, Teodora, 1917–**
Negru I: Istoria medicinii: Sora de ocrotire--Teodora Gându. **Viata Med [Medii Sanit]** 1979 Apr;27(4):89–92

**Gannushkin, Peter Borisovich, 1875–1933**
Lakosina ND: Idei nevroticheskogo razvitiia v trudakh P. B. Gannushkina. **Zh Nevropatol Psikhiatr** 1982;82(11):127–9

**Gantt, William Andrew Horsley, 1892–**
Reese WG: Early history of the Pavlovian Society. Twentyfive plus twentyfive. (W. Horsley Gantt). **Pavlov J Biol Sci** 1982 Oct–Dec;17(4):171–7
Reese WG: 'Don't count the bricks'. Scientific contributions of W. H. Gantt. **Pavlov J Biol Sci** 1982 Jul–Sep;17(3):111–4

**Garciá, Eusebio S.**
Foronda MA: An army doctor in Leyte. **Leyte-Samar Stud** 1980;14(1):1–37

**Gárdi, Jenö, 1886–1944**
Balóné Fleischmann M: A rehabilitáció hazai úttöröje Gárdi Jenö dr. (1886–1944). **Orv Hetil** 1984 Feb 19;125(8):470–2

**Gardiner, Silvester, 1708–1786**
Christianson EH: The colonial surgeon's rise to prominence: Dr. Silvester Gardiner (1707–1786) and the practice of lithotomy in New England. **N Engl Hist Geneal Regist** 1982 Apr;136:104–14

**Gardner, Mary Sewall, 1871-1961**
Kantrov I, Wittenstein K: Mary Sewall Gardner. In: Notable American women. The modern period. Cambridge, Mass., Belknap-Harvard Univ. Press, 1980. 4:262-4.

**Garfield, James Abram, 1831-1881**
Bollet AJ: Wounded presidents: 1981 almost repeats the events of 1881. **Med Times** 1981 Jul;109(7):19-23
Roth N: Tracking by telephone: locating the bullet in President Garfield, 1881. **Med Instrum** 1981 May-Jun;15(3):190

**Gargilius Martialis, Quintus, fl. 220-260**
Riddle JM: Gargilius Martialis as a medical writer. **J Hist Med Allied Sci** 1984 Oct;39(4):408-29

**Garland, Joseph, 1893-**
Bean WB: Occasional notes. My sampler of editors: a Fishbein, a Fox, and a Garland. **N Engl J Med** 1980 Jul 24;303(4):229-33

**Garrison, Fielding Hudson, 1870-1935**
Brieger GH: Fielding H. Garrison: the man and his book. **Trans Stud Coll Physicians Phila** 1981 Mar;3(1):1-21

**Garrison, George Harry, 1898-**
Leitner J: Leaders in medicine--George H. Garrison, MD. **J Okla State Med Assoc** 1981 Sep;74(9):298-304

**Garrod, Alfred Baring, 1819-1907**
Eyman E: Alfred Barring Garrod--pionier badán nad dną (1819--1907). **Reumatologia** 1980;18(2):189-90
Leden I: Doubts about Sandro Botticelli's depiction of juvenile rheumatoid arthritis. **Arthritis Rheum** 1984 Oct;27(10):1197-8

**Garrod, Alfred Henry, 1846-1879**
Lawrence C: Alfred Henry Garrod and the indirect measurement of the isometric period of the heart's contraction. **Med Hist** 1980 Jul;24(3):342-6

**Garrod, Archibald Edward, 1857-1936**
Bearn AG, Miller ED: Archibald Garrod and the development of the concept of inborn errors of metabolism. **Bull Hist Med** 1979 Fall;53(3):315-28
Sinohara H: [Archibald Edward Garrod (1857-1936): a biographical assay (author's transl)] (Jpn). **Seikagaku** 1980 Nov;52(11):1155-72

**Garrod, Paul, 1896?-1979**
Abraham EP: Ernst Chain and Paul Garrod. **J Antimicrob Chemother** 1980 Jul;6(4):423-4

**Garshin, Vladimir Georgievich, 1887-1956**
Bobkov AG, Mikhaĭlov VP: Nauchnaia deiatel'nost' V. G. Garshina (1887-1956) i razvitie nauchnykh kontseptsiĭ v rabotakh sovetskikh morfologov. **Arkh Patol** 1983;45(4):77-80

**Garshin, Vsevolod Mikhailovich, 1855-1888**
Ionov IuV: Meditsinskie temy v proizvedeniiakh V. M. Garshina (k 125-letiiu so dnia rozhdeniia). **Klin Med (Mosk)** 1981 Jan;59(1):110-2

**Gärtner Family, 17-18th cent.**
Graepel PH: Die Calwer Apothekerfamilie Gärtner im Bild. **Beitr Gesch Pharm** 1981;31(12):92-5

**Garzoni, Giovanni, 1419-1505**
Matsen HS: Giovanni Garzoni (1419-1505) to Alessandro Achillini (1463-1512): An unpublished letter and defense. In Edward P Mahoney, ed. Philosophy and humanism: Renaissance essays in honor of Paul Oskar Kristeller. New York: Columbia Univ. Press, 1976. p. 518-530.

**Gasser, Achilles, 1531-1583**
Burmeister KH: Achilles Gasser als Stadtarzt von Feldkirch. **Montfort** 1968;20(3):326-42

**Gasser, Conrad, 1912-1982**
Hitzig WH: Conrad Gasser 1912-1982. **Schweiz Med Wochenschr** 1982 Oct 16;112(42):1486-7

**Gasser, Herbert Spencer, 1888-1963**
Brandt AM: Herbert Spencer Gasser. In Dictionary of American biography, 1961-1965. Suppl. 7, 1981. p. 279-81.

**Gastaut, Henri Jean, 1915-**
Brazier MA: The birth of the International Brain Research Organization: a tribute to Henri Gastaut. **Electroencephalogr Clin Neurophysiol** 1982;35:13-4
Broughton R: A brief outline of the career and accomplishments of Henri Gastaut. **Electroencephalogr Clin Neurophysiol** 1982;35:XII-XV
Henri Gastaut and the Marseilles school's contribution to the neurosciences: Proceedings of the 25th and final Colloque de Marseille. **Electroencephalogr Clin Neurophysiol** 1982;35:1-447
Lambo TA: Professor Gastaut and his contributions to the World Health Organization programme. **Electroencephalogr Clin Neurophysiol** 1982;35:3-6
Lennox MA: Professor Gastaut's contribution to the International League against Epilepsy. **Electroencephalogr Clin Neurophysiol** 1982;35:9-12
Naquet R: Gastaut and the EEG Federation. **Electroencephalogr Clin Neurophysiol** 1982;35:7-8

**Gatch, Willis Dew, 1878-1962**
[Willis Dew Gatch. Includes reprints of three of his articles.]: **Indiana Med Hist Q** 1977;3(3):43-60

**Gates, Reginald Ruggles, 1882-1962**
Roberts JA: Reginald Ruggles Gates. In Dictionary of national biography, 1961-1970. Suppl. 8, 1981. p. 424-5.

**Gatewood, James Duncan, 1857-1924**
Meals RA, Brody GS: Gatewood and the first thenar pedicle. **Plast Reconstr Surg** 1984 Feb;73(2):315-9

**Gatterer, Johann Christoph, 1727-1799**
Rödel V: Johann Christoph Gatterers 'Linnaeismus graphicus'. Klassifikation und Universalismus im 18. Jahrhundert. **Medizinhist J** 1982;17(3):215-38

**Gaucher, Phillipe Charles Ernest, 1854-1918**
Desnick RJ: Gaucher disease (1882-1982): centennial perspectives on the most prevalent Jewish genetic disease. **Mt Sinai J Med (NY)** 1982 Nov-Dec;49(6):443-55

**Gaulard, Pierre Nicolas, 1713-1740**
Besombes A: La triste fin de Pierre-Nicolas Gaulard (1713-1740) 'élève-associé de Fauchard'. **Hist Sci Med** 1980;14(2):213-20

**Gavin, Hector, 1815-1855**
Spriggs EA: Hector Gavin, MD, FRCSE (1815-1855) - his life, his work for the sanitary movement, and his accidental death in the Crimea. **Med Hist** 1984 Jul;28(3):283-92

**Gay-Lussac, Joseph Louis, 1778-1850**
Crosland M: The library of Gay-Lussac. **Ambix** 1981 Nov;28(3):158-70

**Gay Prieto, José, 1905-1979**
Jaqueti G: Profesor José Gay Prieto. Maestro de dermatólogos (1905-1979). **Actas Dermosifiliogr** 1981 Jul-Aug;72(7-8):389-96

**Gazárek, Frantiska, 1912-**
Zivotní jubileum prof. MUDr. Františka Gazárka, CSc: **Cesk Gynekol** 1983 Feb;48(1):75-80

**Gebsattel, Victor Emil von, 1883-1976**
Rattner J: Victor Emil von Gebsattel. In J. Rattner, ed: Wandlungen der Psychoanalyse. Wien, Europaverlag, 1980. p. 257-79.

**Gedner, Christopher Eliasson, 1730-1773**
Schramm E: Linné, Gedner und die biologische Kontrolle. **Medizinhist J** 1984;19(3):244-9

**Geelani, Nizamuddin Ahmed, 1586-1650**
Hussain SA: Hakim Nizamuddin Ahmed Geelani; a physician of Qutub Shahi period. **Bull Indian Inst Hist Med (Hyderabad)** 1979;9:67-73

**Gehlen, Arnold, 1904-**
Pagel G: Narziss und Prometheus: die Theorie der Phantasie bei Freud und Gehlen. Würzburg, Königshausen & Neumann, 1984. 195 p. (Studien zur Anthropologie, Band 8).

**Gehrig, Lou, 1903-1941**
Brady GM: Lou Gehrig: the iron man. **Manuscripts** 1980;32(2):84-9

**Gélineau, Jean Baptiste Edouard, 1828-1906**
Passouant P: Doctor Gelineau (1828-1906): narcolepsy centennial. **Sleep** 1981 Sep;4(3):241-6
Passouant P: Le docteur Gélineau (1828-1906). **Hist Sci Med** 1981;15(2):137-43
Passouant P: La narcolepsie au temps de Gélineau. **Hist Sci Med** 1981;15(2):129-36

**Gelley, Rafael Mihállyal, fl. 1788**
Péterffy I: Híradás két felvilágosodás kori jeles orvosról. **Orv Hetil** 1983 Jul 31;124(31):1895-6

**Genersich, Antal, 1842-1918**
Bugyi B: Genersich Antal vasutépítés orvosakénti tevékenységéröl. **Orv Hetil** 1983 Jul 24;124(30):1825-6

**Geoffroy Saint-Hilaire, Etienne, 1772-1844**
Fischer JL: Etienne Geoffroy Saint-Hilaire (1772-1844) face au problème du déterminisme du sexe. **Hist Philos Life Sci** 1979;1(2):261-83

**Gerard, John, 1545-1612**
Phelps WH: John Gerard, the herbalist. **Library (Lond)** 1980 Mar;2(1):76-85

**Gérard, Pol, 1886-1961**
Dalcq A: Pol Gérard, 1886-1961. In Florilège des Sciences en Belgique - II. Bruxelles, Académie Royale de Belgique, 1980. p. 609-16.

**Gerardus, Cremonensis, 1114-1187**
Jacquart D: Quelques réflexions sur la traduction du Kitab al-Mansuri de Rhazès par Gérard de Crémone. In International Congress of the History of Medicine, 27th, Barcelona, 1980. Actas. Barcelona, Académia de Ciències Médiques de Catalunya i Balears, 1981. p. 264-6.
Lindberg DC, ed: Opticae thesaurus. Alhazeni Arabis libri septem, nuncprimùm editi. Eiusdem liber De Crepusculis et nubium ascensionibus. Item Vitellonis Thuringopoloni libri X. Reprint of the 1572 ed. New York, Johnson Reprint Corp., 1972. xxxiv, 288, 474 p.

**Gerbezius, Marcus, 1658-1718**
Mušič D, Rakovec P, Jagodic A, et al: The first description of syncopal attacks in heart block. **PACE** 1984 Mar;7(2):301-3

**Gerhard, William Wood, 1809–1872**
Smith DC: Gerhard's distinction between typhoid and typhus and its reception in America, 1833–1860. **Bull Hist Med** 1980 Fall; 54(3):368–85

**Gerhardt, Carl, 1833–1902**
Seidler E: Carl Gerhardt und seine Rede: 'Die Aufgaben und Ziele der Kinderheilkunde' (1879). **Monatsschr Kinderheilkd** 1983 Sep;131(9):545–8

**Géricault, Jean Louis André Théodore, 1791–1824**
Fossard J: Faut-il rendre à Gamelin l'Ecorché de Bayonne attribué à Géricault? **Hist Sci Med** 1984;18(2):153–8

**Gerngross, Richard, 1878–1956**
Gerngross R: Ein bayerischer Arzt in China. **MMW** 1980 Jan 25;122(4):141–2

**Gershwin, George, 1898–1937**
Ljunggren B: The case of George Gershwin. **Neurosurgery** 1982 Jun;10(6 Pt 1):733–6

**Gertsen, Petr Aleksandrovich, 1871–1947**
Petrovskiĭ BV: Petr Aleksandrovich Gertsen (k 80-letiiu Moskovskogo nauchno-issledovatel'skogo onkologicheskogo instituta im P. A. Gertsena). **Khirurgiia (Mosk)** 1983 Nov;(11):3–7

**Gerung, Mathias, ca. 1500–ca. 1568**
Grasshoff K: Leibesübungen und Gesellschaft im Gemälde 'Melancolia 1558' des Mathias Gerung. **Stadion** 1977;3(1):44–59

**Gesell, Arnold Lucius, 1880–1961**
Radbill SX: Arnold Lucius Gesell. In Dictionary of American biography, 1961–1965. Suppl. 7, 1981. p. 283–5.

**Gesner, Abraham, 1797–1864**
Sherwood RH: Discovery of kerosene. **NS Hist Q** 1979;9(2):157–64

**Gesner, Konrad, 1516–1565**
Durling RJ: Konrad Gessner's Briefwechsel. In: Schmitz R, Krafft F, ed: Humanismus und Naturwissenschaften. Boppard, Boldt, 1979? p. 101–111. (Beiträge zur Humanismusforschung, Band VI).
Nutton V: Conrad Gesner and the English naturalists. **Med Hist** 1985 Jan;29(1):93–7

**Gessard, Louis-Marie, 1771–1855**
Nauroy J, Bossard E: Louis-Marie Gessard, pharmacien et édile de Saint-Denis. **Rev Hist Pharm (Paris)** 1979 Dec;26(243):235–9

**Gettler, Alexander Oscar, 1883–1968**
Eckert WG, Kaye S: Alexander O. Gettler (1883–1983). A centennial of his birth. **Am J Forensic Med Pathol** 1983 Dec;4(4):297–301
Freimuth HC: Alexander O. Gettler (1883–1968). A reflection. **Am J Forensic Med Pathol** 1983 Dec;4(4):303–5
Sunshine I: Dr. Alexander O. Gettler's documentation of a radiation hazard. **Am J Forensic Med Pathol** 1983 Dec;4(4):307–9

**Geyer, Günther, 1930–1980**
Linss W: Im memoriam Günther Geyer (25. 9. 1930--18. 6. 1980). **Anat Anz** 1981;149(3):193–209

**Ghalib, 1796?–1869**
Siddiqi T: Ghalib and Unani medicine. **Stud Hist Med** 1979 Sep;3(3):181–98

**Ghirlandaio, Domenico, 1449–1494**
Dotz W, Berliner N: Rhinophyma. A master's depiction, a patron's affliction. **Am J Dermatopathol** 1984 Jun;6(3):231–5

**Ghirotti, Gigi, 1920–1973**
Sansoni J: Considerazioni e riflessioni sul libro 'Lungo Viaggio nel Tunnel della Mallattia' di Gigi Ghirotti. **Prof Inferm** 1980 Jan–March;33(1):3–6

**Ghon, Anton, 1886–1936**
Ober WB: Ghon but not forgotten: Anton Ghon and his complex. **Pathol Annu** 1983;18 (pt 2):79–85

**Giacometti, Augusto, 1877–1947**
Meares R: Body feeling in human relations: the possible examples of Brancusi and Giacometti. **Psychiatry** 1980 May;43(2):160–7

**Giard, Louis, 1809–1887**
Audet LP: Louis Giard. In Dictionary of Canadian biography, 1881–1890. 1982;11:345–6.

**Gibbon, Edward, 1737–1794**
Foster WD: Edward Gibbon's health. **Br Med J** 1979 Dec 22–29;2(6205):1633–5

**Gibbon, John Heysham, Jr., 1903–1973**
Dobell AR: John H. Gibbon, Jr. Part II. Personal reminiscenses. **Ann Thorac Surg** 1982 Sep;34(3):342–4
Hill JD: John H. Gibbon, Jr. Part I. The development of the first successful heart-lung machine. **Ann Thorac Surg** 1982 Sep;34(3):337–41

**Gibson, James Jerome, 1904–**
Ben-Zeev A: J. J. Gibson and the ecological approach to perception. **Stud Hist Philos Sci** 1981 Jun;12(2):107–39

**Gibson, Thomas, 1915–**
McGregor IA: Thomas Gibson's contribution to immunology. **Plast Reconstr Surg** 1983 Mar;71(3):440

**Gide, André Paul Guillaume, 1869–1951**
Dimić CA: Gide et la maladie. **Studi Francesi** 1979;23(67):62–75

**Gietzelt, Fritz, 1903–1968**
Dörffel EW, Held F, Oelssner W: Zum 30. Jahrestag der Gründung der Deutschen Demokratischen Republik. Die Bedeutung Fritz Gietzelts für die Radiologie und Geschwulst-bekämpfung. **Radiobiol Radiother (Berl)** 1979 Oct;20(5):621–6
Stahlschmidt S: Professor Dr. med. habil. Fritz Gietzelt--Arzt, Wissenschaftler, Kommunist: ein Lebensbild. Berlin, Humboldt-Universität zu Berlin, 1982. 64 p.

**Gifford, George Edmund, 1930–1981**
Gifford GE: Medicine and science in early America. Being the collected essays of George Edmund Gifford, Jr., 1930–1981. Edited by Dorothy I. Lansing. Devon, Pa., Published by the friends of George E. Gifford, Jr., 1982. ix, 388 p.
Jones GW: George Edmund Gifford, jr. **Proc Am Antiq Soc** 1981;91(1):22–4

**Gil, Francisco, fl. 1784**
Valle RK, Valle AR: La disertacion fisico-médica en la qual se prescribe un método seguro para preservar a los pueblos de viruelas hasta lograr la completa extincion de ellas en todo el reyno, by Dr. Francisco Gil. In International Congress of the History of Medicine, 27th, Barcelona, 1980. Actas. Barcelona, Académia de Ciències Mèdiques de Catalunya i Balears, 1981. p. 217–22.

**Gilbert, William, 1540–1603**
Carter RB: Gilbert and Descartes: the science of conserving the compound body. **Z Allg Wissenschaftstheorie** 1982;13(2):224–33

**Gilbertus Anglicus, 1180?–1250**
Getz FM: Gilbertus Anglicus anglicized. **Med Hist** 1982 Oct;26(4):436–42

**Gilbreth, Lillian Evelyn Moller, 1878–1972**
Cowan RS: Lillian Evelyn Moller Gilbreth. In: Notable American women. The modern period. Cambridge, Mass., Belknap-Harvard Univ. Press, 1980. 4:271–3.

**Gilibert, Jean Emmanuel, 1741–1814**
Ignatovich FI, Semeniuk SI: Zh. E. Zhiliber i ego 'Flora Litvy'. **Sov Zdravookhr** 1981;(11):67–9

**Gill, Richard C., 1901–1958**
Humble RM: The Gill-Merrill expedition: penultimate chapter in the curare story. **Anesthesiology** 1982 Dec;57(6):519–26

**Gillies, Harold Delf, 1882–1960**
Beattie D: Plastic surgery in New Zealand (Sir Harold Gillies). **Ann Plast Surg** 1982 Nov;9(5):358–60

**Giorgione, Giorgio Barbarelli, known as, 1477–1510 or 1511**
Schupbach W: Doctor Parma's medicinal macaronic: poem by Bartolotti, pictures by Giorgione and Titian. [Wellcome MS 461]. **J Warburg Courtauld Inst** 1978;41:147–91, 350

**Girard, G., 1888–**
Coulanges P: Cinquantenaire du vaccin antipesteux EV (Girard et Robic). **Arch Inst Pasteur Madagascar** 1982;50(1):169–84

**Girardot, François, 1773–1831**
Lemaire JF: Le chirurgien-baron François Girardot (1773–1831) un oublié de l'histoire. **Hist Sci Med** 1980;14(1):107–14

**Girdlestone, Gathorne Robert, 1881–1950**
Taylor RG: G. R. Girdlestone, M.D., F.R.C.S. **Clin Orthop** 1983 Mar;(173):125–9

**Gissane, William, 1898–**
Harrison SH: Accident surgery--the life and times of William Gissane. **Injury** 1984 Nov;16(3):145–54
London PS: Inaugural William Gissane Lecture: man and memorial. **Injury** 1982 Nov;14(3):211–34

**Giustiniani, Vincenzo, d. 1570**
Burnett J: The Giustiniani medicine chest. **Med Hist** 1982 Jul;26(3):325–33

**Gladwin, Mary**
Harding PM: A Red Cross nurse in Belgrade: Mary Gladwin saw World War I from the inside of a hospital. Her battles were no easier than those of the soldiers. **Am Hist Illus** 1982;17(1):41–7

**Glanvill, Joseph, 1636–1680**
Jobe TH: The devil in Restoration science: the Glanvill-Webster witchcraft debate. **Isis** 1981 Sep;72(263):343–56

**Glass, David Victor, 1911–1978**
Marshall TH, Laslett P: David Glass: an appreciation. **Br J Sociol** 1979;30(1):1–4

**Glavchev, Vladimir Petrov, 1878–1915**
Altŭnkov P: D-r Vladimir Petrov Glavchev (1878–1915 g.). **Khirurgiia (Sofiia)** 1982;35(6):632

**Gleason, Edward Francis, 1869–1944**
Rogers FB: Dr. Edward F. Gleason (1869–1944) of Hyannis, Massachusetts, and the Cape Cod Hospital and Windmill. **J Hist Med Allied Sci** 1980 Oct;35(4):459–60

**Glenny, Alexander Thomas, 1882–1965**
Evans D: Alexander Thomas Glenny. In Dictionary of national biography, 1961–1970. Suppl 8, 1981. p. 434–5.

**Glinchikov, Vladimir Ignat'evich, 1878–**
Shalaev NF: Terapevt, uchenyĭ i pedagog V.I. Glinchikov. **Klin Med (Mosk)** 1984 Oct;62(10):146–9

**Glinkov, Pavel Faleeviya, 1883–1923**
Nikitin EA: Fel'dsher revoliutsionnogo korablia P. F. Glinkov. **Feldsher Akush** 1982;47(11):36–7

**Glisson, Francis, 1597–1677**
Boss J: Helmont, Glisson, and the doctrine of the common reservoir in the seventeenth-century revolution in physiology. **Br J Hist Sci** 1983 Nov;16(54 Pt 3):261–72
Boss JM: 'Doctrina de circulatione sanguinis haud immutat antiquam Medendi Methodum': an unpublished manuscript (1662) by Francis Glisson (1597–1677) on the implications of Harvey's physiology. **Physis** 1978;20(1–4):309–35
Mani N: Biomedical thought in Glisson's hepatology and in Wepfer's work on apoplexy. With commentary by R. G. Frank, p. 84–8. In Stevenson LG, ed: A celebration of medical history. Baltimore, Johns Hopkins University Press, 1982. (The Henry E. Sigerist supplements to the Bulletin of the History of Medicine; new ser., no. 6). p. 37–63.

**Glotova, Elena Vladimirovna**
Kravchenko AT: Pamiati professora Glotovoĭ Eleny Vladimirovny (k 100-letiiu so dnia rozhdeniia). **Zh Mikrobiol Epidemiol Immunobiol** 1983 Mar;(3):112–3

**Gobineau, Arthur de, 1816–1882**
Seidler E: Die Freiburger Gobineau-Vereinigung und die Verbreitung des Arier-Gedankens in Deutschland. In Seidler E, Schott H, ed: Bausteine zur Medizingeschichte. Stuttgart, Steiner, 1984. p. 121–9.

**Gockel, Eberhard, 1636–1703**
Eisinger J: Lead and wine. Eberhard Gockel and the colica Pictonum. **Med Hist** 1982 Jul;26(3):279–302

**Goddard, Henry Herbert, 1866–1957**
Tyor PL: Henry Herbert Goddard. In Dictionary of American Biography, Suppl. 6, 1956–1960. p. 240–1, 1980.

**Godlee, Rickman John, 1849–1925**
Kirkpatrick DB: The first primary brain-tumor operation. **J Neurosurg** 1984 Nov;61(5):809–13

**Godwin, William**
Ritchey D: The Baltimore theater and the yellow fever epidemic. **Md Hist Mag** 1972;67(3):298–301

**Goebel, Karol, 1845–1891**
Sawicki B, Brońka E: Karol Goebel – pierwszy docent stomatologii w Polsce. **Czas Stomatol** 1979 Aug;32(8):807–9

**Goeppert, Heinrich Robert, 1800–1884**
Sajner J, Geus A: Ueber eine Buchbesprechung von Jan Evangelista Purkyně. **J Soc Bibliogr Nat Hist** 1978 Nov;9(1):53–5

**Goerke, Heinz, 1917–**
Habrich C, Marguth F, Wolf JH, et al: Medizinische Diagnostik in Geschichte und Gegenwart. Festschrift für Heinz Goerke zum sechzigsten Geburtstag. München, Fritsch, 1978. 656 p. Historical contributions by J. Antall, G. Baader, V. Bazala, L. Belloni, G. Bratescu, W. Brendel, L. Burilkova, C. J. Clemedson, K. Goldammer, H. Henne, S. Hofmann, G. Keil, K. P. Killian, W. Klinner, W. Kloppe, M. Knedel, W. Kock, F. Köcher, H. M. Koelbing, K. S. Kolta, E. Kreuzer, V. Krizek, O. Larsen, B. I. Lindskog, N. Mani, V. Møller-Christensen, Y. Otsuka, G. Preiser, L. Premuda, E. Püschel, H. Röhrich, E. Rosner, G. Rudolph, J. Sájner, H. Schadewaldt, H. Schipperges, H. H. Simmer, J. Spielmann, M. Stürzbecher, A. Terzioglu, R. Winau, N. Plovdiv. (Neue Münchner Beiträge zur Geschichte der Medizin und Naturwissenschaften, Medizinhistorische Reihe, Band 7/8).

**Goethe, Johann Wolfgang von, 1749–1832**
Dietsch H: Von der Metamorphose zur Homologie. Zum 150. Todestag Goethes. **Med Welt** 1982 Dec 3;33(48):1767–8
Donat K: Goethe aus ärztlicher Sicht. **Fortschr Med** 1982 May 13;100(18):852–8
Hellmich S, Hellmich J: Der Zwischenkieferknochen und Goethes Mephistopheles. **Laryngol Rhinol Otol (Stuttg)** 1982 Oct;61(10):552–6
Hruby K: Goethes Augenleiden. **Klin Monatsbl Augenheilkd** 1984 Jul;185(1):61–3
Kleeberg J: Goethe und die 'mal de rosa'. **Z Gastroenterol** 1983 May;21(5):241–3
Křížek V: J.W. Goethe a ceské lázně. K 150. výročí básníkovy smrti 22. března 1832. **Cas Lek Cesk** 1982 Jun 4;121(22):695–8
Lacan J: The neurotic's individual myth. **Psychoanal Q** 1979 Jul;48(3):405–25
Neuhauser W: Goethe sprach nie über die Leiden mit seinen Zähnen. **Zahnarztl Mitt** 1982 Aug 16;72(16):1735–43
Sajner J: Goethuv vztah k přírodním vědám, zvláště k lékařství. **Vnitr Lek** 1982 Jun;28(6):615–6
Schachter M: Le malade Johann Wolfgang Goethe (1749–1832) et ses maladies (A l'occasion du 150e anniversaire de sa mort). **Hist Sci Med** 1982;16(2):81–8
Schadewaldt H: Das Badewesen in der Goethezeit. **Therapiewoche** 1982;32:4123–33
Schultz P: Wie Geheimrat von Goethe den Zwischenkiefer-Knochen entdeckte. **Zahnarztl Mitt** 1984 Apr 1;74(7):733–4
Voss H: Goethes Selbstzeugnisse über seine Beschäftigung mit 'organischen Naturen'. II. Briefe (1776 bis 1817). **Gegenbaurs Morphol Jahrb** 1979;125(4):466–518
Voss H: Goethes Selbstzeugnisse über seine Beschäftigung mit 'organischen Naturen'. **Gegenbaurs Morphol Jahrb** 1979;125(5):687–736
Wenzel M: Goethes Morphologie in ihrer Beziehung zum darwinistischen Evolutionsdenken. **Medizinhist J** 1983;18(1–2):52–68

**Goldberger, Joseph, 1874–1929**
Guggenheim YK: [Joseph Goldberger's contributions to pellagra research] (Heb). **Harefuah** 1980;99(5–6):134–6
Health in the southern United States: New York, Arno, 1977. Various paginations. Facsimiles of works by David Ramsay (1790 and 1796), Josiah C. Nott (1847), Edward H. Barton (1851), Wickliffe Rose (1910), Joseph Goldberger (1916).
Schoenberg BS: Plague of pellagra. **South Med J** 1983 Mar;76(3):281–3

**Goldfuss, Georg August, 1782–1848**
Querner H: 'Ein Wort über den Einfluss naturwissenschaftlicher Institute auf humane Bildung' (G. A. Goldfuss 1821). In Seidler E, Schott H, ed: Bausteine zur Medizingeschichte. Stuttgart, Steiner, 1984. p. 86–93.

**Goldhagen, Johann Friedrich Gottlieb, 1742–1788**
Kaiser W: Johann Friedrich Gottlieb Goldhagen (1742–1788) aus Nordhausen, Stadtphysikus und Ordinarius in Halle. **Beitr Heimatkd Stadt Kreis Nordhausen** 1978;(2–3):58–70

**Goldmark, Josephine Clara, 1877–1950**
Matejski MP: Nursing education, professionalism, and autonomy: social constraints and the Goldmark Report. **ANS** 1981;3(3):17–30

**Goldschmidt, Richard Benedict, 1878–1958**
Caspari EW, Allen GE, et al: Controversial geneticist and creative biologist. [Richard B. Goldschmidt] A critical review on his contributions. **Experientia [Suppl]** 1980;Suppl 35:1–154
Piternick LK: Richard Goldschmidt, controversial geneticist and creative biologist: a critical review of his contribution. Basal, Boston, Birkhäuser, 1980. 153 p.

**Goldsmith, Grace Arabell, 1904–1975**
Etheridge EW: Grace Arabell Goldsmith. In: Notable American women. The modern period. Cambridge, Mass., Belknap-Harvard Univ. Press, 1980. 4:283–4.

**Goldsmith, Oliver, 1728–1774**
Miller JM: Poisoning by antimony: a case report (Oliver Goldsmith). **South Med J** 1982 May;75(5):592
Obe JM: Oliver Goldsmith: doctor, poet, writer. **Cent Afr J Med** 1984 Mar;30(3):303–8

**Goldszmit, Henry K., 1878–1942**
Bendiner E: Korczak: pediatrician on the road to hell. **Hosp Pract** 1981 Jul;16(7):125–8, 132–4, 138–9 passim
Klein F: Janusz Korczak--Arzt und Erzieher--Ein Symbol gelebter Menschlichkeit für die heutige medizinische und heilpädagogische Praxis. **Off Gesundheitswes** 1984 May;46(5):244–8
Quintero García P: Janusz Korczac. **Rev Soc Venez Hist Med** 1979;28(42):31–5
Staszyc J: Doktór Janusz Korczak -- lekarz, literat i twórca pedagogicznej koncepcji wychowania. **Ann Univ Mariae Curie Sklodowska [Med]** 1978;33:333–9

**Golgi, Camillo, 1844–1926**
Breathnach CS: Golgi. **Ir Med J** 1983 Jun;76(6):298
Køppe S: The psychology of the neuron: Freud, Cajal and Golgi. **Scand J Psychol** 1983;24(1):1–12
Legée G: Evolution de l'histologie du système nerveux au XIXe siècle; l'impulsion donnée par Camillo Golgi (1844–1926). **Clio Med** 1982 May;17(1):15–32

**Golub, David Moiseevich, 1901?–**
Leontiuk AS, Lobko PI, Novikov II: David Moiseevich Golub (k 80-letiiu so dnia rozhdeniia i 55-letiiu vrachebnoĭ, nauchnoĭ, pedagogicheskoĭ i obshchestvennoĭ deiatel'nosti). **Arkh Anat Gistol Embriol** 1981 Aug;81(8):122–6

**Golubev, Vasilii Zakhar'evich, 1858–**
Mel'man EP, Shutka BV: Issledovanie V. Z. Golubevym mikroangioarkhitektoniki pochki. **Arkh Anat Gistol Embriol** 1983 Dec;85(12):87–9

**Golubkov, Aleksandr Pavlovich, 1880–1945**
Emeksuzian VS: A. P. Golubkov v sibirskoĭ ssylke. **Sov Zdravookhr** 1981;(11):59–62
Idel'chik KI: A. P. Golubkov: 1880–1945. Moskva, Meditsina, 1980. 78 p.
Levitin MN: Stoĭkiĭ bol'shevik-leninets A. P. Golubkov. **Feldsher Akush** 1980;45(11):44–6

**Golubov, Nikolaĭ Fedorovich, 1856–1943**
Kaladze NN: Nikolaĭ Fedorovich Golubov (k 125-letiiu so dnia rozhdeniia). **Klin Med (Mosk)** 1982 Nov;60(11):120–3

**Gómez-Caamaño, José Luis, 1909–1984**
Cornet AM, Sagrera JE de: En memoria de nuestro maestro: José Luis Gómez-Caamaño (1909–1984). **Bol Soc Esp Hist Farm** 1984;35(137):1–22

**Gómez Durán, Manuel, d. 1984**
Matilla Gómez V: Sesión necrológica del Excmo. Sr. D. Manuel Gómez Durán. Día 3 de abril de 1984. **An R Acad Nac Med (Madr)** 1984;101(2):273–88

**Gómez Farias, Valentín, 1781–1858**
Fernández del Castillo F: El expediente médico de Valentín Gómez Farias. **Bol Inst Invest Bibliogr** 1970;(4):125–9
Treviño-Zapata N: Valentín Gómez Farías. Patricio, precursor, médico y político. **Gac Med Mex** 1982 Jan;118(1):39–43

**Gomez Ortega, D. Casimiro, fl. 1788**
Basante Pol RM, Castillo Tello MM: La correspondencia dirigida a D. Casimiro Gomez Ortega, desde Valencia en el periodo comprendido entre 1783–1788. **Bol Soc Esp Hist Farm** 1982 Mar;33(130):131–44
Basante Pol RM, Castillo Tello MM: La correspondencia dirigida a D. Casimiro Gómez Ortega por D. Cándido M.a Trigueros. **Bol Soc Esp Hist Farm** 1981 Sep;32(127):137–47

**Gonthier d'Andernach, Jean, 1497–1574**
Schaff G: Jean Gonthier d'Andernach (1497–1574) et la médecine de son temps. In Livet G, Schaff G, ed: Médecine et assistance en Alsace, XVIe–XXe siècle. Strasbourg, Istra, 1976. p. 21–40.

**Gonzáles de Clavijo, Ruy, d. 1412**
Lindgren U: The problems of being a foreigner: Ruy Gonzáles de Clavijo's journey to Samarkand. **Clio Med** 1980 Jul;14(3–4):225–34

**González Flores, Jesús Mariá, 1857–1947**
Salinas Cantú H: Biografia del Dr. Jesus Ma. González Flores. **Humanitas** 1981;22:201–12

**González, Pedro María, fl. 1789–1805**
Orozco Acuaviva A: Pedro María González y el tratado de las enfermedades de la gente del mar. In International Congress of the History of Medicine, 27th, Barcelona, 1980. Actas. Barcelona, Acadèmia de Ciències Mèdiques de Catalunya i Balears, 1981. p. 394–8.

**González Velasco, Pedro, 1815–1875?**
Uranga E: Un ilustre anatónomo y cirujano con ideas necrofílicas del siglo XIX en Zaragoza. **Bol Real Soc Vascongada Amigos Pais** 1973;29(1–3):375–91

**Good, Robert Alan, 1922–**
Festschrift in honor of Robert A. Good on the occasion of his 60th birthday: **Clin Immunol Immunopathol** 1982 May;23(2):155–61

**Goodenough, Florence Laura, 1886–1959**
Wolf TH: Florence Laura Goodenough. In: Notable American women. The modern period. Cambridge, Mass., Belknap-Harvard Univ. Press, 1980. 4:284–6.

**Goodfellow, George Emery, 1855–1910**
Rehfeldt FC: George Goodfellow: practicing paradoxologist. **Tex Med** 1981;77(3):44–7

**Goodrich, Annie Warburton, 1866–1954**
Tomes N: Annie Warburton Goodrich. In: Notable American women. The modern period. Cambridge., Mass., Belknap-Harvard Univ. Press, 1980. 4:286–8.

**Goodsir, John, 1814–1867**
Jacyna LS: John Goodsir and the making of cellular reality. **J Hist Biol** 1983 Spring;16(1):75–99

**Goodyear, Charles, 1800–1860**
Hagman HC: History: Charles Goodyear. **Dent Lab Rev** 1981 Aug;56(8):33

**Gopalacharyulu, Pandit Divi, 1872–1920**
Purushothamacharyulu G: Pandit D. Gopalacharyulu, regenerator of ayurveda. **Sachitra Ayurved** 1981 Mar;:194–200

**Goraksanātha**
Rama Rao B, Reddy MV: A note on Goraksanātha and his work Yogadipikā. **Bull Indian Inst Hist Med Hyderabad** 1982;12(1–4):34–44

**Gorcy, J. Camille**
Théodoridès J: Les études sur la rage de deux médecins Lorrains: Pierre-Christophe Gorcy (1807–1821) et J. Camille Gorcy (1812). In: Congrès National des Sociétés Savantes, 103e, Nancy, 1978. Comptes Rendus. Paris, 1978. Section des Sciences, Fasc. v. p. 55–69.

**Gorcy, Pierre-Christophe, 1807–1821**
Théodoridès J: Les études sur la rage de deux médecins Lorrains: Pierre-Christophe Gorcy (1807–1821) et J. Camille Gorcy (1812). In: Congrès National des Sociétés Savantes, 103e, Nancy, 1978. Comptes Rendus. Paris, 1978. Section des Sciences, Fasc. v. p. 55–69.

**Gorer, Peter Alfred Isaac, 1907–1961**
Amos DB: Peter Alfred Isaac Gorer. In Dictionary of national biography, 1961–1970. Suppl. 8, 1981. p. 443–5.

**Gorgas, William Crawford, 1854–1920**
Bowen TE: William Crawford Gorgas, physician to the world. **Milit Med** 1983 Dec;148(12):917–20
Ellman MH: William Crawford Gorgas and the American Medical Association. **JAMA** 1980 Feb 15;243(7):659–60

**Gorinevskaia, V. V., 1882–**
Rusakov AB: Zhiznennyĭ i tvorcheskiĭ put' V. V. Gorinevskoĭ (K 100–letiiu so dnia rozhdeniia). **Ortop Travmatol Protez** 1983 Mar;(3):63–5

**Gorka, Sánder, 1878–1944**
Lambrecht M: Gorka Sándor az elsö magyar biológusprofesszor. **Orv Hetil** 1979 Aug 19;120(32):1947–50

**Gorter, Johannes de, 1689–1762**
Püschel E: 'Dictata' zu den Werken von Johannes de Gorter (1689–1762), professor in Harderwijk: medicinae compendium, praxis medicae systema und chirurgia repurgata. **Janus** 1980;67(1–2–3):41–57

**Gortner, Ross Aiken, 1885–1942**
Mann FD: Ross Aiken Gortner and bound water, the water of life. **Perspect Biol Med** 1976 Autumn;20(1):142–4

**Gorup-Besanez, Eugen Franz von, 1817–1878**
Simmer HH: Medizin und Chemie um die Mitte des 19. Jahrhunderts in Erlangen: Eugen Franz Freiherr von Gorup-Besanez (1817–1878). **J Clin Chem Clin Biochem** 1981 Jul;19(7):497–509

**Gottron, Heinrich A., 1890–1974**
Leyh F, Wendt V: Heinrich A. Gottron (1890–1974). **Am J Dermatopathol** 1983 Jun;5(3):241–3
Wendt V: Heinrich A. Gottron: Leben und Werk. Lübeck, Hansisches Verlagskonto H. Scheffler, 1980. 99 p.

**Gotzkirchen, Sigmund, ca. 1410–1475**
Dressendörfer W: Drogeneinkaufsmengen einer Münchener Apotheke um die Mitte des 15. Jahrhunderts. Beiträge zur Geschichte des Arzneimittelhandels im Mittelalter. 1. Mitteilung. **Beitr Gesch Pharm** 1982;31(14):105–7

**Goya y Lucientes, Francisco José, 1746–1828**
Bräutigam W: Die Erkrankung Goyas von 1792. **Nervenarzt** 1980 Apr;51(4):233–8
Chalat NI: Some psychologic aspects of deafness: Beethoven, Goya, and Oscar Wilde. **Am J Otol** 1980 Apr;1(4):240–6

**Goyrand, Jean-Gaspard, 1803–1869**
Charpin J: Goyrand, d'Aix, un académicien de province au XIX siècle (1803–1866). **Bull Acad Natl Med (Paris)** 1982 Jun;166(6):787–90

**Graaf, Reinier de, 1641–1673**
Roger J: Two scientific discoveries: their genesis and destiny. In M. D. Grmek, R. S. Cohen, G. Cimino, ed: On scientific discovery. The Erice Lectures 1977. Dordrecht, D. Reidel, 1981. p. 229–37. (Boston Studies in the Philosophy of Science, v. 34).

**Gradle, Harry Searls, 1883–**
Sugar HS: In appreciation of the contributions of Harry Searls Gradle. **Surv Ophthalmol** 1981 Nov–Dec;26(3):170–3

**Graefe, Albrecht von, 1828–1870**
Bahr G von: Mannen bakom Graefes symtom: dog ung, men ändå ett världsnamn inom oftalmologin. **Lakartidningen** 1984 Mar 21;81(12):1168
Fuhrmeister H: Hallesche Duplikate der Majolikareliefs vom Berliner Albrecht-von-Graefe-Denkmal. **Klin Monatsbl Augenheilkd** 1980 May;176(5):867–9
Münchow W: Albrecht von Graefe (1828–1870) in Memoriam. **Orvostort Kozl** 1979;86(24 no 4):55–64

**Graefe, Carl Ferdinand von, 1787–1840**
Hauben DJ: Carl Ferdinand von Graefe (1787–1840). **Zentralbl Chir** 1984;109(14):950–1

**Gräfenberg, Ernst, 1881–1957**
Ludwig H: Verhütung der Empfängnis--Verhängnis der Verhütung. Die Leistungen Ernst Gräfenbergs und die Reaktion der Gynäkologie seiner Zeit. **Zentralbl Gynakol** 1983;105(18):1197–205
Semm K, Giese KP: Ernst Gräfenberg, das Leben und Werk des Kieler Facharztes. Zum 100. Geburtstag am 26. September 1981. **Geburtshilfe Frauenheilkd** 1981 Jun;41(6):444–8
Semm K, Giese KP: Ernst Gräfenberg: the life and work of the specialist of Kiel on the hundredth anniversary of his birth on 26 September 1881. **Int J Fertil** 1983;28(3):141–8

**Graham, Evarts Ambrose, 1883–1957**
Ackerman LV: Dr. Evarts Graham and surgical pathology. **J Thorac Cardiovasc Surg** 1984 Nov;88(5 Pt 2):851–3
Baue AE: Landmark perspective: Evarts A. Graham and the first pneumonectomy. **JAMA** 1984 Jan 13;251(2):260–4
Breathnach CS: Biographical sketches no. 28 -- Graham. **Ir Med J** 1983 Apr;76(4):167
Brewer LA: The first pneumonectomy. Historical notes. **J Thorac Cardiovasc Surg** 1984 Nov;88(5 Pt 2):810–26
Bricker EM: Evarts A. Graham and the American College of Surgeons. **J Thorac Cardiovasc Surg** 1984 Nov;88(5 Pt 2):834–41
Butcher HR: Evarts Graham and surgical residency education. **J Thorac Cardiovasc Surg** 1984 Nov;88(5 Pt 2):848–50
Cole WH: The development of cholecystography. **J Thorac Cardiovasc Surg** 1984 Nov;88(5 Pt 2):827–33
Eckert C: Evarts A. Graham and the American Board of Surgery.

J Thorac Cardiovasc Surg 1984 Nov;88(5 Pt 2):842–7
Ferguson TB: Evarts A. Graham--the man.
**J Thorac Cardiovasc Surg** 1984 Nov;88(5 Pt 2):803–9
Longmire WP: Two great American surgeons, each with four aces. **Pharos** 1983 Summer;46(3):9–14
Olch PD: Evarts Ambrose Graham. In Dictionary of American Biography, Suppl. 6, 1956–1960. p. 245–7, 1980.
Ternberg JL: Surgical treatment of idiopathic hyperinsulinemic hypoglycemia in children. First successful subtotal pancreatectomy with preservation of spleen reported by Evarts A. Graham (1934). **J Thorac Cardiovasc Surg** 1984 Nov;88(5 Pt 2):898–901
Wynder EL: Some reflections on smoking and lung cancer. **J Thorac Cardiovasc Surg** 1984 Nov;88(5 Pt 2):854–7

**Graham, Sylvester, 1794–1851**
Edwards R: Graham-Kellogg, early American contributors to health education. **J Sch Health** 1981 Nov;51(9):589–91
Nissenbaum S: Sex, diet, and debility in Jacksonian America: Sylvester Graham and health reform. Westport, Connecticut, Greenwood, 1980. 198 p. (Contributions in Medical History, 4).

**Gram, Hans Christian Joachim, 1853–1938**
Jacobson W: Gram's discovery of his staining technique. **J Infect** 1983 Sep;7(2):97–101
Vogt HH: 100 Jahre Gram-Färbung. Ein Forschungsbeitrag aus den Anfängen dieser Zeitschrift. **Fortschr Med** 1984 Apr;102(16):94–5

**Graman, I. I.**
Al'tshular NS, Mikhaĭlov FA: Pervaia otechestvennaia dissertatsiia po tuberkulezu. **Probl Tuberk** 1983 May;(5):70–2

**Grandville, Jean-Ignace-Isidore Gérard, 1803–1847**
Moskow BS: The iconography of the dental profession. Jean-Ignace-Isidore Gérard Grandville (1803–1847). **Quintessence Int** 1984 Oct;15(10):1028–9

**Grant, David Norvell Walker, 1891–1964**
Skinner RE: The making of the air surgeon: the early life and career of David N. W. Grant. **Aviat Space Environ Med** 1983 Jan;54(1):75–82

**Grant, James Frederick, 1887–1946**
Bensley EH: James Grant: ship's surgeon on the ill-fated Empress of Ireland. **Can Med Assoc J** 1982 Feb 1;126(3):318–9

**Grant, Ulysses Simpson, 1822–1885**
Nelson RB: The final victory of General U. S. Grant. **Cancer** 1981 Feb 1;47(3):433–6

**Granville, Augustus Bozzi, 1783–1872**
Sakula A: Augustus Bozzi Granville (1783–1872): London physician-accoucheur and Italian patriot. **J R Soc Med** 1983 Oct;76(10):876–82

**Grasset, Nicole**
Manevy JV: Nicole Grasset, médecin du bout du monde. [Paris?], Balland, 1982. 245 p.

**Gratia, André, 1893–1950**
Welsch M: André Gratia, 1893–1950. In Florilège des Sciences en Belgique - II. Bruxelles, Académie Royale de Belgique, 1980. p. 663–72.

**Graves, Marvin Lee, 1867–1953**
Bowman IA, ed: The care of the insane in Texas. **Bookman** 1984 Mar–Apr;11(2):3–9

**Gray, Andrew Sexton, 1826–1907**
Lowe RF: William R. Wilde, Andrew S. Gray, and two eye and ear hospitals of very similar name. **Aust NZ J Surg** 1981 Dec;51(6):630–6

**Gray, Archibald Montague Henry, 1880–1967**
Goldsmith WN: Sir Archibald Montague Gray. In Dictionary of national biography, 1961–1970. Suppl. 8, 1981. p. 452–3.

**Gray, Louis Harold, 1905–1965**
Loutit JF: Louis Harold Gray. In Dictionary of national biography, 1961–1970. Suppl. 8, 1981. p. 453–5.

**Gréard, Octave**
Sicard A: Un doyen misogyne et un recteur féministe. **Hist Sci Med** 1982;16(1):15–20

**Greatrakes, Valentine, 1629–1683**
Arnold LJ: Valentine Greatrakes, a seventeenth-century 'touch-doctor'. **Eire Irel** 1976;11:3–12
Breathnach CS: Biographical sketches no. 32--Greatrakes. **Ir Med J** 1983 Sep;76(9):402
Kaplan BB: Greatrakes the stroker: the interpretations of his contemporaries. **ISIS** 1982 Jun;73(267):178–85
Steneck NH: Greatrakes the stroker: the interpretations of historians. **ISIS** 1982 Jun;73(267):161–77

**Green, Anne, 1528–1550**
Hughes JT: Miraculous deliverance of Anne Green: an Oxford case of resuscitation in the seventeenth century. **Br Med J [Clin Res]** 1982 Dec 18–25;285(6357):1792–3

**Green, Francis, 1742–1809**
Blakeley PR: Francis Green: 'a suffering loyalist and friend to the British government. **NS Hist Q** 1979;9(1):1–14

**Greene, Edward Lee, 1843–1915**
Greene EL: Landmarks of botanical history. Ed., F. N. Egerton, with contributions by R. P. McIntosh and R. McVaugh. 2 vols. Stanford, Stanford University Press, 1983. 1139 p. (Vol. I first published 1909)

**Greene, Graham, 1904–**
Dirckx JH: Graham Greene's doctors. **Pharos** 1983 Spring;46(2):27–9

**Greenfield, Edward J., 1875–**
Herschfeld JJ: E. J. Greenfield and artificial implants. **Bull Hist Dent** 1984;32(1):33–41

**Greenfield, William Smith, 1846–1919**
Tigertt WD: Anthrax. William Smith Greenfield, M.D., F.R.C.P., Professor Superintendent, the Brown Animal Sanatory Institution (1878–81). Concerning the priority due to him for the production of the first vaccine against anthrax. **J Hyg (Lond)** 1980 Dec;85(3):415–20

**Greenwood, Isaac, 1702–1745**
Leonard DC: Harvard's first science professor: a sketch of Isaac Greenwood's life and work. **Harv Libr Bull** 1981 Apr;29(2):135–68

**Greenwood, John, 1760–1819**
Escoe R: A new look at John Greenwood's denture for George Washington. **Bull Hist Dent** 1981;29(1):37–43

**Greg, William Rathbone, 1809–1881**
Kirsop W: W. R. Greg and Charles Darwin in Edinburgh and after: an antipodean gloss. **Trans Camb Bibliogr Soc** 1979;7(3):376–90

**Gregg, Alan, 1890–1957**
Jones JH: Alan Gregg. In Dictionary of American Biography, Suppl. 6, 1956–1960. p. 252–3, 1980.

**Gregg, Norman McAlister, 1892–1966**
Hertzberg R: Three great ophthalmologists (E. C. Temple-Smith, Norman Gregg, Arthur D'Ombrain). **Med J Aust** 1979 Dec 15;2(12):649–50

**Gregorius, Saint, Bp. of Tours, 538–594**
Janssens PA: Medico-historische gegevens uit de 'Historia Francorum' van Gregorius van Tours. **Hades** 1977;16(30):1–53

**Grekov, Ivan Ivanovich, 1867–1934**
Mirskiĭ MB: Novye dokumenty o zhizni i nauchnoĭ deiatel'nosti I. I. Grekova (1867–1941). **Sov Zdravookhr** 1981;(5):64–7

**Greppi, Enrico, 1896–**
Sicuteri F: The Enrico Greppi International Headache Award. A tribute to the memory of one of medicine's pioneers. **Cephalalgia** 1983 Mar;3(1):11–3

**Grew, Nehemiah, 1641–1712**
Hunter M: Early problems in professionalizing scientific research: Nehemiah Grew (1641–1712) and the Royal Society with an unpublished letter to Henry Oldenburg. **Notes Rec R Soc Lond** 1982 Feb;36(2):189–209

**Grey, Zane, 1872–1939**
Moore RB: Zane Grey: dentist, novelist, baseball player, outdoors man. **Tic** 1982 Jul;41(7):5–7

**Gribov, Stefan A., 1879–1957**
Konin GK: Fel'dsher-revoliutsioner S. A. Gribov. **Feldsher Akush** 1982;47(11):33–5

**Griesinger, Wilhelm, 1817–1868**
Bergener M: Gestalt-wandel in der Psychiatrie. **MMW** 1980 Jan 11;122(2):41–2

**Grigg, Emanuel Radu, 1916–1976**
Kaplan E: E.R.N. Grigg, radiologist-historian. **Semin Nucl Med** 1979 Jul;9(3):149–50

**Grigorenko, Pyotr Grigorevich, 1907–**
Reich W: The case of General Grigorenko: a psychiatric reexamination of a Soviet dissident. **Psychiatry** 1980 Nov;43(4):303–23
Reich W: The case of General Grigorenko: a second opinion. **Encounter (Lond)** 1980;54(4):9–24

**Grinda, Edouard**
Martiny M: Projet de loi présenté le 31 janvier 1923 par le député Edouard Grinda sur les assurances sociales. **Hist Sci Med** 1979;13(4):363–7

**Grinker, Roy Richard, 1900–**
Weinberg J: 'Roy R. Grinker, Sr.' Some biographical notes. **J Am Acad Psychoanal** 1980;8:441–9

**Gripouilleau, Armel-Eugène, 1821–1909**
Huard P: Armel-Eugène Gripouilleau (1821–1909) officier de santé à Montlouis (Indre-et-Loire). In: Congrès National des Sociétés Savantes, 93e, Tours, 1968. Comptes Rendus. Paris, 1971. Section des Sciences, Tome II. p. 189–92.

**Groddeck, Georg Walther, 1866–1934**
Siefert H: Sigmund Freud, Georg Groddeck und die psychosomatische Medizin. **Prax Psychother Psychosom** 1979;24:63–78
Will H: Die Geburt der Psychosomatik: Georg Groddeck, der Mensch und Wissenschaftler. München, Baltimore, Urban & Schwarzenberg, 1984. vi, 231 p.

**Gromashevskiĭ, Lev Vasil'evich, 1887–**
Beliakov VD: Uchenie L. V. Gromashevskogo ob épidemicheskom protsesse i razvitie étogo ucheniia na sovremennom étape. **Zh Mikrobiol Epidemiol Immunobiol** 1984 Jul;(7):115–8
Elkin II: Nauchnyĭ podvig L. A. Gromashevskogo. **Zh Mikrobiol Epidemiol Immunobiol** 1982 Jan;(1):113–7
Favorova LA: Uchenie L. V. Gromashevskogo i problema likvidatsii infekstionnykh bolezneĭ. **Zh Mikrobiol Epidemiol Immunobiol** 1984 Jul;(7):119–23

**Gross, Robert Edward, 1905–**
Allen R: The evolution of pediatric surgery. **J Pediatr Surg** 1980 Dec;15(6):711–8

**Gross, Samuel David, 1805–1884**
Wagner FB: Revisit of Samuel D. Gross, M.D. **Surg Gynecol Obstet** 1981 May;152(5):663–74

**Grosseteste, Robert, 1175?–1253**
McEvoy J: The chronology of Robert Grosseteste's writings on nature and natural philosophy. **Speculum** 1983 July;58(3):614–55

**Grossman, Louis Irving, 1901–**
A tribute to Louis I. Grossman: **J Endod** 1982 Jan;8(Spec issue):S1–48

**Grossman, Morton Irving, 1919–**
Boyle JD: Morton I. Grossman, M.D., Ph.D.: an oral history. **Gastroenterology** 1982 Jul;83(1 Pt 2):285–324

**Grot-Rowecki, Stefan, 1895–1944**
Rudowski W: Ostatnia choroba Generała Stefana Grota-Roweckiego (1895–1944). **Arch Hist Med (Warsz)** 1983;46(4):487–502

**Grotjahn, Alfred, 1869–1931**
Bílek V, Niklíček L: Dílo Alfreda Grotjahna a jeho vliv na vývoj sociálního lékařství v Cechách. Cást I. **Cesk Zdrav** 1982 Apr;30(4):145–56
Dahm I, Schorr R, Niehoff JU: Zum 50. Todestag von Alfred Grotjahn. **Z Arztl Fortbild (Jena)** 1981 Sep 15;75(16):878–81
Labisch A: Alfred Grotjahn (1869–1931) und das gesundheitspolitische Programm der Mehrheitssozialdemokraten von 1922. **MMG** 1983;8:192–7

**Groves, Ernest William Hey, 1872–1944**
Brahma B, Singh M: The man behind the name: Ernest William Hey Groves 1872–1944. **NATNEWS** 1982 Jun;19(6):26
Ratliff AH: Ernest William Hey Groves and his contributions to orthopaedic surgery. **Ann R Coll Surg Engl** 1983 May;65(3):203–6
Ratliff AH: Ernest William Hey Groves and his contributions to orthopaedic surgery. **Bristol Med Chir J** 1983 Jul;98(367):98–103

**Gruby, David, 1810–1898**
Csillag I: David Gruby. **Orvostort Kozl** 1982;28(1–3):177–86

**Gruenfelder, Benno, 1883–1955**
Winter ST, Ginott N: Two pioneer paediatricians in Palestine under the Turks. **Adler Mus Bull** 1983 Nov;Spec issue:58–61

**Grünbaum, Adolf, 1923–**
Cohen RS, Laudan L, ed: Physics, philosophy and psychoanalysis. Essays in honor of Adolf Grünbaum. Dordrecht, D. Reidel, 1983. xviii, 339 p. (Boston Studies in the Philosophy of Science, v. 76).

**Grundy, John Hull**
John Hull Grundy, artist and entomologist: **J Audiov Media Med** 1983 Jan;6(1):17–20

**Grüneberg, Hans, 1907–1982**
Lewis D, Hunt DM: Hans Grüneberg: 26 May 1907–23 October 1982. **Biogr Mem Fellows R Soc** 1984;30:227–47

**Grüneberg, Theodor, 1901–**
Kleine-Natrop HE: Theodor Grüneberg in der Tradition der halleschen Dermatologie. **Dermatol Monatsschr** 1981 Jun;167(6):393–5

**Grünewald, Mathias, d. 1528**
Kierulf H: L'ergotisme chez Bosch et Grünewald. **Nouv Presse Med** 1982 Oct 2;11(38):2803–9
Kierulf H: L'ergotisme chez Bosch et Grünewald. In International Congress of the History of Medicine, 27th, Barcelona, 1980. Actas. Barcelona, Académia de Ciències Médiques de Catalunya i Balears, 1981. p. 81–90.

**Grütz, Otto Julius, 1886–1963**
Schulz EA: Otto Julius Grütz, Leben und Lebenswerk. Diss. Bonn, 1982. 107 p.

**Gudden, Johann Bernhard Aloys von, 1824–1886**
Sărmăşanu-Cortez ML, Cortez P: Bernhard von Gudden şi drama de la lacul Starnberg (1824–1886). **Rev Med Interna [Neurol Psihiatr]** 1983 Jul–Sep;28(3):233–8

**Guérin, Alphonse François Marie, 1816–1875**
Les pansements à la ouate de M. Alphonse Guérin: **Union Med Can** 1981 May;110(5):464

**Guerin, Camille, 1872–1961**
Sakula A: BCG: who were Calmette and Guérin? **Thorax** 1983 Nov;38(11):806–12

**Guerin, Jules, 1801–1886**
Peltier LF: Guerin versus Malgaigne: a precedent for the free criticism of scientific papers. **J Orthop Res** 1983;1(1):115–8

**Guerrero Fernández, J.**
Folch Jou G, Muñoz Calvo S: Un intento de reforma legislativa en la Farmacia Española del siglo XIX: J. Guerrero Fernández y su 'Proyecto de Servicio Farmacéutico'. **Bol Soc Esp Hist Farm** 1980/81 Dec–Mar;31–32(124–5):299–314

**Guesde, Jules, 1845–1922**
Gani L: Jules Guesde, Paul Lafargue et les problèmes de population. **Population** 1979;34(4):1023–1044

**Guggenheim, Markus, 1885–1970**
Klingler M: A glimpse into Roche research: antiparkinson treatment. **Int J Clin Pharmacol Ther Toxicol** 1982 Apr;20(4):190–3

**Guillemin, Roger Charles Louis, 1924–**
Wade N: The Nobel duel. Two scientists' 21-year race to win the world's most coveted research prize. Garden City, Anchor Press/Doubleday, 1981. 321 p.

**Guillerey, Joseph, 1871–1942?**
Fankhauser R: Joseph Guillerey, Porrentruy: premier Dr méd. vét. suisse. Un jubilé passé inaperçu. **Schweiz Arch Tierheilkd** 1983 Dec;125(12):871–5

**Guinefort, Saint**
Schmitt JC: The holy greyhound: Guinefort, healer of children since the thirteenth century. Cambridge, Cambridge University Press; Paris, Editions de la Maison des Sciences de l'Homme, 1983. 215 p. Translation of Le saint lévrier: Guinefort, guérisseur d'enfants depuis le XIIIe siècle, Paris, 1979.

**Guinto, Ricardo S., 1907–1983**
Binford CH, Reich CV: Ricardo S. Guinto, M.D., M.P.H., epidemiologist-leprologist, 1907–1983. In appreciation of 50 years dedicated to research in leprosy. **Int J Lepr** 1983 Dec;51(4):587–91

**Guislain, Joseph, 1797–1860**
Thiry U: Le professeur Joseph Guislain (1797–1860), apôtre des aliénés. **Cah Biloque** 1980;30:35–40

**Gulácsy, Lajos Kálmán, 1882–1932**
Gerevich J: Gulácsy Lajos festömüvész akut pszichózisa (adalék heveny téboly genezisének kérdéséhez). **Orv Hetil** 1981 May 3;122(18):1083–6
Ungvári G: Ujabb adatok Gulácsy Lajos betegségéhez. **Orvostort Kozl** 1982;92(4):113–8

**Gully, James Manby, 1808–1883**
Swinton WE: The hydrotherapy and infamy of Dr. James Gully. **Can Med Assoc J** 1980 Dec 20;123(12):1262–4

**Gumpert, Martin, 1897–1955**
Gumpert M: Hölle im Paradies. Selbstdarstellung eines Arztes. Hildesheim, Gerstenberg, 1983. xxiii, 280 p. (Exilliteratur, Band 17) Reprint of 1939 ed., with new biographical forward by F. Trapp.

**Gunn, John C.**
Dermott R: 'A great black book': East of Eden and Gunn's New family physician. **Am Stud** 1981;22(2):41–57

**Guntrip, Henry James Samuel**
Sutherland JD: The British object relations theorists: Balint, Winnicott, Fairbairn, Guntrip. **J Am Psychoanal Assoc** 1980;28(4):829–60

**Gurney, Ivor, 1890–1937**
Trethowan WH: Ivor Gurney's mental illness. **Music Lett** 1981;62(3–4):300–9

**Gusberg, Saul B., 1913–**
Reproductive immunology. A festschrift in honor of Dr. Saul B. Gusberg.: **Mt Sinai J Med (NY)** 1980 Sep–Oct;47(5):i–vii, 427–560

**Gustek, Marian**
Sikorski J, Kłodiński S: Mjr dr Marian Gustek. **Przegl Lek** 1981;38(1):182–4

**Guthrie, Charles Claude, 1880–1963**
Stephenson HE: Charles Claude Guthrie's contribution to cardiac resuscitation. **Crit Care Med** 1981 May;9(5):428–9

**Guthrie, Douglas James, 1885–1975**
Poynter N: Douglas James Guthrie, M.D., D. Litt., F.R.C.S.E., F.R.C.P.E., F.R.S.E., 8 September 1885 - 8 June 1975. **Med Hist** 1975 Oct;19(4):400–1

**Guthrie, Edwin Ray, Jr., 1886–1959**
Ross B: Edwin Ray Guthrie, Jr. In Dictionary of American Biography, Suppl. 6, 1956–1960. p. 261–3, 1980.

**Gutman, Alexander B., 1902–1973**
Sproul EE: Acid phosphatase and prostate cancer: historical overview. **Prostate** 1980;1(4):411–3

**Gutschy, Ljudevit, 1874–1961**
Tomić-Karović K: Ljudevit Gutschy. In: I simpozij o historiji mikrobiologije i imunologije u Hrvatskoj do 1923. godine. Zagreb, Jugoslavenskoj akademiji, 1973. p. 107–17.

**Gütt, Arthur, 1891–**
Labisch A, Tennstedt F: 50 Jahre Gesetz über Vereinheitlichung des Gesundheitswesens. Dr. med. Arthur Gütt und die Gründung des öffentlichen Gesundheitsdienstes. **Off Gesundheitswes** 1984

Jul;46(7):291-8

**Guttmann, Ludwig, 1899-**
Harris P, Ross JC, et al: [Ludwig Guttmann - special issue]. **Paraplegia** 1979 May;17(1): passim

**Gutzmann, Hermann, 1865-1922**
Wendler J, ed: 75 Jahre Phoniatrie. Festschrift zu Ehren von Hermann Gutzmann sen. Berlin. Humboldt Universität, 1980. 240 p.

**Guy de Chauliac, ca. 1300-ca. 1368**
Amalric P: L'influence de Guy de Chauliac à Toulouse au XVIIe siècle. A propos d'un petit livre inédit. **Bull Soc Ophtalmol Fr** 1980 Jun-Jul;80(6-7):617-8
Barcia Goyanes JJ: Los albores del lenguaje anatómico en las lenguas neolatinos. La traduccion del Inventarium de Guy de Chauliac por Bernat de Casaldovol. **Med Esp** 1980;79:235-49
Wallner B: The Middle English translation of Guy de Chauliac's Treatise on ulcers. Part II. Notes, glossary, marginalia. Book IV of the Great surgery. Edited from Ms. New York Academy of Medicine 12 and related mss. Stockholm, Almqvist & Wiksell International, 1983. 48 p. (Acta Universitatis Lundensis, Sectio I Theologica Juridica Humaniora 44).

**Guyon, René, 1876-1963**
Haeberle EJ: Human rights and sexual rights. The legacy of René Guyon. **Med Law** 1983;2(2):159-72

**Gyger, Ulrich, fl. 1527**
Blaser RH: Ulrich Gyger, sin diener. Versuch einer biographischen Rekonstruktion. **Medizinhist J** 1981;16(1-2):53-66

**Gysi, Alfred, 1865-1957**
Jackle P, Nittenwilm U, Steffens G, et al: Alfred Gysi--ein Pionier der Zahnheilkunde und Zahntechnik. **Dent Labor (Muench)** 1982 Aug;30(8):1153-61
Tanzer G: Professor Dr. Alfred Gysi (1865-1957). **Zahnarzt** 1984 Jun;28(6):447-9

# H

**Haartman, Johan, 1725-1787**
Achté K, Turunen S: Den första psykiatriska artikeln i Finland. **Dan Medicinhist Arbog** 1983;12:74-81

**Haas, Georg, 1886-1971**
Weise M: Experimental and clinical aspects of proteinuria. Introduction. **Contrib Nephrol** 1981;24:VI-IX

**Haass, Friedrich Joseph, 1780-1853**
Kopelev L: Der heilige Doktor Fjodor Petrowitsch: die Geschichte des Friedrich Joseph Haass, Bad Münstereifel 1780-Moskau 1853. 2. Aufl. Hamburg, Hoffmann und Campe, 1984. 231 p.
Müller-Dietz H: Friedrich Joseph Haass als Arzt in Moskau: biographische Skizzen. Berlin, Osteuropa-Institut, 1980. 133 p.
Müller-Dietz HE: Friedrich Joseph Haass, ein deutscher Arzt in Moskau. **Clio Med** 1981 Apr;15(3-4):177-89

**Haberle, Károly, 1764-1832**
Kapronczay K: Haberle Károly (1764-1832) emlékezete. **Orv Hetil** 1982 Nov 14;123(46):2860-1

**Habsburg Family**
Calatrava Páramo L: La llamada enfermedad de los Habsburgo: datos históricos, su tratamiento actual y resultados. **An R Acad Nac Med (Madr)** 1979;96(4):557-74
Loevy HT, Kowitz A: The Habsburgs and the 'Habsburg Jaw'. **Bull Hist Dent** 1982 Apr;30(1):19-23
Lontainé SZ, Susa E, Varga T: A Habsburgok József nádori ágához tartozók vércsoportvizsgálata. **Morphol Igazsagugyi Orv Sz** 1980 Oct;20(4):275-81
Snorrason E: Den Habsburgske underkaebe. **Tandlaegebladet** 1982 May;86(8):277-80

**Hackl, Eduard, 1841-1913**
Slavětínský M: Připomínka prukopníka zestátněnú veřejného zdravotnictví z Moravy na sklonku minulého století. **Cesk Zdrav** 1980 May;28(5):219-20

**Hackmann, Christian Jakob, 1899-1981**
Schubert GE: Christian Jakob Hackmann. **Verh Dtsch Ges Pathol** 1982;66:640-4

**Haddad, Sami I., 1890-1957**
Haddad FS: Arabic medical manuscripts in the Sami I Haddad Memorial Library. **Clio Med** 1981 Dec;16(2/3):123-7
Haddad FS: Arab medical manuscripts in the Sami I. Haddad memorial library. In International Congress of the History of Medicine, 27th, Barcelona, 1980. Actas. Barcelona, Académia de Ciències Médiques de Catalunya i Balears, 1981. p. 253-8.

**Haderup, Victor Frants Nachtegall, 1845-1913**
Pindborg JJ: Victor Haderup. **Tandlaegebladet** 1984 Jun;88(11):411-6

**Hadley, Frederick August, 1873-1961**
Fleming DW: The founders of the college: Western Australia. **Aust NZ J Surg** 1981 Dec;51(6):623-4

**Hadrian, Emperor, 76-138**
Petrakis NL: Diagonal earlobe creases, type A behavior and the death of Emperor Hadrian. **West J Med** 1980 Jan;132(1):87-91

**Hadzi-Nikolic, Nicola, 1855-1915**
Berić B, Rajković D, Babić-Ilić N: Dr Nikola Hadži-Nikolić (1855-1915) prvi akušer-ginekolog u Srbiji i Njegov značaj za razvoj akušerstva i ginekologije u Srbiji. **Jugosl Ginekol Opstet** 1981 Dec;21(5-6):143-8

**Haeckel, Ernst Heinrich Philipp August, 1834-1919**
Bellinazzi P: Panpsichismo e psicologia nel pensiero di Ernst H. Haeckel. **Stor Crit Psicol** 1982 Dec;3(2):281-99
Dose K: Ernst Haeckel's concept of an evolutionary origin of life. **Biosystems** 1981;13(4):253-8
Engelhardt D von: Polemik und Kontroversen um Haeckel. **Medizinhist J** 1980;15(3):284-304
Engelhardt DV: Virchow et Haeckel et la liberté de la science. In Poirier J, Poirier JL, ed: Médecine et philosophie à la fin du XIXe siècle. Paris, Université de Paris XII - Val de Marne, [1980?]. p. 117-25.
Mann G: Ernst Haeckel und der Darwinismus: Popularisierung, Propaganda und Ideologisierung. **Medizinhist J** 1980;15(3):269-83
Mollenhauer D: Die Haeckel-Rezeption durch die Botanik. **Medizinhist J** 1980;15(3):305-36
Oppenheimer JM: Ernst Heinrich Haeckel as an intermediary in the transmutation of an idea. **Proc Am Philos Soc** 1982;126(5):347-55
Rinard RG: The problem of the organic individual: Ernst Haeckel and the development of the biogenetic law. **J Hist Biol** 1981 Fall;14(2):249-76
Szyfman L: Les prétendues falsifications d'Ernst Haeckel et son triomphe sur ses diffamateurs. **Bull Biol Fr Belg** 1980;113(4):375-406
Uschmann G: Haeckel's biological materialism. **Hist Philos Life Sci** 1979;1(1):101-18
Winau R: Ernst Haeckels Vorstellungen von Wert und Werden menschlicher Rassen und Kulturen. **Medizinhist J** 1981;16(3):270-79

**Haffkine, Waldemar Mordecai Wolff, 1860-1930**
Bornside GH: Waldemar Haffkine's cholera vaccines and the Ferran-Haffkine priority dispute. **J Hist Med Allied Sci** 1982 Oct;37(4):399-422
Lutzker E: Some unanswered questions in medical history. In: Congrès international d'histoire de la médecine, XXVe, Québec, 1976. Actes. Québec, 1977. p. 917-27.
Lutzker E, Jochnowitz C: The curious history of Waldemar Haffkine. **Commentary** 1980;69(6):61-4
Lutzker E: Cameron prizewinner: Waldemar M. Haffkine, C.I.E. **Clio Med** 1971 May;13(3-4):269-76
Lutzker E: From Malkowal to Calcutta: an historical appreciation of Haffkine's victorious struggle. In: Science and history: studies in honor of Edward Rosen. (Studia Copernicana, XVI.) Wrocław, Ossolineum, 1978. p. 543-53.
Lutzker E: From Malkowal to Calcutta: an historical appreciation of Haffkine's victorious struggle. **Adler Mus Bull** 1981;7(1):14-8

**Hagedorn, Hans Christian, 1888-1971**
Felig P: Landmark perspective: Protamine insulin. Hagedorn's pioneering contribution to drug delivery in the management of diabetes. **JAMA** 1984 Jan 20;251(3):393-6

**Hagedorn, Werner, 1831-1894**
Neumann A, Heinrich P: Die Bedeutung des Magdeburger Chirurgen Werner Hagedorn (1831 bis 1894) für die Einführung der Antiseptik auf dem europäischen Kontinent. **Zentralbl Chir** 1982;107(11):617-20

**Hagen, Johann Philipp, 1734-1792**
Hofmann-Meier B: Ein Geburtshelfer und Hebammenlehrer des 18. Jahrhunderts. Leben und Werk des Johann Philipp Hagen (1734-1792), Hebammenlehrer und Professor für Entbindungskunst in Berlin. Diss. Bern, 1982. 75 p.

**Haggard, Henry Rider, 1856-1925**
Thomson WA: Rider Haggard and smallpox. **J R Soc Med** 1984 Jun;77(6):506-12

**Hagström, Anders Johan, 1753-1830**
Arenander E: Kirurgi under föranestetisk tid--ur anteckningar efter Anders Johan Hagströms Operations Collegium. **Nord Medicinhist Arsb** 1981;:88-105

**Hahnemann, Christian Friedrich Samuel, 1755-1843**
Barthel I: Arzneimittelversuche des 19.Jahrhunderts am gesunden Menschen im deutschsprachigen Raum. Diss., Universität Düsseldorf. Düsseldorf, 1982. 105 p.
Cook TM: Samuel Hahnemann. The founder of homoeopathic medicine. Wellingborough, Northamptonshire, Thorsons, 1981. 192 p.
Fritsche H: Samuel Hahnemann: Idee und Wirklichkeit der Homöopathie. Göttingen, Verlag für homöopathische Literatur, 1982. 366 p.
Habacher M: Homöopathische Fernbehandlung durch Samuel Hahnemann. **Medizinhist J** 1980;15(4):385-91
Lozowski J: Homeopatia (Samuela Hahnemanna). **Pieleg Polozna** 1982;4-5:16-7
Schwanitz HJ: Homöopathie und Brownianismus 1795-1844. Zwei wissenschaftstheoretische Fallstudien aus der praktischen Medizin. Stuttgart Fischer, 1983. 202 p. (Medizin in Geschichte und Kultur, 15).

**Hai-Thuong**
Huard P, Durand M: Un traité de médecine sino-vietnamienne du XVIIIe siècle: La compréhension intuitive des recettes médicales de Hai-Thuong. **Sci Orient** 1976;:1-24

**Haindorf, Alexander, 1782-1862**
Wunderlich G: Kranheits- und Therapiekonzepte am Anfang der deutschen Psychiatrie (Haindorf, Heinroth, Ideler). Husum, Matthiesen, 1981. 132 p. (Abhandlungen zur Geschichte der Medizin und der Naturwissenschaften, 41).

**Hájek, Tadeás, 1525-1600**
Müller-Jahncke WD: Kleiner Beitrag zum Prioritätenstreit um die Metoposkopie: Hájek contra Cardano. **Sudhoffs Arch** 1982;66(1):79-84

**Halász, Géza, 1816-1888**
Kerekes L: In memoriam Halász Géza (1816-1888). **Orvostort Kozl** 1979;86(24 no 4):113-22

**Halban, Joseph, 1870-1937**
Simmer HH: Innere Sekretion der Ovarien als Ursache der Menstruation. Halbans Falsifikation der Pflügerschen Hypothese. In Ganzinger K, Skopec M, Wyklicky H, ed: Festschrift für Erna Lesky zum 70. Geburtstag. Wien, Brüder Hollinek, 1981. p. 123-48.
Weinzierl S: Frühe Rezeption der Halbanschen Hypothese von der endokrinen Verursachung der Menstruation. Diss. Erlangen-Nürnberg, 1980. 59 p.

**Haldane, John Burdon Sanderson, 1892-1964**
Smith JM: John Burdon Sanderson Haldane. In Dictionary of national biography, 1961-1970. Suppl. 8, 1981. p. 473-5.

**Hálek, Vítězslav, 1835-1874**
Mečíř J: Vítězslav Hálek a jeho obec pomatených. **Cesk Psychiatr** 1983 Feb;79(1):60-3

**Hales, Stephen, 1677-1761**
Earle DP: An eighteenth century suggestion for peritoneal dialysis? **Int J Artif Organs** 1980 Mar;3(2):67-8
Roth N: Hales's hydraulics: measuring blood pressure, 1706. **Med Instrum** 1981 Jan-Feb;15(1):66-7
West JB: Stephen Hales: neglected respiratory physiologist. **J Appl Physiol** 1984 Sep;57(3):635-9
Wilber JA: The founding of Georgia and the discovery of blood pressure. **J Med Assoc Ga** 1981 May;70(5):333

**Haljecka, Eva, 18??-1947**
Berić BM: Dr Eva Haljecka (18??-1947) prva žena akušer-ginekolog u jugoslovenskim zemljama. **Jugosl Ginekol Opstet** 1983 May-Aug;23(3-4):95-9

**Hall, Granville Stanley, 1844-1924**
Averill LA: Recollections of Clark's G. Stanley Hall. **J Hist Behav Sci** 1982 Oct;18(4):341-6
Cole TR: The prophecy of Senescence: G. Stanley Hall and the reconstruction of old age in America. **Gerontologist** 1984 Aug;24(4):360-6

**Hall, Herbert James, 1870-1923**
Hercher GP: The work cure at Devereux Mansion. **Essex Inst Hist Collect** 1980;116(2):101-10

**Hall, John, fl. 1779**
The male midwife.: **Bygone Kent** 1980;1(9):532

**Hall, John Marshall, 1790-1857**
Heywood C: D. H. Lawrence's 'blood consciousness' and the work of Xavier Bichat and Marshall Hall. **Etud Anglaises** 1979;32:397-413
Leys R: Background to the reflex controversy: William Alison and the doctrine of sympathy before Hall. **Stud Hist Biol** 1980;4:1-66
Manuel DE: Marshall Hall, F.R.S. (1790-1857); a conspectus of his life and work. **Notes Rec R Soc Lond** 1980 Dec;35(2):135-66

**Hall, John, 1575-1635**
Richardson RG: Dr. John Hall, Shakespeare's son-in-law. A vignette of Elizabethan medicine. **Practitioner** 1981 Apr;225(1354):593-5

**Hall, Joseph, 1574-1656**
Dallett JB: Paracelsus in Moronia. Bischof Joseph Halls satirische Darstellung von 'Bustius Hohenheimius' und dessen Collegium. Wien, 1976. 20 p. (Salzburger Beiträge zur Paracelsusforschung, 14).

**Hall, Rosetta Sherwood, 1865-1951**
Phillips CJ: Rosetta Sherwood Hall. In: Notable American women. The modern period. Cambridge, Mass., Belknap-Harvard Univ. Press, 1980. 4:299-301.

**Haller, Albin, 1849-1925**
Labrude P: Albin Haller 1849-1925 pharmacien et chimiste. **Rev Hist Pharm (Paris)** 1982 Sep;29(254):207-9

**Haller, Albrecht von, 1708-1777**
Albrecht von Haller, 1708-1777: Zehn Vorträge gehalten am Berner Haller-Symposion vom 6. bis 8. Oktober 1977. Basel, Birkhäuser, 1978. x, 182 p. With contributions by M. Stettler, K. S. Guthke, U. Im Hof, N. Mani, L. Premuda, H. Zoller, R. Toellner, A. Lindt, W. Zimmerli, W. Killy.
Boschung U: Ein Brief Albrecht Hallers über seinen Aufenthalt in Paris und Strassburg (1728). **Physis** 1977;19(1-4):185-96
Duchesneau F: La théorie physiologique de Haller: irritabilité et sensibilité. **Arch Int Hist Idees** 1982;95:141-70
Guthke KS: Haller im Halblicht. Vier Studien. Bern, München, Francke, 1981. 72 p. (Sonderdruck aus Das Abenteuer der Literatur).
Haller alla 'Charité' con Ledran: **Dent Cadmos** 1979 Feb 2;47(2):54-6
Libri e manoscritti di Haller, 1777-1977: Nel II centenario della morte di Albrecht von Haller. Milano, Biblioteca Nazionale Braidense, 1977. 69 p.
Lindeboom GA, ed: Haller in Holland: het dagboek van Albrecht von Haller van zijn verblijf in Holland (1725-1727). Amsterdam, Rodopi, 1979. 122 p.
Mazzolini RG: Sugli studi embriologici di Albrecht von Haller negli anni 1755-1758. **Ann Ist Stor Italo-Ger** 1977;3:183-242
Müller C: Un drame dans la famille d'Albrecht de Haller. **Gesnerus** 1984;41(1/2):133-6
Roe SA: Matter, life, and generation. Eighteenth-century embryology and the Haller-Wolff debate. Cambridge, Cambridge University Press, 1981. 214 p.
Roe SA, ed: The natural philosophy of Albrecht von Haller. New York, Arno, 1981. Various pagings. Reprint of works published 1750-1936.
Schiller J: Les traductions en français des ouvrages scientifiques de Haller. In: Congrès National des Sociétés Savantes, 91e, Rennes, 1966. Comptes Rendus. Paris, 1967. Section des Sciences, Tome 1. p. 241-5.
Schmid-Schönbein H: Die Ursprünge der medizinischen Hämorheologie im 18. Jahrhundert: H. Boerhaave, A. v. Haller und G. van Swieten. **Vasa** 1984;Suppl 12:10-31
Toellner R: Decora Merenti. Glory, merit and science. Haller spellbound by the Newtonian star. **Janus** 1980;67(1-2-3):171-85
Toellner R: Die Bedeutung des physico-theologischen Gottesbeweises für die nachcartesianische Physiologie im 18. Jahrhundert. **Ber Wissenschaftsgesch** 1982;5:75-82

**Haller, Albrecht von, 1758-1823**
Vidal F: La discontinuité de la douleur chez les physiologistes du XVIIIe siècle. **Inf Dent** 1983 Dec 8;65(43):4243-8

**Haller, Karl Johann von, 1749-1781**
Müller C: Un drame dans la famille d'Albrecht de Haller. **Gesnerus** 1984;41(1/2):133-6

**Halliburton, William Dobinson, 1860-1931**
Morgan N: William Dobinson Halliburton, F.R.S. (1860-1931) - pioneer of British biochemistry? **Notes Rec R Soc Lond** 1983 Aug;38(1):129-45

**Hallpike, Charles Skinner, 1900-1979**
Whitteridge D, Merton PA: Charles Skinner Hallpike: 19 July 1900-26 September 1979. **Biogr Mem Fellows R Soc** 1984;30:283-95

**Halpert, Bela, 1896-**
Sparkman RS: 100th anniversary of the first cholecystectomy. **Arch Surg** 1982 Dec;117(12):1525
Török B: Langenbuch és Halpert Béla. Az elsö cholecytektómia centenáriumára. **Orv Hetil** 1983 Jun 26;124(26):1577-81

**Halsted, Caroline Hampton, 1861-1922**
King WH: Caroline Hampton Halsted and her family, revisited. **NC Med J** 1982 Jul;43(7):501-4
Paquet JB: The gloving of a nurse (Caroline Hampton). **Nurs Success Today** 1984 Summer;1(2):44

**Halsted, William Stewart, 1852-1922**
Bland CS: The Halsted mastectomy: present illness and past history. **West J Med** 1981 Jun;134(6):549-55
Colp R Jr: Notes on Dr. William S. Halsted. **Bull NY Acad Med** 1984 Nov;60(9):876-87
Graner JL, Frederick W: William Halsted's cocaine habit. **Arch Ophthalmol** 1984 Dec;102(12):1746
Harvey AM: The influence of William Stewart Halsted's concepts of surgical training. **Johns Hopkins Med J** 1981 May;148(5):215-36
King WH: Caroline Hampton Halsted and her family, revisited. **NC Med J** 1982 Jul;43(7):501-4
Read RD: Marcy's priority in the development of inguinal herniorrphaphy. **Surgery** 1980 Nov;88(5):682-5
Rutkow IM: William Halsted and Rudolph Matas: their unique alliance. **Surgery** 1980 May;87(5):524-38
Rutkow IM: The letters of William Halsted and Anton von Eiselsberg: a very special friendship. **Arch Surg** 1980 Aug;115(8):993-1001
Rutkow IM: The letters of William Halsted and Alexis Carrel. **Surg Gynecol Obstet** 1980 Nov;151(5):676-88
Rutkow IM, Rutkow BG, Ernst CB: Letters of William Halsted and René Leriche: 'Our friendship seems so deep'. **Surgery** 1980 Dec;88(6):806-25

**Halter, Samuel, 1916-1981**
Dhoore L, Halter S: Secretaris-generaal van het Ministerie van Volksgezondheid en van het Gezin, Prof. Dr. S. Halter. **Arch Belg Med Soc** 1981 Jul;39(7)Suppl:1-64
Prof. Dr S. Halter (1916-1981): **Arch Belg** 1984;42(7-8):349-89

**Ham, Thomas Hale, 1905-**
Herbert V: Landmark perspective: An 'extrinsic factor' and pernicious anemia. **JAMA** 1984 Jan 27;251(4):522-3

**Hamarneh, Sami, 1925-**
Anees MA: History of Islamic medicine and pharmacy: contribution

of Sami Hamarneh. **Hamdard** 1983 Apr-Jun;26(2):67-75

**Hamburger, Jenö, 1883-1936**
Kárpáti E: Emlékezés Hamburger Jenöre (1883-1936). **Orv Hetil** 1983 Dec 11;124(50):3063-6

**Hameau, Jean, 1779-1851**
Théodoridès J: Un précurseur girondin de la pathologie infectieuse: Jean Hameau (1779-1851). In: Congrès National des Sociétés Savantes, 104e, Bordeaux, 1979. Comptes Rendus. Paris, 1979. Section des Sciences, Fasc. IV. p. 81-95.

**Hamilton, Alice, 1869-1970**
Freudenberg N: Alice Hamilton 1869-1970. **Women Health** 1976 Sep-Oct;1(5):1-2
Sicherman B: Alice Hamilton. In: Notable American women. The modern period. Cambridge, Mass., Belknap-Harvard Univ. Press, 1980. 4:303-6.

**Hamilton, Frank Hastings, 1813-1886**
Jones OP: A peripatetic surgery in Valhalla (Frank Hastings Hamilton). **Am J Surg** 1982 Mar;143(3):370-3

**Hammond Family**
Bleser C, ed: The Hammonds of Redcliffe. New York, Oxford, Oxford University Press, 1981. xxii, 421 p.

**Hammond, William Alexander, 1828-1900**
Blustein BE: A New York medical man: William Alexander Hammond, M.D. (1828-1900), Neurologist. Ph.D. Diss. University of Pennsylvania. Philadelphia, 1979. 418 leaves.
Zeidenfelt A: Surgeon General William Hammond. **Civ War Times Illus** 1978;17(6):24-32

**Hanaoka, Seishu, 1760-1835**
Matsushita A: [Recent findings in the history of anesthesiology (9); practice of the anesthetic method developed by Seishu Hanaoka] (Jpn). **Masui** 1980 Aug;29(8):828-30

**Hàndel, Georg Friedrich, 1685-1759**
Keynes M: Handel's illnesses. **Lancet** 1980 Dec 20-27;2(8208-8209):1354-5

**Händel, Georg, 1622-1697**
Vértes L: Georg Händel (Händel apja, a 'hallei chirurgus'). **Orv Hetil** 1980 Apr 6;121(14):851-3

**Handler, Philip, 1917-1981**
Jukes TH: Philip Handler (1917-1981). A biographical sketch. **J Nutr** 1983 Jun;113(6):1086-94

**Hann, Fanny, fl. 1918**
Honti J, Szám I: A budapesti Hann Fanny és a Hann syndroma (tranzitoricus diabetes insipidus). **Orv Hetil** 1984 Jun 24;125(26):1581-2

**Hannah, Jason Albert, 1889-1977**
Paterson GR: The Hannah Institute: promoting Canadian history of medicine. **Can Med Assoc J** 1983 Jun 1;128(11):1325-8

**Hannibal, 247?-183 B.C.**
Dirckx JH: Hannibal's ophthalmia. **Pharos** 1983 Fall;46(4):28-30

**Hansel, French Keller, 1893-**
Shambaugh GE: French Keller Hansel and the history of allergy. **Arch Otolaryngol** 1983 Feb;109(2):126-9

**Hansen, Gerhard Henrik Armauer, 1841-1912**
Hansen GA, Watt FB, ed: The memories and reflections of Dr. G. Armauer Hansen. Würzburg, German Leprosy Relief Association, 1976. 135 p.
Harboe M: The work and concepts of Armauer Hansen: how do they stand today? **Ethiop Med J** 1983 Apr;21(2):123-6
Irgens LM: The discovery of Mycobacterium leprae. A medical achievement in the light of evolving scientific methods. **Am J Dermatopathol** 1984 Aug;6(4):337-43

**Hardenberg, Friedrich Leopold von, 1772-1801**
Henkelmann T: Die Struktur des Lebendigen. Die Fragmente zur Physiologie von Novalis. In Seidler E, Schott H, ed: Bausteine zur Medizingeschichte. Stuttgart, Steiner, 1984. p. 45-52.
Schipperges H: Krankwerden und Gesundsein bei Novalis. **Dtsch Vierteljahresschr Lit Wiss Geistesgesch** 1978;226-42
Sohni H: Die Medizin der Frühromantik. Novalis' Bedeutung für den versuch einer Umwertung der 'Romantischen Medizin.' Freiburg, Schulz, 1973. 270 p. (Freiburger Forschungen zur Medizingeschichte, Neue Folge, 2).

**Harder, Johann Jacob, 1656-1711**
Portmann ML: Der Basler Medizinprofessor Johann Jacob Harder (1656-1711) als Geburtshelfer. **Gesnerus** 1983;40(1-2):139-47

**Hardy, Jules 1932-**
Molino-Negro P: Jules Hardy M.D. **Surg Neurol** 1984 Aug;22(2):109-12

**Hare, William**
Douglas H: Burke and Hare. **Br Hist Illus** 1978-79;5(5):32-43

**Hári, Pál, 1869-1933**
Székács I: Hári Pál emléke (1869-1933). **Orv Hetil** 1983 Jul 31;124(31):1889-94

**Harington, John, 1561-1612**
Nelson TG: Death, dung, the devil, and worldly delights: a metaphysical conceit in Harington, Donne, and Herbert. **Stud Philol** 1979 Summer;76(3):272-87

**Al-Harizi, Judah b. Solomon, b. ca. 1170**
Kottek S: Medicine in Hebrew poetry: Judah al-Harizi. **Koroth** 1983 Aug;8(7-8):299-304

**Harless, Johann Christian Friedrich, 1773-1853**
Triebel-Schubert C: Die Anfänge der Bonner akademischen Medizin. Johann Christian Friedrich Harless (1773-1853). **MMW** 1983 Oct 21;125(42):950-2

**Harpestraeng, Henrik, d. 1244**
Hauberg P: Laegebøger med tilknytning til Henrik Harpestraeng. **Theriaca** 1982 Jun;22:1-362

**Harris, Charles Edward, 1868-1947**
Rogers FB: Charles E. Harris (1868-1947) of Hyannis, Massachusetts: family doctor and friend of mankind. **J Hist Med Allied Sci** 1983 Jul;38(3):339-42

**Harris, John, 1798-1849**
Will the real 'father of dental education' please stand up? (John Harris): **Ohio Dent J** 1980 May;54(5):19-20

**Harris, Moses, ca. 1731-ca. 1770**
Waltke R: Moses Harris--inventor of the color wheel. **Dent Lab Rev** 1980 Apr;:24-5

**Harris, Samuel Harry, 1880-1936**
Murphy LJ: Harry Harris and his contribution to suprapubic prostatectomy. **Aust NZ J Surg** 1984 Dec;54(6):579-88

**Harrison, Benjamin**
Kass EH, Carey AB, Kass AM: Thomas Hodgkin and Benjamin Harrison: crisis and promotion in academia. **Med Hist** 1980 Apr;24(2):197-208

**Harrison, Preston E.**
Moore C, Winer JL: Dr. Peterson E. Harrison: pioneer traiblazer for mental health in West Texas. **West Tex Hist Assoc Yearb** 1979;55:49-58

**Harrison, Ross Granville, 1870-1959**
Hamburger V: S. Ramón y Cajal, R. G. Harrison, and the beginnings of neuroembryology. **Perspect Biol Med** 1980;23(4):600-16
Maienschein JA: Ross Harrison's crucial experiment as a foundation for modern American experimental embryology. Ph.D. Diss., Indiana University. Bloomington, 1978. 252 leaves.
Wilens S: Ross Granville Harrison. In Dictionary of American Biography, Suppl. 6, 1956-1960. p. 281-3, 1980.
Witkowski JA: W. T. Astbury and Ross G. Harrison: the search for the molecular determination of form in the developing embryo. **Notes Rec R Soc Lond** 1980 Dec;35(2):195-219

**Harrison, Tinsley Randolph, 1900-**
Morehead RP: The contribution of a great man to Wake Forest University and its Bowman Gray School of Medicine--Tinsley R. Harrison, M.D. **NC Med J** 1983 Dec;44(12):809-11

**Harrower, David, 1857-1937**
Lamping KA, Albert DM, Snyder C, et al: The Harrower collection and its place in the history of ophthalmic pathology. **Surv Ophthalmol** 1983 May-Jun;27(6):374-80

**Hart, Deryl, 1894-**
Sabiston DC: Deryl Hart: leader in the development of the Duke University Medical Center. **NC Med J** 1983 Jul;44(7):441-2

**Hartley, David, 1705-1757**
Webb ME: A reexamination of the inception, development, and 'Newtonianism' of David Hartley's 'Observations on man.' Ph.D. Diss., University of Oklahoma, 1981. ix, 310 p.

**Hartlib, Samuel, d. 1662**
Webster C: Utopian planning and the Puritan revolution. Gabriel Plattes, Samuel Hartlib, and 'Macaria'. Oxford, Wellcome Unit for the History of Medicine, 1979. 89 p. (Research Publications of the Wellcome Unit for the History of Medicine, Oxford, No. II).

**Hartlieb, Johann, d. 1468**
Grubmüller K: Ein Arzt als Literat: Hans Hartlieb. In Honemann V, Ruh K, et al: Poesie und Gebrauchsliteratur im deutschen Mittelalter. Würzburger Colloquium 1978. Tûbingen, Niemeyer, 1979. p. 14-36.
Schmitt W: Magie und Mantik bei Hans Hartlieb. Wien, 1966. 25 p. (Salzburger Beiträge zur Paracelsusforschung, 6).

**Hartmann, Alexis, 1898-1964**
Lee JA: Sydney Ringer (1834-1910) and Alexis Hartmann (1898-1964). **Anaesthesia** 1981 Dec;36(12):1115-21

**Hartmann, Heinz, 1894-1970**
Sanderson ER: Henri Hartmann and the Hartmann operation. **Arch Surg** 1980 Jun;115(6):792-3

**Hartung vom Hoff, Caspar, 16th cent.**
Haage B, ed: Das 'Kunstbüchlein' des Alchemisten Caspar Hartung vom Hoff. Göppingen, Kümmerle, 1975. 141 p.

**Harvey, Edmund Newton, 1887-1959**
Liebenau J: The papers of Edmund Newton Harvey, (1887-1959).

**Surv Sources Newsl** 1977 Nov;6:8-9

**Harvey, Ethel Browne, 1885-1965**

Haraway DJ: Ethel Browne Harvey. In: Notable American women. The modern period. Cambridge, Mass., Belknap-Harvard Univ. Press, 1980. 4:319-21.

**Harvey Family**

Sakula A: The Betchworth Portraits: members of the family of William Harvey. **Med Hist** 1980 Jul;24(3):333-41

**Harvey, Oliver**

McConville E: Oliver Harvey: 'Got to take some risks.' **South Exposure** 6(2):24-8, 1978

**Harvey, Samuel Clark, 1886-1953**

Lindskog GE: Two doctors Harvey: William (1578-1657); Samuel Clark (1886-1953). **Yale J Biol Med** 1979 Sep-Oct;52(5):467-82

**Harvey, Thomas B., 1827-1889**

Bonsett CA: Medical museum notes: Thomas B. Harvey. **J Indiana State Med Assoc** 1983 Jun;76(6):371

**Harvey, William, 1578-1657**

Alsop J: A private consultation by Dr. William Harvey in 1642. **Med Hist** 1980 Jan;24(1):93-8

Alsop JD: A footnote on the circulation of the blood: Joseph Colston and Harvey's discovery in 1642. **J Hist Med Allied Sci** 1981 Jul;36(3):331-4

Andrews BF: William Harvey in perinatal perspective. In Smith GF, Smith PN, Vidyasagar D, ed: Historical review and recent advances in neonatal and perinatal medicine. [Chicago?], Mead Johnson Nutritional Division, 1983. Vol. II. p. 165-78.

Bearn AG, James DG: Dr. William Harvey (1578-1657) and the Harvey Society of New York. **Perspect Biol Med** 1978 Spring;21(3):524-35

Berti-Bock G., et al: Le séjour de William Harvey à Padoue. **Hist Sci Med** 1980;14:317-24

Bloch H: Discovery of blood circulation; Some dependence factors in evolution of a discovery. **NY State J Med** 1979 Nov;79(12):1940-3

Bonnabeau RC, Bonnabeau MM: William Harvey revisited 1578-1978. **Minn Med** 1981 Jan;64(1):28-33

Burchell HB: Mechanical and hydraulic analogies in Harvey's discovery of the circulation. **J Hist Med Allied Sci** 1981 Jul;36(3):260-77

Bylebyl JJ: The growth of Harvey's De Motu Cordis. **Bull Hist Med** 1973 Sep-Oct;47(5):427-70

Bylebyl JJ: Boyle and Harvey on the valves in the veins. **Bull Hist Med** 1982 Fall;56(3):351-67

Bylebyl JJ, ed: William Harvey and his age: the professional and social context of the discovery of the circulation. Baltimore, Johns Hopkins University Press, 1979. xii, 154 p. (Henry E. Sigerist Supplements to the Bulletin of the History of Medicine, n.s., 2). Includes contributions by S. Jarcho, C. Webster, R. G. Frank.

Cohen IB, ed: Studies on William Harvey. New York, Arno Press, 1981. 572 p. in various pagings. (A collection of previously published articles and short works by various authors).

Comtor JH: Harvey's 1651 perfusion of the pulmonary circulation of man. **Circulation** 1982 Jan;65(1):1-3

Frank RG: The physician as virtuoso in seventeenth-century England. In Shapiro, Barbara and Frank, Robert G., Jr. ed: English scientific virtuosi in the 16th and 17th centuries. Los Angeles, William Andrews Clark Memorial Lib., U. of California, 1980. p. 57-114.

Frank RG: Harvey and the Oxford physiologists: scientific ideas and social interaction. Berkeley, University of California Press, 1980. xviii, 368 p.

Gysel C: W. Harvey (1578-1657) et A. van den Spiegel (1578-1625), l'humanisme et l'odontologie. **Rev Belge Med Dent** 1979;34(1):121-6

Gysel C: Umanesimo e odontoiatria: Harvey e Spigelius, due vite parallele. **Dent Cadmos** 1981 Jan;49(1):61-6

Hamburger J: Le journal d'Harvey. Paris, Flammarion, 1983. 339 p.

Hart FD: William Harvey and his gout. **Ann Rheum Dis** 1984 Apr;43(2):125-7

Huard P, Imbault-Huart MJ: Les étapes du traitement des tumeurs par ischémie, priorité de Harvey. **Hist Sci Med** 1980;14(2):171-5

Jucovy PM: Circle and circulation: the language and imagery of William Harvey's discovery. **Perspect Biol Med** 1976 Autumn;20(1):92-107

Keele KD: The life and work of William Harvey. **Endeavour** 1978;2(3):104-7

Knobil E: William Harvey and the physiology of reproduction. **Physiologist** 1981 Feb;24(1):3-7

Leibowitz JO: Early accounts in geriatric pathology (Leonardo, Harvey, James Keill). **Koroth** 1980 Jun;7(11-12):CCLIII-CCLXIV

Lindskog GE: Two doctors Harvey: William (1578-1657); Samuel Clark (1886-1953). **Yale J Biol Med** 1979 Sep-Oct;52(5):467-82

Lipscomb JM: New light on some Harvey portraits, in memoriam Sir Geoffrey Keynes. **Med Hist** 1983 Apr;27(2):197-202

McMichael J: History of atrial fibrillation 1628-1819 Harvey - de Senac - Laënnec. **Br Heart J** 1982 Sep;48(3):193-7

Nikolov G: Uiliam Kharveĭ, otkrivateliat na krŭvoobrashtenieto. Sofiia, Meditsina i fizkultura, 1981. 74 p.

Oppenheimer JM: Harvey, William. Disputations touching the generation of animals: essay review. **Trans Stud Coll Physicians Phila** 1982 Dec;4(4):306-9

Riall CT: Surgical and medical devices and their origins. William Harvey and circulation of the blood. Chapter XVI. **J Oper Room Res Inst** 1982 Nov;2(11):32-6

Schadewaldt H: 'Le génie, c'est une longue patience'. (Teil 1). **Arztl Fortbild** 1982;32(11):12-23

Schadewaldt H: 'Le génie, c'est une longue patience'. (Teil 3). **Arztl Fortbild** 1982;32(13):32-40

Schadewaldt H: 'Le génie, c'est une longue patience'. (Teil 2). **Arztl Fortbild** 1982;32(12):16-8

Schmidtgall H: Zur Rezeption von Harveys Blutkreislaufmodell in der englischen Wirtschaftstheorie des 17. Jahrhunderts. **Sudhoffs Arch** 1973;57(4):416-30

Van Lieburg MJ: De dichter-medicus Daniël Jonctys (1611-1654), zijn strijd tegen het bijgeloof en zijn relatie tot Johan van Beverwijck, William Harvey en Daniël Sennert. **Tijdschr Geschied Geneeskd** 1979;2(4):137-67

Walker W: Harvey's contemporaries--science and society. **Scott Med J** 1981 Oct;26(4):356-63

Wear A: William Harvey and the 'Way of the Anatomists'. **Hist Sci** 1983 Sep;21(53 pt 3):223-49

Whitteridge G: Of the local movement of animals. **Proc R Soc Lond [Biol]** 1979 Nov 30;206(1162):1-13

Whitteridge G: Harvey and sensory neuropathy. **J R Coll Physicians Lond** 1981 Jan;15(1):61-2

**Harwood, Busick, 1745-1814**

Williamson R: Sir Busick Harwood: a reappraisal. **Med Hist** 1983 Oct;27(4):423-33

**Haslam, John, 1764-1844**

Waddington JL: Ventricular enlargement in schizophrenia and the historical studies of John Haslam. **Am J Psychiatry** 1984 Dec;141(12):1640

**Hastings, Charles**

Bator PA: 'The struggle to raise the lower classes': public health reform and the problem of poverty in Toronto, 1910 to 1921. **J Can Stud** 1979;14(1):43-9

**Hastings, Charles, 1794-1866**

Grabham AH: Precepts and practice: Charles Hastings's vision and reality. **Br Med J [Clin Res]** 1982 Dec 18-25;285(6357):1789-92

**Hatvani, István, 1718-1786**

Páal A: Orvostörténeti adatok a 'Magyar Faust', Hatvani istván professzor (1718-1786 ig) tanulmányairól és munkásságáról. **Orv Hetil** 1984 Aug 5;125(32):1957-8, 1961-2

**Hauberg, Poul Richard, 1887-1959**

Jensen VG: Poul Richard Hauberg, 1887-1959. **Theriaca** 1982 Jun;22:xi-xvi

**Hauksbee, Francis, ca. 1666-1713**

Senior JE: Hauksbee's prototypical electrostatic generator. **Med Instrum** 1983 Mar-Apr;17(2):126-7

**Haupt, Alma Cecelia, 1893-1956**

Toppin EA: Alma Cecelia Haupt. In Dictionary of American Biography, Suppl. 6, 1956-1960. p. 283-5, 1980.

**Hauptmann, Carl, 1858-1921**

Walser HH: Ist das Wohl des Landesherrn in Wein zu trinken? Carl und Gerhart Hauptmann bei August Forel in Zürich. **Gesnerus** 1981;38:207-14

**Hauptmann, Gerhart, 1862-1946**

Walser HH: Ist das Wohl des Landesherrn in Wein zu trinken? Carl und Gerhart Hauptmann bei August Forel in Zürich. **Gesnerus** 1981;38:207-14

**Havemann, August Conrad, 1755-1819**

Marx S: Zwei Kollegmitschriften nach den Vorlesungen von August Conrad Havemann, geschrieben 1799 und 1818 an der Tierärztlichen Hochschule Hannover. Diss. Hannover, 1981. 360 p.

**Hawley, Paul Ramsey, 1891-1965**

Schott TE: Paul Ramsey Hawley. In Dictionary of American biography, 1961-1965. Suppl. 7, 1981. p. 328-9.

**Hawthorne, Nathaniel, 1804-1864**

Atropine poisoning in Hawthorne's the Scarlet Letter: **N Engl J Med** 1984 Nov 29;311(22):1438-41

Khan JA: Atropine poisoning in Hawthorne's The Scarlet Letter. **N Engl J Med** 1984 Aug 9;311(6):414-6

Stoehr T: Hawthorne's mad scientists: Pseudoscience and social science in nineteenth-century life and letters. Hamden, Conn., Shoestring Press, 1978. 313 p.

Wygant A: Shelley, Hawthorne, and Wells: images of medicine in early science fiction. **Bookman** 1981 Oct;8(8):3-8

**Hawthorne, Sophia, ca. 1811-1871**

C[one] TE: Mrs. Nathaniel Hawthorne's invalidism, until her marriage at age 31, was attributed to difficult teething in infancy. **Pediatrics** 1981;67:606

**Hayes, Isaac Israel, 1832-1881**

Johnson RE: Isaac Israel Hayes. In Dictionary of Canadian biography, 1881-1890. 1982;11:393-4.

**Hayward, Wally, 1908?-**
Maud PJ, Pollock ML, Foster C, et al: Fifty years of training and competition in the marathon: Wally Hayward, age 70--a physiological profile. **S Afr Med J** 1981 Jan 31;59(5):153-7

**Hazen, Elizabeth Lee, 1885-1975**
Baldwin RS: The fungus fighters: two women scientists and their discovery. Ithaca, Cornell University Press, 1981. 212 p.
Rubin LP: Elizabeth Lee Hazen. In: Notable American women. The modern period. Cambridge, Mass., Belknap-Harvard Univ. Press, 1980. 4:326-8.

**Hazlett, Theodore Lyle, 1885-**
Lauer DJ: T. Lyle Hazlett: his role in industrial medicine, 1920-50. **JOM** 1979 Jun;21(6):403-6

**Healy, William, 1869-1963**
Snodgrass J: William Healy (1869-1963): pioneer child psychiatrist and criminologist. **J Hist Behav Sci** 1984 Oct;20(4):332-9

**Heaton, Leonard D., 1902-**
McLean RB: Leonard D. Heaton--military surgeon. **Milit Med** 1982 Sep;147(9):717-27

**Heberden, William, 1710-1801**
Kligfield P: The frustrated benevolence of 'Dr. Anonymous'. **Am J Cardiol** 1981 Jan;47(1):185-7
Paulshock BZ: When should a physician retire? - William Heberden's view. **Del Med J** 1983;55(6):359-60
Paulshock BZ: William Heberden, M.D., and the end of theriac. **NY State J Med** 1982 Oct;82(11):1612-4
Paulshock BZ: William Heberden and opium--some relief to all. **N Engl J Med** 1983 Jan 6;308(1):53-6

**Hébert, Louis, ca. 1580-1627**
Garner J: Louis Hébert: his pharmaceutical skills helped Canada's first permanent settlement to survive. **Can Pharm J** 1982 Oct;115(10):380-1

**Hebra, Ferdinand von, 1816-1880**
Crissey JT, Parish LC: Ferdinand Hebra: a reexamination of his contributions to dermatology. **Int J Dermatol** 1980 Dec;19(10):585-8
Holubar K: Ferdinand von Hebra und das Allgemeine Krankenhaus in Wien. Uber die Domizilierung der beiden Hautkliniken um die Mitte des 19. Jahrhunderts und ihr Verhältnis zum II. Hof im Allgemeinen Krankenhaus. **Wien Med Wochenschr** 1982 Sep 30;132(18):423-6
Klimpel M: F. von Hebra, Atlas der Hauterkrankungen (1856-1876). Köln, Universität zu Köln, 1980. 322 p. (Kölner medizinhistorische Beiträge, 17) (also Diss.).
Tappeiner J, Holubar K: Ferdinand Ritter von Hebra: Person und Werk (1816 bis 1880). **Wien Klin Wochenschr** 1981 Sep 4;93(16):503-6

**Hecker, August Friedrich, 1763-1811**
Abe HR, Tiedt N: August Friedrich Hecker (1763-1811) und die Anfänge der modernen Pathophysiologie. **Beitr Gesch Univ Erfurt** 1979-83;19:165-85
Kneist W: August Friedrich Heckers 'Die Kunst unsere Kinder zu gesunden Staatsbürgern zu erziehen...' (Erfurt 1805). **Beitr Gesch Univ Erfurt** 1979-83;19:187-204

**Hedin, Sven Gustaf, 1859-1933**
Ljunggren B: Harvey Cushing and Sven Hedin. **Surg Neurol** 1982 Mar;17(3):165-71
Ljunggren B: Cushing och Sven Hedin. **Lakartidningen** 1982 Aug 11;79(32-33):2790-2

**Hedin, Sven, 1865-1952**
Hummel D: Som läkare vid hedinexpeditionen till Kina 1927-31. **Nord Medicinhist Arsbok** 1983;:155-44

**Hegar, Alfred, 1830-1914**
Rihner F: Alfred Hegar--Zum 150. Geburtstag. **Med Welt** 1980 Oct 17;31(42):1522-3

**Hegel, Georg Wilhelm Friedrich, 1770-1831**
Seletskiĭ AI: Gegel' o patologii psikhiki--psikhoze i slaboumii. **Zh Nevropatol Psikhiatr** 1982;82(6):102-5

**Heger, Hans, 1855-1940**
Nowotny O: Hans Heger und seine Bedeutung für die Geschichte der Pharmazie in Oesterreich. In: Vorträge des Internationalen Pharmaziehistorischen Kongresses Innsbruck 1977. Stuttgart, Wissenschaftliche Verlagsgesellschaft, 1979. p. 147-52.

**Heide, Antonius de, b. 1646**
Lindeboom GA: De ontdekking van het trilhaarepitheel door Antonius de Heide (1683). **Ned Tijdschr Geneeskd** 1980 May 24;124(21):839-41
Lindeboom GA: Anton de Heide als proefondervindelijk onderzoeker. **Tijdschr Geschied Geneeskd** 1983;6(3):121-34

**Heidenhain, Rudolf Peter Heinrich, 1834-1897**
Gutt RW: W setna rocznice określenia czynności wydzielniczej komórek błony śluzowej zoładka. **Arch Hist Med (Warsz)** 1978;41(4):479-81

**Heim, Ernst Ludwig, 1747-1834**
Genschorek W: Ernst Ludwig Heim. Das Leben eines Volksarztes. Leipzig, S. Hirzel, 1982. 226 p.

**Heine, Bernhard, 1800-1846**
Huard P, Lefebvre P, Nosny P, et al: La scie ostéotome à chaîne de Bernhard-Franz Heine (1800-1846). **Hist Sci Med** 1983;17(2):147-57
Seufert WD: The chain osteotome by Heine. **J Hist Med Allied Sci** 1980 Oct;35(4):454-9

**Heine, Heinrich, 1797-1856**
Kenéz J: H. Heine betegsége. Egy vita, mely a költ' ó halálának 125. évfordulója után sem zárult le. **Orv Hetil** 1982 May 16;123(20):1246-50

**Heinrich II, Saint, Emperor of Germany, 973-1024**
Valentin P: Mit Brevier und Skalpell. Legendäre Bauchoperation Kaiser Heinrichs II. **Med Welt** 1982 Feb 19;33(7):260-2

**Heinroth, Johann Christian August, 1773-1843**
Fischer W: Der Psychiater Heinroth--eine kritische Betrachtung. **Psychiatr Neurol Med Psychol (Leipz)** 1983 Oct;35(10):623-8
Wunderlich G: Kranheits- und Therapiekonzepte am Anfang der deutschen Psychiatrie (Haindorf, Heinroth, Ideler). Husum, Matthiesen, 1981. 132 p. (Abhandlungen zur Geschichte der Medizin und der Naturwissenschaften, 41).

**Heisler, August, 1881-**
Schneider H: Dr. August Heisler. Erinnerungen an einen grossen Arzt. **ZFA (Stuttgart)** 1983 May 10;59(13):774-6

**Heiss, Hugo Andreas, 1863-1936**
Feige W: Leben und Schaffen des Schlachthofdirektors Oberveterinärrat Dr. med. vet. Hugo Andreas Heiss, Straubing (1863-1936). Diss., Tierärztliche Hochschule. Hannover, 1982. 163 p.

**Heister, Lorenz, 1683-1758**
Boschung U: Iatromechanik and Chirurgie bei Lorenz Heister. **Gesnerus** 1983;40(1-2):31-41
de Moulin D: The value of tobacco smoke in the treatment of intussusception. **Neth J Surg** 1984 Apr;36(2):57-9
Faller A: Welchen Platz nimmt Stensens anatomische Forschung in Lorenz Heisters Chirurgie und Anatomie ein? **Gesnerus** 1983;40(1-2):55-66
Geiger A: Lorenz Heister als Geburtshelfer und gynäkologischer Chirurg. Vergleichende Untersuchung anhand der verschiedenen Auflagen seiner 'Chirurgie'. Zürich, Juris Druck, 1983. 140 p. (Zürcher Medizingeschichtliche Abhandlungen, Neue Reihe, Nr. 162).
Meyer KK, Beck WC: Mastectomy performed by Lawrence Heister in the eighteenth century. **Surg Gynecol Obstet** 1984 Oct;159(4):391-4
Probst J: Lorenz Heister, 1683-1758 Praeceptor Chirurgiae. **Unfallchirurgie** 1984 Feb;10(1):1-8

**Hektoen, Ludvig, 1863-1951**
Beatty WK: Ludvig Hektoen--scientist and counselor. **Proc Inst Med Chic** 1982 Jan-Mar;35(1):7-9

**Held, Jan Theobald, 1770-1851**
Dobíšek K: První čyři primáři pražského ústavu choromyslných. **Cesk Psychiatr** 1980 Aug;76(4):270-5

**Heldman, Anna B.**
Selavan IC: Angel in hell-with-the-lid-off. **Am J Nurs** 1980;80:2064-5

**Hellbridge, Theodor, 1919-**
Halberg E, et al: Forging chronobiology and pediatrics as well as geriatrics - a birthday greeting for Theodor Hellbrugge. **Int J Chronobiol** 1979;6:135-43

**Hellemans, Jan**
Ter herinnering aan professor dr. jan hellemans: **Tijdschr Gerontol Geriatr** 1982 Oct;13(5):171-8

**Heller, Johann Florian, 1813-1871**
Schmalhofer J: Das Werk von Johann Florian Heller mit besonderer Berücksichtigung der Entstehung des ersten pathologisch-chemischen Laboratoriums am Allgemeinen Wiener Krankenhaus und der Ernennung Hellers zum Vorstand des Laboratoriums. Diss. Bonn, 1980. 201 p.

**Heller, John Roderick, 1905-**
Heller SA: A Public Health Service wife. Rockville, Printex, 1978. [144] leaves.

**Heller, Józef, 1896-1982**
Szafrański P, Zagórski W, Filipowicz W: Studies on protein biosynthesis at the Institute of Biochemistry and Biophysics, Polish Academy of Sciences, initiated by Professor J. Heller in 1956. **Acta Biochim Pol** 1984;31(1):9-16
Szarkowski JW, Wierzchowski KL: Professor Józef Heller 1896-1982. **Acta Biochim Pol** 1984;31(1):5-8
Wspomnienie o Profesorze Józefie Hellerze: **Postepy Biochem** 1982;28(4):387-90

**Hellot, Jean, 1685-1766**
Todericiu D: Jean Hellot (1685-1766), savant chimiste, fondateur de la technologie chimique en France au XVIIIe siècle. In: Congrès National des Sociétés Savantes, 105e, Caen. Comptes Rendu, Paris. 1980. Section des Sciences, Fasc. 5. p. 201-11.

**Hellström, Johan, 1859-1941**
Brück C: Tidsbilder kring en läkargeneration för 100 år sedan. Efter

ett föredrag av Johan Hellström 1935. **Nord Medicinhist Arsb** 1984;:141-52

**Helmholtz, Hermann Ludwig Ferdinand von, 1821-1894**
Belloni L: Hermann Helmholtz und Franz Boll. **Medizinhist J** 1982;17(1/2):129-37
Eckhardt G, ed: Zur Geschichte der Psychologie. Berlin, VEB Deutscher Verlag der Wissenschaften, 1979. 128p. Mit Beiträgen von H. Hiebsch, F. Klix, W. Schreier, und L. Sprung.
Enoch JM: To woo a Helmholtz. **Am J Optom Physiol Opt** 1982 Oct;59(10):843
Klauss K: Ein neuentdecktes frühes Dokument zur Geschichte der Erfindung des Augenspiegels durch Hermann v. Helmholtz. **NTM** 1981;18(1):58-61
Klix F: Hermann von Helmholtz' Beitrag zur Theorie der Wahrnehmung--Bleibendes und Vergängliches in einem grossen Lebenswerk. In Eckardt G, ed: Zur Geschichte der Psychologie. Berlin, VEB Deutscher Verlag der Wissenschaften, 1979. p. 45-59.
Sherman PD: Colour vision in the nineteenth century: the Young-Helmholtz-Maxwell theory. Bristol, Adam Hilger, 1981. xiii, 233 p.
Votočková J: 130 let Helmholtzova oftalmoskopu. **Cesk Oftalmol** 1982 Jan;38(1):51-3
Westheimer G: Helmholtz on eye movements. **Hum Neurobiol** 1984;3(3):149-52
Yamaguchi C: [Betrachtungen über die frühesten physiologischen Arbeiten Hermann von Helmholtz, die zu seiner Entdeckung des Gesetzes von der Erhaltung der Energie führen] (Jpn). **Kagakushi Kenkyu** 1984;23(151):169-76

**Helmont, Jean Baptiste van, 1577-1644**
Bloch H: Jan Baptiste Van Helmont, M.D. (1579-1644); religion, mysticism, and science in a century of change. **NY State J Med** 1980 Sep;80(10):1631-3
Boss J: Helmont, Glisson, and the doctrine of the common reservoir in the seventeenth-century revolution in physiology. **Br J Hist Sci** 1983 Nov;16(54 Pt 3):261-72
Debus AG: Thomas Sherley's philosophical essay (1672): Helmontian mechanism as the basis of a new philosophy. **Ambix** 1980 Jul;27(2):124-35
Gysel C: Helmontianisme en odontologie (I). **Rev Belge Med Dent** 1979;34(3):295-312
Gysel C: Jean-Baptiste Van Helmont (1579-1644), le baroque et les dents. **Rev Belge Med Dent** 1979;34(4):397-404
Gysel C: Helmontianisme en odontologie (II). 3. Van Helmont en het nagerslacht. **Rev Belge Med Dent** 1979;34(4):385-96
Halleux R: Gnose et expérience dans la philosophie chimique de Jean-Baptiste Van Helmont. **Bull Cl Sci Acad R Belg** 1979;65:217-27
Pagel W: Joan Baptista Van Helmont: reformer of science and medicine. Cambridge, Cambridge University Press, x, 1982. 219 p. (Cambridge monographs on the history of medicine).
Pagel W: The smiling spleen. In H. Lloyd-Jones, et al., ed: History and imagination: essays in honor of H. R. Trevor-Roper. New York, Holmes & Meier, 1982. p. 81-7.
Skulimowski MM: Jan Baptysta van Helmont (1577-1644) odkrywca dwutlenku węgla (CO2). **Wiad Lek** 1980 Mar 15;33(6):495-7
Todericiu D: Prolongements méconnus de la philosophie chimique de Jean-Baptiste Van Helmont (1578-1644) en Europe centrale et orientale. L'éloge à Van Helmont du savant roumain Démètre Cantémir (1701). **Bull Cl Sci Acad R Belg** 1979;65:228-38
Vandewiele LJ: Van chemiatrie tot iatrochemie--van Paracelsus (1493-1541) tot Van Helmont (1579?-1644). **Farm Tijdschr Belg** 1980;57:25-30

**Helvétius, Claude Adrien, 1715-1771**
Helvétius CA: Anfänge der Erziehung. Claude Adrien Helvétius (1772). **Krankenpfl J** 1984 Mar 1;22(3):30-1

**Hemard, Urban, fl. 1582**
Gysel C: Appréciation d'Urbain Hémard et de sa 'Recherche de la vraye anatomie des dents'. **Actual Odontostomatol (Paris)** 1982;36(139):395-410

**Hemingway, Ernest, 1899-1961**
Allen WR: All the names of death: Walker Percy and Hemingway. **Miss Q** 1982-83;36(1):3-19

**Hench, Philip Showalter, 1896-1965**
Mann R: Philip Showalter Hench. In Dictionary of American biography, 1961-1965. Suppl. 7, 1981. p. 340-341.

**Henderson, Charles, 1923-**
Wilson RK: Charles Henderson-a man stands tall. **J Med Assoc State Ala** 1982 Jun;51(12):41-3

**Henderson, David Willis Wilson, 1903-1968**
Druett H: David Willis Wilson Henderson. In Dictionary of national biography, 1961-1970. Suppl. 8, 1981. p. 504-6.

**Henderson, Lawrence Joseph, 1878-1942**
Recollections & reflections: Lawrence J. Henderson and George Sarton. **Isis** 1984 Mar;75(276):11-32

**Henderson, Virginia**
Nojima Y: [Nursing theory by Henderson. 4. Virginia Henderson and the history of nursing theory] (Jpn) **Kango Tenbo** 1979 Oct;4(10):949-57

**Henle, Jakob, 1809-1885**
Eulner HH, Hoepke H, ed: Der Briefwechsel zwischen Rudolph Wagner und Jacob Henle 1838-1862. Göttingen, Vandenhoeck & Ruprecht, 1979. 115 p. (Arbeiten aus der Niedersächsischen Staats- und Universitätsbibliothek Göttingen, Band 16).
Teulón AA: La constitucion de la histologia celular: Schwann, Henle y Kölliker. **Asclepio** 1978-79;30-31:7-18
Wahl RW: Eponym: the loop of Henle. **South Med J** 1984 Apr;77(4):494-5

**Henley, William Ernest, 1849-1903**
Edwards G: William Ernest Henley: early impressions. **Nurs Mirror** 1981 Jun 17;152(25):33-4

**Henning, Hans, 1885-1946**
Marion P: La polemica tra Henning e Bühler. **Stor Crit Psicol** 1980;1(2):297-310

**Henning, Karl, 1860-1917**
Portele KA: Die Henning-Moulagen des Pathologisch-anatomischen Bundesmuseums in Wien. **Med Lab (Stuttg)** 1979 Feb;32(2):41-3

**Henning, Theodor, 1897-1946**
Portele KA: Die Henning-Moulagen des Pathologisch-anatomischen Bundesmuseums in Wien. **Med Lab (Stuttg)** 1979 Feb;32(2):41-3

**Henry II, King of England, 1133-1189**
Mason E: 'Rocamadour in Quercy above all other churches': the healing of Henry II. In Sheils WJ, ed: The Church and healing. Papers read at the twentieth summer meeting and the twenty-first winter meeting of the Ecclesiastical History Society. Oxford, Basil Blackwell for the Society, 1982. p. 39-54.

**Henry, Joseph, 1797-1878**
Reingold N, ed: The papers of Joseph Henry. Volume 1. December 1797-October 1832. The Albany years. Washington, Smithsonian Institution Press, 1972. xxxix, 496 p.
Reingold N, ed: The papers of Joseph Henry. Volume 2. November 1832-December 1835. The Princeton Years. Washington, Smithsonian Institution Press, 1975. 524 p.

**Henry VI, King of England, 1421-1471**
Theilmann JM: The miracles of King Henri VI of England. **Historian** 1980;42(3):456-71

**Henry VIII, King of England, 1491-1547**
Cohen B: A tale of two paintings. **Ann R Coll Surg Engl** 1982 Jan;64(1):4-12

**Henryson, Robert, 1430?-1506**
Fox D: Henryson's 'Sum Practysis of Medecyne'. **Stud Philol** 1972;69:453-60

**Hensing, Johann Thomas, 1683-1726**
Tower DB: Hensing, 1719. An account of the first chemical examination of the brain and the discovery of phosphorus therein, set against the background of Europe in the 17th and early 18th centuries. A source book in the history of neurochemistry. New York, Raven, 1983. xvi, 407 p.

**Henslow, George, 1835-1925**
Gershenowitz H: George Henslow: true Darwinist. **Indian J Hist Sci** 1979, reçu 1982;14(1):25-30

**Herapath, William, 1796-1868**
Weller RM: Nitrous oxide in Bristol in 1836. A series of lectures by William Herepath (1796-1868). **Anaesthesia** 1983 Jul;38(7):678-82

**Herbart, Johann Friedrich, 1776-1841**
Leary DE: The historical foundation of Herbart's mathematization of psychology. **J Hist Behav Sci** 1980 Apr;16(2):150-63

**Herbert, George, 1593-1633**
Nelson TG: Death, dung, the devil, and worldly delights: a metaphysical conceit in Harington, Donne, and Herbert. **Stud Philol** 1979 Summer;76(3):272-87

**Herculano, Alexandre, 1810-1877**
Machado JT: A doença que vitimou Herculano. **An Acad Port Hist** 1979;26(1):305-34

**Herff, Ferdinand, 1820-1912**
Banks CS: Two pioneer physicians of San Antonio. **Friends P. I. Nixon Med Hist Libr** 1973 Oct;2:2-17

**Herman, Eufemiusz, 1892-**
Prusiński A: Professor dr hab. nauk med. Eufemiusz Herman - nestor polskiej neurologii (w 90 urodziny). **Neurol Neurochir Pol** 1982;(5-6):306-28

**Hermann, Imre, 1889-**
Antal G: Freud in Hungary. An interview with Imre Hermann, the psychoanalyst. **New Hung Q** 1982;23(85):88-95

**Hernández de Gregorio, Manuel, 1771-1833**
Francés C: Manuel Hernández de Gregorio: a Spanish pharmacist dedicated to science and the history of pharmacy. In: Vorträge des Internationalen Pharmaziehistorischen Kongresses Innsbruck 1977. Struttgart, Wissenschaftliche Verlagsgesellschaft, 1979. p. 181-6.

**Hernández, Francisco, ca. 1515-1587**
Fastlicht S: Spain's first scientific expedition to Mexico in the XVI century: the tragic story of Francisco Hernandez. **Bull Hist Dent**

1980 Apr;28(1):3–10
Sanchez Tellez MC, Guerra F, Valverde JL: La doctrina farmacéutica del Renacimiento en la obra de Francisco Hernández, c. 1515–1587. Granada, Universidad de Granada, Hospital Real, 1979. 140 p. (Estudios del Departamento de Historia de la Farmacia y Legislación Farmacéutica, Universidad de Granada, 6).

**Hernández, Francisco, fl. 1734–1786**
Beltrán E: Una polémica sobre Francisco Hernández y su obra en 1785. **An Soc Mex Hist Cienc Tec** 1979;5:49–73

**Hernández Morejón, Antonio, 1773–1836**
Marí Balcells VJ: Tres historiadores de la medicina española: Villalba, Hernandez Morejon y Comenge, e influencia del primero en la obra de los otros dos. In: Sociedad Española de Historia de la Medicina. V Congreso Nacional. Madrid, 1977. **Asclepio** 1977;29:167–76

**Héroard, Jean, d. 1627**
Foisil M: Louis XIII à travers le stethoscope. **Histoire** 1982;42:76–8

**Herodicus**
Vandewiele LJ: Herodikos, de eerste sportarts. **Farm Tijdschr Belg** 1978;55:13–4

**Herodotus, ca. 484–425 B.C.**
Brandenburg D: Medizinisches bei Herodot. Eine literaturhistorische Studie zur antiken Heilkunde. Berlin, Hessling, 1976. 176 p. (Medizingeschichtliche Miniaturen, Band 2).
Kolta KS: Arzt und Hersteller von Heilmitteln im alten Aegypten. **Beitr Gesch Pharm** 1979;31(2):9–12

**Herophilus, 335–280 B.C.**
Pigeaud JM: Du rhythme dans le corps. Quelques notes sur l'interprétation du pouls par le médecin Hérophile. **Bull Assoc Guillaume Bude** 1978;3:258–67

**Herren, Mary, 1858–1887**
Hood B: 'This worry I have': Mary Herren journal. **Oreg Hist Q** 1979;80(3):228–57

**Herrick, James B., 1861–1954**
Hurst JW: Landmark article (JAMA 1912). Clinical features of sudden obstruction of the coronary arteries. By James B. Herrick. **JAMA** 1983 Oct 7;250(13):1757–65
Rhoads PS: James B. Herrick, M.D. Born August 11, 1861--Died March 7, 1954. **Proc Inst Med Chic** 1982 Jan–Mar;35(1):3–6
Ross RS: A parlous state of storm and stress. The life and times of James B. Herrick. **Circulation** 1983 May;67(5):955–9

**Hertig, Arthur Tremain, 1904–**
Acceptance of the Gold Headed Cane Award: **Am J Pathol** 1979 Aug;96(2):368–71
Presentation of the Gold Headed Cane to Arthur T. Hertig: **Am J Pathol** 1979 Aug;96(2):365–8

**Hertwig, Oscar, 1849–1922**
Weindling P: Social concepts in anatomy: theories of the cell state of Oscar Hertwig (1849–1922) and Wilhelm Waldeyer (1836–1921). **Soc Soc Hist Med Bull (Lond)** 1980 Jun;26:15–7

**Hertzen, Aleksandre Ivanovich, 1812–1870**
Arkhangel'skiĭ GV: A. I. Gertsen i S. P. Botkin. **Klin Med (Mosk)** 1982 Nov;60(11):118–20
Vzaimootnosheniia A.I. Gertsena i S. P. Botkina: **Klin Med (Mosk)** 1983 Jun;61(6):108–10

**Herz, Max**
Clarke J: Dr. Max Herz. Sydney, Alternative Publishing Co-operative, 1976. xv, 184 p.

**Herzog, Ferenc, 1879–1952**
Marsovszky P: Herzog Ferenc (1879–1952) emlékezetére. **Orvostort Kozl** 1980;89–91(26 no 1–3):251–6

**Hess, Julius, 1876–1955**
Rambar AC: Julius Hess, M.D. In Smith GF, Smith PN, Vidyasagar D, ed: Historical review and recent advances in neonatal and perinatal medicine. [Chicago?], Mead Johnson Nutritional Division, 1983. Vol. II. p. 161–4.

**Hess, Walter Rudolph, 1881–1973**
Huber A: Walter Rudolf Hess als Ophthalmologe. **Gesnerus** 1982;39(2):287–93
Huber A: W. R. Hess, the ophthalmologist. **Experientia** 1982 Dec 15;38(12):1397–400
Jain KM, Swan KG, Casey KF: Nobel prize winners in surgery. Part 3. (Frederick Grant Banting, Walter Rudolph Hess). **Am Surg** 1982 Jul;48(7):287–90
Jung R: Walter R. Hess (1881–1973). **Rev Physiol Biochem Pharmacol** 1981;88:1–21
Jung R: W. R. Hess und das Ordnungsprinzip in der Physiologie. **Schweiz Arch Neurol Neurochir Psychiatr** 1983;132(2):277–308
Waser PG: Walter Rudolf Hess. Aus seinem Leben und seiner Tätigkeit an der Medizinischen Fakultät der Universität Zürich. **Gesnerus** 1982;39(2):279–86

**Hesse, Friedrich Louis 1849–1906**
Hesse PG: Das erste staatliche zahnärztliche Institut Deutschlands und sein Gründer Friedrich Louis Hesse. **Stomatol DDR** 1983 Dec;33(12):861–3

**Hesse, Ludwig Ferdinand, 1795–1876**
Wunderlich P: Ein Bericht aus dem Jahre 1838 über die Kliniken in Moskau und St. Petersburg. **Z Gesamte Hyg** 1980;26(5):381–2

**Heunert, Hans Henning, 1920–**
Kiermayer O: Werke von Dr. h. c. Hans-Henning Heunert. **Mikroskopie** 1981 Feb;38(1–2):3–12

**Heusinger, Karl Friedrich von, 1792–1883**
Speckner W: Carl Friedrich von Heusinger. Sein Leben und sein Wirken in Würzburg (1824–1829). Diss., Bayerische Julius-Maximilians-Universität, Würzburg, 1981. 154 p.

**Hevesy, George von, 1885–1966**
Iio M: Professor G. V. Hevesy, Doctor Y. Nishina and nuclear medicine in Japan. **Radiat Med** 1983 Jul–Sep;1(3):255–62
Myers WG: Georg Charles de Hevesy: the father of nuclear medicine. **J Nucl Med** 1979 Jun;20(6):590–4

**Hey, William, 1736–1819**
Anning ST: William Hey, F.R.S.: the father of Leeds surgery. **Proc Leeds Philos Lit Soc (Lit Hist Sect)** 1980;17(5):101–11

**Heyer, A. E.**
Heyningen EB van: The mysteries of the scarlet phial: spies and plague in Cape Town in 1907. **Q Bull S Afr Libr** 1979;34(2):53–8

**Heyl, James Bell, 1825 or 6–**
Franke NH: James Bell Heyl, Bermuda's pharmacist-photographer. **Pharm Hist** 1982;24(3):117–9

**Hickman, Henry Hill, 1800–1830**
Nuland SB: The origins of anesthesia: Part III. **Conn Med** 1984 Sep;48(9):597–600

**Hickson, James Moore**
Cunningham RJ: James Moore Hickson and spiritual healing in the American Episcopal church. **Hist Mag Protest Episc Church** 1970;39(1):2 16

**Hidaetullah, Hakeem, fl. 1731**
Azeez Pasha M: Yusrul Ilaj; a Persian medical manuscript compiled in India by Hakeem Hidaetullah, in 1731 A.D. **Bull Inst Hist Med (Hyderabad)** 1973 Oct;3(4):201–6

**Hidalgo de Agüero, Bartholomé, fl. 1604**
Torre E: Las 'Conclusiones' del doctor Estrada de Madrid, contra los 'Avisos particulares' del doctor Hidalgo de Aguero, sevillano. **Asclepio** 1978–79;30–31:389–401

**Hildegard, Saint, 1098?–1178**
Baader G: Naturwissenschaft und Medizin im 12. Jahrhundert und Hildegard von Bingen. **Arch Mittelrheinischen Kirchengesch** 1979;31:33–54
Bork K: Dermatologisches im Werk der Hildegard von Bingen. **Hautarzt** 1980 Jul;31(7):381–3
Hertzka G: Das Wunder der Hildegard-Medizin. Stein am Rhein, Christiana-Verlag, 1984. 236 p.
Hildegard von Bingen: Ursachen und Behandlung der Krankheiten (causae et curae). Ubersetzt von H. Schulz. 4. Auflage. Heidelberg, Haug, 1983. 373 p.
Mueller I: Krankheit und Heilmittel im Werk Hildegards von Bingen. In: Hildegard von Bingen. Festschrift 1179–1979. [1979] pp. 311–349.
Müller I: Die pflanzlichen Heilmittel bei Hildegard von Bingen. Salzburg, D. Müller, 1982. 215 p.
Pereira M: Maternità e sessualità femminile nell' opera di Ildegarda di Bingen. Una proposta di lettura. **Quad Stor** 1980;2
Schipperges H: Der Mensch und seine Welt bei Hildegard von Bingen. **Arzt Christ** 1978–79;1:2–7
Schipperges H: Diätetische Lebensführung nach der 'Regula Benedicti' bei Hildegard von Bingen. **Arzt Christ** 1980;2:87–97
Schipperges H: Die Kardinaltugenden im Weltbild der Hildegard von Bingen. **Grenzgeb Wiss** 1980;29(1):19–34
Schipperges H: Barmherzigkeit als Heilmittel bei Hildegard von Bingen. In Ganzinger K, Skopec M, Wyklicky H, ed: Festschrift für Erna Lesky zum 70. Geburtstag. Wien, Brüder Hollinek, 1981. p. 97–103.

**Hill, Archibald Vivian, 1886–1977**
Miller M: A. V. Hill papers. **Surv Sources Newsl** 1978 Oct;8:8–10

**Hill, Austin Bradford, 1897–**
Austin Bradford Hill: **Stat Med** 1982 Oct–Dec;1(4):305–9
Bibliography: Publications (in English) of Sir Austin Bradford Hill. **Stat Med** 1982 Oct–Dec;1(4):369–75
Doll R: Clinical trials: retrospect and prospect. **Stat Med** 1982 Oct–Dec;1(4):337–44
Fleiss JL: Multicentre clinical trials: Bradford Hill's contributions and some subsequent developments. **Stat Med** 1982 Oct–Dec;1(4):353–9
Himsworth H: Bradford Hill and statistics in medicine. **Stat Med** 1982 Oct–Dec;1(4):301–3
Holland WW, Breeze E, Swan AV: Clinical trials: some reflections. **Stat Med** 1982 Oct–Dec;1(4):361–8
Lilienfeld AM: Bradford Hill's influence on epidemiology. **Stat Med** 1982 Oct–Dec;1(4):325–8
Schilling R: Bradford Hill's contribution to occupational health. **Stat Med** 1982 Oct–Dec;1(4):317–24
Schoolman HM: The clinician and the statistician. **Stat Med** 1982 Oct–Dec;1(4):311–6

**Hill, Christina**
Hill C: On becoming the first woman urologist in Canada. **Can Med Assoc J** 1980 Feb 9;122(3):356

**Hill, David Jayne, 1850–1932**
Brozěk J: David Jayne Hill: between the old and the new psychology. In J. Brozěk, ed: Explorations in the history of psychology in the United States. Lewisburg, Bucknell University Press, 1984. p. 121–47.

**Hill, John, 1714–1775**
Dolman CE: 'That impudent fellow Hill'. **Ann Sci** 1983 May;40(3):281–8
Laundon JR: The date of birth of Sir John Hill (1714–1775). **Arch Nat Hist** 1981 Apr;10(1):65–6
Lemay JA, Rousseau GS: The Renaissance man in the eighteenth century. Papers read at a Clark Library seminar, 9 October 1976. Los Angeles, William Andrews Clark Memorial Library, UCLA, 1978. xi, 139 p.
Rousseau GS: Six new Hill letters. **Med Hist** 1984 Jul;28(3):293–302
Rousseau GS, ed: The letters and papers of Sir John Hill 1714–1775. New York, AMS Press, 1982. li, 208 p.

**Hill, Robert Gardiner, 1811–1878**
Jones K: Robert Gardiner Hill and the non-restraint movement. **Can J Psychiatry** 1984 Mar;29(2):121–4

**Hillebrand, Wilhelm, 1892–1959**
Vollman RF: Pathfinders 2: Wilhelm Hillebrand, first teacher of the sympto-thermic method. **Int Rev Nat Fam Plann** 1979;3:316–21

**Hiller, Lejaren A., 1880–1969**
Skinner RE: Photography, advertising, and the history of medicine: notes on the medico-historical art of Lejaren a Hiller. **Watermark** 1983 Jan;6(2–3):11–2

**Hinckley, Robert, 1853–**
Vandam LD: Robert Hinckley's 'The First operation with ether' **Anesthesiology** 1980 Jan;52(1):62–70

**Hincks, Clarence Meredith, 1885–1964**
Griffin JD: The amazing careers of Hincks and Beers. **Can J Psychiatry** 1982 Dec;27(8):668–71

**Hinshaw, Horton Corwin, 1902–**
Comroe JH: Pay dirt: the story of streptomycin. Part II. Feldman and Hinshaw; Lehmann. **Am Rev Respir Dis** 1978 May;117(5):957–68

**Hippocrates**
Ammar S: Le message hippocratique à travers la médecine arabe. **Tunis Med** 1981 Nov–Dec;59(6):498–504
Anastassiou A: Zur hippokratischen Schrift De locis in homine und zum Hippokratesglossar des Galen. **Rheinisches Mus Philol** 1982;125:193–201
Atallah W: L'intérêt des traductions arabes dans l'édition des textes hippocratiques. In La collection hippocratique et son rôle dans l'histoire de la médecine. Colloque de Strasbourg (23–27 octobre 1972) organisé par le Centre de Recherches sur la Grèce Antique, avec le concours des Facultés de Philosophie et des Langues Classiques. Leiden, E. J. Brill, 1975. p. 19–33.
Aulizio F: Is the Hippocratic oath still uptodate today? In International Congress of the History of Medicine, 27th, Barcelona, 1980. Actas. Barcelona, Académia de Ciències Médiques de Catalunya i Balears, 1981. p. 441–5.
Azeez Pasha M: Bukhrat (Hippocrates); the most famous physician of Yunan (Greece). **Bull Indian Inst Hist Med (Hyderabad)** 1975 Jul;5(3):129–42
Baruk H: La médecine hebraïque face à la médecine hippocratique. In La collection hippocratique et son rôle dans l'histoire de la médecine. Colloque de Strasbourg (23–27 octobre 1972) organisé par le Centre de Recherches sur la Grèce Antique, avec le concours des Facultés de Philosophie et des Langues Classiques. Leiden, E. J. Brill, 1975. p. 291–303.
Belguedj S: La Collection hippocratique et l'embryologie coranique. In La collection hippocratique et son rôle dans l'histoire de la médecine. Colloque de Strasbourg (23–27 octobre 1972) organisé par le Centre de Recherches sur la Grèce Antique, avec le concours des Facultés de Philosophie et des Langues Classiques. Leiden, E. J. Brill, 1975. p. 321–33.
Bonnabeau RC: Hippocratic medicine. **Minn Med** 1984 Jul;67(7):389–91
Bourgey L, Martiny M: Hippokrates und die griechische Medizin des klassischen Zeitalters. In Sournia JC, Martiny M, Poulet J, ed: Illustrierte Geschichte der Medizin. Salzburg, Andreas, 1980. Vol. 1. p. 301–49.
Boylan M: The Galenic and Hippocratic challenges to Aristotle's conception theory. **J Hist Biol** 1984 Spring;17(1):83–112
Brătescu G: Eléments archaïques dans la médecine hippocratique. In La collection hippocratique et son rôle dans l'histoire de la médecine. Colloque de Strasbourg (23–27 octobre 1972) organisé par le Centre de Recherches sur la Grèce Antique, avec le concours des Facultés de Philosophie et des Langues Classiques. Leiden, E. J. Brill, 1975. 41–9.
Braun L: Paracelse, commentateur des Aphroismes d'Hippocrate. In La collection hippocratique et son rôle dans l'histoire de la médecine. Colloque de Strasbourg (23–27 octobre 1972) organisé par le Centre de Recherches sur la Grèce Antique, avec le concours des Facultés de Philosophie et des Langues Classiques. Leiden, E. J. Brill, 1975. p. 335–46.
Bujałowska B: Recepcja poglądów hipokratesa w polsce na tle dziejów medycyny powszechnej. **Pol Tyg Lek** 1983 Aug 15;38(33–34):1063–6
Buschauer W: Homöopathie als Vollendung der Hippokratischen Medizin. Heidelberg, Haug, 1982. Historical sections, p. 9–79.
Byl S: Note sur huit recentiores du livre IV Du régime. **Rev Philol (Paris)** 1978;52:37–49
Calogirou DK: L'Asclêpieion de Cos, Hippocrate et la maladie des coronaires. **Hist Sci Med** 1979;13(4):427–39
Chantraine P: Remarques sur la langue et le vocabulaire du Corpus Hippocratique. In La collection hippocratique et son rôle dans l'histoire de la médecine. Colloque de Strasbourg (23–27 octobre 1972) organisé par le Centre de Recherches sur la Grèce Antique, avec le concours des Facultés de Philosophie et des Langues Classiques. Leiden, E. J. Brill, 1975. p. 35–40.
David M: Critical edition of Hippocrates' Aphorisms translated into Hebrew by J.S. Delmedigo (1591–1655), sections IV, V. **Koroth** 1979 Nov;7(9–10):680–709
David M: Critical edition of Hippocrates' Aphorisms, translated into Hebrew by J. S. Delmedigo (1591–1655), sections VI–VIII (cont. and end). **Koroth** 1980 Jun;7(11–12):764–94
David M: A case of scleroderma mentioned by Hippocrates in his aphorisms. **Koroth** 1981;8(1–2):61–3
Deichgraber K: Die Patienten des Hippokrates. Historisch-prosopographische Beiträge zu den Epidemien des Corpus Hippocraticum. Mainz, Akademie der Wissenschaften und der Literatur, 1982. 41 p. (Abhandlungen der Geistes- und Sozialwissenschaftlichen Klasse, Jahrgang 1982. Nr. 9).
Deichgräber K: Der hippokratische Eid. Text griechisch und deutsch - Interpretation - Nachleben. 4., erweiterte Auflage. Stuttgart, Hippokrates Verlag, 1983. 92 p.
Di Benedetto V: De la maladie au malade particulier: changement de perspective de la médecine du Ve siècle avant Jésus-Christ. In La collection hippocratique et son rôle dans l'histoire de la médecine. Colloque de Strasbourg (23–27 octobre 1972) organisé par le Centre de Recherches sur la Grèce Antique, avec le concours des Facultés de Philosophie et des Langues Classiques. Leiden, E. J. Brill, 1975. p. 51–5.
Diller H: Das Selbstverständnis der griechischen Medizin in der Zeit des Hippokrates. In La collection hippocratique et son rôle dans l'histoire de la médecine. Colloque de Strasbourg (23–27 octobre 1972) organisé par le Centre de Recherches sur la Grèce Antique, avec le concours des Facultés de Philosophie et des Langues Classiques. Leiden, E. J. Brill, 1975. p. 77–93.
Dimopoulos C, Gialas A, Likourinas M, et al: Hippocrates: founder and pioneer of urology. **Br J Urol** 1980 Apr;52(2):73–4
Ducatillon J: Polémiques dans la collection hippocratique. Lille, Atelier de Reproduction des Thèses; Paris, Librairie Honore Champion, 1977. 382 p. (Thèse, Paris, 1976).
Duffy J: An unnoticed copy of Hippocrates' prognosticon. **Scriptorium** 1982;36(1):89–90
Duffy JM: Stephanus the philosopher: lectures on the Prognosticon of Hippocrates. Critical text and translation. Ph. D. Diss., State University of New York, Buffalo, 1975. xxi, 449 p.
Fleissner RF: Putting Falstaff to rest: 'tabulating' the facts. **Shakespeare Stud** 1983;16:57–74
Foster GM, et al: El legado hipocratico latinoamericano: 'caliente' y 'frio' en la medicina popular contemporanea. **Med Tradic** 1979;2(6):5–24
Galen: On the doctrines of Hippocrates and Plato. Edition, translation and commentary by P De Lacy. Second Part: Books VI–IX. Berlin, Akademie Verlag, 1980. p. 361–609. (Corpus Medicorum Graecorum, V, 4, 1, 2).
Gamberale M: La genealogia de Ippocrate di Cos e gli Asclepiadi di Rodi. **Accad Naz Lincei Rome** 1980, Ser 8;35(1–2):109–16, 119
García-Ballester L: Studies on Hippocrates and Galen in modern Spain. **Trans Stud Coll Physicians Phila** 1979 Sep;5(1 No 3):215–29
Grensemann H: Eine jüngere Schicht in den gynäkologischen Schriften. In La collection hippocratique et son rôle dans l'histoire de la médecine. Colloque de Strasbourg (23–27 octobre 1972) organisé par le Centre de Recherches sur la Grèce Antique, avec le concours des Facultés de Philosophie et des Langues Classiques. Leiden, E. J. Brill, 1975. p. 151–69.
Grensemann H: Das 24. Kapitel von 'De aeribus, aquis, locis' und die Einheit der Schrift. **Hermes** 1979;107:423–41
Grensemann H, ed: Hippokratische Gynäkologie. Die gynäkologischen Texte des Autors C nach den pseudohippokratischen Schriften De muliebribus I, II, und De sterilibus. Wiesbaden, Steiner, 1982. 191 p.
Grmek MD: La réalité nosologique au temps d'Hippocrate. In La collection hippocratique et son rôle dans l'histoire de la médecine. Colloque de Strasbourg (23–27 octobre 1972) organisé par le Centre de Recherches sur la Grèce Antique, avec le concours des Facultés de Philosophie et des Langues Classiques. Leiden, E. J. Brill, 1975. p. 239–55.
Grmek MD, ed: Hippocratica. Actes du Colloque hippocratique de Paris (4–9 septembre 1978). Paris, Editions du Centre National de la Recherche Scientifique, 1980. 486 p. (Colloques Internationaux du C.N.R.S., No. 583). Contributions by A. Anastassiou, J. Benedum, J. Bertier, L. Bourgey, G. Brătescu, S. Byl, G. Cambiano, V. Di

Benedetto, J. Ducatillon, M. P. Duminil, L. Garcia-Ballester, D. Gourevitch, H. Grensemann, G. Harig, J. Irigoin, C. Irmer, D. Irmer, R. Joly, J. Jouanna, H. M. Koelbing, V. Langholf, C. Lichtenthaeler, G. Maloney, W. Frohn Villeneuve, J. Mansfeld, P. Manuli, P. Mudry, J. M. Pigeaud, C. Sandulesco, W. D. Smith, A. Thivel, M. Vegetti.

Hanson AE: Hippocrates: Diseases of women. 1. **Signs** 1975;1:567–84

Harig G, Kollesch J: Der hippokratische Eid. **Philologus** 1978;122:157–76

Harig G, Kollesch J: Galen und Hippokrates. In La collection hippocratique et son rôle dans l'histoire de la médecine. Colloque de Strasbourg (23–27 octobre 1972) organisé par le Centre de Recherches sur la Grèce Antique, avec le concours des Facultés de Philosophie et des Langues Classiques. Leiden, E. J. Brill, 1975. p. 257–74.

Hippocrates. Ueber die Krankheiten, III, herausgegeben, übersetzt und erläutert von Paul Potter. Berlin, Akademie Verlag, 1980. 150 p. (Corpus medicorum Graecorum, I, 2, 3). Includes Greek text.

Hippocrates: La nature de l'homme. Edité, traduit, et commenté par Jacques Jouanna. Berlin, Akademie Verlag, 1975. 331 p. (Corpus medicorum Graecorum, I, 1, 3). Includes Greek text.

Hippokrates: Ueber Nachempfängnis, Geburtshilfe, und Schwangerschaftsleiden. Herausgegeben, übersetzt und erläutert von C. Lienau. Berlin, Akademie Verlag, 1973. 143 p. (Corpus Medicorum Graecorum, I, 2, 2).

Irigoin J: Tradition manuscrite et histoire du texte. Quelques problèmes relatifs à la collection hippocratique. In La collection hippocratique et son rôle dans l'histoire de la médecine. Colloque de Strasbourg (23–27 octobre 1972) organisé par le Centre de Recherches sur la Grèce Antique, avec le concours des Facultés de Philosophie et des Langues Classiques. Leiden, E. J. Brill, 1975. p. 3–18.

Joly R: Hippocrates and the school of Cos. Between myth and skepticism. In M. Ruse, ed: Nature animated. Historical and philosophical case studies in Greek medicine, nineteenth-century and recent biology, psychiatry, and psychoanalysis. Volume II. Dordrecht, D. Reidel, 1983. p. 29–47.

Jouanna J: Une forme étymologique retrouvée: omelesis dans le Glossaire hippocratique de Galien et dans le traité hippocratique des Maladies II c, 31. **Rev Philol (Paris)** 1979;53:260–63

Jouanna J: Le traité hippocratique du Régime dans les maladies aiguës: remarques sur la tradition manuscrite et sur le texte. **Rev Hist Textes (Paris)** 1976;6:1–30

Kessel AH: Notes on ps.-Hippocrates De medico. **Mnemosyne** 1978;31:113–33

Kibre P: Hippocrates latinus: repertorium of Hippocratic writings in the Latin Middle Ages. **Traditio** 1977;33:253–95; 1978;34:193–226

Kibre P: Hippocrates latinus: repertorium of Hippocratic writings in the Latin Middle Ages (VIII). **Traditio** 1982;38:169–71

Kibre P: Hippocrates latinus: repertorium of Hippocratic writings in the Latin Middle Ages. (VI). **Traditio** 1980;36:347–72

Kibre P: Hippocrates latinus: repertorium of Hippocratic writings in the Latin Middle Ages (VII). **Zwingliana** 1981;37:267–89

Kozlov AM, Kozlov IA: Filosofskie vzgliady Gippokrata. **Klin Med (Mosk)** 1983 May;61(5):111–5

Kozlov AM: Kliatva Gippokrata i ee vliianie na razvitie vrachebnoĭ étiki. **Sov Med** 1983;(3):79–82

Krakovetskaia GA: Gigienicheskie i lechebnye printsipy antichnoĭ meditsiny. **Gig Sanit** 1984 May;(5):37–40

Kudlien F: Die Bedeutung des Ungeraden in der hippokratischen Krisenarithmetik. **Hermes** 1980;180:200–5

Lain-Entralgo P: Quaestiones hippocraticae disputatae tres. In La collection hippocratique et son rôle dans l'histoire de la médecine. Colloque de Strasbourg (23–27 octobre 1972) organisé par le Centre de Recherches sur la Grèce Antique, avec le concours des Facultés de Philosophie et des Langues Classiques. Leiden, E. J. Brill, 1975. p. 305–19.

Laín Entralgo P: Relieves hipocráticos. **Med Hist (Barc)** 1984;1:1–16

Lebel M: Editions, traductions et lexiques hippocratiques. Le docteur Louis Morin, (1635–1715) et son index des mots d'Hippocrate. In: Congrès international d'histoire de la médecine, XXVe, Québec, 1976. Actes. Québec, 1977. p. 848–65.

Leebron WM: Reflections on Hippocrates. **Am J Proctol Gastroenterol Colon Rectal Surg** 1982 Jun;33(6):7–8, 24

Lichtenthaeler C: Le serment d'Hippocrate: analyse d'ensemble. **Rev Med Suisse Romande** 1980 Dec;100(12):1001 11

Lichtenthaeler C: Chronologische und gedankliche Bezugssysteme in und um 'Ueber die alte Medizin'. XI. Hippokratische Studie. Genève, Droz, 1980. 30 p. (Etudes d'histoire de la médecine, VI).

Lloyd GE: Hippocratic problems. **Classical Rev** 1980;30(2):186–9

Lonie IM: Hippocrates the iatromechanist. **Med Hist** 1981 Apr;25(2):113–50

Lonie IM: The Hippocratic treatises: 'On Generation', 'On the Nature of the Child', 'Diseases IV'. A commentary. Berlin, New York, Walter de Gruyter, 1981. xxxix, 406 p. (Ars medica. II. Abteilung, Griechisch-lateinische Medizin; Bd. 7, 2).

López Férez JA: Algunos datos sobre la influencia de la teoria embriologica de Democrito en el corpus hippocraticum. Gemelos y abortos. **Asclepio** 1981;33:379–90

Maloney G: Les particules dans trois traités d'Hippocrate. In: Mélanges d'études anciennes offerts à Maurice Lebel. St-Jean-Chrysostôme, Québec, 1980. p. 125–34.

Mansfeld J: The historical Hippocrates and the origins of scientific medicine. In M. Ruse, ed: Nature animated. Historical and philosophical case studies in Greek medicine, nineteenth-century and recent biology, psychiatry, and psychoanalysis. Volume II. Dordrecht, D. Reidel, 1983. p. 49–76.

Marketos SG, Ballas CN: Bronchial asthma in the medical literature of Greek antiquity. **J Asthma** 1982;19(4):263–9

Müller CW: Die hippokratischen Schriften. In his: Gleiches zu Gleichem. Ein Prinzip frühgriechischen Denkens. Wiesbaden, Harrassowitz, 1965. p. 112–50. (Klassisch-philologische Studien, 31).

Müller-Rohlfsen I: Die lateinische Ravennatische Uebersetzung der hippokratischen Aphorismen aus dem 5./6. Jahrhundert n. Chr. Textkonstitution auf der Basis der Uebersetzungscodices. Hamburg, Lüdke, 1980. xlviii, 162 p. (Geistes- und Sozialwissenschaftliche Dissertationen, 55).

Ohry A: Respiratory items in Hippocratic medicine. **Koroth** 1980 Jun;7(11–12):CCLXXXV–CCLXLII

Pfohl G: Humanitas Hippocratica. **ZFA (Stuttgart)** 1983 Dec 20;59(35–36):1943–54

Pines S: The oath of Asaph the Physician and Yohanan Ben Zabda: Its relation to the Hippocratic Oath and the Doctrina duarum viarium of the Didaché. **Proc Isr Acad Sci Humanit** 1971–76;5:223–64

Pritchet CD, ed: Iohannis Alexandrini Commentaria in sextum librum Hippocratis Epidemiarum. Leiden, Brill, 1975. xi, 470 p.

Reif AE: Hippocrates and the biomedical scientist: the problems of controlling the dangers of science. **Minerva** 1980 Spring;18(1):29–50

Robert F: Hippocrate, Platon, Aristote et les notions de genre et d'espèce. **Hist Philos Life Sci** 1982;4(2):173–201

Sakula A: In search of Hippocrates: a visit to Kos. **J R Soc Med** 1984 Aug;77(8):682–8

Sandulescu C: Primum non nocere: philological commentaries on a medical aphorism. **Acta Antiq Hung** 1965;13:359–368

Simon I: L'influence hippocratique sur la médecine hébraique, surtout chez Assaph, Isaac Israèli et Maimonide. In La collection hippocratique et son rôle dans l'histoire de la médecine. Colloque de Strasbourg (23–27 octobre 1972) organisé par le Centre de Recherches sur la Grèce Antique, avec le concours des Facultés de Philosophie et des Langues Classiques. Leiden, E. J. Brill, 1975. 275–89.

Sorokina TS: Gippokrat i 'Gippokratov sbornik'. **Feldsher Akush** 1984 Mar;49(3):51–5

Sow M: Des couleurs dans quelques traités de la collection hippocratique. Univ. de Strasbourg, Thèse de 3e cycle, 1979. lxiv, 402 p.

Strohmaier G: Der arabische Hippokrates. Bemerkungen zu einem Aufsatz von Dieter Irmer. **Sudhoffs Arch** 1980;64(3):234–49

Thivel A: Cnide et Cos? Essai sur les doctrines médicales dans la collection hippocratique. Paris, Les Belles Lettres, 1981. 435 p. (Publications de la Faculté des Lettres et des Sciences Humaines de Nice, 21).

Thivel A: Le 'divin' dans la Collection hippocratique. In La collection hippocratique et son rôle dans l'histoire de la médecine. Colloque de Strasbourg (23–27 octobre 1972) organisé par le Centre de Recherches sur la Grèce Antique, avec le concours des Facultés de Philosophie et des Langues Classiques. Leiden, E. J. Brill, 1975. p. 57–76.

Vasilenko VKh: Metod Gippokrata. **Klin Med (Mosk)** 1983 Oct;61(10):3–12

Vetter T: Essai sur la littérature hippocratique au dix-huitième siècle. In La collection hippocratique et son rôle dans l'histoire de la médecine. Colloque de Strasbourg (23–27 octobre 1972) organisé par le Centre de Recherches sur la Grèce Antique, avec le concours des Facultés de Philosophie et des Langues Classiques. Leiden, E. J. Brill, 1975. p. 347–67.

Warren JV: Hippocrates--man and legend. **Forum Med** 1978 May;1(2):18–9

Weisser U: Die hippokratische Lehre von den Siebenmonatskindern bei Galen und Tabit ibn Qurra. **Sudhoffs Arch** 1979;63(3):209–38

Whitteridge G: The Piltdown Hippocrates. **Hist Sci** 1980 Sep;18(41 pt 3):226–30

**Hirsch, August, 1817–1894**

Wagner D: Zu August Hirschs epidemiologischer Reise an die Wolga im Jahre 1879 (ein Beispiel russisch-deutscher Zusammenarbeit auf medizinischem Gebiet. **Z Gesamte Hyg** 1980;26(5):377–8

**Hirsch, Max, 1877–1948**

Schneck P: Max Hirsch (1877–1948)--der Mitbegründer der sozialgynäkologischen Forschungrichtung. **Zentralbl Gynakol** 1983;105(24):1600–4

**Hirsch, Oskar, 1877–1965**

Hamlin H: Oskar Hirsch. **Surg Neurol** 1981 Dec;16(6):391–3

McMurry JF: Oskar Hirsch and surgery for exophthalmos. In Romm S, ed: Symposium on historical perspectives of plastic surgery. Philadelphia, Saunders, 1983. p. 649–52.

**Hirsch, Samson Raphael, 1890–1960**

Schultze-Werninghaus G, Meier-Sydow J: The clinical and pharmacological history of theophylline: first report on the bronchospasmolytic action in man by S. R. Hirsch in Frankfurt (Main) 1922. **Clin Allergy** 1982 Mar;12(2):211–5

**Hirschberg, Julius, 1843–1925**
Hirschberg J: The history of ophthalmology. Translated from the German edition of 1899–1918 by F. C. Blodi. 11 vols. Bonn, Wayenborgh, 1982.
Snyder C: Julius Hirschberg, the neglected historian of ophthalmology. **Am J Ophthalmol** 1981 May;91(5):664–76

**Hirschfeld, J.**
Hirschfeld J: The discovery of the Gc system. **Vox Sang** 1984;46(2):122–4

**Hirschhorn, Thomas, 1410?–1493**
Senger HG: Thomas Hirschhorn: ein Magdeburger Gelehrter des 15. Jahrhunderts. **Hist Jahrb** 1980;100:217–39

**Hirschsprung, Harald, 1830–1916**
Frenckner B: Pionjär för pediatrisk forskning - omtyckt kliniker, mindre värderad föreläsare. **Lakartidningen** 1983 Nov 30;80(48):4664–5
Roed-Petersen K, Madsen CM: Harald Hirschsprung (1830–1916). **Dan Medicinhist Arbog** 1980;:182–99

**Hirshman, Louis Jacob, 1878–1965**
Edgar II: Dr. Louis Jacob Hirshman. **Mich Jew Hist** 1980;20(2):5–10

**Hirszfeld, Ludwig, 1884–1954**
Kucharz E, Stawiarska B: Zycie I Działalność Ludwika Maurycego Hirszfelda. **Wiad Lek** 1982 May 1;35(3–4):261–6
Supady J: Serologia nowotworów w badaniach Ludwika Hirszfelda i jego współpracowników w okresie II Rzeczypospolitej. **Wiad Lek** 1981 Feb 1;34(3):257–62

**His, Wilhelm, Sr., 1831–1904**
Wendler D, Rother P: Wilhelm His sen.--Leben und Wirken des bedeutenden Leipziger Morphologen. **Z Gesamte Inn Med** 1982 Dec;37(23):810–3

**Hispanus, Pedro, b. ca. 1210**
Reis CS, Jans GJ: Sessão comemorativa do 7.o centenário de Pedro Hispano -- 20 de Maio de 1977. **An Inst Hig Med Trop (Lisb)** 1977–1978;5(1–4):3–19

**Hitchcock, Edward, 1828–1911**
Welch JE: Pioneering in health education and services at Amherst College. **J Am Coll Health** 1982 Jun;30(6):289–95

**Hitchcock, Fred A., 1889–1980**
Dean JB: A retrospective look through the camera of Fred A. Hitchcock. **Physiologist** 1984 Jun;27(3):128–30

**Hitler, Adolf, 1889–1945**
Adelman H: Hitler and Gandhi: the will as spirit and as flesh. **Psychoanal Rev** 1980 Winter;67(4):543–61
Ebon M: Why did Hitler hate the Jews? **Midstream** 1979;25(8):19–24
Favazza AR: Hitler's encephalitis? **Am J Psychiatry** 1981 Jul;138(7):999–1000
Favazza AR: Behind the sickness of Hitler. **MD** 1981;25(5):37–8;25(7):15
Heston LL, Heston R: The medical casebook of Adolf Hitler: his illnesses, doctors, and drugs. New York, Stein and Day, 1980. 184 p.
Katz O: Prof. Dr. Med. Theo Morell: Hitlers Leibarzt. Bayreuth, Hestia, 1983. 397 p.
Katz O: Der 'Führer' behandelte sich selbst. Aus jetzt verfügbaren Aufzeichnungen des Leibarztes Theo Morell werden realistische Konturen der geheimnisvollen Krankheiten Adolf Hitlers erkennbar (I). **Fortschr Med** 1984 Oct 4;102(37):70–1
Kenéz J: Hitler patográfiája. Gastrointestinalis panaszok (carcinophobia). **Orv Hetil** 1983 Apr 3;124(14):835–6
Lekisch K: Drugs and politics. **Scalpel Tongs** 1981;25:93–4
Lieberman AN: Adolph Hitler: his diaries and Parkinson's disease. **N Engl J Med** 1983 Aug 11;309(6):375–6
Schöllgen G: Das Problem einer Hitler-Biographie. **Neue Polit Lit** 1978;23(4):421–34
Sognnaes RF: Hitler and Bormann identifications compared by postmortem craniofacial and dental characteristics. **Am J Forensic Med Pathol** 1980 Jun;1(2):105–15
Spann W: Prof. Dr. med. Theo Morell, Hitlers Leibarzt. **MMW** 1983 Jun 17;125(24):534–6
Waite RG: The psychopathic god - Adolf Hitler. New York, Basic Books, 1977. xx, 482 p.

**Hitler, Eva Braun, d. 1945**
Keiser-Nielsen S, Strøm F: The odontological identification of Eva Braun Hitler. **Forensic Sci Int** 1983 Jan–Feb;21(1):59–64

**Hjorth, Niels, 1919–**
Curriculum vitae and writings: Niels Hjorth.: **Acta Derm Venereol [Suppl] (Stockh)** 1979;59(85):5–9

**Hlava, Jaroslav, 1855–1924**
Fingerland A: Iaroslav Glava--osnovatel' chekhoslovatskoĭ shkoly patologoanatomov. **Arkh Patol** 1981;43(10):62–6

**Hobbes, Thomas, 1588–1679**
Heyd D: The place of laughter in Hobbes's theory of emotions. **J Hist Ideas** 1982 Apr–Jun;43(2):285–95

**Hochberg, Julian Edward, 1923–**
Distinguished scientific contribution awards for 1978 (Julian Hochberg, Philip Teitelbaum, Robert B. Zajonc).: **Am Psychol** 1979 Jan;34(1):35–47

**Hodgkin, Dorothy, 1910–**
Cornforth J: Portrait of Dorothy Hodgkin, O.M., F.R.S. **Notes Rec R Soc Lond** 1982 Aug;37(1):1–4
Dodson G, Glusker JP, Sayre D, ed: Structural studies on molecules of biological interest. A volume in honour of Professor Dorothy Hodgkin. Oxford, Clarendon, 1981. xviii, 610 p. Historical and biographical chapters by M. F. Perutz, D. Phillips, D. P. Riley, F. Welch, C. H. Carlisle, L. Pauling, T. You-chi, J. H. Robertson, D. F. Steiner, J. G. White, J. D. Dunitz.

**Hodgkin, Thomas, 1798–1866**
Björkholm M: Mannen bakom syndromet: Thomas Hodgkin. Temperamentsfull föregångare inom patologin och kämpe för rättvisa åt förtryckta folk. **Lakartidningen** 1983 Feb 2;80(5):334–5
Geller SA: Comments on the anniversary of the description of Hodgkin's disease. **J Natl Med Assoc** 1984 Aug;76(8):815–7
Kass AM, Kass EH: Doctors afield. Martin Delany, Thomas Hodgkin, and the Black Nationalist movement. **N Engl J Med** 1981 Sep 17;305(12):682–4
Kass AM: Dr Thomas Hodgkin, Dr Martin Delany, and the 'Return to Africa'. **Med Hist** 1983 Oct;27(4):373–93
Kass AM: Dr. Thomas Hodgkin's friendship with Sir Moses Montefiore. **N Engl J Med** 1984 Feb 9;310(6):401–4
Kass EH, Carey AB, Kass AM: Thomas Hodgkin and Benjamin Harrison: crisis and promotion in academia. **Med Hist** 1980 Apr;24(2):197–208
Nuland SB: The lymphatic contiguity of Hodgkin's disease: a historical study. **Bull NY Acad Med** 1981 Nov;57(9):776–86
Rose M: Curator of the dead: Thomas Hodgkin (1798–1866). London, Owen, 1981 148 p.
Sakula A: Dr. Thomas Hodgkin and Sir Moses Montefiore Bart--the friendship of two remarkable men. **J R Soc Med** 1979 May;72(5):382–7

**Hodgson, Shadworth Hollway, 1832–1912**
High RP: Shadworth Hodgson and William James's formulation of space perception: phenomenology and perceptual realism. **J Hist Behav Sci** 1981 Oct;17(4):466–85

**Hoernigk, Ludwig von, 1600–1667**
Mäder M: Ludwig von Hoernigk: Arzt, Jurist und Bücherkommissar im 17. Jahrhundert. Diss. Bern, 1984. 77 p.

**Hoerr, Normand Louis, 1902–1958**
Bodian D: Normand Louis Hoerr. In Dictionary of American Biography, Suppl. 6, 1956–1960. p. 295–6, 1980.

**Hoff, August, d. 1887**
Johnson A: August Hoff--a Sydney dermatologist of the 1880's. **Australas J Dermatol** 1983 Apr;24(1):37–9

**Hoffa, Albert J., 1859–1907**
Paul U: Das chirurgische Erbe. Albert Hoffa. **Zentralbl Chir** 1981;106(13):901–3

**Hoffmann, Ernst Theodor Amadeus, 1776–1822**
Segebrecht W: Krankheit und Gesellschaft. Zu E.T.A. Hoffmanns Rezeption der Bamberger Medizin. **Dtsch Vierteljahresschr Lit Wiss Geistesgesch** 1978;:267–90

**Hoffmann, Friedrich, 1660–1742**
Duchesneau F: Le système mécaniste de Friedrich Hoffmann. **Arch Int Hist Idees** 1982;95:32–64
Lonie IM: Hippocrates the iatromechanist. **Med Hist** 1981 Apr;25(2):113–50
Scherrer RM: Friedrich Hoffmanns Anweisung zu gesundem langen Leben, verglichen mit Hufelands Makrobiotik. Zürich, Juris, 1984. 47 p. (Zürcher Medizingeschichtliche Abhandlungen, Neue Reihe, Nr. 170)

**Hoffmann, Karl Friedrich, fl. 1761**
Olagüe de Ros G: La epidemia europea de gripe de 1708–1709. Difusión témporo-espacial e interpretaciones contemporáneas: G. M. Lancisi, B. Ramazzini, K. F. Hoffmann. **Dynamis** 1981;1:51–86

**Hogan, Helen**
Pediatric nurse pioneers (Helen Hogan): **Am J Nurs** 1980;80:2084

**Hogarth, William, 1697–1764**
Rodin AE: Infants and gin mania in 18th-century London. **JAMA** 1981 Mar 27;245(12):1237–9

**Hogenberg, Remigius, ca. 1536–**
Corbett M: The emblematic title-page to Stirpium Adversaria nova by Petro Pena and Mathias de L'Obel (1570). **Arch Nat Hist** 1981 Apr;10(1):111–7

**Högyes, Endre, 1847–1906**
Szállási A: Högyes Endre pesti kinevezésének centenáriuma. **Orv Hetil** 1983 Oct 30;124(44):2691–3

**Holbein, Hans, the Elder, ca. 1465–1524**
Roth W: Differentialdiagnostische Erwägungen zu den Hauteffloreszenzen, dargestellt auf dem Sebastiansaltar Hans Holbeins d. A. **Hautarzt** 1980 Dec;31(12):662–4
Virchow R: A painting of lepers by Hans Holbein the Elder. **Am J Dermatopathol** 1984 Aug;6(4):377–8

**Holcombe, Henry Woodruff, 1897–1973**
Holcombe HW: Patent medicine tax stamps. A history of the firms using United States private die proprietary medicine tax stamps. Ed. G. B. Griffenhagen. Lawrence, Quarterman, 1979. xxv, 604 p. Reprinted articles from various journals.

**Holden, Henry Smith, 1887–1963**
Walls HJ: Henry Smith Holden. In Dictionary of national biography, 1961–1970. Suppl. 8, 1981. p. 524–5.

**Hölderlin, Friedrich, 1770–1843**
Bertaux P: Der Wandel der Auffassungen über Hölderlins Krankheit. War Hölderlin geisteskrank? **Med Welt** 1980 Mar 28;31(13):486–90
Fichtner G: Psychiatrie zur Zeit Hölderlins: Ausstellung anlässlich der 63. Jahrestagung der Deutschen Gesellschaft für Geschichte der Medizin, der Naturwissenschaften und Technik in Tübingen, Universitätsbibliothek Tübingen, Bonatzbau 27. September bis 30. Oktober 1980. Tübingen, Universitätsbibliothek, 1980. 99 p.
Peters UH: Hölderlin: Dichter, Kranker--Simulant? **Nervenarzt** 1981 May;52(5):261–8

**Hole, John, 1755–1813**
Houser HR: Wilderness doctor: the life and times of Dr. John Hole. [Centerville, Ohio], Centerville Historical Society, 1980. 32 p.

**Hollaender, Alexander, 1898–**
Fuller MB: Alexander Hollaender Papers (1898– ). **Mendel Newsl** 1984;(24):5–7

**Holland, Eardley Lancelot, 1879–1967**
Peel J: Sir Eardley Lancelot Holland. In Dictionary of national biography, 1961–1970. Suppl. 8, 1981. p. 525–7.

**Holland, Henry Tristram, 1875–1965**
Trevor-Roper PD: Sir Henry Tristram Holland. In Dictionary of national biography, 1961–1970. Suppl. 8, 1981. p. 528–9.

**Holliday, John Henry, 1851–1887**
Barber DN: Doc Holliday, the wildest dentist of the West. **Probe (Lond)** 1984 Mar;25(9):301–2

**Hollier, Thomas, 1609–1690**
Morris GC: A portrait of Thomas Hollier, Pepy's surgeon. **Ann R Coll Surg Engl** 1979 May;61(3):224–9

**Hollós, István, 1872–1957**
Hárdi I: Hollós István (születésének 110-ik évfordulójára). **Orv Hetil** 1982 Dec 12;123(50):3099–100

**Holloway, Thomas, 1800–**
Tring FC: Thomas Holloway and his patent pills. **Pharm Hist (London)** 1977 Dec;7(3):4–5

**Holman, Emile Frederic, 1890–1977**
Olch PD: Some comments on the life of Emile Frederic Holman (1890–1977). **Bull Am Coll Surg** 1981;66(3):22–5

**Holmer, Carl Magnus, 1782–1848**
Stolt CM, Oberg L: En ovariotomi i Borås 1814. **Sydsven Medicinhist Sallsk Arsskr** 1984;21:109–21

**Holmes, Bayard Taylor, 1852–1924**
Beatty WK: Bayard Taylor Holmes--a forgotten man. **Proc Inst Med Chic** 1981 Oct–Dec;34(4):120–3

**Holmes, Edward Morell, 1843–1930**
Shellard EJ: Jaborandi: a note on the contribution of E. M. Holmes to the identification of commercially available Pilocarpus and species. **J Ethnopharmacol** 1979 Dec;1(4):407–10

**Holmes, Gordon Morgan, 1876–1965**
Lepore FE: Neuro-ophthalmology according to Gordon Holmes. **Neurol Clin** 1983 Nov;1(4):789–805
Parsons-Smith BG: Sir Gordon Holmes. In Rose FC, Bynum WF, ed: Historical aspects of the neurosciences. New York, Raven, 1982. p. 357–70.
Penfield W: Sir Gordon Morgan Holmes. In Dictionary of national biography, 1961–1970. Suppl. 8, 1981. p. 534–6.

**Holmes, Oliver Wendell, 1809–1894**
Cash P: Pride, prejudice and politics. **Harv Med Alumni Bull** 1980 Dec;54(6):20–5
Kurth RT, Kurth DJ: Oliver Wendell Holmes, M.D. (1809–1894); medical and literary knowledge intertwined. **NY State J Med** 1980 Jan;80(1):121–4
Schneck JM: S. Weir Mitchell and Oliver Wendell Holmes. A friendship and poetic tribute. **JAMA** 1981 Aug 28;246(9):974–8
Warren R: Oliver Wendell Holmes, H.M.S. '36. **Harv Med Alumni Bull** 1982 Spring;56(2):20–6
White PJ: Medical Leonardo of Boston, Oliver Wendell Holmes, M.D. (1809–1894): an evaluation of versatility. **Perspect Biol Med** 1981 Spring;24(3):411–21

**Holst, Frederik, 1791–1871**
Thuen H: 'Ad denne rent mekaniske vej ...': da tanken om hospitalisering av de sinnssvake kom til Norge. **Hist Tidsskr** 1982;61(4):313–32

**Holter, Norman Jefferis, 1914–1983**
Roberts WC, Silver MA: Norman Jefferis Holter and ambulatory ECG monitoring. **Am J Cardiol** 1983 Oct 1;52(7):903–6

**Holzkamp, Klaus**
Van Ijzendoorn MH, Van der Veer R: Holzkamp's critical psychology and the functional-historical method: a critical appraisal. **Stor Crit Psicol** 1983;4(1):5–26

**Home, Everard, 1756–1832**
Carrillo JL, Olagüe G: La enseñanza de la anatomia comparada en la Inglaterra de comienzos del siglo XIX: a proposito de las Lectures de Everard Home (1756–1832). **Asclepio** 1978–79;30–31:83–8

**Homer**
Grmek M: La vita, la morte, la malattia nel mondo di Omero. **Intersezioni** 1983;3:243–64
Kerkhoff AH: Homerus Herbarius. **Janus** 1980:67(1–2–3):187–90

**Hoobler, Icie Gertrude Macy, 1892–1984**
Hoobler IG: Boundless horizons. Portrait of a pioneer woman scientist. Smithtown, N. Y., Exposition Press, 1982. 197 p.
Williams HH: Icie Gertrude Macy Hoobler (1892–1984). A biographical sketch. **J Nutr** 1984 Aug;114(8):1351–62

**Hood, Arthur James, 1880?–1958**
Myles J, Green E, Hood TK, et al: The doctor who never refused a call: [Arthur James] Hood, M.D. **Northeast Nev Hist Soc Q** 1980;(2):43–58

**Hood, G. J.**
Ketchum LD: An historical account of the development of the calibrated dermatome. **Ann Plast Surg** 1978 Nov;1(6):608–11

**Hood, Humphrey H., d. 1903**
Gegenheimer E: Selected letters of Humphrey Hood, Litchfield physician. **J Ill State Hist Soc** 1979;72:193–212, 243–56

**Hoodless, David Winn**
Guthrie MW: Misi Utu, Dr. D. W. Hoodless and the development of medical education in the South Pacific. Suva, Fiji Institute of Pacific Studies, 1979. vi, 60 p.

**Hooke, Robert, 1635–1703**
Oldroyd DR: Some 'philosophical scribbles' attributed to Robert Hooke. **Notes Rec R Soc Lond** 1980 Jul;35(1):17–32
Pugliese P: The scientific achievement of Robert Hooke: method and mechanics. Ph.D. Diss., Harvard University. Cambridge, 1982. xv, 353 leaves. (Pt. 1).

**Hooker, Worthington, 1806–1867**
Musto DF: Worthington Hooker (1806–1867): physician and educator. **Conn Med** 1984 Sep;48(9):569–74
Young JH: 'The foolmaster who fooled them'. **Yale J Biol Med** 1980 Nov–Dec;53(6):555–66

**Hooper, Philo Oliver, 1833–1902**
Henker FO, Shorey JJ: Dr. P. O. Hooper--father of Arkansas medicine. **J Arkansas Med Soc** 1981 Oct;78(5):189–92

**Hoover, Herbert, 1874–1964**
Giglio JN: Voluntarism and public policy between World War I and the New Deal: Herbert Hoover and the American Child Health Association. **Pres Stud Q** 1983;13(3):430–52
Guth JL: Herbert Hoover, the U. S. Food Administration, and the dairy industry, 1917–1918. **Bus Hist Rev** 1981;55(2):170–87
Johnson JP: Herbert Hoover and David Copperfield: a tale of two childhoods. **J Psychohist** 1980 Spring;7(4):467–75
Johnson JP: Herbert Hoover: the orphan as children's friend. **Prologue J Nat Arch** 1980;12(4):193–206

**Hope, Thomas Charles, 1766–1844**
Doyle WP: Thomas Charles Hope M.D., F.R.S.E., F.R.S. (1766–1844). Edinburgh, University of Edinburgh, 1982. [12 p.] (Scottish Men of Science).

**Hora, Seki, d. 1980?**
Bessho C: [Life of Mrs. Seki Hora, the founder of Japanese public health nursing] (Jpn). **Kango** 1980 Jun;32(6):112–20

**Horemans, Jan Josef, 1682–1859**
Rubin LP: A young woman taken to the doctor by her family. Mezzotint by Johann Andreas Pfeffel after an original painting by Jan Josef Horemans. **J Hist Med Allied Sci** 1981 Oct;36(4):489

**Hörmann, Hans, 1924–1983**
Bosshardt HG: Hans Hörmann (1924–1983). **Arch Psychol (Frankf)** 1983;135(3):163–73

**Horner, Friedrich, 1831–1886**
Ott E: Friedrich Horner, 1831–1886, Leben und Werk. Zürich, Juris, 1980. 54 p. (Zürcher Medizingeschichtliche Abhandlungen, Neue Reihe Nr. 136).

**Horner, Otte E. Friedrich, 1831–1886**
Mannen bakom syndromet: Friedrich Horner. Först att införa antiseptisk behandling i ögonsjukvården. **Lakartidningen** 1984 Mar 21;81(12):1165–7

**Horner, William Edmonds, 1793–1853**
D'Amato NA: William Edmonds Horner: anatomist, educator, author. **Va Med** 1982 Mar;109(3):209–10

**Horney, Karen, 1885–1952**
Buckley NL: Women psychoanalysts and the theory of feminine development: a study of Karen Horney, Helene Deutsch, and Marie

Bonaparte. Ph.D. Diss., University of California. Los Angeles, 1982. 178 p.
Garrison D: Karen Horney and feminism. **Signs** 1981;6(4):672–91
Horney theory and literature: a symposium: **Am J Psychoanal** 1982 Spring;42(1):3–59
Rubins JL: Karen Danielson Horney. In: Notable American women. The modern period. Cambridge, Mass., Belknap-Harvard Univ. Press, 1980. 4:351–4.
Zimmerman J: Transcendent psychology: Erik H. Erikson, Erich Fromm, Karen Horney, Abraham H. Maslow, and Harry Stack Sullivan and the quest for a healthy humanity. Ph.D. Diss., Northwestern University. Evanston, 1982. vi, 498 p.

**Hornschuch, Christian Friedrich, 1793–1850**
Scheele I: Zur Typologie des Botanikers in der ersten Hälfte des 19. Jahrhunderts: Christian Friedrich Hornschuch. **Medizinhist J** 1983;18(3):184–97

**Horsfield, Thomas, 1773–1859**
Ewan J: Five pupils of Benjamin Smith Barton: the men and their minds. **Trans Stud Coll Physicians Phila** 1983 Dec;5(5 no 4):309–20

**Horsley, Victor Alexander Haden, 1857–1916**
Beneš V, Benešová Z: Horsleyv vosk. **Rozhl Chir** 1982 Feb;61(2):141–3
Cooper IS: Sir Victor Horsley: father of modern neurological surgery. In Rose FC, Bynum WF, ed: Historical aspects of the neurosciences. New York, Raven, 1982. p. 235–8.
Walker JB: Charles John Bond of Leicester (1856–1939). **J R Soc Med** 1984 Apr;77(4):316–24

**Horton, Bayard Taylor, 1895–**
Ekbom K, Waldenlind E: Mannen bakom syndromet: Bayard T. Horton. En pionjär inom huvudvärksforskningen. **Lakartidningen** 1982 Sep 15;79(37):3187

**Horwitz, Abraham B., 1910–**
Neghme A: La organización panamericana de la salud en su 75. aniversario. Tributo al Dr. Abraham B. Horwitz. **Rev Med Chil** 1977 Dec;105(12):950–2

**Hotman, François, 1524–1590**
Secret F: Un document oublié sur François Hotman et l'alchimie. **Bibl Hum Renaissance** 1980 May;42(2):435–46

**Houdé, Alfred, 1854–1919**
Gaignault JC: Alfred Houdé. Un bel exemple de fondateur d'une industrie pharmaceutique française au XIXe siècle. **Bull Ordre Natl Pharm** 1980 Dec;239:1816–26

**Houdry, Eugene Jules, 1892–1962**
Stine JK: Eugene Jules Houdry. In Dictionary of American biography, 1961–1965. Suppl. 7, 1981. p. 367–9.

**Houghton, John, 1645–1705**
O'Rourke DT: John Houghton (1645–1705) Journalist, apothecary and F.R.S. **Pharm Hist (London)** 1979 Apr;9(1):2–3

**Houssay, Bernardo Alberto, 1887–1971**
Foglia VG: The history of Bernardo A. Houssay's research laboratory, Instituto de Biologia y Medicina Experimental: the first twenty years, 1944–1963. **J Hist Med Allied Sci** 1980 Oct;35(4):380–96
Pasqualini RQ: Houssay y el serendipismo. **Medicina (B Aires)** 1981;41(6):827–30

**Houstěk, Josef, 1913–**
Hrodek O, Kubát K: Akademik Josef Houštěk sedmdesátiletý. **Cesk Pediatr** 1983 Aug;38(8):496–9

**Howard, Henry, 1815–1887**
Samuel R: Henry Howard. In Dictionary of Canadian biography, 1881–1890. 1982;11:425–6.

**Howard, Robert Palmer, 1823–1889**
Bensley EH: Robert Palmer Howard. In Dictionary of Canadian biography, 1881–1890. 1982;11:428–9.

**Howe, Henry Furbush, 1905–1977**
Hornblower H: Henry Furbush Howe. **Mass Hist Soc Proc** 1977,89:184–6

**Howell, William Henry, 1860–1945**
Fee E: William Henry Howell: physiologist and philosopher of health. **Am J Epidemiol** 1984 Mar;119(3):293–300
Fye WB: Heparin: the contributions of William Henry Howell. **Circulation** 1984 Jun;69(6):1198–203

**Howells, William Dean, 1837–1920**
Crowley JW: Dating Howells' adolescent breakdown. **Old Northwest** 1982;8(1):13–22

**Howley, Thomas, ca. 1840–1889**
Baker M: Thomas Howley. In Dictionary of Canadian biography, 1881–1890. 1982;11:429–30.

**Hoyer, Henryk Fryderyk, 1834–1907**
Nabielek R: Zu den wichtigsten Veröffentlichungen des polnischen Histologen Henryk Fryderyk Hoyer (1834–1907) in deutschen Fachzeitschriften. **Z Mikrosk Anat Forsch** 1983;97(3):393–408

**Hoyt, Ethel Phelps Stokes, 1877–1952**
Powell RC: Mrs. Ethel Phelps Stockes Hoyt (1877–1952) and the Joint Committee on Religion and Medicine (1923–1936): a brief sketch. **J Pastoral Care** 1975 Jun;29(2):99–105

**Hoyt, Henry Franklin, 1854–1930**
Hoyt HF: A frontier doctor. Ed. D. B. Nunis. Chicago, Donnelley -- Lakeside Press, 1979. liii, 518 p.

**Hrabal, Frantisku, d. 1909**
Fröml F: První skolní lékař na Moravě. **Cas Lek Cesk** 1982 Jun 11;121(23):724–5

**Hrodek, Otto, 1922–**
Houštěk J: Professor MUDr. Otto Hrodek, DrSc., šedesátiletý. **Cesk Pediatr** 1983 Jan;38(1):58–60

**Hsüeh, Sheng-pai, 1681–1770**
Wu R: [Xue Shengbai's life and his scholarly method] (Chi). **Chung Hua I Shih Tsa Chih** 1984 Jan;14(1):7–9

**Huard, Pierre Alfonse, 1901–1983**
Brumpt L: Eloge de Pierre Huard (1901–1983). **Bull Acad Natl Med (Paris)** 1984 Jan–Feb;168(1–2):181–7
Imbault-Huart MJ, ed: Table ronde consacrée au recteur Pierre Huard (1901–1983). Contributions by J. L. Flessis, P. M. Niaussat, T. H. Nguyen, J. Théodoridès. **Hist Sci Med** 1983;17(4):381–402

**Huarte de San Juan, Juan, 1529–1588**
Dieckhöfer K: Juan Huarte de San Juan, precursor de la psicologia diferencial. In International Congress of the History of Medicine, 27th, Barcelona, 1980. Actas. Barcelona, Académia de Ciències Médiques de Catalunya i Balears, 1981. p. 64–8.

**Hubbard, Leverett, fl. 1784**
Colonel Leverett Hubbard's address to the Society at their meeting Feby 2d 1784: **Conn Med** 1984 Sep;48(9):557

**Hubble, John Edgar, 1864–1936**
Green MH: John Edgar Hubble, M.D., a rare physician and surgeon. Van Nuys, California, Hoffman, 1979. 61 p.

**Huber, Johann, 1507–1571**
Portmann ML: Der Basler Stadtarzt Johannes Huber (1507–1571). **Gesnerus** 1981;38:81–91

**Hübschmann, Kurt, 1890–**
Danda J: K devadesátým narozeninám prof. MUDr. K. Hübschmanna, DrSc. **Cesk Dermatol** 1980 Oct;55(5):289–94

**Hucbald of St. Amand, ca. 840–930**
Sheerin DJ: A Carolingian cure recovered: Erasmus' citation of Hucbald of St. Amand's Ecloga de caluis. **Bibl Hum Renaissance** 1980 Jan;42(1):167–71

**Hudson, Abraham, fl. 1671**
Oakeley HF: The end of my great ... grandfather's second wife, or chest medicine in Lambeth in 1671. **St Thomas Hosp Gaz** 1981;79:50–1

**Hufeland, Christoph Wilhelm, 1762–1836**
Busse H: Christoph Wilhelm Hufeland: der berühmte Arzt der Goethezeit, Leibarzt der Königin Luise. St. Michael, Bläschke, 1982. 334 p.
Genschorek W: Christoph Wilhelm Hufeland. Der Arzt, der das Leben verlängern half. Leipzig, Hirzel, 1976. 202 p.
Genschorek W: Christoph Wilhelm Hufeland: der Arzt, der das Leben verlängern half. Leipzig, Hirzel, 1982. 215 p.
Scherrer RM: Friedrich Hoffmanns Anweisung zu gesundem langen Leben, verglichen mit Hufelands Makrobiotik. Zürich, Juris, 1984. 47 p. (Zürcher Medizingeschichtliche Abhandlungen, Neue Reihe, Nr. 170)

**Hug-Hellmuth, Hermine von**
Drell MJ: Hermine Hug-Hellmuth, a pioneer in child analysis. **Bull Menninger Clin** 1982 Mar;46(2):139–50

**Huggins, Charles Brenton, 1901–**
Jain KM, Swan KG, Casey KF: Nobel prize winners in surgery. **Am Surg** 1982 Oct;48(10):495–500

**Hughes, David Edward, 1831–1900**
Stephens SD: David Edward Hughes and his audiometer. **J Laryngol Otol** 1979 Jan;93(1):1–6

**Hughes, Matthew Louis, 1867–1899**
Gear JH: The Anglo-Boer War of 1899–1902:enteric fever and Captain Maxwell Louis Hughes. **Adler Mus Bull** 1981;7(1):10–3

**Hugonnai, Vilma, 1847–1922**
Szállási A: 100 éve szerzett oklevelet az elsö magyar orvosnö. **Orv Hetil** 1979 Aug 19;120(32):1950–2
Szekér E: Hugonnaie Vilma balatonfüredi emlékezete. **Orv Hetil** 1982 Mar 7;123(10):611–2

**Hull, Clark Leonard, 1884–**
Triplet RG: The relationship of Clark L. Hull's hypnosis research to his later learning theory: the continuity of his life's work **J Hist Behav Sci** 1982 Jan;18(1):22–31

**Hullihen, Simon P., 1810–1857**
Nodyne KR: Pioneer in oral surgery: Simon P. Hullihen. **J W Va Hist Assoc** 1982;6(1):41–8

**Humboldt, Alexander von, 1769–1859**
Baer KE von: Reden gehalten in wissenschaftlichen Versammlungen und kleinere Aufsätze vermischten Inhalts. With an introduction by

K. B. Sterling. New York, Arno Press, 1978. Three volumes in two. (Reprint. St. Petersburg, 1864/1876/1873).

Biermann KR: Alexander von Humboldt in seinem Verhältnis zur Leopoldina und zu anderen Akademien. **Acta Hist Leopoldina** 1980;13:39–49

Hein WH: Die ephesische Diana als Natursymbol bei Alexander von Humboldt. In Dilg P, et al., ed: Perspektiven der Pharmaziegeschichte. Graz, Austria, Akademische Druck- u. Verlagsanstalt, 1983. p. 131–46.

**Hume, David, 1711–1776**

Force JE: Hume and the relation of science to religion among certain members of the Royal Society. **J Hist Ideas** 1984 Oct–Dec;45(4):517–36

**Hume, John Robert, 1781 or 2–1857**

Hall IS: John Robert Hume: personal physician to the first Duke of Wellington. **J R Coll Surg Edinb** 1980 Jul;25(4):219–32

**Hummel, David, 1893–**

Hummel D: Som läkare vid hedinexpeditionen till Kina 1927–31. **Nord Medicinhist Arsbok** 1983;:155–44

**Hunain ibn Ishak, al-'Ibadi, 809?–873**

Degen R: The Kitab al-Aghdhiya of Hunayn ibn Ishaq. In: International Symposium for the History of Arabic Science, 1st, University of Aleppo, 1976. Proceedings. Aleppo, Syria, 1976. Papers in European Languages, Vol. II. p. 291–9.

Eastwood BS: Cosmology and physiology in Galenic visual theory: Hunayn Ibn Ishaq. **Trans Stud Coll Physicians Phila** 1980 Dec;5(2 no 4):276–83

Eastwood BS: The elements of vision: the micro-cosmology of Galenic visual theory according to Hunayn Ibn Ishaq. Philadelphia, American Philosophical Society, 1982. 59 p. (Transactions of the American Philosophical Society, Vol. 72, pt. 5).

Egri B: Arab triangulum **Orv Hetil** 1981 Jun 28;122(26):1595–600

Ghalioungui P. Hunayn Ibn Ishaq, translator and medical writer. In International Congress of the History of Medicine, 27th, Barcelona, 1980. Actas. Barcelona, Académia de Ciències Médiques de Catalunya i Balears, 1981. p. 245–8.

Hunayn Ibn Ishak, al-Ibadi: Questions on medicine for scholars. Translated into English, with a preface and historical note, by P. Ghalioungui, M.D., from a critical edition by G. M. Moussa, Ph. D., of the ninth century. Arabic text 'Al Masa'il fi al-Tibb lil Muta'allimin.' Cairo, Al-Ahram Center for Scientific Translations, 1980. xlix, 162 p.

Strohmaier G: Der arabische Hippokrates. Bemerkungen zu einem Aufsatz von Dieter Irmer. **Sudhoffs Arch** 1980;64(3):234–49

**Hungate, Robert Edward, 1906–**

Hungate RE: Evolution of a microbial ecologist. **Annu Rev Microbiol** 1979;33:1–20

**Hunn, Anthony, d. 1834**

Weisert JJ: Dr. Anthony Hunn: from storm and stress to tempest and sunshine. **Filson Club Hist Q** 1982;56(2):211–24

**Hunt, Agnes Gwendoline, 1867–1948**

Glupker DF: The yesteryear of orthopaedic nursing (Agnes Hunt). **Orthop Nurs** 1984 Nov–Dec;3(6):48

**Hunt, Ezra Mundy, 1830–1894**

Alewitz S: Ezra Mundy Hunt--physician, writer, humanitarian. **J Med Soc NJ** 1981 May;78(5):381–5

**Hunt, Otis E., 1822–1905**

Barlow W, Powell DO: Ixodes as a source of conflict: Otis E. Hunt vs. J. Mason Warren. **J Hist Med Allied Sci** 1981 Apr;36(2):221–4

**Hunter, Andrew Rennie**

Hunter AR: Anaesthesia for intracranial surgery: an autobiographical view. **Ann R Coll Surg Engl** 1981;63:316–21

**Hunter, Donald, 1898–**

Schilling RS: Donald Hunter--the first editor of the British Journal of Industrial Medicine. **J Cell Biol** 1979 Aug;36(3):243

**Hunter, John, 1728–1793**

Allen E, Cooper JE: A Hunterian account of human rabies. **Vet Hist** 1980/81,n.s.;1:146–8

Asherson N: The age of John Hunter's golden guineas (1763–93). **Ann R Coll Surg Engl** 1982 Jul;64(4):262–5

Breathnach CS: Biographical sketches No. 26--W. Hunter. **Ir Med J** 1983 Feb;76(2):59

Cohen B: John Hunter's application of science to surgery. **Ann R Coll Surg Engl** 1984 Jan;66(1):59–62

Cooper JE: Some aspects of John Hunter's work on the diseases of birds of prey. **Ann R Coll Surg Engl** 1982 Sep;64(5):345–7

Cross SJ: John Hunter, the animal oeconomy, and late eighteenth-century physiological discourse. **Stud Hist Biol** 1981;5:1–110

Forbes TR: John Hunter as expert witness. **Trans Stud Coll Physicians Phila** 1980 Jun;5(2 no 2):75–80

Gray C: The remarkable surgical collection of John Hunter. **Can Med Assoc J** 1983 May 15;128(10):1225–8

Herschfeld JJ: John Hunter and his Practical treatise on diseases of the teeth. **Bull Hist Dent** 1981;29(1):32–6

Jacyna LS: Images of John Hunter in the nineteenth century. **Hist Sci** 1983 Mar;21(51 Pt 1):85–108

Keel O: La pathologie tissulaire de John Hunter. **Gesnerus** 1980;37(1/2):47–61

Keel O: John Hunter et Xavier Bichat: les rapports de leurs travaux en pathologie tissulaire. In International Congress of the History of Medicine, 27th, Barcelona, 1980. Actas. Barcelona, Académia de Ciències Médiques de Catalunya i Balears, 1981. p. 535–49.

Lasky II: John Hunter, the Shakespeare of medicine. **Surg Gynecol Obstet** 1983 Apr;156(4):511–8

Le Fanu W: Natural history drawings collected by John Hunter F.R.S. (1728–1793), at the Royal College of Surgeons of England. **J Soc Bibliogr Nat Hist** 1978;8(4):329–33

Murley R: Peace and strife in Hunter's time. (Part I). **Ann R Coll Surg Engl** 1982 Jan;64(1):20–8

Murley R: Peace and strife in Hunter's time (part II). **Ann R Coll Surg Engl** 1982 Mar;64(2):81–90

Murley R: John Hunter, velvet and vascular surgery. **Ann R Coll Surg Engl** 1984 May;66(3):214–8

Opie LH, Louw JH: John Hunter and angina pectoris. **Am J Cardiol** 1981 Nov;48(5):980

Owen K: John Hunter: a man of his age. **Trans Hunter Soc** 1978–80;37–38:85–97

Pearson AA: John and William Hunter: patrons of the arts. In: Congrès international d'histoire de la médecine, XXVe, Québec, 1976. Actes. Québec, 1977. p. 1053–62.

Qvist G: John Hunter, 1728–1793. London, Heinemann, 1981. xvi, 216 p.

Rains AJ: The continuing message. **Ann R Coll Surg Engl** 1984 May;66(3):151–8

Wilkinson L: 'The other' John Hunter, M.D., F.R.S. (1754–1809): his contributions to the medical literature, and to the introduction of animal experiments into infectious disease research. **Notes Rec R Soc Lond** 1982 Feb;36(2):227–41

Zuck D: John Hunter's treatment of gunshot wounds. **Ann R Coll Surg Engl** 1980 Jan;62(1):74–5

**Hunter, William, 1718–1783**

Breathnach CS: Biographical sketches No. 26--W. Hunter. **Ir Med J** 1983 Feb;76(2):59

Brock CH: Dr. William Hunter's Museum, Glasgow University. **J Soc Bibliogr Nat Hist** 1980 Apr;9(4):403–12

Brock CH: William Hunter, 1718–1783: a memoir. East Kilbride, University of Glasgow Press, 1983. xviii, 81 p.

Different letters from the past: Tobias Smollett to William Hunter. **Ann R Coll Surg Engl** 1980 Mar;62(2):146–9

Pearson AA: John and William Hunter: patrons of the arts. In: Congrès international d'histoire de la médecine, XXVe, Québec, 1976. Actes. Québec, 1977. p. 1053–62.

Thornton JL, Want PC: William Hunter (1718–1783) and his contributions to obstetrics. **Br J Obstet Gynaecol** 1983 Sep;90(9):787–94

**Huray, István, 1827–1911**

Zákonyi F: Dr. Huray István, Balatonfüred föorvosa. **Orv Hetil** 1983 Sep 4;124(36):2192–4

**Hurst, Edward Weston, 1900–1971**

Morton RS: A reappraisal of non-specific genital infection with reference to the work of the late Dr. E. Weston Hurst. **Br J Vener Dis** 1983 Dec;59(6):394–6

**Hutcheson, Francis, 1694–1746**

Brooks GP, Aalto SK: The rise and fall of moral algebra: Frances Hutcheson and the mathematization of psychology. **J Hist Behav Sci** 1981;17:343–56

**Hutchinson, John, 1811–1861**

Gandevia B: Dr. John Hutchinson: the inventor of the spirometer. **Aust Fam Physician** 1981 Jul;10(7):574–8

**Hutchinson, Jonathan, 1828–1913**

Cahn LR: Some notes on Sir Jonathan Hutchinson (1828–1913). **Am J Surg Pathol** 1979 Dec;3(6):563–6

Clemmensen O: Hutchinson's freckle. **Am J Dermatopathol** 1982 Oct;4(5):425–8

Jackson R: Jonathan Hutchinson on syphilis. **Sex Transm Dis** 1980 Apr–Jun;7(2):90–6

Jackson R: Hutchinson on leprosy. **Int J Dermatol** 1982 Dec;21(10):614–9

Swain V: Sir Jonathan Hutchinson 1828–1913: his role in the history of intussusception. **J Pediatr Surg** 1980 Apr;15(2):221–3

**Hutinel, Victor, 1849–1933**

Merger R: Un grand médecin: Victor Hutinel, ancien élève du Collège de Chaumont, professeur de clinique des maladies des enfants (1849–1933).

**Hüttl, Tivadar, 1884–**

Szeleczky G: Hüttl Tivadar centenáriumára. **Orv Hetil** 1984 Aug 19;125(34):2081–2

**Huvé, Claude, 1505–1570**

Renaudie M: Etre généraliste il y a quatre siècles. Réalisme et fiction. **Hist Sci Med** 1984;18(2):173–9

**Huxley, Aldous Leonard, 1894–1963**

Calcraft LG: Aldous Huxley and the Sheldonian hypothesis.

**Ann Sci** 1980 Nov;37(6):657–71

**Huxley, Thomas Henry, 1825–1895**
Altholz JL: The Huxley–Wilberforce debate revisited. **J Hist Med Allied Sci** 1980 Jul;35(3):313–16
Di Gregorio MA: Order or process of nature: Huxley's and Darwin's different approaches to natural sciences. **Hist Philos Life Sci** 1981;3(2):217–41
Di Gregorio MA: The dinosaur connection: a reinterpretation of T. H. Huxley's evolutionary view. **J Hist Biol** 1982 Fall;15(3):397–418
Hall MB: The Royal Society in Thomas Henry Huxley's time. **Notes Rec R Soc Lond** 1984;38(2):153–8
Lucas JR: Wilberforce and Huxley: a legendary encounter. **Hist J (Gt Brit)** 1979;22(2):313–30
Paradis JG: T. H. Huxley, Man's place in nature. Lincoln, University of Nebraska Press, 1978. xi, 226 p.
Ross DA: Neglected bibliographical aspects of the works of Thomas Henry Huxley. **J Soc Bibliogr Nat Hist** 1978;8(4):401–20
Smith JM: Thomas Huxley in Nashville. **Tenn Hist Q** 1974;33(2):191–203;(3):322–41
Wenneker M: Huxley's ethical system: an alternative to evolutionary ethics. **Synthesis** 1980;5(1):13–44

**Huygens, Christiaan, 1629–1695**
Burch CB: Huygens' pulse models as a bridge between phenomena and Huygens' mechanical foundations. **Janus** 1981;68:53–64
Elzinga A: Christiaan Huygens' theory of research. **Janus** 1980;67:281–300
Fournier M: Huygens' microscopical researches. **Janus** 1981;68:199–209
Luyendijk–Elshout AM: Christiaan Huygens en de geneeskunde. **Spiegel Hist** 1979;14(4):230–33
Schneider I: Christiaan Huygens's contribution to the development of a calculus of probabilities. **Janus** 1980;67(4):269–79
Stroup A: Christiaan Huygens & the development of the air pump. **Janus** 1981;68:129–58

**Hwasser, Israel, 1790–1860**
Kock W: Ett filosofiskt tackbrev från Israel Hwasser. **Nord Medicinhist Arsb** 1980;:90–8

**Hyde, Ida Henrietta, 1857–1945**
Johnson EE: Ida Henrietta Hyde: early experiments. **Physiologist** 1981 Dec;24(6):10–1
Sloan JB: The founding of the Naples Table Association for promoting scientific research by women, 1897. **Signs** 1978;4(1):208–16
Tucker GS: Ida Henrietta Hyde: the first woman member of the society. **Physiologist** 1981 Dec;24(6):1–9

**Hyde, James Nevins, 1840–1910**
Beatty WK: James Nevins Hyde: pioneer dermatologist and staunch Navy man. **Proc Inst Med Chic** 1982 Oct–Dec;35(4):139–42

**Hyndman, Charles Robert**
Edwards GA: The mental illness of Captain Hyndman. **Aust NZ J Psychiatr** 1979 Jun;13(2):147–52

**Hynek, Kristiana, d. 1979**
Libánský J: Vývoj hematologie od dob profesora Hynka a její další perspektivy. **Vnitr Lek** 1979 Sep;25(9):915–20

**Hyrtl, Joseph, 1810–1894**
Radbill SX: Josef Hyrtl's Philadelphia connection. **J Hist Med Allied Sci** 1984 Apr;39(2):222–4
Steyer GE: Joseph Hyrtl als komparativer Anatomiker. **Anat Anz** 1980;148(5):462–73
Wolf F: Universitätsprofessor Dr. Josef Hyrtl. **Osterr Gesch Kult** 1965;9(10):531–41

# I

**Iagel'skiĭ, Kas'ian Osipovich, 1736–1774**
Palkin BN: Nastavlenie doktora K. O. Iagel'skogo po profilaktike i lecheniiu chumy. **Zh Mikrobiol Epidemiol Immunobiol** 1982 Jan;(1):117–8

**Iakubovich, Nikolaĭ Martynovich, 1817–1879**
Klishov AA: N. M. Iakubovich––pervyĭ russkiĭ professor–gistolog. **Arkh Anat Gistol Embriol** 1981 Oct;81(10):105–15

**Ianovskiĭ, Mikhail Vladimirovich, 1854–1927**
Borodulin VI, Martynov IV: Uchenie M. V. Ianovskogo o 'perifericheskom serdtse' i razvitie predstavlenii o klinicheskom znachenii sosudistoi periferii. **Klin Med (Mosk)** 1982 May;60(5):9–12

**Iaroshenko, N. A.**
Polenova IV: N. A. Iaroshenko i ucheniki S. P. Botkina. **Klin Med (Mosk)** 1982 Sep;60(9):117–9

**Iavorskiĭ, Ivan Lavrovich, 1853–1920**
Ionov IuV, Ionov AIu: Vrach I. L. Iavorskiĭ – issledovatel' Afganistana. **Sov Zdravookhr** 1983;(12):49–51

**Ibn Abi l–Bayan, 1161–1240**
Valverde JL, Munoz CP, ed: El Formulario de los hospitales De Ibn Abi L–bayan. Introduccion, traduccion espanola y commentarios, con glosarios. Granada, Universidad de Granada, 1981. 256 p. (Cuadernos de historia de la farmacia, 8).
Valverde JL, Peña Muñoz C: El formulario de los hospitales' de Ibn Abi l–Bayan (S. XIII). In International Congress of the History of Medicine, 27th, Barcelona, 1980. Actas. Barcelona, Académia de Ciències Médiques de Catalunya i Balears, 1981. p. 346–51.

**Ibn al–'Ayn Zarbi, d. 1153**
Harmarneh SK: Ibn al–Ayn Zarbi and his definitions of diseases and their diagnoses. In: International Symposium for the History of Arabic Science, 1st, University of Aleppo, 1976. Proceedings. Aleppo, Syria, 1976. Papers in European Languages, Vol. II. p. 305–23.

**Ibn al–Baytar, 1190–1248**
Carrillo JL, Paz Torres M: Ibn Al–Baytar y el arabismo español del XVIII. Edicion trilingüe del prologo de su 'Kitab al–chami.' Benalmádena, Ayuntamiento de Benalmádena, 1982. 57 p.

**Ibn al–Hassa, fl. 13th cent.**
Valverde JL, Peña–Muñoz C: Ibn al–Hassa: Glosario sobre el 'Mansuri' de Razi. **Ars Pharm** 1980;21:317–32

**Ibn al–Khatib, 1313–1374**
Ober WB, Aloush N: The plague at Granada, 1348–1349: Ibn Al–Khatib and ideas of contagion. **Bull NY Acad Med** 1982 May;58(4):418–24
Vazquez de Benito MC, ed: El libro del 'Amal man tabba li–man habba de Muhammad B. 'Abdallah B. Al–Jatib. Salamanca, Universidad de Salamanca, 1972. liii, 86 p. (Acta Salmanticensia, 66).

**Ibn al–Nafis, d. 1288 or 9**
Sliwiński S: Teoria Ibn an–Nafisa (1210–1288) krążenia płucnego krwi. **Wiad Lek** 1981 Mar 15;34(6):531–3

**Ibn al–Quff, 1233–1286**
Hamarneh S: Medical technology in Ibn al–Quff's surgery. In I. El–Sayyad, ed: Papers presented to the First International Conference on Islamic Medicine, celebrating the advent of the fifteenth century hijri. Kuwait, Ministry of Public Health. National Council for Culture, Arts and Letters, 1981. p. 140–7.
Hamarneh SK: Ibn Al–Quff's writings on hygienic regulations and the preservation of health. In A. Hadidi, ed: Studies in the history and archaeology of Jordan. Amman, Department of Antiquities, 1982. p. 373–83.

**Ibn al–Tilmidh, ca. 1073–1165**
Iskandar AZ: Another fragment from the autograph of Ibn Al–Tilmidh's 'Marginal commentary on Ibn Sina's Canon of medicine'. **Bull Sch Orient Afr Stud** 1981;44:253–61

**Ibn Butlan, d. 1068**
Opsomer–Halleux C: La diététique d'Ibn Butlan dans le manuscrit 887 (1041) de l'Université de Liège. Congrès de Comines, 1, 1980. Actes. p. 350.

**Ibn Gabirol, Solomon ben Judah, ca. 1021–ca. 1058**
Rezhabi Y: The disease of Rabbi Solomon ibn Gabirol. **Sinai** 1979;84:1–8

**Ibn Jazlah, d. ca. 1100**
De Marco O, Nebbia G, Pizzoli Mazzacane EM: Ibn Jazla et les connaissances de l'Islam médiéval en sciences naturelles. **Rev Hist Pharm (Paris)** 1979 Dec;26(243):249–58

**Ibn Khaldun, 1332–1406**
Hamarneh SK: Jabir, Jildki and Ibn–Sallum, and Arabic–Islamic Alchemy. **Mesopotamia Q** 1980;8(29,30):110–22, 225–41

**Ibn–Omrane Ishaq, d. 892 or 3**
Ben Milad A: Biographie des médécins arabes: Ishaq Ibn Omrane. **Tunis Med** 1979 Nov–Dec;57(6):378–9

**Ibn Qaiyim al–Gauziya, 1292–1350**
Weisser U: Ibn Quaiyim al–Gauziya über die Methoden der Embryologie. **Medizinhist J** 1981;16(3):227–39

**Ibn Suwadi, d. 1291 or 2**
Ullmann M: Die Tadkira des ibn as–Suwaidi, eine wichtige Quelle zur Geschichte der griechisch–arabischen Medicin und Magie. **Islam** 1977;54:33–65

**Ideler, Carl Wilhelm, 1795–1860**
Wunderlich G: Die psychodynamische Theorie von Ideler (1835). **Z Psychosom Med Psychoanal** 1983;29(3):286–92
Wunderlich G: Kranheits– und Therapiekonzepte am Anfang der deutschen Psychiatrie (Haindorf, Heinroth, Ideler). Husum, Matthiesen, 1981. 132 p. (Abhandlungen zur Geschichte der Medizin und der Naturwissenschaften, 41).

**Imhotep**
Briceño Maaz T: Im–Hotep: dios egipcio de la medicina. **Rev Soc Venez Hist Med** 1969–71;17–19(31–33):75–82

**Imre, József, 1884–1945**
Radnót M: Ifj. Imre József (1884–1945). **Orv Hetil** 1984 Jun 10;125(24):1453–4

**Imshenetskiĭ, Aleksandr Aleksandrovich, 1905–**
Zavarzin GA: Aleksandr Aleksandrovich Imshenetskiĭ. Moskva, Nauka, 1967. 82 p.

**Inagaki, Satorū**
Oguro M: [Late Dr. Satoru Inagaki, a member of the Council of the Japan Society of Clinical Hematology: his life and contributions]

(Jpn) **Rinsho Ketsueki** 1979 Nov;20(11):1532-3

**Indravarman II, 1220-1243?**
Chandler DP: Folk memories of the decline of Angkor in nineteenth-century Cambodia: the legend of the leper king. **J Siam Soc** 1979;67(1):54-62

**Ingenhousz, Jan, 1730-1799**
Smit P: Jan Ingen-Housz (1730-1799): some new evidence about his life and work. **Janus** 1980;67(1-2-3):125-39

**Ingman, Erik, 1810-1858**
Batári G: Erik Ingman finn orvos látogatása Pesten Bugát Pálnál 1847-ben. **Orvostort Kozl** 1981;93-96(27 No 1-4):189-92

**Innocentius XI, Pope, 1611-1689**
Gelabert i Mas A, Gironella i Coll J: El papa Inocencio XI: approximación etiológica a su patología renal. In International Congress of the History of Medicine, 27th, Barcelona, 1980. Actas. Barcelona, Académia de Ciències Médiques de Catalunya i Balears, 1981. p. 506-10.

**Iodocus, fl. 1474**
Pack RA: Magister Iodocus: 'Regule phisonomie'. **Mediaev Stud** 1980;42:212-37

**Ionescu-Mihăesti, C., 1883-1971**
Arion R: Prof. C. Ionescu-Mihăieşti, o personalitate de însemnătate fundamentală în istoria medicinii preventive din România. **Rev Ig [Bacteriol]** 1984 Jan-Mar;29(1):89-95

**Ionescu-Siseşti, Nicolae, 1888-1954**
Alexandru O: Nicolae Ionescu-Siseşti, neurolog, 1888--1954 (91 ani de la naşterea sa). **Rev Med Interna [Neurol Psihiatr]** 1979 Apr-Jun;24(2):143-6

**Iparraguirre, Francisco Fernández, fl. 1883**
Sánchez-Moscoso Hermida A, Alfonso Galán MT: Estudio histórico de una tesis de farmacia juzgada hace 100 años: 'Las divisiones de la naturaleza y de la ciencia', de Francisco Fernández Iparraguirre. **Bol Soc Esp Hist Farm** 1983;34(136):167-84

**Isaacs, Alick, 1921-1967**
Andrewes CH: Alick Isaacs. In Dictionary of national biography, 1961-1970. Suppl. 8, 1981. p. 569-70.

**Isakower, Otto, 1899-1972**
Lothane Z: Listening with the Third Ear as an instrument in psychoanalysis: the contributions of Reik and Isakower. **Psychoanal Rev** 1981-82 Winter;68(4):487-503

**Isamat Vila, Jesús, 1895-**
Rof Carballo MC: Le Dr. Jesús Isamat Vila, premier professeur d'histoire de la pharmacie de l'Université de Barcelone. In: Vorträge des Internationalen Pharmaziehistorischen Kongresses Innsbruck 1977. Stuttgart, Wissenschaftliche Verlagsgesellschaft, 1979. p. 189-94.

**Iscanius, David Lipsius, 17th cent.**
De Poorter DA: David Lipsius Iscanius, 17e-eeuws doctor medicus afkomstig uit Overijse. **Periodiek** 1980;35:16-22

**Iserin von Mazo, Georg, fl. 1527**
Somweber E: Der Zauberer und Hexenmeister Dr. Georg Iserin von Mazo. **Montfort** 1968;20(3):295-325

**Ishaq Ibn 'Imran, 10th cent.**
Milad A ben: Biographie des médécins arabes: Ishaq Ibn Omrane. **Tunis Med** 1979;57:378-9

**Ishibashi, Haya**
[A meeting to commemorate the 100th anniversary of Ms. Haya Ishibashi, a pioneer in psychiatric nursing] (Jpn): **Kango** 1980 Jun;32(6):88

**Israel, James 1848-1926**
Winau R: James Israel, 1848-1926. Wiesbaden, F. Steiner, 1983. 256 p.

**Israeli, Isaac, ca. 832-ca. 932**
Simon I: L'influence hippocratique sur la médecine hébraique, surtout chez Assaph, Isaac Israèli et Maimonide. In La collection hippocratique et son rôle dans l'histoire de la médecine. Colloque de Strasbourg (23-27 octobre 1972) organisé par le Centre de Recherches sur la Grèce Antique, avec le concours des Facultés de Philosophie et des Langues Classiques. Leiden, E. J. Brill, 1975. 275-89.

**Israels, Abraham Hartog, 1822-1883**
Hes-Swartenberg HS: Abraham Hartog Israels, M.D., 1822-1883: Netherlands' first professor in the history of medicine. **NY State J Med** 1979 Aug;79(9):1445-7

**Issekutz, Hugo, 1855-1915**
Kempler K: Hugo Issekutz, der Begründer der ersten ungarischen Universitätsapotheke. In Hein WH, ed: Pharmaziehistorischer Kongress, Budapest, 1981. Stuttgart, Wissenschaftliche Verlagsgesellschaft, 1983. p. 135-9.

**Itard, Jean Marc Gaspard, 1775-1838**
Chalat NI: Jean Marc Gaspard Itard - 1774-1838. **Laryngoscope** 1982 Jun;92(6 Pt 1):627-9
Gineste T, Postel J: J. M. G. Itard et l'enfant connu sous le nom de 'sauvage de l'Aveyron'. **Psychiatr Enfant** 1980;23(1):251-307
Gineste T: Victor de L'Aveyron: dernier enfant sauvage, premier enfant fou. Paris, Le Sycomore, 1981. 327 p.
Lieberman LM: Itard: the great problem solver. **J Learn Disabil** 1982 Nov;15(9):566-8

**Iturbe, Juan, 1883-1962**
Iriarte DR: [Public health in Venezuela]. **Rev Soc Venez Hist Med** 1975-76;23(37):107-21

**Iudin, Sergei Sergeivich**
Fel'berg MV: S. S. Iudin v 'Zakhar'ine'. **Sov Zdravookhr** 1983;(3):71-3

**Iunevich, O. A.**
Makovoz AA: O. A. Iunevich - vidnyĭ zemskiĭ vrach. **Sov Zdravookhr** 1984;(1):64-7

**Ivan IV, the Terrible, Czar of Russia, 1530-1584**
Koretskii VI: Smert' Groznogo Tsaria. **Vopr Istor** 1979;9:93-103

**Ivanchich, Viktor von, 1812-1892**
Vértes L: Dr. Ivanchich Viktor. **Orv Hetil** 1984 Sep 16;125(38):2321-4

**Ivanov, A. V.**
Shtern MI, Karinskaia GS: Zemskiĭ vrach A. V. Ivanov. **Sov Zdravookhr** 1983;(8):64-7

**Ivanovskiĭ, Dmitriĭ Iosifovich, 1864-1920**
Zhdanov VM: Andre L'vov protiv D. I. Ivanovskogo. **Vopr Virusol** 1982 Jul-Aug;27(4):499-502

**Ivy, Andrew Conway, 1893-1978**
Ward PS: 'Who will bell the cat?' Andrew C. Ivy and krebiozen. **Bull Hist Med** 1984 Spring;58(1):28-52

## J

**Jabir ibn Haiyan, al-Tarasusi**
Hamarneh SK: Jabir, Jildki and Ibn Sallum, and Arabic Islamic Alchemy. **Mesopotamia Q** 1980;8(29,30):110-22, 225-41

**Jackson, Andrew, 1767-1845**
Caravati CM: President Andrew Jackson: despite infirmities, a strong leader. **Va Med** 1983 Mar;110(3):194-5
Remini RV: The final days and hours in the life of General Andrew Jackson. **Tenn Hist Q** 1980;39(2):167-77

**Jackson, Arthur Randell, 1877-1944**
Tonge V: Arthur Randell Jackson: 1877-1944. **Br Med J [Clin Res]** 1983 Jul 9;287(6385):97-8

**Jackson, Charles Thomas, 1805-1880**
Campan L: A propos du centenaire de la mort de Charles Thomas Jackson (1805-1880). **Ann Anesthesiol Fr** 1981;22(1):3-7

**Jackson, Chevalier, 1865-1958**
Wechsler HL: Chevalier Jackson. In Dictionary of American Biography, Suppl. 6, 1956-1960. p. 317-18, 1980.

**Jackson, Edward, 1856-1942**
Delaney JJ: Edward Jackson. **Colo Med** 1983 Apr;80(4):116-7
Newell FW: The first editor--Edward Jackson. **Am J Ophthalmol** 1982 Dec;94(6):809-10

**Jackson, Hall, 1739-1797**
Estes JW: Hall Jackson and the purple foxglove: medical practice and research in revolutionary America 1760-1820. Hanover, NH, University Press of New England, 1979. xvi, 291 p.
Estes JW: An account of the foxglove in America. **Bull Hist Med** 1973 Jul-Aug;47(4):394-408

**Jackson, Henry Jr., 1892-1968**
Lemon HM: Motivation in cancer education, with an appreciation of Dr. Henry Jackson, Jr., pioneer medical oncologist-hematologist (1892-1968). **Med Pediatr Oncol** 1980;8(4):407-22

**Jackson, Herbert, d. 1936**
Ramsey LJ: Some notable early contributors to radiography--Thompson, Jackson and Campbell Swinton. **Radiography** 1980 Dec;46(552):289-97

**Jackson, John Hughlings, 1835-1911**
Fullinwider SP: Sigmund Freud, John Hughlings Jackson, and speech. **J Hist Ideas** 1983 Jan-Mar;44(1):151-8
Giannattasio ME, Nencini R: Il mito jacksoniano. **Stor Crit Psicol** 1982 Dec;3(2):315-27
Hamanaka Y: [Jackson's theory of stratification of neurological functions--a controversy involving Broca at a symposium (1868) at Norwich] (Jpn). **No To Shinkei** 1982 Oct;34(10):1018-9
Joynt RJ: The great confrontation: the meeting between Broca and Jackson in 1868. In Rose FC, Bynum WF, ed: Historical aspects of the neurosciences. New York, Raven, 1982. p. 99-102.
Smith CU: Evolution and the problem of mind: part II. John Hughlings Jackson. **J Hist Biol** 1982 Summer;15(2):241-62
Taylor DC, March SM: Hughlings Jackson's Dr Z: the paradigm of temporal lobe epilepsy revealed. **J Neurol Neurosurg Psychiatry** 1980 Sep;43(9):758-67
Tyler KL: Hughlings Jackson: the early development of his ideas on epilepsy. **J Hist Med Allied Sci** 1984 Jan;39(1):55-64

**Jackson, Thomas Jonathan, 1824–1863**
Henry WD: Stonewall Jackson--the soldier eccentric. **Practitioner** 1979 Oct;223(1336):580–7

**Jacobi, Abraham, 1830–1919**
Cone TE: Abraham Jacobi on medical specialization, as viewed in 1880. **Pediatrics** 1981;67:481
Cone TE: Abraham Jacobi on the establishment of systematic instruction in the diseases of childhood in the United States. **Pediatrics** 1981;67:357
Daeschner CW: Education for primary care of children. A report to Abraham and Mary Jacobi. **Am J Dis Child** 1983 Jun;137(6):566–71

**Jacobi, Mary Corinna Putnam, 1842–1906**
Daeschner CW: Education for primary care of children. A report to Abraham and Mary Jacobi. **Am J Dis Child** 1983 Jun;137(6):566–71
Farley F: Two generations of women physicians: the New York Infirmary, 1870–1899. **J Am Med Wom Assoc** 1984 Nov–Dec;39(6):189–91
Morantz RM: Feminism, professionalism, and germs: the thought of Mary Putnam Jacobi and Elizabeth Blackwell. **Amer Q** 1982;34:459–78

**Jacobson, Edith, 1897–**
Kernberg OF: The contributions of Edith Jacobson: an overview. **J Am Psychoanal Assoc** 1979;27(4):793–819

**Jacobson, Edmund, 1888–**
Lehrer PM: How to relax and how not to relax: a re-evaluation of the work of Edmund Jacobson--I. **Behav Res Ther** 1982;20(5):417–28

**Jacobson, Ludwig Lewin, 1783–1843**
Christoffersen JC: L. L. Jacobson (1783–1843). **Invest Urol** 1980;18:227

**Jacopone da Todi, ca. 1230–ca. 1306**
Bazzi F, Panebianco D: Una lauda di interesse medico poco nota di Jacopone da Todi. **Minerva Med** 1981 Nov 14;72(45):3039–43
Bruce-Chwatt LJ: Jacopone da Todi's mystical pathology. **Br Med J [Clin Res]** 1982 Dec 18–25;285(6357):1803–4

**Jacquin, Armand Pierre, 1721–ca. 1790**
Quevauviller A: L'hygiène au XVIIIe siècle d'après l'abbé Jacquin. **Rev Hist Pharm (Paris)** 1980 Mar;27(244):24–38

**Jacquin, Nikolaus Joseph von, 1727–1817**
Bugyi B: N. J. Jacquin, the first medical doctor-chemist in Hungary. **Ther Hung** 1979;27(4):192–3

**Jacquot, François-Félix, 1819–1857**
Huard P, Lefebvre P, Plessis JL: François-Félix Jacquot (1819–1857). **Hist Sci Med** 1983;17(4):403–10

**Jadwiga, Queen of Poland, 1370–1399**
Dawidowicz A, Hornowski J: O wieku królowej Jadwigi. **Arch Hist Med (Warsz)** 1978;41(4):423–46

**Jaeger, Gustav, 1832–1917**
Kaufmann E: Gustav Jaeger, 1832–1917, Arzt, Zoologe und Hygieniker. Zürich, Juris, 1984. 67 p. (Zürcher Medizingeschichtliche Abhandlungen, Neue Reihe, 171)

**Jager, Jacheus de, 1599–1650**
Slenders J: De Anatomische les van Dr. Zacheus de Jager (1640). **Tijdschr Geschied Geneeskd** 1981;4(4):159–67

**Jahn, Theodore Louis, 1905–1979**
Bovee EC: Theodore Louis Jahn. 1905–1979. In memoriam. **J Protozool** 1979 Nov;26(4):527–9

**Jáki, Gyula, 1898–1958**
Zallár A: Huszonöt éve hunyt el jáki Gyula professzor. **Orv Hetil** 1983 Sep 18;124(38):2321–2

**Jakob, Christfried, 1866–1956**
Meyer L: Cristofredo Jakob. A veinticinco años de su muerte. **Acta Psiquiatr Psicol Am Lat** 1981 Mar;27(1):13–4

**Jakóbkiewicz, Józef**
Brodniewicz A: Józef Jakóbkiewicz M.D., pioneer of maritime and tropical medicine in Poland. **Bull Inst Marit Trop Med Gdynia** 1980;31(1–2):5–13

**Jallabert, Jean, 1712–1768**
Benguigui I: La théorie de l'électricité de Nollet et son application en médecine à travers sa correspondance: inédite avec Jallabert. **Gesnerus** 1981;38:225–35

**James, Alice, 1848–1892**
Roth N: Electrotherapy, 19th-century neurasthenia, and the case of Alice James. **Med Instrum** 1981 Mar–Apr;15(2):116

**James Family**
Feinstein HM: The use and abuse of illness in the James family circle: a view of neurasthenia as a social phenomenon. **Psychohist Rev** 1979;8(1–2):6–14
Yeazell RB, Maliszewski B, Constantikes A: An exchange of letters between William and Alice James. **Psychohist Rev** 1979;8(1–2):53–9

**James, Frank Lowber, 1841–1907**
Baird WD, ed: Years of discontent. Doctor Frank L. James in Arkansas, 1877–1878. Memphis, Memphis State University Press, 1977. xxviii, 84 p.

**James, Henry, 1811–1882**
Feinstein HM: The sins of the fathers. **Psychoanal Rev** 1983 Spring;70(1):95–100
Hall R: Henry James: interpreting an obsessive memory. **J Homosex** 1983 Spring–Summer;8(3–4):83–97

**James, Henry, 1843–1916**
Strout C: Henry James's dream of the Louvre, 'The Jolly Corner,' and psychological interpretation. **Psychohist Rev** 1979 Summer–Fall;8(1–2):47–52

**James, Mary**
Anderson JW: In search of Mary James. **Psychohist Rev** 8(1–2):63–70, Summer–Fall 79

**James, Westwood Wallace, d. 1868**
Musick M, ed: 'Glorious war': the diary of Westwood James, 16th Alabama. **Civ War Times Illus** 1978;17(6)34–42

**James, William, 1842–1910**
Anderson JW: In search of Mary James. **Psychohist Rev** 8(1–2):63–70, Summer–Fall 79
Anderson JW: 'The worst kind of melancholy': William James in 1869. **Harv Libr Bull** 1982 Oct;30(4):369–86
Bjork DW: The compromised scientist: William James in the development of American psychology. New York, Columbia University Press, 1983. xiv, 221 p.
Feinstein HM: Family therapy for the historian?--The case of William James. **Fam Process** 1981 Mar;20(1):97–107
Feinstein HM: The 'crisis' of William James: a revisionist view. **Psychohist Rev** 1981;10(2):71–80
Gavin WJ: Vagueness and empathy: a Jamesian view. **J Med Philos** 1981 Feb;6(1):45–65
Gilman SL: Den Geisteskranken sehen: Mackenzie, Kleist, William James. **Confin Psychiatr** 1979;22(3):127–44
High RP: Shadworth Hodgson and William James's formulation of space perception: phenomenology and perceptual realism. **J Hist Behav Sci** 1981 Oct;17(4):466–85
High RP, Woodward WR: William James and Gordon Allport: parallels in their maturing conceptions of self and personality. In R. W. Rieber, K. Salzinger, ed: Psychology: theoretical-historical perspectives. New York, Academic Press, 1980. p. 57–79.
James W: The principles of psychology. Edited and annotated by FH Burkhardt, F. Bowers and I. K. Skrupskelis. 3 vols. Cambridge, Mass. and London, Harvard University Press, 1981. lxviii, 1740 p. (The Works of William James) Introductory historical and biographical essays by G. E. Myers and R. B. Evans.
Karnani C: William James and I. A. Richards. **Indian J Am Stud** 1980;10(1):78–82
Kuo P: Lu-mu-ssu ti ch'e-ti ching-yen lun. **Bull Coll Lib Arts (Taiwan)** 1981;30:207–28
Mackenzie L: William James and the problem of interests. **J Hist Behav Sci** 1980 Apr;16(2):175–85
Rambo LR: Ethics, evolution, and the psychology of William James. **J Hist Behav Sci** 1980 Jan;16(1):50–7
Richards RJ: The personal equation in science: William James's psychological and moral uses of Darwinian theory. **Harv Libr Bull** 1982 Oct;30(4):387–425
Romanell P: Medical history in the religious psychology of William James. In: Congrès international d'histoire de la médecine, XXVe, Québec, 1976. Actes. Québec, 1977. p. 1171–83.
Schwehn MR: Making the world: William James and the life of the mind. **Harv Libr Bull** 1982 Oct;30(4):426–54
Schwehn MR, ed: A William James renaissance: four essays by young scholars. **Harv Libr Bull** 1982 Oct;30(4):367–480
Taylor E: William James on psychopathology: the 1896 Lowell lectures on 'Exceptional mental states'. **Harv Libr Bull** 1982 Oct;30(4):455–79
Woodward WR: William James's psychology of will: its revolutionary impact on American psychology. In J. Brozěk, ed: Explorations in the history of psychology in the United States. Lewisburg, Bucknell University Press, 1984. p. 148–95.

**Jameson, George Chauncey, 1865–1948**
Siddall AC: George Chauncey Jameson, M.D., 1865–1948. From bloodletting to antibiotics. **Northwest Ohio Q** 1980;52(1):168–78

**Jan II Kasimierz Wasa, King of Poland, 1609–1672**
Dudziński W: Choroby i zgon króla Jana Kazimierza. **Wiad Lek** 1980 Jan 1;33(1):61–5

**Janáček, Leos, 1854–1928**
Sajner J: Patografická studie o Leoši Janáckovi. **Vnitr Lek** 1982 Aug;28(8):823–7

**Jančik, J.**
Fröml F: Venkovský lékař a ranhojič na konci 19. století. **Cas Lek Cesk** 1979 May 25;118(21):662–4

**Jancsó, Miklós Sr., 1868–1930**
Lukács D: Id. Jancsó Miklós malária kutatásai. **Orv Hetil** 1981 Jan 25;122(4):224–6

**Janet, Pierre, 1859–1947**
Fusswerk-Fursay J: A propos d'un inédit de Pierre Janet sur les croyances. **Ann Med Psychol (Paris)** 1984 May;142(5):703–10
Girard R: Force et tension psychologique selon Pierre Janet. **Schweiz Arch Neurol Neurochir Psychiatr** 1981;128(1):33–51

**Janicki, Konstanty S., 1876–1932**
Slusarski W: W pięćdziesiątą rocznicę śmierci Konstantego S. Janickiego (1876–1932). **Wiad Parazytol** 1983;28(5–6):507–15

**Janiszewski, Stanisław**
Przychodzki M: Dr Stanislaw Janiszewski. **Przegl Lek** 1981;38(1):180–2, 187–9

**Janiszewski, Tomasz, 1867–1939**
Talewski R: Zakopiański lekarz klimatyczny ministrem zdrowia (w czterdziestą rocznicę śmierci prof. Tomasza Janiszewskiego). **Arch Hist Med (Warsz)** 1980;43(3):331–41

**Janský, Jan, 1907–**
Adamec J: Jan Janský. **Cas Lek Cesk** 1983 Sep 23;122(38):1180–2
Skala E: Kdo objevil krevní skupiny? **Cas Lek Cesk** 1984 Oct 19;123(42):1292–4

**Jarrett, Mary Cromwell, 1877–1961**
Grayson VS: Mary Cromwell Jarrett. In: Notable American women. The modern period. Cambridge, Mass., Belknap-Harvard Univ. Press, 1980. 4:377–9.

**Jaspers, Karl, 1883–1969**
Blankenburg W: Unausgeschöpftes in der Psychopathologie von Karl Jaspers. **Nervenarzt** 1984 Sep;55(9):447–60
Glatzel J: Die Psychopathologie Karl Jaspers' in der Kritik. **Nervenarzt** 1984 Jan;55(1):10–7
Huber G: Die Bedeutung von Karl Jaspers für die Psychiatrie der Gegenwart. **Nervenarzt** 1984 Jan;55(1):1–9
Janzarik W: Jaspers, Kurt Schneider und die Heidelberger Psychopathologie. **Nervenarzt** 1984 Jan;55(1):18–24
López Ibor JJ: Karl Jaspers en su centenario. **Actas Luso Esp Neurol Psiquiatr** 1982 Nov–Dec;10(6):321–30
Nica-Udangiu S: Karl Jaspers (1883–1969). **Rev Med Interna [Neurol Psihiatr]** 1983 Oct–Dec;28(4):311–6
Ojeda Figueroa C: Karl Jaspers: filosofía y psicoterapia. **Acta Luso Esp Neurol Psiquiatr** 1983 Mar–Apr;11(2):181–8
Putscher M: Jaspers und Van Gogh—oder über Krankheit und Kunst. **Janus** 1980;67(1–2–3):157–69
Schmitt W: Grundlinien psychiatrischer Praxis bei Karl Jaspers. In Seidler E, Schott H, ed: Bausteine zur Medizingeschichte. Stuttgart, Steiner, 1984. p. 99–104.
Seidler E, Kindt H, Schaub N: Jaspers und Freud. **Sudhoffs Arch** 1978;62(1):37–63
Taylor FK: On pseudo-hallucinations. **Psychol Med** 1981 May;11(2):265–71

**Jayle, Max Fernand, 1913–**
Hevér O: Max-Fernand Jayle, a haptoglobin felfedezöje. **Orv Hetil** 1979 Aug 26;120(34):2071–2

**al-Jayyānī, Abū 'Abd Allāh Muhammad ibn Mu'ādh**
Lindberg DC, ed: Opticae thesaurus. Alhazeni Arabis libri septem, nuncprimùm editi. Eiusdem liber De Crepusculis et nubium ascensionibus. Item Vitellonis Thuringopoloni libri X. Reprint of the 1572 ed. New York, Johnson Reprint Corp., 1972. xxxiv, 288, 474 p.

**Jean de Dieu, Saint, 1495–1550**
Tessier JF: L'hôpital de Ste-Marguerite de Cadillac et la littérature consacrée à Saint Jean de Dieu et ses disciples en France au XVIIe siècle. **Rev Fr Hist Livre** 1979;23:317–28

**Jeanne d'Arc, Saint, 1412–1431**
Allen C: The schizophrenia of Joan of Arc. **Hist Med (Lond)** 1975 Autumn-Winter;6(3–4):4–9

**Jefferson, Geoffrey, 1886–1961**
Himsworth H: Sir Geoffrey Jefferson. In Dictionary of national biography, 1961–1970. Suppl. 8, 1981. p. 580–1.
Jefferson A: Geoffrey Jefferson 1886–1961. **Surg Neurol** 1984 Jul;22(1):1–4

**Jefferson, Thomas, 1743–1826**
Battle JD Jr: The 'periodical head-achs' of Thomas Jefferson. **Cleve Clin Q** 1984 Fall;51(3):531–9
Cohen IB, ed: Thomas Jefferson and the sciences. New York, Arno Press, 1980. Reprints of various works. Various paginations. (Three Centuries of Science in America).
Dewey FL: Thomas Jefferson's law practice: the Norfolk anti-inoculation riots. **Va Mag Hist Biogr** 1983;91(1):39–53
Greene JC: American science in the age of Jefferson. Ames, Iowa State University Press, 1984. xiv, 484 p.
McCoy DR: Jefferson and Madison on Malthus: population growth in Jeffersonian political economy. **Va Mag Hist Biogr** 1980;88(3):259–76
Ragsdale JS: What did Thomas Jefferson mean by 'I have not yet lost a tooth by age'? **J Am Dent Assoc** 1984 Apr;108(4):643–4
Thorup OA: Thomas Jefferson: founder of two medical schools. **Trans Am Clin Climatol Assoc** 1980;92:16–22

**Jeffries, John, 1745–1819**
Cash P, Pine C: John Jeffries and the struggle against smallpox in Boston (1775–1776) and Nova Scotia (1776–1779). **Bull Hist Med** 1983;57(1):93–7
Gryfe CI: John Jeffries: the first flying physician. **Scalpel Tongs** 1981;25:80–2

**Jejjata, 9th cent.**
Sastry VV, Pandey AN: Jajjata. **Bull Indian Inst Hist Med (Hyderabad)** 1975 Jul;5(3):115–22

**Jelliffe, Smith Ely, 1866–1945**
Burnham JC, McGuire W: Jelliffe: American psychoanalyst and physician & his correspondence with Sigmund Freud and C. G. Jung. Chicago, University of Chicago Press, 1983. xx, 324 p. With contributions by A. R. D'Amore and J. E. Sauer.

**Jendrassik, Ernö, 1858–1921**
Czeizel A: A historical evaluation of the doctrine of heredodegeneration. **Orvostort Kozl** 1979;87–88(25 no 1–2):157–79

**Jenkins, Robert, fl. 1731–1738**
Liston SL: Traumatic amputation of the external ear: the War of Jenkins' Ear and George Washington. **Am J Surg** 1984 Nov;148(5):599–601

**Jenner, Edward, 1749–1823**
Baxby D: Jenner's smallpox vaccine. The riddle of vaccinia virus and its origin. London, Heinemann Educational Books, 1981. xiv, 214 p.
Bendiner E: Jenner: from folklore to scientific triumph. **Hosp Pract [Off]** 1984 Apr;19(4):183–7, 190–1, 196, passim
Bliquez LJ: An unidentified Roman surgical instrument in Bingen. **J Hist Med Allied Sci** 1981 Apr;36(2):219–20
Bonnabeau RC: Edward Jenner and the advent of vaccination. **Minn Med** 1983 May;66(5):331–3
Hammarsten JF, Tattersall W, Hammarsten JE: Who discovered smallpox vaccination? Edward Jenner or Benjamin Jesty? **Trans Am Clin Climatol Assoc** 1979;90:44–55
Kahn A: Highlights of the Adler Museum collections: the Jenner letter. **Adler Mus Bull** 1984 Jun;10(2):15–7
Kligfield P: The early pathophysiolic understanding of angina pectoris (Edward Jenner, Caleb Hillier Parry, Allan Burns). **Am J Cardiol** 1982 Dec;50(6):1433–5
Miller G: Edward Jenner letters in Baltimore, Maryland. In International Congress of the History of Medicine. 26th, Plovdiv, 1978. Actes du Congress. Sofia, 1981. Volume II. p. 157–9.
Miller G, ed: Letters of Edward Jenner and other documents concerning the early history of vaccination. From the Henry Barton Jacobs Collection in the William H. Welch Medical Library. Baltimore, London, Johns Hopkins University Press, 1983. xxix, 145 p. (Henry E. Sigerist Supplements to the Bulletin of the History of Medicine, n.s., no. 8).
Perry CB: Edward Jenner. **Ear Nose Throat J** 1984 Dec;63(12):605–17
Saunders P: Edward Jenner. The Cheltenham years 1795–1823. Being a chronicle of the vaccination campaign. Hanover, London, University Press of New England, 1982. xviii, 469 p.
White PJ, Shackelford PG: Edward Jenner, MD, and the scourge that was. **Am J Dis Child** 1983 Sep;137(9):864–9

**Jennings, Herbert Spencer, 1868–1947**
Pauly PJ: The Loeb-Jennings debate and the science of animal behavior. **J Hist Behav Sci** 1981 Oct;17(4):504–15

**Jensen, Wilhelm, 1837–1911**
Jaffe NC: A second opinion on delusions and dreams. A reading of Freud's interpretation of Jensen. In Jones AH, ed: Images of healers. Albany, State University of New York Press, 1983. p. 101–7.

**Jephson, Henry, 1798–1878**
Baxter EG: Dr. Jephson of Leamington Spa. Edited by J. Lane and R. Bearman. Leamington Spa, Warwickshire Local History Society, 1980. xii, 104 p.

**Jerie, Josef**
Sebek V: Josef Jerie—jeho život, doba, činnost, zásluhy. **Cesk Gynekol** 1980 Feb;45(1):55–68

**Jessen, Peter Willers, 1793–1895**
Hamann P: Peter Willers Jessens ehemaliges Asyl Hornheim in Kiel. Ein Beitrag zur Psychiatriegeschichte Schleswig-Holsteins. **Hist Hosp** 1979–80;13:69–95

**Jessen, Peter Willers, 1832–1912**
Hamann P: Peter Willers Jessens ehemaliges Asyl Hornheim in Kiel. Ein Beitrag zur Psychiatriegeschichte Schleswig-Holsteins. **Hist Hosp** 1979–80;13:69–95

**Jesty, Benjamin, 1737–1816**
Hammarsten JF, Tattersall W, Hammarsten JE: Who discovered smallpox vaccination? Edward Jenner or Benjamin Jesty? **Trans Am Clin Climatol Assoc** 1979;90:44–55
Wallace EM: The first vaccinator. Benjamin Jesty of Yetminster and Worth Matravers and his family. Wareham and Swanage (England), Anglebury-Bartlett, 1981. 20 p.

**Jesus Christ**
Fichtner G: Christus als Arzt: Ursprünge und Wirkungen eines Motivs. **Fruhmittelalt Stud** 1982;16:1–18
Miller VD, Pellicori SF: Ultraviolet fluorescence photography of the Shroud of Turin. **J Biol Photogr** 1981 Jul;49(3):71–85
Rocchietta S: Un 'Christ à la pharmacie' ou 'Les Saints Côme et Damien'? **Rev Hist Pharm (Paris)** 1984 Jun;31(261):131–3

**Jewett, Sarah Orne, 1849–1909**
Crumpacker L: The art of the healer: women in the fiction of Sarah Orne Jewett. **Colby Libr Q** 1983;19(3):155–66

**Jianzhen, fl. 688**
Chen YZ: The courageous and brilliant blind monk Jianshen. **Chin Med J [Engl]** 1980 Feb;93(2):130–3

**Al-Jildaki, d. ca. 1342**
Hamarneh SK: Jabir, Jildki and Ibn-Sallum, and Arabic-Islamic Alchemy. **Mesopotamia Q** 1980;8(29,30):110–22, 225–41

**Jiménez, Miguel Francisco, 1813–1876**
Fournier Villada R: Miguel Jiménez y su contribución al estudio del absceso hepático. In Academia Nacional de Medicina. Libro conmemorativo del primer centenario. México, Comité Editorial de la Comisión Organizadora del Congreso del Centenario, 1964. Tome 2. p. 558–60.

**Jimenez Murillo, Manuel, 1784–1859**
Alegre Pérez E, González García M: Estudio de la vida y obra científica de D. Manuel Jiménez Murillo. **Bol Soc Esp Hist Farm** 1983;34(136):185–201

**Jirsová, Blažena, 1901–1979**
Potměšilová R: RNDr. Blažena Jirsová zemřela první vedoucí redaktorka oddělení lékařských časopisu 6. 6. 1901--3. 9. 1979. **Cas Lek Cesk** 1979 Dec;118(52)1632

**João de Deus, 1618–1684**
Castro F de: Historia da vida e obras de S. Joao de Deus. Translation and notes by Foâo Gameiro, OH. Montemor-O-Novo, Editorial Franciscana, 1982. 166 p.
Filipe NF: S. João de deus um homem que soube amar. 2. edição. Lisboa, Edições Paulistas, [198–?]. 150 p.
Gastão M: S. João de Deus: sua vida-sua obra. Lisboa, Centro do Livro Brasileiro, 1982. 733 p.

**Jobert, Jean Baptiste, 1733–1792**
Desjardins E: Le docteur Jean-Baptiste Jobert (1733--1792). **Union Med Can** 1979 Feb;108(2):200

**Johann Maurits, Prince of Nassau-Siegen, 1604–1679**
De Moulin D: Medizinische und naturwissenschaftliche Aspekte der Regierungszeit des Grafen Johann Moritz von Nassau als Gouverneur in Brasilien (1637–1644). In: Soweit der Erdkreis reicht. J. M. von Nassau-Siegen 1604–1679. Kleve: Städtisches Museum Haus Koekkoek. 1979. pp. 33–46.

**Johannes Aegidius Zamorensis, 1240 or 41–ca. 1316**
Castro M de: Johannes Aegidii Zamorensis, OFM, contra venena et animalia venenosa. Introducción edición y notas. **Arch Iberoam** 1976;36:3–116

**Johannes Damascenus, b. ca. 676**
Rocchietta S: Von der Apothekergilde während des 15. Jahrhunderts gestiftete Glasfenster im Dom von Mailand. **Beitr Gesch Pharm** 1981;31(13):97–100

**Johannes XXI, Pope, d. 1277**
Dirckx JH: Peter Juliani, physician and pope. **Pharos** 1980 Fall;43(4):8–13

**Johannis of Alexandria**
Pritchet CD, ed: Iohannis Alexandrini Commentaria in sextum librum Hippocratis Epidemiarum. Leiden, Brill, 1975. xi, 470 p.

**Johansson, Sven, 1880–**
Bauer G: Sven Johanssons betydelse för höftfrakturernas behandling. **Sydsven Medicinhist Sallsk Arsskr** 1981;:12–29

**John I Albert, King of Poland, 1459–1501**
Dudziński W: Choroby zgon króla Jana Olbrachta. **Wiad Lek** 1981 Jul 1;34(13):1131–5

**Johnson, Frank Chambliss, 1894–1934**
Ström J: Männen bakom syndromet: Albert Stevens och Frank Johnson. Först att beskriva 'okänd infektionssjukdom'--allergi utlöst av läkemedel eller infektion. **Lakartidningen** 1983 Mar 16;80(11):1076–7

**Johnson, Hosmer Allan, 1822–1891**
Friedberg SA: The memorable life of Hosmer A. Johnson, early midwestern laryngologist. **Ann Otol Rhinol Laryngol** 1983 Sep-Oct;92(5 Pt 1):470–2

**Johnson, Robert Wilkinson, Jr., 1854–1930**
Harvey AM: Orthopaedic surgery at Johns Hopkins: a heritage of excellence in clinical practice, training and research. **Johns Hopkins Med J** 1982 Jun;150(6):221–45

**Johnson, Samuel, 1709–1784**
Glaser FB: Samuel Johnson: sometimes abstemious, always intemperate. **J Addict Res Found** 1981;10(9):11
Mulhallen J, Wright DJ: Samuel Johnson: amateur physician. **J R Soc Med** 1983 Mar;76(3):217–22
Murray TJ: Doctor Samuel Johnson's abnormal movements. **Adv Neurol** 1982;35:25–30

**Johnson, Wendell Andrew Leroy, 1906–1965**
Williams DE: Wendell Andrew Leroy Johnson. In Dictionary of American biography, 1961-1965. Suppl. 7, 1981. p. 395–6.

**Johnston, George, 1797–1855**
Binnie GA: George Johnston: 1797-1855. **Br Med J [Clin Res]** 1982 Oct 9;285(6347):1014–6

**Johnston, Harriet Lane, 1833–1903**
Rosenberger HT: Harriet Lane Johnston: pioneer advocate of special care for children with chronic diseases. **J Lanc Cty Hist Soc** 1972;76(1):1–28

**Johnston, Jan, 1603–1675**
Szpilczyński S: Jan Jonston z Szamotuł. Tytaniczny trud barokowego erudyty w świetle wielkiej dydaktyki. **Slaski Kwart Hist Sobotka** 1976;31(2):223–9

**Johnston, William, 1846–1900**
Fraser SM: Dr William Johnston (1846–1900) of Leicester--an unknown Victorian general practitioner. **J R Coll Gen Pract** 1983 Jun;33(251):369–71

**Joliot-Curie, Jean Frédéric, 1900–1958**
Del Regato JA: Jean Frederic Joliot. **Int J Radiat Oncol Biol Phys** 1980 May;6(5):621–40

**Jonas, Hans, 1903–**
Spicker SF, ed: Organism, medicine, and metaphysics. Essays in honor of Hans Jonas on his 75th birthday May 10, 1978. Dordrecht and Boston, Reidel, 1978. xxvii, 330 p. Contributions by A. Lowe, M. Landmann, P. O. Kristeller, O. E. Guttentag, E. J. Cassell, L. R. Kass, M. Grene, C. Hartshorne, S. Donnelley, B. S. Currie, R. Kennington, W. Magnus, M. Greene, R. M. Zaner, J. N. Mohanty, H. Arendt.

**Jonctys, Daniël, 1600–1654**
Moerman AK: Daniël Jonckthys--Dordts dokter en dichter. **Kwartaal Teken** 1979;5(3):5–10
Van Lieburg MJ: De dichter-medicus Daniël Jonctys (1611–1654), zijn strijd tegen het bijgeloof en zijn relatie tot Johan van Beverwijck, William Harvey en Daniël Sennert. **Tijdschr Geschied Geneeskd** 1979;2(4):137–67

**Jones, Calvin, 1775–1846**
Jones TB: Calvin Jones, M.D.: a case study in the practice of early American medicine. **NC Hist Rev** 1972;49(1):56–71

**Jones, Ernest, 1879–1958**
Brome V: Ernest Jones, Freud's alter ego. London, Caliban Books, 1982. 250 p.
D'Amore AR: Ernest Jones: founder of the American Psychoanalytic Association. **Int J Psychoanal** 1979;60(Pt 3)287–90
King P: The contributions of Ernest Jones to the British Psycho-Analytical Society. **Int J Psychoanal** 1979;60(Pt 3):280–4
Leys R: Meyer's dealings with Jones: a chapter in the history of the American response to psychoanalysis. **J Hist Behav Sci** 1981 Oct;17(4):445–65

**Jones, John Kenyon Netherton, 1912–1977**
Szarek WA, Stacey M, Hay GW: John Kenyon Netherton Jones (1912–1977). **Adv Carbohydr Chem Biochem** 1983;41:1–26

**Jones, John Paul, 1747–1792**
Eckert WG: Identification of the remains of John Paul Jones: a look at early methods. **Am J Forensic Med Pathol** 1982 Jun;3(2):143–52
Lasky II: Autopsy of Admiral John Paul Jones 113 years postmortem; historic and forensic aspects. **NY State J Med** 1982 Jun;82(7):1110–5

**Jones, Joseph, 1833–1896**
Breeden JO: Andersonville--a southern surgeon's story. **Bull Hist Med** 1973 Jul–Aug;47(4):317–43

**Jonson, Ben, 1572?–1637**
Drew-Bear A: Face-painting scenes in Ben Jonson's plays. **Stud Philol** 1980 Fall;47(4):338–401

**Jordán, Marcos, b. 1715**
Fernández DW: Marcos Jordan. **Rev Soc Venez Hist Med** 1979;28(42):25–7

**Jordan, Sara Claudia Murray, 1884–1959**
Rosenkrantz BG: Sara Claudia Murray Jordan. In: Notable American women. The modern period. Cambridge, Mass., Belknap-Harvard Univ. Press, 1980. 4:387–8.

**Jordan, Thomás, 1539–1586**
Petrescu AD: D. în secolul XVI, un clujean: medic de faimă europeană. **Mag Istor** 1976;10(12):27

**Jordon, Minnie Evangeline, 1865–1952**
Loevy HT: M. Evangeline Jordon, pioneer in pedodontics. **Bull Hist Dent** 1984;32(1):19–26

**Jores, Arthur, 1901–**
Menzel W: Klinische Rhythmusforschung unter A. Jores. **Dtsch Med Wochenschr** 1981;106:186–9

**Jörg, Johann Christian Gottfried, b. 1779**
Bethge R: Erstes orthopädisches Lehrbuch der Welt für den Gebrauch der Arzte. Zum 200. Geburtstage von Johann Christian Gottfried Jörg. **Beitr Orthop Traumatol** 1979 Sep;26(9):520–4

**Jorgensen, Niels Bjorn, 1894–1974**
Hayden J: Niels Bjorn Jorgensen: painless dentist. **Advent Herit** 1979;6(2):44–8

**Jósa, András, 1834–1918**
Fazekas A: Jósa András 150 éve született (1834. nov. 30.–1918. szept. 6.). **Orv Hetil** 1984 Sep 30;125(40):2444–6

**Joseph ben Meir ibn Zabara, b. ca. 1140**
Kottek SS: Joseph ben Meir ibn Zabara of Barcelona (1140?–?) (his place in the history of medicine). In International Congress of the History of Medicine, 27th, Barcelona, 1980. Actas. Barcelona, Académia de Ciències Mèdiques de Catalunya i Balears, 1981. p. 181–7.
Kottek SS: 'The book of delights' by Joseph ben Meir ibn Zabara of Barcelona (12th cent.). **Koroth** 1981;8(1–2):21–6

**Joseph II, Emperor of Germany, 1741–1790**
Wyklicky H: Förderer der Heilkunde. Medizin und Gesundheitswesen Josephs II. In: Was blieb von Joseph II.? Eine Dokumentation; Internationales Symposion Melk, 1980. [Vienna?], Edition Morgen, 1980. p. 66–76.
Wyklicky H: Maria Theresia und Joseph II. als Reformatoren des Gesundheitswesens in Oesterreich. **Wien Tierarztl Monatsschr** 1981;68(1):3–7
Wyklicky H: Uber die Fürsorge Josephs II. für elternlose und kranke Kinder. **Padiatr Padol** 1982;17(2):437–40

**Joseph, Jacques, 1865–1934**
Hauben DJ: Jacques Joseph (1865–1934). **Laryngol Rhinol Otol (Stuttg)** 1983 Feb;62(2):56–7
Natvig P: Jacques Joseph, surgical sculptor. Philadelphia, Saunders, 1982. xiii, 264 p.

**Joseph, Mother, 1828–1902**
Weiss RE: Mother Joseph: the legendary nun who broke ground for women and men health administrators in the West. **Hosp Forum** 1981 Jan–Feb;24(1):17–8

**Joseph, the Patriarch**
Berger J: New views on the Biblical Joseph. **Am J Psychoanal** 1981 Fall;41(3):277–82

**Joubert, Laurent, 1529–1582**
Ackerman RH: Joubert's 'Erreurs populaires'. An insight into some aspects of sixteenth century health care. In: Congrès international d'histoire de la médecine, XXVe, Québec, 1976. Actes. Québec, 1977. p. 455–60.
Joubert L: Treatise on laughter. Translated and annotated by G. D. de Rocher. University, Alabama, University of Alabama Press, 1980. xv, 155 p.

**Jouvet, Louis, 1887–1951**
Une lettre de Louis Jouvet à la veille d'entreprendre ses études de pharmacie: **Rev Hist Pharm (Paris)** 1981 Jun;28(249):121–4

**Jovanovic-Batut, Milana**
Dragić M: Povodom stogodišnjice osnivanja časopisa 'Zdravlje' dr Milana Jovanović-Batuta. **Srp Arh Celok Lek** 1980 Apr;108(4):391–5

**Joyce, James, 1882–1941**
Foley GP: A treasury of dentistry. **J Am Coll Dent** 1983 Spring;50(1):42–3
Shen WW, Soldo JJ: Symbol hunting in James Joyce's 'syphilizations'. **Arch Intern Med** 1981 Apr;141(5):691–2
Sullivan E: Ocular history of James Joyce. **Surv Ophthalmol** 1984 Mar–Apr;28(5):412–5
Tashjian LD: Aspects of internalization and individuation: James Joyce's Portrait of the artist as a young man. **Adolesc Psychiatry** 1982;10:75–84

**József, Attila, 1905–1937**
Kertész T: Attila József (1905–1937). **Orv Hetil** 1980;121:2207–9
Szállási A: Fábián Dániel és József Attila. **Orv Hetil** 1983 Feb 20;124(8):464–6

**Juan de Alós y Serradora, 1617–1695**
Suñé JM, ed: Pharmacopea cathalana sive antidotarium barcinonense. (Edición Facsímil). Barcelona, Catedra de Historia de la Farmacia y Legislacion Farmaceutica, Universidad de Barcelona, 1975. Various paginations.

**Juan de Dios, Saint, 1495–1550**
Díaz F: Influencia de San Juan de Dios en la enfermería. **Rev Enferm** 1982 Mar;5(45):12–4

**Juchereau de la Ferté, Jeanne-Françoise, 1650–1723**
Campeau L: Jeanne-Françoise Juchereau de la Ferté. In Dictionary of Canadian biography, 1701 to 1740. Volume 2, 1969. p. 302–3.

**Judah ha-Lévi, 1085?–1140?**
Kottek S: Eléments de physiologie dans le 'Kusari' de Juda Halevi (Espagne, 12e siècle). In: Congrès international d'histoire de la médecine, XXVe, Québec, 1976. Actes. Québec, 1977. p. 840–7.

**Juhász, Gyula, 1883–1937**
Péter L: Juhász Gyula betegségtudata. **Orv Hetil** 1983 May 15;124(20):1205–7

**Julliard, Gustave, 1836–1911**
Jost A: Commentaires sur les articles de Gustave Julliard. Fistule pyo-stercorale--laparotomie et suture de l'intestin--guérison par première intention. Hernio-laparotomie--résection de dix-huit centimètres d'intestin--guérison. **Rev Med Suisse Romande** 1980 Dec;100(12):1089–96

**Juncker, Johann, 1679–1759**
Lambrecht M: A magyar klinikai oktatás hallei mint ája. Johann Juncker, az orvospedagógus. **Orv Hetil** 1982 Jul 11;123(28):1745–8

**Jung, Carl Gustav, 1794–1864**
Zimmermann RE: The structure of mythos: on the cultural stability of alchemy. **Ambix** 1984 Nov;31(3):125–37

**Jung, Carl Gustav, 1875–1961**
Barz H: Psychologische Probleme des Unbewussten: C.G. Jung und sein Lebenswerk für die moderne Psychologie. **Universitas (Stuttg)** 1980;35(3):275–82
Burnham JC, McGuire W: Jelliffe: American psychoanalyst and physician & his correspondence with Sigmund Freud and C. G. Jung. Chicago, University of Chicago Press, 1983. xx, 324 p. With contributions by A. R. D'Amore and J. E. Sauer.
Carotenuto A: A secret symmetry: Sabina Spielrein between Jung and Freud. New York, Pantheon Books, 1982. xix, 250 p.
Evans RI: Dialogue with C. G. Jung. New York, Praeger, 1981. xi, 241 p.
Frey-Rohn L: Von Freud zu Jung. Eine vergleichende Studie zur Psychologie des Unbewussten. (2. überarbeitete Ausgabe) Zürich, Daimon Verlag, 1980?. 456 p.
Glaus B: Autographen und Manuskripte zur ETH- und zur Wissenschaftsgeschichte. **Gesnerus** 1982;39(3–4):437–42
Goering JD: Sigmund Freud, Carl Jung and religion. **Mennon Q Rev** 1982;56(1):47–56
Goldwert M: Toynbee and Jung: the historian and analytical psychology--a brief comment. **J Anal Psychol** 1983 Oct;28(4):363–6
Goodheart WB: C. G. Jung's first 'patient': on the seminal emergence of Jung's thought. **J Anal Psychol** 1984 Jan;29(1):1–34
Gras VW: Myth and the reconciliation of opposites: Jung and Lévi-Strauss. **J Hist Ideas** 1981 Jul–Sep;42(3):471–88
Gunter PA: Bergson and Jung. **J Hist Ideas** 1982 Oct–Dec;43(4):635–52
Hermanns LM. John F. Rittmeister und C. G. Jung. **Psyche (Stuttg)** 1982 Nov;36(11):1022–31
Hogenson GB: Jung's struggle with Freud. Notre Dame, London, University of Notre Dame Press, 1983. xi, 180 p.
Iijima E: [Records of hallucination: my attraction to Jung's world of hallucination]. (Jpn) **Kango Kyoiku** 1980 Feb;21(2):74–8
Iselin HK: Zur Entstehung von C. G. Jungs 'Psychologischen Typen.' Der Briefwechsel zwischen C. G. Jung und Hans Schmid-Guisan im Lichte ihrer Freundschaft. Aarau, Sauerländer, 1982. 152 p. (Veröffentlichungen der Schweizerischen Gesellschaft für Geschichte der Medizin und der Naturwissenschaften, Bd. 38).
Jaffé A: Aufsätze zur Psychologie C. G. Jungs. Zürich, Daimon, 1982. 160 p.
Jung CG: The essential Jung. Princeton, Princeton University Press, 1983. 447 p.
Jung CG: Erinnerungen, Träume, Gedanken. Olten, Walter-Verlag, 1984. 419 p.
Jung-Merker L, Ruf E, ed: C. G. Jung: Bibliographie. Olten [Switzerland], Walter-Verlag, 1983. 295 p. (C. G. Jung gesammelte Werke, 19)
Kirsch J: Jung's transference on Freud: its Jewish element. **Am Imago** 1984;41:63–84
Odajnyk VW: Jung and politics. The political and social ideas of C. G. Jung. New York, New York University Press, 1976. xv, 190 p.
Rice JL: Russian stereotypes in the Freud-Jung correspondence. **Slavic Rev** 1982 Spring;41(1):19–34
Rintelen F: Zur Persönlichkeit Karl Gustav Jungs. **Gesnerus** 1982;39(2):237–42
Rodríguez A: Samuel Ramos: influencia de Adler y Jung en su estudio sobre el carácter del Mexicano. **Cuad Hispanoam** 1977;109(326–327):420–30
Rogers FB: The legacy of Carl Jung. **Trans Stud Coll Physicians Phila** 1979 Sep;5(1 No 3):211–14
Rogers FB: Analytical psychology: Carl Jung and his circle. **Trans Stud Coll Physicians Phila** 1980 Dec;5(2 no 4):284–8
Rogers FB: Psychology in practice: a jungian perspective. **Del Med J** 1982 Mar;54(3):179–81
Rogers FB: Carl Jung and self-realization. **Penn Med** 1983 Oct;86(10):30, 32
Scheidhauer M: Un problème épineux entre Freud et Jung: le rêve. **Rev Hist Philos Relig** 1981;61(4):413–25
Sirota M: On the Freud-Jung correspondence. **Mod Stud** 1977;2(3):45–8
Smythies JR: A visit to Dr. Jung. **Ala J Med Sci** 1981 Jan;18(1):93–4
Staude JR: The adult development of C. G. Jung. Boston, Routledge & Kegan Paul, 1981. xxiv, 134 p.
Steele RS, Swinney SV: Freud and Jung: conflicts of interpretation. London, Boston, Routledge and Kegan Paul, 1982. x, 390 p.
Tedeschi G: Jung-Freud: un dilemma inattuale. Roma, Astrolabio, 1979. 88 p.
Thomas DM: Freud and the 'White Hotel'. **Br Med J [Clin Res]** 1983 Dec 24–31;287(6409):1957–60
Ujhely GB: Jungian approach to clinical practice. **ANA Publ** (NP-59):319–32, 1979
Van der Post L: Jung and the story of our time. New York, Vintage Books, 1977. 276 p.
Wallace ER: A commentary on the Freud-Jung letters.

Psychoanal Rev 1980 Spring;67(1):112-37
Wilson C: Lord of the underworld: Jung and the twentieth century. Wellingborough, Northamptonshire, Aquarian Press, 1984. 160 p.
Witten LC, Pachella R, ed: Alchemy and the occult: a catalogue of books and manuscripts from the collection of Paul and Mary Mellon given to Yale University Library. Vols. 3 and 4: Manuscripts 1225-1922. With an introduction by P. Kibre and additional notes by W. McGuire. New Haven, Yale University Library, 1977. 853 p.
Woodman RG: Freud and Jung: the parting of the ways. **Queens Q** 1978;85(1):93-108
Zinsstag: Memories of what mother told about her cousin Carl Gustav Jung. **J Am Soc Psychosom Dent Med** 1980;27(2):42-6

**Jung-Stilling, Johann Heinrich, 1740-1817**
Mehlhose F: Der gottesfürchtige Jung-Stilling. Ein Pionier der Star-Extraktion. Düsseldorf, Triltsch, 1983. 63 p. (Düsseldorfer Arbeiten zur Geschichte der Medizin, Beiheft VII).
Propach G: Johann Heinrich Jung-Stilling (1740-1817) als Arzt. Köln, 1983. 410 p. (Arbeiten der Forschungsstelle des Instituts für Geschichte der Medizin der Universität zu Köln, Band 27).

**Jünger, Ernst, 1895-**
Théodoridès J: Ernst Jünger ou 'l'oeil vivant'. **Gesnerus** 1983;40(1-2):193-202

**Junot, Jean Andoche, 1771-1813**
Poulet J: La mort de Junot. **Rev Inst Napoleon (Paris)** 1972;(123):57-62

**Jurasz, Antoni, 1847-1923**
Ergetowski R: Akta personalne prof. Antoniego Stanisława Jurasza w Heidelbergu i Karlsruhe. **Arch Hist Med (Warsz)** 1983;46(2):215-35
Schwann H: Anton Jurasz's Bedeutung für die Rhinolaryngologie aus heutiger Sicht. **Arch Hist Med (Warsz)** 1979;42(3):317-21

**Jussieu, Antoine de, 1686-1758**
Laissus J: La succession de Le Monnier au Jardin du Roi: Antoine-Laurent de Jussieu et René Louiche-Desfontaines. In: Congrès National des Sociétés Savantes, 91e, Rennes, 1966. Comptes Rendus. Paris, 1967. Section des Sciences, Tome 1. p. 137-52.

**Just, Adolf**
Rothschuh KE: Aus der Geschichte der Naturheilbewegung (VII). Die Heilkräfte von Licht, Luft und Erde. Arnold Rikli, Adolf Just und Pastor Felke. **ZFA (Stuttgart)** 1983 Jun 10;59(16):933-40

## K

**Kabay, János, 1896-1936**
Menner O: Kabay jános emléke képzömüvészeti alkotásokon. **Orvostort Kozl** 1981;93-96(27 No 1-4):237-49

**Kabiruddin, Hakim, 1894-1976**
Siddiqi T: Zubdat al-Hukama Allama Hakim Kabiruddin. **Stud Hist Med** 1981 Jun;5(2):87-132

**Kadanoff, Dimitri, 1900-1984**
Kühnel W, Wassilev W: In memoriam Dimitri Kadanoff. **Anat Anz** 1984;156(2):81-95

**Kadlický, Roman, 1899-1979**
Dienstbier E: Prof. MUDr. Roman Kadlický. Jeho život a dílo. **Cas Lek Cesk** 1980 Aug 22;119(33-34):915-20

**Kadyi, Henryk, 1851-1912**
Ergetowski R: Uzupełniajace studia H. Kadyi'ego w Uniwersytecie Lipskim w 1879 r. **Arch Hist Med (Warsz)** 1979;42(3):309-15
Sokołowska-Pituchowa J: Two monographs on the spinal cord vascularization. **Folia Morphol (Warsz)** 1980;39(1):1-8

**Kaempfer, Engelbert, 1651-1716**
Bonn G: Der wissenschaftliche Nachlass des lippischen Forschungsreisenden Engelbert Kaempfer im Britischen Museum. **Lipp Mitt Gesch Landeskd** 1979;48:69-116
Bowers JZ, Carrubba RW: Exotic antidotes in seventeenth century Asia: two assays from the Amoenitatum Exoticarum of Engelbert Kaempfer. **Clio Med** 1980 May;14(2):129-40
Carrubba RW: The first report of the harvesting of Asafetida in Iran. **Agric Hist** 1979;53(2):451-61
Carrubba RW: The first detailed report on Persian mummy. **Physis** 1981;23(4):461-71
Kaempfer E: Amoenitatum Exoticarum Politico-physico-medicarum. Fasciculi V, Quibus Continentur Variae Relationes, Observationes and Descriptiones Rerum Persicarum and Ulterioris Asiae (Lemgo: Meyeri, 1712). **J Hist Med Allied Sci** 1978 Jul;33(3):320-43

**Kafka, Franz, 1883-1924**
Mecke G: Der Jäger Gracchus, Kafkas Geheimnis. **Psyche (Stuttg)** 1981 Mar;35(3):209-36
Ortega Millán A, García Prieto A, Ocio León S: Acercamiento a la vida y obra de Kafka. **Actas Luso Esp Neurol Psiquiatr** 1982 Jul-Aug;10(4):223-7
Solana RM: Communication, language and family: a communicational analysis of Kafka's letter to his father. **Psychiatry** 1983 Nov;46(4):387-92

**Kagan, Helena, 1889-1978**
Winter ST, Ginott N: Two pioneer paediatricians in Palestine under the Turks. **Adler Mus Bull** 1983 Nov;Spec issue:58-61

**Kagawa, Genetsu, 1700-1777**
Sugitachi G: [Gen-etsu Kagawa and his obstetric practice] (Jpn). **Josanpu Zasshi** 1983 Jun;37(6):484-9

**Kájoni, Joannes, 1629 or 30-1687**
Spielmann J, Spielmann M: L'herbier de Joanus Kájoni. In: Congrès international d'histoire de la médecine, XXVe, Québec, 1976. Actes. Québec, 1977. p. 1301-15.

**Kalinskiĭ, Ossip, 1792-1858**
Zolotnitskiĭ IaI: O knige O. Kalinskogo 'Retseptura ili nastavlenie sochiniat' pravil'nye retsepty dlia studentov imperatorskoĭ mediko-khirurgicheskoĭ akademii'. **Klin Med (Mosk)** 1984 Apr;62(4):151

**Kalkar, Jan Stevenszoon van, 1499?-ca. 1550**
Roth-Woelfle L: Jan Stephen van Kalkar als Illustrator der Anatomie des Andreas Vesal. **Imprimatur** 1980;8:11
Roth-Wölfle L: Jan Stephan von Kalkar als Illustrator der Anatomie des Andreas Vesal. **Imprimatur** 1980;9:86-100

**Kallikak, Deborah, 1889-1978**
Doll EE: Deborah Kallikak: 1889-1978, a memorial. **Ment Retard** 1983 Feb;21(1):30-2

**Kallmann, Franz Josef, 1897-1965**
Gershon ES: The historical context of Franz Kallmann and psychiatric genetics. **Arch Psychiatr Nervenkr** 1981;229(4):273-6

**Kamenetskii, Osep Kirillovich, 1754-1823**
Bawden CR: W. A. Unkrig's correspondence with the British and Foreign Bible Society. A contribution to ... printing in Mongolian. **Zentralasiat Stud** 1980;14(1):65-108

**Kanavel, Allen Buckner, 1874-1938**
Wetzel N: Loyal Davis; Allen Kanavel; surgery, gynecology and obstetrics, and the development of neurosurgery. **Surg Gynecol Obstet** 1983 Aug;157(2):135-9

**Kandinskiĭ, Viktor Khrisanfovich, 1849-1889**
Kelemen G: V. H. Kandinszkij (1849-1889) a pszichopatológia nagy orosz úttörője. **Orv Hetil** 1984 Nov 25;125(48):2943-4, 2947
Taylor FK: On pseudo-hallucinations. **Psychol Med** 1981 May;11(2):265-71

**Kändler, Johannes Joachim, 1706-1775**
Moskow BS: The iconography of the dental profession. Der Zahnbrecher--the toothbreaker. Johannes Joachim Kändler (1706-1775). **Quintessence Int** 1984 Jan;15(1):40-1

**Kanitz, Felix Philipp, 1829-1904**
Bugyi B: Medical topography of Bulgaria and Serbia in the third quarter of the 19th century. **Geogr Med** 1981;11:158-61

**Kanner, Leo, 1894-1981**
Schopler E, Chess S, Eisenberg L: Our memorial to Leo Kanner. **J Autism Dev Disord** 1981 Sep;11(3):257-69
Wilk D: In memoriam Dr. Leo Kanner, 1894-1981. **Koroth** 1982 Aug;8(3/4):213-20

**Kant, Immanuel, 1724-1804**
Dietsch H: Die Altershygiene Kants. **Med Welt** 1982 Apr 16;33(15):570-2
Eckhardt G, ed: Zur Geschichte der Psychologie. Berlin, VEB Deutscher Verlag der Wissenschaften, 1979. 128p. Mit Beiträgen von H. Hiebsch, F. Klix, W. Schreier, und L. Sprung.
Lenoir T: Kant, Blumenbach, and vital materialism in German biology. **Isis** 1980 Mar;71(256):77-108
Löw R: Philosophie des Lebendigen. Der Begriff des Organischen bei Kant, sein Grund und seine Aktualität. Frankfurt am Main, Suhrkamp, 1980. 358 p.
Seidler MJ: Kant and the stoics on suicide. **J Hist Ideas** 1983 Jul-Sep;44(3):429-53
Sprung L: Immanuel Kant in der Geschichte der Psychologie--Aspekte seines Beitrages in der Entwicklung zur Einzelwissenschaft. In Eckardt G, ed: Zur Geschichte der Psychologie. Berlin, VEB Deutscher Verlag der Wissenschaften, 1979. p. 33-42.

**Kantor, Jacob Robert, 1888-**
Delprato DJ: The reactional biography concept: early contribution to a perspective for the psychology of aging. **Hum Dev** 1980;23(5):314-22

**Kaposi, Moriz, 1837-1902**
Braun M: Classics in Oncology. Idipathic multiple pigmented sarcoma of the skin by Kaposi. **CA** 1982 Nov-Dec;32(6):340-7
Frankl J: Adatok Kaposi Móricz professzor magyarságához. **Orv Hetil** 1982 Jan 10;123(2):110-1
Holubar K, Frankl J: Moriz (Kohn) Kaposi. **Am J Dermatopathol** 1981 Winter;3(4):349-54

**Kapsukas, Vincas, 1880-1935**
Bergman A: Pobeg V. S. Mitskevicha-Kapsukasa iz suvalkskoi bol'nitsy v 1906 G. **Vopr Istor** 1965;(3):74-6

**Karafiát, Ferdinand, 1870-1928**
Kraus B: MUDR. Ferdinand Karafiát (1870-1928). Aliis serviendo consumor. **Cas Lek Cesk** 1983 Jul 1;122(26):830-1

**Karll, Agnes, 1868-1927**
Lungershausen M: Unsere Rückblende aus dem Jahr 1952. Agnes Karll (25. 3. 1868 - 12. 2. 1927). **Krankenpflege (Frankfurt)** 1982 Feb;36(2):71-2
Sticker A: Agnes Karll, die Reformerin der deutschen Krankenpflege. Ein Wegweiser für heute zu ihrem 50. Todestag am 12. Februar 1927. Wuppertal, Aussat, 1977. 240 p.

**Karpov, Sergei Petrovich, 1903-**
Iastrebov VK: Nauchnoe nasledie S. P. Karpova v oblasti prirodno-ochagovykh infektsiĭ. **Zh Mikrobiol Epidemiol Immunobiol** 1983 Oct;(10):113-5

**Karwowski, Rowan**
Sienkiewicz H: Wspomnienie pośmiertne o doc. dr. med. Romanie Karwowskim. **Otolaryngol Pol** 1980;34(4):417-9

**Kashchenko, Petr Petrovich, 1859-1920**
Gerish AG: P. P. Kashchenko: 1859-1920. Moskva, Meditsina, 1980. 77 p.

**Kassirskiĭ, Iosif Abramovich, 1898-1972?**
Askarov UA: Znachenie trudov Akademika AMN SSSR I. A. Kassirskogo v nauchnoĭ razrabotke uzlovykh problem kraevoĭ patologii Uzbekistana (k 10-letiiu so dnia smerti). **Ter Arkh** 1982;54(2):150-2
Borob'ev RI: I. A. Kassirskiĭ i razvitie Sovetskoĭ meditsiny. **Ter Arkh** 1982;54(2):148-50
Vorob'ev RI: Istoriko-meditsinskie raboty I. A. Kassirskogo. **Feldsher Akush** 1984 Jul;49(7):44-6
Zhuravleva TV, Vorob'ev RI: Problemy deontologii v trudakh akademika AMN SSSR I. A. Kassirskogo. **Sov Zdravookhr** 1984;(10):56-7

**Kasznicki, Jerzy, 1934-1979**
Fijałek J: Dr. N. Med. Jerzy Kasznicki (3.1.1934--20.VII.1979). **Arch Hist Med (Warsz)** 1980;43(2):121-5

**Katayama, Kunika, 1855-1931**
Ozawa S: Hoigaku shiso Katayama Kunika/G. Tokyo, Shin Jinbutsu Oraisha, Showa 50 nen [1975]. 130 p.

**Katsch, Gerhardt, 1887-**
Dittrich HM: Die Pavlov-Lehre im Forschungsprogramm von Gerhardt Katsch. **Z Gesamte Inn Med** 1983 Apr 1;38(7):230-2

**Kaulbach, Wilhelm von, 1805-1874**
Rothkopf A: 'Das Narrenhaus' von W. Kaulbach und die Deutung des Bildes durch J. A. Schilling 1863. **Confin Psychiatr** 1980;23(1):51-64

**Kavetskiĭ, Rostyslav Ievhenovych**
Diadiusha GF, Turkevich NM, Bulkina ZP: Vklad R. E. Kavetskogo v razvitie onkologii (k 80-letiiu so dnia rozhdeniia). **Vopr Onkol** 1979;25(11):102-10

**Kay-Shuttleworth, James Phillips, 1804-1877**
Pickstone JV: Ferriar's fever and Kay's cholera: disease and social structure in Cottonopolis. **Soc Soc Hist Med Bull (Lond)** 1980;27:19-22
Pickstone JV: Ferriar's fever to Kay's cholera: disease and social structure in cottonopolis. **Hist Sci** 1984 Dec;22(58 pt 4):401-19

**Kayser, Marie-Elise, 1885-1950**
Abe HR, Schmidt H: Dr. med. Marie-Elise Kayser (1885-1950) - ein Leben für die Kinder. **Beitr Gesch Univ Erfurt** 1979-83;19:293-8
Schmidt H: Dr. med Marie-Elise Kayser in ihren Beziehungen zur Sowjetunion. **Beitr Gesch Univ Erfurt** 1979-83;19:299-303

**Kazanjian, Varaztad Hovhonnes, 1879-1974**
Converse JM: The extraordinary career of Doctor Varaztad Hovhannes Kazanjian. **Plast Reconstr Surg** 1983 Jan;71(1):138-43
Deranian HM: The miracle man of the western front: the story of Dr. Varaztad Kazanjian. **Bull Hist Dent** 1984 Oct;32(2):85-103

**Kazinczy, Ferenc, 1759-1831**
Hogye I: Kazinczy Ferenc feljegyzései a betegségekrol. **Orvostort Kozl** 1982;28(1-3):241-3

**Keats, John, 1795-1821**
Dubovsky H: John Keats (1795-1821)--poet, physician and tuberculosis patient. **S Afr Med J** 1981 Jun 6;59(24):875-8
Gittings R: Keats and medicine. **Contemp Rev** 1971;219(1268):138-42
Gittings R: Edward Osler and John Keats. In J. Cule, ed: Wales and medicine. London, British Society for the History of Medicine, 1975. p. 107-11.
Holbrook DM: John Keats: student at the United Hospitals. **St Thomas Hosp Gaz** 1981;79(1):22-4
Smith H: John Keats: poet, patient, physician. **Rev Infect Dis** 1984 May-Jun;6(3):390-404
Walsh W: The Keatsian paradox: the hectic and the healthy. **Ann R Coll Surg Engl** 1984 Mar;66(2):139-44

**Keeling, James Hurd, 1831-1909**
Sakula A: L'histoire du bacille tuberculeux telle qu'il nous la raconte dans 'La Ballade de la Seringue'. **Bull Int Union Tuberc** 1982 Sep-Dec;57(3-4):192-3

**Keen, William Williams, 1837-1932**
Geist DC: William Williams Keen, M.D. (1837-1932), surgeon and author. **Trans Stud Coll Physicians Phila** 1977 Apr;44(4):182-93

**Keen, William Wilson**
Miller M: The Walter Bradford Cannon Papers. **Surv Sources Newsl** 1977 May;5:8-9

**Kehr, Hans, 1862-1916**
Abe HR: Zur Sicherstellung des Nachlasses von Prof. Dr. Hans Kehr. **Beitr Gesch Univ Erfurt** 1979-83;19:259-64
Abe HR: Zur Biographie von Hans Kehr (1862-1916). **Beitr Gesch Univ Erfurt** 1979-83;19:233-40
Abe HR: Der soziale Aspekt im ärztlichen Wirken des grossen deutschen Gallenchirurgen Dr. Hans Kehr. **Beitr Gesch Univ Erfurt** 1979-83;19:241-58

**Keilin, David, 1887-1963**
Hartree EF: David Keilin. In Dictionary of national biography, 1961-1970. Suppl. 8, 1981. p. 604-5.

**Keill, James, 1673-1719**
Boss J: An early eighteenth-century criticism of clinical medicine as experimental philosophy. **Koroth** 1980 Jun;7(11-12):CCLXV-CCLXXV
Leibowitz JO: Early accounts in geriatric pathology (Leonardo, Harvey, James Keill). **Koroth** 1980 Jun;7(11-12):CCLIII-CCLXIV

**Keller, Helen Adams, 1880-1968**
Lash JP: Helen Keller. In: Notable American women. The modern period. Cambridge, Mass., Belknap-Harvard Univ. Press, 1980. 4:389-93.

**Kelley, Florence, 1859-1932**
Cloutier RJ: Florence Kelley and the radium dial painters. **Health Phys** 1980 Nov;39(5):711-6
Harmon SD: Florence Kelley in Illinois. **J Ill State Hist Soc** 1981;74(3):162-78

**Kellogg, John Harvey, 1852-1943**
Edwards R: Graham-Kellogg, early American contributors to health education. **J Sch Health** 1981 Nov;51(9):589-91

**Kells, Charles Edmund, 1856-1928**
Carr JD: The great radiology debate: the letters of C. Edmund Kells and Howard R. Raper. **Bull Hist Dent** 1981 Oct;29(2):69-73
Gardiner JF: C. Edmund Kells: New Orleans' gift to dentistry. **Bull Hist Dent** 1981;29(1):2-7

**Kelly, Howard Atwood, 1858-1943**
Kelly HA: Pre-1933 history of gynecology in Maryland. Part 1. **Md State Med J** 1980 Mar;29(3):81-5

**Kelly, James Gordon, 1930-**
Todd DM, Trickett EJ: The 1978 Division 27 award for distinguished contributions to community psychology and community mental health: James G. Kelly. **Am J Community Psychol** 1979 Jun;7(3):239-61

**Kelso, John Joseph, 1864-1935**
Jones A: In the children's aid: J. J. Kelso and child welfare in Ontario. Toronto, Buffalo, University of Toronto Press, 1981. viii, 210 p.

**Kemp, Tage, 1896-1964**
Czeizel E: Tage Kemp, a nagy dán orvos-genetikus, az elsö gentikai tanácsadó megalapítója. **Orv Hetil** 1980 Jun 15;121(24):1460-2

**Kemper, William Harrison, 1839-1927**
Bonsett CA: Dr. G. W. H. Kemper and his work in indexing the Transactions of the Indiana State Medical Society. **J Indiana State Med Assoc** 1980 Sept;73(9):561
Bonsett CA: G. W. H. Kemper, M.D. (1839-1927), Indiana medical historian. **J Indiana State Med Assoc** 1980 Jul;73(7):424

**Kempner, Walter, 1903-**
Stead EA: Kempner revisited. **NC Med J** 1983 Apr;44(4):237-40

**Kendall, Edward Calvin, 1886-1972**
Nusynowitz ML: The isolation of thyroxine (Edward C Kendall). **JAMA** 1983 Oct 21;250(15):2047-8

**Kennedy, Evory, 1807?-1886**
Pinkerton JH: Evory Kennedy: a master controversial. **Ir Med J** 1984 Mar;77(3):77-81

**Kennedy, John Fitzgerald, 1917-1963**
Berkowitz ED: The politics of mental retardation during the Kennedy Administration. **Soc Sci Q** 1980;61(1):128-43
Reexamination of accoustic evidence in the Kennedy assassination: **Science** 1982 Oct 8;218(4568):127-33

**Kennedy, William, fl. 1845-1866**
C[one] TE: Early viability of the fetus - an extraordinary case (1845). **Pediatrics** 1981;67:903

**Kennicott, John A.**
Ernst EA: John A. Kennicott of the Grove: physician, horticulturist, and journalist in nineteenth-century Illinois. **J Ill State Hist Soc** 1981;74(2):109-18

**Kennon, Uolter, 1871–1945**
IAroshevskiĭ MG: Uolter Kennon (1871–1945). Moskva, Nauka, 1976. 374 p.

**Kenny, Elizabeth, 1880–1952**
Cohn V: Sister Kenny's fierce fight for better polio care. **Smithsonian** 1981;12(8):180–200
Hall EM: In the ward next door to Sister Kenny. **Aust Nurses J** 1981 May;10(10):57–8
Willis E: Sister Elizabeth Kenny and the evolution of the occupational division of labour in health care. **Aust NZ J Sociol** 1979;15(3):30–8

**Kent, Stanley**
Anderson RH, Becker AE: Stanley Ken and accessory atrioventricular connections. **J Thorac Cardiovasc Surg** 1981 May;81(5):649–58

**Kepes Gyula, 1847–**
Szállási A: A fagyvilágmagyar orvosvándora. **Orv Hetil** 1984 Apr 1;125(14):835–7

**Kępiński, Antoni**
Aleksandrowicz JW, Bomba J, Broszkiewicz E, et al: Kępiński jako klinicysta. **Przegl Lek** 1983;40(12):843–8
Drozdowski P, Kokoszka A: Psychoterapia według Antoniego Kępińskiego. **Przegl Lek** 1983;40(12):877–80
Fortuna D, Nieniewska M, Szymusik A: Kępiński jako nauczyciel i wychowawca. **Przegl Lek** 1983;40(12):837–41
Jakubik A: Psychiatria fenomenologiczna w ujęciu Antoniego Kępińskiego. **Psychiatr Pol** 1980 Jul–Aug;14(4):395–401
Jakubik A: Antoni Kępiński -- Twórca psychiatrii aksjologicznej. **Psychiatr Pol** 1980 Jul–Aug;14(4):403–7
Jakubik A: Antoni Kepiński: człowiek i dzieło. Warszawa, Państwowy Zakład Wydawn. Lekarskich, 1981. 426 p.
Leśniak E, Leśniak R, Ryn Z: Nurt oświecimski w twórczości Antoniego Kępińskiego. **Przegl Lek** 1983;40(12):849–54
Maslowski J: Antoni Kepiński w latach 1939–1947. **Przegl Lek** 1981;38(1):126–37
Masłowski J: Reakcje na twórczość Antoniego Kępińskiego. **Przegl Lek** 1983;40(12):861–4
Ryn Z: Antoni Kępiński we wspomnieniach. **Przegl Lek** 1983;40(12):881–4
Struzik T: Metabolizm informacyjny Kępińskiego w świetle teorii informacji. **Przegl Lek** 1983;40(12):865–71
Tischner J: Refleksje nad dziełem Antoniego Kępińskiego. **Przegl Lek** 1983;40(12):855–9
Zadecki J: O Kępińskiego 'Schizofrenii'. **Przegl Lek** 1983;40(12):873–6

**Kepler, Johann, 1571–1630**
Gregory RL: Two pins and a length of string: Kepler's vision. **Perception** 1983;12(4):371–4
Häussler S: Johannes Kepler und die Allgemeinmedizin. **ZFA (Stuttgart)** 1982 May 31;58(15):I–1037–8

**Kern, Ferdo, 1872–1960**
Rapić S: O zivotu i radu Ferde Kerna. In: I simpozij o historiji mikrobiologije i imunologije u Hrvatskoj do 1923. godine. Zagreb, Jugoslavenskoj akademiji, 1973. p. 85–93.

**Kerner, Justinus, 1786–1862**
Weber M: Kerners 'Kleksographien' und Rorschachs 'Psychodiagnostik'. **Gesnerus** 1984;41(1/2):101–9

**Kernohan, James Watson, 1896–1981**
Dahlin DC: James Watson Kernohan: 1896–1981. **Surg Neurol** 1984 Feb;21(2):107–9

**Kerr, Frederick William Lawson, 1923–1983**
Yaksh TL: Obituary for Dr. Frederick W. L. Kerr. **Pain** 1984 Mar;18(3):217–20

**Kersting, Johann Adam, 1727–1784**
Wens HM: Johann Adam Kerstings Neujahrs-Kolleg an der Thierarzney-Schule (TAS), Hannover vom 3. Januar 1784. **DTW** 1981 Jan 5;88(1):35–8

**Ketilsson, Magnús, 1732–1803**
Johnsen B: Islands folkemedicin og Magnus Ketilsson. **Dan Medicinhist Arbog** 1982;:56–70

**Kety, Seymour Solomon, 1915–**
Kety SS: The metamorphosis of a psychobiologist. **Annu Rev Neurosci** 1979;2:1–15

**Keyes, Edward Lawrence, 1843–1924**
The cutaneous punch by Edward L. Keyes (J Cutan Genitourin Dis, March 1887): **Arch Dermatol** 1982 Nov;118(11):940–2

**Keynes, Geoffrey, 1887–**
Keynes G: The gates of memory. Oxford, Clarendon, 1981. xi, 428 p.

**Khavkin, Vladimir Aaronovich**
Karavaev AG, Berenshteĭn GF: Vydaiushchiĭsia épidemiolog (Vladimir Aaronovich Khavkin). **Med Sestra** 1981 Jul;40(7):55–7

**Khodin, Andreĭ Vasil'evich, 1847–**
Volkov VV, Danilichev VF: Professor A.V. Khodin - osnovatel' i pervyĭ redaktor-izdatel' 'Vestnika oftal'mologii' (k 100-letiiu zhurnala). **Vestn Oftalmol** 1984 Nov–Dec;(6):3–4

**Kholodkovskiĭ, Nikolaĭ Aleksandrovich, 1858–1921**
Shcherbina VP, Liashenko NI: Vsia zhizn'--vdokhnovennyĭ trud. **Voen Med Zh** 1983 Mar;3:70–1
Shusterov AK, Shcherbina VP: Nikolaĭ Aleksandrovich Kholodkovskiĭ (K 125-letiiu so dnia rozhdeniia). **Parazitologiia** 1983 Jul–Aug;17(4):322–4

**Khotsianov, Lev Kipricanovich, 1889–**
Shirokov IuG, Lebedeva NV, Koliadich MN: Uchastie L. K. Khotsianova v rabote s'ezdov gigienistov i sanitarnykh vracheĭ. **Gig Sanit** 1983 Feb;(2):31–5

**Khwada**
Matsumoto A: [Recent findings in the history of anesthesiology (10)--Khwada, a celebrated physician at the Han dynasty was a Persian] (Jpn). **Masui** 1980 Sep;29(9):946–8

**Kienboeck, Robert, 1871–1953**
Peltier LF: The classic. Concerning traumatic malacia of the lunate and its consequences: degeneration and compression fractures. **Clin Orthop** 1980 Jun;149:4–8

**Kierkegaard, Søren Aabye, 1813–1855**
Holder FL: Søren Kierkegaard's final illness and death. **Anglican Theol Rev** 1979;61(4):508–14
Smith JH, ed: Kierkegaard's truth: the disclosure of the self. New Haven, London, Yale University, 1981. xvii, 438 p. (Psychiatry and the Humanities. Volume 5.) With contributions by P. L. Holmer, P. B. Armstrong, J. Collins, H. A. Durfee, W. Kerrigan, B. H. Kirmmse, L. H. Mackey, V. A. McCarthy, W. W. Meissner, P. Ricoeur, M. C. Taylor, M Theunissen.

**Kierstede, Hans, d. 1666**
Riker DM: Surgeon Hans Kierstede of New Amsterdam. **Halve Maen** 1983;57(3):11–3, 24

**Kieser, Dietrich Georg, 1779–1862**
Ortmann F: Dietrich Georg Kieser (1779–1862)--nur ein romantischer **Z Gesamte Inn Med** 1979 Sep 1;34(17):486–9

**Kilgore, Harley Martin, 1893–1956**
Maddox RF: The politics of World War II science: Senator Harley M. Kilgore and the legislative origins of the National Science Foundation. **W Va Hist** 1979;41(1):20–39

**Kilmer, Frederick Barnett, 1851–1934**
Bowers RA: Frederick B. Kilmer: a notable New Jersey pharmacist. **J Med Soc NJ** 1984 Sep;81(9):765–8

**Kilner, Thomas Pomfret, 1890–**
As I remember. T. P. Kilner.: **Ann Plast Surg** 1980 Apr;4(4):328–36

**Kimberly, Edmund Stoughton, 1803–1874**
Beatty WK: ESK--a medical original. (Edmund Stoughton Kimberly). **Proc Inst Med Chic** 1980 Apr–Jun;33(2):54–8

**Kimmelstiel, Paul, 1900–1970**
Bergstrand A, Ostman J: Männen bakom syndromet: Paul Kimmelstiel och Clifford Wilson. Tysk och engelsman som möttes vid Harvard - först att beskriva speciell glomerulusskada. **Lakartidningen** 1984 Jan 25;81(4):227–8

**King, Albert Freeman Africanus, 1841–1914**
Chernin E: Two physicians, a landscape architect, and malaria. **Bull NY Acad Med** 1984 Nov;60(9):932–7

**King, Earl Judson, 1901–1962**
Wootton ID: Earl Judson King. In Dictionary of national biography, 1961–1970. Suppl. 8, 1981. p. 612–3.

**King, Frederic Truby, 1858–1938**
Olssen E: Truby King and the Plunket Society: an analysis of a prescriptive ideology. **NZ J Hist** 1981;15(1):3–23

**King, John, 1614–1681**
Birken W: Dr. John King (1614–1681) and Dr. Assuerus Regemorter (1615–1650). Brethren in the Dutch Church and in the Royal College of Physicians of London, with added references to other 'Dutch' congregants in the Royal College, Dr. Baldwin Hamey and Dr. George Ent. **Med Hist** 1976 Jul;20(3):276–95

**King, Thomas Starr, 1824–1864**
Posner RM: Thomas Starr King and the mercy million. **Calif Hist Soc Q** 1964;43(4);291–308

**Kingsley, Norman Williams, 1829–1913**
Herschfeld JJ: Norman W. Kingsley and his pioneering techniques in the correction of cleft palate. **Bull Hist Dent** 1983 Apr;31(1):23–8
Santopolo JL: Norman W. Kingsley. 'He helped the dumb to speak'. **NY State Dent J** 1980;46:606, 608, 610
Walter JD: Charles W. Stearns and Norman W. Kingsley and the development of the artificial velum. **Bull Hist Dent** 1981 Oct;29(2):74–81

**Kinsey, Alfred Charles, 1894–1956**
Christenson CV: Alfred Charles Kinsey. In Dictionary of American Biography, Suppl. 6, 1956–1960. p. 342–4, 1980.

**Kircher, Athanasius, 1602–1680**
Jaeger W: Die Ordnungsprinzipien der Farbsysteme des 17. Jahrhunderts. (Franciscus Aguilonius--Athanasius Kircher--Isaac Newton). **Klin Monatsbl Augenheilkd** 1984 Apr;184(4):321–5

Kaiser W: Athanasius Kircher (1602–1680) und die medizinisch-naturwissenschaftlichen Konzeptionen seiner Zeit. **Z Gesamte Inn Med** 1981 Jul 15;36(14):494–9

**Kirchner, Ernst Ludwig, 1880–1938**
Reiter A: Ernst L. Kirchner--Psychoanalytische Perspektiven der Psychoökonomie seines künstlerischen Schaffens. **Confin Psychiatr** 1980;23(2):118–28

**Kirk, Norman Thomas, 1888–1960**
Williams WH: Norman Thomas Kirk. In Dictionary of American Biography, Suppl. 6, 1956–1960. p. 344–5, 1980.

**Kirkbride, Thomas Story, 1809–1833**
Layne GS: The Kirkbride-Langenheim collaboration: early use of photography in psychiatric treatment in Philadelphia. **Pa Mag Hist Biogr** 1981;105(2):182–202

**Kirschenfeld, J. J., 1919–**
McDonald WH: Country doctor: he can't go home again. **J Med Assoc State Ala** 1982 Oct;52(4):8–9, 12–4, 19–22

**Kirschner, Martin, 1879–1942**
Romm S: The person behind the name: Martin Kirschner. **Plast Reconstr Surg** 1983 Jul;72(1):104–7
Zenker R: Die Chirurgie Martin Kirschners in unserer Zeit. **MMW** 1980 Feb 29;122(9):318–9

**Kitagawa, Otojiro, fl. 1901**
Matsuki A: Nothing new under the sun--a Japanese pioneer in the clinical use of intrathecal morphine. **Anesthesiology** 1983 Mar;58(3):289–90

**Kiter, Aleksandr A., 1813–1884**
Mirskiĭ MB, Verbitskiĭ VM, Khil'chenko MA: K 170–letiiu so dnia rozhdeniia A. A. Kitera. **Akush Ginekol (Mosk)** 1983 Sep;(9):72–3
Mirskiĭ MB, Khil'chenko MA: Professor A. A. Kiter--pervyĭ uchenik Pirogova (k 170–letiiu so dnia rozhdeniia A. A. Kitera). **Sov Zhdravookhr** 1983;(11):68–71

**Kiwisch, Alexander Franz Wilhelm, 1814–1851**
Müller B: Franz Kiwisch, Ritter von Rotterau 1814–1851. Diss. Würzburg, 1980. 111 p.

**Klaesi, Jakob, 1883–**
Haenel T: Jakob Klaesi--Schlafkur und Antieidodiathese. **Gesnerus** 1979;36(3–4):246–65

**Klebs, Arnold Carl, 1870–1943**
Fulton JF: History of medicine-Arnold Klebs and Harvey Cushing at the 1st International Neurological Congress at Berne in 1931. **Int J Neurol** 1980;14(1):103–15

**Klebs, Edwin, 1834–1913**
Thom A: Theorie und Empirie in der Entstehungsgeschichte der Bakteriologie - der Beitrag von Edwin Klebs zur Begründung der bakteriologischen Ara. **Wiss Beitr Martin Luther Univ Halle Wittenberg** 1983;5–R80:71–8

**Klecki, Karol, 1866–1931**
Guzek JW: Professor Karol Klecki 1866–1931. **Przegl Lek** 1981;38(12):873–4
Szymańska R: Karol Klecki (1866–1931) - wybitny patofizjolog i profesor Fakultetu Medycznego w Krakowie (w 50 rocznicę śmierci). **Pol Tyg Lek** 1981 Sep 21;36(38):1487–90

**Klee, Paul, 1879–1940**
Eckstaedt A: 'Mimi überreicht Madam Grenouillet einen Blumenstrauss'. Eine psychoanalytische Studie über den Weg der Phantasie des vierjährigen Paul Klee anhand einer Kinderzeichnung. **Psyche (Stuttg)** 1980 Dec:34(12):1123–44

**Kleegman, Sophia Josephine, 1901–1971**
Dwork D: Sophia Josephine Kleegman. In: Notable American women. The modern period. Cambridge, Mass., Belknap–Harvard Univ. Press, 1980. 4:398–400.

**Klein, George Stuart, 1917–**
Ross JM, Slap JW, Gehrie MJ, et al: George Klein's 'Psychoanalytic theory' in perspective. **Psychoanal Rev** 1980 Summer;67(2):161–216

**Klein, Marc, 1905–1975**
Gusdorf G: Médecine romantique. A la mémoire du Pr Marc Klein. **Etud Philos** 1981;(1):11–23

**Klein, Melanie, 1882–1960**
King PH: The life and work of Melanie Klein in the British Psycho-Analytical Society. **Int J Psychoanal** 1983;64 (Pt 3):251–60
Petot JM: Mélanie Klein: le moi et le bon objet, 1932–1960. [Paris], Dunod, 1982. xvi, 303 p.
Segal H: Klein. Brighton, England, Harvester Press with Fontana Books, 1979. 189 p.
Segal H: Melanie Klein. New York, Viking, 1980. vii, 194 p.

**Kleinwächter, Ludwig, 1839–1906**
Kahle E: Kleinwächter, Ludwig. In Neue Deutsche Biographie 12. 1980. p. 9–10.

**Kleist, Heinrich von, 1777–1811**
Gilman SL: Den Geisteskranken sehen: Mackenzie, Kleist, William James. **Confin Psychiatr** 1979;22(3):127–44

**Kleist, Karl, 1879–**
Barahona Fernándes H: O sentido actual de obra de K. Kleist e as repercusões nos países Ibero-Americanos. **Actas Luso Esp Neurol Psiquiatr** 1979 Nov–Dec;7(6):341–52

**Klinkosch, Joseph Thaddäus, 1734–1778**
Kahle E: Klinkosch, Joseph Thaddäus. In Neue Deutsche Biographie 12. 1980. p. 101–2.

**Kloos, Karlferdinand, 1911–1980**
Karlferdinand Kloos (17. 8. 1911 bis 29. 12. 1980): **Verh Dtsch Ges Pathol** 1981;65:548–59

**Kluyskens, Jozef Frans, 1771–1843**
Quintyn JB: Jozef Frans Kluyskens (1771–1843), eerste voorman van het Vlaams-Belgisch doktersgild. **Sartonia** 1980 Dec;49:1–37

**Knaus, Hermann Hubert, 1892–1970**
Siefert H: Hermann Knaus. **Neue Dtsch Biogr** 1980;12:163–4

**Kneipp, Sebastian, 1821–1897**
Beckmann P, Kirchhoff HW: Heilkunst und Heilkunde am Beispiel des Pfarrers Sebastian Kneipp. **Ther Ggw** 1980 Aug;119(8):945–53
Kolb A: Sebastian Kneipp und Vorarlberg. **Montfort** 1971;23(2):158–62
Mader G: Studien zur Gesundheitsbildung und Ordnungslehre bei Sebastian Kneipp: ein Beitrag zur Frage 'machbarer' Gesundheit. Frankfurt am Main, Haag + Herchen, 1984. 198, 49 p.
Rothschuh KE: Aus der Geschichte der Naturheilbewegung (VI). Zur Fortentwicklung und Pflege der Naturheilverfahren in der zweiten Hälfte des 19. Jahrhunderts. **ZFA (Stuttgart)** 1983 Apr 10;59(10):585–91
Schomburg E: Sebastian Kneipp, 1821–1897. Bad Wörishofen, Kneipp–Verlag, 1976. 154 p.

**Knight, Richard, 1768–1844**
Hunt LB, Buchanan PD: Richard Knight (1768–1844): a forgotten chemist and apparatus designer. **Ambix** 1984 Jul;31(2):57–67

**Knolle, Jan Fryderyk, b. 1740**
Lambert M: Jan Fryderyk Knolle's forgotten dissertation on osseous syphilis, 1763. **Sex Transm Dis** 1984 Jan–Mar;11(1):36–40

**Knorre, Alekseĭ Georgievich, 1914–1981**
Mikhaĭlov VP: Pamiati Alekseia Georgievicha Knorre. **Arkh Anat Gistol Embriol** 1982 Feb;82(2):5–16
Tokin BP, Ivanovo–Kazas OM, Gabaeva NS: Vklad A. G. Knorre v razvitie sovremennoĭ émbriologii. **Arkh Anat Gistol Embriol** 1984 Jul;87(7):92–4

**Knoth, Wilhelm, 1923–1982**
Hundeiker M: Wilhelm Knoth. **Verh Dtsch Ges Pathol** 1982;66:646–52

**Knowlton, Charles, 1800–1850**
Chandrasekhar S: 'A dirty, filthy book.' The writings of Charles Knowlton and Annie Besant on reproductive physiology and birth control and an account of the Bradlaugh–Besant trial. With the definitive texts of Fruits of philosophy by Charles Knowlton; The law of population by Annie Besant; Theosophy and the law of population by Annie Besant. Berkeley, University of California Press, 1981. xi, 217 p.

**Knox, Robert, 1791–1862**
Douglas H: Burke and Hare. **Br Hist Illus** 1978–79;5(5):32–43
Stephen K: Robert Knox, M.D., F.R.S.E. (1791–1862). Edinburgh, University of Edinburgh, [1981]. 11 p. (Scottish men of medicine).

**Kobavashi, Osamu**
Niigata Daigaku Igakubu Shonikagaku Kyoshitsu shi: [Niigata, Japan], Do Iinkai, Showa 52 nen [1977]. 180 p.

**Kobert, Rudolf, 1854–1918**
Jack DB: Dastardly deeds at Dorpat. **Pharm Hist (London)** 1984 Sep;14(3):9–12

**Koblinsky, Albert, fl. 1916**
Heintel H: Ein unbekanntes Porträt des Hirnforschers Oskar Vogt (1870–1959). **Medizinhist J** 1984;19(3):277–9

**Koch, Gerhard, 1913–**
Koch G: Inhaltsreiche Jahre eines Humangenetikers: Mein Lebensweg in Bildern und Dokumenten. Erlangen, Perimed Fachbuchgesellschaft, 1982. 472 p.

**Koch, Richard, 1882–1949**
Rothschuh KE: Richard Hermann Koch (1882–1949): Arzt, Medizinhistoriker, Medizinphilosoph (Biographisches, Ergographisches). 1. Teil. Zur Biographie. **Medizinhist J** 1980;15(1/2):16–43
Rothschuh KE: Richard Hermann Koch (1882–1949). **Medizinhist J** 1980;15(3):223–43
Schwann H: Richard Kochs Beziehungen zum Karl-Sudhoff-Institut. Archivstudie anlässlich seines 100. Geburtstages. **NTM** 1982;19(1):94–103

**Koch, Robert, 1843–1910**
Algeorge G: La 100 de ani de la descoperirea de către Robert Koch a agentului etiologic al tuberculozei. **Rev Ig [Pneumoftiziol]** 1982 Jan–Mar;31(1):13–7
Allen BW, Hinkes WF: Koch's cultivation of tubercle bacilli. **Med Lab Sci** 1983 Jan;40(1):85–7
Allen BW, Hinkes WF: La coloration de Koch pour les bacilles de

la tuberculose. **Bull Int Union Tuberc** 1982 Sep–Dec;57(3–4):194–6

Ananthanarayan R: Robert Koch's contribution to microbiology. **Indian J Pathol Microbiol** 1982 Apr;25(2):169–71

Anastasatu C: Centenarul descoperirii bacilului Koch. **Rev Ig [Pneumoftiziol]** 1982 Jan–Mar;31(1):1–3

Bazanov VA, Schneck P: Robert Koch und die deutsch–russischen Beziehungen auf dem Gebiete der Mikrobiologie. **Z Gesamte Hyg** 1982 Mar;28(3):201–5

Bazanov VA, Schneck P: Nauchnye sviazi Roberta Kokha i ego shkoly s russkimi issledovateliami. **Sov Zdravookhr** 1982;(3)64–7

Bednarski Z: Robert Koch (1843–1910). **Wiad Lek** 1983 Mar 1;36(5):425–7

Bednarski Z: Sto lat od odkrycia prątka gruźlicy (1882–1982) przez Roberta Kocha: szybka reakcja w polskich czasopismach lekarskich. **Pol Tyg Lek** 1983 Mar 28;38(13):419–21

Benison S: Celebration and history: the centenary of Robert Koch's discovery of the tubercle bacillus. **Bull Hist Med** 1982 Summer;56(2):157–9

Blasi A: Der Kochsche Grundversuch und seine gegenwärtigen experimentellen Varianten. **Z Erkr Atmungsorgane** 1983;161(1):51–5

Bretey J: Robert Koch et son bacille. Un reportage. **Bull Acad Natl Med (Paris)** 1982 Mar;166(3):399–406

Bulla A: Reîntîlnire cu opera ştiinţifică a lui Robert Koch. **Rev Ig [Pneumoftiziol]** 1982 Jan–Mar;31(1):5–11

Centennial: Koch's discovery of the tubercle bacillus: **MMWR** 1982 Mar 19;31(10):121–3

Centennial of Koch's bacillus: **NZ Med J** 1982 Jun 9;95(709):384

Ciulei SG: Robert Koch (1843–1910), membru de onoare al Societăţii de Medici şi Naturalişti din Iaşi. **Rev Med Chir Soc Med Nat Iasi** 1983 Jul–Sep;87(3):503–4

Daniel TM: Robert Koch, tuberculosis, and the subsequent history of medicine. **Am Rev Respir Dis** 1982 Mar;125(3 Pt 2):1–3

Döhner L: Die Kochschen Postulate und die Virologie. **Z Erkr Atmungsorgane** 1983;161(1):21–4

Drössler K: Robert Koch--auch ein Pionier der Immunitätsforschung? **Allerg Immunol (Leipz)** 1982;28(1):13–20

Dubb A: Medical philately: Robert Koch (1843–1910) the man, his germ and history. **Adler Mus Bull** 1984 Mar;10(1):16–22

Dubovsky H: Robert Koch (1843–1910)--the man and his work. **S Afr Med J** 1982 Nov 17;Spec No:3–5

Dwork D: Koch and the Colonial Office: 1902–1904; the second South Africa Expedition. **NTM** 1983;20(1):67–74

Etiología de la tuberculosis: Dr. Roberto Koch: **Salud Publica Mex** 1982 May–Jun;24(3):241–57

Eule H: Die Auswirkung der Entdeckung und der Arbeiten Robert Kochs auf die Entwicklung der Therapie der Tuberkulose. **Z Erkr Atmungsorgane** 1982;158(1–2):155–62

Ferrari Sacco A, Oliaro T: A cent'anni dalla scoperta del micobatterio della tbc. (1822–1982). Robert Koch autore della grande scoperta. **Minerva Med** 1982 Sep 8;73(34):2199–202

Findeisen DG: Tuberkulose und Allergie. Erkenntnisschritte von der Entdeckung des Mycobacterium tuberculosis durch Robert Koch (24 März 1882). Zu einer umfassenden Immundiagnostik, Immuntherapie und Immunprophylaxe. **Allerg Immunol (Leipz)** 1982;28(1):3–12

Foreman T, Gordon B, Weese WC: In honor of Robert Koch, M.D. **Ariz Med** 1983 Mar;40(3):149

Freerksen E: Die Atiologie der Tuberkulose--Der Weg dahin und die Folgen. **Prax Klin Pneumol** 1982 Mar;36(3):122–34

Fujita S: Robert Kochs Bedeutung für die japanische Medizin--Tuberkuloseforschung in Japan. **Prax Klin Pneumol** 1983 Oct;37 Suppl 1:423–9

Genschorek W: Robert Koch. Selbstloser Kampf gegen Seuchen und Infektionskrankheiten. Leipzig, Hirzel, 1981. 224 p. (Hervorragende Arzte im Dienste des Menschen).

Girstenbrey W: Robert Koch und sein Erbe. Bedingungen, Konsequenzen und aktuelle Bedeutung einer historischen Leistung für Medizin und Gesundheitspolitik. **Fortschr Med** 1982 Mar 25;100(12):541, 544–6

Grange JM, Bishop PJ: 'Uber Tuberkulose'. A tribute to Robert Koch's discovery of the tubercle bacillus, 1882. **Tubercle** 1982 Mar;63(1):3–17

Grujić M: Stogodišnjica otkrića bacila tuberkuloze. Zivot i delo Roberta Kocha. **Plucne Bolesti Tuberk** 1982 Jan–Jun;34(1–2):5–7

Haase HH: Uber einige Auswirkungen Robert Kochs und seiner Lehre auf die Entwicklung der Allgemeinen und Kommunalen Hygiene. **Z Gesamte Hyg** 1982 Mar;28(3):154–6

Heifets L: Metchnikoff's recollections of Robert Koch. **Tubercle** 1982 Jun;63(2):139–41

Henneberg G: Das Robert Koch–Haus in Wollstein. **Med Welt** 1982 Mar 26;33(12):427

Hidvegi J: Die Resonanz der Kochschen Entdeckung in der medizinischen Fachpresse Ungarns. **Wiss Beitr Martin Luther Univ Halle Wittenberg** 1983;5–R80:87–90

Hillerdal O: Robert Koch och hans 100–årsjubileer. **Nord Medicinhist Arsbok** 1983;:127–34

Howard–Jones N: Robert Koch and the cholera vibrio: a centenary. **Br Med J [Clin Res]** 1984 Feb 4;288(6414):379–81

Jenschorek N: Robert Koch: Leben, Werk, Zeit. 2. durchgesehene Auflage. Leipzig, Hirzel, 1976. 247 p.

Kaiser W: Vor 100 Jahren beschrieb Robert Koch den Tuberkulose–Erreger. **Z Gesamte Inn Med** 1982 Mar 1;37(5):137–44

Kaiser W, Hübner H, ed: Robert Koch (1843–1910). **Wiss Beitr Martin Luther Univ Halle Wittenberg** 1983;5–R80:3–321

Kaiser W: Robert Koch und die Entdeckung des Tuberkulose–Erregers. **Wiss Beitr Martin Luther Univ Halle Wittenberg** 1983;5–R80:31–9

Kalich R: Aktuelle Ergebnisse auf dem Gebiet der Resistenzbestimmung von Mykobakterien. **Z Erkr Atmungsorgane** 1983;161(1):80–5

Karasszon D: Robert Kochs Forschungen zur Rinder–Tuberkulose. **Wiss Beitr Martin Luther Univ Halle Wittenberg** 1983;5–R80:111–6

Knorr M: Das Jahr 1882 – Anfang und Folgen einer neuren medizinischen Methodik um und von Robert Koch. **Zentralbl Bakteriol Mikrobiol Hyg [B]** 1982;176(5–6):413–24

Koch R: Classics in infectious diseases. The etiology of tuberculosis: Robert Koch. Berlin, Germany, 1882. **Rev Infect Dis** 1982 Nov–Dec;4(6):1270–4

Koch T: Gedanken zur 100. Wiederkehr des Tages der Entdeckung des Tuberkuloseerregers durch Robert Koch. **Gegenbaurs Morphol Jahrb** 1982;128(1):1–11

Koch centennial supplement: 100th anniversary of the announcement of the discovery of the tubercle bacillus by Robert Koch, March 24, 1882. **Am Rev Respir Dis** 1982 Mar;125(3 pt 2):1–132

Kochemasova ZN, Dykhno MM, Dorozhkova IR, et al: L–transformatsiia kak odin iz faktorov izmenchivosti vozbuditelia tuberkuleza (k 100–letiiu otkrytiia vozbuditelia tuberkuleza). **Sov Med** 1983;(3):20–3

Kochemasova ZN, Dykhno MM, Dorozhkova IR, et al: 100–letie so dnia otkrytiia R. Kokhom vozbuditelia tuberkuleza. **Klin Med (Mosk)** 1982 Nov;60(11):115–7

Koch's bacillus: **Tubercle** 1982 Mar;63(1):1–2

Krakówka P: W 100–lecie odkrycia prątka gruźlicy. **Pneumonol Pol** 1982 Nov;50(11):557–8

Krause AK: Introduction à l'étiologie de la tuberculose. **Bull Int Union Tuberc** 1981 Sept–Dec;56(3–4):110–4

Krause RM: Koch's postulates and the search for the AIDS agent. **Rev Infect Dis** 1984 Mar–Apr;6(2):270–9

Kreibich H: Betrachtungen zum 100. Jahrestag der Entdeckung des Mycobacterium tuberculosis durch Robert Koch. **Zentralbl Gynakol** 1982;104(5):258–67

Lammel HU: Virchow contra Koch? Neue Untersuchungen zu einer alten Streitfrage. **Z Gesamte Hyg** 1982 Mar;28(3):206–10

Lock W: Robert Koch. Bemerkungen aus heutiger Sicht. **Prax Klin Pneumol** 1982 Mar;36(3):106–10

Lock W: Robert Koch, Leben und Werk. **Prax Klin Pneumol** 1983 Oct;37 Suppl 1:409–11

Marchand H, Müller KP: Der Berufsweg Robert Kochs bis zur Entdeckung des Tuberkelbakteriums. **Wiss Beitr Martin Luther Univ Halle Wittenberg** 1983;5–R80:99–109

Maulitz RC: Robert Koch and American medicine. **Ann Intern Med** 1982 Nov;97(5):761–6

Maulitz RC: Robert Koch in the United States of America. **NTM** 1983;20(1):75–84

Mayer R: Il y a cent ans, à Genève, au 4e Congrès international d'hygiène et de démographie, l''altercation' Pasteur – Koch. **Rev Med Suisse Romande** 1982 Aug;102(8):805–9

Mayer R: Il y a cent ans, Robert Koch découvrait le bacille de la tuberculose. **Rev Med Suisse Romande** 1982 Mar;102(3):199–226

Mecklinger L: Robert Koch. **Bull Int Union Tuberc** 1982 Jun;57(2):109–10

Mecklinger L: Zum 100. Jahrestag der Entdeckung des Tuberkelbakteriums durch Robert Koch. **Z Gesamte Hyg** 1982 Dec 12;28(12):822–6

Meijer J: De tuberkelbacterie een eeuw bekend; 1882 – 24 Maart – 1982 (Heinrich Hermann Robert Koch). **Ned Tijdschr Geneeskd** 1982 Mar 13;126(11):488–9

Mendoza F: Acerca del descubrimiento del bacilo de Koch. **Rev Med Chil** 1983 May;111(5):539–43

Meve EB: Put' iskaniĭ Roberta Kokha. **Klin Med (Mosk)** 1982 Nov;60(11):111–4

Mocek R: Robert Koch und die geistige Situation seiner Zeit. **Wiss Beitr Martin Luther Univ Halle Wittenberg** 1983;5–R80:15–29

Mochmann H, Kohler W: The clarification of the etiology of Asiatic cholera by the German cholera commission under the direction of Robert Koch in the year 1883--1884. **Indian J Public Health** 1983 Jan–Mar;27(1):6–20

Mochmann H: Biographische und literarische Notizen über Robert Koch aus Anlass des 100. Jahrestages -- 24. März 1982 -- seiner Bekanntgabe der Entdeckung des Tuberkelbazillus. **Padiatr Grenzgeb** 1982;21(2):83–112

Mollaret HH: Contribution à la connaissance des relations entre Koch et Pasteur. **NTM** 1983;20(1):57–65

Moskwa Z: W setną rocznic e odkrycia prątka gruźlicy. **Wiad Lek** 1983 May 1;36(9):799–802

Moskwa Z: Tuberkulina. **Wiad Lek** 1983 Jun 15;36(12):1033–5

Nabielek R: Robert Koch und die Begründung des Lehrstuhls für Hygiene an der Berliner Universität. **Z Gesamte Hyg** 1982 Mar;28(3):185–93

Ocklitz HW, Landmann H: Robert Koch und die Kindertuberkulose. **Kinderarztl Prax** 1982 Mar;50(3):117–29

Oliveira JC de: Em louvor de Koch. A propósito da descoberta do bacilo da tuberculose. **Acta Med Port** 1983 Mar;4(3):195–9

Opitz R, Horn H, Heinecke P, et al: Robert Koch. Die Vorgeschichte der Berufung als ersten Ordinarius für Hygiene an die Universität Berlin. **MMW** 1981 Oct 16;123(42):1593–5

Pacheco CR: Con motivo del centenario del descubrimiento del bacilo de la tuberculosis. **Salud Publica Mex** 1982 May–Jun;24(3):231–3

Pacheco CR, Quijano-Pitman F, Kuthy-Porter J, et al: Centenario del descubrimiento del bacilo de la tuberculosis. **Gac Med Mex** 1982 Nov;118(11):439–48

Piechocki W: Robert Kochs Aufenthalt in Halle zur Cholerabekämpfung im Spiegel der Presse (1893). **Wiss Beitr Martin Luther Univ Halle Wittenberg** 1983;5–R80:41–9

Pilipchuk NS, Pilipchuk VN: K stoletiiu otkrytiia Robertom Kokhom vozbuditelia tuberkuleza. **Vrach Delo** 1982 Nov;(11):119–21

Ranasinghe L: Koch and Koch's bacillus: 100 years ago and today. **Ceylon Med J** 1982 Mar;27(1):1–5

Referent Robert Koch: Der Entdecker des Tuberkulose-Erregers als sachverständiger Referent in der ersten Ausgabe der 'Fortschritte der Medicin'. **Fortschr Med** 1982 Jun 3;100(21):1012–3

Robert Koch: **Probl Tuberk** 1982 Mar;(3):8–9

Robert Koch: father of bacteriology and infectious diseases: **Ceylon Med J** 1982 Mar;27(1):6–7

Rothe J, Werner K, Kaiser W: Sozialhygienische Konsequenzen aus der Klärung der Tuberkulose-Atiologie durch Robert Koch. **Z Gesamte Hyg** 1982 Mar;28(3):176–9

Sackmann W: Vor hundert Jahren: Robert Koch entdeckt den Erreger der Tuberkulose. **Schweiz Arch Tierheilkd** 1982 May;124(5):217–25

Sakula A: Robert Koch (1843–1910): founder of the science of bacteriology and discoverer of the tubercle bacillus. A study of his life and work. **Br J Dis Chest** 1979 Oct;73(4):389–94

Sakula A: Robert Koch: centenary of the discovery of the tubercle bacillus, 1882. **Thorax** 1982 Apr;37(4):246–51

Sakula A: Centenary of the discovery of the tubercle bacillus. **Lancet** 1982 Mar 27;1(8274):750

Saueressig H: Die Tuberkulose als Paradigma des Lebensgefühls. **Med Welt** 1982 Mar 26;33(12):428–34

Schadewaldt H: L'histoire de la découverte du bacille de Koch. **Hist Sci Med** 1982;16(4):337–41

Schadewaldt H: Die Entdeckung des Tuberkuloseerregers durch Robert Koch vor 100 Jahren. **Krankenhausarzt** 1983 Mar 3;56:157–66

Schierhorn H: Zur Säkularfeier von Robert Kochs Entdeckung des Tuberkulose-Bakteriums. **Z Mikrosk Anat Forsch** 1982;96(3):377–99

Schmidt G: O znachenii otkrytiĭ Roberta Kokha dlia razvitiia bakteriologii i épidemiologii. **Zh Mikrobiol Epidemiol Immunobiol** 1983 Mar;(3):106–9

Schmidt G: Zur Bedeutung der Entdeckung Robert Kochs für die Entwicklungen der Bakteriologie. **Z Erkr Atmungsorgane** 1983;161(1):15–20

Schmitt W: Robert Koch, Mensch und Werk. **Zentralbl Chir** 1982;107(5–6):251–9

Schneeweiss U: Die Spezifitätslehre Robert Kochs; 100 Jahre Entdeckung der Tuberkelbakterien. **Medizinhist J** 1983;18(1–2):21–32

Schneeweiss U: Die Immunitätslehre im Lichte der Vorstellungen von Robert Koch. **Z Erkr Atmungsorgane** 1983;161(1):46–50

Shapiro E: Robert Koch and his tuberculin fallacy. **Pharos** 1983 Fall;46(4):19–22

Skrobacki A: Robert Koch in Wolsztyn. **Wiss Beitr Martin Luther Univ Halle Wittenberg** 1983;5–R80:51–61

Smith DW: Koch's postulates and the Koch phenomenon, an update. **Indian J Chest Dis Allied Sci** 1982 Apr–Sep;24(2–3):95–100

Solov'eva VA: K 100-letiiu otkrytiia Robertom Kokhom vozbuditelia tuberkuleza (1882–1982). **Sov Med** 1982;(3):120–2

Somolinos Palencia J: Roberto Koch. El descubrimiento del bacilo de la tuberculosis y su primera noticia en México. **Salud Publica Mex** 1982 May–Jun;24(3):237–40

Sönnichsen N: Zum 100. Jahrestag der Entdeckung des Erregers der Tuberkulose durch Robert Koch. **Dermatol Monatsschr** 1982 Mar;168(3):145–6

Steinbruck P: Hommage à Robert Koch, Sa vie et son oeuvre contre la tuberculose. **Bull Int Union Tuberc** 1981 Sep–Dec;56(3–4):115–9

Steinbrück P: Robert Koch und sein Werk. Seine Auswirkungen auf die Tuberkulosebekämpfung. **Z Erkr Atmungsorgane** 1982;158(1–2):5–23

Steinbrück P: Der Erkenntnisprozess in Robert Koch auf seinem Wege zum Begründer der Tuberkulosebekämpfung. **Z Erkr Atmungsorgane** 1983;161(1):6–14

Strubel K: Robert Koch und die Tuberkulose im Spiegel der halleschen Presse im ausgehenden 19. Jahrhundert. **Wiss Beitr Martin Luther Univ Halle Wittenberg** 1983;5–R80:225–42

Süla L: The 100th anniversary of the discovery of Koch's bacillus, the etiologic agent of tuberculosis. **J Hyg Epidemiol Microbiol Immunol** 1982;26(3):227–9

Szabó I: A Koch bacilus 100 éve. **Orv Hetil** 1982 Jan 24;123(4):227–9

Szabó I: The influence of the discovery of Koch's bacterium on the Hungarians. **Indian J Chest Dis Allied Sci** 1982 Apr–Sep;24(2–3):175–8

Takeda Y, Zinnaka Y: [Centenary of the discovery of Vibrio cholerae by Robert Koch] (Jpn) **Nippon Saikingaku Zasshi** 1984 Jul;39(4):709–12

Talewski R: Robert Koch 11.XII.1843--27.V.1910. **Pneumonol Pol** 1982 Nov;50(11):553–5

Tavassoli M: Selected items from the history of pathology - Robert Koch (1843–1910). **Am J Pathol** 1980;101(1):78

Viswanathan R: Robert Koch's contribution to medical science. **Indian J Chest Dis Allied Sci** 1982 Apr–Sep;24(2–3):65–7

Wagner G: Robert Koch--Leistungen für die Menschheit. **Z Arztl Fortbild (Jena)** 1982 Jul 15;75(14):653–5

Weise W: Die Entdeckung des Erregers der Tuberkulose durch Robert Koch vor 100 Jahren. **MMW** 1982 Mar 26;124(12):299–300

Weuffen W: Der Beitrag Robert Koch zur Begründung der Desinfektionslehre und heutige Schwerpunkte der Desinfektionsforschung und -praxis. **Z Gesamte Hyg** 1982 Mar;28(3):167–71

Weuffen W: Der Beitrag Robert Kochs zur Begründung der Desinfektionslehre und heutige Schwerpunkte der Desinfektionsforschung und -praxis. **Z Erkr Atmungsorgane** 1983;161(1):28–35

Wildfuehr G: Robert Koch, Begründer der modernen Mikrobiologie. **Z Gesamte Hyg** 1982 Mar;28(3):145–8

Winter K: Ein historischer Wendepunkt in der Geschichte von Naturwissenschaft und Medizin. Zum 100. Jahrestag der Entdeckung des Mycobacterium tuberculosis durch Robert Koch. **Z Arztl Fortbild (Jena)** 1982 Mar 15;76(6):229–30

Wyklicky H: Zur hundertsten Wiederkehr der ersten Demonstration des Tuberkelbazillus durch Robert Koch (1843–1910). **Osterr Apoth Ztg** 1982 Apr 3;36(14):266–7

Zahradnický J: 100 let od objevu puvodce tuberkulózy Robertem Kochem. **Cesk Epidemiol Mikrobiol Imunol** 1983 Jan;32(1):4–7

Zegaya M: 1882–1982: Robert Koch. Réquisitoire contre la tuberculose. **Tunis Med** 1982 March–Apr;60(2):98–105

Znachenie otkrytiia Roberta Kokha dlia razvitiia bakteriologii tuberkuleza: **Probl Tuberk** 1982 Mar;(3):3–7

Zolyomi ND: Die Kochsche Entdeckung in der Pressburger Tagespresse. **Wiss Beitr Martin Luther Univ Halle Wittenberg** 1983;5–R80:79–84

100 de ani de la descoperirea de către Robert Koch a bacilului tuberculozei: **Rev Ig [Pneumoftiziol]** 1982 Oct–Dec;31(4):289–90

**Kocher, Theodor, 1841–1917**

Tröhler U: Theodor Kocher und die neurotopographische Diagnostik: angewandte Forschung mit grundlegendem Ergebnis um 1900. **Gesnerus** 1983;40(1–2):203–14

**Kočwara, Franz, d. 1791**

Ober WB: The sticky end of Frantisek Koczwara, composer of 'The Battle of Prague'. **Am J Forensic Med Pathol** 1984 Jun;5(2):145–9

**Koebner, Heinrich, 1823–1904**

Waisman M: Historical note: Koebner on the isomorphic phenomenon. **Arch Dermatol** 1981 Jul;117(7):415

**Koelbing, Huldrych M., 1923–**

Boschung U, Rüttimann B: Herrn Professor Dr. med. H. M. Koelbing zum 60. Geburtstag. **Gesnerus** 1983;40(1–2):3–13

**Koffka, Kurt, 1886–1941**

Mecacci L: Koffka e la psicologia sovietica. **Stor Crit Psicol** 1980;1(1):95–109

**Köhler, Wolfgang, 1887–1967**

Windholz G: Pavlov vs. Köhler. Pavlov's little-known primate research. **Pavlov J Biol Sci** 1984 Jan–Mar;19(1):23–31

**Kohman, Emma Anna, 1889–1982**

Bing FC: Emma Kohman and the early history of nutritional edema. **J Am Diet Assoc** 1983 Jun;82(6):605–9

**Kohut, Heinz, 1913–1981**

Harper R: A psychoanalytic geronimo. **Queen Q** 1981;88(2):256–63

Wolf ES: Tomorrow's self: Heinz Kohut's contribution to adolescent psychiatry. **Adolesc Psychiatry** 1980;8:41–50

**Kölcsey, Ferenc, 1790–1838**

Csorba S: Kölcsey Ferenc hibás szemének kérdéséhez. **Orvostort Kozl** 1982;28(1–3):191–9

**Koler, Wacław, d. 1546**

Andrejew A: Wacław Koler, sławny medyk Krakowski w świetle swego inwentarza. **Arch Hist Med (Warsz)** 1984;47(1):39–47

**Köleséri, Samuel, 1663–1732**

Szentgyörgyvölgyi G: Köleséri Sámuel pályája és jelleme. **Orvostort Kozl** 1981;93–96(27 No 1–4):183–7

**Kolletschka, Jacob, 1803–1847**

Silló-Seidl G: Kolletschkas Tod. **Beitr Gerichtl Med** 1979;37:415–7

**Kölliker, Albert von, 1817–1905**

Hildebrand R: Beitrag der Würzburger Anatomie zur Entwicklung des mikroskopisch-anatomischen Unterrichts (1847 Kölliker--Petersen 1940). **Anat Anz** 1984;155(1–5):115–22

Kahle E: Koelliker, Albert Ritter v. In Neue Deutsche Biographie 12. 1980. p. 322–3.

Teulón AA: La constitucion de la histologia celular: Schwann, Henle y Kölliker. **Asclepio** 1978–79;30–31:7–18

**Kolomnin, Sergeĭ Petrovich, 1842–1886**

Iurikhin AP: K 140-letiiu so dnia rozhdeniia Sergeia Petrovicha Kolomnina (1842–1886). **Klin Khir** 1982 Dec;(12):61–3

**Koltson, Alexey Vasilievich, 1809–1842**

Lieber Z: Is there a relationship between illness and creativity? An analysis of the life and poetry of A. V. Koltsov. **Int J Soc Psychiatry** 1980;26(3):212-7

**Koltypin, Aleksandr Alekseevich, 1883-1942**
Vel'tishchev IuE: A. A. Koltypin--uchenyĭ, vrach, obshchestvennyĭ deiatel' (k 100-letiiu so dnia rozhdeniia). **Pediatriia** 1983 Sep;(9):73-4

**Konchalovskii, Maksim Petrovich, 1875-1942**
Bregadze IL: Novoe v pokazaniiakh k khirurgicheskim vmeshatel'stvam pri vnutrennikh zabolevaniiakh (k 40-letiiu so dnia smerti M. P. Konchalovskogo). **Klin Med (Mosk)** 1981;59(10):78-9

**Koncz, Joszef, fl. 1789**
Péterffy I: Híradás két felvilágosodás kori jeles orvosról. **Orv Hetil** 1983 Jul 31;124(31):1895-6

**Kondoidi, Pavel Zakharovich, 1710-1760**
Palkin BN: Pervyĭ karantinnyĭ ustav v Rossii, sostavlennyĭ P. Z. Kondoidi. **Sov Zdravookhr** 1982;(9):63-5

**Kondrat'ev, N. S., 1887-**
Mel'man EP: N. V. Kondrat'ev i ego vklad v anatomiiu vegetativnoĭ nervnoĭ sistemy. **Arkh Anat Gistol Embriol** 1983 Nov;85(11):90-4

**König, Franz, 1832-1910**
Paul U: Das chirurgische Erbe. Franz König (1832-1910)--Weg und Wandel der Chirurgie seiner Zeit. **Zentralbl Chir** 1983;108(22):1451-6

**Konopka, Stanisław, 1896-1982**
Bojczuk H: Stanisław Konopka (1896-1982), historyk medycyny, bibliotekarz i bibliograf, twórca polskiej bibliografii lekarskiej. **Arch Hist Med (Warsz)** 1983;46(4):439-51
Profesor dr med. Stanisław Konopka (1896-1982). Wspomnienie: **Pol Tyg Lek** 1983 Sep 5;38(36):1125-6

**Konrad der Münzmeister, fl. 1400**
Hils HP: Konrad der Münzmeister oder Konrad der Apotheker? Zur Analyse eines spätmittelalterlichen Pesttraktates. **Sudhoffs Arch** 1984;68(1):105-9

**Koppel, Mat, 1890-1916**
Roos A, Boron WF: The buffer value of weak acids and bases: origin of the concept, and first mathematical derivation and application to physico-chemical systems. The work of M. Koppel and K. Spiro (1914). **Respir Physiol** 1980 Apr;40(1):1-32

**Koprowski, Hilary**
Garfield E: W hołdzie Hilaremu Koprowskiemu: uczonemu, muzykowi i przyjacielowi. **Pol Tyg Lek** 1983 Sep 5;38(36):1119-23
Kaplan MM: Three decades of collaboration with Hilary Koprowski. **J Cell Physiol [Suppl]** 1982;2:1-6
Kritchevsky D: Hilary Koprowski and The Wistar Institute. **J Cell Physiol [Suppl]** 1982;2:vi-viii

**Korányi, Frigyes, 1828-1913**
Silló-Seidl G: Korányi Frigyes bécsi ösztöndíja. **Orvostort Kozl** 1979;87-88(25 no 1-2):311-3
Somogyi E: Korányi Frigyes közéleti munkássága. **Orv Hetil** 1984 Apr 29;125(18):1079-82

**Korba-Pribylev, A. P., 1849-1939**
Malozemova AI: Revoliutsionery-mediki Pribylevy. **Sov Zdravookhr** 1984;(8):62-5

**Korchak-Chepurkovskiĭ, Avksentiĭ Vasilevich, 1857-1947**
Belitskaia EIa: O sotsial-gigieniste A. V. Korchake-Chepurkovskom (K 125-letiiu so dnia rozhdeniia). **Sov Zdravookhr** 1982;(6):66-8
Popushoĭ EP, Ioksa VA: Vklad A. V. Korchaka-Chepurkovskogo v razvitie zdravookhraneniia i bor'bu s épidemiiami v Moldavii. **Zh Mikrobiol Epidemiol Immunobiol** 1983 Oct;(10):109-11
Siniak KM, Rudichenko VF: Avksentiĭ Vasil'evich Korchak-Chepurkovskiĭ (k 125-letiiu so dnia rozhdeniia). **Vrach Delo** 1983 Apr;(4):118-21

**Korczynski, Edward, 1844-1905**
Sliwiński S: Edward Korczyński (1844-1905) autor pierwszego opisu klinicznego zawału serca w medycynie polskiej. **Wiad Lek** 1979 Nov 15;32(22):1647-50

**Kornalewski, Joachim, 1850-**
Skrobacki A, Völker A: Lekarz olsztyński, Joachim Kornalewskiijego rozprawa o koltunie z 1897 roku. **Komun Mazursko Warm** 1980;(2):155-67

**Kornev, Petr Georgievich, 1883-1974**
Epifanov NS: Neustannyĭ borets s tiazhelym nedugom (k 100-letiiu so dnia rozhdeniia P. G. Korneval). **Feldsher Akush** 1983 Sep;48(9):37-8
Petrov IN: P.G. Kornev i ego shkola. **Probl Tuberk** 1984 Jul;(7):73-5

**Kornilovich, Aleksandr Osipovich, d. 1833**
Katsnel'bogen AG: Meditsinskaia zapiska dekabrista A. O. Kornilovicha. **Sov Zdravookhr** 1981;(11):62-4

**Korotkoff, Nikolai Sergeevich, 1874-1920**
Korotkoff NS: Experiments for determining the efficiency of arterial collaterals. Preface, biographical notes and editing of translation from Russian by H. N. Segall. Montreal, H. N. Segall, 1980. 265 p. (M. D. Thesis, Imperial Military Medical Academy, 1910).
Laher M, O'Brien E: In search of Korotkoff. **Br Med J [Clin Res]** 1982 Dec 18-25;285(6357):1796-8

**Korotkov, Aleksandr Grigor'evich, 1921-**
Valishin ES: Aleksandr Grigor'evich Korotkov (K 60-letiiu so dnia Rozhdeniia). **Arkh Anat Gistol Embriol** 1981 May;80(5):122-5

**Korotkov, Nikolaj Sergeevich, 1874-1920**
Zivković K: Dr Nikolaj S. Korotkov (13. II. 1874-1920). **Srp Arh Celok Lek** 1983 Jan;111(1):97-9

**Körte, Werner, 1853-1937**
Winkelmann O: Werner Körte. **Neue Dtsch Biogr** 1980;12:395-6

**Koski, Kalevi, 1921-**
Kalevi Koski 60 years: **Proc Finn Dent Soc** 1981;77(1-3):9-16

**Kostanecki, Kazimierz, 1863-**
Kuś J, Miodoński A: Kazimierz Kostranecki i jego uczniowie na tle epoki. **Przegl Lek** 1981;38(12):875-82

**Köstl, Franz, 1811-1882**
Baudiš P: Franz Köstl a jeho práce s epidemiologickým zaměřením. **Cesk Psychiatr** 1979 Apr;75(2):144-7

**Kostlivý, Stanislavý, 1877-**
Moravec R, Tichý M, Moravcová M, et al: Z dejín chirurgie v Bratislave. Profesor Kostlivý a začiatky chirurgickej kliniky na LFUK v Bratislava] **Rozhl Chir** 1984 Jul;63(7):526-31

**Kotnis, D. S.**
Kelkar GS: Kotnis in Kokung. **China Rep (India)** 1979;15(2):97-111

**Kots, Nadezhda Nikolaevna Ladygina, 1890-1963**
Misiti R: Ladygina-Kots and Soviet comparative psychology. **Stor Crit Psicol** 1982 Jun;3(1):109-12

**Kotsovskiĭ, A. D., 1864-1937**
Popushoĭ EP, Spineĭ LV: A.D. Kotsovskiĭ--vidnyĭ predstavitel' obshchestvennoĭ meditsiny Moldavii. **Sov Zdravookhr** 1980;(9):58-61

**Kovács, Ferenc, 1890-1974**
Gyöngyössy A: Kovács Ferenc (1890-1974). **Orv Hetil** 1984 Aug 19;125(34):2085-6

**Kowalczykowa, Janina, 1907-1970**
Urban A: Konspiracyjna działalnść dydaktyczna profesor Janiny Kowalczykowej w okresie okupacji 1939-1944. **Patol Pol** 1980 Apr-Jun;31(2):161-9

**Kozhevnikov, A. Ia.**
Guliaeva SE: K istorii izucheniia épilepsii Kozhevnikova. **Zh Nevropatol Psikhiatr** 1984;84(6):919-29

**Kraepelin, Emil, 1856-1926**
Heimann H: Nosologie und Pathophysiologie in der Psychiatrie--Aspekte der Krankheitslehre Kraepelins heute. **Confin Psychiatr** 1980;23(4):262-74
Heimann H: De Kraepelin au sytème AMDP. **Acta Psychiatr Belg** 1983 Mar-Apr;83(2):147-54
Hippius H: Ziele und Wege der psychiatrischen Forschung. **MMW** 1981 May 8;123(19):770-1
Hoenig J: The concept of Schizophrenia. Kraepelin-Bleuler-Schneider. **Br J Psychiatry** 1983 Jun;142:547-56
James RL, May PR: Diagnosing schizophrenia: Professor Kraepelin and the research diagnostic criteria. **Am J Psychiatry** 1981 Apr;138(4):501-4
Kick H: Der Forschungsansatz Kraepelins aus der Sicht seiner klinischen Praxis. **Fortschr Neurol Psychiatr** 1981 Jul;49(7):259-64
Leonhard K: Psychiatrische Behandlungsmethodik von Kraepelin nach seinen Lebenserinnerungen. **Psychiatr Neurol Med Psychol (Leipz)** 1984 Jul;36(7):395-405
Marchais P: Vers la fin de l'ère Kraepelinienne? **Ann Med Psychol (Paris)** 1980 Nov;138(9):1061-78
Siefert H: Emil Kraepelin. **Neue Dtsch Biogr** 1980;12:639-40

**Krafft, Charles, 1863-1921**
Morer G: La découverte de Charles Krafft. **Hist Sci Med** 1984;18(1):33-40

**Krafft-Ebing, Richard von, 1840-1902**
Salvetti ME: Gefässpsychopathologie bei Richard von Krafft-Ebing (1840-1902). Bern, Huber, 1984. 125 p. (Berner Beiträge zur Geschichte der Medizin und der Naturwissenschaften, Neue Folge, Band 10)

**Krasnogorskiĭ, Nikolaĭ Ivanovich, 1883-**
Kliorin AI: N. I. Krasnogorskiĭ (k 100-letiiu so dnia rozhdeniia). **Pediatriia** 1983 May;5:76-8

**Krassovskiĭ, Anton Iakovlevich, 1821-1898**
Abramenko VV, Gendel' MG: Rol' A. Ia. Krassovskogo v razvitii operativnogo akusherstva. **Akush Ginekol (Mosk)** 1984 Jan;(1):67-9
Mirskiĭ MB, Verbitskiĭ VM, Khil'chenko MA: Vklad A. Ia. Krassovskiĭ v organizatsiiu rodovspomozheniia v Peterburge. **Sov Zdravookhr** 1984;(3):62-4

**Kraus, Friedrich, 1858-1936**
Kenéz J: 125 éve született Friedrich Kraus (1858-1936). **Orv Hetil** 1984 Oct 28;125(44):2691-3

**Kraus, Karl, 1874-1936**
Sherman MH, ed: Psychoanalysis and old Vienna: Freud, Reik, Schnitzler, Kraus. New York, Human Sciences Press, 1978. 192 p.

**Kravchenko, Vladimir Semenovich, 1873–**
Sipukhin IaM: Vladimir Semenovich Kravchenko. K istorii otechestvennoĭ rentgenologii. **Vestn Rentgenol Radiol** 1983 May–Jun;(3):91–2
Zolotarev V: Zapiska starshego vracha kreisera avrora. **Voen Istor Zh** 1976;(1):51–60

**Krebs, Hans Adolf, 1900–1981**
Blaschko H: Hans Krebs: nineteen nineteen and after. **FEBS Lett** 1980 Aug 25;117 Suppl:K11–15
Kornberg H, Williamson DH: Hans Adolf Krebs: 25 August 1900–22 November 1981. **Biogr Mem Fellows R Soc** 1984;30:351–85
Krebs H: Wie ich aus Deutschland vertrieben wurde: Dokumente mit Kommentaren. **Medizinhist J** 1980;15(4):357–77
Krebs H: Reminiscenses and reflections. In collaboration with Anne Martin. Oxford, Clarendon Press, 1981. x, 298 p.
Lipmann F: Hans Krebs and his metabolic cycles. **Naturwiss Rundsch** 1982;35:228–30
Lund P: Sir Hans Krebs (1900–1981). **Clin Sci** 1982 Sep;63(3):225–30

**Krestovskiĭ, Vsevolod Vladimirovich, 1840–1895**
Brzheskiĭ VC: Neskol'ko slov o zabytom prioritete. **Grudn Khir** 1983 May–Jun;3:82–3

**Kretschmer, Ernst, 1888–1964**
Vojáček M: Cíle a úkoly psychoterapie v díle Ernsta Kretschmera. **Cesk Psychiatr** 1979 Feb;75(1):69–72

**Kreutzer, Johann Martin, 1810–1855**
Härtl J: Prof. Dr. phil. et Dr. med. h.c. Johann Martin Kreutzer, märtyrer oder rebell? **Hist Med Vet** 1977;2(4):112–22

**Krichevskiĭ, Il'ia L'vovich, 1883–1943**
Kravchenko AT: Razvitie ideĭ prof. I. L. Krichevskogo o priobretennom immuniteta (k 100–letiiu so dnia rozhdeniia I. L. Krichevskogo). **Zh Mikrobiol Epidemiol Immunobiol** 1984 Feb;(2):110–4

**Kriukov, Adrian Aleksandrovich, 1849–1908**
Krasnov MM: Proshloe v nastoiashchem: Adrian Aleksandrovich Kriukov, redaktor 'Vestnika oftal'mologii' i osnovatel' Moskovskogo oftal'mologicheskogo veshchestva (k 75–letiiu zhurnala). **Vestn Oftalmol** 1984 Nov–Dec;(6):4–6

**Krogh, August, 1874–1949**
Schmidt-Nielsen B: August and Marie Krogh and respiratory physiology. **J Appl Physiol** 1984 Aug;57(2):293–303

**Krogh, Marie (Jorgensen), 1874–1943?**
Schmidt-Nielsen B: August and Marie Krogh and respiratory physiology. **J Appl Physiol** 1984 Aug;57(2):293–303

**Krüche, Arno, 1854–1926**
Schneider HJ, Doberentz D: Zur Geschichte der Jenaer Harnsteinforschung. Mit einem vollständigen Abdruck der Dissertationsschrift Arno Krüches 'Ueber Struktur und Entstehung der Uratsteine' aus dem Jahre 1879. Jena, Friedrich-Schiller-Universität, 1979. 84, 42 p. (Jenaer Reden und Schriften).

**Krumbhaar, Edward Bell, 1882–1966**
Classics in infectious diseases. Letter from Theobald Smith to Edward Krumbhaar: **Rev Infect Dis** 1984 Mar–Apr;6(2):280–1
Smith T: Document: [letter to Dr. Edward B. Krumbhaar]. **Trans Stud Coll Physicians Phila** 1981 Sep;5(3 no 3):214–5

**Krupinski, Andrzej, 1744–1783**
Barg L: Andrzej Krupiński (1744–1783). W dwusetną rocznicę śmierci. **Arch Hist Med (Warsz)** 1983;46(3):347–53

**Krusenstern, Adam Johann von, 1770–1846**
Seidel T: Medizinische Beobachtungen während der Weltumsegelung des Adam Johann von Krusenstern. Diss. Düsseldorf, 1979. 89 p.

**Kruty, Vladislav**
Peňáz J: K úmrtí prof. MUDr. Vladislava Kruty, DrSc. **Cesk Fysiol** 1980 Mar;29(2):159–70

**Krwawicz, Tadensz, 1910–**
Szwarc B: Spis prac Prof. Tadeusza Krwawicza. **Klin Oczna** 1980 Jan;82(1):1–4

**Kübler-Ross, Elisabeth, 1926–**
Germain CP: Nursing the dying: implications of Kübler-Ross' staging theory. **Ann Am Acad Polit Soc Sci** 1980;447:46–58
Gill D: Quest, the life of Elisabeth Kübler-Ross. New York, Harper & Row, 1980. xiv, 329 p.

**Kubokawa, Chukichi**
Matsufuji H: [Chukichi Kubokawa and industrial Hygiene] (Jpn). **Igakushi Kenkyu** 1978;49:14–7

**Kuhlenbeck, Hartwig, 1897–**
Gerlach J: Hartwig Kuhlenbeck--60 Jahre vergleichend neuroanatomische Forschung. **J Hirnforsch** 1979;20(2):107–13

**Kuhn, Franz, 1866–1929**
Franco Grande A, Martinón JM, Pombo MV, et al: Evolución histórica de la intubación tráqueal. A porpósito de Franz Kuhn en el aniversario de su muerte. **Rev Esp Anestesiol Reanim** 1979 May;26(3):243–54

**Kühn, Karl Gottlob, 1754–1840**
Nutton V, ed: Karl Gottlob Kühn and his edition of the works of Galen. Oxford, Oxford Microform Publications, 1976. 35 p. (First published with the microfiche edition of Kühn's edition of The works of Galen, March 1976).

**Kukaĭn, Rita Aleksandrovna, 1922–**
Kocere V: Latvijas PSR Zinātnu akademijas akademike Rita Kukaine: biobibliogrāfiskais rādītājs. Riga, Zinātne, 1982. 129 p.

**Kulczyńska, Teresa**
Krzanowska Z: Nauczycielka najbardziej humanistycznego zawodu. **Pieleg Polozna** 1982;4–5:23–4

**Kumpf, Johann Gottfried, 1781–1862**
Frick K: Dr. Med. Johann Gottfried Kumpf (1781–1862) und die ägyptische Augenkrankheit in Kärnten. **Carinthia** 1966;156:670–712

**Kundrat, Hanns, 1845–1893**
Dieckmann I: Untersuchungen des menschlichen Endometriums durch Hanns Kundrat (1845–1893) und George Julius Engelmann (1847–1903). Diss. Erlangen-Nürnberg, 1980. 73 p.

**Künkel, Fritz, 1889–1956**
Rattner J: Fritz Künkel. In J. Rattner, ed: Wandlungen der Psychoanalyse. Wien, Europaverlag, 1980. p. 141–63.

**Kupalov, Petr Stepanovich, 1888–1964**
Buzsàki G: Situational conditional reflexes. Physiologic studies of the higher nervous activity of freely moving animals: P. S. Kupalov. **Pavlov J Biol Sci** 1983 Jan–Mar;18(1):13–21

**Kupffer, Karl Wilhelm, 1829–1902**
Kahle E: Kupffer. In Neue Deutsche Biographie 13. 1982. p. 319–20.
Szymańska R, Schmidt-Pospuła M: Z historii badań tadeusza Browicza (1847–1928) i Karola Kupffera (1829--1902) nad komórkami siateczkowo-śródbłonkowymi watroby. **Arch Hist Med (Warsz)** 1979;42(3):331–6

**Kuřák, Frantisek, 1801–1868**
První české přednášky na Pražské lékařské fakultě – Kuřákovy přednášky z fysiologie: **Cesk Fysiol** 1983;32(5):467–8

**Kurashov, Sergei Vladimirovich**
Serenko AF, Ermakov VV: S. V. Kurashov--vydaiushchiĭsia deiatel' sovetskogo zdravookhraneniia. **Sov Zdravookhr** 1980;(10):45–8

**Kurliandskiĭ, Veniamin IUr'evich, 1908?–**
Troianskiĭ AN: Vklad prof. V. Iu. Kurliandskogo v razvitie nauchnykh problem ortopedicheskoĭ stomatologii (k 75–letiiu so dnia rozhdeniia). **Stomatologiia (Mosk)** 1983 Nov–Dec;62(6):75–6

**Kurlov, Mikhail Georgievich, 1859–1932**
Egaĭ VS: Razvitie terapii v Sibiri: M. G. Kurlov i ego shkola. M. G. Kurlov i ego shkola. Novosibirsk, Nauka, Sibirskoe otd–nie, 1981. 112 p.

**Kutuzov, Mikhail Illarionovich, 1745–1813**
Gladkikh PF: Zabota M. I. Kutuzova o zdorov'e Russkogo soldata (k 170–letiiu so dnia Borodinskogo srazheniia). **Sov Zdravookhr** 1983;(3):68–70

## L

**La Brosse, Guy de, 1586?–1641**
Howard RC: The family of Guy de la Brosse, founder of the Jardin des Plantes in Paris. In: Conrès international d'histoire de la médecine, XXVe, Québec, 1976. Actes. Québec, 1977. p. 771–89.

**La Condamine, Charles Marie de, 1701–1774**
Hein WH: Zum Curarebericht des Jesuitenpaters Franz Xaver Veigl. **Beitr Gesch Pharm** 1981;11:81–4

**La Forge, Louis de, 1632–1667?**
Vetter T: Louis de la Forge (1632–1667?) angevin et fidèle adepte de la physiologie cartésienne. In: Congrès National des Sociétés Savantes, 93e, Tours, 1968. Comptes Rendus. Paris, 1971. Section des Sciences, Tome II. p. 31–50.

**La Martinière, Germain Pichaut de, 1696–1783**
Lefebvre P: Il y a deux siècles mourait Germain Pichault de la Martinière (1697–1783). **Chirurgie** 1983;109(10):805–8

**La Mettrie, Julien Offray de, 1709–1751**
Cappelletti AJ: Lamettrie medico y filosofo del hombre. **Rev Soc Venez Hist Med** 1972–73;20–21(34–35):211–27
Rudolph G: Iconographie de La Mettrie (1709–1751) à propos de la découverte d'un portrait inconnu du médecin et philosophe breton. In: Congrès National des Sociétés Savantes, 91e, Rennes, 1966. Comptes Rendus. Paris, 1967. Section des Sciences. Tome 1, p. 171–9.
Vartanian A: Le frère de Maupertuis et l'homme machine. **Dix-huit Siecle** 1982;14:305–23

**La Peyronie, François Gigot de, 1678–1747**
Tournier-Lasserve C: La Peyronie et la présence des chirurgiens militaires au sein de l'Académie de Chirurgie. **Chirurgie** 1981;107(9):719–22

**La Rue, Francois A. Hubert, 1833–1881**
Lortie L: François-Alexandre-Hubert La Rue. In Dictionary of Canadian biography, 1881–1890. 1982;11:495–7.

**La Torre, Felice, 1846–1923**
Rocchietta S: Musica e medicina negli scritti di Felice La Torre (1846–1923). **Minerva Ginecol** 1980 Oct;32(10):949–53
Rocchietta S: Musica e medicina negli scritti di Felice La Torre (1846–1923). **Minerva Med** 1980 Jul;71(27):1949–53

**Labadie, Jean de, 1610–1674**
Bordes F: Le livre des remèdes de Labadie. Contribution à l'histoire de la médecine populaire landaise au XVIIIe siècle. **Bull Soc Borda** 1982;107(387):399–412

**Labat, Pierre-Léon-Auguste, 1803–1847**
Ortiz-Monasterio F: Labat and the three-lobed forehead flap. **Plast Reconstr Surg** 1984 Apr;73(4):705

**Laborde, Jean Baptiste Vincent, 1830–1903**
Dubarry JJ: J. Vincent Laborde et son procédé de réanimation par tractions rythmées de la langue; la survie neuro-musculaire après décapitation. **Hist Sci Med** 1980;14(1):77–82

**Lacan, Jacques, 1901–**
Fisher DJ: Lacans's ambiguous impact on French psychoanalysis. **Contemp Fr Civiliz** 1981–82;6(1–2):89–114
Galati D: Lacan: un ritorno a Freud? **Stor Crit Psicol** 1980;1(1):79–91
Gorney JE: The clinical application of Lacan in the psychoanalytic situation. **Psychoanal Rev** 1982 Summer;69(2):241–8
Heinrichs HJ: Bibliographie der Schriften von Jacques Lacan. **Psyche (Stuttg)** 1980 Oct;34(10):958–73
Julien P: Un psychanalyste, Jacques Lacan. **Etudes (Fr)** 1982;357(4):333–46
Lebovici S: Jacques Lacan and French psychiatry. **Psychol Med** 1983 Feb;13(1):9–13
Lemaire A: Jacques Lacan. London and Boston, Rutledge and Kegan Paul, 1977. xxiv, 266 p.
Muller JP: Ego and subject in Lacan. **Psychoanal Rev** 1982 Summer;69(2):234–40
Richardson WJ: Lacan's view of language and being. **Psychoanal Rev** 1982 Summer;69(2):229–33
Schneiderman S: Jacques Lacan, the death of an intellectual hero. Cambridge, Harvard University Press, 1983. vii, 182 p.
Turkle S: Psychoanalytic politics: Freud's French Revolution. Cambridge, MIT Press, 1981, c1978. x, 278 p.
Turkle S: 'Mon oncle de Marienbad: sociobiology comes to the land of the structuralists. **Contemp Fr Civiliz** 1981–82;6(1–2):67–87

**Lacauchie, Adolphe-Euclide, 1806–1853**
Plessis JL: Un anatomiste militaire mort victime du devoir: Adolphe-Euclide Lacauchie (1806–1853), latiniste distingué et inventeur de l'hydrotomie. **Hist Sci Med** 1982;16(3):151–61

**Lacaze-Duthiers, Félix Joseph Henri de, 1821–1901**
Florkin M, Théodoridès J: Henri de Lacaze-Duthiers et Léon Fredericq: correspondance (1876–1900). **Arch Int Physiol Biochim** 1982 Jul;90(2):Suppl 1–94

**Lactantius, Lucius Caecilius Firmianus, ca. 260–ca. 340**
Lactance: L'ouvrage du Dieu créateur. 2 vols. Ed. par M. Perrin. Paris, Editions du Cerf, 1974. 456 p. (Sources Chrétiennes, No. 213, 214).

**Ladd, Anna Coleman, 1878–1939**
Romm S, Zacher J: Anna Coleman Ladd: maker of masks for the facially mutilated. **Plast Reconstr Surg** 1982 Jul;70(1):104–11

**Laehr, Heinrich, 1820–1905**
Kahle E: Laehr, Heinrich. In Neue Deutsche Biographie 13. 1982. p. 396–7.

**Laennec, Guillaume François, 1748–1822**
Saint-Maur PP: Que pensait Laennec de l'anatomie pathologique? **Ann Pathol** 1981;1(4):249–50

**Laennec, René Théophile Hyacinthe, 1781–1826**
Adler C: René Théophile Hyacinthe Laënnec (1781–1826), inventor of the stethoscope. **Adler Mus Bull** 1981;7(2):3–7
Anastasatu C: 200 de ani de la naşterea lui Laennec. **Rev Ig [Pneumoftiziol]** 1981 Oct–Dec;30(4):250–1
Bastholm E: Laennec og stetoskopet. **Dan Medicinhist Arbog** 1982;:112–35
Baumann J: Destinée de la méthode anatomo-clinique. **Bull Acad Natl Med (Paris)** 1981 Feb 17;Spec No:45–50
Bendiner E: A rebellious Breton who revolutionized medicine. **Hosp Pract** 1983 Nov;18(11):205–7, 210–1, 214 passim
Bernard J: Laennec et la médecine moderne. **Nouv Rev Deux Mondes** 1981;4:13–9
Birtalan G: Laennec and Skoda, classics of internal diagnostics. **Orvostort Kozl** 1982;28(1–3):33–41
Bishop PJ: Laennec: a great student of tuberculosis. **Tubercle** 1981 Jun;62(2):129–34
Bishop PJ: Reception of the stethoscope and Laënnec's book. **Thorax** 1981 Jul;36(7):487–92
Boulle L, Grmek MD, Lupovici C, et al: Laennec, Catalogue des manuscrits scientifiques. Paris, Masson, 1982. 316 p.
Bourgeois P: Laennec et son temps. **Sem Hop Paris** 1981 Dec 18–25;57(47–48):2047–56
Charpin J: Laënnec et l'asthme. **Rev Fr Mal Respir** 1981;9(2):151–3
Commémoration du bicentenaire de la naissance de M.T.H. Laennec 1781–1826: **Bull Acad Natl Med (Paris)** 1981 Feb 17;Spec no.:1–61
De Saint-Maur PP: Que pensait Laennec de l'anatomie pathologique? **Ann Pathol** 1981;1(4):249–50
Finot A: Les premiers élèves et collaborateurs (surtout Bretons) de Laennec. In: Congrès National des Sociétés Savantes, 91e, Rennes, 1966. Comptes Rendus. Paris, 1967. Section des Sciences, Tome 1. p. 181–9.
Fox ER: Mrs. Laennec and the stethoscope. **West J Med** 1981 Jan;134(1):73–4
Fréour P: Du pneumo-thorax vu par Th. Laënnec. **Rev Fr Mal Respir** 1981;9(3):265–9
Grassi C: Influence de l'oeuvre de Laénnec sur la médecine italienne. **Rev Fr Mal Respir** 1981;9(5):421–6
Hanngren A: René Théophile Hyacinthe Laennec (1781–1826). **Nord Medicinhist Arsb** 1981;:106–19
Hanngren A: R. T. H. Laënnec, lungmedicinens fader, 1781–1826. **Kvartalsskr Sven Hjart Lungsjukdomor** 1981;76:73–82
Huard P, Grmek MD: Coup d'oeil sur les élèves étrangers de Laennec. In: Congrès National des Sociétés Savantes, 97e, Nantes, 1972. Comptes Rendus. Paris, 1976. Section des Sciences, Tome 1. p. 21–35.
Huard P: Les facettes multiples de René Théophile Laennec (1781–1826). **Bull Acad Natl Med (Paris)** 1981 Feb 17;Spec No:51–6
Keers RY: Laennec: his medical history. **Thorax** 1981 Feb;36(2):91–4
Kerbrat G: Laennec et ses combats (1781–1826). In: Congrès National des Sociétés Savantes, 107e. Brest, 1982. Comptes Rendus, Paris, 1983. Section des Sciences, Fasc. IV. p. 287–98.
Kligfield P: Laennec and the discovery of mediate auscultation. **Am J Med** 1981 Feb;70(2):275–8
Leroy D: Laennec étudiant en médecine. **Bull Acad Natl Med (Paris)** 1979 Nov 6–27;163(8):849–56
McMichael J: History of atrial fibrillation 1628–1819 Harvey - de Senac - Laënnec. **Br Heart J** 1982 Sep;48(3):193–7
Mann RJ, Mann FD: Laennec as a critical pathologist. **J Hist Med Allied Sci** 1981 Oct;36(4):446–54
Mann RJ, Mann FD: Emphysema. Era of Laennec; era of the cigarette. **Minn Med** 1984 Mar;67(3):142, 159–61
Marketos S: [The deep influence of ancient Greek civilization on the work of René Laënnec, inventor of the stethoscope.] (Gre). **Prakt Akad Athenon** 1981;56:132–8
Marketos SG: [René Théophile Laënnec (1781–1826)] (Gre). **Mater Med Greca** 1981;9:1–10
Marketos SG: [The concert for Laënnec's stethoscope] (Gre). **Mater Med Greca** 1981;9:125–34
Marketos S, et al: [René Théophile Laënnec: his relatively unknown research work] (Gre). **Mater Med Greca** 1981;9:249–57
Martiny M: Laënnec et la pensée hippocratique. In La collection hippocratique et son rôle dans l'histoire de la médecine. Colloque de Strasbourg (23–27 octobre 1972) organisé par le Centre de Recherches sur la Grèce Antique, avec le concours des Facultés de Philosophie et des Langues Classiques. Leiden, E. J. Brill, 1975. p. 97–105.
Matteo J di: L'oeuvre cardiologique de Laennec. **Bull Acad Natl Med (Paris)** 1981 Feb 17;Spec No:37–44
Mikhaĭlov FA: Rene Teofil' Giatsint Laénnek (1781–1826). **Klin Med (Mosk)** 1981 Dec;59(12):92–5
Rousseau A: Laennec Celtisant. In: Congrès National des Sociétés Savantes, 97e, Nantes, 1972. Comptes Rendus. Paris, 1976. Section des Sciences, Tome 1. p. 9–19.
Rousselot Y: De quelques influences qui se sont exercées sur R. Théophile Laennec et ce qui en résulta. In: Congrès National des Sociétés Savantes, 97e, Nantes, 1972. Comptes Rendus. Paris, 1976. Section des Sciences, Tome 1. p 37–45.
Sakula A: R.T.H. Laënnec 1781–1826, his life and work: a bicentenary appreciation. **Thorax** 1981 Feb;36(2):81–90
Sakula A: Laennec's influence on some British physicians in the nineteenth century. **J R Soc Med** 1981 Oct;74(10):759–67
Sakula A: In search of Laënnec. **J R Coll Physicians Lond** 1981 Jan;15(1):55–7
Sakula A: Bicentenary of Laennec's birth celebrated in Paris. **Med Hist** 1981;25:320–1
Sakula A: The story of the stethoscope. **Trans Med Soc Lond** 1981–82;98:27–31
Somolinos-Palencia J: René Teófilo Jacinto Laennec, a los 200 años de su nacimiento. **Gac Med Mex** 1981 Mar;117(3):122–6
Trautmann M, Trautmann JC: R. T. H. Laennec 1781–1826. Zum 200. Geburtstag des Autors der Auscultation médiate. **MMW** 1981 Nov 6;123(45):1717–20
Turiaf J: Laennec et la pathologie respiratoire. **Bull Acad Natl Med (Paris)** 1981 Feb 17;Spec No:31–6
Vita a Laennec megemlékezés körül: **Orv Hetil** 1981 Dec 13;122(50):3115–6

**Laestadius, Lars Levi, 1780–1861**
Fagerheim E: Lars Levi Laestadius' teologiske studier. **Nor Teol Tidsskr** 1972;73(1):35–50

**Lafarge, Marie Capelle, 1816–1852**
Lépine P: Un dossier contesté, l'affaire Lafarge. **Lyon Pharm** 1980 Jan 1;31(1):39–44
Lépine P: Le secret de Madame Lafarge (lumières nouvelles sur une affaire célèbre). **Sem Hop Paris** 1983 Dec 22;59(48):3387–94

**Lafargue, Paul, 1842–1911**
Gani L: Jules Guesde, Paul Lafargue et les problèmes de population. **Population** 1979;34(4):1023–1044

Makarenko EM: Molodoi Lafarg. **Vopr Istor** 1981;(6):115–22

**Lafontaine, Franz Leopold de, 1756–1812**
Kaiser W, Pankiewicz H: Zum Leben und Werk Franz Leopold de Lafontaine 1756--1812. **Arch Hist Med (Warsz)** 1979;42(2):231–9

**Laforest, Nicholas Laurent, fl. 1782**
Laforest NL: L'art de soigner les pieds. Fac-simile de l'édition de 1782. Ed. R. Habert. Bruxelles, Caducea, 1979. 257 p.

**Laguna, Andrés de, d. 1560**
Hernando y Ortega T: Dos estudios históricos (vieja y nueva medicina). Madrid, Espasa-Calpe, 1982. 243 p.

**Lahey, Frank Howard, 1880–1953**
Boyd DP: Doctor Lahey and his clinic. **Postgrad Med** 1984 Feb 15;75(3):14–6, 18

**Laín Entralgo, Pedro, 1908–**
Barcia D: La significacion de la antropologia medica de Lain Entralgo para la psiquiatria actual. **Asclepio** 1980;32:19–45
López Piñero JM: El estudio histórico de la medicina en la obra de Laín Entralgo. **Dynamis** 1981;1:231–9
Sociedad Española de Historia de la Medicina: V Congreso Nacional. Homenaje al Profesor Pedro Lain Entralgo. Madrid, 29–30 septiembre-1 octubre 1977. **Asclepio** 1977;29:1–358

**Lains, Ronald David, 1927–**
Evans RI: Dialogue with R. D. Laing. New York, Praeger, 1981. lxxv, 170 p. (Reprint of 1976 ed; with new introduction).

**Lairesse, Gerard de, 1641–1711**
Dumaitre P: La curieuse destinée des planches anatomiques de Gérard de Lairesse, peintre en Hollande - Lairesse, Bidloo, Cowper. Amsterdam, Rodopi, 1982. xvii, 107 p. (Nieuwe Nederlandse Bijdragen tot de Geschiedenis der Geneeskunde en der Natuurwetenschappen, no. 6).

**Lakhovsky, Georges, 1870–1942**
Farrell K: Hyperthermia for malignant disease--a history of medicine note--the work of Georges Lakhovsky. **Adv Exp Med Biol** 1982;157:9–10

**Lakshmipathi, Bhishagratna Achanta, 1880–1964**
Rama Rao B: Bhishagratna Achanta Lakshmipathi, his dedicated service to Ayurveda. **Bull Indian Inst Hist Med (Hyderabad)** 1980;10(1–4):76–83
Shankarashastry V: The eminence of Lakshmipathi. **Bull Indian Inst Hist Med (Hyderabad)** 1980;10(1–4):62–8
Vasanth P: The life and deeds of late Dr. Achanta Lakshmipathi. **Sachitra Ayurved** 1981 Mar;:174–8

**Lam, Wilfredo, 1902–1982**
Golliet P, Binet JL: Deux historiens du sang, ou Réponse de Lucien Lévy-Bruhl et de Wifredo Lam à Jean Bernard. **Nouv Rev Fr Hematol** 1983;25(5):337–41

**Lamarck, Jean Baptiste Pierre Antoine de Monet de, 1744–1829**
Aymonin GG: Lamarck et son herbier. **Hist Nat** 1980–81;17–18:13–7
Aymonin GG: L'herbier de Lamarck. **Rev Hist Sci (Paris)** 1981;34:25–58
Bowler PJ: E. W. MacBride's Lamarckian eugenics and its implications for the social construction of scientific knowledge. **Ann Sci** 1984 May;41(3):245–60
Danchin A: Une révolution lamarckienne en immunologie. **Recherche** 1981;12(118):84–5
Fischer JL: Yves Delage (1854–1920): l'epigenèse néo-lamarckienne contre la prédétermination weismannienne. **Rev Synth (Paris)** 1979;100(95–6):443–61
Gershenowitz H: Napoleon and Lamarck. **Indian J Hist Sci** 1980;15:204–9
López-Fanjul de Argüelles C: El lamarckismo y algo sobre los neolamarckismos. **Arbor** 1982;113(441–2):41–57
Sheets-Johnstone M: Why Lamarck did not discover the principle of natural selection. **J Hist Biol** 1982 Fall;15(3):443–65
Szyfman L: Remarques sur l'ouvrage d'Ernst Mayr: 'Lamarck Revisited'. **Bull Biol Fr Belg** 1977;111(3):209–29

**Lamare-Picquot, Christophe-Augustin, 1785–1873**
Chaigneau M: Christophe-Augustin Lamare-Picquot, pharmacien, naturaliste, explorateur. **Rev Hist Pharm (Paris)** 1982 Mar;29(252):5–26

**Lamarre, Henri, d. 1740**
Moogk PN: Henri Lamarre. In Dictionary of Canadian biography, 1701 to 1740. Volume 2, 1969. p. 339–40.

**Lambe, John, 1546–1628**
Goldstein LM: The life and death of John Lambe. **Guildhall Stud Lond Hist** 1979;4(1):19–32

**Lambert, Edward Howard, 1915–**
Bibliography of Dr. E. H. Lambert: **Muscle Nerve** 1982;5(9S):S166–72
Simpson JA: Electrophysiology of neuromuscular junction disease: an appreciation of the contributions of Edward H. Lambert. **Muscle Nerve** 1982;5(9S):S6–11
Willison RG: Dr. E. H. Lambert's contributions to electromyography. **Muscle Nerve** 1982;5(9S):S2–5

**Lambert, Jean-Henri, 1728–1777**
Jacquel R: Trois Alsaciens et les débuts--modestes--de la médecine sociale en Pologne pendant l'époque des lumières (troisième tiers du XVIIIe siècle). Les médecins strasbourgeois Jacques Reinbold Spielmann (1722–1783) et Jean Boecler (1737–1808) et le savant mulhousien Jean-Henri Lambert (1728–1777). In Livet G, Schaff G, ed: Médecine et assistance en Alsace, XVIe-XXe siècle. Strasbourg, Istra, 1976. p. 155–200.

**Lambie, Mary, 1889–1971**
Campbell H: Mary Lambie: a biography. Wellington, New Zealand Nursing Education and Research Foundation, 1976. x, 100 p.

**Lambotte, Albin, 1866–1955**
de Marneffe R: Albin Lambotte, pionnier de l'ostéosynthèse moderne. **Rev Med Brux** 1982 Sep;3(7):493–5

**Lämmler, Georg, 1925–1981**
Boray JC: Obituary: Georg Lämmler. **Int J Parasitol** 1981 Oct;11(5):335–40

**Lampe, Isadore, 1906–**
del Regato JA: Isadore Lampe. **Int J Radiat Oncol Biol Phys** 1984 Feb;10(2):173–83

**Lancisi, Giovanni Maria, 1654–1720**
Kligfield PD: A survey of variant title page vignettes in Lancisi's De subitaneis mortibus. **J Hist Med Allied Sci** 1983 Jul;38(3):336–9
Olagüe G: El programa de reforma educativa de Giovanni Maria Lancisi: De recta medicorum studiorum ratione instituenda (1715). **Episteme** 1976 Jan–Dec;1–4:180–9
Olagüe G: El discurso de Giovanni Maria Lancisi 'sobre la recta ordenacion de los estudios medicos segun la razon' (1715). **Asclepio** 1981;33:143–62
Olagüe de Ros G: La epidemia europea de gripe de 1708–1709. Difusión témporo-espacial e interpretaciones contemporáneas: G. M. Lancisi, B. Ramazzini, K. F. Hoffmann. **Dynamis** 1981;1;51–86
Olague Ros G: Biografia cientifica de Giovanni Maria Lancisi. **Med Esp** 1980;79:250–60

**Landauer, Walter, 1896–1978**
Oppenheimer JM: Walter Landauer and developmental genetics. In Subtelny S, Abbott U, ed: Levels of genetic control in development. New York, Liss, 1981. p. 1–13.

**Landry, Jean-Etienne, 1815–1884**
Sylvain P: Jean-Etienne Landry. In Dictionary of Canadian biography, 1881–1890. 1982;11:483–6.

**Landsteiner, Karl, 1868–1943**
Mazumdar PM: Karl Landsteiner and the problem of species 1838–1968. Ph.D. Diss., Johns Hopkins University. Baltimore, 1976. 725 leaves.
Schneider WH: Chance and social setting in the application of the discovery of blood groups. **Bull Hist Med** 1983 Winter;57(4):545–62
Speiser P, Smekal FG: Karl Landsteiner, Entdecker der Blutgruppen und Pionier der Immunologie. Biographie eines Nobelpreisträgers aus der Wiener Medizinischen Schule. 2., vollständig überarb. Aufl. Vienna, Hollinek, 1975. 207 p.
Speiser P: Rhesus-Prophylaxe. Zum 40. Todestag von Karl Landsteiner. **Wien Med Wochenschr** 1983 Dec 31;133(23–24):592–4

**Lane, Arbuthnot, 1856?–1943**
Smith JL: Sir Arbuthnot Lane, chronic intestinal stasis, and autointoxication. **Ann Intern Med** 1982 Mar;96(3):365–9

**Lane, Edward, ca. 1823–**
Colp R: Charles Darwin, Dr. Edward Lane, and the 'Singular Trial' of Robinson v. Robinson and Lane. **J Hist Med Allied Sci** 1981 Apr;36(2):205–13

**Lanfranco, of Milan, fl. 1290–1296**
Berg A, ed: Lanfranks 'Chirurgia parva' in der Abschrift Konrad Schrecks von Aschaffenburg. Diss. Würzburg 1975, 145 S. (Altdeutsche Lanfrank-Uebersetzungen III).
Scholle S: Lanfranks 'Chirurgia Parva' in mittelniederfränkischer Ubertragung. Diss. Würzburg, 1978. Pattensen, Horst Wellm Verlag, 1978. 147 p. (Altdeutsche Lanfrank-Ubersetzungen, II, 1).

**Lange, Johannes, 1485–1565**
Nutton V: John Caius und Johannes Lange: medizinischer Humanismus zur Zeit Vesals. **NTM** 1984;21(2):81–7

**Langenbeck, Bernhard von, 1810–1887**
Hauben DJ: Das chirurgische Erbe. Bernhard Rudolf Conrad Langenbeck (1810–1887). **Zentralbl Chir** 1984;109(20):1338–9

**Langenbuch, Carl Johann August, 1846–1901**
Casal MA: Hace cien años: 1882–1982. 'Carl Langenbuch, la primera colecistectomía y breve historia de una polémia famosa. **Acta Gastroenterol Latinoam** 1982;12(2):181–4
Rains AJ: A thought for Carl Langenbuch (1846–1901): a centenary. **Ann R Coll Surg Engl** 1982 Jul;64(4):268–9
Sparkman RS: 100th anniversary of the first cholecystectomy. **Arch Surg** 1982 Dec;117(12):1525
Török B: Langenbuch és Halpert Béla. Az elsö cholecytektómia centenáriumára. **Orv Hetil** 1983 Jun 26;124(26):1577–81

**Langerhans, Paul, 1847–1888**
Ebling FJ: Homage to Paul Langerhans. **J Invest Dermatol** 1980

Jul;75(1):3-5
Ebling FJ, Ebling E: The contribution of Paul Langerhans (1847-1888) to tuberculosis research. **Wiss Beitr Martin Luther Univ Halle Wittenberg** 1983;5-R80:261-72

**Langfeldt, Gabriel, 1895-**
Rousselot Y: La conception de la schizophrénie chez Langfeldt. **Ann Med Psychol (Paris)** 1981;139(8):879-92

**Langie, Adam Marian, 1829-1907**
Gaertner H: Adam Marian Langie. **Klin Oczna** 1982 Apr;84(4):131-4

**Langworthy, Solon Massey, 1868-**
Gibbons RW: Solon Massey Langworthy: keeper of the flame during the 'lost years' of chiropractic. **Chiropr Hist** 1981;1(1):15-21

**Laplace, Pierre Simon de, 1749-1827**
Kurfess JF: The legacy of Laplace. **J Ky Med Assoc** 1980 Apr;78(4):197-202

**Lappe, Christian Theodor, 1802-1877**
Schwarz HD: Christian Theodor Lappe (1802-1877). **Pharm Ztg** 1977;122:338

**Lardizábal, Vicente de, ca. 1746-1814**
Richter T: Das Sargassokraut in Vicente de Lardizábals Werk 'Consuelo de Navegantes' (Madrid 1772). Diss., Universität Düsseldorf. Düsseldorf, 1982. 111 p.

**Larionov, Vladimir Efimovich, 1857-1919**
Arkhangel'skiĭ GV: V. E. Larionov--odin iz osnovopolozhnikov otechestvennoĭ otonevrologii. **Vestn Otorinolaringol** 1984 Mar-Apr;(2):88-93

**Larkey, Sanford Vincent, 1898-1969**
Webster C, ed: Health, medicine and mortality in the sixteenth century. London and New York, Cambridge University Press, 1979. 394 p. In memory of Sanford V. Larkey. Contributions by P. Slack, R. Schofield, E. A. Wrigley, A. B. Appleby, T. R. Forbes, P. Allderidge, M. Pelling, A. Chapman, J. J. Bylebyl.

**Larrey, Dominique Jean, 1766-1842**
Amalric P: De l'Hôpital de la Grave à la Grande Armée. L'ophtalmologie de Dominique Larrey. **Bull Soc Ophtalmol Fr** 1979 Feb;79(2):151-4
Bodemer CW: Baron Dominique Jean Larrey, Napoleon's surgeon. **Bull Am Coll Surg** 1982 Jul;67(7):18-21
Csillag I: Eckstein Ferenc és a hadisebészet a Napóleon elleni háborúban. **Orv Hetil** 1984 Feb 19;125(8):467-70
Demerson P: Le chirurgien Larrey et 'l'invasion française' à l'academie de médecine de Madrid. **Melanges Casa Velasquez** 1973;9:483-501
DiGioia JM, Rocko JM, Swan KG: Baron Larrey. Modern military surgeon. **Am Surg** 1983 May;49(5):226-30
Egeblad K: Militaerkirurgen Dominique Jean Larrey: Om pesten i felttoget til Aegypten og Syrien 1798-1801. **Dan Medicinhist Arbog** 1979;132-59
Hau T: The surgical practice of Dominique Jean Larrey. **Surg Gynecol Obstet** 1982 Jan;154(1):89-94
Hockemeyer H: Die Zeit seiner Schiffsarzttätigkeit in den Memoiren des napoleonischen Chirurgen Dominique-Jean Larrey. Diss., Universität Düsseldorf. Düsseldorf, 1982. 44 p.
Jensen JE: Napoleonic medicine. **Md State Med J** 1981 Jul;30(7):66-8
Lefebvre P, Godon A: Les cendres du baron Larrey. **Nouv Presse Med** 1982 Jan 30;11(4):235-9

**Larsson, Bergljot, 1883-**
Norsk Sykepleierforbund 70-års dag: historisk høytidsstund på Vettre: 'Arhundrets sykepleier' har fått sitt monument. **Sykepleien** 1982 Oct 20;69(18):6-7, 31

**Lasègue, Ernest Charles, 1816-1883**
Biographical sketches no. 31--Lasèque: **Ir Med J** 1983 Aug;76(8):367

**Lashley, Karl Spencer, 1890-1958**
Herrnstein RJ: Karl Spencer Lashley. In Dictionary of American Biography, Suppl. 6, 1956-1960. p. 367-8, 1980.

**Lathrop, Julia Clifford, 1858-1932**
Parker JK, Carpenter EM: Julia Lathrop and the Children's Bureau: the emergence of an institution. **Soc Serv Rev** 1981;55(1):60-77

**Latos, Jan Walenty, 1539-ca. 1610**
Lisiewicz J: Jan Walenty Latos (1539--początek XVII w.) lekarz i astrolog Akademii Krakowskiej. **Wiad Lek** 1982 Dec 15;35(23-24):1589-91

**Latrobe, Benjamin Henry, 1764-1820**
Stapleton DH, Carter EC: 'I have the itch of botany, of chemistry, of mathematics ... strong upon me': the science of Benjamin Henry Latrobe. **Proc Am Philos Soc** 1984 Sep;128(3):173-92

**Lattes, Leone, 1887-**
Giusti GV: Leone Lattes: Italy's pioneer in forensic serology. **Am J Forensic Med Pathol** 1982 Mar;3(1):79-81

**Laughlin, Harry Hamilton, 1880-1943**
Bird RD, Allen G: The J.H.B. Archive report: the papers of Harry Hamilton Laughlin, eugenicist. **J Hist Biol** 1981 Fall;14(2):339-53

**Lautard, Jean-Baptiste, b. 1778**
Alliez J: Jean-Baptiste Lautard et la 'maison des fous' de Marseille. **Marseille** 1981;127:44-9

**Lavalle, Juan Galo de, 1797-1841**
Benencia JA: Los restos del general D. Juan Galo de Lavalle. **Historia (Argentina)** 1965;10(39):84-5

**Lavater, Johann Caspar, 1741-1801**
Goscilo H: Lermontov's debt to Lavater and Gall. **Slav East Eur Rev** 1981;59(4):500-15

**Laveran, Alphonse, 1845-1922**
Beauperthuy de Benedetti R: Laveran y Beauperthuy. **Acta Med Venez** 1981 Jan-Mar;28(1):47-52
Beltrán E: Conmemoración del descubrimiento de uno de los gérmenes patogénicos del paludismo. **Gac Med Mex** 1981 May;117(5):195-201
Bruce-Chwatt LJ: Alphonse Laveran's discovery 100 years ago and today's global fight against malaria. **J R Soc Med** 1981 Jul;74(7):531-6
Brumpt L: L'oeuvre de Laveran en protozoologie et ses conséquences. **Bull Acad Natl Med (Paris)** 1980 Jan;164(1):88-93
Camelin A: Considérations biographiques sur Alphonse Laveran (1845-1922). **Hist Sci Med** 1980;14:377-82
Jarcho S: Laveran's discovery in the retrospect of a century. **Bull Hist Med** 1984 Summer;58(2):215-24
Laveran CL: Classics in infectious diseases: A newly discovered parasite in the blood of patients suffering from malaria. Parasitic etiology of attacks of malaria: Charles Louis Alphonse Laveran (1845-1922). **Rev Infect Dis** 1982 Jul-Aug;4(4):908-11
Lefebvre P: L'hôpital Militaire Laveran de Constantine. **Med Trop (Mars)** 1980 Nov-Dec;40(6):645-9
Lévy A: Alphonse Laveran, initiateur de la pathologie coronaro-myocardique. **Nouv Presse Med** 1981 Mar 21;10(13):1015
Lukács D: Száz éve fedezte fel Charles Alphonse Louis Laveran a malária kórokozóit. **Orv Hetil** 1980 Dec 14;121(50):3076-8
Mollaret P: La découverte, par Alphonse Laveran de l'agent du paludisme. Constantine, 6 Novembre 1880. **Nouv Presse Med** 1980 Nov 1;9(41):3055-63
Nicolle P: Alphonase Laveran et Charles Nicolle. **Arch Inst Pasteur Tunis** 1981 Sep-Dec;58(3):265-79
Nosny P: Alphonse Laveran et la découverte de l'hématozoaire du paludisme. **Bull Acad Natl Med (Paris)** 1980 Jan;164(1):80-7
Pene P: De Laveran aux conséquences médicales, sociales et économiques de sa découverte. **Bull Acad Natl Med (Paris)** 1980 Apr;164(4):382-92
Percebois G: Il y un siècle, Laveran découvrit l'hématozoaire du paludisme. **Ann Med Nancy** 1981;20:549-58
Percebois G: Laveran et le pays messin. **J Med Strasb** 1980;11:311-6
Théodoridès J: La contribution d'A. Laveran à l'étude des Sporozoaires (Hémosporidies exceptées) et des Myxosporidies. **Hist Nat** 1980-81;17-18:77-84
Theodorides J: Célébration du centenaire de la découverte par A. Laveran de l'Hématozoaire du paludisme. Strasbourg, 2-3 mai 1980. **Rev Hist Sci (Paris)** 1980;33(4):351-2

**Lavoisier, Antoine Laurent, 1743-1794**
Abrahams HJ: Lavoisier and his contemporaries debate the supply of water for Paris. **Bull NY Acad Med** 1981 Jun;57(5):355-69
Anderson WC: Translating the language of chemistry: Priestley and Lavoisier. **Eighteenth Cent Theory Interpret** 1981;22(1):21-31
Gouch JB: Lavoisier's memoirs on the nature of water and their place in the chemical revolution. **Ambix** 1983 Jul;30(2):89-106
Kieft L, Willeford BR, ed: Joseph Priestley. Scientist, theologian, and metaphysician. A symposium celebrating the two hundredth anniversary of the discovery of oxygen by Joseph Priestley in 1774. Lewisburg, Bucknell University Press, 1980. 117 p. With contributions by E. N. Hiebert, A. J. Ihde, R. E. Schofield.
Levin A: Venel, Lavoisier, Fourcroy, Cabanis and the idea of scientific revolution: the French political context and the general patterns of conceptualization of scientific change. **Hist Sci** 1984 Sep;22(57 pt 3):303-20
Van Elst H: Jan Baptist Van Mons: aanhanger en verdediger van de leer van Lavoisier. **Farm Tijdschr Belg** 1980;57:145-58

**Lavrentiev, Boris Innokentievich, 1892-1944**
Afanas'ev IuI, Belova TI, Fel'dman NG: Boris Innokent'evich Lavrent'ev (k 90-letiiu so dnia rozhdeniia). **Arkh Anat Gistol Embriol** 1983 Nov;85(11):98-101

**Lawkowicz, Włodzimierz, 1908-1979**
Kłodziński S: Prof. dr Włodzimierz Lawkowicz. **Przegl Lek** 1981;38(1):197-202

**Lawrence, David Herbert, 1885-1930**
Dervin D: Rainbow, phoenix, and plumed serpent: D. H. Lawrence's great composite symbols and their vicissitudes. **Psychoanal Rev** 1980 Winter;67(4):515-41
Gutierrez D: D. H. Lawrence and modern destructiveness. **Suicide Life Threat Behav** 1980 Winter;10(4):219-29
Morowitz HJ: The mating poems of D. H. Lawrence. **Hosp Pract [Off]** 1984 May;19(5):233-5, 238

**Lawrence, John Hundale, 1904-**
Myers WG: Historian's note: early experiences in nuclear medicine by John H. Lawrence, 1956. **J Nucl Med** 1979 Jun;20(6):560-4

**Lawson, Thomas, 1789-1861**
Gillett MC: Thomas Lawson, second Surgeon General of the U. S. Army: a character sketch. **Prologue J Nat Arch** 1982 Spring;14(1):15-24

**Lazarevic, Laza, 1851–1890**
Mijalković D: Doprinos dr Laze K.Lazarevića infektologiji XIX veka. **Srp Arh Celok Lek** 1980 Jan;108(1):77–80

**Lazear, Jesse William, 1866–1900**
Norman C: The unsung hero of yellow fever? **Science** 1984 Mar 30;223(4643):1370–2

**Lazimir, P. E.**
Korsunskiĭ MA: Voennyĭ fel'dsher P. E. Lazimir. **Feldsher Akush** 1980;45(12):41–4

**Le Boë, Frans de, 1614–1672**
Beukers H: Het laboratorium van Sylvius. **Tijdschr Geschied Geneeskd** 1980;3(1):28–36
Beukers H: Mechanistische principes bij Franciscus dele Boë, Sylvius. **Tijdschr Geschied Geneeskd** 1982;5(1):6–15

**Le Dantec, Félix Alexandre, 1869–1917**
Diara A: Sens et definition du mot 'espece' dans l'oeuvre biologique de Felix Le Dantec. **Rev Synth (Paris)** 1981;102(101–102):73–86
Wrotnowska D: Lettres de Le Dantec, disciple de Pasteur. In: Congrès National des Sociétés Savantes, 107e. Brest, 1982. Comptes Rendus, Paris, 1983. Section des Sciences, Fasc. IV. p. 253–64.

**Le Dran, Henri François, 1685–1770**
Haller alla 'Charité' con Ledran: **Dent Cadmos** 1979 Feb 2;47(2):54–6

**Le Fort, Leon**
Higier J: Sto lat sporu o autorstwo (priorytet) operacji pośrodkowego zeszycia pochwy (colpocleisis mediana) 1881–1981. **Ginekol Pol** 1982;53(3)

**Le Goust, Philippe, fl. 1650**
Duchatel F: L'auscultation obstétricale de Philippe Le Goust au monitorage foetal. **Hist Sci Med** 1982;16(1):37–47

**Le Jumeaux de Kergaradec, Jean Alexandre, 1787–1877**
Higier J. J. A. Kergaradec (1787–1877) – zapomniany odkrywca i pionier słuchawki położniczej. **Ginekol Pol** 1982;53(11):817–20
Stofft H: Kergaradec à l'écoute du foetus. **J Gynecol Obstet Biol Reprod (Paris)** 1981;10(6):611–22

**Le Monnier, Louis Guillaume, 1717–1799**
Laissus Y: Lettres inédites de René Desfontaines à Louis-Guillaume le Monnier, conservées à la Bibliothèque centrale du Muséum national d'histoire naturelle. In: Congrès National des Sociétés Savantes, 91e, Rennes, 1966. Comptes Rendus. Paris, 1967. Section des Sciences, Tome 1. p. 153–69.

**Leake, Chauncey Depew, 1896–1978**
Keys TE: Chauncey Depew Leake, 1896–1978: an appreciation. **J Hist Med Allied Sci** 1978 Jul;33(3):428–31

**Leale, Charles Augustus, 1842–1932**
Read H: 'A hand to hold while dying': Dr. Charles A. Leale at Lincoln's side. **Lincoln Her** 1977;79:21–6

**Learmonth, James Rognvald, 1895–1967**
Douglas DM: Sir James Rögnvald Learmonth. In Dictionary of national biography, 1961–1970. Suppl. 8, 1981. p. 638–40.

**Leber, Theodor, 1840–1917**
Perkin GD: Leber's optic atrophy. In Rose FC, Bynum WF, ed: Historical aspects of the neurosciences. New York, Raven, 1982. p. 463–72.
Pinckers AJ: Leber's congenital amaurosis as conceived by Leber. **Ophthalmologica** 1979;179(1):48–51

**Leborgne, 1810–1861**
Signoret JL, Castaigne P, Lhermitte F, et al: Rediscovery of Leborgne's brain: anatomical description with CT scan. **Brain Lang** 1984 Jul;22(2):303–19

**L'Ecluse, Charles de, 1526–1609**
Dodoens R: Histoire des plantes. Traduction française, suivie du Petit recueil, auquel est contenue la description d'aucunes gommes et liqueurs etc., par Charles de l'Escluse (1557). Fac-similé avec introduction, commentaires et la concordance avec la terminologie scientifique moderne, par J.-E. Opsomer. Bruxelles, Centre National d'Histoire des Sciences, 1978. 78, 584 p. (Publications du Centre National d'Histoire des Sciences, V).
Ubrizsy in Savoia A: I rapport fra Carolus Clusius ed i naturalisti italiani del suo tempo. **Physis** 1978;20(1–4):49–68

**LeConte, Joseph, 1823–1901**
Enoch JM: Joseph Le Conte. **Am J Optom Physiol Opt** 1983 Dec;60(12):1003
Stephens LD: Joseph LeConte and the development of the physiology and psychology of vision in the United States. **Ann Sci** 1980 May;37(3):303–21
Stephens LD: Joseph LeConte. Gentle prophet of evolution. Baton Rouge, London, Louisiana State University Press, 1982. xix, 340 p.

**Lederer, Bernd, 1939–1982**
Propst A: Bernd Lederer. **Verh Dtsch Ges Pathol** 1982;66:652–7

**Lee, Lyndon Edmund, 1887–**
Rehm WS: In tribute to a living pioneer: Dr. Lyndon Edmund Lee. **Chiropr Hist** 1981;1(1):47–50

**Lee, Robert Edward, 1807–1870**
Cox MK: Victory through defeat: a character analysis of Robert E. Lee. **Psychoanal Rev** 1980 Winter;67(4):443–63

**Leenhardt, Maurice, 1878–1954**
Leenhardt RH: Un tournant de l'histoire de la nouvelle caledonie: Maurice Leenhardt (1878–1954). **Rev Fr Hist Outre Mer** 1978;65(2):236–52

**Leeuwenhoek, Anthony van, 1632–1723**
Bardell D: The roles of the sense of taste and clean teeth in the discovery of bacteria by Antoni van Leeuwenhoek. **Microbiol Rev** 1983 Mar;47(1):121–6
Bardell D: Antoni van Leeuwenhoek's explanation in 1704 of the function of eyelids. **J Hist Med Allied Sci** 1984 Oct;39(4):464–7
Bendiner E: The man who did not invent the microscope. **Hosp Pract [Off]** 1984 Aug;19(8):139, 144–5, 149 passim
Bibel DJ: The discovery of the oral flora--a 300-year retrospective. **J Am Dent Assoc** 1983 Oct;107(4):569–70
Brazier MA: The problem of neuromuscular action: two 17th century Dutchmen. In Rose FC, Bynum WF, ed: Historical aspects of the neurosciences. New York, Raven, 1982. p. 13–22.
Ford BJ: Leeuwenhoek's specimens discovered after 307 years [news]. **Nature** 1981 Jul 30;292(5822):407
Ford BJ: The van Leeuwenhoek specimens. **Notes Rec R Soc Lond** 1981;36(1):37–59
Ford BJ: Bacteria and cells of human origin on van Leeuwenhoek's sections of 16741,2. **Trans Am Microsc Soc** 1982 Jan;101(1):1–9
Ford BJ: Correlated optical and electron microscopy of Leeuwenhoek's elder-pith sections. **J Microsc** 1982 Nov;128 Pt 2:211–3
Ford BJ: Cytological examination of Leeuwenhoek's first microbial specimens. **Tissue Cell** 1982;14(2):207–17
Ford BJ: Found – van Leeuwenhoek's original specimens. **New Sci** 1981;91:301
Fournier M: 'Ontdeckte onsightbaarheden'. **Spiegel Hist** 1982;17(2):612–8
Houtzager HL: Antonie van Leeuwenhoek. **Eur J Obstet Gynecol Reprod Biol** 1983 Jul;15(3):199–203
Kremer J: The significance of Antoni van Leeuwenhoek for the early development of andrology. **Andrologia** 1979;11:243–9
López-Ochoterena E: La décima octava carta de Leeuwenhoek. (Delft en Holanda, 9 octubre, 1676). **An Soc Mex Hist Cienc Tec** 1979;5:85–90
Lukács D: Háromszázötven éve született Antony van Leeuwenhoek. **Orv Hetil** 1982 Oct 31;123(44):2732–7
Luyendijk-Elshout AM: Antoni van Leeuwenhoek (1632–1723) herdacht. **Ned Tijdschr Geneeskd** 1983 Jun 18;127(25):1111–2
Mikx F: A. van Leeuwenhoek's microscopes: upside down? **Lancet** 1983 Jun 18;1(8338):1387–8
Mikx F: Antoni van Leeuwenhoek--300 sodina oralne mikrobiologije. **Acta Stomatol Croat** 1983;17(4):323–5
Mikx FH: Het tandplaque-onderzoek van Antoni van Leeuwenhoek in 1683. **Ned Tijdschr Tandheelkd** 1983 Sep;90(9):421–4
Palm LC: Van Leeuwenhoek en Swammerdam cartesiaanse microscopisten. **Spiegel Hist** 1979;14(4):223–9
Palm LC, Snelders HA, ed: Antoni van Leeuwenhoek, 1632–1723. Studies on the life and work of the Delft scientist commemorating the 350th anniversary of his birthday. Amsterdam, Rodopi, 1982. 209 p. (Nieuwe Nederlandse Bijdragen tot de Geschiedenis der Geneeskunde en der Natuurwetenschappen, no. 8). Contributions by W. H. van Seters, B. C. Damsteegt, J. van Zuylen, P. Bass, J. E. van Bronswijk, G. A. Lindeboom, P. Smit, K. van Berkel.
Roger J: Two scientific discoveries: their genesis and destiny. In M. D. Grmek, R. S. Cohen, G. Cimino, ed: On scientific discovery. The Erice Lectures 1977. Dordrecht, D. Reidel, 1981. p. 229–37. (Boston Studies in the Philosophy of Science, v. 34).
Ruestow EG: Images and ideas: Leeuwenhoek's perception of the spermatozoa. **J Hist Biol** 1983 Summer;16(2):185–224
Tal M: Periodontal disease and oral hygiene. Described by Antoni van Leeuwenhoek. **J Periodontol** 1980 Nov;51(11):668–9
Van Zuylen J: The microscopes of Antoni van Leeuwenhoek. **J Microsc** 1981 Mar;121(pt 3):309–28
Zuylen J van: On the microscopes of Antoni van Leeuwenhoek. **Janus** 1981;68:159–98

**Lefèvre, Amédée, 1798–1869**
Niaussat P: Les 'coliques sèches' dans la Marine au XIXe siècle: Amédée Lefevre et son combat contre une tenace erreur médicale. In: Congrès National des Sociétés Savantes, 104e, Bordeaux, 1979. Comptes Rendus. Paris, 1979. Section des Sciences, Fasc. IV. p. 183–91.
Valentin M, Niaussat PM: Le rôle fondamental d'Amédée Lefèvre, médecin de la Marine (1798–1869), en médecine du travail et en histoire de la médecine. **Hist Sci Med** 1979;13(4):407–17

**Léger de la Grange, Jean, 1663–ca. 1736**
Lee D: Jean Léger de la Grange. In Dictionary of Canadian biography, 1701 to 1740. Volume 2, 1969. p. 387–8.

**Lehmann, Fritz Erich, 1902–1970**
Bairati A: Ultrastructure of the protoplasm. The 'pioneer' work by A. Bairati and F. E. Lehmann revisited. **J Submicrosc Cytol** 1981 Apr;13(2):117–25

**Lehmann, Jörgen**
Comroe JH: Pay dirt: the story of streptomycin. Part II. Feldman and Hinshaw; Lehmann. **Am Rev Respir Dis** 1978 May;117(5):957–68

**Leibniz, Gottfried Wilhelm von, 1646–1716**
Rudolph G: Les relations entre Denis Papin (1647–1714) et Leibniz (1646–1716). In: Congrès National des Sociétés Savantes, 93e, Tours, 1968. Comptes Rendus. Paris, 1971. Sections des Sciences, Tome II. p. 55–68.
Van der Star P, ed: Fahrenheit's letters to Leibniz and Boerhaave. Amsterdam, Rodopi, 1983. 195 p. (Nieuwe Nederlandse bijdragen tot de geschiedenis der geneeskunde en der natuurwetenschappen, no. 10).

**Leibowitz, Joshua O., 1895–**
Kottek S, Wilk D: Professor Joshua O. Leibowitz; jubilee of his medico-historical activity. **Koroth** 1983 Aug;8(7–8):233–55

**Leiper, Robert Thomson, 1881–1969**
Shortt HE: Robert Thomson Leiper. In Dictionary of national biography, 1961–1970. Suppl. 8, 1981. p. 647–8.

**Leipoldt, Christian Frederik Louis, 1880–1947**
Gilder SS: Leipoldt the editor. **S Afr Med J** 1980 Dec 6;58(23):926–32
Louw JH: Leipoldt the paediatrician. **S Afr Med J** 1980 Dec 6;58(23):915–20
Sandler EM: C. Louis Leipoldt--medical student extraordinary. **Adler Mus Bull** 1981 Oct;7(3):8–14
Shields P: Leipoldt the physician. **S Afr Med J** 1980;58:932–3
Villiers JC de: Leipoldt as geneesheer. **S Afr Med J** 1980 Dec 6;58(23):921–5

**Lelli, Ercole, 1702–1766**
Armoroli M, ed: Le cere anatomiche Bolognesi del settecento. Catalogo della mostra organizzata Settembre–Novembre 1981. Bologna, Università degli Studi di Bologna, Accademia delle Scienze, 1981. 97 p. Contributions by R. A. Bernabeo, L. Bonuzzi, F. Ruggeri.

**Lemnius, Levinus, 1505–1568**
Hoorn CM van: Willem Lemnius [William Lemnius]. **Spiegel Hist** 1980:15(2):111–4

**Lemon, Henry Martyn, 1915–**
Lemon HM: My specialty: oncology. **Nebr Med J** 1979 Aug;64(8):259

**Lenard, Philipp, 1862–1947**
Fischmann E: Retracing Röntgen's discovery. **Diagn Imaging** 1979;48(5):294–303
Kraft E, Finby N: Röntgen's discovery of X-ray and Lenard's priority claim; award of first Nobel Prize in physics in 1901. **NY State J Med** 1980 Sep;80(10):1623–5

**Lencsés György, Váradi, 1530–1593**
Fazekas A: Lencsés György és az elsö magyar nyelvü kéziratos orvosi könyv 1577-böl. **Egeszsegneveles** 1982;23:79–81

**LeNeil, Raynard N., 1908–**
Hodge GP: The drawings of Raynard N. LeNeil. **J Biocommun** 1983 Mar;10(1):24–9

**Lengyel, Dániel, 1815–1884**
Szállási A: Arany János tanártársa Lengyel Dániel doktor. **Orv Hetil** 1983 Apr 3;124(14):833–4

**Lenin, Vladimir Il'ich, 1870–1924**
Akhapkin IA, ed: Leninskie dekrety po zdravookhraneniiu. Moskva, Meditsina, 1980. 510 p.
Asratian EA, Shingarov GKh: Leninskaia teoriia otrazheniia i uchenie I. P. Pavlova o vyssheĭ nervnoĭ deiatel'nosti (k 110-i godovshchine so dnia rozhdeniia V. I. Lenina). **Zh Vyssh Nerv Deiat** 1980 Mar–Apr;30(2):227–34
Bazhan TA: K. Marks ob okhrane zdorov'ia rabochego klassa. **Gig Sanit** 1984 Feb;(2):37–40
Belitskaia EIa: V. I. Lenin on voprosakh narodnonaseleniia. **Sov Zdravookhr** 1980;(4):8–10
Bogoliubov VM: V. I. Lenin i razvitie sanatorno-kurortnogo dela v SSSR. **Vopr Kurortol Fizioter Lech Fiz Kult** 1980 Mar–Apr;(2):1–3
Bokeriia LA: Leninskie dekrety v oblasti zdravookhraneniia. **Anesteziol Reanimatol** 1980 Mar–Apr;(2):3–5
Burenkov SP: Torzhestvo leninskikh ideĭ v zdrakhookhranenii. **Sov Zdravookhr** 1980;(11):3–8
Chechenkina OI: Progress zdravookhraneniia c respublikakh Sredneĭ Azii i Kazakhstane - rezul'tat Leninskoĭ natsional'noĭ politiki. **Sov Zdravookhr** 1982;(11):49–51
Cherkasov SV: Leninskoe uchenie ob istine i probleme kriterii praktiki v diagnostike. **Ter Arkh** 1980;52(7):146–40
Cherkasov SV: Leninskoe uchenie ob istine i problema kriteriia praktiki v diagnostike. **Klin Khir** 1980 Jun;(6):1–6
Chikin SIa: Leninskie printsipy okhrany narodnogo zdorov'ia. **Vestn Akad Med Nauk SSSR** 1980;(4):3–9
Evdokimov PP: Lechashchie vrachi sem'i I.N. Ul'ianova. **Sov Zdravookhr** 1980;(11):64–5
Hudzenko PM: Vtilennia ideĭ V. I. Lenina u spravu okhorony zdorov'ia baterynstva i dyttnstva. **Pediatr Akush Ginekol** 1980 Mar–Apr;(2):3–7
Ivaniushkin AIa: Lenin--kul'tura--meditsina. **Farmakol Toksikol** 1980 May–Jun;43(3):261–5
Krotkov FG: Lenin i sovetskoe zdravookhranenie. **Gig Sanit** 1980 Apr;(4):3–5
Kuznetsov DN, Tikhonov AF: V. I. Lenin i sovetskaia meditsina. **Vestn Khir** 1980 Apr;124(4):3–8
Leninskaia zabota o blage naroda: **Vopr Onkol** 1980;26(4):3–9
Leninskie printsipy v rabote oftal'mologov: **Vestn Oftalmol** 1980 May–Jun;(3):3–5
Levit AZ, Vankhanen NV: V. I. Lenin o sotsial'nykh aspektakh narodnogo pitaniia. **Gig Sanit** 1981 Jan;(1):37–9
Lisitsyn IuP: V. I. Lenin i sovremennye voprosy sotsial'noĭ gigieny. **Zdravookhr Ross Fed** 1980;(4):3–9
Löther R, ed: Philosophische Schriften von Marx, Engels und Lenin und ihre Bedeutung für die Medizin heute. Jena, Fischer, 1979. 127 p. Contributions by U. Körner, I. Löther, P. W. Ruff, R. Stach, G. Straass.
Müller-Dietz HE: Utländska läkare vid Lenins sjukbädd. **Sydsven Medicinhist Sallsk Arsskr** 1984;21:141–56
Novikova ECh: V. I. Lenin i deti. **Vopr Okhr Materin Det** 1980 Apr;25(4):3–7
Petrov BD: Bor'ba s tuberkulezom v SSR, provodimaia v sootvetstvii s ideiami V. I. Lenina. **Probl Tuberk** 1980 Apr;(4):3–6
Poliak VE: Voprosy okhrany zdorov'ia naroda v trudakh V. I. Lenina. **Feldsher Akush** 1980;45(4):5–7
Pomper P: Nečaev, Lenin and Stalin: the psychology of leadership. **Jahrb Gesch Osteur** 1978;26(1):11–30
Portulov BM: Torzhestvo ideĭ V. I. Lenina v meditsine. **Sov Med** 1980;(4):3–9
Potulov BM: Leninskie zavety meditsinskim rabotnikam. **Voen Med Zh** 1980 Jan;(1):11–4
Potulov BM: Leninskaia zabota o zdorov'e naroda. **Sov Zdravookhr** 1980;(3):3–8
Potulov BM: Voprosy bor'by s épidemiiami v trudakh V. I. Lenina. **Zh Mikrobiol Epidemiol Immunobiol** 1980 Apr;(4):3–9
Potulov BM: V. I. Lenin and public health. **Sante Publique (Bucur)** 1981;24(1):3–12
Potulov BM: V. I. Lenin o sotsial'noĭ obuslovlennosti zdorov'ia i zdravookhraneniia. **Sov Zdravookhr** 1984;(4):3–10
Potulov VM: [V. I. Lenin's concern for the health of the soldiers]. (Rus) **Voen Med Zh** 1979 Dec;(12):7–10
Raskin BV: Razrabotka V. I. Leninym programmnykh zadach partii v oblasti zdravookhraneniia. **Zdravookhr Ross Fed** 1980;(4):9–13
Réti E: Lenin, a modern egészségpolitika úttöröje. **Orvostort Kozl** 85(24 No 3):77–84, 1978
Rezanov II: Raboty sanitarnykh vracheĭ v trudakh V. I. Lenina. **Gig Tr Prof Zabol** 1983 Feb;(2):41–3
Romanenko AE: V.I. Lenin i zdravookhranenie Sovetskoĭ Ukrainy. **Vrach Delo** 1980 Mar;(3):1–7
Serdiuk AM: Leninskim putem k novym sversheniiam. **Vrach Delo** 1980 Apr;(4):1–7
Shingarov Gkh: Teoreticheskie nasledie V. I. Lenina i nekotorye metodologicheskie problemy sovremennoĭ meditsiny. **Vestn Akad Med Nauk SSSR** 1980;(4):9–16
Smolenskiĭ VS, Tarasov KE: Znachenie leninskogo ucheniia o dialekticheskoĭ vzaimosviazi ob'ektivnogo i sub'ektivnogo v oschchushcheniiakh dlia diagnostiki. **Klin Med (Mosk)** 1980 Sep;58(9):3–6
Tarasenko NIu: Gigiena truda i okhrana zdorov'ia trudiashchikhsia v rabotakh V. I. Lenina. **Gig Tr Prof Zabol** 1982 Apr;(4):1–3
Ternovoĭ KS: V. I. Lenin i okhrana zdorov'ia naroda. **Klin Khir** 1980 Apr;(4):1–7
Torzhestvo leninskikh ideĭ: **Voen Med Zh** 1980 Apr;(4):3–12
Tsaregorodtsev GI, Anokhin AM: V. I Lenin i problemy okhrany zdorov'ia cheloveka v razvitom sotsialisticheskom obshchestve. **Ter Arkh** 1980;52(4):3–7
V. I. Lenin or razvitii fizicheskoĭ kul'tury i sporta: **Voen Med Zh** 1980 Mar;(3):8–10
Vorontsova EI, Moĭkin IuV: V. I Lenin o profilakticheskom napravlenii sovetskogo zdravookhraneniia (k 110-ĭ godovshchine so dnia rozhdeniia Vladimira Il'icha Lenina). **Gig Tr Prof Zabol** 1980 Apr;(4):1–4
Zuev AI, Sergienko VI: V. I. Lenin--organizator sovetskogo zdravookhraneniia. **Zh Ushn Nos Gorl Bolezn** 1980 Jan–Feb;1:1–6

**Lennander, Karl Gustaf, 1857–1908**
Thorén L: K. G. Lennander och kirurgien i Uppsala kring sekelskiftet. **Nord Medicinhist Arsb** 1984;:153–64

**Lentini Diaz, José**
Lentini J, Taure Gómez C, Leveroni J: Conmemoración de un cincuentenario. In International Congress of the History of Medicine, 27th, Barcelona, 1980. Actas. Barcelona, Académia de Ciències Médiques de Catalunya i Balears, 1981. p. 564–9.

**Lentulo, Henri, 1889–1981**
Amadeo EM: Recordando a un maestro de la odontología internacional y pionero de la endodoncia: Henry Lentulo 1889–1981. **Rev Asoc Odontol Argent** 1983 Sep;71(5):150–2
Verchere L: Henri Lentulo, inventeur du bourre-pâte, 1889–1981. **Rev Odontostomatol (Paris)** 1981 Mar–Apr;10(2):175–7

**Lenz, Fritz, 1887–**
Rissom R: Fritz Lenz und die Rassenhygiene. Husum, Matthiesen, 1983. 143 p. (Abhandlungen zur Geschichte der Medizin und der Naturwissenschaften, 47).

**Leon, R. Jehuda Messer, fl. 1470**
Carpi D: R. Yehuda Messer Lion vepe'ulato kerofe. **Michael Hist Jews Diaspora** 1972;1:277–301

**Leonardo da Vinci, 1452–1519**
Aaron PG, Clouse RG: Freud's psychohistory of Leonardo de Vinci: A matter of being right or left. **J Interdiscip Hist** 1982;13(1):1–16
Axdorph S: Den första 'röntgenblicken' – en studie av Leonardo da Vincis anatomiska bilder. **Lakartidningen** 1983 Dec 21;80(51):5005–8
Baur O, Bott B, Braunfels-Esche S, et al: Leonardo da Vinci Anatomie, Physiognomik, Proportion und Bewegung. Köln, 1984. 343 p. (Kölner medizinhistorische Beiträge: Arbeiten der Forschungsstelle des Instituts für Geschichte der Medizin der Universität zu Köln, Band 23/1)
Belloni L: Zur Deutung zweier pathologischer Stellen (eine mit Zeichnung) aus der Anatomie von Leonardo: Lungenechinococcus, Halslymphdrüsenverkalkung. **Gesnerus** 1980;37(1/2):139–44
DiGeronimo EM, Marraccini P: Body-mind sculpture: battle of the titans. **Plast Reconstr Surg** 1984 Feb;73(2):324–5
Gribanov ED, Sgibova LI: Leonardo da Vinchi kak anatom. **Feldsher Akush** 1982;47(7):43–6
Guggenheim YK: Leonardo da Vinci's views on nutrition. **Koroth** 1981;8(1–2):31–9
Heitz R: Leonardo da Vinci did not invent contact lenses. **CLAO J** 1983 Oct–Dec;9(4):313–6
Iwai H, Morimoto I: Reonarudo to kaibo. Leonardo anatomy. Tokyo, Iwasaki Bijutsusha, 1977. 171 p.
Ladendorf H: Leonardo da Vinci und die Wissenschaften: eine Literaturübersicht. Köln, 1984. 190 p. (Kölner medizinhistorische Beiträge: Arbeiten der Forschungsstelle des Instituts für Geschichte der Medizin der Universität zu Köln, Band 23/2)
Leibowitz JO: Early accounts in geriatric pathology (Leonardo, Harvey, James Keill). **Koroth** 1980 Jun;7(11–12):CCLIII–CCLXIV
Lines D: 15th century ureteric reflux. **Lancet** 1982 Dec 25;2(8313):1473
Pedretti C, Keele K, ed al., ed: Leonardo da Vinci: disegni anatomici dalla Biblioteca Reale di Windsor. Firenze, Barbèra, 1979. 159 p.
Sabin JA, Sanmartín Urchaga P: Estudio comparado de las aportaciones iconográficas, en el sistema muscular, en las obras de Leonardo y Vesalio. In International Congress of the History of Medicine, 27th, Barcelona, 1980. Actas. Barcelona, Académia de Ciències Mèdiques de Catalunya i Balears, 1981. p. 446–53.
Schott GD: Some neurological observations on Leonardo da Vinci's handwriting. **J Neurol Sci** 1979 Aug;42(3):321–9
Todd EM: The neuroanatomy of Leonardo Da Vinci. Ph.D. Diss., University of California, Los Angeles, 1981 xviii, 267 leaves.
Todd EM: The neuroanatomy of Leonardo da Vinci. Santa Barbara, Capra Press, 1983. 189 p.
Woodruff AW: J M W Turner and some of his predecessors and successors, from the viewpoint of medical history. **J R Soc Med** 1980 May;73(5):381–92

**Leonardov, Boris Konstantinovich, 1892–1939**
Leonov IT: Vydaiushchiĭsia organizator meditsinskoĭ sluzhby i voenno-meditsinskogo obrazovaniia (k 90-letiiu so dnia rozhdeniia B. K. Leonardova). **Sov Zdravookhr** 1982;(9):60–2

**Leoniceno, Niccolò, 1428–1524**
Mugnai Carrara D: Fra causalità astrologica e causalità naturale. Gli interventi di Nicolò Leoniceno e della sua scuola sul morbo gallico. **Physis** 1979;21(1–4):37–54

**Leopardi, Giacomo, 1798–1837**
Giulio L: Un tema ricorrente nello Zibaldone: la memoria. **Stor Crit Psicol** 1982 Jun;3(1):27–40

**Leopold, Duke of Albany, 1853–1884**
Whitfield AG: The scholar prince. **J R Coll Physicians Lond** 1984 Jul;18(3):195–7

**Leopoldina, Empress of Brazil, 1797–1826**
Cunha Rodrigues MR da: A morte da Imperatriz Leopoldina (11-XII-1826). **Rev Hist (Brazil)** 1971;43(88):345–52

**Lerche, Martin**
Mayr T: Martin Lerche--in memoriam. **Zentralbl Veterinarmed [A]** 1981;28(1):1–17

**Leriche, René, 1879–1955**
Paul U. Das chirurgische Erbe. René Leriche. **Zentralbl Chir** 1983;108(18):1177–80
Rutkow IM, Rutkow BG, Ernst CB: Letters of William Halsted and René Leriche: 'Our friendship seems so deep'. **Surgery** 1980 Dec;88(6):806–25

**Lermontov, Mikhail Iur'evich, 1814–1841**
Goscilo H: Lermontov's debt to Lavater and Gall. **Slav East Eur Rev** 1981;59(4):500–15
Katsnel'bogen AG: Doktor N. V. Maĭer i dekabristy. **Sov Zdravookhr** 1980;(8):59–62
Konovalov II: A. S. Pushkin i M. Iu. Lermontov na Kavkazskikh Mineral'nykh Vodakh (k 200-letiiu Piatigorska). **Vopr Kurortol Fizioter Lech Fiz Kult** 1980 Sep–Oct;(5):68–70

**Leshaft, Petr Frantsevich, 1837–1909**
Shabunin AV: P. F. Lesgaft i razvitie fel'dshersko-akusherskogo obrazovaniia v Rossii. **Feldsher Akush** 1981;46(4):57–8
Shabunin AV: P. F. Lesgaft, 1837–1909. Moskva, Meditsina, 1982. 75 p.

**Leskov, Nikolaĭ Semenovich, 1831–1895**
Arkhangel'skiĭ GV: N. S. Leskov o problemakh zdravookhraneniia (k 150-letiiu so dnia rozhdeniia pisatelia). **Sov Zdravookhr** 1981;(10):63–5
Arkhangel'skiĭ GV: Vrachi meditsina v tvorchestve N. S. Leskova (k 150-letiiu so dnia rozhdeniia pisatelia). **Klin Med (Mosk)** 1981;59(10):114–7
Morogues IM de: N. S. Leskov: premieres polemiques. janvier 1860–mai 1862. **Cah Monde Russe Sovietique** 1982;23(2):243–55

**Lesky, Erna, 1911–**
Ganzinger K, Skopec M, Wyklicky H, ed: Festschrift für Erna Lesky zum 70. Geburtstag. Wien, Brüder Hollinek, 1981. 212 p.
Risse GB: Erna Lesky and the history of medicine. **Bull Hist Med** 1981 Winter;55(4):575–80
Verzeichnis der wissenschaftlichen Arbeiten von Erna Lesky: In Ganzinger K, Skopec M, Wyklicky H, ed: Festschrift für Erna Lesky zum 70. Geburtstag. Wien, Brüder Hollinek, 1981. p. 193–203.

**Leśniewska, Antonina, 1866–1937**
Roeske W: Antonina Leśniewska, 1866-1937. [Warszawa], Zarzad Główny Polskiego Towarzystwa Farmaceutycznego, 1970. 26 p.

**L'Esperance, Elsie Stang, 1878?–1959**
Dwork D: Elsie Strang L'Esperance. In: Notable American women. The modern period. Cambridge, Mass., Belknap-Harvard Univ. Press, 1980. 4:417–9.

**Lessing, Gotthold Ephraim, 1729–1781**
Leibowitz JO: The final illness of Gotthold Ephraim Lessing. **Janus** 1980;67(1–2–3):21–30

**Lett, Hugh, 1876–1964**
Moore AM: Sir Hugh Lett. In Dictionary of national biography, 1961–1970. Suppl. 8. 1981. p. 650–1.

**Letterman, Jonathan, 1824–1872**
Joy RJ: Jonathan Letterman of Jefferson: medical director of the Army of the Potomac. In Medical-Science colloquium. Special edition of Topic: a journal of the liberal arts. Washington, Pennsylvania, Washington and Jefferson College, 1983. p. 26–38.

**Lettsom, John Coakley, 1744–1815**
James DG: John Coakley Lettsom's Welsh connexions. In J. Cule, ed: Wales and medicine. London, British Society for the History of Medicine, 1975. p. 190–95.
Jones FA: Presidential address. Lettsom, food and fibre. **Trans Med Soc Lond** 1977–78;94:1–14
Marcovich A: Concerning the continuity between the image of society and the image of the human body – an examination of the work of the English physician, J. C. Lettsom (1746–1815). In P. Wright, A. Treacher, ed: The problem of medical knowledge. Examining the social construction of medicine. Edinburgh, Edinburgh University Press, 1982. p. 69–86.

**Leulier, Albert, 1883–1957**
Kalis F: Albert Leulier (1883–1957): a l'occasion du centenaire de sa naissance. Thèse, Univ. Claude-Bernard-Lyon I, U.E.R. de Pharm., 1983. 98 leaves.

**Leuthold, Alfred, 1901–1982**
Fankhauser F: Prof. Dr. Alfred Leuthold, Bern, 1901–1982. **Schweiz Arch Tierheilkd** 1982 Sep;124(9):473–8

**Lev, Adol'f Aronovich, 1923?–**
Vorob'ev VI, Krolenko SA, Rumiantsev PP, et al: Adol'f Aronovich Lev (k 60-letiiu so dnia rozhdeniia). **Tsitologiia** 1983 Jul;25(7):852–9

**Levaditi, Constantin, 1874–1953**
Iftimovici R: Constantin Levaditi, a forerunner of the modern research and interpretation of virus multiplication. **Virologie** 1979 Jul–Sep;30(3):237–42

**Leveuf, Jacques, 1885–1948**
Monod-Broca P: Jacques Leveuf (1885–1948). **Chirurgie** 1980 Jan;106(1):18–25

**Lévi-Strauss, Claude, 1908–**
Gras VW: Myth and the reconciliation of opposites: Jung and Lévi-Strauss. **J Hist Ideas** 1981 Jul Sep;42(3):471 88
Pace D: Claude Lévi-Strauss, the bearer of ashes. Boston, Routledge & Kegan Paul, 1983. x, 263 p.

**Levine, Lena, 1963–1965**
Gordon L: Lena Levine. In: Notable American women. The modern period. Cambridge, Mass., Belknap-Harvard Univ. Press, 1980. 4:419–20.

**Levit, Vladimir Semenovich, 1883–**
Aleksanian IV, Knopov MSh: Vladimir Semenovich Levit (k 100-letiiu so dnia rozhdeniia). **Voen Med Zh** 1983 Jun;6:72–3
Aleksanian IV, Knopov MSh: Vidnyĭ sovetskiĭ khirurg V. S. Levit (k 110-letiiu so dnia rozhdeniia). **Klin Khir** 1983 Jun;6:58–60
Maiat VS: Vladimir Semenovich Levit (K 100-letiiu so dnia rozhdeniia). **Khirurgiia (Mosk)** 1983 Jun;6:111–3

**Levitskiĭ, Grigorii Andreevich, 1873–1943**
Prokof'eva-Bel'govskaia AA: [G. A. Levitskiĭ and Soviet research on chromosome morphology.] (Rus). **Istor Biol Issled** 1978;7:46–64

**Levret, André, 1703–1780**
Dumont M: André Levret et la 'fièvre de lait'. **Nouv Presse Med** 1981 Mar 14;70(12):935–6
Rihner F: André Levert zum 200. Todestag. **MMW** 1980;122:1163–4

**Lévy-Bruhl, Lucien, 1857–1939**
Golliet P, Binet JL: Deux historiens du sang, ou Réponse de Lucien Lévy-Bruhl et de Wifredo Lam à Jean Bernard. **Nouv Rev Fr Hematol** 1983;25(5):337–41

**Lewes, George Henry, 1817–1878**
Bell S: George Henry Lewes: a man of his time. **J Hist Biol** 1981 Fall;14(2):278–98

**Lewicki, Józef, 1882–1942**
Stembrowicz W: Tłumaczenie z jezyka łacińskiego pracy na stopień doktora medycyny z 1829 roku Józefa Lewickiego o osłuchiwaniu i opukiwaniu. **Arch Hist Med (Warsz)** 1984;47(1):49–74

**Lewis, Aubrey Julian, 1900–**
Marley E: Sir Aubrey Lewis: the golden age of a career. **J Psychiatr Res** 1982–83;17(1):93–9
Shepherd M: From social medicine to social psychiatry: the achievement of Sir Aubrey Lewis. **Psychol Med** 1980 May;10(2):211–8
Taylor FK: Sir Aubrey Lewis: Inquiries in Psychiatry; The State of Psychiatry; The Later Papers of Sir Aubrey Lewis. **Br J Psychiatry** 1983 Jul;143:89–93

**Lewis, Dioclesian, 1823–1886**
Wosh PJ: Sound minds and unsound bodies: Massachusetts schools and mandatory physical training. **N Engl Q** 1982;55(1):39–60

**Lewis, Howard Bishop, 1887–1954**
Brandt P: The Howard Bishop Lewis papers. **Surv Sources Newsl** 1976 Dec;4:5–7

**Lewis, John, 1834–**
Colp R: Charles Darwin's coffin, and its maker. **J Hist Med Allied Sci** 1980 Jan;35(1):59–74

**Lewis, Meriwether, 1774–1809**
Kushner HI: The suicide of Meriwether Lewis: a psychoanalytic inquiry. **William Mary Q** 1981;38(3):464–81

**Lewis, Stephen Johnson, 1882–1951**
Dummett CO: Stephen Johnson Lewis and his contributions to American dentistry. **Bull Hist Dent** 1981;29(1):15–23

**Lewis, Thomas, 1881–1945**
Burchell H: Sir Thomas Lewis: his impact on American cardiology. **Br Heart J** 1981 Jul;46(1):1–4
Callahan JA, Key JD, Keys TE: Sir Thomas Lewis: the centennial of a medical human dynamo. **Mayo Clin Proc** 1981 Dec;56(12):749–52
Himsworth H: Thomas Lewis and the development of support for clinical research. **Pharos** 1982 Spring;45(2):15–9
Hollman A: Thomas Lewis--the early years. **Br Heart J** 1981 Sep;46(3):233–44
Hollman A: Sir Thomas Lewis (1881–1945). In J. Cule, ed: Wales and medicine. London, British Society for the History of Medicine, 1975. p. 203–7.
James TN: Sir Thomas Lewis redivivus: from pebbles in a quiet pond to autonomic storms. **Br Heart J** 1984 Jul;52(1):1–23
Rosenbaum MB: Sir Thomas Lewis: a view from the south. **Br Heart J** 1981 Oct;46(4):349–50
Rosol Z: Známý anglický kardiolog Thomas Lewis se narodil před 100 lety. **Vnitr Lek** 1982 Mar;28(3):297–9
Shapiro E: The first textbook of electrocardiography. Thomas Lewis: Clinical Electrocardiography. **J Am Coll Cardiol** 1983 Apr;1(4):1160–1
Sir Thomas Lewis centenary stamp: **Lancet** 1981;ii:378
Snellen HA: Thomas Lewis (1881–1945) and cardiology in Europe. **Br Heart J** 1981 Aug;46(2):121–5
Taylor RC: Thomas Lewis and clinical research. **Br Med J** 1981;282:1976

**Lewkowicz, Ksawery, 1869–1958**
Marzec M: Ksawery Lewkowicz (1869–1958) wybitny pediatra i bakteriolog. **Wiad Lek** 1982 Aug 15;35(13):845–7

**Leydig, Franz von, 1821–1908**
Ober WB, Sciagura C: Leydig, Sertoli, and Reinke: three anatomists who were on the ball. **Pathol Annu** 1981;16 Pt 1:1–13

**Li Ching Chün, 1912–**
Spiess EB: Ching Chun Li, courageous scholar of population on genetics, human genetics, and biostatistics: a living history essay. **Am J Med Genet** 1983 Dec;16(4):603–30

**Li, Shih-chen, 1518–1593**
Li Z: [On Li Shizhen's contributions to the method of systematization of Chinese herbology] (Chi). **Chung Hua I Shih Tsa Chih** 1984 Jan;14(1):35–9

**Liautard, Alexandre François, 1835–1918**
De Wailly P, Crawford LM: The life of Alexandre Liautard. **Hist Med Vet** 1978;3(2):47–9

**Lichtenberg, Alexander von, 1880–1980**
Pérez Castro E: Antologia urologica: Profesor Alexander von Lichtenberg (1880–1980). **Arch Esp Urol** 1980 Nov-Dec;33(6):529–38

**Lichtenberg, Georg Christoph, 1742–1799**
Eulner HH: Zur Geschichte der Meeresheilkunde: Georg Christoph Lichtenberg und das Seebad Cuxhaven. **Medizinhist J** 1982;17(1/2):115–28
Grupe G: Die Identifikation des Skelettes von Georg Christoph Lichtenberg. **Anthropol Anz** 1984 Mar;42(1):1–9

**Lichtenthaeler, Charles, 1915–**
Pfohl G: Medizin und Philologie--Allgemeine humanistische Bildung als Anliegen des Schweizer Medizinhistorikers Charles Lichtenthaeler. **Med Welt** 1980 Nov 7;31(45):1651

**Lichtenthal, Peter, 1780–1853**
Bugyi B: Lichtenthal Péter, egy elfelejtett nagy magyar orvos-zenetudós.

**Liebermeister, Carl, 1833–1901**
Baumberger HR: Carl Liebermeister 1833–1901. Zürich, Juris, 1980. 181 p (Zürcher Medizingeschichtliche Abhandlungen, Neue Reihe, 137).
Wiegand W: Die Antipyretikatherapie bei Carl Liebermeister. Diss. Bonn, 1981. 96 p.

**Liebig, Justus von, 1803–1873**
Brock WH: Liebigiana: old and new perspectives. **Hist Sci** 1981 Sep;19(45 pt 3):201–18
Forbes EG: Liebig in Grossbritannien. **Nachrichtenbl Dtsch Ges Gesch Med Naturwiss Tech** 1983 Winter;33(3):115–33
Götz W: Die Bedeutung Johann Bartholomäus Trommsdorffs für die Entwicklung der Chemie in Deutschland zu Beginn des 19. Jahrhunderts. Ein Versuch anhand seiner Korrespondenz mit Justus von Liebig und Heinrich Emanuel Merck. In Dilg P, et al., ed: Perspektiven der Pharmaziegeschichte. Graz, Austria, Akademische Druck- u. Verlagsanstalt, 1983. p. 97–112.
Habacher M: Auf der suche nach dem 'Od'; Karl Ludwig Freiherr von Reichenbach (1788–1869) und Karl Wilhelm Mayrhofer (1806–1853), zwei Verbündete contra Justus von Liebig. **Clio Med** 1980 May;14(2):105–18
Hall VM: The role of force or power in Liebig's physiological chemistry. **Med Hist** 1980 Jan;24(1):20–59

**Liebling, Friedrich, 1893–1982**
Hug H, ed: Friedrich Liebling, 1893–1982, zum Gedenken: Gedenkfeier vom 28. März 1982. Zürich, Verlag Psychologische Menschenkenntnis, 1983. 140 p.

**Liebow, Averill Abraham**
Smith GJ: Averill Abraham Liebow: contributions to pulmonary pathology. **Yale J Biol Med** 1981 Mar–Apr;54(2):139–46

**Liepmann, Wilhelm, 1875 or 8–1939**
Schneck P: Wilhelm Liepmann (1878–1939) und die soziale Gynäkologie im Spiegel der Aktenbestände des Archivs der Humboldt-Universität zu Berlin. **NTM** 1980;17(2):102–20
Schneck P: Wilhelm Liepmann (1878–1939)--ein Gynäkologenschicksal zwischen Kaiserreich und faschistischer Diktatur. **Zentralbl Gynakol** 1984;106(17):1223–8

**Liesching, Friedrich Ludwig**
Spohr OH: Dr. Med. Friedrich Ludwig Liesching. **Q Bull S Afr Libr** 1968;23(2):45–55

**Liétard, Gustave Alexandre, 1833–1904**
Allan NM: Gustave Alexandre Liétard, orientalist and physician. **Med Hist** 1981 Jan;25(1):85–8

**Lilienfeld, Abraham M., 1920–1984**
Gordis L: Symposium in honor of Abraham M. Lilienfeld. Chronic disease epidemiology at the threshold of a new decade. **Am J Epidemiol** 1980 Aug;112(2):169–77
Hannaway C: Abraham M. Lilienfeld (1920–1984). **Bull Hist Med** 1984 Winter;58(4):558–9
Winkelstein W: A tribute to Abe Lilienfeld. **Am J Epidemiol** 1980 Aug;112(2):178–84

**Lilland, Harvey, 1856–1925**
Westbrooks B: The troubled legacy of Harvey Lillard: the black experience in chiropractic. **Chiropr Hist** 1982;2(1):47–53

**Lillie, Ralph Dougall, 1896–1979**
Kasten FH: Ralph D. Lillie, 1896–1979. **Stain Technol** 1980 Jul;55(4):201–15
Longley JD: Ralph Dougall Lillie. 1896--1979. **J Histochem Cytochem** 1980 Apr;28(4):291–6

**Lilpop, Wacław, 1884–1949**
Milik JR: W XXX rocznicę śmierci Wacława Lilpopa i założenia polskiego towarzystwa urologicznego. **Wiad Lek** 1979 Nov 1;32(21):1569–71

**Limborgh, Jan van, 1900–1884**
Van der Molen HR: Hommage à Jan ven Limborgh (1900–1984). **Phlebologie** 1984 Jul-Sep;37(3):XXV–XXXI

**Lincke, Harold, d. 1977**
Heinrichs HJ: Harold Linckes Versuch einer Vermittlung von Natur- und Geisteswissenschaften. **Psyche (Stuttg)** 1980 Feb;34(2):152–67

**Lincoln, Abraham, 1809–1865**
Fehrenbacher DE: In quest of the psychohistorical Lincoln. **Rev Am Hist** 1983;11(1):12–9
Isacsson A: A study of Louis J. Weichmann. **Lincoln Her** 1978;80(1):25–38
Lattimer JK: Lincoln did not have the Marfan Syndrome; documented evidence. **NY State J Med** 1981 Nov;81(12):1805–13
Massey EW: Dr. Samuel Mudd: justice at last. **South Med J** 1980 Oct;73(10):1375–6
Miller B: The incident. **Lincoln Her** 1980;82(1):342–3
Read H: 'A hand to hold while dying': Dr. Charles A. Leale at Lincoln's side. **Lincoln Her** 1977;79:21–6

**Lincoln, Robert Todd, 1843–1926**
Carson SL: Presidential children: abandonment, hysteria and suicide. **J Psychohist** 1984 Spring;11(4):533–44

**Lind, James, 1716–1794**
Hughes RE: James Lind and the cure of scurvy: an experimental approach. **Med Hist** 1975 Oct;19(4):342–51
Tröhler U: Towards clinical investigation on a numerical basis: James Lind at Haslar Hospital 1758–1783. In International Congress of the History of Medicine, 27th, Barcelona, 1980. Actas. Barcelona, Académia de Ciències Mèdiques de Catalunya i Balears, 1981. p. 414–9.
Winge M: James Lind Grundlaeggeren af den maritime medicin. **Dan Medicinhist Arbog** 1983;12:9–20

**Lind, Jenny, 1820–1887**
Baron JH: James Lind would not have approved. **Lancet** 1982 Jun 5;1(8284):1313
Schein CJ, Koch E: Jenny Lind's concert in Göttingen. Billroth's letter to his mother. **NY State J Med** 1979 Oct;79(11):1786–1891

**Lindbergh, Charles Augustus, 1902–1974**
Eckert WG: The Lindbergh case. A triumph in forensic investigation. **Am J Forensic Med Pathol** 1980 Jun;1(2):151–3
Logan RD: Charles Lindbergh and the 'right stuff'. **Aviat Space Environ Med** 1982 Jul;53(7):708–11

**Lindeboom, Gerrit Arie, 1905–**
De Moulin D: Gerrit Arie Lindeboom and the history of medicine in the Netherlands. **Janus** 1980;67(1–2–3):1–6

**Lindemann, Erich, 1900–1974**
Lindemann E: Beyond grief: studies in crisis intervention. Ed. by E. B. Lindemann. Biographical introduction by B. S. Brown. New York and London, Aronson, 1979. 274 p.
Satin DG: Erich Lindemann: the humanist and the era of community mental health. **Proc Am Philos Soc** 1982 Aug;126(4):327–46
Satin DG: Erich Lindemann as humanist, scientist, and change agent. **Am J Community Psychol** 1984 Oct;12(5):519–27

**Lindner, S., fl. 1879–**
Macmillan MB: Freud and Lindner on pleasure sucking. **Stor Crit Psicol** 1980;1(1):111–43

**Lindsay, John Ralston, 1898–1981**
Fredrickson JM: Otoneurology. **Ann Otol Rhinol Laryngol [Suppl]** 1983 Jan–Feb;102:17–9
Kohut RI: The clinical research of John Lindsay. **Ann Otol Rhinol Laryngol [Suppl]** 1983 Jan–Feb;102:20–2
Mhoon EE, Lanzl EF, ed: John Ralston Lindsay, MD, 1898–1981. Contributions by H. F. Schuknecht, J. M. Fredrickson, R. I. Kohut, C. Fernandez, R. A. Butler, R. F. Naunton. (Supplement 102). **Ann Otol Rhinol Laryngol [Suppl]** 1983 Jan–Feb;92(1 Pt.3):1–36
Naunton RF: Clinical research in otolaryngology at the University of Chicago. **Ann Otol Rhinol Laryngol [Suppl]** 1983 Jan–Feb;102:30–1
Publications by John R. Lindsay: **Ann Otol Rhinol Laryngol [Suppl]** 1983 Jan–Feb;102:33–6

**Lindsay, William A., 1795–1876**
Carmichael AG: The Lindsay-Stipp debate. **Indiana Med Hist Q** 1981;7(4):6–19
McDonell KM: Surgery in early nineteenth century Indiana. **Indiana Med Hist Q** 1980;6(4):3–23
McDonell KM: Women and medicine in early nineteenth century Indiana. **Indiana Med Hist Q** 1980;6(2):3–23
McDonell KM: Dr. William A. Lindsay, innovator, physician, enterpreneur. **Indiana Med Hist Q** 1980;6(1):5–23
McDonell KM: William A. Lindsay in perspective. **Indiana Hist Soc** 1981 Jun;7(2):3–20
McDonell KM: 'One bold incision': Dr. William A. Lindsay's radical cure. **Indiana Med Hist Q** 1980;6(3):3–23

**Ling, Per Henrik, 1776–1839**
Burius A: Lings gymnastik och homeopatien. **Nord Medicinhist Arsb** 1980;:99–123
Janzon B: Idrott och ling-gymnastik i populär-medicinsk belysning. **Nord Medicinhist Arsb** 1980;:124–35

**Lingner, Karl August, 1861–1916**
Hoffmann-Axthelm W: Karl August Lingner und die soziale Zahnmedizin. **Zahnarztl Mitt** 1983 Sep 16;73(18):1981–2, 1987–9

**Link, Goethe, 1879–**
[Goethe Link. Includes text of two of his talks.]: **Indiana Med Hist Q** 1977;3(4):63–71

**Linné, Carl von, 1707–1778**
Frängsmyr T, ed: Linnaeus. The man and his work. Berkeley, University of California Press, 1983. xii, 203 p. With contributions by S. Lindroth, G. Eriksson, G. Broberg.
Goerke H: Linné und die Pharmacopoea Svecica (1775). In Dilg, P, et al., ed: Perspektiven der Pharmaziegeschichte. Graz, Austria, Akademische Druck- u. Verlagsanstalt, 1983. p. 89–96.
Goerke H: Carl von Linné als Marinearzt (1739–1741). In Göpfert W, Otten HH, ed: Metavoeite: wandelt euch durch neues Denken. Düsseldorf, Triltsch, 1983. p. 89–94.
Larson JL: An alternative science, Linnaean natural history in Germany, 1770–1790. **Janus** 1979;66(4):267–83
Leikola A: Zeus Faber--antiikin tarustoa eläinkunnassa. **Hist Arkisto (Finl)** 1978;(73):110–19
Schramm E: Linné, Gedner und die biologische Kontrolle. **Medizinhist J** 1984;19(3):244–9
Sourander P: Linnaeus and Neurology. **Sven Linnesallskap Arsskr** 1978; Commemorative Volume:88–117
Strandell B: Linné och Stockholm. **Sven Farm Tidskr** 1979;83:677–84
Synek VM: Linnaeus--physician and king of flowers. **NZ Med J** 1984 Apr 25;97(754):267–9

**Lipmann, Fritz Albert, 1899–**
Lipmann F: A long life in times of great upheaval. **Annu Rev Biochem** 1984;53:1–33
Novelli G: Personal recollections to Fritz Lipmann during the early years of coenzyme A research. **Mol Biol Biochem Biophys** 1980;32:415–30
Rasmussen L: En forstander og hans assistent. **Dan Medicinhist Arbog** 1981;:130–40

**Lippay, János, 1606–1666**
Szlatky M: Lippay János Posoni Kertjének orvos-botanikai vonatkozásai (1664–1667). **Orvostort Kozl** 1979;87(25 no 1–2):79–90

**Lipps, Theodor, 1851–1914**
Kanzer M: Freud, Theodor Lipps, and 'scientific psychology'. **Psychoanal Q** 1981;50(3):393–410

**Lipsius, David, fl. 1607–1678**
Poorter DA de: David Lipsius Iscanius, 17e-eeuws doctor medicus afkomstig uit Overijse. **Periodiek** 1980;35:16–22

**Lisitsyn, Mikhail Semenovich, 1891–1961**
Mitrofanov VG: K 90-letiiu so dnia rozhdeniia Mikhaila Semenovicha Lisitsyna. **Vestn Khir** 1983 May;130(5):141–2

**Lister, Joseph Jackson, 1786–1869**
Moran HM: Looking back: Lister. **Lamp** 1981 Mar;38(3):57–60

**Lister, Joseph Lister, 1827–1912**
Gelfand M: Joseph Lister. **Cent Afr J Med** 1981 Feb;27(2):31–4
Landes RR, Hall S: A letter from Joseph Lister to Dr. David Walsh. **JAMA** 1984 Jun 15;251(23):3101–3
Ravitch MM: The danger of stating an opinion or the hazards of going on record. **Surg Gynecol Obstet** 1980 Dec;151(6):810–6
Trease GE: Joseph Lister, 1827–1912. **Br J Pharm Pract** 1981;2(10):34, 36

**Lister, Martin, 1638?–1712**
Keynes G: Dr. Martin Lister. A bibliography. Godalming, Surrey, St. Paul's Bibliographies, 1981. xii, 52 p.

**Liston, Robert, 1794–1847**
Hauben DJ: Robert Liston's life and work in the renaissance of plastic surgery. **Ann Plast Surg** 1983 Jun;10(6):502–9

**Liszt, Franz von, 1811–1886**
Vladimirova LB, Gribanov ED: A nagy magyar zeneszerzo, Liszt Ferenc és az ogyesszai gyermekkórház épületének története (orosz nyelven). **Orvostort Kozl** 1982;28(1–3):169–76

**Little, William John, 1810–1894**
Accardo PJ: Deformity and character. Dr. Little's diagnosis of Richard III. **JAMA** 1980 Dec 19;244(24):2746–7

**Littré, Emile, 1801–1881**
Sournia JC: Littré l'Académie de Médecine. **Bull Acad Natl Med (Paris)** 1981 Oct;165(7):941–7

**Livingstone, David, 1813–1873**
Clendennen GW: Livingstone's second book. **Bibliotheck** 1980;10(1):10–9
McDermott WV: Endorphins, I presume. **Lancet** 1980 Dec 20–27;2(8208–8209):1353

**Lizàrdo, César, 1925–**
Mazzei Uzcátegui M: Cesar Lizardo, bondad y corazon. **Rev Soc Venez Hist Med** 1972–73;20–21(34–35):111–27

**Ljungdahl, Malte, 1882–1957**
Oberg L: Malte Ljungdahl 1882–1957. **Sydsven Medicinhist Sallsk Arsskr** 1983;:59–64

**Lloyd George, David, 1863–1945**
Davies J: David Lloyd George and the National Insurance Act of 1911. In J. Cule, ed: Wales and medicine. London, British Society for the History of Medicine, 1975. p. 1–9.

**Llull, Ramón, 1235?–1316?**
Esteva de Sagrera J: Alquimia seudoluliana y medicina. In Congrés

International d'Història de la Medicina Catalana, 2nd, Barcelona, 1975. Llibre d'Actes. Barcelona, Socitra, 1977. p. 301-3.
Esteva de Sagrera J: Influencia decisiva de la biografía y la filosofía de Ramón Llull en su obra médica. In Congrés International d'Historia de la Medicina Catalana, 2nd, Barcelona, 1975. Llibre d'Actes. Barcelona, Socitra, 1977. p. 305-7.
Esteva de Sagrera J: Aplicación del 'Ars' luliana a la medicina. In Congrés International d'Història de la Medicina Catalana, 2nd, Barcelona, 1975. Llibre d'Actes. Barcelona, Socitra, 1977. p. 295-300.
Patai R: An unknown Hebrew medicl alchemist: a medieval treatise on the quinta essentia. **Med Hist** 1984 Jul;28(3):308-23
Rodríguez-Tejerina JM: El pensamiento medico de Ramon Llull en la epoca de Miramar. **Asclepio** 1978-79,30-31:277-82

**Lobato, Rita, 1867-**
Lobo FB: Duas pioneiras-Madame Dubocher, Rita Lobato. **Rev Inst Hist Geogr Bras** 1980;(328):53-6

**L'Obel, Matthias de, 1538-1616**
Corbett M: The emblematic title-page to Stirpium Adversaria nova by Petro Pena and Mathias de L'Obel (1570). **Arch Nat Hist** 1981 Apr;10(1):111-7
Louis A: Mathieu de L'Obel 1538-1616. Episode de l'histoire de la botanique. Ghent/Louvain, Story-Scientia, 1980. 544 p.

**Lobmayer, Antun, 1844-1906**
Berić B, Babić N: Dr. Antun Lobmayer (1844-1906) pionir savremenog akušerstva i školovanja primalja u Hrvatskoj. **Jugosl Ginekol Opstet** 1979;19(1-2):113-8

**Locke, John, 1632-1704**
Eng E: Locke's Tabula Rasa and Freud's 'Mystic writing pad.' **J Hist Ideas** 1980 Jan-Mar;41(1):133-40
Loehlin JC: John Locke and behavior genetics. **Behav Genet** 1983 Jan;13(1):117-21
Petryszak NG: Tabula rasa--its origins and implications. **J Hist Behav Sci** 1981 Jan;17(1):15-27
Romanell P: The scientific and medical genealogy of Locke's 'historical, plain method'. **Trans Stud Coll Physicians Phila** 1983 Dec;5(5 no 4):339-52
Tomaselli S: The first person: Descartes, Locke and mind-body dualism. **Hist Sci** 1984;22(pt 2):185-205
Torgersen J: Medisineren John Locke og demokratiets ideer. **Samtiden (Norway)** 1970;79(1):29-43
Windstrup G: Locke on suicide. **Polit Theory** 1980;8(2):169-82

**Locock, Charles, 1799-1875**
Maulitz RC: Metropolitan medicine and the man-midwife: the early life and letters of Charles Locock. **Med Hist** 1982 Jan;26(1):25-46

**Loder, C. I., 1753-1836**
Katsnel'bogen AG: Obshchestvenno-meditsinskaia deiatel'nost' Kh. I. Lodera. **Klin Med (Mosk)** 1982 Jun;60(6):117-20

**Loeb, Jacques, 1859-1924**
Pauly PJ: The Loeb-Jennings debate and the science of animal behavior. **J Hist Behav Sci** 1981 Oct;17(4):504-15
Pauly PJ: Jacques Loeb and the control of life: an experimental biologist in Germany and America, 1859-1924. Ph.D. Diss., The Johns Hopkins University. Baltimore, 1981. viii, 311 p.
Weissmann G: Loeb and a Gloria. **Hosp Pract [Off]** 1984 Oct;19(10):65-74

**Loeb, Leo, 1869-1959**
Corner GW: Leo Loeb. In Dictionary of American Biography, Suppl. 6, 1956-1960. p. 385-7, 1980.
Witkowski JA: Experimental pathology and the origins of tissue culture: Leo Loeb's contribution. **Med Hist** 1983 Jul;27(3):269-88

**Loeffler, Friedrich, 1852-1915**
Röhrer H: Friedrich Loeffler. Begründer der medizinischen Virusforschung vor 80 Jahren. **Hist Med Vet** 1979;4(2):46-8

**Loeffler, Friedrich, 1885-1967**
Bethge R, Knöfler EW: 30 Jahre Gesellschaft für Orthopädie der DDR--Zur Erinnerung an ihren Mitbegründer und ersten Vorsitzenden Friedrich Loeffler. **Beitr Orthop Traumatol** 1983 May;30(5):233-6

**Loewe, Walter Siegfried, 1884-1963**
Kattermann R: Walter Siegfried Loewe (1884-1963)). Sein Beitrag zur Analytik, Biologie und Pharmakologie der Sexualhormone. **J Clin Chem Clin Biochem** 1984 Aug;22(8):505-14

**Loewel, Henri, 1795-1856**
Schmitt R: Henri Loewel, chimiste alsacien, élève, collaborateur et ami du savant Angevin Michel-Eugène Chevreul. In: Congrès National des Sociétés Savantes, 93e, Tours, 1968. Comptes Rendus. Paris, 1971. Section des Sciences, Tome II. p. 175-88.

**Loewenthal, Leonard Joseph Alphonse, 1903-1983**
Findlay GH: Alphonse Loewenthal (1903-1983)--the uncrowned king of dermatology in Africa. **S Afr Med J** 1983 Dec 24;64(27):1064-7

**Loewi, Otto, 1873-1961**
Van der Kloot W: Otto Loewi. In Dictionary of American biography, 1961-1965. Suppl. 7, 1981. p. 475-7.

**Löfberg, Otto, 1881-1954**
Lindskog BI: Otto Löfberg 1881-1954. **Sydsven Medicinhist Sallsk Arsskr** 1983;:65-76

**Loff, Romão**
Guerra M: Os primeiros passos na clínica de há 70 anos descritos por Romão Loff. **Acta Med Port** 1983 Jul-Aug;4(7-8):379-80

**Loghem, Johannes Jacobus von, 1878-**
Hollán SR: An appreciation: J. J. van Loghem. **Haematologia (Budap)** 1980;13(1-4):5-22

**Löhlein, Walther, 1882-**
Harms H: Zum 100. Geburtstag von Walther Löhlein. **Klin Monatsbl Augenheilkd** 1983 Jun;182(6):585-90

**Löhr, Wilhelm, 1889-**
Schierhorn H: Egas Moniz, Wilhelm Löhr und die cerebrale Angiographie. Ein Streifzug durch die Entdeckungsgeschichte der Hirngefässe. **J Hirnforsch** 1981;22(5):491-515

**Lombroso, Cesare, 1835-1909**
Caffaratto AT: La raccolta di fotografie segnaletiche del Museo di Antropologia Criminale di Torino: la fotografia come documento e testimonianza dell'opera di Cesare Lombroso. **Ann Osp Maria Vittoria Torino** 1980 Jul-Dec;23(7-12):295-332
Peset JL: Cesare Lombroso y la psiquiatría de su tiempo: el caso U.S.A. In International Congress of the History of Medicine, 27th, Barcelona, 1980. Actas. Barcelona, Acadèmia de Ciències Mèdiques de Catalunya i Balears, 1981. p. 134-9.

**Lominskiĭ, F. I., 1857-**
Kvitnitskiĭ-Ryzhov IuN: Zhizn' i deiatel'nost' ukrainskogo gistologa F. I. Lominskogo (k 125-letiiu so dnia rozhdeniia). **Arkh Anat Gistol Embriol** 1982 Apr;82(4):96-101

**Lomonaco, Tomaso, 1901-**
Lomonaco T: Un medico fra gli aviatori. **Riv Med Aeronaut Spaz** 1980;Suppl:1-176

**Lomonosov, Mikhail Vasil'evich, 1711-1765**
Zabludovskiĭ PE: K 200-letiiu knigi 'Nastavlenie narodu v rassuzhdenii ego zdorov'ia'. **Feldsher Akush** 1982;47(4):52-3

**London, Efim Semenovich, 1869-1939**
Prokhorova MI: E. S. London i funktsional'naia neĭrokhimiia. **Nerv Sist** 1982;23:137-42
Romanova NN: E. S. London's contribution to the problem of DNA structure. **Istor Biol Issled** 1983;9:166-75

**London, Jack, 1876-1916**
Spangler GM: Suicide and social criticism: Durkheim, Dreiser, Wharton, and London. **Am Q** 1979;31(4):496-516

**Long, Crawford Williamson, 1815-1878**
Agris J: Stamps commemorating medicine. 'Dr. Crawford Williamson Long' the father of anesthesia. **J Dermatol Surg Oncol** 1980 May;6(5):415
Crawford WM: More on the ether operation. **N Engl J Med** 1984 Feb 23;310(8):534
Letton AH: Pyramids or Parthenons? **J Surg Oncol** 1983 Jun;23(2):63-9
Nuland SB: The origins of anesthesia: Part III. **Conn Med** 1984 Sep;48(9):597-600

**Long, Esmond Ray, 1890-1979**
Binford Ch: Esmond Ray Long, M.D., Ph. D., 1890-1979, Editor, International Journal of Leprosy, 1964-1968. **Int J Lepr** 1980 Sep;48(3):322-6
Stowell RE: Esmond R. Long, MD, 1890-1979. **Am J Pathol** 1980 Aug;100(2):321-5

**Long, Perrin Hamilton, 1899-1965**
Austrian R: Perrin Hamilton Long. In Dictionary of American biography, 1961-1965. Suppl. 7, 1981. p. 477-8.

**Longcope, Warfield Theobald, 1877-1953**
Harvey AM: Science at the bedside: the story of Warfield Theobald Longcope. **Trans Stud Coll Physicians Phila** 1981 Sep;5(3 no 3):161-73

**Longhi, Pietro, 1702-1785**
Julien P: Sur le célèbre 'dentiste' ou 'pharmacien' de Pietro Longhi. **Pharm Weekbl** 1981 Nov 6;116(45):1389-92
Moskow BS: The iconography of the dental profession. Pietro Longhi (1702-1785). **Quintessence Int** 1984 Jul;15(7):728-9

**Longmore, George, ca. 1758-1811**
Tunis B: George Longmore. In Dictionary of Canadian biography, 1801 to 1820. Volume 5, 1983. p. 501-3.

**Longworth, Alice Roosevelt, 1884-1980**
Carson SL: Presidential children: abandonment, hysteria and suicide. **J Psychohist** 1984 Spring;11(4):533-44

**Lönnrot, Elias, 1802-1884**
Heikkinen R: Lönnrot Kajaanin piirin ja linnan lääkärinä. **Duodecim** 1983;99(23-24):1726-9

**Loomis, Horatio N.**
Drachman VG: The Loomis trial: social mores and obstetrics in the mid-nineteenth century. In Reverby S, Rosner D, ed: Health care in America. Philadelphia, Temple University Press, 1979. p. 67-83.

**Loos, Willem de, 1736-1771**
Snelders HA: De chemische voordrachten van Wille de Loos (circa

1770). **Tijdschr Geschied Geneeskd** 1979;2(4):168–75

**Looser, Emil, 1877–1936**
Kis J: Der Knochenpathologe Emil Looser (1877–1936). Zürich, Juris, 1982. 68 p. Zürcher Medizingeschichtliche Abhandlungen, Neue Reihe, 149; also Diss.).

**López Albo, 1889–1944**
Izquierdo Rojo JM: Wenceslao López Albo. **Arch Neurobiol (Madr)** 1983 Mar–Apr;46(2):131–46

**Lopez de Paz, Michel, 1680–1746?**
Loker Z: Docteur Michel Lopez de Paz, médecin et savant de Saint-Domingue. **Rev Hist Med Heb** 1980 Oct;134(33 no 3):55–7
Loker Z: A Franco-Jewish physician--among the pioneers of medicine and science in Central America (Haiti). **Koroth** 1982 Aug;8(3/4):195–7

**Lorenz, Franz, 1805–1883**
Gerhartl G: Dr. med. Franz Lorenz (1805–1883). **Mitt Krems Stadtarch** 1971;11:107–14

**Lorenz, Konrad Zacharias, 1903–**
Kalikow TJ: Konrad Lorenz's ethological theory: explanation and ideology, 1938–1943. **J Hist Biol** 1983 Spring;16(1):39–73
Rossi L: Il concetto di adattamento nella psicologia evoluzionistica di K. Lorenz e nell'epistemologia genetica di J. Piaget. **Stor Crit Psicol** 1984;5(2):301–17
Weinberger C: Wissenschaftstheoretische Anmerkungen zu Konrad Lorenz' 'Vergleichende Verhaltensforschung'. **Z Allg Wissenschaftstheorie** 1980;10(1):147–61

**Lorenzer, Alfred, 1922–**
Neiss R: Alfred Lorenzer. In J. Rattner, ed: Wandlungen der Psychoanalyse. Wien, Europaverlage, 1980. p. 233–56.

**Lorenzini, Carlo, 1826–1890**
Smith RD: The cricket and the marionette. **South Med J** 1982 Jan;75(1):59–60

**Lorry, Anne Charles, 1726–1783**
Everett MA: Anne-Charles Lorry. The first French dermatologist. **Int J Dermatol** 1979 Nov;18(9):762–4

**Loscos Bernal, Francisco, 1823–1886**
Bueno AG: La flora de Aragon: notas a un proyecto de Francisco Loscos y Jose Pardo. **Bol Soc Esp Hist Farm** 1984;35(137):23–33

**Louis, Antoine, 1723–1792**
Huard P, Imbault-Huart MJ: Les papiers d'Antoine Louis (1723–1792). In: Congrès National des Sociétés Savantes, 102e, Limoges, 1977. Comptes Rendus. Paris, 1977. Section des Sciences, Fasc. III. p. 7–14.

**Louis XI, King of France, 1423–1483**
Aron E: Louis XI et ses guérisseurs. Chambray, C. L. D., [1983]. 197 p.
Vally G: Ludovic cel stăruitor si misterioasa sa moarte. **Mag Istor** 1976;10(10):52–4

**Louis XIII, King of France, 1601–1643**
Bernier JJ, Chevallier P, Teysseire D, et al: La maladie de Louis XIII. Tuberculose intestinale ou maladie de Crohn? **Nouv Presse Med** 1981 Jun 20;10(27):2243, 2247–50
Foisil M: Louis XIII à travers le stethoscope. **Histoire** 1982;42:76–8
Goldfischer S, Janis M: A 42-year-old king with a cavitary pulmonary lesion and intestinal perforation. **Bull NY Acad Med** 1981 Mar;57(2):139–43

**Louis XIV, King of France, 1638–1715**
Bodemer CW: France, the fundament, and the rise of surgery. **Dis Colon Rectum** 1983 Nov;26(11):743–50
David T, Dagen G, Gauval VB: Les dents de Louis XIV. **Soc Fr Hist Art Dent** 1979 Sep–Dec;(5–6):6–10
Gérard A: De la gastro-entérologie à la politique: la fistule du Grand Roi. **LARC Med** 1983 May;3(5):341–8

**Louis XV, King of France, 1710–1774**
Flahaut S: Le pharmacien Charles-Louis Cadet de Gassicourt, bâtard de Louis XV, et sa famille. **Rev Hist Pharm (Paris)** 1980 Mar;27(244):53–61

**Louis XVIII, King of France, 1755–1824**
Hillemand P, Gilbrin E: Le père Elisée (1753–1817); premier chirurgien de Louis XVIII. **Hist Sci Med** 1980;14(2):233–40

**Louw, Jan Hendrik, 1915–**
De Villiers JC, Munnik LA, Luyt R, et al: Jan Hendrik Louw. **S Afr Med J** 1980 Mar;57(16):605–12

**Lovejoy, Esther Pohl, 1870–1967**
Thomson EH: Esther Pohl Lovejoy. In: Notable American women. The modern period. Cambridge, Mass., Belknap-Harvard Univ. Press, 1980. 4:424–6.

**Løvset, Jørgen, 1896–1981**
Bergsjø P, Ulstein M: Jørgen Løvset 1896–1981. **Acta Obstet Gynecol Scand** 1982;61(3):193–4

**Lowe, Ronald Francis**
Hertzberg R: Ronald Francis Lowe. **Aust J Ophthalmol** 1980 May;8(2):109–15

**Lower, Richard, 1631–1691**
Nakamura T: T. Willis' and Lower's physiology with special reference to the theory of heart movement. **Jpn Stud Hist Sci** 1977;16:23–41
Rulliere R, Heymans G, Vial F: La version en langue française (1679) du Tractatus de Corde (1669) de Richard Lower. In International Congress of the History of Medicine, 27th, Barcelona, 1980. Actas. Barcelona, Académia de Ciències Mèdiques de Catalunya i Balears, 1981. p. 331–5.

**Lu Liuliang**
Chu Tinxiang: [A sketch of the life of Lu Liuliang.] (Chi). **Chin J Med Hist** 1981;11:89–90

**Lucas, Prosper, 1808–1885**
Biéder J: Un président de la Société Médico-Psychologique: Prosper Lucas (1808–1885). **Ann Med Psychol (Paris)** 1983 Sep–Oct;141(8):908–15

**Lucia, Saint**
Orłowski WJ: Patronka cierpiacych na oczy. **Klin Oczna** 1984 May;86(5):231–5

**Lucio, Rafael, 1819–1886**
Somolinos-Palencia J: El doctor Rafael Lucio y las artes. **Gac Med Mex** 1980;116(9):422–8

**Lucretius Carus, Titus, ca. 96–55 B.C.**
Phillips JH: Lucretius on the inefficiency of the medical arts: 6.1179 and 6.1226–38. **Classical Philol** 1982;77:233–5

**Ludlow, Abraham, fl. 1764**
Chitwood WR: Ludlow's esophageal diverticulum: a preternatural bag. **Surgery** 1979 May;85(5):549–53

**Ludwig, Karl Friedrich Wilhelm, 1816–1895**
Cranefield PF, ed: Two great scientists of the nineteenth century. Correspondence of Emil Du Bois-Reymond and Carl Ludwig. Collected by Estelle Du Bois-Reymond. Foreword, notes, and indexes by Paul Diepgen. Translation of 1927 German ed. Baltimore, London, Johns Hopkins Univ. Press, 1982. xix, 183 p.

**Luke, Saint**
Dirckx JH: Scientific and medical terms and references in the writings of St. Luke. **Am J Dermatopathol** 1983 Oct;5(5):491–9

**Lukomskiĭ, Pavlov Evgen'evich, 1899–**
Tareev EM: P. E. Lukomskiĭ i stanovlenie sovetskoĭ kardiologii. **Kardiologiia** 1982 Feb;22(2):119–25

**Lumière, Auguste M., 1862–**
Aterman K, Grimaud JA: The brothers Lumière. Pioneers in medical photography. **Am J Dermatopathol** 1983 Oct;5(5):479–81

**Lumière, Louis Jean, 1864–1948**
Aterman K, Grimaud JA: The brothers Lumière. Pioneers in medical photography. **Am J Dermatopathol** 1983 Oct;5(5):479–81

**Lumley, John, 1533–1609**
Robb-Smith AH: The quatercentenary of the Lumleian Lecture. **J R Coll Physicians Lond** 1983 Jan;17(1):74–8

**Lunin, Nikolai Ivanovich, 1853–1937**
Efremov VV: K istorii otkrytiia vitaminov N. I. Luninym. **Vopr Pitan** 1982 May–Jun;(3):68–72

**Lupton, Edward**
Jackson WA: Lupton of Levenshulme. **Pharm Hist (London)** 1977 Jul;7(2):2–4

**Lupu, Nicolae Gheorghe, 1884–1966**
Negru I: Prof. dr. Nicolae Gh. Lupu în lumina autobiografică şi a istoriei medicinii româneşti. **Viata Med [Medii Sanit]** 1983 Feb;31(2):45–7

**Luriia, Aleksandr Romanovich, 1902–1977**
Estévez González A: El cerebro frontal y motor, según Luria. Su patologia, síndromes y afasias. **Arch Neurobiol (Madr)** 1981 Mar–Apr;44(2):75–94
Hatfield FM: Analysis and remediation of aphasia in the U.S.S.R: the contribution of A. R. Luria. **J Speech Hear Disord** 1981 Nov;46(4):338–47
Luria AR: The making of mind. A personal account of Soviet psychology. Edited by M. Cole and S. Cole. Cambridge, London, Harvard University Press, 1979. 234 p.

**Lusardi, Christophe Mathieu, 1778–1853**
Pini UA: Cristoforo Matteo Lusardi oculista giramondo. **Arch Stor Prov Parmensi** 1979;31:271–4

**Luther, Martin, 1483–1546**
Becke U: Eine hinterlassene psychiatrische Studie Paul Johann Reiters über Luther. **Z Kirchengesch** 1979;90(1):85–95
Böhmer W, Kirsten F: Reformatorische Ausstrahlungen Martin Luthers auf das Gesundheitswesen seiner Zeit. **Z Gesamte Inn Med** 1983 Oct 15;38(20):546–51
Gaude W: Zur Krankengeschichte Martin Luthers. **Beitr Gesch Univ Erfurt** 1979–83;19:113–63
Hahn S: Martin Luther--was sagt er uns Ärzten heute? **Z Gesamte Inn Med** 1983 Oct 15;38(20):551–4
Kaiser W: Eisleben und das Mansfelder Land im medizinhistorischen Aspekt. Ein Beitrag zum Lutherjahr 1983. **Z Gesamte Inn Med** 1983 Oct 15;38(20):539–46

Kapronczay K: Magyar medikusok a wittenbergi egyetemen Luther és Melanchton korában. **Orv Hetil** 1984 Apr 15;125(16):958–60

Neuhauser W: Martin Luther bat Freund um Fürbitte bei heftigem Zahnschmerz. **Zahnarztl Mitt** 1983 Nov 1;73(21):2361–3

Ozment S: Luther and the family. **Harv Libr Bull** 1984 Winter;32(1):36–53

Völker A: Martin Luther und seine Arzte. Ein Beitrag zum Lutherjahr 1983. **Z Gesamte Inn Med** 1983 Oct 15;38(20):533–9

**Lux, Jakab, 1822–1876**

Bak M: Lux Jakab dr. (1822–1876) munkássága mai orvosi szemléletünkben. **Orv Hetil** 1984 Apr 29;125(18):1082–4

**Luxemburg, Rosa, 1870–1919**

Mullaney MM: Gender and revolution: Rosa Luxemburg and the female revolutionary personality. **J Psychohist** 1984 Spring;11(4):463–76

**Luzsénszky, Alfonz**

Ismét Luzsénszky Talmudja?: **Orv Hetil** 1984 Aug 19;125(34):2086–7

**Lwoff, André, 1902–**

Zhdanov VM: Andre L'vov protiv D. I. Ivanovskogo. **Vopr Virusol** 1982 Jul–Aug;27(4):499–502

**Ly Yanshi**

Chen Menglai: [Ly Yanshi, life and medical achievements.] (Chi). **Chin J Med Hist** 1981;11:93–4

**Lycett, James, 1811–1883**

Cartwright MF: The filthy state of Cape Town in 1858. **Q Bull S Afr Libr** 1978;33(2):53–6

**Lynen, Feodor, 1911–1979**

Block K: Feodor Lynen: Architekt der klassischen Biochemie. **Max Planck Ges Ber Mitt** 1980;2:21–30

**Lyngdoh, Homiwell, 1877–1958**

Lyngdoh MG: Life and works of Dr. Homiwell Lyngdoh. Shillong, Kyknsai M. Warjrie, 1980. 70 p.

**Lyon, Elias Potter, 1867–1937**

Wangensteen OW, ed: Elias Potter Lyon: Minnesota's leader in medical education. St. Louis, Green, 1981. 292 p. Contributions by J. A. Anderson, E. S. Benson, R. A. Good, J. C. Hinsey, C. H. Hodgson, L. P. Leone, R. J. McCollister, J. A. Myers, L. G. Rigler, H. G. Scheie, D. C. Smith, W. W. Spink, M. B. Visscher, J. H. Westerman, L. G. Wilson.

# M

**Maass, Clara Louise, 1876–1901**

Arvy L: Clara Louise Maass (1876-1901) et la fièvre jaune. **Clio Med** 1979 May;13(3–4):277–82

Tigertt HB, Tigertt WD: Clara Louise Maass: a nurse volunteer for yellow fever inoculations--1901. **Milit Med** 1983 Mar;148(3):252–3

**Macallum, Archibald Byron, 1858–1934**

Neelin JM: Archibald Byron Macallum, pioneer of biochemistry in Canada. **Can J Biochem Cell Biol** 1984 Jun;62(6):viii–xi

**McAlmont, John J., 1821–1896**

Clark RB: John J. McAlmont, M.D. 1821–1896. **J Arkansas Med Soc** 1984 Apr;80(11):552

**MacArthur, Douglas, 1880–1964**

Askew M: The health of General Douglas MacArthur. **Practitioner** 1982 Oct;226(1372):1814–5

**MacArthur, William Porter, 1884–1964**

Boyd J: Sir William Porter MacArthur. In Dictionary of national biography, 1961–1970. Suppl. 8, 1981. p. 688–9.

**MacBride, Ernest William, 1866–1940**

Bowler PJ: E. W. MacBride's Lamarckian eugenics and its implications for the social construction of scientific knowledge. **Ann Sci** 1984 May;41(3):245–60

**McBride, John Adam, 1843?–1889**

Smith RN: D. J. A. McBride, MRCVS, 1843?–1889, itinerant professor extraordinary. **Vet Hist** 1981 N.Ser;2(1):3–25

**McCarthy, Daniel Joseph, 1874–1958**

Powell RC: Daniel Joseph McCarthy. In Dictionary of American Biography, Suppl. 6, 1956–1960. p. 402–4, 1980.

**McCaw, James Brown, 1823–1906**

Cullen JP: Chimborazo Hospital: 'That charnal house of living sufferers.' **Civ War Times Illus** 1981;19(9):36–42

**McClintock, Barbara, 1902–**

Keller EF: A feeling for the organism: the life and work of Barbara McClintock. New York, Freeman, 1983. xix, 235 p.

Lengeler J: Barbara McClintock und die Entdeckung der beweglichen Gene. **MMW** 1983 Nov 25;125(47):1095–7

Norrby E: Den medicinska betydelsen av rörliga strukturer i arvsmassan. **Lakartidningen** 1983 Oct 19;80(42):3911–3

Ringertz NR: Upptäckt av 'hoppande gener' hos majs gav 81–årig kvinna hela medicinpriset Barbara McClintock--en unik medicinsk nobelpristagare. **Lakartidningen** 1983 Oct 19;80(42):3908–10

**McCollum, Elmer Verner, 1879–1967**

Bing FC, Prebluda HJ: E. V. McCollum: pathfinder in nutrition investigations and world agriculture. **Agric Hist** 1980;54(1):157–66

Davis DR: Some legacies of nutrition pioneer E. V. McCollum. **Trans Kans Acad Sci** 1979 Aug;82(3):133–45

Day HG, Prebluda HJ: E. V. McCollum: 'lamplighter' in public and professional understanding of nutrition. **Agric Hist** 1980 Jan;54(1):149–56

Day HG: E. V. McCollum and dietitians in nutrition education. **J Am Diet Assoc** 1980 Feb;76(2):126–7

Harper AE: McCollum and directions in the evaluation of protein quality. **J Agric Food Chem** 1981 May–Jun;29(3):429–35

Herriott RM: Life and contributions of Elmer V. McCollum. **Fed Proc** 1980 Aug;39(10):2713–5

Mayer J: The impact of Elmer Verner McCollum on national and global nutritional problems. **Trans Kans Acad Sci** 1982 Aug;85(3):142–51

**MacCormac, William, 1836–1901**

Fraser I: Sir William MacCormac and his times. **Ann R Coll Surg Engl** 1983 Sep;65(5):339–46

**McCormick, Katharine Dexter, 1875–1967**

Reed J: Katharine Dexter McCormick. In: Notable American women. The modern period. Cambridge, Mass., Belknap–Harvard Univ. Press, 1980. 4:440–2.

**McCormick, Richard**

Cahill LS: Within shouting distance: Paul Ramsey and Richard McCormick on method. **J Med Philos** 1979 Dec;4(4):398–417

**McCormick, Robert, 1800–1890**

Johnson RE: Robert McCormick. In Dictionary of Canadian biography, 1881–1890. 1982;11:543–4.

**McCouch, Grayson Prevost, 1888–1979**

Starr I: Concerning Dr. Grayson Prevost McCouch with recollections of the earlier days of physiology in Philadelphia. **Neurol Res** 1983;5(1):1–17

**McCrae, John, 1872–1918**

Prescott JF: The extensive medical writings of soldier-poet John McCrae. **Can Med Assoc J** 1980 Jan 12;122(1):110,113–4

**Macculloch, John, 1773–1835**

Flinn D: John Macculloch, M.D., F.R.S., and his geological map of Scotland: his years in the Ordnance. 1795–1826. **Notes Rec R Soc Lond** 1981;36(1):83–101

**MacDonald, Mary, 1869–1933**

Greenland C, Griffin JD: The Honorable Mary Macdonald: a lesson in attitude. **Can Med Assoc J** 1981 Aug 1;125(3):305–8

O'Carrigan C: Two veteran nurses of World War I days (Sister Mary MacDonald, Sister Mary Vianney). **Med J Aust** 1984 Jun 23;140(13):782–4

**McDonough, David**

Murray AE: Bright delusion: Presbyterians and African colonization. **J Presbyt Hist** 1980;58(3):224–37

**McDowell, Ephraim, 1771–1830**

Agris J: Stamps commemorating medicine: 'Ephraim McDowell' (1771–1830). **J Dermatol Surg Oncol** 1980 Aug;6(8):621

Bernhard CM: Dr. Ephraim McDowell: father of abdominal surgery. **Am Surg** 1980 Jan;46(1):1–5

Graham SD: Ephraim McDowell (1771–1830). The President's lithotomist. **Invest Urol** 1981 Nov;19(3):216–7

Mumey N: Ephraim McDowell, 1771–1830: a frontiersman who advanced the art of surgery. **Denver West Roundup** 1979 Jul–Aug;35:3–20

**McElvain, Samuel Marion, 1897–1973**

Stork G: Samuel Marion McElvain: December 9, 1897–April 11, 1973. **Biogr Mem Natl Acad Sci** 1983;54:221–48

**Macewen, William, 1848–1924**

Brandt L, Pokar H, Schütte H: 100 Jahre Intubationsnarkose. William Macewen, ein Pionier der endotrachealen Intubation. **Anaesthesist** 1983 May;32(5):200–4

Peltier LF: The classic. The growth of bone. Chapter III. Osteogenic power of bone bereft of periosteum. William Macewen, F.R.S. **Clin Orthop** 1983 Apr;(174):5–14

**McGavran, Edward G., 1902–1972**

Barr HH, Barrie FH: Edward G. McGavran: guardian of the body politic. Chapel Hill, School of Public Health, Univ. of North Carolina at Chapel Hill, 1979. xii, 177 p.

**McGavran, Mary Theodora, 1869–1923**

Kaiser RM, Chaff SL, Peitzman SJ: A Philadelphia medical student of the 1890's: the diary of Mary Theodora McGavran **Pa Mag Hist Biogr** 1984 Apr;108(2):217–36

**McGill, Samuel Ford**

Campbell P: Medical education for an African colonist. **Md Hist Mag** 1970;65(2):130–7

**McGuire, Hunter Holmes, 1835–**

Hassler WW: Dr. Hunter Holmes McGuire: surgeon to Stonewall Jackson, the Confederacy, and the Nation. **Va Cavalcade**

1982;32(2):52-61

**Mach, Ernst, 1838-1916**
Henn V: E. Mach on the analysis of motion sensation. **Hum Neurobiol** 1984;3(3):145-8
Kaiser W: Ernst Mach und das Mechanismusproblem in der Biologie. **Medizinhist J** 1982;17(3):179-94

**McHale, Kathryn, 1889-1956**
Susskind JL: Kathryn McHale. In Dictionary of American Biography, Suppl. 6, 1956-1960. p. 412-13, 1980.

**Machalski, Jacek, 1926-1979**
Müldner-Nieckowski P: Dr. Jacek Machalski (2.VI.1926--3.X.1979). **Arch Hist Med (Warsz)** 1980;43(2):117-20

**Macht, David Israel, 1882-1961**
Wilk D: David Israel Macht (1882-1961). **Koroth** 1983 Aug;8(7-8):305-17

**McIntire, Ross, 1889-1959**
Stewart WJ: Ross McIntire. In Dictionary of American Biography, Suppl. 6, 1956-1960. p. 413-14, 1980.

**McIntosh, James Higgins, 1866-1944**
Donald AG: James Higgins Mcintosh, M.D.: an archetype for the family practitioner? **J SC Med Assoc** 1980 May;76(5):245-8

**Mack, Theophilus, 1820-1881**
Godfrey CM: Theophilus Mack. In Dictionary of Canadian Biography, 1881-1890. 1982;11:558-9.

**MacKee, George Miller, 1878-1955**
Pascher F: George Miller MacKee (1878-1955): a memoir. **J Am Acad Dermatol** 1983 Jul;9(1):168-72

**MacKenna, Robert Merttins Bird, 1903-**
MacKenna RM: Robert M. B. MacKenna. **J Am Acad Dermatol** 1982 Jan;6(1):135-44

**MacKenzie, Henry, 1745-1831**
Gilman SL: Den Geisteskranken sehen: Mackenzie, Kleist, William James. **Confin Psychiatr** 1979;22(3):127-44

**Mackenzie, James, 1853-1925**
McCormick JS: James Mackenzie and coronary heart disease. **J R Coll Gen Pract** 1981 Jan;31(222):26-30
McMichael J: Sir James Mackenzie and atrial fibrillation--a new perspective. **J R Coll Gen Pract** 1981 Jul;31(228):402-6
Phillips WR: Sir James Mackenzie and family medicine. **Am Fam Physician** 1981 Jul;23(7):46, 50

**McKenzie, Kenneth George, 1892-**
Botterell EH: Kenneth George McKenzie, M.D., F.R.C.S., 1923-1963. **Surg Neurol** 1982 Feb;17(2):81-9

**Mackenzie, Morell, 1837-1892**
Chalat NI: Sir Morell Mackenzie revisited. **Laryngoscope** 1984 Oct;94(10):1307-10
Lin JI: Virchow's pathological reports on Frederick III's cancer. **N Engl J Med** 1984 Nov 8;311(19):1261-4

**McKenzie, Robert Tait, 1867-1938**
Martin D: Dr. Robert Tait McKenzie: Canada's renaissance man. **Can Med Assoc J** 1984 Sep 1;131(5):493-6

**Mackerras, Ian Murray**
Spratt DM: Dr Ian Murray Mackerras. **Int J Parasitol** 1980 Nov-Dec;10(5-6):329-36

**McKie, Douglas, 1896-1967**
Hartley H: Douglas McKie. In Dictionary of national biography, 1961-1970. Suppl. 8, 1981. p. 695-7.

**Mackieson, John, 1795-1885**
Rogers IL: John Mackieson. In Dictionary of Canadian biography, 1881-1890. 1982;11:565-6.

**McKinley, William, 1843-1901**
Adler S: The operation on President McKinley. In Plesur M, ed.: An American Historian: essays to honor Selig Adler (Buffalo: State U. of N.Y., 1980): 37-49.

**McKinney, Susan Smith, 1847-1918**
Alexander LL: Early medical heroes: Susan Smith McKinney-Steward, M.D., 1847-1918. **Crisis** 1980;87(1):21-3

**Mackintosh, James Macalister, 1891-1966**
Brotherston JH: James Macalister Mackintosh. In Dictionary of national biography, 1961-1970. Suppl. 8, 1981. p. 698-9.

**Macklin, Madge Thurlow, 1893-1962**
Mehler B: Madge Thurlow Macklin. In: Notable American women. The modern period. Cambridge, Mass., Belknap-Harvard Univ. Press, 1980. 4:451-2.

**McLean, Mary Hancock, 1861-1930**
Hunt M: Woman's place in medicine: the career of Dr. Mary Hancock McLean. **Bull Mo Hist Soc** 1980;36(4):255-63

**MacLean, Paul D., 1906-**
Holden C: Paul MacLean and the triune brain. **Science** 1979 Jun 8;204(4397):1066-8

**Macleane, Laughlin, 1728?-1777**
Cordasco F: Laughlin Macleane's Expediency of Inoculation (1756): a checklist of deposit locations. **Am Notes Queries** 1981 Jan-Feb;19(5/6):75

**MacLeod, Colin Munro, 1909-1972**
McDermott W: Colin Munro MacLeod: January 28, 1909-February 11, 1972. **Biogr Mem Natl Acad Sci** 1983;54:183-219

**McLetchie, James Leslie, 1909-1965**
Hackett CJ: McLetchie on mass campaigns. **Trop Doct** 1982 Jan;12(1):35-8

**McLoughlin, John, 1784-1857**
Agris J: 'John McLoughlin' physician, pioneer, fur trader, settler. **J Dermatol Surg Oncol** 1979 Oct;5(10):760
Raines JR: Dr. John McLoughlin. **JAMA** 1982 Mar 19;247(11):1566-7

**McMichael, John, 1904-**
Thirty years of drugs for hypertension: a festschrift for Sir John McMichael: **Br J Clin Pharmacol** 1982 Jan;13(1):5-142

**MacNalty, Arthur Salusbury, 1880-1969**
Godber GE: Sir Arthur Salusbury MacNalty. In Dictionary of national biography, 1961-1970. Suppl. 8, 1981. p. 706-7.

**McNaughton, Daniel, 1813-1865**
Brody M: Trial of Daniel M'Naghten. Insanity defense, and its well-kept secret. **NY State J Med** 1982 Mar;82(3):381-6
Rollin HR: Crime and mental disorder. Daniel McNaughton, a case in point. **Med Leg J** 1982;50(Pt 3):102-13

**McNeil, Charles, 1881-1964**
Tait HP: The McNeil Library and some of its notable volumes. **Univ Edinb J** 1980;29:313-7

**MacNutt, Joseph Scott, 1885-**
Clean water and the health of the cities: New York, Arno, 1977. Various paginations. Facsimile reprints of works by William T. Sedgwick (1893), George C. Whipple (1907), and J. Scott MacNutt (1910).

**Macphail, Andrew, 1864-1938**
Shortt SE: Andrew Macphail: the ideal in nature. In his The search for an ideal: six Canadian intellectuals and their convictions in an age of transition, 1890-1930. Toronto, Buffalo, University of Toronto Press, 1976. p. 12-38.

**Macura, Jiří, d. 1979**
Selected bibliography of Dr. J. Macura: **Folia Microbiol (Praha)** 1980;25(2):81-5

**Maddox, Ernest Edmund, 1860-1933**
Morgan MW: The Maddox classification of vergence eye movements. **Am J Optom Physiol Opt** 1980;57:537-9

**Madison, James, 1751-1836**
McCoy DR: Jefferson and Madison on Malthus: population growth in Jeffersonian political economy. **Va Mag Hist Biogr** 1980;88(3):259-76

**Madsen, Thorvald Johannes Marius, 1870-1957**
Parnas J: Thorvald Madsen 1870-1957. Leader in international public health. **Dan Med Bull** 1981;28(2):82-6

**Maerlant, Jacob van, 1235?-1300**
Vandewiele LJ: Stenen in de Farmacie in de Leer bij Jacob van Maerlant. In Dilg P, et al., ed: Perspektiven der Pharmaziegeschichte. Graz, Austria, Akademische Druck- u. Verlagsanstalt, 1983. p. 419-30.

**Magajna, Bogomir, 1904-1963**
Jan Z: Biografija Bogomira Magajne. **Goriski Letnik** 1979;6:491-502

**Magalhaes, Francisco Bento**
Costa C: Prehistoria de la cátedra de histología de la Universidad de Chile (1872-1881). Parte I. El affaire Magalhaes. **Rev Med Chil** 1980 Apr;108(4):367-73

**Magati, Cesare, 1579-1647**
Kapronczay K: Cesare Magati (1579-1647). **Orv Hetil** 1980 Feb 10;121(6):343-5

**Magendie, François, 1783-1855**
Bonnemain H: François Magendie et ses perspectives pharmacologiques. **Hist Sci Med** 1983;17(4):333-43
Breathnach CS: Biographical sketches No. 34--Magendie. **Ir Med J** 1983 Nov;76(11):471
Dillemann G: L'éloge de Magendie par Claude Bernard. **Hist Sci Med** 1983;17(4):345-9
Gallistel CR: Bell, Magendie, and the proposals to restrict the use of animals in neurobehavioral research. **Am Psychol** 1981 Apr;36(4):357-60
Kenéz J: Forradalmi átalakulás a medicinában a XIX. század elején. **Orv Hetil** 1984 May 27;125(22):1330-3
Laporte Y: La sensibilité récurrente des racines rachidiennes antérieures. **Hist Sci Med** 1983;17(4):351-5
Lazorthes G, Campan L: François Magendie (1783-1855). **Bull Acad Natl Med (Paris)** 1984 Jan-Feb;168(1-2):105-11
Legée G: La place de Magendie dans la physiologie expérimentale du système nerveux. **Hist Sci Med** 1983;17(4):357-66
Lichtenthaeler C: Die sechs Leitgedanken von Magendies

medizinischer Revolution. **Z Arztl Fortbild (Jena)** 1983;77(18):785-8
Théodoridès J: Magendie et la pathologie infectieuse. **Hist Sci Med** 1983;17(4):367-80
Vial F, Rullière R: François Magendie. **Hist Sci Med** 1983;17(4):323-32

**Magill, Ivan Whiteside, 1888-**
Thomas KB: Sir Ivan Whiteside Magill, KCVO, DSc, MB, BCh, BAO, FRCS, FFARCS, (Hon), FFARCSI (Hon), DA. A review of his publications and other references to his life and work. **Anaesthesia** 1978 Jul-Aug;33(7):628-34

**Magil'nitskii, S. G.**
Magil'nitskiĭ SG: Oftal'mologi-revoliutsionery. **Vestn Oftalmol** 1983 Nov-Dec;(6):72-5

**Magitot, Emile, 1843-1897**
Geiser E: Emile Magitot (1834-1897)--ein Lebensbild. **Schweiz Monatsschr Zahnmed** 1984 Sep;94(9):813-20

**Magrath, George Burgess, 1870-1938**
Tedeschi LG: George Burgess Magrath. Tribute to a resting lion. **Am J Forensic Med Pathol** 1980 Jun;1(2):169-72

**Al-Magusi, Ali ibn al-Abbas**
Gewargis AA: Gynäkologisches aus dem Kamil as-Sina a At Tibbiya des Ali ibn Al-Abbas Al-Magusi. Die Abschnitte über Anatomie, Pathologie und konservative Therapie des nichtschwangeren Uterus. Diss. Erlangen-Nürnberg, 1980. 153 p.
Kahle E: Al-Magusi (Haly Abbas) über Kinderkrankheiten im Kamil as-sina'a at-tibbiya. Erlangen, Verlagsbuchhandlung Hannelore Lüling, 1980. 61, [6] p.

**Mahler, Gustav, 1860-1911**
Alonso HO: La enfermedad cardíaca de Gustav Mahler. **Medicina (B Aires)** 1981;41(3):373-7
Collins DT: Gustav Mahler's summer of 1910. **Bull Menninger Clin** 1982 May;46(3):255-79

**Mahoney, John Friend, 1889-1957**
Kennedy JW: Introduction of penicillin in syphilotherapy. **Ariz Med** 1982 Nov;39(11):730, 735
Price DE: John Friend Mahoney. In Dictionary of American Biography, Suppl. 6, 1956-1960. p; 423-4, 1980.

**Maiakovskiĭ, Vladimir Vladimirovich, 1894-1930**
Mozhaev VP: Sanitarnye biulleteni o V. V. Maiakovskom. **Feldsher Akush** 1983 Dec;48(12):36-8

**Maĭer, Nikolai Vasil'evich, 1806-1846**
Katsnel'bogen AG: Doktor N. V. Maĭer i dekabristy. **Sov Zdravookhr** 1980;(8):59-62

**Maillot, François-Clément, 1804-1894**
Larcan A: Le médecin inspecteur F. C. Maillot. In: Congrès National des Sociétés Savantes, 103e, Nancy, 1978. Comptes Rendus. Paris, 1978. Section des Sciences, Fasc. V. p. 19-30.

**Maisonabe, Charles Auguste, 1779-1851**
Izac R: Du Rouergue en Moldavie; note sur Charles Maisonabe (1779-1851). **Hist Sci Med** 1979;13(4):451-8

**Maixner, Emerich, 1847-1920**
Petrásek J, Adamec J: Prof. MUDr. Emerich Maixner 1847--1920, významná osobnost počátku českého vnitřního lékařství. **Cas Lek Cesk** 1980 Jun 13;119(23-24):684-6

**Al-Majusi, d. 994**
Hamarneh SK: Majusi's observations and instructions on medicine and public health. **Hamdard** 1980 Jan-Mar;23(1):3-35

**Maklakov, Aleksei Nikolaevich, 1837-1895**
Krasnikov PG: Vydaiushcheesia izobretenie otechestvennogo oftal'mologa (100 let so vremeni sozdaniia applanatsionnogo tonometra Prof. A.N. Maklakova). **Vestn Oftalmol** 1984 Nov-Dec;(6):70-2

**Makluire, Johne, fl. 1630**
McHarg JF: Dr. Johne Makluire and the 1630 attempt to establish the College. In Passmore R, ed: Proceedings of the Royal College of Physicians of Edinburgh Tercentenary Congress, 1981. Edinburgh, Royal College of Physicians of Edinburgh, 1982. p. 44-58.

**Maksimovich-Ambodik, Nestor, 1744-1812**
Borodiĭ NK: K biografii N. M. Maksimovicha-Ambodika. **Akush Ginekol (Mosk)** 1982;(8):60-1
Dmitriev VG: 'Nauka o babich'em dele' i ee avtor. (N. Maksimovich-Ambodik). **Feldsher Akush** 1984 Feb;49(2):50-1

**Malgaigne, Joseph François, 1806-1865**
Peltier LF: Joseph François Malgaigne and Malgaigne's fracture. **Clin Orthop** 1980 Sep;(151):4-7
Peltier LF: Guerin versus Malgaigne: a precedent for the free criticism of scientific papers. **J Orthop Res** 1983;1(1):115-8

**Malinowski, Bronislaw-Kasper, 1884-1942**
Stocking GW: Contradicting the doctor: Billy Hancock and the problem of baloma. **Hist Anthropol Newsl** 1977;4(1):4-7

**Mallinatha, 15th cent.**
Rama Rao B: References to Ayurveda in the commentaries of Mallinatha. **Bull Indian Inst Hist Med (Hyderabad)** 1979;9:13-20

**Maloët, Pierre Louis Marie, 1730-1810**
[Pigalle's bust of Dr. Maloët acquired by Fitzwilliam Museum, Cambridge, 1979.]: **Burlington Mag** 1980 Jan;122:83

**Malpighi, Marcello, 1628-1694**
Belloni L: Il Morgagni tra il Malpighi e il Cotugno. **Gesnerus** 1982;39(2):195-213
Bendiner E: Marcello Malpighi: a life of passionate exploration. **Hosp Pract** 1980 Jul;15(7):109-36
Busacchi V: Marcello Malpighi (1628-1694), lettore a Bologna, Pisa e Messina, archiatra pontificio. **Strenna Stor Bolognese** 1978;28:81-98
Saraf PG, Cockett AT: Marcello Malpighi--a tribute. **Urology** 1984 Jun;23(6):619-23
Solberg WU: Cotton Mather's indebtedness to Marcello Malpighi. **J Hist Med Allied Sci** 1981 Jul;36(3):326-31

**Malthus, Thomas Robert, 1766-1834**
Berlan JP: The world food problem: Malthus, Marx and their epigones. **Mon Rev** 1980;31(10):20-32
Berntsen B: Fra Malthus til befolkningsåret 1974. **Samtiden (Norway)** 1973;82(4):232-9
Coleman W: Medicine against Malthus: François Mélier on the relation between subsistence and mortality (1843). **Bull Hist Med** 1980 Spring;54(1):23-42
Dupâquier J: Avez-vous lu Malthus? **Population** 1980;35(2):279-90
Dupâquier J, Fauve-Chamoux A, Grebenik E, ed: Malthus past and present. London; New York, Academic Press, 1983. xix, 416 p. Contributions by A. Béjin, Y. Breton, Y. Charbit, L. Devance, A. Digby, M. W. Flinn, R. E. Frisch, M. Godelier, L. Gordon, P. Guillaume, G. Heinsohn, T. H. Hollingsworth, P. A. Jewell, N. Keyfitz, R. Keynes, H. Le Bras, M. Perrot, F. Rausky, M. Rebérioux, R. Remond, F. Ronsin, G. R. Searle, B. Stapleton, O. Steiger, P. Vallin, E. Van de Walle, A. Waterman, J. Wolff, E. A. Wrigley, V. Wynne-Edwards.
Isenburg T: Il dibattito su Malthus e sulla popolazione nell'Italia di fine '800. **Studi Stor** 1977;18(3):41-67
James P: Population Malthus, his life and times. London, Routledge and Kegan Paul, 1979. xv, 524 p.
Llombart V: Anotaciones a la introducción del 'ensayo sobre la población de Malthus en España. **Moneda Credito** 1973;126:79-86
McCoy DR: Jefferson and Madison on Malthus: population growth in Jeffersonian political economy. **Va Mag Hist Biogr** 1980;88(3):259-76
Oguse, D: 'Socialisme et néo-malthusianisme', la Revue Socialiste, t. XLVI, juillet-décembre 1907, p. 27-124. **Ann Demogr Hist (Paris)** 1983;:371-89
Petersen W: Malthus. Cambridge, Mass. Harvard University Press, 1979. vi, 302 p.
Santurri EN: Theodicy and social policy in Malthus' thought. **J Hist Ideas** 1982 Apr-Jun;43(2):315-30
Talmor E, ed: Malthus our contemporary. Contributions by K. W. Back, A. J. Field, L. Murard, P. Zylberman. **Hist Eur Ideas** 1983;4:121-214

**Malvern, Godfrey Martin Huggins, 1883-1971**
Gann LH, Gelfand M: Huggins of Rhodesia. London, Allen & Unwin [1964]. 285 p.

**Manasein, Viacheslav Avksent'evich, 1841-1901**
Estrin GB: Voprosy khirurgii i travmatologii v zhurnale 'Vrach' V. A. Manasseina (1880-1901 gg.). **Vestn Khir** 1981 Oct;127(10):142-4

**Mandryka, P. V., 1884-**
Kapitanenko AM: Talantlivyĭ organizator, iskusnyĭ khirurg (k 100-letiiu so dnia rozhdeniia P. V. Mandryki). **Sov Zdravookhr** 1984;(10):58-60

**Mangold, Hilde, 1898-1924**
Hamburger V: Hilde Mangold, co-discoverer of the organizer. **J Hist Biol** 1984 Spring;17(1):1-11

**Mann, Horace, 1796-1859**
Wosh PJ: Sound minds and unsound bodies: Massachusetts schools and mandatory physical training. **N Engl Q** 1982;55(1):39-60

**Mann, Thomas, 1875-1955**
Finck J: Thomas Mann et la psychanalyse. Précédé de Thomas Mann et l' irrationnel par J-M Palmier. Paris, Société d'Edition 'Les Belles Lettres', 1982. 216 p. (Confluents Psychanalytiques).
Klein P: Die Infektionskrankheit im erzählerischen Werk Thomas Manns. **Medizinhist J** 1980;15(1/2):3-15
Montiel L: El escritor y su enfermedad: patobiografía de Thomas Mann. In International Congress of the History of Medicine, 27th, Barcelona, 1980. Actas. Barcelona, Académia de Ciències Mèdiques de Catalunya i Balears, 1981. p. 586-91.
Montiel L: Freud y el psicoanálisis en dos conferencias de Thomas Mann. In International Congress of the History of Medicine, 27th, Barcelona, 1980. Actas. Barcelona, Académia de Ciències Mèdiques de Catalunya i Balears, 1981. p. 111-5.
Montiel L: El psicoanálisis en la Montaña mágica. In International Congress of the History of Medicine, 27th, Barcelona, 1980. Actas. Barcelona, Académia de Ciències Mèdiques de Catalunya i Balears, 1981. p. 116-20.
Montiel Llorente LE: La ciencia medica en 'La montaña magica' de Thomas Mann. **Asclepio** 1980;32:271-85
Saueressig H: Die Tuberkulose als Paradigma des Lebensgefühls.

**Med Welt** 1982 Mar 26;33(12):428-34
Scherg C: Literatur als Lebenshilfe. Am Beispiel Thomas Manns. **Psyche (Stuttg)** 1982 Jul;36(7):630-61

**Mannagetta, Johann Wilhelm, 1588-1666**
Beck-Mannagetta P: Zum 300. Todestag des Johann Wilhelm Ritter von Mannagetta und seinem Wirken in Niederösterreich. **Unsere Heimat** 1966;37(4-6):125-9

**Mannerheim, Sophie, 1863-1928**
Tallberg M: Sophie Mannerheim: en historisk beskrivning och analys av hennes verksamhet 1904-1928. **Vard Nord Utveckl Forsk** 1983 Spring;3(4):123-30

**Manning, Frederick Norton, 1839-1903**
Edwards GA: Causation of insanity in nineteenth century Australia. **Aust NZ J Psychiatry** 1982 Mar;16(1):53-62

**Manninger, Vilmos, 1876-**
Balogh J, Sükösd L: Manninger Vilmos akadémiai pályadíjának 80 éves évfordulójára. **Orv Hetil** 1983 Oct 30;124(44):2693-5

**Manson, Patrick, 1844-1922**
Chernin E: Sir Patrick Manson: an annotated bibliography and a note on a collected set of his writings. **Rev Infect Dis** 1983 Mar-Apr;5(2):353-86
Chernin E: Sir Patrick Manson's studies on the transmission and biology of filariasis. **Rev Infect Dis** 1983 Jan-Feb;5(1):148-66

**Mantell, Gideon Algernon, 1790-1852**
Dean DR: The Gideon Mantell collection, New Zealand. **J Soc Bibliogr Nat Hist** 1979 Apr;9(2):121-4

**Manzolini, Anna Morandi, 1716-1774**
Armoroli M, ed: Le cere anatomiche Bolognesi del settecento. Catalogo della mostra organizzata Settembre-Novembre 1981. Bologna, Università degli Studi di Bologna, Accademia delle Scienze, 1981. 97 p. Contributions by R. A. Bernabeo, L. Bonuzzi, F. Ruggeri.

**Manzolini, Giovanni, 1700-1755**
Armoroli M, ed: Le cere anatomiche Bolognesi del settecento. Catalogo della mostra organizzata Settembre-Novembre 1981. Bologna, Università degli Studi di Bologna, Accademia delle Scienze, 1981. 97 p. Contributions by R. A. Bernabeo, L. Bonuzzi, F. Ruggeri.

**Mapson, Leslie William, 1907-1970**
Hill R: Leslie William Mapson. In Dictionary of national biography, 1961-1970. Suppl. 8, 1981. p. 721-2.

**Marais, Marin, 1656-1728**
Brøndum N: Et kirurgisk indgreb skildret i musik. **Dan Medicinhist Arbog** 1983;12:170-4
Rocchietta S: Musica e litotomia in una composizione di Marin Marais (1656-1728). **Minerva Med** 1983 Nov 16;74(44):2713

**Marañón, Gregorio, 1887-1960**
Cela CJ: Marañon, el hombre. In Congrés International d'Història de la Medicina Catalana, 2nd, Barcelona, 1975. Llibre d'Actes. Barcelona, Socitra, 1977. p. 59-71.
Costa-Casaretto C: Marañon y los chilenos. **Rev Med Chil** 1980 Mar;108(3):277-81
Gómez-Santos M: Vida de Gregorio Marañón. Esplugas de Llobregat, Plaza & Janés, 1977. 478 p.
Hofmann C: Stimme und Konstitution im Werk Gregorio Marañóns. **Medizinhist J** 1984;19(3):259-66

**Marat, Jean Paul, 1743-1793**
Dotz W: Jean Paul Marat. His life, cutaneous disease, death, and depiction by Jacques Louis David. **Am J Dermatopathol** 1979 Fall;1(3):247-50
Jelinek JE: Jean-Paul Marat. The differential diagnosis of his skin disease. **Am J Dermatopathol** 1979 Fall;1(3):251-2
Rechtman J: Le Dr. J.P. Marat et le secret professionnel. **Soc Fr Hist Art Dent** 1979 Sep-Dec;(5-6):22-5
Rechtman J: Un précurseur génial de la prévention et de la diététique, du bouche à bouche et du massage cardiaque externe de l'asepsie et parrain de J. P. Marat: Le docteur William Buchan (1729-1805). Diss. Paris VII, 1979. 115 p.
Rechtman J: Jean-Paul Marat, ses origines, ses apports à la médecine. Agent secret? **Hist Sci Med** 1980;14:261-70
Schiller F: Reverend Wesley, Doctor Marat and their electric fire. **Clio Med** 1981 Apr;15(3-4):159-76
Sebastiani F: Jean-Paul Marat, l'ami de la nature. **Physis** 1984;26(3):325-59

**Mařatka, Zdeněk**
Pětašedesátiny doc. MUDr. Z. Mařatky, DrSc.: **Cesk Gastroenterol Vyz** 1979 Jun;33(4):236-47

**Marbecke, Roger, 1536-1605**
Whitfield AG: Roger Marbeck--first Registrar. **J R Coll Physicians Lond** 1981 Jan;15(1):59-60

**Marbode, Bp. of Rennes, d. 1123**
Riddle JM: Marbode of Rennes' (1035-1123) De lapidibus, considered as a medical treatise with text, commentary and C. W. King's translation, together with text and translation of Marbode's minor works on stones. Wiesbaden, Steiner, 1977. 144 p. (Sudhoffs Archiv, Beihefte, Heft 20).

**Marcano, Gaspar, 1850-1910**
Alegría C: Doctor Gaspar Marcano; médico y antropólogo de gran prestigio. **Rev Soc Venez Hist Med** 1972-73;20-21(34-35):151-60

**Marcellus Empiricus, 4th-5th cent.**
Merlette B, Vial F, Rulliere R: Le Marcellus de Laon: observations paléographiques et critiques. **Hist Sci Med** 1980;14(1):52-60
Vial F, Merlette B, Paris R, et al: Les recettes retenues par les Laonnois: observations médicales. **Hist Sci Med** 1980;14(1):61-9

**March, Alden, 1795-1869**
Buell FD: Nineteenth century surgeon: Dr. Alden March, founder, Albany Medical College, 1795-1869. Albany, Albany Medical College, 1981. 12 p.

**Marchant, Nicolas-Damas, 1767-1833**
Rivet R: A propos de l'oeuvre médicale du Baron Marchant (1767-1833). In: Congrès National des Sociétés Savantes, 103e, Nancy, 1978. Comptes Rendus. Paris, 1978. Section des Sciences, Fasc. V. p. 125-30.

**Marci von Kronland, Johannes Marcus, 1595-1667**
Servít Z: Počátky české novověké medicíny a biologie. Jan Marek Marci z Kronlandu (Joannes Marcus Marci, 1595-1667). Stručná biografie. **Cesk Fysiol** 1984;33(5):394-413

**Marcinkowski, Karol, 1800-1846**
Jakóbczyk W: Karol Marcinkowski, 1800-1846. Warszawa; Poznań, Państwowe Wydawn. Nauk., Oddz. w Poznaniu, 1981. 189 p.

**Marcus, Carl Friedrich von, 1802-1862**
Wolf R: Das Leben und Wirken von Carl Friedrich von Marcus (1802-1862). Diss. Würzburg, 1980. 141 p.

**Marcuse, Herbert, 1898-**
Malinovich MM: On Herbert Marcuse and the concept of psychological freedom. **Soc Res (NY)** 1982;49(1):158-80

**Marcy, Henry Orlando, 1837-1924**
Read RD: Marcy's priority in the development of inguinal herniorrphaphy. **Surgery** 1980 Nov;88(5):682-5

**Marey, Etienne Jules, 1830-1904**
Baron JB: Etienne-Jules Marey. **Acta Belg Med Phys** 1983 Oct-Dec;6(4):187-97
De Neve M: E. J. Marey, inventieve registrator van de fysiologische fenomenen. **Acta Belg Med Phys** 1983 Oct-Dec;6(4):153-5
Dupuis M: Etienne-Jules Marey, le photographe du mouvement. **Sci Avenir** 1980;400:95-100
Espinosa RE, Vlietstra RE, Mann RJ: J. B. A. Chauveau, E. J. Marey, and their resolution of the apex beat controversy through intracardiac pressure recordings. **Mayo Clin Proc** 1983 Mar;58(3):197-202
Fleckenstein K: Etienne Marey and the electric torpedo fish. **Med Instrum** 1984 Sep-Oct;18(5):288-9
Lequime J: Marey et la cardiologie. **Acta Belg Med Phys** 1983 Oct-Dec;6(4):181-5
Snellen HA: E. J. Marey and cardiology: physiologist and pioneer of technology, 1830-1904: selected writings in facsimile with comments and summaries, a brief history of life and work, and a bibliography. 264 p.

**Maria, Prophetess, 2nd or 3rd cent.**
Patai R: Maria the Jewess--founding mother of alchemy. **Ambix** 1982 Nov;29(3):177-92

**Maria Theresa, Empress of Austria, 1717-1780**
Lesky E: Heilkunde und Gesundheitswesen unter Maria Theresia. **Osterr Apoth Ztg** 1980 May 17;34(20):357-60
Wyklicky H: Maria Theresia und Joseph II. als Reformatoren des Gesundheitswesens in Oesterreich. **Wien Tierarztl Monatsschr** 1981;68(1):3-7

**Mariátegui, José Carlos, 1894-1930**
Alarco F: La psicoterápia dinámica y José Carlos Mariátegui. **Rev Neuropsiquiatr** 1979 Sep-Dec;42(3-4):145-64

**Marie, Pierre, 1853-1940**
Ryckewaert A, Naveau B: Principaux apports de Charcot et de Pierre Marie à la pathologie ostéo-articulaire. **Rev Rhum Mal Osteoartic** 1984 Jul-Sep;51(7-8):405-13

**Marine, David, 1880-1976**
Harvey AM: David Marine: America's pioneer thyroidologist. **Am J Med** 1981 Mar;70(3):483-5
Matovinovic J: David Marine (1880-1976): Nestor of thyroidology. **Perspect Biol Med** 1978 Spring;21(3):565-89

**Marinescu, Gheorghe, 1863-1938**
Marinesco M, Argemi-Lloveras J: Georges Marinescu (Roumanie) et Santiago Ramon y Cajal; deux représentants du génie latin. In International Congress of the History of Medicine, 27th, Barcelona, 1980. Actas. Barcelona, Acadèmia de Ciències Mèdiques de Catalunya i Balears, 1981. p. 570-4.
Marinesco M, Petresco A, Marinesco G: Georges Marinesco et la France. **Hist Sci Med** 1984;18(1):13-8
Marinescu M, Petrescu A: Ecouri contemporane ale operei stiințifice a lui Gh. Marinescu. **Rev Med Interna [Neurol Psihiatr]** 1980 Oct-Dec;25(4):311-4
Negru I: Muzeul memorial 'Prof. dr. Gh. Marinescu'. **Viata Med [Medii Sanit]** 1981 Aug;29(8):187-90

**Marjolin, Jean Nicolas, 1780–1850**
Gutmann RA: Une lettre de Marjolin sur ses rapports avec Dupuytren. **Hist Sci Med** 1981;15(2):123–7
Steffen C: Marjolin's ulcer. Report of two cases and evidence that Marjolin did not describe cancer arising in scars of burns. **Am J Dermatopathol** 1984 Apr;6(2):187–93
Steffen C: Jean-Nicolas Marjolin. **Am J Dermatopathol** 1984 Apr;6(2):163–5

**Markelov, G. I., 1880–**
Arkhangel'skiĭ GV: Vklad Akademika G.I. Markelova v teoriiu otechestvennoĭ nevrologii (k 100–letiiu so dnia rozhdeniia). **Klin Med (Mosk)** 1980 Oct;58(10):114–8

**Markham, Gervase, 1568?–1637**
Best MR: Medical use of a sixteenth-century herbal: Gervase Markham and the Banckes herbal. **Bull Hist Med** 1979 Fall;53(3):449–58

**Markiewicz, Stanisław, 1839–1911**
Demel M: Wysoko jak król Zygmunt. Zycie i dzieło dra Stanisława Markiewicza. Warszawa, Państwowy Zakład Wydawn. Lekarskich, 1977. 102 p.

**Markovic, Svetozar, 1846–1875**
Lukić D: O narodnom zdravlju u delima Svetozara markovića. **Srp Arh Celok Lek** 1981 Apr;109(4):579–86

**Marks, Urban, 1880–1949**
Stuart D: Urban Marks: 1880–1949. **Br Med J [Clin Res]** 1982 Jul 31;285(6338):345–7

**Markusovszky, Lajos, 1815–1893**
Az Orvosi Hetilap múltjából: **Orv Hetil** 1982 Jan 10;123(2):111
Hidvégi J: Az ifjú Markusovszky világa. **Orv Hetil** 1982 Dec 26;123(52):3207–13
Kapronczay K: Markusovszky Lajos utolsó levele Fodor Józsefhez. **Orvostort Kozl** 1980;89–91(26 no 1–3):269–71
Kapronczay K: Markusovszky Lajos utolsó levele Fodor Józsefhez. **Orv Hetil** 1982 Dec 26;123(52):3213–4
Petrányi L: Markusovszky szellemének idézése a 3. évezred küszöbén. **Orv Hetil** 1984 Jun 17;125(25):1487–92

**Marlowe, Christopher, 1564–1593**
Herring H: The self and madness in Marlowe's 'Edward II' and Webster's 'The Duchess of Malfi'. **J Mediev Renaiss Stud** 1979;9:307–23
Kuriyama CB: Hammer or anvil. Psychological patterns in Christopher Marlowe's plays. New Brunswick, Rutgers University Press, 1980. xiv, 240 p.

**Marsh, John**
Stuart R, Stuart W: John Marsh. **Pac Hist** 1980;24(3):369–75

**Marshall, Geoffrey, 1887–**
Marshall G: A doctor in the Great War––an interview with Sir Geoffrey Marshall. **Br Med J [Clin Res]** 1982 Dec 18–25;285(6357):1780–3

**Marsilius van Inghen, d. 1396**
Cadden J: The medieval philosophy and biology of growth: Albertus Magnus, Thomas Aquinas, Albert of Saxony and Masilius of Inghen on Book I, Chapter V, of Aristotle's 'De generatione et corruptione.' With translated texts of Albertus Magnus and Thomas Aquinas. Ph. D. Diss. Indiana University. Bloomington, 1971. vii, 267 leaves.

**Martel, Thierry de, 1875–1940**
Hepp J: Un grand chirurgien du début de ce siècle. **Sem Hop Paris** 1981 Jun 8–15;57(21–24):1049–54
Pecker J: Thierry de Martel, 1875–1940. **Surg Neurol** 1980;13:401–3

**Marti, Manuel, 1663–1737**
Gil L, Buño W: La medicina, los médicos y las enfermedades en el epistolario de Manuel Marti. **Med Esp** 1980;79:261–72

**Martí y Juliá, Domènec, 1861–1917**
Mas i Perera P: Tribut al Doctor Domènec Martí i Julià. **Xaloc** 1972;56:182–5

**Martin, Barthelemy, 1629–1698?**
Gysel C: Bernardin Martin et sa 'dissertation sur les dents' (1679–1979). **Actual Odontostomatol (Paris)** 1980;34(129):59–72

**Martin, Elioner**
Rawlings FH: Two 17th century women apothecaries. **Pharm Hist (London)** 1984 Sep;14(3):7

**Martin, Franklin Henry, 1857–1935**
Ochsner A: To our founder [Franklin H. Martin], with reflections. **Bull Am Coll Surg** 1981;66(5):26–30

**Martin, George M., fl. 1890**
Ciuffreda KJ: Astigmatic amblyopia: George Martin. 1890. Translation. **Am J Optom Physiol Opt** 1978 Feb;55(2):133–6

**Martin, John, 1789–1854**
Woodruff AW: J M W Turner and some of his predecessors and successors, from the viewpoint of medical history. **J R Soc Med** 1980 May;73(5):381–92

**Martin, John, 1904–**
Heirs of Hippocrates: The development of medicine in a catalogue of historic books in the Health Sciences Library, The University of Iowa. Compiled by R. Eimas, E. Holtum, D. Curry. Iowa City, Friends of the University of Iowa Libraries, 1980. xiv, 474 p.

**Martindale, William, 1840–1902**
Wade A: 'Martindale'. The International Use of 'Martindale: the Extra Pharmacopoeia'. **Farm Tid** 1979 Dec 1;89(48):1001–4

**Martineau, Harriet, 1802–1876**
Sanders V: 'No ordinary case of a village apothecary': the doctor as hero in Harriet Martineaus's Deerbrook. **Notes Queries** 1983 Aug;30(4):293–4

**Martínez de Leache, Miguel, fl. 1644–1652**
Sánchez-Moscoso Hermida A: La peligrosidad del medicamento a través del 'Discurso Farmacéutico sobre los Cánones de Mesué', de Miguel Martínez de Leache (1652). **Bol Soc Esp Hist Farm** 1984 Jun;35(138):103–23

**Martland, Harrison Stanford, 1883–1954**
Eckert WG: Dr. Harrison Stanford Martland (1883–1954). **Am J Forensic Med Pathol** 1981 Mar;2(1):83–4

**Martyn, John, 1699–1768**
MacPhail I, Hess WJ: The date of the Linnaean index in John Martyn's Historia plantarum rariorum. **Huntia** 1979;3(2):73–81

**Martynov, Aleksei Vasil'evich, 1868–**
Kotel'nikov VP: Nauchnoe nasledie A. V. Martynova v izuchenii zabolevaniĭ podzheludochnoĭ zhelezy i zhelchevyvodiashchikh puteĭ. **Klin Med (Mosk)** 1983 Apr;61(4):117–9

**Marx, Karl, 1818–1883**
Bazhan TA: K. Marks ob okhrane zdorov'ia rabochego klassa. **Gig Sanit** 1984 Feb;(2):37–40
Berlan JP: The world food problem: Malthus, Marx and their epigones. **Mon Rev** 1980;31(10):20–32
Büttner L, Meyer B: Karl Marx und die Begründung der Gesundheitspolitik der revolutionären Arbeiterbewegung. II. Marx' Aufdeckung des Klasseninhalts der bürgerlichen Gesundheitspolitik. **Z Arztl Fortbild (Jena)** 1983;77(19):819–23
Chikin SIa: Sotsial'no–gigienicheskie idei K. Marksa (k 100–letiiu so dnia smerti). **Sov Med** 1983;(3):75–8
Hidvégi J: Marx Károly betegsége és halála. **Orv Hetil** 1983 Mar 6;124(10):589–91
Kaiser W: Medizinhistorische Impressionen zum Karl–Marx–Jahr 1983. **Z Gesamte Inn Med** 1983 Dec 15;38(24):669–72
Kelley DR: The science of anthropology: an essay on the very old Marx. **J Hist Ideas** 1984 Apr–Jun;45(2):245–62
Kovel J: Marx and Freud. In M. Albin, R. J. Devlin, G. Heeger, ed: New directions in psychohistory. The Adelphi papers in honor of Erik H. Erikson. Lexington, Toronto, D. C. Heath, 1980. p. 21–6.
Kozlov AM, Kel'ner MS, Losev NI: K. Marks is problemy meditsiny (k 165–letiiu so dnia rozhdeniia K. Marksa). **Patol Fiziol Eksp Ter** 1983 May–Jun;3:3–9
Kozlov AM: Genial'nyĭ myslitel', plamennyĭ revoliutsioner i velikiĭ chelovek (k 165–letiiu so dnia rozhdeniia i 100–letiiu so dnia smerti Karla Marksa). **Feldsher Akush** 1983;48(5):3–4
Löhr HG: Ein Vierteljahrhundert gemeinsamen Weges von Karl Marx und Friedrich Engels mit ihrem treuen Freund und Kampfgefährten Carl Schorlemmer. **Pharmazie** 1983 Nov;38(11):768–72
Löther R, ed: Philosophische Schriften von Marx, Engels und Lenin und ihre Bedeutung für die Medizin heute. Jena, Fischer, 1979. 127 p. Contributions by U. Körner, I. Löther, P. W. Ruff, R. Stach, G. Straass.
Marx E: The biography of a great man. **Z Gesamte Hyg** 1983 Oct;29(10):571–2
Spaar H: Die Begründung der Vorzüge des Gesundheitsschutzes im Sozialismus und seiner gesetzmässigen Schranken im Kapitalismus im Lichte der Lehre von Karl Marx. **Z Gesamte Hyg** 1983 Oct;29(10):573–6
Vengrova IV: K. Marks i razvitie sotsial'noĭ gigieny. **Sov Zdravookhr** 1983;6:3–8

**Mary Stuart, Queen of Scots, 1542–1587**
Haeger-Aronsen B, Haeger K: Porfyri hos Mary Stuarts efterkommande: en historisk–medicinsk tvistefråga. **Sydsven Medicinhist Sallsk Arsskr** 1984;21:63–75

**Marzeev, Aleksandr Nikitich, 1883–1956**
Ermolaev MM: Vklad A. N. Marzeeva v stanovlenie i razvitie sanitarnogo prosveshcheniia na Ukraine. **Vrach Delo** 1983 Jan;(1):118–21
Shandala MG: Aleksandr Nikitich Marzeev (k 100–letiiu so dnia rozhdeniia). **Vrach Delo** 1983 May;5:119–21
Shandala MG, Kogan VIa: Ot zemskogo sanitarnogo vracha do akademika (k 100–letiiu so dnia rozhdeniia A. N. Marzeeva). **Gig Sanit** 1983 Oct;(10):43–5
Sivolob NI: Rol' A. N. Marzeeva v razvitii otechestvennoĭ gigieny (k 100–letiiu so dnia rozhdeniia). **Sov Zdravookhr** 1983;(8):54–6

**Marzell, Heinrich, 1885–1970**
Wölfel A: Pflanzen in der Volksmedizin. Die volksmedizinischen Studien von Heinrich Marzell. Diss. Erlangen–Nürnberg, 1983. 117 p.

**Mascagni, Paolo, 1755–1815**
Ciardi RP: Fra pelle e ossa. **Kos** 1984 Mar;1(2):93–117
Dumaitre P: Les planches anatomiques d'Antommarchi. **Clio Med** 1981

Sep;16(1):13-23

**Mascellini, Giovanni**
Vătămanu N: Contribution à l'étude de la vie et de l'oeuvre di Giovanni Mascellini, médecin et secrétaire princier. **Rev Etud Sud Est Eur** 1978;16(2):269-87

**Masdevall, José, d. 1801**
Riera J: José Masdevall y la medicina española ilustrada (Enseñanza, epidemias y guerra a finales del siglo XVIII). Valladolid, Universidad de Valladolid, 1980. 257 p. (Acta Historico-Medica Vallisoletana, Monografias, X)

**Masheter, James William Hall, d. 1943**
Salter AL: Veterinary life in the Boer War 1899-1902. Correspondence of James William Hall Masheter M.R.C.V.S. **Vet Hist** 1984;3(3):87-92

**Mashkilleysson family**
Mashkilleysson NA: Four generations of dermatologists. **Int J Dermatol** 1983 Nov;22(9):546-7

**Maslovskiĭ, Aleksandr Fedorovich**
Borodiĭ NK: A.F. Maslovskiĭ--vydaiushchiĭsia Ukrainskiĭ vrach XVIII v. **Sov Zdravookhr** 1984;(5):70-2

**Maslow, Abraham Harold, 1908-1970**
Zimmerman J: Transcendent psychology: Erik H. Erikson, Erich Fromm, Karen Horney, Abraham H. Maslow, and Harry Stack Sullivan and the quest for a healthy humanity. Ph.D. Diss., Northwestern University. Evanston, 1982. vi, 498 p.

**Mason, James Monroe, Jr., 1871-**
Carmichael JL: Dr. James Monroe Mason, Jr. and his era in medicine. **J Med Assoc State Ala** 1982 May;51(11):30-7

**Mason, Karl Ernest, 1900-1978**
Ames SR: Karl Ernest Mason (1900-1978): a biographical sketch. **J Nutr** 1984 Mar;114(3):463-6
Karl Ernest Mason, 1900-1978.: **Anat Rec** 1980 Sep;198(1):1-12

**Massenhove, Ghislaine van**
In honor of the memory of Ghislaine van Massenhove, international president of CICIAMS: **Nouv Com Int Cathol Infirm Assist Med Soc** 1980;(1):1-24

**Masson, Pierre, 1880-1959**
Cabanne F: Pierre Masson. Précurseur et rénovateur (1880-1959). **Ann Pathol** 1983;3(1):95-7
Cadotte M: Historique du laboratoire de pathologie de l'Hôtel-Dieu de Montréal: de sa création en 1896, à l'arrivée du professeur Pierre Masson en 1928. **Union Med Can** 1979 May;108(5):479-94
Cadotte M: L'héritage scientifique du professeur Pierre Masson. **Union Med Can** 1984 May;113(5):344-5
Michalany I: Masson's contribution to pathology and to histological technique. With special reference to the discovery of argentaffin cells. **Ann Pathol** 1983;3(1):85-93
Michalany J: Masson que j'ai connu: mon maître et mon ami. **Union Med Can** 1984 May;113(5):386-9
Riopelle JL: A la mémoire du Professeur Pierre Masson, Vingt ans après. **Union Med Can** 1979 May;108(5):473-6
Seemayer TA: The life and legacy of Professor Pierre Masson. **Am J Surg Pathol** 1983 Mar;7(2):179-83

**Masterman, Charles Frederick Gurney, 1873-1927**
Mason FM: Charles Masterman and National Health Insurance. **Albion** 1978;10(1):54-75

**Mata, Justo Martinez**
Woodruff HB, Hernandez S, Stapley EO: Evolution of an antibiotic screening programme. A tribute to Justo Martinez Mata. **Hindustan Antibiot Bull** 1979 Feb;21(3):71-84

**Mata y Fontanet, Pedro, 1811-1877**
Bertrán Capella A, Huguet Ramia E: La aportacion de Pedro Mata a la toxicologia. **Asclepio** 1980;32:53-63
Corbella Corbella J, Martí Amengual G: Recuerdo de la obra de Pedro Mata y Fontanet (1811-1877) en su centenario. **Asclepio** 1980;32:111-9
Doménech Llabería E: Las ideas de Pedro Mata en el campo de la psicologia de su tiempo. **Asclepio** 1980;32:137-50
Rodríguez Pazos M, Martí Lloret JB: La aportacion de pedromata al derecho medico de su tiempo. **Asclepio** 1980;32:415-20

**Matas, Rudolph, 1860-1957**
Duffy J: Rudolph Matas. In Dictionary of American Biography, Suppl. 6, 1956-1960. p. 434-5, 1980.
Rich NM, Clagett GP, Salander JM, et al: The Matas/Soubbotitch connection. **Surgery** 1983 Jan;93(1 Pt 1):17-9
Rutkow IM: William Halsted and Rudolph Matas: their unique alliance. **Surgery** 1980 May;87(5):524-38
Tomlinson WK, Perret JJ: Rudolph Matas father of cardiovascular surgery. In International Congress of the History of Medicine, 27th, Barcelona, 1980. Actas. Barcelona, Académia de Ciències Médiques de Catalunya i Balears, 1981. p. 212-6.

**Mather, Cotton, 1663-1728**
Breitwieser MR: Cotton Mather's pharmacy. **Early Am Lit** 1981;16(1):42-9
Solberg WU: Cotton Mather's indebtedness to Marcello Malpighi. **J Hist Med Allied Sci** 1981 Jul;36(3):326-31
Warner MH: Vindicating the minister's medical role: Cotton Mather's concept of the nishmath-chajim and the spiritualization of medicine. **J Hist Med Allied Sci** 1981 Jul;36(3):278-95

**Mathon, Jaroslav, 1867-1953**
Kraus B: MUDr. Jaroslav Mathon - chirurg, umělecký a památkový praukopník. **Cas Lek Cesk** 1983 Sep 30;122(39):1214-5

**Matthiae, Georg M., 1708-1773**
Schwann S: Lekarze polscy w świetle historyczno-medycznego dzieła Grzegorza Matthiasa z XVIII wieku. **Arch Hist Med (Warsz)** 1979;42(2):217-22

**Mattioli, Pietro Andrea, 1500-1577**
Müller-Jahncke WD: Der 'latheinisch aussgestrichene Matthiolus' Landgraf Wilhelms IV von Hessen-Kassel und sein Schicksal. **Pharm Ztg** 1983 Feb 17;128(7):357-61

**Maty, Matthieu, 1718-1776**
Janssens U: Matthieu Maty and the adoption of inoculation for smallpox in Holland. **Bull Hist Med** 1981 Summer;55(2):246-56

**Mátyus, István, 1725-1802**
Spielmann J: Az erdélyi néptáplálkozás kérdései Mátyus István müvében. **Nor Tannlaegeforen Tid** 1982 Jun 13;123(24):1495-8

**Mauchaut, Guillaume de, 1300?-1377**
Cosman MP: Machaut's medical musical world. In Cosman MP, Chandler B, ed: Machaut's world: science and art in the fourteenth century. New York, New York Academy of Sciences, 1978. (Annals of the New York Academy of Sciences, v. 314). p. 1-36.

**Maudsley, Henry, 1835-1918**
Maudsley H: The pathology of mind: a study of its distempers, deformities and disorders. Reprint of 1895 ed. Biographical introduction by A. Lewis. London, Friedmann, 1979. 571 p.

**Mauduyt de la Varenne, Pierre Jean Claude, ca. 1732-1792**
Zelbstein MU: Mauduyt de La Varenne (1733-1792) un médecin au siècle des 'Lumières'. **Hist Sci Med** 1984;18(3):295-306

**Maufils, Marie-Madeleine, d. 1702**
Bernier H: Marie-Madeleine Maufils. In Dictionary of Canadian biography, 1701 to 1740. Volume 2, 1969. p. 466.

**Maugham, William Somerset, 1874-1965**
Szállási A: Csehov és Maugham a Nyugat kedvenc írói. **Orv Hetil** 1980 Jan 27;121(4):226-9

**Maumenee, Alfred Edward, 1913-**
Paton D: The surgery of A. Edward Maumenee. **Am J Ophthalmol** 1979 Sep;88(3 Pt 1):297-302
Patz A: Contributions of A. Edward Maumenee in the field of retinal and choroidal diseases. **Am J Ophthalmol** 1979 Sep;88(3 Pt 1):295-6
Randolph ME: A. Edward Maumenee--an appreciation. **Am J Ophthalmol** 1979 Sep;88(3 Pt 1):289-92
Silverstein AM: Contributions of A. Edward Maumenee to ocular immunology. **Am J Ophthalmol** 1979 Sep;88(3 Pt 1):302-5
To honor A. Edward Maumenee: **Am J Ophthalmol** 1979 Sep;88(3 Pt 1):285, 288-316

**Maumousseau, Françoise, 1657-1704**
Bernier H: Françoise Maumousseau. In Dictionary of Canadian biography, 1701 to 1740. Volume 2, 1969. p. 466-7.

**Maunsell, Henry, 1806-1879**
Blaney R: Henry Maunsell (1806-1879): an early community physician. **Ir J Med Sci** 1984 Jan;153(1):42-3

**Maupertuis, Pierre Louis Moreau de, 1698-1759**
Bednarczyk A: Pierre Louis Moreau de Maupertuis (1698-1759) atomizm biologiczny i panpsychizm. **Kwart Hist Nauki Tech** 1981;26(2):335-62
Hoffheimer MH: Maupertuis and the eighteenth-century critique of preexistence. **J Hist Biol** 1982 Spring;15(1):119-44
Sandler I: Pierre Louis Moreau de Maupertuis - a precursor of Mendel? **J Hist Biol** 1983 Spring;16(1):101-36
Sandler IL: Pierre Louis Moreau de Maupertuis--a precursor of Mendelian genetics?: an inquiry into the biological ideas of Maupertuis, the Mendelian principles of heredity and the nature of the precursor. Ph.D. diss. University of Washington. Seattle, 1979. 265 leaves.
Vartanian A: Le frère de Maupertuis et l'homme machine. **Dix-huit Siecle** 1982;14:305-23

**Maurichaud-Beaupré, Pierre-Jean, 1778-1857**
Peumery JJ: Une grande figure de la médecine et de la chirurgie française: Pierre-Jean Mauricheau-Beaupré (1778-1857). **Hist Sci Med** 1983;17(1):95-104

**Maurocordato, Alexander, ca. 1636-ca. 1710**
Apostolopoulos DG: Alexandros Maurokordatos. **Ellenika** 1976;29:311-5

**Maximinus I, Gaius Julius Verus, 173-238**
Klawans HL: The acromegaly of Maximinus I: the possible influence of a pituitary tumor on the life and death of a Roman emperor. In Rose FC, Bynum WF, ed: Historical aspects of the neurosciences. New York, Raven, 1982. 317-26.
Ljunggren B: En stor man med en sjuk hjärna.

Sydsven Medicinhist Sallsk Arsskr 1984;21:77–85

**Maxwell, James Clerk, 1831–1879**
Sherman PD: Colour vision in the nineteenth century: the Young–Helmholtz–Maxwell theory. Bristol, Adam Hilger, 1981. xiii, 233 p.

**May, Rollo, 1909–**
Rattner J: Rollo May. In J. Rattner, ed: Wandlungen der Psychoanalyse. Wien, Europaverlag, 1980. p. 309–32.

**Mayer, Julius Robert von, 1814–1878**
Mayer JR von: Die Mechanik der Wärme: sämtliche Schriften. In Zusammenarbeit mit dem Stadtarchiv Heilbronn herausgegeben von Hans Peter Münzenmayer. Heilbronn, Stadtarchiv, 1978. 457 p. (Veröffentlichungen des Archivs der Stadt Heilbronn; 22).

**Mayer, Karol, 1882–1946**
Meissner R: Swiatowy priorytet Karola Mayera w dziedzinie radiodiagnostyki--przyczynek do dziejów tomografii. **Kwart Hist Nauki Tech** 1982;27(1):125–37

**Mayer, Rudolph Leopold, 1895–1962**
Scholz A: Rudolph Leopold Mayer, Werk und Persönlichkeit. **Dermatol Monatsschr** 1981 Sep;167(9):582–6

**Mayerne, Theodore Turquet de, 1573–1655**
Paulshock BZ: Dr. Theodore de Mayerne. **JAMA** 1981;245:1732

**Mayersbach, Heinz von**
Reale E: Wissenschaftliche Arbeiten von H. von Mayersbach. **Mikroskopie** 1981;38(3–4):67–77

**Mayerson, Hyman Samuel, 1900–**
Symposium on capillary permeability and mechanism of transport, American Physiological Society, New Orleans, 1979. A salute to Professor Hyman S. Mayerson.: **Physiologist** 1980 Feb;23(1):34–93
Taylor AE: Dr. Mayerson, the scientist. **Physiologist** 1980 Feb;23(1):38–40

**Mayo, Charles Horace, 1865–1939**
Agris J: Stamps commemorating medicine. 'The Doctors William James and Charles Horace Mayo'. **J Dermatol Surg Oncol** 1980 Jul;6(7):523
Carson CC: Charles Horace Mayo (1865-1939). **Invest Urol** 1981;18:313–4
Keys TE: The Mayos: a historical vignette. **Adler Mus Bull** 1984 Nov;10(3):16–24

**Mayo, Elton, 1880–1949**
Garbelotto N: Teoria e politica nella psicosociologia di E. Mayo. **Stor Crit Psicol** 1980;1(1):61–78

**Mayo Family**
Link EP: The Mayo family: a study in changing social ideas. In: Congrès international d'histoire de la médecine, XXVe, Québec, 1976. Actes. Québec, 1977. p. 895–916.
Moerchel J: Sauerbruch und die Mayos. **Dtsch Med Wochenschr** 1980 May 9;105(19):697–9

**Mayo, William James, 1861–1939**
Agris J: Stamps commemorating medicine. 'The Doctors William James and Charles Horace Mayo'. **J Dermatol Surg Oncol** 1980 Jul;6(7):523
Key JD, Callahan JA, Nelson CW: William J. Mayo--centennial notes. **Minn Med** 1982 Oct;65(10):636–8
Keys TE: The Mayos: a historical vignette. **Adler Mus Bull** 1984 Nov;10(3):16–24

**Mayo, William Worrall, 1819–1911**
Hayles AB, Key JD: Adventures of two prairie pioneers. **Minn Med** 1981 Oct;64(10):629–32
Keys TE, Key JD: An overlooked tribute for Dr. William Worrall Mayo. **Minn Med** 1984 Jul;67(7):375–8
Klein R: Little 'hospital' on the prairie. Roughly the first hundred years of Rochester's Mayo Clinic. **Postgrad Med** 1984 Sep 1;76(3):15–6, 19, 22–4

**Mayor, Frank Isaac, 1779–1855**
Waszyński E: W dwusetną rocznicę urodzin Franciszka Izaaka Mayora (1779–1855), odkrywcy tonów serca płodu. **Ginekol Pol** 1980 Aug;51(8):765–6

**Mayor, Mathias, 1775–1847**
Biaudet JC: Mathias Mayor (1775–1847). **Rev Med Suisse Romande** 1984 May;104(5):343–7

**Mayrhofer, Carl, 1837–1882**
Carter KC: Ignaz Semmelweis, Carl Mayrhofer, and the rise of germ theory. **Med Hist** 1985 Jan;29(1):33–53
Carter KC: Semmelweis's possible influence on Karl Mayrhofer and on those who subsequently developed nineteenth century etiological theories. **Orvostort Kozl** 1982;28(1–3):23–31

**Mayrhofer, Karl Wilhelm, 1806–1853**
Habacher M: Auf der suche nach dem 'Od'; Karl Ludwig Freiherr von Reichenbach (1788–1869) und Karl Wilhelm Mayrhofer (1806–1853), zwei Verbündete contra Justus von Liebig. **Clio Med** 1980 May;14(2):105–18

**Mazzei, Filippo, 1730–1816**
Chakravorty RC: Philip Mazzei - physician, statesman, horticulturist, citizen of the world. **Scalpel Tongs** 1981;25:50–1

**Mead, Kate Campbell (Hurd), 1867–1941**
Radbill SX: Remarks on the Kate Hurd Mead lectures. **Trans Stud Coll Physicians Phila** 1977 Apr;44(4):179–81
Stevens R: The changing idea of a medical specialty. **Trans Stud Coll Physicians Phila** 1980 Sep;5(2 no 3):159–77

**Means, James Howard, 1885–1967**
Harvey AM: James Howard Means and his romance with the thyroid gland. **Am J Med** 1981 Jun;70(6):1158–60

**Mechnikov, Il'ia Il'ich, 1845–1916**
Baggiolini M: Phagozyten und Phagozytose hundert Jahre nach Metschnikoff. Ein aktuelles Bild des neutrophilen Leukozyten. **Schweiz Med Wochenschr** 1982 Oct;112(41):1403–11
Bibel DJ: Sternberg, Metchnikoff, and the phagocytes. **Milit Med** 1982 Jul;147(7):550–3
Cooper EL: Prix D'Immunologie Behring–Metschnikoff. **Dev Comp Immunol** 1982 Summer;6(3):389–90
Egri B: Mecsnyikov a cambridge–i Darwin–emlékünnepségekröl. **Orv Hetil** 1982 Nov 14;123(46):2858–60
Elkin II, Frolova VV: Rol' N. I. Pirogova v podgotovke I. I. Mechnikova k nauchnoĭ deiatel'nosti (k 135–letiiu so dnia rozhdeniia I. I. Mechnikova. **Zh Mikrobiol Epidemiol Immunobiol** 1980 Sep;(9):114–8
Heifets L: Metchnikoff's recollections of Robert Koch. **Tubercle** 1982 Jun;63(2):139–41
Heifets L: Centennial of Metchnikoff's discovery. **J Reticuloendothel Soc** 1982 May;31(5):381–91
Karnovsky ML: Metchnikoff in Messina: a century of studies on phagocytosis. **N Engl J Med** 1981 May 7;304(19):1178–80
Klemparskaya NN: 100 years of the phagocytosis doctrine (Ilya Ilyich Mechnikov). **J Hyg Epidemiol Microbiol Immunol** 1983;27(3):249–52
Kosiakov PN: K 100–letniu fagotsitarnoĭ teorii immuniteta I.I. Mechnikova. **Vopr Virusol** 1982 Sep–Oct;27(5):4–9
Kucharz E, Jabłońska D: Illya Illich Miechnikov -- in seventieth anniversary of being awarded the Nobel Prize. **Mater Med Pol** 1978 Oct–Dec;10(4):342–4
Semenov BF: Razvitie ideĭ I.I.Mechnikova v oblasti immunologii. **Zh Mikrobiol Epidemiol Immunobiol** 1984 Jul;(7):50–4
Trease GE: Elie Metchnikoff, 1845–1916. **Br J Pharm Pract** 1981;3(3):26–7
Trubina LM: K 100–letiiu fagotsitarnoĭ teorii I. I. Mechnikova. **Zh Mikrobiol Epidemiol Immunobiol** 1983 Dec;(12):99–101
Vladimirova LB: Voprosy bor'by s infektsionnymi zabolevaniiami na VII s'ezde russkikh estestvoispytateleĭ i vracheĭ (k 100–letiiu teorii fagotsitoza). **Zh Mikrobiol Epidemiol Immunobiol** 1984 Aug;(8):115–8

**Meckel, Johann Friedrich, 1781–1833**
Mullen PC: The commemoration of the Meckel bicentennial: Bozeman 1982. **Am J Med Genet** 1984 Aug;18(4):565–9
Schierhorn H: Johann Friedrich Meckel d. J. als Begründer der wissenschaftlichen Teratologie. **Gegenbaurs Morphol Jahrb** 1984;130(3):399–439
Seidler E: Johann Friedrich Meckel the Younger (1781–1833). **Am J Med Genet** 1984 Aug;18(4):571–86

**Medawar, Peter Brian, 1915–**
Advances in immunology: a meeting in honor of Sir Peter Medawar: **Cell Immunol** 1981 Aug;62(2):233–310
Peter Brian Medawar: **Cell Immunol** 1981 Aug;62(2):235–42

**Medgyessy, Ferenc, 1881–**
Szállási A: Medgyessy Ferenc medikuskori rajzaiból. **Orvostort Kozl** 1979;87–88(25 no 1–2):315–9
Szállási A: Egy medikus müvészi metamorfózisa (100 éve születell Medgyessy Ferenc). **Orv Hetil** 1981 Mar 22;122(12):709–11

**Medici, Francesco de, 1541–1587**
Bencivenni M: Il Principe dello Studiolo. **Kos** 1984 Jul–Aug;1(6):52–78

**Meduna, Ladislas Joseph, 1896–**
Fink M: Meduna and the origins of convulsive therapy. **Am J Psychiatry** 1984 Sep;141(9):1034–41

**Medvedev, Zhores Aleksandrovich, 1925–**
Green D: The Medvedev experience: 1984 and medicine. **Perspect Biol Med** 1976 Autumn;20(1):145–55

**Meek, Walter Joseph, 1878–1963**
Brooks CM: Walter Joseph Meek: August 15, 1878–February 15, 1963. **Biogr Mem Natl Acad Sci** 1983;54:251–68

**Meeker, Edward Franklin, 1943–1980**
Higgs R: Edward Franklin Meeker (1943–1980). **Explor Econ Hist** 1981;18(2):209–10

**Mehliss, John Max, 1868–1927**
Collins TF: John Max Mehliss, M.D. A Transvaal medical pioneer. **S Afr Med J** 1983 Jun 29;Spec No:14–6

**Meiers, Joseph, 1894–**
Meiers J: Joseph Meiers' autobiography 1894--an Adlerian physician's mostly non–medical life story. **J Individ Psychol** 1981 Nov;37(2):205–26

**Meige, Henry, 1866–1940**
Tolosa ES, Klawans HL: Meiges disease: a clinical form of facial

convulsion, bilateral and medical. **Arch Neurol** 1979 Oct;36(10):635-7

**Meister, Georg, 1653-1713**
Muntschick W: Ein Manuskript von Georg Meister, dem Kunst- und Lustgärtner, in der British Library. **Medizinhist J** 1984;19(3):225-32

**Melanchthon, Philipp, 1497-1560**
Kapronczay K: Magyar medikusok a wittenbergi egyetemen Luther és Melanchton korában. **Orv Hetil** 1984 Apr 15;125(16):958-60

**Melancon, Marie-Vénérande, 1754-1817**
Rousseau F: Marie-Vénérande Melançon. In Dictionary of Canadian biography, 1801 to 1820. Volume 5, 1983. p. 587-8.

**Meleney, Frank Lamont, 1889-**
Sandusky WR: Frank L. Meleney: pioneer surgeon-bacteriologist. **Arch Surg** 1983 Feb;118(2):151 5

**Mélier, François, 1798-1866**
Coleman W: Medicine against Malthus: François Mélier on the relation between subsistence and mortality (1843). **Bull Hist Med** 1980 Spring;54(1):23-42

**Mellon Family**
Witten LC, Pachella R, ed: Alchemy and the occult: a catalogue of books and manuscripts from the collection of Paul and Mary Mellon given to Yale University Library. Vols. 3 and 4: Manuscripts 1225-1922. With an introduction by P. Kibre and additional notes by W. McGuire. New Haven, Yale University Library, 1977. 853 p.

**Mel'man, Efim Petrovich, 1913-**
Zeliak VL: Efim Petrovich Mel'man (k 70-letiiu so dnia rozhdeniia). **Arkh Anat Gistol Embriol** 1983 Nov;85(11):102-7

**Mel'nikov-Razvedenkov, Nikolaĭ Fedorovich, 1866-1937**
Onopchenko NA, Gun'ko MA, Eremin VM: Nikolaĭ Fedotovich Mel'nikov-Razvedenkov--zamechatel'nyĭ organizator i vidnyĭ uchenyĭ-patologoanatom. **Arkh Patol** 1983;45(10):78-82

**Meltzer, Samuel James, 1851-1920**
Harvey AM: Samuel J. Meltzer: pioneer catalyst in the evolution of clinical science in America. **Perspect Biol Med** 1978 Spring;21(3):431-40

**Melus, fl. 6th cent.**
Bayliss JH: The earliest British medical practitioner? **Lancet** 1984 Dec 22;2(8417-18):1458

**Menaker, Esther, 1907-**
Lerner L: Esther Menaker. **Psychoanal Rev** 1984 Spring;71(1):iii-viii

**Mendel, Gregor Johann, 1822-1884**
Campbell M: Mendel's theory: its context and plausibility. **Centaurus** 1982;26(1):38-69
Cock AG: Faking and the intent to deceive. **Br Med J** 1980 Nov 1;281(6249):1214-5
Cock AG: William Bateson's pilgrimages to Brno. Cesty Williama Batesona do Brna. **Folia Mendeliana** 1980;65(15):243-50
Cruz-Coke R: Centenario de la muerte de Mendel. **Rev Med Chil** 1984 Jan;112(1):61-4
Frolov IT, Pastushnyi SA: Dialektika istoricheskoi formny i soderzhaniia otkrytiia G. Mendelia. **Vopr Istor Estestvozn Tekh** 1981;(4):20-8
George W: The Mendel enigma, the farmer's son: the key to Mendel's motivation. **Arch Int Hist Sci (Paris)** 1982 Dec;32(109):177-83
Gregor Johann Mendel 1822-1884. In centenary commemoration: **Hereditas** 1984;100(1):2-13
Guédès M: Qu'est-ce qu'un mendélien? **Hist Nat** 1980-81;17-18:69-75
Karp LE: Genetic drift. A question of discovery: Part II. **Am J Med Genet** 1983 Aug;15(4):533-5
Karp LE: Genetic drift. A question of discovery: Part I. **Am J Med Genet** 1983 Jul;15(3):379-81
Loevy HT, Kowitz A: Health science on stamps. **J Am Dent Assoc** 1984 May;108(5):797
MacRoberts MH: L. H. Bailey's citations to Gregor Mendel. **J Hered** 1984 Nov-Dec;75(6):500-1
Matalová A: Published primary sources to Gregor Mendel's biography. Mendelianum of the Moravian Museum, Brno. **Folia Mendeliana** 1981;16:239-51
Matalová A: G. Mendel and the foundation of genetics. **Folia Mendeliana** 1983;18:277-85
Monaghan F, Corcos A: On the origins of the Mendelian laws. **J Hered** 1984 Jan-Feb;75(1):67-9
Oldroyd D: Gregor Mendel: founding-father of modern genetics? **Endeavour** 1984;8(1):29-31
Pilgrim I: The too-good-to-be-true paradox and Gregor Mendel. **J Hered** 1984 Nov-Dec;75(6):501-2
Ríman J: From Mendel to molecular genetics and biotechnologies. **Folia Biol (Praha)** 1983;29(1):1-8
Root-Bernstein RS: Mendel and methodology. **Hist Sci** 1983 Sep;21(53 pt 3):275-95
Sandler IL: Pierre Louis Moreau de Maupertuis--a precursor of Mendelian genetics?: an inquiry into the biological ideas of Maupertuis, the Mendelian principles of heredity and the nature of the precursor. Ph.D. diss. University of Washington. Seattle, 1979. 265 leaves.
Sermonti G: Gregor Mendel (1822-1884). **Riv Biol** 1984 Spring;77(1):105-13
Serre JL: Mendel's rejection of the concept of blending inheritance. **Fundam Sci** 1981;2(1):55-66
Soudek D: Gregor Mendel and the people around him (commemorative of the centennial of Mendel's death). **Am J Hum Genet** 1984 May;36(3):495-8

**Mendeleev, Dmitriĭ Ivanovich, 1824-1907**
Semenova EI: Pervaia detskaia lechebnaia koloniia v Rossii (K 150-letiiu so dnia rozhdeniia D.I. Mendeleeva). **Pediatriia** 1984 Sep;(9):78-9

**Mendeleva, Iuliĭ Aronovich, 1883-1959**
Mikirtichan GL: Iu. A. Mendeleva--vidnyĭ organizator sovetskogo zdravookhraneniia (1883-1959). **Sov Zdravookhr** 1983;(11):59-62

**Mendenhall, Dorothy Reed, 1874-1964**
Robinton ED: Dorothy Reed Mendenhall. In: Notable American women. The modern period. Cambridge, Mass., Belknap-Harvard Univ. Press, 1980. 4:468-70.

**Mendez Alvaro, Francisco, 1803-1883**
Mendez Alvaro F: Historia del periodismo medico y farmacéutico en España. Ed. J. Riera. Valladolid, Universidad de Valladolid, 1978. 179 p. (Acta Historico-Medica Vallisoletana, Monografias, VIII).

**Méndez, Cristóbal, fl. 1517**
Somolinos Palencia J: Cristobal Mendez medico y cientifico del siglo XVI. **Bol Soc Mex Hist Filos Med** 1982 Jun;6(39):43-7

**Menelik II, Emperor of Ethiopia, 1844-1913**
Rosenfeld CP: The medical history of Menilek II, Emperor of Ethiopia (1844-1913): a case of medical diplomacy. **Munger Afr Libr Notes** 1978(45-46):3-43

**Ménétrier, Pierre Eugene, 1859-1935**
Olsson JE, Reichard H: Mannen bakom syndromet: Pierre Ménétrier. Tumörpatolog och mikrobiolog med tidig insikt om precanceröśa förändringar. **Lakartidningen** 1984 Oct 10;81(41):3705-6

**Mengele, Josef, 1911-**
Truck B: Mengele, l'ange de la mort. La vie diabolique du docteur Josef Mengele, médecin-chef du camp d'extermination d'Auschwitz. Paris, Presses de la cité, 1976. 248 p.

**Menière, Prosper, 1799-1862**
Chalat NI: Who was Prosper Menière and why am I still so dizzy? **Am J Otol** 1979 Jul;1(1):52-6
Pappas DG, Galanos AN: Prosper Ménière: beyond the controversial autopsy report. **South Med J** 1982 Apr;75(4):470-2
Rauchfuss A: Zur korrekten Schreibweise des Namens von Prosper Menière und einige Anmerkungen zu Leben und Werk. **Laryngol Rhinol Otol (Stuttg)** 1984 Aug;63(8):381-5

**Mennell, Zebulon, 1876-1959**
Hunter AR: Zebulon Mennell. A pioneer of neurosurgical anaesthesia. **Anaesthesia** 1983 Dec;38(12):1214-6

**Menner, Adolf, 1824-1901**
Menner O: Menner Adolf dr. (1824-1901). **Orv Hetil** 1983 Jun 12;124(24):1451-3

**Menninger, Karl Augustus, 1893-**
Karl Menninger: a literary self-portrait: A celebration issue for his 90th birthday. **Bull Menninger Clin** 1983 Jul;47(4):293-400
Pruyser PW: Religio medici: Karl A. Menninger, Calvinism and the Presbyterian Church. **J Presbyt Hist** 1981;59(1):59-72

**Menten, Maud Leonora, 1879-1960**
Fetterman GH: Maud L. Menten (1879-1960). **Perspect Pediatr Pathol** 1984 Spring;1(1):5-7

**Menzel, Arthur, 1844-1878**
Premuda L: Arthur Menzel (1844-1878), einer der liebsten und tüchtigsten Schüler und der treuesten Freunde Billroths, Primarchirung in Triest. **Gesnerus** 1981;38:191-205

**Mepsche, Rudolf de**
Kooij CG van der: Rudolf de Mepsche en de Faanse processen. **Spiegel Hist** 1979;14(6):358-64

**Mercado, Luis, 1525?-1611**
Ballester R: La utilizacion de los clasicos en la obra pediatrica de Luis Mercado (1525-1611). **Asclepio** 1978-79;30-31:307-18

**Mercator, Gerhardus, 1512-1594**
McKusick VA: The human genome through the eyes of Mercator and Vesalius. **Trans Am Clin Climatol Assoc** 1980;92:66-90

**Mercer, Hugh, ca. 1726-1777**
Trice ER: Hugh Mercer: physician-hero of the American Revolution. **Va Med** 1981 Feb;108(2):104-6

**Merck, George Wilhelm, 1894-1957**
Young JH: George Wilhelm Merck. In Dictionary of American Biography, Suppl. 6, 1956-1960. p. 447-8, 1980.

**Merck, Heinrich Emanuel, 1794-1855**
Götz W: Die Bedeutung Johann Bartholomäus Trommsdorffs für die Entwicklung der Chemie in Deutschland zu Beginn des 19. Jahrhunderts. Ein Versuch anhand seiner Korrespondenz mit Justus von Liebig und Heinrich Emanuel Merck. In Dilg P, et al., ed: Perspektiven der Pharmaziegeschichte. Graz, Austria, Akademische

Druck- u. Verlagsanstalt, 1983. p. 97-112.

**Merkel, Friedrich Sigmund, 1845-1919**
Weissmann A, Camisa C: Friedrich Sigmund Merkel. **Am J Dermatopathol** 1982 Dec;4(6):521-35

**Merle d'Aubigné, Robert, 1900-**
Merle d'Aubigné R: Surfing the wave: fifty years in the growth of French orthopedic surgery. **Clin Orthop** 1982 Nov-Dec;(171):3-23

**Merrick, Joseph Carey, 1862-1890**
Bean WB, Felson B, Dolan KD: A nonletter from the editor and a case for all seasons. **Semin Roentgenol** 1982 Jul;17(3):153-62
Carswell H: 'Elephant Man' had more than neurofibromatosis. **JAMA** 1982 Sep 3;248(9):1032-3
Howell M, Ford P: The true history of the elephant man. Harmondsworth, England, Penguin Books, 1980. 223 p.
Karp LE: The elephant man. **Am J Med Genet** 1981;10(1):1-3
Karp LE: More on the Elephant Man. **Am J Med Genet** 1982 Nov;13(3):355
Riley J: The elephant man: 'Treat me as an equal' (John Merrick, Sir Frederick Treves). **Nurs Mirror** 1979 Nov 8;149(19):24-5

**Merrill, James, 1926-**
White E: The inverted type: homosexuality as a theme in James Merrill's prophetic books. **J Homosex** 1983 Spring-Summer;8(3-4):47-52

**Merritt, Hiram Houston, 1902-1979**
Aring CD: The Boston City Hospital days with Drs. Merritt and Putnam. **Epilepsia** 1983;24 Suppl 1:S1-3
Friedman AP: Houston Merritt. In Rose FC, Bynum WF, ed: Historical aspects of the neurosciences. New York, Raven, 1982. p. 379-82.
Rowland LP: Changing approaches to the management of seizures: pharmacologic considerations. Introduction. **Epilepsia** 1982;23 Suppl 1:S1-4

**Merritt, J. Webster, 1906-1963**
Straight WM: Florida's medical historian--J. Webster Merritt. **J Fla Med Assoc** 1979 Aug;66(8):860-5

**Merskey, Clarence, 1914-1982**
Nossel HL, Spaet TH: Clarence Merskey (1914-1982). **Thromb Res** 1983 Jun 1;30(5):401-5

**Mertens, Charles de, 1737-1788**
Mertens C. de: An account of the plague which raged at Moscow, 1771. Facsimile of London, 1799, edition, with introduction and bibliography by J. Alexander. Newtonville, Mass., Oriental Research Partners, 1977. 39, 6, v, 122 p.

**Meryon, Charles, 1821-1868**
Ackerknecht EH: Charles Meryon and physicians. **J Hist Med Allied Sci** 1984 Oct;39(4):462-4

**Mesmer, Franz Anton, 1734-1815**
Glowatzki G: Der Mesmerismus--und seine Spuren in der heutigen Medizin. **ZFA (Stuttgart)** 1983 Sep 10;59(25):1360-6
Hoffeld DR: Mesmer's failure: sex, politics, personality, and the Zeitgeist. **J Hist Behav Sci** 1980 Oct;16(4):377-86
Josipovici J: Franz Anton Mesmer, magnétiseur, médecin et franc-maçon. Monaco, Editions du Rocher, 1982. 200 p.
Pattie FA: A Mesmer-Paradis myth dispelled. **Am J Clin Hypn** 1979 Jul;22(1):29-31
Schott H: Die Mitteilung des Lebensfeuers. Zum therapeutischen Konzept von Franz Anton Mesmer (1734-1815). **Medizinhist J** 1982;17(3):195-214
Sutton G: The magnetic hands. **Med Instrum** 1984 Jul-Aug;18(4):247

**Messerschmidt, Franz Xaver, 1736-1783**
Glandien O: Franz Xaver Messerschmidt (1736-1783) - Ausdrucksstudien und Charakterköpfe, Köln: 1981. 205 p. (Kölner medizinhistorische Beiträge: Arbeiten der Forschungsstelle des Instituts für Geschichte der Medizin der Universität zu Köln, Band 20).

**Messini, Mariano, 1901-**
Messina B: Mariano Messini, il suo insegnamento: le basi scientifiche della terapia termale. **Clin Ter** 1982 Nov 30:103(4):351-6

**Mesuë, d. 857**
Ibn Masawayh Y: Le livre des axiomes médicaux (aphorismi). Edition du texte arabe et des versions latines avec traduction française et lexique par Danielle Jacquart et Gérard Troupeau. Geneva, Librairie Droz, 1980. iii, 368 p. (Centre de Recherches d'Histoire et de Philologie, II; Hautes Etudes Orientales, 14).
Weisser U: The embryology of Yuhanna ibn Masawaith. **J Hist Arabic Sci** 1980;4(1):9-22

**Mészáros, Kálmán**
Kálmán G: Mészáros Kálmán emlékezete. **Orv Hetil** 1983 Apr;124(16):962-7

**Metcalf, William George, 1847-1885**
Greenland C: William George Metcalf. In Dictionary of Canadian biography, 1881-1890. 1982;11:590-1.

**Metcalfe, John Thomas, 1818-1902**
Chernin E: Two physicians, a landscape architect, and malaria. **Bull NY Acad Med** 1984 Nov;60(9):932-7

**Metcalfe, Samuel Lytler, 1798-1856**
Watanabe M: The caloric theory of S. L. Metcalfe. **Br J Hist Sci** 1984 Jul;17(56 pt 2):210-3

**Metzig, Johann Christian Heinrich, 1804-1868**
Gołebiowski SZ: Niemiecki lekarz Jan Metzig (1804--1868) przyjacielem Polaków. **Arch Hist Med (Warsz)** 1979;42(3):295-301

**Meyer, Adolf, 1866-1950**
Leys R: Meyer's dealings with Jones: a chapter in the history of the American response to psychoanalysis. **J Hist Behav Sci** 1981 Oct;17(4):445-65
Mindham RH: My father knew Adolf Meyer. The currency of Meyer's ideas in British psychiatry. **Br J Psychiatry** 1984 Mar;144:323-5
Neill JR: Adolf Meyer and American psychiatry today. **Am J Psychiatry** 1980 Apr;137(4):460-4
Walser HH: Adolf Meyer--student of the Zurich psychiatric school. **Gesnerus** 1984;41(1/2):49-52

**Meyer-Ahrens, Conrad, 1813-1872**
Ilić D: Conrad Meyer-Ahrens (1813-1872) und sein Werk über die Heilquellen und Kurorte der Schweiz. Zürich, Juris, 1975. 61 p.

**Meynell, Richard, fl. 1663**
Burnby J: Three 17th century London apothecaries; Richard Meynell, Charles Needham, William Booker. **Pharm Hist (London)** 1975 May;5(1):2-3

**Meyssonnier, Lazare, 1602-1672**
Trevisani F: Un corrispondente di Cartesio: alcune note su Lazare Meyssonnier (1611/12-1673), medico e astrologo lionese e sulla sua Belle Magie (1669). **Hist Philos Life Sci** 1979;1(2):285-308

**Miasnikov, Aleksandr Leonidovich**
Borodulin VI: A. L. Miasnikov i ego rol' v formirovanii kardiologii v SSSR. **Kardiologiia** 1979;19(12):99-101

**Michael, Saint**
Devaux G: Saint Michel, patron des apothicaires de Bordeaux et d'autres lieux. **Rev Hist Pharm (Paris)** 1982;29(252):151-9

**Michaelson, Isaac Chesar, 1903-**
Patz A: Retinal neovascularisation: early contributions of Professor Michaelson and recent observations. **Br J Ophthalmol** 1984 Jan;68(1):42-6

**Michelangelo, 1475-1564**
DiGeronimo EM, Marraccini P: Body-mind sculpture: battle of the titans. **Plast Reconstr Surg** 1984 Feb;73(2):324-5
Liebert RS: Michelangelo: a psychoanalytic study of his life and images. New Haven, Yale University Press, 1983. xxii, 447 p.
Rosenzweig W: Disease in art: a case for carcinoma of the breast in Michelangelo's La notte. **Paleopathol Newsl** 1983 Mar;41:8-11
Steinberg L: Michelangelo and the doctors. **Bull Hist Med** 1982;56(4):543-53
Verellen T: Cosmas and Damian in the New Sacristy [Medici Chapel of San Lorenzo, Florence]. **J Warburg Courtauld Inst** 1979;42:274-7

**Michelet, Jules, 1798-1874**
Jordanova LJ: Romantic science? Michelet, morals, and nature. **Br J Hist Sci** 1980 Mar;13(43 pt 1):44-50

**Michelson, M. J., 1912-1978**
Voronov IB, Zeimal EV: Obituary: Professor M. J. Michelson (died 16 August 1978). The contribution of Professor M. J. Michelson to comparative and evolutionary pharmacology. **Comp Biochem Physiol** 1979;62C(1):1-4

**Michon, Louis, 1892-1973**
Monod-Broca P: Louis Michon, 1892-1973. **Chirurgie** 1981;107(1):13-22

**Mickiewicz, Adam, 1798-1855**
Adelsen CE: The last days of Adam Mickiewicz, poet of freedom. **Mankind** 1976;5(5):16-20, 60-1

**Mickle, Samuel, fl. 1793**
Snape WJ, Wolfe EL: Courage, compassion, and providence: Woodbury 1793. **Bull Gloucester Cty Hist Soc** 1984 Dec;19(6):41-4

**Middelburg, Paulus van, 1445-1533**
Sambin P: Il dottorato padovano in medicina di Paolo da Middelburgo (1480). **Quad Stor Univ Padova** 1976-7;9-10:252-6

**Middleton, Peter, d. 1781**
Hershkowitz L: Powdered tin and rose petals: Myer Myers, Goldsmith, and Peter Middleton, physician. **Am Jew Hist** 1981;70(4):462-7

**Mieli, Aldo, 1879-1950**
Babini J: Para una bibliografía de Aldo Mieli. **Physis** 1979;21(1-4):357-424

**Mierzecki, Henryk, 1891-1977**
Mierzecki H: Czasy i klimaty. **Kwart Hist Nauki Tech** 1981;26(3-4):503-32

**Mikhaĭlov, Sergeĭ Sergeevich**
Sergeĭ Sergeevich Mikhailov (k 60-letiiu so dnia rozhdeniia): **Arkh Anat Gistol Embriol** 1980 Mar;78(3):121-5

**Mikulicz von Radecki, Johann, 1850-1905**
Kaiser W, Skrobacki A: Królewieckie listy Jana Mukulicza de Fryderyka Althoffa. **Komun Mazursko Warm** 1975;4(130):455-65

Paul U: Das chirurgische Erbe: Johann von Mikulicz-Radecki. **Zentralbl Chir** 1981;106(7):469–72
Piotrowski E: Jan Mikulicz Radecki we Wrocławiu. **Arch Hist Med (Warsz)** 1979;42(3):351–7

**Miles, Ashley A., 1904–**
Burke JF: Ashley A. Miles and the prevention of infection following surgery. **Arch Surg** 1984 Jan;119(1):17–9

**Mill, James, 1773–1836**
Ball T: Platonism and penology: James Mill's attempted synthesis. **J Hist Behav Sci** 1982 Jul;18(3):222–9

**Mill, John Stuart, 1806–1873**
Kowalewski D: Politics and emotion in the thought of John Stuart Mill. **J Psychohist** 1980 Spring;7(4):455–66
Losee J: Whewell and Mill on the relation between philosophy of science and history of science. **Stud Hist Philos Sci** 1983 Jun;14(2):113–26
Shaw JA: The postadolescent crisis of John Stuart Mill. **Adolesc Psychiatry** 1982;10:85–98

**Miller, Edward, 1760–1812**
Chinard FP: Edward Miller--American physician (1760–1812). **J Med Soc NJ** 1981 Apr;78(4):296–9

**Miller, Hugh**
Pattison FL: The Pattison-Miller quarrel. **Scott Med J** 1980 Jul;25(3):234–40

**Miller, Willoughby Dayton, 1853–1907**
Bowers DF: W. D. Miller: a second pilgrimage to his home. **Ohio Dent J** 1982 Mar;56(3):15–23
Hoffmann-Axthelm W: W. D. Miller - Ein Pionier der wissenschaftlichen Zahnheilkunde. **Quintessenz J** 1983 Oct;13(10):927–30
Künzel W: Willoughby Dayton Miller zur 75. Wiederkehr des Todestages am 29. 7. 1982. **Zahn Mund Kieferheilkd** 1982;70(6):579–83
Marvitz L: Manden bag navnet. **Tidsskr Tandlaeger** 1983 Apr;3:51
Millstein CB: W. D. Miller and the beginnings of occupational hygiene in dentistry. **Bull Hist Dent** 1984 Oct;32(2):135–6
Tanzer G: Willoughby Dayton Miller (1853–1907). **Zahnarzt** 1984 May;28(5):375–6

**Milne, John Alexander, 1920–1977**
McQueen A: John Alexander Milne. **J Cutan Pathol** 1977 Dec;4(6):349–52

**Milner, John, fl. 1805**
Champ JF: Bishop Milner, Holywell, and the cure tradition. In Sheils WJ, ed: The Church and healing. Papers read at the twentieth summer meeting and the twenty-first winter meeting of the Ecclesiastical History Society. Oxford, Basil Blackwell for the Society, 1982. p. 153–64.

**Milton, John, 1608–1674**
Mutschmann H: Milton's eyesight and the chronology of his works. New York, Haskell House, 1971. 50 p.

**Minkowska, Franciszka, 1882–1950**
Ostrowska T: Dr Franciska Minkowska (1882–1950), psychiatra i psychoannalityk, twórca pojęcia gliskroidii. W 100-lecie urodzin. **Arch Hist Med (Warsz)** 1983;46(1):39–44

**Minkowski, Oskar, 1858–1931**
Angeli I: 50 éve halt meg Oskar Minkowski a pancreas-diabetes felfedezöje. **Orv Hetil** 1981 Jul 12;122(28):1726–9
Binet JL: Histoire de la sphèrocytose congénitale. **Nouv Rev Fr Hematol** 1981 Sep;23(3):177–84
Kaiser W, Völker A: Oskar Minkowski (1858–1931). **Z Gesamte Inn Med** 1981 Dec 15;36(24):973–9
Zefirova GS, Lebedev VV: Oskar Minkovskiĭ. **Klin Med (Mosk)** 1983 Apr;61(4):119–20

**Minoka-Hill, Lillie Rosa, 1876–1952**
Apple RD: Lillie Rosa Minoka-Hill. In: Notable American women. The modern period. Cambridge, Mass., Belknap-Harvard Univ. Press, 1980. 4:481–3.

**Minor, Lazar Solomo**
Idel'chik KhI: Problema bor'by s alkogolizmom v nauchnoĭ obshchestvennoĭ deiatel'nosti professora L. S. Minora (k 125-letiiu so dnia rozhdeniia). **Sov Zdravookhr** 1981;(3):63–6

**Minot, George Richards, 1885–1950**
Crosby WH: Landmark perspective. Pernicious anemia. **JAMA** 1983 Dec 23–30;250(24):3336–8

**Minovici Family**
Ioanid N, Angelescu B: Fraţii Minovici. Bucureşti, Editura Ştiinţifică, 1970. 174 p.

**Mira y López, Emilio, 1896–**
Pigem Serra JM: Emilio Mira y López y su entorno. **Arch Neurobiol (Madr)** 1982 Mar–Apr;45(2):135–56

**Miroliubov, V. P., 1870–1947**
Ordina OM: Professor V. P. Miroliubov (k 110-letiiu so dnia rozhdeniia). **Arkh Patol** 1982;44(7):80–3

**Mironescu, Eugene I., 1883–1939**
Marinescu CG: Concepţiile social-politice ale Profesorului Dr. E. I. Mironescu (II). **Rev Med Chir Soc Med Nat Iasi** 1979 Jan–Mar;83(1):159–62

**Mirsky, Alfred Ezra, 1900–1974**
Kopp C: The Alfred E. Mirsky papers at the Rockefeller University Archives. **Mendel Newsl** 1983 Nov;23:1–4

**Missoux, Damien Théodore, 1800–1863**
Pomel ML: La médecine d'autrefois d'après des documents inédits. Le docteur Missoux (1800–1863). Rodez, Editions Subervie, 1979. 162 p.

**Mitchell, John Kearsley, 1798–1858**
Animalcular and cryptogamic theories on the origins of fevers. Reprinted works by John Kearsley Mitchell (1849), John L. Riddell (1836), Josiah Clark Nott (1848). New York, Arno, 1977. Various paginations.:

**Mitchell, Silas Weir, 1829–1914**
Fye WB: S. Weir Mitchell, Philadelphia's 'lost' physiologist. **Bull Hist Med** 1983 Summer;57(2):188–202
Poirier S: The Weir Mitchell rest cure: doctor and patients. **Womens Stud** 1983;10(1):15–40
Schneck JM: S. Weir Mitchell and Oliver Wendell Holmes. A friendship and poetic tribute. **JAMA** 1981 Aug 28;246(9):974–8
Schneck JM: S. Weir Mitchell, M.D. (1829 to 1914) and D. Hayes Agnew, M.D. (1818 to 1892). Neuropsychiatrist's poetic tribute to a surgeon. **NY State J Med** 1982 Jul;82(8):1264–8
Schneck JM: Brain injury, psychiatric sequelae, and surgical intervention in S. Weir Mitchell's Westways. **JAMA** 1983 Dec 9;250(22):3048

**Mitchiner, Philip Henry, 1888–1952**
Gray TC: 'Another side of Mars'. **J R Army Med Corps** 1984 Feb;130(1):3–11

**Mitscherlich, Alexander, 1908–1982**
Alexander Mitscherlich: Zur Dynamik des Wechsels von Depression und organischem Symptom. **Psyche (Stuttg)** 1983 Oct;37(10):905–20
Alexander Mitscherlich: Aus der Analyse eines Gummi-Fetischisten. **Psyche (Stuttg)** 1983 Oct;37(10):867–904
Fetscher I: Alexander Mitscherlich--zur Pathologie der bundesdeutschen Gesellschaft. **Psyche (Stuttg)** 1983 Apr;37(4):298–310
Habermas J: Bemerkungen zu Alexander Mitscherlichs analytischer Socialpsychologie. **Psyche (Stuttg)** 1983 Apr;37(4):352–63
König R: Alexander Mitscherlich: Psychoanalyse und Zeitkritik (1969). **Psyche (Stuttg)** 1983 Oct;37(10):921–60
Loch W: Alexander Mitscherlich und die Wiedergeburt der Psychoanalyse in Deutschland. **Psyche (Stuttg)** 1983 Apr;37(4):336–45
Parin P: Psychoanalyse als Gesellschaftskritik im Werk von Alexander Mitscherlich. **Psyche (Stuttg)** 1983 Apr;37(4):364–73
Rattner J: Alexander Mitscherlich. In J. Rattner, ed: Wandlungen der Psychoanalyse. Wien, Europaverlag, 1980. p. 211–32.
Rosenkötter L: Alexander Mitscherlich als Chef und Lehrer. **Psyche (Stuttg)** 1983 Apr;37(4):346–51
Thomä H: Von der Psychosomatischen Medizin zur Psychoanalyse--Heidelberg 1949–1967. **Psyche (Stuttg)** 1983 Apr;37(4):322–35
Unseld S: Versuch, die Welt besser zu bestehen. **Psyche (Stuttg)** 1983 Apr;37(4):311–21

**Mitskevich, Sergeĭ Ivanovich, 1869–1944**
Idel'chik KhI: Vrachi-bol'sheviki S. I. Mitskevich i S. I. Chernomordik u istokov Tsentral'nogo muzeia revoliutsii SSSR (k 60-letiiu muzeia). **Sov Zdravookhr** 1984;(9):56–9

**Miyahara, Tatsutaro, 1878–1926**
Omuro A: X-sen igakukai no senkusha Miyahara Tatsutaro. Ichihara, Japan. Ichihara-shi Kyoiku Iinkai, Showa 50 nen [1975] 88 p.

**Möbius, Paul Julius, 1853–1907**
Schiller F: A Möbius strip. Fin-de-siècle neuropsychiatry and Paul Möbius. Berkeley, University of California Press, 1982. 134 p.
Theopold W: Paul Julius Möbius (1853–1907). **Medizinhist J** 1983;18(1-2):100–17
Waldeck-Semadeni EK: Paul Julius Moebius, 1853–1907, Leben und Werk. Diss. Bern, 1980. 222 p.

**Moffet, Thomas, 1553–1604**
Selwyn S: The transition from mythology to medical microbiology in 1589. In: Congrès international d'histoire de la médecine, XXVe, Québec, 1976. Actes. Québec, 1977. p. 1262–73.

**Mohammed, the Prophet, ca. 570–632**
Nassimi MN: The achievements of the Arab Prophet in the field of hygiene and preventive medicine. In: International Symposium for the History of Arabic Science, 1st, University of Aleppo, 1976. Proceedings. Aleppo, Syria, 1976. Papers in European Languages. Vol. II. p. 343–5.

**Mohr, Hans Jürgen, 1922–1982**
Hans-Jürgen Mohr (1. 11. 1922 bis 7. 6. 1982): **Verh Dtsch Ges Pathol** 1983;67:762–71

**Mohs, Frederic, 1910–**
The evolution of Mohs' surgery: **J Dermatol Surg Oncol** 1982 Aug;8(8):650–4

**Moir, Andrew, 1806–1844**
Bayliss RA: Andrew Moir: an Aberdeen anatomist. **Scott Med J** 1980;25:315–9

**Moir, Chassar, fl. 1932**
MacDonald RR: Classic illustrations: From St. Anthony's fire to ergometrine (Ergonovine). **Eur J Obstet Gynecol Reprod Biol** 1982 Aug;13(5):325–7

**Moissan, Henri, 1852–1907**
Viel C: Quelques vers et écrits de jeunesse d'Henri Moissan. **Rev Hist Pharm (Paris)** 1984 Mar;31(260):5–12

**Molchanov, Vasiliĭ Ivanovich, 1868–1959**
Lebedev DD, Kovaleva EV, Semenova VN: Nekotorye voprosy revmatizma, éndokrinnykh i nervnykh zabolevaniĭ u deteĭ v trudakh V.I. Molchanova i ego uchenikov (k 110-letiiu so dnia rozhdeniia). **Pediatriia** 1980 Aug;(8):64–7

**Moldovan, Iuliu, 1882–**
Negru I: Profesorul Iuliu Moldovan creatorul primului Institut oncologic în România. **Viata Med [Medii Sanit]** 1982 Dec;30(12):281–6

**Molière, Jean Baptiste Poquelin, 1622–1673**
Jackson R: Raynaud and Molière. **Arch Dermatol** 1983 Mar;119(3):263–6
McBride R: The sceptical view of medicine and the comic vision in Molière. **Studi Francesi** 1979, 23(67):27–42

**Molins, Edward, 1610?–1663**
Morris GC: Which Molins treated Cromwell for stone--and did not prescribe for Pepys? **Med Hist** 1982 Oct;26(4):429–35

**Molins, James, d. 1638**
Morris GC: Which Molins treated Cromwell for stone--and did not prescribe for Pepys? **Med Hist** 1982 Oct;26(4):429–35

**Molins, James, 1631–1687**
Morris GC: Which Molins treated Cromwell for stone--and did not prescribe for Pepys? **Med Hist** 1982 Oct;26(4):429–35

**Moll, Albert, 1862–1939**
Shelley HS: The Moll Collection on hypnotism at Vanderbilt. **Bull Med Libr Assoc** 1977 Jan;65(1):65–6

**Mollar, José Ignacio, fl. 1788**
Jordi González R: Criterios del boticario y academico barcelones Jose Ignacio Mollar sobre la tinta de escribir. **Offarm** 1982;1(9):453–67

**Moloney, Michael, d. c. 1935**
Corrigan D: Irish Ethno-botany by Michael Moloney--an early contribution to the concept of ethnopharmacology. **J Ethnopharmacol** 1981 Nov;4(3):343–5

**Moltke, Helmuth Karl Bernhard von, 1800–1891**
Becker H: Helmuth von Moltke als Beobachter der hygienischen und medizinischen Situation im osmanischen Kaiserreich (1835–39). In Göpfert W, Otten HH, ed: Metavoeite: wandelt euch durch neues Denken. Düsseldorf, Triltsch, 1983. p. 147–59.

**Monakow, Constantin von, 1853–1930**
Tsybul'kin AG: Vklad Konstantina Monakova v izuchenie anatomii mozga. **Arkh Anat Gistol Embriol** 1979 Nov;77(11):115–7

**Monconys, Balthasar de, 1611–1665**
Mistler J: Voyageurs d'autrefois. **Nouv Rev Deux Mondes** 1977;(2):265–75;(3):519–27

**Mondelet, Dominique, ca. 1734–1802**
Janson G: Dominique Mondelet. In Dictionary of Canadian biography, 1801 to 1820. Volume 5, 1983. p. 599–600.

**Monet, Claude, 1840–1926**
Royer J, Haut J, Amalric P: L'opération de la cataracte de Claude Monet, correspondence inédite du peintre et de G.-Clemenceau au docteur Coutela. **Hist Sci Med** 1984;18(2):109–27

**Moniz, Egas, 1874–1955**
López Ibor JJ: Egas Moniz, en su centenario. **Actas Luso Esp Neurol Psiquiatr** 1980 Jul–Aug;8(4):239–46
Schierhorn H: Egas Moniz, Wilhelm Löhr und die cerebrale Angiographie. Ein Streifzug durch die Entdeckungsgeschichte der Hirngefässe. **J Hirnforsch** 1981;22(5):491–515

**Monluc, Blaise de, 1500–1577**
Sournia JC: Le dossier médical du maréchal Blaise de Monluc (1500–1577). **Hist Sci Med**

**Monod, Jacques Lucien, 1910–1976**
Morange M: L'oeuvre scientifique de Jacques Monod. **Fundam Sci** 1982;3:396–404

**Monro, John, 1715–1791**
Illustrations from the Wellcome Institute Library: John Monro MD and Charles James Fox: etching by Thomas Rowlandson. **Med Hist** 1983 Jan;27(1):80–3

**Mons, Jean Baptiste van, 1765–1842**
Van Elst H: Jan Baptist Van Mons: aanhanger en verdediger van de leer van Lavoisier. **Farm Tijdschr Belg** 1980;57:145–58

**Monson, George S., 1869–1933**
Hagman HC: George S. Monson, DDS. **Dent Lab Rev** 1982 Mar;57(3):36

**Montagu, Mary (Pierrepont) Wortley, 1689–1762**
McHenry S: The pox upon her. **Aramco World Mag** 1980, 31(4):13–21
Miller G: Putting Lady Mary in her place: a discussion of historical causation. **Bull Hist Med** 1981 Spring;55(1):2–16
Thomson WA: Rider Haggard and smallpox. **J R Soc Med** 1984 Jun;77(6):506–12

**Montaigne, Michel Eyquem de, 1533–1592**
Bernoulli R: Montaigne: ein Medizinprogramm im sechzehnten Jahrhundert. **Gesnerus** 1981;38:119–26
Bernoulli R: A propos d'une vieille querelle: Montaigne était-il hypocondriaque? **Hist Sci Med** 1982;16(3):145–9
Brunyate M: Montaigne and medicine. In K. Cameron, ed: Montaigne and his age. Univ. of Exeter, 1981. p. 26–38, 170–71.
Nutton V: Medicine in the age of Montaigne. In K. Cameron, ed: Montaigne and his age. Univ. of Exeter, 1981. p. 14–25, 163–70.
Rothschuh KE: Aus der Geschichte der Naturheilbewegung (IV). Hatte die Naturheilbewegung Vorläufer in der Renaissance? Montaigne, Paracelsus, Beobachtungsmedizin, Wasserheilkunde. **ZFA (Stuttgart)** 1981 Jun 10;57(16):1251–9
Starobinski J: D'Agrippa de Nettesheim à Montaigne: l'embarras de médecins devant l'origine de la semence. **Gesnerus** 1983;40(1–2):175–83

**Montalto, Philotheus Elianus, d. 1616**
Woolfson RC: Historical perspective on mental retardation. **Am J Ment Defic** 1984 Nov;89(3):231–5

**Montana de Monserrate, Bernardino, b. ca. 1482**
Rodriguez Maffiotte C: Consideraciones acerca de la obra 'Libro de anathomia del hombre', de Bernardino Montana de Monserrate. **Acta Med Tenerife** 1978;39:87–92

**Montefiore, Moses Haim, 1784–1885**
Kass AM: Dr. Thomas Hodgkin's friendship with Sir Moses Montefiore. **N Engl J Med** 1984 Feb 9;310(6):401–4
Sakula A: Dr. Thomas Hodgkin and Sir Moses Montefiore Bart--the friendship of two remarkable men. **J R Soc Med** 1979 May;72(5):382–7

**Montells y Nadall, Francisco de Paula, 1813–1893**
Fernández González M, Gago Bohórquez R: La medicina en la obra cientifica de Francisco de Paula Montells y Nadal (1813–1893). **Asclepio** 1980;32:151–9

**Montyon, Antoine Jean Baptiste Robert Auget, 1733–1820**
Coleman W: L'hygiène et l'état selon Montyon. **Dix-Huit Siecle** 1977;9:101–8
Crosland M: From prizes to grants in the support of scientific research in France in the nineteenth century: the Montyon legacy. **Minerva** 1979 Autumn;17(3):355–80

**Montz, Lucy Dupuy**
Bogardus CR: Kentucky's first woman dentist (Lucy Dupuy Montz). **Ky Dent J** 1984 Mar–Apr;36(2):23–5

**Moorcroft, William, 1765?–1825**
Alder GJ: Moorcroft's life in England; some new evidence. **Vet Hist** 1979–80;1(3):78–93
Oxford Street memorial to pioneer veterinarian (William Moorcroft): **Vet Rec** 1982 Oct 2;111(14):313

**Moore, Albertus Adair, 1834–1910**
Leland TM: Albertus Adair Moore, M.D. 1834–1910. **J SC Med Assoc** 1984 Jul;80(7):358

**Moore, Andrew Barry, 1771–1848**
Leland TM: 'First Physician in Spartanburg County' Andrew Barry Moore, M.D., 1771–1848. **J SC Med Assoc** 1983 May;79(5):299

**Moore, Austin Merrill, 1903–1957**
McCann W: (Austin) Merrill Moore. In Dictionary of American Biography, Suppl. 6, 1956–1960. p. 461–2, 1980.

**Moore, John William, 1845–1937**
Breathnach CS: John William Moore. **Ir J Med Sci** 1983 Jan;152(1):69–71

**Moore, Joseph Earle, 1892–1957**
Turner TB: Joseph Earle Moore. In Dictionary of American Biography, Suppl. 6, 1956–1960. p, 460–1, 1980.

**Mooren, Albert Clemens, 1828–1899**
Hoss J: Albert Mooren: ein Augenarzt im 19. Jahrhundert. Düsseldorf, Triltsch, 1980. 183 p. (Düsseldorfer Arbeiten zur Geschichte der Medizin, 55).
Schadewaldt H: Albert Clemens Mooren als geschichtliche Persönlichkeit. **Jahrb Univ Dusseld** 1977–78;:259–68

**Mór, Jókai, fl. 1890**
Végh F: Jókai Mór Szájmütétje 1891-ben. **Orvostort Kozl** 1979;86(24 no 4):129–30

**Móra, Ferenc, 1879–1934**
Péter L: Móra Ferenc betegségei. Halálának 50. évfordulójára. **Orv Hetil** 1984 Feb 5;125(6):341–4

**Morán, Pedro, 1771-1840**
Costa-Casaretto C: Presentación del Dr. Pedro Morán (1771-1840). **Rev Med Chil** 1984 Jul;112(7):729-38

**Moravia, Pedro, fl. 1578**
Boianov B: Iubileina godishnina na purvata doktorska disertatsiia v oblastta na stomatologiiata. **Stomatologiia (Sofiia)** 1979 Jul-Aug;61(4):256-9

**More, Thomas, 1478-1535**
Elton GR: The real Thomas More? **Psychol Med** 1980 Nov;10(4):611-7

**Moreau de Saint-Elier, Louis Malo, 1701-1754**
Vartanian A: Le frère de Maupertuis et l'homme machine. **Dix-huit Siecle** 1982;14:305-23

**Moreau, Jacques Joseph (de Tours), 1804-1884**
Nica-Udangiu S: J. Moreau de Tours (1804-1884). **Rev Med Interna [Neurol Psihiatr]** 1984 Jan-Mar;29(1):77-80
Pigeaud JM: Le rôle des passions dans la pensée médicale de Pinel à Moreau de Tours. **Hist Philos Life Sci** 1980;2(1):123-40

**Morel, Benedict-Augustin, 1809-1873**
Ledermann F: La psychiatrie française et les médicaments: Pomme, Pinel, Esquirol, Morel. **Rev Hist Pharm (Paris)** 1982 Sep;29(254):189-206

**Morell, Theodor, 1886-1948**
Katz O: Der 'Führer' behandelte sich selbst. Aus jetzt verfügbaren Aufzeichnungen des Leibarztes Theo Morell werden realistische Konturen der geheimnisvollen Krankheiten Adolf Hitlers erkennbar (I). **Fortschr Med** 1984 Oct 4;102(37):70-1
Katz O: Prof. Dr. Med. Theo Morell: Hitlers Leibarzt. Bayreuth, Hestia, 1983. 397 p.
Spann W: Prof. Dr. med. Theo Morell, Hitlers Leibarzt. **MMW** 1983 Jun 17;125(24):534-6

**Morelli, Giovanni, 1816-1891**
Ginzburg C: Morelli, Freud and Sherlock Holmes: clues and scientific method. **Hist Workshop J** 1980;9:5-36

**Moreno, Jacob Levy, 1892-1974**
Bour P: L'apport de Jacob Lévy Moréno. **Ann Med Psychol (Paris)** 1983 Dec;141(10):1079-87

**Moreno y Maïz, Thomas, fl. 1868**
Siegel RK, Hirschman A: Moreno and the first study on cocaine: a historical note and translation. **J Psychoactive Drugs** 1983 Jul-Sep;15(3):219-20

**Morestin, Hippolyte, 1869-1919**
Rogers BO: Hippolyte Morestin (1869-1919). Part I: A brief biography. **Aesthetic Plast Surg** 1982;6(3):141-7

**Morgagni, Giovanni Battista, 1682-1771**
Arquiola E: La lesión neurologica en 'De sedibus et causis morborum' de Morgagni. In: Congrès international d'histoire de la médecine, XXVe, Québec, 1976. Actes. Québec, 1977. p. 461-8.
Belloni L: Il Morgagni tra il Malpighi e il Cotugno. **Gesnerus** 1982;39(2):195-213
Campan L: Le tricentenaire de Morgagni (1682-1721). **Agressologie** 1982;23(7):291-2
Federspil G, Scandellari C: La malattia da Morgagni a oggi. **Veltro** 1982;26(5-6):417-34
Gamba A: Un ritratto inedito di Giambattista Morgagni. **Acta Med Hist Patav** 1982-83;29:67-74
Giordano A: Morgagni and the first steps of a European pathology. A brief historical report. **Pathol Res Pract** 1984 Jul;178(6):642-3
Honti J: Morgagni kórbonctana. **Orv Hetil** 1983 Jan;124(4):219-20
Lazorthes G, Campan L: Jean-Baptiste Morgagni (1682-1771), initiateur de la méthode anatomo-clinique. **Bull Acad Natl Med (Paris)** 1982 Dec;166(9):1317-21
Lindsten J: Sammanställde fall av kortvuxenhet och bristande ovariefunktion hos flickor. **Lakartidningen** 1983 Jul 13;80(28-29):2755
Ongaro G, Mazzolini RG: Quasi tradens se totum: i manoscritti morgagnani della Biblioteca Palatina di Parma. **Ann Ist Mus Stor Sci Fir** 1983;8(1):101-5
Premuda L, Bonuzzi L: Morgagni e la neuropatologia. **Acta Med Hist Patav** 1982-83;29:75-81
Premuda L: G. B. Morgagni und seine Vorstellungen über die Methodik der Medizin. **Sudhoffs Arch** 1984;68(2):173-81
Sarkisov DS: Dzh. B. Morgan'i (k 300-letiiu so dnia rozhdeniia). **Klin Med (Mosk)** 1983 Jan;61(1):110-4
Thiene G, Pennelli N: Terzo centenario della nascita di Giovanni Battista Morgagni (1682-1982): c'è ancora bisogno dell'autopsia? **G Ital Cardiol** 1983 Oct;13(10):262-4
Valvo JR, Cos LR, Cockett AT: Giovanni Battista Morgagni: his contributions to urology. **Urology** 1983 Oct;22(4):452-7
Yonace AH: Morgagni's letters. **J R Soc Med** 1980 Feb;73(2):145-9

**Morgan, Agnes Fay, 1884-1968**
Raacke ID: Agnes Fay Morgan. In: Notable American women. The modern period. Cambridge, Mass., Belknap-Harvard Univ. Press, 1980. 4:495-7.

**Morgan, John Pierpont, 1837-1913**
Dotz W, Berliner N: Rhinophyma. A master's depiction, a patron's affliction. **Am J Dermatopathol** 1984 Jun;6(3):231-5

**Morgan, John, 1735-1789**
Bluemle LW: John Morgan--the father of American medicine. In Passmore R, ed: Proceedings of the Royal College of Physicians of Edinburgh Tercentenary Congress, 1981. Edinburgh, Royal College of Physicians of Edinburgh, 1982. p. 159-61.

**Morgan, Thomas Hunt, 1866-1945**
Allen G: The transformation of a science: T. H. Morgan and the emergence of a new American biology. In Oleson A, Voss J, ed: The organization of knowledge in modern America, 1860-1920. Baltimore and London, Johns Hopkins University Press, 1979. p. 173-210.
Fuller MB: Thomas Hunt Morgan papers at the American Philosophical Society. **Mendel Newsl** 1981 Nov;21:6-8
Harwood J: The reception of Morgan's chromosome theory in Germany: inter-war debate over cytoplasmic inheritance. **Medizinhist J** 1984;19(1-2):3-32
Oppenheimer JM: Thomas Hunt Morgan as an embryologist: the view from Bryn Mawr. **Am Zool** 1983;23:845-54
Ramage JA: Thomas Hunt Morgan: family influences in the making of a great scientist. **Filson Club Hist Q** 1979;53(1):5-25

**Mori, Ogai, 1862-1922?**
Date K: ['Eisei-Shinpen'--Ogai Mori as a physician (II)] (Jpn). **Igakushi Kenkyu** 1978;51:26-41
Miyamoto S: Mori Ogai no Igakushiso (The medical thought of Ogai Mori). Tokyo, Keiso-shobo, 1979. iii, 264 p.
Okada Y: [Background of Rintaro Mori's debates on statistics] (Jpn). **Igakushi Kenkyu** 1978;49:1-13
Schauwecker D: Aspekte der Medizingeschichte Japans im 16.-19. Jhdt. und der Deutschlandaufenthalt des japanischen Schriftstellers und Mediziners Ogai Mori in den Jahren 1884-1888. **Sudhoffs Arch** 1982;66(4):350-89

**Morii, Josen, 1797-1851**
Yamagata S: [Josen Morii and his medicine.] (Jpn). **Nihon I-Shigaku Zasshi** 1981;27(1):35-46

**Morin, Louis, 1635?-1715**
Lebel M: Editions, traductions et lexiques hippocratiques. Le docteur Louis Morin, (1635-1715) et son index des mots d'Hippocrate. In: Congrès international d'histoire de la médecine, XXVe, Québec, 1976. Actes. Québec, 1977. p. 848-65.

**Morin, Marie, 1649-1730**
Bernier H: Marie Morin. In Dictionary of Canadian biography, 1701 to 1740. Volume 2, 1969. p. 489-92.

**Moritz, Alan Richard, 1899-**
Dutra FR: Electrical burns of the skin. Medicolegal investigation. **Am J Forensic Med Pathol** 1981 Dec;2(4):309-12

**Morpurgo, Samson, 1681-1740**
Benayahu M: Rabbi Samson Morpurgo. **Sinai** 1979;84:134-65

**Morsted, Thomas, ca. 1380-1456**
Russell JR: The three royal doctors of Betchworth. **Practitioner** 1981 Jul;225(1357):1070-1

**Morton, Richard, 1637-1698**
Keers RY: Richard Morton (1637-98) and his Phthisiologia. **Thorax** 1982 Jan;37(1):26-31
Silverman JA: Richard Morton, 1637-1698. Limner of anorexia nervosa: his life and times. A tercentenary essay. **JAMA** 1983 Nov 25;250(20):2830-2

**Morton, Samuel George, 1799-1851**
Spencer F: Samuel George Morton's doctoral thesis on bodily pain: the probable source of Morton's polygenism. **Trans Stud Coll Physicians Phila** 1983 Dec;5(5 no 4):321-38

**Morton, William Thomas Green, 1819-1868**
Secher O: Fra Boston til Amaliegade; anaesthesiens vej til Danmark. **Dan Medicinhist Arbog** 1981;:25-56

**Moscati, Giuseppe, 1880-1927**
Papàsogli G: Giuseppe Moscati, 1880-1927: Leben eines heiligen Arztes. Stein am Rhein [Schweiz], Christiana-Verlag, 1982. 109 p.

**Moses**
Baruk H: Moïse, Freud et le veau d'or. **Rev Hist Med Heb** 1984 Jul;37(2):19-23
Schoental R: A corner of history. Moses and mycotoxins. **Prev Med** 1980 Jan;9(1):159-61

**Moses ben Maimon, 1135-1204**
Abrahams HJ: A medicine for 'Sickness of the spirit.' **Trans Stud Coll Physicians Phila** 1977 Apr;44(4):202-3
Baruch JZ: Maimonides as a physician. **Gesnerus** 1982;39(3-4):347-57
Frank JB: Moses Maimonides: rabbi of medicine. **Yale J Biol Med** 1981 Jan-Feb;54(1):79-88
Krosnick A: Moshe ben Maimon Ha-Sepharti (Maimonides). **J Med Soc NJ** 1979 Aug;76(9):569
Leibowitz JO: The idea of metabolism in the medical works of Maimonides. In: Congrès international d'histoire de la médecine, XXVe, Québec, 1976. Actes. Québec, 1977. p. 881-4.
Maĭmonid kak estestvoispytatel' i vrach: **Ter Arkh** 1982;54(10):137-9
Rosner F: Maimonides the physician: a bibliography. **Clio Med** 1980;15(1/2):75-9

Rosner F: Moses Maimonides' treatise on poisons. **NY State J Med** 1980 Sep;80(10):1627-30
Rosner F: Moses Maimonides' treatise on asthma. **Thorax** 1981 Apr;36(4):245-51
Rosner F: The medical writings of Moses Maimonides. **Clio Med** 1981 Sep;16(1):1-11
Rosner F: Moses Maimonides' Treatise on Asthma. **J Asthma** 1984;21(2):119-29
Russell HM, Weinberg J, ed: The book of knowledge from the Mishnah Torah of Maimonides. Translated from the Hebrew. Edinburgh, Royal College of Physicians of Edinburgh, 1981. xi, 135 p. (Publication No. 55).
Sakula A: Moses Maimonides' treatise on asthma. **Thorax** 1981 Jul;36(7):560
Simon I: L'influence hippocratique sur la médecine hébraique, surtout chez Assaph, Isaac Israëli et Maimonide. In La collection hippocratique et son rôle dans l'histoire de la médecine. Colloque de Strasbourg (23-27 octobre 1972) organisé par le Centre de Recherches sur la Grèce Antique, avec le concours des Facultés de Philosophie et des Langues Classiques. Leiden, E. J. Brill, 1975. 275-89.

**Moses ben Nahman, 1194-1270**
Leibowitz JO: Medical items in the book Torat ha-'Adam of Rabbi Moses ben Nahman (1194-1270). **Koroth** 1983 Aug;8(7-8):257-64
Richler B: Manuscripts of Moses ben Nahman's 'Torat ha-Adam'. **Koroth** 1983 Aug;8(7-8):265-7

**Mosher, Clelia Duel, 1863-1940**
Jacob KA: The Mosher report. **Am Heritage** 1981;32(4):56-64

**Mosher, Eliza Maria, 1846-1928**
Hazzard FW: Eliza Maria Mosher, MD (1846-1928). **Women Health** 1982 Summer;7(2):1-4

**Mott, Valentine, 1785-1865**
Valentine Mott: **Surgery** 1979 Dec;86(6):906-7

**Mougeot, Jean-Baptiste, 1776-1858**
Laissus Y: Les papiers du docteur J.-B. Mougeot (1776-1858): un fonds important pour l'histoire des sciences naturelles en Lorraine. In: Congrés National des Sociétés Savantes, 103e, Nancy, 1978. Comptes Rendus. Paris, 1978. Section des Sciences, Fasc. V. p. 233-40.

**Moule, Henry, 1801-1880**
Kerr B: Henry Moule and cholera in Dorset: nineteenth-century sanitary reform. **Hist Today** 1978;28(10):672-80

**Mounsey, James, 1710?-1773**
Appleby JH: 'Rhubarb' Mounsey and the Surinam toad--a Scottish physician--naturalist in Russia. **Arch Nat Hist** 1982 Oct;11(1):137-52

**Mountin, Joseph Walter, 1891-1952**
Models for action: **J Public Health Policy** 1980;1(2):103-9

**Moutier, François, 1881-1961**
Cornet A: François Moutier médecin et poète (1881-1961). **Hist Sci Med** 1983;17(2):171-9

**Moyer, J. Walter**
Loudon B: Pioneer pharmacist J. Walter Moyer's notes on Crawford and Fort Robinson in the 1890's. **Nebr Hist** 1977;58(1):89-117

**Moynihan, Berkeley George Andrew, 1865-1936**
Platt H: The foundation of the Association of Surgeons of Great Britain and Ireland. **Br J Surg** 1982 Oct;69(10):561-3

**Mozart, Wolfgang Amadeus, 1756-1791**
Barthelme E: Sur la fièvre miliaire ardente, a propos de la mort de Mozart. **Hist Sci Med** 1983;17(1):23-8
Blodi FC: Was Mozart cross-eyed? **Arch Ophthalmol** 1981 May;99(5):823
Böhme G: Medizinische Porträts berühmter Komponisten: Wolfgang Amadeus Mozart, Ludwig van Beethoven, Carl Maria von Weber, Frédéric Chopin, Peter Iljitsch Tschaikowski, Béla Bartók. 2. verbesserte und erweiterte Auflage. Stuttgart, New York, Gustav Fischer Verlag, 1981. xi, 199 p.
Davies PJ: Mozart's illness and death. **J R Soc Med** 1983 Sep;76(9):776-85
Davies PJ: Mozart's illness & death. **Bol Asoc Med PR** 1984 Aug;76(8):355-61
Davies PJ: Mozart's illnesses and death. **J R Soc Med** 1984 Jul;77(7):623
Franken FH: Mozarts Todeskrankheit. **Fortschr Med** 1980 Mar 6;98(9):301-2
Reichsman F: Life experiences and creativity of great composers: a psychosomaticist's view. **Psychosom Med** 1981 Aug;43(4):291-300
Sakula A: 'Amadeus' was Mozart poisoned? **Hist Med (Lond)** 1980 Jan-Feb;8(1):6-9
Schoental R: Mozart's illnesses and death. **J R Soc Med** 1983 Dec;76(12):1079-80

**Mozo, Antonio, 1720-1794**
Sánchez Téllez MC: Remedios filipinos descritos por Fr. Antonio Mozo (1763). **Bol Soc Esp Hist Farm** 1983 Sep;135:95-100

**Mrstík, Norbert, 1867-1905**
Sípek Z: Norbert Mrštík. (1867-1905) Ze života venkovského lékaře na začátku 20. století. **Cas Lek Cesk** 1982 Jul 30;121(30):955-6

**Mudd, Samuel Alexander, 1833-1883**
Dusseau JL: Tertium Quid: a third something in a muddied puzzle. **Perspect Biol Med** 1982 Winter;25(2):238-53
Massey EW: Dr. Samuel Mudd: justice at last. **South Med J** 1980 Oct;73(10):1375-6

**Mudrov, Matveĭ Iakovlevich, 1776-1831**
Brevnov VP: M. Ia. Mudrov v bor'be s kholernoĭ épidemieĭ v Rossii (1830-1831 gg.). **Feldsher Akush** 1981;46(11):54-6
Katsnel'bogen AG: M. Ia. Mudrov i voprosy vrachebnoĭ étiki. **Sov Zdravookhr** 1983;(10):58-61

**Muhammad Akbar Arzani Shah**
Siddiqi T: Hakim Muhammad Akbar Arzani. **Stud Hist Med** 1981 Sep;5(3):167-224

**Muhammad b. 'Abdallah b. al-Jatib, 1313-1374**
Vázquez de Benito C, Herrera MT: Dos capitulos ginecologicos: arabe y castellano. **Asclepio** 1981;33:183-241

**Muhm, Teodoro, 1869-1939**
Croxatto H: Homenaje al Dr. Teodoro Muhm (1869-1939). **Rev Med Chil** 1984 Jan;112(1):81-8

**Muir, John, 1838-1914**
Lyon TJ: John Muir's enlightenment. **Pac Hist** 1981;25(2):50-7

**Mukhamed'iarov, Fatykh Garitovich, 1883?-1950**
Treĭman VV: F. G. Mukhamed'iarov--organizator Sovetskogo zdravookhraneniia v Tatarii. **Sov Zdravookhr** 1983;(7):71-2

**Mulcaster, Richard, 1530?-1611**
Teigen KH: A note on the origin of the term 'nature and nurture': not Shakespeare and Galton, but Mulcaster. **J Hist Behav Sci** 1984 Oct;20(4):363-4

**Mulder, Gerardus Johannes, 1802-1880**
Snelders HA: Het chemisch laboratorium 'de Leeuwenbergh' te Utrecht (1845-1903). **Tijdschr Geschied Geneeskd** 1984;7(3):129-56

**Muldoon, William, 1845-1933**
Pearlman M: Leonard Wood, William Muldoon and the medical profession: public health and universal military training. **N Engl Q** 1979;52(3):326-44

**Müller, August, 1864-1949**
Heitz RF: The invention of contact lenses by August Müller (1887). **CLAO J** 1984 Jan-Mar;10(1):88-95

**Müller, Carl, 1861-**
Aus dem Archiv der Psychoanalyse: Carl Müller-Braunschweig: Psychoanalyse und Weltanschauung. **Psyche (Stuttg)** 1983 Dec;37(12):1136-45
Dahmer H: Kapitulation vor der 'Weltanschauung'. Zu einem Aufsatz von Carl Müller-Braunschweig aus dem Herbst 1933. **Psyche (Stuttg)** 1983 Dec;37(12):1116-35

**Müller, Friedrich von, 1858-1941**
Pfarrwaller-Stieve A: Friedrich von Müller (1858-1941) und seine Stoffwechseluntersuchungen. Zürich, Juris Druck, 1983. 58 p. (Zürcher Medizingeschichtliche Abhandlungen, Neue Reihe, 156).

**Müller, Fritz, 1822-1897**
Dittrich M: Der Darwinist Fritz Müller (1822-1897) und sein Medizinstudium in Greifswald. Analyse der Motive seiner progressiven Haltung. In: International Congress of the History of Medicine, 26th, Plovdiv (Bulgaria), 1978. Actes du Congres, Vol. 1. Sofia, 1980. p. 100-1.

**Muller, Hermann Joseph, 1890-1967**
Carlson EA: Genes, radiation, and society. The life and work of H. J. Muller. Ithaca, Cornell University Press, 1981. xiv, 457 p.

**Müller, Jakob, 1670-1703**
Wittop Koning DA, Van Gelder JB: Die Offizin aus der Meteorologia philosophica-politica des Fr. Reinzer. **Beitr Gesch Pharm** 1984;31(24):210

**Müller, Johannes, 1801-1858**
Belloni L: Leeuwenhoek's Sehversuch am zusammengesetzten Auge und die entsprechende Beobachtung Boll's an der Stäbchenschicht der Netzhaut. **Janus** 1980;67(1-2-3):59-61
Fiks A: Cystosarcoma phyllodes of the mammary gland--Müller's tumor. For the 180th birthday of Johannes Müller. **Virchows Arch [Pathol Anat]** 1981;392(1):1-6
Lohff B: Johannes Müller. 'Jahresberichte zur Physiologie', in Müllers Archiv der Jahre 1834-1838. **Sudhoffs Arch** 1981;65(1):32-78
Sandführ K: Das Verständnis vom Leben und vom Organismus im Werk von Johannes Müller (1801-1858). Die Eigenart des Lebendigen und die Methode seiner Erforschung. Diss, Bonn, 1979. 153 p.

**Müller-Lyer, Franz Carl, 1857-1916**
Day RH, Knuth H: The contributions of F C Müller-Lyer. **Perception** 1981;10(2):126-46

**Müller, Otto Friderich, 1730-1784**
Théodoridès J, Rousset JJ: A propos de la découverte de Trichomonas tenax, Protozoaire parasite de l'homme, par O. F. Müller. **Rev Hist Sci (Paris)** 1980 Apr;33(2):163-4

**Mul'tanovskiĭ, Michail Petrovič, 1895–1972**
Sokolov EI, Suvorova RV, Krechmer MI: M. P. Mul'tanovskiĭ – vidnyĭ sovetskiĭ istorik meditsiny. **Sov Zdravookhr** 1983;(12):46–8

**Mummery, John Howard, 1847–1926**
Hughes SG: The life and work of John Howard Mummery. **Bull Hist Dent** 1983 Oct;31(2):69–81

**Munch, Edvard, 1863–1944**
Warick LH, Warick ER: Transitional process and creativity in the life and art of Edvard Munch. **J Am Acad Psychoanal** 1984 Jul;12(3):413–24
Wylie HW: Edvard Munch. **Am Imago** 1980 Winter;37(4):413–43

**Münchhausen, Karl Friedrich Hieronymus von, 1720–1797**
Ludwig J, Mann RJ: Münchhausen versus Munchausen. **Mayo Clin Proc** 1983 Nov;58(11):767–9

**Mundy, Jaromír, 1822–1894**
Wondrák E: Jaromír Mundy (1822–1894). Jeho podíl na vývoji záchranných služeb. **Cas Lek Cesk** 1982 Jan 29;121(4):116–9

**Muñiz, Francisco Javier, fl. 1849**
Ivern A: Muñiz presidente de la Facultad. (Tercer Congreso Nacional de Historia de la Medicina Argentina, 1973). **Sem Med** 1973;79(Aniversario):238–41
Ivern A: El Muñiz de las Actas. (Tercer Congreso Nacional de Historia de la Medicina Argentina, 1973). **Sem Med** 1973;79(Aniversario):234–8

**Munk, Arthur, 1885?–1955?**
Szállási A: Magyar orvosíró és az orosz forradalom. **Orv Hetil** 1984 Mar 18;125(12):712–5

**Munk, H. A., fl. 1862–1870**
Payne LM, Newman CE: History of the College Library 9: Dr. Munk as Harveian Librarian 2 (1862–1870). **J R Coll Physicians Lond** 1978 Jan;12(2):189–95

**Muñoz, Fernando Oliva, 1825–1876**
Gella Iturriaga J: El médico mayor de la escuadra del pacífico: Oliva Muñoz. **Rev Gen Mar** 1980 Aug;199:3–14

**Munro, William John, 1863–1908**
Johnson A: William John Munro (1863–1908). **Am J Dermatopathol** 1983 Oct;5(5):477–8

**Munson, Letitia, b. ca. 1820**
Richardson G: Letitia Munson. In Dictionary of Canadian biography, 1881–1890. 1982;11:629–30.

**Münsterberg, Hugo, 1863–1916**
Hale M: Psychology and social order: an intellectual biography of Hugo Münsterberg. Ph.D. Diss. University of Maryland. College Park, 1977. ix, 444 leaves.
Hale M: Human science and social order: Hugo Münsterberg and the origins of applied psychology. Philadelphia, Temple University Press, 1980. xii, 239 p.

**Munthe, Axel Martin Fredrik, 1857–1949**
Briceño-Maaz T: Sobre Axel Munthe y su libro 'La Historia de San Michele'. **Rev Soc Venez Hist Med** 1969–71;17–19(31–33):121–30
Al-Dabbagh F: Aksel Mentah, nafsani Suwidi, wa-mu'allif qissat San Mishel. **Al-Arabi** 1973;179:60–3

**Munyon, James Munroe**
Heindel ND, Foster NI: Medicine, music and 'Money' Munyon. **Pa Folklife** 1982;32(1):44–8

**Muralt, Johannes von, 1645–1733**
Boschung U: Johannes von Muralt, 1645–1733: Arzt, Chirurg, Anatom, Naturforscher, Philosoph. Zürich, Rohr, 1983. 105 p.

**Murphy, John Benjamin, 1857–1916**
Siegel IM: John B. Murphy – early American orthopaedic surgeon. **Int Surg** 1979 Jan–Feb;64(1):83–5

**Murphy, William Parry, 1892–**
Crosby WH: Landmark perspective. Pernicious anemia. **JAMA** 1983 Dec 23–30;250(24):3336–8

**Murray, George, 1825–1888**
Beck JM: George Murray. In Dictionary of Canadian biography, 1881–1890. 1982;11:633–4.

**Murray, James Patrick, 1839–**
Elmslie R: The colonial career of James Patrick Murray. **Aust NZ J Surg** 1979 Feb;49(1):154–62

**Murray, Joseph Edward, 1919–**
Murray JE: An interview with Joseph E. Murray, M.D. conducted by Joel M. Noe, M.D. **Ann Plast Surg** 1984 Jan;12(1):84–9

**Musgrave, Samuel, 1732–1780**
Luyendijk-Elshout AM: Samuel Musgrave's attack upon Stahl's and Boerhaave's doctrines in 1763. **Janus** 1980;67(1–2–3):141–56

**Musil, Robert, 1880–1942**
Cremerius J: Robert Musil. Das Dilemma eines Schriftstellers vom Typus 'poeta doctus' nach Freud. **Psyche (Stuttg)** 1979 Aug;33(8):733–72
Legrenzi P: L'uomo senza facoltà: modelli del comportamento in Musil. **Stor Crit Psicol** 1982 Dec;3(2):301–13

**Mussehl, Frank**
Bancroft PM: Rickets and solar radiation – medicine's debt to Professor Frank Mussehl. **Nebr Med J** 1982 Jul;67(7):184–5

**Mussen, Aubrey Thomas, 1873–1975**
Olivier A, Bertrand G, Picard C: Discovery of the first human stereotactic instrument. **Appl Neurophysiol** 1983;46(1–4):84–91
Picard C, Olivier A, Bertrand G: The first human stereotaxic apparatus. The contribution of Aubrey Mussen to the field of stereotaxis. **J Neurosurg** 1983 Oct;59(4):673–6

**Muste, Laurent**
Charmasson T: L'établissement d'un almanach médical pour l'année 1437. In: Congrès National des Sociétés Savantes, 99e, Besançon, 1974. Comptes Rendus. Paris, 1976. Section des Sciences, Fasc. V. p. 217–34.

**Muthmann, Arthur, 1875–**
Amitai M, Cremerius J: Dr. med. Arthur Muthmann. Ein Beitrag zur Frühgeschichte der Psychoanalyse. **Psyche (Stuttg)** 1984 Aug;38(8):738–53

**Myer, Albert James, 1828–1880**
Clary DA, ed: 'I am already quite a Texan': Albert J. Myer's letters from Texas. **Southwest Hist Q** 1978;82(1):25–76
Scheips PJ: Albert James Myer, an army doctor in Texas, 1854–1857. **Southwest Hist Q** 1978;82(1):1–24

**Myers, Arthur Thomas, 1851–1894**
Taylor DC, March SM: Hughlings Jackson's Dr Z: the paradigm of temporal lobe epilepsy revealed. **J Neurol Neurosurg Psychiatry** 1980 Sep;43(9):758–67

**Myers, Myer, 1723–1795**
Hershkowitz L: Powdered tin and rose petals: Myer Myers, Goldsmith, and Peter Middleton, physician. **Am Jew Hist** 1981;70(4):462–7

## N

**Nachet Family**
Maison Nachet: Catalogues de fonds de 1854 à 1910. Facsimile edition. Introduction par G. L'E. Turner. Paris, Brieux, 1979. Various paginations.

**Nadelson, Carol Cooperman, 1936–**
Callan CM: A leader in psychiatry--Carol Nadelson, M.D. **Conn Med** 1981 Aug;45(8):491–2

**Naegeli, Otto, 1871–1938**
Dufek WM: Der Internist Otto Naegeli, 1871–1938. Zürich, Juris Druck, 1983. 76 p. (Zürcher Medizingeschichtliche Abhandlungen, Neue Reihe, Nr. 160).

**Nagarjuna, Siddha**
Filliozat J, ed: Yogaśataka. Texte médical attribué à Nagarjuna. Textes sanskrit et tibétain; traduction française. Pondichéry, Institut Français d'Indologie, 1979. xxxviii, 206 p.
Wujastyk D: An alchemical ghost: the Rasaratnâkara by Nâgârjuna. **Ambix** 1984 Jul;31(2):70–83

**Nakamura, Heizo, 1896–**
Ueno T: [In memory of Prof. Heizo Nakamura] (Jpn) **Dent Outlook** 1980;55(5):921–6

**Napier, Richard, d. 1634**
MacDonald M: Mystical bedlam: madness, anxiety, and healing in seventeenth-century England. Cambridge, Cambridge University Press, 1981. xvi, 323 p.

**Napoleon I, Emperor of the French, 1769–1821**
Bodemer CW: Baron Dominique Jean Larrey, Napoleon's surgeon. **Bull Am Coll Surg** 1982 Jul;67(7):18–21
Dumaitre P: Les planches anatomiques d'Antommarchi. **Clio Med** 1981 Sep;16(1):13–23
Gershenowitz H: Napoleon and Lamarck. **Indian J Hist Sci** 1980;15:204–9
Holmes WR: The illness and death of Napoleon. **J Med Assoc Ga** 1983 Mar;72(3):201–4
Iveson-Iveson J: Medical history. Napoleon: his final years. **Nurs Mirror** 1982 Aug 18;155(7):22–4
Jean R: Communication sur la correspondance du docteur Guillard à sa femme lors du voyage à Sainte-Hélène: retour des cendres de Napoléon. **Hist Sci Med** 1980;14:271–6
Jensen JE: Napoleonic medicine. **Md State Med J** 1981 Jul;30(7):66–8
Jones DE, Ledingham KW: Arsenic in Napoleon's wallpaper. **Nature** 1982 Oct 14;299(5884):626–7
Lewin PK, Hancock RG, Voynovich P: Napoleon Bonaparte--no evidence of chronic arsenic poisoning. **Nature** 1982 Oct 14;299(5884):627–8
Poulet J: Le cas Antommarchi. **Rev Inst Napoleon (Paris)** 1971;(120)131–8
Richardson RG: How sick was Napoleon? **Practitioner** 1981 Jan;225(1351):109–10
Robinson JO: The failing health of Napoleon. **J R Soc Med** 1979 Aug;72(8):621–3

**Napoleon III, Emperor of the French, 1808–1873**
Decaux A: Napoléon III et la chirurgie. **Chirurgie** 1984;110(1):23–8

Ellis H: The bladder stone of the Emperor Napoleon III. **Chirurgie** 1984;110(4):370-1

**Narasaraju Urs, fl. 1883**
Shankara MR, Venkataram BS, Leelavathy S: A 19th century manuscript on traditional medicine. **Bull Indian Inst Hist Med (Hyderabad)** 1979;9:33-7

**Narayan, Jayaprakash, 1901?-**
Fellman G: Leaf in a storm: Jayaprakash Narayan as politician and as saint. **Psychohist Rev** 1981;9(3):183-213

**Narimanov, Nariman N., 1872-1925**
Manafov IT: N. Narimanov--vrach, revoliutsioner, partiĭnyi ĭ gosudarstvennyĭ deiatel'. **Sov Zdravookhr** 1982;(4):58-61

**Nasse, Christian Friedrich, 1778-1851**
Kaiser W, Trenckmann U: Christian Friedrich Nasse (1778-1851). **Wiss Z Martin Luther Univ (Math)** 1980;29(2):65-89
Schipperges H: Der Arzt als Zeuge des Lebens. **Gesnerus** 1981;38:105-18

**Naughton, John L., 1915-**
Kremenak N: John L. Naughton, inventor of the Den-Tal-Ez chair. An Iowa original. **Iowa Dent J** 1984 Oct;70(4):23-5

**Naumberg, Margaret, 1890-1983**
Detre KC, Frank T, Kniazzeh CR, et al: Roots of art therapy. Margaret Naumburg (1890-1983) and Florence Cane (1882-1952). A family portrait. **Am J Art Ther** 1983 Jul;22(4):111-23

**Nazarov, Vasiliĭ Mikhaĭlovich, 1883-1945**
Napalkov PN, Shafer II: Professor Vasiliĭ Mikhaĭlovich Nazarov (k 100-letiiu so dnia rozhdeniia). **Vestn Khir** 1983 Mar;130(3):129-30

**Nechaev, Sergei Dennadievich, 1847-1882**
Pomper P: Nečaev, Lenin and Stalin: the psychology of leadership. **Jahrb Gesch Osteur** 1978;26(1):11-30

**Needham, Charles, ca. 1660-ca. 1707**
Burnby J: Three 17th century London apothecaries; Richard Meynell, Charles Needham, William Booker. **Pharm Hist (London)** 1975 May;5(1):2-3

**Needham, Joseph, 1900-**
Elvin M, et al: The work of Joseph Needham. **Past Present** 1980;87:17-53

**Neff, Mary (Lawson), 1862-**
Hancock V: Women in Arizona medicine: Mary Lawson Neff, M.D. **Ariz Med** 1984 Nov;41(11):750-4; Dec;41(12):819-21

**Neifeld, Ernst Jeremias, 1721-1773**
Kaiser W: Ernst Jeremias Neifeld (1721-1773), Herausgeber der ersten medizinischen Fachzeitschrift in Polen. **Wiss Z Martin Luther Univ (Math)** 1977;26(3):123-31

**Neild, James, 1744-1814**
Neild FG: James Neild (1744-1814) and prison reform. **J R Soc Med** 1981 Nov;74(11):834-40

**Neill, Grace, fl. 1899-1906**
Tennant M: Mrs. Grace Neill in the Department of Asylums, Hospitals and Charitable Institutions. **NZ J Hist** 1978 Apr 12;:3-16

**Neisser, Albert, 1855-1916**
Haneveld GT: Bij het eeuwfeest van de gonokok: het belang van zijn ontdekking en de ontvangst daarvan in Nederland (Ludwig Sigesmund Albert Neisser). **Ned Tijdschr Geneeskd** 1979 Oct 27;123(43):1875-8

**Neiva, Arthur, 1880-1943**
Alves M: Dr. Arthur Neiva. **Rev Inst Hist Geogr Bras** 1979;325:123-31

**Nelson, Horatio, 1758-1805**
Different letters from the past. 4) Horatio, Viscount Nelson to Earl Spencer.: **Ann R Coll Surg Engl** 1980 Sep;62(5):388-9
Rüttimann B: Nelsons Oberarm-Amputation. **Z Orthop** 1982 Feb;120(1):86-8
Taylor B: Health in history. Britain's Admiral Lord Horatio Nelson. **Md State Med J** 1979 Dec;28(12):35-50

**Nelson, Marjorie Maxine, 1909-1962**
Raacke ID: Marjorie Maxine Nelson. In Dictionary of American biography, 1961-1965. Suppl. 7, 1981. p. 568-9.

**Nemesius, Bp. of Emesa, fl. 390-400**
Siclari A: L'antropologia di Nemesio di Emesa. Padova, La Garangola, 1974. 318 p. (Filosofia e religione; 9).

**Németh, László, 1901-**
Szállási A: Németh Lázzló és a Nyugat. **Orv Hetil** 1981 Jan 25;122(4):226-7

**Nemilov, Anton Vitalévich, 1879-1942**
Katsnel'son ZS: Anton Vital'evich Nemilov (1879-1942), ego nauchnoe i pedagogicheskoe tvorchestvo (k 100-letiiu so dnia rozhdeniia). **Arkh Anat Gistol Embriol** 1981 Feb;80(2):108-16

**Nemours, Victoria Augusta Antoinetta de, 1822?-1857**
Langham-Carter RR: The death of the Duchesse de Nemours. **Adler Mus Bull** 1982 Nov;8(2):8-9

**Nencki, Marceli, 1847-1901**
Szwejcerowa A: Marceli Nencki (1847-1901), pionnier de la biochimie. In International Congress of the History of Medicine. 26th, Plovdiv, 1978. Actes du Congress. Sofia, 1981. Volume II. p. 97-9.

**Nendtvich, Károly Miksa, 1811-1892**
Szállási A: Nendtvich Károly orvosvegyész amerikai utazása 1855-ben. **Orv Hetil** 1984 Sep 2;125(36):2205-6, 2209-10

**Neri, Ana, 1815-1880**
Nolding Gaffree A: Ana Neri - la première infirmière militaire au Brésil. In: International Congress of the History of Medicine, 26th, Plovdiv (Bulgaria), 1978. Actes du Congres, Vol. 1. Sofia, 1980. p. 114-5.

**Nesterov, Anatoli Innokentevich, 1895-**
Orlova AN: Vklad A. I. Nesterova v uchenie o mikrotsirkuliatsii (k 85-letiiu so dnia rozhdeniia A. I. Nesterova). **Vopr Revm** 1981 Jan-Mar;(1):58-61

**Netter, Frank Henry, 1906-**
Frank Netter: The man, the artist, the surgeon. **Med Times** 1981;109(1):31-3

**Nettleship, Edward, 1845-1913**
Jay M, Phil M: Nettleship's two pedigrees of retinitis pigmentosa: a historical postscript. **Surv Ophthalmol** 1983 Jan-Feb;27(4):264-8

**Neugebauer, Ludwig Adolf, 1824-1890**
Higier J: Sto lat sporu o autorstwo (priorytet) operacji pośrodkowego zeszycia pochwy (colpocleisis mediana) 1881-1981. **Ginekol Pol** 1982;53(3)

**Neuhold, Richard, 1917-1982**
Richard Neuhold (17. 10. 1917 bis 14. 8. 1982): **Verh Dtsch Ges Pathol** 1983;67:774-7

**Neumann, Erich, 1905-1960**
Alex W: The significance of Erich Neuman in Jungian psychology. **Isr Ann Psychiatry** 1979 Dec;17(4):263-8
Meier-Seethaler C: The child: Erich Neumann's contribution to the psychopathology of child development. **J Anal Psychol** 1982 Oct;27(4):357-79

**Neumann, Ernst, 1834-1918**
Neumann-Redlin von Meding E: Ernst Neumann. Zum 150. Geburtstag des Königsberger Pathologen und Hämatologen am 30.1. 1984. **Pathologe** 1984 Jan;5(1):53-6
Neumann-Redlin von Meding E: Neumann' Zahnscheiden und Tomes' Zahnfasern. Zum 150. Geburtstag des Königsberger Pathologen Ernst Christian Neumann. **Dtsch Zahnarztl Z** 1984 Jan;39(1):65-9

**Neumann, Robert, 1882-**
Gold SI: Robert Neumann: a pioneer in periodontal flap surgery. **J Periodontol** 1982 Jul;53(7):456-9

**Neumann, Salomon, 1819-**
Karbe KH: Ein Leben für die soziale Medizin--Salomon Neumann zu seinem 75. Todestag. **Z Gesamte Hyg** 1983 Nov;29(11):696-8

**Newburgh, Louis Harry, 1883-1956**
Harvey AM: Louis Harry Newburgh: compleat clinical investigator with a passion for measurement. **Am J Med** 1981 Apr;70(4):759-61

**Newell, William Augustus, 1817-1901**
Guthorn PJ: William Augustus Newell, M.D., and the Life Saving Service. **J Med Soc NJ** 1984 Sep;81(9):769-72

**Newell, William Wells, 1839-1907**
Bell MJ: The relation of mentality to race: William Wells Newell and the Celtic hypothesis. **J Am Folkl** 1979;92(363):25-43

**Newton, Isaac, 1642-1727**
Broad WJ: Sir Isaac Newton: mad as a hatter. **Science** 1981 Sep 18;213(4514):1341-2, 1344
Ditchburn RW: Newton's illness of 1692-3. **Notes Rec R Soc Lond** 1980 Jul;35(1):1-16
Guerlac H: Theological voluntarism and biological analogies in Newton's physical thought. **J Hist Ideas** 1983 Apr-Jun;44(2):219-29
Jaeger W: Die Ordnungsprinzipien der Farbsysteme des 17. Jahrhunderts. (Franciscus Aguilonius--Athanasius Kircher--Isaac Newton). **Klin Monatsbl Augenheilkd** 1984 Apr;184(4):321-5
Keynes M: Sir Isaac Newton and his madness of 1692-93. **Lancet** 1980 Mar 8;1(8167):529-30
Laker MR: Newton's malady. **Science** 1982 Mar 5;215(4537):1185-6
Lieb J, Hershman D: Isaac Newton: mercury poisoning or manic depression? **Lancet** 1983 Dec 24-31;2(8365-66):1479-80
Toellner R: Decora Merenti. Glory, merit and science. Haller spellbound by the Newtonian star. **Janus** 1980;67(1-2-3):171-85
Tweney RD: Isaac Newton's two uses of hypothetical reasoning: dual influences on the history of psychology. **Stor Crit Psicol** 1980;1(2):235-59
Westfall RS: Alchemy in Newton's library. **Ambix** 1984 Nov;31(3):97-101

**Nicander, fl. ca. 2nd cent. B.C.**
Crugnola A, ed: Scholia in Nicandri Theriaka, cum glossis. Varese-Milano, Istituto Editoriale Cisalpino, 1971. 329 p.
Geymonat M, ed: Scholia in Nicandri Alexipharmaca, cum glossis. Milan, Cisalpino-Goliardica, 1974. 218 p.

Scarborough J: Nicander: Theriaca 811. **Classical Philol** 1980;75:138–40

**Nicholas of Lynne, fl. 1386**
Benson CD: The astrological medicine of Chaucer's physician and Nicholas of Lynn's Kalendarium. **Am Notes Queries** 1984 Jan–Feb;22(5–6):62–6

**Nicholas, Saint, Bp. of Myra, 4th cent.**
Shaw S: Seasonal foundations: Santa–the saint who founded hospitals. **Nurs Mirror** 1981 Dec 23–30;153(26):30–1

**Nichols Family**
Baldwin J: The Nichols: 100 years of Ohio dentistry. **Ohio Dent J** 1980 May;54(5):22–3

**Nichols, Thomas Low, 1815–1901**
Aspinwall B: Social Catholicism and health: Dr. and Mrs. Thomas Low Nichols in Britain. In Sheils WJ, ed: The Church and healing. Papers read at the twentieth summer meeting and the twenty-first winter meeting of the Ecclesiastical History Society. Oxford, Basil Blackwell for the Society, 1982. p. 249–70.

**Nicolaus Cusanus, Cardinal, 1401–1464**
Kohnen N: Nicolai de Cusa. Liber quasi medicinalis: De staticis experimentis. In Göpfert W, Otten HH, ed: Metavoeite: wandelt euch durch Denken. Düsseldorf, Triltsch, 1983. p. 135–45.
Kuntz FJ: Medizinisches bei Nikolaus Cusanus. **Mitt Forschungsbeitr Cusanus Ges** 1977;12:127–36
Oide S: Der Einfluss der galenischen Pneumatheorie auf die cusanische Spiritustheorie. Eine Anmerkung zu 'De quaerendo deum'. **Mitt Forschungsbeitr Cusanus Ges** 1978;13:198–207
Schultheisz E: On the beginnings of quantitative thinking in medicine. (Nicholas of Cusa and the Idiot). In E. Schultheisz, ed: History of physiology. Oxford, Elmsford, New York, Pergamon, 1981. xvi, 208 p. (Advances in Physiological Sciences. Proceedings of the 28th International Congress of Physiological Sciences, Budapest, 1980. Volume 21) p. 1–7.
Schultheisz E: Beginning of quantification in physiology. **Orvostort Kozl** 1980;89–91(26 no 1–3):209–13
Schultheisz E: The beginning of quantification in physiology. **Clio Med** 1983 Mar;17(4):193–7
Stoll C: Nikolaus von Kues (1401–1464) und seine Bedeutung für die Naturwissenschaft. **Pharm Acta Helv** 1979;54(9–10):311–6

**Nicolle, Charles Jules Henri, 1866–1936**
Nicolle P: Alphonase Laveran et Charles Nicolle. **Arch Inst Pasteur Tunis** 1981 Sep–Dec;58(3):265–79
Nicolle P: Un événement capital dans la vie passionnée de Charles Nicolle: le Prix Nobel de physiologie ou médecine. Souvenirs évoqués par Pierre Nicolle. **Bull Soc Pathol Exot Filiales** 1981 Jan–Feb;74(1):101–18

**Niculescu, Ion T., 1895–1957**
Pretresco A: Dos conmemoraciones. **Rev Neuropsiquiatr** 1980 Jun;43(2):115–23

**Niederhäusern, David von, 1847–1882**
Fankhauser R, Hörning B: Zum hundertsten Todestag David von Niederhäusern's. **Schweiz Arch Tierheilkd** 1982 Feb;124(2):53–68

**Niehans, Paul, 1882–1971**
Fraser I: Steinach operation. **Br Med J [Clin Res]** 1984 Jan 21;288(6412):242

**Nielsen, Johannes Maargaard, 1890–1969**
Wortis J: Johannes Maargaard Nielsen, pioneer. **Biol Psychiatry** 1983 Feb;18(2):135–7

**Nieto y Serrano, Matías, 1813–1902**
Riera J: Matías Nieto y Serrano (1813–1902) y la medicina romántica. **Cuad Invest Hist** 1979;3:275–306
Riera J: [Dr. Matias Nieto y Serrano and Romantic medicine in Spain.] (Spa) **Cuad Invest Hist** 1979;:3
Riera J: Matias Nieto y Serrano (1813–1902) y la medicina romantica. **Asclepio** 1980;32:367–81

**Nietzsche, Friedrich Wilhelm, 1844–1900**
Benedetti G: Die neurotische Lebensproblematik Nietzsches als eine Wirkkraft und eine Grenze seiner Philosophie. **Gesnerus** 1984;41(1/2):111–32
Dieckhöfer K: Menschliches, Allzumenschliches---zur verstehenden Psychologie bei Nietzsche. **Z Klin Psychol Psychother** 1980;28(2):101–5
Gilman SL: The Nietzsche murder case. **New Lit Hist** 1983;14(2):359–72
Hayman R: Nietzsche's madness. **Partisan Rev** 1980;47(1):29–44

**Nightingale, Florence, 1820–1910**
Baly M: A new history of nursing. Three. The nurse élite (Florence Nightingale). **Nurs Times** 1984 Oct 17–23;80(42):55–7
Berentson L: Florence Nightingale: change agent. **RN Id** 1982 Apr–May;6(2):3, 7
Boisvert DJ: Florence Nightingale's cap. **N Engl Galaxy** 1978;20(2):42–51
Clocotici L: Sănătatea este un mod de a exista. **Viata Med [Medii Sanit]** 1981 Nov;29(11):259–60
Cohen IB: Florence Nightingale. **Sci Am** 1984 Mar;250(3):128–37
Cruse P: Florence Nightingale. **Surgery** 1980 Sep;88(3):394–9
Dainton C: The years of reform. **Br Herit** 1981–82;3(1):22–31
Florence Nightingale: the original geriatric nurse. **Okla Nurse** 1980 May;25(4):6
Fraga M, Tenenbaum L: Florence Nightingale--model for today's nurse. **Fla Nurse** 1981 May;29(5):11
Gould ME, Gamlen C: [A woman of parts. Florence Nightingale]. (Jpn) **Sogo Kango** 1980;15(1):95–9
Graham S: Notes on nursing, 1860–1980. Angels of plain speech. **Nurs Times** 1980 Oct 23;76(43):1874
Hebert RG: Florence Nightingale: saint, reformer or rebel? Malabar, Florida, Robert E. Krieger, 1981. 236 p.
Hill AJ: Nightingale, sainte ou diablesse? **Infirm Can** 1980 Nov;(10):34–6
Hosono K: [The logical structure in the 'Notes on Nursing' (Florence Nightingale)] (Jpn). **Sogo Kango** 1982;16(4):51–60
Iveson–Iveson J: Nurses in society: a legend in the breaking (Florence Nightingale). **Nurs Mirror** 1983 May 11;156(19):26–7
Johansson B: 'God bless you, my dear Miss Nightingale.' Letters from Emmy Carolina Rappe to Florence Nightingale 1867–1870. Stockholm, Almqvist & Wiksell International, 1977. 57 p. (Stockholm studies in English, 38).
Kalisch BJ, Kalisch PA: Heroine out of focus: media images of Florence Nightingale. Part I. Popular biographies and stage productions. **Nurs Health Care** 1983 Apr;4(4):181–7
Kanai H: [What Nightingale would have written about summer heat and nursing – a thought in connection with folk remedy] (Jpn). **Kango** 1982 Aug;34(9):4–14
Kaneko M: [An encounter with Nightingale] (Jpn) **Sogo Kango** 1980;15(4):22–8
Kaneko M: [The nature of observation expressed in the 'Observation of the sick' (Florence Nightingale)] (Jpn). **Sogo Kango** 1982;16(4):40–50
Karll A: Florence Nightingale. **Nurs J India** 1983 May;74(5):110
Kawakita Y: [Nightingale in the history of medical philosophy--on the meaning of 'health'] (Jpn). **Kango** 1982 Feb;34(2):39–53
Kodama K: [Scenes associated with Florence Nightingale] (Jpn) **Kango** 1980 Nov;32(11):48–59
Kodama K: [From the old notes on Florence Nightingale] (Jpn) **Sogo Kango** 1980;15(4):12–7
Kodama K: [Care and cure defined in the 'Notes on Nursing' (Florence Nightingale)] (Jpn). **Sogo Kango** 1982;16(4):29–39
Koike A: [Hitherto unknown profile of Florence Nightingale]. (Jpn) **Sogo Kango** 1980;15(1):100–8
Konami Y: [Studies on Nightingale: the role of the matron] (Jpn) **Sogo Kango** 1980;15(4):29–36
Kurumada M: ['Introductory notes on lying-in institutions' and problems of management--hospital management and Florence Nightingale] (Jpn). **Sogo Kango** 1983;18(1):107–19
Makabe G: [Nightingale's expectation on women--an impression of her writings] (Jpn) **Sogo Kango** 1980;15(4):70–2
Makabe G: [A visit at Kaiserwerth. (1) (Florence Nightingale)] (Jpn). **Sogo Kango** 1982;16(4):61–74
Makabe G: [Visit to Kaiserwerth (2) (Florence Nightingale)]. (Jpn). **Sogo Kango** 1982;17(1):59–78
Makabe G: [Foundation of nursing. Letter collection of Florence Nightingale] (Jpn). **Sogo Kango** 1982;17(4):8–34
Nagasawa Y: [Encounter with Nightingale---a discovery of Nightingale in the field of hospital designs] (Jpn) **Sogo Kango** 1980;15(4):59–69
Nauright L: Politics and power: a new look at Florence Nightingale. **Nurs Forum** 1984;21(1):5–7
Ninan R: The lady with the lamp: a profile. **Nurs J India** 1982 Jun;73(6):154–5
Nishida A: [In preparation of the key words for Nightingale's 'Notes on Nursing'--introduction to a humanistic theory] **Sogo Kango** 1980;15(4):46–58
Nishida A: [Understanding of man in the 'Notes on Nursing' (Florence Nightingale)] (Jpn). **Sogo Kango** 1982;16(4):9–22
Nuttall P: The passionate statistician (Florence Nightingale). **Nurs Times** 1983 Sep 28–Oct 4;79(39):25–7
Nuttall P: Miss Florence Nightingale: 'the passionate statistician'. **Nurs J India** 1984 Jun;75(6):128–9
Okada M: [Notes on 'Cassandra'. 1 (Florence Nightingale)] (Jpn) **Sogo Kango** 1984 Aug 15;19(3):63–78
Oliver H: The Shore Smith family library: Arthur Hugh Clough and Florence Nightingale. **Book Collect** 1979;28:521–9
Om dårlige arbeidsrutiner. Med hilsen fra Florence Nightingale: **Sykepleien** 1984 Sep 20;71(16):6–8, 30
Ota S: [Florence Nightingale's expectations on modern nursing--thoughts on nursing science] (Jpn). **Sogo Kango** 1984 May 15;19(2):79–88
Palmer IS: Florence Nightingale and international origins of modern nursing. **Image (IN)** 1981 Jun;13(2):28–31
Palmer IS: Florence Nightingale: the myth and the reality. **Nurs Times** 1983 Aug 3–9;79(31):40–2
Palmer IS: Nightingale revisited. **Nurs Outlook** 1983 Jul–Aug;31(4):229–33
Palmer IS: [Nightingale revisited] (Jpn). **Kango** 1983 Nov;35(12):112–22
Prince J: Education for a profession: some lessons from history (Florence Nightingale). **Int J Nurs Stud** 1984;21(3):153–63
Rains AJ: 'The Nightingale touch'. **J R Army Med Corps** 1982 Feb;128(1):4–17

Rogers P: Florence Nightingale: the myth and the reality. **Nurs Focus** 1982 Jul;3(11):10
Rothrock JC: Nursing diagnosis: in the days of Florence Nightingale. **AORN J** 1984 Aug;40(2):189–90
Schmidt V: Hvad fejlede Florence Nightingale? **Sygeplejersken** 1980 Aug 6;80(31):4–10; Oct 5;67(17):16–21
Shannon R: [Re-evaluation of Florence Nightingale: a review of 'Florence Nightingale: Reputation and Power' by F. B. Smith] (Jpn). **Kango Kyoiku** 1982 Nov;23(11):677–85
Smith FB: Florence Nightingale. Reputation and power. London, Canberra, Croom Helm, 1982. xii, 216 p.
Smith FT: Florence Nightingale: early feminist. **Am J Nurs** 1981 May;81(5):1021–4
Smith FT: [Florence Nightingale: early feminist] (Jpn). **Kango Kyoiku** 1982 Nov;23(11):671–6
Swain V: No plaster saint! **Nurs Times** 1983 Mar 16–22;79(11):62–3
Takahashi M: [On participating in the tour of the 'Areas related to Nightingale' (2)] (Jpn). **Kango Kyoiku** 1981 Apr;22(4):262–7
Takahashi M: [A tour of the areas related to Florence Nightingale. (1)] (Jpn). **Kango Kyoiku** 1981 Jan;22(1):54–60
Takeyama M: [Conclusion of the translation of the 'Life of Florence Nightingale'] (Jpn). **Sogo Kango** 1981 Aug;16(3):76–83
Tamura M: [On research on Florence Nightingale -- a future overview] (Jpn). **Sogo Kango** 1980;15(4):18–21
Teramoto M: [Me and the Florence Nightingale letter collection] (Jpn). **Sogo Kango** 1982;17(4):35–8
Thompson JD: The passionate humanist: from Nightingale to the new nurse. **Nurs Outlook** 1980 May;28(5):290–5
Usui T: [The influence of Nightingale on my nursing activities] (Jpn) **Sogo Kango** 1980;15(4):37–45
Van der Peet R: Florence Nightingale en haar visie op verplegen in relatie tot het leven en werk van Charles Darwin. **Tijdschr Ziekenverpl** 1983 Aug 23;36(17):530–6
Wheeler CE: Viewpoint: essay in response to republication of a biography (Florence Nightingale). **ANS** 1984 Jul;6(4):74–9
Wiewiórowska M: Koncepcja pielęgniarstwa Florencji Nightingale. **Pieleg Polozna** 1981;(7):9–10, 15
Wiewiórowska M: Koncepcja pielegniarstwa Florencji Nightingale. **Pieleg Polozna** 1981;(5):8
Wiewiórowska M: Koncepcja pielęgniarstwa Florencji Nightingale. **Pieleg Polozna** 1981;(6):10–2 contd
Wiewiórowska M: Koncepcja piel egniarstwa Florencji Nightingale. **Pieleg Polozna** 1981;(8):7–8
Woodall ME: Ruolo e identita' dell'infermiere: riscoprire il pensiero di Florence Nightingale. **Prof Inferm** 1980 Oct–Dec;33(4):166–9
Yoshikawa R: [Biography of Nightingale published in the early Meiji era - on 'Self-Help for Women'] (Jpn). **Sogo Kango** 1982;17(1):91–102
Yumaki M: [Nightingale's concept of God] (Jpn). **Sogo Kango** 1982;16(4):23–8
Yumaki M: [50 years of the studies on Florence Nightingale] (Jpn). **Sogo Kango** 1980;15(4):7–11

**Nijinsky, Vaslav, 1890–1950**
Ansbacher HL: Discussion of Alfred Alder's preface to The Diary of Vaslav Nijinsky. **Arch Gen Psychiatry** 1981 Jul;38(7):834–41

**Nikiforov, M. N., 1858–1915**
Serov VV: M. N. Nikiforov i Moskovskaia shkola patologoanatomov (k 125-letiiu so dnia rozhdeniia). **Arkh Patol** 1984;46(2):3–12

**Nikol'skiĭ, Petr Vasil'evich, 1858–1940**
Glukhen'kiĭ TT: Petr Vasil'evich Nikol'skiĭ (k 125-letiiu so dnia rozhdeniia). **Vestn Dermatol Venerol** 1984 Jan;(1):69–70

**Nikonov, S. A.**
Tiukina AP: S. A. Nikonov--vrach-revoliutsioner. **Sov Zdravookhr** 1984;(10):64–7

**Nilsson, Arthur Vitolia, 1896–1983**
Gruber B: Anatomist, scholar and gentleman: Arthur V. Nilsson-a legend in his own time. **Chiropr Hist** 1984;4(1):31–8

**Nin, Anais, 1903–1977**
Spencer S: Delivering the woman artist from the silence of the womb: Otto Rank's influence on Anais Nin. **Psychoanal Rev** 1982 Spring;69(1):111–29

**Nishina, Yoshio, 1890–1951**
Iio M: Professor G. V. Hevesy, Doctor Y. Nishina and nuclear medicine in Japan. **Radiat Med** 1983 Jul–Sep;1(3):255–62

**Nixon, Pat Ireland, 1883–1965**
Everett DE: Dr. Pat Ireland Nixon: letters to and from his book-loving friends. **Friends P. I. Nixon Med Hist Libr** 1974 Oct;3:1–13
Nixon PI: Pat Nixon of Texas. Autobiography of a doctor. Ed. by H. H. Lang. College Station, Texas, and London, Texas A & M University Press, 1979. 288 p.

**Nixon, Richard Milhous, 1913–**
Scalettar R: Presidential candidate disability. **JAMA** 1984 Jun 1;251(21):2811

**Nobel, Alfred Bernhard, 1833–1896**
Nicolle P, Jude A: Réflexions sur les prix Nobel de physiologie ou médecine. **Hist Sci Med** 1980;14(1):83–93

**Noble, Joseph Whittlesey, d. 1949**
Walker RT: Joseph Whittlesey Noble: an American in Hong Kong. **J Am Dent Assoc** 1984 Nov;109(5):757

**Noguchi, Hideyo, 1876–1928**
Bendiner E: Noguchi: many triumphs and a brilliant failure. **Hosp Pract [Off]** 1984 Feb;19(2):222–3, 227, 231 passim
Dolman CE: Hideyo Noguchi (1876–1928): his final effort in West Africa. In: Congrès international d'histoire de la médecine, XXVe, Québec, 1976. Actes. Québec, 1977. p. 603–24.
Masaki T: [Hideyo Noguchi and oral spirochaete]. (Jpn) **Dent Outlook** 1978;51(6):1265
Plesset IR: Noguchi and his patrons. Rutherford, N.J., Fairleigh Dickinson, 1980. 314 p.

**Noguer Molins, Luis, d. 1972**
Novoa Montero D: El Profesor Luis Noguer Molins y la Universidad Venezolana. Nueva ed. Mérida, Venezuela, (The Author), 1980. 84 p.

**Nollet, Jean Antoine, 1700–1770**
Benguigui I: La théorie de l'électricité de Nollet et son application en médecine à travers sa correspondance: inédite avec Jallabert. **Gesnerus** 1981;38:225–35

**Nonnius, Ludovicus, ca. 1555–1645?**
Bruce-Chwatt LJ: Ludovicus Nonnius, M.D., 1553–1645. **Bull NY Acad Med** 1984 Nov;60(9):938–43

**Noorden, Carl Harko Hermann Johannes von, 1858–1944**
Hauk J: Carl Harko Hermann Johannes von Noorden (1858–1944), sein Leben und Werk unter besonderer Berücksichtigung seiner Theorien über die Ursachen des Diabetes mellitus. Diss. Mainz, 1980. 288 p.

**Norin, Anna, 1774–**
Malmstedt J: Hon förlöste vävarnas barn--barnmorskan Anna Norin. **Jordemodern** 1982 Oct;95(10):341–4

**Norlén, Ivar, 1910–**
Francke OC: The dental turbine handpiece, a Swedish invention. **Bull Hist Dent** 1981 Oct;29(2):91–3

**Norris, William, d. 1814**
Paly D: Portrait of William Norris. Broadside, 1815, with etched portrait (1814) entitled 'William Norris: confined in this manner in Bethlem Hospital'; George Arnald, A.R.A., artist, etcher, and publisher. **Radic Hist Rev** 1979 Spring/Summer;Spec:65

**Norris, William, 1792–1877**
Davis NC: William Norris, M.D.: a pioneer in the study of melanoma. **Med J Aust** 1980 Jan 26;1(2):52–4
Silvers DN, Gorham JD: Observations on a melanoma by William Norris, M.D., a country practitioner of the early 19th century. **Am J Dermatopathol** 1982 Oct;4(5):421–4

**Norwood, William Frederick, 1904–**
Numbers RL, ed: The education of American physicians: historical essays. [Preface includes biographical tribute to William F. Norwood]. Berkeley, University of California Press, 1980. xiii, 345 p. Contributions by L. G. Stevenson, M. Kaufman, J. B. Blake, J. H. Warner, J. Whorton, D. L. Cowen, R. C. Maulitz, E. C. Atwater, G. H. Brieger, L. D Longo, J. L. Brand, J. W. Leavitt, C R. Burns, G. Miller

**Nossel, Hymie Louis, 1930–1983**
Blombäck B, Copley AL: Hymie Nossel (11 July 1930–8 October 1983). **Thromb Res** 1984 Apr 1;34(1):1–7

**Notredame, Michel de, 1503–1566**
Simonin M: Michel de Nostredame, Pierre Boaistuau, Chavigny et la peste aixoise de 1546. **Bibl Hum Renaissance** 1983;45(1):127–30

**Nott, Josiah Clark, 1804–1873**
Animalcular and cryptogamic theories on the origins of fevers. Reprinted works by John Kearsley Mitchell (1849), John L. Riddell (1836), Josiah Clark Nott (1848). New York, Arno, 1977. Various paginations.:
Chernin E: Josiah Clark Nott, insects, and yellow fever. **Bull NY Acad Med** 1983 Nov;59(9):790–802
Health in the southern United States: New York, Arno, 1977. Various paginations. Facsimiles of works by David Ramsay (1790 and 1796), Josiah C. Nott (1847), Edward H. Barton (1851), Wickliffe Rose (1910), Joseph Goldberger (1916).

**Novy, Frederick George, 1864–1957**
Garrett CG: Frederick George Novy. In Dictionary of American Biography, Suppl. 6, 1956–1960. p. 481–2, 1980.

**Nowell, John, 1553 or 4–1603?**
Wyman AL: John Nowell, an Elizabethan Fellow of the College of Physicians. **J R Coll Physicians Lond** 1984 Jul;18(3):166–9

**Noyes, John Humphrey, 1811–1886**
Karp LE: Past perfect: John Humphrey Noyes, stirpiculture, and the Oneida community - part II. **Am J Med Genet** 1982 Jun;12(2):127–30

**Noyes, Marcia Crocker, 1869–1946**
Smith BT: Marcia Crocker Noyes, medical librarian: the shaping of a career. **Bull Med Libr Assoc** 1974 Jul;62(3):314–24

**Nunes Garcia, José Maurício, 1808–1857**
Sattamini Duarte O: Dr. José Maurício Nunes Garcia. **Rev Inst Hist Geogr Bras** 1971;291:92–103

**Nürnberger, Woldemar, 1818–1869**
Dallett JB: Woldemar Nürnbergers Paracelsus-Roman. **Salzburger Beitr Paracelsusforsch** 1984;23:50–60

**Nutting, Mary Adelaide, 1858–1948**
Sanborn A: The seed for a dream: M. Adelaide Nutting. **Alumni Mag** 1984 Jul;84(1):3–5

**Nyulas, Ferenc, 1758–1808**
Spielmann J: Nyulas Ferenc emlékezete. **Orv Hetil** 1984 Jun 24;125(26):1578–81

## O

**Obaliński, Alfred, 1843–1898**
Cendrzak E: Alfred Obaliński--prekursor urologii w Polsce. **Arch Hist Med (Warsz)** 1984;47(2):239–48

**Obermann, Rudolf**
Cremona GF: Cenni sullo sviluppo della ginnastica educativa e medica in Italia. **Ann Osp Maria Vittoria Torino** 1981 Jan–Jun;24(1–6):210–6

**Oberto, Juan Bautista, fl. 1774**
Alegría C: Dos medicos en la aurora de la gesta emancipadora de Venezuela. **Rev Soc Venez Hist Med** 1969–71;17–19(31–33):29–48

**Obregia, Alexandrŭ, 1860–1937**
Sărmaşanu-Cortez ML, Cortez P: A great forerunner of the modern sanitary organization, Prof. Dr. Alexandru Obregia (1860–1937). **Sante Publique (Bucar)** 1979;22(4):387–93

**O'Callaghan, Edmund Bailey, 1797–1880**
Durley MS: Dr. Edmund Bailey O'Callaghan, his early years in medicine, Montreal, 1823–1828. **Study Sess Can Cathol Hist Assoc** 1980;47:23–40

**Ochsner, Alton, 1896–1981**
Blum A: Alton Ochsner, MD, 1896 1981. He cleared the air. **NY State J Med** 1983 Dec;83(13):1251

**Ochsner, Edward William Alton, 1896–**
Connaugton D: Alton Ochsner: not as a legend. **Bull Am Coll Surg** 1981;66(5):27, 31–2

**O'Connor, Flannery, 1925–1964**
Coles R: Flannery O'Connor's lupus. A commentary on her collected letters, The habit of being. **JAMA** 1980 Sep 26;244(13):1441–2

**Oertel, Max Joseph, 1835–1897**
Habermann G: Max Joseph Oertel 1835–1897. **Folia Phoniatr (Basel)** 1983;35(1–2):91

**Oever, Jan van den, d. 1728**
Muller CF: 'N blad uit die joernaal van 'n sieketrooster, 1709–1710. **Historia (S Afr)** 1978;23(2):90–8

**Officer, Robert, 1800–1879**
Forster FM: David D. Davis' Obstetric Atlas in Tasmania in 1846. Edmund Bowden's gift to Robert Officer. **Aust NZ J Obstet Gynaecol** 1983 May;23(2):88–92

**Ogden, Robert Morris, 1877–1959**
Henle M: Robert M. Ogden and Gestalt psychology in America. **J Hist Behav Sci** 1984 Jan;20(1):9–19

**Ogston, Alexander, 1844–1929**
Smith G: Ogston's Coccus: 102 years and still going strong. **South Med J** 1982 Dec;75(12):1559–62

**Oguse, Docteur**
Oguse, D: 'Socialisme et néo-malthusianisme', la Revue Socialiste, t. XLVI, juillet-décembre 1907, p. 27–124. **Ann Demogr Hist (Paris)** 1983;:371–89

**O'Halloran, Sylvester, 1728–1807**
Lyons JB: Sylvester O'Halloran's 'Treatise on the Air'. **Ir Med J** 1983 Jan;76(1):37–9

**Okubo, Tekisai**
Matsuki A: [Current view of the studies on the history of anesthesiology (7)--Tekisai Okubo, a pioneer of the pain clinic in Japan] **Masui** 1980 Feb;29(2):182–4

**Okunevskiĭ, IaL, 1877–1940**
Smirnov EI, Garin NS: Znachenie nauchnogo naslediia i deiatel'nosti Ia. L. Okunevskogo dlia sozdaniia dezinfektsionnogo i banno-prachechnogo dela v armii. **Voen Med Zh** 1979 Apr;(4):73–5

**Olai, Benedictus, fl. 1578**
Perret L: Benedictus Olai: een nyttigh Läkere-Book 1578. Ett 400-årsminne. Några synpunkter på 1500-talets läkekonst. **Nord Medicinhist Arsb** 1980;Suppl 6:118–21

**Oldenburg, Henry, 1615?–1677**
Hall AR, Boas Hall M: The first human blood transfusion: priority disputes. **Med Hist** 1980;24(4):461–5

**O'Leary, Paul Arthur, 1891–1955**
Perry HO, Powell FC, Cooper AJ: Paul A. O'Leary--dermatologist and teacher. **J Am Acad Dermatol** 1982 Nov;7(5):705–8

**Oleneva, Elizaveta Nikolaevna, 1924–**
Elizaveta Nikolaevna Oleneva (k 60-letiiu so dnia rozhdeniia): **Arkh Anat Gistol Embriol** 1984 Mar;86(3):107–9

**Oliver, Williams, 1695–1764**
Fraser KJ: Anglo-French contributions to the recognition of rheumatoid arthritis. **Ann Rheum Dis** 1982 Aug;41(4):335–43

**Olivercrona, Herbert, 1891–1980**
Crişan V: Herbert Olivecrona (1891–1980). **Rev Med Interna [Neurol Psihiatr]** 1981 Oct–Dec;26(4):307–10

**Olives, Mariano, fl. 1825–1840**
Tarragó Valentines JF: Un informe sobre el hospital de Santa Maria de Lerida, escrito en el siglo XIX por Marioano Olives. **Asclepio** 1980;32:453–6

**Olivier, Charlotte, 1864–1945**
Favez G: Charlotte Olivier (1864–1945). **Rev Med Suisse Romande** 1984 May;104(5):353–68

**Oller, Francisco, 1785–1831**
Rigau Pérez JG: El Dr. Francisco Oller y el inicio de la salud pública moderna en Puerto Rico, 1790–1831. In International Congress of the History of Medicine, 27th, Barcelona, 1980. Actas. Barcelona, Académia de Ciències Médiques de Catalunya i Balears, 1981. p. 199–202.

**Ollier, Léopold, 1830–1900**
Mirskiĭ MB: L. Oll'e i ego rol' v razvitii khirurgii i transplantologii (k 150-letiiu so dnia rozhdeniia). **Ortop Travmatol Protez** 1981 Oct;(10):75–6
Mourgues G de: Léopold Ollier, 1830–1900, père de la chirurgie orthopédique. **Rev Chir Orthop** 1979;65(11):2–3
Vitoria Ortiz M: Ollier et sa contribution à l'étude de l'appareil locomotor. In International Congress of the History of Medicine, 27th, Barcelona, 1980. Actas. Barcelona, Académia de Ciències Médiques de Catalunya i Balears, 1981. p. 680–9.

**Ollinger, Georg, 1487–1557**
Müller-Jahncke WD: Die 'Magnarum Medicine partium herbariae et zoographiae imagines' von Georg Ollinger und Samuel Quicchelberg. **Beitr Gesch Pharm** 1982;31(17):129–33

**Ollivier, Alexandre François, 1790–**
Huard P, Imbault-Huart MJ: La polémique Percy-Ollivier sur le typhus traumatique en 1822. In: Congrès National des Sociétés Savantes, 99e, Besançon, 1974. Comptes Rendus. Paris, 1976. Section des Sciences, Fasc. V. p. 243–9.

**Olmsted, Frederick Law, 1822–1903**
Bean WB: Frederick Law Olmstead and Vanderbilt's Biltmore estate: the contribution of private wealth to forestry, ecology and climatology. **Trans Am Clin Climatol Assoc** 1979;90:132–9
Chernin E: Two physicians, a landscape architect, and malaria. **Bull NY Acad Med** 1984 Nov;60(9):932–7

**Olombel, Jacques-Samuel, 1760–1850**
Théodoridès J: Claude Bernard et les parasites. (Contribution au centenaire de la mort de Claude Bernard). **Hist Nat** 1979;(14):31–8

**Olóriz y Aguilera, Federico, 1855–1912**
Arquiola E: Anatomía y antropología en la obra de Olóriz. **Dynamis** 1981;1:165–77

**Olszak, Wacław, 1902–**
Sembol J: Dr Wacław Olszak. **Przegl Lek** 1981;38(1):169–73

**Ombredanne, Louis, 1871–1956**
Teimourian B, Adham MN: Louis Ombredanne and the origin of muscle flap use for immediate breast mound reconstruction. **Plast Reconstr Surg** 1983 Dec;72(6):905–10
Weisser C: Der Ombrédannesche Ather-Inhalator. Ein Beitrag zur Geschichte der Ather-Apparatnarkose. **Anaesthesist** 1983 Feb;32(2):51–4

**Oppel, Vladimir Andreyevitch, 1872–1932**
Epifanov NS: Khirurg, uchenyĭ, patriot (k110-letiiu so dnia rozhdeniia V.A. Oppelia). **Khirurgiia (Mosk)** 1982 Nov;(11):101–3
Kotel'nikov VP: V. A. Oppel' i razvitie fiziologicheskoĭ khirurgii. **Klin Med (Mosk)** 1984 May;62(5):145–8

**Orakhelashvili, Ivan Dmitrievich, 1881–1937**
Shalaev NF: Vrach-bol'shevik I. D. Orakhelashvili. **Sov Zdravookhr** 1984;(1):51–3

**Orbeli, Leon Abgarovich, 1882–1958**
Govyrin VA, Grigor'ian RA: Akademik L. A. Orbeli: étapy zhizni i nauchnoĭ deiatel'nosti (k 100-letiiu so dnia rozhdeniia). **Usp Fiziol Nauk** 1982 Jun–Sep;13(3):3–8
Grigori'ian NA: Razvitie ucheniia o vyssheĭ nervnoĭ deiatel'nosti v trudakh L. A. Orbeli. **Zh Vyssh Nerv Deiat** 1982 Nov–Dec;32(6):1011–9
Leĭbson LG: L. A. Orbeli i nekotorye aspekty évoliutsionnoĭ fiziologii. **Zh Evol Biokhim Fiziol** 1983 Jul–Aug;19(4):322–32
Mozzhukhin AS: Rol' L. A. Orbeli v stanovlenii i razrabotke fiziologicheskikh problem radiobiologii. **Fiziol Zh SSSR** 1982 Jul;68(7):914–7
Panchenko DI, Vilenskiĭ IuG: Leon Abgarovich Orbeli v Kieve (k 100-letiiu so dnia rozhdeniia). **Vrach Delo** 1982 Sep;(9):119–22
Svetaĭlo EN: Vydaiuschiĭsia uchenyĭ sovremennosti (k 100-letiiu so dnia rozhdeniia L. A. Orbeli). **Fiziol Zh SSSR** 1983 Feb;69(2):281–3

**Oribasius, fl. 4th cent. A.D.**
Riou YF: Un fragment d'un manuscrit disparu d'Oribase, C. L. A. 116 (Vatican, Urb. lat. 293, ff. 95–96, VIIIe siècle). **Scriptorium** 1979;33:235–7

**Orlowski, Witold Eugenjusz, 1874–1966**
Kałużny J: W 25-lecie redagowania Kliniki Ocznej przez prof. dra Witolda Orowskiego. **Klin Oczna** 1981;83(2):55–8
Mrozowski K: Wkład profesora doktora medycyny Witolda Eugeniusza Orłowskiego w zwalczaniu gruźlicy. **Pol Arch Med Wewn** 1981;65(5):385–9

**Orovecz, Bela, 1909–1967**
Bencze B: Emlékezés Orovecz Bélára az Országos Mentöszolgálat megszervezöjére (1909–1967). **Orv Hetil** 1979 Nov 18;120(46):2819–20

**Orr, H. Winnett, 1877–1956**
Connolly JF: Wound management and the legacy of H. Winnett Orr. **Nebr Med J** 1982 Mar;67(3):60–1

**Orrego Luco, Augusto, 1848–1933**
Pérez-Olea J: Don Augusto Orrego Luco. **Rev Med Chil** 1984 Feb;112(2):193–200

**Országh, Pavol, 1849–1921**
Vilček E: O zdravotnom stave P. O. Hviezdoslava. **Bratisl Lek Listy** 1983;79(1):117–22

**Orticochea, Miguel**
Orticochea M: History of the discovery of the musculocutaneous flap method as a substitute for the delay method. **Ann Plast Surg** 1983 Jul;11(1):63–8

**Ortolff von Bayrlandt**
Crossgrove W: Ein frühes Zeugnis für Ortolfs Arzneibuch. **Z Dtsch Altert Dtsch Lit** 1979;108:234–9
Walther H: Ein Magister Ortolf de Bavaria in Paris. **Sudhoffs Arch** 1978;62(3):294–5

**Orzovenszky, Károly**
Szekér E: Emléktábla-ayató ünnepség Balatonfüreden. **Orv Hetil** 1983 Feb 20;124(8):467–8

**Osborn, Henry Fairfield, 1857–1935**
Rainger R: The Henry Fairfield Osborn Papers at the American Museum of Natural History. **Mendel Newsl** 1980 Jun;(18):8–13

**O'Scanlan, Timoteo, 1726–1800**
Parrilla Hermida M: Biografia del doctor Timoto O'Scalan---1726–1800. **Asclepio** 1980;32:287–93

**O'Shaughnessy, William Brooke, 1809–1889**
Gorman M: Sir William B. O'Shaughnessy, pioneer chemical educator in India. **Ambix** 1983 Jul;30(2):107–16
Gorman M: Sir William Brooke O'Shaughnessy, F.R.S. (1809–1889), Anglo-Indian forensic chemist. **Notes Rec R Soc Lond** 1984 Sep;39(1):51–64

**Oshima, Shiro, 1934–1981**
Uchikawa K: Dr. Shiro Oshima (1934–1981). **Acarologia** 1982 Jun;23(2):99–101

**Osiander, Friedrich Benjamin, 1759–1822**
Winkelmann H: Entbindungswissenschaft und Entbindungskunst bei Friedrich Benjamin Osiander. **Medizinhist J** 1983;18(4):306–12

**Osipov, E. Alexelvich, 1841–1904**
Bazanov VA: E. A. Osipov--odin iz osnovopolozhnikov obshchestvennoĭ meditsiny i sanitarnoĭ statistiki v dorevoliutsionnoĭ Rossii. **Feldsher Akush** 1980;45(9):40–4

**Osler, Edward, 1798–1863**
Gittings R: Edward Osler and John Keats. In J. Cule, ed: Wales and medicine. London, British Society for the History of Medicine, 1975. p. 107–11.

**Osler, Grace, 1854–1928**
Harrell GT: Lady Osler. **Bull Hist Med** 1979 Spring;53(1):81–99
Harrell GT: Grace Revere Osler: a turn of the century professor's wife. **Ann Intern Med** 1980 Sep;93(3):504–5

**Osler, William, 1849–1919**
Altaffer LF: Penis captivus and the mischievous Sir William Osler. **South Med J** 1983 May;76(5):637–41
Altschule MD: Occasional notes. A near miss--Osler's early description of Cushing's syndrome with, regrettably, no post-mortem examination. **N Engl J Med** 1980 May 15;302(20):1153–5
Beauperthuy de Benedetti R: Bref commentaire à un travail de Sir William Osler et sa reconnaissance de la théorie scientifique de Beauperthuy sur la fièvre jaune. In: Congrès international d'histoire de la médecine, XXVe, Québec, 1976. Actes. Québec, 1977. p. 487–92.
Berk SL: Bacterial pneumonia in the elderly: the observations of Sir William Osler in retrospect. **J Am Geriatr Soc** 1984 Sep;32(9):683–5
Bondy PK: What's so special about Osler? **Yale J Biol Med** 1980 May–Jun;53(3):213–7
Brodin MB: William Osler and dermatology, pathology, and dermatopathology. **Am J Dermatopathol** 1981 Fall;3(3):261–4
Cantwell JD: Osler: a role model for today's physician. **J Med Assoc Ga** 1983 Jul;72(7)::493–4
Duffy TP: Sir William Osler revisited. **Yale J Biol Med** 1980 May–Jun;53(3):219–24
Dugan DJ: Aequanimitas revisited. **Am J Surg** 1982 Jul;144(1):3–7
Ebers GC, Stewart J: In defence of Osler. **J R Soc Med** 1982 Dec;75(12):989
Fishman N: John Bell, MD--teacher to William Osler. **Can Med Assoc J** 1981 Nov 1;125(9):1042, 1044
Geyman JP: The Oslerian tradition and changing medical education: a reappraisal. **West J Med** 1983 Jun;138(6):884–8
Girard DE: The history of Osler's Principles and practice of medicine. **Med Times** 1981 Jul;109(7):1s–4s, 13s
Golden RL: Medallic tributes to Sir William Osler and their historical associations. **JAMA** 1979 Dec 28;242(26):2862–7
Golden RL: Osler, 'E. Y. D.,' and hysteria. **JAMA** 1982 May 21;247(19):2698–9
Golden RL: A 'forgotten' clinic of Sir William Osler. **JAMA** 1981 Feb 6;245(5):500–1
Golden RL: Osler and Oriental medicine: a discursive review. Princeton, Science Press Associates, 1982. iii, 93 p.
Graner JL: An introduction to the writings of Egerton Yorrick Davis. **IMJ** 1983 Jul;164(1):47–8
Gruman GJ, ed: The 'Fixed period' controversy: prelude to modern ageism. New York, Arno Press, 1979. Various paginations. Reprint of passages by George M. Beard, William Osler, and James Crichton-Browne.
Harrell GT: Lady Osler. **Bull Hist Med** 1979 Spring;53(1):81–99
Harrell GT: Osler's practice. **Bull Hist Med** 1973 Nov–Dec;47(6):545–68
Harrell GT: Grace Revere Osler: a turn of the century professor's wife. **Ann Intern Med** 1980 Sep;93(3):504–5
Harrell GT: The Osler family. **JAMA** 1982 Jul 9;248(2):203–9
Harrell GT: The Osler-endowed Tudor and Stuart Club. **Pharos** 1984 Summer;47(3):23–6
Howard RP: 'The Chief'--Doctor William Osler. **Iowa Med** 1984 Apr;74(4):155–8
Key JD: Osler's baby on the tracks. **Minn Med** 1983 Aug:66(8):515
Key JD, Rodin AE: William Osler and Arthur Conan Doyle versus the antivivisectionists: some lessons from history for today. **Mayo Clin Proc** 1984 Mar;59(3):189–96
Keys TE, Key JD: Osler and Billings: their friendship and contributions to librarianship. **Am Coll Physicians Obs** 1981 Aug;1(8):1, 4–5
Kingsbury M: Book collector, bibliographer, and benefactor of libraries: Sir William Osler. **J Libr Hist** 1981 Winter;16(1):187–98
Kolisch P deR: Paul Revere and medicine. **JAMA** 1984 Jun 22–29;251(24):3224
Lampert RH: Osler and his publishers. **Trans Stud Coll Physicians Phila** 1983 Sep;5(5 No 3):177–90
Lovell RR: The university medical presence in hospitals seventy years after Flexner and a look ahead. **Aust NZ J Med** 1983 Apr;13(2):187–94
McGill University: The Osler Library. Montreal, McGill University, 1979. 64 p.
Massey RU: Reflections from the Dean's office. The cheerful physicians. **Conn Med** 1979 Nov;43(11):747
Matthews WB: Osler Oration. **J R Soc Med** 1982 May;75(5):307–14
Melzer R: William Osler's connection with South Africa. **S Afr Med J** 1983 Jun 29;Spec No.:8–13
Nation EF, McGovern JP, ed: Student and chief: the Osler-Camac correspondence. Pasadena, Castle Press, 1980. 131 p.
Naylor D: Osler's first medical publications. **Can Med Assoc J** 1984 Oct 1;131(7):800–5
Neghme A: Vida y obra de Sir William Osler (1849–1919) y la fundación de la Escuela de Medicina en la Universidad de Johns Hopkins. **Rev Med Chil** 1983 Jan;111(1):83–92
Nelson RB: Occasional notes. Captains of an American credo: Walt and W. O. **N Engl J Med** 1981 Jul 9;305(2):110–2
Pruitt RD: William Osler and his Gulstonian lectures on malignant endocarditis. **Mayo Clin Proc** 1982 Jan;57(1):4–9
Robb-Smith AH: Osler's influence on haematology. **Blood Cells** 1981;7(3):513–36
Rodin AE: Oslerian pathology: an assessment and annotated atlas of museum specimens. Lawrence, Kansas, Coronado, 1981. xviii, 250 p.
Roland CG: Sir William Osler's dreams and nightmares. **Bull Hist Med** 1980 Fall;54(3):418–46
Roland CG: The palpable Osler: a study in survival. **Perspect Biol Med** 1984;27(2):299–313
Rosenow EC: Osler--continuing education advocate. **Bull Am Coll Physicians** 1975 Aug;16(8):6–8
Scott JW: Osler and the science of medicine. In: Congrès international de la médecine XXVe, Quebec, 1976. Actes. Québec, 1977. p. 1244–52.
Sharma OP, James DG: Did Osler's patient, Hannah W, have sarcoidosis? An historical footnote. **Chest** 1984 Aug;86(2):263–4
Spaulding WB: Osler's roots in Dundas. **Ann R Coll Physicians Surg Can** 1982 May;15(3):219–22
Sternbach G: William Osler: narcotic-induced pulmonary edema. **J Emerg Med** 1983;1(2):165–7
Stevenson LG: Joseph Dietl, William Osler and the definition of therapeutic nihilism. In Ganzinger K, Skopec M, Wyklicky H, ed: Festschrift für Erna Lesky zum 70. Geburtstag. Wien, Brüder

Hollinek, 1981. p. 149–52.
Teigen PM: William Osler and comparative medicine. **Can Vet J** 1984;25:400–5
Teigen PM, ed: Books, manuscripts, and the history of medicine. Essays on the fiftieth anniversary of the Osler Library. New York, Science History Publications, 1982. 112 p. Contributions by L. G. Stevenson, C. G. Roland, R. J. Durling, E. Brodman, G. T. Tanselle, E. J. Freeman.
Tigertt WD: An annotated life of Egerton Yorrick Davis, M.D., an intimate of Sir William Osler. **J Hist Med Allied Sci** 1983 Jul;38(3):259–97
Tucker WS: Osler and sleep apnea. **Arch Intern Med** 1984 May;144(5):1085
Weissmann G. Against Aequanimitas. **Hosp Pract [Off]** 1984 Jun;19(6):159–69
Wooley CF: From irritable heart to mitral valve prolapse: the Osler connection. **Am J Cardiol** 1984 Mar 1;53(6):870–4

**Osterhout, Winthrop John Vanleuven, 1871–1964**
Davis AB: Winthrop John Vanleuven Osterhout. In Dictionary of American biography, 1961–1965. Suppl. 7, 1981. p. 592–3.

**Osvát, Kálmán, 1880–1953**
Szállási A: Aki szerkesztönek született, az orvostudomány sem menti meg. **Orv Hetil** 1981 Apr 5;122(14):837–9

**Otelin, Aleksandr Anatol'evich, 1904–1981**
Pamiati Aleksandra Anatol'evicha Otelina: **Arkh Anat Gistol Embriol** 1981 Sep;81(9):123–6

**Otis, Arthur Sinton, 1886–1964**
Smith HC: Arthur Sinton Otis. In Dictionary of American biography, 1961–1965. Suppl. 7, 1981. p. 594–5.

**Ott, Arnold, 1840–1910**
Winkler-Trachsel E: Arnold Ott (1840–1910). Arzt und Dichter. Sein ärztliches Wirken. Zürich, Juris Druck, 1983. 83 p. (Zürcher Medizingeschichtliche Abhandlungen, Neue Reihe, Nr. 163).

**Ott, Dmitri Oskarovich, 1855–1929**
Danilischina EI, Schneck P: D. O. Ott (1855–1929) und die russisch-deutschen medizinischen Beziehungen. **Z Arztl Fortbild (Jena)** 1981 Oct 1;75(19):924–7

**Ottilia, Saint, d. ca. 720**
Grossmann T: Die hl. Ottilie, Patronin der Augenkranken. Eine ungewöhnliche Abbildung am Gnadenstuhlaltar von Bad Aussee mit Krebsscherenattribut. **Klin Monatsbl Augenheilkd** 1981 Jun;178(6):480–1

**Otto, John Conrad, 1774–1844**
Snape WJ, Wolfe EL: The studies of yellow-fever by Noah Webster and John Conrad Otto at Red Bank, New Jersey. **Bull Gloucester Cty Hist Soc** 1984 Jun;19(4):25–32

**Ovid, 43 B.C.–ca. 17 A.D.**
Dirckx JH: Ovid's dermatologic formulary. **Am J Dermatopathol** 1980 Winter;2(4):327–32
Green P: Ars gratia cultus: Ovid as beautician. **Am J Philol** 1979;100:381–92

**Owen, Isambard, 1850–1927**
Jame DG: Dr. Isambard Owen (1850–1927). In J. Cule, ed: Wales and medicine. London, British Society for the History of Medicine, 1975. p. 96–106.

**Owen, Richard, 1804–1892**
Campbell WC: History of trichinosis: Paget, Owen and the discovery of Trichinella Spiralis. **Bull Hist Med** 1979 Winter;53(4):520–52
Gilbert SF: Owen's vertebral archetype and evolutionary genetics -- a Platonic appreciation. **Perspect Biol Med** 1980 Spring;23(3):475–88
O'Rahilly R: The discovery of the parathyroid glands. **Bull Hist Med** 1982 Summer;56(2):263–4

**Owen, Wilfred, 1893–1918**
Hibberd D: 'Problems A': the solution to Wilfred Owen's 'The Imbecile.' **Notes Queries** 1980 Jun;27(3):232–3

**Oxea, Fernando, fl. 1771**
García Guerra D: La 'Disertacion medica' de Fernando Oxea. Un testimonio de auscultacion inmediata del torax en el siglo XVIII. **Asclepio** 1980;32:201–9

**Ozeki, Chikako**
Takahashi M: [Personalities in the history of nursing. (4). Ms. Chika Ozeki] (Jpn). **Kango Kyoiku** 1981 Sep;22(9)575–82

## P

**Paatero, Yrjö Veli**
Pataky L: Az orthopantomográfia kialakulása Paatero munkásságának tükrében. **Fogory Sz** 1979 Sep;72(9):279–80

**Pachner, Frantisek, 1882–1964**
Kvíz D: Příspěvek k historiografii moravské gynekologie. **Cesk Gynekol** 1980 Mar;45(2):142–52

**Pacini, Filippo, 1812–1883**
Subba Rao M: Original observations of Filippo Pacini on vibrio cholera. **Bull Indian Inst Hist Med (Hyderabad)** 1978;8(1–4):32–8

**Packard, Elizabeth Parsons Ware, 1816–1897**
Himelhoch MS, Shaffer AH: Elizabeth Packard: nineteenth-century crusader for the rights of mental patients. **J Am Stud** 1979;13(3):343–75

**Padgett, Earl Calvin, 1893–**
As I remember Earl C. Padgett: **Ann Plast Surg** 1981 Feb;6(2):142–57
Ketchum LD: An historical account of the development of the calibrated dermatome. **Ann Plast Surg** 1978 Nov;1(6):608–11

**Paevskiĭ, Vladimir Vladislavovich, 1893–1934**
Belitskaia EIa: V. V. Paevskiĭ i ego kniga 'Elementy statistiki' (k 50-letiiu opublikovaniia). **Sov Zdravookhr** 1981;(6):64–6

**Paffenbarger, George Corbly, 1902–**
Forrest WR, Christen AG: Recollections of a dental researcher. Fifty years at the U. S. Bureau of Standards: Interviews with George C. Paffenbarger. Part I. **J Ala Dent Assoc** 1982 Summer;66(3):24–8
Forrest WR, Christen AG: Recollections of a dental researcher. Fifty years at the U.S. National Bureau of Standards: interviews with George C. Paffenbarger, D.D.S., D.Sc. Part II. **J Ala Dent Assoc** 1982 Fall;66(4):36–8
Forrest WR, Christen AG: Recollections of a dental researcher. Fifty years at the U.S. National Bureau of Standards: interviews with George C. Paffenbarger, D.D.S., D.Sc. Part VI. **J Ala Dent Assoc** 1984 Spring;68(2):29–31, 34–7

**Paganini, Niccolo, 1782?–1840**
Schoenfeld MR: Nicolo Paganini--musical magician and Marfan mutant? **Med Times** 1980 Nov, 108(11):117–8, 120, 125
Smith RD: Paganini's hand. **Arthritis Rheum** 1982 Nov;25(11):1385–6

**Pagel, Walter, 1898–1983**
Buess H: Prof. Dr. med. Dr.h.c. Walter Pagel (1898–1983). **Gesnerus** 1984;41(3–4):359–63
Davis AB: Walter Pagel, 14 November 1898–1 April 1983. **ISIS** 1984;75(277):363–5
Debus AG: Walter Pagel (1898–1983). **Bull Hist Med** 1983 Winter;57(4):611–5
Müller-Jahncke WD: In memoriam Walter Pagel (1898–1983). **Ber Wissenschaftsgesch** 1983;6(1–4):165–8

**Paget, James, 1814–1899**
Campbell WC: History of trichinosis: Paget, Owen and the discovery of Trichinella Spiralis. **Bull Hist Med** 1979 Winter;53(4):520–52
Estévez R: Sir James Paget. **Rev Med Chil** 1984 Jul;112(7):740–3
García-Alejo RH: Enfermedad osea de Paget: comentarios a sus primeras descripciones y evolucion historica de su etiopatogenia. **Asclepio** 1982;34:181–97
Goldstein HB: Sir James Paget. **Am J Dermatopathol** 1980 Spring;2(1):27–31
Peltier LF: Ununited fractures in children. James Paget, 1891. **Clin Orthop** 1982 Jun;(166):2–4
Reed K, Grage TB: Our surgical heritage. The Paget tradition revisited. **Am J Surg** 1982 Nov;144(5):498–503
Shaw AB: Paget's diseases. **Practitioner** 1980 Dec;224(1350):1323–7
Shenoy BV, Scheithauer BW: Sir James Paget, F.R.S. **Mayo Clin Proc** 1983 Jan;58(1):51–5

**Paine, Henry James, 1816–**
James DC: Dr. Henry James Paine: medical officer of health for Cardiff 1853–1889. **Public Health** 1981 Jul;95(4):215–21

**Palacios, Felix**
Javier Puerto F, Sanz Diaz L: Las ideas cientificas de Felix Palacios. **Bol Soc Esp Hist Farm** 1982 Mar;33(132):237–47

**Palade, George E., 1912–**
Porter KR: An informal tribute to George E. Palade. **J Cell Biol** 1983 Jul;97(1):D3–7

**Pálfyn, Jan, 1650–1730**
Ferkó S: Pálfyn Johann (1650–1730) a szülészeti fogó egyik feltalálója halálának 250. évfordulójára. **Orv Hetil** 1980 Mar 17;121(10):585–6

**Palicki, Bogusław, 1813–1868**
Gołębiowski SZ: Bogusław palicki, lekarz i działacz społeczny w wielkopolsce (1813–1868). **Arch Hist Med (Warsz)** 1983;46(2):249–53

**Palladius, Rutilius Taurus Aemilianus**
Fischer KD. Palladius, De vet. med. 14. 15, 5. **Liverp Classical Mon** 1979;4:73–4
Richter W: Palladius und sein Columella - Text im Buch über die Tiermedizin. **Wien Stud Z Klass Philol** 1978;12:249–71

**Palm, Kerstin, 1946–**
Loevy HT, Kowitz A: Dentistry on stamps (Dr. Kerstin Palm). **J Am Dent Assoc** 1984 Nov;109(5):755

**Palmer, Bartlett Joshua, 1881–1961**
Weiant CW: B. J. Palmer and the 'German issue:' the crisis in postwar European chiropractic. **Chiropr Hist** 1982;2(1):41–4

**Palmer, Daniel David, 1845–1913**
D. D.'s first book: **Chiropr Hist** 1874;4(1):6–10
Gielow V: Daniel David Palmer: rediscovering the frontier years, 1845–1887. **Chiropr Hist** 1981;1(1):11–3
Lee HK: Honoring the founder in his country: conception and struggle for Canada's Memorial College. **Chiropr Hist** 1981;(1):43–5

**Palmer Family**
Palmer TY, ed: The Palmer physicians. [s. l., s. n.], 1966. vii, 93 p.

**Palmer, Ivar, 1897-**
Eriksson E: Ivar Palmer, a great name in the history of cruciate ligament surgery. **Clin Orthop** 1983 Jan-Feb;(172):3-10

**Palmer, Mabel Heath, 1881-1949**
Ferguson A: The sweetheart of the PSC--Mabel Heath Palmer: the early years. **Chiropr Hist** 1984;4(1):25-8

**Pammachius, d. 410**
Kump WL: The xenodochium of Pammachius. **Minn Med** 1982 Oct;65(10):633

**Panaskerteli-Tsitsishvili, Z.**
Shengeliia GM: 'Lechebnaia kniga--Karabadini' Z. Panaskerteli-Tsitsishvili. **Klin Med (Mosk)** 1981 Jun;59(6):110-2

**Panaskerteli-Tsitsishvili, Zaza, fl. 15th cent.**
Dzhanelidze MB: O 'Lechebnoĭ knige-karabadine' i ee avtore Zaze Panaskerteli-Tsitsishvili (k 550-letiiu so dnia rozhdeniia). **Sov Zdravookhr** 1981;(5):67-8

**Pankok, Otto, 1893-**
Greither A: Otto Pankok und Düsseldorf; der Akademieprofessor Otto Pankok und seine Kunst. **Jahrb Univ Dusseld** 1977-78;:249-57

**Pantoja, Manuel, fl. ca. 1810**
Fernández DW: Manuel Pantoja. **Bol Acad Nac Hist (Caracas)** 1982;65(259):685-8

**Panýrek, Jan Duchoslav, 1867-1903**
Janeček M: [The father of modern academic medicine (Jan D. Panýrek)] (Cze). **Cas Lek Cesk** 1980;119:1446-8

**Pápai Páriz, Ferenc, 1649-1716**
Izsák S: Gondolatok, szempontok és kutatások Pápai Páriz Ferenc 'Pax Corporis'-ával kapcsolatban. **Orv Hetil** 1982 May 30;123(22):1365-8

**Papanicolaou, George Nicholas, 1883-1962**
Breathnach CS: Biographical sketches No. 29--Papanicolaou. **Ir Med J** 1983 May;76(5):220
Carmichael E: Dr. Papanicolaou and the Pap smear. **Ala J Med Sci** 1984 Jan;21(1):101-4
Djordjević S: Dr. George N. Papanicolaou (13. V 1883--19. II 1962). **Srp Arh Celok Lek** 1983 May;111(5):699-703
Dub O: 100 let od narození George N. Papanicolaua. **Cas Lek Cesk** 1983 Oct 28;122(43):1337
Ivić J: Povodom 100-te obljetnice rodenja George N. Papanicolaoua 1883-1983. **Jugosl Ginekol Opstet** 1983 May-Aug;23(3-4):53-4
Malarewicz A: 50 lat cytodiagnostyki ginekologicznej -- George Nicholas Papanicolaou. **Arch Hist Med (Warsz)** 1978;41(4):465-8
Puchkov IuG, Buslaeva MM, Volodina MN: Georg Papanikolau (k 100-letiiu so dnia rozhdeniia). **Vopr Onkol** 1983;29(12):87-9
Riley HD: George Nicholas Papanicolaou. In Dictionary of American biography, 1961-1965. Suppl. 7, 1981. p. 598-9.

**Papez, James Wenceslas, 1883-1958**
Breathnach CS: Biographical sketches no. 33--Papez. **Ir Med J** 1983 Oct;76(10):441
Livingston KE, Hornykiewicz O, ed: Limbic mechanisms. The continuing evolution of the limbic system concept. New York and London, Plenum, 1976. xv, 542 p. Tribute to James W. Papez; biographical contributions by P. D. MacLean, J. B. Angevine, P. I. Yakovlev.

**Papin, Denis, 1647-1712?**
Rudolph G: Les relations entre Denis Papin (1647-1714) et Leibniz (1646-1716). In: Congrès National des Sociétés Savantes, 93e, Tours, 1968. Comptes Rendus. Paris, 1971. Sections des Sciences, Tome II. p. 55-68.

**Pappenheim, Bertha, 1859-1936**
Hollender MH: The case of Anna O.: a reformulation. **Am J Psychiatry** 1980 Jul;137(7):797-800

**Pappenheimer, Alwin Max, Jr., 1908-**
Alwin M. Pappenheimer, Jr: **Cell Immunol** 1982 Jan 1;66(1):3-8
Cohn M: An introduction to 'Le Pap'. **Cell Immunol** 1982 Jan 1;66(1):11-6

**Paquette, Albiny**
Trépanier P: Victor Barbeau et Albiny Paquette. **Action Natl** 1978;68(4):324-30

**Paracelsus, 1493-1541**
Blaser RH: Paracelsus und die Basler Apotheker. **Pharm Acta Helv** 1979;54(9-10):281-5
Blaser RH: Paracelsus in Basel. Festschrift für Professor Dr. Robert-Henri Blaser zum 60. Geburtstag. Herausgegeben von der Schweizerischen Paracelsus-Gesellschaft. Biographical introduction by K. Goldammer. Muttenz/Basel, St. Arbogast Verlag, 1979. 210 p. (Reprint of 7 works by Blaser).
Blaser RH: Ulrich Gyger, sin diener. Versuch einer biographischen Rekonstruktion. **Medizinhist J** 1981;16(1-2):53-66
Blaser RH: Paracelsus und die Dichter. **Salzburger Beitr Paracelsusforsch** 1984;23:9-26
Brann NL: Was Paracelsus a disciple of Trithemius? **Sixteenth Century J** 1979;10(1):71-82
Braun L: Paracelsus und die Philosophiegeschichte. Eine systematische Betrachtung. Wien, 1965. 26 p. (Salzburger Beiträge zur Paracelsusforschung, 5).
Braun L: Nature et philosophie. **Medizinhist J** 1981;16(1-2):140-50
Braun L: Paracelse, commentateur des Aphroismes d'Hippocrate. In La collection hippocratique et son rôle dans l'histoire de la médecine. Colloque de Strasbourg (23-27 octobre 1972) organisé par le Centre de Recherches sur la Grèce Antique, avec le concours des Facultés de Philosophie et des Langues Classiques. Leiden, E. J. Brill, 1975. p. 335-46.
Braun L: Paracelse: nature et philosophie. Strasbourg, Association des Publications près les Universités de Strasbourg, 1981. 176 p.
Braun L: Vom Wesen des Grundes bei Paracelsus. **Salzburger Beitr Paracelsusforsch** 1984;23:27-35
Braun L, et al: Paracelse. Paris, Albin Michel, 1980. 280 p. (Cahiers de l'Hermétisme).
Bresgen C: Homo omnis creatura. Arcimboldo und Paracelsus - eine Gegenüberstellung aus der Sicht des Künstlers. **Salzburger Beitr Paracelsusforsch** 1984;23:36-49
Daems WF: Renward Cysat und Paracelsus. **Gesnerus** 1982;39(3-4):469-72
Dallett JB: Paracelsus in Moronia. Bischof Joseph Halls satirische Darstellung von 'Bustius Hohenheimius' und dessen Collegium. Wien, 1976. 20 p. (Salzburger Beiträge zur Paracelsusforschung, 14).
Dallett JB: Woldemar Nürnbergers Paracelsus-Roman. **Salzburger Beitr Paracelsusforsch** 1984;23:50-60
Debus AG: The Paracelsians in eighteenth century France: a Renaissance tradition in the age of the Enlightenment. **Ambix** 1981 Mar;28(1):36-54
Debus AG: The chemical philosophy. Paracelsian science and medicine in the sixteenth and seventeenth centuries. 2 vols. New York, Science History Publications, 1977. xv, 606 p.
Debus AG: History with a purpose: the fate of Paracelsus. **Pharm Hist** 1984;26(2):83-96
Domandi S: Hohenheims De natura rerum. Eine Einführung in die geistige Welt des Paracelsus. **Salzburger Beitr Paracelsusforsch** 1984;23:61-88
Domandl S: Erziehung und Menschenbild bei Paracelsus. Anfänge einer verantwortungsbewussten Pädagogik. Wien, Notring, 1970. 144 p. (Salzburger Beiträge zur Paracelsusforschung, 9).
Domandl S: Paracelsus und Paracelsustradition in Salzburg (1524-1976). Ein Beitrag zur Kultur- und Zeitgeschichte. Wien, 1977. (Salzburger Beiträge zur Paracelsusforschung, 17), p. 9-44, 48-59. Includes O. Kostenzer: Das Paracelsusgrabmal in Stams, p. 45-48.
Domandl S, ed: Paracelsus im Blickfeld heutiger wissenschaftsgeschichtlicher Betrachtung (ein Rundgespräch). Wien, 1974. 59 p. (Salzburger Beiträge zur Paracelsusforschung, 12). Contributions by L. Braun, A. W. Gutsch, V. Bazala, K. Goldammer, H. Goerke, W. Schneider, R. Blaser, KH Weimann, G. Harrer, A. Dyk.
Gilly C: Zwischen Erfahrung und Spekulation. Theodor Zwinger und die religiöse und kulturelle Krise seiner Zeit. **Basler Z Gesch Altertumskd** 1977;77:57-137
Glesinger L: Der Humanist Andreas Dudith im Kreise der Antiparacelsisten. Wien, 1967. (Salzburger Beiträge zur Paracelsusforschung, 7). p. 3-12.
Goldammer K: Paracelsus in der deutschen Romantik. Eine Untersuchung zur Geschichte der Paracelsus-Rezeption und zu geistesgeschichtlichen Hintergründen der Romantik. Mit einem Anhang über die Entstehung und Entwicklung der Elementargeister-Vorstellungen seit dem Mittelalter. Wien, 1980. 212 p. (Salzburger Beiträge zur Paracelsusforschung, 20).
Goldammer K: Paracelsus, Humanisten und Humanismus. Ein Beitrag zur kultur- und geistesgeschichtlichen Stellung Hohenheims. Wien, 1964. 32 p. (Salzburger Beiträge zur Paracelsusforschung, 4).
Goldammer K: Neues zur Frage der Paracelsischen Spuria. **Sudhoffs Arch** 1984;68(2):235-9
Goldammer K: Zur philosophischen und religiösen Sinngebung von Heilung und Heilmittel bei Paracelsus. In Dilg P, et al., ed: Perspektiven der Pharmaziegeschichte. Graz, Austria, Akademische Druck- u. Verlagsanstalt, 1983. p. 113-29.
Guinsburg AM: Paracelsian magic and theology; a case study of the Matthew commentaries. **Medizinhist J** 1981;16(1-2):125-39
Helmrich HE: Spagyrik. Alter Wein in neuen Schläuchen. Heidelberg, Haug, 1977. 253 p.
Kelecom J: Episodes de la médecine liégeoise. Le souvenir de Paracelse au siècle des lumières. **Rev Med Liege** 1981 Sep 1;36(17):638-46
Klutz M: Die Rezepte in Oswald Crolls Basilica Chymica (1609) und ihre Beziehungen zu Paracelsus. Braunschweig, 1974. 124 p. (Veröffentlichungen aus dem Pharmaziegeschichtlichen Seminar der Technischen Universität Braunschweig, 14).
Kollautz A: Eine Episode aus der Praxis des Paracelsus. **Carinthia** 1967;157:578-87
Lenz HG: Der hessische Paracelsist Johann Thoelde. **Salzburger Beitr Paracelsusforsch** 1984;23:89-99
Mann G: Kreatur und Kosmos. Internationale Beiträge zur Paracelsus-Forschung. **Dtsch Arztebl** 1981;78:1020-2
Meier P: Paracelsus-Reminiszenzen--Arzt und Medizin im Werk von Reinhold Schneider. **Salzburger Beitr Paracelsusforsch** 1984;23:100-17
Midelfort HC: The anthropological roots of Paracelsus' psychiatry.

**Medizinhist J** 1981;16(1-2):67-77
Pagel W: The Paracelsian Elias Artista and the alchemical tradition. **Medizinhist J** 1981;16(1-2):6-19
Pagel W: Paracelsus. An introduction to philosophical medicine in the era of the Renaissance, 2nd, revised edition. Basel, Karger, 1982. xii, 399 p.
Paracelsus-Forschung heute: Bericht über den Jubiläumskongress 1976 und die 25 jährige Geschichte der Gesellschaft, mit Beiträgen von K. Goldammer, A. Dyk, S. Domandl. Wien, 1977. 51 p. (Salzburger Beiträge zur Paracelsusforschung, 15).
Paracelsus in der Tradition: Vorträge, Paracelsustag 1978. Wien, Verband der Wissenschaftlichen Gesellschaften Oesterreichs, 1980. 146p. (Salzburger Beiträge zur Paracelsusforschung, Folge 21). Contributions by W. Pagel, F. Baron, H. Rudolph, R. Dilg-Frank, A. Dyk, W. Schneider, A. Miller-Guinsburg, S. Domandl, L. Braun, H. M. Decker-Hauff.
Paskauskas RA: Paracelsus and mental disorders. In International Congress of the History of Medicine, 27th, Barcelona, 1980. Actas. Barcelona, Académia de Ciències Médiques de Catalunya i Balears, 1981. p. 121-4.
Rosner E: Hohenheims Weg von St. Gallen nach Augsburg (1531-1536). Wien, 1977. 91 p. (Salzburger Beiträge zur Paracelsusforschung, 16).
Rosner E: Hohenheims Bergsuchtmonographie. **Medizinhist J** 1981;16(1-2):20-52
Rothschuh KE: Aus der Geschichte der Naturheilbewegung (IV). Hatte die Naturheilbewegung Vorläufer in der Renaissance? Montaigne, Paracelsus, Beobachtungsmedizin, Wasserheilkunde. **ZFA (Stuttgart)** 1981 Jun 10;57(16):1251-9
Rudolph H: Schriftauslegung und Schriftverständnis bei Paracelsus. **Medizinhist J** 1981;16(1-2):101-24
Scheller, EF: Langlebigkeit mit Paracelsus-Arzneien: Versuch einer Geriatrie nach Paracelsus. Heidelberg, Haug, 1977. 150 p.
Schipperges H: Kranksein und Heilung bei Paracelsus. Wien, Verband der wissenschaftlichen Gesellschaften Oesterreichs, 1978. 32 p. (Salzburger Beiträge zur Paracelsusforschung, 18).
Schipperges H: Paracelsus. Das Abenteuer einer sokratischen Existenz. Freiburg im Breisgau, Aurum Verlag, 1983. 108 p. (Reihe: Sokratische Weisheit, Bd. 3).
Schneider W: Ueber den Liber praeparationum des Paracelsus. **Sudhoffs Arch** 1980;64(1):69-78
Schneider W: Arzneirezepte von Paracelsus. **Medizinhist J** 1981;16(1-2):151-66
Schneider W: Das Lot-Gewicht bei Paracelsus. In Dilg P, et al., ed: Perspektiven der Pharmaziegeschichte. Graz, Austria, Akademische Druck- u. Verlagsanstalt, 1983. p. 325-30.
Skopec M: Uber den 'Ring des Paracelsus'. **Osterr Arzteztg** 1981;36(24):4 pages (Sonderdruck)
Skov H, Bastholm E, ed: Petrus Severinus og hans Idea medicinae philosophicae. En dansk paracelsist. Copenhagen, Odense Universitetsforlag, 1979. 299 p. (Acta Historica Scientiarum et Medicinalium, 32).
Stadler F: Paracelsus und die Musik in Salzburg. **Salzburger Beitr Paracelsusforsch** 1984;23:118-25
Telle J: Die Schreibart des Paracelsus im Urteil deutscher Fachschriftsteller des 16. und 17. Jarhunderts. **Medizinhist J** 1981;16(1-2):78-100
Telle J: Paracelsistische Sinnbildkunst. Bemerkungen zu einer Pseudo-'Tabula smaragdina' des 16. Jahrhunderts. In Seidler E, Schott H, ed: Bausteine zur Medizingeschichte. Stuttgart, Steiner, 1984. p. 129-39.
Thornton NT: The power of Paracelsus. **Hist Med (Lond)** 1980 Jan-Feb;8(1):10-15
Vandewiele LJ: Van chemiatrie tot iatrochemie--van Paracelsus (1493-1541) tot Van Helmont (1579?-1644). **Farm Tijdschr Belg** 1980;57:25-30
Von Paracelsus zu Goethe und Wilhelm von Humboldt: Wien, Verband der Wissenschaftlichen Gesellschaften Osterreichs, 1981. 203 p.
Wehr G: Paracelsus. Freiburg im Breisgau, Aurum, 1979. 112 p. (Fermenta Cognitionis, 6).
Weimann KH: Paracelsus-Lexikographie in vier Jahrhunderten. **Medizinhist J** 1981;16(1-2):167-95
Zaunick R: Der sächsische Paracelsist Georg Forberger. Wiesbaden, Steiner, 1977. xii, 110 p. (Kosmosophie, IV).

**Paradis, Maria Theresia, 1759?-1842?**
Pattie FA: A Mesmer-Paradis myth dispelled. **Am J Clin Hypn** 1979 Jul;22(1):29-31

**Parczewski, Eugeniusz**
Przychodzki M: Płk dr Eugeniusz Parczewski. **Przegl Lek** 1981;38(1):177-9

**Pardo Sastrón, José, 1822-1909**
Bueno AG: La flora de Aragon: notas a un proyecto de Francisco Loscos y Jose Pardo. **Bol Soc Esp Hist Farm** 1984;35(137):23-33

**Paré, Ambroise, 1510?-1590**
Bagwell CE: Ambröise Paré and the renaissance of surgery. **Surg Gynecol Obstet** 1981 Mar;152(3):350-4
Bendiner E: From barbershop to battlefield--Paré and the renaissance of surgery. **Hosp Pract** 1983 Aug;18(8):193-5, 199, 202 passim
Brown P: Couching a cataract. **Med Instrum** 1982 Mar-Apr;16(2):123
Colard A: Evocation du passé: des bons soins que donna Ambroise Paré à un Prince en Hainaut et du succès qu'il en advint. **Rev Med Brux** 1980 Jun;1(6):405-8
Colard A: En chirurgie, Ambroise Paré n'a pas innové la ligature vasculaire. **Rev Med Brux** 1980; NS 1;687-9
Colard A: Evocation du passé en chirugie. Ambroise Paré n'a pas innové la ligature vasculaire. **Rev Med Brux** 1980 Dec;1(10):687-9
Duburcq P: Ambroise Paré et l'odontologie. **Chir Dent Fr** 1982 Mar-Apr;52(151-3):21-38
Duburcq P: Odontoiatria del passato. Ambroise Paré l'odontoiatria. III. **Dent Cadmos** 1982 Aug;50(8):83-5
Duburcq P: Odontoiatria del passato. Ambroise Paré e l'odontoiatria. I. 'Io l'ho curato d Dio l'ha guarito'. **Dent Cadmos** 1982 Jun-Jul;50(6-7):75-9, 87-9
Duburq P: Ambroise Paré et l'odontologie. **Chir Dent Fr** 1982 Mar 18;52(150):41-9 contd.
Paré A: The classic. Compound fracture of leg, Paré's personal care (MII, 328). **Clin Orthop** 1983 Sep;178:3-6
Pare A: On monsters and marvels. Translated with an introduction and notes by J.L. Pallister. Chicago, London, University of Chicago Press, 1982. xxxii, 224 p.
Pédron F: Histoire d'Ambroise, chirurgien du roi. Paris, Orban, 1980. 468 p.
Touati B: Ambroise paré. **Rev Odontostomatol (Paris)** 1983 Mar-Apr;12(2):85

**Parent, Marie-Geneviève, 1740-1804**
Rousseau F: Marie-Geneviève Parent. In Dictionary of Canadian biography, 1801 to 1820. Volume 5, 1983. p. 658-9.

**Parin, Vasiliĭ Vasil'evich, 1903-**
Meerson FZ: Razvitie nekotorykh ideĭ V. V. Parina v fiziologii i patofiziologii krovoobrashcheniia. **Usp Fiziol Nauk** 1983 Apr-Jun;14(2):7-27
Severin SE: V. V. Parin. Zhizn' i deiatel'nost'. **Vestn Akad Med Nauk SSSR** 1984;(4):3-7
Shik LL: Akademik V. V. Parin kak fiziolog. **Vestn Akad Med Nauk SSSR** 1984;(4):12-5

**Park, Roswell, 1852-1914**
Murphy GP: Roswell Park Memorial Institute, Genesis of a cancer center. **Oncology** 1980;37(6):426-8

**Park, William Hallock, 1863-1939**
The carrier state. New York, Arno, 1977. Various paginations. Four reprinted papers on microbiology by William H. Park and George Soper, 1895-1919.:

**Parker, Francis Le Jan, 1836-1913**
Leland TM: Francis Lejan Parker, M.D. 1836-1913. **J SC Med Assoc** 1983 Feb;79(2):99

**Parker, James W., 1822-1907**
Strickland WA: Requiem for a frontier physician: James W. Parker, M.D., doctor to the wagon trains and mountaineers of old Westport. **Mo Med** 1981 Oct;78(10):631-6

**Parkinson, James, 1755-1824**
Nybäck H: Mannen bakom syndromet: James Parkinson. Beskrev 'shaking palsy' 1817--i dag prövas transplantation som behandling. **Lakartidningen** 1982 Dec 29;79(52):4910
Thackray JC: James Parkinson's Organic remains of a former world (1804-1811). **J Soc Bibliogr Nat Hist** 1976;7(4):45-66

**Parkinson, Sydney, 1745?-1771**
Lysaght A: A letter from Sydney Parkinson in Batavia to Dr. John Fothergill. **Notes Rec R Soc Lond** 1981;36(1):79-81

**Parkman, Francis, 1823-1893**
Beaver H: Parkman's crack-up: a Bostonian on the Oregon Trail. **N Engl Q** 1975;48(1):84-103

**Parkman, George, 1781-1849**
Grob GN, ed: The beginnings of American psychiatric thought and practice. Five accounts, 1811-1830. New York, Arno, 1973. Various paginations. Includes Account of the rise and progress of the Asylum . . . near Philadelphia (1814), and works by Theodric Romeyn Beck (1811); Thomas Eddy (1815); George Parkman (1814); and Rufus Wyman (1830).

**Parrenin, Dominique, 1665-1741**
Grover Y: La correspondance scientifique du P. Dominique Parrenin (1665-1741). In: France: Centre de Recherches interdisciplinaires de Chantilly (CERIC). Les rapports entre la Chine Sinologie (16-18 septembre 1977). Chantilly, Paris, Les Belles Lettres, 1980, 83-99.

**Parrot, Jules, 1829-1883**
Thieffry S: La découverte de la syphilis congénitale par Jules Parrot à l'Hospice des Enfants Assistés il y a un siècle. **Bull Acad Natl Med (Paris)** 1980 Nov;164(8):725-9

**Parry, Caleb Hillier, 1755-1822**
Kligfield P: The early pathophysiolic understanding of angina pectoris (Edward Jenner, Caleb Hillier Parry, Allan Burns). **Am J Cardiol** 1982 Dec;50(6):1433-5

**Partington, James Riddick, 1886-1965**
Sheptunova ZI: Dzh R. Partington - vydaiushchiisia istorik khimii. **Vopr Istor Estestvozn Tekh** 1981;3:107-10
Smeaton WA: James Riddick Partington. In Dictionary of national

biography, 1961-1970. Suppl. 8, 1981. p. 822-3.

**Pascal, Blaise, 1623-1662**
Bèttica-Giovannini R: La preghiera di Blaise Pascal per il buon uso delle malattie. **Ann Osp Maria Vittoria Torino** 1979 Jul-Dec;22(7-12):420-5

**Pasch, Joseph Georg, 1738-1795**
Lupinc P: Das zahnärztliche Lehrbuch des Wiener Militärarztes Joseph Georg Pasch 1767. Zürich, Juris Druck, 1984. 80 p. (Zürcher Medizingeschichtliche Abhandlungen, Neue Reihe, Nr. 165).

**Pascoli, Giovanni, 1855-1912**
Dolzani C: Un 'prelievo' di sangue adombrato in una poesia di Giovanni Pascoli? **Acta Med Hist Patav** 1982-83;29:25-8

**Passamán, José, fl. 1829**
Costa-Casaretto C: El Dr. D. Jose de Passamán. **Rev Med Chil** 1984 May;112(5):503-8

**Pasteur, Louis, 1822-1895**
Baudin C: Pasteur: un homme, une oeuvre. **Chir Dent Fr** 1983 Jul 7;53(211):23-5
Cafiso, LM: Storia della teoria sulla generazione spontanea: Redi, Spallanzani, Pasteur. **Cult Sc** 1981;20(80):236-43
Carter KC: Nineteenth-century treatments for rabies as reported in the Lancet. **Med Hist** 1982 Jan;26(1):67-78
Delaunay A, ed: Présence de Pasteur. Paris, Fayard, 1973. 225 p. Includes contributions by P. Bidan, A. Gamet, J. Guillaume, L. Léger, J. Piton, J. De Rosnay, R. Scriban, C. Vago.
Farley J, Geison GL, Ebnöther D: Le débat entre Pasteur et Pouchet: science, politique et génération spontanée, au 19e siècle en France. **Pandore** 1982;special number
Fasquelle R: Pasteur et l'épopée pasteurienne. **Sem Hop Paris** 1983 Dec 22;59(48):3395-404
Galérant G: Deux toulousains et un rouennais contre Pasteur au sujet de la génération spontanée. In: Congrès National des Sociétés Savantes, 96e, Toulouse, 1971. Comptes Rendus. Paris, 1974. Histoire des Sciences, Tome 1. p. 193-200.
Geison GL: Pasteur on vital versus chemical ferments: a previously unpublished paper on the inversion of sugar. **Isis** 1981 Sep;72(263):425-45
Gutina VN: Pasteur's views on the science. **Istor Biol Issled** 1983;9:134-44
Heron JR: Louis Pasteur: the nature of his illness. In Passmore R, ed: Proceedings of the Royal College of Physicians of Edinburgh Tercentenary Congress, 1981. Edinburgh, Royal College of Physicians of Edinburgh, 1982. p. 116-27.
Kler JH: Pasteur. **J Med Soc NJ** 1981 Feb;78(2):121-4
Kostychev SP: Pasteur: his life and achievements. Annotated translation from the Russian by S. A. Wilde. New Delhi, Oxford & IBH Publishing Co., 1978. 96 p.
Léonard J: Pasteur, un vétérinaire qui ira loin. **Histoire** 1979;12:78-80
McCracken D: A link with the past. **Br Med J [Clin Res]** 1981 Mar 21;282(6268):964-6
Martínez Báez M: Pasteur, maestro. **Mem Col Nac (Mex)** 1967-68;6(2-3):115-31
Mayer R: Il y a cent ans, à Genève, au 4e Congrès international d'hygiène et de démographie, l''altercation' Pasteur - Koch. **Rev Med Suisse Romande** 1982 Aug;102(8):805-9
Miles A: Reports by Louis Pasteur and Claude Bernard on the organization of scientific teaching and research. **Notes Rec R Soc Lond** 1982 Aug;37(1):101-18
Mollaret HH: Contribution à la connaissance des relations entre Koch et Pasteur. **NTM** 1983;20(1):57-65
Saenz A, Boisvert H: Trois lettres de Louis Pasteur. **Hist Sci Med** 1981;15(4):327-33
Sourander P: Edelfelts berömda pasteurporträtt - originalet och repliken. **Nord Medicinhist Arsbok** 1983;:149-54
Svarch Scharager N: Obra y vida de Luis Pasteur. **Rev Cubana Med Trop** 1980 Jan-Apr;32(1):79-90
Théodoridès J: 'Paris enragé'. **Rev Hist Pharm (Paris)** 1982;29(252):193-8
Wrotnowska D: Pasteur. Premières recherches sur les fermentations (1855-1857). **Clio Med** 1981 Apr;15(3-4):191-9
Wrotnowska D: Un ami de Pasteur: Charles Chappuis. In: Congrès National des Sociétés Savantes, 99e, Besançon, 1974. Comptes Rendus. Paris, 1976. Section des Sciences, Fasc. V. p. 171-84.
Wrotnowska D: La fièvre jaune. Séjour de Pasteur à Bordeaux, en septembre 1881. In: Congrès National des Sociétés Savantes, 104e, Bordeaux, 1979. Comptes Rendus. Paris, 1979. Section des Sciences, Fasc. IV. p. 109-20.
Wrotnowska D: Pasteur et Victor Feltz de Nancy. Correspondance inédite. In: Congrès National des Sociétés Savantes, 103e, Nancy, 1978. Comptes Rendus. Paris, 1978. Section des Sciences, Fasc. V. p. 131-44.
Wrotnowska D: Pasteur, membre du Comice agricole de l'arrondissement de Lille. In: Congrès National des Sociétés Savantes, 101e, Lille, 1976. Comptes Rendus. Paris, 1976. Section des Sciences, Fasc. III. p. 133-44.
Wrotnowska D: Lettres inédites de Gilbert Déclat à Louis Pasteur. **Hist Sci Med** 1982;16(2):115-23
Wrotnowska D: Pasteur et Ferran y Clua, correspondance inédite. In International Congress of the History of Medicine, 27th, Barcelona, 1980. Actas. Barcelona, Académia de Ciències Médiques de Catalunya i Balears, 1981. p. 699-707.
Wrotnowska D: Maladie des vers à soie: Pasteur s'intéresse à la race perpignanaise. In: Congrès National des Sociétés Savantes, 106e, Perpignan, 1981. Comptes Rendus. Paris, Bibliothèque Nationale, 1982. Fasc. IV. p. 197-208.
Wrotnowska D: Jules Raulin, professeur au Lycée de Caen correspondance avec Pasteur. In: Congrès National des Sociétés Savantes, 105e, Caen, 1980. Comptes Rendus, Paris, 1980. Section des Sciences, Fasc. V. p. 109-120.

**Pastia, Constantin C., 1883-1926**
Marcu N: Viaţa si activitatea doctorului Constantin C. Pastia (1883-1926). **Rev Ig [Bacteriol]** 1983 Jan-Mar;28(1):89-95

**Paszkiewicz, Ludwik, 1878-1967**
Kobuszewska-Faryna M: Rok 1978--rokiem ważnych rocznic dla patomorfologów polskich. **Patol Pol** 1979 Apr-Jun;30(2):153-6

**Pater, Walter Horatio, 1839-1894**
Dellamora R: An essay in sexual liberation, Victorian style: Walter Pater's 'Two early French stories'. **J Homosex** 1983 Spring-Summer;8(3-4):139-50

**Paterson, Philip Y.**
Paterson PY: LT/EAE and the MS quest. Going to the dogs and rats to study the patient. **Cell Immunol** 1983 Nov;82(1):55-74

**Patin, Guy, 1601-1672**
Pecker A: Nicolas Venette (1633?-1698) est-il le fils de Guy Patin. **Hist Sci Med** 1982;16(3):167-74

**Patrick, Mother, 1863-1900**
Tonkin RE: Mother Patrick Cosgrave, O.S.D. 1863-1900. **Zimbabwe Rhod Nurse** 1979;:46-54

**Patterson, Arthur Lindo, 1902-**
Bearman D: A. L. Patterson papers. **Surv Sources Newsl** 1981 Apr;10:9-11

**Patterson, Ellen James, 1873-1965**
Stool SE, Brown SL: Ellen James Patterns, MD. **Arch Otolaryngol** 1983 Jan;109(1):60-1

**Patterson, John H., fl. 1895**
Schleppi JR: 'It pays': John H. Patterson and industrial recreation at the National Cash Register Company. **J Sport Hist** 1979;6(3):20-8

**Pattison, Granville Sharp, 1791-1851**
Pattison FL: The Pattison-Miller quarrel. **Scott Med J** 1980 Jul;25(3):234-40

**Patton, George Smith, 1885-1945**
Askew M: 'I have hay fever: I love you. George.' **Practitioner** 1979 Jun;222(1332):866-8

**Paul, Constantin, 1833-1896**
Huard P: II y a cent ans Constantin Paul présentait à l'Académie de Médecine son stéthoscope autostatique bi-auriculaire. **Bull Acad Natl Med (Paris)** 1981 Nov;165(8):1117-21

**Paul, John Rodman, 1893-1971**
Paul JR, Bunnell WW: Classics in infectious diseases. The presence of heterophile antibodies in infectious mononucleosis by John R. Paul and W. W. Bunnell. American Journal of the Medical Sciences, 1932.
Viseltear AJ: John R. Paul and the definition of preventive medicine. **Yale J Biol Med** 1982 May-Aug;55(3-4):167-72

**Paul of Aegina, 7th cent.**
Rice EF: Paulus Aegineta. In Cranz FE, Kristeller PO, ed: Catalogus translationum et commentariorum: Mediaeval and Renaissance Latin translations and commentaries. Annotated lists and guides. Vol. IV. Washington, D.C., Catholic University of America Press, 1980. p. 145-91.

**Paulescu, Nicolas Constantin, 1869-1931**
Pavel I: The priority of N. C. Paulescu in the discovery of insulin. Bucureşti, Editura Academiei Republicii Socialiste Romania, 1976. 251 p.
Teichman SL, Aldea PA: The other side of the insulin story: Paulescu's contribution. **NY State J Med** 1984 Jun;84(6):312-6
Teichman SL, Aldea PA: Pioneers in pituitary physiology: Harvey Cushing and Nicolas Paulescu. **J Hist Med Allied Sci** 1985 Jan;40(1):68-72

**Pauling, Linus Carl, 1901-**
Goertzel TG, Goertzel MG, Goertzel V: Linus Pauling: the scientist as crusader. **Antioch Rev** 1980;38(3):371-82

**Paulli, Simon, 1603-1680**
Andersen S: Simon Paulli. Betaenkning over en Kongelig Ridehest. **Dan Medicinhist Arbog** 1979;9-97
Andersen S, ed: Simonis Paulli velmenende råd gennem hvilke formedelst Guds hjaelp en højadelig person lykkeligt blev kureret da han i året 1668 i Paris blev ramt af slag. **Dan Medicinhist Arbog** 1982;:73-91

**Paullini, Christian Franz, 1643-1712**
Schienbein H: Die 'Neu-Vermehrte Heylsame Dreck-Apotheke' (1696/1734) des Hof- und Stadtarztes Christian Frantz Paulini. **Quintessenz** 1981 Sep;32(9):1699-1702

**Pavese, Cesare, 1908–1950**
Shneidman ES: The suicidal logic of Cesare Pavese. **J Am Acad Psychoanal** 1982 Oct;10(4):547–63

**Pavlov, Georgi, d. 1949**
Kalŭdov I, et al: Prof. Dr. George Pavlov (a centennial of his birth). **Vet Med Nauki** 1981;18(2):3–89

**Pavlov, Ivan Petrovich, 1849–1936**
Asratian EA, Shingarov GKh: Leninskaia teoriia otrazheniia i uchenie I. P. Pavlova o vyssheĭ nervnoĭ deiatel'nosti (k 110–i godovshchine so dnia rozhdeniia V. I. Lenina). **Zh Vyssh Nerv Deiat** 1980 Mar–Apr;30(2):227–34
Coon DJ: Eponymy, obscurity, Twitmyer, and Pavlov. **J Hist Behav Sci** 1982 Jul;18(3):255–62
Dews PB: Pavlov and psychiatry. **J Hist Behav Sci** 1981;17:246–50
Garmash VIa, Ushmarov AK: Znachenie ucheniia I. P. Pavlova dlia kliniki vnutrennikh bolezneĭ. **Med Sestra** 1981 Feb;40(2):8–10
Gorizontov PD: K 130–letiiu so dnia rozhdeniia I. P. Pavlova (vstupitel'noe slovo k Pervym Pavlovskim chteniiam). **Zh Vyssh Nerv Deiat** 1980 May–Jun;30(3):627–30
Gray JA: Ivan Pavlov. New York, Viking Press, 1979. vii, 153 p.
Grigor'ian NA: I. P. Pavlov o nauke i sotsial'noĭ otvetvennosti uchenogo. **Sov Zdravookhr** 1984;(2):58–61
Iaroshevskiĭ MG: Genezis issledovatel'skoĭ programmy I. P. Pavlova (istoricheskoe znachenie madridskoĭ rechi I. P. Pavlova). **Zh Vyssh Nerv Deiat** 1984 Jan–Feb;34(1):3–13
Kozulin A: The influence of the personality of the scientist on his theorizing: I. P. Pavlov and the concept of human signal systems. **Stud Sov Thought** 1981;22(4):249–56
Merkulov VL: I. P. Pavlov--organizator nauchnykh issledovaniĭ. Moskva, Nauka, Glav. red. vostochnoĭ lit–ry, 1971. 8 p.
Pakovich BI: To commemorate the 80th year since discovery of conditional reflexes. **Pavlov J Biol Sci** 1983 Oct–Dec;18(4):175–80
Pappenheimer JR: Pavlov's contributions to physiology before 1900. **J Hist Behav Sci** 1981;17:239–41
Skinner BF: Pavlov's influence on psychology in America. **J Hist Behav Sci** 1981;17:242–5
Windholz G: Pavlov's position toward American behaviorism. **J Hist Behav Sci** 1983 Oct;19(4):394–407
Windholz G: Pavlov vs. Köhler. Pavlov's little–known primate research. **Pavlov J Biol Sci** 1984 Jan–Mar;19(1):23–31

**Pavlovskiĭ, Evgeniĭ Nikanorovich, 1884–1965**
Chagin KP: Rol' akademika E. N. Pavlovskogo v izuchenii épidemiologii parazitarnykh i transmissivnykh bolezneĭ (k 100–letiiu so dnia rozhdeniia). **Zh Mikrobiol Epidemiol Immunobiol** 1984 Jun;(6):117–20
Laird M: Integrirovannye metody bor'by s perenoschikami i ugroza gemorragicheskoĭ likhoradlki Denge v tropicheskoĭ zone Tikhogo Okeana. **Parazitologiia** 1984 Mar–Apr;18(2):99–105
Pervomaĭskiĭ GS, Podolian VIa, Chagin KP, et al: Rol' akademika Evgeniia Nikanorovicha Pavlovskogo v stanovlenii i razvitii parazitologii v SSSR (k 100–letiiu so dnia rozhdeniia). **Parazitologiia** 1984 Mar–Apr;18(2):89–98
Pololian VIa: Vazhneĭshie étapy sozdaniia ucheniia akademika E.N. Pavlovskogo o prirodnoĭ ochagovosti boleznei. **Vestn Akad Med Nauk SSSR** 1980;(10):10–4
Rosický B: Professor Evgenii Nikonorovich Pavlovsky--100 years since his birth. **J Hyg Epidemiol Microbiol Immunol** 1984;28(2):115–8
Rosický B: Razvitie ideĭ akademika E. N. Pavlovskogo v stranakh Tsentral'noĭ Evropy. **Med Parazitol (Mosk)** 1984 Mar–Apr;(2):21–8
Shcherbina VP, Liashenko NI: Akademik Evgeniĭ Nikanorovich Pavlovskiĭ (k 100–letiiu so dnia rozhdeniia). **Voen Med Zh** 1984 Feb;(2):65–8

**Payen de Noyan, Marie–Catherine, ca. 1730–1818**
Plamondon L: Marie–Catherine Payen de Noyan. In Dictionary of Canadian biography, 1801 to 1820. Volume 5, 1983. p. 661–2.

**Payr, Erwin, 1871–1946**
Becker T: Das chirurgische Erbe. Erwin Payr zum Gedenken. **Zentralbl Chir** 1981;106(23):1563–8

**Peabody, Francis Weld, 1881–1927**
Harvey AM: Francis Weld Peabody: the blending of general internal medicine and clinical science. **Pharos** 1981 Summer;44(3):6–8
Rabin PL, Rabin D: Landmark perspective: The care of the patient Francis Peabody revisited. **JAMA** 1984 Aug 10;252(6):819–20

**Peabody, Nathaniel, 1774–1855**
Willens SH: Dr. Nathaniel Peabody and his book: The art of preserving teeth. **Bull Hist Dent** 1980 Oct;28(2):83–6

**Peabody, Richard Rogers, 1892–1936**
McCarthy K: Early alcoholism treatment: the Emmanuel Movement and Richard Peabody. **J Stud Alcohol** 1984 Jan;45(1):59–74

**Peacock, John, 1761?–1841**
Stout G: Adult hypertrophic pyloric stenosis--a description in 1834? **J R Coll Gen Pract** 1983 Apr;33(249):239–41

**Peacock, Thomas Bevill, 1812–1882**
Leonard JC: Thomas Bevill Peacock and the early history of dissecting aneurysm. **Br Med J** 1979 Jul 28;2(6184):260–2

**Péan, Jules Emile, 1830–1898**
Bornemissza G: [Péan and his accomplishments.] (Hun). **Orv Hetil** 1980;121:2951–2

**Peano, Giuseppe, 1858–1932**
Bèttica–Giovannini R: La sfida di Peano: matematica e paranoia. **Ann Osp Maria Vittoria Torino** 1982 Jul–Dec;25(7–12):241–4

**Pearce, Louise, 1885–1959**
Corner GW: Louise Pearce. In: Notable American women. The modern period. Cambridge, Mass., Belknap–Harvard Univ. Press, 1980. 4:531–2.

**Pearl, Raymond, 1879–1940**
Kingsland S: Raymond Pearl: on the frontier in the 1920's. Raymond Pearl memorial lecture, 1983. **Hum Biol** 1984 Feb;56(1):1–18

**Pearson, Karl, 1857–1936**
Billig M: The origins of race psychology – 1. **Patterns Prejudice** 1982;16(3):3–16
Pearson ES, ed: The history of statistics in the 17th and 18th centuries against the changing background of intellectual, scientific and religious thought. Lectures by Karl Pearson given at University College London during the academic sessions 1921–1933. New York, Macmillan, 1978. xix, 744 p.

**Peck, Harvey, 1937–1981**
Buchin ID, Peck S: Harvey Peck, 1937–1981. **Angle Orthod** 1982 Jan;52(1):3–5

**Peirce, Jeremy**
Fraser KJ: Anglo–French contributions to the recognition of rheumatoid arthritis. **Ann Rheum Dis** 1982 Aug;41(4):335–43

**Pelagonius Salonius**
Fischer KD: The first Latin treatise on horse medicine and its author Pelagonius Saloninus. **Medizinhist J** 1981;16(3):215–26
Fischer KD, ed: Pelagonii Ars Veterinaria. Leipzig, Teubner, 1980. xlv, 203 p. (Bibliotheca Teubneriana).

**Pelikan, Josef, 1900–**
Dobíšek K: První čtyři primáři Pražského ústavu choromyslných. 2. Josef Pelikan. **Cesk Psychiatr** 1981 Dec;77(6):414–9

**Pelletier, Madeleine**
Largillière A: Madeleine Pelletier, femme, médecin, féministe. **Penelope** 1981;(5):68–72

**Pena, Pierre, fl. 1535–1605**
Corbett M: The emblematic title–page to Stirpium Adversaria nova by Petro Pena and Mathias de L'Obel (1570). **Arch Nat Hist** 1981 Apr;10(1):111–7

**Pende, Nicola, 1880–**
Giorgino R: Nicola Pende: medico, ricercatore, maestro. **G Clin Med** 1981 Nov;62(11):747–57

**Penfield, Wilder, 1891–1976**
Feindel W: The contributions of Wilder Penfield to the functional anatomy of the human brain. **Hum Neurobiol** 1982;1(4):231–4
Feindel W: The contributions of Wilder Penfield and the Montreal Neurological Institute to Canadian neurosciences. In Roland CG, ed: Health, disease and medicine. Toronto, Hannah Institute for the History of Medicine, 1984. p. 347–58.

**Pennefather, John Pyn**
Pennefather JP: A surgeon with the Alberta Field Force. **Alberta Hist** 1978;26(4):1–14

**Pennington, Mary Engle, 1872–1952**
Wiser V: Mary Engle Pennington. In: Notable American women. The modern period. Cambridge, Mass., Belknap–Harvard Univ. Press, 1980. 4:532–4.

**Penrose, Charles Bingham, 1862–1925**
Romm S: The persons behind the name: Charles Bingham Penrose. **Plast Reconstr Surg** 1982 Sep;70(3):397–9

**Pepys, Samuel, 1633–1703**
Daly RJ: Samuel Pepys and post–traumatic stress disorder. **Br J Psychiatry** 1983 Jul;143:64–8
Morris GC: A portrait of Thomas Hollier, Pepy's surgeon. **Ann R Coll Surg Engl** 1979 May;61(3):224–9
Morris GC: Which Molins treated Cromwell for stone--and did not prescribe for Pepys? **Med Hist** 1982 Oct;26(4):429–35
Newman C: Nature of Samuel Pepys's 'wind colic'. **Br Med J [Clin Res]** 1980 Dec 20–27;281(6256):1716–7

**Percival, Thomas, 1740–1804**
Gracia D: El orden médico. La ética médica de Thomas Percival. **Asclepio** 1983;35:227–55
Paulshock BZ: When should a physician retire? – William Heberden's view. **Del Med J** 1983;55(6):359–60

**Percy, F. Walker, 1916–**
Allen WR: All the names of death: Walker Percy and Hemingway. **Miss Q** 1982–83;36(1):3–19
Graham PW: A mirror for medicine: Richard Selzer, Michael Crichton, and Walker Percy. **Perspect Biol Med** 1981 Winter;24(2):229–39

**Percy, Pierre François, 1754–1825**
Huard P, Imbault–Huart MJ: Travaux de Percy (1754–1825) sur l'hémostase des artères (1790–1810). In: Congrès National des Sociétés Savantes, 99e, Besançon, 1974. Comptes Rendus. Paris, 1976.

Section des Sciences, Fasc. V. p. 251-7.
Huard P, Imbault-Huart MJ: Percy, vénéréologue. In: Congrès National des Sociétés Savantes, 99e, Besançon, 1974. Comptes Rendus. Paris, 1976. Section des Sciences, Fasc. V. p. 259-64.
Huard P, Imbault-Huart MJ: La polémique Percy-Ollivier sur le typhus traumatique en 1822. In: Congrès National des Sociétés Savantes, 99e, Besançon, 1974. Comptes Rendus. Paris, 1976. Section des Sciences, Fasc. V. p. 243-9.

**Perdomo Bethencourt Cortés, Juan Antonio, 1737-1800**
Alegría C: Dos medicos en la aurora de la gesta emancipadora de Venezuela. **Rev Soc Venez Hist Med** 1969-71;17-19(31-33):29-48

**Pereira, Jonathan, 1804-1853**
Guggenheim YK: Jonathan Pereira's contribution to the science of nutrition. **Koroth** 1982 Aug;8(3/4):123-34

**Pereira, Miguel, 1871-1918**
Sousa L de C: Miguel Pereira: um cidadão exemplar. **Rev Inst Hist Geogr Bras** 1973;298:306-14

**Pereire, Jacobo Rodriguez, 1715-1780**
Kottek SS: [Jacob Rodriguez Pereire (1715-1780): an anniversary] (Heb). **Koroth** 1981;8(1-2):83-7; 79-81 [Engl. abstr.]

**Perera, Ambrosio**
Osuna A: Ambrosio Perera dos historieta relacionadas con su persona la disyuntiva 'Ciencia pura y aplicada'. **Rev Soc Venez Hist Med** 1972-73;20-21(34-35):229-41
Osuna A: Una biografia del Dr. Ambrosio Perera. **Rev Soc Venez Hist Med** 1975-76;23(37):71-85

**Pérez Cascales, Francisco, fl. 1576-1611**
Carreras Panchón A: Perez Cascales y la clinica del garrotillo. **Asclepio** 1978-79;30-31:319-22

**Pérez de Herrera, Cristóbal, 1558-1618?**
Parrilla Hermida M: El doctor Cristobal Perez de Herrera. Presentacion de documentos ineditos. **Asclepio** 1978-79;30-31:371-6

**Pérez de la Muela, Hernán, fl. 1529**
Fortique JR: Hernán Pérez de la Muela, primer médico europeo establecido en Venezuela. **Bol Acad Nac Hist (Caracas)** 1979;62(245):147-58

**Pérez Díaz, Manuel, 1872-1931**
Briceño-Maaz T: Dos nombres en la dermatologia venezolana. **Rev Soc Venez Hist Med** 1972-73;20-21(34-35):87-98

**Pérez Galdós, Benito, 1843-1920**
Rubin W: Galdos y la medicina. **Atlantida** 1970;8(43):68-80

**Pérez Mínguez, Mariano, 1809-1887**
Alegre Perez ME, Santonja R: Delito o previsión de futuro? **Bol Soc Esp Hist Farm** 1980 Mar-Jun;31(121-2):31-7

**Perman, Emil, 1856-1937**
Ráf L: Skandinaviska kirurger först med beskrivning av tecken på appendicit. **Lakartidningen** 1984 Aug 8;81(32-33):2829-30

**Perovskaia, Sof'ia L'vovna, 1854-1881**
Ionov IuV: Narodovolets Sof'ia Perovskaia i ee meditsinskaia deiatel'nost'. **Feldsher Akush** 1982;47(10):41-2
Svistunov RI: Meditsinakaia deiatel'nost' Sof'i Perovskoĭ. **Feldsher Akush** 1984 Feb;49(2):47-50

**Perrault, Claude, 1613-1688**
Schiller N: L'iconographie de Claude Perrault (1613-1688). In: Congrès National des Sociétés Savantes, 91e, Rennes, 1966. Comptes Rendus. Paris, 1967. Section des Sciences, Tome 1. p. 217-34.

**Perrin, Ethel, 1871-1962**
Twin SL: Ethel Perrin. In: Notable American women. The modern period. Cambridge, Mass., Belknap-Harvard Univ. Press, 1980. 4:539-41.

**Perroncito, Edoardo, 1847-1936**
Balbo T: In memória di Edoardo Perroncito nel centenario di fondazione della prima Cattedra di Parassitologia. **Parassitologia** 1980 Dec;22(3):233-7

**Personne, Jacques, 1816-1880**
Courtois JE: Le pharmacien Jacques Personne (1816-1880) pionnier de la chimie analytique. **Rev Hist Pharm (Paris)** 1980 Dec;247(68 no 27):263-71

**Pertik, Ottó, 1852-1913**
Lambrecht M: Virchow és Pertik. **Orvostort Kozl** 1980;89-91(26 no 1-3):233-9

**Perzanowska, Stefania**
Kłodziński S: Dr. Stefania Perzanowska. **Przegl Lek** 1981;38(1):189-97

**Peschier, Jacques, 1769-1832**
Götz W: Die Briefe Jacques Peschiers aus Genf an Joh. Barth. Trommsdorff, Erfurt, als Beispiel für internationale pharmazeutische Kontakte zu Beginn des 19. Jahrhunderts. **Pharm Acta Helv** 1979;54(9-10):303-7

**Peset Llorca, Vicente, 1914-1981**
García Ballester L: In memoriam Dr. Vicente Peset Llorca (1914-1981). **Dynamis** 1981;1:221-2

**Pessneger, Joseph, 1766-1836**
Fröml F: Pod dohledem městského fyzika. **Cas Lek Cesk** 1982 Jan 15;121(2):58-60

**Pestalozzi, Johann Heinrich, 1746-1827**
Burgener L: Pestalozzi et l'education physique. **Paedagog Hist** 1977;17(2):516-18
[Understanding of man in education: (3). 'Dusk of a Hermit' by Pestalozzi] (Jpn).

**Pétain, Henri Philippe, 1856-1951**
Szaluta J: Apotheosis to ignominy: the martyrdom of Marshal Pétain. **J Psychohist** 1980 Spring;7(4):415-53

**Péterfi, Tibor, 1883-1953**
Donáth T: Dr. Péterfi Tibor (1883-1953). **Orv Hetil** 1983 Dec 11;124(50):3061-2

**Petersen, Erst Hans, 1885-1946**
Hildebrand R: Beitrag der Würzburger Anatomie zur Entwicklung des mikroskopisch-anatomischen Unterrichts (1847 Kölliker--Petersen 1940). **Anat Anz** 1984;155(1-5):115-22

**Petrarca, Francesco, 1304-1374**
Benedek TG: A comparison of the medical writings of two humanists: F. Petrarca and W. Pirckheimer. In: Congrès international d'histoire de la médecine, XXVe, Québec, 1976. Actes. Québec, 1977. p. 502-6.

**Petrov, Boris Aleksandrovich, 1898-1973**
Permiakov NK: B. A. Petrov. Moskva, Meditsina, 1982. 170 p.

**Petrov, Nikolaĭ Nikolaevich, 1876-1964**
Napalkov NP, Mishura VI, Merabishvili VM, et al: Razvitie ideĭ N. N. Petrova v oblasti organizatsii protivorakovoĭ bor'by. **Vopr Onkol** 1982;28(5):126-32

**Petrowa, G. K.**
Sluchanko BP: Kerchenskoe meditsinskoe uchilishche im. Geroia Sovetskogo Soiuza glavstarshiny meditsinskoĭ sluzhby G. K. Petrovoĭ. **Med Sestra** 1983 Oct;42(10):56-8

**Petrus de Ebulo, fl. 1196**
Orofino G, Brach CC: Nel nome del bagno. **Kos** 1984 Apr;1(3):33-54

**Petrycy, Sebastian, 1554-1626**
Pielat B: Dur plamisty w poglądach Sebastiana Petrycego i Sebastiana Sleszkowskiego w i Połowie XVII wieku. **Arch Hist Med (Warsz)** 1980;43(4):393-406

**Pettenkofer, Max Joseph von, 1818-1901**
Breyer H: Max von Pettenkofer: Arzt im Vorfeld der Krankheit. Leipzig, Hirzel, 1980. 234 p.
Weispfenning I: Pettenkofers Gesundheitswirtschaftslehre. Ein meilenstein in der Entwicklung des öffentlichen Gesundheitswesens. In Seidler E, Schott H, ed: Bausteine zur Medizingeschichte. Stuttgart, Steiner, 1984. p. 146-54.

**Petty, William, 1623-1687**
Barnard TC: Sir William Petty: his Irish estates and Irish population. **Ir Econ Soc Hist** 1979;6

**Peus, Fritz, 1904-1978**
Eichler W, Jahn I: Fritz Peus 1904--1978. **Angew Parasitol** 1979 Oct;20(3):164-72

**Pevzner, Manuil Isaakovich, 1872-1952**
Soloveĭ MG, Gribanov ED: M. I. Pevzner--krupnyĭ sovetskiĭ terapevt-dietolog. **Feldsher Akush** 1983;48(2):52-3

**Pfaff, Philipp, 1713-1766**
Tanzer G: Philipp Pfaff (1713-1766), seine Zeit und seine Vorgänger. **Zahnarzt** 1984 Feb;28(2):129-31

**Pfahler, George Edward, 1874-1957**
Detlefsen EG: George Edward Pfahler. In Dictionary of American Biography, Suppl. 6, 1956-1960. p. 505-6, 1980.

**Pfannenstiel, Hermann Johannes, 1862-1909**
Easton L: Hermann Johannes Pfannenstiel (1862-1909). **Br J Obstet Gynaecol** 1984 Jun;91(6):538-41

**Pfeffel, Johann Andreas, 1674-1748**
Rubin LP: A young woman taken to the doctor by her family. Mezzotint by Johann Andreas Pfeffel after an original painting by Jan Josef Horemans. **J Hist Med Allied Sci** 1981 Oct;36(4):489

**Pfeiffer, Richard Friedrich Johannes, 1858-1945**
Gröschel DH, Hornick RB: Who introduced typhoid vaccination: Almroth Wright or Richard Pfeiffer? **Rev Infect Dis** 1981 Nov-Dec;3(6):1251-4

**Pflüger, Eduard Friedrich Wilhelm, 1829-1910**
Moschner H: Wissenschaftliche Arbeit und Lehre des Bonner Physiologen Eduard Friedrich Wilhelm Pflüger auf dem Gebiet des tierischen Stoffwechsels. Diss. Bonn, 1981. 233 p.
Simmer HH: Experimentelle Prüfungen der pflügerschen Reflexhypothese der Menstruation im späten 19. Jahrhundert. **Clio Med** 1980 Jul;14(3-4):235-54
Simmer HH: Innere Sekretion der Ovarien als Ursache der Menstruation. Halbans Falsifikation der Pflügerschen Hypothese. In Ganzinger K, Skopec M, Wyklicky H, ed: Festschrift für Erna Lesky zum 70. Geburtstag. Wien, Brüder Hollinek, 1981. p. 123-48.

**Philip, Robert, 1857–1939**
Petrescu G: 125 de ani de la nasterea lui Sir Robert Philip (1856–1939). **Rev Ig [Pneumoftiziol]** 1982 Oct-Dec;31(4):383–4

**Philipps, John, ca. 1736–1801**
Kernaghan LK: John Philipps. In Dictionary of Canadian biography, 1801 to 1820. Volume 5, 1983. p. 670.

**Phillips, Newton D., 1835–1909**
Hammond EA: Dr. Newton D. Phillips, Florida Medical Association's eleventh president. **J Fla Med Assoc** 1982 Aug;69(8):683–7

**Physick, Philip Syng, 1768–1837**
Crellin JK: The surgical teaching of Philip Syng Physick. Durham, Medical History Program and the Trent Collection, Duke University Medical Center, 1981 vi, 101 p.
Trice ER: Philip Syng Physick, father of American surgery. **Va Med** 1981 Jul;108(7):456–9

**Pi i Molist, Emilio, 1824–1892**
Comelles JM: El tratamiento moral en Catalunya (I): el 'Proyecto médico razonado' de Emili Pi i Molist (1860). In International Congress of the History of Medicine, 27th, Barcelona, 1980. Actas. Barcelona, Acadèmia de Ciències Mèdiques de Catalunya i Balears, 1981. p. 48–55.

**Pi Suñer, Augusto, 1879–1955**
Puche J, Folch i Pi A: El Doctor August Pi Sunyer. **Xaloc** 1980;16(105):10–2

**Piaget, Jean, 1896–1980**
Boden MA: Jean Piaget. New York, Viking, 1979. xii, 176 p.
Broughton JM, Leadbeater B, Amsel E, ed: Reflections on Piaget: proceedings of the Jean Piaget Memorial Conference. **Teach Coll Rec** 1981;83(2):151–217
Caramelli N: Introduzione a Piaget. **Stor Crit Psicol** 1981;2(1):5–85
Castorina JA, Lerner BD: Comentarios sobre la investigación clínica en Freud y Piaget. **Acta Psiquiatr Psicol Am Lat** 1983 Jun;29(2):85–95
Evans RI: Dialogue with Jean Piaget. New York, Praeger, 1981. lxi, 189 p. (Dialogues in Contemporary Psychology Series).
Gruber HE: Piaget's mission. **Soc Res (NY)** 1982;49(1):239–64
Kitchener RF: Genetic epistemology, normative epistemology and psychologism. **Synthese** 1980;45(2):257–80
Kitchener RF: The nature and scope of genetic epistemology. **Philos Sci** 1981;48(3):400–15
Marbach E: Jean Piaget (1896–1980). **Z Allg Wissenschaftstheorie** 1981;12(1):1–27
Modgil S, Modgil C, ed: Jean Piaget. Consensus and controversy. New York, Praeger, 1982. 446 p.
Pulaski MS: Understanding Piaget. Revised and expanded ed. New York, Harper & Row, 1980. xvii, 248 p.
Rossi L: Il concetto di adattamento nella psicologia evoluzionistica di K. Lorenz e nell'epistemologia genetica di J. Piaget. **Stor Crit Psicol** 1984;5(2):301–17
Stocking GW: Innovation in the Malinowskian mode: an essay review of long-term field research in social anthropology. **J Hist Behav Sci** 1980 Jul;16(3):281–6
Sullivan EV: The career and legacy of Jean Piaget. **Queens Q** 1981;88(2):341–52
Varma VP, Williams P, ed: Piaget, psychology and education; papers in honour of Jean Piaget. Itasca, Illinois, Peacock, 1976. xiv, 233 p. Biographical chapters by E. A. Lunzer, p. xi–xiv, 3–14.
Vidal F, Buscaglia M, Vonèche JJ: Darwinism and developmental psychology. **J Hist Behav Sci** 1983 Jan;19(1):81–94
Voyat G: In tribute to Piaget: a look at his scientific impact in the United States. In R. W. Rieber, K. Salzinger, ed: Psychology: theoretical-historical perspectives. New York, Academic Press, 1980. p. 305–14.
Wall WD: Jean Piaget - 1896–1979. **J Child Psychol Psychiatry** 1982 Apr;23(2):97–104

**Picart, Bernard, 1673–1733**
Lach E: The circumcision of the child on the eighth day...An anonymous engraving after a design by Bernard Picart. **J Hist Med Allied Sci** 1982 Apr;37(2):221

**Picasso, Pablo, 1881–1973**
Triadan H: Picasso--Pionier der Mundhygiene? **SSO Schweiz Monatsschr Zahnheilkd** 1983 Apr;93(4):250–1

**Pichler, Hans, 1877–1949**
Romm S, Luce EA: Hans Pichler: oral surgeon to Sigmund Freud. **Oral Surg** 1984 Jan;57(1):31–2

**Pickles, William Norman, 1885–1969**
Pickering G: William Norman Pickles. In Dictionary of national biography, 1961–1970. Suppl. 8, 1981. p. 843–4.

**Picot, Constant, 1844–**
Mayer R: Ils étaient trois! Jacques-Louis Reverdin, Jean-Louis Prévost et Constant Picot, fondateurs de la Revue médicale de la Suisse Romande. Evocation de la naissance d'une revue médicale et esquisse biographique de ses premiers rédacteurs. **Rev Med Suisse Romande** 1980 Dec;100(12):1013–41

**Picotte, Susan La Flesche, 1865–1915**
Mathes VS: Susan La Flesche Picotte: Indian physician. **Masterkey Ind Lore Hist** 1983;57(1):10–4
Mathes VS: Susan La Flesche Picotte: Nebraska's Indian physician, 1865–1915. **Nebr Hist** 1982;63(4):502–30

**Pictorius, Georg, ca. 1500–1569**
Pictorius G: Badenfahrtbüchlein. Wie und wo man richtig badet. Nachruck des Werkes aus dem Jahre 1560. U. Becker, ed., Basel and Wien; Herder, Freiburg, 1980. 111 p

**Pienitz, Ernst Gottlob, 1777–1853**
Eichhorn H: Ernst Gottlob Pienitz und die Heil- und Verpflegungsanstalt Sonnenstein. **Psychiatr Neurol Med Psychol (Leipz)** 1982 Jan;34(1):60–3

**Pies Family**
Naal W: Arzt und ärztliche Versorgung auf dem Hunsrück seit dem 30jährigen Krieg beispielhaft dargestellt an der Familie Pies. Diss Düsseldorf, 1979. 198 p.

**Pijper, Adrianus, 1886–1964**
Findlay GH: South African tick-bite fever (1931–1981). **S Afr Med J** 1981 Dec 26;60(26):998–1000

**Pikulin, L. E., 1784–1824**
Anisimov VE: Professor L. E. Pikulin (1784–1824) (k 200-letiiu so dnia rozhdeniia). **Sov Zdravookhr** 1984;(10):75–6

**Pilkington, George, 1854–1895**
Stout G: A ledger stamped 'G.P'. **J R Coll Gen Pract** 1984 Apr;34(261):223–5

**Pillemer, Louis, 1908–1957**
Lepow IH: Louis Pillemer, Properdin, and scientific controversy. **J Immunol** 1980 Aug;125(2):471–5
Ratnoff WD: A war with the molecules: Louis Pillemer and the history of properdin. **Perspect Biol Med** 1980;23(4):638–57

**Pimstone, Bernard Laurence, d. 1979**
Berman MC: The clinical investigator: a tribute to the late Professor Bernard Pimstone. **S Afr Med J** 1983 Mar 5;63(10):366–71

**Pincus, Gregory Goodwin, 1903–1967**
Diczfalusy E: Gregory Pincus and steroidal contraception revisited. **Acta Obstet Gynecol Scand [Suppl]** 1982;105:7–15

**Pindborg, Jens Jørgen, 1921–**
Holmstrup P, et al: [J. J. Pindborg and Danish dentistry]. **Tandlaegebladet** 1981 Aug;85(13):380–408

**Pineda, Antonio María, 1850–**
Silva Alvarez A: Que haria y que no haria hoy Antonio Maria Pineda? **Rev Soc Venez Hist Med** 1980;29(43–44):125–30

**Pinel, Philippe, 1745–1826**
Baruk H: Actualité du traitement moral et de la nosographie de Pinel. **Ann Med Psychol (Paris)** 1982 Apr;140(4):442–7
Bendiner E: Philippe Pinel: reason for the unreasoning. **Hosp Pract** 1981 Jun;16(6):76E–76P
Cavallo C, Cei A: Pinel e il magnetismo animale. **Stor Crit Psicol** 1984 Jun;5(1):91–109
Chabbert P, Mangin P: Les premières publications de Philippe Pinel consacrées à la médecine mentale. In International Congress of the History of Medicine, 27th, Barcelona, 1980. Actas. Barcelona, Acadèmia de Ciències Mèdiques de Catalunya i Balears, 1981. p. 42–7.
Jones C: The 'new treatment' of the insane in Paris: the formation of the lunatic asylum under the French Revolution. **Hist Today** 1980 Oct;30:5–10
Keel O: La généalogie de l'histopathologie; une révision déchirante. Philippe Pinel, lecteur discret de J.-C. Smyth (1741–1821). Paris, Librairie Philosophique J. Vrin, 1979. ii, 135 p. (Histoire des Sciences: Textes et Etudes).
Ledermann F: La psychiatrie française et les médicaments: Pomme, Pinel, Esquirol, Morel. **Rev Hist Pharm (Paris)** 1982 Sep;29(254):189–206
Pigeaud JM: Le rôle des passions dans la pensée médicale de Pinel à Moreau de Tours. **Hist Philos Life Sci** 1980;2(1):123–40
Pinel P: The clinical training of doctors. An essay of 1793. Ed. D. B. Weiner. Baltimore, Johns Hopkins University Press, 1980. 102 p. (Henry E. Sigerist suppl. to the Bull. Hist. Med. N.S. no. 3).
Postel J: Un manuscrit inédit de Philippe Pinel sur 'Les guérisons opérées dans le 7ème emploi' de Bicêtre, en 1794. **Rev Int Hist Psychiatr** 1983;1(1):79–82
Postel J: Les premières expériences psychiatriques de Philippe Pinel à la Maison de santé Belhomme. **Can J Psychiatry** 1983 Nov;28(7):571–6
Rodegra H: Philippe Pinels Ideen von der Befreiung der Irren und ihre Verwirklichung im norddeutschen Raum zu Beginn des 19. Jahrhunderts. **Med Welt** 1981 Feb 6;32(6):199–201
Rodegra H: Philippe Pinels Ideen von der Befreiung der Irren und ihre Verwirklichung im norddeutschen Raum zu Beginn des 19. Jahrhunderts. In International Congress of the History of Medicine, 27th, Barcelona, 1980. Actas. Barcelona, Acadèmia de Ciències Mèdiques de Catalunya i Balears, 1981. p. 140–4.
Weiner DB: Trois moments-clefs dans la vie de Ph. Pinel. In International Congress of the History of Medicine, 27th, Barcelona, 1980. Actas. Barcelona, Acadèmia de Ciències Mèdiques de Catalunya i Balears, 1981. p. 154–61.

**Pinelli, Gian Vincenzo, 1535-1601**
Belloni L: Konsilien von Professoren aus Neapel und Padua gegen die Sehstörungen von G. V. Pinelli. **Gesnerus** 1981;38:135-42

**Pinkham, Lydia Estes, 1819-1883**
Stage S: Female complaints: Lydia Pinkham and the business of women's medicine. New York, Norton, 1979. 304 p.

**Pinkus, Hermann**
Pinkus H: Etiology of an anatomist's discoveries in dermatology. **Am J Dermatopathol** 1982 Apr;4(2):127-35

**Piorry, Pierre Adolphe, 1794-1879**
Sakula A: Pierre Adolphe Piorry (1794-1879): pioneer of percussion and pleximetry. **Thorax** 1979 Oct;34(5):575-81

**Pipelet, Jean-Baptiste, 1759-1823**
Huard P, Théodoridès J: Jean-Baptiste Pipelet (1759-1823), Constance de Théis (1767-1845), Josef de Salm-Dyck (1773-1861) ou le chirurgien, la poétesse et le botaniste. In: Congrès National des Sociétés Savantes, 93e, Tours, 1968. Comptes Rendus. Paris, 1971. Section des Sciences, Tome II. p. 127-36.

**Pirandello, Luigi, 1867-1936**
Bouissy A: Pirandello, 'psychologue de décadence'. **Rev Etud Ital** 1981;26(2-4):173-94

**Pirch, Otto Ferdinand Dubislav, 1799-1832**
Dragić M: Higijenske prilike u Beogradskoj tvrdjavi i Beogradu 1829. godine (prema putopisu Ota Dubislava Pirha). **Srp Arh Celok Lek** 1982 Jul-Aug;110(7-8):951-7

**Pirckheimer, Wilibald, 1470-1530**
Benedek TG: A comparison of the medical writings of two humanists: F. Petrarca and W. Pirckheimer. In: Congrès international d'histoire de la médecine, XXVe, Québec, 1976. Actes. Québec, 1977. p. 502-6.
Benedek TG: The gout of Desiderius Erasmus and Willibald Pirckheimer: medical autobiography and its literary reflections. **Bull Hist Med** 1983 Winter;57(4):526-44

**Pirie, James Hunter Harvey, 1879-1965**
Bernstein RE: Dr Harvey Pirie and the Scottish National Antartic Expedition (1902-4). Scottish science and medicine in the Falklands and Antarctica. **Scott Med J** 1983 Jan;28(1):75-9
Bernstein RE: Historical vignette: Harvey Pirie (1879-1965) and the Falklands. **S Afr Med J** 1983 Jan 29;63(5):169-70
Bernstein RE: Dr. Harvey Pirie: versatile man of science and pioneer explorer of sub-antarctic regions eighty years ago. **Adler Mus Bull** 1984 Mar;10(1):4-10

**Pirodon, Eugene, 1824-1908**
Telson HW: Une leçon du Docteur Charcot à la Salpêtrière. Lithograph by Eugene Pirodon after a painting (1887) by André Brouillet. **J Hist Med Allied Sci** 1980 Jan;35(1):58

**Pirogov, Nikolaĭ Ivanovich, 1810-1881**
Bagdasar'ian SM: Velikiĭ russkiĭ khirurg N. I. Pirogov (k 100-letiiu so dnia smerti). **Klin Med (Mosk)** 1982 Jul;60(7):111-5
Balon LR: N. I. Pirogov--osnovopolozhnik otechestvennoĭ vosstanovitel'noĭ khirurgii. **Vestn Khir** 1983 Jun;130(6):93-7
Berkutov AN: Zavety N. I. Pirogova i sovremennaia khirurgiia. **Vestn Khir** 1982 May;128(5):125-7
Berkutov AN: Das chirurgische Erbe. N.I. Pirogov und die gegenwärtige Chirurgie. **Zentralbl Chir** 1984;109(17):1149-52
Bilyk VD, Klantsa PA, Kul'chitskiĭ KI, et al: Zaslugi N. I. Pirogova v sozdanii i razvitii material'no-tekhnicheskoĭ bazy vysshego meditsinskogo obrazovaniia. **Klin Khir** 1983 Mar;(3):55-7
Brzheskiĭ VCh: O znakakh, uvekovechivaiushchikh imia N. I. Pirogova v strane. **Khirurgiia (Mosk)** 1980 Feb;(2):105-6
Chernyĭ VP: Znamenitye patsienty N. I. Pirogova. **Feldsher Akush** 1983 Sep;48(9):34-7
Dal' MK: Zdorov'e N. I. Pirogova v razlichnom vozraste i ego posledniaia. bolezn'. **Klin Khir** 1981 Mar;(3):59-60
Efimov AE: Neizvestnoe pis'mo N. I. Pirogova. **Sov Zdravookhr** 1983;(8):61-2
Elkin II, Frolova VV: Rol' N. I. Pirogova v podgotovke I. I. Mechnikova k nauchnoĭ deiatel'nosti (k 135-letiiu so dnia rozhdeniia I. I. Mechnikova. **Zh Mikrobiol Epidemiol Immunobiol** 1980 Sep;(9):114-8
Epifanov NS: Nastavnik pervykh russkikh meditsinskikh sester. **Med Sestra** 1983 Mar;42(3):48-50
Galin LL: Publikatsii N. I. Pirogova na stranitsakh 'Voenno--meditsinskogo zhurnala. **Voen Med Zh** 1980 Nov;(11):69-71
Geselvich AM: Letopis' zhizni N.I. Pirogova, 1810-1881. Moskva, Meditsina, 1976. 97 p.
Gol'braĭkh VR: Velikiĭ khirurg N. I. Pirogov--osnovopolozhnik khirurgii cheliustno-litsevoĭ oblasti (k 100-letiiu so dnia smerti). **Stomatologiia (Mosk)** 1982 Jul-Aug;61(4):66-7
Grachev AI: Zainteresovannost' N. I. Pirogova istorieĭ i arkheologieĭ. **Vrach Delo** 1980 Jan;(1):114-6
Grebenev AL: S. P. Botkin o N. I. Pirogove. **Klin Med (Mosk)** 1982 Sep;60(9):108-10
Gribanov ED: Memorial'nye medali N. I. Pirogova (k 100-letiiu so dnia smerti). **Feldsher Akush** 1981;46(12):42-5
Iurikhin AP: N. I. Pirogov, ego ucheniki i posledovateli. **Klin Khir** 1984 May;(5):62-4
Katsnel'bogen AG: Neopublikovannaia rabota N. I. Pirogova. **Sov Zdravookhr** 1982;(11):61-4
Katsnel'bogen AG: N. I. Pirogov i brat'ia Pushchiny. **Sov Zdravookhr** 1983;(9):62-5
Klantsa PA, Sobchuk GS, Fishchenko AIa: Vishenskiĭ period deiatel'nosti N. I. Pirogova. **Khirurgiia (Mosk)** 1980 Feb;(2):106-10
Kolmsee P: Nikolai Iwanowitsch Pirogow - Kriegschirurg und militärmedizinischer Organisator in Russland des 19. Jahrhunderts. **Militaergesch** 1981;20(5):536-45
Korotkikh RV: N. I. Pirogov i voprosy vrachebnoĭ étiki. (K 100-letiiu so dnia smerti). **Sov Zdravookhr** 1981;(12)54-7
Korzh AA, Bondarenko NS: Pamiati N. I. Pirogova (k 100-latiiu so dnia smerti). **Ortop Travmatol Protez** 1982 Apr;(4):56-9
Kozovenko MN: Rol' N. I. Pirogova v organizatsii truda meditsinskikh sester na voĭne. **Voen Med Zh** 1980 Nov;(11);72-3
Kravtsov DE: Prosvetitel'skaia deiatel'nost' N. I. Pirogova v Kieve. **Voen Med Zh** 1982 Nov;(11):65-6
Kul'chitskiĭ KI, Romenskiĭ OIu, Sobchuk GS, et al: Nikolaĭ Ivanovich Pirogov v usad'be 'Vishnia'. **Arkh Anat Gistol Embriol** 1980 Aug;79(8):110-7
Kul'chitskiĭ KI, Klantsa PA, Sobchuk GS: Chestvovanie N.I. Pirogova na ego 50-letnem iubilee. **Vrach Delo** 1981;(6):1-5
Kul'chitskiĭ KI, Klantsa PA, Sobchuk GS: N. I. Pirogov--osnovopolozhnik topograficheskoĭ (prikladnoĭ) anatomii. **Klin Khir** 1981 Nov;(11):73-6
Kul'chitskiĭ KI: N. I. Pirogov v usad'be Vishnia. Kiev, Zdorov'ia, 1981. 99 p.
Kuz'min MK: Velikiĭ Russkiĭ khirurg N. I. Pirogov i sovremennost'. **Sov Med** 1983;(2):117-9
Leonov IT: N. I. Pirogov i voennaia meditsina. **Feldsher Akush** 1981;46(11):51-3
Maiat VS, Kochnova IE: K 100-letiiu so dnia smerti N.I. Pirogova. **Klin Med (Mosk)** 1981 Nov;59(11):114-9
Makovoz AA: [Nikolai Ivanovich Pirogov in the Korovograd District] (Rus). **Sov Zdravookhr** 1981;3:59-60
Mazurik EV: O pedagogicheskoĭ deiatel'nosti N. I. Pirogova v Kamenets--Polol'ske i o ego sviaziakh s Obshchestvom polol'skikh vracheĭ (k 100-letiiu so dnia smerti N. I. Pirogova). **Sov Zdravookhr** 1981;(8):66-8
Mirskiĭ MB: N. I. Pirogov--krupneĭshiĭ khirurg XIX veka. **Feldsher Akush** 1981;46(12):37-40
Novakova LIa: Publikatsii o N. I. Pirogove v khirurgicheskom zhurnale Ukrainy. **Klin Khir** 1982 Feb;(2):49-50
Pendler MB: Muzeĭ-usad'ba N. I. Pirogova (k 100-letiiu so dnia smerti N. I. Pirogova). **Feldsher Akush** 1981;46(12):40-2
Pytel' AIa: Velikiĭ russkiĭ khirurg Nikolaĭ Ivanovich Pirogov (k 100-letiiu so dnia smerti). **Urol Nefrol (Mosk)** 1981 Jan-Feb;(1):3-8
Rusanov GA, Simbirtsev SA, Balanski R: Sto godini ot publikuvaneto na truda na N. I. Pirogov vurkhu opita v meditsinata, pridobit vuv voĭnata za osvobozhdenieto na Bulgariia prez 1877-1878 g. **Khirurgiia (Sofiia)** 1979;32(3):247-53
Savel'ev VS: N. I. Pirogov -- veljkiĭ russkiĭ khirurg i uchenyĭ. **Sov Med** 1981;(11):116-8
Selivanov EF, Kantorovich MM: Relikvii N. I. Pirogova v Noenno-meditsinskom muzee. **Voen Med Zh** 1983 Nov;(11):71-3
Shabunin AV: Uchastie N.I. Pirogova v Obshchestve S.-Peterburgskikh prakticheskikh vracheĭ. **Sov Zdravookhr** 1983;(4):63-5
Skopakov Kh: N. I. Pirogov--genialen khirug i osnovopolozhnik na topografskata anatomiia. **Khirurgiia (Sofiia)** 1982;35(1):99-100
Smol'iannikov AV, Sarkisov DS, Serebrennikov AB: N. I. Pirogov--velikiĭ uchenyĭ, vrach, grazhdanin. **Arkh Patol** 1982;44(9):3-13
Sobchuk GS, Klantsa PA: N. I. Pirogov o nagrazhdenii zarubezhnykh uchenykh Russkimi orderami (Po neopublikovannym materialam). **Sov Zdravookhr** 1983;(4):65-8
Toporov GN: N. I. Pirogov ob usovershenstvovanii meditsinkikh kadrov v Rossii (k 100-letiiu so dnia smerti N. I. Pirogova, 1810-1881 gg). **Sov Zdravookhr** 1982;(2):66-8
Toporov GN: Khirurgiia krovenosnykh sosudov v trudakh N. I. Pirogova (K stoletiiu vykhoda v svet piatogo izdaniia knigi N. I. Pirogova 'Khirurgicheskaia anatomiia arterial'nykh stvolov i fastsiĭ'. CPB, 1881-1882). **Klin Khir** 1982 Nov;(11):71-3
Tret'iak TP, Stetsula TI: Zaslugi N. I. Pirogova v oftal'mologii. **Oftalmol Zh** 1981;36(8):506-8
Velikoretskiĭ AN: Vzgliady N. I. Pirogova na preduprezhdenie zarazheniia ran. **Feldsher Akush** 1979 Sep;44(9):44-6
Vytrishchak VIa: Vklad N. I. Pirogova v razvitie cheliustno-litsevoĭ khirurgii. **Voen Med Zh** 1982 Nov;(11):64-5
Zabludovskiĭ PE: N. I. Pirogov i meditsinskiĭ trud zhenshchin. **Feldsher Akush** 1981;46(11):53-4
Zabludovskiĭ PE: Trudy nauchnykh uchrezhdeniĭ Ukrainskoĭ SSR k Pirogovskoĭ godovshchine. **Vrach Delo** 1983 Feb;(2):121-2

**Pirquet von Cesenatico, Clemens Peter, 1874-1929**
Bendiner E: Baron von Pirquet: the aristocrat who discovered and defined allergy. **Hosp Pract** 1981 Oct;16(10):137, 141, 144 passim
Kallós P: Immunity and concomitant immunity in infectious diseases. Introduction. **Prog Allergy** 1982;31:IX-XV
Wyklicky H: Gedanken zur Geschichte der Allergie. In memoriam Clemens von Pirquet. **Wien Med Wochenschr** 1980 Feb 15;130(3):123-5

**Piso, Willem, 1611-1678**
Pies E: Willem Piso (1611-1678): Begründer der kolonialen Medizin und Leibarzt des Grafen Johann Moritz von Nassau-Siegen in Brasilien: eine Biographie. Düsseldorf, Interma-Orb Verlagsgruppe, 1981. 227 p.

**Pissarro, Camille, 1830-1903**
Schmidt V: Camille Pissarro, hans danske relationer og hans sygdom. **Dan Medicinhist Arbog** 1983;12:144-61

**Pitcairn, William, 1711-1791**
Schneck JM: William Pitcairn (1711-1791) and tne Gold-Headed Cane. **JAMA** 1984 Apr 20;251(15):1952

**Pitcairne, Archibald, 1652-1713**
Appleby JH, Cunningham A: Robert Erskine and Archibald Pitcairne: two Scottish physicians' outstanding libraries. **Bibliotheck** 1982;11:3-16
Freeman FW, Law A: Allan Ramsay's first published poem: the poem to the memory of Dr. Archibald Pitcairne. **Bibliotheck** 1979;9:153-60

**Pitcher, Samuel, 1824-1907**
Rogers FB: Dr. Samuel Pitcher (1824-1907): Cape Cod and Castoria. **J Hist Med Allied Sci** 1982 Jul;37(3):323-5

**Pitré, Giuseppe, 1841-1916**
Morricone A, Pedicino V: Medici e guaritori in Sicilia: spunti di medicina popolare in un'opera diGiuseppe Pitré. In Congrès international d'histoire de la médecine, XXVe, Québec, 1976. Actes. Québec, 1977. p. 992-8.

**Pitts, Robert Franklin, 1908-**
Alexander RS: Pitts and urine acidification. **Physiologist** 1983 Dec;26(6):364-6

**Piuze, Liveright, 1754-1813**
Morin J: Liveright Piuze. In Dictionary of Canadian biography, 1801 to 1820. Volume 5, 1983. p. 676.

**Planck, Max Karl Ernst Ludwig, 1858-1947**
Lüst R: Max Planck und die Max-Planck-Gesellschaft. **Gesch Wiss Unterr** 1979;30(9):527-37
Regato JA del: Max Planck. **Int J Radiat Oncol Bill Phys** 1979 Nov-Dec;5(11-12):2097-111

**Planque, Hugues, fl. 1837**
Febres-Cordero F: Fue Hugues Planque autorizado para ejerceer en Venezuela 'su industria de dentista'? **Acta Odontol Venez** 1982 Jan-Apr;20(1):39-52

**Plato**
Galen: On the doctrines of Hippocrates and Plato. Edition, translation and commentary by P De Lacy. Second Part: Books VI-IX. Berlin, Akademie Verlag, 1980. p. 361-609. (Corpus Medicorum Graecorum, V, 4, 1, 2).
Mann L: The wax block metaphor: Plato's views on learning disabilities. **J Learn Disabil** 1980 Oct;13(8):420-4
Pomeroy SB: Plato and the female physician ('Republic', 454d 2). **Am J Philol** 1978;99:496-500
Robert F: Hippocrate, Platon, Aristote et les notions de genre et d'espèce. **Hist Philos Life Sci** 1982;4(2):173-201

**Platonov, IIa**
Miliavskiĭ VM: K istorii prepodavaniia psikhiatrii v fel'dsherskikh shkolakh. **Feldsher Akush** 1982;47(4):53-4

**Platter, Felix, 1536-1614**
Lenzen W: Mentis Laesiones, Psychopathologie bei Felix Platter (1536-1614). Diss. Bonn, 1982. 151 p.
Mistler J: Voyageurs d'autrefois. **Nouv Rev Deux Mondes** 1977;(2):265-75;(3):519-27
Schiller F: A note on the Pickwickian syndrome and Felix Platter (1536-1614). **J Hist Med Allied Sci** 1985 Jan;40(1):66-7

**Platter, Thomas, 1574-1628**
Mistler J: Voyageurs d'autrefois. **Nouv Rev Deux Mondes** 1977;(2):265-75;(3):519-27

**Plattes, Gabriel, fl. 1638-1643**
Webster C: Utopian planning and the Puritan revolution. Gabriel Plattes, Samuel Hartlib, and 'Macaria'. Oxford, Wellcome Unit for the History of Medicine, 1979. 89 p. (Research Publications of the Wellcome Unit for the History of Medicine, Oxford, No. II).

**Pleadwell, Frank Lester, 1872-1957**
Wilbur DA: The inimitable surgeon Pleadwell. **US Navy Med** 1983 May-Jun;74(3):5-10

**Plenck, Joseph Jacob, 1738-1807**
Gysel C: Anomalies, mélanodontie et orthodontie dans le traité de pathologie dentaire (1778) de Joseph Jakob Plenk (1732-1807). **Orthod Fr** 1979;50:769-88
Holubar K, Frankl J: Joseph Plenck (1735-1807). A forerunner of modern European dermatology. **J Am Acad Dermatol** 1984 Feb;10(2 pt 1):326-32
King DF, King LA: Josef Plenck--grandfather of modern dermatology. **J Am Acad Dermatol** 1984 Jul;11(1):143-6
Terencio de las Aguas J: La lepra en el libro 'Doctrina de morbis cutaneis' de José Jacoba Plenck. **Fontilles** 1980;12:409-14

**Plinius Secundus, C., 23-79**
Classics in infectious diseases: Excerpts from the Natural History of Pliny. **Rev Infect Dis** 1982 Nov-Dec;4(6):1266-9

**Plinius Secundus, C., 23-79 A.D.**
Nauert CG: The author of a Renaissance commentary on Pliny: Rivius, Trithemius or Aquaeus. **J Warburg Courtauld Inst** 1979;42:282-6
Nauert CG: Caius Plinius Secundus. In Cranz FE, Kristeller PO, ed: Catalogus translationum et commentariorum: Mediaeval and Renaissance Latin translations and commentaries. Annotated lists and guides. Vol. IV. Washington, D.C., Catholic University of America Press, 1980. p. 297-422.
Phillips JH: Juxtaposed medical traditions: Pliny HN 27, 131. **Classical Philol** 1981;76(2):130-2
Roemer F: Plinius der Aeltere. (Annotated bibliog. 1964-77.) **Anz Altertumswiss** 1978;31:129-206
Römer F: Plinius der Aeltere. III. Bericht. **Anz Altertumswiss** 1978;31:129-206
Stannard J: Medicinal plants and folk remedies in Pliny, Historia Naturalis. **Hist Philos Life Sci** 1982;4(1):3-23

**Ploegh Family**
Haneveld GT: De ledezetters van Jisp. **Spiegel Hist** 1977;12(100):514-17

**Poe, Edgar Allan, 1809-1849**
Burke GW, Shepard FE: Edgar Allan Poe: Richmond's bright star. **Va Dent J** 1980;57(2):12-8
Kennedy JG: Poe and magazine writing on premature burial. **Stud Am Renaiss** 1977;165-78
Scarlett C: A tale of ratiocination: the death and burial of Edgar Allan Poe. **Md Hist Mag** 1978;73(4):360-74

**Polanyi, Michael, 1891-**
Stephenson W: Micheal Polanyi, science and belief. **Ethics Sci Med** 1980;7(2):97-110
Torrance TF: The place of Michael Polanyi in the modern philosophy of science. **Ethics Sci Med** 1980;7(2):57-95

**Poletika, Ivan Andrejewitsch, 1722-1783**
Borodiĭ NK: I. A. Poletika--vydaiushchiĭsia ukrainskiĭ vrach i uchenyĭ XVIII st. **Mikrobiol Zh** 1982 May-Jun;44(3):90-4

**Polgar, Franz J., 1900-1979**
Gravitz MA, Gerton MI: Polgar as Freud's hypnotist? contrary evidence. **Am J Clin Hypn** 1982 Apr;24(4):272-6

**Polis, Beryl David, 1914-1977**
Cope FW: In memoriam . . . B. David Polis--mitochondrial biochemist, discoverer of polymeric prostaglandin PGBx for prevention and therapy of damaged mitochondrial oxidative phosphorylation. **Physiol Chem Phys** 1980;12(6):541-4

**Pollock, Paul Jackson, 1912-1956**
Rubin W: Pollock as Jungian illustrator: the limits of psychological criticism. **Art Am** 1979;67(7):104-23, (8):72-91

**Pomme, Pierre, 1728-1814**
Ledermann F: La psychiatrie française et les médicaments: Pomme, Pinel, Esquirol, Morel. **Rev Hist Pharm (Paris)** 1982 Sep;29(254):189-206

**Pommerin, Reiner**
Lilienthal G: 'Rheinlandbastarde', Rassenhygiene und das Problem der rassenideologischen Kontinuität. Zur Untersuchung von Reiner Pommerin: 'Sterilisierung der Rheinlandbastarde'. **Medizinhist J** 1980;15(4):426-36

**Ponce de Santa Cruz, Antonio, 1561-1632**
Riera J: El libro de la peste (1600) del doctor Antonio Ponce de Santa Cruz. In: Sociedad Española de Historia de la Medicina. V Congreso Nacional. Madrid, 1977. **Asclepio** 1977;29:319-29

**Pons i Freixa, Francisco de Asís, 1863-1938**
García Peña de Alexander M del P: Nota biográfica sobre el Doctor Francisco de Asís Pons i Freixa. In Congrés Internacional d'Historie de la Medicina Catalana, 1st, Barcelona-Montpellier, 1970. Barcelona, Editorial Scienta, 1971. v 4, p. 81-6.

**Pool, Judith Graham, 1919-1975**
Brinkhous KM: Judith Graham Pool. In: Notable American women. The modern period. Cambridge, Mass., Belknap-Harvard Univ. Press, 1980. 4:553-4.

**Popa, Grigore T., 1859-1930**
Stratone N, Stratone A: Probleme de gnoseologie în lucrările doctorului Grigore T. Popa. **Rev Med Chir Soc Med Nat Iasi** 1979 Oct-Dec;83(4):713-6

**Pope, Amy Elizabeth, 1869-**
Moss C, Marchfield F, Hansen H, et al: A treasury of practice history. (Amy Elizabeth Pope). **Calif Nurse** 1983 Sep;79(3):6-7

**Popescu-Sibiu, Ioan I., 1901-1974**
Sărmăşanu-Cortez ML, Cortez P: Dr. Ioan I. Popescu-Sibiu, promotor al psihanalizei şi neobosit animator al vieţii culturale din Romąnia (1901-1974). **Rev Med Interna [Neurol Psihiatr]** 1982 Oct-Dec;27(4):313-8

**Popielski, Boleslaw**
Raszeja S: Fifty years of the scientific work of Professor Boleslaw

Popielski. **Forensic Sci Int** 1981 Mar-Apr;17(2):97-100

**Popovic, Pavao, 1854-1937**
Plamenac SD: Dr. Pavao Popović (30. X 1854 - 17. X 1937), pionir oftalmologije u Srbiji. **Srp Arh Celok Lek** 1980 Feb;108(2):169-80

**Porta, Luigi, 1800-1875**
Zanobio B: Le osservazioni clinico-anatomiche di Luigi Porta (1800-1875) sulle 'cotilitidi'. **Rend Ist Lomb Accad Sci Lett B** 1978;112:82-98

**Portal, Antoine, 1742-1832**
Berman A: An unpublished letter from Eugene Soubeiran to Antoine Portal, June 3, 1828. **Pharm Hist** 1982;24(1):32-7
Brégeat P: Antoine Portal, fondateur de l'Académie de médecine. **Bull Acad Natl Med (Paris)** 1982 Dec;166(9):1304-16
Lemaire JF: A propos d'Antoine Portal. Le passé de la médecine et le regard de l'historien. **Hist Sci Med** 1980;14:399-406
Sicard A: Hommage rendu au cimetière Saint-Pierre de Montmartre par l'Académie nationale de médecine au baron Antoine Portal, son fondateur, à l'occasion du 150e anniversaire de sa mort. **Hist Sci Med** 1983;17(2):195-8
Théodoridès J: Antoine Portal et la rage (avec des documents inédits). In Ganzinger K, Skopec M, Wyklicky H, ed: Festschrift für Erna Lesky zum 70. Geburtstag. Wien, Brüder Hollinek, 1981. p. 161-5.

**Portal, Paul, 1630-1703**
Duchatel F: Paul Portal (1630? - ler juillet 1703): un accoucheur méconnu du XVIIe siècle. **Hist Sci Med** 1980;14:407-18

**Portaleone, Abraham, 1542-1612**
Kottek S: Abraham Portaleone (1542-1612): an Italian Jewish physician of the Renaissance period. His life and his will; reflections on early burial. **Koroth** 1983 Aug;8(7-8):269-77

**Portales, Diego, 1773-1837**
Costa-Casaretto C: Don Diego Portales y el Dr. Guillermo C. Blest. **Rev Med Chil** 1984 Jun;112(6):625-31

**Porter, Charles, 1864-1934**
Adler C: Dr. Charles Porter. **Adler Mus Bull** 1984 Jun;10(2):9-14

**Porter, John B., fl. 1804-1869**
Aldrete JA, Marron GM, Wright AJ: The first administration of anesthesia in military surgery: on occasion of the Mexican-American War. **Anesthesiology** 1984 Nov;61(5):585-8

**Porter, William Townsend, 1862-1949**
Barger AC: The meteoric rise and fall of William Townsend Porter, one of Carl J. Wigger's 'Old Guard'. **Physiologist** 1982 Oct;25(5):407-13
Benison S, Barger AC, Wolfe EL: Changing of the guard. **Harv Med Alumni Bull** 1982 Spring;56(2):34-41
Fye WB: Acute coronary occlusion always results in death--or does it? The observations of William T. Porter. **Circulation** 1985 Jan;71(1):4-10

**Postell, William Dosité, Sr., 1908-**
Skinner RE: The historical work of William Dosité Postell, Sr. **Watermark** 1983 Fall;7(2):8-10

**Potiralovskiĭ, Petr Petrovich, 1872-1927**
Galin LL: Vklad P. P. Potiralovskogo v razvitie organizatsionnykh voprosov voennoĭ meditsiny. **Voen Med Zh** 1982 Apr;(4):68-70

**Pott, John, 1595-ca.1642**
Given FT: Dr. John Pott: maligned early patriot. **Am J Obstet Gynecol** 1983 Sep 15;147(2):115-20
Horton CE, Horton CE: Dr. John Pott: America's first physician-governor and revolutionary. **Bull NY Acad Med** 1983 Sep;59(7):678-85

**Pott, Percivall, 1714-1788**
Haneveld GT: Pott's disease before Pott. **Neth J Surg** 1980;32(1):2-7

**Potter, Ellen Culver, 1871-1958**
Romanofsky P: Ellen Culver Potter. In Dictionary of American Biography, Suppl. 6, 1956-1960. p. 515-16, 1980.

**Potter, Irving White, 1868-1956**
Bullough VL, Groeger S: Irving W. Potter and internal podalic version: the problems of disciplining a skilled but heretical doctor. **Soc Probl** 1982;30(1):109-16

**Potts, Jonathan, 1745-1781**
Blanco RL: Physician of the American revolution, Jonathan Potts. New York, Garland STPM Press, 1979. xv, 276 p.
Blanco RL: The diary of Jonathan Potts: a Quacker medical student in Edinburgh (1766-67). **Trans Stud Coll Physicians Phila** 1977 Jan;44(3):119-30

**Pouchet, Félix-Archimède, 1800-1872**
Farley J, Geison GL, Ebnöther D: Le débat entre Pasteur et Pouchet: science, politique et génération spontanée, au 19e siècle en France. **Pandore** 1982;special number
Legée G: Lettres inédites des Félix Archimède Pouchet (1800-1872) au physiologiste Pierre Flourens (1794-1867). In International Congress of the History of Medicine. 26th, Plovdiv, 1978. Actes du Congress. Sofia, 1981. Volume II. p. 130-8.

**Pound, Dudley, 1877-1943**
Ljunggren B: The sleepy sea lord who was Churchill's friend. **Surg Neurol** 1982 Nov;18(5):307-19

**Pound, Ezra Loomis, 1885-1972**
Kimpel BD, Eaves TC: More on Pound's prison experience. **Am Lit** 1981;53(3):469-76

**Powers, Samuel R. Jr., 1919-1980**
Festschrift to Dr. Samuel R. Powers, Jr. September 25, 1919 - March 27, 1980: **Arch Surg** 1981 Oct;116(10):1241-1356

**Poznanin, Petr L'vovich, 1881-1943**
Dorosevich AE: Professor Petr L'vovich Poznanin--predstavitel' moskovskoĭ shkoly patologoanatomov. **Arkh Patol** 1983;45(1):79-80

**Prados y Such, Miguel, d. 1969**
Linares Maza A: La psiquiatría andaluza en la primera mitad de nuestro siglo. Personalidades destacadas. I. Miguel Prados Such (Málaga). **Arch Neurobiol (Madr)** 1983 Jan-Feb;46(1):59-66

**Prausnitz-Giles, Carl, 1876-1963**
Beritić T: Carl Prausnitz Giles i saga or reaginima. **Lijec Vjesn** 1981 Jul;103(7):312-4

**Pravdin, Nikolaĭ Sergeevich, 1882-**
Korbakova AI, Ulanova IP: Nauchnaia deiatel'nost' vydaiushchegosia sovetskogo toksikologa N. S. Pravdina i razvitie ego ideĭ v mashi dni. **Gig Tr Prof Zabol** 1983 Feb;(2):44-5
Nikolaĭ Sergeevich Pravdin (k 100-letiiu so dnia rozhdeniia): **Farmakol Toksikol** 1983 May-Jun;46(3):127-8

**Preis, Karl**
Levinger IM, ed: 'Medizinisch-schwierige Talmudstellen' [by Karl Preis]. **Udim** 1977-78;7-8:95-107

**Prescott, Jonathan, 1725-1807**
Punch TM: Jonathan Prescott, M.D.: vincit qui patitur. **NS Hist Q** 1979;9(1):59-80

**Prescott, Samuel Cate, 1872-1962**
Cravens H: Samuel Cate Prescott. In Dictionary of American biography, 1961-1965. Suppl. 7, 1981. p. 629-30.
Goldblith SA: Samuel Cate Prescott: - pioneer food technologist -gifted teacher. **Adv Food Res** 1981;27:1-21

**Preston, Ann, 1813-1872**
Fullard J: Ann Preston: pioneer of medical education and women's rights. **Pa Herlt** 1982;8(1):9-14

**Preuss, Julius, 1861-1913**
Rosner F: Julius Preuss. **Med Hist** 1975 Oct;19(4):376-88

**Prevost, Jean Louis, 1790-1850**
Castellani C: Fra preformismo e epigenesi: le teorie di Prevost e Dumas. **Hist Philos Life Sci** 1980;2(2):253-68
Mayer R: Ils étaient trois! Jacques-Louis Reverdin, Jean-Louis Prévost et Constant Picot, fondateurs de la Revue médicale de la Suisse Romande. Evocation de la naissance d'une revue médicale et esquisse biographique de ses premiers rédacteurs. **Rev Med Suisse Romande** 1980 Dec;100(12):1013-41

**Prevost, Jean-Louis, 1838-1927**
Castellani C: Una rilettura ottocentesca di Spallanzani: la nouvelle théorie de la génération di Prévost e Dumas (1824). **Hist Philos Life Sci** 1979;1(2):215-59

**Preyer, William Thierry, 1841-1897**
Becker KH, Schmidt HD: Uber eine bisher unerschlossene Quelle der Preyer-Forschung. **Z Psychol** 1984;192(2):182-91
Sprung H, Sprung L: William Thkerry Preyer (1841-1897) als Methodologe und Methodiker. **Z Psychol** 1984;192(2):170-81
Tobach E: The relationship between Preyer's concept of psychogenesis and his views of Darwin's theory of evolution. **Z Psychol** 1983;191(4):388-95

**Pribil, Jan, 1781-1866**
Petrov BD: I. A. Pribil' (k 200-letiiu so dnia rozhdeniia). **Zh Mikrobiol Epidemiol Immunobiol** 1983 Oct;(10):108-9

**Pribylev, A. V., 1857-1936**
Malozemova AI: Revoliutsionery-mediki Pribylevy. **Sov Zdravookhr** 1984;(8):62-5

**Price, Derek John de Solla, 1922-1983**
Bedini SA: Derek J. de Solla Price (1922-1983). **Technol Cult** 1984 Jul;25(3):701-5
Bedini SA: Derek J. DeSolla Price. **Ann Ist Mus Stor Sci Fir** 1984;9(1):95-115
Mackay A: Derek John de Solla Price: an appreciation. **Soc Stud Sci** 1984 May;14(2):315-20

**Price, Don Krasher, 1910-**
Dupree AH: The rise and fall of the American establishment. **Minerva** 1984 Spring;22(1):116-24

**Price, Hartley D'Oyley, 1902-**
Fulton MW: Hartley D. Price: his contributions to physical education and gymnastics. Ph.D. Diss., Florida State University. Tallahassee, 1981. xvii, 171 leaves.

**Price, William, 1800-1893**
Cule J: William Price of Llantrisant--1800-1893. **Br Med J [Clin Res]** 1982 Feb 13;284(6314):483-4

## Q



## R

**Rabelais, François, ca. 1490–1553**
Frey EF: The influence of Rabelais on medicine and its reform. **Clio Med** 1980;15(1/2):25–33
Swinton WE: Rabelais' coarse humour was therapy for his patients. **Can Med Assoc J** 1981 Feb 15;124(4):500–4

**Rabs, Mattheus, b. 1652**
Wittop Koning DA: Ein Niederlassungszettel des Chymisten Mattheus Rabs. In Hickel E, Schröder G, ed: Neue Beiträge zur Arzneimittelgeschichte. Festschrift für Wolfgang Schneider zum 70. Geburtstag. Stuttgart, Wissenschaftliche Verlagsgesellschaft, 1982. p. 47–58.

**Racchetti, Vincenzo, 1777–1819**
Armocida G, Ambrosoli C, Majeron MA: Note biografich intorno a Vincenzo Racchetti (1777–1819). Contributo alla storia della neurologia. **Minerva Med** 1980 Apr 21;71(16):1221–6

**Rácz, Sámuel, 1744–1817**
Kötay P: Rácz Sámuel és a magyar orvosi oktatás hajnala. **Orv Hetil** 1982 Jan 10;123(2):103–9

**Radford, John Blair, 1813–1872**
Streitmatter R: John Blair Radford of Arnheim: New River Valley doctor and businessman. **Va Cavalcade** 1979;28(4):180–5

**Rado, Sandor, 1890–1972**
Kobarg I: Das Leben und Werk von Sandor Rado. Diss. Mainz, 1979. 73 p.

**Rafinesque, Constantine Samuel, 1783–1840**
Bloch H: Medical botany; note on Constantine Samuel Refinesque (1784–1841). **NY State J Med** 1979 Sep;79(10):1610–1
Boewe C: Editing Rafinesque's holographs: the case of the short letters. **Filson Club Hist Q** 1980;54(1):37–49
Reynaud G: Un grand naturaliste méconnu: Constantin Samuel Rafinesque (1783–1840). **Marseille** 1978;112:61–70

**Ragg Family**
Burnby J: The Raggs of Edmonton Green. **Pharm Hist (London)** 1975 Dec;5(3):2–3

**Ragoza, Nikolaĭ Ivanovich, 1883–1959**
Matkovskiĭ NI: Vydaiushchiisia Sovetskiĭ terapevt–infektsionist Nikolaĭ Ivanovich Ragoza (k 100–letiiu so dnia rozhdeniia). **Klin Med (Mosk)** 1983 Oct;61(10):136–8
Nikolaĭ Ivanovich Ragoza (K 100–letiiu so dnia rozhdeniia): **Voen Med Zh** 1983 Jul;(7):76

**Raicus, Johann, d. 1631**
Dahlström G: Johannes Raicus' tankar om lungsoten. **Nord Medicinhist Arsb** 1984;:63–70

**Raimon de Castelnou, fl. ca. 1350**
Norwood FE, ed: The fourteenth–century medico–botanical glossary of Raimon de Castelnou. Leeds, W. S. Maney for the Leeds Philosophical and Literary Society, 1974. (Proceedings of the Leeds Philosophical and Literary Society, Literary and Historical Section, Vol. XV, Part VI, pp. 135–225).

**Ramaer, Johannes Nicolaas, 1817–1887**
Lindeboom GA: Geschiedenis der geneeskunde: J. N. Ramaer (1817–1887) en zijn bibliotheek. **Ned Tijdschr Geneeskd** 1982 Aug 14;126(33):1504–10

**Ramazzini, Bernardino, 1633–1714**
Bertelli G, Foà V: Ramazzini, cinquanta anni dopo, su 'la medicina del lavoro'. **Med Lav** 1983 Nov–Dec;74(6):423–5
Brieger GH: The diseases of runners: a view from the eighteenth century--a commentary. **Pharos** 1980 Fall;43(4):29–32
Olagüe de Ros G: La epidemia europea de gripe de 1708–1709. Difusión témporo–espacial e interpretaciones contemporáneas: G. M. Lancisi, B. Ramazzini, K. F. Hoffmann. **Dynamis** 1981;1:51–86
Parmeggiani L: L'opera di Bernadino Ramazzini nel campo della medicina del lavoro. **Med Lav** 1983 Nov–Dec;74(6):426–32
Pericle di Pietro: Le fonti bibliografiche nella 'De morbis artificum diatriba' di Bernardino Ramazzini. **Hist Philos Life Sci** 1981;3(1):95–114
Premuda L: L'istanza sociale in Ramazzini pre–illuminista. **Med Lav** 1983 Nov–Dec;74(6):433–41
Sakula A: Ramazzini's De Morbis Artificum and occupational lung disease. **Br J Dis Chest** 1983 Oct;77(4):349–61

**Ramírez, Carlos María, 1848–1898**
González AD: La mision de Carlos M. Ramirez al Brasil y el convenio sanitario de 1887. **Bol Acad Nac Hist (Argentina)** 1964;35:327–53

**Ramírez de Arellano, Nicolás**
Marcial LD, Gutiérrez Avila JH: La vigilancia epidemiológica un siglo después. Nil novi sub sole? Comentarios al trabajo del Dr. Nicolás Ramírez de Arellano. **Salud Publica Mex** 1982 Sep–Oct;24(5):491–5

**Ramon, Gaston, 1886–1963**
Gilbrin E: Gaston Ramon (1886–1963). Le soixantième anniversaire des anatoxines. **Hist Sci Med** 1984;18(1):53–60

**Ramón y Cajal, Santiago, 1852–1934**
Abarracín Teulón A: Santiago Ramón y Cajal, o la pasión de España. Barcelona, Editorial Labor, [1978?] 319 p.
Albarracín A: Ramón y Cajal entre los poderes y los saberes. **Med Hist (Barc)** 1984;4:1–16
Albarracín Teulón A: Cajal y el problema del conocimiento cientifico. **Asclepio** 1980;32:7–17
Carrato Ibáñez A: Cajal y su Instituto. **Trab Inst Cajal Invest Biol** 1979;70(3):181–94
Hamburger V: S. Ramón y Cajal, R. G. Harrison, and the beginnings of neuroembryology. **Perspect Biol Med** 1980;23(4):600–16
Kock W: Santiago Ramón y Cajal och Nobelpriset. **Nord Medicinhist Arsb** 1981;:151–9
Kock W: Santiago Ramón y Cajal and the Nobel prize. In International Congress of the History of Medicine, 27th, Barcelona, 1980. Actas. Barcelona, Acadèmia de Ciències Mèdiques de Catalunya i Balears, 1981. p. 550–6.
Køppe S: The psychology of the neuron: Freud, Cajal and Golgi. **Scand J Psychol** 1983;24(1):1–12
Lorenzo Velázquez B: Algunos recuerdos sobre Cajal en el XLVII aniversario de su muerte. **An R Acad Nacl Med (Madr)** 1981;98(4):663–88
Marinesco M, Argemi–Lloveras J: Georges Marinescu (Roumanie) et Santiago Ramon y Cajal; deux représentants du génie latin. In International Congress of the History of Medicine, 27th, Barcelona, 1980. Actas. Barcelona, Acadèmia de Ciències Mèdiques de Catalunya i Balears, 1981. p. 570–4.
Nunez D: Anotaciones a un articulo de Ramon y Cajal. ['La sociedad del porvenir'. Vida Socialista, 1912, July '14.]. **Llull (Spain)** 1978;2:106–13
Peltier LF: The classic: qualities of intellectual order which the investigator should possess. Santiago Ramón y Cajal. **Clin Orthop** 1981;(160):2–13
Simmer HH: Santiago Ramón y Cajal und die Typologie des Wissenschaftlers. **Medizinhist J** 1981;16(4):414–23
Szállási A: Ramón y Cajal und die ungarischen Arzte. In International Congress of the History of Medicine, 27th, Barcelona, 1980. Actas. Barcelona, Acadèmia de Ciències Mèdiques de Catalunya i Balears, 1981. p. 632–5.
Valenciano Gayá L: Cajal (recuerdos y reflexiones de uno de sus últimos alumnos). **Arch Neurobiol (Madr)** 1983 Jul–Aug;46(4):272–81

**Ramsay, Allan, 1686–1758**
Freeman FW, Law A: Allan Ramsay's first published poem: the poem to the memory of Dr. Archibald Pitcairne. **Bibliotheck** 1979;9:153–60

**Ramsay, David, 1749–1815**
C[one] TE: On the proper treatment of infants according to David Ramsay of South Carolina (1790). **Pediatrics** 1981;68:353
Friedman LJ, Shaffer AH: History, politics, and health in early American thought: the case of David Ramsay. **J Am Stud** 1979;13(1):37–56
Health in the southern United States: New York, Arno, 1977. Various paginations. Facsimiles of works by David Ramsay (1790 and 1796), Josiah C. Nott (1847), Edward H. Barton (1851), Wickliffe Rose (1910), Joseph Goldberger (1916).
Olson GD: Dr. David Ramsay and Lt. Colonel Thomas Brown: patriot historian and loyalist critic. **SC Hist Mag** 1976;77:256–67

**Ramsbotham, Francis Henry, 1800–1868**
Waserman M: Sir James Y. Simpson and London's 'conservative and so curiously prejudiced' Dr. Ramsbotham. **Br Med J** 1980 Jan 19;280(6208):158–61

**Ramsey, Paul, 1913–**
Cahill LS: Within shouting distance: Paul Ramsey and Richard McCormick on method. **J Med Philos** 1979 Dec;4(4):398–417
Neff DS: "Extraordinary means': healers and healing in 'A Conversation with My Father'. In Jones AH, ed: Images of healers. Albany, State University of New York Press, 1983. p. 118–24.

**Ramusio, Girolamo, 1555–1610**
Lucchetta F: Girolamo Ramusio: profilo biografico. **Quad Stor Univ Padova** 1982;15:1–60

**Ran, Isaac, 1807–1881**
Jacobs F: Issac Ray and the profession of psychiatry. **RI Hist** 1979;38(4):99–111

**Rand, Marie Gertrude, 1886–1970**
Garber E: Marie Gertrude Rand. In: Notable American women. The modern period. Cambridge, Mass., Belknap–Harvard Univ. Press, 1980. 4:565.

**Randall, Alexander, 1858–**
Stool SE: A historical vignette: memoirs of an otologist's European study in 1883. **Am J Otol** 1983 Apr;4(4):346–9
Stool SE, Kemper M, Kemper B: The compleat otolaryngologist: Burton Alexander Randall. **Laryngoscope** 1984 Jan;94(1):16–9

**Rangel, Rafael, 1877–1909**
Carbonell JA: Rafael Rangel. **Rev Soc Venez Hist Med** 1975–76;23(37):129–33
Feldman M: Rafael Rangel y la crisis del medico. **Rev Soc Venez Hist Med** 1979;28(42):13–24
Iriarte DR: [Public health in Venezuela]. **Rev Soc Venez Hist Med** 1975–76;23(37):107–21

**Rank, Otto, 1884–1939**
Baumer G, Greulich G: Otto Rank. In J. Rattner, ed: Wandlungen der Psychoanalyse. Wien, Europaverlag, 1980. p. 31–52.

Klein DB: Jewish origins of the psychoanalytic movement. New York, Praeger, 1981. xvi, 198 p.
Menaker E: Otto Rank: a rediscovered legacy. New York, Columbia University Press, 1982. xvii, 166 p.
Zottl A: Otto Rank: das Lebenswerk eines Dissidenten der Psychoanalyse. München, Kindler, 1982. 316 p.

**Ranouw, Willem van, 1673–1724**
Beukers H: De tijdschriften van Willem van Ranouw. **Ned Tijdschr Geneeskd** 1981 Oct 3;125(40):1613–7

**Ransome, Gordon Arthur**
Works of the man: extracts from research papers written or co-authored by Sir Gordon Arthur Ransome. **Ann Acad Med Singapore** 1979 Jan;8(1):13–26

**Rapaport, David, 1911–1960**
Gill MM: David Rapaport. In Dictionary of American Biography, Suppl. 6, 1956–1960. p. 526–8, 1980.

**Raper, Howard Riley, 1886–1928**
Carr JD: The great radiology debate: the letters of C. Edmund Kells and Howard R. Raper. **Bull Hist Dent** 1981 Oct;29(2):69–73

**Rappe, Emmy Carolina, 1835–1896**
Johansson B: 'God bless you, my dear Miss Nightingale.' Letters from Emmy Carolina Rappe to Florence Nightingale 1867–1870. Stockholm, Almqvist & Wiksell International, 1977. 57 p. (Stockholm studies in English, 38).

**Rasori, Giovanni, 1766–1837**
Cosmacini G: Scienza medica e giacobinismo in Italia: l'impresa politico-culturale di Giovanni Rasori (1796–1799). Milano, F. Angeli, 1982. 130 p.

**Raspail, François-Vincent, 1794–1878**
Duchemin A: F. V. Raspail, l'apôtre du camphre. **Bull Liaison Assoc Amis Mus Pharm Montp** 1979;4:7–14
Hildebrand R: F. V. Raspail, Begründer der Histochemie und Wegbereiter der Zelltheorie, im Spiegel zeitgenössischer Medaillen. **Anat Anz** 1983;154(4):353–8
Raspail S: Raspail, savant et militant. **Histoire** 1978 Dec;7:89–91

**Raspe, Rudolph Erich, 1737–1794**
Iveson-Iveson J: Munchausen's syndrome: fantasy island (Rudolph Raspe). **Nurs Mirror** 1982 Jun 30;154(26):21
Ludwig J, Mann RJ: Münchhausen versus Munchausen. **Mayo Clin Proc** 1983 Nov;58(11):767–9

**Rasputin, Grigorii Efimovich, 1871–1916**
Willbanks OL, Willbanks SE: Femoral neuropathy due to retroperitoneal bleeding. A red herring in medicine complicates anticoagulant therapy and influences the Russian Communist Revolution (Crown Prince Alexis, Rasputin). **Am J Surg** 1983 Feb;145(2):193–8

**Rathbone, William, 1819–1902**
Hardy G: William Rathbone and the early history of district nursing. Ormskirk, Hesketh, 1981. 54 p.

**Raulin, Jules, 1836–1896**
Wrotnowska D: Jules Raulin, professeur au Lycée de Caen correspondance avec Pasteur. In: Congrès National des Sociétés Savantes, 105e, Caen, 1980. Comptes Rendus, Paris, 1980. Section des Sciences, Fasc. V. p. 109–120.

**Ravana**
Meulenbeld GJ: Observations on the Arkaprakaśa, a medical Sanskrit Text ascribed to Ravana. In Mazars G, ed: Les médecines traditionnelles de l'Asie. Strasbourg, Université Louis Pasteur, 1981. p. 111–39.

**Ravizza, Carlo, 1811–**
Bonalumi F: Il medico di Balzac e il curato di Ravizza. **Aevum** 1979;53(3):519–32

**Ray, Cyrus N., 1880–1966**
Hale DK: Cyrus N. Ray: the Abilene man. **West Tex Hist Assoc Yearb** 1979;55:17–36

**Ray, Isaac, 1807–1881**
Hughes JS: In the law's darkness: insanity and the medical-legal career of Isaac Ray, 1707–1881. Ph.D. Diss., Rice University. Houston, 1982. xvii, 393 p.
Payne H, Luthe R: Isaac Ray and forensic psychiatry in the United States. **Forensic Sci Int** 1980 Mar–Apr;15(2):115–27
Quen JM: Remarks on Doctor Isaac Ray (1807–1881). **RI Med J** 1980 Jun;63(6):217–9
Quen JM: Isaac Ray and the development of American psychiatry and the law. **Psychiatr Clin North Am** 1983 Dec;6(4):527–37

**Ray, Kaviraj Gangadhar**
Tripathi RD, Verma KC: Contribution of Kaviraj Gangadhar Ray in the development of ayurvedic education. **Sachitra Ayurved** 1981 Mar;:190–3

**Raynaud, Maurice, 1834–1881**
Jackson R: Raynaud and Molière. **Arch Dermatol** 1983 Mar;119(3):263–6
Merlen JF: Pnénomène de Raynaud. Historique. **Rev Prat** 1981 Dec 1;31(55):3971–2, 3975–6
Roncière J de la, Fiessinger JN: Maurice Raynaud, 1835–1881. **Rev Prat** 1981 Dec 1;31(55):3967–9

**Razetti, Luis, 1862–1932**
Archila R: Discurso de orden pronunciado el 23 de junio de 1982 con motivo del traslado de los restos del Doctor Luis Razetti al Panteón Nacional. Caracas, Miguel Angel Garcia, 1982. 18 p.

**Razumovskiĭ, Vasiliĭ Ivanovich, 1857–1935**
Abdullaev MS: Vklad V. I. Razumovskogo v istoriiu otechestvennoĭ anatomii (k 125-letiiu so dnia rozhdeniia). **Arkh Anat Gistol Embriol** 1982 Aug;83(8):96–100
Aminev AM: 125 let so dnia rozhdeniia Vasiliia Ivanovicha Razumovskogo. **Vestn Khir** 1983 May;130(5):137–9
Epifanov NS: Vasiliĭ Ivanovich Razumovskiĭ (k 125-letiiu so dnia rozhdeniia). **Feldsher Akush** 1982;47(7):42–3
Makarova EP: V. I. Razumovskiĭ--pervyĭ rektor Saratovskogo universiteta. **Vestn Khir** 1983 May;130(5):140–1
Mirskiĭ MB: V. I. Razumovskiĭ kak istorik khirurgii (k 125-letiiu so dnia rozhdeniia). **Sov Zdravookhr** 1983;5:66–70

**Reagan, Ronald Wilson, 1911–**
deMause L: The making of a fearful leader: 'Where's the rest of me?' **J Psychohist** 1984 Summer;12(1):5–21
Keigher SM: Reagan's 'New' federalism and the 1971 California Medi-cal reforms. **Urban Soc Change Rev** 1983;16(2):3–8

**Reagles, James, Jr.**
Roberson JW: A view from Oklahoma, 1866–1868: the diary and letters of Dr. James Reagles, Jr., Assistant Surgeon, U. S. Army. **Red River Val Hist Rev** 1978;3(4):19–46

**Recklinghausen, Friedrich Daniel von, 1833–1910**
Crump T: Translation of case reports in Ueber die multiplen Fibrome der Haut und ihre Beziehung zu den multiplen Neuromen by F. v. Recklinghausen. **Adv Neurol** 1981;29:259–75
Warkany J: Friedrich Daniel von Recklinghausen and his times. **Adv Neurol** 1981;29:251–7

**Redi, Francesco, 1626–1697**
Bacchi W: Su alcune note sperimentali inedite di Francesco Redi. **Ann Ist Mus Stor Sci Fir** 1982;7(1):35–56
Cafiso, LM: Storia della teoria sulla generazione spontanea: Redi, Spallanzani, Pasteur. **Cult Sc** 1981;20(80):236–43
DelChicca S, Tedeschi J: L'insonnia di Galileo in una lettera inedita di Francesco Redi. **Arch Stor Ital** 1979;173(4):615–8
Gottdenker P: Francesco Redi and the fly experiments. **Bull Hist Med** 1979 Winter;53(4):575–92

**Redon, Henri, 1899–1974**
Monod-Broca P: Henri Redon, 1899–1974. **Chirurgie** 1983;109(1):15–22

**Redwitz, Erich, 1883–1964**
Gütgemann A: In Memoriam Freiherr von Redwitz. Bonn, Hanstein, 1966. 40 p.

**Redwood, Theophilus, 1806–1892**
Thomas PH: Professor Theophilus Redwood (1806–92). **Pharm Hist (London)** 1983 Jun;13(2):9–12

**Reed, Walter, 1851–1902**
Bean WB: Walter Reed. A biography. Charlottesville, University Press of Virginia, 1982. 190 p.
Bean WB: Walter Reed and yellow fever. **JAMA** 1983 Aug 5;250(5):659–62
Crosby WH, Haubrich WS: The death of Walter Reed. **JAMA** 1982 Sep 17;248(11):1342–5
Norman C: The unsung hero of yellow fever? **Science** 1984 Mar 30;223(4643):1370–2

**Regaud, Claudius, 1870–1940**
Regaud J: Claudius Regaud, (1870–1940): pionnier de la cancérologie, créateur de la Fondation Curie: chronique de sa vie et son oeuvre. Paris, Maloine, 1982. 233 p.

**Regimorter, Assuerus, 1614–1650**
Birken W: Dr. John King (1614–1681) and Dr. Assuerus Regemorter (1615–1650). Brethren in the Dutch Church and in the Royal College of Physicians of London, with added references to other 'Dutch' congregants in the Royal College, Dr. Baldwin Hamey and Dr. George Ent. **Med Hist** 1976 Jul;20(3):276–95

**Regius, Henricus, 1598–1679**
Farina P: Il corpuscolarismo di Henricus Regius: materialismo e medicina in un cartesiano olandese del Seicento. In: Ricerche sull'atomismo del Seicento. Florence: La Nuova Italia, 1977. p. 119–78.
Gysel C: Cartesianisme en tandheelkunde bij Henricus Regius (1598--1679--1979). **Rev Belge Med Dent** 1979;34(2):213–22

**Reich, Wilhelm, 1897–1957**
Ackerknecht EH: Wilhelm Reich (1897–1957). In Ganzinger K, Skopec M, Wyklicky H, ed: Festschrift für Erna Lesky zum 70. Geburtstag. Wien, Brüder Hollinek, 1981. p. 5–12.
Angelini A: Wilhelm Reich nel dibattito psicoanalitico degli anni Trenta. **Stor Crit Psicol** 1984;5(2):373–88
Mann WE, Hoffman E: The man who dreamed of tomorrow. A conceptual biography of Wilhelm Reich. Los Angeles, Tarcher, 1980. 295 p.

Raditsa L: Some sense about Wilhelm Reich. New York, Philosophical Library, 1978. 126 p.
Sharaf M: Fury on Earth. A biography of Wilhelm Reich. New York, St. Martin's Press/Marek, 1983. xiii, 550 p.
Wilson C: The quest for Wilhelm Reich. Garden City, N.Y., Anchor, 1981. xv, 272 p.

**Reichborn-Kjennerud, Ingjald, 1865-1949**
Tillhagen CH: Ingjald Reichborn-Kjennerud (1865-1949). **Arv** 1969-70;25-26:353-74

**Reichenbach, Karl Ludwig von, 1788-1869**
Habacher M: Auf der suche nach dem 'Od'; Karl Ludwig Freiherr von Reichenbach (1788-1869) und Karl Wilhelm Mayrhofer (1806-1853), zwei Verbündete contra Justus von Liebig. **Clio Med** 1980 May;14(2):105-18

**Reid, Donald Darnley, 1914-1977**
Rose G: Professor D.D. Reid, MD Aberdeen, PHD DSc London, FRCP London. **J Epidemiol Community Health** 1978 Dec;32(4):229-34

**Reid, R. K.**
Gill D: The dueling doctors of Stockton. **Pac Hist** 1981;25(1):52-8

**Reik, Theodor, 1888-1969**
Berlin JB: Richard Beer-Hofmann and Theodor Reik: a letter in exile. **Psychoanal Rev** 1981-82 Winter;68(4):479-86
Gödde G: Theodor Reik. In J. Rattner, ed: Wandlungen der Psychoanalyse. Wien, Europaverlag, 1980. p. 87-113.
Grotjahn M: Remembering Theodor Reik and the third ear. **Psychoanal Rev** 1981-82 Winter;68(4):473-6
Lothane Z: Listening with the Third Ear as an instrument in psychoanalysis: the contributions of Reik and Isakower. **Psychoanal Rev** 1981-82 Winter;68(4):487-503
Rawn ML: Some reflections on the work of Theodor Reik. **Psychoanal Rev** 1981-82 Winter;68(4):477-8
Sherman MH: The paradox of Theodor Reik. **Psychoanal Rev** 1981-82 Winter;68(4):467-72
Sherman MH, ed: Psychoanalysis and old Vienna: Freud, Reik, Schnitzler, Kraus. New York, Human Sciences Press, 1978. 192 p.

**Reil-Bey, Wilhelm, 1820-1880**
Koch HT: Wilhelm Reil-Bey (1820-1880) und die Klimabehandlung der Tuberkulose. **Wiss Beitr Martin Luther Univ Halle Wittenberg** 1983;5-R80:251-60

**Reil, Johann Christian, 1759-1813**
Fischer W: Die Psychiatrie des Mediziners J.C. Reil--eine kritische Betrachtung. **Psychiatr Neurol Med Psychol (Leipz)** 1984 Apr;36(4):229-35
Heller R: Johann Christian Reil's training scheme for medical auxiliaries. **Med Hist** 1975 Oct;19(4):321-32

**Reilly, James Paul Marie, 1887-1974**
Decourt P: L'oeuvre de James Reilly. **Hist Sci Med** 1983;17(1):29-35

**Reimann, Johann Adam, 1690-1770**
Kaiser W: Wissenschaftsgeschichtliche Kooperation am Beispiel der slowakisch-ungarisch-halleschen Gemeinschaftsforschung zu Leben und Werk von Johann Andreas Segner und Johann Adam Reimann. **Wiss Z Martin Luther Univ (Math)** 1975;24(3):89-98

**Reimarus, Johann Albert Heinrich, 1729-1814**
Ort-Wädensweiler L: Johann Melchior Aepli: zur Verbesserung des Medizinalwesens in der Schweiz (1783/88). Zürich, Juris Druck, 1984. 70 p. (Zürcher Medizingeschichtliche Abhandlungen, Neue Reihe, Nr. 167).

**Reimer, Hermann Andreas, 1825-1906**
Heintel H: Hermann Andreas Reimer und seine 1855 eröffnete 'Heilanstalt für Epileptische' in Görlitz. **Medizinhist J** 1982;17(1/2):156-60
Lauschke HP: Der Epileptologe Herrmann Andreas Reimer in Görlitz. **Psychiatr Neurol Med Psychol (Leipz)** 1982 Dec;34(12):745-8

**Reinhold, John Gunther, 1900-**
Reinhold JG: Adventures of a clinical chemist. **Clin Chem** 1982 Nov;28(11):2314-23

**Reinke, Friedrich, 1862-**
Ober WB, Sciagura C: Leydig, Sertoli, and Reinke: three anatomists who were on the ball. **Pathol Annu** 1981;16 Pt 1:1-13

**Reinsberg, Viktor, 1875-1938**
Ozorovský V, Tychý M, Buchvald J, et al: Sociálne aspeckty začiatkov dermatovenerológie v Bratislave po roku 1918 a úloha professora Reinsberga. **Cesk Zdrav** 1982 Jul;30(7):319-25
Tichý M, Ozorovský V, Beniak M, et al: Pôsobenie profesora Reinsberga v akademických funkciách na LFUK v Bratislave (1925-1927). **Cesk Zdrav** 1984 Feb;32(2):68-73

**Reinzer, Franz, 1661-1708**
Wittop Koning DA, Van Gelder JB: Die Offizin aus der Meteorologia philosophica-politica des Fr. Reinzer. **Beitr Gesch Pharm** 1984;31(24):210

**Reitinger, Christopher, 1557?-1612**
Appleby JH: Doctor Christopher Reitinger and a seal of Tsar Boris Godunov. **Oxf Slav Pap** 1979;12:32-9

**Reko, Victor Aloisius, 1880-**
Tyler VE: The case of Victor A. Reko--an unrecognized pioneer writer on New World hallucinogens. **J Nat Prod** 1979 Sep-Oct;42(5):489-95

**Rembrandt, Hermanszoon van Rijn, 1607-1669**
Braithwaite PA, Shugg D: Rembrandt's Bathsheba: the dark shadow of the left breast. **Ann R Coll Surg Engl** 1983 Sep;65(5):337-8
Cremone JC: The anatomy lesson of Dr. Nicolaas Tulp. **J Hand Surg** 1982 Sep;7(5):530
Dymarskiĭ LIu: Taĭna 'Virsavii', kartiny Rembrandta. **Vopr Onkol** 1984;30(10):90-101
Leyh F: Hatte Rembrandt van Rijn eine Nickelallergie? **Hautarzt** 1984 Sep;35(9):472-3
Pytel' AIa: Bol', prishedshaia iz glubiny vekov (k 375-letiiu so dnia rozhdeniia Rembrandta). **Sov Med** 1980;(12):98-9
Schupbach W: The paradox of Rembrandt's 'Anatomy of Dr. Tulp'. London, Wellcome Institute for the History of Medicine, 1982. 110 p. (Medical History, Suppl. No. 2).

**Remington, Frederic, 1861-1909**
Williams GR: A history of appendicitis. With anecdotes illustrating its importance. **Ann Surg** 1983 May;197(5):495-506

**Remsen, Ira, 1846-1927**
Wankmüller A: Die deutschen Lehrbücher von Ira Remsen. **Dtsch Apoth Ztg** 1979 Aug 30;119(35):1381-2

**Renaudot, Théophraste, 1584-1653**
Kneist W: Théophraste Renaudot und die Dispensairebetreuung. **Z Arztl Fortbild (Jena)** 1982 Mar 1;76(5):220-3

**Renoux, André, fl. 1690**
Chaïa J: Contrat d'un chirurgien d'une plantation de Cayenne au XVIIe siècle. In: Congrès National des Sociétés Savantes, 93e, Tours, 1968. Comptes Rendus. Paris, 1971. Section des Sciences, Tome II. p. 51-4.

**Renterghem, Albert Willem van, 1846-1939**
Bulhof IN: From psychotherapy to psychoanalysis: Frederik van Eeden and Albert Willem van Renterghem. **J Hist Behav Sci** 1981;17:209-21

**Retzius, Anders Adolf, 1796-1860**
Retzius' stilling i den svenske patologiske anatomi: **Tandlaegebladet** 1979 Oct;83(18):659

**Retzius, Anders Jahan, 1742-1821**
Bruun NW, Baerentsen K, Jensen VG: Anders Jahan Retzius: 'Fragmentum historiae pharmaceutices veterum'. Med dansk oversaettelse, biografiske noter og kommentarer. **Theriaca** 1981;20:5-151
Retzius AJ: Fragmentum historiae pharmaceutices veterum. Med dansk oversaettelse, biografiske noter og kommentarer, ved N. W. Bruun, K. Baerentsen, V. G. Jensen. København, Dansk Farmacihistorisk Selskab, 1981. 152 p. (Theriaca, 20).

**Reverdin, Jacques Louis, 1842-1929**
Mayer R: Ils étaient trois! Jacques-Louis Reverdin, Jean-Louis Prévost et Constant Picot, fondateurs de la Revue médicale de la Suisse Romande. Evocation de la naissance d'une revue médicale et esquisse biographique de ses premiers rédacteurs. **Rev Med Suisse Romande** 1980 Dec;100(12):1013-41
Mirskiĭ MB: Vklad Revedena v transplantologiiu i khirurgiiu. **Khirurgiia (Mosk)** 1980 Jun;(6):109-10
Schneider S: Commentaires sur l'article de Jacques-Louis Reverdin: 'des opérations modernes de cure radicale des hernies'. **Rev Med Suisse Romande** 1980 Dec;100(12):1097-101

**Revere, Paul, 1735-1818**
Kolisch P deR: Paul Revere and medicine. **JAMA** 1984 Jun 22-29;251(24):3224
Paul Revere, goldsmith: **Dent Lab Rev** 1981 Feb;56(2):40

**Révérend, Alejandro Prospero, 1796-1881**
Mérida F: Semblanzas de Alejandro Prospero Révérend, primicias para calificar su actuacion frente a la ultima enfermedad del Libertador. **Rev Soc Venez Hist Med** 1981;30(47):71-80

**Revers, Wilhelm Josef, 1918-**
Wyss D, Zacher A: W. J. Revers' Bedeutung für die moderne Psychologie. Ein Uberblick. **Z Klin Psychol Psychother** 1983;31(2):137-48

**Reynaud, Claude-Auguste, 1804-1878**
Trocme C: L'atélectasie découverte et délaissée: Claude-Auguste Reynaud et Nicolas Bailly. **Hist Sci Med** 1979;13(4):441-50

**Reynolds, Edward, 1599-1676**
Reynolds E: A treatise of the passions and faculties of the soule of man (1640). Facsimile, with introduction by M. L. Wiley. Gainesville, Florida, Scholars' Facsimiles & Reprints, 1971. 585 p. in various pagings.

**Reynolds, Lawrence, 1889-1961**
Weaver B, Britt MC: Dr. Lawrence Reynolds and his medical history collection. **Ala J Med Sci** 1984 Oct;21(4):441-7
Weaver B, Britt MC: Dr. Lawrence Reynolds and his medical history collection. **Ala J Med Sci** 1984 Jul;21(3):311-7 contd

**Reynolds, Mary, 1785-**
Carlson ET: The history of multiple personality in the United States:

Mary Reynolds and her subsequent reputation. **Bull Hist Med** 1984 Spring;58(1):72-82

**Rhazes, 865-925**
Egri B: Arab triangulum **Orv Hetil** 1981 Jun 28;122(26):1595-600
Jacquart D: Quelques réflexions sur la traduction du Kitab al-Mansuri de Rhazès par Gérard de Crémone. In International Congress of the History of Medicine, 27th, Barcelona, 1980. Actas. Barcelona, Académia de Ciències Médiques de Catalunya i Balears, 1981. p. 264-6.
Kataya S, ed.: Quelle est la différence (Diagnostics Différentiels) de Abou-Bakr Zakaria Al-Razi (Rhazes). Edition Critique et commentaire de S. Kataya. Alep, Université d'Alep, Institut du Patrimoine Scientifique Arabe, 1978.
Soltani A: Ancient Jundi-Shahpour and its role in medicine and pharmaceutical progress. In International Congress of the History of Medicine. 26th, Plovdiv, 1978. Actes du Congress. Sofia, 1981. Volume II. p. 196-202.
Tayab M: Clinical observations of Rāzi. **Stud Hist Med** 1982 Jun;6(2):79-121
Trynková O: Některé metody středověkého léčení podle mistra Rhazesa a mistra Salicettiho. I. Rhazesovo a Salicettiho ranná lékařství a jejich vydavatelé. **Sb Lek** 1981;83(11-12):363-7
Trynková O: Některé metody středověkého léčení podle mistra rhazesa a mistra Salicettiho. III. Výběr z anatomických pojmu užívaných ve středověké medicíně. **Sb Lek** 1982 Feb;84(2):59-63
Trynková O: Některé metody středověkého léčení podle Mistra Rhazesa a Mistra Salicettiho. II. Uspěchy a neúspěchy středověkých léčitelu. **Sb Lek** 1982 Jan;84(1):25-32

**Rheede tot Drakestein, Hendrik Adriaan van, 1637?-1691**
Sastry VV: Hortus Indicus Malabaricus (Garden of Malabar of India). **Bull Indian Inst Hist Med (Hyderabad)** 1975 Jul;5(3):143-9

**Rhijne, Willem ten, 1647-1700**
Carrubba RW: The Latin document confirming the date and institution of Wilhem ten Rhyne's M.D. **Gesnerus** 1982;39(3-4):473-6
Subba Reddy DV: Wilhem Ten Rhyne (Rhijne) and his Treatise on Asiatic Leprosy; a medical classic by a Dutch physician in Java in the last quarter of 17th century. **Bull Indian Inst Hist Med (Hyderabad)** 1975 Jul;5(3):150-61

**Rhine, Joseph Banks, 1895-**
Mauskopf SH, Seymour H, McVaugh MR: The elusive science: origins of experimental psychical research. Baltimore: Johns Hopkins University Press. 1980. xvi, 368 p.

**Rhoads, Cornelius Packard, 1898-1959**
Slocum A: Cornelius Packard Rhoads. In Dictionary of American Biography, Suppl. 6, 1956-1960. p. 537-8. 1980.

**Rhodes, Cecil John, 1853-1902**
Shore MF: Cecil Rhodes and the ego ideal. **J Interdiscip Hist** 1979;10(2):249-65

**Ribeiro, Samuel Nunes**
Barnett RD: Dr. Samuel Nunes Ribeiro and the settlement of Georgia. In: Migration and settlement. London, Jewish Historical Society of England, 1971. p. 63-100.

**Ricardus de Bello, fl. 1276-1312**
Schierhorn H: Die Terata auf der Weltkarte des Richard de Haldingham (um 1280). **Gegenbaurs Morphol Jahrb** 1982;128(2):137-67

**Rice, William Gorham**
Brown GC, ed: With the ambulance service in France: the wartime letters of William Gorham Rice, jr. **Wis Mag Hist** 1981;64(4):278-93

**Rich, John B., 1811-1910**
Foley GP: A treasury of dentistry: John B. Rich, pioneer dental leader. **J Am Coll Dent** 1982 Summer;49(2):28-9

**Richard III, King of Great Britain, 1452-1485**
Accardo PJ: Deformity and character. Dr. Little's diagnosis of Richard III. **JAMA** 1980 Dec 19;244(24):2746-7
Jones EW: Richard III's disfigurement: a medical postscript. **Folklore** 1980;91:211-27

**Richards, Alfred Newton, 1876-1966**
Bearman D: The Alfred Newton Richards papers. **Surv Sources Newsl** 1975 Nov;1(1):9-10

**Richards, Ivor Armstrong, 1893-1979**
Karnani C: William James and I. A. Richards. **Indian J Am Stud** 1980;10(1):78-82

**Richards, Linda Ann Judson, 1841-1930**
Doona ME: At least as well cared for ... Linda Richards and the mentally ill. **Image J Nurs Sch** 1984 Spring;16(2):51-6
Nursing revisited: Linda Richards (1841-1930): **Mass Nurse** 1983 Jul;52(7):8
Tokugawa S: [Encounter with history of nursing: on Linda Richards and others] (Jpn). **Kango Kyoiku** 1982 Sep;23(9):539-43

**Richardson, Benjamin Ward, 1828-1896**
Blamire RV: Meat hygiene: the changing years. **J R Soc Health** 1984 Oct;104(5):180-5

**Richardson, John, 1787-1865**
Houston CS: New light on Dr. John Richardson. **Can Med Assoc J** 1984 Sep 15;131(6):653-4, 656-8, 660

**Richardson, Katherine Berry, 1858-1933**
Lynaugh J: Katherine Berry Richardson, MD (1858-1933). **Women Health** 1982 Spring;7(1):1-3

**Richardson, Maurice Howe, 1851-1912**
Romm S: Maurice Howe Richardson. **Plast Reconstr Surg** 1983 Mar;71(3):432-4

**Richardson, Samuel, 1689-1761**
Peters D: The pregnant Pamela: characterizations and popular medical attitudes in the 18th century. **Eighteenth Cent Stud** 1980-81;14:432-51

**Richter, Christian Friedrich, 1676-1711**
Arndal S: Krop, sjael og ånd Georg Ernst Stahls og Christian Friedrich Richters medicinske antropologi. **Dan Medicinhist Arbog** 1980;:126-66

**Richter, Hugo, 1887-1945**
Kenéz J: Hugó Richter, an outstanding Hungarian neurohistologist (1887--1945). **Ther Hung** 1979;27(2):99-100

**Ricketts, Fanny**
Naisawald LV: Fanny Ricketts, nurse, diarist, devoted wife. **Va Cavalcade** 1972;21(3):14-21

**Ricketts, Howard Taylor, 1871-1910**
Beatty WK, Beatty VL: Howard Taylor Ricketts--imaginative investigator. **Proc Inst Med Chic** 1981 Apr-Jun;34(2):46-8
Mullen PC: Bitterroot enigma: Howard Taylor Ricketts and the early struggle against spotted fever. **Montana** 1983;32(1):2-13

**Riddell, John L., 1807-1865**
Animalcular and cryptogamic theories on the origins of fevers. Reprinted works by John Kearsley Mitchell (1849), John L. Riddell (1836), Josiah Clark Nott (1848). New York, Arno, 1977. Various paginations.:

**Riddle, Mary M., 1856-1936**
Nursing revisited: Mary M. Riddle (1856-1936). **Mass Nurse** 1983 Oct;52(10):4

**Ridgely, Frederick, 1757-1824**
Eberson FW: Kentucky biographical notebook: Dr. Frederick Ridgely, 1757-1824. **Filson Club Hist Q** 1983;57(2):223-5

**Ridgway, Matthew Bunker, 1895-**
Milza P: La guerre froide à Paris: 'Ridgway la peste'. **Histoire** 1980;25:38-47

**Riebeeck, Jan Anthony van, 1618-1677**
DeJong CJ: Een verklaring door Anthony van Riebeeck als scheepschirurgijn in 1636. **Historia (S Afr)** 1973;18(4):231-3

**Riechert, Traugott, 1905-**
Pothoff PC, Schwarz R: Traugott Riechert. **Surg Neurol** 1983 May;19(5):403-5

**Riegel, Klaus F., 1925-1977**
van Ijzendoorn MH, Goossens FA, van der Veer R: Klaus F. Riegel and dialectical psychology: in search for the changing individual in a changing society. **Stor Crit Psicol** 1984 Jun;5(1):5-28

**Riese, Walther, 1890-1976**
Riese W: Selected papers on the history of aphasia. With an introduction by W. Gooddy. Edited with prefatory notes by R. Hoops, Y. Lebrun, E. Buyssens. Amsterdam, Swets and Zeitlinger, 1977. 144 p. (Neurolinguistics, 7).

**Rieutord, Jean-Baptiste, ca. 1733-1818**
Cadotte M, Lessard R: Jean-Baptiste Rieutord. In Dictionary of Canadian biography, 1801 to 1820. Volume 5, 1983. p. 712-3.

**Riggs, Robert, 1896-1969**
Nolan E: Children's ward. Lithograph by Robert Riggs, ca. 1940-45. **J Hist Med Allied Sci** 1982 Jul;37(3):322

**Righi, Augusto, 1850-1920**
Toti A: Augusto Righi precursore della xeroradiografia. **Radiol Med (Torino)** 1979 Sep;65(9):615-6

**Rigler, Gustav, 1868-1930**
Szállási A: [Gusztáv Rigler: prominent figure in Hungarian public health (1868-1930)] (Hun). **Orv Hetil** 1980;121:2209-11

**Rignano, Eugenio, 1870-1930**
Masin SC: Note on Eugenio Rignano as a forerunner of the 'New Look' theory of visual perception. **J Hist Behav Sci** 1980 Oct;16(4):313-6

**Rikli, Arnold, 1823-1906**
Rothschuh KE: Aus der Geschichte der Naturheilbewegung (VII). Die Heilkräfte von Licht, Luft und Erde. Arnold Rikli, Adolf Just und Pastor Felke. **ZFA (Stuttgart)** 1983 Jun 10;59(16):933-40

**Rinaldi, Carlo Bartolomeo, fl. 1655**
Fehringer WT: Studien zum altitalienischen Pferdearzneibuch des Carlo Bartolomeo Rinaldi (1655). Diss. Hannover, 1978, 247 p.

**Rincolini, Ernst Samuel, 1722-1786**
Kroupa J: Lékařský rod Rincolini v osvíceneckém Brně.

**Cas Lek Cesk** 1982 Nov 19;121(46):1429-30

**Rinecker, Franz von, 1811-1883**
Pfeffer R: Professor Franz von Rinecker, 1811-1883. Diss., Bayerische Julius-Maximilians-Universität, Würzburg, 1981. 180 p.

**Ringer, Sydney, 1835-1910**
Breathnach CS: Biographical sketches No. 27--Ringer. **Ir Med J** 1983 Mar;76(3):119
Fye WB: Sydney Ringer, calcium, and cardiac function. **Circulation** 1984 Apr;69(4):849-53
Lee JA: Sydney Ringer (1834-1910) and Alexis Hartmann (1898-1964). **Anaesthesia** 1981 Dec;36(12):1115-21
Nayler WG: Sydney Ringer--physician and scientist. **J Mol Cell Cardiol** 1984 Feb;16(2):113-6

**Ringseis, Johannes Nepomuk von, 1785-1880**
Rehder K, Shampo MA, Kyle RA: Physician's personal in-flight medical kit. **JAMA** 1982 Feb 19;247(7):1011

**Rio, Andrés del, fl. 1794**
Riera J: Los viajes de estudios de Andres del Rio (un documento de 1794). **Asclepio** 1980;32:361-5

**Riolan, Jean, 1580-1657**
Rihner F: Jean Riolan der Jüngere, 1580-1657. **MMW** 1980;122:1341-3
Rihner F: Jean Riolan der Jüngere. **Med Welt** 1981;32:476-8

**Ríos, Jóse Manuel de los, 1826 or 1832-1914**
Alvarez PJ: Doctor J. M. de los Ríos: precursor de la pediatria en Venezuela. **Rev Sos Venez Hist Med** 1972-73;20-21(34-35):15-20

**Risner, Friedrich, d. ca. 1580**
Lindberg DC, ed: Opticae thesaurus. Alhazeni Arabis libri septem, nuncprimùm editi. Eiusdem liber De Crepusculis et nubium ascensionibus. Item Vitellonis Thuringopoloni libri X. Reprint of the 1572 ed. New York, Johnson Reprint Corp., 1972. xxxiv, 288, 474 p.

**Risquez, Jésus Rafael, 1883-**
Iriarte DR: [Public health in Venezuela]. **Rev Soc Venez Hist Med** 1975-76;23(37):107-21

**Risso, Antoine, 1777-1845**
Monod T, Hureau JC: Un pharmacien niçois, Antoine Risso (1777-1845), sa vie et son oeuvre. In their: Antoine Risso, 1777-1845. Nice, Editions du Centre d'Etudes Méditerranéennes, 1977. pp. 9-28 (Annales du Muséum d'Histoire Naturelle de Nice, V, 1977).

**Rittmeister, John F., 1898-1943**
Aus dem Archiv der Psychoanalyse. John F. Rittmeister: Voraussetzungen und Konsequenzen der Jungschen Archetypenlehre: **Psyche (Stuttg)** 1982 Nov;36(11):1032-44
Hermanns LM: John F. Rittmeister und C. G. Jung. **Psyche (Stuttg)** 1982 Nov;36(11):1022-31
Schulz M: Dr. John Rittmeister--Nervenarzt und Widerstandskämpfer. **Psychiatr Neurol Med Psychol (Leipz)** 1979 Apr;31(4):213-6

**Rivers, Thomas Milton, 1888-1962**
Corner GW: Thomas Milton Rivers. In Dictionary of American biography, 1961-1965. Suppl. 7, 1981. p. 648-9.

**Riviera, Diego, 1886-1957**
Rodríguez A: Samuel Ramos: influencia de Adler y Jung en su estudio sobre el carácter del Mexicano. **Cuad Hispanoam** 1977;109(326-327):420-30

**Rivolta, Sebastiano, 1832-1893**
Théodoridès J: Sebastiano Rivolta (1832-1893) parasitologiste et microbiologiste. **Hist Sci Med** 1980;14(2):227-32

**Rizal, José Protacio, 1861-1896**
Barón Fernández J: La faceta medica del gran patriota Filipino Jose Rizal. **Asclepio** 1980;32:47-52
Kohnen N: Nationalheld und Wissenschaftler; der philippinische Arzt José Rizal. **Dtsch Arztebl** 1983 Apr 22;80(16):102-6

**Rizzoli, Francesco, 1809-1880**
Riunione straordinaria dei Consigli Comunale e Provinciale in occasione del 1 centenario della morte di Francesco Rizzoli (24-5-1880) e della nascita di Vittorio Putti (1-3-1880): **Chir Organi Mov** 1979 Jul-Aug;65(4):367-98

**Robb, Isabel Adams Hampton, 1860-1910**
James JW: Isabel Hampton and the professionalization of nursing in the 1890s. In Vogel MJ, Rosenberg CE, ed: The therapeutic revolution. Philadelphia, 1979. p. 201-244.

**Robbins, Frederick Chapman, 1916-**
Bendiner E: Enders, Weller, and Robbins: the trio that 'fished in troubled waters'. **Hosp Pract** 1982 Jan;17(1):163, 169, 174-5 passim

**Roberton, John, 1797-1876**
Cardwell D, Mottram J: Fresh light on John Dalton. **Notes Rec R Soc Lond** 1984 Sep;39(1):29-40
White BM: Medical police. Politics and police: the fate of John Roberton. **Med Hist** 1983 Oct;27(4):407-22

**Roberts, John Bingham, 1852-1924**
Shell DH: John Bingham Roberts: Philadelphia plastic surgeon. **Plast Reconstr Surg** 1982 Jan;69(1):145-54

**Roberts, Lydia Jane, 1879-1965**
Ihde AJ: Lydia Jane Roberts. In: Notable American women. The modern period. Cambridge, Mass., Belknap-Harvard Univ. Press, 1980. 4:580-1.

**Roberts, Mary May, 1877-1959**
Tomes N: Mary May Roberts. In: Notable American women. The modern period. Cambridge, Mass., Belknap-Harvard Univ. Press, 1980. 4:581-3.

**Robertson, Felix, 1781-1865**
Smith B, Robertson RM, Robertson D: An early Southern description of Curschmann's spirals. **Clin Notes Respir Dis** 1982 Summer;21(1):10-2

**Robertson, Graeme**
Hooper R: Graeme Robertson and the golden age of neurology. **Proc Aust Assoc Neurol** 1978;15:1-10

**Robertson, Oswald Hope, 1886-1966**
Allen JG: First blood bank, first blood banker Oswald Hope Robertson, M.D. **Lab World** 1981 Feb;:20-3

**Robertson, William Ford, 1867-1923**
Sturrock RR: William Ford Robertson (1867-1923): his study of neuroglia. **Med Hist** 1975 Oct;19(4):370-5

**Robespierre, Maximilien Marie Isidor de, 1758-1794**
Shulim JI: The birth of a revolutionary: Robespierre in Artois. **Consortium Revolut Eur 1750-1850 Proc** 1977;:22-33

**Robic, J., 1893-1968**
Coulanges P: Cinquantenaire du vaccin antipesteux EV (Girard et Robic). **Arch Inst Pasteur Madagascar** 1982;50(1):169-84

**Robin de Keriavalle, Claude-Marie, 1743-1785**
Théodoridès J: Un correspondant breton de la Société Royale de Médecine: Claude-Marie Robin de Keriavalle (1743-1785). In: Congrès National des Sociétés Savantes, 107e. Brest, 1982. Comptes Rendus, Paris, 1983. Section des Sciences, Fasc. IV. p. 225-39.

**Robin, Pierre, 1725-ca. 1804**
Gélis J: La pratique obstétricale dans la France moderne: les carnets du chirurgien accoucheur Pierre Robin (1770-1797). **Ann Bretagne** 1979;86:191-210

**Robinson, George Canby, 1878-1960**
Harvey AM: George Canby Robinson. In Dictionary of American Biography, Suppl. 6, 1956-1960. p. 546-7, 1980.

**Robinson, Robert A.**
Harvey AM: Orthopaedic surgery at Johns Hopkins: a heritage of excellence in clinical practice, training and research. **Johns Hopkins Med J** 1982 Jun;150(6):221-45

**Robinson, William**
Schlicke CP: The Robinson affair. **Pac Northwest** 1983;27(2):81-93

**Rocha-Lima, Henrique da, 1879-1956**
Sackmann W: Fleckfieber und Fleckfieberforschung zur Zeit des ersten Weltkrieges;zum Gedenken an Henrique da Rocha Lima (1879-1956). **Gesnerus** 1980;37(1/2):113-32

**Rochefoucauld, J. B. de la, 1709-1746**
Bedwell SF: D'Anville's doom--a neurological vignette from historic Halifax. **Can J Neurol Sci** 1980 Feb;7(1):1-8

**Rock, John Charles, 1890-**
McLaughlin L: The pill, John Rock, and the church: the biography of a revolution. Boston, Little, Brown, 1982. 243 p.

**Rockefeller Family**
Brown ER: Rockefeller medicine men. Medicine and capitalism in America. Berkeley, University of California Press, 1979. xii, 283 p.

**Rockefeller, John Davison, 1839-1937**
Brown ER: Exporting medical education: professionalism, modernization and imperialism. **Soc Sci Med [Med Psychol Med Sociol]** 1979 Nov;13A(6):585-95

**Rodrigues, Francisco Victor, d. 1972**
Silva B: Administração e medicina. Goiânia, Goiás Brasil, Editora da Universidade Federal de Goiás, [1979]. 48 p.

**Rodriguez Lafora, Gonzalo, 1887-**
Valenciano Gayá L: El Doctor Lafora y su época. Madrid, Morata, 1977. 226 p.

**Rodriguez-Péreire, Jacob, 1715-1780**
Kottek S: Jacob Rodriguez-Péreire (1715-1780); pionnier de l'éducation des sourds-muets: à l'occasion du 200e anniversaire de sa disparition. **Rev Hist Med Heb** 1981 Mar-Apr;34(1):5-8

**Rodríguez Rivero, Placido Daniel, 1876-1939**
Sociedad Venezolana de Historia de la medicina: En homenaje al Dr. Placido Daniel Rodriguez Rivero en el 100e aniversario de su nacimiento. Revista de la Sociedad Venezolana de Historia de la Medicina, 1977; 26(40), p. 11-85. Contributions by M. Rodríguez Navarro, G. Briceño Romero, D. W. Fernández Pérez, A. Osuna, C. R. Travieso, A. Silva Alvarez, N. Perazo, R. Beauperthuy de Benedetti, M. Granier-Doyaux, R. Caldera.

**Roe, Joseph H., 1892-1967**
Rice EW: Joseh H. Roe (1892-1967): American man of science, pioneer

clinical chemist. **Clin Chem** 1984 Sep;30(9):1575-8

**Roener, L. S. von**
Hekma G: Homoseksualiteit: van zonde tot geaardheid. **Spiegel Hist** 1980;15(9):484-91

**Roepke, W. J., 1917-**
Smits WH: Prof. W.J. Roepke: Forty year link between science and practice. **Vet Q** 1984 Jul;6(3):105-6

**Roeslin, Eucharius, d. 1526**
Rösslin E: Der Swangern Frauwen und hebammen Rosengarten. Facsimile of Strasbourg edition of 1513. Einführung von H. M. Koelbing. Dietikon/Zürich, Stocker, 1976. 137 p.

**Roeslin, Eucharius, d. 1547?**
Belkin J: Eucharius Rösslin des Jüngeren Lebensgeschichte. **Gutenberg Jahrb** 1978;96-105

**Rogalski, Tadeusz, 1881-**
Kuś J: Profesor dr. Tadeusz Rogalski i jego działalność w czasie II wojny światowej (w stulecie jego urodzin). **Przegl Lek** 1982;39(10):683-9

**Roger, Henri, 1809-1891**
Allwork SP: Maladie du Roger 1879: a new translation for the centenary. **Am Heart J** 1979 Sep;98(3):307-11

**Rogers, Carl Ransom, 1902-**
Evans RI: Dialogue with Carl Rogers. New York, Praeger, 1981. lxxxviii, 195 p.
Recent acquisitions of the manuscript division: Carl R. Rogers papers. **Q J Libr Congr** 1978;35-258-9
Stam I, Lahmann F: Carl R. Rogers. In J. Rattner, ed: Wandlungen der Psychoanalyse. Wien, Europaverlag, 1980. p. 165-86.

**Rogers, Frederick Rand, 1894-1972**
Pennington G: Frederick Rand Rogers: educational provocateur (1894-1972). **Can J Hist Sport Phys Educ** 1981;12(1):24-50

**Rogers, Leonard, 1868-1962**
McRobert G: Sir Leonard Rogers. In Dictionary of national biography, 1961-1970. Suppl. 8, 1981. p. 891-3.
Sheppard J: Illustrations from the Wellcome Institute Library: Sir Leonard Rogers, FRS (1868-1962) and his papers. **Med Hist** 1983 Apr;27(2):214-5

**Roget, Peter Mark, 1779-1869**
Swinton WE: The remarkable accomplishments of Dr. Peter Roget. **Can Med Assoc J** 1980 Nov 8;123(9):916-21

**Rojas Paúl, Juan Pablo, 1826-1905**
Silva Alvarez A: Ensayo patobiografico sobre el Dr. Juan Pablo Rojas Paúl. **Bol Acad Nac Hist (Caracas)** 1981;64(256):859-68

**Rokitansky, Karl von, 1804-1878**
Miciotto RJ: Carl Rokitansky: nineteenth-century pathologist and leader of the new Vienna school. Ph.D. diss. Johns Hopkins University, 1979. 301 leaves.

**Rola, Evstatie, 1766-1831**
Sibechi G: Un doctor ieşean de prestigiu: Evstatie Rola. **Rev Med Chir Soc Med Nat Iasi** 1982 Jul-Sep;86(3):436, 440, 504

**Roland Family**
Morel MF: Madame Roland, sa fille et les médecins: prime éducation et médicalisation à l'époque des lumières. **Ann Bretagne** 1979;86(3):211-9

**Roland l'Ecrivain, fl. 1430**
Charmasson T: L'établissement d'un almanach médical pour l'année 1437. In: Congrès National des Sociétés Savantes, 99e, Besançon, 1974. Comptes Rendus. Paris, 1976. Section des Sciences, Fasc. V. p. 217-34.
Charmasson T: Roland l'Ecrivain, médecin des Ducs de Bourgogne. In: Congrès National des Sociétes Savantes, 101e, Lille, 1976. Comptes Rendus. Paris, 1976. Section des Sciences, Fasc. III. p. 21-32.

**Rolfus, Karl, 1819-1907**
Seidler E: Die Behinderten in Herten. **Gesnerus** 1982;39(1):133-40

**Rolle, Józef Apolinary, 1829-1894**
Wacek S: Sytuacja zdrowotna Podola w świetle pism dr med Józefa Apolinarego Rollego. **Arch Hist Med (Warsz)** 1981;44(1):99-110

**Rona, Elizabeth, 1890-1981**
Brucer M: Historical note. Elizabeth Rona 1890-1981. **Health Phys** 1982 Apr;42(4):405-6

**Roncati, Francesco, 1834-1906**
Manzi L: Commento ad un consulto inedito di Francesco Roncati. **Minerva Med** 1982 Jan 28;73(3-4):133-6

**Röntgen, Wilhelm Conrad, 1845-1923**
Berneaud-Kötz G: Wilhelm Conrad Röntgen: aus den Erinnerungen des Schweizer Ophthalmologen Ernst Wölfflin. **Klin Monatsbl Augenheilkd** 1982 Aug;181(2):138-41
Drinnan AJ: Odontophilately. **NY State Dent J** 1980 Feb;46(2):73
Fischmann E: Retracing Röntgen's discovery. **Diagn Imaging** 1979;48(5):294-303
Franke OC: Wilhelm Conrad Roentgen and other X-ray pioneers. **Bull Hist Dent** 1983 Apr;31(1):11-7
Kalok L: Wilhelm Conrad Röntgen in Giessen, 1879-1888: Ausstellung in der Universitätsbibliothek Giessen vom 28. Juni-27. Juli 1979 aus Anlass der Berufung Röntgens nach Giessen vor 100 Jahren: Katalog. Giessen, Universitätsbibliothek, 1979. 34 p.
Klickstein HS: Wilhelm Conrad Röntgen: on a new kind of rays; a bibliographical study. [Philadelphia?], 1966. xvi, 129 p. (Mallinckrodt Classics of Radiology, v. 1).
Kraft E, Finby N: Röntgen's discovery of X-ray and Lenard's priority claim; award of first Nobel Prize in physics in 1901. **NY State J Med** 1980 Sep;80(10):1623-5
Kraft E, Finby N: Beginning of radiology in 1896; first newspaper report of discovery of x-ray. **NY State J Med** 1981 Apr;81(5):805-6
Maurer HJ: Die Entdeckung einer 'neuen Form von Strahlen' durch W. C. Röntgen im Spiegel der Presse. **Med Welt** 1982 Apr 8;33(14):520-4

**Roosevelt, Eleanor, 1884-1962**
Sherman ED: Geriatric profile of Eleanor Roosevelt (1884-1962). **J Am Geriatr Soc** 1983 Jan;31(1):28-33

**Roosevelt, Franklin Delano, 1882-1945**
Gallagher HG: FDR: handicapped American. **Public Welf** 1984 Spring;42(2):6-18
Stewart WJ: Ross McIntire. In Dictionary of American Biography, Suppl. 6, 1956-1960. p. 413-14, 1980.

**Ropes, Hannah Anderson, 1809-1863**
Brumgardt JR, ed: Civil war nurse. The diary and letters of Hannah Ropes. Knoxville, University of Tennessee Press, 1980. 149 p.

**Rorer, Sarah Tyson (Heston), 1849-1937**
Weigley ES: Sarah Tyson Rorer: first American dietitian? **J Am Diet Assoc** 1980 Jul;77(1):11-5

**Rorschach, Hermann, 1884-1922**
Nica-Udangiu S: Hermann Rorschach (1884-1922). **Rev Med Interna [Neurol Psihiatr]** 1984 Jul-Sep;29(3):235-40
Weber M: Kerners 'Kleksographien' und Rorschachs 'Psychodiagnostik'. **Gesnerus** 1984;41(1/2):101-9

**Rosa, Daniele, 1857-1944**
Martucci V: Sviluppo ontogenetico e citologia nell'ologenesi di Daniele Rosa. **Physis** 1980;22(1):73-84

**Roschlaub, Andreas, 1768-1835**
Tsouyopoulos N: Andreas Röschlaub und die Romantische Medizin. Stuttgart, Fischer, 1982. 258 p. (Medizin in Geschichte und Kultur, 14).

**Rose, Jerzy E., 1909-**
Cowan WM: Jerzy E. Rose. **J Comp Neurol** 1980 Aug 1;192(3):401-6

**Rose, Wickliffe, 1862-1931**
Health in the southern United States: New York, Arno, 1977. Various paginations. Facsimiles of works by David Ramsay (1790 and 1796), Josiah C. Nott (1847), Edward H. Barton (1851), Wickliffe Rose (1910), Joseph Goldberger (1916).

**Roselt, Jan Albert, 1714-1785**
Abeele R van den: Jan Albert Roselt, plattelandschirurgijn te Machelen (1714-1785). **Jaarb Kunst Oudheidk Kring Deinze** 1978;:83-117

**Rosen, George, 1910-1977**
George Rosen: In Memoriam: With contributions by S. Benison, E. H. Ackerknecht, J. Z. Bowers, L. A. Falk, G. A. Silver, O. H. Wangensteen, A. J. Viseltear, E. H. Thomson. **J Hist Med Allied Sci** 1978 Jul;33(3):244-317
Susser M: The work of George Rosen: observations on a very small sample. **Int J Health Serv** 1980;10(2):323-8

**Rosen von Rosenstein, Nils, 1706-1773**
Bologa VL: Nils Rosen Rosenstein über die Erbsyphilis. **Acta Hist Rerum Nat Tech** 1972;6:77-82

**Rosenbaum, Julius, 1807-1874**
Koch HT: Julius Rosenbaum (1807-1874) als Medizinhistoriker. **NTM** 1981;18(1):84-90

**Ross, Ronald, 1857-1932**
Lukács D: Száz éve fedezte fel Charles Alphonse Louis Laveran a malária kórokozóit. **Orv Hetil** 1980 Dec 14;121(50):3076-8

**Rossell, Juan Francisco, fl. 1627-1629**
Riera J, Jiménez Muñoz JM: El doctor Rossell y los temores en España por la peste de Milan (1629-1631). In: Sociedad Española de Historia de la Medicina. V Congreso Nacional. Madrid, 1977. **Asclepio** 1977;29:283-307

**Roudier, Juan, fl. 1842**
Beauperthuy de Benedetti R: Un cirujano y un medico de Montpellier en el siglo pasado en Caracas. **Rev Soc Venez Hist Med** 1979;28(42):29-30

**Rouppe, Hendrik Willem, 1765-1816**
Snelders HA: Het fysisch-chemisch werk van de Rotterdamse arts Hendrik Willem Rouppe (1765-1816). **Tijdschr Geschied Geneeskd** 1981;4(1):25-44

**Rous, Francis Peyton, 1879-1970**
Dubos R: Peyton Rous. **J Exp Med** 1979 Oct 1;150(4):735-7
Huggins CB: Peyton Rous and his voyages of discovery. **J Exp Med** 1979 Oct 1;150(4):733-4

Pitot HC: Landmark article (JAMA 1911;56:198). Transmission of a malignant new growth by means of a cell-free filtrate. By Peyton Rous. **JAMA** 1983 Sep 16;250(11):1445-9

**Rousseau, Jean Jacques, 1712-1778**
Clément PP: Quelques aspects de la vie et de l'oeuvre de Jean-Jacques Rousseau: s'oublier--se surveiller--fixer par l'écriture. **Univ Ottawa Q** 1979;49(3-4):292-9
Ito J: [In search of educational humanity (5). Understanding of man in education (2): 'Emile' by Jean Jacques Rousseau] (Jpn). **Kango Kyoiku** 1983 May;24(5):310-4
Rothschuh KE: Aus der Geschichte der Naturheilbewegung (III). 'Vorläufer' des Rousseauschen Naturismus in der römischen Kaiserzeit. Die Philosophie der Stoa und die Methodische Medizin. **ZFA (Stuttgart)** 1981 May 31;57(15):1172-9
Rowe C: Jean-Jacques Rousseau: ce qu'il pensait des médecins. **Bull Soc Hist Protestantisme Fr** 1978;124(4):501-17
Scanlan TM: La fonction de la mort dans la pensée sociale de Rousseau. **Univ Ottawa Q** 1981;51(1):91-7

**Roussy, Gustave, 1874-1948**
Bernoulli R: Un grand méconnu: Gustave Roussy. **Gesnerus** 1980;37(1/2):34-46

**Routley, Thomas Clarence, 1889-**
Stewart B: CMA's Dr. T. Clarence Routley: 34 years of devoted service. **Can Med Assoc J** 1983 Sep 15;129(6):642-3, 645

**Roux, César, 1857-1934**
Saegesser F: César Roux (1857-1934) et son époque. **Rev Med Suisse Romande** 1984 Jun;104(6):403-64

**Roux, Pierre Paul Emile, 1853-1933**
Berndt H: Emile Roux zum 50. Todestag. **Z Arztl Fortbild (Jena)** 1983;77(3):126-7
Saenz A, Boisvert H: Trois lettres de Louis Pasteur. **Hist Sci Med** 1981;15(4):327-33

**Roux, Wilhelm, 1850-1924**
Mocek R: Wilhelm Roux--Hans Driesch. Zur Geschichte der Entwicklungsphysiologie der Tiere ['Entwicklungsmechanik']. Jena, Fischer, 1974. 229 p. (Biographien bedeutender Biologen, Band 1).
Oppenheimer JM: Ernst Heinrich Haeckel as an intermediary in the transmutation of an idea. **Proc Am Philos Soc** 1982;126(5):347-55

**Rovenstine, Emery Andrew, 1895-1960**
Hershey SG: The Rovenstine inheritance--a chain of leadership. **Anesthesiology** 1983 Nov;59(5):453-8
Morris JP: Emery Andrew Rovenstine. In Dictionary of American Biography, Suppl. 6, 1956-1960. p. 553-4, 1980.

**Rovsing, Nils Thorkild, 1862-1927**
Ráf L: Skandinaviska kirurger först med beskrivning av tecken på appendicit. **Lakartidningen** 1984 Aug 8;81(32-33):2829-30

**Rowiński, Ksawery, 1904-1983**
Ostrowska T: Profesor Ksawery Rowiński (1904-1983) i Jego działanść naukowa (Wspomnienie pośmiertne). **Arch Hist Med (Warsz)** 1984;47(3):327-48
Ostrowska T: Ksawery Rowiński (1904-1983) i jego działalność w zakresie historii medycyny. **Kwart Hist Nauki Tech** 1984;29(2):445-66

**Rowlandson, Thomas, 1756-1827**
Illustrations from the Wellcome Institute Library: John Monro MD and Charles James Fox: etching by Thomas Rowlandson. **Med Hist** 1983 Jan;27(1):80-3
Paly D: The antiquaries' last will and testament; an etching with sepia wash by Thomas Rowlandson, 1814. **J Hist Med Allied Sci** 1980 Apr;35(2):215

**Royo, Domingo, fl. 1715-1734**
Crawford LM: Maestro Domingo Royo and the Llave de Albeyteria. **Hist Med Vet** 1977;2(2):33-6

**Roździeński, Walenty, ca. 1560-ca. 1622**
Jonecko A: Drzeworyt ukazujacy amputowane i protezowane produdzie w ślaskim poemacie Roździeńskiego 'Officina Ferraria' z roku 1616. **Arch Hist Med (Warsz)** 1984;47(1):107-16

**Rózsay, József, 1815-1885**
Vértes L: Elsö gerontológusunk: Rózsay József akadémikus. **Orv Hetil** 1983 Oct 16;124(42):2564-8

**Rozsnyay, Mátyás, 1833-1895**
Kempler K: A gyógyszerészeti technológia hazai úttöröje Rozsnyay Mátyás. **Orv Hetil** 1984 Jul 22;125(30):1832-4, 1837

**Ruano, Francisco**
Peset JL, Nuñex D: Filosofía, ciencia y alquimia en la ilustacion española. **Cuad Hispanoam** 1980;120(359):371-93

**Rubakin, Aleksandr Nikolavich, 1889-**
Salnikova GP: Zhizn' i delatel' nost' A.N. Rubakina. **Sov Med** 1981;(2):114-6

**Rubashkin, Vladimir IaKovlevich, 1876-1925**
Klishov AA, Khilova IuK, Pankov EIa, et al: Zhizn' i deiatel'nost' professora V. Ia. Rubashkina. **Arkh Anat Gistol Embriol** 1983 Nov;85(11):94-8

**Rubens, Peter Paul, 1577-1640**
Appelboom T, Boelpaepe C de, Ehrlich GE, et al: Rubens and the question of antiquity of rheumatoid arthritis. **JAMA** 1981 Feb 6;245(5):483-6

**Rubin, Isidor Clinton, 1883-1958**
Hill EC: The Rubin test. **JAMA** 1983 Nov 4;250(17):2366-8
Saffron MH: Isidor Clinton Rubin. In Dictionary of American Biography, Suppl. 6, 1956-1960. p. 554-6, 1980.

**Rudakov, P. A.**
Pal'chikov PA: Oni zhertvovali soboĭ radi pobedy. **Voen Med Zh** 1983 May;(5):68-70

**Rudbeck, Olof, 1630-1702**
Eriksson G: Om ingenting. Olof Rudbeck föreläsningsprogram 1679. **Lychnos** 1979-80;:79-108

**Rüdinger, Nikolaus, 1832-1896**
Schmutz HK: Rüdingers 'Atlas des peripherischen Nervensystems des menschlichen Körpers' mit Photographien von Joseph Albert; zur Frühgeschichte der medizinischen Photographie. **Gesnerus** 1980;37(1/2):83-90

**Rudnev, Georgiĭ Pavlovich, 1899-1970**
Abdullokhodzhaev ZI: G. P. Rudnev: 1899-1970. Moskva, Meditsina, 1981. 70 p.

**Rudnev, M. M., 1831-1878**
Mikhaĭlov VP: Zhurnal Rudneva (poluzabytaia glava v istorii otechestvennoĭ gistologii). **Arkh Anat Gistol Embriol** 1980 Feb;78(2):104-15
Vaĭl' SS: M.M.Rudnev--odin iz osnovopolozhnikov otechestvennoĭ patologicheskoĭ anatomii (k 100-letiiu so dnia smerti). **Klin Med (Mosk)** 1979 Jul;57(7):107-10

**Rudolphi, Karl Asmund, 1771-1832**
Obermajer J: Neznámé dopisy Purkyňova tchána K. A. Rudolphiho J. J. Berzeliovi. **Cas Lek Cesk** 1984 Feb 17;123(7):199-203

**Rufanov, Ivan Gur'evich, 1884-1964**
Struchkov VI: Ivan Gur'evich Rufanov (k 100-letiiu so dnia rozhdeniia). **Sov Med** 1984;(7):114-5

**Rüff, Jakob, 1500-1558**
Funder W: Uber eine bisher unbekannte ophthalmologische Monographie von Jakob Rüff (um 1500-1558). **Klin Monatsbl Augenheilkd** 1981 Oct;179(4):297-8
Houtzager HL: Jacob Rueff. **Eur J Obstet Gynecol Reprod Biol** 1982 Mar;13(2):105-7
Koelbing HM: 'De conceptu et generatione hominis'. Die lateinische Fassung von Jakob Rueffs 'Trostbüchle', Zürich 1554. In International Congress of the History of Medicine, 27th, Barcelona, 1980. Actas. Barcelona, Académia de Ciències Mèdiques de Catalunya i Balears, 1981. p. 271-5.
Koelbing HM: 'De conceptu et generatione hominis' - die lateinische Fassung von Jakob Rueffs 'Trostbüchle', Zürich 1554. **Gesnerus** 1981;38:51-8
Rueff J: Ein schön lustig Trostbüchle von den Empfengknussen und Geburten der Menschen. 2 v. Facsimile of 1554 ed., with Einführung von H. M. Koelbing. Dietikon-Zürich, Verlag Bibliophile Drucke, 1981. 29, cxliii p.

**Ruffini, Angelo, 1864-1929**
Lambertini G: Il pensiero e i trovati di Angelo Ruffini nella sua opera 'Physiogeny'. [Italian and English] Padova, Piccin, 1980. 111 p.

**Rufus, of Ephesus**
Ullmann M: Die arabische Ueberlieferung der Werke des Rufus von Ephesos. In: International Symposium for the History of Arabic Science, 1st, University of Aleppo, 1976. Proceedings. Aleppo, Syria, 1976. Papers in European Languages, Vol. II. p. 348-57
Ullmann M: Die Schrift des Rufus von Ephesos über die Gelbsucht in arabischer und lateinischer Ubersetzung. Göttingen, Vandenhoeck & Ruprecht, 1983. 87 p. (Abhandlungen der Akademie der Wissenschaften in Göttingen, Philologisch-Historische Klass; Folge 3, No. 138).
Ullmann M, ed: Rufus von Ephesos Krankenjournale. Wiesbaden, Harrassowitz, 1978. 128 p.

**Ruge, Carl, 1846-1926**
Becker V: Carl Ruge: 100 Jahre Stückchen-Diagnose. **Arch Gynecol** 1979 Sep;227(3):193-204

**Al Ruhawi, Ishaq ibn Ali, 9th cent.**
Levey M: Medical ethics on medieval Islam with special reference to Al-Ruhawi's 'Practical ethics of the physician.' Philadelphia, American Philosophical Society, 1967. 100 p. (Transactions of the American Philosophical Society, n.s., Vol. 57, Part 3, 1967).

**Ruiz de Luzuriaga, Ignacio Maria, 1763-1822**
Gago R, Carrillo JL: La obra fisiológica de Ignacio María Ruiz de Luzuriaga (1763-1822) y su plagio del cientifico británico Adair Crawford (1748-1795). **Dynamis** 1981;1:87-100

**Ruiz, Hipólito, 1754-1815**
Schultes RE: Peruvian and Chilean psychoactive plants mentioned in Ruiz's Relación (1777-1788). **J Psychoactive Drugs** 1983 Oct-Dec;15(4):303-12

**Ruiz, José Martinez, 1874-1967**
Aznar B: Personalidad biologica de Azorín. Salamanca, Universidad

de Salamanca, 1973. 73p. (Cuadernos de Historia de la Medicina Española, Monografías, 23).

**Rukhadze, N. P., 1880?-**
Maruashvili GM: Istoriia zavoza gambuzii v SSSR (k 100-letiiu so dnia rozhdeniia N. P. Rukhadze). **Med Parazitol (Mosk)** 1980 Jan-Feb;49(1):80-2

**Ruland Family**
Duka Zólyomi N: Ein ärztliches Vademecum der Aerztefamilie Ruland aus dem 16. Jahrhundert. **Sudhoffs Arch** 1977;61(3):281-97

**Rupp, N. János, 1808-1881**
Somogyi E: Rupp N. János. **Orv Hetil** 1983 Nov 13;124(46):2821-2

**Rusby, Henry Hurd, 1855-1940**
Bender GA: Henry Hurd Rusby: scientific explorer, societal crusader, scholastic innovator. **Pharm Hist** 1981;23(2):71-85

**Rusch, Harold P., d. 1979**
Dr. Harold P. Rusch and the Wisconsin Clinical Cancer Center: **Wis Med J** 1979 Jun;78(6):96-7

**Rush, Benjamin, 1745-1813**
Bell WJ, Butterfield LH, ed: My dearest Julia: the love letters of Dr. Benjamin Rush to Julia Stockton. New York, Neale Watson Academic Publications, 1979. xvii, 62 p.
Carlson ET: Benjamin Rush and his friends on human nature. **Psychiatr Q** 1979 Winter;51(4):300-6
Carlson ET: The history of multiple personality in the United States: I: The beginnings. **Am J Psychiatry** 1981 May;138(5):666-8
Carlson ET, Wollock JL, Noel PS, ed: Benjamin Rush's Lectures on the mind. Philadelphia, American Philosophical Society, 1981. xix, 735 p. (Memoirs of the American Philosophical Society, 144).
Davies NE, Davies GH, Sanders ED: William Cobbett, Benjamin Rush, and the death of General Washington. **JAMA** 1983 Feb 18;249(7):912-5
Kittle CF: Benjamin Rush--heritage and hope. **Proc Inst Med Chic** 1981 Apr-Jun;34(2):49-53
Plummer BL: Document: letters of James Durham to Benjamin Rush. **J Negro Hist** 1980;65(3):261-9
Risse GB: A letter to Benjamin Rush. **J Hist Med Allied Sci** 1980 Oct;35(4):461
Schneck JM: Elisha Dick, Benjamin Rush, and George Washington. **JAMA** 1983 Jul 8;250(2):164

**Rushton, Martin A., 1903-1970**
Leatherman GH: Martin Rushton--the man, 1903 to 1970. **Br Dent J** 1983 Nov 5;155(9):315-7

**Rushton, William Albert Hugh, 1901-1980**
Hodgkin AL: Some recollections of William Rushton and his contributions to neurophysiology. (1925-52). **Vision Res** 1982;22(6):623-5
Obituary William Albert Hugh Rushton F.R.S.: **Vision Res** 1982;22(6):611-21

**Rusk, Howard A., 1901-**
Yanes-Hoffman N: Howard Rusk, MD: an equal chance. **JAMA** 1981 Oct 2;246(14):1503-5, 1509-10

**Russel, Jane Anne, 1911-1967**
Raacke ID: Jane Anne Russell. In: Notable American women. The modern period. Cambridge, Mass., Belknap-Harvard Univ. Press, 1980. 4:610-1.

**Russell, Alexander, 1715?-1768**
Roberts KB: Plague in 18th century Syria: the work of Alexander and Patrick Russell. In: Congrès international d'histoire de la médecine, XXVe, Québec, 1976. Actes. Québec, 1977. p. 1157.

**Russell, Bertrand, 1872-1970**
Brink A: Love and conflict in Bertrand Russell's letters. **Queens Q** 1979;86(1):1-15

**Russell, Edward Stuart, 1887-1954**
Roll-Hansen N: E. S. Russell and J. H. Woodger: the failure of two twentieth-century opponents of mechanistic biology. **J Hist Biol** 1984 Fall;17(3):399-428

**Russell, Patrick, 1727-1805**
Roberts KB: Plague in 18th century Syria: the work of Alexander and Patrick Russell. In: Congrès international d'histoire de la médecine, XXVe, Québec, 1976. Actes. Québec, 1977. p. 1157.

**Russell, William, 1852-1940**
King DF, Eisenberg D: Russell's fuchsine body. 'The characteristic organism of cancer.' **Am J Dermatopathol** 1981 Spring;3(1):55-8

**Russkikh, N. A., ca. 1857-**
Selezneva VT: N. A. Russkikh--organizator bor'by s detskoĭ smertnost'iu (k 125-letiiu so dnia rozhdeniia). **Sov Zdravookhr** 1982;(7):64-7

**Rust, Johann Nepomuk, 1775-1840**
Skulimowski M, Sliwiński S: Zwiazki Jana Nepomucena Rusta (1775--1840) z Krakowskim Fakultetem Medycznym. **Arch Hist Med (Warsz)** 1979;42(2):245-9
Wondrak E: Johann Nepomuk Rust (1775-1840): der Lebensweg des Chirurgen und Förderers des jungen J.E. Purkyne. **Acta Univ Palacki Olomuc Fac Med** 1977;83:169-76

**Rusznyák, István, 1889-1977 or 8**
Hollán Z: Rusznyák István utca. **Orv Hetil** 1983 Jun 26;124(26):1575-7

**Rutherford, Ernest, 1871-1937**
Kratochvíl L, Lustig M: K historii tzv. Batemanovy funkce. **Cesk Farm** 1984 Jun;33(5):210-2

**Rutherford, Hiram, 1815-1900**
Hendrick W, Hendrick G, ed: On the Illinois frontier. Dr. Hiram Rutherford 1840-1848. Carbondale and Edwardsville, Southern Illinois University Press, 1981. xxv, 155 p.

**Ruysch, Frederik, 1638-1731**
Houtzager HL: Frederik Ruysch. **Eur J Obstet Gynecol Reprod Biol** 1982 May;13(3):199-201

**Ryan, Cornelius, 1920-1974**
Hawkins A: Two pathographies: a study in illness and literature. **J Med Philos** 1984 Aug;9(3):231-52

**Ryba, Josef Arnošt, 1795-1856**
Kadlecová V, Matoušek O: Deník Dr. Med. Josefa A. Ryby. Překlad z Německého Rukopisu Věra Kadleová. **Cesk Oftalmol** 1981 Sep;37(5):383-8
Kadlecová V, Maloušek O, ed: Deník Dr. Med. Josefa Ryby. Překlad z německého rukopisu. **Cesk Oftalmol** 1981 Jul;37(4):293-6

**Rydygier, Ludwig von, 1850-1920**
Moll J: Das chirurgische Erbe. Ludwik Rydygier (1850-1920). **Zentralbl Chir** 1983;108(23):1532-5

**Ryer, Washington N.**
Gill D: The dueling doctors of Stockton. **Pac Hist** 1981;25(1):52-8

**Ryman, Brenda E.**
Whelan WJ: Use of liposomes in medicine. **Biochem Soc Trans** 1984 Apr;12(2):331-2

**Rymsdyk, Jan van, fl. 1750-1788**
Thornton JL: Jan Van Rymsdyk: medical artist of the eighteenth century. Cambridge, New York, Oleander Press, 1982. ix, 111 p.

**Ryosen, Tezuka, d. 1877**
Fukase Y: [Tezuka Ryosen, army doctor-in-chief of the infantry regiment.] (Jpn). **Nihon I-Shigaku Zasshi** 1981;27(1):21-34

**Rzasnicki, Adolf, 1884-1953**
Kapuścik J: Dr Adolf Rząśnicke - lekarz, uczony, artysta (w 30 rocznicę śmierci). **Arch Hist Med (Warsz)** 1983;46(2):237-48

# S

**Sabin, Albert Bruce, 1906-**
Benison S: International medical cooperation: Dr. Albert Sabin, live poliovirus vaccine and the Soviets. **Bull Hist Med** 1982;56(4):460-83

**Sabin, Florence Rena, 1871-1953**
Brieger GH: Florence Rena Sabin. In: Notable American women. The modern period. Cambridge, Mass., Belknap-Harvard Univ. Press, 1980. 4:614-7.

**Sabina, Maria, 1894-**
Krippner S, Winkelman M: Maria Sabina: wise lady of the mushrooms. **J Psychoactive Drugs** 1983 Jul-Sep;15(3):225-8

**Sabuncuoglu, Serafeddin, fl. 1404-1468**
Dizdar A: Der türkische Arzt Serafeddin Sabuncuoğlu (1385-1472) und seine Verdienste um die Zahnheilkunde. Diss. Würzburg, 1981. 68 p.

**Sacristán, José Miguel, 1887-1956**
Germain J, Solís J: José Miguel Sacristán (1887-1956). **Arch Neurobiol (Madr)** 1982 Jul-Aug;45(4):299-319

**Sade, Donatien Alphonse François de, 1740-1814**
Chasseguet-Smirgel J: De Sade: Der Körper und der Mord an der Realität. **Psyche (Stuttg)** 1981 Mar;35(3):237-52
Farr AD: The Marquis de Sade and induced abortion. **J Med Ethics** 1980 Mar;6(1):7-10

**Safarik, Janko, 1814-1876**
Dragić M: Dr. Janko i hjegove zasluge za nauku, književnost i prosvety u Srbiji. **Srp Arh Celok Lek** 1981 Aug;109(8):1101-8

**Sagar, Johann Baptist Michael, Elder von, 1732? 1813?**
Subrtová A: Johann Bapt. Michael Sagar (1732-1813). **Cas Nar Muz** 1981;150(3-4):153-90

**Sage, Balthasar-Georges, 1740-1824**
Todericiu D: Balthasar-Georges Sage (1740-1824) chimiste et minéralogiste français, fondateur de la première Ecole des Mines (1783). **Rev Hist Sci (Paris)** 1984 Jan;37(1):29-46

**Sahagún, Bernardino de, 1499-1590**
Alarcón-Segovia D: Descriptions of therapeutic arthrocenthesis and of synovial fluid in a Nahuatl text from prehispanic Mexico. **Bol Soc Mex Hist Filos Med** 1979 Sep;4(28):105-12
López Austin A: Textos acerca de las partes del cuerpo humano y de las enfermedades y medicinas en los primeros memoriales de Sahagún. **Estud Cult Nahuatl** 1972;10:129-53

**Sailer, Daniel, 1887-1958**
Gross-Bachmann M: Daniel Sailer, Leben und Wirken eines Idealisten.

Tirol Heimat 1976;40:163–90

**St. Medard, Peter, 1756–1822**
Estes JW: Naval medicine in the age of sail: the voyage of the New York, 1802–1803. **Bull Hist Med** 1982 Summer;56(2):238–53

**Saint-Simon, Claude Henri, 1760–1825**
Schneiderman L: Henri Saint-Simon: his ideology and personality. **Am J Psychoanal** 1980 Winter;40(4):349–64

**Saint-Simon, Louis de Rouvroy, 1675–1755**
Potvliege P: Le syndrome 'de Pickwick'. Priorité de sa description par le duc de Saint-Simon (1675–1755). **Nouv Presse Med** 1982 Jul 3;11(31):2360

**Sakel, Manfred Joshua, 1900–1957**
Powell RC: Manfred Joshua Sakel. In Dictionary of American Biography, Suppl. 6, 1956–1960. p. 563–4, 1980.

**Sakharov, Andrei, 1921–**
Melnick M: Sakharov and genetic science in the Soviet Union [editorial] **J Craniofac Genet Dev Biol** 1984;4(3):171–2
Soyfer V: Andrei Sakharov and the fate of biological science in the USSR. **J Craniofac Genet Dev Biol** 1984;4(3):173–8

**Sakhnovskaia, Anna Akimovna, 1882–1951**
Brzheskiĭ VCh: A. A. Sakhnovskaia (k stoletiiu so dnia rozhdeniia). **Vestn Dermatol Venerol** 1983 May;(5):73–4

**Sala, Antonio, fl. 1788**
Jordi R: Antonio Sala, un boticario barcelon/B//es aficionado a la botánica. **Farm Univers** 1980;13(1,2):10–7,78–82
Jordi González R: Anotaciones a los discursos botánicos del boticario barcelonés Antonio Sala Domènech. **An Med Cir** 1982;60(261):24–45

**Salanter, Israel, 1810–1883**
Goldberg H: An early psychologist of the unconscious. **J Hist Ideas** 1982 Apr–Jun;43(2):269–84

**Sales Laterrière, Pierre de, ca. 1740–1815**
Dufour P, Hamelin J: Pierre de Sales Laterrière. In Dictionary of Canadian biography, 1801 to 1820. Volume 5, 1983. p. 735–8.

**Salicetti, ca. 1210–1275 or 80**
Trynková O: Některé metody středověkého léčení podle mistra rhazesa a mistra Salicettiho. III. Výběr z anatomických pojmu užívaných ve středověké medicíně. **Sb Lek** 1982 Feb;84(2):59–63
Trynková O: Některé metody středověkého léčení podle Mistra Rhazesa a Mistra Salicettiho. II. Uspěchy a neúspěchy středověkých léčitelu. **Sb Lek** 1982 Jan;84(1):25–32
Trynková O: Některé metody středověkého léčení podle mistra Rhazesa a mistra Salicettiho. I. Rhazesovo a Salicettiho ranná lékařství a jejich vydavatelé. **Sb Lek** 1981;83(11–12):363–7

**Salieri, Antonio, 1750–1825**
Sakula A: 'Amadeus' was Mozart poisoned? **Hist Med (Lond)** 1980 Jan–Feb;8(1):6–9

**Salishchev, Erast Gavrilovich, 1851–1901**
Zadorozhnyĭ AA, Saks FF, Dolgikh VP, et al: Erast Gavrilovich Salishchev (k 130-letiiu so dnia rozhdeniia). **Vestn Khir** 1982 Jul;129(7):140–3

**Salk, Jonas Edward, 1914–**
Bendiner E: Salk: adulation, animosity, and achievement. **Hosp Pract** 1983 Jun;18(6):194–6, 200–1, 204–5 passim
Brandt AM: Polio, politics, publicity, and duplicity: ethical aspects in the development of the Salk vaccine. **Conn Med** 1979 Sep;43(9):581–7, 589–90

**Salm-Dyck, Josef von, 1773–1861**
Huard P, Théodoridès J: Jean-Baptiste Pipelet (1759–1823), Constance de Théis (1767–1845), Josef de Salm-Dyck (1773–1861) ou le chirurgien, la poétesse et le botaniste. In: Congrès National des Sociétés Savantes, 93e, Tours, 1968. Comptes Rendus. Paris, 1971. Section des Sciences, Tome II. p. 127–36.

**Salmon, Daniel Elmer, 1850–1914**
Niemi SM: D. E. Salmon and the first bacterin. **Mod Vet Pract** 1981 Dec;62(12):913–7
Stalheim OH: Daniel Elmer Salmon, the National Veterinary College, and veterinary education. **J Am Vet Med Assoc** 1983 Jan 1;182(1):33–6

**Salmon, Urbain-Philippe, 1768–1805**
Mars FL, Théodoridès J: Un savant angevin de l'époque révolutionnaire: Urbain-Philippe Salmon (1768–1805) médecin militaire, géologue et ami de Stendhal. In: Congrès National des Sociétés Savantes, 93e, Tours, 1968. Comptes Rendus. Paris, 1971. Section des Sciences, Tome II. p. 103–25.

**Salomonsz, Andries, fl. 1553–1561**
Bangs JD: Andries Salomonsz, a converted 'Rabbi and Doctor' in Leiden (1553–1561). **Jew Soc Stud** 1978;40(3–4):271–86

**Saltykov-Shchedrin, Mikhail Evgrafovich, 1826–1889**
Arkhangel'skiĭ GV: S. P. Botkin i M. E. Saltykov-Shchedrin. **Klin Med (Mosk)** 1982 Oct;60(10):114–8

**Salvany Lleopart, José**
Parrilla Hermida M: Biografia del doctor Jose Salvany Lleopart. **Asclepio** 1980;32:303–10

**Salzmann, Maximilian, 1862–1954**
Sugar HS, Foster CC: Maximilian Salzmann. Ophthalmic pioneer and artist. **Surv Ophthalmol** 1981 Jul–Aug;26(1):28–30

**Samberger, Frantisek, 1871–1944**
Hübschmann K: Sambergerovi současníci na klinice Janovského. **Cesk Dermatol** 1980 Oct;55(5):349–53

**Samman, Charles Thomas, 1865–1939**
Neild FG: Lieutenant Colonel C. T. Samman, OStJ, MRCS, LSA, DPH, Master of the Society of Apothecaries, 1928–31. **J R Army Med Corps** 1983 Oct;129(3):184–5

**Samoĭlov, Aleksandr Filippovich, 1867–1930**
Chernov AZ: Aleksandr Filippovich Samoĭlov. **Klin Med (Mosk)** 1983 Jan;61(1):116–20

**Samson**
Kleeberg J: A medical study of the story of Samson and Delilah. **Koroth** 1979 Nov;7(9–10):CXCV–CCII(644–9)

**Samson, Paul Curkeet, 1905–1982**
Ellison RG: Paul C. Samson, M.D., 1905–1982. Part I. His contributions to the Society of Thoracic Surgeons. **Ann Thorac Surg** 1983 Nov;36(5):500–1

**Samus', Valeriĭ Nikolaevich**
Pakhomov AF: Peredovoi aviatsionnyi vrach. **Voen Med Zh** 1983 Aug;(8):7–10

**San Martin, José de, 1778–1850**
Beaujón O: La salud y el pensamiento militar y politico del General San Martín. **Bol Acad Nac Hist (Caracas)** 1979;62(245):35–56
Loza Colomer JC, Olascoaga ML: La Sanidad del Ejército de los Andes. In Congreso de Historia de la Medicina Argentina [Transactions], 5th, Mendoza, 1983. p. 7–17.

**Sanabria Bruzual, Jesus, 1867–1950**
Vélez Boza F: Discurso pronunciado con motivo de la colocacion del retrato del Dr. Jesus Sanabria Bruzual en el salon de sesiones de la Sociedad Venezolana de Historia de la Medicina, el 12 de julio de 1978. **Rev Soc Venez Hist Med** 1980;29(43–44):63–71

**Sanchez, Francisco, 1550–1623**
Limbrick E: Franciscus Sanchez 'Scepticus': un médecin philosophe précurseur de Descartes (1550–1623). **Renaiss Reformation** 1982;18:264–72

**Sanchís Banús, José, 1893–1932**
Nieto D: José Sanchís Banús. **Arch Neurobiol (Madr)** 1982 Sep–Oct;45(5):407–16

**Sanctis, Sante de, 1862–1935**
Luccio R: De Sanctis e la psicologia italiana. **Stor Crit Psicol** 1981;2(2):317–68

**Sandifort, Eduard, 1742–1814**
Macpherson AI: Blue babies before Fallot. **J R Coll Surg Edinb** 1984 Jul;29(4):199–204

**Sandritter, Walter, 1920–1980**
Walter Sandritter (7. 7. 1920 bis 12. 11. 1980): **Verh Dtsch Ges Pathol** 1981;65:533–48

**Sandström, Ivar Victor, 1852–1889**
Breimer L, Sourander P: The discovery of the parathyroid glands in 1880: triumph and tragedy of Ivar Sandström. **Bull Hist Med** 1981 Winter;55(4):558–63

**Sanger, Margaret Higgins, 1879–1966**
Aul DJ: Margaret Sanger labeled 'racist'. **Am J Public Health** 1981 Jan;71(1):91
Green D, Murdock ME, ed: The Margaret Sanger Centennial Conference, November 13 & 14, 1979. Northampton, Smith College, 1982. 68 p. Contributions by J. K. Conway, A. Harper, L. Gordon, J. Reed, E. Fee.
Lampé L: Margaret Sanger munkássága és annak hatása a családtervezési mozgalomra. **Orv Hetil** 1984 Jan 22;125(4):221–2
Lindemann C: Margaret Sanger and the birth control movement. **Women Health** 1978 Mar–Apr;3(2):12–13,16–21
Reed J: Margaret Sanger. In: Notable American women. The modern period. Cambridge, Mass., Belknap-Harvard Univ. Press, 1980. 4:623–7.

**Santero y Moreno, Tomas, 1817–1888**
Montiel L: La influencia de la ideologia en la clinica medica del S. XIX español. La obra de Tomas Santero y Moreno (1817–1888). **Asclepio** 1981;33:127–42

**Santorini, Giovanni Domenico, 1681–1737**
Velasco Suárez C: The Santorini valves. **Mt Sinai J Med (NY)** 1981 Mar–Apr;48(2):149–57

**Saraphides, Hector, 1872–1950**
Marinéskou-Chýmou M: Ektor saraphídes: iatrós kaí lógis (1872–1950). **Epet Etaireias Stereoelladikon Meleton** 1974–75;5:547–52

**Sargent, Dudley Allen, 1849–1924**
Makechnie GK: Optimal health: the quest. A history of Boston University's Sargent College of Allied Health Professionals, founded 1881, tendered to Boston University 1929. Boston, Boston University, 1979. x, 228 p.

**Sarngadhara, fl. 13th cent.**
Sharma PV: Contributions of Sarngadhara in the field of materia medica and pharmacy. **Indian J Hist Sci** 1981, reçu 1982;16(1):3-10

**Sarrazin, Michel, 1659-1734**
Rousseau J: Michel Sarrazin. In Dictionary of Canadian biography, 1701 to 1740. Volume 2, 1969. p. 593-600.

**Sarton, George, 1884-1956**
Calcoen R: George Sarton. **Handel Maatsch Geschied Oudheidk Gent** 1980;N.R.,34:181-91
George Sarton's correspondence: **Isis** 1984 Mar;75(276):33-62
Hamarneh S: Sarton (1884-1956) and the Arabic-Islamic legacy. **J Hist Arabic Sci** 1977 Nov;1(2):299-318
Merton RK: George Alfred Léon Sarton. In Dictionary of American Biography, Suppl. 6, 1956-1960. p. 564-6, 1980.
Recollections & reflections: Lawrence J. Henderson and George Sarton. **Isis** 1984 Mar;75(276):11-32

**Sartre, Jean Paul, 1905-1980**
Atwood GE: The pursuit of being in the life and thought of Jean-Paul Sartre. **Psychoanal Rev** 1983 Summer;70(2):143-62
Mitzman A: Sartres Flaubert. **Psyche (Stuttg)** 1981 Mar;35(3):268-98

**Sattamini, Samuel Duarte**
Vasconcellos Pedrosa MX de: O ensino da anatomia no Brasil: saudação a Samuel Duarte Sattamini. **Rev Inst Hist Geogr Bras** 1971;291:83-91

**Sauerbruch, Ernst Ferdinand, 1875-1951**
Abe HR, Kaiser L: Ferdinand Sauerbruch und Erfurt. **Beitr Gesch Univ Erfurt** 1979-83;19:271-81
Kudlien F, Andree C: Sauerbruch und der Nationalsozialismus. **Medizinhist J** 1980;15(3):201-222
Moerchel J: Sauerbruch und die Mayos. **Dtsch Med Wochenschr** 1980 May 9;105(19):697-9
Moerchel J: The introduction of thoracic surgery into America. **Clio Med** 1980;15(1/2):67-73

**Saul, King of Israel**
Littmann SK: King Saul: persecutor or persecuted? **Can J Psychiatry** 1981 Nov;26(7):464-7

**Saunders, William, 1835-1906**
Hyson JM: William Saunders: the United States Army's first dentist--West Point's forgotten man. **Milit Med** 1984 Aug;149(8):435-41

**Savary, M., fl. 1814**
Lever WF: Savary's 1814 article on the history of pemphigus related to contemporary views. **Int J Dermatol** 1979 Sep;18(7):584-5

**Save, Philippe Ignace, 1659-1702**
Jacques E: Médecine et spiritualité: un médecin belge oublié, ami de Port Royal, Philippe Ignace Save (1659-1702). **Rev Hist Eccles** 1980;75(2):322-42

**Sawada, Miki**
Takahashi M: [Nurses in the history of nursing (6). Mrs. Miki Sawada and a home nurse] (Jpn). **Kango Kyoiku** 1981 Nov;22(11):718-24

**Sayn-Wittgenstein, Casimir zu, 1687-1741**
Habrich C: Mediziner und Medizinisches am Hofe des Grafen Casimir zu Sayn-Wittgenstein (1687-1741). **Beitr Gesch Pharm** 1983;31(18/19):138-44

**Sayre, Lewis Albert, 1820-1900**
Il tripode si Sayre: **Chir Organi Mov** 1981;66(2):279-81

**Sazie, Carlos**
Costa-Casaretto C: Sobre el. Dr. Carlos Sazie, primer profesor de neurología y segundo de psiquiatria en la universidad de Chile (1881-1891). **Rev Med Chil** 1980 Aug;108(8):749-56

**Scarborough, Charles, 1615 or 6-1694**
Frank RG: The physician as virtuoso in seventeenth-century England. In Shapiro, Barbara and Frank, Robert G., Jr. ed: English scientific virtuosi in the 16th and 17th centuries. Los Angeles, William Andrews Clark Memorial Lib., U. of California, 1980. p. 57-114.

**Scarlett, Earle Parkhill, 1896-**
Roland CG: Dr. Earl Scarlett: melding tradition and beauty in historical writing. **Can Med Assoc J** 1980 Apr 5;122(7):822-6

**Scellinck, Thomas, fl. 1317-1343**
Tabanelli M: Gli albori della chirurgia nelle Fiandre. Il libro del maestro Thomas Scellinck. Firenze, Leo S. Olschki, 1974. xxxviii, 284 p. (Biblioteca della 'Rivista di Storia delle Scienze Mediche e Naturali', v. 19).

**Schabel, Frank Milton, 1918-**
Dr. Frank M. Schabel Jr. **Cancer** 1984 Sep 15;54(6 Suppl):1132-52

**Schächter, Miksa, 1859-1917**
Szállási A: Rekviem a 'Gyógyászat'--ért Schachter Miksa szerkesztése ürügyén. **Orv Hetil** 1980 Dec 14;121(50):3073-6

**Schadewaldt, Hans, 1923-**
Göpfert W, Otten HH, ed: Metavoeite: wandelt euch durch neues Denken: Festschrift für Professor Hans Schadewaldt zur Vollendung des 60. Lebensjahres. Düsseldorf, Triltsch, 1983. 226 p.

**Schaedler, Gebhard, 1776-1842**
Rheinberger R: Zum 200. Geburtstag von Landesphysikus Gebhard Schaedler. ein Liechtensteinischer Artzt als Pionier der Pockenschutzimpfung. **Jahrb Hist Ver Fuerst Liechtenstein** 1976;76:337-43

**Schaffer, Károly, 1864-1939**
Czeizel A: A historical evaluation of the doctrine of heredodegeneration. **Orvostort Kozl** 1979;87-88(25 no 1-2):157-79

**Schally, Andrew V., 1926-**
Wade N: The Nobel duel. Two scientists' 21-year race to win the world's most coveted research prize. Garden City, Anchor Press/Doubleday, 1981. 321 p.

**Schamberg, Jay Frank, 1870-1934**
Shelley WB, Beerman H: Jay Frank Schamberg (1870-1934). **Am J Dermatopathol** 1984 Oct;6(5):441-4

**Scharandaeus, Johann Jakob, 1630-1682**
Schürmann-Roth J: 'Modus et ratio visendi aegros' des Solothurner Arztes Johann Jakob Scharandaeus (1630-1682). **Gesnerus** 1980;37(1/2):73-82

**Schaudinn, Fritz Richard, 1871-1906**
Hesse PG: Współpraca naukowa Schaudinn--Siedlecki w roku 1897. **Przegl Dermatol** 1983 May-Jun;70(3):307-10
Hesse PG: F. R. Shaudinn i jego dzieło. **Przegl Dermatol** 1983 May-Jun;70(3):303-6

**Scheel, Paul Friedrich, 1883-**
Paul U: Paul Friedrich Scheel zum 100. Geburtstag. **Beitr Orthop Traumatol** 1983 Oct;30(10):505-7

**Scheele, Karl Wilhelm, 1742-1786**
Cassebaum H: Neues über die Entdeckung von Säuren in organischem Material durch C.W. Scheele. **Pharmazie** 1981;36(2):135-8

**Schelenz, Hermann, 1848-1922**
Kraus I: Hermann Schelenz. In Balde JH, Schmiking W, ed: Festschrift zum 86. Deutschen Arztetag in Kassel. Kassel, Arztevereins, 1983. p. 41-9.

**Schemann, Ludwig, 1852-1938**
Seidler E: Die Freiburger Gobineau-Vereinigung und die Verbreitung des Arier-Gedankens in Deutschland. In Seidler E, Schott H, ed: Bausteine zur Medizingeschichte. Stuttgart, Steiner, 1984. p. 121-9.

**Scherer, Maria Theresia, 1825-**
Seidler E: Die Behinderten in Herten. **Gesnerus** 1982;39(1):133-40

**Scherf, Johann Christian Friedrich, 1750-1818**
Ganzinger K: Der Lippe-Detmoldische Leibarzt Johann Christian Friedrich Scherf (1750-1818) als Medizinalpolitiker und Reformator der Pharmazie. **Beitr Gesch Pharm** 1981;31(10):73-8

**Scheuchzer, Johann Jakob, 1672-1733**
Beerli UP: Medizinisches in Scheuchzers Physica sacra oder Kupferbibel. Zürich, Juris, 1980. 89p. (Zürcher medizingeschichtliche Abhandlungen, Neue Reihe, Nr. 143).
Büchi J: Die wiederaufgefundene 'Pharmacia contracta' des Johann Jakob Scheuchzer (1672-1733). **Gesnerus** 1982;39(2):145-69

**Schiff, Moritz, 1823-1896**
Heintel H: Moritz Schiffs gescheiterter Habilitationsversuch an der Universität Göttingen im Jahre 1855. **Medizinhist J** 1980;15(4):378-84

**Schilder, Paul, 1886-1940**
Langer D: Paul Ferdinand Schilder, Leben und Werk. Diss. Mainz, 1979. 259 p.

**Schiller, Johann Christoph Friedrich von, 1759-1805**
Ionov IuV: Raboty Fridrikha Shellera kak vracha, ego meditsinskie dissertatsii i bolezn' (k 175-letiiu so dnia smerti). **Klin Med (Mosk)** 1981 Jun;59(6):112-5
Montiel L: La 'filosofia de la fisiologia' de Federico Schiller. **Asclepio** 1981;33:163-81

**Schilling, Johann August, 1829-1884**
Rothkopf A: 'Das Narrenhaus' von W. Kaulbach und die Deutung des Bildes durch J. A. Schilling 1863. **Confin Psychiatr** 1980;23(1):51-64

**Schilling, Viktor, 1883-1960**
Bast G: Viktor Schilling 1883-1983. Selbstzeugnisse und Erinnerungen an den Altmeister der morphologischen Hämatologie. **Folia Haematol (Leipz)** 1983;110(5):617-29
Krüger M: Uber progressive Traditionen in der haltung bürgerlicher deutscher ärzte der 20er Jahre gegenüber der Sowjetunion und ihrer Medizin am Beispiel des Hämatologen Viktor Schilling. **Wiss Z Univ Rostock** 1971;20(5):329-32
Stobbe H: Viktor Schilling 1883-1983. Sein hämatologisches Lebenswerk unter Bevorzugung der Tätigkeiten in Berlin. **Folia Haematol (Leipz)** 1983;110(5):630-3

**Schimmoler, Lauretta M.**
Skinner RE: The roots of flight nursing: Lauretta M. Schimmoler and the Aerial Nurse Corps of America. **Aviat Space Environ Med** 1984 Jan;55(1):72-7

**Schipperges, Heinrich, b. 1918**
Seidler E, Schott H, ed: Bausteine zur Medizingeschichte. Heinrich Schipperges zum 65. Geburtstag. Stuttgart, Steiner, 1984. 154 p.

(Sudhoffs Archiv, Beihefte, Heft 24)

**Schlatter, Francis, 1856–1896?**
Bullock A: Francis Schlatter: a fool for God. **Palacio** 1975;83(1):38–45
Szasz FM: Francis Schlatter: the healer of the southwest. **NM Hist Rev** 1979;54(2):89–104

**Schleiden, Matthias Jacob, 1804–1881**
Querner H: La cuestion metodologica en la biologia del siglo XIX. **Folia Hum (Barc)** 1981;19(225):595–611

**Schleisner, Peter Anton, 1818–1900**
Johnsen B: Miasmer eller kontagion. Ginklofi (tetanus neonatorum) på Vestmannöerne og dr Peter Anton Schleisners indsats i dens bekaempelse. **Nord Medicinhist Arsb** 1982;:162–70

**Schlickum, Oscar, 1838–1889**
Wankmüller A: Schlickums Lehrbuch für den Apothekerlehrling. **Dtsch Apoth Ztg** 1981 Sep 3;121(36):1921–3

**Schlink, Herbert Henry, 1883–1962**
Maddox K: Schlink of Prince Alfred. A biography of Sir Herbert Schlink. Sydney, Royal Prince Alfred Hospital, 1978. vii, 283 p.

**Schlossmann, Arthur, 1867–1932**
Wunderlich P: Arthur Schlossmann (1867–1932) als Vorbild für unsere Zeit. **Kinderarztl Prax** 1982 Dec;50(12):589–95

**Schmalhausen, Ivan, 1884–1963**
Gall YM: [I. I. Schmalhausen and the problem of the causes of evolution] (Rus). **Istor Biol Issled** 1980;8:106–23

**Schmid-Guisan, Hans, 1881–1932**
Iselin HK: Zur Entstehung von C. G. Jungs 'Psychologischen Typen.' Der Briefwechsel zwischen C. G. Jung und Hans Schmid-Guisan im Lichte ihrer Freundschaft. Aarau, Sauerländer, 1982. 152 p. (Veröffentlichungen der Schweizerischen Gesellschaft für Geschichte der Medizin und der Naturwissenschaften, Bd. 38).

**Schmid, Hans Hermann, 1884–**
Seidenschnur G: Hans Hermann Schmid--Zum 100. Geburtstag. **Zentralbl Gynakol** 1984;106(18):1288–91

**Schmidt, Arno, 1914–**
Drews J: Ein Kratersturz ins Unbewusste. Zur Konstruktion von Traum und Tagtraum [in] Arno Schmidts Roman 'Kaff auch Mare Crisium' (1960). **Psyche (Stuttg)** 1981 Dec;35(12):1103–21

**Schmidt, Béla, 1881–1943**
Batári G: Schmidt Béla és az erdélyi Magyar Népegészségügyi Szemle. **Orv Hetil** 1982 Oct 31;123(44):2737–8

**Schmidtmann, Martha, 1892–1981**
Martha Schmidtmann (4. 8. 1892 bis 28. 4. 1981): **Verh Dtsch Ges Pathol** 1981;65:571–5

**Schmitz, Rudolf 1918–**
Dilg, P, et al., ed: Perspektiven der Pharmaziegeschichte: Festschrift für Rudolf Schmitz zum 65. Geburtstag. Bibliography by F. J. Kühlen. Graz, Austria, Akademische Druck- u. Verlagsanstalt, 1983. xviii, 497 p.

**Schneider, Kurt, 1887–1967**
Hoenig J: Kurt Schneider and Anglophone psychiatry. **Compr Psychiatry** 1982 Sep–Oct;23(5):391–400
Hoenig J: The concept of Schizophrenia. Kraepelin–Bleuler–Schneider. **Br J Psychiatry** 1983 Jun;142:547–56
Janzarik W: Jaspers, Kurt Schneider und die Heidelberger Psychopathologie. **Nervenarzt** 1984 Jan;55(1):18–24
Kröber HL: K. Schneiders Psychopathiebegriff als Hemmnis psychosomatischen Denkens. **Nervenarzt** 1984 Jan;55(1):25–9

**Schneider, Reinhold, 1903–1958**
Meier P: Paracelsus-Reminiszenzen--Arzt und Medizin im Werk von Reinhold Schneider. **Salzburger Beitr Paracelsusforsch** 1984;23:100–17

**Schneider, Wolfgang, 1912–**
Hickel E, Schröder G, ed: Neue Beiträge zur Arzneimittelgeschichte. Festschrift für Wolfgang Schneider zum 70. Geburtstag. Stuttgart, Wissenschaftliche Verlagsgesellschaft, 1982. 285 p. (Veröffentlichungen der Internationalen Gesellschaft für Geschichte der Pharmazie e. V., Neue Folge, Band 51).

**Schnirch, Emil, 1822–1884**
Bugyi B: Akit indokolatlanul elfelejtettek: Schnirch Emil (1822–1884). **Orv Hetil** 1982 Oct 17;123(42):2613–4

**Schnitzler, Arthur, 1862–1931**
Schachter M: L'écrivain-médecin Arthur Schnitzler (1862–1931). **Prov Med** 1979;6/7:347–53
Sherman MH, ed: Psychoanalysis and old Vienna: Freud, Reik, Schnitzler, Kraus. New York, Human Sciences Press, 1978. 192 p.
Szállá A: Arthur Schnitzler és Georges Duhamel a Nyugatban. **Orv Hetil** 1982 Sep 5;123(36):2246–50

**Schoenheimer, Rudolf, 1898–1941**
Kohler RE: Rudolf Schoenheimer, isotopic tracers, and biochemistry in the 1930's. **Hist Stud Phys Sci** 1977;8:257–98

**Schoenmackers, Jakob, 1912–1982**
Jakob Schoenmackers (26. 5. 1912 bis 22. 11. 1982): **Verh Dtsch Ges Pathol** 1983;67:778–85

**Schönfeld, Walter, 1888–1977**
Schipperges H: Walther Schönfeld (1888–1977) und seine Verdienste als Medizinhistoriker. **Hautarzt** 1980 Aug;31(8):441–3

**Schönlein, Johann Lucas, 1793–1864**
Bleker J: Die Naturhistorische Schule 1825–1845. Ein Beitrag zur Geschichte der klinischen Medizin in Deutschland. Stuttgart, New York, Fischer, 1981. ix, 174 p.

**Schopenhauer, Arthur, 1788–1860**
Legée G: Schopenhauer (1788–1860) et les sciences de la nature. **Hist Nat** 1979;(14):39–62
Paskaukas RA: Sigmund Freud and Arthur Schopenhauer reexamined. In International Congress of the History of Medicine, 27th, Barcelona, 1980. Actas. Barcelona, Acadèmia de Ciències Mèdiques de Catalunya i Balears, 1981. p. 125–9.

**Schorlemmer, Carl, 1834–1892**
Löhr HG: Ein Vierteljahrhundert gemeinsamen Weges von Karl Marx und Friedrich Engels mit ihrem treuen Freund und Kampfgefährten Carl Schorlemmer. **Pharmazie** 1983 Nov;38(11):768–72

**Schrakamp, Franz, 1860–1920**
Stürzbecher M: Franz Schrakamp (1860–1920) Stadt- und Kreisarzt in Düsseldorf. **Clin Notes Respir Dis** 1980 May;42(5):289–92

**Schreber, Daniel Paul, 1842–1911**
Chabot CB: Freud on Schreber. Psychoanalytic theory and the critical act. Amherst, University of Massachusetts Press, 1982. 171 p.
Dortmund EK: Daniel Paul Schreber: a case study of private fate as public possibility. **Res Stud** 1978;46(3):141–55
Lipton AA: Was the 'nervous illness' of Schreber a case of affective disorder? **Am J Psychiatry** 1984 Oct;141(10):1236–9
Schweighofer F: Der Fall Schreber. **Psychother Psychosom Med Psychol** 1982 Jan;32(1):4–8

**Schreck von Aschaffenburg, Konrad**
Berg A, ed: Lanfranks 'Chirurgia parva' in der Abschrift Konrad Schrecks von Aschaffenburg. Diss. Würzburg 1975, 145 S. (Altdeutsche Lanfrank-Uebersetzungen III).

**Schröder, Robert, 1884–1959**
Kyank H, Möbius W: Zum 100. Geburtstag von Robert Schröder. **Zentralbl Gynakol** 1984;106(15):1092–8

**Schrödinger, Erwin, 1887–1961**
Morange M: Schrödinger et la biologie moléculaire. **Fundam Sci** 1983;4(3/4):219–33

**Schroeder, Theodore, 1901–1950**
Brudnoy D: An untarnished youth in the gilded age: Theodore Schroeder of Wisconsin and Dakota territory. **ND Hist** 1972;39(4):17–25, 34

**Schroff, Carl Damian, 1802–1887**
Dobíšek K: První čtyři primáři pražského ústavu choromyslných. 3. Karl Damian Schroff, medicinae Doctor et Chirurgae magister. **Cesk Psychiatr** 1982 Feb;78(1):61–6

**Schubert, Franz Peter, 1797–1828**
Reichsman F: Life experiences and creativity of great composers: a psychosomaticist's view. **Psychosom Med** 1981 Aug;43(4):291–300

**Schubert, Gotthilf Heinrich von, 1780–1860**
Schott H: Der versteckte Poet in uns; zur Sprachtheorie in der naturphilosophischen Seelenlehre von Gotthilf Heinrich von Schubert (1780–1860). **Sudhoffs Arch** 1981;65(3):226–50

**Schuch, Ignacy, 1772–1864**
Bec M, Bec A: Ignacy Schuch -- lekarz sandomierski. **Arch Hist Med (Warsz)** 1984;47(3):383–7

**Schullian, Dorothy May, 1906–**
Wilson LG: Dorothy Schullian retires from the Journal. **J Hist Med Allied Sci** 1984 Oct;39(4):457–61

**Schulthess, Wilhelm, 1855–1917**
Rüttimann B: Wilhelm Schulthess (1855–1917) und die Schweizer Orthopädie seiner Zeit. Zürich, Schulthess Polygraphischer Verlag, 1983. xv, 272 p.

**Schultz-Hencke, Harald, 1892–**
Zander E: Was hat Schultz-Hencke uns heute noch zu sagen? **Z Psychosom Med Psychoanal** 1982;28(2):231–8

**Schultz, Jacob, 1681–1766**
Modig M: Karl XII:s siste fältskär. **Sydsven Medicinhist Sallsk Arsskr** 1983;:77–86

**Schultz, Johannes Heinrich, 1884–**
Brede K, Irion U, Lohmann HM, et al: Mitscherlich, Alexander, 1908–19821700 to PresentGermany **Psyche (Stuttg)** 1984 Nov;38(11):1023–52
Schröder C, König W: Die Integration der Psychotherapie in die klinische Medizin in Deutschland--der Beitrag von J. H. Schultz. **Psychiatr Neurol Med Psychol (Leipz)** 1984 Oct;36(10):586–90

**Schultze, Wilhelm, 1840–1924?**
Hesekiel T, ed: Ein deutscher Chirurg und seine Frau in Japan vor 100 Jahren. Briefe von Dr. Wilhelm Schultze und seiner Frau Emma geb. Wegscheider an die Eltern Dr. Wegscheider in Berlin aus Japan 1878–1881. Lübeck, (the author), 1980. 316 p.

**Schulz, David, 1732–1823**
Strandell B: Hur David Schulz von Schulzenheim fick sitt namn. **Nord Medicinhist Arsbok** 1983;:83–7

**Schulze, Curt i.e. Max Curt Gustav, 1881–**
Frielinghaus E: Initiativen des Veterinär-Inspekteurs der deutschen Wehrmacht auf dem Gebiet der Pferdezucht im Kriege 1939–45. **DTW** 1981 Nov 5;88(11):457–61
Zieger W: Zur 100. Wiederkehr des Geburtstages von Generaloberstabsveterinär Professor Dr. Curt Schulze. **DTW** 1981 Nov 5;88(11):449–52

**Schulze, Johann Heinrich, 1687–1744**
Kaiser W, Völker A: Hygiene, Präventiv, und Unfallmedizin in den Schriften des halleschen Ordinarius Johann Heinrich Schulze (1687–1744). **Z Gesamte Hyg** 1981 Oct;27(10):779–84
Kaiser W, Voelker A: Medizingeschichte und Populärwissenschaft bei Johann Heinrich Schulze. **Altertum** 1980;26:243–9

**Schumann, Robert Alexander, 1810–1856**
Andre P: Schumann. Les chants de l'ombre. Paris, Jean-Claude Lattes, 1982. 225 p.

**Schüppach, Michel, 1707–1781**
Julien P: Le 'médecin de la montagne' Michel Schüppach (1707–1781): médecin ou charlatan? In International Congress of the History of Medicine. 26th, Plovdiv, 1978. Actes du Congress. Sofia, 1981. Volume II. p. 116–9.
Meyer-Salzmann M: Michel Schüppach, 1707–1781. Ein Höhepunkt handwerklicher Heilkunst. Bern, Haupt, 1981. 135 p. (Berner Heimatbücher, 126).

**Schuute, Cornelis, d. 1580**
Cockx-Indestege E: Cornelis Schuute en de onlangs ontdekte almanak voor 1551. Biekorf, Westvlaams Archief, 1981. 12 p.

**Schwann, Theodor, 1810–1882**
Hinokida T: T. Schwann's three preliminary articles on 'Cell theory'. **Kagakushi Kenkyu** 1983;22(145):35–43
Kiszely G: Theodor Schwann. **Orv Hetil** 1983 Apr;124(16):959–62
Petlenko VP, Klishov AA: Kletochnaia teoriia i teoriia kletok (k 100-letiiu so dnia smerti T. Shvanna). **Arkh Anat Gistol Embriol** 1982 Nov;83(11):17–27
Pierard GE, Lapiere CM: Liège. The 'Ardent City' of Theodor Schwann and Tchantches. **Am J Dermatopathol** 1984 Feb;6(1):95–7
Teulón AA: La constitucion de la histologia celular: Schwann, Henle y Kölliker. **Asclepio** 1978–79;30–31:7–18
Watermann R: Schwanns mikroskopische Forschungen und die Zellentheorie. Ein Beitrag zu seinem 100. Todestag. **Z Mikrosk Anat Forsch** 1982;96(6):1032–43

**Schwartz, Anselme, 1872–1957**
Monod-Broca P: Anselme Schwartz 1872–1957. **Chirurgie** 1984;110(1):11–21

**Schwartz, Mark**
Jacobs DW: Mark Schwartz and the Biofeedback Certification Institute of America: an appreciation. **Biofeedback Self Regul** 1983 Jun;8(2):279–80

**Schwartze, Hermann, 1837–1910**
Jakobi H: Hermann Schwartze. 100 Jahre Ohrchirurgie in Halle/S. **Wiss Z Martin Luther Univ (Math)** 1976;25(2):109–12

**Schwartzer, Otto, 1853–1913**
Batári G: Schwartzer Ottó mint az orvosi sajtóreferálás kezdeményezöje. **Orv Hetil** 1979 Jul 1;120(26):1586–7

**Schwarz, Ante**
Posinovec J: Histologija i embriologija u djelu dra Ante Schwarza (u povodu 100. obljetnice njegove smrti). **Lijec Vjesn** 1980 Apr;102(4):208–10

**Schwarz, Dragutin, 1868–1917**
Sariić P: Je li Zabrebački kirurg Dragutin Schwarz uradio prvu nefrektomiju u Hrvatskoj? **Lijec Vjesn** 1980 Apr;102(4):205–7

**Schweitzer, Albert, 1875–1965**
Achterberg E: Albert Schweitzer: ein Leben in der Zeitenwende. Hameln, Soltsien, 1968. 88 p.
Kler JH: Medical philately. Missionary medicine. **J Med Soc NJ** 1983 Apr;80(4):302
Lamprecht-Naef E: Albert Schweitzer und die Schweiz. Zurich, Juris Druck, 1982. 116 p. (Zürcher Medizingeschichtliche Abhandlungen, Neue Reihe, Nr. 153).
Luther E: Gedanken zum 100. Geburtstag von Albert Schweitzer. **Wiss Z Martin Luther Univ (Math)** 1975;24(4):81–5
Nossik BM: Albert Schweitzer. Ein Leben fur die Menschlichkeit. Leipzig, S. Hirzel, 1982. 372 p. (Humanisten der Tat. Hervorragende Arzte im Dienste des Menschen).
Pierhal J: Albert Schweitzer. München, Kindler, 1979. 363 p.
Pierhal J: Albert Schweitzer: biographie. München, Fischer, 1979 (1982 printing). 263 p.
Vencovský E: Ceskoslovenský psychiatr spolupracovníkem profesora dr. Alberta Schweitzera v Lambarène. **Cesk Psychiatr** 1984 Apr;80(2):125–8

**Schweninger, Ernst, 1850–1924**
Rothschuh KE: Das Buch 'Der Arzt' (1906) stammt nicht von Ernst Schweninger! **Medizinhist J** 1983;18(1–2):137–44
Rothschuh KE: Ernst Schweninger (1850–1924). Zu seinem Leben und Wirken. Ergänzungen, Korrekturen. **Medizinhist J** 1984;19(3):250–8

**Schwidetzky, Oscar Otto Rudolf, 1874–1963**
Davis AB: Oscar Otto Rudolf Schwidetzky. In Dictionary of American biography, 1961–1965. Suppl. 7, 1981. p. 678–9.

**Scott, Frederick Hughes, 1876–1951**
Blaschko H: Frederick Hughes Scott and his contribution to the early history of the transmitter concept. **Notes Rec R Soc Lond** 1983 Mar;37(2):235–47

**Scott, James, 1770–1848**
Watkins AH: James Scott, the famous surgeon of Bromley, 1770–1848. **Bromley Local Hist** 1979;4:41–7

**Scrini, Basile, 1869–1931**
Théodoridès J: Le docteur Basile Scrini (1869–1931) et la thérapeutique oculaire. **Rev Hist Pharm (Paris)** 1982 Jun;29(253):101–6

**Scudder, Ida Sophia, 1870–1960**
Rabe V: Ida Sophia Scudder. In: Notable American women. The modern period. Cambridge, Mass., Belknap-Harvard Univ. Press, 1980. 4:634–6.

**Scultetus, Joannis, 1595–1645**
Pirsig W: Hals-Nasen-Ohrenheilkunde im Werk des Ulmer Stadtarztes Johannes Scultetus (1595–1645). **HNO** 1984 Apr;32(4):149–54

**Seacole, Mary, 1805–1881**
Dopson L: One hundred years on. **Nurs Times** 1982 May 12–18;78(19):781–2
Iveson-Iveson J: Profile: the forgotten heroine. (Mary Seacole). **Nurs Times** 1983 Sep 7;157(10):44–7
Marshall-Burnett S: A brief reflection on the life of Mary Seacole 1805–1881. **Jamaican Nurse** 1981 Dec;21(2):14–5
Seivwright M: The Florence Nightingale of Jamaica: Mary Seacole. **Jamaican Nurse** 1981 Dec;21(2):16
Smith JP: Mary Jane Seacole 1805–1881: a black British nurse. **J Adv Nurs** 1984 Sep;9(5):427–8

**Seagrave, Gordon Stifler, 1897–1965**
Morris JP: Gordon Stifler Seagrave. In Dictionary of American biography, 1961–1965. Suppl. 7, 1981. 679–81.

**Searcy, George Harris, 1877–**
Carmichael EB: The pellagra story in the United States of America. **J Med Assoc State Ala** 1980 Mar;49(9):23, 31, 33

**Seashore, Carl Emil, 1866–1949**
Linton SJ: The man and the mind: Carl Emil Seashore, a pioneer on two frontiers. **Swed Pioneer Hist Q** 1980;31(2):122–8

**Sechenov, Ivan Mikhaĭlovich, 1829–1905**
Alekseev MA, Person RS: I. M. Sechenov i nekotorye voprosy fiziologii dvizheniĭ. **Usp Fiziol Nauk** 1979 Jul–Sep;10(3):15–25
Bechtereva NP, Bundzen PV, Malyshev VN: [Sechenov's tradition in the development of physiology of mental activity, its origins and perspectives] (Rus). **Istor Biol Issled** 1980;8:163–72
Berezovskiĭ VA: Ivan Mikhaĭlovich Sechenov. Kiev, Nauk. dumka, 1981. 173 p.
Bragin AM: I. M. Sechenov i otechestvennaia meditsina (k 150-letiiu so dnia rozhdeniia. **Klin Med (Mosk)** 1980 Jun;58(6):113–7
Demidova NI: [The role of I. M. Sechenov's school in the development of electrophysiology] (Rus). **Istor Biol Issled** 1980;8:156–62
Grigorian NA: I. M. Sechenov i razvitie nauki v Rossii (k 150-letiiu so dnia rozhdeniia). **Sov Zdravookhr** 1979;(10):50–4
Grigorian NA: [I. M. Sechenov on science and its history] (Rus). **Istor Biol Issled** 1980;8:173–87
Karamian AI: Ivan Mikhaĭlovich Sechenov i evoliutsionnaia neĭrofiziologiia. Leningrad, Nauka, Leningradskoe otd-nie, 1980. 112 p.
Karamyan AI: The importance of I. M. Sechenov's ideas on formation of human nervous and mental activity for evolutionary neurophysiology. **Hum Physiol** 1979 Nov–Dec;5(5):717–23
Makarov VA: Razvitie I. M. Sechenovym ucheniia o edinstve organizma i sredy. **Usp Fiziol Nauk** 1979 Jul–Sep;10(3):5–14
Makarov VA: [I. M. Sechenov and the development of physiology in the Moscow University] (Rus). **Istor Biol Issled** 1980;8:138–55
Medvedev VI: I. M. Sechenov's ideas in modern physiology. **Hum Physiol** 1979 May–Jun;5(3):261–8
Moikin IuV, Tarasenko NIu, Anan'ev BV: Znachenie naslediia I. M. Sechenova dlia razvitiia otechestvennoĭ fiziologii i gigieny truda. **Gig Tr Prof Zabol** 1980 Mar;(3):1–5
Moiseeva NI: The role of I M. Sechenov's ideas in development of modern views on time perception. **Hum Physiol** 1979 Nov–Dec;5(5):723–7
Mozzhukhin AS: [I. M. Sechenov – The founder of the first physiological school in Russia] (Rus). **Istor Biol Issled** 1980;8:124–37
Roitbak AI: The importance of I. M. Sechenov's electrophysiological research. **Acta Neurobiol Exp (Warsz)** 1980;40(2):451–61
Shingarov GKh: Gordost' russkoĭ nauki (k 150-letiiu so dnia rozhdeniia I. M. Sechenova). **Patol Fiziol Eksp Ter** 1979 Nov–Dec;(6):3–8
Tarasenko NIu, Moĭkin IuV, Anan'ev BV: Razvitie ideĭ I. M. Sechenova v sovremennykh issledovaniiakh po gigiene i fiziologii truda. **Vestn Akad Med Nauk SSSR** 1981;(1):3–9

Todes DP: Biological psychology and the Tsarist censor: the dilemma of scientific development. **Bull Hist Med** 1984 Winter;58(4):529-44
Tonkikh AV: K mekhanizmu sechenovskogo tormozheniia. **Zh Vyssh Nerv Deiat** 1980 Sep-Oct;30(5):1037-43
Vorob'ev AI: Ivan Mikhaĭlovich Sechenov. **Klin Med (Mosk)** 1980;58(11):105-8

**Secker, Thomas, 1693-1768**
Guy JR: Archbishop Secker as a physician. In Sheils WJ, ed: The Church and healing. Papers read at the twentieth summer meeting and the twenty-first winter meeting of the Ecclesiastical History Society. Oxford, Basil Blackwell for the Society, 1982. p. 127-35.

**Sedgwick, William Thompson, 1855-1921**
Clean water and the health of the cities: New York, Arno, 1977. Various paginations. Facsimile reprints of works by William T. Sedgwick (1893), George C. Whipple (1907), and J. Scott MacNutt (1910).

**Sedláček, Eva**
Novák A: Doc. MUDr. Eva Sedláčková, csc., a československá foniatrie. **Cesk Otolaryngol** 1982 Apr;31(2):68-71

**Seeger, Rudolf, fl. 1848**
Huter F: Ein tiroler Student erlebt den Beginn der Wiener Märzrevolution. **Tirol Heimat** 1972;36:131-9

**Seegers, Walter H., 1910-**
Henry RL: A recognition of the work of Walter H. Seegers in hemostasis and thrombosis. **Semin Thromb Hemostas** 1980;6(4):325-7

**Seeman, Miloslav, 1892-**
Sedláček K: Sedesáté výrocí založení československé foniatrie prof. MUDr. Miloslavem Seemanem, DrSc. **Cesk Otolaryngol** 1982 Apr;31(2):65-8

**Segall, Harold Nathan, 1897-**
Segall H: Dr. Harold Segall: a pioneer cardiologist reminisces. **Can Med Assoc J** 1982 May 1;126(9):1109-13-7

**Segen, Johan van, fl. 1487?**
Alstermark H: Das Arzneibuch des Johan van Segen. Stockholm, Almquist & Wiksell, 1977. 174 p. (Acta Universitatis Stockholmiensis. Stockholmer germanistische Forschungen, 22)

**Segner, Johann Andreas von, 1704-1777**
Kaiser W: Wissenschaftsgeschichtliche Kooperation am Beispiel der slowakisch-ungarisch-halleschen Gemeinschaftsforschung zu Leben und Werk von Johann Andreas Segner und Johann Adam Reimann. **Wiss Z Martin Luther Univ (Math)** 1975;24(3):89-98

**Séguin, Edward, 1812-1880**
Hänsel D: Die 'Physiologische Erziehung' der Schwachsinningen. Edouard Séguin (1812-1880) und sein Konzept einer medizinischen Pädegogik. Freiburg, Schulz, 1974. 329 p. (Freiburger Forschungen zur Medizinigeschichte, Neue Folge, 3).
Pelicier Y: Edouard Seguin et l'éducation spéciale. **Bull Acad Natl Med (Paris)** 1981 May;165(5):627-30
Pelicier Y, Thuillier G: Edouard Séguin (1812-1880). Nouveaux documents. Nevers, Centre Departemental de Documentation Pedagogique de Nevers, 1981. 211 p.
Pélicier Y, Thuillier G: Le fondateur de l'éducation des idiots: Edouard Séguin (1812-1880). **Paedagog Hist** 1980;20:129-52

**Ségur, Sophie Rostopchine, 1799-1874**
Lanchy F: La comtesse de Ségur et la santé des enfants. **Rev Hist Pharm (Paris)** 1982;29(252):179-85

**Sehestedt, Mogens, 1598-1657**
Vial G: Studien zum ersten altdeutschen Pferdearzneibuch des dänischen Lehnsmannes Mogens Sehestedt (1598-1657). Diss. Hannover, 1978. 272 p.

**Seixas, David G., fl. 1812-1824**
[Notes on David Seixas and education of the deaf in Pennsylvania in the 1820's] In: Myers, S. H. Handcraft to industry: Philadelphia ceramics. Washington, D. C., Smithsonian Institution Press, 1980. pp. 8-12 passim, 83-4.

**Seldinger, Sven-Ivar, 1921-**
Doby T: A tribute to Sven-Ivar Seldinger. **AJR** 1984 Jan;142(1):1-4

**Selig, Arpád, 1880-1929**
Fekete J: Dr. Selig Arpád (1880-1929). **Orv Hetil** 1980 Jan 13;121(2):98-101

**Sellheim, Hugo, 1871-1936**
Spitzbart H: Hugo Sellheim (1871 - 1936). **Zentralbl Gynakol** 1984;106(10):693-5

**Selvaresa, Josef, d. 1805**
Orozco Acuaviva, A: El 'Compendio de medicina práctica' de Josef Salvaresa del Real Colegio de Cirugía de Cádiz. In International Congress of the History of Medicine, 27th, Barcelona, 1980. Actas. Barcelona, Acadèmia de Ciències Mèdiques de Catalunya i Balears, 1981. p. 387-93.

**Selzer, Richard, 1928-**
Carson RA: Selzer's surgeon as seer. **Perspect Biol Med** 1981 Winter;24(2):284-9
Graham PW: A mirror for medicine: Richard Selzer, Michael Crichton, and Walker Percy. **Perspect Biol Med** 1981 Winter;24(2):229-39
Peschel ER: 'Alchemy of the word'--language and 'the knife' a commentary on Richard Selzer's work. **Pharos** 1979 Winter;42(1):25-32
Schuster CI: Passion and pathology: Richard Selzer's philosophy of doctoring. **Perspect Biol Med** 1984 Autumn;28(1):65-74

**Semashko, Nikolai Aleksandrovich, 1874-1949**
Kadyrov AA: N. A. Semashko v Uzbekistane. **Sov Zdravookhr** 1984;(1):49-50
Potulov BM: Vydaiushchiĭsia teoretik i organizator sovetskogo zdravookhraneniia (k 110-ĭ godovshchine so dnia rozhdeniia N. A. Semashko). **Voen Med Zh** 1984 Sep;(9):65-8

**Semmelweis, Ignác Fülöp, 1818-1865**
Antall J: Wien und Budapest im Lebenswerk Semmelweis'. **Wien Med Wochenschr** 1982 Apr 15;132(7):161-7
Antall J: Wien und Budapest im Lebenswerk Semmelweis'. In Ganzinger K, Skopec M, Wyklicky H, ed: Festschrift für Erna Lesky zum 70. Geburtstag. Wien, Brüder Hollinek, 1981. p. 13-23.
Benedek I: Semmelweis. Budapest, Gondolat, 1980. 269 p.
Benedek I: Semmelweis' Krankheit. Budapest, Akadémiai Kiadó, 1983. 110 p. (Hungarian version published 1978 in Communicationes de historia artis medicinae, Nos. 83-84)
Carter KC: Semmelweis and his predecessors. **Med Hist** 1981 Jan;25(1):57-72
Carter KC: Ignaz Semmelweis, Carl Mayrhofer, and the rise of germ theory. **Med Hist** 1985 Jan;29(1):33-53
Carter KC: Semmelweis's possible influence on Karl Mayrhofer and on those who subsequently developed nineteenth century etiological theories. **Orvostort Kozl** 1982;28(1-3):23-31
Csillag I: Elfelejtett kórházak nyomában. Balassa és Semmelweis a régi zsidó kórházban. **Orv Hetil** 1981 Feb 22;122(8):463-5
Epifanov NS: I. F. Zemmel'veĭs. **Med Sestra** 1983 Aug;42(8):50-1
The first report on Semmelweis' discovery of the cause and prevention of childbed fever: Most important experiences about the etiology of puerperal fevers epidemic in birthing institutions. **Infect Control** 1982 Nov-Dec;3(6):478-9
Kenéz J: War Semmelweis geisteskrank? **Med Welt** 1981 Dec 25;32(51-52):1964-6
Miller PJ: Semmelweis. **Infect Control** 1982 Sep-Oct;3(5):405-9
Pytel' AIa: I. F. Zemmel'weis: ego bolezn' i prichina smerti. **Sov Med** 1979 Oct;(10):119-21
Schober KL: Vor etwa hundert Jahren (41). **Zentralbl Chir** 1982;107(23):1538-40
Silló-Seidl G: Kolletschkas Tod. **Beitr Gerichtl Med** 1979;37:415-7
Silló-Seidl G: Die Wahrheit über Semmelweis. Genf, Ariston Verlag, 1978. 214 p.
Szemkeö E: Ein Beitrag zu den letzten Wochen von Semmelweis. **Orvostort Kozl** 1979;87-88(25 no 1-2):291-7
Szemkeö E: Adalék Semmelweis életének utolsó heteihez. **Orv Hetil** 1980 Jul 27;121(30):1837-8
Wyklicky H, Skopec M: Ignaz Philipp Semmelweis, the prophet of bacteriology. **Infect Control** 1983 Sep-Oct;4(5):367-70
Zambon JV: Brugmans, voorloper van Semmelweis. **Ned Tijdschr Geneeskd** 1983 Jun 11;127(24):1060-4

**Semonkeho, Miroslav, 1919-1979**
Tomiček F, Křepelka J, Beran M: In memoriam Doc. Dr. Ing. M. Semonského, DrSc. **Cesk Farm** 1979 Dec;28(9-10):362-6

**Senac, Jean Baptiste, 1693-1770**
McMichael J: History of atrial fibrillation 1628-1819 Harvey - de Senac - Laënnec. **Br Heart J** 1982 Sep;48(3):193-7

**Seneca, Lucius Annaeus**
Dieckhöfer K: Aspekte einer rudimentären Psychologie, Psychopathologie und Psychotherapie bei Seneca. In: Congrès international d'histoire de la médecine, XXVe, Québec, 1976. Actes. Québec, 1977. p. 579-95.

**Seneca, Lucius Annaeus (the Elder)**
Fischer KD: Seneca d. A., Controversiae 10,5,17: ein übersehenes Zeugnis zur Geschichte der antiken Anatomie. **Sudhoffs Arch** 1984;68(1):110-2

**Senguerd, Arnold, 1610-1667**
Gysel C: Arnoldus Senguerdius (1610-1668) en zijn wijsgerige verhandeling 'De Dentibus'. **Ned Tijdschr Tandheelkd** 1978 Nov;85(11):468-70

**Senn, Albert, 1869-1934**
Held AJ: A propos de dentifrices et du Dr Albert Senn (1869-1934)--notice historique. **SSO Schweiz Monatsschr Zahnheilkd** 1981 Apr;91(4):218-20

**Senn, Nicholas, 1844-1908**
Beatty WK: Nicholas Senn -- surgeon and traveler. **Proc Inst Med Chic** 1980 Jan-Mar;33(1):8-9
Brown HM: Reminiscences of Dr. Senn. **Milw Hist** 1981;4(3-4):87-94
Buess H: Nikolaus Senn (1844-1908), ein schweizerischer Pionier der Chirurgie in den USA. **Gesnerus** 1979;36(3-4):238-45

**Sennert, Daniel, 1572-1637**
Brentini P: Die Institutiones medicinae des Daniel Sennert (1572-1637). Zürich, Juris, 1971. 69 p. (Diss., Zürich).
Van Lieburg MJ: De dichter-medicus Daniël Jonctys (1611-1654), zijn strijd tegen het bijgeloof en zijn relatie tot Johan van Beverwijck,

William Harvey en Daniël Sennert. **Tijdschr Geschied Geneeskd** 1979;2(4):137–67

**Sergiev, Petr Grigor'evich, 1893–1983**
Soprunov FF: K 90-letiiu so dnia rozhdeniia Petra Grigor'evicha Sergieva (1893–1983). **Med Parazitol (Mosk)** 1983 Nov–Dec;(6):3–6

**Serre, Johann Jacob Joseph, 1759–1830**
Marvitz L: Nanden bag navnet. Johann Jacob Joseph Serre. **Tidsskr Tandlaeger** 1982 Feb;2(1):35

**Serres, Alexandre, ca. 1732–1812**
Lessard R: Alexandre Serres. In Dictionary of Canadian biography, 1801 to 1820. Volume 5, 1983. p. 752.

**Sertoli, Enrico, 1842–1910**
Ober WB, Sciagura C: Leydig, Sertoli, and Reinke: three anatomists who were on the ball. **Pathol Annu** 1981;16 Pt 1:1–13

**Sertürner, Friedrich Wilhelm, 1783–1841**
Doenicke A: Zum 200. Geburtstag von Friedrich Wilhelm Adam Sertürner. **Anaesthesist** 1983 Jun;32(6):239–41
Kempler K: Az alkaloida-kutatás kezdetei. **Orv Hetil** 1983 Jul 24;124(30):1821–5

**Servan, Joseph Michel Antoine, 1737–1807**
Azouvi F: Irritabilité et magnétisme animal: une lettre inédite de J.-M.-A. Servan. **Dix-huit Siecle** 1982;14:191–7

**Servetus, Michael, 1509 or 11–1553**
Cappelletti AJ: Servet, teologo, filosofo y medico. **Rev Soc Venez Hist Med** 1975–76;23(37):147–61
Corsano A: Medicina e teologia nel pensiero rinascimentale. La fisiologia di Michele Serveto. **G Crit Filos Ital** 1975;6(1):84–8
Donáth T: Egy évforduló ürügyén. **Orv Hetil** 1984 Sep 30;125(40):2441–4
Hirsch EF: Michael Servetus and the neoplatonic tradition: God, Christ and Man. **Bibl Hum Renaissance** 1980 Sep;42(3):561–75
Paglia L: Odontoiatria del passato. Chi era Servet? **Dent Cadmos** 1984 Jan;52(1):79–81
Sliwiński S: Miquel Serveto (1511–1553) -- odkrywca płucnego krążenia krwi. **Wiad Lek** 1980 Apr 1;33(7):589–91
Vidal F: Michel Servet (1511–1553). La découverte de la circulation du sang. **Chir Dent Fr** 1981 Apr;51(110):39–43

**Seutin, Louis Joseph Ghislain, 1793–1862**
Colard A: Evocation du passé: sur le professeur Baron Seutin et sa méthode amovo-inamovible. **Rev Med Brux** 1983 Jan;4(1):39–44
Soeur R: Evocation du passé: le professeur Baron Seutin et sa réaction au bandage plâtré. **Rev Med Brux** 1983 Jun;4(6):447–9

**Sevastopol'skaia, Dasha A.**
Tiuliandin AD: Dasha Sevastopol'skaia--pervaia sestra miloserdiia. **Med Sestra** 1982 Dec;41(12):60–1

**Severino, Marco Aurelio, 1580–1656**
Oliaro T: Marco Aurelio Severino il perseguitato ricreatore della chirurgia italiana (1580–1656). **Minerva Chir** 1980 Sep 30;35(18 Suppl):32–4

**Sévigné, Marie de Rabutin-Chantal, Marquise de, 1626–1696**
Duthoit JP: La Marquise de Sévigné et quelques aspects de la thérapeutique médicale au XVIIe siècle. Lille, 1980. 110, 8 p.

**Sevigny, Anna May, 1895–1979**
Hunter JA, ed: Anna May: eighty-two years in New England. **Northeast Folkl** 1979;20:7–106

**Shadd, Furman Jeremiah, 1852–1908**
Robinson HS: Furman Jeremiah Shadd, MD 1852–1908. **J Natl Med Assoc** 1980 Feb;72(2):151–3

**Shakespeare, William, 1564–1616**
Fleissner RF: Putting Falstaff to rest: 'tabulating' the facts. **Shakespeare Stud** 1983;16:57–74
Fox A: Obstetrics and Gynecology in Macbeth. **Shakespeare Stud** 1979;12:127–41
Junghans RP: Falstaff was drunker than he was fat. **N Engl J Med** 1983 Jun 16;308(24):1483
Kail AC: The bard and the body. 1. Shakespeare' physicians. **Med J Aust** 1983 Oct 1;2(7):338–44
Kail AC: The bard and the body. 5. Disease: its causes, diagnosis and cure. **Med J Aust** 1983 Nov 26;2(11):568–77
Kail AC: Medicine in Shakespeare. The bard and the body. 2. Mental illness. **Med J Aust** 1983 Oct 15;2(8):399–405
Kail AC: The bard and the body. 3. Venereal disease--'the pox'. **Med J Aust** 1983 Oct 29;2(9):445–9
Kail AC: Medicine in Shakespeare. The bard and the body. 6. Therapeutics. **Med J Aust** 1983 Dec 10–24;2(12):657–62
Lawless DS: On Shakespeare's death, funeral, and burial. **Notes Queries** 1980 Apr;27(2):176–7
Lutz LA: Shakespeare on plastic surgery. **Plast Reconstr Surg** 1984 Dec;74(6):841
Porst S: Gynäkologie und Geburtshilfe bei Shakespeare. **Zentralbl Gynakol** 1984;106(12):863–75
Porst S: Gynäkologische, geburtshilfliche, embryologische und teratologische Beschreibungen im Werke Shakespeares. Würzburg, Horst Wellm, 1981. 178 p. (Dissertation, Julius-Maximilians-Universität Würzburg).

**Shakow, David, 1901–1981**
David Shakow, Ph.D., 1901–1981: In Memoriam. **Schizophr Bull** 1981;7(3):383–7

**Shamov, Vladimir Nikolaevich, 1880–1962**
Nechaĭ AI, Sitenko VM: Vladimir Nikolaevich Shamov (k 100-letiiu so dnia rozhdeniia). **Klin Khir** 1982 May;(5):62–4
Samotokin BA, Nechaĭ AI, Sitenko VM, et al: Vladimir Nikolaevich Shamov (k 100-letiiu so dnia rozhdeniia). **Voen Med Zh** 1982 Jun;(6):73–4

**Sharimanian, Stepanos**
Mardzhanian KS: Stepanos Sharimanian. **Patma-Banasirakam Handes. Ist-Filol Zh** 1971;(3):236–46

**Sharland, James Craig, fl. 1870**
Combes RE: J. C. Sharland's pharmacy at Apothecaries' Hall. **J Auckl Waikato Hist Soc** 1979;34:31–4

**Sharpe, Ella Freeman, 1875–1947**
Netzer C: Annals of psychoanalysis: Ella Freeman Sharpe. **Psychoanal Rev** 1982 Summer;69(2):207–19

**Shaw, George Bernard, 1856–1950**
Postlewait T: Bernard Shaw and science: the aesthetics of causality. In Paradis J, Postlewait T, ed: Victorian science and Victorian values: literary perspectives. New York, New York Academy of Sciences, 1981. p. 319–58.

**Shaw, Jon Angus, 1937–**
Esman AH: The study of lives: discussion of Tashjian and Shaw. **Adolesc Psychiatry** 1982;10:99–105

**Sheehan, Joseph Eastman, 1885–1951**
Orenstein HH: How excellent a showman: Joseph Eastman Sheehan, 1885–1951. **Bull NY Acad Med** 1983 Apr;59(3):327–30

**Sheldon, William, 1899–1977**
Calcraft LG: Aldous Huxley and the Sheldonian hypothesis. **Ann Sci** 1980 Nov;37(6):657–71

**Shelley, Mary, 1797–1851**
Baudry FD: Problems in the application of psychoanalysis to Mary Shelley's Frankenstein. **Int J Psychoanal Psychother** 1982–83;9:647–56
Myers WA: Mary Shelley's Frankenstein: creativity and the psychology of the exception. **Int J Psychoanal Psychother** 1982–83;9:625–45
Wygant A: Shelley, Hawthorne, and Wells: images of medicine in early science fiction. **Bookman** 1981 Oct;8(8):3–8

**Shem, Samuel**
Hunter KM: The satiric image: healers in The House of God. In Jones AH, ed: Images of healers. Albany, State University of New York Press, 1983. p. 135–47.

**Sherif, Muzafer, 1905–**
Gorman M: Pre-war conformity research in social psychology: the approaches of Floyd H. Allport and Muzafer Sherif. **J Hist Behav Sci** 1981 Jan;17(1):3–14

**Sherley, Thomas, 1638–1678**
Debus AG: Thomas Sherley's philosophical essay (1672): Helmontian mechanism as the basis of a new philosophy. **Ambix** 1980 Jul;27(2):124–35

**Sherrington, Charles Scott, 1857–1952**
Eccles JC, Gibson WC: Sherrington: his life and thought. Berlin, New York, Springer International, 1979. xv, 269 p.
Jokl E: Sherrington, his life and thought: essay-review. **Trans Stud Coll Physicians Phila** 1980 Sep;5(2 no 3):223–35
McIlwain H: Neurochemistry and Sherrington's enchanted loom. **J R Soc Med** 1984 May;77(5):417–25
Sinclair HM: Sherrington and industrial fatigue. **Notes Rec R Soc Lond** 1984 Sep;39(1):91–104

**Shields, James, 1918–1978**
Gottesman II: James Shields, 1918–1978. **Acta Genet Med Gemellol (Roma)** 1979;28(1):83–90

**Shimanovskiĭ, IuK, 1829–**
Mirskiĭ MB: Iu. K. Shimanovskiĭ i ego rol' v razvitii otechestvennoĭ khirurgii i transplantologii (k 150-letiiu so dnia rozhdeniia). **Klin Khir** 1980 Mar;(3):68–71

**Shippen, William, 1736?–1808**
Jensen JE: Manuscript notes of William Shippen, Jr., MD found in the Faculty Library. **Md State Med J** 1984 Jun;33(6):438–40

**Shmal'gauzen, Ivan Ivanovich, 1884–1963**
Nikitiuk BA, Kozlov AI: Nekotorye spornye polozheniia ucheniia ob antropogeneze v svete predstavlenii o destabiliziruiushchem otbore i dannykh sovremennoĭ paléoendokrinologii (k 100-letiiu so dnia rozhdeniia I. I. Shmal'gauzena). **Arkh Anat Gistol Embriol** 1984 Aug;87(8):5–14
Sokolov VE, Vorob'eva EI: I. I. Shmal'gauzen i évoliutsionnaia morfologiia. **Arkh Anat Gistol Embriol** 1984 Jul;87(7):5–17

**Shor, Vladimir Georgievich, 1872–1948**
Zhuravleva TB: Uchenie G. V. Shora o tanatogeneze i rol' ego shkoly v razvitii sovetskoĭ patologicheskoĭ anatomii (k 110-letiiu so dnia rozhdeniia). **Arkh Patol** 1984;46(3):76–80

**Short, Arthur Rendle, 1880–1952**
Capper WM, Johnson D, ed: The faith of a surgeon. Belief and experience in the life of Arthur Rendle Short. Exeter, England, Paternoster Press, 1976. 156 p.

**Shrapnell, Henry Jones, 1792–1834**
Hellström S, Stenfors LE: The original description of Shrapnell's membrane reviewed in the light of recent experimental studies. **J Laryngol Otol** 1983 Nov;97(11):985–9
McGovern FH: The elusive Henry Jones Shrapnell. **Laryngoscope** 1983 Jul;93(7):903–5

**Shtefko, V. G., 1893–1945**
Strukov AI, Puzik VI, Zemskova ZS, et al: V. G. Shtefko i otechestvennaia shkola patologov-ftiziatrov. **Arkh Patol** 1984;46(2):81–5

**Shumlianskiĭ, Aleksandr Mikhaĭlovich, 1748–1795**
Dudchenko MA: Aleksandr Mikhaĭlovich Shumlianskiĭ. **Klin Med (Mosk)** 1983 Jan;61(1):114–6
Gusakov NI: K 200-letiiu ucheniia A.M. Schumlianskogo o pochke (1782–1982). **Sov Med** 1983;(4):117–8
Suslov VV, Gusakov NI: K 200-letiiu ucheniia A. M. Shumlianskogo o pochke (1782–1982). **Urol Nefrol (Mosk)** 1983 Jan–Feb;(1):61–3

**Shute, Percy George, 1894–1977**
Tiburskaia NA, Dukhanina NN: Pamiati P. G. Shute (issledovaniia P. G. Shute shtammov Plasmodium vivax). **Med Parazitol (Mosk)** 1980 Jan–Feb;49(1):87–90

**Sibbald, Robert, 1641–1722**
Simpson AD: Sir Robert Sibbald--the founder of the College. In Passmore R, ed: Proceedings of the Royal College of Physicians of Edinburgh Tercentenary Congress, 1981. Edinburgh, Royal College of Physicians of Edinburgh, 1982. p. 59–91.

**Sibly, Ebenezer, 1751–1799**
Debus AG: Scientific truth and occult tradition: the medical world of Ebenezer Sibly (1751–1799). **Med Hist** 1982 Jul;26(3):259–77

**Siebeck, Richard, 1883–1965**
Curtius F: Richard Siebeck (1883–1965). **Med Welt** 1983 Mar 18;34(11):347–53

**Siedlecki, Michał,1873–1940**
Hesse PG: Współpraca naukowa Schaudinn--Siedlecki w roku 1897. **Przegl Dermatol** 1983 May–Jun;70(3):307–10

**Siegemund, Justine Dittrich, 1648–1705**
Watanabe N: [On Siegemundine and her 'The most needed training in difficult and abnormal delivery'] (Jpn). **Josanpu Zasshi** 1980 Dec;34(12):812–7

**Siegle, Emil, 1833–1900**
Schwartz RH: The pneumatic otoscope, a new instrument for the examination of the tympanic membrane--E. Siegle. 1984. **Int J Pediatr Otorhinolaryngol** 1980 Sep;2(3):261–3

**Siemens, Hermann Werner, 1891–1969**
Nasemann T: Der Morphologe Hermann Werner Siemens und seine Bemühungen um eine 'Allgemeine Dermatologie'. **Hautarzt** 1983 Nov;34(11):569–73

**Sievert, Rolf Maximilian, 1896–**
Pochin EE: Sieverts and safety. **Health Phys** 1984 Jun;46(6):1173–9

**Sigerist, Henry Ernest, 1891–1957**
Beer FJ: Le souvenir d'Henri-Ernest Sigerist (1891–1957). **Hist Sci Med** 1982;16(1):49–53
Buess H: Henry E. Sigerist (1891–1957) und die erste medizinhistorische Konferenz in Pura (Tessin); zur Erinnerung an den 25./26. März 1950. **Gesnerus** 1980;37(1/2):104–12
Landsberger M: The story of the history of medicine: essay-review. **Trans Stud Coll Physicians Phila** 1980 Dec;5(2 no 4):315–8
Miller G: Henry Ernest Sigerist. In Dictionary of American Biography, Suppl. 6, 1956–1960. p. 580–1, 1980.
Sonnedecker G: The American correspondence between George Urdang and Henry E. Sigerist 1941–1948. In Perspektiven der Pharmaziegeschichte. Festschrift für Rudolf Schmitz zum 65. Geburtstag. Graz, Akademische Druck- u. Verlagsanstalt. p. 343–63.

**Sigismund I, King of Poland, 1467–1548**
Dudziński W: Choroby i zgon króla Zygmunta Starego. **Wiad Lek** 1981 Aug 1;34(15):1317–22

**Sigismund II, Augustus, King of Poland, 1518–1572**
Dudziński W: Choroby i zgon króla Zygmunta Augusta. **Wiad Lek** 1981 Aug 15;34(16):1411–6

**Sigismund III, Vasa, King of Poland, 1566–1632**
Kaczorowski W: Choroba i prawdopodobna przyczyna zgonu Zygmunta III Wazy. **Arch Hist Med (Warsz)** 1982;45(1–4):45–54

**Sigismund, of Austria**
Zwanowetz G: Herzog Sigismund von Osterreich in Gastein. **Mitt Ges Salzburger Landeskd** 1972–73;112–113(2):325–9

**Silikova, A. I., 1908–1980**
Grigor'eva VA: Tvorcheskiĭ vklad v biokhimiiu myshts. **Ukr Biokhim Zh** 1980 Nov–Dec;52(6):783–8

**Silkwood, Karen**
Annas GJ: The case of Karen Silkwood. **Am J Public Health** 1984 May;74(5):516–8

**Silliman, Benjamin, 1779–1864**
Ewan J: Five pupils of Benjamin Smith Barton: the men and their minds. **Trans Stud Coll Physicians Phila** 1983 Dec;5(5 no 4):309–20
Jackman SW: The tribulations of an editor: Benjamin Silliman and the early days of the American Journal of Science and the Arts. **N Engl Q** 1979;52(1):99–106
Wilson LG, ed: Benjamin Silliman and his circle: Studies on the influence of Benjamin Silliman on science in America. Prepared in honor of Elizabeth H. Thomson. New York, Science History Publications, 1979. x, 227 p. Contributions by S. D Beckham, J. C. Greene, L. I. Kuslan, G. Robinson, M. W. Rossiter.

**Silva, Pedro José da, 1834–1878**
Mosch E: Der Apotheker Pedro José da Silva, ein unbekannter Lebenslauf. **Beitr Gesch Pharm** 1980;31(9):65–71

**Silverberg, William Victor, 1897–1967**
Crowley RM: William V. Silverberg as teacher and colleague. **J Am Acad Psychoanal** 1981 Oct;9(4):493–500

**Simka, Ján, 1922–**
K 60. narodeninám doc. MUDr. Jána Simku, CSc: **Cesk Gynekol** 1983 Mar;48(2):151–8

**Simola, Paavo Eevertii, 1902–1961**
Järnefelt J: P. E. Simola ja sitruunahappokierto. **Duodecim** 1981;97(13):928–30

**Simon, Bela, 1892–1965**
Huszár G: Emlékezés Simon Béla professzorra. **Fogorv Sz** 1983 May;76(5):151–5

**Simon, Gustav, 1824–1876**
King DF: Gustav Simon. The father of dermatopathology. **Am J Dermatopathol** 1979 Fall;1(3):225–8

**Simon, Hermann, 1867–1947**
Sărmăşanu-Cortez ML, Cortez P: Dr. Hermann Simon, sitemul Gütersloh şi tratamentul activ al bolilor psihice. **Rev Med Interna [Neurol Psihiatr]** 1980 Oct–Dec;25(4):295–302

**Simone de Cinozzo di Giovanni Cini**
Caroti S: La biblioteca di un medico fiorentino [Simone de Cinozzo di Giovanni Cini]. **Bibliofilia** 1978;80:123–38

**Simoni, Simone, 1532–1602**
Szpilczyński S: Das traditionelle und progressive Gesicht der Medizin in der Renaissance-Epoche im Lichte der Polemik zwischen S. Simonius und N. Buccella nach dem Tode des Königs Stefan Batory. **Organon** 1979;15:229–37

**Simpson, George Gaylord, 1902–**
Gershenowitz H: George Gaylord Simpson and Lamarck. **Indian J Hist Sci** 1978, reçu 1982;13(1):56–61
Laporte LF: Simpson's Tempo and Mode in Evolution revisited. **Proc Am Philos Soc** 1983 Dec 30;127(6):365–417

**Simpson, James Young, 1811–1870**
Classic articles in colonic and rectal surgery: James Young Simpson 1811–1870. **Dis Colon Rectum** 1982 Sep;25(6):611–22
Crider S: Anesthesia. A history of Simpson's discovery of chloroform. **J Kans Med Soc** 1983 Mar;84(3):143–6
Jones IW: Chloroform anaesthesia in Liverpool. **Anaesthesia** 1983 Jun;38(6):578–80
Pinkerton JH: Sir James Young Simpson: Irish influences. **Ir Med J** 1982 Jun;75(6):183–7
Waserman M: Sir James Y. Simpson and London's 'conservative and so curiously prejudiced' Dr. Ramsbotham. **Br Med J** 1980 Jan 19;280(6208):158–61

**Sims, James Marion, 1813–1883**
Breathnach CS: Biographical sketches no. 36 -- Sims. **Ir Med J** 1984 Jan;77(1):27
Dittmer I: James Marion Sims. 1813–1883. **MMW** 1984 Feb 10;126(6):159–60

**Sinan ibn Thabit ibn Qurra, Abu Said, ca. 880–943**
Hajal F: Galen's ethical psychotherapy: its influence on a medieval Near Eastern physician. **J Hist Med Allied Sci** 1983 Jul;38(3):320–33

**Sinasi, d. 1702**
Köhbach M: Europäische Aerzte im Osmanischen Reich am Beginn des 18. Jahrhunderts--der Fall Sinasi. **Sudhoffs Arch** 1980;64(1):79–85

**Singer, Isaac Bashevis, 1904–**
Blinderman A: Isaac Bashevis Singer; medicinal fiction. **NY State J Med** 1981 Aug;81(9):1382–91

**Singer, Israel Jashua, 1893–1944**
Gilman SL: Madness and racial theory in I. J. Singer's The family Carnovsky. **Mod Jud** 1981;1(1):90–100

**Sippy, Bertram Walton, 1866–1924**
Zucker GM, Clayman CB: Landmark perspective: Bertram W. Sippy and ulcer disease therapy. **JAMA** 1983 Oct 28;250(16):2198–202

**Sison, Honoria Acosta, 1888–1970**
Agris J: Stamps commemorating medicine. 'Honoria Acosta Sison'

pioneer gynecologist and obstetrician. **J Dermatol Surg Oncol** 1980 Mar;6(3):178

**Sjöbring, Henrik, 1879–1956**
Essen-Möller E: The psychology and psychiatry of Henrik Sjöbring (1879–1956). **Psychol Med** 1980 May;10(2):201–10
Nielzén S: Sjöbrings tankemodeller för personlighet och psykisk sjukdom. **Sydsven Medicinhist Sallsk Arsskr** 1980;:124–33

**Skakel, Alexander, 1776–1846**
Frost SB: Alexander Skakel, LL.D.: a founder, M.G.H. governor, and a many sided man. **Montreal Gen Hosp News** 1980;18(2):3–5

**Skarżyński, Bolesław, 1901–1963**
Milik JR: W 20 rocznicę śmierci Bolesława Skarżyńskiego o jego zasługach w rozwoju historii medycyny w Polsce. **Wiad Lek** 1983 Sep 15;36(18):1561–2

**Skeggs, Leonard Tucker, 1918–**
Leonard Tucker Skeggs--a multifaceted diamond: **Clin Chem** 1981 Aug;27(8):1465–8

**Skelton, John, 1460?–1529**
Wooden WW: Childhood and death: a reading of John Skelton's Phillip Sparrow. **J Psychohist** 1980 Spring;7(4):403–14

**Skinner, Burrhus Frederic, 1904–**
Evans RI: B. F. Skinner, the man and his ideas: dialogue with B. F. Skinner. New York, Praeger, 1981. xiv, 140 p.
Gantt WH: Review of the shaping of a behaviorism (B.F. Skinner). **Pavlov J Biol Sci** 1980 Jan–Mar;15(1):42–4
Skinner BF: Notebooks. Edited with an introduction by R. Epstein. Englewood Cliffs, Prentice-Hall, 1980. xiii, 386 p.
Skinner BF: The experimental analysis of operant behavior: a history. In R. W. Rieber, K. Salzinger, ed: Psychology: theoretical-historical perspectives. New York, Academic Press, 1980. p. 191–202.
Skinner BF: The shaping of a behaviorist. New York, Knopf, 1979. 373 p.

**Skinner, Edward Hohman, 1881–**
Lang EF: From earlier pages: the position and relationships of fragments in acute fractures. (E.H. Skinner). **AJR** 1980 Jan;134(1):206

**Skoda, Josef, 1805–1881**
Egy történelmi adat pontosításáról és Skoda orvos-beteg kapcsolatáról. **Orv Hetil** 1983 Jan 16;124(3):175–6
Birtalan G: Laennec and Skoda, classics of internal diagnostics. **Orvostort Kozl** 1982;28(1–3):33–41
Sakula A: Joseph Skoda 1805–81: a centenary tribute to a pioneer of thoracic medicine. **Thorax** 1981 Jun;36(6):404–11

**Sköldberg, Sven, 1838–1872**
Kock W: Sven Sköldberg och ovariotomien en pionjärinsats i svensk gynekologi. **Nord Medicinhist Arsbok** 1983;:103–16

**Skvortsov, Mikhail Aleksandrovich, 1876–**
Ivanovskaia TE: Patologicheskaia anatomiia bolezneĭ detskogo vozrasta na sovremennom étape. **Arkh Patol** 1983;45(10):3–8

**Slater, William Kershaw, 1893–1970**
Cox EG: Sir William Kershaw Slater. In Dictionary of national biography, 1961–1970. Suppl. 8, 1981. p. 955–6.

**Sleszkowski, Sebastian, 1569–1648**
Pielat B: Dur plamisty w poglądach Sebastiana Petrycego i Sebastiana Sleszkowskiego w i Połowie XVII wieku. **Arch Hist Med (Warsz)** 1980;43(4):393–406

**Sloane, Hans, 1660–1753**
Cooke AM: Sir Hans Sloane and the Philosophical Transactions. **J R Coll Physicians Lond** 1984 Jul;18(3):170–1

**Slye, Maud Caroline, 1869–1954**
McCoy JJ: The cancer lady: Maud Slye and her heredity studies. Nashville, Nelson, 1977. 191 p.
Parascandola J: Maud Caroline Slye. In: Notable American women. The modern period. Cambridge, Mass., Belknap-Harvard Univ. Press, 1980. 4:651–2.

**Smetana, Bedřich, 1824–1884**
Bořík O, Khel R, Zdichynec B: Několik poznámek k ušnímu onemocnění Bedřicha Smetany. **Cesk Otolaryngol** 1983 Nov;32(6):367–71

**Smith, Adam, 1723–1790**
Mitchell H: The passions according to Adam Smith and Pierre-Jean-Georges-Cabanis. Two sciences of man(1). **Soc Soc Hist Med Bull (Lond)** 1979 Dec;25:20–7

**Smith, David W., 1926–**
Festschrift in honor of David W. Smith: **J Pediatr** 1982 Nov;101(5):797–804

**Smith Family**
Oliver H: The Shore Smith family library: Arthur Hugh Clough and Florence Nightingale. **Book Collect** 1979;28:521–9

**Smith, Frederick, 1857–1929**
Hickman J: Sir Frederick Smith--his life and work. **Equine Vet J** 1984 Sep;16(5):403–10

**Smith, Harry P.,, 1895–1972**
Owen CA: H. P. Smith's place in the history of blood coagulation. **Am J Clin Pathol** 1984 Apr;81(4):424–6

**Smith, Homer William, 1895–1962**
Riley HD: Homer William Smith. In Dictionary of American biography, 1961–1965. Suppl. 7, 1981. p. 699–700.

**Smith, James Edward, 1759–1828**
Allen DE: James Edward Smith and the Natural History Society of Edinburgh. **J Soc Bibliogr Nat Hist** 1978;8(4):483–93

**Smith, Jerome van Crowningshield, 1800–1879**
Garland J: Jerome Van Crowningshield Smith. **N Engl J Med** 1970 Aug 6;283:303–4

**Smith, Joseph, 1805–1844**
Wirthlin LS: Joseph Smith's boyhood operation: an 1813 surgical success. **Brigham Young Univ Stud** 1981;21(2):131–54

**Smith, Margaret G., 1896–1970**
Kissane JM: Founders of Pediatric Pathology. Margaret G. Smith. 1896–1970. **Perspect Pediatr Pathol** 1982;7:v–viii

**Smith, Nathan, 1762–1829**
Wirthlin LS: Joseph Smith's boyhood operation: an 1813 surgical success. **Brigham Young Univ Stud** 1981;21(2):131–54

**Smith, Robert Angus, 1817–1884**
Eyler JM: The conversion of Angus Smith: the changing role of chemistry and biology in sanitary science, 1850–1880. **Bull Hist Med** 1980 Summer;54(2):216–34
Gorham E: Robert Angus Smith, F.R.S., and 'Chemical climatology'. **Notes Rec R Soc Lond** 1982 Feb;36(2):267–72

**Smith, Sydney Alfred, 1883–1969**
Camps F: Sir Sydney Alfred Smith. In Dictionary of national biography, 1961–1970. Suppl. 8, 1981. p. 963–4.

**Smith, Thaddeus Dewey, d. 1917**
Smith R: The first American officer wounded in World War I. **JAMA** 1982 Mar 26;247(12):1743

**Smith, Theobald, 1859–1934**
Classics in infectious diseases. Letter from Theobald Smith to Edward Krumbhaar: **Rev Infect Dis** 1984 Mar–Apr;6(2):280–1
Smith T: Document: [letter to Dr. Edward B. Krumbhaar]. **Trans Stud Coll Physicians Phila** 1981 Sep;5(3 no 3):214–5

**Smith, William, fl. 1784–1803**
Morgan RJ: William Smith. In Dictionary of Canadian biography, 1801 to 1820. Volume 5, 1983. p. 766–7.

**Smollett, Tobias George, 1721–1771**
Different letters from the past: Tobias Smollett to William Hunter. **Ann R Coll Surg Engl** 1980 Mar;62(2):146–9
Nemoianu V: The semantics of Bramble's hypochondria: a connection between illness and style in the eighteenth century. **Clio (US)** 1979;9(1):39–51
Poirier S: Tobias Smollett, M.D.--expert on the body--and the bawdy. **Pharos** 1984 Winter;47(1):17–22

**Smyth, James Carmichael, 1741–1821**
Keel O: La généalogie de l'histopathologie; une révision déchirante. Philippe Pinel, lecteur discret de J.-C. Smyth (1741–1821). Paris, Librairie Philosophique J. Vrin, 1979. ii, 135 p. (Histoire des Sciences: Textes et Etudes).

**Snellen, Herman, 1834–1908**
Brajkovich HL: Dr. Snellen's 20/20: the development and use of the eye chart. **J Sch Health** 1980 Oct;50(8):472–4

**Sniadecki, Jedrzej, 1768–1838**
Chrzęściewski L: Jędrzej śniadecki (1768–1838) – prekursor współczesnej myśli pedagogicznej w medycynie. **Arch Hist Med (Warsz)** 1983;46(1):29–38

**Snow, John, 1813–1858**
Cameron D, Jones IG: John Snow, the broad street pump and modern epidemiology. **Int J Epidemiol** 1983 Dec;12(4):393–6
Leaman A: John Snow MD--his early days. **Anaesthesia** 1984 Aug;39(8):803–5
Lilienfeld AM, Lilienfeld DE: John Snow, the Broad Street pump and modern epidemiology. **Int J Epidemiol** 1984 Sep;13(3):376–8
Matsuki A. [Recent findings in the history of anesthesiology (16) Tracing John Snow's work in London] (Jpn). **Masui** 1982 Mar;31(3):264–9

**Snyder, Laurence Hasbrouck, 1901–**
On the rôle of Laurence H. Synder in the development of human and medical genetics in the United States; an oral history tape interview: **Am J Med Genet** 1981;8(4):449–68

**Sobieszczański, Zbigniew**
Kłodziński S: Lek. Zbigniew Sobieszczański. **Przegl Lek** 1984;41(1):131–6

**Sobolev, Andrei Andreevich, 1904–1966**
Oshmarin AP: Razvitie ékologicheskogo napravleniia v otechestvennoĭ gel'mintologii nauchnoĭ shkoloĭ A. A. Soboleva. **Parazitologiia** 1983 Jul–Aug;17(4):324–8

**Socrates**
Chessick RD: Socrates: first psychotherapist. **Am J Psychoanal** 1982 Spring;42(1):71–83

Fritts HW: Are we Socratic teachers? **Trans Am Clin Climatol Assoc** 1979;90:109–15
Hoffmann WF: Socrates revisited: his relevance today. **J Fam Pract** 1982 Jan;14(1):179–80

**Soemmerring, Detmar Wilhelm, 1793–1891**
Rusch T: Detmar Wilhelm Soemmerring, Leben und Werk. Diss. Mainz, 1981. 126 p.

**Soemmerring, Margarethe Elisabeth Grunelius, 1768–1802**
Rösler HP: Samuel Thomas von Soemmerring (1755–1830), Aquarell, gemalt 1794 von seiner Frau Margarethe Elisabeth, geb. Grunelius (1768–1802), Grösse des Bildovals 12,8 cm (Höhe): 11,5 cm (Breite) (Privatbesitz). **Medizinhist J** 1980;15(4):422–5

**Soemmerring, Samuel Thomas von, 1755–1830**
Bachmann R: Samuel Thomas von Sömmerring - 18. Januar 1755 bis 2. März 1830. Gedenken zum 150. Todestag. **Verh Anat Ges** 1981;75(Pt 1):33–46
Baer KE von: Reden gehalten in wissenschaftlichen Versammlungen und kleinere Aufsätze vermischten Inhalts. With an introduction by K. B. Sterling. New York, Arno Press, 1978. Three volumes in two. (Reprint. St. Petersburg, 1864/1876/1873).
Dumont F: Bericht über das Soemmerring–Symposion 1983. **Ber Wissenschaftsgesch** 1984;7(1):58–64
Roesler HP: Soemmerring--Denkmäler in Frankfurt am Main. **Nat Mus** 1978;108:345–53
Rösler HP: Samuel Thomas von Soemmerring (1755–1830), Aquarell, gemalt 1794 von seiner Frau Margarethe Elisabeth, geb. Grunelius (1768–1802), Grösse des Bildovals 12,8 cm (Höhe): 11,5 cm (Breite) (Privatbesitz). **Medizinhist J** 1980;15(4):422–5
Schierhorn H: Samuel Thomas Soemmerring (1755–1830) als Neuroanatom. **Z Mikrosk Anat Forsch** 1980;94(6):1051–76

**Soiland, Albert, 1873–1946**
Regato JA del: Albert Soiland and the early development of therapeutic radiology in the United States. **Int J Radiat Oncol Biol Phys** 1983 Feb;9(2):243–53

**Sokol, Stanisław, 1911–1968**
Sieńkowski E: Ekslibris lekarski prof. dr Stanisława Sokoła. **Arch Hist Med (Warsz)** 1978;41(4):473–8

**Sokol'nikov, P. N., 1865–**
Pinigin VV: Pervyĭ vrach–iakut P.N. Sokol'nikov. **Sov Zdravookhr** 1979;(8):61–3

**Sokolov, P., 1893?–**
Aleksandrovskiĭ BN, Shchepetova GA: P. H. Sokolov--vidnyĭ organizator zdravookhraneniia Saratova. **Sov Zdravookhr** 1979;(11):55–9
Petr Andreevich Sokolov (k 80–letiiu so dnia rozhdeniia): **Arkh Anat Gistol Embriol** 1980 Jul;79(7):118–20

**Solano, Francisco Antonio, d. 1771**
Morales y Morales A: Francisco Antonio Solano, boticario revalidado. Asentista del Hospital Militar de Santa Cruz de Tenerife (1764–1771). **Bol Soc Esp Hist Farm** 1980 Mar–Jun;3(121–2):109–38

**Soley, Elizabeth Jane, fl. 1860–1893**
Kennedy JE: Jane Soley Hamilton, midwife. **NS Hist Rev** 1982;2(1):6–29

**Solon, 638?–599? B.C.**
Phillips JH: Early Greek medicine and the poetry of Solon. **Clio Med** 1980;15(1/2):1–4

**Solovev, M. N., 1886–1980**
Gol'd E IU: M. N. Solov'ev: 1886–1980. Moskva, Meditsina, 1982. 60 p.

**Solov'ev, Zinoviĭ Petrovich, 1876–1928**
Solov'eva VA, ed: Zhizn' deiatel'nost' Z. P. Solov'eva. Moskva, Meditsina, 1980. 205 p.

**Son, Joseph Mozes, 1818–1884**
Van Cittert–Eymers JG: Joseph Mozes Son (1818–1884), een illuster tandmeester te Utrecht. **Tijdschr Geschied Geneeskd** 1978;2(2):62–9

**Soper, Fred Lowe, 1893–1977**
Duffy J, ed: Ventures in world health; the memoirs of Fred Lowe Soper. Washington, Pan American Health Organization, 1977. 365 p. (Scientific Publ. No. 355).
Vaccarezza RF: Devoción a la causa de la salud: Fred Lower Soper. **Medicina (B Aires)** 1981;41(1):101–6

**Soper, George Albert, 1870–1948**
The carrier state. New York, Arno, 1977. Various paginations. Four reprinted papers on microbiology by William H. Park and George Soper, 1895–1919.:

**Soranus, of Ephesus, 2nd cent.**
Bobbio S: Sorano de Efeso. **Femina** 1979;7:791–6
Raju TN: Soranus of Ephesus: who was he and what did he do? In Smith GF, Smith PN, Vidyasagar D, ed: Historical review and recent advances in neonatal and perinatal medicine. [Chicago?], Mead Johnson Nutritional Division, 1983. Vol. II. p. 179–86.

**Sorapan de Rieros, Juan, 1572–1638**
Moreno Gonzalez JP, Gonzalez Iglesias J: Sorapan de Rieros y la odontologia. **Bol Inf Dent (Madr)** 1979 Sep–Oct;(302):37–44

**Sorbait, Paul de, 1624?–1691**
Gysel C: L'odonto–stomatologie formellement scolastique de Paul de Sorbait (1624–1691). **Rev Belge Med Dent** 1983 Mar;38(2):55–62

**Sørensen, Peder, 1540 or 42–1602**
Koch CH: Petrus Severinus, Francis Bacon og Naturiagttagelsen. **Dan Medicinhist Arbog** 1979;161–72
Skov H, Bastholm E, ed: Petrus Severinus og hans Idea medicinae philosophicae. En dansk paracelsist. Copenhagen, Odense Universitetsforlag, 1979. 299 p. (Acta Historica Scientiarum et Medicinalium, 32).

**Sosberger, Aleksander, 1873–1944**
Berić BM: Prvi ginekolog–akušer u Vojvodini--dr Aleksander Sosberger (1873–1944). **Jugosl Ginekol Opstet** 1984 May–Aug;24(3–4):71–2

**Soubbotitch, V.**
Rich NM, Clagett GP, Salander JM, et al: The Matas/Soubbotitch connection. **Surgery** 1983 Jan;93(1 Pt 1):17–9

**Soubeiran, Eugène, 1797–1858**
Berman A: An unpublished letter from Eugene Soubeiran to Antoine Portal, June 3, 1828. **Pharm Hist** 1982;24(1):32–7

**Soufflot, Jacques Germain, 1713–1780**
Garmier JF: Soufflot et Mâcon: La charité, l'Hotel–Dieu. **Cah Rech Archit** 1980;6–7, Suppl:142–51

**Soulier, Jean Pierre**
Soulier JP: The history of PPSB. **Vox Sang** 1984;46(1):58–61

**Soumande, Louise, 1664–1708**
Paquin M: Louise Soumande. In Dictionary of Canadian biography, 1701 to 1740. Volume 2, 1969. p. 613.

**Soupiran, Simon, 1670–1724**
Moogk PN: Simon Soupiran. In Dictionary of Canadian biography, 1701 to 1740. Volume 2, 1969. p. 613–4.

**Souttar, Henry Sessions, 1875–1964**
Sellors TH: Sir Henry Sessions Souttar. In Dictionary of national biography, 1961–1970. Suppl. 8, 1981. p. 969–70.

**Soyer, Alexis, 1809–1858**
Watkins D: The man who reformed hospital kitchens (Alexis Benoit Soyer). **Nurs Times** 1981 Nov 18–24;77(47):2029

**Soyka, Isidor, 1850–1889**
Steiner I: První popis 'senilního' amyloidu srdce--I. Soyka, 1876, Praha. **Cesk Patol** 1984 Feb;20(1):11–3

**Spallanzani, Lazzaro, 1729–1799**
Altieri Biagi ML: L'episteme stillistica di Lazzaro Spallanzani. **Intersezioni** 1981;1:575–99
Bonilauri F: Museo e città. Le collezioni Spallanzani e chierici a Reggio Emilia. Firenze, Olschki, 1978. 199 p. (Biblioteca della 'Rivista di Storia delle Scienze Mediche e Naturali').
Cafiso, LM: Storia della teoria sulla generazione spontanea: Redi, Spallanzani, Pasteur. **Cult Sc** 1981;20(80):236–43
Castellani C: Una rilettura ottocentesca di Spallanzani: la nouvelle théorie de la génération di Prévost e Dumas (1824). **Hist Philos Life Sci** 1979;1(2):215–59
Castellani C: Appunti per uno studio della biologia post–Spallanazaniana: 1780–1820. **Physis** 1978;20(1–4):5–29
Castellani C: Ontogenesi di una dissertazione: le 'osservazioni e sperienze sui vermicelli spermatici ...' di L. Spallanzani. **Hist Philos Life Sci** 1982;4(1):125–57
Castellani C: Ricognizione di alcuni inediti spallanzaniani, con particolare riguardo agli studi sui pipistrelli (1793–1794). La Memoria sul volo cieco dei pipistrelli dedicata al Senebier nelle due versioni: testo e considerazioni. **Physis** 1984;26(3):433–83
Di Pietro P: La 'storia naturale del mare' di Lazzaro Spallanzani. **Thalassia Salentina** 1978;8:53–62
Spallanzani M: Nuovi studi su Spallanzani e la biologia del '700. **Quad Stor** 1981;16(3):1080–90

**Span von Spanau, Laurentius, 1539–1575**
Wondrák E: Drei Bilder eines Arztes des 16. Jahrhunderts. **Medizinhist J** 1983;18(3):250–55
Wondrák E: Der Arzt und Dichter Laurentius Span (1530–1575). **Medizinhist J** 1983;18(3):238–49

**Spedding, Carlisle, 1695–1755**
Beckett JV: An eighteenth–century case history: Carlisle Spedding 1738. **Med Hist** 1982 Jul;26(3):303–6

**Spemann, Hans, 1869–1941**
Oppenheimer JM: Ernst Heinrich Haeckel as an intermediary in the transmutation of an idea. **Proc Am Philos Soc** 1982;126(5):347–55

**Spencer, George John, 1758–1834**
Different letters from the past. 4) Horatio, Viscount Nelson to Earl Spencer.: **Ann R Coll Surg Engl** 1980 Sep;62(5):388–9

**Spencer, Herbert, 1820–1903**
Churchill FB: The Weismann–Spencer controversy over the inheritance of acquired characters. In Forbes EG, ed: Human implications of scientific advance. Edinburgh, Edinburgh University Press, 1978. p. 451–68.
Freeman D: The evolutionary theories of Charles Darwin and Herbert

Spencer. **Curr Anthropol** 1974;15(3):211–21
Smith CU: Evolution and the problem of mind: part I. Herbert Spencer. **J Hist Biol** 1982 Spring;15(1):55–88
Smith CU: Evolution and the problem of mind: part II. John Hughlings Jackson. **J Hist Biol** 1982 Summer;15(2):241–62

**Speranskiĭ, Georgiĭ Nestorovich, 1873–**
Matveev MP: Slovo o Georgii Nestoroviche Speranskom (K 110-letiiu so dnia rozhdeniia). **Pediatriia** 1983 Feb;(2):3–9

**Spiegel, Adriaan van de, 1578–1625**
Gysel C: De tandheelkunde van Adrianus Spigelius Bruxellensis (1578–1625–1978). **Rev Belge Med Dent** 1979;34(1):99–120
Gysel C: W. Harvey (1578–1657) et A. van den Spiegel (1578–1625), l'humanisme et l'odontologie. **Rev Belge Med Dent** 1979;34(1):121–6
Gysel C: Umanesimo e odontoiatria: Harvey e Spigelius, due vite parallele. **Dent Cadmos** 1981 Jan;49(1):61–6

**Spielmann, Jacob Reinbold, 1722–1783**
Grass U: Zu Leben und Werk von Jakob Reinbold Spielmann (1722–1783). Stuttgart, Deutscher Apotheker, 1983. 254 p. (Quellen und Studien zur Geschichte der Pharmazie, Bd. 20).
Jacquel R: Trois Alsaciens et les débuts--modestes--de la médecine sociale en Pologne pendant l'époque des lumières (troisième tiers du XVIIIe siècle). Les médecins strasbourgeois Jacques Reinbold Spielmann (1722–1783) et Jean Boecler (1737–1808) et le savant mulhousien Jean-Henri Lambert (1728–1777). In Livet G, Schaff G, ed: Médecine et assistance en Alsace, XVIe–XXe siècle. Strasbourg, Istra, 1976. p. 155–200.

**Spilenberg Family**
Kapronczay K: A Spilenberger orvoscsalád. **Orv Hetil** 1980 Jul 27;121(30):1840–3

**Spillmann Family**
Sordet D: Un homme, une famille. Le médecin principal Pierre Spillmann, professeur agrégé du Val-de-Grâce, professeur à l'Ecole préparatoire de Médecine et de Pharmacie d'Alger (1833–1883). Lyon, Association corporative des Etudiants en Médecine de Lyon, 1978. 40 p. (Thèse, Lyon).

**Spillmann, Pierre, 1833–1883**
Sordet D: Un homme, une famille. Le médecin principal Pierre Spillmann, professeur agrégé du Val-de-Grâce, professeur à l'Ecole préparatoire de Médecine et de Pharmacie d'Alger (1833–1883). Lyon, Association corporative des Etudiants en Médecine de Lyon, 1978. 40 p. (Thèse, Lyon).

**Spilsbury, Bernard Henry, 1879–1947**
Eckert WG: The writings of Sir Bernard Spilsbury: Part I. **Am J Forensic Med Pathol** 1984 Sep;5(3):231–8

**Spinks, Alfred, 1917–1982**
Johnson AW, Rose FL, Suckling CW: Alfred Spinks: 25 February 1917–11 February 1982. **Biogr Mem Fellows R Soc** 1984;30:567–94

**Spinoza, Benedictus de, 1632–1677**
Kraemer S: A note on Spinoza's contribution to systemic therapy. **Fam Process** 1982 Sep;21(3):353–7
Matheron A: Spinoza et la sexualité. **G Crit Filos Ital** 1977;56:436–57

**Spiro, Karl, 1867–1932**
Roos A, Boron WF: The buffer value of weak acids and bases: origin of the concept, and first mathematical derivation and application to physico-chemical systems. The work of M. Koppel and K. Spiro (1914). **Respir Physiol** 1980 Apr;40(1):1–32

**Spivak, Charles David, 1861–1927**
Hornbein M: Dr. Charles Spivak of Denver: physician, social worker, Yiddish author. **West States Jew Hist Q** 1979;11(3):195–211

**Spizharnyĭ, Ivan Konstantinovich, 1857–1924**
Epifanov NS: I. K. Spizharnyĭ v Viatskoĭ ssylke (materialy biografii). **Sov Zdravookhr** 1983;(2):70–1

**Spock, Benjamin McLane, 1903–**
Graebner W: The unstable world of Benjamin Spock: social engineering in a democratic culture, 1917–1950. **J Am Hist** 1980 Dec;67(3):612–29

**Spokes, Sidney, 1852–1938**
Donaldson JA: The life and times of Sidney Spokes. **J R Soc Med** 1981 Jul;74(7):537–9

**Sprengel, Kurt Polycarp Joachim, 1766–1833**
Kaiser W: In memoriam Kurt Sprengel (1766–1833)--Zur 150. Wiederkehr seines Todestages am 15. März 1983. **Z Gesamte Inn Med** 1983 Feb 1;38(3):90–7

**Springsfeld, Karl Gottlob, 1714–1772**
Bach I: Karl Gottlob Springsfeld--Arzt, Gelehrter und Akademiemitglied in der Zeit der Aufklärung. **Z Arztl Fortbild (Jena)** 1984;78(19):829–32

**Spurzheim, Johann Christoph, 1776–1832**
Fischer W: Franz Joseph Gall und Johann Kaspar Spurzheim--Vorläufer einer biologischen Psychiatrie. **Psychiatr Neurol Med Psychol (Leipz)** 1984 Jul;36(7):433–7
Gross G: Medizin zwischen Wissenschaft und Spekulation. Die Phrenologie des Dr. Johann Kaspar Spurzheim aus Longwich. **Kurtrier Jahrb** 1977;17:35–52

**Sraga, Dragoljub, 1866–1915**
Djordjević SP: Stampani radovi i prikazi bolesnika prvog otorhinolaringologa u Beogradu i Srbiji dr Dragoljuba Srage. **Srp Arh Celok Lek** 1982 Oct;110(10):1261–6
Djordjević SP: Prvo Otorinolaringološko odeljenje u Srbiji u Opštoj državnoj bolnici u Beogradu, i prvi otorinolaringolog dr Dragoljub Sraga. **Srp Arh Celok Lek** 1982 Oct;110(10):1245–60

**Sreseli, Mikhail Andreevich, b. ca. 1904**
Mikhail Andreevich Sreseli (k 75-letiiu so dnia rozhdeniia): **Arkh Anat Gistol Embriol** 1980 Apr;78(4):122–5

**Srinivasabhatta, fl. 1600**
Venkata Reddy M: Hatharatnavali of Srinivasabhatta, a late medieval treatise on yoga and tantra. **Bull Indian Inst Hist Med (Hyderabad)** 1979;9:74–81

**Stahl, Georg Ernst, 1660–1734**
Arndal S: Krop, sjael og ånd Georg Ernst Stahls og Christian Friedrich Richters medicinske antropologi. **Dan Medicinhist Arbog** 1980;:126–66
Bednarczyk A: Antymechanicyzm w osiemnastowiecznej filozofii medycyny: Georg Ernst Stahl (1659–1734) i animizm. **Arch Hist Med (Warsz)** 1981;44(2):163–87
Duchesneau F: G. E. Stahl: Antimécanisme et physiologie. **Arch Int Hist Sci (Paris)** 1976;26:3–26
Duchesneau F: G. E. Stahl: antimécanisme et concept d'organisme. **Arch Int Hist Idees** 1982;95:1–31
Kaiser W: Georg Ernst Stahl (1659–1734)--Zur 250. Wiederkehr seines Todestages am 14. Mai 1984. **Z Gesamte Inn Med** 1984 Aug 1;39(15):371–6
Luyendijk-Elshout AM: Samuel Musgrave's attack upon Stahl's and Boerhaave's doctrines in 1763. **Janus** 1980;67(1-2-3):141–56

**Stalin, Josef, 1879–1953**
Pomper P: Nečaev, Lenin and Stalin: the psychology of leadership. **Jahrb Gesch Osteur** 1978;26(1):11–30
Tucker RC: A case of mistaken identity: djugashvili-Stalin. **Biography** 1982;5(1):17–24

**Stanford, Jane (Lathrop), 1825–1905**
Ogle G: The mysterious death of Mrs. Leland Stanford. **Pac Hist** 1981 Spring;25:1–7

**Stanisław I, Leszczński, King of Poland, 1677–1766**
Stanisława Leszczyńska nasza patronka: **Pieleg Polozna** 1984;(3):29

**Stanko, Johanne, 1430–1493**
Roeske W: Lexicon Synonymorum Mineralo-Chymico-Pharmaceuticorum Trilingue Latino-Germano-Polonicum Collectum et Conscriptum a Johanne Stanko anno MCDLXXII (1472). In Hickel E, Schröder G, ed: Neue Beiträge zur Arzneimittelgeschichte. Festschrift für Wolfgang Schneider zum 70. Geburtstag. Stuttgart, Wissenschaftliche Verlagsgesellschaft, 1982. p. 29–39.

**Stanley, John, fl. 1687**
Cook LG: A 17th century drug account. **Pharm Hist (London)** 1974 Jul;4(2):2–4

**Stanley, Louise, 1883–1954**
Conable CW: Louise Stanley. In: Notable American women. The modern period. Cambridge, Mass., Belknap-Harvard Univ. Press, 1980. 4:657–9.

**Stanojevi'c, B., d. 1967**
Dürrigl T: Počeci auroterapije u Jugoslaviji. **Reumatizam** 1982;29(2):37–9

**Stanojevic, Vlademir S., 1886–1978**
Djordjević SP: General Prof. Dr. Vladimir S. Stanojević (3. III 1886 – 5. VI 1978. **Srp Arh Celok Lek** 1980 Mar;108(3):281–92

**Stanton, Madeline Earle, 1898–1980**
Ebbert A, et al: [Reminiscences and appreciations of Madeline E. Stanton] Contributions by L. G. Wilson, L. G. Stevenson, T. R. Forbes, S. B. Nuland, F. Gyorgyey, J. Bylebyl, G. L. Geison, W. Le Fanu, G. Robinson. **J Hist Med Allied Sci** 1981 Apr;36(2):129–50
Thomson EH: Madeline Earle Stanton, disciple: the years 1920 to 1941. **J Hist Med Allied Sci** 1981 Apr,36(2):151–67
Wilson LG: Madeline Earle Stanton 1898–1980. **Bull Med Libr Assoc** 1981 Jul;69(3):357–8

**Stark, Karl Wilhelm, 1787–1845**
Bauer A: Das öffentliche Krankenhaus als wissenschaftliche Bildungs-Anstalt. In Seidler E, Schott, ed: Bausteine zur Medizingeschichte. Stuttgart, Steiner, 1984. p. 9–27.
Bleker J: Die Naturhistorische Schule 1825–1845. Ein Beitrag zur Geschichte der klinischen Medizin in Deutschland. Stuttgart, New York, Fischer, 1981. ix, 174 p.

**Starling, Ernest Henry, 1866–1927**
Altschule MD: Invalidity of using so-called Starling curves in clinical medicine. **Perspect Biol Med** 1983 Winter;26(2):171–87
Fye WB: Ernest Henry Starling, his law and its growing significance in the practice of medicine. **Circulation** 1983 Nov;68(5):1145–8

**Staszic, Stanisław, 1755–1826**
Wójcik Z: O Staszciou i nowych taszicianach. **Kwart Hist Nauki Tech** 1981;26:177–86

**Staton, Lycurgus Lafayette, 1849–1921**
Walker LG: L. L. Staton, M.D., and the first successful gastrostomy in America. **Surg Gynecol Obstet** 1984 Apr;158(4):387–8

**Stead, Eugene Anson, 1908–**
Cebe B, Rozear MP, ed: E. A. Stead, Jr.: what this patient needs is a doctor. Durham, N. C., Carolina Academic Press, 1978. xii, 244 p.

**Stead, William Thomas, 1849–1912**
Robson A: The significance of 'The maiden tribute of modern Babylon'. **Victorian Period Newsl** 1978;11(2):50–7

**Stearns, Charles W., 1817–1887**
Walter JD: Charles W. Stearns and Norman W. Kingsley and the development of the artificial velum. **Bull Hist Dent** 1981 Oct;29(2):74–81

**Stearns, William Augustus, 1805–1876**
Welch JE: Pioneering in health education and services at Amherst College. **J Am Coll Health** 1982 Jun;30(6):289–95

**Stebbing, George, 1749–1825**
Van Zwanenberg D: Interesting GPs of the past: George Stebbing: 1749–1825. **Br Med J [Clin Res]** 1981 Dec 5;283(6305):1517–8

**Stefan Batory, King of Poland, 1533–1586**
Szpilczyński S: Das traditionelle und progressive Gesicht der Medizin in der Renaissance-Epoche im Lichte der Polemik zwischen S. Simonius und N. Buccella nach dem Tode des Königs Stefan Batory. **Organon** 1979;15:229–37

**Steffen, August, 1825–1910**
Oehme J: Rückbesinnung zum 100 jährigen Bestehen der Deutschen Gesellschaft für Kinderheilkunde. **Klin Paediatr** 1983 Jan–Feb;195(1):1–3

**Steger, Johann Heinrich, 1767–1842**
Gaberthüel M: Krankengeschichten und Operationsberichte 1784–1811 nach den Aufzeichnungen von Johann Heinrich Steger (1767–1842) und Johann Jakob Steger (1798–1857). Zürich, Juris, 1980. 121 p. (Zürcher Medizingeschichtliche Abhandlungen, Neue Reihe, 140).

**Steger, Johann Jakob, 1798–1857**
Bezel E: Johann Jakob Steger, 1798–1857. Beispiel eines Medizinstudiums im frühen 19. Jahrhundert nach den Briefen an seine Eltern. Zürich Juris, 1981. 156 p. (Zürcher medizingeschichtliche Abhandlungen, Neue Reihe, Nr. 147).
Gaberthüel M: Krankengeschichten und Operationsberichte 1784–1811 nach den Aufzeichnungen von Johann Heinrich Steger (1767–1842) und Johann Jakob Steger (1798–1857). Zürich, Juris, 1980. 121 p. (Zürcher Medizingeschichtliche Abhandlungen, Neue Reihe, 140).

**Steiger, Adolf, 1862–1920**
Sorsby A, Benjamin B, Bennett AG: Steiger on refraction: a reappraisal. **Br J Ophthalmol** 1981 Dec;65(12):805–11

**Stein, Georg Wilhelm, 1773–1870**
Makowski HM: Georg Wilhelm Stein und die frühe Geburtshilfe in Bonn. Diss. Bonn, 1979. 110 p.

**Steinbach, Henry Burr, 1905–**
Bishop DW: H. Burr Steinbach: Prosit! **Soc Gen Physiol Ser** 1981;36:xi–xiv

**Steinbeck, John, 1902–1968**
Dermott R: 'A great black book': East of Eden and Gunn's New family physician. **Am Stud** 1981;22(2):41–57

**Steinhausen, Wilhelm, 1887–1954**
Trincker DE: Wilhelm Steinhausen (1887–1954). **Rev Physiol Biochem Pharmacol** 1980;87:25–32

**Stella, Giulio, 1899–1978**
Pinotti O: Giulio Stella 1899–1978. **Arch Sci Biol (Bologna)** 1978 Jan–Dec;62(1–4):i–xiv

**Steno, Nicolaus, 1638–1686**
Bierbaum M, Faller A: Niels Stensen. Anatom, Geologe und Bischof, 1638–1686. 2d ed. Münster, Aschendorff, 1979. xi, 203 p. Includes Thomasen AL, Der Wandel des Stensenbildes.
Faller A: Die Präparation der weissen Substanz des Gehirns bei Stensen, Willis und Vieussens. **Gesnerus** 1982;39(2):171–93
Faller A: Wertschätzung von Stensens 'Discours sur l'anatomie du cerveau' im Verlaufe von drei Jahrhunderten. Aarau, Verlag Sauerländer, 1981. 96 p. (Veröffentlichungen der Schweizerischen Gesellschaft für Geschichte der Medizin und der Naturwissenschaften, 35).
Faller A: Elemente einer Wissenschaftslehre und einer Wissenschaftskritik in den Schriften von Niels Stensen (1638–1686). **Gesnerus** 1980;37(3/4):169–88
Faller A: Welchen Platz nimmt Stensens anatomische Forschung in Lorenz Heisters Chirurgie und Anatomie ein? **Gesnerus** 1983;40(1–2):55–66
Schirren C: Niels Stensen - ein Pionier der Wissenschaft. **MMW** 1981;123:267–70
Thomasen AL: Fra Trinitatis kirkes Loft til Universitetsbibliotekets 2. afdeling i følgeskab med Niels Stensen. **Ugeskr Laeger** 1983 Jun 27;145 Spec No:78–96

**Stephanopoulos-Vrettos, Basileios, 1908–1980**
Basileios Stephanopoulos-Vrettos: mia alesmonete mneme: **Stomatologia (Athenai)** 1980 Nov–Dec;37(6):5–48

**Stephanus, of Athens, 7th cent.**
Duffy JM: Stephanus the philosopher: lectures on the Prognosticon of Hippocrates. Critical text and translation. Ph. D. Diss., State University of New York, Buffalo, 1975. xxi, 449 p.

**Stephen, Leslie, 1832–1904**
Hyman VR: Concealment and disclosure in Sir Leslie Stephen's mausoleum book. **Biography** 1980;3(2):121–31

**Stephen of Bourbon, ca. 1180–1262**
Schmitt JC: The holy greyhound: Guinefort, healer of children since the thirteenth century. Cambridge, Cambridge University Press; Paris, Editions de la Maison des Sciences de l'Homme, 1983. 215 p. Translation of Le saint lévrier: Guinefort, guérisseur d'enfants depuis le XIIIe siècle, Paris, 1979.

**Stephens, Joanna**
Blum L: An eighteenth century health care provider and medical entrepreneur. **Bull NY Acad Med** 1984 Nov;60(9):944–7

**Stern, Erich, 1889–1959**
Schachter M: Le professeur Erich Stern (1889–1959) psychiatre et psychologue. **Rev Hist Med Heb** 1980 Oct;134(33 no 3):53–4)

**Stern, Kurt Guenter, 1904–1956**
Ihde AJ: Kurt Guenter Stern. In Dictionary of American Biography, Suppl. 6, 1956–1960. p. 595–6, 1980.

**Stern, William, 1871–1938**
Hardesty FP: Louis William Stern: a new view of the Hamburg years. In K. Salzinger, ed: Psychology in progress: an interim report. (Annals of the New York Academy of Sciences, 1976. p. 31–44.

**Sternberg, Erich, 1903–1980**
Huber G: Erich Sternberg 1903–1980. **Arch Psychiatr Nervenkr** 1981;230(1):1–3

**Sternberg, George Miller, 1838–1915**
Bibel DJ: Sternberg, Metchnikoff, and the phagocytes. **Milit Med** 1982 Jul;147(7):550–3

**Sterne, Laurence, 1713–1768**
Rodgers JS: 'Life' in the novel: Tristram Shandy and some aspects of eighteenth-century physiology. **Eighteenth Cent Life** 1980;6(1):1–20
Rogers JS: 'Life' in the novel: Tristram Shandy and some aspects of 18th-century physiology. **Eighteenth Cent Life** 1980;6(1):1–20

**Stevens, Albert Mason, 1884–1945**
Ström J: Männen bakom syndromet: Albert Stevens och Frank Johnson. Först att beskriva 'okänd infektionssjukdom'--allergi utlöst av läkemedel eller infektion. **Lakartidningen** 1983 Mar 16;80(11):1076–7

**Stevenson, Lloyd Grenfell, 1918–**
Thibodeau D, ed: A bibliography of the writings of Lloyd G. Stevenson. **Bull Hist Med** 1983 Summer;57(2):267–79

**Stevenson, Robert Louis, 1850–1894**
Bushnell OA: 'Our good friend Mr. Stevenson'. **Biography** 1982;5(2):118–28

**Stevenson, Sarah Ann Hackett, 1841–1909**
Beatty WK: Sarah Hackett Stevenson--concerned practitioner and social activist. **Proc Inst Med Chic** 1982 Jul–Sep;35(3):99–101

**Stewart, David, 1813–1899**
Allen B: David Stewart: first professor of pharmacy in America. **Md Pharm** 1982 Feb;:4–8

**Stewart, Fred Waldorf, 1894–**
Hutter RV: Classics in Oncology. Lobular carcinoma in situ by Foote and Stewart. **CA** 1982 Jul–Aug;32(4):232–7

**Stewart, Isabel Maitland, 1878–1963**
Austin AL: Isabel Maitland Stewart. In: Notable American women. The modern period. Cambridge, Mass., Belknap-Harvard Univ. Press, 1980. 4:660–2.
Donahue MP: Isabel Maitland Stewart's philosophy of education. **Nurs Res** 1983 May–Jun;32(3):140–6
Donahue MP: [Isabel Maitland Stewart's philosophy of education] (Jpn). **Kango Kyoiku** 1984 Oct;25(10):611–21

**Still, Andrew Taylor, 1828–1917**
Finlayson G: The birth of a profession: osteopathic medicine. **OH** 1984 Sep;28(8):16–7
Mercer SR: America's minority medical profession. In: Congrès international d'histoire de la médecine, XXVe, Québec, 1976. Actes. Québec, 1977. p. 969–79.

**Stilling, Benedict, 1810–1879**
Aumüller G: Benedict Stillings (1810–1879) Untersuchungen über das Rückenmark--ein Wendepunkt in der neuroanatomischen Forschung. **Medizinhist J** 1984;19(1–2):53–69

**Stipp, George W.**
Carmichael AG: The Lindsay-Stipp debate. **Indiana Med Hist Q** 1981;7(4):6–19

**Stock, Charles, 1790–**
Clarke B: Mental illness and rehabilitation in early nineteenth-century Ireland; the case of Charles Stock. **Psychol Med** 1983 Nov;13(4):727–34

**Stockard, Charles Rupert, 1879–1939**
Oppenheimer JM: Basic embryology and clinical medicine: a case history in serendipity. **Bull Hist Med** 1984 Summer;58(2):236–40

**Stocki, Edward, 1909–1978**
Meissner RK: In memoriam: Dr med. Edward Stocki (1909--1978), członek honorowy Polskiego Towarzystwa Historii Medycyny. **Arch Hist Med (Warsz)** 1979;42(2):141–55

**Stockton, Charles G., 1853–**
Adler S. The operation on President McKinley. In Plesur M, ed.. An American Historian: essays to honor Selig Adler (Buffalo: State U. of N.Y., 1980): 37–49.

**Stoddard, Charles Warren, 1843–1909**
Austen R: Stoddard's little tricks in South Sea Idyls. **J Homosex** 1983 Spring–Summer;8(3–4):73–81

**Stoeber, Victor, 1803–1871**
Vetter T: Témoignages du Strasbourgeois Victor Stoeber sur la médecine parisienne (1824–1825). **Gesnerus** 1983;40(1–2):215–22

**Stoeckel, Walter, 1871–1961**
Bayer H: Walter Stoeckel--Leben und Werk. **Zentralbl Gynakol** 1983;105(1):52–5

**Stöhr, Philipp, 1891–1979**
Fleischhauer K: In memoriam Philipp Stöhr jr. **Anat Anz** 1981;150(3):239–47

**Stokes, John Hinchman, 1885–1961**
Beerman H: John Hinchman Stokes, M.D. An appreciation. **J Am Acad Dermatol** 1983 Aug;9(2):321–34

**Stokes, William, 1804–1878**
Pinkerton JH: John Creery Ferguson. Friend of William Stokes and pioneer of auscultation of the fetal heart in the British Isles. **Br J Obstet Gynaecol** 1980 Apr;87(4):257–60

**Stolte, Karl, 1881–1951**
Külz J: Interessantes und Amüsantes aus dem Nachlass von Karl Stolte. **Kinderarztl Prax** 1981 Nov;49(11):583–90
Ocklitz HW, Schmitz HH: Unserem Lehrer Karl Stolte zum 100. Geburtstag. **Kinderarztl Prax** 1981 Nov;49(11):591–5
Ratzmann GW, Jährig K: Karl Stolte in seiner Zeit und für unsere Zeit. **Kinderarztl Prax** 1981 Dec;49(12):617–27

**Stone, Abraham, 1890–1959**
Detlefsen EG: Abraham Stone. In Dictionary of American Biography, Suppl. 6, 1956–1960. p. 602–3, 1980.

**Stone, Irving, 1903–**
Duffy S: The origin of speeches: Inherit the Wind, Irving Stone and the Scopes trial. **Am Notes Queries** 1983 Sep–Oct;22(1–2):14–7

**Stone, William Spencer, 1902–1983**
Simeone FA: Studies of trauma and shock in man: William S. Stone's role in the military effort. **J Trauma** 1984 Mar;24(3):181–7

**Stonescu, Nicolae**
Cernovodeanu D: Din corespondenta inedită a medicului militar Nicolae Stonescu in timpul Războiului de Independenta. **Rev Istor** 1977;30(6):1051–70

**Stopes, Marie Charlotte Carmichael, 1880–1958**
Hall LA: The Stopes collection in the Contemporary Medical Archives Centre at the Wellcome Institute for the History of Medicine. **Soc Soc Hist Med Bull (Lond)** 1983 Jun;32:50–1
Holtzman EM: Marriage, sexuality, and contraception in the British middle class, 1918–1939: the correspondence of Marie Stopes. Ph.D. Diss., Rutgers University, The State Univ. of New Jersey. New Brunswick, 1982. v, 170 p.

**Stopford, John Sebastian Bach, 1888–1961**
Cooper WM, Platt H: John Sebastian Bach Stopford. In Dictionary of national biography, 1961–1970. Suppl. 8, 1981. p. 985–7.

**Störck, Anton, 1731–1803**
Schweppe KW, Probst C: Die Versuche zur medikamentösen Karzinomtherapie des Anton Störck (1731–1803). Ein Beitrag zur Geschichte der experimentellen Arzneimittelforschung in der älteren Wiener medizinischen Schule. **Wien Med Wochenschr** 1982 Mar 15;132(5):107–17
Schweppe KW, Probst C: Die Versuche zur medikamentösen Karzinomtherapie des Anton Störck (1731 bis 1803). Ein Beitrag zur Geschichte der experimentellen Arzneimittelforschung in der älteren Wiener medizinischen Schule. In Ganzinger K, Skopec M, Wyklicky H, ed: Festschrift für Erna Lesky zum 70. Geburtstag. Wien, Brüder Hollinek, 1981. p. 105–22.

**Stouffer, Samuel Andrew, 1900–1960**
Hyman HH: Samuel Andrew Stouffer. In Dictionary of American Biography, Suppl. 6, 1956–1960. p. 604–6, 1980.

**Stout, Arthur Purdy, 1885–1967**
Azar HA: Arthur Purdy Stout (1885–1967). The man and the surgical pathologist. **Am J Surg Pathol** 1984 Apr;8(4):301–7

**Stout, Samuel Hollingsworth, 1822–1903**
Emmons J: The medical career of Samuel H. Stout. **J Med Assoc Ga** 1980 Nov;69(11):904–10, 1981 Mar;80(3):169–77

**Stowe-Gullen, Augusta, 1857–1943**
Smith K: Dr. Augusta Stowe-Gullen: a pioneer of social conscience. **Can Med Assoc J** 1982 Jun 15;126(12):1465–7

**Straatsma, Clarence Ralph, 1896–1974**
As I remember: Clarence R. Straatsma: **Ann Plast Surg** 1981 Oct;7(4):327–32

**Strachey, James, 1887–1967**
Etchegoyen RH: Fifty years after the mutative interpretation. **Int J Psychoanal** 1983;64 ( Pt 4):445–59

**Straet, Jan van der, 1523–1605**
Gariepy TP: Hyacum, et lues venerea. **J Hist Med Allied Sci** 1981 Jul;36(3):325

**Stratz, Carl Heinrich, 1858–1924**
Grimm H: Carl Heinrich Stratz (1858 bis 1924) als Mitbegründer einer ärztlichen Jugendkunde. Zeittafeln zu seinem Leben und seiner Wirksamkeit. **Aerztl Jugendkd** 1979 Jun;70(3):177–92

**Strauss, Anselm Franz, 1780–1830**
Bartels K: Ein vielseitiger Apotheker der ersten Hälfte des 19. Jahrhunderts: Anselm Franz Strauss. **Beitr Gesch Pharm** 1979;31(4):26–30

**Stromayr, Caspar, fl. 1557–1567**
Kuemmel WF: Chirurgie vor 400 Jahren: die Bilderhandschrift des Caspar Stromayr. **Medita** 1980;10, Suppl. (Geschichte der Medizin, f.6:16)
Nover A, Kümmel WF: Der Schnitt- und Augenarzt Caspar Stromayr und die ophthalmologischen Illustrationen in seiner 'Practica copiosa' (1559). **Klin Monatsbl Augenheilkd** 1984 Nov;185(5):321–3

**Stromer, Heinrich, 1476–1542**
Schnelbögl F: Auerbacher Lebensbilder. Zum 500. Geburtsjahr Heinrich Stromers, genannt Auerbach. **Altnurnb Landsch** 1976;25(Sonderh. 1):1–26

**Stromeyer, Louis, 1804–1876**
Machalett G: Ludwig Stromeyer--sein Beitrag zur Entwicklung der Militärmedizin in Deutschland. **Militaergesch** 1975;14(6):694–705

**Strong, Anne Hervey, 1876–1925**
Haggerty L: Nursing revisited: Strong public health nurse leader and educator. **Mass Nurse** 1984 Jul–Aug;54(7):7

**Strübing, Paul, 1852–**
Wilmanns JC: Paroxysmal nocturnal hemoglobinuria first described in 1882 by Paul Strübing: an example of cooperation between clinical and basic research. **Blut** 1982 Dec;45(6):367–73

**Struensee, Johann Friedrich, 1737–1772**
Wallerström A: Johann Friedrich Struensee--en psykologisk gåta. **Nord Medicinhist Arsb** 1981;:74–87
Winkle S: Johann Friedrich Struensee: Arzt, Aufklärer und Staatsmann: Beitrag zur Kultur-, Medizin- und Seuchengeschichte der Aufklärungszeit. Stuttgart, Fischer, 1983. 654 p.

**Strukov, Anatoli Ivanovich**
Razvitic A.I. Strukovym ucheniza o tuberculoza: **Probl Tuberk** 1981 Apr;(4):3–6

**Strümpell, Adolf, 1853–1925**
Thom A: Zur disziplinären Genese der Neurologie im ausgehenden 19. Jahrhundert--aus den Briefen Wilhelm Erbs an Adolf Strümpell. **Z Gesamte Inn Med** 1982 Jun 1;37(11):340–6

**Stuart, James Daniel, 1860–1938**
Stuart RB, ed: Memoirs of a Council Bluffs druggist. **Palimpsest** 1980;61(3):66–79

**Stubbe, Henry, 1631–1676**
Steneck NH: Greatrakes the stroker: the interpretations of historians. **ISIS** 1982 Jun;73(267):161–77

**Suárez, Ramón M., 1895–1981**
Bibliography of the scientific works of Dr. Ramón M. Suárez. **Bol Asoc Med PR** 1983 Nov;75(11):521–5
Busó R: Fundación de Investigaciones Clínicas. (Pro Deus, patriae eus scientia). **Bol Asoc Med PR** 1983 Nov;75(11):500
García Palmieri MR: Observaciones sobre la contribución del Dr. Ramón M. Suárez al reconocimiento de la cardiopatía reumática en el trópico. **Bol Asoc Med PR** 1983 Nov;75(11):503–5
Hernández-Morales F: La contribución del Dr. Ramón M. Suárez a la investigación del esprú. **Bol Asoc Med PR** 1983 Nov;75(11):496–7
Ramírez EA: Comentarios sobre la contribución del Dr. Ramón M. Suárez al estudio de la hipertensión arterial. **Bol Asoc Med PR** 1983 Nov;75(11):498–9
Torres-Gómez JM: Suárez, Ramón M., 1895–19811700 to PresentPuerto Rico **Bol Asoc Med PR** 1983 Nov;75(11):501–2
Torres-Gómez JM, García-Palmieri MR: Datos biográficos del Dr. Ramón M. Suárez Calderón. **Bol Asoc Med PR** 1983 Nov;75(11):490

**Suárez Rodriguez, Antonio, 1807–1907**
Báguena Cervellera J, Gener Galbis C: La triquinosis en la España del siglo XIX a través de la obra de Antonio Suárez: de las trichinas y de la trichinosis en España. **Med Hist (Barc)** 1984;3:1–26

**Sudhoff, Karl Friedrich Jakob, 1853–1938**
Diehl B: Der Wandel der Historiographie von Medizin und Naturwissenschaften in ihrer gesellschaftlichen Bedingtheit. **Sudhoffs Arch** 1982;66(3):276–300
Keil G: Karl-Sudhoff-Gedächtnissitzung. Sudhoffs Sicht vom deutschen medizinischen Mittelalter. **Nachrichtenbl Dtsch Ges Gesch Med Naturwiss Tech** 1981 Dec;31(3):94–129

**Sullivan, Evelyn Erickson**
Hodge GP: Medical illustration: our early years. Student days at Johns Hopkins, Evelyn Erickson Sullivan. **J Biocommun** 1982 Mar;9(1):18–22

**Sullivan, Harry Stack, 1892–1949**
Chapman AH, Vieira e Silva D: Base para uma psiquiatria científica: os conceitos de Harry Stack Sullivan. **Arq Neuropsiquiatr** 1980 Mar;38(1):76–80
Chatelaine KL: Harry Stack Sullivan, the formative years. Washington, D.C., University Press of America, 1981. xxiv, 553 p.
Crowley RM: Harry Stack Sullivan as social critic. **J Am Acad Psychoanal** 1981 Apr;9(2):211–26
Perry HS: Psychiatrist of America. The life of Harry Stack Sullivan. Cambridge, Belknap Press, 1982. 462 p.
Zimmerman J: Transcendent psychology: Erik H. Erikson, Erich Fromm, Karen Horney, Abraham H. Maslow, and Harry Stack Sullivan and the quest for a healthy humanity. Ph.D. Diss., Northwestern University. Evanston, 1982. vi, 498 p.

**Sulzberger, Marion Baldur, 1895–1983**
Baer RL, Kopf AW: Marion B. Sulzberger (1895–1983). **J Am Acad Dermatol** 1984 Jun;10(6):91A–96A
Cohen SG: In memoriam. Marion B. Sulzberger (1895–1983). A dermatologist's contributions to allergy. **J Allergy Clin Immunol** 1984 Dec;74(6):855–60
Sulzberger! Biography, autobiography, iconography. A posthumous festschrift: **Am J Dermatopathol** 1984 Aug;6(4):344–70

**Sumner, Francis Bertody, 1874–1945**
Provine WB: Francis B. Sumner and the evolutionary synthesis. **Stud Hist Biol** 1979;3:211–40

**Sumpter, Grover Cleveland, 1885–1965**
Collins BC: A round of calomel. **J Tenn Med Assoc** 1983 Sep;76(9):609–10

**Sun, Ssu-miao, 581–682**
Miyasita S: Son Shibo no keikenbô. (Sun Ssu-mo's empirical remedies.) **Kampo No Rinsho** 1973;20:544–7
Thomas L: Un manuel d'oculistique chinoise attribué a Sun Si-Miao des tang: le Yin hai jing wei. In Mazars G, ed: Les médecines traditionnelles de l'Asie. Strasbourg, Université Louis Pasteur, 1981. p. 85–92.

**Sun Yat-Sen, 1866–1925**
Dodds WR: From medicine to president [Sun Yat Sen]. **Practitioner** 1981 Sep;225(1359):1342–3

**Sung Tz'u, 1186–1249**
McKnight BE, ed: The washing away of wrongs: forensic medicine in thirteenth-century China. Ann Arbor, Center for Chinese Studies, University of Michigan, 1981. xv, 181 p.

**Supliceau, Théodore, fl. ca. 1835**
Delaveau P: Sur le 'registre pour l'inscription des poisons' d'un pharmacien tourangeau (1833–1841). **Rev Hist Pharm (Paris)** 1984 Jun;31(261):144–50

**Surflet, Richard, ca. 1560–ca. 1605**
Cooke MA: Richard Surflet, translator and practitioner in physic. **Med Hist** 1981 Jan;25(1):41–56

**Susini, Clemente, 1754–1814**
Azzaroli ML, Lanza B: La Venere scomponibile. **Kos** 1984 May;1(4):65–81

**Susruta**
Das S: Shusruta of India, the pioneer in the treatment of urethral stricture. **Surg Gynecol Obstet** 1983 Dec;157(6):581–2
Das S: Shusruta of India: pioneer in vesicolithotomy. **Urology** 1984 Mar;23(3):317–9
Hauben DJ: Sushruta Samhita (Sushruta's Collection) (800–600 B.C.?). Pioneers of plastic surgery. **Acta Chir Plast (Prague)** 1984;26(2):65–8
Singhal GD, Singh RH, Shukla KP: Non-operative considerations in ancient Indian surgery: (based on Susruta Samhita, Cikitsa-Sthana, chapters 24–40). Varanasi, India, Institute of Medical Sciences, Banaras Hindu University, 1971. xlii, 396 p.
Singhal GD, Guru LV: Anatomical and obstetric considerations in ancient Indian surgery: based on Sarirasthana of Susruta Samhita. Varanasi, India, Institute of Medical Sciences, Banaras Hindu University, 1973. L, 241 p.
Sugimoto S: [An interpretation of a syndrome depicted in Buddhist cannon [sic] through Susruta Samhita] (Jpn). **Igakushi Kenkyu** 1980;54:12–7
Wijesinha SS: El Zahrawi (936–1013 AD), the father of operative surgery. **Ann R Coll Surg Engl** 1983 Nov;65(6):423

**Süssmilch, Johann Peter, 1707–1767**
Hecht J: Johann Peter Sussmilch, point alpha ou omega de la science démographique naïve? **Ann Demogr Hist (Paris)** 1979;:101–34

**Sutton, Samuel, fl. 1743**
Zuckerman A: Scurvy and the ventilation of ships in the Royal Navy: Samuel Sutton's contribution. **Eighteenth Cent Stud** 1976/77;10:222–34

**Suzor, François-Michel, 1756–1810**
Lessard R: François-Michel Suzor. In Dictionary of Canadian biography, 1801 to 1820. Volume 5, 1983. p. 788–9.

**Suzuki, Masa**
Takahashi M: [Nurses in the history of nursing. (1) Masa Suzuki] (Jpn). **Kango Kyoiku** 1981 Jun;22(6):399–403

**Svevo, Italo, 1861–1928**
Mahler-Schachter E: Svevo, Trieste and the Vienna Circle: Zeno's analyst analysed. **Eur Stud Rev** 1982;12(1):45–66

**Swain, Clara, 1834–1910**
Lahiri K: Clara Swain, MD (1834–1910) and her work in India. **Women Health** 1983 Spring;8(1):3–6

**Swammerdam, Jan, 1637–1680**
Baer KE von: Reden gehalten in wissenschaftlichen Versammlungen und kleinere Aufsätze vermischten Inhalts. With an introduction by K. B. Sterling. New York, Arno Press, 1978. Three volumes in two. (Reprint. St. Petersburg, 1864/1876/1873).
Brazier MA: The problem of neuromuscular action: two 17th century Dutchmen. In Rose FC, Bynum WF, ed: Historical aspects of the neurosciences. New York, Raven, 1982. p. 13–22.
Fournier M: Jan Swammerdam en de 17e eeuwse microscopie. **Tijdschr Geschied Geneeskd** 1981;4(2)74–86
Gysel C: Jan Swammerdam (1637–1680–1980), zijn Cartesianisme en de fysiologie van het kauwstelsel (II). **Ned Tijdschr Tandheelkd** 1981 Jul–Aug;88(7–8):274–7
Gysel C: Jan Swammerdam (1637– 1680– 1980), zijn Cartesianisme en de fysiologie van het kauwstelsel (SLOT). **Ned Tijdschr Tandheelkd** 1981 Nov;88(11):414–6
Gysel C: Jan Swammerdam (1637–1680–1980), zijn Cartesianism en de fysiologie van het kauwstelsel (I). **Ned Tijdschr Tandheelkd** 1981 Jun;88(6):238–41
Houtzager HL: Jan Swammerdam [Jan Swammerdam]. **Spiegel Hist** 1980;15(5):295–300
Lindeboom GA: De verdiensten van Jan Swammerdam voor de medische wetenschap. **Ned Tijdschr Geneeskd** 1980 Dec 13;124(50):2135–41
Lindeboom GA: Jan Swammerdam als microscopist. **Tijdschr Geschied Geneeskd** 1981;4(2):87–110
Lindeboom GA: Jan Swammerdam (1637–1680) and his Biblia Naturae. **Clio Med** 1982 Dec;17(2–3):113–31
Lindeboom GA, ed: Het cabinet van Jan Swammerdam (1637–1680). Facsimile reprinted from 1681 ed., Amsterdam, Rodopi, 1980. xxiv, 16 p.
Palm LC: Van Leeuwenhoek en Swammerdam cartesiaanse microscopisten. **Spiegel Hist** 1979;14(4):223–9
Palm LC: Bij een beeld van Swammerdam. **Tijdschr Geschied Geneeskd** 1981;4:61–2
Visser RP: Theorie en praktijk van Swammerdams wetenschappelijke methode in zijn entomologie. **Tijdschr Geschied Geneeskd** 1981;4(2):63–72

**Swan, George E.**
Reed LA: Doctor Swan's restorative waters. **Wis Mag Hist** 1980–81;64(2):124–6

**Swedenborg, Emanuel, 1688–1772**
Gejvall NG: Swedenborg--a man with head enough for two. **Ossa** 1978;5:123–31

**Sweetser, William, 1797–1875**
Grob GN, ed: The beginnings of mental hygiene in America. Three selected essays 1833–1850. New York, Arno, 1973. Various paginations. Includes works by Amariah Brigham (1833); William Sweetser (1850); Samuel B. Woodward (1840).

**Swieten, Gerard van, 1700–1772**
Schmid-Schönbein H: Die Ursprünge der medizinischen Hämorheologie im 18. Jahrhundert: H. Boerhaave, A. v. Haller und G. van Swieten. **Vasa** 1984;Suppl 12:10–31

**Swift, Jonathan, 1667–1745**
Powell F: Dean Swift and the Dublin Foundling Hospital. **Studies** 1981;70(278–9):162–70
Smith FN: Swift and cannabis. **Am Notes Queries** 1983 Nov–Dec;22(3–4):37–9

**Switzer, Mary Elizabeth, 1900–1971**
Christie J: Mary Elizabeth Switzer. In: Notable American women. The modern period. Cambridge, Mass., Belknap-Harvard Univ. Press, 1980. 4:669–70.

**Sychugov, Sabbatir Ivanovich, 1841–1902**
Il'in AI: S. I. Sychugov--osnovopolozhnik sanitarnoĭ organizatsii Vladimirskoĭ gubernii. **Gig Sanit** 1983 Nov;:(11):53–5

**Sydenham, Thomas, 1624–1689**
Bates DG: Sydenham and social history. **Soc Soc Hist Med Bull (Lond)** 1980;27:27–9

Borodulin VI: T. Sidengam i razvitie klinicheskoĭ meditsiny (k 300-letiiu opisaniia podagry). **Ter Arkh** 1984;56(1):135-8
Boss J: The relation of clinical to non-clinical medicine according to Thomas Sydenham (1624-1689). In E. Schultheisz, ed: History of physiology. Oxford, Elmsford, New York, Pergamon, 1981. xvi, 208 p. (Advances in Physiological Sciences. Proceedings of the 28th International Congress of Physiological Sciences, Budapest, 1980. Volume 21). p. 9-21.
Day RA: Thomas Sydenham (1624-1689). **Friends P. I. Nixon Med Hist Libr** 1977 Oct;6:3-8
Taylor FK: Sydenham's disease entities. **Psychol Med** 1982 May;12(2):243-50

**Sydow, Frans Edvard von, 1828-1914**
Sydow C von: Notiser från Frans von Sydows utrikes studieresor 1861-1886. **Nord Medicinhist Arsb** 1984;:117-28

**Sykes, William Stanley, 1894-1961**
Sykes WS: Essays on the first hundred years of anaesthesia. 3 vols. Park Ridge, Illinois, Wood Library-Museum of Anesthesiology, 1982. 171, 187, 272 p. (Vols. 1 and 2 are reprints of 1960 ed; Vol. 3 is edited by R. H. Ellis)

**Sysin, Alekseĭ Nikolaevich, 1879-1956**
Mikhaĭlov GN: Voprosy okhrany truda v rabotakh A. N. Sysina. **Gig Tr Prof Zabol** 1982 Oct;(10):41-3
Vasil'ev KG: A. N. Sysin: 1879-1956. Moskva, Meditsina, 1981. 54 p.
Vasil'ev KK: Rol' A. N. Sysina v organizatsii i provendenii vserossiĭskikh (vsesoiuznykh) s'ezdov bakteriologov, épidemiologov i sanitarynykh vracheĭ. **Gig Sanit** 1980 Apr;(4):31-3

**Szasz, Thomas Stephen, 1920-**
Laor N: Szasz, Feuchtersleben, and the history of psychiatry. **Psychiatry** 1982;45(4):316-24
Laor N: Old whig psychiatry: the Szaszian variant. **Isr J Psychiatr Relat Sci** 1982;19(3):215-27
Wiegand R: Thomas S. Szasz. In J. Rattner, ed: Wandlungen der Psychoanalyse. Wien, Europaverlag, 1980. p. 333-68.

**Szechenyi, István, 1791-1860**
Tóth A: Orvosok Széchenyi naplójában. **Orv Hetil** 1981 May 31;122(22):1329-37

**Székely, August von, 1864-1927**
Szállási A: Székey Agoston--a szerkesztöi másodvonalból. **Orv Hetil** 1983 Jan 9;124(2):95-7

**Szentágothai, János, 1912-**
Szentágothai J: Too 'much' and too 'soon'. A lifetime of inquiry into the functional organization of the nervous system. **Acta Biol Acad Sci Hung** 1982;33(2-3):107-26

**Szily, Adolf, 1848-1920**
Bíró I: Szily Adolf, Szily Aurél. **Orv Hetil** 1983 Aug 21;124(34):2065-6

**Szily, Aurel von, 1880-1945**
Bíró I: Szily Adolf, Szily Aurél. **Orv Hetil** 1983 Aug 21;124(34):2065-6

**Szuman, Leon Stanisław, 1852-1920**
Sieńkowski E: Dr med. Leon Stanisław Szuman (1852-1920), chirurg, społecznik, poeta. **Arch Hist Med (Warsz)** 1984;47(1):133-41

**Szumowski, Władisław, 1875-1954**
Chrześciewski L: Filozofia medycyny Wøadysøawa Szumowskiego (1875-1954). **Wiad Lek** 1984 Feb 15;37(4):321-2
Chrześciewski L: Filozofia medycyny Władysława Szumowskiego (1875-1954). **Wiad Lek** 1984 Apr 15;37(8):653-4

**Szwejcerowa-Gruszczyńska, Aniela, 1905-1981**
Ostrowska T: Dr Aniela Szwejcerowa-Gruszczyńska (1905-1981); Wspomnienie pośmiertne. **Arch Hist Med (Warsz)** 1981;44(3/4):227-35

**Szymanowski, Julius von, 1829-1868**
Rogers BO: Julius von Szymanowski (1829--1868). His life and contributions to plastic surgery. **Plast Reconstr Surg** 1979 Oct;64(4):465-78

**Szymonowicz, Władysław, 1869-1939**
Loetzke HH: Die wissenschaftlichen Arbeiten des polnischen Histologen Władysław Szymonowicz während seiner Studienaufenthalte 1895 und 1896 in Berlin. **Arch Hist Med (Warsz)** 1979;42(3):359-64

## T

**Tabit ibn Qurra**
Weisser U: Die hippokratische Lehre von den Siebenmonatskindern bei Galen und Tabit ibn Qurra. **Sudhoffs Arch** 1979;63(3):209-38

**Tadini, fl. 1758-1789**
Fechner PU, Fechner MU: Tadini, the man who invented the artificial lens. **J Am Intraocul Implant Soc** 1979 Jan;5(1):22-3
Fechner PU, Fechner MU, Reis H: Der Okulist Tadini. Zur Geschichte der künstlichen Augenlinse. **Klin Monatsbl Augenheilkd** 1980 Jun;176(6):1003-11

**Taeuber, Irene Barnes, 1906-1974**
Keyfitz N: Irene Barnes Taeuber. In: Notable American women. The modern period. Cambridge, Mass., Belknap-Harvard Univ. Press, 1980. 4:672-3.

**Taft, Jessie, 1882-1960**
Axinn J: Jessie Taft. In: Notable American women. The modern period. Cambridge, Mass., Belknap-Harvard Univ. Press, 1980. 4:673-5.

**Tailhandier, Marien, 1665-1738 or 9**
Lahaise R: Marien Tailhandier. In Dictionary of Canadian biography, 1701 to 1740. Volume 2, 1969. p. 617-8.

**Tainard, fl. 1076**
Karnofsky ES: The vision of Tainard, miraculum de quodam canonico Guatenensi per Sanctum Donatianum curato. In Sheils WJ, ed: The Church and healing. Papers read at the twentieth summer meeting and the twenty-first winter meeting of the Ecclesiastical History Society. Oxford, Basil Blackwell for the Society, 1982. p. 15-24.

**Tait, Robert Lawson, 1845-1899**
Shepherd JA: Lawson Tait, the rebellious surgeon (1845-1899). Lawrence, Kansas, Coronado Press, xv, 249 p.
Shepherd JA: Lawson Tait - disciple of Charles Darwin. **Br Med J [Clin Res]** 1982 May;284(6326):1386-7

**Takagi, Kenji, 1888-1963**
Takagi K: Arthroscope. Kenji Takagi. J. Jap. Orthop. Assoc., 1939. **Clin Orthop** 1982 Jul;(167):6-8

**Takano, Kyo**
Takâhashi M: [Nurses in the history of nursing. (2). Kyo Takano] (Jpn). **Kango Kyoiku** 1981 Jul;22(7):451-6

**Talachon, Marie-Vincent, 1753-1817**
Hillemand P, Gilbrin E, Segal A: Le père Elisée et la réforme des études médicales. **Hist Sci Med** 1981;15(2):159-65
Hillemand P, Gilbrin E: Le Père Elisée, premier chirurgien de Louis XVIII et la création de l'Académie de Médecine. **Bull Acad Natl Med (Paris)** 1981 Jan;165(1):23-6

**Taliaferro, William Hay, 1895-1973**
Talmage DW: William Hay Taliaferro: February 10, 1895-December 21, 1973. **Biogr Mem Natl Acad Sci** 1983;54:375-407

**Tal'iantsev, Anton Ivanovich, 1858-1929**
Tarasonov VM: Vklad A.I. Tal'iantseva v éksperimental'noe issledovanie patologii serdechno-sosudistoĭ sistemy. **Patol Fiziol Eksp Ter** 1980 Mar-Apr;(2):92-3

**Talma, François-Joseph, 1763-1826**
Fouré J: Talma - the dentist who became the greatest French actor of all times. **Bull Hist Dent** 1983 Apr;31(1):3-10

**Talochon, Marie-Vincent (Père Elisée), 1753-1817**
Hillemand P, Gilbrin E: Le père Elisée (1753-1817); premier chirurgien de Louis XVIII. **Hist Sci Med** 1980;14(2):233-40

**Tanaka, Shin, 1920-**
Shima K: [Endless voyage. The life of Ms. Shin Tanaka. 5. Chapter 2.] (Jpn). **Josanpu Zasshi** 1982 Nov;36(11):946-53 (continued regularly)

**Tandler, Julius, 1869-1936**
Sablik K: Julius Tandler: Mediziner und Sozialreformer: eine Biographie. Wien, A. Schendl, 1983. 389 p.

**Taniguchi, Joshiaki**
Inomata H: Yoshiaki Taniguchi, M.D. **Jpn J Ophthalmol** 1983;27(1):1-8

**Tansini, Iginio, 1855-1943**
Maxwell GP: Iginio Tansini and the origin of the latissimus dorsi musculocutaneous flap. **Plast Reconstr Surg** 1980 May;65(5):686-92

**Tao, Lieh**
Hsu K: [Tao Lieh---the pioneer in neurosciences of our country] (Chi). **Sheng Li Ko Hsueh Chin Chan** 1980 Apr;11(4):376-8

**Tardieu, Ambroise Auguste, 1818-1879**
Fernandez D: Francois Carlier, La Prostitution antiphysique (1857). Précédé de La Pederastie (1887) par Ambroise Tardieu. Paris, Le Sycomore, 1981. ix, 250 p.
Gaillard J: Le médecin et l'avortement au XIXe siècle. **Histoire** 1979;16:35-7

**Tarnier, Stéphane, 1828-1897**
Logeay R: Bonheurs et malheurs de la clinique Tarnier. **Hist Sci Med** 1984;18(3):261-70

**Tashjian, Levon Donald, 1934-**
Esman AH: The study of lives: discussion of Tashjian and Shaw. **Adolesc Psychiatry** 1982;10:99-105

**Tatarinov, Alexander Alekseevich, 1817-1886**
Walravens H: Alexander Tatarinov (1817-1886)--russischer Arzt und Sinologe, eine biobibliographische Skizze. **Sudhoffs Arch** 1980;64(4):392-6

**Tatishchev, Vasilii Nikitich, 1686-1750**
Palkin BN: V. N. Tatishchev i zdravookhranenie Astrakhanskoĭ gubernii. **Sov Zdravookhr** 1982;(4):65-8

**Tatum, Edward Lawrie, 1909-1975**
Kopp C: The J. H. B. Archive report; the Edward Lawrie Tatum papers at the Rockefeller University Archives. **J Hist Biol** 1982 Spring;15(1):153-4

Kopp C: The Edward Lawrie Tatum papers. **Mendel Newsl** 1981 Jul;20:1-2
Lederberg J: Edward Lawrie Tatum. **Annu Rev Genet** 1979;13:1-5

**Tauffer, Vilmos, 1851-1934**
Lampé L: Egységes nemzetközi szülészeti adatgyüjtés (Tauffer nyomdokain). **Orv Hetil** 1982 Apr 11;123(15):895-903
Raics J: Tauffer Vilmos mint szülészeti miniszteri biztos. **Orvostort Kozl** 1980;89-91(26 no 1-3):137-55

**Tausk, Victor, 1879-1919**
Eissler KR: Victor Tausk's suicide. New York, International Universities Press, 1983. 322 p.

**Taussig, Helen Brooke, 1898-**
Engle MA: Biographies of great American pediatricians--Helen Brooke Taussig: the mother of pediatric cardiology. **Pediatr Ann** 1982 Jul;11(7):629-31
McNamara DG: Landmark perspective: the Blalock-Taussig operation and subsequent progress in surgical treatment of cardiovascular diseases. **JAMA** 1984 Apr 27;251(16):2139-41

**Tawara, Sunao**
International Symposium on Cardiac Pacing, 5th, Tokyo, 1976: Tawara memorial note. Tokyo, Organizing Committee of the Symposium, 1976. 28 p.

**Taylor, Alfred Swaine, 1806-1880**
Besson A: The Medico-Legal Tracts Collection of Dr. A. S. Taylor, FRCP. **J R Coll Physicians Lond** 1983 Apr;17(2):147-9

**Taylor, Euphemia Jane**
Buckwalter KC, Church OM: Euphemia Jane Taylor: an uncommon psychiatric nurse. **Perspect Psychiatr Care** 1979 May-Jun;17(3):125-31

**Taylor, Harry Pearson, 1862-1945**
Williams S: A 'Taylor made' practice. **Br Med J [Clin Res]** 1984 Jan 14;288(6411):116-8

**Taylor, Lucy Beaman Hobbs, 1833-1910**
Hofer K: Dr. Lucy Hobbs Taylor, first woman dentist. **CAL** 1981 Oct;45(4):13-5, 18
Saltzman BB: Saga of America's first woman dental graduate. **Dent Stud** 1983 Oct;62(1):24-5

**Teggart, Frederick John, 1870-1946**
Karp LE: Genetic drift. A question of discovery: Part II. **Am J Med Genet** 1983 Aug;15(4):533-5

**Tegnér, Esaias, 1782-1846**
Fehrman C: Esaias Tegnér and psychiatry: history of literature from medical view-point. **Sydsven Medicinhist Sallsk Arsskr** 1984;21:47-8

**Teichmann, Ludwik Karol, 1823-1895**
Stahnke J: Häminkristalle--Ludwik Teichmanns Blutnachweis. **Medizinhist J** 1981;16(4):391-413

**Teissler, Viktor, 1883-**
Kukurová E, Sajter V: Osobnost prof. PhDr. Viktora Teisslera a prvých 15 rokov existencie Ustavu lekárskej fyziky Univerzity Komenského v Bratislave. **Bratisl Lek Listy** 1983 Dec;80(6):725-30

**Teitelbaum, Philip, 1928-**
Distinguished scientific contribution awards for 1978 (Julian Hochberg, Philip Teitelbaum, Robert B. Zajonc).: **Am Psychol** 1979 Jan;34(1):35-47

**Teleki, Joseph, 1738-1796**
Csanak DF: Teleki József Szerepe egy XVIII. századi francia tudományos vitaban. **Szazadok** 1974;108(2):406-22

**Teleky, Ludwig, 1872-1957**
Buess H: Der Wiener Sozialmediziner Ludwig Teleky (1872-1957) und seine 'History of factory and mine hygiene'. **Wien Med Wochenschr** 1981 Oct 15;131(19):479-83
Buess H: Der Wiener Sozialmediziner Ludwig Teleky (1872-1957) und seine 'History of Factory and Mine Hygiene'. In Ganzinger K, Skopec M, Wyklicky H, ed: Festschrift für Erna Lesky zum 70. Geburtstag. Wien, Brüder Hollinek, 1981. p. 31-7.
Rodríguez Ocaña E: Aproximacion al concepto y practica de la medicina social en Ludwig Teleky (1872-1957). **Dynamis (Spain)** 1982;2:299-323

**Tellenbach, Hubertus, 1918-**
Kraus A, ed: Leib. Geist. Geschichte. Brennpunkte anthropologischer Psychiatrie. Festschrift zum 60. Geburtstag von Hubertus Tellenbach. With contributions by W. Baeyer, W. Blankenburg, H. G. Gadamer, W. Jacob, B. Kimura, H. Lang, A. Leder, G. Marcel, A Métraux, B. Pauleikhoff, H. Schipperges. Heidelberg, Hüthig, 1978. (Medizin im Wandel).

**Tello y Muñoz, Jorge Francisco, 1880-**
Ricoy JR: In memoriam: J. F. Tello. **Arch Neurobiol (Madr)** 1980 Nov-Dec;43(6):347-52

**Temple-Smith, E. C., d. 1968**
Hertzberg R: Three great ophthalmologists (E. C. Temple-Smith, Norman Gregg, Arthur D'Ombrain). **Med J Aust** 1979 Dec 15;2(12):649-50

**Ter-Arutiuniants, S. M., 1880-**
Belous VI, Mesiats NK: S. M. Ter-Arutiuniants--osnovatel' glaznoĭ sluzhby na Zhitomirshchine. **Oftalmol Zh** 1984;(1):63-4

**Teresa of Avila, Saint, 1515-1582**
Huguet M: Expérience mystique, pathologie mentale et condition féminine. **Penelope** 1983;(8):25-8

**Terman, Lewis Madison, 1877-1956**
Sears RR: Lewis Madison Terman. In Dictionary of American Biography, Suppl. 6, 1956-1960. p. 626-7, 1980.

**Terson, Jean, 1803-1884**
Emerit M: Un curé de l'aude atteint du mal du siècle: Jean Terson. In Congrès National des Sociétés Savantes, 102e, Limoges, 1977. Actes. Paris, 1978. Tome I, p. 351-60.

**Teulon, Giraud, d. 1887**
Amalric P: La naissance et les premiers pas de l'ophtalmoscopie binoculaire. **Bull Soc Ophthalmol Fr** 1982 Nov;82(11):1469-71

**Textor, Cajetan, 1782-1860**
Wirth M: Das Leben und Wirken des Chirurgen Cajetan von Textor. Diss. Würzburg, 1980. 107 p.

**Thalhammer, Otto, 1922-**
Festschrift Otto Thalhammer zum 60. Geburtstag: **Padiatr Padol** 1982;17(2):127-548

**Theiler, Arnold, 1867-1936**
Gutsche T: There was a man. The life and times of Sir Arnold Theiler K.C.M.G. of Onderstepoort. Cape Town, Timmins, 1979. 487 p.

**Theimer, Carl, 1823-1870**
Cižmář J: Botanist Carl Theimer (1823--1870) in the cultural context of Brno during the period of Mendel's research. **Folia Mendeliana** 1979;14:265-70

**Theodore of Sykeon, d. 613**
Horden P: Saints and doctors in the early Byzantine Empire: the case of Theodore of Sykeon. In Sheils WJ, ed: The Church and healing. Papers read at the twentieth summer meeting and the twenty-first winter meeting of the Ecclesiastical History Society. Oxford, Basil Blackwell for the Society, 1982. p. 1-13.

**Theophane Nonno, 10th cent.**
Felici L: L'opera medica die Teofane Nonno in manoscritti inediti. **Acta Med Hist Patav** 1981/82;28:59-74

**Theophrastus**
Longrigg J: Two notes on Theophrastus 'De sensibus.' **Philologus** 1975;119:163-9

**Theotocopuli, Dominico, called El Greco, d. 1614**
Ravin JG: El Greco of Toledo. **Ohio State Med J** 1982 Nov;78(11):745-53

**Thewlis, Malford Wilcox, 1889-1956**
History of the American Geriatrics Society: Malford W. Thewlis, J. Am. Geriatrics Soc. 1: 3, 1953. **J Am Geriatr Soc** 1981 Dec;29(12):544-9

**Thölde, Johann, fl. 1599-1624?**
Lenz HG: Der hessische Paracelsist Johann Thoelde. **Salzburger Beitr Paracelsusforsch** 1984;23:89-99

**Thomas Aquinas, Saint, 1225?-1274**
Cadden J: The medieval philosophy and biology of growth: Albertus Magnus, Thomas Aquinas, Albert of Saxony and Masilius of Inghen on Book I, Chapter V, of Aristotle's 'De generatione et corruptione.' With translated texts of Albertus Magnus and Thomas Aquinas. Ph. D. Diss. Indiana University. Bloomington, 1971. vii, 267 leaves.
Jung R: Sinnesphysiologische Bemerkungen zu Thomas von Aquinos Maxime der Sinneserkenntnis. **Sudhoffs Arch** 1980;64(4):371-84
Ushida N: Etude comparative de la psychologie d'Aristote, d'Avicenne et de St. Thomas d'Aquin. Tokyo, Keio Institute of Cultural and Linguistic Studies, 1968. vi, 231 p. (Studies in the humanities and social relations; v. 11.).

**Thomas, Henry M., 1861-1925**
Golden RL: Osler, 'E. Y. D.,' and hysteria. **JAMA** 1982 May 21;247(19):2698-9
Harvey AM: Henry M. Thomas: Johns Hopkins's first neurologist. **Johns Hopkins Med J** 1982 Jan;150(1):11-21

**Thomas, Lewis, 1913-**
Clyde WA, Fernald GW: Mycoplasmas: the pathogens' pathogens. **Cell Immunol** 1983 Nov;82(1):88-97
Farber SJ: A tribute to Lewis Thomas. **Cell Immunol** 1983 Nov;82(1):21-2
Green H: Some things that happened on Lew Thomas' floor. **Cell Immunol** 1983 Nov;82(1):98-101
Lawrence HS: An appreciation: notes of a Lewis Thomas-Watcher. **Cell Immunol** 1983 Nov;82(1):139-43
Lewis Thomas: **Cell Immunol** 1983 Nov;82(1):3-17
Paterson PY: LT/EAE and the MS quest. Going to the dogs and rats to study the patient. **Cell Immunol** 1983 Nov;82(1):55-74
Thomas L: The youngest science. Notes of medicine-watcher. New York, Viking Press, 1983. xvi, 270 p.
Wannamaker LW: The pathogenesis of rheumatic fever: Lewis Thomas and the Minnesota years. **Cell Immunol** 1983 Nov;82(1):82-7

Weissmann G: From Auden to arachidonate: a tribute and a hypothesis. **Cell Immunol** 1983 Nov;82(1):117-26

**Thomas, Mary Frame Myers, 1816-1888**
Bonsett CA: Mary Frame Thomas, M.D. (1816-1888). **J Indiana State Med Assoc** 1980;73:270

**Thompson, Clara Mabel, 1893-1958**
Perry HS: Clara Mabel Thompson. In: Notable American women. The modern period. Cambridge, Mass., Belknap-Harvard Univ. Press, 1980. 4:680-3.

**Thompson, Isaac, 1775-1852**
Ferry AP, Ferry MK: Dr. Isaac Thompson and his celebrated eye water. **Ophthalmology** 1984 May;91(5):528-37

**Thompson, Mary Harris, 1829-1895**
Beatty WK: Mary Harris Thompson--pioneer surgeon and hospital founder. **Proc Inst Med Chic** 1981 Jul-Sep;34(3):83-6

**Thompson, Silvanus Phillips, 1851-1916**
Boag JW: Silvanus Phillips Thompson--some studies in the 'prehistory' of X rays. **Br J Radiol** 1984 Jan;57(673):1-15
Ramsey LJ: Some notable early contributors to radiography--Thompson, Jackson and Campbell Swinton. **Radiography** 1980 Dec;46(552):289-97

**Thomson, Elihu, 1853-1937**
Carlson WB: Innovation in medical technology: Elihu Thomson, General Electric, and X rays in 1896. **Med Instrum** 1982 Jul-Aug;16(4):218

**Thomson, Elizabeth Harriet, 1907-**
Wilson LG, ed: Benjamin Silliman and his circle: Studies on the influence of Benjamin Silliman on science in America. Prepared in honor of Elizabeth H. Thomson. New York, Science History Publications, 1979. x, 227 p. Contributions by S. D Beckham, J. C. Greene, L. I. Kuslan, G. Robinson, M. W. Rossiter.

**Thomson, Harriet Blackstock**
Thomson LR: Medical illustration: our early years--reminiscing in letters: Harriet Blackstock Thomson to Ranice Crosby. **J Biocommun** 1981 Jul;8(2):13-5

**Thomson, John, 1808-1884**
McGahan EW: John Thomson. In Dictionary of Canadian biography, 1881-1890. 1982;11:878-9.

**Thomson, Samuel, 1769-1843**
Bonnabeau RC: Samuel Thomson and Thomsonian medicine. The near-destruction of American medicine. **Minn Med** 1984 May;67(5):285-7
Wallace DJ: Thomsonians: the people's doctors. **Clio Med** 1980 Jul;14(3-4):169-86

**Thomson, William (Lord Kelvin), 1824-1907**
Merton RK, Sills DL, Stigler SM: The Kelvin dictum and social science: an excursion into the history of an idea. **J Hist Behav Sci** 1984 Oct;20(4):319-31

**Thoreau, Henry David, 1817-1862**
Morowitz HJ: Thoreau as a scientist. **Hosp Pract [Off]** 1984 Nov;19(11):143-6, 151

**Thorek, Max, 1880-1960**
Bush RB: Max Thorek. In Dictionary of American Biography, Suppl. 6, 1956-1960. p. 631-2, 1980.
Ruberg RL, Shah RR: Max Thorek: a surgeon for all seasons. In Romm S, ed: Symposium on historical perspectives of plastic surgery. Philadelphia, Saunders, 1983. p. 611-8.

**Thorndike, Lynn, 1882-1965**
Clagett M: Lynn Thorndike. In Dictionary of American biography, 1961-1965. Suppl. 7, 1981. p. 741-2.

**Threlkeld, Caleb, 1676-1728**
Nelson EC: 'In the Contemplation of Vegetables'--Caleb Threlkeld (1676-1728), his life, background and contribution to Irish botany. **J Soc Bibliogr Nat Hist** 1979 Nov;9(3):257-73

**Thucydides, b. ca. 460 B.C.**
Habs H: Immunologische Begriffe bei Thukydides. **Zentralbl Bakteriol Mikrobiol Hyg [A]** 1982 Jun;252(2):143-6
Lichtenthaeler C: Outé gar iatori èrkoun to proton therapeuontes agnoia. **Hermes** 1979, 1978;107(3):270-86
Longrigg J: Thucydides and the great plague of Athens. In International Congress of the History of Medicine, 27th, Barcelona, 1980. Actas. Barcelona, Académia de Ciències Mèdiques de Catalunya i Balears, 1981. p. 281-8.
Poole JC, Holladay AJ: Thucydides and the plague of Athens. **Classical Q** 1979;29:282-300
Poole JC, Holladay AJ: Thucydides and the plague: a footnote. **Classical Q** 1982;32:235-6
Radt SL: Zu Thukydides' Pestbeschreibung. **Mnemosyne** 1978;31:233-45; 1979;32:163
Thucydides: The plague in Athens. Thucydides. The history of the Peloponnesian War. Translated by Thomas Hobbes. **NC Med J** 1980 Apr;41(4):230-2
Thucydides and the Athenian plague: a reconsideration of the evidence: **Pharm Hist (London)** 1984 Dec;14(4):6-7

**Thudicum, John Louis William, 1829-1901**
Rafaelsen OJ: Thudichum: the founder of neurochemistry. In Rose FC, Bynum WF, ed: Historical aspects of the neurosciences. New York, Raven, 1982. p. 293-305.

**Thunberg, Carl Peter, 1743-1828**
Fodstad H: Carl Peter Thunberg: Swedish pioneer of Occidental medicine in Japan. **Neurol Med Chir (Tokyo)** 1982 Jul;22(7):577-81
Thunberg CP: Ma visite à l'Ecole Vétérinaire d'Alfort en 1771. **Hist Med Vet** 1977;2(4):123-6

**Thurneisser zum Thurn, Leonhard, 1531-1596**
Junkte F: Ueber Leonhard Thurneisser zum Thurn und seine deutschen Kalendar 1572-1584. **Arch Gesch Buchwes** 1978;19:1349-400
Junkte F: Ueber Leonhard Thurneisser zum Thurn und seine Schriften nach seine Flucht aus Berlin (1584). **Arch Gesch Buchwes** 1980;21:679-718
Möhsen JK: Beiträge zur Geschichte der Wissenschaften in der Marke Brandenburg; Leben Leonhard Thurneissers zum Thurn. München, Fritsch, 1976. 226 p.
Morys P: Medizin und Pharmazie in der Kosmologie Leonhard Thurneissers zum Thurn (1531-1596). Husum, Matthiesen, 1982. 179 p. (Abhandlungen zur Geschichte der Medizin und der Naturwissenschaften, 43).

**Tiberio, Vincenzo, 1869-1915**
Daglio P: Vincenzo Tiberio e la scoperta della penicillina. Una grande conquista a cavallo di due secoli. **Minerva Med** 1982 Jul 14;73(28-29):2005-9

**Ticknor, Francis Orray, 1822-1874**
Gay EW: Francis O. Ticknor, 19th century physician-poet--Part I and II. **J Med Assoc Ga** 1981;70(7):499-503, (8):561-4

**Tigerstedt, Robert Adolf Armand, 1853-1923**
Marks LS, Maxwell MH: Tigerstedt and the discovery of renin. An historical note. **Hypertension** 1979 Jul-Aug;1(4):384-8

**Tilt, Archibald Preston, 1854?-1890**
Sakula A: Baroness Burdett-Coutts' garden party: the International Medical Congress, London, 1881. **Med Hist** 1982 Apr;26(2):183-90

**Tilt, Edward John, 1815-1893**
Wilbush J: Historical perspective: Tilt, E. J. and the change of life (1857)--the only work on the subject in the English language. **Maturitas** 1980 Dec;2(4):259-67

**Timakov, Vladimir Dmitrievich, 1905-1977**
Bochkov NP: V. D. Timakov (1905--1977). Moskva, Meditsina, 1982. 62 p.

**Timme, Walter, 1874-1956**
Morris JP: Walter Timme. In Dictionary of American Biography, Suppl. 6, 1956-1960. p. 634-5, 1980.

**Timmermann, Guenter, 1908-1979**
Eichler W: Nachruf auf Günter Timmermann (zugleich eine wissenschaftsgeschichtliche Studie zum Disput um die Fahrenholzsche Regel). **Angew Parasitol** 1981 Feb;22(1):53-6

**Timof'eeff-Ressovsky, Nikolai Wladimirovich, 1900-1981**
Nikolai Wladimirovich Timof'eeff-Ressovsky, (1900-1981): **Genetics** 1982 Jan;100(1):1-5

**Timur, the Great, 1336-1405**
Lindgren U: The problems of being a foreigner: Ruy Gonzáles de Clavijo's journey to Samarkand. **Clio Med** 1980 Jul;14(3-4):225-34

**Tinel, Jules, 1879-1952**
Clark D: Jules Tinel and Tinel's sign. In Romm S, ed: Symposium on historical perspectives of plastic surgery. Philadelphia, Saunders, 1983. p. 627-8.

**Tissot, Clément Joseph, 1747-1826**
Imbroscio C: Tissot e il suo tempo. **Atti Accad Sci Ist Bologna** 1978-1979, reçu 1980;67(1):323-43

**Tissot H.**
Zabludovskiĭ PE: K 200-letiiu knigi 'Nastavlenie narodu v rassuzhdenii ego zdorov'ia'. **Feldsher Akush** 1982;47(4):52-3

**Tissot, Samuel Auguste André David, 1728-1797**
Godonnèche J: La dégradation de la santé des gens de lettres d'après Tissot. In: Congrès National des Sociétés Savantes, 99e, Besançon, 1974. Comptes Rendus. Paris, 1976. Section des Sciences, Fasc. V. p. 235-41.
Jéquier MC: Auguste Tissot (1728-1797). **Rev Med Suisse Romande** 1984 May;104(5):337-41
Portmann ML: Relations d'Auguste Tissot (1728-1797), médecin à Lausanne, avec le patriciat bernois. **Gesnerus** 1980;37(1/2):21-7
Tissot SA: De la santé des gens de lettres; présentation de F. Azouvi. Genève and Paris, Slatkine, 1981. viii, 246 p. Reprint of Lausanne ed., 1768.

**Titchener, Edward Bradford, 1867-1927**
Dazzi N, Ferruzzi F: Wundt, Titchener e la psicologia americana. **Stor Crit Psicol** 1980;1(1):29-52
Evans RB, MacLeod RB: Foreword to Systematic psychology: Prolegomena by Edward Bradford Titchener. Ithaca, London, Cornell University Press, 1972. v-xvi.
Leahey TH: The mistaken mirror: on Wundt's and Titchener's

psychologies. **J Hist Behav Sci** 1981;17:273-82

**Titian, Vecelli, 1477 or 1489-1576**
Putscher M: Ein Totentanz von Tizian. Die 17 grossen Holzschnitte zur Fabrica Vesals (1538-1542). In Göpfert W, Otten HH, ed: Metavoeite: wandelt euch durch neues Denken. Düsseldorf, Triltsch, 1983. p. 23-40.
Schupbach W: Doctor Parma's medicinal macaronic: poem by Bartolotti, pictures by Giorgione and Titian. [Wellcome MS 461]. **J Warburg Courtauld Inst** 1978;41:147-91, 350

**Tito, Josip Broz, 1892-1980**
Dragić D: Drug tito i njegov doprinos razvoju vojnomedicinske misli. **Vojnosanit Pregl** 1980 May;37:54-7

**Todd, John L., 1876-1949**
Fallis AM: John L. Todd: Canada's first professor of parasitology. **Can Med Assoc J** 1983 Sep 1;129(5):486, 488-90

**Todd, Robert Bentley, 1809-1860**
Lyons JB: The neurology of Robert Bentley Todd. In Rose FC, Bynum WF, ed: Historical aspects of the neurosciences. New York, Raven, 1982. p. 137-50.

**Tököly, Imre, 1657-1705**
Vladár I: Thököly Imre fejedelem megrokkanása. **Orv Hetil** 1979 Sep 23;120(38):2317-8

**Toldy (Schedel), Ferenc, 1805-1875**
Antall J, Kapronczay K: Toldy Ferenc az orvos. **Orvostort Kozl** 1979;87-88(25 no 1-2):105-22
Hidvégi L: Toldy Ferenc ceglédi iskolaéveiröl. **Orv Hetil** 1984 Sep 2;125(36):2203-5

**Tolman, Edward Chace, 1886-1959**
Amundson R: E. C. Tolman and the intervening variable: a study in the epistemological history of psychology. **Philos Sci** 1983;50:268-82
Hilgard ER: Edward Chace Tolman. In Dictionary of American Biography, Suppl. 6, 1956-1960. p. 639-41, 1980.

**Tolmie, William Fraser, 1812-1886**
Lamb WK: William Fraser Tolmie. In Dictionary of Canadian biography, 1881-1890. 1982;11:885-8.

**Tolstoĭ, Lev Nikolaevich, 1828-1910**
Dohnány L: L. N. Tolsztoj az egészségügyröl. **Orv Hetil** 1982 Aug 8;123(32):1985-8
Gurevich SA: Lev Tolstoĭ i psikhiatriia. **Zh Nevropatol Psikhiatr** 1981;81(9):1386-9
Schein CJ: The death of Ivan Ilych; an axiomatic hypothesis. **NY State J Med** 1981 Mar;81(3):416
Smyrniw W: Tolstoy's depiction of death in the context of recent studies of the 'experience of dying.' **Can Slavonic Pap** 1979;21(3):367-79

**Tomcsik, József, 1898-1964**
Kenéz J: József Tomcsik. Life and activity of an outstanding Hungarian microbiologist. **Ther Hung** 1980;28(4):189-90

**Tomes, John, 1815-1895**
Herschfeld JJ: Sir John Tomes, dental pioneer. **Bull Hist Dent** 1981 Oct;29(2):94-8

**Tomíček, Oldřich, 1891-**
Votavová J: Prof. PhDr. PhMr. O. Tomíček a jeho analytická škola. **Cesk Farm** 1984 Jun;33(5):213-4

**Tomsa, Vladimir Bogamilowitsch, 1831-**
Trojan S, Trávníčkova E: Přednášky Vladimíra Tomsy. **Cesk Fysiol** 1979;80(5):471-2

**Tönnis, Wilhelm, 1898-1978**
Geiger I: Das Leben und Werk von Wilhelm Tönnis unter besonderer Berücksichtigung seiner Würzburger Zeit. Diss. Würzburg, 1981. 109 p.

**Toole, Harry I., ca. 1899-**
Toole HI: Historical studies. Athens, [s.n.], 1984. 608 p. (Greek with English summaries) Includes a collection of the author's previously published essays, mostly on Greek medicine, with a short autobiographical sketch and bibliography.

**Topchibashev, Mustafa Agaevich, 1895-**
Aĭrapetova RA, Kiazimov RA, ed: M. A. Topchibashev. Baku, Izd-vo Akademii nauk Azerbaĭdzhanskoĭ SSR, 1965. 66 p.

**Topinard, Paul, 1830-1911**
Arquiola E: Topinard: medico y antropologo fisico. **Asclepio** 1978-79;30-31:41-61

**Törne, Frans Vilhelm, 1870-1949**
Gejrot T: Frans Vilhelm Törne. **Sydsven Medicinhist Sallsk Arsskr** 1984;21:129-34

**Toro, Luis de, b. 1532**
Sayans Castaños M: Importante impulso en el conocimiento cientifico dado por un medico placentino del siglo XVI. In: Sociedad Española de Historia de la Medicina. V Congreso Nacional. Madrid, 1977. **Asclepio** 1977;29:343-50

**Torres Estrada, Antonio**
Limón E: Homenaje al doctor Antonio Torres Estrada. **Gac Med Mex** 1984 May;120(5):205-12

**Torrigiani da Corniglio, Flaminio Domenico, 1729-1792**
Pini UA: I medici parmigiani nelle poesie del Frugoni. L'Ippocrate dei mori, Medico freddoloso. **Minerva Med** 1980 Sep 19;71(34):2438-9

**Tortelli, Giovanni, 1400-1466**
Kapronczay K: Két kevéssé ismert 15. századi orvostörténeti munka. **Orv Hetil** 1983 Jul 10;124(28):1701-5

**Tóth, Nep. János, 1833-1865**
Szállási A: 150 éve született Tóth N. János, az elsö dualista magyar szifidológus. **Orv Hetil** 1984 Jun 10;125(24):1457-8

**Tournefort, Joseph Pitton de, 1656-1708**
Tomasi LT: L'isola dei semplici. **Kos** 1984 Jun;1(5):61-84

**Towne, Joseph, 1806-1879**
Atherton DJ: Joseph Towne: wax modeler extraordinary. **J Am Acad Dermatol** 1980 Sep;3(3):311-6

**Townsend, Francis Everett, 1867-1960**
Bennett DH: Francis Everett Townsend. In Dictionary of American Biography, Suppl. 6, 1956-1960. p. 645-7, 1980.

**Toynbee, Arnold Joseph, 1899-1975**
Goldwert M: Toynbee and Jung: the historian and analytical psychology--a brief comment. **J Anal Psychol** 1983 Oct;28(4):363-6

**Tozzetti, Giovanni Targioni, 1712-1783**
Arrigoni T: Fra la curiosità e la scienza. **Kos** 1984 May;1(4):47-64
Knoefel PK: Famine and fever in Tuscany. Eighteenth century Italian concern with the environment. **Physis** 1979;21(1-4):7-35

**Trabucchi, Emilio**
Montorsi W, Pezzuoli G, Guzzon V: Influenza della farmacologia di Emilio Trabucchi nelle discipline chirurgiche e parachirurgiche. **Minerva Med** 1982 May 7;73(19):1255-68

**Trapham, Thomas, d. 1692?**
Ashcroft MT: Tercentenary of the first English book on tropical medicine, by Thomas Trapham of Jamaica. **Br Med J** 1979 Aug 25;2(6188):475-7

**Trapl, Jiří, 1880-**
Dopis prof. J. Trapla prof. L. Havláskovi: **Cesk Gynekol** 1983 Feb;48(1):51-5
Presl J: K stoletému výročí narození prof. MUDr. Jiřího Trapla--zakladatele československé perinatologie. **Cesk Gynekol** 1980 Sep;45(8):611-3

**Trappe, Antoine, 1767-1847**
Delooz F: Petites touches sur le portrait de Saint-Etienne-aux-Clos: Antoine Trappe, médecin (1767-1847). **Lemouzi** 1981;80:411-30

**Treil, Sylvie**
Bornstein S, Bitty L: Essai sur folie et roman: un auteur en quête de psychiatres. **Ann Med Psychol (Paris)** 1983 Nov;141(9):957-67

**Treitz, Václav, 1819-1872**
Dobiás J, Marek J: Dr. Václav Treitz (1819-1872). K 110. výročí úmrtí a 125. výročí vybudování patologickoanatomického ústavu v Praze. **Cas Lek Cesk** 1983 Apr 1;122(13):405-7

**Trélat, Ulysse, 1795-1879**
Biéder J: L'odyssée d'Ulysse Trélat (1795-1879). **Ann Med Psychol (Paris)** 1984 Jan;142(1):128-41

**Tremigliozzi, Gaetano, 1655-1710**
Renaldo JJ: A note on the history of medicine and a debate on Parnassus. **Bull Hist Med** 1979 Winter;53(4):606-13

**Trendelenburg, Friedrich, 1844-1924**
Sabiston DC: Trendelenburg's classic work on the operative treatment of pulmonary embolism. **Ann Thorac Surg** 1983 May;35(5):570-4

**Trethowan, William, 1860-1929**
Fleming DW: The founders of the college: Western Australia. **Aust NZ J Surg** 1981 Dec;51(6):623-4

**Treves, Frederick, 1853-1923**
Howell M, Ford P: The true history of the elephant man. Harmondsworth, England, Penguin Books, 1980. 223 p.
Karp LE: The elephant man. **Am J Med Genet** 1981;10(1):1-3
Riley J: The elephant man: 'Treat me as an equal' (John Merrick, Sir Frederick Treves). **Nurs Mirror** 1979 Nov 8;149(19):24-5
Waldron G: Sir Frederick Treves and the elephant man. **Lancet** 1980 Jul 5;2(8184):42

**Trevisa, John, ca. 1342-1402**
Seymour MC, et al, ed: On the properties of things. John Trevisa's translation of Bartholomaeus Anglicus De proprietatibus rerum. A critical text. 2 vols. Oxford, Oxford University Press, 1975. xix, 1397 p.

**Trigueros, Cándido Maria, fl. 1781**
Basante Pol RM, Castillo Tello MM: La correspondencia dirigida a D. Casimiro Gómez Ortega por D. Cándido M.a Trigueros. **Bol Soc Esp Hist Farm** 1981 Sep;32(127):137-47

**Tristán, Gaspar, fl. 1606**
Carreras Panchón A: El ejercicio profesional segun el testimonio de Gaspar Tristan. **Asclepio** 1980;32:87-92

**Trithemius, 1462–1516**
Brann NL: Was Paracelsus a disciple of Trithemius? **Sixteenth Century J** 1979;10(1):71–82

**Trocsányi, Imre, 1851–1888**
Szentgyörgyvölgyi G: Egy régi hajdúszoboszlói gyógyszerész: Trocsányi Imre és köre. **Orv Hetil** 1982 Nov 28;123(48):2972–3

**Troisier, Charles Emile, 1844–1919**
Morgenstern L: The Virchow–Troisier node: a historical note. **Am J Surg** 1979 Nov;138(5):703

**Trommsdorff, Johann Bartholomäus, 1770–1837**
Götz W: Die Briefe Jacques Peschiers aus Genf an Joh. Barth. Trommsdorff, Erfurt, als Beispiel für internationale pharmazeutische Kontakte zu Beginn des 19. Jahrhunderts. **Pharm Acta Helv** 1979;54(9–10):303–7
Götz W: J. B. Trommsdorffs 'Chemische Receptirkunst'. Bisher unbekannte Ubersetzungen und Ausgaben. **Beitr Gesch Pharm** 1982;31(14):107–10
Götz W: Die Bedeutung Johann Bartholomäus Trommsdorffs für die Entwicklung der Chemie in Deutschland zu Beginn des 19. Jahrhunderts. Ein Versuch anhand seiner Korrespondenz mit Justus von Liebig und Heinrich Emanuel Merck. In Dilg P, et al., ed: Perspektiven der Pharmaziegeschichte. Graz, Austria, Akademische Druck- u. Verlagsanstalt, 1983. p. 97–112.

**Troshin, Afanasiĭ Semenovich, 1913–**
Braun AD, Vereninov AA, Kaulin AB: Afanasiĭ Semenovich Troshin (k 70-letiiu so dnia rozhdeniia). **Tsitologiia** 1983 Jun;25(6):726–32

**Trotsky, Leon, 1879–1940**
Nicolino F: Trotskij e la psicoanalisi. **Nuova Riv Stor** 1978;62(5–6):605–25

**Trotter, Wilfred Batten Lewis, 1872–1935**
Black SP: Wilfred Trotter. **Surg Neurol** 1983 Mar;19(3):199–204

**Trotula de Ruggiero, 12th cent.**
Caffaratto TM: Rilettura e commento dell'opera 'De Mulierum passionibus' di Trotula de Ruggiero, o Trocta Salernitana. **Minerva Med** 1981 Nov 17;72(46):3123–31
Poitras JM: Trotula of Salerno. **Md State Med J** 1980 Apr;29(4):62–4
Rowland B: Exhuming Trotula, sapiens matrona of Salerno. **Florilegium** 1979;1:42–57

**Troup, James Macdonald, 1867–1964**
Findlay GH: South African tick-bite fever (1931–1981). **S Afr Med J** 1981 Dec 26;60(26):998–1000

**Trousseau, Armand, 1801–1867**
Stolinsky DC: Trousseau's phenomenon. **Blood** 1983 Dec;62(6):1304

**Trudeau, James de Berty, 1817?–1887**
Gifford GE: James de Berty Trudeau: physician-naturalist. **Bull Hist Med** 1980 Spring;54(1):78–94

**Trueta Raspall, José, 1897–1977**
Rodrigo A: Doctor Trueta: héroe anónimo de dos guerras. Barcelona, Plaza & Janes, 1978. 294 p.
Strubell M, ed: Trueta: surgeon in war and peace. The memoirs of Joep Trueta. London, Gollancz, 1980. 288 p.

**Truex, Raymond Carl, 1911–**
Ladman AJ: R. C. Truex memorial. **Anat Rec** 1981 Sep;201(1):3–11

**Truman, Harry S., 1884–1972**
Morgan AH: Is there a doctor in the house? or for the house? **Rev Am Hist** 1980;8(1):129–33
Poen MM: Harry S. Truman versus the medical lobby. The genesis of Medicare. Columbia, London, University of Missouri Press, 1979. xii, 260 p.

**Tsái, Ching-feng**
Tsai C: [Retrospect of a physiologist engaged in scientific research and education for 60 years] (Chi). **Sheng Li Ko Hsueh Chin Chan** 1982 Jul;13(3):193–200

**TSarvulanov, Neno, 1876–1925**
Todorov D: D-r Neno TSarvulvanov. Sofiia, Meditsina i fizkultura, 1981. 113 p.

**Tschaikowski, Peter Iljitsch, 1840–1893**
Böhme G: Medizinische Porträts berühmter Komponisten: Wolfgang Amadeus Mozart, Ludwig van Beethoven, Carl Maria von Weber, Frédéric Chopin, Peter Iljitsch Tschaikowski, Béla Bartók. 2. verbesserte und erweiterte Auflage. Stuttgart, New York, Gustav Fischer Verlag, 1981. xi, 199 p.

**Tschirch, Alexander, 1856–1939**
Mitteilung zur Tschirch Biographie: **Schweiz Apoth Ztg** 1979;117:558 (continued irregularly here and in Pharm. Ztg, Dtsch Apoth Ztg, and Oesterr. Apoth Ztg)

**Tsetkin, Maxim, 1883–1965**
Korotkikh RV, Gorelova LE, Shtil'man NL: M. Tsetkin (k 100-letiiu so dnia rozhdeniia). **Sov Zdravookhr** 1983;(11):63–6

**Tsiolkovskii, K. E.**
Kopanev VI: The importance of K. E. Tsiolkovskii's ideas in the formation and development of space medicine. **Biol Bull Acad Sci USSR** 1979 Nov–Dec;6(6):764–71

**Tswett, Mikhail Semenovich, 1872–1919**
Senchenkova EM: [The importance of M. S. Tswett's investigations of the carotinoids.] (Rus). **Istor Biol Issled** 1978;7:65–92

**Tuckwell, Gertrude, fl. 1890–1920**
Morris J: The Gertrude Tuckwell collection (Trades Union Congress, Gt. Russell St., London, W.C.1.). **Hist Workshop J** 1978;5:155–62

**Tucovic, Dimitrije, 1881–1914**
Lukić D: Alkoholizam u vidjenju Dimitrija Tucovića. **Srp Arh Celok Lek** 1983 Mar;111(3):397–402
Lukić D: Gledišta Dimitrija Tucovića o tuberkulozi. **Srp Arh Celok Lek** 1981;109(12):1677–86

**Tulloch, William John, 1887–1966**
Green DM: William John Tulloch. In Dictionary of national biography, 1961–1970. Suppl. 8, 1981. p. 1019–20.

**Tulp, Nicolaas, 1593–1674**
Cremone JC: The anatomy lesson of Dr. Nicolaas Tulp. **J Hand Surg** 1982 Sep;7(5):530
Pytel' AIa: Nicolaus Van Tul'p – vydaiushchiĭsia anatom i khirurg (k 340-letiiu opublikovania ego znamenitoĭ knigi 'Meditsinskie nabliudeniia'). **Khirurgiia (Mosk)** 1980 Aug;(8):117–9
Schupbach W: The paradox of Rembrandt's 'Anatomy of Dr. Tulp'. London, Wellcome Institute for the History of Medicine, 1982. 110 p. (Medical History, Suppl. No. 2).

**Tur, Aleksandr Fedorovich, 1894–1974**
Tarasov OF: A. F. Tur: 1894–1974. Moskva, Meditsina, 1980. 125 p.

**Turchini, Jean, 1894–1979**
Dulieu L: Le doyen Jean Turchini (Nice, 1894 – Montpellier, 1979) et l'histoire de la médecine. **Hist Sci Med** 1979;13(4):339–41

**Turner, Daniel, 1667–1741**
Lyell A: Daniel Turner (1667–1740) LRCP London (1711) M.D. honorary, Yale (1723) surgeon, physician and pioneer dermatologist: the man seen in the pages of his book on the skin. **Int J Dermatol** 1982 Apr;21(3):162–70

**Turner, Genrikh Ivanovich, 1858–1941**
Aleksanian IV, Knopov MSh: K 125-letiiu so dnia rozhdeniia G. I. Turnera. **Khirurgiia (Mosk)** 1984 Jan;(1):154–5
Tkachenko SS, Andrianov VL, Kapitanaki IA: K 125-letiiu so dnia rozhdeniia G. I. Turnera--osnovopolozhnika otechestvennoĭ travmatologii i ortopedii. **Ortop Travmatol Protez** 1984 Jun;(6):68–70

**Turner, George Grey, 1877–1951**
Rank BK: George Grey Turner, F.R.A.C.S. (Hon). **Aust NZ J Surg** 1981 Dec;51(6):627–30

**Turner, Henry Hubert, 1892–1970**
Lindsten J: Sammanställde fall av kortvuxenhet och bristande ovariefunktion hos flickor. **Lakartidningen** 1983 Jul 13;80(28–29):2755

**Turner, Joseph Mallord William, 1775–1851**
Woodruff AW: J M W Turner and some of his predecessors and successors, from the viewpoint of medical history. **J R Soc Med** 1980 May;73(5):381–92

**Turner, Kerenhappuch**
Davis CC: The tribulations of Mrs. Turner: an episode after Guilford Court House. **Md Hist Mag** 1981;76(4):376–9

**Turner, William, 1508–1568**
Pineas R: William Turner's Spirituall physik. **Sixteenth Cent J** 1983;14:387–98

**Tushinskiĭ, Mikhail Dmitrievich, 1882–1962**
Lopatenok AA, Fisher AM: Deiatel'nosti M. D. Tushinskogo v blokirovannom Leningrade. **Klin Med (Mosk)** 1982 Jan;60(1):112–4
Lopatenok AA: M. D. Tushinskiĭ, 1882–1962. Moskva, Meditsina, 1983. 47 p.
Smorodintsev AA: K istorii izucheniia étiologii i vaktsinoprofilaktiki grippa (nauchnyĭ vklad v étu problemu kliniki M. D. Tushinshinskogo). **Klin Med (Mosk)** 1982 Jan;60(1):108–12

**Tutankhamun, fl. ca. 1358 B.C.**
Czeizel A: Life and death [of] Tutankhamun from human genetic aspects. **Ther Hung** 1980;28(1):40–3
Paulshock BZ: Tutankhamun and his brothers. Familial gynecomastia in the Eighteenth Dynasty. **JAMA** 1980 Jul 11;244(2):160–4

**Tutyshkin, Petr Petrovich, 1868–1937**
Popushoĭ EP, Ioksa VA: Progressivnaia rol' vracha-revoliutsionera P. P. Tutyshkina v razvitii nauchnoĭ mysli v Moldavii. **Sov Zdravookhr** 1984;(4):69–71

**Twardowski**
Kuchowicz Z, Ojrzyński J: Czy twardowski był niemcem? **Przegl Hist** 1978;69(2):309–15

**Twitchell, Amos, 1781–1850**
Allison HM: Doctor Amos Twitchell: pioneer surgeon. **Hist NH** 1978;33(2):167–79

**Twitmyer, Edwin Burket, 1873–1943**
Coon DJ: Eponymy, obscurity, Twitmyer, and Pavlov. **J Hist Behav Sci** 1982 Jul;18(3):255–62

**Tyler, John Mason, 1851–1929**
Hawkins H: Transatlantic discipleship: two American biologists and

their German mentor. **Isis** 1980 Jun;71(257):197–210

**Tytler, James, 1747?–1804?**
Swinton WE: Dr. James Tytler: author, balloonist, encyclopedist. **Can Med Assoc J** 1981 Jan 15;124(2):216–23

## U

**Udagawa, Yôan, 1798–1846**
Dôke T: Yôan Udagawa: a pioneer scientist of early 19th century feudalistic Japan. **Jpn Stud Hist Sci** 1973;12:99–120

**Udjahorresnet**
Ghalionungui P: A naval physician in ancient Egypt. In International Congress of the History of Medicine, 27th, Barcelona, 1980. Actas. Barcelona, Académia de Ciències Médiques de Catalunya i Balears, 1981. p. 373–5.

**Ukhtomskiĭ, Aleksei Alekseevich, 1875–1942**
Sokolova LV: Obzor: Problema vzaimodeĭstviia vozbuzhdeniia i tormozheniia pri formirovanii ucheniia A. A. Ukhtomskogo o printsipe dominanty. **Fiziol Zh SSSR** 1981 Jun;67(6):781–6
Sokolova LV: Uchenie A. A. Ukhtomskogo o dominante ka vektore povedeniia. **Nerv Sist** 1982;23:5–13

**Ulezko-Stroganova, Klavdiia Petrovna, 1856–1943**
Khmel'nitskiĭ OK: Klavdiia Petrovna Ulezko-Stroganova (1856–1943). **Arkh Patol** 1981;43(8):72–4

**Ulhoorn, Hendrik, 1692–1749**
de Moulin D: The value of tobacco smoke in the treatment of intussusception. **Neth J Surg** 1984 Apr;36(2):57–9

**Ul'ianov Dmitriĭ Il'ich, 1874–1943**
Evdokimov PP, Kulak VM: [D. I. Ul'ianov in Simbirsk] (Rus). **Med Sestra** 1981;40(1):42–3
Potulov BM: Vrach-bol'shevik (k 110-ĭ godovshchine so dnia rozhdeniia D.I. Ul'ianova). **Voen Med Zh** 1984 Aug;(8):69–70

**Ulrichs, Karl Heinrich, 1825–1895**
Kennedy HC: The 'Third sex' theory of Karl Heinrich Ulrichs. **J Homosex** 1980–81 Fall-Winter;6(1-2):103–11

**Uncumber, Saint**
Lacey JH: Anorexia nervosa and a bearded female saint. **Br Med J [Clin Res]** 1982 Dec 18–25;285(6357):1816–7

**Underwood, Benton J., 1915–**
Underwood BJ: Studies in learning and memory: selected papers. New York, Praeger, 1982. x, 331 p.

**Underwood, Edgar Ashworth, 1899–1980**
Rowbottom ME: Dr. E. Ashworth Underwood (1899–1980). **Med Hist** 1980 Jul;24(3):349–52

**Unger, Ernst, 1875–1938**
Winkler EA: Ernst Unger: a pioneer in modern surgery. **J Hist Med Allied Sci** 1982 Jul;37(3):269–86

**Unkrig, Wilhelm A.**
Bawden CR: W. A. Unkrig's correspondence with the British and Foreign Bible Society. A contribution to ... printing in Mongolian. **Zentralasiat Stud** 1980;14(1):65–108

**Unna, Paul Gerson, 1850–1929**
Brooks HG: A visit to Dr. Unna's clinic in Hamburg. an excerpt: British Journal of Dermatology 1890. **Am J Dermatopathol** 1982 Jun;4(3):225–8
Hollander A: Glimpses at the life and work of P. G. Unna. **Am J Dermatopathol** 1980 Summer;2(2):137–42
Hollander A: Betrachtungen über Paul Gerson Unna. **Z Hautkr** 1984 May 15;59(10):680–7

**Urdang, George, 1882–1960**
Dann G, Higby G: Bibliography of the publications of George Urdang on his birth centenary. **Pharm Hist** 1982;24(3):106–14
Sonnedecker G: The American correspondence between George Urdang and Henry E. Sigerist 1941–1948. In Perspektiven der Pharmaziegeschichte. Festschrift für Rudolf Schmitz zum 65. Geburtstag. Graz, Akademische Druck- u. Verlagsanstalt. p. 343–63.
Wankmüller A: Entstehung des 'Grundriss der Geschichte der deutschen Pharmazie' von Adlung und Urdang. **Pharm Ztg** 1980;125:403–6

**Uredale, Robert, 1642–1722**
Burnby J: Robert Uredale (1642–1722) botanist. **Pharm Hist (London)** 1974 Jul;4(2):4–5

**Urlanis, Boris Tsezarevich, 1906–1981**
Zadneprovski IA, Podol'ski AG: Borisz Cezarevics Urlanisz (1906–1981). **Demografia** 1981;24(4):553–5

**Usteri, Paulus, 1768–1831**
Peter CH: Der Briefwechsel zwischen Paulus Usteri und Melchior Aepli. Zürich, Juris Druck, 1983. 161 p. (Zürcher Medizingeschichtliche Abhandlungen, Neue Reihe, Nr. 155).

**Uvnäs, Börge, 1913–**
Uvnäs B: From physiologist to pharmacologist--promotion or degradation? Fifty years in retrospect. **Annu Rev Pharmacol Toxicol** 1984;24:1–18

**Uzunov, Georgi, 1904–1971**
Kilimov N: Georgi Uzunov. Sofiia, Izd-vo na Bŭlgarskata akademiia na naukite, 1978. 178 p.

## V

**Vacher de Lapouge, Georges, 1854–1936**
Nagel G: Georges Vacher de Lapouge (1854–1936). Ein Beitrag zur Geschichte des Sozialdarwinismus in Frankreich. Freiburg, Schulz, 1975. 109 p. (Freiburger Forschungen zur Medizingeschichte, Neue Folge, 4).

**Vagbhata, son of Nomikumara, ca. 1200**
Gurjar GK, Anand RM: Apurva Vaidya of Vagbhata. **Bull Indian Inst Hist Med (Hyderabad)** 1975 Oct;5(4):207–10

**Vail, Edwin Arnold, 1817–1885**
Whalen JM: Edwin Arnold Vail. In Dictionary of Canadian biography, 1881–1890. 1982;11:896–7.

**Valdizán, Hermilio, 1885–1929**
Mariátegui J: Hermilio Valdizán y la psiquiatriá peruana. **Rev Neuropsiquiatr** 1980 Mar;43(1):1–22
Mariátegui J: Hermilio Valdizán, la psiquiatría comparativa y la medicina folklórica. **Acta Psiquiatr Psicol Am Lat** 1980 Jun;26(2):96–106

**Valentin, Johannes Franz Wilhelm, 1884–1959**
Friedrich C, Seidlein HJ: Beiträge zur Geschichte der Pharmazeutischen Wissenschaft. 11. Mitteilung: Die Bedeutung Johannes (Hans) Valentin für die Entwicklung der Pharmazeutischen Wissenschaft. **Pharmazie** 1984 Apr;39(4):262–9

**Valéry, Paul Ambroise, 1871–1945**
Laurenti H: Une thèse de médecine sur Paul Valéry. **Bull Etud Valeryennes** 1980;(25):5–7
Roucoules L: Paul Valery et l'art de guérir. **Bull Acad Chir Dent (Paris)** 1981–82;27(27):53–64

**Valette, Guillaume, 1902–1982**
Delaby PA: Le doyen Guillaume Valette (1902–1982). **Hist Sci Med** 1982;16(2):65–79
Dillemann G: Le Doyen Guillaume Valette (1902–1982). **Rev Hist Pharm (Paris)** 1982 Jun;29(253):83–6

**Valeur, Amand, 1859–1927**
Bouriez J: Lens, trois savants oubliés: Auguste Behal, Amand Valeur, Raymond Delaby. [France], Société de recherches historiques de la région d'Henin-Carvin, [1981] 69 leaves.

**Valla, Lorenzo, 1407?–1457**
Waswo R: The reaction of Juan Luis Vives to Valla's philosophy of language. **Bibl Hum Renaissance** 1980 Sep;42(3):595–609

**Vallambert, Simon de, d. 1558?**
Simon de Vallambert on the treatment of diarrhea in infants (1565): **Pediatrics** 1982 Feb;69(2):163

**Vallisneri, Antonio, 1661–1730**
Lucchetta PM: Nuovi documenti per la biografia di Antonio Vallisneri. **Quad Stor Univ Padova** 1982;15:131–45
Testoni G: Una lettera di Cestoni a Vallisneri (1710). **Riv Biol** 1983 Spring;76(1):125–31

**Valtolini, Giovambattista, fl. 1790**
Dondi RF: Uno strumento chirurgico dimenticato: le forbici del Valtolini. **Ann Osp Maria Vittoria Torino** 1980 Jul–Dec;23(7-12):289–94

**Valverde, Juan de, ca. 1520–ca. 1588**
Luyendijk-Elshout AM: The introduction of Juan Valverde's and Bartholomy Cabrol's anatomy into Low Countries between 1568–1633. In International Congress of the History of Medicine, 27th, Barcelona, 1980. Actas. Barcelona, Académia de Ciències Médiques de Catalunya i Balears, 1981. p. 298–303.
Riera J: Valverde y la anatomía del Renacimiento. Valladolid, Ediciones de la Universidad de Valladolid, 1981. 63 p.

**Van Bandeloo Family, 1586–1785**
De Backer C: De apothekers Van Baudeloo te Gent, 1586–1785. **Farm Tijdschr Belg** 1980;57:351–5

**Van Blarcom, Carolyn Conant, 1879–1960**
Litoff JB: Carolyn Conant van Blarcom. In: Notable American women. The modern period. Cambridge, Mass., Belknap-Harvard Univ. Press, 1980. 4:703–4.

**Vance, Benjamin M., 1886–1962**
Eckert WG: Dr. Benjamin M. Vance (1886–1962). **Am J Forensic Med Pathol** 1980 Mar;1(1):73–6

**Vandamme, Dominique-René, 1770–1830**
Gerard A, Milot J: Histoire médicale du Camp de Boulogne d'après les papiers du général Vandamme. **Hist Sci Med** 1982;16(1):29–36

**Van der Looy, Cornelis Hendrik, 1813–1895**
Merriënboer FJ: Eene buitenbaarmoederlijke zwangerschap, waar het foetus na 18 Jaren bij de moeder vertoefd te hebben door de anus is ontlast, beschreven door C.H. van der Looy (1850). **Tijdschr Geschied Geneeskd** 1980;3(1):37–40

Van der Paele, G., 1370-1443
Dequeker JV: Polymyalgia rheumatica with temporal arteritis, as painted by Jan van Eyck in 1436. **Can Med Assoc J** 1981 Jun 15;124(12):1597-8

van der Reis, Viktor, 1889-1958
Knoke M: Viktor van der Reis--Wegbereiter der gastrointestinalen Mikroökologie des Menschen. **Nahrung** 1984;28(6-7):593-8

Van der Straet, Jan, 1523-1605
Kleberger E: Fin Brillenfan des 16. Jahrhunderts. **Klin Monatsbl Augenheilkd** 1982 Sep;181(3):223-6

Vanderbilt, George Washington, 1862-1914
Bean WB: Frederick Law Olmstead and Vanderbilt's Biltmore estate: the contribution of private wealth to forestry, ecology and climatology. **Trans Am Clin Climatol Assoc** 1979;90:132-9

Van Eeden, Frederik, 1860-1932
Verkroost CM: A. W. van Renterghem und Frederik van Eeden, zwei holländische Aerzte als Bahnbrecher auf dem Gebiete der psychischen Therapie. **Janus** 1980;67(1-2-3):191-9

Van Gieson, Ransford E.
Burns SB: Early medical photography in America (1839--1883); IV. Early wet-plate era. **NY State J Med** 1979 Nov;79(12):1931-8

Van Gogh, Vincent, 1853-1890
Albert-Puleo M: Van Gogh's vision: thujuone intoxication. **JAMA** 1981 Jul 3;246(1):42
Beeck M: Merkmale epileptischer Bildnerei: mit Pathographie Van Gogh. Bern, Huber, 1982. 134 p.
Haas WH de: Vincent van Gogh, zijn lichamelijke ziekten, verwondingen en zelfmoord. **Ned Tijdschr Geneeskd** 1983 Dec 24;127(52):2390-2
Lee TC: Van Gogh's vision. Digitalis intoxication? **JAMA** 1981 Feb 20;245(7):727-9
Putscher M: Jaspers und Van Gogh--oder über Krankheit und Kunst. **Janus** 1980;67(1-2-3):157-69
Ravin JG: Van Gogh's illness. **Ohio State Med J** 1981 Dec;77(12):699-702
Runyan WM: Why did Van Gogh cut off his ear? The problem of alternative explanations in psychobiography. **J Pers Soc Psychol** 1981 Jun;40(6):1070-7
Southgate MT: Vincent van Gogh, portrait of Dr. Gachet. **JAMA** 1981 Feb 20;245(7):657, 688

Van Hoosen, Bertha, 1863-1952
Batchelor AJ: AMWA's founder--the 'red headed dynamo'. **J Am Med Wom Assoc** 1984 Jul-Aug;39(4):123, 139
Morantz RM: Bertha van Hoosen. In: Notable American women. The modern period. Cambridge, Mass., Belknap Harvard Univ. Prcss, 1980. 4:706-7.

Van Mons, Jean-Baptiste, 1765-1842
Perrin CE: J. B. Van Mons' essai sur les principes de la chimie antiphlogistique: a mystery solved. **Ambix** 1984;31(1):1-5

Van Renterghem, Albert Willem, 1845-1939
Verkroost CM: A. W. van Renterghem und Frederik van Eeden, zwei holländische Aerzte als Bahnbrecher auf dem Gebiete der psychischen Therapie. **Janus** 1980;67(1-2-3):191-9

Van Riper, Paul, 1875-
Van Riper C: My father, Doctor Van. Marquette, Mich., John M. Longyear Research Library, 1982. ix, 74 p.

Van Rippen, Bene, 1882-
Van Reenen JF: Doctor 'Ribbebene' - cobbler, lumberman, dentist, politician and researcher. **Adler Mus Bull** 1983 Nov;Spec issue:53-7

Varrier-Jones, Pendrill Charles, 1883-1941
Bryder L: Papworth Village Settlement--a unique experiment in the treatment and care of the tuberculous? **Med Hist** 1984 Oct;28(4):372-90

Varsányi Borbély, György, fl. 1570
Endrei W: Egy korai magyar nyelvü orvoslevél. **Orvostort Kozl** 1980;89-91(26 no 1-3):267-8

Vasen, Sarah, 1870-1944
Clar R: First Jewish women physician of Los Angeles. **West States Jew Hist Q** 1981;14(1):66-75

Vasil'ev, Stepan Mikhailovich, 1855?-1905?
Tsiklik AM: S. M. Vasil'ev i ego klinicheskoe nasledie (K 125-letiiu so dnia rozhdeniia). **Ter Arkh** 1980;52(7):143-6

Vasiliu, N.
Marinescu CG: Concepţiile progresiste ale Doctorului N. Vasiliu. **Rev Med Chir Soc Med Nat Iasi** 1980 Jul-Sep;84(3)578-80

Vassé, Loys, fl. 1524-1560
Paillard E: Louis Vassé, médecin à Chalôns. **Mem Soc Agric Commer Sci Arts Marne** 1975;90:109-29

Vater, Abraham, 1684-1751
Kaiser W, Völker A: Gedenktage 1980 aus der Geschichte der Medizinischen Fakultät Wittenberg (II): Lehre und Forschung in der Amtsphase von Christian Vater (1651-1732) und Abraham Vater (1684-1751). **Z Gesamte Inn Med** 1981 May 15;36(10):325-32
Suárez CV: Ampulla of Vater---a misnomer. **Mt Sinai J Med (NY)** 1980 Jul-Aug;47(4):373-85

Vater, Christian, 1651-1732
Kaiser W, Völker A: Gedenktage 1980 aus der Geschichte der Medizinischen Fakultät Wittenberg (II): Lehre und Forschung in der Amtsphase von Christian Vater (1651-1732) und Abraham Vater (1684-1751). **Z Gesamte Inn Med** 1981 May 15;36(10):325-32

Vaughan, Henry, 1621-1695
Davies GC: The Welsh doctor as a poet: Henry Vaughan-Silurist. In J. Cule, ed: Wales and medicine. London, British Society for the History of Medicine, 1975. p. 112-18.
Harrison DF: Neurochemistry and Sherrington's enchanted loom. **J R Soc Med** 1984 Aug;77(8):706-7

Vaughan, Thomas, 1622-1666
Newman W: Thomas Vaughan as an interpreter of Agrippa von Nettesheim. **Ambix** 1982 Nov;29(3):125-40

Veber, Jean, 1864-1928
Dentistry in folk art XI: L'arracheuse de dents (The tooth puller): **Bull Hist Dent** 1980 Oct;28(2):87

Vegas, Martín, 1897-
Briceño-Maaz T: Dos nombres en la dermatologia venezolana. **Rev Soc Venez Hist Med** 1972-73;20-21(34-35):87-98

Veigl, Franz Xaver, 1723-1798
Hein WH: Zum Curarebericht des Jesuitenpaters Franz Xaver Veigl. **Beitr Gesch Pharm** 1981;11:81-4

Veit, Gustav von, 1834-1905
Engel C: Leben und Werk des Bonner Frauenarztes Gustav von Veit. Diss., Rheinische Friedrich-Wilhelms-Universität. Bonn, 1983. 141 p.

Velasco, Pedro Gonzalez de, 1815-1882
Puig-Samper Mulero MA: El Doctor Pedro Gonzalez de Velasco y la antropologia española en el siglo XIX. **Asclepio** 1982;34:327-37

Vélez Boza, Fermin, 1916-
Silva Alvarez A: Juicio critico y discurso de contestacion. **Rev Soc Venez Hist Med** 1977;25(39):93-8

Velikovsky, Immanuel, 1895-1979
Iles JD: Velikovsky: psychiatrist, historian and catastrophist. **Can Med Assoc J** 1981 Sept 1;125(5):496-505

Vella, Luigi, 1822-1886
Belloni L: Un circolo bernardiano in Italia: la Società delle Scienze Biologiche in Torino. Luigi Vella de la curaroterapia del tetano. **Physis** 1981;23(3):301-10

Velpeau, Alfred Louis Armand Marie, 1795-1867
Huard P: Velpeau, cancérologue. In: Congrès National des Sociétés Savantes, 93e, Tours, 1968. Comptes Rendus. Paris, 1971 Section des Sciences, Tome II. p. 159-62.

Velthuysen, Lambert van, 1622-1685
Matuschka MM: Lambert van Velthuysens (1622-1685) Menstruationstheorie in ihrer wissenschaftshistorischen Bedeutung. Zur Vorgeschichte der Endokrinologie der Ovarien. Amsterdam, B. M. Israël, 1980. vii, 72 p.

Venel, Gabriel François, 1723-1775
Levin A: Venel, Lavoisier, Fourcroy, Cabanis and the idea of scientific revolution: the French political context and the general patterns of conceptualization of scientific change. **Hist Sci** 1984 Sep;22(57 pt 3):303-20

Venette, Nicolas, ca. 1631-1678
Pecker A: Nicolas Venette (1633?-1698) est-il le fils de Guy Patin. **Hist Sci Med** 1982;16(3):167-74

Ventura, Giovanni de, fl. 1479
Cipolla CM: A plague doctor. In Miskimin HA, et al, ed.: the medieval city. New Haven. Yale Univ. Press, 1977. p. 65-72

Venulet, Franciszek, 1878-1967
Guzek JW: Profesor Franciszek Venulet (1878-1967) w 15 rocznice śmierci. **Arch Hist Med (Warsz)** 1982;45(1-4):27-38

Verbezius, David, 1577-1644
Pajorin K: David Verbec könyvtárának töredéke a Semmelweis orvostörténeti könyvtárban. **Magy Konyvsz** 1978;94(3-4):314-21

Verey, George, ca. 1830-1881
Rasporich AW, Getty IA: George Verey. In Dictionary of Canadian biography, 1881-1890. 1982;11:900-1.

Vergés, Dominique, 1775-1855
Català F: Autour d'une consultation par correspondance sous l'Empire. In Congrés International d'Història de la Medicina Catalana, 2nd, Barcelona, 1975. Llibre d'Actes. Barcelona, Socitra, 1977. p. 133-7.

Verhoeff, Frederick Hermann, 1874-1968
Keeney AH, Keeney VT: Frederick Herman Verhoeff, M. D. **Filson Club Hist Q** 1981;55(2):202-9

Vermeer, Johannes, 1632-1675
Dotz W: Jan Vermeer and his alopecic models. **Am J Dermatopathol** 1983 Jun;5(3):245-8

**Verney, Ernest Basil, 1894–1967**
Pickford M: Ernest Basil Verney. In Dictionary of national biography, 1961–1970. Suppl. 8, 1981. p. 1035.

**Verocay, José, 1876–1928**
Speroni Verner J: Vida y obra de José Verocay. Montevideo, Universidad de la Republica, Division Publicaciones y Ediciones, 1980. 51 p.

**Véron, Louis Désiré, 1798–1867**
Julien P: Le Dr. Véron et Daumier, ou le fabricant de pâté pectorale en proie à la caricature. In: Congrès international d'histoire de la médecine, XXVe, Québec, 1976. Actes. Québec, 1977. p. 807–21.

**Veronin, V. V.**
Natadze TG: O prioritete V. V. Voronina v nekotorykh oblastakh meditsiny i biologii (k 110–letiiu so dnia rozhdeniia V. V. Voronina). **Patol Fiziol Eksp Ter** 1981 May–Jun;(3):53–7

**Verri, Pietro, 1728–1797**
Premuda L: Die Medizin in der Sicht eines italienischen Denkers der Aufklärung. **Gesnerus** 1983;40(3/4):249–56

**Verson, Franz Xaver, 1805–1849**
Premuda L: The revival of the anatomico-clinical method in Padua: the fundamental contribution of F. S. Verson (1805–1849) from Trieste, a disciple of the Vienna School of Medicine. **Janus** 1980;67(1–2–3):31–9

**Vertiz, Ricardo, fl. 1898**
Blodi FC: Ophthalmology and philately: I. Ophthalmologists on stamps--Ricardo Vertiz. **Arch Ophthalmol** 1979 Sep;97(9):1706 (continued periodically)

**Vesalius, Andreas, 1514–1564**
Barcia Goyanes JJ: Las correcciones de Vesalio a la anatomia de Galeno. **Med Esp** 1980;79:1–16
Barcia Goyanes JJ: Los terminos osteologicos de la Fabrica y la evolucion del lenguaje anatomico hebreo en la Edad Media. **Sefarad** 1982;42:299–326
Cavanagh GS: A new view of the Vesalian landscape. **Med Hist** 1983 Jan;27(1):77–9
Clark H: Foiling the pirates: the preparation and publication of Andreas Vesalius's De humani corporis fabrica. **Libr Q** 1981;51(3):301–11
Doornaert JP: Vesalius. **Plast Reconstr Surg** 1984 Nov;74(5):726
Horowitz M, Collins J: A census of copies of the first edition of Andreas Vesalius' De humani corporis fabrica (1543), with a note on the recently discovered variant issue. **J Hist Med Allied Sci** 1984 Apr;39(2):198–221
Huard P, Imbault-Huart MJ: André Vesale, iconographie anatomique (Fabrica, Epitome, Tabulae sex). Paris, Dacosta, 1980. 255 p.
Kottek SS: 'Andre Vesale'. Some remarks on a painting by E. J. C. Hamman. **Koroth** 1982 Aug;8(3/4):135–43
McKusick VA: The human genome through the eyes of Mercator and Vesalius. **Trans Am Clin Climatol Assoc** 1980;92:66–90
Putscher M: Ein Totentanz von Tizian. Die 17 grossen Holzschnitte zur Fabrica Vesals (1538–1542). In Göpfert W, Otten HH, ed: Metavoeite: wandelt euch durch neues Denken. Düsseldorf, Triltsch, 1983. p. 23–40.
Riall CT: Surgical and medical devices and their origins. Chapter XIV. Beginnings of modern surgery (Andreas Vesalius). **J Oper Room Res Inst** 1982 Sep;2(9):30–3
Roth-Woelfle L: Jan Stephen van Kalkar als Illustrator der Anatomie des Andreas Vesal. **Imprimatur** 1980;8:11
Roth-Wölfle L: Jan Stephan von Kalkar als Illustrator der Anatomie des Andreas Vesal. **Imprimatur** 1980;9:86–100
Sabin JA, Sanmartín Urchaga P: Estudio comparado de las aportaciones iconográficas, en el sistema muscular, en las obras de Leonardo y Vesalio. In International Congress of the History of Medicine, 27th, Barcelona, 1980. Actas. Barcelona, Académia de Ciències Mèdiques de Catalunya i Balears, 1981. p. 446–53.
Simeone FA: Andreas Vesalius: anatomist, surgeon, count palatine, and pilgrim. **Am J Surg** 1984 Apr;147(4):432–40
Speransky LS, Bocharov VJ, Goncharov NI: The personages of Jan Stephan van Calcar's frontispiece to Andreas Vesalius' book 'On the Structure of the Human Body'. **Anat Anz** 1983;153(5):465–79

**Vetch, John, 1783–1835**
Feibel RM: John Vetch and the Egyptian ophthalmia. **Surv Ophthalmol** 1983 Sep–Oct;28(2):128–34

**Viader Family**
Jordi Gonzàlez FR: Contribució a la genealogia dels farmacèutics catalans; consideracions sobre Narcís Viader i Font. Barcelona, the author, 1981. p. 4–10.

**Viana Mentesano, Juan de, fl. 1637**
Palma Rodriguez F: Vida y obra de Viana Mentesano. Salamanca, Universidad de Salamanca, 1977. 54 p. (Cuadernos de Historia de la Medicina Española, Monografias, XXXI).

**Vianney, Mary, 1894–**
O'Carrigan C: Two veteran nurses of World War I days (Sister Mary MacDonald, Sister Mary Vianney). **Med J Aust** 1984 Jun 23;140(13):782–4

**Viborg, Erik, 1759–1822**
Excerpt of a letter from veterinary surgeon Haldoe Dahl: from the Diocese of Trondheim to Professor E. Viborg. **Hist Med Vet** 1977;2(1):4–9
Harrison JD: Professor E. Viborg and therapeutic parotid ductal ligation. **Hist Med Vet** 1977;2(2):42–9

**Vicentini, Giuseppe, 1860–**
Lenarduzzi G, Pescarini L, Miotto D: Un precursore dell'esame radiologico del tubo digerente: il prof. G. Vicentini. **Radiol Med (Torino)** 1980 Apr;66(4):263–4

**Vicq-d'Azyr, Félix, 1748–1794**
Chaia J: Vicq d'Azyr, la Société Royale de Médecine et la Guyane. In: Congrès National des Sociétés Savantes, 105e, Caen, 1980. Comptes Rendus, Paris, 1980. Section des Sciences, Fasc. V. p. 9–15.
Huard P, Imbault-Huart MJ: Vicq d'Azyr et la nomenclature moderne des nerfs crâniens. In: Congrès National des Sociétés Savantes, 105e, Caen, 1980. Comptes Rendus, Paris, 1980. Section des Sciences, Fasc. V. p. 61–83.

**Victor de l'Aveyron**
Gineste T: Victor de L'Aveyron: dernier enfant sauvage, premier enfant fou. Paris, Le Sycomore, 1981. 327 p.

**Victoria, Queen of Great Britain, 1819–1901**
Cooke AM: Queen Victoria's medical household. **Med Hist** 1982 Jul;26(3):307–20

**Vieillard, Eugène, fl. 1855–1867**
McKee ME, McKee HS: E. Vieillard et E. Deplanche, deux grands botanistes collecteurs en Nouvelle-Calédonie. **Hist Nat** 1980–81;17–18:49–68

**Vien, Ivan Ivanovich, ca. 1750–1809**
Alexander JT: Ivan Vien and the first comprehensive plague tractate in Russian. **Med Hist** 1980;24(4):419–31

**Viet, David, 1771–1814**
Zondek T: Dr. Med. David Viet (1771–1814), eine Gestalt aus der Emanzipationszeit. **Bull Leo Beck Inst** 1976;15(52):49–7

**Vieussens, Raymond, 1641–1715?**
Amalric P: La naissance de la neuro-ophtalmologie à Montpellier au XVIIme siècle à travers l'oeuvre de Raymond Vieussens et de Guilhem Briggs. **Bull Soc Ophtalmol Fr** 1983 Jan;83(1):83–8
Faller A: Die Präparation der weissen Substanz des Gehirns bei Stensen, Willis und Vieussens. **Gesnerus** 1982;39(2):171–93
Mounier-Kuhn P, Guerrier Y: Vieussens et l'anatomie de l'oreille. **Acta Otorhinolaryngol Belg** 1982;36(6):1029–38

**Villalba, Joaquín de, 1750–1807**
Marí Balcells VJ: Tres historiadores de la medicina española: Villalba, Hernandez Morejon y Comenge, e influencia del primero en la obra de los otros dos. In: Sociedad Española de Historia de la Medicina. V Congreso Nacional. Madrid, 1977. **Asclepio** 1977;29:167–76

**Villanueva y Godoy, Francisco Javier**
López McCabe A: Francisco Javier Villanueva y Godoy: cirujano major de la armada. **Rev Mar** 1981;98(1):72–87

**Villarreal, Juan Joseph de, 17th cent.**
Carreras Panchon A: La obra de Juan de Villarreal y otros estudios historico-medicos. Salamanca, Ediciones Universidad de Salamanca, 1978. 69 p. (Cuadernos de Historia de la Medicina Española, Mongrafias, XXXIII).

**Villemanzy, Jacques de, 1751–1830**
Des Cilleuls J: L'inspecteur général Jacques de Villemanzy, Sénateur et Pair de France (1751–1830). **Hist Sci Med** 1979;13(4):379–81

**Villemin, Jean Antoine, 1827–1892**
Perçebois G: Jean-Antoine Villemin (1827–1892). In: Congrès National des Sociétés Savantes, 103e, Nancy, 1978. Comptes Rendus. Paris, 1978. Section des Sciences, Fasc. V. p. 31–41.
Percebois G: Jean-Antoine Villemin, Vosgien de Prey, et la notion de contagiosité de la tuberculose. **Ann Med Nancy** 1979;18:685–98

**Villermé, Louis-René, 1782–1863**
Maitre AM, Ducable G: Louis-René Villermé et le choléra en 1832. **Hist Sci Med** 1982;16(4):317–25
Plessis JL, Huard P, Lefebvre P, et al: Louis-René Villermé, chirurgien-major à la Grande Armée. **Hist Sci Med** 1982;16(4):305–15
Valentin M: Louis-René Villermé (1782–1863); aperçu biographique. **Hist Sci Med** 1982;16(4):289–304

**Vincent de Paul, Saint, 1581–1660**
Peyresblanques J: Monsieur Vincent, ses maladies, ses médecins. **Hist Sci Med** 1982;16(4):253–61

**Vink, Peter, 1713–1773**
Van Lieburg MJ: The instrument-collection of Peter Vink, a chapter in the development of the surgical profession in the Netherlands during the 18th century. **Janus** 1980:67(1–2–3):207–19

**Vinogradov, Nikolaĭ Andreevich, 1831–1886**
Al'bitskiĭ VIu: K 150–letiiu so dnia rozhdeniia Nikolaia Andreevicha Vinogradova - uchenika S. P. Botkina. **Klin Med (Mosk)** 1982 Sep;60(9):121–3
Anisimov VE: Nikolaĭ Andreevich Vinogradov (k 150–letiiu so dnia rozhdeniia). **Klin Med (Mosk)** 1982 Mar;60(3):118–9

**Virchow, Rudolf Ludwig Karl, 1821–1902**
Bauer A: Rudolf Virchow: der politische Arzt. Berlin, Stapp, 1982. 131 p. (Preussische Köpfe, 6).
Büchner F: Der junge Rudolf Virchow. **Verh Dtsch Ges Pathol** 1981;65:458–61
Eisenberg L: Rudolf Ludwig Karl Virchow, where are you now that we need you? **Am J Med** 1984 Sep;77(3):524–32
Engelhardt DV: Virchow et Haeckel et la liberté de la science. In Poirier J, Poirier JL, ed: Médecine et philosophie à la fin du XIXe siècle. Paris, Université de Paris XII – Val de Marne, [1980?]. p. 117–25.
Figlio K, Weindling P: Was social medicine revolutionary? Rudolf Virchow and the revolutions of 1848. **Soc Soc Hist Med Bull (Lond)** 1984 Jun;34:10–8
Jahn CM: Rudolf Virchow (1821–1902): Auswahlbibliographie. Berlin, Humboldt Universität, 1983. 87 p. (Schriftenreihe der Universitätsbibliothek Berlin, Nr. 42).
Karbe KH: Ueber eine von Rudolf Virchow empfohlene anonyme Schrift aus dem Jahre 1848 zum Hungertyphus in Oberschlesien. **Arch Hist Med (Warsz)** 1979;42(3):291–4
Keil G: Zur Ueberlieferung von Virchows Würzburger Sektionsprotokollen. **Sudhoffs Arch** 1980;64(3):287–97
Kohl EW: Virchow in Würzburg. Pattensen/Han., Wellm, 1976. 129 p. (Diss., Würzburg).
Lambrecht M: Virchow és Pertik. **Orvostort Kozl** 1980;89–91(26 no 1–3):233–9
Lammel HU: Virchow contra Koch? Neue Untersuchungen zu einer alten Streitfrage. **Z Gesamte Hyg** 1982 Mar;28(3):206–10
Lin JI: Virchow's pathological reports on Frederick III's cancer. **N Engl J Med** 1984 Nov 8;311(19):1261–4
Morgenstern L: The Virchow–Troisier node: a historical note. **Am J Surg** 1979 Nov;138(5):703
Trease GE: Rudolf Virchow 1821–1902. **Br J Pharm Pract** 1981;3(1):34–5
Zajusz K, Orłowski J: Rudolf Virchow a problemy niepodległościowe i społeczne narodu polskiego. **Arch Hist Med (Warsz)** 1979;42(3):285–9

**Virgil**
Dirckx JH: Virgil and medicine. **JAMA** 1981 Sep 18;246(12):1326–9
Dirckx JH: Virgil on anthrax. **Am J Dermatopathol** 1981 Summer;3(2):191–5

**Vischer, Adolf Lukas Jacob, 1884–1974**
Djordjević M: [Surgeon and gerontologist Dr. Adolf L. Vischer: a contribution to Serbo–Swiss relations] (Serbo–Croat). **Srp Arh Celok Lek** 1979;107:1079–92

**Vitry, Jacques de, ca. 1165–1240**
Bonenfant–Feytmans AM: Les organisations hospitalières vues par Jacques de Vitry (1225). **Ann Soc Belg Hist Hop** 1980;18:17–45

**Vives, Juan Luis, 1492–1540**
Noreña CG: Juan Luis Vives. The Hague, Nijhoff, 1970. xiii, 327 p.
Trueta J: Els orígens del 'Welfare State' i de les lleis socials: Lluí Vives. In Congrés International d'Història de la Medicina Catalana, 2nd, Barcelona, 1975. Llibre d'Actes. Barcelona, Socitra, 1977. p. 39–47.
Waswo R: The reaction of Juan Luis Vives to Valla's philosophy of language. **Bibl Hum Renaissance** 1980 Sep;42(3):595–609

**Voegen van Engelen, Jacobus**
Lindeboom GA: Jacob Voegen van Engelen, medisch journalist; 'De Surinaamsche Artz'. **Ned Tijdschr Geneeskd** 1981 Jun 27;125(26):1044–9

**Vogt, Alfred, 1879–1943**
Rintelen F: Zum 100. Geburtstag von Alfred Vogt -- Versuch einer Würdigung seines wissenschaftlichen Werkes. **Klin Monatsbl Augenheilkd** 1979 Oct;175(4):439–41
Speiser P: Vogts Lehrbuch und Atlas der Spaltlampenmikroskopie des lebenden Auges. **Gesnerus** 1981:38(3/4):339–45

**Vogt, Oskar, 1870–1959**
Heintel H: Ein unbekanntes Porträt des Hirnforschers Oskar Vogt (1870–1959). **Medizinhist J** 1984;19(3):277–9

**Voiculescu, Vasile, 1884–1963**
Brătescu G: Preocupări epidemiologice ale doctorului V. Voiculescu. **Rev Ig [Bacteriol]** 1980 Jan–Mar;25(1):59–61

**Voĭtkevich, Anatoliĭ Anatol'evich**
Shlykov IP, Dedov II: Anatoliĭ Anatol'evich Voĭtkevich. **Arkh Anat Gistol Embriol** 1979 Dec;77(12):81–4

**Volchenetskiĭ, D. V., 1751–1811**
Makovoz AA: D. V. Volchenetskiĭ--vydaiushchiĭsia vrach Rossii. **Feldsher Akush** 1983;48(4):57–8

**Vol'f, A.M.**
Shabunin AV: K 150–letiiu pervogo v Rossii perelivaniia krovi. **Akush Ginekol (Mosk)** 1982;(8):59–60

**Vol'f, F. B., d. 1854**
Katsnel'bogen AG: Obshchestvenno–politicheskaia deiatel'nost' vracha–dekabrista F. B. Vol'fa. **Sov Zdravookhr** 1981;(1):66–70

**Volhard, Franz, 1872–1950**
Bock HE: Franz Volhard: Erinnerungen. Stuttgart, New York, Schattauer, 1982. xi, 345 p.
Bock HE, ed, Hildebrand KH, ed, Sarre HJ, ed: Franz Volhard, Erinnerungen. Stuttgart and New York, Schattauer, 1982. 345 p.

**Volkenshteĭn, Liudmila Aleksandrovna, 1857–1906**
Miliavskiĭ VM, Ikonnikov MV: Fel'dsheritsa Liudmila Aleksandrovna Volkenshteĭn. **Feldsher Akush** 1983 Oct;48(10):42–3

**Volkmann, Richard von, 1809–1894**
Schober KL: Gedächtnisvorlesung zum 150. Geburtstag von Richard von Volkmann, dem Mit–Gründer der Deutschen Gesellschaft für Chirurgie. **Langenbecks Arch Chir** 1981;355:597–606
Schober KL: Das chirurgische Erbe. Richard von Volkmann zum 150. Geburtstag am 17. 8. 1980. **Zentralbl Chir** 1980;105(24):1635–43

**Volkovich, Nikolaĭ Markiianovich, 1858–1928**
Khokholia VP: Nikolaĭ Markiianovich Volkovich (k 125–letiiu so dnia rozhdeniia). **Klin Khir** 1983 Dec;(12):55–6

**Voltaire, François Marie Arouet de, 1694–1778**
Bréhant J: La médecine dans la vie et l'oeuvre de Voltaire (Première partie). **Bull Acad Natl Med (Paris)** 1980 Oct;164(7):659–64
Bréhant J: La médecine, dans la vie et l'oeuvre de Voltaire (deuxième partie). **Bull Acad Natl Med (Paris)** 1980 Oct;164(7):675–81
Bréhant J: Un visage peu connu de Voltaire: le Voltaire biologiste (ses expériences de décapitation des gastéropodes). **Bull Mem Acad R Med Belg** 1981;136(12):580–8
Bréhant J: Voltaire et la médecine. **Sem Hop Paris** 1982 Dec 23;58(47):2792–801
Dirckx JH: Voltaire on the pox. **Am J Dermatopathol** 1983 Dec;5(6):581–4
Frey EF: Voltaire's relation to the discipline of medicine. **Bookman** 1982 May–Jun;9(5):3–7
Rocchietta S: Medici e speziali in tre romanzi de Voltaire. **Minerva Med** 1982 Feb 11;73(5):219–20
Roche R: L'apoplexie de Voltaire. **Hist Sci Med** 1981;15(2):145–9

**Voors, Antonie Wouter, 1924–**
Paddison RM, Skinner RE, ed: Antonie Wouter Voors, M.D., M.P.H., D.P.H. A biographical sketch and a bibliography of his work. New Orleans: History of Medicine Club of Louisiana State University Medical Center, 1983. 23 p.

**Voronoi, Iu. Iu., 1895–1961**
Hamilton DN, Reid WA: Yu. Yu. Voronoy and the first human kidney allograft. **Surg Gynecol Obstet** 1984 Sep;159(3):289–94
Mirskiĭ MB: Pervaia peresadka pochki v klinike (k 50–letiiu operatsii sovetskogo khirurga Iu. Iu. Voronogo). **Klin Med (Mosk)** 1983 Nov;61(11):147–9

**Votkin, Sergeĭ Petrovich, 1832–1889**
Nasonova VA: Razvitie ideĭ S. P. Botkina v sovremennoĭ revmatologii. **Vestn Akad Med Nauk SSSR** 1983;(3):41–6

**Vries, Hugo de, 1848–1935**
Heimans J: Hugo De Vries and the gene theory. In Forbes EG, ed: Human implications of scientific advance. Edinburgh, Edinburgh University Press, 1978. p. 469–80.
Sinding C: Le concept de gène. Une approche épistémologique. **Arch Fr Pediatr** 1984 Jan;41(1):1–3

**Vrolik, Willem, 1801–1863**
Baljet B: Willem Vrolik als teratoloog. **Ned Tijdschr Geneeskd** 1984 Aug 11;128(32):1530–4

**Vulpien, Alfred, 1826–1887**
Légée G: A. Vulpien (1826–1887), physiologiste élève de P. Flourens (1794–1867). In: Congrès international d'histoire de la médecine, XXVe, Québec, 1976. Actes. Québec, 1977. p. 873–80.

**Vvedenskii, Nikolai Evgenevich, 1852–1922**
Matiushkin DP: Obzor: uchenie N. E. Vvedenskogo o vozbuzhdenii i tormozhenii v svete sovremennoĭ neĭrofiziologii. **Fiziol Zh SSSR** 1981 Mar;67(3):349–56

**Vygotskii, Lev Semenovich, 1896–1934**
Iaroshevski MG, Gurgenidze GS: L. S. Vygotski o prirode psikhiki. **Vopr Filos** 1981;(1):142–54
Mecacci L: Il manifesto della scuola storico–culturale. **Stor Crit Psicol** 1980;1(2):263–95

## W

**Waardenburg, Petrus Johannes, 1886–1979**
Arias S: In connection with the Waardenburg commemoration, Dr. Sergio Arias has submitted the following correspondence. **Am J Med Genet** 1980;7(1):41–5
Opitz JM: In memoriam: Petrus Johannes Waardenburg, 1886–1979. **Am J Med Genet** 1980;7(1):35–9

**Wackenroder, Heinrich Wilhelm Ferdinand, 1798–1854**
Hellmuth H: Heinrich Wilhelm Ferdinand Wackenroder 8. März 1798--14. September 1854. **Pharmazie** 1980;34(5–6):321–3

**Wafer, Lionel, 1660?–1705?**
Forbes TR: When did Lionel Wafer die? **J Hist Med Allied Sci** 1981 Jan;36(1)69–70

**Wagner, Heinz, 1923–**
Staheli LT: A visit with Professor Heinz Wagner: Orthopädische Klinik Wichernhaus Rummelsberg/Nuremberg. **J Pediatr Orthop** 1982 Oct;2(4):448–52

**Wagner-Jauregg, Julius von, 1857–1940**
Beckh-Widmannstetter HA: Zur Geschichte der Individualpsychologie: Julius Wagner-Jauregg über Alfred Adler. **Unsere Heimat** 1965;36(10–12):182–8
Eissler KR: Freud und Wagner-Jauregg vor der Kommission zur Erhebung militärischer Pflichtverletzungen. Wien, Löcker, 1979. 333 p.
Kampmeier RH: Wagner von Jauregg and the treatment of general paresis by fever. **Sex Transm Dis** 1980 Jul–Sep;7(3):142–4

**Wagner, Richard, 1813–1883**
Guillemin J: La maladie de Richard Wagner. Pour le centenaire de sa mort à Venise. **Sem Hop Paris** 1983 May 12;59(19):1493–6
Rather LJ: The dream of self-destruction. Wagner's Ring and the modern world. Baton Rouge, Louisiana State Univ. Press, 1979. xx, 215 p.

**Wagner, Rudolph, 1805–1864**
Eulner HH, Hoepke H, ed: Der Briefwechsel zwischen Rudolph Wagner und Jacob Henle 1838–1862. Göttingen, Vandenhoeck & Ruprecht, 1979. 115 p. (Arbeiten aus der Niedersächsischen Staats- und Universitätsbibliothek Göttingen, Band 16).

**Waksman, Selman Abraham, 1888–1973**
Lechevalier HA: The search for antibiotics at Rutgers University. In J. Parascandola, ed: The history of antibiotics. Madison, American Institute of the History of Pharmacy, 1980. p. 113–23.

**Waldemar IV, At'terdag, 1320?–1375**
Jakobsen J, Jorgensen JB, Kreiborg S, et al: Kong Valdemar Atterdag: antropologiske fund under en odontologisk synsvinkel. **Tandlaegebladet** 1981 Jan;85(1):9–16

**Waldeyer-Hartz, Wilhelm von, 1836–1921**
Weindling P: Social concepts in anatomy: theories of the cell state of Oscar Hertwig (1849–1922) and Wilhelm Waldeyer (1836–1921). **Soc Soc Hist Med Bull (Lond)** 1980 Jun;26:15–7

**Waldie, David, 1813–1889**
Jones IW: Chloroform anaesthesia in Liverpool. **Anaesthesia** 1983 Jun;38(6):578–80

**Waldmeier, Theophilus, 1831–1915**
Katchadourian H: The historical background of psychiatry in Lebanon. **Bull Hist Med** 1980 Winter;54(4):544–53

**Waldron, John, 1744–ca. 1818**
Hancock WG: John Waldron. In Dictionary of Canadian biography, 1801 to 1820. Volume 5, 1983. p. 837–9.

**Walker, Donald Gregory, 1925–**
Kahn AJ, Raisz LG: Dedication to Donald G. Walker. **Metab Bone Dis Relat Res** 1981;3(2):77–80

**Walker, Edwin, 1853–1922**
Wellborn MB: Edwin Walker, M.D., Evansville, Indiana. **Indiana Med Hist Q** 1975;2(2):29–34

**Walker, Mary Edwards, 1832–1919**
Agris J: Stamps commemorating medicine. 'Dr. Mary Edwards Walker' (1832–1919). **J Dermatol Surg Oncol** 1982 Nov;8(11)::926
Lockwood A: Pantsuited pioneer of women's lib, Dr. Mary Walker. **Smithsonian** 1977;7(12):113–9

**Walkhoff, Otto, 1860–1934**
Rezai RF: Tribute to dental pioneer Friedrich Otto Walkhoff. **Quintessence Int** 1984 Jun;15(6):655–7

**Wallace, Alfred Russel, 1823–1913**
Bernstein RE: Darwin's alter ego: co-originator Alfred Wallace. **Perspect Biol Med** 1984;27(2):234–8
Kottler MJ: Darwin, Wallace, and the origin of sexual dimorphism. **Proc Am Philos Soc** 1980 Jun;124(3):203–26

**Wallace, William, 1791–1837**
Kampmeier RH: The introduction of iodine in the treatment of syphilis: the writings of William Wallace, M.D., of Dublin. **Sex Transm Dis** 1980 Jan–Mar;7(1):26–8

**Wallaszkay, János, 1709–1767**
Vallaszky D: Adatok Wallaszkay János, Pest város föorvosa életéhez. **Orvostort Kozl** 1979;87–88(25 no 1–2):249–53

**Wallich, George Charles, 1815–1899**
Rice AL, Burstyn HL, Jones AG: G. C. Wallich M.D.---megalomaniac or mis-used oceanographic genius? **J Soc Bibliogr Nat Hist** 1976;7(4):423–50

**Wallis, Charles Edward, 1869–1927**
Gelbier S, Randall S: Charles Edward Wallis and the rise of London's school dental service. **Med Hist** 1982 Oct;26(4):395–404
Gelbier S, Randall SB: Charles Edward Wallis and London's Toothbrush Clubs: 1909 style. **Dent Health (London)** 1982;21(1):12–5

**Wallon, Henri, 1879–1962**
Léon A: Psychopédagogie scientifique et humanisme dans l'oeuvre d'Henri Wallon (1879–1962). **Paedagog Hist** 1979;19(1):132–45

**Walpole, Horace, 1717–1797**
Viseltear AJ: The last illnesses of Robert and Horace Walpole. **Yale J Biol Med** 1983 Mar–Apr;56(2):131–52

**Walpole, Robert, 1676–1745**
Spriggs EA: The illnesses and death of Robert Walpole. **Med Hist** 1982 Oct;26(4):421–8
Viseltear AJ: The last illnesses of Robert and Horace Walpole. **Yale J Biol Med** 1983 Mar–Apr;56(2):131–52

**Walsh, David, 1852?–1943**
Landes RR, Hall S: A letter from Joseph Lister to Dr. David Walsh. **JAMA** 1984 Jun 15;251(23):3101–3

**Walsh, Frank Burton, 1895–1978**
Coston TO: A personal sketch of Frank Burton Walsh. **Surv Ophthalmol** 1983 Jul–Aug;28(1):50–4

**Walter, Carl Waldemar, 1905–**
Ausman RK, Bellamy D Jr: Problems and resolutions in the development of the flexible plastic blood container (Carl W. Walter). **Am J Surg** 1984 Nov;148(5):559–61
Barger AC: Some of Carl Walter's contributions to Harvard Medical School and Hospitals. **Am J Surg** 1984 Nov;148(5):578–80
Brooks JR: Carl W. Walter, MD: surgeon, inventor, and industrialist. **Am J Surg** 1984 Nov;148(5):555–8
Hufnagel CA, Thorn GW: Observations of a colleague (Carl W. Walter). **Am J Surg** 1984 Nov;148(5):581–3
Kundsin RB: Creative crusader against sepsis (Carl W. Walter). **Am J Surg** 1984 Nov;148(5):573–4
Kunitomo T: Development of new artificial kidney systems (Carl W. Walter). **Am J Surg** 1984 Nov;148(5):594–8
Laufman H: Carl Walter's half century of achievement in asepsis. **Am J Surg** 1984 Nov;148(5):565–70
Lowell JD: The ultraviolet environment in a nutshell (Carl W. Walter). **Am J Surg** 1984 Nov;148(5):575–7
Murphy WP: Carl Walter: a pioneer in shaping the medical device industry. **Am J Surg** 1984 Nov;148(5):590–3
Murray JE, Zollinger RM: Carl Walter Appreciation Day: April 28, 1984. **Am J Surg** 1984 Nov;148(5):552–3
Soutter L, Surgeonor DM: Reflections on blood transfusion (Carl W. Walter). **Am J Surg** 1984 Nov;148(5):562–4
Tilney NL: Carl Walter and the evolution of the Surgical Research Laboratory: 1937 through 1949. **Am J Surg** 1984 Nov;148(5):584–9

**Wang, Shih-hsiung, 1808–1868**
Lu W, et al: [A brief textual research on the life of Wang Shixiong, a renowned physician of Qing Dynasty] (Chi). **Chung Hua I Shih Tsa Chih** 1984 Jan;14(1):10–3

**Wangensteen, Owen Harding, 1898–1981**
Buchwald H: The scientist-surgeon. **Am J Surg** 1981 Aug;142(2):245–6
Classic articles in colonic and rectal surgery. Owen Harding Wangensteen 1899–1981: **Dis Colon Rectum** 1982 Jan–Feb;25(1):65–78
Edlich RF: Reflections on Wangensteen's academic village. **Am J Surg** 1981 May;141(5):601–4
Leonard AS: A tribute to Dr. Owen H. Wangensteen, 'the Chief'. **Surgery** 1981;89:402–6
Lillehei RC: The Wangensteen tradition: what it is and how can we perpetuate it? **Minn Med** 1981 Oct;64(10):626–8
Olch PD: Owen H. Wangensteen (1898–1981). **Bull Hist Med** 1981;55:260–2

**Warbasse, James Peter, 1866–1957**
Saffron MH: James Peter Warbasse. In Dictionary of American Biography, Suppl. 6, 1956–1960. p. 663–5, 1980.

**Warburg, Otto Heinrich, 1883–1970**
Höxtermann E: Ein Halbjahrhundert Fortschritte der Zellphysiologie, Biochemie und Photobiologie - Otto Heinrich Warburg (1883 bis 1970). **NTM** 1983;20(2):1–24
Krebs H: Otto Warburg: Zellphysiologe--Biochemiker--Mediziner---1883–1970. Stuttgart, Wissenschaftliche Verlagsgesellschaft, 1979. 167 p. (Grosse Naturforscher, Band 41).
Krebs H, Schmid R: Otto Warburg: cell physiologist, biochemist, and eccentric. Oxford, Clarendon. 1981. x, 141 p.
Werner P: Zur experimentellen Methode des Biochemikers Otto Heinrich Warburg. **Z Arztl Fortbild (Jena)** 1983;77(22):947–9

**Ward, Henry Baldwin, 1865–1945**
Hawkins H: Transatlantic discipleship: two American biologists and their German mentor. **Isis** 1980 Jun;71(257):197–210

**Waring, Joseph Ioor, 1897–**
Pratt-Thomas HR: Joseph I. Waring, M.D.: the man and his times. **J SC Med Assoc** 1981 Dec;77(12):597–601
Radbill SX: Joseph Ioor Waring, 1897–1977. **J Hist Med Allied Sci** 1978 Jul;33(3):427–8

**Warkany, Josef, 1912–**
Brent RL: Biography of Josef Warkany. **Teratology** 1982 Apr;25(2):137–51

**Warneck, Nicolas**
Mikhaĭlov VP: Nikolaĭ Varnek i Karl Bér. **Arkh Anat Gistol Embriol** 1982 Apr;82(4):86–95

**Warren, John Collins, 1778-1856**
Eavey RD: First operation under ether anesthesia: a correction. **N Engl J Med** 1983 Oct 20;309(16):990-1

**Warren, Jonathan Mason, 1811-1867**
Barlow W, Powell DO: Ixodes as a source of conflict: Otis E. Hunt vs. J. Mason Warren. **J Hist Med Allied Sci** 1981 Apr;36(2):221-4

**Warren, Marjory Winsome, 1897-1960**
Matthews DA: Dr. Marjory Warren and the origin of British geriatrics. **J Am Geriatr Soc** 1984 Apr;32(4):253-8

**Warren, Shields, 1898-1980**
Bowers JZ: Shields Warren's exemplary sanitary survey. **Am J Forensic Med Pathol** 1980 Dec;1(4):365-6
Tedeschi LG: Shields Warren: the legend and the man. **Am J Forensic Med Pathol** 1980 Dec;1(4):297-301
Warren S: Shields Warren, M.D.: Excerpts from 'Medical aspects of the atomic bombings'. 1946. **Am J Forensic Med Pathol** 1980 Dec;1(4):303-7

**Washington, George, 1732-1799**
Adams RR: Dr. James Craik, George Washington's physician and friend. **Record** 1980 May, Sep;1-4,1-3
Agins TC: Collector's item. Americana. **NY J Dent** 1983 Nov;53(7):317
Davies NE, Davies GH, Sanders ED: William Cobbett, Benjamin Rush, and the death of General Washington. **JAMA** 1983 Feb 18;249(7):912-5
Escoe R: A new look at John Greenwood's denture for George Washington. **Bull Hist Dent** 1981;29(1):37-43
Liston SL: Traumatic amputation of the external ear: the War of Jenkins' Ear and George Washington. **Am J Surg** 1984 Nov;148(5):599-601
Scheidemandel HH: Death of General Washington. **JAMA** 1983 Dec 2;250(21):2928
Schneck JM: Elisha Dick, Benjamin Rush, and George Washington. **JAMA** 1983 Jul 8;250(2):164
Sognnaes RF: President Washington's most famous dentures stolen from the Smithsonian. **J Am Dent Assoc** 1983 Feb;106(2):216-8
Sognnaes RF: Preface to professional progress from Washington's old ivory relics to the modern Maryland bridge. **J Md State Dent Assoc** 1983 Aug;26(2):79-86
Spiers CH: The drug suppliers of George Washington and other Virginians. **Pharm Hist (London)** 1977 Mar;7(1):2-3
Thompson WT: Don't just do something.... **Va Med** 1980 Feb;107(2):146-9
Wilcox HG: The president ails: American medicine in retrospect (George Washington). **Eval Program Plann** 1981 Apr;53(4):201-10

**Washington, Lawrence, 1746?-**
Liston SL: Traumatic amputation of the external ear: the War of Jenkins' Ear and George Washington. **Am J Surg** 1984 Nov;148(5):599-601

**Wassermann, August von, 1866-1925**
Fleck L: Genesis and development of a scientific fact. Edited by T. J. Trenn and R. K. Merton. Chicago, Univ. of Chicago Press, 1979. xxviii, 203 p.

**Waters, Samuel C., 1861-1932**
Waters SC: A country doctor of yesteryear: Samuel C. Waters (1861-1932) of Middletown, Indiana. **J Indiana State Med Assoc** 1983 Feb;76(2):144-5

**Waterton, Charles, 1782-1865**
Ellis FR: Waterton's wourali. **Can Anaesth Soc J** 1983 Jan;30(1):110
McDowall DG: The Yorkshire Connection--Priestley and Waterton. **Anaesth Intensive Care** 1982 Feb;10(1):4-8
Maltby JR: Charles Waterton (1782-1865): curare and a Canadian National Park. **Can Anaesth Soc J** 1982 May;29(3):195-202
Proceedings of a symposium held to commemorate the bicentenary of Charles Waterton (1782-1865): **Br J Anaesth** 1983 Mar;55(3):221-33

**Watson, Archibald, d. 1941**
Elmslie RG: Our honoured anatomists. **Aust NZ J Surg** 1981 Oct;51(5):415-9

**Watson, James D., 1928-**
Thirty years of DNA--and after: **Nature** 1983 Apr 14;302(5909):557-8

**Watson, John Broadus, 1878-1958**
Buckley KW: The selling of a psychologist: John Broadus Watson and the application of behavioral techniques to advertising. **J Hist Behav Sci** 1982 Jul;18(3):207-21
Buckley KW: Behaviorism and the professionalization of American psychology: a study of John Broadus Watson, 1878-1958. Ph.D. Diss., University of Massachusetts. Amherst, 1982. vii, 313 p.
Burnham JC: John Broadus Watson. In Dictionary of American Biography, Suppl. 6, 1956-1960. p. 670-3, 1980.
Cohen D: J. B. Watson, the founder of behaviourism: a biography. London, Routledge and Kegan Paul, 1979. vi, 297 p.
Lomax EM, Kagan J, Rosenkrantz BG: Science and patterns of child care. San Francisco, W. H. Freeman, 1978. xiv, 247 p.
Samelson F: A note on an unpublished article by John B. Watson. **J Hist Behav Sci** 1982 Jan;18(1):20-1

**Watson, Robert Irving, 1909-1980**
Brozek J, Evans RB, ed: R. I. Watson's selected papers on the history of psychology. Hanover, University of New Hampshire, 1977. xiii, 393 p.
Robert I. Watson and the development of the history of psychology: a symposium: With contributions by E. S. Mills, E. R. Hilgard, B. Ross, J. Popplestone, M. W. McPherson, R. B. Evans, E. S. Goodman, J. Brožek. **J Hist Behav Sci** 1982 Oct;18(4):307-31
Ross B: In memoriam: Robert I. Watson, Sr. 1909-1980. **J Hist Behav Sci** 1981 Jan;17(1):1-2

**Waugh, Evelyn, 1903-1966**
Hurst DL, Hurst MJ: Bromide psychosis: a literary case. **Clin Neuropharmacol** 1984;7(3):259-64

**Weber, Carl Maria von, 1786-1826**
Böhme G: Medizinische Porträts berühmter Komponisten: Wolfgang Amadeus Mozart, Ludwig van Beethoven, Carl Maria von Weber, Frédéric Chopin, Peter Iljitsch Tschaikowski, Béla Bartók. 2. verbesserte und erweiterte Auflage. Stuttgart, New York, Gustav Fischer Verlag, 1981. xi, 199 p.

**Weber, Max, 1864-1920**
Parson T: The articulation of the personality and the social-action system: Sigmund Freud and Max Weber. In M. Albin, R. J. Devlin, G. Heeger, ed: New directions in psychohistory. The Adelphi papers in honor of Erik H. Erikson. Lexington, Toronto, D. C. Heath, 1980. p. 27-35.

**Webster, John, 1580?-1625?**
Herring H: The self and madness in Marlowe's 'Edward II' and Webster's 'The Duchess of Malfi'. **J Mediev Renaiss Stud** 1979;9:307-23

**Webster, John, 1610-1682**
Jobe TH: The devil in Restoration science: the Glanvill-Webster witchcraft debate. **Isis** 1981 Sep;72(263):343-56

**Webster, Noah, 1758-1843**
Snape WJ, Wolfe EL: The studies of yellow-fever by Noah Webster and John Conrad Otto at Red Bank, New Jersey. **Bull Gloucester Cty Hist Soc** 1984 Jun;19(4):25-32

**Wecker, Johann Jacob, 1528-1586**
Rocchietta S: Sulle edizioni degli 'Antidotari' e di altre opere di J.-J. Wecker. **Minerva Med** 1981 Sep 19;72(34):2297

**Wedgwood, Josiah, 1730-1795**
Chaldecott JA: Wedgwood's ceramic wares for chemical use, production and supply from 1779-1794. **Ambix** 1981 Nov;28(3):184-205
Posner E: Josiah Wedgwood's doctors. **Pharm Hist (London)** 1973 Sep;3(2):2-5

**Wegelius, Juhana, 1693-1764**
Pesonen N: Rovasti Wegelius ja hänen lääkärikirjansa. **Duodecim** 1984;100(2):72-9

**Wehle, Ferdinand Alois, 1820-1860**
Frankl J: Somogy megyei adatok az abszolutizmus orvostörténelméhez. **Orv Hetil** 1982 Aug 22;123(34):2117-20

**Wehrli, Gustav Adolf, 1888-1949**
Boschung U: Gustav Adolf Wehrli (1888-1949), Gründer der Medizinhistorischen Sammlung der Universität Zürich. **Gesnerus** 1980;37(1/2):91-103

**Weichardt, Teodor Tomasz, fl. 1783**
Barg L: O poprawną bio-bibliografię Teodora Tomasza Weichardta kandydata na profesora patologii i terapii akademii krakowskiej w 1783 roku. **Arch Hist Med (Warsz)** 1980;43(3):289-304

**Weichmann, Louis J.**
Isacsson A: A study of Louis J. Weichmann. **Lincoln Her** 1978;80(1):25-38

**Weidman, Frederick Deforest, 1881-1956**
Beerman H: Frederick Deforest Weidman, M.D. **J Am Acad Dermatol** 1983 Sep;9(3):479-86

**Weigel, Christian Ehrenfried von, 1748-1831**
Friedrich C, Langer H, Seidlein HJ: Beiträge zur Geschichte der Pharmazeutischen Wissenschaft 3. Mitteilung: Christian Ehrenfried von Weigel -- Seine Bedeutung für die Entwicklung der Pharmazeutischen Wissenschaft. Teil 1: Herkunft und Entwicklung. **Pharmazie** 1982 Apr;37(4):290-3
Friedrich C, Langer H, Seidlein HJ: Beiträge zur Geschichte der Pharmazeutischen Wissenschaft. 4. Mitteilung: Christian Ehrenfried von Weigel--Seine Bedeutung für die Entwicklung der Pharmazeutischen Wissenschaft. Teil 2: Christian Ehrenfried von Weigel als Hochschullehrer. **Pharmazie** 1982 Jun;37(6):446-50
Friedrich C, Langer H, Seidlein HJ: Beiträge zur Geschichte der Pharmazeutischen Wissenschaft. 5. Mitteilung: Christian Ehrenfried von Weigel--Seine Bedeutung für die Entwicklung der pharmazeutischen Wissenschaft. **Pharmazie** 1982 Jul;37(7):514-7

**Weigert, Carl, 1845-1904**
Lie JT: Carl Weigert (1845-1904), a pathfinder in medicine. **Mayo Clin Proc** 1980 Nov;55(11):716-20

**Weinberg, Wilhelm, 1862–1937**
Pirchner F: Wilhelm Weinberg's contribution to quantitative genetics. **Folia Mendeliana** 1978;13(63):261–6

**Weiner, Herbert M., 1921–**
Ackerman SH: Herbert Weiner 'at home'. **Psychosom Med** 1982 Mar;44(1):5–17
Katz JL: Three studies in psychosomatic medicine revisited: a tribute to the psychobiological perspective of Herbert Weiner. **Psychosom Med** 1982 Mar;44(1):29–42

**Weiner, Hyman J.**
Clarke SS: Hyman J Weiner's use of systems and population approaches: their relevance to social work practice in health care today. **Soc Work Health Care** 1983 Winter;9(2):5–14

**Weiner, Joseph Sidney, 1915–1982**
Harrison G, Collins K: In memoriam Joseph Sydney Weiner (1915–1982). **Ann Hum Biol** 1982 Nov–Dec;9(6):583–92

**Weir, Robert F., 1838–1927**
Classic articles in colonic and rectal surgery. Robert Fulton Weir 1838–1927: An improved method of treating high-seated cancers of the rectum. **Dis Colon Rectum** 1982 Jul–Aug;25(5):503–7
Weir RF: Remarks on the gunshot wounds of the Civil War by Robert F. Weir. New York State Journal of Medicine, April, 1904. **NY State J Med** 1982 Mar;82(3):391–3

**Weismann, August, 1834–1914**
Churchill FB: The Weismann–Spencer controversy over the inheritance of acquired characters. In Forbes EG, ed: Human implications of scientific advance. Edinburgh, Edinburgh University Press, 1978. p. 451–68.
Kirkwood TB, Cremer T: Cytogerontology since 1881: a reappraisal of August Weisman and a review of modern progress. **Hum Genet** 1982;60(2):101–21
Sinding C: Le concept de gène. Une approche épistémologique. **Arch Fr Pediatr** 1984 Jan;41(1):1–3

**Weiss, Ernst, 1882–1940**
Wondrák E: Aerztliches und Arzttum im Werk von Ernst Weiss. In: Bilaterale Germanistenkommission CSSR–DDR. IV. Fachtagung ... 1977. Olomouc, Univerzita Palackého, 1979. pp. 142–54.

**Weissmann, Max**
Fischer JL: Yves Delage (1854–1920): l'epigenèse néo-lamarckienne contre la prédétermination weismannienne. **Rev Synth (Paris)** 1979;100(95–6):443–61

**Welch, Thomas B., 1825–1903**
Church LE: The ancestors we never knew. **J Md State Dent Assoc** 1983 Dec;26(3):122–3

**Welch, William Henry, 1850–1934**
Koudelka JB: The genesis of the William H. Welch Medical Library and the Johns Hopkins Institute of the History of Medicine. In Stevenson LG, ed: A celebration of medical history. Baltimore, Johns Hopkins University Press, 1982. (The Henry E. Sigerist supplements to the Bulletin of the History of Medicine; new ser., no. 6). p. 69–76

**Wellcome, Henry Solomon, 1853–1936**
Duggan AJ: Henry Wellcome: architect of tropical opportunities. **Trans R Soc Trop Med Hyg** 1981;75(4):477–83
Garner J: Burroughs and Wellcome: American architects of a British empire. **Can Pharm J** 1980 Dec;:417–9
Gray C: The Wellcome library: reflection of an insatiable collector. **Can Med Assoc J** 1982 Mar 15;126(6):712, 716–20
Hayles AB, Key JD: Adventures of two prairie pioneers. **Minn Med** 1981 Oct;64(10):629–32
Skinner GM: The Wellcome Museum. **Sydsven Medicinhist Sallsk Arsskr** 1983;:13–22
Turner H: Henry Wellcome: the man, his collection and his legacy. London, Heinemann for the Wellcome Trust, 1980. 96 p.
Vane JR: The research heritage of Henry Wellcome. **Pharm Hist (London)** 1980 Aug;10(2):2–8
Vane JR: The Wellcome centenary. Henry S. Wellcome, his research philosophy and current excitements. **Trans Med Soc Lond** 1980–81;97:41–50

**Weller, Thomas Huckle, 1915–**
Bendiner E: Enders, Weller, and Robbins: the trio that 'fished in troubled waters'. **Hosp Pract** 1982 Jan;17(1):163, 169, 174–5 passim

**Wells, Ben**
Crutcher JC: A memorial lecture for Dr. Ben Wells. **Ala J Med Sci** 1979 Oct;16(4):346–9

**Wells, Calvin, 1908–1978**
Hart GD, ed: Disease in ancient man. An international symposium held in London, 1979. Toronto, Clarke Irwin, 1983. 297 p. Contributions by D. A. Birkett, F. F. Cartwright, R. Cramp, J. Dobson, A. J. Duggan, N. G. Gejvall, P. S. Gooch, C. J. Hackett, P. D. Horne, P. Janssens, B. Knight, A. K. Knowles, N. B. Millet, V. Møller-Christensen, W. J. Moore, R. Perrot, F. D. Pooley, D. F. Rideout, A. Rook, W. M. Russell, P. Slack, W. E. Swinton, H. A. Waldron.

**Wells, Herbert George, 1866–1946**
Wygant A: Shelley, Hawthorne, and Wells: images of medicine in early science fiction. **Bookman** 1981 Oct;8(8):3–8

**Wells, Horace, 1815–1848**
Williams WD: Did Horace Wells stage a newspaper publicity scheme? Some unreported newspaper items. **Bull Hist Dent** 1983 Oct;31(2):93–8

**Wells, Lawrence Herbert, 1908–1980**
Morris AG, Keen EN: Lawrence Herbert Wells and the history of anatomical illustration. **S Afr Med J** 1982 Jan 9;61(2):40–3

**Wells, Thomas Spencer, 1818–1897**
Brahma B, Singh M: What lies behind a name? (Sir Thomas Spencer Wells 1818–1897). **NATNEWS** 1981 Jul;18(7):15
Swain VA: Some portraits of Sir Thomas Spencer Wells (1818–1897). **Ann R Coll Surg Engl** 1983 May;65(3):201–2

**Wells, William Charles, 1757–1817**
Bloch H: William Charles Wells, M.D., F.R.S., 1757–1817. An American physician-scientist America almost forgot. **NY State J Med** 1983 Feb;83(2):248–50
Ono H: On Wells's (1792) law of visual direction. **Percept Psychophys** 1981 Oct;30(4):403–6

**Went, István, 1899–1963**
Varga E: Megemlékezés Went Istvánról. **Orv Hetil** 1983 Sep 18;124(38):2319–20

**Wenzel, Heinrich Karl, 1769–1827**
Asendorf MI: Die gelehrten Arzte Joseph und Karl Wenzel, ihr Leben und Werk in Mainz und Frankfurt am Main. Diss. Mainz, 1981. 269 p.

**Wenzel, Joseph, 1768–1808**
Asendorf MI: Die gelehrten Arzte Joseph und Karl Wenzel, ihr Leben und Werk in Mainz und Frankfurt am Main. Diss. Mainz, 1981. 269 p.

**Wepfer, Johann Jakob, 1620–1695**
Jost M: Die Apoplexielehre Johann Jakob Wepfers (1620–1695). Diss., Rheinische Friedrich-Wilhelms-Universität, Bonn, 1982. 76 p.
Maehle AH: Johann Jakob Wepfer (1620–1695) als Toxikologe. Diss., Rheinische Friedrich-Wilhelms-Universität. Bonn, 1983. 202 p.
Mani N: Biomedical thought in Glisson's hepatology and in Wepfer's work on apoplexy. With commentary by R. G. Frank, p. 84–8. In Stevenson LG, ed: A celebration of medical history. Baltimore, Johns Hopkins University Press, 1982. (The Henry E. Sigerist supplements to the Bulletin of the History of Medicine; new ser., no. 6). p. 37–63.
Mani N: Johann Jakob Wepfers Doktordisputation über das Herzklopfen (1647). **Gesnerus** 1981;38:143–7

**Werdt, Daniel von, 1611–1658**
Jaeschke G, Diesbachs A von: Berner 'Arzneibüchlein' in der Erlacher Fassung Daniel von Werdts (1658). Teil I: Text. Pattensen/Han., Wellm, 1978. 180 p. (Würzburger medizinhistorische Forschungen, Band 16).

**Werle, Eugen, 1902–**
Huber R: E. Werle's kallikrein inactivator, a model in biochemistry and biophysics. **Adv Exp Med Biol** 1983;156:29–36

**Werner, Artur Karol**
Marczyński A: Dr Artur Karol Werner. **Przegl Lek** 1981;38(1):206–9

**Wernher, Adolph Carl Gustav, 1809–1883**
Bijok H: Adolph Carl Gustav Wernher (1809–1883); Sein Leben und Wirken am Giessener Akademischen Hospital. Giessen, Schmitz, 1979. 235 p. (Arbeiten zur Geschichte der Medizin in Giessen, Band 1).

**Wernicke, Carl, 1848–1905**
Eggert GH: Wernicke's works on aphasia. The Hague, New York, Mouton, 1977. xiii, 307 p.

**Wertheim, Th., fl. 1891**
Wertheim T: Peripheral visual acuity: Th. Wertheim. **Am J Optom Physiol Opt** 1980 Dec;57(12):915–24

**Wesley, John, 1703–1791**
Bolander V: A preliminary examination of John Wesley's 'Primitive physick'. **Bookman** 1983 Jul–Aug;10(4):3–10
Ott PW: John Wesley on health: a word for sensible regimen. **Methodist Hist** 1980;18(3):193–204
Ott PW: A corner of history. John Wesley and the non-naturals. **Prev Med** 1980 Jul;9(4):578–84
Schiller F: Reverend Wesley, Doctor Marat and their electric fire. **Clio Med** 1981 Apr;15(3–4):159–76
Wilder F: The remarkable world of John Wesley, pioneer in mental health. Hicksville, Exposition Press, 1978. 192 p.

**West, Charles, 1816–1898**
Besser FS: Notes on Dr. Charles West and his grave in Chislehurst (Kent). **Hist Med (Lond)** 1975 Autumn–Winter;6(3–4):47–50
Lomax E: Charles West (1816–1898) on the mental peculiarieties and disorders of childhood. In International Congress of the History of Medicine, 27th, Barcelona, 1980. Actas. Barcelona, Académia de Ciències Médiques de Catalunya i Balears, 1981. p. 98–102.
Lomax E: A mid-nineteenth century British pediatrician's interpretations of the mental peculiarities and disorders of childhood.

**Clio Med** 1983 Mar;17(4):223-33

**West, Hamilton A., 1849-1903**
Bowman IA: Was it yellow fever? **Bookman** 1981 Feb;8(2):3-4

**Westheimer, Gerald, 1924-**
Alpern M: Presentation of the Procter Medal for Research in vision and Ophthalmology to Gerald Westheimer. **Invest Ophthalmol Vis Sci** 1979 Sep;18(9):883-92

**Weszprémi, István, 1723-1799**
Kótay P: István Weszprémi 1723-1799. **Orvostort Kozl** 1980;89-91(26 no 1-3):215-22

**Wetmore, Charles Hinckley, 1820-1898**
Labor under ether: Hilo, 1850. **Hawaii Med J** 1981 Oct;40(10):291-2

**Wharton, Edith Newbold Jones, 1862-1937**
Spangler GM: Suicide and social criticism: Durkheim, Dreiser, Wharton, and London. **Am Q** 1979;31(4):496-516

**Whetnall, Edith Aileen Mandl**
Beagley HA: Edith Whetnall's contribution to British audiology. **J R Soc Med** 1978 Dec;71(12):870-8

**Whewell, William, 1794-1866**
Losee J: Whewell and Mill on the relation between philosophy of science and history of science. **Stud Hist Philos Sci** 1983 Jun;14(2):113-26

**Whipple, George Chandler, 1866-1924**
Clean water and the health of the cities: New York, Arno, 1977. Various paginations. Facsimile reprints of works by William T. Sedgwick (1893), George C. Whipple (1907), and J. Scott MacNutt (1910).

**Whistler, Daniel, 1619-1684**
Cone TE: A rachitic infant painted by Burgkmair 136 years before Dr. Whistler described rickets. **Clin Pediatr (Phila)** 1980 Mar;19(3):194

**White, Ellen Gould Harmon, 1827-1915**
Shapiro HD: Getting back---and down---to basics. **Rev Am Hist** 1977;5(2):242-48

**White, Gilbert, 1720-1793**
Radford P: Gilbert White: medical and social aspects of his letters. **Bristol Med Chir J** 1984 Apr;99(370):46-7

**White, James Platt, 1811-1881**
Drachman VG: The Loomis trial: social mores and obstetrics in the mid-nineteenth century. In Reverby S, Rosner D, ed: Health care in America. Philadelphia, Temple University Press, 1979. p. 67-83.

**White, John, 1757 or 8-1832**
Gandevia B: A surgeon's view of Cape Town in 1787. **Adler Mus Bull** 1983 Nov;Spec issue:9-12

**White, Park Jerauld, 1891-**
Hunt M: A coming of age with pediatrics: Park Jerauld White, attending physician. **Outlook Mag** 1982 Spring;19(1):18-24

**Whitman, Walt, 1819-1892**
Nelson RB: Occasional notes. Captains of an American credo: Walt and W. O. **N Engl J Med** 1981 Jul 9;305(2):110-2

**Whitton, Charlotte Elizabeth, 1896-1975**
Rooke PT, Schnell RL: Charlotte Whitton and the 'babies for export' controversy, 1947-48. **Alberta Hist** 1982;30(1):11-6

**Wicherkiewicz, Boleslaw, 1847-1915**
Zygulska-Machowa H, Starzycka M: Professor Bolesław Wicherkiewicz jako współtwórca krakowskiej szkoły okulistycznej. **Klin Oczna** 1982 Sep;84(9):245-9

**Wichmann, Johann Ernst, 1740-1802**
Raith L: Johann Ernst Wichmann--ein zu Unrecht wenig bekannter Dermatologe des 18. Jahrhunderts. **Dermatol Monatsschr** 1983;169(11):725-7

**Wickersheimer, Ernest, 1880-1965**
Jacquart D: Le milieu médical en France du XIIe au XVe siècle: en annexe 2e supplément au 'Dictionnaire' d'Ernest Wickersheimer. Genève, Droz; Paris, Champion, 1981. 487 p. (Centre de recherches d'histoire et de philologie de la IVe section de l'Ecole pratique des hautes études. V, Hautes études médiévales et modernes ; 46)

**Wiedmann, Albert, 1901-1970**
Lindemayr W: Die Bedeutung Albert Wiedmanns für die Entwicklung der Dermatologie in Wien nach 1945. **Wien Klin Wochenschr** 1981 Dec 25;93(24):735-9

**Wierzejewski, Ireneusz, 1881-1930**
Dega W: Profesor dr Ireneusz Wierzejewski jako prekursor rehabilitacji. (Z okazji setnej rocznicy jego urodzin). **Chir Narzadow Ruchu Ortop Pol** 1981;46(6):599-602
Labaziewicz L: Pisarstwo naukowe Ireneusza Wierzejewskiego. **Chir Narzadow Ruchu Ortop Pol** 1981;46(6):595-7
Lempicki A: Ireneusz Wierzejewski (1881-1930). **Chir Narzadow Ruchu Ortop Pol** 1981;46(6):589-93

**Wiggers, Carl John, 1883-1963**
Barger AC: The meteoric rise and fall of William Townsend Porter, one of Carl J. Wigger's 'Old Guard'. **Physiologist** 1982 Oct;25(5):407-13

**Wigglesworth, Edward, 1732-1794**
Vinovskis MA: The 1789 life table of Edward Wigglesworth. **J Econ Hist** 1971;31(3):570-90

**Wightman, Henderson, 1791-1823**
Morton G: Henderson Wightman, R. N., 1810-16. **Ir Sword** 1980;14(54):69-72

**Wijerama, Edmund Medonza, 1896-1980**
Mirando EH: Dr E. M. Wijerama. **Ceylon Med J** 1981 Mar;26(1):5-7
Ranasinghe L: The medical writings of Dr. E. M. Wijerama. **Ceylon Med J** 1981 Mar;26(1):1-4

**Wikerhauser, Teodor, fl. 1894**
Saric P: Je li Zabrebački kirurg Dragutin Schwarz uradio prvu nefrektomiju u Hrvatskoj? **Lijec Vjesn** 1980 Apr;102(4):205-7

**Wilberforce, Samuel, 1805-1873**
Altholz JL: The Huxley-Wilberforce debate revisited. **J Hist Med Allied Sci** 1980 Jul;35(3):313-16
Lucas JR: Wilberforce and Huxley: a legendary encounter. **Hist J (Gt Brit)** 1979;22(2):313-30

**Wilde, Oscar, 1854-1900**
Chalat NI: Some psychologic aspects of deafness: Beethoven, Goya, and Oscar Wilde. **Am J Otol** 1980 Apr;1(4):240-6
Robins AH: Did imprisonment ruin Oscar Wilde? **Practitioner** 1981 May;225(1355):773-5
Spencer FJ: The Gay Nineties: Oscar Wilde reconsidered. **MCVQ** 1981;16(3):67-70

**Wilde, William Robert Wills, 1815-1876**
Lowe RF: William R. Wilde, Andrew S. Gray, and two eye and ear hospitals of very similar name. **Aust NZ J Surg** 1981 Dec;51(6):630-6
Pappas DG: Sir William Wilde: a historical review. **Ear Nose Throat J** 1983 Jun;62(6):58, 60-2

**Wilder, Burt Green, 1841-1925**
Marshall LH: More on Burt Green Wilder at Cornell. **Physiologist** 1983 Dec;26(6):361-3

**Wilder, Harris Hawthorne, 1864-1928**
Stewart TD: Pioneer contributions of Harris Hawthorne Wilder, Ph.D., to forensic sciences. **J Forensic Sci** 1982 Oct;27(4):754-62

**Wilder, Russell Morse, 1885-1959**
Roland CG: Russell Morse Wilder. In Dictionary of American Biography, Suppl. 6, 1956-1960. p. 697-8, 1980.

**Wildführ, George, 1904-**
Hiepe T, Odening K, Vater G: Georg Wildführ sen. zum 80. Geburtstag. **Angew Parasitol** 1984 Aug;25(3):117-20

**Wile, Udo Julius, 1882-1965**
Arnold HL: Udo Julius Wile, A.B., M.D., LL.D. (1882-1965). **J Am Acad Dermatol** 1984 Jan;10(1):157-62
Hollander A: Udo Julius Wile. **J Am Acad Dermatol** 1984 Jun;10(6):1071-2
Lederer SE: 'The right and wrong of making experiments on human beings': Udo J. Wile and syphilis. **Bull Hist Med** 1984 Fall;58(3):380-97

**Wiley, Harvey Washington, 1844-1930**
Goyan JE: Dr. Harvey Wiley's brainchild, 75 years later. **J Assoc Off Anal Chem** 1981 Mar;64(2):256-9
Harvey W. Wiley and the Pure Food and Drug Act: **Nutr Hist Notes** 1981;11:2-4
Stutzman RH: Harvey Washington Wiley; a famous Hoosier and 'The father of pure food'. **Indiana Med Hist Q** 1981;7(4):20-1

**Wilgefortis, Saint**
Lacey JH: Anorexia nervosa and a bearded female saint. **Br Med J [Clin Res]** 1982 Dec 18-25;285(6357):1816-7

**Wilhelm, Augustin, 1933-**
Kraft H: Die Zeichnungen des Augustin Wilhelm. Psychopathologische Aspekte und kulturhistorische Vergleiche. **Confin Psychiatr** 1980;23(4):230-49

**Wilkie, James Sterling, 1906-1982**
Crombie AC: James Sterling Wilkie: 1906-1982. **Br J Hist Sci** 1984 Nov;17(57 pt 3):310-1

**Wilks, Samuel, 1824-1911**
García-Alejo RH: Enfermedad osea de Paget: comentarios a sus primeras descripciones y evolucion historica de su etiopatogenia. **Asclepio** 1982;34:181-97

**Willan Family**
Booth CC: Robert Willan and his kinsmen. **Med Hist** 1981 Apr;25(2):181-96

**Willan, Robert, 1757-1812**
Sharma OP: Robert Willan remembered. **J Am Acad Dermatol** 1983 Dec;9(6):971-6

**Willard Family**
Karsh E: Taking the waters at Stafford Springs: the role of the Willard Family of Boston in America's first health spa. **Harv Libr Bull** 1980 Jul;28(3):264-81
Karsh E: Taking the waters at Stafford Springs. The role of the Willard

family in America's first health spa. In: Congrès international d'histoire de la médecine, XXVe, Québec, 1976. Actes. Québec, 1977. p. 822–39.

**Willcox, Walter Francis, 1861–1964**
Aldrich M: Progressive economics, and scientific racism: Walter Willcox and black Americans, 1895–1910. **Phylon** 1979;40(1):1–14

**Wille, Johan Valentin, 1651–1676**
Nansen P: A Danish pathography from the 16th century. **Hist Med Vet** 1979;4(4):73–81
Nansen P: En sygdomsbeskrivelse fra 1600-tallets Danmark. **Nord Vet Med** 1980 Jan;32(1):38–45

**William I, King of Netherlands, 1772–1843**
Haneveld GT: Koning Willem I en de aankoop van anatomische kabinetten. **Spiegel Hist** 1978;13(7–8):488–95

**William I, Prince of Orange, Count of Nassau, 1533–1584**
Pollitt R: The wounding and treatment of William of Orange in 1582. **J Hist Med Allied Sci** 1982 Apr;37(2):135–58

**Williams, Anna Wessels, 1863–1954**
Robinton ED: Anna Wessels Williams. In: Notable American women. The modern period. Cambridge, Mass., Belknap-Harvard Univ. Press, 1980. 4:737–9.

**Williams, Cicely Delphine, 1893–**
Craddock S: Retired except on demand: the life of Dr. Cicely Williams. Oxford, Green College, 1983. 198 p.

**Williams, Daniel Hale, 1858–1931**
Beatty WK: Daniel Hale Williams--pioneer surgeon and hospital administrator. **Proc Inst Med Chic** 1979 Jul–Sep;32(7):156
Dummett CO: Health professional emancipators: examples in excellence. **J Natl Med Assoc** 1984 Sep;76(9):925–30
Olivier AF: In proper perspective: Daniel Hale Williams, M.D. **Ann Thorac Surg** 1984 Jan;37(1):96–7

**Williams, David I.**
De mortuis nil nisi bonum: **J Am Acad Dermatol** 1982 May;6(5):968–76

**Williams, Francis Henry, 1852–1936**
Kaufman JA: Francis H. Williams and the shadows of disease. **Conn Med** 1980 Apr;44(4):229–32
Regato JA del: Francis Henry Williams. **Int J Radiat Oncol Biol Phys** 1983 May;9(5):739–49

**Williams, Henry Willard, 1821–1895**
Wand M, Sewall RB: 'Eyes be blind, heart be still': a new perspective on Emily Dickinson's eye problem. **N Engl Q** 1979;52(3):400–6

**Williams, John Calthrop, 1801–1856**
Bartecchi CE: Historical beginnings of the mitral valve prolapse syndrome. **Am J Cardiol** 1984 Nov 1;54(8):1165–6

**Williams, John Whitridge, 1866–1931**
Longo LD: John Whitridge Williams and academic obstetrics in America. **Trans Stud Coll Physicians Phila** 1981 Dec;5(3 no 4):221–54

**Williams, John, 1840–1926**
Jones EW: Sir John Williams (1840–1926): his background and achievement. In J. Cule, ed: Wales and medicine. London, British Society for the History of Medicine, 1975. p. 86–95.

**Williams, Richard Tecwyn, 1909–1979**
Neuberger A, Smith RL: Richard Tecwyn Williams: the man, his work, his impact. **Drug Metab Rev** 1983;14(3):559–607

**Williams, Thomas, 1818–1865**
Thomas PH: Dr. Thomas Williams of Swansea, 1818–65. In J. Cule, ed: Wales and medicine. London, British Society for the History of Medicine, 1975. p. 196–202.

**Williams, William Carlos, 1883–1963**
Coles R: William Carlos Williams. A writing physician. **JAMA** 1981 Jan 2;245(1):41–2
Graham TR: William Carlos Williams. In Dictionary of American biography, 1961–1965. Suppl. 7, 1981. p. 788–91.
Graham TR: The courage of his diversity: medicine, writing and William Carlos Williams. In Jones AH, ed: Images of healers. Albany, State University of New York Press, 1983. p. 9–20.
Graham TR: William Carlos Williams: biographical note. In Jones AH, ed: Images of healers. Albany, State University of New York Press, 1983. p. 1–2.
Ratzan RM: 'No wreaths please': for William Carlos Williams. **Ann Intern Med** 1982 Dec;97(6):933–7
Stone J: A lifetime of careful listening. A centennial retrospective on the work of William Carlos Williams (1883–1963). **JAMA** 1983 Sep 16;250(11):1421–5
Williams WE: The school physician's notebook: a cameo of William Carlos Williams. In Jones AH, ed: Images of healers. Albany, State University of New York Press, 1983. p. 3–8.

**Williamson, George, 1819–1865**
Acharya AM: The first Indian War of Independence and military surgery. **Bull Indian Inst Hist Med (Hyderabad)** 1975 Oct;5(4):225–39

**Willis, Thomas, 1621–1675**
Dewhurst K: Thomas Willis's Oxford Lectures. Oxford, Sandford, 1980. x, 182 p.
Dewhurst K: Thomas Willis and the foundations of British neurology. In Rose FC, Bynum WF, ed: Historical aspects of the neurosciences. New York, Raven, 1982. p. 327–46.
Dewhurst K, ed: Willis's Oxford casebook (1650–52). Oxford, Sanford, 1981 xi, 199 p.
Faller A: Die Präparation der weissen Substanz des Gehirns bei Stensen, Willis und Vieussens. **Gesnerus** 1982;39(2):171–93
Hughes JT: Spinal cord arteries described by Willis. In Rose FC, Bynum WF, ed: Historical aspects of the neurosciences. New York, Raven, 1982. p. 195–203.
Meier RY: 'Sympathy' in the neurophysiology of Thomas Willis. **Clio Med** 1982 Dec;17(2–3):95–111
Nakamura T: T. Willis' and Lower's physiology with special reference to the theory of heart movement. **Jpn Stud Hist Sci** 1977;16:23–41

**Willits, Mary, 1855–1902**
Peitzman SJ: The quiet life of a Philadelphia medical woman: Mary Willits (1855--1902). **J Am Med Wom Assoc** 1979 Dec;34(12):443–6, 448, 450, passim

**Wilson, Charles, 1804–1884**
Drummond CG: Charles Wilson (1804–1884). In Passmore R, ed: Proceedings of the Royal College of Physicians of Edinburgh Tercentenary Congress, 1981. Edinburgh, Royal College of Physicians of Edinburgh, 1982. p. 199–203.

**Wilson, Clifford, 1906–**
Bergstrand A, Ostman J: Männen bakom syndromet: Paul Kimmelstiel och Clifford Wilson. Tysk och engelsman som möttes vid Harvard - först att beskriva speciell glomerulusskada. **Lakartidningen** 1984 Jan 25;81(4):227–8

**Wilson, Edmund Beecher, 1856–1939**
Baxter AL: E. B. Wilson's 'Destruction' of the germ-layer theory. **Isis** 1977 Sep;68(243):363–74

**Wilson, Edward O., 1929–**
Haraway D: The biological enterprise: sex, mind, and profit from human engineering to sociobiology. **Radic Hist Rev** 1979 Spring/Summer;Spec:206–37

**Wilson, Louis Blanchard, 1866–1943**
Ormsbee RA: A review: 'Studies in Pyroplasmosis hominis ('spotted fever' or 'tick fever' of the Rocky Mountains)' by Louis B. Wilson and William M. Chowning, published in The Journal of Infectious Diseases 1:31–57, 1904. **Rev Infect Dis** 1979 May–Jun;1(3):559–62

**Wilson, Maud Mellish, d. 1933**
Wilson LB: A women pioneer in a new profession, medical editing. **Mayo Alumnus** 1982 Apr;:20–3

**Wilson, Peter, 1791–1863**
Lambert G: Peter Wilson: colonial surgeon. Palmerston North, N.Z., Dunmore Press, 1981. 213 p.

**Wilson, William James Erasmus, 1809–1884**
Calwell HG: W. J. Wilson and the Weil-Felix reaction. **Ulster Med J** 1980;49:169–70

**Wilson, Woodrow, 1856–1924**
Freud S, Bullitt WC: Thomas Woodrow Wilson, twenty-eighth President of the United States: a psychological study. Boston, Houghton Mifflin; and Cambridge, Riverside, 1967. 307 p.
Marmor MF: Wilson, strokes, and zebras. **N Engl J Med** 1982 Aug 26;307(9):528–35
Ross D: Woodrow Wilson and the case for psychohistory. **J Am Hist** 1982;69(3):659–68
Texter JH: The President's dilemma, 1919 (Woodrow Wilson). **Va Med** 1980 Nov;107(11):756–62
Weinstein EA: Woodrow Wilson: a medical and psychological biography. Princeton, Princeton University Press, 1981. xi, 399 p.
Wilson, strokes, and zebras: **N Engl J Med** 1983 Jan 20;308(3):163–4

**Winiwarter, Alexander von, 1848–1917**
Lie JT, Mann RJ, Ludwig J: The brothers von Winiwarter, Alexander (1848–1917) and Felix (1852–1931), and thromboangiitis obliterans. **Mayo Clin Proc** 1979 Dec;54(12):802–7

**Winiwarter, Felix von, 1852–1931**
Lie JT, Mann RJ, Ludwig J: The brothers von Winiwarter, Alexander (1848–1917) and Felix (1852–1931), and thromboangiitis obliterans. **Mayo Clin Proc** 1979 Dec;54(12):802–7

**Winiwarter, Hans de, 1875–1949**
Leplat G: Hans de Winiwarter, 1875–1949. In Florilège des Sciences en Belgique - II. Bruxelles, Académie Royale de Belgique, 1980. p. 587–97.

**Winnicott, Donald Woods, 1896–1971**
Sutherland JD: The British object relations theorists: Balint, Winnicott, Fairbairn, Guntrip. **J Am Psychoanal Assoc** 1980;28(4):829–60

**Winslow, Charles-Edward Amory, 1877–1957**
Four from '44: the Winslow editorials: **J Public Health Policy** 1980 Mar;1(1):15–24
In the spirit of C.-E. A. Winslow: **J Public Health Policy** 1980 Mar;1(1):3–5
Viseltear AJ: Charles-Edward Amory Winslow. In Dictionary of American Biography, Suppl. 6, 1956–1960. p. 701–3, 1980.
Viseltear AJ: 'C.-E.A. Winslow and the early years of public health at Yale, 1915–1925'. **Yale J Biol Med** 1982 Mar–Apr;55(2):137–51

Winslow CE: Health in the twentieth century. New York, Arno, 1977. Reprint of Winslow's The evolution and significance of the modern public health campaign (New Haven, 1923); and Winslow's A city set on a hill: The significance of the health demonstration at Syracuse, New York (Garden City, N. Y., 1934). Various paginations.
The Winslow tradition: **J Public Health Policy** 1984 Sep;5(3):320-6

**Wintrobe, Maxwell Meyer, 1901-**
Wintrobe B: Mrs. Wintrobe writes about her husband. **Med Times** 1979 Nov;107(11):59-64

**Wishard, William Henry, 1816-1913**
Rice TB: One hundred years medicine: Indianapolis, 1820-1920. **Indiana Med Hist Q** 1976;2(3):40-4

**Wishard, William Niles, Sr., 1851-1941**
Rice TB: One hundred years medicine: Indianapolis, 1820-1920. **Indiana Med Hist Q** 1976;2(3):40-4

**Wislocki, George Bernays, 1892-1956**
Amoroso EC: George Bernays Wislocki. In Dictionary of American Biography, Suppl. 6, 1956-1960. p. 703-5, 1980.

**Wiśniowiecki, (Korybut), Michał, King of Poland, d. 1673**
Dudziński W: Choroba i zgon króla Michała Korybuta Wiśniowieckiego. **Wiad Lek** 1979 Jan 1;32(1):55-8

**Witelo, 1230 or 35-ca. 1275**
Lindberg DC, ed: Opticae thesaurus. Alhazeni Arabis libri septem, nuncprimùm editi. Eiusdem liber De Crepusculis et nubium ascensionibus. Item Vitellonis Thuringopoloni libri X. Reprint of the 1572 ed. New York, Johnson Reprint Corp., 1972. xxxiv, 288, 474 p.
Szpilczynski S: La théorie de la vision chez Witelo 'Peri optikes', 1273. In: Congrès international d'histoire de la médecine, XXVe, Québec, 1976. Actes. Québec, 1977. p. 1347-53.
Szpilczyński S: A látás kérdése Witelon (Vitellio) Peri optices (1275) c. munkájában. **Orvostort Kozl** 1979;87 88(25 no 1 2)219 22

**Withering, William, 1741-1799**
Albasanz Gallan JL: La digital, en su segundo centenario. **An R Acad Nac Med (Madr)** 1983;100(2):181-208

**Wittgenstein, Ludwig, 1889-1951**
McGuinness BF: Freud e Wittgenstein. **Ann Sc Norm Super Pisa** 1979;9(1):409-24

**Wittkower, Eric, 1899-**
Minde K: The scientific analyst -- a student's perspective. **Can J Psychiatry** 1979 Aug;24(5):498

**Wittmann, Michael Ferdinand, 1755-1862**
Frick K: Michael Ferdinand Wittmann (1755-1826) Magister und Doktor der Chirurgie, der erste graduierte Chirurg in Kärnten. **Carinthia** 1968;158:643-62

**Wittop Koning, Dirk Arnold, 1911-**
Ahlrichs EL: Dr. D. A. Wittop Koning 70 jaar. **Pharm Weekbl** 1981 Nov 6;116(45):1365-9

**Witzel, Adolf, 1847-1906**
Tanzer G: Adolf Witzel (1847-1906) und die Zahnerhaltung. **Zahnarzt** 1984 Jan;28(1):49-52
Ullmann E: Adolf Witzel--Leben und Werk. **Stomatol DDR** 1981 Jul;31(7):535-41

**Władysław III of Varna, 1424-1444**
Dudziński W: Smierć króla Władysława Warneńczvka. **Wiad Lek** 1981 Jun 1;34(11):953-5

**Władyslaw Jagiełło, 1350-1434**
Dudziński W: Choroby i zgon króla Władysława Jagiełły. **Wiad Lek** 1981 May 15;34(10):859-61

**Wöhler, Friedrich, 1800-1882**
Schmitz R: Der Beginn der organischen Chemie und der Neo-Vitalismus von heute. In Seidler E, Schott H, ed: Bausteine zur Medizingeschichte. Stuttgart, Steiner, 1984. p. 105-11.

**Wolf-Man, 1886-**
Loughman C: Voices of the Wolf Man: the Wolf Man as autobiographer. **Psychoanal Rev** 1984 Sep;71(2):211-25

**Wolfart, Karl Christian, 1778-1832**
Landauer AA: A note on the role of Karl Christian Wolfart (1778-1832) in the study of animal magnetism. **J Hist Behav Sci** 1981;17:206-8

**Wolfe, Thomas, 1900-1938**
Brown CL: Thomas Wolfe: a psychiatric view. **J Med Assoc State Ala** 1981 Oct;51(4):11-5

**Wolff, August Ferdynand, 1768-1846**
Wagner D: August Ferdynand Wolff und die Bedeutung der Semiotik. **Arch Hist Med (Warsz)** 1979;42(2):263-8

**Wolff, Caspar Friedrich, 1733-1794**
Gaĭsinovich AE: K. F. Vol'f i ego rol' v istorii embriologii i anatomii (k 250-letiiu so dnia rozhdeniia). **Arkh Anat Gistol Embriol** 1984 Aug;87(8):90-6
Lukács D: Caspar Friedrick Wolff (1733-1794), a modern fejlödéstan megalapítója. **Orv Hetil** 1984 Aug 5;125(32):1962
Roe SA: Matter, life, and generation. Eighteenth-century embryology and the Haller-Wolff debate. Cambridge, Cambridge University Press, 1981. 214 p.

**Wolff, Christian von, 1679-1754**
Richards RJ: Christian Wolff's prolegomena to empirical and rational psychology: translation and commentary. **Proc Am Philos Soc** 1980 Jun;124(3):227-39

**Wolff, James A.**
Pochedly C: Dr. James A. Wolff. I. Early progress in treatment of Rh hemolytic disease. **Am J Pediatr Hematol Oncol** 1984 Fall;6(3):319-23

**Wölfflin, Ernst, 1873-1959**
Berneaud-Kötz G: Wilhelm Conrad Röntgen: aus den Erinnerungen des Schweizer Ophthalmologen Ernst Wölfflin. **Klin Monatsbl Augenheilkd** 1982 Aug;181(2):138-41

**Wolter, Friedrich, 1863-1944?**
Howard-Jones N: Friedrich Wolter (1893?-1944): the last anticontagionist. **Br Med J** 1980 Feb 9;280(6211):372-3

**Wood, Earl Howard, 1912-**
Burchell HB: The investigator as volunteer subject. **Mayo Clin Proc** 1982 Jul;57 Suppl:28-33

**Wood, Jones Frederic, 1879-1954**
Elmslie RG: Our honoured anatomists. **Aust NZ J Surg** 1981 Oct;51(5):415-9

**Wood, Leonard, 1860-1927**
Chapman RF: Leonard Wood and leprosy in the Philippines: the Culion Leper Colony, 1921-1927. [Washington, D. C.], University Press of America, 1982. xviii, 219 p.
Leonard Wood, M.D.: Some Arizona Territory influences. **Ariz Med** 1982 Sep;39(9):593-6
Ljunggren B: The case of General Wood. **J Neurosurg** 1982 Apr;56(4):471-4
Pearlman M: Leonard Wood, William Muldoon and the medical profession: public health and universal military training. **N Engl Q** 1979;52(3):326-44

**Woodall, John, 1556?-1643**
Appleby JH: New light on John Woodall, surgeon and adventurer. **Med Hist** 1981 Jul;25(3):251-68
Ring ME: Oddments in dental history: what every sea surgeon of around 1600 ought to know concerning treating teeth. **Bull Hist Dent** 1984 Oct;32(2):109-11
Woodall J: The surgions mate. Facsimile of 1617 ed. Ed. J. Kirkup Bath, England, Kingsmead, 1978. xxxiv, 348 p.

**Woodger, Joseph Henry, 1894-1981**
Roll-Hansen N: E. S. Russell and J. H. Woodger: the failure of two twentieth-century opponents of mechanistic biology. **J Hist Biol** 1984 Fall;17(3):399-428

**Woods, Donald Devereux, 1912-1964**
Gale EF: Donald Devereux Woods. In Dictionary of national biography, 1961-1970. Suppl. 8, 1981. p. 1102-3.

**Woodward, Samuel Bayard, 1787-1850**
Grob GN, ed: The beginnings of mental hygiene in America. Three selected essays 1833-1850. New York, Arno, 1973. Various paginations. Includes works by Amariah Brigham (1833); William Sweetser (1850); Samuel B. Woodward (1840).

**Woolf, Virginia (Stephen), 1882-1941**
Feinstein SC: Why they were afraid of Virginia Woolf: perspectives on juvenile manic-depressive illness. **J Adolesc** 1980 Sep;3(3):187-96
Feinstein SC: Why they were afraid of Virginia Woolf: perspectives on juvenile manic-depressive illness. **Adolesc Psychiatry** 1980;8:332-43
Fromm H: Virginia Woolf: art and sexuality. **Va Q Rev** 1979;55(3):441-59
Hyman V: The autobiographical present in 'A Sketch of the Past'. **Psychoanal Rev** 1983 Spring;70(1):24-32
Panken S: 'Working through and the novel. **Psychoanal Rev** 1983 Spring;70(1):4-23
Sherman MH: Psychosensory images from Virginia Woolf's 'A Sketch of the Past'. **Psychoanal Rev** 1983 Spring;70(1):33-9
Southgate MT: A summer's reading: Virginia Woolf and her granddaughters. **Conn Med** 1981 Aug;45(8):483-6
Trombley S: All that summer she was mad: Virginia Woolf and her doctors. **Soc Soc Hist Med Bull (Lond)** 1981 Jun;28:21-5
Trombley S: All that summer she was mad: Virginia Woolf, female victim of male medicine. New York, Continuum, 1982. ix, 338 p.

**Worcester, Noah, fl. 1846**
Weiner AL: The Noah Worcester Dermatological Society. **Int J Dermatol** 1980 Jun;19(5):288-90

**Wordsworth, Dorothy, 1771-1855**
Gibson II: Illness of Dorothy Wordsworth. **Br Med J [Clin Res]** 1982 Dec 18-25;285(6357):1813-5

**Work, Hubert, 1860-1942**
Delaney JJ: Hubert Work. **Colo Med** 1983 Oct;80(10):285-6

**Worm, Johan, 1529-1601**
Hovesen E: Ole Worm og familien i Arhus.

**Dan Medicinhist Arbog** 1981;:9-23

**Worm, Ole, 1588-1654**
Hovesen E: Ole Worm og familien i Arhus. **Dan Medicinhist Arbog** 1981;:9-23
Hovesen E: Ole Worm - aegtemand og husfader. **Dan Medicinhist Arbog** 1982;:93-111

**Worm, Willum, 1563-1629**
Hovesen E: Ole Worm og familien i Arhus. **Dan Medicinhist Arbog** 1981;:9-23

**Wormall, Arthur, 1900-1964**
Morgan WT: Arthur Wormall. In Dictionary of national biography, 1961-1970. Suppl. 8, 1981. p. 1110-1.

**Wright, Almroth Edward, 1861-1947**
Gröschel DH, Hornick RB: Who introduced typhoid vaccination: Almroth Wright or Richard Pfeiffer? **Rev Infect Dis** 1981 Nov-Dec;3(6):1251-4

**Wright, Chauncey, 1830-1875**
Gershenowitz H: Chauncey Wright's views on Lamarck. **Indian J Hist Sci** 1979, reçu 1982:14(1):16-24

**Wright, Christopher A., 1928-1983**
Southgate VR: Obituary. Dr. Christopher A. Wright. **Int J Parasitol** 1984 Jun;14(3):223-7

**Wright, David Hudson, 1881-1948**
McDonald WH: Then and now. 75 years of Alabama medicine by father and son with comments on the birth of malpractice. **J Med Assoc State Ala** 1979 Jan;48(7):16-8

**Wright, Helena, 1887-1981**
Evans B: Freedom to choose: the life and work of Dr. Helena Wright, pioneer of contraception. London, Bodley Head, 1984. 285 p.

**Wright, Norman Charles, 1900-1970**
Hollingsworth DF: Sir Norman Charles Wright. In Dictionary of national biography, 1961-1970. Suppl. 8, 1981. p. 1115-6.

**Wright, Orville, 1871-1948**
Tipton DA, Mohler SR: The Wright brothers: a personality profile. **Aviat Space Environ Med** 1983 Jun;54(6):560-2

**Wright, Sewall, 1889-**
Crow JF: Sewall Wright, the scientist and the man. **Perspect Biol Med** 1982 Winter;25(2):279-94
Opitz JM: Introduction of Sewall Wright on the occasion of receiving the first Meckel medal and prize in mammalian developmental genetics. **Am J Med Genet** 1984 Aug;18(4):587-90

**Wright, Wilbur, 1817-1912**
Tipton DA, Mohler SR: The Wright brothers: a personality profile. **Aviat Space Environ Med** 1983 Jun;54(6):560-2

**Wright, William Thomas, 1927-**
McDonald WH: Then and now. 75 years of Alabama medicine by father and son with comments on the birth of malpractice. **J Med Assoc State Ala** 1979 Jan;48(7):16-8

**Wrzosek, Adam, 1875-1965**
Konopka S: Działalność naukowa, redakcyjna i wydawnicza prof. Adama Wrzoska w świetle jego wypowiedzi i listów nie ogłoszonych w druku. **Arch Hist Med (Warsz)** 1982;45(1-4):11-26

**Wu Hsien, 1893-1959**
Bishop C: Hsien Wu (1893-1959): a biographical sketch. **Clin Chem** 1982 Feb;28(2):378-80

**Wunderlich, Karl Reinhold August, 1815-1877**
Wunderlich CA: Wien und Paris. Ein Beitrag zur Geschichte und Beurteilung der gegenwärtigen Heilkunde in Deutschland und Frankreich, 1841. Herausgegeben und eingeleitet von H. M. Koelbing. Bern, Huber, 1974. 159 p. (Hubers Klassiker der Medizin und der Naturwissenschaften, Bd. 13).

**Wundt, Wilhelm Maximilian, 1832-1920**
Blumenthal AL: Wundt - revisions and reappraisals. In K. Salzinger, ed: Psychology in progress: an interim report. (Annals of the New York Academy of Sciences, vol. 270). New York, New York Academy of Sciences, 1976. p. 21-9.
Blumenthal AL: Wilhelm Wundt and early American psychology: a clash of cultures. In R. W. Rieber, K. Salzinger, ed: Psychology: theoretical-historical perspectives. New York, Academic Press, 1980. p. 25-42.
Bringmann WG, Balk MM: Wilhelm Wundt's publication record: a re-examination. **Stor Crit Psicol** 1983;4(1):61-86
Bringmann WG, Ungerer GA: The establishment of Wilhelm Wundt's Leipzig laboratory. **Stor Crit Psicol** 1980;1(1):11-28
Dazzi N, Ferruzzi F: Wundt, Titchener e la psicologia americana. **Stor Crit Psicol** 1980;1(1):29-52
Eckhardt G, ed: Zur Geschichte der Psychologie. Berlin, VEB Deutscher Verlag der Wissenschaften, 1979. 128p. Mit Beiträgen von H. Hiebsch, F. Klix, W. Schreier, und L. Sprung.
Leahey TH: The mistaken mirror: on Wundt's and Titchener's psychologies. **J Hist Behav Sci** 1981;17:273-82
Marion P: La psicologia del pensiero dalla polemica di Wundt alla Entwicklungspsychologie di Bühler. **Stor Crit Psicol** 1982 Dec;3(2):249-79
Poggi I: Wundt e il linguaggio dei gesti. **Stor Crit Psicol** 1981;2(2):297-314
Rieber RW, ed: Wilhelm Wundt and the making of a scientific psychology. New York, Plenum, 1980. xii, 252 p. Includes contributions by S. Diamond, K. Danziger, A. L. Blumenthal, W. James, S. Feldman, H. K. Haebertin.
Ross HE, Bischof K: Wundt's views on sensations of innervation: a reevaluation. **Perception** 1981;10(3):319-29
Smith R: Wilhelm Wundt resurrected. **Br J Hist Sci** 1982 Nov;15(51 pt 3):285-91
Sprung L: Wilhelm Wundt--Bedenkenswertes und Bedenkliches aus seinem Lebenswerk. In Eckardt G, ed: Zur Geschichte der Psychologie. Berlin, VEB Deutscher Verlag der Wissenschaften, 1979. p. 73-82.
Todes DP: Biological psychology and the Tsarist censor: the dilemma of scientific development. **Bull Hist Med** 1984 Winter;58(4):529-44
Ungerer GA: Wilhelm Wundt als Psychologe und Politiker: Anmerkungen zur Biographie. **Psychol Rundschau** 1980;31:99-110

**Wyeth, John Allan, 1845-1922**
Shell DH, Sparkman RS: John Allan Wyeth, MD. Surgeon, soldier, author and founder of postgraduate medical education in America. **Am J Surg** 1980 Sep;140(3):447-56

**Wyman, Rufus, 1777-1842**
Grob GN, ed: The beginnings of American psychiatric thought and practice. Five accounts, 1811-1830. New York, Arno, 1973. Various paginations. Includes Account of the rise and progress of the Asylum . . . near Philadelphia (1814), and works by Theodric Romeyn Beck (1811); Thomas Eddy (1815); George Parkman (1814); and Rufus Wyman (1830).

**Wynder, Ernest Ludwig, 1922-**
Wynder EL: Some reflections on smoking and lung cancer. **J Thorac Cardiovasc Surg** 1984 Nov;88(5 Pt 2):854-7

# X

**Xue Lizhai**
Shi Changyong: [Life and chronology of Xue Lizhai.] (Chi). **Chin J Med Hist** 1981;11:65-9

# Y

**Yandell, David Wendel, 1826-1898**
Baird ND: David Wendel Yandell, physician of old Louisville. Lexington: University Press of Kentucky, 1978. x, 116 p.

**Yandell, Lunsford P., 1837-1884**
Baird ND: There is no Sunday in the army: Civil War letters of Lunsford P. Yandell, 1861-62. **Filson Club Hist Q** 1979;53(4):317-27

**Yandell, Lunsford Pitts, 1902-**
Baird ND: A Kentucky physician examines Memphis. **Tenn Hist Q** 1978;37(2):190-202

**Yáñez, Agustín, fl. 1831**
Esteva de Sagrera J: Una obra inédita y desconocida de Agustín Yáñez y Girona. **Bol Soc Esp Hist Farm** 1979 Dec;30(120):295-304

**Yang T'iein Hui, fl. 11th-12th cent.**
Guo Chengyu: [Yang Tianhui and his 'Records on Radix aconitinum'] (Chi). **Chin J Med Hist** 1981;11(1):48-50

**Yater, Wallace Mason, 1895-1976**
Luongo EP: A biography of Wallace Mason Yater, M.D. [S.l., s.n.], 1982. iv, 180 p.

**Yates, Horatio, 1821-1882**
Angus MS: Horatio Yates. In Dictionary of Canadian biography, 1881-1890. 1982;11:940-1.

**Yeager, Robert Lee, 1872-1940**
Wygant LJ, ed: The Galveston smallpox quarantine camp in 1899. **Bookman** 1982;9(3):3-8

**Yeats, William Butler, 1865-1939**
Lock S: 'O that I were young again': Yeats and the Steinach operation. **Br Med J [Clin Res]** 1983 Dec 24-31;287(6409):1964-8
Pruitt VD: Yeats, the Mask, and the poetry of old age. **J Geriatr Psychiatry** 1982;15(1):99-112

**Yerena, Jesus Antonio, 1917-**
Velez Boza F: Homenaje a la memoria del Dr. Jesus A. Yerena. **Rev Soc Venez Hist Med** 1975-76;23(37):91-100

**Yerkes, Robert Mearns, 1876-1956**
Cravens H: Robert Mearns Yerkes. In Dictionary of American Biography, Suppl. 6, 1956-1960. p. 717-19, 1980.
Haraway D: The biological enterprise: sex, mind, and profit from human engineering to sociobiology. **Radic Hist Rev** 1979 Spring/Summer;Spec:206-37

**Yersin, Alexandre, 1863-1943**
Bonifas V: Alexandre Yersin (1863-1943). **Rev Med Suisse Romande** 1984 May;104(5):349-51
Butler T: Plague and other Yersinia infections. New York, London, Plenum Medical Book Co., 1983. xii, 220 p. (Current Topics in

Infectious Disease).
Dilg-Frank R: Alexandre Yersin als Medizinstudent in Marburg. **Alma Mater Philipp** 1978-1979;19-23
Moseley JE: Travels of Alexandre Yersin: letters of a pastorian in Indochina, 1890-1894. **Perspect Biol Med** 1981 Summer;24(4):607-18

**Yonge, James, 1647-1721**
Harper E: The sailor's surgeon (James Yonge). **J R Nav Med Serv** 1979 Spring;65(1):35-7
Poynter FN: James Yonge. In Dictionary of Canadian biography, 1701 to 1740. Volume 2, 1969. p. 670-2.

**Youatt, William, 1776-1847**
Carter HE: Historical cases. Illustrations of the distemper of dogs. By William Youatt. **J Small Anim Pract** 1981 Apr;22(4):207-11

**Young, Anne Austin, 1892-**
Klosky BA: Daring venture: a biography of Anne Austin Young, pioneer woman doctor. Columbia, S.C., Bryan, 1978. xiii, 193 p.

**Young, Brigham, 1801-1877**
McCue RJ: Did the word of wisdom become a commandment in 1851? **Dialogue J Mormon Thought** 1981;14(3):66-77

**Young, Thomas, 1773-1829**
Chappert A: L' autobiographical sketch de Thomas Young. **Rev Hist Sci (Paris)** 1981 Apr;34(2):137-8
Laird JD: Thomas Young, M.D. (1773-1829). **Am Heart J** 1980 Jul;100(1):1-8
Sherman PD: Colour vision in the nineteenth century: the Young-Helmholtz-Maxwell theory. Bristol, Adam Hilger, 1981. xiii, 233 p.

**Yperman, Jan, fl. 1310**
Colard A: Evocation du passé. Jehan Yperman et l'éthique médicale. **Rev Med Brux** 1982 Mar;3(3):171-2
Vrebos J: Jehan Yperman, medieval cleft lip surgeon. **Plast Reconstr Surg** 1982 Dec;70(6):762-5

**Ysabeau, A.**
Bazzi F, Bèttica-Giovannini R: L'atlante fisiognomonico e frenologico del sig. Ysabeau tra quelli di Lavater e di Fall e quello di Lombroso. **Ann Osp Maria Vittoria Torino** 1980 Jul-Dec;23(7-12):343-416

# Z

**Zablotskiĭ-Desiatovskiĭ, Paulus, 1814-1883**
Il'in II, Preĭsman BS: P. P. Zablotskiĭ-Desiatovskiĭ i ego rol' v razvitii venerologii v Rossii (k 100-letiiu so dnia smerti). **Vestn Dermatol Venerol** 1983 Dec;(12):59-60

**Zabolotnyĭ, Daniil Kirillovich, 1866-1929**
Mazurik EV: Pervye shagi nauchnoĭ deiatel'nosti D. K. Zabolotnogo. **Zh Mikrobiol Epidemiol Immunobiol** 1983 May;(5):99-101
Smirnov VV, Bilaĭ VI: Zhizn' i deiatel'nost' D. K. Zabolotnogo v Kieve. **Mikrobiol Zh** 1982 May-Jun;44(3):86-90

**Zacchias, Paolo, 1584-1659**
Maeder H: Die Frau im 17. Jahrhundert im Spiegel der 'Quaestiones medico-legales' des Paolo Zacchia (1584-1659). Diss. Bern, 1981. 101 p.

**Záček, Adolf, 1917-**
Významné životné jubileum prof. MUDr. Adolfa Zácka: **Cesk Zdrav** 1982 Dec;30(12):530-6

**Zacutus, Abraham Lusitanus, 1575-1642**
Kottek S: Aperçu sur l' 'introduction à la pratique médicale', (introitus medici ad praxin) de Zacutus Lusitanus, 1575 - 1642. **Rev Hist Med Heb** 1980 Mar-Apr;33(1):13-16
Kottek S: Aperçu sur l''introduction à la pratique médicale', (introitus medici ad praxin) de Zacutus Lusitanus, 1575 - 1642. **Rev Hist Med Heb** 1980 Jul;33(2):35-8

**Zahorski, Karol, 1879-1970**
Brożek K: Dr med. Karol Zahorski (1879--1970) lekarz-społecznik w Zagłębiu Dąbrowskim (w 100-lecie urodzin). **Pol Tyg Lek** 1979 Jun 25;34(26):1057-9

**Zahrádniček, Jan, 1882-1958**
Kubat R, Mřena V: Operatsiia Zagradnicheka pri vrozhdennom vyvikhe bedra segodnia (posviashchaetsia 100-letiiu so dnia rozhdeniia professora Iana Zagradnicheka). **Ortop Travmatol Protez** 1982 Jul;(7):69-71

**Zajonc, Robert B., 1923-**
Distinguished scientific contribution awards for 1978 (Julian Hochberg, Philip Teitelbaum, Robert B. Zajonc).: **Am Psychol** 1979 Jan;34(1):35-47

**Zakhar'in, Grigoriĭ Antonovich, 1829-1897**
Mikhaĭlov FA: Iz rasskazov o G. A. Zakhar'ine. **Klin Med (Mosk)** 1980 Jan;58(1):113-4

**Zakrzewska, Marie Elizabeth, 1829-1902**
Punnett L: Women-controlled medicine--theory and practice in 19th century Boston. **Women Health** 1976 Jul-Aug;1(4)3-11
Punnett L: Marie Elizabeth Zakrzewska 1829-1902. **Women Health** 1976 Jul-Aug;1(4):1-2

**Zambonino da Gazza, d. ca. 1298**
Marangon P: Il trattato 'De conservatione sanitatis' di Zanbonino da Gazzo (d. dopo il 1298). **Quad Stor Univ Padova** 1975;8:1-17

**Zamenhof, Ludwik Lazar, 1859-1917**
Commemorative coin for Dr. Zamenhof: **Newsl Optom Hist Soc** 1981;12(1):6

**Zangger, Rudolf, 1826-1882**
Zerobin K, Senn C: Rudolf Zangger, Direktor der Tierarzneischule in Zürich (26. November 1826-6, März 1882). **Schweiz Arch Tierheilkd** 1982 Mar;124(3):111-9

**Zavadovskiĭ, Mikhail Mikhailovich, 1891-1957**
Oshmarin AP: Gel'mintologicheskie issledovaniia M. M. Zavadovskogo. **Parazitologiia** 1980 May-Jun;14(3):282-7

**Zelenin, Vladimir Filippovich, 1881-1968**
Borodulin VI: Vydaiushchiĭsia terapevt V. F. Zelenin i ego rol' v razvitii sovetskoĭ meditsiny. **Feldsher Akush** 1982;47(3):52-4
Kuz'min MK: V. F. Zelenin i ego rol' v razvitii klinicheskoĭ élektrokardiografii i funktsional'noĭ diagnostike. **Klin Med (Mosk)** 1981 Aug;59(8):115-8
Martynov IV, Borodulin VI: Rol' V.F. Zelenina v otechestvennoĭ kardiologii. **Klin Med (Mosk)** 1981 Aug;59(8):118-20

**Zetkin, Maxim, 1883-1965**
Burmeister KJ, Lange-Pfautsch R: Maxim Zetkin--Kommunist und Arzt (1883-1965). **Z Arztl Fortbild (Jena)** 1983;77(16):695-7
Dobek R, Kolmsee P: Maxim Zetkin--Arzt, Kriegschirurg und Kommunist. **Militaergesch** 1978;17(5):595-603
Eitner S: Das gerontologische Engagement von Maxim Zetkin in seinen späten Lebensjahren. **ZFA** 1984 Jan-Feb;39(1):5-8

**Zhukovskiĭ, Vasiliĭ Andreevich, 1783-1852**
Arkhangel'skiĭ GV: Vrachebnoe okruzhenie vydaiusnchegosia Russkogo poéta V. A. Zhukovskogo (k 200-letiiu so dnia rozhdeniia). **Klin Med (Mosk)** 1984 May;62(5):139-44

**Zielina, Jan**
Kłodziński S: Ppłk lek. med. Jan Zielina. **Przegl Lek** 1981;38(1):202-6

**Ziembicki, Witold, 1874-1949**
Konopka S: Relacje profesorów Wydziału lekarskiego Uniwersytetu Jagiellonskiego o dziejach medycyny polskiej. **Arch Hist Med (Warsz)** 1979;42(1):107-24

**Zilboorg, Gregory, 1890-1959**
Mora G: Gregory Zilboorg. In Dictionary of American Biography, Suppl. 6, 1956-1960. p. 724-5, 1980.

**Zimmermann, Johann Georg, 1728-1795**
Brister L: J. G. Zimmermanns Essay 'Von der Erfahrung in der Arzneikunst': Ein Beitrag zur rationalen Medizin. **Schweiz Med Wochenschr** 1980 Apr 19;110(16):615-9

**Ziurek, Otto Adolph Albert, 1821-1886**
Blum W: Der Apotheker und Chemiker Otto A. Ziurek (1821-1886) und die Apothekenreformbewegung von 1848. Braunschweig, 1980. 110 p. (Veröffentlichungen aus dem Pharmaziegeschichtlichen Seminar der Technischen Universität Braunschweig, 22).

**Zlábek, Karel, 1902-1983**
Kos J: In memoriam Professor Karel Zlábek. **Anat Anz** 1984;156(5):345-50

**Zmeev, Lev Fedorovich, 1832-1901**
Arkhangel'skiĭ GV: L.F. Zmeev-vydaiushchiĭsia otechestvennyĭ istorik meditsiny i bibliograf. **Sov Zdravookhr** 1979;(8):64-7

**Zola, Emile, 1840-1902**
Malinas C, Malinas Y: Emile Zola et la génétique. La nevrose des Rougon-Macquart. **J Genet Hum** 1981 Dec;29(5 Suppl):593-602

**Zubirán, Salvador, 1898-**
XXXVI aniversario de la fundación del Instituto nacional de la nutrición Salvador Zubirán. Homenaje al Dr. Salvador Zubirán: **Rev Invest Clin** 1983 Jan-Mar;35(1):85-103

**Zubku-Kodrianu, N. P., 1850-**
Popushoĭ EP, Ioksa VA: N. P. Zubku-Kodrianu--progressivnyĭ vrach, vidnyĭ uchastnik revoliutsionno-demokraticheskogo dvizheniia. **Sov Zdravookhr** 1979;(3):59-63

**Zuckerkandl, Emil, 1849-1910**
Ober WB: Emil Zuckerkandl and his delightful little organ. **Pathol Annu** 1983;18(Pt 1):103-19

**Zur-mkhar Mnyam-nyid-rdo-rje, 1439-1475**
Bye Ba Rin Bsrel: Instructions of the great Zur-mkhar Mñam-ñid-rdo-rje on medical treatment comprising the Ma yig, Bu yig, and Kha 'thor collections. (Tib) Reproduced from a print from the Tsharon Sman-dgon blocks. Leh, Ladakh, Tashigangpa, 1974. np (Smanrtsis Shesrig Spendzod, Vol. 58).

**Zur Verth, Max, 1874-1941**
Watermann RA: Figures for bone-amputations, introduced by Zur Verth and regarding artificial limbs. In: Congrès international d'histoire de la médecine, XXVe, Québec, 1976. Actes. Québec, 1977. p. 1386-95.

**Zurbarán, Francisco, 1598-1664**
Moskow BS: The iconography of the dental profession. Francisco

Zurbarán (1598-1664). **Quintessence Int** 1984 Aug;15(8):814-5

**Zweig, Stefan, 1881-1942**
Haenel T: Die Suizidproblematik bei Stefan Zweig. **Schweiz Arch Neurol Neurochir Psychiatr** 1981;129(2):297-314

**Zwinger, Théodor, 1533-1588**
Gilly C: Zwischen Erfahrung und Spekulation. Theodor Zwinger und die religiöse und kulturelle Krise seiner Zeit. **Basler Z Gesch Altertumskd** 1977;77:57-137

# CHRONOLOGICAL AND GEOGRAPHICAL SUMMARY OF BIOGRAPHIES

Habsburg Family

**Belgium**

Van Bandeloo Family, 1586–1785

**China**

Dar-mo Sman-ram Blo-bzan-chos-grags

**France**

Spillmann Family

**Germany**

Gärtner Family, 17–18th cent.
Pies Family

**Hungary**

Spilenberg Family

**India**

Dalhana

**Spain**

Viader Family

## BEFORE 500 A.D.

Agatha, Saint
Apollonia of Alexandria, Saint
Ben Zabda, Yohanan
Buddha
Cosmas and Damian, Saints
Eshmun, God of Sidon
Gargilius Martialis, Quintus, fl. 220–260
Jesus Christ
Joseph, the Patriarch
Lucia, Saint
Luke, Saint
Maria, Prophetess, 2nd or 3rd cent.
Michael, Saint
Moses
Nicholas, Saint, Bp. of Myra, 4th cent.
Pelagonius Salonius

**Carthage**

Hannibal, 247?–183 B.C.

**China**

Bao Qianguang, fl. 310–363
Chunyu, Yi, ca. 205–ca. 134 B.C.
Khwada

**Egypt**

Imhotep
Tutankhamun, fl. ca. 1358 B.C.
Udjahorresnet

**Greco-Roman**

Apollonius, of Tyana
Aretaeus of Cappadocia
Galen
Nemesius, Bp. of Emesa, fl. 390–400
Oribasius, fl. 4th cent. A.D.

**Greece**

Aesculapius, God of Medicine
Alcmaeon, of Crotona, fl. 5th cent. B.C.
Alexander the Great, 356–323 B.C.
Aristotle
Democritus, ca. 460–ca. 370 B.C.
Demosthenes, 385?–322 B.C.
Dioscorides, Pedanius, of Anazarbos
Erasistratus, fl. ca. 250 B.C.
Euclid
Herodicus
Herodotus, ca. 484–425 B.C.
Herophilus, 335–280 B.C.
Hippocrates
Homer
Nicander, fl. ca. 2nd cent. B.C.
Plato
Rufus, of Ephesus
Socrates
Solon, 638?–599? B.C.
Soranus, of Ephesus, 2nd cent.
Theophrastus
Thucydides, b. ca. 460 B.C.

**India**

Atreya, Maharshi
Ravana
Susruta

**Israel**

Ezekiel (prophet)
Samson
Saul, King of Israel

**Rome**

Aelius Aristides, 117–180
Asclepiades Bithynus
Aurelianus, Caelius
Calcidius, fl. 400
Cato, Marcus Porcius, 234–149 B.C.
Celsus, Aulus Cornelius
Cicero, Marcus Tullius
Hadrian, Emperor, 76–138
Lactantius, Lucius Caecilius Firmianus, ca. 260–ca. 340
Lucretius Carus, Titus, ca. 96–55 B.C.
Marcellus Empiricus, 4th–5th cent.
Maximinus I, Gaius Julius Verus, 173–238
Ovid, 43 B.C.–ca. 17 A.D.
Palladius, Rutilius Taurus Aemilianus
Pammachius, d. 410
Plinius Secundus, C., 23–79
Plinius Secundus, C., 23–79 A.D.
Seneca, Lucius Annaeus
Seneca, Lucius Annaeus (the Elder)
Virgil

## 500 A.D.–1450

Albertus Magnus, Saint, Bp. of Ratisbon, 1193?–1280
Apuleius Barbarus
Asaph Ha-Yehoudi, 7th cent.
Boniface VIII, Pope, 1235?–1303
Emmeram, Saint, d. ca. 660
Fontana, Giovanni, ca. 1395–ca. 1455
Gilbertus Anglicus, 1180?–1250
Gregorius, Saint, Bp. of Tours, 538–594
Hucbald of St. Amand, ca. 840–930
Israeli, Isaac, ca. 832–ca. 932
Johannes Aegidius Zamorensis, 1240 or 41–ca. 1316
Johannes XXI, Pope, d. 1277
Johannis of Alexandria
Nicholas of Lynne, fl. 1386
Nicolaus Cusanus, Cardinal, 1401–1464
Uncumber, Saint
Wilgefortis, Saint

#### Arabic

Abu Mansur al-Hasan b. Nuh al-Qumri, 10th cent.
Abulcasis, 936?–1013?
Ahmad ibn Ibrāhim, called Ibn al-Jazzār, d. ca. 1009
Alhazen, 965–1039
Alkindus, Jacobus, d. ca. 870
Averroes, 1126–1198
Avicenna, 980?–1037
al-Biruni, 973?–1048
Bukhtishu' ibn Jibrail, d. 870
Costa Ben Luca, fl. 870
Djahiz, 776–868
Dunash ben Tamin, 10th cent.
Duran, R. Simon ben Zemah, 1361–1444
Hunain Ibn Ishak, al-'Ibadi, 809?–873
Ibn Abi l-Bayan, 1161–1240
Ibn al-'Ayn Zarbi, d. 1153
Ibn al-Hassa, fl. 13th cent.
Ibn al-Nafis, d. 1288 or 9
Ibn al-Quff, 1233–1286
Ibn al-Tilmidh, ca. 1073–1165
Ibn Butlan, d. 1068
Ibn Gabirol, Solomon ben Judah, ca. 1021–ca. 1058
Ibn Jazlah, d. ca. 1100
Ibn Khaldun, 1332–1406
Ibn-Omrane Ishaq, d. 892 or 3
Ibn Qaiyim al-Gauziya, 1292–1350
Ibn Suwadi, d. 1291 or 2
Ishaq Ibn 'Imran, 10th cent.
Jabir ibn Haiyan, al-Tarasusi
al-Jayyāni, Abū 'Abd Allāh Muhammad ibn Mu'ādh
Al-Jildaki, d. ca. 1342
Al-Magusi, Ali ibn al-Abbas
Al-Majusi, d. 994
Mesuë, d. 857
Mohammed, the Prophet, ca. 570–632
Moses ben Maimon, 1135–1204
Moses ben Nahman, 1194–1270
Rhazes, 865–925
Al Ruhawi, Ishaq ibn Ali, 9th cent.
Sinan ibn Thabit ibn Qurra, Abu Said, ca. 880–943
Tabit ibn Qurra

#### Asia

Nagarjuna, Siddha
Timur, the Great, 1336–1405

#### Belgium

Eyck, Jan van, ca. 1390–1440
Van der Paele, G., 1370–1443
Yperman, Jan, fl. 1310

#### Byzantium

Aetius, of Amida
Agathias
Theodore of Sykeon, d. 613
Theophane Nonno, 10th cent.

#### Cambodia

Indravarman II, 1220–1243?

#### China

Sun, Ssu-miao, 581–682
Sung Tz'u, 1186–1249
Yang T'iein Hui, fl. 11th–12th cent.

#### Denmark

Harpestraeng, Henrik, d. 1244
Waldemar IV, At'terdag, 1320?–1375

#### France

Astruc de Sestiers, fl. early 15th cent.
Bernard de Gordon, fl. ca. 1283–ca. 1308
Charles VI, King of France, 1368–1422
Despars, Jacques, 1380–1458
Guinefort, Saint
Guy de Chauliac, ca. 1300–ca. 1368
Jeanne d'Arc, Saint, 1412–1431
Louis XI, King of France, 1423–1483
Marbode, Bp. of Rennes, d. 1123
Mauchaut, Guillaume de, 1300?–1377
Muste, Laurent
Raimon de Castelnou, fl. ca. 1350
Roland l'Ecrivain, fl. 1430
Stephen of Bourbon, ca. 1180–1262
Tainard, fl. 1076

#### Germany

Albrant, Meister, fl. 13th cent.
Elizabeth, of Hungary, Saint, 1207–1231
Engelin, Jakob, ca. 1365–1420
Frederick II, Emperor of Germany, 1194–1250
Hartlieb, Johann, d. 1468
Heinrich II, Saint, Emperor of Germany, 973–1024
Hildegard, Saint, 1098?–1178
Konrad der Münzmeister, fl. 1400
Nicolaus Cusanus, Cardinal, 1401–1464
Ortolff von Bayrlandt
Ottilia, Saint, d. ca. 720
Schreck von Aschaffenburg, Konrad

#### Great Britain

Arderne, John, fl. 1307–1370
Bartholomaeus Anglicus, fl. 1230–1250
Bede (the Venerable), 673–735
Bradwardine, Thomas, Abp. of Canterbury, 1290?–1349
Chaucer, Geoffrey, 1344–1400
Cuthbert, Saint, d. 687
Grosseteste, Robert, 1175?–1253
Henry II, King of England, 1133–1189
Melus, fl. 6th cent.
Morsted, Thomas, ca. 1380–1456
Ricardus de Bello, fl. 1276–1312
Trevisa, John, ca. 1342–1402

#### Greece

Johannes Damascenus, b. ca. 676
Paul of Aegina, 7th cent.
Stephanus, of Athens, 7th cent.

#### Hungary

Elizabeth, of Hungary, Saint, 1207–1231

#### India

Diya Muhammad Masud Rashid Zangi Umar Ghaznavi
Fayyad bin Hakim Wahhaj
Gadadhara, 7th and 8th cent.
Goraksanātha
Jejjata, 9th cent.
Mallinatha, 15th cent.
Sarngadhara, fl. 13th cent.
Vagbhata, son of Nomikumara, ca. 1200

#### Italy

Alderotti, Taddeo, 1223–1295?
Benedetto Greco da Salerno, fl. 1401
Benedict of Nursia, Saint, ca. 480–ca. 544
Cesi, Nicolò, fl. 1391
Colonna Egidio, 1247?–1316
Dagomari, Paolo, ca. 1281–1365
Francesco, d'Assisi, Saint, 1182–1226
Francis of Assisi, Saint, 1182–1226
Gerardus, Cremonensis, 1114–1187
Jacopone da Todi, ca. 1230–ca. 1306
Lanfranco, of Milan, fl. 1290–1296
Petrarca, Francesco, 1304–1374
Petrus de Ebulo, fl. 1196
Salicetti, ca. 1210–1275 or 80
Scellinck, Thomas, fl. 1317–1343

Thomas Aquinas, Saint, 1225?–1274
Tortelli, Giovanni, 1400–1466
Trotula de Ruggiero, 12th cent.
Valla, Lorenzo, 1407?–1457
Vitry, Jacques de, ca. 1165–1240
Zambonino da Gazza, d. ca. 1298

### Japan

Jianzhen, fl. 688

### Lebanon

Qustā Ibn Lūqā al-Ba'labakki, ca. 820–912

### Netherlands

Maerlant, Jacob van, 1235?–1300
Marsilius van Inghen, d. 1396

### Poland

Jadwiga, Queen of Poland, 1370–1399
Witelo, 1230 or 35–ca. 1275
Władysław III of Varna, 1424–1444
Władyslaw Jagiełło, 1350–1434

### Portugal

Hispanus, Pedro, b. ca. 1210

### Rome

Cassiodorus, Flavius Magnus Aurelius, ca. 487–ca. 580

### Spain

Abd Al-Malik Ibn Habib al-Sulami al Ilbiri, ca. 790–854
Abu Muhammad 'Ali ibn Hazm, 994–1063
Arnaldus de Villanova, d. 1313?
Avenzoar, d. ca. 1162
Chirino, Alonso, d. 1430?
Clapers, Bernat dez, d. 1311
Gonzáles de Clavijo, Ruy, d. 1412
Al-Harizi, Judah b. Solomon, b. ca. 1170
Ibn al-Baytar, 1190–1248
Ibn al-Khatib, 1313–1374
Joseph ben Meir ibn Zabara, b. ca. 1140
Judah ha-Lévi, 1085?–1140?
Llull, Ramón, 1235?–1316?
Muhammad b. 'Abdallah b. al-Jatib, 1313–1374

### Switzerland

Armengandus Blasii, fl. 1280–1309

### Turkey

Sabuncuoglu, Serafeddin, fl. 1404–1468

### USSR

Panaskerteli-Tsitsishvili, Z.
Panaskerteli-Tsitsishvili, Zaza, fl. 15th cent.

## 1450–1700

Arcimboldo, Giuseppe, 1527?–1593
Augustus II (the Strong), 1670–1733
Columbus, Christopher, 1446–1506
Cornarius, Janus, 1500–1558
Iodocus, fl. 1474
Kalkar, Jan Stevenszoon van, 1499?–ca. 1550
Middelburg, Paulus van, 1445–1533
Moravia, Pedro, fl. 1578
Riebeeck, Jan Anthony van, 1618–1677
Ruland Family
Verbezius, David, 1577–1644
Vesalius, Andreas, 1514–1564
Zacchias, Paolo, 1584–1659

### Austria

Cuefner, Johannes
Gasser, Achilles, 1531–1583
Iserin von Mazo, Georg, fl. 1527
Mannagetta, Johann Wilhelm, 1588–1666
Sigismund, of Austria

### Belgium

Aguilon, François d', 1566–1617
Calcar, Jan Stephan van, 1499–1546?
Helmont, Jean Baptiste van, 1577–1644
Hogenberg, Remigius, ca. 1536–
Iscanius, David Lipsius, 17th cent.
L'Ecluse, Charles de, 1526–1609
Mercator, Gerhardus, 1512–1594
Nonnius, Ludovicus, ca. 1555–1645?
Rubens, Peter Paul, 1577–1640
Save, Philippe Ignace, 1659–1702
Schuute, Cornelis, d. 1580
Sorbait, Paul de, 1624?–1691
Spiegel, Adriaan van de, 1578–1625
Straet, Jan van der, 1523–1605

### Bulgaria

Busbecq, Ogier Ghiselin de, 1522–1592

### Canada

Baudeau, Pierre, 1643–1708
Bourdon, Marguerite, 1642–1706
Bourgeois, Jacques, ca. 1620–1701
Chaudillon, Antoine, 1643–1707
Enault de Barbaucannes, Philippe, 1651–ca. 1708
Forestier, Antoine, 1646–1717
Gallard, Charlotte, 1648–1725
Hébert, Louis, ca. 1580–1627
Juchereau de la Ferté, Jeanne-Françoise, 1650–1723
Maufils, Marie-Madeleine, d. 1702
Maumousseau, Françoise, 1657–1704
Soumande, Louise, 1661–1708

### China

Li, Shih-chen, 1518–1593
Xue Lizhai
Zur-mkhar Mnyam-nyid-rdo-rje, 1439–1475

### Czechoslovakia

Croll, Oswald, ca. 1560–1609
Frederick of Olomouc
Marci von Kronland, Johannes Marcus, 1595–1667
Span von Spanau, Laurentius, 1539–1575

### Denmark

Bartholin, Thomas, 1616–1680
Brahe, Tycho, 1546–1601
Frederick II, King of Denmark, 1534–1588
Paulli, Simon, 1603–1680
Sehestedt, Mogens, 1598–1657
Sørensen, Peder, 1540 or 42–1602
Steno, Nicolaus, 1638–1686
Wille, Johan Valentin, 1651–1676
Worm, Johan, 1529–1601
Worm, Ole, 1588–1654
Worm, Willum, 1563–1629

### France

Anne of Austria, Queen of France, 1601–1666
Aurach, Georges, fl. 1470
Boaistuau, Pierre, d. 1566
Bossuet, Jacques Bénigne, Bp. of Meaux, 1627–1704
Bourdelin, Claude, ca. 1621–1699
Boursier, Louise (Bourgeois), 1563–1636
Cabrol, Barthélemy, b. 1529
Cartier, Jacques, 1491–1557
Champier, Symphorien, 1471 or 2–ca. 1539
Daléchamps, Jacques, 1513–1588
d'Attenhoven, Gerald, d. 1413
Denis, Jean Baptiste, 1640?–1704
Descartes, René, 1596–1650
Du Gardin, Louis, fl. 1617
Duverney, Guichard Joseph, 1648–1730
Fernel, Jean François, 1506 or 7–1558
Ferrier, Auger, 1513–1585
Fleurimont, Sieur de, fl. 1682
Forestier, Thomas, fl. 1485
Fouquet, Marie (de Maupeon), 1590–1681
Franco, Pierre, ca. 1505–ca. 1579
Gonthier d'Andernach, Jean, 1497–1574
Hemard, Urban, fl. 1582
Héroard, Jean, d. 1627
Hotman, François, 1524–1590
Huvé, Claude, 1505–1570

Joubert, Laurent, 1529–1582
La Brosse, Guy de, 1586?–1641
La Forge, Louis de, 1632–1667?
Le Goust, Philippe, fl. 1650
L'Obel, Matthias de, 1538–1616
Louis XI, King of France, 1423–1483
Louis XIII, King of France, 1601–1643
Louis XIV, King of France, 1638–1715
Marais, Marin, 1656–1728
Martin, Barthelemy, 1629–1698?
Meyssonnier, Lazare, 1602–1672
Molière, Jean Baptiste Poquelin, 1622–1673
Monconys, Balthasar de, 1611–1665
Monluc, Blaise de, 1500–1577
Montaigne, Michel Eyquem de, 1533–1592
Morin, Louis, 1635?–1715
Notredame, Michel de, 1503–1566
Papin, Denis, 1647–1712?
Pare, Ambroise, 1510?–1590
Pascal, Blaise, 1623–1662
Patin, Guy, 1601–1672
Pena, Pierre, fl. 1535–1605
Perrault, Claude, 1613–1688
Portal, Paul, 1630–1703
Primrose, James, 1592–1659
Rabelais, François, ca. 1490–1553?
Regius, Henricus, 1598–1679
Renaudot, Théophraste, 1584–1653
Riolan, Jean, 1580–1657
Sévigné, Marie de Rabutin-Chantal, Marquise de, 1626–1696
Tournefort, Joseph Pitton de, 1656–1708
Vallambert, Simon de, d. 1558?
Vassé, Loys, fl. 1524–1560
Venette, Nicolas, ca. 1631–1678
Vieussens, Raymond, 1641–1715?
Vincent de Paul, Saint, 1581–1660

**Germany**

Agrippa von Nettesheim, Heinrich Cornelius, 1486–1535
Albert III, Duke of Saxony, 1443–1500
Bartisch, Georg, 1535–1606
Bohn, Johann, 1640–1718
Brant, Sebastian, 1458–1521
Brunfels, Otto, 1488–1534
Burgkmair, Hans, the Elder, 1473–ca. 1531
Cleyer, Andreas, 1634–1697 or 8
Cranach, Lucas, 1472–1553
Dhur, Lorenz, b. ca.1515
Dürer, Albrecht, 1471–1528
Elsheimer, Adam, 1578–1610
Fabricius von Hilden, Wilhelm, 1560–1634
Forberger, Georg, ca. 1543–ca. 1604
Fuchs, Leonhart, 1501–1566
Fugger, Octavianus Secundus, 1549–1600
Gerung, Mathias, ca. 1500–ca. 1568
Gockel, Eberhard, 1636–1703
Gotzkirchen, Sigmund, ca. 1410–1475
Grünewald, Mathias, d. 1528
Gyger, Ulrich, fl. 1527
Händel, Georg, 1622–1697
Hartlieb, Johann, d. 1468
Hartung vom Hoff, Caspar, 16th cent.
Hirschhorn, Thomas, 1410?–1493
Hoernigk, Ludwig von, 1600–1667
Holbein, Hans, the Elder, ca. 1465–1524
Huber, Johann, 1507–1571
Johann Maurits, Prince of Nassau-Siegen, 1604–1679
Kaempfer, Engelbert, 1651–1716
Kepler, Johann, 1571–1630
Kircher, Athanasius, 1602–1680
Lange, Johannes, 1485–1565
Leibniz, Gottfried Wilhelm von, 1646–1716
Luther, Martin, 1483–1546
Meister, Georg, 1653–1713
Melanchthon, Philipp, 1497–1560
Müller, Jakob, 1670–1703
Ollinger, Georg, 1487–1557
Paullini, Christian Franz, 1643–1712
Pictorius, Georg, ca. 1500–1569
Pirckheimer, Wilibald, 1470–1530
Quicchelberg, Samuel, 1529–1567
Rabs, Mattheus, b. 1652
Reinzer, Franz, 1661–1708
Risner, Friedrich, d. ca. 1580
Roeslin, Eucharius, d. 1526
Roeslin, Eucharius, d. 1547?
Scultetus, Joannis, 1595–1645
Segen, Johan van, fl. 1487?
Sennert, Daniël, 1572–1637
Siegemund, Justine Dittrich, 1648–1705
Stromer, Heinrich, 1476–1542
Thölde, Johann, fl. 1599–1624?
Thurneisser zum Thurn, Leonhard, 1531–1596
Trithemius, 1462–1516

**Great Britain**

Anne Boleyn, Queen, consort of Henry VIII, 1507–1536
Anthony, Francis, 1550–1623
Bacon, Francis, 1561–1626
Badger, John, fl. 1683
Bate, George, 1608–1669
Benion, Samuel, 1673–1708
Bennet, Sara
Biggs, Noah
Blomefylde, Myles, 1525–1603
Blood, Peter, 1653–
Booker, William, fl. 1682
Boyle, Robert, 1627–1691
Briggs, William, ca. 1650–1704
Browne, Edward, 1644–1708
Browne, Thomas, 1605–1682
Burton, Robert, 1577–1640
Burton, William, 1609–1657
Caius, John, 1510–1573
Carew, Richard, b. 1555
Catherine, of Aragon, queen consort of Henry VIII, 1485–1536
Charles I, King of England, 1600–1649
Charles II, King of Great Britain, 1630–1685
Clayton, Robert, 1629–1707
Cogan, Thomas, 1545?–1607
Colston, Joseph, fl. 1664
Connor, Bernard, 1666–1698
Cotta, John, 1575?–1650?
Crane, John, 1571–1652
Cromwell, Oliver, 1599–1658
Culpeper, Nicholas, 1616–1654
Dee, Arthur, 1579–1651
Donne, John, 1573–1631
Dryden, John, 1631–1700
Edwardes, David, fl. 16th cent.
Elyot, Thomas, 1490?–1546
Erskine, Robert, 1677–1718
Fautrart, Thomas, fl. 1670
Fenton, Joseph, fl. 1623–1634
Fludd, Robert, 1574–1637
Gerard, John, 1545–1612
Gilbert, William, 1540–1603
Glanvill, Joseph, 1636–1680
Glisson, Francis, 1597–1677
Green, Anne, 1528–1550
Grew, Nehemiah, 1641–1712
Hall, John, 1575–1635
Hall, Joseph, 1574–1656
Harington, John, 1561–1612
Hartlib, Samuel, d. 1662
Harvey Family
Harvey, William, 1578–1657
Hauksbee, Francis, ca. 1666–1713
Henry VI, King of England, 1421–1471
Henry VIII, King of England, 1491–1547
Henryson, Robert, 1430?–1506
Herbert, George, 1593–1633
Hobbes, Thomas, 1588–1679
Hollier, Thomas, 1609–1690
Hooke, Robert, 1635–1703
Houghton, John, 1645–1705
Hudson, Abraham, fl. 1671
Jonson, Ben, 1572?–1637
King, John, 1614–1681
Lambe, John, 1546–1628
Lister, Martin, 1638?–1712
Locke, John, 1632–1704
Lower, Richard, 1631–1691
Lumley, John, 1533–1609
Makluire, Johne, fl. 1630
Marbecke, Roger, 1536–1605
Markham, Gervase, 1568?–1637
Marlowe, Christopher, 1564–1593
Martin, Elioner
Mary Stuart, Queen of Scots, 1542–1587
Mayerne, Theodore Turquet de, 1573–1655
Meynell, Richard, fl. 1663
Milton, John, 1608–1674
Moffet, Thomas, 1553–1604
Molins, Edward, 1610?–1663
Molins, James, d. 1638
Molins, James, 1631–1687
More, Thomas, 1478–1535
Morton, Richard, 1637–1698
Mulcaster, Richard, 1530?–1611

Napier, Richard, d. 1634
Needham, Charles, ca. 1660–ca. 1707
Newton, Isaac, 1642–1727
Nowell, John, 1553 or 4–1603?
Oldenburg, Henry, 1615?–1677
Pepys, Samuel, 1633–1703
Petty, William, 1623–1687
Pitcairne, Archibald, 1652–1713
Plattes, Gabriel, fl. 1638–1643
Pott, John, 1595–ca. 1642
Regimorter, Assuerus, 1614–1650
Reitinger, Christopher, 1557?–1612
Reynolds, Edward, 1599–1676
Richard III, King of Great Britain, 1452–1485
Scarborough, Charles, 1615 or 6–1694
Shakespeare, William, 1564–1616
Sherley, Thomas, 1638–1678
Sibbald, Robert, 1641–1722
Skelton, John, 1460?–1529
Stanley, John, fl. 1687
Stubbe, Henry, 1631–1676
Surflet, Richard, ca. 1560–ca. 1605
Sydenham, Thomas, 1624–1689
Trapham, Thomas, d. 1692?
Turner, William, 1508–1568
Uredale, Robert, 1642–1722
Vaughan, Henry, 1621–1695
Vaughan, Thomas, 1622–1666
Wafer, Lionel, 1660?–1705?
Webster, John, 1580?–1625?
Webster, John, 1610–1682
Whistler, Daniel, 1619–1684
Willis, Thomas, 1621–1675
Woodall, John, 1556?–1643
Yonge, James, 1647–1721

**Greece**

Maurocordato, Alexander, ca. 1636–ca. 1710

**Hungary**

Bánfihunyadi, János, d. 1646
Batthyány, Boldizar, fl. 1572
Bausner, Bartholomaeus, 1629–1682
Bethlen, Gabor, prince of Transylvania, 1580–1629
Csipkés, György Komáromi, 1628–1678
Dudith, András, Bp. of Pécs, 1533–1589
Köleséri, Samuel, 1663–1732
Lencsés György, Váradi, 1530–1593
Lippay, János, 1606–1666
Pápai Páriz, Ferenc, 1649–1716
Tököly, Imre, 1657–1705
Varsányi Borbély, György, fl. 1570

**India**

Bharadvaja
Geelani, Nizamuddin Ahmed, 1586–1650
Srinivasabhatta, fl. 1600

**Ireland**

Greatrakes, Valentine, 1629–1683

**Italy**

Achillini, Alessandro, 1463–1512
Adelphus, Johannes, fl. 1500–1523
Alberti, Leon Battista, 1404–1472
Aldrovandi, Ulisse, 1522–1605
Alpago, Andrea, d. 1521
Ariosto, Lodovico, 1474–1533
Aubri, Claude, 17th cent.
Baglivi, Giorgio, 1668?–1707?
Bartolotti, Gian Giacomo, ca. 1470–ca. 1530
Beer, Benjamin Ben Elizah Harofe
Borelli, Giovanni Alfonso, 1608–1679
Botticelli, Sandro, 1444 or 45–1510
Buccella, Nicola, d. 1610
Buffi da Bertipaglia, Leonardo, fl. 1448
Campani, Giuseppe, 1635–1715
Cardano, Girolamo, 1501–1576
Cartegni da Bagnone, Giovanbattista, 1559–1624
Casabona, Giuseppe, d. 1595
Cesalpino, Andrea, 1524–1603
Cestoni, Giacinto, 1637–1718
Colombo, Realdo, ca. 1515–1559
Cornelio, Tommaso, 1614–1686
Cortona, Pietro Berrettini, 1596–1669
Cristofano di Giulio, Cessini, d. 1642
Delmedigo, Joseph Solomon, 1591–1655
De Ribera, J., 1588–1656
Divini, Eustachio, 1610–1685
Eustachi, Bartolomeo, d. 1574
Fabricius, Hieronymus, ab Aquapendente, ca. 1533–1619
Ferrari, Antonio de, Galateo, 1444–1517
Ficino, Marsilio, 1433–1499
Filelfo, Francesco, 1398–1481
Fracastoro, Girolamo, 1483–1553
Galilei, Galileo, 1564–1642
Garzoni, Giovanni, 1419–1505
Ghirlandaio, Domenico, 1449–1494
Giorgione, Giorgio Barbarelli, known as, 1477–1510 or 1511
Giustiniani, Vincenzo, d. 1570
Innocentius XI, Pope, 1611–1689
Leon, R. Jehuda Messer, fl. 1470
Leonardo da Vinci, 1452–1519
Leoniceno, Niccolò, 1428–1524
Magati, Cesare, 1579–1647
Malpighi, Marcello, 1628–1694
Mascellini, Giovanni
Mattioli, Pietro Andrea, 1500–1577
Medici, Francesco de, 1541–1587
Michelangelo, 1475–1564
Pinelli, Gian Vincenzo, 1535–1601
Portaleone, Abraham, 1542–1612
Ramazzini, Bernardino, 1633–1714
Ramusio, Girolamo, 1555–1610
Redi, Francesco, 1626–1697
Rinaldi, Carlo Bartolomeo, fl. 1655
Severino, Marco Aurelio, 1580–1656
Simone de Cinozzo di Giovanni Cini
Simoni, Simone, 1532–1602
Titian, Vecelli, 1477 or 1489–1576
Tremigliozzi, Gaetano, 1655–1710
Ventura, Giovanni de, fl. 1479

**Mexico**

Badiano, Juan, fl. 16th cent.
Barrios, Juan de, fl. 1590–1610
Bravo, Francisco, fl. ca. 1553
Esteyneffer, Juan de, 1664–1716
Quiroga, Vasco de, ca. 1470–1565
Sahagún, Bernardino de, 1499–1590

**Netherlands**

Barlaeus, Caspar, 1584–1648
Beverwijck, Johan van, 1594–1647
Bidloo, Govard, 1649–1713
Blankaart, Stephanus, 1650–1702
Blasius, Gerard, 1626–1682
Bosch, Hieronymus van Aken, known as, d. 1516
Brueghel, Jan, the Elder, 1568–1625
Coeuershof, Christiaen, 1596–1659
Dapper, Olfert, 1636 or 37–1689
Dodoens, Rembert, 1517–1585
Erasmus, Desiderius, d. 1536
Graaf, Reinier de, 1641–1673
Heide, Antonius de, b. 1646
Helmont, Jean Baptiste van, 1577–1644
Huygens, Christiaan, 1629–1695
Jager, Jacheus de, 1599–1650
Jonctys, Daniël, 1600–1654
Labadie, Jean de, 1610–1674
Lairesse, Gerard de, 1641–1711
Le Boë, Frans de, 1614–1672
Leeuwenhoek, Anthony van, 1632–1723
Lemnius, Levinus, 1505–1568
Lipsius, David, fl. 1607–1678
Piso, Willem, 1611–1678
Ploegh Family
Regius, Henricus, 1598–1679
Rembrandt, Hermanszoon van Rijn, 1607–1669
Rheede tot Drakestein, Hendrik Adriaan van, 1637?–1691
Rhijne, Willem ten, 1647–1700
Ruysch, Frederik, 1638–1731
Salomonsz, Andries, fl. 1553–1561
Senguerd, Arnold, 1610–1667
Spinoza, Benedictus de, 1632–1677
Swammerdam, Jan, 1637–1680
Tulp, Nicolaas, 1593–1674
Van der Straet, Jan, 1523–1605
Velthuysen, Lambert van, 1622–1685
Vermeer, Johannes, 1632–1675
William I, Prince of Orange, Count of Nassau, 1533–1584
Zacutus, Abraham Lusitanus, 1575–1642

**Pakistan**

Babar, Emperor of Hindostan, 1483–1530

**Peru**

Acarí, Santiago de Parcos de, fl. 1593

**Poland**

Alexander, King of Poland, 1461–1506
Casimir IV, King of Poland, 1427–1492
Copernicus, Nicolaus, 1473–1543
Jan II Kasimierz Wasa, King of Poland, 1609–1672
John I Albert, King of Poland, 1459–1501
Johnston, Jan, 1603–1675
Koler, Wacław, d. 1546
Latos, Jan Walenty, 1539–ca. 1610
Roździeński, Walenty, ca. 1560–ca. 1622
Sigismund I, King of Poland, 1467–1548
Sigismund II, Augustus, King of Poland, 1518–1572
Sigismund III, Vasa, King of Poland, 1566–1632
Stanko, Johanne, 1430–1493
Stefan Batory, King of Poland, 1533–1586
Twardowski
Wiśniowiecki, (Korybut), Michał, King of Poland, d. 1673

**Portugal**

Acosta, Cristavão, ca. 1525–1594
Alvares, Manuel, 1545–1612
Camões, Luis Vaz de, 1524?–1580
Jean de Dieu, Saint, 1495–1550
João de Deus, 1618–1684
Juan de Dios, Saint, 1495–1550
Montalto, Philotheus Elianus, d. 1616

**Romania**

Cantacuzino, Serban, 1640–1688
Jordan, Thomáš, 1539–1586
Kájoni, Joannes, 1629 or 30–1687

**Spain**

Acosta, José, 1539–1600
Aguilar, Francisco, fl. ca. 1590
Alvarez Chanca, Diego, fl. 1493
Bayle, Juan del, fl. 1698
Cardenas, Juan de, 1563–1609
Carlos, Prince of Asturias, 1545–1568
Cervantes Saavedra, Miguel de, 1547–1616
Diaz del Castillo, Bernal, ca. 1498–ca. 1568
Enríquez Jorge, Enrique, fl. 1594
Estrada, Dr., fl. 1584
Fragoso, Juan, d. 1597
Hernández, Francisco, ca. 1515–1587
Hidalgo de Agüero, Bartholomé, fl. 1604
Huarte de San Juan, Juan, 1529–1588
Juan de Alós y Serradora, 1617–1695
Laguna, Andrés de, d. 1560
Martínez de Leache, Miguel, fl. 1644–1652
Méndez, Cristóbal, fl. 1517
Mercado, Luis, 1525?–1611
Montana de Monserrate, Bernardino, b. ca. 1482
Palacios, Felix
Pérez Cascales, Francisco, fl. 1576–1611
Pérez de Herrera, Cristóbal, 1558–1618?
Ponce de Santa Cruz, Antonio, 1561–1632
Rossell, Juan Francisco, fl. 1627–1629
Sanchez, Francisco, 1550–1623
Servetus, Michael, 1509 or 11–1553
Sorapan de Rieros, Juan, 1572–1638
Teresa of Avila, Saint, 1515–1582
Theotocopuli, Dominico, called El Greco, d. 1614
Toro, Luis de, b. 1532
Tristán, Gaspar, fl. 1606
Valverde, Juan de, ca. 1520–ca. 1588
Viana Mentesano, Juan de, fl. 1637
Villarreal, Juan Joseph de, 17th cent.
Vives, Juan Luis, 1492–1540
Zurbarán, Francisco, 1598–1664

**Sweden**

Olai, Benedictus, fl. 1578
Raicus, Johann, d. 1631
Rudbeck, Olof, 1630–1702

**Switzerland**

Bonet, Théophile, 1620–1689
Calvin, John, 1509–1564
Cysat, Renward, 1545–1614
Fatio, Johannes, 1649–1691
Gesner, Konrad, 1516–1565
Harder, Johann Jacob, 1656–1711
Paracelsus, 1493–1541
Platter, Felix, 1536–1614
Platter, Thomas, 1574–1628
Rüff, Jakob, 1500–1558
Scharandaeus, Johann Jakob, 1630–1682
Stromayr, Caspar, fl. 1557–1567
Wecker, Johann Jacob, 1528–1586
Wepfer, Johann Jakob, 1620–1695
Werdt, Daniel von, 1611–1658
Zwinger, Théodor, 1533–1588

**Turkey**

Sinasi, d. 1702

**United States**

Kierstede, Hans, d. 1666
Pott, John, 1595–ca.1642

**USSR**

Graman, I. I.
Ivan IV, the Terrible, Czar of Russia, 1530–1584
Tatishchev, Vasilii Nikitich, 1686–1750

**Venezuela**

Pérez de la Muela, Hernán, fl. 1529

**Yugoslavia**

Hájek, Tadeás, 1525–1600

## 1700 TO PRESENT

Acheson, James Alexander, 1892–1968
Alder, Albert, 1888–1980
Amstein, Johann Georg, 1819–1892
Antommarchi, Francesco A., 1780–1838
Ariss, E. A.
Bateman, Harry, 1882–1946
Bourbon Family
Brighenti, Alberto, 1886–
Butler, Mary Joseph, Mother, 1901–
Chopin, Frédéric François, 1810–1849
Dearborn, J. G., fl. 1886
De Trey, Emil, 1846–1898
Deutsch, Felix, 1884–1964
Donovan, John Charles, d. 1976
Doué, Pierre-Alphonse, 1832–1895
Duncan, James Matthews, 1826–1890
Ehrenfels, Christian von, 1859–1932
Ehrmann, Albert, 1821–1871
Eppinger, Hans, 1879–1946
Fahrenheit, Gabriel Daniel, 1686–1736
Fergusson, William, 1773–1846
Flemming, Walther, 1843–1905
Fougerat, André Jacques
Frankenthal, Käte, 1889–1976
Freud, Sigmund, 1856–1939
Fromm-Reichmann, Frieda, 1889–1957
Fully, Georges, 1926–1973
Galifret-Granjon, Nadine
Gehlen, Arnold, 1904–
Ghon, Anton, 1886–1936
Goldszmit, Henry K., 1878–1942
Grüneberg, Hans, 1907–1982
Gurney, Ivor, 1890–1937
Haartman, Johan, 1725–1787
Haffkine, Waldemar Mordecai Wolff, 1860–1930
Hàndel, Georg Friedrich, 1685–1759
Heller, Jozef, 1896–1982
Hollaender, Alexander, 1898–
Hörmann, Hans, 1924–1983
Horner, Otte E. Friedrich, 1831–1886
Ivanchich, Viktor von, 1812–1892
Kleinwächter, Ludwig, 1839–1906
Klinkosch, Joseph Thaddäus, 1734–1778
Knolle, Jan Fryderyk, b. 1740
Krogh, August, 1874–1949
Kupffer, Karl Wilhelm, 1829–1902
Langie, Adam Marian, 1829–1907

Le Fort, Leon
Liebling, Friedrich, 1893–1982
Liesching, Friedrich Ludwig
Lindner, S., fl. 1879–
Loewe, Walter Siegfried, 1884–1963
Lux, Jakab, 1822–1876
MacBride, Ernest William, 1866–1940
Mayor, Mathias, 1775–1847
Mazzei, Filippo, 1730–1816
Mendel, Gregor Johann, 1822–1884
Ménétrier, Pierre Eugene, 1859–1935
Menten, Maud Leonora, 1879–1960
Merskey, Clarence, 1914–1982
Mertens, Charles de, 1737–1788
Mesmer, Franz Anton, 1734–1815
Munk, Arthur, 1885?–1955?
Neumann, Ernst, 1834–1918
Nürnberger, Woldemar, 1818–1869
Obermann, Rudolf
Osler, William, 1849–1919
Pagel, Walter, 1898–1983
Pasch, Joseph Georg, 1738–1795
Pijper, Adrianus, 1886–1964
Porter, Charles, 1864–1934
Ramírez, Carlos María, 1848–1898
Rank, Otto, 1884–1939
Reimarus, Johann Albert Heinrich, 1729–1814
Révérend, Alejandro Prospero, 1796–1881
Rhoads, Cornelius Packard, 1898–1959
Robin de Keriavalle, Claude-Marie, 1743–1785
Schorlemmer, Carl, 1834–1892
Schultz, Johannes Heinrich, 1884–
Schweitzer, Albert, 1875–1965
Serre, Johann Jacob Joseph, 1759–1830
Ulhoorn, Hendrik, 1692–1749
Urlanis, Boris Tsezarevich, 1906–1981
Valentin, Johannes Franz Wilhelm, 1884–1959
Vetch, John, 1783–1835
Warneck, Nicolas
Weissmann, Max
Wolf-Man, 1886–
Zweig, Stefan, 1881–1942

**Americas**

Bolívar, Simón, 1783–1830

**Argentina**

Bialet Massé, Juan, 1840–1907
Farini, Juan Angel, 1901–
Houssay, Bernardo Alberto, 1887–1971
Jakob, Christfried, 1866–1956
Lavalle, Juan Galo de, 1797–1841
Muñiz, Francisco Javier, fl. 1849
Puiggari, Miguel, 1827–1889
Puiggari, Miguel, 1866–1947
San Martin, José de, 1778–1850
Villanueva y Godoy, Francisco Javier

**Australia**

Asche, Justice
Beaney, James George, 1826–1891
Bennetts, Harold William, 1898–
Blake, I. F.
Bowden, Edmund, 1801–1847
Bowen, Thomas Aubrey, 1837–1893
Box, John, 1863–1934
Box, William, 1905–1982
Cade, John F.
Cade, John Frederick Joseph, d. 1980
Campbell, Alfred Walter, 1868–1937
Chidley, William, 1860–1916
Clubbe, Charles, 1854–1932
D'Ombrain, Arthur, d. 1963
Fawcett, Benjamin, ca. 1817–1890
Flynn, John, 1880–1951
Gray, Andrew Sexton, 1826–1907
Gregg, Norman McAlister, 1892–1966
Hadley, Frederick August, 1873–1961
Harris, Samuel Harry, 1880–1936
Herz, Max
Hoff, August, d. 1887
Hyndman, Charles Robert
Kenny, Elizabeth, 1880–1952
Lowe, Ronald Francis
Mackerras, Ian Murray
Manning, Frederick Norton, 1839–1903
Munro, William John, 1863–1908
Officer, Robert, 1800–1879
Robertson, Graeme
Schlink, Herbert Henry, 1883–1962
Temple-Smith, E. C., d. 1968
Trethowan, William, 1860–1929
Vianney, Mary, 1894–
Watson, Archibald, d. 1941
Wood, Jones Frederic, 1879–1954

**Austria**

Adler, Alfred, 1870–1937
Auenbrugger, Leopold, 1722–1809
Auspitz, Heinrich, 1835–1886
Badurski, Andrzej, 1740–1789
Bárány, Robert, 1876–1936
Beer-Hofmann, Richard, 1866–1945
Boltzmann, Ludwig Edward, 1844–1906
Breuer, Josef, 1842–1925
Bühler, Karl, 1879–1963
Daubrawa, Ferdinand
Economo, Constantin von, 1876–1931
Elfinger, Anton, 1821–1864
Escherich, Theodor, 1857–1911
Feuchtersleben, Ernst von, 1806–1849
Frankl, Viktor Emil, 1905–
Fuchs, Ernst, 1851–1930
Gall, Franz Joseph, 1758–1828
Halban, Joseph, 1870–1937
Hebra, Ferdinand von, 1816–1880
Heger, Hans, 1855–1940
Heller, Johann Florian, 1813–1871
Henning, Karl, 1860–1917
Henning, Theodor, 1897–1946
Hirsch, Oskar, 1877–1965
Hug-Hellmuth, Hermine von
Hyrtl, Joseph, 1810–1894
Isakower, Otto, 1899–1972
Jacquin, Nikolaus Joseph von, 1727–1817
Joseph II, Emperor of Germany, 1741–1790
Kienboeck, Robert, 1871–1953
Knaus, Hermann Hubert, 1892–1970
Kolletschka, Jacob, 1803–1847
Kraus, Karl, 1874–1936
Kumpf, Johann Gottfried, 1781–1862
Kundrat, Hanns, 1845–1893
Lederer, Bernd, 1939–1982
Lesky, Erna, 1911–
Lorenz, Franz, 1805–1883
Mach, Ernst, 1838–1916
Mahler, Gustav, 1860–1911
Maria Theresa, Empress of Austria, 1717–1780
Mayrhofer, Carl, 1837–1882
Menaker, Esther, 1907–
Mendel, Gregor Johann, 1822–1884
Mozart, Wolfgang Amadeus, 1756–1791
Mundy, Jaromír, 1822–1894
Pappenheim, Bertha, 1859–1936
Paradis, Maria Theresia, 1759?–1842?
Payr, Erwin, 1871–1946
Pirquet von Cesenatico, Clemens Peter, 1874–1929
Plenck, Joseph Jacob, 1738–1807
Rokitansky, Karl von, 1804–1878
Sailer, Daniel, 1887–1958
Salzmann, Maximilian, 1862–1954
Schmid, Hans Hermann, 1884–
Schnitzler, Arthur, 1862–1931
Schrödinger, Erwin, 1887–1961
Schubert, Franz Peter, 1797–1828
Seeger, Rudolf, fl. 1848
Störck, Anton, 1731–1803
Tandler, Julius, 1869–1936
Tausk, Victor, 1879–1919
Teleky, Ludwig, 1872–1957
Thalhammer, Otto, 1922–
Veigl, Franz Xaver, 1723–1798
Wagner-Jauregg, Julius von, 1857–1940
Wiedmann, Albert, 1901–1970
Winiwarter, Alexander von, 1848–1917
Winiwarter, Felix von, 1852–1931
Wittmann, Michael Ferdinand, 1755–1862
Zangger, Rudolf, 1826–1882
Zuckerkandl, Emil, 1849–1910

**Barbados**

Cave, Charles J. B., 1879–1939

**Belgium**

Biourge, Philibert, 1864–1942
Bobon, Jean

Bordet, Jules, 1870–1961
Charlotte, Consort of Maximilian, Emperor of Mexico, 1840–1927
Dalcq, Albert, 1893–1973
Debaisieux, Paul, 1886–1978
Ermengem, Emile P. van, 1851–1932
Florkin, Marcel, 1900–1979
Fredericq, Léon, 1851–1935
Gérard, Pol, 1886–1961
Gratia, André, 1893–1950
Halter, Samuel, 1916–1981
Hellemans, Jan
Kluyskens, Jozef Frans, 1771–1843
Lacaze-Duthiers, Félix Joseph Henri de, 1821–1901
Lambotte, Albin, 1866–1955
Massenhove, Ghislaine van
Mons, Jean Baptiste van, 1765–1842
Pálfyn, Jan, 1650–1730
Roselt, Jan Albert, 1714–1785
Seutin, Louis Joseph Ghislain, 1793–1862
Van Mons, Jean-Baptiste, 1765–1842
Winiwarter, Hans de, 1875–1949

**Brazil**

Aragáo, Joáo Moniz Barreto de, 1874–1922
Bandeira, Manuel, 1886–1968
Brethel, Alexandre, 1834–1901
Candau, Marcolino Gomes, 1911–1983
Chagas, Carlos Ribeiro Justiniano, 1879–1934
Costa Barreto, Manuel Alves de, fl. 1797
Cruz Jobim, José Martin da
Cruz, Oswaldo Gonçalves, 1872–1917
Durocher, Marie Josephine, 1809–1894
Fajardo, Francisco de Paula, d. 1906
Ferreira, Luiz Gomes, fl. 1735–1745
Leopoldina, Empress of Brazil, 1797–1826
Lobato, Rita, 1867–
Neiva, Arthur, 1880–1943
Neri, Ana, 1815–1880
Nunes Garcia, José Maurício, 1808–1857
Pereira, Miguel, 1871–1918
Rocha-Lima, Henrique da, 1879–1956
Rodrigues, Francisco Victor, d. 1972
Sattamini, Samuel Duarte

**Bulgaria**

Berovich, Petr, 1799–1871
Chilov, Konstantin, 1898–1955
Chomakov, Stoian, 1819–1893
Glavchev, Vladimir Petrov, 1878–1915
Kadanoff, Dimitri, 1900–1984
Pavlov, Georgi, d. 1949
TSarvulanov, Neno, 1876–1925
Uzunov, Georgi, 1904–1971

**Canada**

Abbott, Albert Clifford, 1897–
Abbott, Anderson Ruffin, 1837–1913
Abbott, Maude Elizabeth Seymour, 1869–1940
Almon, William James, 1755–1817
Ash, John, ca. 1821–1886
Badelard, Philippe-Louis-François, 1728–1802
Banting, Frederick Grant, 1891–1941
Barbeau, Victor, 1896–
Barker, Edward John, 1799–1884
Barrett, Michael, 1816–1887
Beaubien, Pierre, 1796–1881
Beddome, Henry Septimus, ca. 1830–1881
Bell, John, 1845–1878
Bertier, Michel, 1695–1740
Berzins, Elfrida K., 1904–
Best, Charles Herbert, 1899–1978
Bethune, Henry Norman, 1890–1939
Blake, Charles, 1746–1810
Blanchet, François, 1776–1830
Blanchet, Joseph-Godric, 1829–1890
Brouse, William Henry, 1824–1881
Bucke, Richard Maurice, 1837–1902
Calef, John, 1725–1812
Cameron, D. Ewen, 1901–1967
Campbell, George William, 1810–1882
Céloron, Marie-Catherine-Françoise, 1744–1809
Clark, Duncan, ca. 1759–1808
Clinch, John, 1749–1819
Collip, James Bertram, 1892–1965
Compain, Pierre-Joseph, 1740–1806
Cove, John William, 1838–1901
Crevier, Joseph Alexandre, 1824–1889
Davis, Egerton Yorrick, ca.1850–ca.1920
Dawson, William, 1820–1899
Dearin, John Joseph, ca. 1818–1890
Dénéchaud, Jacques, 1728–1810
Dickson, John Robinson, 1819–1882
Dièreville, fl. 1699–1711
Dionne quintuplets
Dizy, Marguerite, 1663–ca. 1730
Dobbs, Harriet, 1808–1887
Douglas, George Mellis, 1809?–1864
Douglas, James, 1800–1886
Dugay, Jacques, ca. 1647–1727
Dussaus, Marie-Angélique, 1737–1809
Earle, Sylvester Zobieski, 1822–1888
Emery-Coderre, Joseph, 1813–1888
Fafard, Théogène, 1855–1890
Fisher, C. Miller, 1913–
Fortin, Pierre-Etienne, 1823–1888
Fulton, John, 1837–1887
Gesner, Abraham, 1797–1864
Giard, Louis, 1809–1887
Grant, James Frederick, 1887–1946
Hannah, Jason Albert, 1889–1977
Hastings, Charles
Hill, Christina
Hincks, Clarence Meredith, 1885–1964
Howard, Henry, 1815–1887
Howard, Robert Palmer, 1823–1889
Howley, Thomas, ca. 1840–1889
Jobert, Jean Baptiste, 1733–1792
Kelso, John Joseph, 1864–1935
La Rue, Francois A. Hubert, 1833–1881
Lamarre, Henri, d. 1740
Landry, Jean-Etienne, 1815–1884
Léger de la Grange, Jean, 1663–ca. 1736
Longmore, George, ca. 1758–1811
Macallum, Archibald Byron, 1858–1934
MacDonald, Mary, 1869–1933
Mack, Theophilus, 1820–1881
McKenzie, Kenneth George, 1892–
McKenzie, Robert Tait, 1867–1938
Mackieson, John, 1795–1885
Macphail, Andrew, 1864–1938
Melancon, Marie-Vénérande, 1754–1817
Metcalf, William George, 1847–1885
Mondelet, Dominique, ca. 1734–1802
Morin, Marie, 1649–1730
Munson, Letitia, b. ca. 1820
Murray, George, 1825–1888
Paquette, Albiny
Parent, Marie-Geneviève, 1740–1804
Payen de Noyan, Marie-Catherine, ca. 1730–1818
Penfield, Wilder, 1891–1976
Pennefather, John Pyn
Philipps, John, ca. 1736–1801
Piuze, Liveright, 1754–1813
Prescott, Jonathan, 1725–1807
Rieutord, Jean-Baptiste, ca. 1733–1818
Routley, Thomas Clarence, 1889–
Sales Laterrière, Pierre de, ca. 1740–1815
Sarrazin, Michel, 1659–1734
Scarlett, Earle Parkhill, 1896–
Segall, Harold Nathan, 1897–
Serres, Alexandre, ca. 1732–1812
Skakel, Alexander, 1776–1846
Smith, William, fl. 1784–1803
Soley, Elizabeth Jane, fl. 1860–1893
Soupiran, Simon, 1670–1724
Stowe-Gullen, Augusta, 1857–1943
Suzor, François-Michel, 1756–1810
Tailhandier, Marien, 1665–1738 or 9
Thomson, John, 1808–1884
Todd, John L., 1876–1949
Tolmie, William Fraser, 1812–1886
Vail, Edwin Arnold, 1817–1885
Verey, George, ca. 1830–1881
Waldron, John, 1744–ca. 1818
Whitton, Charlotte Elizabeth, 1896–1975
Wintrobe, Maxwell Meyer, 1901–
Wittkower, Eric, 1899–
Yates, Horatio, 1821–1882

**Chile**

Alessandri, Hernán, 1900–
Allende, Salvador, 1908–1973
Blest, Guillermo Cunningham, 1800–1884
Bustillos, José Vicente, 1803–1873
Díaz, Eloísa, 1866–1950
Elguero, Jose Ramón, fl. 1862
Fonck, Francisco, 1830–1912
Horwitz, Abraham B., 1910–

Morán, Pedro, 1771–1840
Muhm, Teodoro, 1869–1939
Orrego Luco, Augusto, 1848–1933
Passamán, José, fl. 1829
Portales, Diego, 1773–1837
Sazie, Carlos

**China**

Chao, Hsüeh-min, fl. 1765
Chu, Judy
Hsüeh, Sheng-pai, 1681–1770
Kotnis, D. S.
Lu Liuliang
Ly Yanshi
Sun Yat-Sen, 1866–1925
Tao, Lieh
Tsái, Ching-feng
Wang, Shih-hsiung, 1808–1868
Wu Hsien, 1893–1959

**Colombia**

Bonilla-Naar, Alfonso, 1916–
Campo Posada, Arturo, 1909–
Florén Lozano, Luis, 1913–
Orticochea, Miguel

**Costa Rica**

Cañas, Ricardo Moreno, 1890–1938

**Cuba**

Blackely, Carlos
Castro, Fidel, 1927–
Dumont, Henri Joseph, 1824–1878
Encarnación Valencia, José de la
Figueredo y Diaz, Félix, 1828–1892
Finlay, Carlos Juan, 1833–1915
Lafargue, Paul, 1842–1911
Lam, Wilfredo, 1902–1982

**Czechoslovakia**

Albert, Eduard, 1841–1900
Alexander, Vojtech, 1857–1916
Basch, Samuel von, 1837–1905
Bayer, Karl, fl. 1891
Beneš, Eduard, 1884–1948
Birčák, Ján, 1923–
Bochdalka, Vincence Alexandra, 1801–1883
Boháč, Antonín, 1882–1950
Bolzano, Bernard, 1781–1848
Brdlík, Jiří
Brdlík, Jiří, 1883–1965
Cermák, Josef, 1825–1872
Cerveňanský, Ján, 1905–
Chodounský, Karel, 1843–
Cmunt, Eduard, 1878–
Czermák, Johann Nepomuk, 1828–1873
Dreuschuch, František, 1855–1938
Dvorzhak, Milan, 1929–
Ehrmann, Martin, fl. 1836–1866
Elschnig, Anton, 1863–1939
Felsenfeld, Oscar
Fencl, Zdeněk, 1922–1981
Fischer, Johann Nepomuk, 1777–1847
Friedmann, Richard
Gazárek, Františka, 1912–
Hackl, Eduard, 1841–1913
Hálek, Vítězslav, 1835–1874
Held, Jan Theobald, 1770–1851
Hlava, Jaroslav, 1855–1924
Houštěk, Josef, 1913–
Hrabal, Františku, d. 1909
Hrodek, Otto, 1922–
Hübschmann, Kurt, 1890–
Hynek, Kristiana, d. 1979
Janáček, Leoš, 1854–1928
Jančik, J.
Janský, Jan, 1907–
Jerie, Josef
Jirsová, Blažena, 1901–1979
Kadlický, Roman, 1899–1979
Kafka, Franz, 1883–1924
Karafiát, Ferdinand, 1870–1928
Koczwara, Franz, d. 1791
Köstl, Franz, 1811–1882
Kostlivý, Stanislavý, 1877–
Kruty, Vladislav
Kuřák, František, 1801–1868
Macura, Jiří, d. 1979
Maixner, Emerich, 1847–1920
Mařatka, Zdeněk
Mathon, Jaroslav, 1867–1953
Mrštík, Norbert, 1867–1905
Országh, Pavol, 1849–1921
Pachner, František, 1882–1964
Panýrek, Jan Duchoslav, 1867–1903
Pelikan, Josef, 1900–
Pessneger, Joseph, 1766–1836
Prochaska, Georg, 1749–1820
Purkyně, Jan Evangelista, 1787–1869
Reinsberg, Viktor, 1875–1938
Rincolini, Ernst Samuel, 1722–1786
Ryba, Josef Arnošt, 1795–1856
Sagar, Johann Baptist Michael, Elder von, 1732?–1813?
Samberger, Frantisek, 1871–1944
Schroff, Carl Damian, 1802–1887
Sedláček, Eva
Seeman, Miloslav, 1892–
Semonkeho, Miroslav, 1919–1979
Simka, Ján, 1922–
Skoda, Josef, 1805–1881
Smetana, Bedřich, 1824–1884
Soyka, Isidor, 1850–1889
Teissler, Viktor, 1883–
Theimer, Carl, 1823–1870
Tomíček, Oldřich, 1891–
Tomsa, Vladimir Bogamilowitsch, 1831–
Trapl, Jiří, 1880–
Treitz, Václav, 1819–1872
Záček, Adolf, 1917–
Zahrádniček, Jan, 1882–1958
Zlábek, Karel, 1902–1983

**Denmark**

Aaskow, Urban Bruun, 1742–1806
Andersen, Hans Christian, 1805–1875
Bang, Bernhard, 1848–1932
Bjerrum, Jannik Petersen, 1851–1920
Fibiger, Johannes Andreas Grib, 1867–1928
Finsen, Niels Ryberg, 1860–1904
Fischer, Albert, 1891–1956
Gram, Hans Christian Joachim, 1853–1938
Haderup, Victor Frants Nachtegall, 1845–1913
Hagedorn, Hans Christian, 1888–1971
Hauberg, Poul Richard, 1887–1959
Hirschsprung, Harald, 1830–1916
Hjorth, Niels, 1919–
Jacobson, Ludwig Lewin, 1783–1843
Kemp, Tage, 1896–1964
Kierkegaard, Søren Aabye, 1813–1855
Krogh, Marie (Jorgensen), 1874–1943?
Müller, Otto Friderich, 1730–1784
Pindborg, Jens Jørgen, 1921–
Pissarro, Camille, 1830–1903
Schleisner, Peter Anton, 1818–1900
Viborg, Erik, 1759–1822

**Ethiopia**

Menelik II, Emperor of Ethiopia, 1844–1913

**Finland**

Edelfelt, Albert, 1854–1905
Ingman, Erik, 1810–1858
Koski, Kalevi, 1921–
Lönnrot, Elias, 1802–1884
Mannerheim, Sophie, 1863–1928
Paatero, Yrjö Veli
Simola, Paavo Eevertii, 1902–1961
Tigerstedt, Robert Adolf Armand, 1853–1923
Wegelius, Juhana, 1693–1764

**France**

Achard, François, d. 1853
Albarrán, Joaquin, 1860–1912
Alibert, Jean Louis Marie, 1766?–1837
Amar, Jules, 1879–1935
Ampère, André-Marie, 1775–1836
Andral, Gabriel, 1797–1876
Anel, Dominique, 1679–1730
Anglada, Joseph, 1775–1833
Anglade, Jean, 1698–1764
Antommarchi, Francesco A., 1780–1838
Anzoux, Louis Thomas Jérome, 1797–1880
Apert, Eugène, 1868–1940

Appert, Nicolas, 1749–1841
Aragon, Louis, 1897–1982
Ariès, Philippe, 1914–1984
Armengaud, André, 1920–1980
Arsonval, Asène d', 1851–1940
Artur, Jacques-Français, 1708–1779
Astruc, Jean, 1684–1766
Audibran, Joseph, 1801–1867
Audouard Family
Audouard, Maxence, 1776–1856
Augiéras Family
Babinski, Joseph François Félix, 1857–1932
Bachelard, Gaston, 1884?–1962
Bacq, Zénon M., 1903–1983
Bailly, Nicolas, 1817–1907
Balzac, Honoré de, 1799–1850
Barbot, Jean, 1655–1713
Barrès, Auguste Maurice, 1862–1923
Barthez, Paul Joseph, 1734–1806
Baudelaire, Charles Pierre, 1821–1867
Baudelocque, Jean Louis, 1745?–1810
Baudens, Jean Baptiste Lucien, 1804–1857
Baumé, Antoine, 1728–1804
Baumès, Prosper, 1791–1871
Béchamp, Pierre Jacques Antoine, 1816–1908
Béclaed, Jules
Béclère, Antoine, 1856–1939
Behal, Auguste, 1859–1941
Behr, Georg Heinrich, 1708–1761
Bergson, Henri Louis, 1859–1941
Bernard, Camille, 1802–1879
Bernard, Claude, 1813–1878
Bernard, Jean Jacques, 1888–
Bernay, Paul, fl. 1872
Bernheim, Hippolyte, 1840–1919
Bernou Family
Bert, Paul, 1833–1886
Berthelot, Marcellin Pierre Eugène, 1827–1907
Bertillon family
Bertin, René Joseph Hyacinthe, 1767–1828
Beyle, Marie Henri, 1783–1842
Bichat, Marie François Xavier, 1771–1802
Binet, Alfred, 1857–1911
Blainville, Henri Marie Ducrotay de, 1777–1850
Bocage, André, 1892–1953
Boecler, Jean, 1737–1808
Boillaud, Jean Baptiste, 1796–1887
Bonaparte, Marie, 1882–1962
Bonnafont, Jean-Pierre, 1805–1891
Bory de Saint-Vincent, Jean-Baptiste Marcellin, 1778–1846
Bouchardat, Apollinaire, 1806–1886
Boucher, André, 1903–1980
Bouestard, Jean-Jacques, 1730–1810
Boule, Marcellin, 1861–1942
Bourgelat, Claude, 1712–1779
Bourguet, Julien, 1877–
Bourrus, Josep, 1865–
Bredin, Claude-Julien, 1776–1854
Breton, André, 1896–1966
Bretonneau, Pierre Fidèle, 1778–1862
Briquet, Paul, d. 1882
Broca, Pierre Paul, 1824–1880
Brouillet, André, 1857–1914
Broussais, François Joseph Victor, 1772–1838
Brown-Séquard, Charles Edouard, 1817–1894
Buchan, John, 1769–1847
Buffon, Georges Louis Leclerc, 1707–1788
Cabanis, Pierre Jean Georges, 1757–1808
Cadet de Gassicourt, Charles Louis, 1769–1821
Caillié, René-Auguste, 1799–1838
Calmette, Albert, 1863–1933
Calot, Jean François, 1861–1944
Camus, Albert, 1913–1960
Carlier, Francois
Carnot, Marie François Sadi, 1837–1894
Carrel, Alexis, 1873–1944
Casanova, Danielle, 1909–1943
Caujole, Paul, 1978–1961
Chabbert, Pierre, 1924–1981
Chappuis, Charles, 1822–1897
Charcot, Jean Baptiste, 1867–1936
Charcot, Jean Martin, 1825–1893
Charles, Jacques Alexandre César, 1746–1823
Charvet, A. P., fl. 1826
Chastenet, Armand-Marie, Marquis de Puségur, fl. 1784
Chauffard, Anatole Marie Emile, 1855–1932
Chauveau, Jean Baptiste Auguste, 1827–1917
Chevreul, Michel Eugène, 1786–1889
Chirac, Pierre, 1650–1732
Christophe, Pierre, 1758–1826
Clemenceau, Georges, 1841–1929
Clot, Antoine-Barthélemy, 1793–1868
Cohn, Tobias, 1652–1729
Collomb, Henri, 1913–1979
Colombat, Emile, 1839–1891
Combes, Justin Louis Emile, 1835–1921
Comte, Auguste, 1798–1857
Condillac, Etienne Bonnôt de, 1714–1780
Condorcet, Marie Jean Antoine Nicolas de Coritat, 1743–1794
Constantin, Paul
Corvisart des Marets, Jean Nicolas, 1755–1821
Coste, Jean François, 1741–1819
Cotard, Jules, 1840–1889
Coutela, Charles, 1876–1969
Cruveilhier, Jean, 1791–1874
Cuénot, Lucien, 1866–1951
Curie, Marie Skłodowska, 1867–1934
Curie, Pierre, 1859–1906
Cuvier, George, 1769–1832
Dagonet, Henri
Darier, Jean, 1856–1938
Daubenton, Louis Jean Marie, 1716–1799
Daudet, Alphonse, 1840–1897
Daumier, Honoré, 1808–1879
Davaine, Casimir-Joseph, 1812–1882
David, Jacques Louis, 1748–1825
Daviel, Jacques, 1693–1762
Dax, Gustave, 1815–1893
Dax, Marc, 1770–1837
Dazille, Jean Barthélemy, 1733–1812
De Bap, Jean-César, 1718–1785
Debray, Charles, 1907–1979
Debré, Robert, 1882–1978
Déclat, Gilbert, 1827–1896
Déjerine, Joseph Jules, 1849–1917
Delaby, Raymond, 1891–1958
Delachaux, Armand, 1911–
Delage, Yves, 1854–1920
Delagenière, Henry, 1858–1930
Delaunay, Paul, 1878–1958
Delioux de Savignac, Joseph François, 1812–1876
Delpech, Jacques Matthieu, 1777–1832
Denigès, Georges, 1859–1951
Déplanche, Emile, 1824–1875
Deschiens, Robert, 1893–
Desfontaines, René, 1750?–1833
Desgenettes, René Nicolas Dufriche, 1762–1837
Destot, Etienne Auguste Joseph, 1864–1918
De Théis, Constance Marie, 1767–1845
Dezeimeris, Jean-Eugène, 1799–1852
Diderot, Denis, 1713–1784
Dieulafoy, Georges, 1839–1911
Dionis, Pierre, 1643–1718
Dorvault, François-Laurent-Marie, 1815–1879
Doyen, Eugene Louis, 1859–1916
Dubois de Chemant, Nicolas, 1753–1824
Dubois, J. A., 1765–1848
Dubois, Paul, 1848–1918
Duhamel du Monceau, Henri Louis, 1700–1781?
Duhamel, Georges, 1884–1966
Dumarest, Frédéric, 1862–1951
Dumas, Alexandre, 1802–1870
Dumas, Jean-Baptiste, 1800–1884
Dupuytren, Guillaume, 1777–1835
Durkheim, Emile, 1858–1917
Dutrochet, René Joachim Henri, 1776–1847
Esquirol, Jean Etienne Dominique, 1772–1840
Evrat, Louis-Antoine, 1797–1876
Ey, Henri, 1900–1977
Fallot, Arthur, 1850–1911
Falret, Jean Pierre, 1794–1870
Farabeuf, Louis Hubert, 1841–1910
Fauchard, Pierre, 1678–1761
Feltz, Victor Thimothé, 1835–1893
Feydeau, Georges Léon Jules Marie, 1862–1921
Filliozat, Jean, 1906–1982
Finot, André, 1884–1980
Flaubert, Achille Cléophas, 1784–1846
Flaubert, Gustave, 1821–1880
Flourens, Marie Jean Pierre, 1794–1867
Foix, Charles, 1882–1927
Foucault, Michel Jean Pierre, 1925–
Foucher, Emile, 1823–1867
Fourcroy, Antoine François de, 1755–1809
Fournier de Lempdes, J.-F., 1783–1861
Fournier, Jean Alfred, 1832–1914
Foy, Maximilien-Sebastien, 1775–1825
Fragonard, Jean Honoré, 1732–1806
France, Anatole, 1844–1924
Fusco, Silvain, 1903–1940
Gachet, Paul Fernand, 1828–1909
Gamelin, Jacques, 1738–1803

Gastaut, Henri Jean, 1915-
Gaucher, Phillipe Charles Ernest, 1854-1918
Gaulard, Pierre Nicolas, 1713-1740
Gay-Lussac, Joseph Louis, 1778-1850
Gélineau, Jean Baptiste Edouard, 1828-1906
Geoffroy Saint-Hilaire, Etienne, 1772-1844
Géricault, Jean Louis André Théodore, 1791-1824
Gessard, Louis-Marie, 1771-1855
Gide, André Paul Guillaume, 1869-1951
Girard, G., 1888-
Girardot, François, 1773-1831
Gobineau, Arthur de, 1816-1882
Gorcy, J. Camille
Gorcy, Pierre-Christophe, 1807-1821
Goyrand, Jean-Gaspard, 1803-1869
Grandville, Jean-Ignace-Isidore Gérard, 1803-1847
Grasset, Nicole
Gréard, Octave
Grinda, Edouard
Gripouilleau, Armel-Eugène, 1821-1909
Gruby, David, 1810-1898
Guérin, Alphonse François Marie, 1816-1875
Guerin, Camille, 1872-1961
Guerin, Jules, 1801-1886
Guesde, Jules, 1845-1922
Guillemin, Roger Charles Louis, 1924-
Guislain, Joseph, 1797-1860
Guyon, René, 1876-1963
Haller, Albin, 1849-1925
Hameau, Jean, 1779-1851
Hellot, Jean, 1685-1766
Houdé, Alfred, 1854-1919
Huard, Pierre Alfonse, 1901-1983
Hutinel, Victor, 1849-1933
Itard, Jean Marc Gaspard, 1775-1838
Jacquin, Armand Pierre, 1721-ca. 1790
Jacquot, François-Félix, 1819-1857
Jallabert, Jean, 1712-1768
Janet, Pierre, 1859-1947
Jayle, Max Fernand, 1913-
Joliot-Curie, Jean Frédéric, 1900-1958
Jouvet, Louis, 1887-1951
Junot, Jean Andoche, 1771-1813
Jussieu, Antoine de, 1686-1758
Klein, Marc, 1905-1975
La Condamine, Charles Marie de, 1701-1774
La Martinière, Germain Pichaut de, 1696-1783
La Mettrie, Julien Offray de, 1709-1751
La Peyronie, François Gigot de, 1678-1747
Labat, Pierre-Léon-Auguste, 1803-1847
Laborde, Jean Baptiste Vincent, 1830-1903
Lacan, Jacques, 1901-
Lacauchie, Adolphe-Euclide, 1806-1853
Laennec, Guillaume François, 1748-1822
Laennec, René Théophile Hyacinthe, 1781-1826
Lafarge, Marie Capelle, 1816-1852
Lafargue, Paul, 1842-1911
Laforest, Nicholas Laurent, fl. 1782
Lakhovsky, Georges, 1870-1942
Lamarck, Jean Baptiste Pierre Antoine de Monet de, 1744-1829
Lamare-Picquot, Christophe-Augustin, 1785-1873
Lambert, Jean-Henri, 1728-1777
Laplace, Pierre Simon de, 1749-1827
Larrey, Dominique Jean, 1766-1842
Lasègue, Ernest Charles, 1816-1883
Lautard, Jean-Baptiste, b. 1778
Laveran, Alphonse, 1845-1922
Lavoisier, Antoine Laurent, 1743-1794
Le Dantec, Félix Alexandre, 1869-1917
Le Jumeaux de Kergaradec, Jean Alexandre, 1787-1877
Le Monnier, Louis Guillaume, 1717-1799
Leborgne, 1810-1861
Leenhardt, Maurice, 1878-1954
Lefèvre, Amédée, 1798-1869
Lentulo, Henri, 1889-1981
Leriche, René, 1879-1955
Leulier, Albert, 1883-1957
Levaditi, Constantin, 1874-1953
Leveuf, Jacques, 1885-1948
Lévi-Strauss, Claude, 1908-
Levret, André, 1703-1780
Lévy-Bruhl, Lucien, 1857-1939
Liautard, Alexandre François, 1835-1918
Liétard, Gustave Alexandre, 1833-1904
Littré, Emile, 1801-1881
Loewel, Henri, 1795-1856
Lopez de Paz, Michel, 1680-1746?
Lorry, Anne Charles, 1726-1783
Louis, Antoine, 1723-1792
Louis XV, King of France, 1710-1774
Louis XVIII, King of France, 1755-1824
Lucas, Prosper, 1808-1885
Lumière, Auguste M., 1862-
Lumière, Louis Jean, 1864-1948
Lwoff, André, 1902-
Magendie, Francois, 1783-1855
Magitot, Emile, 1843-1897
Maillot, François-Clément, 1804-1894
Maisonabe, Charles Auguste, 1779-1851
Malgaigne, Joseph François, 1806-1865
Maloët, Pierre Louis Marie, 1730-1810
Marais, Marin, 1656-1728
Marat, Jean Paul, 1743-1793
Marchant, Nicolas-Damas, 1767-1833
Marey, Etienne Jules, 1830-1904
Marie, Pierre, 1853-1940
Marjolin, Jean Nicolas, 1780-1850
Martel, Thierry de, 1875-1940
Martin, George M., fl. 1890
Masson, Pierre, 1880-1959
Mauduyt de la Varenne, Pierre Jean Claude, ca. 1732-1792
Maupertuis, Pierre Louis Moreau de, 1698-1759
Maurichaud-Beaupré, Pierre-Jean, 1778-1857
Meige, Henry, 1866-1940
Mélier, François, 1798-1866
Menière, Prosper, 1799-1862
Merle d'Aubigné, Robert, 1900-
Meryon, Charles, 1821-1868
Michelet, Jules, 1798-1874
Michon, Louis, 1892-1973
Missoux, Damien Théodore, 1800-1863
Moissan, Henri, 1852-1907
Monet, Claude, 1840-1926
Monod, Jacques Lucien, 1910-1976
Montyon, Antoine Jean Baptiste Robert Auget, 1733-1820
Moreau de Saint-Elier, Louis Malo, 1701-1754
Moreau, Jacques Joseph (de Tours), 1804-1884
Morel, Benedict-Augustin, 1809-1873
Morestin, Hippolyte, 1869-1919
Mougeot, Jean-Baptiste, 1776-1858
Moutier, François, 1881-1961
Nachet Family
Napoleon I, Emperor of the French, 1769-1821
Napoleon III, Emperor of the French, 1808-1873
Nemours, Victoria Augusta Antoinetta de, 1822?-1857
Nicolle, Charles Jules Henri, 1866-1936
Nollet, Jean Antoine, 1700-1770
Oguse, Docteur
Ollier, Léopold, 1830-1900
Ollivier, Alexandre François, 1790-
Olombel, Jacques-Samuel, 1760-1850
Ombredanne, Louis, 1871-1956
Parrenin, Dominique, 1665-1741
Parrot, Jules, 1829-1883
Pasteur, Louis, 1822-1895
Paul, Constantin, 1833-1896
Péan, Jules Emile, 1830-1898
Pelletier, Madeleine
Percy, Pierre François, 1754-1825
Pereire, Jacobo Rodriguez, 1715-1780
Personne, Jacques, 1816-1880
Pétain, Henri Philippe, 1856-1951
Picart, Bernard, 1673-1733
Picasso, Pablo, 1881-1973
Pinel, Philippe, 1745-1826
Piorry, Pierre Adolphe, 1794-1879
Pipelet, Jean-Baptiste, 1759-1823
Pirodon, Eugene, 1824-1908
Pomme, Pierre, 1728-1814
Portal, Antoine, 1742-1832
Pouchet, Félix-Archimède, 1800-1872
Proust, Marcel, 1871-1922
Prunelle, Clément Victor François Gabriel, 1777-1853
Rabbinowicz, Israel Michael, 1818-1893
Ramon, Gaston, 1886-1963
Raspail, François-Vincent, 1794-1878
Raulin, Jules, 1836-1896
Raynaud, Maurice, 1834-1881
Redon, Henri, 1899-1974
Regaud, Claudius, 1870-1940
Reilly, James Paul Marie, 1887-1974
Renoux, André, fl. 1690
Reynaud, Claude-Auguste, 1804-1878
Risso, Antoine, 1777-1845
Robespierre, Maximilien Marie Isidor de, 1758-1794
Robic, J., 1893-1968
Robin, Pierre, 1725-ca. 1804
Rochefoucauld, J. B. de la, 1709-1746
Rodriguez-Péreire, Jacob, 1715-1780
Roger, Henri, 1809-1891
Roland Family
Rousseau, Jean Jacques, 1712-1778

Roussy, Gustave, 1874–1948
Roux, Pierre Paul Emile, 1853–1933
Sade, Donatien Alphonse François de, 1740–1814
Sage, Balthasar-Georges, 1740–1824
Saint-Simon, Claude Henri, 1760–1825
Saint-Simon, Louis de Rouvroy, 1675–1755
Salmon, Urbain-Philippe, 1768–1805
Sartre, Jean Paul, 1905–1980
Schwartz, Anselme, 1872–1957
Scrini, Basile, 1869–1931
Ségur, Sophie Rostopchine, 1799–1874
Senac, Jean Baptiste, 1693–1770
Servan, Joseph Michel Antoine, 1737–1807
Soubeiran, Eugène, 1797–1858
Soufflot, Jacques Germain, 1713–1780
Soulier, Jean Pierre
Spielmann, Jacob Reinbold, 1722–1783
Spillmann, Pierre, 1833–1883
Stern, Erich, 1889–1959
Stoeber, Victor, 1803–1871
Supliceau, Théodore, fl. ca. 1835
Talachon, Marie-Vincent, 1753–1817
Talma, François-Joseph, 1763–1826
Talochon, Marie-Vincent (Père Elisée), 1753–1817
Tardieu, Ambroise Auguste, 1818–1879
Tarnier, Stéphane, 1828–1897
Terson, Jean, 1803–1884
Teulon, Giraud, d. 1887
Tinel, Jules, 1879–1952
Tissot, Clément Joseph, 1747–1826
Tissot H.
Topinard, Paul, 1830–1911
Trappe, Antoine, 1767–1847
Treil, Sylvie
Trélat, Ulysse, 1795–1879
Troisier, Charles Emile, 1844–1919
Trousseau, Armand, 1801–1867
Turchini, Jean, 1894–1979
Vacher de Lapouge, Georges, 1854–1936
Valery, Paul Ambroise, 1871–1945
Valette, Guillaume, 1902–1982
Valeur, Amand, 1859–1927
Vandamme, Dominique-René, 1770–1830
Veber, Jean, 1864–1928
Velpeau, Alfred Louis Armand Marie, 1795–1867
Venel, Gabriel François, 1723–1775
Vergés, Dominique, 1775–1855
Véron, Louis Désiré, 1798–1867
Vicq-d'Azyr, Félix, 1748–1794
Victor de l'Aveyron
Vieillard, Eugène, fl. 1855–1867
Villemanzy, Jacques de, 1751–1830
Villemin, Jean Antoine, 1827–1892
Villermé, Louis-René, 1782–1863
Voltaire, François Marie Arouet de, 1694–1778
Vulpien, Alfred, 1826–1887
Wallon, Henri, 1879–1962
Wickersheimer, Ernest, 1880–1965
Zola, Emile, 1840–1902

**Germany**

Abderhalden, Emil, 1877–1950
Abraham, Karl, 1877–1925
Adlung, Alfred, 1875–
Albert, Joseph, 1825–1886
Albinus, Bernard Siegfried, 1697–1770
Altenähr, Eberhard, 1940–1981
Althoff, Friedrich
Anselmino, Otto, 1873–1955
Aubert, Hermann Rudolf, 1826–1892
Axhausen, Georg, 1877–
Bachmann, Christian Ludwig, 1763–1813
Baelz, Erwin, 1849–1913
Balser, Georg Friedrich Wilhelm, 1780–1846
Bardeleben, Karl Heinrich von, 1849–1919
Bargmann, Wolfgang, 1906–1978
Bass, Heinrich, 1690–1754
Baumgärtner, Karl Heinrich, 1798–1886
Beethoven, Ludwig van, 1770–1827
Behring, Emil Adolf von, 1854–1917
Benckiser, Robert, fl. 1831
Benjamin, Georg, 1895–1942
Berger, Hans, 1873–1941
Bergmann, Carl, 1814–1865
Bergmann, Ernst von, 1836–1907
Bernstein, Julius, 1839–1917
Bertalanffy, Ludwig von, 1901–1972
Bertele, Georg, 1767–1818
Beuys, Joseph, 1921–
Bielschowsky, Alfred, 1871–
Bier, August, 1861–1949
Bilharz, Theodor, 1825–1862
Billroth, Theodor, 1829–1894
Bing, R. Abraham, 1752–1841
Binswanger, Ludwig, 1881–1966
Blasius, Ernst, 1802–1875
Block, Dr., d. 1892
Blumenbach, Johann Friedrich, 1752–1840
Boll, Franz, 1849–1879
Bonhoeffer, Karl, 1868–1948
Bormann, Martin, 1900–1945?
Bostroem, Eugen Woldemar, 1850–1928
Brahms, Johannes, 1833–1897
Brass, Arnold, 1854–
Brauer, Ludolph, 1865–1951
Brücke, Ernst Wilhelm von, 1819–1892
Brugsch, Theodor, 1878–1963
Buchner, Eduard, 1860–1917
Bumm, Ernst, 1858–1925
Bunsen, Robert Wilhelm Eberhard, 1811–1899
Burow, Carl August, 1809–1874
Busanny-Caspari, Willi, 1922–1982
Busch, Wilhelm, 1832–1908
Cohn, Ferdinand Julius, 1828–1898
Constantini Family
Correns, Carl Franz Joseph Erich, 1864–1933
Coschwitz, Georg Daniel, 1679–1729
Credé, Carl S. F., 1819–1892
Czerny, Adalbert, 1863–1941
Dann, Georg Edmund, 1898–
Darré, Richard Walther, 1895–1953
Deigendesch, Johannes
Dieck, Wilhelm, 1867–1935
Dieffenbach, Johann Friedrich, 1792–1847
Döblin, Alfred, 1878–1957
Dohrn, Anton, 1840–1909
Dragendorff, Johann Georg Noël, 1836–1898
Driesch, Hans Adolf Eduard, 1867–1941
Drost-Hülshoff, Annette Elizabeth, Freiin von, 1797–1848
Du Bois-Reymond, Emil Heinrich, 1818–1896
Düring, Ernst Eduard Kamille von, 1858–1944
Ebbinghaus, Hermann, 1850–1909
Ehlers, Ernst Heinrich, 1835–1925
Ehrenberg, Christian Gottfried, 1795–1876
Ehrlich, Paul, 1854–1915
Eichhorst, Hermann, 1849–1921
Eiselsberg, Anton von, 1860–1939
Eisenbarth, Johann Andreas, 1663–1727
Eisler, Robert, 1882–1949
Engels, Friedrich, 1820–1895
Erb, Wilhelm Heinrich, 1840–1921
Ertl, Johann von, 1881–
Erxleben, Dorthea Christiana, 1715–1762
Eskuchen, Karl, 1885–1955
Esmarch, Friedrich von, 1823–1908
Euler, Leonhard, 1707–1783
Eulner, Hans-Heinz, 1925–1980
Fechner, Gustav Theodor, 1801–1887
Fehling, Hermann Johannes Karl, 1847–1925
Felixmüller, Conrad, 1897–1977
Felke, Emanuel, 1856–1926
Feuerbach, Ludwig Andreas, 1804–1872
Fikentscher, Richard, 1903–
Finkelnburg, D. C., fl. 1870
Flechsig, Paul Emil, 1847–1929
Fliedner, Theodor, 1800–1864
Fliess, Wilhelm, 1858–1928
Fontane, Theodor, 1819–1898
Formey, Johann Ludwig F., 1766–1823
Forssmann, Werner, 1904–1979
Forster, Georg, 1754–1794
Forster, Johann Reinhold, 1729–1798
Frank, Johann Peter, 1745–1821
Fränkel, Albert, 1864–1938
Fränkel, Moritz Ottomar, 1814–1902
Frederic II, King of Prussia, 1712–1786
Frederick III, Emperor of Germany, 1831–1888
Frey, Heinrich, 1822–1890
Fricke, Johann Karl Georg, 1790–1841
Fries, Jakob Friedrich, 1773–1843
Froriep, Robert Friedrich, 1804–1861
Gaehtgens, Carl, fl. 1881–1898
Gatterer, Johann Christoph, 1727–1799
Gebsattel, Victor Emil von, 1883–1976
Gerhardt, Carl, 1833–1902
Gerngross, Richard, 1878–1956
Geyer, Günther, 1930–1980
Gietzelt, Fritz, 1903–1968
Goerke, Heinz, 1917–
Goethe, Johann Wolfgang von, 1749–1832
Goldfuss, Georg August, 1782–1848

Goldhagen, Johann Friedrich Gottlieb, 1742–1788
Gorup-Besanez, Eugen Franz von, 1817–1878
Gottron, Heinrich A., 1890–1974
Graefe, Albrecht von, 1828–1870
Graefe, Carl Ferdinand von, 1787–1840
Gräfenberg, Ernst, 1881–1957
Griesinger, Wilhelm, 1817–1868
Groddeck, Georg Walther, 1866–1934
Grotjahn, Alfred, 1869–1931
Grüneberg, Theodor, 1901–
Grütz, Otto Julius, 1886–1963
Gudden, Johann Bernhard Aloys von, 1824–1886
Gumpert, Martin, 1897–1955
Gütt, Arthur, 1891
Gutzmann, Hermann, 1865–1922
Gysi, Alfred, 1865–1957
Haas, Georg, 1886–1971
Haass, Friedrich Joseph, 1780–1853
Hackmann, Christian Jakob, 1899–1981
Haeckel, Ernst Heinrich Philipp August, 1834–1919
Hagedorn, Werner, 1831–1894
Hagen, Johann Philipp, 1734–1792
Hahnemann, Christian Friedrich Samuel, 1755–1843
Haindorf, Alexander, 1782–1862
Hardenberg, Friedrich Leopold von, 1772–1801
Harless, Johann Christian Friedrich, 1773–1853
Hauptmann, Carl, 1858–1921
Hauptmann, Gerhart, 1862–1946
Havemann, August Conrad, 1755–1819
Hecker, August Friedrich, 1763–1811
Hegar, Alfred, 1830–1914
Hegel, Georg Wilhelm Friedrich, 1770–1831
Heidenhain, Rudolf Peter Heinrich, 1834–1897
Heim, Ernst Ludwig, 1747–1834
Heine, Bernhard, 1800–1846
Heine, Heinrich, 1797–1856
Heinroth, Johann Christian August, 1773–1843
Heisler, August, 1881–
Heiss, Hugo Andreas, 1863–1936
Heister, Lorenz, 1683–1758
Helmholtz, Hermann Ludwig Ferdinand von, 1821–1894
Henle, Jakob, 1809–1885
Henning, Hans, 1885–1946
Hensing, Johann Thomas, 1683–1726
Herbart, Johann Friedrich, 1776–1841
Hertwig, Oscar, 1849–1922
Hesse, Friedrich Louis 1849–1906
Hesse, Ludwig Ferdinand, 1795–1876
Heunert, Hans Henning, 1920–
Heusinger, Karl Friedrich von, 1792–1883
Hillebrand, Wilhelm, 1892–1959
Hirsch, August, 1817–1894
Hirsch, Max, 1877–1948
Hirsch, Samson Raphael, 1890–1960
Hirschberg, Julius, 1843–1925
Hitler, Adolf, 1889–1945
Hitler, Eva Braun, d. 1945
Hoffa, Albert J., 1859–1907
Hoffmann, Ernst Theodor Amadeus, 1776–1822
Hoffmann, Friedrich, 1660–1742
Hoffmann, Karl Friedrich, fl. 1761
Hölderlin, Friedrich, 1770–1843
Holzkamp, Klaus
Horemans, Jan Josef, 1682–1859
Hornschuch, Christian Friedrich, 1793–1850
Hufeland, Christoph Wilhelm, 1762–1836
Humboldt, Alexander von, 1769–1859
Ideler, Carl Wilhelm, 1795–1860
Israel, James 1848–1926
Jaeger, Gustav, 1832–1917
Jaspers, Karl, 1883–1969
Jensen, Wilhelm, 1837–1911
Jessen, Peter Willers, 1793–1895
Jessen, Peter Willers, 1832–1912
Jores, Arthur, 1901–
Jörg, Johann Christian Gottfried, b. 1779
Joseph, Jacques, 1865–1934
Juncker, Johann, 1679–1759
Jung-Stilling, Johann Heinrich, 1740–1817
Jünger, Ernst, 1895–
Just, Adolf
Kändler, Johannes Joachim, 1706–1775
Kant, Immanuel, 1724–1804
Karll, Agnes, 1868–1927
Katsch, Gerhardt, 1887–
Kaulbach, Wilhelm von, 1805–1874
Kayser, Marie-Elise, 1885–1950
Kehr, Hans, 1862–1916
Kerner, Justinus, 1786–1862
Kersting, Johann Adam, 1727–1784
Kieser, Dietrich Georg, 1779–1862
Kimmelstiel, Paul, 1900–1970
Kirchner, Ernst Ludwig, 1880–1938
Kirschner, Martin, 1879–1942
Kiwisch, Alexander Franz Wilhelm, 1814–1851
Klebs, Edwin, 1834–1913
Kleist, Heinrich von, 1777–1811
Kleist, Karl, 1879–
Kloos, Karlferdinand, 1911–1980
Kneipp, Sebastian, 1821–1897
Knoth, Wilhelm, 1923–1982
Kobert, Rudolf, 1854–1918
Koblinsky, Albert, fl. 1916
Koch, Gerhard, 1913–
Koch, Richard, 1882–1949
Koch, Robert, 1843–1910
Koebner, Heinrich, 1823–1904
Köhler, Wolfgang, 1887–1967
Kölliker, Albert von, 1817–1905
König, Franz, 1832–1910
Koppel, Mat, 1890–1916
Körte, Werner, 1853–1937
Kraepelin, Emil, 1856–1926
Krafft-Ebing, Richard von, 1840–1902
Kraus, Friedrich, 1858–1936
Kretschmer, Ernst, 1888–1964
Kreutzer, Johann Martin, 1810–1855
Krüche, Arno, 1854–1926
Kuhn, Franz, 1866–1929
Kühn, Karl Gottlob, 1754–1840
Künkel, Fritz, 1889–1956
Laehr, Heinrich, 1820–1905
Lämmler, Georg, 1925–1981
Landauer, Walter, 1896–1978
Langenbeck, Bernhard von, 1810–1887
Langenbuch, Carl Johann August, 1846–1901
Langerhans, Paul, 1847–1888
Lappe, Christian Theodor, 1802–1877
Leber, Theodor, 1840–1917
Lenard, Philipp, 1862–1947
Lenz, Fritz, 1887–
Lerche, Martin
Lessing, Gotthold Ephraim, 1729–1781
Leydig, Franz von, 1821–1908
Lichtenberg, Alexander von, 1880–1980
Lichtenberg, Georg Christoph, 1742–1799
Liebermeister, Carl, 1833–1901
Liebig, Justus von, 1803–1873
Liepmann, Wilhelm, 1875 or 8–1939
Lincke, Harold, d. 1977
Lingner, Karl August, 1861–1916
Lipps, Theodor, 1851–1914
Liszt, Franz von, 1811–1886
Loeffler, Friedrich, 1852–1915
Loeffler, Friedrich, 1885–1967
Loewi, Otto, 1873–1961
Löhlein, Walther, 1882–
Löhr, Wilhelm, 1889–
Lorenz, Konrad Zacharias, 1903–
Lorenzer, Alfred, 1922–
Ludwig, Karl Friedrich Wilhelm, 1816–1895
Luxemburg, Rosa, 1870–1919
Lynen, Feodor, 1911–1979
Mangold, Hilde, 1898–1924
Mann, Thomas, 1875–1955
Marcus, Carl Friedrich von, 1802–1862
Marx, Karl, 1818–1883
Marzell, Heinrich, 1885–1970
Matthiae, Georg M., 1708–1773
Mayer, Julius Robert von, 1814–1878
Mayer, Rudolph Leopold, 1895–1962
Mayersbach, Heinz von
Mayrhofer, Karl Wilhelm, 1806–1853
Meckel, Johann Friedrich, 1781–1833
Mengele, Josef, 1911
Menzel, Arthur, 1844–1878
Merck, Heinrich Emanuel, 1794–1855
Merkel, Friedrich Sigmund, 1845–1919
Messerschmidt, Franz Xaver, 1736–1783
Metzig, Johann Christian Heinrich, 1804–1868
Mitscherlich, Alexander, 1908–1982
Möbius, Paul Julius, 1853–1907
Mohr, Hans Jürgen, 1922–1982
Moll, Albert, 1862–1939
Moltke, Helmuth Karl Bernhard von, 1800–1891
Mooren, Albert Clemens, 1828–1899
Morell, Theodor, 1886–1948
Müller, August, 1864–1949
Müller, Carl, 1861–
Müller, Friedrich von, 1858–1941
Müller, Fritz, 1822–1897
Müller, Johannes, 1801–1858

Müller-Lyer, Franz Carl, 1857–1916
Münchhausen, Karl Friedrich Hieronymus von, 1720–1797
Musil, Robert, 1880–1942
Muthmann, Arthur, 1875–
Nasse, Christian Friedrich, 1778–1851
Neisser, Albert, 1855–1916
Neugebauer, Ludwig Adolf, 1824–1890
Neuhold, Richard, 1917–1982
Neumann, Erich, 1905–1960
Neumann, Robert, 1882–
Neumann, Salomon, 1819–
Nietzsche, Friedrich Wilhelm, 1844–1900
Noorden, Carl Harko Hermann Johannes von, 1858–1944
Oertel, Max Joseph, 1835–1897
Osiander, Friedrich Benjamin, 1759–1822
Pankok, Otto, 1893–
Petersen, Erst Hans, 1885–1946
Pettenkofer, Max Joseph von, 1818–1901
Peus, Fritz, 1904–1978
Pfaff, Philipp, 1713–1766
Pfannenstiel, Hermann Johannes, 1862–1909
Pfeffel, Johann Andreas, 1674–1748
Pfeiffer, Richard Friedrich Johannes, 1858–1945
Pflüger, Eduard Friedrich Wilhelm, 1829–1910
Pichler, Hans, 1877–1949
Pienitz, Ernst Gottlob, 1777–1853
Pirch, Otto Ferdinand Dubislav, 1799–1832
Planck, Max Karl Ernst Ludwig, 1858–1947
Pommerin, Reiner
Prausnitz-Giles, Carl, 1876–1963
Preis, Karl
Preuss, Julius, 1861–1913
Preyer, William Thierry, 1841–1897
Prinzhorn, Hans, 1886–1933
Quincke, Heinrich Irenaeus, 1842–1922
Raspe, Rudolph Erich, 1737–1794
Recklinghausen, Friedrich Daniel von, 1833–1910
Redwitz, Erich, 1883–1964
Reichenbach, Karl Ludwig von, 1788–1869
Reil-Bey, Wilhelm, 1820–1880
Reil, Johann Christian, 1759–1813
Reimer, Hermann Andreas, 1825–1906
Reinke, Friedrich, 1862–
Revers, Wilhelm Josef, 1918–
Richter, Christian Friedrich, 1676–1711
Riechert, Traugott, 1905–
Rikli, Arnold, 1823–1906
Rinecker, Franz von, 1811–1883
Ringseis, Johannes Nepomuk von, 1785–1880
Rittmeister, John F., 1898–1943
Rolfus, Karl, 1819–1907
Röntgen, Wilhelm Conrad, 1845–1923
Rorschach, Hermann, 1884–1922
Roschlaub, Andreas, 1768–1835
Rosenbaum, Julius, 1807–1874
Roux, Wilhelm, 1850–1924
Rüdinger, Nikolaus, 1832–1896
Rudolphi, Karl Asmund, 1771–1832
Ruge, Carl, 1846–1926
Rust, Johann Nepomuk, 1775–1840
Rydygier, Ludwig von, 1850–1920
Salm-Dyck, Josef von, 1773–1861
Sandritter, Walter, 1920–1980
Sauerbruch, Ernst Ferdinand, 1875–1951
Sayn-Wittgenstein, Casimir zu, 1687–1741
Schadewaldt, Hans, 1923–
Schaudinn, Fritz Richard, 1871–1906
Scheel, Paul Friedrich, 1883–
Schelenz, Hermann, 1848–1922
Schemann, Ludwig, 1852–1938
Scherf, Johann Christian Friedrich, 1750–1818
Schiff, Moritz, 1823–1896
Schiller, Johann Christoph Friedrich von, 1759–1805
Schilling, Johann August, 1829–1884
Schilling, Viktor, 1883–1960
Schipperges, Heinrich, b. 1918
Schleiden, Matthias Jacob, 1804–1881
Schlickum, Oscar, 1838–1889
Schlossmann, Arthur, 1867–1932
Schmidt, Arno, 1914–
Schmidtmann, Martha, 1892–1981
Schmitz, Rudolf 1918–
Schneider, Kurt, 1887–1967
Schneider, Reinhold, 1903–1958
Schneider, Wolfgang, 1912–
Schoenmackers, Jakob, 1912–1982
Schönfeld, Walter, 1888–1977
Schönlein, Johann Lucas, 1793–1864
Schopenhauer, Arthur, 1788–1860
Schrakamp, Franz, 1860–1920
Schreber, Daniel Paul, 1842–1911
Schröder, Robert, 1884–1959
Schubert, Gotthilf Heinrich von, 1780–1860
Schultz-Hencke, Harald, 1892–
Schultze, Wilhelm, 1840–1924?
Schulze, Curt i.e. Max Curt Gustav, 1881–
Schulze, Johann Heinrich, 1687–1744
Schumann, Robert Alexander, 1810–1856
Schwann, Theodor, 1810–1882
Schwartze, Hermann, 1837–1910
Schweninger, Ernst, 1850–1924
Sellheim, Hugo, 1871–1936
Sertürner, Friedrich Wilhelm, 1783–1841
Siebeck, Richard, 1883–1965
Siegle, Emil, 1833–1900
Sievert, Rolf Maximilian, 1896–
Simon, Gustav, 1824–1876
Simon, Hermann, 1867–1947
Soemmerring, Detmar Wilhelm, 1793–1891
Soemmerring, Margarethe Elisabeth Grunelius, 1768–1802
Soemmerring, Samuel Thomas von, 1755–1830
Spemann, Hans, 1869–1941
Spiro, Karl, 1867–1932
Sprengel, Kurt Polycarp Joachim, 1766–1833
Springsfeld, Karl Gottlob, 1714–1772
Spurzheim, Johann Christoph, 1776–1832
Stahl, Georg Ernst, 1660–1734
Stark, Karl Wilhelm, 1787–1845
Steffen, August, 1825–1910
Steiger, Adolf, 1862–1920
Stein, Georg Wilhelm, 1773–1870
Steinhausen, Wilhelm, 1887–1954
Stern, William, 1871–1938
Sternberg, Erich, 1903–1980
Stilling, Benedict, 1810–1879
Stoeckel, Walter, 1871–1961
Stöhr, Philipp, 1891–1979
Stolte, Karl, 1881–1951
Stratz, Carl Heinrich, 1858–1924
Strauss, Anselm Franz, 1780–1830
Stromeyer, Louis, 1804–1876
Strübing, Paul, 1852–
Struensee, Johann Friedrich, 1737–1772
Strümpell, Adolf, 1853–1925
Sudhoff, Karl Friedrich Jakob, 1853–1938
Süssmilch, Johann Peter, 1707–1767
Szymonowicz, Władysław, 1869–1939
Tellenbach, Hubertus, 1918–
Textor, Cajetan, 1782–1860
Thudicum, John Louis William, 1829–1901
Timmermann, Guenter, 1908–1979
Tönnis, Wilhelm, 1898–1978
Trendelenburg, Friedrich, 1844–1924
Trommsdorff, Johann Bartholomäus, 1770–1837
Ulrichs, Karl Heinrich, 1825–1895
Unger, Ernst, 1875–1938
Unkrig, Wilhelm A.
Unna, Paul Gerson, 1850–1929
van der Reis, Viktor, 1889–1958
Vater, Abraham, 1684–1751
Vater, Christian, 1651–1732
Veit, Gustav von, 1834–1905
Viet, David, 1771–1814
Virchow, Rudolf Ludwig Karl, 1821–1902
Vogt, Oskar, 1870–1959
Volhard, Franz, 1872–1950
Volkmann, Richard von, 1809–1894
Wackenroder, Heinrich Wilhelm Ferdinand, 1798–1854
Wagner, Heinz, 1923–
Wagner, Richard, 1813–1883
Wagner, Rudolph, 1805–1864
Waldeyer-Hartz, Wilhelm von, 1836–1921
Walkhoff, Otto, 1860–1934
Warburg, Otto Heinrich, 1883–1970
Wassermann, August von, 1866–1925
Weber, Carl Maria von, 1786–1826
Weber, Max, 1864–1920
Weigel, Christian Ehrenfried von, 1748–1831
Weigert, Carl, 1845–1904
Weinberg, Wilhelm, 1862–1937
Weismann, August, 1834–1914
Weiss, Ernst, 1882–1940
Wenzel, Heinrich Karl, 1769–1827
Wenzel, Joseph, 1768 1808
Werle, Eugen, 1902–
Wernher, Adolph Carl Gustav, 1809–1883
Wernicke, Carl, 1848–1905
Wertheim, Th., fl. 1891
Wichmann, Johann Ernst, 1740–1802
Wildführ, George, 1904–
Wilhelm, Augustin, 1933–
Witzel, Adolf, 1847–1906

Wöhler, Friedrich, 1800–1882
Wolfart, Karl Christian, 1778–1832
Wolff, Caspar Friedrich, 1733–1794
Wolff, Christian von, 1679–1754
Wolter, Friedrich, 1863–1944?
Wunderlich, Karl Reinhold August, 1815–1877
Wundt, Wilhelm Maximilian, 1832–1920
Zetkin, Maxim, 1883–1965
Ziurek, Otto Adolph Albert, 1821–1886
Zur Verth, Max, 1874–1941

**Great Britain**

Abrahams, Adolpho, 1884
Addenbrooke, John, 1680–1719
Addison, Christopher, 1869–1951
Addison, Thomas, 1795–1860
Adrian, Edgar Douglas, 1889–1977
Albert, Prince Consort, 1819–1861
Alexander, Frederick Matthias, 1869–1955
Alice Maud Mary, Princess of Great Britain, 1843–1878
Alison, William Pulteney, 1790–1859
Allen, William, 1770–1843
Amoroso, Emmanuel Ciprian
Anderson, Elizabeth Garrett, 1836–1917
Angibaud, Charles, fl. 1678–1728
Annan, Ebenezer, fl. 1836–1843
Arbuthnot, John, 1667–1735
Armstrong, Fergus, 1887–
Armstrong, John Richard, 1872–1931
Arnald, George, 1763–1841
Arnott, Neil, 1788–1874
Astbury, William Thomas, 1898–1961
Atkins, Hedley, 1905–
Aykroyd, Wallace Ruddell, 1899–1979
Bach, Edward, 1886–1936
Bacharach, Alfred Louis, 1891–1966
Baillie, Matthew, 1761–1823
Baker, Edward, 1818–1902
Baker, William Morrant, 1839–1896
Balint, Michael, 1896–
Banks, Joseph, 1743–1820
Barcroft, Joseph, 1872–1947
Barlow, Thomas, 1845–1945
Barnardo, Thomas John, 1845–1905
Barry, James, 1795–1865
Bartlett, Frederick Charles, 1886–1969
Bastian, Henry Charlton, 1837–1915
Bateson, William, 1861–1926
Beatson, George Thomas, 1848–1933
Beddoes, Thomas, 1760–1808
Bedson, Samuel Phillips, 1886–1969
Bell, Andrew, 1753–1832
Bell, Charles, 1774–1842
Bell, Joseph, 1837–1911
Bennett, Alexander Hughes, 1848–1901
Bennett, Arnold, 1867–1931
Bentham, Jeremy, 1748–1832
Bentom, Clark, ca. 1774–ca. 1820
Berkeley, George, Bp. of Cloyne, 1685–1753
Bernal, John Desmond, 1901–1971
Besant, Annie, 1847–1933
Beveridge, William, 1879–1963
Bigsby, John Jeremiah, 1792–1881
Black, Joseph, 1728–1799
Blake, William, 1757–1827
Blane, Gilbert, 1749–1834
Blundell, James, 1790–1878
Blyth, Edward, 1810–1873
Bodington, George, 1799–1882
Bond, Charles John, 1856–1939
Booth, William, 1829–1912
Boswell, James, 1740–1795
Bowlby, John Mostyn, 1907–
Boyd, William, 1885–
Bradlaugh, Charles, 1833–1891
Bradshaw, William, 1830–1861
Bragg, William Henry, 1862–1942
Braid, James, 1795–1860
Brain, Walter Russell, 1895–1966
Bramwell, Byrom, 1847–1931
Bramwell, Edwin, 1873–1955
Breese, Frederick, 1866–1945
Brent, Charles Henry, 1862–1929
Brewster, David, 1781–1868
Bright, Richard, 1789–1858
Brodie, Benjamin Collins, 1783–1862
Brown, Isaac Baker, 1812–1873
Brown, John, 1735–1788
Brown, Robert, 1773–1858
Brown, Thomas Graham, 1882–1965
Brown, Thomas, 1778–1820
Brown, William Michael Court, 1918–1968
Brownlee, John, 1868–1927
Brownrigg, William, 1712–1800
Bruce, David, 1855–1931
Bruce, James, 1730–1794
Bruce, John Mitchell, 1846–1929
Bruce, William, 1835–1920
Buchan, William, 1729–1805
Buckley, Wilfred, 1873–1933
Bucknill, John Charles, 1817–1897
Budd, William, 1811–1880
Bumm, Ernst, 1778–1820
Burdett-Coutts, Angelina Georgina, 1814–1906
Burke, Edmund, 1729–1797
Burke, Thomas, 1886–1945
Burke, William, 1792–1829
Burn, Joshua Harold, 1892–1981
Burney, Fanny, 1752–1840
Burns, Allan, 1781–1813
Burns, Robert, 1759–1796
Burroughs, Silas Mainville, 1846–1895
Burt, Cyril, 1883–1971
Byron, George Gordon Noël, 1788–1824
Cadogan, William, 1711–1797
Cairns, Hugh William Bell, 1896–1952
Cameron, Gordon Roy, 1899–1966
Campbell, C. S.
Campbell Swinton, Alan A., d. 1930
Carlyle, Thomas, 1795–1881
Carmichael, Edward Arnold, 1896–
Carpenter, Edward, 1844–1929
Carr-Saunders, Alexander Morris, 1886–1966
Carroll, Lewis, 1832–1898
Carson, James, 1772–1843
Carswell, John, 1856–1931
Carswell, Robert, 1793–1857
Carter, Robert Brudenell, 1828–1918
Catlin, George, 1796–1872
Cavell, Edith Louisa, 1865–1915
Cawthorne, Terence Edward, 1902–1970
Chadwick, Edwin, 1800–1890
Chadwick, Samuel Taylor, 1809–1873
Chain, Ernst Boris, 1906–1979
Chaplin, Charles, 1889–1977
Charlotte Augusta, of Wales, Consort of Prince Leopold of Saxe-Coburg-Saalfeld, 1796–1817
Charnley, John, 1911–1982
Chesterton, Gilbert Keith, 1874–1936
Christie, Agatha, 1891?–1976
Churchill, Randolph, 1849–1895
Cleave, Thomas Latimer, 1906–
Clift, Caroline Amelia, 1801–1873
Clift, William Home, 1803–1832
Clift, William, 1775–1849
Close, Harold George, 1898–
Clough, Arthur Hugh, 1819–1861
Clowes, George Henry Alexander, 1877–1958
Cobbe, Frances Power, 1822–1904
Cobbett, William, 1763–1835
Colebrook, Leonard, 1883–1967
Coleridge, Samuel Taylor, 1772–1834
Collingwood, Edward Foyle, 1900–1970
Collins, Wilkie, 1824–1889
Collins, William, 1721–1759
Conolly, John, 1794–1866
Cook, Albert Ruskin, 1870–1951
Cook, James, 1728–1779
Cookworthy, William, 1705–1780
Cooper, Astley Paston, 1768–1841
Cooper, Thomas Henry, 1813–1881
Coram, Thomas, 1668–1751
Cosslett, Vernon Ellis, 1908–
Cowper, William, 1731–1800
Cox, Alfred, 1866–1954
Craik, Kenneth James Williams, 1914–1945
Crapper, Thomas, 1837–1910
Crawford, Adair, 1748–1795
Crawford, James, 1682–1731
Cree, Edward Hodges, 1814–1901
Crichton, Alexander, 1763–1856
Crick, Francis Harry, 1916–
Critchley, Macdonald, 1900–
Cromwell, Oliver, 1599–1658
Crosse, Andrew, 1784–1855
Cruikshank, George, 1792–1878
Dain, Harry Guy, 1870–1966
Dale, Henry Hallett, 1875–1968
Daley, William Allen, 1887–1969
Dalmahoy, Alexander, ca. 1723–1783
Dalton, John, 1766–1844

Klein, Melanie, 1882–1960
Knight, Richard, 1768–1844
Knowlton, Charles, 1800–1850
Knox, Robert, 1791–1862
Krebs, Hans Adolf, 1900–1981
Lains, Ronald David, 1927–
Lane, Arbuthnot, 1856?–1943
Lane, Edward, ca. 1823–
Lawrence, David Herbert, 1885–1930
Learmonth, James Rognvald, 1895–1967
Leiper, Robert Thomson, 1881–1969
Leopold, Duke of Albany, 1853–1884
Lett, Hugh, 1876–1964
Lettsom, John Coakley, 1744–1815
Lewes, George Henry, 1817–1878
Lewis, Aubrey Julian, 1900–
Lewis, John, 1834–
Lewis, Thomas, 1881–1945
Lind, James, 1716–1794
Lind, Jenny, 1820–1887
Lister, Joseph Jackson, 1786–1869
Lister, Joseph Lister, 1827–1912
Liston, Robert, 1794–1847
Livingstone, David, 1813–1873
Lloyd George, David, 1863–1945
Locock, Charles, 1799–1875
Ludlow, Abraham, fl. 1764
Lupton, Edward
MacArthur, William Porter, 1884–1964
McBride, John Adam, 1843?–1889
MacCormac, William, 1836–1901
McCormick, Robert, 1800–1890
Macculloch, John, 1773–1835
Macewen, William, 1848–1924
MacKenna, Robert Merttins Bird, 1903–
MacKenzie, Henry, 1745–1831
Mackenzie, James, 1853–1925
Mackenzie, Morell, 1837–1892
McKie, Douglas, 1896–1967
Mackintosh, James Macalister, 1891–1966
Macleane, Laughlin, 1728?–1777
McLetchie, James Leslie, 1909–1965
McMichael, John, 1904–
MacNalty, Arthur Salusbury, 1880–1969
McNaughton, Daniel, 1813–1865
McNeil, Charles, 1881–1964
Magill, Ivan Whiteside, 1888–
Malthus, Thomas Robert, 1766–1834
Malvern, Godfrey Martin Huggins, 1883–1971
Manson, Patrick, 1844–1922
Mantell, Gideon Algernon, 1790–1852
Mapson, Leslie William, 1907–1970
Marks, Urban, 1880–1949
Marshall, Geoffrey, 1887–
Martin, John, 1789–1854
Martindale, William, 1840–1902
Martineau, Harriet, 1802–1876
Martyn, John, 1699–1768
Masheter, James William Hall, d. 1943
Masterman, Charles Frederick Gurney, 1873–1927
Maudsley, Henry, 1835–1918
Maugham, William Somerset, 1874–1965
Maxwell, James Clerk, 1831–1879
Medawar, Peter Brian, 1915–
Mennell, Zebulon, 1876–1959
Merrick, Joseph Carey, 1862–1890
Michaelson, Isaac Chesar, 1903–
Miles, Ashley A., 1904–
Mill, James, 1773–1836
Mill, John Stuart, 1806–1873
Miller, Hugh
Milne, John Alexander, 1920–1977
Milner, John, fl. 1805
Mitchiner, Philip Henry, 1888–1952
Moir, Andrew, 1806–1844
Moir, Chassar, fl. 1932
Monro, John, 1715–1791
Montagu, Mary (Pierrepont) Wortley, 1689–1762
Montefiore, Moses Haim, 1784–1885
Moorcroft, William, 1765?–1825
Moule, Henry, 1801–1880
Mounsey, James, 1710?–1773
Moynihan, Berkeley George Andrew, 1865–1936
Mummery, John Howard, 1847–1926
Munk, H. A., fl. 1862–1870
Musgrave, Samuel, 1732–1780
Mussen, Aubrey Thomas, 1873–1975
Myers, Arthur Thomas, 1851–1894
Needham, Joseph, 1900–
Neild, James, 1744–1814
Nelson, Horatio, 1758–1805
Nettleship, Edward, 1845–1913
Nightingale, Florence, 1820–1910
Norris, William, 1792–1877
Ogston, Alexander, 1844–1929
Oliver, Williams, 1695–1764
O'Shaughnessy, William Brooke, 1809–1889
Osler, Edward, 1798–1863
Owen, Isambard, 1850–1927
Owen, Richard, 1804–1892
Owen, Wilfred, 1893–1918
Paget, James, 1814–1899
Paine, Henry James, 1816–
Parkinson, James, 1755–1824
Parkinson, Sydney, 1745?–1771
Parry, Caleb Hillier, 1755–1822
Partington, James Riddick, 1886–1965
Pater, Walter Horatio, 1839–1894
Pattison, Granville Sharp, 1791–1851
Peacock, John, 1761?–1841
Peacock, Thomas Bevill, 1812–1882
Pearson, Karl, 1857–1936
Peirce, Jeremy
Percival, Thomas, 1740–1804
Pereira, Jonathan, 1804–1853
Philip, Robert, 1857–1939
Pickles, William Norman, 1885–1969
Pilkington, George, 1854–1895
Pirie, James Hunter Harvey, 1879–1965
Pitcairn, William, 1711–1791
Pott, Percivall, 1714–1788
Pound, Dudley, 1877–1943
Price, William, 1800–1893
Priestley, Joseph, 1733–1804
Pringle, James Hogarth, 1863–1941
Pulteney, Richard, 1730–1801
Pybus, Frederick Charles, 1883–1975
Ragg Family
Ramsay, Allan, 1686–1758
Ramsbotham, Francis Henry, 1800–1868
Ransome, Gordon Arthur
Rathbone, William, 1819–1902
Redwood, Theophilus, 1806–1892
Reid, Donald Darnley, 1914–1977
Rhodes, Cecil John, 1853–1902
Richards, Ivor Armstrong, 1893–1979
Richardson, Benjamin Ward, 1828–1896
Richardson, John, 1787–1865
Richardson, Samuel, 1689–1761
Ringer, Sydney, 1835–1910
Roberton, John, 1797–1876
Robertson, William Ford, 1867–1923
Rogers, Leonard, 1868–1962
Roget, Peter Mark, 1779–1869
Ross, Ronald, 1857–1932
Rowlandson, Thomas, 1756–1827
Rushton, Martin A., 1903–1970
Rushton, William Albert Hugh, 1901–1980
Russell, Alexander, 1715?–1768
Russell, Bertrand, 1872–1970
Russell, Edward Stuart, 1887–1954
Russell, Patrick, 1727–1805
Russell, William, 1852–1940
Rutherford, Ernest, 1871–1937
Ryman, Brenda E.
Samman, Charles Thomas, 1865–1939
Savary, M., fl. 1814
Schally, Andrew V., 1926–
Scott, James, 1770–1848
Seacole, Mary, 1805–1881
Secker, Thomas, 1693–1768
Sharpe, Ella Freeman, 1875–1947
Shaw, George Bernard, 1856–1950
Sheldon, William, 1899–1977
Shelley, Mary, 1797–1851
Sherrington, Charles Scott, 1857–1952
Shields, James, 1918–1978
Short, Arthur Rendle, 1880–1952
Shrapnell, Henry Jones, 1792–1834
Shute, Percy George, 1894–1977
Sibly, Ebenezer, 1751–1799
Simpson, James Young, 1811–1870
Slater, William Kershaw, 1893–1970
Sloane, Hans, 1660–1753
Smith, Adam, 1723–1790
Smith Family
Smith, Frederick, 1857–1929
Smith, James Edward, 1759–1828
Smith, Robert Angus, 1817–1884
Smith, Sydney Alfred, 1883–1969
Smollett, Tobias George, 1721–1771
Smyth, James Carmichael, 1741–1821

Snow, John, 1813–1858
Souttar, Henry Sessions, 1875–1964
Soyer, Alexis, 1809–1858
Spedding, Carlisle, 1695–1755
Spencer, George John, 1758–1834
Spencer, Herbert, 1820–1903
Spilsbury, Bernard Henry, 1879–1947
Spinks, Alfred, 1917–1982
Spokes, Sidney, 1852–1938
Starling, Ernest Henry, 1866–1927
Stead, William Thomas, 1849–1912
Stebbing, George, 1749–1825
Stephen, Leslie, 1832–1904
Stephens, Joanna
Sterne, Laurence, 1713–1768
Stokes, William, 1804–1878
Stopes, Marie Charlotte Carmichael, 1880–1958
Stopford, John Sebastian Bach, 1888–1961
Strachey, James, 1887–1967
Sutton, Samuel, fl. 1743
Swift, Jonathan, 1667–1745
Sykes, William Stanley, 1894–1961
Tait, Robert Lawson, 1845–1899
Taylor, Alfred Swaine, 1806–1880
Taylor, Harry Pearson, 1862–1945
Thompson, Silvanus Phillips, 1851–1916
Thomson, William (Lord Kelvin), 1824–1907
Tilt, Archibald Preston, 1854?–1890
Tilt, Edward John, 1815–1893
Tomes, John, 1815–1895
Towne, Joseph, 1806–1879
Toynbee, Arnold Joseph, 1899–1975
Treves, Frederick, 1853–1923
Trotter, Wilfred Batten Lewis, 1872–1935
Troup, James Macdonald, 1867–1964
Tuckwell, Gertrude, fl. 1890–1920
Tulloch, William John, 1887–1966
Turner, George Grey, 1877–1951
Turner, Joseph Mallord William, 1775–1851
Tytler, James, 1747?–1804?
Underwood, Edgar Ashworth, 1899–1980
Varrier-Jones, Pendrill Charles, 1883–1941
Verney, Ernest Basil, 1894–1967
Victoria, Queen of Great Britain, 1819–1901
Waldie, David, 1813–1889
Wallace, Alfred Russel, 1823–1913
Wallich, George Charles, 1815–1899
Wallis, Charles Edward, 1869–1927
Walpole, Horace, 1717–1797
Walpole, Robert, 1676–1745
Walsh, David, 1852?–1943
Warren, Marjory Winsome, 1897–1960
Waterton, Charles, 1782–1865
Watson, James D., 1928–
Waugh, Evelyn, 1903–1966
Wedgwood, Josiah, 1730–1795
Weiner, Joseph Sidney, 1915–1982
Wellcome, Henry Solomon, 1853–1936
Wells, Calvin, 1908–1978
Wells, Herbert George, 1866–1946
Wells, Thomas Spencer, 1818–1897
Wells, William Charles, 1757–1817
Wesley, John, 1703–1791
West, Charles, 1816–1898
Whetnall, Edith Aileen Mandl
Whewell, William, 1794–1866
White, Gilbert, 1720–1793
Wilberforce, Samuel, 1805–1873
Wilkie, James Sterling, 1906–1982
Wilks, Samuel, 1824–1911
Willan Family
Willan, Robert, 1757–1812
Williams, Cicely Delphine, 1893–
Williams, David I.
Williams, John Calthrop, 1801–1856
Williams, John, 1840–1926
Williams, Richard Tecwyn, 1909–1979
Williams, Thomas, 1818–1865
Williamson, George, 1819–1865
Wilson, Charles, 1804–1884
Wilson, Clifford, 1906–
Wilson, William James Erasmus, 1809–1884
Winnicott, Donald Woods, 1896–1971
Withering, William, 1741–1799
Wittgenstein, Ludwig, 1889–1951
Woodger, Joseph Henry, 1894–1981
Woods, Donald Devereux, 1912–1964
Woolf, Virginia (Stephen), 1882–1941
Wordsworth, Dorothy, 1771–1855
Wormall, Arthur, 1900–1964
Wright, Almroth Edward, 1861–1947
Wright, Christopher A., 1928–1983
Wright, Helena, 1887–1981
Wright, Norman Charles, 1900–1970
Yonge, James, 1647–1721
Young, Thomas, 1773–1829

### Greece

Basiädes, Erokles
Cohen, Abraham, of Zante, 1678–1722
Saraphides, Hector, 1872–1950
Stephanopoulos-Vrettos, Basileios, 1908–1980
Toole, Harry I., ca. 1899–

### Haiti

Lopez de Paz, Michel, 1680–1746?

### Hungary

Abonyi, Joźsef
Abrahám, Ambrus, 1893–
Ady, Endre, 1877–1919
Arany, János, 1817–1882
Arkövy, József, 1851–1922
Babits, Mihály, 1883–1941
Bacsó, Bálint, 1789–1855
Baintner, Ferenc, 1805–1883
Balassa, János, 1814–1868
Balogh, Kálmán, 1853–1888
Bartók, Béla, 1881–1945
Berzsenyi, Daniel, 1776–1836
Bókay, János, 1858–1937
Brenner, József, 1887–1919
Bugát, Pál, 1793–1865
Csáth, Géza, 1887–1919
Csokonai, Vitéz Mihály, 1773–1805
Csorba, József
Csörsz, Károly, 1892–1935
Diósszilágyi, Samuel, 1882–
Donáth, Gyula
Dudits, Andor, 1866–1944
Eckstein, Ferenc, 1769–1833
Elischer, Gyula, 1846–1909
Entz, Béla, 1877–1959
Faber, Tamás, fl. 1710–1719
Fábián, Daniel
Farkas, Géza, 1872–1934
Ferenczi, Sándor, 1873–1933
Fodor, József, 1843–1901
Földi, János, 1755–1801
Fuszek, Rudolf, 1882–1941
Gálfalvi Domby, Sámuel, 1729–1807
Gárdi, Jenö, 1886–1944
Gelley, Rafael Mihállyal, fl. 1788
Genersich, Antal, 1842–1918
Gorka, Sánder, 1878–1944
Gulácsy, Lajos Kálmán, 1882–1932
Haberle, Károly, 1764–1832
Halász, Géza, 1816–1888
Hamburger, Jenö, 1883–1936
Hann, Fanny, fl. 1918
Hári, Pál, 1869–1933
Hatvani, István, 1718–1786
Hermann, Imre, 1889–
Herzog, Ferenc, 1879–1952
Hevesy, George von, 1885–1966
Högyes, Endre, 1847–1906
Hollós, István, 1872–1957
Hugonnai, Vilma, 1847–1922
Huray, István, 1827–1911
Hüttl, Tivadar, 1884–
Imre, József, 1884–1945
Issekutz, Hugo, 1855–1915
Jáki, Gyula, 1898–1958
Jancsó, Miklós Sr., 1868–1930
Jendrassik, Ernö, 1858–1921
Jósa, András, 1834–1918
József, Attila, 1905–1937
Juhász, Gyula, 1883–1937
Kabay, János, 1896–1936
Kanitz, Felix Philipp, 1829–1904
Kaposi, Moriz, 1837–1902
Kazinczy, Ferenc, 1759–1831
Kepes Gyula, 1847–
Kölcsey, Ferenc, 1790–1838
Koncz, Joszef, fl. 1789
Korányi, Frigyes, 1828–1913
Kovács, Ferenc, 1890–1974
Lengyel, Dániel, 1815–1884
Lichtenthal, Peter, 1780–1853

Luzsénszky, Alfonz
Manninger, Vilmos, 1876-
Markusovszky, Lajos, 1815-1893
Mátyus, István, 1725-1802
Medgyessy, Ferenc, 1881-
Meduna, Ladislas Joseph, 1896-
Menner, Adolf, 1824-1901
Mészáros, Kálmán
Mór, Jókai, fl. 1890
Móra, Ferenc, 1879-1934
Németh, László, 1901-
Nendtvich, Károly Miksa, 1811-1892
Nyulas, Ferenc, 1758-1808
Orovecz, Bela, 1909-1967
Orzovenszky, Károly
Osvát, Kálmán, 1880-1953
Pertik, Ottó, 1852-1913
Péterfi, Tibor, 1883-1953
Rácz, Sámuel, 1744-1817
Reimann, Johann Adam, 1690-1770
Richter, Hugo, 1887-1945
Rigler, Gustav, 1868-1930
Rózsay, József, 1815-1885
Rozsnyay, Mátyás, 1833-1895
Rupp, N. János, 1808-1881
Rusznyák, István, 1889-1977 or 8
Schächter, Miksa, 1859-1917
Schaffer, Károly, 1864-1939
Schmidt, Béla, 1881-1943
Schnirch, Emil, 1822-1884
Schwartzer, Otto, 1853-1913
Segner, Johann Andreas von, 1704-1777
Selig, Arpád, 1880-1929
Semmelweis, Ignác Fülöp, 1818-1865
Simon, Bela, 1892-1965
Szechenyi, István, 1791-1860
Székely, August von, 1864-1927
Szentágothai, János, 1912-
Szily, Adolf, 1848-1920
Szily, Aurel von, 1880-1945
Tauffer, Vilmos, 1851-1934
Teleki, Joseph, 1738-1796
Toldy (Schedel), Ferenc, 1805-1875
Tomcsik, József, 1898-1964
Tóth, Nep. János, 1833-1865
Trocsányi, Imre, 1851-1888
Wallaszkay, János, 1709-1767
Wehle, Ferdinand Alois, 1820-1860
Went, István, 1899-1963
Weszprémi, István, 1723-1799

**Iceland**

Ketilsson, Magnús, 1732-1803

**India**

Aziz al-Din
Bhatia, Sohan Lal, 1891-1981
Chopra, Ram Nath, 1882-
Fezl-e-Ali-Shifa-ee Khan
Gandhi, Mohandas Karamchand, 1869-1948
Ghalib, 1796?-1869
Gopalacharyulu, Pandit Divi, 1872-1920
Hidaetullah, Hakeem, fl. 1731
Kabiruddin, Hakim, 1894-1976
Lakshmipathi, Bhishagratna Achanta, 1880-1964
Lyngdoh, Homiwell, 1877-1958
Muhammad Akbar Arzani Shah
Narasaraju Urs, fl. 1883
Narayan, Jayaprakash, 1901?-
Ray, Kaviraj Gangadhar

**Ireland**

Aikenhead, Mary, 1787-1858
Beckett, Samuel, 1906-
Carnwath, Thomas, 1878-
Colles, Abraham, 1773-1843
Corrigan, Dominic John, 1802-1880
Crawford, Thomas, 1824-1895
Doolin, William, 1887-1962
Ferguson, John Creery, 1802-1865
Joyce, James, 1882-1941
Kennedy, Evory, 1807?-1886
Kernohan, James Watson, 1896-1981
Maunsell, Henry, 1806-1879
Moloney, Michael, d. c. 1935
Moore, John William, 1845-1937
O'Halloran, Sylvester, 1728-1807
O'Scanlan, Timoteo, 1726-1800
Patrick, Mother, 1863-1900
Stock, Charles, 1790-
Threlkeld, Caleb, 1676-1728
Todd, Robert Bentley, 1809-1860
Wallace, William, 1791-1837
Wightman, Henderson, 1791-1823
Wilde, Oscar, 1854-1900
Wilde, William Robert Wills, 1815-1876
Yeats, William Butler, 1865-1939

**Israel**

Ben-Gurion, David, 1886-1973
Buber, Martin, 1878-1965
Dayan, Moshe, 1915-
Gruenfelder, Benno, 1883-1955
Kagan, Helena, 1889-1978
Leibowitz, Joshua O., 1895-

**Italy**

Annaratone, Carlo
Bairati, Angelo, 1901 or 11-
Bassini, Edoardo, 1844-1924
Beccaria, Giovanni Battista, 1715-1781
Bellini, Vincenzo, 1801-1835
Berruti, Giuseppe, 19th cent.
Bizzozero, Giulio Cesare, 1846-1901
Bodio, Luigi, 1840-1920
Bodoni, Giovanni Battista, 1740-1813
Brambilla, Giovanni Alessandro, 1728-1800
Breda, Achille, 1850-1934
Buzzi, Francesco, 1751-1805
Casanova, Giacomo Girolamo, 1725-1798
Casotti, Luigi, 1891-1959
Catalani, Vincenzo, 1769-1843
Cattaneo, Carlo, 1801-1869
Cavina, Cesare, 1888-1935
Cirillo, Domenico, 1739-1799
Cornelio, Vittorio, b. ca. 1760
Cotugno, Domenico, 1736-1822
Devoto, Luigi, 1864-1936
Durante, Francesco, 1844-1934
Erspamer, Vittorio, 1909-
Fabi, Mauritius, 1738-1801
Fermi, Enrico, 1901-1954
Ferrata, Adolfo, 1880-1946
Fontana, Felice, 1730-1805
Fonzi, Giuseppangelo Lucinto, 1768-1840
Forlanini, Carlo, 1847-1918
Frugoni, Carlo Innocenzo, 1692-1768
Ghirotti, Gigi, 1920-1973
Golgi, Camillo, 1844-1926
Greppi, Enrico, 1896-
La Torre, Felice, 1846-1923
Lancisi, Giovanni Maria, 1654-1720
Lattes, Leone, 1887-
Lelli, Ercole, 1702-1766
Leopardi, Giacomo, 1798-1837
Lombroso, Cesare, 1835-1909
Lomonaco, Tomaso, 1901-
Longhi, Pietro, 1702-1785
Lorenzini, Carlo, 1826-1890
Lusardi, Christophe Mathieu, 1778-1853
Manzolini, Anna Morandi, 1716-1774
Manzolini, Giovanni, 1700-1755
Mascagni, Paolo, 1755-1815
Messini, Mariano, 1901-
Mieli, Aldo, 1879-1950
Morelli, Giovanni, 1816-1891
Morgagni, Giovanni Battista, 1682-1771
Morpurgo, Samson, 1681-1740
Moscati, Giuseppe, 1880-1927
Pacini, Filippo, 1812-1883
Paganini, Niccolo, 1782?-1840
Pascoli, Giovanni, 1855-1912
Pavese, Cesare, 1908-1950
Peano, Giuseppe, 1858-1932
Pende, Nicola, 1880-
Perroncito, Edoardo, 1847-1936
Pirandello, Luigi, 1867-1936
Pitré, Giuseppe, 1841-1916
Porta, Luigi, 1800-1875
Pupilli, Giulio Cesare, 1893-1973
Putti, Vittorio, 1880-1940
Racchetti, Vincenzo, 1777-1819
Rasori, Giovanni, 1766-1837
Ravizza, Carlo, 1811-
Righi, Augusto, 1850-1920
Rignano, Eugenio, 1870-1930
Rivolta, Sebastiano, 1832-1893

Rizzoli, Francesco, 1809–1880
Roncati, Francesco, 1834–1906
Rosa, Daniele, 1857–1944
Ruffini, Angelo, 1864–1929
Salieri, Antonio, 1750–1825
Sanctis, Sante de, 1862–1935
Santorini, Giovanni Domenico, 1681–1737
Sertoli, Enrico, 1842–1910
Spallanzani, Lazzaro, 1729–1799
Stella, Giulio, 1899–1978
Susini, Clemente, 1754–1814
Svevo, Italo, 1861–1928
Tadini, fl. 1758–1789
Tansini, Iginio, 1855–1943
Tiberio, Vincenzo, 1869–1915
Torrigiani da Corniglio, Flaminio Domenico, 1729–1792
Tozzetti, Giovanni Targioni, 1712–1783
Trabucchi, Emilio
Vallisneri, Antonio, 1661–1730
Valtolini, Giovambattista, fl. 1790
Vella, Luigi, 1822–1886
Verri, Pietro, 1728–1797
Verson, Franz Xaver, 1805–1849
Vicentini, Giuseppe, 1860–
Ysabeau, A.

**Japan**

Hanaoka, Seishu, 1760–1835
Hora, Seki, d. 1980?
Inagaki, Satorū
Ishibashi, Haya
Kagawa, Genetsu, 1700–1777
Katayama, Kunika, 1855–1931
Kitagawa, Otojiro, fl. 1901
Kobavashi, Osamu
Kubokawa, Chukichi
Miyahara, Tatsutaro, 1878–1926
Mori, Ogai, 1862–1922?
Morii, Josen, 1797–1851
Nakamura, Heizo, 1896–
Nishina, Yoshio, 1890–1951
Noguchi, Hideyo, 1876–1928
Okubo, Tekisai
Oshima, Shiro, 1934–1981
Ozeki, Chikako
Ryosen, Tezuka, d. 1877
Sawada, Miki
Suzuki, Masa
Takagi, Kenji, 1888–1963
Takano, Kyo
Tanaka, Shin, 1920–
Taniguchi, Joshiaki
Tawara, Sunao
Udagawa, Yôan, 1798–1846

**Lebanon**

Haddad, Sami I., 1890–1957

**Liberia**

McGill, Samuel Ford

**Liechtenstein**

Schaedler, Gebhard, 1776–1842

**Martinique**

Fanon, Frantz, 1925–1961

**Mexico**

Aragon, Enrique O., 1880–1942
Barreda, Gabino, 1818–1881
Carmona y Valle, Manuel, 1827–1902
Cendala y Gómez, Isabel, fl. 1805
Chávez, Ignacio, 1897–1979
Del Pozo, Efrén C., 1907–1979
Espinosa de los Reyes, Isidro, 1887–1951
Esteyneffer, Juan de, 1664–1716
Fastlicht, Samuel, 1902–1983
Flores y Troncoso, Francisco de Asis, 1855–1931
Gómez Farías, Valentin, 1781–1858
González Flores, Jesús Mariá, 1857–1947
Jiménez, Miguel Francisco, 1813–1876
Ramírez de Arellano, Nicolás
Reko, Victor Aloisius, 1880–
Riviera, Diego, 1886–1957
Sabina, Maria, 1894–
Torres Estrada, Antonio
Vertiz, Ricardo, fl. 1898
Zubirán, Salvador, 1898–

**Netherlands**

Aletrino, Arnold, 1858–1916
Auzoux, Louis Thomas Jérome, 1797–1880
Barchusen, Johann Conrad, 1666–1723
Barneveld, Willem van, 1747–1826
Benavente, Samuel de Lion, 1643–1723
Bicker, Lambertus, 1732–1801
Boerhaave, Herman, 1668–1738
Brongersma, H. R., 1869–1944
Brugmans, Sebald Instinus, 1763–1819
Burggraaf jr., Johannes Philips, 1700–1775
Camper, Petrus, 1722–1789
Conscience, Hendrik, 1812–1883
Dentz, S. N., Jr., 1817–1872
Deventer, Hendrik van, 1651–1724
Eeden, Frederik van, 1860–1932
Einthoven, Willem, 1860–1927
Fokker, Abraham Peter, 1840–1906
Frank, Anne, 1929–1945
Gorter, Johannes de, 1689–1762
Ingenhousz, Jan, 1730–1799
Israels, Abraham Hartog, 1822–1883
Limborgh, Jan van, 1900–1884
Lindeboom, Gerrit Arie, 1905–
Loghem, Johannes Jacobus von, 1878–
Loos, Willem de, 1736–1771
Maty, Matthieu, 1718–1776
Mepsche, Rudolf de
Mulder, Gerardus Johannes, 1802–1880
Oever, Jan van den, d. 1728
Ramaer, Johannes Nicolaas, 1817–1887
Ranouw, Willem van, 1673–1724
Renterghem, Albert Willem van, 1846–1939
Roener, L. S. von
Roepke, W. J., 1917–
Rouppe, Hendrik Willem, 1765–1816
Rymsdyk, Jan van, fl. 1750–1788
Sandifort, Eduard, 1742–1814
Siemens, Hermann Werner, 1891–1969
Snellen, Herman, 1834–1908
Son, Joseph Mozes, 1818–1884
Swammerdam, Jan, 1637–1680
Swieten, Gerard van, 1700–1772
Van der Looy, Cornelis Hendrik, 1813–1895
Van Eeden, Frederik, 1860–1932
Van Gogh, Vincent, 1853–1890
Van Renterghem, Albert Willem, 1845–1939
Vink, Peter, 1713–1773
Voegen van Engelen, Jacobus
Vries, Hugo de, 1848–1935
Vrolik, Willem, 1801–1863
Waardenburg, Petrus Johannes, 1886–1979
William I, King of Netherlands, 1772–1843
Wittop Koning, Dirk Arnold, 1911–

**New Zealand**

Bakewell, Robert Hall, 1831–1908
Bell, Gordon, 1863–1923
Bennett, Francis Oswald, 1898–1976
Campbell, John Logan, 1817–1912
Esdaile, James, 1808–1859
Fischer, Carl, d. 1893
Gillies, Harold Delf, 1882–1960
King, Frederic Truby, 1858–1938
Lambie, Mary, 1889–1971
Murray, James Patrick, 1839–
Neill, Grace, fl. 1899–1906
Sharland, James Craig, fl. 1870
Wilson, Peter, 1791–1863

**Norway**

Boeck, Caesar, 1845–1917
Dahl, Haldoe Christian, fl. 1800
Eng, Helga Kristine, 1875–
Falkberget, Johan Petter, 1879–1967
Hansen, Gerhard Henrik Armauer, 1841–1912
Holst, Frederik, 1791–1871
Laestadius, Lars Levi, 1780–1861
Langfeldt, Gabriel, 1895–
Larsson, Bergljot, 1883–
Løvset, Jørgen, 1896–1981
Madsen, Thorvald Johannes Marius, 1870–1957
Munch, Edvard, 1863–1944

### Pacific Islands

Hoodless, David Winn

### Peru

Delgado, Honorio
Mariátegui, José Carlos, 1894–1930
Moreno y Maïz, Thomas, fl. 1868
Valdizán, Hermilio, 1885–1929

### Philippines

Garciá, Eusebio S.
Guinto, Ricardo S., 1907–1983
Mozo, Antonio, 1720–1794
Rizal, José Protacio, 1861–1896
Sison, Honoria Acosta, 1888–1970

### Poland

Adamkiewicz, Albert Wojciech, 1850–1921
Andrzejewski, Antoni, 1807–1883
Asratian, Ezras Asratovich, 1903–
Augustus III, King of Poland, 1696–1763
Bandurska, Halina
Bardadin, Tadeusz
Batawia, Stanisław
Beck, Henryk, 1896–1946
Bednarz, Jósef
Biegański, Władysław, 1857–1917
Bierkowski, Ludwig Jożef, 1801–1860
Bilikiewicz, Tadeusz, 1901–1980
Boczoń, Tadeusz
Brodniewicz, Anita Zofia
Browicz, Tadeusz, 1847–1928
Bujwid, Odon, 1857–1942
Bukowiecki, Henryk, 1903–
Bularski, Jan
Chałubiński, Tytus, 1820–1889
Chodźko, Witold, 1875–1954
Cholewa, Leon
Dega, Wiktor, 1897?–
Dietl, Josef, 1804–1878
Długosz, Jan
Dolliner, Jan, 1808–
Dominik, Małgorzata, 1941–1979
Fleck, Ludwik, 1896–1961
Furmaga, Stefan, 1924–1983
Fusek Family
Galka, Jozef
Goebel, Karol, 1845–1891
Goeppert, Heinrich Robert, 1800–1884
Goldszmit, Henry K., 1878–1942
Grot-Rowecki, Stefan, 1895–1944
Gustek, Marian
Heller, Józef, 1896–1982
Herman, Eufemiusz, 1892–
Hirszfeld, Ludwig, 1884–1954
Hoyer, Henryk Fryderyk, 1834–1907
Jakóbkiewicz, Józef
Janicki, Konstanty S., 1876–1932
Janiszewski, Stanisław
Janiszewski, Tomasz, 1867–1939
Jurasz, Antoni, 1847–1923
Kadyi, Henryk, 1851–1912
Karwowski, Rowan
Kasznicki, Jerzy, 1934–1979
Kepinski, Antoni
Klecki, Karol, 1866–1931
Konopka, Stanisław, 1896–1982
Korczynski, Edward, 1844–1905
Kornalewski, Joachim, 1850–
Kostanecki, Kazimierz, 1863–
Kowalczykowa, Janina, 1907–1970
Krupinski, Andrzej, 1744–1783
Krwawicz, Tadensz, 1910–
Kulczyńska, Teresa
Lafontaine, Franz Leopold de, 1756–1812
Lawkowicz, Włodzimierz, 1908–1979
Leśniewska, Antonina, 1866–1937
Lewicki, Józef, 1882–1942
Lewkowicz, Ksawery, 1869–1958
Lilpop, Wacław, 1884–1949
Machalski, Jacek, 1926–1979
Marcinkowski, Karol, 1800–1846
Markiewicz, Stanisław, 1839–1911
Mayer, Karol, 1882–1946
Mickiewicz, Adam, 1798–1855
Mierzecki, Henryk, 1891–1977
Mikulicz von Radecki, Johann, 1850–1905
Minkowska, Franciszka, 1882–1950
Neifeld, Ernst Jeremias, 1721–1773
Nencki, Marceli, 1847–1901
Obaliński, Alfred, 1843–1898
Olszak, Wacław, 1902–
Orlowski, Witold Eugenjusz, 1874–1966
Palicki, Bogusław, 1813–1868
Parczewski, Eugeniusz
Paszkiewicz, Ludwik, 1878–1967
Perzanowska, Stefania
Petrycy, Sebastian, 1554–1626
Popielski, Boleslaw
Przyborowski, Karol Sulima, 1824–1879
Rogalski, Tadeusz, 1881–
Rolle, Jozef Apolinary, 1829–1894
Rowiński, Ksawery, 1904–1983
Rzasnicki, Adolf, 1884–1953
Schuch, Ignacy, 1772–1864
Siedlecki, Michał,1873–1940
Skarżyński, Bolesław, 1901–1963
Sleszkowski, Sebastian, 1569–1648
Sniadecki, Jedrzej, 1768–1838
Sobieszczański, Zbigniew
Sokol, Stanisław, 1911–1968
Stanisław I, Leszczński, King of Poland, 1677–1766
Staszic, Stanisław, 1755–1826
Stocki, Edward, 1909–1978
Szuman, Leon Stanisław, 1852–1920
Szumowski, Władisław, 1875–1954
Szwejcerowa-Gruszczyńska, Aniela, 1905–1981
Teichmann, Ludwik Karol, 1823–1895
Venulet, Franciszek, 1878–1967
Weichardt, Teodor Tomasz, fl. 1783
Werner, Artur Karol
Wicherkiewicz, Bolesław, 1847–1915
Wierzejewski, Ireneusz, 1881–1930
Wolff, August Ferdynand, 1768–1846
Wrzosek, Adam, 1875–1965
Zahorski, Karol, 1879–1970
Zielina, Jan
Ziembicki, Witold, 1874–1949

### Portugal

Andrade, Corino
Cambournac, Francisco, 1903–
Castelo Branco, Camilo, 1825–1890
Danta, Júlio, 1876–1962
De Gama Pinto, M. R., 1853–1945
Herculano, Alexandre, 1810–1877
Loff, Romão
Magalhaes, Francisco Bento
Moniz, Egas, 1874–1955
Silva, Pedro José da, 1834–1878

### Puerto Rico

Betances, Ramón Emeterio, 1830–1898
Oller, Francisco, 1785–1831
Suárez, Ramón M., 1895–1981

### Romania

Aburel, Eugen Bogdan, 1899–1975
Babes, Victor, 1854–1926
Bagdasar, Dimitrie, 1893–1946
Brancusi, Constantin, 1876–1957
Brandt, Josef, 1838–1912
Brascu, Stefan S., 1895–1965
Bruteanu, Mircea, 1882–1957
Cantémir, Demetris, 1673–1723
Ciucă, Mihai, 1883–1969
Combiescu, Dumitru, 1887–1961
Conta, Vasile, 1845–1882
Davila, Carol, 1828–1884
Dosios, Anastase Andrei Periclis, 1900–1974
Felix, Iacob, 1832–
Gându, Teodora, 1917–
Ionescu-Mihăesti, C., 1883–1971
Ionescu-Siseşti, Nicolae, 1888–1954
Lupu, Nicolae Gheorghe, 1884–1966
Marinescu, Gheorghe, 1863–1938
Minovici Family
Mironescu, Eugene I., 1883–1939
Moldovan, Iuliu, 1882–
Niculescu, Ion T., 1895–1957
Obregia, Alexandrŭ, 1860–1937
Pastia, Constantin C., 1883–1926
Paulescu, Nicolas Constantin, 1869–1931
Popa, Grigore T., 1859–1930
Popescu-Sibiu, Ioan I., 1901–1974

Rola, Evstatie, 1766–1831
Stonescu, Nicolae
Vasiliu, N.
Voiculescu, Vasile, 1884–1963
Zubku-Kodrianu, N. P., 1850–

**Scandinavia**

Perman, Emil, 1856–1937
Rovsing, Nils Thorkild, 1862–1927

**South Africa**

Adler, Cyril, 1903–
Brand, Johannes Henricus, 1823–1888
Burgers, Thomas François, 1834?–1881
Crichton, Eric Cuthbert, 1888–1962
Franz Family
Hayward, Wally, 1908?–
Heyer, A. E.
Hughes, Matthew Louis, 1867–1899
Leipoldt, Christian Frederik Louis, 1880–1947
Loewenthal, Leonard Joseph Alphonse, 1903–1983
Louw, Jan Hendrik, 1915–
Lycett, James, 1811–1883
Mehliss, John Max, 1868–1927
Pimstone, Bernard Laurence, d. 1979
Theiler, Arnold, 1867–1936
Van Rippen, Bene, 1882–
Wells, Lawrence Herbert, 1908–1980
White, John, 1757 or 8–1832

**Spain**

Achúcarro, Nicolás, 1880–1918
Alberca Lorente, Roman, 1903–1967
Alcón, Andrés, 1782–1850
Alfonso XII, King of Spain, 1857–1885
Aranguren, Manuel Bernardino de, 1743–1794
Areilza, Enrique de, 1860–1926
Arejula, Juan Manuel de, 1755–1830
Arenal, Concepción, 1820–1893
Baltar Domínguez, Ramón, 1902–1981
Barraquer Roviralta, Lluis, 1855–1928
Batllés y Torres de Amat, Mariano, 1798–1865
Blasco, Manuel, 1899–
Borja de Guzman, Pedro, 1908–
Botey, Ricardo, 1855–1927
Call i Morros, Josep
Calvo Asensio, Pedro, 1821–1863
Carbonell y Bravo, Francisco, 1768–1837
Carlos III, King of Spain, 1716–1788
Carracido, José Rodríguez, 1856–1928
Casal, Gaspar, 1680–1759
Casona, Alejandro, 1903–1965
Castro, Rosalía de, 1837–1885
Cibat, Antonio, 1770–1812
Codorníu y Ferreras, Manuel
Comenge y Ferrer, Luis, 1854–1916
Corachán, Juan Bautista, 1661–1741
Creus y Manso, Juan, 1828–1897
De la Quadra Family
Delgado y Amestoy, Claudio, 1843–1916
Del Río-Hortega, Pío, 1882–1945
Ferran y Clua, Jaime, 1852–1929
Franco, Francisco, 1892–1975
Freixas i Freixas, Joan, 1860–1933
Gay Prieto, José, 1905–1979
Gil, Francisco, fl. 1784
Gómez-Caamaño, José Luis, 1909–1984
Gómez Durán, Manuel, d. 1984
Gomez Ortega, D. Casimiro, fl. 1788
González, Pedro María, fl. 1789–1805
González Velasco, Pedro, 1815–1875?
Goya y Lucientes, Francisco José, 1746–1828
Guerrero Fernández, J.
Hernández de Gregorio, Manuel, 1771–1833
Hernández, Francisco, fl. 1734–1786
Hernández Morejón, Antonio, 1773–1836
Iparraguirre, Francisco Fernández, fl. 1883
Isamat Vila, Jesús, 1895–
Jimenez Murillo, Manuel, 1784–1859
Laín Entralgo, Pedro, 1908–
Lardizábal, Vicente de, ca. 1746–1814
Lentini Diaz, José
López Albo, 1889–1944
Loscos Bernal, Francisco, 1823–1886
Marãnon, Gregorio, 1887–1960
Marti, Manuel, 1663–1737
Martí y Juliá, Domènec, 1861–1917
Masdevall, José, d. 1801
Mata, Justo Martinez
Mata y Fontanet, Pedro, 1811–1877
Mendez Alvaro, Francisco, 1803–1883
Mira y López, Emilio, 1896–
Mollar, José Ignacio, fl. 1788
Montells y Nadall, Francisco de Paula, 1813–1893
Muñoz, Fernando Oliva, 1825–1876
Nieto y Serrano, Matías, 1813–1902
Olives, Mariano, fl. 1825–1840
Olóriz y Aguilera, Federico, 1855–1912
Oxea, Fernando, fl. 1771
Pardo Sastrón, José, 1822–1909
Perdomo Bethencourt Cortés, Juan Antonio, 1737–1800
Pérez Galdós, Benito, 1843–1920
Pérez Mínguez, Mariano, 1809–1887
Peset Llorca, Vicente, 1914–1981
Pi i Molist, Emilio, 1824–1892
Pi Suñer, Augusto, 1879–1955
Pons i Freixa, Francisco de Asís, 1863–1938
Prados y Such, Miguel, d. 1969
Ramón y Cajal, Santiago, 1852–1934
Rio, Andrés del, fl. 1794
Rodriguez Lafora, Gonzalo, 1887–
Royo, Domingo, fl. 1715–1734
Ruano, Francisco
Ruiz de Luzuriaga, Ignacio Maria, 1763–1822
Ruiz, Hipólito, 1754–1815
Ruiz, José Martinez, 1874–1967
Sacristán, José Miguel, 1887–1956
Sala, Antonio, fl. 1788
Salvany Lleopart, José
Sanchís Banús, José, 1893–1932
Santero y Moreno, Tomas, 1817–1888
Selvaresa, Josef, d. 1805
Solano, Francisco Antonio, d. 1771
Suárez Rodriguez, Antonio, 1807–1907
Tello y Muñoz, Jorge Francisco, 1880–
Trigueros, Cándido Maria, fl. 1781
Trueta Raspall, José, 1897–1977
Velasco, Pedro Gonzalez de, 1815–1882
Villalba, Joaquín de, 1750–1807
Yáñez, Agustín, fl. 1831

**Sri Lanka**

Wijerama, Edmund Medonza, 1896–1980

**Sweden**

Acrel, Olof af, 1717–1806
Arrhenius, Svante, 1859–1927
Bergman, Hjalmar Frederik Elgerus, 1883–1931
Bergman, Per, 1874–
Berzelius, Jöns Jacob, 1779–1848
Caspersson, Torbjörn Oskar, 1910–
Dubb, Per, 1750–1834
Ekman, Olof Jacob, 1764–1839
Enghoff, Henrik, 1894–
Erichsen, Johann Gottfried, 1712–1768
Euler, Ulf Svante von, 1905–1983
Forssell, Gösta, 1876–1950
Fredrik I, King of Sweden, 1676–1751
Gedner, Christopher Eliasson, 1730–1773
Hagström, Anders Johan, 1753–1830
Hedin, Sven Gustaf, 1859–1933
Hedin, Sven, 1865–1952
Hellström, Johan, 1859–1941
Hirschfeld, J.
Holmer, Carl Magnus, 1782–1848
Hummel, David, 1893–
Hwasser, Israel, 1790–1860
Johansson, Sven, 1880–
Lehmann, Jörgen
Lennander, Karl Gustaf, 1857–1908
Ling, Per Henrik, 1776–1839
Linné, Carl von, 1707–1778
Ljungdahl, Malte, 1882–1957
Löfberg, Otto, 1881–1954
Munthe, Axel Martin Fredrik, 1857–1949
Nobel, Alfred Bernhard, 1833–1896
Norin, Anna, 1774–
Norlén, Ivar, 1910–
Olivercrona, Herbert, 1891–1980
Palm, Kerstin, 1946–
Palmer, Ivar, 1897–
Rappe, Emmy Carolina, 1835–1896
Reichborn-Kjennerud, Ingjald, 1865–1949
Retzius, Anders Adolf, 1796–1860
Retzius, Anders Jahan, 1742–1821
Rosen von Rosenstein, Nils, 1706–1773
Sandström, Ivar Victor, 1852–1889

Scheele, Karl Wilhelm, 1742–1786
Schultz, Jacob, 1681–1766
Schulz, David, 1732–1823
Seldinger, Sven-Ivar, 1921–
Sjöbring, Henrik, 1879–1956
Sköldberg, Sven, 1838–1872
Swedenborg, Emanuel, 1688–1772
Sydow, Frans Edvard von, 1828–1914
Tegnér, Esaias, 1782–1846
Thunberg, Carl Peter, 1743–1828
Törne, Frans Vilhelm, 1870–1949
Uvnäs, Börge, 1913–

**Switzerland**

Aepli, Johann Melchior, 1744–1813
Appia, Louis, 1818–1898
Attenhofer, Heinrich Ludwig, 1783–1856
Bernhard, Wilhelm, 1920–1978
Bernoulli, Daniel, 1700–1782
Bircher, Willy, 1898–1970
Blaser, Robert Henry
Bleuler, Eugen, 1857–1939
Bleuler, Manfred Eugen, 1902–1983
Bloch, Bruno, 1878–1933
Bonnet, Charles, 1720–1793
Boss, Medard, 1903–
Bräker, Ulrich, 1735–1798
Brenner, Friedrich, 1809–1874
Brun, Rudolf, 1885–1969
Brunner, Alfred, 1890–1972
Brupbacher, Fritz, 1874–1945
Candolle, Alphonse de, 1806–1893
Carro, Jean de, 1770–1857
Christoffel, Hans, 1888–1959
Coindet, Jean-François, 1774–1834
De Quervain, Johann Friedrich, 1868–1940
Diller, Hans, 1905–1977
Dumont, Fritz Ludwig, 1854–1932
Dunant, Jean Henri, 1828–1910
Erisman, Friedrich Huldreich, 1842–1915
Erni, Hans, 1909–
Flournoy, Théodore, 1854–1920
Forel, Auguste Henri, 1848–1931
Fritzsche, Christian Friedrich, 1851–1938
Gasser, Conrad, 1912–1982
Giacometti, Augusto, 1877–1947
Guggenheim, Markus, 1885–1970
Guillerey, Joseph, 1871–1942?
Haller, Albrecht von, 1708–1777
Haller, Albrecht von, 1758–1823
Haller, Karl Johann von, 1749–1781
Hess, Walter Rudolph, 1881–1973
His, Wilhelm, Sr., 1831–1904
Horner, Friedrich, 1831–1886
Julliard, Gustave, 1836–1911
Jung, Carl Gustav, 1794–1864
Jung, Carl Gustav, 1875–1961
Klaesi, Jakob, 1883–
Klebs, Arnold Carl, 1870–1943
Klee, Paul, 1879–1940
Kocher, Theodor, 1841–1917
Koelbing, Huldrych M., 1923–
Krafft, Charles, 1863–1921
Lavater, Johann Caspar, 1741–1801
Le Dran, Henri François, 1685–1770
Lehmann, Fritz Erich, 1902–1970
Leuthold, Alfred, 1901–1982
Lichtenthaeler, Charles, 1915–
Looser, Emil, 1877–1936
Mayor, Frank Isaac, 1779–1855
Meyer-Ahrens, Conrad, 1813–1872
Monakow, Constantin von, 1853–1930
Muralt, Johannes von, 1645–1733
Naegeli, Otto, 1871–1938
Niederhäusern, David von, 1847–1882
Niehans, Paul, 1882–1971
Olivier, Charlotte, 1864–1945
Ott, Arnold, 1840–1910
Peschier, Jacques, 1769–1832
Pestalozzi, Johann Heinrich, 1746–1827
Piaget, Jean, 1896–1980
Picot, Constant, 1844–
Prevost, Jean Louis, 1790–1850
Reverdin, Jacques Louis, 1842–1929
Rorschach, Hermann, 1884–1922
Roux, César, 1857–1934
Scherer, Maria Theresia, 1825–
Scheuchzer, Johann Jakob, 1672–1733
Schmid-Guisan, Hans, 1881–1932
Schulthess, Wilhelm, 1855–1917
Schüppach, Michel, 1707–1781
Senn, Albert, 1869–1934
Sigerist, Henry Ernest, 1891–1957
Steger, Johann Heinrich, 1767–1842
Steger, Johann Jakob, 1798–1857
Tissot, Samuel Auguste André David, 1728–1797
Tschirch, Alexander, 1856–1939
Usteri, Paulus, 1768–1831
Vischer, Adolf Lukas Jacob, 1884–1974
Vogt, Alfred, 1879–1943
Waldmeier, Theophilus, 1831–1915
Wehrli, Gustav Adolf, 1888–1949
Wölfflin, Ernst, 1873–1959
Yersin, Alexandre, 1863–1943
Zimmermann, Johann Georg, 1728–1795

**Tunisia**

Conseil, Ernest Alfred, 1879–

**Turkey**

Adil Mustafa (Adil-Bey), 1871–1904

**United States**

Abbe, Robert, d. 1928
Abbott, Edward Gilbert, 1825–1855
Abel, John Jacob, 1857–1938
Abrams, Albert, 1863–1924
Adams Family
Adams, Scott, 1909–1982
Addams, Jane, 1860–1935
Adler, Kurt A., 1905–
Agassiz, Louis, 1807–1873
Aggrey, James E. Kadwo Kwegyir, 1875–1927
Agnew, David Hayes, 1818–1892
Albright, Fuller, 1900–1969
Alcott, Louisa May, 1832–1888
Alexander, Alexander, 1849–1928
Alexander, Eben, Jr., 1913–
Alexander, Franz Gabriel, 1981–1964
Alexander, Hattie Elizabeth, 1901–1968
Alexander, John, 1891–
Alexander, Samuel, 1888–1952
Allison, William David, 1854–1928
Allport, Floyd Henry, 1890–1978
Allport, Gordon Willard, 1897–1967
Ames, Blanche Ames, 1878–1969
Amesse Family
Andersen, Dorothy Hansine, 1901–1963
Anderson, Charles Henry
Anderson, Elda Emma, 1899–1961
Anderson, Victor Vance, 1879–1960
Anderson, William Wallace
Andrus, Edwin Cowles, 1896–
Angel, John Lawrence
Anger, Hal O., 1920–
Angle, Edward Hartley, 1855–1930
Angrist, Alfred Alvin, 1902–
Angus, Samuel, 1784–1840
Anokhin, Petr Kusmich, 1898–1974
Apgar, Virginia, 1909–1974
Appel, Kenneth Ellwaker, 1896–1979
Arnold, Harry Loren, 1912–
Arnstein, Margaret Gene, 1904–1972
Arthurs, Robert, fl. 1886
Artzybasheff, Boris, 1899–1965
Asch, Morris Joseph, 1833–1902
Ash, James Earle, 1884–1984
Atwater, Wilbur Olin, 1844–1907
Aub, Joseph Charles, 1890–
Avery, Oswald Theodore, 1877–1955
Badger, Robert, 1829–
Badger, Roderick, 1834–1890
Baer, William Stevenson, 1872–1931
Bagley, William Chandler, 1874–1946
Bailey, Harriet
Bailey, Jacob Whitman, 1811–1857
Bailey, Liberty Hyde, 1858–1954
Bailey, Percival Sylvester, 1892–
Baker, Burton Lowell, 1912–1978
Baldwin, James Mark, 1861–1934
Baldwin, William, 1779–1819
Bancroft, Jessie Hubbell, 1867–1952
Barber, Marshall Albert, 1868–1953
Barnes, Djuna, 1892–1982
Barnhill, John Finch, 1865–1943
Barnum, Sanford Christie, 1838–1885
Bartholow, Roberts, 1831–1904
Bartlett, Edwin Lewis, 1904–1968

Bartlett, Josiah, 1729–1795
Barton, Benjamin Smith, 1766–1815
Barton, Clarissa Harlowe, 1821–1912
Barton, Edward Hall, d. 1857?
Barton, William Paul Crillon, 1786–1856
Bartram, John, 1699–1777
Baruch, Simon, 1840–1921
Bass, Charles Cassedy, 1875–1975
Bass, Mary Elizabeth, 1876–1956
Bates, Katharine Lee, 1859–1929
Bateson, Gregory, 1904–
Baxley, H. Willis
Bayne-Jones, Stanhope, 1888–1970
Bean, William Bennett, 1909–
Beanes, William, 1749–1828?
Beard, George Miller, 1839–1883
Beaumont, William, 1785–1853
Beck, Theodric Romeyn, 1791–1855
Beecher, Catharine Esther, 1800–1878
Beers, Clifford Whittingham, 1876–1943
Beilhardt, Jacob, 1846–1908
Bell, Alexander Graham, 1847–1922
Bennet, Jesse, 1769–1842
Bennett, George Eli, 1885–
Bennett, Jesse, 1769–1842
Bensley, Robert Russell, 1867–1956
Bentley, Arthur Fisher, 1870–1957
Bentley, Charles Edwin, 1859–1929
Bentley, Edwin, 1824–1917
Benton, Arthur Lester, 1909–
Berg, Albert Ashton, 1872–
Bergh, Henry, 1811–1888
Bergmann, Max, 1886–1944
Berman, Mones, 1920–1982
Bernfeld, Siegfried, 1892–1953
Bernhisel, John Milton, 1799–1881
Berryhill, Walter Reece, 1900–1979
Bevan, Arthur Dean, 1861–1943
Bickerdyke, Mary Ann Ball, 1817–1901
Bigelow Family
Bigelow, Jacob, 1786–1879
Biggs, Hermann Michael, 1859–1923
Billings, John Shaw, 1838–1913
Bissell, Emily Perkins, 1861–1948
Black, Greene Vardiman, 1836–1915
Black, John Janvier, 1837–1909
Blackburn, Luke Pryor, 1816–1887
Blacklock, Donald Breadalbane, 1879–
Blackwell, Elizabeth, 1821–1910
Blackwell Family, 19th cent.
Blackwood, Thomas
Bláhnik Family
Blake, John Ballard, 1922–
Blalock, Alfred, 1899–1964
Blanchfield, Florence Aby, 1882–1971
Bland, Theodorick, 1777–1846
Blaszkowski, Thomas
Bleyer, Adrian, 1879–1965?
Blos, Peter, 1904–
Blunt, Katharine, 1876–1954
Boardman, Mabel Thorp, 1860–1946
Bobbs, John Stough, 1809–1870
Bodley, Rachel Littler, 1831–1888
Boisen, Anton Theophilus, 1876–1965
Bond, Thomas, 1712–1784
Bonwill, William G. A., 1833–1899
Boone, Levi Day, 1808–1882
Boseman, Benjamin A., Jr., 1840–1881
Bovie, William T., 1882–1958
Bowditch, Henry Pickering, 1840–1911
Bowen, John Templeton, 1857–
Bowers, Jacob, 1841–1922
Boyd, David R.
Boyden, Edward Allen, 1886–
Boylston, Zabdiel, 1680–1766
Brand, Paul Wilson, 1914–
Bratton, James Rufus, 1821–1897
Brauer, John Charles, 1905–
Breckinridge, Mary, 1881–1965
Brenner, Charles, 1913–
Bridgeman, Laura Dewey, 1829–1889
Brigham, Amariah, 1798–1849
Brinkhous, Kenneth Merle, 1909–
Brock, Frederick W.
Bromberg, Walter, 1900–
Bronner, Augusta Fox, 1881–1866
Brooks, Barney, 1884–
Brooks, William Keith, 1848–1908
Brown, Charles Brockden, 1771–1810
Brown, Charles, 1783–1879
Brown, Lucius Polk, 1867–1935
Brown, Rachel, 1898–1980
Brown, Solyman, 1790–1876
Brown, Thomas
Brown, William, 1748–1792
Browne, Charles Albert, 1870–1947
Brush, Clinton E., 1879–1981
Bryant, Louise Frances Stevens, 1885–1959
Buck, Gurdon, 1807–1877
Budden, William Alfred, 1884–1954
Buerger, Leo, 1879–1943
Bühler, Charlotte Bertha, 1893–1974
Bullitt, James Bell, 1874–1964
Bunnell, Sterling, 1882–1957
Bunnell, Walls Willard, 1902–
Burchenal, Elizabeth, 1876?–1959
Burd, Joseph G.
Burgesser, William Slater, 1853–1927
Burlingham, Dorothy, 1891–1979
Burns, Kit
Burns, Louisa, 1870–1958
Burrough, William, fl. 1825–1850
Busby, John
Butler, Harry B., d. 1965
Cabot, Richard Clarke, 1868–1939
Cairns, Thomas
Caldwell, Charles, 1772–1853
Callahan, John Ross, 1853–1918
Camac, Charles Nicoll Bancker, 1868–1940
Camper, John E., d. 1977
Cane, Florence, 1882–1952
Cannon, Claude Clenton
Cannon, Ida Maud, 1877–1960
Cannon, Walter Bradford, 1871–1945
Carli, Christopher, 1811–1887
Carlson, Anton Julius, 1875–1956
Carmichael, John Leslie, 1897–
Carnegie, Andrew, 1835?–1919
Carnegie, Dale, 1888–1955
Carson, Rachel Louise, 1907–1964
Cassel, John C., 1921–1976
Castle, William B., 1897–
Cattell, James McKeen, 1860–1944
Cawker, Lenore Harrison
Chandler, Raymond, 1888–1959
Chang and Eng, 1811–1874
Chapanis, Alphonse Robert Everysta, 1917–
Chapin, Charles Value, 1856–1941
Chapman, Nathaniel, 1780–1853
Chargaff, Erwin, 1905–
Charters, Werrett Wallace, Sr., 1875–1952
Chase, Alvin Wood, 1817–1885
Cheshire, Johnathan Singleton, 1830–1891
Childs, Richard Spencer, 1882–1978
Chisolm, Julian John, 1830–1903
Chivers, Thomas Holley, 1809–1858
Chowning, William M.
Clagett, Horatio C., 1793–1858
Clark, Kenneth Bancroft, 1914–
Clark, William Mansfield, 1884–1964
Clarke, Hans Thacher, 1887–1972
Clemens, Samuel Langhorne, 1835–1910
Cleveland, Grover, 1837–1908
Clyman, Martin J., 1914–1979
Coates, Samuel, 1748–1830
Cobb, David, 1748–1830
Cobb, William Montague, 1904–
Coca, Arthur F., 1875–1959
Codman, Ernest Amory, 1869–1940
Cogswell, Henry D., 1820–
Cohn, Alfred Einstein, 1879–1957
Colden, Cadwallader, 1688–1776
Cole, Warren Henry, 1899–
Coles, Robert Martin, 1929–
Colledge, Thomas Richardson, 1796–1879
Coman, Katharine, 1857–1915
Compton, Arthur Holly, 1892–
Comstock, Oliver E.
Conner, Eugene Hayward, 1921–
Consolazio, Carlo Frank, 1913–1976
Cooke, Elisha, Jr., 1678–1737
Cooke, Robert Anderson, 1880–1960
Cooper, Thomas, 1759–1839
Cope, Freeman Widener, 1930–1982
Copley, Alfred Lewin, 1910–
Cori, Gerty Theresa Radnitz, 1896–1957
Cornelius, Elias, 1758–1823
Corner, George Washington, 1889–1981
Corner, Thomas Cromwell, 1865–1938
Cornfield, Jerome, 1912–1979
Cottam, Nephi, 1883–1966
Cotterman, Charles William, 1914–

Cotzias, George C., 1918–1977
Coues, Elliott, 1842–1899
Councilman, William Thomas, 1854–1933
Couney, Martin A., 1860 or 70–1950
Courville, Cyril Brian, 1900–1968
Cousins, Norman, 1912–
Craig, Winchell McKendree, 1892–1960
Craik, James, 1730–1814
Crane, Caroline Julia Bartlett, 1858–1938
Crichton Browne, James, 1840–1938
Crichton, Michael, 1942–
Crile, George Washington, 1864–1943
Crohn, Burrill Bernard, 1884–
Cromwell, Frances Elisabeth, 1875–1950
Crowe, Samuel James, 1883–1955
Crowell, Edward Payson, 1856–1934
Crowley, Ralph Manning, 1905–
Cummings, Martin Marc, 1920–
Cummins, Harold, 1893–
Cumston, Charles Greene, 1868–1928
Cupples, George H., 1816–1865
Curran, Edward J., 1873–1962
Currey, Richard Owen
Cushing, George Hoppin, 1829–1900
Cushing, Harvey Williams, 1869–1939
Custer, George Armstrong, 1839–1876
Cutler, Elliott Carr, 1888–1947
DaCosta, Jacob Mendez, 1833–1900
Dailey, Ulysses Grant, 1885–1961
Dakin, Henry Drysdale, 1880–1952
Dalton, John Call, 1825–1889
Dandy, Walter Edward, 1886–1946
Darling, Samuel Taylor, 1872–1925
Darlington, William, 1782–1863
DaVega, Columbus, 1830–1882
Davenport, Horace Willard, 1912–
Davidoff, Leo Max, 1898–1975
Davis, Adelle, 1904–1974
Davis, Frances Elliot, 1882?–1965
Davis, John Staige, 1872–1946
Davis, Loyal Edward, 1896–1982
Davis, Mary Ellen, 1840–1924
Davis, Nathan Smith, 1817–1904
Day, Paul Louis, 1899–1980
Dean-Throckmorton, Jeannette, 1883–1963
Dearborn, Henry, 1751–1829
DeBakey, Michael Ellis, 1908–
Delano, Jane Arminda, 1862–1919
Delany, Martin Robinson, 1812–1885
Delbrück, Max, 1906–1981
De Morti, Mark
DePauw, Cornelius
De Schweinitz, Georg Edmund, 1858–1938
Deutsch, Helene, 1884–1982
Diamond, Louis Klein, 1902–
Dibner, Bern
Dick, Elisha, 1762?–1825
Dick, Gladys Rowena Henry, 1881–1963
Dickinson, Emily, 1830–1886
Dickson, Earle Ensign, 1892–1961
Diehl, Harold Sheely, 1891–1973
Disney, Walter E., 1901–1966
Dix, Dorothea Lynde, 1802–1887
Dobzhansky, Theodosius Grigorievich, 1900–1975
Dock, George, 1860–1951
Dock, Lavinia Lloyd, 1858–1956
Dooley, Thomas Anthony, 1927–1961
Doolittle, Hilda, 1886–1961
Dorn, Harold Fred, 1906–1963
Dorsey, John Morris, 1900–1978
Douglass, William, ca. 1691–1752
Doull, James Angus, 1889–1963
Dow, Margaret Cornelius
Dragstedt, Lester Reynold, 1893–
Drake, Daniel, 1785–1852
Drake, John Poad, 1794?–1883
Dreiser, Theodore, 1871–1945
Drew, Charles Richard, 1904–1950
Drinker, Cecil Kent, 1887–1956
Du Vigneaud, Vincent, 1901–1978
DuBois, W. E. B., 1868–1963
Duhring, Louis Adolphus, 1845–1913
Duke, William Waddel, 1882–1946
Dummer, Ethel Sturges, 1866–1954
Dunbar, Helen Flanders, 1902–1959
Dunglison, Robley, 1798–1869
Dunham, Ethel Collins, 1883–1969
Dunn, Charles Wesley, 1885–1959
Durham, James, fl. 1802
Dyer, Charles Volney, 1808–1878
Easlick, Kenneth Alexander, 1893–1979
Eastman, Joseph, 1842–1902
Eddy, Mary Baker, 1821–1910
Eddy, Thomas, 1758–1827
Edwards, Charles Cornell, 1923–
Edwards, Jonathan, 1703–1758
Eisenhower, Dwight David, 1890–1969
Eliot, Charles William, 1834–1926
Elkin, Daniel Collier, 1893–1958
Elkin, William Simpson, 1858–
Elkind, Mortimer Murray, 1922–
Ellis, Calvin, 1826–1883
Elman, Robert, 1897–1956
Eloesser, Leo, 1881?–1976
Elsaesser, Armin Emil, 1875–1952
Elsner, John, 1844–1922
Elvehjem, Conrad Arnold, 1901–1962
Emerson, Haven, 1874–1957
Emerson, Louville Eugene, 1873–1939
Emmens, Stephen H., ca. 1845–
Enders, John Franklin, 1897–
Engel, George Libman, 1913–
Engel, Rudolph, 1904–
Engelmann, George Julius, 1847–1903
Erickson, Milton Hyland, 1901–1980
Erikson, Erik Homburger, 1902–
Erlanger, Joseph, 1874–1965
Estrada, José, fl. 1821
Evans, Alice, 1881–1975
Evans, Amos Alexander, 1785–1848
Evans, Herbert McLean, 1882–1971
Evans, Thomas Wiltberger, 1823–1897
Evans, Warren Felt, 1817–1889
Faget, Jean-Charles, 1818–
Fankuchen, Isidor, 1905–1964
Fantus, Bernard, 1874–1940
Farrell Family
Faulkner, William, 1897–1962
Feldman, William Hugh, 1892–
Felty, Augustus Roi, 1895–
Fenn, Wallace Osgood, 1893–1971
Field, Edward, 1782?–1840
Finfrock, John H., 1836–1893
Fischelis, Robert P., 1891–1981
Fishbein, Morris, 1889–1976
Fisher, George Jackson, 1825–1893
Fisher, Russell Sylvester, 1916–
Fiske, John, 1842–1901
Fitz, Reginal Heber, 1843–1913
Fitzgerald, Alice Louise Florence, 1875–1962
Fitzpatrick, Thomas Bernard, 1919–
Fleming, William, 1728–1795
Fletcher, Horace, 1849–1919
Fletcher, William Baldwin, 1837–1907
Flexner, Abraham, 1866–1959
Flexner, Simon, 1863–1946
Fogarty, John Edward, 1913–1967
Folin, Otto, 1867–1934
Folks, Homer, 1867–1963
Folsom, James Elisha, 1908–
Foote, Edward Bliss, 1829–1906
Foote, Frank William, 1911–
Fortas, Abe, 1910–1982
Foster, Abigail Kelley, 1810–1887
Foster, Stephen Symonds, 1809–1881
Fowler, Russell Story, 1874–1959
Fraiberg, Selma, 1918–
Francke, Donald Eugene, 1910–
Frank, Jerome, 1889–1957
Franklin, Benjamin, 1706–1790
Frantz, Virginia Kneeland, 1896–1967
Freeman, Leonard, 1860–1935
French, Dexter, 1918–1981
Frenkel-Brunswik, Else, 1908–1958
Frick, George, 1793–1870
Friedenwald Family
Friedenwald, Jonas Stein, 1897–
Friedman, Israel, 1906–1980
Froelicher, Hans, Jr.
Fromm, Erich, 1900–
Fromm-Reichmann, Frieda, 1889–1957
Fronczak, Francis Eustace, 1874–1955
Frost, Wade Hampton, 1880–1938
Fryer, Douglas Henry, 1891–1960
Fuller, Margaret, 1810–1850
Fulton, John Farquhar, 1899–1960
Gaines, Walter Lee, 1881–1950
Gajdusek, Daniel Carleton, 1923–
Galbraith, James Garber, 1914–
Gallaudet, Thomas Hopkins, 1787–1851
Gamble, Clarence James, 1894–1966
Gamble, James Lawder, 1883–1959

Thompson, Isaac, 1775–1852
Thompson, Mary Harris, 1829–1895
Thomson, Elihu, 1853–1937
Thomson, Elizabeth Harriet, 1907–
Thomson, Harriet Blackstock
Thomson, Samuel, 1769–1843
Thoreau, Henry David, 1817–1862
Thorek, Max, 1880–1960
Thorndike, Lynn, 1882–1965
Ticknor, Francis Orray, 1822–1874
Timme, Walter, 1874–1956
Titchener, Edward Bradford, 1867–1927
Tolman, Edward Chace, 1886–1959
Townsend, Francis Everett, 1867–1960
Trudeau, James de Berty, 1817?–1887
Truex, Raymond Carl, 1911–
Truman, Harry S., 1884–1972
Turner, Daniel, 1667–1741
Turner, Henry Hubert, 1892–1970
Turner, Kerenhappuch
Twitchell, Amos, 1781–1850
Twitmyer, Edwin Burket, 1873–1943
Tyler, John Mason, 1851–1929
Underwood, Benton J., 1915–
Urdang, George, 1882–1960
Van Blarcom, Carolyn Conant, 1879–1960
Vance, Benjamin M., 1886–1962
Vanderbilt, George Washington, 1862–1914
Van Gieson, Ransford E.
Van Hoosen, Bertha, 1863–1952
Van Riper, Paul, 1875–
Vasen, Sarah, 1870–1944
Velikovsky, Immanuel, 1895–1979
Verhoeff, Frederick Hermann, 1874–1968
Voors, Antonie Wouter, 1924–
Waksman, Selman Abraham, 1888–1973
Walker, Donald Gregory, 1925–
Walker, Edwin, 1853–1922
Walker, Mary Edwards, 1832–1919
Walsh, Frank Burton, 1895–1978
Walter, Carl Waldemar, 1905–
Wangensteen, Owen Harding, 1898–1981
Warbasse, James Peter, 1866–1957
Ward, Henry Baldwin, 1865–1945
Waring, Joseph Ioor, 1897–
Warkany, Josef, 1912–
Warren, John Collins, 1778–1856
Warren, Jonathan Mason, 1811–1867
Warren, Shields, 1898–1980
Washington, George, 1732–1799
Washington, Lawrence, 1746?–
Waters, Samuel C., 1861–1932
Watson, John Broadus, 1878–1958
Watson, Robert Irving, 1909–1980
Webster, Noah, 1758–1843
Weichmann, Louis J.
Weidman, Frederick Deforest, 1881–1956
Weiner, Herbert M., 1921–
Weiner, Hyman J.
Weir, Robert F., 1838–1927
Welch, Thomas B., 1825–1903
Welch, William Henry, 1850–1934
Weller, Thomas Huckle, 1915–
Wells, Ben
Wells, Horace, 1815–1848
West, Hamilton A., 1849–1903
Westheimer, Gerald, 1924–
Wetmore, Charles Hinckley, 1820–1898
Wharton, Edith Newbold Jones, 1862–1937
Whipple, George Chandler, 1866–1924
White, Ellen Gould Harmon, 1827–1915
White, James Platt, 1811–1881
White, Park Jerauld, 1891–
Whitman, Walt, 1819–1892
Wiggers, Carl John, 1883–1963
Wigglesworth, Edward, 1732–1794
Wilder, Burt Green, 1841–1925
Wilder, Harris Hawthorne, 1864–1928
Wilder, Russell Morse, 1885–1959
Wile, Udo Julius, 1882–1965
Wiley, Harvey Washington, 1844–1930
Willard Family
Willcox, Walter Francis, 1861–1964
Williams, Anna Wessels, 1863–1954
Williams, Daniel Hale, 1858–1931
Williams, Francis Henry, 1852–1936
Williams, Henry Willard, 1821–1895
Williams, John Whitridge, 1866–1931
Williams, William Carlos, 1883–1963
Willits, Mary, 1855–1902
Wilson, Edmund Beecher, 1856–1939
Wilson, Edward O., 1929–
Wilson, Louis Blanchard, 1866–1943
Wilson, Maud Mellish, d. 1933
Wilson, Woodrow, 1856–1924
Winslow, Charles-Edward Amory, 1877–1957
Wishard, William Henry, 1816–1913
Wishard, William Niles, Sr., 1851–1941
Wislocki, George Bernays, 1892–1956
Wolfe, Thomas, 1900–1938
Wolff, James A.
Wood, Earl Howard, 1912–
Wood, Leonard, 1860–1927
Woodward, Samuel Bayard, 1787–1850
Worcester, Noah, fl. 1846
Work, Hubert, 1860–1942
Wright, Chauncey, 1830–1875
Wright, David Hudson, 1881–1948
Wright, Orville, 1871–1948
Wright, Sewall, 1889–
Wright, Wilbur, 1817–1912
Wright, William Thomas, 1927–
Wyeth, John Allan, 1845–1922
Wyman, Rufus, 1777–1842
Wynder, Ernest Ludwig, 1922–
Yandell, David Wendel, 1826–1898
Yandell, Lunsford P., 1837–1884
Yandell, Lunsford Pitts, 1902–
Yater, Wallace Mason, 1895–1976
Yeager, Robert Lee, 1872–1940
Yerkes, Robert Mearns, 1876–1956
Youatt, William, 1776–1847
Young, Anne Austin, 1892–
Young, Brigham, 1801–1877
Zajonc, Robert B., 1923–
Zakrzewska, Marie Elizabeth, 1829–1902
Zilboorg, Gregory, 1890–1959

**Uruguay**

Verocay, José, 1876–1928

**USSR**

Abakeliia, Iosif Konstantinovich, 1883–1938?
Adrianov, Nikolai Konstantinovich, 1869–1931
Akhutin, Mikhail Nikiforovich, 1898–1948
Akimovich, V. V., 1912–1968
Aladashvili, Aleksandr Stepanovich
Alekseev, A. A., 1882–1950
Alekseev, Nikolai Aleksandrovich, 1873–
Alexis, Crown Prince of Russia, 1904–1918
Aliev, A. M.
Andreevskii, Stepan Semenovich, 1760–1818
Anokhin, Petr Kusmich, 1898–1974
Aristovskiĭ, Viacheslav Mikhaĭlovich, 1882–
Astaurov, Boris L'vovich, 1904–
Babel, Isaac, 1894–1941
Babmindra, Viktor Petrovich, 1923–
Baer, Karl Ernst von, 1792–1876
Bagration, P. I.
Bashenin, Viktor Andreevich, 1882–
Baten'kov, G. S.
Bekhterev, Vladimir Mikhaĭlovich, 1857–1927
Bekkers, L. A., 1831–
Beklemishev, Vladimir Nikolaevich, 1890–1962
Beletskiĭ, P. K., 1871–
Beliaev, I. V.
Belinskiĭ, Vissarion Grigor'evich, 1811–1848
Belliarminov, Leonid Gorovich, 1859–1930
Belogolovyĭ, Nikolaĭ Andreevich, 1834–1895
Bertenson, Iosef Vasil'evich, 1833–1895
Berzin, Robert Iur'evich, 1887–1950
Bilibin, Aleksandr Fedorovich
Biriukov, Dmitriĭ Andreevich, 1904–1969
Blonski, Pavel Petrovich
Bogdanov, Ivan Luk'ianovich, 1903–
Bogdanovskiĭ, Evstafii Ivanovich
Bogomolets, Aleksandr Aleksandrovich, 1881–1946
Borodin, Aleksandr Porfir'evich, 1833–1887
Borzenkov, Ia A., 1825–1883
Botkin, Sergeĭ Petrovich, 1832–1889
Buchheim, Rudolf, 1820–1879
Buĭnovskiĭ, A. A., 1844–
Burdenko, Nikolai Nilovich, 1876–1946
Catherine II, the Great, of Russia, 1729–1796
Chagovets, Rotislav Vsesolodovich, 1904–1982
Chaliapin, Feodor Ivanovich, 1873–1938
Charukovskiĭ, Prokhor Alekseevich, 1790–1842
Chekhov, Anton Pavlovich, 1860–1904
Chemodanov, Mikhail Mikhailovich, 1856–1908
Cherkinskiĭ, Samuil Naumovich

Chernogubov, A., fl. 1892
Chernomordik, Solomon Isaevich, 1880–1938
Chernorutskiĭ, Mikhail Vasil'evich, 1884–1957
Chetyrkin, Roman Sergeevich, 1797–1865
Chichagov, Leonid Mikhailovich, 1853–1938
Davidenkov, Sergeĭ Nikolaevich, 1880–
Davydovskiĭ, Ippolit Vasil'evich, 1887–
Demich, V. F., 1858–1930
Diad'kovskiĭ, Iustin Evdokimovich, 1784–1841
Diterikhs, Mikhail Konstantinovich, 1874–
Dobroslavin, Alekseĭ Petrovich, 1842–1889
Dogel, Valentin Aleksandrovich, 1882–
Dogiel, Valentin Aleksandrovich, 1882–1955
Domashiavichius, A. I.
Doroshevskiĭ, Nikolaĭ Antonovich, 1857–1910
Dostoevskiĭ, Fedor Mikhaĭlovich, 1821–1881
Dzhanelidze, Iustin Iulianovich, 1883–1950
Elanski, A. N., 1894–1964
Elin, Vladimir Leont'evich, 1883–1962
Eliseev, Aleksandr Vasil'evich, 1858–1895
Elpat'evskiĭ, Sergeĭ IAkovievich, 1854–1933
Evdokimov, Aleksandr Ivanovich, 1883–
Fedorov, Nikolay Aleksandrovich, 1904–
Filatov, Antonin Nikolaevich, 1902–1974
Filipchenko, IuA, 1882–1930
Frenkel', Zakhariĭ Grigor'evich, 1869–1970
Gaaz, Fedor Petrovich, 1780–1853
Gabričevskij, Georgij Norbertovič, 1860–1907
Gamaleia, Nikolai Fedorovich, 1859–1949
Gannushkin, Peter Borisovich, 1875–1933
Garshin, Vladimir Georgievich, 1887–1956
Garshin, Vsevolod Mikhailovich, 1855–1888
Gertsen, Petr Aleksandrovich, 1871–1947
Gilibert, Jean Emmanuel, 1741–1814
Glinchikov, Vladimir Ignat'evich, 1878–
Glinkov, Pavel Faleeviya, 1883–1923
Glotova, Elena Vladimirovna
Golub, David Moiseevich, 1901?–
Golubev, Vasilii Zakhar'evich, 1858–
Golubkov, Aleksandr Pavlovich, 1880–1945
Golubov, Nikolaĭ Fedorovich, 1856–1943
Gorinevskaia, V. V., 1882–
Grekov, Ivan Ivanovich, 1867–1934
Gribov, Stefan A., 1879–1957
Grigorenko, Pyotr Grigorevich, 1907–
Gromashevskiĭ, Lev Vasil'evich, 1887–
Hertzen, Aleksandre Ivanovich, 1812–1870
Iagel'skiĭ, Kas'ian Osipovich, 1736–1774
Iakubovich, Nikolaĭ Martynovich, 1817–1879
Ianovskiĭ, Mikhail Vladimirovich, 1854–1927
Iaroshenko, N. A.
Iavorskiĭ, Ivan Lavrovich, 1853–1920
Imshenetskiĭ, Aleksandr Aleksandrovich, 1905–
Iudin, Sergei Sergeivich
Iunevich, O. A.
Ivanov, A. V.
Ivanovskiĭ, Dmitriĭ Iosifovich, 1864–1920
Kalinskiĭ, Ossip, 1792–1858
Kamenetskii, Osep Kirillovich, 1754–1823
Kandinskii, Viktor Khrisanfovich, 1849–1889
Kapsukas, Vincas, 1880–1935
Karpov, Sergei Petrovich, 1903–
Kashchenko, Petr Petrovich, 1859–1920
Kassirskiĭ, Iosif Abramovich, 1898–1972?
Kavetskiĭ, Rostyslav Ievhenovych
Kennon, Uolter, 1871–1945
Khavkin, Vladimir Aaronovich
Khodin, Andreĭ Vasil'evich, 1847–
Kholodkovskiĭ, Nikolaĭ Aleksandrovich, 1858–1921
Khotsianov, Lev Kipricanovich, 1889–
Kiter, Aleksandr A., 1813–1884
Knorre, Alekseĭ Georgievich, 1914–1981
Kolomnin, Sergeĭ Petrovich, 1842–1886
Koltson, Alexey Vasilievich, 1809–1842
Koltypin, Aleksandr Alekseevich, 1883–1942
Konchalovskii, Maksim Petrovich, 1875–1942
Kondoidi, Pavel Zakharovich, 1710–1760
Kondrat'ev, N. S., 1887–
Korba-Pribylev, A. P., 1849–1939
Korchak-Chepurkovskiĭ, Avksentiĭ Vasil'evich, 1857–1947
Kornev, Petr Georgievich, 1883–1974
Kornilovich, Aleksandr Osipovich, d. 1833
Korotkoff, Nikolai Sergeevich, 1874–1920
Korotkov, Aleksandr Grigor'evich, 1921–
Korotkov, Nikolaj Sergeevich, 1874–1920
Kots, Nadezhda Nikolaevna Ladygina, 1890–1963
Kotsovskiĭ, A. D., 1864–1937
Kozhevnikov, A. Ia.
Krasnogorskiĭ, Nikolaĭ Ivanovich, 1883–
Krassovskiĭ, Anton Iakovlevich, 1821–1898
Kravchenko, Vladimir Semenovich, 1873–
Krestovskiĭ, Vsevolod Vladimirovich, 1840–1895
Krichevskiĭ, Il'ia L'vovich, 1883–1943
Kriukov, Adrian Aleksandrovich, 1849–1908
Krusenstern, Adam Johann von, 1770–1846
Kukaĭn, Rita Aleksandrovna, 1922–
Kupalov, Petr Stepanovich, 1888–1964
Kurashov, Sergei Vladimirovich
Kurliandskiĭ, Veniamin IUr'evich, 1908?–
Kurlov, Mikhail Georgievich, 1859–1932
Kutuzov, Mikhail Illarionovich, 1745–1813
Larionov, Vladimir Efimovich, 1857–1919
Lavrentiev, Boris Innokentievich, 1892–1944
Lazimir, P. E.
Lenin, Vladimir Il'ich, 1870–1924
Leonardov, Boris Konstantinovich, 1892–1939
Lermontov, Mikhail Iur'evich, 1814–1841
Leshaft, Petr Frantsevich, 1837–1909
Leskov, Nikolaĭ Semenovich, 1831–1895
Lev, Adol'f Aronovich, 1923?–
Levit, Vladimir Semenovich, 1883–
Levitskiĭ, Grigorii Andreevich, 1873–1943
Lisitsyn, Mikhail Semenovich, 1891–1961
Loder, C. I., 1753–1836
Lominskiĭ, F. I., 1857–
Lomonosov, Mikhail Vasil'evich, 1711–1765
London, Efim Semenovich, 1869–1939
Lukomskiĭ, Pavlov Evgen'evich, 1899–
Lunin, Nikolai Ivanovich, 1853–1937
Luriia, Aleksandr Romanovich, 1902–1977
Magil'nitskii, S. G.
Maiakovskiĭ, Vladimir Vladimirovich, 1894–1930
Maĭer, Nikolai Vasil'evich, 1806–1846
Maklakov, Aleksei Nikolaevich, 1837–1895
Maksimovich-Ambodik, Nestor, 1744–1812
Manasein, Viacheslav Avksent'evich, 1841–1901
Mandryka, P. V., 1884–
Markelov, G. I., 1880–
Martynov, Aleksei Vasil'evich, 1868–
Marzeev, Aleksandr Nikitich, 1883–1956
Mashkilleysson family
Maslovskiĭ, Aleksandr Fedorovich
Mechnikov, Il'ia Il'ich, 1845–1916
Medvedev, Zhores Aleksandrovich, 1925–
Mel'man, Efim Petrovich, 1913–
Mel'nikov-Razvedenkov, Nikolaĭ Fedorovich, 1866–1937
Mendeleev, Dmitriĭ Ivanovich, 1824–1907
Mendeleva, Iuliĭ Aronovich, 1883–1959
Miasnikov, Aleksandr Leonidovich
Michelson, M. J., 1912–1978
Mikhaĭlov, Sergeĭ Sergeevich
Minkowski, Oskar, 1858–1931
Minor, Lazar Solomo
Miroliubov, V. P., 1870–1947
Mitskevich, Sergeĭ Ivanovich, 1869–1944
Molchanov, Vasiliĭ Ivanovich, 1868–1959
Mudrov, Matveĭ Iakovlevich, 1776–1831
Mukhamed'iarov, Fatykh Garitovich, 1883?–1950
Mul'tanovskiĭ, Michail Petrovič, 1895–1972
Narimanov, Nariman N., 1872–1925
Nazarov, Vasiliĭ Mikhaĭlovich, 1883–1945
Nechaev, Sergei Dennadievich, 1847–1882
Nemilov, Anton Vitalévich, 1879–1942
Nesterov, Anatoli Innokentevich, 1895–
Nijinsky, Vaslav, 1890–1950
Nikiforov, M. N., 1858–1915
Nikol'skiĭ, Petr Vasil'evich, 1858–1940
Nikonov, S. A.
Okunevskiĭ, IaL, 1877–1940
Oleneva, Elizaveta Nikolaevna, 1924–
Oppel, Vladimir Andreyevitch, 1872–1932
Orakhelashvili, Ivan Dmitrievich, 1881–1937
Orbeli, Leon Abgarovich, 1882–1958
Osipov, E. Alexelvich, 1841–1904
Otelin, Aleksandr Anatol'evich, 1904–1981
Ott, Dmitriĭ Oskarovich, 1855–1929
Paevskiĭ, Vladimir Vladislavovich, 1893–1934
Parin, Vasiliĭ Vasil'evich, 1903–
Pavlov, Ivan Petrovich, 1849–1936
Pavlovskiĭ, Evgeniĭ Nikanorovich, 1884–1965
Perovskaia, Sof'ia L'vovna, 1854–1881
Petrov, Boris Aleksandrovich, 1898–1973
Petrov, Nikolaĭ Nikolaevich, 1876–1964
Petrowa, G. K.
Pevzner, Manuil Isaakovich, 1872–1952
Pikulin, L. E., 1784–1824
Pirogov, Nikolaĭ Ivanovich, 1810–1881
Platonov, IIa
Poletika, Ivan Andrejewitsch, 1722–1783
Potiralovskiĭ, Petr Petrovich, 1872–1927
Poznanin, Petr L'vovich, 1881–1943
Pravdin, Nikolaĭ Sergeevich, 1882–

Pribil, Jan, 1781–1866
Pribylev, A. V., 1857–1936
Priselkov, Vasiliĭ Ivanovich, 1828–1894
Prives, Mikhail Grigor'evich
Pukhlev, Aleksi
Pushkin, Aleksandr Sergieevich, 1799–1837
Putiata, Raisa Vasil'evna, 1853–
Ragoza, Nikolaĭ Ivanovich, 1883–1959
Rasputin, Grigorii Efimovich, 1871–1916
Razumovskiĭ, Vasiliĭ Ivanovich, 1857–1935
Rubakin, Aleksandr Nikolavich, 1889–
Rubashkin, Vladimir IaKovlevich, 1876–1925
Rudakov, P. A.
Rudnev, Georgiĭ Pavlovich, 1899–1970
Rudnev, M. M., 1831–1878
Rufanov, Ivan Gur'evich, 1884–1964
Rukhadze, N. P., 1880?–
Russkikh, N. A., ca. 1857–
Sakharov, Andrei, 1921–
Sakhnovskaia, Anna Akimovna, 1882–1951
Salanter, Israel, 1810–1883
Salishchev, Erast Gavrilovich, 1851–1901
Saltykov-Shchedrin, Mikhail Evgrafovich, 1826–1889
Samoĭlov, Aleksandr Filippovich, 1867–1930
Samus', Valeriĭ Nikolaevich
Schmalhausen, Ivan, 1884–1963
Sechenov, Ivan Mikhaĭlovich, 1829–1905
Semashko, Nikolai Aleksandrovich, 1874–1949
Sergiev, Petr Grigor'evich, 1893–1983
Sevastopol'skaia, Dasha A.
Shamov, Vladimir Nikolaevich, 1880–1962
Sharimanian, Stepanos
Shimanovskiĭ, IuK, 1829–
Shmal'gauzen, Ivan Ivanovich, 1884–1963
Shor, Vladimir Georgievich, 1872–1948
Shtefko, V. G., 1893–1945
Shumlianskiĭ, Aleksandr Mikhaĭlovich, 1748–1795
Silikova, A. I., 1908–1980
Skvortsov, Mikhail Aleksandrovich, 1876–
Sobolev, Andrei Andreevich, 1904–1966
Sokol'nikov, P. N., 1865–
Sokolov, P., 1893?–
Solovev, M. N., 1886–1980
Solov'ev, Zinoviĭ Petrovich, 1876–1928
Speranskiĭ, Georgiĭ Nestorovich, 1873–
Spizharnyĭ, Ivan Konstantinovich, 1857–1924
Sraga, Dragoljub, 1866–1915
Sreseli, Mikhail Andreevich, b. ca. 1904
Stalin, Josef, 1879–1953
Strukov, Anatoli Ivanovich
Sychugov, Sabbatir Ivanovich, 1841–1902
Sysin, Alekseĭ Nikolaevich, 1879–1956
Szymanowski, Julius von, 1829–1868
Tal'iantsev, Anton Ivanovich, 1858–1929
Tatarinov, Alexander Alekseevich, 1817–1886
Ter-Arutiuniants, S. M., 1880–
Timakov, Vladimir Dmitrievich, 1905–1977
Timof'eeff-Ressovsky, Nikolai Wladimirovich, 1900–1981
Tolstoĭ, Lev Nikolaevich, 1828–1910
Topchibashev, Mustafa Agaevich, 1905–
Troshin, Afanasiĭ Semenovich, 191
Trotsky, Leon, 1879–1940
Tschaikowski, Peter Iljitsch, 1840–189
Tsetkin, Maxim, 1883–1965
Tsiolkovskii, K. E.
Tswett, Mikhail Semenovich, 1872–1919
Tur, Aleksandr Fedorovich, 1894–1974
Turner, Genrikh Ivanovich, 1858–1941
Tushinskiĭ, Mikhail Dmitrievich, 1882–1962
Tutyshkin, Petr Petrovich, 1868–1937
Ukhtomskiĭ, Aleksei Alekseevich, 1875–1942
Ulezko-Stroganova, Klavdiia Petrovna, 1856–1943
Ul'ianov Dmitriĭ Il'ich, 1874–1943
Vasil'ev, Stepan Mikhailovich, 1855?–1905?
Veronin, V. V.
Vien, Ivan Ivanovich, ca. 1750–1809
Vinogradov, Nikolaĭ Andreevich, 1831–1886
Voĭtkevich, Anatoliĭ Anatol'evich
Volchenetskiĭ, D. V., 1751–1811
Vol'f, A.M.
Vol'f, F. B., d. 1854
Volkenshteĭn, Liudmila Aleksandrovna, 1857–1906
Volkovich, Nikolaĭ Markiianovich, 1858–1928
Voronoĭ, Iu. Iu., 1895–1961
Votkin, Sergeĭ Petrovich, 1832–1889
Vvedenskii, Nikolai Evgenevich, 1852–1922
Vygotskii, Lev Semenovich, 1896–1934
Zablotskiĭ-Desiatovskiĭ, Paulus, 1814–1883
Zabolotnyĭ, Daniil Kirillovich, 1866–1929
Zakhar'in, Grigoriĭ Antonovich, 1829–1897
Zamenhof, Ludwik Lazar, 1859–1917
Zavadovskiĭ, Mikhail Mikhailovich, 1891–1957
Zelenin, Vladimir Filippovich, 1881–1968
Zhukovskiĭ, Vasiliĭ Andreevich, 1783–1852
Zmeev, Lev Fedorovich, 1832–1901

**Venezuela**

Alvarado, Lisandro
Baptista, José María, 1908–
Beauperthuy, Louis Daniel, 1807–1871
Benítez, José María, 1790–1855
Bonavita, Juan María, fl. 1832
Cadet, Sócrate, 1808–1879
Carvallo, Temislocles, 1885–1964
Díaz Rodríguez, Manuel, 1871–1927
Durant, Sálvano Velasco, 1833–1905
Fébres-Cordero, Focion, 1910–
Iturbe, Juan, 1883–1962
Jordán, Marcos, b. 1715
Lizàrdo, César, 1925–
Marcano, Gaspar, 1850–1910
Noguer Molins, Luis, d. 1972
Oberto, Juan Bautista, fl. 1774
Pantoja, Manuel, fl. ca. 1810
Perera, Ambrosio
Pérez Díaz, Manuel, 1872–1931
Pineda, Antonio María, 1850–
Planque, Hugues, fl. 1837
Rangel, Rafael, 1877–1909
Razetti, Luis, 1862–1932
Ríos, Jóse Manuel de los, 1826 or 1832–1914
Risquez, Jésus Rafael, 1883–
Rodríguez Rivero, Placido Daniel, 1876–1939
Rojas Paúl, Juan Pablo, 1826–1905
Roudier, Juan, fl. 1842
Sanabria Bruzual, Jesus, 1867–1950
Vegas, Martín, 1897–
Vélez Boza, Fermin, 1916–
Yerena, Jesus Antonio, 1917–

**Vietnam**

Hai-Thuong

**Yugoslavia**

Andrić, Ivo, 1892–
Arsenijević, Milan, 1901–1981
Bogišić, Baltazar, 1834–1908
Borić, Dušan, 1889–1978
Botteri, Albert, 1879–1955
Budisavljević, Julije, 1882–1981
Burijan, Richard
Dordevic, Vladan, 1844–1930
Florschütz, Vatroslav, 1876–1967
Gerbezius, Marcus, 1658–1718
Gutschy, Ljudevit, 1874–1961
Hadzi-Nikolić, Nicola, 1855–1915
Haljecka, Eva, 18??–1947
Jovanović-Batut, Milana
Kern, Ferdo, 1872–1960
Lazarevic, Laza, 1851–1890
Lobmayer, Antun, 1844–1906
Magajna, Bogomir, 1904–1963
Marković, Svetozar, 1846–1875
Popović, Pavao, 1854–1937
Pupin, Michael Idvorsky, 1858–1935
Safarik, Janko, 1814–1876
Schwarz, Ante
Schwarz, Dragutin, 1868–1917
Sosberger, Aleksander, 1873–1944
Soubbotitch, V.
Sraga, Dragoljub, 1866–1915
Stanojevi'c, B., d. 1967
Stanojević, Vlademir S., 1886–1978
Tito, Josip Broz, 1892–1980
Tucović, Dimitrije, 1881–1914
Wikerhauser, Teodor, fl. 1894

# PART II. SUBJECT INDEX

## AEROSPACE MEDICINE

### 1700 to Present

Colin J: Geschichte der Luftfahrtmedizin. In Sournia JC, Martiny M, Poulet J, ed: Illustrierte Geschichte der Medizin. Salzburg, Andreas, 1980. Vol. 8. p. 3025–51.
Engle EK, Lott AS: Man in flight: biomedical achievements in aerospace. Annapolis, Md., Leeward, 1979. xxvii, 396 p.
Harding RM, Mills FJ: Special form of flight. I. Balloons, gliders, and hang gliders. **Br Med J [Clin Res]** 1983 Jul 23;287(6387):277–8
Hill IR: The historical background to aerospace pathology. **Aviat Space Environ Med** 1982 Jan;53(1):1–5
Jones DR: Aeromedical transportation of psychiatric patients: historical review and present management. **Aviat Space Environ Med** 1980 Jul;51(7):709–16
Lozina-Lozinsky LK, Zaar EI: [To the history of the rise of exobiology] (Rus). **Istor Biol Issled** 1980;8:3–32
Sparvieri F: Teorie freudiane e psicologia aeronautica. **Riv Med Aeronaut Spaz** 1980 Jan–Jun;43(1–2):81–103

#### France

Perdriel G: La médecine aéronautique dans l'armée de l'air. **Med Armees** 1980;8(10)spec:813–6
Pesquiès-Courbier S: Le renouveau de la médecine aéronautique en France de 1945 à 1950. **Rev Hist Armees** 1982;3:102–9

#### Germany

Lauschner EA: The beginnings of aviation medicine in Germany. **Aviat Space Environ Med** 1984 May;55(5):355–7
Püschel E: Die Seenotverbände der Deutschen Luftwaffe und ihr Sanitätsdienst 1939–1945. Düsseldorf, Droste, 1978. 180 p. ((Schriftenreihe Erfahrungen des deutschen Sanitätsdienst im zweiten Weltkrieg, 1).
Reimer T: Die Entwicklung der Flugmedizin in Deutschland. Köln, 1979. 282 p. (Kölner medizinhistorische Beiträge, Band 13)

#### Great Britain

Howard P: From Concorde to the cosmos. **Trans Hunter Soc** 1978–80;37–38:37–48
Iveson-Iveson J: History of nursing in the Air Force: string, sealing wax and individual daring. **Nurs Mirror** 1981 Jul 15;153(3):27–8
James T: A history of the medical branch of the Royal Air Force: part II aviation medicine. **Adler Mus Bull** 1984 Nov;10(3):2–7
James T: A history of the Medical Branch of the Royal Air Force, part 1. **Adler Mus Bull** 1984 Jun;10(2):3–8
Mackenzie Hume WG: Aviation medicine? **Br Med J [Clin Res]** 1983 Dec 24–31;287(6409):1950–2
Maxwell VB: The first 2 years--a brief history of the British Association of Aviation Medical Examiners. **Aviat Space Environ Med** 1983 May;54(5):xiii–xiv
Nicholson AN: Long-range air capability and the South Atlantic Campaign. **Aviat Space Environ Med** 1984 Apr;55(4):269–70
Reid DD: The historical background to wartime research in psychology and psychiatry in the Royal Air Force. In Dearnaley EJ, Warr PB, ed: Aircrew stress in wartime operations. London, New York, Academic Press, 1979. p. 1–8.

#### Israel

Glazer I: A brief history of the Israel Society of Aerospace Medicine--a 1981 affiliate of the Aerospace Medical Association. **Aviat Space Environ Med** 1983 Apr;54(4):371–2

#### Italy

Lomonaco T: Un medico fra gli aviatori. **Riv Med Aeronaut Spaz** 1980;Suppl:1–176

#### Poland

Rudnicki J: Słuzba zdrowia 1 Polskiej Samodzielnej Brygady Spadochronowej w operacji 'Market-Garden'--relacje uczestników. **Arch Hist Med (Warsz)** 1984;47(1):127–31

#### Spain

Guardia y Pascual del Pobil R de la: Los servicios de sanidad de la Armada en la Aeronautica Naval. **Rev Gen Mar** 1978 Aug–Sep;195:109–23

#### United States

Barger J: Origin of flight nursing in the United States Army Air Forces. **Aviat Space Environ Med** 1979 Nov;50(11):1176–8
Collins WE, Boone JO, VanDeventer AD: The selection of air traffic control specialists: history and review of contributions by the Civil Aeromedical Institute, 1960–80. **Aviat Space Environ Med** 1981 Apr;52(4):217–40
Eckert WG: Fatal commercial air transport crashes, 1924–1981. Review of history and information on fatal crashes. **Am J Forensic Med Pathol** 1982 Mar;3(1):49–56
Eckert WG: The Rockne crash. American commercial air crash investigation in the early years. **Am J Forensic Med Pathol** 1982 Mar;3(1):17–27
Logan RD: Charles Lindbergh and the 'right stuff'. **Aviat Space Environ Med** 1982 Jul;53(7):708–11
Meiling RL: The United States Air Force medical service: tumultuous years of heritage and history. **Aviat Space Environ Med** 1984 Jul;55(7):642–56
Mills JG, Jones DR: The adaptability rating for military aeronautics: an historical perspective of a continuing problem. **Aviat Space Environ Med** 1984 Jun;55(6):558–62
Skinner RE: The making of the air surgeon: the early life and career of David N. W. Grant. **Aviat Space Environ Med** 1983 Jan;54(1):75–82
Skinner RE: The roots of flight nursing: Lauretta M. Schimmoler and the Aerial Nurse Corps of America. **Aviat Space Environ Med** 1984 Jan;55(1):72–7
Skinner RE: The U. S. flight nurse: a supplementary bibliography. **Aviat Space Environ Med** 1983 Aug;54(8):735–7
Skinner RE: The U. S. flight nurse: an annotated historical bibliography. **Aviat Space Environ Med** 1981 Nov;52(11 pt 1):707–12

#### USSR

Babin VP: O travmaticheskikh povrezhdeniiakh u lits letnogo sostava v period Velikoĭ Otechestvennoĭ voĭny. **Voen Med Zh** 1980 Jul;(7):19–21
Gazenko OG, Genin AM, Gurovskiĭ NN, et al: Pervyĭ kosmicheskiĭ polet cheloveka. **Kosm Biol Aviakosm Med** 1981 Mar–Apr;15(2):5–7
Khlebnikov GF: Mediko-biologicheskaia podgotovka kosmonavtov (istoriia, soderzhanie, étpy, évoliustsiia i tendentsii razvitiia). **Kosm Biol Aviakosm Med** 1981 Mar–Apr;15(2):8–14
Kopanev VI: [Role of the scientists of the S. M. Kirov Military Medical Academy in the development of aviation medicine]. (Rus) **Voen Med Zh** 1979 Dec;(12):63–5
Kopanev VI: The importance of K. E. Tsiolkovskii's ideas in the formation and development of space medicine. **Biol Bull Acad Sci USSR** 1979 Nov–Dec;6(6):764–71
Pakhomov AF: Peredovoi aviatsionnyi vrach. **Voen Med Zh** 1983 Aug;(8):7–10
Platonov KK: K istorii otechestvennoĭ aviatsionnoĭ psikhologii: dokumenty i materialy. Moskva, Meditsina, 1981. 316 p.

## AEROSPACE MEDICINE

Rudnyĭ NM: Opyt meditsinskogo obespecheniia Voenno-Vozdushnykh Sil v Velikuiu Otechestvennuiu voĭnu. **Voen Med Zh** 1980 May;(5):34-7

Tolmachev EP: Nachal'nyĭ period razvitiia kosmonavtiki v SSSR (1917-1945). **Kosm Biol Aviakosm Med** 1982 Nov-Dec;16(6):7-15

**Yugoslavia**

Dželajlija S, Debijadi R: Razvoj sanitetske službe u RV i PVO. **Vojnosanit Pregl** 1982 Nov-Dec;39(6):408-11

Stojan D, Petrović M: Razvoj sanitetske opreme u Ratnom vazduhoplovstvu. **Vojnosanit Pregl** 1981 Jan-Feb;38(1):37-40

## ANATOMY

See also **Cytology; Histology**

Barcia Goyanes JJ: Las correcciones de Vesalio a la anatomia de Galeno. **Med Esp** 1980;79:1-16

Barcia Goyanes JJ: Los albores del lenguaje anatómico en las lenguas neolatinos. La traduccion del inventarium de Guy de Chauliac por Bernat de Casaldovol. **Med Esp** 1980;79:235-49

Barcia Goyanes JJ: Los arabismos en las ediciones latinas del libro I del Colliget de Averroes. **Med Esp** 1984 Jan-Feb;83:9-29

Barcia Goyanes JJ: Onomatologia anatomica nova: historia del lenguaje anatomico. Tomo VI. Nares-Profundus. Valencia, Universidad de Valencia, 1983. 467 p.

Barcia Goyanes JJ: Onomatologia anatomica nova; historia del lenguaje anatómico. Tomos I-III. Valencia, Universidad de Valencia, 1978.

Barcia Goyanes JJ: Un extraño nombre del apendice xifoides: 'malum punicum'; a strange name of the xiphoid process: 'malum punicum'. **Med Esp** 1981;80:105-11

Baumann HU: Ueber Mehrfachentdeckungen. Eine Darstellung des allgemeinen Problems mit Beispielen aus drei Teilgebieten der theoretischen Medizin. Diss. Münster, 1972. 133 p.

Belloni L: Il Morgagni tra il Malpighi e il Cotugno. **Gesnerus** 1982;39(2):195-213

Benjamin JA, Tobin CE: The fasciae of the genito-urinary organs: historical, anatomical, and clinical aspects. **Trans Stud Coll Physicians Phila** 1981 Dec;5(3 no 4):264-79

Binet JL: Dessins et traités d'anatomie. Paris, Chêne, 1980. 247 p.

Boschung U: Medizinische Lehrmodelle. **Medita** 1980;10(Geschichte der Medizin, 4):xv

Bouchet A, Masson JL: Les localisations anatomiques de l'âme au cours des siècles. **Hist Sci Med** 1980;14(1):95-106

Bowman IA: Anatomical illustrations with superimposed flaps. **Bookman** 1981 Jul-Aug;9(6):3-7

Busnardo AC, DiDio LJ, Tidrick RT, et al: History of the pancreas. **Am J Surg** 1983 Nov;146(5):539-50

Darmon P: Les vols de cadavres et la science (XVIIe-XIXe siècles). **Histoire** 1982;48:30-7

Delmas A: Geschichte der Anatomie. In Sournia JC, Martiny M, Poulet J, ed: Illustrierte Geschichte der Medizin. Salzburg, Andreas, 1980. Vol. 3. p. 871-929.

Delmas A: L'anatomiste devant les problèmes du langage. **Bull Assoc Anat (Nancy)** 1980;64:313-47

Doerr W: Evolutionstheorie und pathologische Anatomie. **Verh Dtsch Ges Pathol** 1983;67:663-84

Donáth T: Nagy anatómusok jubileuma. **Orv Hetil** 1984 Feb 5;125(6):344-6

Dumaitre P: La curieuse destinée des planches anatomiques de Gérard de Lairesse, peintre en Hollande - Lairesse, Bidloo, Cowper. Amsterdam, Rodopi, 1982. xvii, 107 p. (Nieuwe Nederlandse Bijdragen tot de Geschiedenis der Geneeskunde en der Natuurwetenschappen, no. 6).

French RK: An origin for the bone text of the 'five-figure series'. **Sudhoffs Arch** 1984;68(2):143-56

Glenn WW: The lymphatic system. Some surgical considerations. **Arch Surg** 1981 Aug;116(8):989-95

Hinton RJ: Relationships between mandibular joint size and craniofacial size in human groups. **Arch Oral Biol** 1983 Jan;28(1):37-43

Hixson J: The history of the human body. A 5000 year old mystery. New York, Cooper Square Publisher, 1966. 128 p.

Huard P: El problema de la representación del cuerpo humano. Su evolución en Eurasia. **Nueva Enferm** 1979 Dec;(7):3-6

Jalil A: Mermas and acupuncture points, a comparative study. **Stud Hist Med** 1981 Mar;5(1):18-34

Jayatilaka AD: Historical review of the study of anatomy. **Cent Afr J Med** 1983 Jul;29(7):147-53

Kronick DA: Artists and anatomists, some notes for an exhibit of anatomical atlases. **Friends P. I. Nixon Med Hist Libr** 1978 Oct;7:1-7

Lantos PL: Changing images of the brain. **Psychol Med** 1983 May;13(2):255-6

L'homme et son corps dans la société traditionelle: Paris, Ministère de la culture et de la communication, Editions de la Réunion des musées nationaux, 1978. 144 p.

Light TR: Hands on stamps. **J Hand Surg** 1982 Jan;7(1):20

Macdonald AA: Studies on the anatomy and physiology of the pig fetus and placenta: an historical review. In E. Schultheisz, ed: History of physiology. Oxford, Elmsford, New York, Pergamon, 1981. xvi, 208 p. (Advances in Physiological Sciences. Proceedings of the 28th International Congress of Physiological Sciences, Budapest, 1980. Volume 21). p. 53-60.

Morris AG, Keen EN: Lawrence Herbert Wells and the history of anatomical illustration. **S Afr Med J** 1982 Jan 9;61(2):40-3

O'Neill YV: Ossa mandibulae inferioris duo. **Clio Med** 1980 May;14(2):97-104

Premuda L: Considerazioni sull'illustrazione anatomica dall'antichità all'Ottocento. **Acta Med Hist Patav** 1980-81;27:31-40

Puma FA: El significado historico de la anatomia. **Rev Soc Venez Hist Med** 1969-71;17-19(31-33):91-108

Rassengeschichte der Menscheit: 7 vols. Vol. 1 ed. by K. Saller; Vols. 2-7 ed. by I. Schwidetzky. München und Wien, R. Oldenbourg Verlag, 1968-1979. Continuing.

Reynolds F: [Grave robbing]. **Indiana Med Hist Q** 1978;4(1):5-13

Rodriguez Maffiotte C: Consideraciones acerca de la obra 'Libro de anathomia del hombre', de Bernardino Montana de Monserrate. **Acta Med Tenerife** 1978;39:87-92

Saban R: Les sinus veineux méningés à travers les traités d'anatomie du XVe au XIXe siècle. In: Congrès National des Sociétés Savantes, 106e, Perpignan, 1981. Comptes Rendus. Paris, Bibliothèque Nationale, 1982. Fasc. IV. p. 119-31.

Tinkelenberg J: On the morphology of creative forms and art. **Acta Morphol Neerl Scand** 1983 Mar;21(1):83-95

Wackenheim A: Die Entwicklung der menschlichen Hand in der Kunst. **Radiologe** 1982 May;22(5):195-8

Wayman A: The human body as microcosm in India, Greek cosmology, and sixteenth-century Europe. **Hist Relig** 1982;22(2):172-90

Wright A: Scanning electron microscopy of the human organ of Corti. **J R Soc Med** 1983 Apr;76(4):269-78

Zhang Baochang: [Knowledge of the human body displayed in inscriptions on bone and tortoise shell.] (Chi). **Chin J Med Hist** 1981;11:235-40

Znamenatel'nye i jubileĭnye daty istorii morfologii v 1983 godu: **Arkh Anat Gistol Embriol** 1982 Oct;83(10):109-10

**Americas**

Corruccini RS, Handler JS: Temporomandibular joint size decrease in American Blacks: evidence from Barbados. **J Dent Res** 1980 Sep;59(9):1528

**Asia**

Rassengeschichte der Menschheit: 8. Lieferung. Asien I: Japan, Indonesien, Ozeanien. München and Wien, Oldenbourg, 1981. 166 p. Contributions by H. Suzuki, S. Watanabe, J. Glinka, W. W. Howells, I. Schwidetzky.

**Brazil**

Vasconcellos Pedrosa MX de: O ensino da anatomia no Brasil: saudação a Samuel Duarte Sattamini. **Rev Inst Hist Geogr Bras** 1971;291:83-91

**Denmark**

Christensen OS: Modellen af Domus Anatomica. **Dan Medicinhist Arbog** 1980;:169-79

**Germany**

Huppertz A: Die Vertreter der Anatomie und des anatomischen Unterrichts in Giessen von 1702-1748. Giessen, Schmitz, 1982. 283 p. (Arbeiten zur Geschichte der Medizin in Giessen, 4).

**Great Britain**

Goose DH: Changes in human face breadth since the Mediaeval period in Britain. **Arch Oral Biol** 1981;26(9):757-8

**Hungary**

Izsák S: Gondolatok, szempontok és kutatások Pápai Páriz Ferenc 'Pax Corporis'-ával kapcsolatban. **Orv Hetil** 1982 May 30;123(22):1365-8

**Italy**

Sinha DN: Status of anatomy in the University of Bologna (13th to 18th century). **Stud Hist Med** 1982 Jun;6(3):141-6

**Netherlands**

Houtzager HL: Frederik Ruysch. **Eur J Obstet Gynecol Reprod Biol** 1982 May;13(3):199-201

Witkam HJ: Catalogues of all the chiefest rarities in the Publick Anatomie Hall of the University of Leyden. Leiden, Witkam, 1980. xv, 86 leaves.

**Turkey**

Demirhan A: The development of education of pathology and anatomy in Ottoman Turks. **Stud Hist Med** 1981 Jun;5(2):160–6

Kâhya E: Bízde díseksíyon ne zaman ve nasil başladi? **Belleten (Turk)** 1979;43(172):739–59

Kahya E: Quand et comment la dissection a commencé chez nous. **Bell Turk Tarie Kürümü** 1979;43(172):739–60

**USSR**

Derums VIa, Pfafrod GO, Vilks IuK: Dinamika strukturnykh i biomekhanicheskikh izmeneniï bedrennoï. **Arkh Anat Gistol Embriol** 1980 Aug;79(8):78–84

**Before 500 A.D.**

Haensch WG: Die menschlichen statuetten des mittleren Jungpaläolithikums aus der sicht der Somatischen Anthropologie. Bonn, Habelt, 1982. 294 p. (Antiquitas, 2).

Lewis OJ: The joints of the evolving foot. Part III. The fossil evidence. **J Anat** 1980 Sep;131(Pt 2):275–98

Louis R: The anatomy of antiquity. **Anat Clin** 1983;5(3):139–40

Manuli P, Vegetti M: Cuore, sangue e cervello. Biologia e antropologia nel pensiero antico. Milano, Episteme, 1977. 241 p.

Murthy CK: Origin and slow progress of study of anatomy in ancient times. **Bull Indian Inst Hist Med (Hyderabad)** 1978;8(1–4):24–5

Oxnard CE, Lisowski FP: Functional articulation of some hominoid foot bones: implications for the Olduvai (hominid 8) foot. **Am J Phys Anthropol** 1980 Jan;52(1):107–17

**Asia**

Riehm K: Die Schädelstruktur des Frühmenschen als Ausdruck seines Waldlebens und seiner weiteren Entwicklung. **Gegenbaurs Morphol Jahrb** 1980;126(6):884–99

**Australia**

Thorne AG, Wolpoff MH: Regional continuity in Australasian Pleistocene hominid evolution. **Am J Phys Anthropol** 1981 Jul;55(3):337–49

**Babylon**

Adamson PB: Anatomical and pathological terms in Akkadian. **J R Asiat Soc GB Irel** 1974;102–6: 1979;2–8: 1981;125–32.

**Brazil**

Pereira CB, Galvao CA, Evans WG, et al: A cephalometric evaluation of a Brazilian pre-historic man. **Tydskr Tandheelkd Ver S Afr** 1983 Oct;38(10):627–31

**China**

Zheng GZ, Feng WH, Boa YH, et al: Microscopic and submicroscopic studies on the peripheral nerve and the skeletal muscle of the female. Cadaver found in the Han Tomb No. 1. **Sci Sin** 1979 Sep;22(9):1095–8

**Ecuador**

Ubelaker DH: Skeletal evidence for kneeling in prehistoric Ecuador. **Am J Phys Anthropol** 1979 Nov;51(4):679–86

**Ethiopia**

Kimbel WH, White TD, Johanson DC: Cranial morphology of Australopithecus afarensis: a comparative study based on a composite reconstruction of the adult skull. **Am J Phys Anthropol** 1984 Aug;64(4):337–88

**France**

Hammond M: The expulsion of the Neanderthals from human ancestry: Marcellin Boule and the social context of scientific research. **Soc Stud Sci** 1982 Feb;12(1):1–36

Wildgoose M, Hadingham E, Hooper A: The prehistoric hand pictures at Gargas: attempts at simulation. **Med Hist** 1982 Apr;26(2):205–7

**Great Britain**

Seddon RP: A cephalometric study of the Romano-British. **Eur J Orthod** 1984 Nov;6(4):303–12

**Greco-Roman**

Cheng Zhifan: [Galen's thought, physiology and anatomy as taught by him] (Chi). **Chin J Med Hist** 1980;10:92–5

French RK, Lloyd GE: Greek fragments of the lost books of Galen's Anatomical procedures. **Sudhoffs Arch** 1978;62(3):235–49

Siclari A: L'antropologia di Nemesio di Emesa. Padova, La Garangola, 1974. 318 p. (Filosofia e religione; 9).

**Greece**

Abdullaev MS: Anatomiia v trudakh Aristotelia. **Arkh Anat Gistol Embriol** 1984 Mar;86(3):95–9

Coulomb J: Les Minoens et l'anatomie humaine. **Hist Sci Med** 1981;15(1):81–9

Kullmann W: Aristoteles' Grundgedanken zu Aufbau und Funktion der Körpergewebe. **Sudhoffs Arch** 1982;66(3):209–38

Rousselle A: Observation féminine et idéologie masculine: le corps de la femme d'après les médecins grecs. **Ann Econ Soc Civilis** 1980;35:1089–115

Smith WD: Erasistratus's dietetic medicine. **Bull Hist Med** 1982 Fall;56(3):398–409

Van Praagh R, Van Praagh S: Aristotle's 'triventricular' heart and the relevant early history of the cardiovascular system. **Chest** 1983 Oct;84(4):462–8

**India**

Murthy CK: Sculpture of fasting Buddha; artist's knowledge of anatomy in ancient India. **Bull Inst Hist Med (Hyderabad)** 1973 Oct;3(4):186–8

**Pakistan**

Pilbeam D: New hominoid skull material from the Miocene of Pakistan. **Nature** 1982 Jan 21–27,295(5846).232–4

**Peru**

Selmanowitz VJ: Impressions of Sechnin. Anatomy by slaughter. **NY State J Med** 1980 Dec;80(13):2016–21

**Rome**

Fischer KD: Seneca d. A., Controversiae 10,5,17: ein übersehenes Zeugnis zur Geschichte der antiken Anatomie. **Sudhoffs Arch** 1984;68(1):110–2

Goss CM, Chodkowski EG: 'On Bones for Beginners' by Galen of Pergamon: a translation with commentary. **Am J Anat** 1984 Jan;169(1):59–74

**500 A.D.–1450**

Barcia Goyanes JJ: Dos nombres enigmaticos del trocanter mayor: tharuca y carchametra; two enigmatic names of the greater trochanter: tharuca and carchametra. **Med Esp** 1980 Nov–Dec;79:1–11

Barcia Goyanes JJ: Los terminos osteologicos de la Fabrica y la evolucion del lenguaje anatomico hebreo en la Edad Media. **Sefarad** 1982;42:299–326

Brown EA: Death and the human body in the later Middle Ages: the legislation of Boniface VIII on the division of the corpse. **Viator** 1981;12:221–70

Louis R: The anatomy of the Middle Ages. **Anat Clin** 1984;6(1):1–2

Maragi M: Le glossaire latin-allemand d'anatomie de Walfridus Strabo (IXème siècle). In International Congress of the History of Medicine, 27th, Barcelona, 1980. Actas. Barcelona, Académia de Ciències Médiques de Catalunya i Balears, 1981. p. 304–15.

O'Neill YV: An anatomical mystery with global dimensions. In: Congrès international d'histoire de la médecine, XXVe, Québec, 1976. Actes. Québec, 1977. p. 1031–44.

Steudel K: New estimates of early hominid body size. **Am J Phys Anthropol** 1980 Jan;52(1):52–63

Trynková O: Některé metody středověkého léčení podle mistra rhazesa a mistra Salicettiho. III. Výběr z anatomických pojmu užívaných ve středověké medicíně. **Sb Lek** 1982 Feb;84(2):59–63

**Arabic**

Brahmaji Rao U: Avicenna's contribution to the understanding of anatomy and pathology of heart. **Bull Indian Inst Hist Med (Hyderabad)** 1981;1–4:91–4

Rahman SA: Avicenna on digestion of food. **Bull Indian Inst Hist Med (Hyderabad)** 1981;1–4:59–63

Vajda G: La structure du corps humain d'après le commentaire de Dunash ben Tamin sur le 'Livre de la Création'. **J Semit Stud** 1978;23(1):88–94

**Byzantium**

Bliquez LJ, Kazhdan A: Four testimonia to human dissection in Byzantine times. **Bull Hist Med** 1984 Winter;58(4):554–7

# ANATOMY

**Great Britain**

Getz FM: Anatomia del medioevo. **Kos** 1984 May;1(4):33–46

**Iran**

Kupriianov VV: Vydaiushcheesia znachenie trudov Avitsenny dlia iatorii anatomii (k tysiacheletiiu so dnia rozhdeniia Ibn Siny). **Arkh Anat Gistol Embriol** 1980 Sep;79(9):109–11

**Italy**

Aiken J: Leon Battista Alberti's system of human proportions. **J Warburg Courtauld Inst** 1980;43:68–96

**1450–1700**

Gysel C: Thomas Bartholinus (1616–1680–1980), zijn nederlandse relaties en de tandheelkunde (II). **Ned Tijdschr Tandheelkd** 1982 Oct;89(10):414–9

Horowitz M, Collins J: A census of copies of the first edition of Andreas Vesalius' De humani corporis fabrica (1543), with a note on the recently discovered variant issue. **J Hist Med Allied Sci** 1984 Apr;39(2):198–221

Huard P, Imbault-Huart MJ: André Vesale, iconographie anatomique (Fabrica, Epitome, Tabulae sex). Paris, Dacosta, 1980. 255 p.

Light TR: Hands on stamps. **J Hand Surg** 1981 Sep;6(5):441

Luyendijk-Elshout AM: The introduction of Juan Valverde's and Bartholomy Cabrol's anatomy into Low Countries between 1568–1633. In International Congress of the History of Medicine, 27th, Barcelona, 1980. Actas. Barcelona, Acadèmia de Ciències Mèdiques de Catalunya i Balears, 1981. p. 298–303.

Putscher M: Ein Totentanz von Tizian. Die 17 grossen Holzschnitte zur Fabrica Vesals (1538–1542). In Göpfert W, Otten HH, ed: Metavoeite: wandelt euch durch neues Denken. Düsseldorf, Triltsch, 1983. p. 23–40.

Roth-Woelfle L: Jan Stephen van Kalkar als Illustrator der Anatomie des Andreas Vesal. **Imprimatur** 1980;8:11

Roth-Wölfle L: Jan Stephan von Kalkar als Illustrator der Anatomie des Andreas Vesal. **Imprimatur** 1980;9:86–100

Sawday J: The Leiden Anatomy Theatre as a source for Davenant's 'Cabinet of death' in Gondibert. **Notes Queries** 1983 Oct;30(5):437–9

Sedler MJ: Amendments to the Presidential papers. **Am J Psychiatry** 1982 Jan;139(1):136–7

Simeone FA: Andreas Vesalius: anatomist, surgeon, count palatine, and pilgrim. **Am J Surg** 1984 Apr;147(4):432–40

Trevisani F: 'Ratio' und 'Experimentum': Johannes Bohn (1640–1718) und die italienische Experimentalphysiologie. **Clio Med** 1983 Mar;17(4):199–206

**Belgium**

Doornaert JP: Vesalius. **Plast Reconstr Surg** 1984 Nov;74(5):726

**Denmark**

Bierbaum M, Faller A: Niels Stensen. Anatom, Geologe und Bischof, 1638–1686. 2d ed. Münster, Aschendorff, 1979. xi, 203 p. Includes Thomasen AL, Der Wandel des Stensenbildes.

Faller A: Welchen Platz nimmt Stensens anatomische Forschung in Lorenz Heisters Chirurgie und Anatomie ein? **Gesnerus** 1983;40(1–2):55–66

**France**

Ahlström CG, Ekström P, Persson O: Cartesius' kranium. **Sydsven Medicinhist Sallsk Arsskr** 1983;:23–50

Mounier-Kuhn P, Guerrier Y: Vieussens et l'anatomie de l'oreille. **Acta Otorhinolaryngol Belg** 1982;36(6):1029–38

Schaff G: Jean Gonthier d'Andernach (1497–1574) et la médecine de son temps. In Livet G, Schaff G, ed: Médecine et assistance en Alsace, XVIe–XXe siècle. Strasbourg, Istra, 1976. p. 21–40.

**Germany**

Kaiser W: Athanasius Kircher (1602–1680) und die medizinisch-naturwissenschaftlichen Konzeptionen seiner Zeit. **Z Gesamte Inn Med** 1981 Jul 15;36(14):494–9

**Great Britain**

Mani N: Biomedical thought in Glisson's hepatology and in Wepfer's work on apoplexy. With commentary by R. G. Frank, p. 84–8. In Stevenson LG, ed: A celebration of medical history. Baltimore, Johns Hopkins University Press, 1982. (The Henry E. Sigerist supplements to the Bulletin of the History of Medicine; new ser., no. 6). p. 37–63.

Rook A, Newbold M: David Edwardes: his activities at Cambridge. **Med Hist** 1975 Oct;19(4):389–92

Wear A: William Harvey and the 'Way of the Anatomists'. **Hist Sci** 1983 Sep;21(53 pt 3):223–49

**Italy**

Axdorph S: Den första 'röntgenblicken' – en studie av Leonardo da Vincis anatomiska bilder. **Lakartidningen** 1983 Dec 21;80(51):5005–8

Baur O, Bott B, Braunfels-Esche S, et al: Leonardo da Vinci Anatomie, Physiognomik, Proportion und Bewegung. Köln, 1984. 343 p. (Kölner medizinhistorische Beiträge: Arbeiten der Forschungsstelle des Instituts für Geschichte der Medizin der Universität zu Köln, Band 23/1)

Belloni L: Ancora sul manoscritto 'De dissensionibus, et controversis anatomicis' di Bartolomeo Eustachi. **Physis** 1981;23(4):581–7

Belloni L: Bartolomeo Eustachi, anatomico del cinquecento, al lume di recenti ricerche. **Arch Int Hist Sci (Paris)** 1979 Jun–Dec;29(104):5–10

Bendiner E: Marcello Malpighi: a life of passionate exploration. **Hosp Pract** 1980 Jul;15(7):109–36

Donáth T: Egy évforduló ürügyén. **Orv Hetil** 1984 Sep 30;125(40):2441–4

Duhme L: Die Tabulae anatomicae des Pietro Berrettini da Cortona. Köln, Universität zu Köln, 1980. 185 p. (Kölner medizinhistorische Beiträge, 18) (also Diss.).

Gribanov ED, Sgibova LI: Leonardo da Vinchi kak anatom. **Feldsher Akush** 1982;47(7):43–6

Herschfeld JJ: Bartholomeus Eustachius--the first great dental anatomist. **Bull Hist Dent** 1982 Oct;30(2):123–8

Iwai H, Morimoto I: Reonarudo to kaibo. Leonardo anatomy. Tokyo, Iwasaki Bijutsusha, 1977. 171 p.

Karlan MS: An anatomic plate from Bartolomeo Eustachi. **J Hist Med Allied Sci** 1980 Jul;35(3):316–18

Pedretti C, Keele K, ed al., ed: Leonardo da Vinci: disegni anatomici dalla Biblioteca Reale di Windsor. Firenze, Barbèra, 1979. 159 p.

Roberts KB: Eustachius and his anatomical plates. **Newsl Can Soc Hist** 1979 Apr;:9–13

Speransky LS, Bocharov VJ, Goncharov NI: The personages of Jan Stephan van Calcar's frontispiece to Andreas Vesalius' book 'On the Structure of the Human Body'. **Anat Anz** 1983;153(5):465–79

Todd EM: The neuroanatomy of Leonardo Da Vinci. Ph.D. Diss., University of California, Los Angeles, 1981 xviii, 267 leaves.

Velasco Suárez C: The Santorini valves. **Mt Sinai J Med (NY)** 1981 Mar–Apr;48(2):149–57

**Netherlands**

Alting MP, Waterbolk TW: New light on the anatomical errors in Rembrandt's Anatomy Lesson of Dr. Nicolass Tulp. **J Hand Surg** 1982 Nov;7(6):632–4

Burch CB: Huygens' pulse models as a bridge between phenomena and Huygens' mechanical foundations. **Janus** 1981;68:53–64

Cremone JC: The anatomy lesson of Dr. Nicolaas Tulp. **J Hand Surg** 1982 Sep;7(5):530

Houtzager HL: Dieren in Delft. **Tijdschr Geschied Geneeskd** 1979;2(2):52–61

Houtzager HL: Medicyns, Vroedwyfs en Chirurgyns. Schets van de gezondheidszorg in Delft en beschrijving van het Theatrum Anatomicum aldaar in de 16e en 17e eeuw. Amsterdam, Rodopi, 1979. 133 p. (Serie-nitgave van het Genootschap Delfia Batavorum, 5).

Lindeboom GA: De ontdekking van het trilhaarepitheel door Antonius de Heide (1683). **Ned Tijdschr Geneeskd** 1980 May 24;124(21):839–41

Lindeboom GA: Jan Swammerdam (1637–1680) and his Biblia Naturae. **Clio Med** 1982 Dec;17(2–3):113–31

Lindeboom GA, ed: Het cabinet van Jan Swammerdam (1637–1680). Facsimile reprinted from 1681 ed., Amsterdam, Rodopi, 1980. xxiv, 16 p.

Pagel W: The smiling spleen. In H. Lloyd-Jones, et al., ed: History and imagination: essays in honor of H. R. Trevor-Roper. New York, Holmes & Meier, 1982. p. 81–7.

Pytel' AIa: Nicolaus Van Tul'p – vydaiushchiĭsia anatom i khirurg (k 340-letiiu opublikovania ego znamenitoĭ knigi 'Meditsinskie nabliudeniia'). **Khirurgiia (Mosk)** 1980 Aug;(8):117–9

Roger J: Two scientific discoveries: their genesis and destiny. In M. D. Grmek, R. S. Cohen, G. Cimino, ed: On scientific discovery. The Erice Lectures 1977. Dordrecht, D. Reidel, 1981. p. 229–37. (Boston Studies in the Philosophy of Science, v. 34).

Schupbach W: The paradox of Rembrandt's 'Anatomy of Dr. Tulp'. London, Wellcome Institute for the History of Medicine, 1982. 110 p. (Medical History, Suppl. No. 2).

Slenders J: De Anatomische les van Dr. Zacheus de Jager (1640). **Tijdschr Geschied Geneeskd** 1981;4(4):159–67

**Spain**

Riera J: Valverde y la anatomía del Renacimiento. Valladolid, Ediciones de la Universidad de Valladolid, 1981. 63 p.

**Switzerland**

Clark H: Foiling the pirates: the preparation and publication of Andreas Vesalius's De humani corporis fabrica. **Libr Q** 1981;51(3):301–11

### 1700 to Present

Aleksandrowicz R: From the history of the Polish Anatomical Society and the International Federation of Anatomical Societies. **Folia Morphol (Warsz)** 1980;39(4):393-5
Aterman K: Connective tissue: an eclectic historical review with particular reference to the liver. **Histochem J** 1981 May;13(3):341-96
Balan B: L'ordre et le temps. L'anatomie comparée et l'histoire des vivants au XIXe siècle. Paris, Vrin, 1979. 610 p.
Barone R: L'Association Mondiale des Anatomistes Vétérinaires: 1955-1980. **Anat Histol Embryol** 1980;9(3):280-8
Delon M: Le prétexte anatomique. **Dix-Huit Siecle** 1980;12:35-48
Dumaitre P: Les planches anatomiques d'Antommarchi. **Clio Med** 1981 Sep;16(1):13-23
Hahn von Dorsche H: Die Nomenklaturen der Anatomen. Ein historischer Uberblick. **Anat Anz** 1981;150(1-2):11-43
Hilloowala R: Illustrations from the Wellcome Institute Library: the origin of the Wellcome anatomical waxes Albinus and the Florentine collection at La Specola. **Med Hist** 1984 Oct;28(4):432-7
Himes JH: An early hand-wrist atlas and its implications for secular change in bone age. **Ann Hum Biol** 1984 Jan-Feb;11(1):71-5
Imhof AE, ed: Leib und Leben in der Geschichte der Neuzeit: Vorträge eines internationalen Colloquiums. Berlin, Duncker & Humblot, 1983. 266 p. Text in German and French. (Berliner Historische Studien, Bd. 9. Einzelstudien 2).
Jordanova L: La donna di cera. **Kos** 1984 May;1(4):82-9
Karl Ernest Mason, 1900-1978.: **Anat Rec** 1980 Sep;198(1):1-12
Keel O: John Hunter et Xavier Bichat: les rapports de leurs travaux en pathologie tissulaire. In International Congress of the History of Medicine, 27th, Barcelona, 1980. Actas. Barcelona, Académia de Ciències Mèdiques de Catalunya i Balears, 1981. p. 535-49.
Kermorvan F: Les sirènes existent, l'histoire les a rencontrées. **Histoire** 1980;24:76-8
McHenry LC: L'idea e la mano. **Kos** 1984 Jul-Aug;1(6):79-90
Megvinov LS: Izgotovlenie anatomicheskikh muzeĭnykh preparatov s sokhraneniem ikh tsveta i konsistentsii. **Arkh Patol** 1981;43(8):71-2
Meredith HV, Spurgeon JH, Meredith EM: Early seriatim research on human somatic growth. **Growth** 1981 Autumn;45(3):151-67
Net echt!: De anatomische wereld van Dr. Auzoux. [Exhibition, Museum Boerhaave, Leiden.] **Tijdschr Geschied Geneeskd** 1981;4(1):50-2
Ober WB, Sciagura C: Leydig, Sertoli, and Reinke: three anatomists who were on the ball. **Pathol Annu** 1981;16 Pt 1:1-13
Oliaro A: La chirurgia cento anni or sono. L'Anatomia Chirurgica del dott. **Minerva Chir** 1982 Dec 15-31;37(23-24):2159-79
O'Rahilly R: Plain words on planes and sections. **Radiol Technol** 1981 May-Jun;52(6):615-7
Puymèges D: Les anatomies mouvantes. **Milieux** 1981-82;7-8:62-9
Raskin SP: The pulmonary acinus: historical notes. **Radiology** 1982 Jul;144(1):31-4
Saunders JB, Lee FR, ed: The Manchu anatomy and its historical origin. Taipei, Li Ming Cultural Enterprise Co., 1981. 8, 180 p. English and Chinese.
Zacharias KL: The construction of a primate order: taxonomy and comparative anatomy in establishing the human place in nature, 1735-1916. Ph.D. diss. The Johns Hopkins University. Baltimore, 1980. 464 leaves.

### Australia

Elmslie RG: Our honoured anatomists. **Aust NZ J Surg** 1981 Oct;51(5):415-9

### Austria

Portele KA: Die Henning-Moulagen des Pathologisch-anatomischen Bundesmuseums in Wien. **Med Lab (Stuttg)** 1979 Feb;32(2):41-3
Radbill SX: Josef Hyrtl's Philadelphia connection. **J Hist Med Allied Sci** 1984 Apr;39(2):222-4
Sablik K: Julius Tandler: Mediziner und Sozialreformer: eine Biographie. Wien, A. Schendl, 1983. 389 p.
Steyer GE: Joseph Hyrtl als komparativer Anatomiker. **Anat Anz** 1980;148(5):462-73

### Brazil

Sattamini Duarte O: Dr. José Maurício Nunes Garcia. **Rev Inst Hist Geogr Bras** 1971;291:92-103

### Bulgaria

Kühnel W, Wassilev W: In memoriam Dimitri Kadanoff. **Anat Anz** 1984;156(2):81-95

### Canada

Persaud TV: A brief history of anatomy at the University of Manitoba. **Anat Anz** 1983;153(1):3-31

### China

Grover Y: La correspondance scientifique du P. Dominique Parrenin (1665-1741). In: France: Centre de Recherches interdisciplinaires de Chantilly (CERIC). Les rapports entre la Chine Sinologie (16-18 septembre 1977). Chantilly, Paris, Les Belles Lettres, 1980, 83-99.

### Cuba

Rivero de la Calle M, Collado Lopez O: Reporte sobre las primeras mediciones craneometricas de tipo comparativo realizadas en Cuba. [H. J. Dumont.]. **Cienc Habana Ser 9** 1976;6:3-27

### Czechoslovakia

Dobiás J, Marek J: Dr. Václav Treitz (1819-1872). K 110. výročí úmrtí a 125. výročí vybudování patologickoanatomického ústavu v Praze. **Cas Lek Cesk** 1983 Apr 1;122(13):405-7
Kos J: In memoriam Professor Karel Zlábek. **Anat Anz** 1984;156(5):345-50
Wondrák E: Ceský anatom a patolog V. A. Bochdalek--100 let od smrti. **Cas Lek Cesk** 1983 Oct 28;122(43):1334-7

### France

Antoine JP: 'Les horreurs' anatomiques de Florence. **Histoire** 1980;26:96-8
Arquiola E: Anatomia y antropologia en el positivismo frances. **Asclepio** 1978-79;30-31:19-32
Delmas A: Paul Broca (1824-1880). Esquisse biographique. Le chirurgien et l'anatomiste. **Cah Anthropol** 1980;1-2:15-45
Ellenberger M: Fragonard, l'anatomiste. **Pour Sci** 1982;53:98-108
Fossard J: Faut-il rendre à Gamelin l'Ecorche de Bayonne attribué à Géricault? **Hist Sci Med** 1984;18(2):153-8
Guarner V: El pequeño farabeuf, aquel gigante de mi vida estudiantil. **Bol Soc Mex Hist Filos Med** 1982 Mar;6(38):15-22
Guarner V: Louis-Hubert Farabeuf (1841-1910). **Gac Med Mex** 1982 Dec;118(12):505-8
Gysel C: Daubenton (1716-1800) et ses recherches sur le trou occipital. **Orthod Fr** 1979;50:377-92
Huard P: Claude Bernard et la morphologie. In: Congrès National des Sociétés Savantes, 107e. Brest, 1982. Comptes Rendus, Paris, 1983. Section des Sciences, Fasc. IV. p. 273-9.
Huard P: Paul Broca anatomiste. **Chirurgie** 1980;106(10):774-6
Mulder WJ: De 'Anatomie clastique' van Dr. L. T. J. Anzoux. **Tijdschr Geschied Geneeskd** 1981:4(3):133-43
Peltier LF: Joseph Guichard Duverney (1648-1730). Champion of applied comparative anatomy. **Clin Orthop** 1984 Jul-Aug;(187):308-11
Plessis JL: Un anatomiste militaire mort victime du devoir: Adolphe-Euclide Lacauchie (1806-1853), latiniste distingué et inventeur de l'hydrotomie. **Hist Sci Med** 1982;16(3):151-61
Rocko JM, Di Gioia JM: Calot's triangle revisited. **Surg Gynecol Obstet** 1981 Sep;153(3):410-4
Schiller J: Henri Dutrochet et la terminologie scientifique. In: Congrès National des Sociétés Savantes, 97e, Nantes, 1972. Comptes Rendus. Paris, 1976. Section des Sciences, Tome 1. p. 83-9.
Theunissen B: Theorie en praktijk van Cuviers Recherches sur les ossemens fossiles. **Tijdschr Geschied Geneeskd** 1983;6(1):1-17

### Germany

Bachmann R: Samuel Thomas von Sömmerring - 18. Januar 1755 bis 2. März 1830. Gedenken zum 150. Todestag. **Verh Anat Ges** 1981;75(Pt 1):33-46
Breathnach CS: Biographical sketches No. 18--Flemming. **Ir Med J** 1982 Jun;75(6):177
Dietsch H: Von der Metamorphose zur Homologie. Zum 150. Todestag Goethes. **Med Welt** 1982 Dec 3;33(48):1767-8
Ergetowski R: Uzupełniajace studia H. Kadyi'ego w Uniwersytecie Lipskim w 1879 r. **Arch Hist Med (Warsz)** 1979;42(3):309-15
Eulner HH, Hoepke H, ed: Der Briefwechsel zwischen Rudolph Wagner und Jacob Henle 1838-1862. Göttingen, Vandenhoeck & Ruprecht, 1979. 115 p. (Arbeiten aus der Niedersächsischen Staats- und Universitätsbibliothek Göttingen, Band 16).
Fleischhauer K: In memoriam Wolfgang Bargmann. **Anat Anz** 1979;146(8):209-34
Froriep R: Aspects of tongue (1828). Original Latin text edited and translated by C. Garton, J. D. Gerencser, A. J. Drinnan. Buffalo, Dept. of Classics, State University of N. Y., 1982. xix, 109, 108a p. (Arethusa Monographs IX).
Gaĭsinovich AE: K. F. Vol'f i ego rol' v istorii embriologii i anatomii (k 250-letiiu so dnia rozhdeniia). **Arkh Anat Gistol Embriol** 1984 Aug;87(8):90-6
Hildebrand R: Beitrag der Würzburger Anatomie zur Entwicklung des mikroskopisch-anatomischen Unterrichts (1847 Kölliker--Petersen 1940). **Anat Anz** 1984;155(1-5):115-22
Hoepke H: Aus der Geschichte der Heidelberger Anatomie. **Ruperto Carola (Germany)** 1978;30(61):23-31
Kahle E: Klinkosch, Joseph Thaddäus. In Neue Deutsche Biographie 12.

1980. p. 101–2.
Kahle E: Koelliker, Albert Ritter v. In Neue Deutsche Biographie 12. 1980. p. 322–3.
Kahle E: Kupffer. In Neue Deutsche Biographie 13. 1982. p. 319–20.
Linss W: Im memoriam Günther Geyer (25. 9. 1930--18. 6. 1980). **Anat Anz** 1981;149(3):193–209
Linss W: Karl von Bardeleben--der Begründer des 'Anatomischen Anzeigers'. **Anat Anz** 1981;150(1–2):5–10
Mullen PC: The commemoration of the Meckel bicentennial: Bozeman 1982. **Am J Med Genet** 1984 Aug;18(4):565–9
Roesler HP: Soemmerring--Denkmäler in Frankfurt am Main. **Nat Mus** 1978;108:345–53
Rösler HP: Samuel Thomas von Soemmerring (1755–1830), Aquarell, gemalt 1794 von seiner Frau Margarethe Elisabeth, geb. Grunelius (1768–1802), Grösse des Bildovals 12,8 cm (Höhe): 11,5 cm (Breite) (Privatbesitz). **Medizinhist J** 1980;15(4):422–5
Schierhorn H: Die Hirnanatomie im Spiegel der ersten 50 Bände des Anatomischen Anzeigers. **Anat Anz** 1981;150(1–2):77–118
Schierhorn H: Die Multinationalität der Anatomischen Gesellschaft und die Mehrsprachigkeit ihrer Versammlungen. **Anat Anz** 1980;148(2):168–206
Seidler E: Johann Friedrich Meckel the Younger (1781–1833). **Am J Med Genet** 1984 Aug;18(4):571–86
Voss H: Goethes Selbstzeugnisse über seine Beschäftigung mit 'organischen Naturen'. II. Briefe (1776 bis 1817). **Gegenbaurs Morphol Jahrb** 1979;125(4):466–518
Wahl RW: Eponym: the loop of Henle. **South Med J** 1984 Apr;77(4):494–5
Wendler D, Rother P: Wilhelm His sen.--Leben und Wirken des bedeutenden Leipziger Morphologen. **Z Gesamte Inn Med** 1982 Dec;37(23):810–3

### Great Britain

Atherton DJ: Joseph Towne: wax modeler extraordinary. **J Am Acad Dermatol** 1980 Sep;3(3):311–6
Bayliss RA: Andrew Moir: an Aberdeen anatomist. **Scott Med J** 1980;25:315–9
Breathnach CS: Biographical sketches No. 26--W. Hunter. **Ir Med J** 1983 Feb;76(2):59
Carrillo JL, Olagüe G: La enseñanza de la anatomia comparada en la Inglaterra de comienzos del siglo XIX: a proposito de las Lectures de Everard Home (1756–1832). **Asclepio** 1978–79;30–31:83–8
Cave AJ: A constellation of conservators. **Ann R Coll Surg Engl** 1980 Jan;62(1):66–70
Cooper WM, Platt H: John Sebastian Bach Stopford. In Dictionary of national biography, 1961–1970. Suppl. 8, 1981. p. 985–7.
Crainz F: The editions and translations of Dr. Matthew Baillie's Morbid Anatomy. **Med Hist** 1982 Oct;26(4):443–52
Donnelly FK: The destruction of the Sheffield School of Anatomy in 1835: a popular response to class legislation. **Trans Hunter Archaeol Soc** 1975;10:167–72
Douglas H: Burke and Hare. **Br Hist Illus** 1978–79;5(5):32–43
Fee E: Nineteenth-century craniology: the study of the female skull. **Bull Hist Med** 1979 Fall;53(3):415–33
Forbes TR: 'To be dissected and anatomized.' **J Hist Med Allied Sci** 1981 Oct;36(4):490–2
Fozzard JA: Professors of anatomy in the University of Cambridge: the first two hundred and sixty-one years of the Cambridge University Department of Anatomy, 1707–1968. Cambridge, FOSSLIA, 1983. 87 p.
Gilbert SF: Owen's vertebral archetype and evolutionary genetics -- a Platonic appreciation. **Perspect Biol Med** 1980 Spring;23(3):475–88
Loudon IS: Sir Charles Bell and the anatomy of expression. **Br Med J [Clin Res]** 1982 Dec 18–25;285(6357):1794–6
Qvist G: John Hunter, 1728–1793. London, Heinemann, 1981. xvi, 216 p.
Rains AJ: The continuing message. **Ann R Coll Surg Engl** 1984 May;66(3):151–8
Richardson R: A dissection of the Anatomy Act. **Soc Soc Hist Med Bull (Lond)** 1980 Jun;26:38–9
Stephen K: Robert Knox, M.D., F.R.S.E. (1791–1862). Edinburgh, University of Edinburgh, [1981]. 11 p. (Scottish men of medicine).
Williamson R: Sir Busick Harwood: a reappraisal. **Med Hist** 1983 Oct;27(4):423–33

### Hungary

Bugyi B: A hazai anthropológia néhány korai írása. **Orvostort Kozl** 1979;87–88(25 no 1–2):261–8

### Italy

Armoroli M, ed: Le cere anatomiche Bolognesi del settecento. Catalogo della mostra organizzata Settembre–Novembre 1981. Bologna, Università degli Studi di Bologna, Accademia delle Scienze, 1981. 97 p. Contributions by R. A. Bernabeo, L. Bonuzzi, F. Ruggeri.
Azzaroli ML, Lanza B: La Venere scomponibile. **Kos** 1984 May;1(4):65–81
Ciardi RP: Fra pelle e ossa. **Kos** 1984 Mar;1(2):93–117
Knoefel PK: Felice Fontana: light thrown on his character by the case of the 'spazzino' Guidetti. **Med Secoli** 1981 May–Aug;18(2):229–42
Ongaro G, Mazzolini RG: Quasi tradens se totum: i manoscritti morgagnani della Biblioteca Palatina di Parma. **Ann Ist Mus Stor Sci Fir** 1983;8(1):101–5
Premuda L: The revival of the anatomico-clinical method in Padua: the fundamental contribution of F. S. Verson (1805–1849) from Trieste, a disciple of the Vienna School of Medicine. **Janus** 1980;67(1–2–3):31–9
Thiene G, Pennelli N: Terzo centenario della nascita di Giovanni Battista Morgagni (1682–1982): c'è ancora bisogno dell'autopsia? **G Ital Cardiol** 1983 Oct;13(10):262–4
Zanobio B: Le osservazioni clinico-anatomiche di Luigi Porta (1800–1875) sulle 'cotilitidi'. **Rend Ist Lomb Accad Sci Lett B** 1978;112:82–98

### Netherlands

Gysel C: Conférence autour de Camper (1722–1789) et de 'son' angle facial. **Orthod Fr** 1980;51:LIX–XCVII
Haneveld GT: Koning Willem I en de aankoop van anatomische kabinetten. **Spiegel Hist** 1978;13(7–8):488–95
Thornton JL: Jan Van Rymsdyk: medical artist of the eighteenth century. Cambridge, New York, Oleander Press, 1982. ix, 111 p.
Woerdeman MW: The pre-constitutional years of the Dutch anatomical society. **Acta Morphol Neerl Scand** 1983 Mar;21(1):7–8

### New Zealand

Abel GB: The subapical segment: a historical note. **NZ Med J** 1980 Jul 9;92(663):24–6

### Poland

Kucharz E, Stawiarska B: Zycie I Działalność Ludwika Maurycego Hirszfelda. **Wiad Lek** 1982 May 1;35(3–4):261–6
Kuś J, Miodoński A: Kazimierz Kostranecki i jego uczniowie na tle epoki. **Przegl Lek** 1981;38(12):875–82
Lasiński W: Achievements of the Polish morphology in 35 years of the Polish People's Republic. **Folia Morphol (Warsz)** 1981;40(3):205–16
Sokołowska-Pituchowa J: Two monographs on the spinal cord vascularization. **Folia Morphol (Warsz)** 1980;39(1):1–8
Wyrost P: A hundred years of Lvov-Wrocxaw veterinary anatomy (1881–1981). **Folia Morphol (Warsz)** 1982;41(1):5–16

### Romania

Achievements in the normal and pathological morphology in Romania: **Morphol Embryol (Bucur)** 1981 Apr–Jun;27(2):105–8

### Spain

Arquiola E: Anatomía y antropología en la obra de Olóriz. **Dynamis** 1981;1:165–77
Arquiola E: Anatomia y antropologia fisica en el positivismo español. **Asclepio** 1981;33:3–22
Orozco Acuaviva A: Apuntes para la historia de la anatomia gaditana del siglo XIX. **Asclepio** 1978–79;30–31:99–116
Uranga E: Un ilustre anatónomo y cirujano con ideas necrofilicas del siglo XIX en Zaragoza. **Bol Real Soc Vascongada Amigos Pais** 1973;29(1–3):375–91

### Sweden

Broberg G: Homo sapiens; Linnaeus's classification of man. In Frängsmyr T, ed: Linnaeus, the man and his work. Berkeley, University of California Press, 1983. p. 156–94.

### Switzerland

Albrecht von Haller, 1708–1777: Zehn Vorträge gehalten am Berner Haller-Symposion vom 6. bis 8. Oktober 1977. Basel, Birkhäuser, 1978. x, 182 p. With contributions by M. Stettler, K. S. Guthke, U. Im Hof, N. Mani, L. Premuda, H. Zoller, R. Toellner, A. Lindt, W. Zimmerli, W. Killy.
Boschung U: Ein Brief Albrecht Hallers über seinen Aufenthalt in Paris und Strassburg (1728). **Physis** 1977;19(1–4):185–96
Boschung U: Johannes von Muralt, 1645–1733: Arzt, Chirurg, Anatom, Naturforscher, Philosoph. Zürich, Rohr, 1983. 105 p.
Töndury G: Anatomie in Zürich. **Gesnerus** 1980;37(3/4):271–87

### United States

Amoroso EC: George Bernays Wislocki. In Dictionary of American Biography, Suppl. 6, 1956–1960. p. 703–5, 1980.
Bell WJ: George W. Corner (1889–1981): historian. **Bull Hist Med** 1982 Spring;56(1):93–8
Bodian D: Normand Louis Hoerr. In Dictionary of American Biography,

Suppl. 6, 1956–1960. p. 295–6, 1980.
Brieger GH: Florence Rena Sabin. In: Notable American women. The modern period. Cambridge, Mass., Belknap-Harvard Univ. Press, 1980. 4:614–7.
D'Amato NA: William Edmonds Horner: anatomist, educator, author. **Va Med** 1982 Mar;109(3):209–10
Falk D: Primate neuroanatomy: an evolutionary perspective. In F. Spencer, ed: A history of American physical anthropology, 1930–1980. New York, Academic Press, 1982. 75–103.
Garrett CG: Robert Russell Bensley. In Dictionary of American Biography, Suppl. 6, 1956–1960. p. 53–4, 1980.
Gruber B: Anatomist, scholar and gentleman: Arthur V. Nilsson–a legend in his own time. **Chiropr Hist** 1984;4(1):31–8
Holtz W: Bankrobbers, burkers and bodysnatchers. **Mich Q Rev** 1967;6(2):90–8
Kaplan MM: Three decades of collaboration with Hilary Koprowski. **J Cell Physiol [Suppl]** 1982;2:1–6
Kaufman M, Hanawalt LL: Body snatching in the Midwest. **Mich Hist** 1971;55(1):23–40
Kritchevsky D: Hilary Koprowski and The Wistar Institute. **J Cell Physiol [Suppl]** 1982;2:vi–viii
Ladman AJ: R. C. Truex memorial. **Anat Rec** 1981 Sep;201(1):3–11
Marvin HN: Anatomy in Arkansas' Medical College 1879–1979. The history of a department. (continued) **J Arkansas Med Soc** 1980 Dec;77(7):253–64; 1981;77(8,9,10):305–12, 347–52, 386–419
Riley HD: George Nicholas Papanicolaou. In Dictionary of American biography, 1961–1965. Suppl. 7, 1981. p. 598–9.
Savitt TL: The use of Blacks for medical experimentation and demonstration in the Old South. **J South Hist** 1982 Aug;48(3):331–48
Spady JG: Dr. W. Montague Cobb: anatomist, physician, physical anthropologist, editor emeritus of the Journal of the National Medical Association, and first black president of NAACP. **J Natl Med Assoc** 1984 Jul;76(7):739–44
Spencer F, ed: A history of American physical anthropology, 1930–1980. New York, Academic Press, 1982. xvi, 495 p.

### USSR

Abdullaev MS: Vklad V. I. Razumovskogo v istoriiu otechestvennoĭ anatomii (k 125-letiiu so dnia rozhdeniia). **Arkh Anat Gistol Embriol** 1982 Aug;83(8):96–100
Bobrik II, Chernyshenko LV: Istoriia anatomicheskikh muzeev na Ukraine i ikh znachenie dlia ateisticheskoĭ propagandy i populiarizatsii dostizheniĭ nauki. **Vrach Delo** 1984 Feb;(2):119–22
Bobrik II, Chernyshenko LV: Istoriia anatomii na Ukraine v gody Sovetskoĭ vlasti. **Arkh Anat Gistol Embriol** 1983 Jan;84(1):95–8
Bobrik II, Chernyshenko LV: 140 let kafedry anatomii Kievskogo meditsinskogo instituta. **Vrach Delo** 1982 Feb;(2):1–2
Brzheskiĭ VCh: Uvekovechennye imena otechestvennykh uchenykh--morfologov. **Arkh Anat Gistol Embriol** 1981 Jan;80(1):108–9
Dyskin EA, Klishov AA: O roli Voenno-meditsinskoĭ akademii im. S. M. Kirova v podgotovke vysokokvalifitsirovannykh kadrov anatomov i gistologov SSSR. **Arkh Anat Gistol Embriol** 1983 Mar;84(3):90–6
Dyskin EA: Stanovlenie i razvitie prepodavaniia anatomii v Peterburge v XVIII v. **Arkh Anat Gistol Embriol** 1984 Feb;86(2):96–101
Elizaveta Nikolaevna Oleneva (k 60-letiiu so dnia rozhdeniia): **Arkh Anat Gistol Embriol** 1984 Mar;86(3):107–9
Ibragimova ZI, Burak GG, Ol'shannikova VV, et al: 50 let kafedre anatomii cheloveka Vitebskogo meditsinskogo instituta. **Arkh Anat Gistol Embriol** 1984 Jul;87(7):95–6
Katsnel'bogen AG: Obshchestvenno-meditsinskaia deiatel'nost' Kh. I. Lodera. **Klin Med (Mosk)** 1982 Jun;60(6):117–20
Korotkov AG, Valishin ES: K 175-letiiu kafedry normal'noĭ anatomii cheloveka Kazanskogo meditsinskogo instituta. **Arkh Anat Gistol Embriol** 1982 Jan;82(1):110–4
Kul'chitskiĭ KI, Klantsa PA, Sobchuk GS: N. I. Pirogov--osnovopolozhnik topograficheskoĭ (prikladnoĭ) anatomii. **Klin Khir** 1981 Nov;(11):73–6
Kupriianov VV: Otechestvennaia anatomiia na etapakh istorii. Moskva, Meditsina, 1981. 319 p.
Kurdiumov NA, Novikova TP: Kafedra normal'noĭ anatomii Dagestanskogo meditsinskogo instituta (k 50-letnemu iubileiu). **Arkh Anat Gistol Embriol** 1983 Dec;85(12):90–2
Kvitnitskiĭ-Ryzhov IuN: O nekotorykh aktual'nykh voporosakh istorii morfologii (po povodu stateĭ V. Ch. Brzheskogo i V. P. Mikhaĭlova). **Arkh Anat Gistol Embriol** 1981 Aug;81(8):97–101
Leontiuk AS, Lobko PI, Novikov II: David Moiseevich Golub (k 80-letiiu so dnia rozhdeniia i 55-letiiu vrachebnoĭ, nauchnoĭ, pedagogicheskoĭ i obshchestvennoĭ deiatel'nosti). **Arkh Anat Gistol Embriol** 1981 Aug;81(8):122–6
Mel'man EP, Shutka BV: Issledovanie V. Z. Golubevym mikroangioarkhitektoniki pochki. **Arkh Anat Gistol Embriol** 1983 Dec;85(12):87–9
Mel'man EP: N. V. Kondrat'ev i ego vklad v anatomiiu vegetativnoĭ nervnoĭ sistemy. **Arkh Anat Gistol Embriol** 1983 Nov;85(11):90–4
Mikhail Andreevich Sreseli (k 75-letiiu so dnia rozhdeniia): **Arkh Anat Gistol Embriol** 1980 Apr;78(4):122–5
Mikhail Grigor'evich Prives (k 75-letiiu so dnia rozhdeniia): **Arkh Anat Gistol Embriol** 1980 Mar;78(3):120–1
Mikhaĭlov VP: Delo bol'shogo obshchestvennogo znacheniia (po povodu stat'i V. Ch. Brzheskogo). **Arkh Anat Gistol Embriol** 1981 Jan;80(1):109–13
Mikhaĭlov VP: Pamiati Alekseia Georgievicha Knorre. **Arkh Anat Gistol Embriol** 1982 Feb;82(2):5–16
Morfologiia v SSSR: **Arkh Anat Gistol Embriol** 1982 Dec;83(12):9–35
Pamiati Aleksandra Anatol'evicha Otelina: **Arkh Anat Gistol Embriol** 1981 Sep;81(9):123–6
Petr Andreevich Sokolov (k 80-letiiu so dnia rozhdeniia): **Arkh Anat Gistol Embriol** 1980 Jul;79(7):118–20
Sergeĭ Sergeevich Mikhailov (k 60-letiiu so dnia rozhdeniia): **Arkh Anat Gistol Embriol** 1980 Mar;78(3):121–5
Shabunin AV: P. F. Lesgaft, 1837–1909. Moskva, Meditsina, 1982. 75 p.
Skopakov Kh: N. I. Pirogov--genialen khirug i osnovopolozhnik na topografskata anatomiia. **Khirurgiia (Sofiia)** 1982;35(1):99–100
Sokolov VE, Vorob'eva EI: I. I. Shmal'gauzen i évoliutsionnaia morfologiia. **Arkh Anat Gistol Embriol** 1984 Jul;87(7):5–17
Speranskiĭ VS, Burdeĭ GD, Iudin KA: Muzeĭ i biblioteka kafedry anatomii cheloveka Saratovskogo. **Arkh Anat Gistol Embriol** 1980 Jun;78(6):115–9
Stepanov PF, Romanov NA: Istoriko-leksikologicheskiĭ aspekt russkoĭ anatomicheskoĭ terminologii. **Arkh Anat Gistol Embriol** 1980 Jun;78(6):111–5
Stepanov PF, Romanov NA: O russkoĭ osteologicheskoĭ terminologii XVIII v. **Arkh Anat Gistol Embriol** 1983 May;84(5):93–6
Valishin ES: Aleksandr Grigor'evich Korotkov (K 60-letiiu so dnia Rozhdeniia). **Arkh Anat Gistol Embriol** 1981 May;80(5):122–5
Zagrebin AM: Kafedre anatomii cheloveka Izhevskogo meditsinskogo instituta 50 let. **Arkh Anat Gistol Embriol** 1984 Apr;86(4):91–5
Zeliak VL: Efim Petrovich Mel'man (k 70-letiiu so dnia rozhdeniia). **Arkh Anat Gistol Embriol** 1983 Nov;85(11):102–7
Zeligman SB, Kir'iakulov GS: 50 let kafedre anatomii cheloveka Donetskogo meditsinskogo instituta im. M. Gor'kogo. **Arkh Anat Gistol Embriol** 1981 Apr;80(4):102–4

## ANESTHESIOLOGY

See also **Surgery**

Akupunktur--en framtidsmetod med gamla anor: **Odontol Foren Tidskr** 1980 Nov;44(4):47–50
Bonnabeau RC: The development of inhalation anesthesia. **Minn Med** 1984 Sep;67(9):507–8
Bossy J: Acupuncture et organisation nerveuse periphérique, segmentaire et intersegmentaire. In Mazars G, ed: Les médecines traditionnelles de l'Asie. Strasbourg, Université Louis Pasteur, 1981. p. 41–8.
Cook D: The story of inhalation anaesthesia. **Br Dent Surg Assist** 1981 Sep–Oct;40(5):103–5; Nov–Dec;40(6):111–3
Crul JF: [History of anesthesiology]. (Ita) **Minerva Anestesiol** 1979 Sep;45(9):721–9
Davis AB: The development of anesthesia. **Am Sci** 1982 Sep–Oct;70(5):522–8
Enjoubault: Petite histoire de l'anesthésie. **Infirm Fr** 1982 Jul;(237):27–30
Gibson HB: Pain and its conquest. London, Boston, Peter Owen, 1982. 224 p.
Gravenstein JS: A perspective on science. The language and history of anesthesia. **Ala J Med Sci** 1984 Jul;21(3):304–10
Gravenstein JS: The history of drug inhalation: a brief overview. **Anesth Analg (Cleve)** 1980 Feb;59(2):140–5
Hossli G: Die historische Entwicklung der intravenösen Narkose. **Klin Anaesthesiol Intensivther** 1981;23:1–7
Ivanov VI: O sochetannom primenenii akupunktury i medikamentoznoĭ terapii. **Voen Med Zh** 1982 Feb;(2):49–51
Jenkins MT: History of sequestered edema associated with surgical operations and trauma. **Contemp Anesth Pract** 1983;6:1–31
Lecomte J: L'acupuncture: approche historique et applications. **Cah Clio** 1981;67:17–21
Martiny M: Geschichte der Akupunktur. In Sournia JC, Martiny M, Poulet J, ed: Illustrierte Geschichte der Medizin. Salzburg, Andreas, 1980. Vol. 8. p. 3081–91.
Matsuki A: [Recent findings in the history of anesthesiology] (Jpn). **Masui** 1981 Oct;30(10):1142–6 (continued regularly)
Matsuki A: [Recent findings in the study of anesthesiologic history (21). An etymological study of 'masui'.] (Jpn). **Masui** 1983 Aug;32(8):1012–7
Nuland SB: The origins of anesthesia. **Conn Med** 1984 Mar;48(3):171–4 contd
Ohry A: A short history of anaesthesia. **Koroth** 1983 Aug;8(7–8):281–3
Rolls R: Bark, blisters and the bathe: some problems of pain relief in former times. **J R Soc Med** 1982 Oct;75(10):812–9
Stahnke J: Geschichtliches zur Lokalanästhesie. **MMW** 1980 Sept 5;122(36):1236–8
Vaksman IA, Popugaĭlo VM: Istoriia anesteziologii i reanimatsii v filatelii. **Anesteziol Reanimatol** 1984 Mar–Apr;(2):75–7
Vidal F: Les anodins dans le traitement des douleurs dentaires aux XVIIe et XVIIIe siècles. **Inf Dent** 1982 Feb 25;64(8):695–703
Vidal F: Odontoiatria del passato. Gli 'anodini' nel trattamento del mal

di denti nel XVII e nel XVIII secolo. **Dent Cadmos** 1982 Jan;50(1):57–61
Vidal F: Un anesthésique vieux de 19 siècles: la mandragore. **Chir Dent Fr** 1982 Oct 7;52(173):21–6

**China**

Jonecko A, Stasienko J, Jonecko U: Historia akupunktury chińskiej w średniowieczu i w czasach nowożytnych. **Wiad Lek** 1982 Dec 15;35(23–24):1593–601
Soulie de Morant G: Acuponcture. (Communications 1929–1951). Avant-propos par N. Soulié de Morant. Paris, Guy Trédaniel, 1979. 234 p.

**Germany**

Arnold HJ: Die Geschichte der Akupunktur in Deutschland. Heidelberg Haus, 1976. 128 p.
Holtkamp P: Narkosen mit 'Weingenuss bis zum Nasenbluten'. **Quintessenz J** 1981 Nov;11(11):995–6

**Great Britain**

Harris R: An excursion in serendipity--the conquest of pain. **Ann R Australas Coll Dent Surg** 1979 Nov;6:103–11

**Hong Kong**

Lett Z: Anaesthesia in Hong Kong: evolution and present position. [Hong Kong], Centre of Asian Studies, University of Hong Kong, 1982. 36 p.

**Lebanon**

Haddad FS: Gleanings of anaesthesia in Lebanon. **Middle East J Anaesthesiol** 1980 Oct;5(8):553–6

**Before 500 A.D.**

**China**

Matsumoto A: [Recent findings in the history of anesthesiology (10)--Khwada, a celebrated physician at the Han dynasty was a Persian] (Jpn). **Masui** 1980 Sep;29(9):946–8

**500 A.D.–1450**

**Arabic**

Hijazi AR: L'anesthésie chez Avicenne et les techniques anesthésiques au XIe siècle. **Ann Fr Anesth Reanim** 1984;3(1):76–8
Jasser MT: Anaesthesia and resuscitation in the history of Arabic medicine. In: International Symposium for the History of Arabic Science, 1st, University of Aleppo, 1976. Proceedings. Aleppo, Syria, 1976. Papers in European Languages, Vol. II. p. 324–5.

**1450–1700**

Schmitz R, Kuhlen FJ: Anästhesie und Arzneimittelmissbrauch in peinlichen Gerichtsverfahren des 16. und 17. Jahrhunderts. In Göpfert W, Otten HH, ed: Metavoeite: wandelt euch durch neues Denken. Düsselfort, Triltsch, 1983. p. 189–99.

**1700 to Present**

Baraka A: Anesthesiology is the 'Critical Care of the Surgical Patient'. **Middle East J Anaesthesiol** 1982 Jun;6(5):237–9
Baraka A: Evolution of anaesthesia circuits **Middle East J Anaesthesiol** 1979 Jun;5(4):225–7
Bendixen HH: Respirators and respiratory care. **Acta Anaesthesiol Scand** 1982 Jun;26(3):279–86
Bonica JJ: History, current status and future of regional anesthesia. **Ann Chir Gynaecol** 1984;73(3):108–17
Boulton TB: The rise and fall of general anaesthesia in the dental chair. **SAAD Dig** 1980 Jul;4(7):156–65
Bradley BE: The historic use of diazepam in dentistry. **Anesth Prog** 1981 Mar–Apr;28(2):38–40
Buffat JJ, Thonnier C, Bourdais A, et al: Anesthésie et odonto-stomatologie. **Actual Odontostomatol (Paris)** 1982;36(139)303–13
Curelaru I, Sandu L: Eugen Bogdan Aburel (1899–1975). The pioneer of regional analgesia for pain relief in childbirth. **Anaesthesia** 1982 Jun;37(6):663–9
Dundee JW, McIlroy PD: The history of barbiturates. **Anaesthesia** 1982 Jul;37(7):726–34
Farr AD: Religious opposition to obstetric anaesthesia: a myth? **Ann Sci** 1983 Mar;40(2):159–77
Feldman SA: Anesthesia's debt to science and its contribution to medicine. **Acta Anaesthesiol Belg** 1979;30 Suppl:13–21
Fitz-Hugh GS: Anesthesia in otolaryngology: historical overview. **Otolaryngol Clin North Am** 1981 Aug;14(3):467–81
Goldberg MF: Cocaine: the first local anesthetic and the 'third scourge of humanity'. A centennial melodrama. **Arch Ophthalmol** 1984 Oct;102(10):1443–7
Gray TC: 'Another side of Mars'. **J R Army Med Corps** 1984 Feb;130(1):3–11
Greene NM: Anesthesia and the development of surgery (1846–1896). **Middle East J Anaesthesiol** 1979 Oct;5(5):309–23
Hall LW: Equine anaesthesia: discovery and rediscovery. **Equine Vet J** 1983 Jul;15(3):190–5
Helliwell PJ: The Association of Anaesthetists of Great Britain and Ireland. **Anaesthesia** 1982 Sep;37(9):913–23
Henschel WF, Kljucar S: Intravenous anesthesia. Its development towards its position in today's anesthesia. **Acta Anaesthesiol Belg** 1980;31(3):195–205
Jaffe M: The evolution of ambulatory anesthesiology in dentistry **Anesth Prog** 1980 May–Jun;27(3):76–84
Keown KK: A brief history of anesthesia and surgery of the heart and great vessels. **Can Anaesth Soc J** 1982 Jul;29(4):325–9
Knight N: Early moral and medical opposition to inhalation anesthesia and childbirth. In The history and sociology of technology: Proceedings of the 24th annual meeting of the Society for the History of Technology. Milwaukee, Milwaukee Public Museum, 1982. p. 29–37.
Kunegel JM, Limoge A, Debras C: Historique de l'électroanesthésie. **Inf Dent** 1982 Nov 18:64(40):3919–24
L'acide barbiturique: **Pour Sci** 1982;61:6
Landauer B: Inhalationsanästhesie heute. Teil 1: Historische Entwicklung, allgemeine Tatsachen. **Fortschr Med** 1983 May 5;101(17):796–802
Lasagna L: Analgesic methodology: a brief history and commentary. **J Clin Pharmacol** 1980 May–Jun;20(5–6 Pt 2):373–6
Mason AH: Crime and anaesthesia -- robbery. **Hist Med (Lond)** 1980 Jan–Feb;8(1):18–19,32
Matsuki A: [Current findings on the studies of the history of anesthesiology (8) -- Erwin Von Baelz and obstetrical anesthesia] (Jpn). **Masui** 1980 Mar;29(3):287–90
Matsumoto A: [Current findings in the history of anesthesiology (12)] (Jpn) **Masui** 1980 Nov;29(12):1541–6
Newman JL: Acupuncture, anaesthesia, and all that. **NZ Med J** 1982 Jan 13;95(699):22
Nuland SB: The origins of anesthesia: part II. **Conn Med** 1984 Jun;48(6):379–83 contd
Nuland SB: The origins of anesthesia: Part III. **Conn Med** 1984 Sep;48(9):597–600
Paiement B, Boulanger M, Taillefer J, et al: Anesthésie et cardiopathie: évolution des concepts et perspectives. **Union Med Can** 1979 Oct;108(10):1158–66
Pantaleoni M: Perfezionamenti tecnici e metodologici ed apparecchiature per anestesia generale. **Minerva Anestesiol** 1982 Dec;48(12):879–86
Papper EM, Mark LC, Ngai SH: Anesthesiology: progress since 1940. Coral Gables, Fla., Univ. of Miami Press, [1973]. 192 p.
Papper EM: The fiftieth anniversary of the use of thiopentone in man. **Anaesthesia** 1984 Jun;39(6):517–9
Payne JP: Anaesthetic deaths. **Br J Hosp Med** 1983 Dec;30(6):411–4
Pierce EC: Analysis of anesthetic mishaps. Historical perspectives. **Int Anesthesiol Clin** 1984 Summer;22(2):1–16
Secher O: Fra Boston til Amaliegade; anaesthesiens vej til Danmark. **Dan Medicinhist Arbog** 1981;:25–56
Senior JE: The elusive search for electroanesthesia. **Med Instrum** 1984 Jan–Feb;18(1):86–7
Silvay G, Griffin R: The history and development of cardiovascular monitoring during anesthesia. **Mt Sinai J Med (NY)** 1984 Sep;51(5):560–3
Sykes WS: Essays on the first hundred years of anaesthesia. 3 vols. Park Ridge, Illinois, Wood Library-Museum of Anesthesiology, 1982. 171, 187, 272 p. (Vols. 1 and 2 are reprints of 1960 ed; Vol. 3 is edited by R. H. Ellis)
Vandam LD: Anesthesiologists as clinicians. **Anesthesiology** 1980 Jul;53(1):40–8
Vandam LD: Intravenous anesthesia--history, currency, prospects. **Mt Sinai J Med (NY)** 1983 Jul–Aug;50(4):316–22
Wawersik J: Die Geschichte des Narkoseapparates in Grundzügen. **Anaesthesist** 1982 Oct;31(10):541–8
Whitby JD: Alcohol in anaesthesia and surgical resuscitation. **Anaesthesia** 1980 May;35(5):502–5
Wildsmith JA, Strichartz GR: Local anaesthetic drugs--an historical perspective. **Br J Anaesth** 1984 Sep;56(9):937–9
Zuck D: Early opposition to obstetric anasthesia [letter] **Anaesthesia** 1981 May;36(5):538–42

**Australia**

Cole WH: Some ether anecdotes. **Anaesth Intensive Care** 1981 May;9(2):174–6
Wilson G: The first anaesthetic in Australia. **Anaesth Intensive Care** 1980 Aug;8(3):378–9
Wilson G: The pioneering anaesthetists of Australia. **Anaesth Intensive Care** 1979 Nov;7(4):311–21

**Burma**

Mitchell JV: Burma revisited. **Anaesthesia** 1979 Sep;34(8):811-21

**Canada**

Gordon RA: Forty years onward. **Can Anaesth Soc J** 1983 Sep;30(5):460-5

**China**

Johnson DA: History and the understanding of acupuncture anesthesia. **South Med J** 1983 Apr;76(4):497-8

**France**

Courtine JC: L'Armée d'Afrique et l'anesthésie-réanimation: de Baudens (1853) au Corps expéditionnaire française à la Première Armée (1942-1945) et à la guerre d'Algérie. **Hist Sci Med** 1983;17(4):411-17
Jullien Y: Histoire des benzodiazépines. **Ann Fr Anesth Reanim** 1984;3(3):153-4
Picard JM, Aussedat M: Historique de l'anesthésie par hypnose à Nancy. In: Congrès National des Sociétés Savantes, 103e, Nancy, 1978. Comptes Rendus. Paris, 1978. Section des Sciences, Fasc. V. p. 95-8.

**Germany**

Doenicke. A: Zum 200. Geburtstag von Friedrich Wilhelm Adam Sertürner. **Anaesthesist** 1983 Jun;32(6):239-41
Lewerenz-Steinsiepe M: Fritz Ludwig Dumont: ein moderner Anaesthesist. **Anaesthesist** 1982 Jun;31(6):302-5
Weisser C: Der Braunsche Apparat zur Äther-Chloroform-Mischnarkose. Ein Beitrag zur Frühgeschichte der Kombinationsnarkose. **Anaesthesist** 1983 Aug;32(8):369-73
Weisser C: Der Ombrédannesche Äther-Inhalator. Ein Beitrag zur Geschichte der Äther-Apparatnarkose. **Anaesthesist** 1983 Feb;32(2):51-4
Zenker R: Die Chirurgie Martin Kirschners in unserer Zeit. **MMW** 1980 Feb 29;122(9):318-9

**Great Britain**

Brandt L, Pokar H, Schütte H: 100 Jahre Intubationsnarkose. William Macewen, ein Pionier der endotrachealen Intubation. **Anaesthesist** 1983 May;32(5):200-4
Crider S: Anesthesia. A history of Simpson's discovery of chloroform. **J Kans Med Soc** 1983 Mar;84(3):143-6
Defalque RJ: The first experiment in obstetrical anesthesia. **Anesth Analg (Cleve)** 1983 Dec;62(12):1136
Edmonds-Seal J, Mitchell JV: The Oxford training scheme in anaesthesia and other matters. **Anaesthesia** 1979 Sep;34(8):776-83
Farr AD: Early opposition to obstetric anaesthesia. **Anaesthesia** 1980 Sept;35(9):896-907
Helliwell PJ: Henry Walter Featherstone, first President of the Association of Anesthetists of Great Britain and Ireland (1932-34). **Anaesthesia** 1982 Apr;37(4):394-7
Hunter AR: Zebulon Mennell. A pioneer of neurosurgical anaesthesia. **Anaesthesia** 1983 Dec;38(12):1214-6
Jones IW: Chloroform anaesthesia in Liverpool. **Anaesthesia** 1983 Jun;38(6):578-80
Leaman A: John Snow MD--his early days. **Anaesthesia** 1984 Aug;39(8):803-5
Lee JA: Anaesthesia. **Br Med J** 1979 Nov 10;2(6199):1192-4
McDowall DG: The Yorkshire Connection--Priestley and Waterton. **Anaesth Intensive Care** 1982 Feb;10(1):4-8
Matsuki A: [Current findings in the history of anesthesiology (17)--the first anesthesia-related fatalities in the world] (Jpn). **Masui** 1982 Apr;31(4):408-14
Matsuki A: [Current findings on the history of anesthesiology (11)--the Hannah Greener incident (1)] (Jpn). **Masui** 1980 Oct;29(10):1070-4
Matsuki A: [Recent findings in the history of anesthesiology (16) Tracing John Snow's work in London] (Jpn). **Masui** 1982 Mar;31(3):264-9
Padfield A, Alderson JD: Early days of anaesthesia in Sheffield. **Ann R Coll Surg Engl** 1984 Jul;66(4):293-6
Proceedings of a symposium held to commemorate the bicentenary of Charles Waterton (1782-1865): **Br J Anaesth** 1983 Mar;55(3):221-33
Smith WD: Under the influence. A history of nitrous oxide and oxygen anaesthesia. London, Macmillan, 1982. xxviii, 188 p.
Thomas KB: Sir Ivan Whiteside Magill, KCVO, DSc, MB, BCh, BAO, FRCS, FFARCS, (Hon), FFARCSI (Hon), DA. A review of his publications and other references to his life and work. **Anaesthesia** 1978 Jul-Aug;33(7):628-34
Waserman M: Sir James Y. Simpson and London's 'conservative and so curiously prejudiced' Dr. Ramsbotham. **Br Med J** 1980 Jan 19;280(6208):158-61
Weller RM: Nitrous oxide in Bristol in 1836. A series of lectures by William Herepath (1796-1868). **Anaesthesia** 1983 Jul;38(7):678-82

**Hong Kong**

Lett Z: Anaesthesia in Hong Kong. Its history and present position. **Anaesthesia** 1980 Oct;35(10):993-8

**Hungary**

Földes F: Az aneaesthesiológia szerepe a betegellátásban, orvosképzésben és az orvostudomány fejlödéséven **Orv Hetil** 1981 Feb 15;122(7):375-9
Giacinto M: A modern anaesthesia kialakuklása, jelene és perspektívái. **Orv Hetil** 1979 Oct 28;120(43):2593-7
Széll K: A regionalis érzéstelenités helye a korszerü anaesthesiológiában. **Orv Hetil** 1982 Jul 4;123(27):1651-8

**Italy**

Bellucci G: Storia della Società Italiana di Anestesia ed Analgesia, Società Italiana di Anestesiologia, Società Italiana di Anestesia e Rianimazione, Società Italiana di Anestesiologia, Analgesia, Rianimazione e Terapia Intensiva. **Minerva Anestesiol** 1980 Jul;46(7):733-56
Evoluzione dell'anestesiologia in Italia: **Minerva Anestesiol** 1984 Jun;50(6):285-92

**Japan**

Matsuki A: [Current view of the studies on the history of anesthesiology (7)--Tekisai Okubo, a pioneer of the pain clinic in Japan] **Masui** 1980 Feb;29(2):182-4
Matsuki A: [Erwin von Baelz as a pioneer in obstetrical anaesthesia in Japan.] (Jpn). **Nihon I-Shigaku Zasshi** 1981;27(1):47-55
Matsuki A: Nothing new under the sun--a Japanese pioneer in the clinical use of intrathecal morphine. **Anesthesiology** 1983 Mar;58(3):289-90
Matsuki A: [Recent findings in the history of anesthesiology (20) Discovery of muscle relaxant, magnocuraine in Japan. (Jpn). **Masui** 1982 Dec;31(12):1414-9
Matsushita A: [Recent findings in the history of anesthesiology (9); practice of the anesthetic method developed by Seishu Hanaoka] (Jpn). **Masui** 1980 Aug;29(8):828-30

**Lebanon**

Haddad FS: History of anesthesia in Lebanon 1800-1914. **Middle East J Anaesthesiol** 1982 Jun;6(5):241-80
Muallem M: Anesthesiology in the American University of Beirut 1922-1970. **Middle East J Anaesthesiol** 1982 Jun;6(5):281-8

**Mexico**

Bandera B: La Academia Nacional de Medicina y la evolución de la anestesia en México. In Academia Nacional de Medicina. Libro conmemorativo del primer centenario. México, Comité Editorial de la Comisión Organizadora del Congreso del Centenario, 1964. Tome 2. p. 546-52.
Salinas Cantú H: Biografia del Dr. Jesus Ma. González Flores. **Humanitas** 1981;22:201-12

**Netherlands**

Wolff JD: Over chloroform-narcose en een Nederlandse pionier (S.N. Dentz Jr.). **Ned Tijdschr Geneeskd** 1981 Oct 17;125(42):1719-22

**Poland**

Wajs S: Sposoby znieczulenia stosowane przy usuwaniu zebow przed stu laty. **Czas Stomatol** 1979 Dec;32(12):1211-3

**Spain**

Franco Grande A, Ginesta Galán F, Martinón Sanchez JM: Primeras tesis doctorales sobre anestesia en lengua castellana. **Rev Esp Anestesiol Reanim** 1980 Jul;27(4):337-61
Miguel Martínez J, Cabarrocas Gafarot E: Bodas de plata de la associació catalana d'anestesiologia i reanimació (1953-1978). **Rev Esp Anestesiol Reanim** 1981 Mar;28(2):51-110

**Switzerland**

1952-1982, 30e anniversaire de la Société suisse d'anesthésiologie et de réanimation: [Switzerland: s.n., 1982?]. 72 p.

**United States**

Agris J: Stamps commemorating medicine. 'Dr. Crawford Williamson Long' the father of anesthesia. **J Dermatol Surg Oncol** 1980 May;6(5):415
Aldrete JA, Marron GM, Wright AJ: The first administration of anesthesia in military surgery: on occasion of the Mexican-American War. **Anesthesiology** 1984 Nov;61(5):585-8

## ANESTHESIOLOGY

Bellagarda M, Trisoglio M: Il contributo della scienza e dell'odontostomatologia in particolare alla scoperta ed al progresso dell'anestesia. **Minerva Med** 1981 Apr 7;72(14):897–902
Calmes SH: Virginia Apgar: a woman physician's career in a developing specialty. **J Am Med Wom Assoc** 1984 Nov–Dec;39(6):184–8
Campan L: A propos du centenaire de la mort de Charles Thomas Jackson (1805–1880). **Ann Anesthesiol Fr** 1981;22(1):3–7
Chow EP: Acupuncture: its history and educational significance to health practices in the United States. Ph.D. Diss., The Fielding Institute. Santa Barbara, 1975. 156 leaves.
Crawford WM: More on the ether operation. **N Engl J Med** 1984 Feb 23;310(8):534
Duncalf D: History of anesthesia for pediatric cardiac surgery. **Int Anesthesiol Clin** 1980 Spring;18(1):1–3
Dundee JW: Fifty years of thiopentone. **Br J Anaesth** 1984 Mar;56(3):211–3
Eavey RD: First operation under ether anesthesia: a correction. **N Engl J Med** 1983 Oct 20;309(16):990–1
Hershey SG: The Rovenstine inheritance--a chain of leadership. **Anesthesiology** 1983 Nov;59(5):453–8
Johnson CS: Anesthesia and photography. **Harv Mag** 1980 Jul–Aug;82(6):57
Labor under ether: Hilo, 1850. **Hawaii Med J** 1981 Oct;40(10):291–2
Leavitt JW: Birthing and anesthesia: the debate over twilight sleep. **Signs** 1980;6(1):147–64
Leland TM: Anesthesiology in the Civil War (Dr. Julian John Chisolm). **J SC Med Assoc** 1981 Nov;77(11):524
Little DM: The founding of the specialty boards. **Anesthesiology** 1981 Sep;55(3):317–21
Miller LG: Pain, parturition, and the profession: twilight sleep in America. In Reverby S, Rosner D, ed: Health care in America. Philadelphia, Temple University Press, 1979. p. 19–44.
Morris JP: Emery Andrew Rovenstine. In Dictionary of American Biography, Suppl. 6, 1956–1960. p. 553–4, 1980.
Nuland SB: Ingelfinger rule violated in 1846. **N Engl J Med** 1983 Apr 14;308(15):907
Pernick MS: A calculus of suffering: pain, anesthesia, and utilitarian professionalism in nineteenth-century American medicine. Ph.D. Diss. Columbia University. New York, 1979.
Pullen JJ: Gentleman, this is no humbug. **Am Heritage** 1979;30(5):80–96
Stork G: Samuel Marion McElvain: December 9, 1897–April 11, 1973. **Biogr Mem Natl Acad Sci** 1983;54:221–48
Vandam L, Volpitto PP: The Genesis of contemporary American anesthesiology. Springfield, Thomas, 1982. xvi, 246 p.
Vandam LD, Abbott JA: Edward Gilbert Abbott: enigmatic figure of the ether demonstration. **N Engl J Med** 1984 Oct 11;311(15):991–4
Vandam LD: Impressions of anesthetics past. **Transplant Proc** 1981 Mar;13(1):61–4
Vandam LD: Robert Hinckley's 'The First operation with ether'. **Anesthesiology** 1980 Jan;52(1):62–70
Waldinger RJ: Virginia Apgar. In: Notable American women. The modern period. Cambridge, Mass., Belknap-Harvard Univ. Press, 1980. 4:27–8.
Williams WD: Did Horace Wells stage a newspaper publicity scheme? Some unreported newspaper items. **Bull Hist Dent** 1983 Oct;31(2):93–8
Young DM: Eugene H. Conner, M.D., KMA historian. **J Ky Med Assoc** 1982 Apr;80(4):224–6

**Uruguay**

Pernin A, Vega DE: Historia de la anestesia en el Uruguay. Montevideo, Roche, 1981. n. p.

**USSR**

Altschuller GI, Keenan WA: History of the development of painless surgery in Russia. **Bull NY Acad Med** 1982 Jun;58(5):493–502
Broder LIa: K istorii primeneniia zakisi azota v Rossii. **Anesteziol Reanimatol** 1983 Mar–Apr;(2):f73
Poliakov VA: K stoletiiu otkrytiia mestnoĭ anestezii. **Ortop Travmatol Protez** 1981 Sep;(9):65–8
Shabunin AV: Efirnyĭ narkoz v pervyĭ god ego primeneniia v Rossii. **Sov Zdravookhr** 1983;8:62–4

**Venezuela**

Wikinski JA: Apuntes para una historia de la anestesiologia venezolana. **Rev Soc Venez Hist Med** 1981;30(45–46):25–55

## ANIMALS

See also **Veterinary Medicine**

Baker J: Animal diseases in archaeology. London, New York, Academic Press, 1980. ix, 235 p.
Blaxter K: Cervinus annos vivere: an account of opinion about the length of life of the deer. **Br Vet J** 1979 Nov–Dec;135(6):591–9
Brewer NR, et al: The origins of laboratory animal science and medicine: proceedings of a symposium ... American Association for Laboratory Animal Science ... 1979. **Lab Anim Sci** 1980;30:737–800
Castro M de: Johannes Aegidii Zamorensis, OFM, contra venena et animalia venenosa. Introducción edición y notas. **Arch Iberoam** 1976;36:3–116
Cooper T, Stucki JC: Commentary on 'animal research - for and against: a philosophical, social, and historical perspective'. **Perspect Biol Med** 1983 Autumn;27(1):18–21
Cunningham SG, Mitchell PH: The use of animals in nursing research. **ANS** 1982 Jul;4(4):72–84
Espinosa y León VM: Reseña histórica de los roedores domésticos. **Salud Publica Mex** 1984 Jan–Feb;26(1):77–81
Gow CE: The dentitions of the Tritheledontidae (therapsida: cynodontia). **Proc R Soc Lond [Biol]** 1980 Jul 17;208(1173):461–81
Hahn U: Die Entwicklung des Tierschutzgedankens in Religion und Geistesgeschichte. DMV Diss. Hannover, 1980. 192 p.
Hall DL: Why do animals breathe? New York, Arno Press, 1981. xviii, 296 p.
Hovesen E: Slangen i laegekunsten. **Dan Medicinhist Arbog** 1983;12:105–21
Leclercq-Kadaner J: Physiologus de naturis animalium et bestiarum. Fédération des Cercles d'Archéologie et d'Histoire de Belgique. 44e session. Congrès de Huy, 1976. Annales. Tielt, 1978. p. 790–5
McCullagh KG, Silver IA: The actual cautery -- myth and reality in the art of firing. **Equine Vet J** 1981 Apr;13(2):81–4
Macdonald AA: Studies on the anatomy and physiology of the pig fetus and placenta: an historical review. In E. Schultheisz, ed: History of physiology. Oxford, Elmsford, New York, Pergamon, 1981. xvi, 208 p. (Advances in Physiological Sciences. Proceedings of the 28th International Congress of Physiological Sciences, Budapest, 1980. Volume 21). p. 53–60.
Markl H: Tiere als Automaten oder als Verwandte? Descartes oder Darwin. **MMW** 1982 Nov 5;124(44):973–6
Mittwoch U: Whistling maids and crowing hens--hermaphroditism in folklore and biology. **Perspect Biol Med** 1981 Summer;24(4):595–606
Payton BW: An historical survey of illustrations of the medicinal leech. **J Audiov Media Med** 1984 Jul;7(3):105–12
Rousselle R: Comparative psychohistory: snake-handling in Hellenistic Greece and the American South. **J Psychohist** 1984 Spring;11(4):477–89
Rowan AN, Rollin BE: Animal research - for and against: a philosophical, social, and historical perspective. **Perspect Biol Med** 1983 Autumn;27(1):1–17
Schwabe CW: Cattle, priests, and progress in medicine. Minneapolis, University of Minnesota Press, 1978. xiii, 277 p.
Teaford MF, Walker A: Quantitative differences in dental microwear between primate species with different diets and a comment on the presumed diet of Sivapithecus. **Am J Phys Anthropol** 1984 Jun;64(2):191–200
Tillhagen CH: Vögel in der Volksmedizin. **Ethnomedizin** 1978–79;5(3–4):263–86
Trowell HC: Ants distinguish diabetes mellitus from diabetes insipidus. **Br Med J [Clin Res]** 1982 Jul 17;285(6336):217
Wells EB: The disease horse. **Factotum** 1981;12:14

**France**

Schmitt JC: The holy greyhound: Guinefort, healer of children since the thirteenth century. Cambridge, Cambridge University Press; Paris, Editions de la Maison des Sciences de l'Homme, 1983. 215 p. Translation of Le saint lévrier: Guinefort, guérisseur d'enfants depuis le XIIIe siècle, Paris, 1979.

**Spain**

Saiz Moreno L: Antiguas vías de circulación del ganado. La trashumancia del ganado merino en España y las epizootias. **Rev Sanid Hig Publica (Madr)** 1983 Nov–Dec;57(11–12):1229–53

**United States**

Henderson RW, ed: Early American sport: a checklist of books by American and foreign authors published prior to 1860, including sporting songs. Third edition revised and enlarged. Rutherford, New Jersey, Fairleigh Dickinson University Press, 1977. 309 p.

**Before 500 A.D.**

Osborn JW, Hillman J: Enamel structure in some therapsids and mesozoic mammals. **Calcif Tissue Int** 1979 Nov;29(1):47–61
Oxnard CE, Lisowski FP: Functional articulation of some hominoid foot bones: implications for the Olduvai (hominid 8) foot. **Am J Phys Anthropol** 1980 Jan;52(1):107–17
Prager EM, Wilson AC, Lowenstein JM, et al: Mammoth albumin. **Science** 1980 Jul 11;209(4453):287–9
Swinton WE: Brains of dinosaurs. In Rose FC, Bynum WF, ed: Historical aspects of the neurosciences. New York, Raven, 1982. p. 473–9.
Symposium: adaptive grades in the evolution of primates: **Z Morphol Anthropol** 1980;71(2):113–227
Szalay FS: A critique of some recently proposed paleogene primate taxa

and suggested relationships. **Folia Primatol (Basel)** 1982;37(3-4):153-62

**Brazil**

Araújo AJ, Confalonieri UE, Ferreira LF: Oxyurid infestations in small animals from 9,000 B.P. in Brazil. **Paleopathol Newsl** 1980 Sep;(31):13-14

**Great Britain**

Singer R, Wolff RG, Gladfelter BG, et al: Pleistocene Macaca from Hoxne, Suffolk, England. **Folia Primatol (Basel)** 1982;37(3-4):141-52

**Greco-Roman**

Bodson L: Des animaux parmi les hommes. L'ethnozoologie appliquée à l'Antiquité gréco-romaine. **Cah Clio** 1979;:9-16

Dierauer U: Tier und Mensch im Denken der Antike: Studien zur Tierpsychologie, Anthropologie, und Ethik. Amsterdam, Grüner, 1977. xvii, 320 p. (Studien zur antiken Philosophie, 6.).

**Greece**

Bodson L: Aristotle's statement on the reproduction of sharks. **J Hist Biol** 1983 Fall;16(3):391-407

Hidiroglou M: The form and structure of the horse in Greek sculpture. **Hist Med Vet** 1977;2(2):37-41

Hidiroglou M: The horse in the low reliefs of the Parthenon. **Hist Med Vet** 1977;2(4):102-5

Kung J: Aristotle's De motu animalium and the separability of the sciences. **J Hist Philos** 1982;20:65-76

**United States**

Neiburger EJ: Lesions in a prehistoric bear: differential diagnosis. **Paleopathol Newsl** 1984 Dec;(48):8-11

**USSR**

Barnhart MI, Barmatoski SP, Goodman M, et al: Tissue vestiges of an ancient Magadan mammoth calf. **Scan Electron Microsc** 1980;(pt 2):163-70

Reyman TA, Goodman M: The histology of ancient mammoth tissue. **Paleopathol Newsl** 1981 Jan;33:13-5

**500 A.D.-1450**

Henkel N: Studien zum Physiologus im Mittelalter. Tübingen, Max Niemeyer, 1976. xi, 227 p. (Hermaea Germanistische Forschungen, N. F. xi, Bd. 38).

Steudel K: New estimates of early hominid body size. **Am J Phys Anthropol** 1980 Jan;52(1):52-63

**Arabic**

Bel-Haj Mahmoud N: La psychologie des animaux chez les arabes, notamment à travers le kitab al-hayawan de Djahiz. Paris, Klincksieck, 1977. xxiii, 231 p. (Etudes arabes et islamiques, Série 3; Etudes et documents, 8).

Faruqi AH: Use of leeches in Greco-Arab medicine. **Stud Hist Med** 1982 Jun;6(2):137-40

**1450-1700**

**Great Britain**

Oppenheimer JM: Harvey, William. Disputations touching the generation of animals: essay review. **Trans Stud Coll Physicians Phila** 1982 Dec;4(4):306-9

Whitteridge G: Of the local movement of animals. **Proc R Soc Lond [Biol]** 1979 Nov 30;206(1162):1-13

**Italy**

Gottdenker P: Francesco Redi and the fly experiments. **Bull Hist Med** 1979 Winter;53(4):575-92

**Netherlands**

Houtzager HL: Dieren in Delft. **Tijdschr Geschied Geneeskd** 1979;2(2):52-61

**1700 to Present**

Betteridge KJ: An historical look at embryo transfer. **J Reprod Fertil** 1981 May;62(1):1-13

Chang MC: [History and background of research on fertilization in mammals] (Chi). **Sheng Li Ko Hsueh Chin Chan** 1983 Oct;14(4):289-93

Continenza B, Gagliasso E: Ricerche pre-etologiche sul comportamento sociale animale e umano. **Physis** 1980;22(3-34):355-78

Fenner F: Mousepox (infectious ectromelia): past, present, and future. **Lab Anim Sci** 1981 Oct;31(5 Pt 2):553-9

Gallistel CR: Bell, Magendie, and the proposals to restrict the use of animals in neurobehavioral research. **Am Psychol** 1981 Apr;36(4):357-60

Jonas AM: The mouse in biomedical research. **Physiologist** 1984 Oct;27(5):330-46

Kenyon J: Brain stimulation and affective behavior: a note on an early demonstration of a 'reward center'. **J Hist Behav Sci** 1981;17:174-5

Key JD, Rodin AE: William Osler and Arthur Conan Doyle versus the antivivisectionists: some lessons from history for today. **Mayo Clin Proc** 1984 Mar;59(3):189-96

Lippert GP: Xenogener Uretterersatz in Tierversuch unter besonderer Berücksichtigung der historischen Entwicklung von Ureterbioprothesen. Diss. Mainz, 1979. 43 p.

Ribnick R: A short history of primate field studies: old world monkeys and apes. In F. Spencer, ed: A history of American physical anthropology, 1930-1980. New York, Academic Press, 1982. p. 49-73.

Roth N: Animal electricity. **Med Instrum** 1980 Jul-Aug;14(4):228

Roth N: Bugs and blasphemy: Andrew Crosse and the Acarus electricus. **Med Instrum** 1979 Nov-Dec;13(6):357

Schurig V: Die Eingliederung des Begriffs 'Ethologie' in das System der Biowissenschaften im 19. Jahrhundert. **Sudhoffs Arch** 1984;68(1):94-104

Sechzer JA: The ethical dilemma of some classical animal experiments. **Ann NY Acad Sci** 1983;406:5-12

Turner J: Reckoning with the beast. Animals, pain, and humanity in the Victorian mind. Baltimore, London, Johns Hopkins University Press, 1980. xii, 190 p. (The Johns Hopkins University Studies in Historical and Political Science; 98th ser., no. 2).

Turner JC: Kindness to animals: The animal-protection movement in England and America during the 19th century. Ph.D. diss., Harvard University. Cambridge, 1976.

**Africa**

McMartin DA, MacOwan KJ, Swift LL: A century of classical contagious caprine pleuropneumonia: from original description to aetiology. **Br Vet J** 1980 Sep-Oct;136(5):507-15

**France**

Charroppin P: L'escargot contre la hernie? **Rev Hist Pharm (Paris)** 1983 Sep;30(258):215-9

Fleckenstein K: Etienne Marey and the electric torpedo fish. **Med Instrum** 1984 Sep-Oct;18(5):288-9

Vidal F: Les drogues tirées du corps des animaux dans la matière médicale du XVIIIe siècle. **Chir Dent Fr** 1984 Feb 2;54(235):21-9

**Germany**

Hofschulte B: Die Geschichte des Schlacht- und Viehhofes der Stadt Karlsruhe bis zum Jahre 1927. Diss., Tierärzliche Hochschule Hannover. Hannover, 1983. 226 p.

Moschner H: Wissenschaftliche Arbeit und Lehre des Bonner Physiologen Eduard Friedrich Wilhelm Pflüger auf dem Gebiet des tierischen Stoffwechsels. Diss. Bonn, 1981. 233 p.

**Great Britain**

Bendiner E: Jenner: from folklore to scientific triumph. **Hosp Pract [Off]** 1984 Apr;19(4):183-7, 190-1, 196, passim

Cooper JE: Some aspects of John Hunter's work on the diseases of birds of prey. **Ann R Coll Surg Engl** 1982 Sep;64(5):345-7

Radford P: Gilbert White: medical and social aspects of his letters. **Bristol Med Chir J** 1984 Apr;99(370):46-7

Wilkinson L: 'The other' John Hunter, M.D., F.R.S. (1754-1809): his contributions to the medical literature, and to the introduction of animal experiments into infectious disease research. **Notes Rec R Soc Lond** 1982 Feb;36(2):227-41

**Ireland**

Niven Mackay IM: The relationship between human and animal health in nineteenth century Dublin. **Vet Hist** 1984;3(3):110-4

**Italy**

Azzone GF: L'opinione di studiosi sulla vivisezione. **Minerva Med** 1980 May 7;71(18):1334-5

**Japan**

Tajima Y: [30 years of research using experimental animals--transition from bacteriology to the study of experimental animals] (Jpn). **Nippon Saikingaku Zasshi** 1984 Jul;39(4):739-43

# ANIMALS

**Netherlands**

Bardell D: Antoni van Leeuwenhoek's explanation in 1704 of the function of eyelids. **J Hist Med Allied Sci** 1984 Oct;39(4):464–7

**Sweden**

Ahlström CG: Om spansk fluga och dess medicinska användning i Lund. **Sydsven Medicinhist Sallsk Arsskr** 1984;21:49–61

**United States**

Bayer RA: Q fever as an occupational illness at the National Institutes of Health. **Public Health Rep** 1982 Jan–Feb;97(1):58–60
Brewer NR: Personalities in the early history of laboratory animal science and medicine. **Lab Anim Sci** 1980 Aug;30(4 pt 2):741–58
Burrows GE: Lead toxicosis in domestic animals: a review of the role of lead mining and primary lead smelters in the United States. **Vet Hum Toxicol** 1981 Oct;23(5):337–43
Clarkson TB: Evolution and history of training and academic programs in laboratory animal medicine. **Lab Anim Sci** 1980 Aug;30(4 pt 2):790–2
Dunlap TR: DDT: scientists, citizens, and public policy. Princeton, Princeton University Press, 1981. 318 p.
Flynn RJ: The founding and early history of the American Association for Laboratory Animal Science. **Lab Anim Sci** 1980 Aug;30(4 pt 2):765–79
Foster HL: The history of commercial production of laboratory rodents. **Lab Anim Sci** 1980 Aug;30(4 pt 2):793–8
Goldhaft TM: Historical note on the origin of the LaSota strain of Newcastle disease virus. **Avian Dis** 1980 Apr–Jun;24(2):297–301
Grafton TS: The founding and early history of the National Society for Medical Research. **Lab Anim Sci** 1980 Aug;30(4 pt 2):759–64
Hill BF: The founding and early history of the Institute of Laboratory Animal Resources. **Lab Anim Sci** 1980 Aug;30(4 pt 2):780–5
Kaufman M, Kaufman HJ: Henry Bergh, Kit Burns, and the sportsmen of New York. **NY Folkl Q** 1972;28(1):15–29
Koucky RW: The buffalo disaster of 1882. **ND Hist** 1983;50(1):23–30
Lederer SE: 'The right and wrong of making experiments on human beings': Udo J. Wile and syphilis. **Bull Hist Med** 1984 Fall;58(3):380–97
Loew FM: Animal experimentation. **Bull Hist Med** 1982 Spring;56(1):123–6
McClary A: 'Swat the Fly': popular magazines and the anti-fly campaign. **Prev Med** 1982 May;11(3):373–8
McPherson CW: The origins of laboratory animal science at the National Institutes of Health. **Lab Anim Sci** 1980 Aug;30(4 pt 2):786–9
Midkiff VC: The history of feed analysis, as chronicled in the development of AOAC official methods, 1884–1984. **J Assoc Off Anal Chem** 1984 Sep–Oct;67(5):851–60
Miller M: The Walter Bradford Cannon Papers. **Surv Sources Newsl** 1977 May;5:8–9
The origins of laboratory animal science and medicine: proceedings of a symposium presented at the 30th annual session of the American Association for Laboratory Animal Science, Atlanta, 16–21 September 1979.: **Lab Anim Sci** 1980 Aug;30(4 pt 2):737–800
Palmer VA: Lenore H. Cawker, the animals' friend. **Milw Hist** 1979;2(2):43–8
Pauly PJ: The Loeb–Jennings debate and the science of animal behavior. **J Hist Behav Sci** 1981 Oct;17(4):504–15
Salem J: Coon dog graveyard. **South Exposure** 1979;7(3):27–9
Sechzer JA: Historical issues concerning animal experimentation in the United States. **Soc Sci Med [F]** 1981 Mar;15F(1):13–7
Sechzer JA: The use of animals for experimentation in the United States. **Psychopharmacol Bull** 1981 Apr;17(2):88–91
Stockton JJ, ed: A century of service. Veterinary medicine in Indiana, 1884–1984. Indianapolis, Indiana Veterinary Medical Association, 1984. 199 p.
Worth D, Beck AM: Multiple ownership of animals in New York City. **Trans Stud Coll Physicians Phila** 1981 Dec;5(3 no 4):280–300

**USSR**

Maruashvili GM: Istoriia zavoza gambuzii v SSSR (k 100–letiiu so dnia rozhdeniia N. P. Rukhadze). **Med Parazitol (Mosk)** 1980 Jan–Feb;49(1):80–2

# ART

See also **Exhibits; Medical Illustration; Photography; Portraits; Symbolism and Heraldry**

Appels A: Cultural aspects of coronary prone behavior. An approach from the history of art. **Adv Cardiol** 1982;29:32–6
Bartels M, ed: Mensch und Tod: Totentanzsammlung der Universität Düsseldorf. Eine Ausstellung. Düsseldorf, Goethe–Museum, [1978?] 111 p. Einführung von H. Schadewaldt.
Benedum J, Michler M: Das Siegel der Medizinischen Fakultät Giessen. Giessen, Universitätsbibliothek, 1982. 47 p., [18 leaves]. (Berichte und Arbeiten aus der Universitätsbibliothek Giessen, no. 35).
Bonuzzi L: Per l'iconologia della melancolia. **Acta Med Hist Patav** 1980–81;27:55–80
Boussel P, Bonnemain H, Bove FJ: Histoire de la pharmacie et de l'Industrie pharmaceutique. Paris, Editions de la Porte Verte, 1982. 287 p.
Brinkman AA: Chemie in de Kunst. Amsterdam, Rodopi, 1975. 69 p.
Brinkman AA: De alchemist in de prentkunst. Amsterdam, Rodopi, 1982. 69 p. Reprint of several articles. (Nieuwe Nederlandse Bijdragen tot de Geschiedenis der Geneeskunde en der Natururwetenschappen, no. 5).
Burgess R: The dance of Death. An iconographic interpretation of the popular theme of death through five centuries. **Soc Soc Hist Med Bull (Lond)** 1980 Jun;26:25–37
Carstensen G: Die Chirurgie in der Kunst. Düsseldorf, Econ, 1983. 206 p.
Cohen IB: From Leonardo to Lavoisier 1450–1800. New York, Scribner's, 1980. xiii. 298 p. (Album of Science).
Cone TE: A rachitic infant painted by Burgkmair 136 years before Dr. Whistler described rickets. **Clin Pediatr (Phila)** 1980 Mar;19(3):194
Dotz W, Berliner N: Rhinophyma. A master's depiction, a patron's affliction. **Am J Dermatopathol** 1984 Jun;6(3):231–5
Dotz W: St. Anthony's fire. **Am J Dermatopathol** 1980 Fall;2(3):249–53
Duff W: An essay on original genius and its various modes of exertion in philosophy and the fine arts, particularly in poetry (1767). Facsimile. Ed. by J. L. Mahoney. Delmar, New York, Scholars' Facsimiles and Reprints, 1978. ix, 296 p.
Dumaitre P: La curieuse destinée des planches anatomiques de Gérard de Lairesse, peintre en Hollande – Lairesse, Bidloo, Cowper. Amsterdam, Rodopi, 1982. xvii, 107 p. (Nieuwe Nederlandse Bijdragen tot de Geschiedenis der Geneeskunde en der Natuurwetenschappen, no. 6).
Dustmann HO, Ebel V: Darstellungen von Fussdeformierungen und deren Behandlung in der Kunst. In KF Schlegel, ed: Der Körperbehinderte in Mythologie und Kunst. Stuttgart, New York, Thieme, 1983. p. 41–56.
Dustmann HO: Das Bildnis des Amputierten in der Kunst. In KF Schlegel, ed: Der Körperbehinderte in Mythologie und Kunst. Stuttgart, New York, Thieme, 1983. p. 57–87.
Emmerson JS, ed: Catalogue of the Pybus collection of medical books, letters and engravings, 15th–20th centuries, held in the University Library, Newcastle upon Tyne. Newcastle Upon Tyne, Manchester University Press, for the University Library, 1981. xiv, 270 p.
Fulton T: Through the artist's eyes. **Ulster Med J** 1982;51(1):1–22
Furukawa A: [The rod of Asklepios and Hygieia's cup--medico-dental and pharmacological symbols] (Jpn). **Shikai Tenbo** 1981 Nov;58(5):977–86
Gicklhorn R, Göpfert W, Müller I, et al: Bemerkungen zur Geschichte und Ikonographie des Drachenbaumes. **Dtsch Apoth Ztg** 1980 Jul 3;120(27):1260–6
Gilman SL: Seeing the insane: a cultural history of madness and art in the western world, showing how the portrayal of stereotypes has both reflected and shaped the perception and treatment of the mentally disturbed. New York, Wiley; Brunner/Mazel, 1982. xiii, 241 p.
Gribanov ED: Emblemy meditsiny. Tbilisi, Sabchota Sakartvelo, 1979. 111 p.
Hausmann W: Weibliche Fruchtbarkeitssymbole der Quanchen und Tarasken. **Tierarztl Prax** 1983;11(3):417–20
The healing art: **Am Heritage** 1981;32(4):16–27
Hovesen E: Slangen i laegekunsten. **Dan Medicinhist Arbog** 1983;12:105–21
Huard P: El problema de la representación del cuerpo humano. Su evolución en Eurasia. **Nueva Enferm** 1979 Dec;(7):3–6
Huard P, Laplane R: Histoire illustrée de la puériculture: aspects diététiques, socio–culturels et ethnologiques. Paris, Les Editions Roger Dacosta, 1979?, 196 p.
Illustrations from the Wellcome Institute Library: A note on the botanical prints and drawings.
Jacobs N: Les dents et la peinture classique et contemporaine. **Actual Odontostomatol (Paris)** 1981;136:631–51
Jago JD: Early dental charlatans and quacks. **Bull Hist Dent** 1984 Oct;32(2):118–25
Kallinich G, Schmidt–Glassner H: Schöne alte Apotheken. 2. Auflage. München, Callwey, 1977. 251 p.
Kemper R: Zur Syphillis–Erkrankung des Conrad Celtis zum 'Vaticinium' Ulsens und zum sogenannten 'Pestbild' Dürers. **Arch Kulturgesch** 1977;59:99–118
Kierulf H: L'ergotisme chez Bosch et Grünewald. **Nouv Presse Med** 1982 Oct 2;11(38):2803–9
Kronick DA: Artists and anatomists, some notes for an exhibit of anatomical atlases. **Friends P. I. Nixon Med Hist Libr** 1978 Oct;7:1–7
La médicine populaire: Exposition, 27 mars – 17 mai 1981. Bruxelles, Galerie CGER, 1981. 109 p.
Ladendorf H: Der alte Mensch in der Kunst. In Göpfert W, Otten HH, ed: Metavoeite: wandelt euch durch neues Denken. Düsseldorf, Triltsch, 1983. p. 55–68.
Lénárt G, László G: Das Erleben der Verstümmelung in der alten Kunst. In KF Schlegel, ed: Der Körperbehinderte in Mythologie und Kunst. Stuttgart, New York, Thieme, 1983. p. 29–39.
Leon L: Cos'è un ex libris. **Kos** 1984 Jun;1(5):112–6
Lorenz B: Il medico bibliofilo. **Kos** 1984 Jun;1(5):101–11
Loux F: L'ogre et la dent. Pratiques et savoirs populaires relatifs aux dents. Paris, Berger–Levrault, 1981. 186 p.

McHenry LC: Neurology and Art. In Rose FC, Bynum WF, ed: Historical aspects of the neurosciences. New York, Raven, 1982. p. 481–519.
Meurer-Keldenich M: Medizinische Literatur zur Bildnerei von Geisteskranken. Köln, 1979. 327 p. (Kölner medizinhistorische Beiträge, Band 14)
Modig M: The allegory of Christ in a pharmacy. **Pharm Hist** 1984;26(1):44–5
Moray G, Moray N: A note on the basis of reversed perspective. **Perception** 1982;10(6):703–5
Ober WB: Bottoms up! The fine arts and flagellation. Part I. **Am J Dermatopathol** 1984 Oct;6(5):451–60
Ober WB: Can the leper change his spots? The iconography of leprosy. Part I. **Am J Dermatopathol** 1983 Feb;5(1):43–58
Ouvrard J: Perception de l'angoisse et de l'anxiété par quelques artistes à travers les siècles. **Actual Odontostomatol (Paris)** 1983 Dec;144:593–622
Poulet W: Atlas on the history of spectacles. Volume Two. The arts and spectacles over five centuries. Bonn-Bad Godesberg, Wayenborgh, 1980. 505 p.
Raddatz FJ: Der Zahn, behandelt durch den Künstler. **Zahnarztl Mitt** 1983 Dec 1;73(23):2603–32
Reimers D: Tuberkulose und Kunst. **Med Welt** 1982 Mar 26;33(12):435–41
Schadewaldt H: Der Zahnarzt in der Kunst. **Zahnarztl Mitt** 1983 Dec 16;73(24):2760, 2762–4, 2768–70
Schadewaldt H: Kunst und Ophthalmologie. **Ber Zusammenkunft Dtsch Ophthalmol Ges** 1979;76:9–16
Schadewaldt H: Totentanz und Heilberufe. **Jahrb Univ Dusseld** 1980/81;:171–84
Schlegel KF: Der Körperbehinderte in Mythologie und Kunst. Stuttgart; New York, Thieme, 1983. 125 p.
Schlegel KF: Luzifer - ein orthopädischer Patient. In KF Schlegel, ed: Der Korperbehinderte in Mythologie und Kunst. Stuttgart, New York, Thieme, 1983. p. 19–27.
Schlegel KF, ed: Der Körperbehinderte in Mythologie und Kunst. Stuttgart, New York, Georg Thieme Verlag, 1983. 125 p.
Scholz A: Von kleinen und grossen Tumoren in der Kunst. **Hautarzt** 1982 Nov;33(11):598–604
Schuster E: Arzt, Apotheker und Tod in den Totentanzdarstellungen. **Apoth J** 1984;7:47–52
Schuster E: Erbauungsbilder in der Totentanzsammlung (Mensch und Tod) der Universität Düsseldorf. In Göpfert W, Otten HH, ed: Metavoeite: wandelt euch durch neues Denken. Düsseldorf, Triltsch, 1983. p. 41–54.
Silverman FN: De l'art du diagnostic des nanismes et du diagnostic des nanismes dans l'art. **J Radiol** 1982 Feb;63(2):133–40
Simon P, Seifert E: Rollende Hilfsmittel fur Körperbehinderte als Gegenstand in der bildenden Kunst. In KF Schlegel, ed: Der Körperbehinderte in Mythologie und Kunst. Stuttgart, New York, Thieme, 1983. p. 89–125.
Skvortsov VIa, Skvortsova AI: Obrazy vracheĭ v proizvedeniiakh literatury i iskusstva. **Sov Zdravookhr** 1984;(9):59–62
Smith DB: The science of medicine and the art of hypnosis. **Pharos** 1980 Winter;43(1):6–9
Sournia JC, Martiny M, Poulet J, et al., ed: Illustrierte Geschichte der Medizin. Salzburg, Andreas, 1980. 9 vols. (Transl. of Histoire de la médecine de la pharmacie, de l'art dentaire, et de l'art vétérinaire, Paris, 1978).
Sullivan EJ: Depictions of skin ailments in Western European and American art from the Middle Ages to the 20th century. **Am J Dermatopathol** 1982 Aug;4(4):343–52
Talbott JH: Medical maladies as seen by the artist. **JAMA** 1981 Feb 6;245(5):497–8
Theopold W: Das Kind in der Votivmalerei. Munich, Karl Thiemig, 1981.
Thomasen AL: Fra Trinitatis kirkes Loft til Universitetsbibliotekets 2. afdeling i følgeskab med Niels Stensen. **Ugeskr Laeger** 1983 Jun 27;145 Spec No:78–96
Tinkelenberg J: On the morphology of creative forms and art. **Acta Morphol Neerl Scand** 1983 Mar;21(1):83–95
Vega Diaz F: El corazón en la simbología y en la iconografía profana y religiosa. In Academia Nacional de Medicina. Libro conmemorativo del primer centenario. México, Comité Editorial de la Comisión Organizadora del Congreso del Centenario, 1964. Tome 2. p. 78–82.
Vogt H: Das Bild des Kranken. Die Darstellung äusserer Veränderungen durch innere Leiden und ihrer Heilmassnahmen von der Renaissance bis in unsere Zeit. 2d. ed. München, Bergmann, 1980. 384 p.
Wackenheim A: Die Entwicklung der menschlichen Hand in der Kunst. **Radiologe** 1982 May;22(5):195–8
Wells EB: The disease horse. **Factotum** 1981;12:14
Woodruff AW: J M W Turner and some of his predecessors and successors, from the viewpoint of medical history. **J R Soc Med** 1980 May;73(5):381–92
Wüger HJ: Die Darstellung des Schmerzes in der bildenden Kunst. **Ther Umsch** 1983 Aug;40(8):679–82
Zglinicki F von: Die Uroskopie in der bildenden Kunst: eine kunst- und medizinhistorische Untersuchung über die Harnschau. Darmstadt, G-I-T Verlag Giebeler, 1982. 173 p.
Zhang Baochang: [Knowledge of the human body displayed in inscriptions on bone and tortoise shell.] (Chi). **Chin J Med Hist** 1981;11:235–40

### Africa

Cervenka J: African mask with cleft lip and palate. **Cleft Palate J** 1984 Jan;21(1):38–40
Schechter DC: Medical motifs in West African sculptures. **NY State J Med** 1980 May;80(6):1000–12

### Americas

Robicsek F: The smoking gods; tobacco in Maya art, history, and religion. Norman, Oklahoma, Univ. of Oklahoma Press, 1978. xxv, 233 p.

### Belgium

Homblé AG: Het keisnijden. Kwakzalverij of werkelijkheid? **Oostvlaam Zanten** 1980;55:105–14

### China

Winder M: Il Buddha della medicina. **Kos** 1984 Apr;1(3):55–74

### Denmark

Kofod H: Danish contributions to the unicorn story. **Beitr Gesch Pharm** 1979;31(2):12–15

### France

Garnot NS, Simon N: Parigi degli ospedali. **Kos** 1984 May;1(4):95–114
Julien P: Deux saints médecins et pharmaciens, Côme et Damien. **Bull Liaison Assoc Amis Mus Pharm Montp** 1982;:(7):13–35
Patrimoine hospitalier de la Bourgogne: [Dijon], Ministère de la Culture et de la Communication; Direction Régionale des Affaires Culturelles de Bourgogne, 1980. 163 p. Contributions by E. Pommier, J. Gaillard, S. Deyts, J. Richard, M. Guillaume, C. Lamarre-Tainturier.

### Germany

Dobras W: Cosmas und Damian in oberbayerischen Kirchen. **Pharm Ztg** 1981 Dec 24;126(52-53):2715–6
Völksen W: Die Stuckbilder der Berg-Apotheke in Clausthal-Zellerfeld. **Beitr Gesch Pharm** 1984;31(23):197–203

### Great Britain

McWilliam CE: The college buildings and their architects. In Passmore R, ed: Proceedings of the Royal College of Physicians of Edinburgh Tercentenary Congress, 1981. Edinburgh, Royal College of Physicians of Edinburgh, 1982. p. 92–102.

### Hungary

Benko F: Die Gemälde der Apotheke zum Goldenen Einhorn im Debrecziner Déri Museum. In Hein WH, ed: Pharmaziehistorischer Kongress, Budapest, 1981. Stuttgart, Wissenschaftliche Verlagsgesellschaft, 1983. p. 85–96.
Fleishmann-Bánó M, Zalai K: St. Cosmas and St. Damian relics in Hungary. **Ther Hung** 1981;29(3):142–6

### Italy

Rocchietta S: Due raffigurazioni di santa Apollonia. (sec. XVI e sec. XVIII). **Minerva Med** 1983 Oct 6;74(38):2245–6
Rocchietta S: Iconografia statuaria e pittorica di Santa Apollonia nel Duomo di Milano. **Minerva Med** 1981 Jan 14;72(1):45–9
Roth W: Lentigo maligna und Sclerodermia circumscripta auf Olgemälden der Uffizien. **Hautarzt** 1982 Apr;33(4):229–30

### Japan

Homma K: On the toothpick. In International Congress of the History of Medicine. 26th, Plovdiv, 1978. Actes du Congress. Sofia, 1981. Volume II. p. 111–4.

### Mexico

Fuente JR de la, Alarcón-Segovia D: Depression as expressed in pre-Columbian Mexican art. **Am J Psychiatry** 1980 Sep;137(9):1095–8

### Netherlands

Haneveld GT: Oude medische gebouwen van Nederland. Amsterdam, Meesters, 1976. 218 p.
Schenk J: Homoseksualiteit in de Nederlandse beeldende kunst voor 1800. **Spiegel Hist** 1982;17(11):576–83

# ART

### Peru

Dobkin de Rios M, Cardenas M: Plant hallucinogens, shamanism and Nazca ceramics. **J Ethnopharmacol** 1980 Sept;2(3):233–46
Doig FK: Sexualverhalten im alten Peru. Lima, Kompaktos, 1979. 189 p.
Kauffmann Doig F: Comportamiento sexual en el antiguo Perú. Lima, Kompaktos G. S., [1978]. 189 p.

### Poland

Roeske W: Freski z dawnych polskich aptek. **Arch Hist Med (Warsz)** 1980;43(2):191–7

### United States

Gerdts WH: The art of healing: medicine and science in American art. [Birmingham, Alabama], Birmingham Museum of Art, 1981. 119 p. (Exhibit, Birmingham, 1981).
Pontius AA: Face representation linked with literacy level in colonial American tombstone engravings and Third World preliterates' drawings. Toward a cultural-evolutional neurology. **Experientia** 1982 May 15;38(5):577–81

### USSR

Murav'eva EF: Meditsinskie temy v ékspozitsii Gosudarstvennogo Ermitazha. **Sov Zdravookhr** 1984;(9):62–5
Schmidt-Voigt J: Russische Ikonmalerei und Medizin. München, Thiemig. 1980. 168 p.
Skvortsov VIa: O nekotorykh aspektakh istoricheskoĭ vzaimosviazi meditsiny i iskusstva. **Vestn Akad Med Nauk SSSR** 1982;(4):57–65

## Before 500 A.D.

Campillo D, Viñas R: Contribución a la paleopatología a través del arte rupestre. In International Congress of the History of Medicine, 27th, Barcelona, 1980. Actas. Barcelona, Académia de Ciències Médiques de Catalunya i Balears, 1981. p. 462–71.
Haensch WG: Die menschlichen statuetten des mittleren Jungpaläolithikums aus der sicht der Somatischen Anthropologie. Bonn, Habelt, 1982. 294 p. (Antiquitas, 2).
Kiss A: Medizinal-kultische Darstellungen und Hinweise altertümlicher Mosaiken. **Orvostort Kozl** 1981;93–96(27 No 1–4):79–82
Marí VJ: El martirio de Santa Agatha, un precedente de la mastectomia. Représentacion artistica con especial referencia a una coleccion de tallas. In International Congress of the History of Medicine. 26th, Plovdiv, 1978. Actes du Congress. Sofia, 1981. Volume II. p. 150–7.
Niederland WG: Morbid conditions expressed in prehistoric art. **Am J Psychiatry** 1981 Jan;138(1):126–7
Pontius AA: Icono-diagnosis, a medical-humanistic approach, detecting Crouzon's malformation in Cook Islands' prehistoric art. **Perspect Biol Med** 1983 Autumn;27(1):107–20
Schadewaldt H: Orthopädische Aspekte der Mythologie. In KF Schlegel, ed: Der Körperbehinderte in Mythologie und Kunst. Stuttgart, New York, Thieme, 1983. p. 1–18.
Schumacher HR, Alarcon-Segovia D: Osteoarthritic knees in a Pre-Columbian ceramic figure. **J Rheumatol** 1980 May–Jun;7(3):381–2
Sermonti G: Orpheus in Perugia. **Riv Biol** 1981 Winter;74(4):453–8

### Asia

Hausmann W: Der Becher des Gudea. **Tierarztl Prax** 1979;7(2):141–3

### Colombia

Torres CM: Evidence for snuffing in the prehispanic stone sculpture of San Agustín, Colombia. **J Psychoactive Drugs** 1981 Jan–Mar;13(1):53–60

### Egypt

Reeves C: Illustrations of medicine in ancient Egypt. **J Audiov Media Med** 1980 Jan;3(1):4–13

### Europe

Grimm H: Weibliche Figurinen als Zeugnisse vorgeschichtlicher Jugendweihe-Riten? **Aerztl Jugendkd** 1982 Mar;73(1):40–3

### France

Hooper A: Further information on the prehistoric representations of human hands in the cave of Gargas. **Med Hist** 1980 Apr;24(2):214–16
Wildgoose M, Hadingham E, Hooper A: The prehistoric hand pictures at Gargas: attempts at simulation. **Med Hist** 1982 Apr;26(2):205–7

### Greco-Roman

Sandyk R: Brain development and the phylogenesis of writing and drawing direction. **S Afr Med J** 1982 Jul 10;62(2):43–4

### Greece

Callmer C: Tre bilder av grekiska läkare. **Sydsven Medicinhist Sallsk Arsskr** 1981;:30–8
Hidiroglou M: The form and structure of the horse in Greek sculpture. **Hist Med Vet** 1977;2(2):37–41
Hidiroglou M: The horse in the low reliefs of the Parthenon. **Hist Med Vet** 1977;2(4):102–5
Smith NW: Illusions and counter-illusions or aesthetic effects in Greek temples? **Stor Crit Psicol** 1983 Dec;4(2):157–70

### India

Murthy CK: Sculpture of fasting Buddha; artist's knowledge of anatomy in ancient India. **Bull Inst Hist Med (Hyderabad)** 1973 Oct;3(4):186–8

### Italy

Marsili A, Bregante-Marsili D, Santoni-Rugiu P: The horned hand: an acquired deformity, or just another Etruscan mystery? **Br J Plast Surg** 1980 Jan;33(1):56–60

### Mexico

Martínez Marañón R: Urna olmeca que podría representar la leishmaniasis tegumentaria diseminada. **Salud Publica Mex** 1982 Sep–Oct;24(5):497–507

### Peru

Dobkin de Rios M: Plant hallucinogens, sexuality and shamanism in the ceramic art of ancient Peru. **J Psychoactive Drugs** 1982 Jan–Jun;14(1–2):81–90
Selmanowitz VJ: Impressions of Sechnin. Anatomy by slaughter. **NY State J Med** 1980 Dec;80(13):2016–21

### Rome

Benedum J: Die Augenanomalie an einem römischen Bildnis. **Medizinhist J** 1981;16(4):446–52
Petrakis NL: Diagonal earlobe creases, type A behavior and the death of Emperor Hadrian. **West J Med** 1980 Jan;132(1):87–91

### Spain

Bernard J, Wintrobe M, Faure E, et al: Le sang d'Altamira ou la naissance de l'hématologie. **Nouv Rev Fr Hematol** 1981;23(4):249–51

### USSR

Moriyama N: [Controversies on the Kul-Oba vase and its relation to the ancient Scythian dentistry (author's transl)] (Jpn). **Shikwa Gakuho** 1980 Apr;80(4):597–602

## 500 A.D.–1450

Friedman JB: The monstrous races in medieval art and thought. Cambridge, London, Harvard University Press, 1981. xiii, 268 p.
Lenhardt F: Zur Ikonographie der Blutschau. **Medizinhist J** 1982;17(1/2):63–77
Nutton V: Galeno salvato dalle acque. **Kos** 1984 Mar;1(2):33–50
Ober WB: Can the leper change his spots? The iconography of leprosy. Part II. **Am J Dermatopathol** 1983 Apr;5(2):173–86
Plant M, Hueston JT: Hands before faces-- the evolution of gesture in fourteenth-century frescoes. **Ann Plast Surg** 1982 Nov;9(5):436–44

### Americas

Björnberg A: Ansiktsmutilationer inom Mochicakonsten. **Sydsven Medicinhist Sallsk Arsskr** 1982;19:32–44

### Arabic

Hein WH: Ein arabisches Apothekeninterieur vom Jahre 1222. **Pharm Ztg** 1979 Jan 4;124(1):3–4

### Belgium

Dequeker JV: Polymyalgia rheumatica with temporal arteritis, as painted by Jan van Eyck in 1436. **Can Med Assoc J** 1981 Jun 15;124(12):1597–8

**France**

Cosman MP: Machaut's medical musical world. In Cosman MP, Chandler B, ed: Machaut's world: science and art in the fourteenth century. New York, New York Academy of Sciences, 1978. (Annals of the New York Academy of Sciences, v. 314). p. 1-36.

**Germany**

Hühns E: Der Berliner Totentanz. **Dtsch Jahrb Volkskd** 1968;14(2):235-46
Valentin P: Mit Brevier und Skalpell. Legendäre Bauchoperation Kaiser Heinrichs II. **Med Welt** 1982 Feb 19;33(7):260-2

**Great Britain**

Foley GP: A treasury of dentistry. The dental attraction of the Wells Cathedral. **J Am Coll Dent** 1983 Fall;50(3):16-7
Schierhorn H: Die Terata auf der Weltkarte des Richard de Haldingham (um 1280). **Gegenbaurs Morphol Jahrb** 1982;128(2):137-67

**Hungary**

Vida M: Az orvosi gyakorlat és a gyógyítószentek ikonográfiája a XIII-XIV. századi magyarországi falfestészetben. **Orvostort Kozl** 1979;87-88(25 no 1-2):13-63

**Italy**

Eramo S: L'odontoiatria nell'arte. Su un affresco raffigurante S. Apollonia nella Basilica di Santa Maria di Collemaggio a l'Aquila. **Dent Cadmos** 1984 Apr;52(4):135-7
Jones P: Secreta Salernitana. **Kos** 1984 Feb;1(1):33-50
Orofino G, Brach CC: Nel nome del bagno. **Kos** 1984 Apr;1(3):33-54

**Netherlands**

Iveson-Iveson J: Joined in parenthood. **Nurs Mirror** 1982 Sep 15;155(11):24

**Peru**

Heck J: Leishmaniasis und Fruchtbarkeitskult. **Dtsch Med Wochenschr** 1982 Jun 4;107(22):872-4

**Thailand**

Kohnen N: 'Ein und dasselbe ist Lebendiges und Totes ...'. Die enthaupteten Mutterschaftsfiguren aus Sawankhalok. **Dtsch Arztebl** 1982 Nov 5;79(44):83-7

**Yugoslavia**

Dolenc A: Medizinische Fragen und Aspekte des mittelalterlichen Totentanzes (Ein Beitrag aus Jugoslawien). **Beitr Gerichtl Med** 1980;38:347-52

**1450-1700**

Cavanagh GS: A new view of the Vesalian landscape. **Med Hist** 1983 Jan;27(1):77-9
Hofmann B: Kranker und Krankheit um 1500. Die Darstellung des Kranken im Zusammenhang mit den spätgotischen Bildnissen der Heiligen Elisabeth. Herzogenrath, Verlag Murken-Altrogge, 1983. 226 p. (Studien zur Medizin-, Kunst- und Literaturgeschichte, Bd. 3).
Huard P, Imbault-Huart MJ: André Vesale, iconographie anatomique (Fabrica, Epitome, Tabulae sex). Paris, Dacosta, 1980. 255 p.
Kierulf H: L'ergotisme chez Bosch et Grünewald. In International Congress of the History of Medicine, 27th, Barcelona, 1980. Actas. Barcelona, Académia de Ciències Médiques de Catalunya i Balears, 1981. p. 81-90.
Massironi M: Considerazioni psicologiche su alcuni fenomeni della visione descritti nei trattati di prospettiva dei secoli XV-XVII. **Stor Crit Psicol** 1983 Dec;4(2):171-214
Parker RG: Academy of fine arts; print from a copper engraving, 1578, by Cornelis Cort after a drawing by Jan Van Der Straet, 1573. **J Hist Med Allied Sci** 1983 Jan;38(1):76-7
Sabin JA, Sanmartín Urchaga P: Estudio comparado de las aportaciones iconográficas, en el sistema muscular, en las obras de Leonardo y Vesalio. In International Congress of the History of Medicine, 27th, Barcelona, 1980. Actas. Barcelona, Académia de Ciències Médiques de Catalunya i Balears, 1981. p. 446-53.
Sullivan EJ: Art in dermatopathology. Jusepe de Ribera. An interpreter of the skin through art. **Am J Dermatopathol** 1979 Summer;1(2):159-62

**Austria**

Grossmann T: Die hl. Ottilie, Patronin der Augenkranken. Eine ungewöhnliche Abbildung am Gnadenstuhlaltar von Bad Aussee mit Krebsscherenattribut. **Klin Monatsbl Augenheilkd** 1981 Jun;178(6):480-1

**Belgium**

Gariepy TP: Hyacum, et lues venerea. **J Hist Med Allied Sci** 1981 Jul;36(3):325

**Ethiopia**

Pankhurst R: Le piaghe d'Etiopia. **Kos** 1984 Jul-Aug;1(6):33-50

**Germany**

Calagan JL: The conjoined twins born near Worms, 1495. **J Hist Med Allied Sci** 1983 Oct;38(4):450-1
Dotz W: Albrecht Dürer. Depictions of facies as expressions of personality. **Am J Dermatopathol** 1981 Spring;3(1):59-65
Eberle MW: Lucas Cranach's cupid as honey thief paintings: allegories of syphilis? **Com J Mediev Renaiss Stud** 1979-80;10:21-30
Grasshoff K: Leibesübungen und Gesellschaft im Gemälde 'Melancolia 1558' des Mathias Gerung. **Stadion** 1977;3(1):44-59
Jaeger W: Symbolische Augendarstellungen in einer Ars Memorandi des 16. Jahrhunderts. **Klin Monatsbl Augenheilkd** 1983 Apr;182(4):337-40
Kraft H: Die Zeichnungen des Augustin Wilhelm. Psychopathologische Aspekte und kulturhistorische Vergleiche. **Confin Psychiatr** 1980;23(4):230-49
Roth W: Differentialdiagnostische Erwägungen zu den Hauteffloreszenzen, dargestellt auf dem Sebastiansaltar Hans Holbeins d. A. **Hautarzt** 1980 Dec;31(12):662-4
Schupbach WM: Elsheimer il malinconico. **Kos** 1984 Jun;1(5):85-100
Tschassovnikarov D, Markov G: Personologische Untersuchungen über einige Urbilder im Schaffen von Hieronymus Bosch. **Psychiatr Neurol Med Psychol (Leipz)** 1980 Oct;32(10):623-30
Virchow R: A painting of lepers by Hans Holbein the Elder. **Am J Dermatopathol** 1984 Aug;6(4):377-8
Wirth J: La jeune fille et la mort: recherches sur les themes macabres dans l'art germanique de la Renaissance. Genève, Droz, 1979. 194 p., 64 p. of plates. (Centre de recherches d'histoire et de philologie de la IVe section de l'Ecole pratique des hautes études. V, Hautes études médiévales et modernes; 36).

**Great Britain**

Cohen B: A tale of two paintings. **Ann R Coll Surg Engl** 1982 Jan;64(1):4-12
Stromquist DL: The true portraiture of a Roman youth; etching by Wenceslaus Hollar, 1641. New Haven, Yale Medical Library, Clements C. Fry Collection. **J Hist Med Allied Sci** 1983 Apr;38(2):176-7

**Italy**

Baur O, Bott B, Braunfels-Esche S, et al: Leonardo da Vinci Anatomie, Physiognomik, Proportion und Bewegung. Köln, 1984. 343 p. (Kölner medizinhistorische Beiträge: Arbeiten der Forschungsstelle des Instituts für Geschichte der Medizin der Universität zu Köln, Band 23/1)
Bencivenni M: Il Principe dello Studiolo. **Kos** 1984 Jul-Aug;1(6):52-78
Dequeker J: Arthritis in the paintings of Sandro Botticelli. **Arthritis Rheum** 1984 Oct;27(10):1196-7
DiGeronimo EM, Marraccini P: Body-mind sculpture: battle of the titans. **Plast Reconstr Surg** 1984 Feb;73(2):324-5
Goldman L: Portrait of an elderly woman with a nodular eruption. What was it? **Am J Dermatopathol** 1982 Aug;4(4):353
Hein WH: Sur le frontispice de la Pharmacopée de Milan de 1698. **Rev Hist Pharm (Paris)** 1982 Jun;29(253):87-90
Jensen JE: More treasures. **Md State Med J** 1982 Nov;31(11):26-9
Kleberger E: Ein Brillenfan des 16. Jahrhunderts. **Klin Monatsbl Augenheilkd** 1982 Sep;181(3):223-6
Leden I: Doubts about Sandro Botticelli's depiction of juvenile rheumatoid arthritis. **Arthritis Rheum** 1984 Oct;27(10):1197-8
Liebert RS: Michelangelo: a psychoanalytic study of his life and images. New Haven, Yale University Press, 1983. xxii, 447 p.
Lines D: 15th century ureteric reflux. **Lancet** 1982 Dec 25;2(8313):1473
Manzi L: I santi protettori degli artisti dello studio bolognese... Santi Cosma e Damiano. **Strenna Stor Bolognese** 1977;27:179-93
Putscher M: Ein Totentanz von Tizian. Die 17 grossen Holzschnitte zur Fabrica Vesals (1538-1542). In Göpfert W, Otten HH, ed: Metavoeite: wandelt euch durch neues Denken. Düsseldorf, Triltsch, 1983. p. 23-40.
Rocchietta S: Von der Apothekergilde während des 15. Jahrhunderts gestiftete Glasfenster im Dom von Mailand. **Beitr Gesch Pharm** 1981;31(13):97-100
Rosenzweig W: Disease in art: a case for carcinoma of the breast in Michelangelo's La notte. **Paleopathol Newsl** 1983 Mar;41:8-11
Roth W: Atherom auf einem Olgemälde Pinakothek in Brescia. **Hautarzt** 1983 Aug;34(8):407-8
Schott GD: Some neurological observations on Leonardo da Vinci's handwriting. **J Neurol Sci** 1979 Aug;42(3):321-9
Schupbach W: Doctor Parma's medicinal macaronic: poem by Bartolotti, pictures by Giorgione and Titian. [Wellcome MS 461].

J Warburg Courtauld Inst 1978;41:147–91, 350
Speransky LS, Bocharov VJ, Goncharov NI: The personages of Jan Stephan van Calcar's frontispiece to Andreas Vesalius' book 'On the Structure of the Human Body'. **Anat Anz** 1983;153(5):465–79
Steinberg L: Michelangelo and the doctors. **Bull Hist Med** 1982;56(4):543–53
Todd EM: The neuroanatomy of Leonardo Da Vinci. Ph.D. Diss., University of California, Los Angeles, 1981 xviii, 267 leaves.
Todd EM: The neuroanatomy of Leonardo da Vinci. Santa Barbara, Capra Press, 1983. 189 p.
Verellen T: Cosmas and Damian in the New Sacristy [Medici Chapel of San Lorenzo, Florence]. **J Warburg Courtauld Inst** 1979;42:274–7

**Korea**

Lee S: Vitiligo auf einem historischen Porträt. **Hautarzt** 1982 Jun;33(6):335–6

**Mexico**

Bárcena A, Barrera A, Ruiz E, et al: Interpretación etnobotánica de la iconografía del Códice de la Cruz-Badiano. **An Soc Mex Hist Cienc Tec** 1979;5:35–48

**Netherlands**

Alting MP, Waterbolk TW: New light on the anatomical errors in Rembrandt's Anatomy Lesson of Dr. Nicolass Tulp. **J Hand Surg** 1982 Nov;7(6):632–4
Appelboom T, Boelpaepe C de, Ehrlich GE, et al: Rubens and the question of antiquity of rheumatoid arthritis. **JAMA** 1981 Feb 6;245(5):483–6
Braithwaite PA, Shugg D: Rembrandt's Bathsheba: the dark shadow of the left breast. **Ann R Coll Surg Engl** 1983 Sep;65(5):337–8
Cremone JC: The anatomy lesson of Dr. Nicolaas Tulp. **J Hand Surg** 1982 Sep;7(5):530
Dixon LS: Alchemical imagery in Bosch's Garden of Delights. Ann Arbor, UMI Research Press, 1981. xxii, 225 p. (Studies in the Fine Arts: Iconography, no. 2).
Dotz W: Jan Vermeer and his alopecic models. **Am J Dermatopathol** 1983 Jun;5(3):245–8
Dymarskiĭ LIu: Taĭna 'Virsavii', kartiny Rembrandta. **Vopr Onkol** 1984;30(10):90–101
Hoppe B: Darstellung der Alchemie in Gemälden von Jan Brueghel d. A. (1568–1625). **Beitr Gesch Pharm** 1983;31(18/19):144–9
Leyh F: Hatte Rembrandt van Rijn eine Nickelallergie? **Hautarzt** 1984 Sep;35(9):472–3
Peck S, Peck H: Prosperity and decay: a portrait of the Dutch golden age. **Dent Abstr** 1980 Mar;25(3):116–8
Pytel' AIa: Bol', prishedshaia iz glubiny vekov (k 375-letiiu so dnia rozhdeniia Rembrandta). **Sov Med** 1980;(12):98–9
Schupbach W: The paradox of Rembrandt's 'Anatomy of Dr. Tulp'. London, Wellcome Institute for the History of Medicine, 1982. 110 p. (Medical History, Suppl. No. 2).
Slenders J: De Anatomische les van Dr. Zacheus de Jager (1640). **Tijdschr Geschied Geneeskd** 1981;4(4):159–67

**Poland**

Jonecko A: Drzeworyt ukazujący amputowane i protezowane podudzie w śląskim poemacie Roździeńskiego 'Officina ferraria' a roku 1612. **Wiad Lek** 1983 Jun 15;36(12):1025–31
Jonecko A: Drzeworyt ukazujacy amputowane i protezowane produdzie w ślaskim poemacie Roździeńskiego 'Officina Ferraria' z roku 1616. **Arch Hist Med (Warsz)** 1984;47(1):107–16

**Spain**

Moskow BS: The iconography of the dental profession. Francisco Zurbarán (1598–1664). **Quintessence Int** 1984 Aug;15(8):814–5
Ravin JG: El Greco of Toledo. **Ohio State Med J** 1982 Nov;78(11):745–53

**Yugoslavia**

Rudelić I: Glagolijski grafiti kao svjedočanstva socijalnih i zdravstvenih prilka u Istri. **Lijec Vjesn** 1984 Jun;106(6):261–4

**1700 to Present**

Ansbacher HL: Discussion of Alfred Alder's preface to The Diary of Vaslav Nijinsky. **Arch Gen Psychiatry** 1981 Jul;38(7):834–41
Beeck M: Merkmale epileptischer Bildnerei: mit Pathographie Van Gogh. Bern, Huber, 1982. 134 p.
Berenbrinker A: Die zahnmedizinische Karikatur I: 1780–1840. Köln, 1982. 227 p. (Arbeiten der Forschungsstelle des Instituts für Geschichte der Medizin der Universität zu Köln, Band 25).
Bresgen C: Homo omnis creatura. Arcimboldo und Paracelsus – eine Gegenüberstellung aus der Sicht des Künstlers. **Salzburger Beitr Paracelsusforsch** 1984;23:36–49
Crellin JK, Helfand WH: Medical care in the 20th century. Facets of change illustrated by American and British postcards. Durham, Duke University Medical Center, 1982. 106 p. (Readings and Perspectives in Medicine, Booklet Number 3).
Dubovsky H: Tuberculosis and art. **S Afr Med J** 1983 Nov 12;64(21):823–6
Feller I: Die zahnmedizinische Karikatur II: 1840–1880. Köln, 1983. 284 p. (Arbeiten der Forschungsstelle des Instituts für Geschichte der Medizin der Universität zu Köln, Band 26).
Fields K, Kontrovitz M: An invisible art blazes into life under microscope. **Smithsonian** 1980;11(7):109–13
Forschbach G: Tuberculosis and creative man. **Bull Int Union Tuberc** 1984 Mar–Jun;59(1–2):104–7
Helfand WH, Crellin JK: The pharmacy in comic postcards. **Pharm Hist** 1981;23(3):107–13
Hügelow M: Original-Lithographien speziell für Pharmazeuten: Historische Apothekergeräte und Heilpflanzen. **Pharm Unserer Zeit** 1984 Jul;13(4):97–101
Iveson-Iveson J: The art of observation. 2. Shock treatment. **Nurs Mirror** 1982 Sep 1;155(9):26
Julien P: Sur le célèbre 'dentiste' ou 'pharmacien' de Pietro Longhi. **Pharm Weekbl** 1981 Nov 6;116(45):1389–92
Koning A: Die Pharmazie in der holländischen politischen Karikatur. **Pharm Acta Helv** 1979;54(9–10):308–10
Kottek SS: 'Andre Vesale'. Some remarks on a painting by E. J. C. Hamman. **Koroth** 1982 Aug;8(3/4):135–43
Lanthony P: Daltonisme et peinture. **Bull Soc Ophtalmol Fr** 1982 Apr;82(4):509–13
Lanthony P: Daltonisme et peinture. **J Fr Ophtalmol** 1982;5(6–7):373–85
Lesky E: Meilensteine der Wiener Medizin. Grosse Arzte Osterreichs in drei Jahrhunderten. Wien, Wilhelm Maudrich, 1981. 251 p.
McCall N: The statue of the Christus Consolator at the Johns Hopkins Hospital: its acquisition and historic origins. **Johns Hopkins Med J** 1982 Jul;151(1):11–9
Meares R: Body feeling in human relations: the possible examples of Brancusi and Giacometti. **Psychiatry** 1980 May;43(2):160–7
Menner O: Kabay jános emléke képzömüvészeti alkotásokon. **Orvostort Kozl** 1981;93–96(27 No 1–4):237–49
Murken AH, Rodegra H: Krankenhausrundbauten in Vergangenheit und Gegenwart. Zur historischen Entwicklung von kreisförmigen Bettenhäusern und panoptisch angelegten Krankensälen. **Hist Hosp** 1979–80;13:197–216
Putscher M: Jaspers und Van Gogh--oder über Krankheit und Kunst. **Janus** 1980;67(1–2–3):157–69
Ross D: Vision and the artist. **Occup Health (Lond)** 1980 Feb;32(2):68–73
Rubin LP: A young woman taken to the doctor by her family. Mezzotint by Johann Andreas Pfeffel after an original painting by Jan Josef Horemans. **J Hist Med Allied Sci** 1981 Oct;36(4):489
Salmon P: Psychosociologie du collectionneur. **Rev Inst Sociol** 1977;2:271–87
Sandblom P: Skapande och Sjukdom. Hur lidande påverkar litteratur, konst och musik. Södertälje, Fingraf Tryckeri, 1983. 142 p. (Nordisk Medicinhistorisk Arsbok, Supplementum IX).
Schiffczyk D: Vom Therapiekonzept zur Architekturform. Betrachtungen über das Terrassenkrankenhaus. **Hist Hosp** 1979–80;13:177–96
Slatter EM: Illustrations from the Wellcome Institute Library: the new lazaretto at Siros (Syra), Greece, in 1840. **Med Hist** 1984 Jan;28(1):73–80
Southgate MT: Vincent van Gogh, portrait of Dr. Gachet. **JAMA** 1981 Feb 20;245(7):657, 688
Sullivan EJ: Beauty marks or pigmented skin lesions? **Am J Dermatopathol** 1981 Fall;3(3):311–2
Vogt H: Medizinische Karikaturen von 1800 bis zur Gegenwart. 5th ed. München, Bergmann, 1980. 184 p.

**Austria**

Poch-Kalous M, Till R: Cajetan. Ein Wiener Mediziner und Karikaturist um die Mitte des 19. Jahrhunderts. **Wien Geschichtsbl** 1967;22(3):220–4
Sugar HS, Foster CC: Maximilian Salzmann. Ophthalmic pioneer and artist. **Surv Ophthalmol** 1981 Jul–Aug;26(1):28–30

**Canada**

Bensley EH: John Poad Drake (1794–1883), the first artist to portray the Hospital. **Montreal Gen Hosp News** 1981;19(1):8–9
Krosnick A: The art of Banting. **J Med Soc NJ** 1984 Feb;81(2):138–9

**Europe**

Kiessling W: Der Tierarzt in der bildenden Kunst seit Gründung der tierärztlichen Bildungsstätten. Diss. Hannover, 1981. 385 p.

**Finland**

Sourander P: Edelfelts berömda pasteurporträtt – originalet och repliken. **Nord Medicinhist Arsbok** 1983;:149–54

### France

Ackerknecht EH: Charles Meryon and physicians. **J Hist Med Allied Sci** 1984 Oct;39(4):462–4
Cantarel-Besson Y: Les morts exemplaires dans la peinture militaire sous le consulat et l'empire. **Rev Inst Napoleon (Paris)** 1977;(133):97–105
Dentistry in folk art XI: L'arracheuse de dents (The tooth puller): **Bull Hist Dent** 1980 Oct;28(2):87
Dotz W: Jean Paul Marat. His life, cutaneous disease, death, and depiction by Jacques Louis David. **Am J Dermatopathol** 1979 Fall;1(3):247–50
Ellenberger M: Fragonard, l'anatomiste. **Pour Sci** 1982;53:98–108
Ferrières M: Les Donatifs Comtadins: une iconographie hospitalière méconnue. **Bull Soc Fr Hist Hop** 1980;(40):23–8
Fossard J: Faut-il rendre à Gamelin l'Ecorché de Bayonne attribué à Géricault? **Hist Sci Med** 1984;18(2):153–8
Gagnière S, Julien P: Panneaux peints de la pharmacie de l'hôpital de Valréas. **Rev Hist Pharm (Paris)** 1981;28(248):21–4
Garmier JF: Soufflot et Mâcon: La charité, l'Hotel-Dieu. **Cah Rech Archit** 1980;6–7, Suppl:142–51
Godonnèche J: La Doulou: auto-observation d'Alphonse Daudet. **Hist Sci Med** 1981;15(4):321–5
Handelsman A: Le médecin hydropathe---color lithograph by Honoré Daumier. **J Hist Med Allied Sci** 1981 Jan;36(1)63
Julien P: Le Dr. Véron et Daumier, ou le fabricant de pâté pectorale en proie à la caricature. In: Congrès international d'histoire de la médecine, XXVe, Québec, 1976. Actes. Québec, 1977. p. 807–21.
Medaer R: Classics in neurology. Etching showing Claude Bernard doing an experiment surrounded by his colleagues. **Neurology** 1982 Oct;32(10):1145
Moskow BS: Dentistry in folk art XV: Decamps--le dentiste. **Bull Hist Dent** 1982 Oct;30(2):128
Moskow BS: The dental cartoons of Honoré Daumier (1808–1879). **J Am Dent Assoc** 1981 Jan;102(1):82–6
Moskow BS: The iconography of the dental profession. **Quintessence Int** 1983 Oct;14(10):1072–3
Moskow BS: The iconography of the dental profession. **Quintessence Int** 1983 Nov;14(11):1184–5
Moskow BS: The iconography of the dental profession. **Quintessence Int** 1983 Dec;14(12):1278–9
Moskow BS: The iconography of the dental profession. **Quintessence Int** 1984 Apr;15(4):406–7
Moskow BS: The iconography of the dental profession. Jean-Ignace-Isidore Gérard Grandville (1803–1847). **Quintessence Int** 1984 Oct;15(10):1028–9
Mulder WJ: De 'Anatomie clastique' van Dr. L. T. J. Anzoux. **Tijdschr Geschied Geneeskd** 1981:4(3):133–43
Ness DE: C'est fini. . . .le pouls ne bat plus! Drawn by Paul Bernay, for Le Charivari, in 1872. **J Hist Med Allied Sci** 1980 Jul;35(3):312
Rocchietta S: Caricature di Daumier correlate alla medicina in una mostra commemorativa. **Minerva Med** 1981 May 7;72(18):1157–8
Royer J, Haut J, Amalric P: L'opération de la cataracte de Claude Monet, correspondence inédite du peintre et de G.-Clemenceau au docteur Coutela. **Hist Sci Med** 1984;18(2):109–27
Schmidt V: Camille Pissarro, hans danske relationer og hans sygdom. **Dan Medicinhist Arbog** 1983;12:144–61
Signoret JL: Une leçon clinique a la Salpêtrière (1887) par André Brouillet. **Rev Neurol (Paris)** 1983;139(12):687–701
Simeoni CE, Mouren MC, Aulas JJ: Psychose et créativité. Réflexions à propos d'un peintre autiste: Sykvain Fusco. **Confin Psychiatr** 1980;23(3):151–63
Telson HW: Une leçon du Docteur Charcot à la Salpêtrière. Lithograph by Eugene Pirodon after a painting (1887) by André Brouillet. **J Hist Med Allied Sci** 1980 Jan;35(1):58
Vogt DD, Montagne M: Absinthe: behind the emerald mask. **Int J Addict** 1982 Aug;17(6):1015–29
Wechsler J: A human comedy. Physiognomy and caricature in 19th century Paris. Chicago, University of Chicago Press, 1982. 208 p.

### Germany

Fuhrmeister H: Hallesche Duplikate der Majolikareliefs vom Berliner Albrecht-von-Graefe-Denkmal. **Klin Monatsbl Augenheilkd** 1980 May;176(5):867–9
Gercke H, Jarchov I, ed: Die Prinzhorn-Sammlung. Bilder, Skulpturen, Texte aus psychiatrischen Anstalten (ca. 1890–1920). Königstein/Taunus, Athenäum Verlag, 1980. 312 p.
Glandien O: Franz Xaver Messerschmidt (1736–1783) – Ausdrucksstudien und Charakterköpfe, Köln: 1981. 205 p. (Kölner medizinhistorische Beiträge: Arbeiten der Forschungsstelle des Instituts für Geschichte der Medizin der Universität zu Köln, Band 20).
Greither A: Otto Pankok und Düsseldorf; der Akademieprofessor Otto Pankok und seine Kunst. **Jahrb Univ Dusseld** 1977–78;:249–57
Keene BE: Portrait of a man protected against cholera. **J Hist Med Allied Sci** 1982 Oct;37(4):439
Korting GW: Atherom auf einem Olgemälde der Pinakothek in Brescia. **Hautarzt** 1984 Jun;35(6):321
Moskow BS: The iconography of the dental profession. Der Zahnbrecher--the toothbreaker. Johannes Joachim Kändler (1706–1775). **Quintessence Int** 1984 Jan;15(1):40–1
Murken AH: Joseph Beuys und die Medizin. Münster, Coppenrath, 1979. 160 p. German and English.
Murken AH, ed: Kind, Krankheit und Krankenhaus im Bilderbuch von 1900 bis 1982. (Studien zur Medizin-, Kunst- und Literaturgeschichte. Band 5.). Herzogenrath, Verlag Murken-Altrogge, 1982. 238 p.
Reiter A: Ernst L. Kirchner--Psychoanalytische Perspektiven der Psychoökonomie seines künstlerischen Schaffens. **Confin Psychiatr** 1980;23(2):118–28
Rothkopf A: 'Das Narrenhaus' von W. Kaulbach und die Deutung des Bildes durch J. A. Schilling 1863. **Confin Psychiatr** 1980;23(1):51–64
Schellmann B: Kunst und Pathologie: Joseph Beuys--'zeige deine Wunde'. **Pathologe** 1983 Nov;4(6):325–7
Schulze W: Conrad Felixmüller 1897 - 1977--ein Maler der Tierärzte. **Hist Med Vet** 1977;2(2):51–5
Tschinkel A: Unser Bild. - Das 'Licht der Natur' [A. Tschinkel, 1964]. **Medizinhist J** 1981;16(1/2):196–8
Wittop Koning DA, Van Gelder JB: Die Offizin aus der Meteorologia philosophica-politica des Fr. Reinzer. **Beitr Gesch Pharm** 1984;31(24):210

### Great Britain

Atherton DJ: Joseph Towne: wax modeler extraordinary. **J Am Acad Dermatol** 1980 Sep;3(3):311–6
Austin F, Jones B: The Clifts and the arts. **Ann R Coll Surg Engl** 1984 Jan;66(1):63–70
Carty MA: The examination of a young surgeon. Hand-colored etching by George Cruikshank, from The Scourge, 1811. **J Hist Med Allied Sci** 1981 Apr;36(2):214
Doughty J: The dentist in comic postcards. **Br Dent J** 1984 Mar 10;156(5):186–7
Illustrations from the Wellcome Institute Library: John Monro MD and Charles James Fox: etching by Thomas Rowlandson. **Med Hist** 1983 Jan;27(1):80–3
Illustrations from the Wellcome Institute library: The last moments of H. R. H. the Prince Consort. **Med Hist** 1982 Jul;26(3):321–4
Iveson-Iveson J: The art of observation, 3. Attitudes to mental health. **Nurs Mirror** 1982 Sep 8;155(10):17
Lee RV: The generalist: a jaundiced view. **Am J Med** 1983 Dec;75(6):902–5
Loudon IS: Sir Charles Bell and the anatomy of expression. **Br Med J [Clin Res]** 1982 Dec 18–25;285(6357):1794–6
Moskow BS: Dentistry in folk art, XIII: The dentist. **Bull Hist Dent** 1981 Oct;29(2):99
Paly D: Portrait of William Norris. Broadside, 1815, with etched portrait (1814) entitled 'William Norris: confined in this manner in Bethlem Hospital'; George Arnald, A.R.A., artist, etcher, and publisher. **Radic Hist Rev** 1979 Spring/Summer;Spec:65
Paly D: The antiquaries' last will and testament; an etching with sepia wash by Thomas Rowlandson, 1814. **J Hist Med Allied Sci** 1980 Apr;35(2):215
Pearson AA: John and William Hunter: patrons of the arts. In: Congrès international d'histoire de la médecine, XXVe, Québec, 1976. Actes. Québec, 1977. p. 1053–62.
Rodin AE: Infants and gin mania in 18th-century London. **JAMA** 1981 Mar 27;245(12):1237–9
Sakula A: Baroness Burdett-Coutts' garden party: the International Medical Congress, London, 1881. **Med Hist** 1982 Apr;26(2):183–90
Short AL: Portraits, paintings and caricatures. **Pharm Hist (London)** 1970 Jun;1(5):10–11
Swain V: No plaster saint! **Nurs Times** 1983 Mar 16–22;79(11):62–3
Wahrman A: The Philadelphia physician-factory. **J Hist Med Allied Sci** 1983 Jul;38(3):334–5

### Hungary

Gerevich J: Gulácsy Lajos festömüvész akut pszichózisa (adalék heveny téboly genezisének kérdéséhez). **Orv Hetil** 1981 May 3;122(18):1083–6
Monsées Y: 'Klinisches Ambulatorium' von Andor Dudits, 1890. **Medizinhist J** 1981;16(4):454–8
Szállási A: Egy medikus müvészi metamorfózisa (100 éve születell Medgyessy Ferenc). **Orv Hetil** 1981 Mar 22;122(12):709–11
Szállási A: Id. Elischer Gyula élete--a mügyüjtés apológiája. **Orv Hetil** 1984 Oct 14;125(42):2567–9
Szállási A: Medgyessy Ferenc medikuskori rajzaiból. **Orvostort Kozl** 1979;87–88(25 no 1–2):315–9

### Italy

Armoroli M, ed: Le cere anatomiche Bolognesi del settecento. Catalogo della mostra organizzata Settembre–Novembre 1981. Bologna, Università degli Studi di Bologna, Accademia delle Scienze, 1981. 97 p. Contributions by R. A. Bernabeo, L. Bonuzzi, F. Ruggeri.
Azzaroli ML, Lanza B: La Venere scomponibile. **Kos** 1984 May;1(4):65–81
Gamba A: Un ritratto inedito di Giambattista Morgagni. **Acta Med Hist Patav** 1982–83;29:67–74
Moskow BS: The iconography of the dental profession. Pietro Longhi

(1702–1785). **Quintessence Int** 1984 Jul;15(7):728–9
Rocchietta S: Un 'Christ à la pharmacie' ou 'Les Saints Côme et Damien'? **Rev Hist Pharm (Paris)** 1984 Jun;31(261):131–3

**Japan**

Telson H: An explanation of the charm against measles. **J Hist Med Allied Sci** 1978 Jul;33(3):408

**Mexico**

Pérez Gallardo R: El monumento del Dr. Manuel Carmona y Valle. **Bol Soc Mex Hist Filos Med** 1981 Mar;5(34):147–58
Somolinos-Palencia J: El doctor Rafael Lucio y las artes. **Gac Med Mex** 1980;116(9):422–8

**Netherlands**

Albert-Puleo M: Van Gogh's vision: thujuone intoxication. **JAMA** 1981 Jul 3;246(1):42
Haas WH de: Vincent van Gogh, zijn lichamelijke ziekten, verwondingen en zelfmoord. **Ned Tijdschr Geneeskd** 1983 Dec 24;127(52):2390–2
Lee TC: Van Gogh's vision. Digitalis intoxication? **JAMA** 1981 Feb 20;245(7):727–9
Ravin JG: Van Gogh's illness. **Ohio State Med J** 1981 Dec;77(12):699–702
Runyan WM: Why did Van Gogh cut off his ear? The problem of alternative explanations in psychobiography. **J Pers Soc Psychol** 1981 Jun;40(6):1070–7

**Norway**

Warick LH, Warick ER: Transitional process and creativity in the life and art of Edvard Munch. **J Am Acad Psychoanal** 1984 Jul;12(3):413–24
Wylie HW: Edvard Munch. **Am Imago** 1980 Winter;37(4):413–43

**Poland**

Jaworska J: Henryka Becka 'Bunkier 1944 roku'. Wrocław, Zakład Narodowy im. Ossolińskich, 1982. 119 p.
Pabis-Braunstein M: Aptekarstwo w Bieczu. Dzieje rodziny Fusków. **Arch Hist Med (Warsz)** 1984;47(2):191–206

**Portugal**

De Maar FE: The toothpick carvers of Lorvao. **Bull Hist Dent** 1980 Apr;28(1):11–15

**Spain**

Bräutigam W: Die Erkrankung Goyas von 1792. **Nervenarzt** 1980 Apr;51(4):233–8
Jordi R: Humor colérico. **Circ Farm** 1981 Apr;12(137):61–71
Jordi R: Manuel Blasco, pintor, escritor y bohemio. **Circ Farm** 1981 Mar;12(136):83–8

**Switzerland**

Eckstaedt A: 'Mimi überreicht Madam Grenouillet einen Blumenstrauss'. Eine psychoanalytische Studie über den Weg der Phantasie des vierjährigen Paul Klee anhand einer Kinderzeichnung. **Psyche (Stuttg)** 1980 Dec:34(12):1123–44
Rogers BO: Hans Erni: humanistic and aesthetic artist. **Aesthetic Plast Surg** 1983;7(1):51–67

**Thailand**

Matics KI: Medical arts at Wat Phra Chetuphon: various Rishi statues. **J Siam Soc** 1977;65(2):145–52

**United States**

Astrow A: Anxiety - frustration - repressed hostility. An original drawing, painted in gouache, by Boris Artzybasheff. **J Hist Med Allied Sci** 1980 Oct;35(4):453
Bonsett CA: Medical museum notes. **J Indiana State Med Assoc** 1981 Dec;74(12):770
Borowitz HO: A medical tour through The Cleveland Museum of Art. **Cleve Clin Q** 1983 Winter;50(4):417–38
Detre KC, Frank T, Kniazzeh CR, et al: Roots of art therapy. Margaret Naumburg (1890–1983) and Florence Cane (1882–1952). A family portrait. **Am J Art Ther** 1983 Jul;22(4):111–23
Gibbs RC: Portrait of a dermatologist as an artist. **Am J Dermatopathol** 1984 Feb;6(1):73–9
Helfand WH, Cowen DL: American pharmaceutical posters. In W.H. Hein, G. Schramm, ed: Die Vorträge des Internationalen Pharmaziehistorischen Kongresses Basel 1979. Stuttgart, Wissenschaftliche Verlagsgesellschaft, 1981. (Veröffentlichungen der Internationalen Gesellschaft für Geschichte der Pharmazie e.V., Neue Folge, Bd. 50).
Keys TE, Key JD: An overlooked tribute for Dr. William Worrall Mayo. **Minn Med** 1984 Jul;67(7):375–8
Kramer ES: The history of art therapy in a large mental hospital. **Am J Art Ther** 1982 Apr;21(3):75–84
Nolan E: Children's ward. Lithograph by Robert Riggs, ca. 1940–45. **J Hist Med Allied Sci** 1982 Jul;37(3):322
Rubin W: Pollock as Jungian illustrator: the limits of psychological criticism. **Art Am** 1979;67(7):104–23, (8):72–91
Skinner RE: Photography, advertising, and the history of medicine: notes on the medico-historical art of Lejaren a Hiller. **Watermark** 1983 Jan;6(2–3):11–2
Szczepaniak AS: Thomas Cromwell Corner, Baltimore Portrait artist. **Md State Med J** 1980 Apr;29(4):78–9
[The caricature of the teacher]: **Indiana Med Hist Q** 1977;3(2):23–37
Vandam LD: Robert Hinckley's 'The First operation with ether'. **Anesthesiology** 1980 Jan;52(1):62–70

**USSR**

Arkhangel'skii GV: S. P. Botkin i otechestvennye deiateli muzykal'noĭ i khudozhestvennoĭ kul'tury. **Klin Med (Mosk)** 1982 May;60(5):112–7
Murav'eva EF: Unikal'nyĭ al'bom. **Sov Zdravookhr** 1980;(9):67–72
Polenova IV: N. A. Iaroshenko i ucheniki S. P. Botkina. **Klin Med (Mosk)** 1982 Sep;60(9):117–9

# AWARDS AND PRIZES

**1700 to Present**

Costa-Casaretto C: Por que se les otorgo el Premio Nobel de medicina y fisiologia a Ehrlich y a Metchnikoff en 1908? **Rev Med Chil** 1980;108:775–6
Diamant H: Robert Bárány och Nobel-priset. **Sydsven Medicinhist Sallsk Arsskr** 1984;21:123–8
Jain KM, Swan KG, Casey KF: Nobel Prize winner in surgery. Part 2. **Am Surg** 1982 May;48(5):191–6
Lutzker E: Cameron prizewinner: Waldemar M. Haffkine, C.I.E. **Clio Med** 1971 May;13(3–4):269–76
Nicolle P, Jude A: Réflexions sur les prix Nobel de physiologie ou médecine. **Hist Sci Med** 1980;14(1):83–93
Nobel lectures in molecular biology, 1933–1975: New York, Elsevier, 1977. ix, 534 p.
Sicuteri F: The Enrico Greppi International Headache Award. A tribute to the memory of one of medicine's pioneers. **Cephalalgia** 1983 Mar;3(1):11–3
Solomon-Bayet C: L'interprétation historique des archives du Comité Nobel de Médecine, 1901–1920. **Soc Sci Inf** 1983;22:487–510
Wade N: The Nobel duel. Two scientists' 21-year race to win the world's most coveted research prize. Garden City, Anchor Press/Doubleday, 1981. 321 p.

**Denmark**

Kock W: Nordens första medicinska Nobelpris. **Nord Medicinhist Arsb** 1982;:110–21

**France**

Crosland M: From prizes to grants in the support of scientific research in France in the nineteenth century: the Montyon legacy. **Minerva** 1979 Autumn;17(3):355–80
Nicolle P: Un événement capital dans la vie passionnée de Charles Nicolle: le Prix Nobel de physiologie ou médecine. Souvenirs évoqués par Pierre Nicolle. **Bull Soc Pathol Exot Filiales** 1981 Jan–Feb;74(1):101–18
Société française d'histoire des hôpitaux: [1978–79 prizes in hospital history]: **Bull Soc Fr Hist Hop** 1980;(40):4–22

**Germany**

Garnerus K: Die Versammlungen Deutscher Narturforscher und Arzte--Medaillen berichten. **Naturwissenschaften** 1982 Apr;69(4):158–61
Kraft E, Finby N: Röntgen's discovery of X-ray and Lenard's priority claim; award of first Nobel Prize in physics in 1901. **NY State J Med** 1980 Sep;80(10):1623–5
Roth JK: Verleihung des Ehrendoktors der Johann-Wolfgang-Goethe-Universität an Anna Freud. **Psyche (Stuttg)** 1982 Oct;36(10):951–3

**Great Britain**

Smith DC: William Budd manuscript at the National Library of Medicine. **J Hist Med Allied Sci** 1980 Jul;35(3):318–19
Smith DC, ed: 'On the causes of fevers' (1839) by William Budd. Baltimore and London, Johns Hopkins University Press, 1984. xi, 164 p. (Henry E. Sigerist Supplements to the Bulletin of the History of Medicine, n.s.,

no. 9)

**Portugal**

Sessão solene de homenagem ao Prof. Dr. Francisco Cambournac, por ocasião da atribuição do prémio e medalha da Fundação Léon Bernard pela Organização Mundial de Saúde--22 de Junho de 1978: **An Inst Hig Med Trop (Lisb)** 1977-1978;5(1-4):37-53

**Spain**

Kock W: Santiago Ramón y Cajal and the Nobel prize. In International Congress of the History of Medicine, 27th, Barcelona, 1980. Actas. Barcelona, Académia de Ciències Médiques de Catalunya i Balears, 1981. p. 550-6.
Kock W: Santiago Ramón y Cajal och Nobelpriset. **Nord Medicinhist Arsb** 1981;:151-9

**United States**

Acceptance of the Gold Headed Cane Award: **Am J Pathol** 1979 Aug;96(2):368-71
Ayvasian LF: American Thoracic Society: the fifty-five Trudeau medalists (1926-1980): a seventy-fifty anniversary review. **Am Rev Respir Dis** 1980 Apr;121(4):753-75
Dew WC: John Ross Callahan: a man, a memorial, an award. **Ohio Dent J** 1982 Jul-Aug;56(7-8):46-52
Jain KM, Swan KG, Casey KF: Nobel prize winners in surgery. **Am Surg** 1982 Oct;48(10):495-500
National Institute of General Medical Sciences. Office of Research Reports: Nobel prize laureates. [Bethesda, Md.], National Institutes of Health, Dept. of Health, Education, and Welfare. [1978]. 24 p.
Palermo DS: The history of the Boyd R. McCandless Young Scientist Awards: the first recipients. **Adv Child Dev Behav** 1982;16:1-6
Perlmutter G: History of the Achievement Medal. **Alpha Omegan** 1982 Sep;75(3):24-9
Premio Abraham Horwitz. Dr. Martin M. Cummings: **Bol Of Sanit Panam** 1984 Jan;96(1):73-8
Presentation of the Gold Headed Cane to Arthur T. Hertig: **Am J Pathol** 1979 Aug;96(2):365-8
Williams JE, Johns RB, Evans P: The Gold-Headed Cane award of the Taylor-Jones County Medical Society. **Tex Med** 1981 Nov;77(11):50-1
Yalow R: Science and technology: problems and perceptions. In Cohen EP, ed: Medicine in transition. [Chicago], University of Illinois College of Medicine, 1981. p. 53-63.

**USSR**

Kucharz E, Jablońska D: Illya Illich Miechnikov -- in seventieth anniversary of being awarded the Nobel Prize. **Mater Med Pol** 1978 Oct-Dec;10(4):342-4
Sobchuk GS, Klantsa PA: N. I. Pirogov o nagrazhdenii zarubezhnykh uchenykh Russkimi orderami (Po neopublikovannym materialam). **Sov Zdravookhr** 1983;(4):65-8

## BALNEOLOGY, HYDROTHERAPY, AND HEALTH RESORTS

Bankhofer H: Die grossen Naturheiler. Ihr Leben - ihre Lehren. Frankfurt, Ullstein, 1982. 359 p.
Brödner E: Zur Entwicklungsgeschichte des Bades, 2. Teil. **Antike Welt** 1978;9(1):47-57
Heischkel-Artelt E: Kurort, Patient und Badearzt in ihrem Zusammenwirken, gezeigt an historischen Beispielen. **Z Angew Bader Klimaheilkd** 1978;25:318-25
Jaltel M: La santé par les eaux. 2000 ans de thermalisme. Orleans, L'Instant Durable, 1983. 176 p.
Kersley GD: The history and effects of spa treatment. **Rev Environ Health** 1982;4(1):57-62
Rothschuh KE: Aus der Geschichte der Naturheilbewegung (III). 'Vorläufer' des Rousseauschen Naturismus in der römischen Kaiserzeit. Die Philosophie der Stoa und die Methodische Medizin. **ZFA (Stuttgart)** 1981 May 31;57(15):1172-9
Rudolph G: Zwei Beiträge zur Geschichte der Balneologie. Die kulturgeschichtlichen und medizinischen Wurzeln des Bäderwesens. 100 Jahre wissenschaftliche Balneologie. Kassel, Meister, 1982. 132 p. (Schriftenreihe des Deutschen Bäderverbandes e.V., Heft 45).

**Austria**

Ogris A: Zur Geschichte des Badens. Mit einem Exkurs über Warmbad Villach. **Wien Geschichtsbl** 1978;33(2):87-9

**Byzantium**

Hunger H: Zum Badewesen in byzantinischen Klöstern. **Sitzungsber Oesterr Akad Wiss Philos Hist Kl** 1980;367:353-64
Lumpe A: Zur Kulturgeschichte des Bades in der byzantinischen Ara. **Byzantinische Forsch** 1979;6:151-66

**France**

Dupré P: Les stations bainéaires de la côte du Calvados: Genèse et développement. **Ann Normandie** 1983;33(3):239-58
Tanneau Y: L'ancienneté des bains de mer à Douarnenez. **Cah Iroise** 1979;26(2):78-81

**Germany**

Kreyes E: Die Geschichte der Wasserversorgung der Stadt Würzburg. Diss. Würzburg, 1969. 67 p.
Rothschuh KE: Aus der Geschichte der Naturheilbewegung (V). Welche Umstände begünstigten die Entstehung der deutschen Naturheilbewegung im 19. Jahrhundert? **ZFA (Stuttgart)** 1981 Jun 20;57(17):1310-20
Wegner E: Leo von Klenzes Badehaus im Staatsbad Brückenau. **Mainfraenk Jarb** 1979;31:143-51
Wehsarg FK: Bad Aachen-Burtscheid: Geschichte und Bedeutung. Stuttgart, New York, Schattauer, 1979. 79 p.
Woeber K: Uber die historische Bedeutung der Bad Aachener Heilquellen für die Dermato-Venerologie. **Rehabilitation (Bonn)** 1981;34(3-4):17-25

**Great Britain**

Anderson AB: Vanishing spas. Dorchester, [Eng.], Friary Press, 1974. 103 p.
Ford JM: Medical indications for taking the waters of Tunbridge Wells. **J R Soc Med** 1984 Nov;77(11):955-9
Harley D: Religious and professional interests in northern spa literature, 1625-1775. **Soc Soc Hist Med Bull (Lond)** 1984 Dec;35:14-6
Lewis TH: Richard Carew on the treatment of a 'Franticke person' in Medieval Cornwall. **J Hist Med Allied Sci** 1981 Jan;36(1)64-6
Little B: Cheltenham: a gently sited town. **Contemp Rev** 1980;237(1377):191-3
Rolls R: The rise and fall of the Bath waters. **Soc Soc Hist Med Bull (Lond)** 1984 Dec;35:17-20
Sakula A: The waters of Epsom Spa. **J R Coll Physicians Lond** 1982 Apr;16(2):124-8

**Italy**

Bèttica-Giovannini R: Terra di Castagneto Po e acqua di San Genesio presso Chivasso. **Ann Osp Maria Vittoria Torino** 1981 Jan-Jun;24(1-6):217-27
Eschebach H: Schola labri. Die Entwicklung der Schola labri in den Vesuvstädten, dargestellt am Labrum des Männercaladariums der Stabianer Thermen in Pompeji. **Cron Pompeiane** 1977;3:156-76

**Sweden**

Bergmark M: Medevi 300 år. Ett nytt blad i vår svenska hydroterapis historia. **Nord Medicinhist Arsb** 1980;Suppl 6:122-8

**USSR**

Shavianidze ON, Shavianidze GO: Kurort Tskhaltubo. **Vopr Kurortol Fizioter Lech Fiz Kult** 1984 Jul-Aug;(4):53-5

**Before 500 A.D.**

Broedner E: Zur Entwicklungsgeschichte des Bades. **Antike Welt** 1977;8(4):45-56
Naidenov G, Konaréva N, Nikiforov N: Hissar - station thermale de l'Antiquité jusqu'à nos jours. In International Congress of the History of Medicine. 26th, Plovdiv, 1978. Actes du Congress. Sofia, 1981. Volume II. p. 217-9.
Zahlhaas G: Die Fresken des römischen Thermengebäudes von Schwangau. **Antike Welt** 1978;9(4):13-23

**Greece**

Papalas AJ: Medicinal bathing in mineral springs in fifth century B. C. Greece. **Clio Med** 1981 Dec;16(2/3):81-2

**Israel**

Gichon M: Roman baths, Erets, Israel. (Heb) **Qadmoniot** 1978;11(2-3):37-53

### 500 A.D.–1450

#### Arabic

Estestvennye i preformirovannye fizicheskie faktory vo vrachebnoĭ deiatel'nosti Abu-Ali Ibn-Siny (k 1000-letiiu so dnia rozhdneiia): **Vopr Kurortol Fizioter Lech Fiz Kult** 1981 Jan-Feb;(1):64-6

#### Italy

Orofino G, Brach CC: Nel nome del bagno. **Kos** 1984 Apr;1(3):33-54

### 1450–1700

Rothschuh KE: Aus der Geschichte der Naturheilbewegung (IV). Hatte die Naturheilbewegung Vorläufer in der Renaissance? Montaigne, Paracelsus, Beobachtungsmedizin, Wasserheilkunde. **ZFA (Stuttgart)** 1981 Jun 10;57(16):1251-9

#### Austria

Zwanowetz G: Herzog Sigismund von Osterreich in Gastein. **Mitt Ges Salzburger Landeskd** 1972-73;112-113(2):325-9

#### Germany

Pictorius G: Badenfahrtbüchlein. Wie und wo man richtig badet. Nachruck des Werkes aus dem Jahre 1560. U. Becker, ed., Basel and Wien; Herder, Freiburg, 1980. 111 p

### 1700 to Present

Coley NG: The preparation and uses of artificial mineral waters (ca. 1680-1825). **Ambix** 1984;31(1):32-48

#### Austria

Charbusky K: Zur Geschichte des Vöslauer Thermalbades. **Jahrb Landeskd Niederoesterr** 1964;36:425-44

Kolb A: Sebastian Kneipp und Vorarlberg. **Montfort** 1971;23(2):158-62

Waldhauser H: Zur Kur in Oesterreich, 'wo heilsam Wasser durch die Klüfte schleicht.' St. Pölten, Verlag Niederösterreichisches Pressehaus, 1980. 160 p.

#### Belgium

Trente années d'existence: Alsemberg, La Fondation, [1977?]. 23 p.

#### Czechoslovakia

Ambrus O: Historie a přehled lázeňské péče v psychiatrii v Ceskoslovensku. **Fysiatr Reumatol Vestn** 1982 Apr;60(2):105-7

Křížek V: J.W. Goethe a ceské lázně. K 150. výročí básníkovy smrti 22. března 1832. **Cas Lek Cesk** 1982 Jun 4;121(22):695-8

Křižek V, Nevoral V: Jöns Jacob Berzelius a české minerální vody. **Fysiatr Reumatol Vestn** 1980 Aug;58(4):238-42

Novák J: Stočtyřicet let od narození prof. MUDr. Karla Chodounského. **Cas Lek Cesk** 1983 May 13;122(19):600-1

Skodáček P: Prof. MUDr Eduard Cmunt, prvý slovanský balneológ v Piešťanoch. **Fysiatr Reumatol Vestn** 1984 Feb;62(1):44-6

Steifl A: Die Braunkohle und das Egerer Becken. **Bohemia Jahrb Coll Caronium (Ger)** 1978;19:309-20

Vendl L: Dvacet let Detské nefrologické léčebny Miramonte v Mariánských Láznich. **Cesk Pediatr** 1982 Jul;37(7):419

#### France

Burrus O: Les aventures d'un curiste..de Napoléon III à la Belle Epoque. **Rev Infirm** 1982 Mar;32(6):26-8

Cosma-Muller P: Entre science et commerce: les eaux minerales en France a la fin de l'ancien regime. **Hist Reflect** 1982;9(1-2):249-62

Godonnèche J: Médecins hydrologues à Châtelguyon au XIXe siècle. In: Congrès National des Sociétés Savantes, 93e, Tours, 1968. Comptes Rendus. Paris, 1971. Section des Sciences, Tome II. p. 193-200.

Handelsman A: Le médecin hydropathe---color lithograph by Honoré Daumier. **J Hist Med Allied Sci** 1981 Jan;36(1)63

Loustaud JP, Reboul G, Viroulet JJ: Les thermes de la place de Jacobins à Limoges. **Archeologia** 1981;157:30-34

#### Germany

Baatz D: Das Badegebäude des Limeskastells Walldürn (Odenwaldkreis). **Saalburg Jahrb** 1978;35:61-107

Eulner HH: Zur Geschichte der Meeresheilkunde: Georg Christoph Lichtenberg und das Seebad Cuxhaven. **Medizinhist J** 1982;17(1/2):115-28

Mader G: Studien zur Gesundheitsbildung und Ordnungslehre bei Sebastian Kneipp: ein Beitrag zur Frage 'machbarer' Gesundheit. Frankfurt am Main, Haag + Herchen, 1984. 198, 49 p.

Petrova L: Die Bedeutung des Wassers in den volkstümlichen Bräuchen und in der Volksmedizin. In International Congress of the History of Medicine, 27th, Barcelona, 1980. Actas. Barcelona, Académia de Ciències Mèdiques de Catalunya i Balears, 1981. p. 603-9.

Schadewaldt H: Das Badewesen in der Goethezeit. **Therapiewoche** 1982;32:4123-33

Schomburg E: Sebastian Kneipp, 1821-1897. Bad Wörishofen, Kneipp-Verlag, 1976. 154 p.

Thiele F: Zur Notwendigkeit von Kuren--Definition, Indikation, Erfolgsaussichten, Wiederholung. **Off Gesundheitswes** 1982 Mar;44(3):169-75

Wehsarg FK: Die Quecksilber-Schmierkur in Bad Aachen als einstmalige Syphilistherapie. **Rehabilitation (Bonn)** 1981;34(3-4):26-32

#### Great Britain

Annear MW: Some healing and holy wells of Wales. In J. Cule, ed: Wales and medicine. London, British Society for the History of Medicine, 1975. p. 185-89.

Brown PS: Some treatments of skin disease in eighteenth century Bath. **Int J Dermatol** 1982 Nov;21(9):555-9

Coley NG: Physicians and the chemical analysis of mineral waters in eighteenth-century England. **Med Hist** 1982 Apr;26(2):123-44

Hyde A: Hospital life: a breath of good sea air. **Health Soc Serv J** 1980 Jan 18;90(4676):78-9

Mowat AG: Strathpeffer Spa: Dr. William Bruce and polymyalgia rheumatica. **Ann Rheum Dis** 1981 Oct;40(5):503-6

Price R: Hydropathy in England 1840-70. **Med Hist** 1981 Jul;25(3):269-80

Smith HG: Architecture, form and conservation in a spa town. **R Soc Health J** 1982 Oct;102(5):196-200

Steen P: Spas: pleasure of penance? **Hist Today** 1981 Sep;31:21-6

Swinton WE: The hydrotherapy and infamy of Dr. James Gully. **Can Med Assoc J** 1980 Dec 20;123(12):1262-4

When Harrogate was a spa: **Nurs Times** 1982 Apr 21-27;78(16):suppl 11-3

#### Hungary

Péterffy I: Híradás két felvilágosodás kori jeles orvosról. **Orv Hetil** 1983 Jul 31;124(31):1895-6

Szekér E: Emléktábla-ayató ünnepség Balatonfüreden. **Orv Hetil** 1983 Feb 20;124(8):467-8

Tóth A: Hévízi érmek. **Orv Hetil** 1982 Jul 11;123(28):1751-3

Zákonyi F: Dr. Huray István, Balatonfüred föorvosa. **Orv Hetil** 1983 Sep 4;124(36):2192-4

#### Italy

Messina B: Mariano Messini, il suo insegnamento: le basi scientifiche della terapia termale. **Clin Ter** 1982 Nov 30:103(4):351-6

#### Poland

Ryn Z: Zakopiańskie placówki słyzby zdrowia podczas okupacji hitlerowskiej. **Przegl Lek** 1981;38(1):114-21

Skulimowski M, Sliwiński S: Z przeszłości uzdrowiskowej Krzeszowic. **Wiad Lek** 1979 Nov 15;32(22):1651-4

#### Romania

Pîrvulescu M, Pîrvulescu A: Slănic Moldova, în documente ale trecutului. **Rev Med Chir Soc Med Nat Iasi** 1983 Oct-Dec;87(4):659-60

#### South Africa

Langham-Carter RR: The Caledon baths. **Adler Mus Bull** 1984 Jun;10(2):18-9

#### Spain

Ustrell Torrent JM: El balneario de Vallfogona de Riucorb. **Asclepio** 1980;32:467-84

#### Sweden

Ericsson R: Mineralvatten på svenska apotek--en svunnen epok. **Nord Medicinhist Arsb** 1980;Suppl 6:129-38

Nevoral V, Křižek V: J. J. Berzelius jako analytik minerálních vod. **Fysiatr Reumatol Vestn** 1980 Aug;58(4):244-7

#### Switzerland

Ilić D: Conrad Meyer-Ahrens (1813-1872) und sein Werk über die Heilquellen und Kurorte der Schweiz. Zürich, Juris, 1975. 61 p.

**United States**

DeMark JL: Chasing the cure--a history of healthseekers to Albuquerque, 1902–1940. **J West** 1982 Jul;21(3):49–58
Gittings CL: Arizona's reputation as a health spa. **Ariz Med** 1983 Mar;40(3):150–3
Johnson JM: The water cure at 'the San.' **NY Folkl Q** 1966;22(3):201–5
Jones WB: Mineral springs and medicine in North Carolina. **NC Med J** 1983 Sep;44(9):593–5
Karsh E: Taking the waters at Stafford Springs. The role of the Willard family in America's first health spa. In: Congrès international d'histoire de la médecine, XXVe, Québec, 1976. Actes. Québec, 1977. p. 822–39.
Karsh E: Taking the waters at Stafford Springs: the role of the Willard Family of Boston in America's first health spa. **Harv Libr Bull** 1980 Jul;28(3):264–81
Lawrence HW: Southern spas: source of the American resort tradition. **Landscape** 1983;27(2):1–12
Meeks HA: Stagnant, smelly and successful: Vermont's mineral springs. **Vt Hist** 1979;47(1):5–20
Miller LE: San Diego's early years as a health resort. **J San Diego Hist** 1982;28(4):232–47
Moerchel J: Simon Baruch (1840–1921) und die öffentliche Gesundheitspflege in New York. **Medizinhist J** 1982;17(1/2):138–47
Pond N: Tennesse's Tyree Springs: the most celebrated watering place in the State. **Ky Folkl Rec** 1978;24(3–4):64–73
Reed LA: Doctor Swan's restorative waters. **Wis Mag Hist** 1980–81;64(2):124–6
Shane KD: New Mexico: salubrious El Dorado. **NM Hist Rev** 1981;56(4):387–99
Stielow F: Health and pleasure seekers at the springs of Indiana: pamphlet literature in the Library of Congress. **Indiana Med Hist Q** 1982;8(1):4–7
Thorne CB: The watering spas of middle Tennessee. **Tenn Hist Q** 1970–71;29(4):321–59
Vining JW: Slater Burgesser and his famous spring. **West Ill Reg Stud** 1982;5(2):184–95
Vining JW: Versailles Mineral Springs: an historical geography. **Pioneer Am Soc Trans** 1982;5:37–43

**USSR**

Arkhangel'skiĭ GV: Moskovskiĭ vrach-gumanist Fedor Petrovich Gaaz (1780–1853) i ego znachenie v razvitii otechestvennoĭ meditsiny. **Klin Med (Mosk)** 1981 Feb;59(2):118–20
Artiukhov SA: Sochinskaia gospital'naia baza v gody Velikoĭ Otechestvennoĭ voĭny. **Sov Zdravookhr** 1981;(9):66–7
Bogoliubov VM: V. I. Lenin i razvitie sanatorno-kurortnogo dela v SSSR. **Vopr Kurortol Fizioter Lech Fiz Kult** 1980 Mar–Apr;(2):1–3
Bogoliubov VM: Vklad russkikh uchenykh v razvitie kurortologii v Gruzii. **Vopr Kurortol Fizioter Lech Fiz Kult** 1984 Mar–Apr;(2):5–9
Derbenev NE: Zdravnitsa dlia ranenykh voinov. **Voen Med Zh** 1980 Jul;(7):21–2
Fokina EN: Fedor Petrovich Gaaz i ego issledovaniia po izucheniiu lechebnykh mineral'nykh istochnikov Kavkaza. **Vopr Kurortol Fizioter Lech Fiz Kult** 1980 Sep–Oct;(5):65–6
Gorbunov VP: 50 let na strazhe zdorov'ia voĭnov. **Voen Med Zh** 1984 Aug;(8):76–8
Gorchakova GA: Osnovnye vekhi razvitiia nauchnykh issledovaniĭ po kurortologii v USSR. **Vopr Kurortol Fizioter Lech Fiz Kult** 1982 Nov–Dec;(6):16–8
Gulida MV: Razvitie sanatorno-kurortnogo lecheniia bol'nykh tuberkulezom na iuzhnom beregu Kryma. **Probl Tuberk** 1981;(7):65–8
Gurauskas VB, Miashka VA: Razvitie kurortologii v Litve za gody Sovetskoĭ vlasti. **Vopr Kurortol Fizioter Lech Fiz Kult** 1982 Nov–Dec;(6):18–20
Konovalov II: A. S. Pushkin i M. Iu. Lermontov na Kavkazskikh Mineral'nykh Vodakh (k 200-letiiu Piatigorska). **Vopr Kurortol Fizioter Lech Fiz Kult** 1980 Sep–Oct;(5):68–70
Kozlov II: Dostizheniia kurortnogo dela v SSSR. **Vopr Kurortol Fizioter Lech Fiz Kult** 1982 Nov–Dec;(6):1–6
Krivobokov NG: Shestidesiatiletie Piatigorskogo instituta kurotologii i fizioterapii. **Vopr Kurortol Fizioter Lech Fiz Kult** 1980 May–Jun;(3):67–8
Makovskiĭ ChN, Terent'eva LA, Ermolaev GT: Kurorty Latviiskoĭ SSR. **Vopr Kurortol Fizioter Lech Fiz Kult** 1982 Nov–Dec;(6):21–2
Mekhtyev MM: K 50-letiiu kurorta 'Baĭram-Ali'. **Vopr Kurortol Fizioter Lech Fiz Kult** 1984 Jan–Feb;(1):66–8
Obrosov AN: Dostizheniia i perspektivy razvitiia nauchnoĭ kurortologii i fizioterapii. **Vopr Kurortol Fizioter Lech Fiz Kult** 1982 Nov–Dec;(6):6–12
Odonchiméd L, Baklykov LI: Razvite sanatorno-kurortnogo dela v Mongol'skoĭ Narodnoĭ Respublike. **Vopr Kurortol Fizioter Lech Fiz Kult** 1984 Jul–Aug;(4):40–3
Orzheshkovskiĭ VV, Chopchik DI: 20-letie Ukrainskogo respublikanskogo nauchnogo obshchestva fizioterapevtov i kurortologov. **Vopr Kurortol Fizioter Lech Fiz Kult** 1979 Sep–Oct;(5):69–70
Semenova EI: Pervaia detskaia lechebnaia koloniia v Rossii (K 150-letiiu so dnia rozhdeniia D.I. Mendeleeva). **Pediatriia** 1984 Sep;(9):78–9
Shukurov AK, Pulatov RP: [Development of health resort science and physiotherapy in Uzbekistan]. (Rus) **Vopr Kurortol Fizioter Lech Fiz Kult** 1979 Nov–Dec;(6):7–11
Starikov NM: K 60-letiiu Tomskogo nauchno-issledovatel'skogo instituta kurortologii Minzdrava RSFSR. **Vopr Kurortol Fizioter Lech Fiz Kult** 1982 Jul–Aug;(4):66–7
V. I. Lenin'i stanovlenie sanatorno-kurortnogo dela v nasheĭ strane: **Voen Med Zh** 1980 Fev;(2):7–9
Viksna D: Kurortpilsetas Jurmala galvenas attistibas linijas socialisma celtniecibas posma (1940–1959). **Latv PSR Zinat Akad Vestis** 1979;6:9–20
Zheleznikov IG, Khomniuk VF: Dostizheniia kurortologov Kazakhstana za gody Sovetskoĭ vlasti. **Vopr Kurortol Fizioter Lech Fiz Kult** 1982 Nov–Dec;(6):22–3

**Yugoslavia**

Majsec M, Manestar M: Od kupališnog lječilišta do bolnice za reumatske bolesti i rehabilitaciju Krapinske Toplice. **Reumatizam** 1979;26(3):73–6

# BIOLOGY

See also **Biophysics; Cytology; Microbiology; Molecular Biology**

Abbott D: The biographical dictionary of scientists: biologists. London and New York, Blond Educational and Bedrick, 1984. 182 p.
Asimov I: A short history of biology. Westport, Conn., Greenwood Press, 1980. ix, 189 p.
Baer KE von: Reden gehalten in wissenschaftlichen Versammlungen und kleinere Aufsätze vermischten Inhalts. With an introduction by K. B. Sterling. New York, Arno Press, 1978. Three volumes in two. (Reprint. St. Petersburg, 1864/1876/1873).
Baumel HB: Biology: its historical development. New York, Philosophical Library, 1978. 101 p.
Bernard J: Les progrès de la biologie et la définition de l'homme. **Rev Med Suisse Romande** 1984 Mar;104(3):239–48
Bernier R: Aux sources de la biologie. 1. Les vingt premiers siècles. La classification. Montrèal, Presses de l'Université du Québec - Paris, Masson, 1975. xii, 264 p.
Borms J, Hebbelinck M, Venerando A, ed: Women and sport: an historical, biological, physiological and sportsmedical approach. Basel, Karger, 1981. 229 p. (Medicine and sport, Vol. 14)
Bridson GD, Phillips VC, Harvey AP, ed: Natural history manuscript resources in the British Isles. London, Mansell; New York, Bowker, 1980. xxxiv, 473 p.
Carter RB: Gilbert and Descartes: the science of conserving the compound body. **Z Allg Wissenschaftstheorie** 1982;13(2):224–33
Cherry R: Biology and sociology and economics: an historical analysis. **Rev Soc Econ** 1980;38(2):141–54
Costa O: Storie sommerse di biologia e medicina. **Scientia** 1980;115:215–25
Davis C: La sociobiologie et son explication de l'humanité. **Ann Econ Soc Civilis** 1981;36:531–71
Gershenowitz H: Chauncey Wright's views on Lamarck. **Indian J Hist Sci** 1979, reçu 1982:14(1):16–24
Gershenowitz H: Gavin De Beer and the Neo-Lamarckians. **Indian J Hist Sci** 1978, reçu 1982;13(1):23–7
Gershenowitz H: George Gaylord Simpson and Lamarck. **Indian J Hist Sci** 1978, reçu 1982;13(1):56–61
Gershenowitz H: George Henslow: true Darwinist. **Indian J Hist Sci** 1979, reçu 1982;14(1):25–30
Glushakova TI: Razvitie predstavleniĭ ob individual'nosti khromosom. Moskva, Nauka, 1983. 119 p.
Haraway DJ: In the beginning was the word: the genesis of biological theory. **Signs** 1981;6(3):469–81
Hoppe B: Arbeit und Gesundheit; historische Aspekte ihrer gegenseitigen Beziehungen. Bericht über eine Tagung der 'International School of History of Biological Sciences' in Ischia/Neapel vom 29. Juni bis 12. Juli 1980. **Ber Wissenschaftsgesch** 1980;3(3–4):214–20
Hoppe B: Biologie, Wissenschaft von der belebten Materie von der Antike zur Neuzeit. Biologische Methodologie und Lehren von der stofflichen Zusammensetzung der Organismen. Wiesbaden, Steiner, 1976. vii, 368 p. (Sudhoffs Archiv, Beihefte, Heft 17)
Katchalsky-Katzir A: Some thoughts on the physics and biology of time. **Adv Biol Med Phys** 1977;16:289–322
Leclercq-Kadaner J: Physiologus de naturis animalium et bestiarum. Fédération des Cercles d'Archéologie et d'Histoire de Belgique. 44e session. Congrès de Huy, 1976. Annales. Tielt, 1978. p. 790–5
Lenoir T: A history of biology: an essay review. **J Hist Med Allied Sci** 1983 Jul;38(3):348–51
Lewontin R, Rose S, Kamin L: Bourgeois ideology and the origins of biological determinism. **Race Cl** 1982;24(1):1–16
Mayr E: The growth of biological thought. Diversity, evolution, and inheritance. Cambridge, London, Harvard University Press, 1982. 974 p.
Savodnik I, ed: Concept and explanation in biology. Oceanside, Dabor, 1977. xvii, 240 p.
Savodnik I, ed: The origins of structure in biology. Oceanside, Dabor, 1977. xvi, 154 p.
Schiller J: La notion d'organisation dans l'histoire de la biologie. Paris,

Maloine, 1978. 133 p.
Shamin AN: Issledovaniia po istorii biologii. **Vopr Istor Estestvozn Tekh** 1981;2:38–45
Sheynin OB: On the history of the statistical method in biology. **Arch Hist Exact Sci** 1980;22(4):323–71
Sichel G: Considerazioni sulla origine storica della biologia generale. **Med Secoli** 1981;17:163–87
Simon HR: Die Bibliographie der Biologie. Eine analytische Darstellung unter wissenschaftshistorischen und informationstheoretischen Gesichtspunkten. Stuttgart, Hiersemann, 1977. x, 315 p. (Bibliothek des Buchwesens, Bd. 4).
Thomasen AL: 'Historia animalium' contra 'Gynaecia' in der Literatur des Mittelalters. **Clio Med** 1980;15(1/2):5–23
Törö I: Service in biological sciences.... **Acta Biol Acad Sci Hung** 1980;31(1–3):5–12
Wuketits FM: Wissenschaftsgeschichte und gegenwärtige Theoriendiskussion in der Biologie. **Nat Mus** 1980;110:175–81

**Americas**

Harper AB, Laughlin WS: Inquiries into the peopling of the new world: development of ideas and recent advances. In F. Spencer, ed: A history of American physical anthropology, 1930–1980. New York, Academic Press, 1982. p. 281–304.

**Great Britain**

Guerlac H: Theological voluntarism and biological analogies in Newton's physical thought. **J Hist Ideas** 1983 Apr–Jun;44(2):219–29

**Italy**

Frassetto F: Le cose son numeri. **Riv Biol** 1981 Autumn;74(3):402–8

**Mexico**

Beltrán E: Reflexiones sobre historiografía de la biología en México. **An Soc Mex Hist Cienc Tec** 1979;5:1–19

**Netherlands**

Palm LC, Snelders HA, ed: Antoni van Leeuwenhoek, 1632–1723. Studies on the life and work of the Delft scientist commemorating the 350th anniversary of his birthday. Amsterdam, Rodopi, 1982. 209 p. (Nieuwe Nederlandse Bijdragen tot de Geschiedenis der Geneeskunde en der Natuurwetenschappen, no. 8). Contributions by W. H. van Seters, B. C. Damsteegt, J. van Zuylen, P. Bass, J. E. van Bronswijk, G. A. Lindeboom, P. Smit, K. van Berkel.

**United States**

Hughes AF: The American biologist through four centuries. Springfield, Ill., Thomas, 1982. xvii, 386 p.

**Yugoslavia**

Tartalja H: [Doctors and biologists in Dubrovník.] (SCC) **Dubrovnik** 1975;18(3–4):5–51

**Before 500 A.D.**

Grmek M: Les ruses de guerre biologiques dans l'antiquité. **Rev Etud Grec** 1979;92:142–63
Manuli P, Vegetti M: Cuore, sangue e cervello. Biologia e antropologia nel pensiero antico. Milano, Episteme, 1977. 241 p.

**Greece**

Barnes J: Aristotle's de Motu Animalium. **Classical Rev** 1980;30(2):222–6
Bodson L: Aristotle's statement on the reproduction of sharks. **J Hist Biol** 1983 Fall;16(3):391–407
Boylan M: Mechanism and teleology in Aristotle's biology. **Apeiron** 1981, reçu 1982;15(2):96–102
Boylan M: The Galenic and Hippocratic challenges to Aristotle's conception theory. **J Hist Biol** 1984 Spring;17(1):83–112
Kádár Z: Survivals of Greek zoological illuminations in Byzantine manuscripts. Budapest, Akadémiai Kiadó. 1978. 138 p. (With 232 half-tone illustrations and 10 color plates).
Kruk R: Aristoteles semitico-latinus. The Arabic version of Aristotle's Parts of animals. Book XI–XIV of the Kitab al-Hayawan. A critical edition with introduction and selected glossary. Amsterdam, Oxford, North-Holland Publishing Co., 1979. 96 [107] p.
Nussbaum MC, ed: Aristotle's De motu animalium. Text with translation, commentary, and interpretive essays. Princeton, Princeton University Press, 1978. xxiii, 430 p.
Oppenheimer JM: Aristotle as a biologist. **Scientia** 1971;65(106):649–58
Pratt V: Aristotle and the essence of natural history. **Hist Philos Life Sci** 1982;4(2):203–23
Roussel M: Physique et biologie dans la 'Génération des animaux' d'Aristote. **Rev Etud Grec** 1980, reçu 1981:93(440–441):42–71

**500 A.D.–1450**

Cadden J: The medieval philosophy and biology of growth: Albertus Magnus, Thomas Aquinas, Albert of Saxony and Masilius of Inghen on Book I, Chapter V, of Aristotle's 'De generatione et corruptione.' With translated texts of Albertus Magnus and Thomas Aquinas. Ph. D. Diss. Indiana University. Bloomington, 1971. vii, 267 leaves.
Goldstein-Préaud T: Albert le Grand et les questions du XIIIe siècle sur le De animalibus d'Aristote. **Hist Philos Life Sci** 1981;3(1):61–71

**Arabic**

Hamarneh SK: Al-Biruni, the father of Arabic pharmacy and marine biology as demonstrated in al-Saydanah. In: International Congress held in Pakistan on the occasion of Millenary of Abu Raihan Muhammad ibn Ahmad al-Biruni (973–ca 1051 A.D.) November 26, 1973 thru December 12, 1973. Proceedings. Karachi, Hamdard National Foundation, 1979. p. 479–500.

**1450–1700**

Slaughter MM: Universal languages and scientific taxonomy in the seventeenth century. Cambridge, Cambridge University Press, 1982. x, 277 p.

**Czechoslovakia**

Servít Z: Počátky české novověké medicíny a biologie. Jan Marek Marci z Kronlandu (Joannes Marcus Marci, 1595–1667). Stručná biografie. **Cesk Fysiol** 1984;33(5):394–413

**Italy**

Barcaro U: Galileo e il mondo biologico. **Physis** 1982;24(3):357–79

**Netherlands**

Lindeboom GA: Jan Swammerdam (1637–1680) and his Biblia Naturae. **Clio Med** 1982 Dec;17(2–3):113–31
Ruestow EG: Images and ideas: Leeuwenhoek's perception of the spermatozoa. **J Hist Biol** 1983 Summer;16(2):185–224

**1700 to Present**

Allen GE: Essay review: the roots of biological determinism. **J Hist Biol** 1984 Spring;17(1):141–5
Allen GE: Morphology and twentieth-century biology: a response. **J Hist Biol** 1981 Spring;14(1):159–76
Armelagos GJ, Carlson DS, Van Gerven DP: The theoretical foundations and development of skeletal biology. In F. Spencer, ed: A history of American physical anthropology, 1930–1980. New York, Academic Press, 1982. p. 305–28.
Baev AA: Sovremennaia biologiia kak sotsial'noe iavlenie. **Vopr Filos** 1981;3:17–26
Baker PT: Human population biology: a viable transdisciplinary science. **Hum Biol** 1982 May;54(2):203–20
Balner H, Marquet RL: Transplantation biology--past and present: reappraisal of 'breakthroughs' since 1955. **Transplant Proc** 1981 Mar;13(1 pt 1):13–8
Bartley RL, Kucewicz WP: 'Yellow rain' and the future of arms agreements. **Foreign Aff** 1983;61(4):805–26
Beatty J: Essay review: life science in the twentieth century. **Ann Sci** 1981;38(2):207–16
Benavente Barreda JM: Evolución biológica y herencia natural. **Arbor** 1982;113(441–2):111–25
Bowler PJ: Biology and social thought. **Can Rev Am Stud** 1980;11(1):87–94
Campbell M: The concepts of dormancy, latency, and dominance in nineteenth-century biology. **J Hist Biol** 1983 Fall;16(3):409–31
Cardiel JR: Sociobiología. La última forma de darwinismo. **Arbor** 1982;113(441–2):87–98
Cavanha AO: La revolucion biologica. **CERON** 1980 Dec;5(3):29–32
Charles Darwin, 1809–1882; Anton Dohrn, 1840–1909: Correspondence. Napoli, Macchiaroli, 1982. 118 p.
Cock AG: Chauvinism and internationalism in science: The International Research Council, 1919–1926. **Notes Rec R Soc Lond** 1983 Mar;37(2):249–88
Conry Y: L'idée d'une 'marche de la nature' dans la biologie prédarwinienne au XIXe siècle. **Rev Hist Sci (Paris)** 1980 Apr;33(2):97–149
Davis BD: Frontiers of the biological sciences. **Science** 1980 Jul 4;209(4452):78–89
Delaporte F: Theories of osteogenesis in the eighteenth century. **J Hist Biol** 1983 Fall;16(3):343–60

Diara A: Sens et definition du mot 'espece' dans l'oeuvre biologique de Felix Le Dantec. **Rev Synth (Paris)** 1981;102(101-102):73-86
Dixon B: Spontaneous generation. **New Sci** 1981;91:553
Durant JR: Innate character in animals and man: a perspective on the origins of ethology. In C. Webster, ed: Biology, medicine and society 1840-1940. Cambridge, Cambridge University Press, 1981. p. 157-92.
Dustin P: Cinquante années de progrès des sciences biologiques. **Rev Med Brux** 1984 Mar;5(3):115-9
Edgar RS: Max Delbrück. **Annu Rev Genet** 1982;16:501-5
Farley J: Gametes & spores. Ideas about sexual reproduction, 1750-1914 Baltimore, London, Johns Hopkins University Press, 1982. x, 299 p.
Fischer JL: L'hybridologie et la zootaxi du Siècle des Lumières à l'Origine des espèces. **Rev Synth (Paris)** 1981;102(101-102):47-72
Foerster I, Kirschke S: Soziobiologie oder Biosoziologie? **Wiss Z Martin Luther Univ (Math)** 1984;33(4):51-67
Geneste B: La biotechnologie: un domaine de recherche particulièrement fécond et porteur d'espoir. **Rev Palais Decouv** 1983;11(107):18-45
Gershenowitz H: The treatment of Lamarckism as found in forty-one college textbooks. **Indian J Hist Sci** 1978, reçu 1982;13(2):144-50
Gilbert SF, Greenberg JP: Intellectual traditions in the life sciences. II. Stereocomplementarity. **Perspect Biol Med** 1984 Autumn;28(1):18-34
Gould SJ: Ever since Darwin. Reflections in natural history. New York, W. W. Norton, 1977. 285 p.
Graham LR: Between science and values. New York, Columbia University Press, 1981. x, 449 p.
Groeben C, ed: Guida alla Mostra allestita nella Sala degli Affreschi della Stazione Zoologica nella Villa Comunale (6 luglio - 30 settembre 1982) su Charles Darwin e la Stazione Zoologica di Napoli.
Grundy JH: The evolution and impact of medical entomology. In Burgess NR, ed: John Hull Grundy's Arthropods of medical importance. Watch Cottage, Chilbolton, Hampshire, Noble Books, 1981. p. 13-25.
Hagen JB: Experimental taxonomy, 1930-1950: the impact of cytology, ecology, and genetics on ideas of biological classification. Ph.D. Diss., Oregon State University. Corvallis, 1982. 226 leaves.
Halberg F, Halberg E: Circadian rhythms in the mammalian central nervous system, blood pressure and parasites - hobbies of Rudolf Engel. **Int J Chronobiol** 1979;7(1):1-16
Hamrum CL, ed: Darwin's legacy. Nobel Conference XVIII, Gustavus Adolphus College. St. Peter, Minnesota, held October 5-6, 1982. San Francisco, Harper & Row, 1983. 125 p. Contributions by S. J. Gould, I. Stone, R. E. Leakey, P. B. Medawar, E. O. Wilson, J. Pelikan.
Hawkins H: Transatlantic discipleship: two American biologists and their German mentor. **Isis** 1980 Jun;71(257):197-210
Hoppe B: Biologische und technische Bewegungslehre. **Forschungsunternehm Fritz Thyssen Stift Stud Naturwiss Tech Wirtsch Neunzehn Jahrhundert** 1976;2:186-206
Hoppe B: Chemophysiologie zwischen vitalistischer und mechanistischer Biologie im 19. Jahrhundert. **Medizinhist J** 1983;18(3):163-83
Kaiser W: Ernst Mach und das Mechanismusproblem in der Biologie. **Medizinhist J** 1982;17(3):179-94
Kohn A: Errors, fallacies, or deception? **Perspect Biol Med** 1978 Spring;21(3):420-30
MacKenzie D: Sociobiologies in competition: the biometrician-Mendelian debate. In C. Webster, ed: Biology, medicine and society 1840-1940. Cambridge, Cambridge University Press, 1981. p. 243-88.
Malter R: Schopenhauer und die Biologie: Metaphysik der Lebenskraft auf empirischer Grundlage. **Ber Wissenschaftsgesch** 1983;6(1-4):43-58
Manier E: History, philosophy and sociology of biology: a family romance. **Stud Hist Philos Sci** 1980 Mar;11(1):1-24
Meagher LR: The influence of Darwinian theory upon biological research of the late nineteenth century. Ph.D. Diss., Duke University. Durham, 1979. xii, 329 leaves.
Michod RE: Positive heuristics in evolutionary biology. **Br J Philos Sci** 1981;32(1):1-36
Mirzoîan EN: [Some trends in the development of biology in the XXth century] (Rus). **Istor Biol Issled** 1978:7:3-24
Muzrukova HB: Chemistry and biology in the history of cellular's study. **Istor Biol Issled** 1983;9:51-65
Nierhaus G: Ludwig von Bertalanffy 1901-1972. **Sudhoffs Arch** 1981;65(2):144-72
Nilius B: Heuristische Aspekte im Verhältnis zwischen Philosophie und Einzelwissenschaft. **Wiss Z Martin Luther Univ (Math)** 1984;33(2):134-42
Ota J: [History of biology and the current status of molecular biology] (Jpn). **Kango Gijutsu** 1981 Apr;27(6):700-7
Paul DB: A war on two fronts: J. B. S. Haldane and the response to lysenkoism in Britain. **J Hist Biol** 1983 Spring;16(1):1-37
Pauly PJ: Jacques Loeb and the control of life: an experimental biologist in Germany and America, 1859-1924. Ph.D. Diss., The Johns Hopkins University. Baltimore, 1981. viii, 311 p.
Querner H: La cuestion metodologica en la biologia del siglo XIX. **Folia Hum (Barc)** 1981;19(225):595-611
Regelmann JP: Struktur des Arguments als Struktur der Geschichte?--oder: Paradigm lost! **Medizinhist J** 1982;17(1/2):37-53
Rheinberger HJ: Naudin, Darwin, Nägeli: Bemerkungen zu den Vererbungsvorstellungen des 19. Jahrhunderts. **Medizinhist J** 1983;18(3):198-212
Richards RJ: The emergence of evolutionary biology of behaviour in the early nineteenth century. **Br J Hist Sci** 1982 Nov;15(51 pt 3):241-80
Roger J: The living world. In G. S. Rousseau, R. Porter, ed. The ferment of knowledge. Studies in the historiography of eighteenth-century science. Cambridge, Cambridge University Press, 1980. p. 255-83.
Roth RR: The foundation of bionics. **Perspect Biol Med** 1983 Winter;26(2):229-42
Smirnov IN: Problema integratsii znaniia v sovremennoi biologii. **Vopr Filos** 1981;11:38-50
Smith TF, Morowitz HJ: Between history and physics. **J Mol Evol** 1982;18(4):265-82
Strojnowski J: Orientacja biologiczna a orientacja społeczna w medycynie w ujeciu historycznym. **Arch Hist Med (Warsz)** 1984;47(1):25-37
Suppan W: Biologische und kulturelle Bedingungen des Musikgebrauches. **Universitas (Stuttg)** 1982;37(12):1279-84
Szyfman L: Remarques sur l'ouvrage d'Ernst Mayr: 'Lamarck Revisited'. **Bull Biol Fr Belg** 1977;111(3):209-29
Toro Ibáñez MA: Altruismo y cooperación: una interpretación darwinista. **Arbor** 1982;113(441-2):101-9
van Hoorn W: Psychoanalysis, romanticism and biology. **Stor Crit Psicol** 1982 Jun;3(1):5-25
Webster G, Goodwin B: History and structure in biology. **Perspect Biol Med** 1981 Autumn;25(1):39-62
Webster C, ed: Biology, medicine and society 1840-1940. Cambridge, Cambridge University Press, 1981. 344 p. (Past and Present Publications).
Yonemoto S: [Progress in life science and humanity--historical changes in the ideological background and the present status of life science] (Jpn). **Kango Gijutsu** 1981 Apr;27(6):739-44
Zacharias KL: The construction of a primate order: taxonomy and comparative anatomy in establishing the human place in nature, 1735-1916. Ph.D. diss. The Johns Hopkins University. Baltimore, 1980. 464 leaves.

#### Americas

Harrison GA: The past fifty years of human population biology in North America: an outsider's view. In F. Spencer, ed: A history of American physical anthropology, 1930-1980. New York, Academic Press, 1982. p. 467-72.

#### Belgium

Brachet J: Esquisse d'une histoire de la biochimie de la biologie cellulaire et de la biologie moléculaire en Belgique. In Florilège des Sciences en Belgique - II. Bruxelles, Académie Royale de Belgique, 1980. p. 289-314.
Dalcq A: Pol Gérard, 1886-1961. In Florilège des Sciences en Belgique - II. Bruxelles, Académie Royale de Belgique, 1980. p. 609-16.
Demal J: Paul Debaisieux, 1886-1978. In Florilège des Sciences en Belgique - II. Bruxelles, Académie Royale de Belgique, 1980. p. 617-23.
Fautrez J: Les Archives de Biologie, les fondateurs et les éditeurs de la revue. **Arch Biol (Liege)** 1980;91(2):133-40
Leplat G: Hans de Winiwarter, 1875-1949. In Florilège des Sciences en Belgique - II. Bruxelles, Académie Royale de Belgique, 1980. p. 587-97.
Mulnard J: Les vingt premières années des Archives de Biologie. **Arch Biol (Liege)** 1980;91(2):285-95
Poll M, Herlant-Meewis H: Esquisse de l'histoire de la zoologie et de la biologie animale en Belgique depuis 1920. In Florilège des Sciences en Belgique - II. Bruxelles, Académie Royale de Belgique, 1980. p. 249-69.

#### Canada

Cornell JF: From creation to evolution: Sir William Dawson and The idea of design in the nineteenth century. **J Hist Biol** 1983 Spring;16(1):137-70

#### Chile

Brncic D: El desarrollo de la biología general en la Facultad de Medicina y su impacto en la actividad científica nacional. **Rev Med Chil** 1982 Aug;110(8):801-5
Pérez Olea J: Influencia de la biología en la medicina chilena. **Rev Med Chil** 1982 May;110(5):487-90

#### Czechoslovakia

Janisch R: 60 let Ceskoslovenské biologické společnosti při CSAV v Brně. **Cas Lek Cesk** 1982 Nov;121(47):1467-8

#### Denmark

Rasmussen L, Wheatley DN: The Biological Institute of the Carlsberg foundation: international centre for cell biology for 50 years. **Cell Biol Int Rep** 1983 Dec;7(12):1071-9

#### France

Bednarczyk A: Pierre Louis Moreau de Maupertuis (1698-1759) atomizm

biologiczny i panpsychizm. **Kwart Hist Nauki Tech** 1981;26(2):335–62
Bréhant J: Un visage peu connu de Voltaire: le Voltaire biologiste (ses expériences de décapitation des gastéropodes). **Bull Mem Acad R Med Belg** 1981;136(12):580–8
Buican D: Milestones in the philosophic and historical framework of the development of biology in France. **Scientia** 1982;117(9–12):609–21
Eddy JH: Buffon, organic alterations, and man. **Stud Hist Biol** 1984;7:1–45
Farley J, Geison GL, Ebnöther D: Le débat entre Pasteur et Pouchet: science, politique et génération spontanée, au 19e siècle en France. **Pandore** 1982;special number
Legée G: Lettres inédites des Félix Archimède Pouchet (1800–1872) au physiologiste Pierre Flourens (1794–1867). In International Congress of the History of Medicine. 26th, Plovdiv, 1978. Actes du Congress. Sofia, 1981. Volume II. p. 130–8.
Limoges C: The development of the Muséum d'Histoire Naturelle of Paris, c. 1800–1914. In R. Fox, G. Weisz, ed: The organization of science and technology in France 1808–1914. Cambridge, Cambridge University Press, 1980. p. 211–40.
Mikulinskij SR, Markova LA, Starostin BA: Alphonse de Candolle (1806–1893). Jena, Fischer, 1980. 224 p. (Biographien bedeutender Biologen, Band 3).
Pineau H: Paul Broca. L'anthropologiste et le biologiste. **Cah Anthropol** 1980;1–2:47–93
Sandler I: Pierre Louis Moreau de Maupertuis – a precursor of Mendel? **J Hist Biol** 1983 Spring;16(1):101–36

**Germany**

Cappelletti V: Aspects of German biology. From Virchow to Driesch. **Riv Biol** 1981 Winter;74(4):479–502
Engelhardt D von: Polemik und Kontroversen um Haeckel. **Medizinhist J** 1980;15(3):284–304
Hamburger V: Hilde Mangold, co-discoverer of the organizer. **J Hist Biol** 1984 Spring;17(1):1–11
Heinrich WL: Richard Walther Darré und der Hegehofgedanke. Diss. Mainz, 1980. 161 p.
Hinokida T: T. Schwann's three preliminary articles on 'Cell theory'. **Kagakushi Kenkyu** 1983;22(145):35–43
Höxtermann E: Ein Halbjahrhundert Fortschritte der Zellphysiologie, Biochemie und Photobiologie – Otto Heinrich Warburg (1883 bis 1970). **NTM** 1983;20(2):1–24
Kaiser W, Völker A: Die naturwissenschaftlichen Disziplinen im halleschen medizinischen Kollegeprogramm des 18. und 19. Jahrhunderts. **Z Gesamte Inn Med** 1983 Jul 15;38(14):375–82
Kalikow TJ: Konrad Lorenz's ethological theory: explanation and ideology, 1938–1943. **J Hist Biol** 1983 Spring;16(1):39–73
Lenoir T: Kant, Blumenbach, and vital materialism in German biology. **Isis** 1980 Mar;71(256):77–108
Lenoir T: The strategy of life: teleology and mechanics in nineteenth century German biology. Dordrecht, Holland; Boston, Reidel, 1982. xii, 314 p.
Löw R: Philosophie des Lebendigen. Der Begriff des Organischen bei Kant, sein Grund und seine Aktualität. Frankfurt am Main, Suhrkamp, 1980. 358 p.
Rinard RG: The problem of the organic individual: Ernst Haeckel and the development of the biogenetic law. **J Hist Biol** 1981 Fall;14(2):249–76
Scheele I: Zur Typologie des Botanikers in der ersten Hälfte des 19. Jahrhunderts: Christian Friedrich Hornschuch. **Medizinhist J** 1983;18(3):184–97
Siesser WG: Christian Gottfried Ehrenberg: Founder of micropaleontology. **Centaurus** 1981;25(3):166–88
Uschmann G: Haeckel's biological materialism. **Hist Philos Life Sci** 1979;1(1):101–18
Voss H: Goethes Selbstzeugnisse über seine Beschäftigung mit 'organischen Naturen'. **Gegenbaurs Morphol Jahrb** 1979;125(5):687–736
Weinberger C: Wissenschaftstheoretische Anmerkungen zu Konrad Lorenz' 'Vergleichende Verhaltensforschung'. **Z Allg Wissenschaftstheorie** 1980;10(1):147–61
Weindling P: Theories of the cell state in Imperial Germany. In C. Webster, ed: Biology, medicine and society 1840–1940. Cambridge, Cambridge University Press, 1981. p. 99–155.
Wenzel M: Goethes Morphologie in ihrer Beziehung zum darwinistischen Evolutionsdenken. **Medizinhist J** 1983;18(1–2):52–68
Winau R: Ernst Haeckels Vorstellungen von Wert und Werden menschlicher Rassen und Kulturen. **Medizinhist J** 1981;16(3):270–79

**Great Britain**

Cain AJ: Zoological ideas 1831–1981. **Nature** 1981 Sep 3;293(5827):15–6
Cock AG: William Bateson's rejection and eventual acceptance of chromosome theory. **Ann Sci** 1983 Jan;40:19–59
Colp R: [Charles Darwin: Essay–Review] **Trans Stud Coll Physicians Phila** 1983 Dec;5(5 no 4):353–75
Di Gregorio MA: In search of the natural system: problems of zoological classification in Victorian Britain. **Hist Philos Life Sci** 1982;4(2):225–54
Di Gregorio MA: Order or process of nature: Huxley's and Darwin's different approaches to natural sciences. **Hist Philos Life Sci** 1981;3(2):217–41
Evans LT: Darwin's use of the analogy between artificial and natural selection. **J Hist Biol** 1984 Spring;17(1):113–40
Eyler JM: The conversion of Angus Smith: the changing role of chemistry and biology in sanitary science, 1850–1880. **Bull Hist Med** 1980 Summer;54(2):216–34
George W: Darwin. Glasgow, Fontana Paperbacks, 1982. 160 p.
Jacyna LS: John Goodsir and the making of cellular reality. **J Hist Biol** 1983 Spring;16(1):75–99
Jacyna LS: The romantic programme and the reception of cell theory in Britain. **J Hist Biol** 1984 Spring;17(1):13–48
Jenkins EW: The development of school biology, 1918–1945. **Hist Educ** 1979;8(1):59–73
Le Fanu W: Natural history drawings collected by John Hunter F.R.S. (1728–1793), at the Royal College of Surgeons of England. **J Soc Bibliogr Nat Hist** 1978;8(4):329–33
Márquez-Monter H: Conmemoración del centenario de la muerte de Charles R. Darwin. **Gac Med Mex** 1983 May;119(5):212–8
Novák VJ: Zakladatel moderní biologie. Sto let od smrti Ch. R. Darwina. **Cas Lek Cesk** 1982 Apr 16;121(15):449–50
Ospovat D: The development of Darwin's theory: natural history, natural theology, and natural selection, 1838–1859. Cambridge, New York, Cambridge University Press, 1981. xii, 301 p.
Paradis JG: T. H. Huxley, Man's place in nature. Lincoln, University of Nebraska Press, 1978. xi, 226 p.
Roll-Hansen N: E. S. Russell and J. H. Woodger: the failure of two twentieth-century opponents of mechanistic biology. **J Hist Biol** 1984 Fall;17(3):399–428
Secord JA: Nature's fancy: Charles Darwin and the breeding of pigeons. **Isis** 1981;72:163–86
Smith DG: The voyage of the challenger. **Bookman** 1983 Apr;10(2):3–9
Spear JL: Filaments, females, families and social fabric: Carlyle's extension of a biological analogy. In Paradis J, Postlewait T, ed: Victorian science and Victorian values: literary perspectives. New York, New York Academy of Sciences, 1981. p. 69–84.
Sulloway FJ: Further remarks on Darwin's spelling habits and the dating of Beagle voyage manuscripts. **J Hist Biol** 1983 Fall;16(3):361–90

**Hungary**

Csillik B: Prof. Dr. Ambrus Abrahám. **Acta Biol Acad Sci Hung** 1983;34(2–3):131–5
Donáth T: Dr. Péterfi Tibor (1883–1953). **Orv Hetil** 1983 Dec 11;124(50):3061–2
Lambrecht M: Gorka Sándor az elsö magyar biológusprofesszor. **Orv Hetil** 1979 Aug 19;120(32):1947–50
Sztanyik BL: A sugárbiológia negyedszázada. **Orv Hetil** 1983 Sep 11;124(37):2223–32

**Italy**

Belloni L: Un circolo bernardiano in Italia: la Società delle Scienze Biologiche in Torino. Luigi Vella de la curaroterapia del tetano. **Physis** 1981;23(3):301–10
Castellani C: Appunti per uno studio della biologia post-Spallanazaniana: 1780–1820. **Physis** 1978;20(1–4):5–29
Castellani C: Ontogenesi di una dissertazione: le 'osservazioni e sperienze sui vermicelli spermatici ...' di L. Spallanzani. **Hist Philos Life Sci** 1982;4(1):125–57
Cremona GF: La bioclimatologia medica: aspetti dell'evoluzione storica, con particolare riguardo al contributo degli scienziati piemontesi. **Ann Osp Maria Vittoria Torino** 1982 Jul–Dec;25(7–12):245–58
Cremona GF: Studi di biologia e medicina nell'opera del fisico piemontese G. B. Beccaria. **Ann Osp Maria Vittoria Torino** 1982 Jul–Dec;25(7–12):259–68
Di Pietro P: La 'storia naturale del mare' di Lazzaro Spallanzani. **Thalassia Salentina** 1978;8:53–62
Fischer JL: L'aspect social et politique des relations épistolaires entre quelques savants français et la Station zoologique de Naples de 1878 à 1912. **Rev Hist Sci (Paris)** 1980 Jul;33(3):225–51
Lucchetta PM: Nuovi documenti per la biografia di Antonio Vallisneri. **Quad Stor Univ Padova** 1982;15:131–45
Marbach JU: Domenico Cirillo; ein Lebenslauf, 1739–1799. **Gesnerus** 1980;37(3/4):257–69
Partsch KJ: Die zoologische Station in Neapel: Modell internationaler Wissenschaftszusammenarbeit. Göttingen, Vandenhoeck & Ruprecht, 1980. 369 p.
Partsch KJ: Die Zoologische Station in Neapel. Modell internationaler Wissenschaftszusammenarbeit. Gottingen, Vandenhoeck & Ruprecht, 1980. 369 p. (Studien zu Naturwissenschaft, Technik und Wirtschaft im Neunzehnten Jahrhundert, Bd. 11).
Spallanzani M: Nuovi studi su Spallanzani e la biologia del '700. **Quad Stor** 1981;16(3):1080–90
Spirito A: Breve istoria della 'rivista di biologia' con particolare riguardo all'ultimo trentennio. **Riv Biol** 1979 Jan–Jun;72(1–2):3–10

**Japan**

Uchikawa K: Dr. Shiro Oshima (1934–1981). **Acarologia** 1982 Jun;23(2):99–101

**Poland**

Brennan JF, Zieliński K: Science in Poland. The Nencki Institute of Experimental Biology. **Pavlov J Biol Sci** 1981 Apr–Jun;16(2):118–23
Feliksiakowa J: Stand der biologischen Bibliographie in Polen in den Jahren 1945–1970. **Hist Philos Life Sci** 1981;3(1):115–31
Kuźnicke L: The Section of Biological Science of the Polish Academy of Sciences over the last 25 years. **Rev Pol Acad Sci (Warsz)** 1978;23:21–35
Kuźnicki L, Radziwiłł M: The section of biological science of the Polish Academy of Sciences over the last 25 years. **Rev Pol Acad Sci (Warsz)** 1978;23(1):21–35
Zieliński K: Sixty years of the Nencki Institute of Experimental Biology. **Rev Pol Acad Sci (Warsz)** 1978;23(4):47–74

**Romania**

Jitariu P: Societatea de Medici si Naturalisti si dezvoltarea stiintelor biologicie. **Rev Med Chir Soc Med Nat Iasi** 1980 Oct–Dec;84(4):636–42

**Spain**

Sala Catalá J: Cambio de paradigma y polemica cientifica entre los biologos españoles (1860–1922). **Asclepio** 1982;34:239–63
Sala Catalá J: El evolucionismo en la practica cientifica de los biologos españoles del siglo XIX (1860–1907). **Asclepio** 1981;33:81–125

**Sweden**

Schramm E: Linné, Gedner und die biologische Kontrolle. **Medizinhist J** 1984;19(3):244–9

**Switzerland**

Marx J: Charles Bonnet contre les Lumières. 2 v. Oxford, Voltaire Foundation at the Taylor Institution, 1976. 782 p.

**Tanzania**

Beck A: Priorities in biological research at Amani, 1902–1914. **Tanzan Notes Rec** 1981;(86–87):13–6

**United States**

Allen G: The transformation of a science: T. H. Morgan and the emergence of a new American biology. In Oleson A, Voss J, ed: The organization of knowledge in modern America, 1860–1920. Baltimore and London, Johns Hopkins University Press, 1979. p. 173–210.
Benson KR: William Keith Brooks (1848–1908): a case study in morphology and the development of American biology. Ph.D. Diss. Oregon State University. Corvallis, 1979. 356 leaves.
Benson KR: 'William Keith Brooks (1848–1908): primary resource material'. **Mendel Newsl** 1983 Nov;23:7–11
Blustein BE: The Philadelphia Biological Society, 1857–61: a failed experiment? **J Hist Med Allied Sci** 1980 Apr;35(2):188–202
Byrne R: Keynote address--50th anniversary BPA meeting, Boston, Massachusetts. **J Biol Photogr** 1981 Apr;49(2):39–44
Churchill FB: In search of the new biology: an epilogue. **J Hist Biol** 1981 Spring;14(1):177–91
Gibson HL: The Biological Photographic Association, its half century. The era of maturation, 1965–1980. **J Biol Photogr** 1980 Apr;48(2):41–86
Haas JD: The development of research strategies for studies of biological variation in living human populations. In F. Spencer, ed: A history of American physical anthropology, 1930–1980. New York, Academic Press, 1982. 435–46.
Haraway D: The biological enterprise: sex, mind, and profit from human engineering to sociobiology. **Radic Hist Rev** 1979 Spring/Summer;Spec:206–37
Kaplan MM: Three decades of collaboration with Hilary Koprowski. **J Cell Physiol [Suppl]** 1982;2:1–6
Kingsland S: Raymond Pearl: on the frontier in the 1920's. Raymond Pearl memorial lecture, 1983. **Hum Biol** 1984 Feb;56(1):1–18
Kohler RE: Rudolf Schoenheimer, isotopic tracers, and biochemistry in the 1930's. **Hist Stud Phys Sci** 1977;8:257–98
Kritchevsky D: Hilary Koprowski and The Wistar Institute. **J Cell Physiol [Suppl]** 1982;2:vi–viii
Liebenau J: The papers of Edmund Newton Harvey, (1887–1959). **Surv Sources Newsl** 1977 Nov;6:8–9
Little MA: The development of ideas on human ecology and adaptation. In F. Spencer, ed: A history of American physical anthropology, 1930–1980. New York, Academic Press, 1982. p. 405–33.
Lovejoy CO, Mensforth RP, Armelagos GJ: Five decades of skeletal biology as reflected in the American Journal of Physical Anthropology. In F. Spencer, ed: A history of American physical anthropology, 1930–1980. New York, Academic Press, 1982. p. 329–36.
Pauly PJ: The appearance of academic biology in late nineteenth-century America. **J Hist Biol** 1984 Fall;17(3):369–97
Piternick LK: Richard Goldschmidt, controversial geneticist and creative biologist: a critical review of his contribution. Basal, Boston, Birkhäuser, 1980. 153 p.
Rainger R: The Henry Fairfield Osborn Papers at the American Museum of Natural History. **Mendel Newsl** 1980 Jun;(18):8–13
Rall JE: Mones Berman--the man and his legacy to quantitative biology. **Am J Physiol** 1983 Nov;245(5 Pt 1):R618–9
Smith KC: History of American Society for Photobiology (ASP). The first 10 years, and before. **Photochem Photobiol** 1982 May;35(5):597–614
Thomas L: The right track. **Wilson Q** 1980;4(2):87–98
Wilens S: Ross Granville Harrison. In Dictionary of American Biography, Suppl. 6, 1956–1960. p. 281–3, 1980.

**USSR**

Adams MB: Biology after Stalin: a case study. **Survey** 1977–78;23(1):53–80
Bliakher LI: Ia. A. Borzenkov–istorik biologii. **Vopr Istor Estestvozn Tekh** 1982;1:36–44
Gusev AV: 150 Jahre Zoologisches Institut der Akademie der Wissenschaften der UdSSR. **Angew Parasitol** 1982 May;23(2):109–11
Mikhaĭlov VP: Nikolaĭ Varnek i Karl Bér. **Arkh Anat Gistol Embriol** 1982 Apr;82(4):86–95
Prokof'eva-Bel'govskaïa AA: [G. A. Levitskiĭ and Soviet research on chromosome morphology.] (Rus). **Istor Biol Issled** 1978;7:46–64
Soyfer V: Andrei Sakharov and the fate of biological science in the USSR. **J Craniofac Genet Dev Biol** 1984;4(3):173–8
Sytnik KM, Dyshlebyi PS: Dialektika revoliutsii v estestvoznanii. **Vopr Filos** 1981;(3):42–56
Zhurnalu 'Uspekhi sovremennoĭ biologii'--50 let:

**Venezuela**

Beauperthuy de Benedetti R: Beauperthuy. La herpetología y Venuzuela. In International Congress of the History of Medicine, 27th, Barcelona, 1980. Actas. Barcelona, Académia de Ciències Mèdiques de Catalunya i Balears, 1981. p. 454–7.

# BIOPHYSICS

**1700 to Present**

Beynon JH: The history of mass spectrometry and the search for zero. **Biomed Mass Spectrom** 1981 Sep;8(9):380–3
Blahd WH: History of external counting procedures. **Semin Nucl Med** 1979 Jul;9(3):159–63
Blaufox MD, Constable AR: Antique hazards: a latter day encounter with radium. **J Nucl Med** 1983 Jan;24(1):79–82
Brucer M: Historical note. Elizabeth Rona 1890–1981. **Health Phys** 1982 Apr;42(4):405–6
Donato L: Twenty-five years of nuclear medicine. **J Nucl Med Allied Sci** 1981 Oct–Dec;25(4):195–200
Edwards CL: Tumor-localizing radionuclides in retrospect and prospect. **Semin Nucl Med** 1979 Jul;9(3):186–9
Fisenne IM, Keller HW: A short history of ZnS on Mylar as an alpha-scintillation detector. **Health Phys** 1981 May;40(5):739–41
Freedman GS: Radionuclide tomography. **Semin Nucl Med** 1979 Jul;9(3):201–2
Hawkins HB, Cinti DC: Magnetic resonance imaging. Where did it come from? What is it? Where is it going? Part I. History and physical principles. **Conn Med** 1984 Sep;48(9):575–7
Holland NN: Freud, physics, and literature. **J Am Acad Psychoanal** 1984 Jul;12(3):301–20
Hör G, Munz DL: Nuklearmedizin--einst und jetzt. Folge 1: Entwicklung, Aufgabenspektrum, Radiopharmazeutika, Messtechnik, Klinische Indikationen. **Fortschr Med** 1983 Mar 17;101(10):415–22
The interaction of acoustical and electromagnetic fields with biological systems: A collection of papers from the symposium honoring Professor Herman P. Schwan on the occasion of his 65th birthday. Philadelphia, November 24 and 25, 1980. **Prog Clin Biol Res** 1982;86:1–183
Johns HE: The physicist in cancer treatment and detection. **Int J Radiat Oncol Biol Phys** 1981 Jun;7(6):801–8
Loken MK, Williams LE: A history of computers in nuclear medicine. **Semin Nucl Med** 1979 Jul;9(3):197–200
Myers WG: Georg Charles de Hevesy: the father of nuclear medicine. **J Nucl Med** 1979 Jun;20(6):590–4
Myers WG: PET = positrin+electron transmutation. **JNM** 1980;21:1200
Ram PC, Fordham EW: An historical survey of bone scanning. **Semin Nucl Med** 1979 Jul;9(3):190–6
Regato JA del: Enrico Fermi. **Int J Radiat Oncol Biol Phys** 1982 Aug;8(8):1393–416
Richards P, Tucker WD, Srivastava SC: Technetium-99m: an historical perspective. **Int J Appl Radiat Isot** 1982 Oct;33(10):793–9

## BIOPHYSICS

Taplin GV: The history of lung imaging with radionuclides. **Semin Nucl Med** 1979 Jul;9(3):178-85
Taylor DM: Blutzellmarkierung: Rückblick und Ausblick. **Wien Klin Wochenschr** 1984 Feb 3;96(3):89-92
Taylor LS: Who is the father of health physics? **Health Phys** 1982 Jan;42(1):92-2
Thakur ML, Sinzinger H, Höfer R: Radioisotopenmarkierung menschlicher Blutzellen--ein historischer Uberblick. **Wien Klin Wochenschr** 1984 Feb 3;96(3):87-8
Ziemer PL, Kathren RL, ed: Health physics: a backward glance. New York, Pergamon Press, 1980. 237 p.

**Bulgaria**

Kardashev TD, Velkov DL: On the historical development of biophysics in Bulgaria. In International Congress of the History of Medicine. 26th, Plovdiv, 1978. Actes du Congress. Sofia, 1981. Volume II. p. 216.

**Czechoslovakia**

Dienstbier Z: Třicet let Ustavu biofyziky a nukleární medicíny FVL KU. **Sb Lek** 1983 Mar;85(3):65-7
Dienstbier Z: 25 let Ceskoslovenské společnosti nukleární medicíny a radiační hygieny. **Cas Lek Cesk** 1981 Aug 13;120(31-32):963-7
Dienstbier Z: 25 years of the Czechoslovak Society for Nuclear Medicine and Radiation Hygiene. **Czech Med** 1981;4(3):97-106
Hradečná Z: Pódíl Biofyzikálního ústavu CSAV na začátcích biofyzikálního výzkumu v CSSR. **Bratisl Lek Listy** 1984 Jan;81(1):106-8
Kapitola J: Dvacet let provozu radioizotopového oddělení III. interní kliniky FVL KU v Praze. **Sb Lek** 1983 Sep;85(7-8):211-5
Kukurová E, Sajter V: Osobnost prof. PhDr. Viktora Teisslera a prvých 15 rokov existencie Ustavu lekárskej fyziky Univerzity Komenského v Bratislave. **Bratisl Lek Listy** 1983 Dec;80(6):725-30
Tichý M, Kukurová E, Beniak M, et al: Historické okolnosti vzniku Ustavu pre lekársku fyziku. **Bratisl Lek Listy** 1984 Feb;81(2):235-9

**Germany**

Regato JA del: Max Planck. **Int J Radiat Oncol Bill Phys** 1979 Nov-Dec;5(11-12):2097-111
Schreier W: Ueber historische Wurzeln von Fechners Psychophysik. In Eckardt G, ed: Zur Geschichte der Psychologie. Berlin, VEB Deutscher Verlag der Wissenschaften, 1979. p. 61-71.

**Great Britain**

Del Regato JA: William Henry Bragg. **Int J Radiat Oncol Biol Phys** 1981 Jan;7(1):83-97
Mallard J, Trott NG: Some aspects of the history of nuclear medicine in the United Kingdom. **Semin Nucl Med** 1979 Jul;9(3):203-17
Miller H: 40 years of development in radioisotope non-imaging techniques. **Phys Med Biol** 1984 Feb;29(2):157-61
Ross WM, Day MJ: Mullard 4 MV linear accelerator at Newcastle upon Tyne. **Br J Radiol** 1981 Sep;54(645):819

**Japan**

Iio M: Professor G. V. Hevesy, Doctor Y. Nishina and nuclear medicine in Japan. **Radiat Med** 1983 Jul-Sep;1(3):255-62
Yamaguchi C, Yamanaka Y, Tateno Y: Kakuigaku : kanri to hokisei. Institutional requirements and history of nuclear medicine. Tokyo, Jitsugyo Kohosha, Showa 53 nen. [1978]. 269 p.

**United States**

A. L. Copley: curriculum vitae and publications: **Biorheology** 1981;18(3-6):703--23
Andrew ER: A historical review of NMR and its clinical applications. **Br Med Bull** 1984 Apr;40(2):115-9
Beatty WK: William T. Bovie. In Dictionary of American Biography, Suppl. 6, 1956-1960. p. 69-70, 1980.
Brucer M, Harris CC, MacIntyre WJ, et al: The heritage of nuclear medicine. Commemorating the 25th anniversary of the Society of Nuclear Medicine, 1954-1979. New York, Society of Nuclear Medicine, 1979. xxvi, 167 p. Reprints of various articles.
Brumley WC, Sphon JA: Regulatory mass spectrometry. **Biomed Mass Spectrom** 1981 Sep;8(9):390-6
'Health Physics': 25th anniversary issue commemorating the founding of the Health Physics Society 1955-1980.: **Health Phys** 1980 Jun;38(6):883-1209
Heckelsberg LF: Historical note: thermoluminescent dosimetry (LiF) 1950-51. **Health Phys** 1980 Sep;39(3):391-3
Kathren RL: Elda Emma Anderson. In: Notable American women. The modern period. Cambridge, Mass., Belknap-Harvard Univ. Press, 1980. 4:20-1.
Llaurado JG: Role of the biomedical engineer in nuclear medicine. **J Clin Eng** 1981 Oct-Dec;6(4):269-76
Myers WG: Historian's note: early experiences in nuclear medicine by John H. Lawrence, 1956. **J Nucl Med** 1979 Jun;20(6):560-4
Perspectives in biorheology: Festschrift for A. L. Copley. **Biorheology** 1981;18(3-6):305-729
Powell MR: H.O. Anger and his work at the Donner Laboratory. **Semin Nucl Med** 1979 Jul;9(3):164-8
Schwan HP: Physical properties of biological matter: some history, principles, and applications. **Bioelectromagnetics** 1982;3(1):3-8
Simberloff D: Entropy, information and life: biophysics in the novels of Thomas Pynchon. **Perspect Biol Med** 1978 Spring;21(3):617-25

## BIRTH CONTROL

See also **Statistics and Demography**

Declaración sobre el aborto provocado: Sagrada Congregación para la Doctrina de la Fe **Rev Med Univ Navarra** 1982 Dec;26(4):255-60
Döring GK: Ist das Kondom heute besser als sein Ruf? **Fortschr Med** 1980 Jan 31;98(4):113-7
Fairbanks B, Scharfman B: The cervical cap: cap and current experience. **Women Health** 1980 Fall;5(3):61-80
Grenon-Plante D: La contraception: oui, mais à quel prix? **Infirm Can** 1982 Nov;24(10):27-31
Guyotjeannin C: A propos des préservatifs. **Monit Pharm Lab** 1983;37(1566):2364-5
Hoffer PC, Hull NE: Murdering mothers: infanticide in England and New England 1558-1803. New York and London, New York University Press, 1981. xxii, 211 p. (New York University School of Law Series in Legal History, 2).
Käser O: Zur Geschichte der Kontrazeption und ein Blick in die Zukunft. **Geburtshilfe Frauenheilkd** 1983 Jun;43 Suppl 1:2-7
Kass N: Abortion in Jewish law. **Koroth** 1983 Aug;8(7-8):323-31
Kuznetsov VK, Baranova EV: Istoriia i sovremennoe sostoianie zakonodatel'stv ob absorte v stranakh mira. **Feldsher Akush** 1980;45(8):3-6
Linhard J: Aspectos sociales de los métodos naturales. **Reproduccion** 1981 Apr-Jun;5(2):95-104
Matuschka ME: Gynäkologische Sterilisationen zur Zeit des Hexenwahns. Eine Studie zur Geschichte der Human- und Veterinärmedizin sowie des zeitgenössischen Rechtsdenkens. Graz, Akademische Druck- u. Verlagsanstalt, 1981. 69 p.
Musallam BF: Why Islam permitted birth control. **Arab Stud Q** 1981;3(2):181-97
Piga Sánchez-Morate B: Aspectos médico-legales del aborto. **An R Acad Nac Med (Madr)** 1982;99(1):51-70
Saidi MH, Zainie CM: Contraception and sterilization, a brief history. In their: Female sterilization, a handbook for women. New York, Garland, 1980. p. 1-14.
Schadewaldt H: Die Geschichte der Kontrazeption. **Mod Med (Stuttg)** 1980;8:527-8
Tatum HJ, Connell-Tatum EB: Barrier contraception: a comprehensive overview. **Fertil Steril** 1981 Jul;36(1):1-12

**Australia**

Cowlishaw G: Infanticide in aboriginal Australia. **Oceania** 1978;48:262-83

**Chile**

Romero H: Población y planificación de familia. **Rev Med Chil** 1977 Dec;105(12):946-50

**Denmark**

Manniche E: [History of induced abortion in Denmark from 1200 to 1979] (Jpn). **Josanpu Zasshi** 1982 Oct;36(10):842-7

**France**

Avellano E, Bedault M, Bedrani R, et al: Un mémoire sur la contraception. **Soins Gynecol Obstet Pueric Pediatr** 1982 Jul-Aug;(14-15):55-61

**Japan**

Obayashi M: [Historical background of the acceptance of induced abortion] (Jpn). **Josanpu Zasshi** 1982 Dec;36(12):1011-6

**Mexico**

Aguirre Zozaya F, Iglesias M, Reyes RM, et al: Aspectos históricos, culturales, legales, psicosociales y educativos del aborto inducido. **Ginecol Obstet Mex** 1980 Aug;48(286):111-35

**Netherlands**

De Bruijn J: Geschiedenis van de abortus in Nederland. Een analyse van opvattingen en discussies, 1600-1979. Amsterdam, Van Gennep, 1979.

330 p.

**Sweden**

Högberg U: Mylingar, arsenik, fosfor och sonder--om aborter under gångna århundraden. **Lakartidningen** 1981 Aug 26;78(35):2951-2

**United States**

Acevedo Z: Abortion in early America. **Woman Health** 1979 Summer;4(2):121-33
Kantrow L: Philadelphia gentry: fertility and family limitation among an American aristocracy. **Popul Stud** 1980 Mar;34(1):21-30
Leavitt JW, ed: Women and health in America: historical readings. Madison, University of Wisconsin Press, 1984. ix, 526 p. (Previously published articles by various authors)

**Before 500 A.D.**

Peto M: A népességnövekedés szabályozása az ókorban. **Orvostort Kozl** 1982;28(1-3):131-9
Preus A: Biomedical techniques for influencing human reproduction in the fourth century B.C. **Arethusa** 1975;8:237-63

**Egypt**

Diener L: Från antikonception till amning - om tillökning i familjen i det faraoniska Egypten. **Nord Medicinhist Arsbok** 1983;:41-58

**Greco-Roman**

Engels D: The problem of female infanticide in the Greco-Roman world. **Classical Philol** 1980;75:112-20
Fontanille MT: Avortement et contraception dans la médecine gréco-romaine. Paris, Laboratoires Searle, 1977. 233 p.
Hendriks IH, Vries PA de: Anticonceptie en abortus provocatus in de Grieks-Romeinse oudheid. **Groniek** 1978 Dec;60:1-11, 18

**Greece**

Carrick PJ: Ancient Greek ethical perspectives on abortion and euthanasia. Ph.D. Diss., Temple University. Philadelphia, 1982. vii, 346 p.

**1450-1700**

**Great Britain**

Wrigley EA: Marital fertility in seventeenth century Colyton. **Econ Hist Rev** 1978;31(3):429-36

**1700 to Present**

Abbott P, Wertheimer R: Philosophers and the abortion question. **Polit Theory** 1978;6(3):313-44
Bullough VL: A brief note on rubber technology and contraception: the diaphragm and the condom. **Technol Cult** 1981;22(1):104-11
Chandrasekhar S: 'A dirty, filthy book.' The writings of Charles Knowlton and Annie Besant on reproductive physiology and birth control and an account of the Bradlaugh-Besant trial. With the definitive texts of Fruits of philosophy by Charles Knowlton; The law of population by Annie Besant; Theosophy and the law of population by Annie Besant. Berkeley, University of California Press, 1981. xi, 217 p.
Fijałkowski W: 50 lat naturalnego planowania rodziny. **Ginekol Pol** 1979 Nov;50(11):909-16
Franz MM, Chiba M: Abortion, contraception, and motherhood in post-war Japan and the United States. **Int J Womens Stud** 1980;3(1):66-75
Genné WH: Sex, marriage and family: an update from Amsterdam. **J Ecumenical Stud** 1979;16(1):154-60
Goldsmith A, Edelman DA: Métodos anticonceptivos de barrera. **Reproduccion** 1982 Jul-Dec;6(3-4):185-92
Huusen AH: Geboortenregeling in de moderne tijd. **Spiegel Hist** 1981;16(2):66-70
Kay CR: James Mackenzie Lecture 1979. The happiness pill? **J R Coll Gen Pract** 1980 Jan;30(210):8-19
McLaren A: Contraception and its discontents: Sigmund Freud and birth control. **J Soc Hist** 1979;12(4):513-29
Mazur DP: Procreation and new definitions in the role of women in a Soviet bloc country: the case of Poland. Yedlin Tova, ed. Women in Eastern Europe and the Soviet Union. New York, Praeger, 1980. p. 226-38.
Miringoff ML: The impact of population policy upon social welfare. **Soc Serv Rev** 1980;54(3):301-16
Pototschnig F: Entwicklungstendenzen im kanonischen Ehe- und Eheprozessrecht. **Osterr Arch Kirchenr** 1978;29(1-2):52-81
Rose H: The social determinants of reproduction science and technology. In Knorr KD, et al, ed: Determinants and controls of scientific development. Dordrecht, Boston, D. Reidel, 1975. (Theory and decision library, v. 10). p. 407-30.
Serlin R: Contraceptives: back to the barriers. **New Sci** 1981;91:281-4
Sloan DG: The extent of contraceptive use and the social paradigm of modern demography. **Sociology** 1983;17(3):380-7
Valencia-Villa H: Derecho y aborto: una relación de poder. **Cuad Filos Let** 1980;3(2):79-84
Vasilev D: Izmenenie na zakonodatelstvoto, koeto regulira pravniia rezhim na izkustveniia abort v sveta prez poslednite 10 godini. **Akush Ginekol (Sofiia)** 1981;20(4):269-75
Vollman RF: Pathfinders 2: Wilhelm Hillebrand, first teacher of the sympto-thermic method. **Int Rev Nat Fam Plann** 1979;3:316-21
Weiner NF: Of feminism and birth control propaganda (1790-1840). **Int J Womens Stud** 1980;3(5):411-30
Wells RV: Birth control: different conceptions. **J Interdiscip Hist** 1979;10(3):511-6

**Africa**

Grosse SD: The politics of family planning in the Maghrib. **Stud Comp Int Dev** 1982;17(1):22-48
Perova M: V poiskakh resheniia demograficheskikh problem. **Aziia Afr Segodnia** 1981;5:31-3

**Americas**

Randall M: La penetración imperialista y sus consecuencias para la mujer Latinoamericana. **Santiago (Cuba)** 1974;(15):227-47
Weaver JL: The politics of Latin American family-planning policy. **J Dev Areas** 1978;12(4):415-37

**Belgium**

Leboutte R: L'infanticide dans l'est de la Belgique aux XVIIIe-XIXe siècles: une réalité. **Ann Demogr Hist (Paris)** 1983;:163-92

**Brazil**

Monteiro LA: Population policy and the press: the example of Brazil. **Contemp Rev** 1975;226(1309):76-81

**Canada**

Collins LD, Higgins D, ed: The politics of abortion: trends in Canadian fertility policy. **Atlantis** 1982;7(2):2-20
DeValk A: Understandable but mistaken: law, morality and the Canadian Catholic Church 1966-1969. **Can Cathol Hist Assoc Study Sess** 1982;49:87-109
Lamoureux D: La lutte pour le droit à l'avortement (1969-1981). **Rev Hist Am Fr** 1983;37(1):81-90
McLaren A: 'What has this to do with working class women?': Birth control and the Canadian left, 1900-1939. **Soc Hist (Canada)** 1981;14(28):435-54

**Chile**

Romero H: La planificación de familia en Chile, 1952-1977. **Rev Med Chil** 1977 Oct;105(10):724-30

**China**

Bianco L: Birth control in China: local data and their reliability. **China Q** 1981;(85):119-37
Bianco L: Voyage en Chine. **Esprit** 1973; (4):595-604
Lin SP: Family planning in Taiwan: its problems and solutions. **She Hui K'ohsueh Lun Ts'ung** 1978;27:109-51
Loraine JA: Population and birth control in China. **Contemp Rev** 1981;239(1388):126-130
Maloney JM: Recent developments in China's population planning: notes and comments. **Pac Aff** 1981;54(1):100-14
Verma A: Birth control and planned parenthood in China. **China Rep (India)** 1971;7(2):41-8
Wülker G: Das grösste Volk der Erde: Bevölkerungsprobleme und Bevölkerungspolitik der Volksrepublik China. **Eur Arch** 1972;27(8):285-94
Yuan Tien H: Induced fertility transition: impact of population planning and socio-economic change in the People's Republic of China. **Popul Stud** 1984 Nov;38(3):385-400

**Colombia**

Sanz de Santamaría MC de, Salas Sánchez M, Sabogal F: Aspectos psicosociales del aborto (mesa redonda). **Cuad Filos Let** 1980;3(2):85-105

**Egypt**

Calabrese MC: La politica di planificazione familiare in Egitto fino al 1977. **Oriente Mod** 1978;58(1-3):97-107

# BIRTH CONTROL


**France**

Ariès P: La contraception autrefois. **Histoire** 1978;1:36-44
Collomb P: La diffusion des méthodes contraceptives modernes en France de 1971 à 1978. **Population** 1979;34(6):1045-65
Dumont GF, Legrand J: Evolution récente du nombre des décès déclarés dus à l'avortement. **Population** 1981;36(2):410-14
D'une révolte à une lutte: 25 ans d'histoire du planning familial. Paris, Tierce, 1982. 506 p.
Dupâquier J, Lachiver M: Du contresens à l'illusion technique, suivi d'une réponse de John Knodel à Jacques Dupâquier. **Ann Econ Soc Civilis** 1981;36(3):489-92
Farr AD: The Marquis de Sade and induced abortion. **J Med Ethics** 1980 Mar;6(1):7-10
Fine-Souriac A: La limitation des naissances dans le sud-ouest de la France: fécondité, allaitement et contraception au pays de Sault du milieu du XVIIIe siècle à 1914. **Ann Midi** 1978;90(2):155-88
Gaillard J: Le médecin et l'avortement au XIXe siècle. **Histoire** 1979;16:35-7
Guillat JC: La contraception: introduction. **Soins Gynecol Obstet Pueric Pediatr** 1982 Jul-Aug;(14-15):3-4
Guillat JC: L'histoire de la contraception à travers les textes officiels. **Soins Gynecol Obstet Pueric Pediatr** 1982 Jul-Aug;(14-15):53-4
McLaren A: Abortion in nineteenth-century France. **Fr Hist Stud** 1978;10
Olivier-Friguet G: Les femmes du nord face à l'avortement (de 1975 à nos jours). **Rev Nord** 1981;63(250):775-800
Ronsin F: La classe ouvrière et le néo-Malthusianisme: l'exemple français avant 1914. **Mouvement Soc** 1979;106:85-117
Van de Walle E: Motivation and technology in the decline of French fertility. In R. Wheaton, T. K. Hareven, ed: Family and sexuality in French history. Philadelphia, University of Pennsylvania Press, 1980. p. 135-78.

**Germany**

Arendt HJ: Eine demokratische Massenbewegung unter Führung der KPD im Frühjahr 1931. **Z Geschichtswiss** 1971;19(2):212-23
Deneke JF: Vorbeugende Massnahmen gegen Kindesmord im 19. Jahrhundert. **Krankenpfl J** 1984 May 1;22(5):36-8
Engel K: Der Gräfenberg-Ring. Zu seiner Vorgeschichte, Entwicklung, Anwendung und frühen Rezeption. Diss. Erlangen-Nürnberg, 1979. 137 p.
Khalatbari P, Müllen K, Strohbach E: Népesedéspolitikai problémák a német demokratikus köztársaságban. **Demografia** 1972;15(2):184-94
Knodel J: Espacement des naissances et planification familiale: une critique de la méthode Dupâquier-Lachiver. **Ann Econ Soc Civilis** 1981;36(3):473-88
Knodel J: From natural fertility to family limitation: the onset of fertility transition in a sample of German villages. **Demography** 1979 Nov;16(4):493-521
Ludwig H: Verhütung der Empfängnis--Verhängnis der Verhütung. Die Leistungen Ernst Gräfenbergs und die Reaktion der Gynäkologie seiner Zeit. **Zentralbl Gynakol** 1983;105(18):1197-205
Neuman RP: Working class birth control in Wilhelmine Germany. **Comp Stud Soc Hist** 1978;20(3):408-28
Pfäfflin F, Gross J: Involuntary sterilization in Germany from 1933 to 1945 and some consequences for today. **Int J Law Psychiatry** 1983;5(3-4):419-23
Pommerin R: The fate of mixed blood children. **Ger Stud Rev** 1982;5(3):315-23
Rodegra H: Kindestötung und Verheimlichung der Schwangerschaft: eine sozialgeschichtliche und medizinsoziologische Untersuchung mit Einzelfallanalysen. Herzogenrath [Germany], Murken-Altrogge, 1981. 68 p.
Simmer HH: Die Anfänge der hormonalen Kontrazeption und die Münchener Medizinische Wochenschrift. **MMW** 1982 May 21;124(20):499-503

**Ghana**

Tiberini ES: Note sull'aborto e la contraccezione tra gli Nzema del Ghana. **Africa (Italy)** 1980;35(2):159-70

**Great Britain**

Clarke K: Infanticide, illegitimacy and the medical profession in nineteenth century England. **Soc Soc Hist Med Bull (Lond)** 1980 Jun;26:11-14
Dupâquier J, Fauve-Chamoux A, Grebenik E, ed: Malthus past and present. London; New York, Academic Press, 1983. xix, 416 p. Contributions by A. Béjin, Y. Breton, Y. Charbit, L. Devance, A. Digby, M. W. Flinn, R. E. Frisch, M. Godelier, L. Gordon, P. Guillaume, G. Heinsohn, T. H. Hollingsworth, P. A. Jewell, N. Keyfitz, R. Keynes, H. Le Bras, M. Perrot, F. Rausky, M. Rebérioux, R. Remond, F. Ronsin, G. R. Searle, B. Stapleton, O. Steiger, P. Vallin, E. Van de Walle, A. Waterman, J. Wolff, E. A. Wrigley, V. Wynne-Edwards.
Evans B: Freedom to choose: the life and work of Dr. Helena Wright, pioneer of contraception. London, Bodley Head, 1984. 285 p.
Hall LA: The Stopes collection in the Contemporary Medical Archives Centre at the Wellcome Institute for the History of Medicine. **Soc Soc Hist Med Bull (Lond)** 1983 Jun;32:50-1
Hansen E: 'Overlaying' in 19th-century England: infant mortality in infanticide? **Hum Ecol** 1979;7:333-52
Holtzman EM: Marriage, sexuality, and contraception in the British middle class, 1918-1939: the correspondence of Marie Stopes. Ph.D. Diss., Rutgers University, The State Univ. of New Jersey. New Brunswick, 1982. v, 170 p.
Lewis J: The ideology and politics of birth control in inter-war Britain. **Womens Stud** 1979;2(l)
Muñoz-Perez F: Douze ans d'avortement légal en Angleterre-Galles. **Population** 1981;36(6):1105-38
Peel J: Changing patterns of contraception. **Proc Annu Symp Eugen Soc** 1981;16:41-8
Schall JV: The rarest of all revolutions: G. K. Chesterton on the relation of human life to Christian doctrine. **Am Benedictine Rev** 1981;32(4):304-27
Siegler AM, Grunebaum A: The 100th anniversary of tubal sterilization. **Fertil Steril** 1980 Dec;34(6):610-3
Soloway RA: Birth control, and the population question in England, 1877-1930. Chapel Hill, University of North Carolina Press, 1982. xix, 418 p.

**Hungary**

Andorka R: Birth control in the eighteenth and nineteenth centuries in some Hungarian villages. **Local Popul Stud (Matlock)** 1979;22:38-43
Mikolás M: Gesztációs folyamatokra vonatkozó matematikai statisztikai vizsgálatok (Magyarország, 1931-1978). **Demografia** 1980;23(2-3):163-207
Molmár ES: Birth control, abortion and public opinion. **New Hung Q** 1982;23(85):125-30
Sas M: A hormonalis anticonceptio 25 éve. **Orv Hetil** 1982 Jan 24;123(4):195-200

**India**

Verkuyl J: Bezinning op family-planning in India. **Wereld Zending** 1973;2(5):328-36
Vicziany M: Coercion in a soft state: the family planning program of India. **Pac Aff** 1982;55(3):373-402;(4):557-92

**Israel**

Yisai Y: Abortion in Israel: social demand and political responses. **Policy Stud J** 1978;7(2):270-90

**Italy**

Detragiache D: Un aspect de la politique demographique de l'Italie fasciste: la repression de l'avortement. **Melanges Archeol Hist Ec Fr Rome** 1980;92(2):691-735

**Korea**

Rindfuss RR, Bumpass LL, Palmore JA, et al: The transformation of Korean child-spacing practices. **Popul Stud** 1982 Mar;36(1):87-104

**Netherlands**

Bruijn J: Abortus in de 19de eeuw. **Spiegel Hist** 1980;15(9):463-5
Praag P van: Het nieuw-malthusianisme in Vlaanderen en Holland. **Spiegel Hist** 1978;13(11):662-8

**New Zealand**

Brookes B: Housewives' depression: the debate over abortion and birth control in the 1930's. **NZ J Hist** 1981;15(2):115-34
Gluckman LK: Abortion in the nineteenth century Maori: a historical and ethnopsychiatric review. **NZ Med J** 1981 Jun 10;93(685):384-6

**Norway**

Sogner S: Om barnebegrensning i Norge ved sluten av 1800-tallet. **Heimen** 1981;18(9):577-85

**Poland**

Kasperek S: Przymusowe sterylizacje w rejencji opolskiej 1934-1938. **Przegl Lek** 1980;37(1):33-9
Skarżyński Z: Z problematyki przerywania clazy. **Panstwo Prawo** 1981;36(9-12):96-106

**Puerto Rico**

Mass B: Puerto Rico: a case study of population control.

**Lat Am Perspect** 1977;4(4):66–82
Ramírez de Arellano AB: Colonialism, Catholicism, and contraception: a history of birth control in Puerto Rico. Chapel Hill, University of North Carolina Press, 1983. xii, 219 p.

**Romania**

Moskoff W: Pronatalist policies in Romania. **Econ Dev Cult Change** 1980;28(3):597–614

**Sweden**

Hagenfeldt K: Dramatiskt minskad mödramortalitet. Framsynta åsikter i abortfrågan. **Lakartidningen** 1983 Nov 9;80(45):4299–302

**Thailand**

Krannich RL, Krannich CR: Initiating a population revolution in Thailand: politics, bureaucracy, and social change. **Asian Profile** 1982;10(2):173–92

**Turkey**

Ozbay F, Shorter FC: Türkiye'de Aile plânlamasi uygulamalarinda 1963 ve 1968 yillari arasinda görülen degismeler. **Hacettepe Sosyal Bilimler Derg** 1970;2(2):194–211

**United States**

Aul DJ: Margaret Sanger labeled 'racist'. **Am J Public Health** 1981 Jan;71(1):91
Barnartt SN, Harris RJ: Recent changes in predictors of abortion attitudes. **Sociol Soc Res** 1982;66(3):320–34
Bond JR, Johnson CA: Implementing a permissive policy: hospital abortion services after Roe V. Wade. **Am J Pol Sci** 1982;26(1):1–24
Bullough VL: Female physiology, technology and women's liberation. In Trescott, Martha Moore, ed. Dynamos and Virgins revisited: Women and technological change in history. Metuchen, N. J., Scarecrow Pr., 1979. p. 236–51.
Cates W: Abortion attitudes of black women. **Women Health** 1979 Nov–Dec;2(3):3–9
Cirillo VJ: Edward Bliss Foote: pioneer American advocate of birth control. **Bull Hist Med** 1973 Sep–Oct;47(5):471–9
Combs MW, Welch S: Blacks, Whites, and attitudes toward abortion. **Public Opin Q** 1982;46(4):510–20
D'Antonio WV, Stack S: Religion, ideal family size, and abortion: extending Renzi's hypothesis. **J Sci Stud Relig** 1980;19(4):397–408
Davis KS: The story of the pill. **Am Heritage** 1978;29(5):80–91
Dawson DA, Meny DJ, Ridley JC: Fertility control in the United States before the contraceptive revolution. **Fam Plann Perspect** 1980 Mar–Apr;12(2):76–86
DelCastillo AR: Sterilization: an overview. In Mora, Magdalena and DelCastillo, Adelaida R., ed. Mexican Women in the United States: Struggles past and present. Los Angeles, U. of California Chicano Studies Res. Center, 1980. p. 65–70.
Detlefsen EG: Abraham Stone. In Dictionary of American Biography, Suppl. 6, 1956–1960. p. 602–3, 1980.
Diczfalusy E: Gregory Pincus and steroidal contraception revisited. **Acta Obstet Gynecol Scand [Suppl]** 1982;105:7–15
Dixon RB: Hallelujah the pill? **Trans Action** 1970;8(1/2):44–9, 92
Fee E, Wallace M: The history and politics of birth control: a review essay. **Feminist Stud** 1979;5(1):201–15
Francome C: Abortion politics in the United States. **Polit Stud** 1980;28(4):613–21
Friedell JN: Blanche Ames Ames. In: Notable American women. The modern period. Cambridge, Mass., Belknap–Harvard Univ. Press, 1980. 4:15–6.
Goldzieher JW: Estrogens in oral contraceptives: historical perspectives. **Johns Hopkins Med J** 1982 May;150(5):165–9
Gordon L: The long struggle for reproductive rights. **Radic Am** 1981;15(1–2):75–88
Gould KH: Family planning and abortion policy in the United States. **Soc Serv Rev** 1979;53(3):452–63
Green D, Murdock ME, ed: The Margaret Sanger Centennial Conference, November 13 & 14, 1979. Northampton, Smith College, 1982. 68 p. Contributions by J. K. Conway, A. Harper, L. Gordon, J. Reed, E. Fee.
Green E: U. S. population policies, development, and the rural poor of Africa. **J Mod Afr Stud** 1982;20(1):45–67
Guillory F: Family planning in Louisiana. **New South** 1971;26(4):29–34
Hansen SB: State implementation of supreme court decision: abortion rates since Roe v. Wade. **J Polit** 1980;42(2):372–95
Harper JP: Be fruitful and multiply: origins of legal restrictions on planned parenthood in nineteenth-century America. In Berkin, C. R., Norton, M. B. ed: Women of America: a history. Boston, Houghton Mifflin, 1979: 245–69.
Harper JP: 'Be fruitful and multiply': the reaction to family limitation in nineteenth-century America. Ph.D. Dis., Columbia University, New York, 1975. 273 leaves.
Hayler B: Abortion. **Signs** 1979;5(2):307–23
Hellman LM: A history and reminiscence of the office of the Deputy Assistant Secretary for Population Affairs, Department of Health, Education and Welfare, 1969–1977. **Bull Hist Med** 1982 Spring;56(1):77–87
Johnson CA, Bond JR: Policy implementation and community linkages: hospital abortion services after Roe V. Wade. **West Polit Q** 1982;35(3):385–405
Kennedy DM: Decrease and stultify: contraception and abortion in American society. **Rev Am Hist** 1979;7(1):18–25
Klos SF: Reform initiatives in American maternal health services: 1900–1940. Ed. D. Diss., Harvard University. Cambridge, 1979, vi, 182 p.
Lampé L: Margaret Sanger munkássága és annak hatása a családtervezési mozgalomra. **Orv Hetil** 1984 Jan 22;125(4):221–2
Lane AJ: The politics of birth control. **Marx Perspect** 1979;2(3):160–9
Leahy PJ, Mazur A: The rise and fall of public opposition in specific social movements. **Soc Stud Sci** 1980 Aug 3;10(3):259–84
Lindemann C: Margaret Sanger and the birth control movement. **Women Health** 1978 Mar–Apr;3(2):12–13,16–21
McFalls JA, Masnick GS: Birth control and the fertility of the U. S. Black population, 1880 to 1980. **J Fam Hist** 1981 Spring;6(1):89–106
McLaughlin L: The pill, John Rock, and the church: the biography of a revolution. Boston, Little, Brown, 1982. 243 p.
Margolis M, Neary K: Pressure politics revisited: the anti-abortion campaign. **Policy Stud J** 1980;8(5):698–716
Milbauer B, Obrentz BN: The law giveth: legal aspects of the abortion controversy. New York, Atheneum, 1983. 363 p.
Polenberg R: The second victory of Anthony Comstock? **Society** 1982;19(4):32–8
Reed J: Doctors, birth control, and social values, 1830–1970. In Vogel MJ, Rosenberg CE, ed: The therapeutic revolution. Philadelphia, 1979. p. 109–133.
Reed J: Katharine Dexter McCormick. In: Notable American women. The modern period. Cambridge, Mass., Belknap–Harvard Univ. Press, 1980. 4:440–2.
Reed J: Margaret Sanger. In: Notable American women. The modern period. Cambridge, Mass., Belknap–Harvard Univ. Press, 1980. 4:623–7.
Ryan MP: Reproduction in American history. **J Interdiscip Hist** 1979;10(2):319–32
Sanderson WC: Quantitative aspects of marriage, fertility and family limitation in nineteenth century America: another application of the Coale specifications. **Demography** 1979 Aug;16(3):339–58
Sands D: Using oral history to chart the course of illegal abortions in Montana. **Frontiers** 1983;7(1):32–7
Sernett MC: The rights of personhood: the Dred Scott case and the question of abortion. **Relig Life** 1980;49(4):461–76
Swierenga RP: Physicians and abortion reform in the nineteenth century: social control as the new orthodoxy. **Fides Et Hist** 1979;11(2):51–9
Tedrow LM, Mahoney ER: Trends in attitudes toward abortion: 1972–76. **Public Opin Q** 1979;43(2):181–9
Ten year progress report of the Center for Population Research: [Bethesda], The Center, 1978. 73 p.
Velez-I CG: Se me acabó la canción: an ethnography of non-consenting sterilizations among Mexican women in Los Angeles. Mora, Magdalena and Del Castillo, Adelaida R., ed. Mexican Women in the United States: Struggles past and present. Los Angeles, U. of California Chicano Studies Res. Center, 1980 p. 71–91.
Wardell D: Margaret Sanger: birth control's successful revolutionary. **Am J Public Health** 1980 Jul;70(7):736–42
We walk the line: the struggle at preterm.: **Radic Am** 1979;13(2):8–24
Williams D, Williams G: Every child a wanted child. Clarence James Gamble, M.D., and his work in the birth control movement. Ed. E. P. Flint. Boston, Harvard University Press for Countway Library of Medicine, 1978. xvii, 445 p.

**Yugoslavia**

Kožuh-Novak M: Kliničko istraživački rad Instituta za planiranje porodice na području intrauterine kontracepcije od 1964. do 1980. **Jugosl Ginekol Opstet** 1981 Jan–Apr;21(1–2):54–7
Ograjenšek Z: Raxvoj Instituta za planiranje porodice u Ljubljani. **Jugosl Ginekol Opstet** 1981 Jan–Apr;21(1–2):50–3

**Zimbabwe**

Lovel H, Mkandla M, Morley D: Birth spacing in Zimbabwe a generation ago. **Lancet** 1983 Jul 16;2(8342):161–2

## BLACKS

Cohn RL, Jensen RA: The determinants of slave mortality rates on the middle passage. **Explor Econ Hist** 1982;19(3):269–82
Kiple K, Kiple V: The African connection: slavery, disease and racism. **Phylon** 1980;41(3):211–22
Marr JJ: Merchants of death: the role of slave trade in the transmission

of disease from Africa to the Americas. **Pharos** 1982 Winter;45(1):31–5

**Africa**

Ransford O: 'Bid the sickness cease': disease in the history of black Africa. London, John Murray, 1983. x, 235 p.

**Americas**

Corruccini RS, Handler JS: Temporomandibular joint size decrease in American Blacks: evidence from Barbados. **J Dent Res** 1980 Sep;59(9):1528

Puckrein G: Climate, health and black labor in the English Americas. **J Am Stud** 1979;13(2):179–93

**Barbados**

Corruccini RS, Handler JS, Mutaw RJ, et al: Osteology of a slave burial population from Barbados, West Indies. **Am J Phys Anthropol** 1982 Dec;59(4):443–59

**Colombia**

Chandler DL: Health and slavery in colonial Colombia. New York, Arno Press, 1981. iv, 307 p. (Ph.D. Diss., Tulane 1972).

**United States**

Baer HA: Toward a systematic typology of black folk healers. **Phylon** 1982;43(4):327–43

Cooper R: A note on the biologic concept of race and its application in epidemiologic research. **Am Heart J** 1984 Sep;108(3 Pt 2):715–22

Kuna RR: Hoodoo: the indigenous medicine and psychiatry of the black American. **Ethnomedizin** 1974–75;3(3–4):273–94

Robinson SA: A historical development of midwifery in the black community: 1600–1940. **J Nurse Midwife** 1984 Jul–Aug;29(4):247–50

Rutman DB, Wetherell C, Rutman AH: Rhythms of life: black and white seasonality in the early Chesapeake. **J Interdiscip Hist** 1980;11(1):29–53

Smith WD, et al: Reflections on black psychology. Washington, University Press of America, 1979. ix, 528 p.

Sullivan LW: The education of black health professionals. **Phylon** 1977;38(2):181–93

**1700 to Present**

Cameron S, Falk LA: Some black medical history: Dr. Martin R. Delany's Canadian years as medical practitioner and abolitionist (1856–1864). In: Congrès international d'histoire de la médecine, XXVe, Québec, 1976. Actes. Québec, 1977. p. 537–45.

Kass AM, Kass EH: Doctors afield. Martin Delany, Thomas Hodgkin, and the Black Nationalist movement. **N Engl J Med** 1981 Sep 17;305(12):682–4

Littlefield DC: Plantations, paternalism, and profitability: factors affecting African demography in the old British Empire. **J South Hist** 1981;47(2):167–82

Murray AE: Bright delusion: Presbyterians and African colonization. **J Presbyt Hist** 1980;58(3):224–37

Sheridan RB: The Guinea surgeons on the middle passage: the provision of medical services in the British slave trade. **Int J Afr Hist Stud** 1981;14(4):601–25

Stein R: Mortality in the eighteenth-century French slave trade. **J Afr Hist** 1980, 21(1):35–41

Stewart L: The edge of utility: slaves and smallpox in the early eighteenth century. **Med Hist** 1985 Jan;29(1):54–70

**Africa**

Northrup D: African mortality in the suppression of the slave trade: the case of the bight of Biafra. **J Interdiscip Hist** 1978;9(1):47–64

**Americas**

Fogel RW, Engerman SL: Recent findings in the study of slave demography and family structure. **Sociol Soc Res** 1979;63(3):566–89

Johansen HC: Slave demography of the Danish West Indian Islands. **Scand Econ Hist Rev** 1981;29(1):1–20

**Canada**

Richardson G: Letitia Munson. In Dictionary of Canadian biography, 1881–1890. 1982;11:629–30.

**Caribbean**

Kiple KF, Kiple VH: Deficiency diseases in the Caribbean. **J Interdiscip Hist** 1980 Autumn;11(2):197–215

Reusch C: Die medizinische Versorgung auf den französischen Westindischen Inseln im 18. Jhd. im Spiegel des Werkes von J.B. Dazille 'Les Maladies des Nègres, leurs causes, leur traitement, et les moyens de les prévenir.' Diss., Universität Düsseldorf. Düsseldorf, 1982. 117 p.

**Cuba**

Deschamps Chapeaux P: El negro en la economía Habanera del siglo XIX. Flebotomianos y dentistas. **Rev Bibl Nac Jose Marti** 1971;13(1):75–86

Iglesias F: Características de la población cubana en 1862. **Rev Bibl Nac Jose Marti** 1980;22(3):89–110

**France**

Butts HF: Frantz Fanon's contribution to psychiatry: the psychology of racism and colonialism. **J Natl Med Assoc** 1979 Oct;71(10):1015–8

**Guyana**

Boisanger B de, Cudennec Y, Buffe P: Aperçu sur la médecine de soins et la médecine du travail, dans une plantation de Guyane au XVIIIe siècle. **Hist Sci Med** 1984;18(3):215–21

**Jamaica**

Smith JP: Mary Jane Seacole 1805–1881: a black British nurse. **J Adv Nurs** 1984 Sep;9(5):427–8

**South Africa**

Barker A: A Zulu contribution. **Trans R Soc Trop Med Hyg** 1979;73(4):364–5

**Trinidad**

Friedman GC: The heights of slaves in Trinidad. **Soc Sci Hist** 1982;6(4):482–515

**United States**

Agris J: Stamps commemorating medicine. 'Dr. Charles R. Drew'. **J Dermatol Surg Oncol** 1982 Feb;8(2):96

Aldrich M: Progressive economics, and scientific racism: Walter Willcox and black Americans, 1895–1910. **Phylon** 1979;40(1):1–14

Alexander LL: Early medical heroes: Susan Smith McKinney-Steward, M.D., 1847–1918. **Crisis** 1980;87(1):21–3

Baer HA: Prophets and advisors in black spiritual churches: therapy, palliative, or opiate? **Cult Med Psychiatry** 1981 Jun;5(2):145–70

Beardsley EH: Making separate, equal: black physicians and the problems of medical segregation in the pre-World War II South. **Bull Hist Med** 1983 Fall;57(3):382–96

Blount M: Surpassing obstacles: black women in medicine. **J Am Med Wom Assoc** 1984 Nov–Dec;39(6):192–5

Boone MS: A socio-medical study of infant mortality among disadvantaged Blacks. **Hum Organ** 1982;41(3):227–36

Breed W: The Negro and fatalistic suicide. **Pac Sociol Rev** 1970;13(3):156–62

Brown SE: Sexuality and the slave community. **Phylon** 1981;42(1):1–10

Brunswick AF: Social meanings and developmental needs: perspectives on black youth's drug abuse. **Youth Soc** 1980;11(4):449–73

Cahn JD: A doctor's legacy: Dr. John E. T. Camper and the MeDeSo. **J Natl Med Assoc** 1980 Mar;72(3):283–7

Campbell P: Medical education for an African colonist. **Md Hist Mag** 1970;65(2):130–7

Carnegie ME: Nurses and war. Black nurses at the front. **Am J Nurs** 1984 Oct;84(10):1250–2

Cash P: Pride, prejudice and politics. **Harv Med Alumni Bull** 1980 Dec;54(6):20–5

Cates W: Abortion attitudes of black women. **Women Health** 1979 Nov–Dec;2(3):3–9

Chakravorty RC: Charles Richard Drew (1904–1950). **Scalpel Tongs** 1981;25:69–70

Cobb WM: Forward--the only way. **J Natl Med Assoc** 1984 May;76(5):487–97

Cobb WM: The Black American in medicine. **J Natl Med Assoc** 1981 Dec;73 Suppl:1185–244

Cody CA: Slave demography and family formation: a community study of the Ball Family plantations, 1720–1896. Ph.D. Diss., University of Minnesota. Minneapolis, 1982. xiv, 429 p.

Combs MW, Welch S: Blacks, Whites, and attitudes toward abortion **Public Opin Q** 1982;46(4):510–20

Cutright P, Shorter E: The effects of health on the completed fertility of nonwhite and white U.S. women born from 1867 through 1935. **J Soc Hist** 1979;13(2):191–218

Davidson AT: The role of the historic black colleges in the training of black professionals. **J Natl Med Assoc** 1983 Oct;75(10):1019–22

Davis R: Black suicide and social support systems: an overview and some implications for mental health practitioners. **Phylon** 1982;43(4):307–14

Davis R: Suicide among young blacks: trends and perspectives. **Phylon** 1980;41(3):223–9
Downey-Anderson C: The 'Coggins Affair': desegregation and Southern mores in Madison County, Florida. **Fla Hist Q** 1981 Apr;59:464–72
Drew GR: The Dr. Charles R. Drew stamp. **J Afro-Am Hist Geneol Soc** 1981;2(4):139–42
Dummett CO: Charles Edwin Bentley: a genuine emancipator. **Crisis** 1979;86(4):133–5
Dummett CO: Contributions of Afro-Americans to American dentistry. **J Ala Dent Assoc** 1984 Fall;68(4):42–6
Dummett CO: Dental education for Afro-Americans. **J Tenn Dent Assoc** 1982 Oct;61(4):14–6
Dummett CO: Health professional emancipators: examples in excellence. **J Natl Med Assoc** 1984 Sep;76(9):925–30
Dummett CO: Historical notes on dental education for Afro-Americans. **J DC Dent Soc** 1981 Fall;56(1):35–9
Dummett CO: Stephen Johnson Lewis and his contributions to American dentistry. **Bull Hist Dent** 1981;29(1):15–23
Elmore JA: Frances Elliott Davis. In: Notable American women. The modern period. Cambridge, Mass., Belknap-Harvard Univ. Press, 1980. 4:180–2.
Engerman SL: Changes in black fertility, 1880–1940. In T. K. Hareven and M. A. Vinovskis, ed: Family and population in nineteenth-century America. Princeton, Princeton University Press, 1978. p. 126–53.
Falk LA: Black Abolitionist doctors and healers, 1810–1885. **Bull Hist Med** 1980 Summer;54(2):258–72
Foster GM: The limitations of federal health care for freed men, 1862–1868. **J South Hist** 1982;48(3):349–72
Galishoff S: Germs know no color line: black health and public policy in Atlanta, 1900–1918. **J Hist Med Allied Sci** 1985 Jan;40(1):22–41
Gatz M, Gease EI, Tyler FB, et al: Psychosocial competence characteristics of black and white women: the constraining effects of 'triple jeopardy'. **Black Scholar** 1982;13(1):5–12
Hansen AC: Black Americans in medicine. **J Natl Med Assoc** 1984 Jul;76(7):693–5
Hasson GS: Health and welfare of freedmen in reconstruction Alabama. **Ala Rev** 1982;35(2):94–110
Hasson GS: The medical activities of the Freedmen's Bureau in Reconstruction Alabama, 1865–1868. Ph.D. Diss, University of Alabama, University, 1982. 252 p.
Hine DC: From hospital to college: black nurse leaders and the rise of collegiate nursing schools. **J Negro Educ** 1982 Summer;51:222–37
Hine DC: The Ethel Jones Report: black women in the nursing profession, 1925. **J Negro Hist** 1982 Fall;67:212–28
Hine WC: Dr. Benjamin A. Boseman, Jr.: Charleston's black physician-politician. In Rabinowitz HN, ed: Southern Black leaders of the reconstruction era. Urbana, University of Illinois Press, 1982. p. 335–62.
Holmes L: Alabama granny midwife. **J Med Soc NJ** 1984 May;81(5):389–91
Jackson JS, Chatters LM, Neighbors HW: The mental health status of older black Americans: a national study. **Black Scholar** 1982;13(1):21–35
Jacobs SE: 'Our babies shall not die': a community's response to medical neglect. **Hum Organ** 1979;38(2):120–33
Jerrido MJ: In recognition of...early black women physicians. **Women Health** 1980 Fall;5(3):1–3
Johnson MP: Smothered slave infants; were slave mothers at fault? **J South Hist** 1981;47(4):493–520
Johnson NE: Minority-group status and the fertility of black Americans, 1970: a new look. **Am J Sociol** 1979;84(6):1386–1400
Jones JH: Bad blood: the Tuskegee syphilis experiment. New York, Free Press; London, Collier Macmillan; 1981. xii, 272 p.
Joseph A: Intelligence, IQ, and race: When, how, and why they became associated. San Francisco, R & E Research Associates, 1977. vii, 142 p.
Kass AM: Dr Thomas Hodgkin, Dr Martin Delany, and the 'Return to Africa'. **Med Hist** 1983 Oct;27(4):373–93
Kaufman M: Medicine and slavery: an essay review. **Ga Hist Q** 1979;64(3):380–90
Kidd F, ed: Profile of the Negro in American dentistry. Washington, Howard University Press, 1979. viii, 211 p.
Kiple KF, King VH. Another dimension to the black diaspora: diet, disease, and racism. Cambridge, Cambridge University Press, 1981. 295 p.
Kiple KF, Kiple VH: Black tongue and black men: pellagra and slavery in the Antebellum South. **J South Hist** 1977 Aug;43(3):411–28
Kiple KF, Kiple VH: Slave child mortality: some nutritional answers to a perennial puzzle. **J Soc Hist** 1977 Mar;10(3):284–309
Kiple KF, Kiple VH: The African connection: slavery, disease and racism. **Phylon** 1980 Fall;41(3):211–22
Kiple KL, Kiple VH: Black yellow fever immunities, innate and acquired, as revealed in the American South. **Soc Sci Hist** 1977;1(4):419–36
Lee AS, Lee ES: The health of slaves and the health of freedmen: a Savannah study. **Phylon** 1977;38(2):170–80
Lichello R: Pioneer in blood plasma; Dr. Charles Richard Drew. New York, Messner, [1968]. 190 p.
Lyles MR, Carter JH: Myth and strengths of the black family: a historical and sociological contribution to family therapy. **J Natl Med Assoc** 1982 Nov;74(11):1119–23
McFalls JA, Masnick GS: Birth control and the fertility of the U. S. Black population, 1880 to 1980. **J Fam Hist** 1981 Spring;6(1):89–106
Margo RA, Steckel RH: The heights of American slaves: new evidence on slave nutrition and health. **Soc Sci Hist** 1982;6(4):516–38
Maultsby MC: A historical view of Blacks' distrust of psychiatry. In Turner SM, Jones RT, ed: Behavior modification in Black populations; psychosocial issues and empirical findings. New York, Plenum, 1982. p. 39–55.
Miles DE: The growth of suicide among black Americans. **Crisis** 1979;86(10):430–3
Morrison LR: 'Nearer to the brute creation': the scientific defense of American slavery before 1830. **South Stud** 1980;19(3):228–42
Odegaard CE: Minorities in medicine. From receptive passivity to positive action 1966–76. New York, Josiah Macy, Jr. Foundation, 1977. vii, 164 p.
Olivier AF: In proper perspective: Daniel Hale Williams, M.D. **Ann Thorac Surg** 1984 Jan;37(1):96–7
Palmer CA: Public health in the South. **Rev Am Hist** 1982;10(2):229–33
Plummer BL: Document: letters of James Durham to Benjamin Rush. **J Negro Hist** 1980;65(3):261–9
Pollard LJ: Aging and slavery: gerontological perspective. **J Negro Hist** 1981 Fall;66:228–34
Powers BA: The use of orthodox and black American folk medicine. **ANS** 1982 Apr;4(3):35–47
Ram B: Regional-sub-cultural explanations of black fertility in the United States. **Popul Stud** 1976;30(3):553ff
Reid JD, Jedlicka D, Lee ES, et al: Trends in black health. **Phylon** 1977;38(2):105–16
Richardson L: Breakthrough to nursing: the black nurse's story. **Imprint** 1981 Dec;28(5):27, 60, 73
Robinson HS: Furman Jeremiah Shadd, MD 1852–1908. **J Natl Med Assoc** 1980 Feb;72(2):151–3
Robinson HS: Robert and Roderick Badger, pioneer Georgia dentists. **Negro Hist Bull** 1961;24(4):77–80
Ruffin CB: Records of the Sellers Funeral Home, Chambersburg, Pennsylvania, relating to the black families of Franklin County, 1866–1933. **J Afro-Am Hist Geneal Soc** 1982;3(4):165–82; 1983;4(1):32–4
Savit TL: The use of blacks for medical experimentation and demonstration in the old South. **J South Hist** 1982;48(3):331–48
Savitt TL: Lincoln University Medical Department--a forgotten 19th century black medical school. **J Hist Med Allied Sci** 1985 Jan;40(1):42–65
Savitt TL: Medicine and slavery: the diseases and health care of blacks in antebellum Virginia. Urbana, University of Illinois Press, 1978. 332 p.
Savitt TL: Slave life insurance in Virginia and North Carolina. **J South Hist** 1977 Nov;43(4):583–600; 1978 Feb;44(1):163
Savitt TL: The invisible malady: sickle cell anemia in America, 1910–1970. **J Natl Med Assoc** 1981 Aug;73(8):739–46
Savitt TL: The use of Blacks for medical experimentation and demonstration in the Old South. **J South Hist** 1982 Aug;48(3):331–48
Sernett MC: The rights of personhood: the Dred Scott case and the question of abortion. **Relig Life** 1980;49(4):461–76
Shick TW: Race, class, and medicine: 'Bad Blood' in twentieth-century America. **J Ethn Stud** 1982;10(2):97–105
Sorenson AA: Black Americans and the medical profession, 1930–1970. **J Negro Educ** 1972;41(4):337–42
Spady JG: Dr. W. Montague Cobb: anatomist, physician, physical anthropologist, editor emeritus of the Journal of the National Medical Association, and first black president of NAACP. **J Natl Med Assoc** 1984 Jul;76(7):739–44
Steckel RH: Slave height profiles from coastwise manifests. **Explor Econ Hist** 1979;16(4):363–80
Steckel RH: Slave marriage and the family. **J Fam Hist** 1980 Winter;5(4):406–21
Steckel RH: The fertility of American slaves. **Res Econ Hist** 1982;7:239–86
Steiner PE: Medical history of a Civil War regiment: disease in the sixty-fifth United States colored infantry. Clayton, Mo., Institute of Civil War Studies, 1977. xxii, 137 p.
Stewart JB: The political economy of black male suicides. **J Black Stud** 1980;11(2):249–61
Sullivan OR: Who's testing black children and youth in the public schools? **Freedomways** 1981;21(2):114–8
Summerville J: Educating black doctors: a history of Meharry Medical College. University, Ala., University of Alabama Press, 1983. xiii, 279 p.
Summerville J: Formation of a black medical profession in Tennessee, 1880–1920. **J Tenn Med Assoc** 1983 Oct;76(10):644–6
Takaki R: Aesculapius was a white man: antebellum racism and male chauvinism at Harvard Medical School. **Phylon** 1978;39(2):128–34
Taylor CM: W. E. B. Dubois's challenge to scientific racism. **J Black Stud** 1981;11(4):449–60
Tolnay SE: Black fertility in decline: urban differentials in 1900. **Soc Biol** 1980 Winter;27(4):249–60
Tolnay SE: Fertility of southern black farmers in 1900: evidence and speculation. **J Fam Hist** 1983 Winter;8(4):314–32
Tolnay SE: Trends in total and marital fertility for black Americans, 1886–1899. **Demography** 1981 Nov;18(4):443–63

## BLACKS

Tomashevich GV, ed: Some of the incidents in the life of Mark De Mortie. **Afro-Am NY Life Hist** 1979;3(1):61-71
Ward RD, Rogers WW: Racial inferiority, convict labor, and modern medicine: a note on the Coalburg affair. **Ala Hist Q** 1982;44(3-4):203-10
Webb H, Rhodes LC: The book of presidents: leaders of organized dentistry. [s.l., s.n.] 1977. [63] p.
Westbrooks B: The troubled legacy of Harvey Lillard: the black experience in chiropractic. **Chiropr Hist** 1982;2(1):47-53
Whitten DO: Medical care of slaves: Louisiana sugar region and South Carolina rice district. **South Stud** 1977;16:153-80
Wynes CE: Dr. James Durham, mysterious eighteenth-century black physician: man or myth? **Pa Mag Hist Biogr** 1979;103(3):325-33
Yancey AG: US postage stamp issued in honor of Charles R. Drew, MD, MDSc. **J Natl Med Assoc** 1982 Jun;74(6):561-5

## BLOOD TRANSFUSION

See also **Cardiology and Circulatory System**

Dawson RB: Preservation of red blood cells for transfusion. **Hum Pathol** 1983 Mar;14(3):213-7
Diamond LK: Milestones in blood transfusion and blood banking. **Pharos** 1982 Spring;45(2):7-10
Farsund O: Fra hjerte til hjerte: om blod og blodoverføring. **Sykepleien** 1980 Jun 5;67(10):11-5
Gervin AS, Fischer RP: Resuscitation of trauma patients with type-specific uncrossmatched blood. **J Trauma** 1984 Apr;24(4):327-31
Hylland RG: Further evidence for plasmapheresis. **Arthritis Rheum** 1980 Jan;23(1):129
Müller N: Zur Entwicklung der Transfusionsmedizin. **MMW** 1979 Nov 9;121(45):1485-8
Orr MD: Autotransfusion: intraoperative scavenging. **Int Anesthesiol Clin** 1982 Winter;20(4):97-119
Reyment RA: Moors and Christians: an example of multivariate analysis applied to human blood-groups. **Ann Hum Biol** 1983 Nov-Dec;10(6):505-21
Shimizu K: [Blood transfusion--practice at Komagome Municipal Hospital. 12. Progress in blood transfusion]. (Jpn) **Kangogaku Zasshi** 1979 Dec;43(12):1313-6

#### France

Bernard J: Hématologie et transfusion sanguine. **Nouv Rev Fr Hematol** 1982;24(5):277-9

#### United States

Kuhns WJ: Blood letting and early blood transfusion in the Carolinas. **NC Med J** 1983 Jun;44(6):385-8

### 1450-1700

Farr AD: The first human blood transfusion. **Med Hist** 1980 Apr;24(2):143-62
Hall AR, Boas Hall M: The first human blood transfusion: priority disputes. **Med Hist** 1980;24(4):461-5

#### Great Britain

Krantz JC: An architect designs a needle. **W Va Med J** 1980 Apr;76(4):84-5

### 1700 to Present

Clarke JM: Surgery in Jehovah's witnesses. **Br J Hosp Med** 1982 May;27(5):497-500
Curtis CH: Autotransfusion in gynecologic hemoperitoneum. **Am J Obstet Gynecol** 1983 Jul 1;146(5):501-4
Glover JL, Broadi TA: Intraoperative autotransfusion. **Prog Clin Biol Res** 1982;108:151-70
Isbister JP: Direct blood transfusion. **Med J Aust** 1980 Feb 9;1(3):136
Jamróg-Cendrzak A, Cendrzak E: 100-lecie prac doświadczalnych nad dootrzewnowym przetaczaniem krwi. **Arch Hist Med (Warsz)** 1982;45(1-4):55-9
Lindgren FT: The plasma lipoproteins: historical developments and nomenclature. **Ann NY Acad Sci** 1980;348:1-15
Lontainé SZ, Susa E, Varga T: A Habsburgok József nádori ágához tartozók vércsoportvizsgálata. **Morphol Igazsagugyi Orv Sz** 1980 Oct;20(4):275-81
Mollison PL: The introduction of acidified citrate-glucose solutions as red cell preservatives. **Vox Sang** 1983;45(6):449-50
Muller A, Garretta M, Hebert M: Groupamatic system: overview, history of development and evaluation of use. **Vox Sang** 1981;40(3):201-13
Rechsteiner J, Lockyer WJ, Friedman LI: Overview, history, evaluation and future developments of the AutoGrouper 16-C. **Vox Sang** 1981;40(3):192-200
Rex-Kiss B: A vércsoportkutatás rövid története. **Orv Hetil** 1980 Sep 21;121(38):2335-9
Rex-Kiss B: Short history of blood group research. **Ther Hung** 1982;30(3):144-9
Rosenfield RE: Immunobiology of the erythrocyte: perspectives since 1945. **Prog Clin Biol Res** 1980;43:13-7
Soulier JP: The history of PPSB. **Vox Sang** 1984;46(1):58-61
Speiser P, Smekal FG: Karl Landsteiner, Entdecker der Blutgruppen und Pionier der Immunologie. Biographie eines Nobelpreisträgers aus der Wiener Medizinischen Schule. 2., vollständig überarb. Aufl. Vienna, Hollinek, 1975. 207 p.
Speiser P: Rhesus-Prophylaxe. Zum 40. Todestag von Karl Landsteiner. **Wien Med Wochenschr** 1983 Dec 31;133(23-24):592-4
Walsh RJ: Adverse reactions to blood transfusion: introduction -- historical overview. **Anaesth Intensive Care** 1980 May;8(2):112-4

#### Australia

McLean JA: Direct blood transfusion. Its history, with special reference to the Alfred Hospital, Melbourne. **Med J Aust** 1979 Dec 15;2(12):625-8
Verso ML: Fifty years of the Red Cross Blood Transfusion Service in Victoria. **Victorian Hist J** 1980;51(4):218-36

#### China

Renkonen KO: Old Chinese observation correlated to ABO groups. **Hum Genet** 1980;55(2):279

#### Czechoslovakia

Dobrý E: 35 let transfúzní služby v CSSR. **Vnitr Lek** 1984 Sep;30(9):833-5
Hrubiško M: 30 rokov národnej transfúznej služby v CSSR. **Vnitr Lek** 1980 Feb;26(2):105-6

#### France

Dausset J: The birth of MAC. **Vox Sang** 1984;46(4):235-7
van Rood JJ: Discovery of 4a and 4b. **Vox Sang** 1984;46(4):238-42

#### Great Britain

Dodd BE: First tests with anti-human globulin on the red cells of patients suffering from haemolytic anaemia. **Vox Sang** 1984;46(3):183-4
Farr AD: Treatment of haemophilia by transfusion: the first recorded case. **J R Soc Med** 1981 Apr;74(4):301-5
Race RR, Sanger R: Fisher's contribution to Rh. **Vox Sang** 1982;43(6):354-6
Race RR, Sanger R: Some early and surprising blood group findings. **Vox Sang** 1983;44(2):126-8

#### Hungary

Rex-Kiss B: A vérátömlesztés története hazánkban - történeti elozmények és visszaemlékezés. **Orvostort Kozl** 1982;28(1-3):87-105
Rex-Kiss B: A vitás származás vércsoport-vizsgálatokkal való tisztázásának története hazánkban. **Orvostort Kozl** 1979;86(24 no 4):39-54

#### Spain

Martín Villar J: Esfuerzos realizados en el pasado. **Sangre (Barc)** 1980;25(5C):930-46

#### Sweden

Hirschfeld J: The discovery of the Gc system. **Vox Sang** 1984;46(2):122-4

#### Switzerland

Hässig A: 40 Jahre Blutspendedienst des Schweizerischen Roten Kreuzes. **Ther Umsch** 1984 Aug;41(8):533-5

#### United States

Allen JG: First blood bank, first blood banker Oswald Hope Robertson, M.D. **Lab World** 1981 Feb;:20-3
Ausman RK, Bellamy D Jr: Problems and resolutions in the development of the flexible plastic blood container (Carl W. Walter). **Am J Surg** 1984 Nov;148(5):559-61
Brooks JR: Carl W. Walter, MD: surgeon, inventor, and industrialist. **Am J Surg** 1984 Nov;148(5):555-8
Camp FR: Forensic serology in the United States. I. Blood grouping and blood transfusion--historical aspects. **Am J Forensic Med Pathol** 1980 Mar;1(1):47-55
Diamond LK: The Rh problem: (an example of the tsunami phenomenon in medicine). **Turk J Pediatr** 1982 Jan-Mar;24(1):35-47
Drew GR: The Dr. Charles R. Drew stamp. **J Afro-Am Hist Geneol Soc** 1981;2(4):139-42
Edsall JT: Stabilization of serum albumin to heat, and inactivation of the hepatitis virus. **Vox Sang** 1984;46(5):338-40
Hardin RC: An Iowa contribution to blood banking. **J Iowa Med Soc**

1983 Oct;73(10):399–404
Hooper GS: A regional blood program for Florida. **J Fla Med Assoc** 1980 Feb;67(2):146–8
Lichello R: Pioneer in blood plasma; Dr. Charles Richard Drew. New York, Messner, [1968]. 190 p.
Myhre BA: Landmark perspective: the significance of Dr. Fantus' report. **JAMA** 1984 Feb 3;251(5):650–2
Oberman HA: The crossmatch. A brief historical perspective. **Transfusion** 1981 Nov–Dec;21(6):645–51
Schmidt PJ: Blood transfusion in the South before the war between the states. **South Med J** 1979 Dec;72(12):1587–9
Soutter L, Surgeonor DM: Reflections on blood transfusion (Carl W. Walter). **Am J Surg** 1984 Nov;148(5):562–4
Van Loghem JJ: Introduction to a historical paper. An unusual case of intra-group agglutination by Philip Levine and Rufus E. Stetson. **Vox Sang** 1980;38(5):297–300
Wain SL: The controversy of unmodified versus citrated blood transfusion in the early 20th century. **Transfusion** 1984 Sep–Oct;24(5):404–7
Windsor HM: Direct blood transfusion. **Med J Aust** 1980 Feb 9;1(3):136
Yancey AG: US postage stamp issued in honor of Charles R. Drew, MD, MDSc. **J Natl Med Assoc** 1982 Jun;74(6):561–5

**USSR**

Fedorov NA, Movshed BE: Teoriia A. A. Bogomol'tsa o kolloidoklazii v mekhanizme deĭstviia perelivaniia krovi i ee sovremennoe razvitie. **Probl Gematol Pereliv Krovi** 1981 May;26(5):5–13
Fedorova ZD: Osnovnye napravleniia rabot A. N. Filatova po probleme svertyvaniia krovi. **Vestn Khir** 1982 Oct;129(10):13–6
Fedotenkov AG, Agranenko VA: Sluzhba krovi i transfuziologiia k 60–letiiu obrazovaniia SSSR. **Probl Gematol Pereliv Krovi** 1982 Dec;27(12):3–11
Golovin GV, Depp ME, Dutkevich IG: Vydaiushchiĭsia sovetskiĭ khirurg i transfuziolog (k 80–letiiu so dnia rozhdeniia A. N. Filatova). **Vestn Khir** 1982 Oct;129(10):3–8
Goznyĭ AD: K istorii perelivaniia posmertnoĭ krovi. **Feldsher Akush** 1980;45(12):58–9
Kirsanov NA, Razumov VI: Iz istorii organizatsii massovogo donorskogo dvizheniia v gody velikoi otechestvennoi voiny. **Vestn Mosk Univ Ser 8 Istor** 1980;(5):32–41
Kolomiĭchenko MI: Materialy X plenuma Nauchnogo obshchestva khirurgov USSR. Kiev, Zdorov'ia, 1967. 157 p.
Koziner VB, Iarochkin VS: Razvitie problemy krovezameniteleĭ v trudakh akademika N. A. Fedorova i ego shkoly. **Gematol Transfuziol** 1984 Jan;29(1):12–6
Movshev BE: Razvitie ucheniia A. A. Bogomol'tsa o mekhanizme deĭstviia perelivaniia krovi. **Gematol Transfuziol** 1984 Jan;29(1):6–12
Shabunin AV: K 150–letiiu pervogo v Rossii perelivaniia krovi. **Akush Ginekol (Mosk)** 1982;(8):59–60
Shabunin AV: Novye svedeniia o pervom perelivanii krovi v Rossii. **Sov Zdravookhr** 1982;(5):69–70
Shabunin AV: Pervomu v Rossii perelivaniiu krovi––150 let. **Probl Gematol Pereliv Krovi** 1982 Aug;27(8):56–8
Terekhov NT: Razvitie idei akademika A. A. Bogomol'tsa v sovremennoĭ transfuziologii. **Fiziol Zh** 1981 May–Jun;27(3):384–7

**Yugoslavia**

Milić N: Imunoproliferativne bolesti. Uvod. **Lijec Vjesn** 1983 Feb–Mar;105(2–3):105–6
Radović M, Taseski J: Služba za transfuziju krvi i ratovi. **Vojnosanit Pregl** 1979 Sep–Oct;36(5):359–64
Stručno–znanstveni sastanak u povodu tridesete obljetnice o snutka sekcije za hematologiju i transfuziologiju ZLH (1948–1978): **Lijec Vjesn** 1981;103(3):105–30

# BOTANY

See also **Herbals**

Adly A, ed: The history of medicinal and aromatic plants. Proceedings of the Second International Congress organised by The Arab Society for the History of Pharmacy in co–operation with The World Union of Societies of the History of Pharmacy, Alexandria - Egypt, December 15th to 19th, 1980. Karachi, Hamdard Foundation Press, 1982. 216 p.
Bock HE: Pflanzen und Pflanzliches in Geschichte und Gegenwart der Medizin. **Universitas (Stuttg)** 1981;4
Boussel P, Bonnemain H, Bove FJ: Histoire de la pharmacie et de l'Industrie pharmaceutique. Paris, Editions de la Porte Verte, 1982. 287 p.
Crellin JK, ed: Plants in medicine: from yesterday to today. Durham, Duke University Medical Center, 1982. 114 p. Readings and Perspectives in Medicine, Booklet Number 2.
Daems WF: Heilpflanzenkunde in Vergangenheit, Gegenwart und Zukunft. **Drei Z Wiss Kunst Soz Leben** 1978;11:642–57
Delaveau P: Histoire et renouveau des plantes médicinales. Paris, Albin Michel, 1982. 354 p.
Girre L: La médecine par les plantes, à travers les âges. Rennes, Ouest–France. 1981, 187 p.
Greene EL: Landmarks of botanical history. Ed., F. N. Egerton, with contributions by R. P. McIntosh and R. McVaugh. 2 vols. Stanford, Stanford University Press, 1983. 1139 p. (Vol. I first published 1909)
Hünemörder C: Aims and intentions of botanical and zoological classification in the Middle Ages and Renaissance. **Hist Philos Life Sci** 1983;5(1):53–67
Illustrations from the Wellcome Institute Library: A note on the botanical prints and drawings.
Jüttner G: Der Dialog in Pharmazie, Chemie und Botanik. Zum Anteil einer literarischen Gattung in der Darstellung, Vermittlung und im Unterricht der Naturwissenschaften. **Ber Wissenschaftsgesch** 1980;3(1–2):23–34
Kerkhoff AH: Homerus Herbarius. **Janus** 1980:67(1–2–3):187–90
Morton AG: History of botanical science. An account of the development of botany from ancient times to the present day. London, New York, N. Y., Academic Press, 1981. xii, 474 p.
Nauert CG: Caius Plinius Secundus. In Cranz FE, Kristeller PO, ed: Catalogus translationum et commentariorum: Mediaeval and Renaissance Latin translations and commentaries. Annotated lists and guides. Vol. IV. Washington, D.C., Catholic University of America Press, 1980. p. 297–422.
Stafleu FA, Cowan RS: Taxonomic literature. A selective guide to botanical publications and collections with dates, commentaries and types. Second edition. Utrecht; Bohn, Scheltema and Holkema; The Hague, Junk; Vol. II, 1979, 991 p; Vol. III, 1981, xii, 980 p.
Stafleu FA, Cowan RS, ed: Taxonomic literature. A selective guide to botanical publications and collections with dates, commentaries and types. Volume I: A–G. Second edition. Utrecht, Bohn, Scheltema and Holkema, 1976. xl, 1136 p.
Stearn WT: From Theophrastus and Dioscorides to Sibthorp and Smith: the background and origin of the 'Flora Graeca'. **Biol J Linn Soc Lond** 1976;8:285–98
Stieber MT, Karg AL, Connelly DM, et al: Guide to the botanical records and papers in the archives of the Hunt Institute. **Huntia** 1981;4(1):3–89

**Americas**

Erichsen–Brown C: Use of plants for the past 500 years. Aurora, Ont., Breezy Creeks Press, 1980, xxii, 512 p.
Hirschhorn HH: Botanical remedies of South and Central America, and the Caribbean: an archival analysis. Pt. 1. **J Ethnopharmacol** 1981;4:129–58

**Arabic**

Carrillo JL, Paz Torres M: Ibn Al–Baytar y el arabismo español del XVIII. Edicion trilingüe del prologo de su 'Kitab al–chami.' Benalmádena, Ayuntamiento de Benalmádena, 1982. 57 p.
Fleurentin J, Mazars G, Pelt JM: Cultural background of the medicinal plants of Yemen. **J Ethnopharmacol** 1983 Mar;7(2)183–203

**Bolivia**

Bastien JW: Pharmacopeia of Qollahuaya Andeans. **J Ethnopharmacol** 1983 Jul;8(1):97–111

**China**

Hu SY: An enumeration of Chinese materia medica. Hong Kong, Chinese University Press, 1980. 287 p.
Lama S, Santra SC: Development of Tibetan plant medicine. **Sci Cult** 1979;45(7):262–5
Li Z: [On Li Shizhen's contributions to the method of systematization of Chinese herbology] (Chi). **Chung Hua I Shih Tsa Chih** 1984 Jan;14(1):35–9

**France**

Bygoo E: Les médecins de Montpellier et le Jardin du Roi à Paris. **Hist Nat** 1979;(14):3–29

**Great Britain**

Rosser A: Midsummer magic. **Nurs Times** 1983 Jun 22–9;79(25):50–1

**India**

Singh AN, Pathak SK, Singh RS: Non–plant Vedic epithets in the Sanskrit nomenclature of Indian economic plants. **Stud Hist Med** 1982 Sep;6(3):225–30

**Italy**

Azzi Visentini M: Il giardino dei semplici die Padova: un prodotto della cultura del Rinascimento. **Comunita** 1980;34(182):259–338

# BOTANY

### Mexico

Lozoya X: Fuentes bibliograficas de la herbolaria medicinal mexicana. **Med Tradic** 1980;3(10):69–71

Lozoya X: La herbolaria medicinal en Mexico y el Doctor Del Pozo. **Bol Soc Mex Hist Filos Med** 1980 Mar;5(30):11–6

### Poland

Bernardi L: La diaspora dotanique polonaise. **Mus Geneve** 1981;216:11–6

### United States

Gomberg SJ: Colonial cultivation and concoctions. **MCVQ** 1981;16(3):113–7

Tierney GD: Botany and witchcraft. **Palacio** 1974;80(2):44–50

### USSR

Galaziĭ GI: Istoriia botanicheskikh issledovaniĭ na Baĭkale: itogi i perspektivy ekologo-botanicheskikh rabot. Novosibirsk, Nauka, Sibirskoe otd-nie, 1982. 152 p.

Rowell M: Russian medical botany before the time of Peter the Great. **Sudhoffs Arch** 1978;62(4):339–58

### Yemen

Fleurentin J, Mazars G, Pelt JM: Additional information on the cultural background of drugs and medicinal plants of Yemen. **J Ethnopharmacol** 1983 Sep;8(3):335–44

## Before 500 A.D.

Mazal O: Pflanzen, Wurzeln, Säfte, Samen: antike Heilkunst in Miniaturen des Wiener Dioskurides. Graz, Akademische Druck- u. Verlagsanstalt, 1981. 103 p.

### India

Meulenbeld GJ: Observations on the Arkaprakaśa, a medical Sanskrit Text ascribed to Ravana. In Mazars G, ed: Les médecines traditionnelles de l'Asie. Strasbourg, Université Louis Pasteur, 1981. p. 111–39.

Singh R, Singh AN: Socio-economic and trade relations of ancient India with the western world as reflected in plant names with particular reference to saffron (Kunkum/Kesara). **Stud Hist Med** 1981 Sep;5(3):228–32

Singh RS, Singh AN: On the identity and economico-medicinal uses of hastikarnapalasa (Leea macrophylla Roxb., family: Ampelidaceae) as evinced in the ancient (Sanskrit) texts and traditions. **Indian J Hist Sci** 1981;16(2):219–22

### Rome

Phillips JH: Juxtaposed medical traditions: Pliny HN 27, 131. **Classical Philol** 1981;76(2):130–2

Roemer F: Plinius der Aeltere. (Annotated bibliog. 1964–77.) **Anz Altertumswiss** 1978;31:129–206

Römer F: Plinius der Aeltere. III. Bericht. **Anz Altertumswiss** 1978;31:129–206

Stannard J: Medicinal plants and folk remedies in Pliny, Historia Naturalis. **Hist Philos Life Sci** 1982;4(1):3–23

## 500 A.D.–1450

Daems WF: Synonymenvielfalt und Deutungstechnik bei den nomina plantarum medievalia. In Dilg P, et al., ed: Perspektiven der Pharmaziegeschichte. Graz, Austria, Akademische Druck- u. Verlagsanstalt, 1983. p. 29–37.

### France

Norwood FE, ed: The fourteenth-century medico-botanical glossary of Raimon de Castelnou. Leeds, W. S. Maney for the Leeds Philosophical and Literary Society, 1974. (Proceedings of the Leeds Philosophical and Literary Society, Literary and Historical Section, Vol. XV, Part VI, pp. 135–225).

### Germany

Müller I: Die pflanzlichen Heilmittel bei Hildegard von Bingen. Salzburg, D. Müller, 1982. 215 p.

### Great Britain

Bierbaumer P: Der botanische Wortschatz des Altenglischen. 1. Teil: Das Laeceböc. Bern, Herbert Lang; Frankfurt, Peter Lang, 1975. xv, 168 p. (Grazer Beiträge zur Englischen Philologie, Bd. 1).

### India

Singh BN: Contribution of Madanapala Nighantu to the knowledge of Indian materia medica with particular reference to fig [Anjira] **Indian J Hist Sci** 1981, reçu 1982;16(1):89–94

Singh RS: Contribution of Unani materia medicas to the identification of Vedic plants with special reference to Usana. **Indian J Hist Sci** 1981, reçu 1982;16(1):41–6

## 1450–1700

Corbett M: The emblematic title-page to Stirpium Adversaria nova by Petro Pena and Mathias de L'Obel (1570). **Arch Nat Hist** 1981 Apr;10(1):111–7

Kraft ES: Andreas Cleyer. In Balde JH, Schmiking W, ed: Festschrift zum 86. Deutschen Arztetag in Kassel. Kassel, Arztevereins, 1983. p.40.

Le Traité de matière médicale de Dioscoride à la Renaissance: Exposition d'exemplaires des XVe et XVIe siecles. Du 11 au 24 février 1984 à Louvain-en-Woluwe à la Bibliothèque de la Faculté de Médecine de l'U.C.L. Louvain, Université Catholique de Louvain, Centre d'Histoire de la Pharmacie et du Médicament, 1984. 40 p.

Louis A: Mathieu de L'Obel 1538–1616. Episode de l'histoire de la botanique. Ghent/Louvain, Story-Scientia, 1980. 544 p.

### Asia

Flaumenhaft E: Asian medicinal plants in 17th century French literature. **Econ Bot** 1982;36:147–62

Muntschick W: Ein Manuskript von Georg Meister, dem Kunst- und Lustgärtner, in der British Library. **Medizinhist J** 1984;19(3):225–32

### France

Howard R: Medical politics and the founding of the Jardin des Plantes in Paris. **J Soc Bibliogr Nat Hist** 1980 Apr;9(4):395–402

Howard RC: The family of Guy de la Brosse, founder of the Jardin des Plantes in Paris. In: Conrès international d'histoire de la médecine, XXVe, Québec, 1976. Actes. Québec, 1977. p. 771–89.

### Great Britain

Burnby J: Robert Uredale (1642–1722) botanist. **Pharm Hist (London)** 1974 Jul;4(2):4–5

Hunter M: Early problems in professionalizing scientific research: Nehemiah Grew (1641–1712) and the Royal Society with an unpublished letter to Henry Oldenburg. **Notes Rec R Soc Lond** 1982 Feb;36(2):189–209

Potterton D: Alternative medicine: Culpeper and his cure-alls. **Health Soc Serv J** 1983 Feb 3;93(4832):145–6

### Greece

Tomasi LT: L'isola dei semplici. **Kos** 1984 Jun;1(5):61–84

### India

Sastry VV: Hortus Indicus Malabaricus (Garden of Malabar of India). **Bull Indian Inst Hist Med (Hyderabad)** 1975 Jul;5(3):143–9

### Italy

Morton AG: Marginalia to Andrea Cesalpino's work on botany. **Arch Nat Hist** 1981 Apr;10(1):31–6

Müller-Jahncke WD: Der 'latheinisch aussgestrichene Matthiolus' Landgraf Wilhelms IV von Hessen-Kassel und sein Schicksal. **Pharm Ztg** 1983 Feb 17;128(7):357–61

Palmer R: The influence of botanical research on pharmacists in sixteenth century Venice. **NTM** 1984;21(2):69–80

Tongiorgi Tomasi L: Inventari della galleria e attivita iconografica dell'orto dei semplici dello studio pisano tra Cinque e Seicento. **Ann Ist Mus Stor Sci Fir** 1979;4(2):21–7

### Mexico

Beltrán E: Una polémica sobre Francisco Hernández y su obra en 1785. **An Soc Mex Hist Cienc Tec** 1979;5:49–73

Comas J: Influencia de la farmacopea y terapéutica indígenas de Nueva España en la obra de Juan de Barrios (1607). **An Antropol** 1971;8:125–50

López Austín A: De las plantas medicinales y de otras cosas medicinales. **Estud Cult Nahuatl** 1971;9:125–230

### Netherlands

Vandewiele LJ: De ruime bijdrage van de Nederlandstalige botanisten op het gebied van de geneeskundige kruidenleer voor 1600. **Farm Tijdschr Belg** 1980;57:441–7

### Sri Lanka

Gunawardena DC: Medicinal and economic plants of the Musaeum Zeylanicum of Paul Hermann. **J Sri Lanka Branch R Asiat Soc** 1975;19:33–48

### 1700 to Present

Appleby JH: Robert Erskine--Scottish pioneer of Russian natural history. **Arch Nat Hist** 1982 Apr;10(3):377–98
Delaporte F: Nature's second kingdom. Explorations of vegetality in the eighteenth century. Cambridge, London, MIT Press, 1982. xii, 266 p. (Originally published in France under the title Le second règne de la nature, 1979).
Eisnerova V: The anatomy of plants and its contribution to the origin of cellular theory in the early 19th century. **Acta Hist Rerum Nat Tech** 1971;5:269–333
Johnson DE: A concordance of abbreviations used in references to reviews in botanical bibliographies by Cobres (1782), Bohmer (1787), and Militz (1829). **Huntia** 1979;3(2):103–14
Kapronczay K: Haberle Károly (1764–1832) emlékezete. **Orv Hetil** 1982 Nov 14;123(46):2860–1
Reynaud G: Un grand naturaliste méconnu: Constantin Samuel Rafinesque (1783–1840). **Marseille** 1978;112:61–70
Sajner J, Geus A: Ueber eine Buchbesprechung von Jan Evangelista Purkyně. **J Soc Bibliogr Nat Hist** 1978 Nov;9(1):53–5

### Belgium

Dons R: Projet d'établissement d'un jardin botanique à Saint-Gilles-Bruxelles en 1789. **Folkl Brabancon** 1980;227–228:310–22

### China

Walravens' H: Alexander Tatarinov (1817–1886)--russischer Arzt und Sinologe, eine biobibliographische Skizze. **Sudhoffs Arch** 1980;64(4):392–6

### Czechoslovakia

Cižmář J: Botanist Carl Theimer (1823--1870) in the cultural context of Brno during the period of Mendel's research. **Folia Mendeliana** 1979;14:265–70

### France

Aymonin GG: Lamarck et son herbier. **Hist Nat** 1980–81;17–18:13–7
Aymonin GG: L'herbier de Lamarck. **Rev Hist Sci (Paris)** 1981;34:25–58
Dejussieu J: Note sur le jardin botanique de la Marine à Rochefort-sur-Mer. In: Congrès National des Sociétés Savantes, 91e, Rennes, 1966. Comptes Rendus. Paris, 1967. Section des Sciences, Tome 1. p. 129–33.
Duquénois P: Devenir des plantes médicinales et des médications végétales aux XVIIIe et XIXe siècles sous l'influence de la chimie moderne. In Livet G, Schaff G, ed: Médecine et assistance en Alsace, XVIe–XXe siècle. Strasbourg, Istra, 1976. p. 227–39.
Guéguen E: Les jardins botaniques de Bretagne aux XVIIIe et XIXe siècles. In: Congrès National des Sociétés Savantes, 97e, Nantes, 1972. Comptes Rendus. Paris, 1976. Section des Sciences, Tome 1. p. 377–83.
Huard P, Théodoridès J: Jean-Baptiste Pipelet (1759–1823), Constance de Théis (1767–1845), Josef de Salm-Dyck (1773–1861) ou le chirurgien, la poétesse et le botaniste. In: Congrès National des Sociétés Savantes, 93e, Tours, 1968. Comptes Rendus. Paris, 1971. Section des Sciences, Tome II. p. 127–36.
Huard P, Lacombe C, Théodoridès J: Marine et botanique aux XVIIIe et XIXe siècles; les jardins botaniques de la Marine. In: Congrès National des Sociétés Savantes, 91e, Rennes, 1966. Comptes Rendus. Paris, 1967. Section des Sciences, Tome 1. p. 109–27.
Laissus J: La succession de Le Monnier au Jardin du Roi: Antoine-Laurent de Jussieu et René Louiche-Desfontaines. In: Congrès National des Sociétés Savantes, 91e, Rennes, 1966. Comptes Rendus. Paris, 1967. Section des Sciences, Tome 1. p. 137–52.
Laissus Y: Lettres inédites de René Desfontaines à Louis-Guillaume le Monnier, conservées à la Bibliothèque centrale du Muséum national d'histoire naturelle. In: Congrès National des Sociétés Savantes, 91e, Rennes, 1966. Comptes Rendus. Paris, 1967. Section des Sciences, Tome 1. p. 153–69.
McKee ME, McKee HS: E. Vieillard et E. Deplanche, deux grands botanistes collecteurs en Nouvelle-Calédonie. **Hist Nat** 1980–81;17–18:49–68

### Germany

Hein WH: Die ephesische Diana als Natursymbol bei Alexander von Humboldt. In Dilg P, et al., ed: Perspektiven der Pharmaziegeschichte. Graz, Austria, Akademische Druck- u. Verlagsanstalt, 1983. p. 131–46.
Mollenhauer D: Die Haeckel-Rezeption durch die Botanik. **Medizinhist J** 1980;15(3):305–36
Scheele I: Zur Typologie des Botanikers in der ersten Hälfte des 19. Jahrhunderts: Christian Friedrich Hornschuch. **Medizinhist J** 1983;18(3):184–97
Wölfel A: Pflanzen in der Volksmedizin. Die volksmedizinischen Studien von Heinrich Marzell. Diss. Erlangen-Nürnberg, 1983. 117 p.

### Great Britain

Allen DE: The plagiarisms of Thomas Henry Cooper. **J Soc Bibliogr Nat Hist** 1979 Nov;9(3):275–9
Binnie GA: George Johnston: 1797–1855. **Br Med J [Clin Res]** 1982 Oct 9;285(6347):1014–6
Brock CH: James Douglas (1675–1742), botanist. **J Soc Bibliogr Nat Hist** 1979 Apr;9(2):137–45
Brockway LH: Science and colonial expansion. The role of the British Royal Botanic Gardens. New York, Academic Press, 1979. 215 p. (Studies in Social Discontinuity).
Brown PS: Herbalists and medical botanists in mid-nineteenth-century Britain with special reference to Bristol. **Med Hist** 1982 Oct;26(4):405–20
Brown PS: The vicissitudes of herbalism in late nineteenth- and early twentieth-century Britain. **Med Hist** 1985 Jan;29(1):71–92
Browne J: Darwin's botanical arithmetic and the 'principle of divergence,' 1854–1858. **J Hist Biol** 1980 Spring;13(1):53–89
Harrod DC: Chelsea physic garden tercentenary. **Pharm Hist (London)** 1974 Jan;4(1):4–5
Hatfield G: Robert Brown A.M., F.R.S.E. (1773–1858). Edinburgh, History of Medicine and Science Unit, University of Edinburgh, [1981?]. [11] p.
Lysaght A: A letter from Sydney Parkinson in Batavia to Dr. John Fothergill. **Notes Rec R Soc Lond** 1981;36(1):79–81
Lyte C: Sir Joseph Banks, 18th century explorer, botanist and entrepreneur. London, David & Charles, 1980. 248 p.
MacPhail I, Hess WJ: The date of the Linnaean index in John Martyn's Historia plantarum rariorum. **Huntia** 1979;3(2):73–81
Morgan N: The development of biochemistry in England through botany and the brewing industry (1870–1890). **Hist Philos Life Sci** 1980;2(1):141–66
Roberts JA: Reginald Ruggles Gates. In Dictionary of national biography, 1961–1970. Suppl. 8, 1981. p. 424–5.
Smith E: The life of Sir Joseph Banks. New York, Arno Press, 1975. xvi, 348 p.
Waldron HA: Richard Pulteney (1730–1801): Linnean botanist and cardiologist. **Trans Stud Coll Physicians Phila** 1980 Mar;5(2 no 1):31–40

### Hungary

Lugosi MM: Die im Pray-Codex beschriebenen Heilpflanzen im späteren botanischen Lehrstoff der ersten ungarischen medizinischen Fakultät. In Hein WH, ed: Pharmaziehistorischer Kongress, Budapest, 1981. Stuttgart, Wissenschaftliche Verlagsgesellschaft, 1983. p. 97–9.

### Ireland

Corrigan D: Irish Ethno-botany by Michael Moloney--an early contribution to the concept of ethnopharmacology. **J Ethnopharmacol** 1981 Nov;4(3):343–5
Nelson EC: 'In the Contemplation of Vegetables'--Caleb Threlkeld (1676–1728), his life, background and contribution to Irish botany. **J Soc Bibliogr Nat Hist** 1979 Nov;9(3):257–73
Nelson EC: The influence of Leiden on botany in Dublin in the early eighteenth century. **Huntia** 1982;4(2):133–46

### Japan

Fodstad H: Carl Peter Thunberg: Swedish pioneer of Occidental medicine in Japan. **Neurol Med Chir (Tokyo)** 1982 Jul;22(7):577–81

### Mexico

Cervantes V: 'Ensayo a la materia medica vegetal de Mexico' (Introduccion). **Med Tradic** 1982;3(11):34–6

### South Africa

Spohr OH: Dr. Med. Friedrich Ludwig Liesching. **Q Bull S Afr Libr** 1968;23(2):45–55

### Spain

Bueno AG: La flora de Aragon: notas a un proyecto de Francisco Loscos y Jose Pardo. **Bol Soc Esp Hist Farm** 1984;35(137):23–33
Elósegui J: Un guipuzcoano benemérito del siglo XVIII, Manuel Bernardino de Aranguren, médico (1743–1794). **Bol Real Soc Vascongada Amigos Pais** 1973;29(1–3):171–91
Jordi R: Antonio Sala, un boticario barcelon/B//es aficionado a la botánica. **Farm Univers** 1980;13(1,2):10–7,78–82

## BOTANY

Puente Veloso S: Aportación de la botánica a la medicina en el reinado de Carlos III. **An R Acad Nac Med (Madr)** 1982;99(3):437-501

Valverde López JL, Vidal Casero MC: Notas sobre médicos y cirujanos que trabajaron para el Jardín Botánico de Madrid. In International Congress of the History of Medicine, 27th, Barcelona, 1980. Actas. Barcelona, Acadèmia de Ciències Mèdiques de Catalunya i Balears, 1981. p. 650-5.

Vidal Casero MC: Aportacion a la historia del Jardin de Aclimatacion de San Lucard de Barrameda. **Bol Soc Esp Hist Farm** 1981 Dec;32(128):235-49

Vidal Casero MC: Plantas medicinales cultivadas en el Jardín Botánico con destino a las reales boticas de los hospitales militares del Campo de San Roque establecido en Algeciras. In International Congress of the History of Medicine, 27th, Barcelona, 1980. Actas. Barcelona, Acadèmia de Ciències Mèdiques de Catalunya i Balears, 1981. p. 656-62.

Vidal Casero MC, Aguilera Guirao A: Plantas medicinales cultivadas en el Jardín Botánico del Monasterio de Nuestra Señora de Carracido. In International Congress of the History of Medicine, 27th, Barcelona, 1980. Actas. Barcelona, Acadèmia de Ciències Mèdiques de Catalunya i Balears, 1981. p. 663-8.

**Sweden**

Eriksson G: Linnaeus the botanist. In Frängsmyr T, ed: Linnaeus, the man and his work. Berkeley, University of California Press, 1983. p. 63-109.

Leikola A: Zeus Faber--antiikin tarustoa eläinkunnassa. **Hist Arkisto (Finl)** 1978;(73):110-19

Ljungdell J: Juglans regia L. - i den svenska farmakopéen och annorstädes. **Sydsven Medicinhist Sallsk Arsskr** 1982;19:54-62

Söderström N: Infusum amarum alkalinum militare; en arabesk kring ett gammalt amarum. **Sydsven Medicinhist Sallsk Arsskr** 1982;19:137-43

Synek VM: Linnaeus--physician and king of flowers. **NZ Med J** 1984 Apr 25;97(754):267-9

**United States**

Berkeley E, Berkeley DS: The life and travels of John Bartram: from Lake Ontario to the River St. John. Tallahassee, University Presses of Florida, 1982. xvi, 376 p.

Bloch H: Medical botany; note on Constantine Samuel Refinesque (1784-1841). **NY State J Med** 1979 Sep;79(10):1610-1

Boewe C: Editing Rafinesque's holographs: the case of the short letters. **Filson Club Hist Q** 1980;54(1):37-49

Cowen DL: The trustees' garden at Savannah. **Ga Pharm Q** 1983 Spring;60(2):5-3

Gifford GE: The medical botany of the New England area, 1782-1842. **Proc Camb Mass Hist Soc 1973-5** [1980];43:127-40

Rudolph ED: The introduction of the Natural System of classification of plants to nineteenth century American students. **Arch Nat Hist** 1982 Apr;10(3):461-8

Stuckey RL: Dr. William Darlington's botanical contacts on the western American frontier. **Trans Stud Coll Physicians Phila** 1983 Sep;5(5 No 3):213-43

Stuckey RL: Medical botany in the Ohio Valley (1800-1850). **Trans Stud Coll Physicians Phila** 1978 Jul;45(5):262-79

Whittet TD: Botanic garden of the trustees of the Georgia colony at Savannah. **Pharm J** 1983;231:770-1

Wolfe RJ: Jacob Bigelow's American medical botany 1817-1821. An examination of the origin, printing, binding and distribution of America's first color plate book. With special emphasis on the manner of making and printing its colored plates. North Hills, Pennsylvania, and Boston, Bird & Bull Press and Boston Medical Library, 1979. 121 p.

**USSR**

Ignatovich FI, Semeniuk SI: Zh. E. Zhiliber i ego 'Flora Litvy'. **Sov Zdravookhr** 1981;(11):67-9

Mardzhanian KS: Stepanos Sharimanian. **Patma-Banasirakam Handes. Ist-Filol Zh** 1971;(3):236-46

**Venezuela**

Vélez Boza F: Licenciado Jose Maria Benitez; maestro en artes, médico y botánico. **Rev Soc Venez Hist Med** 1977;25(39):71-92

## CARDIOLOGY AND CIRCULATORY SYSTEM

See also **Blood Transfusion; Surgery-Cardiovascular**

Agostoni G, Berti Bock G, Favero GA: Il concetto di miocardite nell'Ottocento. **Acta Med Hist Patav** 1979-80;26:9-27

Bearn AG, James DG: Dr. William Harvey (1578-1657) and the Harvey Society of New York. **Perspect Biol Med** 1978 Spring;21(3):524-35

Bell BA: A history of the study of the cerebral circulation and the measurement of cerebral blood flow. **Neurosurgery** 1984 Feb;14(2):238-46

Brewer LA: Sphygmology through the centuries. Historical notes. **Am J Surg** 1983 Jun;145(6):696-702

Chávez I: Historia de la cardiologia, raíces, desarrollo y perspectivas. **Bol Soc Mex Hist Filos Med** 1980 Jun;5(31):25-35

Chávez I: Reflexiones de un clinico en torno de los momentos culminantes de la cardiologia. **Bol Soc Mex Hist Filos Med** 1980 Jun;5(31):37-55

Chevalier PA, ed: The heart and circulation. Stroudsburg, Pennsylvania, Dowden, Hutchinson & Ross, 1976. xix, 385 p. (Benchmark Papers in Human Physiology, 8).

DeBard ML: The history of cardiopulmonary resuscitation. **Ann Emerg Med** 1980 May;9(5):273-5

Degeorges M: De l'auscultation médiate à l'auscultation intra-cardiaque. Les avatars de la découverte de Laennec. **Rev Palais Decouv** 1981;10(92):17-8

Fich S, Li JK: Aorto-ventricular dynamics: theories, experiments, and instrumentation. **Crit Rev Biomed Eng** 1983;9(3):245-85

Fishman AP, Richards DW: Circulation of the blood: men and ideas. Bethesda, American Physiological Society, 1982. xx, 859 p.

Furkalo NK: Osnovnye étapy razvitiia kardiologii. **Vrach Delo** 1980 Aug;(8):5-9

Gawel M: The development of concepts concerning cerebral circulation. In Rose FC, Bynum WF, ed: Historical aspects of the neurosciences. New York, Raven, 1982. p. 171-8.

Harthorne JW: Historic milestones of electrotherapy and cardiac pacing. **Prog Cardiovasc Dis** 1981 May-Jun;23(6):389-92

Hirzel HO: Der Weg zur modernen Kardiologie. **Praxis** 1983 Nov 29;72(48):1521-8

Ježek V: Historický vývoi a současný stav výzkumu vztahu mezi plicní a systémovou cirkulací a funkcí obou srdečních komor. **Cesk Fysiol** 1981;30(2):103-6

Kaiser W, Trenckmann U: Aus der Frühgeschichte der kardiologischen Diagnostik. **Z Gesamte Inn Med** 1980 Jun 1;35(11):454-62

Kawai S, Kanoh T, Okada R: [History of the etiological studies of myocardial infarction and angina pectoris] (Jpn). **Nippon Rinsho** 1983;41(2):265-70

Lara-Terrazas A, Ortega A, Gutiérrez A, et al: El fenómeno de acoplamiento-excitación-contracción y relajacion cardíaca. Análisis retrospectivo. **Arch Inst Cardiol Mex** 1983 Jul-Aug;53(4):373-8

Legee G: P. Flourens, historien des sciences: valeur de son histoire de la découverte de la circulation du sang. In: Congrès National des Sociétés Savantes, 107e. Brest, 1982. Comptes Rendus, Paris, 1983. Section des Sciences, Fasc. IV. p. 313-31.

Lind J: Researches in perinatal circulation. In Smith GF, Smith PN, Vidyasagar, D, ed: Historical review and recent advances in neonatal and perinatal medicine. [Chicago?], Mead Johnson Nutritional Division, 1983. Vol. II. p. 1-20.

McMichael J: History of atrial fibrillation 1628-1819 Harvey - de Senac - Laënnec. **Br Heart J** 1982 Sep;48(3):193-7

Neuhausen T: Das Cholesterin. Vorstellungen über seine Rolle im Körper. Köln, Universität zu Köln, 1977. 187 p. (Kölner medizinhistorische Beiträge, 6).

Pfannkuche K, Schadewaldt H: Die Bedeutung der Blutgefässe im Laufe der Entwicklung der Medizin. In Müller-Wiefel H, et. al., ed: Mikrozirkulation und Blutrheologie. Therapie der peripheren arteriellen Verschlusskrankheit. Baden-Baden, New York, Witzstrock, 1980. p. 4-9.

Rapson H: The circulation of blood: a history. London, F. Muller, 1982. 132 p.

Rashkind WJ, ed: Congenital heart disease. Stroudsburg, Pennsylvania, Hutchinson Ross, 1982. xv, 390 p. (Benchmark papers in human physiology, 16).

Reichert P: A history of the development of cardiology as a medical specialty. **Clin Cardiol** 1978 Apr;1(1):5-15

Richardson JP: Surgeons, physicians, and cardiology. **Aust NZ J Surg** 1980 Dec;50(6):668-71

Rullière R: Die Kardiologie bis zum Ende des 18. Jahrhunderts. In Sournia JC, Martiny M, Poulet J, ed: Illustrierte Geschichte der Medizin. Salzburg, Andreas, 1980. Vol. 3. p. 1075-123.

Schölmerich P: Historische Anmerkungen zum Begriff Myokarditis - Kardiomypathie. **Med Welt** 1984 Jan 13;35(1-2):109-13

Schott A: Historical notes on the mechanism of closure of the atrioventricular valves. **Med Hist** 1980 Apr;24(2):163-84

Simon I: Les notions de cardiologie bibliques et talmudiques. **Rev Hist Med Heb** 1984;37(1):3-6

Simon I: Les notions de cardiologie bibliques et talmudiques. **Rev Hist Med Heb** 1984 Jul;37(2):26-30

Skalak R, Chien S: Capillary flow: history, experiments and theory. **Biorheology** 1981;18(3-6):307-30

Trocme C: Esquisse d'une histoire de la pléthore, de la volémie et du retour veineux. **Hist Sci Med** 1981;15(1):69-80

Vega Diaz F: El corazón en la simbología y en la iconografía profana y religiosa. In Academia Nacional de Medicina. Libro conmemorativo del primer centenario. México, Comité Editorial de la Comisión Organizadora del Congreso del Centenario, 1964. Tome 2. p. 78-82.

Warren JV, ed: Cardiovascular physiology. Stroudsburg, Pennsylvania, Dowden, Hutchinson & Ross, 1975. xvi, 441 p. (Benchmark Papers in Human Physiology, 4).

Whitteridge G: The Piltdown Hippocrates. **Hist Sci** 1980 Sep;18(41 pt 3):226-30

**China**

Dakpa N: La Sphygnologie tibétaine. In Mazars G, ed: Les médecines traditionnelles de l'Asie. Strasbourg, Université Louis Pasteur, 1981. p. 23–9.

Meyer F: Le système canalaire et la sphygmologie en médecine tibétaine d'après le rgyud-bži et son commentaire le Vaidurya snon-po (1). In Mazars G, ed: Les médecines traditionnelles de l'Asie. Strasbourg, Université Louis Pasteur, 1981. p. 30–40.

**Egypt**

Ghalioungui P: Four landmarks of Egyptian cardiology. **J R Coll Physicians Lond** 1984 Jul;18(3):182–6

**Vietnam**

Nguyen-Tran-Huan: La sphygmologie dans la médecine vietnamienne traditionnelle. Contribution à l'étude du traité 'Bin hú mài xué' de Lĭ Shí Zhen. In Mazars G, ed: Les médecines traditionnelles de l'Asie. Strasbourg, Université Louis Pasteur, 1981. p. 13–22.

**Yugoslavia**

Mušič D, Rakovec P, Jagodic A, et al: The first description of syncopal attacks in heart block. **PACE** 1984 Mar;7(2):301–3

**Before 500 A.D.**

**Egypt**

Bonnabeau RC: The school at Alexandria and the vascular system. The circulation near miss. **Minn Med** 1983 Feb;66(2):100–1

**Greco-Roman**

Nickel D: Galens Untersuchungen zur embryonalen Blutbewegung. **Orvostort Kozl** 1981;93–96(27 No 1–4):25–35

**Greece**

Boylan M: The digestive and 'circulatory' systems in Aristotle's biology. **J Hist Biol** 1982 Spring;15(1):89–118

**500 A.D.–1450**

Lenhardt F: Zur Ikonographie der Blutschau. **Medizinhist J** 1982;17(1/2):63–77

**Arabic**

Durrany KS, Uddin Siddiqui T: Al-Adwiyat al-Qalbiya. **Stud Hist Med** 1980 Mar;4(1):29–38

Gracia D, Vidal JL: Avicena, sobre el corazón. In International Congress of the History of Medicine, 27th, Barcelona, 1980. Actas. Barcelona, Académia de Ciències Médiques de Catalunya i Balears, 1981. p. 711–22.

Katsenovich RA, Mirzaev NL: Kardiologicheskoe nasledie Abu Ali Ibn-Siny (k 1000-letiu so dnia rozhdeniia). **Kardiologiia** 1980 Nov;20(11):120–2

Micheli A de: Los balbuceos de la cardiologia en la medicina islamica. **Bol Soc Mex Hist Filos Med** 1982 Mar;6(38):5–13

Micheli A de: Tópicos cardiológicos en la antigua medicina islámica. **Arch Inst Cardiol Mex** 1981 Sep–Oct;51(5):497–500

Sliwiński S: Teoria Ibn an-Nafisa (1210–1288) krążenia płucnego krwi. **Wiad Lek** 1981 Mar 15;34(6):531–3

Uddinahmed R: Single drugs mentioned by Avicenna for cardiac ailments in his canon and Kitab-Ul-Adwiyyah Qalbiyyah. **Bull Indian Inst Hist Med (Hyderabad)** 1979;9:46–66

**USSR**

Shengeliia GM: 'Lechebnaia kniga--Karabadini' Z. Panaskerteli-Tsitsishvili. **Klin Med (Mosk)** 1981 Jun;59(6):110–2

**1450–1700**

Bloch H: Discovery of blood circulation; Some dependence factors in evolution of a discovery. **NY State J Med** 1979 Nov;79(12):1940–3

Mani N: Biomedical thought in Glisson's hepatology and in Wepfer's work on apoplexy. With commentary by R. G. Frank, p. 84–8. In Stevenson LG, ed: A celebration of medical history. Baltimore, Johns Hopkins University Press, 1982. (The Henry E. Sigerist supplements to the Bulletin of the History of Medicine; new ser., no. 6). p. 37–63.

Schouten J, Goltz D: James Primrose und sein Kampf gegen die Theorie vom Blutkreislauf. **Sudhoffs Arch** 1977;61(4):331–52

Toellner R: Logical and psychological aspects of the discovery of the circulation of the blood. In M. D. Grmek, R. S. Cohen, G. Cimino, ed: On scientific discovery. The Erice Lectures 1977. Dordrecht, D. Reidel, 1981. p. 239–59. (Boston Studies in the Philosophy of Science, v. 34).

Vetter T: Un siècle d'histoire de la circulation du sang, 1564–1664. [Bâle, Geigy, 1965]. 6 pts. in 1 v.

**Great Britain**

Alsop JD: A footnote on the circulation of the blood: Joseph Colston and Harvey's discovery in 1642. **J Hist Med Allied Sci** 1981 Jul;36(3):331–4

Andrews BF: William Harvey in perinatal perspective. In Smith GF, Smith PN, Vidyasagar D, ed: Historical review and recent advances in neonatal and perinatal medicine. [Chicago?], Mead Johnson Nutritional Division, 1983. Vol. II. p. 165–78.

Bonnabeau RC, Bonnabeau MM: William Harvey revisited 1578–1978. **Minn Med** 1981 Jan;64(1):28–33

Boss JM: 'Doctrina de circulatione sanguinis haud immutat antiquam Medendi Methodum': an unpublished manuscript (1662) by Francis Glisson (1597–1677) on the implications of Harvey's physiology. **Physis** 1978;20(1–4):309–35

Burchell HB: Mechanical and hydraulic analogies in Harvey's discovery of the circulation. **J Hist Med Allied Sci** 1981 Jul;36(3):260–77

Bylebyl JJ: Boyle and Harvey on the valves in the veins. **Bull Hist Med** 1982 Fall;56(3):351–67

Bylebyl JJ: The growth of Harvey's De Motu Cordis. **Bull Hist Med** 1973 Sep–Oct;47(5):427–70

Bylebyl JJ, ed: William Harvey and his age: the professional and social context of the discovery of the circulation. Baltimore, Johns Hopkins University Press, 1979. xii, 154 p. (Henry E. Sigerist Supplements to the Bulletin of the History of Medicine, n.s., 2). Includes contributions by S. Jarcho, C. Webster, R. G. Frank.

Cohen IB, ed: Studies on William Harvey. New York, Arno Press, 1981. 572 p. in various pagings. (A collection of previously published articles and short works by various authors).

Comtor JH: Harvey's 1651 perfusion of the pulmonary circulation of man. **Circulation** 1982 Jan;65(1):1–3

Huard P, Imbault-Huart MJ: Les étapes du traitement des tumeurs par ischémie, priorité de Harvey. **Hist Sci Med** 1980;14(2):171–5

Hughes JT: Spinal cord arteries described by Willis. In Rose FC, Bynum WF, ed: Historical aspects of the neurosciences. New York, Raven, 1982. p. 195–203.

Jucovy PM: Circle and circulation: the language and imagery of William Harvey's discovery. **Perspect Biol Med** 1976 Autumn;20(1):92–107

Keele KD: The life and work of William Harvey. **Endeavour** 1978;2(3):104–7

Rulliere R, Heymans G, Vial F: La version en langue française (1679) du Tractatus de Corde (1669) de Richard Lower. In International Congress of the History of Medicine, 27th, Barcelona, 1980. Actas. Barcelona, Académia de Ciències Médiques de Catalunya i Balears, 1981. p. 331–5.

Schadewaldt H: 'Le génie, c'est une longue patience'. (Teil 1). **Arztl Fortbild** 1982;32(11):12–23

Schadewaldt H: 'Le génie, c'est une longue patience'. (Teil 2). **Arztl Fortbild** 1982;32(12):16–8

Schadewaldt H: 'Le génie, c'est une longue patience'. (Teil 3). **Arztl Fortbild** 1982;32(13):32–40

Schmidtgall H: Zur Rezeption von Harveys Blutkreislaufmodell in der englischen Wirtschaftstheorie des 17. Jahrhunderts. **Sudhoffs Arch** 1973;57(4):416–30

Wear A: William Harvey and the 'Way of the Anatomists'. **Hist Sci** 1983 Sep;21(53 pt 3):223–49

**Greece**

Apostolopoulos DG: Alexandros Maurokordatos. **Ellenika** 1976;29:311–5

**Italy**

Donáth T: Egy évforduló ürügyén. **Orv Hetil** 1984 Sep 30;125(40):2441–4

Pariente L: Le De venarum ostiolis de Jerome Fabrice d'Acquapendente: sa place dans l'histoire de la découverte de la circulation du sang. Paris, Louis Pariente, 1981. 2 volumes.

**Mexico**

Torre JM: La cardiologia en Nueva España durante el siglo XVI. **Bol Soc Mex Hist Filos Med** 1982 Sep;6(40):57–9

Torre JM: La contribución de Nueva España a la cardiología. **Arch Inst Cardiol Mex** 1980 Sep–Oct;50(5):623–9

Torre JM: Los balbuceos de la cardiologia mexicana. **Bol Soc Mex Hist Filos Med** 1980 Sep–Dec;5(32–33):109–22

Torre JM: Los balbuceos de la cardiología mexicana. **Prensa Med Mex** 1979 May–Jun;44(5–6):105–11

# CARDIOLOGY AND CIRCULATORY SYSTEM

**Spain**

Paglia L: Odontoiatria del passato. Chi era Servet? **Dent Cadmos** 1984 Jan;52(1):79–81

Sliwiński S: Miquel Serveto (1511–1553) -- odkrywca płucnego krążenia krwi. **Wiad Lek** 1980 Apr 1;33(7):589–91

Vidal F: Michel Servet (1511–1553). La découverte de la circulation du sang. **Chir Dent Fr** 1981 Apr;51(110):39–43

**Switzerland**

Mani N: Johann Jakob Wepfers Doktordisputation über das Herzklopfen (1647). **Gesnerus** 1981;38:143–7

**1700 to Present**

Albasanz Gallan JL: La digital, en su segundo centenario. **An R Acad Nac Med (Madr)** 1983;100(2):181–208

Anderson RH, Becker AE: Stanley Ken and accessory atrioventricular connections. **J Thorac Cardiovasc Surg** 1981 May;81(5):649–58

Anger P, Wenz W: Aus der Pionierzeit der Arteriographie. **Radiologe** 1981 Feb;21(2):65–71

Antoszewski Z: Krótki rys historyczny rozwoju pozaustrojowego krażenia krwi i niektórych aparatórych aparatów sztuczne 'płuco-serce'. **Przegl Lek** 1979;36(12):869–72

Bartecchi CE: Cardiopulmonary resuscitation--an element of sophistication in the 18th century. **Am Heart J** 1980 Oct;100(4):580–1

Belic N, Gardin JM: Implantable cardiac pacemakers--an overview. **Int J Dermatol** 1982 Nov;21(9):543–50

Besterman E: Waller before Einthoven in the clinical development of noninvasive ECG. **Am Heart J** 1982 Apr;103(4 pt 1):572

Burchell HB: The QT interval historically treated. **Pediatr Cardiol** 1983 Apr–Jun;4(2):139–48

Callaghan JC: Early experiences in the study and development of an artificial electrical pacemaker for standstill of the heart: view from 1949. **PACE** 1980 Sep;3(5):618–9

Carlson PA: Three contributors to cardiac catheterization. **J Thorac Cardiovasc Surg** 1980 May;79(5):782–8

Chang S, Chang JK: A historical review of echocardiographic detection of pericardial effusion. **Jpn Heart J** 1981 Sep;22(5):789–800

Cleghorn RA: Cardiovascular failure in experimental adrenal insufficiency: a historical rivival. **Perspect Biol Med** 1983 Autumn;27(1):135–55

Comroe JH: Exploring the heart: discoveries in heart disease and high blood pressure. New York, Norton, 1983. 348 p.

Doby T: History of cardiovascular catheterization. In: Congrès international d'histoire de la médecine, XXVe, Québec, 1976. Actes. Québec, 1977. p. 596–602.

Dolabjian ZL: The International Congress on Electrocardiography: a brief history. **J Electrocardiol** 1984 Jul;17(3):307–8

Ecker A: The discovery of human cerebral arterial spasm in angiograms: an autobiographical note.. **Neurosurgery** 1982 Jan;10(1):90

Favaloro RG: The present era of myocardial revascularization--some historical landmarks. **Int J Cardiol** 1983 Oct;4(3):331–44

Fleckenstein K: The early ECG in medical practice. **Med Instrum** 1984 May–Jun;18(3):191–2

Freimanis I, Starr A: The unnatural history of valvular heart disease: late results with silastic ball valve prostheses. **J Cardiovasc Surg (Torino)** 1984 May–Jun;25(3):191–8

Fye WB: Coronary arteriography--it took a long time! **Circulation** 1984 Nov;70(5):781–7

García-Argüelles R: De la digital de ayer a los lanatosidos de hoy. Una breve historia de los cardiotonicos. **Asclepio** 1980;32:195–9

Gathiram P, Katzeff IE, Edwards H, et al: Dynamic electrocardiography IV. The 'imaginary cardiac vector' hypothesis: the evolution of the vectorcardiographic inverse solution. **Med Hypotheses** 1981 Jul;7(7):825–62

Gold RD: Cardiac pacing--from then to now. **Med Instrum** 1984 Jan–Feb;18(1):15–21

Green AF: The discovery of bretylium and bethanidine. **Br J Clin Pharmacol** 1982 Jan;13(1):25–34

Grosse-Brockhoff F: Herzbehandlung mit dem 'Fingerhut' einst und jetzt. Opladen, Westdeutscher Verlag, 1980. 58 p. (Rheinisch-Westfälische Akademie der Wissenschaften; Natur-, Ingenieur- und Wirtschaftswissenschaften, Vorträge N 293).

Howell JD: Early perceptions of the electrocardiogram: from arrhythmia to infarction. **Bull Hist Med** 1984 Spring;58(1):83–98

Inguaggiato B: Evoluzione tecnologica del pace-maker. **Minerva Med** 1980 Oct 6;71(38):2793–6

James TN: The development of ideas concerning the conduction system of the heart. **Ulster Med J** 1982;51(2):81–97

Kyrge KKh: K istorii transtorakal'nogo massazha serdtsa. **Klin Med (Mosk)** 1981 Jun;59(6):109–10

Lagergren H: Den implanterbara pacemakern 25 år. Utveckling och erfarenheter. **Lakartidningen** 1983 Oct 5;80(40):3688–91

Laham J: Le concept de bloc de branche. Evolution des idées (1910–1982). **Ann Cardiol Angeiol (Paris)** 1983 Jul–Sep;32(5):343–50

Laragh JH: Concept of anti-renin system therapy. Historic perspective. **Am J Med** 1984 Aug 20;77(2A):1–6

Lavenne F: L'electrocardiographie et vectocardiographie. **Rev Inst Hyg Mines (Hasselt)** 1980;35(3):133–4

Leatham A: Auscultation of the heart since Laënnec. **Thorax** 1981 Feb;36(2):95–8

Leme C de A: Desenvolvimento histórico da eletrocardiografia. **Rev Hosp Clin Fac Med Sao Paulo** 1980 Aug;35(4):205–17

Leonard JC: Thomas Bevill Peacock and the early history of dissecting aneurysm. **Br Med J** 1979 Jul 28;2(6184):260–2

Lur'e GO, Savel'ev SA, Iushkov MA: Iskusstvennoe krovoobrashchenie v usloviiakh giperbaricheskoĭ oksigenatsii. **Anesteziol Reanimatol** 1982 Nov–Dec;(6):63–7

Luyendijk W: The arteries of the spinal cord. The history of a paradigmal shift. **Acta Neurochir (Wien)** 1982;61(1–3):25–41

MacAlpin RN: Coronary arterial spasm: a historical perspective. **J Hist Med Allied Sci** 1980 Jul;35(3):288–311

McNamara DG: Twenty-five years of progress in the medical treatment of pediatric and congenital heart disease. **J Am Coll Cardiol** 1983 Jan;1(1):264–73

Marquis RM: The continuous murmur of persistence of the ductus arteriosus---an historical review. **Eur Heart J** 1980 Dec;1(6):465–78

Menárguez Carretero L: Los avances de la cardiología en lo que va de siglo. **An R Acad Nac Med (Madr)** 1982;99(2):297–309

Mezzetti MG: Il massaggio cardiaco agli albori della tecnica. Uno strumento di dubbia utilità. **Minerva Anestesiol** 1981 Mar;47(3):123–5

Moe GK: Oscillating concepts in arrhythmia research; a personal account. **Int J Cardiol** 1984 Jan;5(1):109–13

Pariente L, ed: Les appareils de mesure du pouls et de la pression artérielle. Paris, L. Pariente, 1979. 113 p.

Piccolo E: L'elettrocardiografia a una svolta semeiologica. **G Ital Cardiol** 1981;11(1):1–3

Postnov IuV: Popytka opisaniia gipertonicheskoĭ bolezni bolee 200 let nazad. **Kardiologiia** 1983 Dec;23(12):89

Pruitt RD: Symptoms, signs, signals, and shadows. The pathophysiology of angina pectoris--a historical perspective. **Mayo Clin Proc** 1983 Jun;58(6):394–8

Rabinovich RS, Serdiuk GV, Egorysheva IV, et al: Znamenatel'nye i iubileĭnye daty istorii kardiologii 1984. **Kardiologiia** 1984 Feb;24(2):124–5

Radner S: Den selektiva angiografins bakgrund och begynnelse. **Sydsven Medicinhist Sallsk Arsskr** 1982;19:109–18

Reis DJ: The brain and hypertension: reflections on 35 years of inquiry into the neurobiology of the circulation. **Circulation** 1984 Nov;70(5 Pt 2):III31–45

Rijlant P: The coming of age of electrophysiology and electrocardiography. **NTM** 1980;17(1):108–23

Rosenbaum MB: Sir Thomas Lewis: a view from the south. **Br Heart J** 1981 Oct;46(4):349–50

Ruhdorfer UE: Die klinische Blutdruckmessung - rund 100 Jahre alt. **Osterr Arzteztg** 1982;37(4):193

Rullière R: Geschichte der Kardiologie im 19. und 20. Jahrhundert. In Sournia JC, Martiny M, Poulet J, ed: Illustrierte Geschichte der Medizin. Salzburg, Andreas, 1980. Vol. 4. p. 1251–309.

Salvetti ME: Gefässpsychopathologie bei Richard von Krafft-Ebing (1840–1902). Bern, Huber, 1984. 125 p. (Berner Beiträge zur Geschichte der Medizin und der Naturwissenschaften, Neue Folge, Band 10)

Sapira JD: Quincke, de Musset, Duroziez, and Hill: some aortic regurgitations. **South Med J** 1981 Apr;74(4):459–67

Scheld HH, Mulch J, Schaper J, et al: Myokardprotektion im Wandel der letzten 20 Jahre. **Med Welt** 1982 May 21;33(20):746–9

Schmid-Schönbein H: Die Ursprünge der medizinischen Hämorheologie im 18. Jahrhundert: H. Boerhaave, A. v. Haller und G. van Swieten. **Vasa** 1984;Suppl 12:10–31

Schuur KH: Radiological visualization of the portal venous system. A historical review. **Diagn Imag Clin Med** 1984;53(4):173–6

Segall H: Dr. Harold Segall: a pioneer cardiologist reminisces. **Can Med Assoc J** 1982 May 1;126(9):1109–13–7

Seipel L, Breithardt G, Borggrefe M: Die Entwicklung der klinischen Elektrophysiologie. Indikation, Komplikationen und Ergebnisse von 1296 invasiven elektrophysiologischen Untersuchungen 1971 bis 1981 in Düsseldorf. **Z Kardiol** 1984 Apr;73(4):194–8

Senning A: Cardiac pacing in retrospect. **Am J Surg** 1983 Jun;145(6):733–9

Silvay G, Griffin R: The history and development of cardiovascular monitoring during anesthesia. **Mt Sinai J Med (NY)** 1984 Sep;51(5):560–3

Skerritt PW: Anxiety and the heart--a historical review. **Psychol Med** 1983 Feb;13(1):17–25

Smith HL: [Development of] heart transplantation. In Reich WT, et al, ed: Encyclopedia of bioethics, v. 2. New York, Free Press, 1978. p. 654–60.

Snellen HA, Dunning AJ, Arntzenius AC, ed: History and perspectives of cardiology. Catheterization, angiography, surgery and concepts of circular control. The Hague, Leiden University Press, 1981. 204 p. Major historical contributions by L. Dexter, H. L. Abrams, H. Swan, A. C. Guyton, J. Sonolet.

Tota B: The importance of comparative cardiology. **Comp Biochem Physiol [A]** 1983;76(3):401–3

Van der Molen HR: Le développement de la phlébologie au cours des 30 dernières années (1948–1978). **Phlebologie** 1981 Jul–Sep;34(3):313–32

Weidmann S: Cardiac electrophysiology and its contribution to cardiology. **Mayo Clin Proc** 1982 Jul;57 Suppl:2-5
Weinberg SL: The patient with heart diseases and the cardiovascular physician and surgeon: 1958-1983. **J Am Coll Cardiol** 1983 Jan;1(1):6-12
Wooley CF: From the 'irritable heart' of DaCosta to mitral valve prolapse: the development of medical thought about a constitutional, neuroendocrine cardiovascular process. **J Cardiogr** 1984 Oct;14 Suppl 5:9-10
Woschick E: Die kontrollierte Hypotension--Vergangenheit und Gegenwart. Eine Ubersicht. **Zentrabl Neurochir** 1984;45(1):1-10
Yechezkel M, Deviri E, Levy MJ: [Prosthetic heart valves--historical review] (Heb). **Harefuah** 1984 May 15;106(10):475-6
Zimmerman AN, Hülsmann WC: The calcium paradox: historical remarks. **Eur Heart J** 1983 Dec;4 Suppl H:3-4

**Australia**

Mond HG, Sloman JG, Edwards RH: The first pacemaker. **PACE** 1982 Mar;5(2):278-82

**Brazil**

Leme C de A: História da eletrocardiografia no Brasil. **Rev Hosp Clin Fac Med Sao Paulo** 1981 Aug;36(4):179-83

**Bulgaria**

Petkova M: Naukometrichna kharakteristika na publikanoto nauchno tvorchestvo na akad. Aleksi Pukhlev. **Vutr Boles** 1982;21(3):92-100

**Canada**

Bourassa MG, Goulet C: L'évolution de la recherche à l'Institut de Cardiologie de Montréal. **Union Med Can** 1979 Oct;108(10):1128-38
Hopps JA: The development of the pacemaker. **PACE** 1981 Jan;4(1):106-8

**Czechoslovakia**

Křížek V: Samuel von Basch. Sto let od vynálezu nekrvavého měření krevního tlaku. **Cas Lek Cesk** 1980 Nov 28;119(48):1322-5
Reiniš Z: Padesát let Ceskoslovenské kardiologické společnosti. **Cas Lek Cesk** 1979 Nov 9;118(45):1404-7
Reiniš Z: Přehled 50 leté činnosti Cs. kardiologické spolčnosti. **Vnitr Lek** 1980 Apr;26(4):306-9
Reiniš Z, Gvozdják J, Widimský J, et al: The fiftieth anniversary of the Czechoslovak Society of Cardiology. **Cor Vasa** 1979;21(6):445-9

**Europe**

Snellen HA: Birth and growth of the European Society of Cardiology. **Eur Heart J** 1980 Feb;1(1):5-7
Snellen HA: Thomas Lewis (1881-1945) and cardiology in Europe. **Br Heart J** 1981 Aug;46(2):121-5

**France**

Borodulin VI: Klinicheskaia shkola Korvizara i ee rol' v razvitii ucheniia o bolezniakh serdtsa (k 100-letiiu so dnia smerti Zhana Batista Buĭo). **Kardiologiia** 1982 Jan;22(1):113-5
Bouvrain Y: La thérapeutique cardiologique au XIXe siècle. **Ann Cardiol Angeiol (Paris)** 1983 Mar-Apr;32(2):79-82
Di Matteo J: Les Archives des maladies du coeur et des vaisseaux. **Arch Mal Coeur** 1980 Jun;73(6):563-84
Espinosa RE, Vlietstra RE, Mann RJ: J. B. A. Chauveau, E. J. Marey, and their resolution of the apex beat controversy through intracardiac pressure recordings. **Mayo Clin Proc** 1983 Mar;58(3):197-202
Higier J: J. A. Kergaradec (1787-1877) - zapomniany odkrywca i pionier słuchawki położniczej. **Ginekol Pol** 1982;53(11):817-20
Huard P: Claude Bernard et le système vasculaire. In: Congrès National des Sociétés Savantes, 107e. Brest, 1982. Comptes Rendus, Paris, 1983. Section des Sciences, Fasc. IV. p. 281-6.
Lequime J: Marey et la cardiologie. **Acta Belg Med Phys** 1983 Oct-Dec;6(4):181-5
Matteo J di: Les 'Archives des Maladies du Coeur et des Vaisseaux'. Three-quarters of a century of cardiology. **Arch Mal Coeur** 1980;73:563-84
Matteo J di: L'oeuvre cardiologique de Laennec. **Bull Acad Natl Med (Paris)** 1981 Feb 17;Spec No:37-44
Roth N: Capturing the heart, 1880: Marey's cardiac tongs. **Med Instrum** 1980 Sep-Oct;14(5):285
Snellen HA: E. J. Marey and cardiology: physiologist and pioneer of technology, 1830-1904: selected writings in facsimile with comments and summaries, a brief history of life and work, and a bibliography. 264 p.

**Germany**

Biadała E: Sztuczne oddychanie metodą usta-usta i pobudzanie prądem elektrycznym akcji serca opisane przed 200 laty. **Wiad Lek** 1981 Sep 1;34(17):1471-7
Blömer H: 20 Jahre Herzschrittmacher-therapie. **ZFA (Stuttgart)** 1982 Jan 10;58(1):19-25
Bock HE: Franz Volhard: Erinnerungen. Stuttgart, New York, Schattauer, 1982. xi, 345 p.
Bock HE, ed, Hildebrand KH, ed, Sarre HJ, ed: Franz Volhard, Erinnerungen. Stuttgart and New York, Schattauer, 1982. 345 p.
Greeff K: Zur 48. Jahrestagung der Deutschen Gesellschaft für Herz- und Kreislaufforschung. Eröffnungsansprache. **Verh Dtsch Ges Herz Kreislaufforsch** 1982;48:XI-XX
Howard-Jones N: Cardiac catheterization, a historical note. **Bull Hist Med** 1973 Sep-Oct;47(5):524-6
Michel D: 100 Jahre 'Fortschritte der Medizin'--100 Jahre Kardiologie. **Fortschr Med** 1982 Dec 16;100(47-48):2191-3
Steckelberg JM, et al: Werner Forssmann (1904-1979) and his unusual success story. **Conn Med** 1981;45(2):110-2

**Great Britain**

Callahan JA, Key JD, Keys TE: Sir Thomas Lewis: the centennial of a medical human dynamo. **Mayo Clin Proc** 1981 Dec;56(12):749-52
Fye WB: Ernest Henry Starling, his law and its growing significance in the practice of medicine. **Circulation** 1983 Nov;68(5):1145-8
Hollman A: Thomas Lewis--the early years. **Br Heart J** 1981 Sep;46(3):233-44
James TN: Sir Thomas Lewis redivivus: from pebbles in a quiet pond to autonomic storms. **Br Heart J** 1984 Jul;52(1):1-23
Kligfield P: The early pathophysiolic understanding of angina pectoris (Edward Jenner, Caleb Hillier Parry, Allan Burns). **Am J Cardiol** 1982 Dec;50(6):1433-5
Kligfield P: The frustrated benevolence of 'Dr. Anonymous'. **Am J Cardiol** 1981 Jan;47(1):185-7
Laird JD: Thomas Young, M.D. (1773-1829). **Am Heart J** 1980 Jul;100(1):1-8
Lawrence C: Alfred Henry Garrod and the indirect measurement of the isometric period of the heart's contraction. **Med Hist** 1980 Jul;24(3):342-6
McMichael J: Sir James Mackenzie and atrial fibrillation--a new perspective. **J R Coll Gen Pract** 1981 Jul;31(228):402-6
Pinkerton JH: John Creery Ferguson. Friend of William Stokes and pioneer of auscultation of the fetal heart in the British Isles. **Br J Obstet Gynaecol** 1980 Apr;87(4):257-60
Rosol Z: Známý anglický kardiolog Thomas Lewis se narodil před 100 lety. **Vnitr Lek** 1982 Mar;28(3):297-9
Roth N: Hales's hydraulics: measuring blood pressure, 1706. **Med Instrum** 1981 Jan-Feb;15(1):66-7
Shapiro E: The first textbook of electrocardiography. Thomas Lewis: Clinical Electrocardiography. **J Am Coll Cardiol** 1983 Apr;1(4):1160-1
Waldron HA: Richard Pulteney (1730-1801): Linnean botanist and cardiologist. **Trans Stud Coll Physicians Phila** 1980 Mar;5(2 no 1):31-40

**Hungary**

Robicsek F, Littmann L: The first reported case of external heart massage (János Balassa). **Clin Cardiol** 1983 Nov;6(11):569, 571

**Ireland**

O'Brien E: Corrigan's disease. **J Ir Coll Physicians Surg** 1980 Jul;10(1):32-7
O'Brien ET: The man behind the eponym: Sir Dominic John Corrigan (1802-1880). **N Engl J Med** 1981 Feb 5;304(6):365-6

**Italy**

Masoni A: Continuita' e novita'. **G Ital Cardiol** 1979;9(1):1-3
Rovelli F: Il 'giornale italiano di cardiologia': 10 anni di storia della cardiologia in Italia. **G Ital Cardiol** 1981;11 Suppl 1:1-7

**Japan**

International Symposium on Cardiac Pacing, 5th, Tokyo, 1976: Tawara memorial note. Tokyo, Organizing Committee of the Symposium, 1976. 28 p.

**Mexico**

Aceves S: Contribuciones de México a la cardiología. Breve síntesis de la historia de la cardiología mexicana. In Academia Nacional de Medicina. Libro conmemorativo del primer centenario. México, Comité Editorial de la Comisión Organizadora del Congreso del Centenario, 1964. Tome 2. p. 535-46.
Torre JM: Publicaciones periódicas sobre cardiología en la actualidad. **Arch Inst Cardiol Mex** 1980 Nov-Dec;50(6):725-32
40 aniversario del Institute Nacional de Cardiología de México: **Arch Inst Cardiol Mex** 1984 Jul-Aug;54(4):411-26

# CARDIOLOGY AND CIRCULATORY SYSTEM

### Netherlands

Lamas GA, Koller LR, Antman EM, et al: Electrocardiogram by Einthoven 63 years earlier. **Am J Cardiol** 1984 Nov 1;54(8):1163-5

Macpherson AI: Blue babies before Fallot. **J R Coll Surg Edinb** 1984 Jul;29(4):199-204

Meijler FL: Vijftig jaar Nederlandse Vereniging voor Cardiologie of, Nederland, debakermat van de elektrocardiografie. **Ned Tijdschr Geneeskd** 1984 Mar 24;128(12):571-3

### Poland

Aleksandrow D, Aleksandrow W: Osiagni ecia i niepowodzenia intensywnej terapii kardiologicznej za okres 13 lat (doświadczenia własne). **Kardiol Pol** 1980;23(2):103-10

Rijlant P: Results and perspectives in electrocardiology. **Adv Cardiol** 1981;28:1-8

Sliwiński S: Edward Korczyński (1844-1905) autor pierwszego opisu klinicznego zawału serca w medycynie polskiej. **Wiad Lek** 1979 Nov 15;32(22):1647-50

### Puerto Rico

Bibliography of the scientific works of Dr. Ramón M. Suárez. **Bol Asoc Med PR** 1983 Nov;75(11):521-5

García Palmieri MR: Observaciones sobre la contribución del Dr. Ramón M. Suárez al reconocimiento de la cardiopatía reumática en el trópico. **Bol Asoc Med PR** 1983 Nov;75(11):503-5

Ramírez EA: Comentarios sobre la contribución del Dr. Ramón M. Suárez al estudio de la hipertensión arterial. **Bol Asoc Med PR** 1983 Nov;75(11):498-9

Torres-Gómez JM, García-Palmieri MR: Datos biográficos del Dr. Ramón M. Suárez Calderón. **Bol Asoc Med PR** 1983 Nov;75(11):490

Torres-Gómez JM: Suárez, Ramón M., 1895-19811700 to PresentPuerto Rico **Bol Asoc Med PR** 1983 Nov;75(11):501-2

### South Africa

Torrington M, Botha JL, Pilcher GJ, et al: Association between familial hypercholesterolaemia and church affiliation. Is this the result of sociocultural isolation of migrant farmers in 19th-century South Africa? **S Afr Med J** 1984 May 12;65(19):762-7

### Sweden

Elmqvist R: Review of early pacemaker development. **PACE** 1978 Oct;1(4):535-6

### Switzerland

Waszyński E: W dwusetną rocznicę urodzin Franciszka Izaaka Mayora (1779-1855), odkrywcy tonów serca płodu. **Ginekol Pol** 1980 Aug;51(8):765-6

### Tunisia

Calo AA: Notes on a bygone practice in a North African country. **J Med Soc NJ** 1981 Aug;78(9):606-10

### United States

Alexander RS: History of the Cardiovascular Section. **Physiologist** 1984 Apr;27(2):67-8

Battocletti JH, Halbach RE, Salles-Cunha SX, et al: The NMR blood flowmeter--theory and history. **Med Phys** 1981 Jul-Aug;8(4):435-43

Bernstein BJ, et al: The artificial heart program. **Cent Mag** 1981;14(3):22-41

Blake TM: Myocardial infarction and electrocardiography in historical perspective. **South Med J** 1983 Dec;76(12):1470-2

Braunwald E: Thirty-five years of progress in cardiovascular research. **Circulation** 1984 Nov;70(5 Pt 2):III8-25

Brooks CM: Walter Joseph Meek: August 15, 1878-February 15, 1963. **Biogr Mem Natl Acad Sci** 1983;54:251-68

Burchell H: Sir Thomas Lewis: his impact on American cardiology. **Br Heart J** 1981 Jul;46(1):1-4

Burchell HB: Important events in cardiology, 1940-1982 a retrospective view. **JAMA** 1983 Mar 4;249(9):1197-200

Chardack WM: Recollections--1958-1961. **PACE** 1981 Sep;4(5):592-6

Criley JM, Niemann JT, Rosborough JP: Cardiopulmonary resuscitation research 1960-1984: discoveries and advances. **Ann Emerg Med** 1984 Sep;13(9 Pt 2):756-8

Davis JO, Freeman RH: Historical perspectives on the renin-angiotensin-aldosterone system and angiotensin blockade. **Am J Cardiol** 1982 Apr 21;49(6):1385-9

Engle MA: Biographies of great American pediatricians--Helen Brooke Taussig: the mother of pediatric cardiology. **Pediatr Ann** 1982 Jul;11(7):629-31

Fye WB: Heparin: the contributions of William Henry Howell. **Circulation** 1984 Jun;69(6):1198-203

Fye WB: Sydney Ringer, calcium, and cardiac function. **Circulation** 1984 Apr;69(4):849-53

Josephson ME: The AJC in March 1959. **Am J Cardiol** 1984 Mar 1;53(6):803-4

Knoebel SB: On the occasion of the 25th year of the Journal of the American College of Cardiology. **J Am Coll Cardiol** 1983 Jan;1(1):1-2

Miller BJ: The development of heart lung machines. **Surg Gynecol Obstet** 1982 Mar;154(3):403-14

Murphy WP: Carl Walter: a pioneer in shaping the medical device industry. **Am J Surg** 1984 Nov;148(5):590-3

Page IH: A history of the Council for High Blood Pressure research. Past imperfect, present indicative, and future perfect. **Hypertension** 1984 Mar-Apr;6(2 pt 2):208-10

Rahimtoola SH: The twenty-fifth anniversary of valve replacement: a time for reflection. **Circulation** 1985 Jan;71(1):1-3

Ramsey EM: The story of spiral arteries. **J Reprod Med** 1981 Aug;26(8):393-9

Reddy CP, Surawicz B: Terminology of tachycardias: historical background and evolution. **PACE** 1983 Sep;6(5 Pt 2):1123-42

Roberts WC, Silver MA: Norman Jefferis Holter and ambulatory ECG monitoring. **Am J Cardiol** 1983 Oct 1;52(7):903-6

Roberts WC, Warnes CA: The AJC in December 1958. **Am J Cardiol** 1983 Dec 1;52(10):1355

Ross RS: A parlous state of storm and stress. The life and times of James B. Herrick. **Circulation** 1983 May;67(5):955-9

Scheinman MM: The AJC in September 1959. **Am J Cardiol** 1984 Sep 1;54(6):702-3

Scherlag BJ: The development of the His bundle recording technique. **PACE** 1979 Mar;2(2):230-3

Strauss MJ: The political history of the artificial heart. **N Engl J Med** 1984 Feb 2;310(5):332-6

Taussig HB: Little choice and a stimulating environment. **J Am Med Wom Assoc** 1981 Feb;36(2):43-4

Thomas HD: Fifty years of cardiology in Alabama. **J Med Assoc State Ala** 1981 Jul;51(1):19-20

A tribute: Michael E. DeBakey, M.D. **Compr Ther** 1984 Feb;10(2):3-5

Wilber JA: The founding of Georgia and the discovery of blood pressure. **J Med Assoc Ga** 1981 May;70(5):333

Wooley CF: Jacob Mendez DaCosta: medical teacher, clinician, and clinical investigator. **Am J Cardiol** 1982 Nov;50(5):1145-8

### USSR

Al'bitskiĭ VIu: K 150-letiiu so dnia rozhdeniia Nikolaia Andreevicha Vinogradova - uchenika S. P. Botkina. **Klin Med (Mosk)** 1982 Sep;60(9):121-3

Andreeva VN, Kosmachevskaia EA: Ocherk razvitiia fiziologii krovoobrashcheniia v laboratoriiakh Mediko-khirurgicheskoĭ (Voenno-meditsinskoĭ) akademii v XIX veke (K istorii vzaimosviazi teorii i praktiki v issledovatel'skoĭ rabote). **Fiziol Zh SSSR** 1981 Jun;67(6):934-50

Borodulin VI: A. L. Miasnikov i ego rol' v formirovanii kardiologii v SSSR. **Kardiologiia** 1979;19(12):99-101

Borodulin VI: Stanovlenie kardiologii v SSSR. **Kardiologiia** 1982 Dec;22(12):96-9

Borodulin VI, Martynov IV: Uchenie M. V. Ianovskogo o 'perifericheskom serdtse' i razvitie predstavleniĭ o klinicheskom znachenii sosudistoi periferii. **Klin Med (Mosk)** 1982 May;60(5):9-12

Carlisle R: Arterial sounds by phases: an object lesson in terminological confusion? **J R Soc Med** 1981 Mar;74(3):212-8

Ianushkevichus ZI: Razvitie ideĭ i rabot S. P. Botkina i ego shkoly v kardiologii i klinicheskoĭ farmakologii. **Vestn Akad Med Nauk SSSR** 1983;(3):14-7

Karpov RS: Vklad tomskikh uchenykh v razvitie otechestvennoĭ kardiologii. **Vestn Akad Med Nauk SSSR** 1981;(9):63-6

Kavtaradze VG: O razvitii i sostoianii kardiologicheskoĭ pomoshchi v Gruzinskoĭ SSR. **Kardiologiia** 1982 Dec;22(12):16-8

Korotkoff NS: Experiments for determining the efficiency of arterial collaterals. Preface, biographical notes and editing of translation from Russian by H. N. Segall. Montreal, H. N. Segall, 1980. 265 p. (M. D. Thesis, Imperial Military Medical Academy, 1910).

Kuz'min MK: V. F. Zelenin i ego rol' v razvitii klinicheskoĭ élektrokardiografii i funktsional'noĭ diagnostike. **Klin Med (Mosk)** 1981 Aug;59(8):115-8

Martynov IV, Borodulin VI: Rol' V.F. Zelenina v otechestvennoĭ kardiologii. **Klin Med (Mosk)** 1981 Aug;59(8):118-20

Meerson FZ: Razvitie nekotorykh ideĭ V. V. Parina v fiziologii i patofiziologii krovoobrashcheniia. **Usp Fiziol Nauk** 1983 Apr-Jun;14(2):7-27

Oganov RG: Istoriia vsemirnykh kongressov kardiologov i uchastie v nikh sovetskikh uchenykh. **Kardiologiia** 1982 May;22(5):7-9

Orlova AN: Vklad A. I. Nesterova v uchenie o mikrotsirkuliatsii (k 85-letiiu so dnia rozhdeniia A. I. Nesterova). **Vopr Revm** 1981 Jan-Mar;(1):58-61

Orlova NV, Pariĭskaia TV, Vorob'ev AS: 20 Let raboty po usovershenstvovaniiu znaniĭ pediatrov v oblasti kardiorevmatologii.

**Pediatriia** 1982 Jun;(6):59-61
Ostapiuk FE: Prepodavanie kardiologii v Tsentral'nom Institute Usovershenstvovaniia Vracheĭ (k 50-letiiu so dnia osnovaniia Instituta). **Kardiologiia** 1981;21(1):117-8
Segall H: N. C. Korotkoff and how he, a surgeon, discovered the sounds for measuring arterial pressure. In: Cóngrès international d'histoire de la médecine, XXVe, Québec, 1976. Actes. Québec, 1977. p. 1253-8.
Shik LL: Akademik V. V. Parin kak fiziolog. **Vestn Akad Med Nauk SSSR** 1984;(4):12-5
Shul'tsev GP: Razvitie kardiologii v trudakh uchenykh Tsentral'nogo instituta usovershenstvovaniia vracheĭ (k 50-letiiu Tsentral'nogo instituta usovershentsvovaniia vracheĭ. **Sov Med** 1980;(11):120-1
Smirnov-Kamenskiĭ EA: K 60-letiiu kardiologicheskoĭ kliniki im. V.I. Lenina v Kislovodske. **Vopr Kurortol Fizioter Lech Fiz Kult** 1983 Jan-Feb;(1):66-8
Tarasonov VM: Vklad A.I. Tal'iantseva v éksperimental'noe issledovanie patologii serdechno-sosudistoĭ sistemy. **Patol Fiziol Eksp Ter** 1980 Mar-Apr;(2):92-3
Tareev EM: P. E. Lukomskiĭ i stanovlenie sovetskoĭ kardiologii. **Kardiologiia** 1982 Feb;22(2):119-25

**Yugoslavia**

Vukadinović S: Razvoj i zadaci pedijatrijske kardiologije. **Lijec Vjesn** 1979 Dec;101(12):733-6

## CHEMISTRY AND BIOCHEMISTRY

See also **Drugs and Chemicals; Pharmacy**

Ardry R: Alchimie, une odeur de soufre. **Rev Hist Pharm (Paris)** 1984 Mar;31(260):13-7
Astrup P: Blutgase und medizinische Säure-Basen-Chemie einst und jetzt. I. Blutgase. **Z Med Lab Diagn** 1984;25(6):299-306
Bardeau F: Les clefs secrètes de la chimie des anciens. Paris, Laffont, 1975. 204 p.
Barraco RA: Paleobiochemistry. In A. Cockburn, E. Cockburn, ed: Mummies, disease, and ancient cultures. Cambridge, Cambridge University Press, 1980. p. 312-26.
Baumann HU: Ueber Mehrfachentdeckungen. Eine Darstellung des allgemeinen Problems mit Beispielen aus drei Teilgebieten der theoretischen Medizin. Diss. Münster, 1972. 133 p.
Bearman D, Edsall JT, ed: Archival sources for the history of biochemistry and molecular biology. A reference guide and report. Boston, American Academy of Arts and Sciences, Philadelphia, American Philosophical Society, 1980. 338 p. plus microfiche. Contributions by M. Miller, M. Konopka
Belloni L: Zur Entdeckung des Eisens im Organismus. In Ganzinger K, Skopec M, Wyklicky H, ed: Festschrift für Erna Lesky zum 70. Geburtstag. Wien, Brüder Hollinek, 1981. p. 25-30.
Berger RL, Clem TR, Harden VA, et al: Historical development and newer means of temperature measurement in biochemistry. **Methods Biochem Anal** 1984;30:269-331
Bernus A von: Alchymie und Heilkunst. Nürnberg, Carl, 1981. 243 p.
Beswick FW: Chemical agents used in riot control and warfare. **Hum Toxicol** 1983 Apr;2(2):247-56
Brandenburg D: Medizin und Magie. Heilkunde und Geheimlehre des islamischen Zeitalters. Berlin, Hessling, 1975. 159 p. (Medizingeschichtliche Miniaturen, Band 1).
Brinkman AA: Chemie in de Kunst. Amsterdam, Rodopi, 1975. 69 p.
Brinkman AA: De alchemist in de prentkunst. Amsterdam, Rodopi, 1982. 69 p. Reprint of several articles. (Nieuwe Nederlandse Bijdragen tot de Geschiedenis der Geneeskunde en der Natururwetenschappen, no. 5).
Buettner J: Why the history of our discipline should be discussed in this journal. **J Clin Chem Clin Biochem** 1981;19:309-10
Bykov GV, Trifonov DN: Issledovaniia po istorii khimii. **Vopr Istor Estestvozn Tekh** 1981;2:33-8
Dallett JB: Woldemar Nürnbergers Paracelsus-Roman. **Salzburger Beitr Paracelsusforsch** 1984;23:50-60
Fenner ET: Rasayana Siddhi: medicine and alchemy in the Buddhist tantras. Ph.D. diss. University of Wisconsin. Madison, 1979. 272 leaves.
Franz ML von: Alchemy: an introduction to the symbolism and the psychology. Toronto, Inner City Books, 1980. 280 p. (Studies in Jungian Psychology, 5).
Gettings F: Dictionary of occult, hermetic and alchemical sigils. London, Routledge & Kegan Paul, 1981. 410 p.
Glass E: Chemistry and physiology in their historical and philosophical relations. Delft, Delft University Press, 1979. xiii, 199 p.
Grossinger R, ed: Alchemy; pre-Egyptian legacy, millennial promise. Richmond, California, North Atlantic Books, 1979. 253 p.
Halleux R: Les textes alchimiques. Turnhout, Brepols, 1979. 153 p. (Typologie des sources du Moyen Age occidental, fasc. 32).
Halleux R: Marcellin Berthelot, historien de l'alchimie. In: Congrès National des Sociétés Savantes, 104e, Bordeaux, 1979. Comptes Rendus. Paris, 1979. Section des Sciences, Fasc. IV. p. 169-80.
Jüttner G: Alchemie und Sympathielehre in der Therapie der frühen Neuzeit. In: Der Uebergang zur Neuzeit und die Wirkung von Traditionen. VortrAB/age, gehalten auf der Tagung der Joachim-Jungius-Gesellschaft der Wissenschaften, Hamburg, am 13. und 14. Oktober 1977. Göttingen, Vandenhoeck & Ruprecht, 1978. p. 130-140.
Jüttner G: Der Dialog in Pharmazie, Chemie und Botanik. Zum Anteil einer literarischen Gattung in der Darstellung, Vermittlung und im Unterricht der Naturwissenschaften. **Ber Wissenschaftsgesch** 1980;3(1-2):23-34
Mahdihassan S: Alchemy and its fundamental terms in Greek, Arabic, Sanskrit and Chinese. **Indian J Hist Sci** 1981;16(1):64-76
Mahdihassan S: Alembic and ambix as Sino-Arabic terms with an explanation of Mary's bath. **Stud Hist Med** 1980 Mar;4(1):39-43
Manuscripta alchemica der Sammlung Mellon: Bemerkungen zum Katalog: **Sudhoffs Arch** 1981;65(1):79-96
Neuhausen T: Das Cholesterin. Vorstellungen über seine Rolle im Körper. Köln, Universität zu Köln, 1977. 187 p. (Kölner medizinhistorische Beiträge, 6).
Ochoa S: The thrill of discovery. **Comp Biochem Physiol** 1980;67B:359-65
Pritchard A: Alchemy: a bibliography of English-language writings. London, Routledge & Kegan Paul jointly with The Library Association, 1980. 439 p.
Ron M: Catalog of the Sidney M. Edelstein Collection of the history of chemistry, dyeing and technology. Jerusalem, The Jewish National and University Library, 1981. 182 p.
Schadewaldt H: Zur Geschichte des Fermentbegriffes. In: Festschrift der Kali-Chemie Aktiengesellschaft Hannover. Hannover, Kali-Chemie Aktiengesellschaft, n.d. 40 p.
Sheptunova ZI: Dzh R. Partington - vydaiushchiisia istorik khimii. **Vopr Istor Estestvozn Tekh** 1981;3:107-10
Snelders HA: Hoofdstukken uit de geschiedenis van de scheikunde. 2e vermmerderde druk. Amsterdam, Rodopi, 1979. 175 p.
Teich M: A history of biochemistry. **Hist Sci** 1980;18(1):46-67
Telle J: Manuscripta alchemica der Sammlung Mellon. Bemerkungen zum Katalog. **Suddtsch Opt Ztg** 1981;65(1):79-96
Todericiu D: Prolongements méconnus de la philosophie chimique de Jean-Baptiste Van Helmont (1578-1644) en Europe centrale et orientale. L'éloge à Van Helmont du savant roumain Démètre Cantémir (1701). **Bull Cl Sci Acad R Belg** 1979;65:228-38
Ullman AH: Analytical chemists on postage stamps. **Anal Chem** 1982 Jun;54(7):780A-785A
Witten LC, Pachella R, ed: Alchemy and the occult: a catalogue of books and manuscripts from the collection of Paul and Mary Mellon given to Yale University Library. Vols. 3 and 4: Manuscripts 1225-1922. With an introduction by P. Kibre and additional notes by W. McGuire. New Haven, Yale University Library, 1977. 853 p.
Zimmermann RE: The structure of mythos: on the cultural stability of alchemy. **Ambix** 1984 Nov;31(3):125-37

**China**

Johnson OS: A study of Chinese alchemy. New York, Arno, 1974. xi, 156 p.

**France**

Secret F: Réforme et alchimie. **Bull Soc Hist Protestantisme Fr** 1978;124:173-86

**Germany**

Kaiser W, Völker A: Gedenktage 1980 aus der Geschichte der Medizinischen Fakultät Wittenberg (I): Die Chemie im medizinischen Ausbildungsprogramm des 17. und 18. Jahrhunderts. **Z Gesamte Inn Med** 1981 Feb 15;36(4):114-22

**India**

Mahdihassan S: Indian alchemy or Rasayana in the light of asceticism [and] geriatrics. New Delhi, Vikas, 1979. x, 139 p.
Sikdar JC: Jaina alchemy. **Indian J Hist Sci** 1980 May;15(1):6-17
Wujastyk D: An alchemical ghost: the Rasaratnâkara by Nâgârjuna. **Ambix** 1984 Jul;31(2):70-83

**Before 500 A.D.**

**China**

Benfey OT: Spinach is an alchemical antidote to heavy metal poisoning. **Kagakushi Kenkyu** 1981;15:8-12
Mahdihassan S: Chinese alchemy in the light of its fundamental terms. **Am J Chin Med** 1980 Winter;8(4):307-12

**Egypt**

Patai R: Maria the Jewess--founding mother of alchemy. **Ambix** 1982 Nov;29(3):177-92

# CHEMISTRY AND BIOCHEMISTRY

**Greece**

Halleux R: Les alchimistes grecs. Tome I. Papyrus de Leyde, Payrus de Stockholm, Fragments de Recettes. Paris. Les Belles Lettres, 1981. xv, 235 p.
Plass P: A Greek alchemical formula. **Ambix** 1982 Jul;29(2):69–73

**India**

Mahdihassan S: The tradition of alchemy in India. **Am J Chin Med** 1981 Spring;9(1):23–33

**500 A.D.–1450**

Escudero Mendo A, Sagrera JE de: El Rosario de los filósofos: una copia en castellano del siglo XIII (I). **Bol Soc Esp Hist Farm** 1983;34(136):151–66
Hutin S: La vie quotidienne des alchimistes au moyen âge. Paris, Hachette, 1977. 254 p.
Kibre P: Albertus Magnus on alchemy. In Weisheipl JA, ed: Albertus Magnus and the sciences. Toronto, Pontifical Institute of Mediaeval Studies 1980. p. 187–202.
Pereira M: Alchimia medievale: alcuni studi recenti. **Ann Ist Mus Stor Sci Fir** 1984;9(2):89–98
Schipperges H: Handschriftliche Funde zu den 'verdrängten Wissenschaften' in der Frühen Neuzeit. **Ber Wissenschaftsgesch** 1981;4(1/2):31–40

**Arabic**

Debus AG: The Arabic tradition in the medical chemistry of the scientific revolution. In: International Symposium for the History of Arabic Science, 1st, University of Aleppo, 1976. Proceedings. Aleppo, Syria, 1976. Papers in European Languages, Vol. II. p. 275–90.
Folch Jou G: Medicamentos empleados por los arabes y su posible influencia en la introduccion de la quimica en la Farmacia. **Asclepio** 1978–79;30–31:177–86
Hamarneh SK: Arabic-Islamic alchemy--three intertwined stages. **Ambix** 1982 Jul;29(2):74–87
Hamarneh SK: Jabir, Jildki and Ibn-Sallum, and Arabic-Islamic Alchemy. **Mesopotamia Q** 1980;8(29,30):110–22, 225–41

**Spain**

Esteva de Sagrera J: Alquimia seudoluliana y medicina. In Congrés International d'Història de la Medicina Catalana, 2nd, Barcelona, 1975. Llibre d'Actes. Barcelona, Socitra, 1977. p. 301–3.
Patai R: An unknown Hebrew medicl alchemist: a medieval treatise on the quinta essentia. **Med Hist** 1984 Jul;28(3):308–23

**1450–1700**

Ardry R: Alchimie, une odeur de soufre. **Rev Hist Pharm (Paris)** 1984 Jun;31(261):121–30
Bosch K: Zur Vorgeschichte chemiatrischer Pharmakopöepräparate im 16./17. Jahrhundert. Braunschweig, 1980. 223 p. (Veröffentlichungen aus dem Pharmaziegeschichtlichen Seminar der Technischen Universität Braunschweig, 21).
Christie JR, Golinski JV: The spreading of the word: new directions in the historiography of chemistry 1600–1800. **Hist Sci** 1982 Dec;50(4):235–66
Dallett JB: Paracelsus in Moronia. Bischof Joseph Halls satirische Darstellung von 'Bustius Hohenheimius' und dessen Collegium. Wien, 1976. 20 p. (Salzburger Beiträge zur Paracelsusforschung, 14).
Debus AG: The chemical philosophy. Paracelsian science and medicine in the sixteenth and seventeenth centuries. 2 vols. New York, Science History Publications, 1977. xv, 606 p.
Dubois CG: Isomorphisme de deux constructions imaginaires: le grand oeuvre alchmique et la grand oeuvre de Dieu. **Aust J Fr Stud** 1980;17(1):73–85
Goldammer K: Neues zur Frage der Paracelsischen Spuria. **Sudhoffs Arch** 1984;68(2):235–9
Kapronczay K: Einige alchimistische Werke aus der Raritätensammlung der Semmelweis-Bibliothek für Geschichte der Medizin. In Hein WH, ed: Pharmaziehistorischer Kongress, Budapest, 1981. Stuttgart, Wissenschaftliche Verlagsgesellschaft, 1983. p. 57–72.
Linden SJ: Alchemy and eschatology in seventeenth-century poetry. **Ambix** 1984 Nov;31(3):102–24
Nowotny O: De auro potabili. Wien, 1967. (Salzburger Beiträge zur Paracelsusforschung, 7). p. 13–23.
Pagel W: The Paracelsian Elias Artista and the alchemical tradition. **Medizinhist J** 1981;16(1–2):6–19
Secret F: Palingenesis, alchemy and metempsychosis in Renaissance medicine. **Ambix** 1979 Jul;26(2):81–92
Secret F: Un document oublié sur François Hotman et l'alchimie. **Bibl Hum Renaissance** 1980 May;42(2):435–46
Telle J: Paracelsistische Sinnbildkunst. Bemerkungen zu einer Pseudo-'Tabula smaragdina' des 16. Jahrhunderts. In Seidler E, Schott H, ed: Bausteine zur Medizingeschichte. Stuttgart, Steiner, 1984. p. 129–39.
Vandewiele LJ: Van chemiatrie tot iatrochemie--van Paracelsus (1493–1541) tot Van Helmont (1579?–1644). **Farm Tijdschr Belg** 1980;57:25–30

**Belgium**

Halleux R: Gnose et expérience dans la philosophie chimique de Jean-Baptiste Van Helmont. **Bull Cl Sci Acad R Belg** 1979;65:217–27
Pagel W: Joan Baptista Van Helmont: reformer of science and medicine. Cambridge, Cambridge University Press, x, 1982. 219 p. (Cambridge monographs on the history of medicine).

**Denmark**

Skov H, Bastholm E, ed: Petrus Severinus og hans Idea medicinae philosophicae. En dansk paracelsist. Copenhagen, Odense Universitetsforlag, 1979. 299 p. (Acta Historica Scientiarum et Medicinalium, 32).

**Europe**

Secret F: Situation de la littérature alchimique en Europe, a la fin du XVIe et au début du XVIIe siècle. **Dix-Sept Siecle** 1978;30(3):135–44

**France**

Aurach G: Le jardin de richesses. Texte calligraphié et préface par B. Biebel. Neuilly-sur-Seine, Arma Artis, 1978. xix, 83 p.
Husson B, ed: Trois textes alchimiques inédits du XVIIe siècle. L'or potable des anciens; Lettres philosophiques; Le testament d'or. Paris, Librairie de Médicis, 1979. 101 p.

**Germany**

Haage BD: Das alchemistische Bildgedicht vom 'Nackten Weib' in seiner bisher ältesten Uberlieferung. **Centaurus** 1982–3;26(2–3):204–14
Haage B, ed: Das 'Kunstbüchlein' des Alchemisten Caspar Hartung vom Hoff. Göppingen, Kümmerle, 1975. 141 p.
Klutz M: Die Rezepte in Oswald Crolls Basilica Chymica (1609) und ihre Beziehungen zu Paracelsus. Braunschweig, 1974. 124 p. (Veröffentlichungen aus dem Pharmaziegeschichtlichen Seminar der Technischen Universität Braunschweig, 14).
Möhsen JK: Beiträge zur Geschichte der Wissenschaften in der Marke Brandenburg; Leben Leonhard Thurneissers zum Thurn. München, Fritsch, 1976. 226 p.
Morys P: Medizin und Pharmazie in der Kosmologie Leonhard Thurneissers zum Thurn (1531–1596). Husum, Matthiesen, 1982. 179 p. (Abhandlungen zur Geschichte der Medizin und der Naturwissenschaften, 43).
Zaunick R: Der sächsische Paracelsist Georg Forberger. Wiesbaden, Steiner, 1977. xii, 110 p. (Kosmosophie, IV).

**Great Britain**

Baker DC, Murphy JL: Myles Blomefylde, Elizabethan physician, alchemist and book collector: a sketch of a life. **Bodleian Libr Rec** 1982 Nov;11(1):35–46
Debus AG: Thomas Sherley's philosophical essay (1672): Helmontian mechanism as the basis of a new philosophy. **Ambix** 1980 Jul;27(2):124–35
Gömöri G: Bejegyzések Bánfihunyadi János oxfordi bibliájában és adalekok Angliai múködéséhez. **Magyar Könyvsz** 1978;94(1):93–9
Newman W: Thomas Vaughan as an interpreter of Agrippa von Nettesheim. **Ambix** 1982 Nov;29(3):125–40
Nicholl C: The chemical theatre. London, Boston, Routledge and Kegan Paul, 1980. ix, 292 p.
Schuler RM: Some spiritual alchemies of seventeenth-century England. **J Hist Ideas** 1980;41(2):293–318
Westfall RS: Alchemy in Newton's library. **Ambix** 1984 Nov;31(3):97–101

**Hungary**

Barlay OS: Boldizsár Batthyány und sein Humanisten-Kreis. Die ersten Jahrzehnten der Güssinger Bibliothek. **Magy Konyvsz** 1979;95(3):231–51

**Netherlands**

Beukers H: Het laboratorium van Sylvius. **Tijdschr Geschied Geneeskd** 1980;3(1):28–36
Beukers H: Mechanistische principes bij Franciscus dele Boë, Sylvius. **Tijdschr Geschied Geneeskd** 1982;5(1):6–15
Dixon LS: Alchemical imagery in Bosch's Garden of Delights. Ann Arbor, UMI Research Press, 1981. xxii, 225 p. (Studies in the Fine Arts: Iconography, no. 2).
Hoppe B: Darstellung der Alchemie in Gemälden von Jan Brueghel d.

A. (1568-1625). **Beitr Gesch Pharm** 1983;31(18/19):144-9
Skulimowski MM: Jan Baptysta van Helmont (1577-1644) odkrywca dwutlenku węgla (CO2). **Wiad Lek** 1980 Mar 15;33(6):495-7

### Spain

Gago R, Olagüe G, Carrillo JL: Aportación al estudio del movimiento novator en España: el Laboratorio Químico del Palacio Real (1694) y la obra del boticario aragonés Juan del Bayle (fl. 1698). **Bol Soc Esp Hist Farm** 1981 Jun;32(126):95-107

### Switzerland

Braun L: Paracelse: nature et philosophie. Strasbourg, Association des Publications près les Universités de Strasbourg, 1981. 176 p.
Helmrich HE: Spagyrik. Alter Wein in neuen Schläuchen. Heidelberg, Haug, 1977. 253 p.
Koelbing HM: Paracelsus. **Praxis** 1982 Dec 21;71(51):1973-6
Pagel W: Paracelsus. An introduction to philosophical medicine in the era of the Renaissance, 2nd, revised edition. Basel, Karger, 1982. xii, 399 p.
Schipperges H: Paracelsus. Das Abenteuer einer sokratischen Existenz. Freiburg im Breisgau, Aurum Verlag, 1983. 108 p. (Reihe: Sokratische Weisheit, Bd. 3).

### 1700 to Present

Abir-Am P: From biochemistry to molecular biology: DNA and the acculturated journey of the critic of science Erwin Chargaff. **Hist Philos Life Sci** 1980;2(1):3-60
Ahlquist RP: Historical perspective. Classification of adrenoreceptors. **J Auton Pharmacol** 1980 Nov;1(1):101-6
American Academy of Arts and Sciences, American Philosophical Society: Survey of sources for the history of biochemistry and molecular biology. **Surv Sources Newsl** 1975-1981;1(1-10):various pagings
Anderson WC: Translating the language of chemistry: Priestley and Lavoisier. **Eighteenth Cent Theory Interpret** 1981;22(1):21-31
Baguenier-Desormeaux L: Henry Drysdale Dakin à Compiègne, en 1915. **Rev Hist Pharm (Paris)** 1981 Jun;28(249):79-88
Banga I: Az izomkutatás eredményei. **Orv Hetil** 1983 Oct 2;124(40):2440-3
Barciszewski J: Transferowe kwasy rybonukleinowe--dwadzieścia pieć lat badań. **Postepy Biochem** 1983;29(3-4):255-60
Bartley RL, Kucewicz WP: 'Yellow rain' and the future of arms agreements. **Foreign Aff** 1983;61(4):805-26
Bay A: Chemical warfare: perspectives and potentials. **Strategy Tactics** 1980;81:23-33
Bennett HS: A perception of histochemistry. **J Histochem Cytochem** 1983 Jan;31(1A Suppl):127-30
Bindra JS, Lednicer D, ed: Chronicles of drug discovery. Volume 1. New York, John Wiley & Sons, 1982. xiii, 283 p.
Blanco MA, Melnikov VP: On the history of application of isotopes in biochemical research. **Istor Biol Issled** 1983;9:85-98
Blaschko H: Hans Krebs: nineteen nineteen and after. **FEBS Lett** 1980 Aug 25;117 Suppl:K11-15
Braunstein AY: The main stages of enzymatic transfer of amino groups studies. **Istor Biol Issled** 1983;9:16-50
Büttner J: Evolution of clinical enzymology. **J Clin Chem Clin Biochem** 1981 Aug;19(8):529-38
Büttner J: From chemistry of life to chemistry of disease: the rise of clinical biochemistry. **Clin Biochem** 1980 Oct;13(5):232-5
Büttner J: Interrelationships between clinical medicine and clinical chemistry, illustrated by the example of the German-speaking countries in the late 19th century. **J Clin Chem Clin Biochem** 1982 Jun;20(6):465-71
Büttner J, ed: History of clinical chemistry. Berlin, New York, Walter de Gruyter, 1983. 91 p. Various reprints from the Journal of Clinical Chemistry and Clinical Biochemistry. Contributions by N. Mani, J.S. Fruton, E. Hickel, H.H. Simmer, W.T. Caraway.
Caraway WT: Major developments in clinical chemical instrumentation. **J Clin Chem Clin Biochem** 1981 Jul;19(7):491-6
Cartwright FF: Pneumatic medicine. **Pharm Hist (London)** 1970 Jun;1(5):4-6
Cheshko VT: The development of ideas on nature of heterosis in biochemical genetics (1940-1970). **Istor Biol Issled** 1983;9:186-90
Cowen DL: A note on pharmaceutical literature and the introduction of the new chemical nomenclature. **Beitr Gesch Pharm** 1981;11:84-5
Crick F: Crick looks back on DNA. **Science** 1979 Nov 9;206(4419):667
Crosland M: Chemistry and the chemical revolution. In G. S. Rousseau, R. Porter, ed: The ferment of knowledge. Studies in the historiography of eighteenth-century science. Cambridge, Cambridge University Press, 1980. p. 389-416.
Davenport HW: The early days of research on carbonic anhydrase. **Ann NY Acad Sci** 1984;429:4-9
Dodson G, Chothia C: Fifty years of pepsin crystals [news] **Nature** 1984 May 24-30;309(5966):309
Edsall JT: Some perspectives on carbonic anhydrase since 1960. **Ann NY Acad Sci** 1984;429:18-25
Edsall JT: The forgotten paper on buffer values: Koppel and Spiro, 1914. **Surv Sources Newsl** 1981;10:11
Erspamer V: Half a century of comparative research on biogenic amines and active peptides in amphibian skin and molluscan tissues. **Comp Biochem Physiol [C]** 1984;79(1):1-7
Euler US von: Chemical neurotransmission--yesterday and today. **Ciba Found Symp** 1982;(91):3-12
Fantini B: Chemical and biological classification of proteins. **Hist Philos Life Sci** 1983;5(1):3-32
Florkin M: A history of biochemistry. Part IV. Early studies of biosynthesis. Amsterdam, Elsevier, 1977. xx, 362 p. (Comprehensive biochemistry, Vol. 32).
Fruton JS: A bio-bibliography for the history of the biochemical sciences since 1800. Philadelphia, American Philosophical Society, 1982. xiii, 885 p.
Fruton JS: Biochemistry and clinical chemistry--a retrospect. **J Clin Chem Clin Biochem** 1982 Apr;20(4):243-52
Fuwa K: Metallothionein: historical aspects of trace spectrochemical. **Dev Toxicol Environ Sci** 1982;9:1-10
Ganzinger K: Zur Geschichte der chemischen Nomenklatur in den amtlichen Arzneibüchern. **Beitr Gesch Pharm** 1980;31(5):33-7
Gilbert SF, Greenberg JP: Intellectual traditions in the life sciences. II. Stereocomplementarity. **Perspect Biol Med** 1984 Autumn;28(1):18-34
Glas E: Chemistry and physiology in their historical and philosophical relations. Delft, Delft University Press, 1979. 199 p.
Godtfredsen E: Forbraendigens forudsaetninger i medicinsk-historisk lys. **Dan Medicinhist Arbog** 1981;:142-56
Gorevic PD, Cleveland AB, Franklin EC: The biologic significance of amyloid. **Ann NY Acad Sci** 1982;389:380-94
Götz W: J. B. Trommsdorffs 'Chemische Receptirkunst'. Bisher unbekannte Uebersetzungen und Ausgaben. **Beitr Gesch Pharm** 1982;31(14):107-10
Hickel E: The emergence of clinical chemistry in the 19th century: presuppositions and consequences. **J Clin Chem Clin Biochem** 1982 Jul;20(7):521-30
Holmes FL: The history of biochemistry: a review of the literature of the field. **Spec Collect** 1982;1(2):7-15
Hoppe B: Chemophysiologie zwischen vitalistischer und mechanistischer Biologie im 19. Jahrhundert. **Medizinhist J** 1983;18(3):163-83
Ihde AJ: Kurt Guenter Stern. In Dictionary of American Biography, Suppl. 6, 1956-1960. p. 595-6, 1980.
Isbell HS: Development of concepts of ring conformation and neighboring group effects prior to 1940. In Harmon RE, ed: Asymmetry of carbohydrates. New York, Dekker, 1979. p 1-14.
Janko J: From physiological chemistry to biochemistry. **Acta Hist Rerum Nat Tech** 1977;9:223-79
Joyce RM: Frontiers in Chemistry. **Science** 1980 Jul 4;209(4452):89-95
Kleber BE, Birdsell D: The unused weapon. **Milit Rev** 1965;45(1):54-62
Kohler RE: From medical chemistry to biochemistry: the making of a biomedical discipline. Cambridge, New York, Cambridge University Press, 1982. ix, 399 p.
Kornberg A: Biochemistry evolving. **Can J Biochem** 1980 Feb;58(2):93-6
Lipmann F: Hans Krebs and his metabolic cycles. **Naturwiss Rundsch** 1982;35:228-30
Löw R: Pflanzenchemie zwischen Lavoisier und Liebig. Straubing und München, Donau Verlag, 1979. 404, 75 p. (Münchener Hochschulschriften, Reihe: Naturwissenschaften, 1).
Mani N: Physiologische und medizinische Chemie zwischen 1800 und 1850. **Pharm Acta Helv** 1979;54(9-10):273-80
Mani N: The historical background of clinical chemistry. **J Clin Chem Clin Biochem** 1981 Jun;19(6):311-22
Maren TH: Carbonic anhydrase: the middle years, 1945-1960, and introduction to pharmacology of sulfonamides. **Ann NY Acad Sci** 1984;429:10-7
Mazumdar PM: Karl Landsteiner and the problem of species 1838-1968. Ph.D. Diss., Johns Hopkins University. Baltimore, 1976. 725 leaves.
Meinel C: Nationalismus und Internationalismus in der Chemie des 19. Jahrhunderts. In Dilg P, et al., ed: Perspektiven der Pharmaziegeschichte. Graz, Austria, Akademische Druck- u. Verlagsanstalt, 1983. p. 225-42.
Meinel C: Theory or practice? The eighteenth-century debate on the scientific status of chemistry. **Ambix** 1983 Nov;30(3):121-32
Meselson M: Gas warfare and the Geneva protocol of 1945. **Bull At Sci** 1972;28(2):33-7
Mommaerts WF: Gondolatok az izomkutatás történetéről (A. Katschalsky-Katzir professzor emlékezetére). **Orv Hetil** 1983 Oct 2;124(40):2436-40
Mothes K: Zur Geschichte unserer Kenntnisse über die Alkaloide. **Pharmazie** 1981 Mar;36(3):199-209
Muzrukova HB: Chemistry and biology in the history of cellular's study. **Istor Biol Issled** 1983;9:51-65
Ostrowski WS: Zarys rozwoju badań nad metaloporfirynami. **Postepy Biochem** 1983;29(3-4):247-53
Puchtler H, Meloan SN: On Schiff's bases and aldehyde-fuchsin: a review from H. Schiff to R. D. Lillie. **Histochemistry** 1981;72(3):321-32
Racker E: Resolution and reconstitution of biological pathways from 1919 to 1984. **Fed Proc** 1983 Sep;42(12):2899-909
Rinsler MG: Spectroscopy, colorimetry, and biological chemistry in the nineteenth century. **J Clin Pathol** 1981 Mar;34(3):287-91
Rosenfeld L: Origins of clinical chemistry: the evolution of protein analysis.

New York, Academic Press, 1982. xviii, 366 p.

Rubin LP: Styles in scientific explanations: Paul Ehrlich and Svante Arrhenius on immunochemistry. **J Hist Med Allied Sci** 1980 Oct;35(4):397–425

Sackmann W: Der Arzt und Biochemiker Emil Abderhalden (1877–1950) und seine Beziehungen zur Tiermedizin. **Schweiz Arch Tierheilkd** 1982 Jan;124(1):1–10

Schmidt V: Klinisk kemi--medicinsk eller kemisk subspeciale? **Nord Med** 1983;98(1):26–7

Schmitz R: Der Beginn der organischen Chemie und der Neo-Vitalismus von heute. In Seidler E, Schott H, ed: Bausteine zur Medizingeschichte. Stuttgart, Steiner, 1984. p. 105–11.

Schroeder WA: The background of our knowledge of the mutant hemoglobins. **Tex Rep Biol Med** 1980–81;40:137–42

Smith RE: Contributions of histochemistry to the development of the proteolytic enzyme detection system in diagnostic medicine. **J Histochem Cytochem** 1983 Jan;31(1A Suppl):199–209

Stoffregen M: Zur Rolle histochemischer Phänomene bei der Erforschung und Systematisierung des chromaffinen Gewebes. **Medizinhist J** 1984;19(3):191–209

Stokstad EL: Early work with folic acid. **Fed Proc** 1979 Dec;38(13):2696–8

Strbánová S: Biochemical journals and their profile in 1840–1930. **Acta Hist Rerum Nat Tech** 1981;16:149–95

Sunderman FW: Trends in clinical science. **Ann Clin Lab Sci** 1980 Sep–Oct;10(5):361–7

Swann JP: The search for synthetic penicillin during World War II. **Br J Hist Sci** 1983 Jul;16(53 Pt 2):154–90

Teich M: Ferment or enzyme: what's in a name? **Hist Philos Life Sci** 1981;3(2):193–215

Trumpener U: The road to Ypres: the beginnings of gas warfare in World War I. **J Mod Hist** 1975;47(3):460–8

Vallee BL: Metallothionein: historical review and perspectives. **Experientia [Suppl]** 1979;34:19–39

Van der Star P, ed: Fahrenheit's letters to Leibniz and Boerhaave. Amsterdam, Rodopi, 1983. 195 p. (Nieuwe Nederlandse bijdragen tot de geschiedenis der geneeskunde en der natuurwetenschappen, no. 10).

Weisser U: Künstliches Adrenalin. Der mühevolle Weg zur ersten Hormonsynthese. **Med Welt** 1980 Jan 4;31(1):40–4

Welch AD: Folic acid: discovery and the exciting first decade. **Perspect Biol Med** 1983 Autumn;27(1):64–75

Wootton ID: Earl Judson King. In Dictionary of national biography, 1961–1970. Suppl. 8, 1981. p. 612–3.

Yamakawa T: Wonders in glycolipids--a historical view. **Adv Exp Med Biol** 1984;174:3–13

**Austria**

Schmalhofer J: Das Werk von Johann Florian Heller mit besonderer Berücksichtigung der Entstehung des ersten pathologisch-chemischen Laboratoriums am Allgemeinen Wiener Krankenhaus und der Ernennung Hellers zum Vorstand des Laboratoriums. Diss. Bonn, 1980. 201 p.

**Belgium**

Bacq ZM: Marcel Florkin, 1900–1979. In Florilège des Sciences en Belgique - II. Bruxelles, Académie Royale de Belgique, 1980. p. 675–78.

Brachet J: Esquisse d'une histoire de la biochimie de la biologie cellulaire et de la biologie moléculaire en Belgique. In Florilège des Sciences en Belgique - II. Bruxelles, Académie Royale de Belgique, 1980. p. 289–314.

Edsall JT: Marcel Florkin, August 15, 1900--May 3, 1979. **Isis** 1980 Jun;71(257):286–8

Florkin M: L'Ecole Liégeoise de Physiologie et son Maître Léon Fredericq (1851–1935), pionnier de la zoologie chimique. Liège, Vaillant-Carmanne, 1979. 211 p. (Publication des Archives Internationales de Physiologie et de Biochimie, Médecine et Médicins au Pays de Liège, IV).

Fruton JS: Marcel Florkin, 1900–1979, historian of biochemistry. **Hist Philos Life Sci** 1980;2(1):167–71

Perrin CE: J. B. Van Mons' essai sur les principes de la chimie antiphlogistique: a mystery solved. **Ambix** 1984;31(1):1–5

Schoffeniels E: In memoriam Marcel Florkin (Liège, 15 août 1900–3 mai 1979). Les chênes qu'on abat. **Rev Med Liege** 1979 Jun 1;34(11):481–7

Schoffeniels E: Marcel Florkin et les aspects molecularies de la biologie. **Bull Mem Acad R Med Belg** 1979 Nov 24;134(10):604–16

Schoffeniels E: Marcel Florkin: founding father of comparative biochemistry. **Comp Biochem Physiol** 1980;67B:353–8

Théodoridès J: Marcel Florkin (1900–1979). **Hist Sci Med** 1980;14(2):145–50

Van Elst H: Jan Baptist Van Mons. aanhanger en verdediger van de leer van Lavoisier. **Farm Tijdschr Belg** 1980;57:145–58

**Burma**

Shi NC: Forensic laboratory work in Burma (with special reference to the Office of the Chemical Examiner, Burma). **Am J Forensic Med Pathol** 1980 Jun;1(2):173–6

**Canada**

Kates M: Adventures in membrane land. **Univ Ottawa Q** 1982;52(2):167–80

Lortie L: François-Alexandre-Hubert La Rue. In Dictionary of Canadian biography, 1881–1890. 1982;11:495–7.

Neelin JM: Archibald Byron Macallum, pioneer of biochemistry in Canada. **Can J Biochem Cell Biol** 1984 Jun;62(6):viii–xi

**China**

Bishop C: Hsien Wu (1893–1959): a biographical sketch. **Clin Chem** 1982 Feb;28(2):378–80

**Czechoslovakia**

Homolka J: Ze začátku historie Společnosti klinické biochemie. **Cas Lek Cesk** 1981 Jun 11;120(23):713–5

Obermajer J: Neznámé dopisy Purkyňova tchána K. A. Rudolphiho J. J. Berzeliovi. **Cas Lek Cesk** 1984 Feb 17;123(7):199–203

Tomiček F, Křepelka J, Beran M: In memoriam Doc. Dr. Ing. M. Semonského, DrSc. **Cesk Farm** 1979 Dec;28(9–10):362–6

Votavová J: Prof. PhDr. PhMr. O. Tomíček a jeho analytická škola. **Cesk Farm** 1984 Jun;33(5):213–4

**Denmark**

Rasmussen L: En forstander og hans assistent. **Dan Medicinhist Arbog** 1981;:130–40

With TK: Thirty years with biochemistry and clinic of porphyrias in man and animals. **Int J Biochem** 1980;12(5–6):985–8

**France**

Albury WR: French nosologies around 1800 and their relationship with chemistry. In Forbes EG, ed: Human implications of scientific advance. Edinburgh, Edinburgh University Press, 1978. p. 502–17.

Albury WR: Going beyond the introduction: Claude Bernard scholarship in the 1970s, an essay review. **Bull Hist Med** 1982 Summer;56(2):271–5

Berman A: An unpublished letter from Eugene Soubeiran to Antoine Portal, June 3, 1828. **Pharm Hist** 1982;24(1):32–7

Casaux-Bussière M: Georges Denigès (1859–1951). Essai biographique. Thèse, Bordeaux II, 1981. 374 leaves.

Courtois JE: Le pharmacien Jacques Personne (1816–1880) pionnier de la chimie analytique. **Rev Hist Pharm (Paris)** 1980 Dec;247(68 no 27):263–71

Crosland M: The library of Gay-Lussac. **Ambix** 1981 Nov;28(3):158–70

Debus AG: The Paracelsians in eighteenth century France: a Renaissance tradition in the age of the Enlightenment. **Ambix** 1981 Mar;28(1):36–54

Decourt P: Les zymases ou ferments solubles de Béchamp à la lumière des connaissances du XXe siècle. **Hist Sci Med** 1984;18(2):147–51

Delaunay A, ed: Présence de Pasteur. Paris, Fayard, 1973. 225 p. Includes contributions by P. Bidan, A. Gamet, J. Guillaume, L. Léger, J. Piton, J. De Rosnay, R. Scriban, C. Vago.

Duquénois P: Devenir des plantes médicinales et des médications végétales aux XVIIIe et XIXe siècles sous l'influence de la chimie moderne. In Livet G, Schaff G, ed: Médecine et assistance en Alsace, XVIe–XXe siècle. Strasbourg, Istra, 1976. p. 227–39.

Geison GL: Pasteur on vital versus chemical ferments: a previously unpublished paper on the inversion of sugar. **Isis** 1981 Sep;72(263):425–45

Gouch JB: Lavoisier's memoirs on the nature of water and their place in the chemical revolution. **Ambix** 1983 Jul;30(2):89–106

Granger R: Histoire de la chimie organique à la Faculté de Pharmacie de Montpellier. **Trav Soc Pharm Montp** 1978;38:301–8

Hevér O: Max-Fernand Jayle, a haptoglobin felfedezöje. **Orv Hetil** 1979 Aug 26;120(34):2071–2

Kalugai I: Michel-Eugène Chevreul, 1786–1889. **Koroth** 1980 Jun;7(11–12):796–802

Kursanova TA: A. F. Fourcroy and zoochemistry in France at the beginning of the XIXth century. **Istor Biol Issled** 1983;9:176–86

Labrude P: Albin Haller 1849–1925 pharmacien et chimiste. **Rev Hist Pharm (Paris)** 1982 Sep;29(254):207–9

Le Grand HE: Chemistry in a provincial context: the Montpellier Société Royale des Sciences in the eighteenth century. **Ambix** 1982 Jul;29(2):88–105

Llana JW: Elements in eighteenth century French chemistry. Ph.D. diss. Indiana University. Bloomington, 1979. 226 leaves.

Morange M: L'oeuvre scientifique de Jacques Monod. **Fundam Sci** 1982;3:396–404

Neville RG, Smeaton WA: Macquer's Dictionnaire de Chymie: a bibliographical study. **Ann Sci** 1981;38(6):613–62

Nonclercq M: Antoine Béchamp 1816–1908: l'homme et le savant originalité et fécondité de son oeuvre. Preface et note documentaire par le Docteur Philippe Decourt. Paris, Maloine, 1982. 249 p.

Rocchietta S: Alchimia e medicina nel romanzo 'La rosticceria della regina Pedoca' di Anatole France. **Minerva Med** 1980 Oct 31;71(42):3091–2

Schmitt R: Henri Loewel, chimiste alsacien, élève, collaborateur et ami du savant Angevin Michel-Eugène Chevreul. In: Congrès National des

Sociétés Savantes, 93e, Tours, 1968. Comptes Rendus. Paris, 1971. Section des Sciences, Tome II. p. 175–88.
Sutton G: The physical and chemical path to vitalism: Xavier Bichat's Physiological Researches on Life and Death. **Bull Hist Med** 1984 Spring;58(1):53–71
Todericiu D: Jean Hellot (1685–1766), savant chimiste, fondateur de la technologie chimique en France au XVIIIe siècle. In: Congrès National des Sociétés Savantes, 105e, Caen. Comptes Rendu, Paris. 1980. Section des Sciences, Fasc. 5. p. 201–11.
Viel C: Quelques vers et écrits de jeunesse d'Henri Moissan. **Rev Hist Pharm (Paris)** 1984 Mar;31(260):5–12
Wrotnowska D: Pasteur. Premières recherches sur les fermentations (1855–1857). **Clio Med** 1981 Apr;15(3–4):191–9

**Germany**

Babushkin A: Razvedka khimicheskikh sredstv protivnika (po opytu v 1944–1945 gg.). **Voen Istor Zh** 1973;(1):85–9
Bäumler E: Paul Ehrlich, Forscher für das Leben. Frankfurt, Societäts-Verlag, 1979. 370 p.
Block K: Feodor Lynen: Architekt der klassischen Biochemie. **Max Planck Ges Ber Mitt** 1980;2:21–30
Blum W: Der Apotheker und Chemiker Otto A. Ziurek (1821–1886) und die Apothekenreformbewegung von 1848. Braunschweig, 1980. 110 p. (Veröffentlichungen aus dem Pharmaziegeschichtlichen Seminar der Technischen Universität Braunschweig, 22).
Brock WH: Liebigiana: old and new perspectives. **Hist Sci** 1981 Sep;19(45 pt 3):201–18
Forbes EG: Liebig in Grossbritannien. **Nachrichtenbl Dtsch Ges Gesch Med Naturwiss Tech** 1983 Winter;33(3):115–33
Götz W: Die Bedeutung Johann Bartholomäus Trommsdorffs für die Entwicklung der Chemie in Deutschland zu Beginn des 19. Jahrhunderts. Ein Versuch anhand seiner Korrespondenz mit Justus von Liebig und Heinrich Emanuel Merck. In Dilg P, et al., ed: Perspektiven der Pharmaziegeschichte. Graz, Austria, Akademische Druck- u. Verlagsanstalt, 1983. p. 97–112.
Groehler O: Die Entwicklung der technischen Mittel des chemischen Krieges im imperialistischen Deutschland 1915–1945. **Militaergesch** 1976;15(6):718–28
Hall VM: The role of force or power in Liebig's physiological chemistry. **Med Hist** 1980 Jan;24(1):20–59
Haschen RJ: Entwicklung der Forschung auf dem Gebiet der Pathologischen und Klinischen Biochemie. **Z Med Lab Diagn** 1983;24(7):381–6
Hermann A, Wankmüller A: Physik, Physiologische Chemie und Pharmazie an der Universität Tübingen. Tübingen, J.C.B. Mohr, 1980. 181 p. (Contubernium, Bd. 21).
Höxtermann E: Ein Halbjahrhundert Fortschritte der Zellphysiologie, Biochemie und Photobiologie - Otto Heinrich Warburg (1883 bis 1970). **NTM** 1983;20(2):1–24
Huber R: E. Werle's kallikrein inactivator, a model in biochemistry and biophysics. **Adv Exp Med Biol** 1983;156:29–36
Hufbauer K: The formation of the German chemical community (1720–1795). Berkeley, University of California Press, 1982. viii, 312 p.
Kaiser W: Georg Ernst Stahl (1659–1734)--Zur 250. Wiederkehr seines Todestages am 14. Mai 1984. **Z Gesamte Inn Med** 1984 Aug 1;39(15):371–6
Kempler K: Az elemek rendszerezésének kezdetei (Megemlékezés Johann Wolfgang Döbereiner születésének 200. évfordulóján). **Orv Hetil** 1981 Jan 11;122(2):101–3
Krebs H, Schmid R: Otto Warburg: cell physiologist, biochemist, and eccentric. Oxford, Clarendon. 1981. x, 141 p.
Krebs H: Otto Warburg: Zellphysiologe--Biochemiker--Mediziner---1883–1970. Stuttgart, Wissenschaftliche Verlagsgesellschaft, 1979. 167 p. (Grosse Naturforscher, Band 41).
Krebs H: Wie ich aus Deutschland vertrieben wurde: Dokumente mit Kommentaren. **Medizinhist J** 1980;15(4):357–77
Meinel C: Die Chemie an der Universität Marburg seit Beginn des 19. Jahrhunderts. Ein Beitrag zu ihrer Entwicklung als Hochschulfach. Marburg, Elwert, 1978. xvi, 669 p. (Academia Marburgensis. Herausgegeben von der Philipps-Universität Marburg, Band 3).
Parascandola J: The theoretical basis of Paul Ehrlich's chemotherapy. **J Hist Med Allied Sci** 1981 Jan;36(1)19–43
Rafaelsen OJ: Thudichum: the founder of neurochemistry. In Rose FC, Bynum WF, ed: Historical aspects of the neurosciences. New York, Raven, 1982. p. 293–305.
Reale E: Wissenschaftliche Arbeiten von H. von Mayersbach. **Mikroskopie** 1981;38(3–4):67–77
Reichelt D: Zur Entwicklung des Informationswesens im Fachgebiet und in der Gesellschaft. **Z Med Lab Diagn** 1983;24(7):408–14
Roos A, Boron WF: The buffer value of weak acids and bases: origin of the concept, and first mathematical derivation and application to physico-chemical systems. The work of M. Koppel and K. Spiro (1914). **Respir Physiol** 1980 Apr;40(1):1–32
Schachter M: Kallikreins and kinins, an overview: some thoughts old and new. **Adv Exp Med Biol** 1983;156:13–27
Scheuch DW, Hoffmann H: 20 Jahre Gesellschaft für Klinische Chemie und Laboratoriumsdiagnostik der DDR. **Z Med Lab Diagn** 1983;24(7):371–80
Schmidt V: Emil Abderhalden. Laege, professor, Geheimrat, kolonihavemand, afholdsmand -- og glemt! **Dan Medicinhist Arbog** 1979;116–29
Simmer HH: Medizin und Chemie um die Mitte des 19. Jahrhunderts in Erlangen: Eugen Franz Freiherr von Gorup-Besanez (1817–1878). **J Clin Chem Clin Biochem** 1981 Jul;19(7):497–509
Sinohara H: [Eduard Buchner (1860–1917): a biographical essay] (Jpn). **Seikagaku** 1981;53(10):1139–60
Stahnke J: Häminkristalle--Ludwik Teichmanns Blutnachweis. **Medizinhist J** 1981;16(4):391–413
Tower DB: Hensing, 1719. An account of the first chemical examination of the brain and the discovery of phosphorus therein, set against the background of Europe in the 17th and early 18th centuries. A source book in the history of neurochemistry. New York, Raven, 1983. xvi, 407 p.
Wankmüller A: Anfänge des Chemie- und Pharmaziestudiums in Stuttgart unter Professor Hermann Fehling. **Dtsch Apoth Ztg** 1982 Sep 9;122(36):1805–6
Werner P: Zur experimentellen Methode des Biochemikers Otto Heinrich Warburg. **Z Arztl Fortbild (Jena)** 1983;77(22):947–9
Wiegert J: Anfangsprobleme der Nahrungsmittelchemie in Deutschland unter besonderer Berücksichtigung pharmazeutischer Verhältnisse. Braunschweig, 1975. 180 p. (Veröffentlichungen aus dem Pharmaziegeschichtlichen Seminar der Technischen Universität Braunschweig, Band 15).

**Great Britain**

Buchanan WW, Brown DH: Joseph Black (1728–1799): Scottish physician and chemist. **Practitioner** 1980 Jun;224(1344):663–6
Chaldecott JA: Wedgwood's ceramic wares for chemical use, production and supply from 1779–1794. **Ambix** 1981 Nov;28(3):184–205
Cocker W: A history of the university chemical laboratory, Trinity College, Dublin. **Hermathena** 1978;124:58–76
Cohen SS: Two refugee chemists in the United States, 1794: how we see them. **Proc Am Philos Soc** 1982 Aug;126(4):301–15
Coley NG: Physicians and the chemical analysis of mineral waters in eighteenth-century England. **Med Hist** 1982 Apr;26(2):123–44
Cox EG: Sir William Kershaw Slater. In Dictionary of national biography, 1961–1970. Suppl. 8, 1981. p. 955–6.
Doyle WP: James Crawford (1682–1731), M. D. Edinburgh, University of Edinburgh, [1981]. 10 p. (Scottish men of science).
Doyle WP: Thomas Charles Hope M.D., F.R.S.E., F.R.S. (1766–1844). Edinburgh, University of Edinburgh, 1982. [12 p.] (Scottish Men of Science).
Eyler JM: The conversion of Angus Smith: the changing role of chemistry and biology in sanitary science, 1850–1880. **Bull Hist Med** 1980 Summer;54(2):216–34
Forgan S, ed: Science and the sons of genius: studies on Humphry Davy. London, Science Reviews, 1980. xii, 247 p. Contributions by M. Neve, T. H. Levere, J. Z. Fullmer, M. Crosland, J. H. Brooke, R. Siegfried, D. Knight, E. B. Smith.
Gale EF: Donald Devereux Woods. In Dictionary of national biography, 1961–1970. Suppl. 8, 1981. p. 1102–3.
Garg NK, Nigam SK: Interaction in chemistry and medicine between India and Europe in 18th–19th century. **Indian J Hist Sci** 1981;16(2):145–55
Gorham E: Robert Angus Smith, F.R.S., and 'Chemical climatology'. **Notes Rec R Soc Lond** 1982 Feb;36(2):267–72
Gorman M: Sir William Brooke O'Shaughnessy, F.R.S. (1809–1889), Anglo-Indian forensic chemist. **Notes Rec R Soc Lond** 1984 Sep;39(1):51–64
Griffith WP: Priestley in London. **Notes Rec R Soc Lond** 1983 Aug;38(1):1–16
Hamlin C: Edward Frankland's early career as London's official water analyst, 1865–1876: the context of 'previous sewage contamination'. **Bull Hist Med** 1982 Spring;56(1):56–76
Hartley H: Humphry Davy. London, Nelson, 1966. viii, 160 p.
Hill R: Leslie William Mapson. In Dictionary of national biography, 1961–1970. Suppl. 8, 1981. p. 721–2.
Hunt LB, Buchanan PD: Richard Knight (1768–1844): a forgotten chemist and apparatus designer. **Ambix** 1984 Jul;31(2):57–67
Johnson AW, Rose FL, Suckling CW: Alfred Spinks: 25 February 1917–11 February 1982. **Biogr Mem Fellows R Soc** 1984;30:567–94
Kieft L, Willeford BR, ed: Joseph Priestley. Scientist, theologian, and metaphysician. A symposium celebrating the two hundredth anniversary of the discovery of oxygen by Joseph Priestley in 1774. Lewisburg, Bucknell University Press, 1980. 117 p. With contributions by E. N. Hiebert, A. J. Ihde, R. E. Schofield.
Knight DM: Chemistry, physiology and materialism in the romantic period. **Durham Univ J** 1972;64(2):139–45
Kornberg H, Williamson DH: Hans Adolf Krebs: 25 August 1900–22 November 1981. **Biogr Mem Fellows R Soc** 1984;30:351–85
Krebs H: Reminiscenses and reflections. In collaboration with Anne

Martin. Oxford, Clarendon Press, 1981. x, 298 p.
Levere TH: Dr. Thomas Beddoes at Oxford: radical politics in 1788–1793 and the fate of the Regius Chair in Chemistry. **Ambix** 1981 Jul;28(2):61–9
Levere TH: Dr. Thomas Beddoes: the interaction of pneumatic and preventive medicine with chemistry. **Interdiscip Sci Rev** 1982;7:137–47
Levere TH: Humphry Davy and the idea of glory. **Trans R Soc Can** 1980;18:247–61
Lund P: Sir Hans Krebs (1900–1981). **Clin Sci** 1982 Sep;63(3):225–30
McIlwain H: Neurochemistry and Sherrington's enchanted loom. **J R Soc Med** 1984 May;77(5):417–25
Morgan N: The development of biochemistry in England through botany and the brewing industry (1870–1890). **Hist Philos Life Sci** 1980;2(1):141–66
Morgan N: William Dobinson Halliburton, F.R.S. (1860–1931) – pioneer of British biochemistry? **Notes Rec R Soc Lond** 1983 Aug;38(1):129–45
Morgan WT: Arthur Wormall. In Dictionary of national biography, 1961–1970. Suppl. 8, 1981. p. 1110–1.
Nuttall RH: The Department of Pure and Applied Chemistry: a history 1830–1980. Glasgow, University of Strathclyde, 1980. 16 p.
Parascandola J: Chemistry and pharmacology in Britain 1840–1916. **Pharm Hist (London)** 1976 May;6(1):2
Parkes AS: Sydney John Folley. In Dictionary of national biography, 1961–1970. Suppl. 8, 1981. p. 375–6.
Perrin CE: A reluctant catalyst: Joseph Black and the Edinburgh reception of Lavoisier's chemistry. **Ambix** 1982 Nov;29(3):141–76
Roberts GK: The establishment of the Royal College of Chemistry: an investigation of the social context of early-Victorian chemistry. **Hist Stud Phys Sci** 1976;7:437–85
Roberts GK: The liberally-educated chemist: chemistry in the Cambridge Natural Science Tripos, 1851–1914. **Hist Stud Phys Sci** 1980;11(1):157–83
Scott-Moncrieff R: The classical period in chemical genetics; recollections of Muriel Wheldale Onslow, Robert and Gertrude Robinson and J. B. S. Haldane. **Notes Rec R Soc Lond** 1981;36(1):125–54
Smeaton WA: James Riddick Partington. In Dictionary of national biography, 1961–1970. Suppl. 8, 1981. p. 822–3.
Sporn MB: Edward Charles Dodds: diethylstilbestrol. **Cancer Res** 1983 Sep;43(9):preceding 3981
Szabadváry F: Joseph Priestley születésének 250. évfordulójára. **Orv Hetil** 1983 Oct 16;124(42):2563–4
Szarek WA, Stacey M, Hay GW: John Kenyon Netherton Jones (1912–1977). **Adv Carbohydr Chem Biochem** 1983;41:1–26
Whelan WJ: Use of liposomes in medicine. **Biochem Soc Trans** 1984 Apr;12(2):331–2

### Hungary

Bugyi B: N. J. Jacquin, the first medical doctor-chemist in Hungary. **Ther Hung** 1979;27(4):192–3
Spielmann J: Nyulas Ferenc emlékezete. **Orv Hetil** 1984 Jun 24;125(26):1578–81
Szállási A: Farkas Géza-akinek élete volt a főmüve. **Orv Hetil** 1984 Sep 16;125(38):2324–7
Szállási A: Nendtvich Károly orvosvegyész amerikai utazása 1855-ben. **Orv Hetil** 1984 Sep 2;125(36):2205–6, 2209–10
Székács I: Hári Pál emléke (1869–1933). **Orv Hetil** 1983 Jul 31;124(31):1889–94

### India

Gorman M: Sir William B. O'Shaughnessy, pioneer chemical educator in India. **Ambix** 1983 Jul;30(2):107–16

### Ireland

Lyons JB: Sylvester O'Halloran's 'Treatise on the Air'. **Ir Med J** 1983 Jan;76(1):37–9

### Italy

Colapinto L: Il Nobile Collegio Chimico Farmaceutico Romano. Cenni storici. Roma, Stomygen, 1979, 30 p.

### Korea

Cowdrey AE: 'Germ warfare' and public health in the Korean conflict. **J Hist Med Allied Sci** 1984 Apr;39(2):153–72

### Netherlands

Scopa JP: Boerhaave on alchemy. **Synthesis** 1979;4(4):24–37
Snelders HA: De chemische voordrachten van Wille de Loos (circa 1770). **Tijdschr Geschied Geneeskd** 1979;2(4):168–75
Snelders HA: De natuur- en scheikundige wetenschappen in de medische tijdschriften. **Ned Tijdschr Geneeskd** 1981 Apr 25;125(17):668–73
Snelders HA: Het chemisch laboratorium 'de Leeuwenbergh' te Utrecht (1845–1903). **Tijdschr Geschied Geneeskd** 1984;7(3):129–56
Snelders HA: Het fysisch-chemisch werk van de Rotterdamse arts Hendrik Willem Rouppe (1765–1816). **Tijdschr Geschied Geneeskd** 1981;4(1):25–44
Snelders HA: Het Gezelschap der Hollandsche Scheikundigen. Amsterdamse chemici uit het einde van de achttiende eeuw. Amsterdam, Rodopi, 1980. 111 p. (Nieuwe Nederlandse Bijdragen tot de Geschiedenis der Geneeskunde en der Natuurwetenschappen, no. 4).
Snelders HA: Lambertus Bicker (1732–1801). An early adherent of Lavoisier in the Netherlands. **Janus** 1980;67(1–2–3):101–23
Snelders HA: The Amsterdam pharmacist Willem van Barneveld (1747–1826) and the discovery of photosynthesis (1778). **Janus** 1981;68:1–14
Van Kampen EJ, Jijlstra WG: Haemoglobinometry: from estimation to reference method. **J Clin Chem Clin Biochem** 1981 Aug;19(8):517–9

### Poland

Kasprzyk Z: Irena Chmielewska. **Acta Biochim Pol** 1982;29(1–2):3–5
Kucharz E: Herman Fudakowski--pierwszy kierownik katedry chemii lekarskiej w Warszawie. **Wiad Lek** 1980 Jun 1;33(11):931–4
Ostrowski W: The work of the Committee on Biochemistry and Biophysics during twenty five years of the Polish Academy of Sciences. **Rev Pol Acad Sci (Warsz)** 1978;23(2):101–12
Pabis-Stachoń M: Gremia aptekarskie w latach 1802–1939 na obszarach byłej Galicji Zachodniej. **Arch Hist Med (Warsz)** 1980;43(3):311–15
Sarnecka-Keller M: Biochemia na Uniwersytecie Jagiellońskim: Przesyłość i terazniejszość. **Stud Mater Dziejow Nauk Pol** 1981;25:87–105
Szarkowski JW, Wierzchowski KL: Professor Józef Heller 1896–1982. **Acta Biochim Pol** 1984;31(1):5–8
Szwarczyński W: Rozwój badań w dziedzinie oryginalnego polskiego leku syntetycznego. **Arch Hist Med (Warsz)** 1984;47(3):443–6
Szwejcerowa A: Marceli Nencki (1847–1901), pionnier de la biochimie. In International Congress of the History of Medicine. 26th, Plovdiv, 1978. Actes du Congress. Sofia, 1981. Volume II. p. 97–9.
Wspomnienie o Profesorze Józefie Hellerze: **Postepy Biochem** 1982;28(4):387–90

### Portugal

Mosch E: Der Apotheker Pedro José da Silva, ein unbekannter Lebenslauf. **Beitr Gesch Pharm** 1980;31(9):65–71

### Romania

Popa LM, Repanovici R, Iliescu R: Investigations in the field of recombinant DNA technology performed in the 'Stefan S. Nicolau' Institute of Virology. **Virologie** 1984 Oct–Dec;35(4):315–22

### Spain

Beya Alonso E: 'Los ingenieros industriales como Analistas Clínicos'. **Bol Soc Esp Hist Farm** 1981 Jun;32(126):91–3
Carmona Cornet AM, Gómez Caamaño JL: Historia de la Cátedra de técnica física aplicada a la Farmacia y análisis químico y en particular de los alimentos, medicamentos y venenos de la Facultad de Farmacia de la Universidad de Barcelona (1886–1936). **Bol Soc Esp Hist Farm** 1984 Jun;35(138):125–37
Carrillo JL, Gago R: Memoria sobre una nueva y metodica clasificacion de los fluidos elasticos permanentes y gaseosos de Juan Manuel de Arejula (1755–1830). Introduccion, transcripcion y notas. Malaga, Universidad de Malaga, 1980. 47 p.
Gago R, Olagüe G, Carrillo JL, et al: El plan de estudios del rector Blasco (1786) y la renovacion de las disciplinas cientificas en la Universidad de Valencia: la quimica y la enseñanza clinica. **Estudis** 1977;6:157–65
Muñoz Calvo S, Turegano Lopez A: El control de alimentos del Laboratorio Químico Municipal de Madrid en el siglo XIX: contribución a su estudio. **Bol Soc Esp Hist Farm** 1981 Sep;32(127):149–67
Peset JL, Nuñex D: Filosofía, ciencia y alquimia en la ilustacion española. **Cuad Hispanoam** 1980;120(359):371–93
Puerto Sarmiento FJ: Andrés Alcón (1782–1850), farmacéutico, político y profesor de Química. **Bol Soc Esp Hist Farm** 1984 Sep;35(139):143–64
Puerto Sarmiento FJ, Cobo Cobo J: La evolucion de la quimica farmaceutica durante el siglo XVIII. **Bol Soc Esp Hist Farm** 1983 Mar–Jun;34(133–134):25–33
Rof Carballo MC: Biografía y labor docente de Francisco Carbonell y Bravo. Diss. Barcelona, Facultad de Farmacia, Universidad de Barcelona, 1975. 189 p. (Publicaciones del Seminario de Historia de la Farmacia).
Sanchez-Moscoso A: José Rodríguez Carracido. **Bol Soc Esp Hist Farm** 1971 Jun;22(86):54–84

### Sweden

Cassebaum H: Neues über die Entdeckung von Säuren in organischem Material durch C.W. Scheele. **Pharmazie** 1981;36(2):135–8
Ekström S: Jöns Jacob Berzelius--ett 200-årsminne. **Sven Farm Tidskr** 1979;83:635–51
Gutt RW: Jöns Jacob Berzelius (1779–1848) i poczatki chemii fizjologicznej). **Arch Hist Med (Warsz)** 1979;42(1):83–92
Krook H: Jacob Berzelius privat. **Nord Medicinhist Arsb** 1980;:81–9

Marks LS, Maxwell MH: Tigerstedt and the discovery of renin. An historical note. **Hypertension** 1979 Jul-Aug;1(4):384-8

Melhado EM: Jacob Berzelius. The emergence of his chemical system. Stockholm, Almqvist & Wiksell International; Madison, University of Wisconsin Press, 1981. 357 p. (Also published as 'Studies and sources published by the Swedish History of Science Society No. 34').

Nevoral V, Křížek V: J. J. Berzelius jako analytik minerálních vod. **Fysiatr Reumatol Vestn** 1980 Aug;58(4):244-7

Trofast J: Jöns Jacob Berzelius och djurkemien. **Svdsven Medicinhist Sallsk Arsskr** 1981;:170-84

**Switzerland**

Jonecko A: Uwagi o podręczniku histochemii Freya z roku 1870 na tle osiągnięć histochemicznych połowy XIX wieku. **Wiad Lek** 1979 Dec 15;32(24):1811-4

Picco C: Das Biochemische Institut der Universität Zürich 1931-1981. Aarau, Verlag Sauerländer, 1981. 62 p. (Veröffentlichungen der Schweizerischen Gesellschaft für Geschichte der Medizin und der Naturwissenschaften, 37).

Prijs B: Chymia Basiliensis: Episoden aus der Basler Chemiegeschichte. Basel; New York, Karger, 1983. x, 125 p.

**United States**

Andrews WH: A perspective review of the development of AOAC microbiological methods. **J Assoc Off Anal Chem** 1984 Jul-Aug;67(4):661-73

Austrian R: Perrin Hamilton Long. In Dictionary of American biography, 1961-1965. Suppl. 7, 1981. p. 477-8.

Bendiner E: Avery: making sense of a 'stupid tetranucleotide'. **Hosp Pract** 1982 Oct;17(10):195, 199, 202-3 passim

Bing FC: Vincent du Vigneaud (1901-1978): a biographical sketch. **J Nutr** 1982 Aug;112(8):1463-73

Bodian D: Normand Louis Hoerr. In Dictionary of American Biography, Suppl. 6, 1956-1960. p. 295-6, 1980.

Briscoe AM: Diary of a mad feminist chemist. **Int J Womens Stud** 1981;4(4):420-30

Brown BI: Gerty Theresa Radnitz Cori. In Dictionary of American Biography, Suppl. 6, 1956-1960. p. 126-7, 1980.

Carroll PT: Academic chemistry in America, 1876-1976: diversification, growth, and change. Ph.D. Diss., University of Pennsylvania. Philadelphia, 1982. xviii, 551 p.

Carter HE: Identification and synthesis of threonine. **Fed Proc** 1979 Dec;38(13):2684-6

Cope FW: In memoriam . . . B. David Polis--mitochondrial biochemist, discoverer of polymeric prostaglandin PGBx for prevention and therapy of damaged mitochondrial oxidative phosphorylation. **Physiol Chem Phys** 1980;12(6):541-4

Damadian R: In memoriam--Freeman Widener Cope--1930-1982. **Physiol Chem Phys** 1982;14(5):411-4

Edsall JT: The Journal of Biological Chemistry after seventy-five years. **J Biol Chem** 1980 Oct 10;255(19):8939-51

Edsall JT: The William Mansfield Clark papers: a second installment. **Surv Sources Newsl** 1981;10:1

Heidelberger M: A 'pure' organic chemist's downward path: chapter 3--'retirement'. **Perspect Biol Med** 1981 Summer;24(4):619-36

Ihde AJ: Conrad Arnold Elvehjem. In Dictionary of American biography, 1961-1965. Suppl. 7, 1981. p. 223-4.

Irwin LN: Fulfillment and frustration: the confessions of a behavioral biochemist. **Perspect Biol Med** 1978 Spring;21(3):476-91

Jacobson LO: From atom to eve. **Perspect Biol Med** 1981 Winter;24(2):195-216

Jones DP: American chemists and the Geneva protocol. **Isis** 1980 Sep;71(258):426-40

Kanaoka Y: [The chemist in a biomedical environment: personal reflections on a quarter century of research at NIH] (Jpn) **Tanpakushitsu Kakusan Koso** 1979;24(14):1521-30

Kasten FH: Ralph D. Lillie, 1896-1979. **Stain Technol** 1980 Jul;55(4):201-15

Kauffman GB: The mystery of Stephen H. Emmens: successful alchemist or ingenious swindler?. **Ambix** 1983 Jul;30(2):65-88

Kohler RE: Medical reform and biomedical science: biochemistry -- a case study. In Vogel MJ, Rosenberg CE, ed: The therapeutic revolution. Philadelphia, 1979. p. 27-66.

Kohler RE: Rudolf Schoenheimer, isotopic tracers, and biochemistry in the 1930's. **Hist Stud Phys Sci** 1977;8:257-98

Kopp C: The Edward Lawrie Tatum papers. **Mendel Newsl** 1981 Jul;20:1-2

Kopp C: The J. H. B. Archive report; the Edward Lawrie Tatum papers at the Rockefeller University Archives. **J Hist Biol** 1982 Spring;15(1):153-4

Lechevalier HA: The search for antibiotics at Rutgers University. In J. Parascandola, ed: The history of antibiotics. Madison, American Institute of the History of Pharmacy, 1980. p. 113-23.

Leonard Tucker Skeggs--a multifaceted diamond: **Clin Chem** 1981 Aug;27(8):1465-8

Lipmann F: A long life in times of great upheaval. **Annu Rev Biochem** 1984;53:1-33

McCarty M: Historical perspective on C-reactive protein. **Ann NY Acad Sci** 1982;389:1-10

McDermott W: Colin Munro MacLeod: January 28, 1909-February 11, 1972. **Biogr Mem Natl Acad Sci** 1983;54:183-219

Mann FD: Ross Aiken Gortner and bound water, the water of life. **Perspect Biol Med** 1976 Autumn;20(1):142-4

Meites S: Otto Folin's decade in Minnesota, 1882-1892: a brief review. **Clin Chem** 1982 Oct;28(10):2173-7

Meites S: The first call for clinical chemists in the United States. **Clin Chem** 1983 Oct;29(10):1852-3

Novelli G: Personal recollections to Fritz Lipmann during the early years of coenzyme A research. **Mol Biol Biochem Biophys** 1980;32:415-30

Nusynowitz ML: The isolation of thyroxine (Edward C Kendall). **JAMA** 1983 Oct 21;250(15):2047-8

Ochoa S: The thrill of discovery. **Boll Soc Ital Biol Sper** 1980 Sep 30;56(18 Pt 2):17-40

Parascandola J: Gerty Theresa Radnitz Cori. In: Notable American women. The modern period. Cambridge, Mass., Belknap-Harvard Univ. Press, 1980. 4:165-7.

Pazur JH: Dexter French 1918-1981. **Adv Carbohydr Chem Biochem** 1984;42:1-13

Pittman W: Chemical regulation in Mississippi: the State Laboratory (1882- ). **J Miss Hist** 1979;41(2):133-53

Raacke ID: Agnes Fay Morgan. In: Notable American women. The modern period. Cambridge, Mass., Belknap-Harvard Univ. Press, 1980. 4:495-7.

Raacke ID: Jane Anne Russell. In: Notable American women. The modern period. Cambridge, Mass., Belknap-Harvard Univ. Press, 1980. 4:610-1.

Raacke ID: Marjorie Maxine Nelson. In Dictionary of American biography, 1961-1965. Suppl. 7, 1981. p. 568-9.

Ratnoff WD: A war with the molecules: Louis Pillemer and the history of properdin. **Perspect Biol Med** 1980;23(4):638-57

Reinhold JG: Adventures of a clinical chemist. **Clin Chem** 1982 Nov;28(11):2314-23

Rice EW: Joseh H. Roe (1892-1967): American man of science, pioneer clinical chemist. **Clin Chem** 1984 Sep;30(9):1575-8

Sinohara H: [James Batcheller Sumner (1887-1955): a biographical essay] **Seikagaku** 1979 Dec;51(12):1301-21

Smith EK: History of the Pacific Northwest Section, AACC 1961-1981. **Clin Chem** 1981 May;27(5):762-4

Sproul EE: Acid phosphatase and prostate cancer: historical overview. **Prostate** 1980;1(4):411-3

Stork G: Samuel Marion McElvain: December 9, 1897-April 11, 1973. **Biogr Mem Natl Acad Sci** 1983;54:221-48

Stutzman RH: Harvey Washington Wiley; a famous Hoosier and 'The father of pure food'. **Indiana Med Hist Q** 1981;7(4):20-1

Watanabe M: The caloric theory of S. L. Metcalfe. **Br J Hist Sci** 1984 Jul;17(56 pt 2):210-3

Winsten S, Sideman L: History of the Philadelphia Section, American Association for Clinical Chemistry. **Clin Chem** 1981 Jan;27(1):192-4

Wiser V: Mary Engle Pennington. In: Notable American women. The modern period. Cambridge, Mass., Belknap-Harvard Univ. Press, 1980. 4:532-4.

Young JH: George Wilhelm Merck. In Dictionary of American Biography, Suppl. 6, 1956-1960. p. 447-8, 1980.

**USSR**

Berezin IV, Osipova TA, Figurovsky NA: The development of investigation of immobilized enzymes in the USSR. **Istor Biol Issled** 1983;9:113-26

Boldyrev AA: 55 let otechestvennoĭ biokhimii. **Biol Nauki** 1982;(5):107-8

Grigor'eva VA: Tvorcheskiĭ vklad v biokhimiiu myshts. **Ukr Biokhim Zh** 1980 Nov-Dec;52(6):783-8

Ionov IuV, Ionov AIu: A. P. Borodin - vrach, khimik, pedagog (k 150-letiiu so dnia rozhdeniia). **Sov Zdravookhr** 1984;(1):61-4

Khaidarov A: On the isolation of crystalline oxidase in 1906. **Istor Biol Issled** 1983;9:158-66

Khalmuradov AG, Rybina AA: Tvorcheskiĭ vklad akademika AN USSR R. V. Chagovtsa v razvitie biokhimii. **Ukr Biokhim Zh** 1984 Sep-Oct;56(5):576-86

Liashenko NI: Aleksandr Porfir'evich Borodin (k 150 letiiu so dnia rozhdeniia). **Voen Med Zh** 1983 Nov;(11):66-9

Prokhorova MI: E. S. London i funktsional'naia neĭrokhimiia. **Nerv Sist** 1982;23:137-42

Shamin AN: Studies on the history of biochemistry. **Istor Biol Issled** 1983;9:4-15

Shul'tsev GP: Aleksandr Porfir'evich Borodin (k 150-letiiu so dnia rozhdeniia). **Klin Med (Mosk)** 1984 Jul;62(7):144-7

# CHILD HEALTH

See also **Human Development and Growth; Pediatrics; Public Health**

Battin J: Le sentiment de l'enfance. In: Congrès National des Sociétés Savantes, 104e, Bordeaux, 1979. Comptes Rendus. Paris, 1979. Section des Sciences, Fasc. IV. p. 319-27.

# CHILD HEALTH

Boswell JE: Expositio and oblatio: the abandonment of children and the ancient and medieval family. **Am Hist Rev** 1984;89(1):10–33

Brodie B: Children: a glance at the past. **MCN** 1982 Jul–Aug;7(4):219–25

Cain LP: Child abuse: historical precedent and legal ramifications. **Health Soc Work** 1980 Aug;5(3):61–7

Calhoun D: On the psychohistory of childhood. **Hist Educ Q** 1974;14(3):371–7

Child abuse: historical perspective: In D. N. Jones, J. Pickett, M. R. Oates, P. R. Barbor, ed: Understanding child abuse. Kent, Hodder and Stoughton, 1982. p. 38–50.

Cohn J: Misbruk og mishandling av barn – før og nå. **Dan Medicinhist Arbog** 1981;:158–68

Cone TE: History of infant and child feeding: from the earliest years through the development of scientific concepts. In Bond JT, et. al., ed: Infant and child feeding. New York, Academic Press, 1981. p. 3–34.

Ende A: Children in history: a personal review of the past decade's published research. **J Psychohist** 1983 Summer;11(1):65–88

Fildes V: The early history of the infant feeding bottle. **Nurs Times** 1981 Jan 15 and 22;77(3–4):128, 168–9

Fildes V: Weaning: on the bottle again. **Nurs Mirror** 1980;151(24):18–21

Fox VC, Quitt MH, ed: Loving, parenting and dying: the family cycle in England and America, past and present. New York, Psychohistory Press, 1980. v, 488 p. Includes original essays by the editors, by M. A. Glendon, and A. Macfarlane. Also includes numerous previously published articles by various other authors.

Franciosi RA: Evolution of SIDS diagnosis. **Minn Med** 1983 Jul;66(7):411–3

Huard P, Laplane R: Histoire illustrée de la puériculture: aspects diététiques, socio-culturels et ethnologiques. Paris, Les Editions Roger Dacosta, 1979?, 196 p.

Jackson BS: Historical aspects of legal drafting in the light of modern theories of cognitive development. **Int J Law Psychiatry** 1980;3(4):349–69

Kahn A: Highlights of the Adler Museum collections. **Adler Mus Bull** 1984 Nov;10(3):25–9

Kloë E: Hysterie im Kindesalter. Zur Entwicklung des kindlichen Hysteriebegriffes. Freibug, Schulz, 1979. 181 p. (Freiburger Forschungen zur Medizingeschichte, Neue Folge, 9).

Larsen O: Fårlig a vaere barneår og livesjanser. [Dangers of childhood--life prospects] (Nor). **Forskningsnytt (Norway)** 1979;24(4):14–9

Means RK: Historical perspectives on school health. Thorofare, New Jersey, Slack, 1975. 253 p.

Merritt DH, ed: Infant nutrition. Stroudsburg, Pennsylvania, Dowden, Hutchinson & Ross, 1976. xv, 431 p. (Benchmark Papers in Human Physiology, 7).

Mössmer A: Säuglingsflaschen aus Holz. In Göpfert W, Otten HH, ed: Metavoeite: wandelt euch durch neues Denken. Düsseldorf, Triltsch, 1983. p. 201–8.

Navarro P: Lactancia mercenaria: hipocresía y exploitación. **Asclepio** 1983;35:375–87

Pernick MS: Childhood death and medical ethics: an historical perspective on truth-telling in pediatrics. **Prog Clin Biol Res** 1983;139:173–88

Radbill SX: Infant feeding through the ages. **Clin Pediatr (Phila)** 1981 Oct;20(10):613–21

Riordan J, Countryman BA: Basics of breastfeeding. Part I: Infant feeding patterns past and present. **JOGN Nurs** 1980 Jul–Aug;9(4):207–10

Robin M: Sheltering arms: the roots of child protection. In E. H. Newberger, ed: Child abuse. Boston, Little, Brown and Company, 1982. p. 1–21.

Rothman BK: In labor. Women and power in the birthplace. New York, London, W.W. Norton, 1982. 320 p.

Savitt TL: The social and medical history of crib death. **J Fla Med Assoc** 1979 Aug;66(8):853–9

Schadewaldt H: 'Schulmedizin--Aussenseitermethoden'; eine Betrachtung aus historischer Sicht. **Rheinisches Arztebl** 1980;8:225–30

Smith GF, Smith PN, Vidyasagar D, ed: Historical review and recent advances in neonatal and perinatal medicine. 2 vols. [Chicago?], Mead Johnson Nutritional Division, 1983. xxii, 212 p.; viii, 189 p. Historical contributions by B. F. Andrews, L. Ballowitz, L. J. Butterfield, V. Chernick, T. E. Cone, R. L. Day, M. L. Duxbury, D. Dye, L. M. Gartner, P. J. Goldstein, M. H. Greenberg, L. Johnson, A. Kaul, J. O. Klein, J. Lind, L. O. Lubchenco, N. M. Nelson, K. C. Pringle, T. N. Raju, A. C. Rambar, R. Sosa, M. T. Stahlman, L. Stern, K. Tarpey, A. Zipursky.

Stahl A: Swaddling: its disappearance as an illustration of the process of cultural change. **Koroth** 1983 Aug;8(7–8):285–98

Theopold W: Das Kind in der Votivmalerei. Munich, Karl Thiemig, 1981.

Utrilla PN: Lactancia mercenaria: otra expresion de la doble moral burguesa. **Asclepio** 1982;34:33–70

Weber HG, Stickl H: Auswirkungen der Urbanisation auf das Kind. **Off Gesundheitswes** 1982 Sep;44(9):560–5

Zglinicki F von: Die Wiege: volkskundlich, kulturgeschichtlich, kunstwissenschaftlich, medizinhistorisch. Regensburg, Pustet, 1979. 419 p.

**Belgium**

Vandenbroeke C: Zuigelingensterfte, bevallingsstoornissen en kraambedsterfte (17–19de eeuw). **Bijdr Geschied Geneeskd** 1977;60:133–63

**Chile**

Mardones F: Historia y situación actual de la lactancia materna en Chile. **Rev Med Chil** 1979 Aug;107(8):750–60

Santander FM: Marco histórico para el análisis de las causas del descenso en la práctica de la lactancia materna. **Rev Chil Pediatr** 1982 Nov–Dec;53(6):607–14

**Europe**

Imhof AE: Säuglingssterblichkeit im europäischen Kontext, 17.–20 Jahrhundert. Ueberlegungen zu einem Buch von Anders Brändström. Umeå, Umeå University, 1984. 73 p. (Demographic Data Base, Newsletter No. 2)

**France**

Exposition 'enfants des montagnes' au musée dauphinois à Grenoble: **Bull Soc Fr Hist Hop** 1980;(41):32–5

Gélis J: La Pierre et le saint: recours populaires pour la guérison des petits enfants (XVIIe–XIXe siècles). **Asclepio** 1983;35:129–58

Gélis J: Miracle et medecine aux siècles classiques: le corps medical et le retour temporaire a la vie des mort-nes. **Hist Reflect** 1982;9(1–2):85–101

Les enfants du Rouergue: **Bull Soc Fr Hist Hop** 1980;(41):36

Morel MF: Les parents devant la maladie de leurs enfants dans la France moderne (XVIe–XVIIIe siècles). **Asclepio** 1983;35:359–74

Regards sur la condition enfantine – XVIe–XXe siècles: **Bull Soc Fr Hist Hop** 1980;(41):29–31

Roubert J: L'adoption des enfants par des particuliers à Lyon sous l'ancien régime. **Bull Soc Fr Hist Hop** 1978;(36–37):41–67

Schmitt JC: The holy greyhound: Guinefort, healer of children since the thirteenth century. Cambridge, Cambridge University Press; Paris, Editions de la Maison des Sciences de l'Homme, 1983. 215 p. Translation of Le saint lévrier: Guinefort, guérisseur d'enfants depuis le XIIIe siècle, Paris, 1979.

Vigarello G: L'eau: Un imaginaire pédagogique dans la médecine des enfants aux XVIe–XVIIe et XVIIIe siècles. **Hist Philos Life Sci** 1981;3(2):171–91

**Germany**

Rodegra H: Zur Geschichte der Gesundheitserziehung in deutschen Schulen. **Med Welt** 1979 Oct 26;30(43):1615–20

**Great Britain**

Fildes V: The age of weaning in Britain 1500–1800. **J Biosoc Sci** 1982 Apr;14(2):223–40

Finlay R: Differential child mortality in pre-industrial England: the example of Cartmel, Cumbria, 1600–1750. **Ann Demogr Hist (Paris)** 1981;:67–80

Matossian MK: Mold poisoning: an unrecognized English health problem, 1550–1800. **Med Hist** 1981 Jan;25(1):73–84

**Italy**

Bellettini A, Samoggia A: Evolution différentielle et mouvement saisonnier de la mortalité infantile et enfantine dans la banlieue de Bologne (XVIIe–XIXe siècles). **Ann Demogr Hist (Paris)** 1983;:195–207

**Japan**

Sawada K: [History of breast feeding in Japan]. (Jpn) **Josanpu Zasshi** 1979 Sep;33(9):596–604

**Poland**

Dembińska M: Pożywienie dziecka w polskich żródlach historycznych. **Kwart Hist Kultury Mater** 1980;28(4):481–99

**Spain**

Ballester R: Factores biológicos y actitudes vigentes frente a la infancia en la sociedad española del antiguo régimen. **Asclepio** 1983;35:343–57

**Before 500 A.D.**

Grimm H: Was wissen wir über ur- und frühgeschichtliche Kindernahrung? **Aerztl Jugendkd** 1981;72(3):170–3

### Egypt

Diener L: Från antikonception till amning - om tillökning i familjen i det faraoniska Egypten. **Nord Medicinhist Arsbok** 1983;:41–58

### Israel

Brian VA: Infant welfare in the Bible. **Nurs Times** 1980 Dec 18–25;76(51):2230–1

### 500 A.D.–1450

Shahar S: Infants, infant care, and attitudes toward infancy in the medieval Lives of Saints. **J Psychohist** 1983 Winter;10(3):281–309

### Arabic

Kahle E: Al-Magusi (Haly Abbas) über Kinderkrankheiten im Kamil as-sina'a at-tibbiya. Erlangen, Verlagsbuchhandlung Hannelore Lüling, 1980. 61, [6] p.
Kahle E: Avicenna (Ibn Sina) über Kinderkrankheiten im Kinderregimen seines Qanun. Erlangen, Verlagsbuchhandlung Hannelore Lüling, 1979. 53, [14] p.
Kahle E: Das Ammenregimen des Avicenna (Ibn Sina) in seinem Qanun. Erlangen, Verlagsbuchhandlung Hannelore Lüling, 1980. 45, [13] p.

### Italy

Klapisch-Zuber C: Parents de sang, parents de lait: la mise en nourrice à Florence (1300–1530). **Ann Demogr Hist (Paris)** 1983;:33–64

### 1450–1700

### Americas

Cone TE: The nursing bottle caries syndrome. **JAMA** 1981 Jun 12;245(22):2334

### Europe

Ozment S: The family in Reformation Germany: the bearing and rearing of children. **J Fam Hist** 1983 Summer;8(2):159–76

### Germany

Heintel H: Die Fallhaube: eine Erfindung des 16. Jahrhunderts? **Medizinhist J** 1984;19(3):273–6

### Great Britain

Wooden WW: Childhood and death: a reading of John Skelton's Phillip Sparrow. **J Psychohist** 1980 Spring;7(4):403–14

### Italy

Dequeker J: Arthritis in the paintings of Sandro Botticelli. **Arthritis Rheum** 1984 Oct;27(10):1196–7
Klapisch-Zuber C: Genitori naturali e genitori di latte nella Firenze del quattrocento. **Quad Stor** 1980;15(2):543–63
Leden I: Doubts about Sandro Botticelli's depiction of juvenile rheumatoid arthritis. **Arthritis Rheum** 1984 Oct;27(10):1197–8

### Spain

Carreras Panchon A: El problema del niño exposito en la España ilustrada. Salamanca, 1977. 94 p. (Cuadernos de Historia de la Medicina Española, Monografias, 32).

### 1700 to Present

Bowman IA, ed: Child health on postage stamps. **Bookman** 1982 Feb;9(2):3–7
Brickman JP: Mother love - mother death. Maternal and infant care: social class and the role of government. Ph.D. Diss., City University of New York. New York, 1978. vii, 750 leaves. (2 v.).
Brügelmann J: Medikalisierung von Säuglings- und Erwachsenenalter in Deutschland zu Beginn des 19. Jahrhunderts aufgrund von medizinischen Topographien. In Imhof AE, ed.: Leib und Leben in der Geschichte der Neuzeit. Berlin, Duncker & Humblot, 1983. p. 177–92.
Buchanan I: Infant mortality and social policy: the eugenists and the social amelioratore, 1900–1914. **Soc Soc Hist Med Bull (Lond)** 1980;27:5–7
Bullough VL: Bottle feeding: an amplification. **Bull Hist Med** 1981 Summer;55(2):257–9
Calame A: Etre prématuré: hier, aujourd'hui, demain. **Rev Med Suisse Romande** 1983 Apr;103(4):319–31
English PC, Grossman H: Radiology and the history of child abuse. **Pediatr Ann** 1983 Dec;12(12):870–4
Ewerbeck H: Die Gesundheit des Kindes im Laufe des 20. Jahrhunderts. **Off Gesundheitswes** 1979 Sep;41 Suppl 1:1–6
Fegersten S: Crude death rate and infant mortality (1840–1900) in Norway, Sweden, Denmark, England and Wales with particular attention to the relationship between mortality and population density-urbanisation. **Scand Popul Stud** 1979;5:83–97
Flegg AT: Inequality of income, illiteracy and medical care as determinants of infant mortality in underdeveloped countries. **Popul Stud** 1982 Nov;36(3):441–58
Fuster P: Análisis bibliográfico de las psicosis infantiles. **Asclepio** 1980;32:171–94
Gerlach LP: The flea and the elephant: infant formula controversy. **Society** 1980;17(6):51–7
Jenny J: An historic parallel: 19th century education, 20th century dental care. **J Public Health Dent** 1979 Fall;39(4):295–7
Kapronczay K: Adatok koraszülöttek inkubátoros ápolásának kezdeteiröl. **Orv Hetil** 1982 Oct 3;123(40):2487–90
Kern SR: Freud and the emergence of child psychology. [New York, s. n.], 1973. 3, vii, 415 leaves.
Kett JF: The search for a science of infancy. **Hastings Cent Rep** 1984 Apr;14(2):34–9
Lehning JR: The history of wet-nursing and the history of the family. **Peasant Stud** 1982;9(4):250–7
Lévy C: La mortalité par accident des enfants et des adolescents dans huit pays développés. **Population** 1980;35(2):291–319
Lithell UB: Breast-feeding habits and their relation to infant mortality and marital fertility. **J Fam Hist** 1981;6:182–94
Lomax EM, Kagan J, Rosenkrantz BG: Science and patterns of child care. San Francisco, W. H. Freeman, 1978. xiv, 247 p.
Macmillan MB: Freud and Lindner on pleasure sucking. **Stor Crit Psicol** 1980;1(1):111–43
Meindl RS: Components of longevity: developmental and genetic responses to differential childhood mortality. **Soc Sci Med** 1982;16(2):165–74
Peutillot A: Petite histoire de la vulgarisation en puériculture. **Soins Gynecol Obstet Pueric** 1982 Feb;(9):47–50
Phillilps S: Psychoanalysis and childhood education: a historical review. **Paedagog Hist** 1977;17(2):378–85
Quintero García P: Janusz Korczac. **Rev Soc Venez Hist Med** 1979;28(42):31–5
Reese WJ: After bread, education: nutrition and urban school children, 1890–1920. **Teach Coll Rec** 1980;81(4):496–525
Rollet C: Variole et mortalité des enfants au XVIIIe siècle. **Cah Hist** 1978;23(4):417–36
Stainback S, Stainback W: Historical development of treatments for maladaptive behavior. In their: Educating children with severe maladaptive behaviors. New York, Grune & Stratton, 1980. p. 36–60.
Vandenbroeke C, Van Poppel F, Van Der Woude AM: Le développement séculaire de la mortalité aux jeunes âges dans le territoire du Bénélux. **Ann Demogr Hist (Paris)** 1983;:257–89
Van Eys J: Nutritional therapy in childhood malignancies--a historical perspective. In Van Eys J, Seelig MS, Nichols BL, ed: Nutrition and cancer. New York and London, SP, 1979. P. 91–110.
Weiner PS: The study of childhood language disorders in the nineteenth century. **ASHA** 1984 Apr;26(4):35–8
Ziegler CR: The image of the physically handicapped in children's literature. New York, Arno, 1980. 156 p. (Also Ed. D. Diss. Philadelphia, Temple University, 1971).

### Australia

Gandevia B: Childhood mortality in Australia from 1788. In International Congress of the History of Medicine. 26th, Plovdiv, 1978. Actes du Congress. Sofia, 1981. Volume II. p. 100–3.
Lewis M: Milk, mothers, and infant welfare. In J. Roe, ed: Twentieth century Sydney: studies in urban and social history. Sydney, Hale & Iremonger for the Sydney Hist. Group, 1980. p. 193–207.
Lewis M: Some infant health problems in Sydney, 1880–1939. **J R Aust Hist Soc** 1982;68(1):67–73
Lewis M: The problem of infant feeding: the Australian experience from the mid-nineteenth century to the 1920s. **J Hist Med Allied Sci** 1980 Apr;35(2):174–87
Lewis MJ: Populate or perish: aspects of infant and maternal health in Sydney, 1870–1939. [S.l.:s.n.], 1976. xx, 365 p.
The rights of the child: **Aust Paediatr J** 1982 Mar;18(1):6–12

### Austria

Wyklicky H: Uber die Fürsorge Josephs II. für elternlose und kranke Kinder. **Padiatr Padol** 1982;17(2):437–40

### Belgium

André R, Gyselings R: Variation saisonnière de la mortalité infantile en Belgique. **Rev Inst Sociol** 1970;3:587–97
Leboutte R: L'infanticide dans l'est de la Belgique aux XVIIIe-XIXe siècles: une réalité. **Ann Demogr Hist (Paris)** 1983;:163–92
Masuy-Stroobant G: La surmortalité infantile des Flandres au cours de

la deuxième moitié du XIXe siècle: mode d'alimentation ou mode de développement? **Ann Demogr Hist (Paris)** 1983;:231–56
Verheyen H: De zorg voor het gevonden kind te Antwerpen (1830–1870). **Ann Soc Belg Hist Hop** 1978;16:87–109

**Brazil**

Abreu Fialho S de: O Instituto Imperial dos Meninos Cegos. **Rev Inst Hist Geogr Bras** 1977;315:201–31
Goldberg HI, Rodrigues W, Thome AM, et al: Infant mortality and breast-feeding in North-Eastern Brazil. **Popul Stud** 1984 Mar;38(1):105–15
Wood CH: Infant mortality trends and capitalist development in Brazil: the case of Sao Paulo and Belo Horizonte. **Lat Am Perspect** 1977:4(4):56–65

**Bulgaria**

Vutov M, Ivanova K: Stomatologichnata pomost na podrastvastoto pokolenie u nas do September 9, 1944 godina. **Stomatologiia (Sofiia)** 1979 Nov–Dec;61(6):400–5

**Canada**

Buckley S: Efforts to reduce infant maternity mortality in Canada between the two world wars. **Atlantis** 199;2 (2 pt 2):76–84
Delage J: Cinquante ans de pédopsychiatrie à Quebec. De l'Ecole La Jemmerais à la Chaire de Psychiatrie infantile et juvénile (Hôtel-Dieu du Sacré-Coeur). **Neuropsychiatr Enfance Adolesc** 1980 Jun;28(6):239–41
Jones A: In the children's aid: J. J. Kelso and child welfare in Ontario. Toronto, Buffalo, University of Toronto Press, 1981. viii, 210 p.
McLeod K: Hallmarks of reform: social change and the new education in Canada. **Hist Educ Q** 1980;20(3):369–75
Rooke PT, Schnell RL: Charlotte Whitton and the 'babies for export' controversy, 1947–48. **Alberta Hist** 1982;30(1):11–6
Rooke PT, Schnell RL: Child welfare in English Canada. **Soc Serv Rev** 1981;55(3):484–506
Siegel LS: Child health and development in English Canada, 1790–1850. In Roland CG, ed: Health, disease and medicine. Toronto, Hannah Institute for the History of Medicine, 1984. p. 360–80.
Sutherland N: 'To create a strong and healthy race': school children in the public health movement, 1880–1914. **Hist Educ Q** 1972;12(3):304–33
Ward WP, Ward PC: Infant birth weight and nutrition in industrializing Montreal. **Am Hist Rev** 1984;89(2):324–45

**Chile**

Kaempffer AM: Evolución de la salud materno infantil en Chile, 1952–1977. **Rev Med Chil** 1977 Oct;105(10):680–6
Monckeberg F: Lucha contra la desnutrición del niño en Chile, 1952–1977. **Rev Med Chil** 1977 Oct;105(10):687–95

**Czechoslovakia**

Březina Z: Péče o děti v CSSR před dvaceti lety. **Cesk Zdrav** 1984 Feb;32(2):92–3
Fröml F: První skolní lékař na Moravě. **Cas Lek Cesk** 1982 Jun 11;121(23):724–5
Mišurcová V: K 150. výročí institucí předškolní výchovy. **Cesk Pediatr** 1983 Mar;38(3):177–9
Navrátil M: Padesát let Kojeneckého ústavu v Ostravě. **Cesk Pediatr** 1981 Aug;36(8):475–6
Slavětinský M: List z historie severomoravského zdravotnictví. **Vnitr Lek** 1979 Dec;25(12):1219–21
Slosarová V, Tomanová M: 100 let školího lékařství v Praze. **Cesk Pediatr** 1984 Jul;39(7):420–4

**Denmark**

Ryssing E: Historien om Børnehospitalet i Rigensgade og Dronning Louises Børnehospital. **Dan Medicinhist Arbog** 1981;:58–92

**Europe**

Lebrun F: Quand un enfant sur deux mourait. **Histoire** 1982;42:78–81
Ströder J, Schuster J: Estudio comparativo de la mortalidad infantil entre los niños Judios y no Judios en Europa Central y Oriental a finales del siglo diecinueve y principios del veinte. **Folia Hum (Barc)** 1983;21(240):1–10

**Finland**

Lithell UB: Infant mortality rate and standards of living in the past. **Scand J Hist** 1981;6(4):297–315
Turpeinen O: Infant mortality in Finland 1749–1865. **Scand Econ Hist Rev** 1979;27(1):1–21,67
Ylppö A: Lapsen arvostuksesta vuosisatojen aikana. **Duodecim** 1981;97(6):300–5

**France**

Achard A: 'La nourrice sur place'. **Ann Demogr Hist (Paris)** 1984;:259–68
Aron JP: Le régime des nourrices au début du XIXe siècle à Paris. In: Congrès National des Sociétés Savantes, 93e, Tours, 1968. Actes. Paris, 1971. Section d'Histoire Moderne et Contemporaine, Tome 1. p. 207–15.
Bideau A: Variables familiales de la mortalité infantile. In Imhof AE, ed: Mensch und Gesundheit in der Geschichte. Husum, Matthiesen, 1980. p. 223–50.
Brison M: L'école et l'enfant à Lyon: le problème de l'alimentation dans les cantines scolaires. **Rev Hist Deuxieme Guerre Mond** 1982;32(125):37–71
Constantin-Lhuillery A: Les enfants du bureau des pauvres de Chartres (1693–1715). Mém. de maîtrise. Univ. de Tours, 1976, 213 p
Delmas J: Le travail des enfants dans les manufactures de 1841 à 1914. **Bull Soc Fr Hist Hop** 1980;(41):17–25
Dumazet A: 'Au pays des nourrices'. **Ann Demogr Hist (Paris)** 1984;:279–84
Dupré J: Les enfants abandonnés à l'hospice civil et militaire de Châteauroux de 1805 à 1820 inclusivement. **Bull Soc Fr Hist Hop** 1980;(41):9–16
Engrand C: Les abandons d'enfants à Amiens vers la fin de l'Ancien Régime. **Rev Nord** 1982;64(252):73–92
Fay-Sallois F: Les nourrices à Paris au XIXe siècle. Paris, Payot, 1980. 284 p.
Lamarre C: Vivre de charité à l'hôpital de Dijon au XVIIIe siècle: les secours aux enfants et aux viellards. **Bull Soc Fr Hist Hop** 1981;(42):25–35
Lanchy F: La comtesse de Ségur et la santé des enfants. **Rev Hist Pharm (Paris)** 1982;29(252):179–85
Lecomte MC: Les enfants trouvés d'après les archives du bureau des pauvres de Chartres, de 1780 à 1792. Mém. de Maîtrise, Univ. de Tours, 1976. vii, 195 p.
L'Exposition Universelle de 1889: Recherche des réponses au questionnaire et d'objets. **Bull Soc Fr Hist Hop** 1979;(39):19–21
Loux F: Recours convergents à la médecine officielle et à la médecine parallèle en matière de soins aux enfants en France (XIXe–XXe siècles). In Imhof AE, ed: Mensch und Gesundheit in der Geschichte. Husum, Matthiesen, 1980. p. 315–21.
Martin-Fugier A: La fin des nourrices. **Mouvement Soc** 1978 Oct–Dec;11–32
Morel MF: Health and illness in traditional rural France in the 18th and 19th centuries: the example of wet-nurses. **Soc Soc Hist Med Bull (Lond)** 1983 Dec;33:24–6
Morel MF: L'élevage des nourrissons dans la France d'autrefois XVIIIe–XIXe siècles. **Neuropsychiatr Enfance Adolesc** 1982 Apr–May;30(4–5):271–3
Morel MF: Mère, enfant, médecin: la médicalisation de la petite enfance en France (XVIIIe–XIXe siècles). In Imhof AE, ed: Mensch und Gesundheit in der Geschichte. Husum, Matthiesen, 1980. p. 301–13.
Morel MF: Mères et nourrices au XVIIIe siècle: les soins aux jeunes enfants. **Penelope** 1981;(5):29–32
Pelicier Y, Thuillier G: Pour une histoire de l'education des enfants idiots en France (1830–1914). **Rev Hist (Paris)** 1979;261(1):99–130
Perrot M: De la nourrice à l'employée. Travaux de femmes dans la France du XIXe siècle. **Mouvement Soc** 1978 Oct–Dec;3–10
Perrot M: Sur la ségrégation de l'enfance au XIX siècle. **Psychiatr Enfant** 1982;25(1):179–206
Pihet C: Les enfants abandonnés à Poitiers dans la seconde moitié du XVIIIe siècle (1755–1789). Maîtrise, Univ. de Poitiers, 1976, XII, 222 p.
Pollet M: Naissances illégitimes, filles-mères et enfants trouvés à Grasse au XVIIIe siècle, 1751–1789. **Bull Inf Soc Demogr Hist** 1979;:5–21
Roche D: L'amour paternel à Paris au XVIIIe siècle. **Ann Demogr Hist (Paris)** 1983;:73–80
Rollet C: L'allaitement artificiel des nourrissons avant Pasteur. **Ann Demogr Hist (Paris)** 1983;:81–92
Rollet C: Nourrices et nourrissons dans le département de la Seine et en France de 1880 à 1940. **Population** 1982;37(3):573–604
Senior N: Aspects of infant feeding in 18th-century France. **Eighteenth Cent Stud** 1983;16:367–88
Simon N: 1979, au musée de l'Assistance publique de Paris. **Bull Soc Fr Hist Hop** 1980;(41):26–8
Sussman GD: Selling mother's milk. The wet-nursing business in France, 1715–1914. Urbana, University of Illinois Press, 1982. xi, 210 p.
Sussman GD: The end of the wet-nursing business in France, 1874–1914. In R. Wheaton, T. K. Hareven, ed: Family and sexuality in French history. Philadelphia, University of Pennsylvania Press, 1980. p. 224–52.
Thieffry S: Avec Parrot, il y a un siècle, à l'Hospice des Enfants Assistés. **Ann Pediatr (Paris)** 1981 Jan;28(1):63–71

**Germany**

Abe HR, Schmidt H: Dr. med. Marie-Elise Kayser (1885–1950) – ein Leben für die Kinder. **Beitr Gesch Univ Erfurt** 1979–83;19:293–8
Becker KH, Schmidt HD: Uber eine bisher unerschlossene Quelle der Preyer-Forschung. **Z Psychol** 1984;192(2):182–91

Cieślawski M: Z przezyć dzieci i matek-robotnic przymusowych na Pomorzu Zachodnim. **Przegl Lek** 1981;38(1):121-4

Gieger G: Schwachsinnigenfürsorge und Hilfe für das geistig behinderte Kind. Eine Analyse der 'Zeitschrift für das Idiotenwesen' (1880-1934). Freiburg, Schulz, 1977. 245 p. (Freiburger Forschungen zur Medizingeschichte, Neue Folge, 6).

Helvétius CA: Anfänge der Erziehung. Claude Adrien Helvètius (1772). **Krankenpfl J** 1984 Mar 1;22(3):30-1

Kalcher J: Ambrosius war kein Dinosaurier--dem Hansischen Jugendbund nachträglich zum Geburtstag. Versuch einer Deutung. **Prax Kinderpsychol Kinderpsychiatr** 1979 Aug-Sep;28(6):212-24

Kneist W: Arzte als Gesundheitserzieher von Kindern. **Z Gesamte Hyg** 1982 Apr;28(4):256-9

Knodel J, Hermalin AI: Effects of birth rank, maternal age, birth interval, and sibship size on infant and child mortality: evidence from 18th and 19th century reproductive histories. **Am J Public Health** 1984 Oct;74(10):1098-106

Knodel J: Seasonal variation in infant mortality: an approach with applications. **Ann Demogr Hist (Paris)** 1983;:208-30

Kreis R: The history of childhood through German literature: a psychogenic model. **J Psychohist** 1982 Winter;9(3):311-9

Lindemann M: Love for hire: the regulation of the wet-nursing business in eighteenth-century Hamburg. **J Fam Hist** 1981 Winter;6(4):379-95

Marcusson H: Zusammenhang zwischen Sozialpolitik und Gesundheitsschutz für Mutter und Kind--Ein Rückblick über 80 Jahre. **Z Gesamte Hyg** 1979 Oct;25(10):775-80

Murken AH, ed: Kind, Krankheit und Krankenhaus im Bilderbuch von 1900 bis 1982. (Studien zur Medizin-, Kunst- und Literaturgeschichte. Band 5.). Herzogenrath, Verlag Murken-Altrogge, 1982. 238 p.

Pankoke KT: Im wilhelminischen Preussen nahm man sie ernst. Zur Geschichte der Jugendzahnpflege in Deutschland. **Zahnarzt** 1984 Aug;28(8):619-21

Spree R: Die Entwicklung der differentiellen Säuglingssterblichkeit in Deutschland seit der Mitte des 19. Jahrhunderts. (Ein Versuch zur Mentalitäts-Geschichte). In Imhof AE, ed: Mensch und Gesundheit in der Geschichte. Husum, Matthiesen, 1980. p. 251-78.

Sprung H, Sprung L: William Thkerry Preyer (1841-1897) als Methodologe und Methodiker. **Z Psychol** 1984;192(2):170-81

Stephan P: Geburtlichkeit und Kindersterblichkeit in einem Dorf im 17. und 18. Jahrhundert. **Arztl Jugendkd** 1984 Jun;75(3):178-89

Teubel S: Schulhygiene in der Zeit von 1870 bis 1900. Diss. Bonn, 1981. 149 p.

Wunderlich P: Die Anfänge der Staatlichen Waisen-Fürsorge in Sachsen unter August dem Starken (Waldheim 1716). **Kinderarztl Prax** 1984 Nov;52(11):510-20

### Ghana

Ofosu-Amaah S: The maternal and child health services in Ghana (their origins and future). **J Trop Med Hyg** 1981 Dec;84(6):265-9

### Great Britain

Behlmer GK: Child abuse and moral reform in England, 1870-1908. Stanford, Stanford University Press, 1982. viii, 320 p.

Bloor DU: The certifying surgeons. **J R Coll Gen Pract** 1981 Jan;31(222):33-7

Bound JP, Harvey PW, Brookes DM, et al: The incidence of anencephalus in the Fylde peninsula 1956-76 and changes in water hardness. **J Epidemiol Community Health** 1981 Jun;35(2):102-5

C[one] TE: A plea to give weakly children a fair chance, by William Farr (1865). **Pediatrics** 1981;68:49

Cameron N: The growth of London schoolchildren 1904-1966: an analysis of secular trend and intra-county variation. **Ann Hum Biol** 1979 Nov-Dec;6(6):505-25

Checkland O: Maternal and child welfare. In Checkland O, Lamb M, ed: Health care as social history; the Glasgow case. Aberdeen, Aberdeen University Press, 1982. p. 117-33.

Dyhouse C: Working-class mothers and infant mortality in England, 1895-1914. **J Soc Hist** 1978;12(2):248-67

Dyhouse C: Working-class mothers and infant mortality in England, 1895-1914. In C. Webster, ed: Biology, medicine and society 1840-1940. Cambridge, Cambridge University Press, 1981. p. 73-98.

Feinstein SC: Why they were afraid of Virginia Woolf: perspectives on juvenile manic-depressive illness. **Adolesc Psychiatry** 1980;8:332-43

Fildes V: Neonatal feeding practices and infant mortality during the 18th century. **J Biosoc Sci** 1980 Jul;12(3):313-24

Fildes V: Weaning the Elizabethan child. **Nurs Times** 1980 July-Aug 7;76:31-32:1357-9,1402-3

Fisch L: Development of school screening audiometry. **Br J Audiol** 1981 May;15(2):87-95

Gelbier S: Frederick Breese and London's first school dental clinic. **Br Dent J** 1981 Nov 3;151(9):309-11

Goldstein J: Anna Freud in law. **Psychoanal Study Child** 1984;39:3-13

Hallett GE: Progress of children's dentistry. **Br Dent J** 1980 Jul 1;149(1):13-6

Hansen E: 'Overlaying' in 19th-century England: infant mortality in infanticide? **Hum Ecol** 1979;7:333-52

Hare EH, Moran PA, Macfarlane A: The changing seasonality of infant deaths in England and Wales 1912-78 and its relation to seasonal temperature. **J Epidemiol Community Health** 1981 Jun;35(2):77-82

Herzka HS, Otti L: Geschichte der Kindheit--zum Belspiel: Industrialisierung. **Acta Paedopsychiatr (Basel)** 1984 May;50(1):5-6

Heywood JS: Childhood and society a hundred years ago. London, [1969]. 72 p.

Hirst JD: A failure 'without parallel': the School Medical Service and the London County Council 1907-12. **Med Hist** 1981 Jul;25(3):281-300

Jordan TE: Lancashire lasses and Yorkshire lads: childhood in the early nineteenth century. **R Soc Health J** 1982 Feb;102(1):14-20

Knox PL: Convergence and divergence in regional patterns of infant mortality in the United Kingdom from 1949-51 to 1970-72. **Soc Sci Med** 1981;15(3):323-8

Langford CM: A consideration of some retrospective data on breast-feeding in Great Britain. **J Biosoc Sci** 1978;10:389-400

Leavy BF: Fathering and the British Mother's Magazine, 1845-1864. **Victorian Period Rev** 1980;13(1-2):10-7

Lewis IC: The years of children. Part I. **Aust Nurses J** 1980 Jul;10(1):46-9

Lewis J: The politics of motherhood: child and maternal welfare in England, 1900-1939. London, Croom Helm, 1980. 235 p.

Lomax E: Charles West (1816-1898) on the mental peculiarieties and disorders of childhood. In International Congress of the History of Medicine, 27th, Barcelona, 1980. Actas. Barcelona, Acadèmia de Ciències Mèdiques de Catalunya i Balears, 1981. p. 98-102.

McClure RK: Coram's children, the London Foundling Hospital in the eighteenth century. New Haven, Yale University Press, 1981. xiii, 321 p.

Montague L: Ambassadors of the king. **Nurs Times** 1983 Dec 14-20;79(50):57-60

Pharoah PO, Alberman ED: Mortality of low birthweight infants in England and Wales 1953 to 1979. **Arch Dis Child** 1981 Feb;56(2):86-9

Riley D: 'The free mothers': pronatalism and working women in industry at the end of the last war in Britain. **Hist Workshop J** 1981;11:59-118

Rodin AE: Infants and gin mania in 18th-century London. **JAMA** 1981 Mar 27;245(12):1237-9

Solnit AJ, Newman LM: Anna Freud: the child expert. **Psychoanal Study Child** 1984;39:45-63

Wallerstein RS: Anna Freud: radical innovator and staunch conservative. **Psychoanal Study Child** 1984;39:65-80

Watterson P: Environmental factors in infant and early childhood mortality decline in England and Wales, 1895 to 1910. **Soc Soc Hist Med Bull (Lond)** 1984 Dec;35:37-40

Wilson AF: The Enlightenment and infant care. **Soc Soc Hist Med Bull (Lond)** 1979 Dec;25:44-7

### Haiti

Wallace CE, Marshall FN, Robinson C: A retrospective review of maternal and child health services at the Albert Schweitzer Hospital in rural Haiti. **Bull Pan Am Health Organ** 1982;16(1):7-16

### India

Bagley C: Social policy and development: the case of child welfare, health and nutritional services in India. **Plural Soc** 1979;10(1):3-26

### Indonesia

Bracher MD, Santow G: Breast-feeding in Central Java. **Popul Stud** 1982 Nov;36(3):413-29

### Italy

Bèttica-Giovannini R: Giuseppe Berruti e l'Ospizio Marino Piemontese per ragazzi scrofolosi poveri con una nota su la fondazione dell'Ospedale Maria Vittoria di Torino (1887). **Ann Osp Maria Vittoria Torino** 1977 Jul-Dec;20(7-12):227-340

Della Peruta F: Infanzia e famiglia nella prima metà dell'ottocento. **Studi Stor** 1979;20(3):473-91

### Japan

Fukuyama Y: A quarter-century of the Japanese Society of Child Neurology. **Brain Dev** 1984;6(2):109-18

Koba F: [History of school health nursing] (Jpn). **Kango** 1984 Jun;36(7):38-46

Matsumoto S: [Maternal and child health in Japan during last 80 years (author's transl)] (Jpn). **Nippon Sanka Fujinka Gakkai Zasshi** 1980 Sep;32(9):1171-9

### Malaysia

Manderson L: Bottle feeding and ideology in colonial Malaya: the production of change. **Int J Health Serv** 1982;12(4):597-616

# CHILD HEALTH

### Mexico

Espinosa de los Reyes V: El doctor Isidro Espinosa de los Reyes y los inicios de la atención materno-infantil en México. **Gac Med Mex** 1981 Feb;117(2):81-7

Frenk S: Historia reciente de la asistencia materno-infantil en México. **Salud Publica Mex** 1983 Sep-Oct;25(5):513-7

Malvido E: El abandono de los hijos--una forma de control del tamaño la familia y del trabajo indígena--Tula (1683-1730). **Hist Mex** 1980;29:521-61

Mina VA: Estimaciones de los niveles, tendencias y diferenciales de la mortalidad infantil y en los primeros años de vida en México, 1940-77. **Demogr Econ** 1981;15(1):85-142

### Netherlands

Knecht, van Eekelen A de: Bakerboekjes in de 19e eeuw: en aanvulling. **Tijdschr Geschied Geneeskd** 1981;4(1):45-7

### New Zealand

Olssen E: Truby King and the Plunket Society: an analysis of a prescriptive ideology. **NZ J Hist** 1981;15(1):3-23

### Poland

Felchner A, Pepłowska E: Polski Komitet Pomocy Sanitarnej jednym z prekursorów świeckiego pielegniarstwa w Polsce. **Arch Hist Med (Warsz)** 1984;47(1):91-7

Jaroszewski Z, Tarmanowska B: Dzieci w Instytucie Higieny Psychicznej (w Warszawie, 1943-1944). **Przegl Lek** 1981;38(1):152-5

Radiukiewicz S: Opieka nad matką i dzieckiem. **Pieleg Polozna** 1981;(6):1-3

Sosińska-Trawińska M: Zalecenia lecznicze w chorobach dzieci zawarte w wybranych czasopismach nielekarskich XVIII w w Polsce. **Arch Hist Med (Warsz)** 1983;46(3):285-94

Supady J: Wpływ wychowania i nauczania domowego oraz szkolnego na psychofizyczny rozwój młodzieży szlacheckiej w Polsce w XVIII w. **Wiad Lek** 1981 May 1;34(9):789-98

### Portugal

André R, Pereira-Roque J: La mortalité infantile au Portugal. **Rev Inst Sociol** 1972;3:573-91

### Romania

Lucaşciuc A: Din istoricul ocrotirii mamei şi copilului în România (II). **Viata Med [Medii Sanit]** 1979 Oct;27(10):235-7

Negru I: 'Secolul copilului' in discuţia congreselor medicale din România (1919 şi 1925). **Viata Med [Medii Sanit]** 1982 Feb;30(2):45-7

Ploeşteanu I: Aspecte ale activitătii de ocrotire a mamei şi copilului în România, în perioada dintre cele două războaie mondiale. **Viata Med [Medii Sanit]** 1981 Jan;29(1):21-3

### Spain

Bouza Brey F: Las enfermedades infantiles de Rosalia de Castro y los ritos de medicina magica en Galicia. **Cuad Estud Gallegos** 1967;22(67):183-97

### Sweden

Brändström A, Broström G, Persson LA: The impact of feeding patterns on infant mortality in a nineteenth century Swedish parish. **J Trop Pediatr** 1984 Jun;30(3):154-9

Hedenvind A: Födelseår 1903. **Arbetarrörel Arsb** 1975;:32-42

Källén B, Löfkvist E: Time trends of spina bifida in Sweden 1947-81. **J Epidemiol Community Health** 1984 Jun;38(2):103-7

Mattsson V: Ammor och barnafödande i Malmö 1750-1850. **Scandia** 1980;46(2):173-98

### Switzerland

Caramelli N: Introduzione a Piaget. **Stor Crit Psicol** 1981;2(1):5-85

Eckstaedt A: 'Mimi überreicht Madam Grenouillet einen Blumenstrauss'. Eine psychoanalytische Studie über den Weg der Phantasie des vierjährigen Paul Klee anhand einer Kinderzeichnung. **Psyche (Stuttg)** 1980 Dec:34(12):1123-44

Pulaski MS: Understanding Piaget. Revised and expanded ed. New York, Harper & Row, 1980. xvii, 248 p.

### Thailand

Frenzen PD, Hogan DP: The impact of class, education, and health care on infant mortality in a developing society: the case of rural Thailand. **Demography** 1982 Aug;19(3):391-408

### United States

Apple RD: 'How shall I feed my baby?' Infant feeding in the United States, 1870-1940. Ph. D. Diss., University of Wisconsin. Madison, 1981. xxxiii, 428 p.

Apple RD: 'To be used only under the direction of a physician': commercial infant feeding and medical practice, 1870-1940. **Bull Hist Med** 1980 Fall;54(3):402-17

Baumgartner L: Two hundred years of children. **Trans Stud Coll Physicians Phila** 1977 Apr;44(4):165-78

Berger LR, Johansson SR: Child health in the workplace: the Supreme Court in Hammer v. Dagenhart (1918). **J Health Polit Policy Law** 1980 Spring;5(1):81-97

Berkelhamer JE, Noyes EJ, Chen RT: Child health policy-an overview of federal involvement. **Adv Pediatr** 1982;29:211-8

Boone MS: A socio-medical study of infant mortality among disadvantaged Blacks. **Hum Organ** 1982;41(3):227-36

Brown DC: Health of farm children in the South, 1900-1950. **Agric Hist** 1979;53(1):170-87

Buser BN: The evolution of school health services: New York and nationwide. **J Sch Health** 1980 Oct;50(8):475-7

C[one] TE: The appalling industrial hazards to which American working children were exposed in 1900. **Pediatrics** 1981;68:378

Children's Bureau studies: Introduction by W. M. Schmidt. New York, Arno, 1974. Reprinted works by various authors.

Cone TE: On dressing the American newborn infant a century ago. **Pediatrics** 1981;67:268

Davoren E: The profession of social work and the protection of children. In E. H. Newberger, ed: Child abuse. Boston, Little, Brown and Company, 1982. p. 257-73.

Enarson HL: Perspectives on college health in the 80's: a president's view. **J Am Coll Health Assoc** 1981 Aug;30(1):11-3

English PC: Pediatrics and the unwanted child in history: foundling homes, disease, and the origins of foster care in New York City, 1860 to 1920. **Pediatrics** 1984 May;73(5):699-711

Figa'Talamanca I, Galmacci G: Infant mortality and economic stability. An analysis of the last century. **Nuovi Ann Ig Microbiol** 1979 Mar-Apr;30(2):107-26

Giglio JN: Voluntarism and public policy between World War I and the New Deal: Herbert Hoover and the American Child Health Association. **Pres Stud Q** 1983;13(3):430-52

Gordon S: Motherhood is powerful. **Work Pap Mag** 1982;9(2):15-9

Graebner W: Doing the world's unhealthy work: the fiction of free choice. **Hastings Cent Rep** 1984 Aug;14(4):28-37

Hannemann EA: Little Laura and others like her. Health care of American Colonial children. **Indiana Med** 1984 Jan;77(1):48-52

The health of women and children. New York, Arno, 1977. Varius paginations. Five reprinted articles by various authors, 1909-1953.:

Hedderson J, Daudistel HC: Infant mortality of the Spanish surname population. **Soc Sci J** 1982;19(4):67-78

Hefner LL: The National Women's Relief Society and the U.S. Sheppard-Towner Act. **Utah Hist Q** 1982;50(3):255-67

Heins M: Landmark perspective: The 'battered child' revisited. **JAMA** 1984 Jun 22-29;251(24):3295-300

Hirschman C, Butler M: Trends and differentials in breast feeding: an update. **Demography** 1981 Feb;18(1):39-54

Hoekelman RA: Well-child visits revisited. **Am J Dis Child** 1983 Jan;137(1):17-20

Ihde AJ: Lydia Jane Roberts. In: Notable American women. The modern period. Cambridge, Mass., Belknap-Harvard Univ. Press, 1980. 4:580-1.

Jackson DJ: Contributions to the history of psychology: XXXV. Dorothy Burlingham. **Psychol Rep** 1984 Jun;54(3):855-63

Jacobs SE: 'Our babies shall not die': a community's response to medical neglect. **Hum Organ** 1979;38(2):120-33

Johnson JP: Herbert Hoover: the orphan as children's friend. **Prologue J Nat Arch** 1980;12(4):193-206

Johnson MP: Smothered slave infants; were slave mothers at fault? **J South Hist** 1981;47(4):493-520

Johnson MP, Hufbauer K: Sudden infant death syndrome as a medical research problem since 1945. **Soc Probl** 1982;30(1):65-81

Kett JF: Rites of passage. Adolescence in America, 1790 to the present. New York, Basic Books, 1977. ix, 327 p.

Kiple KF, Kiple VH: Slave child mortality: some nutritional answers to a perennial puzzle. **J Soc Hist** 1977 Mar;10(3):284-309

Levin H: Conservatism of social work. **Soc Serv Rev** 1982;56(4):605-15

Loevy HT: M. Evangeline Jordon, pioneer in pedodontics. **Bull Hist Dent** 1984;32(1):19-26

McConnell NF, Dore MM: Crittenton services, the first century, 1883-1983. Washington, D.C., National Florence Crittenton Mission, 1983. vi, 95 p.

Mason LB: Babies hospital, 1920-1978. **NC Med J** 1984 Jan;45(1):53-6

Mennel RM: Ethel Sturges Dummer. In: Notable American women. The modern period. Cambridge, Mass., Belknap-Harvard Univ. Press, 1980. 4:208-10.

Orme JG, Stuart P: The Habit Clinics: behavioral social work and prevention in the 1920s. **Soc Serv Rev** 1981;55(2):242-56

Page SL: The law, the lawyer, and medical aspects of child abuse. In

E. H. Newberger, ed: Child abuse. Boston, Little, Brown and Company, 1982. p. 105–35.
Parker JK, Carpenter EM: Julia Lathrop and the Children's Bureau: the emergence of an institution. **Soc Serv Rev** 1981;55(1):60–77
Peck DL, Bharadwaj LK: Personal stress and fatalism as factors in college suicide. **Soc Sci** 1980;55(1):19–24
Remley ML: Jessie Hubbell Bancroft. In: Notable American women. The modern period. Cambridge, Mass., Belknap–Harvard Univ. Press, 1980. 4:46–7.
Rhodes SL: Trends in child development research important to day–care policy. **Soc Serv Rev** 1979;53(2):285–94
Robinton ED: Dorothy Reed Mendenhall. In: Notable American women. The modern period. Cambridge, Mass., Belknap–Harvard Univ. Press, 1980. 4:468–70.
Salkever DS: Effects of children's health on maternal hours of work: a preliminary analysis. **South Econ J** 1980;47(1):156–66
Sharma OP, James DG: Did Osler's patient, Hannah W, have sarcoidosis? An historical footnote. **Chest** 1984 Aug;86(2):263–4
Siefert K: An exemplar of primary prevention in social work: the Sheppard–Towner Act of 1921. **Soc Work Health Care** 1983 Fall;9(1):87–103
Silverman WA: Incubator–baby side shows (Dr. Martin A. Couney). **Pediatrics** 64(2):127–41, Aug 79
Snodgrass J: William Healy (1869–1963): pioneer child psychiatrist and criminologist. **J Hist Behav Sci** 1984 Oct;20(4):332–9
Takanishi R: Childhood as a social issue: historical roots of contemporary child advocacy movements. **J Soc Issues** 1978;34(2):8–28
Tank RM: Young children, families, and society in America since the 1820s: the evolution of health, education, and child care programs for preschool children. Ph.D. Diss., University of Michigan. Ann Arbor, 1980. v, 471 leaves.
Thompson HC: 20th–century US child health care. Past, present, future. **Am J Dis Child** 1984 Sep;138(9):804–9
Trattner WI: Homer Folks. In Dictionary of American biography, 1961–1965. Suppl. 7, 1981. p. 250–2.
Twin SL: Ethel Perrin. In: Notable American women. The modern period. Cambridge, Mass., Belknap–Harvard Univ. Press, 1980. 4:539–41.
Waserman MJ: The emergence of modern child health care: pediatrics, public health, and the federal government. Ph.D. Diss., The Catholic University of America, Washington, D. C., 1982. v, 232 p.
Weissman MB: Elizabeth Burchenal. In: Notable American women. The modern period. Cambridge, Mass., Belknap–Harvard Univ. Press, 1980. 4:121–2.
Wheeler R: Health and human resources. **New South** 1971;26(4):2–16
Williams WE: The school physician's notebook: a cameo of William Carlos Williams. In Jones AH, ed: Images of healers. Albany, State University of New York Press, 1983. p. 3–8.
Wilson RK: Charles Henderson–a man stands tall. **J Med Assoc State Ala** 1982 Jun;51(12):41–3
Zelizer VA: The price and value of children: the case of children's insurance. **AJS** 1981;86(5):1036–1056

#### USSR

Beloborodova NL: Moskovskiĭ vospitatel'nyĭ dom i ego rol' v istorii zdravookhraneniia Rossii. **Sov Zdravookhr** 1984;(7):58–61
Borisenko NF, Slepushkina II, Rakitskaia TV: Stanovlenie i razvitie sanitarnoĭ sluzhby po gigiene deteĭ i podrostkov na Ukraine (1919–1938 gg.). **Gig Sanit** 1983 Aug;(8):38–41
Borisenko NF, Slepushkina II, Proklina TL, et al: Stanovlenie i razvitie sanitarnoĭ sluzhby po gigiene deteĭ i podrostkov na Ukraine (1938–1945 gg.). **Gig Sanit** 1984 Aug;(8):44–8
Chesnais JC: La hausse de la mortalité infantile en Union Sovietique. **Population** 1981;36(6):1176–80
Chokin AR, Ibragimov NG: Okhrana materinstva i detstva v Kazakhstane i Bashkirii v pervoe desiatiletie Sovetskoĭ vlasti. **Sov Zdravookhr** 1984;(3):55–9
Danilishina EI: Razvitie okhrany materinstva i detstva v SSSR. **Sov Zdravookhr** 1983;(1):61–4
Danilishina EI: Rol' Narkomzdrava RSFSR v stanovlenii okhrany zdorov'ia materi i rebenka. **Sov Zdravookhr** 1983;(7):59–63
Daniushevskiĭ SM: Leninskaia zabota o detiakh. **Sov Zdravookhr** 1980;(4):10–4
Davis C, Feshbach M: Rising infant mortality in the USSR in the 1970's. Washington, U. S. Dept. of Commerce, Bureau of the Census, 1980. 33 p. (International population reports. Series P–95, no. 74).
Davydov MI: Zabota o detiakh iz istorii deiatel'–nosti Soveta zashchity detei v 1918–1920 godakh. **Istor SSSR** 1979;5:163–71
Démant F: Vplyv Vel'kej októbrovej socialistickej revolúcie na starostlivost' o diet'a ZSSR. **Cesk Pediatr** 1979 Dec;34(12):697–8
Dement'ev IuG: V. M. Velichkina (Bonch–Bruevich)--organizator sluzhby okhrany materinstva i detstva. **Pediatriia** 1979 Nov;(11):53–4
Druzhinina LV: Razvitie detskikh doshkol'nykh uchrezhdeniĭ v SSSR. **Pediatriia** 1982;(9):3–7
Frieden NM: Child care: medical reform in a traditionalist culture. In Ransel DL, ed: The family in Imperial Russia: new lines of historical research. Urbana, University of Illinois Press, 1978. p. 236–59.
Gracheva AG: Sistema okhrany zdorov'ia deteĭ v Rossiiskoĭ Federatsii. **Pediatriia** 1982 Dec;(12):9–11
Granat NE: K 40–letiiu Ukaza Prezidiuma Verkhovnogo Soveta SSSR ob okhrane materinstva i detstva. **Med Sestra** 1984 Jun;43(6):6–10
Hudzenko PM: Vtilennia ideĭ V. I. Lenina u spravu okhorony zdorov'ia baterynstva i dyttnstva. **Pediatr Akush Ginekol** 1980 Mar–Apr;(2):3–7
Ibragimov NG: Uchastie obshchestvennosti v organizatsii okhrany zdorov'ia deteĭ v Bashkirii v pervoe desiatiletie Sovetskoĭ vlasti. **Sov Zdravookhr** 1979;(12):44–7
Kiriushchenkov AP: Zabota Sovetskogo gosudarstva ob okhrane zdorov'ia materi i rebenka. **Feldsher Akush** 1982;47(8):3–9
Mečíř J: Z počátku sovětské dětské psychiatrie. **Cesk Psychiatr** 1979 Dec;75(6):402–7
Muchiev GS, Frolova OG: Okhrana zdorov'ia ploda i novorozhdennogo v SSSR. Moskva, Meditsina, 1979. 207 p.
Nikonchik OK: Razvitie sistemy okhrany materinstva i detstva v SSSR (1922–1982). **Akush Ginekol (Mosk)** 1982;(7):3–7
Novikova ECh: Okhrana zdorov'ia zhenshchin i deteĭ v strane v 60–iu godovshchinu obrazovaniia Soiuza Sovetskikh Sotsialisticheskikh Respublik. **Pediatriia** 1982 Dec;(12):3–8
Novikova ECh: V. I. Lenin i deti. **Vopr Okhr Materin Det** 1980 Apr;25(4):3–7
Radchenko VV: Osoboe vnimanie podrastaiushchemu pokoleniiu (1917–1926 gg). **Sov Arkh** 1979(2):43–6
Romanenko AE: Okhrana zdorov'ia materi i rebenka v Ukrainskoĭ SSR. **Pediatriia** 1982 Dec;(12):11–4
Savchenko NE: Okhrana zdorov'ia deteĭ v Belorusskoĭ SSR. **Pediatriia** 1982 Dec;(12):15–8
Schmidt H: Dr. med Marie–Elise Kayser in ihren Beziehungen zur Sowjetunion. **Beitr Gesch Univ Erfurt** 1979–83;19:299–303
Selezneva VT: N. A. Russkikh--organizator bor'by s detskoĭ smertnost'iu (k 125–letiiu so dnia rozhdeniia). **Sov Zdravookhr** 1982;(7):64–7
Semenova EI: Pervaia detskaia lechebnaia koloniia v Rossii (K 150–letiiu so dnia rozhdeniia D.I. Mendeleeva). **Pediatriia** 1984 Sep;(9):78–9
Shakhmet AV: Deiatel'nost' zhenotdelov Leningrada po okhrane materinstva i detstva (1926--1929). **Sov Zdravookhr** 1980;(4):64–6
Sharmanov TSh: Dostizheniia okhrany materinstva i detstva v Kazakhskoĭ SSR. **Pediatriia** 1982 Dec;(12):18–22
Shereshkov GM, Leont'ev PA: Velikiĭ podvig sovetskogo naroda. **Vopr Okhr Materin Det** 1980 May;25(5):3–6
Shishkin AP: Bor'ba s detskoĭ smertnost'iu v pervye gody Sovetskoĭ vlasti. **Sov Zdravookhr** 1981;(12):46–50
Stahnke J: Skizzen zur Geschichte des russischen Findelhauswesens. Erläutert am St. Petersburger Erziehungshaus. Pattensen (Han.), Wellm, 1983. ix, 628 p. (Würzburger medizinhistorische Forschungen, ix, Bd. 28).
Studenikin MI, Ryleeva RN: Pervyĭ nauchnyĭ tsentr okhrany materinstva idetstva v SSSR. **Pediatriia** 1982 Oct;(10):3–7
Tabolkina NM: Okhrana materinstva i detstva v poslevoennom Leningrade (1945–1948). **Sov Zdravookhr** 1983;(7):67–9
Tambovtsev PD: K istorii organizatsii i razvitiia sanatornoĭ pomoshchi detiam. **Pediatriia** 1983 Sep;:(9):71–3
Ustinovich AK: 50–letie Belorusskogo nauchno–issledovatel'skogo instituta okhrany materinstva i detstva. **Pediatriia** 1982 Jul;(7):74–6
Vengrova IV, Danilishina EI: Sotsial'no–gigienicheskie issledovaniia organizovannogo detskogo naseleniia v 20–e gody v Sibiri i Dal'nem Vostoke. **Sov Zdravookhr** 1981;(4):63–6
Vodop'ianova ZK: 'Nedelia rebenka' v Respublike Sovetov. **Vopr Istor** 1979;11:175–9
Zhukova LA: Narkomzdrav RSFSR v bor'be s detskoĭ besprizornost'iu (1917--1935). **Sov Zdravookhr** 1980;(4):61–3

#### Yugoslavia

Dugački V: Povijesni pregled zaštite vida školske djece i omladine u Hrvatskoj. **Lijec Vjesn** 1979 Aug;101(8):503–5
Nikolić D: Razvoj neonatalne službe bolnice u Vršcu (34–godišnji period: 1947–1981). **Med Pregl** 1982;35(9–10):383–5
Purkov J: Razvoj neonatološke službe u Zrenjaninu. **Med Pregl** 1983 Jan;36(1–2):61–4

## CHIROPRACTIC

### 1700 to Present

Baer HA: A historical overview of British and European chiropractic. **Chiropr Hist** 1984;4(1):11–5
Peper W: Der Chiropraktische Report. Heidelberg, Haug, 1978. 208 p.
Weiant CW: B. J. Palmer and the 'German issue:' the crisis in postwar European chiropractic. **Chiropr Hist** 1982;2(1):41–4

#### Canada

Boase J: Regulation and the paramedical professions: an interest group study. **Can Public Adm** 1982;25(3):332–53
Lee HK: Honoring the founder in his country: conception and struggle for Canada's Memorial College. **Chiropr Hist** 1981;(1):43–5

## CHIROPRACTIC

**United States**

Alloway WJ, Ronkin ME: The social anthropology of chiropractic in Washington, D.C.: project DC/DC. **Chiropr Hist** 1982;2(1):7–11
Anderson RA: Chiropractic in American history: the ins and outs of museums. **Chiropr Hist** 1982;2(1):15–9
Blair WG: The chiropractic story. [s.l., s.n.], 1973. 17 p.
Chiropractors -- healers or quacks? Part 1: The 80-year war with science: **Consum Rep** 1975 Sep;40(9):542–7
Cottam C, Smith EM: The roots of cranial manipulation: Nephi Cottam and 'craniopathy'. **Chiropr Hist** 1981;1(1):31–5
Crisp KA: Chiropractic lyceums: the colorful origins of chiropractic continuing education. **Chiropr Hist** 1984;4(1):17–22
D. D.'s first book: **Chiropr Hist** 1874;4(1):6–10
Ferguson A: The sweetheart of the PSC--Mabel Heath Palmer: the early years. **Chiropr Hist** 1984;4(1):25–8
Gatterman MI: W. A. Budden: the transition through proprietary education, 1924–1954. **Chiropr Hist** 1982;2(1):21–5
Gibbons RW: Chiropractic in America: the historical conflicts of cultism and science. **J Pop Cult** 1977;10:720–31
Gibbons RW: Forgotten parameters of general practice: the chiropractic obstetrician. **Chiropr Hist** 1982;2(1):27–33
Gibbons RW: Physician-chiropractors: medical presence in the evolution of chiropractic. **Bull Hist Med** 1981 Summer;55(2):233–45
Gibbons RW: Solon Massey Langworthy: keeper of the flame during the 'lost years' of chiropractic. **Chiropr Hist** 1981;1(1):15–21
Gielow V: Daniel David Palmer: rediscovering the frontier years, 1845–1887. **Chiropr Hist** 1981;1(1):11–3
Gilliand E: The legalization of chiropractic in the state of Louisiana. **North La Hist Assoc J** 1981;12(2–3):104–10
Gromala T: Broadsides, epigrams, and testimonials: the evolution of chiropractic advertising. **Chiropr Hist** 1984;4(1):41–5
Miller L: The role of a Braucher-chiropractor in an Amish community. **Mennon Q Rev** 1981;55(2):157–71
Napolitano EG, Gruber B: The struggle for accreditation in chiropractic: a unique history of educational bootstrapping. **Chiropr Hist** 1981;1(1):23–4
Patzwald GA: Discovering and recording chiropractic history: for a systematic program in the profession. **Chiropr Hist** 1981;1(1):5–9
Ransom JF: The origins of chiropractic physiological therapeutics: Howard, Forester and Schulze. **Chiropr Hist** 1984;4(1):47–52
Rehm WS: In tribute to a living pioneer: Dr. Lyndon Edmund Lee. **Chiropr Hist** 1981;1(1):47–50
Rosenthal MJ: The structural approach to chiropractic: from Willard Carver to present practice. **Chiropr Hist** 1981;1(1):25–8
Walden DM: Rebels among dissenters: a local history of chiropractic in Provo, Utah. **Chiropr Hist** 1984;4(1):55–61
Wardwell WI: The cutting edge of chiropractic recognition: prosecution and legislation in Massachusetts. **Chiropr Hist** 1982;2(1):55–65
Westbrooks B: The troubled legacy of Harvey Lillard: the black experience in chiropractic. **Chiropr Hist** 1982;2(1):47–53

## CLIMATE

Lundquist SB: Blixtens inverkan på människan - magi och vetenskap. **Sydsven Medicinhist Sallsk Arsskr** 1981;:98–113
Pelling M: Social history of medicine and the geographers--a bibliography. **Soc Soc Hist Med Bull (Lond)** 1984 Dec;35:55–8
Sargent F: Hippocratic heritage. A history of ideas about weather and human health. New York, Pergamon, 1982. xlii, 581 p. (Pergamon International Library of Science, Technology, Engineering and Social Studies).
Swantes HJ, Lamsfuss J: Historische Beobachtungen über den Wetter- und Klimaeinfluss auf Krankheiten diskutiert aus heutiger Sicht. **Med Welt** 1981 Nov 20;32(47):1802–7

**Africa**

Miller JC: The significance of drought, disease and famine in the agriculturally marginal zones of West-Central Africa. **J Afr Hist** 1982;23(1):17–61

**Americas**

Puckrein G: Climate, health and black labor in the English Americas. **J Am Stud** 1979;13(2):179–93

**1450–1700**

Dobson MJ: Environments of disease and mortality in the New World and the Old World. **Soc Soc Hist Med Bull (Lond)** 1984 Dec;35:7–10

**Americas**

Wear A: Perceptions of health and environment in the settlement of North America in the early seventeenth century. **Soc Soc Hist Med Bull (Lond)** 1984 Dec;35:11–3

**United States**

Earle C: Environment, disease and mortality in early Virginia. **J Hist Geogr** 1979;5(4):365–90

**1700 to Present**

Black LT: Volcanism as a factor in human ecology: the Aleutian case. **Ethnohistory** 1981;28(4):313–40
Schnitzler H, Lieth H: 25 year activities of the International Society of Biometeorology and 25 year publication index. **Int J Biometeorol** 1983 Dec;27(4):287–434

**Argentina**

Semorile A: Aspectos sanitarios del terremoto de Mendoza de 1861. In Congreso de Historia de la Medicina Argentina [Transactions], 5th, Mendoza, 1983. p. 19–32.

**France**

Comiti VP: La géographie médicale de la Corse à la fin du XVIIIe siècle. Genève, Droz, 1980. 142 p. (Centre de Recherches d'Histoire et de Philologie de la IVe Section de l'Ecole pratique des Hautes Etudes; Hautes Etudes Médiévales et Modernes, 41).
Desaive JP: Médecins, climat et épidémies à la fin du XVIIIe siècle. Paris, Mouton, [1972]. 254 p.
Favre R: De 'médico-topographique' à Lyon en 1783. **Dix-Huit Siecle** 1977;9:151–9
Houdaille J: Mouvement saisonnier des conceptions en France de 1740 à 1829. **Population** 1979;34(2):452–57

**Great Britain**

Craig P: Medical topography. **Soc Soc Hist Med Bull (Lond)** 1984 Dec;35:33–4
Gorham E: Robert Angus Smith, F.R.S., and 'Chemical climatology'. **Notes Rec R Soc Lond** 1982 Feb;36(2):267–72
Hare EH, Moran PA, Macfarlane A: The changing seasonality of infant deaths in England and Wales 1912–78 and its relation to seasonal temperature. **J Epidemiol Community Health** 1981 Jun;35(2):77–82
Read MB: A 19th-century weatherman, Dr. George Henry [sic] Fielding of Grove House, Tonbridge. **Cantium** 1972;3,4(4):99–100
Watterson P: Environmental factors in infant and early childhood mortality decline in England and Wales, 1895 to 1910. **Soc Soc Hist Med Bull (Lond)** 1984 Dec;35:37–40

**Italy**

Cremona GF: La bioclimatologia medica: aspetti dell'evoluzione storica, con particolare riguardo al contributo degli scienziati piemontesi. **Ann Osp Maria Vittoria Torino** 1982 Jul-Dec;25(7–12):245–58

## COLD

Bru Villaseca L: Física del frío y medicina. **An R Acad Nac Med (Madr)** 1983;100(2):243–78
Daněk K: Skiing in and through the history of medicine. **Nord Medicinhist Arsb** 1982;:86–100
Shepherd J, Dawber RP: The historical and scientific basis of cryosurgery. **Clin Exp Dermatol** 1982 May;7(3):321–8

**1700 to Present**

Alfredsson JH, Gudmundsson SP, Snaedal G: Artificial insemination by donor with frozen semen. **Obstet Gynecol Surv** 1983 Jun;38(6):305–13
Francis TJ: Non freezing cold injury: a historical review. **J R Nav Med Serv** 1984 Winter;70(3):134–9
Okamura H, Kito O, Sakamoto T, et al: [History and prospect of hypothermia] (Jpn). **Rinsho Kyobu Geka** 1983 May;3(3):321–30
Templin DW: Some historical aspects of the treatment of hypothermia. **Alaska Med** 1984 Jan-Mar;26(1):13
Zingg W: Historical use of hypothermia for cancer. **Can J Surg** 1983 Mar;26(2):97–8

**Great Britain**

Craig RP: Military cold injury during the war in the Falkland Islands 1982: an evaluation of possible risk factors. **J R Army Med Corps** 1984 Jun;130(2):89–96

**USSR**

Matusov AL: Iz istorii meditsinskogo obespecheniia russkikh morskikh i poliarnykh ekspeditsiĭ. Leningrad, Gidrometeoizdat, 1972. 118 p.

**Yugoslavia**

Zimolo A: Kongelacije s naročitim osvrtom na preventivne mjere. **Lijec Vjesn** 1979 Nov;101(11):710–3

## COMMUNICABLE DISEASE CONTROL

See also **Preventive Medicine; Public Health**

Chase A: Magic shots: a human and scientific account of the long and continuing struggle to eradicate infectious diseases by vaccination. New York, Morrow, 1982. 576 p.
Gepts-Friedenreich E: Ziekenhuishygiëne vroeger en nu. **FNIB** 1981 Apr;59(2):7–15
Grundy JH: The evolution and impact of medical entomology. **J R Army Med Corps** 1980 Oct;126(3):140–50
Prindle RF: Disinfection--yesterday and today. **Resid Staff Physician** 1977 Dec;23(12):suppl 1s–5s, 10s–11s
Radovi sa Medunarodnog simpozija u povodu sestote obljetnice Dubrovacke karantene: Dubrovnik, 29. i 30. rujna 1977. Zagreb, Jugoslavenska Akademija Znanosti i Umjetnosti, 1980. 173 p.
Schadewaldt H: Infektionskrankheiten in Kunstdarstellungen. In Ganzinger K, Skopec M, Wyklicky H, ed: Festschrift für Erna Lesky zum 70. Geburtstag. Wien, Brüder Hollinek, 1981. p. 87–96.
Walters EM: Infection control up to the Renaissance. **Nurs Times** 1981 Sep 2;77 Supp(36):JICN16–8
Weiss MM: Fumigated mail. **J Ky Med Assoc** 1981 Jan;79(1):19–22
Winslow CE: The conquest of epidemic disease: a chapter in the history of ideas. Madison, University of Wisconsin Press, 1980 printing, c1971. viii, 411 p.

**Canada**

Canada's amazing health history: let's murder the medical officer: **Can J Public Health** 1984 Sep–Oct;75(5):344–7

**France**

Hildesheimer F: Le Bureau de la Santé de Marseille sous l'Ancien Régime. Le renfermement de la contagion. Marseille, Fédération historique de Provence, 1980. 256 p.
Huard P, Comiti VP: Quarantaine et lazarets en France. In Radovi sa Medunarodnog simpozija u povodu sestote obljetnice Dubrovacke karantene. Dubrovnik, 29 i 30. rujna 1977. Zagreb, 1980. p. 121–34.

**Germany**

Schadewaldt H: Die Entwicklung der Quarantäne in Deutschen Seehäfen. In Radovi sa Medunarodnog simpozija u povodu sestote obljetnice Dubrovacke karantene. Dubrovnik, 29 i 30. rujna 1977. Zagreb, 1980. p. 137–50.

**Italy**

Anselmi S, Sorcinelli P: Epidemie e rivalità commerciali nelle piazze maritime marchigiane (secoli XVI–XIX). **Econ Stor** 1977;24(3):293–310
Premuda L: Storia della quarantena nei porti italiani. In Radovi sa Medunarodnog simpozija u povodu sestote obljetnice Dubrovacke karantene. Dubrovnik, 29 i 30. rujna 1977. Zagreb, 1980. p. 107–18.

**Malta**

Püschel E: Die Quarantäne auf Malta. Geschichte--Lazarettos und Hospital--Vorschriften. In Göpfert W, Otten HH, ed: Metavoeite: wandelt euch durch neues Denken. Düsseldorf, Triltsch, 1983. p. 95–105.

**Romania**

Barbu G: Din istoria combaterii epidemiilor în țara noastră. (I). Frățiile milosteniei. **Rev Ig [Bacteriol]** 1984 Apr–Jun;29(2):189–92

**United States**

Hinman AR: Prospects for disease eradication or elimination. **NY State J Med** 1984 Oct;84(10):502–6
Smith CM: Control of tuberculosis in Delaware: an historical perspective on joint public and private involvement. **Del Med J** 1983 Oct;55(10):593–7

**Yugoslavia**

Glesinger L: Der Ursprung der Pestepidemien und deren Vorbeugungsmethoden im Alten Dubrovnik. In Radovi sa Medunarodnog simpozija u povodu sestote obljetnice Dubrovacke karantene. Dubrovnik, 29 i 30. rujna 1977. Zagreb, 1980. p. 93–102.
Tartalja H: Pomorska zdravstvena zaštita u narodnooslobodilackoj borbi. In Radovi sa Medunarodnog simpozija u povodu sestote obljetnice Dubrovacke karantene. Dubrovnik, 29 i 30. rujna 1977. Zagreb, 1980. p. 153–71.

**500 A.D.–1450**

Carmichael AG: Plague legislation in the Italian Renaissance. **Bull Hist Med** 1983 Winter;57(4):508–25

**Yugoslavia**

Mitić I: Utjecaj kopnene trgovine na osnivanje dubrovačke karantene u XIV. In Radovi sa Medunarodnog simpozija u povodu sestote obljetnice Dubrovacke karantene. Dubrovnik, 29 i 30. rujna 1977. Zagreb, 1980. p. 85–90.

**1450–1700**

Walters EM: Infection control and the Renaissance. **Nurs Times** 1982 Feb 17–23;78(7):suppl 8

**Italy**

Cipolla CM: Fighting the plague in seventeenth-century Italy. Madison, University of Wisconsin Press, 1981, xi, 123 p. (Merle Curti Lectures, 1978).

**Switzerland**

Waldis V: Hospitalisation und Absonderung in Pestzeiten--die Schweiz im Vergleich zu Oberitalien. **Gesnerus** 1982;39(1):71–8

**Yugoslavia**

Grmek MD: Le concept d'infection dans l'Antiquité et au Moyen Age, les anciennes mesures sociales contre les maladies contagieuses et la fondation de la première quarantaine à Dubrovnik (1377). In Radovi sa Medunarodnog simpozija u povodu sestote obljetnice Dubrovacke karantene. Dubrovnik, 29 i 30. rujna 1977. Zagreb, 1980. p. 9–54.

**1700 to Present**

Agafonov VI: Nekotorye uroki iz opyta Velikoĭ Otechestvennoĭ voĭny 1941–1945 gg. i zadachi po dal'neĭshemu sovershenstvovaniiu protivoépidemicheskoĭ raboty. **Zh Mikrobiol Epidemiol Immunobiol** 1980 May;(5):3–6
Altemeier WA: Sepsis in surgery. **Arch Surg** 1982 Feb;117(2):107–12
Brück C: Vaccination och smittskoppor--ett livs erfarenhet. **Nord Medicinhist Arsb** 1982;:122–36
Bugyi I: Az antisepsistöl a hyperasepsisig. **Orv Hetil** 1981 Feb 8;122(6):345–7
Christol D: Historique et définitions de l'antisepsie et de la désinfection. Leurs frontières. Position actuelle du problème. **Rev Prat** 1980 Jun 11;30(33):2159–65
Collins JJ: The contribution of medical measures to the decline of mortality from respiratory tuberculosis: an age-period-cohort model. **Demography** 1982 Aug;19(3):409–27
Doberneck RC, Kleinman R: The surgical garb. **Surgery** 1984 Jun;95(6):694–8
Harrison G: Mosquitoes, malaria, and man: A history of the hostilities since 1880. New York, Dutton, 1978. 314 p.
Henderson DA: The deliberate extinction of a species. **Proc Am Philos Soc** 1982 Dec 17;126(6):461–71
Howard-Jones N: Prelude to modern preventive medicine. In Stanley NF, Joske RA, ed: Changing disease patterns and human behaviour. London, New York, Academic Press, 1980. p. 69–80.
Marwick CS: Managing viral diseases--two centuries of progress. **Am Pharm** 1982 Apr;22(4):36–44
Miller PJ: Semmelweis. **Infect Control** 1982 Sep–Oct;3(5):405–9
Raska K: How the smallpox programme began. **World Health Forum** 1981;2:290–1
Siniak KM: Epidemicheskie posledstviia vremennoĭ fashistskoĭ okkupatsii Ukrainskoĭ SSR i mery po ikh preodoleniiu. **Zh Mikrobiol Epidemiol Immunobiol** 1982 May;(5):11–4
Wagner D: Einige Aspekte von den Anfängen der experimentellen Desinfektionslehre. **Z Gesamte Hyg** 1982 Mar;28(3):172–6
White FM: Nosocomial infection control: scope and implications for health care--historical view. **Am J Infect Control** 1981 Aug;9(3):61–9
Zemskov MV: Protivoépidemicheskoe obespechenie Iassko-Kisshinevskoĭ operatsii. **Zh Mikrobiol Epidemiol Immunobiol** 1980 May;(5):21–5

**Africa**

Eyckmans L: Le problème du choléra en Afrique de l'Est. **Bull Seances Acad R Sci Outre Mer** 1979;(3):445–50
Lyons M: Death camps in the Congo: administrative responses to sleeping sickness 1903–1911. **Soc Soc Hist Med Bull (Lond)** 1984 Jun;34:28–31

# COMMUNICABLE DISEASE CONTROL

**Australia**

Dawson B: Sanitary condition of Melbourne, 1888–1891: a study. **Anu Hist J** 1979–80;14:37–49
Feery B: Impact of immunization on disease patterns in Australia. **Med J Aust** 1981 Aug 22;2(4):172–6
Loaring K, Wards M: Brief history of Northfield. **Australas Nurses J** 1981 Apr;10(4):5–6, 8

**Austria**

Negru I: Carantinele Austriei şi rolul lor pe frontiera Dunării (Sec. XVIII-XIX). **Viata Med [Medii Sanit]** 1982 Jun;30(6):139–42

**Brazil**

Gusmão HH: Indústria e Comércio de Minérios S.A.--ICOMI, Rio de Janeiro, Brazil. **Am J Trop Med Hyg** 1982 Jul;31(4):705–10

**Canada**

Craig B: Smallpox in Ontario: public and professional perceptions of disease, 1884–1885. In Roland CG, ed: Health, disease and medicine. Toronto, Hannah Institute for the History of Medicine, 1984. p. 215–49.
McCuaig K: 'From social reform to social service': the changing role of volunteers: the anti-tuberculosis campaign, 1900–30. **Can Hist Rev** 1980;61(4):480–501
Spaulding WB: Smallpox control in the Ontario wilderness, 1880–1910. In Roland CG, ed: Health, disease and medicine. Toronto, Hannah Institute for the History of Medicine, 1984. p. 194–214.
Trent B: Grosse Ile: island of the dead. **Can Med Assoc J** 1984 Oct 15;131(8):960–8
Tunis B: Public vaccination in Lower Canada, 1815–1823: controversy and a dilemma. **Hist Reflect** 1982;9(1–2):264–78

**Chile**

Borgoño JM: Control de las enfermedades transmisibles. Chile, 1952–1977. **Rev Med Chil** 1977 Oct;105(10):696–700
Costa-Casaretto C: Primeros proyectos de organización sanitaria y de campaña antivenerea después de la emancipación politica de Chile. **Rev Med Chil** 1980 Dec;108(12):1161–9

**China**

Haide M: Leprosy control in China 1981. **East Horiz** 1981;20(9):18–21

**France**

Hildesheimer F: La protection sanitaire des côtes françaises au XVIIIe siècle. **Rev Hist Mod Contemp** 1980 Jul–Sep;27:443–67
Hildesheimer F: Prévention de la peste et attitudes mentales en France au XVIIIe siècle. **Rev Hist (Paris)** 1981;265(1):65–79
Knibiehler Y: La 'lutte antituberculeuse,' instrument de la médicalisation des classes populaires (1870–1930). **Ann Bretagne** 1979;86(3):321–36
Lert F: Emergence et devenir du système de prise en charge de la tuberculose en France entre 1900 et 1940. **Soc Sci Med** 1982;16(23):2073–82
Stofft H: Bouestard, médecin des épidémies à Morlaix. **Hist Sci Med** 1984;18(3):223–45

**Germany**

Haase HH: Uber einige Auswirkungen Robert Kochs und seiner Lehre auf die Entwicklung der Allgemeinen und Kommunalen Hygiene. **Z Gesamte Hyg** 1982 Mar;28(3):154–6
Heckmann G: Anzeigepflichtige Tierseuchen in der Bundesrepublik Deutschland von 1950 bis 1983, unter besonderer Darstellung des Zeitabschnittes von 1970 bis 1983 in Zahlen und Grafiken. Berlin, Parey, 1984. 123 p.
Schadewaldt H: Le développement de la quarantaine dans les ports allemands. In International Congress of the History of Medicine, 27th, Barcelona, 1980. Actas. Barcelona, Acadèmia de Ciències Mèdiques de Catalunya i Balears, 1981. p. 408–13.
Stembrowicz W: Pruski kordon sanitarny w okresie wojny Polsko-Rosyjskiej (1830–1831). **Arch Hist Med (Warsz)** 1982;45(1–4):39–44
Taddey G: Pockenschutz in Hohenlohe. **Medizinhist J** 1983;18(4):313–23
Voss HJ: Beitrag zur Seuchenlage in den Pferdebeständen einer Armee 1940/41 und zur Erfahrung als Leiter eines Seuchenlazarettes für Pferde. **DTW** 1981 Nov 5;88(11):483–6
Weuffen W: Der Beitrag Robert Koch zur Begründung der Desinfektionslehre und heutige Schwerpunkte der Desinfektionsforschung und -praxis. **Z Gesamte Hyg** 1982 Mar;28(3):167–71

**Great Britain**

Duggan AJ: Henry Wellcome: architect of tropical opportunities. **Trans R Soc Trop Med Hyg** 1981;75(4):477–83
Gelfand M: Joseph Lister. **Cent Afr J Med** 1981 Feb;27(2):31–4
Hamilton M: Opposition to the Contagious Diseases Act, 1864–1886. **Albion** 1978;10:14–27
Jones GR: The King Edward VII Welsh National Memorial Association, 1912–1948. In J. Cule, ed: Wales and medicine. London, British Society for the History of Medicine, 1975. p. 30–41.
Kerr B: Henry Moule and cholera in Dorset: nineteenth-century sanitary reform. **Hist Today** 1978;28(10):672–80
McHugh PF: The campaign against the Contagious Diseases Act: Some organizational aspects, 1869–1886. Ph.D thesis, Oxford Univ, 1976.

**Greece**

Marketos LJ: [Recent data on the inoculation against smallpox in the Ionian Islands] (Gre). **Mater Med Greca** 1981;9:104–9

**India**

Hughes E: The fight against cholera: India 1812 - 1912. **Hist Med (Lond)** 1975 Autumn-Winter;6(3–4):68–74
Naidis M: 'Ants, muskeetoes, flies and stinking chints': the British battle against disease in India. **West Hum Rev** 1964;17(1):39–47

**Ivory Coast**

Khromov AS, Kutuzova EP: Istoriia i sostoianie organizatsii bor'by protiv éndemicheskikh bolezneĭ v Respublike Bereg Slonovoĭ Kosti. **Med Parazitol (Mosk)** 1979 Nov–Dec;48(6):64–8

**Netherlands**

Schneeloch NH: 'Praecautien tegens de pest'. Pestgefahr in den Vereinigten Niederlanden 1720–1722. **Econ Soc Hist Jaarb** 1977;40:26–47

**Panama**

Guardia CA: Salud pública y saneamiento en la Zona del Canal de Panamá: un recuento histórico, 1880–1915. **Bol Of Sanit Panam** 1983 Jul;95(1):62–73

**Poland**

Bec M, Bec A: Ignacy Schuch -- lekarz sandomierski. **Arch Hist Med (Warsz)** 1984;47(3):383–7
Krysa-Leszczyńska D: Przyczynek do powstania szpitala zakaźnego w Sandomierzu. **Wiad Lek** 1979 Jul 15;32(14):1039–42

**Romania**

Barbu G: Din istoria luptei antiepidemice în România (II). Completări la istoricul spitalului Dudeşti. **Rev Ig [Bacteriol]** 1984 Jul–Sep;29(3):283–7
Brătescu C, Gheorghiu E: Vizita unei misiuni austriece la carantinele româneşti în 1849. **Rev Ig [Bacteriol]** 1982 Jul–Sep;27(3):217–21
Brătescu G, Gheorghiu E: Vizita unei misiuni austriece la carantinele româneşti in 1849. **Rev Ig [Bacteriol]** 1982 Jan–Mar;27(1):53–7
Franche M: Omagiu Profesorului Mihai Ciucă, la 100 ani de la naştere. Profesorul Mihai Ciucă şi spitalul clinic de boli contagioase 'izolarea' Iaşi. **Rev Med Chir Soc Med Nat Iasi** 1983 Oct–Dec;87(4):726–8

**Spain**

Rodríguez Ocaña E: El cólera de 1834 en Granada. Enfermedad catastrófica y crisis social. Granada, Universidad de Granada, 1983. 170 p. (Colección Monográfica Universidad de Granada, 81).
Schadewaldt H: Le lazaret de quarantaine à Mahón (Minorque). In: Congrès National des Sociétés Savantes, 97e, Nantes, 1972. Comptes Rendus. Paris, 1976. Section des Sciences, Tome 1. p. 215–26.

**United States**

Bernstein BJ: On mass inoculation, who should be heard? **Cent Mag** 1981;14(5):56–61
Bernstein BJ: The swine flu vaccination campaign of 1976: politics, science, and the public. **Congr Pres J Cap Stud** 1983;10(1):95–103
Castle M, Klimek JJ: From newsletter to journal: a 10-year review. **Am J Infect Control** 1982 Aug;10(3):79–83
Cornesco M: American-Romanian cooperation in the study of and fight against scarlet fever. In International Congress of the History of Medicine, 27th, Barcelona, 1980. Actas. Barcelona, Acadèmia de Ciències Mèdiques de Catalunya i Balears, 1981. p. 499–502.
Duffy J: School vaccination: the precursor to school medical inspection. **J Hist Med Allied Sci** 1978 Jul;33(3):344–55
Ensley PC: Indiana and the influenza pandemic of 1918.

**Indiana Med Hist Q** 1983 Dec;9(4):3–15
Foege WH: Centers for disease control. **J Public Health Policy** 1981 Mar;2(1):8–18
McDermott W, Rogers DE: Social ramifications of control of microbial disease. **Johns Hopkins Med J** 1982 Dec;151(6):302–12
Pearson EF, Miles W: Disinfection of mail in the United States. **Bull Hist Med** 1980 Spring;54(1):111–24
Sabin TD: The Penikese Hospital: a Massachusetts hospital for the treatment of Hansen's disease. **N Engl J Med** 1981 Jun 25;304(26):1610–2
Wygant LJ, ed: The Galveston smallpox quarantine camp in 1899. **Bookman** 1982;9(3):3–8
Zanjani SS: George Springmeyer and the quarantine rebellion of 1902: student revolt reaches the University of Nevada. **Nev Hist Soc Q** 1980;23(4):283–9

**USSR**

Agafonov VI, Perepelkin VS: Opyt protivoépidemicheskoĭ raboty v gody voĭny i ego znachenie v sovremennykh usloviiakh. **Voen Med Zh** 1980 May;(5):57–60
Aleksanian IV, Kulish IM: Sanitarno-gigienicheskoe i protivoé pidemicheskoe obespechenie voĭsk v gody Velikoĭ Otechestvennoĭ voĭny.
Alexander JT: Communicable disease, anti-epidemic policies, and the role of medical professionals in Russia, 1725–62. **Can Am Slav Stud** 1978;12(1):154–69
Borodiĭ NK: Karantinnaia sluzhba i protivoépidemicheskie meropriiatiia na Ukraine v XVIII veke. **Zh Mikrobiol Epidemiol Immunobiol** 1980 May;(5):117–20
Burgasov PN: Itogi i perspektivy profilaktiki infektsionnykh bolezneĭ. **Zh Mikrobiol Epidemiol Immunobiol** 1982 Dec;(12):3–7
Deviatova LN: Itogi profilaktiki infektsionnykh zabolevaniĭ i bor'by s infektsiiami v SSSR. **Feldsher Akush** 1982;47(12):9–13
Elkin II: Voenno-épidemicheskaia doktrina (po opytu protivoépidemicheskoĭ zashchity voĭsk v Velikuiu Otechestvennuiu voinu 1941–1945). **Zh Mikrobiol Epidemiol Immunobiol** 1980 May;(5):11–7
Favorova LA: Uchenie L. V. Gromashevskogo i problema likvidatsii infekstionnykh bolezneĭ. **Zh Mikrobiol Epidemiol Immunobiol** 1984 Jul;(7):119–23
Gol'd EIu, Ladnyĭ ID: S. V. Suvorov i ego rol' v istorii sovetskoĭ protivochumnoĭ organizatsii. **Zh Mikrobiol Epidemiol Immunobiol** 1979 Nov;(11):106–9
Ivashchenko IK: Organizatsiia sanitarno-protivoépidemicheskikh meropriiatiĭ v voĭskakh Sibirskogo voennogo okruga v gody voĭny. **Voen Med Zh** 1981 Mar;(3):11–2
Kalankhodzhaev AA: Istoriia organizatsii i razvitiia protivotuberkuleznoĭ sluzhby v Uzbekistane. **Probl Tuberk** 1983 Jul;(7):71–3
Kosareva AA, Kondrat'ev IM: 'Babii bunt' 1830 goda. **Vopr Istor** 1980;8:180–3
Kupriianova ES, Detinova TS, Anufrieva VN, et al: Osnovnye napravleniia rabot V. N. Baklemisheva v oblasti meditsinskoĭ éntomologii i ikh znachenie v épidemiologii i profilaktike transmissivnykh bolezneĭ. **Med Parazitol (Mosk)** 1982 Jan–Feb;51(1):33–9
Lebedev NI: Epidemicheskie posledstviia nemetsko-fashistkoĭ okkupatsii Belorussii v 1941–1944 gg. i mery po ikh likvidatsii. **Zh Mikrobiol Epidemiol Immunobiol** 1982 Jul;(7):106–10
Lebedev NI: Istoricheskie preimushchestva sovetskoĭ épidemiologii v teorii i praktike profilaktiki infektsionnykh bolezneĭ. **Zh Mikrobiol Epidemiol Immunobiol** 1981 Feb;(2):3–6
Maruashvili GM: Istoriia zavoza gambuzii v SSSR (k 100-letiiu so dnia rozhdeniia N. P. Rukhadze). **Med Parazitol (Mosk)** 1980 Jan–Feb;49(1):80–2
Palkin BN: Pervyĭ karantinnyĭ ustav v Rossii, sostavlennyĭ P. Z. Kondoidi. **Sov Zdravookhr** 1982;(9):63–5
Pavlov AV: Dostizheniia v bor'be infektsionnymi bolezniami v Ukrainskoĭ SSR za gody desiatŏi piatiletki i dal'neĭshie zadachi po ikh profilaktike. **Zh Mikrobiol Epidemiol Immunobiol** 1982 Apr;(4):3–7
Pavlov AV: Istoricheskie preimushchestva sotsialisticheskogo zdravookhraneniia v oblasti profilaktiki infektsionnykh zabolevaniĭ. **Zh Mikrobiol Epidemiol Immunobiol** 1980 Aug;(8):3–8
Popushoĭ EP, Ioksa VA: Vklad A. V. Korchaka-Chepurkovskogo v razvitie zdravookhraneniia i bor'bu s épidemiiami v Moldavii. **Zh Mikrobiol Epidemiol Immunobiol** 1983 Oct;(10):109–11
Potulov BM: Voprosy bor'by s épidemiiami v trudakh V. I. Lenina. **Zh Mikrobiol Epidemiol Immunobiol** 1980 Apr;(4):3–9
Pozyvaĭ TT: Organizatsiia protivoépidemicheskoĭ zashchity voĭsk na Zapadnom (3-m Belorusskom) fronte. **Voen Med Zh** 1980 Aug;(8):20–1
Pozyvaĭ TT: Protivoépidemicheskaia rabota sredi naseleniia v polose boevykh deĭstvii Zapadnogo (3-go Belorusskogo) fronta. **Zh Mikrobiol Epidemiol Immunobiol** 1980 May;(5):17–21
Skovránek V: From the beginnings of infectious diseases control in USSR (a few notes on important jubilees). **J Hyg Epidemiol Microbiol Immunol** 1982;26(3):225–6
Smirnov EI, Garin NS: Voĭna i protivoépidemicheskaia zashchita. **Zh Mikrobiol Epidemiol Immunobiol** 1980 May;(5):6–10
Verenkina TN, Markina LZ, Bashtanova LV: Istoriia razvitiia bor'by s tuberkulezom v Sevastopole. **Probl Tuberk** 1984 Jan;(1):70–2
Vladimirova LB: Voprosy bor'by s infektsionnymi zabolevaniiami na VII s'ezde russkikh estestvoispytateleĭ i vracheĭ (k 100-letiiu teorii fagotsitoza). **Zh Mikrobiol Epidemiol Immunobiol** 1984 Aug;(8):115–8
Zhamba G, Gorin OZ, Avilov EN, et al: Itogi bor'by s infektsionnymi zabolevaniiami v Mongol'skoĭ Narodnoĭ Respublike za 60 let narodnoĭ vlasti. **Zh Mikrobiol Epidemiol Immunobiol** 1982 Jun;(6):23–6
Zhdanov VM: 60 Let bor'by s infektsionnymi bolezniami. **Vopr Virusol** 1982 Nov–Dec;27(6):645–9

**Yugoslavia**

Rasuhin J: Epidemiologija i profilaksa zaraznih bolesti u partizanskim prilikama. **Lijec Vjesn** 1979 Nov;101(11):714–6
Snajder D: Pola veka rada na eradikaciji difterije u našoj zemlji. **Srp Arh Celok Lek** 1983 Feb;111(2):239–48

# CONGRESSES

**USSR**

Ocherki istorii fiziologicheskikh nauk v SSSR: Istoki i osobennosti razvitiia: materialy Pervoĭ Vsesoiuznoĭ konferentsii po istorii fiziologicheskikh nauk, Tartu, 1981. Leningrad, Nauka, Leningradskoe otd-nie, 1984. 287 p.

**1700 to Present**

Dolabjian ZL: The International Congress on Electrocardiography: a brief history. **J Electrocardiol** 1984 Jul;17(3):307–8
Francis J: International (World) Veterinary Congress. **Aust Vet J** 1983 Aug;60(8):249–50
Fulton JF: History of medicine–Arnold Klebs and Harvey Cushing at the 1st International Neurological Congress at Berne in 1931. **Int J Neurol** 1980;14(1):103–15
Idel'chik KhI, Shtil'man NL: Vazhnyĭ étap v razvitii russko-nemetskikh meditsinskikh sviazeĭ. **Sov Zdravookhr** 1982;(6):72–5
International Congress of the History of Medicine, 27th, Barcelona, 1980: XXVII Congreso Internacional de Historia de la Medicina, 31 agosto – 6 septiembre 1980: Actas. Barcelona, Acadèmia de Ciències Mèdique de Catalunya i Balears, 1981. 2 Vol., 799 p.
Léonard J: Le premier Congrès international d'eugénique (Londres, 1912) et ses conséquences françaises. **Hist Sci Med** 1983;17(2):141–6
Parish LC: The history of tropical dermatology and the 1907 International Congress of Dermatology. **Int J Dermatol** 1980 Oct;19(8):474–7

**Asia**

Nagaishi C: A brief history of the Asia-Pacific Congress on Diseases of the Chest. **Chest** 1984 Nov;86(5):656–7

**Australia**

Fay FR: History of medical congresses in Tasmania. **Med J Aust** 1980 May 3;1(9):414–6, 437

**Austria**

Ganzinger K, ed: Die Vorträge des Internationalen Pharmaziehistorischen Kongresses Innsbruck 1977. Stuttgart, Wissenschaftliche Verlagsgesellschaft, 1979. 213 p. (Veröffentlichungen der Internationalen Gesellschaft für Geschichte der Pharmazie, Neue Folge, 47).

**Brazil**

González AD: La mision de Carlos M. Ramirez al Brasil y el convenio sanitario de 1887. **Bol Acad Nac Hist (Argentina)** 1964;35:327–53

**Bulgaria**

Pŭrvi Natsionalen kongres po istoriia na meditsinata: Shumen, 9–11 oktomvri 1981 god: reziumeta. Bulgaria], Nauch. druzhestvo po istoriia na meditsinata v Bŭlgariia, [1981?]. 146 p.

**Canada**

Congrès international d'histoire de la médecine, XXVe, Québec, 1976: Actes. Québec, 1977. 3 vols. 1403 p.

**Chile**

Costa-Casaretto C: Nonagésimo aniversario del primer Congreso Médico Chileno. **Rev Med Chil** 1979 Sep;107(9):865–75

**Czechoslovakia**

Málek P: První sjezd ćeských lékařuv a přírodozpytcuv v Praze o letnicích roku 1880. **Cas Lek Cesk** 1980 Nov;119(45):1225
Zadina R: První sjezd českých lékařu a přírodozpytcu v Praze roku 1880.

## CONGRESSES

**Cas Lek Cesk** 1980 Jan 11;119(2):64

**France**

Bourquelot L: Le congrès médical de France: défense d'und profession libérale sous la Monarchie de Juillet. **Ann Bretagne** 1979,86(3):301-12
Grmek MD, ed: Hippocratica. Actes du Colloque hippocratique de Paris (4-9 septembre 1978). Paris, Editions du Centre National de la Recherche Scientifique, 1980. 486 p. (Colloques Internationaux du C.N.R.S., No. 583). Contributions by A. Anastassiou, J. Benedum, J. Bertier, L. Bourgey, G. Brătescu, S. Byl, G. Cambiano, V. Di Benedetto, J. Ducatillon, M. P. Duminil, L. Garcia-Ballester, D. Gourevitch, H. Grensemann, G. Harig, J. Irigoin, C. Irmer, D. Irmer, R. Joly, J. Jouanna, H. M. Koelbing, V. Langholf, C. Lichtenthaeler, G. Maloney, W. Frohn Villeneuve, J. Mansfeld, P. Manuli, P. Mudry, J. M. Pigeaud, C. Sandulesco, W. D. Smith, A. Thivel, M. Vegetti.

**Germany**

Buslaeva MM, Volodina MN: Pervaia Mezhdunarodnia konferentsiia po izucheniiu raka (k 75-letiiu so dnia provedeniia). **Vopr Onkol** 1981;27(11):90-2
Hamelmann H: Zur Geschichte der Vereinigung Nordwestdeutscher Chirurgen: zur 125. Tagung 12.-14. Juni 1980. Lübeck, Wullenwever, 1980?. 103 p.
Rothschuh KE, Krafft F: Forschungsberichte und Spezial-Bibliographien. **Ber Wissenschaftsgesch** 1978;1(3-4):201-15
Schierhorn H: Die Multinationalität der Anatomischen Gesellschaft und die Mehrsprachigkeit ihrer Versammlungen. **Anat Anz** 1980;148(2):168-206
Troschke J von: Möglichkeiten und Grenzen ärztlicher Gesundheitsberatung. Freiburg, Gesomed, 1981. 373 p.
Wyatt F: Erinnerungen vom ersten psychoanalytischen Kongress in Wiesbaden 1932. **Psyche (Stuttg)** 1984 Apr;38(4):360-7

**Great Britain**

Cule J, ed: Wales and medicine. An historical survey from papers given at the Ninth British Congress on the History of Medicine at Swansea & Cardiff, 4-8th September, 1973. London, British Society for the History of Medicine, 1975. xi, 249 p.
Forbes EG, ed: Human implications of scientific advance. Proceedings of the XVth International Congress of the History of Science, Edinburgh 10-15 August 1977. Edinburgh, Edinburgh University Press, 1978. 596 p. (This volume includes papers delivered at ten special symposia)
Lindskog BI: Europeisk musei-konferens. **Sydsven Medicinhist Sallsk Arsskr** 1984;21:11-4
Sakula A: Baroness Burdett-Coutts' garden party: the International Medical Congress, London, 1881. **Med Hist** 1982 Apr;26(2):183-90

**Italy**

Hoppe B: Arbeit und Gesundheit; historische Aspekte ihrer gegenseitigen Beziehungen. Bericht über eine Tagung der 'International School of History of Biological Sciences' in Ischia/Neapel vom 29. Juni bis 12. Juli 1980. **Ber Wissenschaftsgesch** 1980;3(3-4):214-20

**Panama**

Vasco Núñez P: El primer Congreso Médico Internacional efectuado en la República de Panamá. **Rev Med Panama** 1984 May;9(2):164-71

**Poland**

Berezowski S: Ceský vědecký přínos v programech sjezdu polských lékařu a přírodovědcu 100. Výročí prvního sjezdu polských lékařu a přírodovědcu. **Cas Lek Cesk** 1979 Nov 23;118(47):1463-5
Orłowski WJ: W stulecie polskich zjazdów okulistycznych. **Klin Oczna** 1981 Oct-Dec;83(10-12):465-6
Supady J: Udział lekarzy polskich w krajowych i międzynarodowych zjazdach onkologicznych w latach 1918-1938. **Nowotwory** 1979 Oct-Dec;29(4):315-20

**Spain**

Sociedad Española de Historia de la Medicina: V Congreso Nacional. Homenaje al Profesor Pedro Lain Entralgo. Madrid, 29-30 septiembre-1 octubre 1977. **Asclepio** 1977;29:1-358

**Switzerland**

Berges PH, ed: Internationaler Kongress für Geschichte der Pharmazie in Basel/Lausanne, vom 13. bis 19. Juni 1979. [Summary of events plus abstracts of papers] Sonderdruck aus: Deutsche Apotheker Zeitung 119 (1979): 973-976, 1081-1084, 1133-1138, 1170-1173.
Buess H: Henry E. Sigerist (1891-1957) und die erste medizinhistorische Konferenz in Pura (Tessin); zur Erinnerung an den 25./26. März 1950. **Gesnerus** 1980;37(1/2):104-12
Lochmann EH: Das 16. Internationale Symposion der Welt-Gesellschaft für Geschichte der Veterinärmedizin, 21.-24. Mai 1980 in Bärau, Schweiz. **Ber Wissenschaftsgesch** 1980;3(3-4):207-13
Mayer R: Il y a cent ans, à Genève, au 4e Congrès international d'hygiène et de démographie, l''altercation' Pasteur - Koch. **Rev Med Suisse Romande** 1982 Aug;102(8):805-9

**United States**

Benjamin LT, Jones MR: From motivational theory to social cognitive development: twenty-five years of the Nebraska Symposium. **Nebr Symp Motiv** 1978;26:ix-xix
Braude RM: Medical librarians and the White House Conference: from complacency, to concern, to commitment. **Bull Med Libr Assoc** 1981 Apr;62(2):231-5
Cohen EP, ed: Medicine in transition: the centennial of the University of Illinois College of Medicine: a symposium in Chicago, October 1-2, 1981. [Chicago], University of Illinois College of Medicine, and University of Illinois Press, 1981. 340 p.
Doona ME: Nursing revisited: the 1903 convention. **Mass Nurse** 1984 Jun;54(6):6
Duncan CP: A note on the 1929 International Congress of Psychology. **J Hist Behav Sci** 1980 Jan;16(1):1-5
Ebert RV: The First Aspen Conference in retrospect. **Chest** 1984 Jun;85(6 Suppl):2S-3S
Mann G: The Third International Eugenics Congress, 1932. **Medizinhist J** 1980;15(3):338-9
Petty TL: 25 years of Aspen Lung Conferences. **Chest** 1984 Jun;85(6 Suppl):1S

**USSR**

Charkviani LI: Zakavlazskie konferentsii onkologov. **Vopr Onkol** 1981;27(9):48-52
Chertok L: La riabilitazione dell'inconscio in Unione Sovietica: il Convegno internazionale di Tbilisi. **Stor Crit Psicol** 1982 Jun;3(1):41-62
Dionesov SM: Stranitsa iz istorii Pervogo s'ezda Russkogo soiuza psikhiatrov i nevropatologov. **Zh Nevropatol Psikhiatr** 1981;(5):744-5
Evdokimov PP, Kulak VM: Pervye s'ezdy vracheĭ v Povolzh'e. **Sov Zdravookhr** 1983;9:70-2
Granat NE: O 1-ĭ obshchegorodskoĭ nauchno-prakticheskoĭ konferentsii akusherok i meditsinskikh sester akushersko-ginekologicheskikh uchrezhdeniĭ Leningrada (1939 g.). **Med Sestra** 1980 Jun;39(6):40-2
Kanep VV: Aktual'nye voprosy muzeevedeniia: iz opyta raboty Muzeia istorii meditsiny im. P. Stradynia : tezisy dokladov. Riga, Ministerstvo zdravookhraneniia Latviĭskoĭ SSR, 1982. 195 p.
Knel'ts VF: Pervyĭ s'ezd zemskikh vracheĭ i ego rol' v razvitii zdravookhraneniia Udmurtii. **Sov Zdravookhr** 1981;(7):62-3
Kogan VIa, Petrova LF: Sanitarnye s'ezdy USSR i ikh sotsial'no-gigienicheskaia napravlennost'. **Sov Zdravookhr** 1983;(3):58-61
Kulak VM, Evdokimov PP: S'ezdy vracheĭ Povolzh'ia v sovetskoe vremia. **Sov Zdravookhr** 1984;(6):68-9
Nechiporuk VM, Boliukh BA: Iz istorii s'ézdov khirurgov USSR. **Klin Khir** 1979 Nov;(11):61-4
Neĭman IM: K 50-letiiu sozyva I Vsesoiuznogo s'ezda onkologov (iz vospominaniĭ uchastnika). **Vopr Onkol** 1981;27(11):88-9
Tikotin MA: Voprosy obshchestvennoĭ gigieny na s'ezdakh russkikh estestvoispytateleĭ i vracheĭ. **Gig Sanit** 1981 Oct;(10):55-8
Vasil'ev KK: Rol' A. N. Sysina v organizatsii i provendenii vserossiĭskikh (vsesoiuznykh) s'ezdov bakteriologov, épidemiologov i sanitarynykh vracheĭ. **Gig Sanit** 1980 Apr;(4):31-3
Vasil'ev KK: Rol' nauchnykh s'ezdov v nauchnoĭ meditsinskoĭ informatsii (iz istorii vserossiĭskikh i vsesoiuznykh s'ezdov bakteriologov, épidemiologov i sanitarnykh vracheĭ, 1918-1928 gg.) **Sov Zdravookhr** 1980;(6):58-60
Vasil'ev KK: S'ezd, zalozhivshiĭ osnovy sanitarno-épidemiologicheskoĭ sluzhby SSSR (k 60-letiiu VI Vserossiĭskogo c'ezda bakteriologov i épidemiologov). **Zh Mikrobiol Epidemiol Immunobiol** 1982 Dec;(12):102-3
Vasil'ev KK: 60 let VII Vserossi ĭskogo s'ézda bakteriologov, épidemiologov i sanitarnykh vracheĭ. **Zh Mikrobiol Epidemiol Immunobiol** 1983 Oct;(10):111-3
Vladimirova LB: Sotsial'nye problemy meditsiny i gigieny na VII s'ezde russkikh estestvoispytateleĭ i vracheĭ. **Sov Zdravookhr** 1984;(1):54-7
Vladimirova LB: Voprosy bor'by s infektsionnymi zabolevaniiami na VII s'ezde russkikh estestvoispytateleĭ i vracheĭ (k 100-letiiu teorii fagotsitoza). **Zh Mikrobiol Epidemiol Immunobiol** 1984 Aug;(8):115-8
Zikeev PD. Chrezvychaĭnyĭ kholernyĭ s'ezd Obshchestva russkikh vracheĭ v pamiat' N. I. Pirogova. **Sov Zdravookhr** 1981;(11):56-9

**Yugoslavia**

Prvi kongres liječnika Narodnooslobodilačke Fronte Hrvatske: Glina--Topusko--Slunj, 24--27. Veljače 1944. **Lijec Vjesn** 1979 Nov;101(11):686-90
Zarković G: Historijsko značenje prvog kongresa liječnika partizana NOF

Hrvatske. **Lijec Vjesn** 1979 Nov;101(11):654–5
Zimolo A: Rad i značenje prvog kongresa liječnika Narodnooslobodilačke Fronte Hrvatske 24–27. 2. 1944. **Lijec Vjesn** 1979 Nov;101(11):674–8

# CYTOLOGY

See also **Anatomy; Biology; Molecular Biology**

Brinkmann A: Streiftog i cellehistorie. **Tidsskr Nor Laegeforen** 1981 Jan 20;101(2):147–50
Schulz-Schaeffer J: History of cytogenetics. In his: Cytogenetics--plants, animals, humans. New York, Springer, 1980. p. 2–29.

### 1450–1700

#### Netherlands

Ford BJ: Cytological examination of Leeuwenhoek's first microbial specimens. **Tissue Cell** 1982;14(2):207–17

### 1700 to Present

Aterman K: The development of the concept of lysosomes. A historical survey, with particular reference to the liver. **Histochem J** 1979 Sep;11(5):503–41
Bainton DF: The discovery of lysosomes. **J Cell Biol** 1981 Dec;91(3 pt 2):66s–76s
Bechtel W: The evolution of our understanding of the cell: a study in the dynamics of scientific progress. **Stud Hist Philos Sci** 1984 Dec;15(4):309–56
Binet JL: Aspect des cellules sanguines au XIXe siècle. **Clio Med** 1982 Dec;17(2–3):133–44
Brachet J: Un demi siècle de recherches en embryologie et en cytologie. **Comp Biochem Physiol** 1980;67B:367–72
Carmichael SW: The adrenal chromaffin vesicle: an historical perspective. **J Auton Nerv Syst** 1983 Jan;7(1):7–12
Chayen Y, Bitensky L: Modern cytological techniques in biological and medical research. **Acta Med Pol** 1982;23(3–4):127–39
De Duve C: Le développement de centrifugeuses à haute vitesse et leurs applications au fractionnement cellulaire. Un demi-siècle de collaboration entre la Belgique et l'Institut Rockefeller. **Bull Cl Sci Acad R Belg** 1980;5(66):470–2
Duplenko IûK: Die russisch-deutschen naturwissenschaftlichen Kontakte in der Diskussion über die Zellmechanismen des Alterns und der Lebensdauer. **Z Alternsforsch** 1980;35:239–43
Duve C de: Le lysosome: essai d'une esquisse historique et évolutive. **Arch Biol (Liege)** 1980;91(2):175–91
Eisnerova V: The anatomy of plants and its contribution to the origin of cellular theory in the early 19th century. **Acta Hist Rerum Nat Tech** 1971;5:269–333
Grunze H, Spriggs AI: History of clinical cytology: a selection of documents. Darmstadt, Giebeler, 1980. 185 p.
Kepner GR, ed: Cell membrane permeability and transport. Stroudsburg, Pa., Dowden, Hutchinson & Ross, 1979. xiii, 410 p. (Benchmark Papers in Human Physiology, 12).
Kirkwood TB, Cremer T: Cytogerontology since 1881: a reappraisal of August Weisman and a review of modern progress. **Hum Genet** 1982;60(2):101–21
Koss LG: Analytical and quantitative cytology. A historical perspective. **Anal Quant Cytol** 1982 Dec;4(4):251–6
Koulu L, Jansén C: Epidermiksen Langerhansin solu--ajankohtainen satavuotias. **Duodecim** 1980;96(23–24):1587–91
Miczbán I: A sejtkép szemléletének alakulása a XX. században. **Orvostort Kozl** 1982;92(4):9–16
Pan Chengxiang: Origin and development of cytobilogy. (Chi) **Chin J Med Hist** 1981;11(1):11–7
Porter KR: The cytomatrix: a short history of its study. **J Cell Biol** 1984 Jul;99(1 Pt 2):3s–12s
Szymańska R, Schmidt-Pospuła M: Z historii badań tadeusza Browicza (1847–1928) i Karola Kupffera (1829--1902) nad komórkami siateczkowo-śródbłonkowymi watroby. **Arch Hist Med (Warsz)** 1979;42(3):331–6
Tavassoli M: The cell theory: a foundation to the edifice of biology. **Am J Pathol** 1980 Jan;98(1):44
Taylor DM: Blutzellmarkierung: Rückblick und Ausblick. **Wien Klin Wochenschr** 1984 Feb 3;96(3):89–92
Thakur ML, Sinzinger H, Höfer R: Radioisotopenmarkierung menschlicher Blutzellen--ein historischer Uberblick. **Wien Klin Wochenschr** 1984 Feb 3;96(3):87–8
Waddington CH, Thom R: On cell differentiation. **Riv Biol** 1981;74(1–2):213–27
Witkowski JA: Dr. Carrel's immortal cells. **Med Hist** 1980 Apr;24(2):129–42

#### France

Hildebrand R: F. V. Raspail, Begründer der Histochemie und Wegbereiter der Zelltheorie, im Spiegel zeitgenössischer Medaillen. **Anat Anz** 1983;154(4):353–8
Stanguennec A: Le scalpel contre le microscope: Auguste Comte et la théorie cellulaire. **Sci Tech Perspect** 1981–82;1:11.1–.12

#### Germany

Krebs H, Schmid R: Otto Warburg: cell physiologist, biochemist, and eccentric. Oxford, Clarendon. 1981. x, 141 p.
Krebs H: Otto Warburg: Zellphysiologe--Biochemiker--Mediziner---1883–1970. Stuttgart, Wissenschaftliche Verlagsgesellschaft, 1979. 167 p. (Grosse Naturforscher, Band 41).
Petlenko VP, Klishov AA: Kletochnaia teoriia i teoriia kletok (k 100–letiiu so dnia smerti T. Shvanna). **Arkh Anat Gistol Embriol** 1982 Nov;83(11):17–27
Siefert G, Stöckl T: Die Entdeckung der Mastzellen durch den Freiburger Medizinstudenten Paul Ehrlich. **Medizinhist J** 1983;18(3):227–37
Teulón AA: La constitucion de la histologia celular: Schwann, Henle y Kölliker. **Asclepio** 1978–79;30–31:7–18
Watermann R: Schwanns mikroskopische Forschungen und die Zellentheorie. Ein Beitrag zu seinem 100. Todestag. **Z Mikrosk Anat Forsch** 1982;96(6):1032–43
Weindling P: Social concepts in anatomy: theories of the cell state of Oscar Hertwig (1849–1922) and Wilhelm Waldeyer (1836–1921). **Soc Soc Hist Med Bull (Lond)** 1980 Jun;26:15–7

#### Great Britain

Doll R: William Michael Court Brown. In Dictionary of national biography, 1961–1970. Suppl. 8, 1981. p. 152–3.
Roberts JA: Reginald Ruggles Gates. In Dictionary of national biography, 1961–1970. Suppl. 8, 1981. p. 424–5.

#### Greece

Breathnach CS: Biographical sketches No. 29--Papanicolaou. **Ir Med J** 1983 May;76(5):220

#### Hungary

Kiszely G: Theodor Schwann. **Orv Hetil** 1983 Apr;124(16):959–62

#### Italy

Bairati A: Ultrastructure of the protoplasm. The 'pioneer' work by A. Bairati and F. E. Lehmann revisited. **J Submicrosc Cytol** 1981 Apr;13(2):117–25
Martucci V: Sviluppo ontogenetico e citologia nell'ologenesi di Daniele Rosa. **Physis** 1980;22(1):73–84

#### Poland

Malarewicz A: 50 lat cytodiagnostyki ginekologicznej -- George Nicholas Papanicolaou. **Arch Hist Med (Warsz)** 1978;41(4):465–8

#### Sweden

Klein G, Klein E: Torbjörn Caspersson: some personal perspectives. **Cytometry** 1984 Jul;5(4):318
Mayall BH: Torbjörn Oskar Caspersson: curriculum vitae and selected publications. **Cytometry** 1984 Jul;5(4):314–7

#### United States

De Duve C, Beaufay H: A short history of tissue fractionation. **J Cell Biol** 1981 Dec;91(3 pt 2):293s–99s
Garrett CG: Robert Russell Bensley. In Dictionary of American Biography, Suppl. 6, 1956–1960. p. 53–4, 1980.
Hadju SI: A note on the history of Carbowax in cytology **Acta Cytol (Baltimore)** 1983 Mar-Apr;27(2):204–6
Koss LG: On the history of cytology. **Acta Cytol (Baltimore)** 1980 Nov-Dec;24(6):475–7
Porter KR: An informal tribute to George E. Palade. **J Cell Biol** 1983 Jul;97(1):D3–7
Porter KR, Bennett HS: Introduction: recollections on the beginnings of the Journal of Cell Biology. **J Cell Biol** 1981 Dec;91(3 pt 2):IX–XI

#### USSR

Baglaĭ EB: [The first attempt to prove the dominant role of the nucleus in heredity.] (Rus). **Istor Biol Issled** 1978;7:156–62
Braun AD, Vereninov AA, Kaulin AB: Afanasiĭ Semenovich Troshin (k 70–letiiu so dnia rozhdeniia). **Tsitologiia** 1983 Jun;25(6):726–32
Klemparskaya NN: 100 years of the phagocytosis doctrine (Ilya Ilyich Mechnikov). **J Hyg Epidemiol Microbiol Immunol** 1983;27(3):249–52
Kunitsa LK, Mel'nik AN, Loboda VI: K istorii razvittia metoda

tsitologicheskoĭ diagnostiki. **Vrach Delo** 1981 Jul;(7):123-5

Mikhaĭlov VP: Nikolaĭ Varnek i Karl Bér. **Arkh Anat Gistol Embriol** 1982 Apr;82(4):86-95

Vorob'ev VI, Krolenko SA, Rumiantsev PP, et al: Adol'f Aronovich Lev (k 60-letiiu so dnia rozhdeniia). **Tsitologiia** 1983 Jul;25(7):852-9

# DEATH

See also **Mortuary Practice**

[A century of euthanasia] (Dut): **Geneeskd Gids** 1978;141:150-60

Ariès P: L'homme devant la mort. Paris, Seuil, 1977. 641 p.

Ariès P: The hour of our death. New York, Knopf, 1981. xvii, 651 p.

Bartels M, ed: Mensch und Tod: Totentanzsammlung der Universität Düsseldorf. Eine Ausstellung. Düsseldorf, Goethe-Museum, [1978?] 111 p. Einführung von H. Schadewaldt.

Bennahum DA: Intimations of mortality reconsidered: terminal care. **Am J Med** 1980 Oct;69(4):488-90

Białowąs M: Z rozmyślaño śmierci. **Wiad Lek** 1981 Sep 15;34(18):1581-3

Burgess R: The dance of Death. An iconographic interpretation of the popular theme of death through five centuries. **Soc Soc Hist Med Bull (Lond)** 1980 Jun;26:25-37

Chorover SL: From genesis to genocide. The meaning of human nature and the power of behavior control. Cambridge, Mass., MIT Press, 1979. xiii, 238 p.

Cockburn A, Cockburn E, ed: Mummies, disease, and ancient cultures. Cambridge, Cambridge University Press, 1980. x, 340 p.

deWachter MA: Is death and dying merely an ethical issue? **Ann Am Acad Polit Soc Sci** 1980;447:78-88

Feggetter G: Suicide in opera. **Br J Psychiatry** 1980 Jun;136:552-7

Fitzpatrick JJ: Suicidology and suicide prevention: historical perspectives from the nursing literature. **J Psychosoc Nurs Ment Health Serv** 1983 May;21(5):20-8

Fleissner RF: Putting Falstaff to rest: 'tabulating' the facts. **Shakespeare Stud** 1983;16:57-74

Fox VC, Quitt MH, ed: Loving, parenting and dying: the family cycle in England and America, past and present. New York, Psychohistory Press, 1980. v, 488 p. Includes original essays by the editors, by M. A. Glendon, and A. Macfarlane. Also includes numerous previously published articles by various other authors.

Friel PB: Death and dying. **Ann Intern Med** 1982 Nov;97(5):767-71

Haenel T: Die Bewertung des Suizides im Laufe der Geschichte. **Medizinhist J** 1983;18(3):213-26

Hoffer PC, Hull NE: Murdering mothers: infanticide in England and New England 1558-1803. New York and London, New York University Press, 1981. xxii, 211 p. (New York University School of Law Series in Legal History, 2).

Hogenson GB: Depth psychology, death and the hermeneutic of empathy. **J Med Philos** 1981 Feb;6(1):67-89

Hollingsworth TH: A preliminary suggestion for the measurement of mortality crises. In Charbonneau H, Larose A, ed: The great mortalities: methodological studies of demographic crises in the past. Liège, Belgium, Ordina Editions, 1980. p. 21-8.

Hudson RP: Suicide: madness or the noble Roman way? **Pharos** 1982 Fall;45(4):14-7

Jensenius H: Eutanasi -- historisk og aktuelt. **Dan Medicinhist Arbog** 1979;100-13

Koch G: Euthanasie, Sterbehilfe. Eine dokumentierte Bibliographie. Erlangen, Palm und Enke, 1984. xvi, 300 p. (Bibliographica genetica medica, Vol. 18).

Lindeboom GA: Euthanasie in Historisch Perspectief. Amsterdam, Rodopi, 1978. 47 p.

Lithner K: Bilden i ögat. **Sydsven Medicinhist Sallsk Arsskr** 1983;:51-8

Maman C: Comment établir le moment de la mort. **Rev Hist Med Heb** 1980 Jul;33(2):27-34

Monory B: Euthanasia - a pro és contra nézetek tükrében. **Orvostort Kozl** 1982;28(1-3):107-26

Ness DE: C'est fini. . . .le pouls ne bat plus! Drawn by Paul Bernay, for Le Charivari, in 1872. **J Hist Med Allied Sci** 1980 Jul;35(3):312

Pałasz M: Eutanazja w świetle refleksji deontologicznej. **Pol Tyg Lek** 1981 Apr 27;36(17):611-13

Pârvu E, Russo G: Une approche psychosociologique de lat tentative de suicide. **Sante Publique (Bucur)** 1981;24(1):61-5

Pernick MS: Childhood death and medical ethics: an historical perspective on truth-telling in pediatrics. **Prog Clin Biol Res** 1983;139:173-88

Peschel RE, Peschel ER: 'But what if she should die?'--case histories, literary histories: a discussion of maternal death in childbirth. **Pharos** 1981 Winter;44(1):11-8

Peschel RE, Peschel ER: Ritual and the death certificate: case histories, literary histories. **Pharos** 1983 Spring;46(2):11-6

Plaza Izquierdo F: Enfermedad final de Francisco Franco, a proposito de los que mueren en el poder. **Rev Soc Venez Hist Med** 1980;29(43-44):95-124

Porter R: Death and the doctors. **Med Hist** 1982 Jul;26(3):335-41

Robin M: Sheltering arms: the roots of child protection. In E. H. Newberger, ed: Child abuse. Boston, Little, Brown and Company, 1982. p. 1-21.

Roth N: Life-and-death decisions: electrodiagnosis and premature burial. **Med Instrum** 1980 Nov-Dec;14(6):322

Schadewaldt H: Totentanz und Heilberufe. **Jahrb Univ Dusseld** 1980/81;:171-84

Schuster E: Arzt, Apotheker und Tod in den Totentanzdarstellungen. **Apoth J** 1984;7:47-52

Schuster E: Erbauungsbilder in der Totentanzsammlung (Mensch und Tod) der Universität Düsseldorf. In Göpfert W, Otten HH, ed: Metavoeite: wandelt euch durch neues Denken. Düsseldorf, Triltsch, 1983. p. 41-54.

Seidler MJ: Kant and the stoics on suicide. **J Hist Ideas** 1983 Jul-Sep;44(3):429-53

Shanley E: The medicalisation of dying - 1. **Nurs Times** 1982 Aug 11-17;78(32):1360-2

Stoessel I: Scheintod und Todesangst. Aeusserungsformen der Angst in ihren geschichtlichen Wandlungen (17.-20. Jahrhundert). Köln, 1983. 247 p. (Kölner medizinhistorische Beiträge, Band 30)

Vovelle M: Rediscovery of death since 1960. **Ann Am Acad Polit Soc Sci** 1980;447:89-99

Vovelle M: The history of mankind in the mirror of death. **Proc Annu Meet West Soc Fr Hist** 1978;6:91-109

Whaley J: Mirrors of mortality: studies in the social history of death. New York, St. Martin's Press, 1982. viii, 252 p.

Wilson S: Death and the social historians: some recent books in French and English. **Soc Hist (Lond)** 1980;5(3):435-51

**Canada**

Cliche MA: Les attitudes devant la mort d'après les clauses testamentaires dans le gouvernement de Québec sous le régime français. **Rev Hist Am Fr** 1978;32(1):57-94

**Europe**

Ariès P: Døden i historien. **Samtiden (Norway)** 1980;89(3):7-14

Cohen J: Death and the Danse Macabre. **Hist Today** 1982 Aug;32:35-40

Myíri JK: Philosophy and suicide--statistics in Austria-Hungary. **East Cent Eur** 1978;5(1):69-89

**Finland**

Achté K: Döden i den fornfinska kulturen. Tron påsjälens odödlighet. **Dan Medicinhist Arbog** 1983;12:82-90

**France**

Dinet D: Mourir en religion aux dix-septième et dix-huitième siècles; la mort dans quelques couvents des dioceses d'Auxerre, Langres et Dijon. **Rev Hist (Paris)** 1978;259(3):29-54

Meyer J: Pierre Chaunu: la mort à Paris, XVIe, XVIIe, XVIIIe siècles. **Rev Hist (Paris)** 1980;263(2):403-16

Mitchell A: Philippe Ariès and the French way of death. **Fr Hist Stud** 1978;10(4):684-95

**Germany**

Schimming I, Mann H: Zur historischen Bedingtheit der Qualität ärztlicher Bewahrungspflicht für das menschliche Leben sowie der Betreuung Sterbender. **Z Arztl Fortbild (Jena)** 1984;78(16):693-4

**India**

Thomas C: Inde: le pays du suicide? **Histoire** 1981;(30):81-3

**Japan**

Pinguet M: 'Harakiri': L'art de l'éventrement au Japon. **Histoire** 1981;(31):10-8

**Netherlands**

Wachter MA de: Is death and dying dying merely an ethical issue? **Ann Am Acad Polit Soc Sci** 1980;447:78-88

**Spain**

López de Guerenñu G: Muerte, entierro y funerales in algunos lugares de Alava. **Bol Inst Sancho Sabio** 1978;22:189-242

**United States**

Cole T: The ideology of old age and death in American history. **Am Q** 1979;31(2):223-31

Hijiya J: American gravestones and attitudes toward death: a brief history. **Proc Am Philos Soc** 1983 Oct;127(5):339-63

## Before 500 A.D.

### Australia

Pounder DJ, Prokopec M, Pretty GL: A probable case of euthanasia amongst prehistoric aborigines at Roonka, South Australia. **Forensic Sci Int** 1983 Nov–Dec;23(2–3):99–108

### Egypt

Thomas C: First suicide note? **Br Med J** 1980 Jul 26;281(6235):284–5

### Greco–Roman

Robinson PA: The conception of death in Judaism in the Hellenistic and early Roman period. Ph.D. Diss., University of Wisconsin. Madison, 1978. ix, 176 leaves.

### Greece

Carrick PJ: Ancient Greek ethical perspectives on abortion and euthanasia. Ph.D. Diss., Temple University. Philadelphia, 1982. vii, 346 p.

## 500 A.D.–1450

Brown EA: Death and the human body in the later Middle Ages: the legislation of Boniface VIII on the division of the corpse. **Viator** 1981;12:221–70

Guillemain B, Chaunu P, et al.: La mort au moyen âge. Colloque de l'Association des Historiens médiévistes fraçais rèunis à Strasbourg en Juin 1975 au Palais Universitaire. Strasbourg, Istra, 1975. 152 p. Contributions by J. Le Goff, J. P. Sodini, P. C. Timbal, L. Buchet, C. Lorren, J. C. Schmitt, F. Rapp, M. Berthe, P. Vaillant, P. Paravy, H. Martin, C. Beaune, F. Thiriet.

Sutto C, ed: Le sentiment de la mort au Moyen Age. Etudes présentées au Cinquième colloque de l'Institut d'études médiévales de l'Université de Montréal. Quebec, L'Aurore, 1979. Contributions by M. Hébert, R. Lavoie, B. Saint-Pierre, C. Dolan-Leclerc, B. Roy, R. M. Kully, A. Chené-Williams, P. Boglioni, G. H. Allard, E. Schulze-Busacker, D. Smoje.

### Germany

Hühns E: Der Berliner Totentanz. **Dtsch Jahrb Volkskd** 1968;14(2):235–46

### Yugoslavia

Dolenc A: Medizinische Fragen und Aspekte des mittelalterlichen Totentanzes (Ein Beitrag aus Jugoslawien). **Beitr Gerichtl Med** 1980;38:347–52

## 1450–1700

Putscher M: Ein Totentanz von Tizian. Die 17 grossen Holzschnitte zur Fabrica Vesals (1538–1542). In Göpfert W, Otten HH, ed: Metavoeite: wandelt euch durch neues Denken. Düsseldorf, Triltsch, 1983. p. 23–40.

### Austria

Jäger-Sunstenau H: Auswärtige in einem wiener Totenbuch 1687–1690. **Adler** 1967;7(13–14):205–8

### France

Demoulin B: Bossuet et la Mort. In Congrès National des Sociétés Savantes, 102e, Limoges, 1977. Actes. Paris, 1978. Tome I, p. 263–79.

### Germany

Wirth J: La jeune fille et la mort: recherches sur les themes macabres dans l'art germanique de la Renaissance. Geneve, Droz, 1979. 194 p., 64 p. of plates. (Centre de recherches d'histoire et de philologie de la IVe section de l'Ecole pratique des hautes études. V, Hautes études médiévales et modernes; 36).

### Great Britain

Attreed LC: Preparation for death in sixteenth-century northern England. **Sixteenth Century J** 1982;13(3):37–66

Marshall R: Bereavement: attitudes to death in seventeenth century Scotland. **Nurs Mirror** 1983 Nov 9;157(19):xiii–vi

Windstrup G: Locke on suicide. **Polit Theory** 1980;8(2):169–82

Wooden WW: Childhood and death: a reading of John Skelton's Phillip Sparrow. **J Psychohist** 1980 Spring;7(4):403–14

## 1700 to Present

Alexander M: 'The rigid embrace of the narrow house': premature burial & the signs of death. **Hastings Cent Rep** 1980 Jun;10(3):25–31

Ariès P: Invisible Death. **Wilson Q** 1981;5(1):105–15

Blumenthal-Barby K: Gedanken zu Sterben und Tod in der Belletristik. **ZFA** 1983 Sep–Oct;38(5):395–8

Burg BR: The sick and the dead: the development of psychological theory on necrophilia from Krafft-Ebing to the present. **J Hist Behav Sci** 1982 Jul;18(3):242–54

Burkhardt C: Euthanasie – 'Vernichtung lebensunwerten Lebens' im Spiegel der Diskussionen zwischen Juristen und Medizinern von 1900 bis 1940. Diss., Johannes-Gutenberg-Universität. Mainz, 1981. 221 p.

Cremerius J: Freuds Sterben--Die Identität von Denken, Leben und Sterben. **Psychother Psychosom Med Psychol** 1983 Sep;33(5):163–6

Friedsam HJ: The coming on of years: social science perspectives on aging and death. **Soc Sci Q** 1970;51(1):120–8

Germain CP: Nursing the dying: implications of Kübler-Ross' staging theory. **Ann Am Acad Polit Soc Sci** 1980;447:46–58

Imhof AE: The analysis of eighteenth-century causes: some methodological considerations. **Hist Methods Newsl** 1978;2(1):3–36

Lifton RJ: On the consciousness of holocaust. **Psychohist Rev** 1980;9(1):3–22

Morris JP: Historical, medical, and social perspectives on the public's view of death. In Dempsey D., et al, ed: Death, the press, and the public. New York, Arno Press, 1982. p. 10–22.

Nyiri JK: Philosophy and suicide--statistics in Austria-Hungary. **East Cent Eur** 1978;5(1):69–89

Pallis C: From brain death to brain stem death. **Br Med J [Clin Res]** 1982 Nov 20;285(6353):1487–90

Phillips DP: The influence of suggestion on suicide: substantive and theoretical implications of the Werther effect. **Am Sociol Rev** 1974;39(3):340–54

Seidel-Aprin H: Zum Selbstmordgeschehen in der Bundesrepublik und den sozialistischen Staaten Osteuropas. Diss. Bonn, 1980. 94 p.

Spangler GM: Suicide and social criticism: Durkheim, Dreiser, Wharton, and London. **Am Q** 1979;31(4):496–516

Vallaud D: Infanticide et folie au XIX siècle. **Penelope** 1983;(8):51–3

Van der Sluis I: Het recht om grootmoeder te doden. Korte geschiedenis van de euthanasiebeweging sinds 1870. Amsterdam, Buijten & Schipperheijn, 1977. 90 p.

### Austria

Haenel T: Die Suizidproblematik bei Stefan Zweig. **Schweiz Arch Neurol Neurochir Psychiatr** 1981;129(2):297–314

### Brazil

Cassorla RM: Suicídio e adolescência. I--Incidência, histórico e fatores suicidógenos. **Acta Psiquiatr Psicol Am Lat** 1979 Dec;25(4):288–95

### Canada

Cumming E, Lazer C: Kinship structure and suicide: a theoretical link. **Can Rev Sociol Anthropol** 1981;18(3):271–82

### France

Baumont M: Maurice Barrès et les morts de la guerre de 1914–18. **Inf Hist** 1969;31(1):30–5

Cantarel-Besson Y: Les morts exemplaires dans la peinture militaire sous le consulat et l'empire. **Rev Inst Napoleon (Paris)** 1977;(133):97–105

Coleman W: Death is a social disease. Public health and political economy in early industrial France. Madison, University of Wisconsin Press, 1982. xxi, 322 p. (Wisconsin Publications in the History of Science and Medicine, 1).

Favre R: La mort dans la littérature et la pensée française au siècle des lumières. Lyon, Presses universitaires de Lyon, 1978. 640 p.

McManners J: Death and the Enlightenment. Changing attitudes to death among Christians and unbelievers in eighteenth-century France. Oxford, Clarendon Press; New York, Oxford University Press; 1981. vii, 619 p.

Peset JL: La sociedad enferma: algunas reflexiones sobre la muerte del presidente Carnot (1894). **Asclepio** 1983;35:177–88

Scanlan TM: La fonction de la mort dans la pensée sociale de Rousseau. **Univ Ottawa Q** 1981;51(1):91–7

### Germany

Cohen CB: 'Quality of life' and the analogy with the Nazis. **J Med Philos** 1983 May;8(2):113–35

Hahn L: 'Was tut denn der noch da?' Ein Beitrag zum Thema 'Euthanasie'. **Krankenpfl J** 1982 Jan 15;20(1):11

Klee E: 'Euthanasie' im NS-Staat: die 'Vernichtung lebensunwerten Lebens'. Frankfurt am Main, S. Fischer, 1983. 502 p.

Kulessa C, Böhme K: Ursprung und Entwicklung der

Selbstmordverhütung in der deutschsprachigen Psychiatrie. **Fortschr Neurol Psychiatr** 1980 Dec;48(12):629–42
Lifton RJ: Medicalized killing in Auschwitz. **Psychiatry** 1982;45(4):283–97
Przyboś A: Smierć wieźnia Stefana Przybosia w Mauthausen. **Przegl Lek** 1984;41(1):97–9
Rodegra H: Kindestötung und Verheimlichung der Schwangerschaft: eine sozialgeschichtliche und medizinsoziologische Untersuchung mit Einzelfallanalysen. Herzogenrath [Germany], Murken-Altrogge, 1981. 68 p.
Rückleben H: Deportation und Tötung von Geisteskranken aus den badischen Anstalten der Inneren Mission Kork und Mosbach. Karlsruhe, Evangelischer Presseverband für Baden, 1981. 104 p. (Veröffentlichungen des Vereins für Kirchengeschichte in der evangelischen Landeskirche in Baden, Band 33).
Scharfetter C: Ein Anliegen der Menschheitserziehung: Delegierte Destruktivität. Massenmord an Psychiatriepatienten in Hitler-Deutschland. **Schweiz Arch Neurol Neurochir Psychiatr** 1984;134(2):279–93
Volk L: Episkopat und Kirchenkampf im Zweiten Weltkrieg. Lebensvernichtung und Klostersturm 1939–1941. **Stimmen Zeit** 1980;198(9):597–611

**Great Britain**

Anderson O: Did suicide increase with industrialization in Victorian England? **Past Present** 1980;86:149–73
Anderson O: Suicide in Victorian London; an urban view. **Soc Soc Hist Med Bull (Lond)** 1980 Jun;26:18–21
Barrow L: Deviants in death? Plebeian secularists and spiritualists c. 1860–1910. **Soc Soc Hist Med Bull (Lond)** 1980 Jun;26:22–4
Cecil R: Holy dying: evangelical attitudes to death. **Hist Today** 1982 Aug;32:30–4
Gates BT: Suicide and the Victorian physicians. **J Hist Behav Sci** 1980 Apr;16(2):164–74
Goldin G: A protohospice at the turn of the century: St. Luke's House, London, from 1893 to 1921. **J Hist Med Allied Sci** 1981 Oct;36(4):383–415
Gutierrez D: D. H. Lawrence and modern destructiveness. **Suicide Life Threat Behav** 1980 Winter;10(4):219–29
Hunnisett RF, ed: Wiltshire coroners' bills, 1752–1796. Devizes, Wiltshire Record Society, 1981. liv, 239 p. (Wiltshire Record Society, v. 36).
Lerner JC: The public and private management of death in Britain, 1890–1930. Ph.D. Diss., Columbia University. New York, 1981. iv, 309 leaves.
Low AA, Farmer RD, Jones DR, et al: Suicide in England and Wales: an analysis of 100 years, 1876–1975. **Psychol Med** 1981 May;11(2):359–68
Paly D: The antiquaries' last will and testament; an etching with sepia wash by Thomas Rowlandson, 1814. **J Hist Med Allied Sci** 1980 Apr;35(2):215
Richardson R: Old people's attitudes to death in the twentieth century. **Soc Soc Hist Med Bull (Lond)** 1984 Jun;34:48–51
Saunders C: A pioneering approach to the dying [interview by Laurence Dopson] **Nurs Times** 1984 Mar 28–Apr 3;80(13):16–8
Smith R: Trial by medicine. Insanity and responsibility in Victorian trials. Edinburgh, Edinburgh University Press, 1981. ix, 238 p.
Walker RG: Public death in the eighteenth century. **Res Stud** 1980;48(1):11–24

**Guyana**

Baechler J: Mourir à Jonestown. **Eur J Sociol** 1979;20(2):173–210

**Hungary**

Böszörményi E: Hódmezövásárhelyi öngyilkosságok. **Tort Stat Tanulm** 1977;3:237–304
Valenti R: Ongyilkosságok Budapesten 1881–82-ben. Egykorú boncjegyzökönyvek összehasonlító vizsgálata. **Morphol Igazsagugyi Orv Sz** 1982 Jan;22(1):67–70

**Italy**

Beer M: Suicidio e inettitudine: nota sui romanzi femminili Italiani del ventennio 1880–1890. **Mem Riv Stor Donne** 1981;(2):76–88
Kligfield PD: A survey of variant title page vignettes in Lancisi's De subitaneis mortibus. **J Hist Med Allied Sci** 1983 Jul;38(3):336–9
Shneidman ES: The suicidal logic of Cesare Pavese. **J Am Acad Psychoanal** 1982 Oct;10(4):547–63

**Japan**

Fusé T: Modernization and suicide in Japan: a comparative approach. **Cult Dev** 1980;12(1):45–80
Lifton RJ, Kato S, Reich MR: Six lives, six deaths. Portraits from modern Japan. New Haven and London, Yale University Press, 1979. xiii, 305 p.

**Netherlands**

Cohen LA: Een curieus geval van schijndood in 1857. **Ned Tijdschr Geneeskd** 1983 Dec 10;127(50):2304
Haas WH de: Vincent van Gogh, zijn lichamelijke ziekten, verwondingen en zelfmoord. **Ned Tijdschr Geneeskd** 1983 Dec 24;127(52):2390–2

**Norway**

Christensen AL: 'Og så gjekk me og så på lik'. **Samtiden (Norway)** 1980;89(3):23–9

**Poland**

Bogusz J: Uwagi lekarza o martyrologii Zydów polskich. **Przegl Lek** 1984;41(1):54–62
Jarosz M: Le suicide en Pologne. **Rev Etud Comp Est Ouest** 1978;9(4):65–101
Marek Z, Kołodziej J: Samobójstwa w Krakowie w latach 1881–1980. **Przegl Lek** 1982;39(11):709–14
Meclewski E: Der faschistische völkermord in polen. **Dtsch Aussenpolit** 1967;12(2):169–76
Monkiewicz W, Kretowski J: Los chorych psychicznie, kalek i starców w okupowanym Białostockiem. **Przegl Lek** 1984;41(1):80–4
Wyziembło M: Losy polaków ... **Zesz Hist** 1974;(30):16–23

**Spain**

Uranga E: Un ilustre anatónomo y cirujano con ideas necrofílicas del siglo XIX en Zaragoza. **Bol Real Soc Vascongada Amigos Pais** 1973;29(1–3):375–91

**United States**

Allen WR: All the names of death: Walker Percy and Hemingway. **Miss Q** 1982–83;36(1):3–19
Ames KL: Ideologies in stone: meanings in Victorian gravestones. **J Pop Cult** 1981;14(4):641–56
Barrick ME: Cumberland county death lore. **Pa Folklife** 1979;28(4):37–46
Barton M: Painful duties: art, character, and culture in Confederate letters of condolence. **South Q** 1979;17(2):123–34
Bollen KA, Phillips DP: Imitative suicides: a national study of the effects of television news stories. **Am Sociol Rev** 1982;47(6):802–9
Boor M: Effects of United States presidential elections on suicide and other causes of death. **Am Sociol Rev** 1981;46(5):616–8
Breed W: The Negro and fatalistic suicide. **Pac Sociol Rev** 1970;13(3):156–62
Capron AM: Death and the law: a decade of change. **Soundings** 1980;63(3):290–320
Carson SL: Presidential children: abandonment, hysteria and suicide. **J Psychohist** 1984 Spring;11(4):533–44
Davis R: Black suicide and social support systems: an overview and some implications for mental health practitioners. **Phylon** 1982;43(4):307–14
Davis R: Suicide among young blacks: trends and perspectives. **Phylon** 1980;41(3):223–9
Dundes A: The dead baby joke cycle. **West Folkl** 1979;38(3):145–57
Eckert WG: Catastrophes et morts collectives. Recent American experiences in mass deaths. **Am J Forensic Med Pathol** 1980 Mar;1(1):77–9
Engel BF: Why so doleful? The funereal poetry of the early Midwest. **Old Northwest** 1981;7(2):147–59
Farrell JJ: Inventing the American way of death, 1830–1920. Philadelphia, Temple University Press, 1980 viii, 287 p.
Farrell JJ: The dying of death: the meaning and management of death in America, 1830–1920. Ph.D. diss. University of Illinois, Urbana, Ill., 1980. 329 p.
Fox RC: The sting of death in American society. **Soc Serv Rev** 1981;55(1):42–59
Holden C: The hospice movement and its implications. **Ann Am Acad Polit Soc Sci** 1980;447:59–63
Johnson MP: Smothered slave infants; were slave mothers at fault? **J South Hist** 1981;47(4):493–520
Johnson MP, Hufbauer K: Sudden infant death syndrome as a medical research problem since 1945. **Soc Probl** 1982;30(1):65–81
Joynt RJ: Landmark perspective: A new look at death. **JAMA** 1984 Aug 3;252(5):680–2
Kennedy JG: Poe and magazine writing on premature burial. **Stud Am Renaiss** 1977;165–78
King DR: The brutalization effect: execution publicity and the incidence of homicide in South Carolina. **Soc Forces** 1978;57(2):683–7
Kushner HI: The suicide of Meriwether Lewis: a psychoanalytic inquiry. **William Mary Q** 1981;38(3):464–81
Lane R: Suicide and the city. **Society** 1980;17(2):74–82
Lane R: Violent death in the city: suicide, accident, and murder in nineteenth-century Philadelphia. Cambridge, Mass., Harvard University Press, 1979. xiii, 193 p.
Levy JE, Kunitz SJ, Everett M: Navajo criminal homicide.

Southwest J Anthropol 1969;25(2):124–52
Marshall JR: Political integration and the effect of war on suicide: United States, 1933–76. **Soc Forces** 1981;59(3):771–85
Miles DE: The growth of suicide among black Americans. **Crisis** 1979;86(10):430–3
Morris JP: Historical perspectives on educating the medical student in thanatology. In Schoenberg B., et al, ed: Educating medical students in thanatology. New York, Arno Press, 1981. p. 18–28.
Ostheimer JM: The polls: changing attitudes toward euthanasia. **Public Opin Q** 1980;44(1):123–8
Patrick JW: Personal faith and the fear of death among divergent religious populations. **J Sci Stud Relig** 1979;18(3):298–305
Peck DL, Bharadwaj LK: Personal stress and fatalism as factors in college suicide. **Soc Sci** 1980;55(1):19–24
Plews JH: Charles Darwin and Hawaiian sex ratios, or, genius is a capacity for making compensating errors. **Hawaii J Hist** 1980;14:24–49
Rado L: Death redefined: social and cultural influences on legislation. **J Commun** 1971;31(1):41–7
Remes NR: The rural cemetery. **Nineteenth Century Fict** 1979;5(4):52–5
Remini RV: The final days and hours in the life of General Andrew Jackson. **Tenn Hist Q** 1980;39(2):167–77
Ridlen SS: Funerary art in the 1890's: a reflection of culture. **Pioneer Am Soc Trans** 1983;6:27–35
Rowe WF: Discussion of 'George Armstrong Custer and the Battle of the Little Bighorn: homicide or mass suicide'. **J Forensic Sci** 1984 Jul;29(3):696–9
Stack S: The effect of the decline in institutionalized religion on suicide, 1954–1978. **J Sci Stud Relig** 1983;22(3):239–52
Steele TJ: The death cart: it's place among the Santos of New Mexico. **Colo Mag** 1978;55(1):1–14
Stein J: The bioethicists: facing matters of life and death. **Smithsonian** 1979;9(10):107–15
Stewart JB: The political economy of black male suicides. **J Black Stud** 1980;11(2):249–61
Thomas L: Dying as failure. **Ann Am Acad Polit Soc Sci** 1980;447:1–4
Uhlenberg P: Death and the family. **J Fam Hist** 1980 Fall;5(3):313–20
Veatch RM, Tai E: Talking about death: patterns of lay and professional change. **Ann Am Acad Polit Soc Sci** 1980;447:29–45
Vovelle M: A century and one-half of American epitaphs (1660–1813): toward the study of collective attitudes about death. **Comp Stud Soc Hist** 1980;22(4):534–47
Wilkenson F: Spotsylvania: reflections. How men die in battle. **Civ War Times Illus** 1983;22(2):16–8
Zelizer VA: Human values and the market: the case of life insurance and death in 19th-century America. **AJS** 1978 Nov;84(3):591–610

**USSR**

Gaïev A: Suicides d'écrivains sovietiques. **Contrat Soc** 1968;12(4):237–41
Smyrniw W: Tolstoy's depiction of death in the context of recent studies of the 'experience of dying.' **Can Slavonic Pap** 1979;21(3):367–79
Zhuravleva TB: Uchenie G. V. Shora o tanatogeneze i rol' ego shkoly v razvitii sovetskoĭ patologicheskoĭ anatomii (k 110-letiiu so dnia rozhdeniia). **Arkh Patol** 1984;46(3):76–80

**Yugoslavia**

Purić J, Obradović M: Radovi Stevana Koturovića i Bogoljuba Jovanovića o samoubistvima u Srbiji od 1845. do 1884. i od 1898. do 1907 godine. **Srp Arh Celok Lek** 1983 Apr;111(4):513–9
Striković J: Analiza jednog samoubistva u delu Ive Andrića 'Na Drini Cuprija'. **Srp Arh Celok Lek** 1979 Sep;107(9):477–82

**Zimbabwe**

Cockcroft IG: They did not leave the valley. **Nada** 1969;10(1):50–3

## DENTISTRY

Andrik P, Stukovský R. K otázkám terminálnej redukcie chrupu. **Cesk Stomatol** 1980 Jul;80(4):242–5
Arnold G: Breve storia delle estrazioni dentarie dall'antichità ai nostri giorni. **Dent Cadmos** 1980 Dec;48(12):61–3
Baume LG, Treccani A: La biologia della polpa dentaria e della dentina: storia delle scoperte istologiche (parte I). **Riv Ital Stomatol** 1983 Oct;52(10):799–803
Baume LJ: Evolution de la médecine dentaire opératoire. **Rev Belge Med Dent** 1983 Mar;38(2):33–7
Besombes A: Die Zahnheilkunde vom Mittelalter bis zum achtzehnten Jahrhundert. In Sournia JC, Martiny M, Poulet J, ed: Illustrierte Geschichte der Medizin. Salzburg, Andreas, 1980. Vol. 6. p. 2045–73.
Bromage TG, Horne PD: Stafne defect: a histological approach. **Paleopathol Newsl** 1981 Jan;33:7–9
Brown KS: Evolution and development of the dentition. **Birth Defects** 1983;19(1):29–66
Brulin F, Doual A, Gysel C: Evolution des rapports de la psychologie et de l'odontologie. **Orthod Fr** 1980;51:197–202
Burns PE: Log-linear analysis of dental caries occurrence in four skeletal series. **Am J Phys Anthropol** 1979 Nov;51(4):637–47
Calatrava Páramo DL: La boca en lo social, la salud, la enfermedad y lo legal. **An R Acad Nac Med (Madr)** 1982;99(1):91–108
Campbell JM: Dentistry then and now. Revised and enlarged Third edition of From a trade to a profession. [S.l. : s.n.], 1981 (Glasgow: Bell & Bain). xvi, 395 p.
Cislaghi: Storia dei denti artificiali. Analisi dei materiali e delle tecniche di costruzione dai Fenici agli attuali orientamenti biomeccanici. Pisa, Mariotti, 1968. 84 p. (Clinica Odonto-Protesica Stomatologica, Monografie, 1; Supplemento alla Rivista Clinica Odonto-Protesica Stomatologica, 14, 1968).
Cook DC: Koniag Eskimo tooth ablation: was Hrdlička right after all? **Curr Anthropol** 1981;22(2):159–63
Covert HH, Kay RF: Dental microwear and diet: implications for determining the feeding behaviors of extinct primates, with a comment on the dietary patterns of Sivapithecus. **Am J Phys Anthropol** 1981 Jul;55(3):331–6
Croxson LJ: The dentist and society: a symbiosis? **Ann R Australas Coll Dent Surg** 1977 Jun;5:109–17
Cruse WP, Bellizzi R: A historic review of endodontics, 1689–1963, part 1–3. **J Endod** 1980;6(3–5):495–9,532–5,576–80
Cundey B: Artificial teeth: a bit of a mouthful. **Nurs Mirror** 1981 Apr 9;152(15):30–2
Cunin OE: Femmes dentistes, femmes de dentistes. **Hist Sci Med** 1980;14(2):207–12
Drinnan AJ: Odontophilately. **NY State Dent J** 1980 Apr;46(4):173
Emling RC: Historical overview of causes and treatment of dental hypersensitivity. **Compend Contin Educ Dent** 1982;(Suppl 3):S92–4
Febres-Cordero F: Acerca de la 'Desmonopolizacion' en odontologia. **Acta Odontol Venez** 1979 May–Dec;17(2–3):3–11
Febres-Cordero F: Cirujanos y odontologos proceden de los barberos medievales? **Acta Odontol Venez** 1981 Sep–Dec;19(3):283–304
Febres-Cordero F: Incorrecciones en el lenguaje de medicos y odontologos. Trabajo presentado en el X Congreso Venezolano de Ciencias Medicas. Caracas, 8 de marzo de 1983. 19 p.
Febres-Cordero F: La odontologia andina prehispanica. **Acta Odontol Venez** 1984;22(1):39–73
Febres-Cordero F: La odontologia, es una 'profesion' o un oficio? **Acta Odontol Venez** 1980 May–Aug;18(2):337–52
Foley GP: A treasury of dentistry. Royal extractions. **J Am Coll Dent** 1984 Fall;51(3):22–3
Gantt DG: A method of interpreting enamel prism patterns. **Scan Electron Microsc** 1979;(3):491–6
Gelbier S: Some early dental history. **Dent Health (London)** 1982;21(6):6–7
Glazer J: Ancestors. **J Am Dent Assoc** 1984 Jul;109(1):17
Gow CE: The dentitions of the Tritheledontidae (therapsida: cynodontia). **Proc R Soc Lond [Biol]** 1980 Jul 17;208(1173):461–81
Guerini V: Historia tes odontiatrikes. **Odontostomatol Proodos** 1981 Nov–Dec;35(6):198–204 contd
Hagman HC: History of partial dentures, part 1. **Dent Lab Rev** 1980;55(8):28–9
Hagman HC: 3,000 years of dental gold. **Dent Lab Rev** 1979 Jun;54(7):28–30
Hargreaves AS: Old bones are brittle. **Dent Tech** 1980 Sept;33(9):5–9
Hasegawa M: [Changes in oral (endodontic) treatment] (Jpn). **Shikwa Gakuho** 1983 May;83(5):587–97
Hernández PH: Cronología odontológica. **Rev Odontol PR** 1981 Feb–Apr;18(1):13–20 contd
Hine MK: The status of the teaching of dental history: 1980. **Bull Hist Dent** 1981 Oct;29(2):102–4
Hoffmann-Axthelm W: History of dentistry. Chicago, Quintessence, 1981. 435 p. (Translation of Die Geschichte der Zahnheilkunde.).
Holland MR: Chronology of dental history. **Northwest Dent** 1983 Mar–Apr;62(2):72–81
Hugly C: L'argent dans la relation thérapeutique. **Rev Odontostomatol (Paris)** 1981 May–Jun;10(3):239–44
Jacobs N: Les dents et la peinture classique et contemporaine. **Actual Odontostomatol (Paris)** 1981;136:631–51
Jago JD: Early dental charlatans and quacks. **Bull Hist Dent** 1984 Oct;32(2):118–25
Johnson DL, Stratton RJ: Introduction to removable partial dentures. **Quintessence Int** 1979;10(10):55–62
Kanterman CB: Touch the tooth of a hanged man. **Tic** 1984 Oct;43(10):12–4
Kowitz A: You don't have anything, do you? The historical resources of the American Dental Association. **Bull Hist Dent** 1980 Oct;28(2):69–75
Kramer MG: Professionalism and principles of ethics--changing concepts for dentistry. **Pediatr Dent** 1980 Sep;2(3):245–51
Little DA: The relevance of prosthodontics and the science of dental materials to the practice of dentistry. **J Dent** 1982 Dec;10(4):300–10
Loevy HT, Kowitz A: Dentistry on stamps. **J Am Dent Assoc** 1980 Jun;100(6):917, 924
Loevy HT, Kowitz A: Dentistry on stamps. **J Am Dent Assoc** 1981 Jul;103(1):143
Loevy HT, Kowitz A: Dentistry on stamps. **J Am Dent Assoc** 1983 Oct;107(4):618 (continued periodically)
Loevy HT, Kowitz A: Health science on stamps. **J Am Dent Assoc** 1980 Jan;100(1):86

# DENTISTRY

Loevy HT, Kowitz A: The Habsburgs and the 'Habsburg Jaw'. **Bull Hist Dent** 1982 Apr;30(1):19-23
Loux F: L'ogre et la dent. Pratiques et savoirs populaires relatifs aux dents. Paris, Berger-Levrault, 1981. 186 p.
Ludlow MO: A brief history of endodontics. **Chronicle** 1983 Mar;46(3):50-1
Maire M: Une mini histoire de la presse dentaire. **Chir Dent Fr** 1979 Dec 13;49(44):53-7
Mandel ID: Dental caries. **Am Sci** 1979 Nov-Dec;67(6):680-8
Manski RJ: A synopsis of recent literature concerning the dental implant. **J Oral Implantol** 1982;10(2):275-88
Marić D: Stomatologija--medicinska disciplina. **Med Pregl** 1981;34(1-2):91-4
Markens IS: Een historisch overzicht van de ontwikkeling van de orthodontie tot aan de Middeleeuwen. **Ned Tijdschr Tandheelkd** 1983 Mar;90(3):154-60
Marmasse A: Soins de canaux de Fauchard à aujourd'hui. **Actual Odontostomatol (Paris)** 1980;34(129):37-49
Martin MW: Stamping out dentistry. **Tic** 1979;38(7):11;(9):5
May BR: Barbers, 'quacks,' and other early 'dentists'. **CAL** 1983 Feb;46(8):25-7
Moore WJ: The role of sugar in the aetiology of dental caries. 1. Sugar and the antiquity of dental caries. **J Dent** 1983 Sep;11(3):189-90
Nally JN: Développement scientifique de la prothèse dentaire et éthique médicale. **Schweiz Monatsschr Zahnmed** 1984 Jan;94(1):23-8
Naujoks R: Zivilisation und Zahnheilkunde. **Dtsch Zahnarztl Z** 1980 Feb;35(2):156-61
Neiburger EJ: The evolution of human occlusion (II). **Quintessence Int** 1979 Jul;10(7):75-84
Novak DE: Dental auxiliary evolution: a historical perspective. **Dent Assist** 1984 Sep-Oct;53(5):17-22
Ott W: Abriss zur Geschichte der Zahnheilkunde. **Zahnarztebl Baden Wurttemb** 1980 May;(5):108-11
Pastinszky I: A száj müködése: harapás, evés, nevetés, beszéd, ízlelés a klasszikus közmondásokban és idézetekben. **Fogorv Sz** 1984 Jul;77(7):217-8
Pastinszky I: Stomatologia a klasszikus kózmondásokban és idézetekben. **Fogorv Sz** 1984 May;77(5):139-41
Pirmann F: Fachkunde der Zahntechnik. **Zahntechnik (Geneve)** 1983;41(5):431-4, 436-8, 440-6 contd
Proskauer C: A pictorial history of dentistry. **Tic** 1979 May;38(5):13-4 (continued periodically
Proskauer C: A pictorial history of dentistry. Part 1 -- prehistoric, Egyptian, Assyrian. **Tic** 1979 Feb;38(2):8-10 (continued periodically)
Raddatz FJ: Der Zahn, behandelt durch den Künstler. **Zahnarztl Mitt** 1983 Dec 1;73(23):2603-32
Rosen J: Of serpents and symbols. **J Am Dent Assoc** 1984 Apr;108(4):534
Rudowska I: Kosmetyka zębów w starożytności. **Czas Stomatol** 1980 Aug;33(8):476-50
Schadewaldt H: Der Zahnarzt in der Kunst. **Zahnarztl Mitt** 1983 Dec 16;73(24):2760, 2762-4, 2768-70
Schipperges H: Die Zähne und das Schöne im Wandel der Zeiten. **Dtsch Zahnarztl Z** 1981;36(7):406-13
Schulz HH: Zur Geschichte der Prothetik. **Dent Labor (Muench)** 1979 Mar;27(3):394-8 (contd regularly)
Sebban: Esquisse historique de la pratique dentaire populaire sous la Renaissance. **Soc Fr Hist Art Dent** 1979 Mar-Jun;(3-4):9-22
Sugden K: Glimpses of medical history. **Br Dent J** 1981;150(3):75-6
Swanson BZ: A dental Notgeld note. **Bull Hist Dent** 1982 Apr;30(1):27-30
Tanitsu M: [Medico-dental and pharmacological history--miscellaneous records (7)] (Jpn) **Dent Outlook** 1980;(7):114-5 (continued periodically)
Teaford MF, Walker A: Quantitative differences in dental microwear between primate species with different diets and a comment on the presumed diet of Sivapithecus. **Am J Phys Anthropol** 1984 Jun;64(2):191-200
Vidal F: Les anodins dans le traitement des douleurs dentaires aux XVIIe et XVIIIe siècles. **Inf Dent** 1982 Feb 25;64(8):695-703
Vidal F: Odontoiatria del passato. Gli 'anodini' nel trattamento del mal di denti nel XVII e nel XVIII secolo. **Dent Cadmos** 1982 Jan;50(1):57-61
Vidal F: Odontoiatria del passato. Salasso e mal di denti nel XVII e nel XVIII sécolo. **Dent Cadmos** 1981 Mar;49(3):59-63
Wójciak L, Maćkowiak K: Problemy stomatologii wieku rozwojowego w aspekcie rozwoju historycznego. **Czas Stomatol** 1979 Nov;32(11):1063-8
Wolff M, Osborne JW, Hanson AL: Mercury toxicity and dental amalgam. **Neurotoxicology (Park Forest Il)** 1983 Fall;4(3):201-4
Yazu M: [Medico-dental and pharmacological history--miscellaneous records (1)] **Dent Outlook** 1980 Jan;(1):130-1 (contd. regularly)
Yazu M: [Teeth and toothache in the history of dentistry] (Jpn) **Dent Outlook** 1978;51(5):993-5
Yonkers AJ: My specialty: otorhinolaryngology and maxillofacial surgery. **Nebr Med J** 1981 Jan;66(1):4-5

**Americas**

Anjard R: Mayan dental wonders. **J Oral Implantol** 1981;9(3):423-6
Perzigian AJ: Allometric analysis of dental variation in a human population. **Am J Phys Anthropol** 1981 Mar;54(3):341-5

**Asia**

Bergemann H: Zahnheilkunde zwischen Magie und Grobschmied. **Zahnarztl Mitt** 1981 Jul;71(14):856-7

**Austria**

Snorrason E: Den Habsburgske underkaebe. **Tandlaegebladet** 1982 May;86(8):277-80

**China**

Kao i ya i hsüeh hsi ch'eng li 20 chou nien t'e k'an: Kaohsiung: Kao-hsiung i hsüeh yüan Ya i hsüeh hsi K'ou ch'iang i hsüeh hui Ting she, Min Kuo 66 nien, [1977]. 315 p.
Schlissel CH: A short history of dentistry in China from earliest times through 1900. **Bull Hist Dent** 1984;32(1):52-6
Tsao TF: Endodontic treatment in China. **Int Endod J** 1984 Jul;17(3):163-75

**Cuba**

Mena CA: Historia de la odontologia en Cuba. I. La colonia (1492-1898). Miami, Ediciones Universal, 1981. xxii, 395 p.

**France**

Cecconi: Le Marais et le mal de dents. **Soc Fr Hist Art Dent** 1979 Sep-Dec;(5-6):18-21
Gysel C: Cartesianisme en tandheelkunde bij Henricus Regius (1598--1679--1979). **Rev Belge Med Dent** 1979;34(2):213-22
Gysel C: Il dentista Fauchard. **Dent Cadmos** 1980 Jan;48(1):61-3. Feb;48(2):49-52
Gysel C: Un tricentenaire: la prophylaxie dentaire du Sieur de Fleurimont (1682-1982) (I). **Med Hyg (Geneve)** 1983 Jul 15;41(1525):2549-50; Jul 30;41(1526):2622-3
Vidal F: [Bloodletting and dentistry in the 17th and 18th centuries.] (Fre). **Inf Dent** 1980;62:4059-64
Vidal F: Odontoiatria del passato. L''Edit Royal' del maggio 1699. L''Editto' del 1699 y quello del 1768. **Dent Cadmos** 1982 Jan, Feb;50(1,2):57-63, 67-74

**Germany**

Holtkamp P: Narkosen mit 'Weingenuss bis zum Nasenbluten'. **Quintessenz J** 1981 Nov;11(11):995-6
Müller E: Die geschichtliche Entwicklung der Zahnheilkunde im Grossherzogtum Hessen-Darmstadt--einschliesslich seiner Vorgänger- und Nachfolgeterritorien--unter besonderer Berücksichtigung seiner Universitätsstadt Giessen. Giessen, Schmitz, 1981. 120 p. (Arbeiten zur Geschichte der Medizin in Giessen, 3).

**Great Britain**

Wickes HL: The Royal Army Dental Corps. **Br Dent J** 1980 Jun 3-17;148(11-12):269-70

**Italy**

Rocchietta S: Due raffigurazioni di santa Apollonia. (sec. XVI e sec. XVIII). **Minerva Med** 1983 Oct 6;74(38):2245-6
Rocchietta S: Iconografia statuaria e pittorica di Santa Apollonia nel Duomo di Milano. **Minerva Med** 1981 Jan 14;72(1):45-9

**Japan**

Brace CL, Nagai M: Japanese tooth size: past and present. **Am J Phys Anthropol** 1982 Dec;59(4):399-411
Dentistry in Japan: **Br Dent J** 1983 Aug 20;155(4):136
Hasegawa M: [History of endodontics (1)] (Jpn). **Nippon Shika Hyoron** 1983 Feb;(484):135-45
Inoue N, Kuo CH, Ito G, et al: [Dental caries in Japanese remains (author's transl)] (Jpn). **Koku Eisei Gakkai Zasshi** 1981 Jul;31(2):90-7
Japan and dentistry: **CAL** 1983 Jul;47(1):1, 3-4
Motoyama S: [Dental clinics in the Edo period] (Jpn). **Shikai Tenbo** 1984 Aug;64(2):353-61

**Mexico**

Fastlicht S: Tooth mutilations and dentistry in pre-Columbian Mexico. Berlin, Buch- und Zeitschriften-Verlag 'Die Quintessenz', 1976. 164 p.
Sanfilippo J: Bibliografía histórico-odontológica del Dr. Samuel Fastlicht. **Bol Soc Mex Hist Filos Med** 1984 Jun;7(47):317-24

**Pacific Islands**

Beecher DM: The history of dental health on Guam. **Bull Hist Dent** 1983

Oct;31(2):108-12

**Peru**

Sawyer DR, Allison MJ, Pezzia A, et al: Crown dimensions of deciduous teeth from pre-Columbian Peru. **Am J Phys Anthropol** 1982 Dec;59(4):373-6

Sawyer DR, Logan WW, Oleru UG, et al: The effect of attrition on the pre-Columbian Indian arch length. **J Dent** 1983 Jun;11(2):154-8

**Puerto Rico**

Hernández PH: Breve historia de la odontologia en Puerto Rico. **Rev Odontol PR** 1979 Nov-1980 May;17(1):2-15

**South Africa**

Dreyer WP: The history of periodontology in South Africa. **Tydskr Tandheelkd Ver S Afr** 1981 Apr;36(4):271-2, 274-5

**Spain**

Iglesias JG: Origenes y evolucion de la odontoestomatologia en España. **Acta Odontol Venez** 1981 Sep-Dec;19(3):305-12

Pérez PJ, Arsuaga JL, Bermudez de Castro JM: Atypical toothwear in fossil man. **Paleopathol Newsl** 1982 Sep;39:11-3

**Syria**

Drinnan AJ: Odontophilately (Abul Kasim). **NY State Dent J** 1979 Aug-Sep;45(7):332

**United States**

Costa RL: Periodontal disease in the prehistoric Ipiutak and Tigara skeletal remains from Point Hope, Alaska. **Am J Phys Anthropol** 1982 Sep;59(1):97-110

Goodman AH, Armelagos GJ, Rose JC: The chronological distribution of enamel hypoplasias from prehistoric Dickson Mounds populations. **Am J Phys Anthropol** 1984 Nov;65(3):259-66

Hinton RJ: Differences in interproximal and occlusal tooth wear among prehistoric Tennessee Indians: implications for masticatory function. **Am J Phys Anthropol** 1982 Jan;57(1):103-15

**Venezuela**

Febres-Cordero F: Bibliografía Odontólogica Venezolana. **Acta Odontol Venez** 1982 Sep-Dec;20(3):183-91

**Before 500 A.D.**

Davidson M: Ancient references to dentistry and 'Biblical bites'. **Bull Hist Dent** 1983 Apr;31(1):30-1

Deutsch-Kasimir M: Die Heilige Apollonia. **Quintessenz J** 1982 Nov;12(11):1025-6

Gingerich PD: Dental and cranial adaptations in Eocene Adapidae. **Z Morphol Anthropol** 1980;71(2):135-42

Graham EE: A probable submandibular gland defect in a prehistoric mandible. **Oral Surg** 1980 Aug;50(2):187-9

Jaworski Z: Abrazja z ebów a zmiany w budowie anatomicznej żuchwy ludzi sprzed 3.000 lat z okolic Tarnobrzega. **Protet Stomatol** 1983 Jan-Feb;33(1):59-66

Levers BG, Darling AI: Continuous eruption of some adult human teeth of ancient populations. **Arch Oral Biol** 1983;28(5):401-8

McHenry HM: Relative cheek-tooth size in Australopithecus. **Am J Phys Anthropol** 1984 Jul;64(3):297-306

Maringer J: Menschliche Unterkiefer und Zähne im Brauch und Glauben der vorgeschichtlichen Menschen. **Anthropol Anz** 1980 May;38(1):69-73

Moorhead TF: Chirurgia, medicina, dentrifricium. A brief trip into antiquity. **Br Dent J** 1983 May 21;154(10):340-2

Nardoux M, Montarnal: Carie--abrasion--dimension. Dents de la préhistoire. **Ligament (Montp)** 1980;137:88-91

Neuhauser W: Zur Zeit der Bibel war der Zahn so viel wert wie das Leben selbst. **Zahnarztl Mitt** 1984 Apr 1;74(7):729-33

Osborn JW, Hillman J: Enamel structure in some therapsids and mesozoic mammals. **Calcif Tissue Int** 1979 Nov;29(1):47-61

Puech PF, Prone A, Albertini H: Reproduction expérimentale des processus d'altération de la surface dentaire par friction non abrasive et non adhésive: application à l'étude de l'alimentation de l'homme fossile. **C R Seances Acad Sci [III]** 1981 Nov 9;293(9):497-502

Puech PF, Prone A: Reproduction expérimentale des processus d'usure dentaire par abrasion: implications paléoécologiques chez l'homme fossile. **C R Acad Sci [D] (Paris)** 1979 Nov 19;289(13):895-8

Ramsey WO: Hermetic sealing of root canals--the Greeks had a name for it. **J Endod** 1982 Mar;8(3):100

Rouot J: Die Zahnheilkunde in der Antike. In Sournia JC, Martiny M, Poulet J, ed: Illustrierte Geschichte der Medizin. Salzburg, Andreas, 1980. Vol. 2. p. 523-37.

Rudney JD, Katz RV, Brand JW: Interobserver reliability of methods for paleopathological diagnosis of dental caries. **Am J Phys Anthropol** 1983 Nov;62(3):243-8

Sakai T: [Morphology of premolar in primitive anthropoidea] (Jpn). **Shikai Tenbo** 1983 Jan;61(1):81-90

Setoguchi T: [Paleontological view points on the morphological characteristics of human molar teeth. I (author's transl)] (Jpn). **Shikai Tenbo** 1981;(7):31-8

Setoguchi T: [Paleontological view points on the morphological characteristics of human molar teeth. II, III (author's transl)] (Jpn). **Shikai Tenbo** 1981;(8,9):319-25,441-8

Walker A: Diet and teeth. Dietary hypotheses and human evolution. **Philos Trans R Soc Lond [Biol]** 1981 May 8;292(1057):57-64

Williams JA: Fourier analysis and homology of the first molars of the Palaeocene primate family Picrodontidae. **Arch Oral Biol** 1981;26(2):111-6

Wood BA, Abbott SA, Graham SH: Analysis of the dental morphology of Plio-Pleistocene hominids. II. Mandibular molars--study of cusp areas, fissure pattern and cross sectional shape of the crown. **J Anat** 1983 Sep;137(Pt 2):287-314

Wood BA: Tooth size and shape and their relevance to studies of hominid evolution. **Philos Trans R Soc Lond [Biol]** 1981 May 8;292(1057):65-76

Yamada M, Horibe H, Fujimori K, et al: Paleobiophysical studies on tooth tisues by microfluorometry and Raman-spectrometry. **Cell Mol Biol** 1979;25(3):167-72

Yinyun Z: Variability and evolutionary trends in tooth size of Gigantopithecus blacki. **Am J Phys Anthropol** 1982 Sep;59(1):21-32

**Africa**

Wood BA, Abbott SA: Analysis of the dental morphology of Plio-pleistocene hominids. I. Mandibular molars: crown area measurements and morphological traits. **J Anat** 1983 Jan;136 (Pt 1):197-219

**Americas**

Cook DC: Hereditary enamel hypoplasia in a prehistoric Indian child. **J Dent Res** 1980 Sep;59(9):1522

**Arabic**

Højgaard K: Dentition on Umm an-Nar (Trucial Oman), 2500 B.C. **Scand J Dent Res** 1980 Oct;88(5):355-64

**Argentina**

Hershkovitz P: Comparative anatomy of platyrrhine mandibular cheek teeth dpm4, pm4, ml with particular reference to those of Homunculus (Cebidae), and comments on platyrrhine origins. **Folia Primatol (Basel)** 1981;35(2-3)179-217

**Asia**

Hojgaard K: Dilmun-tidens taender. Umm an-Nar (2500 f.v.t.). Al-Bahrain (2000 f.v.t.). **Tandlaegebladet** 1980 Sep;84(16):548

**Austria**

Nicola M, Stiebitz R: Morphologische und pathologische Befunde von Zähnen und Kiefern aus der Mittleren Bronzezeit (Pitten, Niederösterreich). **Anthropol Anz** 1979 Oct;37(3):182-203

**Bahrain**

Højgaard K: Dentition on Bahrain, 2000 B.C. **Scand J Dent Res** 1980 Dec;88(6):467-75

**Chile**

Turner CG, Bird J: Dentition of Chilean paleo-Indians and peopling of the Americas. **Science** 1981 May 29;212(4498):1053-5

**China**

Pindborg JJ: Nyt om Peking-manden og hans forgaengere. **Tandlaegebladet** 1981 Feb;85(3):82-5

Tode I: [Significance of the letter 'u' in ancient Chinese. Did it mean caries or tooth?] (Jpn). **Shikai Tenbo** 1983 Nov;62(5):975-81

**Cyprus**

Taramides G: Ta dontia ton Kyprios tes neolithikos epoches (5800-3000 P.Ch.). **Odontostomatol Proodos** 1983 Jul-Aug;37(4):213-8

# DENTISTRY

**Denmark**

Sct Apollonia og dansk odontologi: **Tandlaegebladet** 1984 Jan;88(1):5-8

**Egypt**

Leek FF: Palaeodontology of the Nile Valley. **Paleopathol Newsl** 1981 Jan;33:9-12
Lipton JS: Oral surgery in Ancient Egypt as reflected in the Edwin Smith Papyrus. **Bull Hist Dent** 1982 Oct;30(2):108-14
Mann P: Taking a look at 3,000-year-old teeth. **Br Dent J** 1980 Jul 15;149(2):57-8
Peluso A: Patologia orale in una antica popolazione egiziana. **Dent Cadmos** 1980 Dec;48(12):9-28
Tronnberg G: S:ta Apollonia av Alexandra--tandlakarnas skyddshelgon. **Odontol Foren Tidskr** 1980 Dec;44(5):22-8

**Europe**

Scholz F, Rossiwall B: Taurodontismus: Eine anthropologische Streitfrage und ein Mikrosymptom für genetische Störungen. **Osterr Z Stomatol** 1981 Oct;78(10):373-8

**France**

Tillier AM: Evolution de la région symphysaire chez les homo sapiens juvéniles du paléolithique moyen: pech de l'azé 1, roc de marsal et la chaise 13. **C R Seances Acad Sci** [III] 1981 Nov 9;293(9):493-5
Tillier AM, Genet-Varcin E: La plus ancienne mandibule d'enfant découverte en France dans le gisement de La Chaise de Vouthon (Abri Suard) en Charente. **Z Morphol Anthropol** 1980;71(2):196-214

**Germany**

Jaworski Z: Morfologia zębów stałych z dziecięcych grobów ciałopalnych kultury łuzyckiej. **Czas Stomatol** 1981 May;34(5):487-92
Jaworski Z: Przyżyciowe braki zębowe w szczatkach kostnych z grobów ciałopalnych kultury łużyckiej. **Czas Stomatol** 1981 Oct;34(10):969-74
Jaworski Z: Szczątki szczęk i żuchw Prasłowian z grobów ciałopalnych kultury łużychiej. **Czas Stomatol** 1981 Sep;34(9):897-907

**Great Britain**

Ivanhoe F: Interglovular dentine in first and third molars: relation to hours of sunshine during growth in two archeological populations from England. **Calcif Tissue Int** 1982 Mar;34(2):136-44
Newman HN, Levers BG: Tooth eruption and function in an early Anglo-Saxon population. **J R Soc Med** 1979 May;72(5):341-50
Whittaker DK, Molleson T, Bennett RB, et al: The prevalence and distribution of dental caries in a Romano-British population. **Arch Oral Biol** 1981;26(3):237-45
Whittaker DK, Parker JH, Jenkins C: Tooth attrition and continuing eruption in a Romano-British population. **Arch Oral Biol** 1982;27(5):405-9

**Greco-Roman**

Deeley WS: Greeks, Romans applied science to knowledge of the oral cavity. **Dent Stud** 1976 Jun;54(9):38-40

**Greece**

Iskander Z, Harris J, Shafik Farid: Further evidence of dental prothesis in ancient Egypt. **Ann Serv Antiq Egypte** 1979;63(spécial);Mélanges Selim Hassan II:103-13

**India**

Bergemann H: Drachenzähne und Opfergaben. **Zahnarztl Mitt** 1980 May 16;70(10):655-7
Lukacs JR: Crown dimensions of deciduous teeth from prehistoric India. **Am J Phys Anthropol** 1981 Jun;55(2):261-6

**Italy**

Gavazzi C: Odontoiatria del passato. I denti umani fossili di Salto (Valle Orco). **Dent Cadmos** 1981 Oct, Nov;49(10,11):59-63 contd, 71-9
Lassig HE: Etruskische Zahnärzte entwickelten eine sehr beachtliche Prothetik. **Zahnarztl Mitt** 1984 Sep 16;74(18):2015-9
Nihlen B: Fenomenala tandläkare - för 2500 år sedan! **Tandlakartidningen** 1982 Sep 15;74(18):999-1000

**Japan**

Sugimoto S: [Man-yo-shu and dentistry] (Jpn). **Rinsho Shika** 1982;(304):22-4

**Nigeria**

Fraudet JR: La pression antéro-postérieure des lèvres sur l'arcade dentaire inférieure à l'époque néolithique. **Rev Stomatol Chir Maxillofac** 1984;85(5):438-40

**Peru**

Miura F, Soma K, Hatate M: [The orthodontic observation of ancient Peruvian calvaria--orthopedically induced deformity of the skull]. (Jpn) **Kokubyo Gakkai Zasshi** 1979 Sep;46(3):220-7

**Poland**

Biedowa J: Morfologia zębów trzonowych na tle ich tendencji ewolucyjnych. **Czas Stomatol** 1980 Mar;33(3):191-6

**Rome**

Brøndum N: Tandforhold i det klassiske Rom. **Dan Medicinhist Arbog** 1983;12:164-8
Pujol F: L'odontologie à la fin de l'empire romain: Caelius Aurelianus. **Chir Dent Fr** 1984 May 31;54(252):21-5
Smith P, Tau S: Dental pathology in the period of the Roman Empire: a comparison of two populations. **Ossa** 1978;5:35-41
Vidal F: Caelius Aurelianus et la douleur dentaire: 'de dolore dentium'. **Inf Dent** 1984 Jul 12-19;66(28-29):2875-88
Vidal F: La pharmacologie bucco-dentaire au temps d'Auguste. **Chir Dent Fr** 1983 Mar 10;53(194):21-30

**South Africa**

Tobias PV: The natural history of the helicoidal occlusal plane and its evolution in early Homo. **Am J Phys Anthropol** 1980 Aug;53(2):173-87

**Spain**

Castro JM de: Etude anthropologique de la denture de la population préhispanique de l'Ile de Grande Canarie. **Bull Group Int Rech Sci Stomatol Odontol** 1984 Jan;27(1):11-29

**United States**

Cook DC, Buikstra JE: Health and differential survival in prehistoric populations: prenatal dental defects. **Am J Phys Anthropol** 1979 Nov;51(4):649-64
Goodman AH, Armelagos GJ, Rose JC: Enamel hypoplasias as indicators of stress in three prehistoric populations from Illinois. **Hum Biol** 1980 Sept;52(3):515-28
Hinton RJ, Smith MO, Smith FH: Tooth size changes in prehistoric Tennessee Indians. **Hum Biol** 1980 May;52(2):229-45

**USSR**

Moriyama N: [Controversies on the Kul-Oba vase and its relation to the ancient Scythian dentistry (author's transl)] (Jpn). **Shikwa Gakuho** 1980 Apr;80(4):597-602

**Zimbabwe**

Koritzer RT, St. Hoyme LE: Extensive caries in early man circa 110,000 years before present. **J Am Dent Assoc** 1979 Oct;99(4):642-3

**500 A.D.-1450**

Bowers DF: Return of the worm. **Ohio Dent J** 1984 Sep;58(9):9-10
Larsson E: Malocclusions in a juvenile medieval skull material. **Swed Dent J** 1983;7(5):185-90
May BR: Curious dental practices of the Middle Ages. **CAL** 1979 Mar;42(9):23-4
Sigron G: Zahnmedizin im Frühmittelalter. **Schweiz Monatsschr Zahnmed** 1984 Jan;94(1):49-56

**Arabic**

Belolapotkova AV: Voprosy stomatologii v 'Kanone vrachebnoĭ nauki' Ibn-Siny. **Stomatologiia (Mosk)** 1980 Nov-Dec;59(6):69-70

**Austria**

Stiebitz R, Teschler-Nicola M: Pathologische Befunde am Kauapparat eines Schädels aus dem 6. Jh. n. Chr., Fundort: Schwechat, Niederösterreich. **Wien Klin Wochenschr** 1981 Nov 27;93(22):703-7

**Bulgaria**

Kadunkov D: Niakoi danni za meditsinata zubolechenito prez vtoroto bulgarsko tsarstvo i srednovekov neto. **Stomatologiia (Sofiia)** 1979 Jan–Feb;61(1):68–9

**Denmark**

Helm S, Prydsö U: Assessment of age-at-death from mandibular molar attrition in medieval Danes. **Scand J Dent Res** 1979 Apr;87(2):79–90

Helm S, Prydsö U: Prevalence of malocclusion in medieval and modern Danes contrasted. **Scand J Dent Res** 1979 Apr;87(2):91–7

Jakobsen J, Jorgensen JB, Kreiborg S, et al: Kong Valdemar Atterdag: antropologiske fund under en odontologisk synsvinkel. **Tandlaegebladet** 1981 Jan;85(1):9–16

Klafstad J: Odontopathology of a Norwegian medieval population--a pilot study. **Ossa** 1978;5:43–55

**Dominican Republic**

Garcia-Godoy F: Caries dental en cráneos primitivos de la Isla Santo Domingo. **Rev Asoc Odontol Argent** 1978 Jul–Sep;66(3):147–50

**Germany**

Scheiper R: Zahnerkrankungen unserer Vorfahren, der Alamannen. **Zahnarztl Mitt** 1984 Feb 16;74(4):363–4, 367–8

**Great Britain**

Claxton AC: An early dental identification of a corpse. **Br Dent J** 1984 Aug 25;157(4):122

Foley GP: A treasury of dentistry. The dental attraction of the Wells Cathedral. **J Am Coll Dent** 1983 Fall;50(3):16–7

**Hungary**

Kocsis SG, Marcsik A: Zománcképzödmények a VII–VIII. századból származó koponýak fogain. **Fogorv Sz** 1981 Mar;74(3):89–93

**Italy**

Eramo S: L'odontoiatria nell'arte. Su un affresco raffigurante S. Apollonia nella Basilica di Santa Maria di Collemaggio a l'Aquila. **Dent Cadmos** 1984 Apr;52(4):135–7

Sigron G: Zahnheilkunde und Kieferchirurgie in Salerno. **SSO Schweiz Monatsschr Zahnheilkd** 1983 Jun;93(6):449–53

**Japan**

Inoue N: [Dental diseases in Kamakura period (author's transl)] (Jpn). **Shikai Tenbo** 1980;(12):1009–18

Ito G: [Tooth to denture base discrepancy among Japanese during the Middle Ages] (Jpn). **Shikai Tenbo** 1980;(11):825–33

**Peru**

Sawyer DR, Nwoku AL, Elzay RP, et al: Two probable cases of a depression in the mandible caused by the submandibular salivary gland in Pre-Columbian Peruvians. **J Maxillofac Surg** 1981 Aug;9(3):194–6

**Sweden**

Bergman LE, Hansson T: Hard tissue changes of the temporomandibular joint in an archaeo-osteological material from the 11th century. **Swed Dent J** 1979;3(5):149–55

Mohlin B, et al: The frequency of malocclusion and the craniofacial morphology in a medieval population in southern Sweden. **Ossa** 1978;5:57–84

**Switzerland**

Roulet JF, Ulrich-Bochsler S: Zahnärztliche Untersuchung frühmittelalterlicher Schädel aus Biel-Mett. **SSO Schweiz Monatsschr Zahnheilkd** 1979 Jun;89(6):526–40

Wiederkehr M, Roulet JF, Ulrich-Bochsler S: Zahnärztliche Untersuchung mittelalterlicher Schädel aus drei Regionen des Kantons Bern. **SSO Schweiz Monatsschr Zahnheilkd** 1982 Feb;92(2):127–36

**Turkey**

Dizdar A: Der türkische Arzt Serafeddin Sabuncuoğlu (1385–1472) und seine Verdienste um die Zahnheilkunde. Diss. Würzburg, 1981. 68 p.

**United States**

Gregg JB, Zimmerman L, Clifford S, et al: Craniofacial anomalies in the Upper Missouri River over a millennium: archeological and clinical evidence. **Cleft Palate J** 1981 Jul;18(3):210–22

**1450–1700**

Gysel C: Arnoldus Senguerdius (1610–1668) en zijn wijsgerige verhandeling 'De Dentibus'. **Ned Tijdschr Tandheelkd** 1978 Nov;85(11):468–70

Gysel C: Dentistry and Cartesianism (1637–1650). **Dent Cadmos** 1980;48(3):53–5

Gysel C: Jan Swammerdam (1637–1680–1980), zijn Cartesianism en de fysiologie van het kauwstelsel (I). **Ned Tijdschr Tandheelkd** 1981 Jun;88(6):238–41

Gysel C: Les implications cartésiennes de la nosologie bucco-dentaire de Pierre Fauchard (1678–1761–1978). **Rev Belge Med Dent** 1979;34(3):313–20

Gysel C: L'odonto-stomatologie d'après les 'vrais et solides fondements de la médecine', établis par Louis du Gardin, professeur à l'université de Douai, sous le règne d'Albert et d'Isabelle. **Rev Belge Med Dent** 1982 Jul;37(4):164–71

Gysel C: Odontologie et cartesianisme naissant (1637--1650). **Rev Belge Med Dent** 1979;34(2):223–30

Gysel C: Thomas Bartholinus (1616–1680–1980), zijn nederlandse relaties en de tandheelkunde (II). **Ned Tijdschr Tandheelkd** 1982 Oct;89(10):414–9

Gysel C: Umanesimo e odontoiatria: Harvey e Spigelius, due vite parallele. **Dent Cadmos** 1981 Jan;49(1):61–6

Gysel C: W. Harvey (1578–1657) et A. van den Spiegel (1578–1625), l'humanisme et l'odontologie. **Rev Belge Med Dent** 1979;34(1):121–6

Markens IS: De orthondontice ten tijde van de Renaissance. **Ned Tijdschr Tandheelkd** 1984 Sep;91(9):362–4

**Americas**

Cone TE: The nursing bottle caries syndrome. **JAMA** 1981 Jun 12;245(22):2334

**Belgium**

Gysel C: De tandheelkunde van Adrianus Spigelius Bruxellensis (1578–1625–1978). **Rev Belge Med Dent** 1979;34(1):99–120

Gysel C: Helmontianisme en odontologie (I). **Rev Belge Med Dent** 1979;34(3):295–312

Gysel C: Helmontianisme en odontologie (II). 3. Van Helmont en het nagerslacht. **Rev Belge Med Dent** 1979;34(4):385–96

Gysel C: Jean-Baptiste Van Helmont (1579–1644), le baroque et les dents. **Rev Belge Med Dent** 1979;34(4):397–404

**Denmark**

Gysel C: Thomas Bartholinus (1616–1680–1980), zijn Zederlandse relaties en de tandheelkunde (I). **Ned Tijdschr Tandheelkd** 1982 Jan;89(1):39–43

**Europe**

Muratori G: Odontoiatria del passato. I tumori della lingua. **Dent Cadmos** 1981 Apr;49(4):68–9

Muratori G: Odontoiatria del passato. I tumori odontogeni. **Dent Cadmos** 1981 Apr;49(4):65–7

Schienbein G, Schienbein H: 'Der Zähn stincken verbessern'--Zahnheilkunde in einem Kräuterbuch von 1602 (I, II). **Quintessenz** 1980 Jun–Jul;31(6,7):133–40, 165–70

**France**

David T, Dagen G, Gauval VB: Les dents de Louis XIV. **Soc Fr Hist Art Dent** 1979 Sep–Dec;(5–6):6–10

Duburcq P: Ambroise Paré et l'odontologie. **Chir Dent Fr** 1982 Mar–Apr;52(151–3):21–38

Duburcq P: Odontoiatria del passato. Ambroise Paré e l'odontoiatria. I. 'Io l'ho curato d Dio l'ha guarito'. **Dent Cadmos** 1982 Jun–Jul;50(6–7):75–9, 87–9

Duburcq P: Odontoiatria del passato. Ambroise Paré l'odontoiatria. III. **Dent Cadmos** 1982 Aug;50(8):83–5

Duburq P: Ambroise Paré et l'odontologie. **Chir Dent Fr** 1982 Mar 18;52(150):41–9 contd.

Gauval VB: Détails piquants sur la vie d'un des praticiens du Roi et de ses honoraires. **Soc Fr Hist Art Dent** 1979 Sep–Dec;(5–6):11–14

Gysel C: Appréciation d'Urbain Hémard et de sa 'Recherche de la vraye anatomie des dents'. **Actual Odontostomatol (Paris)** 1982;36(139):395–410

Gysel C: Bernardin Martin et sa 'dissertation sur les dents' (1679–1979). **Actual Odontostomatol (Paris)** 1980;34(129):59–72

Gysel C: L'odontologie à la fin de la Renaissance, sous le règne de Galien et des deux Riolan. **Actual Odontostomatol (Paris)** 1981;(135):373–90

Gysel C: Odontoiatria del passato. L'odontostomatologia nel contesto delle 'vere e solide fondamenta della medicine', definite da Louis Du Gardin, Professore all'Universitá di Douai, sotto il regno di Alberto ed Isabella. **Dent Cadmos** 1983 Apr;51(4):91–5 contd

Gysel G: Odontoiatria del passato. L'odontostomatologia nel contesto delle 'vere e solide fondamenta della medicina', definite da Louis Du Gardin, Professore all'Università di Douai, sotto il regno di Alberto ed Isabella.

II. **Dent Cadmos** 1983 May;51(5):107–9, 112
'Le chirurgien-dentiste' di Pierre Fauchard, I and II: **Dent Cadmos** 1980 May;48(5):57–60, (6):53–7
Vidal F: L'Edit Royal de mai 1699––une date capitale pour l'odontologie. **Chir Dent Fr** 1981 Sep 3;51(123):25–37

**Germany**

Riethe P, Czarnetzki A: Amalgam- und Goldfolienfüllung Anno Domini 1601. **Dtsch Zahnarztl Z** 1983 Jun;38(6):610–6

**Great Britain**

Ring ME: Oddments in dental history: what every sea surgeon of around 1600 ought to know concerning treating teeth. **Bull Hist Dent** 1984 Oct;32(2):109–11

**Italy**

Herschfeld JJ: Bartholomeus Eustachius––the first great dental anatomist. **Bull Hist Dent** 1982 Oct;30(2):123–8
Scarano GB: Le malattie della bocca e dei denti nell'opera di Girolamo Fabrizio d'Acquapendente. **Med Secoli** 1982 Jan–Apr;19(1):101–23

**Japan**

Yatsu M: [Miscellaneous records of medico-dental and pharmacological history (49). 'Jinrinkinmozui', a publication dated 1690 (3)] (Jpn). **Shikai Tenbo** 1984 Jan;63(1):194–5

**Netherlands**

Gysel C: Een vulgarisator van de anatomie van het kauwstelsel: Gerard Blasius (1626–1682–1982). **Ned Tijdschr Tandheelkd** 1984 Jun;91(6):153–8
Mikx F: Antoni van Leeuwenhoek––300 sodina oralne mikrobiologije. **Acta Stomatol Croat** 1983;17(4):323–5
Mikx FH: Het tandplaque-onderzoek van Antoni van Leeuwenhoek in 1683. **Ned Tijdschr Tandheelkd** 1983 Sep;90(9):421–4
Peck S, Peck H: Prosperity and decay: a portrait of the Dutch golden age. **Dent Abstr** 1980 Mar;25(3):116–8
Tal M: Periodontal disease and oral hygiene. Described by Antoni van Leeuwenhoek. **J Periodontol** 1980 Nov;51(11):668–9

**Spain**

Moreno Gonzalez JP, Gonzalez Iglesias J: Sorapan de Rieros y la odontologia. **Bol Inf Dent (Madr)** 1979 Sep–Oct;(302):37–44
Moskow BS: The iconography of the dental profession. Francisco Zurbarán (1598–1664). **Quintessence Int** 1984 Aug;15(8):814–5

**Yugoslavia**

Hadžiomeragić M: Prvi zubni lijecnik kod nas (1493. god.). **Stomatol Vjesn** 1978;7(3–4):89–92

**1700 to Present**

Als die Zahnheilkunde ihre Lehrzeit absolvierte: **Zahnarztl Mitt** 1983 Dec 16;73(24):2766–7
Aurel D: De l'histoire des relations médicales franco-roumaines –– au 120e anniversaire de la mort de François Achard –– l'activité de François Achard en Roumanie. **Soc Fr Hist Art Dent** 1979 Sep–Dec;(5–6):30–3
Bates JD: The extraction debate of 1911. **New Dent** 1980 Jan;10(5):36–7
Beeching BW: Historical background to radiation safety of dental x-ray sets in the English speaking countries. **Dentomaxillofac Radiol** 1981;10(2):85–92
Berenbrinker A: Die zahnmedizinische Karikatur I: 1780–1840. Köln, 1982. 227 p. (Arbeiten der Forschungsstelle des Instituts für Geschichte der Medizin der Universität zu Köln, Band 25).
Besombes A: Die Zahnmedizin vom 18. Jahrhundert bis zur Gegenwart. In Sournia JC, Martiny M, Poulet J, ed: Illustrierte Geschichte der Medizin. Salzburg, Andreas, 1980. Vol. 8. p. 3053–79.
Bethmann W, Hampel H, Knöfler W: Zur Problematik der stomatologischen Implantation. Die historische Betrachtung der Implantologie-Forschung mit dem Versuch einer Periodizierung nach wissenschaftlichen Gesichtspunkten. **Stomatol DDR** 1981;31(2):100–7
Bird PD: The development of dental radiology. The realisation of a scientific dream. **Br Dent J** 1981 Jul 7;151(1):28–30
Boulton TB: The rise and fall of general anaesthesia in the dental chair. **SAAD Dig** 1980 Jul;4(7):156–65
Bradley BE: The historic use of diazepam in dentistry. **Anesth Prog** 1981 Mar–Apr;28(2):38–40
Buffat JJ, Thonnier C, Bourdais A, et al: Anesthésie et odonto-stomatologie. **Actual Odontostomatol (Paris)** 1982;36(139)303–13
Carr MW: Thomas W. Evans: his life and influence on the development of dentistry as a learned profession. **J Am Coll Dent** 1979 Apr;46(2):87–100
Cawson RA, Stocker IP: The early history of fluorides as anti-caries agents. **Br Dent J** 1984 Dec 8;157(11):403–4
The changing look of dental assisting: **Dent Assist** 1984 Sep–Oct;53(5):23–6
Christen AG: The oral history interview: a treasurehouse for present and future dental historiographers. **Bull Hist Dent** 1981;29(1):8–14
Cohen LK: Dentistry and the behavioral/social sciences: an historical overview. **J Behav Med** 1981 Sep;4(3):247–56
Cooke BE: History of oral medicine. **Br Dent J** 1981 Jul 7;151(1):11–3
Dale JG: Orthodontics: past, present and future? **Can Dent Assoc J** 1982 Mar;48(3):180–2
Dewel BF: Orthodontics: midcentury recollections. **Eur J Orthod** 1981;3(2):77–87
Dietz G: Abriss der Entwicklung der Endodontie. **Zahnarzt** 1983 Dec;27(12):780–4
Donaldson JA: Ars scientia mores. **Br Dent J** 1980 Dec 2;149(11):335–6
Feller I: Die zahnmedizinische Karikatur II: 1840–1880. Köln, 1983. 284 p. (Arbeiten der Forschungsstelle des Instituts für Geschichte der Medizin der Universität zu Köln, Band 26).
The first fifty years 1931–1981: **Dent Assist** 1981 Jan–Feb;50(1):24–6
Fischer CH: Die Entwicklung der japanisch-deutschen Beziehungen aus zahnärztlicher Sicht. **Zahnarztl Mitt** 1981;71(5):292–4
Foley GP: A treasury of dentistry. Early offices were a dangerous place to practice. **J Am Coll Dent** 1983 Summer;50(2):24–5
Fox B, Maddick I: A century of dental myths and messages. **Soc Soc Hist Med Bull** 1980;27:47–53
Fox BW: Turn of the century dentistry. **CAL** 1983 Aug;47(2):18–9, 21–4
Franke OC: Wilhelm Conrad Roentgen and other X-ray pioneers. **Bull Hist Dent** 1983 Apr;31(1):11–7
Gold SI: Early origins of hydrogen peroxide use in oral hygiene. A historical note. **J Periodontol** 1983 Apr;54(4):247
Hagman HC: Gnathology and its originators. **Dent Lab Rev** 1982 Jul;57(7):20–1
Haller JS: The foul tongue: a 19th century index of disease. **West J Med** 1982 Sep;137(3):258–64
Harris CD: Dental electrosurgery. **Georgetown Dent J** 1979 Jul;53(2):45–53
Harsch OM: Philatelistisch-Odontologises Panopticum. **Zahnarztl Mitt** 1983 Jul 1;73(13):1470–1 contd
Häussermann E: Für den Zahnarzt im Dichter-Schloss nur ein kleines Mansarden-Zimmer. **Zahnarztl Mitt** 1983 Sep 16;73(18):1990, 1993–4
Helöe LA, Haugejorden O: 'The rise and fall' of dental caries: some global aspects of dental caries epidemiology. **Community Dent Oral Epidemiol** 1981 Dec;9(6):294–9
Heydt H: 30th year reunion of four scientists marks less tooth decay around the world––the monofluorophosphate story. **J Dent Assoc S Afr** 1980 Dec;35(12):837–9
Hilderbrand RM: Dental remedies of the past. **Alumni Bull Sch Dent Indiana Univ** 1982 Spring;:25–31, 87
Hoffman JH: Dentistry is quack-less. **CAL** 1982 Apr;45(10):18–21
Hoffman W: Der Zahnarzt in dieser Welt––gestern, heute und morgen. **Zahnarztliche Mitteilungen** 1980 Sep 1;70(17):1080–6
Hoffmann-Axthelm W: W. D. Miller - Ein Pionier der wissenschaftlichen Zahnheilkunde. **Quintessenz J** 1983 Oct;13(10):927–30
Holtkamp P: Ringwerke––die erste Brückenprothetik. **Quintessenz Zahntech** 1981 Apr;7(4):401–3
Hunstadbråten K: Fluor i kariesprofylaksen omkring århundriskiftet. **Nor Tannlaegeforen Tid** 1981 May;91(7):227–31
Hunstadbråten K: Fluor in der Kariesprophylaxe der Jahrhundertwende. **Quintessenz J** 1984 Feb;14(2):147–51
Hunstadbraten K: Fluoride in caries prophylaxis at the turn of the century. **Bull Hist Dent** 1982 Oct;30(2):117–20
Hunstadbraten K: Kariesprophylaxe durch Fluoride um die Jahrhundertwende. **Zahnarztl Mitt** 1982 Nov 16;72(22):2537–9
Jackle P, Nittenwilm U, Steffens G, et al: Alfred Gysi––ein Pionier der Zahnheilkunde und Zahntechnik. **Dent Labor (Muench)** 1982 Aug;30(8):1153–61
Jaffe M: The evolution of ambulatory anesthesiology in dentistry **Anesth Prog** 1980 May–Jun;27(3):76–84
Janson I: Kieferorthopädie gestern und heute. **Zahnarztl Prax** 1979 May 11;30(5):203–14
Jenkins GN: A century of oral physiology. **Br Dent J** 1981 Jul 7;151(1):6–10
Jenny J: An historic parallel: 19th century education, 20th century dental care. **J Public Health Dent** 1979 Fall;39(4):295–7
Julien P: Sur le célèbre 'dentiste' ou 'pharmacien' de Pietro Longhi. **Pharm Weekbl** 1981 Nov 6;116(45):1389–92
Jung T: X-rays in dentistry. **J Am Dent Assoc** 1982 Apr;104(4):438
Karnoff EM: Fifty years of the same thing. **NY J Dent** 1980 May;50(5):189–90
Kogge D: Zur geschichtlichen Entwicklung der Behandlungsmassnahmen bei Lippen-Kiefer-Gaumenspalten. Diss. Bonn, 1981. 84 p.
Kunegel JM, Limoge A, Debras C: Historique de l'électroanesthésie. **Inf Dent** 1982 Nov 18:64(40):3919–24
Kurashima K: [Angle's orthodontics: a critical review. I. Angle's quest for science, and his classification of malocclusion] (Jpn). **Nippon Kyosei Shika Gakkai Zasshi** 1983 Sep;42(3):379–84
Lange J: Humant spyt og auxiner––et historisk tilbagekig. **Tandlaegebladet** 1982 Oct;86(17):595
Leatherman GH: 80 Jahre FDI––eine Chronik moderner

Gesundheitspolitik. **Zahnarztliche Mitteilungen** 1980 Sep 1;70(17):1070–9
Leatherman GH: 80 Jahre FDI-- 'Erntejahre' 1962–1980. **Zahnarztliche Mitteilungen** 1980 Nov 1;70(21):1392–7 concl
Leatherman GH: 80 Jahre FDI--1900–1980. Aktivitäten der Kommissionen 1962–1979. **Zahnarztliche Mitteilungen** 1980 Oct 16;70(2):1313–7 contd
Leatherman GH: 80 Jahre FDI--1900–1980. Die Zeit des Wiederaufbaus und der Reformen. **Zahnarztliche Mitteilungen** 1980 Sep 16;70(18):1172–8 contd
Löe HA: Scientific revolutions in dentistry. **J Dent Res** 1979 Nov;58(Spec Issue D):2164–8
Martin LR: The history of endodontics. **J Miss Dent Assoc** 1981 Summer;37(2):30–2
Marvitz L: Manden bag navnet. **Tidsskr Tandlaeger** 1983 Apr;3:51
Marvitz L: Nanden bag navnet. Johann Jacob Joseph Serre. **Tidsskr Tandlaeger** 1982 Feb;2(1):35
Meinke H: A short history of dental advertising. **Bull Hist Dent** 1983 Apr;31(1):36–42
Mikhail M, Rosen H: History and etiology of myofascial paindysfunction syndrome. **J Prosthet Dent** 1980;44:438–44
Miller GH: A drill in either hand. **CAL** 1981 Mar;44(9):14–5, 18–9
Moriyama N: The origin of the immediate root-canal filling. **Bull Hist Dent** 1982 Apr;30(1):34–9
Muratori G: Odontoiatria del passato. I tumori delle labbra e della mucosa orale. **Dent Cadmos** 1981 May;49(5):71–2
Myers ML: Centric relation records--historical review. **J Prosthet Dent** 1982 Feb;47(2):141–5
Nortjé CJ: Kefaloröntgenografie: 'n historiese literatuuroorsig. **Tydskr Tandheelkd Ver S Afr** 1979 Jun;34(6):327–33
Odontoiatria del passato: Dei campanelli di Loreto. **Dent Cadmos** 1981 Jul;49(7):59–60
Odontoiatria del passato: La storia di De Trey. **Dent Cadmos** 1983 Mar;51(3):75–81
Ostrander FD: Some musings on past and present endodontics. **J Endod** 1980 Oct;6(10):766–8
Paffenbarger GC: Important accomplishments in dentistry, 1930–1980: a personal appraisal. **NY J Dent** 1980 May;50(5):190–1
Pankey LD: Evolution of a philosophy. **Continuum** 1980;:1–9
Pankey LD: The PMS technique: an historical perspective. **Continuum** 1981;:5–11
Pickard HM: Conservative dentistry in the past century. **Br Dent J** 1980 Jul 1;149(1):5–8
Pinkham JR: The dentist and child-patient encounter: an Adlerian analysis. **ASDC J Dent Child** 1982 Jul–Aug;49(4):266–72
Povey DW: Historical perspectives of mucogingival surgery. **Can Dent Assoc J** 1983 Oct;49(10):721–3
Premuda L: I fondamenti storici dell'ortognatodonzia. **Mondo Ortod** 1980 Mar–Apr;5(2):35–42
Premuda L, Gasparini F: La protesi dentaria: breve excursus storico. **G Stomatol Ortognatodonzia** 1982 Dec;1(4):7–10
Reis e Almeida FS: Estomatologia sofrologia. **Rev Port Estomatol Cir Maxilofac** 1983 Apr–Jun;24(2):183–97
Ricketts RM: Perspectives in the clinical application of cephalometrics. The first fifty years. **Angle Orthod** 1981 Apr;51(2):115–50
Ring M: Dentures: the restoration of choice in the 1920s. **Dent Lab Rev** 1982 Aug;57(8):27, 34
Ring M: The age of cosmetic dentistry. **Dent Lab Rev** 1982 Nov;57(11):36
Ring ME: Fagan implant. **NY J Dent** 1984 Jun–Aug;54(5):194
Ring ME: Oddments in dental history. **Bull Hist Dent** 1980 Apr;28(1):19–20 (continued periodically)
Rizzuti A: Il dolore dei denti. **Dent Cadmos** 1981 May;49(5):75–6
Romm S, Luce EA: Hans Pichler: oral surgeon to Sigmund Freud. **Oral Surg** 1984 Jan;57(1):31–2
Ross PJ: The history of hypnosis in dentistry. **Bull Hist Dent** 1981;29(1):24–8
Ruel-Kellermann M: Repères historiques de l'évolution du recours de l'odonto-stomatologie à la psychologie. **Inf Dent** 1981 Oct 1;63(33):3071–83
Schweitzer JM: An evaluation of 50 years of reconstructive dentistry. Part I: Jaw relations and occlusion. **J Prosthet Dent** 1981 Apr;45(4):383–8
Schweitzer JM: An evaluation of 50 years of reconstructive dentistry. Part II: Effectiveness. **J Prosthet Dent** 1981 May;45(5):492–8
Smollon JF: A review and history of endosseous implant dentistry. **Georgetown Dent J** 1979 Jan;63(1):33–45
Szymanski B, Hieke M: Zur Geschichte der Dentitionsforschung unter dem Gesichtspunkt der Entwicklungsdiagnostik. **Aerztl Jugendkd** 1981;72(5):304–26
Teething troubles, 1921--1971. Part twelve: **Dent Tech** 1980 Jan;33(1):11–2 (continued periodically)
Teplitsky PE, Grieman R: History of formocresol pulpotomy. **Can Dent Assoc J** 1984 Aug;50(8):629–34
Topelius C: Om tandvärk och löständer. **Tandlakartidningen** 1981 May 15;73(10):565–9
Witkop CJ: History of genetics in dentistry. **Birth Defects** 1980;16(5):13–26
Zambito RF: A history of hospital dental practice. Part I and II. **New Dent** 1979 Oct–Nov;10(2–3):31–3, 35–8

#### Americas

Canelon JS: Hacia una historia social de la odontológia latinoamericana. **Acta Odontol Venez** 1982 Jan–Apr;20(1):55–63
Febres-Cordero F: Datos sobre el estado de la salud dentaria del Libertador. Caracas, 1983. [2 p.]
Mérida F: Las enfermedades odontologicas y dermatologicas del Libertador. **Rev Soc Venez Hist Med** 1981;30(47):81–7
Mérida MT: Las enfermedades odontológicas y dermatológicas del Liberatador. **Acta Odontol Venez** 1983 May–Aug;21(2):154–61

#### Argentina

Amadeo EM: Recordando a un maestro de la odontología internacional y pionero de la endodoncia: Henry Lentulo 1889–1981. **Rev Asoc Odontol Argent** 1983 Sep;71(5):150–2
Muñoz Al, Hernández Sánchez FA, Bagur DB, et al: Jerarquización de la profesión odontológica. **Salud Bucal** 1981 Jun–Jul;8(44):23–38

#### Australia

Anderson DA: Dental health services and the Northern Territory of Australia. A short review of people, places, and programmes to 1981. **Aust Dent J** 1982 Dec;27(6):345–51
Barnard PD: Review of activities and progress, 1962–1972, Dental Health Education and Research Foundation. Sydney, Dental Health Education and Research Foundation, Univ. of Sydney, [1972?] 30 p.
Brown KA: The identification of Linda Agostini: the significance of dental evidence in the Albury Pyjama Girl case. **Am J Forensic Med Pathol** 1982 Jun;3(2):131–41
Heithersay GS: Endodontic treatment in Australia. **Int Endod J** 1984 Jul;17(3):125–38

#### Austria

Gysel C: Anomalies, mélanodontie et orthodontie dans le traité de pathologie dentaire (1778) de Joseph Jakob Plenk (1732–1807). **Orthod Fr** 1979;50:769–88
Lupinc P: Das zahnärztliche Lehrbuch des Wiener Militärarztes Joseph Georg Pasch 1767. Zürich, Juris Druck, 1984. 80 p. (Zürcher Medizingeschichtliche Abhandlungen, Neue Reihe, Nr. 165).

#### Belgium

Gysel C: De ontwikkeling van de tandheelkunde in België van 1830 tot 1930. **Rev Belge Med Dent** 1981;36(3):103–10
Gysel C: Un siècle d'ephémérides médico-dentaires belges (1830–1930). **Rev Belge Med Dent** 1981;36(3):124–7

#### Bulgaria

Kadankov D: Usuvurshenstvuvane na Bulgarskite zubolekari (1890–1930). **Stomatologiia (Sofiia)** 1979 Jul–Aug;61(4):273–5
Kadunkov D: Diplomirovani zubolekari v Bulgariia ot 1905 do 1914 g. **Stomatologiia (Sofiia)** 1979;(3):201–3
Kadŭnkov D: Njakoi danni za zubloekarstvoto v Bulgarija (1911–1930). **Stomatologiia (Sofiia)** 1979 Sep–Oct;61(5):328–31
Kadunkov D: Purvite obstestveni zubolekarski kabineti v Bulgarija (1907–1971). **Stomatologiia (Sofiia)** 1979 Nov–Dec;61(6):405–8
Kadunkov D: Zubolecenieto v bulgariia prez bulgarskoto vuzrazdane do osvobozdenieto na bulgariia. **Stomatologiia (Sofiia)** 1979 Mar–Apr;61(2):130–3
Vutov M, Krumova E: Razvitie na stomatologicnata pomost i obrazovanie v bulgariia. **Stomatologiia (Sofiia)** 1979 Mar–Apr;61(2):133–6
Vutov M, Ivanova K: Stomatologichnata pomost na podrastvastoto pokolenie u nas do September 9, 1944 godina. **Stomatologiia (Sofiia)** 1979 Nov–Dec;61(6):400–5

#### Canada

McComb F, Gray AS: Dental public health in British Columbia. **Can J Public Health** 1984 Sep–Oct;75(5):368–9
MacEntee MI: The denturist movement in Canada. Part I: Growth and development in the western provinces. **Can Dent Assoc J** 1981 Aug;47(8):521–4

#### Colombia

Mallarino Paz A: Sintesis historica de los programas de personal auxiliar de odontologia en Colombia. **Rev Fac Odontol Univ Nac Colomb** 1980 Jan–Mar;27(132):50–2

#### Cuba

Deschamps Chapeaux P: El negro en la economía Habanera del siglo XIX. Flebotomianos y dentistas. **Rev Bibl Nac Jose Marti** 1971;13(1):75–86

# DENTISTRY

**Cyprus**

Rosenzweig KA: Dental health service in the Cyprus detention camps, 1946–1948. **Bull Hist Dent** 1982 Oct;30(2):92–5

**Denmark**

Britze N: Da en kvindelig tandlaege kun behandlede kvinder og børn. **Tandlaegebladet** 1982 Nov;86(20):714–5
Dyrskjøt I: Familien Friis har haft tandklinik i Hjørring i 100 år. **Tandlaegebladet** 1983 Jan;87(1):29–32
Holmstrup P, et al: [J. J. Pindborg and Danish dentistry]. **Tandlaegebladet** 1981 Aug;85(13):380–408
Marvitz L, Rasmussen EG: Tandlaegeskaebner fra perioden 1790–1850. **Dan Medicinhist Arbog** 1983;12:23–36
Pindborg JJ: Victor Haderup. **Tandlaegebladet** 1984 Jun;88(11):411–6

**Europe**

Held AJ: Un demi-siècle de parodontologie. **Rev Belge Med Dent** 1983 Mar;38(2):30–3
Koller M: Kinderzahnmedizin im 18. und 19. Jahrhundert. **Swiss Dent** 1980 Dec;1(12):32–3
Leatherman GH: 80 years of the FDI. **Probe (Lond)** 1981 Aug;23(2):53–4 contd.

**Finland**

Kalevi Koski 60 years: **Proc Finn Dent Soc** 1981;77(1–3):9–16

**France**

Angot JL: Pierre Fauchard (1677?–1761). Expert pour les dents, et maître chirurgien de Saint-Côme de Paris. **Clio Med** 1983 Mar;17(4):207–21
Aron JP: Odontoiatria del passato. Mutamenti del 'potere medico' in Francia dalla rivoluzione ad oggi. **Dent Cadmos** 1982 Mar;50(3):65–9
Besombes A: La triste fin de Pierre-Nicolas Gaulard (1713–1740) 'élève-associé de Fauchard'. **Hist Sci Med** 1980;14(2):213–20
Carson G: The dentist and the empress. The adventures of Dr. Tom Evans in gas-lit Paris. Boston, Houghton Mifflin, 1983. xiii, 222 p.
Clement A: André Boucher. **Bull Acad Chir Dent (Paris)** 1981–82;27(27):99–102
Dechaume M, Huard P: Paul Broca (1824–1880). Stomatologiste ou la stomatologie du siècle dernier. **Actual Odontostomatol (Paris)** 1980;(132):537–43
Dentistry in folk art XI: L'arracheuse de dents (The tooth puller): **Bull Hist Dent** 1980 Oct;28(2):87
Droz R: Aperçu sur les dentistes strasbourgeois aux XVIIIe et XIXe siècles. In Livet G, Schaff G, ed: Médecine et assistance en Alsace, XVIe–XXe siècle. Strasbourg, Istra, 1976. p. 209–23.
Droz R: Dentistes et dentisteries à Strasbourg au XVIIIe siècle. **Annu Soc Amis Vieux Strasb** 1977;7:29–51
Fouré J: A French woman dentist who gave her life as a freedom fighter against the Nazis. **Bull Hist Dent** 1984 Oct;32(2):133–4
Fouré J: Talma – the dentist who became the greatest French actor of all times. **Bull Hist Dent** 1983 Apr;31(1):3–10
Geiser E: Emile Magitot (1834–1897)--ein Lebensbild. **Schweiz Monatsschr Zahnmed** 1984 Sep;94(9):813–20
Hagman HC: History roots. **Dent Lab Rev** 1981 Jul;56(7):30
Huard P, Imbault-Huart MJ: La stomatologie navale au XVIIIe siècle. In: Congrès National des Sociétés Savantes, 101e, Lille, 1976. Comptes Rendus. Paris, 1976. Section des Sciences, Fasc. III. p. 145–56. (also in 97e Congrès National des Sociétés Savantes, Nantes, 1972, Sciences, Tome I, p. 167–9).
Moskow BS: Dentistry in folk art XV; Decamps--le dentiste. **Bull Hist Dent** 1982 Oct;30(2):128
Moskow BS: The dental cartoons of Honoré Daumier (1808–1879). **J Am Dent Assoc** 1981 Jan;102(1):82–6
Moskow BS: The iconography of the dental profession. **Quintessence Int** 1983 Oct;14(10):1072–3
Moskow BS: The iconography of the dental profession. **Quintessence Int** 1983 Nov;14(11):1184–5
Moskow BS: The iconography of the dental profession. **Quintessence Int** 1983 Dec;14(12):1278–9
Moskow BS: The iconography of the dental profession. **Quintessence Int** 1984 Apr;15(4):406–7
Moskow BS: The iconography of the dental profession. Jean-Ignace-Isidore Gérard Grandville (1803–1847). **Quintessence Int** 1984 Oct;15(10):1028–9
Premuda L: Significativi ritorni: Pierre Fauchard (1690–1761). **G Stomatol Ortognatodonzia** 1982 Apr–Jun;1(1):5–9
Rechtman J: Le Dr. J.P. Marat et le secret professionnel. **Soc Fr Hist Art Dent** 1979 Sep–Dec;(5–6):22–5
Richard A: L'évolution de la condition militaire des chirurgiens-dentistes. **Bull Acad Chir Dent (Paris)** 1979–1980;25(25):59–69
Sugden KC: Dentists in the rare books. Joseph Audibran and incorruptible artificial teeth. **Br Dent J** 1983 Dec 24;155(12):420
Tanzer G: Aus der Geschichte der Zahnheilkunde. Pierre Fauchard. **Zahnarzt** 1983 Nov;27(11):713–7
1879–1979 – centenaire de la bibliothèque de l'Ecole Dentaire de Paris, Centre Français de Documentation Odonto-stomatologique.: **Rev Odontostomatol (Paris)** 1980 Mar–Apr;9(2):13–5

**Germany**

Alt K: In der Weimarer Zeit war der Rundfunk ein beliebtes Fortbildungs-Instrument. **Zahnarztl Mitt** 1984 Oct 16;74(20):2325–6
Andrä A: Zur Entwicklung der Kieferchirurgie in Rostock. **Zahn Mund Kieferheilkd** 1982;70(1):4–9
Axthelm H: Fortbildung aus der Sicht einer 50 jährigen Praxistätigkeit. **Zahnarztl Mitt** 1984 Feb 1;74(3):227–30, 235
Froriep R: Aspects of tongue (1828). Original Latin text edited and translated by C. Garton, J. D. Gerencser, A. J. Drinnan. Buffalo, Dept. of Classics, State University of N. Y., 1982. xix, 109, 108a p. (Arethusa Monographs IX).
Gangler P: Endodontic treatment in the GDR. **Int Endod J** 1984 Jul;17(3):152–62
Guter P: Die Krankenversicherung. Vertrags- und Honorarsituation seit 1935. **Zahnarzt** 1980 Jan;24(1):12–20 contd.
Hampel H, Knöfler W: Stand und Entwicklung der stomatologischen enossalen Hemiimplantologie an der Karl-Marx-Universität Leipzig. **Stomatol DDR** 1980 Jul;30(7):457–61
Hantsche HJ: Die Entwicklung der wissenschaftlichen Zahnheilkunde in Halle/Saale vor 100 Jahren. **Zahntechnik (Berl)** 1983 Oct;24(10):415–6
Hoffmann-Axthelm: 'Machtergreifung' vor 50 Jahren: Ein ausserst unerfreuliches Jubilaum. **Zahnarztl Mitt** 1983 Nov 16;73(22):2499–500, 2503
Hoffmann-Axthelm W: Karl August Lingner und die soziale Zahnmedizin. **Zahnarztl Mitt** 1983 Sep 16;73(18):1981–2, 1987–9
Hoffmann-Axthelm W: Wilhelm Dieck--Lehrer, Forscher und Standespolitiker. **Quintessenz** 1984 Feb;35(2):365–9
Jarmer K: Die Kurierfreiheit der Zahnärzte seit der Gewerbeordnung von 1869 und die Kämpfe der Zahnärzte mit ihren Konkurrenten. Teil I: Vorbemerkung und die Freigabe der Zahnheilkunde an jedermann. **Stomatol DDR** 1981;31(1):1–5
Jarmer K: I. Die Freigabe der Zahnheilkunde an jedermann. Fortsetzung von 'Die Kurierfreiheit der Zahnärzte...', siehe Heft 2/81, S. 119. 3. Die Freigabe der Zahnheilkunde an die eingewanderten Amerikaner, DDS. **Stomatol DDR** 1981 Mar;31(3):194–7
Keiser-Nielsen S, Strøm F: The odontological identification of Eva Braun Hitler. **Forensic Sci Int** 1983 Jan–Feb;21(1):59–64
Kimmel K, Steinkrüger F: Der deutsche dental-medizinische Fachhandel (II). Geschichte--Aufgaben--Strukturen. **Dent Echo (Heidelb)** 1982 Feb;52(1):18–37
Kimmel K, Steinkruger F: Der deutsche dental-medizinische Fachhandel (III). Geschichte--Aufgaben--Strukturen. **Dent Echo (Heidelb)** 1982 Mar;52(2):14–33
Kimmel K, Steinkruger F: Der deutsche dental-medizinische Fachhandel. (IV). Geschichte--Aufgaben--Strukturen. **Dent Echo (Heidelb)** 1982 May;52(3):11–6, 18–21
Kimmel K, Steinkrüger F: Der deutsche dental-medizinische Fachhandel (V). Geschichte – Aufgaben – Strukturen. **Dent Echo (Heidelb)** 1982 Jun;52(4):36–52
Kimmel K, Steinkrüger F: Der deutsche dental-medizinische Fachhandel (VI). Geschichte – Aufgaben – Strukturen. **Dent Echo (Heidelb)** 1982 Aug;52(5):72–7, 80–2
Kimmel K, Steinkrüger F: Der deutsche dental-medizinische Fachhandel (VII). Geschichte – Aufgaben – Strukturen. **Dent Echo (Heidelb)** 1982 Nov;52(7):15–6, 19–20, 22–4 passim
Kimmel K, Steinkrüger F: Die Geschichte des deutschen dental-medizinischen Fachhandels. Geschichte--Aufgaben--Strukturen (I). **Dent Dienst** 1982 Feb;(2):8–9
Kimmel K, Steinkrüger F: Die Geschichte des deutschen dental-medizinischen Fachhandels (II). 1882–1939: Eine stürmische Epoche. **Dent Dienst** 1982 Mar;(3):14–7
Konrad M, Bleker J: Der Dr. med. dent. und die Medizingeschichte--Uber 1000 Dissertationen zur Geschichte der Zahnheilkunde seit 1919. **Dtsch Zahnarztl Z** 1983 May;38(5):590–1
Künzel W: 20 Jahre Trinkwasserfluoridierung in der Deutschen Demokratischen Republik. **Stomatol DDR** 1979;29(10):743–52
Mit Stücken von Silberteller füllte Zahnarzt kranke Zähne: **Niedersachs Zahnarztebl** 1982 Sep;17(9):403
Mitscherlich A: Vor etwa 100 Jahren (7). Die Replantation und die Transplantation der Zähne. **Zentralbl Chir** 1979;104(9):612–4
Moskow BS: The iconography of the dental profession. Der Zahnbrecher--the toothbreaker. Johannes Joachim Kändler (1706–1775). **Quintessence Int** 1984 Jan;15(1):40–1
Neumann-Redlin von Meding E: Neumann' Zahnscheiden und Tomes' Zahnfasern. Zum 150. Geburtstag des Königsberger Pathologen Ernst Christian Neumann. **Dtsch Zahnarztl Z** 1984 Jan;39(1):65–9
Pankoke KT: Im wilhelminischen Preussen nahm man sie ernst. Zur Geschichte der Jugendzahnpflege in Deutschland. **Zahnarzt** 1984 Aug;28(8):619–21
Rezai RF: Tribute to dental pioneer Friedrich Otto Walkhoff.

Quintessence Int 1984 Jun;15(6):655-7

Schmitt WM: Die Sozialversicherung von 1883 bis 1962. **Zahnarzt** 1980 Jan;24(1):7-11

Schneider HG, Witte B: Die Zeitschrift 'Deutsche Stomatologie/Stomatologie der DDR' in den Jahren 1961-1980. Eine Analyse ihrer Beiträge hinsichtlich Inhalt, Form und thematischer Trends. **Stomatol DDR** 1982 Jan;32(1):2-9

Schultz P: Wie Geheimrat von Goethe den Zwischenkiefer-Knochen entdeckte. **Zahnarztl Mitt** 1984 Apr 1;74(7):733-4

Schwann H: Zur Gestaltung spezieller Vorlesungen 'Geschichte der Zahnheilkunde' für Stomatologie-Studenten. **Stomatol DDR** 1982 Mar;32(3):229-33

Sognnaes RF: Hitler and Bormann identifications compared by postmortem craniofacial and dental characteristics. **Am J Forensic Med Pathol** 1980 Jun;1(2):105-15

Spranger H: Daten und Fakten zur Entwicklung der Parodontologie in der Bundesrepublik Deutschland. **Dtsch Zahnarztl Z** 1981;36(7):445-8

Tanzer G: Adolf Witzel (1847-1906) und die Zahnerhaltung. **Zahnarzt** 1984 Jan;28(1):49-52

Tanzer G: Philipp Pfaff (1713-1766), seine Zeit und seine Vorgänger. **Zahnarzt** 1984 Feb;28(2):129-31

Tanzer G: Willoughby Dayton Miller (1853-1907). **Zahnarzt** 1984 May;28(5):375-6

Ullmann E: Adolf Witzel--Leben und Werk. **Stomatol DDR** 1981 Jul;31(7):535-41

### Great Britain

Bowles G: National Health Dental Services 1948-1955. **Soc Soc Hist Med Bull (Lond)** 1981 Dec;29:1-6

Centenary issue: 1880-1980.: **Br Dent J** 1980 Jul 1;149(1):1-36

Corbett ME, Hardwick JL: The investigation of dental disease in exhumed remains. **J Dent** 1981 Dec;9(4):302-10

Coventry JB: The dental estimates board. Thirty-three years at Eastbourne. **Br Dent J** 1981 Jul 7;151(1):33-4

Donaldson JA: The life and times of Sidney Spokes. **J R Soc Med** 1981 Jul;74(7):537-9

Doughty J: The dentist in comic postcards. **Br Dent J** 1984 Mar 10;156(5):186-7

Dussault G, Sheiham A: Medical theories and professional development. The theory of focal sepsis and dentistry in early twentieth century Britain. **Soc Sci Med** 1982;16(15):1405-12

Emslie RD: A century of British periodontology. **Br Dent J** 1980 Jul 1;149(1):3-4

Extracts from the last century: Dental preventive medicine. **Br Dent J** 1981 Jul 7;151(1):23

Fox B, Maddick I: A hundred years of dental health education. **Br Dent J** 1980 Jul 1;149(1):28-32

Gardner of Parkes: 'Fair to the fair'. **Br Dent J** 1982 Aug 3;153(3):117-9

Gelbier S, Randall SB: Charles Edward Wallis and London's Toothbrush Clubs: 1909 style. **Dent Health (London)** 1982;21(1):12-5

Gelbier S, Randall S: Charles Edward Wallis and the rise of London's school dental service. **Med Hist** 1982 Oct;26(4):395-404

Gelbier S: Frederick Breese and London's first school dental clinic. **Br Dent J** 1981 Nov 3;151(9):309-11

Hallett GE: Progress of children's dentistry. **Br Dent J** 1980 Jul 1;149(1):13-6

Hardy JH: Royal Army Dental Corps diamond jubilee (1921-1981). **Br Dent J** 1981 Nov 17;151(10):351-2

Harty FJ: Endodontic treatment in England. **Int Endod J** 1984 Jul;17(3):106-12

Herschfeld JJ: John Hunter and his Practical treatise on diseases of the teeth. **Bull Hist Dent** 1981;29(1):32-6

Herschfeld JJ: Joseph Fox - pioneer dental investigator and author of The Natural History of the Human Teeth. **Bull Hist Dent** 1983 Oct;31(2):101-7

Herschfeld JJ: Sir John Tomes, dental pioneer. **Bull Hist Dent** 1981 Oct;29(2):94-8

Hindley-Smith D: The general dental council. Twenty-five years on. **Br Dent J** 1981 Jul 7;151(1):31-2

Hindley-Smith D: The General Dental Council. Twenty-five years on. **Probe (Lond)** 1981 Jul;23(1):29-30, 32

Hughes SG: The life and work of John Howard Mummery. **Bull Hist Dent** 1983 Oct;31(2):69-81

James PM: One hundred years of dental public health. **Br Dent J** 1981 Jul 7;151(1):20-3

Kowitz A: The earliest use of dental evidence in a courtroom: His Majesty's Advocate vs. Pattison et al, High Court of Justiciary, Edinburgh, Scotland, June 6-7, 1814. **Bull Hist Dent** 1981 Oct;29(2):82-7

Leatherman GH: Dentistry as I have seen it--1920 to 1984. **Br Dent J** 1984 Aug 25;157(4):141-6

Leatherman GH: Martin Rushton--the man, 1903 to 1970. **Br Dent J** 1983 Nov 5;155(9):315-7

Leighton BD, Howard RD: Orthodontics--the last hundred years. **Br Dent J** 1981 Jul 7;151(1):14-9

Marvitz L: Therapia antiqua. **Tidsskr Tandlaeger** 1983 Jun;3(2-3):24

Morrant GA: Eastman Dental Hospital/Institute of Dental Surgery. **Apex** 1979 Winter;11(3):80-4

Morrant GA: The Eastman reaches its half century. **Br Dent J** 1980 Oct 21;149(8):237-8

Moskow BS: Dentistry in folk art, XIII: The dentist. **Bull Hist Dent** 1981 Oct;29(2):99

Pedley CE: A personal record of dentistry. **Tydskr Tandheelkd Ver S Afr** 1984 Jan;39(1):11-20

Poyton HG: Reminiscenses of the hygiene pilot programme. **Dent Health (London)** 1983;22(2):14, 16

Rechtman J: Un précurseur génial de la prévention et de la diététique, du bouche à bouche et du massage cardiaque externe de l'asepsie et parrain de J. P. Marat: Le docteur William Buchan (1729-1805). Diss. Paris VII, 1979. 115 p.

Reichart PA: Toothpastes containing betel nut (Areca catechu L.) from England of the nineteenth century. **J Hist Med Allied Sci** 1984 Jan;39(1):65-79

Richards ND: Morals and molars. Physical deterioration and the beginnings of the School Dental Service 1878 to 1921. **Br Dent J** 1982 Jul 6;153(1):35-6

Seward M: More than a century of change. **Br Dent J** 1980 Jul 1;149(1):35-6

Spencer EM: Notes on the history of dental dispensaries. **Med Hist** 1982 Jan;26(1):47-66

Tonge CH: Oral anatomy--progress of a discipline. **Br Dent J** 1981 Jul 7;151(1):3-5

Waltke R: Moses Harris--inventor of the color wheel. **Dent Lab Rev** 1980 Apr;:24-5

Ward T: A century of achievement in oral surgery. **Br Dent J** 1980 Jul 1;149(1):25-7

### Hong Kong

Walker RT: Joseph Whittlesey Noble: an American in Hong Kong. **J Am Dent Assoc** 1984 Nov;109(5):757

### Hungary

Bánóczy J, Borós S: A Semmelweis Orvostudományi Egyetem Konzerváló Fogászati Klinika negyedszázados története és munkássága. **Fogorv Sz** 1984 Nov;77(11):321-3

Dénes J: A Semmelweis Orvostudományi Egyetem Gyermekfogászati és Fogszabályozási Klinikájának negyedszázados története és munkássága. **Fogorv Sz** 1984 Sep;77(9):258-9

Fábián T: A Semmelweis OTE fogpótlástani klinikájának negyedszázados története és munkássága. **Fogorv Sz** 1984 Oct;77(10):289-91

Fábián T: 75 éves a Fogorvosi Szemle. **Fogorv Sz** 1982 Jan;75(1):1-3

Huszár G: A magyar fogászat feilódése Arkövytól napjainkig. **Orv Hetil** 1982 May 16;123(20):1243-6

Huszár G: A parodontológia magyar úttöröi. **Fogorv Sz** 1984 Apr;77(4):109-14

Huszár G: Abonyi József, a hazai protetika úttörője. **Fogorv Sz** 1980 Jun;73(6):187-91

Huszár G: Ady Endre fogbántalmairól. **Orv Hetil** 1984 Oct 14;125(42):2575-6

Huszár G: Az önéletrajzok, mint fogorvostörténelmünk forrásai. **Orvostort Kozl** 1980;89-91(26 no 1-3):157-74

Huszár G: Emlékezés Simon Béla professzorra. **Fogorv Sz** 1983 May;76(5):151-5

Lovász A: A konzerváló fogászati ellátás fejlödése az állami fogbetegellátásban 1951 és 1981 között a Központi Stomtologiai Intézet munkásságának tükrében. **Fogorv Sz** 1982;75(8):247-53

Orsós S: A megyei 'fogász-föorvostól' a stomatologus felügyelö szakföorvosig. **Fogorv Sz** 1984 Jun;77(6):165-9

Orsós S, Bodó L: Változások a fogorvosi szolgálat 25 éves dokumentációjában. **Forgorv SZ** 1982 May;75(5):135-9

Percze E: A fogszabályozási ellátás megszervezése és kiépítése során szerzett 10 éves tapasztalatok, eredmények értékelése Bács-Kiskun megyében. **Fogorv Sz** 1982 Nov;75(11):338-41

Tóth P: A gyermekfogászat oktatásának 25 éve. **Fogorv Sz** 1980 Dec;73(12):377-8

Végh F: Jókai Mór Szájmütétje 1891-ben. **Orvostort Kozl** 1979;86(24 no 4):129-30

Zelles T: A fogorvosi elméleti kutatás húsz éve és perspektívái a Semmelweis Orvostudományi Egyetem Kórélettani Intézetében, a Fogorvostudományi Kar Orálbiológiai Csoportjának létrejötte és jelenlegi tevékenysége. **Fogorv Sz** 1980 Dec;73(12):378-80

### Ireland

Casey A: A history of dentistry in Northern Ireland 1920-1973. Part I. **J Ir Dent Assoc** 1982 May-Jun;28(3):53-7

Casey AJ: A history of dentistry in Northern Ireland 1920-1973. Part II. **J Ir Dent Assoc** 1982 Sep-Oct;28(5):113-5

Casey AJ: A history of dentistry in Northern Ireland 1920-1973. Part IV. **J Ir Dent Assoc** 1983 Jan-Feb;29(1):9-11

# DENTISTRY

**Israel**

Tagger M: Endodontic treatment in Israel. **Int Endod J** 1984 Jul;17(3):113-24

**Italy**

Bellagarda M, Bellagarda G: L'attività storico-scientifica di Luigi Casotti (1891-1959). **Minerva Med** 1984 Nov 17;75(44):2695-704
Favero GA: Odontoiatria del passato. La stomatologia nelle opere di Cessare Cavina (1888-1935). **Dent Cadmos** 1982 Oct;50(10):83-91
Moskow BS: The iconography of the dental profession. Pietro Longhi (1702-1785). **Quintessence Int** 1984 Jul;15(7):728-9
Robetti I, Iorio M: Università degli Studi di Torino, Istituto di Medicina Legale e delle Assicurazioni. **Minerva Stomatol** 1981 Jul-Aug;30(4):321-30
Sugden KC: Dentists in the rare books. 2. Vittorio Cornelio. **Br Dent J** 1983 Oct 22;155(8):278
Tanzer G: Aus der Geschichte der Zahnheilkunde. Giuseppangelo Fonzi, 13.7.1768-31.8.1840. **Zahnarzt** 1983 Dec;27(12):765-9

**Japan**

Fusayama T: [Progress in operative dentistry in the past 30 years] (Jpn). **Shikai Tenbo** 1982 Jun;59(7):1375-85
Kikuchi S: [The progress of 'Shigaku' in the past 70 years] (Jpn). **Shigaku** 1982 Jun;70(1):iii-ix
Shimoosa T: [History of dental prothesis and dental engineering] (Jpn). **Shikai Tenbo** 1982 Oct;60(4):731-44
Ueno T: [In memory of Prof. Heizo Nakamura] (Jpn) **Dent Outlook** 1980;55(5):921-6

**Mexico**

Díaz y de Ovando C: Odontología y publicidad en la prensa mexicana del siglo XIX. **Bol Soc Mex Hist Filos Med** 1984 Jun;7(47):325-46
Sanfilippo J: Homenaje a los fundadores de la odontologia en México. **ADM** 1980 Mar-Apr;37(2):82-4
Sanfilippo J: Semblanza del doctor Samuel Fastlicht. **Bol Soc Mex Hist Filos Med** 1984 Jun;7(47):309-15
Sanfilippo J: The life and accomplishments of Dr. Samuel Fastlicht. **Bull Hist Dent** 1983 Oct;31(2):87-92
Sanfilippo B. J: Bibliografia historia de la odontologia en Mexico. [Mexico City, Sociedad de la Historia y Filosofia de la Medicina], 1984. 23 p.

**Netherlands**

Van Cittert-Eymers JG: Joseph Mozes Son (1818-1884), een illuster tandmeester te Utrecht. **Tijdschr Geschied Geneeskd** 1978;2(2):62-9

**New Zealand**

Hanan R: A dentist at large. Christchurch, N. Z. Merivale, 1977. 181 p.
New Zealand Dental Journal. Seventy-fifth jubilee issue: **NZ Dent J** 1980 Jul;76(345):107-48
Pack AR: Women in New Zealand dentistry, 1880-1980. **NZ Dent J** 1981 Jan;77(347):19-25
Stockwell RF: Personalities of importance in the early days of New Zealand dentistry. **NZ Dent J** 1981 Jul;77(349):102-5

**Nigeria**

Akpata ES: Endodontic treatment in Nigeria. **Int Endod J** 1984 Jul;17(3):139-51

**Philippines**

Leonard AG: Three score years and fifteen in the Philippines. **Br Dent J** 1983 Oct 22;155(8):284

**Poland**

Pawela T, Przepiórkowska E: Przypadki schorzeń stomatologicznych leczonych w klinice chirurgicznej UJ w latach 1924-1939. **Czas Stomatol** 1983 Nov-Dec;36(11-12):869-74
Stefański K, Chudańska T, Jakubiak J, et al: Przekrój działalności leczniczej Kliniki Chirurgii Szczękowej SS CMKP w Toruniu w latach 1972-1977. **Czas Stomatol** 1981 Mar;34(3):303-8
Stypułkowska J: 25 lat Kliniki Chirurgii Stomatologicznej AM w Krakowie. Historia i kierunki działalności. **Czas Stomatol** 1981 Jan;34(1):51-6
Wajs S: O pierwszym zabiegu uranoplastyki w Polsce. **Czas Stomatol** 1980 Nov;33(11):1043-6
Wajs S: Sposoby znieczulenia stosowane przy usuwaniu zebow przed stu laty. **Czas Stomatol** 1979 Dec;32(12):1211-3
Waszyński E: O mechanizmie żucia w 'Primitiae Physico-Medicae...' (1750-1753), pierwszym w Polsce czasopiśmie medycznym. **Czas Stomatol** 1984 Mar;37(3):227-32
Wilczyńska M: Działalność Warszawskiej Podsekcji Ortodontycznej w latach 1956-78. **Czas Stomatol** 1980 May;33(5):475-8

**Portugal**

Cunha AS: Algumas considerações sobre medicina dentária forense e o seu início em Portugal. **Rev Port Estomatol Cir Maxilofac** 1980 Apr-Jun;22(2):187-200

**Scandinavia**

Afseth J: 20 Jahre skandinavische Plaquepharmakologie. **Schweiz Monatsschr Zahnmed** 1984 Jan;94(1):86-90

**South Africa**

Van Reenen JF: Doctor 'Ribbebene' - cobbler, lumberman, dentist, politician and researcher. **Adler Mus Bull** 1983 Nov;Spec issue:53-7

**Spain**

Gonzalez Iglesias J: Los Borbones y el desarrollo de la odontologia en Espãna. **Bol Inf Dent (Madr)** 1978;Spec no:63-92
Gonzalez Iglesias J: Los dentistas Catalanes de finales del siglo XIX. Su influencia en el desarrollo de la odonto-estomatologia en España. **Rev Esp Estomatol** 1979 May-Jun;27(3):164-82
Huertas Garcia G: Bosquejo hist/BC/orico sobre endodoncia. **Rev Esp Endodoncia** 1983 Dec;1(3):123-33

**Sweden**

Loevy HT, Kowitz A: Dentistry on stamps (Dr. Kerstin Palm). **J Am Dent Assoc** 1984 Nov;109(5):755
Molin C: Karolinska sjukhusets avdelning för tand--och käksjukdomar--en tillbakablick efter fyrtio år. **Nord Medicinhist Arsb** 1981;:183-92
Thuréus S: Historiska glimtar och synpunkter på stomato-odontologi. **Nord Medicinhist Arsb** 1981;:176-82

**Switzerland**

Held AJ: A propos de dentifrices et du Dr Albert Senn (1869-1934)--notice historique. **SSO Schweiz Monatsschr Zahnheilkd** 1981 Apr;91(4):218-20
Held AJ: Une gestation longue et un enfantement laborieux: la médecine dentaire d'aujourd'hui en Swisse. **SSO Schweiz Monatsschr Zahnheilkd** 1981 Oct;91(10):769-857
Hobi F: Zahnärztliche Röntgenologie von den Anfängen bis zum Jahre 1914: ihre Entwicklung in der Schweiz unter Berücksichtigung der im Ausland geschaffenen Voraussetzungen im Rahmen der Zahnheilkunde jener Zeit. Zürich, Juris, 1981. 126 p. (Zürcher medizingeschichtliche Abhandlungen, Neue Reihe, 145).
Mühlemann HR: 25 Jahre Schweizer Plaque-Pharmakologie. **Schweiz Monatsschr Zahnmed** 1984 Jan;94(1):91-101
Sigron G: Die Geschichte der Zahnmedizin in Graubünden. Zürich, Juris, 1981. 138 p. (Zürcher medizingeschichtliche Abhandlungen, Neue Reihe, 148).
Tanzer G: Professor Dr. Alfred Gysi (1865-1957). **Zahnarzt** 1984 Jun;28(6):447-9

**United States**

History, information, and examination requirements of the American Board of Prosthodontics. **J Prosthet Dent** 1984 Aug;52(2):281-7
ADA historical report--dental insurance: how it started and where it is today: **Employ Benefit Plan Rev** 1978 Nov;33(5):94, 96
Agins TC: Collector's item. Americana. **NY J Dent** 1983 Nov;53(7):317
Agins TC: Year of the twenty-dollar gold piece. **NY J Dent** 1980 Apr;50(4):123-6
American Dental Association 1859-1880: **J Am Dent Assoc** 1984 Apr;108(4):479-89, 492
American Dental Association 1881-1917: **J Am Dent Assoc** 1984 Apr;108(4):497-510
American Dental Association 1918-1928: **J Am Dent Assoc** 1984 Apr;108(4):515-9, 522
American Dental Association 1929-1945: **J Am Dent Assoc** 1984 Apr;108(4):527-33, 535-6
American Dental Association 1946-1962: **J Am Dent Assoc** 1984 Apr;108(4):541-51, 554-6
American Dental Association 1963-1984: **J Am Dent Assoc** 1984 Apr;108(4):561-71, 574-9
Asbell MB: The dental art and its practitioners in colonial Philadelphia. **Bull Phila Cty Dent Soc** 1981 Mar;46(6):6-11
Baldwin J: The Nichols: 100 years of Ohio dentistry. **Ohio Dent J** 1980 May;54(5):22-3
Barber DN: Doc Holliday, the wildest dentist of the West. **Probe (Lond)** 1984 Mar;25(9):301-2
Bellagarda M, Trisoglio M: Il contributo della scienza e

dell'odontostomatologia in particolare alla scoperta ed al progresso dell'anestesia. **Minerva Med** 1981 Apr 7;72(14):897–902
Berndt T: Bite mark science. Forensic dentistry's hottest frontier. **Fla Dent J** 1982 Spring;53(1):22–4, 42–3
Besombes A: Odonto-stomatologie et diplomatie de l'Impératrice Eugénie à Clemenceau. **Hist Sci Med** 1983;17(1):13–22
Bogardus CR: Kentucky's first woman dentist (Lucy Dupuy Montz). **Ky Dent J** 1984 Mar–Apr;36(2):23–5
Bowers DF: W. D. Miller: a second pilgrimage to his home. **Ohio Dent J** 1982 Mar;56(3):15–23
Buchin ID, Peck S: Harvey Peck, 1937–1981. **Angle Orthod** 1982 Jan;52(1):3–5
Burt BA: The epidemiological basis for water fluoridation in the prevention of dental caries. **J Public Health Policy** 1982 Dec;3(4):391–407
Carr JD: The great radiology debate: the letters of C. Edmund Kells and Howard R. Raper. **Bull Hist Dent** 1981 Oct;29(2):69–73
Charles AD: History of dentistry in South Carolina. Greenville, S.C., [s.n.], 1982. viii, 124 p.
Charles AD: History of dentistry in South Carolina. Ph.D. Diss., University of South Carolina. Columbia, 1981. v, 222 leaves.
Christen AG: Charles C. Bass, M.D.--1875–1975: that cantankerous genius of preventive dentistry. **Bull Hist Dent** 1982 Apr;30(1):8–18
Church LE: The ancestors we never knew. **J Md State Dent Assoc** 1983 Dec;26(3):122–3
Dammann GE: Dental care during the Civil War. **Ill Dent J** 1984 Jan–Feb;53(1):12–7
The Dental Corps of the United States Navy: Washington, Bureau of Medicine and Surgery, Navy Dept. 73 p.
Dentistry--for music's sake. I. How dental 'miracles' helped jazz greats with their careers (Buck Clayton). **Tic** 1979 Dec;38(12):1–3
Deranian HM: An historical overview of American dentistry. **Compend Contin Educ Dent** 1984 Jul–Aug;5(7):592–9
Deranian HM: The miracle man of the western front: the story of Dr. Varaztad Kazanjian. **Bull Hist Dent** 1984 Oct;32(2):85–103
Dew WC: John Ross Callahan: a man, a memorial, an award. **Ohio Dent J** 1982 Jul–Aug;56(7–8):46–52
Doyle CC: The power of not thinking: a jocular toothache cure. **Ky Folkl Rec** 1983;29(1–2):24–9
Dummett CO: Charles Edwin Bentley: a genuine emancipator. **Crisis** 1979;86(4):133–5
Dummett CO: Contributions of Afro-Americans to American dentistry. **J Ala Dent Assoc** 1984 Fall;68(4):42–6
Dummett CO: Dentistry's immediate past is prologue. **NY J Dent** 1980 Apr;50(4):128–30
Dummett CO: Prevention began early: Charles Edwin Bentley, DDS 1859–1929. **J Natl Med Assoc** 1983 Dec;75(12):1235–6
Dummett CO: Stephen Johnson Lewis and his contributions to American dentistry. **Bull Hist Dent** 1981;29(1):15–23
Dunn WE: Dentistry and society in late 1800s and early 1900s in South Dakota. **Northwest Dent** 1983 Jul–Aug;62(4):23–7
Dunn WE: Fight for fluoridation. **Northwest Dent** 1983 Jul–Aug;62(4):34–6
Dunn WE: The busy years. **Northwest Dent** 1983 Jul–Aug;62(4):30–1
Dunn WE: The devastating thirties. **Northwest Dent** 1983 Jul–Aug;62(4):28–9
Escoe R: A new look at John Greenwood's denture for George Washington. **Bull Hist Dent** 1981;29(1):37–43
Establishment of the American Board of Oral and Maxillofacial Radiology.: **Oral Surg** 1980 Jun;49(6):549–51
Fershee NF: Dental hygiene in Michigan--our 'roots'. **Bull Mich Dent Hyg Assoc** 1984 Sep;14(3):4–7
Foley GP: A treasury of dentistry. Henry Cogswell. **J Am Coll Dent** 1984 Summer;51(2):20–1
Foley GP: A treasury of dentistry: John B. Rich, pioneer dental leader. **J Am Coll Dent** 1982 Summer;49(2):28–9
Forrest WR, Christen AG: Recollections of a dental researcher. Fifty years at the U. S. Bureau of Standards: Interviews with George C. Paffenbarger. Part I. **J Ala Dent Assoc** 1982 Summer;66(3):24–8
Forrest WR, Christen AG: Recollections of a dental researcher. Fifty years at the U.S. National Bureau of Standards: interviews with George C. Paffenbarger, D.D.S., D.Sc. Part II. **J Ala Dent Assoc** 1982 Fall;66(4):36–8
Francke OC: Tandbehandling för 100 år sedan och Mark Twain som patient. **Nord Medicinhist Arsb** 1984;:137–40
Fraundorf KC: Organized dentistry and the pursuit of entry control. **J Health Polit Policy Law** 1984 Winter;8(4):759–81
Galginaitis C: An analysis of dental practice from 1952 to 1976. Council on Dental Practice and Bureau of Economic and Behavioral Research. **J Am Dent Assoc** 1980 Jan;100(1):89–96
Gardiner JF: C. Edmund Kells: New Orleans' gift to dentistry. **Bull Hist Dent** 1981;29(1):2–7
Gardiner JF: Solyman Brown and his epic poem 'Dentologia'. **Bull Hist Dent** 1984;32(1):44–51
Gold SI: Robert Neumann: a pioneer in periodontal flap surgery. **J Periodontol** 1982 Jul;53(7):456–9
Gottsegen R: Periodontics 1950–1980 **NY J Dent** 1980 Apr;50(4):132–3
Grossman LI: A personal history of dental practice: 1920–1980. **J Am Dent Assoc** 1981;102:360–5
Grossman LT: A personal history of dental practice: 1920–1980. **J Am Dent Assoc** 1981 Mar;102(3):360–5
Hamilton WA, Hamilton PR: Sex and the dental practice: a reinterpretation of the history of dental hygienists. **Bull Hist Dent** 1980 Oct;28(2):64–8
Harada M: A brief history of hospital dentistry in the United States. **Bull Hist Dent** 1982 Apr;30(1):46–54
Hastreiter RJ: Fluoridation conflict: a history and conceptual synthesis. **J Am Dent Assoc** 1983 Apr;106(4):486–90
Herschfeld JJ: G. V. Black and the search for a better amalgam. **Bull Hist Dent** 1980 Oct;28(2):76–82
Herschfeld JJ: Norman W. Kingsley and his pioneering techniques in the correction of cleft palate. **Bull Hist Dent** 1983 Apr;31(1):23–8
Hitchcock HP: Contributions of orthodontists to organized dentistry. **J Am Dent Assoc** 1980 Jan;100(1):76–8
Hofer K: Dr. Lucy Hobbs Taylor, first woman dentist. **CAL** 1981 Oct;45(4):13–5, 18
Hollander FP: A giant step forward: dentistry in Connecticut a century ago. **Bull Hist Dent** 1980 Apr;28(1):35–7
Hyson JM: William Saunders: the United States Army's first dentist--West Point's forgotten man. **Milit Med** 1984 Aug;149(8):435–41
Johnson BH: Doctors, druggists and dentists in the Oklahoma Territory, 1889–1907. **Ariz West** 1977;19:121–34
The Journal's 30th anniversary: **J Prosthet Dent** 1980 Jan;43(1):4–8
Kaltenbach RF, Smith AA: History of the Organization of Teachers of Dental Practice Administration. **J Dent Pract Adm** 1984 Jan–Mar;1(1):6–7
Kidd F, ed: Profile of the Negro in American dentistry. Washington, Howard University Press, 1979. viii, 211 p.
Knudson KG: Walt Disney, dentistry and the armed forces during World War II. **Bull Hist Dent** 1984 Oct;32(2):112–7
Kowitz A: Dentists of Chicago before the great fire. **Bull Hist Dent** 1984 Oct;32(2):126–30
Künzel W: Willoughby Dayton Miller zur 75. Wiederkehr des Todestages am 29. 7. 1982. **Zahn Mund Kieferheilkd** 1982;70(6):579–83
Kuttler SL: Dental hygiene: 70 years of growth and change taking a look at yesterday, today, and tomorrow. **Iowa Dent J** 1983 Oct;69(4):31–5
Leahy PJ, Mazur A: The rise and fall of public opposition in specific social movements. **Soc Stud Sci** 1980 Aug 3;10(3):259–84
Loevy HT: M. Evangeline Jordon, pioneer in pedodontics. **Bull Hist Dent** 1984;32(1):19–26
McCauley HB: Professional dentistry and the University of Maryland at Baltimore. **Bull Hist Dent** 1982 Oct;30(2):73–91
McCauley HB: The Maryland State Board of Dental Examiners. In the beginning. **J Md State Dent Assoc** 1984 Apr;27(1):22–9
McGonagle RR: Our golden age of orthodontics revisited. **Am J Orthod** 1980 Apr;77(4):461–4
Mann WV: G. V. Black revisited. **J Dent Educ** 1981 Jun;45(6):338–9
Massachusetts Dental Society: The story of dentistry in Massachusetts presented by the Massachusetts Dental Society on the occasion of its centennial, 1864–1964. Boston, The Society, 1964. 63 p.
Miller GH: I remember Mama, too: a dentist's wife--circa 1900. **Tic** 1982 Mar;41(3):1–4
Millstein PL, Howe E: A hundred years of dental history in a Boston building. **J Am Dent Assoc** 1984 Apr;108(4):641–2
Moloney F, Worthington P: The origin of the Le Fort I maxillary osteotomy: Cheever's operation. **J Oral Surg** 1981 Oct;39(10):731–4
Moore RB: Zane Grey: dentist, novelist, baseball player, outdoors man. **Tic** 1982 Jul;41(7):5–7
Mosteller JH: 'Practices dentistry in Fayette, Alabama'. A tardy but sincere tribute to Claude Clenton Cannon. **J Ala Dent Assoc** 1977 Oct;61(4):19–24
Murphey GT: A Navy dentist's diary: from Okinawa to Viet Nam. (Griffin T. Murphey). **Dent Stud** 1979 Oct;58(2):52–4, 59, 67
Nodyne KR: Pioneer in oral surgery: Simon P. Hullihen. **J W Va Hist Assoc** 1982;6(1):41–8
Nordstrom WR: How a dental museum - built and staffed by dental students - helps generate interest in dental history. **Bull Hist Dent** 1983 Apr;31(1):18–22
Odrich J, Stanaland J: Early development of dental hygiene. **NY J Dent** 1982 Apr;52(4):127 contd.
Pappas CN: The life and times of G. V. Black. Chicago, Quintessence Pub. Co., 1983. 128 p.
Penland L: A decade of dental health education: review of the 1970s. **Dent Hyg (Chic)** 1982 Sep;56(9):16–8, 20–2
Pike JS, Ireland RL: Pioneers in pedodontics. Kenneth Alexander Easlick, 1893–1979. **Pediatr Dent** 1982 Sep;4(3):268–9
Ragsdale JS: What did Thomas Jefferson mean by 'I have not yet lost a tooth by age'? **J Am Dent Assoc** 1984 Apr;108(4):643–4
Ring ME: Nothing new under the sun: an examination of newly discovered inventions and techniques. **J Am Dent Assoc** 1980 Jan;100(1):22–5
Ring ME: Oddments in dental history: a case of tooth implantation by the patient. **Bull Hist Dent** 1983 Apr;31(1):29
Ring ME: Oddments in dental history: the advertising, cut-rate dentist: a prophesy of a century ago. **Bull Hist Dent** 1982 Oct;30(2):115–6
Robinson HS: Robert and Roderick Badger, pioneer Georgia dentists. **Negro Hist Bull** 1961;24(4):77–80
Rothman MA: Unfinished business. **NY J Dent** 1980 Apr;50(4):134–5
Saltzman BB: Saga of America's first woman dental graduate. **Dent Stud** 1983 Oct;62(1):24–5

## DENTISTRY

Scholle RH: The best of American dentistry. **J Am Dent Assoc** 1982 Jun;104(6):962
Schweitzer J: Sixty-two years of practice. **NY J Dent** 1980 Apr;50(4):135–7
Skillman K: The struggle to save a dental shrine. **Ohio Dent J** 1983 May;57(3):44–6
Sognnaes RF: Preface to professional progress from Washington's old ivory relics to the modern Maryland bridge. **J Md State Dent Assoc** 1983 Aug;26(2):79–86
Sognnaes RF: President Washington's most famous dentures stolen from the Smithsonian. **J Am Dent Assoc** 1983 Feb;106(2):216–8
Srisopark SS: [Who blocked the inferior alveolar nerve first?] **J Dent Assoc Thai** 1982 Nov–Dec;32(6):249–55
Stahl SS: Fiftieth year. **NY J Dent** 1980 Apr;50(4):137
Suyehiro H, Asahino SN, Uesato G: [The development of orthodontic treatment in America, the past, present, future] (Jpn). **Nippon Kyosei Shika Gakkai Zasshi** 1982 Mar;41(1):1–8
The symposium, part I: Fifty years of change. **NY J Dent** 1980 Apr;50(4):127–37
Thoburn R, ed: One hundred years of dentistry in Florida. Tampa, Florida Dental Education Foundation, 1983. xxxix, 412 p.
A tribute to Louis I. Grossman: **J Endod** 1982 Jan;8(Spec issue):S1–48
Watson WG: Dentofacial orthopedics: fifty years of concern. **Am J Orthod** 1981 Nov;80(5):561–3
Watson WG: The journal––a record of professional transition and progress. **Am J Orthod** 1981 Feb;79(2):219–22
Webb H, Rhodes LC: The book of presidents: leaders of organized dentistry. [s.l., s.n.] 1977. [63] p.
Willens SH: Dr. Nathaniel Peabody and his book: The art of preserving teeth. **Bull Hist Dent** 1980 Oct;28(2):83–6
Williams WD: Did Horace Wells stage a newspaper publicity scheme? Some unreported newspaper items. **Bull Hist Dent** 1983 Oct;31(2):93–8

**USSR**

Arzhantsev PZ: Etapy razvitiia spetsializirovannoĭ stomatologicheskoĭ pomoshchi v GVKG imeni N. N. Burdenko. **Voen Med Zh** 1980 Feb;(2):78–80
Chepulis SP, Tertsionas PV: Nekotorye aspekty razvitiia stomatologii v Litve. **Stomatologiia (Mosk)** 1982;(6):10–1
Danilevskiĭ NF, Sakharchuk IM: Druzhba narodov SSSR––reshaiushchiĭ faktor vosstanovleniia stomatologicheskikh kadrov na Ukraine. **Stomatologiia (Mosk)** 1982;(6):7–10
Gol'braĭkh VR: Velikiĭ khirurg N. I. Pirogov––osnovopolozhnik khirurgii cheliustno-litsevoĭ oblasti (k 100-letiiu so dnia smerti). **Stomatologiia (Mosk)** 1982 Jul–Aug;61(4):66–7
Gruzdev NA, Gol'braĭkh VR: Voprosy istorii klinicheskoĭ stomatologicheskoĭ anatomii. **Stomatologiia (Mosk)** 1981 May–Apr;60(2):59–60
Kozlov VA, Iarchuk NI, Kotov GA: Razvitie cheliustno-litsevoĭ khirurgii c SSSR. **Vestn Khir** 1982 Nov;129(11):9–12
Norovpil TS, Avilov EN, Barer GM: Razvitie stomatologicheskoĭ pomoshchi i podgotovka vracheĭ-stomatologov v Mongol'skoĭ Narodnoĭ Respublike. **Stomatologiia (Mosk)** 1981 Jan–Feb;60(1):91–2
Osnovipolozhnik sovetskoĭ stomatologii (k 100-letiiu so dnia rozhdeniia Aleksandra Ivanovicha Evdokimova): **Stomatologiia (Mosk)** 1984 Jan–Feb;63(1):4–6
Rol' nauchnykh meditsinskikh obshchestv stomatologov v razvitii sovetskoĭ stomatologii: **Stomatologiia (Mosk)** 1982;(6):4–6
Rudenko AT: Kafedre cheliustno-litsevoĭ khirurgii so stomatologieĭ VMA imeni S. M. Kirova––50 let. **Voen Med Zh** 1980 Mar;(3):77
Troianskiĭ AN: Vklad prof. V. Iu. Kurliandskogo v razvitie nauchnykh problem ortopedicheskoĭ stomatologii (k 75-letiiu so dnia rozhdeniia). **Stomatologiia (Mosk)** 1983 Nov–Dec;62(6):75–6
Troianskiĭ GN, Krechmer MI: A. I. Evdokimov––odin iz osnovopolozhnikov sovetskoĭ stomatologii. **Sov Zdravookhr** 1984;(10):60–4

**Vatican**

Rizzuti A: Odontoiatria del passato. 'Matricole' di Dentista rilasciate nello Stato Pontificio. **Dent Cadmos** 1982 Nov;50(11):75–7

**Venezuela**

Canelón JS: Dos artículos odontológicos en la 'Gaceta Cientifica de Venezuela' de 1877. **Acta Odontol Venez** 1980 Jan–Apr;18(1):87–95
Caricote N: Formacion odontopediatrica del odontologo general en la UCV. **Acta Odontol Venez** 1980 Jan–Apr;18(1):69–85
Febres-Cordero F: Fue Hugues Planque autorizado para ejerceer en Venezuela 'su industria de dentista'? **Acta Odontol Venez** 1982 Jan–Apr;20(1):39–52
Fébres-Cordero F: Hoja de servicios (1929–1979). Datos biográficos, actividades, labor intelectual y algunos juicios y comentarios sobre la obra realizada. Caracas, Publicaciones del Consejo de Profesores Universitarios Jubilados, 1979. 256 p.
Febres Cordero F: La odontologia venezolana ante la historia. **Acta Odontol Venez** 1980 Jan–Apr;18(1):175–90
Febres-Cordero F: Publicaciones periodicas odontologicas de Venezuela. **Acta Odontol Venez** 1983;21(2):129–47; 21(3):237–59
Sardi M: Modelos de ejercicio de la odontologia en Venezuela desde Los años cuarenta. **Acta Odontol Venez** 1980 Jan–Apr;18(1):37–66
Saturno Canelón J: Dos articulos odontologicos en la Gaceta Cientifica de Venezuela de 1877. **Acta Odontol Venez** 1980 Jan–Apr;18(1):87–95

**Yugoslavia**

Andelić P, Balević M, Nikolin P, et al: Razvoj stomatološke službe u regionu istočnog Srema. **Med Pregl** 1982;35(11–12):495–6
Branovački D, Marić D: Razvoj stomatološke delatnosti na teritoriji SAP Vojvodine posle II svetskog rata. **Med Pregl** 1980;33(11–12):447–8
Farcnik F, Vrbic V: Stomatološka klinika včeraj, danes, jutri. **Zobozdrav Vestn** 1981 Summer;36(3–4):81–7
Posinovec J: O hrvatskom stomatološkom nazivlju u drugoj polovici XIX. stoljeća. **Lijec Vjesn** 1980 May;102(5):282–3
Protić M, Sarac V, Pilja M, et al: Stomatologija Vojvodine: razvojni put, stanje i perspektiva. **Med Pregl** 1982;35(11–12):499–502
Sarac S, Lalić R, Jovanović L, et al: Stogodišnjica stomatologije u Somboru (1881–1981). **Med Pregl** 1982;35(11–12):497–8

### EDUCATION

**Brazil**

Madeira AA, Rosa JE: [Historical background of dentistry teaching in the state of Santa Catarina] (Por). **Rev Catarinense Odontol** 1977;4(2):5–10

**Europe**

Farmer ED: Dental education in Europe. **J R Soc Med** 1984 Jun;77(6):452–8

**Japan**

Kobe Daigaku Igakubu Shika Koko Geka gojisshunen kinen gyoseki shu: Kobe, Japan, Do Geka, [1977]. 93 p.

**United States**

Clarke JH: Increased student participation in a dental history course after changing the grading method. **Bull Hist Dent** 1980 Apr;28(1):44–6

**1450–1700**

Boianov B: Iubileina godishnina na purvata doktorska disertatsiia v oblastta na stomatologiiata. **Stomatologiia (Sofiia)** 1979 Jul–Aug;61(4):256–9

**Belgium**

Gysel C: L'odonto-stomatologie formellement scolastique de Paul de Sorbait (1624–1691). **Rev Belge Med Dent** 1983 Mar;38(2):55–62

**1700 to Present**

Rizzuti A: Instituzione ed evoluzione dell'insegnamento dell'odontoiatria e genesi del dentista moderno. **Dent Cadmos** 1981 Jul;49(7):25–30

**Australia**

Lester KS: A short history of Westmead Centre Dental Clinical School. **Aust Dent J** 1981 Oct;26(5):321–7
Marlay E: A history of dental education in Queensland, 1863–1964. Brisbane, University of Queensland, 1979. xi, 226 p.

**Belgium**

Boute P: De ontwikkeling van de tandheelkunde aan de VUB – van 1950–'68 in het kader van de unitaire ULB – van 1969–heden: als zelfstandige universiteit. **Rev Belge Med Dent** 1981;36(3):120–3
De Boever J: Vijftig jaar universitaire opleiding in de tandheelkunde: een historisch overzicht. **Rev Belge Med Dent** 1981;36(3):101–2
De Bondt J: Historische overzicht van de dienst stomatologie en tandheelkunde aan de Katholieke Universiteit te Leuven. **Rev Belge Med Dent** 1981;36(3):111–4
Eisenring R: La médecine dentaire à l'Université de Liège. **Rev Belge Med Dent** 1981;36(3):137–40
Mayer R: L'enseignement de la médecine dentaire à l'Université Libre de Bruxelles. **Rev Belge Med Dent** 1981;36(3):130–6
Vanderdonck R: De ontwikkeling van de tandheelkunde aan de RUG sinds 1930. **Rev Belge Med Dent** 1981;36(3):115–9
Vermeersch AG: L'enseignement de la médecine dentaire à l'Universitè Catholique de Louvain. **Rev Belge Med Dent** 1981;36(3):128–9

**Brazil**

Faculdade de Odontologia da Universidade de São Paulo, 1934–1974: São Paulo, Faculdade, [1974?]. 60 p.
Madeira AA, Rosa JE: O curso de odontologia da Faculdade de Farmacia e Odontologia de Santa Catarina. **Rev Catarinense Odontol** 1979 Jul–Dec;6(2):9–20
Madeira AA, Rosa JE: O curso de odontologia do Instituto Polytechnico. **Rev Catarinense Odontol** 1978 Jan–Jun;5(2):7–17
Rosa JE, Madeira AA: A fundação da faculdade de farmácia e odontologia de Santa Catarina antecedentes e funcionamento. **Rev Catarinense Odontol** 1979 Jan–Jun;6(1):7–20
Rosa JE, Madeira AA: Instituto Polytechnico--primeira instituição de ensino superior no Estado de Santa Catarina. **Rev Catarinense Odontol** 1978;5(1 Spec No):30–40

**Canada**

Teteruck WR, Boyd MA, Teteruck L: The history of the dental aptitude test program in Canada. **Can Dent Assoc J** 1979 Aug;45(8):400–2

**Colombia**

Ordosgoitia Yarzagaray E, Viaña Olaya R, Buelvas Acosta E: Proceso historico de la Universidad de Carsagena. **Rev Fed Odontol Colomb** 1979 Jan–Mar;25(128):31–40

**Czechoslovakia**

Sícha V, Velková A: K 25. výročí vzniku stomatologické katedry II.F. **Cesk Stomatol** 1981 Mar;81(2):81–5
Velgos S: Rozvoj stomatologichej vetvy lekárskej fakulty Univerzity Komensk'ho v Bratislave. **Cas Lek Cesk** 1979 Dec 21;118(51):1586–8

**Denmark**

Holst JJ: Tandlaegeskolen - Stormgade 17. **Tandlaegebladet** 1982 Dec;86(22):771–9

**Dominican Republic**

Brea Tavárez CA: 80 años de instruccion odontologica en la Universidad Autonoma de Santo Domingo. Primera parte. **Rev Dent (St Domingo)** 1979 Jun–Dec;22(1–2):35–45

**France**

Rizzuti A: Odontoiatria del passato. Chirurgia e Medicina nel '700: nascita della Università moderna. **Dent Cadmos** 1982 Dec;50(12):59–61

**Germany**

Künzel W: Stomatologie - eine neue Grundstudieneinrichtung an der Medizinischen Akademie Erfurt (1975–1980). **Beitr Gesch Univ Erfurt** 1979–83;19:305–37

**Great Britain**

Cegielka L: A sound investment. The Department of Dental Science at the Royal College of Surgeons of England. **Br Dent J** 1983 Jul 9;155(1):30–1
Leighton BC: The Dental Education Advisory Council: 50 years. **Br Dent J** 1980 Nov 4;149(9):267–8

**Hungary**

Bánóczy J: Visszapillantás. **Fogorv Sz** 1980 Dec;73(12):354–5
Huszár G: A budapesti Fogorvostudományi Kar negyedszázados története. **Fogorv Sz** 1980 Dec;73(12):356–8
Sugár L: Morelli Gusztáv munkássága és szerepe a magyar parodontológiai oktatás kialakulásában. **Fogorv Sz** 1981 Feb;74(2):33–6

**Poland**

Dominik K: Dwusetna rocznica rozpoczecia na ziemiach polskich uniwersyteckich wykładów ze stomatologii. **Arch Hist Med (Warsz)** 1984;47(3):395–401
Sawicki B, Brońka E: Karol Goebel - pierwszy docent stomatologii w Polsce. **Czas Stomatol** 1979 Aug;32(8):807–9
Wajs S: Sześćdziesięcioletcie Państwowego Instytutu Dentystycznego. **Czas Stomatol** 1981 Aug;34(8):823–35

**Singapore**

Masaki T: [Department of dentistry at Singapore University during the war] (Jpn). **Dent Outlook** 1978;52(2):277

**Switzerland**

Baume LJ: Centenaire de l'Ecole dentaire de Genève. La biologie pulpo-dentinaire au temps de la création d l'Ecole dentaire de Genève (21 octobre 1881). **Swiss Dent** 1981 Dec;2(12):16–8, 20–2
Held AJ: Chronique des Ecoles universitaires suisses de médecine dentaire. **SSO Schweiz Monatsschr Zahnheilkd** 1982 Aug;92(8):711–9
Held AJ: L'enseignement de la médecine dentaire à Genève. A la recherche d'une voie. **Med Hyg (Geneve)** 1981 Oct 7;39(1440):3282–95
Held AJ: 100e anniversaire de la fondation de l'Ecole de Médecine dentaire de l'Université de Genève (1881–1981). Sommaire bilan d'un premier siècle. **SSO Schweiz Monatsschr Zahnheilkd** 1981 Oct;91(10):764–8
100 anniversaire de la fondation de l'Ecole de Médecine dentaire de l'Université de Genève (1881–1981): **SSO Schweiz Monatsschr Zahnheilkd** 1981 Oct;91(10):755–63

**United States**

Allen DL: The history and current status of curriculum length in the United States dental schools. **J Dent Educ** 1981 Oct;45(10):702–5
Baylor College of Dentistry.: **Dent Radiogr Photogr** 1980;53(3):inside front cover, 57–9
Carr JD: History of dental education in Indiana. **Indiana Med Hist Q** 1978;4(3):4–20
A century of dental education in Indiana. 1879–1979: **Alumni Bull Sch Dent Indiana Univ** 1979 Spring;:5–146
Cramer CH: The story of dentistry and the school in University Circle. Cleveland, School of Dentistry, Case Western Reserve University, 1982. x, 235 p.
Dummett CO: Dental education for Afro-Americans. **J Tenn Dent Assoc** 1982 Oct;61(4):14–6
Dummett CO: Historical notes on dental education for Afro-Americans. **J DC Dent Soc** 1981 Fall;56(1):35–9
Dunning JM: The Harvard School of Dental Medicine: phase two in the development of a university dental school. [Boston], Harvard School of Dental Medicine, 1981. viii, 141 p.
Fox BW: Dental school circa 1920. **CAL** 1983 Dec;47(6):9–11, 21
Hayden J: Niels Bjorn Jorgensen: painless dentist. **Advent Herit** 1979;6(2):44–8
Historical sketch: Loma Linda University School of Dentistry.: **New Dent** 1979 Feb;9(3):28–9
Histories of present dental schools in the United States: **Dent Radiogr Photogr** 1981;54(4):Inside front cover, 79, 87–8 (continued regularly)
Histories of present dental schools in the United States: **Dent Radiogr Photogr** 1983;56(1):inside front cover, 19–20
Histories of present dental schools in the United States: Loma Linda University School of Dentistry. **Dent Radiogr Photogr** 1981;54(2),2,39–40
Holland MR: University of Minnesota School of Dentistry: a proud and productive history. **Northwest Dent** 1983 Mar–Apr;62(2):68–71
Knudtzon K, Crandell CE, ed: From quonset hut to number one and beyond. A history of the UNC School of Dentistry. Chapel Hill, Univ. of North Carolina Dental Alumni Association, 1982. xxv, 426 p.
Kremenak N: A centennial scrapbook. **Iowa Dent J** 1983 Jan;69(1):28–46
Loveland LW: A short history of continuing education in New York State dentistry. **NY State Dent J** 1984 Nov;50(9):614, 616
McCauley HB: The century old Dental Department of the University of Maryland at Baltimore. **J Md State Dent Assoc** 1982 Dec;25(3):96–102
Santangelo MV: The history and development of United States dental education. **J Dent Educ** 1981 Oct;45(10):619–27
Savopoulos NM, ed: The Baltimore College of Dental Surgery: heritage and history. Baltimore, Baltimore College of Dental Surgery, 1980?. 22 p.
Schoen WP: The modern history of Loyola University Dental School. **CDS Rev** 1983 Jun;76(5):18–24
The University of Iowa College of Dentistry.: **Dent Radiogr Photogr** 1980;53(1):preceding 1, 19–20
University of North Carolina at Chapel Hill School of Dentistry: **Dent Radiogr Photogr** 1981;54(1):preceding 1, 19–20
Vanes JM: The Indiana University School of Dentistry in times of war. **Bull Hist Dent** 1980 Oct;28(2):91–5
Will the real 'father of dental education' please stand up? (John Harris): **Ohio Dent J** 1980 May;54(5):19–20
Winslow JE, Warren GB: Dental school capitation--an historical perspective. **J Dent Educ** 1981 Nov;45(11):759–62
75 years of dental hygiene education.: **Dent Hyg (Chic)** 1980 Mar;54(3):115–7

**USSR**

Gol'braĭkh VR: U istokov stomatologicheskogo obrazovaniia (k 100-letiiu pervoĭ zubovrachebnoĭ shkoly v Rossii). **Stomatologiia (Mosk)** 1982 Jul–Aug;61(4):64–5
Shabunin AV: Sto let otechestvennomu zubovrachebnomu obucheniiu. **Sov Zdravookhr** 1981;(11):52–3
Vorob'ev IuI, Veretennikova VP: 25 let kafedry rentgenologii i radiologii Moskovskogo meditsinskogo stomatologicheskogo instituta im. N. A.

Semashko. **Vestn Rentgenol Radiol** 1980 Sep-Oct;(5):88-9

**Venezuela**

Febres-Cordero F: Acerca de la fundacion de la Escuela Dental en Venezuela. **Acta Odontol Venez** 1980 Jan-Apr;18(1):7-35
Febres-Cordero F: La creacion de la Facultad de Odontologia. **Acta Odontol Venez** 1980 May-Aug;18(2):293-305
Febres-Cordero F: La enseñanza en Venezuela de la historia de la odontologia. **Acta Odontol Venez** 1979 May-Dec;17(2-3):210-11

**INSTRUMENTS AND EQUIPMENT**

Burningham RL: The evolution of the dental office. **Bull Hist Dent** 1980 Apr;28(1):21-8
Casado Llopmart JR: La microfusion como principio de los colados en protesis estomatologica. **Rev Esp Estomatol** 1982 Mar-Apr;30(2):113-22
Castagnola L, Garberoglio U: Breve cronistoria dei materiali e delle metodiche di impronta. **Riv Odontoiatr Amici Brugg** 1983 Apr-Jun;2(2):101-2
Donaldson JA: The use of gold in dentistry: an historical overview. **Gold Bull** 1980;13(3):117-24; (4),160-5
Downing J: An outline of the history of dental mechanics (1). **Dent Tech** 1984 Mar;37(3):17-8 (cont)
Greener EH: Amalgam -- yesterday, today, and tomorrow. **Oper Dent** 1979 Winter;4(1):24-35
Hagman HC: History of crown and bridgework, part I. **Dent Lab Rev** 1980 May;55(5):20-4
Hagman HC: Prosthetic memoirs, part III. **Dent Lab Rev** 1979 Dec;54(13):22-6
Hagman HC: The history of dentures. **Dent Lab Rev** 1979 Mar;54(3):24-9 (continued periodically)
Hoffmann-Axthelm W: Zur Geschichte des Gaumenobturators. **Quintessenz Zahntech** 1980 Mar-Apr;6(3,4):85-93, 97-100
Holtkamp P: Die Entwicklung der Bohrmaschine. **Quintessenz Zahntech** 1981 May;7(5):507-9
Rechtman J: La brosse à dents et son histoire (1780-1980). **Hist Sci Med** 1980;14(2):221-5
Rice RW: Computers in dentistry. Part 1. **Chronicle** 1982 Sep;45(7):130-2
Rickenbacher B: Die Zahntechnik, von der Vergangenheit zur Gegenwart. **Zahntechnik (Geneve)** 1983;41(2):124-6
Riethe P: Geschichtliche Entwicklung der Amalgame. **Dtsch Zahnarztl Z** 1980;35(4):443-9
Rizzuti A: Odontoiatria del passato. Storia dell'amalgama dentale (I). **Dent Cadmos** 1983 Aug;51(8):69-73
Schütter R: Die Namen der Metalle. Herkunt und Bedeutung. **Zahnarzt** 1984 Sep;28(9):726-30
Sumii T: [History of casting]. (Jpn) **Nippon Shika Ishikai Zasshi** 1979;32(4):367-73
Swanson BZ: Spain's private dental museum. **Bull Hist Dent** 1984;32(1):27-30

**Germany**

Loevy HT, Kowitz A: Dentistry on stamps. **J Am Dent Assoc** 1982 Jun;104(6):890

**Italy**

Aulizio F: Come si estraevano i denti un tempo. Lo strumentario dentistico della Fondazione Putti ... Bologna. **Strenna Stor Bolognese** 1979;29:29-41

**Before 500 A.D.**

**Rome**

Longfield-Jones GM: A set of silver dental instruments from the New Milton Collection. **Med Hist** 1984 Jan;28(1):42-8

**500 A.D.-1450**

**Americas**

Gwinnett AJ, Gorelick L: Inlayed teeth of ancient Mayans: a tribological study using the SEM. **Scan Electron Microsc** 1979:(3);575-80

**1700 to Present**

Adjusting the dental chair: **J Am Dent Assoc** 1984 Apr;108(4):490-1
Ahlin JH: The historical development of Maxillofacial orthopedic technique. **Bull Hist Dent** 1982 Oct;30(2):96-107
Baum L: Gold foil. **Oper Dent** 1984 Spring;9(2):42-9
Berenholc C, Martin C: Du rotatif au manuel. Considerations sur l'utilisation du mouvement en endodontie. **Chir Dent Fr** 1982 Oct 7;52(173):29-33
Berenholc C: L'amalgame d'argent, obturation provisoire de longue durée. **Chir Dent Fr** 1981 Feb;51(98):37-42 contd.
The bright side of dentistry: **J Am Dent Assoc** 1984 Apr;108(4):520-1
Charles AD: The story of dental amalgam. **Bull Hist Dent** 1982 Apr;30(1):2-7
Cohen RA: Cyrus Fay, a pioneer in forceps design. **Bull Hist Dent** 1983 Apr;31(1):32-3
Dewel BF: The ribbon arch. Its influence in the development of orthodontic appliances. **Angle Orthod** 1981 Oct;51(4):263-8
Endres L: Entwicklung der Artikulatoren. **Zahntechnik (Geneve)** 1980;38(4):334-5
Geppert W, Hartmann E, Hennis I, et al: Die Entwicklung dentaler Technologien, dargestellt am Bestand einer historischen Sammlung. (II). **Quintessenz Zahntech** 1982 Nov;8(11):1261-70
Geppert W, Hartmann E, Hennis I, et al: Die Entwicklung dentaler Technologien, dargestellt am Bestand einer historischen Sammlung (III). **Quintessenz** 1983 Mar;34(3):543-9
Glendinning V: A gentle probe into dentistry 1770-1970. **Dent Tech** 1980 Feb;33(2):9-12
Grossman LI: In the interest of historical fact. **J Endod** 1984 Apr;10(4):168
Hagman HC: Artic-u-logic. **Dent Lab Rev** 1981 Feb;56(2):18-21
Hagman HC: History of articulators. **Dent Lab Rev** 1980 Feb;55(2):28-31
Hagman HC: History of ceramics, part II. **Dent Lab Rev** 1980 Dec;55(3):34-6
Hagman HC: History of ceramics, part 1. **Dent Lab Rev** 1980 Nov;:34, 36
Hagman HC: The elusive condyles, part I. **Dent Lab Rev** 1982 Oct;57(10):33
Hagman HC: The evolution of dental castings. **Dent Lab Rev** 1979 Jul;54(8):28-33
Hagman HS: History of partical dentures, part 1. **Dent Lab Rev** 1980 Jul;55(8):28-9
Hansson O, Eklund J: A historical review of hydrocolloids and an investigation of the dimensional accuracy of the new alginates for crown and bridge impressions when using stock trays. **Swed Dent J** 1984;8(2):81-95
Hargreaves AS: The development of denture design. **Br Dent J** 1981 Aug 4;151(3):101-2
Harvey WL, Hatch R: Articulators--a perspective: wristolator to robots. **J Colo Dent Assoc** 1981 Nov-Dec;60(3):3-5
Hein JW: The industrial contribution to safe and effective dentifrices. **Community Dent Oral Epidemiol** 1980;8(5):230-6
Hohmann E: 100 years of equipment technology for the practice of dentistry. **Dent Echo (Heidelb)** 1981 May;50(3):89-109
Holtkamp P: Fortschritte in der zahnärztlichen Prothetik durch die Einführung der Gusstechnik. **Quintessenz J** 1983 Jun;13(6):571-9
Llistosella Alberti R: Evolucion historica de la ceramica. **Rev Esp Estomatol** 1983 Jan-Feb;31(1):27-30
Lopez Lozano JF: Articuladores. **Rev Esp Estomatol** 1980 May-Jun;28(3):145-54
Martinez Ramos JM: Articuladores: su influencia en la evolución de la propedeutica y terapeutica prostodoncica. **Estodont Press** 1983;1(1):32-5
Marvitz L: Therapia antiqua. **Tidsskr Tandlaeger** 1982 Dec;2(6):30
Marvitz L: Therapia antiqua. **Tidsskr Tandlaeger** 1983 Apr;3:48
Marvitz L: Therapia antiqua. **Tidsskr Tandlaeger** 1983 Dec;3(4):23
Miller GM, Kreuzer DW: The modified Hawley appliance: part I. **Int J Periodontics Restorative Dent** 1981;1(6):8-21
A review of dental radiography: **J Am Dent Assoc** 1984 Apr;108(4):552-3
Rodriguez Arroyo JL, Ivich Treviño MP: Historia de la porcelana. **ADM** 1980 Jan-Feb;37(1):26-7
Schmid R, Barbakow F, Mühlemann H, et al: Amine fluoride and monofluorophosphate: I. Historical review of fluoride dentifrices. **ASDC J Dent Child** 1984 Mar-Apr;51(2):99-103
Schmidt A: Die Geschichte der Methakrylate in der Stomatologie. **Zahntechnik (Berl)** 1978 Oct;19(10):436-44
Schmuth GP: Milestones in the development and practical application of functional appliances. **Am J Orthod** 1983 Jul;84(1):48-53
A short history of the dental drill: **J Am Dent Assoc** 1984 Apr;108(4):572-3
Smith DC: Dental materials today. Part 1: perspectives - past and present. **Ont Dent** 1980 Dec;57(12):16-9
Sugden KC: Nicolas Dubois de Chemant and the disputed invention of mineral teeth. **Br Dent J** 1983 Sep 24;155(6):202
Sugimoto S: [Makers of wooden denture bases] (Jpn). **Rinsho Shika** 1982;303:15-8
Sugimoto S: [Wooden denture bases] (Jpn). **Rinsho Shika** 1982;(304):19-21
Williams DF: In search of perfect dental materials. **Br Dent J** 1981 Jul 7;151(1):24-7
Zinner ID, Sherman H: An analysis of the development of complete denture impression techniques. **J Prosthet Dent** 1981 Sep;46(3):242-9

**Denmark**

Marvitz L: Theraphia antiqua. **Tidsskr Tandlaeger** 1981 Dec;1(3):36
Marvitz L: Therapia antiqua. **Tidsskr Tandlaeger** 1984 Jun;4(3):24

**France**

Baron A, Baron P: Du charlatan au chirurgien-dentiste. **Inf Dent** 1983 Jan 13;65(2):123-4
Herschfeld JJ: Nicholas Dubois de Chemant and the invention of mineral

teeth. **Bull Hist Dent** 1982 Apr;30(1):40-3
Maire M: L'or du temps. Le musée de la chirurgie dentaire de la faculté d'odontologie de Lyon. **Chir Dent Fr** 1979 May 31;49(22):25-30
Verchere L: Henri Lentulo, inventeur du bourre-pâte, 1889-1981. **Rev Odontostomatol (Paris)** 1981 Mar-Apr;10(2):175-7

**Germany**

Hohmann E: 100 Jahre Ausrüstungstechnik für die zahnärztliche Berufsarbeit. **Dent Echo (Heidelb)** 1980 Aug;50(5):36-58
Kimmel K, Steinkrüger F: Der deutsche dental-medizinische Fachhandel. Geschichte--Aufgaben--Strukturen. **Dent Echo (Heidelb)** 1981 Dec;51(8):10-32
Kimmel K: Was ist daraus geworden? (I) Ein Milchsauger und ein Kieferformer 25 Jahre nach ihrer Einführung. **ZWR** 1980 Feb;89(2):62-7

**Great Britain**

Grant AA: A century of change in prosthetic dentistry. **Br Dent J** 1980 Jul 1;149(1):9-12

**Japan**

Nihon Shika Kigyo Kyogikai, Gyokaishi Henshu Iinkai: Nihon shika gyokai shi. Tokyo, Nihon Shika Kigyo Kyogikai, Showa 52, 1977- v.

**Sweden**

Francke OC: The dental turbine handpiece, a Swedish invention. **Bull Hist Dent** 1981 Oct;29(2):91-3

**United States**

Abrams RA, Drake CW, Segal H: Dr. Sanford C. Barnum and the invention of the rubber dam. **Gen Dent** 1982 Jul-Aug;30(4):320-2
A dental laboratory's catalog: from before the turn of the century. **Bull Hist Dent** 1980 Apr;28(1):47-8
Fifty years of cephalometric radiography: **Angle Orthod** 1981 Apr;51(2):88-171
Forrest WR, Christen AG: Recollections of a dental researcher. Fifty years at the U.S. National Bureau of Standards: interviews with George C. Paffenbarger, D.D.S., D.Sc. Part VI. **J Ala Dent Assoc** 1984 Spring;68(2):29-31, 34-7
Hagman HC: George S. Monson, DDS. **Dent Lab Rev** 1982 Mar;57(3):36
Hagman HC: History: Charles Goodyear. **Dent Lab Rev** 1981 Aug;56(8):33
Hagman HC: Prosthetic memoirs. **Dent Lab Rev** 1979 Sep-Oct;54(10-11):12-3, 54; 40-2
Herschfeld JJ: E. J. Greenfield and artificial implants. **Bull Hist Dent** 1984;32(1):33-41
Herschfeld JJ: W.G.A. Bonwill and the 'anatomical articulator.' **Bull Hist Dent** 1980 Apr;28(1):29-34
Jackson E: Treasures from the national collections. **Bull Hist Dent** 1982 Oct;30(2):121-2
Kremenak N: John L. Naughton, inventor of the Den-Tal-Ez chair. An Iowa original. **Iowa Dent J** 1984 Oct;70(4):23-5
Millstein CB: W. D. Miller and the beginnings of occupational hygiene in dentistry. **Bull Hist Dent** 1984 Oct;32(2):135-6
Paul Revere, goldsmith: **Dent Lab Rev** 1981 Feb;56(2):40
Ring ME: The rubber denture murder case: the true story of the vulcanite litigations. **Bull Hist Dent** 1984;32(1):3-18
Walter JD: Charles W. Stearns and Norman W. Kingsley and the development of the artificial velum. **Bull Hist Dent** 1981 Oct;29(2):74-81

**SOCIETIES**

**Japan**

Toyohashi-shi Shika Ishikai shi: Toyohashi, Japan, Toyohashi-shi Shika Ishikai, Showa 52 nen. [1977]. 755 p.

**1700 to Present**

**Americas**

Muller E: Bosquejo histórico de la Asociación Panamericana de Periodontología. **Acta Odontol Venez** 1983 May-Aug;21(2):173-9
Muñoz AL, Hernández Sánchez FA: 3 de Octubre: fecha rememorativa de la odontología y de la Confraternidad Odontológica Latinoamericana. **Salud Bucal** 1981 Oct-Nov;8(46):10-4, 73-7

**Argentina**

Bagur D: Sociedad odontologica del Rio de la Plata, periodo 1897-98. **Rev Asoc Odontol Argent** 1980 Nov;68(7):464-7
Bagur DB: Sociedad odontologica del Rio de la Plata: periodo 1899-1902. **Rev Asoc Odontol Argent** 1981 May;69(3):147-50

**Belgium**

Klees L: Quelques souvenirs des debuts du G.I.R.S.O. **Bull Group Int Rech Sci Stomatol Odontol** 1981 Jun;24(2):75-80

**Colombia**

Qué es la Federación Odontológica Colombiana: **Rev Fed Odontol Colomb** 1982 Jul-Sep;31(142):97-113

**Europe**

Leatherman GH: 80 years of the FDI. **Probe (Lond)** 1981 Oct;23(4):155-6, 161, Nov;23(5):203, 205-6, 208

**Germany**

Breustedt A: 30 Jahre DDR--30 Jahre Mitarbeit der stomatologisch-wissenschaftlichen Gesellschaften bei der Gestaltung des sozialistischen Gesundheitswesens in der DDR. **Stomatol DDR** 1979;29(10):729-34
Die Deutsche Gesellschaft für Zahn-, Mund- und Kieferheilkunde: Vom Zentralverein 1859 bis heute; ein weiter und erfolgreicher Weg. **ZWR** 1981 Apr;90(4):10-6
Kottenkamp W: 75 Jahre Niederrheinische Zahnärztliche Gesellschaft. **Dtsch Zahnarztl Z** 1981 Oct;36(10):610-3
Künzel W: Die Gesellschaft für Stomatologie der DDR, 1964-1984. Leipzig, J. A. Barth, 1984. 187 p.

**Great Britain**

Cohen RA, et al: The British Dental Association. The advance of the dental profession; a centenary history 1880-1980. London, British Dental Association, 1979. ix, 289 p.
Harris R: Centenary of the British Dental Association. **Aust Dent J** 1980 Jun;25(3):169-70
Leatherman GH: The FDI: 1900-1980. **Probe (Lond)** 1981 Jul;23(1):5-10 (continued)
Pearson G: Yorkshire dentists in the formative years of the B.D.A. **Br Dent J** 1981 Apr 21;150(8):231-2
Watson RM, Harty FJ: A coming of age. The British Endodontic Society. **Br Dent J** 1984 Jan 21;156(2):66-7
Western Countries Branch centenary celebrations: **Br Dent J** 1979 Dec 4;147(11):315-6

**Greece**

Basileios Stephanopoulos-Vrettos: mia alesmonete mneme: **Stomatologia (Athenai)** 1980 Nov-Dec;37(6):5-48

**Japan**

Gojunen no kaiko: Tokyo, Do Dosokai, Showa 53 nen. [1978]. 2 v.
Moriyama N, Takazoe I: The historical relationship between Japanese dentistry and the Fédération Dentaire Internationale. **Bull Hist Dent** 1984 Oct;32(2):104-8

**New Zealand**

The jubilee year: **NZ Dent J** 1980 Apr;76(344):47-8

**Poland**

Kościukiewicz-Michiewicz I: Działalność i osiągnięcia Sekcji Ortodontycznej Polskiego Towarzystwa Stomatologicznego W latach 1951-1977. **Czas Stomatol** 1980 Jun;33(6):567-70
Orlik-Grzybowska A: Geneza powstania Sekcji Ortodontycznej Polskiego Tow. Stomat. i jej początkowa działalność w latach 1950-1955. **Czas Stomatol** 32(9):909-13, Sep 79

**Sweden**

Francke OC: Svenska Tandläkare-Sällskapets samlingar. **Nord Medicinhist Arsb** 1980;Suppl 6:143-6
Historik: Svenska Tandteknikerförbundet: **Tandteknikern** 1981 Oct;50(10):500-23

**Switzerland**

Baume LJ: Vers le centenaire de notre Société. **Schweiz Monatsschr Zahnmed** 1984 Oct;94(10):1061-2
Stutz GM: Zur Geschichte der Zürcher Zahnärztegesellschaft. Zürich, Juris, 1984. 76 p. (Zürcher Medizingeschichtliche Abhandlungen, Neue Reihe, Nr. 172)

## DENTISTRY

**United States**

Founding of the American Academy of Dental Group Practice. **J Dent Pract Adm** 1984 Jan-Mar;1(1):8
The American Dental Association in 1982: **Tic** 1982 Nov;41(11):1-3
Berkey LG: History of the Ninth District Dental Society, 1909-1984. **Bull Ninth Dist Dent Soc** 1984 Jun;68(6):11pp
Early history of the South Dakota Dental Society: **Northwest Dent** 1983 Jul-Aug;62(4):17-22
Ecker HA, Epsteen CM: The American Society of Maxillofacial Surgeons. Williamsport, Pa., Grit Pub. Co., 1978. 69 p.
Gordon B: Maryland section's ACD day. **J Am Coll Dent** 1984 Summer;51(2):27-32
Holland MR: The Minnesota Dental Association: 1958-1983. **Northwest Dent** 1983 Mar-Apr;62(2):23-44
McCauley HB: The Maryland State Dental Association: in the beginning. **J Md State Dent Assoc** 1983 Aug;26(2):74-8
Perlmutter G: History of the Achievement Medal. **Alpha Omegan** 1982 Sep;75(3):24-9
Pioneers in pedodontics: influential leaders of the past (John C. Brauer): **Pediatr Dent** 1982 Jun;4(2):143-4
The presidents: **J Am Dent Assoc** 1979 Oct;99(4):601 (continued periodically)
The presidents: **J Am Dent Assoc** 1983 Oct;107(4):690 (continued periodically)
The presidents. George Hoppin Cushing, 1871-1872: **J Am Dent Assoc** 1979 Dec;99(6):956
Reflections of the past: **J Md State Dent Assoc** 1983 Aug;26(2):62-73
Starkey VL: The way we were--Ohio State Dental Society, 1866. **Ohio Dent J** 1980 May;54(5):17-9
Stinaff R, Hollander L: Origins of the American Academy of Dental Practice Administration. **J Dent Pract Adm** 1984 Jan-Mar;1(1):4-5

**USSR**

Akhmedov AA: K istorii organizatsii Azerbaĭdzhanskogo nauchnogo obshchestva stomatologov. **Stomatologiia (Mosk)** 1980 Jun;59(3):89-91

## DERMATOLOGY

Basset A, Burgun R: Geschichte der Dermatologie. In Sournia JC, Martiny M, Poulet J, ed: Illustrierte Geschichte der Medizin. Salzburg, Andreas, 1980. Vol. 4. p. 1547-73.
Foussereau J: History of epicutaneous testing: the blotting-paper and other methods. **Contact Dermatitis** 1984 Oct;11(4):219-23
Huckbody E: Dermatology throughout the dark ages. The interchange of experience. **Int J Dermatol** 1980 Jul-Aug;19(6):344-7
King JM: Historical review of early dermatology by J. M. King, MD, Nashville, Tenn. Originally published May 1927. **South Med J** 1983 Apr;76(4):426-36
Lyell A: Daniel Turner (1667-1740) LRCP London (1711) M.D. honorary, Yale (1723) surgeon, physician and pioneer dermatologist: the man seen in the pages of his book on the skin. **Int J Dermatol** 1982 Apr;21(3):162-70
Parish LC, Crissey JT: Bibliography of secondary sources on the history of dermatology. III. Books, monographs, and chapters in English supplemented through 1980. **Int J Dermatol** 1981 Jun;20(5):390-2
Portele KA: Die Moulagensammlung des Pathologisch-Anatomischen Bundesmuseums in Wien. [Wien, Pathologisch-Anatomisches Bundesmuseum in Wien], 1977. 84 p.
Tsankov N, Puissant A: Les dermatologistes bulgares à l'hôpital Saint-Louis et leurs relations avec la dermatologie française. **Hist Sci Med** 1980;14:349-56
Zanca A, Tagliavini R: Iconografia dermatologica e venereologica: ieri e oggi. **Acta Med Hist Patav** 1980-81;27:81-97
Zimmermann R, Zimmermann K: Antike Tätowierungen aus heutiger Sicht. **Hautarzt** 1981 Jun;32(6):324-30

**China**

Chuan-Kui H, Da-Ding F, Gan-Yun Y: Some sketches on the history of Chinese dermatology. **Arch Dermatol Res** 1982;272(1-2):185-90

**France**

Wachs GN: The French school of dermatology. **Int J Dermatol** 1982 Jun;21(5):277-9

**Great Britain**

Waisman M: Concepts of acne of the British school of dermatology prior to 1860. **Int J Dermatol** 1983 Mar;22(2):126-9

**México**

Latapí F, Ortiz Y: Historia de la dermatología en México. In Academia Nacional de Medicina. Libro conmemorativo del primer centenario. México, Comité Editorial de la Comisión Organizadora del Congreso del Centenario, 1964. Tome 2. p. 565-92.
Vérut DD: PreColombian dermatology and cosmetology in Mexico. [S.1]: Schering Corp. USA, 1973. [107 p].

**Spain**

Carreras Verdaguer A: La dermatología en la medicina catalana. Su contribución a la medicina mundial. **Actas Dermosifiliogr** 1980 Nov-Dec;71(11-12):487-94

**Sri Lanka**

Uragoda CG: Some historical aspects of dermatology in Sri Lanka. **Int J Dermatol** 1984 Jan-Feb;23(1):78-80

**Thailand**

Terwiel BJ: Tattooing in Thailand's history. **J R Asiat Soc GB Irel** 1979;156-66

**Before 500 A.D.**

**Rome**

Dirckx JH: Dermatologic terms in the De Medicina of Celsus. **Am J Dermatopathol** 1983 Aug;5(4):363-9
Dirckx JH: Ovid's dermatologic formulary. **Am J Dermatopathol** 1980 Winter;2(4):327-32
Laur WE: Shave and a haircut--two sesterces: a brief account of men and their hair in Imperial Rome. **Int J Dermatol** 1981 Sep;20(7U):504-5

**500 A.D.-1450**

**Arabic**

Belova LV, Mirakhmedov UM: Vklad Abu Ali ibn-Sina v dermato-venerologiiu. **Vestn Dermatol Venerol** 1983 Dec;(12):60-4

**1450-1700**

Bartsocas CS: Paleodermatoglyphics. **Prog Clin Biol Res** 1982;84:139-43
Sullivan EJ: Art in dermatopathology. Jusepe de Ribera. An interpreter of the skin through art. **Am J Dermatopathol** 1979 Summer;1(2):159-62

**Poland**

Rudowska I, Rudzki E: Dermatologiczna analiza ziołowych surowców kosmetycznych zalecanych w zielniku Falimirza z roku 1534. **Przegl Dermatol** 1983 Jul-Aug;70(4):429-37

**1700 to Present**

Bernhard JD, Elliot AD: A letter from Darier to Bowen on the naming of Bowen's disease. **Arch Dermatol** 1983 Mar;119(3):261-2
Bluefarb SM: Dermatologists on postage stamps (Hulusi Behçet, Ruzar Briffa). **Int J Dermatol** 1982 Jan-Feb;21(1):54
Brodin MB: William Osler and dermatology, pathology, and dermatopathology. **Am J Dermatopathol** 1981 Fall;3(3):261-4
Caplan RM: The circumstances of the missing biographer or why Watson didn't narrate these four Sherlock Holmes stories. **J Am Acad Dermatol** 1982 Jun;6(6):1112-4
Civatte J: Jean Darier: a memoir. **Am J Dermatopathol** 1979 Spring;1(1):57-60
Crissey JT, Parish LC: The dermatology and syphilology of the nineteenth century. New York, Praeger, 1981. viii, 439 p.
Curtis AC, Owens BB: Centennial paper: Beta dimethylaminoethyl benzhydryl ether hydrochloride (benadryl) in treatment of urticaria by Arthur C. Curtis and Betty Brechner Owens. **Arch Dermatol** 1983 May;119(5):438-41
Frank SB: International Society of Tropical Dermatology in perspective. **Int J Dermatol** 1981 Jan-Feb;20(1):69-71
Holubar K: The influence of the British School of Dermatology on the Vienna School in the first half of the 19th century. **Int J Dermatol** 1982 May;21(4):224-6
Kalis JB, Malkinson FD: Landmark perspective: Dermatitis herpetiformis. A commentary. **JAMA** 1983 Jul 8;250(2):217-21
Katz SI: 'Sulfoxone (Diasone) sodium for dermatitis herpetiformis' by Cornbleet, December 1951. Commentary: Sulfoxone (Diasone) in the treatment of dermatitis herpetiformis. **Arch Dermatol** 1982 Oct;118(10):805-12
Klasen HJ: History of free skin grafting--knowledge or empiricism? Berlin, New York, Springer, 1981. 190 p.
Köster W: Medizin-historische Studie über die Weiterführung der Vorstellungen von P. G. Unna in der Therapie und Biochemie von Hautkrankheiten in der Gegenwart. Therapie und Biochemie von Hautkrankheiten nach P. G. Unna. Berlin, Grosse, 1977. 161 p.
Koulu L, Jansén C: Epidermiksen Langerhansin solu--ajankohtainen

satavuotias. **Duodecim** 1980;96(23-24):1587-91
Lever WF: Savary's 1814 article on the history of pemphigus related to contemporary views. **Int J Dermatol** 1979 Sep;18(7):584-5
Lyell A: The staphylococcal scalded skin syndrome in historical perspective: emergence of dermopathic strains of Staphylococcus aureus and discovery of the epidermolytic toxin. A review of events up to 1970. **J Am Acad Dermatol** 1983 Aug;9(2):285-94
Parish LC, Crissey JT: Bibliography of secondary sources on the history of dermatology. **Int J Dermatol** 1981 Oct;20(8):555-61
Parish LC: The history of tropical dermatology and the 1907 International Congress of Dermatology. **Int J Dermatol** 1980 Oct;19(8):474-7
Pinkus H: Etiology of an anatomist's discoveries in dermatology. **Am J Dermatopathol** 1982 Apr;4(2):127-35
Plato CC, Wertelecki W: Changing trends in dermatoglyphic research. **Prog Clin Biol Res** 1982;84:1-11
Pochi PE: 'Effect of androgen on the sebaceous glands of human skin' by Rony and Zakon, December 1943. Commentary: Androgen effects on human sebaceous glands. **Arch Dermatol** 1982 Oct;118(10):799-804
Scholz A: Rudolph Leopold Mayer, Werk und Persönlichkeit. **Dermatol Monatsschr** 1981 Sep;167(9):582-6
Shelley WB: Commentary: antihistamines and the treatment of urticaria. **Arch Dermatol** 1983 May;119(5):442-4
Sulzberger MB: My companions on the International Committee of Dermatology. **J Am Acad Dermatol** 1982 Feb;6(2):179-94
Waisman M: Historical note: Koebner on the isomorphic phenomenon. **Arch Dermatol** 1981 Jul;117(7):415

**Australia**

Johnson A: August Hoff--a Sydney dermatologist of the 1880's. **Australas J Dermatol** 1983 Apr;24(1):37-9
Johnson A: William John Munro (1863-1908). **Am J Dermatopathol** 1983 Oct;5(5):477-8
Weedon D: Conception, birth, and growth of the Australian Dermatopathology Society. **Am J Dermatopathol** 1984 Apr;6(2):159-60

**Austria**

Braun M: Classics in Oncology. Idipathic multiple pigmented sarcoma of the skin by Kaposi. **CA** 1982 Nov-Dec;32(6):340-7
Crissey JT, Parish LC: Ferdinand Hebra: a reexamination of his contributions to dermatology. **Int J Dermatol** 1980 Dec;19(10):585-8
Holubar K: Die Dermatologie in Wien und die Deutsche Dermatologische Gesellschaft (DDG). Eine historische Perspektive. **Hautarzt** 1983;34(Suppl 6):xvii-xviii
Holubar K: Ferdinand von Hebra und das Allgemeine Krankenhaus in Wien. Über die Domizilierung der beiden Hautkliniken um die Mitte des 19. Jahrhunderts und ihr Verhältnis zum II. Hof im Allgemeinen Krankenhaus. **Wien Med Wochenschr** 1982 Sep 30;132(18):423-6
Holubar K, Frankl J: Joseph Plenck (1735-1807). A forerunner of modern European dermatology. **J Am Acad Dermatol** 1984 Feb;10(2 pt 1):326-32
Kerl H, Konrad K, Holubar K: The Austrian Society of Dermatopathology. **Am J Dermatopathol** 1984 Jun;6(3):221-2
King DF, King LA: Josef Plenck--grandfather of modern dermatology. **J Am Acad Dermatol** 1984 Jul;11(1):143-6
King DF: Modern textbooks of dermatopathology and acantholysis of Auspitz. **J Am Acad Dermatol** 1984 Aug;11(2 Pt 1):301-3
Klimpel M: F. von Hebra, Atlas der Hauterkrankungen (1856-1876). Köln, Universität zu Köln, 1980. 322 p. (Kölner medizinhistorische Beiträge, 17) (also Diss.).
Lindemayr W: Die Bedeutung Albert Wiedmanns für die Entwicklung der Dermatologie in Wien nach 1945. **Wien Klin Wochenschr** 1981 Dec 25;93(24):735-9
Tappeiner J, Holubar K: Ferdinand Ritter von Hebra: Person und Werk (1816 bis 1880). **Wien Klin Wochenschr** 1981 Sep 4;93(16):503-6

**Belgium**

Pierard GE, Lapiere CM: Liège. The 'Ardent City' of Theodor Schwann and Tchantches. **Am J Dermatopathol** 1984 Feb;6(1):95-7

**Czechoslovakia**

Danda J: K devadesátým narozeninám prof. MUDr. K. Hübschmanna, DrSc. **Cesk Dermatol** 1980 Oct;55(5):289-94
Hübschmann K: History of Dermatology and Venerology from 1848 to the end of 1944 in Prague, Czechoslovakia. **Int J Dermatol** 1982 Jul-Aug;21(6):356-60
Hübschmann K: Sambergerovi současníci na klinice Janovského. **Cesk Dermatol** 1980 Oct;55(5):349-53
Ozorovský V, Tychý M, Buchvald J, et al: Sociálne aspeckty začiatkov dermatovenerológie v Bratislave po roku 1918 a úloha professora Reinsberga. **Cesk Zdrav** 1982 Jul;30(7):319-25
Pospíšil L: K prioritě objevu specifické imobilizace treponém. **Cesk Dermatol** 1981 Oct;56(5):346-8

**Denmark**

Bonnevie P: Dermatologi og dermatologer - før og nu. **Dan Medicinhist Arbog** 1982;:137-52
Bonnevie P: Dermatology in Denmark. **Int J Dermatol** 1983 Apr;22(3):193-200
Curriculum vitae and writings: Niels Hjorth.: **Acta Derm Venereol [Suppl] (Stockh)** 1979;59(85):5-9

**France**

Dahm S: Frühe Krankenbildnisse: Alibert Esquirol Baumgartner. Köln, 1981. (Kölner medizinhistorische Beiträge; Arbeiten der Forschungsstelle des Instituts für Geschichte der Medizin der Universität zu Köln, Band 21).
Everett MA: Anne-Charles Lorry. The first French dermatologist. **Int J Dermatol** 1979 Nov;18(9):762-4
Everett MA: Jean Louis Alibert. The father of French dermatology. **Int J Dermatol** 1984 Jun;23(5):351-6
Goldwyn RM: Keloid. **Plast Reconstr Surg** 1981 Oct;68(4):640-1
Prosper Baumès, dermatologist of Lyon 1791-1871 and the Willan-Alibert controversy: **Br J Dermatol** 1981 Dec;105(6):727-31

**Germany**

Braun-Falco O: 50 Jahre Dermatologie im Städtischen Krankenhaus Thalkirchnerstrasse - Rückblick und Ausblick. **Hautarzt** 1980 Jan;31(1):37-41
Brooks HG: A visit to Dr. Unna's clinic in Hamburg. an excerpt: British Journal of Dermatology 1890. **Am J Dermatopathol** 1982 Jun;4(3):225-8
Hollander A: Betrachtungen über Paul Gerson Unna. **Z Hautkr** 1984 May 15;59(10):680-7
Hollander A: Glimpses at the life and work of P. G. Unna. **Am J Dermatopathol** 1980 Summer;2(2):137-42
Hollander A: P. G. Unna revisited. **Am J Dermatopathol** 1981 Summer;3(2):187-9
Hundeiker M: Wilhelm Knoth. **Verh Dtsch Ges Pathol** 1982;66:646-52
King DF: Gustav Simon. The father of dermatopathology. **Am J Dermatopathol** 1979 Fall;1(3):225-8
King DF, King LA: Jews in dermatology. **Am J Dermatopathol** 1984 Aug;6(4):415-6
Klaschka F, Rauhut K, ed: 100 Jahre Dermatologie in Berlin. Beiträge und Aufzeichnungen anlässlich der Festsitzung der Berliner Dermatologischen Gesellschaft am 12. und 13 Februar 1982. Berlin, Grosse Verlag, 1984. 152 p.
Kleine-Natrop HE: Theodor Grüneberg in der Tradition der halleschen Dermatologie. **Dermatol Monatsschr** 1981 Jun;167(6):393-5
Lever WF: Reminiscences about dermatopathology. **Am J Dermatopathol** 1979 Winter;1(4):313-7
Leyh F, Wendt V: Heinrich A. Gottron (1890-1974). **Am J Dermatopathol** 1983 Jun;5(3):241-3
Müller W: Geschichte der Universitätshautklinik Essen. **Hautarzt** 1982 Jan;33(1):26-9
Pfister R: 100 Jahre Dermatologie. **Fortschr Med** 1982 Dec 16;100(47-48):2214-21
Raith L: Johann Ernst Wichmann--ein zu Unrecht wenig bekannter Dermatologe des 18. Jahrhunderts. **Dermatol Monatsschr** 1983;169(11):725-7
Rothschuh KE: Ernst Schweninger (1850-1924). Zu seinem Leben und Wirken. Ergänzungen, Korrekturen. **Medizinhist J** 1984;19(3):250-8
Schreier J, Haustein UF, Karbe KH: Zur Geschichte der Dermatologie an der Universität Leipzig. **Dermatol Monatsschr** 1984;170(1):1-14
Schulz EA: Otto Julius Grütz, Leben und Lebenswerk. Diss. Bonn, 1982. 107 p.
Weiss J: Die Universitätshautklinik Hamburg-Eppendorf im Wandel der Zeit. **Hautarzt** 1981 Jan;32(1):28-32
Weissmann A, Camisa C: Friedrich Sigmund Merkel. **Am J Dermatopathol** 1982 Dec;4(6):521-35
Wendt V: Heinrich A. Gottron: Leben und Werk. Lübeck, Hansisches Verlagskonto H. Scheffler, 1980. 99 p.

**Great Britain**

Alsop JD: Two letters on the cuticular glove: keratolysis of 1769. **J Hist Med Allied Sci** 1984 Apr;39(2):224-5
Atherton DJ: Joseph Towne: wax modeler extraordinary. **J Am Acad Dermatol** 1980 Sep;3(3):311-6
De mortuis nil nisi bonum: **J Am Acad Dermatol** 1982 May;6(5):968-76
Goldsmith WN: Sir Archibald Montague Gray. In Dictionary of national biography, 1961-1970. Suppl. 8, 1981. p. 452-3.
Hershman MJ: William Morrant Baker (1839-1896). **Int J Dermatol** 1980 Sep;19(7):409-12
MacKenna RM: Robert M. B. MacKenna. **J Am Acad Dermatol** 1982 Jan;6(1):135-44
McQueen A: John Alexander Milne. **J Cutan Pathol** 1977 Dec;4(6):349-52
Manson-Bahr PE, Willmott S: Dermatology and the Royal Society of Tropical Medicine and Hygiene. **Int J Dermatol** 1981

Jul-Aug;20(6):429-30
Rook A: William Tilbury Fox (1836-1879): his contribution to tropical dermatology. **Int J Dermatol** 1981 Mar;20(2):140-2
Sharma OP: Robert Willan remembered. **J Am Acad Dermatol** 1983 Dec;9(6):971-6
White IR, MacDonald DM: Thomas Addison, M.D. First dermatologist at Guy's Hospital. **J Am Acad Dermatol** 1982 Mar;6(3):426-30

**Hungary**

Holubar K, Frankl J: Moriz (Kohn) Kaposi. **Am J Dermatopathol** 1981 Winter;3(4):349-54

**Japan**

Fukuyama K, Yasuda T: Outstanding contributions by Japanese dermatologists. **J Am Acad Dermatol** 1982 Feb;6(2):173-8

**Netherlands**

Nasemann T: Der Morphologe Hermann Werner Siemens und seine Bemühungen um eine 'Allgemeine Dermatologie'. **Hautarzt** 1983 Nov;34(11):569-73

**Norway**

Epstein WL: 'Multiple benign sarkoid of the skin' by Boeck, December 1899. Commentary: What begot Boeck? **Arch Dermatol** 1982 Oct;118(10):711-22
Fyrand O: The history of Norwegian dermato-venereology during the last two centuries. **Int J Dermatol** 1983 Dec;22(10):593-7

**Poland**

Skrobacki A, Völker A: Lekarz olsztyński, Joachim Kornalewskiijego rozprawa o koltunie z 1897 roku. **Komun Mazursko Warm** 1980;(2):155-67

**Romania**

Costea V: Cîteva date din activitatea primilor trei profesori titulari ai clinicii dermato-venerologice: Gh. Demetriade, E. I. Mironescu şi Gh. Nastase (1901-1962). **Rev Med Chir Soc Med Nat Iasi** 1983 Jan-Mar;87(1):149-55
Dobrescu AL: Dermato-venerologia ieşeană in ultimii 20 de ani (1962-1982). **Rev Med Chir Soc Med Nat Iasi** 1983 Jan-Mar;87(1):156-66
Munteanu M: Inflinţaree clinicii dermato-venerologice din Iaşi şi activitatea desfăşurată în perioada suplinirilor (1882-1901). **Rev Med Chir Soc Med Nat Iasi** 1983 Jan-Mar;87(1):141-8

**South Africa**

Findlay GH: Alphonse Loewenthal (1903-1983)--the uncrowned king of dermatology in Africa. **S Afr Med J** 1983 Dec 24;64(27):1064-7

**Spain**

Jaqueti G: Profesor José Gay Prieto. Maestro de dermatólogos (1905-1979). **Actas Dermosifiliogr** 1981 Jul-Aug;72(7-8):389-96

**Switzerland**

Storck H: De genio loci dermatologiae Turicensis. **Hautarzt** 1980 Sep;31(9):505-9
Sulzberger MB: Three lessons learned in Bloch's clinic. **Am J Dermatopathol** 1980 Winter;2(4):321-5

**United States**

Arndt KA: Archives of Dermatology. Second century. **Arch Dermatol** 1984 Jan;120(1):42-3
Arnold HL: Udo Julius Wile, A.B., M.D., LL.D. (1882-1965). **J Am Acad Dermatol** 1984 Jan;10(1):157-62
Baer RL, Kopf AW: Marion B. Sulzberger (1895-1983). **J Am Acad Dermatol** 1984 Jun;10(6):91A-96A
Bauriedel K: Early continuing medical education in dermatology. **Int J Dermatol** 1981 Nov;20(9):614-5
Beatty WK: James Nevins Hyde: pioneer dermatologist and staunch Navy man. **Proc Inst Med Chic** 1982 Oct-Dec;35(4):139-42
Beerman H: Frederick Deforest Weidman, M.D. **J Am Acad Dermatol** 1983 Sep;9(3):479-86
Beerman H: John Hinchman Stokes, M.D. An appreciation. **J Am Acad Dermatol** 1983 Aug;9(2):321-34
Beerman H: My half century in dermatopathology (1928-1978). **Am J Dermatopathol** 1979 Fall;1(3):237-43
Burnett JW: Reflections of a dermatology professor. **Cutis** 1984 May;33(5):471-4
Callaway JL: Saga of a North Carolina dermatologist. An autobiographical experience. **J Am Acad Dermatol** 1980 Nov;3(5):544-50
Cohen SG: In memoriam. Marion B. Sulzberger (1895-1983). A dermatologist's contributions to allergy. **J Allergy Clin Immunol** 1984 Dec;74(6):855-60
Crissey JT: William Allen Pusey. **J Am Acad Dermatol** 1984 Oct;11(4 Pt 1):702-8
Curriculum vitae: Thomas Bernard Fitzpatrick. **J Invest Dermatol** 1983 Jun;80 Suppl:6s-11s
The cutaneous punch by Edward L. Keyes (J Cutan Genitourin Dis, March 1887): **Arch Dermatol** 1982 Nov;118(11):940-2
Freeman RG: History of the American Society of Dermatopathology. **Am J Dermatopathol** 1984 Feb;6(1):25-33
Gibbs RC: Portrait of a dermatologist as an artist. **Am J Dermatopathol** 1984 Feb;6(1):73-9
Gifford GE: Magdeleine of Martinique. **Int J Dermatol** 1980 Mar;19(2):107-10
Hollander A: Udo Julius Wile. **J Am Acad Dermatol** 1984 Jun;10(6):1071-2
Kenney JA: The Department of Dermatology of the Howard University College of Medicine. **Cutis** 1983 Oct;32(4):336, 341
Livingood CS: History of the American Board of Dermatology, Inc. (1932-1982). **J Am Acad Dermatol** 1982 Dec;7(6):821-50
Lund HZ: It was a long way to dermatopathology. **J Cutan Pathol** 1984 Apr;11(2):81-7
Parish LC: Amerikanische dermatologische Zeitschriften und die New Yorker Dermatologische Gesellschaft. **Hautarzt** 1981 Mar;32(3):136-8
Parish LC, Crissey JT: Bibliography of secondary sources on the history of dermatology: II. obituaries and biographies in English journals supplemented through 1980. **Int J Dermatol** 1981 Sep;20(7U):497-503
Parrish JA: Festschrift: Thomas B. Fitzpatrick--a powerful difference. **J Invest Dermatol** 1983 Jun;80 Suppl:3s-5s
Pascher F: George Miller MacKee (1878-1955): a memoir. **J Am Acad Dermatol** 1983 Jul;9(1):168-72
Pearson RW: The Archives of Dermatology: the first hundred years. **Arch Dermatol** 1982 Oct;118(10):699-709
Perry HO: Department of Dermatology, Mayo Clinic. **Cutis** 1984 Sep;34(3):237-8
Perry HO, Powell FC, Cooper AJ: Paul A. O'Leary--dermatologist and teacher. **J Am Acad Dermatol** 1982 Nov;7(5):705-8
Resnik SS: The making of dermatologic surgeons. The first decade of the American Society for Dermatologic Surgery. **J Dermatol Surg Oncol** 1980 Dec;6(12):993-5
Rife DC, et al: Dr. Harold Cummins and dermatoglyphics. **Birth Defects** 1979;15(6):1-797, passim
Shelley WB, Beerman H: Jay Frank Schamberg (1870-1934). **Am J Dermatopathol** 1984 Oct;6(5):441-4
Smith EB, Head ES, Raimer SS: Dermatology on Galveston Island at the turn of the century. **Int J Dermatol** 1981 Jul-Aug;20(6):449-54
Sulzberger! Biography, autobiography, iconography. A posthumous festschrift: **Am J Dermatopathol** 1984 Aug;6(4):344-70
Weiner AL: The Noah Worcester Dermatological Society. **Int J Dermatol** 1980 Jun;19(5):288-90
Zivković K: Sečanje na prof. Dr. Luisa A. Djuringa (23. XII 1854 - 8. V 1913). **Srp Arh Celok Lek** 1982 Apr;110(4):523-4

**USSR**

Buranchiev AB, Sizov IE: K 40-letiiu kafedry kozhnykh i venericheskikh bolezneĭ Kirgizskogo meditsinskogo instituta. **Vestn Dermatol Venerol** 1980 Nov;(11):27-9
Glukhen'kiĭ TT: Petr Vasil'evich Nikol'skiĭ (k 125-letiiu so dnia rozhdeniia). **Vestn Dermatol Venerol** 1984 Jan;(1):69-70
Gus'kov EN, Mustaev RK: Dostizheniia dermato-venerologicheskoĭ sluzhby v Mordovskiĭ ASSR za 50 let. **Vestn Dermatol Venerol** 1980;(5):35-6
Mashkilleysson NA: Four generations of dermatologists. **Int J Dermatol** 1983 Nov;22(9):546-7
Mirakhmedov UM: K 60-letiiu kafedry kozhnykh i venericheskikh bolezneĭ Tashkentskogo meditsinskogo instituta. **Vestn Dermatol Venerol** 1981 Nov;(11):74-6
Ovchinnikov NM, Timchenko GF: Dvadtsatiletniĭ opyt raboty Tsentral'nogo nauchno-issledovatel'skogo kozhnovenerologicheskogo instituta Minzdrava SSR po kontroliu i uluchsheniiu kachestva serologicheskikh laboratorii dermatovenerologicheskikh uchrezhdeniĭ SSSR. **Lab Delo** 1981;(2):120-2
Skripkin IuK, Turanov NM, Mordovtsev VN, et al: Tsentral'nomu nauchno-issledovatel'skomu kozhno-venerologicheskomu institut--60 let. **Vestn Dermatol Venerol** 1981 Dec;(12):4-10
Sosnovskiĭ AT, Eremenko SA, Korsun VF: K 60-letiiu kafedry kozhnykh i venericheskikh bolezneĭ Minskogo meditsinskogo instituta. **Vestn Dermatol Venerol** 1984 Jan;(1):66-9
Stoianov BG, Selisskiĭ GD: Sostoianie dermatologicheskoĭ pomoshchi v gorodakh dorevoliutsionnoĭ Rossii. **Vestn Dermatol Venerol** 1981 May;(5):22-5

**Venezuela**

Briceño-Maaz T: Dos nombres en la dermatologia venezolana.

**Rev Soc Venez Hist Med** 1972–73;20–21(34–35):87–98
Mazzei Uzcátegui M: Cesar Lizardo, bondad y corazon. **Rev Soc Venez Hist Med** 1972–73;20–21(34–35):111–27

# DIAGNOSIS

Beyer C: Temperaturmessung. **Pharm Unserer Zeit** 1983 Jul;12(4):97–110
Blum L, Slater S, Reuben D, et al: A consideration of current clinical thermometry. **Bull NY Acad Med** 1982 Oct;58(7)621–7
Drummer F: Uroskopi–föregångare till vår tids laboratorieundersökningar. **Nord Med** 1981 Dec;96(12):325
Degeorges M: De l'auscultation médiate à l'auscultation intra–cardiaque. Les avatars de la découverte de Laennec. **Rev Palais Decouv** 1981;10(92):17–8
Duffy JM: Stephanus the philosopher: lectures on the Prognosticon of Hippocrates. Critical text and translation. Ph. D. Diss., State University of New York, Buffalo, 1975. xxi, 449 p.
Eich W, Seidler E: Historische Modelle der Prognostik in der Heilkunde. **Internist (Berlin)** 1981 Mar;22(3):118–23
Feldmann H: Development of diagnostic hearing tests. **Audiology** 1983;22(4):393–403
Franciosi RA: Evolution of SIDS diagnosis. **Minn Med** 1983 Jul;66(7):411–3
Habrich C, Marguth F, Wolf JH, et al: Medizinische Diagnostik in Geschichte und Gegenwart. Festschrift für Heinz Goerke zum sechzigsten Geburtstag. München, Fritsch, 1978. 656 p. Historical contributions by J. Antall, G. Baader, V. Bazala, L. Belloni, G. Bratescu, W. Brendel, L. Burilkova, C. J. Clemedson, K. Goldammer, H. Henne, S. Hofmann, G. Keil, K. P. Killian, W. Klinner, W. Kloppe, M. Knedel, W. Kock, F. Köcher, H. M. Koelbing, K. S. Kolta, E. Kreuzer, V. Krizek, O. Larsen, B. I. Lindskog, N. Mani, V. Møller–Christensen, Y. Otsuka, G. Preiser, L. Premuda, E. Püschel, H. Röhrich, E. Rosner, G. Rudolph, J. Sájner, H. Schadewaldt, H. Schipperges, H. H. Simmer, J. Spielmann, M. Stürzbecher, A. Terzioglu, R. Winau, N. Plovdiv. (Neue Münchner Beiträge zur Geschichte der Medizin und Naturwissenschaften, Medizinhistorische Reihe, Band 7/8).
Kampmeier RH: Medicine as an art: the history and physical examination. **South Med J** 1982 Feb;75(2):203–10
Laín Entralgo P: Los orígenes del diagnóstico medico. **Dynamis** 1981;1:3–15
Llewelyn DE, Anderson J: The historical development of the concepts of diagnosis and prognosis and their relationship to probabilistic inference. **Med Inf (Lond)** 1980 Oct–Dec;5(4):267–80
Ness DE: C'est fini. . . .le pouls ne bat plus! Drawn by Paul Bernay, for Le Charivari, in 1872. **J Hist Med Allied Sci** 1980 Jul;35(3):312
Reinstein H: Laboratory medicine––then and now. **Am J Med Technol** 1982 Jun;48(6):427–9
Roth N: Life–and–death decisions: electrodiagnosis and premature burial. **Med Instrum** 1980 Nov–Dec;14(6):322
Segal A: Les progrès de l'exploration visuelle des organes aux XVIIe et XVIIIe siècles. **Hist Sci Med** 1979;13(4):395–406

**China**

Dakpa N: La Sphygnologie tibétaine. In Mazars G, ed: Les médecines traditionnelles de l'Asie. Strasbourg, Université Louis Pasteur, 1981. p. 23–9.
Meyer F: Le système canalaire et la sphygmologie en médecine tibétaine d'après le rgyud–bži et son commentaire le Vaidurya snon–po (1). In Mazars G, ed: Les médecines traditionnelles de l'Asie. Strasbourg, Université Louis Pasteur, 1981. p. 30–40.
Veith I: The history of medicine dolls and foot–binding in China. **Clio Med** 1980 Jul;14(3–4):255–67
Yang D: [10 kinds of symptom and sign of the pharynx and throat in ancient Chinese historical materials] (Chi). **Chung Hua I Shih Tsa Chih** 1984 Jan;14(1):4–6

**Iceland**

Steffensen J: Islandske medicinhistoriske kilder, der ikke har påviselige forbilleder i samtidens Europa. **Nord Medicinhist Arsb** 1980;Suppl 6:94–105

**Vietnam**

Nguyen–Tran–Huan: La sphygmologie dans la médecine vietnamienne traditionnelle. Contribution à l'étude du traité 'Bin hú mài xué' de Lĭ Shí Zhen. In Mazars G, ed: Les médecines traditionnelles de l'Asie. Strasbourg, Université Louis Pasteur, 1981. p. 13–22.

**Before 500 A.D.**

Cockburn A, Cockburn E: Autopsies in mummies. **N Engl J Med** 1981 Dec 17;305(25):1534
Kuttner RE: Protohistoric hepatomancy: an oracular form of pathology. **Proc Inst Med Chic** 1982 Jan–Mar;35(1):14



**Greco–Roman**

Nutton V, ed: Galen On prognosis. Berlin, Akademie–Verlag, 1979. 262 p. (Corpus Medicorum Graecorum, vol. 5, pt. 8, fasc. 1).
Oberhelman SM: Galen, On Diagnosis from Dreams. **J Hist Med Allied Sci** 1983 Jan;38(1):36–47

**Rome**

García Ballester L: Experiencia y especulación en el diagnóstico galénico. **Dynamis** 1981;1:203–23

**500 A.D.–1450**

Knoedler F: De egestionibus. Texte und Untersuchungen zur spätmittelalterlichen Koproskopie. Diss., Würzburg. Pattensen/Han, Horst Wellm Verlag, 1979. 107 p. (Würzburger medizinhistorische Forschungen, Band 18).
Lenhardt F: Zur Ikonographie der Blutschau. **Medizinhist J** 1982;17(1/2):63–77
Weisser C: Das Krankheitslunar aus medizinhistorischer Sicht. Ein Beitrag zur iatromathematisch–astrologischen Fachliteratur des Mittelalters. **Sudhoffs Arch** 1981;65(4):390–400

**Arabic**

Harmarneh SK: Ibn al–Ayn Zarbi and his definitions of diseases and their diagnoses. In: International Symposium for the History of Arabic Science, 1st, University of Aleppo, 1976. Proceedings. Aleppo, Syria, 1976. Papers in European Languages, Vol. II. p. 305–23.
Petrov BD: Diagnostika v sisteme meditsinskikh vzgliadov Ibn Siny. **Klin Med (Mosk)** 1979 Dec;57(12):91–6
Tayab M: Clinical observations of Rāzi. **Stud Hist Med** 1982 Jun;6(2):79–121

**India**

Rai NP, Tiwari SK, Upadhya SD, et al: The origin and development of pulse examination in Medieval India. **Indian J Hist Sci** 1981, reçu 1982;16(1):77–88

**1450–1700**

**Belgium**

Cockx–Indestege E: Cornelis Schuute en de onlangs ontdekte almanak voor 1551. Biekorf, Westvlaams Archief, 1981. 12 p.

**Great Britain**

Fleissner RF: Putting Falstaff to rest: 'tabulating' the facts. **Shakespeare Stud** 1983;16:57–74

**1700 to Present**

Berk RN: Gallstones: diagnostic imaging in historical perspective. **Pharos** 1983 Winter;46(1):30–4
Birtalan G: Laennec and Skoda, classics of internal diagnostics. **Orvostort Kozl** 1982;28(1–3):33–41
Bishop PJ: Evolution of the stethoscope. **J R Soc Med** 1980 Jun;73(6):448–56
Bishop PJ: Reception of the stethoscope and Laënnec's book. **Thorax** 1981 Jul;36(7):487–92
Buttermann G: Lungenszintigraphie. Entwicklung, gegenwärtiger Stand und Zukunftsperspektiven. **Fortschr Med** 1983 Mar 17;101(10):403–8
Buus S, Florentine M, Redden RB: The SISI test: a review. Part I. **Audiology** 1982;21(4):273–93
Carmichael E: Dr. Papanicolaou and the Pap smear. **Ala J Med Sci** 1984 Jan;21(1):101–4
Chrościcki A: Osłuchiwanie serca––od stetoskopu do ultradźwi eków. **Pediatr Pol** 1979 Oct;54(10):1095–100
Clark G, White E, White D, et al: Bibliography of biomedical ultrasound from 1 January 1971, No. 20. **Ultrasound Med Biol** 1980;6(1):63–85
Clark WD, Quinn FB: Erroneous reporting of errors. **JAMA** 1984 Jul 13;252(2):207–8
Comiti VP: Histoire des maladies et diagnostic médical historique. **Gaz Med Fr** 1981 Jun 5;88(21):3087–90
Cormack AM: Early two–dimensional reconstruction and recent topics stemming from it. **Science** 1980 Sep 26;209(4464):1482–6
Cormack AM: Recollections of my work with computer assisted tomography. **Mol Cell Biochem** 1980 Sep 15;32(2):59–61
Cunha BA: Typhoid fever, the typhus–like disease: historical perspective. **NY State J Med** 1982 Mar;82(3):321–4
Darius J: Radiography of the living brain. **Nature** 1984 Mar 15–21;308(5956):225
Dondelinger R: La tomodensitométrie des années 80. **Bull Soc Sci Med Grand Duche Luxemb** 1980;117(2):23–7

# DIAGNOSIS

Eich W: 18th and 19th century medical semiotics; a contribution to medical theory. In International Congress of the History of Medicine, 27th, Barcelona, 1980. Actas. Barcelona, Académia de Ciències Médiques de Catalunya i Balears, 1981. p. 503-5.
Engelhardt HT: Clinical judgement. **Metamedicine** 1981;2:301-17
Freedman GS: Radionuclide tomography. **Semin Nucl Med** 1979 Jul;9(3):201-2
Goldman L: Diagnostic advances v the value of the autopsy, 1912-1980. **Arch Pathol Lab Med** 1984 Jun;108(6):501-5
Gow JG: The evolution of modern endoscopic photography. **Eur Urol** 1984;10(2):133-8
Guncheon KF: Diagnostic imaging: an inside look. **Hospitals** 1981 Jan 1;55(1):86-8, 95
Habeck JO, Habeck C: Die Auskultation der Darmgeräusche -- Geschichte und Entwicklungsmöglichkeiten. **Z Arztl Fortbild (Jena)** 1980 Jun 15;74(12):596-9
Haight V: A brief history of hemoglobinometry. **Am J Med Technol** 1983 Feb;49(2):127-8
Haller JS: The foul tongue: a 19th century index of disease. **West J Med** 1982 Sep;137(3):258-64
Hammer B: Die Geschichte der Computertomographie (anlässlich von 10 Jahren klinischer Computertomographie). **Computertomographie** 1982 Jun;2(2):59-61
Hawkins HB, Cinti DC: Magnetic resonance imaging. Where did it come from? What is it? Where is it going? Part I. History and physical principles. **Conn Med** 1984 Sep;48(9):575-7
Hör G, Munz DL: Nuklearmedizin--einst und jetzt. Folge 1: Entwicklung, Aufgabenspektrum, Radiopharmazeutika, Messtechnik, Klinische Indikationen. **Fortschr Med** 1983 Mar 17;101(10):415-22
Howell JD: Early perceptions of the electrocardiogram: from arrhythmia to infarction. **Bull Hist Med** 1984 Spring;58(1):83-98
Huard P, Niaussat P: L'évolution du stéthoscope. In: Congrès National des Sociétés Savantes, 106e, Perpignan, 1981. Comptes Rendus. Paris, Bibliothèque Nationale, 1982. Fasc. IV. p. 91-104.
Jeanmart L: Le radiodiagnostic de Roentgen à Hounsfield. **Flash Inf** 1983 May-Jun;:3-7
Jeffery T: Mass-observation. **Soc Soc Hist Med Bull** 1980;27:8-14
Johns HE: The physicist in cancer treatment and detection. **Int J Radiat Oncol Biol Phys** 1981 Jun;7(6):801-8
Kallee E: Anamnese des Radioimmunassays. Eine historische Reminiszenz. **MMW** 1984 Jan 27;126(4):97-101
Kaltreider S: Tapping the tube. **MCVQ** 1981;16(3):106-12
Kampmeier RH: The demonstration of the immobilizing antibody for treponema pallidum (TPI test). **Sex Transm Dis** 1983 Oct-Dec;10(4):205-7
Kampmeier RH: The evolution of the flocculation screening test for syphilis. **Sex Transm Dis** 1983 Jul-Sep;10(3):156-9
Lanteri Laura G: L'hystérie. Matrice de la sémiologie neurologique. In Poirier J, Poirier JL, ed: Médecine et philosophie à la fin du XIXe siècle. Paris, Université de Paris XII - Val de Marne, [1980?]. p. 141-8.
Larsen O: Eighteenth century diseases. Diagnostical trends and mortality. **Scand Popul Stud** 1979;5
Leatham A: Auscultation of the heart since Laënnec. **Thorax** 1981 Feb;36(2):95-8
Loudon I: The consultation. **Br Med J [Clin Res]** 1983 Dec 24-31;287(6409):1970-1
McIntosh K: Sense and nonsense in viral diagnosis--past, present, and future. **Curr Top Microbiol Immunol** 1983;104:1-6
May LA, ed: Classic descriptions of physical signs in medicine. Oceanside, N.Y., Dabor Science Publications, 1977. ix, 273 p.
Murphy RL: Auscultation of the lung: past lessons, future possibilities. **Thorax** 1981 Feb;36(2):99-107
Nice CM: Medical images: past, present, and future. **CRC Crit Rev Diagn Imaging** 1980;14(1):73-109
Nicholson P: Problems encountered by early endoscopists. **Urology** 1982 Jan;19(1):114-9
Pilarska-Machowicz A: Rozwój diagnostyki bronchoskopowej. **Wiad Lek** 1982 Nov 1;35(19-20):1265-70
Pilarska-Machowik A: Rozwój diagnostyki bronchoskopowej. **Pieleg Polozna** 1983;(5):16-7
Power KT: The Romanowsky stains: a review. **Am J Med Technol** 1982 Jun;48(6):519-23
Radner S: Den selektiva angiografins bakgrund och begynnelse. **Sydsven Medicinhist Sallsk Arsskr** 1982;19:109-18
Ram PC, Fordham EW: An historical survey of bone scanning. **Semin Nucl Med** 1979 Jul;9(3):190-6
Rubin LP: A young woman taken to the doctor by her family. Mezzotint by Johann Andreas Pfeffel after an original painting by Jan Josef Horemans. **J Hist Med Allied Sci** 1981 Oct;36(4):489
Schwan HP: Ultrasound and electromagnetic radiation in hyperthermia--a historical perspective. **Br J Cancer** 1982 Mar;45(5)Suppl:84-92
Smith DC: The rise and fall of typhomalarial fever: II. decline and fall. **J Hist Med Allied Sci** 1982 Jul;37(3):287-321
Steiner W: Fortschritte in der endoskopischen Larynxdiagnostik. **Ther Umsch** 1980 Dec;37(12):1021-8
Szymanski B, Hieke M: Zur Geschichte der Dentitionsforschung unter dem Gesichtspunkt der Entwicklungsdiagnostik. **Aerztl Jugendkd** 1981;72(5):304-26
Taplin GV: The history of lung imaging with radionuclides. **Semin Nucl Med** 1979 Jul;9(3):178-85

### Austria

Hurst LC: What was wrong with Anna O? **J R Soc Med** 1982 Feb;75(2):129-31
Landsberger M: Percussion discovered. **Trans Stud Coll Physicians Phila** 1981 Dec;5(3 no 4):255
Sakula A: Joseph Skoda 1805-81: a centenary tribute to a pioneer of thoracic medicine. **Thorax** 1981 Jun;36(6):404-11

### Belgium

Burke J, Mortelmans J: Rol van België in de strijd tegen de slaapziekte en de dierlijke trypanosomiases en hun studie. **Bull Seances Acad R Sci Outre Mer** 1980 Suppl.;1:111-35

### France

Bastholm E: Laennec og stetoskopet. **Dan Medicinhist Arbog** 1982;:112-35
Bishop PJ: Laennec: a great student of tuberculosis. **Tubercle** 1981 Jun;62(2):129-34
Finot A: Les premiers élèves et collaborateurs (surtout Bretons) de Laennec. In: Congrès National des Sociétés Savantes, 91e, Rennes, 1966. Comptes Rendus. Paris, 1967. Section des Sciences, Tome 1. p. 181-9.
Fox ER: Mrs. Laennec and the stethoscope. **West J Med** 1981 Jan;134(1):73-4
Hanngren A: René Théophile Hyacinthe Laennec (1781-1826). **Nord Medicinhist Arsb** 1981;:106-19
Huard P: II y a cent ans Constantin Paul présentait à l'Académie de Médecine son stéthoscope autostatique bi-auriculaire. **Bull Acad Natl Med (Paris)** 1981 Nov;165(8):1117-21
Huard P, Niaussat PM: L'évolution du stéthoscope de Laennec à nos jours; son influence dans certains domaines des transmissions acoustiques. **Hist Sci Med** 1981;15(2):173-87
Kerbrat G: Laennec et ses combats (1781-1826). In: Congrès National des Sociétés Savantes, 107e. Brest, 1982. Comptes Rendus, Paris, 1983. Section des Sciences, Fasc. IV. p. 287-98.
Kligfield P: Laennec and the discovery of mediate auscultation. **Am J Med** 1981 Feb;70(2):275-8
Meindl JL, Meindl CO: Tuberculous meningitis in the 1830s. **Lancet** 1982 Mar 6;1(8271):554-5
Obermajer J: Endoskopie jako výtvarný motiv. **Cesk Gastroenterol Vyz** 1980 Jan;34(1):51-4
Sakula A: Acceuil du livre 'De l'auscultation médiate' et du stéthoscope par les médecins de Grande-Bretagne. **Rev Palais Decouv** 1981 Aug;22:280-90
Sakula A: In search of Laënnec. **J R Coll Physicians Lond** 1981 Jan;15(1):55-7
Sakula A: Pierre Adolphe Piorry (1794-1879): pioneer of percussion and pleximetry. **Thorax** 1979 Oct;34(5):575-81
Sakula A: R.T.H. Laënnec 1781-1826, his life and work: a bicentenary appreciation. **Thorax** 1981 Feb;36(2):81-90
Sakula A: The story of the stethoscope. **Trans Med Soc Lond** 1981-82;98:27-31
Somolinos-Palencia J: René Teófilo Jacinto Laennec, a los 200 años de su nacimiento. **Gac Med Mex** 1981 Mar;117(3):122-6
Sternbach G: Joseph Babinski: the phenomenon of the toes. **J Emerg Med** 1984;1(3):263-6
Stofft H: Kergaradec à l'écoute du foetus. **J Gynecol Obstet Biol Reprod (Paris)** 1981;10(6):611-22
Trautmann M, Trautmann JC: R. T. H. Laennec 1781-1826. Zum 200. Geburtstag des Autors der Auscultation médiate. **MMW** 1981 Nov 6;123(45):1717-20
Turiaf J: Laennec et la pathologie respiratoire. **Bull Acad Natl Med (Paris)** 1981 Feb 17;Spec No:31-6
Vita a Laennec megemlékezés körül: **Orv Hetil** 1981 Dec 13;122(50):3115-6

### Germany

Cranach M von: Die Münchner Klinik und die psychiatrische Diagnostik. **MMW** 1981 May 8;123(19):777-80
Dahm S: Frühe Krankenbildnisse: Alibert Esquirol Baumgartner. Köln, 1981. (Kölner medizinhistorische Beiträge; Arbeiten der Forschungsstelle des Instituts für Geschichte der Medizin der Universität zu Köln, Band 21).
Egger E: Die Standardisierungskonzeption diagnostischer Laboratoriumsmethoden in der DDR. **Z Med Lab Diagn** 1983;24(7):401-7
Mohr HJ: Medizinische und legislatorische Probleme der inneren Leichenschau. **Pathologe** 1981 Jun;2(3):134-43
Scheuch DW, Hoffmann H: 20 Jahre Gesellschaft für Klinische Chemie und Laboratoriumsdiagnostik der DDR. **Z Med Lab Diagn** 1983;24(7):371-80

**Great Britain**

Colp R: Dr. Erasmus Darwin consults with another physician. **Radic Hist Rev** 1979 Spring/Summer;Spec:66–71
Hounsfield GN: Computed medical imaging. **Med Phys** 1980 Jul–Aug;7(4):283–90
John Mitchell Bruce (1846–1929): **Practitioner** 1982 Apr;226(1366):800
Mayberry JF: The history of a hospital and its diagnostic index. **Public Health** 1979 Sep;93(5):311–6
Mourant AE: The discovery of the anti-globulin test. **Vox Sang** 1983;45(2):180–3
Pinkerton JH: John Creery Ferguson. Friend of William Stokes and pioneer of auscultation of the fetal heart in the British Isles. **Br J Obstet Gynaecol** 1980 Apr;87(4):257–60
Sakula A: Laennec's influence on some British physicians in the nineteenth century. **J R Soc Med** 1981 Oct;74(10):759–67

**Hungary**

Kenéz J: A fizikális mellkasvizsgálat és hazai úttörői. **Orv Hetil** 1982 Oct 3;123(40):2483–7

**Ireland**

Pinkerton JH: John Creery Ferguson 1802–1865: Physician and fetologist. **Ulster Med J** 1981;50(1):10–20

**Italy**

Grassi C: Influence de l'oeuvre de Laénnec sur la médecine italienne. **Rev Fr Mal Respir** 1981;9(5):421–6

**Netherlands**

Falke TH, Ziedses des Plantes BG, Voorthuisen AE van: The Netherlands' initial experience with NMR imaging. **Diagn Imaging** 1984;53(1):43–52
Moulin D de: Microscopie en kankerdiagnostiek in de eerste helft van de negentiende eeuw. **Tijdschr Geschied Geneeskd** 1983;6(2):99–107

**Poland**

Malarewicz A: 50 lat cytodiagnostyki ginekologicznej -- George Nicholas Papanicolaou. **Arch Hist Med (Warsz)** 1978;41(4):465–8
Meissner R: Swiatowy priorytet Karola Mayera w dziedzinie radiodiagnostyki--przyczynek do dziejów tomografii. **Kwart Hist Nauki Tech** 1982;27(1):125–37
Stembrowicz W: Tłumaczenie z jezyka łacińskiego pracy na stopień doktora medycyny z 1829 roku Józefa Lewickiego o osłuchiwaniu i opukiwaniu. **Arch Hist Med (Warsz)** 1984;47(1):49–74
Wagner D: August Ferdynand Wolff und die Bedeutung der Semiotik. **Arch Hist Med (Warsz)** 1979;42(2):263–8

**Portugal**

Veiga-Pires JA, Grainger RG: Pioneers in angiography: The Portuguese School of Angiography. Lancaster, Boston, MTP Press, 1982. 131 p.

**Singapore**

Khoo FY, Chow KW: The development of diagnostic radiology in Singapore. **Ann Acad Med Singapore** 1982 Jul;11(3):444–6

**Spain**

García Guerra D: La 'Disertacion medica' de Fernando Oxea. Un testimonio de auscultacion inmediata del torax en el siglo XVIII. **Asclepio** 1980;32:201–9

**Sweden**

Doby T: A tribute to Sven-Ivar Seldinger. **AJR** 1984 Jan;142(1):1–4

**Switzerland**

Nica-Udangiu S: Hermann Rorschach (1884–1922). **Rev Med Interna [Neurol Psihiatr]** 1984 Jul–Sep;29(3):235–40

**United States**

Blake TM: Myocardial infarction and electrocardiography in historical perspective. **South Med J** 1983 Dec;76(12):1470–2
Charap MH: The periodic health examination: genesis of a myth. **Ann Intern Med** 1981 Dec;95(6):733–5
Cormack AM: Early two-dimensional reconstruction and recent topics stemming from it. **Med Phys** 1980 Jul–Aug;7(4):277–82
Davis AB: Life insurance and the physical examination: a chapter in the rise of American medical technology. **Bull Hist Med** 1981;55(3):392–406
Holmes JH: Diagnostic ultrasound during the early years of A.I.U.M. **JCU** 1980 Aug;8(4):299–308
Jacobson HG, Stern WZ: Landmark perspective: The Graham–Cole 'test' revisited. The oral cholecystogram today. **JAMA** 1983 Dec 2;250(21):2977–82
Kaplan B: 'Peopleware' and medical informatics. **JAMA** 1983 Feb 4;249(5):574–6
Murphy BE, Grigg ER: Radioassays. **Semin Nucl Med** 1979 Jul;9(3):169–72
Rife DC, et al: Dr. Harold Cummins and dermatoglyphics. **Birth Defects** 1979;15(6):1–797, passim
Roberts WC, Silver MA: Norman Jefferis Holter and ambulatory ECG monitoring. **Am J Cardiol** 1983 Oct 1;52(7):903–6
Rytand DA: Sutton's or Dock's law? **N Engl J Med** 1980 Apr 24;302(17):972
Smith DC: The rise and fall of typhomalarial fever: I. origins. **J Hist Med Allied Sci** 1982 Apr;37(2):182–220
Wilson JG: The evolution of teratological testing. **Teratology** 1979 Oct;20(2):205–11

**USSR**

Agamova KA: Razvitie tsitologicheskoĭ diagnostiki opukholĭ cheloveka. **Sov Med** 1982;(6):65–9
Cherkasov SV: Leninskoe uchenie ob istine i problema kriteriia praktiki v diagnostike. **Klin Khir** 1980 Jun;(6):1–6
Cherkasov SV: Leninskoe uchenie ob istine i probleme kriterii praktiki v diagnostike. **Ter Arkh** 1980;52(7):146–40
Kunitsa LK, Mel'nik AN, Loboda VI: K istorii razvittia metoda tsitologicheskoĭ diagnostiki. **Vrach Delo** 1981 Jul;(7):123–5
Kuz'min MK: V. F. Zelenin i ego rol' v razvitii klinicheskoĭ élektrokardiografii i funktsional'noĭ diagnostike. **Klin Med (Mosk)** 1981 Aug;59(8):115–8
Morozova VT: Istoriia kafedry laboratornoĭ klinicheskoĭ diagnostiki Tsentral'nogo instituta usovershenstvovaniia vracheĭ. **Lab Delo** 1981;(6):375–8
Sheĭman' IB, Petrovskaia EG, Pomianskaia NIu, et al: Stanovlenie tsitologicheskoĭ diagnostiki vo L'vovskoĭ oblasti. **Lab Delo** 1984;(1):52–4
Smolenskiĭ VS, Tarasov KE: Znachenie leninskogo ucheniia o dialekticheskoĭ vzaimosviazi ob'ektivnogo i sub'ektivnogo v oschchushcheniiakh dlia diagnostiki. **Klin Med (Mosk)** 1980 Sep;58(9):3–6

# DISEASES AND INJURIES

See also **Communicable Disease Control; Epidemiology; Pathology**

Ackerknecht EH: Diathesis: the word and the concept in medical history. **Bull Hist Med** 1982 Fall;56(3):317–25
Aker F, Cecil JC: The influence of disease upon European history. **Milit Med** 1983 May;148(5):441–6
Beeson PB: Some diseases that have disappeared. **Am J Med** 1980 Jun;68(6):806–11
Bloch H: Man's reasoning about diseases. Time and place. **NY State J Med** 1980 Nov;80(12):1888–91
Boncompagni R: Problemi relativi all'interpretazione e alla composizione del Regime delle malattie acute (Acut.). In La collection hippocratique et son rôle dans l'histoire de la médecine. Colloque de Strasbourg (23–27 octobre 1972) organisé par le Centre de Recherches sur la Grèce Antique, avec le concours des Facultés de Philosophie et des Langues Classiques. Leiden, E. J. Brill, 1975. p. 195–207.
Charbonneau H, Larose A, ed: The great mortalities: methodological studies of demographic crises in the past. Liège, Belgium, Ordina Editions, [1980]. 373 p. Includes contributions by A. Appleby, S. Sogner, J. N. Biraben. Text in English or French.
Comiti VP: Les maladies d'autrefois. **Recherche** 1980 Oct;115:1044–51
Dube CB, Kansal CM: Diseases due to deficiencies of vital principles in the body. **Indian J Hist Sci** 1981;16(1):104–7
Engelhardt HT: Philosophical perspectives [of health and disease]. In Reich WT, et al, ed: Encyclopedia of bioethics, v. 2. New York, Free Press, 1978. p. 599–605.
Felts JH: On epidemics, metaphors and madness. **NC Med J** 1980 Apr;41(4):221–3
Grmek MD: Le concept d'infection dans l'Antiquité et au Moyen Age, les anciennes mesures sociales contre les maladies contagieuses et la fondation de la première quarantaine à Dubrovnik (1377). In Radovi sa Medunarodnog simpozija u povodu sestote obljetnice Dubrovacke karantene. Dubrovnik, 29 i 30. rujna 1977. Zagreb, 1980. p. 9–54.
Hartmann F: Homo patiens. Zur ärztlichen Anthropologie von Leid und Mitleid. In Seidler E, Schott H, ed: Bausteine zur Medizingeschichte. Stuttgart, Steiner, 1984. p. 35–44.
Histoire culturelle de la maladie: Toulouse, Privat, 1980. xvi. 454 p. Contributions by M. Sendrail, G. Baudot, G. Mazars, P. Huard, J. Bossy, P. Theil, P. Hillemand, E. Gilbrin, E. Aron, P. Freour.
Horstmanhoff HF, ed: [Ancient and medieval pestilences]. Includes contributions by R. A. Tybout, M. van Raalte, S. van der Lee, C. G. van Leijenhorst, E. J. Bakker, E. J. Schoten. **Hermeneus Tijdschr Antieke Cult** 1979;51(2):58–157
Hudson RP: Disease and its control. The shaping of modern thought.

Westport, London, Greenwood Press, 1983. xvii, 259 p. (Contributions in Medical History, no. 12).
Jones AH: A commentary on 'Two pathographies: a study in illness and literature'. **J Med Philos** 1984 Aug;9(3):257-9
Kemper R: Zur Syphillis-Erkrankung des Conrad Celtis zum 'Vaticinium' Ulsens und zum sogenannten 'Pestbild' Dürers. **Arch Kulturgesch** 1977;59:99-118
Kilburn KH: Chronic disease in the workplace and the environment. Lung disease: lessons from the past--keys to the future. **Arch Environ Health** 1984 May-Jun;39(3):139-43
Kiple K, Kiple V: The African connection: slavery, disease and racism. **Phylon** 1980;41(3):211-22
Kupferschmidt HG: 'Exotische' Krankheiten--einst und heute. **Z Arztl Fortbild (Jena)** 1983;77(1):33-6
Risse GB: History of the concepts [of health and disease]. In Reich WT, et al, ed: Encyclopedia of bioethics, v. 2. New York, Free Press, 1978. p. 579-85.
Risse GB: La ecología de la enfermedad: tema de estudio médico-histórico. **Bol Soc Mex Hist Filos Med** 1984 Mar;7(46):289-304
Savitt TL: The social and medical history of crib death. **J Fla Med Assoc** 1979 Aug;66(8):853-9
Shelp EE: The experience of illness: integrating metaphors and the transcendence of illness. **J Med Philos** 1984 Aug;9(3):253-6
Stiker HJ: Corps infirmes et sociétés. Paris, Aubier Montaigne, 1982. 250 p.
Talbott JH: Medical maladies as seen by the artist. **JAMA** 1981 Feb 6;245(5):497-8
Temkin O: Some moral implications of the concept of disease. In Ganzinger K, Skopec M, Wyklicky H, ed: Festschrift für Erna Lesky zum 70. Geburtstag. Wien, Brüder Hollinek, 1981. p. 153-60.
Wilken H: Intrauterine und neonatale Infektionen. Geschichtlicher Rückblick. **Zentralbl Gynakol** 1983;105(16):1035-40

**Africa**

Davies JN: Pestilence and disease in the history of Africa. Johannesburg, Witwatersrand University Press, for The Institute for the Study of Man in Africa, 1979. 20 p.
Ransford O: 'Bid the sickness cease': disease in the history of black Africa. London, John Murray, 1983. x, 235 p.

**Austria**

Schwendinger K: Krankheiten und Seuchen bei Mensch und Tier. **Montfort** 1965;17(3):308-12

**Canada**

Larocque R: L'introduction de maladies européennes chez les autochtones des XVIIe et XVIIIe siècles. **Rech Amerindiennes Que Bull Inf** 1982;12(1):13-24

**China**

Li WB: [History of epidemics in ancient China] (Chi). **Chung Hua Liu Hsing Ping Hsueh Tsa Chih** 1983 Oct;4(5):316-9

**Egypt**

Jacobson H: The Egyptian plagues in the Palaea Historica. **Byzantion** 1977;47-363

**Germany**

Wilken U: Zur Geschichte von Einstellungsdeterminanten gegen über Körperbehinderten. **Rehabilitation (Stuttg)** 1984 May;23(2):81-3

**Great Britain**

Barker DJ: Geographical variations in disease in Britain. **Br Med J** 1981;283:398-400

**Peru**

Gade DW: Inca and colonial settlement, coca cultivation and endemic disease in the tropical forest. **J Hist Geogr** 1979 Jul;5:263-80

**Spain**

Marset Campos P, Chacón Jiménez F, Lemeunier G, et al: La sociedad murciana y cartagenera y las epidemias durante los siglos XVII, XVIII y XIX. In: Sociedad Española de Historia de la Medicina. V Congreso Nacional. Madrid, 1977. **Asclepio** 1977;29:177-208

**United States**

Cates GL: 'The seasoning': disease and death among the first colonists of Georgia. **Ga Hist Q** 1980;64(2):146-58
Larocque R: Les maladies chez les Iroquoiens pré-historique. **Rech Amerindiennes Que Bull Inf** 1980;10(3):165-80
Simpson HN: Invisible armies. The impact of disease on American history. Indianapolis, Bobbs-Merrill, 1980. xi, 239 p.

**Before 500 A.D.**

Di Benedetto V: De la maladie au malade particulier: changement de perspective de la médecine du Ve siècle avant Jésus-Christ. In La collection hippocratique et son rôle dans l'histoire de la médecine. Colloque de Strasbourg (23-27 octobre 1972) organisé par le Centre de Recherches sur la Grèce Antique, avec le concours des Facultés de Philosophie et des Langues Classiques. Leiden, E. J. Brill, 1975. p. 51-5.
Kaplan AS, Garfinkel PE: Bulimia in the Talmud. **Am J Psychiatry** 1984 May;141(5):721
Kokaska CJ, Woodward S, Tyler L: Disabled people in the Bible. **Rehabil Lit** 1984 Jan-Feb;45(1-2):20-1
Niederland WG: Morbid conditions expressed in prehistoric art. **Am J Psychiatry** 1981 Jan;138(1):126-7

**Egypt**

Sandison AT: Diseases in ancient Egypt. In A. Cockburn, E. Cockburn, ed: Mummies, disease, and ancient cultures. Cambridge, Cambridge University Press, 1980. p. 29-44.

**Greco-Roman**

Bourgey L: La relation du médecin au malade dans les écrits de l'Ecole de Cos. In La collection hippocratique et son rôle dans l'histoire de la médecine. Colloque de Strasbourg (23-27 octobre 1972) organisé par le Centre de Recherches sur la Grèce Antique, avec le concours des Facultés de Philosophie et des Langues Classiques. Leiden, E. J. Brill, 1975. p. 209-27.
Gourevitch D, Gourevitch M: Chronique anachronique III. Simulation. **Evol Psychiatr (Paris)** 1981;46(1):205-9
Jouanna J: Le schéma d'exposition des maladies et ses déformations dans les traités dérivés des Sentences cnidiennes. In La collection hippocratique et son rôle dans l'histoire de la médecine. Colloque de Strasbourg (23-27 octobre 1972) organisé par le Centre de Recherches sur la Grèce Antique, avec le concours des Facultés de Philosophie et des Langues Classiques. Leiden, E. J. Brill, 1975. p. 129-50.
Robert E: Les adresses de malades dans les Epidémies II, IV et VI. In La collection hippocratique et son rôle dans l'histoire de la médecine. Colloque de Strasbourg (23-27 octobre 1972) organisé par le Centre de Recherches sur la Grèce Antique, avec le concours des Facultés de Philosophie et des Langues Classiques. Leiden, E. J. Brill, 1975. p. 173-94.

**Greece**

Jouanna J: Le traité hippocratique du Régime dans les maladies aiguës: remarques sur la tradition manuscrite et sur le texte. **Rev Hist Textes (Paris)** 1976;6:1-30
Pritchet CD, ed: Iohannis Alexandrini Commentaria in sextum librum Hippocratis Epidemiarum. Leiden, Brill, 1975. xi, 470 p.

**500 A.D.-1450**

**Americas**

Björnberg A: Ansiktsmutilationer inom Mochicakonsten. **Sydsven Medicinhist Sallsk Arsskr** 1982;19:32-44

**Yugoslavia**

Dolenc A: Medizinische Fragen und Aspekte des mittelalterlichen Totentanzes (Ein Beitrag aus Jugoslawien). **Beitr Gerichtl Med** 1980;38:347-52

**1450-1700**

Appleby AB: Epidemics and famine in the little ice age 1550-1700. **J Interdiscip Hist** 1980;10:643-63

**France**

Bèttica-Giovannini R: La preghiera di Blaise Pascal per il buon uso delle malattie. **Ann Osp Maria Vittoria Torino** 1979 Jul-Dec;22(7-12):420-5

**Great Britain**

Kail AC: The bard and the body. 5. Disease: its causes, diagnosis and cure. **Med J Aust** 1983 Nov 26;2(11):568-77
Taylor FK: Sydenham's disease entities. **Psychol Med** 1982 May;12(2):243-50

**Mexico**

Berthe JP: Les epidémies au Mexique au XVIe siècle. **Asclepio** 1983;35:257-63

**Spain**

Dedieu H: Notes sur les pertes humaines subies par les communautés religieuses de Séville durant l'epidémie de 1649. **Arch Franciscanum Hist** 1978;71(3-4):462-68
Vincent B: Las epidemias en Andalucia durante el siglo XVI. In: Sociedad Española de Historia de la Medicina. V Congreso Nacional. Madrid, 1977. **Asclepio** 1977;29:351-8

**1700 to Present**

Astor G: The disease detectives. Deadly medical mysteries and the people who solved them. New York, Scarborough, Ont., NAL Books, 1983. 216 p.
Bogdan R, Biklen D, Shapiro A, et al: The disabled: media's monster. **Soc Policy** 1982;13(2):32-5
Bower EM, ed: The handicapped in literature. A psychosocial perspective. Denver, Love, 1980. xi, 407 p.
Comiti VP: Histoire des maladies et diagnostic médical historique. **Gaz Med Fr** 1981 Jun 5;88(21):3087-90
Dahm S: Frühe Krankenbildnisse: Alibert Esquirol Baumgartner. Köln, 1981. (Kölner medizinhistorische Beiträge; Arbeiten der Forschungsstelle des Instituts für Geschichte der Medizin der Universität zu Köln, Band 21).
Johns OR: Essence of peppermint, a history of the medicine and its bottle. **Hist Archaeol** 1981;15(2):1-57
Loraine JA: Future patterns of disease: maladies of development. **Contemp Rev** 1983;242(1409):298-302
Orosz L, Veress O: Lassai levél... **Orv Hetil** 1980 Nov 2;121(44):2711-5
Pomponi F: En amont de la mort: médecine et morbidité en Corse au XIXe siécle. **Etud Corses** 1979;7(12-13):251-73
Wilson LG: Fevers and science in early nineteenth century medicine. **J Hist Med Allied Sci** 1978 Jul;33(3):386-407
Ziegler CR: The image of the physically handicapped in children's literature. New York, Arno, 1980. 156 p. (Also Ed. D. Diss. Philadelphia, Temple University, 1971).

**Africa**

Brown JS: Of battle and disease: the East African Campaign of 1914-18. **Parameters** 1982;12(2):16-24
Patterson KD: Infectious diseases in twentieth-century Africa: a bibliography of their distribution and consequences. Waltham, Crossroads Press, 1979. xiii, 251 p.
Patterson KD, ed: Infectious diseases in twentieth-century Africa: a bibliography of their distribution and consequences. Waltham, Mass., Crossroads Press of African Studies Association, 1979. xiii, 251 p.
Sabben-Clare EE, Bradley DJ, Kirkwood K, ed: Health in tropical Africa during the colonial period: based on the proceedings of a symposium held at New College, Oxford, 21-23 March 1977. Oxford, Clarendon, 1980. ix, 276 p.

**Asia**

Learmonth AT: Reflections of the regional geography of disease in late colonial South Asia. **Soc Sci Med [Med Geogr]** 1980 Sep;14D(3):271-6

**Canada**

Moss JB: Pathological images in the Quebec novel. **Am Rev Can Stud** 1980;10(1):39-47
Taylor JH: Disease, fire and water in the nineteenth century city: a bibliography. **Urban Hist Rev** 1979;8(1):113-5

**Caribbean**

Reusch C: Die medizinische Versorgung auf den französischen Westindischen Inseln im 18. Jhd. im Spiegel des Werkes von J.B. Dazille 'Les Maladies des Nègres, leurs causes, leur traitement, et les moyens de les prévenir.' Diss., Universität Düsseldorf. Düsseldorf, 1982. 117 p.

**France**

Azemar R: Les causes de décès à La Roque-Sainte-Marguerite, en sud-Rouergue, de 1721 à 1742. **Ann Demogr Hist (Paris)** 1984;:239-58
Levy C: Essai d'estimation de la population handicapée en France. (Handicap sevère). **Population** 1983;38(1):178-84
Musset J: L'intervention de l'administration en matière d'épidémie au XVIIIe siècle: l'élection de Saint-Lô en 1785. **Ann Normandie** 1978 Dec;28:344-6
Rullière R: Les morts subites à la Cour de Louis XIV de 1690 à 1709, d'après Pierre Dionis. **Hist Sci Med** 1984;18(1):19-24
Weiner DB: Les handicapés et la révolution française: aspects de médecine sociale. In: Congrès international d'histoire de la médecine, XXVe, Québec, 1976. Actes. Québec, 1977. p. 333-70.
Wrotnowska D: Maladie des vers à soie: Pasteur s'intéresse à la race perpignanaise. In: Congrès National des Sociétés Savantes, 106e, Perpignan, 1981. Comptes Rendus. Paris, Bibliothèque Nationale, 1982. Fasc. IV. p. 197-208.

**Germany**

Faber-Castell, K von: Arzt, Krankheit und Tod im erzählerischen Werk Theodor Fontanes. Zürich, Juris Druck, 1983. 97 p. (Zürcher Medizingeschichtliche Abhandlungen, Neue Reihe, Nr. 157).
Schachter M: Le malade Johann Wolfgang Goethe (1749-1832) et ses maladies (A l'occasion du 150e anniversaire de sa mort). **Hist Sci Med** 1982;16(2):81-8

**Great Britain**

Cooper JE: Some aspects of John Hunter's work on the diseases of birds of prey. **Ann R Coll Surg Engl** 1982 Sep;64(5):345-7
Loudon IS: Leg ulcers in the eighteenth and early nineteenth centuries. **J R Coll Gen Pract** 1981 May;31(226):263-73
Luckin B: Death and survival in the city: approaches to the history of disease. **Urban Hist Yearb** 1980;:53-62
Qvist G: John Hunter, 1728-1793. London, Heinemann, 1981. xvi, 216 p.
Shaw AB: Paget's diseases. **Practitioner** 1980 Dec;224(1350):1323-7
Williams G, Stretton TB, Leonard JC: AIDS in 1959? **Lancet** 1983 Nov 12;2(8359):1136

**Hungary**

Ungvári G: Ujabb adatok Gulácsy Lajos betegségéhez. **Orvostort Kozl** 1982;92(4):113-8

**Mexico**

Laurell AC, et al: Enfermedad y desarrollo: análisis sociológico de la morbilidad en dos pueblos mexicanos. **Rev Mex Cienc Polit Soc** 1976;22(84):131-58

**Pacific Islands**

Crawford RJ: Missionary accounts of fofo mo'omo'o. **J Polynesian Soc** 1977;86(4):531-4
Lesson PA: Notes sur les maladies des indigènes des iles Marquises en 1844. Manuscrit inédit. **Bull Soc Etud Oceaniennes** 1981;18(216):915-43

**Poland**

Basinski J: Zachorowalność i obrazenia wojenne w Powstaniu Wielkopolskim. Czas od 27.12.1918 do 13.11.1919 roku. **Arch Hist Med (Warsz)** 1979;42(2):177-87
Skrzypek W: Przypadek wyleczenia nosacizny u człowieka w 1828 r. **Arch Hist Med (Warsz)** 1983;46(3):325-32

**South Africa**

Brain JB, Brain P: Nostalgia and alligator bite--morbidity and mortality among Indian migrants to Natal, 1884-1911. **S Afr Med J** 1984 Jan 21;65(3):98-102

**Spain**

García Guerra D: Epidemiologia gallega del siglo XVIII. Su repercusión sobre el Hospital Real de Santiago. In: Sociedad Española de Historia de la Medicina. V Congreso Nacional. Madrid, 1977. **Asclepio** 1977;29:147-65
Peset JL: Epidemias y sociedad en la España del fin del antiguo regimen. In: Sociedad Española de Historia de la Medicina. V Congreso Nacional. Madrid, 1977. **Asclepio** 1977;29:37-65
Rodríguez Galdo MX: Hambre, epidemia y crisis demográfica en la Galicia litoral a mediados del siglo XIX. **Asclepio** 1983;35:53-68
Rodríguez Galdo MX: Hambre y enfermedad en Galicia a mediados del siglo XIX. In: Sociedad Española de Historia de la Medicina. V Congreso Nacional. Madrid, 1977. **Asclepio** 1977;29:331-41

**United States**

Anderson RJ, Reed WG, Hillis LD, et al: History, epidemiology, and medical complications of nasal inhaler abuse. **J Toxicol Clin Toxicol** 1982 Mar;19(1):95-107
Curtis J, Curtis B: Illness and the Victorian lady: the case of Jeannie Sumner. **Int J Womens Stud** 1981;4(5):527-43
Ehrlich GE: Landmark perspective. Diffuse collagen disease. **JAMA** 1984 Mar 23-30;251(12):1595-6

# DISEASES AND INJURIES

Kiple KF, Kiple VH: The African connection: slavery, disease and racism. **Phylon** 1980 Fall;41(3):211–22
Klevay LM: Changing patterns of disease: some nutritional remarks. **J Am Coll Nutr** 1984;3(2):149–58
Kriegel L: The wolf in the pit in the zoo. **Soc Policy** 1982;13(2):16–23
Levin BS: Women and medicine. Metuchen, N. J., London, Scarecrow, 1980. vii, 257 p.
Montella M: La malattia del Legionario: analisi descrittiva di un nuovo evento morboso. **Arch Monaldi** 1978 Sep–Dec;33(5–6):35–40
Sunseri AR: The hazards of the trail. **Palacio** 1975;81(3):29–39
Wagner BM: Connective tissue disease--historical perspective. **Monogr Pathol** 1983;24:1–3
Wendler M van Voorhis: Doctors and diseases on the Ohio frontier. **Ohio Hist** 1980;89(2):222–42
Wylie MS: Images of sickness and health in American medical thought: 1776–1800 and 1835–1865. Ph.D. Diss. American University. Washington, 1981. 541 p.

**USSR**

Lieber Z: Is there a relationship between illness and creativity? An analysis of the life and poetry of A. V. Koltsov. **Int J Soc Psychiatry** 1980;26(3):212–7
Shul'tsev GP: Vnutrennie bolezni v 'Klinicheskoĭ meditsine' za 1970–1979 gg. (obzor materialov.). **Klin Med (Mosk)** 1980 Aug;58(8):112–6
Wheatcroft SG: Famine and epidemic crises in Russia, 1918–1922: the case of Saratov. **Ann Demogr Hist (Paris)** 1983;:329–52

## ABDOMINAL

### 1700 to Present

**Ireland**

Fielding J: Corrigan on abdominal disease. **J Ir Coll Physicians Surg** 1980 Jul;10(1):41–3

**USSR**

Avdeeva TA, Khazenson LB: Osnovnye itogi 60–letnykh issledovaniĭ Leningradskogo instituta épidemiologii i mikrobiologii imeni Pastera po ostrym kishechnym infektsiiam (1923–1983). **Zh Mikrobiol Epidemiol Immunobiol** 1984 Jan;(1):115–9

## ABNORMALITIES

Calatrava Páramo L: La llamada enfermedad de los Habsburgo: datos históricos, su tratamiento actual y resultados. **An R Acad Nac Med (Madr)** 1979;96(4):557–74
DeVries PA: The surgery of anorectal anomalies: its evolution, with evaluations of procedures. **Curr Probl Surg** 1984 May;21(5):1–75
Duke M: Whose tetralogy is it? A short history of the tetralogy of Fallot. **Conn Med** 1984 Feb;48(2):103–4
Faller A: Die 'Tetralogie von Fallot'; zur geschichtlichen Entwicklung von Diagnose und Therapie eines kongenitalen Herzsyndroms von Niels Stensen bis zur modernen Herzchirurgie. **Gesnerus** 1982;39(3–4):321–46
Harper RG, Kenigsberg K, Sia CG, et al: Xiphopagus conjoined twins: a 300–year review of the obstetric, morphopathologic, neonatal, and surgical parameters. **Am J Obstet Gynecol** 1980 Jul 1;137(5):617–29
Lénárt G, László G: Das Erleben der Verstümmelung in der alten Kunst. In KF Schlegel, ed: Der Körperbehinderte in Mythologie und Kunst. Stuttgart, New York, Thieme, 1983. p. 29–39.
Loevy HT, Kowitz A: The Habsburgs and the 'Habsburg Jaw'. **Bull Hist Dent** 1982 Apr;30(1):19–23
Ramzin MS: Teratogene Wirkung von Medikamenten. **Gynakologe** 1982 Sep;15(3):136–42
Schlegel KF: Der Körperbehinderte in Mythologie und Kunst. Stuttgart; New York, Thieme, 1983. 125 p.
Smith GF: Congenital abnormalities and genetic concepts in neonatology. In Smith GF, Smith PN, Vidyasagar D, ed: Historical review and recent advances in neonatal and perinatal medicine. [Chicago?], Mead Johnson Nutritional Division, 1983. Vol. II. p. 73–83.
Thurer S: Disability and monstrosity: a look at literary distortions of handicapping conditions. **Rehabil Lit** 1980 Jan–Feb;41(1–2):12–5
Warkany J: Prevention of congenital malformations. **Curr Probl Pediatr** 1983 May;13(7):1–26

**Austria**

Snorrason E: Den Habsburgske underkaebe. **Tandlaegebladet** 1982 May;86(8):277–80

**Dominican Republic**

Jarcho S: The Siamese twins of Santo Domingo. **Trans Stud Coll Physicians Phila** 1979 Jun;5(1 no 2):145–7

**Great Britain**

Levine D: Siamese twins in the Parish Registers of Shepshed, Leicestershire. **Local Popul Stud (Matlock)** 1981 Spring;26:44–5

**United States**

Houck PW: A vanishing tribe: the Monacan Indians of Virginia. **Va Med** 1983 May;110(5):332–4

### Before 500 A.D.

**France**

Hooper A: Further information on the prehistoric representations of human hands in the cave of Gargas. **Med Hist** 1980 Apr;24(2):214–16

**Italy**

Marsili A, Bregante-Marsili D, Santoni-Rugiu P: The horned hand: an acquired deformity, or just another Etruscan mystery? **Br J Plast Surg** 1980 Jan;33(1):56–60

### 500 A.D.–1450

**Spain**

Parellada Feliu J: Un text i vuit dibuixos teratològics d'un manuscrit català de l'any 1399. In Congrés International d'Història de la Medicina Catalana, 2nd, Barcelona, 1975. Llibre d'Actes. Barcelona, Socitra, 1977. p. 197–221.

**United States**

Gregg JB, Zimmerman L, Clifford S, et al: Craniofacial anomalies in the Upper Missouri River over a millennium: archeological and clinical evidence. **Cleft Palate J** 1981 Jul;18(3):210–22

### 1450–1700

Park K, Daston LJ: Unnatural conceptions: the study of monsters in sixteenth- and seventeenth-century France and England. **Past Present** 1981;(92):20–54
Schärli AF: Kinder mit Missbildungen in der Renaissance (nach den Aufzeichnungen von Fabricius Hildanus, 1560–1634). **Z Kinderchir** 1984 Oct;39(5):296–301

**Belgium**

Jacques E: Médecine et spiritualité: un médecin belge oublié, ami de Port Royal, Philippe Ignace Save (1659–1702). **Rev Hist Eccles** 1980;75(2):322–42

**Europe**

Niccoli O: 'Menstruum quasi monstruum': parti mostruosi e tabù mestruale nel '500. **Quad Stor** 1980;15(2):402–8

**France**

Pare A: On monsters and marvels. Translated with an introduction and notes by J.L. Pallister. Chicago, London, University of Chicago Press, 1982. xxxii, 224 p.

**Great Britain**

Accardo PJ: Deformity and character. Dr. Little's diagnosis of Richard III. **JAMA** 1980 Dec 19;244(24):2746–7
Barker AE: The Kelsale wonder. **Local Popul Stud (Matlock)** 1981 Spring;26:43
Jones EW: Richard III's disfigurement: a medical postscript. **Folklore** 1980;91:211–27
Porst S: Gynäkologische, geburtshilfliche, embryologische und teratologische Beschreibungen im Werke Shakespeares. Würzburg, Horst Wellm, 1981. 178 p. (Dissertation, Julius-Maximilians-Universität Würzburg).

### 1700 to Present

Brent RL: Comments on the history of teratology. **Teratology** 1979 Oct;20(2):199–200
Eskes TK: Classic illustration. Figure showing the relationship between malformations of the thalidomide type and the sales of thalidomide. **Eur J Obstet Gynecol Reprod Biol** 1984 Jan;16(5):365
Höcht B: Operative Behandlung des Hodenhochstandes. Ein Rückblick auf die historische Entwicklung. **MMW** 1983 May 6;125(18):381–4
Klein D: Historical background and evidence for dominant inheritance

of the Klein-Waardenburg syndrome (type III). **Am J Med Genet** 1983 Feb;14(2):231-9
Lugli T: Hand diseases in early photographs. **Hand** 1980 Feb;12(1):97-104
Morte PD: Neurologic aspects of human anomalies. **West J Med** 1983 Aug;139(2):250-6
Palmer AK, Cozens DD: Comments on the history of teratology testing. **Teratology** 1980 Apr;21(2):260
Rhys Evans PH: Prominent ears and their surgical correction. **J Laryngol Otol** 1981 Sep;95(9):9881-92
Tort P: L'Ordre et le monstres. Le débat sur l'origine des déviations anatomiques au XVIIIe siècle. Paris, Sycomore, 1980. 264 p.
Ulfelder H: The stilbestrol disorders in historical perspective. **Cancer** 1980 Jun 15;45(12):3008-11
Warkany J: The medical profession and congenital malformations (1900-1979). **Teratology** 1979 Oct;20(2):201-4
Zirnstein G: Die Erforschung und Bewertung der Lebenserscheinung 'Variabilität' in der Biologie vor 1859. **NTM** 1981;18(2):58-78

**Austria**

Pemmer H: Schaustellungen von Abnormalitäten in Wien von der Mitte des 18. Jahrhunderts an. **Wien Geschichtsbl** 1968;23(1):265-70

**Brazil**

Freire-Maia A: Historical note: the extraordinary handless and footless families of Brazil--50 years of acheiropodia. **Am J Med Genet** 1981;9(1):31-41

**France**

A propos du syndrome de Turner: **LARC Med** 1981 Oct;1(1):63

**Germany**

Schierhorn H: Johann Friedrich Meckel d. J. als Begründer der wissenschaftlichen Teratologie. **Gegenbaurs Morphol Jahrb** 1984;130(3):399-439

**Great Britain**

Howell M, Ford P: The true history of the elephant man. Harmondsworth, England, Penguin Books, 1980. 223 p.
Lundström B: Medicinska aspekter på Lord Byron. **Sydsven Medicinhist Sallsk Arsskr** 1980;:112-23

**Italy**

Phelps PD, Lloyd GA, Windle-Taylor PC, et al: Mondini dysplasia. **Ann Otol Rhinol Laryngol** 1982 Mar-Apr;91(2 Pt 1):254

**Japan**

Smith AM: Mercury poisoning and birth defects in Japan. **Women Health** 1978 Mar-Apr;3(2):9-12

**Netherlands**

Arias S: In connection with the Waardenburg commemoration, Dr. Sergio Arias has submitted the following correspondence. **Am J Med Genet** 1980;7(1):41-5
Baljet B: Willem Vrolik als teratoloog. **Ned Tijdschr Geneeskd** 1984 Aug 11;128(32):1530-4
Opitz JM: In memoriam: Petrus Johannes Waardenburg, 1886-1979. **Am J Med Genet** 1980;7(1):35-9

**Poland**

Jonecko A: Wkład uczonych polskich do badań nad branchiogennymi odchyleniami rozwojowymi szyi na przełomie XIX i XX wieku. **Pol Przegl Chir** 1979 Sep;51(9):921-26

**United States**

Brent RL: Biography of Josef Warkany. **Teratology** 1982 Apr;25(2):137-51
Hertig AT: Early concepts of dysplasia and carcinoma in situ (a backward glance at a forward process). A brief historical review. **Obstet Gynecol Surv** 1979 Nov;34(11):795-803
Massey EW: North Carolina medical curiosities. **NC Med J** 1981 Apr;42(4):278-9
Raacke ID: Marjorie Maxine Nelson. In Dictionary of American biography, 1961-1965. Suppl. 7, 1981. p. 568-9.
Wilson JG: The evolution of teratological testing. **Teratology** 1979 Oct;20(2):205-11

**Venezuela**

Vélez Boza F: Estudio epidemiologico de la mortalidad por malformaciones congenitas letales en Venezuela, de 1950 a 1974. **Rev Soc Venez Hist Med** 1980;29(43-44):73-80

### ADRENAL GLAND

Altschule MD: Occasional notes. A near miss--Osler's early description of Cushing's syndrome with, regrettably, no post-mortem examination. **N Engl J Med** 1980 May 15;302(20):1153-5

**1700 to Present**

**Chile**

Vargas Fernández L: En torno al primer caso de enfermedad de Addison descrito en Chile (1878). **Rev Med Chil** 1979 Jul;107(7):675-8

**United States**

Heerden JA van: First encounters with pheochromocytoma. The story of Mother Joachim. **Am J Surg** 1982 Aug;144(2):277-9
Moore TJ: Credit for describing Cushing's syndrome. **N Engl J Med** 1983 Sep 22;309(12):735

### ALCOHOLISM

Fernández Felgueroso E, Torcida Valiente I, Rodero Vicente B: Alcoholismo y sociedad. **Rev Sanid Hig Publica (Madr)** 1981 Nov-Dec;55(11-12):1277-94
Glaser FB: The origins of the drug-free therapeutic community. **Br J Addict** 1981 Mar;76(1):13-25
Sandmaier M: Bacchantic maidens and temperance daughters: a historical perspective on female alcohol use. **Alcohol Health Res World** 1980 Summer;4(4):41-51
Vejnoska J: Voluntarism: rich heritage of the alcohol field. **Alcohol Health Res World** 1982 Spring;6(3):4-7, 36-40

**Americas**

Stevens SM: Alcohol and world view. A study of Passamaquoddy alcohol use. **J Stud Alcohol [Suppl]** 1981 Jan;9:122-42

**Great Britain**

Higgs EJ: Research into the history of alcohol use and control in England and Wales: the available sources in the Public Record Office. **Br J Addict** 1984 Mar;79(1):41-7

**Mexico**

Wasserman M: Alcohol, no! Gambling, yes: a matter of survival in Aztec society. **Br J Addict** 1982 Sep;77(3):283-6

**Poland**

Bielewicz A: Przemiany struktury spożycia napojów alkoholowych w Polsce. **Psychiatr Pol** 1983 Mar-Apr;17(2):171-8

**United States**

Gomberg ES: Historical and political perspective: women and drug use. **J Soc Issues** 1982;38(2):9-23
Lender ME: Dictionary of American temperance biography: from temperance reform to alcohol research, the 1600s to the 1980s. Westport, Conn., Greenwood Press, 1984. xiv, 572 p.
Lender ME, Martin JK: Drinking in America: a history. New York, Free Press, London, Collier Macmillan, 1982. xv, 222 p.
Levine HG: The alcohol problem in America: from temperance to alcoholism. **Br J Addict** 1984 Mar;79(1):109-19
Proctor RC: History of drinking in America. **South Med J** 1984 Jul;77(7):886-92

**USSR**

Grigorash FF, Tsudechkis LM, Grigor'ev IuP: K istorii bor'by alkogolizmom v Latvii. **Sov Zdravookhr** 1981;(6):58-60

**Before 500 A.D.**

Villard P: Pathologie et thérapeutique de l'ivresse dans l'Antiquité classique. **Hist Sci Med** 1982;16(3):193-8

**Egypt**

el-Guebaly N, el-Guebaly A: Alcohol abuse in ancient Egypt: the recorded evidence. **Int J Addict** 1981 Oct;16(7):1207-21

**1450-1700**

**Denmark**

Karker A: Kong Frederik 2.s dod. **Jyske Saml** 1964;6(3):252-81

**Great Britain**

Junghans RP: Falstaff was drunker than he was fat. **N Engl J Med** 1983 Jun 16;308(24):1483

**Mexico**

Gruzinski S: La mère dévorante: alcoolisme, sexualité et déculturation chez les mexicas (1500-1550). **Cah Am Lat** 1979;20:5-36

**1700 to Present**

Bynum WF: Alcoholism and degeneration in 19th century European medicine and psychiatry. **Br J Addict** 1984 Mar;79(1):59-70
Dunbar-Miller RA: Alcohol and the fighting man--an historical review. **J R Army Med Corps** 1984 Jun;130(2):117-21
Gottheil E: An introduction to the evaluation of alcoholism outcome studies. **Curr Alcohol** 1979;7:275-85
Israelstam S, Lambert S: Homosexuality as a cause of alcoholism: a historical review. **Int J Addict** 1983 Dec;18(8):1085-107
Kurtz E: Why A.A. works; the intellectual significance of Alcoholics Anonymous. **J Stud Alcohol** 1982 Jan;43(1):38-80
Lomax E: Changing attitudes during the past century as to the hazards of parental alcoholism to the progeny. In International Congress of the History of Medicine. 26th, Plovdiv, 1978. Actes du Congress. Sofia, 1981. Volume II. p. 144-7.
Otero Chulian E, Vergara de Campos A: Miocardiopatía alcohólica (I). Evolución histórica de su conocimiento. **Rev Clin Esp** 1983 Feb 28;168(4):229-31

**Americas**

Jilek-Aall L: Acculturation, alcoholism and Indian-style Alcoholics Anonymous. **J Stud Alcohol [Suppl]** 1981 Jan;9:143-58
Menéndez EL: Socioantropología del proceso de alcoholización en América Latina, 1970-1980 (Primera parte). **Acta Psiquiatr Psicol Am Lat** 1983 Dec;29(4):247-56
Thomas RK: The history of North American Indian alcohol use as a community-based phenomenon. **J Stud Alcohol [Suppl]** 1981 Jan;9:29-39

**Canada**

Barron FL: The American origins on the temperance movement in Ontario, 1828-1850. **Can Rev Am Stud** 1980;11(2):131-50
Mitchinson W: The Woman's Christian Temperance Union: a study in organization. **Int J Womens Stud** 1981;4(2):143-56

**Denmark**

Kramp P, Hemmingsen R: Age distribution of patients with delirium tremens in Denmark 1836-1978. **Acta Psychiatr Scand** 1981 Mar;63(3):253-61

**Finland**

Partanen J: Potreblenie alkogol'nykh napitkov i ego gosudarstvennoe regulirovanie. **Sotsiol Issled** 1981;1:178-86

**France**

Barrows S: After the commune: alcoholism, temperance, and literature in the early Third Republic. In Merriman, John M., ed: Consciousness and class experience in nineteenth-century Europe. New York, Holmes and Meier, 1979. p. 205-18.
Prestwich PE: French workers and the temperance movement. **Int Rev Soc Hist** 1980;25(1):35-52
Prestwich PE: Temperance in France: the curious case of absinth. **Hist Reflect** 1979;6(2):301-19
Richou H, Chanoit PF: Une expérience française: la loi sur les alcooliques présumés dangereux. **Drug Alcohol Depend** 1983 Aug;12(1):61-8
Vogt DD, Montagne M: Absinthe: behind the emerald mask. **Int J Addict** 1982 Aug;17(6):1015-29

**Great Britain**

Crellin JK: Alcoholism and drug addiction in the 'nineties: an American in London. **Br J Addict** 1980 Jun;75(2):153-62
Dunbar-Miller RA: Alcohol and the fighting man--an historical review. **J R Army Med Corps** 1984 Feb;130(1):12-5
Glaser FB: Samuel Johnson: sometimes abstemious, always intemperate. **J Addict Res Found** 1981;10(9):11
Gutzke DW: 'The cry of the children': the Edwardian medical campaign against maternal drinking. **Br J Addict** 1984 Mar;79(1):71-84
Loraine JA: Alcoholism: a new pandemic. **Contemp Rev** 1981;238(1381):75-81
McCandless P: 'Curses of civilization': insanity and drunkenness in Victorian Britain. **Br J Addict** 1984 Mar;79(1):49-58
Rodin AE: Infants and gin mania in 18th-century London. **JAMA** 1981 Mar 27;245(12):1237-9
Weir RB: Obsessed with moderation: the drink trades and the drink question (1870-1930). **Br J Addict** 1984 Mar;79(1):93-107

**Hungary**

Szállási A: Fontos adalék a Tanácsköztársaság alkoholellenes küzdelméhez. **Orv Hetil** 1980 Aug 10;121(32):1955-6

**Mexico**

Scardaville MC: Alcohol abuse and tavern reform in late colonial Mexico City. **Hisp Am Hist Rev** 1980;60(4):643-71

**Poland**

Jaroszewski Z: Działalność profesora Stanisława Batawii na polu alkohologii i walki z alkoholizmem. **Psychiatr Pol** 1979 Sep-Oct;13(5):445-9
Zmudzki A, Morawski J: 25 lat przymusowego leczenia alkoholików w Polsce. **Psychiatr Pol** 1983 Mar-Apr;17(2):147-57

**Polynesia**

Apeldoorn J: Cook Islanders' attitude toward excessive drinking of alcohol. **Int J Addict** 1983 May;18(4):583-7

**Sweden**

Aman A: Det sociala tvånget. **Sven Tidskr** 1979;66(1):30-3

**United States**

Blumberg LU: The significance of the alcohol prohibitionists for the Washington temperance societies; with special reference to Paterson and Newark, New Jersey. **J Stud Alcohol** 1980 Jan;41(1):37-77
Breitenbach W: Sons of the fathers: temperance reformers and the legacy of the American Revolution. **J Early Repub** 1983;3(1):69-82
Conrad B: Genius and intemperance. **Horizon** 1980;23(12):33-40
Delahousse J: Gregory Bateson et les Alcooliques Anonymes. **Soins** 1984 Jan;(421-422):52-3
Earle RM: Prevention of alcoholism in the United States and the National Council on Alcoholism: 1944-1950. **Int J Addict** 1982 May;17(4):679-702
Fagan RW, Mauss AL: Padding the revolving door: an initial assessment of the uniform alcoholism and intoxication treatment act in practice. **Soc Probl** 1978;26(2):232-47
Fennel ML, Rodin MB, Kantor GK: Problems in the work setting, drinking, and reasons for drinking. **Soc Forces** 1981;60(1):114-32
Grob GN, ed: Nineteenth-century medical attitudes toward alcoholic addiction: six studies, 1814-1867. New York, Arno. 1981. various pagings (Reprinted works).
Hampel RL: Diversity in early temperance reform; another look at the Massachusetts Society for the Suppression of Intemperance, 1813-1825. **J Stud Alcohol** 1982 May;43(5):453-68
Hodges HE, Lowe GD: Race and change in rates of treatment and deaths due to alcoholism in a southern state: 1970-1974. **Phylon** 1977;38(2):152-9
Kett JF: Temperance and intemperance as historical problems. **J Am Hist** 1981;67(4):878-85
Lender ME: Women alcoholics: prevalence estimates and their problems reflected in turn-of-the-century institutional data. **Int J Addict** 1981 Apr;16(3):443-8
McBride DC, Page JB: Adolescent Indian substance abuse: ecological and sociocultural factors. **Youth Soc** 1980;11(4):475-92
McCarthy K: Early alcoholism treatment: the Emmanuel Movement and Richard Peabody. **J Stud Alcohol** 1984 Jan;45(1):59-74
Poikolainen K: Alcoholism: a social construct. **Scand J Soc Med [Suppl]** 1982;31:73-8

**USSR**

Hutchinson JF: Science, politics, and the alcohol problem in post-1905 Russia. **Slav East Eur Rev** 1980;58(2):232-54
Idel'chik KhI: Problema bor'by s alkogolizmom v nauchnoĭ obshchestvennoĭ deiatel'nosti professora L. S. Minora (k 125-letiiu so dnia rozhdeniia). **Sov Zdravookhr** 1981;(3):63-6

**Yugoslavia**

Lukić D: Alkoholizam u vidjenju Dimitrija Tucovića. **Srp Arh Celok Lek** 1983 Mar;111(3):397–402

### ALTITUDE SICKNESS

Houston CS: The quest to understand high altitude. A trip back in time and a look ahead. **Postgrad Med** 1983 Jun;73(6):307–10, 313–4

**Americas**

Ryn L: Los Andes y la medicina. **Actas Luso Esp Neurol Psiquiatr** 1981 May–Jun;9(3):213–30, Jul–Aug;9(4):315–24

**Before 500 A.D.**

**China**

Gilbert DL: The first documented report of mountain sickness: the China or Headache Mountain story. **Respir Physiol** 1983 Jun;52(3):315–26

**1450–1700**

**Peru**

Gilbert DL: The first documented description of mountain sickness: the Andean or Pariacaca story. **Respir Physiol** 1983 Jun;52(3):327–47

### ANEMIA

Baserga A: Le anemie: passato, presente e futuro. **Recenti Prog Med** 1983 Jan;74(1):1–10
Bessis M, Delpech G: Sickle cell shape and structure: images and concepts (1840–1980). **Blood Cells** 1982;8(2):359–435
Bonard EC: L'anémie du Saint-Gothard. **Rev Med Suisse Romande** 1980 Dec;100(12):1055–60
Grmek MD: La légende et la réalité de la nocivité des fèves. **Hist Philos Life Sci** 1980;2(1):61–121
Guggenheim KY: Nutrition and nutritional diseases. The evolution of concepts. Lexington, Massachusetts, Toronto, D.C. Heath and Company, 1981. xii, 378 p.
Hart GD: Anemia in ancient times. **Blood Cells** 1981;7(3):485–93
Loudon I: The diseases called chlorosis. **Psychol Med** 1984 Feb;14(1):27–36
Loudon IS: Chlorosis, anaemia, and anorexia nervosa. **Br Med J [Clin Res]** 1980 Dec 20–27;281(6256):1669–75

**France**

Starobinski J: Chlorosis--the 'green sickness'. **Psychol Med** 1981 Aug;11(3):459–68

**Italy**

Menini C: Rapporto tra storia della medicina e medicina pratica: un contributo paradigmatico in tema di talassemia e favismo nella popolazione ferrarese. **Acta Med Hist Patav** 1978–79;25:40–54

**United States**

El-Najjar MY, Andrews J, Moore JG, et al: Iron deficiency anemia in two prehistoric American Indian skeletons: a dietary hypothesis. **Plains Anthropol** 1982;27(97):205–9
Von Endt DW, Ortner DJ: Amino acid analysis of bone from a possible case of prehistoric iron deficiency anemia from the American Southwest. **Am J Phys Anthropol** 1982 Dec;59(4):377–85

**1700 to Present**

Lehmann H: Sickle cell anemia 35 years ago: reminiscence of early African studies. **Am J Pediatr Hematol Oncol** 1984 Spring;6(1):72–6
Lehmann H: The gradual understanding of thalassemia. **Prog Clin Biol Res** 1984;165:121–36
Siddall AC: Chlorosis--etiology reconsidered. **Bull Hist Med** 1982 Summer;56(2):254–60

**France**

Bernard J: Lasthénie de Ferjol, Marie de Saint-Vallier, Emilie de Tourville ou le romancier et l'anémie. **Nouv Rev Fr Hematol** 1982;24(1):43–4
Binet JL: Histoire de la sphèrocytose congénitale. **Nouv Rev Fr Hematol** 1981 Sep;23(3):177–84
Starobinski J: Sur la chlorose. **Romantisme** 1981;31:113–30

**Germany**

Wilmanns JC: Paroxysmal nocturnal hemoglobinuria first described in 1882 by Paul Strübing: an example of cooperation between clinical and basic research. **Blut** 1982 Dec;45(6):367–73

**United States**

Brecher G: A further note on red cell discoveries. William B. Castle's contribution to the discovery of hemoglobin S. **Blood Cells** 1982;8(2):471–2
Brumberg JJ: Chlorotic girls, 1870–1920: a historical perspective on female adolescence.
Crosby WH: Landmark perspective. Pernicious anemia. **JAMA** 1983 Dec 23–30;250(24):3336–8
Darby WJ: Folic acid and macrocytic anemias. **South Med J** 1983 Nov;76(11):1341–3
Herbert V: Landmark perspective: An 'extrinsic factor' and pernicious anemia. **JAMA** 1984 Jan 27;251(4):522–3
Kampmeier RH: Pernicious anemia. **South Med J** 1983 Feb;76(2):151–4
Lehmann H: The history of thalassemia. **Birth Defects** 1982;18(7):1–11
Savitt TL: The invisible malady: sickle cell anemia in America, 1910–1970. **J Natl Med Assoc** 1981 Aug;73(8):739–46
Scott RB: Historical review of legislative and national initiatives for sickle cell disease. **Am J Pediatr Hematol Oncol** 1983 Winter;5(4):346–51

### ANTHRAX

**Before 500 A.D.**

**Rome**

Dirckx JH: Virgil on anthrax. **Am J Dermatopathol** 1981 Summer;3(2):191–5

**1700 to Present**

**Cyprus**

Crowther RW, Gambles RM: Anthrax eradication in Cyprus: an historical survey. **Trop Anim Health Prod** 1983 May;15(2):103–5

**Great Britain**

Cunningham W: The control of woolsorter's disease. **Pharm Hist (London)** 1975 May;5(1):4–5
Tigertt WD: Anthrax. William Smith Greenfield, M.D., F.R.C.P., Professor Superintendent, the Brown Animal Sanatory Institution (1878–81). Concerning the priority due to him for the production of the first vaccine against anthrax. **J Hyg (Lond)** 1980 Dec;85(3):415–20

**United States**

Brachman PS: Inhalation anthrax. **Ann NY Acad Sci** 1980;353:83–93

**USSR**

Bardell D: An 1898 report by Gamaleya for a lytic agent specific for Bacillus anthracis. **J Hist Med Allied Sci** 1982 Apr;37(2):222–5

### APPENDICITIS

Williams GR: A history of appendicitis. With anecdotes illustrating its importance. **Ann Surg** 1983 May;197(5):495–506

**1700 to Present**

Berry J Jr, Malt RA: Appendicitis near its centenary. **Ann Surg** 1984 Nov;200(5):567–75
Gundersen A: Appendicitis. **Wis Med J** 1981 Dec;80(12):23–8
Morer G: Naissance d'un vocable. **Hist Sci Med** 1984;18(2):165–71
Seal A: Appendicitis: a historical review. **Can J Surg** 1981 Jul;24(4):427–33

**France**

Morer G: La découverte de Charles Krafft. **Hist Sci Med** 1984;18(1):33–40

**Scandinavia**

Ráf L: Skandinaviska kirurger först med beskrivning av tecken på appendicit. **Lakartidningen** 1984 Aug 8;81(32–33):2829–30

**United States**

Crosby WH, Haubrich WS: The death of Walter Reed. **JAMA** 1982 Sep 17;248(11):1342–5

### ARTHRITIS AND RHEUMATISM

Benedek TG, Rodnan GP: A brief history of the rheumatic diseases.

**Bull Rheum Dis** 1982;32(6):59–68
Brooks PM: Anti-rheumatic therapy through the ages. **Australas Nurses J** 1980 Mar;9(4):19–20
d'Eshougues JR: Gicht und Rheumatismus. In Sournia JC, Martiny M, Poulet J, ed: Illustrierte Geschichte der Medizin. Salzburg, Andreas, 1980. Vol. 6. p. 2319–49.
Domen RE: Paleopathological evidence of rheumatoid arthritis. **JAMA** 1981 Oct 23–30;246(17):1899
Fraser KJ: Anglo-French contributions to the recognition of rheumatoid arthritis. **Ann Rheum Dis** 1982 Aug;41(4):335–43
Kahn MF: L'agent étiologique de la polyarthrite rhumatoïde: une hypothèse. **Rev Rhum Mal Osteoartic** 1979 Jul–Sep;46(7–9):510–1
Kean WF, Buchanan WW: Rheumatoid arthritis: some personal considerations on aetiology and treatment. Part 1. **Br J Clin Pract** 1983 Jan;37(1):4–15
Leden I: Ledgångsreumatism och gikt - en historisk återblick. **Sydsven Medicinhist Sallsk Arsskr** 1981;:65–97
Leden I: Reumatologisk farmakoterapi ur historiskt/filatelistiskt perspektiv. **Lakartidningen** 1980 Dec 24;77(52):4943–6
Minugh NS: A brief survey of osteoarthritis outside of modern human populations. **J Am Podiatry Assoc** 1982 May;72(5):217–21
Schadewaldt H: Der Rheumatismus und seine Behandlung im Wandel der Zeiten. **Z Rheumatol** 1983 Jul–Aug;42(4):139–44
Seror P: Le rhumatisme blennorragique ancêtre des arthrites réactionnelles? **Presse Med** 1984 May 26;13(22):1359–63

**Great Britain**

Rogers J, Watt I, Dieppe P: Arthritis in Saxon and mediaeval skeletons. **Br Med J [Clin Res]** 1981 Dec 19;283(6307)1668–70

**Before 500 A.D.**

Schumacher HR, Alarcon-Segovia D: Osteoarthritic knees in a Pre-Columbian ceramic figure. **J Rheumatol** 1980 May–Jun;7(3):381–2

**Great Britain**

Thould AK, Thould BT: Arthritis in Roman Britain. **Br Med J [Clin Res]** 1983 Dec 24–31;287(6409):1909–11

**500 A.D.–1450**

**Belgium**

Dequeker JV: Polymyalgia rheumatica with temporal arteritis, as painted by Jan van Eyck in 1436. **Can Med Assoc J** 1981 Jun 15;124(12):1597–8

**1450–1700**

**Austria**

Zwanowetz G: Herzog Sigismund von Osterreich in Gastein. **Mitt Ges Salzburger Landeskd** 1972–73;112–113(2):325–9

**Italy**

Alarcón-Segovia D, Laffón A, Alcocer-Varela J: Probable depiction of juvenile arthritis by Sandro Botticelli. **Arthritis Rheum** 1983 Oct;26(10):1266–8
Dequeker J: Arthritis in the paintings of Sandro Botticelli. **Arthritis Rheum** 1984 Oct;27(10):1196–7
Leden I: Doubts about Sandro Botticelli's depiction of juvenile rheumatoid arthritis. **Arthritis Rheum** 1984 Oct;27(10):1197–8

**Mexico**

Alarcón-Segovia D: Descriptions of therapeutic arthrocenthesis and of synovial fluid in a Nahuatl text from prehispanic Mexico. **Bol Soc Mex Hist Filos Med** 1979 Sep;4(28):105–12

**Netherlands**

Appelboom T, Boelpaepe C de, Ehrlich GE, et al: Rubens and the question of antiquity of rheumatoid arthritis. **JAMA** 1981 Feb 6;245(5):483–6

**1700 to Present**

Benedek TG: Subcutaneous nodules and the differentiation of rheumatoid arthritis from rheumatic fever. **Semin Arthritis Rheum** 1984 May;13(4):305–21
Bollet AJ: A report of reactive arthritis following dysentery in 1743. **Arthritis Rheum** 1981 Jun;24(6):860
Champion GD: Gold compounds in rheumatic diseases--1. **Med J Aust** 1984 Jan 21;140(2):73–7
Goodwin JS, Goodwin JM: Failure to recognize efficacious treatments: a history of salicylate therapy in rheumatoid arthritis. **Perspect Biol Med** 1981 Autumn, 25(1):78–92
Kersley GD: The scope of rheumatology. **Ann Rheum Dis** 1981 Dec;40(6):631–2
Reynolds MD: The development of the concept of fibrositis. **J Hist Med Allied Sci** 1983 Jan;38(1):5–35
Scarano GB: Considerazioni storiche sull'uso dei sali d'oro nell'artrite reumatoide. **Med Secoli** 1982 May–Aug;19(2):175–91
Sèze S de: Un demi siècle de rhumatologie: 1930–1980. **Bull Acad Natl Med (Paris)** 1980 Dec;164(9):807–21
Weissmann G: The introduction is over. **Arthritis Rheum** 1983 Nov;26(11):1297–302

**Americas**

Gordon DA: The growth of rheumatology. **J Rheumatol** 1981 Jan–Feb;8(1):4–5

**Czechoslovakia**

Ulrich J: Revmatická horečka na Mostecku--kdysi a dnes. **Vnitr Lek** 1983 Dec;29(12):1176–82

**Europe**

Vainio K: History of surgery of rheumatoid arthritis in Europe. **Scand J Rheumatol** 1983;12(2):65–8

**Germany**

Schattenkirchner M: Rheumatologie heute. **Fortschr Med** 1982 Sep 23;100(36):1633–4

**Great Britain**

Hart ED: Conan Doyle as rheumatologist. **Ann Rheum Dis** 1982 Aug;41(4):437–8
Hart FD: The British rheumatological journals. **Br J Rheumatol** 1984 Aug;23(3):164–5
Mowat AG: Strathpeffer Spa: Dr. William Bruce and polymyalgia rheumatica. **Ann Rheum Dis** 1981 Oct;40(5):503–6

**Hungary**

Vladár I: Thököly Imre fejedelem megrokkanása. **Orv Hetil** 1979 Sep 23;120(38):2317–8

**Ireland**

Cassidy M, Jacobs A, Bresnihan B: The use of unproven remedies for rheumatoid arthritis in Ireland. **Ir Med J** 1983 Nov;76(11):464–5

**Poland**

Luft S: Rys historyczny Instytutu Reumatologicznego. I. Lata 1948–1961. **Reumatologia** 1981;19(2):109–17
Małdyk E: Osiągniecia zakładu anatomii patologicznej IR w zakresie patomorfologii chorób układu ruchu. **Reumatologia** 1981;19(2):123–9
Małdyk E, Luft S: Rys historyczny Instytutu Reumatologicznego II (lata 1962–1980). **Reumatologia** 1982;20(1–2):1–6
Małdyk E: 25 lat działalności Instytutu Rheumatologicznego. **Nauka Pol** 1976;24(9–10):77–83
Małdykowa H: Osiągnięcia Instytutu w zakresie diagnostyki i leczenia układowych chorób tkani łącznej. **Reumatologia** 1981;19(2):119–22

**United States**

Hedfors E: Mannen bakom syndromet: Augustus Roi Felty. Fann ovanlig symtomkonstellation: artrit, splenomegali, leukopeni. **Lakartidningen** 1983 Sep 14;80(37):3281
McCarty DJ: The American Rheumatism Association and the Arthritis Foundation: commentary on 14 years of a happy union. **Arthritis Rheum** 1979 Dec;22(12):1394–5
Mann R: Philip Showalter Hench. In Dictionary of American biography, 1961–1965. Suppl. 7, 1981. p. 340–341.
Tucker EL: A new letter by Thomas Holley Chivers. **Ga Hist Q** 1971;55(4):582–8

**USSR**

Agababov SV, Savinov VA: Vklad russkikh uchenykh XIX veka v sozdanie i razvitie ucheniia o revmatizme. **Ter Arkh** 1983;55(11):139–44
Anokhin VN: K 20-letiiu zhurnala 'Voprosy revmatizma'. **Vopr Revm** 1981 Apr–Jun;(2):3–4
Borob'ev RI: I. A. Kassirskiĭ i razvitie Sovetskoĭ meditsiny. **Ter Arkh** 1982;54(2):148–50
Bunchuk NV, Vasil'ev VI, Trusova TM: Razvitie otechestvennoĭ revmatologii za gody sovetskoĭ vlasti. **Vestn Akad Med Nauk SSSR**

1981;(6):4–7

Lebedev DD, Kovaleva EV, Semenova VN: Nekotorye voprosy revmatizma, éndokrinnykh i nervnykh zabolevaniĭ u deteĭ v trudakh V.I. Molchanova i ego uchenikov (k 110-letiiu so dnia rozhdeniia). **Pediatriia** 1980 Aug;(8):64–7

Nasonova VA: Razvitie ideĭ S. P. Botkina v sovremennoĭ revmatologii. **Vestn Akad Med Nauk SSSR** 1983;(3):41–6

Tareev EM: Kollagenozy: évoliutsiia ucheniia i sovremennye kontseptsii. **Vopr Revm** 1982 Jul–Sep;(3):15–22

Tsitlanadze VG, Tskhomelidze NF, Melikishvili MN, et al: K istorii razvitiia revmatologii v Gruzii. **Vopr Revm** 1982 Jul–Sep;(3):13–5

**Yugoslavia**

Dürrigl T: Počeci auroterapije u Jugoslaviji. **Reumatizam** 1982;29(2):37–9

Majsec M, Manestar M: Od kupališnog lječilišta do bolnice za reumatske bolesti i rehabilitaciju Krapinske Toplice. **Reumatizam** 1979;26(3):73–6

### ASPHYXIA

Goldstein PJ: Birth asphyxia. In Smith GF, Smith PN, Vidyasagar D, ed: Historical review and recent advances in neonatal and perinatal medicine. [Chicago?], Mead Johnson Nutritional Division, 1983. Vol. I. p. 177–84.

### ASTHMA

Furness DA: Asthma -- a note on its history. **Hist Med (Lond)** 1980 Jan–Feb;8(1):26

Gabbay J: Asthma attacked? Tactics for the reconstruction of a disease concept. In P. Wright, A. Treacher, ed: The problem of medical knowledge. Examining the social construction of medicine. Edinburgh, Edinburgh University Press, 1982. p. 23–48.

McFadden ER: Qualifying factors in the classification of asthma: how valuable they are to the clinician. **J Asthma** 1983;20 Suppl 1:5–8

Weissmann G: Proust in khaki. **Hosp Pract** 1983 Apr;18(4):56, 58, 62 passim

**Before 500 A.D.**

**Greece**

Marketos SG, Ballas CN: Bronchial asthma in the medical literature of Greek antiquity. **J Asthma** 1982;19(4):263–9

**500 A.D.-1450**

**Arabic**

Rosner F: Moses Maimonides' treatise on asthma. **Thorax** 1981 Apr;36(4):245–51

Rosner F: Moses Maimonides' Treatise on Asthma. **J Asthma** 1984;21(2):119–29

Sakula A: Moses Maimonides' treatise on asthma. **Thorax** 1981 Jul;36(7):560

**1450–1700**

**Great Britain**

Sakula A: Sir John Floyer's A Treatise of the Asthma (1698). **Thorax** 1984 Apr;39(4):248–54

**1700 to Present**

Roe W: 'Science' in the practice of medicine: its limitations and dangers as exemplified by a study of the natural history of acute bronchial asthma in children. **Perspect Biol Med** 1984 Spring;27(3):386–400

Smith JM: The recent history of the treatment of asthma: a personal view. **Thorax** 1983 Apr;38(4):244–53

**France**

Charpin J: Laënnec et l'asthme. **Rev Fr Mal Respir** 1981;9(2):151–3

**Germany**

Schultze-Werninghaus G, Meier-Sydow J: The clinical and pharmacological history of theophylline: first report on the bronchospasmolytic action in man by S. R. Hirsch in Frankfurt (Main) 1922. **Clin Allergy** 1982 Mar;12(2):211–5

**Great Britain**

Viniaker H: L'asthme et son environnement selon Sir John Floyer (1649–1734). **Hist Sci Med** 1984;18(1):77–82

**United States**

Smith B, Robertson RM, Robertson D: An early Southern description of Curschmann's spirals. **Clin Notes Respir Dis** 1982 Summer;21(1):10–2

**USSR**

Mendelson G, Mendelson D: Psychological aspects of bronchial asthma in the writings of Isaac Babel. **Isr J Psychiatr Relat Sci** 1981;18(1):31–9

### BERIBERI

Guggenheim KY: Nutrition and nutritional diseases. The evolution of concepts. Lexington, Massachusetts, Toronto, D.C. Heath and Company, 1981. xii, 378 p.

**Asia**

Wong M: Contribution à l'histoire des carences en Extrême-Orient: le béribéri. In: Congrès National des Sociétés Savantes, 93e, Tours, 1968. Comptes Rendus. Paris, 1971. Section des Sciences, Tome II. p. 9–15.

**1700 to Present**

Majoor CL, Hafkenscheid JC, Van Dijk C: Enkele kernpunten uit de geschiedenis van cardiale beriberi, die voor de praktisch werkzame arts van betekenis lijken. **Ned Tijdschr Geneeskd** 1982 Apr 24;126(17):771–5

Martin W: The beriberi analogy to myocardial infarction. **Med Hypotheses** 1983 Feb;10(2):185–98

**Japan**

Okada Y: [The incidence of Kakke-disease (beriberi) in pre-war mental hospitals] (Jpn). **Nihon I-Shigaku Zasshi** 1981;27:95–111

### BILIARY TRACT

Longmire WP: Historic landmarks in biliary surgery. **South Med J** 1982 Dec;75(12):1548–50, 1552

Shehadi WH: The biliary system through the ages. **Int Surg** 1979 Nov–Dec;64(6):63–78

**1700 to Present**

An ancient art revived: **Gastrointest Endosc** 1979 Feb;25(1):28–9

### BITES AND STINGS

Castro M de: Johannes Aegidii Zamorensis, OFM, contra venena et animalia venenosa. Introducción edición y notas. **Arch Iberoam** 1976;36:3–116

**Sri Lanka**

De Silva A, Uragoda CG: Traditional methods of snake-bite treatment in Sri Lanka. **Ceylon Med J** 1983 Sep;28(3):170–4

**Before 500 A.D.**

**Greece**

Zapfe H: Ein Schädel von Mesopithecus mit Biss-Spuren. **Folia Primatol (Basel)** 1981;35(4):248–58

**1700 to Present**

Robinson T: Baroque medicine: how a cup of Aunt Ida's hot air rescued a sailor. **Nurs Mirror** 1982 Jul 21;155(3):25

**United States**

Barlow W, Powell DO: Ixodes as a source of conflict: Otis E. Hunt vs. J. Mason Warren. **J Hist Med Allied Sci** 1981 Apr;36(2):221–4

Berndt T: Bite mark science. Forensic dentistry's hottest frontier. **Fla Dent J** 1982 Spring;53(1):22–4, 42–3

Marshall J: The madstone: its origins and application in Barlow, Ballard County, Kentucky. **Ky Folkl Rec** 1978;24(2):42–8

### BLOOD

**1700 to Present**

Levine P: The discovery of Rh hemolytic disease. **Vox Sang** 1984;47(2):187–90

Nossel HL, Spaet TH: Clarence Merskey (1914–1982). **Thromb Res** 1983 Jun 1;30(5):401–5

Prince AM: Detection of the relation between the Australia antigen and

hepatitis B virus. **Vox Sang** 1984;47(3):257-60
Zipursky A: The rise and fall of Rh disease. In Smith GF, Smith PN, Vidyasagar D, ed: Historical review and recent advances in neonatal and perinatal medicine. [Chicago?], Mead Johnson Nutritional Division, 1983. Vol. I. p. 99-106.

**Africa**

Roberts RS: The first description of idiopathic thrombocytopaenic purpura and onyalai in Southern Africa? **Cent Afr J Med** 1980 Dec;26(12):257-8

**United States**

Bithell TC: Hereditary dysfibrinogenemia--the first 25 years. **Acta Haematol (Basel)** 1984;71(3):145-9
Diamond LK: The Rh problem: (an example of the tsunami phenomenon in medicine). **Turk J Pediatr** 1982 Jan-Mar;24(1):35-47
Pochedly C: Dr. James A. Wolff. I. Early progress in treatment of Rh hemolytic disease. **Am J Pediatr Hematol Oncol** 1984 Fall;6(3):319-23
Reynolds WA: Late report of the first case of plasmapheresis for Waldenström's macroglobulinemia [1956] **JAMA** 1981;245:606-7

## BONE

Borišev V, Savić K, Jovanović D: Spina bifida sa istorijskog aspekta. **Med Pregl** 1984;37(1-2):75-6
Grimm H: Neue Hinweise auf ur- und frühgeschichtliches sowie mittelalterliches Vorkommen der Rachitis und ähnlicher Mineralisationsstörungen. **Arztl Jugendkd** 1984 Jun;75(3):168-77
Kelley MA: Intervertebral osteochondrosis in ancient and modern populations. **Am J Phys Anthropol** 1982 Nov;59(3):271-9
Lambert M: Jan Fryderyk Knolle's forgotten dissertation on osseous syphilis, 1763. **Sex Transm Dis** 1984 Jan-Mar;11(1):36-40
Spencer DG, Sturrock RD, Buchanan WW: Ankylosing spondylitis: yesterday and today. **Med Hist** 1980 Jan;24(1):60-9
Waldron HA: Lead in bones: a cautionary tale. **Ecol Dis** 1982;1(2-3):191-6
Wells C, Woodhouse N: Paget's disease in an Anglo-Saxon. **Med Hist** 1975 Oct;19(4):396-400

**Before 500 A.D.**

Walker A, Zimmerman MR, Leakey RE: A possible case of hypervitaminosis A in Homo erectus. **Nature** 1982 Mar 18;296(5854):248-50

**Americas**

Allison MJ, Gerszten E, Munizaga J, et al: Metastatic tumor of bone in a Tiahuanaco female. **Bull NY Acad Med** 1980 Jul-Aug;56(6):581-7

**Greece**

Bartsocas CS: An introduction to ancient Greek genetics and Skeletal Dysplasias. **Prog Clin Biol Res** 1982;104:3-13

**United States**

Gregg JB, Reed A: Monostotic fibrous dysplasia in the temporal bone: a late prehistoric occurrence. **Am J Phys Anthropol** 1980 May;52(4):587-93

**500 A.D.-1450**

Scheidegger S: Gelenkerkrankungen bei Skelettfunden aus dem Mittelalter. **Aktuel Gerontol** 1980 Nov;10(11):509-10

**Germany**

Schultz M: Aseptic bone necrosis found in the skeletal material from the Merovingian cemetery of Kleinlangheim, Southern Germany. **Paleopathol Newsl** 1981 Jun;34:7-9

**Switzerland**

Ulrich-Bochsler S, Glowatzki G: Ossäre Folgezustände einer langzeitig unbehandelten osteomyelitis. Fallbeschreibung an einem mittelalterlichen Skelett. **Anthropol Anz** 1982 Mar;40(1):1-18
Ulrich-Bochsler S, Glowatzki G, Zeltner T: Ossäre Folgezustände einer unbehandelten Osteomyelitis. **Praxis** 1981 Oct;70(43):1913-8

**1450-1700**

**Poland**

Dudziński W: Choroby i zgon króla Zygmunta Starego. **Wiad Lek** 1981 Aug 1;34(15):1317-22
Dudziński W: Smierć króla Kazimierza Jagiellończyka. **Wiad Lek** 1981 Jun 15;34(12):1041-4

**USSR**

Zakharov BI, Zakharov NP: Priznaki ankiloziruiushchego spondiloartrita na iskopaemykh kostiakh liudeĭ, zhivshikh na territorii Sibiri. **Ortop Travmatol Protez** 1980 Apr;(4):46-7

**1700 to Present**

Blönningen J: Die Osteomalazie als Indikation für eine bilaterale Oophorektomie im späten 19. und frühen 20. Jahrhundert. Ergebnisse und Erklärungsversuche. Diss. Erlangen-Nürnberg, 1980. 113 p.
McCarthy EF: Aseptic necrosis of bone. An historic perspective. **Clin Orthop** 1982 Aug;(168):216-21
McCarthy EF: Giant-cell tumor of bone: an historical perspective. **Clin Orthop** 1980 Nov-Dec;(153):14-25
Ram PC, Fordham EW: An historical survey of bone scanning. **Semin Nucl Med** 1979 Jul;9(3):190-6
Schönwetter HP: Zur Geschichte der Akromegalie; mit besonderer Berücksichtigung der Frühgeschichte im Kanton Glarus. **Gesnerus** 1982;39(3-4):369-93
Weil UH: Osteogenesis imperfecta: historical background. **Clin Orthop** 1981 Sep;159:6-10

**France**

Ryckewaert A, Naveau B: Les affections ostéo-articulaires de J.M. Charcot à nos jours. **Rev Neurol (Paris)** 1982;138(12):997-1008
Ryckewaert A, Naveau B: Principaux apports de Charcot et de Pierre Marie à la pathologie ostéo-articulaire. **Rev Rhum Mal Osteoartic** 1984 Jul-Sep;51(7-8):405-13

**Germany**

Grupe G: Die Identifikation des Skelettes von Georg Christoph Lichtenberg. **Anthropol Anz** 1984 Mar;42(1):1-9

**Great Britain**

McGivering NJ: View from childhood. **Br Med J** 1979 Oct 13;2(6195):909
Park WM, Mourad K: Ossification and calcification of the posterior longitudinal ligament of the spine. **Br J Radiol** 1980 Apr;53(628):375-6

**Sweden**

Peltier LF: The classic: congenital osteomalacia. Olaus Jacob Ekman. **Clin Orthop** 1981 Sep;159:3-5

**Switzerland**

Kis J: Der Knochenpathologe Emil Looser (1877-1936). Zürich, Juris, 1982. 68 p. Zürcher Medizingeschichtliche Abhandlungen, Neue Reihe, 149; also Diss.).

**United States**

Cowell HR: Osteomyelitis revisited: a 19th century case report. **Del Med J** 1982 May;54(5):263-5
Gordan GS: Fuller Albright and postmenopausal osteoporosis: a personal appreciation. **Perspect Biol Med** 1981 Summer;24(4):547-60
Kahn AJ, Raisz LG: Dedication to Donald G. Walker. **Metab Bone Dis Relat Res** 1981;3(2):77-80
Wirthlin LS: Joseph Smith's boyhood operation: an 1813 surgical success. **Brigham Young Univ Stud** 1981;21(2):131-54

**USSR**

Petrov IN: P.G. Kornev i ego shkola. **Probl Tuberk** 1984 Jul;(7):73-5

## BOTULISM

**1700 to Present**

Gunn RA: Botulism: from van Ermengem to the present. A comment. **Rev Infect Dis** 1979 Jul-Aug;1(4):720-1

**Germany**

Biadała E: Opis zatrucia jadem kiełbasianym z 1822 roku. **Wiad Lek** 1981 Jul 15;34(14):1223-5

BRUCELLOSIS

500 A.D.-1450

France

Soulié R: Brucellosis: a case report dating from 650-700 A.D. **Paleopathol Newsl** 1982 Jun;38:7-10

1700 to Present

Great Britain

Vella EE: Brucellosis (the Corps disease). **J R Army Med Corps** 1983 Jun;129(2):97-100

Williams E: The history of brucellosis in Wales. In J. Cule, ed: Wales and medicine. London, British Society for the History of Medicine, 1975. p. 75-85.

Mexico

León AP: La brucelosis en México. In Academia Nacional de Medicina. Libro conmemorativo del primer centenario. México, Comité Editorial de la Comisión Organizadora del Congreso del Centenario, 1964. Tome 2. p. 527-32.

United States

O'Hern EM: Alice Catherine Evans. In: Notable American women. The modern period. Cambridge, Mass., Belknap-Harvard Univ. Press, 1980. 4:219-21.

Wise RI: Brucellosis in the United States. Past, present, and future. **JAMA** 1980 Nov 21;244(20):2318-22

BURNS

Robinson DW: The care of burns. Early history to present. **J Arkansas Med Soc** 1984 Apr;80(11):517-25

Watt J: The burns of seafarers under oars, sail and steam. **Injury** 1980 Jul;12(1):69-81

Cuba

Sol A del: Ensayo histórico sobre las quemaduras en Cuba. La Habana, Editorial Científico-Técnica, 1979. 92 p.

Denmark

Thomsen M: The history of burns treatment in Denmark. **Scand J Plast Reconstr Surg** 1984;18(1):7-9

Before 500 A.D.

Scarborough J: On medications for burns in classical antiquity. In Romm S, ed: Symposium on historical perspectives of plastic surgery. Philadelphia, Saunders, 1983. p. 603-610.

1700 to Present

Steffen C: Marjolin's ulcer. Report of two cases and evidence that Marjolin did not describe cancer arising in scars of burns. **Am J Dermatopathol** 1984 Apr;6(2):187-93

Argentina

Benaim F: Thirty years at the service of the burned in Argentina and South America. **J Trauma** 1981 May;21(5):356-63

Denmark

Thomsen M: The Opera fire in Copenhagen. **Scand J Plast Reconstr Surg** 1984;18(1):3-5

France

Steffen C: Jean-Nicolas Marjolin. **Am J Dermatopathol** 1984 Apr;6(2):163-5

Sweden

Arturson G: The history of burns treatment in Sweden. **Scand J Plast Reconstr Surg** 1984;18(1):11-20

United States

Dutra FR: Electrical burns of the skin. Medicolegal investigation. **Am J Forensic Med Pathol** 1981 Dec;2(4):309-12

USSR

Filippova LF: K stanovleniiu kombustiologii na Ukraine. **Klin Khir** 1980 May;(5):72-3

CATARACT

1450-1700

France

Brown P: Couching a cataract. **Med Instrum** 1982 Mar-Apr;16(2):123

1700 to Present

Trevor-Roper PD: Sir Henry Tristram Holland. In Dictionary of national biography, 1961-1970. Suppl. 8, 1981. p. 528-9.

CEREBROVASCULAR

Bell BA: A history of the study of cerebral edema. **Neurosurgery** 1983 Dec;13(6):724-8

Jarcho S: Some lost, obsolete, or discontinued diseases: Serous apoplexy, incubus, and retrocedent ailments. **Trans Stud Coll Physicians Phila** 1980 Dec;5(2 no 4):241-66

Ljunggren B, Säveland H: Hjärnpulsåderbråckens medicinska historia - ett långtifrån avslutat kapitel. **Sydsven Medicinhist Sallsk Arsskr** 1982;19:63-98

1450-1700

Poland

Dudziński W: Choroby i zgon króla Aleksandra Jagiellończyka. **Wiad Lek** 1981 Jul 15;34(14):1227-32

Kaczorowski W: Choroba i prawdopodobna przyczyna zgonu Zygmunta III Wazy. **Arch Hist Med (Warsz)** 1982;45(1-4):45-54

Switzerland

Jost M: Die Apoplexielehre Johann Jakob Wepfers (1620-1695). Diss., Rheinische Friedrich-Wilhelms-Universität, Bonn, 1982. 76 p.

1700 to Present

France

Gautier JC: Accidents vasculaires. **Rev Neurol (Paris)** 1982;138(12):939-51

Heron JR: Louis Pasteur: the nature of his illness. In Passmore R, ed: Proceedings of the Royal College of Physicians of Edinburgh Tercentenary Congress, 1981. Edinburgh, Royal College of Physicians of Edinburgh, 1982. p. 116-27.

Roche R: L'apoplexie de Voltaire. **Hist Sci Med** 1981;15(2):145-9

Sternbach G: Joseph Babinski: the phenomenon of the toes. **J Emerg Med** 1984;1(3):263-6

Great Britain

Langham-Carter RR: The death of the Duchesse de Nemours. **Adler Mus Bull** 1982 Nov;8(2):8-9

Murray TJ: The neurology of Alice in Wonderland. **Can J Neurol Sci** 1982 Nov;9(4):453-7

Poland

Dudziński W. Choroba i zgon króla Augusta III Sasa. **Wiad Lek** 1981 Sep 1;34(17):1479-84

United States

Marmor MF: Wilson, strokes, and zebras. **N Engl J Med** 1982 Aug 26;307(9):528-35

Wilson, strokes, and zebras: **N Engl J Med** 1983 Jan 20;308(3):163-4

USSR

Müller-Dietz HE: Utländska läkare vid Lenins sjukbädd. **Sydsven Medicinhist Sallsk Arsskr** 1984;21:141-56

CHEST

1700 to Present

Asia

Nagaishi C: A brief history of the Asia-Pacific Congress on Diseases of the Chest. **Chest** 1984 Nov;86(5):656-7

# DISEASES AND INJURIES

**France**

Sakula A: R.T.H. Laënnec 1781-1826, his life and work: a bicentenary appreciation. **Thorax** 1981 Feb;36(2):81-90

**Great Britain**

Douglas A: Promises to keep. **Thorax** 1984 Jul;39(7):481-6

**United States**

Ayvasian LF: American Thoracic Society: the fifty-five Trudeau medalists (1926-1980): a seventy-fifty anniversary review. **Am Rev Respir Dis** 1980 Apr;121(4):753-75
Boyd DP: A half century of publishing. **Chest** 1984 Nov;86(5):654-5
Olsen AM: ACCP International--'The world is our classroom'. **Chest** 1984 Nov;86(5):655-6

## CHICKENPOX

**1700 to Present**

Lerman SJ: Why is chickenpox called chickenpox? **Clin Pediatr (Phila)** 1981 Feb;20(2):111-2

## CHOLERA

Leavesley J: Cholera. **Med J Aust** 1984 Nov 10;141(10):659-61

**1700 to Present**

Bornside GH: Waldemar Haffkine's cholera vaccines and the Ferran-Haffkine priority dispute. **J Hist Med Allied Sci** 1982 Oct;37(4):399-422
Cameron D, Jones IG: John Snow, the broad street pump and modern epidemiology. **Int J Epidemiol** 1983 Dec;12(4):393-6
Carpenter CC: Myths, mandarins and molecules: the cautionary tale of cholera. **Trans Am Clin Climatol Assoc** 1980;92:167-93
Chen W: [A history of the discovery of cholera pathogen] (Chi). **Chung Hua I Shih Tsa Chih** 1984;14(2):104-6
Dodin A: Pourquoi les pandémies cholériques? **Bull Soc Pathol Exot Filiales** 1984 Mar-Apr;77(2):127-34
Jusatz HJ: 150 Jahre pandemische Ausbreitung der asiatischen Cholera von 1831 bis 1981. **Zentralbl Bakteriol Mikrobiol Hyg [A]** 1982 Jun;252(2):257-67
Keene BE: Portrait of a man protected against cholera. **J Hist Med Allied Sci** 1982 Oct;37(4):439
Pierce J: A dreaded disease. **Nurs Times** 1983 Jan 26-Feb 1;79(4):57-61
Pratt EL: Development of parenteral fluid therapy. **J Pediatr** 1984 Apr;104(4):581-4
Prayer composed during cholera epidemic outbreak 1831 and 1847?: by R. Abraham Bing of Würzburg. **Koroth** 1979 Nov;7(9-10):719-20
Raj N: The homoeopathic treatment of cholera; a historical study. **Bull Indian Inst Hist Med (Hyderabad)** 1978;8(1-4):39-43
Rische H: Moderne epidemiologische und pathogenetische Erkenntnisse, dargestellt am Beispiel der Cholera. **Z Erkr Atmungsorgane** 1983;161(1):65-73
Seal SC: Centenary of discovery of cholera vibrio. **Indian J Public Health** 1983 Jan-Mar;27(1):1-5
Seal SC: Centenary of discovery of cholera vibrio. **J Indian Med Assoc** 1983 Dec;81(11-12):210-2
Shortt SE: Cholera: doctors' dilemma, historians' delight. **Queens Q** 1981;88(1):130-4
Stembrowicz W: Pruski kordon sanitarny w okresie wojny Polsko-Rosyjskiej (1830-1831). **Arch Hist Med (Warsz)** 1982;45(1-4):39-44
Swan P: Cholera: a visitation on Victorian society. **Nurs Mirror** 1983 Oct 12;157(15):30-4
Unver AS: Les épidémies de choléra dans les terres balkaniques aux XVIIIe et XIXe siècles. **Etud Balk** 1973:4:89-97

**Africa**

Eyckmans L: Le problème du choléra en Afrique de l'Est. **Bull Seances Acad R Sci Outre Mer** 1979;(3):445-50

**Arabic**

Gallagher N: Late contributions to Arabic medicine: a treatise on cholera. In: International Symposium for the History of Arabic Science, 1st, University of Aleppo, 1976. Proceedings. Aleppo, Syria, 1976. Papers in European Languages, Vol. II. p. 300-3.

**Argentina**

Crespo Cossio P: Aportes acerca de la incidencia de la epidemia de cólera de 1867 en el Departamento Totoral y población del mismo nombre. **Rev Fac Cien Med Univ Nac Cordoba** 1980;38(1-4):41-2, 45

**Belgium**

Delannoy Y: Une épidémie de choléra à Enghien (1849). **Ann Cerc Archeol Enghien** 1977;18:279-307
Falise C: Le choléra à Bruxelles en 1866. **Ann Soc Belg Hist Hop** 1979;17:81-104
Lafosse A: Les hôpitaux temporaires à Verviers durant les épidémies de choléra. **Ann Soc Belg Hist Hop** 1979;17:71-9
Van der Haegen H, De Vos R: De cholera-epidemie te Leuven in 1849. **Driemaand Tijdschr Gemeentekrediet Belg** 1980;:197-210

**Canada**

Bilson G: A darkened house: cholera in nineteenth century Canada. Toronto, Buffalo, University of Toronto Press, 1980. 222 p.
Bilson G: Canadian doctors and the cholera. **Hist Pap Can Hist Assoc** 1977:104-19
Bilson G: Cholera and public health in Canada. **Can J Public Health** 1984 Sep-Oct;75(5):352-5
Dechêne L, Robert JC: Le choléra de 1832 dans le Bas-Canada: mesure des inegalités devant la mort. In Charbonneau H, Larose A, ed: The great mortalities: methodological studies of demographic crises in the pase. Liège, Belgium, Ordina Editions, 1980. p. 229-56.
Kennedy E: Immigrants, cholera and the Saint John Sisters of Charity, 1854-64. **Can Cathol Hist Assoc Study Sess** 1977;44:25-44

**Costa Rica**

Tjarks G, Fernández FM, Espinosa JC, et al: La epidemia del cólera de 1856 en el valle central: analysis y consecuencias demográficas. **Rev Hist (Costa Rica)** 1976;2(3):81-129

**France**

Adelsen CE: The last days of Adam Mickiewicz, poet of freedom. **Mankind** 1976;5(5):16-20, 60-1
Maitre AM, Ducable G: Louis-René Villermé et le choléra en 1832. **Hist Sci Med** 1982;16(4):317-25

**Germany**

Breyer H: Max von Pettenkofer: Arzt im Vorfeld der Krankheit. Leipzig, Hirzel, 1980. 234 p.
Dorsz-Szteke E, Maciejewska-Dorsz K: O cholerze w Szczecinie w i poł. xix wieku. **Wiad Lek** 1981 Oct 1;34(19):1657-9
Helm D: Die Cholera in Lübeck. Epidemieprophylaxe und -bekämpfung im 19. Jahrhundert. Neumünster, Wachholtz, 1979. 81 p. (Kieler Beiträge zur Geschichte der Medizin und Pharmazie, 16).
Howard-Jones N: Cardiac catheterization, a historical note. **Bull Hist Med** 1973 Sep-Oct;47(5):524-6
Howard-Jones N: Robert Koch and the cholera vibrio: a centenary. **Br Med J [Clin Res]** 1984 Feb 4;288(6414):379-81
Mochmann H, Kohler W: The clarification of the etiology of Asiatic cholera by the German cholera commission under the direction of Robert Koch in the year 1883--1884. **Indian J Public Health** 1983 Jan-Mar;27(1):6-20
Piechocki W: Robert Kochs Aufenthalt in Halle zur Cholerabekämpfung im Spiegel der Presse (1893). **Wiss Beitr Martin Luther Univ Halle Wittenberg** 1983;5-R80:41-9
Stollenwerk A: Die Cholera im Regierungsbezirk Koblenz [1832]. **Jahrb Westdtsch Landesgesch** 1979;5:241-72
Takeda Y, Zinnaka Y: [Centenary of the discovery of Vibrio cholerae by Robert Koch] (Jpn) **Nippon Saikingaku Zasshi** 1984 Jul;39(4):709-12

**Great Britain**

Durey M: The return of the plague. British society and the cholera 1831-2. Dublin, Gill and Macmillan, 1979. 269 p.
Janet RJ: Providence, prayer and cholera: the English general fast of 1832. **Hist Mag Protest Episc Church** 1982;51(3):297-317
Kearns G: Cholera and public health reform in nineteenth-century England and Wales: interpreting the geographical patterns. **Soc Soc Hist Med Bull (Lond)** 1984 Dec;35:30-2
Kerr B: Henry Moule and cholera in Dorset: nineteenth-century sanitary reform. **Hist Today** 1978;28(10):672-80
Lilienfeld AM, Lilienfeld DE: John Snow, the Broad Street pump and modern epidemiology. **Int J Epidemiol** 1984 Sep;13(3):376-8
Parfit J: The Oxford Board of Health 1831-1833. **Public Health** 1982 Jan;96(1):25-30
Roberts A: Down the drain: cholera in Britain. **Nurs Times** 1984 Oct 10-16;80(41):40-3
Smith CE: The Broad Street pump revisited. **Int J Epidemiol** 1982 Jun;11(2):99-100

**Greece**

Degleris NE, Rozos BP: [Public health, medical education and social care of Ionian Isles in the middle of the 19th century (press documents)] (Gre). **Arch Hyg** 1980;:90–101

**Hungary**

Blázy A: Az 1855. évi kolerajárvány hatása Zala megye lakosságára. [Effect of the 1855 cholera epidemic on the population of Zala county.] (Hun) MTA Pécsi es Veszpremi Akademiai Bizottságának Értesítője. (Proceeding of the Conference on the History of Settlements, Székeféhérvár 24–25 May, 1978). 1978; 3:105–113.
Mészárosné Varga M: Az 1831-es kolerajárvány Veszprém megyei története. **Orv Hetil** 1980 Jan 27;121(4):223–6
Rákóczi T: Adatok az 1831. évi kolerajárvány Moson megyei történetéhez. Tanulmányok Györ és vidéke történetéböl (Gecsényi L., ed.), Györ, Györ-Sopron megyei l.sz. Levéltár, 1978, p. 71–8.
Szállási A: Egy kolera-kiadvány 1831-böl. **Orvostort Kozl** 1979;87–88(25 no 1–2):307–9
Szüts T: Ujabb adatok az 1831. Evi kolerajárvány történetéhez. **Orvostort Kozl** 1979;87–88(25 no 1–2):255–9

**India**

Hughes E: The fight against cholera: India 1812 – 1912. **Hist Med (Lond)** 1975 Autumn-Winter;6(3–4):68–74
Klein I: Cholera: theory and treatment in nineteenth century India. **J Indian Hist** 1980;58(1–3):35–51
Lutzker E: Some unanswered questions in medical history. In: Congrès international d'histoire de la médecine, XXVe, Quebec, 1976. Actes. Québec, 1977. p. 917–27.

**Italy**

Belloni L: Un circolo bernardiano in Italia: la Società delle Scienze Biologiche in Torino. Luigi Vella de la curaroterapia del tetano. **Physis** 1981;23(3):301–10
Mercolli C: Il Ticion del XIX. secolo ed il colera. **Krankenpflege (Bern)** 1982 Aug;(8):85–7
Messina AF: Societa' ed epidemia. Il colera a Napoli nel 1836. Milano, Angeli, 1979. 174 p;
Pontuale L: L'urbanistica 'risanatrice' a Napoli: meglio il colera? **Comunita** 1975;29(174):128–65
Subba Rao M: Original observations of Filippo Pacini on vibrio cholera. **Bull Indian Inst Hist Med (Hyderabad)** 1978;8(1–4):32–8
Vetro C: Il colera del 1837 in provincia di Agrigento. **Arch Stor Sicil** 1975;4(1):57–90

**Japan**

Kikuchi K: Edo jidai ni okeru korera-byô – ne ryûkô – jiin kakochô ni yoru jisshô. **Jimbun Chiri** 1978;30(5):63–77
Yamamoto SI: Cholera in Japan. In Ogawa T, ed: Public health. Tokyo, Saikon, 1981. p. 169–89.

**Poland**

Chojna JW: Piśmiennictwo lekarskie związane z epidemia cholery na ziemiach polskich w czasie powstania listopadowego. **Arch Hist Med (Warsz)** 1981;44(2):143–55

**Romania**

Sibechi G: Unele ştiri despre epidemia de holeră din Moldova anului 1848. **Rev Med Chir Soc Med Nat Iasi** 1983 Jul-Sep;87(3):406, 458, 470

**Spain**

Bornside GH: Jaime Ferran and preventive inoculation against cholera. **Bull Hist Med** 1981 Winter;55(4):516–32
Fernández García A: Enfermedad y sociedad: la epidemia de cólera de 1865 en Madrid. **Cuad Invest Hist** 1979;3:155–86
Fernández García A: Repercusiones sociales de las epidemias de colera del siglo XIX. In: Sociedad Española de Historia de la Medicina. V Congreso Nacional. Madrid, 1977. **Asclepio** 1977;29:127–45
Jiménez MR: La epidemia de colera de 1834 en Zaragoza y su provincia. **Asclepio** 1982;34:3–31
Jordi R: Humor colérico. **Circ Farm** 1981 Apr;12(137):61–71
Rodríguez Ocaña E: El cólera de 1834 en Granada. Enfermedad catastrófica y crisis social. Granada, Universidad de Granada, 1983. 170 p. (Colección Monográfica Universidad de Granada, 81).
Rodriguez Ocaña E: Higiene y terapeutica anticolericas en la primera epidemia de colera en España, 1833–1835. **Asclepio** 1982;34:71–100
Rodriguez Ocaña E: La dependencia social de un comportamiento científico: los medicos españoles y el cólera de 1833–35. **Dynamis** 1981;1:101–30
Ruíz de Loyzaga S: La epidemia de cólera de 1855 en Valdegovía. **Bol Inst Sancho Sabio** 1977;21:441–50
Urquijo y Goitia JR de: Madrid ante la epidemia de cólera de 1854–56. **Asclepio** 1983;35:27–51
Zubiri Vidal F, Zubiri de Salinas R: Las epidemias de peste y cólera morbo-asiático en Aragón (Zaragoza, 1652 y 1885; Caspe, 1834; Alcañiz y Jaca, 1885). Zaragoza, Diputacion Provincial, Institucion 'Fernando el Catolico', [1980]. 195 p. (Temas Aragoneses, 32).

**United States**

Beatty WK: When cholera scourged Chicago. **Chic Hist** 1982;11(1):2–13
Brill RE: The Sabbath-day summer: Madison, Indiana, and the 1849 cholera epidemic. **Indiana Hist Soc** 1982 Sep;8(3):3–16
Cotter JV, Patrick LL: Disease and ethnicity in an urban environment. **Ann Assoc Am Geogr** 1981;71(1):40–9
Divett RT: His chastening rod: cholera epidemics and the Mormons. **Dialogue J Mormon Thought** 1979;12(3):6–15
Kanter DM: The invisible monster. Investigations into the 1833 cholera epidemic in Southern Indiana. **Indiana Med Hist Q** 1978;4(4):4–13
Phaneuf MM: Sanitation and cholera: Springfield and the 1866 epidemic. **Hist J West Mass** 1980;8(1):26–36
Pyle GF: The diffusion of cholera in the United States in the nineteenth century. **Geogr Anal** 1969;1:59–75
Sturm J: Winds from the east – the cholera of '32. **Chronicle** 1982;4:24–7
Thomison JB: Disease in Nashville: a short history. **J Tenn Med Assoc** 1983 Mar;76(3):151–5
Weissmann G: Cholera at the Harvey. **Hosp Pract** 1982 Feb;17(2):129–31, 135–6

**USSR**

Brevnov VP: M. Ia. Mudrov v bor'be s kholernoĭ épidemieĭ v Rossii (1830–1831 gg.). **Feldsher Akush** 1981;46(11):54–6
Dolgova SP: Zapiski ochevidtsa o chumnom bunte v Moskve v 1771 godu. **Sov Arkh** 1976;(6):66–70
Kosareva AA, Kondrat'ev IM: 'Babii bunt' 1830 goda. **Vopr Istor** 1980;8:180–3
Zikeev PD: Chrezvychaĭnyĭ kholernyĭ s'ezd Obshchestva russkikh vracheĭ v pamiat' N. I. Pirogova. **Sov Zdravookhr** 1981;(11):56–9

**Yugoslavia**

Belicza B: Zagreb u borbi protiv kolere. In: I simpozij o historiji mikrobiologije i imunologije u Hrvatskoj do 1923. godine. Zagreb, Jugoslavenskoj akademiji, 1973. p. 17–29.
Jovin S: Kolera u prošlosti Novog Sada. **Med Pregl** 1981;34(7–8):349–54

**Zaire**

Schyns C, Fossa A, Colaert J: L'épidémie de choléra dans le Sud-Kivu. **Bull Seance Acad R Sci Outre Mer** 1979;(3):451–65

## CLEFT PALATE

Hauben D: Die Geschichte der gespaltenen Gaumen. **Z Plast Chir** 1981 Dec;5(4):228–33
Hoffmann-Axthelm W: Zur Geschichte des Gaumenobturators. **Quintessenz Zahntech** 1980 Mar-Apr;6(3,4):85–93, 97–100

**Africa**

Cervenka J: African mask with cleft lip and palate. **Cleft Palate J** 1984 Jan;21(1):38–40

**1450–1700**

Walter JD: More on 'hare-lip'. **Cleft Palate J** 1984 Jan;21(1):44

**1700 to Present**

Kogge D: Zur geschichtlichen Entwicklung der Behandlungsmassnahmen bei Lippen-Kiefer-Gaumenspalten. Diss. Bonn, 1981. 84 p.

**Poland**

Wajs S: O pierwszym zabiegu uranoplastyki w Polsce. **Czas Stomatol** 1980 Nov;33(11):1043–6
Wajs S: Obturatory stosowane w leczeniu protetycznym rozszczepów wrodzonych lub nabytych podniebienia twardego i miękkiego. Czesc III. **Nov Med Tekh** 1979 May-Jun;29(3):211–8

**United States**

Herschfeld JJ: Norman W. Kingsley and his pioneering techniques in the correction of cleft palate. **Bull Hist Dent** 1983 Apr;31(1):23–8
Potter J: Cleft palate—fifty years on. **Ann Plast Surg** 1983 Jan;10(1):12–4

# DISEASES AND INJURIES

### CLUBFOOT

Dustmann HO, Ebel V: Darstellungen von Fussdeformierungen und deren Behandlung in der Kunst. In KF Schlegel, ed: Der Körperbehinderte in Mythologie und Kunst. Stuttgart, New York, Thieme, 1983. p. 41–56.

**1700 to Present**

**France**

Vigliani F, Vigliani MC: La strefopodia nella fantasia e nell'arte di Gustave Flaubert. **Chir Organi Mov** 1980 Jul–Aug;66(4):533–43

### CRETINISM

**Americas**

Benítez RF: Historia de la deficiencia mental endemica en la region Andina. **Asclepio** 1982;34:339–76

### CYSTIC FIBROSIS

Kollberg H: 1000 års erfarenhet av cystisk fibros--ett samlat 'testamente'. **Lakartidningen** 1981 Sep 16;78(38):3258–60

**1450–1700**

Hollander DH: Etiogenesis of the European cystic fibrosis polymorphism: heterozygote advantage against veneral syphilis? **Med Hypotheses** 1982 Feb;8(2):191–7

### CYSTS

**1700 to Present**

**Great Britain**

Kessler RK, Kessler WB, Constantine J, et al: Sclerosis of thyroid cysts. **Arch Intern Med** 1984 Aug;144(8):1693, 1697

**Sweden**

Stolt CM, Oberg L: En ovariotomi i Borås 1814. **Sydsven Medicinhist Sallsk Arsskr** 1984;21:109–21

### DECOMPRESSION SICKNESS

Gunby P: 'Air therapy' history offers lessons for clinicians today. **JAMA** 1981 Sep 4;246(10):1064, 1066

**1700 to Present**

**Great Britain**

Donald KW: Submarine escape breathing air. A review and analysis of animal and human experiments by the Royal Navy. **Bull Physiopathol Respir (Nancy)** 1979 Sep–Oct;15(5):739–54

### DENGUE

**1450–1700**

**Panama**

McSherry JA: Some medical aspects of the Darien scheme: was it dengue? **Scott Med J** 1982 Apr;27(2):183–4

**1700 to Present**

Laird M: Integrirovannye metody bor'by s perenoschikami i ugroza gemorragicheskoĭ likhoradlki Denge v tropicheskoĭ zone Tikhogo Okeana. **Parazitologiia** 1984 Mar–Apr;18(2):99–105

**Americas**

Acuña HR: Aedes aegypti, dengue y fiebre amarilla. **Bol Of Sanit Panam** 1982 Dec:93(6):503–5

**Greece**

Halstead SB, Papaevangelou G: Transmission of dengue 1 and 2 viruses in Greece in 1928. **Am J Trop Med Hyg** 1980 Jul;29(4):635–7

**Indonesia**

Guzmán Tirado MG: Dengue. I. Antecedentes históricos; agentes etiológicos; cuadro clínico. **Rev Cubana Med Trop** 1980 May–Aug;32(2):123–30

**Spain**

Orozco Acuaviva A: La primera epidemia de 'Dengue' en España. In: Sociedad Española de Historia de la Medicina. V Congreso Nacional. Madrid, 1977. **Asclepio** 1977;29:209–15

### DIABETES

Brillante C, Laffi GC: Profilo storico-sintetico della malattia diabetica (dal papiro di Ebers a Banting e Best. **Minerva Med** 1982 Apr 21;73(17):1087–106
Drury MI: Diabetes in pregnancy--Matthews Duncan revisited. **Ir J Med Sci** 1984 Apr;153(4):144–51
Kudva BT: On diabetes mellitus. **J Assoc Physicians India** 1984 Apr;32(4):320, 375
Labhart A: Diskursives Denken und Intuition in der medizinischen Forschung. **Helv Chir Acta** 1981 Feb;47(6):859–72
Lozoya M: Antecedentes historicos de la diabetes Mellitus. **Med Tradic** 1980;3(10):5–9
Ney D, Hollingsworth DR: Nutritional management of pregnancy complicated by diabetes: historical perspective. **Diabetes Care** 1981 Nov–Dec;4(6):647–55
Tratner E: A new Talmudic source on the history of diabetes (late onset). **Koroth** 1982 Aug;8(3/4):205–12
Trowell HC: Ants distinguish diabetes mellitus from diabetes insipidus. **Br Med J [Clin Res]** 1982 Jul 17;285(6336):217
Wang Zhipu: [Brief history of consumption-thirst syndrome (diabetes mellitus)] (Chi). **Chin J Med Hist** 1980;10:79–82

**China**

Miyasita S: An historical analysis of Chinese drugs in the treatment of hormonal diseases, goitre and diabetes mellitus. **Am J Chin Med** 1980 Spring–Summer;8(1–2):17–25

**1450–1700**

**Poland**

Dudziński W: Choroba i zgon króla Michała Korybuta Wiśniowieckiego. **Wiad Lek** 1979 Jan 1;32(1):55–8

**1700 to Present**

Bliss M: The aetiology of the discovery of insulin. In Roland CG, ed: Health, disease and medicine. Toronto, Hannah Institute for the History of Medicine, 1984. p. 333–46.
Dérot M: Perspectives en diabétologie (d'hier à demain). **Bull Mem Acad R Med Belg** 1981;136(8–9):435–42
Kolář J, Michalková D: Sedesát roku používání inzulínu v léčbě diabetes mellitus. **Cesk Pediatr** 1983 Jan;38(1):55–7
Luft R: Lysande upptäckter, men djup klyfta mellan forskningen och de sjukas situation. **Lakartidningen** 1984 Jun 27;81(26–27):2586–94
Whitehouse FW: Classification and pathogenesis of the diabetes syndrome: a historical perspective. **J Am Diet Assoc** 1982 Sep;81(3):243–6

**Canada**

Burrow GN, Hazlett BE, Phillips MJ: A case of diabetes mellitus. **N Engl J Med** 1982 Feb 11;306(6):340–3
Dr. Frederick Banting getting out of town: **Can Med Assoc J** 1984 May 1;130(9):1215–23
Marliss EB: Insulin: sixty years of use. **N Engl J Med** 1982 Feb 11;306(6):362–4
Sunday ME: Canada's Best. **Harv Med Alumni Bull** 1980 Dec;54(6):10–15

**Czechoslovakia**

Syllaba J: Rozvoj československé diabetologie v posledních 60 letech. **Vnitr Lek** 1984 Apr;30(4):401–5

**France**

Federspil G: Lo sviluppo delle teorie sulla glicogenesi e il diabete in Claude Bernard e oggi. **Med Secoli** 1979 Jan–Apr;16(1):31–50
Pyke DA: Claude Bernard et l'étiologie du diabète. **Journ Annu Diabetol Hotel Dieu** 1981;:153–61

**Germany**

Bibergeil H: Vom Diabetikerheim zum Diabetes-Forschungsinstitut--50 jähriges Jubiläum im Zentralinstitut für Diabetes 'Gerhardt Katsch' Karlsburg. **Z Gesamte Inn Med** 1981 Jan 1;36(1):1–3
Dorsche HH von, Dittrich HM: Die Diabetesforschung in Greifswald im 19. Jahrhundert und am Beginn des 20. Jahrhunderts in ihrer Bedeutung

für die Diabetologie. **Anat Anz** 1982;152(5):435–48
Hauk J: Carl Harko Hermann Johannes von Noorden (1858–1944), sein Leben und Werk unter besonderer Berücksichtigung seiner Theorien über die Ursachen des Diabetes mellitus. Diss. Mainz, 1980. 288 p.
Kaiser W, Völker A: Oskar Minkowski (1858–1931). **Z Gesamte Inn Med** 1981 Dec 15;36(24):973–9

**Great Britain**

McLetchie NG: Alloxan diabetes: the sorcerer and his apprentice. **Diabetologia** 1982 Jul;23(1):72–5

**Hungary**

Honti J, Szám I: A budapesti Hann Fanny és a Hann syndroma (tranzitoricus diabetes insipidus). **Orv Hetil** 1984 Jun 24;125(26):1581–2

**New Zealand**

Watson MH: The early days of insulin in New Zealand. **NZ Med J** 1981 May 27;93(684):347–50

**Romania**

Teichman SL, Aldea PA: The other side of the insulin story: Paulescu's contribution. **NY State J Med** 1984 Jun;84(6):312–6

**Sweden**

Carlström S: Första insulinbehandlingen av diabetes i Lund--ett beriktigande. **Sydsven Medicinhist Sallsk Arsskr** 1980;:49–51

**United States**

A case of diabetes mellitus: **N Engl J Med** 1982 Jul 8;307(2):127–8

**USSR**

Angeli I: 50 éve halt meg Oskar Minkowski a pancreas-diabetes felfedezöje. **Orv Hetil** 1981 Jul 12;122(28):1726–9

**Yugoslavia**

Spasić B, Spasić S: Razvoj službe za brigu o obolelim od dijabetesa u Surdulici. **Srp Arh Celok Lek** 1982 Nov;109(11):1519–26

## DIARRHEA

**1450–1700**

**France**

Simon de Vallambert on the treatment of diarrhea in infants (1565): **Pediatrics** 1982 Feb;69(2):163

**1700 to Present**

Pratt EL: Development of parenteral fluid therapy. **J Pediatr** 1984 Apr;104(4):581–4

## DIGESTIVE SYSTEM

Ballantyne GH: Review of sigmoid volvulus: history and results of treatment. **Dis Colon Rectum** 1982 Jul–Aug;25(5):494–501
Ballantyne GH: The meaning of ileus. Its changing definition over three millennia. **Am J Surg** 1984 Aug;148(2):252–6
Beal JM: Historical perspective of gallstone disease. **Surg Gynecol Obstet** 1984 Feb;158(2):181–9
de Moulin D: The value of tobacco smoke in the treatment of intussusception. **Neth J Surg** 1984 Apr;36(2):57–9
Gonvers JJ: L'ulcère: un passé célèbre, un avenir incertain? **Rev Med Suisse Romande** 1984 May;104(5):387–94
Loudon IS: Chlorosis, anaemia, and anorexia nervosa. **Br Med J [Clin Res]** 1980 Dec 20–27;281(6256):1669–75
Puigvert A, Mallo N: El sindrome próstato-hemorroidal. **Rev Clin Esp** 1983 Feb 15;168(3):217–9
Spicer RD: Infantile hypertrophic pyloric stenosis: a review. **Br J Surg** 1982 Mar;69(3):128–35

**France**

Gérard A: De la gastro-entérologie à la politique: la fistule du Grand Roi. **LARC Med** 1983 May;3(5):341–8

**Before 500 A.D.**

Schoental R: Mycotoxins and the Bible. **Perspect Biol Med** 1984 Autumn;28(1):117–20

**500 A.D.–1450**

**Arabic**

Hadžiomeragić M: Prikaz znanja o bolestima jezika prije 1000 godina. **Stomatol Vjesn** 1983;12(3–4):147–51
Hajal F: Psychological treatment of anorexia: a case from the ninth century. **J Hist Med Allied Sci** 1982 Jul;37(3):325–8

**France**

Wallner B: The Middle English translation of Guy de Chauliac's Treatise on ulcers. Part II. Notes, glossary, marginalia. Book IV of the Great surgery. Edited from Ms. New York Academy of Medicine 12 and related mss. Stockholm, Almqvist & Wiksell International, 1983. 48 p. (Acta Universitatis Lundensis, Sectio I Theologica Juridica Humaniora 44).

**1450–1700**

**France**

Bernier JJ, Chevallier P, Teysseire D, et al: La maladie de Louis XIII. Tuberculose intestinale ou maladie de Crohn? **Nouv Presse Med** 1981 Jun 20;10(27):2243, 2247–50
Goldfischer S, Janis M: A 42-year-old king with a cavitary pulmonary lesion and intestinal perforation. **Bull NY Acad Med** 1981 Mar;57(2):139–43
Rudolph G: Histoire mémorable d'une fille d'Anjou laquelle a été quatre ans sans user d'aucune nourriture que de peu d'eau commune; anorexie mentale (?) au XVIe siècle. In: Congrès National des Sociétés Savantes, 93e, Tours, 1968. Comptes Rendus. Paris, 1971. Section des Sciences, Tome II. p. 17–29.

**Germany**

Eisinger J: Lead and wine. Eberhard Gockel and the colica Pictonum. **Med Hist** 1982 Jul;26(3):279–302

**Great Britain**

Newman C: Nature of Samuel Pepys's 'wind colic'. **Br Med J [Clin Res]** 1980 Dec 20–27;281(6256):1716–7

**1700 to Present**

Berk RN: Gallstones: diagnostic imaging in historical perspective. **Pharos** 1983 Winter;46(1):30–4
Habel G: Zur Geschichte der Säuglingspylorusstenose. **Padiatr Grenzgeb** 1983;22(2–3):203–5
Rosenberg D: Evolução do tratamento cirúrgico da úlcera duodenal. **Rev Hosp Clin Fac Med Sao Paulo** 1980 Oct;35(5):247–54
Thiébaud M: Traitement de l'ulcère gastro-duodénal. Point de vue du chirurgien. **Rev Med Suisse Romande** 1984 May;104(5):373–7
Westaby D, Williams R: The history injection sclerotherapy for esophageal varices. **Gastrointest Endosc** 1983 Nov;29(4):303–7

**France**

Grebeneva LS: K 150-letiiu opisaniia Kruivel'e prostoĭ khronicheskoĭ iazvy zheludka. **Klin Med (Mosk)** 1981 May;59(5):112–4
Niaussat P: Les 'coliques sèches' dans la Marine au XIXe siècle: Amédée Lefevre et son combat contre une tenace erreur médicale. In: Congrès National des Sociétés Savantes, 104e, Bordeaux, 1979. Comptes Rendus. Paris, 1979. Section des Sciences, Fasc. IV. p. 183–91.

**Germany**

Katz O: Der 'Führer' behandelte sich selbst. Aus jetzt verfügbaren Aufzeichnungen des Leibarztes Theo Morell werden realistische Konturen der geheimnisvollen Krankheiten Adolf Hitlers erkennbar (I). **Fortschr Med** 1984 Oct 4;102(37):70–1

**Great Britain**

Chitwood WR: Ludlow's esophageal diverticulum: a preternatural bag. **Surgery** 1979 May;85(5):549–53
Fielding JH: Crohn's disease in London in the latter half of the nineteenth century. **Ir J Med Sci** 1984 Jun;153(6):214–20
Smith JL: Sir Arbuthnot Lane, chronic intestinal stasis, and autointoxication. **Ann Intern Med** 1982 Mar;96(3):365–9
Stout G: Adult hypertrophic pyloric stenosis--a description in 1834? **J R Coll Gen Pract** 1983 Apr;33(249):239–41

**Norway**

Ostensen H, Burhol PG, Bonnevie O, et al: Changes in the pattern of peptic ulcer disease in the northern part of Norway between 1946 and 1981. **Scand J Gastroenterol** 1982 Nov;17(8):1073-6

**Poland**

Horbowska-Marzec H, Grodzicka-Królak H, Wielopolska H: Enterowirusy w przypadkach limfocytarnego zapalenia opon mózgowordzeniowych w Warszawie w latach 1963-1976. **Przegl Epidemiol** 1979;33(4):461-6

Rudowski W: Ostatnia choroba Generała Stefana Grota-Roweckiego (1895-1944). **Arch Hist Med (Warsz)** 1983;46(4):487-502

Sobień-Kopczyńska S, Gęsicka T, Rybus B, et al: Epidemiologia choroby Wrzodowej u dzieci w latach 1968-1978 w dzielnicy Lódź-Bałuty. **Pediatr Pol** 1980 Apr;55(4):487-93

**Spain**

Basas M: La epidemia del cólera morbo de 1854-1855 en Bilbao y otras noticias de este tiempo. **Estud Duesto** 1969;17:135-73

**United States**

Janowitz HD: Crohn and his disease. **Lancet** 1983 Nov 12;2(8359):1140

Kirsner JB: Landmark perspective. Crohn's disease. **JAMA** 1984 Jan 6;251(1):80-1

Kovalcik PJ: Early history of regional enteritis. **Curr Surg** 1982 Nov-Dec;39(6):395-400

Thompson WT: Don't just do something.... **Va Med** 1980 Feb;107(2):146-9

Zucker GM, Clayman CB: Landmark perspective: Bertram W. Sippy and ulcer disease therapy. **JAMA** 1983 Oct 28;250(16):2198-202

**USSR**

Kotel'nikov VP: Nauchnoe nasledie A. V. Martynova v izuchenii zabolevaniĭ podzheludochnoĭ zhelezy i zhelchevyvodiashchikh puteĭ. **Klin Med (Mosk)** 1983 Apr;61(4):117-9

## DIPHTHERIA

### 1700 to Present

Alberti PW: Tracheotomy versus intubation. A 19th century controversy. **Ann Otol Rhinol Laryngol** 1984 Jul-Aug;93(4 Pt 1):333-7

**France**

Gilbrin E: Gaston Ramon (1886-1963). Le soixantième anniversaire des anatoxines. **Hist Sci Med** 1984;18(1):53-60

**Germany**

Schadewaldt H: Emil von Behring und die Entwicklung der deutschen Immunologie. **Med Welt** 1979;30(48):1795-801

**Great Britain**

Mann RJ, Key JD: Joseph Bell, M.D., F.R.C.S.: 'notes on a case of paralysis following diphtheria'. **Pharos** 1982 Spring;45(2):27-9

Whitfield AG: The kiss of death (Princess Alice). **Ann R Coll Surg Engl** 1979 Sep;61(5):390-2

**Netherlands**

de Knecht-van Eekelen A: Abraham Pieter Fokker (1840-1906) en de serumtherapie bij difterie. **Tijdschr Geschied Geneeskd Natuurwet Wiskd Tech** 1984;7(4):161-71

**United States**

Cohn M: An introduction to 'Le Pap'. **Cell Immunol** 1982 Jan 1;66(1):11-6

Collier RJ: From Pap to ApUp. **Cell Immunol** 1982 Jan 1;66(1):17-23

Matossian MK: The throat distemper reappraised. **Bull Hist Med** 1980 Winter;54(4):529-43

Robinton ED: Anna Wessels Williams. In: Notable American women. The modern period. Cambridge, Mass., Belknap-Harvard Univ. Press, 1980. 4:737-9.

**USSR**

Kokhan AI, Miliavskiĭ VM: Sestry miloserdiia v bor'be s épidemieĭ difterii. **Med Sestra** 1983 Oct;42(10):48-9

**Yugoslavia**

Snajder D: Pola veka rada na eradikaciji difterije u našoj zemlji. **Srp Arh Celok Lek** 1983 Feb;111(2):239-48

## DISLOCATIONS

### 500 A.D.-1450

**Poland**

Gładykowska-Rzeczycka J: Dislocation of the hip joint (probably congenital) in the woman from the mediaeval burial ground in Poland. **Folia Morphol (Warsz)** 1980;39(2):211-4

## DRUG ADDICTION

Kramer JC: Opium rampant: medical use, misuse and abuse in Britain and the West in the 17th and 18th centuries. **Br J Addict** 1979 Dec;74(4):377-89

Palmer C, Horowitz M, ed: Shaman woman, mainline lady: women's writings on the drug experience. New York, Morrow, 1982. 285 p.

Way EL: History of opiate use in the Orient and the United States **Ann NY Acad Sci** 1982;398:12-23

**Japan**

Inque H: Le problème de l'opium durant la période Jiaqing et Daoguang. **Toyoschi Kenkyu** 1982;41(1):58-83, 3-4

**United States**

Gomberg ES: Historical and political perspective: women and drug use. **J Soc Issues** 1982;38(2):9-23

### 1450-1700

Kaempfer E: Amoenitatum Exoticarum Politico-physico-medicarum. Fasciculi V, Quibus Continentur Variae Relationes, Observationes and Descriptiones Rerum Persicarum and Ulterioris Asiae (Lemgo: Meyeri, 1712). **J Hist Med Allied Sci** 1978 Jul;33(3):320-43

### 1700 to Present

Hurst DL, Hurst MJ: Bromide psychosis: a literary case. **Clin Neuropharmacol** 1984;7(3):259-64

Jeziorski K, Matsumoto H: Leczenie opiatowych zespołów odstawiennych (rys historyczny). **Pol Tyg Lek** 1984 Oct 22;39(43):1433-6

McClary A: The medicated woman: 1880. **Pharos** 1984 Summer;47(3):8-10

Moriarty KM, Alagna SW, Lake CR: Psychopharmacology. An historical perspective. **Psychiatr Clin North Am** 1984 Sep;7(3):411-33

Pharmacology of leadership: **Practitioner** 1980 Feb;224(1340):119

Pittman WE: The noble crusade: Richmond P. Hobson and the struggle to limit the international narcotics trade, 1920-1925. **Ala Hist Q** 1972;34(3-4):181-93

Sardi PA: Epidemiologia della tossicodipendenza e cicli storici di altri disturbi psichici. **Minerva Med** 1981 Sep 26;72(36):2447-52

Trebach AS: The heroin solution. New Haven, London, Yale University Press, 1982.

**Americas**

Walker WO: Drug control in the Americas. Albuquerque, University of New Mexico Press, 1981. xvi, 287 p.

**Austria**

Tschofen H: Die Drogenszene in Vorarlberg. Entwicklung und Abwehrmassnahmen. **Montfort** 1981;33(2):151-8

**Great Britain**

Berridge V: Opiate use in England, 1800-1926. **Ann NY Acad Sci** 1982;398:1-11

Cone TE: Overdosing with opium, a serious pediatric problem in England a century and a half ago. **Pediatrics** 1981;68:86

Crellin JK: Alcoholism and drug addiction in the 'nineties: an American in London. **Br J Addict** 1980 Jun;75(2):153-62

Edwards G, Busch C: Drug problems in Britain: a review of ten years. London, Academic Press, 1981. 333 p.

Miller WH: The habit of Sherlock Holmes. **Trans Stud Coll Physicians Phila** 1978 Jul;45(5):252-7

Pargas K: Bishop Charles Henry Brent (1862-1929)--a retrospective. 'That damned opium mess has started again'. **J Addict Res Found** 1979;8(9):7

Parssinen TM, Kerner K: Development of the disease model of drug addiction in Britain, 1870-1926. **Med Hist** 1980 Jul;24(3):275-96

Peters D: The British medical response to opiate addiction in the nineteenth

century. **J Hist Med Allied Sci** 1981 Oct;36(4):455–88
Schiller F: Thomas de Quincey's lifelong addiction. **Perspect Biol Med** 1976 Autumn;20(1):131–41

**Ireland**

Macken U: Drug abuse in Ireland. Cork [Ire.]. Mercier Press, 1975. 132 p.

**Mexico**

Gereffi G: Drug firms and dependency in Mexico: the case of the steroid hormones industry. **Int Organ** 1978;32:237–86

**Philippines**

Gamez GL: Drug abuse: an overview. **Unitas** 1972;45(3):11–23

**United States**

Brunswick AF: Social meanings and developmental needs: perspectives on black youth's drug abuse. **Youth Soc** 1980;11(4):449–73
Colp R Jr: Notes on Dr. William S. Halsted. **Bull NY Acad Med** 1984 Nov;60(9):876–87
Courtwright D: Opiate addiction in the American West, 1850–1920. **J West** 1982 Jul;21(3):23–31
Courtwright DT: Dark paradise: opiate addiction in America before 1940. Cambridge, London, Harvard Univ. Press, 1982. 270 p.
Courtwright DT, Joseph H, Des Jarlais DC: Memories from the street: oral histories of elderly methadone patients. **Oral Hist Rev** 1981;9:47–64
Courtwright DT: Opiate addiction as a consequence of the Civil War. **Civ War Hist** 1978;24(2):101–11
Courtwright DT: The female opiate addict in 19th-century America. **Essays Arts Sci** 1982;10:161–72
Courtwright DT: The hidden epidemic: opiate addiction and cocaine use in the South, 1860–1920. **J South Hist** 1983;49(1):57–72
Gerstein DR: Cultural action and heroin addiction. **Sociol Inq** 1981;51(3-4):355–70
Graner JL, Frederick W: William Halsted's cocaine habit. **Arch Ophthalmol** 1984 Dec;102(12):1746
Grob GN, ed: American perceptions of drug addiction: five studies, 1872–1912. New York, Arno Press, 1981. 1 v. (various pagings).
Grob GN, ed: Epidemiology of drug addiction: three studies, 1924–1926. New York, Arno, 1981 various pagings. Reprinted works.
Grob GN, ed: Narcotic addiction and American foreign policy: seven studies, 1924–1938. New York, Arno Press, 1981. 276 p. in various pagings. (Reprinted works).
Grob GN, ed: Origins of medical attitudes toward drug addiction in America: eight studies, 1791–1858. New York, Arno Press, 1981. 1 v. (various pagings).
Grob GN, ed: Public policy and the problem of addiction: four studies, 1914–1924. New York, Arno Press, 1981. 1 v. (various pagings).
Grob GN, ed: The medical professions and drug addiction: six studies, 1882–1832. New York, Arno, 1981. various pagings. Reprinted works.
Jaffe A: Addiction reform in the progressive age: scientific and social responses to drug dependence in the United States, 1870–1930. New York, Arno, 1981. vii, 358 p.
Kleber HD, Riordan CE: The treatment of narcotic withdrawal: a historical review. **J Clin Psychiatry** 1982 Jun;43(6 Pt 2):30–4
Lessard S: Busting our mental blocks on drugs and crime. **Wash Mon** 1971;3(4):6–18
McBride DC, Page JB: Adolescent Indian substance abuse: ecological and sociocultural factors. **Youth Soc** 1980;11(4):475–92
Maibaum M, López G: Drug abuse in the East Los Angeles Health District. **Aztlan** 1981;12(1):139–55
March JC: Public issues and private problems: women and drug use. **J Soc Issues** 1982;38(2):153–65
Marsh JC: Help seeking among addicted and nonaddicted women of low socioeconomic status. **Soc Serv Rev** 1980;54(2):239–48
Martin WR, Isbell H, ed: Drug addiction and the U. S. Public Health Service. Proceedings of symposium commemorating the 40th anniversary of the Addiction Research Center at Lexington, Ky. Rockville, Md., National Institute on Drug Abuse, 1978. xiv, 325 p. Historical contributions by R. H. Felix, C. K. Himmelsbach, J. W. Sloan, C. G. Eades, J. F. Maddux, R. L. DuPont, J. H. Jaffe, E. L. May.
Morgan HW, ed: Yesterday's addicts. American society and drug abuse 1865–1920. Norman, University of Oklahoma Press, 1974. viii, 220 p. Collected documents.
Nurco DN: Narcotic addiction over a quarter of a century in a major American city. Rockville, Md., U. S. Alcohol, Drug Abuse, and Mental Health Administration, 1979. vi, 92 p.
Preston W: Fear and loathing in addicted America. **Rev Am Hist** 1975;3(1):123–8
Sandos JA: Prostitution and drugs: the United States Army on the Mexican-American border, 1916–1917. **Pac Hist Rev** 1980;49(4):621–45
Stelle CC: Americans and the China opium trade in the nineteenth century. New York, Arno Press, 1981. 154 p. (Also Diss, Chicago, 1938).
Tamony P: Tripping out from San Francisco. **Am Speech** 1981;56(2):98–103
Vyhnanek L: 'Muggles,' 'Inchy,' and 'Mud': illegal drugs in New Orleans during the 1920's. **La Hist** 1981;22(3):253–79
Way EL: Hooked for thirty years: tales of an investigation. **Natl Inst Drug Abuse Res Monogr Ser** 1979;27:1–10
Whiteside HO: The drug habit in nineteenth-century Colorado. **Colo Mag** 1978;55(1):46–68
Winfree LT, Theis HE, Griffiths CT: Drug use in rural America: a cross-cultural examination of complementary social deviance theories. **Youth Soc** 1981;12(4):465–89

**Vietnam**

Pisztora F: A kábítószer--fogyasztás a régi Vietnámban. Az ellene folytatott harc mai formái. **Orv Hetil** 1984 Oct 14;125(42):2569–72, 2575

**DWARFISM**

Silverman FN: De l'art du diagnostic des nanismes et du diagnostic des nanismes dans l'art. **J Radiol** 1982 Feb;63(2):133–40

**DYSENTERY**

**Belgium**

Meulemans A: Dysenterie te Leuven in de XVIIe en de XVIIIe eeuw. **Farm Tijdschr Belg** 1979;56:267–77

**1700 to Present**

Dollct AJ. A report of reactive arthritis following dysentery in 1743. **Arthritis Rheum** 1981 Jun;24(6):860

**France**

Lebrun F: La grande dysenterie de 1779. **Histoire** 1981;39:17–24
Niaussat PM: Delioux de Savignac et le traitement des dysenteries. In: Congrès National des Sociétés Savantes, 107e. Brest, 1982. Comptes Rendus, Paris, 1983. Section des Sciences, Fasc. IV. p. 299–309.

**Netherlands**

Bruneel C: L'epidemie de dysenterie de 1779 dans les Pays-Bas autrichiens. **Bull Comm R Hist** 1979;145(3-4):191–395
Eerenbeemt HF van den: De 'Rode dood' in stad en meierij van 's-Hertogenbosch: een dysenterie-epidemie in de jaren 1779–1783. **Econ Soc Hist Jaarb** 1973;36:75–101

**United States**

Harvey AM: Amebic dysentery gets its name: the story of William Thomas Councilman. **Johns Hopkins Med J** 1980 May;146(5):185–92, 199–201

**EAR**

Stephens SD: The treatment of tinnitus--a historical perspective. **J Laryngol Otol** 1984 Oct;98(10):963–72

**United States**

Titche LL, Coulthard SW, Wachter RD, et al: Prevalence of mastoid infection in prehistoric Arizona Indians. **Am J Phys Anthropol** 1981 Nov;56(3):269–73

**Before 500 A.D.**

Ashby JK: De aurium doloris et vitium curis or concerning the care of pain and troubles of the ears. **J Speech Hear Disord** 1980 Aug;45(3):424–5

**Rome**

Petrakis NL: Diagonal earlobe creases, type A behavior and the death of Emperor Hadrian. **West J Med** 1980 Jan;132(1):87–91

**500 A.D.–1450**

**United States**

Titche LL, Wachter RD, Coulthard SW, et al: Mastoiditis in prehistoric Arizona Indians. **Ariz Med** 1981 Sep;38(9):712–4

**1700 to Present**

Black NA: Is glue ear a modern phenomenon? A historical review of the medical literature. **Clin Otolaryngol** 1984 Jun;9(3):155–63
Liston SL: Traumatic amputation of the external ear: the War of Jenkins' Ear and George Washington. **Am J Surg** 1984 Nov;148(5):599–601

Portmann M, Bebear JP, Bagot D'Arc M: L'histoire de l'otosclérose du XIXe siècle à 1952. **Acta Otorhinolaryngol Belg** 1982;36(2):297-305

**France**

Portmann G: The old and new in Meniere's disease -- over 60 years in retrospect and a look to the future. **Otolaryngol Clin North Am** 1980 Nov;13(4):567-75

Rauchfuss A: Zur korrekten Schreibweise des Namens von Prosper Menière und einige Anmerkungen zu Leben und Werk. **Laryngol Rhinol Otol (Stuttg)** 1984 Aug;63(8):381-5

**Germany**

Milstein S: Otosclerosis. **Am J Otol** 1981 Jan;2(3):283-5

### EDEMA

Trocmé C: Eléments pour une histoire de l'oedème pulmonaire. **Hist Sci Med** 1983;17(1):71-84

**1700 to Present**

Sternbach G: William Osler: narcotic-induced pulmonary edema. **J Emerg Med** 1983;1(2):165-7

Torack RM: Historical aspects of normal and abnormal brain fluids. III. Cerebral edema. **Arch Neurol** 1982 Jun;39(6):355-7

**United States**

Bing FC: Emma Kohman and the early history of nutritional edema. **J Am Diet Assoc** 1983 Jun;82(6):605-9

### ENCEPHALITIS

**Africa**

Lambrecht FL: Palaeoecology of Tsetse flies and sleeping sickness in Africa. **Proc Am Philos Soc** 1980 Oct 10;124(5):367-85

**1700 to Present**

**Africa**

Lyons M: Death camps in the Congo: administrative responses to sleeping sickness 1903-1911. **Soc Soc Hist Med Bull (Lond)** 1984 Jun;34:28-31

**Australia**

Kratochvil O: 'X' disease in Australia (a historical story of medical detection). **Geogr Med** 1982;12:1-6

**Germany**

Favazza AR: Behind the sickness of Hitler. **MD** 1981;25(5):37-8;25(7):15

Favazza AR: Hitler's encephalitis? **Am J Psychiatry** 1981 Jul;138(7):999-1000

**United States**

Reeves WC, Emmons RW, Hardy JL: Historical perspectives on California encephalitis virus in California. **Prog Clin Biol Res** 1983;123:19-29

**USSR**

Beklemishev VN: Problemy épidemiologii i épizootologii kleshchevogo éntsefalita (po neopublikovannym materialam iz arkhiva V. N. Beklemisheva). **Med Parazitol (Mosk)** 1983 Jan-Feb;52(1):66-74

Khodos KhG: Epidemicheskiĭ éntsefalit Ekonomo--nereshennaia nevrologicheskaia problema (k 60-letiiu opisaniia éntsefalita Ekonomo sovetskimi nevropatologami). **Zh Nevropatol Psikhiatr** 1981;81(2):124-7

### ENDOCRINE

**Before 500 A.D.**

**Rome**

Klawans HL: The acromegaly of Maximinus I: the possible influence of a pituitary tumor on the life and death of a Roman emperor. In Rose FC, Bynum WF, ed: Historical aspects of the neurosciences. New York, Raven, 1982. 317-26.

Ljunggren B: En stor man med en sjuk hjärna. **Sydsven Medicinhist Sallsk Arsskr** 1984;21:77-85

**1450-1700**

Rodger NW, Paulseth JE: Hazards in managing diabetic acidosis. **Can Med Assoc J** 1981 Aug 15;125(4):335

**1700 to Present**

Geller SA: Brown's (Cushing's) syndrome. **N Engl J Med** 1983 Jun 9;308(23):1425

**Canada**

Harrison RC, Mills F: Canadian contributions toward the comprehension of hyperinsulinism: the first successful excision of an insulinoma. **Can J Surg** 1980 Jul;23(4):401-3

**United States**

Ternberg JL: Surgical treatment of idiopathic hyperinsulinemic hypoglycemia in children. First successful subtotal pancreatectomy with preservation of spleen reported by Evarts A. Graham (1934). **J Thorac Cardiovasc Surg** 1984 Nov;88(5 Pt 2):898-901

**USSR**

Lebedev DD, Kovaleva EV, Semenova VN: Nekotorye voprosy revmatizma, éndokrinnykh i nervnykh zabolevaniĭ u deteĭ v trudakh V.I. Molchanova i ego uchenikov (k 110-letiiu so dnia rozhdeniia). **Pediatriia** 1980 Aug;(8):64-7

### EPILEPSY

Bergamini L, Benna P: Social aspects of epilepsy. **Prog Clin Biol Res** 1983;124:325-30

Fouquet C: Le cas de l'épilepsie. **Penelope** 1983;(8):10-2

Melville ID: The medical treatment of epilepsy: a historical review. In Rose FC, Bynum WF, ed: Historical aspects of the neurosciences. New York, Raven, 1982. p. 127-36.

Rektor I, Svejdová M, Hrazdira CL: Epilepsie a sociální problematika epileptiku v minulosti. **Cas Lek Cesk** 1983 Feb 4;122(5):153-4

Vasconcelos D: La enfermedad sagrada. Aspectos históricos y situación actual. **Gac Med Mex** 1982 Jan;118(1):35-7

**Malaysia**

Peng KL: A Malay cultural explanation for epilepsy. **Aust NZ J Psychiatry** 1983 Dec;17(4):397-9

**USSR**

Berman IW: Musicogenic epilepsy. **S Afr Med J** 1981 Jan 10;59(2):49-52

**Before 500 A.D.**

**Rome**

Disertori B, Piazza M: L'epilettologia di Apuleio. **Ann Osp Maria Vittoria Torino** 1977 Jul-Dec;20(7-12):341-53

Dolzani C: Un 'prelievo' di sangue adombrato in una poesia di Giovanni Pascoli? **Acta Med Hist Patav** 1982-83;29:25-8

**500 A.D.-1450**

**France**

Lesný I: Sílenství francouzského krále Karla VI. **Cas Lek Cesk** 1982 May 14;121(19):597-600

**1450-1700**

**Denmark**

Andersen S, ed: Simonis Paulli velmenende råd gennem hvilke formedelst Guds hjaelp en højadelig person lykkeligt blev kureret da han i året 1668 i Paris blev ramt af slag. **Dan Medicinhist Arbog** 1982;:73-91

**1700 to Present**

Beeck M: Merkmale epileptischer Bildnerei: mit Pathographie Van Gogh. Bern, Huber, 1982. 134 p.

Berrios GE: Epilepsy and insanity during the early 19th century. A conceptual history. **Arch Neurol** 1984 Sep;41(9):978-81

A brief history of the European meetings on electroencephalography and epileptology better known as the 'Colloques de Marseille': **Electroencephalogr Clin Neurophysiol** 1982;(35):VIII-XI

Miksanek T: Dostoevsky's The Idiot and psychic disorders in epilepsy. **Perspect Biol Med** 1982 Winter;25(2):231-7

Pasternak JL: An analysis of social perceptions of epilepsy: increasing rationalization as seen through the theories of Comte and Weber. **Soc Sci Med [Med Psychol Med Sociol]** 1981;15(3):223-9
Smith DB, Delgado Escueta AV, Cramer JA, et al: Historical perspective on the choice of antiepileptic drugs for the treatment of seizures in adults. **Neurology** 1983 Mar;33(3 Suppl 1):2-7
Vizioli R, De Rosa A: Medical education and epilepsy. **Prog Clin Biol Res** 1983;124:361-70

**France**

Gastaut H, Gastaut Y, Broughton R: Gustave Flaubert's illness: a case report in evidence against the erroneous notion of psychogenic epilepsy. **Epilepsia** 1984 Oct;25(5):622-37
Gastaut H, Gastaut Y: La maladie de Gustave Flaubert. **Rev Neurol (Paris)** 1982;138(6-7):467-92
Henri Gastaut and the Marseilles school's contribution to the neurosciences: Proceedings of the 25th and final Colloque de Marseille. **Electroencephalogr Clin Neurophysiol** 1982;35:1-447
Lennox MA: Professor Gastaut's contribution to the International League against Epilepsy. **Electroencephalogr Clin Neurophysiol** 1982;35:9-12

**Germany**

Heintel H: Hermann Andreas Reimer und seine 1855 eröffnete 'Heilanstalt für Epileptische' in Görlitz. **Medizinhist J** 1982;17(1/2):156-60
Lauschke HP: Der Epileptologe Herrmann Andreas Reimer in Görlitz. **Psychiatr Neurol Med Psychol (Leipz)** 1982 Dec;34(12):745-8
Müller H: Die Anstalt in Kork (Baden). Von der 'Heil- und Pflegeanstalt für epileptische Kinder' zum 'Epilepsiezentrum Kork'. Freiburg, Schulz, 1979. 190 p. (Freiburger Forschungen zur Medizingeschichte, Neue Folge, 10).

**Great Britain**

Taylor DC, March SM: Hughlings Jackson's Dr Z: the paradigm of temporal lobe epilepsy revealed. **J Neurol Neurosurg Psychiatry** 1980 Sep;43(9):758-67
Tyler KL: Hughlings Jackson: the early development of his ideas on epilepsy. **J Hist Med Allied Sci** 1984 Jan;39(1):55-64

**Poland**

Bilikiewicz A: Problematyka psychiatryczna w polskiej epileptologii ostatniego 35-lecia. **Psychiatr Pol** 1981 Mar-Apr;15(2):189-93

**United States**

Lewis JA: Petit mal epilepsy. An early American report. **NY State J Med** 1983 Jul-Sep;83(8-10):1051-2
Massey EW, Brannon WL, Riley TL: The 'jerks': mass hysteria or epilepsy? **South Med J** 1981 May;74(5):607-9
Massey JM, Massey EW: Ergot, the 'jerks,' and revivals. **Clin Neuropharmacol** 1984;7(1):99-105
Rowland LP: Changing approaches to the management of seizures: pharmacologic considerations. Introduction. **Epilepsia** 1982;23 Suppl 1:S1-4
Swinyard EA: History of the antiepileptic drugs. **Adv Neurol** 1980;27:1-9
Van Allen MW: Landmark perspective: introduction of sodium diphenyl hydantoinate. **JAMA** 1984 Feb 24;251(8):1068-9
Walker AE: The past four decades--experimental epilepsy. **Res Publ Assoc Res Nerv Ment Dis** 1983;61:1-17

**USSR**

Arkhangel'skiĭ GV: K prioritetu opisaniia akademikom V. M. Bekhterevym khoreicheskoĭ paducheĭ. **Zh Nevropatol Psikhiatr** 1981;81(6):929-30
Briskman AM: O 'khoreicheskoĭ paducheĭ' Bekhtereva i mioklonus-épilepsii. **Zh Nevropatol Psikhiatr** 1984;84(1):122-5
Gastaut H: New comments on the epilepsy of Fyodor Dostoevsky. **Epilepsia** 1984 Aug;25(4):408-11
Guliaeva SE: K istorii izucheniia épilepsii Kozhevnikova. **Zh Nevropatol Psikhiatr** 1984;84(6):919-29
Gurevich SA: Problemy épileptologii v otechestvennoĭ psikhiatrii XIX veka (po materialam pervykh psikhiatricheskikh zhurnalov). **Zh Nevropatol Psikhiatr** 1983;83(6):914-7
Retamal P: Consideraciones psicopatológicas sobre el diagnóstico de la enfermedad de Fedor Dostoyevski. **Actas Luso Esp Neurol Psiquiatr** 1983 May-Jun;11(3):231-4
Rice JL: Dostoevsky's medical history: diagnosis and dialectic. **Russ Rev** 1983;42(2):131-61
Voskuil PH: The epilepsy of Fyodor Mikhailovitch Dostoevsky (1821-1881). **Epilepsia** 1983 Dec;24(6):658-67

**Yugoslavia**

Hajnšek F: Osnivanje i razvitak antiepileptičke službe u SR Hrvatskoj (1956-1981). **Lijec Vjesn** 1982 May;104(5):212-4

**ERGOTISM**

Dotz W: St. Anthony's fire. **Am J Dermatopathol** 1980 Fall;2(3):249-53
Haller JS: Smut's dark poison: ergot in history and medicine. **Trans Stud Coll Physicians Phila** 1981 Mar;3(1):62-79
Kierulf H: L'ergotisme chez Bosch et Grünewald. **Nouv Presse Med** 1982 Oct 2;11(38):2803-9
Kierulf H: L'ergotisme chez Bosch et Grünewald. In International Congress of the History of Medicine, 27th, Barcelona, 1980. Actas. Barcelona, Académia de Ciències Mèdiques de Catalunya i Balears, 1981. p. 81-90.
Schramm A, Sperling M: Ergotamin-Schäden einst und heute. Vom Antoniusfeuer zum Medikamentenschaden. **MMW** 1983 Jun 10;125(23):492-4

**France**

Percebois G: Le feu Saint-Antoine et les Antonins dans nos provinces de l'Est. **Acad Soc Lorraines Sci** 1978;17(1):19-36

**1450-1700**

**Great Britain**

Matossian MK: Bewitched or intoxicated? The etiology of witch persecution in early modern England. **Medizinhist J** 1983;18(1-2):33-42

**United States**

Matossian MK: Ergot and the Salem witchcraft affair. **Am Sci** 1982 Jul-Aug;70(4):355-7
Spanos NP: Ergotism and the Salem witch panic: a critical analysis and an alternative conceptualization. **J Hist Behav Sci** 1983 Oct;19(4):358-69

**1700 to Present**

**Great Britain**

Suffolk horror story re-told: **East Anglican Dly Times** 1980 Aug 27

**United States**

Massey JM, Massey EW: Ergot, the 'jerks,' and revivals. **Clin Neuropharmacol** 1984;7(1):99-105

**EYE**

Bouffard P: Historique du strabisme et de la vision binoculaire. Paris, Editions du C.E.R.E.S., 1983. 64 p.
Cornand G: Trachome et armées. **Rev Int Trach Pathol Ocul Trop Subtrop** 1979;56(3-4):99-110
Kampmeier RH: Infection with Chlamydia trachomatis (TRIC agent). **Sex Transm Dis** 1984 Jul-Sep;11(3):169-72
Montandon D: History of plastic surgery of the orbital region. In S. J. Aston, et al., ed: Third international symposium of plastic and reconstructive surgery of the eye and adnexa. Baltimore, London, Williams & Wilkins, 1982. p. 2-10.
Orłowski WJ: Patronka cierpiacych na oczy. **Klin Oczna** 1984 May;86(5):231-5
Ravin JG: Lethal ocular injuries. **J Pediatr Ophthalmol Strabismus** 1980 Jan-Feb;17(1):53-4
Rogers BO: History of cosmetic blepharoplasty. In S. J. Aston, et al., ed: Third international symposium of plastic and reconstructive surgery of the eye and adnexa. Baltimore, London, Williams & Wilkins, 1982. p. 276-81.

**China**

Chen YZ: A brief introduction to the ancient history of eye injuries in China. **Chin Med J [Engl]** 1980 Mar;93(3):164-8

**Before 500 A.D.**

Dirckx JH: Hannibal's ophthalmia. **Pharos** 1983 Fall;46(4):28-30

**Greece**

Marketos SG, Eftychiadis A, Koutras DA: The first recognition of the association between goiter and exophthalmos. **J Endocrinol Invest** 1983 Oct;6(5):401-3

**Rome**

Benedum J: Die Augenanomalie an einem römischen Bildnis. **Medizinhist J** 1981;16(4):446-52

# DISEASES AND INJURIES

500 A.D.-1450

**Switzerland**

Bischoff P, Speiser P: Mittelalterliche Augenheilkunde im Kloster St. Gallen. **Gesnerus** 1982;39(1):47-52

1450-1700

**Austria**

Grossmann T: Die hl. Ottilie, Patronin der Augenkranken. Eine ungewöhnliche Abbildung am Gnadenstuhlaltar von Bad Aussee mit Krebsscherenattribut. **Klin Monatsbl Augenheilkd** 1981 Jun;178(6):480-1

**Italy**

Belloni L: Konsilien von Professoren aus Neapel und Padua gegen die Sehstörungen von G. V. Pinelli. **Gesnerus** 1981;38:135-42

1700 to Present

Bonnin P, Lavat P: A propos d'un cas d'épithéliopathie en plaques de Gass en 1860. **Bull Soc Ophtalmol Fr** 1983 Jan;83(1):49-52
Evens L: History of strabismus treatment. **Bull Soc Belge Ophtalmol** 1981;195:19-52
Figlio K: How does illness mediate social relations? Workmen's compensation and medico-legal practices, 1890-1940. In P. Wright, A. Treacher, ed: The problem of medical knowledge. Examining the social construction of medicine. Edinburgh, Edinburgh University Press, 1982. p. 174-224.
Lepore FE: Toward a definition of papilledema: a historical review, 1851-1911. **Surg Neurol** 1982 Mar;17(3):178-80
Miller S: Glaucoma--then and now. **Trans Ophthalmol Soc UK** 1980 Apr;100(pt 1):17-9
Newell FW: Centenary of Credé prophylaxis. **Am J Ophthalmol** 1980 Dec;90(6):874-5
Offret G: Souvenirs sur une pathologie oculaire en voie d'extinction. **Bull Soc Ophtalmol Fr** 1980 Jan;80(1):43-5
Ryan SJ, Mittl RN, Maumenee AE: The disciform response: an historical perspective. **Albrecht Von Graefes Arch Klin Exp Ophthalmol** 1980;215(1):1-20

**Austria**

Blodi FC: Was Mozart cross-eyed? **Arch Ophthalmol** 1981 May;99(5):823
Frick K: Dr. Med. Johann Gottfried Kumpf (1781-1862) und die ägyptische Augenkrankheit in Kärnten. **Carinthia** 1966;156:670-712

**France**

Le Fichoux Y, Marty P, Denis G, et al: Un ca d'ophtalmomyiase externe à oestrus ovis, linné, 1758 contractée sur la plage de Nice. **Acta Trop (Basel)** 1981 Dec;38(4):461-8
Schmidt V: Camille Pissarro, hans danske relationer og hans sygdom. **Dan Medicinhist Arbog** 1983;12:144-61

**Germany**

Fehlmann HR: 'Herrn Adams äusseres Augenmittel.' Eine Frankfurter Merkwürdigkeit aus dem Jahre 1794. **Pharm Ztg** 1980;125:407-8
Hruby K: Goethes Augenleiden. **Klin Monatsbl Augenheilkd** 1984 Jul;185(1):61-3
Kibel MA: Silver nitrate and the eyes of the newborn--a centennial. **S Afr Med J** 1981 Dec 26;60(26):979-80
Meyer-Schwickerath G: Das Annette von Droste-Hülshoff-Syndrom. **Klin Monatsbl Augenheilkd** 1984 Jun;184(6):574-7
Meyer-Schwickerath G: Die Geschichte der Photokoagulation und die Behandlung der intraocularen Tumoren mit dieser Methode. **Klin Oczna** 1981;83(2):59-61
Romanchuk KG: Fluorescein. Physiochemical factors affecting its fluorescence. **Surv Ophthalmol** 1982 Mar-Apr;26(5):269-83

**Great Britain**

Jay M, Phil M: Nettleship's two pedigrees of retinitis pigmentosa: a historical postscript. **Surv Ophthalmol** 1983 Jan-Feb;27(4):264-8
Jones BR: Changing concepts of trachoma and its control. **Trans Ophthalmol Soc UK** 1980 Apr;100(pt 1):25-9

**Hungary**

Csorba S: Kölcsey Ferenc hibás szemének kérdéséhez. **Orvostort Kozl** 1982;28(1-3):191-9

**Ireland**

Sullivan E: Ocular history of James Joyce. **Surv Ophthalmol** 1984 Mar-Apr;28(5):412-5

**Italy**

Guidotti A: Frequencies of cribra orbitalia in central Italy (19th century) under special consideration of their degrees of expression. **Anthropol Anz** 1984 Mar;42(1):11-6

**Pacific Islands**

Kluxen G, Bernsmeier H: Die endemischen Augenkrankheiten in Samoa 1910 bis 1913. **Klin Monatsbl Augenheilkd** 1979 Dec;175(6):841-5
Kluxen G, Bernsmeier H: Endemic ocular infections of the South Seas in the German colonial era. **Papua New Guinea Med J** 1980 Dec;23(4):197-9

**Romania**

Rosin A: Date de istoria medicinii privitoare la glaucom. **Viata Med [Medii Sanit]** 1980 Oct;28(10):233-5

**United States**

Ferry AP, Ferry MK: Dr. Isaac Thompson and his celebrated eye water. **Ophthalmology** 1984 May;91(5):528-37
McDonald PR: Evolution of cataract surgery since the deSchweinitz era. **Ophthalmic Surg** 1979 May;10(5):44-52
Wand M, Sewall RB: 'Eyes be blind, heart be still': a new perspective on Emily Dickinson's eye problem. **N Engl Q** 1979;52(3):400-6

**Yugoslavia**

Dugacki V: Le traitement des maladies oculaires dans la medecine populaire yougoslave. In International Congress of the History of Medicine. 26th, Plovdiv, 1978. Actes du Congress. Sofia, 1981. Volume II. p. 85-8.

## FEVER

Atkins E: Fever: its history, cause, and function. **Yale J Biol Med** 1982 May-Aug;55(3-4):283-9
Atkins E: Fever: the old and the new. **J Infect Dis** 1984 Mar;149(3):339-48
Comiti VP: La fièvre et les fièvres. **Doc Hist Vocab Sci** 1983;(5):91-5

1450-1700

**France**

Comiti VP: La fièvre à la fin du XVIIe siècle. **Gaz Med Fr** 1980;87:2159-60

1700 to Present

Popp L: Die Fleckfieber-Epidemie in Kulmbach im Jahre 1793. **Medizinhist J** 1981;16(3):257-69
Schwan HP: Ultrasound and electromagnetic radiation in hyperthermia--a historical perspective. **Br J Cancer** 1982 Mar;45(5)Suppl:84-92

**Germany**

Wiegand W: Die Antipyretikatherapie bei Carl Liebermeister. Diss. Bonn, 1981. 96 p.

**Great Britain**

Colp R: Dr. Erasmus Darwin consults with another physician. **Radic Hist Rev** 1979 Spring/Summer;Spec:66-71
Smith G: The physiology of air: eighteenth-century fever therapy in the advice literature. **Soc Soc Hist Med Bull (Lond)** 1984 Dec;35:21-3

**Ireland**

Doyle JS: Corrigan on fever. **J Ir Coll Physicians Surg** 1980 Jul;10(1):44-5

**Italy**

Knoefel PK: Famine and fever in Tuscany. Eighteenth century Italian concern with the environment. **Physis** 1979;21(1-4):7-35

**Spain**

Mociño JM: Disertación de la fiebre epidémica que padeció Cádiz, Sevilla y la mayor parte de Andalucía desde el año 1800 y principalmente Ecixa el año 1804. México, Sociedad Mexicana de Historia y Filosofía de la Medicina, 1982. xxvi, 234 p.

**United States**

Animalcular and cryptogamic theories on the origins of fevers. Reprinted works by John Kearsley Mitchell (1849), John L. Riddell (1836), Josiah Clark Nott (1848). New York, Arno, 1977. Various paginations.:

### FILARIASIS

**1700 to Present**

**Great Britain**

Chernin E: Sir Patrick Manson's studies on the transmission and biology of filariasis. **Rev Infect Dis** 1983 Jan-Feb;5(1):148-66

**Mexico**

Davies JB: Onchocerciasis vector control--50 years ago. **Trans R Soc Trop Med Hyg** 1983;77(1):139-40

### FOOT AND MOUTH

**1700 to Present**

**United States**

Spear DP: California besieged: the foot-and-mouth epidemic of 1924. **Agric Hist** 1982;56(3):528-41

### FRACTURES

Austin RT: Treatment of broken legs before and after the introduction of gypsum. **Injury** 1983 Mar;14(5):389-94

Ray JM: The fractured hip: the historical development of fracture management. **Friends P. I. Nixon Med Hist Libr** 1980 Oct;9:1-9

Ungethüm M, Kolb W: Elektro-Osteo-Stimulation, Teil 1. Historische Entwicklung und 'Stimulations'-Hypothesen. **Biomed Tech (Berlin)** 1982 Jun;27(6):130-5

Verheyden CN: The history of Dupuytren's contracture. In Romm S, ed: Symposium on historical perspectives of plastic surgery. Philadelphia, Saunders, 1983. p. 619-25.

**Finland**

Lindholm RV: Küntscher bone nailing in Finland. Oulu, Finland, Univ. of Oulu, 1979. 35 p..

**Before 500 A.D.**

Grimm M: Frakturen und Frakturheilung in der Ur- und Frühgeschichte. **Beitr Orthop Traumatol** 1982 Feb;29(2):61-70

**Greco-Roman**

Daly LW: Miltiades. Aratus and compound fractures. **Am J Philol** 1980;101:59-60

**500 A.D.-1450**

Ladegaard Jakobsen AL: A cripple from the late Middle Ages. **Ossa** 1978;5:17-24

**1450-1700**

**France**

Paré A: The classic. Compound fracture of leg, Paré's personal care (MII, 328). **Clin Orthop** 1983 Sep;178:3-6

**1700 to Present**

Peltier LF: A brief historical note on the use of electricity in the treatment of fractures. **Clin Orthop** 1981 Nov-Dec;161:4-7

Peltier LF: Fractures of the distal end of the radius. An historical account. **Clin Orthop** 1984 Jul-Aug;(187):18-22

Romm S: Fritz Steinmann and the pin that bears his name. **Plast Reconstr Surg** 1984 Aug;74(2):306-10

Watson-Jones R, Coltart WD: The classic. Slow union of fractures with a study of 804 fractures of the shafts of the tibia and femur. **Clin Orthop** 1982 Aug;(168):2-16

Willenegger H, Bandi W: Werdegang und Aufgabe der AO-International. Teil 2. **Unfallchirurgie** 1984 Jun;10(3):107-9

**Austria**

Galle P: Fortschritte in der operativen Behandlung hüftgelenksnaher Frakturen seit W. Denk. **Wien Klin Wochenschr** 1982 Apr 2;94(7):185-9

**Brazil**

Ribeiro de Araujo A: O ensaio sobre as fracturas do cirurgiao Manuel Alves da Costa Barreto. **Rev Inst Hist Geogr Bras** 1977;317:100-31

**France**

Evans PE: Cerclage fixation of a fractured humerus in 1775. Fact or fiction? **Clin Orthop** 1983 Apr;(174):138-42

Peltier LF: Joseph François Malgaigne and Malgaigne's fracture. **Clin Orthop** 1980 Sep;(151):4-7

**Great Britain**

Elliott CK: Bonesetters. **Practitioner** 1981 Feb;225(1352):253-5

Peltier LF: Ununited fractures in children. James Paget, 1891. **Clin Orthop** 1982 Jun;(166):2-4

**Ireland**

Strmeň J: Abraham Colles (1773-1843) a ním v roku 1814 popísaná zlomenina radia. **Rozhl Chir** 1984 Oct;63(10):701-4

**Sweden**

Bauer G: Sven Johanssons betydelse för höftfrakturernas behandling. **Sydsven Medicinhist Sallsk Arsskr** 1981;:12-29

**United States**

Lang EF: From earlier pages: the position and relationships of fragments in acute fractures. (E.H. Skinner). **AJR** 1980 Jan;134(1):206

### GIGANTISM

**Before 500 A.D.**

**Rome**

Ljunggren B: En stor man med en sjuk hjärna. **Sydsven Medicinhist Sallsk Arsskr** 1984;21:77-85

**1700 to Present**

Hayles AB: Gigantism. **Pediatr Ann** 1980 Apr;9(4):163-9

**Ireland**

Landolt AM, Zachmann M: The Irish giant: new observations concerning the nature of his ailment. **Lancet** 1980 Jun 14;1(8181):1311-2

### GOITER

Freire-Maia DV: Bócio endêmico: classificação e histórico. **AMB** 1981 Mar;27(3):111-2

Guggenheim KY: Nutrition and nutritional diseases. The evolution of concepts. Lexington, Massachusetts, Toronto, D.C. Heath and Company, 1981. xii, 378 p.

Stahnke J: Geschichte der Kropfchirurgie. **MMW** 1981 Feb 20;123(8):315-6

**Americas**

Benítez RF: Historia de la deficiencia mental endemica en la region Andina. **Asclepio** 1982;34:339-76

**China**

Miyasita S: An historical analysis of Chinese drugs in the treatment of hormonal diseases, goitre and diabetes mellitus. **Am J Chin Med** 1980 Spring-Summer;8(1-2):17-25

**Before 500 A.D.**

**Greece**

Marketos SG, Eftychiadis A, Koutras DA: The first recognition of the association between goiter and exophthalmos. **J Endocrinol Invest** 1983 Oct;6(5):401-3

**1700 to Present**

**Finland**

Wahlberg P: Tyreoidologi i Finland under 150 år. **Nord Medicinhist Arsb** 1984;:105-16

**Switzerland**

Rentchnick P: Iode et goitre. A propos du 150e anniversaire de la mort du Dr Jean-François Coindet (12 juillet 1774–11 février 1834). **Med Hyg (Geneve)** 1984 Feb 15;42(1551):465–6, 469–70, 472–4, 477–8

Wiener JD: Ueber Kropf, Hypertyreose und Jodbehandlung. **Schweiz Med Wochenschr** 1980 Nov 22;110(47):1784–7

**United States**

Matovinovic J: David Marine (1880–1976): Nestor of thyroidology. **Perspect Biol Med** 1978 Spring;21(3):565–89

## GONORRHEA

**1700 to Present**

Starzycki Z: W 40 rocznice wprowadzenia penicyliny do leczenia kiły i rzeżaczki. **Przegl Lek** 1984;41(6):453–7

**Germany**

Sons HU: Geschlechtskrankheiten während der Nachkriegszeit. Eine Untersuchung zur Epidemiologie der Gonorrhö und Lues und zur Reorganisation der Fürsorgeeinrichtungen in Nordrhein-Westfalen in den Jahren 1945–1949. **Med Welt** 1983 Oct 7;34(40):1124–6

**Great Britain**

Howie J: Gonorrhoea--a question of tactics. **Br Med J** 1979 Dec 22–29;2(6205):1631–2

**Netherlands**

Haneveld GT: Bij het eeuwfeest van de gonokok: het belang van zijn ontdekking en de ontvangst daarvan in Nederland (Ludwig Sigesmund Albert Neisser). **Ned Tijdschr Geneeskd** 1979 Oct 27;123(43):1875–8

**Poland**

Stapiński A: Kształtowanie się zapadalności na kiłę i rzeżączkęw Polsce w trzydziestoleciu 1948–1978. **Przegl Dermatol** 1979 Sep–Oct;66(5):507–12

Stapiński A: Powojenny wyż demograficzny a zapadalność na kiłę i rzeżączkę w Polsce. **Przegl Dermatol** 1979 Nov–Dec;66(6):667–72

**United States**

Kampmeier RH: Introduction of sulfonamide therapy for gonorrhea. **Sex Transm Dis** 1983 Apr–Jun;10(2):81–4

## GOUT

Benedek TG: A comparison of the medical writings of two humanists: F. Petrarca and W. Pirckheimer. In: Congrès international d'histoire de la médecine, XXVe, Québec, 1976. Actes. Québec, 1977. p. 502–6.

Bernabeo R: La gotta. Presupposti storici alle concezioni moderne. **Minerva Med** 1980 Oct 6;71(38):2739–43

d'Eshougues JR: Gicht und Rheumatismus. In Sournia JC, Martiny M, Poulet J, ed: Illustrierte Geschichte der Medizin. Salzburg, Andreas, 1980. Vol. 6. p. 2319–49.

Fraser KJ: Anglo-French contributions to the recognition of rheumatoid arthritis. **Ann Rheum Dis** 1982 Aug;41(4):335–43

Jarcho S: Some lost, obsolete, or discontinued diseases: Serous apoplexy, incubus, and retrocedent ailments. **Trans Stud Coll Physicians Phila** 1980 Dec;5(2 no 4):241–66

Leden I: Ledgångsreumatism och gikt - en historisk återblick. **Sydsven Medicinhist Sallsk Arsskr** 1981;:65–97

Michler M: Aus der Geschichte der Gicht. **Orthop Prax** 1978;14(5):341–51

Porter GA: Gouty nephropathy: fact or fiction? **Am J Kidney Dis** 1983 Mar;2(5):553–4

Talbott JH: Gout therapy throughout the ages. **Med Times** 1981 Jan;109(1):2s–8s

**Great Britain**

Christophers BE: Gout and its sufferers. **Med J Aust** 1979 Sep 22;2(6):311

**Before 500 A.D.**

Rosner F: Earliest description of gout. **Arthritis Rheum** 1983 Feb;26(2):236

**Rome**

Gaebel RE: Saturnine gout among Roman aristocrats. **N Engl J Med** 1983 Aug 18;309(7):431

Mertz DP: 'Bleigicht': Ursache oder Folge des Verfalls des Römischen Weltreiches? **Med Welt** 1983 Oct 14;34(41):1158–9

Nriagu JO: Saturnine gout among Roman aristocrats. Did lead poisoning contribute to the fall of the Empire? **N Engl J Med** 1983 Mar 17;308(11):660–3

**1450–1700**

Benedek TG: The gout of Desiderius Erasmus and Willibald Pirckheimer: medical autobiography and its literary reflections. **Bull Hist Med** 1983 Winter;57(4):526–44

**Great Britain**

Borodulin VI: T. Sidengam i razvitie klinicheskoĭ meditsiny (k 300-letiiu opisaniia podagry). **Ter Arkh** 1984;56(1):135–8

Eamon W: The tale of Monsieur Gout. **Bull Hist Med** 1981 Winter;55(4):564–7

Hart FD: William Harvey and his gout. **Ann Rheum Dis** 1984 Apr;43(2):125–7

**Italy**

Tateo F: L'esperienza scientifica di A. de Ferrariis Galateo: Osservazioni sul De podagra. In S. Bertelli, G. Ramakus, ed: Essays presented to Myron P. Gilmore. Vol. 1. Florence, La Nuova Italia, 1978.

**1700 to Present**

Mertz DP: 100 Jahre Gicht: Von Scharlatanerie und Hypotheses zur gezielten Therapie. **Fortschr Med** 1982 Apr 15;100(14):636–44

Wedeen RP: 'Punch cures the gout'. **J Med Soc NJ** 1981 Mar;78(3):201–6

**Brazil**

Corrêa JV: Podagra--uma tese de 1788. **Rev Hosp Clin. Fac Med Sao Paulo** 1981 Feb;36(1):1–6

**France**

Rocchietta S: Una ricetta contro la gotta trascritta da Stendhal in italiano. **Minerva Med** 1981 Feb 25;72(6):305

**Great Britain**

Beckett JV: Illness and amputation in the eighteenth century: the case of Sir James Lowther (1673–1755). **Med Hist** 1980 Jan;24(1):88–92

Eyman E: Alfred Barring Garrod--pionier badán nad dną (1819--1907). **Reumatologia** 1980;18(2):189–90

Hart ED: Conan Doyle as rheumatologist. **Ann Rheum Dis** 1982 Aug;41(4):437–8

Nemoianu V: The semantics of Bramble's hypochondria: a connection between illness and style in the eighteenth century. **Clio (US)** 1979;9(1):39–51

Viseltear AJ: The last illnesses of Robert and Horace Walpole. **Yale J Biol Med** 1983 Mar–Apr;56(2):131–52

**United States**

Mann R: Philip Showalter Hench. In Dictionary of American biography, 1961–1965. Suppl. 7, 1981. p. 340–341.

## GYNECOLOGIC

**1700 to Present**

Darga LL, Klauenberg S, Davis KF: The cultural model of the menstrual cycle. **Mich Acad** 1981;13(4):475–84

Look back to 1927: The use of milk injections in pelvic inflammation. **East Afr Med J** 1980 Feb;57(2):71

Shorter E: Women's diseases before 1900. In M. Albin, R. J. Devlin, G. Heeger, ed: New directions in psychohistory. The Adelphi papers in honor of Erik H. Erikson. Lexington, Toronto, D. C. Heath, 1980. p. 183–208.

Thiery M: Classic illustration. **Eur J Obstet Gynecol Reprod Biol** 1982 Dec;14(3):205–6

**United States**

Khademol-Reza L: Theories of dysmenorrhea. An historical review from 1850 to 1979. **J Kans Med Soc** 1983 Jun;84(6):335–40, 355–6

## HAY FEVER

### 1700 to Present

#### United States

Askew M: 'I have hay fever: I love you. George.' **Practitioner** 1979 Jun;222(1332):866-8

## HEADACHE

### 1700 to Present

Sicuteri F: The Enrico Greppi International Headache Award. A tribute to the memory of one of medicine's pioneers. **Cephalalgia** 1983 Mar;3(1):11-3

#### United States

Battle JD Jr: The 'periodical head-achs' of Thomas Jefferson. **Cleve Clin Q** 1984 Fall;51(3):531-9
Ekbom K, Waldenlind E: Mannen bakom syndromet: Bayard T. Horton. En pionjär inom huvudvärksforskningen. **Lakartidningen** 1982 Sep 15;79(37):3187

## HEARING DISORDERS

Guy A: Donner corps à la voix. **Esprit** 1982;2:200-5
McEntee MK: The right to heritage: the teaching of deaf history. **Am Ann Deaf** 1981 Jun;126(4):402-3
Markides A: Some unusual cures of deafness. **J Laryngol Otol** 1982 Jun;96(6):479-90
Stephens SD, Goodwin JC: Non-electric aids to hearing: a short history. **Audiology** 1984;23(2):215-40
Taylor IG: History and current practice in rehabilitation of deaf children. **Int Rehabil Med** 1983;5(2):82-5
Vernon J: The history of masking as applied to tinnitus. **J Laryngol Otol** 1981;4 Suppl:76-9

### 500 A.D.-1450

Perelló J: Un trauma acústico en el siglo XI. **An Otorrinolaringol Ibero Am** 1980;7(1):53-6

### 1700 to Present

Arnold P: The education of the deaf child: for integration or autonomy? **Am Ann Deaf** 1984 Feb;129(1):29-37
Baldwin K: 'The lumberjack and the deaf tree': images of the deaf in folk narrative. **Ky Folkl Rec** 1982;28(1-2):6-11
Beales PH: Otosclerosis-past and present. **J R Soc Med** 1979 Aug;72(8):553-61
Buus S, Florentine M, Redden RB: The SISI test: a review. Part I. **Audiology** 1982;21(4):273-93
Chalat NI: Some psychologic aspects of deafness: Beethoven, Goya, and Oscar Wilde. **Am J Otol** 1980 Apr;1(4):240-6
Chalat NI: Who was Prosper Menière and why am I still so dizzy? **Am J Otol** 1979 Jul;1(1):52-6
Czeizel A: Ludwig van Beethoven. **Ther Hung** 1982;30(1):43-7
Hoogland GA: Some historical remarks on acoustic neuroma. **Adv Otorhinolaryngol** 1984;34:3-7
Kottek SS: [Jacob Rodriguez Pereire (1715-1780): an anniversary] (Heb). **Koroth** 1981;8(1-2):83-7; 79-81 [Engl. abstr.]
Krömer S: Lärm als medizinisches Problem im 19. Jahrhundert. Diss. Mainz, 1981. 83 p.
Mester AF, Stephens SD: Development of the audiometer and audiometry. **Audiology** 1984;23(2):206-14
Schuknecht HF: The Siamese twins, Eng and Chang: their lives and their hearing losses. **Arch Otolaryngol** 1979 Dec;105(12):737-40

#### Australia

Burke JA: The Dominican nun's school for the deaf and dumb in New South Wales. **J R Aust Hist Soc** 1973;59(4):270-85

#### Austria

Zagarra MJ: Ludwig van Beethoven: hipótesis sobre su sordera. **CERON** 1979 Dec;4(3):7-9

#### Czechoslovakia

Bořík O, Khel R, Zdichynec B: Několik poznámek k ušnímu onemocnění Bedřicha Smetany. **Cesk Otolaryngol** 1983 Nov;32(6):367-71

#### France

Kottek S: Jacob Rodriguez-Péreire (1715-1780); pionnier de l'éducation des sourds-muets: à l'occasion du 200e anniversaire de sa disparition. **Rev Hist Med Heb** 1981 Mar-Apr;34(1):5-8
Lafon JC: Le sourd et muet au XIXe siècle. **Bull Audiophonol** 1980;11(2):1-142
Matsuda K: L'enseignement des sourds-muets et les philosophes au siècle de Lumières. **Zinbun** 1979;15:141-74

#### Germany

Schwann H, Wilke J: 'Erbliche Taubheit' im Faschismus. **Z Gesamte Hyg** 1984 Apr;30(4):232-4

#### Great Britain

Beagley HA: Edith Whetnall's contribution to British audiology. **J R Soc Med** 1978 Dec;71(12):870-8
Blakeley PR: Francis Green: 'a suffering loyalist and friend to the British government. **NS Hist Q** 1979;9(1):1-14
Stephens SD: Centenary of British audiometry. London, Royal National Institute for the Deaf in collaboration with the British Society of Audiology, 1979. 40 p.
Stephens SD: The British medical profession and the first audimeters. **J Laryngol Otol** 1981 Dec;95(12):1223-35
Stephens SD: The role of the state in hearing health care. **Br J Audiol** 1982 Nov;16(4):255-63

#### United States

Boatner EB: Captioned films of the deaf. **Am Ann Deaf** 1981 Aug;126(5):520-5
Burns LS: Noise. **Horizon** 1977;20(1):66-9
Fernandes JJ: Thomas Hopkins Gallaudet on language and communication: a reassessment. **Am Ann Deaf** 1983 Aug;128(4):467-73
Gannon JR: Deaf heritage. A narrative history of deaf America. Silver Spring, National Associaton of the Deaf, 1981. xxxi, 483 p.
Lash JP: Helen Keller. In: Notable American women. The modern period. Cambridge, Mass., Belknap-Harvard Univ. Press, 1980. 4:389-93.
[Notes on David Seixas and education of the deaf in Pennsylvania in the 1820's] In: Myers, S. H. Handcraft to industry: Philadelphia ceramics. Washington, D. C., Smithsonian Institution Press, 1980. pp. 8-12 passim, 83-4.
Pappas DG: Alexander Graham Bell: teacher of the deaf. **Am J Otol** 1983 Jan;4(3):263-5
Studebaker GA: Fifty years of hearing aid research: an evaluation of progress. **Ear Hear** 1980 Mar-Apr;1(2):57-62

#### Yugoslavia

Jakopič B: Ob 80-letnici Centra za Rehabilitacijo Sluha in Govora v Ljubljani. **Kronika (Yugosl)** 1980;28(3):212-17
Jakopič B: Slušno in govorno prizadeti in gledališče. **Kronika (Yugosl)** 1978;26(2):100-3
Jakopič B: Zgodovina učnih načrtov in programov šol za gluhe na slovenskem. **Kronika (Yugosl)** 1979;27(3):185-92

## HEART

Appels A: Cultural aspects of coronary prone behavior. An approach from the history of art. **Adv Cardiol** 1982;29:32-6
Barba J, Arrieta JA, Perugachi C, et al: Espasma arterial coronario. Antecedentes históricos. **Rev Med Univ Navarra** 1982 Jun;26(2):12-3
Brest AN, Goldberg S: Coronary thrombosis: historic aspects. **Cardiovasc Clin** 1983;14(1):5-8
Brewer LA: The failing myocardium. Historical notes. **Am J Surg** 1984 Jun;147(6):712-8
Duke M: Whose tetralogy is it? A short history of the tetralogy of Fallot. **Conn Med** 1984 Feb;48(2):103-4
Greeff K, Schadewaldt H: Introduction and remarks on the history of cardiac glycosides. In Greeff K, ed: Handbook of experimental pharmacology. Berlin, Springer, 1981. p. 1-12 (Vol. 56/I).
Horan MJ, Kennedy HL: Ventricular ectopy. History, epidemiology, and clinical implications. **JAMA** 1984 Jan 20;251(3):380-6
Huttmann A: Eine imaginäre Krankheit: der Polyp des Herzens. **Medizinhist J** 1983;18(1-2):43-51
Jarcho S: The concept of heart failure from Avicenna to Albertini. Cambridge, Mass., and London, Harvard Univ. Press, 1980. 407 p.
Johansson BW: Hjärtinfarkt--gammal sjukdom med nytt namn. **Sydsven Medicinhist Sallsk Arsskr** 1980;:57-79
Kawai S, Kanoh T, Okada R: [History of the etiological studies of myocardial infarction and angina pectoris] (Jpn). **Nippon Rinsho** 1983;41(2):265-70
Rashkind WJ: Historical aspects of surgery for congenital heart disease. **J Thorac Cardiovasc Surg** 1982 Oct;84(4):619-25
Rashkind WJ, ed: Congenital heart disease. Stroudsburg, Pennsylvania,

Hutchinson Ross, 1982. xv, 390 p. (Benchmark papers in human physiology, 16).
Schölmerich P: Historische Anmerkungen zum Begriff Myokarditis – Kardiomypathie. **Med Welt** 1984 Jan 13;35(1-2):109-13
Weintraub WS, Helfant RH: Coronary artery spasm: historic aspects. **Cardiovasc Clin** 1983;14(1):1-4

**China**

Chen KJ: Certain progress in the treatment of coronary heart disease with traditional medicinal plants in China. **Am J Chin Med** 1981 Autumn;9(3):193-6

**Yugoslavia**

Mušič D, Rakovec P, Jagodic A, et al: The first description of syncopal attacks in heart block. **PACE** 1984 Mar;7(2):301-3

**Before 500 A.D.**

**Greece**

Calogirou DK: L'Asclêpieion de Cos, Hippocrate et la maladie des coronaires. **Hist Sci Med** 1979;13(4):427-39
Kudlien F: A new testimony for Erasistratus? **Clio Med** 1981 Apr;15(3-4):137-42

**Rome**

Petrakis NL: Diagonal earlobe creases, type A behavior and the death of Emperor Hadrian. **West J Med** 1980 Jan;132(1):87-91

**500 A.D.-1450**

**Arabic**

Brahmaji Rao U: Avicenna's contribution to the understanding of anatomy and pathology of heart. **Bull Indian Inst Hist Med (Hyderabad)** 1981;1-4:91-4
Said HM: Greco-Arab concepts on cardiovascular diseases. Karachi, Pakistan, Hamdard Foundation Press, 1983. 201 p.

**Germany**

Farrar WE: Parzival's pericardial puncture. **Ann Intern Med** 1980 May;92(5):640

**1450-1700**

**Spain**

Carreras Panchón A: Perez Cascales y la clinica del garrotillo. **Asclepio** 1978-79;30-31:319-22

**1700 to Present**

Cantwell JD: Angina: from Heberden to Prinzmetal. **South Med J** 1984 Jul;77(7):896-9
Chrościcki A: Osłuchiwanie serca--od stetoskopu do ultradźwi eków. **Pediatr Pol** 1979 Oct;54(10):1095-100
Cole RB: Noonan's syndrome: a historical perspective. **Pediatrics** 1980 Sep;66(3):468-9
Comroe JH: Exploring the heart: discoveries in heart disease and high blood pressure. New York, Norton, 1983. 348 p.
García MM: History and design of artifical heart valves. **Bol Asoc Med PR** 1981 Nov;73(11):567-73
Greeff K: Therapie der Myokardinsuffizienz, gestern und heute. **Z Kardiol** 1982 Mar;71(3):139-41
Krikler DM: Wolff-Parkinson-White syndrome: long follow-up and an Anglo-American historical note. **J Am Coll Cardiol** 1983 Dec;2(6):1216-8
Muller JE: Coronary artery thrombosis: historical aspects. **J Am Coll Cardiol** 1983 Mar;1(3):893-6
Rashkind WJ: Tricuspid atresia: a historical review. **Pediatr Cardiol** 1982;2(1):85-8
Schechter DC: Flashbacks: ventricular fibrillation, part I. **PACE** 1979 Jul;2(4):490-504

**Austria**

Alonso HO: La enfermedad cardíaca de Gustav Mahler. **Medicina (B Aires)** 1981;41(3):373-7

**Czechoslovakia**

Steiner I: První popis 'senilního' amyloidu srdce--I. Soyka, 1876, Praha. **Cesk Patol** 1984 Feb;20(1):11-3

**France**

Allwork SP: Maladie du Roger 1879: a new translation for the centenary. **Am Heart J** 1979 Sep;98(3):307-11
Bjarke B: Mannen bakom syndromet: Arthur Fallot. En medicinens 'doldis'--fransmannen vars namn alla känner men få vet någonting om. **Lakartidningen** 1984 Oct 24;81(43):3934-5
Heron JR: Louis Pasteur: the nature of his illness. In Passmore R, ed: Proceedings of the Royal College of Physicians of Edinburgh Tercentenary Congress, 1981. Edinburgh, Royal College of Physicians of Edinburgh, 1982. p. 116-27.
Lévy A: Alphonse Laveran, initiateur de la pathologie coronaro-myocardique. **Nouv Presse Med** 1981 Mar 21;10(13):1015

**Germany**

Guillemin J: La maladie de Richard Wagner. Pour le centenaire de sa mort à Venise. **Sem Hop Paris** 1983 May 12;59(19):1493-6

**Great Britain**

Bartecchi CE: Historical beginnings of the mitral valve prolapse syndrome. **Am J Cardiol** 1984 Nov 1;54(8):1165-6
Bartley M: Coronary heart disease: a disease of affluence or a disease of industry? **Soc Soc Hist Med Bull (Lond)** 1983 Dec;33:50-1
Connolly DC, Mann RJ: Dominic J. Corrigan (1802-1880) and his description of the pericardial knock. **Mayo Clin Proc** 1980 Dec;55(12):771-3
Honeyman WP: Myocardial infarction in Carlisle in 1783. **Br Med J [Clin Res]** 1982 Apr 10;284(6322):1113-4
McCormick JS: James Mackenzie and coronary heart disease. **J R Coll Gen Pract** 1981 Jan;31(222):26-30
Opie LH, Louw JH: John Hunter and angina pectoris. **Am J Cardiol** 1981 Nov;48(5):980
Proudfit WL: Origin of concept of ischaemic heart disease. **Br Heart J** 1983 Sep;50(3):209-12
Pruitt RD: William Osler and his Gulstonian lectures on malignant endocarditis. **Mayo Clin Proc** 1982 Jan;57(1):4-9

**Ireland**

Horgan J: Corrigan on cardiac disease. **J Ir Coll Physicians Surg** 1980 Jul;10(1):27-31

**Norway**

Bang HO, Dyerberg J: Personal reflections on the incidence of ischaemic heart disease in Oslo during the Second World War. **Acta Med Scand** 1981;210(4):245-8

**Sweden**

Johansson BW, Nicol P: A Swedish report on acute myocardial infarction in 1859. **Br Med J [Clin Res]** 1982 Mar 20;284(6319):888-9

**United States**

Blake TM: Myocardial infarction and electrocardiography in historical perspective. **South Med J** 1983 Dec;76(12):1470-2
Bond GR, et al: Mended hearts: a self-help case study. **Soc Policy** 1979;9(4):50-7
Edmunds LH: A historical review of shunts for cyanotic heart disease. In B. L. Tucker, G. G. Lindesmith, ed: First clinical conference on congenital heart disease. New York, Grune & Stratton, 1979. p. 207-17.
Estes JW: Hall Jackson and the purple foxglove: medical practice and research in revolutionary America 1760-1820. Hanover, NH, University Press of New England, 1979. xvi, 291 p.
Feinleib M: History of the genetic epidemiology of coronary heart disease. **Prog Clin Biol Res** 1984;147:1-7
Fye WB: Acute coronary occlusion always results in death--or does it? The observations of William T. Porter. **Circulation** 1985 Jan;71(1):4-10
Fyler DC: The history of treatment of patent ductus arteriosus. In B. L. Tucker, G. G. Lindesmith, ed: First clinical conference on congenital heart disease. New York, Grune & Stratton, 1979. p. 3-11.
Hurst JW: Landmark article (JAMA 1912). Clinical features of sudden obstruction of the coronary arteries. By James B. Herrick. **JAMA** 1983 Oct 7;250(13):1757-65
Lellouch A: Histoire de l'angine de poitrine et du spasme artériel coronaire au travers de l'oeuvre de Prinzmetal. **Coeur Med Interne** 1980 Jan-Mar;19(1):85-90
McNamara DG: Landmark perspective: the Blalock-Taussig operation and subsequent progress in surgical treatment of cardiovascular diseases. **JAMA** 1984 Apr 27;251(16):2139-41
Reddy CP, Surawicz B: Terminology of tachycardias: historical background and evolution. **PACE** 1983 Sep;6(5 Pt 2):1123-42
Sladen A: Landmark perspective: Closed-chest massage, Kouwenhoven, Jude, Knickerbocker. **JAMA** 1984 Jun 15;251(23):3137-40

Warren R: Landmark perspective: patent ductus arteriosus. **JAMA** 1984 Mar 2;251(9):1203–7
Wing ES: First American description of calcific aortic stenosis. **RI Med J** 1983 Jun;66(6):243–5
Wooley CF: From irritable heart to mitral valve prolapse: the Osler connection. **Am J Cardiol** 1984 Mar 1;53(6):870–4

**USSR**

Cooper R: Rising death rates in the Soviet Union. The impact of coronary heart disease [1960–77]. **N Engl J Med** 1981;304:1259–65

### HELMINTHIASIS

**Brazil**

Ferreira LF, Araújo AJ de, Confalonieri UE: The finding of helminth eggs in a Brazilian mummy. **Trans R Soc Trop Med Hyg** 1983;77(1):65–7

**Before 500 A.D.**

Africa TW: Worms and the death of kings: a cautionary note on disease and history. **Classical Antiq** 1982;1(1):1–17

**Brazil**

Ferreira LF, Aráujo AJ de, Confalonieri UE: The finding of eggs and larvae of parasitic helminths in archaeological material from Unai, Minas Gerais, Brazil. **Trans R Soc Trop Med Hyg** 1980;74(6):798–800

**1700 to Present**

Rim HJ: Therapy of fluke infections in the past. A review. **Arzneimittelforsch** 1984;34(9B):1127–9

**Great Britain**

Shortt HE: Robert Thomson Leiper. In Dictionary of national biography, 1961–1970. Suppl. 8, 1981. p. 647–8.

**United States**

Brock CH: Dr. Thomas Bond of Philadelphia and his 'Worm'. **Trans Stud Coll Physicians Phila** 1981 Sep;5(3 no 3):209–13
Govier WM: A helminthic tale. **Perspect Biol Med** 1984 Autumn;28(1):104–6

**USSR**

Filatov VG: Gistoricheskie i évoliutsionnye predposylki stanovleniia landshaftnoĭ épidemiologii gel'mintozov. **Parassitologia** 1981 Jan–Feb;15(1):3–9

### HEMOPHILIA

Rosner F: Ancient descriptions of hemophilia and preconception gender selection. **JAMA** 1984 Aug 17;252(7):900

**1700 to Present**

Grobler SA: Hemofilie--'n koninklike siekte. **S Afr Med J** 1981 Jul 25;60(4):143–4

**Germany**

Egli H: The situation of the haemophiliac: yesterday and today. **Haemostasis** 1981;10 Suppl 1:1–10

**Great Britain**

Farr AD: Treatment of haemophilia by transfusion: the first recorded case. **J R Soc Med** 1981 Apr;74(4):301–5
Whitfield AG: The scholar prince. **J R Coll Physicians Lond** 1984 Jul;18(3):195–7

**USSR**

Willbanks OL, Willbanks SE: Femoral neuropathy due to retroperitoneal bleeding. A red herring in medicine complicates anticoagulant therapy and influences the Russian Communist Revolution (Crown Prince Alexis, Rasputin). **Am J Surg** 1983 Feb;145(2):193–8

### HEMORRHAGE

Sparacia A: Dal cerusico all'intensivoterapeuta (rassegna storica dell'emostasi). **Minerva Anestesiol** 1980 Jul;46(7):759–71

**1700 to Present**

Henry RL: A recognition of the work of Walter H. Seegers in hemostasis and thrombosis. **Semin Thromb Hemostas** 1980;6(4):325–7
Jaques LB: The hemostasis paradigm in 1934 and in 1980. **Ann NY Acad Sci** 1981;370:1–4
Ljunggren B, Säveland H, Brandt L: Aneurysmal subarachnoid hemorrhage--historical background from a Scandinavian horizon. **Surg Neurol** 1984 Dec;22(6):605–16

**Sweden**

Myhrman G: Möte med en ny sjukdom--nephropathia epidemica. **Nord Medicinhist Arsb** 1984;:175–9

**United States**

Mathisen DA: Whatever happened to human body glue? **Reason** 1980;12(1):20–7
Sherry S: A tribute to Kenneth M. Brinkhous, M.D. **Thromb Haemost** 1979 Feb 28;40(1):3–23

### HERNIA

Berjón Rufes JJ: Cómo vio el siglo XX nacer y evolucionar a una nueva enfermedad: la hernia hiatal. **Rev Esp Enferm Apar Dig** 1982 Feb;61(2):169–81
Read RC: The development of inguinal herniorrhaphy. **Surg Clin North Am** 1984 Apr;64(2):185–96

**1700 to Present**

Bettex M, Oesch I: The hiatus hernia saga. Ups and downs in gastroesophageal reflux: past, present, and future perspectives. **J Pediatr Surg** 1983 Dec;18(6):670–80
Read RD: Marcy's priority in the development of inguinal herniorrphaphy. **Surgery** 1980 Nov;88(5):682–5

**Czechoslovakia**

Duda M, Serý Z: Historie a současnost chirurgie hiátových hernií a refluxní nemoci jícnu. **Cesk Gastroenterol Vyz** 1979 Sep;33(6):332–41

**France**

Charroppin P: L'escargot contre la hernie? **Rev Hist Pharm (Paris)** 1983 Sep;30(258):215–9

### HERPES

**Italy**

Caffaratto TM: Una pagina di storia per l'herpes progenitalis. **Minerva Med** 1984 May 7;75(19):1159–61

### HOOKWORM INFECTION

**1700 to Present**

Belloni L: The discovery of duodenal ancylostoma and of its pathogenic power. In M. D. Grmek, R. S. Cohen, G. Cimino, ed: On scientific discovery. The Erice Lectures 1977. Dordrecht, D. Reidel, 1981. p. 261–79. (Boston Studies in the Philosophy of Science, v. 34).

**Americas**

Garcia JC: The laziness disease. **Hist Philos Life Sci** 1981;3(1):31–59

**Switzerland**

Peduzzi R, Piffaretti JC: Ancylostoma duodenale and the Saint Gothard anaemia. **Br Med J [Clin Res]** 1983 Dec 24–31;287(6409):1942–5

**United States**

Eberson F: Eradication of hookworm disease in Florida. **J Fla Med Assoc** 1980 Aug;67(8):736–42
Ettling J: The germ of laziness. Rockefeller philanthropy and public health in the new South. Cambridge, Harvard, 1981. x, 263 p.
Farmer HF: The germ of laziness: a Florida historical perspective. **J Fla Med Assoc** 1983 Aug;70(8):659–62
House RV: A brief history of hookworm disease in North Carolina. **NC Med J** 1982 Nov;43(11):765–8

### HYPERSENSITIVITY

Harper DS: Footnotes on allergy. Uppsala, Pharmacia AB, 1980. 103 p.

## DISEASES AND INJURIES

Schadewaldt H: Geschichte der Allergie, in 4 Bänden. Band I. München-Diesenhofen, Dustri Verlag, 1979. xv, 426 p.
Schadewaldt H: Idiosynkrasie, Anaphylaxie, Allergie, Atopie--ein Beitrag zur Geschichte der Ueberempfindlichkeitskrankheiten. Opladen, Westdeutscher Verlag, 1981. 48 p. (Rheinisch-Westfälische Akademie der Wissenschaften; Geisteswissenschaften; Vorträge, G 251).

**Mexico**

Cueva J, Ramírez Oviedo A: Historia de la alergia en México. In Academia Nacional de Medicina. Libro conmemorativo del primer centenario. México, Comité Editorial de la Comisión Organizadora del Congreso del Centenario, 1964. Tome 2. p. 552-8.

**1450-1700**

**Netherlands**

Leyh F: Hatte Rembrandt van Rijn eine Nickelallergie? **Hautarzt** 1984 Sep;35(9):472-3

**1700 to Present**

Bendiner E: Baron von Pirquet: the aristocrat who discovered and defined allergy. **Hosp Pract** 1981 Oct;16(10):137, 141, 144 passim
Breneman JC: Overview of food allergy: historical perspective. **Ann Allergy** 1983 Aug;51(2 Pt 2):220-1
Cazort AG, Gordon VH: History of allergy. University of Arkansas School of Medicine. **J Arkansas Med Soc** 1980 Oct;77(5):197-8
Matsuhashi N: [Introduction to immunology--history] (Jpn). **Shikai Tenbo** 1982 Jan;59(1):169-76
May CD: Food allergy: lessons from the past. **J Allergy Clin Immunol** 1982 Mar;69(3):255-9
Richerson HB: Hypersensitivity pneumonitis--pathology and pathogenesis. **Clin Rev Allergy** 1983 Dec;1(4):469-86

**Austria**

Wyklicky H: Gedanken zur Geschichte der Allergie. In memoriam Clemens von Pirquet. **Wien Med Wochenschr** 1980 Feb 15;130(3):123-5

**Great Britain**

Caplan RM: 'The Lion's Mane'. Concerning the diagnostic acumen of Sherlock Holmes. **Am J Dermatopathol** 1983 Dec;5(6):577-9

**Italy**

Karnovsky ML: Metchnikoff in Messina: a century of studies on phagocytosis. **N Engl J Med** 1981 May 7;304(19):1178-80

**Poland**

Pačes V: Uvahy o nemoci Fryderyka Chopina. **Vnitr Lek** 1980 Oct;26(10):1027-31

**United States**

Buckley RH: Presidential address. Reflections on the 1970s and a look to the future. **J Allergy Clin Immunol** 1980 Dec;66(6):432-7
Chase MW: Irreverent recollections from Cooke and Coca, 1928-1978. **J Allergy Clin Immunol** 1979 Nov;64(5):306-20
Cohen SG: In memoriam. Marion B. Sulzberger (1895-1983). A dermatologist's contributions to allergy. **J Allergy Clin Immunol** 1984 Dec;74(6):855-60
Hast A: Robert Anderson Cooke. In Dictionary of American Biography, Suppl. 6, 1956-1960. p. 123-4, 1980.
Licorish KA: Hypersensitivity pneumonitis--economic and legal aspects. **Clin Rev Allergy** 1983 Dec;1(4):487-96
Shambaugh GE: French Keller Hansel and the history of allergy. **Arch Otolaryngol** 1983 Feb;109(2):126-9
Tuft L: Allergy Practice during the early years. **Ann Allergy** 1982 Oct;49(4):238-43

**USSR**

Ado AD: A. A. Bogomolets i sovremennaia allergologiia. **Patol Fiziol Eksp Ter** 1981 Mar-Apr;(2): 70-3
Ado AD: Razvitie ideĭ A. A. Bogomol'tsa v sovremennoĭ allergologii. **Fiziol Zh** 1981 May-Jun;27(3):354-7
Berezhnaia NM: Uchenie o reaktivnosti A. A. Bogomolets i razvitie sovremennoĭ allergologii. **Fiziol Zh** 1981 May-Jun;27(3):358-68

### IATROGENIC

**1450-1700**

**Great Britain**

Madsen V: Medicine in history. Dryden on the doctors and the death of Charles II. **J Dermatol Surg Oncol** 1981 May;7(5):366-9

### INFECTIOUS

Butler T: Plague and other Yersinia infections. New York, London, Plenum Medical Book Co., 1983. xii, 220 p. (Current Topics in Infectious Disease).
Classics of infectious diseases: **Rev Infect Dis** 1981 Mar-Apr;3(2):372-95 (continued regularly)
Fenner F: Sociocultural change and environmental diseases. In Stanley NF, Joske RA, ed: Changing disease patterns and human behaviour. London, New York, Academic Press, 1980. p. 7-26.
Horstmanhoff HF, et al: The plague and other pestilences in antiquity and the Middle Ages. Contributions by R. A. Tybout, M. van Raalte, S. van der Lee, C. G. van Leijenhorst, E. J. Bakker, E. J. Schoten. **Hermeneus Tijdschr Antieke Cult** 1979;51(2):58-117, 140-157
Kumate J: Aparición declinación y reaparición de las enfermedades infecciosas del hombre. **Mem Col Nac (Mex)** 1979;9(2):19-41
McNeill WH: Migration patterns and infection in traditional societies. In Stanley NF, Joske RA, ed: Changing disease patterns and human behaviour. London, New York, Academic Press, 1980. p. 27-36.
Matumoto M: [Ancient history of viral diseases in man] (Jpn). **Uirusu** 1983 Dec;33(2):79-86
Micoud M: Die ansteckenden Krankheiten. In Sournia JC, Martiny M, Poulet J, ed: Illustrierte Geschichte der Medizin. Salzburg, Andreas, 1980. Vol. 6. p. 2243-93.
Mims C: The emergence of new infectious diseases. In Stanley NF, Joske RA, ed: Changing disease patterns and human behaviour. London, New York, Academic Press, 1980. p. 231-50.
Murrell TG: A history of enteritis necroticans. **Papua New Guinea Med J** 1979 Mar;22(1):5-17
Riley RL: Airborne contagion. Historical background. **Ann NY Acad Sci** 1980;353:3-9
Risse GB: Epidemics and medicine: the influence of disease on medical thought and practice. **Bull Hist Med** 1979 Winter;53(4):505-19
Schadewaldt H: Infektionskrankheiten in Kunstdarstellungen. In Ganzinger K, Skopec M, Wyklicky H, ed: Festschrift für Erna Lesky zum 70. Geburtstag. Wien, Brüder Hollinek, 1981. p. 87-96.
Shoshan A: Rift Valley Fever and its relation to the 4th plague. **Koroth** 1980 Jun;7(11-12):810-3
Wilkinson L: Veterinary cross-currents in the history of ideas on infectious disease. **J R Soc Med** 1980 Nov;73(11):818-27

**Americas**

Milner GR: Epidemic disease in the postcontact southeast: a reappraisal. **Midcont J Archaeol** 1980;5(1):39-56

**Netherlands**

Raalte M van, et al: Epidemieën in Oudheid en Middeleeuwen. **Hermeneus Tijdschr Antieke Cult** 1979;51(2):57-169

**Before 500 A.D.**

Hayman J: Mycobacterium ulcerans: an infection from Jurassic time? **Lancet** 1984 Nov 3;2(8410):1015-6
Koch HA: Zum Nachweis einiger mikrobiologischer Probleme im Buch Leviticus (3. Buch Mose) des Alten Testamentes. **Mykosen** 1983 Mar;26(3):159-62

**Americas**

Fragoso Uribe R: Algunas observaciones que apoyan el origen precolombino de la 'enfermedad de Robles' en América. **SPM** 1979 Nov-Dec;21(6):697-706

**Rome**

Andre JM: La notion de Pestilentia à Rome: du tabou religieux à l'interprétation pré-scientifique. **Latomus** 1980;39:2-16
Classics in infectious diseases: Excerpts from the Natural History of Pliny. **Rev Infect Dis** 1982 Nov-Dec;4(6):1266-9

**500 A.D.-1450**

**Arabic**

Carreras Panchón A: Sobre el concepto de pestilencia (WABA') en el Canon de Avicena. **Asclepio** 1981;33:265-73

### 1450–1700

**Mexico**

Prem HJ: Seuchengeschichte von Zentralmexiko im 16. Jahrhundert. Ein Modell für die heutige weltweite Seuchensituation? **Fortschr Med** 1981 Sep 24;99(36):1421–2

**Morocco**

Rosenberger B, Triki H: Famines et épidémies au Maroc aux XVIe et XVIIe siècles. **Hesperis Tamuda** 1973;14:109–75

### 1700 to Present

Baguenier-Desormeaux L: Henry Drysdale Dakin à Compiègne, en 1915. **Rev Hist Pharm (Paris)** 1981 Jun;28(249):79–88

Crosskey RW, Post RJ: Which cytospecies of the Simulium damnosum complex did Blacklock incriminate in the transmission of Onchocerca volvulus? **Ann Trop Med Parasitol** 1981 Oct;75(5):569–71

Fenner F: Mousepox (infectious ectromelia): past, present, and future. **Lab Anim Sci** 1981 Oct;31(5 Pt 2):553–9

Fernández de Castro J: Historia de la oncocercósis. **SPM** 1979 Nov–Dec;21(6):683–96

Finland M: Empiric therapy for bacterial infections: the historical perspective. **Rev Infect Dis** 1983 Mar–Apr;5 Suppl 1:S2–8

Gonçalves J: Endocardite infecciosa. Sete décadas de evolução. **Acta Med Port** 1979 Mar–Apr;1(2):267–77

Hoare CA: Comparative aspects of human babesiosis. **Trans R Soc Trop Med Hyg** 1980;74(2):143–8

Howard-Jones N: Prelude to modern preventive medicine. In Stanley NF, Joske RA, ed: Changing disease patterns and human behaviour. London, New York, Academic Press, 1980. p. 69–80.

Ignatov D: Istoricheski danni po vŭprosa za lechenieto na peritonita. **Probl Khig** 1980;8:154–63

Imperato PJ: A historical overview of amebiasis. **Bull NY Acad Med** 1981 Apr;57(3):175–87

Kirshenblat IaD: K istorii otkrytiia i izucheniia vozbuditelia adiaspiromikoza. **Mikrobiol Zh** 1980 Nov–Dec;42(6):781–2

Klein JO: Infectious diseases of the newborn infant--historical perspectives. In Smith GF, Smith PN, Vidyasagar D, ed: Historical review and recent advances in neonatal and perinatal medicine. [Chicago?], Mead Johnson Nutritional Division, 1983. Vol. I. p. 185–96.

Klein P: Die Infektionskrankheit im erzählerischen Werk Thomas Manns. **Medizinhist J** 1980;15(1/2):3–15

Marwick CS: Managing viral diseases--two centuries of progress. **Am Pharm** 1982 Apr;22(4):36–44

Meissner K, Meiser G: Primary open wound management after emergency laparotomies for conditions associated with bacterial contamination. Reappraisal of a historical tradition. **Am J Surg** 1984 Nov;148(5):613–7

Rechtman J: De l'asepsie... ou un siècle avant Semmelweis. **Hist Sci Med** 1980;14(2):165–70

Rechtman J: L'asepsie et son histoire; le Dr Buchan précède le Dr Semmelweis de plus d'un siècle (1769–1847). **Soc Fr Hist Art Dent** 1979 Sep–Dec;(5–6):15–17

Scientific essays on infectious diseases in honor of Dorothy M. Horstmann, M.D.: **Yale J Biol Med** 1982 May–Aug;55(3–4):161–389

Vidon DJ: Actualité des streptocoques un siècle après leur découverte. **Lyon Pharm** 1981 Apr;32(3):151–4

**Australia**

Young CM: Epidemics of infectious diseases in Australia prior to 1914. In Charbonneau H, Larose A, ed: The great mortalities: methodological studies of demographic crises in the past. Liège, Belgium, Ordina Editions, 1980. p. 207–27.

**Austria**

Franken FH: Mozarts Todeskrankheit. **Fortschr Med** 1980 Mar 6;98(9):301–2

Wyklicky H: The role of the Vienna Medical School in the investigation and treatment of infectious diseases. In [The Vienna Medical School]. Produced under a grant from the Squibb Institute for Medical Research, [1983]. p. 6–20.

**Belgium**

Bruneel C: Un problème de gouvernement: le pouvoir face à l'epidémie de fièvre putride à Bruxelles en 1772–1773. In Imhof AE, ed: Mensch und Gesundheit in der Geschichte. Husum, Matthiesen, 1980. p. 199–221.

**France**

Decourt P: Les zymases ou ferments solubles de Béchamp à la lumière des connaissances du XXe siècle. **Hist Sci Med** 1984;18(2):147–51

Guyotjeannin C, Lehuenen J: Contribution à l'étude de la pathologie aux îles Saint-Pierre-et-Miquelon (XIXe siècle - début du XXe siècle). **Hist Sci Med** 1984;18(1):61–5

Nicolle P: Un événement capital dans la vie passionnée de Charles Nicolle: le Prix Nobel de physiologie ou médecine. Souvenirs évoqués par Pierre Nicolle. **Bull Soc Pathol Exot Filiales** 1981 Jan–Feb;74(1):101–18

Théodoridès J: Magendie et la pathologie infectieuse. **Hist Sci Med** 1983;17(4):367–80

Théodoridès J: Un précurseur girondin de la pathologie infectieuse: Jean Hameau (1779–1851). In: Congrès National des Sociétés Savantes, 104e, Bordeaux, 1979. Comptes Rendus. Paris, 1979. Section des Sciences, Fasc. IV. p. 81–95.

**Great Britain**

Wilkinson L: 'The other' John Hunter, M.D., F.R.S. (1754–1809): his contributions to the medical literature, and to the introduction of animal experiments into infectious disease research. **Notes Rec R Soc Lond** 1982 Feb;36(2):227–41

**Iceland**

Bjarnason O: Epidemics in Iceland in the 18th century. **Nord Medicinhist Arsb** 1980;Suppl 6:76–81

Cliff A, Haggett P: Island epidemics. **Sci Am** 1984 May;250(5):138–47

**Malagasy Republic**

Zeller H, Coulanges P: Les entérovirus à Madagascar. Bilan de vingt ans d'activité du laboratoire de virologie de l'Institut Pasteur de Madagascar. **Arch Inst Pasteur Madagascar** 1980;47(1):121–69

**Nigeria**

Hackett CJ: Private medical practice and anti-yaws campaigns in South Eastern Nigeria 1925–1950. **Trop Doct** 1980 Jul;10(3):129–32

**Pacific Islands**

Lange R: Plagues and pestilence in Polynesia: the nineteenth-century Cook Islands experience. **Bull Hist Med** 1984 Fall;58(3):325–46

**Panama**

Filós-Díaz JA: Histoplasmosis en Panamá. Revisión histórica y nota de actualización. **Rev Med Panama** 1984 Jan;9(1):8–21

**South Africa**

Findlay GH: South African tick-bite fever (1931–1981). **S Afr Med J** 1981 Dec 26;60(26):998–1000

**Spain**

Riera J: José Masdevall y la medicina española ilustrada (Enseñanza, epidemias y guerra a finales del siglo XVIII). Valladolid, Universidad de Valladolid, 1980. 257 p. (Acta Historico-Medica Vallisoletana, Monografías, X)

**Sweden**

Myhrman G: Möte med en ny sjukdom--nephropathia epidemica. **Nord Medicinhist Arsb** 1984;:175–9

Thulin KE: Infektionernas förändrade sjukdomspanorama under 40 år. **Sydsven Medicinhist Sallsk Arsskr** 1981;:151–69

**Switzerland**

Gubéran E: Tendances de la mortalité en Suisse. 2. Maladies infectieuses 1876–1977. **Schweiz Med Wochenschr** 1980 Apr 12;110(15):574–83

**United States**

Bayer RA: Q fever as an occupational illness at the National Institutes of Health. **Public Health Rep** 1982 Jan–Feb;97(1):58–60

Corner GW: Thomas Milton Rivers. In Dictionary of American biography, 1961–1965. Suppl. 7, 1981. p. 648–9.

Finland M: Gaps in therapy for infectious diseases: a historical perspective. **J Infect Dis** 1982 Mar;145(3):401–7

Goertzel TG, Goertzel MG, Goertzel V: Linus Pauling: the scientist as crusader. **Antioch Rev** 1980;38(3):371–82

Koucky RW: The buffalo disaster of 1882. **ND Hist** 1983;50(1):23–30

Krause RM: Koch's postulates and the search for the AIDS agent. **Public Health Rep** 1984 May–Jun;99(3):291–9

Lattimer GL: Legionnaires' disease legacies. **JAMA** 1980 Nov 28;244(21):2416

Lowell JD: The ultraviolet environment in a nutshell (Carl W. Walter). **Am J Surg** 1984 Nov;148(5):575–7

# DISEASES AND INJURIES

North E: Classics in infectious diseases. Concerning the epidemic of spotted fever in New England: Elisha North, 1811. **Rev Infect Dis** 1980 Sep–Oct;2(5):811–6
Pomerantz MB, Marr JS, Goldman WD: Amebiasis in New York City 1958--1978: identification of the male homosexual high risk population. **Bull NY Acad Med** 1980 Mar;56(2):232–44
Riley HD: The history of histoplasmosis. **J Okla State Med Assoc** 1983 Feb;76(2):31–40
Roşca T: Legioneloza (pneumonia veteranilor). **Rev Med Interna [Med Interna]** 1980 Jul–Aug;32(4):301–6
Schmidt CG: The group-fantasy origins of AIDS. **J Psychohist** 1984 Summer;12(1):37–78
Sherlock S: Landmark perspective: Landmarks in viral hepatitis. **JAMA** 1984 Jul 20;252(3):402–6
Sutliff WD: Histoplasmosis in Veterans Administration hospitals in middle America. **Mycopathologia** 1983;83(1):57–62
Tatlock H: Clarification of the cause of Fort Bragg fever (pretibial fever) - January 1982. **Rev Infect Dis** 1982 Jan–Feb;4(1):157–8
Thomas G, Morgan-Witts M: Anatomy of an epidemic. Garden City, N. Y., Doubleday, 1982. xv, 366 p.

**USSR**

Chagin KP: Rol' akademika E. N. Pavlovskogo v izuchenii épidemiologii parazitarnykh i transmissivnykh bolezneĭ (k 100-letiiu so dnia rozhdeniia). **Zh Mikrobiol Epidemiol Immunobiol** 1984 Jun;(6):117–20
Nosov SD: O nekotorykh tak nazyvaemykh novykh infektsionnykh bolezniakh. **Feldsher Akush** 1980;45(8):7–10
Shuvalova EP: Razvitie ideĭ S. P. Botkina v klinike infektsionnykh bolezneĭ. **Vestn Akad Med Nauk SSSR** 1983;(3):35–40
Vladimirova LB: Voprosy bor'by s infektsionnymi zabolevaniiami na VII s'ezde russkikh estestvoispytateleĭ i vracheĭ (k 100-letiiu teorii fagotsitoza). **Zh Mikrobiol Epidemiol Immunobiol** 1984 Aug;(8):115–8

**Yugoslavia**

Mijalković D: Doprinos dr Laze K.Lazarevića infektologiji XIX veka. **Srp Arh Celok Lek** 1980 Jan;108(1):77–80

## INFECTIOUS MONONUCLEOSIS

**1700 to Present**

**United States**

Paul JR, Bunnell WW: Classics in infectious diseases. The presence of heterophile antibodies in infectious mononucleosis by John R. Paul and W. W. Bunnell. American Journal of the Medical Sciences, 1932.

## INFLUENZA

Pacheco CR: Influenza. **Gac Med Mex** 1982 Feb;118(2):78–82

**Great Britain**

Hope-Simpson RE: Recognition of historic influenza epidemics from parish burial records: a test of prediction from a new hypothesis of influenzal epidemiology. **J Hyg (Lond)** 1983 Oct;91(2):293–308

**1700 to Present**

Shdanov VM: Molekularbiologie und Okologie der Virusgrippe. **Z Erkr Atmungsorgane** 1983;161(1):74–9
Stevens KM: The pathophysiology of influenzal pneumonia in 1918. **Perspect Biol Med** 1981 Autumn;25(1):115–25
Wyss E: Erinnerungen an die Grippeepidemie im Aktivdienst 1918. **Berner Z Gesch Heimatkd** 1977;39:118–30

**Botswana**

Spears JV: An epidemic among the Kgatla: the influenza of 1918. **Botsw Notes Rec** 1979;11:69–76

**Canada**

McGinnis JP: A city faces an epidemic. **Alberta Hist** 1976;24(4):1–11
McGinnis JP: The impact of epidemic influenza, Canada, 1918–1919. **Hist Pap Can Hist Assoc** 1977;120–41
McGinnis JP: The impact of epidemic influenza: Canada, 1918–1919. **Can Hist Assoc Hist Pap** 1977;:121–40

**Europe**

Olagüe de Ros G: La epidemia europea de gripe de 1708–1709. Difusión témporo-espacial e interpretaciones contemporáneas: G. M. Lancisi, B. Ramazzini, K. F. Hoffmann. **Dynamis** 1981;1:51–86

**Great Britain**

Andrewes CH: Alick Isaacs. In Dictionary of national biography, 1961–1970. Suppl. 8, 1981. p. 569–70.
Kapsenberg JG: Een halve eeuw modern influenza-onderzoek. **Ned Tijdschr Geneeskd** 1983 Sep 24;127(39):1780–1
Wilson A: Oddity remembered: 1918 influenza epidemic. **Br Med J** 1981;282:1766

**New Zealand**

Bryder L: 'Lessons' of the 1918 influenza epidemic in Auckland. **NZ J Hist** 1982;16(2):97–121
Wright-St Clair RE: Influenza in New Zealand and the doctors who died from it. **NZ Med J** 1983 Oct 12;96(741):765–8

**Nigeria**

Ohadike DC: The influenza pandemic of 1918–19 and the spread of cassava cultivation on the lower Niger: a study in historical linkages. **J Afr Hist** 1981;22(3):380–91

**Pacific Islands**

Boyd M: Coping with Samoan restistance after the 1918 influenza epidemic: Colonel Tate's problems and perplexities. **J Pac Hist** 1980;15(3):155–74

**South Africa**

Gear JH: The 1918 influenza epidemic. **Adler Mus Bull** 1983 Nov;Spec issue:13–20

**Switzerland**

Nussbaum W: Die Grippe-Epidemie 1918/1919 in der schweizerischen Armee. **Gesnerus** 1982;39(2):243–59

**United States**

Bernstein BJ: On mass inoculation, who should be heard? **Cent Mag** 1981;14(5):56–61
Burch M: 'I don't know only what we hear': the soldiers' view of the 1918 influenza epidemic. **Indiana Med Hist Q** 1983 Dec;9(4):23–7
Cumberland WH: Epidemic! Iowa battles the Spanish influenza. **Palimpsest** 1981;62(1):26–32
Ensley PC: Indiana and the influenza pandemic of 1918. **Indiana Med Hist Q** 1983 Dec;9(4):3–15
Grist NR: Pandemic influenza 1918. **Br Med J** 1979 Dec 22–29;2(6205):1632–3
Hutchens KS: The Indianapolis influenza epidemic of 1918. **Indiana Hist Soc** 1979 Dec;5(4):4–16
Impact of swine non-flu: **Lancet** 1982 Nov 6;2(8306):1029
McLaurin A: The influenza epidemic of 1918 in Shreveport. **North La Hist Assoc J** 1982;13(1):1–14
Melzer R: A dark and terrible moment: the Spanish flu epidemic of 1918 in New Mexico. **NM Hist Rev** 1982;57(3):213–36
Sanford WL: The influenza epidemic of 1918 and its effects on the military. **Indiana Med Hist Q** 1983 Dec;9(4):16–22
South A: What Camp Custer brought to Battle Creek. **Chronicle** 1982;18(4):28–30
Straight WM: Florida and the Spanish flu. **J Fla Med Assoc** 1981 Aug;68(8):644–54
Thomison JB: Disease in Nashville: a short history. **J Tenn Med Assoc** 1983 Mar;76(3):151–5
Walters KA: Mclean County and the influenza epidemic of 1918–1919. **J Ill State Hist Soc** 1981;74(2):130–44
Wolfe RJ: Alaska's great sickness, 1900: an epidemic of measles and influenza in a virgin soil population. **Proc Am Philos Soc** 1982;126(1):91–121

**USSR**

Smorodintsev AA: K istorii izucheniia étiologii i vaktsinoprofilaktiki grippa (nauchnyĭ vklad v étu problemu kliniki M. D. Tushinshinskogo). **Klin Med (Mosk)** 1982 Jan;60(1):108–12

**Yugoslavia**

Dragić M. Zdravstvene prilike u Beogradu za vreme okupacije u prvom svetskom ratu i spanski grip 1918–1919. godine. **Srp Arh Celok Lek** 1980 Sep;108(9):969–74

## JAUNDICE

Gartner LM: Neonatal jaundice: a selected retrospective. In Smith GF, Smith PN, Vidyasagar D, ed: Historical review and recent advances in neonatal and perinatal medicine. [Chicago?], Mead Johnson Nutritional

Division, 1983. Vol. I. p. 87–97.

**Before 500 A.D.**

**Greece**

Ullmann M: Die Schrift des Rufus von Ephesos über die Gelbsucht in arabischer und lateinischer Übersetzung. Göttingen, Vandenhoeck & Ruprecht, 1983. 87 p. (Abhandlungen der Akademie der Wissenschaften in Göttingen, Philologisch-Historische Klass; Folge 3, No 138)

**1700 to Present**

Pavel I: Aperçu historique de l'existence du rôle du shunt disse-canalicule biliaire dans la sécrétion biliaire et dans la pathogénie de certains ictères. **Med Interne** 1981 Oct–Dec;19(4):389–96

### KIDNEY

Giampalmo A: Patologia renale. Riferimenti e riflessioni. **Pathologica** 1983 Sep–Oct;75(1039):607–18
Gordon DB, ed: Hypertension: the renal basis. Stroudsburg, Pa, Dowden, Hutchinson & Ross, 1980. xvi, 432 p. (Benchmark Papers in Human Physiology, 13).
Hirsch B: Geschichte der Nierentuberkulose. Köln, 1983. 183 p. (Kölner medizinhistorische Beiträge, Band 28)
Wedeen RP: The role of lead in renal failure. **Clin Exp Dial Apheresis** 1982;6(2–3):113–46

**1450–1700**

**Italy**

Gelabert i Mas A, Gironella i Coll J: El papa Inocencio XI: approximación etiológica a su patología renal. In International Congress of the History of Medicine, 27th, Barcelona, 1980. Actas. Barcelona, Académia de Ciències Médiques de Catalunya i Balears, 1981. p. 506–10.

**1700 to Present**

Bergstrand A, Ostman J: Männen bakom syndromet: Paul Kimmelstiel och Clifford Wilson. Tysk och engelsman som möttes vid Harvard – först att beskriva speciell glomerulusskada. **Lakartidningen** 1984 Jan 25;81(4):227–8
Black D: The story of nephrology. **J R Soc Med** 1980 Jul;73(7):514–8
Brod J: Nephrology in the past, in the present and perspectives in the future. **Minerva Nefrol** 1983 Jan–Mar;30(1):1–6
Butkus DE: Post-traumatic acute renal failure in combat casualties: a historical review. **Milit Med** 1984 Mar;149(3):117–24
Calne RY: The development of immunosuppressive therapy. **Transplant Proc** 1981 Mar;13(1):44–9
Dimitrov TS: Istoricheski danni za balkanskata endemichna nefropatiia. **Vutr Boles** 1982;21(2):74–7
Hansen H, Susser M: Historic trends in death from chronic kidney disease in the United States and Britain. **Am J Epidemiol** 1971 Jun;93:413–24
Kolff WJ: Past, present, and future of artificial kidneys. **Transplant Proc** 1981 Mar;13(1):35–40
Merrill JP: Early days of the artificial kidney and transplantation. **Transplant Proc** 1981 Mar;13(1):4–8
Nicholls A: Atherosclerosis in chronic renal failure: a historical perspective. **Scott Med J** 1983 Jul;28(3):270–5
Patev E: Peritonealna dializa––minalo, nastoiashte i budeshte. **Vutr Boles** 1980;19(1):7–11
Timio M: Il rene artificiale: la storia di uno strumento per una vita semiartificiale. **Med Secoli** 1982;19(3):273–301
Válek A, Wing AJ: Development of dialysis and transplant activity in the world during the seventies of the 20th century. **Z Exp Chir Transplant Kunstliche Organe** 1984;17(2):69–78

**France**

Mirouze J: Les transformations en un quart de siècle de l'insuffisance rénale aiguë. **Nephrologie** 1981;2(1):20–2

**Germany**

Bach H: Die Entwicklung der künstlichen Niere aus Hydrodiffusion und Hämodialyse, von J. A. Nollet bis G. Haas. Der Ursprung des ersten Künstlichen inneren Organs. Giessen, Schmitz, 1983. 334 p. (Arbeiten zur Geschichte der Medizin in Giessen, Bd. 7)
Sarre HJ: Glomerulonephritis im Wandel der Zeit. Gedanken zu 40 Jahren Nephrologie. **Fortschr Med** 1982 Mar 4;100(9):364–73

**Great Britain**

Boss J: Richard Bright's Reports of Medical Cases (1827): a sesquicentennial note. **Bristol Med Chir J** 1978 Jan–Apr;93(345–346):5–6, 18
Hakulinen E: Mannen bakom syndromet: Richard Bright. En av de stora inom njurforskningen––hans 'Reports of medical cases' epokgörande. **Lakartidningen** 1984 Apr 25;81(17):1722–3
McGeown MG: Twenty-first birthday of the Renal Unit at the Belfast City Hospital. **Ulster Med J** 1981;50(Suppl 1):2–3
McWhinnie DL, Hamilton DN: The rise and fall of surgery for the 'floating' kidney. **Br Med J [Clin Res]** 1984 Mar 17;288(6420):845–7
Peitzman SJ: Bright's disease and Bright's generation––toward exact medicine at Guy's Hospital. **Bull Hist Med** 1981;55(3):307–21
Spriggs EA: The illnesses and death of Robert Walpole. **Med Hist** 1982 Oct;26(4):421–8

**Italy**

Vercellone A: Vent'anni di nefrologia italiana. **Minerva Nefrol** 1979 Oct–Dec;26(4):443–8

**Netherlands**

Hamburger J: Past, present, and future of transplantation. **Transplant Proc** 1981 Mar;13(1):41–3

**Scandinavia**

Groth CG: Kidney transplantations in the Nordic countries 1956–1980. **Scand J Urol Nephrol** 1981;64:12–5

**United States**

Dammin GJ: Transplantation, 1950s. **Transplant Proc** 1981 Mar;13(1):16–23
Gardner KD: Looking upon the water: in which we return to the Civil War. **Am J Kidney Dis** 1984 Sep;4(2):101–2
Goodwin WE: Recollections: early experiences in kidney transplantation. **Transplant Proc** 1981 Mar;13(1):29–31
Gutman RA: Renal dialysis for kidney failure in North Carolina: history, practice, and lessons. **NC Med J** 1984 Jun;45(6):359–63
Hufnagel CA, Thorn GW: Observations of a colleague (Carl W. Walter). **Am J Surg** 1984 Nov;148(5):581–3
Kunitomo T: Development of new artificial kidney systems (Carl W. Walter). **Am J Surg** 1984 Nov;148(5):594–8
Murphy WP: Carl Walter: a pioneer in shaping the medical device industry. **Am J Surg** 1984 Nov;148(5):590–3
Murray JE: Remembrances of the early days of renal transplantation. **Transplant Proc** 1981 Mar;13(1):9–15
Panel on dialysis: **Transplant Proc** 1981 Mar;13(1):67–71
Rettig RA: Health care technology. Lessons learned from the end-stage renal disease experience. Santa Monica, Rand Corp., 1976. 36 p.
Terreros DA, Grantham JJ: Marshall Barber and the origins of micropipette methods. **Am J Physiol** 1982 Mar;242(3):F293–6
Thorn GW: A 50th anniversary celebration. **Transplant Proc** 1981 Mar;13(1):24–8
Vandam LD: Impressions of anesthetics past. **Transplant Proc** 1981 Mar;13(1):61–4

**USSR**

Hamilton DN, Reid WA: Yu. Yu. Voronoy and the first human kidney allograft. **Surg Gynecol Obstet** 1984 Sep;159(3):289–94
Mirski MB: [The history of the problem of kidney transplantation in Soviet medicine (Rus). **Orvostort Kozl** 1980;89–91(26 no 1–3):125–36
Pyrig LA, Mel'man NIa, Nemirovich LI: K istorii nauchnykh issledovaniĭ po nefrologii v nefrologii v Ukrainskoĭ SSR. **Vrach Delo** 1983 Dec;(12):1–5

### LEISHMANIASIS

Goldman L: Pre-Columbian leishmaniasis. **Arch Dermatol** 1983 Jul;119(7):540

**Egypt**

Morsy TA: Cutaneous leishmaniasis in Egypt. Historical background and current knowledge. **J Egypt Soc Parasitol** 1983 Dec;13(2):597–611

**Italy**

Pampiglione S, Bettini S: Bibliografia Italiana delle leishmaniosi dalle origini al 1980. **Ann Ist Super Sanita** 1981;17(1):1–150

**Before 500 A.D.**

**Mexico**

Martínez Marañón R: Urna olmeca que podría representar la leishmaniasis tegumentaria diseminada. **Salud Publica Mex** 1982 Sep–Oct;24(5):497–507

# DISEASES AND INJURIES

### 500 A.D.-1450

#### Peru

Heck J: Leishmaniasis und Fruchtbarkeitskult. **Dtsch Med Wochenschr** 1982 Jun 4;107(22):872-4

### 1700 to Present

#### Africa

Desjeux P, Waroquy L, Dedet JP: La leishmaniose cutanée humaine en Afrique de l'ouest. **Bull Soc Pathol Exot Filiales** 1981 Jul-Aug;74(4):414-25

#### India

Gibson ME: The identification of kala azar and the discovery of Leishmania donovani. **Med Hist** 1983 Apr;27(2):203-13

#### Italy

Pampiglione S: Il contributo di Achille Breda alla conoscenza della leishmaniosi muco-cutanea americana. **Parassitologia** 1979 Dec;21(1-3):35-58

#### Panama

Christensen HA, Fairchild GB, Herrer A, et al: The ecology of cutaneous leishmaniasis in the Republic of Panama. **J Med Entomol** 1983 Oct 5;20(5):463-84

#### USSR

Fonareva KS: K istorii izucheniia kozhnogo leĭshmanioza v Rossii. **Med Parazitol (Mosk)** 1983 Mar-Apr;52(2):84-6

## LEPROSY

Browne SG: How old is leprosy? **Int J Dermatol** 1980 Nov;19(9):530-2
González Galván A: Aspectos sociales de la lepra. **Prensa Med Mex** 1978 Sep-Oct;43(9-10):261-3
Griffin RJ: New approaches to an ancient disease: leprosy. **Am Pharm** 1981 Sep;21(9):18-23
Ober WB: Can the leper change his spots? The iconography of leprosy. Part I. **Am J Dermatopathol** 1983 Feb;5(1):43-58
Prioleau E: Leprosy. Reality and metaphor in literature. **Am J Dermatopathol** 1983 Aug;5(4):377-80
Quiroga MI: La lepra, pasado y presente. Buenos Aires, Lopez, 1974. 195 p.
Rees RJ: An appraisal of medical research in the treatment and control of leprosy. **Lepr India** 1982 Oct;54(4):783-800
Reverte Coma JM: La lepra en la historia. **Fontilles** 1980;12:565-92
Tokunaga S: [Scenes with illness. 8. Tragic past of the leprosy patients] (Jpn). **Kango Kyoiku** 1980 Aug;21(8):519-24
Trautman JR: A brief history of Hansen's disease. **Bull NY Acad Med** 1984 Sep;60(7):689-95

#### Africa

Grainger CR: Leprosy in the Seychelles. **Lepr Rev** 1980;51(1):43-9
Hunter JM, Thomas MO: Hypothesis of leprosy, tuberculosis and urbanization in Africa. **Soc Sci Med** 1984;19(1):27-57

#### Belgium

Marechal G: De leprozen in de kwartieren Brugge en het Brugse Vrije. Nieuwe cijfers. **Ann Soc Emulation Bruges** 1979;116:147-62
Maurissen AW: De leprozerie van Molenbeek. **Eigen Schoon Brabander** 1979;62:29-40
Pirotte F: Note sur l'évolution de la ladrerie de la Hesse à Tohogne. Du moyen âge à la fin de l'ancien régime. **Ann Inst Archeol Luxemb** 1975-76:106-7:163-81

#### Brazil

Belda W: Aspectos da hanseníase na área urbana do município de São Paulo - Hanseníase indiferenciada, 1963-1977. **Hansenol Int** 1981 Jun;6(1):23-50

#### Cambodia

Chandler DP: Folk memories of the decline of Angkor in nineteenth-century Cambodia: the legend of the leper king. **J Siam Soc** 1979;67(1):54-62

#### Ethiopia

Pankhurst R: Le piaghe d'Etiopia. **Kos** 1984 Jul-Aug;1(6):33-50
Pankhurst R: The history of leprosy in Ethiopia to 1935. **Med Hist** 1984 Jan;28(1):57-72

#### Europe

Hörger H: Krankheit und religiöses Tabu--die Lepra in der mittelalterlich-frühneuzeitlichen Gesellschaft Europas. **Gesnerus** 1982;39(1):53-70
Palmer R: The Church, leprosy and plague in medieval and early modern Europe. In Sheils WJ, ed: The Church and healing. Papers read at the twentieth summer meeting and the twenty-first winter meeting of the Ecclesiastical History Society. Oxford, Basil Blackwell for the Society, 1982. p. 79-99.

#### France

Burgun R: Mesures de protection contre la lèpre et la syphilis à Strasbourg au cours des siècles. In Livet G, Schaff G, ed: Médecine et assistance en Alsace, XVIe-XXe siècle. Strasbourg, Istra, 1976. p. 53-67.
Guy Y: Sur les origines possibles de la ségrégation des Cagots. **Hist Sci Med** 1983;17(1):85-93

#### Great Britain

Mortimer R: The Prior of Butley and the lepers of West Somerton. **Bull Inst Hist Res** 1980;53:99-103

#### India

Banerjee B, Hazra J: Geo-ecology of leprosy with special reference to West Bengal. **Geogr Med** 1982;12:26-58

#### Italy

Terencio de las Aguas J: La lepra en el reino de Valencia. **Fontilles** 1977;11:237-40

#### Japan

Kikuchi Keifuen, Koshi, Japan: Kanja Jichikai. Jichikai 50-nenshi Hensan Iinkai. Jichikai 50-nenshi. Koshimachi, Japan, Kikuchi Keifuen Kanja Jichikai, [1976]. 49, 228 p.

#### Korea

Shin JS: Leprosy in Korea. **Nippon Rai Gakkai Zasshi** 1982 Oct-Dec;51(4):211-6

#### Mexico

Saúl A, Latapí F: La lepra en México. In Academia Nacional de Medicina. Libro conmemorativo del primer centenario. México, Comité Editorial de la Comisión Organizadora del Congreso del Centenario, 1964. Tome 2. p. 89-99.

#### Netherlands

Maréchal G: Lepra in Vlaanderen. **Spiegel Hist** 1980;15(3):137-41

#### Norway

Zirinsky L: The Leprosy Museum of Bergen. **St Mary Hosp Gaz** 1979 Autumn;85:23

#### Spain

Juncà i Ramon JM: L'Hospital de Sant Llàtzer: notes històriques. [S.l.]: J. M. Juncà Ramon, 1982. 47 p.

#### United States

Hudson T, Genesse J: Hansen's Disease in the United States. **Soc Sci Med** 1982;16(9):997-1004

### Before 500 A.D.

Freilich AR: Tzaraat--'biblical leprosy'. **J Am Acad Dermatol** 1982 Jan;6(1):131-4
Stettler A: Lepra und Pest in der Antike. **Antike Welt** 1977;8(4):42-4

#### China

Skinsnes OK: Leprosy in archeologically recovered bamboo book in China. **Int J Lepr** 1980 Sept;48(3):333

#### Egypt

Dzierzykray-Rogalski T: Un cas de la lèpre à un stade avancé découvert dans la nécropole musulmane de Kôm El-Dikka, à Alexandrie. **Afr Bull** 1978;28:140–6

### 500 A.D.–1450

Barber M: Lepers, Jews and Moslems: the plot to overthrow Christendom in 1321. **History** 1981;66:1–17

Ober WB: Can the leper change his spots? The iconography of leprosy. Part II. **Am J Dermatopathol** 1983 Apr;5(2):173–86

Terencio de las Aguas J: La lepra en el libro 'Doctrina de morbis cutaneis' de José Jacoba Plenck. **Fontilles** 1980;12:409–14

#### Arabic

Abdullaev AKh, Sharafiddinov TA: Abu Ali Ibn-Sina (Avitsenna) o lepre. **Vestn Dermatol Venerol** 1981 May;(5):76–9

Dols MW: The leper in medieval Islamic society. **Speculum** 1983 Oct;58(4):891–916

#### Belgium

De Keyzer W: L'évolution de la léproserie Saint-Ladre de Mons aux XIIIe et XIVe siècles. Fédération des Cercles d'Archéologie et d'Histoire de Belgique. 44e session. Congrès de Huy, 1976. Annales. Tielt, 1978. p. 174–6.

De Spiegeler P: La léproserie de Cornillon et la cité de Liège (XIIe–XVe siècle). **Ann Soc Belg Hist Hop** 1980;18:3–16

Marechal G: De leprozen in de kwartieren Brugge en het Brugse vrije. Nieuwe cijfers. **Ann Soc Emulation Bruges** 1979;116:147–62

#### Denmark

Jensen KR, Tkocz I: Skeletmaterialet fra udgravningen af St. Jørgensgården i Odense. En foreløbig rapport. **Dan Medicinhist Arbog** 1983;12:52–64

Nielsen E: Udgravningen af Odenses St. Jørgensgård. Foreløbige resultater. **Dan Medicinhist Arbog** 1983;12:39–51

#### France

Touati FO: Une approche de la maladie et du phénomène hospitalier aux XIIe et XIIIe siècles: la léproserie du Grand-Beaulieu à Chartres. **Hist Sci Med** 1980;14:419–24

#### Spain

Terencio de las Aguas J: La lepra en el Reino de Valencia. **Fontilles** 1979;12(1):5–10

### 1450–1700

#### Belgium

Marechal G: Het gebouw van de Brugse Leprozorie in de XVIe eeuw. **Biekorf** 1979;79:316–22

#### France

Vally G: Ludovic cel stăruitor si misterioasa sa moarte. **Mag Istor** 1976;10(10):52–4

#### Germany

Virchow R: A painting of lepers by Hans Holbein the Elder. **Am J Dermatopathol** 1984 Aug;6(4):377–8

#### Indonesia

Subba Reddy DV: Wilhem Ten Rhyne (Rhijne) and his Treatise on Asiatic Leprosy; a medical classic by a Dutch physician in Java in the last quarter of 17th century. **Bull Indian Inst Hist Med (Hyderabad)** 1975 Jul;5(3):150–61

### 1700 to Present

Arnold HL: How 'indeterminate' leprosy got its name. **Int J Dermatol** 1981 Jun;20(5):393–5

Brandt AM: James Angus Doull. In Dictionary of American biography, 1961–1965. Suppl. 7, 1981. p. 194–5.

Cochrane RG: Notes concerning the formation of the International Leprosy Association. **Int J Lepr** 1981 Mar;49(1):67–71

Contreras Dueñas F: La lepra se cura cada vez con mayor frecuencia. De acuerdo con los recientes progresos científicos tienen que terminar todas las enfermedades incurables.

Klokke AH: Antibakterielle Behandlung der erregerreichen Lepra. **Hautarzt** 1983 May;34(5):203–8

Lechat MF: The International Leprosy Association at 50 years. **Int J Lepr** 1981 Mar;49(1):60–4

Siqueira LF, de Almeida RG, Belda W: Métodos tintoriais utilizados na identificação do Mycobacterium leprae. Revisão histórica. **Rev Saude Publica** 1984 Jun;18(3):246–58

Thoire V de: L'Ordre Souverain de Malte au secours des lépreux. Vingt-cinq ans d'activité du CIOMAL 1958–1983. **Acta Leprol (Geneve)** 1983 Oct–Dec;(93):191–203

#### Americas

Kalisch PA: Tracadie and Penikese leprosaria: a comparative analysis of societal response to leprosy in New Brunswick, 1844–1880, and Massachusetts, 1904–1921. **Bull Hist Med** 1973 Sep–Oct;47(5):480–512

#### Argentina

Quiroga M: Juan Angel Farini, medico. **Bol Acad Nac Hist (Argentina)** 1967;40:348–53

#### Australia

Davidson WS: Havens of refuge. Nedlands, Univ. of Western Australia Press, 1978. xii, 188 p.

#### Canada

McGinnis JD: 'Unclean, unclean': Canadian reaction to lepers and leprosy In Roland CG, ed: Health, disease and medicine. Toronto, Hannah Institute for the History of Medicine, 1984. p. 250–75.

#### China

Haide M: Leprosy control in China 1981. **East Horiz** 1981;20(9):18–21

#### France

Basset A: Aperçu sur l'épidémiologie de la lèpre en France au cours de ces cinquante dernières années. **Bull Mem Acad R Med Belg** 1984;139(2):156–64

#### Great Britain

Grainger CR: Leprosy and Curieuse Island. **Lepr Rev** 1981 Jun;52(2):151–4

Jackson R: Hutchinson on leprosy. **Int J Dermatol** 1982 Dec;21(10):614–9

#### India

Acworth GW: Acworth Leprosy Hospital, Bombay. **Lepr Rev** 1984 Mar;55(1):77–8

#### Iran

Assefi V: Le lèpre en Iran. **Acta Leprol (Geneve)** 1982 Nov–Dec;(89):53–60

#### Mali

Saint André P: The Marchoux Institute. **Lepr Rev** 1980 Mar;51(1):35–42

#### Norway

Forsdahl A, Dahl T: Spedalske i brønnøy legedistrikt i forrige århundre. **Tidsskr Nor Laegeforen** 1983 Oct 30;103(30):2024–7

Hansen GA, Watt FB, ed: The memories and reflections of Dr. G. Armauer Hansen. Würzburg, German Leprosy Relief Association, 1976. 135 p.

Harboe M: The work and concepts of Armauer Hansen: how do they stand today? **Ethiop Med J** 1983 Apr;21(2):123–6

Irgens LM: The discovery of Mycobacterium leprae. A medical achievement in the light of evolving scientific methods. **Am J Dermatopathol** 1984 Aug;6(4):337–43

Refsum S: Some aspects of the history of neurology in Norway. In Rose FC, Bynum WF, ed: Historical aspects of the neurosciences. New York, Raven, 1982. p. 415–33.

#### Philippines

Binford CH, Reich CV: Ricardo S. Guinto, M.D., M.P.H., epidemiologist-leprologist, 1907–1983. In appreciation of 50 years dedicated to research in leprosy. **Int J Lepr** 1983 Dec;51(4):587–91

Chapman RF: Leonard Wood and leprosy in the Philippines: the Culion Leper Colony, 1921–1927. [Washington, D. C.], University Press of America, 1982. xviii, 219 p.

# DISEASES AND INJURIES

**Spain**

Terencio de las Aguas J: La lepra en el Reino de Valencia (sigo XX). **Fontilles** 1978;11:465-6

**United States**

Binford Ch: Esmond Ray Long, M.D., Ph. D., 1890-1979, Editor, International Journal of Leprosy, 1964-1968. **Int J Lepr** 1980 Sep;48(3):322-6
Bushnell OA: 'Our good friend Mr. Stevenson'. **Biography** 1982;5(2):118-28
Judd CS Jr: Leprosy in Hawaii, 1889-1976. **Hawaii Med J** 1984 Sep;43(9):328-9, 333-4
Michael JM: The Public Health Service leprosy investigation station on Molokai, Hawaii, 1909-13 -- an opportunity lost. **Public Health Rep** 1980 May-Jun;95(3):203-9
Sabin TD: The Penikese Hospital: a Massachusetts hospital for the treatment of Hansen's disease. **N Engl J Med** 1981 Jun 25;304(26):1610-2
Skinsnes AV, Binford CH: Leprosy research and the Public Health Service -- a brief chronological résumé. **Public Health Rep** 1980 May-Jun;95(3):210-2
Wilson DC: Ten fingers for God: [the complete biography of Dr. Paul Brand]. Nashville, Nelson Publ, 1983. vii, 275 p.

**USSR**

Palkin BN: Iz istorii issledovaniia lepry v Astrakhanskoĭ gubernii v XVIII veke. **Vestn Dermatol Venerol** 1982 Aug;(8):72-4

**Zaire**

Dubois A: La lèpre au Congo avant les sulfones. **Bull Seances Acad R Sci Outre Mer** 1965;11(2):640-51

### LEPTOSPIROSIS

**1700 to Present**

Gsell O: The history of leptospirosis: 100 years. **Zentralbl Bakteriol Mikrobiol Hyg [A]** 1984 Sep;257(4):473-8

**Mexico**

Ruiloba J: Listeriosis, toxoplasmosis y leptospirosis. In Academia Nacional de Medicina. Libro conmemorativo del primer centenario. México, Comité Editorial de la Comisión Organizadora del Congreso del Centenario, 1964. Tome 2. p. 532-5.

**Poland**

Bluszcz G, Ciszek Z: Leptospirozt w materiale chorych oddziału zakaźnego w Raciborzu w latach 1966-1977. **Przegl Epidemiol** 1979;33(4):515-8

### LEUKEMIA

**1450-1700**

**Japan**

Hino S, Konoshita K, Kitamura T: HTLV and the propagation of Christianity in Nagasaki. **Lancet** 1984 Sep 8;2(8402):572-3

**1700 to Present**

Bessis M, Bernard J: Remissions after exchange transfusions in acute leukemia. On the possible antileukemic properties of normal blood. Historical notes and recent reflections. **Blood Cells** 1983;9(1):75-82
Fleming AF: HTLV from Africa to Japan. **Lancet** 1984 Feb 4;1(8371):279
Johnson FL: Marrow transplantation in the treatment of acute childhood leukemia. Historical development and current approaches. **Am J Pediatr Hematol Oncol** 1981 Winter;3(4):389-95
Kerner D: Béla Bartóks Tod in New York. Zu seinem 100. Geburtstag am 25. März 1981. **MMW** 1981 Mar 27;123(13):525-9
Seufert W, Seufert WD: The recognition of leukemia as a systemic disease. **J Hist Med Allied Sci** 1982 Jan;37(1):34-50

**Poland**

Janicki K: Charakterystyka zachorowalności na białaczki w regionie krakowskim w latach 1961-1968 w świetle oceny prawdopodobieństwa według rozkładu Poissona. Doniesienie I: Analiza rozkładu częstości białaczek w 18 powiatowych jednostkach administracyjnych, przy założeniu równomiernego rozrzutu w całym regionie krakowskim. **Folia Med Cracov** 1979;21(2):275-94

**United States**

Miller RW, McKay FW: Decline in US childhood cancer mortality. 1950 through 1980. **JAMA** 1984 Mar 23-30;251(12):1567-70

**USSR**

Evdokimov PP: K istorii bolezni F. I. Shaliapina. **Klin Med (Mosk)** 1983 May;61(5):115-6

### LIVER

Heer K de: Zur Pathogenität der Galle. Historisches und neue experimentelle Ergebnisse. **Med Welt** 1981 Aug 28;32(35):1292-6
Kuehn HA: Virushepatitis - Rückblick und Ausblick. **Leber Magen Darm** 1980;10:131-8
Renger FG: Zur Geschichte der Hepatologie von Galen bis Frerichs. **Dtsch Z Verdau Stoffwechselkr** 1982;42(5):193-202

**Arabic**

Said HM: Diseases of the liver: Greco-Arab concepts. Karachi, Hamdard Foundation Press, 1982. 131 p.

**Austria**

Popper H: Vienna and the liver. **Gastroenterology** 1984 May;86(5 Pt 1):982-6

**500 A.D.-1450**

**Arabic**

Arzumetov IuS: Voprosy gepatologii v 'Kanone vrachebnoĭ nauki' Ibn-Sina. **Sov Zdravookhr** 1980;(5):67-9

**1450-1700**

**Great Britain**

Mani N: Biomedical thought in Glisson's hepatology and in Wepfer's work on apoplexy. With commentary by R. G. Frank, p. 84-8. In Stevenson LG, ed: A celebration of medical history. Baltimore, Johns Hopkins University Press, 1982. (The Henry E. Sigerist supplements to the Bulletin of the History of Medicine; new ser., no. 6). p. 37-63.

**1700 to Present**

Brzozowski R, Piątkiewicz W: Sztuczna wątroba--historia idzień dzisiejszy. **Pol Arch Med Wewn** 1980 Nov;64(5):457-65
McCollum RW: Some observations on viral hepatitis. **Yale J Biol Med** 1982 May-Aug;55(3-4):247-50
Valencia-Parparcen J: Cirrosis hepática. **GEN** 1981 Jan-Jun;35(1-2):43-97

**Australia**

Hussey HH: The hepatitis B saga. **JAMA** 1981 Apr 3;245(13):1317-8

**Czechoslovakia**

Hořejší J: Jak u nás začínal a rozvíjel se výzkum jaterních chorob, zejména hepatitidy a její prevence. Retrospektivní pohled. **Cas Lek Cesk** 1981 Oct 1;120(39):1174-7

**Germany**

Lehmann H: Zur Geschichte der parenteralen Uebertragung der akuten ikterischen Virushepatitis. **Dtsch Med Wochenschr** 1981 Apr 17;106(16):517
Renger F: Razvitie na khepatologiiata v GDR. **Vutr Boles** 1980;19(6):2-6
Wildhirt E: Dreissig Jahre Hepatologie in Kassel. In Balde JH, Schmiking, W, ed: Festschrift zum 86. Deutschen Arztetag in Kassel. Kassel, Arztevereins, 1983. p. 99-104.

**Great Britain**

Whelton MJ: Perspective in liver disease: an Irish experience. **Ir J Med Sci** 1979 May-Jun;148(5-6):161-7

**Mexico**

Fournier Villada R: Miguel Jiménez y su contribución al estudio del absceso hepático. In Academia Nacional de Medicina. Libro conmemorativo del primer centenario. México, Comité Editorial de la Comisión Organizadora del Congreso del Centenario, 1964. Tome 2. p. 558-60.

**Romania**

Babeş VT: Recent research on viral hepatitis performed in the 'Stefan S. Nicolau' Institute of Virology. **Virologie** 1984 Oct-Dec;35(4):251-7

**United States**

Popper H: History of the American Association for the Study of Liver Diseases. **Hepatology** 1982 Nov-Dec;2(6):874-8
Sherlock S: Landmark perspective: Landmarks in viral hepatitis **JAMA** 1984 Jul 20;252(3):402-6

**USSR**

Shliakhtenko LI, Kryga LN, Liamtseva GA, et al: Evoliutsiia épidemicheskogo protsessa virusnogo gepatita v Leningrade za 30 let. **Tr Inst Pastera** 1982;57:43-5

### LYMPHATIC

Fraikor AL: Fiddling on a drifting roof: genetic implications of Jewish settlement patterns and life style. **Prog Clin Biol Res** 1982;95:535-47
Gregl A, Heyden D von, Muschter R: Diagnostik peripherer Odeme in der Praxis und in der Klinik. **Z Lymphol** 1982 Jun;6(1):25-32

**1700 to Present**

Desnick RJ: Gaucher disease: a century of delineation and understanding. **Prog Clin Biol Res** 1982;95:1-30
Gaucher disease: A century of delineation and research. **Prog Clin Biol Res** 1982;95:1-740

**Great Britain**

Geller SA: Comments on the anniversary of the description of Hodgkin's disease. **Mt Sinai J Med (NY)** 1982 Jul-Aug;49(4):308-10

**Japan**

Shigematsu I, ed, Kawasaki T, ed, Kusakawa S, ed: Kawasakibyo (MCLS) kenkyu no ayumi. Tokyo, Kindai Shuppan, 1976. ix, 224 p.
Suchi T: The changing concept and classification of malignant lymphomas. **Jpn J Med** 1984 Feb;23(1):74-6

**United States**

Desnick RJ: Gaucher disease (1882-1982): centennial perspectives on the most prevalent Jewish genetic disease. **Mt Sinai J Med (NY)** 1982 Nov-Dec;49(6):443-55

### MALARIA

De Zulueta J: La introducción del 'Plasmodium falciparum' en la Europa del Mediterráneo: passado y presente. **Rev Sanid Hig Publica (Madr)** 1982 Jul-Aug;56(7-8):693-8
Earle DP: A history of malaria and its ironies. **Trans Am Clin Climatol Assoc** 1979;90:1-26
Garnham PC: The present state of malaria research: an historical survey. **Experientia** 1984 Dec 15;40(12):1305-10
Leavesley J: Malaria. **Med J Aust** 1984 Oct 13;141(8):523-5
Leden I: Antimalarial drugs--350 years. **Scand J Rheumatol** 1981;10(4):307-12
Martínez-Báez M: Conmemoración del descubrimiento de uno de los gérmens patogénicos del paludismo. III. La contribución de la ciencia al conocimiento y dominio del paludismo. **Gac Med Mex** 1981 May;117(5):209-14
Metcalf CD: CAPS jottings on malaria. **Cent Afr J Med** 1979 Sep;25(9):207-11 (continued periodically)
Pitzilis A: Le origini della malaria. **Minerva Med** 1983 Sep 22;74(36):2103-12

**Europe**

Bruce-Chwatt LJ, Zulueta J de: The rise and fall of malaria in Europe; a historico-epidemiological study. Oxford, Oxford University Press, 1980, xvi, 240 p.

**Great Britain**

Dobson M: Marsh fever: the geography of malaria in England. **J Hist Geogr** 1980;6(4):357-89

**Sri Lanka**

Wickramasinghe MB: Malaria and its control in Sri Lanka. **Ceylon Med J** 1981 Sep;26(3):107-15

**1450-1700**

**Great Britain**

Bruce-Chwatt LJ: Myth of quartan malaria. **Trans R Soc Trop Med Hyg** 1982;76(1):133-4

**Sudan**

Kaba L: Archers, musketeers, and mosquitoes: the Moroccan invasion of the Sudan and the Songhay resistance (1591-1612). **J Afr Hist** 1981;22(4):457-75

**1700 to Present**

Beauperthuy de Benedetti R: Laveran y Beauperthuy. **Acta Med Venez** 1981 Jan-Mar;28(1):47-52
Beltrán E: Conmemoración del descubrimiento de uno de los gérmenes patogénicos del paludismo. **Gac Med Mex** 1981 May;117(5):195-201
Bruce-Chwatt LJ: Man against malaria: conquest or defeat. **Trans R Soc Trop Med Hyg** 1979;73(6):605-17
Chapin G, Wasserstrom R: Pesticide use and malaria resurgence in Central America and India. **Soc Sci Med** 1983;17(5):273-90
Downs WG: A new look at yellow fever and malaria. **Am J Trop Med Hyg** 1981 May;30(3):516-22
Durnin E: Cancels unite world against malaria. **Scalpel Tongs** 1981;25:49
Hall AP: Exotic infectious diseases: malaria. **R Soc Health J** 1980 Apr;100(2):57-61
Harrison G: Mosquitoes, malaria, and man: A history of the hostilities since 1880. New York, Dutton, 1978. 314 p.
Smith DC: The rise and fall of typhomalarial fever: II. decline and fall. **J Hist Med Allied Sci** 1982 Jul;37(3):287-321
Zasukhin DN: 100-letie otkrytiia vozbuditelia maliarii. **Parazitologiia** 1981 May-Jun;15(3):298-301

**Africa**

Carlson DG: African fever, a study of British science, technology, and politics in West Africa, 1787-1864. New York, Science History Pub., 1981.
Moretti G, Bosredon J: Le paludisme nautique tropical de la côte d'Afrique, hier et aujourd'hui. In: Congrès National des Sociétés Savantes, 104e, Bordeaux, 1979. Comptes Rendus. Paris, 1979. Section des Sciences, Fasc. IV. p. 309-17.
Nicolle P: Alphonase Laveran et Charles Nicolle. **Arch Inst Pasteur Tunis** 1981 Sep-Dec;58(3):265-79
Wirz A: Malaria-Prophylaxe und kolonialer Städtebau: Fortschritt als Rückschritt? **Gesnerus** 1980;37(3/4):215-34

**Algeria**

Laveran CL: Classics in infectious diseases: A newly discovered parasite in the blood of patients suffering from malaria. Parasitic etiology of attacks of malaria: Charles Louis Alphonse Laveran (1845-1922). **Rev Infect Dis** 1982 Jul-Aug;4(4):908-11

**Belgium**

Bouckaert A: Le paludisme, maladie professionnelle du soldat belge avant 1900. **Rev Belge Hist Milit** 1980;23:525-8

**Canada**

Roland CG: 'Sunk under the taxation of nature': malaria in Upper Canada. In Roland CG, ed: Health, disease and medicine. Toronto, Hannah Institute for the History of Medicine, 1984. p. 154-70.

**China**

Rosner E: 'Gewöhnung' an die Malaria in chinesischen Quellen des 18. Jhdts. **Sudhoffs Arch** 1984;68(1):43-60

**Denmark**

Andersen O: A malaria epidemic in Denmark. In Charbonneau H, Larose A, ed: The great mortalities: methodological studies of demographic crises in the past. Liège, Belgium, Ordina Editions, 1980. p. 33-49.

**France**

Bruce-Chwatt LJ: Alphonse Laveran's discovery 100 years ago and today's global fight against malaria. **J R Soc Med** 1981 Jul;74(7):531-6
Jarcho S: Laveran's discovery in the retrospect of a century. **Bull Hist Med** 1984 Summer;58(2):215-24
Lukács D: Száz éve fedezte fel Charles Alphonse Louis Laveran a malária kórokozóit. **Orv Hetil** 1980 Dec 14;121(50):3076-8
Mollaret P: La découverte, par Alphonse Laveran de l'agent du paludisme.

Constantine, 6 Novembre 1880. **Nouv Presse Med** 1980 Nov 1;9(41):3055–63
Nosny P: Alphonse Laveran et la découverte de l'hématozoaire du paludisme. **Bull Acad Natl Med (Paris)** 1980 Jan;164(1):80–7
Pene P: De Laveran aux conséquences médicales, sociales et économiques de sa découverte. **Bull Acad Natl Med (Paris)** 1980 Apr;164(4):382–92
Percebois G: Il y un siècle, Laveran découvrit l'hématozoaire du paludisme. **Ann Med Nancy** 1981;20:549–58
Theodorides J: Célébration du centenaire de la découverte par A. Laveran de l'Hématozoaire du paludisme. Strasbourg, 2–3 mai 1980. **Rev Hist Sci (Paris)** 1980;33(4):351–2

**Great Britain**

Tiburskaia NA, Dukhanina NN: Pamiati P. G. Shute (issledovaniia P. G. Shute shtammov Plasmodium vivax). **Med Parazitol (Mosk)** 1980 Jan–Feb;49(1):87–90

**Hungary**

Lorincz F: A malária elleni küzdelem hazánkban az elso világháború után - visszaemlékzés. **Orvostort Kozl** 1982;28(1-3):251–4
Lukács D: Id. Jancsó Miklós malária kutatásai. **Orv Hetil** 1981 Jan 25;122(4):224–6

**India**

Seal SC: Hundred years of malarial research. **J Indian Med Assoc** 1980 Apr 16;74(8):156–7

**Israel**

Kohn D, Weiss Z, Flatau E: The history of malaria in the Jezreel Valley in the years 1922–1928 in En Harod. **Koroth** 1982 Aug;8(3/4):177–86

**Malaysia**

Reid JA: Was Anopheles Donaldi a vector of malaria in Kuala Lumpur, Malaysia, in the past? **Trans R Soc Trop Med Hyg** 1980;74(3):337–9

**Pacific Islands**

Nelson HE: Disease, demography, and the evolution of social structure in Highland New Guinea. **J Polynesian Soc** 1971;80(2):204–16

**Panama**

Chaves-Carballo E: Samuel T. Darling: studies on malaria and the Panama Canal. **Bull Hist Med** 1980 Spring;54(1):95–100
Guardia CA: Salud pública y saneamiento en la Zona del Canal de Panamá: un recuento histórico, 1880–1915. **Bol Of Sanit Panam** 1983 Jul;95(1):62–73

**Romania**

Negru I: Primele campanii antimalarice în România. **Viata Med [Medii Sanit]** 1982 Mar;30(3):71–2
Ungureanu EM: Contribuţia Academicianului Mihai Ciucă pe plan naţional şi internaţional în domeniul combaterii malariei. **Rev Med Chir Soc Med Nat Iasi** 1983 Oct–Dec;87(4):729–30

**Spain**

Perez Moreda V: El paludismo en España a fines del siglo XVIII: la epidemia de 1786. **Asclepio** 1982;34:295–316

**United States**

Chernin E: Two physicians, a landscape architect, and malaria. **Bull NY Acad Med** 1984 Nov;60(9):932–7
McClary A: Don't go to Michigan, that land of ills. **Mich Hist** 1983;67(1):46–8
Smith DC: The rise and fall of typhomalarial fever: I. origins. **J Hist Med Allied Sci** 1982 Apr;37(2):182–220
Strickland WA: Quinine pills, manufactured on the Missouri frontier (1832–1862). **Pharm Hist** 1983;25(2):61–8
Wyler DJ: Landmark perspective: The ascent and decline of chloroquine. **JAMA** 1984 May 11;251(18):2420–2

**USSR**

Arkhangel'skiĭ GV: K istorii izucheniia neĭromalariii i soliarnogo sindroma. **Zh Nevropatol Psikhiatr** 1982;82(7):128–30
Conroy MS: Malaria in late Tsarist Russia. **Bull Hist Med** 1982 Spring;56(1):41–55
Maruashvili GM: Istoriia zavoza gambuzii v SSSR (k 100–letiiu so dnia rozhdeniia N. P. Rukhadze). **Med Parazitol (Mosk)** 1980 Jan–Feb;49(1):80–2

**Venezuela**

Gabaldon A: Malaria eradication in Venezuela: doctrine, practice, and achievements after twenty years. **Am J Trop Med Hyg** 1983 Mar;32(2):203–11

**Yugoslavia**

Nežić E: Historijat endemske malarije u Dalmaciji do 1923. g. In: I simpozij o historiji mikrobiologije i imunologije u Hrvatskoj do 1923. godine. Zagreb, Jugoslavenskoj akademiji, 1973. p. 71–9.

### MARFAN'S SYNDROME

**1700 to Present**

**Italy**

Schoenfeld MR: Nicolo Paganini--musical magician and Marfan mutant? **Med Times** 1980 Nov, 108(11):117–8, 120, 125

**United States**

Lattimer JK: Lincoln did not have the Marfan Syndrome; documented evidence. **NY State J Med** 1981 Nov;81(12):1805–13

### MEASLES

**Americas**

Measles and Indians: **Br Med J [Clin Res]** 1982 Dec 18–25;285(6357):1762–3

**Mexico**

Carrada Bravo T: Datos para la epidemiología del sarampión en la República Mexicana. Investigación preliminar. **SPM** 1979 Sep–Oct;21(5):497–519
Carrada Bravo T, Velázquez Díaz G: El impacto del sarampión en México. **Salud Publica Mex** 1981 Jul–Aug;22(4):359–408

**1700 to Present**

Anderson CM: Measles mortality and ethnic groups. **S Afr Med J** 1982 Jul 17;62(3):86–8

**Finland**

Turpeinen O: Die Sterblichkeit an Pocken, Masern und Keuchhusten in Finnland in den Jahren 1751 bis 1865. In Imhof AE, ed: Mensch und Gesundheit in der Geschichte. Husum, Matthiesen, 1980. p. 135–61.

**Japan**

Telson H: An explanation of the charm against measles. **J Hist Med Allied Sci** 1978 Jul;33(3):408

**Pacific Islands**

Ofcansky TP: British colonial administration in the Fiji Islands during the 1875 measles epidemic. **Adler Mus Bull** 1984 Mar;10(1):23–7

**Poland**

Jastrzębowski Z: Występowanie epidemii odry w Królestwie Polskim W XIX wieku (1815–1870). **Wiad Lek** 1983 Jul 1;36(13):1121–5

**Romania**

Rujeola în judeţul Iaşi: 1951–1979: **Rev Med Chir Soc Med Nat Iasi** 1980 Jul–Sep;84(3):406, 420, 436

**United States**

Wolfe RJ: Alaska's great sickness, 1900: an epidemic of measles and influenza in a virgin soil population. **Proc Am Philos Soc** 1982;126(1):91–121

### MENINGITIS

**1700 to Present**

Bastin R: Méningites purulentes. Rappel historique. **Rev Prat** 1981 Jun 11;31(33):2343–4, 2347

**France**

Meindl JL, Meindl CO: Tuberculous meningitis in the 1830s. **Lancet** 1982 Mar 6;1(8271):554–5

**United States**

Danielson L, Mann E: The first American account of cerebrospinal meningitis. **Rev Infect Dis** 1983 Sep–Oct;5(5):969–72
Scheld WM, Mandell GL: Landmark perspective. Sulfonamides and meningitis. **JAMA** 1984 Feb 10;251(6):791–4
Täuber MG, Sande MA: Landmark perspective: the impact of penicillin on the treatment of meningitis. **JAMA** 1984 Apr 13;251(14):1877–80

## MENTAL DISORDERS

Ackerknecht EH: The history of the drug treatment of mental diseases. **Trans Stud Coll Physicians Phila** 1979 Sep;5(1 No 3):161–70, Sep 79
Azouvi F: La peste, la mélancolie et le diable, ou l'imaginaire réglé. **Diogenes** 1979 Oct–Dec
Berrios GE: Stupor: a conceptual history. **Psychol Med** 1981 Nov;11(4):677–88
Berrios GE: Tactile hallucinations: conceptual and historical aspects. **J Neurol Neurosurg Psychiatry** 1982 Apr;45(4):285–93
Bliss EL: History of anorexia nervosa. In Gross M, ed: Anorexia nervosa. A comprehensive approach. Lexington, D. C. Heath, 1982. p. 5–7.
Bonuzzi L: Per l'iconologia della melancolia. **Acta Med Hist Patav** 1980–81;27:55–80
Chandrasena RD: Phenomenology and nosology of schizophrenia: historical review. **Psychiatr J Univ Ottawa** 1983 Jun;8(2):17–24
Cronholm B: Från långbad och isolering till farmakoterapi och rehabilitering. **Nord Medicinhist Arsb** 1981;:133–50
Daněk K: The many facets of nostalgia in the history of medicine. **Nord Medicinhist Arsb** 1984;:71–81
De Leo D, Arisi F, Magni G: Difficoltà interpretative e problemi terapeuti nella neurastenia. Rassegna storica. **Minerva Psichiatr** 1982 Apr–Jun;23(2):75–81
Doerner K: Madmen and the bourgeoisie. A social history of insanity and psychiatry. (First published in German as Bürger und Irre, 1969.) Oxford, Basil Blackwell, 1981 vi, 361 p.
Ellis PS: The origins of the war neuroses. **J R Nav Med Serv** 1984 Winter;70(3):168–77 contd
Georgotas A, Gershon S: Historical perspectives and current highlights on lithium treatment in manic-depressive illness. **J Clin Psychopharmacol** 1981 Jan;1(1):27–31
Gerevich J: Az elemebeteggé minősítés szépirodalmi modelljei. **Orv Hetil** 1982 Nov 28;123(48):2971–2
Giedke A: Die Liebeskrankheit in der Geschichte der Medizin. Diss., Universität Düsseldorf, Düsseldorf, 1983. 205 p.
Gilman SL: Seeing the insane: a cultural history of madness and art in the western world, showing how the portrayal of stereotypes has both reflected and shaped the perception and treatment of the mentally disturbed. New York, Wiley; Brunner/Mazel, 1982. xiii, 241 p.
Gorog F, Leguil F: Histoire de l'hystérie. **Soins Psychiatr** 1983 Jan;(27):3–6
Halpert BP: Development of the term 'senility' as a medical diagnosis. **Minn Med** 1983 Jul;66(7):421–4
Heggelbacher O: Geisteskrankheit und kirchenrechtliche Verantwortlichkeit. **Osterr Arch Kirchenr** 1967;18(1):3–16
Howells JG, Osborn ML: A reference companion to the history of abnormal psychology. Westport, Conn., Greenwood Press, 1984. 2 v. xviii, 1141 p.
Hurst LC: Freud and the great neurosis: discussion paper. **J R Soc Med** 1983 Jan;76(1):57–61
Ishii A: Seishin igaku shippeishi. Tokyo, Kongo Shuppan, [1981]. 161 p.
Israel L: Le corps hystérique. **Soins Psychiatr** 1983 Jan;(27):15–9
Jackson SW: Melancholia and the waning of the humoral theory. **J Hist Med Allied Sci** 1978 Jul;33(3):367–76
Karwat J: Dręczyciele upośledzonych. **Psychiatr Pol** 1980 Jul–Aug;14(4):430–4
Kloë E: Hysterie im Kindesalter. Zur Entwicklung des kindlichen Hysteriebegriffes. Freibug, Schulz, 1979. 181 p. (Freiburger Forschungen zur Medizingeschichte, Neue Folge, 9).
Kloë E, Kindt H: Zur Entstehung und Entwicklung des kindlichen Hysteriebegriffes. **Gesnerus** 1981;38(3/4):281–300
Laxenaire M, Marchand P: L'anorexie mentale a-t-elle changé? **Ann Med Psychol (Paris)** 1982 Apr;140(4):448–53
Lipton MA: The evolution of the biological understanding of affective and schizophrenic disorders. In M. R. Zales, ed: Affective and schizophrenic disorders: new approaches to diagnosis and treatment. New York, Brunner/Mazel, 1983. p. 5–28.
López Piñero JM: Historical origins of the concept of neurosis. Cambridge, New York, Cambridge University Press, 1983. xi, 107 p.
Loudon I: The diseases called chlorosis. **Psychol Med** 1984 Feb;14(1):27–36
Masters A: Bedlam, London, Michael Joseph, 1977. 206 p.
Merskey H: Hysteria: the history of an idea. **Can J Psychiatry** 1983 Oct;28(6):428–33
Meurer-Keldenich M: Medizinische Literatur zur Bildnerei von Geisteskranken. Köln, 1979. 327 p. (Kölner medizinhistorische Beiträge, Band 14)
Pauchard D: Neurasthénie, psychasthénie: evolution des concepts. **Rev Med Suisse Romande** 1982 Jun;102(6):621–7
Porter R: Shutting people up. **Soc Stud Sci** 1982 Aug 3;12(3):467–76
Richard M, Roy R: La folie à travers les temps. **Infirm Can** 1983 Jun;25(6):17–20
Rojo Sierra M: La vida de hoy y los trastornos psíquicos. **Actas Luso Esp Neurol Psiquiatr** 1983 Nov–Dec;11(6):433–41
Schoeneman TJ: Criticisms of the psychopathological interpretation of witch hunts: a review. **Am J Psychiatry** 1982 Aug;139(8):1028–32
Screech MA: A new look at 'Melencolia I'. **J Warburg Courtauld Inst** 1980;43:257–62
Sheehan DV, Sheehan KH: The classification of anxiety and hysterical states. Part I. Historical review and empirical delineation. **J Clin Psychopharmacol** 1982 Aug;2(4):235–44
Singh P: The evolution of anxiety. In: Congrès international d'histoire de la médecine, XXVe, Québec, 1976. Actes. Québec, 1977. p. 1274–88.
Smith SM: Competency. **Psychiatr Clin North Am** 1983 Dec;6(4):635–50
Spanos NP, Gottlieb J: Demonic possession, mesmerism, and hysteria: a social psychological perspective on their historical interrelations. **J Abnorm Psychol** 88(5):527–46, Oct 79
Stoessel I: Scheintod und Todesangst. Aeusserungsformen der Angst in ihren geschichtlichen Wandlungen (17.–20. Jahrhundert). Köln, 1983. 247 p. (Kölner medizinhistorische Beiträge, Band 30)
Tellenbach H: Zwang-Wahn-Schwermut-Melancholie: Dekompositionen normativer Seinsweisen. In Seidler E, Schott H, ed: Bausteine zur Medizingeschichte. Stuttgart, Steiner, 1984. p. 139–46.
Torrey EF: Schizophrenia and civilization. New York, Aronson, 1980. ix, 230 p.
The two manias: **Br J Psychiatry** 1981 Sep;139:258–61
Wajeman G: Le Maître et l'hystérique. Paris, Navarin Editeur, 1982. 286 p. (Bibliothèque des Analytica).
Weissmann G: Foucault and the bag lady. **Hosp Pract** 1982 Aug;17(8):28–9, 33–4, 39
Wermut W: Rodowody literackie niektórych zespołów klinicznych. **Psychiatr Pol** 1980 Jan–Feb;14(1):69–76
Wesley GR: A history of hysteria. Washington, D. C., University Press of America, 1979. 172 p.
Willmuth LR: Medical views of depression in the elderly: historical notes. **J Am Geriatr Soc** 27(11):495–9, Nov 79

**Americas**

Benítez RF: Historia de la deficiencia mental endemica en la region Andina. **Asclepio** 1982;34:339–76

**Belgium**

Villa R: Le famiglie di Gheel: utopia, tradizione e storia nel trattamento della follia. **Studi Stor** 1980;21(3):503–26

**Byzantium**

Eftychiadis AC, Marketos SG: [The treatment of mental disorders ... in Byzantium.] (Gre). **Mater Med Greca** 1981;9:221–5

**Canada**

Frankenburg FR: The history of the confinement of the mentally ill in Ontario. **Psychiatr J Univ Ottawa** 1982 Dec;7(4):240–3
Goudreault L: Naissance de la statistique alieniste au Canada jusqu'en 1867. In: Congrès international d'histoire de la médecine, XXVe, Québec, 1976. Actes. Québec, 1977. p. 706–26.

**China**

Ng VW: Ch'ing laws governing the insane: an historical survey. **Ch'ing-Shih Wen-t'i** 1980;4(4):55–89

**France**

Andrieu L: Les fous de Saint-Aubin-la-Campagne. In Congrès National des Sociétés Savantes, 102e, Limoges, 1977. Actes. Paris, 1978. Tome I, p. 9–21.
Brann NL: Melancholy and the divine frenzies in the French Pléiade: their conflicting roles in the art of 'beaux exercices spirituels.' **J Mediev Renaiss Stud** 1979;9:81–100

**Great Britain**

Lewis TH: Richard Carew on the treatment of a 'Franticke person' in Medieval Cornwall. **J Hist Med Allied Sci** 1981 Jan;36(1)64–6
MacDonald M: Insanity and the realities of history in early modern England. **Psychol Med** 1981 Feb;11(1):11–25
Skultans V: English madness. Ideas on insanity, 1580–1890. London, Routledge & Kegan Paul, 1979. ix, 158 p.

**Italy**

Accati L: Lo spirito della fornicazione: virtù dell'anima e virtù del corpo in Friuli, fra '600 e '700. **Quad Stor** 1979;14(2):644–72

**Mexico**

Fuente JR de la, Alarcón-Segovia D: Depression as expressed in pre-Columbian Mexican art. **Am J Psychiatry** 1980 Sep;137(9):1095–8

**Netherlands**

Jansen JC: Waanzin en verstoring der maatschappelijke orde. **Spiegel Hist** 1980;15(7–8):415–20

**Puerto Rico**

Ahearn FL: Puerto Ricans and mental health: some socio-cultural considerations. **Urban Soc Change Rev** 1979;12(2):4–9

**Romania**

Nicolau A: Practici empirice 'pentru aflarea şi tămăduirea boalelor minţii' în trecutul medicinii româneşti. **Rev Med Interna [Neurol Psihiatr]** 1983 Apr–Jun;28(2):153–60

Petrescu A: Simptoame neuropsihice consemnate în cronici şi vechi însemnări Româneşti. **Rev Med Interna [Neurol Psihiatr]** 1983 Apr–Jun;28(2):149–52

**United States**

Bell LV: Treating the mentally ill: from colonial times to the present. New York, Praeger, 1980. xi, 245 p.

King JO: The iron of melancholy: structures of spiritual conversion in America from the Puritan conscience to Victorian neurosis. Middletown, Conn., Wesleyan University Press, 1983. ix, 456 p.

**Before 500 A.D.**

Bron B: Depression und Glaube bei Hiob. **Schweiz Arch Neurol Neurochir Psychiatr** 1983;133(1):159–74

Littmann SK: King Saul: persecutor or persecuted? **Can J Psychiatry** 1981 Nov;26(7):464–7

Pélicier Y: Beständigheit im Sinngehalt des lateinischen Vokabulars für 'La folie' (Verrücktheit). **Z Klin Psychol Psychother** 1982;30(1):68–76

**China**

Dakpa N: La folie d'après un commentaire du Rgyud-bži, les quatre tantra. **Sci Orient** 1979;16:31–9

**Egypt**

Okasha A: Mental disorders in Pharaonic Egypt. **J Egypt Med Assoc** 1978;61(Suppl 1–2):3–12

**Greco-Roman**

Rabel RJ: Diseases of soul in Stoic psychology. **Greek Roman Byz Stud (Cambridge, Mass.)** 1981;22:385–93

Ullmann M, ed: Rufus von Ephesos Krankenjournale. Wiesbaden, Harrassowitz, 1978. 128 p.

**Greece**

La Croce E: El concepto de locura en Grecia clásica. **Acta Psiquiatr Psicol Am Lat** 1981 Sep–Nov;27(4–5):285–91

**India**

Haldipur CV: Madness in ancient India: concept of insanity in Charaka Samhita (1st century A.D.). **Compr Psychiatry** 1984 May–Jun;25(3):335–44

Stork H: Principes de base des traitements psychiatriques dans l'Ayurveda. **Sci Orient** 1979;16:21–9

**Rome**

Pearcy LT: Melancholy rhetoricians and melancholy rhetoric: 'black bile' as a rhetorical and medical term in the second century A.D. **J Hist Med Allied Sci** 1984 Oct;39(4):446–56

**500 A.D.–1450**

Abrahams HJ: A medicine for 'Sickness of the spirit.' **Trans Stud Coll Physicians Phila** 1977 Apr;44(4):202–3

Jackson SW: Acedia the sin and its relationship to sorrow and melancholia in medieval times. **Bull Hist Med** 1981 Summer;55(2):172–85

Jacquart D: Un jalon dans l'histoire du syndrome hystérique. La 'suffocation de la matrice' dans la tradition médicale médiévale. **Penelope** 1983;(8):7–9

Kroll J, Bachrach B: Visions and psychopathology in the Middle Ages. **J Nerv Ment Dis** 1982 Jan;170(1):41–9

Lacey JH: Anorexia nervosa and a bearded female saint. **Br Med J [Clin Res]** 1982 Dec 18–25;285(6357):1816–7

Rutkowska-Płachcińslak A: Dżuma w Europie Zachodniej w XIV w. straty demograficzne i stutki psychiczne. **Przegl Hist** 1978;69(1):75–102

**Americas**

Rodríguez E: Las enfermedades mentales en la América precolombina. **Rev Enferm** 1984 Mar;7(67):73–5

**Arabic**

Hajal F: Psychological treatment of anorexia: a case from the ninth century. **J Hist Med Allied Sci** 1982 Jul;37(3):325–8

**Europe**

Kroll J, Bachrach B: Sin and mental illness in the Middle Ages. **Psychol Med** 1984 Aug;14(3):507–14

Maher WB, Maher B: The ship of fools. Stultifera Navis or ignis fatuus? **Am Psychol** 1982 Jul;37(7):756–61

**France**

Allen C: The schizophrenia of Joan of Arc. **Hist Med (Lond)** 1975 Autumn–Winter;6(3–4):4–9

Lesný I: Sílenství francouzského krále Karla VI. **Cas Lek Cesk** 1982 May 14;121(19):597–600

**Spain**

Linage Conde A: Ibn Hazm de Cordoba y la neurosis. **Asclepio** 1981;33:349–77

**1450–1700**

Delumeau J: L'age d'or de la melancolie. **Histoire** 1982;42:28–37

Midelfort HC: Madness and civilization in early modern Europe: a reappraisal of Michel Foucault. In Malament, Barbara C., ed. After the Reformation: Essays in honor of J. H. Hexter, Philadelphia; U. of Pennsylvania Press, 1980. p. 247–65.

Midelfort HC: Madness and the problems of psychological history in the sixteenth century. **Sixteenth Century J** 1981;12(1):5–12

Neugebauer R: Application of a capture-recapture method (the Bernoulli census) to historical epidemiology. **Am J Epidemiol** 1984 Oct;120(4):626–34

**Canada**

Griffin JD, Greenland C: Manifestations of madness in New France. In: Congrès international d'histoire de la médecine, XXVe, Québec, 1976. Actes. Québec, 1977. p. 727–45.

**Germany**

Kraft H: Die Zeichnungen des Augustin Wilhelm. Psychopathologische Aspekte und kulturhistorische Vergleiche. **Confin Psychiatr** 1980;23(4):230–49

Schupbach WM: Elsheimer il malinconico. **Kos** 1984 Jun;1(5):85–100

**Great Britain**

Brink A: Depression and loss: a theme in Robert Burton's 'Anatomy of melancholy' (1621). **Can J Psychiatry** 1979 Dec;24(8):767–72

Broad WJ: Sir Isaac Newton: mad as a hatter. **Science** 1981 Sep 18;213(4514):1341–2, 1344

Daly RJ: Samuel Pepys and post-traumatic stress disorder. **Br J Psychiatry** 1983 Jul;143:64–8

Ditchburn RW: Newton's illness of 1692–3. **Notes Rec R Soc Lond** 1980 Jul;35(1):1–16

Faulkner TC: Computer applications for an edition of Robert Burton's The anatomy of melancholy: a system for scholarly publishing. **Comput Hum** 1981 Nov;15(3):163–82

Herring H: The self and madness in Marlowe's 'Edward II' and Webster's 'The Duchess of Malfi'. **J Mediev Renaiss Stud** 1979;9:307–23

Heyd M: Robert Burton's sources on enthusiasm and melancholy: from a medical tradition to religious controversy. **Hist Eur Ideas** 1984;5:17–44

Kail AC: Medicine in Shakespeare. The bard and the body. 2. Mental illness. **Med J Aust** 1983 Oct 15;2(8):399–405

Keynes M: Sir Isaac Newton and his madness of 1692–93. **Lancet** 1980 Mar 8;1(8167):529–30

Lieb J, Hershman D: Isaac Newton: mercury poisoning or manic depression? **Lancet** 1983 Dec 24–31;2(8365–66):1479–80

MacDonald M: Mystical bedlam: madness, anxiety, and healing in seventeenth-century England. Cambridge, Cambridge University Press, 1981. xvi, 323 p.

Shaw AB: Sir Thomas Browne: the man and the physician. **Br Med J [Clin Res]** 1982 Jul 3;285(6334):40–2

Silverman JA: Richard Morton, 1637–1698. Limner of anorexia nervosa: his life and times. A tercentenary essay. **JAMA** 1983 Nov 25;250(20):2830–2

**Switzerland**

Bouwsma WJ: John Calvin's anxiety. **Proc Am Philos Soc** 1984 Sep;128(3):252–6

Lenzen W: Mentis Laesiones, Psychopathologie bei Felix Platter (1536–1614). Diss. Bonn, 1982. 151 p.

Paskauskas RA: Paracelsus and mental disorders. In International Congress of the History of Medicine, 27th, Barcelona, 1980. Actas. Barcelona, Académia de Ciències Médiques de Catalunya i Balears, 1981. p. 121–4.

**United States**

Kupperman KO: Apathy and death in early Jamestown. **J Am Hist** 1979;66(1):24–40

**1700 to Present**

Ansbacher HL: Discussion of Alfred Alder's preface to The Diary of Vaslav Nijinsky. **Arch Gen Psychiatry** 1981 Jul;38(7):834–41

Barondess JA: The doctor, the patient, and the system: reflections on education for clinical careers. **Perspect Biol Med** 1983 Winter;26(2):205–18

Bennett AE: Historical development of somatic therapies in affective disorders. **Int Pharmacopsychiatry** 1979;14(2):85–93

Ber A: Les avatars d'une recherche sur l'hystérie. **Penelope** 1983;(8):15–19

Bercherie P: Le concept de folie hystérique avant Charcot. **Rev Int Hist Psychiatr** 1983;1(1):47–58

Berrios GE: Delirium and confusion in the 19th century: a conceptual history. **Br J Psychiatry** 1981 Nov;139:439–49

Berrios GE: Epilepsy and insanity during the early 19th century. A conceptual history. **Arch Neurol** 1984 Sep;41(9):978–81

Bleuler M: Eugen Bleuler and schizophrenia. **Br J Psychiatry** 1984 Mar;144:327–8

Bornstein S, Bitty L: Essai sur folie et roman: un auteur en quête de psychiatres. **Ann Med Psychol (Paris)** 1983 Nov;141(9):957–67

Burger G: Nerven- und Geisteskrankheiten als Indikationen für eine bilaterale Oophorektomie im späten 19. Jahrhundert. Diss. Erlangen-Nürnberg, 1984. 185 p.

Carter KC: Infantile hysteria and infantile sexuality in late nineteenth-century German-language medical literature. **Med Hist** 1983 Apr;27(2):186–96

Charuty G: La folie féminine dans la société languedocienne traditionnelle. Les effets de la psychiatrisation. **Penelope** 1983;(8):36–9

Conn JH: Unusual features of Anna O. 's illness. **Am J Psychiatry** 1980 Jan;138(1):123

Decker HS: Freud and Dora: constraints on medical progress. **J Soc Hist** 1981;14(3):445–64

Decker HS: The historical evolution of dementia praecox. In Fann, et al, ed: Phenomenology and treatment of schizophrenia. New York, Spectrum, 1978. p. 301–309.

Delion P: Aperçu historico-clinique sur la schizophrénie. Etat des différentes recherches à son sujet. **Soins Psychiatr** 1981 Dec;(14):3–5

D'où nous viennent la d'emence précoce et la schizophrénie?: **Acta Psychiatr Belg** 1982 May–Jun;82(3):243–76

Elliott FA: Biological roots of violence. **Proc Am Philos Soc** 1983 Apr 20;127(2):84–94

Erickson RC, Hyerstay BJ: Historical perspectives on the treatment of the mentally ill. In Gibbs M, et al., ed: Community psychology: theoretical and empirical approaches. New York, Gardner, 1980. p 29–63.

Feinberg M, Pegeron JP, Steiner M: The effect of morphine on symptoms of endogenous depression. **Natl Inst Drug Abuse Res Monogr Ser** 1983 Apr;43:245–50

Fuster P: Análisis bibliográfico de las psicosis infantiles. **Asclepio** 1980;32:171–94

Gibelli A: La guerra laboratorio: eserciti e igiene sociale verso la guerra totale. **Mov Operaio Soc** 1982;5(3):335–49

Gilman SL: Zur Physiognomie des Geisteskranken in Geschichte und Praxis, 1800–1900. **Sudhoffs Arch** 1978;62(3):209–34

Golden RL: Osler, 'E. Y. D.,' and hysteria. **JAMA** 1982 May 21;247(19):2698–9

Gómez EA: El problema del enfermo mental crónico indigente: un análisis histórico. **Acta Psiquiatr Psicol Am Lat** 1983 Sep;29(3):213–22

Gordon E, Kraiuhin C, Kelly P, et al: The development of hysteria as a psychiatric concept. **Compr Psychiatry** 1984 Sep–Oct;25(5):532–7

Guggenbühl-Craig A: Geschichtliche Entwicklung des Begriffes der Psychopathie. In his: Seelenwüsten. Betrachtungen über Eros und Psychopathie. Zürich, Schweizer Spiegel Verlag, 1980. p. 50–68.

Hachinski V: Cerebral arteriosclerosis and dementia: evolution of a misconception. In: Congrès international d'histoire de la médecine, XXVe, Québec, 1976. Actes. Québec, 1977. p. 755–60.

Haffter C: Die Entstehung des Begriffs der Zivilisationskrankheiten. **Gesnerus** 1979;36(3–4):228–37

Halpern AL: Elimination of the exculpatory insanity rule. A modern societal need. **Psychiatr Clin North Am** 1983 Dec;6(4):611–27

Hare E: The two manias: a study of the evolution of the modern concept of mania. **Br J Psychiatry** 1981 Feb;138:89–99

Hausmann J: Die Syndrome 'Manie' und 'Melancholie' an der Wende zum 18. Jahrhundert. Dargestellt an zwei zeitgenössischen Dissertationen. Diss., Rheinische Friedrich-Wilhelms-Universität. Bonn, 1982. 148 p.

Hurst DL, Hurst MJ: Bromide psychosis: a literary case. **Clin Neuropharmacol** 1984;7(3):259–64

Ingraham LH, Manning FJ: Psychiatric battle casualties: the missing column in a war without replacements. **Milit Rev** 1980;60(8):18–29

Inkster I: Lunacy and the Industrial Revolution. Programme notes. **Soc Soc Hist Med Bull** 1980;27:43–6

Iveson-Iveson J: Munchausen's syndrome: fantasy island (Rudolph Raspe). **Nurs Mirror** 1982 Jun 30;154(26):21

Jackson SW: Melancholia and mechanical explanation in eighteenth-century medicine. **J Hist Med Allied Sci** 1983 Jul;38(3):298–319

Jarosz M: Manfred Bleuler i inni o wyst epowaniu prawidłowych stanów psychicznych u chorych na schizofrenię. **Psychiatr Pol** 1981 Jul–Dec;15(4–6):403–9

Jones DR: Aeromedical transportation of psychiatric patients: historical review and present management. **Aviat Space Environ Med** 1980 Jul;51(7):709–16

Kaplan HS: Sexual medicine. A progress report. **Arch Intern Med** 1980 Dec;140(12):1575–6

Knight IF: Freud's 'Project': a theory for Studies on Hysteria. **J Hist Behav Sci** 1984 Oct;20(4):340–58

Koehler K, Sass H: Der Maniebegriff seit Kraepelin. **Nervenarzt** 1981 Jan;52(1):19–25

Krömer S: Lärm als medizinisches Problem im 19. Jahrhundert. Diss. Mainz, 1981. 83 p.

Laclé A: La falsa ciclotimia de Bolivar. **Rev Soc Bolivar Venez** 1979;36(121):71–3

Lanteri Laura G: L'hystérie. Matrice de la sémiologie neurologique. In Poirier J, Poirier JL, ed: Médecine et philosophie à la fin du XIXe siècle. Paris, Université de Paris XII - Val de Marne, [1980?]. p. 141–8.

Leighton AH: A recurrent millennium: the cure and prevention of mental illnesses. **Can Ment Health** 1982 Jun;30(2):2–5

Leighton AH: Caring for mentally ill people. Psychological and social barriers in historical context. Cambridge, Cambridge University Press, 1982. x, 277 p.

Lipton AA: Was the 'nervous illness' of Schreber a case of affective disorder? **Am J Psychiatry** 1984 Oct;141(10):1236–9

Livianos Aldana L, Rojo Moreno L, Rojo Moreno J, et al: La nosología psiquiátrica y las taxonomías numéricas. **Actas Luso Esp Neurol Psiquiatr** 1984 Jan–Feb;12(1):63–72

Lovaas OI: Contrasting illness and behavioral models for the treatment of autistic children: a historical perspective. **J Autism Dev Disord** 1979 Dec;9(4):315–23

Mai FM: Hysteria--100 years after Briquet. **Can J Psychiatry** 1983 Oct;28(6):417

Martin E: Mothers, madness, and the middle class in The bell jar and Les mots pour le dire. **Fr Am Rev** 1981;5(1):24–47

Matthews JH: Surrealism, insanity, and poetry. Syracuse, Syracuse University Press, 1982. xii, 154 p.

Meadow R, Lennert T: Munchausen by proxy or Polle syndrome: which term is correct? **Pediatrics** 1984 Oct;74(4):554–6

Mitchinson W: Gynecological operations on the insane. **Archivaria** 1980 Summer;10:125–44

Moriarty KM, Alagna SW, Lake CR: Psychopharmacology. An historical perspective. **Psychiatr Clin North Am** 1984 Sep;7(3):411–33

Neale JM, Oltmanns TF: Schizophrenia. New York, Wiley, 1980. Historical section, p. 2–16.

Pisztora F: A születési arisztokrácia súlya és a származási téveszmék gyakorisága a Monarchia társadalmában. **Orv Hetil** 1981 Jun 28;122(26):1593–5

Płaźnik A, Kostowski W, Puciłowski O: Historia i postepy współczesnej psychofarmakologii. **Pol Tyg Lek** 1983 Dec 19–26;38(51–52):1633–7

Postel J: Les névroses. Evolution historique du concept de 1769 à nos jours. **Soins Psychiatr** 1982 Feb;(16):13–9

Price HH: The Falklands: rate of British psychiatric combat casualties compared to recent American wars. **J R Army Med Corps** 1984 Jun;130(2):109–13

Putscher M: Jaspers und Van Gogh--oder über Krankheit und Kunst. **Janus** 1980;67(1-2-3):157–69

Ramas M: Freud's Dora, Dora's hysteria: the negation of a woman's rebellion. **Feminist Stud** 1980;6(3):472–510

Rousselot Y: La conception de la schizophrénie chez Langfeldt. **Ann Med Psychol (Paris)** 1981;139(8):879–92

Rubinstein BB: Freud's early theories of hysteria. In R.S. Cohen, L.

Laudan, ed: Physics, philosophy and psychoanalysis. Dordrecht, D. Reidel, 1983. p. 169–90.
Ryalls J: Where does the term 'aphasia' come from? **Brain Lang** 1984 Mar;21(2):358–63
Sardi PA: Epidemiologia della tossicodipendenza e cicli storici di altri disturbi psichici. **Minerva Med** 1981 Sep 26;72(36):2447–52
Schings HJ: Melancholie und Aufklärung. Melancholiker und ihre Kritiker in Erfahrungsseelenkunde und Literatur des 18. Jahrhunderts. Stuttgart, Metzler, 1977. x, 476 p.
Schmidt-Degenhard M: Melancholie und Depression: zur Problemgeschichte der depressiven Erkrankungen seit Beginn des 19. Jahrhunderts. Stuttgart, Kohlhammer, 1983. 169 p.
Scull A: The domestication of madness. **Med Hist** 1983 Jul;27(3):233–48
Shorter E: Women's diseases before 1900. In M. Albin, R. J. Devlin, G. Heeger, ed: New directions in psychohistory. The Adelphi papers in honor of Erik H. Erikson. Lexington, Toronto, D. C. Heath, 1980. p. 183–208.
Simpson GM: A brief history of depot neuroleptics. **J Clin Psychiatry** 1984 May;45(5 pt 2):3–4
Skerritt PW: Anxiety and the heart--a historical review. **Psychol Med** 1983 Feb;13(1):17–25
Smith R: Scientific thought and the boundary of insanity and criminal responsibility. **Psychol Med** 1980 Feb;10(1):15–23
Sommer R, Osmond H: A bibliography of mental patients' autobiographies, 1960–1982. **Am J Psychiatry** 1983 Aug;140(8):1051–4
Strauss JS: The evolution of psychotherapeutic approaches for affective and schizophrenic disorders. In M. R. Zales, ed: Affective and schizophrenic disorders: new approaches to diagnosis and treatment. New York, Brunner/Mazel, 1983. p. 163–77.
Swain G: Les métamorphoses de l'hystérie à la fin du XIX siècle. **Penelope** 1983;(8):13–4
Taylor FK: On pseudo-hallucinations. **Psychol Med** 1981 May;11(2):265–71
Treher W: Jean-Jacques Rousseau oder die Anatomie eines Pulverfasses mit Betrachtungen über Georg Wilhelm Friedrich Hegel und Adolf Hitler verbunden zu einer Vergleichenden Psychopathologie der Funktionsschizophrenie. Emmendigen, W. Treher, 1982. 208 p.
Trethowan WH: Ivor Gurney's mental illness. **Music Lett** 1981;62(3–4):300–9
Widlocher D: L'hystérie, cent ans après. **Rev Neurol (Paris)** 1982;138(12):1053–60

**Australia**

Davies B: The first patient to receive lithium. **Aust NZ J Psychiatry** 1983 Dec;17(4):366–8
Edwards GA: Causation of insanity in nineteenth century Australia. **Aust NZ J Psychiatry** 1982 Mar;16(1):53–62
Edwards GA: The mental illness of Captain Hyndman. **Aust NZ J Psychiatr** 1979 Jun;13(2):147–52
Krupinski J, Alexander L: Patterns of psychiatric morbidity in Victoria, Australia, in relation to changes in diagnostic criteria 1848–1978. **Soc Psychiatry** 1983;18(2):61–7
Lithium salts in the treatment of psychotic excitement: John F Cade: **Aust NZ J Psychiatry** 1982 Sep;16(3):129–33
Rodgers GF: A question of policy: is provision of special schools for defectives to be undertaken by this department? **Anzhes J** 1980;9(2):42–54

**Austria**

Hollender MH: The case of Anna O.: a reformulation. **Am J Psychiatry** 1980 Jul;137(7):797–800
Hurst LC: What was wrong with Anna O? **J R Soc Med** 1982 Feb;75(2):129–31
James RL, May PR: Diagnosing schizophrenia: Professor Kraepelin and the research diagnostic criteria. **Am J Psychiatry** 1981 Apr;138(4):501–4
Pisżtora F: Tipikus társadalmi konfliktusok és reaktív neurosisok-psychosisok a Monarchia idöszakában hazánkban. **Orv Hetil** 1980 Aug 10;121(32):1956–9

**Brazil**

Lisanti L: Urbanisation et folie São Paulo, 1852–1929. **Jahrb Gesch Staat Wirtsch Ges Lateinam** 1980;17:297–315

**Bulgaria**

Petrowa L: Volksheilverfahren für Nervenkrankheiten im Bezirk Warna. In International Congress of the History of Medicine. 26th, Plovdiv, 1978. Actes du Congress. Sofia, 1981. Volume II. p. 71–2.

**Canada**

Mitchinson W: Gynecological operations on insane women: London, Ontario, 1895–1901. **J Soc Hist** 1982;15(3):467–84
Smandych R, Verdun-Jones SN: Catch-22 in the nineteenth century: the evolution of the therapeutic confinement for the criminally insane in Canada, 1840–1900. **Crim Justice Hist** 1981;2:85–108

**Denmark**

Kramp P, Hemmingsen R: Age distribution of patients with delirium tremens in Denmark 1836–1978. **Acta Psychiatr Scand** 1981 Mar;63(3):253–61

**France**

Ackerknecht EH: Charles Meryon and physicians. **J Hist Med Allied Sci** 1984 Oct;39(4):462–4
Cathelin M: Les insensés au XVIIIe siècle: naissance de la solution asilaire. **Bull Soc Fr Hist Hop** 1983;46:21–35
Chertok L: On the centenary of Charcot: hysteria, suggestibility and hypnosis. **Br J Med Psychol** 1984 Jun;57(Pt 2):111–20
Didi-Huberman G: Invention de l'hystérie: Charcot et l'iconographie photographique de la Salpêtrière. Paris, Macula, 1982. 303 p.
Dongier M: Briquet and Briquet's syndrome viewed from France. **Can J Psychiatry** 1983 Oct;28(6):422–7
Emerit M: Un curé de l'aude atteint du mal du siècle: Jean Terson. In Congrès National des Sociétés Savantes, 102e, Limoges, 1977. Actes. Paris, 1978. Tome I, p. 351–60.
Gineste T: Victor de L'Aveyron: dernier enfant sauvage, premier enfant fou. Paris, Le Sycomore, 1981. 327 p.
Goldstein J: The hysteria diagnosis and the politics of anticlericalism in late nineteenth-century France. **J Mod Hist** 1982;54(2):209–39
Kreiser BR: Miracles, convulsions, and ecclesiastical politics in early eighteenth-century Paris. Princeton, Princeton University Press, 1978. xvii, 485 p.
Lefebvre P, Barbas S: L'hystérie de guerre. Etude comparative de ses manifestations au cours des deux derniers conflits mondiaux. **Ann Med Psychol (Paris)** 1984 Feb;142(2):262–6
Mai FM, Merskey H: Briquet's concept of hysteria: an historical perspective. **Can J Psychiatry** 1981 Feb;26(1):57–63
Maire CL: Les convulsionnaires à Paris au XVIII siècle. **Penelope** 1983;(8):29–34
Maire CL: Les possédées de Morzine (1857–1873). Lyon, Presses Universitaires, 1981. 134 p.
Petit JG: Folie, langage, pouvoirs en Maine-et-Loire, 1800–1841. **Rev Hist Mod Contemp** 1980 Oct-Dec;27:529–64
Petitjean F, Bonnefoy JP, Caroli F, et al: Le secteur et la loi du 30 juin 1838. **Ann Med Psychol (Paris)** 1982;140(3):301–19
Picheau P: Diagnostika i klassifikatsiia psikhicheskikh rasstroĭstv vo Frantsii (istoriia, sovremennye vzgliady i terminologicheskie sopostavleniia). **Zh Nevropatol Psikhiatr** 1982;82(8):103–10
Pigeaud JM: Le rôle des passions dans la pensée médicale de Pinel à Moreau de Tours. **Hist Philos Life Sci** 1980;2(1):123–40
Postel J: Un manuscrit inédit de Philippe Pinel sur 'Les guérisons opérées dans le 7ème emploi' de Bicêtre, en 1794. **Rev Int Hist Psychiatr** 1983;1(1):79–82
Rappard P: La folie et l'Etat: aliénation mentale et aliénation sociale. Toulouse, Privat, 1981. 261 p.
Raynaud P: L'education specialisée en France, 1882–1982. **Esprit** 1982;5:79–99
Rossier A: Une jalousie mortelle (Honoré de Balzac). **Ann Pediatr (Paris)** 1981 Apr;28(4):298–300
Simeoni CE, Mouren MC, Aulas JJ: Psychose et créativité. Réflexions à propos d'un peintre autiste: Sykvain Fusco. **Confin Psychiatr** 1980;23(3):151–63
Swain Gladys: Une logique de l'inclusion: les infirmes du signe. **Esprit** 1982;5:61–75

**Germany**

Aulas JJ: La folie dans le cinéma allemand (1913–1933). **Ann Med Psychol (Paris)** 1980;138(8):925–38
Bertaux P: Der Wandel der Auffassungen über Hölderlins Krankheit. War Hölderlin geisteskrank? **Med Welt** 1980 Mar 28;31(13):486–90
Dorsz-Szteke E, Maciejewska-Dorsz K: O opiece nad psychicznie chorymi w Szczecinie w XIX wieku. **Wiad Lek** 1980 Sep 15;33(18):1509–10
Gilman SL: The Nietzsche murder case. **New Lit Hist** 1983;14(2):359–72
Hayman R: Nietzsche's madness. **Partisan Rev** 1980;47(1):29–44
Heimann H: Nosologie und Pathophysiologie in der Psychiatrie--Aspekte der Krankheitslehre Kraepelins heute. **Confin Psychiatr** 1980;23(4):262–74
Lauter H, Meyer JE: Mercy killing without consent. Historical comments on a controversial issue. **Acta Psychiatr Scand** 1982 Feb;65(2):134–41
Ludwig J, Mann RJ: Münchhausen versus Munchausen. **Mayo Clin Proc** 1983 Nov;58(11):767–9
Peters UH: Hölderlin: Dichter, Kranker--Simulant? **Nervenarzt** 1981 May;52(5):261–8
Propping P: Genetic disorders presenting as 'schizophrenia'. Karl Bonhoeffer's early view of the psychoses in the light of medical genetics. **Hum Genet** 1983;65(1):1–10
Rogoll H, Späte HF: Zur gesellschaftlichen Stellung des psychisch Kranken im Spiegel der Geschichte gesetzlicher Regelungen zur Einweisung in stationäre Einrichtungen. **Z Gesamte Hyg** 1983 Jan;29(1):37–9

Rückleben H: Deportation und Tötung von Geisteskranken aus den badischen Anstalten der Inneren Mission Kork und Mosbach. Karlsruhe, Evangelischer Presseverband für Baden, 1981. 104 p. (Veröffentlichungen des Vereins für Kirchengeschichte in der evangelischen Landeskirche in Baden, Band 33).
Sărmăşanu-Cortez ML, Cortez P: Dr. Hermann Simon, sitemul Gütersloh şi tratamentul activ al bolilor psihice. **Rev Med Interna [Neurol Psihiatr]** 1980 Oct-Dec;25(4):295-302
Scharfetter C: Ein Anliegen der Menschheitserziehung: Delegierte Destruktivität. Massenmord an Psychiatriepatienten in Hitler-Deutschland. **Schweiz Arch Neurol Neurochir Psychiatr** 1984;134(2):279-93
Schmidt PO: Asylierung oder psychiatrische Familienpflege? Die Diskussionen in den Irrenärzteverbänden um die psychiatrische Versorgungsstruktur im 19. Jahrhundert. **Psychiatr Prax** 1983 Mar;10(2):56-9

**Great Britain**

Bernstein RE: What was Charles Darwin's illness? **S Afr Med J** 1982 Jun 19;61(25):939
Brody M: Trial of Daniel M'Naghten. Insanity defense, and its well-kept secret. **NY State J Med** 1982 Mar;82(3):381-6
Burrows A, Schumacher I: Doktor Diamonds Bildnisse von Geisteskranken. Transl. of Doctor Diamond's portraits of the insane. Frankfurt am Main, Syndikat, 1979. 159 p.
Dickson P: Passage of the lines. **Army Q Def J** 1982;112(2):199-204
Feinstein SC: Why they were afraid of Virginia Woolf: perspectives on juvenile manic-depressive illness. **J Adolesc** 1980 Sep;3(3):187-96
Feinstein SC: Why they were afraid of Virginia Woolf: perspectives on juvenile manic-depressive illness. **Adolesc Psychiatry** 1980;8:332-43
Gilbert AN: Masturbation and insanity: Henry Maudsley and the ideology of sexual repression. **Albion** 1980;12(3):268-82
Hare E: Was insanity on the increase? The fifty-six Maudsley Lecture. **Br J Psychiatry** 1983 May;142:439-55
Hyman VR: Concealment and disclosure in Sir Leslie Stephen's mausoleum book. **Biography** 1980;3(2):121-31
Kane A, Carlson ET: A different drummer: Robert B. Carter and Nineteenth Century hysteria. **Bull NY Acad Med** 1982 Sep;58(6):519-34
Lomax E: A mid-nineteenth century British pediatrician's interpretations of the mental peculiarities and disorders of childhood. **Clio Med** 1983 Mar;17(4):223-33
Lomax E: Charles West (1816-1898) on the mental peculiarieties and disorders of childhood. In International Congress of the History of Medicine, 27th, Barcelona, 1980. Actas. Barcelona, Académia de Ciències Mèdiques de Catalunya i Balears, 1981. p. 98-102.
McCandless P: 'Curses of civilization': insanity and drunkenness in Victorian Britain. **Br J Addict** 1984 Mar;79(1):49-58
Mellett DJ: The prerogative of asylumdom: social, cultural, and administrative aspects of the institutional treatment of the insane in nineteenth-century Britain. New York, Garland Pub. Co., 1982. 257 p.
Menza AJ: Compulsoary commitment of the mentally ill: a study of the English law. **State Gov** 1977;50(4):255-61
Meyer JE, Meyer R: Selbstschilderungen eines Depressiven--Zur Pathobiographie William Cowper's. **Fortschr Neurol Psychiatr** 1984 Apr;52(4):107-12
Patton MA: An early case of battle hysteria. **Br J Psychiatry** 1981 Feb 1;138:182-3
Porter R: Being mad in Georgian England. **Hist Today** 1981 Dec;31:42-8
Porter R: Le prospettive della 'follia': scienza, medicina, e letteratura nell'Inghilterra dell '700. **Intersezioni** 1982;2:55-76
Rollin HR: Crime and mental disorder. Daniel McNaughton, a case in point. **Med Leg J** 1982;50(Pt 3):102-13
Scull A: Was insanity increasing? A response to Edward Hare. **Br J Psychiatry** 1984 Apr;144:432-6
Showalter E: Victorian women and insanity. **Victorian Stud** 1980;23(2):157-81
Smith R: Trial by medicine. Insanity and responsibility in Victorian trials. Edinburgh, Edinburgh University Press, 1981. ix, 238 p.
Thomas KB: Attitudes to psychological illness in general practice. A historical cycle complete. **Br Med J [Clin Res]** 1981 Oct 31;283(6300):1157-8
Trombley S: All that summer she was mad: Virginia Woolf and her doctors. **Soc Soc Hist Med Bull (Lond)** 1981 Jun;28:21-5
Trombley S: All that summer she was mad: Virginia Woolf, female victim of male medicine. New York, Continuum, 1982. ix, 338 p.
Waddington JL: Ventricular enlargement in schizophrenia and the historical studies of John Haslam. **Am J Psychiatry** 1984 Dec;141(12):1640

**Hungary**

Gerevich J: Gulácsy Lajos festömüvész akut pszichózisa (adalék heveny téboly genezisének kérdéséhez). **Orv Hetil** 1981 May 3;122(18):1083-6
Kenéz J: War Semmelweis geisteskrank? **Med Welt** 1981 Dec 25;32(51-52):1964-6
Orzóy R: Néphit elemek idegbetegek kórképeiben. **Orvostort Kozl** 1982;92(4):101-12
Péter L: Juhász Gyula betegségtudata. **Orv Hetil** 1983 May 15;124(20):1205-7
Pisztora F: A schizophrenia és a paranoid kórformák gyógyítási kísérletei a Monarchia korabeli Magyarország különféle psychiátriai intézményeiben. **Orvostort Kozl** 1982;92(4):53-87
Szemkeö E: Adalék Semmelweis életének utolsó heteihez. **Orv Hetil** 1980 Jul 27;121(30):1837-8

**Ireland**

Clarke B: Mental illness and rehabilitation in early nineteenth-century Ireland; the case of Charles Stock. **Psychol Med** 1983 Nov;13(4):727-34
Finnane M: Insanity and the insane in post-famine Ireland. London, Croom Helm; and Totowa, New Jersey, Barnes & Noble, 1981. 241 p.

**Italy**

Bèttica-Giovannini R: La sfida di Peano: matematica e paranoia. **Ann Osp Maria Vittoria Torino** 1982 Jul-Dec;25(7-12):241-4
Gibelli A: Emarginati e classi lavoratrici: le ragioni di un nodo storiografico. **Mov Operaio Soc** 1980;3(4):361-7
Lanzavecchia P, Lingua P, Sinigaglia G: La popolazione manicomiale di Alessandria nella seconda metà dell'ottocento. **Mov Operaio Soc** 1980;3(4):405-22

**Japan**

Furukawa F, Bourgeois M: Délires de possession par le renard au Japon (ou délire de Kitsune-Tsuki). **Ann Med Psychol (Paris)** 1984 May;142(5):677-87
Matsuda H: [Madness described in essays during the Edo period] (Jpn). **Igakushi Kenkyu** 1980;53:1-9

**Mexico**

Müller C: Historische Reminiszenz: die schizophrene Psychose der Kaiserin von Mexiko. **Fortschr Neurol Psychiatr** 1979 Oct;47(10):550-2

**Netherlands**

Binneveld JM: Van bewaarplaats tot geneeskundig gesticht. **Spiegel Hist** 1981;16(5):267-73
Dieckhöfer K: Der flämische Schriftsteller Hendrik Conscience (1812-1883) und die psychisch Kranken von Geel. **Z Psychosom Med Psychoanal** 1984;30(2):179-90
Van der Esch P: Geschiedenis van het Staatstoezicht op Krankzinningen. 's-Gravenhage, Ministerium van Volksgezondheit en Milieuhygiene, 1975-1980. 3 volumes in 1.

**Norway**

Festy M: Les internements psychiatriques en Norvège. **Population** 1981;36(2):317-36
Thuen H: 'Ad denne rent mekaniske vej ...': da tanken om hospitalisering av de sinnssvake kom til Norge. **Hist Tidsskr** 1982;61(4):313-32
Wylie HW: Edvard Munch. **Am Imago** 1980 Winter;37(4):413-43

**Poland**

Monkiewicz W, Kretowski J: Los chorych psychicznie, kalek i starców w okupowanym Białostockiem. **Przegl Lek** 1984;41(1):80-4
Skrobacki A, Völker A: Lekarz olsztyński, Joachim Kornalewskiijego rozprawa o koltunie z 1897 roku. **Komun Mazursko Warm** 1980;(2):155-67
Zabłotniak R: Towarzystwo opieki nad nerwowo i umysłowo chorymi żydami w Warszawie (1906-1939). **Biul Zydowskiego Inst Hist Pol** 1981;1:37-44

**Spain**

Espinosa Iborra J: El enfermo mental al final del Antiguo Régimen. **Asclepio** 1983;35:277-85
Simón Palmer M del C: Las neurosis femeninas y la educación española. **Asclepio** 1983;35:327-42

**Sweden**

Fehrman C: Esaias Tegnér and psychiatry: history of literature from medical view-point. **Sydsven Medicinhist Sallsk Arsskr** 1984;21:47-8

**Switzerland**

Ernst K: Geisteskrankheit ohne Institution. Eine Feldstudie im Kanton Fribourg aus dem Jahr 1875. **Schweiz Arch Neurol Neurochir Psychiatr** 1983;133(2):239-62
Hitomi K: [Historical progress and the present interpretation of

schizophrenic theory held by Bleuler's school] (Jpn). **Seishin Shinkeigaku Zasshi** 1982;84(10):735–42
Hoenig J: The concept of Schizophrenia. Kraepelin-Bleuler-Schneider. **Br J Psychiatry** 1983 Jun;142:547–56

**United States**

Anderson DL, Anderson GT: Nostalgia and malingering in the military during the Civil War. **Perspect Biol Med** 1984 Autumn;28(1):156–66
Astrow A: Anxiety - frustration - repressed hostility. An original drawing, painted in gouache, by Boris Artzybasheff. **J Hist Med Allied Sci** 1980 Oct;35(4):453
Beaver H: Parkman's crack-up: a Bostonian on the Oregon Trail. **N Engl Q** 1975;48(1):84–103
Bowman IA, ed: The care of the insane in Texas. **Bookman** 1984 Mar–Apr;11(2):3–9
Carlson ET: The history of multiple personality in the United States: I: The beginnings. **Am J Psychiatry** 1981 May;138(5):666–8
Crowley JW: Dating Howells' adolescent breakdown. **Old Northwest** 1982;8(1):13–22
David Shakow, Ph.D., 1901–1981: In Memoriam. **Schizophr Bull** 1981;7(3):383–7
Derogatis LR, et al: The Hopkins symptom checklist (HSCL): a self-report symptom inventory. **Behav Sci** 1974;19(1):1–15
Downs F, Meshad S, Krieger D: The anguish of the veterans. **Cent Mag** 1979;12(4):27–36
Felton BJ, Shinn M: Ideology and practice of deinstitutionalization. **J Soc Issues** 1981;37(3):158–72
Fullinwider SP: Technicians of the finite. The rise and decline of the schizophrenic in American thought 1840–1960. Westport, Conn., Greenwood, 1982. ix, 253 p. (Contributions in Medical History, 9).
Gambill J: Potential problems of detecting and treating psychosis in the White House. Potential psychosis in the White House. **Int J Soc Psychiatry** 1980;26(4):255–62
Gordon S: Motherhood is powerful. **Work Pap Mag** 1982;9(2):15–9
Greenstone JD: Dorothea Dix and Jane Addams: from transcendentalism to pragmatism in American social reform. **Soc Serv Rev** 1979;53(4):527–59
Grob GN: Mental illness and American society, 1875–1940. Princeton, Princeton University Press, 1983. xiii, 428 p.
Grob GN, ed: Public policy and mental illness. Four investigations, 1915–1939. New York, Arno, 1980. Separate paginations.
Hamowy R: Medicine and the crimination of sin: 'self-abuse' in the 19th century America. **J Libert Stud** 1977;1(3):229–70
Hollander R: Mental health policy in Washington territory, 1853–1875. **Pac Northwest Q** 1980;71(4):152–61
Hughes JS: In the law's darkness: insanity and the medical-legal career of Isaac Ray, 1707–1881. Ph.D. Diss., Rice University. Houston, 1982. xvii, 393 p.
Isacsson A: A study of Louis J. Weichmann. **Lincoln Her** 1978;80(1):25–38
Kenyon FE: Mary Baker Eddy, founder of Christian Science; the sublime hysteric. **Hist Med (Lond)** 1975 Autumn-Winter;6(3–4):29–46
Kimpel BD, Eaves TC: More on Pound's prison experience. **Am Lit** 1981;53(3):469–76
Langley HD: Respect for civilian authority: the tragic career of Captain Angus. **Am Neptune** 1980;40(1):23–37
McFarlane W: Beyond bedlam. **Work Pap Mag** 1982;9(2):10–4
Maj M: Evolution of the American concept of schizoaffective psychosis. **Neuropsychobiology** 1984;11(1):7–13
Marshall JR, Dowdall GW: Employment and mental hospitalization: the case of Buffalo, New York, 1914–55. **Soc Forces** 1982;60(3):843–53
Martin J: Psychic epidemics and American literary history: literature, neurosis, and cultural change. **Amerikastudien** 1983;28(3):265–77
Massad PM, Sales BD: Guardianship: an acceptable alternative to institutionalization? **Am Behav Sci** 1981;24(6):755–70
Massey EW, Brannon WL, Riley TL: The 'jerks': mass hysteria or epilepsy? **South Med J** 1981 May;74(5):607–9
Peck DL, Bharadwaj LK: Personal stress and fatalism as factors in college suicide. **Soc Sci** 1980;55(1):19–24
Peszke MA: The historic antecedents to the current polemics on involuntary psychiatric hospitalization. **Compr Psychiatry** 1984 Mar–Apr;25(2):238–46
Plaut EA, Rubenstein S: State care for the mentally ill: a brief history. **State Gov** 1977;50(4):192–7
Roazen P: Anorexia nervosa: Helene Deutsch, M.D. **Bull Menninger Clin** 1981 Nov;45(6):499–501
Roazen P: Two cases of induced insanity. Helene Deutsch, Cambridge, Mass. **Int J Psychoanal** 1981;62(pt 2):139–50
Robison DW: Wisconsin and the mentally ill. A history of the 'Wisconsin Plan' of state and county care 1860–1915. New York, Arno Press, 1980. ix, 322 p. (Historical Issues in Mental Health).
Rosenkrantz BG: Mad and bad in California. **Rev Am Hist** 1980;8(2):258–63
Rothman DJ: The limits of benevolence. **Soc Policy** 1981;12(1):24–8, 37–8
Sato M: Concept of shame and the mental health of Pacific Asian Americans. **Explor Ethnic Stud** 1980;3(1):3–12
Schopler E, Chess S, Eisenberg L: Our memorial to Leo Kanner. **J Autism Dev Disord** 1981 Sep;11(3):257–69
Scull A: A new trade in lunacy: the recommodification of the mental patient. **Am Behav Sci** 1981;24(6):741–54
Scull A: Deinstitutionalization and the rights of the deviant. **J Soc Issues** 1981;37(3):6–20
Smith-Rosenberg C: The new woman and the psycho-historian: a modest proposal. **Group Psychol Hist Newsl** 1975;4(3):4–11
Srole L, Fischer AK: The Midtown Manhattan longitudinal study vs 'the mental paradise lost' doctrine. A controversy joined. **Arch Gen Psychiatry** 1980 Feb;37(2):209–21
Sternbach H: Puerperal psychosis in America--1847. **Arch Gen Psychiatry** 1982 Feb;39(2):235–6
Tigbe JA: 'Be it ever so little': reforming the insanity defense in the Progressive Era. **Bull Hist Med** 1983 Fall;57(3):397–411
Tomes N: The domesticated madman: changing concepts of insanity at the Pennsylvania Hospital, 1780–1830. **Pa Mag Hist Biogr** 1982;106(2):271–86
Warren CA: New forms of social control: the myth of deinstitutionalization. **Am Behav Sci** 1981;24(6):724–40
Wolkinson BW, Barton D: Arbitration and the rights of mentally handicapped workers. **Mon Labor Rev** 1980;103(4):41–7

**USSR**

Bochkov NP: Vklad s. n. Davidenkova v razrabotku probelmy nasledstvennykh nervynkh i psikhicheskikh zabolevaniĭ. **Zh Nevropatol Psikhiatr** 1982;82(3):1–4
Grigorewitsch A: Prinzipien in der Behandlung Geisteskranker im Russland des 19. Jahrhunderts. **Psychiatr Neurol Med Psychol (Leipz)** 1980 Jul;32(7):424–9
Reich W: The case of General Grigorenko: a psychiatric reexamination of a Soviet dissident. **Psychiatry** 1980 Nov;43(4):303–23

## MENTAL RETARDATION

Scheerenberger RC: A history of mental retardation. Baltimore, Brookes, 1983. xvii, 311 p.

**1450–1700**

**Great Britain**

Wolfensberger W: Eulogy for a mentally retarded jester. **Ment Retard** 1982 Dec;20(6):269–70

**Portugal**

Woolfson RC: Historical perspective on mental retardation. **Am J Ment Defic** 1984 Nov;89(3):231–5

**1700 to Present**

Hänsel D: Die 'Physiologische Erziehung' der Schwachsinningen. Edouard Séguin (1812–1880) und sein Konzept einer medizinischen Pädegogik. Freiburg, Schulz, 1974. 329 p. (Freiburger Forschungen zur Medizinigeschichte, Neue Folge, 3).
Ulmer L: Mental retardation: evolution of care. **J Miss State Med Assoc** 1984 Feb;25(2):31–5

**Canada**

Anglin B: Twenty-five years of growing together. A history of the Ontario Association for the Mentally Retarded, 1978. 92, x p.
Simmons HG: From asylum to welfare. Downsview, Ont., National Institute on Mental Retardation, 1982. xv, 355 p.

**France**

Gineste T, Postel J: J. M. G. Itard et l'enfant connu sous le nom de 'sauvage de l'Aveyron'. **Psychiatr Enfant** 1980;23(1):251–307
Pélicier Y, Thuillier G: Le fondateur de l'éducation des idiots: Edouard Séguin (1812–1880). **Paedagog Hist** 1980;20:129–52
Pelicier Y, Thuillier G: Pour une histoire de l'education des enfants idiots en France (1830–1914). **Rev Hist (Paris)** 1979;261(1):99–130
Raynaud P: L'education specialisée en France, 1882–1982. **Esprit** 1982;5:79–99

**Germany**

Gieger G: Schwachsinnigenfürsorge und Hilfe für das geistig behinderte Kind. Eine Analyse der 'Zeitschrift für das Idiotenwesen' (1880 1934). Freiburg, Schulz, 1977. 245 p. (Freiburger Forschungen zur Medizingeschichte, Neue Folge, 6).
Meyer D: Erforschung und Therapie der Oligophrenien in der ersten Hälfte des 19. Jahrhunderts. Berlin-Charlottenburg, Marhold, 1973. 174 p.
Seidler E: Die Behinderten in Herten. **Gesnerus** 1982;39(1):133–40
Wolfensberger W: The extermination of handicapped people in World War II Germany. **Ment Retard** 1981 Feb;19(1):1–7

Great Britain

Davey H: The law relating to the mentally defective. The Mental Deficiency Act, 1913. 2nd ed. Reprint of 1914 ed., with a new introduction by C. Bahn. New York, Da Capo, 1981. x, xxvii, 568 p.
Hibberd D: 'Problems A': the solution to Wilfred Owen's 'The Imbecile.' **Notes Queries** 1980 Jun;27(3):232–3
Woodhouse J: Eugenics and the feeble-minded: the Parliamentary debates of 1912–14. **Hist Educ** 1982;11:127–37

United States

Bair B: The parents council for retarded children and social change in Rhode Island, 1951–1970. **RI Hist** 1981;40(4):144–59
Berkowitz ED: The politics of mental retardation during the Kennedy Administration. **Soc Sci Q** 1980;61(1):128–43
Cobb HV, Gray MZ, et al: Mental retardation: past and present. Washington, President's Committee on Mental Retardation, 1977. viii, 276 p.
Devine P: Mental retardation: an early subspecialty in psychiatric nursing. **J Psychosoc Nurs Ment Health Serv** 1983 Mar;21(3):21–30
Doll EE: Deborah Kallikak: 1889–1978, a memorial. **Ment Retard** 1983 Feb;21(1):30–2
Duffy JT, et al: 'Days of darkness – days of hope' [special issue on the mentally retarded]. **RI Hist** 1981 Nov;40:107–59
Friedberger M: The decision to institutionalize: families with exceptional children in 1900. **J Fam Hist** 1981 Winter;6(4):396–409
Marchetti AG: Wyatt v. Stickney: a historical perspective. **Appl Res Ment Retard** 1983;4(3):189–206
Merges RC: Checking the cycle: the decline of community-based residential programs in New York State 1925 to 1950. **Ment Retard** 1982 Aug;20(4):180–2
Schneider EC: Mental retardation, state policy, and the Ladd School, 1908–1970. **RI Hist** 1981;40(4):133–43
Sigelman L, Roeder PW, Sigelman CK: Social service innovation in the American states: deinstitutionalization of the mentally retarded. **Soc Sci Q** 1982;62(3):503–15
Sloan W, Stevens HA: A century of concern: a history of the American Association on Mental Deficiency 1876–1976. Washington, American Association on Mental Deficiency, 1976, viii, 310p.
Tyor PL, Bell LV: Caring for the retarded in America: a history. Westport, Conn., Greenwood, 1984. 215 p. (Contributions in Medical History, no. 15)
Zainaldin JS, Tyor PL: Asylum and society: an approach to institutional change. **J Soc Hist** 1979;13(1):23–48

USSR

Simmons HG: Explaining social policy: the English Mental Deficiency Act of 1913. **J Soc Hist** 1978;11(3):387–403

## METABOLIC

1700 to Present

Puerto Rico

Hernández-Morales F: La contribución del Dr. Ramón M. Suárez a la investigación del esprú. **Bol Asoc Med PR** 1983 Nov;75(11):496–7

United States

Ternberg JL: Surgical treatment of idiopathic hyperinsulinemic hypoglycemia in children. First successful subtotal pancreatectomy with preservation of spleen reported by Evarts A. Graham (1934). **J Thorac Cardiovasc Surg** 1984 Nov;88(5 Pt 2):898–901

## METABOLISM, INBORN ERRORS

1700 to Present

Great Britain

Bearn AG, Miller ED: Archibald Garrod and the development of the concept of inborn errors of metabolism. **Bull Hist Med** 1979 Fall;53(3):315–28

## MILK SICKNESS

1700 to Present

United States

Snively WD: 'We war perplext by a disease cald milksick'; the story of the pioneers' most dreaded plague. **Indiana Med Hist Q** 1974;1(2):31–5

## MOTION SICKNESS

1700 to Present

United States

Brinnin JM: The sway of the grand saloon: queasy come, queasy go. **Am Heritage** 1971;22(6):16–9, 98–9

## MUSCULOSKELETAL

Dubowitz V: History of muscle disease. In Rose FC, Bynum WF, ed: Historical aspects of the neurosciences. New York, Raven, 1982. p. 213–22.
Ehni G: Seeking the hidden flaw. **Spine** 1981 Jul–Aug;6(4):369–74
Loevy HT, Kowitz A: The Habsburgs and the 'Habsburg Jaw'. **Bull Hist Dent** 1982 Apr;30(1):19–23
Rüttimann B: Hippokratische 'Wirbelverrenkung'. **Gesnerus** 1983;40(1–2):159–66
Stensman R: The paraplegic Viking and the one-armed pianist--some well known persons with locomotor disability. **Scand J Rehabil Med [Suppl]** 1983;9:82–7

Austria

Snorrason E: Den Habsburgske underkaebe. **Tandlaegebladet** 1982 May;86(8):277–80

Germany

Seidel K: Vergleichende Untersuchungen über die Häufigkeit des Auftretens degenerativer Wirbelsäulen-veränderungen bei Menschen des Neolitikums, des Mittelalters und der Jetztzeit. **Z Gesamte Inn Med** 1981 Mar;36(5):159–62

500 A.D.–1450

Peru

Canalis RF, Aragon RM, Cabieses F, et al: Fibrous dysplasia: findings in a pre-Columbian skull. **Am J Otolaryngol** 1980 Feb;1(2):131–5

1700 to Present

Accardo PJ: An early case report of muscular dystrophy. A footnote to the history of neuromuscular disorders. **Arch Neurol** 1981 Mar;38(3):144–6
Bonduelle M: Sclérose latérale amyotrophique. **Rev Neurol (Paris)** 1982;138(12):1027–39
Buchanan WW, Kraag GR, Palmer DG, et al: The first recorded case of osteitis fibrosa cystica. **Can Med Assoc J** 1981 Mar 15;124(6):812–5
Byrne E: Historical and current concepts in mitochondrial myopathies. **Aust NZ J Med** 1983 Jun;13(3):299–305
Bywaters EG: Historical aspects of ankylosing spondylitis. **Rheumatol Rehabil** 1979 Nov;18(4):197–203
Churg J: Diffuse collagen disease. **JAMA** 1984 Nov 16;252(19):2702
De Quervain's stenosing tenovaginitis: Fritz de Quervain, 1868–1940: **Orthop Nurs** 1982 Sep–Oct;1(5):24–5
Pearn J: The discovery of neuronopathy and neuropathy as a cause of progressive paralysis in childhood. The historical origins of modern differential diagnosis in neuromuscular disease. **J Neurol Sci** 1984 Apr;64(1):99–107
Tolo VT: Progression in scoliosis. A 360 degrees change in 75 years. **Spine** 1983 May–June;8(4):373–7

France

Hubault A: Arthropathies nerveuses. **Rev Neurol (Paris)** 1982;138(12):1009–17
Lugnegård H: Mannen bakom dupuytrens kontraktur: 'vilddjuret vid Seine' – sin tids mest namnkunnige kirurg. **Lakartidningen** 1983 Dec 28;80(52):5068–9
Ryckewaert A, Naveau B: Les affections ostéo-articulaires de J.M. Charcot à nos jours. **Rev Neurol (Paris)** 1982;138(12):997–1008
Ryckewaert A, Naveau B: Principaux apports de Charcot et de Pierre Marie à la pathologie ostéo-articulaire. **Rev Rhum Mal Osteoartic** 1984 Jul–Sep;51(7–8):405–13
Sorrel-Dejerine Y, Fardeau M: Naissance et métamorphoses de la myopathie atrophique progressive de Landouzy et Déjerine. **Rev Neurol (Paris)** 1982;138(12):1041–51

Great Britain

Bound JP, Harvey PW, Brookes DM, et al: The incidence of anencephalus in the Fylde peninsula 1956–76 and changes in water hardness. **J Epidemiol Community Health** 1981 Jun;35(2):102–5
Sternbach G: C.S. Campbell: Gamekeeper's thumb. **J Emerg Med**

1984;1(4):345–7

**Italy**

Smith RD: Paganini's hand. **Arthritis Rheum** 1982 Nov;25(11):1385–6

**Switzerland**

Brühlmann-Jecklin E: Zehn Jahre Gesellschaft für Muskelkrankheiten. Fachleute und Betroffene am gleichen Strick. **Krankenpflege Soins Infirm** 1984 Jun;77(6):34–6

**United States**

Rainer JK: Cervical disc surgery--a historical review. **J Tenn Med Assoc** 1984 Jan;77(1):12–6

Wallace DJ: Fibromyalgia: unusual historical aspects and new pathogenic insights. **Mt Sinai J Med (NY)** 1984 Apr;51(2):124–31

Zellweger H, Simpson J, Ionasescu V: Twenty years--Iowa muscle clinic: reminiscences and prospects. **Eur J Pediatr** 1982 Feb;138(1):17–22

## NEOPLASMS

Ackerknecht EH: Zur Geschichte der Krebsbehandlung. **Gesnerus** 1980;37(3/4):189–97

Barthelmé E: Histoire de la notion du cancer. **Hist Sci Med** 1981;15(2):167–72

Bernasconi M, Carminati A, Tamburini C: Panorama storico sulla patalogia del cancro. Lotta tra due vite. **Krankenpflege (Bern)** 1983 Nov;76(11):70–1

Borit A: History of tumors of the pineal region. **Am J Surg Pathol** 1981 Sep;5(6):613–20

Brewer LA: Historical notes on lung cancer before and after Graham's successful pneumonectomy in 1933. **Am J Surg** 1982 Jun;143(6):650–9

Cabanne F, Gérard-Marchant R, Destaing F: Geschichte des Krebses. In Sournia JC, Martiny M, Poulet J, ed: Illustrierte Geschichte der Medizin. Salzburg, Andreas, 1980. Vol. 8. p. 2849–79.

Crouch HE: History of basal cell carcinoma and its treatment. **J R Soc Med** 1983 Apr;76(4):302–6

Deeley TJ: A brief history of cancer. **Clin Radiol** 1983 Nov;34(6):597–608

Delarue NC: Lung cancer in historical perspective: lessons from the past, implications of present experience, challenges for the future. **Can J Surg** 1980 Nov;23(6):549–57

Dymarskiĭ LIu: K istorii razvitiia khirurgicheskogo lecheniia raka molochnoĭ zhelezy, nachinaia s drevnego Egipta i do nashikh dneĭ. **Khirurgiia (Mosk)** 1981 Apr;(4):111–6

Harington JS, McGlashan ND: Migrant workers and cancer patterns in South Africa. **J South Afr Stud** 1976;3(1):92–101

Hutter RV: Classics in Oncology. Lobular carcinoma in situ by Foote and Stewart. **CA** 1982 Jul–Aug;32(4):232–7

Jackson R: How caustics were used to treat skin cancer. **J Dermatol Surg Oncol** 1979 Dec;5(12):949–50

López de la Osa Garcés L: Estudio histórico de la evolución del tratamiento del carcinoma de cuello uterino. **Rev Esp Oncol** 1981;28(4):569–90

Meyer JL: Hyperthermia as an anticancer modality--a historical perspective. **Front Radiat Ther Oncol** 1984;18:1–22

Miké V: Clinical studies in cancer: a historical perspective. In V. Miké, K. E. Stanley, ed: Statistics in medical research. Methods and issues, with applications in cancer research. New York, John Wiley & Sons, 1982. p. 111–55.

Moulin D de: A short history of breast cancer. Boston, Martinus Nijhoff, 1983. xiii, 124 p.

Muir CS: Nasopharyngeal cancer--a historical vignette. **CA** 1983 May–Jun;33(3):180–5

Raven RW: The surgeon and oncology. **Clin Oncol** 1984 Dec;10(4):311–8

Scholz A: Von kleinen und grossen Tumoren in der Kunst. **Hautarzt** 1982 Nov;33(11):598–604

Sears HF: Soft tissue sarcoma: a historical overview. **Semin Oncol** 1981 Jun;8(2):129–32

Senn HJ: Die medizinische Onkologie--eine fachliche und menschliche Herausforderung. **Wien Med Wochenschr** 1981;131(22):541–50

Storm FK, Morton DL: Localized hyperthermia in the treatment of cancer. **CA** 1983 Jan–Feb;33(1):44–56

Vaeth JM: Role of the pharmacist in cancer care throughout history. **Front Radiat Ther Oncol** 1980;15:1–4

Waldron HA: A brief history of scrotal cancer. **Br J Ind Med** 1983 Nov;40(4):390–401

Waldron HA: On the history of scrotal cancer. **Ann R Coll Surg Engl** 1983 Nov;65(6):420–2

Zanca A, Zanca A: Istituti Ospedalieri di Mantova, Mantova, Italy. **Int J Dermatol** 1980 Jan–Feb;19(1):55–8

**Germany**

Wilde J: Historische Aspekte zum Schneeberger Lungenkrebs. **Z Arztl Fortbild (Jena)** 1982 Feb;76(3):118–20

**Netherlands**

Moulin D de: Historical notes on breast cancer, with emphasis on The Netherlands. II. Pathophysiological concepts, diagnosis and therapy in the 18th century. **Neth J Surg** 1981 Oct;33(4):206–16

**Sweden**

Ahlström CG: Uppfattningen om cancer i äldre tider; en översikt med särskild hänsyn till Sverige. **Sydsven Medicinhist Sallsk Arsskr** 1980;:10–39

**Before 500 A.D.**

Steinfeld AD, McDuff HC: An ancient report of a dermoid cyst of the vagina. **Surg Gynecol Obstet** 1980 Jan;150(1):95–6

**Americas**

Allison MJ, Gerszten E, Munizaga J, et al: Metastatic tumor of bone in a Tiahuanaco female. **Bull NY Acad Med** 1980 Jul–Aug;56(6):581–7

**Arabic**

Aslam M, Bano H, Vohora SB: Sartan (cancer) and its treatment in Unami Medicine. **Am J Chin Med** 1981 Summer;9(2):95–107

**Rome**

Klawans HL: The acromegaly of Maximinus I: the possible influence of a pituitary tumor on the life and death of a Roman emperor. In Rose FC, Bynum WF, ed: Historical aspects of the neurosciences. New York, Raven, 1982. 317–26.

Ljunggren B: En stor man med en sjuk hjärna. **Sydsven Medicinhist Sallsk Arsskr** 1984;21:77–85

**United States**

Lagier R, Baud CA, Arnaud G, et al: Lesions characteristic of infection or malignant tumor in Paleo-Eskimo skulls. An anatomical and radiological study of two specimens. **Virchows Arch [Pathol Anat]** 1982;395(3):237–43

**500 A.D.–1450**

**Arabic**

Musaev TM: Vzgliady Abu Ali Ibn Siny (Avitsenny) na opukholevye zabolevaniia. **Vopr Onkol** 1980;26(9):72–4

**Great Britain**

Arderne J: A fourteenth-century description of rectal cancer. **World J Surg** 1983 Mar;7(2):304–7

**1450–1700**

**Denmark**

Karker A: Kong Frederik 2.s dod. **Jyske Saml** 1964;6(3):252–81

**Europe**

Muratori G: Odontoiatria del passato. I tumori della lingua. **Dent Cadmos** 1981 Apr;49(4):68–9

Muratori G: Odontoiatria del passato. I tumori odontogeni. **Dent Cadmos** 1981 Apr;49(4):65–7

**France**

Ayer E, Montandon D: Pierre Franco (1506–1580) and the treatment of a cheek ulcer. **Chir Plast** 1980;5(4):289–93

Kleinmann R: Facing cancer in the seventeenth century: the last illness of Anne of Austria, 1664–1666. **Adv Thanatol** 1978;4:37–55

**Great Britain**

Huard P, Imbault-Huart MJ: Les étapes du traitement des tumeurs par ischémie, priorité de Harvey. **Hist Sci Med** 1980;14(2):171–5

**Italy**

Rosenzweig W: Disease in art: a case for carcinoma of the breast in Michelangelo's La notte. **Paleopathol Newsl** 1983 Mar;41:8–11

### Netherlands

Braithwaite PA, Shugg D: Rembrandt's Bathsheba: the dark shadow of the left breast. **Ann R Coll Surg Engl** 1983 Sep;65(5):337–8

De Moulin D: Historical notes on breast cancer, with emphasis on the Netherlands. I. Pathological and therapeutic concepts in the seventeenth century. **Neth J Surg** 1980;32(4):129–34

Dymarskiĭ LIu: Taĭna 'Virsavii', kartiny Rembrandta. **Vopr Onkol** 1984;30(10):90–101

### 1700 to Present

Ackerman LV: H. P. Smith Award lecture. Tumor pathologists I have known. **Am J Clin Pathol** 1982 Apr;77(4):385–90

Bartecchi CE: Primary cardiac tumors: historically elusive lesions. **South Med J** 1982 Oct;75(10):1249–50

Becker V: Carl Ruge: 100 Jahre Stückchen-Diagnose. **Arch Gynecol** 1979 Sep;227(3):193–204

Bode UK: Frühe histologische Krebsforschung in Deutschland, Frankreich und Oesterreich. Köln, 1979. 208 p. (Kölner medizinhistorische Beiträge. Arbeiten der Forschungsstelle des Instituts für Geschichte der Medizin der Universität zu Köln, Band 12).

Bogdan TT: Poluvekovoĭ opyt khirurgii raka legkogo. **Vestn Khir** 1984 Apr;132(4):69–71

Borch-Johnsen K: Byliv og lungecancer. En kvantitativ og kvalitativ vurdering af den urbane faktor. **Ugeskr Laeger** 1982 Jun 7;144(23):1713–8

Braverman IM: 'Cutaneous manifestations of internal malignant tumors' by Becker, Kahn and Rothman, June 1942. Commentary: Migratory necrolytic erythema. **Arch Dermatol** 1982 Oct;118(10):784–98

Breen RE, Garnjobst W: Surgical procedures for carcinoma of the rectum. A historical review. **Dis Colon Rectum** 1983 Oct;26(10):680–5

Burkitt DP: The discovery of Burkitt's lymphoma. **Cancer** 1983 May 15;51(10):1777–86

Carmichael E: Dr. Papanicolaou and the Pap smear. **Ala J Med Sci** 1984 Jan;21(1):101–4

Clark WD, Quinn FB: Erroneous reporting of errors. **JAMA** 1984 Jul 13;252(2):207–8

Clarkson BD: The elusive goal. **Cancer Res** 1981 Dec;41(12 pt 1):4865–84

Clemmesen J: Johannes Fibiger. Copenhagen, Munksgaard, 1978. 13 p.

Dreznik A, Falk RE, Howard V, et al: Hyperthermia as a treatment for neoplasia. **Can J Surg** 1982 Nov;25(6):603–8

Evans AE: Leukemia: historical development of cancer therapy. The first battle is won. **Front Radiat Ther Oncol** 1981;16:18–29

Fiks A: Cystosarcoma phyllodes of the mammary gland--Müller's tumor. For the 180th birthday of Johannes Müller. **Virchows Arch [Pathol Anat]** 1981;392(1):1–6

Fitzgerald RH: What is the Dukes' system for carcinoma of the rectum? **Dis Colon Rectum** 1982 Jul–Aug;25(5):474–7

García-Alejo RH: Enfermedad osea de Paget: comentarios a sus primeras descripciones y evolucion historica de su etiopatogenia. **Asclepio** 1982;34:181–97

Golub S: Coping with cancer: Freud's experiences. **Psychoanal Rev** 1981 Summer;68(2):191–200

Gómez P, Rosado A: Unidad de Investigación Clínica, Hospital de Oncología, Centro Médico Nacional, IMSS. **Arch Invest Med (Mex)** 1981;12(3):361–75

Gross R, Claus O: Chemotherapie von Tumorleiden: Vergangenheit und Gegenwart. **Med Welt** 1982 Nov 5;33(44):1531–8

Homburger F: Carcinogenesis bioassay in historical perspective. **Prog Exp Tumor Res** 1983;26:182–6

Hoogland GA: Some historical remarks on acoustic neuroma. **Adv Otorhinolaryngol** 1984;34:3–7

Hughes ES: The development of a restorative operation for carcinoma of the rectum. **Aust NZ J Surg** 1981;51:117–9

Hutt MS: Historical introduction, Burkitt's lymphoma, nasopharyngeal carcinoma and Kaposi's sarcoma. **Trans R Soc Trop Med Hyg** 1981;75(6):761–5

Jensen EV: Steroid receptors in breast cancer: historical perspective. **Cancer** 1980 Dec 15;46(12 Suppl):2759–61

Johns HE: The physicist in cancer treatment and detection. **Int J Radiat Oncol Biol Phys** 1981 Jun;7(6):801–8

King DF: Chronic atypical epithelial proliferation of Bowen. A historical and biographical note. **Am J Dermatopathol** 1984 Feb;6(1):35–8

Lawrence W Jr: The scope of surgical oncology. **Aust NZ J Surg** 1982 Aug;52(4):325–30

Lederman M: The early history of radiotherapy: 1895–1939. **Int J Radiat Oncol Biol Phys** 1981 May;7(5):639–48

Levin S: Mongolian spot; Afro-Asian stain; sacral stain. **S Afr Med J** 1981 Jul 25;60(4):123–4

Luce EA: The ordeal of Sigmund Freud. In Romm S, ed: Symposium on historical perspectives of plastic surgery. Philadelphia, Saunders, 1983. p. 715–6.

McCarthy EF: Giant-cell tumor of bone: an historical perspective. **Clin Orthop** 1980 Nov–Dec;(153):14–25

Marbach JU: Wilhelm Bernhard, 1920–1978. **Gesnerus** 1979;36(3–4):303–11

Meerwein P: Der Krebspatient und sein Arzt im 19. Jahrhundert. Ursprünge der Psychoonkologie? Zürich, Juris, 1980. 97 p. (Zürcher Medizingeschichtliche Abhandlungen, Neue Reihe, 139).

Mendelson BC: The evolution of breast reconstruction. **Med J Aust** 1982 Jan 9;1(1):7–8

Mercer AJ: Risk of dying from tuberculosis or cancer: further aspects of a possible association. **Int J Epidemiol** 1981 Dec;10(4):377–80

Michel J: Recherches historiques sur la découverte des maladies des sinus, le XIXe siècle. **J Fr Otorhinolaryngol** 1979 Nov;28(9):577–90

Missotten FE: Historical review of pharyngo-oesophageal reconstruction after resection for carcinoma of pharynx and cervical oesophagus. **Clin Otolaryngol** 1983 Oct;8(5):345–62

Monteil RA, Knoche JF: Etude de l'évolution du terme odontome depuis sa création jusqu'au concept anatomo-patholgique actuel. **Actual Odontostomatol (Paris)** 1980;(132):583–95

Muratori G: I tumori delle ghiandole salivari. **Dent Cadmos** 1981 May;49(5):73–4

Muratori G: Odontoiatria del passato. I tumori delle labbra e della mucosa orale. **Dent Cadmos** 1981 May;49(5):71–2

Nauts HC: Bacterial products in the treatment of cancer: past, present and future. In Jeljaszewicz J, Pulverer G, Roszkowski W, ed: Bacteria and cancer. London; New York, Academic Press, 1982. p. 1–25.

Onuigbo WI: Historical notes on cancer in married couples. **Neth J Surg** 1984 Aug;36(4):112–5

Peller S: Cancer research since 1900. New York, Philosophical Library, 1979. xv, 394 p.

Polglase AL: Rectal excision for cancer 1880 to 1980. **Med J Aust** 1981 Jan 10;1(1):3–4

Potter VR: Physiological adaptation at the molecular level: the frontier where research on differentiation and malignancy meet. **Perspect Biol Med** 1981 Summer;24(4):525–42

Pressman D: The development and use of radiolabeled antitumor antibodies. **Cancer Res** 1980 Aug;40(8 Pt 2):2960–4

Romm S: The oral cancer of Sigmund Freud. In Romm S, ed: Symposium on historical perspectives of plastic surgery. Philadelphia, Saunders, 1983. p. 709–14.

Rosen PP: Specimen radiography and the diagnosis of clinically occult mammary carcinoma. A brief historical review. **Pathol Annu** 1980;15(pt 1):225–37

The rubber industry: Historical overview. In IARC monographs on the evaluation of the carcinogenic risk of chemicals to humans. (Volume 28: The rubber industry). [Geneva], International Agency for Research on Cancer, 1982. p. 31–46.

Rywlin AM: Non-Hodgkin's malignant lymphomas. Brief historical review and simple unifying classification. **Am J Dermatopathol** 1980 Spring;2(1):17–25

Satoh O: [Transsphenoidal surgery for pituitary tumors: historical review and present trends] (Jpn). **No Shinkei Geka** 1984 Jan;12(1):7–26

Schechter DC: Flashbacks: containment of tumors through electricity. **PACE** 1979 Jan;2(1):100–14

Scott WW: Historical overview of the treatment of prostatic cancer. **Prostate** 1983;4(5):435–40

Shimkin MB, ed: Some classics of experimental oncology. 50 selections, 1775–1965. Bethesda, National Institutes of Health, 1980. 739 p. (NIH Publication No. 80–2150).

Sontag S: Illness as metaphor. New York, Farrar, Straus and Giroux, 1978. 87 p.

Stallworthy J: Progress in gynecologic oncology: a personal retrospective view. **Gynecol Oncol** 1979 Dec;8(3):253–64

Steffen C: Marjolin's ulcer. Report of two cases and evidence that Marjolin did not describe cancer arising in scars of burns. **Am J Dermatopathol** 1984 Apr;6(2):187–93

Streuli RA, Ultmann JE: Non-Hodgkin's lymphomas: historical perspective and future prospects. **Semin Oncol** 1980 Sep;7(3):223–33

Studer KE, Chubin DE: The cancer mission. Social contexts of biomedical research. Beverly Hills, London, Sage, 1980. 319 p. (Sage Library of Social Research, V. 103).

Vaeth JM: Historical aspects of tylectomy and radiation therapy in the treatment of cancer of the breast. **Front Radiat Ther Oncol** 1983;17:1–10

Van Eys J: Nutritional therapy in childhood malignancies--a historical perspective. In Van Eys J, Seelig MS, Nichols BL, ed: Nutrition and cancer. New York and London, SP, 1979. P. 91–110.

Vázquez Albaladejo G, Sospedra Ferrer R: Evolución de las técnicas quirúrgicas en el cáncer de mama. **Rev Esp Oncol** 1981;28(1):83–94

Wright JC: Cancer chemotherapy: past, present, and future--Part I. **J Natl Med Assoc** 1984 Aug;76(8):773–84

Zingg W: Historical use of hypothermia for cancer. **Can J Surg** 1983 Mar;26(2):97–8

Zubrod CG: The cure of cancer by chemotherapy - reflections on how it happened. (The fifth Myron Karon Memorial Lecture). **Med Pediatr Oncol** 1980;8:107–14

Zülch KJ: Historical development of the classification of brain tumours and the new proposal of the World Health Organization (WHO). **Neurosurg Rev** 1981;4(3):123–7

Zülch KJ: Reflections on the surgery of the pineal gland (a glimpse into the past). Gleanings from medical history. **Neurosurg Rev** 1981;4(3):159–63

# DISEASES AND INJURIES

**Austria**

Braun M: Classics in Oncology. Idipathic multiple pigmented sarcoma of the skin by Kaposi. **CA** 1982 Nov–Dec;32(6):340–7
Schober KL: Das chirurgische Erbe. Theodor Billroth und die Karzinomchirurgie des Intestinaltraktes. **Zentralbl Chir** 1981;106(10):693–9
Schreiber HW: Wo steht die Carcinom-Chirurgie des Magens 100 Jahre nach der ersten erfolgreichen Magenresektion durch Theodor Billroth? **Langenbecks Arch Chir** 1982;358:53–5
Schweppe KW, Probst C: Die Versuche zur medikamentösen Karzinomtherapie des Anton Störck (1731 bis 1803). Ein Beitrag zur Geschichte der experimentellen Arzneimittelforschung in der älteren Wiener medizinischen Schule. In Ganzinger K, Skopec M, Wyklicky H, ed: Festschrift für Erna Lesky zum 70. Geburtstag. Wien, Brüder Hollinek, 1981. p. 105–22.
Schweppe KW, Probst C: Die Versuche zur medikamentösen Karzinomtherapie des Anton Störck (1731–1803). Ein Beitrag zur Geschichte der experimentellen Arzneimittelforschung in der älteren Wiener medizinischen Schule. **Wien Med Wochenschr** 1982 Mar 15;132(5):107–17

**Canada**

Harrison RC, Mills F: Canadian contributions toward the comprehension of hyperinsulinism: the first successful excision of an insulinoma. **Can J Surg** 1980 Jul;23(4):401–3
Hill GB: Counting cancers. **Can Med Assoc J** 1983 Dec 15;129(12):1262–3

**Denmark**

Jensen OM, Larsen A: Blaerecancer i Danmark 1943–1977. Kraeftstatistik 4. **Ugeskr Laeger** 1982 Nov 15;144(46):3458–60
Sell A, Madsen CB: Radiumstationen in Aarhus from 1962 to 1984. **Acta Radiol [Oncol]** 1984;23(2–3):85–90

**France**

Bernoulli R: Un grand méconnu: Gustave Roussy. **Gesnerus** 1980;37(1/2):34–46
Denoix P: Paul Broca. L'anatomie pathologique, le cancer, la statistique. **Chirurgie** 1980;106(10):787–90
Firmin F: Cancer de la joue et autoplastie en l'an 1838. Opération de génioplastie pratiquée par M. Roux de Brignolles. **Ann Chir Plast** 1982;27(1):91–3
Holmes WR: The illness and death of Napoleon. **J Med Assoc Ga** 1983 Mar;72(3):201–4
Huard P: Velpeau, cancérologue. In: Congrès National des Sociétés Savantes, 93e, Tours, 1968. Comptes Rendus. Paris, 1971 Section des Sciences, Tome II. p. 159–62.
Iveson-Iveson J: Medical history. Napoleon: his final years. **Nurs Mirror** 1982 Aug 18;155(7):22–4
Olsson JE, Reichard H: Mannen bakom syndromet: Pierre Ménétrier. Tumörpatolog och mikrobiolog med tidig insikt om precanceröa förändringar. **Lakartidningen** 1984 Oct 10;81(41):3705–6
Pérel L: Conception pathogénique et traitement du cancer du sein au 18ème siècle. In: Congrès international d'histoire de la médecine, XXVe, Québec, 1976. Actes. Québec, 1977. p. 1073–80.
Regaud J: Claudius Regaud, (1870–1940): pionnier de la cancérologie, créateur de la Fondation Curie: chronique de sa vie et son oeuvre. Paris, Maloine, 1982. 233 p.
Steffen C: Jean-Nicolas Marjolin. **Am J Dermatopathol** 1984 Apr;6(2):163–5
Stolinsky DC: Trousseau's phenomenon. **Blood** 1983 Dec;62(6):1304
Voldman D: Guérir du cancer et mourir de vieillesse: histoire de l'hospice Paul-Brousse de 1905 à 1975. **Asclepio** 1983;35:317–26
Zorgniotti AW: Bladder cancer in the pre-cystoscopic era. **Prog Clin Biol Res** 1984;162A:1–9

**Germany**

Buslaeva MM, Volodina MN: Pervaia Mezhdunarodnia konferentsiia po izucheniiu raka (k 75-letiiu so dnia provedeniia). **Vopr Onkol** 1981;27(11):90–2
Dörffel EW, Held F, Oelssner W: Zum 30. Jahrestag der Gründung der Deutschen Demokratischen Republik. Die Bedeutung Fritz Gietzelts für die Radiologie und Geschwulst-bekämpfung. **Radiobiol Radiother (Berl)** 1979 Oct;20(5):621–6
Imanaga H: [Honoring Theodor Billroth by attaining a hundred years since his first success in gastric cancer resection (author's transl)] (Jpn). **Nippon Gan Chiryo Gakkai Shi** 1981 Jun 20;16(3):405–8
Korting GW: Atherom auf einem Olgemälde der Pinakothek in Brescia. **Hautarzt** 1984 Jun;35(6):321
Kyank H, Schwarz R: Ergebnisse der Behandlung des Zervixkarzinoms an der Universitäts-Frauenklinik Rostock von 1959 bis 1972. **Zentralbl Gynakol** 1980;102(9):481–5
Lin JI: Virchow's pathological reports on Frederick III's cancer. **N Engl J Med** 1984 Nov 8;311(19):1261–4

Meyer KK, Beck WC: Mastectomy performed by Lawrence Heister in the eighteenth century. **Surg Gynecol Obstet** 1984 Oct;159(4):391–4
Meyer-Schwickerath G: Die Geschichte der Photokoagulation und die Behandlung der intraocularen Tumoren mit dieser Methode. **Klin Oczna** 1981;83(2):59–61
Ober WB: History of the Brenner tumor of the ovary. **Pathol Annu** 1979;14 Pt 2:107–24
Wyk AJ: Medisyne uit Suid-Afrika vir die Keiser. **Historia (S Afr)** 1979;24(1):63–5

**Great Britain**

Bean WB, Felson B, Dolan KD: A nonletter from the editor and a case for all seasons. **Semin Roentgenol** 1982 Jul;17(3):153–62
Boyland E: The history and future of chemical carcinogenesis. **Br Med Bull** 1980 Jan;36(1):5–10
Carswell H: 'Elephant Man' had more than neurofibromatosis. **JAMA** 1982 Sep 3;248(9):1032–3
Clemmensen O: Hutchinson's freckle. **Am J Dermatopathol** 1982 Oct;4(5):425–8
Davis NC: William Norris, M.D.: a pioneer in the study of melanoma. **Med J Aust** 1980 Jan 26;1(2):52–4
Geller SA: Comments on the anniversary of the description of Hodgkin's disease. **J Natl Med Assoc** 1984 Aug;76(8):815–7
Greenwood RD: Surgical treatment for facial hemangioma, 1834. **Ala Med** 1984 Sep;54(3):27
King DF, Eisenberg D: Russell's fuchsine body. 'The characteristic organism of cancer.' **Am J Dermatopathol** 1981 Spring;3(1):55–8
Kirkpatrick DB: The first primary brain-tumor operation. **J Neurosurg** 1984 Nov;61(5):809–13
Logan WP: Cancer mortality by occupation and social class 1851–1971. **IARC Sci Publ** 1982;(36):1–253
Nuland SB: The lymphatic contiguity of Hodgkin's disease: a historical study. **Bull NY Acad Med** 1981 Nov;57(9):776–86
The Paterson Laboratories, Manchester, England.: **Oncology** 1981;38(1):59–61
Pearce JM: The first attempts at removal of brain tumors. In Rose FC, Bynum WF, ed: Historical aspects of the neurosciences. New York, Raven, 1982. p. 239–42.
Pruitt RD: William Osler and his Gulstonian lectures on malignant endocarditis. **Mayo Clin Proc** 1982 Jan;57(1):4–9
Ross WM: Carcinoma of the breast in the section of radiology. **J R Soc Med** 1980 Oct;73(10):734–8
Silvers DN, Gorham JD: Observations on a melanoma by William Norris, M.D., a country practitioner of the early 19th century. **Am J Dermatopathol** 1982 Oct;4(5):421–4
Stockwell S: Classics in oncology. George Thomas Beatson, M.D. (1848–1933). **CA** 1983 Mar–Apr;33(2):105–21

**Hungary**

Gyenes G: Adatok a magyarországi Hodgkin-kór kutatáshoz. **Orv Hetil** 1979 Nov 18;120(46):2812–4
Madai L: Le premier enregistrement statistique des malades cancereux dans l'annee 1904, en hongrie. **Genus** 1981;37(3–4):227–40
Péter L: Móra Ferenc betegségei. Halálának 50. évfordulójára. **Orv Hetil** 1984 Feb 5;125(6):341–4

**Ireland**

Walsh BM: Health education and the demand for tobacco in Ireland, 1953–76: a note. **Econ Soc Rev (Irel)** 1980;11(2):147–51

**Italy**

Giuffré R: Successful radical removal of an intracranial meningioma in 1835 by Professor Pecchioli of Siena. **J Neurosurg** 1984 Jan;60(1):47–51

**Japan**

Kageyama K, Mikata A, Harigaya K: [Studies of Hodgkin's disease in Japan: a historical survey] (Jpn). **Nippon Rinsho** 1983 Nov;41(11):2432–8

**Netherlands**

Moulin D de: Historical notes on breast cancer, with emphasis on The Netherlands; III. The growth of scientific surgery in the 19th century. **Neth J Surg** 1982 Dec;34(5):193–200
Moulin D de: Microscopie en kankerdiagnostiek in de eerste helft van de negentiende eeuw. **Tijdschr Geschied Geneeskd** 1983;6(2):99–107

**Poland**

Gadomska H: Ocena częstości wyst ępowania osteosarcoma na tle innych postaci nowotdworów złośliwych kości, Warszawa 1963–1974. **Nowotwory** 1979;Suppl:13–21
Gierek T, Namysłowski G, Kondracka E: Nowotwory złośliwe ucha

leczone w i klinice ORL Sląskiej Akademii Medycznej w okresie od 1967 do 1977 r. **Otolaryngol Pol** 1980;34(1):11-6
Jonecko A: Wkład uczonych polskich do badań nad branchiogennymi odchyleniami rozwojowymi szyi na przełomie XIX i XX wieku. **Pol Przegl Chir** 1979 Sep;51(9):921-26
Kasperski A: Występowanie raka krtani u chorych na obszarze byłego województwa bydgoskiego w latach 1955-1975 z uwzględnieniem niektórych czynników epidemiologicznych. **Otolaryngol Pol** 1980;34(1):125-6
Koszarowski T: Udział Instytutu Onkologii im. Marii Skłodowskiej-Curie w rozwoju społecznej walki z chorobami nowotworowymi w Polsce w latach 1945-1982. **Nowotwory** 1983 Jan-Mar;33(1):7-12
Krawczyk K: Rak płuc wśród chorych leczonych w oddziałach chorób płuc krakowskiego szpitala specjalistycznego im. dr Anki w latach 1956-1977. **Pneumonol Pol** 1979 Aug-Sep;47(7-8):573-80
Olakowski T, Rudzińska H, Gadomska H, et al: Epidemiologia raka płuca w Polsce do roku 1977. **Pneumonol Pol** 1979 Aug-Sep;47(7-8):553-64
Sieiński W, Dąbska M: Mięsaki kościotwórcze w materiale Zakładu Patologii Nowotworów Instytutu Onkologii w Warszawie w latach 1948-1977. **Nowotwory** 1979;Suppl:47-52
Supady J: Ankieta statystyczna z 1931 r. na temat występowania nowotworów złośliwych w populacji II Rzeczypospolitej. **Wiad Lek** 1981 Feb 15;34(4):351-5
Supady J: Doświadczalne badania lekarzy polskich nad rakotwórczym działaniem smoły pogazowej i jej pochondnych (do 1939 r.). **Pol Tyg Lek** 1981 Mar 2;36(9):357-9
Supady J: Działalność Wileńskiego Komitetu do Zwalczania Raka w latach 1931--1936. **Nowotwory** 1979 May-Jun;29(2):151-6
Supady J: Powstanie i działalność stowarzyszenia 'Polski Instytut Przeciwrakowy' we Lwowie (1929-1939). **Wiad Lek** 1982 Nov 1;35(19-20):1301-3
Supady J: Serologia nowotworów w badaniach Ludwika Hirszfelda i jego współpracowników w okresie II Rzeczypospolitej. **Wiad Lek** 1981 Feb 1;34(3):257-62
Supady J: Udział lekarzy polskich w krajowych i międzynarodowych zjazdach onkologicznych w latach 1918-1938. **Nowotwory** 1979 Oct-Dec;29(4):315-20
Werner-Brzezińska H: Pierwotne mi ęsaki kościopochodne leczone w Instytucie Onkologii w latach 1947-1970. **Nowotwory** 1979;Suppl;117-21
50-lecie Zakładu Radiodiagnostyki Instytutu Onkologii im. Marii Skłodowskiej-Curie w Warszawie: **Pol Przegl Radiol (Warszawa)** 1983 Jul-Aug;47(4):261-2

**Romania**

Negru I: Momente remarcabile din trecutul luptei împortriva cancerului în România. **Viata Med [Medii Sanit]** 1980 Sep;28(9):213-5
Negru I: Profesorul Iuliu Moldovan creatorul primului Institut oncologic în România. **Viata Med [Medii Sanit]** 1982 Dec;30(12):281-6

**Scandinavia**

Kjellgren O: The development of gynecological oncology in Scandinavia during the last 50 years. **Acta Obstet Gynecol Scand [Suppl]** 1984;120:27-34

**Sweden**

Ljunggren B: Reflexioner kring en hjärnsvulst hos 'En förnäm herre af 30 år'. **Sydsven Medicinhist Sallsk Arsskr** 1983;:87-102

**United States**

Dr. Frank M. Schabel Jr. **Cancer** 1984 Sep 15;54(6 Suppl):1132-52
Baker HW: The general surgeon and cancer. **Am J Surg** 1980 May;139(5):606-7
Barber D: Secret operation on US president. **Probe (Lond)** 1982 May;23(11):415-6
Barclay WR: Landmark perspective: Asbestos. An industrial asset with a health cost. **JAMA** 1984 Jul 6;252(1):96
Breslow L: From cancer research to cancer control. **Prog Clin Biol Res** 1983;120:1-19
Brewer LA: The first pneumonectomy. Historical notes. **J Thorac Cardiovasc Surg** 1984 Nov;88(5 Pt 2):810-26
Brooks JJ, Enterline HT, Aponte GE: The final diagnosis of President Cleveland's lesion. **Trans Stud Coll Physicians Phila** 1980 Mar;(2 no 1):1-25
Classic articles in colonic and rectal surgery. Robert Fulton Weir 1838-1927: An improved method of treating high-seated cancers of the rectum. **Dis Colon Rectum** 1982 Jul-Aug;25(5):503-7
Corner GW: Leo Loeb. In Dictionary of American Biography, Suppl. 6, 1956-1960. p. 385-7, 1980.
Crile G: Breast cancer. A personal perspective. **Surg Clin North Am** 1984 Dec;64(6):1145-9
Cross W, Moses J: 'My God, sir, I think the president is doomed!' [Grover Cleveland's cancer surgery] **Am Hist Illus** 1982 Nov;17:40-5
Dr. Harold P. Rusch and the Wisconsin Clinical Cancer Center: **Wis Med J** 1979 Jun;78(6):96-7
The evolution of Mohs' surgery: **J Dermatol Surg Oncol** 1982 Aug;8(8):650-4
Fath H: A dream come true: the story of St. Jude Children's Research Hospital and ALSAC. Memphis, TN, ALSAC, 1983. 214 p.
Fournier GA, Albert DM, Bachrach A, et al: Symbol of Boston's Museum of Science has eye tumor. **N Engl J Med** 1983 Mar 31;308(13):782-3
Frei E: Intramural therapeutic research at the National Cancer Institute, Department of Medicine: 1955-1965. **Cancer Treat Rep** 1984 Jan;68(1):21-30
Freireich E: Landmark perspective: Nitrogen mustard therapy. **JAMA** 1984 May 4;251(17):2262-3
Garfinkel L: Asbestos: historical perspective. **CA** 1984 Jan-Feb;34(1):44-7
Gillespie B, Eva D, Johnston R: Carcinogenic risk assessment in the United States and Great Britain: the case of Aldrin/Dieldrin. **Soc Stud Sci** 1979;9(3):265-301
Greenberg ER, Colton T, Bagne C: Measurement of cancer incidence in the United States: sources and uses of data. **JNCI** 1982 May;68(5):743-50
Greenberg MR: A note on the changing geography of cancer mortality within metropolitan regions of the United States. **Demography** 1981 Aug;18(3):411-20
Greenwood RD: 19th century medicine in Indiana. An 1869 clinical report by J. S. Bobbs. **Indiana Med** 1984 Jun;77(6):476
Hawkins A: Two pathographies: a study in illness and literature. **J Med Philos** 1984 Aug;9(3):231-52
Heerden JA van: First encounters with pheochromocytoma. The story of Mother Joachim. **Am J Surg** 1982 Aug;144(2):277-9
Henson PM: Harold Fred Dorn. In Dictionary of American biography, 1961-1965. Suppl. 7, 1981. p. 191-3.
Hertig AT: Early concepts of dysplasia and carcinoma in situ (a backward glance at a forward process). A brief historical review. **Obstet Gynecol Surv** 1979 Nov;34(11):795-803
Hilkemeyer R: A historical perspective in cancer nursing. **Oncol Nurs Forum** 1982 Spring;9(2):47-56
Huggins CB: Peyton Rous and his voyages of discovery. **J Exp Med** 1979 Oct 1;150(4):733-4
Janssen WF: Cancer quackery: past and present. **FDA Consum** 1977 Jul-Aug;11(6):27-32
Jaques DA: The fraternity of strangers. **Am J Surg** 1984 Oct;148(4):426-7
Kardinal CG: Laetrile in historical perspective. **Mo Med** 1980 Sep;77(9):564-9
Laszlo J: Two long-range clinical data bases are terminated: bang, whimper, or ripple? **J Clin Oncol** 1984 May;2(5):532-3
Lemon HM: Motivation in cancer education, with an appreciation of Dr. Henry Jackson, Jr., pioneer medical oncologist-hematologist (1892-1968). **Med Pediatr Oncol** 1980;8(4):407-22
Lemon HM: My specialty: oncology. **Nebr Med J** 1979 Aug;64(8):259
Lerner IJ: The whys of cancer quackery. **Cancer** 1984 Feb 1;53(3 Suppl):815-9
Ljunggren B: The case of George Gershwin. **Neurosurgery** 1982 Jun;10(6 Pt 1):733-6
McCoy JJ: The cancer lady: Maud Slye and her heredity studies. Nashville, Nelson, 1977. 191 p.
Markle GE, Petersen JC, ed: Politics, science, and cancer: the laetrile phenomenon. Boulder, Westview Press, for the American Association for the Advancement of Science, 1980. xiii, 190 p. (AAAS Selected Symposium, v. 46). Contributions by JH Young, RD Smith, RF Rich, GP Monaco, Al Caplan, D Nelkin.
Miller NJ, Howard-Ruben J: Unproven methods of cancer management part I: background and historical perspectives. **Oncol Nurs Forum** 1983 Fall;10(4):46-52
Miller RW, McKay FW: Decline in US childhood cancer mortality. 1950 through 1980. **JAMA** 1984 Mar 23-30;251(12):1567-70
Molino-Negro P: Jules Hardy M.D. **Surg Neurol** 1984 Aug;22(2):109-12
Morris N: The cancer blackout: exposing the official blacklisting of beneficial cancer research, treatment and prevention. Los Angeles, Regent House, 1977. ix, 206 p.
Murphy GP: Landmark perspective: Bladder neoplasms. **JAMA** 1983 Sep 9;250(10):1326
Murphy GP: Roswell Park Memorial Institute, Genesis of a cancer center. **Oncology** 1980;37(6):426-8
Nelson RB: The final victory of General U. S. Grant. **Cancer** 1981 Feb 1;47(3):433-6
Parascandola J: Maud Caroline Slye. In: Notable American women. The modern period. Cambridge, Mass., Belknap-Harvard Univ. Press, 1980. 4:651-2.
Petersen JC, Markle GE: Politics and science in the laetrile controversy. **Soc Stud Sci** 1979;9(2):139-66
Pillsbury DM: General Eisenhower's 'melanoma'. **J Am Acad Dermatol** 1981 May;4(5):631-2
Pitot HC: Landmark article (JAMA 1911;56:198). Transmission of a malignant new growth by means of a cell-free filtrate. By Peyton Rous. **JAMA** 1983 Sep 16;250(11):1445-9
Riley HD: George Nicholas Papanicolaou. In Dictionary of American biography, 1961-1965. Suppl. 7, 1981. p. 598-9.
Russel ES: A century of mammalian genetics and cancer, 1929-2029, a view at midpassage. **Prog Clin Biol Res** 1981;45:xi-xiv

Salsburg D, Heath A: When science progresses and bureaucracies lag: the case of cancer research. **Public Interest** 1981;65:30-9
Schneiderman MA: Trends in cancer mortality and incidence in the United States: is the future clear or clouded? In V. Miké, K. E. Stanley, ed: Statistics in medical research. Methods and issues, with applications in cancer research. New York, John Wiley & Sons, 1982. p. 71-107.
Selikoff IJ, Churg J, Hammond EC: Classics in oncology: asbestos exposure and neoplasia. **CA** 1984 Jan-Feb;34(1):48-56
Slocum A: Cornelius Packard Rhoads. In Dictionary of American Biography, Suppl. 6, 1956-1960. p. 537-8. 1980.
Sproul EE: Acid phosphatase and prostate cancer: historical overview. **Prostate** 1980;1(4):411-3
Stephenson GW: The Commission on Cancer: an historical review. **Bull Am Coll Surg** 1979 Sep;64(9):7-13
Stine JK: Eugene Jules Houdry. In Dictionary of American biography, 1961-1965. Suppl. 7, 1981. p. 367-9.
Weinhouse S: Prometheus and Pandora--cancer research on our Diamond Anniversary: American Association for Cancer Research. **Cancer Res** 1982 Sep;42(9):3471-4
Weisburger EK: History of the Bioassay Program of the National Cancer Institute. **Prog Exp Tumor Res** 1983;26:187-201
Witkowski JA: Experimental pathology and the origins of tissue culture: Leo Loeb's contribution. **Med Hist** 1983 Jul;27(3):269-88
Wynder EL: Some reflections on smoking and lung cancer. **J Thorac Cardiovasc Surg** 1984 Nov;88(5 Pt 2):854-7
Young JH: Laetrile in historical perspective. **Conn Med** 1979 Aug;43(8):497-500
Young JH: Laetrile in historical perspective. In Markle GE, Petersen JC, ed: Politics, science and cancer: the laetrile phenomenon. Boulder, CO. Westview Press, for American Association for the Advancement of Science, Washington, D. C., 1980. p. 11-60.
Zubrod CG: Origins and development of chemotherapy research at the National Cancer Institute. **Cancer Treat Rep** 1984 Jan;68(1):9-19

#### USSR

Agamova KA: Razvitie tsitologicheskoĭ diagnostiki opukholĭ cheloveka. **Sov Med** 1982;(6):65-9
Blokhin NN, Napalkov NP: Razvitie onkologii v SSSR. **Vopr Onkol** 1982;28(12):3-9
Blokhin NN, Trapeznikov NN, Chaklin AV, et al: Vsesoiuznomu onkologicheskomu naushnomu tsentru AMN SSSR 30 let. **Vopr Onkol** 1981;27(12):81-7
Bogovski P: Historical perspectives of occupational cancer. **J Toxicol Environ Health** 1980 Sep-Nov;6(5-6):921-39
Bramberga VM: Stanovlenie, sovremennoe sostoianie i perspektivy razvitiia onkologii v Latviĭskoĭ SSR. **Vopr Onkol** 1982;28(10):8-13
Charkviani LI: Zakavlazskie konferentsii onkologov. **Vopr Onkol** 1981;27(9):48-52
Chissov Vi, Demidov VP, Kapatsinskiĭ EV, et al: Rol' Moskovskogo nauchno-issledovatel'skogo instituta im. P. A. Gertsena Minzdrava RSFSR v razvitii otechestvennoĭ onkologii. **Vopr Onkol** 1983;29(11):3-7
Demin VN: 50 let prepodavaniia onkologii v ordena Lenina Gosudarstvennom institute dlia usovershenstvovaniia vracheĭ im. S. M. Kirova. **Vopr Onkol** 1981;27(4):98-100
Diadiusha GF, Turkevich NM, Bulkina ZP: Vklad R. E. Kavetskogo v razvitie onkologii (k 80-letiiu so dnia rozhdeniia). **Vopr Onkol** 1979;25(11):102-10
Iarmonenko SP: Klinicheskaia radiobiologiia--nauchnaia osnova luchevoĭ terapii opukholeĭ. **Med Radiol (Mosk)** 1982 Mar;27(3):6-9
Kapatsinskiĭ EV, Kozlova EV: Rol' Moskovskogo nauchno-issledovatel'skogo onkologicheskogo instituta im. P. A. Gertsena v razvitii organizatsionnykh osnov onkologii. **Sov Zdravookhr** 1981;(11):50-2
Kuiatkhanov BA: O stanovlenii onkologicheskoĭ sluzhby v Turkmenskoĭ SSR. **Vopr Onkol** 1982;28(12):25-8
Napalkov NP, Mishura VI, Merabishvili VM, et al: Razvitie ideĭ N. N. Petrova v oblasti organizatsii protivorakovoĭ bor'by. **Vopr Onkol** 1982;28(5):126-32
Neĭman IM: K 50-letiiu sozyva I Vsesoiuznogo s'ezda onkologov (iz vospominaniĭ uchastnika). **Vopr Onkol** 1981;27(11):88-9
Perevodchikova NI, Garin AM: Osnovnye étapy razvitiia klinicheskoĭ khimioterapii opukholeĭ v SSSR. **Vopr Onkol** 1982;28(5):31-8
Pinchuk VG: Razvitie ideĭ A. A. Bogomolets v oblasti izucheniia reaktivnosti organizma pri opukholevom protsesse. **Fiziol Zh** 1981 May-Jun;27(3):327-31
Pozmogov AI, Demin VT, Arendarevskiĭ LF: Kievskomu nauchno-issledovatel'skomu rentgenoradiologicheskomu i onkologicheskomu institutu 60 let. **Vestn Rentgenol Radiol** 1980 May-Jun;(3):78-80
Savchenko NE, Shitikov BD: Ob uspekhakh i tendentsiiakh razvitiia onkologicheskoĭ sluzhby v Belorusskoĭ SSR. **Vopr Onkol** 1982;28(12):13-20
Shevchenko IT: K istorii protivorakovoĭ bor'by na Ukraine. **Klin Khir** 1982 May;(5):67-70
Shtern RD: O prioritete opredeleniia limfomatoza zheludka otechestvennymi issledovateliami. **Arkh Patol** 1983;45(5):66-8
Suleĭmenov AA, Balmukhanov SB, Abdrakhimov BE: Onkologicheskaia sluzhba Kazakhstana za 60 let SSSR. **Vopr Onkol** 1982;28(9):3-7
Telichenas AI, Gritsiute LA, Skarulis RI, et al: Istoriia razvitiia onkologicheskoĭ sluzhby v Litovskoĭ SSR. **Vopr Onkol** 1982;28(11):8-11

### NERVOUS SYSTEM

Aarli JA: History of myasthenia gravis. In Rose FC, Bynum WF, ed: Historical aspects of the neurosciences. New York, Raven, 1982. p. 223-34.
Ballantine HT: 'Sciatica' and the neurosurgeon: historical perspectives and personal reminiscenses. **Clin Neurosurg** 1980;27:541-52
Behrman S: Congestion of the brain. In Rose FC, Bynum WF, ed: Historical aspects of the neurosciences. New York, Raven, 1982. p. 179-84.
Dubowitz V: History of muscle disease. In Rose FC, Bynum WF, ed: Historical aspects of the neurosciences. New York, Raven, 1982. p. 213-22.
Hachinski V: Transient cerebral ischemia: a historical sketch. In Rose FC, Bynum WF, ed: Historical aspects of the neurosciences. New York, Raven, 1982. p. 185-93.
History of writing and its relevance in dyslexia: **J R Soc Med** 1982 Nov;75(11):917-8
Levin HS, Peters BH, Hulkonen DA: Early concepts of anterograde and retrograde amnesia. **Cortex** 1983 Dec;19(4):427-40
Robinson JS: Sciatica and the lumbar disk syndrome: a historic perspective. **South Med J** 1983 Feb;76(2):232-8
Russel G: Writing and dyslexia--an historical analysis. **J Child Psychol Psychiatry** 1982 Oct;23(4):383-400
Shapiro AK, Shapiro E: Tourette syndrome: history and present status. **Adv Neurol** 1982;35:17-23
Trimble MR: Functional diseases. **Br Med J [Clin Res]** 1982 Dec 18-25;285(6357):1768-70

#### Canada

Barbeau A, Sadibelouiz M, Roy M, et al: Origin of Friedreich's disease in Quebec. **Can J Neurol Sci** 1984 Nov;11(4 Suppl):506-9

#### Romania

Petrescu A: Simptoame neuropsihice consemnate în cronici şi vechi însemnări Româneşti. **Rev Med Interna [Neurol Psihiatr]** 1983 Apr-Jun;28(2):149-52

#### United States

Devor EJ, Cordell LS: Neural-tube defects in a prehistoric south-western Indian population. **Ann Hum Biol** 1981 Jan-Feb;8(1):65-75

#### Before 500 A.D.

#### Greco-Roman

Sider D, McVaugh M: Galen On tremor, palpitation, spasm, and rigor; Galeni De tremore, palpitatione, convulsione, et rigore. **Trans Stud Coll Physicians Phila** 1979 Sep;5(1 No 3):183-210

#### Middle East

Russell GF: History of writing and its relevance for the linguistic disorder in dyslexia: discussion paper. **J R Soc Med** 1982 Aug;75(8):631-40

#### 500 A.D.-1450

Kottek SS: 'Mater puerorum'. A medieval naming for an enigmatic children's disease. **Eur J Pediatr** 1981 Sep;137(1):75-9
Medaer R: Does the history of multiple sclerosis go back as far as the 14th century? **Acta Neurol Scand** 1979 Sep;60(3):189-92

#### 1450-1700

#### Great Britain

Alsop JD: The fatal illness of the antiquary William Burton (1609-57). **Notes Queries** 1979 Oct;26(5):424-5

#### Italy

DelChicca S, Tedeschi J: L'insonnia di Galileo in una lettera inedita di Francesco Redi. **Arch Stor Ital** 1979;173(4):615-8

#### Switzerland

Mani N: Biomedical thought in Glisson's hepatology and in Wepfer's work on apoplexy. With commentary by R. G. Frank, p. 84-8. In Stevenson LG, ed: A celebration of medical history. Baltimore, Johns Hopkins

University Press, 1982. (The Henry E. Sigerist supplements to the Bulletin of the History of Medicine; new ser., no. 6). p. 37–63.

### 1700 to Present

Accardo PJ: Freud on diplegia. Commentary and translation. **Am J Dis Child** 1982 May;136(5):452–6
Adour KK, Diamond C: Decompression of the facial nerve in Bell's palsy: a historical review. **Otolaryngol Head Neck Surg** 1982 Jul–Aug;90(4):453–60
Aman MG: Hyperactivity: nature of the syndrome and its natural history. **J Autism Dev Disord** 1984 Mar;14(1):39–56
Bujosa i Homar F: La afasia y su historiografía. **Dynamis** 1981;1:131–63
Bujosa i Homar F: Reconsiderations on the history of aphasia. In International Congress of the History of Medicine, 27th, Barcelona, 1980. Actas. Barcelona, Académia de Ciències Médiques de Catalunya i Balears, 1981. p. 27–38.
Burger G: Nerven- und Geisteskrankheiten als Indikationen für eine bilaterale Oophorektomie im späten 19. Jahrhundert. Diss. Erlangen–Nürnberg, 1984. 185 p.
Foster JB: History of syringomyelia. In Rose FC, Bynum WF, ed: Historical aspects of the neurosciences. New York, Raven, 1982. p. 205–7.
Goetz CG, Klawans HL: Gilles de la Tourette on Tourette syndrome. **Adv Neurol** 1982;35:1–16
Gustavson KH: Mannen bakom syndromet: John Down. Banade väg för den kliniska kromosomforskningen. **Lakartidningen** 1984 May 30;81(22):2261–3
Güttler F: Fölling's sygdom: 50 år og stadig katalysator for nye medicinske opdagelser. **Nord Med** 1984;99(3):78–81
Hécaen H: Storia dell'afasia. **Kos** 1984 Mar;1(2):118–27
Henderson VW: Jules Dejerine and the third alexia. **Arch Neurol** 1984 Apr;41(4):430–2
Kampmeier RH: Establishment of Treponema pallidum as the etiologic agent in general paralysis. **Sex Transm Dis** 1980 Oct–Dec;7(4):197–8
Kampmeier RH: Wagner von Jauregg and the treatment of general paresis by fever. **Sex Transm Dis** 1980 Jul–Sep;7(3):142–4
Keppel Hesselink JM: Some historical aspects of Parkinson's disease. The progression of insights in the period 1817–1868. **Janus** 1983;70(3–4):263–79
Lenský P: Sclerosis multiplex. Nosologická identifikace před 150 lety. **Cas Lek Cesk** 1984 Jul 27;123(30):937–8
McDonald WI: Attitudes to the treatment of multiple sclerosis. **Arch Neurol** 1983 Oct 21;40(11):667–70
Matthews WB: Osler Oration. **J R Soc Med** 1982 May;75(5):307–14
Nicolai JP: Facial paralysis -- 100 years of treatment. **Arch Chir Neerl** 1979;31(3):159–69
Nybäck H: Mannen bakom syndromet: James Parkinson. Beskrev 'shaking palsy' 1817--i dag prövas transplantation som behandling. **Lakartidningen** 1982 Dec 29;79(52):4910
Parkes D: History of narcolepsy. In Rose FC, Bynum WF, ed: Historical aspects of the neurosciences. New York, Raven, 1982. p. 151–63.
Pearn J: The discovery of neuronopathy and neuropathy as a cause of progressive paralysis in childhood. The historical origins of modern differential diagnosis in neuromuscular disease. **J Neurol Sci** 1984 Apr;64(1):99–107
Perkin GD, Handler CE: Wernicke–Korsakoff syndrome. **Br J Hosp Med** 1983 Nov;30(5):331, 333–4
Sèze S de: Histoire de la sciatique. **Rev Neurol (Paris)** 1982;138(12):1019–25
Struck HG, Fuchs C: Zum Frühbild des Morbus Recklinghausen vorwiegend im Augenbereich in Verbindung mit Skelettveränderungen und einer Hypospadia glandis. **Wiss Z Martin Luther Univ (Math)** 1976;25(3):93–9
Sutherland JM: Multiple sclerosis: fifty years on. **Clin Exp Neurol** 1983;19:1–12
Tarsy D: History and definition of tardive dyskinesia. **Clin Neuropharmacol** 1983 Jun;6(2):91–9
Todd J: The history of the syndrome of Capgras. In Rose FC, Bynum WF, ed: Historical aspects of the neurosciences. New York, Raven, 1982. p. 117–25.
Tyler KL: Classics in neurology. Fragments of neurologic history: 'Tetanoid Chorea' and progressive lenticular degeneration. **Neurology** 1983 Apr;33(4):461–2

### Australia

Parkes D, Schachter M: Meige, Brueghel or Blake? **Aust Nurses J** 1981 Feb;10(7):32–5

### Canada

Greenland C, Griffin JD: The Honorable Mary Macdonald: a lesson in attitude. **Can Med Assoc J** 1981 Aug 1;125(3):305–8

### France

Alajouanine T, Signoret JL: Paul Broca et l'aphasie. **Bull Acad Natl Med (Paris)** 1980;164(6):545–51
Bibliographie des travaux de P. Broca consacrés à l'aphasie.: **Rev Neurol (Paris)** 1980;136(10):663–4
Cambier J: Le syndrome de Déjerine–Roussy. **Rev Neurol (Paris)** 1982;138(12):979–88
Escourolle R, Gray F, Hauw JJ: Les atrophies cérébelleuses. **Rev Neurol (Paris)** 1982;138(12):953–65
Lapresle J: La dystasie aréflexique héréditaire de Roussy–Lévy. Ses rapports historiques avec la maladie de Friedreich, l'atrophie Charcot–Marie=Tooth et la névrite hypertrophique de Dejerine–Sottas; l'état actuel de la famille originale; la place nosologique de cette entité. **Rev Neurol (Paris)** 1982;138(12):967–78
Lhermitte F, Signoret JL: L'aphasie de J. M. Charcot à Th. Alajouanine. **Rev Neurol (Paris)** 1982;138(12):893–919
Malinas C, Malinas Y: Emile Zola et la génétique. La nevrose des Rougon–Macquart. **J Genet Hum** 1981 Dec;29(5 Suppl):593–602
Monod–Broca P: Paul Broca (1824–1880). Le chirurgien, l'homme. **Bull Acad Natl Med (Paris)** 1980;164(6):536–44
Passouant P: La narcolepsie au temps de Gélineau. **Hist Sci Med** 1981;15(2):129–36
Passouant P: Le docteur Gélineau (1828–1906). **Hist Sci Med** 1981;15(2):137–43
Rascol A, Clanet M: La sclérose en plaques. De Charcot et Vulpian à nos jours. **Rev Neurol (Paris)** 1982;138(12):921–30
Ryckewaert A, Naveau B: Principaux apports de Charcot et de Pierre Marie à la pathologie ostéo–articulaire. **Rev Rhum Mal Osteoartic** 1984 Jul–Sep;51(7–8):405–13
Schiller F: Paul Broca and the history of aphasia. **Neurosci Behav Physiol** 1983 May;33(5):667
Schott B: Histoire du syndrome de Guillain et Barré. **Rev Neurol (Paris)** 1982;138(12):931–8
Signoret JL: La création de la chaire de Charcot. **Rev Neurol (Paris)** 1982;138(12):887–92
Signoret JL, Castaigne P, Lhermitte F, et al: Rediscovery of Leborgne's brain: anatomical description with CT scan. **Brain Lang** 1984 Jul;22(2):303–19

### Germany

Crump T: Translation of case reports in Ueber die multiplen Fibrome der Haut und ihre Beziehung zu den multiplen Neuromen by F. v. Recklinghausen. **Adv Neurol** 1981;29:259–75
Lieberman AN: Adolph Hitler: his diaries and Parkinson's disease. **N Engl J Med** 1983 Aug 11;309(6):375–6
Perkin GD: Leber's optic atrophy. In Rose FC, Bynum WF, ed: Historical aspects of the neurosciences. New York, Raven, 1982. p. 463–72.

### Great Britain

Carswell H: 'Elephant Man' had more than neurofibromatosis. **JAMA** 1982 Sep 3;248(9):1032–3
Howard–Jones N: Fake! **Br Med J [Clin Res]** 1982 Feb 13;284(6314):511
Karp LE: More on the Elephant Man. **Am J Med Genet** 1982 Nov;13(3):355
Karp LE: The elephant man. **Am J Med Genet** 1981;10(1):1–3
Mann RJ, Key JD: Joseph Bell, M.D., F.R.C.S.: 'notes on a case of paralysis following diphtheria'. **Pharos** 1982 Spring;45(2):27–9
Murray TJ: Doctor Samuel Johnson's abnormal movements. **Adv Neurol** 1982;35:25–30
Myers–Levin A: Cerebral palsy: the early years of occupational therapy in Scotland. Edingburgh, Scottish Council for Spastics, 1978. xv, 131 p.
Pearce JM: The first attempts at removal of brain tumors. In Rose FC, Bynum WF, ed: Historical aspects of the neurosciences. New York, Raven, 1982. p. 239–42.
Perkin GD: Arnold Bennett and medicine: with particular reference to his description of dressing apraxia. **Br Med J [Clin Res]** 1981 Dec 19;283(6307):1666–8
Riley J: The elephant man: 'Treat me as an equal' (John Merrick, Sir Frederick Treves). **Nurs Mirror** 1979 Nov 8;149(19):24–5
Robinson GA: The National Hospitals for Nervous Diseases, 1948–1982. London, The Board of Governors of the National Hospitals for Nervous Diseases, 1982. xvii, 133 p.
Rodin AE, Key JD: Arthur Conan Doyle's thesis on tabes dorsalis. **JAMA** 1982 Feb 5;247(5):646–50
Schmidt V: Hvad fejlede Florence Nightingale? **Sygeplejersken** 1980 Aug 6;80(31):4–10; Oct 5;67(17):16–21
Sturrock RR: William Ford Robertson (1867–1923): his study of neuroglia. **Med Hist** 1975 Oct;19(4):370–5
Sugar O: Doyle on tabes dorsalis. **JAMA** 1982 May 21;247(19):2659–60
Waddington JL: Ventricular enlargement in schizophrenia and the historical studies of John Haslam. **Am J Psychiatry** 1984 Dec;141(12):1640
Waldron G: Sir Frederick Treves and the elephant man. **Lancet** 1980 Jul 5;2(8184):42
Wilkinson M: Elizabeth Garrett Anderson and migraine. In Rose FC, Bynum WF, ed: Historical aspects of the neurosciences. New York, Raven, 1982. p. 165–9.

## DISEASES AND INJURIES

**Hungary**

Benedek I: Semmelweis' Krankheit. Budapest, Akadémiai Kiadó, 1983. 110 p. (Hungarian version published 1978 in Communicationes de historia artis medicinae, Nos. 83–84)

**New Guinea**

Farquhar J, Gajdusek DC, ed: Kuru: Early letters and field notes from the collection of D. Carleton Gajdusek. New York, Raven Press, 1981. xxviii, 338 p.
Gajdusek DC: Journal of further explorations in the Kuru region and in the Kukukuku country, eastern highlands of eastern New Guinea and of a return to West New Guinea, December 25, 1963 to May 4, 1964. Bethesda, National Institutes of Health, 1980. [36 leaves], 235 p.

**Pacific Islands**

Scrimgeour EM: Possible introduction of Huntington's chorea into Pacific Islands by New England whalemen. **Am J Med Genet** 1983 Aug;15(4):607–13

**South Africa**

Hayden MR, Hopkins HC, Macrea M, et al: The origin of Huntington's chorea in the Afrikaner population of South Africa. **S Afr Med J** 1980 Aug 2;58(5):197–200

**Sweden**

Källén B, Löfkvist E: Time trends of spina bifida in Sweden 1947–81. **J Epidemiol Community Health** 1984 Jun;38(2):103–7

**United States**

Brady GM: Lou Gehrig: the iron man. **Manuscripts** 1980;32(2):84–9
Burbick J: Emily Dickinson and the revenge of the nerves. **Womens Stud** 1980;7(1–2):95–109
Dalessio DJ: Trigeminal neuralgia, Cushing. **JAMA** 1983 Jul 22–29;250(4):529–31
Feinstein HM: The use and abuse of illness in the James family circle: a view of neurasthenia as a social phenomenon. **Psychohist Rev** 1979;8(1–2):6–14
Hercher GP: The work cure at Devereux Mansion. **Essex Inst Hist Collect** 1980;116(2):101–10
Karp LE: Adrien Bleyer: in the right place at the wrong time. **Am J Med Genet** 1981;10(3):209–11
Poirier S: The Weir Mitchell rest cure: doctor and patients. **Womens Stud** 1983;10(1):15–40
Roth N: Electrotherapy, 19th-century neurasthenia, and the case of Alice James. **Med Instrum** 1981 Mar–Apr;15(2):116
Simpson JA: Electrophysiology of neuromuscular junction disease: an appreciation of the contributions of Edward H. Lambert. **Muscle Nerve** 1982;5(9S):S6–11
Tang LC: A personal and scientific biography of Dr. George C. Cotzias. **Neurotoxicology (Park Forest Il)** 1984 Spring;5(1):5–12
Wallman LJ: Shunting for hydrocephalus: an oral history. **Neurosurgery** 1982 Aug;11(2):308–13
Warkany J: Laissez-faire in research. **J Am Coll Nutr** 1984;3(2):177–81
Weinstein EA: Woodrow Wilson: a medical and psychological biography. Princeton, Princeton University Press, 1981. xi, 399 p.
Yeazell RB, Maliszewski B, Constantikes A: An exchange of letters between William and Alice James. **Psychohist Rev** 1979;8(1–2):53–9

**USSR**

Arkhangel'skiĭ GV: K istorii izucheniia neĭromaliarii i soliarnogo sindroma. **Zh Nevropatol Psikhiatr** 1982;82(7):128–30
Bochkov NP: Vklad s. n. Davidenkova v razrabotku probelmy nasledstvennykh nervynkh i psikhicheskikh zabolevaniĭ. **Zh Nevropatol Psikhiatr** 1982;82(3):1–4
Lebedev DD, Kovaleva EV, Semenova VN: Nekotorye voprosy revmatizma, ėndokrinnykh i nervnykh zabolevaniĭ u deteĭ v trudakh V.I. Molchanova i ego uchenikov (k 110–letiiu so dnia rozhdeniia). **Pediatriia** 1980 Aug;(8):64–7

### OBESITY

Kryger MH: Sleep apnea. From the needles of Dionysius to continuous positive airway pressure. **Arch Intern Med** 1983 Dec;143(12):2301–3

**1450–1700**

**Switzerland**

Schiller F: A note on the Pickwickian syndrome and Felix Platter (1536–1614). **J Hist Med Allied Sci** 1985 Jan;40(1):66–7

**1700 to Present**

Buchwald H, Rucker RD: The history of metabolic surgery for morbid obesity and a commentary. **World J Surg** 1981 Nov;5(6):781–7
Howard AN: The historical development, efficacy and safety of very-low-calorie diets. **Int J Obes** 1981;5(3):195–208
MacLean LD, Rhode BM: The history of surgery for morbid obesity. **Can J Surg** 1984 Mar;27(2):126–7

**United States**

Massey EW: The heaviest man on record. **NC Med J** 1981 Mar;42(3):181–2

### ORAL

Calatrava Páramo DL: La boca en lo social, la salud, la enfermedad y lo legal. **An R Acad Nac Med (Madr)** 1982;99(1):91–108
Cohen B: An inquiry into the decay of teeth. **Ann R Coll Surg Engl** 1982 Nov;64(6):375–82
Mandel ID: Caries through the ages: a worm's eye view. **J Dent Res** 1983 Aug;62(8):926–9
Schroder FW: Karies – ein Preis der Zivilisation. **Quintessenz J** 1983 Jan;13(1):37–9

**Mexico**

Fastlicht S: Tooth mutilations and dentistry in pre-Columbian Mexico. Berlin, Buch- und Zeitschriften-Verlag 'Die Quintessenz', 1976. 164 p.

**Sweden**

Nihlén B: Folkliga föreställningar om tandvärk och tandvård. **Tandlakartidningen** 1983 Mar 15;75(6):328, 330

**United States**

Costa RL: Periodontal disease in the prehistoric Ipiutak and Tigara skeletal remains from Point Hope, Alaska. **Am J Phys Anthropol** 1982 Sep;59(1):97–110

**Before 500 A.D.**

**China**

Zhang YZ: Dental disease of neolithic age skulls excavated in Shaanxi Province. **Chin Med J [Engl]** 1982 Jun;95(6):391–6

**Egypt**

Harris JE, Ponitz PV: Dental health in ancient Egypt. In A. Cockburn, E. Cockburn, ed: Mummies, disease, and ancient cultures. Cambridge, Cambridge University Press, 1980. p. 45–51.

**Germany**

Jaworski Z: Sito zębodołowe a budowa żuchwy i choroby przyzębia u prasłowian. Część II. **Czas Stomatol** 1983 May;36(5):333–8
Jaworski Z: Sito zębodołowe w szczątkach żuchw prasłowian z popielnicowych grobów ciałopalnych kultury łużyckiej. Część I. **Czas Stomatol** 1983 Apr;36(4):257–64

**500 A.D.–1450**

Nihlén B: Medeltidsfynd avslöjär: 55 av 100 människor led av tandsjukdomar. **Tandlakartidningen** 1982 Dec 15;74(24):1436–8

**1450–1700**

**Germany**

Neuhauser W: Martin Luther bat Freund um Fürbitte bei heftigem Zahnschmerz. **Zahnarztl Mitt** 1983 Nov 1;73(21):2361–3

**1700 to Present**

Bredy E, Baugut G: Der offene Biss – eine historische Betrachtung. **Fortschr Kieferorthop** 1982 Apr;43(2):110–26
Hangorsky C: Juvenile periodontitis/periodontosis: historical overview and update. **Dent Hyg (Chic)** 1982 Jun;56(6):29–32, 34
Luce EA: The ordeal of Sigmund Freud. In Romm S, ed: Symposium on historical perspectives of plastic surgery. Philadelphia, Saunders, 1983. p. 715–6.
Norman JE, Painter DM: Hyperplasia of the mandibular condyle. A historical review of important early cases with a presentation and analysis of twelve patients. **J Maxillofac Surg** 1980 Aug;8(3):161–75
Povey DW: Historical perspectives of mucogingival surgery. **Can Dent Assoc J** 1983 Oct;49(10):721–3

Romm S: The oral cancer of Sigmund Freud. In Romm S, ed: Symposium on historical perspectives of plastic surgery. Philadelphia, Saunders, 1983. p. 709–14.
Saxby MS: Juvenile periodontitis: an historical review. **J Oral Rehabil** 1982 Sep;9(5):451–68
Topelius C: Om tandvärk och löständer. **Tandlakartidningen** 1981 May 15;73(10):565–9
Van Rensburg BG: Odontalgia--'n oorsig van die literatuur 1971–1980. **Tydskr Tandheelkd Ver S Afr** 1981 Dec;36(12):847–51
Vidal F: Vers et carie dentaire chez les dentistes du XVIIIe siècle. **Chir Dent Fr** 1983 Jul 14–21;53(212–213):13–8

**Germany**

Neuhauser W: Goethe sprach nie über die Leiden mit seinen Zähnen. **Zahnarztl Mitt** 1982 Aug 16;72(16):1735–43

**South Africa**

Richardson BD: The historical background of research on diet and dental caries in South Africa. **Tydskr Tandheelkd Ver S Afr** 1982 May;37(5):327–33

### PARASITIC

**Argentina**

Zimmerman MR: Enterobiasis in precolumbian America. **Paleopathol Newsl** 1983 Jun;42:8

**China**

Li Y: [The discovery of paragonimiasis in Fujian Province] (Chi). **Chung Hua I Shih Tsa Chih** 1984 Jan;14(1):19–24

**Before 500 A.D.**

**China**

Yang WY, Wei DX, Song GF, et al: Parasitologische Untersuchung einer alten Leiche aus der Chu-Dynastie der Streitenden Reiche aus dem Mazhuan-Grab Nr. 1, Kreis Jiangling, Provinz Hubei. **Acta Acad Med Wuhan** 1984;4(1):23–7

**1700 to Present**

**Yugoslavia**

Perin J: Depedikulacija u uslovima partizanskog rata. **Lijec Vjesn** 1979 Nov;101(11):716–7

### PELLAGRA

Guggenheim KY: Nutrition and nutritional diseases. The evolution of concepts. Lexington, Massachusetts, Toronto, D.C. Heath and Company, 1981. xii, 378 p.

**Kenya**

Jansen AA, Horelli HT: Pellagra in Kenya. Past and present. **East Afr Med J** 1984 Mar;61(3):220–6

**1700 to Present**

Johnson RB: Pellagra, an historical review. **J Okla State Med Assoc** 1981 Dec;74(12):396–8
Roe DA: Attempts at the eradication of pellagra: a historical review. In Lilienfeld AM, ed: Times, places, and persons. Baltimore, London, Johns Hopkins Univ. Press, 1980. (Sigerist suppl. to the Bull Hist Med, n.s., no 4) p. 62–78.
Roe DA: The insect theory of pellagra. **Fed Proc** 1981 Apr;40(5):1523–6
Sebrell WH: History of pellagra. **Fed Proc** 1981 Apr;40(5):1520–2

**Austria**

Lupo O: Sozialmedizin im alten Osterreich. Die Bekämpfung der Pellagra in der Bukowina zu Beginn dieses Jahrhunderts. **Osterr Osthefte** 1971;13(4):343–8

**Germany**

Kleeberg J: Goethe und die 'mal de rosa'. **Z Gastroenterol** 1983 May;21(5):241–3

**Spain**

Albarracín A: Gaspar Casal y el concepto moderno de especie morbosa. **Asclepio** 1983;35:189–95

**United States**

Bean WB: Personal reflections on clinical investigations. **Annu Rev Nutr** 1982;2:1–20
Carmichael EB: The pellagra story in the U.S. **J Med Assoc State Ala** 1980 Jan;49(7):11–7
Carmichael EB: The pellagra story in the United States of America. **J Med Assoc State Ala** 1980 Mar;49(9):23, 31, 33
Guggenheim YK: [Joseph Goldberger's contributions to pellagra research] (Heb). **Harefuah** 1980;99(5–6):134–6
Kiple KF, Kiple VH: Black tongue and black men: pellagra and slavery in the Antebellum South. **J South Hist** 1977 Aug;43(3):411–28
Sandifer SH: Pellagra in South Carolina. **J SC Med Assoc** 1981 Dec;77(12):602–4
Schoenberg BS: Plague of pellagra. **South Med J** 1983 Mar;76(3):281–3
Shepherd M: La découverte de la nature de la pellagre. Leçons d'une recherche épidémiologique et psychiatrique remarquable. **Acta Psychiatr Belg** 1983 May–Jun;83(3):295–303

### PLAGUE

Appleby AB: The disappearance of plague: a continuing puzzle. **Econ Hist Rev** 1980;33(2):161–73
Azouvi F: La peste, la mélancolie et le diable, ou l'imaginaire réglé. **Diogenes** 1979 Oct–Dec
Butler T: Plague and other Yersinia infections. New York, London, Plenum Medical Book Co., 1983. xii, 220 p. (Current Topics in Infectious Disease).
Caffaratto TM: La più grande nemica del genere umano: la peste. **Minerva Ginecol** 1980 Oct;32(10):945–7
Horstmanhoff HF, ed: [Ancient and medieval pestilences]. Includes contributions by R. A. Tybout, M. van Raalte, S. van der Lee, C. G. van Leijenhorst, E. J. Bakker, E. J. Schoten. **Hermeneus Tijdschr Antieke Cult** 1979;51(2):58–157
Horstmanhoff HF, et al: The plague and other pestilences in antiquity and the Middle Ages. Contributions by R. A. Tybout, M. van Raalte, S. van der Lee, C. G. van Leijenhorst, E. J. Bakker, E. J. Schoten. **Hermeneus Tijdschr Antieke Cult** 1979;51(2):58–117, 140–157
Kollmeier K: Leben und Sterben in Pestzeiten. **Med Welt** 1983 Feb 11;34(6):186–91
Ladurie EL: Un concept: l'unification microbienne du monde (XIVe–XVIIe siècles). **Schweiz Z Gesch** 1973;23(4):627–94
Pastore A: Peste e società. **Studi Stor** 1979;4:857–73
Steel D: Plague writing: from Boccaccio to Camus. **J Eur Stud** 1981;11(2):88–110

**Asia**

Dols MW: The second plague pandemic and its recurrences in the Middle East: 1347–1894. **J Econ Soc Hist Orient (Netherl)** 1979;22(2):162–89

**Belgium**

Jacquet-Ladrier F: L'hôpital Saint-Roch et la lutte contre la peste à Namur, aux XVIIe et XVIIIe siècles. **Ann Soc Belg Hist Hop** 1980;18:59–70

**Egypt**

Shoshan B: Notes sur les épidemies de peste en Egypte. **Ann Demogr Hist (Paris)** 1981;:387–404

**Europe**

Flinn MW: Plague in Europe and the Mediterranean countries. **J Eur Econ Hist** 1979;8(1):131–48
Palmer R: The Church, leprosy and plague in medieval and early modern Europe. In Sheils WJ, ed: The Church and healing. Papers read at the twentieth summer meeting and the twenty-first winter meeting of the Ecclesiastical History Society. Oxford, Basil Blackwell for the Society, 1982. p. 79–99.
Slack P: The disappearance of plague: an alternative view. **Econ Hist Rev** 1981;34(3):469–76

**France**

Angers D: La vicomté de Bayeux au bas Moyen-Age: esquisse d'histoire démographique. **Francia** 1979;7:141–72
Biraben JN: Les hommes et la peste en France et dans les pays européens et méditeranéens. Tome II. Les hommes face à la peste. Paris, Mouton, 1976. 416 p.
Canard J: Les pestes en Beaujolais, Forez, Jarez, Lyonnais; du XIVème au XVIIIème siècle. [France: s.n.], 1979. (Règny, Imprimerie de l'Abbaye de Pradines). 121, A–I p.
Mouton P: La mort est venue de la mer. Paris, Pen Duick, 1982. 184 p.

# DISEASES AND INJURIES

**Germany**

Guest C: The Pied Piper of Hamelin. **Lancet** 1984 Dec 22;2(8417–18):1454–5

**Great Britain**

Bayliss JH: The extinction of bubonic plague in Britain. **Endeavour** 1980;4(2):58–66
Bradford DE: Viral haemorrhagic fevers. **J R Army Med Corps** 1983 Jun;129(2):120–1
Roberts A: A history of the plague in England. **Nurs Times** 1979;75:777–9
Roberts A: The plague in England. **Hist Today** 1980 Apr 30;:29–34
Shewsbury JD: A history of bubonic plague in the British Isles. Cambridge, University Press, 1970. xi, 661 p.
Swales RJ: Plague, population and ecology in early modern England. **Can J Hist** 1979;14(2):257–66

**Hungary**

Fazekas A: Szabolcsi adatok a pestisjárványok történetéhez. **Orvostort Kozl** 1979;86(24 no 4):91–106

**Italy**

Petraccone C: La difesa contro la peste: prevenzione e controllo dell'epidemia nelle pestilenze di Terra di Bari (1690–1692) e Noja (1815–1816). **Arch Stor Prov Napol** 1977;95:253–80

**Spain**

Ballesteros Rodríguez J: La peste en Córdoba. Córdoba, Excma. Diputación Provincial de Córdoba, Servicio de Publicaciones, 1982. 238 p.
Zubiri Vidal F, Zubiri de Salinas R: Las epidemias de peste y cólera morbo-asiático en Aragón (Zaragoza, 1652 y 1885; Caspe, 1834; Alcañiz y Jaca, 1885). Zaragoza, Diputacion Provincial, Institucion 'Fernando el Catolico', [1980]. 195 p. (Temas Aragoneses, 32).

**Switzerland**

Bucher S: Die Pest in der Ostschweiz. St. Gallen [Switzerland], Historischer Verein des Kantons St. Gallen, 1979. 90 p.

**USSR**

Zguta R: The one-day votive church: a religious response to the black death in early Russia. **Slavic Rev** 1981;40(3):423–32

**Before 500 A.D.**

Stettler A: Lepra und Pest in der Antike. **Antike Welt** 1977;8(4):42–4

**Asia**

Archi A: La peste presso gli Ittiti. **Parola Passato** 1978;179:81–9

**Greco-Roman**

Thüry G: Zur Infektkette der Pest in hellenistisch-römischer Zeit. In: 75 Jahre Anthropologische Staatssammlung München. Munich: Anthropologische Staatssammlung, 1977. p. 275–83.

**Greece**

Lichtenthaeler C: Outé gar iatori èrkoun to proton therapeuontes agnoia. **Hermes** 1979, 1978;107(3):270–86
Longrigg J: The great plague of Athens. **Hist Sci** 1980 Sep;18(41 pt 3):209–25
Longrigg J: Thucydides and the great plague of Athens. In International Congress of the History of Medicine, 27th, Barcelona, 1980. Actas. Barcelona, Académia de Ciències Mèdiques de Catalunya i Balears, 1981. p. 281–8.
Poole JC, Holladay AJ: Thucydides and the plague: a footnote. **Classical Q** 1982;32:235–6
Poole JC, Holladay AJ: Thucydides and the plague of Athens. **Classical Q** 1979;29:282–300
Radt SL: Zu Thukydides' Pestbeschreibung. **Mnemosyne** 1978;31:233–45; 1979;32:163
Thucydides: The plague in Athens. Thucydides. The history of the Peloponnesian War. Translated by Thomas Hobbes. **NC Med J** 1980 Apr;41(4):230–2
Thucydides and the Athenian plague: a reconsideration of the evidence: **Pharm Hist (London)** 1984 Dec;14(4):6–7
Wylie JA, Stubbs HW: The plague of Athens, 430–428 B.C.: epidemic and epizoötic. **Classical Q** 1983;33:6–11

**500 A.D.–1450**

Brossollet J: Quelques aspects religieux de la grande peste du XIVe siècle. **Rev Hist Philos Relig** 1984 Jan–Mar;64(1):53–66
Bulst N: Der Schwarze Tod. Demographische, wirtschafts- und kulturgeschichtliche Aspekte der Pestkatastrophe von 1347–1352. Bilanz der neueren Forschung. **Saeculum (Freiburg)** 1979;30(1):45–67
Carmichael AG: Plague legislation in the Italian Renaissance. **Bull Hist Med** 1983 Winter;57(4):508–25
Ell SR: Interhuman transmission of medieval plague. **Bull Hist Med** 1980 Winter;54(4):497–510
Ell SR: Some evidence for interhuman transmission of medieval plague. **Rev Infect Dis** 1979 May–Jun;1(3):563–6
Griffiths RA: The interaction of war and plague in the later middle ages. In J. Cule, ed: Wales and medicine. London, British Society for the History of Medicine, 1975. p. 127–40.
Rutkowska-Płachcińslak A: Dźuma w Europie Zachodniej w XIV w. straty demograficzne i stutki psychiczne. **Przegl Hist** 1978;69(1):75–102

**Belgium**

Marechal G: De zwarte dood te Brugge (1349–1351). **Biekorf** 1980;80:377–392

**Byzantium**

Bratton TL: The identity of the plague of Justinian [part II]. **Trans Stud Coll Physicians Phila** 1981 Sep;5(3 no 3):174–80

**Europe**

Gottfried RS: The black death. Natural and human disaster in Medieval Europe. New York, London, Free Press, 1983. xvii, 203 p.
Werthmann-Haas G: Altdeutsche Ubersetzungen des Prager 'Sendbriefs' ('Missum imperatori') (= Untersuchungen zur mittelalterlichen Pestliteratur, I). Pattensen (Han.), Wellm, 1983. 317 p. (Würzburger medizinhistorische Forschungen, Bd. 27).

**Germany**

Bergmann H: Neufunde zum Pesttraktat Jakob Engelins von Ulm. **Sudhoffs Arch** 1978;62(3):282–93
Dirckx JH: The pied piper of Hamelin. A medical-historical interpretation. **Am J Dermatopathol** 1980 Spring;2(1):39–45
Hils HP: Konrad der Münzmeister oder Konrad der Apotheker? Zur Analyse eines spätmittelalterlichen Pesttraktates. **Sudhoffs Arch** 1984;68(1):105–9
Hühns E: Der Berliner Totentanz. **Dtsch Jahrb Volkskd** 1968;14(2):235–46

**Great Britain**

Cule J: Pestis flava: y fad felen. In J. Cule, ed: Wales and medicine. London, British Society for the History of Medicine, 1975. p. 141–55.
Poos LR: Plague mortality and demographic depression in later medieval England. **Yale J Biol Med** 1981 May–Jun;54(3):227–34
Rackham J: Rattus rattus: the introduction of the black rat into Britain. **Antiquity** 1979;53:112–20
Sloan AW: The Black Death in England. **S Afr Med J** 1981 Apr 25;59(18):646–50

**Spain**

Contreras Mas A: Legislacion frente a la peste en Mallorca bajomedieval 'Ordinations; capitols del morbo de la ciutat e regna de Mallorques'. **Asclepio** 1978–79;30–31:167–76
Gyug R: The effects and extent of the Black Death of 1348: new evidence for clerical mortality in Barcelona. **Mediaev Stud** 1983;45:385–98
Ober WB, Aloush N: The plague at Granada, 1348–1349: Ibn Al-Khatib and ideas of contagion. **Bull NY Acad Med** 1982 May;58(4):418–24

**USSR**

Langer LN: Plague and the Russian countryside: monastic estates in the late fourteenth and fifteenth centuries. **Can Am Slav Stud** 1976;10:351–68

**1450–1700**

Burri R: Die Delfter Pest von 1557 nach den Beobachtungen von Petrus Forestus. Zürich, Juris Druck, 1982. III, 219 p. (Zürcher Medizingeschichtliche Abhandlungen, Neue Reihe Nr. 151).
Hils HP: Die Pestrezepte der Basler Handschrift D II 30. **Sudhoffs Arch** 1983;67(2):210–7

**Austria**

Olbort F: Die Pestepidemie von 1653–1657 in Niederösterreich. **Unsere Heimat** 1974;45(1):11–23

Olbort F: Pestebild und Pestbekämpfung im Niederösterreich des 17. Jahrhunderts. **Unsere Heimat** 1977;48(1):13–29
Olbort F: 'Vergessene' Pestjahre. Die Seuche von 1653 bis 1656 in Wien. **Wien Geschichtsbl** 1973;28(1):10–14
Schretter B: Die Pest in Tirol 1611–1612: ein Beitrag zur Medizin–, Kultur– und Wirtschaftsgeschichte der Stadt Innsbruck und der übrigen Gerichte Tirols. Innsbruck, Stadtmagistrat Innsbruck, 1982. 628 p. (Veröffentlichungen des Innsbrucker Stadtarchivs, Neue Folge, Band 12/13)
Spreitzer H: Pestjahre in Mistelbach. **Unsere Heimat** 1970;41(3):132–6

**Belgium**

Bauwens P: La peste à Huy au XVIIe siècle. Fédération des Cercles d'Archéologie et d'Histoire de Belgique. 44e session. Congrès de Huy, 1976. Annales. Tielt, 1978. p. 235–9.
Helin E: A la recherche d'une mesure de la léthalité des épidémies: les désignations de tuteurs pour les orphelins servent–elles d'indicateur? **Ann Demogr Hist (Paris)** 1980;:67–78
Jacquet–Ladrier F: Les épidémies de peste à Namur aux XVIe et XVIIe siècles. Congrès de Comines, 1, 1980. Actes. p. 326–7.
Meeus M: La peste à Tessenderlo au XVIIe siècle. Congrès de Comines, 1, 1980. Actes. p. 329–30.

**Czechoslovakia**

Cáňová E: Mor v čechách v roce 1680. **Sb Arch Pr** 1981;31(2):265–339

**Europe**

Roque MC: As pestes medievais europeias e o 'regimento proucytoso contra ha pestencça': Lisboa, Valentim Fernandes, 1495–1496: tentativa de interpretação à luz dos conhecimentos pestológicos actuais. Paris, Fundação Calouste Gulbenkian, Centro Cultural Português, 1979.
Waldis V: Der 'Stich' von 1564 – eine primäre Lungenpest. **Gesnerus** 1983;40(1–2):223–8

**France**

Dubois E: How to face the plague: some seventeenth–century practices. **Newsl Soc 17th Century Fr Stud** 1980;2:29–36
Kerherve J: La peste à Moncontour en 1500. **Ann Bretagne** 1983;90(4):603–6
Marain Y, Ducourtioux JC: Un 'règlement de police pour la maladie contagieuse' à Saint–Dizier en 1668. **Cah Haut Marnais** 1979;139:162–8
Simonin M: Michel de Nostredame, Pierre Boaistuau, Chavigny et la peste aixoise de 1546. **Bibl Hum Renaissance** 1983;45(1):127–30

**Germany**

Graeser F, Keil G: Die Pestrezepte des Fuldaer Kodex Aa 129. **Z Dtsch Altert Dtsch Lit** 1980;109(1):72–85
Knorre G von, Paasch S: Die Pest in Mitteldeutschland im 17. Jahrhundert. **Z Gesamte Inn Med** 1981 Aug 1;36(15):528–33

**Great Britain**

Barker R: The local study of plague. **Local Hist** 1981;14(6):332–40
Cone TE: Daniel Defoe on the deplorable effect of the great London plague of 1665 on women with child. **Pediatrics** 1981;67:221
Doolittle IG: The effects of the Plague on a provincial town in the sixteenth and seventeenth centuries. **Med Hist** 1975 Oct;19(4):333–41
Finlay R: Population and metropolis. The demography of London, 1580–1650. Cambridge, New York, Cambridge University Press, 1981. xii, 188 p.
Herlan RW: Aspects of population history in the London parish of St. Olave, Old Jewry, 1645–1667. **Guildhall Stud Lond Hist** 1980;4(3):133–40
Skinner J: Plague mortality in Buckinghamshire in the seventeenth century. **Rec Bucks** 1979;20(3):
Wrigley EA: Marital fertility in seventeenth century Colyton. **Econ Hist Rev** 1978;31(3):429–36

**Hungary**

Bugyi B: Bausner Bertalan (1629–1682). **Orv Hetil** 1984 Jul 22;125(30):1831–2
Prickler H: Die Pestepidemie des Jahres 1600. **Burgenl Heimatbl** 1971;33(3):109–16

**Italy**

Calvi G: L'oro, il fuoco, le forche: la peste napoletana del 1656. **Arch Stor Ital** 1981;139(3):405–58
Cipolla C: Peste del 1630––31 nell' Empolese. **Arch Stor Ital** 1978;136:469–81
Cipolla CM: A plague doctor. In Miskimin HA, et al, ed.: the medieval city. New Haven. Yale Univ. Press, 1977. p. 65–72
Cipolla CM: Cristofano e la peste. Bologna, Il Mulino, 1976. 157 p.
Cipolla CM: Faith, reason and the plague in seventeenth–century Tuscany. Ithaca, Cornell University Press, 1979. 113 p.
Cipolla CM: Fighting the plague in seventeenth–century Italy. Madison, University of Wisconsin Press, 1981, xi, 123 p. (Merle Curti Lectures, 1978).
Cipolla CM: Peste del 1630–31 nel'Empolese. **Arch Stor Ital** 1978;136(3–4):469–82
Corsini CA, Delille G: La peste de 1656 dans le diocese de Salerne quelques resultats et problemes. In Charbonneau H, Larose A, ed: The great mortalities: methodological studies of demographic crises in the past. Liège, Belgium, Ordina Editions, 1980. p. 51–60.
Lombardi D: 1629–1631: crisi e peste a Firenze. **Arch Stor Ital** 1979;137(1):3–50
Preto P: Peste e società a Venezia nel 1576. Vicenza, Neri Pozza Editore, 1978. 230 p.
Schupbach WM: A Venetian 'Plague Miracle' in 1464 and 1576. **Med Hist** 1976 Jul;20(3):312–6

**Netherlands**

Alter G: Plague and the Amsterdam annuitant: a new look at life annuities as a source for historical demography. **Popul Stud** 1983 Mar;37(1):23–41

**Portugal**

David–Peyre Y: Manuel Alvares, ou la synthèse de la littérature médicale sur la préservation contre la peste. **Bull Etud Port Bres** 1965;26:67–87

**Spain**

Balaguer Perigüell E, Ballester Añón R: Repercusiones de la epidemia de peste de Zaragoza de 1652. In: Sociedad Española de Historia de la Medicina. V Congreso Nacional. Madrid, 1977. **Asclepio** 1977;29:67–72
Carreras Panchón A: Las epidemias de peste en la España del Renacimiento. In: Sociedad Española de Historia de la Medicina. V Congreso Nacional. Madrid, 1977. **Asclepio** 1977;29:5–15
Castellanos J, Reguero MA: La peste en la Malaga del siglo XVII (1637): approximacion a su historia social. In: Sociedad Española de Historia de la Medicina. V Congreso Nacional. Madrid, 1977. **Asclepio** 1977;29:101–18
Granjel LS: Las epidemias de peste en la España del siglo XVII. In: Sociedad Española de Historia de la Medicina. V Congreso Nacional. Madrid, 1977. **Asclepio** 1977;29:17–36
Maza Zorilla E: [Population and plague of Vallalón 16–17 centuries.] (Spa) **Cuad Invest Hist** 1978;2
Maza Zorrilla E: Villalón de Campos y la peste de 1599. Estudio demografico. **Cuad Invest Hist** 1978;2:363–86
Nadal J: L'última pandèmia de pesta a Catalunya, 1650–1654. In Congrés International d'Història de la Medicina Catalana, 2nd, Barcelona, 1975. Llibre d'Actes. Barcelona, Socitra, 1977. p. 19–38.
Palma Rodriguez F: Vida y obra de Viana Mentesano. Salamanca, Universidad de Salamanca, 1977. 54 p. (Cuadernos de Historia de la Medicina Española, Monografias, XXXI).
Peset JL, Arquiola E, Peset M, et al: Los medicos y la peste de Valencia de 1647–1648. In: Sociedad Española de Historia de la Medicina. V Congreso Nacional. Madrid, 1977. **Asclepio** 1977;29:217–41
Peset M, La Parra S, Mancebo MF, et al: Gobierno y poder politico en la peste de Valencia de 1647–1648. In: Sociedad Española de Historia de la Medicina. V Congreso Nacional. Madrid, 1977. **Asclepio** 1977;29:243–63
Peset M, La Parra S, Mancebo MF, et al: Los bandoleros y la peste de Valencia de mediados del siglo XVII. In: Sociedad Española de Historia de la Medicina. V Congreso Nacional. Madrid, 1977. **Asclepio** 1977;29:265–82
Riera J, Jiménez Muñoz JM: El doctor Rossell y los temores en España por la peste de Milan (1629–1631). In: Sociedad Española de Historia de la Medicina. V Congreso Nacional. Madrid, 1977. **Asclepio** 1977;29:283–307
Riera J: El libro de la peste (1600) del doctor Antonio Ponce de Santa Cruz. In: Sociedad Española de Historia de la Medicina. V Congreso Nacional. Madrid, 1977. **Asclepio** 1977;29:319–29

**Switzerland**

Bucher S: Die Pest in der Ostschweiz. In: Historischer Verein des Kantons St. Gallen, 119. Neujahrsblatt. St. Gallen, Stehle, 1979. p. 7–58.
Eckert EA: Seasonality of plague in early modern Europe: Swiss epidemic of 1628–1630. **Rev Infect Dis** 1980 Nov–Dec;2(6):952–9
Eckert EA: Spatial and temporal distribution of plague in a region of Switzerland in the years 1628 and 1629. **Bull Hist Med** 1982 Summer;56(2):175–94
Mattmüller M: Die Pest in Liestal. Notizen zu den demographischen Implikationen der frühneuzeitlichen Epidemien. **Gesnerus** 1983;40(1–2):119–28
Perrenoud A: Les mécanismes de récupération d'une population frappée par la peste: L'épidémie de 1636–1640 à Genève. **Schweiz Z Gesch**

1978;28(3):265–88
Waldis V: Hospitalisation und Absonderung in Pestzeiten--die Schweiz im Vergleich zu Oberitalien. **Gesnerus** 1982;39(1):71–8
Waldis V: Obrigkeitliche Massnahmen gegen die Pest in Stadt und Herrschaft Rheinfelden im 16. und 17. Jahrhundert. **Gesnerus** 1979;36(3–4):206–27
Zurfluh A: A propos de la peste dans les Alpes: le canton d'Uri en 1629. **Ann Demogr Hist (Paris)** 1983;:353–68

**Yugoslavia**

Glesinger L: Der Ursprung der Pestepidemien und deren Vorbeugungsmethoden im Alten Dubrovnik. In Radovi sa Medunarodnog simpozija u povodu sestote obljetnice Dubrovacke karantene. Dubrovnik, 29 i 30. rujna 1977. Zagreb, 1980. p. 93–102.
Supuk A: Sibenski onomastikon nakon kuge od 1649 godine. **Arh Vjesn** 1978–79;21–22:123–79

**1700 to Present**

Coulanges P: Cinquantenaire du vaccin antipesteux EV (Girard et Robic). **Bull Soc Pathol Exot Filiales** 1983 Mar–Apr;76(2):114–20
Coulanges P: Cinquantenaire du vaccin antipesteux EV (Girard et Robic). **Arch Inst Pasteur Madagascar** 1982;50(1):169–84
Egeblad K: Militaerkirurgen Dominique Jean Larrey: Om pesten i felttoget til Aegypten og Syrien 1798–1801. **Dan Medicinhist Arbog** 1979;132–59
Lutzker E: From Malkowal to Calcutta: an historical appreciation of Haffkine's victorious struggle. In: Science and history: studies in honor of Edward Rosen. (Studia Copernicana, XVI.) Wrocław, Ossolineum, 1978. p. 543–53.

**Asia**

Pryor EG: The great plague of Hong Kong. **J Hong Kong Branch R Asiat Soc** 1975;15:61–70

**Europe**

Marcadé J: La 'peste' de Lisbonne en 1757 et ses conséquences dans le bas Poitou. **Bull Soc Antiq Quest Mus Poitiers** 1977;14:201–8

**France**

Billioud J: Les Saints de la Peste. Une grande page de solidarité. **Marseille** 1983;(132–133):56–63
Blasco A: Berre et la peste de 1720. Berre-L'Etang, Association sciences et culture, 1983. 114 p.
Figarella J: La Provence et la peste de 1720. **Marseille** 1978;112:13–23
Gueniot-Le Minor G: La peste des chiffonniers à Paris en 1920. Diss. Paris, 1980. 83 lv.
Héritier J: La peste des chiffonniers. **Histoire** 1982;51:97–9
Hildesheimer F: Prévention de la peste et attitudes mentales en France au XVIIIe siècle. **Rev Hist (Paris)** 1981;265(1):65–79
Montiel L: La enfermedad como símbolo: la peste en la obra de Albert Camus. **Asclepio** 1983;35:171–6

**Greece**

Slatter EM: Illustrations from the Wellcome Institute Library: the new lazaretto at Siros (Syra), Greece, in 1840. **Med Hist** 1984 Jan;28(1):73–80

**Hungary**

Bolyki J: Komáromi Csipkés György: Pestis pestise (1664). **Orvostort Kozl** 1979;86(24 no 4):81–9
Ila B: Contribution à l'histoire de la peste en Hongrie au XVIIIe siècle. In Charbonneau H, Larose A, ed: The great mortalities: methodological studies of demographic crises in the past. Liège, Belgium, Ordina Editions, 1980. p. 133–8.
Nagy L: Az 1713, évi pécsi pestisjárvány. **Orv Hetil** 1981 Oct 4;122(40):2488–90

**India**

Lutzker E: Cameron prizewinner: Waldemar M. Haffkine, C.I.E. **Clio Med** 1971 May;13(3–4):269–76
Lutzker E: Some unanswered questions in medical history. In: Congrès international d'histoire de la médecine, XXVe, Québec, 1976. Actes. Québec, 1977. p. 917–27.

**Malagasy Republic**

Esoavelomandroso F: Résistance à la médecine en situation coloniale: la peste à Madagascar. **Ann Econ Soc Civilis** 1981;36(2):168–90

**Netherlands**

Schneeloch NH: 'Praecautien tegens de pest'. Pestgefahr in den Vereinigten Niederlanden 1720–1722. **Econ Soc Hist Jaarb** 1977;40:26–47

**Romania**

Sibechi G: Un doctor ieşean de prestigiu: Evstatie Rola. **Rev Med Chir Soc Med Nat Iasi** 1982 Jul–Sep;86(3):436, 440, 504

**South Africa**

Heyningen EB van: The mysteries of the scarlet phial: spies and plague in Cape Town in 1907. **Q Bull S Afr Libr** 1979;34(2):53–8
Mitchell FK: The plague in Cape Town in 1901 and its subsequent establishment as an endemic disease in South Africa. **S Afr Med J** 1983 Jun 29;Spec No:17–9

**Switzerland**

Bonifas V: Alexandre Yersin (1863–1943). **Rev Med Suisse Romande** 1984 May;104(5):349–51

**Syria**

Roberts KB: Plague in 18th century Syria: the work of Alexander and Patrick Russell. In: Congrès international d'histoire de la médecine, XXVe, Québec, 1976. Actes. Québec, 1977. p. 1157.

**United States**

Tomich PQ, Barnes AM, Devick WS, et al: Evidence for the extinction of plague in Hawaii. **Am J Epidemiol** 1984 Feb;119(2):261–73

**USSR**

Alexander JT: Bubonic plague in early modern Russia; public health & urban disaster. Baltimore and London, Johns Hopkins University Press, 1980. xviii, 385 p.
Alexander JT: Ivan Vien and the first comprehensive plague tractate in Russian. **Med Hist** 1980;24(4):419–31
Borodiĭ NK: Karantinnaia sluzhba i protivoépidemicheskie meropriiatiia na Ukraine v XVIII veke. **Zh Mikrobiol Epidemiol Immunobiol** 1980 May;(5):117–20
Gol'd EIu, Ladnyĭ ID: S. V. Suvorov i ego rol' v istorii sovetskoĭ protivochumnoĭ organizatsii. **Zh Mikrobiol Epidemiol Immunobiol** 1979 Nov;(11):106–9
Kahan A: Social aspects of the plague epidemics in eighteenth-century Russia. **Econ Dev Cult Change** 1979;27(2):255–66
Mertens C. de: An account of the plague which raged at Moscow, 1771. Facsimile of London, 1799, edition, with introduction and bibliography by J. Alexander. Newtonville, Mass., Oriental Research Partners, 1977. 39, 6, v, 122 p.
Palkin BN: Nastavlenie doktora K. O. Iagel'skogo po profilaktike i lecheniiu chumy. **Zh Mikrobiol Epidemiol Immunobiol** 1982 Jan;(1):117–8
Veispak T: Rakvere elanikkonna suurus ja sotsiaalnestruktuur 17. sajandi lõpust 1780. Aastateni. **Eesti NSV Tead Akad Toim** 1981;30(2):169–78
Wagner D: Zu August Hirschs epidemiologischer Reise an die Wolga im Jahre 1879 (ein Beispiel russisch-deutscher Zusammenarbeit auf medizinischem Gebiet. **Z Gesamte Hyg** 1980;26(5):377–8

**Yugoslavia**

Pecinjački S: Podaci o kugi 1738. Godine u Bečkereku, Deski i Djali. **Naucni Sastanak Zb Rad Naucno Drus Istor Zdrav Kult Jugosl** 1975;(11):111–17
Pejčić M: Hadži Nešina buna, i kuga u Pirotu 1836–1837. godine. **Srp Arh Celok Lek** 1981 Sep;109(9):1223–31

## PNEUMOCONIOSIS

Posner E: Milestones in the history of mineral dust pneumoconioses. In J. Cule, ed: Wales and medicine. London, British Society for the History of Medicine, 1975. p. 42–53.
Rüttner JR: Staublungenforschung in der Schweiz einst und jetzt. **Schweiz Med Wochenschr [Suppl]** 1983;15:51–61
van Oye E: Enkele mijlpalen in de geschiedenis van de pneumoconiosen. **Arch Belg** 1984;42(5–6):289–93

**Great Britain**

Batty Shaw A: Knappers' rot; silicosis in East Anglian flint-knappers. **Med Hist** 1981 Apr;25(2):151–68

**1700 to Present**

Kerr LE: Black lung. **J Public Health Policy** 1980 Mar;1(1):50–63

**Great Britain**

Greenberg M: Classical syndromes in occupational medicine: the Montague Murray case. **Am J Ind Med** 1982;3(3):351-6

**United States**

Aldrich M: Mortality from byssinosis among New England cotton mill workers. 1905-1912. **J Occup Med** 1982 Dec;24(12):977-80
Banks DE, Barkman HW: Silicosis epidemic reported in 1900. **JAMA** 1984 Jan 13;251(2):217
Banks A, ed: Monumental stone. Barre, Vermont, 1939 and 1940. In her: First-person America. New York, Knopf, 1980. p. 93-119.
Corn JK: Byssinosis--an historical perspective. **Am J Ind Med** 1981;2(4):331-52
Eisenbud M: Origins of the standards for control of beryllium disease (1947-1949). **Environ Res** 1982 Feb;27(1):79-88
Garfinkel L: Asbestos: historical perspective. **CA** 1984 Jan-Feb;34(1):44-7
Kalin J: Flintknapping and silicosis. **Flintknappers Exch** 1981;4(2):2-9
Pappagianis D: Dangerous dust. **Nat Hist** 1983;92(3):36-40
Smith BE: Black lung: the social production of disease. **Int J Health Serv** 1981;11(3):343-59
Stoeckle JD, Oliver LC, Hardy HL: Women with asbestosis in a medical clinic: under reported women workers, delayed diagnosis and smoking. **Women Health** 1982 Spring;7(1):31-6
Yandle B: A social regulation controversy: the cotton dust standard. **Soc Sci Q** 1982;63(1):58-69

### PNEUMONIA

Gsell O: Geschichte der Pneumonie. **Sudhoffs Arch** 1984;68(2):182-216

**500 A.D.-1450**

**Poland**

Dudziński W: Choroby i zgon króla Władysława Jagiełły. **Wiad Lek** 1981 May 15;34(10):859-61

**1700 to Present**

Austrian R: Pneumococcus: the first one hundred years. **Rev Infect Dis** 1981 Mar-Apr;3(2):183-9
Austrian R: Pneumonia in the later years. **J Am Geriatr Soc** 1981 Nov;29(11):481-9
Berk SL: Bacterial pneumonia in the elderly: the observations of Sir William Osler in retrospect. **J Am Geriatr Soc** 1984 Sep;32(9):683-5
Gsell O: Die Geschichte der Pneumonien--Wandel vom 19. zum 21. Jahrhundert. **Prax Klin Pneumol** 1984 Sep;38(9):379-88
Gsell O: Geschichte und Bedeutung der Pneumonie im hohen Alter. **Z Gerontol** 1982 Nov-Dec;15(6):325-31
Steege MM: Creating the pneumococcal pneumonia vaccine: a hundred-year story. **Conn Med** 1979 Nov;43(11):717-20
Stevens KM: The pathophysiology of influenzal pneumonia in 1918. **Perspect Biol Med** 1981 Autumn;25(1):115-25
Zhdanova LG: K 100-letiiu otkrytiia pnevmokokka. **Zh Mikrobiol Epidemiol Immunobiol** 1981 Dec;(12):3-9

**Africa**

McMartin DA, MacOwan KJ, Swift LL: A century of classical contagious caprine pleuropneumonia: from original description to aetiology. **Br Vet J** 1980 Sep-Oct;136(5):507-15

**France**

Peter JP: Reparar el desorden del mundo: la medicina ilustrada ante la enfermedad epidemica (Bas-Poitou, 1784-1785). **Asclepio** 1983;35:3-26

**Germany**

Hein J: Ludolph Brauer--Der Wegbereiter der modernen Pneumologie. **Prax Klin Pneumol** 1984 Oct;38(10):471-3
Szállási A: 100 éve ismert a Pneumococcus pathogén természete. **Orv Hetil** 1984 Dec 9;125(50):3059-62

**Great Britain**

Stout G: The 1888 pneumonia in Middlesbrough. **J R Soc Med** 1980 Sep;73(9):664-8

**United States**

Denny FW: Atypical pneumonia and the Armed Forces Epidemiological Board. **J Infect Dis** 1981 Mar;143(3):305-16
Levin S: Landmark perspective: the atypical pneumonia syndrome. **JAMA** 1984 Feb 17;251(7):945-8
Small WE: Pneumococcal pneumonia vaccine--strange success story. **Am Pharm** 1979 Dec;19(13):39

### POISONING

Burchell HB: Digitalis poisoning: historical and forensic aspects. **J Am Coll Cardiol** 1983 Feb;1(2 Pt 1):506-16
Castro M de: Johannes Aegidii Zamorensis, OFM, contra venena et animalia venenosa. Introducción edición y notas. **Arch Iberoam** 1976;36:3-116
Curran AS: Lead poisoning: a historical overview. **NY State J Med** 1984 Sep;84(9):437-8
Eckert WG: Historical aspects of poisoning and toxicology. **Am J Forensic Med Pathol** 1981 Sep;2(3):261-4
Fischer-Homberger E: Vergiftungen in der Gerichtsmedizin vom 16. bis zum 18. Jahrhundert. **Schweiz Aerzteztg** 1980;61(51):3399-406
Girard P: Toxiques et poisons dans le passé pharmaceutique de la Savoie. **Rev Hist Pharm (Paris)** 1983 Dec;71(30):287-95
Morris E: Lead poisoning: an historic view. **Occup Health (Lond)** 1980 Sep;32(9):449-59
Stefănescu P: Drama otrăvirilor: dosare celebre. Bucuresti, Editura Medicală, 1980. 292 p.
Waldron HA: Lead in bones: a cautionary tale. **Ecol Dis** 1982;1(2-3):191-6
Walker RE: Malleus and podagra: lead poisoning in horse and man. **Vet Hist** 1980/81, n.s.;1:118-36

**China**

Bisset NG: Arrow poisons in China. Part I. **J Ethnopharmacol** 1979 Dec;1(4):325-84

**Great Britain**

Matossian MK: Mold poisoning: an unrecognized English health problem, 1550-1800. **Med Hist** 1981 Jan;25(1):73-84

**Before 500 A.D.**

**China**

Benfey OT: Spinach is an alchemical antidote to heavy metal poisoning. **Kagakushi Kenkyu** 1981;15:8-12

**Greco-Roman**

Crugnola A, ed: Scholia in Nicandri Theriaka, cum glossis. Varese-Milano, Istituto Editoriale Cisalpino, 1971. 329 p.

**Greece**

Geymonat M, ed: Scholia in Nicandri Alexipharmaca, cum glossis. Milan, Cisalpino-Goliardica, 1974. 218 p.
Thucydides and the Athenian plague: a reconsideration of the evidence: **Pharm Hist (London)** 1984 Dec;14(4):6-7

**Rome**

Nriagu JO: Saturnine gout among Roman aristocrats. Did lead poisoning contribute to the fall of the Empire? **N Engl J Med** 1983 Mar 17;308(11):660-3
Scarborough J: The myth of lead poisoning among the Romans: an essay review. **J Hist Med Allied Sci** 1984 Oct;39(4):469-75

**500 A.D.-1450**

Rosner F: Moses Maimonides' treatise on poisons. **NY State J Med** 1980 Sep;80(10):1627-30

**Switzerland**

Daems WF: Ermengald Blasius' Tabellen zum 'Antidotarium Nicolai'. **Pharm Acta Helv** 1979;54(4):101-5

**1450-1700**

**Great Britain**

Broad WJ: Sir Isaac Newton: mad as a hatter. **Science** 1981 Sep 18;213(4514):1341-2, 1344
Laker MR: Newton's malady. **Science** 1982 Mar 5;215(4537):1185-6
Lakie MH, Cook G, MacMurray D: A 17th century poisoning case. **Pharm Hist (London)** 1976 Aug;6(2):2-3
Lieb J, Hershman D: Isaac Newton: mercury poisoning or manic depression? **Lancet** 1983 Dec 24-31;2(8365-66):1479-80

**Hungary**

Szilágyi I: Bethlen Gábor betegsége és halála. **Orv Hetil** 1984 May 13;125(20):1205–10

**USSR**

Koretskii VI: Smert' Groznogo Tsaria. **Vopr Istor** 1979;9:93–103

**1700 to Present**

Crompton R, Gall D: Georgi Markov--death in a pellet. **Med Leg J** 1980;48(2):51–62
Fabre M, Boudet F, Boe M, et al: Intoxications par le phosgène. **Toxicol Eur Res** 1983 Jul;5(4):185–8
Gädeke R: Ein medizingeschichtliches Panorama der akuten Eisenvergiftung. **Klin Paediatr** 1979 Sep;191(5):442–6
Saddique A, Peterson CD: Thallium poisoning: a review. **Vet Hum Toxicol** 1983 Feb;25(1):16–22

**Austria**

Sakula A: 'Amadeus' was Mozart poisoned? **Hist Med (Lond)** 1980 Jan–Feb;8(1):6–9

**France**

Delahaye MC: L'absinthe. Histoire de la fée verte. Paris, Berger-Levrault, 1983. 128 p.
Lépine P: Un dossier contesté, l'affaire Lafarge. **Lyon Pharm** 1980 Jan 1;31(1):39–44
Lewin PK, Hancock RG, Voynovich P: Napoleon Bonaparte--no evidence of chronic arsenic poisoning. **Nature** 1982 Oct 14;299(5884):627–8

**Great Britain**

Paulshock BZ: William Heberden, M.D., and the end of theriac. **NY State J Med** 1982 Oct;82(11):1612–4
Prescott LF: The Regional Poisoning Treatment Centre, Edinburgh. In Passmore R, ed: Proceedings of the Royal College of Physicians of Edinburgh Tercentenary Congress, 1981. Edinburgh, Royal College of Physicians of Edinburgh, 1982. p. 211–20.
Waldron HA: Did the Mad Hatter have mercury poisoning? **Br Med J [Clin Res]** 1983 Dec 24–31;287(6409):1961

**Japan**

Smith AM: Mercury poisoning and birth defects in Japan. **Women Health** 1978 Mar–Apr;3(2):9–12

**Poland**

Dorczak W: Ostre zatrucia w latach 1972--1977 we Wrocławiu. **Pol Tyg Lek** 1979 Aug 13;34(33):1309–10

**United States**

Arena JM: The pediatrician's role in the poison control movement and poison prevention. **Am J Dis Child** 1983 Sep;137(9):870–3
Aronson SM: Lead and the demon rum in colonial America. **RI Med J** 1983 Jan;66(1):37–40
Atropine poisoning in Hawthorne's the Scarlet Letter: **N Engl J Med** 1984 Nov 29;311(22):1438–41
Burrows GE: Lead toxicosis in domestic animals: a review of the role of lead mining and primary lead smelters in the United States. **Vet Hum Toxicol** 1981 Oct;23(5):337–43
Khan JA: Atropine poisoning in Hawthorne's The Scarlet Letter. **N Engl J Med** 1984 Aug 9;311(6):414–6

## POLIOMYELITIS

Melnick JL: Toward eradication of poliomyelitis by combined use of killed and liver vaccines. **Cardiovasc Res Cent Bull** 1982 Jan–Mar;20(3):49–60
Ohry A: A history of poliomyelitis research. **Koroth** 1979 Nov;7(9–10):CCXI–CCXVIII(668–679)

**1700 to Present**

Hinman AR: Mass vaccination against polio. **JAMA** 1984 Jun 8;251(22):2994–6
Wyatt HV: Provocation poliomyelitis: neglected clinical observations from 1914 to 1950. **Bull Hist Med** 1981 Winter;55(4):543–57

**Australia**

Cohn V: Sister Kenny's fierce fight for better polio care. **Smithsonian** 1981;12(8):180–200
Hall EM: In the ward next door to Sister Kenny. **Aust Nurses J** 1981 May;10(10):57–8
Willis E: Sister Elizabeth Kenny and the evolution of the occupational division of labour in health care. **Aust NZ J Sociol** 1979;15(3):30–8

**Germany**

Wyatt HV: Did thalidomide promote poliomyelitis following oral poliovirus vaccination in West Berlin in 1960? **Perspect Biol Med** 1983 Autumn;27(1):93–106

**Israel**

Goldblum N, Swartz T, Gerichter CB, et al: The natural history of poliomyelitis in Israel, 1949–1982. **Prog Med Virol** 1984;29:115–23

**Poland**

Losiowski Z: Sanatorium w Zagórzu i jego rola w lecznictwie neurologicznym dzieci. **Pediatr Pol** 1980 Mar;55(3):379–84

**United States**

Alexander ER: Inactivated poliomyelitis vaccination. Issues reconsidered. **JAMA** 1984 May 25;251(20):2710–2
Bendiner E: Salk: adulation, animosity, and achievement. **Hosp Pract** 1983 Jun;18(6):194–6, 200–1, 204–5 passim
Brandt AM: Polio, politics, publicity, and duplicity: ethical aspects in the development of the Salk vaccine. **Conn Med** 1979 Sep;43(9):581–7, 589–90
Brown RW, Henderson JH: The mass production and distribution of HeLa cells at Tuskegee Institute, 1953–55. **J Hist Med Allied Sci** 1983 Oct;38(4):415–31
Gallagher HG: FDR: handicapped American. **Public Welf** 1984 Spring;42(2):6–18
Nathanson N, Martin JR: The epidemiology of poliomyelitis: enigmas surrounding its appearance, epidemicity, and disappearance. **Am J Epidemiol** 1979 Dec;110(6):672–92
Salk J: The virus of poliomyelitis. From discovery to extinction. **JAMA** 1983 Aug 12;250(6):808–10
Spector B: The great Salk vaccine mess. **Antioch Rev** 1980;38(3):291–303

**USSR**

Benison S: International medical cooperation: Dr. Albert Sabin, live poliovirus vaccine and the Soviets. **Bull Hist Med** 1982;56(4):460–83

## POLYPS

**1700 to Present**

**France**

Huard P, Wong M: Ablation d'un polype naso-pharyngien à la Trinité en 1812. In: Congrès National des Sociétés Savantes, 91e, Rennes, 1966. Comptes Rendus. Paris, 1967. Section des Sciences, Tome 1. p. 99–102.

## PORPHYRIA

Hurst LC: Porphyria revisited. **Med Hist** 1982 Apr;26(2):179–82

**Great Britain**

Haeger-Aronsen B, Haeger K: Porfyri hos Mary Stuarts efterkommande: en historisk-medicinsk tvistefråga. **Sydsven Medicinhist Sallsk Arsskr** 1984;21:63–75

**1700 to Present**

With TK: A short history of porphyrins and the porphyrias. **Int J Biochem** 1980;11(3–4):189–200

**Denmark**

With TK: Thirty years with biochemistry and clinic of porphyrias in man and animals. **Int J Biochem** 1980;12(5–6):985–8

## PUERPERAL INFECTION

**1700 to Present**

Antall J: Wien und Budapest im Lebenswerk Semmelweis'. **Wien Med Wochenschr** 1982 Apr 15;132(7):161–7
Benedek I: Semmelweis. Budapest, Gondolat, 1980. 269 p.
Carter KC: Semmelweis and his predecessors. **Med Hist** 1981 Jan;25(1):57–72
Miller PJ: Semmelweis. **Infect Control** 1982 Sep–Oct;3(5):405–9

**Austria**

Carter KC: Ignaz Semmelweis, Carl Mayrhofer, and the rise of germ theory. **Med Hist** 1985 Jan;29(1):33–53
Carter KC: Semmelweis's possible influence on Karl Mayrhofer and on those who subsequently developed nineteenth century etiological theories. **Orvostort Kozl** 1982;28(1–3):23–31
The first report on Semmelweis' discovery of the cause and prevention of childbed fever: Most important experiences about the etiology of puerperal fevers epidemic in birthing institutions. **Infect Control** 1982 Nov Dec;3(6):478–9

**Finland**

Teramo K: Savusaunasta monitoroituun synnytyssaliin. **Duodecim** 1981;97(20):1682–9

**France**

Dumont M: André Levret et la 'fièvre de lait'. **Nouv Presse Med** 1981 Mar 14;70(12):935–6
Wrotnowska D: Pasteur et Victor Feltz de Nancy. Correspondance inédite. In: Congrès National des Sociétés Savantes, 103e, Nancy, 1978. Comptes Rendus. Paris, 1978. Section des Sciences, Fasc. V. p. 131–44.

**Great Britain**

Abraham EP: Leonard Colebrook. In Dictionary of national biography, 1961–1970. Suppl. 8, 1981. p. 230–2.

**Hungary**

Schober KL: Vor etwa hundert Jahren (41). **Zentralbl Chir** 1982;107(23):1538–40
Wyklicky H, Skopec M: Ignaz Philipp Semmelweis, the prophet of bacteriology. **Infect Control** 1983 Sep–Oct;4(5):367–70

**Sweden**

Höfberg U: 'Jungfru Mariae nycklar' och mödradödligheten genom två sekler. **Lakartidningen** 1982 Sep 1;79(35):2977–9

**United States**

Lansing DI, Penman WR, Davis DJ: Puerperal fever and the Group B beta hemolytic streptococcus. **Bull Hist Med** 1983;57(1):70–80
Sternbach H: Puerperal psychosis in America--1847. **Arch Gen Psychiatry** 1982 Feb;39(2):235–6

## RABIES

The last word: Rabies control in olden times. **Mod Vet Pract** 1981 Dec;62(12):962
Olsen O, Barker P: Rabies archaeologorum. **Antiquity** 1980;54(210):15–20
Soubiran A, Théodoridès J: Guillotin et la rage: un mémoire inédit. **Hist Sci Med** 1982;16(4):227–36
Théodoridès J: Saints in medical history (a complement). **Clio Med** 1980 Jul;14(3–4):269–70
Théodoridès J: Utilisation du sel et de l'eau de mer dans le traitement ancien de la rage. In: Congrès National des Sociétés Savantes, 99e, Besançon, 1974. Comptes Rendus. Paris, 1976. Section des Sciences, Fasc. V. p. 117–22.

**China**

Wei J: [History of the prevention and treatment of rabies by acupuncture and moxibustion, a review and prospect] (Chi). **Chung Hua I Shih Tsa Chih** 1984 Jan;14(1):14–5

**500 A.D.–1450**

**Arabic**

Théodoridès J: Ibn Sina et la rage. In International Congress of the History of Medicine, 27th, Barcelona, 1980. Actas. Barcelona, Académia de Ciències Médiques de Catalunya i Balears, 1981. p. 756–60.
Théodoridès J: Rabies in Arabian medicine. **Stud Hist Med** 1980 Mar;4(1):13–22

**Byzantium**

Théodoridès J: Quelle était la maladie décrite par l'historien Agathias (VIe siècle A.D.)? **Hist Sci Med** 1981;15(2):153–8

**1700 to Present**

Boisvert H: Etudes sur la rage (1925–1935). **Hist Sci Med** 1984;18(2):129–35
McCracken D: A link with the past. **Br Med J [Clin Res]** 1981 Mar 21;282(6268):964–6
Prunet P: Nouvelles technologies et vaccination antirabique. **Arch Inst Pasteur Tunis** 1982 March;59(1):115–20
Théodoridès J: Les recherches histologiques sur la rage au 19e siècle. **Clio Med** 1981 Dec;16(2/3):83–92

**France**

Saenz A, Boisvert H: Trois lettres de Louis Pasteur. **Hist Sci Med** 1981;15(4):327–33
Théodoridès J: Antoine Portal et la rage (avec des documents inédits). In Ganzinger K, Skopec M, Wyklicky H, ed: Festschrift für Erna Lesky zum 70. Geburtstag. Wien, Brüder Hollinek, 1981. p. 161–5.
Théodoridès J: L'abbé de Bap, curé de Sommières, et son prétendu remède antirabique. **Rev Hist Pharm (Paris)** 1979 Dec;26(243):269–79
Théodoridès J: Les études sur la rage de deux médecins Lorrains: Pierre-Christophe Gorcy (1807–1821) et J. Camille Gorcy (1812). In: Congrès National des Sociétés Savantes, 103e, Nancy, 1978. Comptes Rendus. Paris, 1978. Section des Sciences, Fasc. v. p. 55–69.
Théodoridès J, Ming Wong: Les médecins nantais et l'histoire de la rage. In: Congrès National de Sociétés Savantes, 97e Nantes, 1972. Comptes Rendus. Paris, 1976. Section des Sciences, Tome 1. p. 91–7.
Théodoridès J: 'Paris enragé'. **Rev Hist Pharm (Paris)** 1982;29(252):193–8

**Great Britain**

Allen E, Cooper JE: A Hunterian account of human rabies. **Vet Hist** 1980/81,n.s.;1:146–8
Carter KC: Nineteenth-century treatments for rabies as reported in the Lancet. **Med Hist** 1982 Jan;26(1):67–78
Walton JK: Mad dogs and Englishmen: the conflict over rabies in late Victorian England. **J Soc Hist** 1979;13:219–39

**Hungary**

Frankl J, Bodosi M: Csorba József emlékezete. **Orv Hetil** 1984 Aug 19;125(34):2087–9

**Malagasy Republic**

Coulanges P, Rakotonirina-Randriambeloma PJ: Epidémiologie de la rage à Madagascar. **Arch Inst Pasteur Tunis** 1982 Mar;59(1):47–74

**Nigeria**

Umoh JU, Belino ED: Rabies in Nigeria. A historical review. **Int J Zoonoses** 1979 Jun;6(1):41–8

**USSR**

Levitin NN: Iz istorii bor'by s beshenstvom v Rossii. **Feldsher Akush** 1980;45(7):53–5

## RADIATION INJURY

**1700 to Present**

Taylor LS: Technical accuracy in historical writing. **Health Phys** 1981 May;40(5):595–9
Templeton WL: Artificial radionuclides in the oceans. In Sears M, Merriman D, ed: Oceanography, the past. New York, Springer, 1980. p. 420–37.
Ziemer PL, Kathren RL, ed: Health physics: a backward glance. New York, Pergamon Press, 1980. 237 p.

**Canada**

Doern GB: Science and technology in the nuclear regulatory process: the case of Canadian uranium miners. **Can Public Adm** 1978;21(1):51–82

**Japan**

Atomic Bomb Casualty Commission: The Atomic Bomb Casualty Commission, 1947–1975. [Hiroshima?] The Commission, [1978?] vi, 240 p.
Warren S: Shields Warren, M.D.: Excerpts from 'Medical aspects of the atomic bombings'. 1946. **Am J Forensic Med Pathol** 1980 Dec;1(4):303–7

**United States**

Cloutier RJ: Florence Kelley and the radium dial painters. **Health Phys** 1980 Nov;39(5):711–6
Evans RD: Inception of standards for internal emitters, radon and radium. **Health Phys** 1981 Sep;41(3):437–48
Kathren RL: Elda Emma Anderson. In: Notable American women. The modern period. Cambridge, Mass., Belknap-Harvard Univ. Press, 1980.

4:20-1.
Kopp C: The origins of the American Scientific debate over fallout hazards. **Soc Stud Sci** 1979;9(4):403-22
Mazur A: The journalists and technology: reporting about Love Canal and Three Mile Island. **Minerva** 1984 Spring;22(1):45-66
Parker HM: Invited paper delivered at the 25th Annual Meeting of the Health Physics Society. Protection programs of the Plutonium Project. **Health Phys** 1981 Oct;41(4):571-6
Pochin EE: Sieverts and safety. **Health Phys** 1984 Jun;46(6):1173-9
Steneck NH, Cook HJ, Vander AJ, et al: The origins of U.S. safety standards for microwave radiation. **Science** 1980 Jun 13;208(4449):1230-7
Taylor LS: The development of radiation protection standards (1925-1940). **Health Phys** 1981 Aug;41(2):227-32
Tokuhata GK, Smith MW: History of health studies around nuclear facilities: a methodological consideration. **Environ Res** 1981 Jun;25(1):75-85
U. S. Bureau of Radiological Health: Legislative history of Radiation control for health and safety act of 1968. Bureau of Radiological Health; Washington: for sale by the Supt. of Docs., U. S. Govt. Print. Off., 1975. 2 v. (ix, 1494 p.).

## REITER'S DISEASE

### 1450-1700

Allison DJ: Christopher Columbus: first case of Reiter's disease in the Old World? **Lancet** 1980 Dec 13;2(8207):1309
Shizusawa K: [Columbus as the 1st known patient with Reiter's disease?] (Jpn). **Kango** 1981 Apr;33(4):83

### 1700 to Present

Good AE: Reiter's disease: modern concepts. **Cutis** 1979 Nov;24(5):514-23

#### United States

McSherry JA: Reiter's syndrome and the American revolutionary war. **Practitioner** 1982 Apr;226(1366):794-5

## RESPIRATORY TRACT

Bollinelli R, Carles P: Geschichte der Lungenheilkunde. In Sournia JC, Martiny M, Poulet J, ed: Illustrierte Geschichte der Medizin. Salzburg, Andreas, 1980. Vol. 8. p. 2795-825.
Kryger MH: Sleep apnea. From the needles of Dionysius to continuous positive airway pressure. **Arch Intern Med** 1983 Dec;143(12):2301-3
Lee DH, Selikoff IJ: Historical background to the asbestos problem. **Environ Res** 1979 Apr;18(2):300-14

### Before 500 A.D.

#### Greece

Ohry A: Respiratory items in Hippocratic medicine. **Koroth** 1980 Jun;7(11-12):CCLXXXV-CCLXLII

### 1450-1700

#### Italy

Sakula A: Ramazzini's De Morbis Artificum and occupational lung disease. **Br J Dis Chest** 1983 Oct;77(4):349-61

### 1700 to Present

Emanuel DA, Kryda MJ: Farmer's lung disease. **Clin Rev Allergy** 1983 Dec;1(4):509-32
Lavie P: Nothing new under the moon. Historical accounts of sleep apnea syndrome. **Arch Intern Med** 1984 Oct;144(10):2025-8
Le Tacon J: La pleuroscopie. Rappel historique. **Poumon Coeur** 1981 Jan-Feb;37(1):5-6
Mann RJ, Mann FD: Emphysema. Era of Laennec; era of the cigarette. **Minn Med** 1984 Mar;67(3):142, 159-61
Murphy RL: Auscultation of the lung: past lessons, future possibilities. **Thorax** 1981 Feb;36(2):99-107
Pilarska-Machowicz A: Rozwój diagnostyki bronchoskopowej. **Wiad Lek** 1982 Nov 1;35(19-20):1265-70
Pirsig W: Historical notes and actual observations on the nasal septal abscess especially in children. **Int J Pediatr Otorhinolaryngol** 1984 Oct;8(1):43-54
Tucker WS: Osler and sleep apnea. **Arch Intern Med** 1984 May;144(5):1085
Völker A: Die Schwindsucht im halleschen Schrifttum des 18. Jahrhunderts. **Wiss Beitr Martin Luther Univ Halle Wittenberg** 1983;5-R80:203-10

#### Austria

Michel J: Recherches historiques sur la découverte des maladies des sinus--le XIXe siècle. 2e partie: Les affections inflammatoires des sinus. **J Fr Otorhinolaryngol** 1979 Dec;28(10):669-85

#### Belgium

Darquenne R: Controverses sur la nocivité du charbon de terre (18e-19e siècles). **Ann Soc Belg Hist Hop** 1981;:33-45

#### France

Fréour P: Du pneumo-thorax vu par Th. Laënnec. **Rev Fr Mal Respir** 1981;9(3):265-9
Potvliege P: Le syndrome 'de Pickwick'. Priorité de sa description par le duc de Saint-Simon (1675-1755). **Nouv Presse Med** 1982 Jul 3;11(31):2360
Trocme C: L'atélectasie découverte et délaissée: Claude-Auguste Reynaud et Nicolas Bailly. **Hist Sci Med** 1979;13(4):441-50

#### Germany

Ganguin HG: Beitrag der medizinisch-wissenschaftlichen Gesselschaft für Bronchopneumonologie der DDR und ihrer Sektionen zur Entwicklung des Fachgebietes Bronchopneumonologie. **Z Erkr Atmungsorgane** 1979 Apr;153(11):5-13
Scharkoff H: 25 Jahre Gesellschaft für Bronchopneumonologie und Tuberkulose der DDR. **Z Erkr Atmungsorgane** 1983;160(3):199-200

#### Great Britain

Scadding JG: Maurice Davidson 1883-1967--progress in respiratory medicine since his time. **Postgrad Med J** 1984 Mar;60(701):178-82
Wright DS: Man-made mineral fibres: a historical note. **J Soc Occup Med** 1980 Oct;30(4):138-40

#### Iceland

Eliasson Orn: Farmer's lung disease: a new historical perspective from Iceland. **J Hist Med Allied Sci** 1982 Oct;37(4):440-4

#### Ireland

Counihan HE: Corrigan on pulmonary disease. **J Ir Coll Physicians Surg** 1980 Jul;10(1):38-40

#### Italy

Grassi C: Influence de l'oeuvre de Laénnec sur la médecine italienne. **Rev Fr Mal Respir** 1981;9(5):421-6

#### Romania

Lazăr C, Ionescu C: Istoricul chirurgiei toraco-pulmonare din Moldova. **Rev Med Chir Soc Med Nat Iasi** 1980 Jul-Sept;84(3):575-7

#### Spain

Cornudella J: L'obra mèdica del Dr. Joan Freixas i Freixas. In Congrés Internacional d'Historie de la Medicina Catalana, 1st, Barcelona-Montpellier, 1970. Llibr d'Actes. Barcelona, Editorial Scientia, 1971. v 4, p. 362-5.

#### United States

Brewer LA: A historical account of the 'wet lung of trauma' and the introduction of intermittent positive-pressure oxygen therapy in World War II. **Ann Thorac Surg** 1981 Apr;31(4):386-93
Cassedy JH: An American clerical crisis: ministers' sore throat 1830-1860 (the Fielding H. Garrison Lecture). **Bull Hist Med** 1979 Spring;53(1):23-38
Fox DM, Stone JF: Black lung: miners' militancy and medical uncertainty, 1968-1972. **Bull Hist Med** 1980 Spring;54(1):43-63
Smith GJ: Averill Abraham Liebow: contributions to pulmonary pathology. **Yale J Biol Med** 1981 Mar-Apr;54(2):139-46
Sweeney RE, Castleman B: Asbestos disease and compensation. **Ann NY Acad Sci** 1979;330:273-80

## RHEUMATIC FEVER

### 1700 to Present

Benedek TG: Subcutaneous nodules and the differentiation of rheumatoid arthritis from rheumatic fever. **Semin Arthritis Rheum** 1984 May;13(4):305-21

United States

Wannamaker LW: The pathogenesis of rheumatic fever: Lewis Thomas and the Minnesota years. **Cell Immunol** 1983 Nov;82(1):82–7

## RICKETS

Cone TE: A rachitic infant painted by Burgkmair 136 years before Dr. Whistler described rickets. **Clin Pediatr (Phila)** 1980 Mar;19(3):194
Frenk S: Raquitismo, una enfermedad social **Bol Med Hosp Infant Mex** 1984 Mar;41(3):129–39
Frenk SF: El raquitismo: un hito en la historia de la pediatria. **Bol Soc Mex Hist Filos Med** 1982 Dec;6(41):89–104
Grimm H: Neue Hinweise auf ur- und frühgeschichtliches sowie mittelalterliches Vorkommen der Rachitis und ähnlicher Mineralisationsstörungen. **Arztl Jugendkd** 1984 Jun;75(3):168–77
Guggenheim KY: Nutrition and nutritional diseases. The evolution of concepts. Lexington, Massachusetts, Toronto, D.C. Heath and Company, 1981. xii, 378 p.

Before 500 A.D.

Great Britain

Ivanhoe F: Interglovular dentine in first and third molars: relation to hours of sunshine during growth in two archeological populations from England. **Calcif Tissue Int** 1982 Mar;34(2):136–44

1700 to Present

United States

Bancroft PM: Rickets and solar radiation - medicine's debt to Professor Frank Mussehl. **Nebr Med J** 1982 Jul;67(7):184–5
Warkany J: Laissez-faire in research. **J Am Coll Nutr** 1984;3(2):177–81

## ROCKY MOUNTAIN SPOTTED FEVER

1700 to Present

United States

Beatty WK, Beatty VL: Howard Taylor Ricketts--imaginative investigator. **Proc Inst Med Chic** 1981 Apr–Jun;34(2):46–8
Hammarsten JF: The contributions of Idaho physicians to knowledge of Rocky Mountain Spotted Fever. **Trans Am Clin Climatol Assoc** 1982;94:27–43
Marx RS: Rocky mountain spotted fever. **Compr Ther** 1983 May;9(5):43–8
Mullen PC: Bitterroot enigma: Howard Taylor Ricketts and the early struggle against spotted fever. **Montana** 1983;32(1):2–13
North E: Classics in infectious diseases. Concerning the epidemic of spotted fever in New England: Elisha North, 1811. **Rev Infect Dis** 1980 Sep–Oct;2(5):811–6
Ormsbee RA: A review: 'Studies in Pyroplasmosis hominis ('spotted fever' or 'tick fever' of the Rocky Mountains)' by Louis B. Wilson and William M. Chowning, published in The Journal of Infectious Diseases 1:31–57, 1904. **Rev Infect Dis** 1979 May–Jun;1(3):559–62

## RUBELLA

1700 to Present

Lundström R: Rubella under graviditet--historik och nomenklatur. **Lakartidningen** 1979 Oct 10;76(41):3512–3

## SARCOIDOSIS

1700 to Present

Chrétien J, Marsac J: La sarcoïdose. Rappel historique et évolution des concepts. **Rev Prat** 1983 Sep 11;33(39):2011–4, 2017–9
Chrétien J: La sarcoïdose un siècle après Besnier: de l'approche descriptive à l'approche pathogénique. **Ann Med Interne (Paris)** 1984;135(2):89–90
Young RC Jr, Rachal RE, Cowan CL Jr: Sarcoidosis--the beginning: historical highlights of personalities and their accomplishments during the early years. **J Natl Med Assoc** 1984 Sep;76(9):887–96

Norway

Epstein WL: 'Multiple benign sarkoid of the skin' by Boeck, December 1899. Commentary: What begot Boeck? **Arch Dermatol** 1982 Oct;118(10):711–22

United States

Sharma OP, James DG: Did Osler's patient, Hannah W, have sarcoidosis? An historical footnote. **Chest** 1984 Aug;86(2):263–4

## SCABIES

1700 to Present

Italy

Testoni G: Una lettera di Cestoni a Vallisneri (1710). **Riv Biol** 1983 Spring;76(1):125–31

## SCARLET FEVER

1700 to Present

Romania

Cornesco M: American-Romanian cooperation in the study of and fight against scarlet fever. In International Congress of the History of Medicine, 27th, Barcelona, 1980. Actas. Barcelona, Académia de Ciències Médiques de Catalunya i Balears, 1981. p. 499–502.

United States

C[one] TE: William Douglass on the first reported cases of scarlet fever in New England, 1736. **Pediatrics** 1981;68:230
Harvey AM: The conquest of scarlet fever: some Johns Hopkins contributions. **Johns Hopkins Med J** 1980 Aug;147(2):53–63
Matossian MK: The throat distemper reappraised. **Bull Hist Med** 1980 Winter;54(4):529–43
Rubin LP: Gladys Rowena Henry Dick. In: Notable American women. The modern period. Cambridge, Mass., Belknap-Harvard Univ. Press, 1980. 4:191–2.
Stollerman GH: Landmark perspective: The historical role of the Dick test. **JAMA** 1983 Dec 9;250(22):3097–9

## SCHISTOSOMIASIS

Brazil

da Silva LJ: Sobre a antigüidade de alguns focos de esquistossomose do Estado de São Paulo. **Rev Bras Malariol Doencas Trop** 1983;35:73–8

China

Li Yousong: [Exploration of the relationship between defeating Cao Cao in Chibi and schistosomiasis.] (Chi). **Chin J Med Hist** 1981;11:87–8

1700 to Present

Sandbach FR: The history of schistosomiasis research and policy for its control. **Med Hist** 1976 Jul;20(3):259–75
Shortt HE: Robert Thomson Leiper. In Dictionary of national biography, 1961–1970. Suppl. 8, 1981. p. 647–8.

China

Reed JH: Brass butterflies or the thoughts of Mao Tse Tung: the sociology of schistosomiasis control in China. Ithaca, N.Y., Cornell U. Press. 1979. 280 p.

Dominican Republic

Hillyer GV: Schistosomiasis in the Dominican Republic: a review. **Bol Asoc Med PR** 1983 Mar;75(3):114–7

Egypt

Althoff A: Wissenschaftlicher Briefwechsel von und mit Theodor Bilharz. Düsseldorf, Triltsch, 1980. 133 p. (Düsseldorfer Arbeiten zur Geschichte der Medizin, 56; also Diss.) **Dusseld Arb Gesch Med Hefte** 1980;56:1–133
Classics in infectious diseases: A contribution to human helminthology: Theodore Bilharz (1825–1862). **Rev Infect Dis** 1982 May–Jun;4(3):727–32

Germany

Pytel' AIa: Ob otkrytii Bil'gartsem vozbuditelia urinarnogo shistosomoza. **Urol Nefrol (Mosk)** 1980 May–Jun;(3):67–70

## SCROFULA

1700 to Present

Great Britain

Ellis CG: The king's evil. A case of scrofula. **Practitioner** 1981 Oct;225(1360):1519

# DISEASES AND INJURIES

### SCURVY

Carré A: Scorbut marin historique et biologie moderne. In: Congrès National des Sociétés Savantes, 104e, Bordeaux, 1979. Comptes Rendus. Paris, 1979. Section des Sciences, Fasc. IV. p. 219-30.
Dickman SR: The search for the specific factor in scurvy. **Perspect Biol Med** 1981;24:382-95
Gauval VB, Vidal F: Etiologie et pathogénie du mal scorbutique chez les médecins des XVIIe et XVIIIe siècles. **Chir Dent Fr** 1984 Jul 12-19;54(258-259):23-8
Guggenheim KY: Nutrition and nutritional diseases. The evolution of concepts. Lexington, Massachusetts, Toronto, D.C. Heath and Company, 1981. xii, 378 p.
Huard P, Imbault-Huart MJ: A propos du scorbut. In: Congrès National des Sociétés Savantes, 101e, Lille, 1976. Comptes Rendus. Paris, 1976. Section des Sciences, Fasc. III. p. 157-72.
Orozco Acuaviva A: Historia de una enfermedad de los navegantes: el escorbuto. **An R Acad Med Cir Cadiz** 1979;15(1):7-30
Schadewaldt H: Das Sargassokraut als Antiskorbutikum. In Dilg P, et al., ed: Perspektiven der Pharmaziegeschichte. Graz, Austria, Akademische Druck- u. Verlagsanstalt, 1983. p. 281-94.
Schadewaldt H: Skorbut. **Zahnarztl Prax** 1980 Jul 11;31(7):297-301
Watt J: Nutrition in adverse environments, 1. Forgotten lessons of maritime nutrition. **Hum Nutr Appl Nutr** 1982 Feb;36(1):35-45

**Japan**

Matsuki A: [Prevalence of scurvy among soldiers of the Hirosake feudal clan in Yezo area.] (Jpn). **Nihon I-Shigaku Zasshi** 1981;27(1):56-63

**1450-1700**

**France**

Cadotte M: A propos de la description par Jacques Cartier d'une 'grosse maladie' survenue au cours de son deuxième voyage au Canada. **Union Med Can** 1984 Aug;113(8):651-5

**Portugal**

Reis CS: A 'Doença crua e feia' em 'os lusíadas'. **An Inst Hig Med Trop (Lisb)** 1977-1978;5(1-4):127-69

**1700 to Present**

Craig D: History of medicine: observation and theory: some reflections occasioned by reading Nansen's 'Farthest North'. **Practitioner** 1980 Feb;224(1340):219-22
Norris J: The 'scurvy disposition': heavy exertion as an exacerbating influence on scurvy in modern times. **Bull Hist Med** 1983 Fall;57(3):325-38
Stone I: Eight decades of scurvy. **Australas Nurses J** 1979 Sep;8(11):28-30
Watt J: Lettsomian lectures. Medical perspectives of some voyages of discovery. **Trans Med Soc Lond** 1979;95:61-91

**Great Britain**

Baron JH: James Lind would not have approved. **Lancet** 1982 Jun 5;1(8284):1313
Evans PR: Infantile scurvy: the centenary of Barlow's disease. **Br Med J [Clin Res]** 1983 Dec 17;287(6408):1862-3
Hughes RE: James Lind and the cure of scurvy: an experimental approach. **Med Hist** 1975 Oct;19(4):342-51
Leach RD: Sir Gilbert Blane, Bart, MD FRS (1749-1832). **Ann R Coll Surg Engl** 1980 May;62(3):232-9
Lee RV: Scurvy: a contemporary historical perspective (3). **Conn Med** 1984 Jan;48(1):33-5
Lloyd C: Cook and scurvy. **Mar Mirror** 1979 Feb;65:23-8
Tilghman RC: Captain James Cook (1728-1779). **Trans Am Clin Climatol Assoc** 1980;92:1-15
Zuckerman A: Scurvy and the ventilation of ships in the Royal Navy: Samuel Sutton's contribution. **Eighteenth Cent Stud** 1976/77;10:222-34

**Hungary**

Marsovszky P: Egy közel 200 éves orvosi disszertáció a skorbutról. **Orvostort Kozl** 1979;87-88(25 no 1-2):303-5

**Spain**

Richter T: Das Sargassokraut in Vicente de Lardizábals Werk 'Consuelo de Navegantes' (Madrid 1772). Diss., Universität Düsseldorf. Düsseldorf, 1982. 111 p.

**United States**

Lee RV: Scurvy: a contemporary historical perspective. **Conn Med** 1983 Oct;47(10):629-32

### SEX DISORDERS

Janda LH, Klenke-Hamel KE: Human sexuality. New York, Van Nostrand, 1980. xv, 475 p.

**500 A.D.-1450**

**Great Britain**

Rowland B: Chaucer's idea of the pardoner. **Chaucer Rev** 1979-80;14(2):138-54

**Iceland**

Orner R, Hipwell J: Njal's Saga: a 1000 year old record of premature ejaculation. **J Am Soc Psychosom Dent Med** 1980;27(1):10-2

**1700 to Present**

Hanafy HM: Sex aids: 'energising ring' and 'surgical splints' for treatment of impotence. **Urology** 1980 May;15(5):478E, 478F
Kaplan HS: Sexual medicine. A progress report. **Arch Intern Med** 1980 Dec;140(12):1575-6

**Canada**

Altaffer LF: Penis captivus and the mischievous Sir William Osler. **South Med J** 1983 May;76(5):637-41

**Czechoslovakia**

Ober WB: The sticky end of Frantisek Koczwara, composer of 'The Battle of Prague'. **Am J Forensic Med Pathol** 1984 Jun;5(2):145-9

**Poland**

Godlewski G: Chopin génie asexué. **Sem Hop Paris** 1979 Dec 18-25;55(43-44):2051-63

### SHOCK

Bollet AJ: Toxic shock syndrome: a new disease but an old phenomenon. **Conn Med** 1981 Apr;45(4):223-4

**1700 to Present**

Lillehei RC: History of vasodilation in treating shock and low flow states. **Adv Shock Res** 1978;1:1-17
Simeone FA: Studies of trauma and shock in man: William S. Stone's role in the military effort. **J Trauma** 1984 Mar;24(3):181-7

**Canada**

Brown T: Shell shock in the Canadian Expeditionary Force, 1914-1918: Canadian psychiatry in the Great War. In Roland CG, ed: Health, disease and medicine. Toronto, Hannah Institute for the History of Medicine, 1984. p. 308-32.

**United States**

English PC: Shock, physiological surgery, and George Washington Crile. Medical innovation in the Progressive era. Westport, Connecticut, and London, Greenwood, 1980. xi, 271 p. (Contributions in medical history, 5)

**USSR**

Milashkin AG: Nauchno-issledovatel'skaia rabota po voprosam travmaticheskogo shoka v gody Velikoĭ Otechestvennoĭ voĭny. **Voen Med Zh** 1983 Aug;(8):74-5

### SKIN

Blotzer JW: Systemic lupus erythematosus I: historical aspects. **Md State Med J** 1983 Jun;32(6):439-41
Dotz W, Berliner N: Rhinophyma. A master's depiction, a patron's affliction. **Am J Dermatopathol** 1984 Jun;6(3):231-5
Jackson R: Historical outine of attempts to classify skin diseases. In: Congrès international d'histoire de la médecine, XXVe, Québec, 1976. Actes. Québec, 1977. p. 798-806.
Jackson R: How caustics were used to treat skin cancer. **J Dermatol Surg Oncol** 1979 Dec;5(12):949-50
Jarcho S: Some lost, obsolete, or discontinued diseases: Serous apoplexy, incubus, and retrocedent ailments. **Trans Stud Coll Physicians Phila** 1980 Dec;5(2 no 4):241-66

Shelley WB: Experimental disease in the skin of man. A review. **Acta Derm Venereol [Suppl] (Stockh)** 1982;108:1-38
Sullivan EJ: Depictions of skin ailments in Western European and American art from the Middle Ages to the 20th century. **Am J Dermatopathol** 1982 Aug;4(4):343-52
Wright RC, Goldman L: Contact dermatitis: a historical perspective. **Int J Dermatol** 1979 Oct;18(8):665-8

**Italy**

Roth W: Lentigo maligna und Sclerodermia circumscripta auf Olgemälden der Uffizien. **Hautarzt** 1982 Apr;33(4):229-30

**Before 500 A.D.**

Forrai G: Noah or the legend of albinism. **Ther Hung** 1980;28(2):87-9
Freilich AR: Tzaraat--'biblical leprosy'. **J Am Acad Dermatol** 1982 Jan;6(1):131-4

**Egypt**

Paulshock BZ: Tutankhamun and his brothers. Familial gynecomastia in the Eighteenth Dynasty. **JAMA** 1980 Jul 11;244(2):160-4
Zimmermann MR: A possible histiocytoma in an Egyptian mummy. **Arch Dermatol** 1981 Jun;117(6):364-5

**Greece**

David M: A case of scleroderma mentioned by Hippocrates in his aphorisms. **Koroth** 1981;8(1-2):61-3

**500 A.D.-1450**

Sheerin DJ: A Carolingian cure recovered: Erasmus' citation of Hucbald of St. Amand's Ecloga de caluis. **Bibl Hum Renaissance** 1980 Jan;42(1):167-71
Stephanos S: Zur Problematik des omnipotenten Objekts - eine psychoanalytische Studie über Psoriasis. Ein Fall aus dem Jahre 802. **Krankenpfl J** 1984 Mar 1;22(3):20-3

**Americas**

Speck FL, Wheeland RG: Cutaneous histopathology of southwestern American Indian mummies. **Int J Dermatol** 1984 Sep;23(7):487-92

**Germany**

Bork K: Dermatologisches im Werk der Hildegard von Bingen. **Hautarzt** 1980 Jul;31(7):381-3

**1450-1700**

Columbus: was it Reiter's disease?: **Lancet** 1981 Jan 10;1(8211):94-5
Goldwyn RM: Port wine stain. **Plast Reconstr Surg** 1980 Oct;66(4):647

**Germany**

Roth W: Differentialdiagnostische Erwägungen zu den Hauteffloreszenzen, dargestellt auf dem Sebastiansaltar Hans Holbeins d. A. **Hautarzt** 1980 Dec;31(12):662-4

**Great Britain**

Felts JH: Browne spots. **NC Med J** 1982 Aug;43(8):591

**Italy**

Goldman L: Portrait of an elderly woman with a nodular eruption. What was it? **Am J Dermatopathol** 1982 Aug;4(4):353

**Korea**

Lee S: Vitiligo auf einem historischen Porträt. **Hautarzt** 1982 Jun;33(6):335-6

**Netherlands**

Dotz W: Jan Vermeer and his alopecic models. **Am J Dermatopathol** 1983 Jun;5(3):245-8

**1700 to Present**

Benedek TG, Rodnan GP: The early history and nomenclature of scleroderma and of its differentiation from sclerema neonatorum and scleroedema. **Semin Arthritis Rheum** 1982 Aug;12(1):52-67
Blank H: 'The treatment of dermatomycoses with orally administered griseofulvin' by Blank and Roth, March 1959. Commentary: Treatment of dermatomycoses with griseofulvin. **Arch Dermatol** 1982 Oct;118(10):827-36
Braverman IM: 'Cutaneous manifestations of internal malignant tumors' by Becker, Kahn and Rothman, June 1942. Commentary: Migratory necrolytic erythema. **Arch Dermatol** 1982 Oct;118(10):784-98
Hjorth N: Geschichte der Kontaktdermatitis und ihr Einfluss auf die heutige Arbeitsdermatologie. **Hautarzt** 1980 Nov;31(11):621-6
Holubar K: Terminology and iconography of lupus erythematosus. A historical vignette. **Am J Dermatopathol** 1980 Fall;2(3):239-42
Howell JB, Anderson DE. 'The basal-cell nevus' by Howell and Caro, January 1959. Commentary: The nevoid basal cell carcinoma syndrome. **Arch Dermatol** 1982 Oct;118(10):813-26
Jordon RE: 'An unusual type of pemphigus combining feature of lupus erythematosus' by Senear and Usher, June 1926. Commentary: Pemphigus erythematosus, a unique member of the pemphigus group. **Arch Dermatol** 1982 Oct;118(10):723-42
King DF: Chronic atypical epithelial proliferation of Bowen. A historical and biographical note. **Am J Dermatopathol** 1984 Feb;6(1):35-8
Levin S: Mongolian spot; Afro-Asian stain; sacral stain. **S Afr Med J** 1981 Jul 25;60(4):123-4
Lutzner MA: The human papillomaviruses. A review. **Arch Dermatol** 1983 Aug;119(8):631-5
Marmasse J: Les ulcères de jambe d'origine veineuse et leur évolution aux environs de l'année 1955. **Phlebologie** 1984 Jul-Sep;37(3):333-6
Mathews-Roth MM: Carotenoid pigments and protection against photosensitization: how studies in bacteria suggested a treatment for a human disease. **Perspect Biol Med** 1984 Autumn;28(1):127-39
Menzel I: Vive la berloque. Etymologische Betrachtungen zur Berlocke-Dermatitis. **Hautarzt** 1980 Oct;31(10):558-9
Michel B: 'Familial benign chronic pemphigus' by Hailey and Hailey, April 1939. Commentary: Hailey-Hailey disease, familial benign chronic pemphigus. **Arch Dermatol** 1982 Oct;118(10):774-83
Newell LM, Malkinson FD: 'Pyoderma (ecthyma) gangrenosum' by Brunsting, Goeckerman and O'Leary, October 1930. Commentary: Pyoderma gangrenosum. **Arch Dermatol** 1982 Oct;118(10):743-73
Pierard GE, Lapière CM: Les corticostéroïdes à usage externe. Trente années d'utilisation et perspectives d'avenir. **Rev Med Liege** 1984 Feb 15;39(4):156-9
Scadding JG: The eponymy of sarcoidosis. **J R Soc Med** 1981 Feb;74(2):147-57
Steigleder GK: Ixodes-ricinus-Spirochäten: wahrscheinlich Ursache der Acrodermatitis chronica atrophicans Herxheimer. **Dtsch Med Wochenschr** 1984 Jan 6;109(1):3-5
Sullivan EJ: Beauty marks or pigmented skin lesions? **Am J Dermatopathol** 1981 Fall;3(3):311-2
Tuffanelli DL: 'Clinical significance of autoantibodies in pemphigus' by Chorzelski, Von Weiss and Lever, May 1966. Commentary: Clinical importance of autoantibodies in pemphigus. **Arch Dermatol** 1982 Oct;118(10):837-45
Van Scott EJ, Yu RJ: 'Ichthyosiform dermatoses' by Frost and Van Scott, August 1966. **Arch Dermatol** 1982 Oct;118(10):846-61
Voorhees JJ: 'Psoriasis as a possible defect of the adenyl cyclase-cyclic AMP Cascade' by Voorhees and Duell, October 1971. Commentary: Cyclic adenosine monophosphate regulation of normal and psoriatic epidermis. **Arch Dermatol** 1982 Oct;118(10):862-74

**Americas**

Mérida F: Las enfermedades odontologicas y dermatologicas del Libertador. **Rev Soc Venez Hist Med** 1981;30(47):81-7
Mérida MT: Las enfermedades odontológicas y dermatológicas del Liberatador. **Acta Odontol Venez** 1983 May-Aug;21(2):154-61

**Austria**

Skopec M: Anton Elfinger (1821-1864)--a forgotten medical illustrator. **Int J Dermatol** 1983 May;22(4):256-9

**Denmark**

Zachariae H: Changes in disease pattern in a skin clinic 1947 to 1977. **Acta Derm Venereol [Suppl] (Stockh)** 1979;59(85):199-205

**France**

Doby JM, Le Duigou D, Guiguen C, et al: Le favus en Bretagne. Etude historique à propos d'un cas autochtone. **Ann Dermatol Venereol** 1983;110(11):925-31
Dotz W: Jean Paul Marat. His life, cutaneous disease, death, and depiction by Jacques Louis David. **Am J Dermatopathol** 1979 Fall;1(3):247-50
Fanti PA, Varotti C: 'Les eczématides'. Historical review of the term. **Am J Dermatopathol** 1984 Oct;6(5):437-40
Jelinek JE: Jean-Paul Marat. The differential diagnosis of his skin disease. **Am J Dermatopathol** 1979 Fall;1(3):251-2
Patterson JA: The tale of the psorosperm. **Am J Dermatopathol** 1979 Fall;1(3):229-35

## DISEASES AND INJURIES

**Great Britain**

Brown PS: Some treatments of skin disease in eighteenth century Bath. **Int J Dermatol** 1982 Nov;21(9):555–9
Clemmensen O: Hutchinson's freckle. **Am J Dermatopathol** 1982 Oct;4(5):425–8
Hodgson GA: The history of coal miners' skin diseases. In J. Cule, ed: Wales and medicine. London, British Society for the History of Medicine, 1975. p. 54–67.
Loudon IS: Leg ulcers in the eighteenth and early nineteenth centuries. II. Treatment. **J R Coll Gen Pract** 1982 May;32(238):301–9
Rosser EM: Campbell De Morgan and his spots. **Ann R Coll Surg Engl** 1983 Jul;65(4):266–8
Silvers DN, Gorham JD: Observations on a melanoma by William Norris, M.D., a country practitioner of the early 19th century. **Am J Dermatopathol** 1982 Oct;4(5):421–4

**Poland**

Grzegorczyk L: Uwagi na temat sytuacji epidemiologicznej w zakresie chorób zawodowych skóry w Polsce w latach 1971–1977. **Przegl Dermatol** 1980 Jul–Aug;67(4):455–7
Kieć-Swierczyńska M: Uczuleniowy zawodowy wyprysk skóry rozpoznany w Instytucie Medycyny Pracy w Lodzi w latach 1972–1978. **Przegl Dermatol** 1980 Jul–Aug;67(4):449–53

**United States**

Coles R: Flannery O'Connor's lupus. A commentary on her collected letters, The habit of being. **JAMA** 1980 Sep 26;244(13):1441–2
King DF: A foot note to 'The tale of the psorosperm'. **Am J Dermatopathol** 1982 Aug;4(4):313–4
Muller SA, Perry HO: The Goeckerman treatment in psoriasis: six decades of experience at the Mayo Clinic. **Cutis** 1984 Sep;34(3):265–8, 270
Pillsbury DM: General Eisenhower's 'melanoma'. **J Am Acad Dermatol** 1981 May;4(5):631–2

**USSR**

Denko CW: Chernogubov's syndrome: a translation of the first modern case report of the Ehlers-Danlos syndrome. **J Rheumatol** 1978 Fall;5(3):347–52
Sheliuzhenko A: Ekonomicheskie posledstviia poteri rabochego vremeni v sviazi s netrudosposobnost'iu po bolezni. **Ekon Sov Ukr** 1972;14(3):63–6
Sosnovskiĭ AT, Eremenko SA, Korsun VF: K 60-letiiu kafedry kozhnykh i venericheskikh bolezneĭ Minskogo meditsinskogo instituta. **Vestn Dermatol Venerol** 1984 Jan;(1):66–9

**Yugoslavia**

Vukas A: Organizacija borbe protiv kožnih i spolnih bolesti i dosadašnji nedostaci u tom pogledu. **Lijec Vjesn** 1979 Nov;101(11):718–9

### SMALLPOX

Behbehani AM: The smallpox story: life and death of an old disease. **Microbiol Rev** 1983 Dec;47(4):455–509
Behbehani AM: The smallpox story: man finally defeats an old adversary. **J Kans Med Soc** 1980 Oct;81(10):447–56, 474
Bloch H: Smallpox: a disease that disappeared. **Clin Pediatr (Phila)** 1984 May;23(5):290–1
Kostrzewski J: Swiat wolny od ospy. **Przegl Epidemiol** 1980;34(4):365–72
Rosner E: Zur Geschichte der Pocken in Innerasien. **Asiat Forsch** 1980;71:72–6
Smallpox exhibit: **Bull Hist Med** 1981 Spring;55(1):108–10
Stöcklin WH: Sakpata, ein Beitrag Afrikanischer Medizinmänner zur Pockeneradikation. **Gesnerus** 1982;39(3–4):405–15
Strassburg MA: The global eradication of smallpox. **Am J Infect Control** 1982 May;10(2):53–9

**China**

Needham J: China and the origins of immunology. **East Horiz** 1980;19(1):6–12
Serruys H: Smallpox in Mongolia during the Ming and Ching dynasties. **Zentralasiat Stud** 1980;14:41–63

**India**

Nicholas RW: The goddess Sitala and epidemic smallpox in Bengal. **J Asian Stud** 1981;41(1):21–45

**Netherlands**

Braekman WL: Recepten en pokkentraktaat uit een Middelnederlands handschrift. **Volkskunde** 1977;78:177–98

**Puerto Rico**

Rigau-Pérez JG: Smallpox epidemics in Puerto Rico during the prevaccine era (1518–1803). **J Hist Med Allied Sci** 1982 Oct;37(4):423–38

**Switzerland**

Perrenoud A: Contribution à l'histoire cyclique des maladies. Deux cents ans de variole à Genève (1580–1810). In Imhof AE, ed: Mensch und Gesundheit in der Geschichte. Husum, Matthiesen, 1980. p. 175–98.

**Before 500 A.D.**

**Egypt**

Zuckerman AJ: Palaeontology of smallpox. **Lancet** 1984 Dec 22;2(8417–18):1454

**1450–1700**

Zhu BZ: [History of the vaccination of human pox] (Chi). **Chung Hsi I Chieh Ho Tsa Chi** 1982 Oct;2(4):247–8

**Canada**

Jackes MK: Osteological evidence for smallpox: a possible case from seventeenth century Ontario. **Am J Phys Anthropol** 1983 Jan;60(1):75–81

**Switzerland**

Guess HA: Bernoulli's cost-benefit analysis of smallpox immunization. **N Engl J Med** 1981 Aug 6;305(6):347

**USSR**

Petrov BD: Trekhsotletie ukaza ob ospe (stranitsa istorii épidemiologii). **Zh Mikrobiol Epidemiol Immunobiol** 1981 Jun;(6):117–8

**1700 to Present**

Cambier J: De la mort de Louis XV à la vaccination du roi de Rome. **Nouv Presse Med** 1980 Jun 7;9(25):1746
Dittmann S: Die Welt ist pockenfrei--Durchführung und Erfolg eines grandiosen Programms. **Z Gesamte Inn Med** 1980 Dec 15;35(24):858–63
Fenner F: Smallpox and its eradication. In Stanley NF, Joske RA, ed: Changing disease patterns and human behaviour. London, New York, Academic Press, 1980. p. 215–29.
Ferrone V: Il dibattito su probabilità e scienze sociali nel secolo XVIII. **Physis** 1980;22(1):27–71
The global eradication of smallpox: Final report of the Global Commission for the certification of smallpox eradication, Geneva, December 1979. Geneva, World Health Organization, 1980. 122 p.
Hammarsten JF, Tattersall W, Hammarsten JE: Who discovered smallpox vaccination? Edward Jenner or Benjamin Jesty? **Trans Am Clin Climatol Assoc** 1979;90:44–55
Henderson DA: The deliberate extinction of a species. **Proc Am Philos Soc** 1982 Dec 17;126(6):461–71
Henderson DA: The history of smallpox eradication. In Lilienfeld AM, ed: Times, places, and persons. Baltimore, London, Johns Hopkins Univ. Press, 1980. (Sigerist suppl. to the Bull Hist Med. n.s., no 4) p. 99–108.
Keller F, Kirn A: Eradicazione mondiale del vaiolo. Da Sarah Nelmes a Ali Maow Maalin. **Minerva Med** 1980 Oct 20;71(40):2935–40
Nicol W: Exotic infectious diseases: smallpox. **R Soc Health J** 1980 Apr;100(2):41–7
Raska K: How the smallpox programme began. **World Health Forum** 1981;2:290–1
Ray JW, Polk HC: The history of smallpox: an old story of current significance. **J Ky Med Assoc** 1980 Apr;78(4):206–12
Rollet C: Variole et mortalité des enfants au XVIIIe siècle. **Cah Hist** 1978;23(4):417–36
Smeur EW, Smeur FA: 'Krijg de pokken' -- een overwonnen verwensing. **Tijdschr Ziekenverpl** 1980 May 20;33(11):515–7
Wehrle PF: A reality in our time--certification of the global eradication of smallpox. **J Infect Dis** 1980 Oct;142(4):636–8
White PJ, Shackelford PG: Edward Jenner, MD, and the scourge that was. **Am J Dis Child** 1983 Sep;137(9):864–9
Zhdanov VM, Slepushkin AN: Programma likvidatsii ospy vo vsem mire (istoriia razvitiia i rol' Sovetskogo Soiuza). **Vopr Virusol** 1980 Jul–Aug;(4):395–9
150e année: La variole et son éradication. Contributions by L. Justin-Besançon, R. Fasquelle, J. Fasquelle, L. Jacques. **J Med Chir Prat** 1979 Sep;17–18:629–708

**Africa**

Stewart L: The edge of utility: slaves and smallpox in the early eighteenth century. **Med Hist** 1985 Jan;29(1):54–70

Tulloch JL: The last 50 years of smallpox in Africa. **WHO Chron** 1980 Nov;34(11):407-12

**Asia**

Greenough PR: Variolation and vaccination in South Asia, c. 1700-1865: a preliminary note. **Soc Sci Med [Med Geogr]** 1980 Sep;14D(3):345-7

**Australia**

Campbell J: Smallpox in aboriginal Australia, 1829-31. **Hist Stud** 1983;20:536-56

**Canada**

Beahen W: Mob law could not prevail. **Alberta Hist** 1981;29(3):1-7
Bedford J: Prostitution in Calgary 1905-1914. **Alberta Hist** 1981;29(2):1-11
Craig B: Smallpox in Ontario: public and professional perceptions of disease, 1884-1885. In Roland CG, ed: Health, disease and medicine. Toronto, Hannah Institute for the History of Medicine, 1984. p. 215-49.
Gibson JR: Smallpox on the Northwest Coast. **BC Stud** 1982-83;(56):61-81
Spaulding WB: Smallpox control in the Ontario wilderness, 1880-1910. In Roland CG, ed: Health, disease and medicine. Toronto, Hannah Institute for the History of Medicine, 1984. p. 194-214.
Tunis B: Inoculation for smallpox in the Province of Quebec, a re-appraisal. In Roland CG, ed: Health, disease and medicine. Toronto, Hannah Institute for the History of Medicine, 1984. p. 171-93.
Tunis B: Public vaccination in Lower Canada, 1815-1823: controversy and a dilemma. **Hist Reflect** 1982;9(1-2):264-78

**Chile**

Casaretto CC: Juan Ignacio Molina (Huaraculén 1740 - Bolonia 1829), fundador de la patografia y de la autopatografia en Chile. **Rev Med Chil** 1979 Nov;107(11):1053-61
Costa-Casaretto C: La descripción de la viruela--su viruela--por el estudiante jesuita Juan Ignacio Molina (1761). **Rev Med Chil** 1979 Dec;107(12):1141-51

**Czechoslovakia**

Duka-Zólyomi N: Pozsonyi himlöjárványok és himlöhalálozaśok a 18. század végén (1786-1800). **Tort Stat Tanulm** 1977;3:325-48
Slavětínský M: Z historie poslední epidemie neštovic našich zemích. **Cesk Zdrav** 1980 Apr;28(4):172-4

**Europe**

Emch-Dériaz AS: L'inoculation justifiee-or was it? **Eighteenth Cent Life** 1982;7(2):65-72

**Finland**

Turpeinen O: Die Sterblichkeit an Pocken, Masern und Keuchhusten in Finnland in den Jahren 1751 bis 1865. In Imhof AE, ed: Mensch und Gesundheit in der Geschichte. Husum, Matthiesen, 1980. p. 135-61.

**France**

Beauchamp C: Les mécomptes d'un bienfait: sur la pratique de la vaccination au XIXe s. l'exemple du Loir-et-Cher. **Asclepio** 1983;35:389-402
Biraben JN: La diffusion de la vaccination en France au 19e siècle. **Ann Bretagne** 1979;86(3):265-76
Kaufmann C: La question de l'inoculation déférée à l'Eglise. **Asclepio** 1983;35:403-11
Peter JP: Les médecins français face au problème de l'inoculation variolique et de sa diffusion (1750-1790). **Ann Bretagne** 1979;86(3):251-64

**Germany**

Abe HR: Aus der Frühgeschichte der deutschen Impfgesetzgebung. **Z Gesamte Hyg** 1980;26(5):373-4

**Great Britain**

Baxby D: A death from inoculated smallpox in the English Royal Family. **Med Hist** 1984 Jul;28(3):303-7
Baxby D: Jenner's smallpox vaccine. The riddle of vaccinia virus and its origin. London, Heinemann Educational Books, 1981. xiv, 214 p.
Bendiner E: Jenner: from folklore to scientific triumph. **Hosp Pract [Off]** 1984 Apr;19(4):183-7, 190-1, 196, passim
Bonnabeau RC: Edward Jenner and the advent of vaccination. **Minn Med** 1983 May;66(5):331-3
Charlton C: The fight against vaccination: the Leicester demonstration of 1885. **Local Popul Stud (Matlock)** 1983 Spring;30:60-66
Cordasco F: Laughlin Macleane's Expediency of Inoculation (1756): a checklist of deposit locations. **Am Notes Queries** 1981 Jan-Feb;19(5/6):75
Fraser SM: Leicester and smallpox: the Leicester method **Med Hist** 1980 Jul;24(3):315-32
Gill M: Smallpox. **Midwife Health Visit Community Nurse** 1982 Nov;18(11):491-2
Guest-Gornall RG: Good servants are scarce. **Br Med J [Clin Res]** 1981 Dec 19;283(6307):1674-5
Hardy A: Smallpox in London: factors in the decline of the disease in the nineteenth century. **Med Hist** 1983 Apr;27(2):111-38
Kahn A: Highlights of the Adler Museum collections: the Jenner letter. **Adler Mus Bull** 1984 Jun;10(2):15-7
Luckin B: The decline of small pox and the demographic revolution of the eighteenth century. **Soc Hist (Lond)** 1977;(6):793-97
McHenry S: The pox upon her. **Aramco World Mag** 1980, 31(4):13-21
Macrae AD: Laboratory diagnosis of smallpox: role of the Virus Reference Laboratory, Colindale, 1947-70. **J Hyg (Lond)** 1982 Dec;89(3):399-407
Miller G: Edward Jenner letters in Baltimore, Maryland. In International Congress of the History of Medicine. 26th, Plovdiv, 1978. Actes du Congress. Sofia, 1981. Volume II. p. 157-9.
Miller G: Putting Lady Mary in her place: a discussion of historical causation. **Bull Hist Med** 1981 Spring;55(1):2-16
Perry CB: Edward Jenner. **Ear Nose Throat J** 1984 Dec;63(12):605-17
Razzell P: The conquest of smallpox: the impact of inoculation on smallpox mortality in eighteenth century England. Firle, Sussex, Caliban Books, 1977. x, 190 p.
Silverstein AM, Miller G: History of immunology. The royal experiment on immunity: 1721-1722. **Cell Immunol** 1981 Jul 1;61(2):437-47
Thomson WA: Rider Haggard and smallpox. **J R Soc Med** 1984 Jun;77(6):506-12
Wallace EM: The first vaccinator. Benjamin Jesty of Yetminster and Worth Matravers and his family. Wareham and Swanage (England), Anglebury-Bartlett, 1981. 20 p.

**Greece**

Marketos LJ: [Recent data on the inoculation against smallpox in the Ionian Islands] (Gre). **Mater Med Greca** 1981;9:104-9

**Hungary**

Csanak DF: Teleki József Szerepe egy XVIII. századi francia tudományos vitaban. **Szazadok** 1974;108(2):406-22
Réthy L: Medico-historical background of the possibility of introducing the compulsory and nation-wide immunization with combined vaccines in Hungary. **Ann Immunol hung** 1984;24:13-38

**India**

Reaching 'target zero': The story of smallpox eradication in India. **WHO Chron** 1979 Oct;33(10):359-63

**Italy**

Imerti AD: Vincenzo Catalani, Neapolitan Jacobin, jurist, reformer (1769-1843), with an appendix containing a translation of his work 'A digression on vaccination.' Lawrence, Kansas, Coronado Press, 1976. 155 p.

**Kenya**

Dawson MH: II. Disease and social change. Smallpox in Kenya, 1880-1920. **Soc Sci Med [Med Anthropol]** 1979 Dec;13B(4):245-50

**Liechtenstein**

Rheinberger R: Zum 200. Geburtstag von Landesphysikus Gebhard Schaedler. ein Liechtensteinischer Artzt als Pionier der Pockenschutzimpfung. **Jahrb Hist Ver Fuerst Liechtenstein** 1976;76:337-43

**Mexico**

Micheli A de: La viruela en la Nueva España. **Prensa Med Mex** 1979 Sep-Oct;44(9-10):201-7
Price R: Estado, iglesia, caridad y viruela: una crisis epidémica en la Ciudad de México 1797-98. **Bol Soc Mex Hist Filos Med** 1984 Mar;7(46):269-87
Price R: State church charity and smallpox: an epidemic crisis in the City of Mexico 1797-98. **J R Soc Med** 1982 May;75(5):356-7

**Netherlands**

Janssens U: Matthieu Maty and the adoption of inoculation for smallpox in Holland. **Bull Hist Med** 1981 Summer;55(2):246-56
Steendijk-Kuypers J: De Hoornse Geneeskundige Genootschappen en hun ijver ten aanzien van de vaccinatie in de 19de EEUW. **Tijdschr Geschied Geneeskd** 1982;5(3):105-14

**Spain**

Dowling J: Smallpox and literature in eighteenth-century Spain. **Stud Eighteenth Cent Cult** 1979;9:59–77
Riera J: Noticia de una epidemia segoviana de viruela (1740–1741). In: Sociedad Española de Historia de la Medicina. V Congreso Nacional. Madrid, 1977. **Asclepio** 1977;29:309–17

**Sudan**

Hartwig GW: Smallpox in the Sudan. **Int J Afr Hist Stud** 1981;14(1):5–33

**Sweden**

Brück C: Vaccination och smittskoppor--ett livs erfarenhet. **Nord Medicinhist Arsb** 1982;:122–36
Thulin L: 'Om koppors ympande'--ett vaccinationens förstadium i 1700-talets Sverige. **Nord Medicinhist Arsb** 1981;59–73

**Switzerland**

Bonard EC: Variole. **Rev Med Suisse Romande** 1980 Dec;100(12):1051–4

**United States**

Brasseaux CA: Acadians, Creoles, and the 1787 Lafourche smallpox outbreak. **Rev Louisiane-LA Rev** 1979;8(1):55–58
Cash P, Pine C: John Jeffries and the struggle against smallpox in Boston (1775–1776) and Nova Scotia (1776–1779). **Bull Hist Med** 1983;57(1):93–7
Cohen IB, ed: The life and scientific and medical career of Benjamin Waterhouse: with some account of the introduction of vaccination in America. 2 vols. New York, Arno Press, 1980. Reprints of various works. Various paginations.
Hauptman LM: Smallpox and American Indian; depopulation in colonial New York. **NY State J Med** 1979 Nov;79(12):1945–9
Kinney EL: Smallpox in Provincetown, Massachusetts, 1872–73. **J Hist Med Allied Sci** 1981 Jul;36(3):334–6
Michael JM, Bender TR: Fighting smallpox on the Texas border: an episode from PHS's proud past. **Public Health Rep** 1984 Nov–Dec;99(6):579–82
Morris JP: Smallpox inoculation in the American colonies, 1763–1783. **Md Hist** 1977;8:47–58
Moses RJ: Smallpox immunization in Alta California: a story based on José Estrada's 1821 postscript. **South Calif Q** 1979;61(2):125–45
Retsinas J: Smallpox vaccination: a leap of faith. **RI Hist** 1979;38(4):113–24
Schaeffer CE: Plains Kutenai: an ethnological evaluation. **Alberta Hist** 1982;30(4):1–9
Watterson J, ed: Poetic justice; or, an illfated epic by Thomas Burke. **NC Hist Rev** 1978;55(3):339–46
Wilson CE: The Boston inoculation controversy: a revisionist interpretation. **Journalism Hist** 1980;7(1):16–9, 40
Wygant LJ, ed: The Galveston smallpox quarantine camp in 1899. **Bookman** 1982;9(3):3–8
Zanjani SS: George Springmeyer and the quarantine rebellion of 1902: student revolt reaches the University of Nevada. **Nev Hist Soc Q** 1980;23(4):283–9

**USSR**

Griffiths J: Doctor Thomas Dimsdale, and smallpox in Russia. The variolation of the Empress Catherine the Great. **Bristol Med Chir J** 1984 Jan;99(369):14–6
Vasil'ev KG, Vasil'ev KK: K istorii likvidatsii natural'noĭ ospy v SSSR. **Vopr Virusol** 1982 Jan–Feb;(1):113–6

**Yugoslavia**

Kraljević M, Rasuhin-Vekić N, Weisz-Maleček R, et al: O razvoju vakcine i vakcinacije protiv variole (1890–1923). In: I simpozij o historiji mikrobiologije i imunologije u Hrvatskoj do 1923. godine. Zagreb, Jugoslavenskoj akademiji, 1973. p. 63–70.

## SPEECH DISORDERS

O'Neill YV: Speech and speech disorders in Western thought before 1600. Westport, Connecticut, Greenwood, 1980. xii, 246 p. (Contributions in medical history, No. 3).

### 1450–1700

Sheerin DJ: A Carolingian cure recovered: Erasmus' citation of Hucbald of St. Amand's Ecloga de caluis. **Bibl Hum Renaissance** 1980 Jan;42(1):167–71

### 1700 to Present

Rochford EB: Stutterers' practices: folk remedies and therapeutic intervention. **J Commun Disord** 1983 Sep;16(5):373–84
Wendler J, ed: 75 Jahre Phoniatrie. Festschrift zu Ehren von Hermann Gutzmann sen. Berlin. Humboldt Universität, 1980. 240 p.

**Czechoslovakia**

Krahulec I, Ambrušová L, Dresslerová I, et al: Desat rokov činnosti Foniatrického pracoviska na otolaryngologickej klinike FN v Bratislave. **Cesk Otolaryngol** 1984 Jun;33(3):195–9
Mátiková M: 30 rokov logopédie v zdravotníctve v Stredoslovenskom kraji. **Cesk Otolaryngol** 1984 Sep;33(5):313–5
Novák A: Doc. MUDr. Eva Sedláčková, csc., a československá foniatrie. **Cesk Otolaryngol** 1982 Apr;31(2):68–71
Sedláček K: Sedesáté výrocí založení československé foniatrie prof. MUDr. Miloslavem Seemanem, DrSc. **Cesk Otolaryngol** 1982 Apr;31(2):65–8

**France**

Michel J: Notice historique sur la création de l'orthophonie et de la phonologie par M. Colombat de l'Isère (1828). **J Fr Otorhinolaryngol** 1981 May;30(5):281–3

**Germany**

Becker KP, Sovák M: Lehrbuch der Logopädie. 2. Auflage. Königstein/Ts., Verlagsgruppe Athenäum, Hain, Scriptor, Hanstein, 1979. Historical section, p. 31–48.
Eggert GH: Wernicke's works on aphasia. The Hague, New York, Mouton, 1977. xiii, 307 p.

**Great Britain**

Rockey D: Speech disorder in nineteenth century Britain: the history of stuttering. London, Cromm Helm, 1980. 280 p.

**United States**

Bloom L: Notes for a history of speech pathology: an addendum. **Folia Phoniatr (Basel)** 1982 Nov–Dec;34(6):296–9
Matthews J: Twenty five years of Asha. **ASHA** 1984 Sep;26(9):39–40
Williams DE: Wendell Andrew Leroy Johnson. In Dictionary of American biography, 1961–1965. Suppl. 7, 1981. p. 395–6.
Zimmermann G, Liljeblad S, Frank A, et al: The Indians have many terms for it: stuttering among the Bannock-Shoshoni. **J Speech Hear Res** 1983 Jun;26(2):315–8

**USSR**

Hatfield FM: Analysis and remediation of aphasia in the U.S.S.R: the contribution of A. R. Luria. **J Speech Hear Disord** 1981 Nov;46(4):338–47

**Yugoslavia**

Jakopič B: Ob 80-letnici Centra za Rehabilitacijo Sluha in Govora v Ljubljani. **Kronika (Yugosl)** 1980;28(3):212–17

## SPONTANEOUS COMBUSTION

Harrison M: Fire from heaven: a study of spontaneous combustion in human beings. Rev. ed. New York, Methuen, 1978. xvi, 295 p.

### 1700 to Present

Moulin D de: Spontaneous human combustion. In: Congrès international d'histoire de la médecine, XXVe, Québec, 1976. Actes. Quebec, 1977. p. 570–8.

## SWEATING SICKNESS

### 1450–1700

**Austria**

Kühnel H: Das Auftreten des 'Englischen schweisses' in Osterreich 1529/30. **Jahrb Landeskd Niederoesterr** 1968–70;38:339–43

**Belgium**

Müller-Jahncke WD: Agrippa von Nettesheim in Antwerpen. Ein Beitrag zur Geschichte des 'Englischen Schweiss'. In Dilg P, et al., ed: Perspektiven der Pharmaziegeschichte. Graz, Austria, Akademische Druck- u. Verlagsanstalt, 1983. p. 243–68.

**Great Britain**

Walton MT: Stinking air, corrupt water, and the English Sweat: a footnote to the quality of life in fifteenth-century London.

**J Hist Med Allied Sci** 1981 Jan;36(1):67-8
Walton MT: Thomas Forestier and the 'False Lechys' of London. **J Hist Med Allied Sci** 1982 Jan;37(1):71-3
Wylie JA, Linn IJ: Observations upon the distribution and spread of the English sweating sickness (sudar anglicus) in Devon in 1551. **Devon Assoc Adv Sci** 1980;112:97-111
Wylie JA, Collier LH: The English sweating sickness (Sudor Anglicus): a reappraisal. **J Hist Med Allied Sci** 1981 Oct;36(4):425-45

### SYPHILIS

Corbin A: L'hérédosyphilis ou l'impossible rédemption: contribution à l'histoire de l'hérédité morbide. **Romantisme** 1981;31:131-49
Crosby AW: The early history of syphilis: a reappraisal. **Am Anthropol** 1969;71(2):218-27
Lambert M: Jan Fryderyk Knolle's forgotten dissertation on osseous syphilis, 1763. **Sex Transm Dis** 1984 Jan-Mar;11(1):36-40
Moeller DD: The odyssey of guaiac. **Am J Gastroenterol** 1984 Mar;79(3):236-7
Negru I: Informaţii asupra apariţiei şi răspîndirii luesului pe teritoriul Europei apusene. **Viata Med [Medii Sanit]** 1982 Jan;30(1):21-4
Schönfeld J: Zum Ursprung der Krankheitsbezeichnung 'Syphylis'. **Off Gesundheitswes** 1984 Feb;46(2):104-5
Tsouyopoulos N: Auf der Suche nach einer adäquaten Methode für die Geschichte und Theorie der Medizin. Auseinandersetzung mit Ludwik Flecks 'Entstehung und Entwicklung einer wissenschaftlichen Tatsache'. **Medizinhist J** 1982;17(1/2):20-36

**Europe**

Andreski S: The syphilitic shock: puritanism, capitalism, and a medical factor. **Encounter (Lond)** 1980;55(4):76-81

**France**

Burgun R, Laugier P: Die Geschichte der Syphilis in Strassburg. In Sournia JC, Martiny M, Poulet J, ed: Illustrierte Geschichte der Medizin. Salzburg, Andreas, 1980. Vol. 4. p. 1517-45.
Burgun R: Mesures de protection contre la lèpre et la syphilis à Strasbourg au cours des siècles. In Livet G, Schaff G, ed: Médecine et assistance en Alsace, XVIe-XXe siècle. Strasbourg, Istra, 1976. p. 53-67.

**Germany**

Heidel G: Zur wahrscheinlich ältesten deutschen Ubersetzung des Syphilisgedichtes von Girolamo Fracastoro. **Dermatol Monatsschr** 1983;169(2):130-5
Woeber K: Uber die historische Bedeutung der Bad Aachener Heilquellen für die Dermato-Venerologie. **Rehabilitation (Bonn)** 1981;34(3-4):17-25

**Italy**

Panconesi E, Mazzi MS: The day syphilis came. **Int J Dermatol** 1984 May;23(4):284-6
Waugh MA: Role played by Italy in the history of syphilis. **Br J Vener Dis** 1982 Apr;58(2):92-5

**Netherlands**

Van Lieburg MJ: De syfilitische patiënt in de geschiedenis van het Nederlandse ziekenhuiswezen vóór 1900. **Tijdschr Soc Geschied** 1982;8:156-79

#### 500 A.D.-1450

**Arabic**

Guerra F: The description of syphilis in Avicenna. In International Congress of the History of Medicine, 27th, Barcelona, 1980. Actas. Barcelona, Acadèmia de Ciències Mèdiques de Catalunya i Balears, 1981. p. 731-3.

#### 1450-1700

Andreski S: The syphilitic shock: a new explanation of the 'great witch craze' of the 16th and 17th centuries in the light of medicine and psychiatry. **Encounter (Lond)** 1982;58(5):7-26
Gariepy TP: Hyacum, et lues venerea. **J Hist Med Allied Sci** 1981 Jul;36(3):325
Vidal F: Le Gayac, panacée du XVIe siècle. **Chir Dent Fr** 1983 Nov 24;53(226):37-42
Zanca A: Il Mal Francese. **Kos** 1984 Feb;1(1):77-92

**Germany**

Eberle MW: Lucas Cranach's cupid as honey thief paintings: allegories of syphilis? **Com J Mediev Renaiss Stud** 1979-80;10:21-30

**Great Britain**

Kail AC: The bard and the body. 3. Venereal disease--'the pox'. **Med J Aust** 1983 Oct 29;2(9):445-9

**Italy**

Graziani R: Fracastoro's 'syphilis' and Priapus. **Clio Med** 1981 Dec;16(2/3):93-9
Mugnai Carrara D. Fra causalità astrologica e causalità naturale. Gli interventi di Nicolò Leoniceno e della sua scuola sul morbo gallico. **Physis** 1979;21(1-4):37-54

**Poland**

Dudziński W: Choroby zgon króla Jana Olbrachta. **Wiad Lek** 1981 Jul 1;34(13):1131-5

#### 1700 to Present

Crissey JT, Parish LC: The dermatology and syphilology of the nineteenth century. New York, Praeger, 1981. viii, 439 p.
Kampmeier RH: The continuous treatment of early syphilis by arsphenamin and heavy metals. **Sex Transm Dis** 1981 Jul-Sep;8(3):224-6
Kampmeier RH: The evolution of the flocculation screening test for syphilis. **Sex Transm Dis** 1983 Jul-Sep;10(3):156-9
Kampmeier RH: The introduction of penicillin for the treatment of syphilis. **Sex Transm Dis** 1981 Oct-Dec;8(4):260-5
Malamani A: Notizie sul mal francese e gli ospedali degli incurabili in età moderna. **Crit Stor** 1978,15.193-216
Rufli T: Lues-Serologie--gestern, heute und morgen. **Dermatologica** 1982 Oct;165(4):221-31
Starzycki Z: W 40 rocznice wprowadzenia penicyliny do leczenia kiły i rzeżaczki. **Przegl Lek** 1984;41(6):453-7

**Australia**

Gandevia B, Clasen U: James George Beaney: his authorship. **Med J Aust** 1981 Aug 8;2(3):160

**Bulgaria**

Goodman N: Congenital syphilis in the Burgas area in Bulgaria about 1930. A suppressed report of the health organisation of the League of Nations. In International Congress of the History of Medicine. 26th, Plovdiv, 1978. Actes du Congress. Sofia, 1981. Volume II. p. 168-70.

**Canada**

Leblond S: Le mal de la baie était-il syphilis? In: Congrès international d'histoire de la médecine, XXVe, Québec, 1976. Actes. Québec, 1977. p. 866-72.
Roland CG: Dr. James Bowman vs Canada: a struggle to obtain payment for government service. In: Congrès international d'histoire de la médecine, XXVe, Québec, 1976. Actes. Québec, 1977. p. 1158-69.

**France**

Dirckx JH: Voltaire on the pox. **Am J Dermatopathol** 1983 Dec;5(6):581-4
Kampmeier RH: Syphilis and marriage by Alfred Fournier. **Sex Transm Dis** 1981 Jan-Mar;8(1):29-32
Poulet J: La mort de Junot. **Rev Inst Napoleon (Paris)** 1972;(123):57-62
Studnitsin AA, Rukavishnikova VM: K 150-letiiu Zhana Al'freda Furn'e. **Vestn Dermatol Venerol** 1982 Apr;(4):75-7
Thieffry S: La découverte de la syphilis congénitale par Jules Parrot à l'Hospice des Enfants Assistés il y a un siècle. **Bull Acad Natl Med (Paris)** 1980 Nov;164(8):725-9

**Germany**

Fleck L: Genesis and development of a scientific fact. Edited by T. J. Trenn and R. K. Merton. Chicago, Univ. of Chicago Press, 1979. xxviii, 203 p.
Hayman R: Nietzsche's madness. **Partisan Rev** 1980;47(1):29-44
Kampmeier RH: Clarification of the systemic manifestations of syphilis, especially in the tertiary stage. **Sex Transm Dis** 1981 Apr-Jun;8(2):82-4
Kenéz J: H. Heine betegsége. Egy vita, mely a költ' ó halálának 125. évfordulója után sem zárult le. **Orv Hetil** 1982 May 16;123(20):1246-50
Klingmüller G: Treponema pallidum oder Spirochaeta pallida? **Hautarzt** 1983 Dec;34(12):628-31
Ovchinnikov NM: K 75-letiiu otkrytiia vozbuditelia sifilisa. **Vestn Dermatol Venerol** 1980 Mar;(3):74-8
Sons HU: Geschlechtskrankheiten während der Nachkriegszeit. Eine Untersuchung zur Epidemiologie der Gonorrhö und Lues und zur Reorganisation der Fürsorgeeinrichtungen in Nordrhein-Westfalen in den Jahren 1945-1949. **Med Welt** 1983 Oct 7;34(40):1124-6
Thorburn AL: Paul Ehrlich: pioneer of chemotherapy and cure by arsenic

(1854–1915). **Br J Vener Dis** 1983 Dec;59(6):404–5
Wehsarg FK: Die Quecksilber-Schmierkur in Bad Aachen als einstmalige Syphilistherapie. **Rehabilitation (Bonn)** 1981;34(3–4):26–32

**Great Britain**

Jackson R: Jonathan Hutchinson on syphilis. **Sex Transm Dis** 1980 Apr–Jun;7(2):90–6

**Hungary**

Szállási A: 150 éve született Tóth N. János, az elsö dualista magyar szifidológus. **Orv Hetil** 1984 Jun 10;125(24):1457–8

**India**

Sidkar JC: Phirangíroga (syphillis) and its management as described in Vaidyaka Samgraka, an old Gujarati manuscript of an unknown author (18th century A.D.). **Indian J Hist Sci** 1982;17(1):132–53

**Ireland**

Kampmeier RH: The introduction of iodine in the treatment of syphilis: the writings of William Wallace, M.D., of Dublin. **Sex Transm Dis** 1980 Jan–Mar;7(1):26–8
Shen WW, Soldo JJ: Symbol hunting in James Joyce's 'syphilizations'. **Arch Intern Med** 1981 Apr;141(5):691–2

**Mexico**

Arias O: Evolución natural de la sífilis y del mal del pinto. In Academia Nacional de Medicina. Libro conmemorativo del primer centenario. México, Comité Editorial de la Comisión Organizadora del Congreso del Centenario, 1964. Tome 2. p. 83–6.

**Poland**

Stapiński A: Kształtowanie się zapadalności na kiłę i rzeżączkęw Polsce w trzydziestoleciu 1948–1978. **Przegl Dermatol** 1979 Sep–Oct;66(5):507–12
Stapiński A: Powojenny wyż demograficzny a zapadalność na kiłę i rzeżączkę w Polsce. **Przegl Dermatol** 1979 Nov–Dec;66(6):667–72

**Spain**

Bräutigam W: Die Erkrankung Goyas von 1792. **Nervenarzt** 1980 Apr;51(4):233–8

**Sweden**

Bologa VL: Nils Rosen Rosenstein über die Erbsyphilis. **Acta Hist Rerum Nat Tech** 1972;6:77–82
Wikström-Haugen I: Syphilis in Sweden about 1800. In International Congress of the History of Medicine, 27th, Barcelona, 1980. Actas. Barcelona, Académia de Ciències Médiques de Catalunya i Balears, 1981. p. 690–9.

**United States**

Arnold HL: Landmark perspective: penicillin and early syphilis. **JAMA** 1984 Apr 20;251(15):2011–2
Fiumara NJ: A restrospective approach to syphilis in the 1970s. **Int J Dermatol** 1982 Sep;21(7):400–3
Jones JH: Bad blood: the Tuskegee syphilis experiment. New York, Free Press; London, Collier Macmillan; 1981. xii, 272 p.
Kennedy JW: Introduction of penicillin in syphilotherapy. **Ariz Med** 1982 Nov;39(11):730, 735
Lederer SE: 'The right and wrong of making experiments on human beings': Udo J. Wile and syphilis. **Bull Hist Med** 1984 Fall;58(3):380–97
Shick TW: Race, class, and medicine: 'Bad Blood' in twentieth-century America. **J Ethn Stud** 1982;10(2):97–105
Turner TB: Joseph Earle Moore. In Dictionary of American Biography, Suppl. 6, 1956–1960. p, 460–1, 1980.

### TETANUS

**Americas**

Bergoglio RM: Tétanos neonatorum. Intentos históricos de su prevención en América Latina. **Medicina (B Aires)** 1982;42 Suppl 1:77–81

**1450–1700**

**Denmark**

Andersen S: Simon Paulli. Betaenkning over en Kongelig Ridehest. **Dan Medicinhist Arbog** 1979;9–97

**1700 to Present**

Collacott RA: Neonatal tetanus in St. Kilda. **Scott Med J** 1981 Jul;26(3):224–7

**Denmark**

Johnsen B: Miasmer eller kontagion. Ginklofi (tetanus neonatorum) på Vestmannöerne og dr Peter Anton Schleisners indsats i dens bekaempelse. **Nord Medicinhist Arsb** 1982;:162–70

**France**

Gilbrin E: Gaston Ramon (1886–1963). Le soixantième anniversaire des anatoxines. **Hist Sci Med** 1984;18(1):53–60

**Poland**

Caban J: Znaczenie badań nad tężcem J. K. Kostrzewskiego po dwudziestu latach. **Przegl Epidemiol** 1980;34(2):191–2

**United States**

Miller EB: Comparative medicine: American experience with equine tetanus - from Benjamin Rush to Toxoid. **Bull Hist Med** 1983;57(1):81–92

### THYROID

Ljunggren JG: Vem var mannen bakom syndromet: ismail al-jurjani, testa, flagani, parry, graves eller basedow? **Lakartidningen** 1983 Aug 10;80(32–33):2902

**1700 to Present**

Landau RL: Landmark perspective: treatment of hyperthyroidism. **JAMA** 1984 Apr 6;251(13):1747–8
Maluf NS: Owen's gland. **Sudhoffs Arch** 1980;64(1):25–54

**Finland**

Wahlberg P: Tyreoidologi i Finland under 150 år. **Nord Medicinhist Arsb** 1984;:105–16

**Great Britain**

Carter L: Snatching the thyroid. **Nurs Times** 1984 Mar 7–13;80(10):38
Kessler RK, Kessler WB, Constantine J, et al: Sclerosis of thyroid cysts. **Arch Intern Med** 1984 Aug;144(8):1693, 1697

**United States**

Harvey AM: David Marine: America's pioneer thyroidologist. **Am J Med** 1981 Mar;70(3):483–5

### TONSILLITIS

**500 A.D.–1450**

**Arabic**

Kataye S: L'amygdalectomie dans la médecine arabe. **Hist Sci Med** 1979;13(4):419–25

**1700 to Present**

**Denmark**

Agård S: Mandlernes historie 1953–1983. **Sygeplejersken** 1984 Mar 21;84(12):23–4

**France**

Herrera Casado A: Aportación francesa a la amigdalectomiá. **An Otorrinolaringol Ibero Am** 1981;8(6):487–94

**United States**

Catlin FI: Pulmonary complications of tonsillectomy as originally described by Samuel J. Crowe, M.D. **Laryngoscope** 1981 Jan;91(1):52–61

### TOXOPLASMOSIS

**1700 to Present**

**Africa**

Leyva Corzo A: Toxoplasmosis: resumen histórico y revisión bibliográfica.

Rev Cubana Med Trop 1979 May-Aug;31(2):141-58

**Mexico**

Ruiloba J: Listeriosis, toxoplasmosis y leptospirosis. In Academia Nacional de Medicina. Libro conmemorativo del primer centenario. México, Comité Editorial de la Comisión Organizadora del Congreso del Centenario, 1964. Tome 2. p. 532-5.

## TREPONEMAL INFECTIONS

**United States**

Elting JJ, Starna WA: A possible case of pre-Columbian treponematosis from New York State. **Am J Phys Anthropol** 1984 Nov;65(3):267-73

### Before 500 A.D.

El-Najjar MY: Human treponematosis and tuberculosis: evidence from the New World. **Am J Phys Anthropol** 1979 Nov;51(4):599-618

### 500 A.D.-1450

**United States**

Gregg JB, et al: Possible treponematosis in fourteenth century Dakota territory: a progress report. **Paleopathol Newsl** 1981 Jun;34:5-6

### 1700 to Present

Kampmeier RH: The demonstration of the immobilizing antibody for treponema pallidum (TPI test). **Sex Transm Dis** 1983 Oct-Dec;10(4):205-7

**Czechoslovakia**

Pospíšil L: K prioritě objevu specifické imobilizace treponém. **Cesk Dermatol** 1981 Oct;56(5):346-8

**Zambia**

Lowenthal MN: The yaws notebook of Dr. Acheson. **Trans R Soc Trop Med Hyg** 1982;76(5):627-9

## TRICHINOSIS

### 1700 to Present

**Great Britain**

Campbell WC: History of trichinosis: Paget, Owen and the discovery of Trichinella Spiralis. **Bull Hist Med** 1979 Winter;53(4):520-52

**Poland**

Adonajło A: Włośnica. **Przegl Epidemiol** 1980;34(2):213-5

**Spain**

Báguena Cervellera J, Gener Galbis C: La triquinosis en la España del siglo XIX a través de la obra de Antonio Suárez: de las trichinas y de la trichinosis en España. **Med Hist (Barc)** 1984;3:1-26

## TRYPANOSOMIASIS

### 1700 to Present

**Africa**

Ford J: Ideas which have influenced attempts to solve the problems of African trypanosomiasis. **Soc Sci Med [Med Anthropol]** 1979 Dec;13B(4):269-75

Lambrecht FL: Notes on the history of sleeping sickness. **Botsw Notes Rec** 1968;1:41-9

Musambachime MC: The social and economic effects of sleeping sickness in Mweru-Luapula 1906-1922. **Afr Econ Hist** 1981;10:151-73

Saragba M: Histoire de la trypanosomiase ou maladie du sommeil en Oubangui-Chari (R. C. A.) de 1910 à 1950. 2 tomes. Thèse de doct., 3e cycle. Université de Provence, 1983. 630, 85 p.

**Americas**

Brumpt L: Epidémiologie de la maladie de Chagas. **Bull Acad Natl Med (Paris)** 1980 Nov;164(8):782-5

**Brazil**

Bergoglio RM: En el centenario del nacimiento de Carlos Chagas. **Rev Fac Cien Med Univ Nac Cordoba** 1981 Jan-Dec;39(1-4):87-9

Lewinsohn R: Carlos Chagas and the discovery of Chagas' disease (American trypanosomiasis). **J R Soc Med** 1981 Jun;74(6):451-5

**Burundi**

Perich P: Les foyers de trypanosomiase humaine africaine à Trypanosoma rhodesiense (vecteur Glossina morsitans) au Burundi. Aspects historiques et actuels. **Med Trop (Mars)** 1982 Jan-Feb;42(1):33-41

**Great Britain**

Bernstein RE: Darwin's illness: Chagas' disease resurgens. **J R Soc Med** 1984 Jul;77(7):608-9

Castagnino HE, Thompson AC: Sufrió Darwin la enfermedad de Chagas? **Medicina (B Aires)** 1981;41(2):263-4

**Ivory Coast**

Domergue D: La lutte contre la trypanosomiase en Côte d'Ivoire, 1900-1945. **J Afr Hist** 1981;22(1):63-72

**Zaire**

Burke J, Mortelmans J: Rol van België in de strijd tegen de slaapziekte en de dierlijke trypanosomiases en hun studie. **Bull Seances Acad R Sci Outre Mer** 1980 Suppl.;1:111-35

## TUBERCULOSIS

Addison NV: Abdominal tuberculosis--a disease revived. **Ann R Coll Surg Engl** 1983 Mar;65(2):105-11

Arnold E: La lutte contre la tuberculose. **Rev Med Swisse Romande** 1982 Mar;102(3):231-9

Geschichte der Tuberkulose - philatelistisch illustriert: **MMW** 1982 Apr 23;124(16):92-3

Hahn S: Der 'Lübecker Totentanz' (1930), ein Beispiel für ethische Debatten zum Problem der Tuberkulose. **Wiss Beitr Martin Luther Univ Halle Wittenberg** 1983;5-R80:91-8

Haneveld GT: Pott's disease before Pott. **Neth J Surg** 1980;32(1):2-7

Hirsch B: Geschichte der Nierentuberkulose. Köln, 1983. 183 p. (Kölner medizinhistorische Beiträge, Band 28)

Kalich R: Aktuelle Ergebnisse auf dem Gebiet der Resistenzbestimmung von Mykobakterien. **Z Erkr Atmungsorgane** 1983;161(1):80-5

Kühne W: Probleme der Pathogeneses und der Pathologie der Tuberkulose einst und jetzt. **Z Erkr Atmungsorgane** 1982;158(1-2):36-46

Oury M: Geschichte der Tuberkulose. In Sournia JC, Martiny M, Poulet J, ed: Illustrierte Geschichte der Medizin. Salzburg, Andreas, 1980. Vol. 8. p. 2827-47.

Pacheco CR, Quijano-Pitman F, Kuthy-Porter J, et al: Centenario del descubrimiento del bacilo de la tuberculosis. **Gac Med Mex** 1982 Nov;118(11):439-48

Reimers D: Tuberkulose und Kunst. **Med Welt** 1982 Mar 26;33(12):435-41

Sersiron G: La croix à double barre, symbole de l'UICT. Quelques informations sur ses origines. **Bull Int Union Tuberc** 1982 Sep-Dec;57(3-4):196-9

Warring FC: A brief history of tuberculosis. **Conn Med** 1981 Mar;45(3):177-85

Yáñez A, Vargas M: La tuberculosis en el mundo, historia antigua, problema actual. **Salud Publica Mex** 1982 May-Jun;24(3):261-7

**Africa**

Hunter JM, Thomas MO: Hypothesis of leprosy, tuberculosis and urbanization in Africa. **Soc Sci Med** 1984;19(1):27-57

**Americas**

Pfeiffer S: Paleopathology in an Iroquoian ossuary, with special reference to tuberculosis. **Am J Phys Anthropol** 1984 Oct;65(2):181-9

**Germany**

Koch T: Gedanken zur 100. Wiederkehr des Tages der Entdeckung des Tuberkuloseerregers durch Robert Koch. **Gegenbaurs Morphol Jahrb** 1982;128(1):1-11

**Great Britain**

Batty Shaw A: Knappers' rot; silicosis in East Anglian flint-knappers. **Med Hist** 1981 Apr;25(2):151-68

## DISEASES AND INJURIES

**Japan**

Iwasaki T: [History of tuberculosis in Japan--tuberculosis transmitted by Europeans?] (Jpn). **Kekkaku** 1981 Aug;56(8):407–22

**South Africa**

Collins TF: The history of southern Africa's first tuberculosis epidemic. **S Afr Med J** 1982 Nov 13;62(21):780–8

**United States**

Smith CM: Control of tuberculosis in Delaware: an historical perspective on joint public and private involvement. **Del Med J** 1983 Oct;55(10):593–7

**Before 500 A.D.**

El-Najjar MY: Human treponematosis and tuberculosis: evidence from the New World. **Am J Phys Anthropol** 1979 Nov;51(4):599–618

**Americas**

Buikstra JE: Prehistoric tuberculosis in the Americas. Evanston, Northwestern University, Archeological Program, 1981. xii, 182 p.

**500 A.D.–1450**

**Arabic**

Sharma OA: Avicenna's description of tuberculosis. **Bull Indian Inst Hist Med (Hyderabad)** 1981;1–4:83–6

**Switzerland**

Ulrich-Bochsler S, Schäublin E, Zeltner TB, et al: Invalidisierende Wirbelsäulenverkrümmung an einem Skelettfund aus dem Frühmittelalter (7./8. bis Anfang 9. Jh.). Ein Fall einer wahrscheinlichen Spondylitis tuberculosa. **Schweiz Med Wochenschr** 1982 Sep 18;112(38):1318–23

**1450–1700**

Rosner E: Hohenheims Bergsuchtmonographie. **Medizinhist J** 1981;16(1–2):20–52

**France**

Bernier JJ, Chevallier P, Teysseire D, et al: La maladie de Louis XIII. Tuberculose intestinale ou maladie de Crohn? **Nouv Presse Med** 1981 Jun 20;10(27):2243, 2247–50

Goldfischer S, Janis M: A 42-year-old king with a cavitary pulmonary lesion and intestinal perforation. **Bull NY Acad Med** 1981 Mar;57(2):139–43

**Great Britain**

Keers RY: Richard Morton (1637–98) and his Phthisiologia. **Thorax** 1982 Jan;37(1):26–31

**Poland**

Dudziński W: Choroby i zgon króla Zygmunta Augusta. **Wiad Lek** 1981 Aug 15;34(16):1411–6

**Sweden**

Dahlström G: Johannes Raicus' tankar om lungsoten. **Nord Medicinhist Arsb** 1984;:63–70

**USSR**

Al'tshular NS, Mikhaĭlov FA: Pervaia otechestvennaia dissertatsiia po tuberkulezu. **Probl Tuberk** 1983 May;(5):70–2

**1700 to Present**

Bignall JR: A century of treating tuberculosis. **Tubercle** 1982 Mar;63(1):19–22

Bulla A: Revue de la morbidité et de la mortalité par tuberculose d'après les données officiellement rapportées dans le monde (1967–1971–1977). **Bull Int Union Tuberc** 1981 Sep–Dec;56(3–4):122–8

Burke G, Richardson P: The profits of death: a comparative study of miners' phthisis in Cornwall and the Transvaal, 1876–1918. **J South Afr Stud** 1978;4(2):147–71

Collins JJ: The contribution of medical measures to the decline of mortality from respiratory tuberculosis: an age-period-cohort model. **Demography** 1982 Aug;19(3):409–27

Dubb A: Medical philately: Robert Koch (1843–1910) the man, his germ and history. **Adler Mus Bull** 1984 Mar;10(1):16–22

Dubovsky H: Tuberculosis and art. **S Afr Med J** 1983 Nov 12;64(21):823–6

Forschbach G: Tuberculosis and creative man. **Bull Int Union Tuberc** 1984 Mar–Jun;59(1–2):104–7

Genschorek W: Robert Koch. Selbstloser Kampf gegen Seuchen und Infektionskrankheiten. Leipzig, Hirzel, 1981. 224 p. (Hervorragende Arzte im Dienste des Menschen).

Girstenbrey W: Robert Koch und sein Erbe. Bedingungen, Konsequenzen und aktuelle Bedeutung einer historischen Leistung für Medizin und Gesundheitspolitik. **Fortschr Med** 1982 Mar 25;100(12):541, 544–6

Grange JM: Koch's Tubercle Bacillus - a centenary reappraisal. **Zentralbl Bakteriol Mikrobiol Hyg [A]** 1982 Mar;251(3):297–307

Grellet I, Kruse C: Histoires de la tuberculose. Les fièvres de l'âme 1800–1940. Paris, Ramsay, 1983. 333 p.

Hinshaw HC: The dawn of chemotherapy of tuberculosis. **Indian J Chest Dis Allied Sci** 1982 Apr–Sep;24(2–3):179–83

Kaiser W, Hübner H, ed: Robert Koch (1843–1910). **Wiss Beitr Martin Luther Univ Halle Wittenberg** 1983;5–R80:3–321

Kanai O: [Chemotherapy for tuberculosis--experimental studies over the past 100 years. (1) Development of chemotherapy] (Jpn) **Kekkaku** 1982 Dec;57(12):643–51

Kenéz J: Results in drug treatment of tuberculosis (historical survey). **Ther Hung** 1982;30(3):151–5

Knolle H: Zur Pathomorphologie der Tuberkulose Erwachsener in der Gegenwart. **Wiss Beitr Martin Luther Univ Halle Wittenberg** 1983;5–R80:129–44

Kunovskiĭ BV, Bachinskiĭ IuS, Soroka AN: K 100-letiiu otkrytiia vozbuditelia tuberkuleza. **Med Sestra** 1983 Feb;42(2):54–6

Lambrecht G: Die Perikarditis-tuberkulosa-Diagnostik im ausgehenden 19. Jahrhundert. **Wiss Beitr Martin Luther Univ Halle Wittenberg** 1983;5–R80:117–22

Landi S: Production and standardization of tuberculin (a brief history). **Indian J Chest Dis Allied Sci** 1982 Apr–Sep;24(2–3):78–87

Leff A, Lester TW, Addington WW: Tuberculosis. A chemotherapeutic triumph but a persistent socioeconomic problem. **Arch Intern Med** 1979 Dec;139(12):1375–7

Lock W: Die Schwerpunktbekämpfung der Tuberkulose im endemischen Stadium. **Z Erkr Atmungsorgane** 1983;161(1):100–2

Mercer AJ: Risk of dying from tuberculosis or cancer: further aspects of a possible association. **Int J Epidemiol** 1981 Dec;10(4):377–80

Michetti D: L'évolution des traitements de la tuberculose. **Rev Med Swisse Romande** 1982 Mar;102(3):227–9

Middlebrook G: Tuberculosis and medical science. **Am Rev Respir Dis** 1982 Mar;125(3 pt 2):4–7

Murken AH: Heilanstalten für Tuberkulöse. Zur Geschichte der Lungensanatorien und ihrer Therpiekonzeption im 19. Jahrhundert. In Göpfert W, Otten HH, ed: Metavoeite: wandelt euch durch neues Denken. Düsseldorf, Triltsch, 1983. p. 107–24.

Németh T, Nyárády I, Vadász I: A gümökór epidemiológiai helyzete a világban és hazánkban (1882–1982). **Orv Hetil** 1983 May 29;124(22):1309–12

Ober WB: Ghon but not forgotten: Anton Ghon and his complex. **Pathol Annu** 1983;18 (pt 2):79–85

Reimers D: Die interne Behandlung der Tuberkulose. **Prax Klin Pneumol** 1982 Nov;36(11):475–8

Riley RL: The contagiosity of tuberculosis. **Schweiz Med Wochenschr** 1983 Jan 22;1113(3):75–9

Rothe J, Werner K, Kaiser W: Sozialhygienische Konsequenzen aus der Klärung der Tuberkulose-Atiologie durch Robert Koch. **Z Gesamte Hyg** 1982 Mar;28(3):176–9

Rouillon A: The International Union against Tuberculosis. **Tubercle** 1982 Dec;63(4):247–53

Saueressig H: Die Tuberkulose als Paradigma des Lebensgefühls. **Med Welt** 1982 Mar 26;33(12):428–34

Schadewaldt H, Naumann P, Dopp C: 100 Jahre Tuberkelbakterien-Färbung. **Dtsch Med Wochenschr** 1982 Jun 25;107(25):963–6

Schneeweiss U: Die Bedeutung der Entdeckung der Tuberkelbakterien für die Immunitäts- und Krankheitslehre. **Padiatr Grenzgeb** 1982;21(2):127–40

Schoefer G: Die chirurgische Behandlung der Lungentuberkulose. **Zentralbl Chir** 1982;107(5–6):285–94

Shimamura K: [Chronological review of TB research - from a clinical viewpoint.] (Jpn). **Kekkaku** 1980;55:383–8

Sighart H: Die Behandlung der Tuberkulose vor Einführung der Chemotherapie. Pulmologisches Zentrum Stadt Wien/Osterreich. **Z Erkr Atmungsorgane** 1983;161(1):56–60

Sontag S: Illness as metaphor. New York, Farrar, Straus and Giroux, 1978. 87 p.

Tait HP: Two tuberculosis anniversaries. **Practitioner** 1980 Oct;224(1348):1101–3

Tetzner W: Die Prognose und Behandlung der Tuberkulose in der vorchemotherapeutischen Ara. **Z Erkr Atmungsorgane** 1982;158(1–2):149–54

Weingärtner L: Die Tuberkulose im Kindesalter -- Rückblick und

Ausblick (100 Jahre seit Entdeckung der Tuberkelbakterien) durch Robert Koch. **Padiatr Grenzgeb** 1982;21(2):113–26
Wurbs W: Zur Klinik der Tuberkulose Erwachsener in der Gegenwart. **Wiss Beitr Martin Luther Univ Halle Wittenberg** 1983;5–R80:145–59

### Algeria

Ait Khaled N, Oussedik N, Chaulet P: Evolution du coût des médicaments antituberculeux de 1964 à 1980; son influence dans le choix d'une politique de traitement de la tuberculose en Algérie. **Bull Int Union Tuberc** 1981 Sep–Dec;56(3–4):170–4

### Australia

Walker R: The struggle against pulmonary tuberculosis in Australia, 1788–1950. **Hist Stud** 1983;20:439–61

### Austria

Ebner H: Die Lungenabteilung des Pflegeheimes der Stadt Wien–Lainz im Wandel der Zeit. **Wien Med Wochenschr** 1980 Feb 29;130(4):147–8
Hurst LC: What was wrong with Anna O? **J R Soc Med** 1982 Feb;75(2):129–31

### Brazil

Montenegro TH: A tuberculose na vida e obra de Manuel Bandeira. **Interam Rev Bibliogr** 1969;19(3):278–300

### Canada

Gale GL: The changing years. The story of Toronto Hospital and the fight against tuberculosis. Toronto, West Park Hospital, 1979. xvii, 134 p.
Gale GL: Tuberculosis in Canada: a century of progress. **Can Med Assoc J** 1982 Mar 1;126(5):526–9
Hidgson C: The social and political implications of tuberculosis among native Canadians. **Can Rev Sociol Anthropol** 1982;19(4):502–12
McCuaig K: 'From social reform to social service': the changing role of volunteers: the anti-tuberculosis campaign, 1900–30. **Can Hist Rev** 1980;61(4):480–501
McCuaig K: Tuberculosis: the changing concepts of the disease in Canada 1900–1950. In Roland CG, ed: Health, disease and medicine. Toronto, Hannah Institute for the History of Medicine, 1984. p. 296–307.
McGinnis JP: Records of tuberculosis in Calgary. **Archivaria** 1980;10:173–89
McGinnis JP: The white plague in Calgary: sanatarium care in southern Alberta. **Alberta Hist** 1980;28(4):1–15

### Chile

Edwards A, Yerkovic L, Santamaría J: La tuberculosis y el Hospital San José de Santiago. **Rev Med Chil** 1983 Mar;111(3):315–9

### China

Hsu-Yu H: 100 Jahre Bekämpfung der Tuberkulose in China. Eine historische Kurzübersicht. **Prax Klin Pneumol** 1982 Mar;36(3):116–21

### Czechoslovakia

Beniak M: Sociálna podmienenost tuberkulózy na Slovensku pred prvou svetovou vojnou. **Bratisl Lek Listy** 1984 Mar;81(3):376–81
Feuereisl R: 30 years of the Research Institute of Tuberculosis and Respiratory Diseases in Prague. **Czech Med** 1983;6(4):193–5
Fox W: Přerušovaná chemoterapie plicní tuberkulózy. Se zvláštním zřetelem k přínosu Střediska SZO spolupracujícím na chemoterapii tuberkulózy v Praze. **Cas Lek Cesk** 1984 Feb 10;123(6):153–7
Linkesch W, Urge L, Lukac J, et al: Zur Geschichte der Tuberkulosebekämpfung in der CSSR: die ost-slowakischen Mykobakteriologie–Tbk–Seminare in Vysne Hagy und in Presov. **Wiss Beitr Martin Luther Univ Halle Wittenberg** 1983;5–R80:287–99
Slavětínský M: Poznámky k minulosti boje s TBC na Moravě. **Vnitr Lek** 1980;26(5):515–6

### Denmark

Holder FL: Søren Kierkegaard's final illness and death. **Anglican Theol Rev** 1979;61(4):508–14

### Europe

Styblo K, Sutherland I: Epidémiologie de la tuberculose chez l'enfant. **Bull Int Union Tuberc** 1982 Jun;57(2):134–41

### France

Anastasatu C: 200 de ani de la naşterea lui Laennec. **Rev Ig [Pneumoftiziol]** 1981 Oct–Dec;30(4):250–1
Bishop PJ: Laennec: a great student of tuberculosis. **Tubercle** 1981 Jun;62(2):129–34
Ferru M: La faillite du BCG. Poitiers, Ferru, 1977. 274 p.
Knibiehler Y: La 'lutte antituberculeuse,' instrument de la médicalisation des classes populaires (1870–1930). **Ann Bretagne** 1979;86(3):321–36
Lert F: Emergence et devenir du système de prise en charge de la tuberculose en France entre 1900 et 1940. **Soc Sci Med** 1982;16(23):2073–82
Meindl JL, Meindl CO: Tuberculous meningitis in the 1830s. **Lancet** 1982 Mar 6;1(8271):554–5
Mikhaĭlov FA: Rene Teofil' Giatsint Laénnek (1781–1826). **Klin Med (Mosk)** 1981 Dec;59(12):92–5
Pascal JN: Bordeu, Bouvart et Rostain: trois médecins face à la tuberculose in 1772 (documents inédits). In J. Proust, ed: Recherches nouvelles sur quelques érivains des lumières (II). Montpellier, Univ. Paul Valéry, 1979. p. 63–71.
Percebois G: Jean-Antoine Villemin, Vosgien de Prey, et la notion de contagiosité de la tuberculose. **Ann Med Nancy** 1979;18:685–98
Roda JJ: Histoire de la fondation du premier sanatorium populaire français. Ses origines et ses vingt-cinq premières années d'existence (Sanatorium Mangini Hauteville). Thèse. Lyon I, 1976. 85 p.

### Germany

Algeorge G: La 100 de ani de la descoperirea de către Robert Koch a agentului etiologic al tuberculozei. **Rev Ig [Pneumoftiziol]** 1982 Jan–Mar;31(1):13–7
Allen BW, Hinkes WF: La coloration de Koch pour les bacilles de la tuberculose. **Bull Int Union Tuberc** 1982 Sep–Dec;57(3–4):194–6
Anastasatu C: Centenarul descoperirii bacilului Koch. **Rev Ig [Pneumoftiziol]** 1982 Jan–Mar;31(1):1–3
Benison S: Celebration and history: the centenary of Robert Koch's discovery of the tubercle bacillus. **Bull Hist Med** 1982 Summer;56(2):157–9
Centennial: Koch's discovery of the tubercle bacillus: **MMWR** 1982 Mar 19;31(10):121–3
Centennial of Koch's bacillus: **NZ Med J** 1982 Jun 9;95(709):384
Daniel TM: Robert Koch, tuberculosis, and the subsequent history of medicine. **Am Rev Respir Dis** 1982 Mar;125(3 Pt 2):1–3
Ebling FJ, Ebling E: The contribution of Paul Langerhans (1847–1888) to tuberculosis research. **Wiss Beitr Martin Luther Univ Halle Wittenberg** 1983;5–R80:261–72
Etiología de la tuberculosis: Dr. Roberto Koch: **Salud Publica Mex** 1982 May–Jun;24(3):241–57
Eule H: Die Auswirkung der Entdeckung und der Arbeiten Robert Kochs auf die Entwicklung der Therapie der Tuberkulose. **Z Erkr Atmungsorgane** 1982;158(1–2):155–62
Ferrari Sacco A, Oliaro T: A cent'anni dalla scoperta del micobatterio della tbc. (1822–1982). Robert Koch autore della grande scoperta. **Minerva Med** 1982 Sep 8;73(34):2199–202
Findeisen DG: Tuberkulose und Allergie. Erkenntnisschritte von der Entdeckung des Mycobacterium tuberculosis durch Robert Koch (24 März 1882). Zu einer umfassenden Immundiagnostik, Immuntherapie und Immunprophylaxe. **Allerg Immunol (Leipz)** 1982;28(1):3–12
Freerksen E: Die Atiologie der Tuberkulose--Der Weg dahin und die Folgen. **Prax Klin Pneumol** 1982 Mar;36(3):122–34
Grange JM, Bishop PJ: 'Uber Tuberkulose'. A tribute to Robert Koch's discovery of the tubercle bacillus, 1882. **Tubercle** 1982 Mar;63(1):3–17
Hahn S: Schwerpunkte ethischer Diskussionsentwicklung um die Tuberkulose-Bekämpfung in fachwissenschaftlichen Veröffentlichungen von 1900 bis 1932. **Z Gesamte Hyg** 1982 Mar;28(3):193–201
Hanson LA, Kallós P: Host parasite relationships in gram-negative infections. **Prog Allergy** 1983;33:1–8
Henderson AR: A centennial remembrance of Koch's discovery of the tubercle bacillus. **Md State Med J** 1982 May;31(5):47–51
Hidvégi J: Marx Károly betegsége és halála. **Orv Hetil** 1983 Mar 6;124(10):589–91
Hillerdal O: Robert Koch och hans 100–årsjubileer. **Nord Medicinhist Arsbok** 1983;:127–34
Kaiser W: Robert Koch und die Entdeckung des Tuberkulose-Erregers. **Wiss Beitr Martin Luther Univ Halle Wittenberg** 1983;5–R80:31–9
Kaiser W: Vor 100 Jahren beschrieb Robert Koch den Tuberkulose-Erreger. **Z Gesamte Inn Med** 1982 Mar 1;37(5):137–44
Karasszon D: Robert Kochs Forschungen zur Rinder-Tuberkulose. **Wiss Beitr Martin Luther Univ Halle Wittenberg** 1983;5–R80:111–6
Kattentidt B: Erinnerungen eines alten Tuberkulosearztes. **Prax Klin Pneumol** 1982 Sep;36(9):404–7
Koch HT: Wilhelm Reil-Bey (1820–1880) und die Klimabehandlung der Tuberkulose. **Wiss Beitr Martin Luther Univ Halle Wittenberg** 1983;5–R80:251–60
Koch R: Classics in infectious diseases. The etiology of tuberculosis: Robert Koch. Berlin, Germany, 1882. **Rev Infect Dis** 1982 Nov–Dec;4(6):1270–4
Koch centennial supplement: 100th anniversary of the announcement of

the discovery of the tubercle bacillus by Robert Koch, March 24, 1882. **Am Rev Respir Dis** 1982 Mar;125(3 pt 2):1-132
Kochemasova ZN, Dykhno MM, Dorozhkova IR, et al: L-transformatsiia kak odin iz faktorov izmenchivosti vozbuditelia tuberkuleza (k 100-letiiu otkrytiia vozbuditelia tuberkuleza). **Sov Med** 1983;(3):20-3
Kochemasova ZN, Dykhno MM, Dorozhkova IR, et al: 100-letie so dnia otkrytiia R. Kokhom vozbuditelia tuberkuleza. **Klin Med (Mosk)** 1982 Nov;60(11):115-7
Koch's bacillus: **Tubercle** 1982 Mar;63(1):1-2
Krause AK: Introduction à l'étiologie de la tuberculose. **Bull Int Union Tuberc** 1981 Sept-Dec;56(3-4):110-4
Kreibich H: Betrachtungen zum 100. Jahrestag der Entdeckung des Mycobacterium tuberculosis durch Robert Koch. **Zentralbl Gynakol** 1982;104(5):258-67
Kühne W: Die Pathologie der Tuberkulose vor 100 Jahren und ihre heutige Bedeutung als Todesursache. **Zentralbl Allg Pathol** 1982;126(3-4):211-8
Lammel HU: Virchow contra Koch? Neue Untersuchungen zu einer alten Streitfrage. **Z Gesamte Hyg** 1982 Mar;28(3):206-10
Landmann H: Die Entwicklung der Tuberkulose in den letzten 100 Jahren unter besonderer Berücksichtigung der epidemiologischen Situation in der Deutschen Demokratischen Republik.
Lukas W: Epidemiologie der Tuberkulose. Entwicklung seit Entdeckung des Erregers, gegenwärtige Situation in der Bundesrepublik und voraussichtliche Weiterentwicklung. **Med Welt** 1982 Mar 26;33(12):442-9
Marchand H, Müller KP: Der Berufsweg Robert Kochs bis zur Entdeckung des Tuberkelbakteriums. **Wiss Beitr Martin Luther Univ Halle Wittenberg** 1983;5-R80:99-109
Mayer R: Il y a cent ans, Robert Koch découvrait le bacille de la tuberculose. **Rev Med Suisse Romande** 1982 Mar;102(3):199-226
Mecklinger L: Zum 100. Jahrestag der Entdeckung des Tuberkelbakteriums durch Robert Koch. **Z Gesamte Hyg** 1982 Dec 12;28(12):822-6
Meijer J: De tuberkelbacterie een eeuw bekend; 1882 - 24 Maart - 1982 (Heinrich Hermann Robert Koch). **Ned Tijdschr Geneeskd** 1982 Mar 13;126(11):488-9
Mendoza F: Acerca del descubrimiento del bacilo de Koch. **Rev Med Chil** 1983 May;111(5):539-43
Mochmann H: Die Entdeckung des Tuberkelbazillus vor 100 Jahren. **Kinderarztl Prax** 1982 Mar;50(3):113-6
Montiel Llorente LE: La ciencia medica en 'La montaña magica' de Thomas Mann. **Asclepio** 1980;32:271-85
Moskwa Z: Tuberkulina. **Wiad Lek** 1983 Jun 15;36(12):1033-5
Moskwa Z: W setną rocznic e odkrycia prątka grużlicy. **Wiad Lek** 1983 May 1;36(9):799-802
Ocklitz HW, Landmann H: Robert Koch und die Kindertuberkulose. **Kinderarztl Prax** 1982 Mar;50(3):117-29
Pacheco CR: Con motivo del centenario del descubrimiento del bacilo de la tuberculosis. **Salud Publica Mex** 1982 May-Jun;24(3):231-3
Pilipchuk NS, Pilipchuk VN: K stoletiiu otkrytiia Robertom Kokhom vozbuditelia tuberkuleza. **Vrach Delo** 1982 Nov;(11):119-21
Reimer H: Robert Koch und die Rindertuberkulose. **Z Gesamte Hyg** 1982 Mar;28(3):156-60
Robert Koch: **Probl Tuberk** 1982 Mar;(3):8-9
Sackmann W: Vor hundert Jahren: Robert Koch entdeckt den Erreger der Tuberkulose. **Schweiz Arch Tierheilkd** 1982 May;124(5):217-25
Sakula A: Centenary of the discovery of the tubercle bacillus. **Lancet** 1982 Mar 27;1(8274):750
Sakula A: Robert Koch: centenary of the discovery of the tubercle bacillus, 1882. **Thorax** 1982 Apr;37(4):246-51
Sakula A: Robert Koch (1843-1910): founder of the science of bacteriology and discoverer of the tubercle bacillus. A study of his life and work. **Br J Dis Chest** 1979 Oct;73(4):389-94
Schadewaldt H: Die Entdeckung des Tuberkuloseerregers durch Robert Koch vor 100 Jahren. **Krankenhausarzt** 1983 Mar 3;56:157-66
Schierhorn H: Zur Säkularfeier von Robert Kochs Entdeckung des Tuberkulose-Bakteriums. **Z Mikrosk Anat Forsch** 1982;96(3):377-99
Schliesser T: Die Rindertuberkulose im Wandel der letzten 100 Jahre (1882-1982). **Prax Klin Pneumol** 1982 Mar;36(3):151-6
Schliesser T: Zur Geschichte und Entwicklung der Rindertuberkulose-Bekämpfung. **Zentralbl Bakteriol Mikrobiol Hyg [A]** 1982 Mar;251(3):326-40
Schmid PC: Zur Epidemiologie und Ätiologie der Tuberkulose seit Robert Koch. Komplexes Ursachengefüge erfordert komplexe Strategien der Tuberkulose-Bekämpfung. **Fortschr Med** 1982 Mar 25;100(12):499-503
Schneeweiss U: Die Immunitätslehre im Lichte der Vorstellungen von Robert Koch. **Z Erkr Atmungsorgane** 1983;161(1):46-50
Schneeweiss U: Die Spezifitätslehre Robert Kochs; 100 Jahre Entdeckung der Tuberkelbakterien. **Medizinhist J** 1983;18(1-2):21-32
Shapiro E: Robert Koch and his tuberculin fallacy. **Pharos** 1983 Fall;46(4):19-22
Smith DW: Koch's postulates and the Koch phenomenon, an update. **Indian J Chest Dis Allied Sci** 1982 Apr-Sep;24(2-3):95-100
Solov'eva VA: K 100-letiiu otkrytiia Robertom Kokhom vozbuditelia tuberkuleza (1882-1982). **Sov Med** 1982;(3):120-2
Sönnichsen N: Zum 100. Jahrestag der Entdeckung des Erregers der Tuberkulose durch Robert Koch. **Dermatol Monatsschr** 1982 Mar;168(3):145-6
Steinbrück P: Der Erkenntnisprozess in Robert Koch auf seinem Wege zum Begründer der Tuberkulosebekämpfung. **Z Erkr Atmungsorgane** 1983;161(1):6-14
Steinbruck P: Hommage à Robert Koch, Sa vie et son oeuvre contre la tuberculose. **Bull Int Union Tuberc** 1981 Sep-Dec;56(3-4):115-9
Steinbrück P: Robert Koch und sein Werk. Seine Auswirkungen auf die Tuberkulosebekämpfung. **Z Erkr Atmungsorgane** 1982;158(1-2):5-23
Strubel K: Robert Koch und die Tuberkulose im Spiegel der halleschen Presse im ausgehenden 19. Jahrhundert. **Wiss Beitr Martin Luther Univ Halle Wittenberg** 1983;5-R80:225-42
Sŭla L: The 100th anniversary of the discovery of Koch's bacillus, the etiologic agent of tuberculosis. **J Hyg Epidemiol Microbiol Immunol** 1982;26(3):227-9
Szabó I: A Koch bacilus 100 éve. **Orv Hetil** 1982 Jan 24;123(4):227-9
Tetzner W: Erfolgreiche Tuberkulosebekämpfung in der DDR. **Wiss Z Martin Luther Univ (Math)** 1976;25(2):99-103
Völker A: Die Schwindsucht im halleschen Schrifttum des 18. Jahrhunderts. **Wiss Beitr Martin Luther Univ Halle Wittenberg** 1983;5-R80:203-10
Weingärtner L: Zum Problem der BCG-Impfung. **Wiss Beitr Martin Luther Univ Halle Wittenberg** 1983;5-R80:161-73
Weise W: Die Entdeckung des Erregers der Tuberkulose durch Robert Koch vor 100 Jahren. **MMW** 1982 Mar 26;124(12):299-300
Werner K: Sozialhygienische Aspekte in der frühen Ara der Tuberkulose-Therapie. **Wiss Beitr Martin Luther Univ Halle Wittenberg** 1983;5-R80:273-7
Winter K: Ein historischer Wendepunkt in der Geschichte von Naturwissenschaft und Medizin. Zum 100. Jahrestag der Entdeckung des Mycobacterium tuberculosis durch Robert Koch. **Z Arztl Fortbild (Jena)** 1982 Mar 15;76(6):229-30
Wyklicky H: Zur hundertsten Wiederkehr der ersten Demonstration des Tuberkelbazillus durch Robert Koch (1843-1910). **Osterr Apoth Ztg** 1982 Apr 3;36(14):266-7
Zahradnický J: 100 let od objevu puvodce tuberkulózy Robertem Kochem. **Cesk Epidemiol Mikrobiol Imunol** 1983 Jan;32(1):4-7
Zegaya M: 1882-1982: Robert Koch. Réquisitoire contre la tuberculose. **Tunis Med** 1982 March-Apr;60(2):98-105
Znachenie otkrytiia Roberta Kokha dlia razvitiia bakteriologii tuberkuleza: **Probl Tuberk** 1982 Mar;(3):3-7
Zureck A: 30 Jahre BCG-Impfung in der DDR - 20 Jahre BCG-Impfstoff aus Jena. **Z Erkr Atmungsorgane** 1982;158(1-2)168-84

**Great Britain**

Bryder L: Papworth Village Settlement--a unique experiment in the treatment and care of the tuberculous? **Med Hist** 1984 Oct;28(4):372-90
Bryder L: Tuberculosis, silicosis, and the slate industry in North Wales: Medical examinations of the high tuberculosis death rates in the North Wales slate mining and quarrying districts, 1927-1939. **Soc Soc Hist Med Bull (Lond)** 1983;33:43-6
Dubovsky H: John Keats (1795-1821)--poet, physician and tuberculosis patient. **S Afr Med J** 1981 Jun 6;59(24):875-8
Jones GR: The King Edward VII Welsh National Memorial Association, 1912-1948. In J. Cule, ed: Wales and medicine. London, British Society for the History of Medicine, 1975. p. 30-41.
Keers RY: Two forgotten pioneers. James Carson and George Bodington. **Thorax** 1980 Jul;35(7):483-9
Lunt R: Bone and joint tuberculosis. **Br Med J** 1979 Oct 13;2(6195):907-9
McGivering NJ: View from childhood. **Br Med J** 1979 Oct 13;2(6195):909
Pennington C: Tuberculosis. In Checkland O, Lamb M, ed: Health care as social history; the Glasgow case. Aberdeen, Aberdeen University Press, 1982. p. 86-99.
Petrescu G: 125 de ani de la nasterea lui Sir Robert Philip (1856-1939). **Rev Ig [Pneumoftiziol]** 1982 Oct-Dec;31(4):383-4
Sakula A: L'histoire du bacille tuberculeux telle qu'il nous la raconte dans 'La Ballade de la Seringue'. **Bull Int Union Tuberc** 1982 Sep-Dec;57(3-4):192-3
Scadding JG: Maurice Davidson 1883-1967--progress in respiratory medicine since his time. **Postgrad Med J** 1984 Mar;60(701):178-82
Smith H: John Keats: poet, patient, physician. **Rev Infect Dis** 1984 May-Jun;6(3):390-404
Weindling PJ: Die Anfänge der Tuberkulose-Fürsorgestellen in Grossbritannien. **Wiss Beitr Martin Luther Univ Halle Wittenberg** 1983;5-R80:243-9
Worboys M: The development of the sanatorium treatment for consumption in Britain, 1880-1914. **Soc Soc Hist Med Bull (Lond)** 1984 Dec;35:41-3

**Hungary**

Balla J: 50 éves a mátraházai gyógyintézet. **Orv Hetil** 1983 Mar 20;124(12):712-3
Balóné Fleischmann M: A rehabilitáció hazai úttörője Gárdi Jenö dr. (1886-1944). **Orv Hetil** 1984 Feb 19;125(8):470-2
Schweiger O: A tbc-elleni küzdelem eredményei Magyarországon 100 évvel a mycobacterium felfedezése után. **Orv Hetil** 1983 Jul 10;124(28):1667-70
Szabó I: The influence of the discovery of Koch's bacterium on the

Hungarians. **Indian J Chest Dis Allied Sci** 1982 Apr–Sep;24(2–3):175–8

**Iceland**

Sigurosson S: Tuberkulosens forkomst i Island. **Nord Medicinhist Arsbok** 1983;:135–48

**Italy**

Berti Bock G, Vial F, Heymans G, et al: Considerazioni critiche sull'opera di Carlo Forlanini (1847–1918). **Minerva Med** 1980 Jun 30;71(26):1879–83
Bèttica-Giovannini R: Giuseppe Berruti e l'Ospizio Marino Piemontese per ragazzi scrofolosi poveri con una nota su la fondazione dell'Ospedale Maria Vittoria di Torino (1887). **Ann Osp Maria Vittoria Torino** 1977 Jul–Dec;20(7–12):227–340
Manzi L: Commento ad un consulto inedito di Francesco Roncati. **Minerva Med** 1982 Jan 28;73(3–4):133–6
Sakula A: Carlo Forlanini, inventor of artificial pneumothorax for treatment of pulmonary tuberculosis. **Thorax** 1983 May;38(5):326–32

**Japan**

Fujita S: Die Bedeutung Robert Kochs für die japanische Medizin--Tuberkuloseforschung in Japan. **Prax Klin Pneumol** 1982 Mar;36(3):111–5
Iwasaki T: [Historical perspective on problems of the therapy, diagnosis and prevention of tuberculosis in Japan since 1886. (1)] (Jpn). **Kekkaku** 1982 Jun–Jul;57(6–7):357–62, 399–407

**Mexico**

Somolinos Palencia J: Roberto Koch. El descubrimiento del bacilo de la tuberculosis y su primera noticia en México. **Salud Publica Mex** 1982 May–Jun;24(3):237–40
Verduzco Guerrero E: La mortalidad por tuberbulosis en la República Mexicana durante el periodo 1963–1974. **SPM** 1980 Mar–Apr;22(2):191–28

**Netherlands**

Sutherland I, Svandová E, Radhakrishna S: The development of clinical tuberculosis following infection with tubercle bacilli. 1. A theoretical model for the development of clinical tuberculosis following infection, linking from data on the risk of tuberculous infection and the incidence of clinical tuberculosis in the Netherlands. **Tubercle** 1982 Dec;63(4):255–68
Sutherland I, Bleiker MA, Meijer J, et al: The risk of tuberculous infection in The Netherlands from 1967 to 1979. **Tubercle** 1983 Dec;64(4):241–53

**New Guinea**

Wigley SC: The first hundred years of tuberculosis in New Guinea. In Winslow JH, ed: The Melanesian environment, Canberra, Anu Press, 1977, p. 471–84.

**Poland**

Glinski J: 70 lat walki z gruźliça w Rudce. **Pneumonol Pol** 1980 Jul;48(7):491–2
Janowiec M, Pichulowa K: Rozwój mikrobiologicznej diagnostyki gruźlicy w Polsce. **Pneumonol Pol** 1982 Nov;50(11):559–62
Maisel W: Plany Hitlerowskie w odniesieniu do chorych na gruźlicę Polaków w Wartegau. **Przegl Zachod** 1981;37(3–4):99–106
Moskwa Z: Opieka społeczna nad chorymi gruźliczymi na śląsku w latach 1928–1929. **Wiad Lek** 1983 Oct 1;36(19):1645–7
Mrozowski K: Wkład profesora doktora medycyny Witolda Eugeniusza Orłowskiego w zwalczaniu gruźlicy. **Pol Arch Med Wewn** 1981;65(5):385–9
Pačes V: Uvahy o nemoci Fryderyka Chopina. **Vnitr Lek** 1980 Oct;26(10):1027–31
Szpunar W: Zgony z powodu gruźlicy w Lańcucie i okolicy w latach 1786–1970. Próba oceny epidemii. **Pneumonol Pol** 1981 Jul;49(7):527–35

**Romania**

Anastasatu C: Aportul lui Iacob Felix la combaterea tuberculozei în ţara noastră (cu acasia aniversarii a 150 de ani de la naştere). **Rev Ig [Pneumoftiziol]** 1983 Oct–Dec;32(4):379–80
Calciu M: La 125 de ani de la naşterea lui V. Babes (1854–1979). contribuţiile lui Victor Babes la edificarea ftiziologiei ştiinţifice. **Rev Ig [Pneumoftiziol]** 1979 Jul–Sep;28(3):187–91
Negru I: Spitalul de tuberculoză de la 'Filaret' şi doctorul Stefan Irimescu. **Viata Med [Medii Sanit]** 1983 Mar;31(3):68–72
Sturdza SA: The activity of the Cantacuzino Institute in the field of tuberculosis. A review. **Arch Roum Pathol Exp Microbiol** 1982 Jul–Sep;41(3):195–204

**Singapore**

Teo SK, Chew CH: Tuberculosis chemotherapy--developments in Singapore from 1957–1982. **Ann Acad Med Singapore** 1982 Jul;11(3):366–9

**Switzerland**

Bernische Liga gegen die Tuberkulose 1930–1980: Festschrift zum 50jährigen Jubiläum 20. Juni 1980 in Bern. Bern, 1980? 72 p. Contributions by S. Weiss, E. R. Mordasini, E. Arnold, R. Keller.
Favez G: Charlotte Olivier (1864–1945). **Rev Med Suisse Romande** 1984 May;104(5):353–68
Mottier G: Histoire de l'Infirmerie de Lausanne et de La Source. **Krankenpflege (Bern)** 1983 Dec;76(12):27–30

**United States**

DeMark JL: Chasing the cure--a history of healthseekers to Albuquerque, 1902–1940. **J West** 1982 Jul;21(3):49–58
Faler K: The conquest of tuberculosis. A contribution of American veterinary medicine to human welfare. **Mod Vet Pract** 1984 Jan;65(1):51–3
Gittings CL: Arizona's reputation as a health spa. **Ariz Med** 1983 Mar;40(3):150–3
Higgins A: John Janvier Black (1837–1909): an ornament to his profession. **Del Med J** 1982 Apr;54(4):233–7
Hood B: 'This worry I have': Mary Herren journal. **Oreg Hist Q** 1979;80(3):228–57
Leake ES: The Henry Phipps Institute: recollections of a foreign research fellow. **Trans Stud Coll Physicians Phila** 1981 Dec;5(3 no 4):256–63
Maulitz RC: Robert Koch and American medicine. **Ann Intern Med** 1982 Nov;97(5):761–6
Melick DW: Surgical therapy of pulmonary tuberculosis--a rare necessity of the 1980's. An historical review. **Ariz Med** 1983 Mar;40(3):158–9
Mooney EC: The white plague. **Am Heritage** 1979;30(2):54–9
Price JE: Tuberculosis in west Texas, 1870–1940. Ph.D. Diss., University of Texas Grad Sch. of Biomed Sci. Galveston, 1982. x, 418 p.
Shane KD: New Mexico: salubrious El Dorado. **NM Hist Rev** 1981;56(4):387–99
Thomison JB: Disease in Nashville: a short history. **J Tenn Med Assoc** 1983 Mar;76(3):151–5
Wilson JL: American Thoracic Society--five great teachers in the field of tuberculosis. **Am Rev Respir Dis** 1981 May;123(5):571–5
Wilson JL: 'The daily sanatorium routine was the treatment.' **Am Lung Assoc Bull** 1982 Mar;68(2):7–10

**USSR**

Al'tshuler NS: Iz istorii razvitiia bor'by s tuberkulezom v SSSR (1918–1924). **Probl Tuberk** 1980 May;(5):72–4
Al'tshuler NS: Voprosy bor'by s tuberkulezom v deiatel'nosti peredovoĭ meditsinskoĭ obshchestvennosti v dorevoliutsionnoĭ Rossii. **Probl Tuberk** 1979 Dec;(12):62–5
Batiashvili OG: I. K. Abakeliia--osnovopolozhnik ftiziatrii i organizator bor'by s tuberkulezom v Gruzii (k 100-letiiu dnia rozhdeniia). **Probl Tuberk** 1983 Jul;(7):73–4
Bedrin AV, Medvinskaia KG: Sverdlovskomu nauchno-issledovatel'skomu institutu tuberkuleza 50 let. **Probl Tuberk** 1982 May;(5):75–8
Bodarev VKh: Tuberkulez vchera i segodnia (material dlia besed). **Feldsher Akush** 1979 Oct;44(10):13–6
Bogush LK: Razvitie i dostizheniia khirurgii tuberkuleza legkikh v SSSR. **Probl Tuberk** 1983 Oct;10:3–7
Brzheskiĭ VCh, Evdokimov PP: K istorii bolezni V.G. Belinskogo. **Klin Med (Mosk)** 1984 Aug;62(8):150–2
Dzhamadze ShV: Tuberkuleznomu sanatoriiu im. V. I. Lenina v Gul'ripshi - 80 let. **Probl Tuberk** 1983 Feb;(2):73–4
Epifanov NS: Neustannyĭ borets s tiazhelym nedugom (k 100-letiiu so dnia rozhdeniia P. G. Korneval). **Feldsher Akush** 1983 Sep;48(9):37–8
Goregliad KhS, Tuzova RV: K istorii bor'by s tuberkulezom sel'skokhoziaistvennykh zhivotnykh. **Probl Tuberk** 1983 Nov;(11):71–3
Gulida MV: Ialtinskomu protivotuberkuleznomu dispanseru 60 let. **Probl Tuberk** 1984 Mar;(3):71–2
Gulida MV: Razvitie sanatorno-kurortnogo lecheniia bol'nykh tuberkulezom na iuzhnom beregu Kryma. **Probl Tuberk** 1981;(7):65–8
Kalankhodzhaev AA: Istoriia organizatsii i razvitiia protivotuberkuleznoĭ sluzhby v Uzbekistane. **Probl Tuberk** 1983 Jul;(7):71–3
Kariev TM: Razvitie khirurgicheskikh metodov lecheniia tuberkuleza legkikh v Uzbekskoĭ SSR. **Probl Tuberk** 1984 Jun;(6):69–71
Karpenko VS, Kamyshan IS, Kobiakova LF: Razvitie ftiziourologii na Ukraine (1922–1982). **Probl Tuberk** 1984 Jul;(7):75–8
Molotkov VN: Rol' Kievskogo ordena Trudovogo Krasnogo Znameni nauchno-issledovatel'skogo instituta tuberkuleza i grudnoĭ khirurgii im. F. G. Ianovskogo v razvitii ftiziatrii i pul'monologii. **Probl Tuberk** 1982 Dec;(12):18–22
Nikulina TD, Ivanov IV: Kuĭbyshevskoĭ oblastnoĭ tuberkuleznoĭ bol'nitse im. Z. P. Solov'eva 125 let. **Probl Tuberk** 1983 Apr;(4):69–71
Pavluchkova AV: Pervye sovetskie dispansery po bor'be s tuberkulezom

u deteĭ (k Mezhdunarodnomu godu rebenka). **Probl Tuberk** 1979 Dec;(12):11-5
Petrov BD: Bor'ba s tuberkulezom v SSR, provodimaia v sootvetstvii s ideiami V. I. Lenina. **Probl Tuberk** 1980 Apr;(4):3-6
Petrov IN: P.G. Kornev i ego shkola. **Probl Tuberk** 1984 Jul;(7):73-5
Poletaev SD, Sumbatov GA, Chausovskaia MM, et al: Deiatel'nost' kafedry tuberkuleza Tsentral'nogo instituta usovershenstvovaniia vracheĭ v period 1931-1980 gg. **Probl Tuberk** 1980 Dec;(12):3-6
Razvitic A.I. Strukovym ucheniza o tuberculoza: **Probl Tuberk** 1981 Apr;(4):3-6
Safarov RN, Shtern MI, Fel'berg MB: K istorii tuberkuleznoĭ bol'nitsy 'Zakhar'ino'. **Probl Tuberk** 1983 Feb;(2):70-3
Strukov AI, Puzik VI, Zemskova ZS, et al: V. G. Shtefko i otechestvennaia shkola patologov-ftiziatrov. **Arkh Patol** 1984;46(2):81-5
Tsentral'nomu institutu tuberkuleza Ministerstva zdravookhraneniia SSSR 60 let: **Probl Tuberk** 1982 May;(5):3-7
Ulitskaia NIa: Istoriia sovetskoiĭ ftiziatrii. **Med Sestra** 1979 Oct;38(10)):48-9
Verenkina TN, Markina LZ, Bashtanova LV: Istoriia razvitiia bor'by s tuberkulezom v Sevastopole. **Probl Tuberk** 1984 Jan;(1):70-2

**Yugoslavia**

Lukić D: Gledišta Dimitrija Tucovića o tuberkulozi. **Srp Arh Celok Lek** 1981;109(12):1677-86

## TULAREMIA

**1700 to Present**

**United States**

Murphy JA: Tularemia and report of a case by Jerome A. Murphy. N. Y. State J. Med. 1928. **NY State J Med** 1983 Jul-Sep;83(8-10):1062
Sanford JP: Landmark perspective: Tularemia. **JAMA** 1983 Dec 16;250(23):3225-6

## TYPHOID

**1700 to Present**

Bockemühl J: Die Typhus-Schutzimpfung gestern und heute. **Immun Infekt** 1983 Jan;11(1):16-22
Cunha BA: Typhoid fever, the typhus-like disease: historical perspective. **NY State J Med** 1982 Mar;82(3):321-4
Gröschel DH, Hornick RB: Who introduced typhoid vaccination: Almroth Wright or Richard Pfeiffer? **Rev Infect Dis** 1981 Nov-Dec;3(6):1251-4
Milhomem AM, Suassuna I: A imunidade na febre tifóide. I. A vacinação anti-tifoídica de Wright, 1896 a 1979. **Mem Inst Oswaldo Cruz** 1982 Jan-Mar;77(1):93-120
Stevenson LG: Exemplary disease: the typhoid pattern. **J Hist Med Allied Sci** 1982 Apr;37(2):159-81

**Canada**

Lloyd S: The Ottawa typhoid epidemics of 1911 and 1912: a case study of disease as a catalyst for urban reform. **Urban Hist Rev** 1979;8(1):66-89
Norris J: Typhoid in the Rockies: epidemiology in a constrained habitat, 1883-1939. In Roland CG, ed: Health, disease and medicine. Toronto, Hannah Institute for the History of Medicine, 1984. p. 276-95.

**France**

Goubert JP: Ordre et désordre: l'origine aquatique de la fièvre typhoïde. **Asclepio** 1983;35:161-70

**Great Britain**

Smith DC: William Budd manuscript at the National Library of Medicine. **J Hist Med Allied Sci** 1980 Jul;35(3):318-19
Smith DC, ed: 'On the causes of fevers' (1839) by William Budd. Baltimore and London, Johns Hopkins University Press, 1984. xi, 164 p. (Henry E. Sigerist Supplements to the Bulletin of the History of Medicine, n.s., no. 9)

**Poland**

Jastrzebowski Z: Epidemie duru w Królestwie Polskim w latach 1815--1870. **Arch Hist Med (Warsz)** 1980;43(2):179-90

**South Africa**

Gear JH: The Anglo-Boer War of 1899-1902:enteric fever and Captain Maxwell Louis Hughes. **Adler Mus Bull** 1981;7(1):10-3

**United States**

Claman G: A typhoid fever epidemic and the power of the press in Denver in 1879. **Colo Mag** 1979 Summer-Fall;56:143-60
Huch RK: 'Typhoid' Truelsen, water and politics in Duluth, 1896-1900. **Minn Hist** 1981;47(5):189-99
Smith DC: Gerhard's distinction between typhoid and typhus and its reception in America, 1833-1860. **Bull Hist Med** 1980 Fall; 54(3):368-85
Smith DC: The rise and fall of typhomalarial fever: I. origins. **J Hist Med Allied Sci** 1982 Apr;37(2):182-220

**USSR**

Sergiev VP, Nikonova VA: Raschet tendentsiĭ zabolevaemosti briushnym tifom na raznykh territoriiakh strany. **Zh Mikrobiol Epidemiol Immunobiol** 1980 Oct;(10):14-7
Zakharova LV: Osobennosti klinicheskogo techeniia briushnogo tifa za 20 let (1959-1978). **Klin Med (Mosk)** 1981;59(7):98-103

## TYPHUS

**500 A.D.-1450**

**Germany**

Dirckx JH: The pied piper of Hamelin. A medical-historical interpretation. **Am J Dermatopathol** 1980 Spring;2(1):39-45

**1450-1700**

**Great Britain**

Hawkins A: Two pathographies: a study in illness and literature. **J Med Philos** 1984 Aug;9(3):231-52

**1700 to Present**

Cunha BA: Typhoid fever, the typhus-like disease: historical perspective. **NY State J Med** 1982 Mar;82(3):321-4
Smith DC: The rise and fall of typhomalarial fever: II. decline and fall. **J Hist Med Allied Sci** 1982 Jul;37(3):287-321

**Belgium**

Gadeyne G: Oostvlaamse medici en parochiepriesters, slachtoffers van de tyfusepidemie, 1847-48: een episode uit de sociale geschiedenis. **Handel Maatsch Geschied Oudheidk Gent** 1980;34:167-79

**Canada**

Swinton WE: George Mellis Douglas: typhus and tragedy. **Can Med Assoc J** 1981 Dec 1;125(11):1284-6

**Czechoslovakia**

Bárdoš V, Schulz F: Výskyt škvrnitého týfu na východnom Slovensku v rokoch 1939-1945. **Bratisl Lek Listy** 1982 Aug;78(2):235-42

**Europe**

Sackmann W: Fleckfieber und Fleckfieberforschung zur Zeit des ersten Weltkrieges;zum Gedenken an Henrique da Rocha Lima (1879-1956). **Gesnerus** 1980;37(1/2):113-32

**France**

Bykhovskaia-Pavlovskaia IE: Istoriia otkrytiia Sharlem Nikollem puti zarazheniia sypnym tifom. **Parassitologia** 1981 Jan-Feb;15(1):87-91
Huard P, Imbault-Huart MJ: La polémique Percy-Ollivier sur le typhus traumatique en 1822. In: Congrès National des Sociétés Savantes, 99e, Besançon, 1974. Comptes Rendus. Paris, 1976. Section des Sciences, Fasc. V. p. 243-9.

**Mexico**

Varela G: El tifo exantemático en México. In Academia Nacional de Medicina. Libro conmemorativo del primer centenario. México, Comité Editorial de la Comisión Organizadora del Congreso del Centenario, 1964. Tome 2. p. 524-7.

**Poland**

Foster GM: Typhus disaster in the wake of war: the American-Polish relief expedition, 1919-1920. **Bull Hist Med** 1981 Summer;55(2):221-32
Karbe KH: Ueber eine von Rudolf Virchow empfohlene anonyme Schrift aus dem Jahre 1848 zum Hungertyphus in Oberschlesien. **Arch Hist Med (Warsz)** 1979;42(3):291-4
Pielat B: Dur plamisty w poglądach Sebastiana Petrycego i Sebastiana Sleszkowskiego w i Połowie XVII wieku. **Arch Hist Med (Warsz)** 1980;43(4):393-406

Weissmann G: In quest of Fleck: science from the holocaust. **Hosp Pract** 1980 Oct;15(10):48–9, 52, 54–5 passim

Zajusz K, Ornowski J: Rudolf Virchow a problemy niepodległościowe i społeczne narodu polskiego. **Arch Hist Med (Warsz)** 1979;42(3):285–9

**South Africa**

Gear JH: Studies of the rickettsial diseases at the South African Institute for Medical Research: epidemic louse-borne typhus fever. **Adler Mus Bull** 1984 Nov;10(3):8–15

**Sweden**

Nordbring F, Vahlquist B: En sentida kommentar till en berättelse om en svår farsot i Uppsala 1742–1743. **Lakartidningen** 1979 Dec 19;76(51):4714–7

**United States**

Beatty WK, Beatty VL: Howard Taylor Ricketts--imaginative investigator. **Proc Inst Med Chic** 1981 Apr–Jun;34(2):46–8

Mullen PC: Bitterroot enigma: Howard Taylor Ricketts and the early struggle against spotted fever. **Montana** 1983;32(1):2–13

Smith DC: Gerhard's distinction between typhoid and typhus and its reception in America, 1833–1860. **Bull Hist Med** 1980 Fall; 54(3):368–85

Tatge RO: A quarantine quandary; ship fever and yellow fever in Providence, Rhode Island, 1797. **Am Neptune** 1980;40(3):192–210

**USSR**

Vasil'ev KK: Rol' pervykh Vserossiĭskikh sezdov bakteriologov i épidemiologov v bor'be s épidemiiami parazitarnykh tifov (k 60–letiiu IV sezda). **Zh Mikrobiol Epidemiol Immunobiol** 1981 Apr;(4):106–9

## URINARY CALCULI

Andersson L, Kinn AC: Njursten och blåssten--en medicinhistorisk översikt. **Nord Medicinhist Arsb** 1982;:76–85

Ellis H: A history of bladder stone. **J R Soc Med** 1979 Apr;72(4):248–51

Ellis H: Cutting for the stone. **Aust NZ J Surg** 1980 Feb;50(1):4–7

Griffith DP: Urolithiasis. **J Urol** 1981 Oct;126(4):431

Modlin M: A history of urinary stone. **S Afr Med J** 1980 Oct 18;58(18):652–5

Otten HH: Pedra de mijada, der Pinkelstein. Medizinhistorische Betrachtung zur Lithotherapie. **Med Welt** 1981 May 8;32(19):765–6

Otten HH: Zur Geschichte der Lithotripsie und Litholapaxie. **Med Welt** 1983 May 6;34(18):557–61

**Germany**

Schneider HJ, Doberentz D: Zur Geschichte der Jenaer Harnsteinforschung. Mit einem vollständigen Abdruck der Dissertationsschrift Arno Krüches 'Ueber Struktur und Entstehung der Uratsteine' aus dem Jahre 1879. Jena, Friedrich-Schiller-Universität, 1979. 84, 42 p. (Jenaer Reden und Schriften).

**Great Britain**

Shaw AB: East Anglian bladder stone. **J R Soc Med** 1979 Mar;72(3):222–8

**Before 500 A.D.**

**United States**

Streitz JM, Aufderheide AC, El Najjar M, et al: A 1,500–year–old bladder stone. **J Urol** 1981 Oct;126(4):452–3

**500 A.D.-1450**

**Arabic**

Kâhya E: Renal calculi and their treatment in Ibn Sina. In International Congress of the History of Medicine, 27th, Barcelona, 1980. Actas. Barcelona, Acadèmia de Ciències Mèdiques de Catalunya i Balears, 1981. p. 734–8.

**Germany**

Valentin P: Mit Brevier und Skalpell. Legendäre Bauchoperation Kaiser Heinrichs II. **Med Welt** 1982 Feb 19;33(7):260–2

**1450–1700**

**Great Britain**

Morris GC: Which Molins treated Cromwell for stone--and did not prescribe for Pepys? **Med Hist** 1982 Oct;26(4):429–35

**Netherlands**

Kerner S: Samuel de Lion Benavente; chirurgien et lithotomiste (1643–1723). **Rev Hist Med Heb** 1981 Jul;34(2):29–30

**1700 to Present**

Cifuentes Delatte L: Historia del estudio microscópico de los cálculos del aparato urinario en el siglo XIX. **Arch Esp Urol** 1981 Sep–Oct;34(5):375–84

**France**

Brøndum N: Et kirurgisk indgreb skildret i musik. **Dan Medicinhist Arbog** 1983;12:170–4

Ellis H: The bladder stone of the Emperor Napoleon III. **Chirurgie** 1984;110(4):370–1

**Germany**

Schneider HJ, Seiyfarth HH: Die mikroskopische Harnsteinanalyse von den Anfängen 1879 bis zur Gegenwart. Jena, Friedrich-Schiller-Universität, 1980. 81 p.

**Great Britain**

Blum L: An eighteenth century health care provider and medical entrepreneur. **Bull NY Acad Med** 1984 Nov;60(9):944–7

Penfold JB: East Anglian bladder stone. **J R Soc Med** 1979 Sep;72(9):710–1

Viseltear AJ: The last illnesses of Robert and Horace Walpole. **Yale J Biol Med** 1983 Mar–Apr;56(2):131–52

**Spain**

Torres Ramírez C, Aguilar Ruíz J, Zuluaga Gómez A, et al: La cristalografía aplicada al análisis de los cálculos urinarios en España. Revisión histórica de la aportacion española al tema. **Arch Esp Urol** 1980 May–Jun;33(3):241–50

Zuluaga Gómez A, Torres Ramírez C, Rodríguez Rebollo T, et al: Análisis cristalográfico de lithiasis vesicales del siglo XIX. **Arch Esp Urol** 1982 Jul–Aug;35(4):234–45

**United States**

Graham SD: Ephraim McDowell (1771–1830). The President's lithotomist. **Invest Urol** 1981 Nov;19(3):216–7

## UROGENITAL SYSTEM

Farkas G: Eclampsia in the course of times. In: Congrès international d'histoire de la médecine, XXVe, Québec, 1976. Actes. Québec, 1977. p. 650–3.

Kirshen AJ, Cape RD: A history of urinary incontinence: or, 400 years of incontinence--are we any drier? **J Am Geriatr Soc** 1984 Sep;32(9):686–8

**Netherlands**

Haneveld GT: Early Dutch contributions on Peyronie's disease. **Arch Chir Neerl** 1979;31(3):123–9

**1450–1700**

**Italy**

Lines D: 15th century ureteric reflux. **Lancet** 1982 Dec 25;2(8313):1473

**1700 to Present**

Mowrer OH: Enuresis: the beginning work--what really happened. **J Hist Behav Sci** 1980 Jan;16(1):25–30

**Austria**

Davies PJ: Mozart's illnesses and death. **J R Soc Med** 1984 Jul;77(7):623

**France**

Jolidon C, Zephir D, Ybert G: Considérations historiques sur la maladie de La Peyronie. Peu de choses ont changé! **J Urol (Paris)** 1984;90(5):365–6

**United States**

Texter JH: The President's dilemma, 1919 (Woodrow Wilson). **Va Med** 1980 Nov;107(11):756–62

# DISEASES AND INJURIES

## VASCULAR

Fenn JE: Some observations on the evolution of current aortic aneurysm management. **Conn Med** 1979 Dec;43(12):783-9
Gordon DB, ed: Hypertension: the renal basis. Stroudsburg, Pa, Dowden, Hutchinson & Ross, 1980. xvi, 432 p. (Benchmark Papers in Human Physiology, 13).
Sanderson CJ, Cote RJ, Levett JM, et al: Acute aortic dissection. An historical review. **J R Coll Surg Edinb** 1982 Jul;27(4):195-9
Schadewaldt H: Zur Geschichte des Bluthochdrucks. **Med Welt** 1984;35:62--8
Stossel JP: Wie entsteht Arteriosklerose? **Med Klin** 1980 May 9;75(10):349-57
Tolins SH: Treatment of varicose veins. An update. **Am J Surg** 1983 Feb;145(2):248-52

### 500 A.D.-1450

**Arabic**

Said HM: Greco-Arab concepts on cardiovascular diseases. Karachi, Pakistan, Hamdard Foundation Press, 1983. 201 p.

### 1450-1700

**Italy**

Roth W: Atherom auf einem Olgemälde Pinakothek in Brescia. **Hautarzt** 1983 Aug;34(8):407-8

### 1700 to Present

Curry R, Johnston L: Percutaneous transluminal angioplasty. **Ulster Med J** 1982;51(1):59-66
Dotter CT: Two decades of transluminal angioplasty. An overview. **J Mal Vasc** 1982;7 Suppl 4:357-61
Genest J: A satellite view of hypertension. **Clin Invest Med** 1983;6(3):229-41
Guillerot E: Réflexion historique sur le traitement préventif des phlébites des membranes inférieurs selon Nard et Chalier. **Phlebologie** 1984 Jan-Mar;37(1):13-6
Hachinski V: Cerebral arteriosclerosis and dementia: evolution of a misconception. In: Congrès international d'histoire de la médecine, XXVe, Québec, 1976. Actes. Québec, 1977. p. 755-60.
Henry RL: A recognition of the work of Walter H. Seegers in hemostasis and thrombosis. **Semin Thromb Hemostas** 1980;6(4):325-7
Laine E: Histoire de la chirurgie des anévrysmes cérébraux. **Bull Mem Acad R Med Belg** 1983;138(12):576-86
Lévy A: Le rendez-vous manqué de la connaissance immédiate et du hasard. Contribution à l'historie de l'hypertension artérielle. **Coeur Med Interne** 1979 Oct-Dec;18(4):567-70
Nicholls A: Atherosclerosis in chronic renal failure: a historical perspective. **Scott Med J** 1983 Jul;28(3):270-5
Postnov IuV: Popytka opisaniia gipertonicheskoĭ bolezni bolee 200 let nazad. **Kardiologiia** 1983 Dec;23(12):89
Seegers WH: A personal perspective on hemostasis and thrombosis (1937-1981). **Semin Thromb Hemostas** 1981 Dec;7(3-4):177-307
Warren R: Behavior of venous thrombi: historical observations. **Arch Surg** 1980 Oct;115(10):1151-4

**Austria**

Lie JT, Mann RJ, Ludwig J: The brothers von Winiwarter, Alexander (1848-1917) and Felix (1852-1931), and thromboangiitis obliterans. **Mayo Clin Proc** 1979 Dec;54(12):802-7

**France**

Merlen JF: Pnénomène de Raynaud. Historique. **Rev Prat** 1981 Dec 1;31(55):3971-2, 3975-6
Roncière J de la, Fiessinger JN: Maurice Raynaud, 1835-1881. **Rev Prat** 1981 Dec 1;31(55):3967-9

**Germany**

Sabiston DC: Trendelenburg's classic work on the operative treatment of pulmonary embolism. **Ann Thorac Surg** 1983 May;35(5):570-4
Weidenbach H, Massmann J: Der Beitrag des Pathologischen Instituts Leipzig zu den gegenwärtigen Vorstellungen über die Atiopathogenese der Arteriosklerose. **Zentralbl Allg Pathol** 1982;126(3-4):253-9

**Great Britain**

Attwood HD: Matthew Baillie--a possible early description of amniotic fluid embolism. **Aust NZ J Obstet Gynaecol** 1979 Aug;19(3):176-7
Gibson II: Illness of Dorothy Wordsworth. **Br Med J [Clin Res]** 1982 Dec 18-25;285(6357):1813-5
Macpherson AI: Portal hypertension: a pilgrim's progress. **J R Coll Surg Edinb** 1979 Nov;24(6):317-35
Thirty years of drugs for hypertension: a festschrift for Sir John McMichael: **Br J Clin Pharmacol** 1982 Jan;13(1):5-142

**Italy**

Di Giacomo V: A case of Takayasu's disease occurred over two hundred years ago. **Angiology** 1984 Nov;35(11):750-4

**Netherlands**

Van der Molen HR: Hommage à Jan ven Limborgh (1900-1984). **Phlebologie** 1984 Jul-Sep;37(3):XXV-XXXI

**Switzerland**

Hahnloser P, Pugin P: La formation des thromboses et des embolies paradoxales par un shunt interauriculaire. Commentaires sur les articles de F. Wilh. Zahn: de la formation des thrombus, état actuel de cette question. Thrombose de plusieurs branches de la veine cave inférieure avec embolies consécutives dans les artères pulmonaire, splénique, rénale et iliaque droite. **Rev Med Suisse Romande** 1980 Dec;100(12):1103-8
Schettler G: Atherosclerosis during periods of food deprivation following World Wars I and II. **Prev Med** 1983 Jan;12(1):75-83

**United States**

Fagrell B: Först med stort patientmaterial på rökbetingad allergi. **Lakartidningen** 1982 Oct 13;79(41):3669-7
Finn R: Salt and hypertension: discussion paper. **J R Soc Med** 1983 Oct;76(10):853-8
Greenwood RD: Operation for Aneurism of the Axillae'--1834, a historical notation. **J Med Assoc State Ala** 1982 May;51(11):57
Schechter DC: Flashbacks: electrical treatment of aneurysms. **PACE** 1979 Mar;2(2):234-45
Stead EA: Kempner revisited. **NC Med J** 1983 Apr;44(4):237-40
Taylor W, Wasserman D, Behrens V, et al: Effect of the air hammer on the hands of stonecutters. The limestone quarries of Bedford, Indiana, revisited. **Br J Ind Med** 1984 Aug;41(3):289-95

## VENEREAL

Kampmeier RH: Herpes genitalis: a clinical puzzle for two centuries. **Sex Transm Dis** 1984 Jan-Mar;11(1):41-5
Laugier P, Burgun R: Die Geschichte der Geschlechtskrankheiten. In Sournia JC, Martiny M, Poulet J, ed: Illustrierte Geschichte der Medizin. Salzburg, Andreas, 1980. Vol. 4. p. 1483-516.
Roberts A: The pox and the people: a history of venereal diseases and sexual attitudes. **Nurs Times** 1982 Jul 14-20;78(28):1177-85
Schönfeld J: Zur Geschichte der Geschlechtskrankheiten. **Off Gesundheitswes** 1982 Oct;44(10):660-3
Verveen G: Venerologie auf Briefmarken; Philatelistisch illustrierte Geschichte der Venerologie. **Z Hautkr** 1981 Feb 15;56(4):227-33

**Chile**

Costa-Casaretto C: Las enfermedades venéreas en Chile desde el descubrimiento hasta la colonia. **Rev Med Chil** 1980 Oct;108(10):969-76

**France**

Malterre-Barthes A: Un service bien particulier: les dispensaires antivénériens. **Soins Gynecol Obstet Pueric** 1981 Sep;(6):37-46

### 500 A.D.-1450

**Arabic**

Belova LV, Mirakhmedov UM: Vklad Abu Ali ibn-Sina v dermato-venerologiiu. **Vestn Dermatol Venerol** 1983 Dec;(12):60-4

### 1700 to Present

Adams P: Health of the state. New York, N.Y., Praeger, 1982. x, 198 p.
Catterall RD: The emergence of a specialty. **Sex Transm Dis** 1983 Apr-Jun;10(2):85-92
Kampmeier RH: The genito-anal-rectal syndrome: late manifestations of lymphogranuloma inguinale. **Sex Transm Dis** 1983 Jan-Mar;10(1):47-50
Packer H: Memoirs of a venereologist. **J Tenn Med Assoc** 1979 Oct;72(10):731-8
Pastinszky I: A dermatovenerológia Hebrától napjainkig. **Orv Hetil** 1982 Apr 18;123(16):987-90

**Austria**

Biliński Z: Przyczynek do poznania zjawiska szerzenia się chorób wenerycznych-w oparciu o problem występowania prostytucji w Jarosławiu w okresie zaboru austriackiego (1895–1916). **Przegl Dermatol** 1982 Jan–Apr;69(1–2):113–5

**Canada**

Buckley S, McGinnis JD: Venereal disease and public health reform in Canada. **Can Hist Rev** 1982;63(3):337–54
Pierson RR: The double bind of the double standard: VD control and CWAC in World War II. **Can Hist Rev** 1981;62(1):31–58

**Chile**

Costa-Casaretto C: Primeros proyectos de organización sanitaria y de campaña antivenerea después de la emancipación politica de Chile. **Rev Med Chil** 1980 Dec;108(12):1161–9

**Czechoslovakia**

Hübschmann K: History of Dermatology and Venerology from 1848 to the end of 1944 in Prague, Czechoslovakia. **Int J Dermatol** 1982 Jul–Aug;21(6):356–60
Ozorovský V, Tychý M, Buchvald J, et al: Sociálne aspeckty začiatkov dermatovenerológie v Bratislave po roku 1918 a úloha professora Reinsberga. **Cesk Zdrav** 1982 Jul;30(7):319–25

**France**

Huard P, Imbault-Huart MJ: Percy, vénéréologue. In: Congrès National des Sociétés Savantes, 99e, Besançon, 1974. Comptes Rendus. Paris, 1976. Section des Sciences, Fasc. V. p. 259–64.
Lellouch A, Rullière R: René Joseph Hyacinthe Bertin (1767–1827). **Hist Sci Med** 1980;14:325–36

**Germany**

Hollander A: Geschichtliches aus vergangener Zeit: Politische Bekämpfung der Geschlechtskrankheiten? **Fortschr Med** 1981 Jun 25;99(24):927–8
Schulz EA: Otto Julius Grütz, Leben und Lebenswerk. Diss. Bonn, 1982. 107 p.
Wendt V: Heinrich A. Gottron: Leben und Werk. Lübeck, Hansisches Verlagskonto H. Scheffler, 1980. 99 p.
Winkelmann O: Zur Erinnerung an Ernst von Düring-Pascha (1858–1944). In: First International Congress on the History of Turkish-Islamic Science and Technology, ITU 14–18 September 1981. Proceedings Vol. IV, p. 32–44.
Wozniak KD: Zur Bekämpfung der Geschlechtskrankheiten und der Berufsdermatosen in der DDR. **Wiss Z Martin Luther Univ (Math)** 1976;25(2):105–8

**Great Britain**

Adler MW: Academic Department of Genitourinary Medicine, Middlesex Hospital Medical School, London. **Br Med J** 1980 Jul 19;281(6234):206–11
Adler MW: History of the development of a service for the venereal diseases. **J R Soc Med** 1982 Feb;75(2):124–8
De mortuis nil nisi bonum: **J Am Acad Dermatol** 1982 May;6(5):968–76
McHugh P: Prostitution and Victorian social reform. New York, St. Martin's Press, 1980. 306 p.
Morton RS: A reappraisal of non-specific genital infection with reference to the work of the late Dr. E. Weston Hurst. **Br J Vener Dis** 1983 Dec;59(6):394–6
Robson A: The significance of 'The maiden tribute of modern Babylon'. **Victorian Period Newsl** 1978;11(2):50–7
Smith FB: Ethics and disease in the later nineteenth century: the Contagious Diseases Acts. **Hist Stud** 1971;15(57):118–35
Towers BA: Health education policy 1916–1926: venereal disease and the prophylaxis dilemma. **Med Hist** 1980 Jan;24(1):70–87
Walkowitz JR: Prostitution and Victorian society. Women, class, and the state. Cambridge, New York, Cambridge University Press, 1980. ix, 347 p.
Willcox RR: The international venereological scene as viewed by Harrison and St Mary's. **Br J Vener Dis** 1982 Apr;58(2):72–85
Wright DJ: John Hunter and venereal disease. **Ann R Coll Surg Engl** 1981 May;63(3):198–202

**India**

Kaminsky AP: Morality legislation and British troops in late nineteenth century India. **Milit Aff** 1979;43(2):78–83

**Netherlands**

Stemvers FA: Geslachtsziektenbestrijding 1850–1880. **Tijdschr Geschied Geneeskd** 1981;4(1):1–24

**Poland**

Michalowski R: Spital für Geschlechtskranke in Lublin 1832 bis 1982. **Dermatol Monatsschr** 1984;170(4):268–73

**Romania**

Negru I: Istoricul bolilor venerice in studiile clasice ale istoricilor medicinii ramâneşti. **Viata Med [Medii Sanit]** 1981 Dec;29(12):281–5

**Singapore**

Lee YK: Prostitution and venereal disease in early Singapore (1819–1889). **Singapore Med J** 1980;21:720–31
Lee YK: Prostitution and venereal disease in early Singapore (1819–1889)--Part II. **Singapore Med J** 1980 Dec;21(6):781–90

**United States**

Bowman IA: Prostitution and the medical profession in the nineteenth century. **Bookman** 1982 Jan;9(1):3–9
Imber M: The First World War, sex education, and the American Social Hygiene Association's campaign against venereal disease. **J Educ Adm Hist** 1984;16(1):47–56
Kampmeier RH: History of the American Venereal Disease Association. **Sex Transm Dis** 1984 Jul–Sep;11(3 Suppl):185–265
Kampmeier RH: The establishment of lymphogranuloma inguinale (lymphopathia venereum) as a sexually transmitted disease. **Sex Transm Dis** 1982 Jul–Sep;9(3):146–8
Kampmeier RH: Venereal disease in the United States Army: 1775–1900. **Sex Transm Dis** 1982 Apr–Jun;9(2):100–3
Pivar DJ: Cleansing the nation: the war on prostitution, 1917–21. **Prologue J Nat Arch** 1980;12(1):29–40
Price DE: John Friend Mahoney. In Dictionary of American Biography, Suppl. 6, 1956–1960. p; 423–4, 1980.
Sandos JA: Prostitution and drugs: the United States Army on the Mexican-American border, 1916–1917. **Pac Hist Rev** 1980;49(4):621–45
Van Patten HG: The Arkansas Venereal Disease Program historical sketch and current trends. **J Arkansas Med Soc** 1984 Jan;80(8):365–6

**USSR**

Brzheskiĭ VCh: A. A. Sakhnovskaia (k stoletiiu so dnia rozhdeniia). **Vestn Dermatol Venerol** 1983 May;(5):73–4
Gus'kov EN, Mustaev RK: Dostizheniia dermato-venerologicheskoĭ sluzhby v Mordovskiĭ ASSR za 50 let. **Vestn Dermatol Venerol** 1980;(5):35–6
Il'in II, Preĭsman BS: P. P. Zablotskiĭ-Desiatovskiĭ i ego rol' v razvitii venerologii v Rossii (k 100-letiiu so dnia smerti). **Vestn Dermatol Venerol** 1983 Dec;(12):59–60
Mirakhmedov UM: K 60-letiiu kafedry kozhnykh i venericheskikh bolezneĭ Tashkentskogo meditsinskogo instituta. **Vestn Dermatol Venerol** 1981 Nov;(11):74–6
Mirakian ME: K istorii nauchnykh issledovaniĭ v oblasti otechestvennoĭ venerologii (XIX vek). **Vestn Dermatol Venerol** 1984 Jul;(7):72–5
Ovchinnikov NM, Timchenko GF: Dvadtsatiletniĭ opyt raboty Tsentral'nogo nauchno-issledovatel'skogo kozhnovenerologicheskogo instituta Minzdrava SSR po kontroliu i uluchsheniiu kachestva serologicheskikh laboratoriĭ dermatovenerologicheskikh uchrezhdeniĭ SSSR. **Lab Delo** 1981;(2):120–2

**Yugoslavia**

Vukas A: Organizacija borbe protiv kožnih i spolnih bolesti i dosadašnji nedostaci u tom pogledu. **Lijec Vjesn** 1979 Nov;101(11):718–9

## VISION DISORDERS

Marg E: Is the animal model for stimulus deprivation amblyopia in children valid or useful? **Am J Optom Physiol Opt** 1982 Jun;59(6):451–64
Mawas LJ, Mawas E, Weiss JB: Dix siècles de diplopie physiologique d'al Hazen à nos jours (presentation d'instruments). **Bull Soc Ophtalmol Fr** 1981 Mar;81(3):281–6
Pinckers AJ: Leber's congenital amaurosis as conceived by Leber. **Ophthalmologica** 1979;179(1):48–51

**United States**

Koestler FA: The unseen minority: a social history of blindness in the United States. New York, McKay, 1976. 559 p.

# DISEASES AND INJURIES

### 500 A.D.–1450

**China**

Chen YZ: The courageous and brilliant blind monk Jianshen. **Chin Med J [Engl]** 1980 Feb;93(2):130–3

**Italy**

Casanovas J: La enfermedad ocular de Francisco de Asís. **Klin Oczna** 1980 May;82(5):243–4

### 1450–1700

**Great Britain**

Mutschmann H: Milton's eyesight and the chronology of his works. New York, Haskell House, 1971. 50 p.

**Spain**

Ravin JG: El Greco of Toledo. **Ohio State Med J** 1982 Nov;78(11):745–53

### 1700 to Present

Bonneval G: Prévention réele de l'amblyopie strabique. Historique et perspectives. **Bull Soc Ophtalmol Fr** 1982 Mar;82(3):345–8
Jay M: The Eisdell pedigree. Congenital stationary night-blindness with myopia. **Trans Ophthalmol Soc UK** 1983;103(Pt 2):221–6
Lanthony P: Daltonisme et peinture. **Bull Soc Ophtalmol Fr** 1982 Apr;82(4):509–13
Lanthony P: Daltonisme et peinture. **J Fr Ophtalmol** 1982;5(6–7):373–85
Levi F: La cecita nella cultura. **Belfagor** 1982;37(5):569–80

**Austria**

Stepak S: Z dziejów Zakładu Wychowawczego dla Niewidomych we Lwowie w latach 1851–1918. **Klin Oczna** 1984 Apr;86(4):181–3

**Brazil**

Abreu Fialho S de: O Instituto Imperial dos Meninos Cegos. **Rev Inst Hist Geogr Bras** 1977;315:201–31

**Canada**

Sherwood RH: Discovery of kerosene. **NS Hist Q** 1979;9(2):157–64

**France**

Lafon JC: Le sourd et muet au XIXe siècle. **Bull Audiophonol** 1980;11(2):1–142

**Netherlands**

Albert-Puleo M: Van Gogh's vision: thujuone intoxication. **JAMA** 1981 Jul 3;246(1):42
Lee TC: Van Gogh's vision. Digitalis intoxication? **JAMA** 1981 Feb 20;245(7):727–9

**South Africa**

Vaughan VH, Vaughan L: Fifty years of service: The S. A. National Council for the Blind, 1929–1979. The story of the South African National Council for the Blind. Pretoria. S. A. National Council for the Blind, 1979. xii, 468 p.

**United States**

Lash JP: Helen Keller. In: Notable American women. The modern period. Cambridge, Mass., Belknap-Harvard Univ. Press, 1980. 4:389–93.
Litoff JB: Carolyn Conant van Blarcom. In: Notable American women. The modern period. Cambridge, Mass., Belknap-Harvard Univ. Press, 1980. 4:703–4.
Treolo J: Seeing fingers: the ministry of the Christian Record Braille Foundation. **Advent Herit** 1982;7(2):28–37

**USSR**

Shafranov BV: Iz istorii gigieny promyshlennogo osveshcheniia v SSSR. **Gig Tr Prof Zabol** 1980 Jul;(7):46–7

**Yugoslavia**

Dugački V: Počeci organizirane skrbi za slijepe u Hrvatskoj. Prosvećeno Međunarondoj godini invalida. **Lijec Vjesn** 1981 Nov;103(11):531–3

## WHOOPING COUGH

### 1700 to Present

**Australia**

Hamilton DG: Whooping cough immunization. **Med J Aust** 1979 Dec 15;2(12):651

**Finland**

Turpeinen O: Die Sterblichkeit an Pocken, Masern und Keuchhusten in Finnland in den Jahren 1751 bis 1865. In Imhof AE, ed: Mensch und Gesundheit in der Geschichte. Husum, Matthiesen, 1980. p. 135–61.

**Great Britain**

Jones C: The coughing disease. **Health Visit** 1982 Dec;55(12):648–50

**Mexico**

Carrada Bravo T, Gómez Orozco J, Luna Martínez J, et al: La tosferina y la vacunación antitosferinosa. Trabajo para conmemorar el 40 aniversario de la vacunación antitosferinosa en México, Junio 13 de 1940. **Salud Publica Mex** 1982 Jul–Aug;24(4):399–465

## WOUND INFECTION

Majno G: Inflammation and infection: historic highlights. **Monogr Pathol** 1982;(23):1–17

### 1700 to Present

Zambon JV: Brugmans, voorloper van Semmelweis. **Ned Tijdschr Geneeskd** 1983 Jun 11;127(24):1060–4

**United States**

Altemeier WA: Perspectives in surgical infections. **Surg Clin North Am** 1980 Feb;60(1):5–13

**USSR**

Milashkin AG: Ispol'zovanie mazi Vishnevskogo v gody Velikoĭ Otechestvennoĭ voĭny. **Voen Med Zh** 1982 Feb;(2):76
Velikoretskiĭ AN: Vzgliady N. I. Pirogova na preduprezhdenie zarazheniia ran. **Feldsher Akush** 1979 Sep;44(9):44–6

## WOUNDS AND INJURIES

Adams DB: Abdominal gunshot wounds in warfare: a historical review. **Milit Med** 1983 Jan;148(1):15–20
Aker F, Schroeder DC, Baycar RS: Cause and prevention of maxillofacial war wounds: a historical review. **Milit Med** 1983 Dec;148(12):921–7
Alawneh I: Historische Bemerkungen über Gallenwegtrauma. **Aktuel Traumatol** 1981 Dec;11(6):231–3
Bibbings J: Honey, lizard dung and pigeons' blood. **Nurs Times** 1984 Nov 28–Dec 4;80(48):36–8
Flamm ES: The decline of osteology and the rise of surgical neurology in the management of head injuries. In Rose FC, Bynum WF, ed: Historical aspects of the neurosciences. New York, Raven, 1982. p. 243–53.
Forrest RD: Development of wound therapy from the Dark Ages to the present. **J R Soc Med** 1982 Apr;75(4):268–73
Forrest RD: Early history of wound treatment. **J R Soc Med** 1982 Mar;75(3):198–205
Gervin AS, Fischer RP: Resuscitation of trauma patients with type-specific uncrossmatched blood. **J Trauma** 1984 Apr;24(4):327–31
Jalil A: Mermas and acupuncture points, a comparative study. **Stud Hist Med** 1981 Mar;5(1):18–34
Ober WB: Bottoms up! The fine arts and flagellation. Part I. **Am J Dermatopathol** 1984 Oct;6(5):451–60
Ragsdale BD: Gunshot wounds: a historical perspective. **Milit Med** 1984 Jun;149(6):301–15
Schwanitz HJ: Vom Ausgestossenen zum Gesichtsversehrten – Ein Beispiel sozialer Diskriminierung aus der Geschichte der Medizin. **Hautarzt** 1984 Jan;35(1):45–9
Vander Elst E: Die Geschichte der Orthopädie und der Traumatologie. In Sournia JC, Martiny M, Poulet J, ed. Illustrierte Geschichte der Medizin. Salzburg, Andreas, 1980. Vol. 5. p. 1655–1721.
Watt J: Doctors in the wars. **J R Soc Med** 1984 Apr;77(4):265–7
West CG: A short history of the management of penetrating missile injuries of the head. **Surg Neurol** 1981 Aug;16(2):145–9

**Great Britain**

Cannell H: Struck by lightning -- the effects upon the men and the ships of HM Navy. **J R Nav Med Serv** 1979;65(3):165-70

**Spain**

Guerra F: Las heridas de guerra. Contribución de los cirujanos Españoles en la evolución de su tratamiento. Santander, Catedra de Historia de la Medicina, Universidad de Santander, 1981. XVI, 237 p.

**Switzerland**

Fischer-Homberger E: Die gerichtsmedizinische Wundbegutachtung vom 16. zum 18. Jahrhundert. **Gesnerus** 1983;40(1-2):75-80

**Before 500 A.D.**

Barton NJ: Hand markings of the Shroud of Turin. **Hand** 1980;12:323

**France**

Hooper A: Further information on the prehistoric representations of human hands in the cave of Gargas. **Med Hist** 1980 Apr;24(2):214-16

**Iraq**

Trinkaus E, Zimmerman MR: Trauma among the Shanidar Neandertals. **Am J Phys Anthropol** 1982 Jan;57(1):61-76

**Italy**

Massey EW: An interpretation of the hand and arm markings of the shroud of Turin. **Hand** 1980 Feb;12(1):75-80

**USSR**

Dérums VIa: Rentgenomorfologicheskaia kharakteristika travmaticheskikh povrezhdeniĭ i raneniĭ kosteĭ zhiteleĭ drevneĭ Pribaltiki. **Arkh Patol** 1980;42(2):64-8

**500 A.D.-1450**

**Arabic**

Shvabe IuIa: Lechenie travmaticheskikh povrezhdeniĭ v trudakh Ibn-Siny (Avitsenny) (k 1000-letiiu so dnia rozhdeniia Abu Ali Ibn-Siny). **Feldsher Akush** 1980;45(8):47-8

Shvabe IuIa: Voprosy travmatologii v trudakh Ibn-Siny (Avitsenny). **Ortop Travmatol Protez** 1979 Sep;(9):68-70

**India**

Thakral KK: Techniques for extraction of foreign bodies from war wounds in medieval India. **Indian J Hist Sci** 1981, reçu 1982;16(1):11-6

**Yugoslavia**

Zivanović S: Povrede i prelomi kostiju u Srpskog srednjovekovnog stanoviništva iz nekropole Vajuga na Dunavu kod Kladova. **Srp Arh Celok Lek** 1982 Mar;110(3):273-89

**1450-1700**

**Belgium**

Colard A: Evocation du passé: des bons soins que donna Ambroise Paré à un Prince en Hainaut et du succès qu'il en advint. **Rev Med Brux** 1980 Jun;1(6):405-8

**Germany**

Heintel H: Die Fallhaube: eine Erfindung des 16. Jahrhunderts? **Medizinhist J** 1984;19(3):273-6

**Netherlands**

Pollitt R: The wounding and treatment of William of Orange in 1582. **J Hist Med Allied Sci** 1982 Apr;37(2):135-58

**1700 to Present**

Allgöwer M, Border JR: Advances in the care of the multiple trauma patient--introduction. **World J Surg** 1983 Jan;7(1):1-3

Bousigue JY: Les lésions axiales du traumatisme crânien. Evolution des idées depuis un siècle. **Neurochirurgie** 1983;29(5):365-9

Francis TJ: Non freezing cold injury: a historical review. **J R Nav Med Serv** 1984 Winter;70(3):134-9

Lévy C: La mortalité par accident des enfants et des adolescents dans huit pays développés. **Population** 1980;35(2):291-319

Modlin HC: Traumatic neurosis and other injuries. **Psychiatr Clin North Am** 1983 Dec;6(4):661-82

Simeone FA: Studies of trauma and shock in man: William S. Stone's role in the military effort. **J Trauma** 1984 Mar;24(3):181-7

Wallerström A: Levande tärd av maskar--terapeutisk användning av fluglarver. **Nord Medicinhist Arsb** 1980;:136-46

**Brazil**

Cunha Rodrigues MR da: A morte da Imperatriz Leopoldina (11-XII-1826). **Rev Hist (Brazil)** 1971;43(88):345-52

**Canada**

Bercuson DJ: Tragedy at Bellevue: anatomy of a mine disaster. **Labour** 1978;3:221-31

**Czechoslovakia**

Kroupa J: Dvacet pět let výzkumného ústavu traumatologického v brně. **Rozhl Chir** 1979;58(10):675-80

Kroupa J: 30 let trvání Výzkumného ústavu traumatologického v Brně. **Cas Lek Cesk** 1984 Jul 20;123(29):904-6

Kroupa J: 50 let od otevření úrazové nemocnice v Brně a 30 let činnosti Výzkumného ústavu traumatologického v Brně. **Rozhl Chir** 1984 Oct;63(10):633-42

**Ethiopia**

Hulin I: Háborús koponyasérülések. Tapasztalatok az ogadeni és eritreai háborúkból. I. rész. Neurotraumatológiai sérültek statisztikája. **Magy Traumatol Orthop Helyreallito Sebesz** 1982;25(4):273-9

**France**

Colas des Francs G: L'oeuvre de Jules Amar entre 1914 et 1918. Thèse, Université René-Descartes, Faculté Cochin-Port-Royal. Paris, 1984. 21, 29, 7, 70 p.

**Germany**

Ebon M: Why did Hitler hate the Jews? **Midstream** 1979;25(8):19-24

**Great Britain**

Cannell H: Struck by lightning--the effects upon the men and the ships of HM Navy. **J R Nav Med Serv** 1980 Summer;66(2):152-6

Harrison SH: Accident surgery--the life and times of William Gissane. **Injury** 1984 Nov;16(3):145-54

Owen-Smith MS: A computerized data retrieval system for the wounds for war: the Northern Ireland casualties. **J R Army Med Corps** 1981 Feb;127(1):31-54

Ramsey LJ: Bullet wounds and X-Rays in Britain's little wars. **J Soc Army Hist Res** 1982 Summer;:91-102

Zuck D: John Hunter's treatment of gunshot wounds. **Ann R Coll Surg Engl** 1980 Jan;62(1):74-5

**Italy**

Campiglio L: La dinamica degli infortuni sul lavoro nel periodo 1951-1970. **Riv Int Sci Sociali** 1973;81(1-2):134-65

**Norway**

Irgens LM: Trafikkulykkenes epidemiologi: årsaksforhold og forebyggelse fra medisinsk synsvinkel. **Tidsskr Samfunnsforskning** 1981;22(1):17-38

**Poland**

Cyprian T: Problem Karalności zagrożenia w sprawach o wypadki drogowe. **Panstwo Prawo** 1965;20(2):273-9

**Switzerland**

Zanobio B: Je le pansai, Dieu le guérit. Gli aforismi di chirurgia militare di Louis Appia (1818-1898) sulla cura delle ferite d'armi da fuoco. **G Accad Med Torino** 1980;143(Spec No):7-95

**United States**

Bollet AJ: Wounded presidents: 1981 almost repeats the events of 1881. **Med Times** 1981 Jul;109(7):19-23

Chelius JR: Economic and demographic aspects of the occupational injury problem. **Q Rev Econ Bus** 1979;19(2):65-70

Christianson EH: Wound management advice in antebellum America. In Romm S, ed: Symposium on historical perspectives of plastic surgery. Philadelphia, Saunders, 1983. p. 671-7.

Connolly JF: Wound management and the legacy of H. Winnett Orr. **Nebr Med J** 1982 Mar;67(3):60–1
Eastman JW: 'Doctors' orders': the American medical profession and the origins of automobile design for crash protection, 1930–1955. **Bull Hist Med** 1981;55(3):407–24
Eckert WG: The St. Valentine's Day massacre. **Am J Forensic Med Pathol** 1980 Mar;1(1):67–70
Gersuny C: New England mill casualties: 1890–1910. **N Engl Q** 1979;52(4):467–82
Greisman HC: Wound management and medical organization in the Civil War. **Surg Clin North Am** 1984 Aug;64(4):625–38
Kalisch PA: Ordeal of the Oklahoma coal miners: coal mine disasters in the Sooner state, 1886–1945. **Chron Okla** 1979;48(3):331–40
Lane R: Violent death in the city: suicide, accident, and murder in nineteenth-century Philadelphia. Cambridge, Mass., Harvard University Press, 1979. xiii, 193 p.
McGrath MH: Scalping: the savage and the surgeon. In Romm S, ed: Symposium on historical perspectives of plastic surgery. Philadelphia, Saunders, 1983. p. 679–88.
Reexamination of accoustic evidence in the Kennedy assassination: **Science** 1982 Oct 8;218(4568):127–33
Roth N: Tracking by telephone: locating the bullet in President Garfield, 1881. **Med Instrum** 1981 May–Jun;15(3):190
Smith R: The first American officer wounded in World War I. **JAMA** 1982 Mar 26;247(12):1743
Weir RF: Remarks on the gunshot wounds of the Civil War by Robert F. Weir. New York State Journal of Medicine, April, 1904. **NY State J Med** 1982 Mar;82(3):391–3
Wilkins EW: Designation or dedication: seven men in the evolution of a trauma center. **Am J Surg** 1982 Apr;143(4):399–403
Yankauer A: Deregulation and the right to life. **Am J Public Health** 1981 Aug;71(8):797–8

**USSR**

Babin VP: Iz opyta organizatsii lecheniia legkoranenykh v mediko-sanitarnom batal'one mekhanizirovannogo korpusa v gody Velikoĭ Otechestvennoĭ voĭny. **Voen Med Zh** 1981 Jun;(6):73–4
Babin VP: O travmaticheskikh povrezhdeniiakh u lits letnogo sostava v period Velikoĭ Otechestvennoĭ voĭny. **Voen Med Zh** 1980 Jul;(7):19–21
Bragin AI, Ivanov NM: Evakuatsiia ranenykh i grazhdanskogo naseleniia iz Leningrada v tyl strany v period blokady (1941–1943 gg.). **Zdravookhr Ross Fed** 1980;(5):9–11
Estrin GB: Voprosy khirurgii i travmatologii v zhurnale 'Vrach' V. A. Manasseina (1880–1901 gg.). **Vestn Khir** 1981 Oct;127(10):142–4
Gladkikh PF, Galin LL: K istorii teoreticheskoi razrabotki sistemy étapnogo lecheniia ranenykh i bol'nykh. **Voen Med Zh** 1984 May;(5):74–5
Kolontaĭ IuIu, Kondrashov AN, Kolod'ko ED: 50 let kafedre travmatologii, ortopedii i voenno-polevoĭ khirurgii Dnepropetrovskogo ordena Trudovogo Krasnogo Znameni meditsinskogo instituta. **Ortop Travmatol Protez** 1980 Mar;(3):76–7
Pavlov AS: Epidemiia travmatizma na fabrikakh i zavodakh Peterburga perioda kapitalizma. **Ortop Travmatol Protez** 1979 Jul;(7):64–5
Petrovskiĭ BV: Ranenie na duéli i smert' A. S. Pushkina. **Klin Med (Mosk)** 1983 Apr;61(4):109–17
Popov MIa: Ranenie i smert' bagrationa. **Vopr Istor** 1975;(3):211–4
Shumada IV, Gorodniaia VN: K istorii Kievskogo obshchestva travmatologov-ortopedov. **Ortop Travmatol Protez** 1984 Aug;(8):69–73
Sukhanov NV: Meditsinakaia i trudovaia reabilitatsiia ranenykh v gospitaliakh Zapadnoĭ Sibiri v period Velikoĭ Otechestvennoĭ voiny. **Voen Med Zh** 1981;(7):72–4
Tepun PD: Deiatel'nost' partiĭnykh organizatsiĭ i naseleniia Severnogo Kavkaza po okazaniiu pomoshchi ranenym v gody Velikoĭ Otechestvennoĭ voĭny. **Sov Zdravookhr** 1980;(5):61–3
Volkov MV: Tsentral'nomu institutu travmatologii i ortopedii im. N. N. Priorova--60 let. **Ortop Travmatol Protez** 1981;(4):1–5

## YELLOW FEVER

### 1700 to Present

Arvy L: Clara Louise Maass (1876–1901) et la fièvre jaune. **Clio Med** 1979 May;13(3–4):277–82
Beauperthuy de Benedetti R: Bref commentaire à un travail de Sir William Osler et sa reconnaissance de la théorie scientifique de Beauperthuy sur la fièvre jaune. In: Congrès international d'histoire de la médecine, XXVe, Québec, 1976. Actes. Québec, 1977. p. 487–92.
Beauperthuy de Benedetti R: Informe sobre la publicacion del señor Cesar Rodriguez Exposito. **Rev Soc Venez Hist Med** 1972–73;20–21(34–35):141–50
Beauperthuy de Benedetti R: Laveran y Beauperthuy. **Acta Med Venez** 1981 Jan–Mar;28(1):47–52
Bowers JZ, King EE: The conquest of yellow fever: the Rockefeller Foundation. **J Med Soc NJ** 1981 Jul;78(7):539–41
Downs WG: A new look at yellow fever and malaria. **Am J Trop Med Hyg** 1981 May;30(3):516–22
Downs WG: History of epidemiological aspects of yellow fever. **Yale J Biol Med** 1982 May–Aug;55(3–4):179–85
Franklin J, Sutherland J, del Regato JA: Yellow fever research. **Science** 1984 Jun 8;224(4653):1043–4, 1128
Osuna A: Beuperthuy 'Descubridor'. **Rev Soc Venez Hist Med** 1972–73;20–21(34–35):197–201
Wrotnowska D: La fièvre jaune. Séjour de Pasteur à Bordeaux, en septembre 1881. In: Congrès National des Sociétés Savantes, 104e, Bordeaux, 1979. Comptes Rendus. Paris, 1979. Section des Sciences, Fasc. IV. p. 109–20.

**Africa**

Dolman CE: Hideyo Noguchi (1876–1928): his final effort in West Africa. In: Congrès international d'histoire de la médecine, XXVe, Québec, 1976. Actes. Québec, 1977. p. 603–24.

**Americas**

Acuña HR: Aedes aegypti, dengue y fiebre amarilla. **Bol Of Sanit Panam** 1982 Dec:93(6):503–5
Leonard J: The ghost of Yellow Jack. **Harv Mag** 1981 Mar–Apr;83(4):20–7
Yellow fever studies. New York, Arno, 1977. Various paginations. Four reprinted articles by various authors, 1814–1915.:

**Argentina**

Beauperthuy de Benedetti R: Repercusion en la Argentina en 1871 del descubrimiento del vector de la fiebre amarilla realizado por Beauperthuy en Venezuela. **Rev Soc Venez Hist Med** 1980;29(43–44):87–93

**Brazil**

Vasconcellos I de: Francisco de Paula Candido et son 'Rapport sur des mesures d'assainissement réclamées par cité de Rio de Janeiro et sur la fièvre jaune en particulier' - Typographie Nationale - Rio de Janeiro, 1854. In: Congrès international d'histoire de la médecine, XXVe, Québec, 1976. Actes. Québec, 1977. p. 1382–4.

**Cuba**

Belozerov VN: 150-letie so dnia rozhdeniia Karlosa Kh. Finleia. **Parazitologiia** 1983 Nov–Dec;17(6):498–9
Blodi FC: Ophthalmology and philately: II. Ophthalmologists who became famous in other areas of endeavor--Carlos Finlay (1833–1915). **Arch Ophthalmol** 1980 Oct;98(10):1763
Centenario del descubrimiento del agente trasmisor de la fiebre amarilla: **Rev Cubana Med Trop** 1981 Jan–Apr;33(1):3–7
Echemendia V: Zum 100. Jahrestag der Entdeckung des Vektors des Gelbfiebers durch den kubanischen Gelehrten Carlos J. Finlay. **Z Gesamte Hyg** 1983 Jan;29(1):35–6
Finlay Seiglie A: Datos interesantes y anecdóticos sobre el sabio cubano Carlos J. Finlay, descubridor del agente trasmisor de la fiebre amarilla. **Rev Cubana Med Trop** 1981 Jan–Apr;33(1):8–12
Martínez-Fortún y Foyo O: Dr. Claudio Delgado y su aportación al estudio de la fiebre amarilla. La Habana [Consejo Cíentifico, Ministerio de la Salud Pública] 1967. 130 p.

**Europe**

Rupp JP: Gelbfieberabwehr in Mitteleuropa. Düsseldorf, Triltsch, 1981. 49 p. **Dusseld Arb Gesch Med Beihefte** 1981;6:1–49

**France**

Arvy L, Rivet R: Dupuytren (1777–1835) face à l'énigme qu'était la fièvre jaune en 1826. In: Congrès National des Sociétés Savantes, 102e, Limoges, 1977. Comptes Rendus. Paris, 1977. Section des Sciences, Fasc. III. p. 27–32.

**Panama**

Guardia CA: Salud pública y saneamiento en la Zona del Canal de Panamá: un recuento histórico, 1880–1915. **Bol Of Sanit Panam** 1983 Jul;95(1):62–73

**Spain**

Angolotti E: La fiebre amarilla. Historia y situación actual. La fiebre amarilla en la Barcelona de 1821. **Rev Sanid Hig Publica (Madr)** 1980 Jan–Feb;54(1–2):89–102
Carrillo JL, Castellanos J, Ramos MD: Enfermedad y sociedad en la Malaga de Comienzos del siglo XIX: el Diálogo de los muertos en la epidemia de Málaga (c. 1803). Introducción y Transcripción. Málaga, Universidad de Málaga, 1980. 41 p.
Carrillo JL, Garcia-Ballester L: Enfermedad y sociedad en la Málaga de los siglos XVIII y XIX. I. La fiebre amarilla (1741–1821). Málaga, Universidad de Málaga, 1980. 199 p.

Carrillo JL: La dialectica ciencia--creencia y su manifestacion en la Malaga de 1803: el conflicto del cierre de los templos. **Jabega (Malaga)** 1979;26(2):3–8

Carrillo JL, García Ballester L: Repercusiones sociales de la epidemia de fiebre amarilla de Malaga (1803–1804): posturas tradicionales e ilustradas en el estamento eclesiastico. In: Sociedad Española de Historia de la Medicina. V Congreso Nacional. Madrid, 1977. **Asclepio** 1977;29:73–99

Danón J: Un brote de fiebre amarilla en el puerto de Barcelona, en 1803. In: Sociedad Española de Historia de la Medicina. V Congreso Nacional. Madrid, 1977. **Asclepio** 1977;29:119–25

Gutmann R: Une lettre signée de Larrey, Desgenettes, Coste et Parmentier, à propos d'une épidémie de fièvre jaune en Espagne. **Hist Sci Med** 1980;14:337–41

Hermosilla Molina A: Epidemia de fiebre amarilla en Sevilla en el año 1800. Sevilla, Talleres Gráficos 'OIGA', 1978.

**United States**

Bean WB: Walter Reed. A biography. Charlottesville, University Press of Virginia, 1982. 190 p.

Bean WB: Walter Reed and yellow fever. **JAMA** 1983 Aug 5;250(5):659–62

Bowen TE: William Crawford Gorgas, physician to the world. **Milit Med** 1983 Dec;148(12):917–20

Bowman IA: Was it yellow fever? **Bookman** 1981 Feb;8(2):3–4

Bruesch SR: Yellow fever in Tennessee in 1878. Part I. **J Tenn Med Assoc** 1978 Dec;71(12):887–96

Chernin E: Josiah Clark Nott, insects, and yellow fever. **Bull NY Acad Med** 1983 Nov;59(9):790–802

Davis JH: Two martyrs of the yellow fever epidemic of 1878. **West Tenn Hist Soc Pap** 1972;26:20–39

Deaths associated with yellow fever experiments. **JAMA** 1983 Mar 4;249(9):1150–1

Ellman MH: William Crawford Gorgas and the American Medical Association. **JAMA** 1980 Feb 15;243(7):659–60

Farley MF: Stranger's fever. **SC Hist Illus** 1970;1(1):54–61

Ferguson RA: Yellow fever and Charles Brockden Brown: the contest of the emerging novelist. **Early Am Lit** 1979–80;14(3):293–305

Harvey AM: Johns Hopkins and yellow fever: a story of tragedy and triumph. **Johns Hopkins Med J** 1981 Jul;149(1):25–39

Honley SA: A history of the 1873 yellow fever epidemic in Shreveport, Louisiana. **North La Hist Assoc** 1982;13(2–3):90–6

Kiple KL, Kiple VH: Black yellow fever immunities, innate and acquired, as revealed in the American South. **Soc Sci Hist** 1977;1(4):419–36

Moe C: Yellow fever in 19th century New Orleans: Necropolis of the South. Monticello, Illinois, Vance Bibliographies, 1979. (Public Administration Series: no. P–375).

Norman C: The unsung hero of yellow fever? **Science** 1984 Mar 30;223(4643):1370–2

Ritchey D: The Baltimore theater and the yellow fever epidemic. **Md Hist Mag** 1972;67(3):298–301

Robbins P: Alas, Memphis! **Am Hist Illus** 1982;16(9):38–46

Shannon GW, Cromley RG: Philadelphia and the yellow fever epidemic of 1798. **Urban Geogr** 1982 Oct–Dec;3:355–70

Snape WJ, Wolfe EL: Courage, compassion, and providence: Woodbury 1793. **Bull Gloucester Cty Hist Soc** 1984 Dec;19(6):41–4

Snape WJ, Wolfe EL: Preliminary report of yellow fever during the 18th century. **J Med Soc NJ** 1984 Sep;81(9):731–3

Snape WJ, Wolfe EL: The studies of yellow-fever by Noah Webster and John Conrad Otto at Red Bank, New Jersey. **Bull Gloucester Cty Hist Soc** 1984 Jun;19(4):25–32

Stickle DF: Death and class in Baltimore: the yellow fever epidemic of 1800. **Md Hist Mag** 1979;74(3):282–99

Tatge RO: A quarantine quandary; ship fever and yellow fever in Providence, Rhode Island, 1797. **Am Neptune** 1980;40(3):192–210

Tigertt HB, Tigertt WD: Clara Louise Maass: a nurse volunteer for yellow fever inoculations--1901. **Milit Med** 1983 Mar;148(3):252–3

Tomlinson WK, Perret JJ: Jean-Charles Faget and the yellow fever controversy in New Orleans. In: Congrès international d'histoire de la médecine, XXVe, Québec, 1976. Actes. Québec, 1977. p. 1361–73.

Walls E: Observations on the New Orleans yellow-fever epidemic, 1878. **La Hist** 1982 Winter;23:60–7

Woodward TE: Yellow fever: from colonial Philadelphia and Baltimore to the mid-twentieth century. In Lilienfeld AM, ed: Times, places, and persons. Baltimore, London, Johns Hopkins Univ. Press, 1980. (Sigerist suppl. to the Bull Hist Med, n.s., no 4) p. 115–31.

Workman M: Medical practice in Philadelphia at the time of the yellow fever epidemic, 1793. **Pa Folklife** 1978;27(4):33–9

**Venezuela**

Beaujón O: La fiebre amarilla y los capitulares de Coro. **Rev Soc Venez Hist Med** 1981;30(45–46):111–4

Beauperthuy de Benedetti R: Resonancia del descurbrimiento del agente transmisor de la fiebre amarilla que hizo Beauperthuy en Venezuela. **Rev Soc Venez Hist Med** 1972–73;20–21(34–35):67–77

## DRUGS AND CHEMICALS

See also **Chemistry and Biochemistry; Pharmacology; Pharmacy; Therapeutics**

Ackerknecht EH: The history of the drug treatment of mental diseases. **Trans Stud Coll Physicians Phila** 1979 Sep;5(1 No 3):161–70, Sep 79

Albert-Puleo M: The obstetrical use in ancient and early modern times of Convolvulus scammonia or Scammony: another non-fugal source of ergot alkaloids? **J Ethnopharmacol** 1979 Apr;1(2):193–5

Bibbings J: Honey, lizard dung and pigeons' blood. **Nurs Times** 1984 Nov 28–Dec 4;80(48):36–8

Brøndegaard VJ: Ethnomedizinische Cusucuta - Applikationen. **Ethnomedizin** 1978–79;5(1–2):47–56

Chilton WS, Bigwood J, Jensen RE: Psilocin, bufotenine and serotonin: historical and biosynthetic observations. **J Psychedelic Drugs** 1979 Jan–Jun;11(1–2):61–9

Clark EW: A brief history of lanolin. **Pharm Hist (London)** 1980 Dec;10(3):5–6

Crul JF: Relaxant drugs: from native drugs to the selective agents of today. **Acta Anaesthesiol Scand** 1982 Aug;26(4):409–15

Daems WF: Radix Ratanhiae, die Droge mit einer gesicherten Geschichte. **Dtsch Apoth Ztg** 1981 Jan 8;121(2):46–52

Fehlmann HR: Ceratum Galeni. Zur Geschichte von Unguentum leniens. In Dilg P, et al., ed: Perspektiven der Pharmaziegeschichte. Graz, Austria, Akademische Druck- u. Verlagsanstalt, 1983. p. 65–77.

Ferroni G: Nota sull' Erbolato. **Rass Lett Ital** 1979;7(1–2):202–14

Glaser FB: The origins of the drug-free therapeutic community. **Br J Addict** 1981 Mar;76(1):13–25

Haas H: History of antipyretic analgesic therapy. **Am J Med** 1983 Nov 14;75(5A):1–3

Haller JS: Aconite: a case study in doctrinal conflict and the meaning of scientific medicine. **Bull NY Acad Med** 1984 Nov;60(9):888–904

Hightower CE: Plants that kill and cure. **Vet Hum Toxicol** 1979 Oct;21(5):360–2

Jackson R: How caustics were used to treat skin cancer. **J Dermatol Surg Oncol** 1979 Dec;5(12):949–50

Jepson E: Medicine from plants. **Trans Med Soc Lond** 1981–82;98:1–10

Jordi González R: Chocolate. De la taza a la farmacia. **Circ Farm** 1980 Jun;12(127):57–62

Leden I: Antimalarial drugs--350 years. **Scand J Rheumatol** 1981;10(4):307–12

Opsomer C: Quelques somnifères de l'antiquité et du moyen âge. Fédération des Cercles d'Archéologie et d'Histoire de Belgique. 44e session. Congrès de Huy, 1976. Annales. Tielt, 1978. p. 589–92.

Palmer C, Horowitz M, ed: Shaman woman, mainline lady: women's writings on the drug experience. New York, Morrow, 1982. 285 p.

Pasqualini RQ: La vigencia de los remedios. **Medicina (B Aires)** 1983;43(4):463–5

Ramzin MS: Teratogene Wirkung von Medikamenten. **Gynakologe** 1982 Sep;15(3):136–42

Rosenthal F: Cannabis and alcohol: the green and the red. **Adv Biosci** 1978 Jul 22–23;22–23:739–45

Rothschuh KE: Medizinische Kulturgeschichte des Wassers. **ZFA (Stuttgart)** 1983 Mar 31;59(9):485–90

Schadewaldt H: Das Sargassokraut als Antiskorbutikum. In Dilg P, et al., ed: Perspektiven der Pharmaziegeschichte. Graz, Austria, Akademische Druck- u. Verlagsanstalt, 1983. p. 281–94.

Schadewaldt H: Die Nebenwirkungen der Heilmittel aus medizinhistorischer Sicht. **Med Welt** 1981 Feb 13;32(7):207–9

Schmitz R: 'Arzneimittelklassiker'. **Med Welt** 1983 Jul 15;34(28):799–803

Théodoridès J: Considerations on the medical uses of marine invertebrates. In Sears M. Merriman D, ed: Oceanography, the past. New York, Springer, 1980. p. 734–49.

Vidal F: Les anodins dans le traitement des douleurs dentaires aux XVIIe et XVIIIe siècles. **Inf Dent** 1982 Feb 25;64(8):695–703

Wijbenga A, Hutzinger O: Chemicals, man and the environment: a historic perspective of pollution and related topics. **Naturwissenschaften** 1984 May;71(5):239–46

**Americas**

Rosengarten F: A neglected Mayan galactagogue, Ixbut (Euphorbia lancifolia). **Bot Mus Leafl Harv Univ** 1978;26:277–309

**China**

Lin CC, Chen JY: [Development of natural crude drug resources from Taiwǎn (I). Pharmacognostical studies on the Chinese crude drug 'Hàn-lián-cǎo (1). The herbological studies] (Jpn). **Yakushigaku Zasshi** 1983;18(2):65–72

Miyasita S: An historical analysis of Chinese drugs in the treatment of hormonal diseases, goitre and diabetes mellitus. **Am J Chin Med** 1980 Spring–Summer;8(1–2):17–25

Swiderski RM: Chinese-American patent medicines. **Ethnomedizin** 1978–79;5(1–2):97–126

Xiong T: [Preliminary exploration on the materia medica from the localities inhabited by ancient China's minority nationalities] (Chi). **Chung Hua I Shih Tsa Chih** 1984;14(2):112-6

**France**

Gandilhon R: La bouse de vache. Etude d'ethnologie. **Mem Soc Agric Commer Sci Arts Marne** 1978;271-306

**India**

Mitra R: Bakula, a reputed drug of Ayurveda, its history, uses in Indian medicine. **Indian J Hist Sci** 1981;16(2):169-80

Singh AN, Singh RS: On the identity of and Indo-Greek relation reflected in the plant-names and uses evinced in the Kautiliya Arthaśastra with particular reference to 'Kiratatikta' of 'Katuvarga' (group of spices). **Indian J Hist Sci** 1983 Nov;18(2):172-5

Singh RS, Singh LB: Aconites (Visas) in the Ayurvedic therapy (origin, sources, classification and historical antecedents). **Stud Hist Med** 1982 Jun;6(2):147-59

Singh RS, Vyas VD: The identity and critical appraisal of the basis of nomenclature and ancient socio-cultural and geographico-historical reflections evinced with the Paninian perfume-plant/plant-part 'Kisara' (Panini IV. IV. 53). **Indian J Hist Sci** 1983 Nov;18(2):166-71

**Japan**

Hamada T, Namba T: [Pharmacognostical studies on the molluscan drugs (14). Historical and herbological investigations on 'Tianluo' and 'Luosi'] (Jpn). **Yakushigaku Zasshi** 1983;18(2):53-64

Miyazaki M: [On 'Chindoku' a toxicant in the oriental tradition] (Jpn). **Yakushigaku Zasshi** 1983;18(2):101-6

Okazaki K: Kusuri no rekishi. Tokyo, Kodansha, Showa 51 nen, [1976]. 324 p.

**Spain**

Esteva de Sagrera J, Espinosa Ramos E: Los trociscos de vibrora en la obra de Luís de Oviedo, Gerónimo de la Fuente Piérola y Félix Palacios. **Unifarma** 1980 Jun 13;:244-51

**Before 500 A.D.**

Scarborough J: On medications for burns in classical antiquity. In Romm S, ed: Symposium on historical perspectives of plastic surgery. Philadelphia, Saunders, 1983. p. 603-610.

**Americas**

Litzinger WJ: Ceramic evidence for prehistoric datura use in North America. **J Ethnopharmacol** 1981 Jul;4(1):57-74

**China**

Benfey OT: Spinach is an alchemical antidote to heavy metal poisoning. **Kagakushi Kenkyu** 1981;15:8-12

**Egypt**

Emboden WA: Transcultural use of narcotic water lilies in ancient Egyptian and Maya drug ritual. **J Ethnopharmacol** 1981 Jan;3(1):39-83

Youtie LC: [Eye-salves.] **Bull Am Soc Papyrologists** 1979;16:149-51

**Greco-Roman**

Curtis RI: Salted fish products in ancient medicine. **J Hist Med Allied Sci** 1984 Oct;39(4):430-45

**Greece**

Winkler L: Galens Schrift 'De Antidotis'. Ein Beitrag zur Geschichte von Antidot und Theriak. Diss. rer. nat. Marburg, 1980. 390 p.

**India**

Ranade HG: A note on 'Pata in Atharvaveda 2.27'. **Stud Hist Med** 1981 Sep;5(3):225-7

**500 A.D.-1450**

Jenkins M: Medicine and spices, with special reference to medieval monastic accounts. **Gard Hist** 1976;4:47-9

Rosner F: Moses Maimonides' treatise on poisons. **NY State J Med** 1980 Sep;80(10):1627-30

**Arabic**

Durrany KS, Uddin Siddiqui T: Al-Adwiyat al-Qalbiya. **Stud Hist Med** 1980 Mar;4(1):29-38

Folch Jou G: Medicamentos empleados por los arabes y su posible influencia en la introduccion de la quimica en la Farmacia. **Asclepio** 1978-79;30-31:177-86

Johnstone P: Aconite and its antidote in Arabic writings. **J Hist Arabic Sci** 1977 May;1(1):65-71

Mohaghegh M: The title of a work of Razi with reference to al-Tin al-Nishaburi. In: International Symposium for the History of Arabic Science, 1st, University of Aleppo, 1976. Proceedings. Aleppo, Syria, 1976. Papers in European Languages, Vol. II. p. 338-40.

Uddinahmed R: Single drugs mentioned by Avicenna for cardiac ailments in his canon and Kitab-Ul-Adwiyyah Qalbiyyah. **Bull Indian Inst Hist Med (Hyderabad)** 1979;9:46-66

Vazquez C: Sobre la cosmetica (zina) del S. XIV en Al-Andalus. **Bol Soc Esp Hist Farm** 1982 Mar;33(129):9-48

**China**

Guo Chengyu: [Yang Tianhui and his 'Records on Radix aconitinum'] (Chi). **Chin J Med Hist** 1981;11(1):48-50

**Great Britain**

Sass LJ: Religion, medicine, politics and spices. **Appetite** 1981 Mar;2(1):7-13

**Italy**

Russo A: I 'semplici' nella Scuola Salernitana (Nota preliminare). **Rend Atti Accad Sci Med Chir** 128:55-75

**1450-1700**

Kaempfer E: Amoenitatum Exoticarum Politico-physico-medicarum. Fasciculi V, Quibus Continentur Variae Relationes, Observationes and Descriptiones Rerum Persicarum and Ulterioris Asiae (Lemgo: Meyeri, 1712). **J Hist Med Allied Sci** 1978 Jul;33(3):320-43

Schmitz R, Kuhlen FJ: Anästhesie und Arzneimittelmissbrauch in peinlichen Gerichtsverfahren des 16. und 17. Jahrhunderts. In Göpfert W, Otten HH, ed: Metavoeite: wandelt euch durch neues Denken. Düsselfort, Triltsch, 1983. p. 189-99.

**France**

Duthoit JP: La Marquise de Sévigné et quelques aspects de la thérapeutique médicale au XVIIe siècle. Lille, 1980. 110, 8 p.

**Great Britain**

Kail AC: The bard and the body. 4. Drugs, herbs and poisons. **Med J Aust** 1983 Nov 12;2(10):515-9

**Iran**

Carrubba RW: The first detailed report on Persian mummy. **Physis** 1981;23(4):461-71

**Netherlands**

Leyh F: Hatte Rembrandt van Rijn eine Nickelallergie? **Hautarzt** 1984 Sep;35(9):472-3

**Spain**

Sánchez-Moscoso Hermida A: La peligrosidad del medicamento a través del 'Discurso Farmacéutico sobre los Cánones de Mesué', de Miguel Martínez de Leache (1652). **Bol Soc Esp Hist Farm** 1984 Jun;35(138):103-23

**1700 to Present**

Barber GO: The diverse uses of glycerine in pre-antibiotic days. **MIMS Mag** 1981 Apr 15;:46-7

Bennett AE: Historical development of somatic therapies in affective disorders. **Int Pharmacopsychiatry** 1979;14(2):85-93

Bindra JS, Lednicer D, ed: Chronicles of drug discovery. Volume 1. New York, John Wiley & Sons, 1982. xiii, 283 p.

Broome JD: L-Asparaginase: discovery and development as a tumor-inhibitory agent. **Cancer Treat Rep** 1981;65 Suppl 4:111-4

Cheung WY: Discovery and recognition of calmodulin: a personal account. **J Cyclic Nucleotide Res** 1981;7(2):71-84

Crellin JK: Internal antisepsis or the dawn of chemotherapy? **J Hist Med Allied Sci** 1981 Jan;36(1):9-18

Crompton R, Gall D: Georgi Markov--death in a pellet. **Med Leg J** 1980;48(2):51-62

Dauber LG: Compound X given intravenously. On the history of the nitrogen mustards. **NY State J Med** 1984 Mar;84(3 pt 1):122-4

De Haen P: New drug parade: a historical minireview, 1954–1982. Englewood, Colo., Paul de Haen International, 1983. 36 p.
Diczfalusy E: The early history of estriol. **J Steroid Biochem** 1984 Apr;20(4B):945–53
Domino EF, ed: PCP (phencyclidine): historical and current perspectives. Ann Arbor, Mich., NPP Books, 1981. xx, 537 p. Historical chapters by V. H. Maddox and D. A. McCarthy.
Dorkins HR: Suxamethonium--the development of a modern drug from 1906 to the present day. **Med Hist** 1982 Apr;26(2):145–68
Duke M: The story of nitroglycerine. An old favorite with new tricks. **Conn Med** 1983 Aug;47(8):495
Dundee JW, McIlroy PD: The history of barbiturates. **Anaesthesia** 1982 Jul;37(7):726–34
Dworkin AG, Stephen RC: Mexican-American adolescent inhalant abuse: a proposed Model. **Youth Soc** 1980;11(4):493–506
Fieve RR, Jamison KR: Rubidium: overview and clinical perspectives. **Mod Probl Pharmacopsychiatry** 1982;18:145–63
García-Argüelles R: De la digital de ayer a los lanatosidos de hoy. Una breve historia de los cardiotonicos. **Asclepio** 1980;32:195–9
Goodwin JS, Goodwin JM: Failure to recognize efficacious treatments: a history of salicylate therapy in rheumatoid arthritis. **Perspect Biol Med** 1981 Autumn, 25(1):78–92
Goodwin LG: New drugs for old diseases. **Trans R Soc Trop Med Hyg** 1980;74(1):1–7
Haller JS: Hypodermic medication; early history. **NY State J Med** 1981 Oct;81(11):1671–9
Herrerias Gutiérrez JM: Promesas y realidades de la cimetidina. **Rev Esp Enferm Apar Dig** 1979 Oct;56(4):373–80
Hügelow M: Original-Lithographien speziell für Pharmazeuten: Historische Apothekergeräte und Heilpflanzen. **Pharm Unserer Zeit** 1984 Jul;13(4):97–101
Hurst DL, Hurst MJ: Bromide psychosis: a literary case. **Clin Neuropharmacol** 1984;7(3):259–64
Isaac O, Kristen G: Alte und neue Wege der Kamillentherapie. Die Kamille als Beispiel für moderne Arzneipflanzenforschung. **Med Welt** 1980 Aug 8;31(31–32):1145–9
Kenéz J: Results in drug treatment of tuberculosis (historical survey). **Ther Hung** 1982;30(3):151–5
Knapp DA, Knapp DE, Brooks GE: Drug use in Australia and the United States as reflections of legislation and social attitudes. **Drug Intell Clin Pharm** 1977 May;11(5):298–303
Knoll J: Deprenyl (selegiline): the history of its development and pharmacological action. **Acta Neurol Scand [Suppl]** 1983;95:57–80
Laragh JH: Concept of anti-renin system therapy. Historic perspective. **Am J Med** 1984 Aug 20;77(2A):1–6
Laurence DR: Medicines then and now. **Nature** 1981 Sep 3;293(5827):13–5
Leff A, Lester TW, Addington WW: Tuberculosis. A chemotherapeutic triumph but a persistent socioeconomic problem. **Arch Intern Med** 1979 Dec;139(12):1375–7
Lillehei RC: History of vasodilation in treating shock and low flow states. **Adv Shock Res** 1978;1:1–17
Madrid Arias JL: Evolución histórica de los agentes neurolíticos utilizados para tratamiento del dolor crónico. **Rev Esp Anestesiol Reanim** 1984 Sep–Oct;31(5):197–204
Mayrhofer VO: Die Geschichte der Muskelvelaxanzien. **Klin Anaesthesiol Intensivther** 1980;22:1–9
Miller JA, Miller EC: Some historical aspects of N-aryl carcinogens and their metabolic activation. **Environ Health Perspect** 1983 Mar;49:3–12
Modestin J: 30 Jahre Neuroleptika--Zeit zur kritischen Auseinandersetzung. **Dtsch Med Wochenschr** 1983 Sep 23;108(38):1446–51
Newell FW: Centenary of Credé prophylaxis. **Am J Ophthalmol** 1980 Dec;90(6):874–5
Nitroglycerin--the first hundred years: **Lancet** 1979 Dec 22–29;2(8156–8157):1340–1
Pierard GE, Lapière CM: Les corticostéroïdes à usage externe. Trente années d'utilisation et perspectives d'avenir. **Rev Med Liege** 1984 Feb 15;39(4):156–9
Rim HJ: Therapy of fluke infections in the past. A review. **Arzneimittelforsch** 1984;34(9B):1127–9
Schütz H: Benzodiazepine--Entdeckung, Entwicklung und Zukunftsperspektiven. **Pharm Unserer Zeit** 1982 Nov;11(6):161–76
Settle EC, Ayd FJ: Haloperidol: a quarter century of experience. **J Clin Psychiatry** 1983 Dec;44(12):440–8
Simpson GM: A brief history of depot neuroleptics. **J Clin Psychiatry** 1984 May;45(5 pt 2):3–4
Smith PB: Chemical glimpses of paradise. Springfield, Illinois, Charles C. Thomas, 1972. ix, 92 p.
Sternbach G: William Osler: narcotic-induced pulmonary edema. **J Emerg Med** 1983;1(2):165–7
Sternbach LH: The benzodiazepine story. **J Psychoactive Drugs** 1983 Jan–Jun;15(1–2):15–7
Ulfelder H: The stilbestrol disorders in historical perspective. **Cancer** 1980 Jun 15;45(12):3008–11
Weismann G: A fashion in metals. **Hosp Pract** 1982 Apr;17(4):33–4, 38, 42
Whiteside T: The pendulum and the toxic cloud. The course of dioxin contamination. New Haven, London, Yale University Press, 1979. 205 p.
Wildsmith JA, Strichartz GR: Local anaesthetic drugs--an historical perspective. **Br J Anaesth** 1984 Sep;56(9):937–9
Woschick E: Die kontrollierte Hypotension--Vergangenheit und Gegenwart. Eine Ubersicht. **Zentrabl Neurochir** 1984;45(1):1–10
Wright JC: Cancer chemotherapy: past, present, and future--Part I. **J Natl Med Assoc** 1984 Aug;76(8):773–84

**Americas**

Walker WO: Drug control in the Americas. Albuquerque, University of New Mexico Press, 1981. xvi, 287 p.

**Austria**

Mutschlechner G: Erde als Heilmittel für Mensch und Tier. **Tirol Heimatbl** 1974;49(1):23–7

**Belgium**

Aernouts R: L'eau de Lourdes est-elle un médicament? **Rev Hist Pharm (Paris)** 1980 Mar;27(244):5–7

**Czechoslovakia**

Rumpf-Lehmann B: Seltene Drogen von 'Dr. Dittrich aus Prag' in der Wigandschen Drogensammlung der Universität Marburg. **Beitr Gesch Pharm** 1982;31(16):123–6

**France**

Chertok L: 30 ans après. La petite histoire de la découverte des neuroleptiques. **Ann Med Psychol (Paris)** 1982 Nov;140(9):971–6
Guyotjeannin C: Les médicaments de Marcel Proust. **Monit Pharm** 1983 Sep 10;37(1577):3423, 3425, 3427; 1983 Oct 15;37(1582):3987–8
Guyotjeannin C, Lehuenen J: Quelques documents inédits concernant les thérapeutiques utilisées aux îles Saint-Pierre-et-Miquelon (XIXe siècle - début XXe siècle). **Hist Sci Med** 1984;18(2):159–64
Théodoridès J: L'abbé de Bap, curé de Sommières, et son prétendu remède antirabique. **Rev Hist Pharm (Paris)** 1979 Dec;26(243):269–79

**Germany**

Barthel I: Arzneimittelversuche des 19.Jahrhunderts am gesunden Menschen im deutschsprachigen Raum. Diss., Universität Düsseldorf. Düsseldorf, 1982. 105 p.
Kleeberg J: Uber Ehrlichs Benzaldehyd-Reaktion (auf Urobilinogen) nach 80 Jahren. **Z Gastroenterol** 1982 Aug;20(8):424–8

**Great Britain**

Berridge V: Drugs and social policy: the establishment of drug control in Britain 1900–30. **Br J Addict** 1984 Mar;79(1):17–29
Duncan WA, Parsons ME: Reminiscences of the development of cimetidine. **Gastroenterology** 1980 Mar;78(3):620–5
Houston RA: Colliers with colic? **Local Popul Stud (Matlock)** 1979;22:57–9
Prescott LF: The Regional Poisoning Treatment Centre, Edinburgh. In Passmore R, ed: Proceedings of the Royal College of Physicians of Edinburgh Tercentenary Congress, 1981. Edinburgh, Royal College of Physicians of Edinburgh, 1982. p. 211–20.
Rodin AE: Autoexperimentation with a drug by Arthur Conan Doyle. **J Hist Med Allied Sci** 1980 Oct;35(4):426–30
Thirty years of drugs for hypertension: a festschrift for Sir John McMichael: **Br J Clin Pharmacol** 1982 Jan;13(1):5–142

**Hungary**

Rádóczy G: A Magyarországon Hivatalos gyógyszernormatívumok. **Orvostort Kozl** 1981;93–96(27 No 1–4):123–53

**Italy**

Di Marco A, Cassinelli G, Arcamone F: The discovery of daunorubicin. **Cancer Treat Rep** 1981;65 Suppl 4:3–8

**Japan**

Matsuyama K, Ogawa S: [A historical study on expansive use of chloroquine] (Jpn). **Igakushi Kenkyu** 1980;53:22–29
Yasue M: [On the ancient manuscript named 'A Togoku-ohayashi-ninjin'] (Jpn). **Yakushigaku Zasshi** 1983;18(2):87–94

**South Africa**

Wyk AJ: Medisyne uit Suid-Afrika vir die Keiser. **Historia (S Afr)** 1979;24(1):63–5

# DRUGS AND CHEMICALS

**Spain**

de Andrés Turrión ML: Medicacíon vegetal para el rey Alfonso XII. **Bol Soc Esp Hist Farm** 1984 Sep;35(139):187–98
Esteva de Sagrera J: Una obra inédita y desconocida de Agustín Yáñez y Girona. **Bol Soc Esp Hist Farm** 1979 Dec;30(120):295–304
Figuerola JE, Figuerola I: La cuenta de medicinas administradas a la hija del Marques de la Quadra. **Bol Soc Esp Hist Farm** 1980 Mar–Jun;3(121–2)

**Sweden**

Ljungdell J: Juglans regia L. – i den svenska farmakopéen och annorstädes. **Sydsven Medicinhist Sallsk Arsskr** 1982;19:54–62

**United States**

Arata LA: Nostalgia: the medicine show. **J Indiana State Med Assoc** 1980 Jun;73(6):353
Atropine poisoning in Hawthorne's the Scarlet Letter: **N Engl J Med** 1984 Nov 29;311(22):1438–41
Baker HC: Patent medicine in Pennsylvania before 1906: a history through advertising. **Pa Folklife** 1977–78;27(2):20–33
Bell C: Implementing safety and health regulations for women in the workplace. **Feminist Stud** 1979;5(2):286–301
Brinnin JM: The sway of the grand saloon: queasy come, queasy go. **Am Heritage** 1971;22(6):16–9, 98–9
Burger A: Drug development: challenges and hurdles. **Va Q Rev** 1981;57(3):420–39
Caen JP: Heparin: a 70 year history from 1914 to 1984. **Nouv Rev Fr Hematol** 1984;26(4):209–10
Courtwright D: Opiate addiction in the American West, 1850–1920. **J West** 1982 Jul;21(3):23–31
Estes JW: Naval medicine in the age of sail: the voyage of the New York, 1802–1803. **Bull Hist Med** 1982 Summer;56(2):238–53
Ferry AP, Ferry MK: Dr. Isaac Thompson and his celebrated eye water. **Ophthalmology** 1984 May;91(5):528–37
Freireich E: Landmark perspective: Nitrogen mustard therapy. **JAMA** 1984 May 4;251(17):2262–3
Fye WB: Heparin: the contributions of William Henry Howell. **Circulation** 1984 Jun;69(6):1198–203
Goyan JE: FDA at 75--failure, symbiosis, convergence. In Young JH, ed: The early years of federal food and drug control. Madison, American Institute of the History of Pharmacy, 1982. p. 53–60.
Hornbrook MC: Medicinal drugs: risks and regulations. **Curr Hist** 1980;78(457):201–5, 223–6
Jones OR: Essense of peppermint: history of the medicine and its bottle. **Hist Archaeol** 1981;15(2):1–57
Khan JA: Atropine poisoning in Hawthorne's The Scarlet Letter. **N Engl J Med** 1984 Aug 9;311(6):414–6
Levin BS: Women and medicine. Metuchen, N. J., London, Scarecrow, 1980. vii, 257 p.
Mathisen DA: Whatever happened to human body glue? **Reason** 1980;12(1):20–7
Perkins JH: Reshaping technology in wartime: the effect of military goals on entomological research and insect-control practices. **Technol Cult** 1978 Apr;19(2):169–86
Rogers FB: Dr. Samuel Pitcher (1824–1907): Cape Cod and Castoria. **J Hist Med Allied Sci** 1982 Jul;37(3):323–5
Shapiro LJ, Angorn RA, McCormick WC: Look-alike prescription drugs. A historical perspective of the legal issues. **Am Pharm** 1982 Aug;22(8):26–30
Sonnedecker G: Drug standards become official. In Young JH, ed: The early years of federal food and drug control. Madison, American Institute of the History of Pharmacy, 1982. p. 28–39.
Swinyard EA: History of the antiepileptic drugs. **Adv Neurol** 1980;27:1–9
Thomasson WA: Deadly legacy: dioxin and the Vietnam veteran. **Bull At Sci** 1979;35(5):15–19
Tyler VE: Three proprietaries and their claim as American 'Indian' remedies. **Pharm Hist** 1984;26(3):146–9
Van Allen MW: Landmark perspective: introduction of sodium diphenyl hydantoinate. **JAMA** 1984 Feb 24;251(8):1068–9
Vyhnanek L: 'Muggles,' 'Inchy,' and 'Mud': illegal drugs in New Orleans during the 1920's. **La Hist** 1981;22(3):253–79
Ward PS: 'Who will bell the cat?' Andrew C. Ivy and krebiozen. **Bull Hist Med** 1984 Spring;58(1):28–52
Wyler DJ: Landmark perspective: The ascent and decline of chloroquine. **JAMA** 1984 May 11;251(18):2420–2
Young JH: American health quackery: an historical view. **Ga J Sci** [1979?];38:33–40

**USSR**

Miagkaia IP: Antiretikuliarnaia tsitotoksicheskaia syvorotka A. A. Bogomol'tsa kak sredstvo patogeneticheskoĭ terapii razlichnykh zabolevaniĭ. **Patol Fiziol Eksp Ter** 1981 Mar–Apr;(2):39–46
Miagkaia IP: Sovremennye predstavleniia o mekhanizme deĭstviia antiretikuliarnoĭ tsitotoksicheskoĭ syvorotki Bogomol'tsa. **Fiziol Zh** 1981 May–Jun;27(3):347–53
Ovchinnikov NM, Timchenko GF: Dvadtsatiletniĭ opyt raboty Tsentral'nogo nauchno-issledovatel'skogo kozhnovenerologicheskogo instituta Minzdrava SSR po kontroliu i uluchsheniiu kachestva serologicheskikh laboratorii dermatovenerologicheskikh uchrezhdeniĭ SSSR. **Lab Delo** 1981;(2):120–2
Senchenkova EM: [The importance of M. S. Tswett's investigations of the carotinoids.] (Rus). **Istor Biol Issled** 1978;7:65–92

## ABSINTHE

### 1700 to Present

**France**

Delahaye MC: L'absinthe. Histoire de la fée verte. Paris, Berger-Levrault, 1983. 128 p.
Prestwich PE: Temperance in France: the curious case of absinth. **Hist Reflect** 1979;6(2):301–19
Vogt DD: Absinthium: a nineteenth-century drug of abuse. **J Ethnopharmacol** 1981 Nov;4(3):337–42

## ACIDS

### 1700 to Present

Abir-Am P: From biochemistry to molecular biology: DNA and the acculturated journey of the critic of science Erwin Chargaff. **Hist Philos Life Sci** 1980;2(1):3–60
Krehl WA: Discovery of the effect of tryptophan on niacin deficiency. **Fed Proc** 1981;40:1527–30
Welch AD: Folic acid: discovery and the exciting first decade. **Perspect Biol Med** 1983 Autumn;27(1):64–75

**United States**

Darby WJ: Folic acid and macrocytic anemias. **South Med J** 1983 Nov;76(11):1341–3

## ALCOHOL

Maret F: Der Wein in der Medizingeschichte. **ZFA (Stuttgart)** 1980 May 10;56(13):887–97

**Germany**

Holtkamp P: Narkosen mit 'Weingenuss bis zum Nasenbluten'. **Quintessenz J** 1981 Nov;11(11):995–6

**Great Britain**

Higgs EJ: Research into the history of alcohol use and control in England and Wales: the available sources in the Public Record Office. **Br J Addict** 1984 Mar;79(1):41–7

**United States**

Ezell MD: Early attitudes toward alcoholic beverages in the South. **Red River Val Hist Rev** 1982;7(1):64–70
Lender ME: Dictionary of American temperance biography: from temperance reform to alcohol research, the 1600s to the 1980s. Westport, Conn., Greenwood Press, 1984. xiv, 572 p.
Proctor RC: History of drinking in America. **South Med J** 1984 Jul;77(7):886–92

### Before 500 A.D.

**China**

Mahdihassan S: Chinese origin of the word alcohol. **Am J Chin Med** 1980 Autumn;8(3):239–44

**Greece**

Preiser G: Wein im Urteil der griechischen Antike. In Völger G, ed: Rausch und Realität. Drogen im Kulturvergleich. Teil 1. Köln, Raufenstrauch-Joest-Museum für Völkerkunde der Stadt Köln, 1981. p. 296–303 (Materialienband zu einer Ausstellung 7. Aug. bis 11. Okt. 1981).
Ruck CA: The wild and the cultivated: wine in Euripides' Bacchae. **J Ethnopharmacol** 1982 May;5(3):231–70

**Rome**

Preiser G: Wein im Urteil der Römer. In Völger G, ed: Rausch und Realität. Drogen im Kulturvergleich. Teil 1. Köln, Raufenstrauch-Joest-Museum für Völkerkunde der Stadt Köln, 1981.

p. 304–8 (Materialienband zu einer Ausstellung 7. Aug. bis 11. Okt. 1981).

**1700 to Present**

Malcolm MT: Foetal alcohol syndrome: historical aspects. **Alcohol Alcohol** 1984;19(3):261–2
Whitby JD: Alcohol in anaesthesia and surgical resuscitation. **Anaesthesia** 1980 May;35(5):502–5

**Australia**

Hicks R: Rum regulation and riches. Sydney, Australian Hospital Association, 1981. vii, 231 p.

**France**

Rivet R: Usage médical du vin de Bordeaux au XVIIIe siècle. In: Congrès National des Sociétés Savantes, 104e, Bordeaux, 1979. Comptes Rendus. Paris, 1979. Section des Sciences, Fasc. IV. p. 121–31.

**Germany**

Robert JS: Drink and industrial work discipline in 19th century Germany. **J Soc Hist** 1981;15(1):25–38

**Great Britain**

Warner JH: Physiological theory and therapeutic explanation in the 1860s: the British debate on the medical use of alcohol. **Bull Hist Med** 1980 Summer;54(2):235–57
Weir RB: Obsessed with moderation: the drink trades and the drink question (1870–1930). **Br J Addict** 1984 Mar;79(1):93–107

**United States**

Bernard J: The American drinking tradition. **Rev Am Hist** 1980;8(2):206–14
Currie R, Driedger L, Linden R: Abstinence and moderation: mixing Mennonite drinking norms. **Mennon Q Rev** 1979;53(4):263–81
Dannenbaum J: The crusade against drink. **Rev Am Hist** 1981;9(4):497–502
Leader JP: The Pottawatomies and alcohol: an illustration of the illegal trade. **Kans Hist** 1979;2(3):157–65
Williams SE: The use of beverage alcohol as medicine, 1790–1860. **J Stud Alcohol** 1980 May;41(5):543–66

## ALOE

**Spain**

Carmen Frances M del: El aloes en las farmacopeas nacionales Espanolas. In Hickel E, Schröder G, ed: Neue Beiträge zur Arzneimittelgeschichte. Festschrift für Wolfgang Schneider zum 70. Geburtstag. Stuttgart, Wissenschaftliche Verlagsgesellschaft, 1982. p. 149–57.

**Before 500 A.D.**

**Greco-Roman**

Scarborough J: Roman pharmacy and the eastern drug trade. **Pharm Hist** 1982;24(4):135–43

## AMBERGRIS

Dannenfeldt KH: Ambergris: the search for its origin. **Isis** 1982 Sep;73(268):382–97

## AMPHETAMINE

**1700 to Present**

**Germany**

Lekisch K: Drugs and politics. **Scalpel Tongs** 1981;25:93–4

## ANGIOTENSIN

Moore AF: A review of the renin-angiotensin system: historical and methodological perspectives. **Methods Find Exp Clin Pharmacol** 1979;1(1):23–44

## ANTHRACENES

**1700 to Present**

Ashton RE, Andre P, Lowe NJ, et al: Anthralin: historical and current perspectives. **J Am Acad Dermatol** 1983 Aug;9(2):173–92

**Poland**

Supady J: Doświadczalne badania lekarzy polskich nad rakotwórczym działaniem smoły pogazowej i jej pochondnych (do 1939 r.). **Pol Tyg Lek** 1981 Mar 2;36(9):357–9

## ANTIBIOTICS

**1700 to Present**

Cowen DL, Segelman AB, ed: Antibiotics in historical perspective. [Rahway, New Jersey], Merck, Sharp & Dohme, 1981. 225 p.
Hirsch JG: The greatest success story in the history of medicine. **Med Times** 1980 Sep;108(9):36–43
Parascandola J, ed: The history of antibiotics. Madison, Wis., 1980. vi, 136 p. (Publication/American Institute of the History of Pharmacy. new series, no. 5)
Rhoades ER: A seminar on antibiotics. **J Okla State Med Assoc** 1980 Jun;73(6):176–9
Synge RL: Early work on Gramicidin S. In J. Parascandola, ed: The history of antibiotics. Madison, American Institute of the History of Pharmacy, 1980. p. 97–100.
Ward PS: Antibiotics and international relations at the close of World War II. In J. Parascandola, ed: The history of antibiotics. Madison, American Institute of the History of Pharmacy, 1980. p. 101–12.

**Australia**

Blum A: Fleeting hopes and promises of advertising. **Med J Aust** 1982 May 29;1(11):485

**Great Britain**

Abraham EP: Ernst Chain and Paul Garrod. **J Antimicrob Chemother** 1980 Jul;6(4):423–4

**Japan**

Yagisawa Y: Early history of antibiotics in Japan. In J. Parascandola, ed: The history of antibiotics. Madison, American Institute of the History of Pharmacy, 1980. p. 69–90.

**Spain**

Woodruff HB, Hernandez S, Stapley EO: Evolution of an antibiotic screening programme. A tribute to Justo Martinez Mata. **Hindustan Antibiot Bull** 1979 Feb;21(3):71–84

**United States**

Lechevalier HA: The search for antibiotics at Rutgers University. In J. Parascandola, ed: The history of antibiotics. Madison, American Institute of the History of Pharmacy, 1980. p. 113–23.
Thomas L: The right track. **Wilson Q** 1980;4(2):87–98

**USSR**

Gause GF: Gramicidin S and early antibiotic research in the Soviet Union. In J. Parascandola, ed: The history of antibiotics. Madison, American Institute of the History of Pharmacy, 1980. p. 91–5.
Navashin SM, Fomina IP: Nauka ob antibiotikakh v SSSR – istoriia i perspektivy razvitiia. **Antibiotiki** 1982;27(12):5–9
Zhurnalu 'Antibiotiki' chetvert' veka: **Antibiotiki** 1981;26(8):564–6

## ANTIMONY

Daems WF: Stimmi, Stibium, Antimon: eine substanzhistorische Betrachtung. Arlesheim (Schweiz), Weleda, 1976. 35 p.
Ercoli N: L'antimonio da Basilio Valentino all'anno duemila. **Acta Med Hist Patav** 1979–80;26:47–61
Müller I: Zur Theorie und Praxis der Antimontherapie. In Göpfert W, Otten HH, ed: Metavoeite: wandelt euch durch neues Denken. Düsseldorf, Triltsch, 1983. p. 173–88.
Wietschoreck H: Aethiops---eine neue Arzneimittelgruppe der Nachchemiatrie---und ihre Bedeutung in Verbindung mit anderen Antimon-Präparaten. (Ein Beispiel für den Einsatz chemischer Untersuchungen bei der Bearbeitung arzneimittelgeschichtlicher Fragen). In: Vorträge des Internationalen Pharmaziehistorischen Kongresses Innsbruck 1977. Stuttgart, Wissenschaftliche Verlagsgesellschaft, 1979. p. 49–55.

**1450–1700**

Fischer H: Der Streit um das Arzneimittel im Spiegel frühzeitlicher Antimonliteratur. **Beitr Gesch Pharm** 1983;31(18/19):150–4

# DRUGS AND CHEMICALS

**1700 to Present**

**Great Britain**

Miller JM: Poisoning by antimony: a case report (Oliver Goldsmith). **South Med J** 1982 May;75(5):592

**APHRODISIACS**

Bose AK: Aphrodisiacs - a psychosocial perspective. **Indian J Hist Sci** 1981;16(1):100-3
Rosen IL: Aphrodisiacs in the kitchen. **J La State Med Soc** 1980 Oct;132(10):155-9

**Before 500 A.D.**

Rosner F: Mandrakes and other aphrodisiacs in the Bible & Talmud. **Koroth** 1980 Jun;7(11-12):CCLXXVII-CCLXXXIV

**500 A.D.-1450**

Cosman MP: A feast for Aesculapius: historical diets for asthma and sexual pleasure. **Annu Rev Nutr** 1983;3:1-33

**ARECA**

**500 A.D.-1450**

**China**

Netolitzky A: Marginalien über die Arecanuss im mittelalterlichen China. **Asiat Forsch** 1980;71:60-5

**1700 to Present**

**Great Britain**

Reichart PA: Toothpastes containing betel nut (Areca catechu L.) from England of the nineteenth century. **J Hist Med Allied Sci** 1984 Jan;39(1):65-79

**ARSENIC**

**Asia**

Emmerick RE: Arsenic and sida. In Mazars G, ed: Les médecines traditionnelles de l'Asie. Strasbourg, Université Louis Pasteur, 1981. p. 93-102.

**Before 500 A.D.**

**Greece**

Thucydides and the Athenian plague: a reconsideration of the evidence: **Pharm Hist (London)** 1984 Dec;14(4):6-7

**1450-1700**

**Hungary**

Szilágyi I: Bethlen Gábor betegsége és halála. **Orv Hetil** 1984 May 13;125(20):1205-10

**1700 to Present**

**France**

Jones DE, Ledingham KW: Arsenic in Napoleon's wallpaper. **Nature** 1982 Oct 14;299(5884):626-7
Lépine P: Un dossier contesté, l'affaire Lafarge. **Lyon Pharm** 1980 Jan 1;31(1):39-44
Lewin PK, Hancock RG, Voynovich P: Napoleon Bonaparte--no evidence of chronic arsenic poisoning. **Nature** 1982 Oct 14;299(5884):627-8

**Germany**

Thorburn AL: Paul Ehrlich: pioneer of chemotherapy and cure by arsenic (1854-1915). **Br J Vener Dis** 1983 Dec;59(6):404-5

**ARSPHENAMINES**

**1700 to Present**

Kampmeier RH: The continuous treatment of early syphilis by arsphenamin and heavy metals. **Sex Transm Dis** 1981 Jul-Sep;8(3):224-6

**Germany**

Bäumler E: Paul Ehrlich, Forscher für das Leben. Frankfurt, Societäts-Verlag, 1979. 370 p.

**Hungary**

Szállási A: A salvarsan felfedezésének visszhangja a Nyugat-ban. **Orv Hetil** 1980 Apr 20;121(16):966-7

**United States**

Ward PS: The American reception of Salvarsan. **J Hist Med Allied Sci** 1981 Jan;36(1)44-62

**ARTEMESIA**

Thakur RS, Singh SB: Artemisia: the sagebrush plant - a review. **Curr Res Med Aromat Plant** 1979;1:90-108

**ASAFETIDA**

**1450-1700**

**Iran**

Carrubba RW: The first report of the harvesting of Asafetida in Iran. **Agric Hist** 1979;53(2):451-61

**ASPIRIN**

**1700 to Present**

Girstenbrey W: Soll und Haben eines pharmazeutischen Evergreens. **Fortschr Med** 1983 Jul 28;101(27-28):1294-7
Krantz JC, White JM: Aspirin: four score and more. **South Med J** 1980 Dec;73(12):1630-4
Tucker L: Aspirin--more roles for America's most widely used drug. **Am Pharm** 1979 Dec;19(13):26-7

**Germany**

Aspirin-bewährt: **Krankenpfl J** 1982 Oct 15;20(10):14-5

**BARBITURATES**

**1700 to Present**

Hollister LE: The pre-benzodiazepine era. **J Psychoactive Drugs** 1983 Jan-Jun;15(1-2):9-13

**CACAO**

**1700 to Present**

Burnby JG: Pharmacy and the cocoa bean. **Pharm Hist (London)** 1984 Jun;14(2):9-12

**CALCIUM**

**1700 to Present**

Zimmerman AN, Hülsmann WC: The calcium paradox: historical remarks. **Eur Heart J** 1983 Dec;4 Suppl H:3-4

**Great Britain**

Fye WB: Sydney Ringer, calcium, and cardiac function. **Circulation** 1984 Apr;69(4):849-53

**CAMPHOR**

**1700 to Present**

**France**

Duchemin A: F. V. Raspail, l'apôtre du camphre. **Bull Liaison Assoc Amis Mus Pharm Montp** 1979;4:7-14

**CANNABIS**

Abel EL: Marihuana. The first twelve thousand years. New York, London, Plenum Press, 1980. xi, 289 p.
Hindmarch I: A social history of the use of cannabis sativa. **Contemp Rev** 1972;220(1276):252-7

#### Arabic

Nahas GG: Hashish in Islam 9th to 18th century. **Bull NY Acad Med** 1982 Dec;58(9):814–31

#### Asia

Touw M: The religious and medicinal uses of Cannabis in China, India and Tibet. **J Psychoactive Drugs** 1981 Jan–Mar;13(1):23–34

#### India

Vetschera T, Pillai A: The use of hemp and opium in India. **Ethnomedizin** 1978–79;5(1–2):11–23

### Before 500 A.D.

#### Greco–Roman

Brunner TF: Marijuana in ancient Greece and Rome? the literary evidence. **Bull Hist Med** 1973 Jul–Aug;47(4):344–55

### 500 A.D.–1450

Van Winter JM: Het gebruik van cannabis in twee 15e-eeuwse kookboeken. **Farm Tijdschr Belg** 1980;57:411–9

#### India

Chaturvedi GN, Tiwari SK, Rai NP: Medicinal use of opium and cannabis in Medieval India. **Indian J Hist Sci** 1981, reçu 1982;16(1):31–5

### 1700 to Present

#### Great Britain

Smith FN: Swift and cannabis. **Am Notes Queries** 1983 Nov–Dec;22(3–4):37–9

#### Panama

Abel EL: Marijuana on trial: the Panama Canal Zone Report. **Int J Addict** 1982 May;17(4):667–78

#### United States

Himmelstein JL: The strange career of marihuana: politics and ideology of drug control in America. Westport, Greenwood, 1983. xii, 179 p.
Lasagna LC, Lindzey G: Marijuana policy and drug mythology. **Society** 1983;20(2):67–78
Scigliano JA: THC therapeutic research by independent and state-sponsored investigators: a historical review. **J Clin Pharmacol** 1981 Aug–Sept;21(8–9 Suppl):113S–121S
Shepherd RG: Science news of controversy: the case of marijuana. **Journalism Monogr** 1979;62:1–36
Shepherd RG: Selectivity of sources: reporting the marijuana controversy. **J Commun** 1981;31(2):129–37

## CARBON MONOXIDE

### 1700 to Present

#### United States

Morandi M, Eisenbud M: Carbon monoxide exposure in New York City: a historical overview. **Bull NY Acad Med** 1980 Nov–Dec;56(9):817–28

## CHLORAL HYDRATE

Inciardi JA: The changing life of Mickey Finn: some notes on chloral hydrate down through the ages. **J Pop Cult** 1977;11(3):591–6

## CHLOROFORM

### 1700 to Present

#### Great Britain

Crider S: Anesthesia. A history of Simpson's discovery of chloroform. **J Kans Med Soc** 1983 Mar;84(3):143–6
Defalque RJ: The first experiment in obstetrical anesthesia. **Anesth Analg (Cleve)** 1983 Dec;62(12):1136
Jones IW: Chloroform anaesthesia in Liverpool. **Anaesthesia** 1983 Jun;38(6):578–80

#### Netherlands

Wolff JD: Over chloroform-narcose en een Nederlandse pionier (S.N. Dentz Jr.). **Ned Tijdschr Geneeskd** 1981 Oct 17;125(42):1719–22

## COCA

Deschamps A: Aspects de la coca. **Decouv Civilis** 1974 Dec;7–8:31–46
Nicholi AM: Historical perspective––the long and colorful history of Erythoxylon coca. **J Am Coll Health** 1984 Jun;32(6):252–7

#### Americas

La Peña Begué R de: El uso de la coca en América. Según la legislación colonial y republicana. **Rev Esp Antropol Am** 1971;6:179–204
Romano R: Cocamania e cocainomania. **Belfagor** 1982;37(6):661–74

#### Peru

Gade DW: Inca and colonial settlement, coca cultivation and endemic disease in the tropical forest. **J Hist Geogr** 1979 Jul;5:263–80
Gagliano JA: La medicina popular y la coca en el Perú: un análisis histórico de actitudes. **Am Indig** 1978;38(4):789–805

### 500 A.D.–1450

#### Americas

Naranjo P: Social function of coca in pre-Columbian America. **J Ethnopharmacol** 1981 Mar–May;3(2–3):161–72

### 1700 to Present

Caceres B: La coca, el mundo andino y los extirpadores de idolatrías de siglo XX. **Am Indig** 1978;38(4):769–85
Holmstedt B, Fredga A: Sundry episodes in the history of coca and cocaine. **J Ethnopharmacol** 1981 Mar–May;3(2–3):113–47

#### United States

Grinspoon L, Bakalar JB: Coca and cocaine as medicines: an historical review. **J Ethnopharmacol** 1981 Mar–May;3(2–3):149–59

## COCAINE

Siegel RK: Cocaine smoking. **J Psychoactive Drugs** 1982 Oct–Dec;14(4):271–359

#### Americas

Romano R: Cocamania e cocainomania. **Belfagor** 1982;37(6):661–74

### 1700 to Present

Campan L: Naissance, vie, mort et survie de la cocaíne. **Agressologie** 1979;20(3):135–47
Goldberg MF: Cocaine: the first local anesthetic and the 'third scourge of humanity'. A centennial melodrama. **Arch Ophthalmol** 1984 Oct;102(10):1443–7
Holmstedt B, Fredga A: Sundry episodes in the history of coca and cocaine. **J Ethnopharmacol** 1981 Mar–May;3(2–3):113–47
Lebzeltern G: S. Freud und das Kokain. **Wien Klin Wochenschr** 1983 Nov 11;95(21):765–9
Thornton EM: Freud and cocaine: the Freudian fallacy. London, Blond & Briggs, 1983. 340 p.

#### Great Britain

Miller WH: The habit of Sherlock Holmes. **Trans Stud Coll Physicians Phila** 1978 Jul;45(5):252–7

#### Peru

Siegel RK, Hirschman A: Moreno and the first study on cocaine: a historical note and translation. **J Psychoactive Drugs** 1983 Jul–Sep;15(3):219–20

#### United States

Colp R Jr: Notes on Dr. William S. Halsted. **Bull NY Acad Med** 1984 Nov;60(9):876–87
Courtwright DT: The hidden epidemic: opiate addiction and cocaine use in the South, 1860–1920. **J South Hist** 1983;49(1):57–72
Gay GR: You've come a long way, baby! Coke time for the new American lady of the Eighties. **J Psychoactive Drugs** 1981 Oct–Dec;13(4):297–318
Graner JL, Frederick W: William Halsted's cocaine habit. **Arch Ophthalmol** 1984 Dec;102(12):1746

# DRUGS AND CHEMICALS

Grinspoon L, Bakalar JB: Coca and cocaine as medicines: an historical review. **J Ethnopharmacol** 1981 Mar–May;3(2–3):149–59
Thornton EM: Images of cocaine. **Lancet** 1984 Jan 7;1(8367):46

### COLCHICUM

Weinberger A, Pinkhas J: The history of colchicine. **Koroth** 1980 Jun;7(11–12):760–3

### COSMETICS

Simon G: Kosmetische Präparate vom 16. bis 19. Jahrhundert. Braunschweig, Deutscher Apotheker Verlag, 1983. 396 p. (Braunschweiger Veröffentlichungen zur Geschichte der Pharmazie und der Naturwissenschaften, Bd. 27).

#### Before 500 A.D.

##### Egypt

Diener L: Skönhet, skönhetsvård och skönhetsmedel i det faraoniska Egypten. **Nord Medicinhist Arsb** 1980;:38–52
Rudowska I: Zródła kosmetyki leczniczej i upiększającej w starozytnym Egipcie. **Przegl Dermatol** 1981 Jan–Feb;68(1):123–8

##### Rome

Dirckx JH: Ovid's dermatologic formulary. **Am J Dermatopathol** 1980 Winter;2(4):327–32
Green P: Ars gratia cultus: Ovid as beautician. **Am J Philol** 1979;100:381–92

#### 500 A.D.–1450

##### Arabic

Belova LV: Vklad Abu Ali ibn-Siny v kosmetologiiu. **Sov Zdravookhr** 1984;(9):53–6

#### 1450–1700

##### Great Britain

Drew-Bear A: Face-painting scenes in Ben Jonson's plays. **Stud Philol** 1980 Fall;47(4):338–401

##### Poland

Rudowska I, Rudzki E: Dermatologiczna analiza ziołowych surowców kosmetycznych zalecanych w zielniku Falimirza z roku 1534. **Przegl Dermatol** 1983 Jul–Aug;70(4):429–37

### CURARE

#### 1700 to Present

Earles MP: Four eighteenth century experimental studies of crude curare. In Hickel E, Schröder G, ed: Neue Beiträge zur Arzneimittelgeschichte. Festschrift für Wolfgang Schneider zum 70. Geburtstag. Stuttgart, Wissenschaftliche Verlagsgesellschaft, 1982. p. 175–84.
Ellis FR: Waterton's wourali. **Can Anaesth Soc J** 1983 Jan;30(1):110
Hein WH: Zum Curarebericht des Jesuitenpaters Franz Xaver Veigl. **Beitr Gesch Pharm** 1981;11:81–4
Maltby JR: Charles Waterton (1782–1865): curare and a Canadian National Park. **Can Anaesth Soc J** 1982 May;29(3):195–202
Marini Bettolo GB: Recent advances in the research on curare. **Verh K Acad Geneeskd Belg** 1981;43(3):185–212

##### Ecuador

Humble RM: The Gill-Merrill expedition: penultimate chapter in the curare story. **Anesthesiology** 1982 Dec;57(6):519–26

##### Great Britain

Proceedings of a symposium held to commemorate the bicentenary of Charles Waterton (1782–1865): **Br J Anaesth** 1983 Mar;55(3):221–33
West R: An excursion into pharmacology: curare in medicine. **Med Hist** 1984 Oct;28(4):391–405

##### Italy

Belloni L: Un circolo bernardiano in Italia: la Società delle Scienze Biologiche in Torino. Luigi Vella de la curaroterapia del tetano. **Physis** 1981;23(3):301–10

### DDT

#### 1700 to Present

##### United States

Dunlap TR: DDT: scientists, citizens, and public policy. Princeton, Princeton University Press, 1981. 318 p.

### DIGITALIS

Burchell HB: Digitalis poisoning: historical and forensic aspects. **J Am Coll Cardiol** 1983 Feb;1(2 Pt 1):506–16
Chamorro G: Uso y abuso de la digital. **Rev Med Chil** 1982 Apr;110(4):361–7
Greeff K, Schadewaldt H: Introduction and remarks on the history of cardiac glycosides. In Greeff K, ed: Handbook of experimental pharmacology. Berlin, Springer, 1981. p. 1–12 (Vol. 56/I).
Haustein KO: Digitalis. **Pharmacol Ther** 1982;18(1):1–89
Normand J: Histoire d'une thérapeutique: la thérapeutique digitalique hier et aujourd'hui. **Ann Cardiol Angeiol (Paris)** 1982 Mar–Apr;31(2):89–95

#### 1700 to Present

Albasanz Gallan JL: La digital, en su segundo centenario. **An R Acad Nac Med (Madr)** 1983;100(2):181–208
Berghaus A: Die Entwicklung der Methoden zur physiologischen Wertbestimmung von Digitalispräparaten. Husum, Matthiesen, 1982. 135 p. (Abhandlungen zur Geschichte der Medizin und der Naturwissenschaften, 42).
Berghaus A, Winau R: Probleme der Standardisierung von Digitalispräparaten. In Hickel E, Schröder G, ed: Neue Beiträge zur Arzneimittelgeschichte. Festschrift für Wolfgang Schneider zum 70. Geburtstag. Stuttgart, Wissenschaftliche Verlagsgesellschaft, 1982. p. 265–79.
Grosse-Brockhoff F: Herzbehandlung mit dem 'Fingerhut' einst und jetzt. Opladen, Westdeutscher Verlag, 1980. 58 p. (Rheinisch-Westfälische Akademie der Wissenschaften; Natur-, Ingenieur- und Wirtschaftswissenschaften, Vorträge N 293).
Le Winn EB: The steroidal actions of digitalis. **Perspect Biol Med** 1984;27(2):183–99
McMichael J: Digitalis in the last half century. **Eur Heart J** 1982 Dec;3 Suppl D:3–4

##### Great Britain

Drury VW: Foxglove and chips. **J R Coll Gen Pract** 1984 Mar;34(260):129–39

##### Netherlands

Lee TC: Van Gogh's vision. Digitalis intoxication? **JAMA** 1981 Feb 20;245(7):727–9

##### United States

Estes JW: An account of the foxglove in America. **Bull Hist Med** 1973 Jul–Aug;47(4):394–408
Estes JW: Hall Jackson and the purple foxglove: medical practice and research in revolutionary America 1760–1820. Hanover, NH, University Press of New England, 1979. xvi, 291 p.

### DIMETHYL SULFOXIDE

#### 1700 to Present

Jacob SW, Herschler R: Dimethyl sulfoxide after twenty years. **Ann NY Acad Sci** 1983;411:xiii–xvii

### DNA

#### 1700 to Present

Hoagland M: Discovery, the search for DNA's secrets. Boston, Houghton Mifflin, 1981. xiv, 198 p.
Krimsky S: Genetic alchemy. The social history of the Recombinant DNA controversy. Cambridge, London, MIT Press, 1982. xiii, 445 p.
Newmark P: Thirty years of DNA. **Nature** 1983 Sep 29–Oct 5;305(5933):383–4
Romanova NN: E. S. London's contribution to the problem of DNA structure. **Istor Biol Issled** 1983;9:166–75
Thirty years of DNA--and after: **Nature** 1983 Apr 14;302(5909):557–8
Zalesova ZG: The history of the establishment of the genetic role of DNA. **Istor Biol Issled** 1983;9:66–84

**United States**

Sullivan DJ: Biological engineering. **Thought** 1981;56(221):199-211

### ERGOT

**1700 to Present**

Parascandola J: The search for the active oxytocic principle of ergot: laboratory science and clinical medicine in conflict. In Hickel E, Schröder G, ed: Neue Beiträge zur Arzneimittelgeschichte. Festschrift für Wolfgang Schneider zum 70. Geburtstag. Stuttgart, Wissenschaftliche Verlagsgesellschaft, 1982. p. 205-27.

**Great Britain**

MacDonald RR: Classic illustrations: From St. Anthony's fire to ergometrine (Ergonovine). **Eur J Obstet Gynecol Reprod Biol** 1982 Aug;13(5):325-7

### ETHER

**1700 to Present**

**Australia**

Cole WH: Some ether anecdotes. **Anaesth Intensive Care** 1981 May;9(2):174-6

**Denmark**

Secher O: Fra Boston til Amaliegade; anaesthesiens vej til Danmark. **Dan Medicinhist Arbog** 1981;:25-56

**Germany**

Weisser C: Der Ombrédannesche Ather-Inhalator. Ein Beitrag zur Geschichte der Ather-Apparatnarkose. **Anaesthesist** 1983 Feb;32(2):51-4

**Great Britain**

MacLaglan D: The ether song, 1850. With an introduction and notes by K. G. Huston. First printed in Edinburgh and now reprinted in Los Angeles, 1982. [12 p.].

**United States**

Crawford WM: More on the ether operation. **N Engl J Med** 1984 Feb 23;310(8):534

Eavey RD: First operation under ether anesthesia: a correction. **N Engl J Med** 1983 Oct 20;309(16):990-1

Labor under ether: Hilo, 1850. **Hawaii Med J** 1981 Oct;40(10):291-2

**USSR**

Altschuller GI, Keenan WA: History of the development of painless surgery in Russia. **Bull NY Acad Med** 1982 Jun;58(5):493-502

Shabunin AV: Efirnyĭ narkoz v pervyĭ god ego primeneniia v Rossii. **Sov Zdravookhr** 1983;8:62-4

### FATTY ACIDS

**1700 to Present**

Burr GO: The essential fatty acids fifty years ago. **Prog Lipid Res** 1981;20:xxvii-xxix

### FLUORIDES

**1700 to Present**

Cawson RA, Stocker IP: The early history of fluorides as anti-caries agents. **Br Dent J** 1984 Dec 8;157(11):403-4

Heydt H: 30th year reunion of four scientists marks less tooth decay around the world--the monofluorophosphate story. **J Dent Assoc S Afr** 1980 Dec;35(12):837-9

Hunstadbråten K: Fluor i kariesprofylaksen omkring århundriskiftet. **Nor Tannlaegeforen Tid** 1981 May;91(7):227-31

Hunstadbråten K: Fluor in der Kariesprophylaxe der Jahrhundertwende. **Quintessenz J** 1984 Feb;14(2):147-51

Hunstadbraten K: Fluoride in caries prophylaxis at the turn of the century. **Bull Hist Dent** 1982 Oct;30(2):117-20

Hunstadbraten K: Kariesprophylaxe durch Fluoride um die Jahrhundertwende. **Zahnarztl Mitt** 1982 Nov 16;72(22):2537-9

The monofluorophosphate story: **Br Dent J** 1981 May 19;150(10):285-6

Schmid R, Barbakow F, Mühlemann H, et al: Amine fluoride and monofluorophosphate: I. Historical review of fluoride dentifrices. **ASDC J Dent Child** 1984 Mar-Apr;51(2):99-103

White WE: Monofluorophosphate--its beginning. **Caries Res** 1983;17 Suppl 1:2-8

**Germany**

Künzel W: 20 Jahre Trinkwasserfluoridierung in der Deutschen Demokratischen Republik. **Stomatol DDR** 1979;29(10):743-52

**United States**

Hastreiter RJ: Fluoridation conflict: a history and conceptual synthesis. **J Am Dent Assoc** 1983 Apr;106(4):486-90

Leahy PJ, Mazur A: The rise and fall of public opposition in specific social movements. **Soc Stud Sci** 1980 Aug 3;10(3):259-84

### GARLIC

Bolton S, Null G, Troetel WM: The medical uses of garlic--fact and fiction. **Am Pharm** 1982 Aug;22(8):40-3

**Hungary**

Oláh A: Zwiebel und Knoblauch in der Volksmedizin; das ungarische Theriak und Mithridaticum früher und heute. **Ethnomedizin** 1981-82;7(1-4):333-48

### GINSENG

Appleby JH: Ginseng and the Royal Society. **Notes Rec R Soc Lond** 1983 Mar;37(2):121-45

**Asia**

Delaveau P: Le ginseng, drogue ancestrale d'Extrême Orient, devant la critique expérimentale. In Mazars G, ed: Les médecines traditionnelles de l'Asie. Strasbourg, Université Louis Pasteur, 1981. p. 75-84.

**China**

Unschuld PU: Ginseng und 'Kostendämpfung im Gesundheitswesen'. Beiträge zu einer Diskussion im China der Kaiserzeit. **Asiat Forsch** 1980;71:128-32

### GOLD

Hagman HC: 3,000 years of dental gold. **Dent Lab Rev** 1979 Jun;54(7):28-30

**1450-1700**

Nowotny O: De auro potabili. Wien, 1967. (Salzburger Beiträge zur Paracelsusforschung, 7). p. 13-23.

**1700 to Present**

Champion GD: Gold compounds in rheumatic diseases--1. **Med J Aust** 1984 Jan 21;140(2):73-7

Keers RY: The gold rush 1925-35. **Thorax** 1980 Dec;35(12):884-9

Scarano GB: Considerazioni storiche sull'uso dei sali d'oro nell'artrite reumatoide. **Med Secoli** 1982 May-Aug;19(2):175-91

**United States**

Higby GJ: Gold in medicine: a review of its use in the West before 1900. **Gold Bull** 1982;15(4):130-40

**Yugoslavia**

Dürrigl T: Počeci auroterapije u Jugoslaviji. **Reumatizam** 1982;29(2):37-9

### GUAIAC

Moeller DD: The odyssey of guaiac. **Am J Gastroenterol** 1984 Mar;79(3):236-7

**1450-1700**

Gariepy TP: Hyacum, et lues venerea. **J Hist Med Allied Sci** 1981 Jul;36(3):325

Vidal F: Le Gayac, panacée du XVIe siècle. **Chir Dent Fr** 1983 Nov 24;53(226):37-42

### HALLUCINOGENS

Ortegón Páez R: Vorágine alucinante en la historia de las drogas. Bogotá, Columbia, Ediciones Tercer Mundo, 1981. 417 p.

## DRUGS AND CHEMICALS

**Americas**

Emboden WA: The mushroom and the water lily: literary and pictorial evidence for Nymphaea as a ritual psychotogen in Mesoamerica. **J Ethnopharmacol** 1982 Mar;5(2):139–48
Keewaydinoquay: The legend of Miskwedo. **J Psychedelic Drugs** 1979 Jan–Jun;11(1–2):29–31
Sangirardi J: O índio e as plantas alucinógenas: tribos das 3 Américas e civilizações pré-colombianas. [S.l.], Alhambra, 1983. 207 p.
Wasson RG: Traditional use in North America of Amanita muscaria for divinatory purposes. **J Psychedelic Drugs** 1979 Jan–Jun;11(1–2):25–8

**Europe**

Czigány LG: The use of hallucinogens and the shamanistic tradition of the Finno-Ugrian people. **Slav East Eur Rev** 1980;58(2):212–7

**Mexico**

McGuire TM: Ancient Maya mushroom connections: a transcendental interaction model. **J Psychoactive Drugs** 1982 Jul–Sep;14(3):221–38

**Peru**

Dobkin de Rios M, Cardenas M: Plant hallucinogens, shamanism and Nazca ceramics. **J Ethnopharmacol** 1980 Sept;2(3):233–46

**United States**

Tierney GD: Botany and witchcraft. **Palacio** 1974;80(2):44–50

**Before 500 A.D.**

**Greece**

Ruck CA: Mushrooms and philosophers. **J Ethnopharmacol** 1981 Sep;4(2):179–205

**Peru**

Dobkin de Rios M: Plant hallucinogens, sexuality and shamanism in the ceramic art of ancient Peru. **J Psychoactive Drugs** 1982 Jan–Jun;14(1–2):81–90

**1700 to Present**

Cornacchia P, et al: I funghi magici: farmacologia, tossicologia e tecnologia dell'estasi chimica. Milano, Editiemme, 1980. 174 p.
Moriarty KM, Alagna SW, Lake CR: Psychopharmacology. An historical perspective. **Psychiatr Clin North Am** 1984 Sep;7(3):411–33
Protiva M: Wývoj chemie psychofarmak za posledních 20 let. **Cesk Psychiatr** 1978 Dec;74(6):337–49
Schultes RE: Hallucinogenic plants: their earliest botanical descriptions. **J Psychedelic Drugs** 1979 Jan–Jun;11(1–2):13–24

**Americas**

Schultes RE: Evolution of the identification of the myristicaceous hallucinogens of South America. **J Ethnopharmacol** 1979 Oct;1(3):211–39
Schultes RE: The beta-carboline hallucinogens of South America. **J Psychoactive Drugs** 1982 Jul–Sep;14(3):205–20

**Asia**

Solomon R: The rise and fall of the Laotian and Vietnamese opiate trades. **J Psychedelic Drugs** 1979 Jul–Sep;11(3):159–71

**Mexico**

Tyler VE: The case of Victor A. Reko--an unrecognized pioneer writer on New World hallucinogens. **J Nat Prod** 1979 Sep–Oct;42(5):489–95

### HEMLOCK

**Hungary**

Szentgyörgyölgyi G: 'Foltos' bürök. **Orv Hetil** 1981 Nov 1;122(44):2733–4

**Before 500 A.D.**

Wittern R: Das Gift der frommen Denkart - Zur Pharmakologie des Schierlings in der Antike. In Hickel E, Schröder G, ed: Neue Beiträge zur Arzneimittelgeschichte. Festschrift für Wolfgang Schneider zum 70. Geburtstag. Stuttgart, Wissenschaftliche Verlagsgesellschaft, 1982. p. 15–28.

### HEROIN

Way EL: History of opiate use in the Orient and the United States **Ann NY Acad Sci** 1982;398:12–23

**1700 to Present**

Trebach AS: The heroin solution. New Haven, London, Yale University Press, 1982.

**United States**

Courtwright DT: Dark paradise: opiate addiction in America before 1940. Cambridge, London, Harvard Univ. Press, 1982. 270 p.
Gerstein DR: Cultural action and heroin addiction. **Sociol Inq** 1981;51(3–4):355–70

### HORMONES

Peart WS: Humors and hormones. **Harvey Lect** 1979;73:259–90

**1700 to Present**

Matsuo Y: [History and status of study on gastrointestinal hormones] (Jpn). **Nippon Naika Gakkai Zasshi** 1982 Mar 10;71(3):275–85

**United States**

Catchpole HR: Growth hormone. **JAMA** 1980 Feb 15;243(7):652

### INSULIN

**1700 to Present**

Bliss M: The discovery of insulin. Chicago, University of Chicago Press, 1982. 304 p.
Bliss M, ed: Banting's, Best's, and Collip's accounts of the discovery of insulin. **Bull Hist Med** 1982;56(4):554–68
Dérot M: Perspectives en diabétologie (d'hier à demain). **Bull Mem Acad R Med Belg** 1981;136(8–9):435–42
Khardori R: The insulin controversy. **Ann Intern Med** 1980 Feb;92(2 Pt 1):267–8
Kolář J, Michalková D: Sedesát roku používání inzulínu v léčbě diabetes mellitus. **Cesk Pediatr** 1983 Jan;38(1):55–7
Luft R: Lysande upptäckter, men djup klyfta mellan forskningen och de sjukas situation. **Lakartidningen** 1984 Jun 27;81(26–27):2586–94
Mirouze J: L'insuline: hier, aujourd'hui. **Rev Deux Mondes** 1982;10:81–98
Peterson CM: Symposium on optimal insulin delivery. Introduction: History and goals of insulin treatment. **Diabetes Care** 1982 May–Jun;5 Suppl 1:1–5
Scoville AB: Insulin. **South Med J** 1983 Sep;76(9):1085–7
Soltakhanov RM: Iz istorii otkrytiia insulina. **Klin Med (Mosk)** 1982 Jul;60(7):118–20

**Canada**

Bliss M: The aetiology of the discovery of insulin. In Roland CG, ed: Health, disease and medicine. Toronto, Hannah Institute for the History of Medicine, 1984. p. 333–46.
Burrow GN, Hazlett BE, Phillips MJ: A case of diabetes mellitus. **N Engl J Med** 1982 Feb 11;306(6):340–3
Dr. Frederick Banting getting out of town: **Can Med Assoc J** 1984 May 1;130(9):1215–23
Katz S: A new, informal glimpse of Dr. Frederick Banting. **Can Med Assoc J** 1983 Dec 1;129(11):1229–32
Marliss EB: Insulin: sixty years of use. **N Engl J Med** 1982 Feb 11;306(6):362–4
Quinn KF: Banting and his biographers: maker of miracles, makers of myth. **Queens Q** 1982;89(2):243–59
Shortt SE: Banting, insulin and the question of simultaneous discovery. **Queens Q** 1982;89(2):260–73
Sunday ME: Canada's Best. **Harv Med Alumni Bull** 1980 Dec;54(6):10–15
Vipond M: A Canadian hero of the 1920s: Dr. Frederick G. Banting. **Can Hist Rev** 1982;63(4):461–86

**Denmark**

Felig P: Landmark perspective: Protamine insulin. Hagedorn's pioneering contribution to drug delivery in the management of diabetes. **JAMA** 1984 Jan 20;251(3):393–6

**Great Britain**

Pitt B: Insulin. **Br Herit** 1981;2(3):28–38

**New Zealand**

Watson MH: The early days of insulin in New Zealand. **NZ Med J** 1981 May 27;93(684):347–50

**Romania**

Pavel I: The priority of N. C. Paulescu in the discovery of insulin. Bucureşti, Editura Academiei Republicii Socialiste Romania, 1976. 251 p.
Teichman SL, Aldea PA: The other side of the insulin story. Paulescu's contribution. **NY State J Med** 1984 Jun;84(6):312–6

**Sweden**

Carlström S: Första insulinbehandlingen av diabetes i Lund--ett beriktigande. **Sydsven Medicinhist Sallsk Arsskr** 1980;:49–51

**United States**

Thomas L: The right track. **Wilson Q** 1980;4(2):87–98

**IODINE**

**1700 to Present**

**Ireland**

Kampmeier RH: The introduction of iodine in the treatment of syphilis: the writings of William Wallace, M.D., of Dublin. **Sex Transm Dis** 1980 Jan Mar;7(1):26 8

**Switzerland**

Rentchnick P: Iode et goitre. A propos du 150e anniversaire de la mort du Dr Jean-François Coindet (12 juillet 1774–11 février 1834). **Med Hyg (Geneve)** 1984 Feb 15;42(1551):465–6, 469–70, 472–4, 477–8
Wespi HJ: Die Salzjodierung als Vorläufer der Salzfluoridierung. **SSO Schweiz Monatsschr Zahnheilkd** 1982 Apr;92(4):273–89
Wiener JD: Ueber Kropf, Hypertyreose und Jodbehandlung. **Schweiz Med Wochenschr** 1980 Nov 22;110(47):1784–7

**United States**

Chapman EM: History of the discovery and early use of radioactive iodine. **JAMA** 1983 Oct 21;250(15):2042–4

**IPECAC**

**1700 to Present**

**United States**

Smith B, Robertson RM, Robertson D: An early Southern description of Curschmann's spirals. **Clin Notes Respir Dis** 1982 Summer;21(1):10–2

**IRON**

Belloni L: Zur Entdeckung des Eisens im Organismus. In Ganzinger K, Skopec M, Wyklicky H, ed: Festschrift für Erna Lesky zum 70. Geburtstag. Wien, Brüder Hollinek, 1981. p. 25–30.
Stout G: Any old iron. **MIMS Mag** 1981 Sept 1;:48–9

**1700 to Present**

Gädeke R: Ein medizingeschichtliches Panorama der akuten Eisenvergiftung. **Klin Paediatr** 1979 Sep;191(5):442–6

**LAETRILE**

**1700 to Present**

**United States**

Arseneau JC, Thigpen JT: The new quack--pseudoscience, public relations and politics. **J Miss State Med Assoc** 1981 Aug;22(8):202–7
Kardinal CG: Laetrile in historical perspective. **Mo Med** 1980 Sep;77(9):564–9
Markle GE, Petersen JC, ed: Politics, science, and cancer: the laetrile phenomenon. Boulder, Westview Press, for the American Association for the Advancement of Science, 1980. xiii, 190 p. (AAAS Selected Symposium, v. 46). Contributions by JH Young, RD Smith, RF Rich, GP Monaco, Al Caplan, D Nelkin.
Petersen JC, Markle GE: Politics and science in the laetrile controversy. **Soc Stud Sci** 1979;9(2):139–66
Young JH: Laetrile in historical perspective. **Conn Med** 1979 Aug;43(8):497–500
Young JH: Laetrile in historical perspective. In Markle GE, Petersen JC, ed: Politics, science and cancer: the laetrile phenomenon. Boulder, CO. Westview Press, for American Association for the Advancement of Science, Washington, D. C., 1980. p. 11–60.

**LEAD**

Curran AS: Lead poisoning: a historical overview. **NY State J Med** 1984 Sep;84(9):437–8
Morris E: Lead poisoning: an historic view. **Occup Health (Lond)** 1980 Sep;32(9):449–59
Waldron HA: Lead in bones: a cautionary tale. **Ecol Dis** 1982;1(2–3):191–6
Walker RE: Malleus and podagra: lead poisoning in horse and man. **Vet Hist** 1980/81, n.s.;1:118–36
Wedeen RP: The role of lead in renal failure. **Clin Exp Dial Apheresis** 1982;6(2–3):113–46

**United States**

Aufderheide AC, Neiman FD, Wittmers LE, et al: Lead in bone II: skeletal-lead content as an indicator of lifetime lead ingestion and the social correlates in an archaeological population. **Am J Phys Anthropol** 1981 Jul;55(3):285–91

**Before 500 A.D.**

**Greco-Roman**

Nriagu JO: Occupational exposure to lead in ancient times. **Sci Total Environ** 1983 Nov;31(2):105–16

**Rome**

Gaebel RE: Saturnine gout among Roman aristocrats. **N Engl J Med** 1983 Aug 18;309(7):431
Mertz DP: 'Bleigicht': Ursache oder Folge des Verfalls des Römischen Weltreiches? **Med Welt** 1983 Oct 14;34(41):1158–9
Scarborough J: The myth of lead poisoning among the Romans: an essay review. **J Hist Med Allied Sci** 1984 Oct;39(4):469–75

**500 A.D.–1450**

**Great Britain**

Barry PS, Connolly R: Lead concentrations in mediaeval bones. **Int Arch Occup Environ Health** 1981;48(2):173–7

**1450–1700**

**Germany**

Eisinger J: Lead and wine. Eberhard Gockel and the colica Pictonum. **Med Hist** 1982 Jul;26(3):279–302

**1700 to Present**

**United States**

Aronson SM: Lead and the demon rum in colonial America. **RI Med J** 1983 Jan;66(1):37–40
Burrows GE: Lead toxicosis in domestic animals: a review of the role of lead mining and primary lead smelters in the United States. **Vet Hum Toxicol** 1981 Oct;23(5):337–43
Collingridge D, Douglas J: Three models of policymaking: expert advice in the control of environmental lead. **Soc Stud Sci** 1984 Aug;14(3):343–70

**LITHIUM**

Georgotas A, Gershon S: Historical perspectives and current highlights on lithium treatment in manic-depressive illness. **J Clin Psychopharmacol** 1981 Jan;1(1):27–31

**1700 to Present**

Johnson FN, Amdisen A: The first era of lithium in medicine. An historical note. **Pharmacopsychiatria** 1983 Mar;16(2):61–3
Schou M: Lithium perspectives. **Neuropsychobiology** 1983;10(1):7–12
Strobusch AD, Jefferson JW: The checkered history of lithium in medicine. **Pharm Hist** 1980;22(2):72–6

**Australia**

Davies B: The first patient to receive lithium. **Aust NZ J Psychiatry** 1983 Dec;17(4):366–8
Lithium salts in the treatment of psychotic excitement: John F Cade: **Aust NZ J Psychiatry** 1982 Sep;16(3):129–33

## DRUGS AND CHEMICALS

### LSD

#### 1700 to Present

Livingston M: LSD--a generation later. **Hawaii Med J** 1982 Dec;41(12):462, 464, 466 passim

Toy EV: The conservative connection: the chairman of the board took LSD before Timothy Leary. **Am Stud** 1980;21(2):65-77

**Switzerland**

Hofmann A: How LSD originated. **J Psychedelic Drugs** 1979 Jan-Jun;11(1-2):53-60

### MANDRAGORA

Ober WB: Reuben's mandrakes: infertility in the Bible. **Int J Gynecol Pathol** 1984;3(3):299-317

Vidal F: Un anesthésique vieux de 19 siècles: la mandragore. **Chir Dent Fr** 1982 Oct 7;52(173):21-6

#### Before 500 A.D.

Rosner F: Mandrakes and other aphrodisiacs in the Bible & Talmud. **Koroth** 1980 Jun;7(11-12):CCLXXVII-CCLXXXIV

### MERCURY

Wolff M, Osborne JW, Hanson AL: Mercury toxicity and dental amalgam. **Neurotoxicology (Park Forest Il)** 1983 Fall;4(3):201-4

**India**

Damodar Joshi: Mercury in Indian medicine. **Stud Hist Med** 1979 Dec;3(4):234-97

Murthy SR: An occurrence of cinnabar in Rasarnavakalpa. **Indian J Hist Sci** 1979 Nov;14(2):83-6

#### 1450-1700

**Great Britain**

Broad WJ: Sir Isaac Newton: mad as a hatter. **Science** 1981 Sep 18;213(4514):1341-2, 1344

Laker MR: Newton's malady. **Science** 1982 Mar 5;215(4537):1185-6

Lieb J, Hershman D: Isaac Newton: mercury poisoning or manic depression? **Lancet** 1983 Dec 24-31;2(8365-66):1479-80

#### 1700 to Present

**Germany**

Wehsarg FK: Die Quecksilber-Schmierkur in Bad Aachen als einstmalige Syphilistherapie. **Rehabilitation (Bonn)** 1981;34(3-4):26-32

**Great Britain**

Waldron HA: Did the Mad Hatter have mercury poisoning? **Br Med J [Clin Res]** 1983 Dec 24-31;287(6409):1961

**Japan**

Smith AM: Mercury poisoning and birth defects in Japan. **Women Health** 1978 Mar-Apr;3(2):9-12

Suzuki T, Hongo T, Yamamoto R: Hair mercury levels of Japanese women during the period 1881 to 1968. **J Appl Toxicol** 1984 Apr;4(2):101-4

### MESCALINE

La Barre W: Peyotl and mescaline. **J Psychedelic Drugs** 1979 Jan-Jun;11(1-2):33-9

### METHADONE

#### 1700 to Present

**United States**

Courtwright DT, Joseph H, Des Jarlais DC: Memories from the street: oral histories of elderly methadone patients. **Oral Hist Rev** 1981;9:47-64

### MINERAL WATERS

#### 1700 to Present

Coley NG: The preparation and uses of artificial mineral waters (ca. 1680-1825). **Ambix** 1984;31(1):32-48

**Great Britain**

Campbell WA: Joseph Priestley's soda water. **Endeavour** 1983;7(3):141-3

### MOLY

#### Before 500 A.D.

**Greece**

Plaitakis A, Duvoisin RC: Homer's moly identified as Galanthus nivalis L.: physiologic antidote to stramonium poisoning. **Clin Neuropharmacol** 1983 Mar;6(1):1-5

### MORPHINE

Way EL: History of opiate use in the Orient and the United States **Ann NY Acad Sci** 1982;398:12-23

#### 1700 to Present

Feinberg M, Pegeron JP, Steiner M: The effect of morphine on symptoms of endogenous depression. **Natl Inst Drug Abuse Res Monogr Ser** 1983 Apr;43:245-50

Jack DB, Laugher SJ: The earliest demonstration of the placental passage of morphine? **Pharm Hist (London)** 1982 Aug;12(2):7-8

**Germany**

Friedrich C, Seidlein HJ: Beiträge zur Geschichte der Pharmazeutischen Wissenschaft. **Pharmazie** 1984 May;39(5):340-5

**Japan**

Matsuki A: Nothing new under the sun--a Japanese pioneer in the clinical use of intrathecal morphine. **Anesthesiology** 1983 Mar;58(3):289-90

**United States**

Courtwright DT: Dark paradise: opiate addiction in America before 1940. Cambridge, London, Harvard Univ. Press, 1982. 270 p.

Musto DF, Ramos MR: Notes on American medical history: a follow-up study of the New Haven morphine maintenance clinic of 1920. **N Engl J Med** 1981 Apr 30;304(18):1071-7

### MUSHROOMS

**Americas**

Emboden WA: The mushroom and the water lily: literary and pictorial evidence for Nymphaea as a ritual psychotogen in Mesoamerica. **J Ethnopharmacol** 1982 Mar;5(2):139-48

Wasson RG: The wondrous mushroom. Mycolatry in Mesoamerica. New York, McGraw-Hill, 1980. xxvi, 248 p.

**Mexico**

McGuire TM: Ancient Maya mushroom connections: a transcendental interaction model. **J Psychoactive Drugs** 1982 Jul-Sep;14(3):221-38

#### 1700 to Present

**Mexico**

Krippner S, Winkelman M: Maria Sabina: wise lady of the mushrooms. **J Psychoactive Drugs** 1983 Jul-Sep;15(3):225-8

### NICKEL

#### 1700 to Present

**Great Britain**

Morgan JG: The place of nickel in the history of industrial disease. In J. Cule, ed: Wales and medicine. London, British Society for the History of Medicine, 1975. p. 68-74.

### NITROUS OXIDE

#### 1700 to Present

**Great Britain**

Smith WD: Under the influence. A history of nitrous oxide and oxygen anaesthesia. London, Macmillan, 1982. xxviii, 188 p.

Weller RM: Nitrous oxide in Bristol in 1836. A series of lectures by William Herepath (1796-1868). **Anaesthesia** 1983 Jul;38(7):678-82

USSR

Broder LIa: K istorii primeneniia zakisi azota v Rossii. **Anesteziol Reanimatol** 1983 Mar-Apr;(2):f73

### OILS

Caffaratto TM: Elogio dell'olio medicinale. **Minerva Med** 1983 Mar 31;74(13):747-55
Czygan FC: Atherische Ole und Duft kulturhistorisch betrachtet. **Pharm Unserer Zeit** 1981 Jul:10(4):109-21
Galan V: 'Seneca oil'. **Rev Ig [Pneumoftiziol]** 1980 Apr-Jun;29(2):127-8

Austria

Kostenzer O: Das Katharinenöl, ein altes Heilmittel. **Tirol Heimatbl** 1974;49(2):77-80

Before 500 A.D.

Bubis M: Petroleum in Talmudic sources. **Koroth** 1981;8(1-2):41-4

1700 to Present

Austria

Mutschlechner G: Vom Olbrennen und Olhandel im Zillertal. **Tirol Heimatbl** 1971;46(7-9):71-4

### OPIUM

Baraka A: Historical aspects of opium. **Middle East J Anaesthesiol** 1982 Jun;6(5):289-302
Kramer JC: Opium rampant: medical use, misuse and abuse in Britain and the West in the 17th and 18th centuries. **Br J Addict** 1979 Dec;74(4):377-89
Latimer D, Goldberg J: Flowers in the blood; the story of opium. New York, Franklin Watts, 1981. 306 p.
Way EL: History of opiate use in the Orient and the United States **Ann NY Acad Sci** 1982;398:12-23

India

Vetschera T, Pillai A: The use of hemp and opium in India. **Ethnomedizin** 1978-79;5(1-2):11-23

Japan

Inque H: Le problème de l'opium durant la période Jiaqing et Daoguang. **Toyoschi Kenkyu** 1982;41(1):58-83, 3-4

Sri Lanka

Uragoda CG: History of opium in Sri Lanka. **Med Hist** 1983 Jan;27(1):69-76

500 A.D.-1450

India

Chaturvedi GN, Tiwari SK, Rai NP: Medicinal use of opium and cannabis in Medieval India. **Indian J Hist Sci** 1981, reçu 1982;16(1):31-5

1700 to Present

Kramer JC: The metapsychology of opium. **J Psychoactive Drugs** 1981 Jan-Mar;13(1):71-9
Stäuble-Lipman Wulf, M: De Quincey, Baudelaire, e i 'Paradisi artificiali'. **Nuova Antologia** 1972;514(2054):245-54

China

Man-hung L: Ch'ing mo pen kuo ya p'ien chih t'i tai chin k'ou ya p'ien (1858-1906). **Bull Inst Mod Hist Acad Sin** 1980;9:385-432
Wang Shu-huai: Ya p'ien tu hai-kuang hsü erh shih san nien wen chüan tiao ch'a fen hsi. **Bull Inst Mod Hist Acad Sin** 1980;9:183-200
Waung WS: Introduction of opium cultivation to China. **J Chin Univ Hong Kong** 1979;5(1):207-21

France

Siegel RK, Hirschman AE: Charvet and the first psychopharmacological studies on opium: a historical note and translation. **J Psychoactive Drugs** 1983 Oct-Dec;15(4):323-9

Great Britain

Berridge V: Opiate use in England, 1800-1926. **Ann NY Acad Sci** 1982;398:1-11
Berridge V: Opium and oral history. **Oral Hist** 1979;7(2):48-58
Berridge V, Edwards G: Opium and the people. Opiate use in nineteenth-century England. London and New York; Allen Lane and St. Martin's Press; 1981. 369 p.
Berridge V: Victorian opium eating: response to opiate use in nineteenth century England. **Victorian Stud** 1978;21(4):437-61
Cone TE: Overdosing with opium, a serious pediatric problem in England a century and a half ago. **Pediatrics** 1981;68:86
Pargas K: Bishop Charles Henry Brent (1862-1929)--a retrospective. 'That damned opium mess has started again'. **J Addict Res Found** 1979;8(9):7
Paulshock BZ: William Heberden and opium--some relief to all. **N Engl J Med** 1983 Jan 6;308(1):53-6
Peters D: The British medical response to opiate addiction in the nineteenth century. **J Hist Med Allied Sci** 1981 Oct;36(4):455-88

Philippines

Taylor AH: American confrontation with opium traffic in the Philippines. **Pac Hist Rev** 1967;36(3):307-24

United States

Courtwright DT: Dark paradise: opiate addiction in America before 1940. Cambridge, London, Harvard Univ. Press, 1982. 270 p.
Courtwright DT: Opiate addiction as a consequence of the Civil War. **Civ War Hist** 1978;24(2):101-11
Courtwright DT: The hidden epidemic: opiate addiction and cocaine use in the South, 1860-1920. **J South Hist** 1983;49(1):57-72
Stelle CC: Americans and the China opium trade in the nineteenth century. New York, Arno Press, 1981. 154 p. (Also Diss, Chicago, 1938).

### OXYGEN

1700 to Present

Guillerme J: Oxygène et thérapeutique. **Dix-huit Siecle** 1982;14:27-43

Belgium

Colard A: Evocation du passé: les débuts de l'oxygénothérapie. **Rev Med Brux** 1983 Feb;4(2):98-100

Great Britain

Kieft L, Willeford BR, ed: Joseph Priestley. Scientist, theologian, and metaphysician. A symposium celebrating the two hundredth anniversary of the discovery of oxygen by Joseph Priestley in 1774. Lewisburg, Bucknell University Press, 1980. 117 p. With contributions by E. N. Hiebert, A. J. Ihde, R. E. Schofield.
Smith WD: Under the influence. A history of nitrous oxide and oxygen anaesthesia. London, Macmillan, 1982. xxviii, 188 p.

United States

White LW: Adapting commercial oxygen for medical use. **Respir Ther** 1979 Jan-Feb;9(1):30-2

### PENICILLIN

Udelhoven P: Die klassischen Penizilline halten die Stellung. **Med Welt** 1983 Dec 9;34(49):3

1700 to Present

Abraham EP: Fleming's discovery. **Rev Infect Dis** 1980 Jan-Feb;2(1):129-140
Carter L: Down Memory Lane: debut of a drug. **Nurs Mirror** 1982 Nov 3;155(18):21-2
Chain E: A short history of the penicillin discovery from Fleming's early observations in 1929 to the present time. In J. Parascandola, ed: The history of antibiotics. Madison, American Institute of the History of Pharmacy, 1980. p. 15-29.
Costa-Casaretto C: Cincuentenario de la penicilina. **Rev Med Chil** 1979 Jun;107(6):549-56
Dalhoff A: Fünfzig Jahre Penicilline. Eine Ubersicht über Struktur-Wirkungsbeziehungen der Beta-Laktamantibiotika und ihre mikrobiologische sowie klinische Relevanz. **Infection** 1979;7(6):294-302
Fernandes L, Berry H, Hamilton E: Historical perspectives on penicillamine. **Cah Haut Marnais** 1980;14(2):130-6
Fielding J: History of penicillin. **Lancet** 1980 Jan 5;1(8158):43-4
Kampmeier RH: The introduction of penicillin for the treatment of syphilis. **Sex Transm Dis** 1981 Oct-Dec;8(4):260-5
McAllister TA: Penicillins in perspective. **Scott Med J** 1982;27 Spec

No.:S39–47
McEwin R: Florey and Cairns--early work on penicillin. **Med J Aust** 1982 Jan 9;1(1):12–3
Maizumi H: [Early days of antibiotics] (Jpn). **Dent Outlook** 1979;53(2):307–12
Milders JW: Taking a look at the invisible. **Hindustan Antibiot Bull** 1982 Aug–Nov;24(3–4):93–6
Plamenac SD: Fifty years since the discovery of penicillin. In International Congress of the History of Medicine. 26th, Plovdiv, 1978. Actes du Congress. Sofia, 1981. Volume II. p. 88–90.
Plamenac SD: Pojam antibioze i otkriće penicilina (I–II). **Srp Arh Celok Lek** 1981;108(6):675–87;(7–8):823–33
Selwyn S: Pencillin pioneers. **J Antimicrob Chemother** 1980 Jan;6(1):151
Selwyn S: The evolution of the broad-spectrum penicillins. **J Antimicrob Chemother** 1982 Feb;9 Suppl B:1–10
Selwyn S: The first studies on the antibacterial effect of penicillium moulds between 1870 and 1876. In International Congress of the History of Medicine. 26th, Plovdiv, 1978. Actes du Congress. Sofia, 1981. Volume II. p. 192–5.
Sheehan JC: The enchanted ring. The untold story of penicillin. Cambridge, Mass., London, MIT Press, 1982. xvi, 224 p.
Starzycki Z: W 40 rocznice wprowadzenia penicyliny do leczenia kiły i rzeżaczki. **Przegl Lek** 1984;41(6):453–7
Swann JP: The search for synthetic penicillin during World War II. **Br J Hist Sci** 1983 Jul;16(53 Pt 2):154–90
Tovarova II, Shamin AN: Istoriia penitsillinov (k 100-letiiu so dnia rozhdeniia Aleksandra Eleminga). **Vopr Istor Estestvozn Tekh** 1981;3:65–75
Travers R: Florey and Cairns--early work on penicillin. **Med J Aust** 1982 Jul 10;2(1):10–1

**Australia**

Dey DL: Penicillin in Australia. **Med J Aust** 1982 Aug 21;2(4):172
Money R: Early work on penicillin. **Med J Aust** 1982 May 1;1(9):367

**Great Britain**

Burdon JG, Kramer H: Early history of penicillin. **Med J Aust** 1982 Dec 11–25;2(12):555–6
Fleming y la penicilina: **Rev Col Nac Enferm** 1979 Aug–Dec;26(105):16–8
Hankiss J: A tudományos teljesítmény értékelése. Fleming felfedezése tükrében. **Orv Hetil** 1980 Jan 13;121(2):95–8
Kempler K: Tervszerü kutatás, vagy véletlen? Gondolatok Fleming születésének centenáriumán. **Orv Hetil** 1981 Nov 29;122(48):2967–9
Macfarlane RG: Alexander Fleming: the man and the myth. London, Chatto & Windus, The Hogarth Press, 1984. xiv, 304 p.
Macfarlane RG: Howard Florey; the making of a great scientist. Oxford and New York, Oxford University Press, 1979. xvi, 396 p.
Macfarlane RG: Howard Walter Florey. In Dictionary of national biography, 1961–1970. Suppl. 8, 1981. p. 370–4.

**Italy**

Daglio P: Vincenzo Tiberio e la scoperta della penicillina. Una grande conquista a cavallo di due secoli. **Minerva Med** 1982 Jul 14;73(28–29):2005–9

**Japan**

Tsunoda F: Hekiso, Nihon penishirin monogatari. Tokyo, Shinchosha, Showa 53 nen. [1978]. 237 p.

**Switzerland**

Ettlinger L: Wartime research on penicillin in Switzerland and antibiotic screening. In Parascandola J, ed: The history of antibiotics. Madison, American Institute of the History of Pharmacy, 1980. p. 57–67.

**United States**

Adams DP: The penicillin mystique and the popular press (1935–1950). **Pharm Hist** 1984;26(3):134–42
Arnold HL: Landmark perspective: penicillin and early syphilis. **JAMA** 1984 Apr 20;251(15):2011–2
Helfand WH, Woodruff HB, Coleman KM, et al: Wartime industrial development of penicillin in the United States. In Parascandola J, ed: The history of antibiotics. Madison, American Institute of the History of Pharmacy, 1980. p. 31–56.
Kennedy JW: Introduction of penicillin in syphilotherapy. **Ariz Med** 1982 Nov;39(11):730, 735
Täuber MG, Sande MA: Landmark perspective: the impact of penicillin on the treatment of meningitis. **JAMA** 1984 Apr 13;251(14):1877–80

### PEPSIN

**1700 to Present**

Dodson G, Chothia C: Fifty years of pepsin crystals [news] **Nature** 1984 May 24–30;309(5966):309

### PESTICIDES

**1700 to Present**

Chapin G, Wasserstrom R: Pesticide use and malaria resurgence in Central America and India. **Soc Sci Med** 1983;17(5):273–90

**United States**

Gillespie B, Eva D, Johnston R: Carcinogenic risk assessment in the United States and Great Britain: the case of Aldrin/Dieldrin. **Soc Stud Sci** 1979;9(3):265–301
Whitaker AH: Pesticide use in early twentieth century animal disease control. **Agric Hist** 1980;54(1):71–81

### PHENOL

**1700 to Present**

Hugo WB: Phenols: a review of their history and development as antimicrobial agents. **Microbios** 1978;23(92):83–5

### PHOSPHORUS

**1700 to Present**

Felton JS: Classical syndromes in occupational medicine: Phosphorus necrosis--a classical occupational disease. **Am J Ind Med** 1982;3(1):77–120

**Germany**

Tower DB: Hensing, 1719. An account of the first chemical examination of the brain and the discovery of phosphorus therein, set against the background of Europe in the 17th and early 18th centuries. A source book in the history of neurochemistry. New York, Raven, 1983. xvi, 407 p.

**Great Britain**

Matsufuji G: [Phosphor-poisoning in match factories and the Salvation Army General Booth] (Jpn). **Igakushi Kenkyu** 1980;54:1–6

### PLANT

Adly A, ed: The history of medicinal and aromatic plants. Proceedings of the Second International Congress organised by The Arab Society for the History of Pharmacy in co-operation with The World Union of Societies of the History of Pharmacy, Alexandria - Egypt, December 15th to 19th, 1980. Karachi, Hamdard Foundation Press, 1982. 216 p.
Delaveau P: Histoire et renouveau des plantes médicinales. Paris, Albin Michel, 1982. 354 p.
Holtkamp P: 'Pastillen des Cosmus' zur Erhaltung wohlriechenden Atems. **Quintessenz J** 1981 Jun;11(6):559–61
Wollman L: Herbs and drugs. **J Am Soc Psychosom Dent Med** 1982;29(4):110

**Brazil**

Holmstedt B, Wassén SH, Schultes RE: Jaborandi: an interdisciplinary appraisal. **J Ethnopharmacol** 1979 Jan;1(1):3–21

**China**

Bisset NG: Arrow poisons in China. Part I. **J Ethnopharmacol** 1979 Dec;1(4):325–84

**Europe**

Brøndegaard VJ: Das Wurzelstechen. **Sudhoffs Arch** 1983;67(2):199–209

**Italy**

Coccanari MA: Les plantes et leur action sur le cerveau et sur la psiche: science et magie. **Med Secoli** 1982 May–Aug;19(2):215–9

**Mexico**

Gallegos AJ: The zoapatle I--a traditional remedy from Mexico emerges to modern times. **Contraception** 1983 Mar;27(3):211–25

1700 to Present

Schultes RE: Peruvian and Chilean psychoactive plants mentioned in Ruiz's Relación (1777-1788). **J Psychoactive Drugs** 1983 Oct-Dec;15(4):303-12

Great Britain

Shellard EJ: Jaborandi: a note on the contribution of E. M. Holmes to the identification of commercially available Pilocarpus and species. **J Ethnopharmacol** 1979 Dec;1(4):407-10

Spain

Richter T: Das Sargassokraut in Vicente de Lardizábals Werk 'Consuelo de Navegantes' (Madrid 1772). Diss., Universität Düsseldorf. Düsseldorf, 1982. 111 p.

### PROSTAGLANDINS

1700 to Present

Euler US von: History and development of prostaglandins. **Gen Pharmacol** 1983;14(1):3-6

Euler US von: Prostaglandin, historical remarks. **Prog Lipid Res** 1981;20:xxxi-xxxv

Sweden

Ottoson D: Ulf von Euler. Tre milstolpar inom medicinen: substans P, prostaglandin och noradrenalin. **Lakartidningen** 1983 Apr 13;80(15):1579-82

### PROTEINS

1700 to Present

Fantini B: Chemical and biological classification of proteins. **Hist Philos Life Sci** 1983;5(1):3-32

Interferon: twenty-five years on: **Philos Trans R Soc Lond [Biol]** 1982 Sep 24;299(1094):1-144

Lindenmann J: From interference to interferon: a brief historical introduction. **Philos Trans R Soc Lond [Biol]** 1982 Sep 24;299(1094):3-6

United States

Merigan TC: Interferon-the first quarter century. **JAMA** 1982 Nov 19;248(19):2513-6

### QUININE

Leden I: Kinabark--en historisk återblick. **Sydsven Medicinhist Sallsk Arsskr** 1980;:80-93

1450-1700

Spain

Hernando y Ortega T: Dos estudios históricos (vieja y nueva medicina). Madrid, Espasa-Calpe, 1982. 243 p.

1700 to Present

United States

Strickland WA: Quinine pills, manufactured on the Missouri frontier (1832-1862). **Pharm Hist** 1983;25(2):61-8

### RHUBARB

1700 to Present

Great Britain

Appleby JH: 'Rhubarb' Mounsey and the Surinam toad--a Scottish physician--naturalist in Russia. **Arch Nat Hist** 1982 Oct;11(1):137-52

Burnby J: Medals for British rhubarb. **Pharm Hist (London)** 1971 Dec;2(3):6-7

### ROSEMARY

500 A.D.-1450

Zimmermann V: Der Rosmarin als Heilpflanze und Wunderdroge; ein Beitrag zu den mittelalterlichen Drogenmonographien. **Sudhoffs Arch** 1980;64(4):351-70

### SACCHARIN

1700 to Present

United States

Priebe PM, Kauffman GB: Making governmental policy under conditions of scientific uncertainty: a century of controversy about saccharin in Congress and the laboratory. **Minerva** 1980 Winter;18(4):556-74

### SALTS

Meyer P: L'homme et le sel. Réflexions sur l'histoire humaine et l'évolution de la médecine. Paris, Fayard, 1982. 171 p.

Théodoridès J: Utilisation du sel et de l'eau de mer dans le traitement ancien de la rage. In: Congrès National des Sociétés Savantes, 99e, Besançon, 1974. Comptes Rendus. Paris, 1976. Section des Sciences, Fasc. V. p. 117-22.

### SILVER NITRATE

1700 to Present

Germany

Kibel MA: Silver nitrate and the eyes of the newborn--a centennial. **S Afr Med J** 1981 Dec 26;60(26):979-80

### SODIUM CHLORIDE

1700 to Present

France

Cottet J: Evolution de la consommation du sel en France. **Bull Mem Acad R Med Belg** 1981;136(11):556-65

Switzerland

Wespi HJ: Die Salzjodierung als Vorläufer der Salzfluoridierung. **SSO Schweiz Monatsschr Zahnheilkd** 1982 Apr;92(4):273-89

United States

Finn R: Salt and hypertension: discussion paper. **J R Soc Med** 1983 Oct;76(10):853-8

### SQUILL

Stearn WT: Mediterranean and Indian species of Drimia (Liliaceae): a nomenclatural survey with special reference to the medicinal squill, D. maritima (syn. Urginea maritima). **Ann Mus Goulandris** 1978;4:199-210

### STEROIDS

1700 to Present

Pramik MJ, ed: Norethindrone: the first three decades. Palo Alto, Syntex Laboratories, 1978. ix, 100 p.

United States

Yocum WS: The cholesterol debates: some reminiscences on Dr. Irvine H. Page. **J Indiana State Med Assoc** 1980;73:567-8

### STONES AND MINERALS

Otten HH: Pedra de mijada, der Pinkelstein. Medizinhistorische Betrachtung zur Lithotherapie. **Med Welt** 1981 May 8;32(19):765-6

500 A.D.-1450

Riddle JM, Mulholland JA: Albert on stones and minerals. In Weisheipl JA, ed: Albertus Magnus and the sciences. Toronto, Pontifical Institute of Mediaeval Studies. 1980. p. 203-34.

France

Riddle JM: Marbode of Rennes' (1035-1123) De lapidibus, considered as a medical treatise with text, commentary and C. W. King's translation, together with text and translation of Marbode's minor works on stones. Wiesbaden, Steiner, 1977. 144 p. (Sudhoffs Archiv, Beihefte, Heft 20).

Netherlands

Vandewiele LJ: Stenen in de Farmacie in de Leer bij Jacob van Maerlant. In Dilg P, et al., ed: Perspektiven der Pharmaziegeschichte. Graz,

Austria, Akademische Druck- u. Verlagsanstalt, 1983. p. 419–30.

1450–1700

Halleux R: L'usage des pierres précieuses dans la thérapeutique aux XVIe et XVIIe siècles. In International Congress of the History of Medicine. 26th, Plovdiv, 1978. Actes du Congress. Sofia, 1981. Volume II. p. 106–8.

1700 to Present

Vallee BL: Metallothionein: historical review and perspectives. **Experientia [Suppl]** 1979;34:19–39

France

Bonnaud L: Pierre ophtalmiques en Haut-Limousin. **Bull Soc Archeol Hist Limousin** 1978;105:164–70

United States

Marshall J: The madstone: its origins and application in Barlow, Ballard County, Kentucky. **Ky Folkl Rec** 1978;24(2):42–8

**STREPTOMYCIN**

1700 to Present

Comroe JH: Pay dirt: the story of streptomycin. Part II. Feldman and Hinshaw; Lehmann. **Am Rev Respir Dis** 1978 May;117(5):957–68

**SUGAR**

Mahdihassan S: A comparative study of the word sugar and of its equivalents in Hindustani as traceable to Chinese. **Am J Chin Med** 1981 Autumn;9(3):187–92
Mintz SW: Time, sugar and sweetness. **Marx Perspect** 1979–80;2(4):56–73
Moore WJ: The role of sugar in the aetiology of dental caries. 1. Sugar and the antiquity of dental caries. **J Dent** 1983 Sep;11(3):189–90

**SULFONAMIDES**

1700 to Present

Maren TH: Carbonic anhydrase: the middle years, 1945–1960, and introduction to pharmacology of sulfonamides. **Ann NY Acad Sci** 1984;429:10–7
Meyle E: Sulfonamidtherapie gestern und heute. **Pharm Unserer Zeit** 1984 Nov;13(6):177–86

United States

Austrian R: Perrin Hamilton Long. In Dictionary of American biography, 1961–1965. Suppl. 7, 1981. p. 477–8.
Ballentine C: Taste of raspberries, taste of death: the 1937 elixir sulfanilamide incident. **FDA Consum** 1981 Jun;15(5):18–21
Kampmeier RH: Introduction of sulfonamide therapy for gonorrhea. **Sex Transm Dis** 1983 Apr–Jun;10(2):81–4
Petersdorf RG: Landmark perspective: sulfadiazine. **JAMA** 1984 Mar 16;251(11):1475–6
Scheld WM, Mandell GL: Landmark perspective. Sulfonamides and meningitis. **JAMA** 1984 Feb 10;251(6):791–4

**TAR WATER**

1700 to Present

Great Britain

Gaustad ES: George Berkeley in America. New Haven, Yale University Press, 1979. xi, 225 p.

**THALIDOMIDE**

1700 to Present

Eskes TK: Classic illustration. Figure showing the relationship between malformations of the thalidomide type and the sales of thalidomide. **Eur J Obstet Gynecol Reprod Biol** 1984 Jan;16(5):365
Folb PI: The thalidomide disaster and its impact on modern medicine. Cape Town, Univ. of Cape Town, 1977. 11 p.
Knightley P, Evans H, Potter E, et al: Suffer the children: the story of thalidomide. New York, Viking Press, 1979. vi, 309 p.

Germany

Wyatt HV: Did thalidomide promote poliomyelitis following oral poliovirus vaccination in West Berlin in 1960? **Perspect Biol Med** 1983 Autumn;27(1):93–106

United States

Thalidomide: 20 years on: **Lancet** 1981 Sep 5;2(8245):510–1

**THEOPHYLLINE**

1700 to Present

Germany

Schultze-Werninghaus G, Meier-Sydow J: The clinical and pharmacological history of theophylline: first report on the bronchospasmolytic action in man by S. R. Hirsch in Frankfurt (Main) 1922. **Clin Allergy** 1982 Mar;12(2):211–5

**THERIAC**

Brandenburg D: Theriak. Ein Beitrag zur Arzneimittellehre des europäischen und orientalischen Mittelalters. **Med Welt** 1982 Aug 20;33(33):1137–40
Demirhan A: The theriacs in the history of medicine. **Med Bull Istanbul Med Fac** 1976;9:151–8
Vidal F: La thériaque--panacée des XVIe, XVIIe, et XVIIIe siècles. **Chir Dent Fr** 1984 Apr 26;54(247):27–32 contd
Vidal F: La thériaque--panacée des XVIe, XVIIe et XVIIIe siècles. **Chir Dent Fr** 1984 May 3;54(248):33–9 contd

Germany

Holste T, Keil G: Tierheilkundliches im altdeutschen Theriak-Traktat. **Hist Med Vet** 1979;4(1):18–21

Hungary

Zolyomi ND: Ein Beitrag zur Entwicklung der Apothekenvisitationen in Ungarn des 17. und 18. Jahrhunderts. Von den Theriakvorführungen zur wissenschaftlich fundierten Apothekenvisitation. **Pharm Acta Helv** 1979;54(4):114–6

Before 500 A.D.

Greco-Roman

Crugnola A, ed: Scholia in Nicandri Theriaka, cum glossis. Varese–Milano, Istituto Editoriale Cisalpino, 1971. 329 p.

Greece

Scarborough J: Nicander: Theriaca 811. **Classical Philol** 1980;75:138–40
Winkler L: Galens Schrift 'De Antidotis'. Ein Beitrag zur Geschichte von Antidot und Theriak. Diss. rer. nat. Marburg, 1980. 390 p.

1450–1700

Italy

Olmi G: Farmacopea antica e medicina moderna: la disputa sulla teriaca nel cinquecento Bolognese. **Physis** 1977;19(1–4):197–246

1700 to Present

Great Britain

Paulshock BZ: William Heberden, M.D., and the end of theriac. **NY State J Med** 1982 Oct;82(11):1612–4

Spain

Folch Jou G, Muñoz Calvo S: Datos para la historia del Colegio de Boticarios de Madrid. Actos con motivo de la preparacion de la Triaca en el siglo XVIII. **An R Acad Farm (Madr)** 1979;45(4):599–606

**TOBACCO**

Christen AG, Swanson BZ, Glover ED, et al: Smokeless tobacco: the folklore and social history of snuffing, sneezing, dipping, and chewing. **J Am Dent Assoc** 1982 Nov;105(5):821–9
de Moulin D: The value of tobacco smoke in the treatment of intussusception. **Neth J Surg** 1984 Apr;36(2):57–9
Edelman F: Nicotiana, les botanistes et le tabac, des premiers herbiers à nos jours. **Flammes Fumees** 1977;(79):65–128
Kneist W: Rauchen oder Gesundheit. Ein kulturhistorischer Rückblick. **Z Gesamte Hyg** 1981;27(6):477–80
Rival N: Tabac, miroir du temps. Paris, Librairie Academique Perrin, 1981. 282 p.

Shor RE, Shor MB, Williams DC: The distinction between the antismoking and nonsmokers' rights movements. **J Psychol** 1980 Sep;106(First Half):129–46
Stepney R: The Indians' revenge or drunk without drinking. **Practitioner** 1980 Jan;224(1339):109–11

**Americas**

Barbachano AE: Datos prehispanicos del tabaquismo en America. **Bol Soc Mex Hist Filos Med** 1982 Jun;6(39):29–42
Elferink JG: The narcotic and hallucinogenic use of tobacco in Pre-Columbian Central America. **J Ethnopharmacol** 1983 Jan;7(1):111–22
Robicsek F: The smoking gods; tobacco in Maya art, history, and religion. Norman, Oklahoma, Univ. of Oklahoma Press, 1978. xxv, 233 p.

**Bolivia**

Bruhn JG, et al: The tobacco from Niño Korin: identification of nicotine in a Bolivian archaeological collection. **Goteb Ethnogr Mus** 1976;:45–8

**Switzerland**

Trümpy H: Volkskundliche Uberlegungen zum Rauchen. **Ther Umsch** 1983 Feb;40(2):165–8

**United States**

Ethridge RF: Tobacco among the Cherokees. **J Cherokee Stud** 1978;3(2):77–86

**Before 500 A.D.**

**Colombia**

Torres CM: Evidence for snuffing in the prehispanic stone sculpture of San Agustín, Colombia. **J Psychoactive Drugs** 1981 Jan–Mar;13(1):53–60

**1450–1700**

**Mexico**

Anderson JR: Acayatl, ancient Aztec sorcerer. **Ala Med** 1984 Feb;53(8):14, 17–8, 20

**1700 to Present**

Mann RJ, Mann FD: Emphysema. Era of Laennec; era of the cigarette. **Minn Med** 1984 Mar;67(3):142, 159–61

**Great Britain**

Budnick LD: The spirit of Chadwick. **NY State J Med** 1983 Dec;83(13):1345–6
Walker RB: Medical aspects of tobacco smoking and the anti-tobacco movement in Britain in the nineteenth Century. **Med Hist** 1980;24(4):391–402

**Hungary**

Frankl J: 150 éves orvosi vélemény a dohányzásról. **Orv Hetil** 1980 Dec 14;121(50):3078–9

**Ireland**

Walsh BM: Health education and the demand for tobacco in Ireland, 1953–76: a note. **Econ Soc Rev (Irel)** 1980;11(2):147–51

**United States**

Blum A: Alton Ochsner, MD, 1896–1981. He cleared the air. **NY State J Med** 1983 Dec;83(13):1251
Burney LE: Policy over politics. The first statement on smoking and health by the Surgeon General of the United States Public Health Service. **NY State J Med** 1983 Dec;83(13):1252–3
Christen AG: Orally used smokeless tobacco as advertised in the metamorphic trade cards of 1870–1900. **Bull Hist Dent** 1983 Oct;31(2):82–6
Doll R: Smoking and death rates. **JAMA** 1984 Jun 1;251(21):2854–7
Garfinkel L: A tribute to Harold S. Diehl (1891–1973) - changing patterns of smoking and disease. **CA** 1981;31:114–9
Koplin AN: Anti-smoking legislation: the New Jersey experience. **J Public Health Policy** 1981;2(3):247–55
Lutschg JH: Why Uncle Sam is still smoking. **NY State J Med** 1983 Dec;83(13):1278–9
Ring ME: Oddments in dental history: down with toothbrushes - up with tobacco! **Bull Hist Dent** 1984;32(1):31–2
Steinfeld JL: Women and children last? Attitudes toward cigarette smoking and nonsmokers' rights, 1971. **NY State J Med** 1983 Dec;83(13):1257–8
Stewart WH: A warning against complacency. **NY State J Med** 1983 Dec;83(13):1256
Terry LL: The Surgeon General's first report on smoking and health. A challenge to the medical profession. **NY State J Med** 1983 Dec;83(13):1254–5
When 'more doctors smoked Camels': Cigarette advertising in the Journal. **NY State J Med** 1983 Dec;83(13):1347–52
Wynder EL: Some reflections on smoking and lung cancer. **J Thorac Cardiovasc Surg** 1984 Nov;88(5 Pt 2):854–7

## TOXINS

**1700 to Present**

**United States**

Baur FJ, Parker WA: The aflatoxin problem: industry–FDA–USDA cooperation. **J Assoc Off Anal Chem** 1984 Jan–Feb;67(1):3–7
Fischbach H: Coping with the aflatoxin problem in the early years. **J Assoc Off Anal Chem** 1984 Jan–Feb;67(1):1–3

## TURPENTINE

Haller JS: Sampson of the terebinthinates: medical history of turpentine. **South Med J** 1984 Jun;77(6):750–4

## VITAMINS

Sharman IM: Symposium on 'Vitamin A in nutrition and disease.' Historical introduction. **Proc Nutr Soc** 1983 Jan;42(1):1–5

**Before 500 A.D.**

Walker A, Zimmerman MR, Leakey RE: A possible case of hypervitaminosis A in Homo erectus. **Nature** 1982 Mar 18;296(5854):248–50

**1700 to Present**

Jukes TH: A biochemical adventure--the hunt for vitamin D. **J Appl Biochem** 1983 Jun;5(3):147–8
Pawson BA: History of retinoids. **J Am Acad Dermatol** 1982 Apr;6(4 Pt 2 Suppl):577–82
Sharman IM: Vitamins: essential dietary constituents discovered. **Endeavour** 1977;1(3–4):97–102
Shils ME: Historical aspects of minerals and vitamins in parenteral nutrition. **Fed Proc** 1984 Apr;43(5):1412–6

**Germany**

Hoppe B: Adolf Windaus, Heinrich Wieland, Richard Kuhn, Leopold Ružička, Alexander Todd und Adolf Bunenandt. Die Erforschung der Vitamine und der Hormone. In: Die Grossen der Weltgeschichte. Zürich, Kindler, 1978. p. 336–81.

**Italy**

Chiacone FM: Appunti per uno studio sulla vitaminologia in Italia. **Acta Vitaminol Enzymol** 1979;1(1–6):33–109

**United States**

Davis AB: The rise of the vitamin-medicinal as illustrated by vitamin D. **Pharm Hist** 1982;24(2):59–72
Davis DR: Some legacies of nutrition pioneer E. V. McCollum. **Trans Kans Acad Sci** 1979 Aug;82(3):133–45
Goertzel TG, Goertzel MG, Goertzel V: Linus Pauling: the scientist as crusader. **Antioch Rev** 1980;38(3):371–82
Ihde AJ: Conrad Arnold Elvehjem. In Dictionary of American biography, 1961–1965. Suppl. 7, 1981. p. 223–4.

**USSR**

Efremov VV: K istorii otkrytiia vitaminov N. I. Luninym. **Vopr Pitan** 1982 May–Jun;(3):68–72
Lavrov BA: Ocherki po istorii sovetskoĭ vitaminologii, 1917–1967. Moskva, Meditsina, 1980. 199 p.

## ZINC

**Belgium**

Leboutte R: Les métaux et l'hygiène alimentaire: la vaisselle en zinc de l'abbé Dony. **Bull Soc R Vieux Liege** 1977–79;9:311–3

## ECOLOGY

See also **Sanitation; Public Health**

Egerton FN: The history of ecology: achievements and opportunities, part one. **J Hist Biol** 1983 Summer;16(2):259–310
Eisenbud M: Environment, technology, and health: human ecology in historical perspective. New York, New York University Press, 1978. x, 384 p.
Kilburn KH: Chronic disease in the workplace and the environment. Lung disease: lessons from the past--keys to the future. **Arch Environ Health** 1984 May–Jun;39(3):139–43
Klinkenberg HM: Die historische Dimension der Umwelt. **Clio Med** 1980 Jul;14(3–4):187–211
Lee DH, Selikoff IJ: Historical background to the asbestos problem. **Environ Res** 1979 Apr;18(2):300–14
Merchant C: The death of nature. Women, ecology, and the scientific revolution. San Francisco, Harper & Row, 1980. xx, 348 p.
Pelling M: Social history of medicine and the geographers--a bibliography. **Soc Soc Hist Med Bull (Lond)** 1984 Dec;35:55–8
Simoons F: Effects of culture: geographical and historical approaches. **Int J Obes** 1980;4(4):387–94
Wijbenga A, Hutzinger O: Chemicals, man and the environment: a historic perspective of pollution and related topics. **Naturwissenschaften** 1984 May;71(5):239–46

**Great Britain**

Swales RJ: Plague, population and ecology in early modern England. **Can J Hist** 1979;14(2):257–66

**United States**

Capper J, Power G, Shivers FR: Chesapeake waters. Pollution, public health, and public opinion, 1607–1972. Centreville, Maryland, Tidewater Publishers, 1983. xii, 201 p.

**Before 500 A.D.**

Kottek SS, Seligman H: Ecology in Talmudic sources. In H. Shuval, ed: Developments in arid zone ecology and environment quality. Philadelphia, Balaban ISS, 1981. p. 119–26.

**Greece**

Kullmann W: Aristoteles' Grundgedanken zu Aufbau und Funktion der Körpergewebe. **Sudhoffs Arch** 1982;66(3):209–38

**1450–1700**

Dobson MJ: Environments of disease and mortality in the New World and the Old World. **Soc Soc Hist Med Bull (Lond)** 1984 Dec;35:7–10
Hiller I: Betrachtungen zu medizinischen Aspekten des Umweltschutzes im 17. Jahrhundert. **Z Gesamte Hyg** 1983 Sep;29(9):560–3
Pagel W: Mother nature and the scientific revolution. **Hist Sci** 1981 Jun:19(44 pt 2):148–53

**Americas**

Wear A: Perceptions of health and environment in the settlement of North America in the early seventeenth century. **Soc Soc Hist Med Bull (Lond)** 1984 Dec;35:11–3

**United States**

Earle C: Environment, disease and mortality in early Virginia. **J Hist Geogr** 1979;5(4):365–90

**1700 to Present**

Black LT: Volcanism as a factor in human ecology: the Aleutian case. **Ethnohistory** 1981;28(4):313–40
Hulse FS: Habits, habitats, and heredity: a brief history of studies in human plasticity. **Am J Phys Anthropol** 1981 Dec;56(4):495–501
Luten DB: Ecological optimism in the social sciences: the question of limits of growth. **Am Behav Sci** 1980;24(1):125–51

**Bulgaria**

Bugyi B: Medical topography of Bulgaria and Serbia in the third quarter of the 19th century. **Geogr Med** 1981;11:158–61

**France**

Guillerme A: Medical topography and the rebuilding of Le Mans. **Soc Soc Hist Med Bull (Lond)** 1984 Dec;35:26–7

**Great Britain**

Craig P: Medical topography. **Soc Soc Hist Med Bull (Lond)** 1984 Dec;35:33–4
Kearns G: Cholera and public health reform in nineteenth-century England and Wales: interpreting the geographical patterns. **Soc Soc Hist Med Bull (Lond)** 1984 Dec;35:30–2
Viniaker H: L'asthme et son environnement selon Sir John Floyer (1649–1734). **Hist Sci Med** 1984;18(1):77–82

**United States**

Bean WB: Frederick Law Olmstead and Vanderbilt's Biltmore estate: the contribution of private wealth to forestry, ecology and climatology. **Trans Am Clin Climatol Assoc** 1979;90:132–9
Brooks P: Rachel Louise Carson. In: Notable American women. The modern period. Cambridge, Mass., Belknap-Harvard Univ. Press, 1980. 4:138–41.
Dunlap TR: DDT: scientists, citizens, and public policy. Princeton, Princeton University Press, 1981. 318 p.
Etzioni A: How much is a life worth? **Soc Policy** 1979;9(5):4–8
Fox SD: Healing, imagination, and New Mexico. **NM Hist Rev** 1983;58(3):213–37
Shipek FE: A native American adaptation to drought: the Kumeyaay as seen in the San Diego Mission records, 1770–1798. **Ethnohistory** 1981;28(4):295–312

**USSR**

Kurchishvili IB, Asatiani DK, Chomakhashvili AI: Istoki meditsinskoĭ geografii v Gruzii. **Sov Zdravookhr** 1983;(12):51–3
Makarov VA: Razvitie I. M. Sechenovym ucheniia o edinstve organizma i sredy. **Usp Fiziol Nauk** 1979 Jul–Sep;10(3):5–14
Shandala MG: Ozdorovlenie okruzhaiushcheĭ sredy--put' k obshchestvennomu zdorov'iu (k 50-letiiu Kievskogo NII obshcheĭ i kommunal'noĭ gigieny im. A. N. Marzeeva). **Vrach Delo** 1981 Sep;(9):1–5
Weiner DR: Community ecology in Stalin's Russia: 'socialist' and 'bourgeois' science. **ISIS** 1984 Dec;75(279):684–96

## ECONOMICS, MEDICAL

See also **Ethics, Medical; Licensure and Regulation; State Medicine**

Cherry R: Biology and sociology and economics: an historical analysis. **Rev Soc Econ** 1980;38(2):141–54
Fox DM: Economists and health care. From reform to relativism. With commentaries. New York, Prodist, 1979.
Geerts A, Kornblith BA, Urmson WJ: Compensation for bodily harm. L'indemnisation des lésions corporelles à travers les siècles. Brussels, Fernand Nathan, Labor, 1977. 213 p.
Hugly C: L'argent dans la relation thérapeutique. **Rev Odontostomatol (Paris)** 1981 May–Jun;10(3):239–44
Marr JJ: Merchants of death: the role of slave trade in the transmission of disease from Africa to the Americas. **Pharos** 1982 Winter;45(1):31–5
Navarro P: Lactancia mercenaria: hipocresía y exploitación. **Asclepio** 1983;35:375–87
Portwood D, Fielding A: Privilege and the professions. **Sociol Rev** 1981 Nov;29(4):749–73
Sauvy A: Science médicale et science économique. **Ann Med Interne (Paris)** 1982;133(3):216–21
Swanson BZ: A dental Notgeld note. **Bull Hist Dent** 1982 Apr;30(1):27–30

**Americas**

Fogel RW, et al: The economics of mortality in North America, 1650–1910: a description of a research project. **Hist Methods Newsl** 1978;11(2):75–108

**Belgium**

Vandenbroeke C: De medische konsumptie sinds de 16e eeuw. **Handel Maatsch Geschied Oudheidk Gent** 1980;34:143–65

**Colombia**

Chandler DL: Health and slavery in colonial Colombia. New York, Arno Press, 1981. iv, 307 p. (Ph.D. Diss., Tulane 1972).

**France**

Coudurier P: Les prix de journée: détermination et contentieux. Nancy, Berger-Levrault, 1978. 225 p.
Grenier JY: Quelques éléments pour une étude des liens entre conjoncture économique et conjoncture démographique aux XVIIe et XVIIIe siècles. **Ann Demogr Hist (Paris)** 1984;:175–99

**Germany**

Probst J: Unfallmedizin und Lebensversicherungsmedizin. **Lebensversicherungsmedizin** 1982 Nov 25;34(9):193–4

**Great Britain**

Crawford P: Printed advertisements for women medical practitioners in London, 1670–1710. **Soc Soc Hist Med Bull (Lond)** 1984 Dec;35:66–70
Patterson TJ: The medical practice of the East India Company. **Soc Soc Hist Med Bull (Lond)** 1980 Jun;26:40–3
Roy I, Porter S: The social and economic structure of an early modern suburb: the Tything at Worcester. **Bull Inst Hist Res** 1980;53:203–17

**Italy**

Anselmi S, Sorcinelli P: Epidemie e rivalità commerciali nelle piazze maritime marchigiane (secoli XVI–XIX). **Econ Stor** 1977;24(3):293–310

**Poland**

Zajusz K: Z dziejów spółek Brackich. **Arch Hist Med (Warsz)** 1979;42(1):33–43

**South Africa**

Louw NS: Hoe word die dokter betaal? **S Afr Med J** 1983 Jun 29;Spec No:40–2

**Before 500 A.D.**

**India**

Singh R, Singh AN: Socio-economic and trade relations of ancient India with the western world as reflected in plant names with particular reference to saffron (Kunkum/Kesara). **Stud Hist Med** 1981 Sep;5(3):228–32

**500 A.D.–1450**

Jenkins M: Medicine and spices, with special reference to medieval monastic accounts. **Gard Hist** 1976;4:47–9

**Arabic**

Biesterfeldt HH: Some opinions on the physician's remuneration in medieval Islam. **Bull Hist Med** 1984 Spring;58(1):16–27

**France**

La Coste-Messelière R de, Jugnot G, Treuille H: Fonda des XVIIe–XVIIIe siècles et sources de l'histoire hospitalière médiévale XIIe–XIVe siècle. Toulouse, E. Privat, 1978. 283–318 p.

**Germany**

Dressendörfer W: Spätmittelalterliche Arzneitaxen des Münchner Stadtarztes Sigmund Gotzkircher aus dem Grazer Codex 311. Ein Beitrag zur Frühgeschichte des süddeutschen Apothekenwesens. Pattensen/Hannover, Wellm, 1978. 327 p. (Würzburger medizinhistorische Forschungen, 15). Also Diss. (Pharm) München.

**Great Britain**

Cosman MP: The medieval medical third party: compulsory consultation and malpractice insurance. **Ann Plast Surg** 1982 Feb;8(2):152–62

**1450–1700**

**France**

Kubler M: A propos de deux contrats médicaux à la fin du Moyen Age. In Livet G, Schaff G, ed: Médecine et assistance en Alsace, XVIe–XXe siècle. Strasbourg, Istra, 1976. p. 41–50.

**Great Britain**

Pelling M: Occupational diversity: barbersurgeons and the trades of Norwich, 1550–1640. **Bull Hist Med** 1982;56(4):484–511
Pelling M: Old people and poverty in early modern towns. **Soc Soc Hist Med Bull (Lond)** 1984 Jun;34:42–7
Schmidtgall H: Zur Rezeption von Harveys Blutkreislaufmodell in der englischen Wirtschaftstheorie des 17. Jahrhunderts. **Sudhoffs Arch** 1973;57(4):416–30

**Italy**

Grossi Turchetti ML: La dotazione libraria di un collegio universitario del Quattrocento. **Physis** 1980;22(3–4):463–75
Lombardi D: 1629–1631: crisi e peste a Firenze. **Arch Stor Ital** 1979;137(1):3–50

**Spain**

Jiménez Muñoz JM: Salarios de medicos y cirujanos (I) (II). (Nóminas de Corte 1538–1629). **Asclepio** 1981;33:315–47
Jordi González R: Duedas y cuentas de boticarios: una reivindicación histórica obligada. [Barcelona], Réal Academía de Farmacía de Barcelona, 1985. 63 p.

**1700 to Present**

Arouca AS: El trabajo médico, la producción capitalista y la viabilidad del proyecto de prevención. **Rev Mex Cienc Polit Soc** 1976;22(84):33–56
Battistella R, Eastaugh SR: Health cost containment. **Proc Acad Polit Sci** 1980;33(4):192–205
Berliner H: Medical modes of production. In P. Wright, A. Treacher, ed: The problem of medical knowledge. Examining the social construction of medicine. Edinburgh, Edinburgh University Press, 1982. p. 162–73.
Blardone G: Rapports entre alimentation et types de développements. **Acquis Med Recent** 1981;198:35–55
Bullock MB: An American transplant: the Rockefeller Foundation and Peking Union Medical College. Berkeley, University of California Press, 1980. xxvii, 280 p.
Ellacuría I. Seguridad social y solidaridad humana: aproximacion filosofica al fenomeno de la seguridad social. **Estud Cent Am** 1969;24(253):357–66
Eskes TK: Classic illustration. Figure showing the relationship between malformations of the thalidomide type and the sales of thalidomide. **Eur J Obstet Gynecol Reprod Biol** 1984 Jan;16(5):365
Figlio K: How does illness mediate social relations? Workmen's compensation and medico-legal practices, 1890–1940. In P. Wright, A. Treacher, ed: The problem of medical knowledge. Examining the social construction of medicine. Edinburgh, Edinburgh University Press, 1982. p. 174–224.
Gish O: The political economy of primary care and 'health by the people': an historical exploration. **Soc Sci Med** 1979 Dec;13C(4):203–11
Harris SE: History of health insurance. In his: The economics of health care; finance and delivery. Berkeley, McCutchan, 1975. p. 333–92.
Hynes J: The remunerative advantages of ineffective medicines. **MIMS Mag** 1981 May 15;:70–3
Ledermann F: El precio de los medicamentos en el canton de Neuchatel y en Suiza: 1930–1960. **Bol Soc Esp Hist Farm** 1982 Sep;33(131):163–72
Loraine JA: Future patterns of disease: maladies of development. **Contemp Rev** 1983;242(1409):298–302
Loraine JA: The economics of fertility. **Midwife Health Visit Community Nurse** 1982 Jan;18(1):6–8
Meinke H: A short history of dental advertising. **Bull Hist Dent** 1983 Apr;31(1):36–42
Muller M: The health of nations. A North-South investigation. London, Faber and Faber, 1982. 255 p.
Numbers RL, ed: Compulsory health insurance. The continuing American debate. Westport, Connecticut, London, Greenwood Press, 1982. xv, 172 p. With contributions by A. J. Viseltear, G. Land, T. R. Marmor, M. M. Poen, P. Starr, R. Lubove, W. J. Cohen. (Contributions in medical history, no. 11).
Reinhardt UE: Health insurance and cost-containment policies: the experience abroad. **Am Econ Rev** 1980;70(2):149–56
Riesenfeld SA: [The development of] health insurance. In Reich WT, et al, ed: Encyclopedia of bioethics, v. 2. New York, Free Press, 1978. p. 637–42.
Rosales VJ: The medicotrophic syndrome: an acute modern phenomenon. **Unitas** 1970;43(4):30–59
Sindelar JL: Differential use of medical care by sex. **J Polit Econ** 1982;90(5):1003–19
Steckel RH: Height and per capita income. **Hist Methods** 1983;16(1):1–7

**Africa**

Hartwig GW: Economic consequenses of long-distance trade in East-Africa: the disease factor. **Afr Stud Rev** 1975;18(2):63–77

**Algeria**

Ait Khaled N, Oussedik N, Chaulet P: Evolution du coût des médicaments antituberculeux de 1964 à 1980; son influence dans le choix d'une politique de traitement de la tuberculose en Algérie. **Bull Int Union Tuberc** 1981 Sep–Dec;56(3–4):170–4

**Americas**

Garcia JC: The laziness disease. **Hist Philos Life Sci** 1981;3(1):31–59
Zschock DK: Health care financing in Central America and the Andean

Region: a workshop report. **Lat Am Res Rev** 1980;15(3):149–68

**Australia**

Bates EM: A consumer's view of the Australian experience in health insurance. **Lancet** 1980 Jul 5;2(8184):26–8
Blum A: Fleeting hopes and promises of advertising. **Med J Aust** 1982 May 29;1(11):485

**Austria**

Sablik K: Die Finanzierung des Wiener Allgemeinen Krankenhauses (gegründet 1784) durch Kaiser Joseph II. In Schmidtchen V, Jäger E, ed: Wirtschaft, Technik und Geschichte. Beiträge zur Erforschung der Kulturbeziehungen in Deutschland und Osteuropa. Festschrift für Albrecht Timm. Berlin, Verlag Ulrich Camen, 1980. p. 241–50.

**Belgium**

Masuy-Stroobant G: La surmortalité infantile des Flandres au cours de la deuxième moitié du XIXe siècle: mode d'alimentation ou mode de développement? **Ann Demogr Hist (Paris)** 1983;:231–56

**Brazil**

Wood CH: Infant mortality trends and capitalist development in Brazil: the case of Sao Paulo and Belo Horizonte. **Lat Am Perspect** 1977:4(4):56–65

**Canada**

Armstrong C: Federalism and government regulation: the case of the Canadian insurance industry, 1927–34. **Can Public Adm** 1976;19(1):88–101
Black E: Dealing with the doctors: the Canadian experience. **Mon Rev** 1981;33(4):27–35
Chapman ID, Farina C: Accountability and the science research board. **J Can Stud** 1982–83;17(4):3–9
Genest J: L'assureur-vie dans la cité. **Action Natl** 1981;70(7):601–12
LaBerge R: Medicare is not the health charter for Canadians. **Can Labour** 1969;14(9):14–9
Naylor CD: Canadian doctors and state health insurance, 1911–1918. **RSTC** 1982;22,6(3):127–50
Roland CG: Dr. James Bowman vs Canada: a struggle to obtain payment for government service. In: Congrès international d'histoire de la médecine, XXVe, Québec, 1976. Actes. Québec, 1977. p. 1158–69.
Shipley M, Agass M, Bell A, et al: The Quebec Medicare Programme. **R Soc Health J** 1982 Feb;102(1):37–8, 43
Soderstrom L: The Canadian experience. **Proc Acad Polit Sci** 1980;33(4):224–38
Walters V: State, capital, and labour: the introduction of Federal-Provincial insurance for physician care in Canada. **Can Rev Sociol Anthropol** 1982;19(2):157–72
Ward WP, Ward PC: Infant birth weight and nutrition in industrializing Montreal. **Am Hist Rev** 1984;89(2):324–45

**Chile**

Valdivieso R: La ley de medicina curativa para empleados y el Formulario Nacional de Medicamentos. **Rev Med Chil** 1977 Oct;105(10):663–7

**Europe**

Blanpain J, Delesie L, Nys H: National health insurance and health resources. Cambridge, Harvard Univ. Press, 1978. xiv, 294 p.
Lesthaeghe R, Wilson C: Les modes de production, la laïcisation et le rythme de la baisse de la fécondité en Europe de l'Ouest de 1870 à 1930. **Population** 1982;37(3):623–45

**France**

Cosma-Muller P: Entre science et commerce: les eaux minerales en France a la fin de l'ancien regime. **Hist Reflect** 1982;9(1–2):249–62
Dillemann G: Les cumuls d'emplois en 1821. **Rev Hist Pharm (Paris)** 1981 Jun;28(249):109–11
McQuillan K: Modes of production and demographic patterns in nineteenth-century France. **AJS** 1984;89(6):1324–46
Martiny M: Projet de loi présenté le 31 janvier 1923 par le député Edouard Grinda sur les assurances sociales. **Hist Sci Med** 1979;13(4):363–7
Oberlé R: Société et assistance à Mulhouse à la fin du XVIIIe siècle. In Livet G, Schaff G, ed: Médecine et assistance en Alsace, XVIe–XXe siècle. Strasbourg, Istra, 1976. p. 117–34.

**Germany**

Becker K: 100 Jahre gesetzliche Krankenversicherung. Entwicklung, Krise, Lösungsansätze in der Krankenversicherung der Rentner. (Mit einem Beitrag von Jens Jessen, Programmierter Kollaps der GKV?) Mainz, MPS, 1980. 74 p.
Eisenberg L: Rudolf Ludwig Karl Virchow, where are you now that we need you? **Am J Med** 1984 Sep;77(3):524–32
Guter P: Die Krankenversicherung. Vertrags- und Honorarsituation seit 1935. **Zahnarzt** 1980 Jan;24(1):12–20 contd.
Hell W: Research on monocular depth perception between 1884 and 1914: influence of the German Unfallversicherungsgesetz and of the jurisdiction of the Reichsversicherungsamt. **Perception** 1982;10(6):683–94
Labisch A: Gleiche Chance der medizinischen Versorgung; historischer Abriss über ein Leitmotiv in der Entwicklung der gesetzlichen Krankenversicherung. In Hauss, F., Naschold, F., Rosenbrock, R., ed: Schichtenspezifische Versorgungsprobleme im Gesundheitswesen. Bonn, Der Bundesminister für Arbeit und Sozialordnung, 1981. p. 32–50.
Machtan L: Workers' insurance versus protection of the workers. Remarks on state social policy in the early Kaiserreich. **Soc Soc Hist Med Bull (Lond)** 1983 Dec;33:33
Marburger H: 100 Jahre Kaiserliche Botschaft--zur Entwicklung des Leistungsrechts der Krankenversicherung von seinen Anfängen bis heute. **Off Gesundheitswes** 1982 Apr;44(4):247–51
Possehl I: Die Arzneitaxe--auch im 19. Jahrhundert ein Problem. **Beitr Gesch Pharm** 1980;8:61–3
Possehl T: Probleme der Arzneipreisgestaltung im 19. Jahrhundert. **Medizinhist J** 1981;16(4):358–90
Schmidt H: Zur Kostenfreiheit ärztlicher Hilfeleistung; eine Betrachtung aus Anlass des 90. Jahrestages des Erfurter Programms der SPD. **Beitr Gesch Univ Erfurt** 1979–83;19:265–70
Schmitt WM: Die Sozialversicherung von 1883 bis 1962. **Zahnarzt** 1980 Jan;24(1):7–11

**Great Britain**

Asherson N: The age of John Hunter's golden guineas (1763–93). **Ann R Coll Surg Engl** 1982 Jul;64(4):262–5
Bartrip P: Workmen's compensation in British law, society and politics, 1897–1946. **Soc Soc Hist Med Bull (Lond)** 1983 Dec;33:30–2
Blackden S: The Poor Law and wealth: a survey of parochial medical aid in Glasgow, 1845–1900. In: The search for wealth and stability. Ed. by T. C. Smout. London, Macmillan, 1979.
Brown PS: The venders of medicines advertised in eighteenth-century Bath newspapers. **Med Hist** 1975 Oct;19(4):352–69
Butler JR, Boddy FA: The evolution of health services research in Britain. **Community Med** 1983 Aug;5(3):192–9
Davies J: David Lloyd George and the National Insurance Act of 1911. In J. Cule, ed: Wales and medicine. London, British Society for the History of Medicine, 1975. p. 1–9.
Dupâquier J, Fauve-Chamoux A, Grebenik E, ed: Malthus past and present. London; New York, Academic Press, 1983. xix, 416 p. Contributions by A. Béjin, Y. Breton, Y. Charbit, L. Devance, A. Digby, M. W. Flinn, R. E. Frisch, M. Godelier, L. Gordon, P. Guillaume, G. Heinsohn, T. H. Hollingsworth, P. A. Jewell, N. Keyfitz, R. Keynes, H. Le Bras, M. Perrot, F. Rausky, M. Rebérioux, R. Remond, F. Ronsin, G. R. Searle, B. Stapleton, O. Steiger, P. Vallin, E. Van de Walle, A. Waterman, J. Wolff, E. A. Wrigley, V. Wynne-Edwards.
Eder NR: Medical opinion and the first year of national health insurance in Britain. **Albion** 1979;11(2):157–71
Eder NR: National health insurance, social politics and medical practice in Britain, 1913–1939. Ph.D. diss. University of Illinois. Chicago, 1980. 375 leaves.
Gaffney R: Poor law hospitals 1845–1914. In Checkland O, Lamb M, ed: Health care as social history; the Glasgow case. Aberdeen, Aberdeen University Press, 1982. p. 44–58.
Hambridge RA: 'Empiricomany, or an infatuation in favour of Empiricism or Quackery': the socio-economics of eighteenth-century quackery. In S. Soupel, R. A. Hambridge: Literature and science and medicine. Los Angeles, William Andrews Clark Memorial Library, UCLA, 1982. p. 45–102.
Hart H: Some notes on the sponsoring of patients for hospital treatment under the voluntary system. **Med Hist** 1980;24(4):447–60
Hollingsworth DF: Rationing and economic constraints on food consumption in Britain since the Second World War. **World Rev Nutr Diet** 1983;42:191–218
Honigsbaum F: The BMA-TUC alliance and the Beveridge report. **Soc Soc Hist Med Bull (Lond)** 1983 Jun;32:19
Jones IH: Wages through the ages. **Nurs Times** 1980 Jul 17;76(29):1279–80
Loudon IS: A doctor's cash book: the economy of general practice in the 1830s. **Med Hist** 1983 Jul;27(3):249–68
Mason FM: Charles Masterman and National Health Insurance. **Albion** 1978;10(1):54–75
Takei Y: [Administrative reform in 19th-century England, a result of the public health problem] (Jpn). **Shakai Keizai Shigaku** 1976;42(3):1–21
Thomas EG: The old Poor Law and medicine. **Med Hist** 1980 Jan;24(1):2–19
Torrens PR: Health insurance in the United States: implications for the United Kingdom. **Lancet** 1980 Jan 5;1(8158):27–31
Whiteside N: Central control and the approved societies: access to social support under the interwar health insurance scheme. **Soc Soc Hist Med Bull (Lond)** 1983 Jun;32:14–8

Wilson HD: A hundred years of the Ettles scholarship at the University of Edinburgh or 'Whatever happened to the likely lads (and lasses)?' **Med Educ** 1981 Nov;15(6):359–62

**Hungary**

Bartos I: Társadalombiztosításunk 30 éve. **Orv Hetil** 1981 Mar 22;122(12):679–80

The development of social insurance in Hungary over three decades. [Budapest?], The Administration, [1975?]. 114 p.:

**India**

Ram R, Schultz TW: Life span, health, savings, and productivity. **Econ Dev Cult Change** 1979;27(3):399–421

**Japan**

Hasegawa A: [Social events in the history of nursing after World War II. I. Hospital and nurses on strike] (Jpn). **Kango** 1984 Aug;36(9):126–44

Ishikawa no kokuho yonjunen: [Kanazawa, Japan], Ishikawa-ken, Showa 53 nen. [1978]. 221 p.

Steslicke WE: Development of health insurance policy in Japan. **J Health Polit Policy Law** 1982 Spring;7(1):197–26

Suzuki S: Kenko hoken kumiai hattatsu shi. Tokyo, Kitamura Shakai Hoken Shuppan, Showa 51 nen [1976]. 15, 362 p.

**Mexico**

Sepúlveda B: La medicina en la seguridad social. In Academia Nacional de Medicina. Libro conmemorativo del primer centenario. México, Comité Editorial de la Comisión Organizadora del Congreso del Centenario, 1964. Tome 2. p. 678–83.

**Netherlands**

Juffermans P: Economic crisis and health policy in the Netherlands. **Int J Health Serv** 1984;14(1):147–58

**New Zealand**

New Zealand Dept. of Health: Health expenditures in New Zealand -- trends and growth patterns. Wellington, Management Services and Research Unit, Department of Health, 1979. 62 p.

**Norway**

Kringlen E: Legemidler for behov eller profitt. **Samtiden (Norway)** 1970;79(9):546–63

**Poland**

Czeley-Wybieralska M: O ogłoszeniach lekarskich w Polsce. **Arch Hist Med (Warsz)** 1983;46(3):315–23

Jeśman C: Organizacja niemieckiej Izby Aptekarskiej i gospodarka lekami w tzw. Generalnym Gubernatorstwie w latach 1939–1945. **Arch Hist Med (Warsz)** 1984;47(3):403–15

**Scandinavia**

Ito H: Health insurance policy development in Denmark and Sweden 1860--1950. **Soc Sci Med** 1979 Oct;13C(3):143–60

**Spain**

Figuerola JE, Figuerola I: La cuenta de medicinas administradas a la hija del Marques de la Quadra. **Bol Soc Esp Hist Farm** 1980 Mar–Jun;3(121–2)

**Sweden**

Engel A: Halsan fore fodelsen. Prenatal forskning i Sverige. Stockholm, 1981. 128 p. (Nordisk Medicinhistorisk Arsbok, Supplementum, VIII).

Kahlson G: Upprustning av naturvetenskaplig och medicinsk forskning. **Sydsven Medicinhist Sallsk Arsskr** 1981;:44–52

**Tunisia**

L'assistance médicale pendant 50 ans de Protectorat: Dr Mahmoud El Matri: 'La Voie due Tunisien' le 11 mars 1931. **Tunis Med** 1982 Nov–Dec;60(6):378–9

**United States**

ADA historical report--dental insurance: how it started and where it is today: **Employ Benefit Plan Rev** 1978 Nov;33(5):94, 96

Albritton RB, Bahry D: Effects of public and private sector decisions on health care costs. **Policy Stud J** 1979;7(4):762–9

Aldrich M: Progressive economics, and scientific racism: Walter Willcox and black Americans, 1895–1910. **Phylon** 1979;40(1):1–14

Altman D: Health care for the poor. **Ann Am Acad Polit Soc Sci** 1983;(468):103–21

ANA's economic and general welfare program: a historical perspective: **ANA Publ** 1981;(EC–143):1–10

Ashcraft ML, Berki SE: Health maintenance organizations as Medicaid providers. **Ann Am Acad Polit Soc Sci** 1983;(468):122–31

Baker HC: Patent medicine in Pennsylvania before 1906: a history through advertising. **Pa Folklife** 1977–78;27(2):20–33

Banta HD, Burns AK, Behney CJ: Policy implications of the diffusion and control of medical technology. **Ann Am Acad Polit Soc Sci** 1983;(468):165–81

Bennett DH: Francis Everett Townsend. In Dictionary of American Biography, Suppl. 6, 1956-1960. p. 645–7, 1980.

Berkowitz ED: The historian as policy analyst: the challenge of HEW. **Public Hist** 1979;1(3):17–25

Berney B: The rise and fall of the UMW Fund. **South Exposure** 6(2):95–102, 1978

Blair RD, Vogel RJ: A survivor analysis of commercial health insurers. **J Bus** 51(3):521–9, 1978

Blicksilver J: Kinship and friendship in the emergence of a family–controlled southern enterprise: Life Insurance Company of Georgia, 1891–1950. In: Greenfield, Sidney M.; Strickon, Arnold; Aubey, Robert T., ed. Entrepreneurs in Cultural Context. Albuquerque, U. of New Mexico Pr., 1979. p. 9–121.

Bonsett CA: Physician ads of yesteryear lacked scruples. **J Indiana State Med Assoc** 1983 Apr;76(4):229, 246

Boyd TJ: 70 years of NHI. **Hosp Financ Manage** 1976 Oct;30(10):20–2, 24, 26 passim

Bradley JP: Shaping administrative policy with the aid of congressional oversight: the Senate Finance Committee and Medicare. **West Polit Q** 1980;33(4):492–501

Brown ER: He who pays the piper: foundations, the medical profession, and medical education. In Reverby S, Rosner D, ed: Health care in America. Philadelphia, Temple University Press, 1979. p. 132–54.

Brown ER: Rockefeller medicine men. Medicine and capitalism in America. Berkeley, University of California Press, 1979. xii, 283 p.

Brown LD: Competition and health care policy: experience and expectations. **Ann Am Acad Polit Soc Sci** 1983;(468):48–59

Buckley KW: The selling of a psychologist: John Broadus Watson and the application of behavioral techniques to advertising. **J Hist Behav Sci** 1982 Jul;18(3):207–21

Bulgaro PJ, Webb AY: Federal–state conflicts in cost control. **Proc Acad Polit Sci** 1980;33(4):93–110

Burstein SS: Prepaid health care in the United States. **IMJ** 1981 Aug;160(2):83–5

Cangi EC: Abraham Flexner's philanthrophy: the full–time system in the department of surgery at the University of Cincinnati College of Medicine, 1910–1930. **Bull Hist Med** 1982 Summer;56(2):160–74

Canon BC, Jaros D: The impact of changes in judicial doctrine: the abrogation of charitable immunity. **Law Soc Rev** 1979;13(4):969–86

Caplan RL: Pasteurized patients and profits: the changing nature of self–care in American medicine. Ph.D. Diss., University of Massachusetts. Amherst, 1981. xi, 463 p.

Chernomas R: A comparative view of the relationship between the business cycle and mortality, 1871–1900. **Int J Health Serv** 1984;14(1):127–46

Christen AG: Orally used smokeless tobacco as advertised in the metamorphic trade cards of 1870–1900. **Bull Hist Dent** 1983 Oct;31(2):82–6

David SI: To lift a heavy burden: the story of the Medicare and Medicaid law. Ph.D. Diss., City University of New York. New York, 1982. viii, 312 p.

Davis AB: Life insurance and the physical examination: a chapter in the rise of American medical technology. **Bull Hist Med** 1981;55(3):392–406

Drake DF: The cost of hospital regulation. **Proc Acad Polit Sci** 1980;33(4):45–59

Driver WJ: Forty–fifth anniversary of social security. **Soc Secur Bull** 1980;43(8):3–5

Emerson RM, Rochford EB, Shaw LL: Economics and enterprise in Board and Care Homes for the mentally ill. **Am Behav Sci** 1981;24(6):771–85

Engquist–Seidenberg G: The States' role in health care cost containment. **Policy Stud Rev** 1981;1(2):275–87

Etzioni A: How much is a life worth? **Soc Policy** 1979;9(5):4–8

Falk IS: Some lessons from the fifty years since the CCMC final report, 1932. **J Public Health Policy** 1983 Jun;4(2):135–61

Feldman R, Scheffler R: The union impact on hospital wages and fringe benefits. **Ind Labor Relat Rev** 1982;35(2):196–206

Figa'Talamanca I, Galmacci G: Infant mortality and economic stability. An analysis of the last century. **Nuovi Ann Ig Microbiol** 1979 Mar–Apr;30(2):107–26

Fisher D: The role of philanthropic foundations in the reproduction and production of hegemony: Rockefeller foundations and the social sciences. **Sociology** 1983;17(2):206–33

Fox DM: The decline of historicism: the case of compulsory health insurance in the United States. **Bull Hist Med** 1983 Winter;57(4):596–610

Francis WR, Gammill CG, Braucher CL: The MAC concept: a historical

perspective. **Med Mark Media** 1980 Sep;15(9):56–68
Friedman BL: Productivity gains in the drugstore industry, 1958–79. **Mon Labor Rev** 1980;103(11):18–22
Ginzberg E: How many physicians are enough? **Ann Am Acad Polit Soc Sci** 1983;(468)::205–15
Ginzberg E: The public stake in health policy. **J Med Soc NJ** 1979 Aug;76(9):599–601
Grace E: House-staff officers: collective bargaining in the health care system. **J Leg Med (Chicago)** 1981 Sep;2(3):415–31
Graebner W: Doing the world's unhealthy work: the fiction of free choice. **Hastings Cent Rep** 1984 Aug;14(4):28–37
Gromala T: Broadsides, epigrams, and testimonials: the evolution of chiropractic advertising. **Chiropr Hist** 1984;4(1):41–5
Gussow JD: Who pays the piper? **Teach Coll Rec** 1980;81(4):448–66
Hall TD, Lindsay CM: Medical schools: producers of what? sellers to whom? **J Law Econ** 1980;23(1):55–80
Hamowy R: The early development of medical licensing laws in the United States, 1875-1900. **J Libert Stud** 1979;3(1):73–119
Helfand WH, Cowen DL: American pharmaceutical posters. In W.H. Hein, G. Schramm, ed: Die Vorträge des Internationalen Pharmaziehistorischen Kongresses Basel 1979. Stuttgart, Wissenschaftliche Verlagsgesellschaft, 1981. (Veröffentlichungen der Internationalen Gesellschaft für Geschichte der Pharmazie e.V., Neue Folge, Bd. 50).
Helfand WH, Woodruff HB, Coleman KM, et al: Wartime industrial development of penicillin in the United States. In Parascandola J, ed: The history of antibiotics. Madison, American Institute of the History of Pharmacy, 1980. p. 31–56.
A history of South Dakota Blue Shield: **SD J Med** 1981 May;34(5):69
History of the provisions of the old-age, survivors, disability, and health insurance program: **Soc Secur Bull** 1980;Suppl:19–40
History of the provisions of the Supplemental Security Income program for the aged, blind, and disabled: **Soc Secur Bull** 1980;Suppl:43–6
History of the rising costs of the Medicare and Medicaid programs and attempts to control these costs: Washington, U. S. General Accounting Office, 1976. iii, 126 p.
Holcombe HW: Patent medicine tax stamps. A history of the firms using United States private die proprietary medicine tax stamps. Ed. G. B. Griffenhagen. Lawrence, Quarterman, 1979. xxv, 604 p. Reprinted articles from various journals.
Hope RB: Pioneering in the delivery of health care. **Forum Med** 1979 Mar;2(3):218–22
Hornbrook MC: Allocative medicine: efficiency, disease severity, and the payment mechanism. **Ann Am Acad Polit Soc Sci** 1983;(468):12–29
Ingram J, Fischenich J: Physician reimbursement. **Top Health Care Financ** 1982 Fall;9(1):32–52
Keigher SM: Reagan's 'New' federalism and the 1971 California Medi-cal reforms. **Urban Soc Change Rev** 1983;16(2):3–8
Keisling P: Old soldiers never die: can we pay for the VA's version of the baby boom? **Wash Mon** 1982;14(1):20–9
Keith SN: Collective bargaining and strikes among physicians. **J Natl Med Assoc** 1984 Nov;76(11):1117–21
Kennedy L: Health planning in an age of austerity. **Policy Stud J** 1980–81;9(2):232–41
King LS: Medicine in the USA: historical vignettes. XXII. Medical practice: making a living. **JAMA** 1984 Apr 13;251(14):1887–92
Krizay J: Medicine and the market place. **Society** 1982;19(2):46–51
Kunitz SJ: Efficiency and reform in the financing and organization of American medicine in the progressive era. **Bull Hist Med** 1981 Winter;55(4):497–515
Kutner NG: Cost-benefit issues in U. S. national health legislation: the case of the end-stage renal disease program. **Soc Probl** 1982;30(1):51–64
Lave JR, Silverman HA: Financing the health care of the aged. **Ann Am Acad Polit Soc Sci** 1983;(468):149–64
Legge D: Peer review in the U.S.A.: an historical perspective. **Med J Aust** 1981 Jun 27;1(13):709–11
Lemann N: Let the nurses do it. **Wash Mon** 1979;11(2):29–36
Liebenau JM: Medical science and medical industry, 1890–1929: a study of pharmaceutical manufacturing in Philadelphia. Ph. D. Diss., University of Pennsylvania. Philadelphia, 1981. vii, 489 p.
Liu B: The costs of air quality deterioration and benefits of air pollution control: estimates of mortality costs for two pollutants in 40 U.S. metropolitan areas. **Am J Econ Sociol** 1979;38(2):187–95
MacKay M: The regulation of health insurance. **Proc Acad Polit Sci** 1980;33(4):81–91
McPherson MP: 'On the same terms precisely': the women's medical fund and the John Hopkins School of Medicine. **J Am Med Wom Assoc** 1981 Feb;36(2):37–40
Markowitz GE, Rosner D: Doctors in crisis: medical education and medical reform during the Progressive era, 1895-1915. In Reverby S, Rosner D, ed: Health care in America. Philadelphia, Temple University Press, 1979. p. 185–205.
Massey DS: Residential segregation and spatial distribution of a non-labor force population: the needy elderly and disabled. **Econ Geogr** 1980;56(3):190–200
Mathews GS: Contract medicine in Rhode Island. **RI Med J** 1983 Aug;66(8):323–6
Mennel RM: Ethel Sturges Dummer. In: Notable American women. The modern period. Cambridge, Mass., Belknap-Harvard Univ. Press, 1980. 4:208–10.
Miller MD: Health care. **Proc Acad Polit Sci** 1979;33(3):82–90
Morison RS: The Foundation interest. In Stevenson LG, ed: A celebration of medical history. Baltimore, Johns Hopkins University Press, 1982. (The Henry E. Sigerist supplements to the Bulletin of the History of Medicine; new ser., no. 6). p. 212–21.
Numbers RL: Almost persuaded. American physicians and compulsory health insurance, 1912–1920. Baltimore and London, Johns Hopkins University Press, 1978. 158 p. (Henry E. Sigerist Supplements to the Bulletin of the History of Medicine, n.s., 1).
Numbers RL: Compulsory health insurance: the continuing American debate. Westport, Greenwood Press, 1982. xv, 172 p.
Numbers RL: Public protection and self-interest: medical societies in Wisconsin. In Numbers RL, Leavitt JW, ed: Wisconsin medicine. Historical perspectives. Madison, University of Wisconsin Press, 1981. p. 75–104.
Numbers RL: The third party: health insurance in America. In Vogel MJ, Rosenberg CE, ed: The therapeutic revolution. Philadelphia, 1979. p. 177–200.
Peroff K, Podolak-Warren M: Does spending on defence cut spending on health? A time-series analysis of the U. S. economy 1929–74. **Br J Polit Sci** 1979;9(1):21–39
Poen MM: Harry S. Truman versus the medical lobby. The genesis of Medicare. Columbia, London, University of Missouri Press, 1979. xii, 260 p.
Pollard MR: Fostering competition in health care. **Proc Acad Polit Sci** 1980;33(4):158–67
Pond MA: Block grants for health: a brief history of presidential initiatives. **Health Policy Q** 1982 Fall–Winter;2(3–4):180–98
Reed J: Katharine Dexter McCormick. In: Notable American women. The modern period. Cambridge, Mass., Belknap-Harvard Univ. Press, 1980. 4:440–2.
Robins L: A short history of the modern struggle for national health insurance. **J Health Hum Resour Adm** 1983 Winter;5(3):252–65
Rosner D: Business at the bedside: health care in Brooklyn, 1890–1915. In Reverby S, Rosner D, ed: Health care in America. Philadelphia, Temple University Press, 1979. p. 117–31.
Rosner D: Gaining control: reform, reimbursement and politics in New York's community hospitals, 1890--1915. **Am J Public Health** 1980 May;70(5):533–42
Russet B: Defense expenditures and national well-being. **Am Pol Sci Rev** 1982;76(4):767–77
Sabo MO: National health insurance and the states. **Publius** 1978;891):55–62
Saffron MH: James Peter Warbasse. In Dictionary of American Biography, Suppl. 6, 1956–1960. p. 663–5, 1980.
Savitt TL: Slave life insurance in Virginia and North Carolina. **J South Hist** 1977 Nov;43(4):583–600; 1978 Feb;44(1):163
Silverman M, Lee PR, Lydecker M: Pills and the public purse: the routes to national drug insurance. Berkeley, University of California Press, 1981. xviii, 232 p.
Silverman WA: Medical inflation. **Perspect Biol Med** 1980 Summer;23(4):617–37
Skinner RE: Photography, advertising, and the history of medicine: notes on the medico-historical art of Lejaren a Hiller. **Watermark** 1983 Jan;6(2–3):11–2
Sloan FA, Steinwald B: Effects of regulation on hospital costs and input use. **J Law Econ** 1980;23(1):81–109
Smith DG: Federal health grants and regional health politics. **Publius** 1982;12(2):63–77
Stage S: Female complaints: Lydia Pinkham and the business of women's medicine. New York, Norton, 1979. 304 p.
Starr P, Esping-Anderson G: Passive intervention. **Work Pap New Soc** 1979;7(2):15–25
Starr P: Transformation of defeat: the changing objectives of national health insurance, 1915–1980. **Am J Public Health** 1982 Jan;72(1):78–88
Stevens R: Sweet charity: state aid to hospitals in Pennsylvania, 1870–1910. **Bull Hist Med** 1984 Winter;58(4):474–95
Stevens R: Sweet charity: state aid to hospitals in Pennsylvania, 1870–1910. **Bull Hist Med** 1984 Fall;58(3):287–314
Sweeney RE, Castleman B: Asbestos disease and compensation. **Ann NY Acad Sci** 1979;330:273–80
Thomas SJ: Nostrum advertising and the image of woman as invalid in late Victorian America. **J Am Cult** 1982 Fall;5(3):104–12
Torrens PR: Health insurance in the United States: implications for the United Kingdom. **Lancet** 1980 Jan 5;1(8158):27–31
Underhill D: Government health insurance: an analysis of division. **Mich J Polit Sci** 1981;1(1):26–38
Uphoff MJ, Uphoff WH, Lewis RK: Group Health: an American success story in prepaid health care. Minneapolis, Dillon Press, 1980. xvii, 173 p.
Walker FA: Americanism versus Sovietism: a study of the reaction to the committee on the costs of medical care. **Bull Hist Med** 1979 Winter;53(4):489–504
Walls E: The introduction of prepayment medicine to Arkansas: the Trinity Hospital experience. **Arkansas Hist Q** 1983;42(1):3–26

Waring JI: A community fee bill for physicians, 1844. **J Hist Med Allied Sci** 1978 Jul;33(3):416–21
Watson S: Blue Cross idea began in Texas. **Tex Hosp** 1979 Jun;35(1):22–3
When 'more doctors smoked Camels': Cigarette advertising in the Journal. **NY State J Med** 1983 Dec;83(13):1347–52
Whitten DO: Medical care of slaves: Louisiana sugar region and South Carolina rice district. **South Stud** 1977;16:153–80
Wimberley T: Toward national health insurance in the United States: an historical outline, 1910–1979. **Soc Sci Med [Med Econ]** 1980 Mar;14(1):13–25
Yoder D, ed: Advertisements of urban healers. **Pa Folklife** 1978;27(3):44–8
Zelizer VA: Human values and the market: the case of life insurance and death in 19th-century America. **AJS** 1978 Nov;84(3):591–610
Zelizer VA: The price and value of children: the case of children's insurance. **AJS** 1981;86(5):1036–1056
Zelten RA: Consequences of increased third-party payments for health care services. **Ann Am Acad Polit Soc Sci** 1979;443:25–40
Zook CJ, Moore FD, Zeckhauser RJ: 'Catastrophic' health insurance: a misguided prescription? **Public Interest** 1981;(62):66–81

**USSR**

Shaternikov VA, Konyshev VA: 50–ia godovshchina pervogo piatiletnego plana razvitiia narodnogo khoziaĭstva SSSR i nauka o pitanii v nasheĭ strane. **Vopr Pitan** 1979 Sep–Oct;(5):3–7

**Yugoslavia**

Dyck RG: Health care planning in Slovenia. **Pap Slov Stud** 1977;105–23
Mitrović M: Uticaj zdravsvenih prilika na privredni razvitak Pančeva 1792–1815. **Zb Istor** 1978;18:109–24

# EDUCATION, MEDICAL

Acuña HR: Etica médica y educación médica. **Bol Of Sanit Panam** 1981 Jun;90(6):471–7
Anderson NE: The historical development of American nursing education. **JNE** 1981 Jan;20(1):18–36
Beering SC: 'The spark within.' **J Indiana State Med Assoc** 1982 Jan;75(1):22–4
Bondurant S: Some means by which medical schools adapt to changing needs. **Bull NY Acad Med** 1984 Apr;60(3):271–80
Boschung U: Medizinische Lehrmodelle. **Medita** 1980;10(Geschichte der Medizin, 4):xv
Caffaratto TM: Le antiche radici della riforma sanitaria. **Minerva Med** 1982 Jun 30;73(27):1905–16
Cameron N: Ceremony of presentation of diplomates. **Ann R Coll Surg Engl** 1981 Nov;63(6):447–9
Ell SR: Five hundred years of specialty certification and compulsory continuing medical education. Venice 1300–1801. **JAMA** 1984 Feb 10;251(6):752–3
Ellis J: The responsibility of medical schools for teaching hospitals and the provision of clinical services. **Med Educ** 1981 May;15(3):171–83
Jakobovits I: Medical education––a Jewish perspective. **Isr J Med Sci** 1984 Jan;20(1):2–7
Kaiser W, Völker A: Zur Geschichte der ärztlichen Fortbildung auf der Ebene regionaler Vereine und Gesellschaften. **Z Gesamte Inn Med** 1983 Jul 1;38(13):348–58
Maulitz RC, Poses RM, Young MJ: Medical history as an introduction to clinical reasoning. **J Med Educ** 1983 May;58(5):427–9
Oliaro T: La funzione storica e didattica della Stampa Medica. **Minerva Med** 1983 Dec 15;74(47–48):2801–2
Oliaro T: La funzione storica e didattica della stampa medica. **Minerva Stomatol** 1984 May–Jun;33(3):536–7
Pfohl G: Das philosophisch-philologische Element in der medizinischen Fakultät. Ein Beitrag der Medizingeschichte, mehr zu formen als zu informieren. I, II. **Med Welt** 1980 Apr 25, May 9;(17,19):644–6,730–3
Richter W: Der Anteil des Griechischen an den vorklinischen Nomenklaturen und die didaktischen Konsequenzen für die fachsprachliche Ausbildung von Medizinstudenten. **Wiss Z Univ Rostock** 1979;28(3):145–50
Rosoff L: Roger Bacon, William of Occam and Lord Houghton: guides for the perplexed physician. **Am J Surg** 1981 Jan;141(1):2–9
Seidler E: Wie wird man Arzt? Historische Grundformen der medizinischen Ausbildung. In R. Wittern, ed: Jahrbuch des Instituts für Geschichte der Medizin der Robert Bosch Stiftung. Stuttgart, Hippokrates Verlag, 1984. Bd. 1. p. 28–41.

**Austria**

Borisov PU: Die Wiener medizinische Fakultät und die Arzte im ehemaligen Krain. **Wien Med Wochenschr** 1981;131(13–14):357–61
Ganzinger K: Zur Geschichte der Universitätsapotheke. In Dilg P, et al., ed: Perspektiven der Pharmaziegeschichte. Graz, Austria, Akademische Druck- u. Verlagsanstalt, 1983. p. 79–88.
Gracey DR, DeRemee RA: The University of Vienna Medical School. **Mayo Clin Proc** 1981 Oct;56(10):634–8
Skopec M: The Vienna Medical School. Vienna, Institute of the History of Medicine at the University of Vienna, [1983?]. 20 p.

**Belgium**

Elaut LJ: Een epos: het Gentse Akademisch Ziekenhuis. Antwerpen, Nederlandsche Boekhandel, 1977. 83 p. (VVA monografie; 3).

**China**

Ren M: [The therapeutic custom handed down from the Meng He School] (Chi). **Chung Hua I Shih Tsa Chih** 1984;14(2):72–4

**Czechoslovakia**

Brod J: The history of medicine at Charles University. **J R Coll Physicians Lond** 1982 Jul;16(3):195–8
Kapronczay K: Adatok a prágai egyetem magyar orvosi vonatkozásaihoz (1348–1850). **Orvostort Kozl** 1980;89–91(26 no 1–3):223–31
Koerting W: Die Deutsche Universität in Prag. München, Bayerische Landesärztekammer, 1968. 300 p.
Niederland TR: Doterajší vývoj a perspektíva predklinických odborov na lekárskej fakulte Univerzity Komenského v Bratislave. **Cas Lek Cesk** 1979 Dec 21;118(51):1574–6
Pacovský V: Universita a lékařská fakulta. **Cas Lek Cesk** 1983 Oct 14;122(41):1261–4
Tichý M, Kántorová V: Vznik lekárskej fakulty UK v Bratislave. 1. Možnosti štúdia medicíny na území slovenského etnika pred rokom 1918. **Bratisl Lek Listy** 1980 Apr;73(4):515–21

**Denmark**

Behnke O, Wieth JO: Laegeuddannelsen i København 1479–1979. **Nord Med** 1979 Dec;94(12):321–4
Behnke O: Review of the history of the University of Copenhagen and the Faculty of Medicine. **Dan Med Bull** 1980 May;27(Suppl 1):1–4
Christensen OS: Modellen af Domus Anatomica. **Dan Medicinhist Arbog** 1980;:169–79
Laeger i Sønderjylland indtil 1864: **Dan Medicinhist Arbog** 1980;:11–65
Melchior JC, et al, ed: Københavns Universitet 1479–1979. Bind VII. Det laegevidenskabelige Fakultet. København, Københavns Universitet, 1979. xi, 519 p.

**Egypt**

Iskandar AZ: An attempted reconstruction of the late Alexandrian medical curriculum. **Med Hist** 1976 Jul;20(3):235–58
Puma A: La Escuela de Alejandria y nuestro Occidente. **Med Secoli** 1981;17:237–44

**Finland**

Perret L: Medicin och medicinare vid Abo akademi under 1600–och 1700–talen. **Nord Medicinhist Arsbok** 1983;:71–81

**France**

Brygoo E: Les médecins de Montpellier et le Jardin du Roi à Paris. **Hist Nat** 1979;(14):3–29
Curet M, Carre A, Henaff R: Les écoles de chirurgie et de médecine navales. **Med Armees** 1980;8(10)spec:797–800
Duka Zolyomi N: Les relations médicales entre la Hongrie et la France jusqu'à la fin du XVIIIe siècle. **Hist Sci Med** 1983;17(2):189–94
Ehrhardt JP: L'Ecole du Service de Santé de la Marine de Bordeaux des origines à nos jours. In Congrès National des Sociétés Savantes, 103e, Nancy–Metz, 1978. Actes. Paris, 1979. Tome I, p. 9–21.
Lefebvre P: Tradition de l'enseignement dans le Service de santé de l'armée de terre. **Med Armees** 1980;8(10)spec:827–44

**Germany**

Abe HR: Die Medizinische Akademie Erfurt und ihre progressiven Traditionen. **Beitr Gesch Univ Erfurt** 1979–83;19:9–51
Benedum J, Michler M: Das Siegel der Medizinischen Fakultät Giessen. Giessen, Universitätsbibliothek, 1982. 47 p., [18 leaves]. (Berichte und Arbeiten aus der Universitätsbibliothek Giessen, no. 35).
Benedum J, Giese C: Die Professoren der Medizin in der giessener Gemäldegalerie. Giessen, Schmitz, 1983. 230 p. (Arbeiten zur Geschichte der Medizin in Giessen, Bd. 5)
Benedum J: 375 Jahre Medizin in Giessen: eine Bild- und Textdokumentation: Katalog zur Ausstellung anlässlich der 375 - Jahrfeier im Institut für Anatomie und Zytobiologie, vom 11.5.–30.6. 1982. Giessen, Schmitz, 1982. 186 p.
Buchholz R: Famous physicians and scientists in the history of the Medical School of Marburg. **Birth Defects** 1979;15(4):1–4
Güthert H, Abe HR: Zur Entstehungsgeschichte der Medizinisch-wissenschaftlichen Gesellschaft an der Medizinischen

Akademie Erfurt - Gedanken, Reflexionen, Erinnerungen. **Beitr Gesch Univ Erfurt** 1979-83;19:339-59

Kaiser W, Völker A: Gedenktage 1980 aus der Geschichte der Medizinischen Fakultät Wittenberg (I): Die Chemie im medizinischen Ausbildungsprogramm des 17. und 18. Jahrhunderts. **Z Gesamte Inn Med** 1981 Feb 15;36(4):114-22

Kaiser W, Völker A: Universität und Physikat in der Frühgeschichte des Amtsarztwesens. Halle, Martin-Luther-Universität, 1980. 95 p. (Beiträge zur Universitätsgeschichte: Wissenschaftliche Beiträge der Martin-Luther-Universität Halle-Wittenberg, 1980/53, T 39).

Kaiser W: Zur Geschichte des präakademischen medizinischen Unterrichts: Das Gymnasium illustre in Zerbst und das Philanthropinum in Dessau. **Z Gesamte Inn Med** 1983 Jan 1;38(1):22-9

Killian H: Meister der Chirurgie und die Chirurgenschulen im gesamten deutschen Sprachraum. 2., neubearbeitete Auflage. Stuttgart, Thieme, 1980. xii, 492 p.

Pielmeyer K: Statuten der deutschen medizinischen Fakultäten im Mittelalter. Ein Beitrag zur Geschichte des medizinischen Unterrichts an deutschen Universitäten anhand der Statuten der ersten 16 deutschen medizinischen Fakultäten von ihrer Gründung bis zum Ende des 16. Jahrhunderts. Diss. Bonn, 1981. 101 p.

Schneider HJ, Doberentz D: Zur Geschichte der Jenaer Harnsteinforschung. Mit einem vollständigen Abdruck der Dissertationsschrift Arno Krüches 'Ueber Struktur und Entstehung der Uratsteine' aus dem Jahre 1879. Jena, Friedrich-Schiller-Universität, 1979. 84, 42 p. (Jenaer Reden und Schriften).

**Great Britain**

Gibson WC: Oxford revisited. **JAMA** 1980 Aug 8;244(6):577-9

Howie WB: Samuel Benion--Glasgow University's first Doctor of Medicine. **Scott Med J** 1979 Jan;24(1):76-9

**Hungary**

Süle T: Az Erzsébet Tudományegyetem Orvosi Kara, az önálló Pécsi Orvostudományi Egyetem rövid története és numizmatikai emlékei. **Orvostort Kozl** 1982;28(1-3):227-39

**India**

Kirschke G: Die Ausbildung der Aerzte in Hyderabad (Indien). Köln, 1983. 213 p. (Kölner medizinhistorische Beiträge, Band 29)

**Italy**

Chandler ET, Bloomfield RL: Salernitan wisdom. **South Med J** 1983 Jul;76(7):913-5

Lambertini G: Die Schule von Salerno und die Universitäten von Bologna und Padua. In Sournia JC, Martiny M, Poulet J, ed: Illustrierte Geschichte der Medizin. Salzburg, Andreas, 1980. Vol. 2. p. 731-53.

Paravicini Bagliani A: A proposito dell'insegnamento di medicina allo Studium Curiae. In A. Maieru, A. Paravicini Bagliani, ed: Studi sul XIV secolo in memoria di Anneliese Maier. Rome, Storia e Letteratura, 1981. p. 395-413.

Sinha DN: Status of anatomy in the University of Bologna (13th to 18th century). **Stud Hist Med** 1982 Jun;6(3):141-6

**Mexico**

Micheli A de: Libros médicos italianos en la antigua Universidad de México. **Prensa Med Mex** 1979;44:152-6

Rivero-Serrano O: Restauración de la antigua Escuela de Medicina. **Gac Med Mex** 1980;116:429-30

Torre JM: Panorama actual de la enseñanza de la medicina en México. In Academia Nacional de Medicina. Libro conmemorativo del primer centenario. México, Comité Editorial de la Comisión Organizadora del Congreso del Centenario, 1964. Tome 2. p. 702-5.

**Netherlands**

Lieburg MJ van: Het medisch Onderwijs te Rotterdam (1467-1967): een kort historisch Overzicht. Amsterdam, Rodopi, 1978. 111 p.

Witkam HJ: Catalogues of all the chiefest rarities in the Publick Anatomie Hall of the University of Leyden. Leiden, Witkam, 1980. xv, 86 leaves.

**Spain**

Rodríguez Tejerina JM: El doctorado en medicina en la Universidad de Mallorca. In Congrés International d'Història de la Medicina Catalana, 2nd, Barcelona, 1975. Llibre d'Actes. Barcelona, Socitra, 1977. p. 147-56.

**Turkey**

Demirhan A: The development of education of pathology and anatomy in Ottoman Turks. **Stud Hist Med** 1981 Jun;5(2):160-6

Sayili A: Bizde tip ögretimi üzerine. **Belleten (Turk)** 1971;35(138):229-34

**United States**

Carroll DG: Medical education in Maryland: cottage industry to university. **Md State Med J** 1980 Feb;29(2):21-5

Cordasco F, Alloway DN: Medical education in the United States. A guide to information sources. Detroit, Gale Research, 1980. xx, 393 p. (Education Information Guide Series, v. 8).

King LS: Medicine in the USA: Historical vignettes. II. Medical education: the early phases. **JAMA** 1982 Aug 13;248(6):731-4

Lindskog GE: Three generations of Doctors Bigelow at Harvard. **Conn Med** 1983 Dec;47(12):763-9

Wilcox HG: A difficult pregnancy: embryologic development of American medical education. **Ala J Med Sci** 1981 Jan;18(1):86-92

**USSR**

Ashmianskas IuI: Prepodavanie gigieny pitaniia v Vil'niusskom universitete. **Gig Sanit** 1980 Jan;(6):42-3

Biziuliavichius SK, Galvonaĭte AL: Razvitie meditsiny v Vil'niusskom Universitete (k 200-letiiu vysshego meditsinskogo obrazovaniia v Litve). **Sov Zdravookhr** 1982;(4):54-8

Borodulin VI, Gogin EE, Martynov IV, et al: Iz istorii klinicheskogo prepodavaniia (k 275-letiiu Glavnogo voennogo klinicheskogo gospitalia im. N. N. Burdenko). **Klin Med (Mosk)** 1984 Feb;62(2):141-4

Kalnin VV: U istokov nauchnoĭ meditsiny v Tartuskom universitete. **Sov Zdravookhr** 1982;(11):57-61

**Before 500 A.D.**

**Greece**

Fritts HW: Are we Socratic teachers? **Trans Am Clin Climatol Assoc** 1979;90:109-15

Hausmann WO: Die medizinische Höhlenschule des Cheiron. **Berl Munch Tierarztl Wochenschr** 1982 Mar 1;95(5):94-5

**500 A.D.-1450**

Kibre P: Arts and medicine in the universities of the later Middle Ages. In Ijsewijn J, Paquet J, ed: The universities in the late Middle Ages. Leuven University Press, 1978. p. 213-27.

**Arabic**

Hau FR: Die Bildung des Arztes im Islamischen Mittelalter. **Clio Med** 1979 Jul;14(1):7-33

Leiser G: Medical education in Islamic lands from the seventh to the fourteenth century. **J Hist Med Allied Sci** 1983 Jan;38(1):48-75

**France**

Demaitre LE: Doctor Bernard de Gordon: professor and practitioner. Toronto, Pontifical Institute of Mediaeval Studies, 1980. xii, 236 p.

Shatzmiller J: Livres médicaux et éducation médicale: à props d'un contrat de Marseille en 1316. **Mediaev Stud** 1980;42:463-70

Turchini J: Die französischen Schulen im Mittelalter. In Sournia JC, Martiny M, Poulet J, ed: Illustrierte Geschichte der Medizin. Salzburg, Andreas, 1980. Vol. 2. p. 767-92.

**Hungary**

Schultheisz E: Mediaeval universities in Hungary with special relations to Cracow. **Orvostort Kozl** 1980;89-91(26 no 1-3):17-23

**Italy**

Siraisi NG: Taddeo Alderotti and his pupils. Two generations of Italian medical learning. Princeton, Princeton University Press, 1981. xxiii, 461 p.

**Yugoslavia**

Katić RV: Srpske medicinske škole u srednjem veku. **Srp Arh Celok Lek** 1980 Nov;108(11):1193-1201

**1450-1700**

Blaser RH: Ulrich Gyger, sin diener. Versuch einer biographischen Rekonstruktion. **Medizinhist J** 1981;16(1-2):53-66

**Austria**

Beck-Mannagetta P: Zum 300. Todestag des Johann Wilhelm Ritter von Mannagetta und seinem Wirken in Niederösterreich. **Unsere Heimat** 1966;37(4-6):125-9

**Finland**

Leikola A: The problem of generation in the 17th century Finnish university. A study in peripheralism. In International Congress of the History of Medicine, 27th, Barcelona, 1980. Actas. Barcelona, Académia de Ciències Médiques de Catalunya i Balears, 1981. p. 560–3.

**France**

Brockliss LW. Medical teaching at the University of Paris, 1600–1720. **Ann Sci** 1978;35-221–51

Gysel C: Odontoiatria del passato. L'odontostomatologia nel contesto delle 'vere e solide fondamenta della medicine', definite da Louis Du Gardin, Professore all'Universitá di Douai, sotto il regno di Alberto ed Isabella. **Dent Cadmos** 1983 Apr;51(4):91–5 contd

Howard R: Medical politics and the founding of the Jardin des Plantes in Paris. **J Soc Bibliogr Nat Hist** 1980 Apr;9(4):395–402

**Germany**

Gundel HG, ed: Die ältesten Statuten der Giessener Medizinischen Fakultät: Leges et Statuta Collegii Medici. Giessen, Universitätsbibliothek, 1979. 32 p.

Kapronczay K: Magyar medikusok a wittenbergi egyetemen Luther és Melanchton korában. **Orv Hetil** 1984 Apr 15;125(16):958–60

Richter W: Janus Cornarius, ein 'philologischer Mediziner' des 16. Jahrhunderts, und seine Beziehungen zur Rostocker Universität. **Wiss Z Univ Rostock** 1978;27(3):181–9

Schnelbögl F: Auerbacher Lebensbilder. Zum 500. Geburtsjahr Heinrich Stromers, genannt Auerbach. **Altnurnb Landsch** 1976;25(Sonderh. 1):1–26

**Great Britain**

Dewhurst K: Thomas Willis's Oxford Lectures. Oxford, Sandford, 1980. x, 182 p.

Frank RG: Harvey and the Oxford physiologists: scientific ideas and social interaction. Berkeley, University of California Press, 1980. xviii, 368 p.

Harrison DF: Neurochemistry and Sherrington's enchanted loom. **J R Soc Med** 1984 Aug;77(8):706–7

**Italy**

Lucchetta F: Girolamo Ramusio: profilo biografico. **Quad Stor Univ Padova** 1982;15:1–60

Pagni U: Giovanbattista Cartegni da Bagnone lettore di medicina nello Studio di Pisa. **Arch Stor Prov Parmensi** 1979;31:91–102

Pesenti Marañgon T: 'Professores chirurgie', 'medici ciroici' e 'barbitonsores' a Padova nell' età di Leonardo Buffi da Bertipaglia (dopo il 1448). Quad. Stor Univ. Padova, 1978;11:1–38.

Sambin P: Il dottorato padovano in medicina di Paolo da Middelburgo (1480). **Quad Stor Univ Padova** 1976–7;9–10:252–6

**Netherlands**

Slenders J: De Anatomische les van Dr. Zacheus de Jager (1640). **Tijdschr Geschied Geneeskd** 1981;4(4):159–67

**Poland**

Andrejew A: Wacław Koler, sławny medyk Krakowski w świetle swego inwentarza. **Arch Hist Med (Warsz)** 1984;47(1):39–47

**Spain**

Ferrer D: Las ordenanzas de la Universidad del Estudio General de la ciudad de Barcelona, 1596. **Asclepio** 1978–79;30–31:339–58

**1700 to Present**

Armas Cruz R: Alguna meditaciones sobre la medicina actual. **Rev Med Chil** 1980 Apr;108(4):338–50

Barkley S: A nurse who made a difference. **Pulse** 1984 May;20(5):1–2

Bezel E: Johann Jakob Steger, 1798–1857. Beispiel eines Medizinstudiums im frühen 19. Jahrhundert nach den Briefen an seine Eltern. Zürich Juris, 1981. 156 p. (Zürcher medizingeschichtliche Abhandlungen, Neue Reihe, Nr. 147).

Boschung U: Medizinstudium im Zeitalter der Aufklärung. **Schweiz Rundsch Med Prax** 1983 Dec 20;72(51–52):1607–15

Brieger GH: The history of health and disease for health professionals: the case study approach. With a commentary by G.B. Risse. In J. J. Bylebyl, ed: Teaching the history of medicine at a medical center. Baltimore, London, Johns Hopkins University Press, 1982. (The Henry E. Sigerist supplements to the Bulletin of the History of Medicine; new ser., no. 7). p. 13–30.

Burns CR: Medical history and medical humanities: some new styles of learning and teaching. With a commentary by T.L. Savitt. In J. J. Bylebyl, ed: Teaching the history of medicine at a medical center. Baltimore, London, Johns Hopkins University Press, 1982. (The Henry E. Sigerist supplements to the Bulletin of the History of Medicine; new ser., no. 7). p. 31–45.

Bylebyl JJ, ed: Teaching the history of medicine at a medical center. Baltimore, London, Johns Hopkins University Press, 1982. 162 p. (The Henry E. Sigerist supplements to the Bulletin of the History of Medicine; new ser., no. 7).

Chessick RD: Freud teaches psychotherapy. Indianapolis, Cambridge, Hackett, 1980. viii, 342 p.

Costa-Casaretto C: Los primeros becarios chilenos en Europa (1874). Alborada de la docencia y la práctica médicas actuales. **Rev Med Chil** 1979 May;107(5):432–7

Cristoffanini AP: El internado en los estudios médicos. **Educ Med Salud** 1982;16(2):134–50

Do JP, Lacombe M: Approche philosophique et historique à un enseignement des droits de l'homme. **Acta Med Leg Soc (Liege)** 1980;30(1):233–40

Dubarry JJ: Le curriculum universitaire d'un étudiant en médecine en U.R.S.S. **Hist Sci Med** 1980;14:383–6

Ermakov VV, Devyatova LN: The experience and the stages of development in USSR of the WHO English International Courses for epidemiology (1969–1978). **Sante Publique (Bucur)** 1980;23(1):3–14

The faculty of medicine at Harvard College: **N Engl J Med** 1983 Feb 3;308(5):288–9

Forum: the place of prevention in medical education: past, present, and future: **Prev Med** 1981 Nov;10(6):661–740

Golden RL: A 'forgotten' clinic of Sir William Osler. **JAMA** 1981 Feb 6;245(5):500–1

Guarner V: El conocimiento de la historia de la medicina en la educacion del cirujano. **Bol Soc Mex Hist Filos Med** 1979 Mar;4(26):73–87

Harrell GT: The Osler family. **JAMA** 1982 Jul 9;248(2):203–9

Hickel E: The emergence of clinical chemistry in the 19th century: presuppositions and consequences. **J Clin Chem Clin Biochem** 1982 Jul;20(7):521–30

Holubar K: The influence of the British School of Dermatology on the Vienna School in the first half of the 19th century. **Int J Dermatol** 1982 May;21(4):224–6

Howard RP: 'The Chief'--Doctor William Osler. **Iowa Med** 1984 Apr;74(4):155–8

Jordanova L: La donna di cera. **Kos** 1984 May;1(4):82–9

Joy RJ: Occupying the visual cortex: using slides to teach the history of medicine. In J. J. Bylebyl, ed: Teaching the history of medicine at a medical center. Baltimore, London, Johns Hopkins University Press, 1982. (The Henry E. Sigerist supplements to the Bulletin of the History of Medicine; new ser., no. 7). p. 103–14.

King LS: The British background for American medicine. **JAMA** 1982 Jul 9;248(2):217–20

Lejman K: Andrzej Badurski (1740–1789) jako założyciel szpitala akademickiego i inicjator klinicznego nauczania meydycyny. **Przegl Lek** 1981;38(7):567–70

Lovell RR: The university medical presence in hospitals seventy years after Flexner and a look ahead. **Aust NZ J Med** 1983 Apr;13(2):187–94

Maulitz RC: Disciplinary perspectives in the history of medicine: a view from the 1980s. With a commentary by R.P. Hudson. In J. J. Bylebyl, ed: Teaching the history of medicine at a medical center. Baltimore, London, Johns Hopkins University Press, 1982. (The Henry E. Sigerist supplements to the Bulletin of the History of Medicine; new ser., no. 7). p. 46–61.

Mazumdar PM: The history of medicine in a medical context. With a commentary by E. C. Atwater. In J. J. Bylebyl, ed: Teaching the history of medicine at a medical center. Baltimore, London, Johns Hopkins University Press, 1982. (The Henry E. Sigerist supplements to the Bulletin of the History of Medicine; new ser., no. 7). p. 91–102.

Nelken LE: Reminiscences of my medical education (1916–1933) before emigrating to Palestine. **Koroth** 1981;8(1–2):51–6

Osorio RA: Reflexión con madurez. Reseña histórica del propósito y origen de la ceremonia del 'capping' (coronamiento). **Bol Col Prof Enferm PR** 1983 Jun;9(34):26–7

Pernow B: Problem inom dagens medicinska högskola. **Sven Tidskr** 1981,68(7).338–44

Sokal MM, ed: An education in psychology: James McKeen Cattell's journal and letters from Germany and England. 1880–1888. Cambridge, Mass., MIT Press, 1981, xxvii, 372 p.

Vizioli R, De Rosa A: Medical education and epilepsy. **Prog Clin Biol Res** 1983;124:361–70

Wangensteen OH: The University of Glasgow and the Johns Hopkins schools of surgery. **Am J Surg** 1980 Jun;139(6):870–5

**Americas**

Desrosiers G: Evolution de la médecine et répercussion sur la formation médicale en Amérique du Nord. **Union Med Can** 1981 Sep;110(9):817–20

**Argentina**

Aznarez EP: Historia de la Facultad de Ciencias Médicas de Córdoba. **Medicina (B Aires)** 1982;42(2):204–12

## EDUCATION, MEDICAL

Ivern A: Muñiz presidente de la Facultad. (Tercer Congreso Nacional de Historia de la Medicina Argentina, 1973). **Sem Med** 1973;79(Aniversario):238–41

**Australia**

Coppleson VM: Australian Postgraduate Federation in Medicine. The development of graduate education with particular reference to Australia. [s.l.: s.n.], 1964. 46 leaves.

Fleming DW: The founders of the college: Western Australia. **Aust NZ J Surg** 1981 Dec;51(6):623–4

Howard RN: The founders of the College Victoria. **Aust NZ J Surg** 1981 Apr;51(2):227–38

Leggett CA: The founders of the College. **Aust NZ J Surg** 1981 Oct;51(5):508–12

McDonald IA, Cope I, Forster FM: Super Ardua. The Royal College of Obstetricians and Gynaecologists in Australia, 1929–1979. Melbourne, Australian Council RCOG, 1981. iv, 107 p.

Place J: A summary of nurse training at the Royal Women's Hospital, Melbourne. **Aust Nurses J** 1981 Aug;11(2):2–4

Rank BK: George Grey Turner, F.R.A.C.S. (Hon). **Aust NZ J Surg** 1981 Dec;51(6):627–30

Russell RL: We worked hard, but we enjoyed it! General nurse training in NSW--the first 50 years. **Lamp** 1981 May;38(5 Suppl):57–63

Stanley NF: Faculty of Medicine, The University of Western Australia: the first quarter century (1957–1982). Nedlands, W.A., Faculty of Medicine, The University of Western Australia, 1982. xvi, 175 p.

Williams HE: My four teachers. **Med J Aust** 1977 Dec 15;2(12):650–1

Wright-St Clair RE: The medical qualifications of Sir John Logan Campbell. **NZ Med J** 1983 Mar 23;96(728):212–3

**Austria**

Berezowski S: Jan Dolliner--chirurg bocheński (przyczynek do historii zdobywania doktoratów chirurgii w Uniwersytecie Jagiellońskim). **Pol Tyg Lek** 1979 Aug 27;34(35):1403–5

Egglmaier HH: Das medizinisch-chirurgische Studium in Graz. Ein Beispiel für den Wandel staatlicher Zielvorstellungen im Bildungs- und Medizinalwesen. Diss. Graz. 1980. xi, 599 p. (Dissertationen der Universität Graz, 50).

Fellner R, Höflechner W: Die Augenheilkunde an der Universität Graz. Graz, Akademische Druck- u. Verlagsanstalt, 1973. ix, 180 p. (Publikationen aus dem Archiv der Universität Graz, Bd. 2).

Huter F: Die Wiedererrichtung des medizinisch-chirurgischen Studiums zu Innsbruck nach 1814. **Tirol Heimat** 1967–68;31–32:57–77

Huter F: Ein tiroler Student erlebt den Beginn der Wiener Märzrevolution. **Tirol Heimat** 1972;36:131–9

Kapronczay K: Magyar medikusok a bécsi egyetemen (1770–1848). **Orv Hetil** 1980 Oct 5;121(40):2467–9

Lesky E: Die Wiener Medizinische Schule im 19. Jahrhundert. Graz-Köln, Böhlaus, 1978. 660 p. (Studien zur Geschichte der Universität Wien, Band VI).

Lesky E: Die Wiener Medizinische Schule und die Donauländer. In Congress of History, Health, Culture of the Danubian Countries. 1. Novi Sad, 1975. p. 31–6.

Mitterstiller S: 100 Jahre Chirurgische Klinik in Innsbruck. **Tirol Heimat** 1970;34:17–38

Rüden AD von: Medicina Graecensis. Das medizinisch-chirurgische Studium in Graz (1782–1862). Diss. Technischen Universität München, 1978. 195 p.

Spitzy KH, ed, Lau I, ed: Van Swietens Erbe: die Wiener Medizinische Schule heute in Selbstdarstellungen. Wien, Maudrich, 1982. 400 p.

Stepak S: Z dziejów Zakładu Wychowawczego dla Niewidomych we Lwowie w latach 1851–1918. **Klin Oczna** 1984 Apr;86(4):181–3

Wyklicky H: The role of the Vienna Medical School in the investigation and treatment of infectious diseases. In [The Vienna Medical School]. Produced under a grant from the Squibb Institute for Medical Research, [1983]. p. 6–20.

Wyklicky H: Uber einige Aufgaben des medizinhistorischen Unterrichtes. **Wien Klin Wochenschr** 1981 Nov 13;93(21):660–5

Wyklicky H: 175 Jahre Hygiene an Oesterreichs Universitäten. **Zentralbl Bakteriol [B]** 1981;172(6):441–53

**Belgium**

Dickstein-Bernard C: Genèse del'hôpital universitaire, 1834–1935. **Rev Med Brux** 1984 May;5(5):315–8

Ossieur EG: Studenten en hun examens in de Faculteit Geneeskunde R.U.G., 1829–1835. **Vlaam Stam** 1978;14:385–403

**Belize**

Hermann EK: Belizean nursing education in the 19th century. **Belizean Stud** 1979;7(4):16–24

**Brazil**

Carvalho AC de: Escola de Enfermagem da Universidade de São Paulo. Resumo histórico 1942–1980. **Rev Esc Enferm USP** 1980 Aug;14 Suppl:1–271

Corrêa JV: Podagra--uma tese de 1788. **Rev Hosp Clin Fac Med Sao Paulo** 1981 Feb;36(1):1–6

Lobo FB: Os professores de medicina e as conferencias da Gloria. **Rev Inst Hist Geogr Bras** 1980;(328):105–10

Lobo FB: Uma sede para a Faculdade de Medicina do Rio de Janeiro. **Rev Inst Hist Geogr Bras** 1977;315:158–88

Rezende de Castro Monteiro A: 'Hypnotisme'. Analyse de la thèse présentée à la Faculté de Médecine de Rio de Janeiro par Francisco de Paula Fajardo Junior, en vue d'obtenir le grade de docteur en médecine - Rio de Janeiro, 1888. In: Congrès international d'histoire de la médecine, XXVe, Québec, 1976. Actes. Québec, 1977. p. 980–91.

Veras RP, Ribeiro LD, Lima JC: Notas sobre a evolução da escola médica no Brasil. **Educ Med Salud** 1983;17(4):398–413

**Bulgaria**

Apostolov MA: Pervaia Bolgarskaia khirurgicheskaia shkola. **Klin Med (Mosk)** 1984 Oct;62(10):149–51

Dochev D: Razvitie i segashno sŭstoianie na Katedrata po klinichna laboratoriia. **Vutr Boles** 1981;20(6):15–22

Furnadzhiev G: Razvitie i segashno sŭstoianie na Katedrata p farmakologiia i fitoterapiia. **Vutr Boles** 1981;20(6):22–6

Georgiev I: Development and scientific research activity achievements in the higher medical institute 'I. P. Pavlov' - Plovdiv. **Folia Med (Plovdiv)** 1981;23(3–4):5–23

Ivanov S: Razvitie i segashno sŭstoianie na Instituta po vŭtreshni bolesti. **Vutr Boles** 1981;20(6):1–6

Koĭchev K: Po-vazhni momenti ot istoriiata i razvitieto na Katedrata po propodevtika na vŭtreshni bolesti. **Vutr Boles** 1981;20(6):12–5

Popv A: Razvitie i segashno sŭstoianie na Katedrata po vŭtreshni bolesti. **Vutr Boles** 1981;20(6):6–11

Shestdeset godini Vissh veterinarnomeditsinski institut: **Vet Med Nauki** 1984;21(1):3–5

**Canada**

Barr ML: A century of medicine at Western. A centennial history of the Faculty of Medicine, University of Western Ontario. London, Canada, University of Western Ontario, 1977. xiv, 672 p.

Bates DG: Teaching medical history to medical students: the McGill experience, 1966–1981. With a commentary by L.G. Stevenson. In J. J. Bylebyl, ed: Teaching the history of medicine at a medical center. Baltimore, London, Johns Hopkins University Press, 1982. (The Henry E. Sigerist supplements to the Bulletin of the History of Medicine; new ser., no. 7). p. 121–38.

Bélanger LF: On a nickel and a prayer. Ottawa, University of Ottawa Press, 1978. 146 p.

Bensley EH: Robert Palmer Howard. In Dictionary of Canadian biography, 1881–1890. 1982;11:428–9.

Bernier J: La standardisation des études médicales et la consolidation de la profession dans la deuxième moitié du XIXe siècle. **Rev Hist Am Fr** 1983;37(1):51–65

Bonin M: Depuis l'Institut Marguerite-d'Youville, 50 ans d'études supérieures au Québec. **Infirm Can** 1984 Oct;26(9):31–4

Cleghorn RA: The emergence of psychiatry at McGill. **Can J Psychiatry** 1984 Nov;29(7):551–6

Fishman N: John Bell, MD--teacher to William Osler. **Can Med Assoc J** 1981 Nov 1;125(9):1042, 1044

Frost SB: Science education in the 19th century: The Natural History Society of Montreal, 1827–1925. **McGill J Educ** 1982;17(1):31–48

Gaucher D: La formation des hygiénistes à l'Université de Montréal, 1910–1975: de la santé publique à la médecine préventive. **Rech Sociogr** 1979;20(1):59–85

Godfrey CM: Theophilus Mack. In Dictionary of Canadian Biography, 1881–1890. 1982;11:558–9.

Howell CD: Reform and the monopolistic impulse: the professionalization of medicine in the Maritimes. **Acadiensis** 1981;11(1):3–22

Knowles V: Leaving with a red rose. A history of the Ottawa Civic Hospital School of Nursing. Ottawa, Ottawa Civic Hospital School of Nursing Alumnae Association, 1981. vi, 218 p.

Lee HK: Honoring the founder in his country: conception and struggle for Canada's Memorial College. **Chiropr Hist** 1981;(1):43–5

Persaud TV: A brief history of anatomy at the University of Manitoba. **Anat Anz** 1983;153(1):3–31

Sylvain P: Jean-Etienne Landry. In Dictionary of Canadian biography, 1881–1890. 1982;11:483–6.

Tunis B: Medical education and medical licencing in Lower Canada. **Soc Hist (Canada)** 1981;14(27):67–91

Williams HB: The McGill University plastic surgery program. **Ann Plast Surg** 1984 Nov;13(5):362–5

Wood V: Nursing education: the move from hospital schools of nursing--an historical perspective. **Int J Nurs Stud** 1984;21(3):183–92

Wright MJ: History of academic psychology in Canada. Toronto, Hogrefe, 1982. x, 260 p.

**Chile**

Brncic D: El desarrollo de la biología general en la Facultad de Medicina y su impacto en la actividad científica nacional. **Rev Med Chil** 1982 Aug;110(8):801-5
Costa C: Prehistoria de la cátedra de histología de la Universidad de Chile (1872-1881). Parte I. El affaire Magalhaes. **Rev Med Chil** 1980 Apr;108(4):367-73
Costa C: Prehistoria de la cátedra de histología de la Universidad de Chile (1872-1881) Parte II. Microscopio e histología en Chile antes de 1873. **Rev Med Chil** 1980 May;108(5):463-9
Costa-Casaretto C: Centenario del título de profesor extraordinario de la Universidad de Chile. **Rev Med Chil** 1980 Feb;108(2):161-71
Costa-Casaretto C: Dra. Eloísa Díaz. Centenario del ingreso de la mujer chilena al estudio de las profesiones universitarias. **Rev Med Chil** 1981 Apr;109(4):355-66
Costa-Casaretto C: El 'origen real' de la enseñanza para graduados en la Facultad de Medicina de la Universidad de Chile. **Rev Med Chil** 1981 Oct;109(10):1013-23
Costa-Casaretto C: Enseñanza libre contra estado docente: un episodio de la historia educacional chilena (1972-73). **Rev Med Chil** 1981 Jun;109(6):573-81
Costa-Casaretto C: La cátedra de neuropsiquiatría de la Universidad de Chile desde 1891 hasta 1906. **Rev Med Chil** 1980 Sep;108(9):855-62
Costa-Casaretto C: La enseñanza para graduados en la Facultad de Medicina de la Universidad de Chile. I. Antecedentes próximos y no tan próximos. **Rev Med Chil** 1981 Jan;109(1):73-80
Costa-Casaretto C: Nonagésimo aniversario de la Escuela de Medicina de la Avenida Independencia. Testimonios de una odisea. **Rev Med Chil** 1979 Aug;107(8):761-70
Costa-Casaretto C: Presentacion del Dr. Guillermo C. Blest. **Rev Med Chil** 1983 Apr;111(4):364-7
Costa-Casaretto C: Presentación del Dr. Lorenzo Sazié. **Rev Med Chil** 1983 Dec;111(12):1289-98
Costa-Casaretto C: Sobre el. Dr. Carlos Sazie, primer profesor de neurología y segundo de psiquiatria en la universidad de Chile (1881-1891). **Rev Med Chil** 1980 Aug;108(8):749-56
Croxatto H: Homenaje al Dr. Teodoro Muhm (1869-1939). **Rev Med Chil** 1984 Jan;112(1):81-8
Cruz-Coke R: El plan Garretón-Alessandri. **Rev Med Chil** 1980 Nov;108(11):1073-5
Cruz-Coke R: Los profesores de la Escuela de Medicina y la historia política nacional (1833-1983). **Rev Med Chil** 1983 Apr;111(4):380-7
Goić A: 150 años de educación médica formal en Chile (1833-1983). **Rev Med Chil** 1983 Apr;111(4):343-9
Laval E: Los alumnos del curso de medicina de 1833. **Rev Med Chil** 1984 Jan;112(1):65-71
Neghme A: La educación médica y el Servicio Nacional de Salud. **Rev Med Chil** 1977 Oct;105(10):668-73
Neghme A: Significado de la investigación biomédica en el desarrollo académico de una escuela de medicina. Remembranzas de un pasado no tan remoto. **Rev Med Chil** 1981 Sep;109(9):878-84
Quintana C: Cincuentenario de la Facultad de Medicina de la Pontificia Universidad Católica de Chile. **Rev Med Chil** 1980 Jul;108(7):645-8
Toro C: Sesquicentenario de la enseñanza médica. **Rev Chil Pediatr** 1983 Mar-Apr;54(2):81-2

**China**

Brown ER: Exporting medical education: professionalism, modernization and imperialism. **Soc Sci Med [Med Psychol Med Sociol]** 1979 Nov;13A(6):585-95
Bullock MB: An American transplant: the Rockefeller Foundation and Peking Union Medical College. Berkeley, University of California Press, 1980. xxvii, 280 p.
Huang CS: Medical education in China: historical background, present status, and further development. **Am J Surg** 1982 Jun;143(6):660-3
Huang H: [On the formation and development of the Meng He School of Jiangsu Province in traditional Chinese medicine] (Chi). **Chung Hua I Shih Tsa Chih** 1984;14(2):65-71
New PK, Cheung YW: Harvard Medical School of China, 1911--1916: an expanded footnote in the history of western medical education in China. **Soc Sci Med** 1982;16(12):1207-15
Shi Yuanyi: [Advanced medical education in north-east China before the Liberation] (Chi). **Chung Hua I Shih Tsa Chih** 1981;11:70-4
Shipp JC: To serve the people: medical education and care in the People's Republic of China. **Ann Intern Med** 1982 Aug;97(2):277-9
Sun Y: [The historical materials of modern medical education in Nantong city: an early medical school solely established by Chinese] (Chi). **Chung Hua I Shih Tsa Chih** 1984;14(2):90-103

**Colombia**

Serpa-Flores R: La enseñanza de la historia de la medicina en la formación del médico. **Educ Med Salud** 1983;17(4):423-32

**Cuba**

Perspectivas de desarrollo del Instituto de Medicina Tropical 'Pedro Kourí': **Rev Cubana Med Trop** 1979 Sep-Dec;31(3):161-3

**Czechoslovakia**

Adamec J, Petrasek J: Reforma lékařského studia v roce 1953 a okolnosti jejího vzniku. **Cesk Zdrav** 1981 Dec;29(12):508-14
Adamec J: Z historie výuky I. interní kliniky v Praze. **Cas Lek Cesk** 1981;120(49):1475-7
Balaš V: I. chirurgická klinika a její vliv na rozvoj chirurgie v Ceskoslovensku. **Rozhl Chir** 1983 Apr;62(4):289-307
Bek V: Postgraduální výchovně vzdělávací proces v klinické onkologii. Přehled činnosti katedry klinické onkologie u příležitosti 30. výročí Institutu pro další vzdělávání lékařu a farmaceutu v Praze. **Cas Lek Cesk** 1983 Nov 25;122(47):1457-60
Boguszaková J: Třicet let oftalmologické katedry institutu pro další vzdělávání lékařu a farmaceutu v Praze. **Cesk Oftalmol** 1983 May;39(3):145-8
Bolecek O: Protifašistický odboj na zdravotnické frontě. Vzpomínky na ilegální činnost za okupace na Bulovce. **Cas Lek Cesk** 1980 May 9;119(19):538-42
Chlumský J: Třicet let Institutu pro další vzdělávání lékařu a farmaceutu. **Cesk Gastroenterol Vyz** 1983 Nov;37(6-7):361-3
Cierny G: O vývoji a dalších perspektívach teoretických medicínskych odborov lekárskej fakulty Univerzity Komenského v Bratislave. **Cas Lek Cesk** 1979 Dec 21;118(51):1571-3
Dobiáš J, Marek J: Patologická anatomie na pražské univerzitě před rokem 1882. **Cesk Patol** 1984 Feb;20(1):1-10
Dunovský J: Třicet let katedry pediatrie ILF a její další činnost. **Cesk Pediatr** 1983 Oct;38(10):629-32
Filip M: 25 rokov katedry sociálneho lekárstva Lekárskej fakulty UPJS v Košiciach. **Cesk Zdrav** 1980 Oct;28(10):397-402
Fingerland A: 100. Výroči rozděleni Karlovy univerzity na českou a německou. Následný vliv na československou patologii. **Cesk Patol** 1983 Aug;19(3):129-32
Havránek J: Ustavení České university a její lékařské fakulty v letech 1882 a 1883. **Cas Lek Cesk** 1983 Feb 18;122(7):193-5
Heinl E: Třicet let výchovně vzdělávací činnosti Institut pro další vzdělávání lékařu a farmaceutu. **Cas Lek Cesk** 1983 Oct 21;122(42):1286-90
Hlaváčková L: Budování klinických pracovišt české lékařské fakulty v době rozdělení pražské univerzity. II. Snahy o vybudování českých klinických pracovišt' před rozdělením univerzity. **Sb Lek** 1983 Apr;85(4):105-15
Hlaváckové L: Budování klinických pracovišt Ceské Lékařské Fakulty v době rozdělení Pražské Univerzity. III. Budování českých klinických pracovišt' po rozdělení univerzity a lékařské fakulty. **Sb Lek** 1983 May;85(5):147-59
Hlaváčková L: Casopis lékařu českých a Spolek českých lékařu v boji za českou universitu a lékařskou fakultu. **Cas Lek Cesk** 1982 Dec 23;121(51):1569-73
Hlaváčková L: K stému výročí české výuky na I. interní klinice v. Praze. **Cas Lek Cesk** 1981 Nov 26;120(47):1478-82
Hlaváčková L, Adamec J: Sto let od zahájení výuky na české lékařské fakultě. **Cas Lek Cesk** 1983 Oct 14;122(41):1250-3
Horák J, Chrástek J, Novotný V, et al: 30 let práce Ustavu tělovýchovného lékařství fakulty všeobecného lékařství University Karlovy v Praze. **Sb Lek** 1980 Jan;82(1):30-2
Hromádková J: Medici v boji za českou universitu a lékařskou fakultu. **Cas Lek Cesk** 1983 Oct 14;122(41):1254-60
Hromádková J: Medici v boji za českou universitu a lékařskou fakultu. I. Medici a národnostní otázka v revolučních letech 1848-1849 a v období činnosti Klubu mediku českých (do roku 1868). **Sb Lek** 1983 Oct;85(9-10):277-84
Hromádková J: Medici v boji za Ceskou Univerzitu a Lékařskou Fakultu. II. Spolek českých mediku a jeho úloha v boji za českou lékařskou fakultu. **Sb Lek** 1984 Apr;86(4):119-28
Jeřábek J: 22 let trvání Katedry posudkového lékařství. **Cesk Zdrav** 1983 Sep;31(8-9):396-9
Jirouš J: Třicetiletá bilance a perspektivy Katedry sociálního lékařství a organizace zdravotnictví Institutu pro další vzdělávání lékařu a farmaceutu Praha. **Cesk Zdrav** 1983 Sep;31(8-9):360-7
Junas J: Prostredie štúdií a spoločenská aktivita slovenských medikov v 19. storočí. **Cas Lek cesk** 1980 Jul 25;119(29-30):820-2
Kolařik J, Jorda V: Thirty-five years of the Faculty of Medicine at the reestablished university in Olomouc. **Acta Univ Palacki Olomuc Fac Med** 1982;103:7-21
Kotek V, Nikliček L, Stein K: K historii snah o postgraduální vzdělávání lékařu v Ceskoslovensku před rokem 1945. **Cas Lek Cesk** 1983 Oct 21;122(42):1308-12
Kunčar K: Olomoucká psychiatrická klinika očima bývalých studentu. **Cesk Psychiatr** 1981 Oct;77(5):346-7
Kvasnička J: Sest' desat'ročí Univerzity Komenského v Bratislave.

Cas Lek Cesk 1979 Dec 21;118(51):1569-70
Macúch P: K 30. výročí činnosti Institutu pro další vzdělávání lékařu a farmaceutu v Praze. **Cesk Zdrav** 1983 Sep;31(8-9):337-45
Macúch P: Třicet let činnosti Institutu pro další vzdělávání lékařu a farmaceutu v Praze--integrální součást vývoje socialistického zdravotnictví v Ceskoslovensku. **Cas Lek Cesk** 1983 Oct 21;122(42):1281-4
Makovický E: Desat rokov Katedry metodiky a plánovania dalšieho vzdelávania Inštitútu pre dalšie vzdelávanie lekárov a farmaceutov Praha. **Cesk Zdrav** 1983 Sep;31(8-9):346-9
Málek P: Stoleté výroči obnovení činnosti české lékařské fakulty v Praze. **Cas Lek Cesk** 1984 Apr 6;123(14):425-8
Michaličková J: Vývoj a dalšie perspektívy rozvoja pediatrických odborov na lekárskej fakulte Univerzity Komenského v Bratislave. **Cas Lek Cesk** 1979 Dec 21;118(51):1581-3
Moravec R, Tichý M, Moravcová M, et al: Z dejín chirurgie v Bratislave. Profesor Kostlivý a začiatky chirurgickej kliniky na LFUK v Bratislava] **Rozhl Chir** 1984 Jul;63(7):526-31
Müller C, Niklíček L: K postavení sociálního lékařství v historii systému výuky a výchovy lékařu na Univerzitě Karlově. **Cesk Zdrav** 1982 Jan;30(1):22-33
Müller C, Niklícek L: Třicet let lékařské fakulty hygienické Univerzity Karlovy. **Cesk Zdrav** 1982 Oct;30(10):402-7
Niklíček L, Stein K, Kotek V: K historii postgraduální výchovy lékařu--zaměstnancu státní zdravotní správy v Ceskoslovensku před rokem 1938. **Cesk Zdrav** 1983 Dec;31(12):502-12
Ondrejička M: 60 rokov internej medicíny na jubilujúcej lekárskej fakulte University Komenského v Bratizlave. **Vnitr Lek** 1979 Dec;25(12):1145-7
Ondrejička M: 60 rokov internistických disciplín na lekárskej fakulte University Komenského v Bratislave. **Cas Lek Cesk** 1979 Dec 21;118(51):1576-80
Porubčinová Z: Pokrokové tradice katedry sociálního lékařstvílékařské faculty UJEP v Brně. **Cesk Zdrav** 1983 Feb;31(2):71-6
Remišová M, Janec M, Bruchác D, et al: Medici v Slovenskom národnom povstaní. **Bratisl Lek Listy** 1984 Sep;82(3):1142-52
Rybová J: Vývoj ideové výchovné práce Institutu pro další vzdělávání lékařu a farmaceutu. **Cas Lek Cesk** 1983 Oct 21;122(42):1291-4
Santavý F: Prof. Dr. chem. PhMr. Martin Ehrmann a jeho pusobení na medicínskochirurgickém učilišti v Olomouci v letech 1836--1866. **Cesk Farm** 1979 Jun;28(5):221-2
Sídlo R: Příspěvek k významu a metodice výuky dějin lékařství a zdravotnictví na lékařské fakultě. **Sb Ved Pr Lek Fak Univ Karlovy** 1979;22(5 Suppl):579-82
Simon F: Latinčinár ako historik medicíny. **Cas Lek Cesk** 1984 Oct 12;123(40-41):1250
Slavětínský M: Jak se kdysi v Olomouci vzdělávali zdravotničtí pracovníci. **Cesk Gynekol** 1981 May;46(4):321-2
Slavětínský M: K dvoustému výroči vzniku lékařsko-chirurgického studia v Olomouci (1782-1875). **Cesk Zdrav** 1981 Oct;29(10):426-31
Svejcar J: Vznik a vývoj Ceskoslovenské spolupráce na poli doškolování pediatru. **Cesk Zdrav** 1983 Oct;31(10):401-7
Tamáska P: Az orvostörténet oktatásának és müvelésének története Csehorszàgban. **Orv Hetil** 1984 Aug 5;125(32):1963-4
Tichý M, Ozorovský V, Beniak M, et al: Pôsobenie profesora Reinsberga v akademických funkciách na LFUK v Bratislave (1925-1927). **Cesk Zdrav** 1984 Feb;32(2):68-73
Tichý M, Kántorová V: Vznik lekárskej fakulty UK Bratislave. 3. Nová situácia. **Bratisl Lek Listy** 1980 Dec;74(6):686-91
Tichý M, Kántorová V: Vznik lekárskej fakulty UK v Bratislave. 2. Usilie o založenie národnej univerzity a nové prúdy medzi lekármi. **Bratisl Lek Listy** 1980 Aug;74(2):234-40
Tichý M, Kántorová V: Vznik lekárskej fakulty UK v Bratislave. 4. Iniciatíva Hynkovej skupiny. **Bratisl Lek Listy** 1981 Jan;75(1):92-7
Tichý M, Kántorová V: Vznik lekárskej fakulty UK v Bratislave. 5. Misia dobrej vôle z Prahy. **Bratisl Lek Listy** 1981 Mar;75(3):372-8
Tichý M, Kántorová V: Vznik lekárskej fakulty UK v Bratislave. 6. Rokovanie V parlamente. **Bratisl Lek Listy** 1981;75(4):496-502
Tichý M, Dedek J, Ozorovský V: Začiatky lekárskej fakulty UK v Bratislave. **Cesk Zdrav** 1983 Feb;31(2):49-54
Tichý M: Začiatky lekárskej fakulty UK v Bratislave. 1. Prvý profesorský zbor. **Bratisl Lek Listy** 1982 Feb;77(2):235-40
Tichy M: Začiatky lekárskej fakulty UK v Bratislave. 3. Lekári a začiatky Univerzity Komenského. **Bratisl Lek Listy** 1982 Apr;77(4):488-94
Tichý M, Dedek J, Krekáň J, et al: Začiatky lekárskej fakulty UK v Bratislave. 4. Co predchádzalo vzniku Bratislavských lekárskych listov. **Bratisl Lek Listy** 1983;79(4):500-4
Tichý M: Začiatky lekárskej fakulty UK v Bratslave. 2. Prípravy na začatie výučby. **Bratisl Lek Listy** 1982 Mar;77(3):359-65
Trojan S: 100 let od obnovení činnosti Ceské Lékařské fakulty. **Cesk Fysiol** 1982;31(6):481-2
Vacek Z: Fakulta všeobechného lékařství současnosti. **Cas Lek Cesk** 1983 Oct 14;122(41):1265-8
Vlček J: K historii stoletého trvání I. české chirurgické kliniky v Praze. **Cas Lek Cesk** 1983 Jul 15;122(28):865-70
Vojtíšek V: Historie chirurgické kliniky lékařské fakulty hygienické Univerzity Karlovy v Praze. **Rozhl Chir** 1983 Jul;62(7):533-8
Wondrák E: Die Anfänge der chirurgischen und geburtshilflichen Ausbildung in Mähren. In Ganzinger K, Skopec M, Wyklicky H, ed: Festschrift für Erna Lesky zum 70. Geburtstag. Wien, Brüder Hollinek, 1981. p. 185-92.
Zvara V: O vývoji a dalších perspektívach rozvoja chirurgických disciplín na lekárskej fakulte Univerzity Komenského v Bratislave. **Cas Lek Cesk** 1979 Dec 21;118(51):1583-5

**Egypt**

Ghoneim M: Antoine-Barthelemy Clot créateur de l'école de médecine. **Cah Hist** 1969;11:125-36

**Europe**

Costa-Casaretto C: Los primeros becarios chilenos en Europa (1874). **Rev Med Chil** 1979 Sep;107(9):886
Olesińska-Serafin A: Europejskie Stowarzyszenie Kształcenia Medycznego i jego wpływ na rozwój dydaktyki medycznej. **Pol Tyg Lek** 1984 Mar 26;39(13):453-5
Sydow C von: Notiser från Frans von Sydows utrikes studieresor 1861-1886. **Nord Medicinhist Arsb** 1984;:117-28

**Finland**

Klatt CH: Die ersten Doktoranden der Veterinärmedizin in Finnland. **DTW** 1981 Apr 5;88(4):142-3

**France**

Biserte G: L'Histoire de la Faculté Mixte de Médecine et de Pharmacie de Lille. (2 vols). Vol I. Lille, l'Association Corporative des Etudiants en Médecine de Lille, 1975. 169 p.
Blin PC: Bourgelat, founder of veterinary teaching, 1712-1779. **Comp Immunol Microbiol Infect Dis** 1980;3(1-2):xiii-xvi
Bloch H: Guillaume Dupuytren, M.D. (1777-1835). Surgeon of Hôtel Dieu and his American students. **NY State J Med** 1981 Feb;81(2):259-60
Bolzinger R, Beau A: L'hôpital militaire d'instruction de Metz. In: Congrès national des Sociétés Savantes, 103e, Nancy, 1978. Comptes rendus. Paris, Section des Sciences, Fasc. V. p. 11-8.
Bruce-Chwatt LJ: 'Ecole du Pharo' in Marseille. **Trans R Soc Trop Med Hyg** 1981;75(1):131-2
Casaux-Bussière M: Georges Denigès (1859-1951). Essai biographique. Thèse, Bordeaux II, 1981. 374 leaves.
Courtois D: Naissance de l'Institut de Médecine Tropicale du Service de Santé des Armées. **Med Trop (Mars)** 1980 Nov-Dec;40(6):631-4
Debré M: Robert Debré, réformateur. **Bull Acad Natl Med (Paris)** 1982 Dec;166(9):1295-303
Dejussieu J: Note sur le jardin botanique de la Marine à Rochefort-sur-Mer. In: Congrès National des Sociétés Savantes, 91e, Rennes, 1966. Comptes Rendus. Paris, 1967. Section des Sciences, Tome 1. p. 129-33.
Delaunay P: Médecins de jadis et d'aujourd'hui; souvenirs des hôpitaux et de la Faculté de Paris de 1895 à 1905. **Hist Sci Med** 1981;15(4):307-20
Dulieu L: Les relations entre la Bulgarie et la faculté de médecine de Montpellier (1878-1944). In: International Congress of the History of Medicine, 26th, Plovdiv (Bulgaria), 1978. Actes du Congres, Vol. 1. Sofia, 1980. p. 102-10.
Dulieu L: Un projet d'Ecole de santé de la Marine à Montpellier. In: Congrès National des Sociétés Savantes, 91e, Rennes, 1966. Comptes Rendus. Paris, 1967. Section des Sciences, Tome 1. p. 103-7.
Finot A: Les premiers élèves et collaborateurs (surtout Bretons) de Laennec. In: Congrès National des Sociétés Savantes, 91e, Rennes, 1966. Comptes Rendus. Paris, 1967. Section des Sciences, Tome 1. p. 181-9.
Fontaine-Levent P: Prunelle et la bibliothèque de la Faculté de médecine de Montpellier. **Hist Sci Med** 1980;14(2):241-3
Gelfand T: The hospice of the Paris College of Surgery (1774-1793), 'a unique and invaluable institution.' **Bull Hist Med** 1973 Jul-Aug;47(4):375-93
Godonnèche J: A propos d'une thèse de médecine à Paris en 1809. In: Congrès National des Sociétés Savantes, 97e, Nantes, 1972. Comptes Rendus. Paris, 1976. Section des Sciences, Tome 1. p. 331-6.
Goubert JP: L'hygiène de l'eau dans la France contemporaine d'après le thèses de doctorat de la Faculté de Médecine de Paris (1830-1940). In Imhof AE, ed: Mensch und Gesundheit in der Geschichte. Husum, Matthiesen, 1980. p. 59-78.
Grivaux M: Soixante-quinzième anniversaire de l'Associaton d'Enseignement médical des Hôpitaux de Paris (1907-1982). **Sem Hop Paris** 1983 Mar 31;59(13):865-7
Hillemand P, Gilbrin E, Segal A: Le père Elisée et la réforme des études médicales. **Hist Sci Med** 1981;15(2):159-65
Huard P, Grmek MD: Coup d'oeil sur les élèves étrangers de Laennec. In: Congrès National des Sociétés Savantes, 97e, Nantes, 1972. Comptes Rendus. Paris, 1976. Section des Sciences, Tome 1. p. 21-35.
Huard P, Niaussat PM: Die Medizinisch-Chirurgische Schule der Marine in Brest. **Hist Hosp** 1979-80;13:147-52
Kayser C: Note historique sur l'évolution de la chaire de physiologie de la Faculté de Médecine. In Livet G, Schaff G, ed: Médecine et assistance

en Alsace, XVIe-XXe siècle. Strasbourg, Istra, 1976. p. 303-19.
Livet JM: Les années terribles: l'Ecole libre de Médecine de Strasbourg de 1870 à 1872. In Livet G, Schaff G, ed: Médecine et assistance en Alsace, XVIe-XXe siècle. Strasbourg, Istra, 1976. p. 265-86.
Martínez Báez M: Pasteur, maestro. **Mem Col Nac (Mex)** 1967-68;6(2-3):115-31
Morel MF: Madame Roland, sa fille et les médecins: prime éducation et médicalisation à l'époque des lumières. **Ann Bretagne** 1979;86(3):211-9
Mulder WJ: De 'Anatomie clastique' van Dr. L. T. J. Anzoux. **Tijdschr Geschied Geneeskd** 1981:4(3):133-43
Pellcler Y: Edouard Seguin et l'éducation speciale. **Bull Acad Natl Med (Paris)** 1981 May;165(5):627-30
Percebois G: Les Bulgares et la Faculté de Médecine de Nancy à la fin du XIXe siècle et au début du XXe siècle. In International Congress of the History of Medicine. 26th, Plovdiv, 1978. Actes du Congress. Sofia, 1981. Volume II. p. 179-82.
Pinel P: The clinical training of doctors. An essay of 1793. Ed. D. B. Weiner. Baltimore, Johns Hopkins University Press, 1980. 102 p. (Henry E. Sigerist suppl. to the Bull. Hist. Med. N.S. no. 3).
Poirier JL: La réorganisation des études médicales selon Auguste Comte. In Poirier J, Poirier JL, ed: Médecine et philosophie à la fin du XIXe siècle. Paris, Université de Paris XII - Val de Marne, [1980?]. p. 47-59.
Rivet R: Quelques aspects sanitaires de la Bretagne vus à travers les thèses des Facultés de médecine de Paris et de Strasbourg de l'an VII (1798) à 1870. In: Congrès National des Sociétés Savantes, 107e. Brest, 1982. Comptes Rendus, Paris, 1983. Section des Sciences, Fasc. IV. p. 241-52.
Saumande P: Une collection d'instruments scientifiques anciens au Laboratoire de Physique pharmaceutique de la Faculté de Médecine et de Pharmacie de Limoges. **Bull Soc Archeol Hist Limousin** 1981;108:157-8
Sicard A: Un doyen misogyne et un recteur féministe. **Hist Sci Med** 1982;16(1):15-20
Voelckel J: L'école du Pharo. Tradition-permanence-avenir. **Med Trop (Mars)** 1980 Nov-Dec;40(6):635-8
Weisz G: Reform and conflict in French medical education, 1870-1914. In R. Fox, G. Weisz, ed: The organization of science and technology in France 1808-1914. Cambridge, Cambridge University Press, 1980. p. 61-94.

**Germany**

Abe HR, Kaiser L: Ferdinand Sauerbruch und Erfurt. **Beitr Gesch Univ Erfurt** 1979-83;19:271-81
Ash MG: Academic politics in the history of science: experimental psychology in Germany, 1879-1941. **Cent Eur Hist** 1980;13(3):255-86
Behrens H: Geschichte und Aufgaben der deutschen Tiergesundheitsämter. **DTW** 1981 Aug 5;88(8):325-32
Bräutigam W: Rückblick auf das Jahr 1942. Betrachtungen eines psychoanalytischen Ausbildungskandidaten des Berliner Instituts der Kriegsjahre. **Psyche (Stuttg)** 1984 Oct;38(10):905-14
Diehl B: Der Wandel der Historiographie von Medizin und Naturwissenschaften in ihrer gesellschaftlichen Bedingtheit. **Sudhoffs Arch** 1982;66(3):276-300
Dilg-Frank R: Alexandre Yersin als Medizinstudent in Marburg. **Alma Mater Philipp** 1978-1979;19-23
Dillemann G: Les écoles de médecine des départements annexés de l'an XI (1803) à 1814. Le cas de l'école de Mayence. **Hist Sci Med** 1984;18(1):45-51
Dittrich M: Der Darwinist Fritz Müller (1822-1897) und sein Medizinstudium in Greifswald. Analyse der Motive seiner progressiven Haltung. In: International Congress of the History of Medicine, 26th, Plovdiv (Bulgaria), 1978. Actes du Congres, Vol. 1. Sofia, 1980. p. 100-1.
Efkes F: Entstehung und Entwicklung der studentischen Korporationen an der Tierärztlichen Hochschule Hannover im 19. Jahrhundert. Diss. Hannover, 1978. 227 p.
Ergetowski R: Uzupełniajace studia H. Kadyi'ego w Uniwersytecie Lipskim w 1879 r. **Arch Hist Med (Warsz)** 1979;42(3):309-15
Erxleben DC: Gründliche Untersuchung der Ursachen, die das weibliche Geschlecht vom Studieren abhalten. Reprint of the Berlin, 1742, ed., mit einem Nachwort von G. Rechenberg. Hildesheim, New York, Olms, 1977. [68], 250 p.
Ganzinger K: Johann Peter Frank und die Apothekerordnung für die österreichische Lombardei. In Ganzinger K, Skopec M, Wyklicky H, ed: Festschrift für Erna Lesky zum 70. Geburtstag. Wien, Brüder Hollinek, 1981. p. 39-47.
Hambsch K, Treutler H, Pietruschka WD: Profil und Aufgabenstellung einer medizinischen Universitätspoliklinik in Vergangenheit und Gegenwart am Beispiel des Medizinisch-Poliklinischen Institutes der Karl-Marx-Universität Leipzig. **Z Gesamte Inn Med** 1981 Mar 15;36(6):186-9
Harig G: Bemerkungen zum medizinhistorischen Unterricht in der DDR. **Z Gesamte Hyg** 1980;26(5):383-5
Hawkins H: Transatlantic discipleship: two American biologists and their German mentor. **Isis** 1980 Jun;71(257):197-210
Heintel H: Moritz Schiffs gescheiterter Habilitationsversuch an der Universität Göttingen im Jahre 1855. **Medizinhist J** 1980;15(4):378-84
Heller R: Johann Christian Reil's training scheme for medical auxiliaries. **Med Hist** 1975 Oct;19(4):321-32
Hesse PG: Das erste staatliche zahnärztliche Institut Deutschlands und sein Gründer Friedrich Louis Hesse. **Stomatol DDR** 1983 Dec;33(12):861-3
Hoepke H: Aus der Geschichte der Heidelberger Anatomie. **Ruperto Carola (Germany)** 1978;30(61):23-31
Hofmann-Meier B: Ein Geburtshelfer und Hebammenlehrer des 18. Jahrhunderts. Leben und Werk des Johann Philipp Hagen (1734-1792), Hebammenlehrer und Professor für Entbindungskunst in Berlin. Diss. Bern, 1982. 75 p.
Horn H, Winkler H: 25 Jahre Institut für Allgemeine Hygiene der Medizinischen Akademie Erfurt. **Z Gesamte Hyg** 1984 Sep;30(9):529-30
Hungerland H: Deutsche Universität einst und jetzt. **Med Welt** 1981 Apr 24;32(17):672-4
Johannes A: Zur Geschichte der Tierärztlichen Hochschule Hannover während der ersten 200 Jahre ihres Bestehens. II. Die Klinik für Geburtshilfe und Gynäkologie des Rindes und ihre Vorläufer. Diss. Hannover, 1983. 148 p.
Kahle E, Stupp JA: Hochschulschriften zur Geschichte der Medizin, Pharmazie, und Naturwissenschaften der Friedrich-Alexander-Universität Erlangen-Nürnberg 1885-1975. Erlangen, Verlagsbuchhandlung Hannelore Lüling, 1980. 94 p. (Medizinhistorische Materialien, 2).
Kahle E: Hochschulschriften zur Geschichte der Medizin Pharmazie und Naturwissenschaften der Julius-Maximilians-Universität Würzburg, 1885-1970. Medizinhistorische Materialien - 1. Erlangen, Verlagsbuchhandlung, 1979. 48 p.
Kaiser W, Piechocki W: Das hallesche Collegium Orientale und seine Ausstrahlung auf die medizinische Arabistik des 18. Jahrhunderts. **Wiss Z Martin Luther Univ (Math)** 1978;27(5):111-32
Kaiser W: Die ersten promovierten Aerztinnen. Zum 225. Jahrestag der halleschen Graduierung von Dorothea Christian Erxleben (1715-1762). **Z Gesamte Inn Med** 1980 Feb 15;35(4):176-83
Kaiser W, Simon A: Die Geschichte der Gerichtsmedizin an der Universität Halle-Wittenberg. Halle, Martin-Luther-Universität Halle-Wittenberg, 1978. 81 p. (Beiträge zur Universitätsgeschichte, Nr. 12, Tome 25).
Kaiser W, Völker A: Die naturwissenschaftlichen Disziplinen im halleschen medizinischen Kollegeprogramm des 18. und 19. Jahrhunderts. **Z Gesamte Inn Med** 1983 Jul 15;38(14):375-82
Kaiser W: Dokumente zur halleschen Promotion polnischer Mediziner in den Jahren 1791 und 1792. **Wiss Z Martin Luther Univ (Math)** 1976;25(6):75-81
Kaiser W, Völker A: Gedenktage 1980 aus der Geschichte der Medizinischen Fakultät Wittenberg (II): Lehre und Forschung in der Amtsphase von Christian Vater (1651-1732) und Abraham Vater (1684-1751). **Z Gesamte Inn Med** 1981 May 15;36(10):325-32
Kaiser W: In memoriam Kurt Sprengel (1766-1833)---Zur 150. Wiederkehr seines Todestages am 15. März 1983. **Z Gesamte Inn Med** 1983 Feb 1;38(3):90-7
Kaiser W, Völker A: Johann Reinhold Forster (1729-1798) als Ordinarius in Halle. **Wiss Z Martin Luther Univ (Math)** 1981;30(2):61-79
Kaiser W: Medizinisches Grundlagenstudium im frühen 18. Jahrhundert. Zur 300. Wiederkehr des Geburtstages von Georg Daniel Coschwitz (1679-1729). **Z Gesamte Inn Med** 1979 Aug 1;34(15):419-28
Kaiser W, Skrobacki A: Resonanz des polnischen Novemberaufstandes (1831) an der Königsberger Universität. **Arch Hist Med (Warsz)** 1979;42(3):281-4
Kaiser W: 100 Jahre Universitätsklinikum Halle. Die Entwicklung der halleschen Universitätskliniken in den ersten Jahrzehnten ihres Bestehens. **Z Gesamte Inn Med** 1982 Jun 15;37(12):354-68
Karbe KH: Die 'Woche der Sowjet-Medizin' zu Berlin (28. November bis 2. Dezember 1932). **Z Gesamte Hyg** 1981 Oct;27(10):784-8
Klix F: Hermann Ebbinghaus---Ursprünge und Anfang psychologischer Forschungen an der Berliner Universität. In Eckardt G, ed: Zur Geschichte der Psychologie. Berlin, VEB Deutscher Verlag der Wissenschaften, 1979. p. 85-109.
Krumholz W: Eugen Woldemar Bostroem (1850-1928), Lehrer der Bathologie und Förderer der Medizin in Giessen. Giessen, Schmitz, 1983. 311 p. (Arbeiten zur Geschichte der Medizin in Giessen, Bd. 8)
Lambert M: Udział niemieckich ośrodków naukowych w kształtowaniu polskiej myśli medycznej w czasach saskich (1697-1763). **Arch Hist Med (Warsz)** 1979;42(2):223-30
Linde E: Ernst von Bergmann. Rückblick auf das Leben anlässlich der Einweihung der Sanitätsakademie in München. **MMW** 1981 May 1;123(18):751-2
Lindemann M, Cesnokova S: Wissenschaftliche Schulen in Deutschland im XIX. Jahrhundert und ihre Rolle für die Entwicklung der Physiologie in der Welt. In International Congress of the History of Medicine. 26th, Plovdiv, 1978. Actes du Congress. Sofia, 1981. Volume II. p. 140-3.
Mader FH: Zur Geschichte der Famulatur bei Praktischen Aerzten. **ZFA (Stuttgart)** 1980 Aug 20;56(23):1415-8
Marx S: Zwei Kollegmitschriften nach den Vorlesungen von August Conrad Havemann, geschrieben 1799 und 1818 an der Tierärztlichen Hochschule Hannover. Diss. Hannover, 1981. 360 p.
Meinel C: Die Chemie an der Universität Marburg seit Beginn des 19. Jahrhunderts. Ein Beitrag zu ihrer Entwicklung als Hochschulfach.

Marburg, Elwert, 1978. xvi, 669 p. (Academia Marburgensis. Herausgegeben von der Philipps-Universität Marburg, Band 3).
Meyer A: Zur Geschichte der Tierärztlichen Hochschule Hannover während der ersten 200 Jahre ihres Bestehens. I. Die Entwicklung der pathologischen Thematik und des Institutes für Pathologie. Diss. Hannover 1980. 207 p.
Moschke G: Zur Bedeutung des SMAD-Befehls Nr. 234 für die Entwicklung der Lehre über Sozialhygiene an der Leipziger Universität in den Jahren 1948 bis 1952. **Z Gesamte Hyg** 1983 Oct;29(10):620-3
Müller W: Vom Wöchnerinnenasyl zum Universitätsklinikum. Die Geschichte des Städtischen Krankenhauswesens in Essen. Münster, Murken-Altrogge, 1981. 364 p. (Studien zur Geschichte des Krankenhauswesens, 15)
Nabielek R: Robert Koch und die Begründung des Lehrstuhls für Hygiene an der Berliner Universität. **Z Gesamte Hyg** 1982 Mar;28(3):185-93
Niemann H, Wiezorek WD: Zur Geschichte der medizinischen Hochschulbildung in der Deutschen Demokratischen Republik. Teil I und II. **Z Arztl Fortbild (Jena)** 1980 Feb 1;74(3,4):115-22, 178-81
Opitz R, Horn H, Heinecke P, et al: Robert Koch. Die Vorgeschichte der Berufung als ersten Ordinarius für Hygiene an die Universität Berlin. **MMW** 1981 Oct 16;123(42):1593-5
Ostermann E: 25 Jahre Auslandsbeziehungen der Tierärztlichen Hochschule Hannover. Bericht über den Zeitraum von 1958-1983. Diss. Hannover, 1984. 123 p.
Pfohl G: Das philosophisch-philologische Element in der medizinischen Fakultät. **Med Welt** 1980 May 16;31(20):775-8
Querner H: 'Ein Wort über den Einfluss naturwissenschaftlicher Institute auf humane Bildung' (G. A. Goldfuss 1821). In Seidler E, Schott H, ed: Bausteine zur Medizingeschichte. Stuttgart, Steiner, 1984. p. 86-93.
Reimann R: Das Bildungszentrum Essen des DBfK besteht zehn Jahre. **Krankenpflege (Frankfurt)** 1984 Jul-Aug;38(7-8):222-4
Renker K: 30 Jahre Sozialhygiene an der Universität Halle. **Z Gesamte Hyg** 1980;26(2):116-21
Schipperges H: Struktur und Funktion eines Instituts für Gesundheitsbildung. In R. Wittern, ed: Jahrbuch des Instituts für Geschichte der Medizin der Robert Bosch Stiftung. Stuttgart, Hippokrates Verlag, 1984. Bd. 1. p. 42-69.
Schreier J, Haustein UF, Karbe KH: Zur Geschichte der Dermatologie an der Universität Leipzig. **Dermatol Monatsschr** 1984;170(1):1-14
Sendler P: Von der Krüppelheilanstalt zum Universitätsklinikum: die 'Hüfferstiftung' in Münster in Westfalen. Herzogenrath, Murken-Altrogge, 1984. 188 p. (Studien zur Geschichte des Krankenhauswesens, 17)
Seyda B: O nauczaniu historii medycyny w RFN. **Arch Hist Med (Warsz)** 1982;45(1-4):107-10
Stembrowicz W: Lekarze berlińscy pierwszej Połowy XIX wieku w relacjach lekarzy polskich. **Arch Hist Med (Warsz)** 1979;42(3):273-9
Stollenwerk M: Der Fakultätsneubau der Medizin in Aachen-Melaten. Versuch einer Deutung. In Göpfert W, Otten HH, ed: Metavoeite: wandelt euch durch neues Denken. Düsseldorf, Triltsch, 1983. p. 125-34.
Triebel-Schubert C: Die Anfänge der Bonner akademischen Medizin. Johann Christian Friedrich Harless (1773-1853). **MMW** 1983 Oct 21;125(42):950-2
Uerckwitz J: Zur Geschichte der Hygiene an der Universität Rostock. **Z Gesamte Hyg** 1981 Jul 7;27(7):501-3
Usbeck W: 25 Jahre Medizinische Akademie Erfurt -- ihre Traditionen und ihr Weg. Begrüssungsansprache anlässlich der 12. Erfurter Konferenz über Hämostase und Thrombose. **Folia Haematol (Leipz)** 1979;106(5-6):653-5
Vieten B: Medizinstudenten in Münster. Universität, Studentenschaft und Medizin 1905 bis 1945. Köln, Pahl-Rugenstein, 1982. 367 p.
Wilhelm Ebel, ed: Göttinger Universitätsreden aus zwei Jahrhunderten (1737-1934). Göttingen, Vandenhoeck & Ruprecht, 1978. 650 p. (Reprinted lectures by various individuals).
Winter E: Das Dekanatsbuch der Tübinger Medizinischen Fakultät 1808-1858 (Teil 1: 1808-1816). Text und Kommentar. Tübingen, Universitätsarchiv, 1979. 221 p.
Wussing H: 75 Jahre Karl-Sudhoff-Institut für Geschichte der Medizin und der Naturwissenschaften am Bereich Medizin der Karl-Marx-Universität. **NTM** 1981;18(1):2-3

**Great Britain**

Abse D, ed: My medical school. London, Robson, 1978. 211 p.
Anning ST, Walls WK: A history of the Leeds School of Medicine: one and a half centuries, 1831-1981. [Leeds], Leeds University Press, 1982. xiv, 170 p.
Archibald RM: A short historical note on the Conjoint DIH. **J Soc Occup Med** 1984 Aug;34(3):80
Arton M: The development of psychiatric nursing education in England and Wales. **Nurs Times** 1981 Jan 15;77(3):124-7
Baly M: A new history of nursing. Three. The nurse élite (Florence Nightingale). **Nurs Times** 1984 Oct 17-23;80(42):55-7
Blanco RL: The diary of Jonathan Potts: a Quacker medical student in Edinburgh (1766-67). **Trans Stud Coll Physicians Phila** 1977 Jan;44(3):119-30
Bowen P: The early days of postgraduate medical television in London. **J Audiov Media Med** 1980 Oct;3(4):134-5
Carrillo JL, Olagüe G: La enseñanza de la anatomia comparada en la Inglaterra de comienzos del siglo XIX: a proposito de las Lectures de Everard Home (1756-1832). **Asclepio** 1978-79;30-31:83-8
Chitnis AC: Universities, medicine and science. In his: The Scottish Enlightenment: a social history. 279 pp. London: Croom Helm; Totawa, N.J.: Rowman & Littlefield, 1976. p. 124-94.
Cocker W: A history of the university chemical laboratory, Trinity College, Dublin. **Hermathena** 1978;124:58-76
Davies C: Past and present in nursing education. **Nurs Times** 1980 Sep 25;76(39):1703-7
Doll R: Green College, Oxford: its contribution to clinical medicine. **Br Med J [Clin Res]** 1982 Dec 18-25;285(6357):1805-6
Donnelly FK: The destruction of the Sheffield School of Anatomy in 1835: a popular response to class legislation. **Trans Hunter Archaeol Soc** 1975;10:167-72
Douglas H: Burke and Hare. **Br Hist Illus** 1978-79;5(5):32-43
Elliott A, Freeling P, Owen J: District nurse training. **J R Coll Gen Pract** 1980 Feb;30(211):69-74
Farr AD: Learn, that you may improve: the history of the Institute of Medical Laboratory Sciences. Sussex, Denley Instruments, 1982. xi, 214 p.
Forbes TR: 'To be dissected and anatomized.' **J Hist Med Allied Sci** 1981 Oct;36(4):490-2
Fozzard JA: Professors of anatomy in the University of Cambridge: the first two hundred and sixty-one years of the Cambridge University Department of Anatomy, 1707-1968. Cambridge, FOSSLIA, 1983. 87 p.
Garralda Hualde ME: El modelo inglés de formación en psiquiatría infantil. **Actas Luso Esp Neurol Psiquiatr** 1981 Mar-Apr;9(2):103-12
Hermelin R: A law to last the century? **Spec Educ Forward Trends** 1981 Dec;8(4):6-7
Heron JR: Louis Pasteur: the nature of his illness. In Passmore R, ed: Proceedings of the Royal College of Physicians of Edinburgh Tercentenary Congress, 1981. Edinburgh, Royal College of Physicians of Edinburgh, 1982. p. 116-27.
Horder JP, Swift G: The history of vocational training for general practice. **J R Coll Gen Pract** 1979 Jan;29(198):24-32
Jenkins EW: The development of school biology, 1918-1945. **Hist Educ** 1979;8(1):59-73
Jones AT: The new medical centre and the development of medical education in Wales. In J. Cule, ed: Wales and medicine. London, British Society for the History of Medicine, 1975. p. 23-29.
Jones EW: Addysg feddygol i ferched: cyfraniadau o gymru at agor y cyndyn ddorau. **Cylchgrawn Llyfrgell Genedlaethol Cymru** 1976;19(3):249-92
Koblenzer PJ: Edinburgh's influence on medicine in the new world. In Passmore R, ed: Proceedings of the Royal College of Physicians of Edinburgh Tercentenary Congress, 1981. Edinburgh, Royal College of Physicians of Edinburgh, 1982. p. 143-58.
Lenoir T: The Göttingen School and the development of transcendental Naturphilosophie in the Romantic Era. **Stud Hist Biol** 1981;5:111-205
Levere TH: Dr. Thomas Beddoes at Oxford: radical politics in 1788-1793 and the fate of the Regius Chair in Chemistry. **Ambix** 1981 Jul;28(2):61-9
MacLeod R, Moseley R: Fathers and daughters: reflections on women, science, and Victorian Cambridge. **Hist Educ** 1979;8:321-33
McMichael J: Sir Francis Richard Fraser. In Dictionary of national biography, 1961-1970. Suppl. 8, 1981. p. 393-4.
Maulitz RC: Channel crossing: the lure of French pathology for English medical students, 1816-36. **Bull Hist Med** 1981 Winter;55(4):475-96
Mazumdar PM: Anatomical physiology and the reform of medical education: London, 1825-1835. **Bull Hist Med** 1983 Summer;57(2):230-46
Nuttall RH: The Department of Pure and Applied Chemistry: a history 1830-1980. Glasgow, University of Strathclyde, 1980. 16 p.
Ostromęcka H: Z badań nad dziejami polskiego wydziału lekarskiego przy Uniwersytecie w Edynburgu. **Kwart Hist Nauki Tech** 1982;27(2):291-311
Pearson ES, ed: The history of statistics in the 17th and 18th centuries against the changing background of intellectual, scientific and religious thought. Lectures by Karl Pearson given at University College London during the academic sessions 1921-1933. New York, Macmillan, 1978. xix, 744 p.
Peterson MJ: Gentlemen and medical men: the problem of professional recruitment. **Bull Hist Med** 1984 Winter;58(4):457-73
Prince J: Education for a profession: some lessons from history (Florence Nightingale). **Int J Nurs Stud** 1984;21(3):153-63
Roberts GK: The establishment of the Royal College of Chemistry: an investigation of the social context of early-Victorian chemistry. **Hist Stud Phys Sci** 1976;7:437-85
Stewart J: Women pioneers of medicine. **Midwife Health Visit Community Nurse** 1983 Jun;20(6):240, 242
Swift G: Recollections and reflections: general practice since 1946. **J R Coll Gen Pract** 1982 Aug;32(241):471-9
Thomson DM: General practice and the Edinburgh Medical School: 200 years of teaching, care and research. **J R Coll Gen Pract** 1984 Jan;34(258):9-12
Tomaszewski W: The Polish School of Medicine at the University of

Edinburgh: an album. Edinburgh, W. Tomaszewski, 1983. 164 p.
Weaver JA: A hospital for all seasons. **Ulster Med J** 1984;53(1):18–32
Wilson C: Sir Arthur William Mickle Ellis. In Dictionary of national biography, 1961–1970. Suppl. 8, 1981. p. 330–2.
Wilson HD: A hundred years of the Ettles scholarship at the University of Edinburgh or 'Whatever happened to the likely lads (and lasses)?' **Med Educ** 1981 Nov;15(6):359–62

**Greece**

Degleris N, Rozos B: L'Academie Ionienne, la première faculté de médecine dans les Balkans. Athènes, Université d'Athènes, Chaire de l'Histoire de la Médecine, 1979. 24 p.
Degleris NE, Rozos BP: [Public health, medical education and social care of Ionian Isles in the middle of the 19th century (press documents)] (Gre). **Arch Hyg** 1980;:90–101

**Hungary**

Hidvégi L: Toldy Ferenc ceglédi iskolaéveiröl. **Orv Hetil** 1984 Sep 2;125(36):2203–5
Kosáry D: Akadémiai tervek a 18. századi magyarországon. **Tortenelmi Sz** 1979;22(2):341–54
Kötay P: Rácz Sámuel és a magyar orvosi oktatás hajnala. **Orv Hetil** 1982 Jan 10;123(2):103–9
Lambrecht M: A magyar klinikai oktatás hallei mint ája. Johann Juncker, az orvospedagógus. **Orv Hetil** 1982 Jul 11;123(28):1745–8
Marsovszky P: Egy közel 200 éves orvosi disszertáció a skorbutról. **Orvostort Kozl** 1979;87–88(25 no 1–2):303–5
Néhány F: Farkas Géza professzorról a tanítványai. **Orv Hetil** 1984 Nov 11;125(46):2817
Réti E: Idées d'avant-garde dans les thèses hongroises séculaires. **Orvostort Kozl** 1979;86(24 no 4):73–9
Szílási A: A magyar nyelvü belgyógyászati oktatás kezdete. **Orv Hetil** 1979 Oct 7;120(40):2435–7

**India**

Chatterjee PK: Medical education in India since independence. **J Indian Med Assoc** 1981 Sep;77(5–6):91–5
Subba Reddy DV: Prelude to upgraded Department of History of Medicine, Hyderabad. **Bull Indian Inst Hist Med Hyderabad** 1982;12(1–4):92–9

**Ireland**

Bendiner E: The Dublin school: from poverty, a rich legacy. **Hosp Pract [Off]** 1984 Jun;19(6):221–47
Froggatt P: The resignation of Robert Little from the chair of midwifery at Inst [Academical Institution, Belfast] **Ulster Med J** 1979;48(1):19–31
Murphy T: The changing university. **Ir Med J** 1981 Jul;74(7):184–7
Widdess JD: The Royal College of Surgeons in Ireland and its medical school, 1784–1984. Third edition. Dublin, Royal College of Surgeons in Ireland, 1984. x, 194 p.

**Italy**

Armoroli M, ed: Le cere anatomiche Bolognesi del settecento. Catalogo della mostra organizzata Settembre–Novembre 1981. Bologna, Università degli Studi di Bologna, Accademia delle Scienze, 1981. 97 p. Contributions by R. A. Bernabeo, L. Bonuzzi, F. Ruggeri.
Azzaroli ML, Lanza B: La Venere scomponibile. **Kos** 1984 May;1(4):65–81
Balbo T: In memoria di Edoardo Perroncito nel centenario di fondazione della prima Cattedra di Parassitologia. **Parassitologia** 1980 Dec;22(3):233–7
Dondi RF: Vicende dell'Universita' degli Studi di Ferrara nella seconda meta' dell'ottocento. **Ann Osp Maria Vittoria Torino** 1980 Jul–Dec;23(7–12):333–42
L'Istituto di Storia della Medicina dell'Università di Padova: Un triennio di attività (Anni Acc. 1976–77/77–78/78–79). Padova, Tipografia 'La Garangola,' 1979. 23 p.
Olagüe G: El discurso de Giovanni Maria Lancisi 'sobre la recta ordenacion de los estudios medicos segun la razon' (1715). **Asclepio** 1981;33:143–62
Olagüe G: El programa de reforma educativa de Giovanni Maria Lancisi: De recta medicorum studiorum ratione instituenda (1715). **Episteme** 1976 Jan–Dec;1–4:180–9
Premuda L: G. B. Morgagni und seine Vorstellungen über die Methodik der Medizin. **Sudhoffs Arch** 1984;68(2):173–81
Premuda L: The revival of the anatomico–clinical method in Padua: the fundamental contribution of F. S. Verson (1805–1849) from Trieste, a disciple of the Vienna School of Medicine. **Janus** 1980;67(1–2–3):31–9
Squartini F: L'Instituto di Anatomia Patologica di Perugia dall'anno accademico 1941–42 all'anno accademico 1977–78. **Pathologica** 1983 Nov–Dec;75(1040):763–74

**Japan**

Chiba Daigaku Igakubu Hyakushunen Kinenshi Henshu Iinkai: Chiba Daigaku Igakubu hyakushunen kinenshi. Chiba, Japan, Chiba Daigaku Hyakushunen Kinenkai, Showa 53 nen, 1978. xv, 686 p.
Ishigaki Y, Uzawa Y: [Historical review of continuing education in Hokkaido University Hospital] (Jpn). **Kango Tenbo** 1984 Nov;9(11):1021–32
Kishi Y, Uzawa Y, Hanashima T: [Postwar transitions in the theories of nursing education: with special reference to the period between 1945 to 1955] (Jpn) **Kango Kyoiku** 1984 Sep;25(9):541–60
Nakagawa Y: [Medical history in the medical education] (Jpn). **Igakushi Kenkyu** 1978;50:2–10
Nakazato T: [The early days of modern nursing in Japan--the Kyoto School of Nursing] (Jpn). **Kango** 1981 Jan;33(1):70–83
Sapporo Ika Daigaku Soki 30–nenshi Henshu Iinkai: Sapporo Ika Daigaku soki 30–nenshi (Showa 20 nen–Showa 50 nen). Sapporo, Japan, Sapporo Ika Daigaku Soki Sanjunenshi Kankokai, Showa 50 nen, 1975. 488 p.
Tagochi T: [Nursing and nursing education in the past 35 years since the end of the Second World War. (1)] (Jpn) **Kango Kyoiku** 1981 Jan;22(1):34–40
Takada M: [Children who do not know Florence Nightingale: teaching of nursing history at a nursing school] (Jpn). **Kango Kyoiku** 1984 Dec;25(12):725–7

**Lebanon**

Fawaz G: Whither AUB? An excursion through the campus lasting five–score years and ten. **Middle East J Anaesthesiol** 1983 Feb–Jun;7(1 2):9 19
Zablotniak R: Polscy studenci medycyny i farmcji w uniwersytetach bejruckich (1941–1945). **Przegl Lek** 1981;38(1):124–5

**Mexico**

Arreguín E: Datos historicos sobre la fundacion de la escuela medica de Michoacan. **Bol Soc Mex Hist Filos Med** 1980 Sep–Dec;5(32–33):57–65
Frenk J, Hernández–Llamas H, Alvarez–Klein L: Análisis histórico del internado rotatorio de pregrado en México. **Gac Med Mex** 1983 Feb;119(2):87–96
Izquierdo JJ: Los laboratorios para la investigación, la formación y la especialización del profesorado, en la nueva Facultad de Medicina. In Academia Nacional de Medicina. Libro conmemorativo del primer centenario. México, Comité Editorial de la Comisión Organizadora del Congreso del Centenario, 1964. Tome 2. p. 561–5.
Lomnitz L: Hierarchy and peripherality: the organisation of a Mexican research institute. **Minerva** 1979 Winter;17(4):527–48
Micheli A de: El sesquicentenario de la facultad de Medicina de la Universidad Nacional de México (la. parte: 1833–1859). **Arch Inst Cardiol Mex** 1983 May–Jun;53(3):271–6
Micheli A de: El sesquicentenario de la Facultad de Medicina de la Universidad Nacional de México (2a. parte: 1859–1945). **Arch Inst Cardiol Mex** 1983 Jul–Aug;53(4):379–84
Peña Páez I de la, Viesca Treviño C, Casales Ortiz G: Presencia de la cirugía española en México en el siglo XVIII. (Real Colegio de Cirugía). In International Congress of the History of Medicine, 27th, Barcelona, 1980. Actas. Barcelona, Acadèmia de Ciències Mèdiques de Catalunya i Balears, 1981. p. 195–8.
Ramírez Almanza MA: La formación de los médicos y su utilización en el área rural. **Salud Publica Mex** 1983 Sep–Oct;25(5):533–9
Ramos P: El aprendizaje de la gastroenterología. **Rev Gastroenterol Mex** 1982 Jan–Mar;47(1):35–7
Somolinas Palencia J, Campillo Sainz C, Kumate J: Conmemoración del sesquicentenario de la fundación del Establecimiento de Ciencias Médicas. **Gac Med Mex** 1983 Nov;119(11):471–4
Somolinos–Palencia J, Martínez–Cortés F, Sepúlveda B, et al: Etapas de la educación médica en México. **Gac Med Mex** 1984 Jun;120(6):213–28
Somolinos–Palencia J: Gabino Barreda, el educador. **Gac Med Mex** 1981 Sep;117(9):377–81
Somolinos–Palencia J, Corvera–Bernardelli J: Las casas de la Academia. **Gac Med Mex** 1982 Oct;118(10):403–17
Urzais Jimenez C: Reseña historica de la enseñanza medica en Yucatan. **Bol Soc Mex Hist Filos Med** 1984 Dec;7(49):417–30
Véjar–Lacave C: El maestro Ignacio Chávez, la medicina y los problemas educacionales. **Gac Med Mex** 1980 Jan;116(1):43–6

**Nepal**

Shah M: Tribhuvan University Institute of Medicine, Nepal. **Public Health Pap** 1980;2(71):81–96

**Netherlands**

Bool PH: 75 Jaar Centraal Diergeneeskundig Instituut. **Tijdschr Diergeneeskd** 1980 Aug 1;105(15):583–6
Haneveld GT: Koning Willem I en de aankoop van anatomische kabinetten. **Spiegel Hist** 1978;13(7–8):488–95

Heller S: Boerhaaves Schweizer Studenten: ein Beitrag zur Geschichte des Medizinstudiums. Zürich, Juris, 1984. 111 p. (Zürcher Medizingeschichtliche Abhandlungen, Neue Reihe, Nr. 169)
Hes-Swartenberg HS: Abraham Hartog Israels, M.D., 1822-1883: Netherlands' first professor in the history of medicine. **NY State J Med** 1979 Aug;79(9):1445-7
Kegel-Brinkgreve E, Luyendijk-Elshout AM, ed: Boerhaave's orations. Leiden, Leiden University Press, 1983. vi, 374 p.
Lieburg MJ van: De microscopie in het onderwijs van de klinische scholen in Nederland (1824-1865). **Tijdschr Geschied Geneeskd** 1983;6(2):82-98
Mees LF: Kennis en wijsheid, herinneringen aan leermeesters. **Ned Tijdschr Geneeskd** 1980 Aug 9;124(32):1354-6
Püschel E: 'Dictata' zu den Werken von Johannes de Gorter (1689-1762), professor in Harderwijk: medicinae compendium, praxis medicae systema und chirurgia repurgata. **Janus** 1980;67(1-2-3):41-57
Steendijk-Kuypers J: De geneeskundige school te Hoorn (1825-1865). **Tijdschr Geschied Geneeskd** 1980;3(2):49-73
Van Bekkum JG: 75 jaar C. D. I. Ter introduktie. **Tijdschr Diergeneeskd** 1980 Aug 15;105(16):631-5

**New Zealand**

Kinross NJ: Nursing education in New Zealand: a developmental perspective. **Int J Nurs Stud** 1984;21(3):193-9

**Norway**

Fagermoen MS: From apprenticeship to study--the development of nursing education in Norway. **Int J Nurs Stud** 1984;21(3):165-75

**Pacific Islands**

Guthrie MW: Misi Utu, Dr. D. W. Hoodless and the development of medical education in the South Pacific. Suva, Fiji Institute of Pacific Studies, 1979. vi, 60 p.
Penington AH: The Fiji School of Medicine--a brief history. **Hawaii Med J** 1984 Sep;43(9):314, 316, 318

**Poland**

Brzeziński T: Problemy nauczania historii medycyny w Polsce. **Arch Hist Med (Warsz)** 1979;42(3):379-82
Ceypek T: Uzupełnienie do artykułu pt. 'Klinika Laryngologii w 30-leciu Slaskiej Akademii Medycznej'. **Otolaryngol Pol** 1979;33(6):671-2
Chrzęściewski L: Jędrzej śniadecki (1768-1838) - prekursor współczesnej myśli pedagogicznej w medycynie. **Arch Hist Med (Warsz)** 1983;46(1):29-38
Chyrek-Borowska S: XXX lat Akademii Medycznej im. J. Marchlewskiego w Białymstoku. Białystok, Krajowa Agencja Wydawnicza, 1980. 87 p.
Dabrowski S: Wspomnienia z okresu studiów na wydziale lekarskim uniwersytetu poznańskiego (1935-1945). **Arch Hist Med (Warsz)** 1983;46(1):67-90
Dawidowicz A: Tajne nauczanie medycyny i farmacji w latach 1939-1945. Warszawa, Państwówy Zakład Wydawn. Lekarskich, 1977. 398 p.
Dorsz-Szteke E: Nauczanie medycyny na Pomorzu Zachodnim w i poł. XVIII wieku. **Arch Hist Med (Warsz)** 1980;43(3):305-16
Ginalska A: 35 lat mineło. Szkole Pielegniarstwa w Chełmie. **Pieleg Polozna** 1984;(4):26-8
Góral R: Akademia Medyczna w Poznaniu--osiągniecia i perspektywy rozwoju. **Nauka Pol** 1977;25(4):55-72
Heimrath T, Smereka J: Lekarze polscy wykształceni we wrocławskiej Klinice Kobiecej w latach 1811--1918. **Arch Hist Med (Warsz)** 1979;42(3):345-9
Iwankiewicz S, Kossowski S: Klinika Otolaryngologiczna AM we Wrocławiu (1948-1978). **Otolaryngol Pol** 1980;34(2-3):141-65
Kapronczay K: A krakkói orvosi kar 200 éves reformja. **Orv Hetil** 1980 Oct 19;121(42):2596-8
Kapronczay K: Az orvostörténelem oktatása a krakkói egyetemen. **Orv Hetil** 1979 Sep 23;120(38):2315-7
Kielanowski T: Powstanie i organizacja Akademii Medycznej w Białymtoku. **Kwart Hist Nauki Tech** 1980;25(2):299-318
Konopka S: Relacje profesorów Wydziału lekarskiego Uniwersytetu Jagiellonskiego o dziejach medycyny polskiej. **Arch Hist Med (Warsz)** 1979;42(1):107-24
Krus S: Sylwetki niektórych profesorów Warszawskiej Akademii Medycznej. Wystapienie na posiedzeniu Towarzystwa Lekarskiego Warszawskiego w dniu 24 IV 1980 r. **Pol Tyg Lek** 1980 Dec 15;35(50):1981-4
Kruś S: Tradycje historyczne Warszawskiej Akademii Medycznej. **Pol Tyg Lek** 1981 Jul 20;36(29):1123-7
Kucharz E: Herman Fudakowski--pierwszy kierownik katedry chemii lekarskiej w Warszawie. **Wiad Lek** 1980 Jun 1;33(11):931-4
Leszczak M: 200 lat. **Pieleg Polozna** 1984;(3):30-1
Pacyńska M, Kedzia A, Smereka J: Tematy neurologiczne w pracach doktorskich polaków studiujacych we Wrocławiu w XIX wieku. **Arch Hist Med (Warsz)** 1980;43(2):199-204
Rybak J: Tradycje Krakowskiej Szkoły Połżnych. **Pieleg Polozna** 1980;(3):25-7
Sarnecka-Keller M: Biochemia na Uniwersytecie Jagiellońskim: Przesylość i terazniejszość. **Stud Mater Dziejow Nauk Pol** 1981;25:87-105
Schneck P: Die medizinische Fakultät an der Universität Krakau zur Zeit des Herzogtums Warschau (1809-1815). **Arch Hist Med (Warsz)** 1979;42(2):251-5
Skulimowski M, Sliwiński S: Zwiazki Jana Nepomucena Rusta (1775--1840) z Krakowskim Fakultetem Medycznym. **Arch Hist Med (Warsz)** 1979;42(2):245-9
Smereka J: Rozprawy doktorskie obronione przez lekarzy polskich we Wrocławskiej Klinice Okulistycznej przed r. 1918. **Klin Oczna** 1979 Nov;81(11):635-6
Sosińska-Trawińska M, Sródka A: O utworzeniu Wydziałów Lekarskich W polskich instytucjach naukowych. I. Polska Akademia Umiejętności (PAU). **Arch Hist Med (Warsz)** 1981;44(3/4):363-7
Sródka A, Sosińska-Trawińska M: O utworzeniu Wydziałow Lekarskich w polskich instytucjach naukowych. II. Towarzystwo Naukowe Warszawskie (TNW). **Arch Hist Med (Warsz)** 1982;45(1-4):81-4
Stanisława Leszczyńska nasza patronka: **Pieleg Polozna** 1984;(3):29
Stembrowicz W: Tłumaczenie z jezyka łacińskiego pracy na stopień doktora medycyny z 1829 roku Józefa Lewickiego o osłuchiwaniu i opukiwaniu. **Arch Hist Med (Warsz)** 1984;47(1):49-74
Szymańska R: Karol Klecki (1866-1931) - wybitny patofizjolog i profesor Fakultetu Medycznego w Krakowie (w 50 rocznicę śmierci). **Pol Tyg Lek** 1981 Sep 21;36(38):1487-90
Szymczykiewicz K: XXX lat działalności Instytutu Medycyny Pracy w Sosnowcu. **Med Pr** 1981;32(5):309-15
Tkaczewski W: Dwudziestopi ęciolecie Wojskowej Akademii Medycznej im. gen. dyw. prof. Bolesława Szareckiego. **Pol Tyg Lek** 1983 Jul 11-18;38(28-29):857-9
Urban A: Konspiracyjna działalnść dydaktyczna profesor Janiny Kowalczykowej w okresie okupacji 1939-1944. **Patol Pol** 1980 Apr-Jun;31(2):161-9
Wadecki Z: Nadgraniczny jubileusz. **Pieleg Polozna** 1984;(2):27
Wunderlich P: Zur Geschichte der Universitäts-Kinderklinik in Breslau unter Adalbert Czerny (1863--1941) von 1894--1910. **Arch Hist Med (Warsz)** 1979;42(3):337-43

**Portugal**

Guerra M: Origens do ensino da história da medicina em Portugal. **Acta Med Port** 1980 Sep-Dec;2(5-6):335-6
Ses MO de: As dissertações finais centenárias da Escola Médico-Cirurgica do Porto - 1967. **Arch Hist Med Port** 1968-70;3(1-4):35-50

**Puerto Rico**

Cruz Dones A: Escuela de Enfermería de la Clínica Díaz García. **Bol Col Prof Enferm PR** 1982 Sep;8(31):23

**Romania**

Bratescu G: Des préliminaires de la création des Facultés de Médecine de Bucarest et de Jassy. **Noesis** 1981;7:63-7
Centenarul Institutului de Medicină şi Farmacie din Iaşi (1879-1979): **Rev Med Chir Soc Med Nat Iasi** 1979 Oct-Dec;83(4):727-32
Costea V: Cîteva date din activitatea primilor trei profesori titulari ai clinicii dermato-venerologice: Gh. Demetriade, E. I. Mironescu şi Gh. Nastase (1901-1962). **Rev Med Chir Soc Med Nat Iasi** 1983 Jan-Mar;87(1):149-55
Cotrău M: Procesful cottorului Carol Davila (Iaşi, 1872). **Rev Med Chir Soc Med Nat Iasi** 1980 Apr-Jun;84(2):325-6
Diculescu I, Onicescu D: At the hundredth anniversary of the Department of Histology of the Bucharest Faculty of Medicine. **Morphol Embryol (Bucur)** 1980 Jul-Sep;26(3):199-204
Munteanu A, Dobrescu G, Cotuţiu C, et al: The 100th anniversary of the Jassy Faculty of Medicine and an historical approach to the evolution of its department of histology. **Morphol Embryol (Bucur)** 1980 Oct-Dec;26(4):371-3
Negru I: O şcoală de surori de ocrotire mai puţin cunoscută-şcoala din Timişoara (septembrie 1939-februarie 1942). **Viata Med [Medii Sanit]** 1984 Jul;32(7):163-6
Scripcaru G: Traditia si actualitatea relatiei dintre învătămîntul medical si Societatea de Medici si Naturalisti. **Rev Med Chir Soc Med Nat Iasi** 1980 Oct-Dec;84(4):629-35
Scripcaru G: Un secol de învătămînt medical universitar la Iaşi. **Rev Med Chir Soc Med Nat Iasi** 1979 Oct-Dec;83(4):557-63

**Singapore**

Lee YK: The founding of the medical school in Singapore (Part I). **Singapore Med J** 1980 Jun;21(3):544-55
Lee YK: The founding of the medical school in Singapore (Part II). **Singapore Med J** 1980 Aug;21(4):666-76
Ratnam SS, Karim SM, Ng CS, et al: Research and development in obstetrics and gynaecology in the Department of Obstetrics and Gynaecology at the National University of Singapore. **Ann Acad Med Singapore** 1982 Jul;11(3):313-21

Tan NC: The Academy of Medicine of Singapore. **Ann Acad Med Singapore** 1982 Jul;11(3):307–8

Wong HB: Postgraduate medical education in Singapore. **Ann Acad Med Singapore** 1982 Jul;11(3):473–7

### South Africa

Daubenton F: Professor Cuthbert Crichton--the man and his times. **S Afr Med J** 1979 Dec 15;56(25):1064–75

Louw JH: A brief history of the Medical Faculty, University of Cape Town. **S Afr Med J** 1979 Nov 24;56(22):864–70

Louw JH: Professor Eric Cuthbert Crichton's contribution to the medical school. **S Afr Med J** 1979 Dec 15;56(25):1075–84

Luyt R: The Medical School of the University of Cape Town. **S Afr Med J** 1979 Nov 24;56(22):861–2

McKenzie D: Die mediese fakulteit van die universiteit van Kaapstad. **S Afr Med J** 1979 Nov 24;56(22):862–3

Nel CJ: Die departement chirurgie, universiteit van die oranje-vrystaat--die eerste tien jaar. **S Afr J Surg** 1980 Sep;19(3):81–6

Retief FP: The Medical University of Southern Africa after 5 years. **S Afr Med J** 1982 Nov 27;62(23)841–5

Sandler EM: C. Louis Leipoldt--medical student extraordinary. **Adler Mus Bull** 1981 Oct;7(3):8–14

Sharp RG: Tribute to a great teacher. **S Afr Med J** 1979 Dec 15;56(25):1059–64

Sloan AW: Highlights of physiological research at the University of Cape Town, 1912–1978. **S Afr Med J** 1979 Nov 24;56(22):974–6

### Spain

Arques J, Suñe JM: Razones que motivaron la individualizacion de la Catedra de Historia de la Farmacia de la Universidad Central, en 1896. **Bol Soc Esp Hist Farm** 1983 Mar–Jun;34(133–134):3–10

Balaguer Perigüell E, Ballester Añon R: El colegio di cirugía de Zaragoza, intento de renovación de las instituciones médicas aragonesas. 2. Jornadas sobre el estado actual de los Estudios sobre Aragón, diciembre de 1979, Esp. 1980: 713–8.

Ferrer D: Dictamen solicitando la erección de los actuales edificios de la Facultad de Medicina y Hospital Clínico de Barcelona. In Congrés International d'Història de la Medicina Catalana, 2nd, Barcelona, 1975. Llibre d'Actes. Barcelona, Socitra, 1977. p. 249–58.

Ferrer D: Representación para el establecimiento de un Colegio de Ciruxia en Barcelona a la manera del de Cádiz (1759). In Congrés International d'Història de la Medicina Catalana, 2nd, Barcelona, 1975. Llibre d'Actes. Barcelona, Socitra, 1977. p. 259–61.

Franco Grande A, Ginesta Galán F, Martinón Sanchez JM: Primeras tesis doctorales sobre anestesia en lengua castellana. **Rev Esp Anestesiol Reanim** 1980 Jul;27(4):357–61

Gago R, Olagüe G, Carrillo JL, et al: El plan de estudios del rector Blasco (1786) y la renovacion de las disciplinas cientificas en la Universidad de Valencia: la quimica y la enseñanza clinica. **Estudis** 1977;6:157–65

García del Carrizo San Millán MG: Breve apunte sobre los estudios histologicos en el departamento de anatomia de San Carlos hasta la creacion de la catedra de histologia. **Asclepio** 1978–79;30–31:89–97

Garcia Gonzalez R, Prieto Cantero A: Licenciados en medicina y cirugia graduados en la Universidad de Valladolid (1871–1936). Vallodolid, Universidad de Valladolid, 1979. 383 p. (Acta Historico-Medica Vallisoletana, Monografias, IX)

García Guerra D: La 'Disertacion medica' de Fernando Oxea. Un testimonio de auscultacion inmediata del torax en el siglo XVIII. **Asclepio** 1980;32:201–9

Jaqueti G: Profesor José Gay Prieto. Maestro de dermatólogos (1905–1979). **Actas Dermosifiliogr** 1981 Jul–Aug;72(7–8):389–96

Kagan RL: From trade to profession: surgical education in eighteenth-century Spain. **Hist Educ Q** 1978;18(2):195–200

Montiel L: La influencia de la ideologia en la clinica medica del S. XIX español. La obra de Tomas Santero y Moreno (1817–1888). **Asclepio** 1981;33:127–42

Navarro Brotóns V: Juan Bautista Corachán y la enseñanza universitaria. In: Estudios de historia de Valencia. Valencia, Universidad, Facultad de Derecho, 1978. p. 279–92

Peset M, Mancebo MF, Peset JL: Estudiantes medicos en Valencia durante la primera mitad del XVIII. **Asclepio** 1980;32:311–25

Riera J: Antonio Cibat y la catedra de fisica experimental de Barcelona (un proyecto de 1807). **Asclepio** 1980;32:383–8

Riera J: Los viajes de estudios de Andres del Rio (un documento de 1794). **Asclepio** 1980;32:361–5

Ruiz-Falcó López F: Escuela Nacional de Sanidad. Problemática pasada, actual y futura. **Rev Sanid Hig Publica (Madr)** 1983 Mar–Apr;57(3–4):359–72

Vitoria M: Universidad Padre Vitoria. Facultad de Medicina de Bilbao 1936–1937. **Gac Med Bilbao** 1981;78:1–54

### Sweden

Ahlström CG: Patologisk anatomi i Lund, 1668–1962. Lund, 1983. 155 p. (Sydsvenska Medicinhistoriska Sällskapets Arsskrift, Suppl. 2, 1983).

Erikson B: Sjuksköterskeutbildningen i Sverige genom tiderna. **Nord Medicinhist Arsb** 1980;Suppl 6:69–75

Fagerheim E: Lars Levi Laestadius' teologiske studier. **Nor Teol Tidsskr** 1972;73(1):35–50

Gejrot T: Medikofilosofisk examen; om medikofilare och medikofilen. **Sydsven Medicinhist Sallsk Arsskr** 1982;19:45–53

Kahlson G: Upprustning av naturvetenskaplig och medicinsk forskning. **Sydsven Medicinhist Sallsk Arsskr** 1981;:44–52

Kock W: Ett filosofiskt tackbrev från Israel Hwasser. **Nord Medicinhist Arsb** 1980;:90–8

Kock W: Från Sjukwakterska till sjuksköterska. **Nord Medicinhist Arsb** 1984;:129–35

Larsson J: Kirurgi och medicinsk teori vid Lunds Universitet under 1700–talet. En medicinhistorisk studie. (Supplementum nr 1). **Sydsven Medicinhist Sallsk Arsskr** 1982;Suppl V:1–262

Schramm E: Linné, Gedner und die biologische Kontrolle. **Medizinhist J** 1984;19(3):244–9

Westin M: Så var det då. **Sjukskoterskan** 1984 Apr;:17–20

### Switzerland

Boyer M: Hier et aujourd'hui: l'école d'infirmières de La Source. **Krankenpflege Soins Infirm** 1984 May;77(5):38–43

Cramer M, Starobinski J, ed, Barblan MA: Centenaire de la Faculté de Médecine de l'Université de Genève. Genève, Editions Médecine et hygiène, 1978. xvi, 165 p.

Fankhauser R, Hörning B: 175 Jahre tierärztliche Lehranstalt zu Bern. **Schweiz Arch Tierheilkd** 1980 Feb;122(2):57–94

Jucker-Wannier E: Zum Jubiläumsjahr der Ingenbohler Schwestern. Ein Rückblick auf Festfeiern und Ausstellung an der Schule für allgemeine Krankenpflege des Instituts Ingenbohl am St.-Clara-Spital Basel. **Krankenpflege (Bern)** 1980 Aug;(8):406–7

Koelbing HM: Akademische Medizin und Offentlichkeit. Rektoratsreden von Zürcher Medizinern seit 1933. In Ganzinger K, Skopec M, Wyklicky H, ed: Festschrift für Erna Lesky zum 70. Geburtstag. Wien, Brüder Hollinek, 1981. p. 49–55.

Leisibach M: Das Medizinisch-chirurgische Institut in Zürich, 1782–1833: Vorläufer der Medizinischen Fakultät der Universität Zürich. Zürich, Rohr, 1982. 136, [39] p.

Miéville C: Fortbildungskurs der Schweizerischen Gesellschaft für Psychiatrie. Biologische Aspekte der Psychiatrie. Eröffnung. **Schweiz Arch Neurol Neurochir Psychiatr** 1979;125(2):187–91

Mordacq C: Ecoles et soignants d'hier à demain, ou les sources du renouvellement d'une institution d'enseignement professionnel. **Krankenpflege (Bern)** 1981 Feb;(2):15–9

Morscher E: Entwicklungen in der Chirurgie: das Department Chirurgie der Universität Basel 1967–1983. Basel, Schwabe, 1983. 192 p.

Pfohl G: Medizin und Philologie--Allgemeine humanistische Bildung als Anliegen des Schweizer Medizinhistorikers Charles Lichtenthaeler. **Med Welt** 1980 Nov 7;31(45):1651

Picco C: Das Biochemische Institut der Universität Zürich 1931–1981. Aarau, Verlag Sauerländer, 1981. 62 p. (Veröffentlichungen der Schweizerischen Gesellschaft für Geschichte der Medizin und der Naturwissenschaften, 37).

Rintelen F: Geschichte der Medizinischen Fakultät in Basel 1900–1945. Basel/Stuttgart, Schwabe, 1980. 454 p.

Terrier G: Louis Secrétan et les débuts de l'enseignement de l'ORL en Suisse Romande. **Acta Otorhinolaryngol Belg** 1982;36(2):306–10

Töndury G: Anatomie in Zürich. **Gesnerus** 1980;37(3/4):271–87

Waser PG: Walter Rudolf Hess. Aus seinem Leben und seiner Tätigkeit an der Medizinischen Fakultät der Universität Zürich. **Gesnerus** 1982;39(2):279–86

### Thailand

Goldstein MS, Donaldson PJ: Exporting professionalism: a case study of medical education. **J Health Soc Behav** 1979 Dec;20(4):322–37

### Tunisia

Ben Yedder W: Enseignement para médical en Tunisie. L'école professionnelle de la santé publique de Tunis 'Avicenne'. **Tunis Med** 1981 Jan–Feb;59(1):874–5

### Turkey

Gençer AI: Istanbul tersansesinde acilan ilk tib mektebi **Tarih Dergesi (Turkey)** 1977;31:301–16

Kâhya E: Bízde díseksíyon ne zaman ve nasil başladi? **Belleten (Turk)** 1979;43(172):739–59

Uyer G: Nursing education in Turkey: past and present. **Int J Nurs Stud** 1984;21(3):209–19

### United States

Alsobrook DE: Mobile v. Birmingham: the Alabama Medical College controversy, 1912–1920. **Ala Rev** 1983;36(1):37–56

Annegers JH: Department of Physiology Northwestern University Medical School. **Physiologist** 1983 Jun;26(3):120-1
Antler J: Medical women and social reform--a history of the New York Infirmary for Women and Children. **Women Health** 1976 Jul-Aug;1(4):11-15,18
Arena JM: Medical student life at Duke fifty years ago. **NC Med J** 1983 Apr;44(4):235-7
At the turn-of-the-decade: **J Iowa Med Soc** 1980 Apr;70(4):144-58
Atwater EC: 'Making fewer mistakes': a history of students and patients. **Bull Hist Med** 1983 Summer;57(2):165-87
Austin AL: Isabel Maitland Stewart. In: Notable American women. The modern period. Cambridge, Mass., Belknap-Harvard Univ. Press, 1980. 4:660-2.
Baird WD: Medical education in Arkansas, 1879-1978. Memphis, Memphis State University Press, 1979. 505 p.
Baker GL: The medical curriculum--from the 70's into the 80's. **J Iowa Med Soc** 1980 Apr;70(4):159-60
Balog CE: History, medicine, and culture: history for science students. **Indiana Soc Stud Q** 1980-81;33(3):53-62
Barger AC: Some of Carl Walter's contributions to Harvard Medical School and Hospitals. **Am J Surg** 1984 Nov;148(5):578-80
Barker WH, Jonas S: The teaching of preventive medicine in American medical schools, 1940-1980. **Prev Med** 1981 Nov;10(6):674-88
Barlow W, Powell DO: A case for medical coeducation in the 1870s. **J Am Med Wom Assoc** 1980 Dec;35(12):285-8
Barlow W, Powell DO: Homeopathy and sexual equality: the controversy over coeducation at Cincinnati's Pulte Medical College, 1873-1879. **Ohio Hist** 1981 Spring;90(2):101-13
Barnhill JF: An epoch of medical education. **Indiana Med Hist Q** 1975;3(1):53-63
Barrow MV, Stetson CA: Origin and development of University of Florida College of Medicine. **J Fla Med Assoc** 1980 Mar;67(3):279-82
Baserga SJ: The early years of coeducation at the Yale University School of Medicine. **Yale J Biol Med** 1980 May-Jun;53(3):181-90
Bauriedel K: Early continuing medical education in dermatology. **Int J Dermatol** 1981 Nov;20(9):614-5
Beatty WK: Bayard Taylor Holmes--a forgotten man. **Proc Inst Med Chic** 1981 Oct-Dec;34(4):120-3
Beatty WK: Nathan Smith Davis: observer, motivator, and doer. **Proc Inst Med Chic** 1980 Jul-Sep;33(3):88-90
Beebe RT: Albany Medical College and Albany Hospital: a history, 1839-1982. Albany, N. Y., New Art Printing, 1983. xxv, 458 p.
Behn RD, Sperduto K: Medical Schools and the 'entitlement ethic'. **Public Interest** 1979;57:48-68
Beljan JR: Medical education: historical perspectives and future directions. **Aviat Space Environ Med** 1979 Nov;50(11):1161-5
Bendiner E: Past and present: Elizabeth Blackwell: 'heresy with intelligence'. **Hosp Pract** Jun;15(6):1821-1910
Benison S, Barger AC, Wolfe EL: Changing of the guard. **Harv Med Alumni Bull** 1982 Spring;56(2):34-41
Bennett JL: Room M-112: Medical Sciences Building. **J Fla Med Assoc** 1980 Mar;67(3):251-7
Bergen SS: Medical education of New Jersey: the development of UMDNJ. **J Med Soc NJ** 1984 Sep;81(9):791-7
Bingham M: Medical education at Hartford Hospital: an historical review. **Conn Med** 1979 Nov;43(11):683-6
Bixler RH: The Psychology Department at the University of Louisville, 1907-1953. **Filson Club Hist Q** 1983;57(3):253-69
Blain D, Barton M: The history of American psychiatry: a teaching and research guide. Washington, American Psychiatric Association, 1979. iv, 44 p. Contributions by D. F. Musto, G. Mora, E. T. Carlson.
Bluemle LW: Jefferson College and Thomas Jefferson University. In Medical-Science colloquium. Special edition of Topic: a journal of the liberal arts. Washington, Pennsylvania, Washington and Jefferson College, 1983. p. 39.
Blythe WB, et al: Walter Reece Berryhill. **NC Med J** 1984 Oct;45(10):615-29
Bonsett CA: Mystery photo: why was it shown to med students? **J Indiana State Med Assoc** 1980 Mar;73(3):123
Bowers JZ: A note on the history of medical education in the United States. **Dan Med Bull** 1980 May;27(Suppl 1):4-5
Bowman IA, ed: UTMB: eighty years ago. **Bookman** 1983 May-Jun;10(3):3-10
Brandt AM: Virginia Kneeland Frantz. In: Notable American women. The modern period. Cambridge, Mass., Belknap-Harvard Univ. Press, 1980. 4:247-8.
Brandt EN: Medical education: the past 80 years. **Tex Med** 1980 May;76(5):4-5
Bridgforth LR: Medical education in Mississippi. Ph.D. Diss., Memphis State University. Memphis, 1982. vii, 400 p.
Brieger GH: 'Fit to study medicine': notes for a history of pre-medical education in America. **Bull Hist Med** 1983;57(1):1-21
Brieger GH: Medical education in the Far West. **J West** 1982 Jul;21(3):42-8
Brodie B: One long step: Virginia nursing moves into the university setting. **Va Nurse** 1983 Winter;51(4):201-4
Brown ER: He who pays the piper: foundations, the medical profession, and medical education. In Reverby S, Rosner D, ed: Health care in America. Philadelphia, Temple University Press, 1979. p. 132-54.
Brown JM: History of masters education in nursing in the United States, 1945-1969. Ed.D. Diss., Columbia University. New York, 1979. 225 leaves.
Brown M: History of the formation of the UW School of Veterinary Medicine. **J Vet Med Educ** 1982;8:105-8
Brozěk J: David Jayne Hill: between the old and the new psychology. In J. Brozěk, ed: Explorations in the history of psychology in the United States. Lewisburg, Bucknell University Press, 1984. p. 121-47.
Bryant BJ: The Harvard residency program in otolaryngology: an overview. **Am J Otol** 1979 Jul;1(1):60-3
Bryant BJ: The residency program in otolaryngology at Baylor College of Medicine. **Am J Otol** 1979 Oct;1(2):132-4
Buell FD: Nineteenth century surgeon: Dr. Alden March, founder, Albany Medical College, 1795-1869. Albany, Albany Medical College, 1981. 12 p.
Bullough B, Bullough V: Education problems in a woman's profession. **JNE** 1981 Sep;20(7):6-17
Bulmer M: The early institutional establishment of social science research: the local community research committee at the University of Chicago, 1923-30. **Minerva** 1980 Spring;18(1):51-110
Burke CB: American collegiate population: a test of the traditional view. New York, London, New York Univ. Press, 1982. ix, 373 p.
Burnett JW: Reflections of a dermatology professor. **Cutis** 1984 May;33(5):471-4
Butcher HR: Evarts Graham and surgical residency education. **J Thorac Cardiovasc Surg** 1984 Nov;88(5 Pt 2):848-50
Campbell P: Medical education for an African colonist. **Md Hist Mag** 1970;65(2):130-7
Cangi EC: Abraham Flexner's philanthrophy: the full-time system in the department of surgery at the University of Cincinnati College of Medicine, 1910-1930. **Bull Hist Med** 1982 Summer;56(2):160-74
Carroll D: The contribution of the Johns Hopkins University School of Medicine. **Md State Med J** 1981 Oct;30(10):76-8
Carroll D: The University of Maryland School of Medicine, 1807-1920. **Md State Med J** 1981 Jun;30(6):35-50
Cash P: Pride, prejudice and politics. **Harv Med Alumni Bull** 1980 Dec;54(6):20-5
Castaing L, Chapman C, Rooker C, et al: This I remember...An informal history of Louisiana State University School of Medicine. New Orleans, Louisiana State University School of Medicine, 1983. xi, 83 p.
Cebe B, Rozear MP, ed: E. A. Stead, Jr.: what this patient needs is a doctor. Durham, N. C., Carolina Academic Press, 1978. xii, 244 p.
Christianson EH: The conditions for science in the academic department of Transylvania University, 1799-1857. **Regist Ky Hist Soc** 1981;79(4):305-25
Christy TE: Clinical practice as a function of nursing education: an historical analysis. **Nurs Outlook** 1980 Aug;28(8):493-7
Clark D, Hyde GL: A brief history of the University of Kentucky Department of Surgery. **J Ky Med Assoc** 1984 Jul;82(7):343-7
Clarkson TB: Evolution and history of training and academic programs in laboratory animal medicine. **Lab Anim Sci** 1980 Aug;30(4 pt 2):790-2
Cobb WM: Forward--the only way. **J Natl Med Assoc** 1984 May;76(5):487-97
Cooper T, Olimpio NA: Medical education. **Proc Acad Polit Sci** 1980;33(4):32-44
Crawford S: Health sciences libraries in the United States: II. Medical school libraries, 1960-1980. **Bull Med Libr Assoc** 1983 Jan;71(1):21-9
Crisp KA: Chiropractic lyceums: the colorful origins of chiropractic continuing education. **Chiropr Hist** 1984;4(1):17-22
Crowley RM: William V. Silverberg as teacher and colleague. **J Am Acad Psychoanal** 1981 Oct;9(4):493-500
Curran JA: Founders of the Harvard School of Public Health, with biographical notes, 1909-1946. New York, Josiah Macy, Jr. Foundation, 1970. xviii, 294 p.
D'Amato NA: William Edmonds Horner: anatomist, educator, author. **Va Med** 1982 Mar;109(3):209-10
Davidson AT: The role of the historic black colleges in the training of black professionals. **J Natl Med Assoc** 1983 Oct;75(10):1019-22
Day HG: E. V. McCollum and dietitians in nutrition education. **J Am Diet Assoc** 1980 Feb;76(2):126-7
Dishong A: Highlights of twenty years' research at the University of Florida College of Medicine. **J Fla Med Assoc** 1980 Mar;67(3):288-93
Dockery JL, Deal WB, Cuppy D, et al: The University of Florida College of Medicine's alumni during the school's first twenty years. **J Fla Med Assoc** 1980 Mar;67(3):283-7
Donahue MP: [Isabel Maitland Stewart's philosophy of education] (Jpn). **Kango Kyoiku** 1984 Oct;25(10):611-21
Donatucci CF: In anticipation of Flexner. **Trans Stud Coll Physicians Phila** 1978 Jul;45(5):280-9
Dorsey JM: University Professor John M. Dorsey. Detroit, Wayne State University Press, 1980. 282 p.
Dowling HF: City hospitals. The undercare of the underprivileged. Cambridge, Mass., London, Harvard University Press, 1982. vii, 245 p.
Drachman VG: The Loomis trial: social mores and obstetrics in the mid-nineteenth century. In Reverby S, Rosner D, ed: Health care in America. Philadelphia, Temple University Press, 1979. p. 67-83.

Edlich RF: Reflections on Wangensteen's academic village. **Am J Surg** 1981 May;141(5):601–4

Eliot's farewell address, May 1, 1909: **Harv Med Alumni Bull** 1982 Spring;56(2):14–6

Elizondo RS, Jacobs N, Moore WW: Physiology at Indiana University–Bloomington. A history. **Physiologist** 1984 Oct;27(5):319–24

Etheridge EW: Grace Arabell Goldsmith. In: Notable American women. The modern period. Cambridge, Mass., Belknap–Harvard Univ. Press, 1980. 4:283–4.

Etzkowitz H: Entrepreneurial scientists and entrepreneurial universities in American academic science. **Minerva** 1983 Summer–Autumn;21(2–3):198–233

Evans RB, Talmadge P: Dial access: a history of the Southern Medical Association's newest contribution to continuing medical education. **South Med J** 1980 Apr;73(4):489–96

Evans RB: The origins of American academic psychology. In J. Brozěk, ed: Explorations in the history of psychology in the United States. Lewisburg, Bucknell University Press, 1984. p. 17–60.

Fee E: Competition for the first school of hygiene and public health. **Bull Hist Med** 1983 Fall;57(3):339–63

Finland M, Castle WB: The Harvard Medical Unit at Boston City Hospital. Boston, Harvard Medical School: Distributed by the University Press of Virginia for The Francis A. Countway Library of Medicine, 1982–83. 2 volumes in 3.

Fondiller SH: The entry dilemma: the National League for Nursing and the higher education movement, 1952–1972, with an epilogue to 1983. New York, N.Y., National League for Nursing, 1983. vii, 136 p.

Forbes TR: Books and broadsides: what Colonial physicians read. **Conn Med** 1984 Sep;48(9):566–8

Fox DM: Abraham Flexner's unpublished report: foundations and medical education, 1909–1928. **Bull Hist Med** 1980 Winter;54(4):475–96

Freymann JG: The origins of disease orientation in American medical education. **Prev Med** 1981 Nov;10(6):663–73

Fullard J: Ann Preston: pioneer of medical education and women's rights. **Pa Herit** 1982;8(1):9–14

Gellhorn A: The evolving post–Flexnerian model of medical education. In: Congrès international d'histoire de la médecine, XXVe, Québec, 1976. Actes. Québec, 1977. p. 141–59.

Gerhardt RE: The first teaching hospital. **N Engl J Med** 1983 May 19;308(20):1230

Geyman JP: The Oslerian tradition and changing medical education: a reappraisal. **West J Med** 1983 Jun;138(6):884–8

Golbeck AL: Quantification in ethnology and its appearance in regional culture trait distribution studies (1888 to 1939). **J Hist Behav Sci** 1980 Jul;16(3):225–7

Goldblith SA: Samuel Cate Prescott: – pioneer food technologist –gifted teacher. **Adv Food Res** 1981;27:1–21

Gray L, Rodriguez K, Dale DC: University of Washington School of Medicine. **West J Med** 1984 May;140(5):803–11

Gross EG, Long JP: Pharmacology at Iowa 1920–1980. **Life Sci** 1980 Dec 22–29;27(25–26):2423–6

Gruber B: Anatomist, scholar and gentleman: Arthur V. Nilsson–a legend in his own time. **Chiropr Hist** 1984;4(1):31–8

Hadley GG: Loma Linda University School of Medicine. **West J Med** 1983 May;138(5):742–5

Hall TD, Lindsay CM: Medical schools: producers of what? sellers to whom? **J Law Econ** 1980;23(1):55–80

Hare HJ: First graduate––USD School of Medicine. Lyle Hare, M.D., family practitioner. **SD J Med** 1981 May;34(5):70–1

Harmon MD: The evolution of nursing education in the U.S. **Nev Rnformation** 1984 May;:6

Harrell GT: Pediatrics in an academic health center. **J Fla Med Assoc** 1984 Mar;71(3):163–6

Harrell GT: The early years at Bowman Gray. **NC Med J** 1983 Dec;44(12):805–7

Harrell GT: The first years of the University of Florida College of Medicine. **J Fla Med Assoc** 1980 Mar;67(3):247–50

Harris MR: Abraham Flexner. In Dictionary of American Biography, Suppl. 6, 1956–1960. p. 207–9, 1980.

Hart AW: Religion and education: the Scopes controversy in Utah. **Utah Hist Q** 1983;5(2):183–98

Harvey AM: George Canby Robinson. In Dictionary of American Biography, Suppl. 6, 1956–1960. p. 546–7, 1980.

Harvey AM: Henry Mills Hurd: the first superintendent of the Johns Hopkins Hospital and the first professor of psychiatry. **Johns Hopkins Med J** 1981 Mar;148(3):135–48

Harvey AM: Johns Hopkins and yellow fever: a story of tragedy and triumph. **Johns Hopkins Med J** 1981 Jul;149(1):25–39

Harvey AM: Johns Hopkins's pioneer venture into international medicine: the commission to the Philippine Islands. **Johns Hopkins Med J** 1980 Jul;147(1):13–27

Harvey AM: Orthopaedic surgery at Johns Hopkins: a heritage of excellence in clinical practice, training and research. **Johns Hopkins Med J** 1982 Jun;150(6):221–45

Harvey AM: Research and discovery in medicine. Contributions from Johns Hopkins. Baltimore and London, Johns Hopkins University Press, 1981. xiii, 322 p. [Collected historical papers reprinted from various journals].

Harvey AM: Science at the bedside. Clinical research in American medicine, 1905–1945. Baltimore, London, Johns Hopkins University Press, 1981. xix, 554 p.

Harvey AM: Science at the bedside: the footprints of Yale and Johns Hopkins. **Yale J Biol Med** 1979 Nov–Dec;52(6):569–79

Harvey AM: The influence of William Stewart Halsted's concepts of surgical training. **Johns Hopkins Med J** 1981 May;148(5):215–36

Heindel ND, Foster NI: The Allentown Academy: America's first German medical school. **Pa Folklife** 1980;30(1):2–8

Herman JK: Home of BUMED: a hilltop in Foggy Bottom. Where medical college left off. The U.S. Naval Medical School and Naval Hospital 1902–1917. **US Navy Med** 1983 Jan–Feb;74(1):8–17 contd

Hiestand WC: Midwife to nurse–midwife: a history. The development of nurse–midwifery education in the continental United States to 1965. Ed. D. Diss., Columbia University. New York, 1976. 294 p.

Hine MK: The status of the teaching of dental history: 1980. **Bull Hist Dent** 1981 Oct;29(2):102–4

Hipskind MM: A doctor's fifty year perspective. **Indiana Med Hist Q** 1983 Sep;9(3):4–15

History of accreditation of medical education programs: **JAMA** 1983 Sep 23–30;250(12):1502–8

Hodge GP: Medical illustration: our early years. Student days at Johns Hopkins, Evelyn Erickson Sullivan. **J Biocommun** 1982 Mar;9(1):18–22

Hodgson ER: Did early Spokane have a medical school? **Pac Northwest** 1983;27(2):93–6

Holtz W: Bankrobbers, burkers and bodysnatchers. **Mich Q Rev** 1967;6(2):90–8

Huggins CG: The first decade. **J Med Assoc State Ala** 1983 Feb;52(8):9–17

Jarcho S: Some experiences with seminars in the history of medicine. In J. J. Bylebyl, ed: Teaching the history of medicine at a medical center. Baltimore, London, Johns Hopkins University Press, 1982. (The Henry E. Sigerist supplements to the Bulletin of the History of Medicine; new ser., no. 7). p. 115–20.

Jensen JE: Manuscript notes of William Shippen, Jr., MD found in the Faculty Library. **Md State Med J** 1984 Jun;33(6):438–40

Jones JH: Alan Gregg. In Dictionary of American Biography, Suppl. 6, 1956–1960. p. 252–3, 1980.

Jordan CA: Graduate medical education in Mobile 1859–1981. **J Med Assoc State Ala** 1981 Oct;51(4):16, 18, 24–9

Joy RJ: Starting from scratch: installing a history of medicine program in a new medical school. With a commentary by L.G. Stevenson. In J. J. Bylebyl, ed: Teaching the history of medicine at a medical center. Baltimore, London, Johns Hopkins University Press, 1982. (The Henry E. Sigerist supplements to the Bulletin of the History of Medicine; new ser., no. 7). p. 139–51.

Kaiser RM, Chaff SL, Peitzman SJ: A Philadelphia medical student of the 1890's: the diary of Mary Theodora McGavran. **Pa Mag Hist Biogr** 1984 Apr;108(2):217–36

Kampmeier RH: Women in medical school. **South Med J** 1984 Sep;77(9):1217

Kaufman M, Hanawalt LL: Body snatching in the Midwest. **Mich Hist** 1971;55(1):23–40

Kettel LJ: University of Arizona, College of Medicine. **West J Med** 1983 Sep;139(3):395–9

Kiefer JH, Wittman E: University of Illinois College of Medicine centennial. **IMJ** 1981 Aug;160(2):92–5

King LS: Medical education: the decade of massive change. **JAMA** 1984 Jan 13;251(2):219–24

King LS: Medicine in the USA: Historical vignettes. VII. The painfully slow progress in medical education. **JAMA** 1983 Jan 14;249(2):270–4

King LS: Medicine in the USA: historical vignettes. XV. Clinical science gets enthroned. Part I. **JAMA** 1983 Sep 2;250(9):1169–72

King LS: Medicine in the USA: historical vignettes. XVII. Medical education: elitisms and reform. **JAMA** 1983 Nov 11;250(18):2457–61

King LS: Medicine in the USA: historical vignettes. XVIII. Medical education: the problems intensify. **JAMA** 1983 Dec 9;250(22):3100–4

King LS: Medicine in the USA: historical vignettes. XX. The Flexner report of 1910. **JAMA** 1984 Feb 24;251(8):1079–86

King LS: VI. Medical education: the AMA surveys the problems. **JAMA** 1982 Dec 10;248(22):3017–21

Kinnaird DW: Kentucky's Doctors Elkin contributions to growth of Emory's medical school. **J Ky Med Assoc** 1984 Jun;82(6):291–3

Koudelka JB: The genesis of the William H. Welch Medical Library and the Johns Hopkins Institute of the History of Medicine. In Stevenson LG, ed: A celebration of medical history. Baltimore, Johns Hopkins University Press, 1982. (The Henry E. Sigerist supplements to the Bulletin of the History of Medicine; new ser., no. 6). p. 69–76

Kraus S: Stanford University School of Medicine. **West J Med** 1983 Aug;139(2):244–7

Laufman H: Loyal Davis and the young surgeon. **Surg Gynecol Obstet** 1983 Aug;157(2):123–8

Learning to deal with life and death: the story of becoming a doctor in Texas.: **Tex Med** 1980 May;76(5):53–68

Lemann N: Let the nurses do it. **Wash Mon** 1979;11(2):29–36

Lemon HM: Motivation in cancer education, with an appreciation of Dr. Henry Jackson, Jr., pioneer medical oncologist–hematologist

(1892–1968). **Med Pediatr Oncol** 1980;8(4):407–22
Leopold LA: Radiology at the University of Pennsylvania 1890–1975. Philadelphia, University of Pennsylvania Press, 1981. xvi, 163 p.
Lepore MJ: Death of the clinician, requiem or reveille? Springfield, Thomas, 1982. xviii, 359 p.
Linton SJ: The man and the mind: Carl Emil Seashore, a pioneer on two frontiers. **Swed Pioneer Hist Q** 1980;31(2):122–8
Liston SE, Fetgatter GL: The general essentials of accredited residencies in graduate medical education. **JAMA** 1982 Jun 4;247(21):3002–3
Lobeck C: UMC four-year medical school observes 25th anniversary. **Mo Med** 1981 Jun;78(6):293, 297
Loew ER: Departmental history. Department of Physiology. Boston University School of Medicine (1873–1948). **Physiologist** 1984 Feb;27(1):4–12
Longmire WP: Changing patterns of surgical training and practice. **Am J Surg** 1981 Jun;141(6):632–7
Longmire WP: Surgical upbringing in America. **Bull Am Coll Surg** 1978 Sep;63(9):6–11
Longo LD: John Whitridge Williams and academic obstetrics in America. **Trans Stud Coll Physicians Phila** 1981 Dec;5(3 no 4):221–54
Lostetter JO, Chapman JE: The participation of the United States government in providing financial support for medical education. **Health Policy Educ** 1979 Spring;1(1):27–65
Loughry CW: Fifty years of surgical education at Akron City Hospital. **Ohio State Med J** 1982 Oct;78(10):723–6
Ludmerer KM: Reform at Harvard Medical School, 1869–1909. **Bull Hist Med** 1981;55(3):343–70
Ludmerer KM: Reform of medical education at Washington University. **J Hist Med Allied Sci** 1980 Apr;35(2):149–73
Ludmerer KM: The plight of clinical teaching in America. **Bull Hist Med** 1983 Summer;57(2):218–29
Ludmerer KM: The rise of the teaching hospital in America. **J Hist Med Allied Sci** 1983 Oct;38(4):389–414
McDougall IR: Stanford University Medical School. **Scott Med J** 1979 Apr;24(2):159–62
McPherson MP: 'On the same terms precisely': the women's medical fund and the John Hopkins School of Medicine. **J Am Med Wom Assoc** 1981 Feb;36(2):37–40
Makechnie GK: Optimal health: the quest. A history of Boston University's Sargent College of Allied Health Professionals, founded 1881, tendered to Boston University 1929. Boston, Boston University, 1979. x, 228 p.
Malinsky BJ: The (Woman's) Medical College of Pennsylvania. **Women Health** 1979 Fall;4(3):217–21
Manhart GB: The Indiana Central Medical College, 1849–1852. **Indiana Hist Soc** 1982 Dec;8(4):3–13
Mannion RA: Indiana medical history--the medical school at LaPorte. **Indiana Med Hist Q** 1975;2(1):70–1
Markowitz GE, Rosner D: Doctors in crisis: medical education and medical reform during the Progressive era, 1895–1915. In Reverby S, Rosner D, ed: Health care in America. Philadelphia, Temple University Press, 1979. p. 185–205.
Marvin HN: Anatomy in Arkansas' Medical College 1879–1979. The history of a department. (continued) **J Arkansas Med Soc** 1980 Dec;77(7):253–64; 1981;77(8,9,10):305–12, 347–52, 386–419
Medical school reformer: **MD** 1978 Jul;22(7):133–8
Miciotto RJ: Anniversary 50: the birth and development of the LSU School of Medicine. The Murmur: LSU Medical Center Yearbook 1981 Fall; 13:34–41, 302–3.
Miller EB: Nonacademic influences on education of the veterinarian in the United States, 1887–1921. **J Am Vet Med Assoc** 1979 Nov 15;175(10):1106–10
Miller EB: Private veterinary colleges in the United States, 1852–1927. **J Am Vet Med Assoc** 1981 Mar 15;178(6):583–93
Miller RM: Admission of foreign medical graduates to the U.S. **INS Rep** 1979;27(4):6–11
Moore FD: The changing mission and status of surgery 1780 to 1980. **Arch Surg** 1983 Sep;118(9):1013–8
Moore FD: Two hundred years ago: origins and early years of the Harvard Medical School. **Ann Surg** 1982 Nov;196(5):525–35
Moore JT: Battle for the Medical College: physicians, politicians, and the courts, 1882–1883. **Va Cavalcade** 1982;31(3):158–67
Morehead RP: The contribution of a great man to Wake Forest University and its Bowman Gray School of Medicine--Tinsley R. Harrison, M.D. **NC Med J** 1983 Dec;44(12):809–11
Morison RS: The Foundation interest. In Stevenson LG, ed: A celebration of medical history. Baltimore, Johns Hopkins University Press, 1982. (The Henry E. Sigerist supplements to the Bulletin of the History of Medicine; new ser., no. 6). p. 212–21.
Morris JP: Historical perspectives on educating the medical student in thanatology. In Schoenberg B., et al, ed: Educating medical students in thanatology. New York, Arno Press, 1981. p. 18–28.
Mottus JE: New York Nightingales: the emergence of the nursing profession at Bellevue and New York Hospital, 1850–1920. Ann Arbor, Mich., UMI Research Press, 1981. xvii, 277 p. (Ph.D. Diss., New York University, 1980.
Murphy LP, McNair EW: Summer program in medical school environment for undergraduate students: an evaluation. **J Negro Educ** 1981;50(4):407–14
Murray AE: Bright delusion: Presbyterians and African colonization. **J Presbyt Hist** 1980;58(3):224–37
Musto DF: Worthington Hooker (1806–1867): physician and educator. **Conn Med** 1984 Sep;48(9):569–74
Napodano RJ, Young LE: The University of Rochester Associated Hospitals Programs in internal medicine. Seven years experience with an innovative city-wide residency for preparation of general internists. **Am J Med** 1982 Jun;72(6):945–50
Napolitano EG, Gruber B: The struggle for accreditation in chiropractic: a unique history of educational bootstrapping. **Chiropr Hist** 1981;1(1):23–4
Neghme A: Vida y obra de Sir William Osler (1849–1919) y la fundación de la Escuela de Medicina en la Universidad de Johns Hopkins. **Rev Med Chil** 1983 Jan;111(1):83–92
Noore FD: In medicina, veritas; the British and turbulent youth of the faculty of medicine and Harvard College. **N Engl J Med** 1982 Oct 7;307(15):917–25
Norwood WF: The CME School of Medicine: its struggle for recognition and status, 1905–1915. **Advent Herit** 1979;6(2):15–24
Numbers RL: A note on medical education in Wisconsin. In Numbers RL, Leavitt JW, ed: Wisconsin medicine. Historical perspectives. Madison, University of Wisconsin Press, 1981. p. 177–84.
Numbers RL, ed: The education of American physicians: historical essays. [Preface includes biographical tribute to William F. Norwood]. Berkeley, University of California Press, 1980. xiii, 345 p. Contributions by L. G. Stevenson, M. Kaufman, J. B. Blake, J. H. Warner, J. Whorton, D. L. Cowen, R. C. Maulitz, E. C. Atwater, G. H. Brieger, L. D Longo, J. L. Brand, J. W. Leavitt, C R. Burns, G. Miller
Odegaard CE: Minorities in medicine. From receptive passivity to positive action 1966–76. New York, Josiah Macy, Jr. Foundation, 1977. vii, 164 p.
Olch PD: Evarts Ambrose Graham. In Dictionary of American Biography, Suppl. 6, 1956–1960. p. 245–7, 1980.
The old pathology building (The Pathological Department of the Central Indiana Hospital for the Insane): **Indiana Med Hist Q** 1974;1(1):7–10
Olsen AM: ACCP International--'The world is our classroom'. **Chest** 1984 Nov;86(5):655–6
Ono J: Legacies of Jefferson men to Japanese medicine. **Ann Otol Rhinol Laryngol [Suppl]** 1981 Sep–Oct;90(5 pt 2 Suppl 87):1–10
Oppenheimer JM: Thomas Hunt Morgan as an embryologist: the view from Bryn Mawr. **Am Zool** 1983;23:845–54
Oral history abstract catalog: Interviews 1969–1978. St. Louis, Archives Section, Washington Univ. School of Medicine Library, 1979. 15 p:
Parascandola J: John J. Abel and the early development of pharmacology at the Johns Hopkins University. **Bull Hist Med** 1982;56(4):512–27
Pauly PJ: The appearance of academic biology in late nineteenth-century America. **J Hist Biol** 1984 Fall;17(3):369–97
Peitzman SJ: Lecturing in American medical schools. Tenacious tradition. **Arch Intern Med** 1983 Aug;143(8):1593–6
Peitzman SJ: 'Thoroughly practical': America's polyclinic medical schools. **Bull Hist Med** 1980 Summer;54(2):166–87
Pennington TG: The history of medical education in Nashville. **J Tenn Med Assoc** 1983 Jul;76(7):445–9
Petersdorf RG: The evolution of departments of medicine. **N Engl J Med** 1980 Aug 28;303(9):489–96
Petrisko TW: Schism and suppression: the elimination of medical protest schools, 1846–1939. **Chiropr Hist** 1982;2(1):35–9
Petty CS: The medical examiner and medical education (Russell S. Fisher). **Hum Pathol** 1980 Mar;11(2):101–3
Pittman JA: Medical education in Alabama: Part I, the early years. **J Med Assoc State Ala** 1982 Apr;51(10):22–9
Profile: four academic pioneers who stayed to help the Health Center grow. **J Fla Med Assoc** 1980 Mar;67(3):298–301
Quinn J: Medical education in Mississippi. **J Miss State Med Assoc** 1981 Dec;22(12):325–9
Rambar AC: Julius Hess, M.D. In Smith GF, Smith PN, Vidyasagar D, ed: Historical review and recent advances in neonatal and perinatal medicine. [Chicago?], Mead Johnson Nutritional Division, 1983. Vol. II. p. 161–4.
Ransom JF: The origins of chiropractic physiological therapeutics: Howard, Forester and Schulze. **Chiropr Hist** 1984;4(1):47–52
Raphelson AC: Psychology at Michigan: the Pillsbury years, 1897–1947. **J Hist Behav Sci** 1980 Oct;16(4):301–12
Raphelson AC: The history course as the capstone of the psychology curriculum. **J Hist Behav Sci** 1982 Jul;18(3):279–85
Reed K, Perakis CR: Medical historiography: its place in osteopathic medicine. Parts I and II. **J Am Osteopath Assoc** 1984 Jun;83(10):738–44
Reese WG: Academic psychiatry in Arkansas. **J Arkansas Med Soc** 1981 Nov;78(6):220–33
Reitman N: The history of medicine and medical care in New Brunswick. **J Med Soc NJ** 1984 Sep;81(9):737–9
Relman AS: The Harvard Medical School Bicentennial. **N Engl J Med** 1982 Oct 7;307(15):943–4
Reynolds KJ: Early days of Loma Linda.....and even before. **Advent Herit** 1975;2(1):42–50
Richards EL: 50 years ago--blazing the trail. **Alumni Mag** 1984;84(2):9–12

Rising JD: Rambling recollections about the 'Postgraduate Department' -- now the Division of Continuing Education of the College of Health Sciences. **J Kans Med Soc** 1980 Mar;81(3):102, 156-8

Robert I. Watson and the development of the history of psychology: a symposium: With contributions by E. S. Mills, E. R. Hilgard, B. Ross, J. Popplestone, M. W. McPherson, R. B. Evans, E. S. Goodman, J. Brožek. **J Hist Behav Sci** 1982 Oct;18(4):307-31

Rosenberg CE: Inward vision and outward glance: the shaping of the American hospital, 1880-1914. **Bull Hist Med** 1979 Fall;53(3):346-91

Rosenfeld LM: Physiology at Jefferson Medical College (1842-1982). **Physiologist** 1984 Jun;27(3):113-27

Rosenow EC: Osler--continuing education advocate. **Bull Am Coll Physicians** 1975 Aug;16(8):6-8

Rosenthal PA, Eaton J: Women MDs in America: 100 years of progress and backlash. **J Am Med Wom Assoc** 1982 May;37(5):129-33

Ruhe CH: Seventy-five years of American medical education: perceptions and reflections. **Conn Med** 1980 Feb;44(2):95-9

Ryan TA: Psychology at Cornell after Titchener: Madison Bentley to Robert Macleod, 1928-1948. **J Hist Behav Sci** 1982 Oct;18(4):347-69

Sabiston DC: Deryl Hart: leader in the development of the Duke University Medical Center. **NC Med J** 1983 Jul;44(7):441-2

Sandson JI: Medical education: past, present, and future. **RI Med J** 1984 Dec;67(12):537-42

Savitt TL: Lincoln University Medical Department--a forgotten 19th century black medical school. **J Hist Med Allied Sci** 1985 Jan;40(1):42-65

Savitt TL: The use of Blacks for medical experimentation and demonstration in the Old South. **J South Hist** 1982 Aug;48(3):331-48

Schor I: The continuing nursing education and adult education movements in the United States. **Nurs Forum** 1981;20(1):87-101

Schuknecht HF: Harvard Medical School and the Massachusetts Eye and Ear Infirmary. **Adv Otorhinolaryngol** 1983;31:1-7

Selkurt EE: Physiology at Indiana University School of Medicine-Indianapolis. **Physiologist** 1984 Oct;27(5):325-9

Shearer AW: A commitment to excellence: a history of the School of Nursing, College of Allied Health Sciences, Thomas Jefferson University, 1891-1982. Wynnewood, Pa., Heden-Livingston, 1982. x, 148 p.

Shearer J: History of the Department of Nursing Education at the North Dakota State Hospital. **Prairie Rose** 1984 Oct-Dec;53(4):20-1

Shell DH, Sparkman RS: John Allan Wyeth, MD. Surgeon, soldier, author and founder of postgraduate medical education in America. **Am J Surg** 1980 Sep;140(3):447-56

Shortt SE: History in the medical curriculum. A clinical perspective. **JAMA** 1982 Jul 2;248(1):79-81

Skinner RE, Marcotte JM: Bibliographic instruction in the health sciences: an historical review. **Med Ref Serv Q** 1982 Summer;1(2):53-76

Smith BL: The brain drain re-emergent: foreign medical graduates in American medical schools. **Minerva** 1979 Winter;17(4):483-503

Smith DC: The emergence of organized clinical instruction in the nineteenth century American cities of Boston, New York and Philadelphia. Ph.D. Diss. University of Minnesota. Minneapolis, 1979. 357 leaves.

Sorenson AA: Black Americans and the medical profession, 1930-1970. **J Negro Educ** 1972;41(4):337-42

Spalding P: Women in the Medical College of Georgia. **South Med J** 1981 Feb;74(2):221-4

Stephenson LW: Reflections on the military involvement of a medical school. **Surg Gynecol Obstet** 1982 Jun;154(6):888-96

Stetten D: High-powered research and the microscopic viewpoint. **J Med Educ** 1981 Jan;56(1):3-7

Stevenson LG: Cushion into launching pad; the fiftieth anniversary of the Institute of the History of Medicine. **Bull Hist Med** 1979 Winter;53(4):487-88

Stevenson LG, ed: A celebration of medical history. The fiftieth anniversary of The Johns Hopkins Institute of the History of Medicine and The Welch Medical Library. Baltimore and London, Johns Hopkins University Press, 1982. vi, 228 p. (Henry E. Sigerist Supplements to the Bulletin of the History of medicine, new ser., no. 6)

Stinson JM: Department of Physiology, Meharry Medical College, Nashville, Tennessee. **Physiologist** 1983 Jun;26(3):119-20

Sullivan LW: The education of black health professionals. **Phylon** 1977;38(2):181-93

Sullivan LW: The Morehouse School of Medicine: a state of mind, of mission, and of commitment. **J Natl Med Assoc** 1983 Aug;75(8):837-9

Sullivan LW: The school of medicine at Morehouse College: status in 1979 and plans for the future. **J Med Assoc Ga** 1980 Aug;69(8):673-4

Summerville J: Educating black doctors: a history of Meharry Medical College. University, Ala., University of Alabama Press, 1983. xiii, 279 p.

Takaki R: Aesculapius was a white man: antebellum racism and male chauvinism at Harvard Medical School. **Phylon** 1978;39(2):128-34

Taylor E: Louville Eugene Emerson: psychotherapy, Harvard, and the early Boston scene. **Harv Med Alumni Bull** 1982 Spring;56(2):42-8

[The caricature of the teacher]: **Indiana Med Hist Q** 1977;3(2):23-37

Thomas CB: Fulfilling the promise: Hopkins women before World War II. **J Am Med Wom Assoc** 1981 Feb;36(2):40-3

Thompson JA, Kronenfeld MR: Graefenberg Medical Institute. **Ala J Med Sci** 1979 Oct;16(4):350-2

Thorup OA: Thomas Jefferson: founder of two medical schools. **Trans Am Clin Climatol Assoc** 1980;92:16-22

Tipton R: Continued controversy: the Rutgers Medical School and the Library of Science and Medicine. **J Rutgers Univ Libr** 1983;45(1):1-24

Tomes N: Annie Warburton Goodrich. In: Notable American women. The modern period. Cambridge., Mass., Belknap-Harvard Univ. Press, 1980. 4:286-8.

Tyler HR, Tyler KL: Charles Edouard Brown-Séquard: professor of physiology and pathology of the nervous system at Harvard Medical School. **Neurology** 1984 Sep;34(9):1231-6

Tyndall RM: A history of the Bellevue School for midwives 1911-1936. Diss (Ed D), Columbia University. New York, 1978. xi, 260 p.

Van Buskirk EL: Fort Wayne College of Medicine. Includes The practice of medicine in the Fort Wayne area written in 1889 by B. S. Woodworth. **Indiana Med Hist Q** 1977;3(2):4-6

Van Buskirk EL: The Fort Wayne Medical Schools 1876-1905 and the Union with Purdue University. **Indiana Med Hist Q** 1976 Summer;3(1):55-66

Vermeulen CW: For the greatest good to the largest number. A history of the Medical Center, the University of Chicago. Chicago, Univ. of Chicago, 1977. x, 129 p.

Viseltear AJ: 'C.-E.A. Winslow and the early years of public health at Yale, 1915-1925'. **Yale J Biol Med** 1982 Mar-Apr;55(2):137-51

Viseltear AJ: Looking back at tomorrow. Commencement address delivered at the Yale University School of Medicine, New Haven, Connecticut, May 24, 1981. **Yale J Biol Med** 1981 May-Jun;54(3):219-25

Wahrman A: The Philadelphia physician-factory. **J Hist Med Allied Sci** 1983 Jul;38(3):334-5

Walker JD: Family Medicine Education. A Kansas historical review, 1967-1982. **J Kans Med Soc** 1983 Mar;84(3):138-42

Walsh MR: The rediscovery of the need for a feminist medical education. **Harv Educ Rev** 1979;49(4):447-66

Wangensteen OH: Mandated celibacy in the academic arena. **Surg Gynecol Obstet** 1980 May;150(5):739-45

Wangensteen OH: Reflections on life's odyssey for medical school graduates. **Minn Med** 1980 May;63(5):341-5

Wangensteen OW, ed: Elias Potter Lyon: Minnesota's leader in medical education. St. Louis, Green, 1981. 292 p. Contributions by J. A. Anderson, E. S. Benson, R. A. Good, J. C. Hinsey, C. H. Hodgson, L. P. Leone, R. J. McCollister, J. A. Myers, L. G. Rigler, H. G. Scheie, D. C. Smith, W. W. Spink, M. B. Visscher, J. H. Westerman, L. G. Wilson.

Ward PS: An experiment in medical education: or How the College of Physicians and Surgeons of Chicago became The University of Illinois College of Medicine. In Cohen EP, ed: Medicine in transition. [Chicago], University of Illinois College of Medicine, 1981. p. 27-51.

Ward PS: 100 years: a history [of the University of Illinois College of Medicine.] **Scope** 1981-82 centennial special;8(3):4-42

Warner JH: A Southern medical reform: the meaning of the Antebellum argument for Southern medical education. **Bull Hist Med** 1983 Fall;57(3):364-81

Weaver B: Should women be admitted to medical school? The issue in the late 19th century. **South Med J** 1984 May;77(5):623-5

Weigley ES: Sarah Tyson Rorer: first American dietitian? **J Am Diet Assoc** 1980 Jul;77(1):11-5

Wickwar H, Bryan CS: Broussais in Columbia, South Carolina - 1831. **J SC Med Assoc** 1981 Dec;77(12):615-22

[Wilson L]: The education of historians of medicine. **J Hist Med Allied Sci** 1982 Jul;37(3):265-8

Wintrobe MM: Medical education in Utah. **West J Med** 1982 Apr;136(4):357-66

Wiseman H: Graduate medical education in Mobile. **J Med Assoc State Ala** 1983 Feb;52(8):43-9

Wolfe EL: Calvin Ellis, the forgotten dean. **Harv Med Alumni Bull** 1982 Spring;56(2):27-31

Ziem G: Medical education since Flexner. **Health PAC Bull** 1977;(76):8-14, 23

## USSR

Abramov ShI: Iubileĭ pervoĭ kafedry. **Vestn Rentgenol Radiol** 1980 Jan-Feb;(1):89-91

Aĭdaraliev AA: Kirgizskomu gosudartsvennomu meditsinskomu institutu--40 let. **Zdravookhr Kirg** 1980;(1):3-6

Alikhanian SI: Kafedra genetiki Moskovskogo gosudartsvennogo universiteta imeni M. V. Lomonosova--1930-1948 gg. **Genetika (Moskva)** 1981;17(7):1320-7

Al'zhanov AG: Iz istorii podgotovki fel'dsherov v dorevoliutsionnom Kazakhstane. **Feldsher Akush** 1982;47(12):38-40

Anton'ev AA, Milich VM, Suvorova KN: K 50-letiiu tsentral'nogo ordena Lenina instituta usovershenstvovaniia vracheĭ. **Vestn Dermatol Venerol** 1980 Aug;(8):33-8

Antonov AM: Kafedre patologicheskoĭ anatomii Saratovskogo ordena Trudovogo Krasnogo Znameni meditsinskogo instituta 70 let (1911-1981). **Arkh Patol** 1981;43(7):80-3

Batuev AS: Fiziologicheskaia nauchnaia shkola Leningradskogo universiteta. **Fiziol Zh SSSR** 1984 Oct;70(10):1353-60

# EDUCATION, MEDICAL

Belitskaia EIa, Zhuravleva KI: K 60-letiiu Kafedry sotsial'noĭ gigieny i organizatsii zdravookhraneniia Leningradskogo sanitarno-gigienicheskogo meditsinskogo instituta. **Sov Zdravookhr** 1982;(7):61-3

Bilyk VD, Klantsa PA, Kul'chitskiĭ KI, et al: Zaslugi N. I. Pirogova v sozdanii i razvitii material'no-tekhnicheskoĭ bazy vysshego meditsinskogo obrazovaniia. **Klin Khir** 1983 Mar;(3):55-7

Bobrik II, Chernyshenko LV: 140 let kafedry anatomii Kievskogo meditsinskogo instituta. **Vrach Delo** 1982 Feb;(2):1-2

Brzheskiĭ VCh: K istorii pervoĭ v mire kafedry oftal'mologii. **Vestn Oftalmol** 1981 Sep-Oct;(5):69-70

Buranchiev AB, Sizov IE: K 40-letiiu kafedry kozhnykh i venericheskikh bolezneĭ Kirgizskogo meditsinskogo instituta. **Vestn Dermatol Venerol** 1980 Nov;(11):27-9

Chernenko VD, Shtel'makh NI: K 100-letiiu osnovaniia kafedry propevtiki vnutrennikh bolezneĭ lechebnogo fakul'teta Khar'kovskogo meditsinskogo instituta. **Vrach Delo** 1984 Aug;(8):119-21

Dagurov VG, Miazdrikova AA: Stanovlenie farmakologii v Moskovskom universitete. **Farmakol Toksikol** 1981 Nov-Dec;;44(6):733-7

Demidova NI: [The role of I. M. Sechenov's school in the development of electrophysiology] (Rus). **Istor Biol Issled** 1980;8:156-62

Demin VN: 50 let prepodavaniia onkologii v ordena Lenina Gosudarstvennom institute dlia usovershenstvovaniia vracheĭ im. S. M. Kirova. **Vopr Onkol** 1981;27(4):98-100

D'iachkov VI: Revoliutsionnoe proshloe pervogo meditsinskogo uchebnogo zavedeniia v Sibiri (o Tobol'skoĭ povival'noĭ shkole). **Feldsher Akush** 1984 Mar;49(3):55-6

Dionesov SM: K istorii zhenskogo meditsinskogo obrazovaniia v Rossii. **Feldsher Akush** 1983 Dec;48(12):44-5

Dionesov SM: Zhenskie vrachebnye kursy pri Peterburgskom nikolaevskom voennom gospitale. **Sov Med** 1982;(6):117-9

Dobin MA: Veterinarnoe obrazovanie v Rossii. **Veterinariia** 1980 Jan;(1):76-7

Dogel' LV, Shalagina TL: S. N. Davidenkov v Leningradskom gosudarstvennom institute usovershenstvovaniia vracheĭ. **Zh Nevropatol Psikhiatr** 1982;82(3):107-9

Dolgoleev NF: Brianskoe meditsinskoe uchilishche No. 1. **Feldsher Akush** 1983 Sep;48(9):41-2

Dyskin EA: Stanovlenie i razvitie prepodavaniia anatomii v Peterburge v XVIII v. **Arkh Anat Gistol Embriol** 1984 Feb;86(2):96-101

Evdokimov PP: Uchastie studentov-medikov Kazani v revoliutsionnom dvizhenii 1870-1880 gg. **Sov Zdravookhr** 1981;(1):60-2

Fel' II, Truman GL: Meditsinskiĭ fakul'tet Bakinskogo (Azerbaĭdzhanskogo) universiteta i rol' russkikh uchenykh v stanovlenii i razvitii vyshego meditsinskogo obrazovaniia i meditsinskoĭ nauki v Sovetskom Azerbaĭdzhane (k 60-letiiu obrazovaniia Azerbaĭdzhanskoĭ SSR). **Sov Zdravookhr** 1980;(5):64-7

Gan'zha SV: U istokov zhenskogo meditsinskogo obrazovaniia. **Med Sestra** 1984 Feb;43(2):45-7

Gladkikh PF: Perestroĭka sistemy podgotovki voenno-meditsinskikh kadrov v tridtsatye gody. **Voen Med Zh** 1983 Sep;9:70-2

Golda DM, Berdyshev GD: Prepodavanie genetiki v Kievskom universitete (k 150-letiiu KGU). **Tsitol Genet** 1984 Sep-Oct;18(5):393-4

Grando AA, Makarenko IM, Polianskiĭ AA: Kafedre sotsial'noĭ gigieny i organizatsii zdravookhraneniia Kievskogo meditsinskogo instituta--60 let. **Sov Zdravookhr** 1984;(3):52-3

Gribanov ED: Rol' Tsentral'nogo instituta usovershenstvovaniia vracheĭ v podgotovke kadrov istorikov meditsiny. **Sov Zdravookhr** 1979;(10):60-1

Grigorian NA: Rol' uchenykh Kazanskogo universiteta v razvitii obshchestvennoĭ meditsiny. **Sov Zdravookhr** 1981;(7):48-51

Iaremchuk AIâ, et al: [Importance of museums in optimizing the academic process and academic research work of students in a department of surgery.] (Rus). **Klin Khir** 1981;2:47-9

Iarovinskiĭ MIa: Rol' istorii meditsiny v deontologicheskoĭ podgotovke meditsinskikh rabotnikov. **Sov Zdravookhr** 1982;(4):51-3

Ibragimov NG: Iz istorii podgotovki meditsinskikh sester v nasheĭ strane. **Med Sestra** 1982 Feb;41(02):55-7

Ibragimova ZI, Burak GG, Ol'shannikova VV, et al: 50 let kafedre anatomii cheloveka Vitebskogo meditsinskogo instituta. **Arkh Anat Gistol Embriol** 1984 Jul;87(7):95-6

Idel'chik KhI: Iz istorii meditsinskogo fakul'teta Moskovskogo universiteta. **Sov Zdravookhr** 1981;(2):60-4

Ionov IuV, Ionov AIu: A. P. Borodin - vrach, khimik, pedagog (k 150-letiiu so dnia rozhdeniia). **Sov Zdravookhr** 1984;(1):61-4

Ivanov NG: Znachenie opyta Velikoĭ Otechestvennoĭ Voĭny dlia podgotovki voenno-meditsinskikh kadrov. **Voen Med Zh** 1980 May;(5):21-4

Johanson C: Autocratic politics, public opinion, and women's medical education during the reign of Alexander II, 1855-1881. **Slavic Rev** 1979;38(3):426-43

Käbin I: Medicinska fakulteten vid universitetet i Dorpat (Tartu) 1802-1940. **Nord Medicinhist Arsb** 1984;:91-103

Kadyrov AA, Madakhanov AS: Pervyĭ meditsinskiĭ institut Uzbekistana. **Sov Zdravookhr** 1980;(6):57-8

Kadyrov AA, Asliddinov IF: Razvitie vysshego meditsinskogo obrazovaniia v respublikakh Sovetskogo Vostoka. **Sov Zdravookhr** 1984;(3):50-1

Kafedre genetiki Moskovskogo gosudarstvennogo universiteta imeni M. V. Lomonosova--50 let: **Genetika (Moskva)** 1981;17(7):1318-20

Kalnin VV, Al'bitskiĭ VIu: Iz istorii Tartuskogo i Kazanskogo universitetov. **Klin Med (Mosk)** 1981 Jan;59(1):108-10

Khromchenko OM, Sapegina AV: Dvadtsatipiatletniĭ opyt usovershenstvovaniia rukovodiashchikh kadrov sanitarno-épidemiologicheskoĭ sluzhby v Tsentral'nom institute usovershenstvovaniia vracheĭ. **Gig Sanit** 1981 Mar;(3):51-3

Kirilenko TG: Rol' Akademii meditsinskikh nauk SSSR v podgotovke mauchnykh kadrov. **Sov Zdravookhr** 1980;(2):64-7

Kishkovskiĭ AN, Tiutin LA: K 50-letiiu kafedry rentgenologii i radiologii VMA imeni S.M. Kirov. **Voen Med Zh** 1980 Sep;(9):76-8

Kochemasova ZN, Dykhno MM: 60 let kafedre mikrobiologii i Moskovskogo meditsinskogo instituta im. I. M. Sechenova. **Zh Mikrobiol Epidemiol Immunobiol** 1981 May;(5):113-6

Kokoska U: Johann Georg Noël Dragendorff (20.4.1836 - 7.4.1898): Sein Beitrag zur Gerichtsmedizin, Pharmakologie und Pharmazie an der Universität Dorpat. Diss. Berlin, 1983. 234 p.

Konovalov AN, Iartsev VV: 50-letie Nauchno-issledovatel'skogo ordena Trudovogo Krasnogo Znameni instituta neĭrokhirurgii im. akad. N. N. Burdenko AMN SSSR. **Zh Vopr Neirokhir** 1981 Nov-Dec;(6):3-9

Kopanev VI: [Role of the scientists of the S. M. Kirov Military Medical Academy in the development of aviation medicine]. (Rus) **Voen Med Zh** 1979 Dec;(12):63-5

Korol'kov AA: Iz istorii pervykh gigienicheskikh kafedr v Rossii. **Zdravookhr Ross Fed** 1980;(5):19-22

Korostelev NB: Osnovanie pervykh gigienicheskikh kafedr v Rossii. **Gig Sanit** 1984 Feb;(2):40-4

Korotkov AG, Valishin ES: K 175-letiiu kafedry normal'noĭ anatomii cheloveka Kazanskogo meditsinskogo instituta. **Arkh Anat Gistol Embriol** 1982 Jan;82(1):110-4

Kovaleva EP, Deviatova LN, Kasparova TIu, et al: K 50-letiiu kafedry épidemiologii Tsentral'nogo instituta usovershenstvovaniia vracheĭ. **Zh Mikrobiol Epidemiol Immunobiol** 1981 Jun;(6):113-7

Kovrigina MD: Tsentral'nomu ordena Lenina institutu usovershenstvovaniia vracheĭ 50 let. **Sov Zdravookhr** 1980;(11):13-6

Kovrigina MD: 50-letie Tsentral'nogo Instituta Usovershenstvovaniia Vracheĭ. **Klin Med (Mosk)** 1981 Jan;59(1):4-7

Kravtsov DE: Prosvetitel'skaia deiatel'nost' N. I. Pirogova v Kieve. **Voen Med Zh** 1982 Nov;(11):65-6

Krivobokov NG: Shestidesiatiletie Piatigorskogo instituta kurotologii i fizioterapii. **Vopr Kurortol Fizioter Lech Fiz Kult** 1980 May-Jun;(3):67-8

Kurdiumov NA, Novikova TP: Kafedra normal'noĭ anatomii Dagestanskogo meditsinskogo instituta (k 50-letnemu iubileiu). **Arkh Anat Gistol Embriol** 1983 Dec;85(12):90-2

Kuz'min MK, Rumiantsev GI: Razvitie osnovnykh napravleniĭ profilakticheskoĭ meditsiny na sanitarno-gigienicheskom fakul'tete (1930-1980). **Sov Med** 1981;(5):115-9

Kvitnitskiĭ-Ryzhov IuN: Iz istorii pervoĭ Kievskoĭ gistologicheskoĭ shkoly. **Arkh Anat Gistol Embriol** 1980 May;78(5):107-11

Lavrik SS: Podgotovka vrachebnykh kadrov v Kievskom meditsinskom institute. **Vrach Delo** 1982 Jun;(6):5-9

Lavrik SS, Pogrebinskiĭ MB: Traditsii vuza i formirovanie kachestv sovetskogo vracha. **Sov Zdravookhr** 1981;(2):46-51

Leonov IT: Bol'sheviki-lenintsy--vospitanniki Voenno-meditsinskoĭ akademii. **Voen Med Zh** 1984 Oct;(10):62-5

Levit MM: Metodologiia i metodika prepodavaniia istorii meditsiny. **Sov Zdravookhr** 1980;(3):54-7

Liepa A: Ikh imena nosiat meditsinskie uchilischcha. **Med Sestra** 1980 Sep;37(9):54-6

Lindenbraten LD: Voprosy prepodavaniia i podgotovki kadrov po rentgenologii i radiologii na stranitsakh zhurnala 'Meditsinskaia Radiologiia' (1956-1981). **Med Radiol (Mosk)** 1981;26(10):49-53

Lobanov GP, Zhuravskiĭ VA: Nekotorye voprosy organizatsii spetsial'noĭ podgotovki lichnogo sostava voenno-meditsinskoĭ sluzhby v period Voĭny. **Voen Med Zh** 1980 May;(5):28-33

Lotsmanov IuA, Safin MS: Bashkirskomu meditsinskomu institutu 50 let. **Sov Zdravookhr** 1982;(6):62-4

Makarov VA: [I. M. Sechenov and the development of physiology in the Moscow University] (Rus). **Istor Biol Issled** 1980;8:138-55

Makarov VA: 50 let kafecre normal'noĭ fiziologii l-go Moskovskogo meditsinskogo instituta im. I. M. Sechenova (1930-1980). **Fiziol Zh SSSR** 1980 Dec;66(12):1860-4

Makarova EP: V. I. Razumovskiĭ--pervyĭ rektor Saratovskogo universiteta. **Vestn Khir** 1983 May;130(5):140-1

Makhmudov M: Tashkentskiĭ meditsinskiĭ institut. **Sov Zdravookhr** 1980;(7):54-6

Makovický E: Pätdesiat rokov Centrálneho inštitútu pre dalšie vzdelávanie lekárov, nositel'a Radu Lenina, v Moskve. **Vnitr Lek** 1981 May;27(5):417-20

Matveev MP, Klaĭshevich GI, Gavriushova LP, et al: Rol' kafedry pediatrii v sisteme poslediplomnogo obucheniia pediatrov (k 50-letiiu Tsentral'nogo ordena V. I. Lenina instituta usovershenstvovaniia vracheĭ. **Pediatriia** 1981 Jul;(7):77-8

Mazurenko MD, Porksheian OKh, Servatinskiĭ GL, et al: K 100-letiiu Leningradskogo Gosudarstvennogo ordena Lenina instituta usovershenstvovaniia vracheĭ im. S. M. Kirova i 60-letiiu kafedry

sudebnoĭ meditsiny. **Sud Med Ekspert** 1984 Oct–Dec;27(4):57–9
Mazurik EV: O pedagogicheskoĭ deiatel'nosti N. I. Pirogova v Kamenets--Polol'ske i o ego sviaziakh s Obshchestvom polol'skikh vracheĭ (k 100–letiiu so dnia smerti N. I. Pirogova). **Sov Zdravookhr** 1981;(8):66–8
Mendrina GI: 100–letie Tomskogo universiteta. **Sov Zdravookhr** 1981;(2):64–7
Miliavskiĭ VM: K istorii prepodavaniia psikhiatrii v fel'dsherskikh shkolakh. **Feldsher Akush** 1982;47(4):53–4
Mirakhmedov UM: K 60–letiiu kafedry kozhnykh i venericheskikh bolezneĭ Tashkentskogo meditsinskogo instituta. **Vestn Dermatol Venerol** 1981 Nov;(11):74–6
Moteiunas LI: Meditsinskiĭ fakul'tet Vil'niusskogo universiteta na poroge tret'ego stoletiia. **Zh Mikrobiol Epidemiol Immunobiol** 1983 Jan;(1):115–7
Mozzhukhin AS: [I. M. Sechenov - The founder of the first physiological school in Russia] (Rus). **Istor Biol Issled** 1980;8:124–37
Murav'ev MV: K istorii stanovleniia sistemy usovershenstvovaniia vracheĭ v nasheĭ strane. **Sov Zdravookhr** 1980;(11):60–3
Murav'ev MV: K istorii vyezdnykh tsiklov--progressivnoĭ formy provysheniia kvalifikatsii vracheĭ. **Sov Zdravookhr** 1981;(4):59–63
Natadse R: Die Rolle der Universität Tbilisi bei der entwicklung der Psychologie in Georgien. **Wiss Z Friedrich Schiller Univ (Gesellsch)** 1973;22(3):497–509
Ostapiuk FE: Prepodavanie kardiologii v Tsentral'nom Institute Usovershenstvovaniia Vracheĭ (k 50–letiiu so dnia osnovaniia Instituta). **Kardiologiia** 1981;21(1):117–8
Palkin BN: Reformy kontsa XVIII--nachala XIX stoletiia v oblasti meditsinskogo obrazovaniia v Rossii. **Sov Zdravookhr** 1981;(8):71–4
Piaĭ LT, Kalnin VV: Razvitie terapii v Tartuskom universitete. **Ter Arkh** 1984;56(3):44–6
Piatak OA, Perekhrestenko PM, Sadovskaia AG: Programma issledonvaniĭ po istorii meditsiny i ee znachenie dlia dal'neĭshego razvitiia zdravookhraneniia, meditsinskogo obrazovaniia i meditsinskoĭ nauki v USSR. **Vrach Delo** 1981;(4):7–10
Poletaev SD, Sumbatov GA, Chausovskaia MM, et al: Deiatel'nost' kafedry tuberkuleza Tsentral'nogo instituta usovershenstvovaniia vracheĭ v period 1931–1980 gg. **Probl Tuberk** 1980 Dec;(12):3–6
Ponomareva PA, Kuznetsova AI: K 50–letiiu klinicheskikh pediatricheskikh kafedr II Moskovskogo meditsinskogo instituta im. N. I. Pirogova. **Pediatriia** 1981 Dec;(12):61–3
Retnev VM: 60 let kafedre gigieny truda i professional'nykh bolezneĭ. **Gig Tr Prof Zabol** 1984 May;(5):34–7
Roshchin AV, Kozik IV, Arkhangel'skaia LN, et al: Piatidesiatiletie kafedry promyshlennoĭ gigeny Tsentral'nogo ordena Lenina instituta usovershenstvovaniia vracheĭ. **Gig Tr Prof Zabol** 1981 Aug;(8):37–41
Rosliakov AG, Konstantinov AA: Pervyĭ meditsinskiĭ vuz na Sovetskom Dal'nem Vostoke. **Sov Zdravookhr** 1980;(4):67–70
Rudenko AT: Kafedre cheliustno–litsevoĭ khirurgii so stomatologieĭ VMA imeni S. M. Kirova--50 let. **Voen Med Zh** 1980 Mar;(3):77
Rumiantsev GI, Korostelev NB: Osnovanie kafedry gigieny v Moskovskom universitete (K 100–letiiu kafedry). **Gig Sanit** 1984 Aug;(8):41–4
Saarma IuM: 100–letie kafedry i kliniki psikhiatrii v Tartu. **Zh Nevropatol Psikhiatr** 1981;81(11):1716–20
Selivanov EF: Meditsinskie muzei i vospitanie sovetskogo vracha. **Sov Med** 1982;(7):82–5
Shabunin AV: Kalinkinskiĭ khirurgicheskiĭ institut (k 200–letiiu so dnia osnovaniia). **Sov Zdravookhr** 1983;(11):66–7
Shabunin AV: P. F. Lesgaft i razvitie fel'dshersko–akusherskogo obrazovaniia v Rossii. **Feldsher Akush** 1981;46(4):57–8
Shalaev NF: Uchastie studentov Voenno–meditsinskoĭ akademii v revoliutsii 1905–1907 gg. **Sov Zdravookhr** 1980;(8):53–6
Shereshevskiĭ AM: Organizatsiia usovershenstvovaniia vracheĭ–psikhiatrov v Rossii. **Zh Nevropatol Psikhiatr** 1980;80(8):1230–4
Shostak NA, Gorelova LE: Kafedra fakul'tetskoĭ terapii II Moskovskogo meditsinskogo instituta im. I. N. Pirogova (k 70–letiiu so dnia osnovaniia). **Vopr Revm** 1980 Jan–Mar;(1):66–9
Shul'pina NB, Krasnov ML, Shmeleva VV: Postdiplomnoe usovershenstvovanie oftal'mologov (k 50–letiiu Tsentral'nogo instituta usovershenstvovaniia vracheĭ). **Vestn Oftalmol** 1980 Sep–Oct;(5):7–10
Shul'tsev GP: Razvitie kardiologii v trudakh uchenykh Tsentral'nogo instituta usovershenstvovaniia vracheĭ (k 50–letiiu Tsentral'nogo instituta usovershentsvovaniia vracheĭ. **Sov Med** 1980;(11):120–1
Shul'tsev GP: Vklad uchenykh Tsentral'nogo ordena Lenina instituta usovershenstvovaniia vracheĭ v razvitie sovetskoĭ terapii (k 50–letiiu instituta). **Klin Med (Mosk)** 1980 Jun;58(6):8–11
Shyp NA: Z istorii rozvytku medychnoi osvity v Rosii i na Ukraini v druhii polovyni 18 st. **Ukr Istor Zb** 1975;(11):97–104
Siudikas VP, Kutorga VV, Stalioraĭtite EI, et al: Patologiia i ee prepodavanie v Vil'niusskom universitete (k 400–letiiu Vil'niusskogo universiteta i 200–letiiu meditsinskogo fakul'teta ėtogo universiteta). **Arkh Patol** 1980;42(9):70–5
Smol'iannikov AV: Kafedre patologicheskoĭ anatomii Tsentral'nogo ordena Lenina instituta usovershenstvovannia vracheĭ 50 let. **Arkh Patol** 1980;42(12):59–61
Sobchuk GS, Klantsa PA: N. I. Pirogov o nagrazhdenii zarubezhnykh uchenykh Russkimi orderami (Po neopublikovannym materialam). **Sov Zdravookhr** 1983;(4):65–8
Sokolov IuN, Rozenshtraukh LS: Kafedre rentgenologii Tsentral'nogo instituta usovershenstvovaniia vracheĭ 50 let (kratkiĭ istoricheskiĭ ocherk). **Vestn Rentgenol Radiol** 1980 May–Jun;(3):75–8
Solokhin AA: K istorii poslediplomnogo obazovaniia sudebno–meditsinskikh ėkspertov v SSSR (istoki, razvitie, stanovlenie). **Sud Med Ekspert** 1983 Apr–Jun;26(2):55–8
Sosnin VV: Iaroslavskomu meditsinskomu uchilishchu--110 let. **Med Sestra** 1983 Sep;42(9):52–3
Sukharev AG, Fokina NS, Telenchi VI: Kafedre Gigieny Deteĭ i Podrostkov Tsentral'nogo Ordena Lenina Instituta Usovershenstvovaniia Vracheĭ 50 let. **Gig Sanit** 1984 Aug;(8):38–40
Suvorov VIu, Bliumel' NF, Levtova KZ: 50 Let Kafedre ėpidemiologii I Moskovskogo meditsinskogo instituta im. I. M. Sechenova. **Zh Mikrobiol Epidemiol Immunobiol** 1982 Jul;(7):102–6
Suvorova RV, Mikirtichan GL: Metodicheskie voprosy prepodavaniia istorii meditsiny na pediatricheskikh fakul'tetakh. **Sov Zdravookhr** 1982;(1):58–61
Tarasenko NIu: Rol' sanitarno–gigienicheskogo fakul'teta v podgotovke vracheĭ profilakticheskoĭ meditsiny i v razvitii gigieny truda (k 50–letiiu obrazovaniiu sanitarno–gigienicheskogo fakul'teta I Moskovskogo meditsinskogo instituta im I. M. Sechenova). **Gig Tr Prof Zabol** 1980 Oct;(10):29–32
Tikotin MA: Peterburgskiĭ zhenskiĭ meditsinskiĭ institut v revoliutsionnom dvizhenii. **Sov Zdravookhr** 1981;(7):51–4
Timofeeva GA, Valenkevich LN: O podgotovke pediatricheskikh kadrov v SSSR. **Pediatriia** 1980;(1):3–5
Tiurin EI, Kovachev VI: Kafedre rentgenologii i radiologii voenno–meditsinskoĭ akademii im. S. M. Kirova. **Vestn Rentgenol Radiol** 1981 Mar–Apr;(2):87–9
Toporov GN: N. I. Pirogov ob usovershenstvovanii meditsinkikh kadrov v Rossii (k 100–letiiu so dnia smerti N. I. Pirogova, 1810–1881 gg). **Sov Zdravookhr** 1982;(2):66–8
Trubnikov VF: K 60–letiiu osnovanii kafedry ortopedii, travmatologii i voenno–polevoi khirurgii Khar'kovskogo meditsinskogo instituta. **Ortop Travmatol Protez** 1981 Sep;(9):68–70
Valatkene R: Kaunasskoe meditsinskoe uchilishche im. P. Mazhilisa. **Med Sestra** 1981 Apr;40(4):55–6
Vasil'ev KG, Vasil'ev KK: Rol' I. P. Franka a razvitii vysshego meditsinskogo obrazovaniia v Rossii. **Sov Zdravookhr** 1980;(10):62–5
Veselkin PN: K 100–letiiu kafedry patologicheskoĭ fiziologii ordena Lenina Krasnoznamennoĭ voenno–meditsinskoĭ akademii im. S. M. Kirova. **Patol Fiziol Eksp Ter** 1980;(4):3–11
Viduta VK: Tobol'skaia fel'dsherskaia shkola i ee rol' v formirovanii revoliutsionerov. **Sov Zdravookhr** 1984;(8):57–9
Zabłotniak R: Polacy studiujący medycynę i farmację w Kownie (1940–1944). **Przegl Lek** 1980;37(1):101–4
Zagrebin AM: Kafedre anatomii cheloveka Izhevskogo meditsinskogo instituta 50 let. **Arkh Anat Gistol Embriol** 1984 Apr;86(4):91–5
Zaĭko NN: A. A. Bogomolets kak pedagog. **Patol Fiziol Eksp Ter** 1981 Mar–Apr;(2):9–16
Zeligman SB, Kir'iakulov GS: 50 let kafedre anatomii cheloveka Donetskogo meditsinskogo instituta im. M. Gor'kogo. **Arkh Anat Gistol Embriol** 1981 Apr;80(4):102–4
Zhuravleva AI: Role' kafedry lechebnoĭ fizkul'tury i vrachebnogo kontrolia Tsentral'noho instituta usovershenstvovaniia vracheĭ v razvitii nauchnykh osnov spetsial'nosti. **Vopr Kurotal Fizioter Lech Fiz Kult** 1982 Sept–Oct;(5):50–2
Zolotnitskiĭ IaI: O knige O. Kalinskogo 'Retseptura ili nastavlenie sochiniat' pravil'nye retsepty dlia studentov imperatorskoĭ mediko–khirurgicheskoĭ akademii'. **Klin Med (Mosk)** 1984 Apr;62(4):151
Zorina LA, Rashevskaia AM: Postdiplomnoe obuchenie vracheĭ na kafedre profpatologii (k 50–letiiu iubileiu Tsentral'nogo instituta usovershenstvovaniia vracheĭ). **Gig Tr Prof Zabol** 1980 Oct;(10):32–4

**Venezuela**

Algería C: 'El vejamen' y 'El hucusque' en la universidad colonial. **Rev Soc Venez Hist Med** 1972–73;20–21(34–35):29–34
Novoa Montero D: El Profesor Luis Noguer Molins y la Universidad Venezolana. Nueva ed. Mérida, Venezuela, (The Author), 1980 84 p.

**Yugoslavia**

Berić B, Babić N: Dr. Antun Lobmayer (1844–1906) pionir savremenog akušerstva i školovanja primalja u Hrvatskoj. **Jugosl Ginekol Opstet** 1979;19(1–2):113–8
Godišen zbornik na medicinskiot fakultet vo Skopje: **God Zb Med Fak Skopje** 1979 Jan;25:1–536
Kostić AD: Osvrt na ličnost prof. dr. Riharda Burijana i na vreme osnivanja medicinskog fakulteta univerziteta u Beogradu. **Srp Arh Celok Lek** 1982 Mar;110(3):387–98
Nikulin A: U povodu 35–godišnjice rada Medicinskog fakulteta u Sarajevu. **Med Arh** 1981;35(5–6):245–7
Popović M: Razvoj Instituta za pomorsku medicinu Ratne mornarice. **Vojnosanit Pregl** 1980 Sep–Oct;37(5):319–26
1947–1977: po povod zo godini na medidžinskiot fakultet Skopje: **God Zb Med Fak Skopje** 1979 Jan;25:5–126

# EMBRYOLOGY

See also **Generation and Reproduction; Obstetrics**

Girod C: Geschichte der Embryologie. In Sournia JC, Martiny M, Poulet J, ed: Illustrierte Geschichte der Medizin. Salzburg, Andreas, 1980. Vol. 5. p. 1939–87.
Kottek SS: Embryology in Talmudic and Midrashic literature. **J Hist Biol** 1981 Fall;14(2):299–315
Pisanó A: El determinante germinal en la dinámica embriológica. **Acta Physiol Lat Am** 1979;29(1):7–13
Thomasset C: Quelques principes de l'embryologie médiévale (de Salerne à la fin du 13e siècle). **Senefiance** 1980;9:107–21

**France**

Duchatel F: L'auscultation obstétricale de Philippe Le Goust au monitorage foetal. **Hist Sci Med** 1982;16(1):37–47

**Before 500 A.D.**

**Greco–Roman**

Nickel D: Galens Untersuchungen zur embryonalen Blutbewegung. **Orvostort Kozl** 1981;93–96(27 No 1–4):25–35

**Greece**

Lonie IM: The Hippocratic treatises: 'On Generation', 'On the Nature of the Child', 'Diseases IV'. A commentary. Berlin, New York, Walter de Gruyter, 1981. xxxix, 406 p. (Ars medica. II. Abteilung, Griechisch-lateinische Medizin; Bd. 7, 2).
López Férez JA: Algunos datos sobre la influencia de la teoria embriologica de Democrito en el corpus hippocraticum. Gemelos y abortos. **Asclepio** 1981;33:379–90
López Férez JA: Ideas embriologicas de Democrito. **Asclepio** 1982;34:317–26
Roussel M: Ether et chaleur dans l'embryologie aristotélienne: influences archaïques. In: Mélanges d'études anciennes offerts à Maurice Lebel. St-Jean-Chrysostôme, Québec, 1980. p. 157–60.

**500 A.D.–1450**

Demaitre L, Travill AA: Human embryology and development in the works of Albertus Magnus. In Weisheipl JA, ed: Albertus Magnus and the sciences. Toronto, Pontifical Institute of Mediaeval Studies, 1980. p. 405–40.

**Arabic**

Weisser U: Ibn Quaiyim al-Gauziya über die Methoden der Embryologie. **Medizinhist J** 1981;16(3):227–39
Weisser U: The embryology of Yuhanna ibn Masawaith. **J Hist Arabic Sci** 1980;4(1):9–22

**Great Britain**

Hargreaves H: 'De spermate hominis': a Middle English poem on human embryology. [Nat. Libr. Scotland, Advocates' MS. 23.7.11]. **Mediaev Stud** 1977;39:506–10

**Rome**

Houtzager HL: Giles of Rome. **Eur J Obstet Gynecol Reprod Biol** 1981 Aug;12(2):127–9

**1450–1700**

**Great Britain**

Porst S: Gynäkologische, geburtshilfliche, embryologische und teratologische Beschreibungen im Werke Shakespeares. Würzburg, Horst Wellm, 1981. 178 p. (Dissertation, Julius-Maximilians-Universität Würzburg).

**Italy**

Belloni L: Claudius Aubrius a Francesco M. Fiorentini sull'assunzione di latte da parte del feto nell'utero. **Physis** 1977;19(1–4):378–82

**1700 to Present**

Brachet J: Un demi siècle de recherches en embryologie et en cytologie. **Comp Biochem Physiol** 1980;67B:367–72
Hamburger V: S. Ramón y Cajal, R. G. Harrison, and the beginnings of neuroembryology. **Perspect Biol Med** 1980;23(4):600–16
Hirschhorn K: Overview and historical perspective of prenatal diagnosis. **Methods Cell Biol** 1982;26:1–9
Jack DB, Laugher SJ: The earliest demonstration of the placental passage of morphine? **Pharm Hist (London)** 1982 Aug;12(2):7–8
Lukács D: Caspar Friedrick Wolff (1733–1794), a modern fejlödéstan megalapítója. **Orv Hetil** 1984 Aug 5;125(32):1962
Oppenheimer JM: Asymmetry revisited. **Am Zool** 1974 Summer;14(3):867–79
Oppenheimer JM: Ernst Heinrich Haeckel as an intermediary in the transmutation of an idea. **Proc Am Philos Soc** 1982;126(5):347–55
Richards E: The German romantic concept of embryonic repetition and its role in evolutionary theory in England up to 1859. Ph. D. Diss. University of New South Wales, 1976.
Roe SA: Matter, life, and generation. Eighteenth-century embryology and the Haller–Wolff debate. Cambridge, Cambridge University Press, 1981. 214 p.
Sloan PR: Ontogeny and phylogeny. **Br J Hist Sci** 1980;13(1):50–5
Stephens TD: The Wolffian ridge: history of a misconception. **ISIS** 1982 Jun;73(267):254–9
Weets J, Picard JJ: L'élaboration des conceptions sur la gamétogenèse, la fécondation et le développement embryonnaire précoce à la fin du 19e siècle. **Arch Biol (Liege)** 1980;91(2):297–304
Willier BH, Oppenheimer JM, ed: Foundations of experimental embryology. 2nd ed., enlarged and with a new introduction, by J. M. Oppenheimer. New York, Hafner, 1974. xx, 277 p. Selections from various authors.
Witkowski JA: W. T. Astbury and Ross G. Harrison: the search for the molecular determination of form in the developing embryo. **Notes Rec R Soc Lond** 1980 Dec;35(2):195–219
Wolff E: Le développement de la biologie du développement. **Bull Assoc Anat (Nancy)** 1980 Jun;64(185):135–42

**Czechoslovakia**

Cech S: Milan Dvorzhak (k 50-letiiu so dnia rozhdeniia). **Arkh Anat Gistol Embriol** 1980 Jul;79(7):121–5

**Europe**

Skreb N, McKenzie J: The early days of European Developmental Biology Organisation (E.D.B.O.). **Anat Anz** 1981;150(4):443–8

**France**

Castellani C: Fra preformismo e epigenesi: le teorie di Prevost e Dumas. **Hist Philos Life Sci** 1980;2(2):253–68
Fischer JL: Etienne Geoffroy Saint-Hilaire (1772–1844) face au problème du déterminisme du sexe. **Hist Philos Life Sci** 1979;1(2):261–83
Fischer JL, Smith J: French embryology and the 'Mechanics of development' from 1887 to 1910: L. Chabry, Y. Delage & E. Bataillon. **Hist Philos Life Sci** 1984;6(1):25–39
Hoffheimer MH: Maupertuis and the eighteenth-century critique of preexistence. **J Hist Biol** 1982 Spring;15(1):119–44

**Germany**

Gaĭsinovich AE: K. F. Vol'f i ego rol' v istorii embriologii i anatomii (k 250-letiiu so dnia rozhdeniia). **Arkh Anat Gistol Embriol** 1984 Aug;87(8):90–6

**Great Britain**

Roll-Hansen N: E. S. Russell and J. H. Woodger: the failure of two twentieth-century opponents of mechanistic biology. **J Hist Biol** 1984 Fall;17(3):399–428

**Switzerland**

Mazzolini RG: Sugli studi embriologici di Albrecht von Haller negli anni 1755–1758. **Ann Ist Stor Italo-Ger** 1977;3:183–242

**United States**

Baxter AL: E. B. Wilson's 'Destruction' of the germ-layer theory. **Isis** 1977 Sep;68(243):363–74
Benson KR: Problems of individual development: descriptive embryological morphology in America at the turn of the century. **J Hist Biol** 1981 Spring;14(1):115–28
C[one] TE: Early viability of the fetus – an extraordinary case (1845). **Pediatrics** 1981;67:903
Corner GW: The seven ages of a medical scientist, an autobiography. Philadelphia, University of Pennsylvania Press, 1981. xi, 411 p.
Haraway DJ: Ethel Browne Harvey. In: Notable American women. The modern period. Cambridge, Mass., Belknap-Harvard Univ. Press, 1980. 4:319–21.
Maienschein J: Shifting assumptions in American biology: embryology, 1890–1910. **J Hist Biol** 1981 Spring;14(1):89–113
Maienschein JA: Ross Harrison's crucial experiment as a foundation for

modern American experimental embryology. Ph.D. Diss., Indiana University. Bloomington, 1978. 252 leaves.
Oppenheimer JM: Basic embryology and clinical medicine: a case history in serendipity. **Bull Hist Med** 1984 Summer;58(2):236–40
Oppenheimer JM: Thomas Hunt Morgan as an embryologist: the view from Bryn Mawr. **Am Zool** 1983;23:845–54
Werdinger J: Embryology at Woods Hole: the emergence of a new American biology. Ph.D. Diss., Indiana University. Bloomington, 1980. xii, 640 leaves.
Wilens S: Ross Granville Harrison. In Dictionary of American Biography, Suppl. 6, 1956–1960. p. 281–3, 1980.

**USSR**

Baglaĭ EB: Formirovanie predstavleniĭ o prichinakh individual'nogo razvitiia: istoricheskiĭ ocherk. Moskva, Nauka, 1979. 152 p.
Bogdanov OV: Vklad D. A. Biriukova v émbriofiziologiiu i dal'neĭshee razvitie ego ideĭ. **Fiziol Zh SSSR** 1984 Sep;70(9):1248–55
Tokin BP: O nekotorykh problemakh émbriologii i teoreticheskoĭ biologii. **Arkh Anat Gistol Embriol** 1980 Dec;79(12):5–18
Tokin BP, Ivanovo-Kazas OM, Gabaeva NS: Vklad A. G. Knorre v razvitie sovremennoĭ émbriologii. **Arkh Anat Gistol Embriol** 1984 Jul;87(7):92–4

**Yugoslavia**

Posinovec J: Histologija i embriologija u djelu dra Ante Schwarza (u povodu 100. obljetnice njegove smrti). **Lijec Vjesn** 1980 Apr;102(4):208–10

# EMERGENCY MEDICAL SERVICES

See also **Red Cross; Resuscitation; Transportation of Patients**

Medical emergencies: **MD** 1978 Nov;22(11):101–13
Schmidt J: Individuelle Rettungsmittel für Seenotfälle. In Göpfert W, Otten HH, ed: Metavoeite: wandelt euch durch neues Denken. Düsseldorf, Triltsch, 1983. p. 79–87.
Stewart RD: Prehospital emergency care: historical foundations. **Top Emerg Med** 1979 Jul;1(2):11–5

**Germany**

Gögler E: Notarztsysteme in der Bundesrepublik Deutschland. Geschichtlicher Rückblick. **MMW** 1982 Dec 3;124(48):1083–6

**1700 to Present**

**Argentina**

Semorile A: Aspectos sanitarios del terremoto de Mendoza de 1861. In Congreso de Historia de la Medicina Argentina [Transactions], 5th, Mendoza, 1983. p. 19–32.

**Austria**

Spängler H, Galle P: 70 Jahre Unfallchirurgie an den Wiener Kliniken. **Wien Klin Wochenschr** 1981 Jun 26;93(13):423–8

**Belgium**

Askenasi R: Plaidoyer pour une nouvelle spécialité. **Acta Clin Belg** 1983;38(4):265–70

**Canada**

Keenan M: St. John Ambulance 1883–1983. **Can Anaesth Soc J** 1983 Sep;30(5):466–8
Stevenson AL: The Canadian Medic-Alert Foundation. **Can Anaesth Soc J** 1983 Nov;30(6):573–4

**Chile**

Costa-Casaretto C: Septuagésimo aniversario de la asistencia pública de Santiago. **Rev Med Chil** 1981 Aug;109(8):795–803

**Czechoslovakia**

Wondrák E: Jaromír Mundy (1822–1894). Jeho podíl na vývoji záchranných služeb. **Cas Lek Cesk** 1982 Jan 29;121(4):116–9

**France**

Cara M: Le Service d'Aide Médicale Urgente (SAMU) de Paris. **Bull Acad Natl Med (Paris)** 1981 Mar;165(3):365–72

**Germany**

Kaiser W, Völker A: Hygiene, Präventiv, und Unfallmedizin in den Schriften des halleschen Ordinarius Johann Heinrich Schulze (1687–1744). **Z Gesamte Hyg** 1981 Oct;27(10):779–84
Sefrin P: Notfall-Medizin heute. **Fortschr Med** 1982 Jul 22;100(27–28):1273–5

**Great Britain**

Fletcher I: Aid, first and foremost: a brief outline history of the St John Ambulance Association and Brigade. **Injury** 1979 Nov;11(2):104–9
London PS: Inaugural William Gissane Lecture: man and memorial. **Injury** 1982 Nov;14(3):211–34

**Hungary**

Bencze B: Emlékezés Orovecz Bélára az Országos Mentöszolgálat megszervezöjére (1909–1967). **Orv Hetil** 1979 Nov 18;120(46):2819–20

**Spain**

Lorenzo Velázquez B: Presentación de dos formularios: 'Formulario de Terapéutica Clínica' (XV edición) y 'Formulario de Urgénica' (XVII edicion). **An R Acad Nac Med (Madr)** 1981;98(2):211–26

**United States**

History and use of Public Health Service Commissioned Corps: hearing before the Subcommittee on Health and the Environment of the Committee on Energy and Commerce, House of Representatives, Ninety-seventh Congress, session, June 14, 1982. Washington, GPO, 1982. iii, 141 p.
The ACT Foundation: ten years of service to EMS: **J Emerg Med Serv JEMS** 1981 Oct;6(10):35–7
Boyd DR: The conceptual development of EMS systems in the United States, Part I. **Emerg Med Serv** 1982 Jan–Feb;11(1):19–23
Doerner WG: Why does Johnny Reb die when shot? The impact of medical resources upon lethality. **Sociol Inq** 1983;53(1):1–15
Dolphin J: Private ambulance. **Emerg Med Serv** 1977 Nov–Dec;6(6):155–6
Fitzgerald RH: Disaster relief after the Charleston earthquake of 1886. **J SC Med Assoc** 1981 Dec;77(12):607–8
Guthorn PJ: William Augustus Newell, M.D., and the Life Saving Service. **J Med Soc NJ** 1984 Sep;81(9):769–72
Hirschman JC, Nagel EL: Prehospital mobile emergency care in Miami, Florida. An historical commentary. **J Fla Med Assoc** 1981 Aug;68(8):624–34
Jelenko C, Matthews JB, Matthews JC: Emergency medicine in colonial America: Revolutionary War casualties. **Ann Emerg Med** 1982 Jan;11(1):73–6
Johnson JC: Emergency medicine in Indiana: past, present and future. **J Indiana State Med Assoc** 1980 Jun;73(6):354–6
Stephenson GW: The Committee on Trauma: its men and its mission. **Bull Am Coll Surg** 1979 Oct;64(10):17–8, 22–6
Wiegenstein JG: Emergency medicine. **JAMA** 1980 Jun 6;243(21):2182–3
Wilkins EW: Designation or dedication: seven men in the evolution of a trauma center. **Am J Surg** 1982 Apr;143(4):399–403

**USSR**

Bogdanov EA: 50 Let travmatologicheskomu punktu Moskovskogo raĭona Leningrada. **Ortop Travmatol Protez** 1982 Dec;(12):61–3
Chaplinskiĭ VV, Iatsekevich IaE: L'vovskomu nauchnomu obshchestvu travmatologov–ortopedov 25 let. **Ortop Travmatol Protez** 1982 Dec;(12):60–1
Dumbrov DA, Ivanenko AN, Zhalkovskiĭ BV, et al: Stantsii skoroĭ meditsinskoĭ pomoshchi Odessy--80 let. **Sov Zdravookhr** 1983;8:67–9
Dusmuratov MD, Semeniuta AIa: Travmatologiia i ortopediia v Uzbekskoĭ SSR (istoriia, sostoianie i perspektivy razvitiia). **Ortop Travmatol Protez** 1982 Dec;(12):4–7
Grachev AI, Zhalkovskiĭ BV: Istoriia sozdaniia i deiatel'nosti Odesskoĭ stantsii skoroĭ meditsinskoĭ pomoshchi. **Klin Khir** 1983 Dec;(12):56–8
Komarov BD, Bognitskaia TN, Umanskaia VV: Razvitie nauchnykh osnov neotlozhnoĭ khirurgii v Sovetskom Soiuze za 60 let. **Vestn Khir** 1982 Dec;129(12):10–3
Komarov BD, Kustova EA: 60 let skoroĭ meditsinskoĭ pomoshchi. **Sov Med** 1982;(12):25–9
Korol' GG, Denisova TP, Naumenko AM: Iz istorii instituta im. N. V. Sklifosovskogo. **Sov Zdravookhr** 1984;(10):53–5
Lubegina ZP: K 50-letiiu Sverdlovskogo nauchno-issledovatel'skogo instituta travmatologii i ortopedii. **Ortop Travmatol Protez** 1981 Dec;(12):58–61
Stamatin SI, Marin IM: Rol'kafedry meditsinskogo instituta v razvitii ortopedii i travmatologii v Moldavskoĭ SSR. **Ortop Travmatol Protez** 1982 Jul;(7):64–6
Volkov MV, Mattis ER: Osnovnye itogi napravleniia razvitiia Sovetskoĭ travmatologii i ortopedii. **Vestn Khir** 1982 Nov;129(11):3–9

# EMERGENCY MEDICAL SERVICES

Zhalkovskiĭ BV: O pervykh pravilakh vyzova skoroĭ meditsinskoĭ pomoshchi v Odesse. **Sov Zdravookhr** 1984;(7):73-4
Zhalkovskiĭ BV: Osobye sluchai v praktike vyezdnykh vracheĭ Odesskoĭ stantsii skoroĭ medpomoshchi v pervye gody ee deiatel'nosti. **Sov Zdravookhr** 1984;(4):58-9

# ENDOCRINOLOGY

Borit A: History of tumors of the pineal region. **Am J Surg Pathol** 1981 Sep;5(6):613-20
Castro-Vázquez A: The dawn of neuroendocrinology: conquest and heroes. **Acta Physiol Lat Am** 1981;31(3):151-9
Kappers JA: Short history of pineal discovery and research. **Prog Brain Res** 1979;52:3-22
Lindsten J: Sammanställde fall av kortvuxenhet och bristande ovariefunktion hos flickor. **Lakartidningen** 1983 Jul 13;80(28-29):2755
Medvei VC: A history of endocrinology. Lancaster, Boston, MTP Press, 1982. xviii, 913 p.
Medvei VC: Some notes on the history of neuroendocrinology. In Rose FC, Bynum WF, ed: Historical aspects of the neurosciences. New York, Raven, 1982. p. 307-15.
Nedvei VC: A history of endocrinology. Lancaster, Boston, MTP Press, 1982. xviii, 913 p.
Serrano P: Avances en endocrinología. **Gac Med Mex** 1980 Oct;116(10):459-62
Stoffregen M: Nebennieren Anmerkungen zur vorendokrinologischen Ara. **Med Welt** 1980 Feb;31(8):295-301

**1450-1700**

Matuschka MM: Lambert van Velthuysens (1622-1685) Menstruationstheorie in ihrer wissenschaftshistorischen Bedeutung. Zur Vorgeschichte der Endokrinologie der Ovarien. Amsterdam, B. M. Israël, 1980. vii, 72 p.

**France**

Perret L: René Descartes--drottning Kristinas Cartesius--filosof, matematiker och medicinsk läromästare. **Nord Medicinhist Arsb** 1981;:52-8

**1700 to Present**

Beach FA: Historical origins of modern research on hormones and behavior. **Horm Behav** 1981 Dec;15(4):325-76
Butenandt O: 100 Jahre Endokrinologie. **Fortschr Med** 1982 Dec 16;100(47-48):2194-8
Cady B, Sedgwick CE: History of thyroid and parathyroid surgery. **Major Probl Clin Surg** 1980;15:1-5
Dixon B: Tissue therapy. **Br J Hosp Med** 1979 Nov;22(5):512
Gooddy W: Charles Edward Brown-Séquard. In Rose FC, Bynum WF, ed: Historical aspects of the neurosciences. New York, Raven, 1982. p. 371-8.
Gooddy W: Dr. Brown-Sequard in space and time. **Trans Hunter Soc** 1978-80;37-38:153-9
Karlson P: Was sind Hormone? Der Hormonbegriff in Geschichte und Gegenwart. **Naturwissenschaften** 1982 Jan;69(1):3-14
Kattermann R: Walter Siegfried Loewe (1884-1963)). Sein Beitrag zur Analytik, Biologie und Pharmakologie der Sexualhormone. **J Clin Chem Clin Biochem** 1984 Aug;22(8):505-14
Laws ER: Functional pituitary tumors. The neurosurgeon and neuroendocrinology. **Clin Neurosurg** 1980;27:3-18
Maluf NS: Owen's gland. **Sudhoffs Arch** 1980;64(1):25-54
Mattar E: Reminiscênias históricas da endocrinologia. Uma introdução à neuroendocrinologia e suas fronteiras. **Rev Hosp Clin Fac Med Sao Paulo** 1980 Aug;35(4):218-22
Money J: The genealogical descent of sexual psychoneuroendocrinology from sex and health theory: the eighteenth to the twentieth centuries. **Psychoneuroendocrinology** 1983;8(4):391-400
Simmer HH: Zur Geschichte der hormonalen Auslösung einer echten Menstruation. Versuche an menstruierenden Affen und an Frauen in den frühen dreissiger Jahren unseres Jahrhunderts. In Göpfert W, Otten HH, ed: Metavoeite: wandelt euch durch neues Denken. Düsseldorf, Triltsch, 1983. p. 161-71.
Sowers JR: Hypothalamic hormones. Stroudsburg, Pennsylvania, Dowden, Hutchinson & Ross, 1980. xviii, 342 p. (Benchmark Papers in Human Physiology, 14).
Teichman SL, Aldea PA: Pioneers in pituitary physiology: Harvey Cushing and Nicolas Paulescu. **J Hist Med Allied Sci** 1985 Jan;40(1):68-72
Vague J: Die Geschichte der Endokrinologie bis zum Zweiten Weltkrieg. In Sournia JC, Martiny M, Poulet J, ed: Illustrierte Geschichte der Medizin. Salzburg, Andreas, 1980. Vol. 7. p. 2749-70.
Vague J: Geschichte der Endokrinologie nach dem Zweiten Weltkrieg. In Sournia JC, Martiny M, Poulet J, ed: Illustrierte Geschichte der Medizin. Salzburg, Andreas, 1980. Vol. 8. p. 3141-79.
Völker A: Markierungspunkte in der Geschichte der Parathyreoideaforschung. **Z Gesamte Inn Med** 1983 Aug 1;38(15):386-7
Wade N: The Nobel duel. Two scientists' 21-year race to win the world's most coveted research prize. Garden City, Anchor Press/Doubleday, 1981. 321 p.
Yamagata S: [Studies of the pancreas -- historical survey]. (Jpn) **Nippon Rinsho** 1980;38(1):4-8

**Austria**

Ober WB: Emil Zuckerkandl and his delightful little organ. **Pathol Annu** 1983;18(Pt 1):103-19
Weinzierl S: Frühe Rezeption der Halbanschen Hypothese von der endokrinen Verursachung der Menstruation. Diss. Erlangen-Nürnberg, 1980. 59 p.

**Belgium**

Herlant M: Travaux consacrés aux glandes endocrines parus dans les Archives de Biologie entre 1880 et 1931. **Arch Biol (Liege)** 1980;91(2):243-65

**Canada**

Barr ML: James Bertram Collip (1892-1965): a Canadian pioneer in endocrinology. In: Congrès international d'histoire de la médecine, XXVe, Québec, 1976. Actes. Québec, 1977. p. 469-76.

**Czechoslovakia**

Macho L, Langer P: 30 years of the Institute of Experimental Endocrinology. **Endocrinol Exp (Bratisl)** 1982 Nov;16(3-4):147-9
Podoba J: Tridsat rokov od založenia endokrinologického ústavu v Bratislave. **Bratisl Lek Listy** 1982;78(4):489-99

**Finland**

Wahlberg P: Tyreoidologi i Finland under 150 år. **Nord Medicinhist Arsb** 1984;:105-16

**France**

Role A: La vie étrange d'un grand savant: le professeur Brown-Sequard, 1817-1894. Paris, Plon, 1977. 219 p.

**Germany**

Ebling FJ: Homage to Paul Langerhans. **J Invest Dermatol** 1980 Jul;75(1):3-5
Hoppe B: Adolf Windaus, Heinrich Wieland, Richard Kuhn, Leopold Ružička, Alexander Todd und Adolf Bunenandt. Die Erforschung der Vitamine und der Hormone. In: Die Grossen der Weltgeschichte. Zürich, Kindler, 1978. p. 336-81.

**Great Britain**

O'Rahilly R: The discovery of the parathyroid glands. **Bull Hist Med** 1982 Summer;56(2):263-4
Tait JF, Tait SA: Recent perspectives on the history of the adrenal cortex. **J Endocrinol** 1979 Oct;83(1):3P-24P
Zuckerman L: The launching of the Journal of Endocrinology and the founding of the Society for Endocrinology. **J Endocrinol** 1984 Jan;100(1):1-5

**Italy**

Giorgino R: Nicola Pende: medico, ricercatore, maestro. **G Clin Med** 1981 Nov;62(11):747-57
Mutt V: An appreciation of the work of Vittorio Erspamer. **Peptides (Fayetteville)** 1981;2(Suppl 2):3-6

**Romania**

Milcu SM: Brief history of Romanian endocrinology. Bucharest, Medical Pub. House, 1981. 51 p.
Milcu Sm: The contributions made by Romanian physicians to the development of endocrinology. **Endokrinologie** 1981 Apr-Jun;19(2):81-6

**South Africa**

Berman MC: The clinical investigator: a tribute to the late Professor Bernard Pimstone. **S Afr Med J** 1983 Mar 5;63(10):366-71

**Spain**

Hofmann C: Stimme und Konstitution im Werk Gregorio Marañóns. **Medizinhist J** 1984;19(3):259-66

**Sweden**

Breimer L, Sourander P: The discovery of the parathyroid glands in 1880: triumph and tragedy of Ivar Sandström. **Bull Hist Med** 1981 Winter;55(4):558–63
Kock W: 80-talet: da å upptäcktes bisköldkörtlarna och då gjorde bakterierna sin entré. **Lakartidningen** 1979 Dec 19;76(51):4697–9

**United States**

Catchpole HR: Growth hormone. **JAMA** 1980 Feb 15;243(7):652
Corner GW: Leo Loeb. In Dictionary of American Biography, Suppl. 6, 1956–1960. p. 385–7, 1980.
Fisher DA: The Endocrine Society: past and present. **J Clin Endocrinol Metab** 1984 Dec;59(6):1229–33
Grumbach MM: Herbert McLean Evans, revolutionary in modern endocrinology: a tale of great expectations. **J Clin Endocrinol Metab** 1982 Dec;55(6):1240–7
Harvey AM: James Howard Means and his romance with the thyroid gland. **Am J Med** 1981 Jun;70(6):1158–60
Howard JE: Fuller Albright: the endocrinologists' clinical endocrinologist. **Perspect Biol Med** 1981 Spring;24(3):374–81
Knigge KM: Burton Lowell Baker 1912–1978. **Am J Anat** 1980 Aug;158(4):391–4
Kroc RL: Relaxin--a perspective, or personal anecdotal recollections. **Ann NY Acad Sci** 1982;380:1–5
Morris JP: Walter Timme. In Dictionary of American Biography, Suppl. 6, 1956–1960. p. 634–5, 1980.
Raacke ID: Jane Anne Russell. In: Notable American women. The modern period. Cambridge, Mass., Belknap-Harvard Univ. Press, 1980. 4:610–1.

**USSR**

Bondar PN: O role uchenykh Kievskogo meditsinskogo instituta v razvitii éndokrinologii. **Vrach Delo** 1981 Aug;(8):124–5
Iudaev NA: Sostoianie i puti razvitiia sovetskoĭ éndokrinologii. **Sov Med** 1982;(12):41–6
Komissarenko PV: Znachenie issledovaniĭ A. A. Bogomol'tsa v razvitii sovremennoĭ ĕndokrinologii. **Fiziol Zh** 1981 May–Jun;27(3):388–93
Komissarenko VP: Idei A. A. Bogomol'tsa v razvitii sovremennoĭ éndokrinologii. **Patol Fiziol Eksp Ter** 1981 Mar–Apr;(2):82–9
Leibson L: Endocrinology evolution and evolutionary endocrinology. **Perspect Biol Med** 1979 Autumn;23(1):25–43
Nikitiuk BA, Kozlov AI: Nekotorye spornye polozheniia ucheniia ob antropogeneze v svete predstavleniĭ o destabiliziruiushchem otbore i dannykh sovremennoĭ paléoendokrinologii (k 100–letiiu so dnia rozhdeniia I. I. Shmal'gauzena). **Arkh Anat Gistol Embriol** 1984 Aug;87(8):5–14
Shurygin DIa: Razvitie ideĭ S. P. Botkina v oblasti épidemiologii. **Klin Med (Mosk)** 1982 Apr;60(4):112–5

# EPIDEMIOLOGY

See also **Climate; Communicable Disease Control; Diseases and Injuries; Preventive Medicine; Public Health; Statistics and Demography; International Health**

Black FL: Modern isolated pre-agricultural populations as a source of information on prehistoric epidemic patterns. In Stanley NF, Joske RA, ed: Changing disease patterns and human behaviour. London, New York, Academic Press, 1980. p. 37–54.
Comiti VP: Intoxications non microbiennes et epidemies infectieuses historiques. In International Congress of the History of Medicine, 27th, Barcelona, 1980. Actas. Barcelona, Académia de Ciències Mèdiques de Catalunya i Balears, 1981. p. 495–8.
Herzlich C: Malades d'hier, malades d'aujourd'hui: de la mort collective au devoir de guérison. Paris, Payot, 1984. 295 p.
Inglis B: The diseases of civilisation. London, Hodder and Stoughton, 1981. xi, 371 p.
Knorr M, Schadewaldt H: Infektiöse Erkrankungen im Wandel. Jahreszeitliche und säkulare Rhythmik von Infektionskrankheiten. Seasonal und periodic rhythms of infectious diseases. **Zentralbl Bakteriol [Orig B]** 1979;168(1–2):1–17
Lilienfeld AM, Lilienfeld DE: Threads of epidemiologic history. In their: Foundations of epidemiology. 2d ed. New York and Oxford, Oxford University Press, 1980. p. 23–45.
Luckin B: States and epidemic threats. **Soc Soc Hist Med Bull (Lond)** 1984 Jun;34:25–7
McNeill WH: Historical patterns of migration. **Curr Anthropol** 1979;20(1):94–8
Marr JJ: Merchants of death: the role of slave trade in the transmission of disease from Africa to the Americas. **Pharos** 1982 Winter;45(1):31–5
Mercier C: L'épidémiologie et la population. **Infirm Fr** 1983 Jun;(246):3–6
Pérez PJ, Arsuaga JL de: Estudio paleoepidemiológico y paleodemográfico de la necrópolis de Mirmad (Argin-Sur, Nubia sudanesa). In International Congress of the History of Medicine, 27th, Barcelona, 1980. Actas. Barcelona, Académia de Ciències Mèdiques de Catalunya i Balears, 1981. p. 596–602.
Risse GB: La ecología de la enfermedad: tema de estudio médico-histórico. **Bol Soc Mex Hist Filos Med** 1984 Mar;7(46):289–304
Siniak KM, Davidenko OS: Materialisticheskoe ponimanie razvitiia épidemiologii. **Zh Mikrobiol Epidemiol Immunobiol** 1980 Sep;(9):12–7
Verso ML: Airs, waters and places. **Victorian Hist J** 1977 Feb;48(1):6–21
Winslow CE: The conquest of epidemic disease: a chapter in the history of ideas. Madison, University of Wisconsin Press, 1980 printing, c1971. viii, 411 p.

**Africa**

Miller JC: The significance of drought, disease and famine in the agriculturally marginal zones of West-Central Africa. **J Afr Hist** 1982;23(1):17–61

**Americas**

Benítez RF: Historia de la deficiencia mental endemica en la region Andina. **Asclepio** 1982;34:339–76

**Great Britain**

Barker DJ: Geographical variations in disease in Britain. **Br Med J** 1981;283:398–400
Hope-Simpson RE: Recognition of historic influenza epidemics from parish burial records: a test of prediction from a new hypothesis of influenzal epidemiology. **J Hyg (Lond)** 1983 Oct;91(2):293–308

**India**

Jaggi OP: Western medicine in India: epidemics and other tropical diseases. Delhi, Atma Ram, 1979. xii, 331 p.

**Italy**

Jarcho S: Some Italian broadsides and passports of epidemiologic interest (1618–1723). **Trans Stud Coll Physicians Phila** 1981;Ser.5 3(1):40–52

**Romania**

Barbu G: Din istoria combaterii epidemiilor în ţara noastră. (I). Frăţiile milosteniei. **Rev Ig [Bacteriol]** 1984 Apr–Jun;29(2):189–92

**United States**

Cooper R: A note on the biologic concept of race and its application in epidemiologic research. **Am Heart J** 1984 Sep;108(3 Pt 2):715–22
Simpson HN: Invisible armies. The impact of disease on American history. Indianapolis, Bobbs-Merrill, 1980. xi, 239 p.

**Before 500 A.D.**

**Greece**

Habs H: Die sogenannte Pest des Thukydides: Versuch einer epidemiologischen Analyse. Berlin, New York, Springer-Verlag, 1982. 46 p.
Longrigg J: Thucydides and the great plague of Athens. In International Congress of the History of Medicine, 27th, Barcelona, 1980. Actas. Barcelona, Académia de Ciències Mèdiques de Catalunya i Balears, 1981. p. 281–8.

**500 A.D.–1450**

**Great Britain**

Cule J: Pestis flava: y fad felen. In J. Cule, ed: Wales and medicine. London, British Society for the History of Medicine, 1975. p. 141–55.

**1450–1700**

Neugebauer R: Application of a capture-recapture method (the Bernoulli census) to historical epidemiology. **Am J Epidemiol** 1984 Oct;120(4):626–34

**Italy**

Jarcho S: Some early Italian epidemiological maps. **Imago Mundi** 1983;35:9–19

**Mexico**

Prem HJ: Seuchengeschichte von Zentralmexiko im 16. Jahrhundert. Ein Modell für die heutige weltweite Seuchensituation? **Fortschr Med** 1981 Sep 24;99(36):1421–2

# EPIDEMIOLOGY

**1700 to Present**

Aleksandrovskiĭ BN, Shchetova GA: K istorii russko-nemetskikh nauchnykh sviazeĭ v oblasti épidemiologii i gigieny. **Sov Zdravookhr** 1982;(1):61–5
Bleker J: Die historische Pathologie, Nosologie und Epidemiologie im 19. Jahrhundert. **Medizinhist J** 1984;19(1–2):33–52
Brandt AM: James Angus Doull. In Dictionary of American biography, 1961–1965. Suppl. 7, 1981. p. 194–5.
Butler T: Plague and other Yersinia infections. New York, London, Plenum Medical Book Co., 1983. xii, 220 p. (Current Topics in Infectious Disease).
Cameron D, Jones IG: John Snow, the broad street pump and modern epidemiology. **Int J Epidemiol** 1983 Dec;12(4):393–6
Desowitz RS: New Guinea tapeworms and Jewish grandmothers. Tales of parasites and people. New York, London, W. W. Norton, 1981. 224 p.
Ermakov VV, Devyatova LN: The experience and the stages of development in USSR of the WHO English International Courses for epidemiology (1969–1978). **Sante Publique (Bucur)** 1980;23(1):3–14
The history of the International Epidemiological Association brought up to date: **Int J Epidemiol** 1984 Jun;13(2):139–41
Krause RM: A matter of opportunity. **J Allergy Clin Immunol** 1982 Jul;70(1):2–3
Krause RM: The restless tide. The persistent challenge of the microbial world. Washington, D. C., National Foundation for Infectious Diseases, 1981. 152 p.
Lilienfeld AM: Ceteris Paribus: the evolution of the clinical trial. (The Fielding H. Garrison Lecture). **Bull Hist Med** 1982 Spring;56(1):1–18
Lilienfeld AM: Epidemiology and health policy: some historical highlights. **Public Health Rep** 1984 May–Jun;99(3):237–41
Lilienfeld AM, Lilienfeld DE: 'The epidemiologic fabric'. I--Weaving the threads. **Int J Epidemiol** 1980 Sep;9(3):199–206
Lilienfeld AM, ed: Times, places, and persons. Aspects of the history of epidemiology. Baltimore and London, Johns Hopkins University Press, 1980. 144 p. (Sigerist Supplements to the Bulletin of the History of Medicine, n.s., no. 4).
Paddison RM, Skinner RE, ed: Antonie Wouter Voors, M.D., M.P.H., D.P.H. A biographical sketch and a bibliography of his work. New Orleans: History of Medicine Club of Louisiana State University Medical Center, 1983. 23 p.
Pickstone JV: Ferriar's fever and Kay's cholera: disease and social structure in Cottonopolis. **Soc Soc Hist Med Bull (Lond)** 1980;27:19–22
Ravenholt RT, Foege WH: 1918 influenza, encephalitis lethargica, parkinsonism. **Lancet** 1982 Oct 16:2(8303):860–4
Rische H: Moderne epidemiologische und pathogenetische Erkenntnisse, dargestellt am Beispiel der Cholera. **Z Erkr Atmungsorgane** 1983;161(1):65–73
Rothman KJ: The rise and fall of epidemiology, 1950–2000 A.D. **N Engl J Med** 1981 Mar 5;304(10):600–2
Siniak KM: Epidemicheskie posledstviia vremennoĭ fashistskoĭ okkupatsii Ukrainskoĭ SSR i mery po ikh preodoleniiu. **Zh Mikrobiol Epidemiol Immunobiol** 1982 May;(5):11–4
Wilson LG: Fevers and science in early nineteenth century medicine. **J Hist Med Allied Sci** 1978 Jul;33(3):386–407

**Africa**

Ofcansky TP: The 1889–97 rinderpest epidemic and the rise of British and German colonialism in eastern and southern Africa. **J Afr Stud** 1981;8(1):31–8
Tymowski M: Famines et épidémies à Oualata et à Tichit au XIXe siècle. **Afr Bull** 1978;27:35–53

**Americas**

Garrafa V: Epidemiología: desarrollo histórico de su concepto. **CERON** 1979 Apr;4(1):23–7
Garrafa V: Epidemiologia: desenvolvimento histórico do seu conceito. **Rev Assoc Paul Cir Dent** 1980 May–Jun;34(3):196–202

**Angola**

Dias JR: Famine and disease in the history of Angola, C. 1830–1930. **J Afr Hist** 1981;22(3):349–78

**Canada**

Carley CD: Historical and archaeological evidence of 19th century fever epidemics and medicine at Hudson's Bay Company's Fort Vancouver. **Hist Archaeol** 1981;15(1):19–35
Farley M, Keel O, Limoges C: Les commencements de l'administration montréalaise de la santé publique (1865–1885). **HSTC** 1982 May;21(6 no 2):85–109
Mathieu J, Cyr C, Dinel G, et al: Les alliances matrimoniales exogames dans le gouvernement de Québec 1700–1760. **Rev Hist Am Fr** 1981;35(1):3–32

**Cuba**

Lopez Sanchez J: Carlos J. Finlay and the conception of contagion. **Indian J Hist Sci** 1981;16(2):156–68
López Sánchez J: Karlos KH. Finlai i teoriia peredachi infektsii. **Vopr Istor Estestvozn Tekh** 1981;(4):29–34

**Czechoslovakia**

Baudiš P: Franz Köstl a jeho práce s epidemiologickým zaměřením. **Cesk Psychiatr** 1979 Apr;75(2):144–7
Kyntera F: Přínos vojenské epidemiologie za období 25leté existence Vojenského lékařského výzkumného a doškolovacího ústavu Jana Evangelisty Purkyně v Hradci Králové. **Cesk Epidemiol Mikrobiol Imunol** 1984 Jan;33(1):53–5
Petrov BD: I. A. Pribil' (k 200–letiiu so dnia rozhdeniia). **Zh Mikrobiol Epidemiol Immunobiol** 1983 Oct;(10):108–9
Skovránek V: Naše epidemiologie a mikrobiologie v posledních třiceti letech. **Cesk Epidemiol Mikrobiol Imunol** 1982 May;31(3):132–4
Skovránek V: Thirty years of the Czechoslovak sanitary and epidemiological service--1952–1982. **J Hyg Epidemiol Microbiol Immunol** 1982;26(4):329–33

**Denmark**

Lamblin-Robert J, Lecomte D, Lathrop M, et al: Epidemies virales et rapport de masculinité des naissances: des données divergentes. **Population** 1983;38(1):162–5

**France**

Desaive JP: Médecins, climat et épidémies à la fin du XVIIIe siècle. Paris, Mouton, [1972]. 254 p.
Stofft H: Bouestard, médecin des épidémies à Morlaix. **Hist Sci Med** 1984;18(3):223–45

**Germany**

Howard-Jones N: Friedrich Wolter (1893?–1944): the last anticontagionist. **Br Med J** 1980 Feb 9;280(6211):372–3
Schmidt G: O znachenii otkrytiĭ Roberta Kokha dlia razvitiia bakteriologii i épidemiologii. **Zh Mikrobiol Epidemiol Immunobiol** 1983 Mar;(3):106–9
Wagner D: Die Epidemiologie in der Berliner medizinhistorischen Forschung des 19. Jahrhunderts. **Z Gesamte Hyg** 1980;26(12):920–3

**Great Britain**

Fine PE: John Brownlee and the measurement of infectiousness: an historical study in epidemic theory. **J R Stat Soc** 1979;142:347–62
Leaman A: John Snow MD--his early days. **Anaesthesia** 1984 Aug;39(8):803–5
Lilienfeld AM: Bradford Hill's influence on epidemiology. **Stat Med** 1982 Oct–Dec;1(4):325–8
Lilienfeld AM, Lilienfeld DE: Epidemiology and the public health movement: a historical perspective. **J Public Health Policy** 1982 Jun;3(2):140–9
Lilienfeld AM, Lilienfeld DE: John Snow, the Broad Street pump and modern epidemiology. **Int J Epidemiol** 1984 Sep;13(3):376–8
Lilienfeld AM, Lilienfeld DE: 'The epidemiologic fabric'. II. The London Bridge--it never fell. **Int J Epidemiol** 1980 Dec;9(4):299–304
Lilienfeld DE: Epidemiology 101: III. A 19th century example. **Int J Epidemiol** 1981 Mar;10(1):69–72
Lloyd O: Epidemiology: some early lessions. **Occup Health (Lond)** 1981 Jan;33(1):27–36
McLaren D: Disease and dirty water in West Somerset in the late nineteenth century. **Soc Soc Hist Med Bull (Lond)** 1974 Dec;35:35–6
Pickering G: William Norman Pickles. In Dictionary of national biography, 1961–1970. Suppl. 8, 1981. p. 843–4.
Richards T: Farr sighted. **Br Med J [Clin Res]** 1983 May 28;286(6379):1736–7
Rose G: Professor D.D. Reid, MD Aberdeen, PHD DSc London, FRCP London. **J Epidemiol Community Health** 1978 Dec;32(4):229–34
Sheppard J: Illustrations from the Wellcome Institute Library: Sir Leonard Rogers, FRS (1868–1962) and his papers. **Med Hist** 1983 Apr;27(2):214–5
Smith CE: The Broad Street pump revisited. **Int J Epidemiol** 1982 Jun;11(2):99–100

**India**

Gibson ME: The identification of kala azar and the discovery of Leishmania donovani. **Med Hist** 1983 Apr;27(2):203–13
Lardinois R: Une conjoncture de crise démographique en Indé du Sud au XIXe siècle: la famine de 1876–1878. **Population** 1982;37(2):371–404

**Ireland**

O'Brien W: The fevers of the Great Famine.

**J Ir Coll Physicians Surg** 1980 Jul;10(1):46-9

### Italy

Sorcinelli P: Miseria e malattie nel XIX secolo. I ceti popolari nell'Italia centrale fra tifo petecchiale e pellagra. Milano, Franco Angeli, 1979. 285 p.

### Mexico

Jackson RH: Epidemic disease and population decline in the Baja California Missions, 1697-1834. **South Calif Q** 1981;63(4):308-46

Marcial LD, Gutiérrez Avila JH: La vigilancia epidemiológica un siglo después. Nil novi sub sole? Comentarios al trabajo del Dr. Nicolás Ramírez de Arellano. **Salud Publica Mex** 1982 Sep-Oct;24(5):491-5

### Netherlands

Palm LC: De paalwormepidemie van 1730. **Spiegel Hist** 1980;15(5):266-72

### Poland

Jastrzebowski Z: Epidemie a rozwój ludności Królestwa Polskiego w latach 1815-1870. **Arch Hist Med (Warsz)** 1984;47(3):355-74

Kieć E, et al: Prof. Dr. Leon Cholewa. **Przegl Lek** 1984;41(7):465-76

### Romania

Brătescu G: Preocupări epidemiologice ale doctorului V. Voiculescu. **Rev Ig [Bacteriol]** 1980 Jan-Mar;25(1):59-61

Sibechi G: Un doctor ieşean de prestigiu: Evstatie Rola. **Rev Med Chir Soc Med Nat Iasi** 1982 Jul-Sep;86(3):436, 440, 504

### South Africa

Ibrahim MA, Kaplan BH, Patrick RC, et al: The legacy of John C. Cassel. **Am J Epidemiol** 1980 Jul;112(1):1-7

Marks S, Andersson N: Epidemics and social control in twentieth-century South Africa. **Soc Soc Hist Med Bull (Lond)** 1984 Jun;34:32-4

### Tunisia

Gallagher NE: Medicine and power in Tunisia, 1780-1900. Cambridge; New York, Cambridge University Press, 1983. xii, 145 p.

Gaumer B: Contribution de Ernest Conseil à la naissance de l'épidémiologie en Tunisie. **Arch Inst Pasteur Tunis** 1983 Mar-Sep;60(1-2):49-64

### United States

Bean WB: Walter Reed. A biography. Charlottesville, University Press of Virginia, 1982. 190 p.

Buchanan AV, Weiss KM, Schwartz RJ, et al: Reconstruction of genealogies from vital records: the Laredo Epidemiology Project. **Comput Biomed Res** 1984 Aug;17(4):326-51

Denny FW: Atypical pneumonia and the Armed Forces Epidemiological Board. **J Infect Dis** 1981 Mar;143(3):305-16

Gordis L: Symposium in honor of Abraham M. Lilienfeld. Chronic disease epidemiology at the threshold of a new decade. **Am J Epidemiol** 1980 Aug;112(2):169-77

Greenhouse SW: Jerome Cornfield's contributions to epidemiology. **Biometrics** 1982 Mar;38 Suppl:33-45

Hannaway C: Abraham M. Lilienfeld (1920-1984). **Bull Hist Med** 1984 Winter;58(4):558-9

Henson PM: Harold Fred Dorn. In Dictionary of American biography, 1961-1965. Suppl. 7, 1981. p. 191-3.

Levison CH, Hastings DW, Harrison JN: The epidemiologic transition in a frontier town--Manti, Utah, 1849-1977. **Am J Phys Anthropol** 1981 Sep;56(1):83-93

Lilienfeld AM: Wade Hampton Frost: contributions to epidemiology and public health. **Am J Epidemiol** 1983 Apr;117(4):379-83

Putney DT: Fighting the scourge: American Indian morbidity and federal policy, 1897-1928. Ph.D. Diss., Marquette University. Milwaukee, 1980. 355 leaves.

Schwartz RJ, Weiss KM, Buchanan AV: Looking into the black box: practical approaches to record linkage. **Ann Demogr Hist (Paris)** 1984;:119-28

Skolnick MH, Bean LL, Mineau GP, et al: Etudes génétiques et démographiques et base de données généalogiques de l'Utah. **Ann Demogr Hist (Paris)** 1984;:103-13

Terris M: The complex tasks of the second epidemiologic revolution. **J Public Health Policy** 1983 Mar;4(1):8-24

Terris M: The epidemiologic tradition. **Public Health Rep** 1979 Jun;94(3):203-9

Thomas G, Morgan-Witts M: Anatomy of an epidemic. Garden City, N. Y., Doubleday, 1982. xv, 366 p.

Winkelstein W: A tribute to Abe Lilienfeld. **Am J Epidemiol** 1980 Aug;112(2):178-84

### USSR

Beliakov VD: Uchenie L. V. Gromashevskogo ob épidemicheskom protsesse i razvitie étogo ucheniia na sovremennom étape. **Zh Mikrobiol Epidemiol Immunobiol** 1984 Jul;(7):115-8

Borodiĭ NK: I. A. Poletika--vydaiushchiĭsia ukrainskiĭ vrach i uchenyĭ XVIII st. **Mikrobiol Zh** 1982 May-Jun;44(3):90-4

Chaĭka NA: Deiatel'nost' Leningradskogo nauchno-issledovatel'skogo instituta épidemiologii i mikrobiologii im. Pastera v gody Velikoĭ Otechestvennoĭ voĭny. **Sov Zdravookhr** 1980;(8):47-51

Dekhtsunian KM: Nauchnaia deiatel'nost' Armianskogo ordena Trudovogo Krasnogo Znameni NII épidemiologii, virusologii i meditsinskoĭ parazitologii im. A. B. Aleksaniana (k 60-letiiu so dnia osnovaniia instituta). **Zh Mikrobiol Epidemiol Immunobiol** 1984 Feb;(2):114-7

Elkin II: Leninskiĭ étap v razvitii épidemiologii. **Zh Mikrobiol Epidemiol Immunobiol** 1981 Jan;(1):3-8

Elkin II: Nauchnyĭ podvig L. A. Gromashevskogo. **Zh Mikrobiol Epidemiol Immunobiol** 1982 Jan;(1):113-7

Favorova LA: Uchenie L. V. Gromashevskogo i problema likvidatsii infekstionnykh bolezneĭ. **Zh Mikrobiol Epidemiol Immunobiol** 1984 Jul;(7):119-23

Gol'd E IU: M. N. Solov'ev: 1886-1980. Moskva, Meditsina, 1982. 60 p.

Ivan Luk'ianovich Bogdanov (k 80-letiiu so dnia rozhdeniia): **Vrach Delo** 1983 Aug;(8):125-6

Karavaev AG, Berenshteĭn GF: Vydaiushchiĭsia épidemiolog (Vladimir Aaronovich Khavkin). **Med Sestra** 1981 Jul;40(7):55-7

Kas'ianenko AM: Sanitarno-épidemiologicheskaia sluzhba Sovetskoĭ Ukrainy. **Vrach Delo** 1983 Jan;(1):1-6

Kaulen DR: Itogi i perspektivy deiatel'nosti nauchno-issledovatel'skogo instituta épidemiologii i mikrobiologii im. N. F. Gamalei AMN SSSR (k 90-letiiu so dnia osnovaniia). **Zh Mikrobiol Epidemiol Immunobiol** 1982 May;(5):116-20

Konin GK: Fel'dsher-revoliutsioner S. A. Gribov. **Feldsher Akush** 1982;47(11):33-5

Kovaleva EP, Deviatova LN, Kasparova TIu, et al: K 50-letiiu kafedry épidemiologii Tsentral'nogo instituta usovershenstvovaniia vracheĭ. **Zh Mikrobiol Epidemiol Immunobiol** 1981 Jun;(6):113-7

Kurchishvili IB, Asatiani DK, Chomakhashvili AI: Istoki meditsinskoĭ geografii v Gruzii. **Sov Zdravookhr** 1983;(12):51-3

Lebedev NI: Epidemicheskie posledstviia nemetsko-fashistkoĭ okkupatsii Belorussii v 1941-1944 gg. i mery po ikh likvidatsii. **Zh Mikrobiol Epidemiol Immunobiol** 1982 Jul;(7):106-10

Lebedev NI: Istoricheskie preimushchestva sovetskoĭ épidemiologii v teorii i praktike profilaktiki infektsionnykh bolezneĭ. **Zh Mikrobiol Epidemiol Immunobiol** 1981 Feb;(2):3-6

Mazurik EV: Pervye shagi nauchnoĭ deiatel'nosti D. K. Zabolotnogo. **Zh Mikrobiol Epidemiol Immunobiol** 1983 May;(5):99-101

Medzhidov BF: Istoriia Nauchno-issledovatel'skogo instituta virusologii, mikrobiologii i gigieny imeni G. M. Musabekova. Baku, Azerbaidzhanskoe gos. izd-vo, 1968. 183 p.

Podolyan VY: Development of medico-geographical ideas in the epoch of the developed socialism and scientific and technological progress. **Geogr Med** 1984;14:284-93

Pololian VIa: Vazhneĭshie étapy sozdaniia ucheniia akademika E.N. Pavlovskogo o prirodnoĭ ochagovosti bolezneĭ. **Vestn Akad Med Nauk SSSR** 1980;(10):10-4

Rykushin IuP, Smorodintsev AA, Shliakhtenko LI, et al: Professor V. A. Bashenin--odin iz osnovopolozhnikov otechestvennoĭ épidemiologii. **Zh Mikrobiol Epidemiol Immunobiol** 1983 Apr;(4):112-6

Sanzharov BN: Deiatel'nost' glavnykh épidemiologov frontov v 1941-1945 gg. **Voen Med Zh** 1980;(12):13-4

Selezneva VT: N. A. Russkikh--organizator bor'by s detskoĭ smertnost'iu (k 125-letiiu so dnia rozhdeniia). **Sov Zdravookhr** 1982;(7):64-7

Shipitsina NK: Vliianie issledovaniĭ V. N. Beklemisheva v oblasti obshcheĭ biologii, parazitologii i épidemiologii transmissivnykh bolezneŭ na razvitie étikh otrasleĭ nauki (k 90-letiiu so dnia rozhdeniia). **Med Parazitol (Mosk)** 1982 Mar-Apr;60(2):86-8

Shirokov IuG, Lebedeva NV, Koliadich MN: Uchastie L. K. Khotsianova v rabote s'ezdov gigienistov i sanitarnykh vracheĭ. **Gig Sanit** 1983 Feb;(2):31-5

Shliakhtenko LI, Kryga LN, Liamtseva GA, et al: Evoliutsiia épidemicheskogo protsessa virusnogo gepatita v Leningrade za 30 let. **Tr Inst Pastera** 1982;57:43-5

Siniak KM, Rudichenko VF: Avksentiĭ Vasil'evich Korchak-Chepurkovskiĭ (k 125-letiiu so dnia rozhdeniia). **Vrach Delo** 1983 Apr;(4):118-21

Skobulovich GV: Itogi deiatel'nosti Amursjkogo otdeleniia Nauchnogo obshchestva épidemiologov, mikrobiologov i parazitologov za 25 let (1957-1982). **Zh Mikrobiol Epidemiol Immunobiol** 1984 Feb;(2):117-9

Smirnov EI, Garin NS: S. P. Botkin o variabel'nosti klinicheskogo techeniia infektsionnykh bolezneĭ i épidemiologicheskikh aspektakh étoĭ problemy (K 150-letiiu so dnia rozhdeniia). **Vestn Akad Med Nauk SSSR** 1982;(10):3-9

Smirnov EI, Garin NS: Vklad S. P. Botkina v razvitie épidemiologii (k 150-letiiu so dnia rozhdeniia). **Zh Mikrobiol Epidemiol Immunobiol** 1982 May;(5):109-15

Suvorov VIu, Bliumel' NF, Levtova KZ: 50 Let Kafedre épidemiologii

# EPIDEMIOLOGY

I Moskovskogo meditsinskogo instituta im. I. M. Sechenova. **Zh Mikrobiol Epidemiol Immunobiol** 1982 Jul;(7):102-6

Vasil'ev KG: Metodologischeskie voprosy izucheniia otechestvennoi epidemiologii. **Zh Mikrobiol Epidemiol Immunobiol** 1982 Feb;(2):114-6

Vasil'ev KK: Rol' pervykh Vserossiĭskikh sezdov bakteriologov i épidemiologov v bor'be s épidemiiami parazitarnykh tifov (k 60-letiiu IV sezda). **Zh Mikrobiol Epidemiol Immunobiol** 1981 Apr;(4):106-9

Vasil'ev KK: S'ezd, zalozhivshiĭ osnovy sanitarno-épidemiologicheskoĭ sluzhby SSSR (k 60-letiiu VI Vserossiĭskogo c'ezda bakteriologov i épidemiologov). **Zh Mikrobiol Epidemiol Immunobiol** 1982 Dec;(12):102-3

Vasil'ev KK: 60 let VII Vserossi ĭskogo s'ézda bakteriologov, épidemiologov i sanitarnykh vracheĭ. **Zh Mikrobiol Epidemiol Immunobiol** 1983 Oct;(10):111-3

# ETHICS, MEDICAL

See also **Economics, Medical; Licensure and Regulation**

Acuña HR: Etica médica y educación médica. **Bol Of Sanit Panam** 1981 Jun;90(6):471-7

Aulizio F: Is the Hippocratic oath still uptodate today? In International Congress of the History of Medicine, 27th, Barcelona, 1980. Actas. Barcelona, Acadèmia de Ciències Mèdiques de Catalunya i Balears, 1981. p. 441-5.

Brody H: Placebos and the philosophy of medicine: clinical, conceptual and ethical issues. Chicago and London, University of Chicago Press, 1980. vii, 164 p.

Brody H: The lie that heals: the ethics of giving placebos. **Ann Intern Med** 1982 Jul;97(1):112-8

Chapman CB: The importance of being ethical. **Perspect Biol Med** 1981 Spring;24(3):422-39

Curran WJ: An historical perspective on the law of personality and status with special regard to the human fetus and the rights of women. **Milbank Mem Fund Q** 1983 Winter;61(1):58-75

Doerr W: Bedürfen wir einer Bio-Ethik? In Seidler E, Schott H, ed: Bausteine zur Medizingeschichte. Stuttgart, Steiner, 1984. p. 18-26.

Dunstan GR: The moral status of the human embryo: a tradition recalled. **J Med Ethics** 1984 Mar;10(1):38-44

Fischer-Homberger E: Aerztliche Ethik und ärztliche Standespolitik--ein Aspekt der Geschichte der ärztlichen Ethik. **Bull Schweiz Akad Med Wiss** 1980 Nov;36(4-6):395-410

Frankel DA: Human experimentation: codes of ethics. **Leg Med Q** 1977 Mar;1(1):7-14

Giuseppe Capailla D: El psiquiatra frente a los derechos del hombre. **An R Acad Nac Med (Madr)** 1981;98(3):463-72

Glantz LH: The role of personhood in treatment decisions made by courts. **Milbank Mem Fund Q** 1983 Winter;61(1):76-100

Green LC: War law and the medical profession. **Leg Med Q** 1979;3(3):175-96

Hartree EF: Ethics for authors: a case history of acrosin. **Perspect Biol Med** 1976 Autumn;20(1):82-91

Howard-Jones N: Expérimentation humaine et déontologie: une interprétation historique. In: Médicine et expérimentation. Québec, Les Presses de l'Université Laval, 1982. p. 39-65. (Cahiers de Bioethique, 4).

Jensenius H: Eutanasi -- historisk og aktuelt. **Dan Medicinhist Arbog** 1979;100-13

Jonsen AR, Sagan L: Torture and the ethics of medicine. **Man Med** 1978;3(1):33-49

Kleeberg J, ed: Eide und Bekenntnisse in der Medizin, eine Anthologie. Basel, München, Karger, 1979. 81 p.

Kozlov AM: Kliatva Gippokrata i ee vliianie na razvitie vrachebnoĭ étiki. **Sov Med** 1983;(3):79-82

Kramer MG: Professionalism and principles of ethics--changing concepts for dentistry. **Pediatr Dent** 1980 Sep;2(3):245-51

Kuthy-Porter J, Corvera-Bernardelli J, Martínez-Palomo A, et al: Etica en la investigación clínica. **Gac Med Mex** 1983 Mar;119(3):97-112

Lee RV: The generalist: a jaundiced view. **Am J Med** 1983 Apr;74(4):532-4

Lindeboom GA: Euthanasie in Historisch Perspectief. Amsterdam, Rodopi, 1978. 47 p.

McCullough LB: Justice and health care: historical perspectives and precedents. In E. E. Shelp, ed: Justice and health care. Dordrecht, Reidel, 1981. (Philosophy and medicine, Vol. 8), p. 51-71.

MacIntyre A: Why is the search for the foundations of ethics so frustrating? **Hastings Cent Rep** 9(4):16-22, Aug 79

Maman C: Comment établir le moment de la mort. **Rev Hist Med Heb** 1980 Jul;33(2):27-34

Medicine and the law: **Am Med News** 1981 Apr 17;24(15):3, 10

Nally JN: Développement scientifique de la prothèse dentaire et éthique médicale. **Schweiz Monatsschr Zahnmed** 1984 Jan;94(1):23-8

Pałasz M: Eutanazja w świetle refleksji deontologicznej. **Pol Tyg Lek** 1981 Apr 27;36(17):611-13

Pernick MS: Childhood death and medical ethics: an historical perspective on truth-telling in pediatrics. **Prog Clin Biol Res** 1983;139:173-88

Phillips WR: Patients, pills, and professionals: the ethics of placebo therapy. **Pharos** 1981 Winter;44(1):21-5

Piga Sánchez-Morate B: Aspectos médico-legales del aborto. **An R Acad Nac Med (Madr)** 1982;99(1):51-70

Pines S: The oath of Asaph the Physician and Yohanan Ben Zabda: Its relation to the Hippocratic Oath and the Doctrina duarum viarium of the Didaché. **Proc Isr Acad Sci Humanit** 1971-76;5:223-64

Rachels J: Can ethics provide answers? **Hastings Cent Rep** 1980 Jun;10(3):32-40

Ramos P: Etica médica en la era pretecnológica. **Gac Med Mex** 1980 Mar;116(3):102-8

Reif AE: Hippocrates and the biomedical scientist: the problems of controlling the dangers of science. **Minerva** 1980 Spring;18(1):29-50

Reiser SJ: Words as scalpels: transmitting evidence in the clinical dialogue. **Ann Intern Med** 1980 Jun;92(6):837-42

Rosenbaum M, ed: Ethics and values in psychotherapy: a guidebook. New York, Free Press; London, Collier Macmillan; 1982. xvi, 464 p. Historical chapter by J. F. Drane.

Rosner F, Bleich JD, ed: Jewish bioethics. New York, Sanhedrin Press, 1979. xix, 424 p.

Rowan AN, Rollin BE: Animal research - for and against: a philosophical, social, and historical perspective. **Perspect Biol Med** 1983 Autumn;27(1):1-17

Schipperges H: Vindication of the doctor's decisions. **Hexagon Roche** 1981;9(3):1-8

Schwarz S: Asklepios a Temida. **Ginekol Pol** 1983 Oct;54(10):585-98

Temkin O, Frankena WK, Kadish SH: Respect for life in medicine, philosophy, and the law. (Thalheimer lectures, 1975). Baltimore: Johns Hopkins Univ. Press, 1977. ix, 107 p.

Temkin O: Some moral implications of the concept of disease. In Ganzinger K, Skopec M, Wyklicky H, ed: Festschrift für Erna Lesky zum 70. Geburtstag. Wien, Brüder Hollinek, 1981. p. 153-60.

Thom A: Ethische Prinzipien und moralische Normen ärztlichen Handelns--ihre Quellen, Begründungen und praktischen Funktionen. **Stomatol DDR** 1983 Feb;33(2):124-9

Veith I: On privileged communication: a comparative study of several medical cases. **West J Med** 1983 Mar;138(3):437-40

Vilter RW: The evolution of medical ethics. **Forum Med** 1980 Sep;3(9):576-80

Vries A de: The essence of medical ethics. **Biomed Pharmacother** 1982 Jan;36(1):59-65

Wilson W: Old ethics: new dilemmas. **Ulster Med J** 1982;51(1):23-34

**Arabic**

Ammar S: Le message hippocratique à travers la médecine arabe. **Tunis Med** 1981 Nov-Dec;59(6):498-504

Hameed A: Medical ethics in Islam. **Stud Hist Med** 1981 Jun;5(2):133-59

**China**

Unschuld PU: Medical ethics in imperial China: a study in historical anthropology. Berkeley, University of California Press, 1979. viii, 141 p. (Comparative Studies of Health Systems and Medical Care, 2).

**Germany**

Schimming I, Mann H: Zur historischen Bedingtheit der Qualität ärztlicher Bewahrungspflicht für das menschliche Leben sowie der Betreuung Sterbender. **Z Arztl Fortbild (Jena)** 1984;78(16):693-4

Zimmermann V: Ein besonderer Eid für die jüdischen Arzte und Wundärzte in Preussen. Ein Beitrag zur Geschichte der jüdischen Arzte in Deutschland. **Medizinhist J** 1982;17(1/2):78-88

**Greco-Roman**

Ferngren GB: A Roman declamation on vivisection. **Trans Stud Coll Physicians Phila** 1982 Dec;5(4 no 4):272-90

**Mexico**

Chávez I: La moral médica frente a la medicina de nuestro tiempo. In Academia Nacional de Medicine. Libro conmemorativo del primer centenario. México, Comité Editorial de la Comisión Organizadora del Congreso del Centenario, 1964. Tome 2. p. 668-73.

**Before 500 A.D.**

Harig G: Soziale Aspekte der antiken medizinischen Deontologie. **Orvostort Kozl** 1981;93-96(27 No 1-4):37-45

**Greece**

Deichgräber K: Der hippokratische Eid. Text griechisch und deutsch - Interpretation - Nachleben. 4., erweiterte Auflage. Stuttgart, Hippokrates Verlag, 1983. 92 p.

Harig G, Kollesch J: Der hippokratische Eid. **Philologus** 1978;122:157-76

Lichtenthaeler C: Le serment d'Hippocrate: analyse d'ensemble. **Rev Med Suisse Romande** 1980 Dec;100(12):1001-11

Sandulescu C: Primum non nocere: philological commentaries on a medical aphorism. **Acta Antiq Hung** 1965;13:359-368
Seidler MJ: The medical paradigm in Aristotelian ethics. **Thomist** 1978;42:400-33

**India**

Chakravorty RC: Medical ethics in ancient India. In International Congress of the History of Medicine, 27th, Barcelona, 1980. Actas. Barcelona, Acadèmia de Ciències Mèdiques de Catalunya i Balears, 1981. p. 486-9.

**500 A.D.-1450**

Amundsen DW: Casuistry and professional obligations: the regulation of physicians by the court of conscience in the late Middle Ages. Part II. **Trans Stud Coll Physicians Phila** 1981 Jun;3(2):93-112
Crisciani C: Valeurs éthiques et savoir médical entre le XIIe et le XIVe siècle. Problèmes et thèmes d'une recherche. **Hist Philos Life Sci** 1983;5(1):33-52

**Arabic**

Haddad FS: Arab medical ethics. **Stud Hist Med** 1982 Jun;6(2):122-36
Hameed A: Medical ethics in Medieval Islam. **Stud Philos Med** 1977 Mar;1(1):108-24
Hau FR: Die Bildung des Arztes im Islamischen Mittelalter. **Clio Med** 1979 Jul;14(1):7-33
Lauer HH: Ethik und ärztliches Denken im arabischen Mittelalter. In Seidler E, Schott H, ed: Bausteine zur Medizingeschichte. Stuttgart, Steiner, 1984. p. 72-86.
Levey M: Medical ethics on medieval Islam with special reference to Al-Ruhawi's 'Practical ethics of the physician.' Philadelphia, American Philosophical Society, 1967. 100 p. (Transactions of the American Philosophical Society, n.s., Vol. 57, Part 3, 1967).
Mukhitdinov BN: Eticheskie printsipy Abu Ali Ibn-Siny (Avitsenny) i voprosy sovremennoĭ deontologii (k 1000-letiiu so dnia rozhdeniia). **Vestn Rentgenol Radiol** 1980 May-Jun;(3):80-2
Nuralev IuN: Abu Ali Ibn-Sina i voprosy vrachebnoĭ étiki. **Klin Med (Mosk)** 1980 Oct;58(10):112-4

**Germany**

Schipperges H: Die Kardinaltugenden im Weltbild der Hildegard von Bingen. **Grenzgeb Wiss** 1980;29(1):19-34

**1450-1700**

**France**

Lemaire JF: 1696, l'irresponsabilité médicale momentanément consacrée. **Hist Sci Med** 1984;18(1):41-3

**Germany**

Hahn S: Martin Luther--was sagt er uns Arzten heute? **Z Gesamte Inn Med** 1983 Oct 15;38(20):551-4
Kottek S: An oath taken by Jewish community physicians at Frankfort on Main, 1656. **Koroth** 1979 Nov;7(9-10):CCIII-CCVIII(650-7).

**1700 to Present**

Bean WB: 'A testament of duty' revisited. **J Lab Clin Med** 1981 Dec;98(6):795-806
Bugyi B: Az orvosi sajtó etikájáról--hetven évvel ezelött. **Orv Hetil** 1979 Dec 30;120(52):3184-6
Burkhardt C: Euthanasie - 'Vernichtung lebensunwerten Lebens' im Spiegel der Diskussionen zwischen Juristen und Medizinern von 1900 bis 1940. Diss., Johannes-Gutenberg-Universität. Mainz, 1981. 221 p.
Carroll MA, Humphrey RH: Moral problems in nursing: case studies. Washington, University Press of America, 1979. Historical chapters, p. 6-28.
Concepcion R: Medical ethics in connection with torture of prisoners and other persons under some form of detention. **Unitas** 1976;49(4):542-92
Fletcher JC: The evolution of the ethics of informed consent. **Prog Clin Biol Res** 1983;128:187-228
Fox RC, Swazey JP: Medical morality is not bioethics--medical ethics in China and the United States. **Perspect Biol Med** 1984 Spring;27(3):336-60
Graham LR: Between science and values. New York, Columbia University Press, 1981. x, 449 p.
Howard-Jones N: Human experimentation in historical and ethical perspectives. **Soc Sci Med** 1982;16(15):1429-48
Hynes J: The remunerative advantages of ineffective medicines. **MIMS Mag** 1981 May 15;:70-3
Isambert FA: Bio-éthique et techniques biomédicales. **Soc Sci Inf** 1983;22(1):125-37
Jonsen AR: Ethics as immunotherapy. **Forum Med** 1978 Oct;1(7):50-2
Kepler MO: Medical stewardship: fulfilling the Hippocratic legacy. Westport, London, Greenwood Press, 1981. xviii, 280 p.
Knight N: Early moral and medical opposition to inhalation anesthesia and childbirth. In The history and sociology of technology: Proceedings of the 24th annual meeting of the Society for the History of Technology. Milwaukee, Milwaukee Public Museum, 1982. p. 29-37.
Korarev II: Evoliutsiia meditsinskogo éticheskogo kodeksa v SSSR i za rubezhom (printsipy i ikh realizatsiia). **Vestn Akad Med Nauk SSSR** 1980;(4):47-52
Loudon I: How it strikes a historian. **Br Med J [Clin Res]** 1984 Jan 14;288(6411):125-6
Luther E: Humanismus und gesellschaftliche Verantwortung. **Wiss Z Martin Luther Univ (Math)** 1984;33(2):122-7
Roth G: Ad salutem et prosperitatem hominum. Zur Entwicklung der ärztlichen Gelöbnisse in mittel- und osteuropäischen Staaten. In Ganzinger K, Skopec M, Wyklicky H, ed: Festschrift für Erna Lesky zum 70. Geburtstag. Wien, Brüder Hollinek, 1981. p. 67-73.
Sarro R: Razon y sinrazon de las heterodoxias psicoanaliticas. **Asclepio** 1980;32:421-32
Sechzer JA: The ethical dilemma of some classical animal experiments. **Ann NY Acad Sci** 1983;406:5-12
Van der Sluis I: Het recht om grootmoeder te doden. Korte geschiedenis van de euthanasiebeweging sinds 1870. Amsterdam, Buijten & Schipperheijn, 1977. 90 p.
Wondrák E: Lékaři hanby. **Cas Lek Cesk** 1984 Aug 3;123(31):969-72

**Canada**

Naylor CD: The CMA's first code of ethics: medical morality or borrowed ideology? **J Can Stud** 1982-83;17(4):20-32

**Czechoslovakia**

Adamec J: Lékařská na stránkách Casopisu lékařu českých v prvním pulstoletí jeho existence. **Cas Lek Cesk** 1981;120(52):1589-93

**France**

Colard A: Evocation du passé. Jehan Yperman et l'éthique médicale. **Rev Med Brux** 1982 Mar;3(3):171-2

**Germany**

Bogusz J: Wpływ norymberskiego procesu lekarzy hitlerowskich na kształtowanie sie pojeć o dokonywaniu badań na ludziach. **Przegl Lek** 1981;38(1):72-9
Boozer JS: Children of Hippocrates: doctors in Nazi Germany. **Ann Am Acad Polit Soc Sci** 1980;450:83-97
Brand U: Aerztliche Ethik im 19. Jahrhundert. Der Wandel ethischer Inhalte im medizinischen Schrifttum. Ein Beitrag zum Verständnis der Arzt-Patient-Beziehung. Freiburg, Schulz, 1977. 224 p. (Freiburger Forschungen zur Medizingeschichte, Neue Folge, 5).
Cohen CB: 'Quality of life' and the analogy with the Nazis. **J Med Philos** 1983 May;8(2):113-35
Hahn S: Die Herausbildung progressiver bürgerlicher Auffassungen zur lebensbewahrenden Aufgabe der Medizin und zur Betreuung Sterbender zu Beginn des 19. Jahrhunderts in Deutschland. **Z Gesamte Inn Med** 1982 Dec 15;37(24):857-62
Hahn S: Schwerpunkte ethischer Diskussionsentwicklung um die Tuberkulose-Bekämpfung in fachwissenschaftlichen Veröffentlichungen von 1900 bis 1932. **Z Gesamte Hyg** 1982 Mar;28(3):193-201
Lauter H, Meyer JE: Mercy killing without consent. Historical comments on a controversial issue. **Acta Psychiatr Scand** 1982 Feb;65(2):134-41
Luther E: Theodor Brugsch und das ärztliche Ethos. **Wiss Z Martin Luther Univ (Math)** 1980;29(2):91-6
Moe K: Should the Nazi research data be cited? **Hastings Cent Rep** 1984 Dec;14(6):5-7
Mück H: Die rechtliche Entwicklung des Arzt-Patient-Verhältnisses in der DDR; vom Dienstvertrag zum medizinischen Betreuungsverhältnis. Köln, 1982. 322 p. (Kölner medizinhistorische Beiträge, Band 24)
Sass HM: Reichsrundschreiben 1931: Pre-Nuremberg German regulations concerning new therapy and human experimentation. **J Med Philos** 1983 May;8(2):99-111
Schneck P: Zum Wandel ärztlich-ethischer und deontologischer Auffassungen auf dem Gebiete der Frauenheilkunde während des ersten Drittels des 20. Jahrhunderts. **Z Gesamte Hyg** 1984 Apr;30(4):246-8
Toellner R: The historical preconditions for the origin of medical ethics committees in West Germany. **Metamedicine** 1981;2:275-82
Wolfensberger W: The extermination of handicapped people in World War II Germany. **Ment Retard** 1981 Feb;19(1):1-7
Wondrák E: Medicína na scestí. **Cas Lek Cesk** 1982 Jul;121(28):882-5

**Great Britain**

Gracia D: El orden médico. La ética médica de Thomas Percival. **Asclepio** 1983;35:227-55
Lock S: A question of confidence. An editor's view.

**Br Med J [Clin Res]** 1984 Jan 14;288(6411):123–5
Paulshock BZ: When should a physician retire? – William Heberden's view. **Del Med J** 1983;55(6):359–60
Shinebourne EA: Ethics of innovative cardiac surgery. **Br Heart J** 1984 Dec;52(6):597–601
Smith FB: Ethics and disease in the later nineteenth century: the Contagious Diseases Acts. **Hist Stud** 1971;15(57):118–35
Soffer RN: Ethics and society in England: the revolution in the social sciences, 1870–1914. Berkeley, University of California Press, 1978. ix, 325 p.
Wenneker M: Huxley's ethical system: an alternative to evolutionary ethics. **Synthesis** 1980;5(1):13–44

**Japan**

Okamura A: [Hospice and human rights movement. (2)] (Jpn). **Kango Kyoiku** 1983 May;24(5):294–302

**Poland**

Podgórska-Klawe Z: Nieznane polskie teksty deontologiczne z pierwszej połowy XIX wieku. **Arch Hist Med (Warsz)** 1978;41(4):469–72

**Switzerland**

Anner E: Gelöbnisse der Medizinalpersonen im Kanton Zürich seit 1798. Zürich, Juris, 1979. 76 p. (Zürcher Medizingeschichtliche Abhandlungen, Neue Reihe Nr. 135).

**United States**

Bazzi F, Bèttica-Giovannini R: Di un codice deontologico medico Newyorkese del 1823: commento critico storico e attuale. **Ann Osp Maria Vittoria Torino** 1982 Jan–Jun;25(1–6):85–96
Brandt AM: Polio, politics, publicity, and duplicity: ethical aspects in the development of the Salk vaccine. **Conn Med** 1979 Sep;43(9):581–7, 589–90
Burchell HB: The investigator as volunteer subject. **Mayo Clin Proc** 1982 Jul;57 Suppl:28–33
Cahill LS: Within shouting distance: Paul Ramsey and Richard McCormick on method. **J Med Philos** 1979 Dec;4(4):398–417
Carmen IH: The constitution in the laboratory: recombinant DNA research as 'free expression.' **J Polit** 1981;43(3):737–62
Cavanaugh G: The corruptions of science. **Dissent** 1981;28(2):195–202
Deaths associated with yellow fever experiments: **JAMA** 1983 Mar 4;249(9):1150–1
Drachman VG: The Loomis trial: social mores and obstetrics in the mid-nineteenth century. In Reverby S, Rosner D, ed: Health care in America. Philadelphia, Temple University Press, 1979. p. 67–83.
Gill D: The dueling doctors of Stockton. **Pac Hist** 1981;25(1):52–8
Green HP: The recombinant DNA controversy: a model of public influence. **Bull At Sci** 1978;34(9):12–16
Jones JH: Bad blood: the Tuskegee syphilis experiment. New York, Free Press; London, Collier Macmillan; 1981. xii, 272 p.
King LS: IX. The AMA gets a new code of ethics. **JAMA** 1983 Mar 11;249(10):1338–42
King LS: The 'old code' of medical ethics and some problems it had to face. **JAMA** 1982 Nov 12;248(18):2329–33
Knepper JD: Use of human subjects in experimentation: a review of legal and ethical issues. **J Am Med Rec Assoc** 1982 Aug;53(4):62–7 contd.
Lear J: Recombinant DNA: the untold story. New York, Crown, 1978. 280 p.
Lederer SE: 'The right and wrong of making experiments on human beings': Udo J. Wile and syphilis. **Bull Hist Med** 1984 Fall;58(3):380–97
Morrow CK: Sick doctors: the social construction of professional deviance. **Soc Probl** 1982;30(1):92–108
Page SL: The law, the lawyer, and medical aspects of child abuse. In E. H. Newberger, ed: Child abuse. Boston, Little, Brown and Company, 1982. p. 105–35.
Parsons W: Uninformed consent in 1942. **N Engl J Med** 1984 May 24;310(21):1397
Physician murderers and criminals: **Forensic Sci Int** 1982 Jul–Aug;20(1):101–6
Proceedings of the State Medical Convention, held in Raleigh, April, 1849, and Constitution and Medical Ethics of the Medical Society of the State of North Carolina, then adopted: **NC Med J** 1982 Mar;43(3):212–21
Rothman DJ: Conscience and convenience. The asylum and its alternatives in progressive America. Boston, Toronto, Little, Brown and Company, 1980. xii, 464 p.
Schlicke CP: The Robinson affair. **Pac Northwest** 1983;27(2):81–93
Sechzer JA: Historical issues concerning animal experimentation in the United States. **Soc Sci Med [F]** 1981 Mar;15F(1):13–7
Sechzer JA: The use of animals for experimentation in the United States. **Psychopharmacol Bull** 1981 Apr;17(2):88–91
Sernett MC: The rights of personhood: the Dred Scott case and the question of abortion. **Relig Life** 1980;49(4):461–76
Stein J: The bioethicists: facing matters of life and death. **Smithsonian** 1979;9(10):107–15
Swierenga RP: Physicians and abortion reform in the nineteenth century: social control as the new orthodoxy. **Fides Et Hist** 1979;11(2):51–9
Ward PS: 'Who will bell the cat?' Andrew C. Ivy and krebiozen. **Bull Hist Med** 1984 Spring;58(1):28–52

**USSR**

Belov SI: Vrachebnaia étika v kurse istorii meditsiny. **Sov Med** 1981;(6):116–7
Graham L: Biomedicine and the politics of science in the USSR. **Sov Union** 1981;8(2):147–58
Iarovinskiĭ MIa: Rol' istorii meditsiny v deontologicheskoĭ podgotovke meditsinskikh rabotnikov. **Sov Zdravookhr** 1982;(4):51–3
Katsnel'bogen AG: M. Ia. Mudrov i voprosy vrachebnoĭ étiki. **Sov Zdravookhr** 1983;(10):58–61
Korotkikh RV: N. I. Pirogov i voprosy vrachebnoĭ étiki. (K 100-letiiu so dnia smerti). **Sov Zdravookhr** 1981;(12)54–7
Korotkikh RV: Vklad A. F. Bilibina v razvitie problwm meditsinskoĭ deontologii. **Ter Arkh** 1982;54(10):103–6
Kuz'min MK: O proiskhozhdenii 'Prisiagi vracha Sovetskogo Soiuza'. **Sov Med** 1984;(8):117–9
Zhuravleva TV, Vorob'ev RI: Problemy deontologii v trudakh akademika AMN SSSR I. A. Kassirskogo. **Sov Zdravookhr** 1984;(10):56–7

**Zimbabwe**

Gelfand M: The N'anga, the guardian of the Shona way of life, its ethics and behaviour. **Cent Afr J Med** 1981 Jul;27(7):146–8

## EVOLUTION

Busvine JR: The evolution and mutual adaptation of insects, microorganisms and man. In Stanley NF, Joske RA, ed: Changing disease patterns and human behaviour. London, New York, Academic Press, 1980. p. 55–68.
Cronin JE, Boaz NT, Stringer CB, et al: Tempo and mode in hominid evolution. **Nature** 1981 Jul 9;292(5819):113–22
Doerr W: Evolutionstheorie und pathologische Anatomie. **Verh Dtsch Ges Pathol** 1983;67:663–84
Eldredge N, Tattersall I: The myths of human evolution. New York, Columbia University Press, 1982. 197 p.
Fenner F: Sociocultural change and environmental diseases. In Stanley NF, Joske RA, ed: Changing disease patterns and human behaviour. London, New York, Academic Press, 1980. p. 7–26.
Irsigler FJ: Evolution and hominization. **Mankind Q** 1981 Spring;21(3):211–26
Johnston FE, Selby H: Anthropology: the biocultural view. Dubuque, Iowa, Brown, 1978. Historical sections, p. 73–80, 125–213, 270–275.
Jope EM: The emergence of man: information from protein systems. **Philos Trans R Soc Lond [Biol]** 1981 May 8;292(1057):121–31
Lewis RW: Evolution: a system of theories. **Perspect Biol Med** 1980;23(4):551–72
Masters J, Lambert D, Paterson H: Scientific prejudice, reproductive isolation, and apartheid. **Perspect Biol Med** 1984 Autumn;28(1):107–16
Mayr E: The growth of biological thought. Diversity, evolution, and inheritance. Cambridge, London, Harvard University Press, 1982. 974 p.
Shapiro HL: Peking man. London, George Allen & Unwin, 1976. 190 p.
Stebbins GL: Darwin to DNA, molecules to humanity. San Francisco, Freeman, 1982. xiv, 491 p.
Van der Hammen L: Type-concept, higher classification and evolution. **Acta Biotheor (Leiden)** 1981;30(1):3–48
Vora E: Evolution of race: a synthesis of social and biological concepts. **J Black Stud** 1981;12(2):182–91
Wassermann GD: On the nature of the theory of evolution. **Philos Sci** 1981;48(3):416–37
Wuketits FM: Das Kausalitätsproblem in der Evolutionslehre. Ein Beitrag zur Strukturgeschichte der Biologie. **Medizinhist J** 1980;15(4):392–402

**Americas**

Harper AB, Laughlin WS: Inquiries into the peopling of the new world: development of ideas and recent advances. In F. Spencer, ed: A history of American physical anthropology, 1930–1980. New York, Academic Press, 1982. p. 281–304.
Laughlin WS, Harper AB, ed: The first Americans: origins, affinities, and adaptations. New York and Stuttgart, Fischer, 1979. xi, 340 p.

**Before 500 A.D.**

Pilbeam D: The descent of hominoids and hominids. **Sci Am** 1984 Mar;250(3):84–96
Symposium: adaptive grades in the evolution of primates: **Z Morphol Anthropol** 1980;71(2):113–227
Walker A: Diet and teeth. Dietary hypotheses and human evolution. **Philos Trans R Soc Lond [Biol]** 1981 May 8;292(1057):57–64

Wood BA: Tooth size and shape and their relevance to studies of hominid evolution. **Philos Trans R Soc Lond [Biol]** 1981 May 8;292(1057):65–76

### Asia

Riehm K: Die Schädelstruktur des Frühmenschen als Ausdruck seines Waldlebens und seiner weiteren Entwicklung. **Gegenbaurs Morphol Jahrb** 1980;126(6):884–99

### Australia

Thorne AG, Wolpoff MH: Regional continuity in Australasian Pleistocene hominid evolution. **Am J Phys Anthropol** 1981 Jul;55(3):337–49

### France

Tillier AM: Evolution de la région symphysaire chez les homo sapiens juvéniles du paléolithique moyen: pech de l'azé 1, roc de marsal et la chaise 13. **C R Seances Acad Sci [III]** 1981 Nov 9;293(9):493–5

### Hungary

Kretzoi M: The significance of the Rudabánya prehominid finds in hominization research. **Acta Biol Acad Sci Hung** 1980;31(4):503–6

## 1700 to Present

Adams MB: From 'Gene Fund' to 'Gene Pool': on the evolution of evolutionarylanguage. **Stud Hist Biol** 1979;3:241–85

Armelagos GJ, Carlson DS, Van Gerven DP: The theoretical foundations and development of skeletal biology. In F. Spencer, ed: A history of American physical anthropology, 1930–1980. New York, Academic Press, 1982. p. 305–28.

Arquiola E: Darwinism in the Société d'Anthropologie de Paris. **Clio Med** 1980 May;14(2):119–28

Aulie RP: Evolution and special creation: historical aspects of the controversy. **Proc Am Philos Soc** 1983 Dec 30;127(6):418–62

Beloff M: Dr. Darlington's provocative work: the genetic approach to world history. **Encounter (Lond)** 1970;35(4):85–8

Benavente Barreda JM: Evolución biológica y herencia natural. **Arbor** 1982;113(441–2):111–25

Bendall DS, ed: Evolution from molecules to men. Cambridge, Cambridge University Press, 1983. xiii, 594 p.

Blanckaert C: Réflexions sur la détermination de l'espèce en anthropologie (XVIII–XIX siècles). **Doc Hist Vocab Sci** 1983;(4):43–80

Blinderman CS: Unnatural selection: creationism and evolutionism. **J Church State** 1982;24(1):73–86

Bowler PJ: E. W. MacBride's Lamarckian eugenics and its implications for the social construction of scientific knowledge. **Ann Sci** 1984 May;41(3):245–60

Campbell DT: On the conflicts between biological and social evolution and between psychology and moral tradition. **Zygon** 1976;11:167–208

Campbell EK: Beyond anthropocentrism. **J Hist Behav Sci** 1983 Jan;19(1):54–67

Campbell M: Mendel's theory: its context and plausibility. **Centaurus** 1982;26(1):38–69

Castrodeza C: La importancia práctica del darwinismo. **Arbor** 1982;113(441–2):127–36

Churchill FB: The Weismann–Spencer controversy over the inheritance of acquired characters. In Forbes EG, ed: Human implications of scientific advance. Edinburgh, Edinburgh University Press, 1978. p. 451–68.

Crook DP: Darwinism – the political implications. **Hist Eur Ideas** 1981;5:99–139

Gall YM: [I. I. Schmalhausen and the problem of the causes of evolution] (Rus). **Istor Biol Issled** 1980;8:106–23

Gershenowitz H: The treatment of Lamarckism as found in forty-one college textbooks. **Indian J Hist Sci** 1978, reçu 1982;13(2):144–50

Gould SJ: Darwinism and the expansion of evolutionary theory. **Science** 1982 Apr 23;216(4544):380–7

Gould SJ: Ever since Darwin. Reflections in natural history. New York, W. W. Norton, 1977. 285 p.

Greene JC: Science, ideology, and world view: essays in the history of evolutionary ideas. Berkeley/Los Angeles, Univ. of California Press, 1981. x, 202 p.

Hamrum CL, ed: Darwin's legacy. Nobel Conference XVIII, Gustavus Adolphus College. St. Peter, Minnesota, held October 5–6, 1982. San Francisco, Harper & Row, 1983. 125 p. Contributions by S. J. Gould, I. Stone, R. E. Leakey, P. B. Medawar, E. O. Wilson, J. Pelikan.

Iarygin VN: Nekotorye problemy darvinizma na sovremonnom étape. **Arkh Anat Gistol Embriol** 1982 Nov;83(11):7–17

Jurmain R: Human evolution: a century of research. **San Jose Stud** 1982;8(3):40–50

Kolchinskiĭ EI: [Development of the idea of transformation in evolution] (Rus). **Istor Biol Issled** 1978;7:25–45

Laporte LF: Simpson's Tempo and Mode in Evolution revisited. **Proc Am Philos Soc** 1983 Dec 30;127(6):365–417

McKinney HL, ed: Lamarck to Darwin: contributions to evolutionary biology 1809–1859. Contributions by J. B. Lamarck, W. C. Wells, P. Matthew, C. Lyell, E. Blyth, R. Chambers, A. R. Wallace, C. Darwin. Lawrence, Kansas, Coronado, 1971, 3rd printing R 75, 122 p.

Mann G: Teleologie und Evolutionslehre. **Ber Wissenschaftsgesch** 1982;5:83–96

Mayr E, Provine WB, ed: The evolutionary synthesis: perspectives on the unification of biology. Cambridge, Mass., and London, England, Harvard University Press, 1980. xi, 487 p. Contributions by M. B. Adams, G. E. Allen, E. Boesiger, R. W. Burkhardt, H. L. Carson, F. B. Churchill, W. Coleman, C. D. Darlington, T. Dobzhansky, E. B. Ford, M. T. Ghiselin, S. J. Gould, V. Hamburger, R. C. Lewontin, C. Limoges, B. Rensch, D. Shapere, G. L. Stebbins, A. Weinstein.

Neel JV: Human evolution: many small steps, but not punctuated equilibria. **Perspect Biol Med** 1984 Autumn;28(1):75–103

Oldroyd DR: Darwinian impacts. An introduction to the Darwinian revolution. Atlantic Highlands, N. J., Humanities Press, 1980. xiv, 399 p.

Plews JH: Charles Darwin and Hawaiian sex ratios, or, genius is a capacity for making compensating errors. **Hawaii J Hist** 1980;14:24–49

Prevost A: La selección natural en la evolución biológica. **Arbor** 1982;113(441–2):21–40

Rhodes FH: Gradualism, punctuated equilibrium and the Origin of Species. **Nature** 1983 Sep 22–28;305(5932):269–72

Richards E: The German romantic concept of embryonic repetition and its role in evolutionary theory in England up to 1859. Ph. D. Diss. University of New South Wales, 1976.

Ridley M: Coadaptation and the inadequacy of natural selection. **Br J Hist Sci** 1982 Mar;15((1 no 1):45–68

Schwarz H: Darwinism between Kant and Haeckel. **J Am Acad Relig** 1980;48(4):581–602

Sermonti G: L'evoluzione e il metodo delle scienze biologiche. **Med Secoli** 1981 May–Aug;18(2):193–208

Sloan PR: Ontogeny and phylogeny. **Br J Hist Sci** 1980;13(1):50–5

Thaler L: La génétique des populations dans la théorie moderne de l'évolution. In Actes du Colloque R.A. Fisher.... Paris, 5–6 déc. 1979. p. 351–79. **Rev Synth (Paris)** 1981;102(103–104)

Tobach E: The relationship between Preyer's concept of psychogenesis and his views of Darwin's theory of evolution. **Z Psychol** 1983;191(4):388–95

Valderas JM: Vuelve el lamarckismo? **Folia Hum (Barc)** 1981;19(216):57–65

Wallace ER: Freud and anthropology. A history and reappraisal. New York, International Universities Press, 1983. xi, 306 p. (Psychological Issues, Monograph 55).

Washburn SL: Fifty years of studies of human evolution. **Bull At Sci** 1982;38(5):37–43

Winsor MP: Louis Agassiz and the species question. **Stud Hist Biol** 1979;3:89–138

Wuketits FM: Evolutionsmodelle in der Erklärung menschlicher Denkstrukturen im 19. Jahrhundert. **Ber Wissenschaftsgesch** 1983;6(1–4):115–22

Zirnstein G: Die Erforschung und Bewertung der Lebenserscheinung 'Variabilität' in der Biologie vor 1859. **NTM** 1981;18(2):58–78

Zirnstein G: Zur gesellschaftlichen Stellung der Wissenschaftler in der Geschichte von Evolutionstheorie und Vererbungsforschung. **Rostocker Wiss Hist Manuskripte** 1981;6:57–60

### Austria

Broda E: Ludwig Boltzmann als evolutionistischer Philosoph. **Ber Wissenschaftsgesch** 1983;6(1–4):103–14

### Canada

Berger C: Science, God, and nature in Victorian Canada. Toronto; Buffalo, University of Toronto Press, 1983. xiv, 92 p.

Cornell JF: From creation to evolution: Sir William Dawson and The idea of design in the nineteenth century. **J Hist Biol** 1983 Spring;16(1):137–70

Pighetti C: L'antievoluzionismo nel Canada ottocentesco. **Physis** 1983;25(3):433–79

### France

Buican D: Histoire de la génétique et de l'évolutionnisme en France. Paris, Presse universitaires de France, 1984. 421 p.

Buican D: La génétique classique en France devant le neo-lamarckisme tardif. **Arch Int Hist Sci (Paris)** 1983 Dec;33(111):300–24

Fischer JL: Yves Delage (1854–1920): l'epigenèse néo-lamarckienne contre la prédétermination weismannienne. **Rev Synth (Paris)** 1979;100(95–6):443–61

López-Fanjul de Argüelles C: El lamarckismo y algo sobre los neolamarckismos. **Arbor** 1982;113(441–2):41–57

Nagel G: Georges Vacher de Lapouge (1854–1936). Ein Beitrag zur Geschichte des Sozialdarwinismus in Frankreich. Freiburg, Schulz, 1975. 109 p. (Freiburger Forschungen zur Medizingeschichte, Neue Folge, 4).

Sheets-Johnstone M: Why Lamarck did not discover the principle of

natural selection. **J Hist Biol** 1982 Fall;15(3):443–65
Szyfman L: Remarques sur l'ouvrage d'Ernst Mayr: 'Lamarck Revisited'. **Bull Biol Fr Belg** 1977;111(3):209–29

**Germany**

Dose K: Ernst Haeckel's concept of an evolutionary origin of life. **Biosystems** 1981;13(4):253–8
Engelhardt DV: Virchow et Haeckel et la liberté de la science. In Poirier J, Poirier JL, ed: Médecine et philosophie à la fin du XIXe siècle. Paris, Université de Paris XII - Val de Marne, [1980?]. p. 117–25.
Kelly A: The descent of Darwin: the popularization of Darwinism in Germany, 1860–1914. Chapel Hill, University of North Carolina Press, 1981. 185 p.
Mann G: Ernst Haeckel und der Darwinismus: Popularisierung, Propaganda und Ideologisierung. **Medizinhist J** 1980;15(3):269–83
Szyfman L: Les prétendues falsifications d'Ernst Haeckel et son triomphe sur ses diffamateurs. **Bull Biol Fr Belg** 1980;113(4):375–406
Wenzel M: Goethes Morphologie in ihrer Beziehung zum darwinistischen Evolutionsdenken. **Medizinhist J** 1983;18(1–2):52–68

**Great Britain**

Altholz JL: The Huxley-Wilberforce debate revisited. **J Hist Med Allied Sci** 1980 Jul;35(3):313–16
Ayala FJ: Darwin y la idea de progreso. **Arbor** 1982;113(441–2):59–75
Beatty J: What's in a word? Coming to terms in the Darwinian revolution. With a comment by D. Hull. In M. Ruse, ed: Nature animated. Historical and philosophical case studies in Greek medicine, nineteenth-century and recent biology, psychiatry, and psychoanalysis. Volume II. Dordrecht, D. Reidel, 1983. p. 79–111.
Bendiner E: The descent of man and the ascent of the Darwins. **Hosp Pract** 1982 Dec;17(12):160, 165, 173–4 passim
Bernstein RE: Darwin's alter ego: co-originator Alfred Wallace. **Perspect Biol Med** 1984;27(2):234–8
Browne J: Essay review: new developments in Darwins studies? **J Hist Biol** 1982 Summer;15(2):275–80
Colp R: [Charles Darwin: Essay-Review] **Trans Stud Coll Physicians Phila** 1983 Dec;5(5 no 4):353–75
Colp R: Charles Darwin's reprobation of nature. 'Clumsy, wasteful, blundering low and horribly cruel.' **NY State J Med** 1981 Jun;81(7):1116–9
Colp R: 'I was born a naturalist': Charles Darwin's 1838 notes about himself. **J Hist Med Allied Sci** 1980 Jan;35(1):8–39
Colp R: The Darwin exhibition at the Cambridge University Library. **Bull NY Acad Med** 1983 Jun;59(5):526–8
Cornell JF: Analogy and technology in Darwin's vision of nature. **J Hist Biol** 1984 Fall;17(3):303–44
Darwin CR: The descent of man, and selection in relation to sex. 2 vols in 1. Reprint of 1871 ed, with historical introduction by J. T. Bonner and R. M. May. Princeton, Princeton University Press, 1981. xli, 475, x, p.
Diamond P: The natural theologians and Darwin: a case of divergent evolution in the history of ideas. **Aust J Polit Hist** 1980;26(2):204–11
Di Gregorio MA: Order or process of nature: Huxley's and Darwin's different approaches to natural sciences. **Hist Philos Life Sci** 1981;3(2):217–41
Di Gregorio MA: The dinosaur connection: a reinterpretation of T. H. Huxley's evolutionary view. **J Hist Biol** 1982 Fall;15(3):397–418
Dupâquier J, Fauve-Chamoux A, Grebenik E, ed: Malthus past and present. London; New York, Academic Press, 1983. xix, 416 p. Contributions by A. Béjin, Y. Breton, Y. Charbit, L. Devance, A. Digby, M. W. Flinn, R. E. Frisch, M. Godelier, L. Gordon, P. Guillaume, G. Heinsohn, T. H. Hollingsworth, P. A. Jewell, N. Keyfitz, R. Keynes, H. Le Bras, M. Perrot, F. Rausky, M. Rebérioux, R. Remond, F. Ronsin, G. R. Searle, B. Stapleton, O. Steiger, P. Vallin, E. Van de Walle, A. Waterman, J. Wolff, E. A. Wrigley, V. Wynne-Edwards.
Egozcue J: Darwin y el origen del hombre. **Arbor** 1982;113(441–2):77–86
Eiseley L: Darwin and the mysterious Mr. X: new light on the evolutionists. New York and London, Harcourt Brace Jovanovich, 1981. xii, 278 p.
Evans LT: Darwin's use of the analogy between artificial and natural selection. **J Hist Biol** 1984 Spring;17(1):113–40
Freeman D: The evolutionary theories of Charles Darwin and Herbert Spencer. **Curr Anthropol** 1974;15(3):211–21
Freeman RB: The works of Charles Darwin: an annotated bibliographical handlist. 2d. ed. Folkestone, England, Dawson, 1977. 235 p.
George W: Darwin. Glasgow, Fontana Paperbacks, 1982. 160 p.
Gilbert SF: Owen's vertebral archetype and evolutionary genetics -- a Platonic appreciation. **Perspect Biol Med** 1980 Spring;23(3):475–88
Gruber HE: Darwin on man: a psychological study of scientific creativity. 2d. ed. Chicago, University of Chicago Press, 1981. xxvii, 310 p.
Gruber HE: Darwin on psychology and its relation to evolutionary thought. In R. W. Rieber, K. Salzinger, ed: Psychology: theoretical-historical perspectives. New York, Academic Press, 1980. p. 145–74.
Haugen LK: Darwin, evolusjonen og medisinen. **Tidsskr Nor Laegeforen** 1982 Dec 10;102(34–36):1835–8
Herbert S, ed: The red notebook of Charles Darwin. Ithaca and London, Cornell University Press and British Museum (Natural History), 1980. 164 p.
Howard J: Darwin. New York, Hill and Wang, 1982. viii, 101 p.
K 100-letiiu so dnia smerti Charlza Darvina: **Arkh Anat Gistol Embriol** 1982 Nov;83(11):5–6
Kinch MP: Geographical distribution and the origin of life: the development of early nineteenth-century British explanations. **J Hist Biol** 1980 Spring;13(1):91–119
Kleiner SA: Problem solving and discovery in the growth of Darwin's theories of evolution. **Synthese** 1981;47(1):119–62
Kohn D, Stauffer RC, Smith S: New light on The foundations of the origin of species: A reconstruction of the archival record. **J Hist Biol** 1982 Fall;15(3):419–42
Kohn D: Theories to work by: rejected theories, reproduction, and Darwin's path to natural selection. **Stud Hist Biol** 1980;4:67–70
Kottler MJ: Darwin, Wallace, and the origin of sexual dimorphism. **Proc Am Philos Soc** 1980 Jun;124(3):203–26
Lewin R: Darwin died at a most propitious time. **Science** 1982 Aug 20;217(4561):717–8
Lucas JR: Wilberforce and Huxley: a legendary encounter. **Hist J (Gt Brit)** 1979;22(2):313–30
Márquez-Monter H: Conmemoración del centenario de la muerte de Charles R. Darwin. **Gac Med Mex** 1983 May;119(5):212–8
Maynard-Smith J: The century since Darwin. **Nature** 1982 Apr 15;296(5858):599–601
Norton B: Fisher and the neo-Darwinian synthesis. In Forbes EG, ed: Human implications of scientific advance. Edinburgh, Edinburgh University Press, 1978. p. 481–94.
Obál F: Emlékezés Charles Robert Darwin-ra (1809–1882) halála centenáriuma alkalmából. **Orv Hetil** 1982 Nov 14;123(46):2857–8
Ospovat D: God and natural selection: the Darwinian idea of design. **J Hist Biol** 1980 Fall;13(2):169–94
Ospovat D: The development of Darwin's theory: natural history, natural theology, and natural selection, 1838–1859. Cambridge, New York, Cambridge University Press, 1981. xii, 301 p.
Rabasa SL: Dificultades del neo-darwinismo a los 100 años de la muerte de Darwin (19-IV-1882). **Medicina (B Aires)** 1982;42(2):213–6
Rheinberger HJ, McLaughlin P: Darwin's experimental natural history. **J Hist Biol** 1984 Fall;17(3):345–68
Richards RJ: Instinct and intelligence in British natural theology: some contributions to Darwin's theory of the evolution of behavior. **J Hist Biol** 1981 Fall;14(2):193–230
Richards RJ: Why Darwin delayed, or interesting problems and models in the history of science. **J Hist Behav Sci** 1983 Jan;19(1):45–53
Ruffié J: Darwin, cent ans après. **Biomed Pharmacother** 1982;36(3):170–3
Ruse M: Charles Darwin and group selection. **Ann Sci** 1980;37(6):615–30
Ruse M: Ought philosophers consider scientific discovery? A Darwinian case-study. In T. Nickles, ed: Scientific discovery: case studies. Dordrecht, D. Reidel, 1980. (Boston Studies in the Philosophy of Science, v. 60). p. 131–49.
Schweber SS: Darwin and the political economists: divergence of character. **J Hist Biol** 1980 Fall;13(2):195–289
Sheets-Pyenson S: Darwin's data: his reading of natural history journals, 1837–1842. **J Hist Biol** 1981 Fall;14(2):231–48
Smith CU: Evolution and the problem of mind: part I. Herbert Spencer. **J Hist Biol** 1982 Spring;15(1):55–88
Smith CU: Evolution and the problem of mind: part II. John Hughlings Jackson. **J Hist Biol** 1982 Summer;15(2):241–62
Sulloway FJ: Darwin's conversion: the Beagle voyage and its aftermath. **J Hist Biol** 1982 Fall;15(3):325–96
Sulloway FJ: Geographic isolation in Darwin's thinking: the vicissitudes of a crucial idea. **Stud Hist Biol** 1979;3:23–65
Templado J: Darwin: ayer y hoy. **Arbor** 1982;113(441–2):7–20
Wenneker M: Huxley's ethical system: an alternative to evolutionary ethics. **Synthesis** 1980;5(1):13–44
Yates F: Sir Ronald Aylmer Fisher. In Dictionary of national biography, 1961–1970. Suppl. 8, 1981. p. 361–2.

**Italy**

Martucci V: Sviluppo ontogenetico e citologia nell'ologenesi di Daniele Rosa. **Physis** 1980;22(1):73–84

**Netherlands**

Heimans J: Hugo De Vries and the gene theory. In Forbes EG, ed: Human implications of scientific advance. Edinburgh, Edinburgh University Press, 1978. p. 469–80.

**Spain**

Sala Catalá J: El evolucionismo en la practica cientifica de los biologos españoles del siglo XIX (1860–1907). **Asclepio** 1981;33:81–125

**Syria**

Leavitt DM: Darwinism in the Arab world: the Lewis affair at the Syrian Protestant College. **Muslim World** 1981;71(2):85-98

**United States**

Baker AL: The San Francisco evolution debates: June 13-14, 1925. **Advent Herit** 1975;2(2):23-32
Cartmill M: Basic primatology and prosimian evolution. In F. Spencer, ed: A history of American physical anthropology, 1930-1980. New York, Academic Press, 1982. p. 147-86.
Cravens H: The triumph of evolution: American scientists and the heredity-environment controversy 1900-1941. [Philadelphia], University of Pennsylvania Press, 1978. xvi, 351 p.
Dexter RW: The impact of evolutionary theories on the Salem group of Agassiz zoologists (Morse, Hyatt, Packard, Putnam). **Essex Inst Hist Collect** 1979;115(3):144-71
Duffy S: The origin of speeches: Inherit the Wind, Irving Stone and the Scopes trial. **Am Notes Queries** 1983 Sep-Oct;22(1-2):14-7
Fleagle JG, Jungers WL: Fifty years of higher primate phylogeny. In F. Spencer, ed: A history of American physical anthropology, 1930-1980. New York, Academic Press, 1982. p. 187-230.
Goodman M, Cronin JE: Molecular anthropology: its development and current directions. In F. Spencer, ed: A history of American physical anthropology, 1930-1980. New York, Academic Press, 1982. p. 105-46.
Hart AW: Religion and education: the Scopes controversy in Utah. **Utah Hist Q** 1983;5(2):183-98
Hatch CE: New Jersey's Reaction to the Tennesse evolution trial. **NJ Hist** 1972;90(4):226-41
Ingraham RL: Evolution in context. **San Jose Stud** 1982;8(3):4-19
Lester JF: John Fiske's philosophy of science: the union of science and religion through the principle of evolution. Ph.D. Diss., Oregon State University, Corvallis, 1979. 275 leaves.
Mayr E: Reflections on human paleontology. In F. Spencer, ed: A history of American physical anthropology, 1930-1980. New York, Academic Press, 1982. p. 231-37.
Provine WB: Francis B. Sumner and the evolutionary synthesis. **Stud Hist Biol** 1979;3:211-40
Rambo LR: Ethics, evolution, and the psychology of William James. **J Hist Behav Sci** 1980 Jan;16(1):50-7
Smith JM: Thomas Huxley in Nashville. **Tenn Hist Q** 1974;33(2):191-203;(3):322-41
Spencer F, ed: A history of American physical anthropology, 1930-1980. New York, Academic Press, 1982. xvi, 495 p.
Stephens LD: Joseph LeConte. Gentle prophet of evolution. Baton Rouge, London, Louisiana State University Press, 1982. xix, 340 p.

**USSR**

Esakov VD: Soobshcheniie N. M. Tulaikova ob otkrytii N. I. Vavilovym Zakona gomologicheskikh riadov. **Vopr Istor Estestvozn Tekh** 1981;4:111-3
Gaissinovitch AE: The origins of Soviet genetics and the struggle with Lamarckism, 1922-1929. **J Hist Biol** 1980 Spring, 13(1):1-51
Kokina NN: P. K. Anokhin's concept of systems genesis and its subsequent development. **Neurosci Behav Physiol** 1980 Mar-Apr;10(2):142-6
Leibson L: Endocrinology evolution and evolutionary endocrinology. **Perspect Biol Med** 1979 Autumn;23(1):25-43
Nikitiuk BA, Kozlov AI: Nekotorye spornye polozheniia ucheniia ob antropogeneze v svete predstavlenii o destabiliziruiushchem otbore i dannykh sovremennoĭ paléoendokrinologii (k 100-letiiu so dnia rozhdeniia I. I. Shmal'gauzena). **Arkh Anat Gistol Embriol** 1984 Aug;87(8):5-14
Sokolov VE, Vorob'eva EI: I. I. Shmal'gauzen i évoliutsionnaia morfologiia. **Arkh Anat Gistol Embriol** 1984 Jul;87(7):5-17

# EXHIBITS

See also **Libraries; Museums**

**France**

Les enfants du Rouergue: **Bull Soc Fr Hist Hop** 1980;(41):36

**Germany**

Benedum J: 375 Jahre Medizin in Giessen: eine Bild- und Textdokumentation: Katalog zur Ausstellung anlässlich der 375 - Jahrfeier im Institut für Anatomie und Zytobiologie, vom 11.5.-30.6. 1982. Giessen, Schmitz, 1982. 186 p.

**500 A.D.-1450**

**Germany**

Czarnetzki A: Menschen des Frühen Mittelalters im Spiegel der Anthropologie und Medizin: Begleitheft zur Ausstellung. Stuttgart, Würtemmbergisches Landesmuseum Stuttgart, 1982. 103 p.

**1700 to Present**

**Austria**

Bauerndoktor und Volksmedizin. 1. Ausstellung anlässlich des 800-jährigen Bestehens von Stainz. Sonderausstellung: Juni bis Okt. 1977. Katalog: Nr. 3. Maria Kundegraber, unter Mitarb. v. Bernd Mader. Steiermark, Landesmuseum Joanneum, 1977. 63 p.:
Leitner H: Die jüdischen Arzte in Osterreich und ihr Beitrag zur medizinischen Wissenschaft. In K. Lohrmann, ed: 1000 Jahre Osterreichisches Judentum. Ausstellungskatalog. Eisenstadt, 1982. p. 161-92.

**Canada**

Gray C: Travelling archives depict early days in Canadian medicine. **Can Med Assoc J** 1980 Sep 6;123(5):426, 430, 432

**France**

Cotinat L: Les vases de pharmacie à l'exposition de faïences françaises du Grand-Palais (juin-août 1980). **Rev Hist Pharm (Paris)** 1981;28(248):49-53
Exposition 'enfants des montagnes' au musée dauphinois à Grenoble: **Bull Soc Fr Hist Hop** 1980;(41):32-5
Julien P: Trois expositions. **Rev Hist Pharm (Paris)** 1980 Dec;247(68 no 27):272-6
Le Traité de matière médicale de Dioscoride à la Renaissance: Exposition d'exemplaires des XVe et XVIe siecles. Du 11 au 24 février 1984 à Louvain-en-Woluwe à la Bibliothèque de la Faculté de Médecine de l'U.C.L. Louvain, Université Catholique de Louvain, Centre d'Histoire de la Pharmacie et du Médicament, 1984. 40 p.
L'Exposition Universelle de 1889: Recherche des réponses au questionnaire et d'objets. **Bull Soc Fr Hist Hop** 1979;(39):19-21
L'homme et son corps dans la société traditionelle: Paris, Ministère de la culture et de la communication, Editions de la Réunion des musées nationaux, 1978. 144 p.
Regards sur la condition enfantine - XVIe-XXe siècles: **Bull Soc Fr Hist Hop** 1980;(41):29-31
Simon N: 1979, au musée de l'Assistance publique de Paris. **Bull Soc Fr Hist Hop** 1980;(41):26-8

**Germany**

Bartels M, ed: Mensch und Tod: Totentanzsammlung der Universität Düsseldorf. Eine Ausstellung. Düsseldorf, Goethe-Museum, [1978?] 111 p. Einführung von H. Schadewaldt.
Fichtner G: Psychiatrie zur Zeit Hölderlins: Ausstellung anlässlich der 63. Jahrestagung der Deutschen Gesellschaft für Geschichte der Medizin, der Naturwissenschaften und Technik in Tübingen, Universitätsbibliothek Tübingen, Bonatzbau 27. September bis 30. Oktober 1980. Tübingen, Universitätsbibliothek, 1980. 99 p.
Gercke H, Jarchov I, ed: Die Prinzhorn-Sammlung. Bilder, Skulpturen, Texte aus psychiatrischen Anstalten (ca. 1890-1920). Königstein/Taunus, Athenäum Verlag, 1980. 312 p.
Telle J: Pharmazie und der gemeine Mann: Hausarznei und Apotheke in deutschen Schriften der frühen Neuzeit: Ausstellung der Herzog August Bibliothek Wolfenbüttel in der Halle des Zeughauses vom 23. August 1982 bis März 1983. Wolfenbüttel, Herzog August Bibliothek, 1982. 144 p.

**Great Britain**

Across the channel: catalogue of an exhibition. London, Royal College of Physicians of London, 1982. iii, 24 p.

**Hungary**

Kapronczay K: A Magyar Vöröskereszt száz éve--idöszaki kiállítás a Semmelweis Orvostörténeti Múzeumban. **Orv Hetil** 1981 Nov 1;122(44):2732-3

**Ireland**

Mills R, O'Brien E: Memorabilia and letters of Dominic Corrigan: catalogue of an exhibition. **J Ir Coll Physicians Surg** 1980 Jul;10(1):55-7

**Israel**

Kottek SS: 'Medicina in Nummis': an exhibition of medical medals in the Hebrew University Hadassah Medical School--Jerusalem (May-June 1979). **Koroth** 1979 Nov;7(9-10):CCXXXI-CCXXXIV(722-3)

# EXHIBITS

**Italy**

Armoroli M, ed: Le cere anatomiche Bolognesi del settecento. Catalogo della mostra organizzata Settembre-Novembre 1981. Bologna, Università degli Studi di Bologna, Accademia delle Scienze, 1981. 97 p. Contributions by R. A. Bernabeo, L. Bonuzzi, F. Ruggeri.
Groeben C, ed: Guida alla Mostra allestita nella Sala degli Affreschi della Stazione Zoologica nella Villa Comunale (6 luglio - 30 settembre 1982) su Charles Darwin e la Stazione Zoologica di Napoli.

**Netherlands**

Net echt!: De anatomische wereld van Dr. Auzoux. [Exhibition, Museum Boerhaave, Leiden.] **Tijdschr Geschied Geneeskd** 1981;4(1):50-2

**Poland**

Dutkiewicz M, Felchner A, Kuna M: Wystawa czasowa 'Starodruki medyczne w zbiorach łodzkich bibliotek naukowych' zorganizowana w dziesieciolecie Muzeum Polskiej Wojskowej Słuzby Zdrowia WAM. **Arch Hist Med (Warsz)** 1982;45(1-4):93-100

**Sweden**

Clemedson CJ: Berömda svenska böcker inom medicin och farmaci. **Nord Medicinhist Arsb** 1980;Suppl 6:35-51

**United States**

Boisvert DJ: Florence Nightingale's cap. **N Engl Galaxy** 1978;20(2):42-51
Cassedy JH: Highlights in the development of medical history in the United States. (Materials from an exhibit). Bethesda, National Library of Medicine, 1984. 30 p.
Gerdts WH: The art of healing: medicine and science in American art. [Birmingham, Alabama], Birmingham Museum of Art, 1981. 119 p. (Exhibit, Birmingham, 1981).
Krivatsy P: Medical incunabula and the diffusion of scientific knowledge. Incunabula in the National Library of Medicine. Published in conjunction with an exhibit at the National Library of Medicine, May-Oct. 1984. [Bethesda, National Library of Medicine, 1984.] 14 p.
Liberti L, Coyle G, Der Marderosian A: Historical pharmaceutical exhibits at PCP&S. **Pharm Hist** 1980;22(3):115-18
McDonell KM: Medicine in antebellum Indiana: conflict, conservatism, and change. Indianapolis, Indiana Historical Society, 1984. 58 p. (Publications in Indiana Medical History, No. 1).
Sammis S, Dummett E: On display: the science and art of healing. **J Med Soc NJ** 1984 Sep;81(9):747-57
Smallpox exhibit: **Bull Hist Med** 1981 Spring;55(1):108-10

# FAMOUS PERSONS

See also **Art; Literature; Music; Politics; Specific persons under Biographies**

Abbott EC: Composers and tuberculosis: the effects on creativity. **Can Med Assoc J** 1982 Mar 1;126(5):534, 536-8, 543-4
Foley GP: A treasury of dentistry. Royal extractions. **J Am Coll Dent** 1984 Fall;51(3):22-3
Hurst LC: Porphyria revisited. **Med Hist** 1982 Apr;26(2):179-82
Levin MJ: Psychology. A biographical approach. New York, McGraw-Hill, 1978. 662 p.
Loevy HT, Kowitz A: The Habsburgs and the 'Habsburg Jaw'. **Bull Hist Dent** 1982 Apr;30(1):19-23
Plaza Izquierdo F: Enfermedad final de Francisco Franco, a proposito de los que mueren en el poder. **Rev Soc Venez Hist Med** 1980;29(43-44):95-124
Runyan WM: Life histories and psychobiography. Explorations in theory and method. New York, Oxford, Oxford University Press, 1982. xiii, 288 p.
Stefănescu P: Drama otrăvirilor: dosare celebre. Bucuresti, Editura Medicală, 1980. 292 p.
Veith I: On privileged communication: a comparative study of several medical cases. **West J Med** 1983 Mar;138(3):437-40

**Great Britain**

Carlton C: Three British revolutions and the personality of kingship. In Pocock, JG. ed: Three British revolutions: 1641, 1688, 1776. Princeton, N.J., Princeton U. Press, 1980. p. 165-207.
Dewhurst J: Royal confinements. **Ala J Med Sci** 1982 Oct;19(4):445-52
Haeger-Aronsen B, Haeger K: Porfyri hos Mary Stuarts efterkommande: en historisk-medicinsk tvistefråga. **Sydsven Medicinhist Sallsk Arsskr** 1984;21:63-75
Russell JR: The three royal doctors of Betchworth. **Practitioner** 1981 Jul;225(1357):1070-1

**Sweden**

Diener L: Osteologi och historia--röntgenologiska aspekter. **Nord Medicinhist Arsb** 1980;Suppl 6:112-7

**Before 500 A.D.**

Africa TW: Worms and the death of kings: a cautionary note on disease and history. **Classical Antiq** 1982;1(1):1-17

**Egypt**

Timmons CF: Genetics of the eighteenth dynasty. **JAMA** 1981 Apr 17;245(15):1525

**Greco-Roman**

Callmer C: Ur arkiater-titelns historia. **Sydsven Medicinhist Sallsk Arsskr** 1980;:40-80

**500 A.D.-1450**

**France**

Charmasson T: Roland l'Ecrivain, médecin des Ducs de Bourgogne. In: Congrès National des Sociétes Savantes, 101e, Lille, 1976. Comptes Rendus. Paris, 1976. Section des Sciences, Fasc. III. p. 21-32.

**1450-1700**

**Austria**

Beck-Mannagetta P: Zum 300. Todestag des Johann Wilhelm Ritter von Mannagetta und seinem Wirken in Niederösterreich. **Unsere Heimat** 1966;37(4-6):125-9

**Czechoslovakia**

Wondrák E: Olomoucký Mistr Fridrich--zapomenutý lékař králuv a císařuv. **Cas Lek Cesk** 1984 May 4;123(18):551-2

**Great Britain**

Fraser A: King Charles II, 'The Father of His People'. In Passmore R, ed: Proceedings of the Royal College of Physicians of Edinburgh Tercentenary Congress, 1981. Edinburgh, Royal College of Physicians of Edinburgh, 1982. p. 23-43.

**Romania**

Vătămanu N: Contribution à l'étude de la vie et de l'oeuvre di Giovanni Mascellini, médecin et secrétaire princier. **Rev Etud Sud Est Eur** 1978;16(2):269-87

**1700 to Present**

Beeck M: Merkmale epileptischer Bildnerei: mit Pathographie Van Gogh. Bern, Huber, 1982. 134 p.
Cambier J: De la mort de Louis XV à la vaccination du roi de Rome. **Nouv Presse Med** 1980 Jun 7;9(25):1746
L'Etang H: Fit to lead? London, Heinemann, 1980. 211 p.
Lontainé SZ, Susa E, Varga T: A Habsburgok József nádori ágához tartozók vércsoportvizsgálata. **Morphol Igazsagugyi Orv Sz** 1980 Oct;20(4):275-81
Meyer A: The search for a morphological substrate in the brains of eminent persons including musicians: a historical review. In Critchley M, Henson RA, ed: Music and the brain: studies in the neurology of music. London, Heinemann, 1977. p. 255-81.
Pharmacology of leadership: **Practitioner** 1980 Feb;224(1340):119
Pisztora F: A születési arisztokrácia súlya és a származási téveszmék gyakorisága a Monarchia társadalmában. **Orv Hetil** 1981 Jun 28;122(26):1593-5
Vega H: Así sufrieron. Barcelona, Argos Vergara, 1981. 204 p.

**Americas**

Plaza Izquierdo F: Medicos presidentes de America. **Rev Soc Venez Hist Med** 1976;24(38):19-36

**Brazil**

Cunha Rodrigues MR da: A morte da Imperatriz Leopoldina (11-XII-1826). **Rev Hist (Brazil)** 1971;43(88):345-52

**Germany**

Meyer-Schwickerath G: Das Annette von Droste-Hülshoff-Syndrom.

**Klin Monatsbl Augenheilkd** 1984 Jun;184(6):574–7

**Great Britain**

Baxby D: A death from inoculated smallpox in the English Royal Family. **Med Hist** 1984 Jul;28(3):303–7
Whitfield AG: The scholar prince. **J R Coll Physicians Lond** 1984 Jul;18(3):195–7

**Spain**

Gonzalez Iglesias J: Los Borbones y el desarrollo de la odontologia en Espãna. **Bol Inf Dent (Madr)** 1978;Spec no:63-92

**United States**

Brown P: National celebrities brought cheer to young patients at Riley Hospital (I. U. Medical Center) in the 1930's. **Indiana Med Hist Q** 1976;2(4):65–9
Carson SL: Presidential children: abandonment, hysteria and suicide. **J Psychohist** 1984 Spring;11(4):533–44
Gambill J: Potential problems of detecting and treating psychosis in the White House. Potential psychosis in the White House. **Int J Soc Psychiatry** 1980;26(4):255–62
Graham SD: Ephraim McDowell (1771–1830). The President's lithotomist. **Invest Urol** 1981 Nov;19(3):216–7
Pond MA: Presidential initiatives in organizing health affairs: from Harding to Roosevelt. **Pres Stud Q** 1983;13(3):417–29
Robins RS, Rothschild H: Hidden health disabilities and the presidency: medical management and political consideration. **Perspect Biol Med** 1981 Winter;24(2):240–53
Stern MB, comp: A phrenological dictionary of nineteenth-century Americans. Westport, Conn., Greenwood Press, 1982. xx, 430 p.

**USSR**

Chernyĭ VP: Znamenitye patsienty N. I. Pirogova. **Feldsher Akush** 1983 Sep;48(9):34–7

# FOLK AND POPULAR MEDICINE

See also **Hygiene; Magic and Occult; Primitive Medicine; Quackery; Religion and Medicine; Therapeutic Cults**

Coin rubbing and related folk medicine: **JAMA** 1981 May 8;245(18):1819
Hand WD: Magical medicine: the folkloric component of medicine in the folk belief, custom, and ritual of the peoples of Europe and America: selected essays. Berkeley, University of California Press, 1980. xxvii, 345 p.
Hand WD: Medical science's legacy of outmoded doctrines to folk and primitive medicine. In International Congress of the History of Medicine, 27th, Barcelona, 1980. Actas. Barcelona, Acadèmia de Ciències Mèdiques de Catalunya i Balears, 1981. p. 517–21.
Homblé AG: De echel of bloedzuiger in de volksgeneeskunde. **Oostvlaam Zanten** 1980;55(1):1–32
Joannis C: Santé et sagesse traditionnelle. Le Puy, France, Bonneton, 1981. 127 p.
Jünemann J: Nachlese zu Rillen und Näpfchen auf sakralen Denkmalen (2). **Beitr Gesch Pharm** 1980;31(7):49–54
Kanei H: [The role of women and nursing – a lesson in folk medicine. 3]. **Sogo Kango** 1982;17(1):79–89
La médicine populaire: Exposition, 27 mars – 17 mai 1981. Bruxelles, Galerie CGER, 1981. 109 p.
L'homme et son corps dans la société traditionelle: Paris, Ministère de la culture et de la communication, Editions de la Réunion des musées nationaux, 1978. 144 p.
Meigs JA: Choosing your baby's sex – now and in the sixteenth century. **Tenn Folkl Soc Bull** 1982;48(4):111–6
Mittwoch U: Whistling maids and crowing hens--hermaphroditism in folklore and biology. **Perspect Biol Med** 1981 Summer;24(4):595–606
Schlegel KF: Der Körperbehinderte in Mythologie und Kunst. Stuttgart; New York, Thieme, 1983. 125 p.
Tillhagen CH: Vögel in der Volksmedizin. **Ethnomedizin** 1978–79;5(3–4):263–86

**Afghanistan**

Penkala D: 'Hot' and 'cold' in the traditional medicine of Afghanistan. **Ethnomedizin** 1980;6(1–4):201–28

**Africa**

Ademuwagun ZA, et al, ed: African therapeutic systems. Waltham, Massachusetts, Crossroads Press of the African Studies Association, 1979. vii, 273 p.
Elom-Ntouzo'o E: Médecine, pharmacopées traditionelles et développement en Afrique. **Presence Afr** 1978;108:38–49
Kerharo J: Die traditionelle Medizin in Schwarzafrika. In Sournia JC, Martiny M, Poulet J, ed: Illustrierte Geschichte der Medizin. Salzburg, Andreas, 1980. Vol. 6. p. 2351–82.
Moersch E: Psychiatrie in Afrika zwischen Tradition und Moderne. **Psyche (Stuttg)** 1984 Aug;38(8):673–95

**Americas**

Foster GM, et al: El legado hipocratico latinoamericano: 'caliente' y 'frio' en la medicina popular contemporanea. **Med Tradic** 1979;2(6):5–24
Hand WD, ed: American folk medicine; a symposium. Berkeley, University of California Press, 1976. viii, 347 p. Contributions by C. H. Talbot, T. R. Forbes, S. X. Radbill, J. Puhvel, D. B. Price, D. J. Hufford, B. Gebhard, B. G. Myerhoff, L. J. Bean, V. J. Vogel, R. I. Ford, W. A. Emboden, F. Guerra, J. S. Graham, B. H. Granger, L. Lacourcière, E. Brandon, D. Yoder, J. A. Hostetler, B. Jackson, A. E. Fife, L. E. Barrett, M. O. Jones, J. Q. Anderson.
Johannessen CL: Folk medicine uses of melanotic Asiatic chickens as evidence of early diffusion to the New World. **Soc Sci Med [D]** 1981 Nov;15D(4):427–34
Ryn L: Los Andes y la medicina. **Actas Luso Esp Neurol Psiquiatr** 1981 May–Jun;9(3):213–30, Jul–Aug;9(4):315–24
Wendorf de Sejas M, Sejas García R: Medicina y psicologia tradicional de la region andina: bibliografía comentada. **Nuevos Libros** 1980;23–24:1–23

**Asia**

Mazars G, ed: Les médecines traditionnelles de l'Asie. Actes du colloque de Paris 11–12 Juin 1979. Strasbourg, Université Louis Pasteur, 1981. 162 p. (Publication du Séminaire sur les Sciences et les Techniques en Asie).

**Austria**

Bauerndoktor und Volksmedizin. 1. Ausstellung anlässlich des 800–jährigen Bestehens von Stainz. Sonderausstellung: Juni bis Okt. 1977. Katalog: Nr. 3. Maria Kundegraber, unter Mitarb. v. Bernd Mader. Steiermark, Landesmuseum Joanneum, 1977. 63 p.:
Hölzl N: Zauberbücher, Vampire und einige vernünftige Köpfe. **Tirol Heimatbl** 1972;47(1–3):35–8
Kostenzer O: Das Katharinenöl, ein altes Heilmittel. **Tirol Heimatbl** 1974;49(2):77–80

**Belgium**

Homble AG: De medecijn Winckel van den verstandigen hovenier. **Brabantse Folkl** 1979 Sept;223:287–324

**Canada**

Dulong G: Médecine populaire au Canada français. In: Congrès international d'histoire de la médecine, XXVe, Québec, 1976. Actes. Québec, 1977. p. 625–33.

**China**

Liu X: Psychiatry in traditional Chinese medicine. **Br J Psychiatry** 1981 May;138:429–33
Schiffeler JW: Chinese folk medicine: a study of the Shan-hai Ching. **Asian Folkl Stud** 1980;39(2):41–83
Wong M: Histoire du massage en Chine. In M. Wong: Les massages en médecine traditionnelle chinoise. Paris, Masson, 1984. p. 7–29.

**Czechoslovakia**

Zolyomi ND: L'acceptation des remèdes populaires par les médecins érudits. In: Congrès international d'histoire de la médecine, XXVe, Québec, 1976. Actes. Québec, 1977. p. 1396–1402.

**Denmark**

Brade AE: The Danish folk medicine. A research project. In International Congress of the History of Medicine, 27th, Barcelona, 1980. Actas. Barcelona, Acadèmia de Ciències Mèdiques de Catalunya i Balears, 1981. p. 458–61.

**Ecuador**

Bernand C: El caso Manuel: enfermedad y fatalidad en los Andes. **Asclepio** 1983;35:265–73

**Ethiopia**

Abebe W: Traditional pharmaceutical practice in Gondar region, northwestern Ethiopia. **J Ethnopharmacol** 1984 Jun;11(1):33–47

# FOLK AND POPULAR MEDICINE

**Europe**

Brøndegaard VJ: Das Wurzelstechen. **Sudhoffs Arch** 1983;67(2):199–209
Czigány LG: The use of hallucinogens and the shamanistic tradition of the Finno-Ugrian people. **Slav East Eur Rev** 1980;58(2):212–7

**Finland**

Strandberg H, ed: Folk medicine in Finland. A bibliography. (In Finnish, English and German). Helsingin, Nordiskt Folkmedicinmuseum, 1977. 15 p. (Meddelanden Nr. 1).

**France**

Gandilhon R: La bouse de vache. Etude d'ethnologie. **Mem Soc Agric Commer Sci Arts Marne** 1978;271–306
Gélis J: La Pierre et le saint: recours populaires pour la guérison des petits enfants (XVIIe–XIXe siècles). **Asclepio** 1983;35:129–58
Guyotjeannin C: Remèdes d'autrefois aux îles Saint-Pierre-et-Miquelon. **Rev Hist Pharm (Paris)** 1984 Jun;31(261):115–20
Raphaël F: La médecine populaire juive en Alsace. In Livet G, Schaff G, ed: Médecine et assistance en Alsace, XVIe–XXe siècle. Strasbourg, Istra, 1976. p. 287–302.
Schmitt JC: The holy greyhound: Guinefort, healer of children since the thirteenth century. Cambridge, Cambridge University Press; Paris, Editions de la Maison des Sciences de l'Homme, 1983. 215 p. Translation of Le saint lévrier: Guinefort, guérisseur d'enfants depuis le XIIIe siècle, Paris, 1979.

**Germany**

Belke I: Die Begründung der Völkerpsychologie in Deutschland: Eine Alternative zur etablierten Geschichtswissenschaft? **Riv Filos** 1982;73:192–233
Holtkamp P: Narkosen mit 'Weingenuss bis zum Nasenbluten'. **Quintessenz J** 1981 Nov;11(11):995–6
Schienbein H: Die 'Neu-Vermehrte Heylsame Dreck-Apotheke' (1696/1734) des Hof- und Stadtarztes Christian Frantz Paulini. **Quintessenz** 1981 Sep;32(9):1699–1702

**Great Britain**

Lewis TH: Richard Carew on the treatment of a 'Franticke person' in Medieval Cornwall. **J Hist Med Allied Sci** 1981 Jan;36(1)64–6

**Hungary**

Fazekas A: A magyar nyelvu herbárium irodalomról. **Orvostort Kozl** 1982;28(1–3):43–64
Oláh A: Althergebrachte Tierheilpraktiken im Komitat Békés, Ungarn. **Ethnomedizin** 1978–79;5(3–4):301–18
Oláh A: Zwiebel und Knoblauch in der Volksmedizin; das ungarische Theriak und Mithridaticum früher und heute. **Ethnomedizin** 1981–82;7(1–4):333–48

**India**

Bhattacharyya NN: Indian puberty rites. Second edition, revised and enlarged. New Delhi, Munshiram Manoharlal, 1980. 124 p.
Gangadharam V, Sudhakara Reddy P, Subba Reddy BV: Concept of disease and folk therapy in a village of Andhra Pradesh. **Bull Indian Inst Hist Med (Hyderabad)** 1978;8(1–4):44–50
Kakar S: Shamans, mystics, and doctors: a psychological inquiry into India and its healing traditions. New York, Knopf, 1982. x, 306 p.

**Italy**

Celant E: L'empirico dei mali e dei rimedi. Palermo, 'Il Vespro', 1979. 173 p.
Coccanari MA: Les plantes et leur action sur le cerveau et sur la psiche: science et magie. **Med Secoli** 1982 May–Aug;19(2):215–9
Sacino G: Singolari figure della tradizione medica popolare remota e recente nell'appennino centro-meridionale d'Italia: 'le janare', 'le masciare'. In: Congrès international d'histoire de la médecine, XXVe, Québec, 1976. Actes. Québec, 1977. p. 1196–207.

**Japan**

Ishigoro T: [Historical background of the 'hara-obi' (a piece of cloth wrapped around the abdomen of a pregnant woman) and the origin of its name] (Jpn). **Josanpu Zasshi** 1984;38(4):336–9; (5):437–40; (6):519–23

**Peru**

Gagliano JA: La medicina popular y la coca en el Perú: un análisis histórico de actitudes. **Am Indig** 1978;38(4):789–805
Ryn L: Medicina popular andina. **Actas Luso Esp Neurol Psiquiatr** 1982 Jan–Feb;10(1):33–42

**Romania**

Farkas G, Farkas G Jr: People's customs related to pregnancy and delivery in former Transylvania. In: Congrès international d'histoire de la médecine, XXVe, Québec, 1976. Actes. Québec, 1977. p. 654–8.
Neagu I, Neagu M: Vieux médicament utilisé dans la thérapeutique populaire de Roumanie. In: Congrès international d'histoire de la médecine, XXVe, Québec, 1976. Actes. Québec, 1977. p. 1015–25.

**Scandinavia**

Strandberg H: Nordiskt seminarium om folkmedicin på Kilen i Sideby, Kristinestad, Finland. **Nord Medicinhist Arsb** 1980;Suppl 6:139–42

**Spain**

Deloncle J: Sobre la terapèutica a través dels sants a Catalunya Nord. In Congrés International d'Història de la Medicina Catalana, 2nd, Barcelona, 1975. Llibre d'Actes. Barcelona, Socitra, 1977. p. 129–32.
García Ramos JA: Datos originales del folklore medico almeriense. **Asclepio** 1981;33:275–314
Zubiri Vidal F, Zubiri de Salinas R: Refranes médicos oidos en Aragón. **Cuad Aragon Hist Med Cienc (A)** 1978, 1980;2:1–99

**Sri Lanka**

De Silva A, Uragoda CG: Traditional methods of snake-bite treatment in Sri Lanka. **Ceylon Med J** 1983 Sep;28(3):170–4

**Sweden**

Högberg U: Allmogens förlossningsställningar. **Jordemodern** 1982 Jun;95(6):199–202

**United States**

Baer HA: Toward a systematic typology of black folk healers. **Phylon** 1982;43(4):327–43
Hand WD, Casetta A, Thiederman SB, ed: Popular beliefs and superstitions. A compendium of American folklore from the Ohio Collection of Newbell Niles Puckett. 3 volumes. Boston, G. K. Hall, 1981.
Kuna RR: Hoodoo: the indigenous medicine and psychiatry of the black American. **Ethnomedizin** 1974–75;3(3–4):273–94

**USSR**

Maslov AA: Iz istorii narodnoĭ meditsiny Kabardiono-Balkarii. **Vopr Kurortol Fizioter Lech Fiz Kult** 1980 Sep–Oct;(5):66–8

**Before 500 A.D.**

Kudlien F: Zur Erforschung archaisch-griechischer 'Zeugungslehren'. **Medizinhist J** 1981;16(4):323–39

**Rome**

Stannard J: Medicinal plants and folk remedies in Pliny, Historia Naturalis. **Hist Philos Life Sci** 1982;4(1):3–23

**500 A.D.–1450**

Gerhardt C: Kröte und Igel in schwankhafter Literatur des späten Mittelalters. **Medizinhist J** 1981;16(4):340–57
Hirth W: Popularisierungstendenzen in der mittelalterlichen Fachliteratur. **Medizinhist J** 1980;15(1/2):70–89
Jordi González R: Fórmulas medicinales populares y supersticiosas pertenecientes a la primera mitad del siglo XV (1417–1459). **Circ Farm** 1981 Oct–Dec;39(273):469–82
Pinto LB: The folk practice of gynecology and obstetrics in the Middle Ages. **Bull Hist Med** 1973 Sep–Oct;47(5):513–23
Stannard J: Folkloristic elements in medieval herbalism. In International Congress of the History of Medicine. 26th, Plovdiv, 1978. Actes du Congress. Sofia, 1981. Volume II. p. 203–5.
Weisser C: Studien zum mittelalterlichen Krankheitslunar. Ein Beitrag zur Geschichte laienastrologischer Fachprosa. Pattensen/Hannover, Horst Wellm, 1982. 468 p. (Würzburger medizinhistorische Forschungen, 21).

**Arabic**

Kuz'min MK, Bukharov PL: Ibn-Sina (Avitsenna) i narodnaia meditsina. **Feldsher Akush** 1981;46(3):50–2

**Germany**

Hirth W: Corpusbildung in der deutschsprachigen medizinischen Fachliteratur des Mittelalters. **Suhoffs Arch** 1982;66(3):239–75

**Great Britain**

Mooney LR: A middle English verse compendium of astrological medicine. **Med Hist** 1984 Oct;28(4):406–19

**Iceland**

Orner R, Hipwell J: Njal's Saga: a 1000 year old record of premature ejaculation. **J Am Soc Psychosom Dent Med** 1980;27(1):10–2

**Italy**

Rowland B: Exhuming Trotula, sapiens matrona of Salerno. **Florilegium** 1979;1:42–57

**USSR**

Dzhanelidze MB: O 'Lechebnoĭ knige-karabadine' i ee avtore Zaze Panaskerteli-Tsitsishvili (k 550-letiiu so dnia rozhdeniia). **Sov Zdravookhr** 1981;(5):67–8

**1450–1700**

Bergamaschi MT, et al: Streghe e raccoglitrici di bambori: al confine tra la medicina colta, empiria e pratiche magiche (XV-XVI secolo). **Mem Riv Stor Donne** 1981,(1):106–13

Horsley RA: Who were the witches? The social roles of the accused in the European witch trials. **J Interdiscip Hist** 1979;9(4):689–715

**Europe**

Niccoli O: 'Menstruum quasi monstruum': parti mostruosi e tabù mestruale nel '500. **Quad Stor** 1980;15(2):402–8

**Germany**

Dilg P: Examen pharmacopoeorum vulgare. Aus einer Handschrift des Laurentius Blumentrost d. A. (1619–1705). In Dilg P, et al., ed: Perspektiven der Pharmaziegeschichte. Graz, Austria, Akademische Druck- u. Verlagsanstalt, 1983. p. 39–64.

**Great Britain**

Walton MT: Thomas Forestier and the 'False Lechys' of London. **J Hist Med Allied Sci** 1982 Jan;37(1):71–3

**Ireland**

Arnold LJ: Valentine Greatrakes, a seventeenth-century 'touch-doctor'. **Eire Irel** 1976;11:3–12

**Poland**

Gomołka B: On the authorship of an astrologico-medical calendar for 1474. (Pol) **Biul Bibl Jagiellon** 1978;28(1–2)

**Spain**

Jordi Gonzáles R: Curiosas formulas de medicina popular pertenecientes al ultimo cuarto del siglo XV. **Offarm** 1982;1(4):239–46

Jordi González R: Formulas de medicina popular y supersticiosa pertenecientes a la primera mitad del siglo XVI (1504–1568). **Circ Farm** 1983;281:283–309

**1700 to Present**

Albanese CL: The poetics of healing: root metaphors and rituals in nineteenth-century America. **Soundings** 1980;63(4):381–406

Baasher T: Promotion and development of research in traditional medicine: the WHO role in countries of the Eastern Mediterranean Region. **J Ethnopharmacol** 1980 Mar;2(1):75–9

Kermorvan F: Les sirènes existent, l'histoire les a rencontrées. **Histoire** 1980;24:76–8

Maclean V: A short-title catalogue of household and cookery books published in the English tongue 1701–1800. London, Prospect, 1981. 197 p.

Morley P, Wallis R, et al: Culture and curing. Anthropological perspectives on traditional medical beliefs and practices. London, Owen, 1978. vii, 190 p.

Robinson T: Baroque medicine: how a cup of Aunt Ida's hot air rescued a sailor. **Nurs Mirror** 1982 Jul 21;155(3):25

Rochford EB: Stutterers' practices: folk remedies and therapeutic intervention. **J Commun Disord** 1983 Sep;16(5):373–84

Rosner F: Therapeutic efficacy of chicken soup. **Chest** 1980;78:672–4

Schröder E: 'Der Mensch und sein Körper' aus der Sicht des Ethnomediziners. In Imhof AE, ed: Leib und Leben in der Geschichte der Neuzeit. Berlin, Duncker & Humblot, 1983. p 77–86.

Sequeira MM: A medicina moderna e os curandeiros. **Acta Med Port** 1980 Sep-Dec;2(5–6):439–41

Valdivia Ponce O: Bases dinámicas de la psicoterapia tradicional. **Rev Neuropsiquiatr** 1979 Mar;42(1):31–46

Weismann G: A fashion in metals. **Hosp Pract** 1982 Apr;17(4):33–4, 38, 42

Werner R: Medicine men (traditional medical practitioners) in primary health care and the role of traditional medicine towards modern medicine. **Off Gesundheitswes** 1980;42(9):637–56

**Africa**

Kiernan J: Saltwater and ashes: instruments of curing among some Zulu zionists. **J Relig Afr** 1978;9:27–32

**Americas**

Kay MA: The Florilegio Medicinal: source of Southwest ethnomedicine. **Ethnohistory** 1977;24(3):251–9

**Austria**

Dolenc M: 'Nova Gronat-Jabuka'-rokopisne ljudskomedicinske bukve iz 1751. leta. **Cas Zgodovino Narodop** 1980;16(2):311–21

Mutschlechner G: Erde als Heilmittel für Mensch und Tier. **Tirol Heimatbl** 1974;49(1):23–7

**Belgium**

Havelange C: Médecine traditionnelle ou exerçice illégal de l'art de guérir? Les empiriques liégeois au dix-neuvième siècle. **Rev Med Liege** 1983 Nov 15;38(22):860–8

**Bulgaria**

Marinow W: Uber einige irrationale psychotherapeutische Heilmittel der Volksmedizin. In International Congress of the History of Medicine. 26th, Plovdiv, 1978. Actes du Congress. Sofia, 1981. Volume II. p. 80–1.

**Cambodia**

Chandler DP: Folk memories of the decline of Angkor in nineteenth-century Cambodia: the legend of the leper king. **J Siam Soc** 1979;67(1):54–62

**Canada**

Brunel G, Morissette L: Guérison et ethno-étiologie populaire. **Anthropologica** 1979;21(1):43–72

Nadeau J: La médecine populaire dans quatre paroisses du comté de Bellechasse. **Rev Ethnol Que** 1976;2(1):51–104

Richardson G: Letitia Munson. In Dictionary of Canadian biography, 1881–1890. 1982;11:629–30.

**Costa Rica**

Low SM: Dr. Moreno Cañas: a symbolic bridge to the demedicalization of healing. **Soc Sci Med** 1982;16(5):527–31

**Finland**

Hänninen O, Vaskilampi T: Cupping as a part of living Finnish traditional healing. A remedy against pain. **Acupunct Electrother Res** 1982;7(1):39–50

**France**

Bachoffner P: Vulgarisation thérapeutique à travers la 'Materia Medica' de Georges-Henri Behr, médecin strasbourgeois. In Livet G, Schaff G, ed: Médecine et assistance en Alsace, XVIe–XXe siècle. Strasbourg, Istra, 1976. p. 145–53.

Bordes F: Le livre des remèdes de Labadie. Contribution à l'histoire de la médecine populaire landaise au XVIIIe siècle. **Bull Soc Borda** 1982;107(387):399–412

Fournier R: La médicine ancienne dans le centre-ouest. Coutumes populaires disparues et survivances. Poitiers, Brissaud, 1979. 170 p.

Léonard J: Les guérisseurs en France au XIXe siècle. **Rev Hist Mod Contemp** 1980 Jul-Sep;27:501–16

Loux F: Recours convergents à la médecine officielle et à la médecine parallèle en matière de soins aux enfants en France (XIXe-XXe siècles). In Imhof AE, ed: Mensch und Gesundheit in der Geschichte. Husum, Matthiesen, 1980. p. 315–21.

Ramsey M: Popular medicine and medical power in France, 1707–1830.

Ph.D. Diss. Harvard University. Cambridge, Mass., 1979.
Ramsey M: Sous le régime de la législation de 1803: trois enquêtes sur les charlatans au XIVe siècle. **Rev Hist Mod Contemp** 1980 Jul-Sept;27:485-500
Religion et médecine populaires: **Lemouzi** 1979;71:235-367
Spears J: Folk medicine and popular attitudes toward disease in the High Alps, 1780-1870. **Bull Hist Med** 1980 Fall;54(3):303-36
Wilson LB: Les maladies des femmes: women, charlatanry, and professional medicine in eighteenth-century France. Ph.D. Diss., Stanford University. Palo Alto, 1982. vi, 449 p.

**Germany**

Buck MR: Medicinischer Volksglauben u. Volksaberglauben aus Schwaben. Eine kulturgeschichtliche Skizze. 4. Auflage. (Reprint, originally published 1865.) Riedlingen, Ulrich, 1981. vi, 72 p.
Petrova L: Die Bedeutung des Wassers in den volkstümlichen Bräuchen und in der Volksmedizin. In International Congress of the History of Medicine, 27th, Barcelona, 1980. Actas. Barcelona, Académia de Ciències Médiques de Catalunya i Balears, 1981. p. 603-9.
Wölfel A: Pflanzen in der Volksmedizin. Die volksmedizinischen Studien von Heinrich Marzell. Diss. Erlangen-Nürnberg, 1983. 117 p.
Wyklicky H: Warum sich ein Arzt mit Volkskunde beschäftigte. **Osterr Arzteztg** 1982 Jan 25;2

**Ghana**

Tiberini ES: Note sull'aborto e la contraccezione tra gli Nzema del Ghana. **Africa (Italy)** 1980;35(2):159-70

**Great Britain**

Harkness B: Greene's old-fashioned remedy in the heart of the matter. **Am Notes Queries** 1982 Mar-Apr;20(7-8):115-6
Jackson WA: The Carbolic smoke ball. **Pharm Hist (London)** 1984;14(1):9-10
Kanai H: [What Nightingale would have written about summer heat and nursing - a thought in connection with folk remedy] (Jpn). **Kango** 1982 Aug;34(9):4-14
Moskow BS: Dentistry in folk art, XIII: The dentist. **Bull Hist Dent** 1981 Oct;29(2):99
Pickstone JV: Medical botany (self-help medicine in Victorian England). **Mem Proc Manch Lit Philos Soc** 1976-77;119:85-95
Rechtman J: Un précurseur génial de la prévention et de la diététique, du bouche à bouche et du massage cardiaque externe de l'asepsie et parrain de J. P. Marat: Le docteur William Buchan (1729-1805). Diss. Paris VII, 1979. 115 p.
Sigsworth EM, Swan P: Para-medical provision in the West Riding. **Soc Soc Hist Med Bull (Lond)** 1981 Dec;29:37-9
Wilder F: The remarkable world of John Wesley, pioneer in mental health. Hicksville, Exposition Press, 1978. 192 p.

**Hungary**

Bugyi B: Az elsö 'népszerü orvostan' föiskolai tanszék (1834-1852) történetéböl. **Orvostort Kozl** 1981;93-96(27 No 1-4):225-35
Hörcsik E, Pisztora F: Ritkuló és halványuló babonás hiedelmek valamint széles körben elterjedt technikai ismeretek napjaink pszichiátriai kórképeiben. **Orvostort Kozl** 1982;92(4):93-9
Orzóy R: Néphit elemek idegbetegek kórképeiben. **Orvostort Kozl** 1982;92(4):101-12

**Iceland**

Johnsen B: Islands folkemedicin og Magnus Ketilsson. **Dan Medicinhist Arbog** 1982;:56-70

**Ireland**

Buckley AD: Unofficial healing in Ulster. **Ulster Folklife** 1980;26:15-34
Corrigan D: Irish Ethno-botany by Michael Moloney--an early contribution to the concept of ethnopharmacology. **J Ethnopharmacol** 1981 Nov;4(3):343-5

**Italy**

Morricone A, Pedicino V: Medici e guaritori in Sicilia: spunti di medicina popolare in un'opera diGiuseppe Pitré. In Congrès international d'histoire de la médecine, XXVe, Québec, 1976. Actes. Québec, 1977. p. 992-8.

**Ivory Coast**

Handloff R: Prayers, amulets and charms: health and social control. **Afr Stud Rev** 1982;25(2-3):185-94

**Kenya**

Meschig R, Schadewaldt H: Uvulektomie--ein Initiationsritus? **MMW** 1981;123(11):437-40

**Libya**

Abu-Shwairb 'Abd al-Karim: Mushahadati haul al-tib al-sha'bi fi Fazan (tarjamah wa-taqdim limushahadat tabib Turki). **Majallat al-Puhuth al-Tarikhiya (Lybia)** 1979;1(2):37-50

**Nigeria**

Nwokedike A: Folkmedicine in Iboland/Nigeria. Diss. Düsseldorf, 1980. 58 p.

**Pacific Islands**

Howard A: The power to heal in colonial Rotuma. **J Polynesian Soc** 1979;88(3):243-75
Stocking GW: Contradicting the doctor: Billy Hancock and the problem of baloma. **Hist Anthropol Newsl** 1977;4(1):4-7

**Peru**

Mariátegui J: Hermilio Valdizán, la psiquiatría comparativa y la medicina folklórica. **Acta Psiquiatr Psicol Am Lat** 1980 Jun;26(2):96-106

**Romania**

Ionescu C: Des 'remèdes' appliqués dans le district Prahova, par la médecine populaire, à fin du XIX siècle et le début du XX siècle. In: Congrès international d'histoire de la médecine, XXVe, Québec, 1976. Actes. Québec, 1977. p. 790-7.
Vulcanescu R: Les chevaux fantastiques et la psychothérapie populaire. In International Congress of the History of Medicine. 26th, Plovdiv, 1978. Actes du Congress. Sofia, 1981. Volume II. p. 83-5.

**Sweden**

Diener L, et al: Nutida folkmedicin. **Nord Medicinhist Arsb** 1981;:193-202
Janzon B: Idrott och ling-gymnastik i populär-medicinsk belysning. **Nord Medicinhist Arsb** 1980;:124-35
Tillhagen CH: Ingjald Reichborn-Kjennerud (1865-1949). **Arv** 1969-70;25-26:353-74

**United States**

Agogino GA, Ferguson B: Curanderismo: the folk healer in the Spanish-speaking community. **Masterkey Ind Lore Hist** 1983;57(3):101-6
Barlow J, Richardson C: China doctor of John Day. Portland, Bonford & Mort, 1979. ix, 118 p.
Barrow MV: Self-treatment practices in North Florida. **J Fla Med Assoc** 1979 Aug;66(8):840-4
Batchen LS: La curandera. **Palacio** 1975;81(1):20-5
Boudreaux AM: Les remèdes du vieux temps: remedies and cures of the Kaplan area in southwestern Louisiana. **South Folkl Q** 1971;35(2):121-40
Burnham JC: Change in the popularization of health in the United States. **Bull Hist Med** 1984 Summer;58(2):183-97
Carey GG: Folklore from the printed sources of Essex County, Massachusetts. **South Folkl Q** 1968;32(1):17-43
Colbert L: Amish attitudes and treatment of illness. **Pa Folklife** 1980;30(1):9-15
Dieffenbach VC: Powwowing among the Pennsylvania Germans. **Pa Folklife** 1975-76;25(2):29-46
Doyle CC: The power of not thinking: a jocular toothache cure. **Ky Folkl Rec** 1983;29(1-2):24-9
Dundes A: The dead baby joke cycle. **West Folkl** 1979;38(3):145-57
Fellman AC, Fellman M: Making sense of self. Medical advice literature in late nineteenth-century America. Philadelphia, University of Pennsylvania Press, 1981. 198 p.
Fiedler LA: Images of the nurse in fiction and popular culture. In Jones AH, ed: Images of healers. Albany, State University of New York Press, 1983. p. 79-90.
Herman BL: Folk medical recipes in nineteenth-century American farm journals. **Pa Folklife** 1976;25(4):16-25
Japp PM: Pioneer medicines: doctors, nostrums, and folk cures. **J West** 1982 Jul;21(3):15-22
Jaskoski H: 'My heart will go out': healing songs of native American women. **Int J Womens Stud** 1981;4(2):118-34
Jenner CL, ed: The Vi-Ton-Ka medicine show. American Place Theatre, 1983. 36 p. Contributions by B. McNamara, G. Hinson, F. F. Bloodgood, A. Dargan, C. Wolfe, J. H. Young, W. Helfand.
Jordan TG: 'The roses so red and the lilies so fair': southern folk cemeteries in Texas. **Southwest Hist Q** 1980;83(3):227-58
Krell R: At a children's hospital; a folklore survey. **West Folkl** 1980;39(3):223-31

Labarbera M: An ounce of prevention, and grandma tried them all. **NY Folkl Q** 1964;20(2):126-9
McIntosh K: Folk obstetrics, gynecology, and pediatrics in Utica, New York. **NY Folkl** 1978;4(1-4):49-59
Marshall J: The madstone: its origins and application in Barlow, Ballard County, Kentucky. **Ky Folkl Rec** 1978;24(2):42-8
Pocius GL: Veterinary folk medicine in Susquehanna County, Pennsylvania. **Pa Folklife** 1976;25(4):2-15
Powers BA: The use of orthodox and black American folk medicine. **ANS** 1982 Apr;4(3):35-47
Reimensnyder B: Annotated bibliography of Pennsylvania folk medicine. **Pa Folklife** 1977;27(1):40-8
Roeder BA: Health care beliefs and practices among Mexican Americans: a review of the literature. **Aztlan** 1982;13(1-2):223-56
Sawyer DJ: The lady with the snake in her. **NY Folkl Q** 1969;25(4):299-305
Snow LF: Con men and conjure men: a ghetto image. In Jones AH, ed: Images of healers. Albany, State University of New York Press, 1983. p. 45-78.
Stewart S: Rational powwowing: an examination of choice among medical alternatives in rural York County, Pennsylvania. **Pa Folklife** 1976;26(1):12-7
Studer GC: Powwowing: folk medicine or white magic? **Pa Mennon Heritage** 1980;3(3):17-23
Waller T, Killion G: Georgia folk medicine. **South Folkl Q** 1972;36(1):71-92
Warner JH: 'Exploring the inner labyrinths of creation': popular microscopy in nineteenth-century America. **J Hist Med Allied Sci** 1982 Jan;37(1):7-33
Wilson G: Swallow it or rub it on: more mammoth cave remedies. **South Folkl Q** 1967;31(4):296-303
Yoder D, ed: Advertisements of urban healers. **Pa Folklife** 1978;27(3):44-8

**USSR**

Kvitnitskiĭ-Ryzhov IN: Vydaiushchiĭsia issledovatel' otechestvennoĭ narodnoĭ meditsiny V. F. Demich (1858-1930). **Sov Zdravookhr** 1982;7:70-4

**Venezuela**

Pollak-Eltz A: Folk-medicine in Venezuela. **Acta Ethnol Linguist** 1982;53:1-231

**Yugoslavia**

Dugacki V: Le traitement des maladies oculaires dans la medecine populaire yougoslave. In International Congress of the History of Medicine. 26th, Plovdiv, 1978. Actes du Congress. Sofia, 1981. Volume II. p. 85-8.
Pejčić M: O nekim lekarima, apotekarima, i narodonoj medicini u Nišu za vreme Turaka (XIX vek). **Srp Arh Celok Lek** 1981 Oct;109(10):1405-12

**Zimbabwe**

Gelfand M: The N'anga, the guardian of the Shona way of life, its ethics and behaviour. **Cent Afr J Med** 1981 Jul;27(7):146-8

## FOODS AND FOOD SUPPLY

See also **Nutrition and Diet; Public Health**

Bender AE: The future of our food supplies. **R Soc Health J** 1981 Aug;101(4):158-62
Borman SA: Origins of risk assessment. **Anal Chem** 1983 Dec;55(14):1438A-1440A
Forster R, Ranum O, ed: Food and drink in history. Selections from the Annales economies, sociétés, civilisations. Volume 5. Baltimore, London, Johns Hopkins University Press, 1979. xiii, 173 p. Reprinted articles by M. Aymard, M. Morineau, J. Revel, JJ. Hémardinquer, W. Frijhoff, JC. Bonnet, R. Barthes, D. Julia, J. Leclant, J.P. Aron, G. Thuillier, J. Soler.
Grmek MD: La légende et la réalité de la nocivité des fèves. **Hist Philos Life Sci** 1980;2(1):61-121
James EO: Cultural and religious taboos related to food. **Prog Food Nutr Sci** 1979;3(3):67-77
Little AC: The eyes have it. **J Am Diet Assoc** 1980 Dec;77(6):688-91
Maret F: Der Wein in der Medizingeschichte. **ZFA (Stuttgart)** 1980 May 10;56(13):887-97
Navarro P: Lactancia mercenaria: hipocresía y exploitación. **Asclepio** 1983;35:375-87
Rosen IL: Aphrodisiacs in the kitchen. **J La State Med Soc** 1980 Oct;132(10):155-9

**Africa**

Miller JC: The significance of drought, disease and famine in the agriculturally marginal zones of West-Central Africa. **J Afr Hist** 1982;23(1):17-61

**Belgium**

Leboutte R: Les métaux et l'hygiène alimentaire: la vaisselle en zinc de l'abbé Dony. **Bull Soc R Vieux Liege** 1977-79;9:311-3

**Brazil**

Fish WR: Changing food use patterns in Brazil. **Luso-Braz Rev** 1978;15(1):69-89

**China**

Lee J: Food supply and population growth in southwest China, 1250-1850. **J Asian Stud** 1982;41(4):711-46
Li LM: Food and famine in China. **Soc Sci Res Counc Items** 1981;35(1-2):11-4
Li LM: Workshop on food and famine in Chinese history. **Ch'ing-Shih Wen-t'i** 1980;4(4):90-100

**France**

Amiot M, Béguinot P: L'alimentation en eau potable de la ville de Dijon et son assainnissement. **Mem Acad Sci Arts B-Lett Dijon** 1977;122:551-602
Nauroy J: L'équipement technique et le ravitaillement. **Med Armees** 1980;8(10)spec:845-50

**Great Britain**

Matossian MK: Mold poisoning: an unrecognized English health problem, 1550-1800. **Med Hist** 1981 Jan;25(1):73-84
Walker B: Meat preservation in Scotland. **R Soc Health J** 1981 Feb;101(1):19-28

**Morocco**

Meyers AR: Famine relief and imperial policy in early modern Morocco: the political functions of public health. **Am J Public Health** 1981 Nov;71(11):1266-73
Rosenberger B: Cultures complémentaires et nourritures de substitution au Maroc (XVe-XVIIIe siècle). **Ann Econ Soc Civilis** 1980;35(3-4):477-503

**United States**

Lender ME: Dictionary of American temperance biography: from temperance reform to alcohol research, the 1600s to the 1980s. Westport, Conn., Greenwood Press, 1984. xiv, 572 p.
Maas J: Plant pathology: contributions in improving the American food supply. **J NAL Assoc** 1980;5(3-4):76-8
McMahon SF: 'A comfortable subsistence': a history of diet in New England, 1630-1850. Ph.D. Diss., Brandeis University. Waltham, 1982. v, 351 p.

**Before 500 A.D.**

**China**

Benfey OT: Spinach is an alchemical antidote to heavy metal poisoning. **Kagakushi Kenkyu** 1981;15:8-12

**Greco-Roman**

Curtis RI: Salted fish products in ancient medicine. **J Hist Med Allied Sci** 1984 Oct;39(4):430-45

**Greece**

Preiser G: Wein im Urteil der griechischen Antike. In Völger G, ed: Rausch und Realität. Drogen im Kulturvergleich. Teil 1. Köln, Raufenstrauch-Joest-Museum für Völkerkunde der Stadt Köln, 1981. p. 296-303 (Materialienband zu einer Ausstellung 7. Aug. bis 11. Okt. 1981).

**India**

Sharma PV: Fruits and vegetables in ancient India. Varanasi and Delhi, Chaukhambha Orientalia, 1979. xxvl, 188 p. (Jaikrishnadas Ayurveda Series, No. 28).

**Rome**

Loposzko T: La famine à Rome en 57 avant J-Ch. **Quad Stor** 1979 Jul-Dec;5
Preiser G: Wein im Urteil der Römer. In Völger G, ed: Rausch und Realität. Drogen im Kulturvergleich. Teil 1. Köln, Raufenstrauch-Joest-Museum für Völkerkunde der Stadt Köln, 1981.

p. 304–8 (Materialienband zu einer Ausstellung 7. Aug. bis 11. Okt. 1981).

### 500 A.D.–1450

#### Europe

Bowman IA: Ottoman and European diet in the fifteenth century **Bookman** 1981 Mar;8(3):3–9
Henisch BA: Fast and feast: food in medieval society. University Park, Pennsylvania State University Press, 1976. 279 p.

#### Great Britain

Sass LJ: Religion, medicine, politics and spices. **Appetite** 1981 Mar;2(1):7–13

### 1450–1700

Appleby AB: Epidemics and famine in the little ice age 1550–1700. **J Interdiscip Hist** 1980;10:643–63

#### China

Shu-Yuen Yim: Famine relief statistics as a guide to the population of sixteenth-century China: a case-study of Honan province. **Ch'ing-Shih Wen-t'i** 1978;3(9):1–30
Yim SY: Famine relief statistics as a guide to the population of sixteenth century China: a case study of Honan Province. **Ch'ing-Shih Wen-t'i** 1978 Nov;3:1–30

#### France

Kaplan SL: Les subsistances et l'Ancien Régime: l'oeuvre de Jean Meuvret. **Ann Econ Soc Civilis** 1981;36(2):294–300

#### Germany

Eisinger J: Lead and wine. Eberhard Gockel and the colica Pictonum. **Med Hist** 1982 Jul;26(3):279–302

#### Great Britain

Appleby AB: Famine in Tudor and Stuart England. Stanford, Stanford Univ. Press, 1978. 250 p.
Dymond D: The famine of 1527 in Essex. **Local Popul Stud (Matlock)** 1981 Spring;26: 29–40

#### Italy

Guenzi A: Processo popolare in Piazza Maggiore: la carestia del 1648 a Bologna. **Archiginnasio (Italy)** 1979;74:161–80

#### Morocco

Rosenberger B, Triki H: Famines et épidémies au Maroc aux XVIe et XVIIe siècles. **Hesperis Tamuda** 1973;14:109–75

### 1700 to Present

Berlan JP: The world food problem: Malthus, Marx and their epigones. **Mon Rev** 1980;31(10):20–32
Blardone G: Rapports entre alimentation et types de développements. **Acquis Med Recent** 1981;198:35–55
Coppock JB: Food technology [in the twentieth century]. In Williams TI, ed: A history of technology. Vol. VII. The twentieth century, ca. 1900 to ca. 1950. Part II. Oxford, Clarendon, 1978. p. 1399–445.
Eberstadt N: America and world hunger. **Wilson Q** 1981;5(3):138–46
Gerlach LP: The flea and the elephant: infant formula controversy. **Society** 1980;17(6):51–7
May CD: Food allergy: lessons from the past. **J Allergy Clin Immunol** 1982 Mar;69(3):255–9
Pratt EL: Historical perspectives: food, feeding, and fancies. **J Am Coll Nutr** 1984;3(2):115–21
Prokhorova G: Prodovol'stvennaia problema kapitalizma. **Mirovaia Ekon Mezhdunar Otnosheniia** 1981;(9):81–91
Rutkowska I: Ludność świata i jej wyżywienie-kierunki zmian po kryzysie żywnościowym lat siedemdziesiątych. **Ekonomista** 1979;(2):445–63
Schubert JN: The impact of food aid on world malnutrition. **Int Organ** 1981;35(2):329–54
Sen A: Ingredients of famine analysis: availability and entitlements. **Q J Econ** 1981;96(3):433–64

#### Africa

Chauleur P: Développement et problèmes démographiques Africains. **Etudes (Fr)** 1981;354(4):437–49
Eicher CK: Facing up to Africa's food crisis. **Foreign Aff** 1982;61(1):151–74

#### Americas

González AD: La mision de Carlos M. Ramirez al Brasil y el convenio sanitario de 1887. **Bol Acad Nac Hist (Argentina)** 1964;35:327–53

#### Angola

Dias JR: Famine and disease in the history of Angola, C. 1830–1930. **J Afr Hist** 1981;22(3):349–78

#### Australia

Lewis M: Milk, mothers, and infant welfare. In J. Roe, ed: Twentieth century Sydney: studies in urban and social history. Sydney, Hale & Iremonger for the Sydney Hist. Group, 1980. p. 193–207.

#### Canada

Rick AM: Analysis of animal remains from the Old Fort Point site, northern Alberta. **Can Hist Sites** 1981;(26):269–89
Stieb EW: Three centennials: a retrospective view of Canada's pure food and drug legislation. In: Congrès international d'histoire de la médecine, XXVe, Québec, 1976. Actes. Québec, 1977. p. 1327–40.
Williams D, Young R: Canadian food aid: surplus and hunger. **Int J** 1981;36(2):335–52

#### China

Bandyopadhyaya K: The Chinese food-grain crisis: 1959–61--some explanations. **China Rep (India)** 1971;7(3):16–25
Buck DD: Imperially inspired philanthropy in the Ch'ing: the case of granaries in the eighteenth century. **Bull Inst Mod Hist Acad Sin** 1982;11:225–50
Smil V: Communist China's food: still a long way to go. **Issues Stud** 1980;16(4):37–44
Will PE: Chine: la terre des grandes famines. **Histoire** 1982;44:26–37

#### Europe

Sobczak T: Rozmiary spozycia mięsa i przetworów zbożowych w większych miastach Poznańskiego Pomorza i śląska w latach 1831–1861. **Kwart Hist Kultury Mater** 1979;27(1):17–30

#### France

Achard A: 'La nourrice sur place'. **Ann Demogr Hist (Paris)** 1984;:259–68
Brison M: L'école et l'enfant à Lyon: le problème de l'alimentation dans les cantines scolaires. **Rev Hist Deuxieme Guerre Mond** 1982;32(125):37–71
Coleman W: Medicine against Malthus: François Mélier on the relation between subsistence and mortality (1843). **Bull Hist Med** 1980 Spring;54(1):23–42
Delaunay A, ed: Présence de Pasteur. Paris, Fayard, 1973. 225 p. Includes contributions by P. Bidan, A. Gamet, J. Guillaume, L. Léger, J. Piton, J. De Rosnay, R. Scriban, C. Vago.
Dumazet A: 'Au pays des nourrices'. **Ann Demogr Hist (Paris)** 1984;:279–84
Goubert JP: A 'quiet revolution': the coming of pure water to contemporary France. **Soc Soc Hist Med Bull (Lond)** 1984 Dec;35:28–9
Goubert JP: Ordre et désordre: l'origine aquatique de la fièvre typhoïde. **Asclepio** 1983;35:161–70
Graham JC: The French connection in the early history of canning. **J R Soc Med** 1981 May;74(5):374–81
Molinier A: Une arme contre la famine: les greniers à blé du XVIIIe siècle. **Histoire** 1979;17:70–2
Panouillé JP: Et les Français prirent gout a l'absinthe! **Histoire** 1983;(52):50–9
Rollet C: L'allaitement artificiel des nourrissons avant Pasteur. **Ann Demogr Hist (Paris)** 1983;:81–92
Senior N: Aspects of infant feeding in 18th-century France. **Eighteenth Cent Stud** 1983;16:367–88
Tijm W: L'évolution de la consommation du fromage dans les hôpitaux de Clermont-Ferrand (1818–1952). **Cah Hist** 1979;24(1):71–8

#### Germany

Hofschulte B: Die Geschichte des Schlacht- und Viehhofes der Stadt Karlsruhe bis zum Jahre 1927. Diss., Tierärzliche Hochschule Hannover. Hannover, 1983. 226 p.

#### Great Britain

Blamire RV: Meat hygiene: the changing years. **J R Soc Health** 1984 Oct;104(5):180–5
Dewey PE: Food production and policy in the United Kingdom, 1914–1918. **Trans R Hist Soc** 1980;(30):71–89
Hardy A: Water and the search for public health in London in the eighteenth and nineteenth centuries. **Med Hist** 1984 Jul;28(3):250–82

Hollingsworth DF: Rationing and economic constraints on food consumption in Britain since the Second World War. **World Rev Nutr Diet** 1983;42:191–218

Lance D: Meals on the mess deck: from canteen messing to professional catering. **Hist Today** 1978;28(7):476–9

Sheail P: Hampshire man [Wilfred Buckley] and the quest for clean milk. **Hampshire** 1981 Mar;:60–2

Thomas B: Feeding England during the Industrial Revolution: a view from the Celtic fringe. **Agric Hist** 1982;56(1):328–42

Watkins D: The man who reformed hospital kitchens (Alexis Benoit Soyer). **Nurs Times** 1981 Nov 18–24;77(47):2029

**Hungary**

Spielmann J: Az erdélyi néptáplálkozás kérdései Mátyus István müvében. **Nor Tannlaegeforen Tid** 1982 Jun 13;123(24):1495–8

Várhidy I: Adatok a Budapesti központi tejesarnok szövetkezet szerepéröl a föváros tejellátásában (1883–1916). **Agrartort Sz** 1978;20(1–2):172–80

**India**

Ahmed M: Bengal famine of 1943: British responsibility and social consequences. **Dacca Univ Stud [A]** 1978;(28):68–80

Greenough PR: Indian famines and peasant victims: the case of Bengal in 1943–44. **Mod Asian Stud** 1980;14(2):205–35

Lardinois R: Une conjoncture de crise démographique en Indé du Sud au XIXe siècle: la famine de 1876–1878. **Population** 1982;37(2):371–404

Sur N: The Bihar famine of 1770. **Indian Econ Soc Hist Rev** 1976;13(4):525–31

**Ireland**

Donnelly B: The great famine and the literary imagination. **Studies** 1980;69(275–6):260–72

Gráda CO: The population of Ireland 1700–1900: a survey. **Ann Demogr Hist (Paris)** 1979;:281–99

O'Brien W: The fevers of the Great Famine. **J Ir Coll Physicians Surg** 1980 Jul;10(1):46–9

O'Farrel P: Whose reality?: The Irish famine in history and literature. **Hist Stud** 1982;20(78):1–13

Sarbaugh TJ: A moral spectacle: American relief and the famine, 1845–1849. **Eire Irel** 1980;15(4):6–14

Woodham-Smith CB: The great hunger, Ireland 1845–9. London, New England Library, 1979. 429 p.

**Italy**

Knoefel PK: Famine and fever in Tuscany. Eighteenth century Italian concern with the environment. **Physis** 1979;21(1–4):7–35

**Japan**

Kitahara I: 'Kyoho' kikin to machikata segyo. **Nihonshi Kenkyu** 1981;228:1–38

Omameuda M: 1920 (sen-kyuhyaku niju) nen-dai ni okeru shokuryo seisaku no tenkai: kome-sodo-go no zosan seisaku to beikokuho. **Shigaku Zasshi** 1982;91(10):40–73

**Mexico**

Coatsworth JH: Anotaciones sobre la producción de alimentos durante el Porfiriato. **Hist Mex** 1976;26(2):167–87

Super JC: Pan, alimentación y política en Querétaro a fines del siglo XVIII. **Hist Mex** 1980;30(2):247–72

**Middle East**

Askari H, Cummings J: Food shortages in the Middle East. **Middle East Stud** 1978;14(3):326–51

**Netherlands**

Van Logtestijn JG: 60 jaren V.V.D.O.---10 jaren afdeling technologie. **Tijdschr Diergeneeskd** 1980 Nov 1;105(21):883–4

**Poland**

Dembińska M: Z badań nad dziennymi racjami żywnościowymi rabotników przemysłowych w królestwie polskim w drugiej poł. XIX w. (próba interpretacji zródeł). **Kwart Hist Kultury Mater** 1979;27(2):145–56

Frenk S: Non omnis moriar. A cuarenta años de distancia de las investigaciones clínicas sobre el hambre realizadas en 1942 en el gueto de Varsovia. **Gac Med Mex** 1982 Dec;118(12):509–13

Karbe KH: Ueber eine von Rudolf Virchow empfohlene anonyme Schrift aus dem Jahre 1848 zum Hungertyphus in Oberschlesien. **Arch Hist Med (Warsz)** 1979;42(3):291–4

Ryn Z, Kłodziński S: Głód w obozie koncentracyjnym. **Przegl Lek** 1984;41(1):21–37

**Spain**

Carmona Cornet AM, Gómez Caamaño JL: Historia de la Cátedra de técnica física aplicada a la Farmacia y análisis químico y en particular de los alimentos, medicamentos y venenos de la Facultad de Farmacia de la Universidad de Barcelona (1886–1936). **Bol Soc Esp Hist Farm** 1984 Jun;35(138):125–37

Enríquez Morales MJ, Gelabert González JE: Un aspecto del consumo alimentico en la España de la secunda mitad del siglo XIX. **Hispania** 1978;38(140):617–35

Grande Covian F: Vitamin deficiencies during the Spanish Civil War in Madrid: a reminiscence. **Acta Vitaminol Enzymol** 1982;4(1–2):99–103

Rodríguez Galdo MX: Hambre, epidemia y crisis demográfica en la Galicia litoral a mediados del siglo XIX. **Asclepio** 1983;35:53–68

Rodríguez Galdo MX: Hambre y enfermedad en Galicia a mediados del siglo XIX. In: Sociedad Española de Historia de la Medicina. V Congreso Nacional. Madrid, 1977. **Asclepio** 1977;29:331–41

**United States**

Andrews WH: A perspective review of the development of AOAC microbiological methods. **J Assoc Off Anal Chem** 1984 Jul–Aug;67(4):661–73

Apple RD: 'To be used only under the direction of a physician': commercial infant feeding and medical practice, 1870–1940. **Bull Hist Med** 1980 Fall;54(3):402–17

Baur FJ, Parker WA: The aflatoxin problem: industry-FDA-USDA cooperation. **J Assoc Off Anal Chem** 1984 Jan–Feb;67(1):3–7

Black EF, Libby LM: Commercial food irradiation. **Bull At Sci** 1983;39(6):48–50

Bruce J: Of sugar and salt and things in the cellar and sun: food preservation in Jackson County in the 1850's. **Mo Hist Rev** 1981;75(4):417–47

Brumley WC, Sphon JA: Regulatory mass spectrometry. **Biomed Mass Spectrom** 1981 Sep;8(9):390–6

Conlins J: Beans, bacon, and galantine truffles: the food of the Western miners. **Ariz West** 1981;23(1):29–52

Darby WJ: A perspective on food legislation. **Nutr Rev** 1981 Nov;39(11):413–6

Dourson ML, Stara JF: Regulatory history and experimental support of uncertainty (safety) factors. **Regul Toxicol Pharmacol** 1983 Sep;3(3):224–38

Fischbach H: Coping with the aflatoxin problem in the early years. **J Assoc Off Anal Chem** 1984 Jan–Feb;67(1):1–3

Goldblith SA: Samuel Cate Prescott: - pioneer food technologist -gifted teacher. **Adv Food Res** 1981;27:1–21

Goodger WJ, Ruppanner R: Historical perspective on the development of dairy practice. **J Am Vet Med Assoc** 1982 Jun 1;180(11):1294–7

Gussow JD: Who pays the piper? **Teach Coll Rec** 1980;81(4):448–66

Guth JL: Herbert Hoover, the U. S. Food Administration, and the dairy industry, 1917–1918. **Bus Hist Rev** 1981;55(2):170–87

Hammer SN, ed: Symposium for the 75th Anniversary of the Food, Drug & Cosmetic Act, Meat Inspection Act, 1906–1981. Monday, June 8, 1981. Washington, D.C. **Food Drug Cosmet Law J** 1982 Jan;37(1):3–149

Harvey W. Wiley and the Pure Food and Drug Act: **Nutr Hist Notes** 1981;11:2–4

Hayes AH: Food and drug regulation after 75 years. **JAMA** 1981 Sep 11;246(11):1223–6

Hochheiser S: Synthetic food colors in the United States: a history under regulation. Diss. University of Wisconsin. [Madison, Wis.?: s.n.], 1982. v. 232 p.

Hochheiser S: The evolution of U. S. food color standards, 1913–1919. **Agric Hist** 1981;55(4):385–91

Hutt PB: Food and drug law: a strong and continuing tradition. In Hammer SN, ed: Symposium for the 75th Anniversary of the Food, Drug & Cosmetic Act, Meat Inspection Act, 1906–1981. Monday, June 8, 1981. Washington, D.C. **Food Drug Cosmet Law J** 1982 Jan;37(1):123–37

Ihde AJ. Food controls under the 1906 act. In Young JH, ed: The early years of federal food and drug control. Madison, American Institute of the History of Pharmacy, 1982. p. 40–50.

Janssen WF: FDLI's unforgettable character: Charles Wesley Dunn. **Food Drug Cosmet Law J** 1982 Oct;37(4):446–56

Janssen WF: Food and Drug Administration celebrates 75 years of consumer protection -- an album from the archives. **Public Health Rep** 1981 Nov–Dec;96(6):487–94

Janssen WF: The story of the laws behind the labels. **FDA Consum** 1981 Jun;15(5):32–45

Johnson DR: The history of the 1906 Pure Food and Drugs Act and the Meat Inspection Act. In Hammer SN, ed: Symposium for the 75th Anniversary of the Food, Drug & Cosmetic Act, Meat Inspection Act, 1906–1981. Monday, June 8, 1981. Washington, D.C. **Food Drug Cosmet Law J** 1982 Jan;37(1):5–9

Lambert EI: The United States labeling regulations for vegetable proteins: an historical perspective. **J Am Oil Chem Soc** 1979 Mar;56(3):234–7

Litman RC, Litman DS: Protection of the American consumer: the

congressional battle for the enactment of the First Federal Food and Drug Law in the United States. **Food Drug Cosmet Law J** 1982 Jul;37(3):310–29
Matossian MK: The throat distemper reappraised. **Bull Hist Med** 1980 Winter;54(4):529–43
Midkiff VC: The history of feed analysis, as chronicled in the development of AOAC official methods, 1884–1984. **J Assoc Off Anal Chem** 1984 Sep–Oct;67(5):851–60
Perkins JH: Insects, food, and hunger: the paradox of plenty for U. S. entomology, 1920–1970. **Environ Rev** 1983;7(1):71–96
Rothschild L: FDA's changing role in food safety. **FDA Consum** 1981 Jun;15(5):28–31
Taylor MR: History of cosmetic color additive regulation: creative maneuvering by FDA bodes well for the future. **Food Drug Cosmet Law J** 1982 Apr;37(2):152–62
Theophano J: Feast, fast, and time. **Pa Folklife** 1978;27(3):25–32
Welsh SO, Marston RM: Review of trends in food use in the United States, 1909 to 1980. **J Am Diet Assoc** 1982 Aug;81(2):120–8
Wiser V: Mary Engle Pennington. In: Notable American women. The modern period. Cambridge, Mass., Belknap-Harvard Univ. Press, 1980. 4:532–4.
Wolfe MR: Lucius Polk Brown and progressive food and drug control. Tennessee and New York City 1908–1920. Lawrence, Regents Press of Kansas, 1978. 194 p.
Woodruff NE: The failure of relief during the Arkansas drought of 1930–1931. **Arkansas Hist Q** 1980;39(4):301–13
Young JH: The early years of federal food and drug control. Madison, Wis., 1982. 60 p. (Publication/American Institute of the History of Pharmacy. new series, no. 7)
Young JH: The long struggle for the 1906 law. **FDA Consum** 1981 Jun;15(5):12–7
Young JH: 'This greasy counterfeit': butter versus oleomargarine in the United States Congress, 1886 (the Fielding H. Garrison Lecture). **Bull Hist Med** 1979 Fall;53(3):392–414
Young JH: Three southern food and drug cases. **J South Hist** 1983:49(1):3–36

**USSR**

Aleksentsev AI: Otchet o deiatel'nosti prodovol'stvennoi armii za pervyi god ee sushchestvovaniia. **Sov Arkh** 1981;5:33–8
Chemerisski IA: Kommunisticheskaia partiia: organizator bor'by s golodom (1921–1922 gg). **Vopr Istor KPSS** 1971;11:42–53
Edmondson CM: An enquiry into the termination of Soviet famine relief programmes and the renewal of grain export, 1922–23. **Sov Stud** 1981;33(3):370–85
Edmondson CM: The politics of hunger: the Soviet response to famine. **Sov Stud** 1977;29(4):506–18
Giesinger A: Conditions in the Volga region 1919–1922. **J Am Hist Soc Ger Russ** 1982;5(1):7–10
The great famine in Ukraine: a journalist's eyewitness account: **Ukr Rev (Lond)** 1979;27(2):87–97
Hoch SL: Serf diet in nineteenth-century Russia. **Agric Hist** 1982;56(2):391–414
Konev A: Krasnaia gvardiia v bor'be za khleb. **Voen Istor Zh** 1978;3:78–83
Landa LM: Pomoshch' trudiashchikhsia turkestana golodaiushchemu naseleniiu RSFSR v 1921–1922 gg. **Istor SSSR** 1971;2:136–40
Laverychev VI: Gosudarstvenno-monopolisticheskie tendentsii pri organizatsii prodovol'stvennogo dela v Rossii (1914–fevral' 1917 g). **Istor Zap Acad Nauk SSSR** 1978;101:100–59
Laverychev VI: Krupnaia burzhuaziia i prodovol'stvennyi vopros v 1917 g. **Istor Filol Zh** 1977;99:312–21
Mikoian AI: Prodovol'stvie frontu. **Voen Istor Zh** 1978;1:63–71
Petrovskiĭ KS: Razvitie sanitarnogo nadzora po gigiene pitaniia v SSSR za 60 let. **Gig Sanit** 1982 Sep;(9):21–3
Pol'ski MP: K istorii organizatsii prodovol'stvennogo snabzhenia naseleniia v pervye gody sovetskoi vlasti. **Istor SSSR** 1974;6:149–62
Prokop M: Pro vorkutu, holod ta problemy samooborony narodu. **Sucasnist** 1980;(3):48–56
Strizhkov IK, Suslov AI: Noveishaia istoricheskaia literatura o bor'be na prodovol' stvennom fronte v gody grazhdanskoi voiny. **Vopr Istor** 1980;2:118–27
Vasilev D: Borbata na BKP v pomosht na gladuvashtite v Suvestska Rusiia. **Izv Inst Istor BKP** 1968;18:339–65
Vodop'ianova ZK: 'Nedelia rebenka' v Respublike Sovetov. **Vopr Istor** 1979;11:175–9
Wheatcroft SG: Famine and epidemic crises in Russia, 1918–1922: the case of Saratov. **Ann Demogr Hist (Paris)** 1983;:329–52
Yaremovich AJ: Collectivization through famine. **Ukr Q** 1978;34(4):349–62

**Yugoslavia**

Peričić S: Oskudica i glad u dalmaciji u XIX i početkom XX stoljeća. **Rad Inst Hrvat Povij** 1980;13(1):1–31

# FORENSIC MEDICINE

Ackner D: The crime of incest. **Med Leg J** 1980;48(pt 3):79–91
Ander Z: Quo vadis medicina legalis? In: International Congress of the History of Medicine, 26th, Plovdiv (Bulgaria), 1978. Actes du Congres, Vol. 1. Sofia, 1980. p. 82–3.
Berg S: Die Bedeutung der Rechtsmedizin für die Archäologie. **Beitr Gerichtl Med** 1982;40:287–96
Brody BA: Law and morality [in bioethics]. In Reich WT, et al, ed: Encyclopedia of bioethics, v. 2. New York, Free Press, 1978. p. 817–21.
Burchell HB: Digitalis poisoning: historical and forensic aspects. **J Am Coll Cardiol** 1983 Feb;1(2 Pt 1):506–16
Cameron JM: The medico-legal expert--past, present and future. **Med Sci Law** 1980 Jan;20(1):3–13
Emerson RS, Schwartz RM: Professional liability. **NY State J Med** 1983 Jan;83(1):69–74
Fischer-Homberger E: Vergiftungen in der Gerichtsmedizin vom 16. bis zum 18. Jahrhundert. **Schweiz Aerzteztg** 1980;61(51):3399–406
Földes V, Kósa F, Virágos-Kis E, et al: Atomabsorptions-spektrophotometrische Untersuchung des Gehaltes an anorganischen Substanzen von Skelettbefunden zur Ermittlung der Dauer des Begrabenseins in der Erde. **Arch Kriminol** 1980 Sep–Oct;166(3–4):105–11
Goldberg BA: Horseshoers, doctors and judges and the law on medical competence. **Spec Law Dig Health Care (Mon)** 1980 May;2(3):3–41
Hoeger K: Medicinare som mördare. **Sydsven Medicinhist Sallsk Arsskr** 1981;:39–43
Hoffer PC, Hull NE: Murdering mothers: infanticide in England and New England 1558–1803. New York and London, New York University Press, 1981. xxii, 211 p. (New York University School of Law Series in Legal History, 2).
Jackson BS: Historical aspects of legal drafting in the light of modern theories of cognitive development. **Int J Law Psychiatry** 1980;3(4):349–69
Karwat J: Dręczyciele upośledzonych. **Psychiatr Pol** 1980 Jul–Aug;14(4):430–4
Mallach HJ: Gibt es Ansätze zur Gerichtlichen Medizin in Friedrichs II. von Hohenstaufen Konstitutionen von Melfi? **Beitr Gerichtl Med** 1982;40:463–72
Mukherjee JB: History of forensic medicine. In his Forensic medicine and toxicology. Volume One. Calcutta, New Delhi, Academic Publishers, 1981. p. 1–6.
Nanetti L: Su alcuni rapporti tra storia e medicina legale. **Acta Med Hist Patav** 1978–79;25:105–28
Quen JM: Forensic psychiatry. **JAMA** 1980 Jan 4;243(1):30
Rieber RW, Green M, ed: Milestones in the history of forensic psychology and psychiatry; a book of readings. New York, Da Capo, 1981. xi, 271 p.
Rodegra H: Arztlicher Kunstfehler und Arzthaftung aus medizinhistorischer Sicht. **Med Welt** 1982 Sep 17;33(37):1256–61
Smith JC, Weisstub DN: The evolution of Western legal consciousness. **Int J Law Psychiatry** 1979;2(2):215–34
Smith SM: Competency. **Psychiatr Clin North Am** 1983 Dec;6(4):635–50
Temkin O, Frankena WK, Kadish SH: Respect for life in medicine, philosophy, and the law. (Thalheimer lectures, 1975). Baltimore: Johns Hopkins Univ. Press, 1977. ix, 107 p.

**Canada**

Boissonnault CM: Antoine Forestier. In Dictionary of Canadian biography, 1701 to 1740. Volume 2, 1969. p. 226.

**China**

Bodde D: Forensic medicine in pre-imperial China. **J Am Orient Soc** 1982;102:1–15

**France**

Kurz C: De l'enfermement au secteur. **Soins Psychiatr** 1982 Feb;(16):2

**Germany**

Fischer-Homberger E: Medizin vor Gericht: Gerichtsmedizin von der Renaissance bis zur Aufklärung. Bern, H. Huber, 1983. 487 p.

**Great Britain**

Eigen JP: Historical developments in psychiatric forensic evidence: the British experience. **Int J Law Psychiatry** 1983;6(3–4):423–9
Reed FA: The fingermark. The prime piece of scientific evidence. **J Forensic Sci Soc** 1981 Jan;21(1):9–13

**Hungary**

Somogyi E: Az orvosszakértöi felülvéleményezés történetéböl. 25 éves az ETT Igazs agügyi Bizottsága. **Orv Hetil** 1981 Nov 15;122(46):2851–3

**Switzerland**

Fischer-Homberger E: Die gerichtsmedizinische Wundbegutachtung vom 16. zum 18. Jahrhundert. **Gesnerus** 1983;40(1-2):75-80

**United States**

Lansing DI: The coroner system and some ot its coroners in early Pennsylvania. **Trans Stud Coll Physicians Phila** 1977 Jan;44(3):135-40

**Before 500 A.D.**

**Rome**

Amundsen DW, Ferngren GB: The forensic role of physicians in Roman Law. **Bull Hist Med** 1979 Spring;53(1):39-56

**500 A.D.-1450**

**China**

McKnight BE, ed: The washing away of wrongs: forensic medicine in thirteenth-century China. Ann Arbor, Center for Chinese Studies, University of Michigan, 1981. xv, 181 p.

**Great Britain**

Chapman CB: Stratton vs. Swanlond: the fourteenth-century ancestor of the law of malpractice. **Pharos** 1982 Fall;45(4):20-4

Claxton AC: An early dental identification of a corpse. **Br Dent J** 1984 Aug 25;157(4):122

**Yugoslavia**

Dolenc A: Medizinische Fragen und Aspekte des mittelalterlichen Totentanzes (Ein Beitrag aus Jugoslawien). **Beitr Gerichtl Med** 1980;38:347-52

**1450-1700**

Fischer-Homberger E: The medicalization of demonology--the contribution of forensic medicine to early modern psychiatry. In International Congress of the History of Medicine, 27th, Barcelona, 1980. Actas. Barcelona, Académia de Ciències Médiques de Catalunya i Balears, 1981. p. 69-73.

Schmitz R, Kuhlen FJ: Anästhesie und Arzneimittelmissbrauch in peinlichen Gerichtsverfahren des 16. und 17. Jahrhunderts. In Göpfert W, Otten HH, ed: Metavoeite: wandelt euch durch neues Denken. Düsselfort, Triltsch, 1983. p. 189-99.

**France**

Billich A: Un procès de sorcellerie à Turckheim en 1628. In: Congrès National des Sociétés Savantes, 104e, Bordeaux, 1979. Actes. Paris, 1981. Histoire Moderne et Contemporaine, Tome 2. p. 407-10.

Lemaire JF: 1696, l'irresponsabilité médicale momentanément consacrée. **Hist Sci Med** 1984;18(1):41-3

**Great Britain**

Burg BR: Ho hum, another work of the devil. Buggery and sodomy in early Stuart England. **J Homosex** 1980-81 Fall-Winter;6(1-2):69-78

Geis G, Bunn I: Sir Thomas Browne and witchcraft: a cautionary tale for contemporary law and psychiatry. **Int J Law Psychiatry** 1981;4(1-2):1-11

Lakie MH, Cook G, MacMurray D: A 17th century poisoning case. **Pharm Hist (London)** 1976 Aug;6(2):2-3

**Italy**

Maeder H: Die Frau im 17. Jahrhundert im Spiegel der 'Quaestiones medico-legales' des Paolo Zacchia (1584-1659). Diss. Bern, 1981. 101 p.

**Spain**

Carreras Panchon A: La obra de Juan de Villarreal y otros estudios historico-medicos. Salamanca, Ediciones Universidad de Salamanca, 1978. 69 p. (Cuadernos de Historia de la Medicina Española, Mongrafias, XXXIII).

Corbella Corbella J: El crecimiento del saber medico legal en España en el siglo XVI. **Asclepio** 1978-79;30-31:323-37

**United States**

Oaks RF: Defining sodomy in seventeenth-century Massachusetts. **J Homosex** 1980-81 Fall-Winter;6(1-2):79-83

**1700 to Present**

Altchek ED: Plus ça change. **Plast Reconstr Surg** 1980 Jun;65(6):849-50

Belanger M: Une nouvelle branche du droit international: le droit international de la sante. **Etud Int** 1982;13(4):611-32

Burkhardt C: Euthanasie - 'Vernichtung lebensunwerten Lebens' im Spiegel der Diskussionen zwischen Juristen und Medizinern von 1900 bis 1940. Diss., Johannes-Gutenberg-Universität. Mainz, 1981. 221 p.

Camp J: One hundred years of medical murder. London, Bodley Head, 1982. 221 p.

Camps F: Sir Sydney Alfred Smith. In Dictionary of national biography, 1961-1970. Suppl. 8, 1981. p. 963-4.

Crompton R, Gall D: Georgi Markov--death in a pellet. **Med Leg J** 1980;48(2):51-62

Do JP, Lacombe M: Approche philosophique et historique à un enseignement des droits de l'homme. **Acta Med Leg Soc (Liege)** 1980;30(1):233-40

Eckert WG: Identification of the remains of John Paul Jones: a look at early methods. **Am J Forensic Med Pathol** 1982 Jun;3(2):143-52

Eckert WG: Physician crimes and criminals. The historical and forensic aspects. **Am J Forensic Med Pathol** 1982 Sep;3(3):221-30

Eckert WG, Garland N: The history of the forensic applications in radiology. **Am J Forensic Med Pathol** 1984 Mar;5(1):53-6

Emson HE: The case of Emmett-Dunne. A personal reminiscence. **Am J Forensic Med Pathol** 1983 Sep;4(3):255-8

Halpern AL: Elimination of the exculpatory insanity rule. A modern societal need. **Psychiatr Clin North Am** 1983 Dec;6(4):611-27

Lasky II: Autopsy of Admiral John Paul Jones 113 years postmortem; historic and forensic aspects. **NY State J Med** 1982 Jun;82(7):1110-5

Lloyd-Bostock SM: Psychology and the law: a critical review of research and practice. **Br J Law Soc** 1981;8(1):1-28

Mason AH: Crime and anaesthesia -- robbery. **Hist Med (Lond)** 1980 Jan-Feb;8(1):18-19,32

O'Brien M: Legal implications of the use of vaccines. **Med Leg J** 1979;47(4):152-9

Schneider WH: Chance and social setting in the application of the discovery of blood groups. **Bull Hist Med** 1983 Winter;57(4):545-62

Smith R: Scientific thought and the boundary of insanity and criminal responsibility. **Psychol Med** 1980 Feb;10(1):15-23

Wright RK, Tate LG: Forensic pathology. Last stronghold of the autopsy. **Am J Forensic Med Pathol** 1980 Mar;1(1):57-60

**Australia**

Brown KA: The identification of Linda Agostini: the significance of dental evidence in the Albury Pyjama Girl case. **Am J Forensic Med Pathol** 1982 Jun;3(2):131-41

Edwards GA, Hall W: The case of William Chidley: a study in psychiatry, morality and lunacy law. **Aust NZ J Psychiatry** 1980 Jun;14(2):133-9

Edwards GA: The mental illness of Captain Hyndman. **Aust NZ J Psychiatr** 1979 Jun;13(2):147-52

Pounder DJ: Death investigation in early colonial South Australia, 1839-40. **Med Sci Law** 1984 Oct;24(4):273-82

**Austria**

Silló-Seidl G: Kolletschkas Tod. **Beitr Gerichtl Med** 1979;37:415-7

**Burma**

Shi NC: Forensic laboratory work in Burma (with special reference to the Office of the Chemical Examiner, Burma). **Am J Forensic Med Pathol** 1980 Jun;1(2):173-6

**Canada**

Powell M: Public health litigation in Ontario, 1884-1920. In Roland CG, ed: Health, disease and medicine. Toronto, Hannah Institute for the History of Medicine, 1984. p. 412-35.

Weisstub DN, ed: Law and psychiatry in the Canadian context. New York, Pergamon Press, 1980. xlvi, 911 p.

**Czechoslovakia**

Kokavec M, Tichý M, Porubský V, et al: Vznik Ustavu súdneho lekárstva v Bratislave. **Soud Lek** 1983;28(1):1-6

Tesař J: Sto let českeho ústavu pro soudní lékařství v Praze. **Soud Lek** 1984 Aug;29(3):33-9

Tesař J: Sto let od vydání první učebnice soudního lékařství Josafem Reinsbergrem. **Cesk Patol** 1983 Aug;19(3):45-6

Tesšar J: Rozvoj soudniho lékařatví na Karlově Univerzitě. **Soud Lek** 1979;24(4):49-50

**France**

Erzinçlioğlu YZ: The application of entomology to forensic medicine. **Med Sci Law** 1983 Jan;23(1):57-63

Julien P: Les 'Eléments de pharmacie' de Baumé et la contrefaçon. **Rev Hist Pharm (Paris)** 1981 Jun;28(249):103–6
Lépine P: Le secret de Madame Lafarge (lumières nouvelles sur une affaire célèbre). **Sem Hop Paris** 1983 Dec 22;59(48):3387–94
Marx P: Un procès médical en Normandie en 1730. **Hist Sci Med** 1981;15(4):293–8
Stewart TD: A tribute to the French forensic anthropologist Georges Fully (1926–1973). **J Forensic Sci** 1979 Oct;24(4):916–24

**Germany**

Eriksson B: A lesbian execution in Germany, 1721: the trial records. **J Homosex** 1980–81 Fall–Winter;6(1–2):27–40
Kaiser W, Simon A: Die Geschichte der Gerichtsmedizin an der Universität Halle-Wittenberg. Halle, Martin-Luther-Universität Halle-Wittenberg, 1978. 81 p. (Beiträge zur Universitätsgeschichte, Nr. 12, Tome 25).
Keiser-Nielsen S, Strøm F: The odontological identification of Eva Braun Hitler. **Forensic Sci Int** 1983 Jan–Feb;21(1):59–64
Kohlhausen K: 30 Jahre Bundesverband der Vertrauensärzte (jetzt: Bundesverband der Vertrauens- und Rentenversicherungsärzte e.V.). **Off Gesundheitswes** 1982 Apr;44(4):205–8
Krauland W: Die Deutsche Gesellschaft für Rechtsmedizin im Spiegel ihrer Tagungen. **Beitr Gerichtl Med** 1982;40:9–20
Mai A: Diagnosestellung niedergelassener Arzte bei der Leichenschau im Vergleich zu den Ergebnissen der gerichtlichen Obduktion. Diss., Johannes Gutenberg - Universität in Mainz. Mainz, 1982. 143 p.
Mohr HJ: Medizinische und legislatorische Probleme der inneren Leichenschau. **Pathologe** 1981 Jun;2(3):134–43
Rodegra H: Zur Problematik des ärztlichen Kunstfehlers im 19. Jahrhundert. Arzthaftung im Beziehungsgeflecht von Recht und Medizin. **Med Welt** 1981 Mar 13;32(11):370–4
Sognnaes RF: Hitler and Bormann identifications compared by postmortem craniofacial and dental characteristics. **Am J Forensic Med Pathol** 1980 Jun;1(2):105–15
Stahnke J: Häminkristalle--Ludwik Teichmanns Blutnachweis. **Medizinhist J** 1981;16(4):391–413
Weber W: Gerichtsärztlicher Beitrag zur Rekonstruktion eines Tötungs-deliktes zu Aachen 1734. **Beitr Gerichtl Med** 1984;42:373–8

**Great Britain**

Aronson ME: Sherlock Holmes, father of forensic pathology. **Trans Stud Coll Physicians Phila** 1978 Jul;45(5):258–61
Besson A: The Medico-Legal Tracts Collection of Dr. A. S. Taylor, FRCP. **J R Coll Physicians Lond** 1983 Apr;17(2):147–9
Brody M: Trial of Daniel M'Naghten. Insanity defense, and its well-kept secret. **NY State J Med** 1982 Mar;82(3):381–6
Colp R: Charles Darwin, Dr. Edward Lane, and the 'Singular Trial' of Robinson v. Robinson and Lane. **J Hist Med Allied Sci** 1981 Apr;36(2):205–13
Corbett ME, Hardwick JL: The investigation of dental disease in exhumed remains. **J Dent** 1981 Dec;9(4):302–10
Davey H: The law relating to the mentally defective. The Mental Deficiency Act, 1913. 2nd ed. Reprint of 1914 ed., with a new introduction by C. Bahn. New York, Da Capo, 1981. x, xxvii, 568 p.
Eckert WG: The Whitechapel murders: the case of Jack the Ripper. **Am J Forensic Med Pathol** 1981 Mar;2(1):53–60
Eckert WG: The writings of Sir Bernard Spilsbury: Part I. **Am J Forensic Med Pathol** 1984 Sep;5(3):231–8
Forbes TR: Coroners' inquisitions on the deaths of prisoners in the hulks at Portsmouth, England, in 1817–27. **J Hist Med Allied Sci** 1978 Jul;33(3):356–66
Forbes TR: Early forensic medicine in England: the Angus murder trial. **J Hist Med Allied Sci** 1981 Jul;36(3):296–309
Forbes TR: John Hunter as expert witness. **Trans Stud Coll Physicians Phila** 1980 Jun;5(2 no 2):75–80
Forbes TR: 'To be dissected and anatomized.' **J Hist Med Allied Sci** 1981 Oct;36(4):490–2
Gilbert AN: Sodomy and the law in eighteenth- and early nineteenth-century Britain. **Societas** 1978;8(3):225–41
Goldstein J: Anna Freud in law. **Psychoanal Study Child** 1984;39:3–13
Gorman M: Sir William Brooke O'Shaughnessy, F.R.S. (1809–1889), Anglo-Indian forensic chemist. **Notes Rec R Soc Lond** 1984 Sep;39(1):51–64
Greenwald GI, Greenwald MW: Medicolegal progress in inquest of felonious deaths: Westminster, 1761–1866. **J Leg Med (Chicago)** 1981 Jun;2(2):193–264
Hailsham: The British Academy of Forensic Sciences. The Inaugural Lund Lecture: legal aid. **Med Sci Law** 1982 Jul;22(3):169–77
Heritage J: The background to a royal commission. **Med Leg J** 1981;49(pt 2):58–71
Kowitz A: The earliest use of dental evidence in a courtroom: His Majesty's Advocate vs. Pattison et al, High Court of Justiciary, Edinburgh, Scotland, June 6–7, 1814. **Bull Hist Dent** 1981 Oct;29(2):82–7
Murphy GK: The case of Stanley Setty. **Am J Forensic Med Pathol** 1980 Sep;1(3):245–7
Smith R: Criminal insanity: from a historical point of view. **Bull Am Acad Psychiatry Law** 1983;11(1):27–34
Smith R: Trial by medicine. Insanity and responsibility in Victorian trials. Edinburgh, Edinburgh University Press, 1981. ix, 238 p.
Swan M: Fitness to plead. **Br J Hosp Med** 1981 Nov;26(5):503, 505–9
Taylor JL: A backward glance; a forward view. **Med Leg J** 1981;49(pt 4):128–38
Thomson WA: Presidential address to the British Academy of Forensic Sciences: an Edinburgh quintet. **Med Sci Law** 1982 Jul;22(3):154–67
Walls HJ: Henry Smith Holden. In Dictionary of national biography, 1961–1970. Suppl. 8, 1981. p. 524–5.

**Hungary**

Fazekas A: 100 éve volt az eszlári per -nem ölték meg, a tiszának ment Solymosi Eszter-. **Orv Hetil** 1982 Jul 25;123(30):1870–2
Somogyi E: A tiszaeszlári vérvád a 100. évfordulóra. **Orv Hetil** 1982 Sep 5;123(36):2243–5
Somogyi E: Rupp N. János. **Orv Hetil** 1983 Nov 13;124(46):2821–2

**Iraq**

Ali WM: The establishment and practice of forensic medicine in Iraq. **Am J Forensic Med Pathol** 1980 Mar;1(1):81–4

**Ireland**

McQuitty JL: The old Irish Bar and Bench. **Med Leg J** 1982;50(Pt 1):5–18
Smith BA: Irish prison doctors--men in the middle, 1865–90. **Med Hist** 1982 Oct;26(4):371–94

**Italy**

Giusti GV: Leone Lattes: Italy's pioneer in forensic serology. **Am J Forensic Med Pathol** 1982 Mar;3(1):79–81
Robetti I, Iorio M: Università degli Studi di Torino, Istituto di Medicina Legale e delle Assicurazioni. **Minerva Stomatol** 1981 Jul–Aug;30(4):321–30

**Japan**

Ozawa S: Hoigaku shiso Katayama Kunika/G. Tokyo, Shin Jinbutsu Oraisha, Showa 50 nen [1975]. 130 p.

**Netherlands**

Bakker-van der Kooij C: Honderd jaar krankzinnigheid. **Tijdschr Ziekenverpl** 1984 Aug 21;37(17):545–8
Boon LJ: 'Utrechtenaren': de sodomieprocessen in Utrecht, 1730–1732. **Spiegel Hist** 1982;17(11):553–8

**Poland**

Czeley-Wybieralska M: Nieznana relacja obdukcyjna (visum repertum) z 1853 r. zachowana w aktach państwowego Archiwum w Lublinie. **Arch Hist Med (Warsz)** 1981;44(1):111–3
Kieć E, et al: Prof. Dr. Leon Cholewa. **Przegl Lek** 1984;41(7):465–76
Markiewicz J: Institute of Forensic Research in Cracow (Poland). Its history, organisation and activity. **Acta Med Leg Soc (Liege)** 1979;29(1):85–92
Raszeja S: Fifty years of the scientific work of Professor Boleslaw Popielski. **Forensic Sci Int** 1981 Mar–Apr;17(2):97–100
Traunfellner Z: Polska medycyna sadowa drugiej połowy XIX wieku. **Arch Hist Med (Warsz)** 1979;42(1):45–60
Uszkiewiczowa L: Działalność profesora Stanisława Batawii w dziedzinie psychiatrii sądowej. **Psychiatr Pol** 1979 Sep–Oct;13(5):441–3

**Portugal**

Cunha AS: Algumas considerações sobre medicina dentária forense e o seu início em Portugal. **Rev Port Estomatol Cir Maxilofac** 1980 Apr–Jun;22(2):187–200

**Romania**

Cotrău M: Procesful cottorului Carol Davila (Iaşi, 1872). **Rev Med Chir Soc Med Nat Iasi** 1980 Apr–Jun;84(2):325–6
Ioanid N, Angelescu B: Fraţii Minovici. Bucareşti, Editura Ştiinţifică, 1970. 174 p.
Scripcaru: A century of forensic teachings research and medicolegal assistance in Iasi-Romania. **Am J Forensic Med Pathol** 1983 Dec;4(4):371–2

**Singapore**

Chao TC: Coroner's practice in Singapore. **Ann Acad Med Singapore** 1982 Jul;11(3):469–72

**Spain**

Aznar B: Personalidad biologica de Azorín. Salamanca, Universidad de Salamanca, 1973. 73p. (Cuadernos de Historia de la Medicina Española, Monografias, 23).
Rodríguez Pazos M, Martí Lloret JB: La aportacion de pedromata al derecho medico de su tiempo. **Asclepio** 1980;32:415–20

**Turkey**

Salaçin S: Forensic medicine in Turkey. **Am J Forensic Med Pathol** 1982 Jun;3(2):179–80

**United States**

Abraham HJ: Religion, medicine, and the state: reflections on some contemporary issues. **J Church State** 1980;22(3):423–36
Benson F: Blood tests showing nonpaternity–conclusive or rebuttable evidence? The Chaplin case revisited. **Am J Forensic Med Pathol** 1981 Sep;2(3):221–3
Berndt T: Bite mark science. Forensic dentistry's hottest frontier. **Fla Dent J** 1982 Spring;53(1):22–4, 42–3
Camp FR: Forensic serology in the United States. I. Blood grouping and blood transfusion--historical aspects. **Am J Forensic Med Pathol** 1980 Mar;1(1):47–55
Chase A: Jerome Frank and American psychoanalytic jurisprudence. **Int J Law Psychiatry** 1979;2(1):29–54
Diamond BL: The psychiatrist as expert witness. **Psychiatr Clin North Am** 1983 Dec;6(4):597–609
Dutra FR: Electrical burns of the skin. Medicolegal investigation. **Am J Forensic Med Pathol** 1981 Dec;2(4):309–12
Eckert WG: Advances in American forensic sciences. California's role. **Am J Forensic Med Pathol** 1981 Jun;2(2):155–61
Eckert WG, Kaye S: Alexander O. Gettler (1883–1983). A centennial of his birth. **Am J Forensic Med Pathol** 1983 Dec;4(4):297–301
Eckert WG: American forensic sciences 1776–1976. **Am J Forensic Med Pathol** 1982 Mar;3(1):57–62
Eckert WG: Dr. Benjamin M. Vance (1886–1962). **Am J Forensic Med Pathol** 1980 Mar;1(1):73–6
Eckert WG: Dr. Harrison Stanford Martland (1883–1954). **Am J Forensic Med Pathol** 1981 Mar;2(1):83–4
Eckert WG: Fatal commercial air transport crashes, 1924–1981. Review of history and information on fatal crashes. **Am J Forensic Med Pathol** 1982 Mar;3(1):49–56
Eckert WG: History of the U.S. Army Graves Registration Service (1917–1950s). **Am J Forensic Med Pathol** 1983 Sep;4(3):231–43
Eckert WG: Medicolegal investigation in New York City. History and activities 1918–1978. **Am J Forensic Med Pathol** 1983 Mar;4(1):33–54
Eckert WG: The Lindbergh case. A triumph in forensic investigation. **Am J Forensic Med Pathol** 1980 Jun;1(2):151–3
Eckert WG: The murder masquerade. The Domer case. **Am J Forensic Med Pathol** 1980 Mar;1(1):71–2
Eckert WG: The Rockne crash. American commercial air crash investigation in the early years. **Am J Forensic Med Pathol** 1982 Mar;3(1):17–27
Eckert WG: The St. Valentine's Day massacre. **Am J Forensic Med Pathol** 1980 Mar;1(1):67–70
Flowers RB: Freedom of religion versus civil authority in matters of health. **Ann Am Acad Polit Soc Sci** 1979;446:149–61
Freimuth HC: Alexander O. Gettler (1883–1968). A reflection. **Am J Forensic Med Pathol** 1983 Dec;4(4):303–5
Goddard CH: A history of firearms identification to 1930. **Am J Forensic Med Pathol** 1980 Jun;1(2);155–68
Gravitz MA: An early case of investigative hypnosis: a brief communication. **Int J Clin Exp Hypn** 1983 Oct;31(4):224–6
Helpern M: History of the methods of detecting murder. **Am J Forensic Med Pathol** 1981 Mar;2(1):61–5
Hirschhorn B: Richard Spencer Childs (1882–1978). His role in modernization of medicolegal investigation in America. **Am J Forensic Med Pathol** 1983 Sep;4(3):245–54
Hughes JS: In the law's darkness: insanity and the medical-legal career of Isaac Ray, 1707–1881. Ph.D. Diss., Rice University. Houston, 1982. xvii, 393 p.
Konopka AF: Problems, history, and dilemma. A case for science law. **Ala J Med Sci** 1981 Oct;18(4):352–3
Laurence JR, Perry C: Forensic hypnosis in the late nineteenth century. **Int J Clin Exp Hypn** 1983 Oct;31(4):266–83
Milbauer B, Obrentz BN: The law giveth: legal aspects of the abortion controversy. New York, Atheneum, 1983. 363 p.
Moritz AR: Classical mistakes in forensic pathology. **Am J Forensic Med Pathol** 1981 Dec;2(4):299–308
Murphy GK: Death in the desert. The sabotage–derailment of 'The City of San Francisco'. **Am J Forensic Med Pathol** 1983 Jun;4(2):145–8
Niyogi SK: Historic development of forensic toxicology in America up to 1978. **Am J Forensic Med Pathol** 1980 Sept;1(3):249–64
Oaks R: Perceptions of homosexuality by justices of the peace in colonial Virginia. **J Homosex** 1979–80 Fall–Winter;5(1–2):35–41
Page SL: The law, the lawyer, and medical aspects of child abuse. In E. H. Newberger, ed: Child abuse. Boston, Little, Brown and Company, 1982. p. 105–35.
Payne H, Luthe R: Isaac Ray and forensic psychiatry in the United States. **Forensic Sci Int** 1980 Mar–Apr;15(2):115–27
Petty CS: The medical examiner and medical education (Russell S. Fisher). **Hum Pathol** 1980 Mar;11(2):101–3
Physician murderers and criminals: **Forensic Sci Int** 1982 Jul–Aug;20(1):101–6
Powell RC: Daniel Joseph McCarthy. In Dictionary of American Biography, Suppl. 6, 1956–1960. p. 402–4, 1980.
Reexamination of accoustic evidence in the Kennedy assassination: **Science** 1982 Oct 8;218(4568):127–33
Ring ME: The rubber denture murder case: the true story of the vulcanite litigations. **Bull Hist Dent** 1984;32(1):3–18
Ritchey FJ: Medical rationalization, cultural lag, and the malpractice crisis. **Hum Organ** 1981;40(2):97–112
Rothman DJ: Conscience and convenience. The asylum and its alternatives in progressive America. Boston, Toronto, Little, Brown and Company, 1980. xii, 464 p.
Schlicke CP: The Robinson affair. **Pac Northwest** 1983;27(2):81–93
Schroeder O: Toxicology and law--1980. **Leg Med** 1980;:91–110
Stewart TD: Essentials of forensic anthropology, especially as developed in the United States. Springfield, Ill, Thomas, 1979. xvii, 300 p.
Stewart TD: Pioneer contributions of Harris Hawthorne Wilder, Ph.D., to forensic sciences. **J Forensic Sci** 1982 Oct;27(4):754–62
Sunshine I: Dr. Alexander O. Gettler's documentation of a radiation hazard. **Am J Forensic Med Pathol** 1983 Dec;4(4):307–9
Tedeschi LG: George Burgess Magrath. Tribute to a resting lion. **Am J Forensic Med Pathol** 1980 Jun;1(2):169–72
Tedeschi LG: The Massachusetts Medico-Legal Society. The early years. **Am J Forensic Med Pathol** 1981 Sep;2(3):257–60
Thompson DD: Forensic anthropology. In F. Spencer, ed: A history of American physical anthropology, 1930–1980. New York, Academic Press, 1982. p. 357–69.
Tigbe JA: 'Be it ever so little': reforming the insanity defense in the Progressive Era. **Bull Hist Med** 1983 Fall;57(3):397–411
Unusual blood evidence in a homicide a century ago: **Am J Forensic Med Pathol** 1982 Sep;3(3):231–9
Young JH, Stitt RS: Nutrition quackery. Upholding the right to criticize. **Food Technol** 1981 Dec;:42–7

**USSR**

Akopov VI, Akopov AI: Iz istorii otechestvennykh sudebno-meditsinskikh zhurnalov. **Sud Med Ekspert** 1982 Jan–Mar;25(1):53–5
Ciucura TB: Dissent, law and psychiatry in the Soviet Union. **Can Slavonic Pap** 1979;21(1):98–108
Gromov AP, Panov IE, Panfilenko OA: Razvitie sudebno-meditsinskoĭ sluzhby v SSSR. **Sud Med Ekspert** 1982 Oct–Dec;25(4):6–9
Kapustin AV, Panfilenko OA: Osnovnye itogia nauchnoĭ deiatel'nosti Nauchno-issledovatel'skogo instituta sudebnoĭ meditsiny za 50 let. **Sud Med Ekspert** 1981 Oct–Dec;24(4):7–10
Kokoska U: Johann Georg Noël Dragendorff (20.4.1836 – 7.4.1898): Sein Beitrag zur Gerichtsmedizin, Pharmakologie und Pharmazie an der Universität Dorpat. Diss. Berlin, 1983. 234 p.
Lukash AA: 30 let deiatel'nosti Estonskogo otdeleniia Vsesouiznogo nauchnogo obshchestva sudebnykh medikov. **Sud Med Ekspert** 1982 Apr–Jun;25(2):57–9
Mazurenko MD, Porksheian OKh, Servatinskiĭ GL, et al: K 100-letiiu Leningradskogo Gosudarstvennogo ordena Lenina instituta usovershenstvovaniia vracheĭ im. S. M. Kirova i 60-letiiu kafedry sudebnoĭ meditsiny. **Sud Med Ekspert** 1984 Oct–Dec;27(4):57–9
Petrovskiĭ BV: Ranenie na duéli i smert' A. S. Pushkina. **Klin Med (Mosk)** 1983 Apr;61(4):109–17
Savich VI, Maksimov SS, Gusakov IuA: 50 let sudebno-meditsinskoĭ sluzhby Belorussii. **Sud Med Ekspert** 1980;23(3):57–8
Solokhin AA: K istorii poslediplomnogo obazovaniia sudebno-meditsinskikh ékspertov v SSSR (istoki, razvitie, stanovlenie). **Sud Med Ekspert** 1983 Apr–Jun;26(2):55–8

## GASTROENTEROLOGY AND DIGESTIVE SYSTEM

See also **Surgery–Abdominal**

Alawneh I: Historische Bemerkungen über Gallenwegtrauma. **Aktuel Traumatol** 1981 Dec;11(6):231–3
Antepowicz J: Historia leczenia przetoki okołloodbytniczej. **Wiad Lek** 1981 May 15;34(10):863–6
Bravo JL: Bosquejo histórico de la cirugía de la ulcera péptica. **Rev Gastroenterol Mex** 1981 Apr–Jun;46(2):63–70
Classic articles in colonic and rectal surgery: **Dis Colon Rectum** 1981 Jul–Aug;24(5):408–10 (continued periodically)
DeVries PA: The surgery of anorectal anomalies: its evolution, with evaluations of procedures. **Curr Probl Surg** 1984 May;21(5):1–75

## GASTROENTEROLOGY AND DIGESTIVE

Graney MJ, Graney CM: Colorectal surgery from antiquity to the modern era. **Dis Colon Rectum** 1980 Sep;23(6):432–41

Grucci J de: Consideraciones sobre Historia de la Gastroenterologia. (Tercer Congreso Nacional de Historia de la Medicina Argentina, 1973). **Sem Med** 1973;79(Aniversario):251–6

Hillemand P: Geschichte der Magen-Darm-Heilkunde. In Sournia JC, Martiny M, Poulet J, ed: Illustrierte Geschichte der Medizin. Salzburg, Andreas, 1980. Vol. 5. p. 1829–75.

Knežević S: Gastroenterologija i njena povijest kao povod za razmišljanje o stanju suvremene medicinske znanosti. **Lijec Vjesn** 1981 Oct;103(10):421–4

Lerut T: Groei en ontwekkeling van de slokdarmchirurgie. **Verh K Acad Geneeskd Belg** 1984;46(3):161–82

Lick RF: Geschichte der Magenchirurgie. **MMW** 1980 May 9;122(19):720–2

Sanjeeva Rao I: Surgical treatment of Fistula-in-Ano. Historical evolution of a technique. **Bull Inst Hist Med (Hyderabad)** 1973 Oct;3(4):169–72

#### Poland

Antepowicz J: Historia leczenia przetoki okołoodbytniczej w piśmiennictwie polskim. **Wiad Lek** 1981 Jun 1;34(11):957–61

### Before 500 A.D.

#### Greco-Roman

Moszyński J: Galenus - De victu attenuante. **Arch Hist Med (Warsz)** 1982;45(1–4):61–75

#### Greece

Boylan M: The digestive and 'circulatory' systems in Aristotle's biology. **J Hist Biol** 1982 Spring;15(1):89–118

### 500 A.D.–1450

Knoedler F: De egestionibus. Texte und Untersuchungen zur spätmittelalterlichen Koproskopie. Diss., Würzburg. Pattensen/Han, Horst Wellm Verlag, 1979. 107 p. (Würzburger medizinhistorische Forschungen, Band 18).

Leibowitz JO: The idea of metabolism in the medical works of Maimonides. In: Congrès international d'histoire de la médecine, XXVe, Québec, 1976. Actes. Québec, 1977. p. 881–4.

#### Arabic

Usmanova RA: Fiziologiia pishchevareniia v trudakh Ibn Siny. **Fiziol Zh SSSR** 1980 Sep;66(9):1424–8

### 1450–1700

Eberhardt-Müller R: Pankreasforschung im XVII. Jahrhundert. Diss., Bonn. Hatten, 1982. 151 p.

Gysel C: Jan Swammerdam (1637-1680-1980), zijn Cartesianisme en de fysiologie van het kauwstelsel (II). **Ned Tijdschr Tandheelkd** 1981 Jul–Aug;88(7–8):274–7

Kler JH: Along the path of modern medicine. **J Med Soc NJ** 1983 Jul;80(7):552

### 1700 to Present

Buchwald H, Rucker RD: The history of metabolic surgery for morbid obesity and a commentary. **World J Surg** 1981 Nov;5(6):781–7

Downing R: Historical review of pancreatic islet transplantation. **World J Surg** 1984 Apr;8(2):137–42

Habeck JO, Habeck C: Die Auskultation der Darmgeräusche -- Geschichte und Entwicklungsmöglichkeiten. **Z Arztl Fortbild (Jena)** 1980 Jun 15;74(12):596–9

Herrington JL, Sawyers JL: Surgical management of alkaline reflux gastritis and esophagitis. **Surg Annu** 1981;13:341–59

Lindell P: Gastrostomi--enkel metod med många fördelar. **Lakartidningen** 1981 Jun 17;78(25):2473–5

Lux G, Demling L: 100 Jahre Gastroskopie. **Fortschr Med** 1983 Jan 27;101(4):107–12

Matsuo Y: [History and status of study on gastrointestinal hormones] (Jpn). **Nippon Naika Gakkai Zasshi** 1982 Mar 10;71(3):275–85

Morrissey JF: Gastrointestinal endoscopy--20 years of progress. **Gastrointest Endosc** 1983 Feb;29(1):53–6

Ottenjann R: Gastroenterologie: Ein Stück Geschichte. **Med Welt** 1983 Jun 24;34(25–26):suppl 3

Polglase AL: Rectal excision for cancer 1880 to 1980. **Med J Aust** 1981 Jan 10;1(1):3–4

Poll M: Die Entwicklung der Gastroskopie. In M. Poll, ed: Gastro-Duodenoskopie. Grundlagen und Hinweise für die Praxis. Weinheim, Edition Medizin, 1982. p. 13–20.

Rusanov AA: K stoletiiu rezektsii zheludka. **Vestn Khir** 1981 Sep;127(9):13–42

Stoecklin WH: Die Erfindung der Magensonde. Ein ethnomedizinischer Beitrag zur Prioritätsfrage. **Gesnerus** 1981;38:237–46

Vara López R: Teodoro Billroth (con motivo del centenario de la primera gastrectomía). **An R Acad Nac Med (Madr)** 1981;98(2):283–310

Veltheer W: History: the dawn of gastric resection. **Neth J Surg** 1981 Aug;33(3):107–14

Wolf S: The psyche and the stomach. A historical vignette. **Gastroenterology** 1981 Mar;80(3):605–14

Wondrák E: Ke 100. výročí velkého výkonu v chirurgii žaludku. **Cas Lek Cesk** 1981 May 28;120(21):646–50

#### Austria

Casal A: Hace cien años, 1881-1981--Billroth y la primera gastrectomía. **Acta Gastroenterol Latinoam** 1981;11(2):326–8

Schober KL: Das chirurgische Erbe. Theodor Billroth und die Karzinomchirurgie des Intestinaltraktes. **Zentralbl Chir** 1981;106(10):693–9

Wyklicky H: Vor hundert Jahren. Billroths erste Pylorusresektion, seine diesbezüglichen Publikationen in der 'Wiener Medizinischen Wochenschrift' und ein Rückblick auf seine Zeit. **Wien Med Wochenschr** 1981 Jan 15;131(1):1–13

#### Canada

Beck IT: Canadian gastroenterology: yesterday, today and tomorrow. **Clin Invest Med** 1982;5(2–3):93–107

#### Czechoslovakia

Pětašedesátiny doc. MUDr. Z. Mařatky, DrSc.: **Cesk Gastroenterol Vyz** 1979 Jun;33(4):236–47

#### France

Roux M: Eloge de Charles Debray, 1907–1979. **Bull Acad Natl Med (Paris)** 1979 Dec;163(9):897–906

Ségal A: Le médecin principal de 1re classe Jean-Pierre Bonnafont (1805–1891); sa place prépondérante dans l'histoire de l'endoscopie aus XIXe siècle. **Hist Sci Med** 1983;17(1):63–70

#### Germany

Dittrich HM: Die Pavlov-Lehre im Forschungsprogramm von Gerhardt Katsch. **Z Gesamte Inn Med** 1983 Apr 1;38(7):230–2

Imanaga H: [Honoring Theodor Billroth by attaining a hundred years since his first success in gastric cancer resection (author's transl)] (Jpn). **Nippon Gan Chiryo Gakkai Shi** 1981 Jun 20;16(3):405–8

Knoke M: Endotoxine in der Gastroenterologie--Ein medizinhistorischer Abriss. **Dtsch Z Verdau Stoffwechselkr** 1984;44(3):109–17

Knoke M: Viktor van der Reis--Wegbereiter der gastrointestinalen Mikroökologie des Menschen. **Nahrung** 1984;28(6–7):593–8

Koelsch KA: Die Entwicklukng der gastroenterologischen Endoskopie in der DDR während der letzten 10 Jahre, alte und neue Probleme. **Z Arztl Fortbild (Jena)** 1979 Oct 1;73(19–20):981–3

Schober KL: Das chirurgische Erbe. Vor etwa hundert Jahren (27). **Zentralbl Chir** 1981;106(4):255–8 (continued periodically)

Suárez CV: Ampulla of Vater---a misnomer. **Mt Sinai J Med (NY)** 1980 Jul–Aug;47(4):373–85

#### Great Britain

Doll R: The controlled trial. **Postgrad Med J** 1984 Nov;60(709):719–24

Earle DP: An eighteenth century suggestion for peritoneal dialysis? **Int J Artif Organs** 1980 Mar;3(2):67–8

Sircus W: Medical-surgical collaboration in the practice of gastroenterology. **Postgrad Med J** 1984 Nov;60(709):725–32

Swain V: Sir Jonathan Hutchinson 1828–1913: his role in the history of intussusception. **J Pediatr Surg** 1980 Apr;15(2):221–3

#### Italy

Lenarduzzi G, Pescarini L, Miotto D: Un precursore dell'esame radiologico del tubo digerente: il prof. G. Vicentini. **Radiol Med (Torino)** 1980 Apr;66(4):263–4

#### Japan

Matsunaga F: [80 years of the Japanese Society of Gastroenterology] (Jpn). **Nippon Shokakibyo Gakkai Zasshi** 1983 Jul;80(7):1395–409

#### Mexico

Olarte J: La bacteriología intestinal en México. In Academia Nacional de Medicina. Libro conmemorativo del primer centenario. México, Comité Editorial de la Comisión Organizadora del Congreso del

Centenario, 1964. Tome 2. p. 521-3.
Ramos P: Crónica. La Asociación Mexicana de Gastroenterología. **Rev Gastroenterol Mex** 1981 Apr-Jun;46(2):71-3 contd.
Ramos P: El aprendizaje de la gastroenterología. **Rev Gastroenterol Mex** 1982 Jan-Mar;47(1):35-7

**Poland**

Gutt RW: W setna rocznice określenia czynności wydzielniczej komórek błony śluzowej zoładka. **Arch Hist Med (Warsz)** 1978;41(4):479-81
Tabeński Z: Wkład polskich chirurgów w rozwój leczenia chorobv Hirschsprunga u dzieci. **Pediatr Pol** 1981 Jun;56(6):695-7

**Spain**

Lentini J, Taure Gómez C, Leveroni J: Conmemoración de un cincuentenario. In International Congress of the History of Medicine, 27th, Barcelona, 1980. Actas. Barcelona, Académia de Ciències Médiques de Catalunya i Balears, 1981. p. 564-9.
Ramón Baltar Domínguez: **Rev Esp Enferm Apar Dig** 1981 Oct;60(4):413-5

**United States**

Bonsett CA: The world's first gall bladder surgeon was a Hoosier. **J Indiana State Med Assoc** 1980 Apr;73(4):201
Boyle JD: Morton I. Grossman, M.D., Ph.D.: an oral history. **Gastroenterology** 1982 Jul;83(1 Pt 2):285-324
Classic articles in colonic and rectal surgery. Owen Harding Wangensteen 1899-1981: **Dis Colon Rectum** 1982 Jan-Feb;25(1):65-78
Classic articles in colonic and rectal surgery. Robert Fulton Weir 1838-1927: An improved method of treating high-seated cancers of the rectum. **Dis Colon Rectum** 1982 Jul-Aug;25(5):503-7
Cole WH: The development of cholecystography. **J Thorac Cardiovasc Surg** 1984 Nov;88(5 Pt 2):827-33
Crispell KR: Beaumont and Dunglison: who was Dunglison? **Trans Am Clin Climatol Assoc** 1980;92:194-8
Dreiling DA: The first fifty years--a history of evolution of the American College of Gastroenterology as a Society for Clinical Gastroenterology. **Am J Gastroenterol** 1983 Mar;78(3):138-9
Fiftieth anniversary: American College of Gastroenterology. Reprints. The American Journal of Gastroenterology celebrates the Golden Anniversary of the College. **Am J Gastroenterol** 1982 Oct;77(10):701-832
Higgins GA: Problems in clinical trials: lessons from the 'tuck uppers'. **Cancer** 1981;47:2167-71
Johnson LR: A footnote to modern gastroenterology. **Gastroenterology** 1982 Jun;82(6):1293-4
Lightdale CJ: Notes on the development of the American Society for Gastrointestinal Endoscopy. **Gastrointest Endosc** 1983 Feb;29(1):51-3
Myer JS: William Beaumont: a pioneer American physiologist. New ed. of his: Life and letters of Dr. William Beaumont. With historical introductions by E. Brodman and R. E. Shank. Includes reprint of 1833 ed. of Beaumont's Experiments and observations on the gastric juice and the physiology of digestion. St. Louis, Mosby, 1981. xi, 394 p.
Mysh VG: L. R. Dragstedt (vklad v uchenie o patogeneze i lechenii iazvennoi bolezni). **Khirurgiia (Mosk)** 1983 Jul;7:140-1
Numbers RL, Orr WJ: William Beaumont's reception at home and abroad. **Isis** 1981 Dec;72(264):590-612
Rausch VL, Freier EF: Liver function tests. **Am J Med Technol** 1983 May;49(5):367-8
Rosenkrantz BG: Sara Claudia Murray Jordan. In: Notable American women. The modern period. Cambridge, Mass., Belknap-Harvard Univ. Press, 1980. 4:387-8.
Veidenheimer MC: Presidential address. Who dug your well? **Dis Colon Rectum** 1982 Mar;25(2):85-9
Woodward ER: Dr. Dragstedt's first vagotomy. **World J Surg** 1983 Jul;7(4):554

**USSR**

Kryshen' PF: Razvitie gastroénterologii na Ukraine za gody desiatoĭ piatiletki. **Vrach Delo** 1981 Dec;(12):1-7
Shtern RD: O prioritete opredeleniia limfomatoza zheludka otechestvennymi issledovateliami. **Arkh Patol** 1983;45(5):66-8
Soloveĭ MG, Gribanov ED: M. I. Pevzner--krupnyĭ sovetskiĭ terapevt-dietolog. **Feldsher Akush** 1983;48(2):52-3

# GENERAL PRACTICE

Leavesley J: A history of general practice. **Med J Aust** 1984 Jul 21;141(2):107-9
Phillips TJ: The intellectual roots of family practice. **Pharos** 1981 Winter;44(1):26-31

**Denmark**

Laeger i Sønderjylland indtil 1864: **Dan Medicinhist Arbog** 1980;:11-65

**Great Britain**

Cule J: A doctor for the people: 2000 years of general practice in Britain. London and Boston, Update, 1980. 145 p.

**1450-1700**

**France**

Renaudie M: Etre généraliste il y a quatre siècles. Réalisme et fiction. **Hist Sci Med** 1984;18(2):173-9

**Great Britain**

Sawyer RC: Ordinary medicine for ordinary people: illness and its treatment in the East Midlands, 1600-1630. **Soc Soc Hist Med Bull (Lond)** 1983 Dec;33:20-3

**1700 to Present**

Curtis P: Three hundred years of family health care: some perspectives. **J Fam Pract** 1981 Feb;12(2):323-7
Illich I: Medicalization and primary care. **J R Coll Gen Pract** 1982 Aug;32(241):463-70
Loudon I: The concept of the family doctor. **Bull Hist Med** 1984 Fall;58(3):347-62

**Australia**

Humphries SV: Medical practice in the Australian outback 25 years ago. **Cent Afr J Med** 1982 Feb;28(2):45-7
Royal Australian College of General Practitioners: The Royal Australian College of General Practioners, 1958-1978. [Sydney?] The College, [1979?] 130 p.

**Canada**

Norris J: The country doctor in British Columbia: 1887-1975. **BC Stud** 1981;(49):15-39
Shortt SE: 'Before the age of miracles': the rise, fall, and rebirth of general practice in Canada, 1890-1940. In Roland CG, ed: Health, disease and medicine. Toronto, Hannah Institute for the History of Medicine, 1984. p. 123-52.

**France**

Rochefort R, Devevey J: Les jeunes médecins libéraux. Evolution de 1979 à 1982. **Cah Sociol Demogr Med** 1984 Apr-Jun;24(2):97-123

**Germany**

Braun RN: Allgemeinmedizin zwischen gestern und morgen. **Fortschr Med** 1983 Mar 10;101(9):343-4
Mader FH: Zur Geschichte der Famulatur bei Praktischen Aerzten. **ZFA (Stuttgart)** 1980 Aug 20;56(23):1415-8
Mitzscherling R: Die Entwicklung der Allgemeinmedizin in der Deutschen Demokratischen Republik. **Z Arztl Fortbild (Jena)** 1983;77(6):268-71
Schneider H: Dr. August Heisler. Erinnerungen an einen grossen Arzt. **ZFA (Stuttgart)** 1983 May 10;59(13):774-6

**Great Britain**

Binnie GA: George Johnston: 1797-1855. **Br Med J [Clin Res]** 1982 Oct 9;285(6347):1014-6
Cule J: William Price of Llantrisant--1800-1893. **Br Med J [Clin Res]** 1982 Feb 13;284(6314):483-4
Felstein I, Naqvi N: Samuel Taylor Chadwick: 1809-73. **Br Med J [Clin Res]** 1983 Jun 25;286(6383):2031-2
Fraser SM: Dr William Johnston (1846-1900) of Leicester--an unknown Victorian general practitioner. **J R Coll Gen Pract** 1983 Jun;33(251):369-71
Fry J, Hunt JH, Pisent RJ, ed: A history of the Royal College of General Practitioners. The first 25 years. Lancaster, Boston, MTP Press, 1983. xiii, 270 p.
Fry J, Hunt JH, Pinsent RJ: The Royal College of General Practitioners: the first 25 years.
Gibson R: The family doctor: his life and history. London, Boston, Allen & Unwin, 1981. xv, 214 p.
Harris CM: The GP and the medical student. The background. **Br Med J [Clin Res]** 1983 Jan 8;286(6359):111-2
Hewetson J: Before and after the 'appointed day'. **Br Med J [Clin Res]** 1983 Oct 29;287(6401):1271-2
Horder J: The origin of the Royal College of General Practitioners. **Soc Soc Hist Med Bull (Lond)** 1983 Dec;33:13-4
Horder JP, Swift G: The history of vocational training for general practice. **J R Coll Gen Pract** 1979 Jan;29(198):24-32
Jefferys M, Sachs H: Re-thinking general practice: some issues of policy

and practice in the 1970s illustrated by case study. **Soc Soc Hist Med Bull (Lond)** 1983 Dec;33:17-9
Lewis J, Brookes B: The Peckham Health Centre, 'Pep', and the concept of General practice during the 1930s and 1940s. **Med Hist** 1983 Apr;27(2):151-61
Loudon I: The nature of provincial medical practice in eighteenth-century England. **Med Hist** 1985 Jan;29(1):1-32
Loudon I: Two thousand medical men in 1847. **Soc Soc Hist Med Bull (Lond)** 1983 Dec;33:4-8
Loudon IS: A doctor's cash book: the economy of general practice in the 1830s. **Med Hist** 1983 Jul;27(3):249-68
Loudon IS: The origin of the general practitioner. **J R Coll Gen Pract** 1983 Jan;33(246):13-23
Marks J: The Conference of Local Medical Committees and its executive: an historical review. [London?], Trustees of the General Medical Services Defence Trust, 1979. 32 p.
Phillips WR: Sir James Mackenzie and family medicine. **Am Fam Physician** 1981 Jul;23(7):46, 50
Pickering G: William Norman Pickles. In Dictionary of national biography, 1961-1970. Suppl. 8, 1981. p. 843-4.
Robinson K: The crisis in general practice--1965. **Soc Soc Hist Med Bull (Lond)** 1983 Dec;33:15-6
Stevenson D: Sir Harry Guy Dain. In Dictionary of national biography, 1961-1970. Suppl. 8, 1981. p. 262.
Stout G: A ledger stamped 'G.P'. **J R Coll Gen Pract** 1984 Apr;34(261):223-5
Stuart D: Urban Marks: 1880-1949. **Br Med J [Clin Res]** 1982 Jul 31;285(6338):345-7
Swift G: Recollections and reflections: general practice since 1946. **J R Coll Gen Pract** 1982 Aug;32(241):471-9
Thomas KB: Attitudes to psychological illness in general practice. A historical cycle complete. **Br Med J [Clin Res]** 1981 Oct 31;283(6300):1157-8
Thomson DM: General practice and the Edinburgh Medical School: 200 years of teaching, care and research. **J R Coll Gen Pract** 1984 Jan;34(258):9-12
Tonge V: Arthur Randell Jackson: 1877-1944. **Br Med J [Clin Res]** 1983 Jul 9;287(6385):97-8
Van Zwanenberg D: Interesting GPs of the past: George Stebbing: 1749-1825. **Br Med J [Clin Res]** 1981 Dec 5;283(6305):1517-8
Wand S: After the first world war. **Br Med J [Clin Res]** 1983 Oct 1;287(6397):952-3
Watts CA: General practice. **Br Med J** 1979 Oct 27;2(6197):1055-6
Webster C: General practice under the panel - the last phase. **Soc Soc Hist Med Bull (Lond)** 1983 Jun;32:20-3
Williams S: A 'Taylor made' practice. **Br Med J [Clin Res]** 1984 Jan 14;288(6411):116-8
Wilson C: Horace Evans. In Dictionary of national biography, 1961-1970. Suppl. 8, 1981. p. 336-7.

**Ireland**

Blaney R: Henry Maunsell (1806-1879): an early community physician. **Ir J Med Sci** 1984 Jan;153(1):42-3
Casey M: 50 years of general practice. **Ir Med J** 1981 Jun;74(6):155-8

**Poland**

Michalczak W, Lisiewicz J: Antoni Andrzejewski (1807-1883) -- lekarz powiatu kieleckiego. **Przegl Lek** 1980;37(10):717-8

**South Africa**

Schaffer R: Country practice in the 1920s. **S Afr Med J** 1983 Jun 29;Spec No:27-9

**United States**

Amundson LH: The roots of family practice in South Dakota. **SD J Med** 1981 May;34(5):43-8
Baker PQ: Memories of medicine. **Nebr Med J** 1983 Oct;68(10):338-9
Collins BC: A round of calomel. **J Tenn Med Assoc** 1983 Sep;76(9):609-10
Donald AG: James Higgins Mcintosh, M.D.: an archetype for the family practitioner? **J SC Med Assoc** 1980 May;76(5):245-8
Hare HJ: First graduate--USD School of Medicine. Lyle Hare, M.D., family practitioner. **SD J Med** 1981 May;34(5):70-1
Harstad PT: Frontier medicine in the Territory of Wisconsin. In Numbers RL, Leavitt JW, ed: Wisconsin medicine. Historical perspectives. Madison, University of Wisconsin Press, 1981. p. 13-23.
Hornbein M: Dr. John Elsner, a Colorado pioneer. **West States Jew Hist Q** 1981;13(4):291-302
Leland TM: 'First Physician in Spartanburg County' Andrew Barry Moore, M.D., 1771-1848. **J SC Med Assoc** 1983 May;79(5):299
McDonald WH: Country doctor: he can't go home again. **J Med Assoc State Ala** 1982 Oct;52(4):8-9, 12-4, 19-22
Palmieri A, Humberson C: Medical incidents in the life of Dr. John H. Finfrock. **Ann Wyo** 1981;53(2):64-9
Rosenthal R: Dr. Christopher Carli, pioneer physician of Minnesota. **Minn Med** 1982 Dec;65(12):765-8
Stewart FH: The doctor who practiced in Miami. **J Fla Med Assoc** 1982 Aug;69(8):702-5
Van Buskirk EL: Fort Wayne College of Medicine. Includes The practice of medicine in the Fort Wayne area written in 1889 by B. S. Woodworth. **Indiana Med Hist Q** 1977;3(2):4-6
Waters SC: A country doctor of yesteryear: Samuel C. Waters (1861-1932) of Middletown, Indiana. **J Indiana State Med Assoc** 1983 Feb;76(2):144-5
Wendler M van Voorhis: Doctors and diseases on the Ohio frontier. **Ohio Hist** 1980;89(2):222-42
Young DM: Eugene H. Conner, M.D., KMA historian. **J Ky Med Assoc** 1982 Apr;80(4):224-6

**USSR**

Shtern MI, Karinskaia GS: Zemskiĭ vrach A. V. Ivanov. **Sov Zdravookhr** 1983;(8):64-7

**Yugoslavia**

Dragić M: Dr. Janko i hjegove zasluge za nauku, književnost i prosvety u Srbiji. **Srp Arh Celok Lek** 1981 Aug;109(8):1101-8

## GENERATION AND REPRODUCTION

See also **Birth Control; Embryology; Genetics and Heredity; Gynecology; Obstetrics; Sex Behavior**

Bullough VL: Age at menarche: a misunderstanding. **Science** 1981 Jul 17:209(4505):365-6
Cafiso, LM: Storia della teoria sulla generazione spontanea: Redi, Spallanzani, Pasteur. **Cult Sc** 1981;20(80):236-43
Gebbie DA: Reproductive anthropology--descent through woman. New York, Wiley, 1981. 371 p.
Hartree EF: Ethics for authors: a case history of acrosin. **Perspect Biol Med** 1976 Autumn;20(1):82-91
Macdonald AA: Studies on the anatomy and physiology of the pig fetus and placenta: an historical review. In E. Schultheisz, ed: History of physiology. Oxford, Elmsford, New York, Pergamon, 1981. xvi, 208 p. (Advances in Physiological Sciences. Proceedings of the 28th International Congress of Physiological Sciences, Budapest, 1980. Volume 21). p. 53-60.
Meigs JA: Choosing your baby's sex - now and in the sixteenth century. **Tenn Folkl Soc Bull** 1982;48(4):111-6
Valdiserri RO: Menstruation and medical theory: an historical overview. **J Am Med Wom Assoc** 1983 May-Jun;38(3):66-70

**Americas**

Viel B: Fertility policies in the Latin American continent. **Proc Annu Symp Eugen Soc** 1981;16:15-22

**Belgium**

Gutmann MR, Wyrick R: Adapting methods to needs: studying fertility and nuptiality in seventeenth- and eighteenth-century Belgium. **Hist Methods** 1981;14(4):163-71

**Spain**

Ott S: Aristotle among the Basques: the 'cheese analogy' of conception. **Man** 1979;14:699-711

**Before 500 A.D.**

Hausmann W: Der Stier als Fruchtbarkeitssymbol. Ein Bericht über Funde aus mehreren Ländern. **DTW** 1982 Feb 5:89(2):86-8
Kass N: Sex determination--medically and in the Talmud. **Koroth** 1980 Jun;7(11-12):CCLXLIII-CCCI
Kudlien F: Zur Erforschung archaisch-griechischer 'Zeugungslehren'. **Medizinhist J** 1981;16(4):323-39

**Greece**

Lennox J: Teleology, chance, and Aristotle's theory of spontaneous generation. **J Hist Philos** 1981;19:219-38
Lonie IM: The Hippocratic treatises: 'On Generation', 'On the Nature of the Child', 'Diseases IV'. A commentary. Berlin, New York, Walter de Gruyter, 1981. xxxix, 406 p. (Ars medica. II. Abteilung, Griechisch-lateinische Medizin; Bd. 7, 2).
Plass P: A Greek alchemical formula. **Ambix** 1982 Jul;29(2):69-73

**India**

Corcos AF: Reproduction and heredity beliefs of the Hindus based on their sacred books. **J Hered** 1984 Mar-Apr;75(2):152-4

Guttman FM, Guttman HA: Historical note on embryo transfer: 599 B. C (with apologies to drs. Steptoe and Edwards). **Fertil Steril** 1980 Nov;34(5):513-5

### 500 A.D.-1450

Jacquart D, Thomasset C: Albert le Grand et les problèmes de la sexualité. **Hist Philos Life Sci** 1981;3(1):73-93
Lemay H: The stars and human sexuality: some medieval scientific views. **Isis** 1980 Mar; 71(256):127-37
Rowland D, Jennings M. Medieval multiple birth. **Neuphilol Mitt** 1980;81:169-73
Wood CT: The doctors' dilemma: sin, salvation, and the menstrual cycle in medieval thought. **Speculum** 1981;56(4):710-27

### 1450-1700

Matuschka MM: Lambert van Velthuysens (1622-1685) Menstruationstheorie in ihrer wissenschaftshistorischen Bedeutung. Zur Vorgeschichte der Endokrinologie der Ovarien. Amsterdam, B. M. Israël, 1980. vii, 72 p.
Secret F: Palingenesis, alchemy and metempsychosis in Renaissance medicine. **Ambix** 1979 Jul;26(2):81-92

#### Europe

Niccoli O: 'Menstruum quasi monstruum': parti mostruosi e tabù mestruale nel '500. **Quad Stor** 1980;15(2):402-8

#### Germany

Calagan JL: The conjoined twins born near Worms, 1495. **J Hist Med Allied Sci** 1983 Oct;38(4):450-1

#### Great Britain

Crawford P: Attitudes to menstruation in seventeenth-century England. **Past Present** 1981;91:47-73
Knobil E: William Harvey and the physiology of reproduction. **Physiologist** 1981 Feb;24(1):3-7
Oppenheimer JM: Harvey, William. Disputations touching the generation of animals: essay review. **Trans Stud Coll Physicians Phila** 1982 Dec;4(4):306-9

#### Italy

Gottdenker P: Francesco Redi and the fly experiments. **Bull Hist Med** 1979 Winter;53(4):575-92

#### Netherlands

Kremer J: The significance of Antoni van Leeuwenhoek for the early development of andrology. **Andrologia** 1979;11:243-9

### 1700 to Present

Alfredsson JH, Gudmundsson SP, Snaedal G: Artificial insemination by donor with frozen semen. **Obstet Gynecol Surv** 1983 Jun;38(6):305-13
Betteridge KJ: An historical look at embryo transfer. **J Reprod Fertil** 1981 May;62(1):1-13
Billingham RE, Beer AE: Reproductive immunology: past, present, and future. **Perspect Biol Med** 1984;27(2):259-75
Castellani C: Una rilettura ottocentesca di Spallanzani: la nouvelle théorie de la génération di Prévost e Dumas (1824). **Hist Philos Life Sci** 1979;1(2):215-59
Chang MC: [History and background of research on fertilization in mammals] (Chi). **Sheng Li Ko Hsueh Chin Chan** 1983 Oct;14(4):289-93
Chang MC: The meaning of sperm capacitation. A historical perspective. **J Androl** 1984 Mar-Apr;5(2):45-50
Churchill FB: Sex and the single organism: biological theories of sexuality in mid-nineteenth century. **Stud Hist Biol** 1979,3.139-77
Darga LL, Klauenberg S, Davis KF: The cultural model of the menstrual cycle. **Mich Acad** 1981;13(4):475-84
Dieckmann I: Untersuchungen des menschlichen Endometriums durch Hanns Kundrat (1845-1893) und George Julius Engelmann (1847-1903). Diss. Erlangen-Nürnberg, 1980. 73 p.
Eskes TK: Classic illustrations: Researches on prenatal life. **Eur J Obstet Gynecol Reprod Biol** 1981 May;11(6):435-6
Farley J: Gametes & spores. Ideas about sexual reproduction, 1750-1914. Baltimore, London, Johns Hopkins University Press, 1982. x, 299 p.
Holle S: Die Widerlegung des Postulates von der Gleichzeitigkeit der Ovulation und Menstruation bei der Frau. Klinische und histologische Untersuchungen im frühen 20. Jahrhundert. Diss. Erlangen-Nürnberg, 1984. 100 p.
Mosek C: Nutrition and fertility: a review essay. **Hist Methods** 1981;14(1):43-6
Raboch J: Historický vývoj lékařské sexuologie. **Cesk Psychiatr** 1982 Oct;78(5):353-7
Zirnstein G: Die Erforschung und Bewertung der Lebenserscheinung 'Variabilität' in der Biologie vor 1859. **NTM** 1981;18(2):58-78

#### Austria

Weinzierl S: Frühe Rezeption der Halbanschen Hypothese von der endokrinen Verursachung der Menstruation. Diss. Erlangen-Nürnberg, 1980. 59 p.

#### Denmark

Manniche E: Age at menarche: Nicolai Edvard Ravn's data on 3385 women in mid-19th century Denmark. **Ann Hum Biol** 1983 Jan-Feb;10(1):79-82

#### France

Arvy L: Jean-Baptiste Marcellin Bory de Saint-Vincent (1778-1846) et les 'Animaux Spermatiques'. In: Congrès National des Sociétés Savantes, 104e, Bordeaux, 1979. Comptes Rendus. Paris, 1979. Section des Sciences, Fasc. IV. p. 21-5.
Galérant G: Deux toulousains et un rouennais contre Pasteur au sujet de la génération spontanée. In: Congrès National des Sociétés Savantes, 96e, Toulouse, 1971. Comptes Rendus. Paris, 1974. Histoire des Sciences, Tome 1. p. 193-200.
McLaren A: Sexuality and social order: the debate over the fertility of women and workers in France, 1770-1920. New York, Holmes & Meier, 1982.
Shorter E: L'âge des premières règles en France, 1750-1950. **Ann Econ Soc Civilis** 1981;36(3):495-511

#### Germany

Simmer HH: Experimentelle Prüfungen der pflügerschen Reflexhypothese der Menstruation im späten 19. Jahrhundert. **Clio Med** 1980 Jul;14(3-4):235-54
Simmer HH: Innere Sekretion der Ovarien als Ursache der Menstruation. Halbans Falsifikation der Pflügerschen Hypothese. In Ganzinger K, Skopec M, Wyklicky H, ed: Festschrift für Erna Lesky zum 70. Geburtstag. Wien, Brüder Hollinek, 1981. p. 123-48.

#### Great Britain

Kohn D: Theories to work by: rejected theories, reproduction, and Darwin's path to natural selection. **Stud Hist Biol** 1980;4:67-70

#### Mexico

Shedlin MG, Hollerbach PE: Modern and traditional fertility regulation in a Mexican community: the process of decision making. **Stud Fam Plann** 1981 Jun-Jul:12(6-7):278-96

#### Pacific Islands

Stocking GW: Contradicting the doctor: Billy Hancock and the problem of baloma. **Hist Anthropol Newsl** 1977;4(1):4-7

#### South Africa

Ibrahim MA, Kaplan BH, Patrick RC, et al: The legacy of John C. Cassel. **Am J Epidemiol** 1980 Jul;112(1):1-7

#### United States

Benson F: Blood tests showing nonpaternity-conclusive or rebuttable evidence? The Chaplin case revisited. **Am J Forensic Med Pathol** 1981 Sep;2(3):221-3
Breeden JO: 'The case of the miraculous bullet' revisited. **Milit Aff** 1981;45(1):23-6
Chavkin W: Occupational hazards to reproduction: a review essay and annotated bibliography. **Feminist Stud** 1979,5(2).310-25
Jacob KA: The Mosher report. **Am Heritage** 1981;32(4):56-64
Michel D: Corps sauvages, corps étranges. **Dix-Huit Siecle** 1977;9:27-38
Namboodiri NK: On factors affecting fertility at different stages in the reproduction history: an exercise in cohort analysis. **Soc Forces** 1981;59(4):114-29
Plews JH: Charles Darwin and Hawaiian sex ratios, or, genius is a capacity for making compensating errors. **Hawaii J Hist** 1980;14:24-49
Ramsey EM: The story of spiral arteries. **J Reprod Med** 1981 Aug;26(8):393-9
Sloane DM: Sex of privious children and intentions for further birth in the United States, 1965-1976. **Demography** 1983 Aug;20(3):353-67
Van Horn SH: Women's roles: work and fertility for American women between 1900 and 1980. Ph.D. Diss., Carnegie-Mellon University. Pittsburgh, 1980. 344 leaves.
Wright A: An ethnography of the Navajo reproductive cycle. **Am Indian Q** 1982;6(1-2):52-70

## GENERATION AND REPRODUCTION

**Zaire**

Romaniuk A: Increase in natural fertility during the early stages of modernization: evidence from an African case study, Zaire. **Popul Stud** 1980;34(2):293–310

## GENETICS AND HEREDITY

See also **Generation and Reproduction**

Bideau A, et al: Démographie historique et génétique des populations: la concentration géographique d'une maladie héréditaire rare. **Ann Econ Soc Civilis** 1979;34:85–105

Corbin A: L'hérédosyphilis ou l'impossible rédemption: contribution à l'histoire de l'hérédité morbide. **Romantisme** 1981;31:131–49

Czeizel E: A genetika fejlödésének belsö ellentmondása. **Orv Hetil** 1982 Feb 7;123(6):349–57

Fraikor AL: Fiddling on a drifting roof: genetic implications of Jewish settlement patterns and life style. **Prog Clin Biol Res** 1982;95:535–47

Glushakova TI: Razvitie predstavlenii ob individual'nosti khromosom. Moskva, Nauka, 1983. 119 p.

Karp LE: Eutelegenesis: a historical perspective. **Am J Med Genet** 1980;5(4):327–9

Motulsky AG: Impact of genetic manipulation on society and medicine. **Science** 1983 Jan 14;219(4581):135–40

Norton B: La situation intellectuelle au moment des débuts de Fisher en génétique des populations. In Actes du Colloque R.A. Fisher.... Paris, 5–6 déc. 1979. p. 231–50. **Rev Synth (Paris)** 1981;102(103–104)

Regelmann JP: Die Geschichte des Lyssenkoismus. Frankfurt/Main, G. Fischer, 1980. 353 p.

Rosner F: Ancient descriptions of hemophilia and preconception gender selection. **JAMA** 1984 Aug 17;252(7):900

Rothschild H: Diseases of the Jews. In his: Biocultural aspects of disease. New York, Academic Press, 1981. p. 531–55.

Schulz-Schaeffer J: History of cytogenetics. In his: Cytogenetics--plants, animals, humans. New York, Springer, 1980. p. 2–29.

Smith GF: Congenital abnormalities and genetic concepts in neonatology. In Smith GF, Smith PN, Vidyasagar D, ed: Historical review and recent advances in neonatal and perinatal medicine. [Chicago?], Mead Johnson Nutritional Division, 1983. Vol. II. p. 73–83.

Stebbins GL: Darwin to DNA, molecules to humanity. San Francisco, Freeman, 1982. xiv, 491 p.

**Americas**

Laughlin WS, Harper AB, ed: The first Americans: origins, affinities, and adaptations. New York and Stuttgart, Fischer, 1979. xi, 340 p.

**Ireland**

Relethford JH: Genetic structure and population history of Ireland: a comparison of blood group and anthropometric analyses. **Ann Hum Biol** 1983 Jul–Aug;10(4):321–33

**Italy**

Pettener D: Inbreeding secular changes in the Riomaggiore and Silla Valleys, Italy, from 1565 to 1980. **Acta Anthropogenet** 1981;5(4):271–8

**Sweden**

Hed H: Opportunity for selection during the 17th–19th centuries in the diocese of Linköping as estimated with Crow's index in a population of clergymen's wives. **Hum Hered** 1984;34(6):378–87

**West Indies**

Mayer FM, Lavoie Y: Généalogie, démographie et génétique; étude d'un cas: Saint-Barthélemy. **Ann Demogr Hist (Paris)** 1984;:89–102

**Before 500 A.D.**

Yinyun Z: Variability and evolutionary trends in tooth size of Gigantopithecus blacki. **Am J Phys Anthropol** 1982 Sep;59(1):21–32

**Australia**

Thorne AG, Wolpoff MH: Regional continuity in Australasian Pleistocene hominid evolution. **Am J Phys Anthropol** 1981 Jul;55(3):337–49

**Egypt**

Czeizel A: Life and death [of] Tutankhamun from human genetic aspects. **Ther Hung** 1980;28(1):40–3

Timmons CF: Genetics of the eighteenth dynasty. **JAMA** 1981 Apr 17;245(15):1525

**Greece**

Bartsocas CS: An introduction to ancient Greek genetics and Skeletal Dysplasias. **Prog Clin Biol Res** 1982;104:3–13

**India**

Corcos AF: Reproduction and heredity beliefs of the Hindus based on their sacred books. **J Hered** 1984 Mar–Apr;75(2):152–4

**500 A.D.–1450**

Bouchard CB: Consanguinity and noble marriages in the tenth and eleventh centuries. **Speculum** 1981 Apr;56(2):268–87

**1450–1700**

**Belgium**

McKusick VA: The human genome through the eyes of Mercator and Vesalius. **Trans Am Clin Climatol Assoc** 1980;92:66–90

**Great Britain**

Loehlin JC: John Locke and behavior genetics. **Behav Genet** 1983 Jan;13(1):117–21

**1700 to Present**

Adams MB: From 'Gene Fund' to 'Gene Pool': on the evolution of evolutionarylanguage. **Stud Hist Biol** 1979;3:241–85

Allen GE: Naturalists and experimentalists: the genotype and the phenotype. **Stud Hist Biol** 1979;3:179–209

Beloff M: Dr. Darlington's provocative work: the genetic approach to world history. **Encounter (Lond)** 1970;35(4):85–8

Bowler PJ: E. W. MacBride's Lamarckian eugenics and its implications for the social construction of scientific knowledge. **Ann Sci** 1984 May;41(3):245–60

Buchanan I: Infant mortality and social policy: the eugenists and the social ameliorators, 1900–1914. **Soc Soc Hist Med Bull (Lond)** 1980;27:5–7

Burkhardt RW: Closing the door on Lord Morton's mare: the rise and fall of telegony. **Stud Hist Biol** 1979;3:1–21

Campbell A: Some general questions about movable elements and their implications. **Cold Spring Harbor Symp Quant Biol** 1980;45(1):1–9

Campbell M: Mendel's theory: its context and plausibility. **Centaurus** 1982;26(1):38–69

Carles J: Monogenisme ou polygenisme: les leçons de la génétique. **Etudes (Fr)** 1983;358(3):355–66

Chase A: The legacy of Malthus: the social costs of the new scientific racism. Urbana, University of Illinois Press, 1980. xxix, 686, xviii p.

Cheshko VT: The development of ideas on nature of heterosis in biochemical genetics (1940–1970). **Istor Biol Issled** 1983;9:186–90

Churchill FB: Sex and the single organism: biological theories of sexuality in mid-nineteenth century. **Stud Hist Biol** 1979;3:139–77

Churchill FB: The Weismann–Spencer controversy over the inheritance of acquired characters. In Forbes EG, ed: Human implications of scientific advance. Edinburgh, Edinburgh University Press, 1978. p. 451–68.

Cock AG: William Bateson's pilgrimages to Brno. Cesty Williama Batesona do Brna. **Folia Mendeliana** 1980;65(15):243–50

Cruz-Coke R: Centenario de la muerte de Mendel. **Rev Med Chil** 1984 Jan;112(1):61–4

Fancher RE: Alphonse de Candolle, Francis Galton, and the early history of the nature-nurture controversy. **J Hist Behav Sci** 1983 Oct;19(4):341–52

Fantini B: La genetica classica. Torino, Loescher, 1979. 293 p. (Storia della Scienza, 5).

Friesen JD: The emergence of the new genetics. In J. G. Little, ed: Prospects for man: genetic engineering. Toronto, Centre for Research on Environmental Quality, Faculty of Science, York University, 1979. p. 1–23.

Frolov IT, Pastushnyi SA: Dialektika istoricheskoi formny i soderzhaniia otkrytiia G. Mendelia. **Vopr Istor Estestvozn Tekh** 1981;(4):20–8

Glass B: The preservation of historical materials in genetics. **Bull Hist Med** 1983;57(1):98–105

Gluecksohn-Waelsch S: Fifty years of developmental genetics. **Trans NY Acad Sci** 1983;41:243–51

Graham LR: Between science and values. New York, Columbia University Press, 1981. x, 449 p.

Guédès M: Qu'est-ce qu'un mendélien? **Hist Nat** 1980–81;17–18:69–75

Hagerman RJ, McBogg P, Hagerman PJ: The fragile X syndrome: history, diagnosis, and treatment. **JDBP** 1983 Jun;4(2):122–30

Hilts VL: Obeying the laws of hereditary descent: phrenological views on inheritance and eugenics. **J Hist Behav Sci** 1982 Jan;18(1):62–77

Hoagland M: Discovery, the search for DNA's secrets. Boston, Houghton Mifflin, 1981. xiv, 198 p.

Hulse FS: Habits, habitats, and heredity: a brief history of studies in human

plasticity. **Am J Phys Anthropol** 1981 Dec;56(4):495–501
Huppert J: Somatic cell hybrids. **Folia Biol (Praha)** 1983;29(1):56–64
Jacobs PA: Human population cytogenetics: the first twenty-five years. **Am J Hum Genet** 1982 Sep;34(5):689–98
Jacquard A: De la génétique des populations à la sociobiologie. In Actes du Colloque R.A. Fisher.... Paris, 5–6 déc. 1979. p. 405–31. **Rev Synth (Paris)** 1981;102(103–104)
Jörgensen G: Spiel und Sport aus genetisch-phylogenetischer Sicht. **MMW** 1981 Jun 19;123(25):1039–42
Kevles DJ: Genetics in the United States and Great Britain, 1890–1930: a review with speculations. **Isis** 1980 Sep;71(258):441–55
Kevles DJ: Genetics in the United States and Great Britain 1890–1930: a review with speculations. In C. Webster, ed: Biology, medicine and society 1840–1940. Cambridge, Cambridge University Press, 1981. p. 193–215.
Kimbrough SO: On the reduction of genetics to molecular biology. **Philos Sci** 1979;46:389–406
Kirkwood TB, Cremer T: Cytogerontology since 1881: a reappraisal of August Weisman and a review of modern progress. **Hum Genet** 1982;60(2):101–21
Krimsky S: Genetic alchemy. The social history of the Recombinant DNA controversy. Cambridge, London, MIT Press, 1982. xiii, 445 p.
Léonard J: Le premier Congrès international d'eugénique (Londres, 1912) et ses conséquences françaises. **Hist Sci Med** 1983;17(2):141–6
Lewontin RC, Moore JA, Provine WB, et al: Dobzhansky's genetics of natural populations, I–XLIII. New York, Columbia University Press, 1981. xiv, 942 p. Includes Provine WB: Origins of the Genetics of natural populations series, p. 1–76.
L'Héritier P: Souvenirs d'un généticien. In Actes du Colloque R.A. Fisher.... Paris, 5–6 déc. 1979. p. 331–350. **Rev Synth (Paris)** 1981;102(103–104)
Loevy HT, Kowitz A: Health science on stamps. **J Am Dent Assoc** 1984 May;108(5):797
Lomax E: Changing attitudes during the past century as to the hazards of parental alcoholism to the progeny. In International Congress of the History of Medicine. 26th, Plovdiv, 1978. Actes du Congress. Sofia, 1981. Volume II. p. 144–7.
MacKenzie D: Sociobiologies in competition: the biometrician–Mendelian debate. In C. Webster, ed: Biology, medicine and society 1840–1940. Cambridge, Cambridge University Press, 1981. p. 243–88.
MacRoberts MH: L. H. Bailey's citations to Gregor Mendel. **J Hered** 1984 Nov–Dec;75(6):500–1
Mann G: The Third International Eugenics Congress, 1932. **Medizinhist J** 1980;15(3):338–9
Matalová A: Published primary sources to Gregor Mendel's biography. Mendelianum of the Moravian Museum, Brno. **Folia Mendeliana** 1981;16:239–51
Mayr E, Provine WB, ed: The evolutionary synthesis: perspectives on the unification of biology. Cambridge, Mass., and London, England, Harvard University Press, 1980. xi, 487 p. Contributions by M. B. Adams, G. E. Allen, E. Boesiger, R. W. Burkhardt, H. L. Carson, F. B. Churchill, W. Coleman, C. D. Darlington, T. Dobzhansky, E. B. Ford, M. T. Ghiselin, S. J. Gould, V. Hamburger, R. C. Lewontin, C. Limoges, B. Rensch, D. Shapere, G. L. Stebbins, A. Weinstein.
Mazumdar PM: Karl Landsteiner and the problem of species 1838–1968. Ph.D. Diss., Johns Hopkins University. Baltimore, 1976. 725 leaves.
Michod, RE: Positive heuristics in evolutionary biology. **Br J Philos Sci** 1981;32:1–36
Monaghan F, Corcos A: On the origins of the Mendelian laws. **J Hered** 1984 Jan–Feb;75(1):67–9
Müntzing A: Analysen av människans kromosomer. **Sydsven Medicinhist Sallsk Arsskr** 1981;:116–31
Nathans D: The new genetics. **Trans Am Clin Climatol Assoc** 1979;91:75–97
Neel JV: Human evolution: many small steps, but not punctuated equilibria. **Perspect Biol Med** 1984 Autumn;28(1):75–103
Nobel lectures in molecular biology, 1933–1975: New York, Elsevier, 1977. ix, 534 p.
Norton B: Psychologists and class. In C. Webster, ed: Biology, medicine and society 1840–1940. Cambridge, Cambridge University Press, 1981. p. 289–314.
Olby R: La théorie génétique de la sélection naturelle vue par un historien. **Rev Synth (Paris)** 1981;102(103–104):251–89
Oppitz R: Freiherr von Ehrenfels (1859–1932) und die Entwicklung des 'Neuen Menschen' zu Beginn des 20. Jahrhunderts. Diss. Mainz, 1980. 256 p.
Paul D: Eugenics and the Left. **J Hist Ideas** 1984 Oct–Dec;45(4):567–90
Peters DS: Das Biogenetische Grundgesetz––Vorgeschichte und Folgerungen. **Medizinhist J** 1980;15(1/2):57–69
Petit C: Problèmes actuels de la génétique des populations. In Actes du Colloque R.A. Fisher.... Paris, 5–6 déc. 1979. p. 351–79. **Rev Synth (Paris)** 1981;102(103–104)
Pisztora F: A születési arisztokrácia súlya és a származási téveszmék gyakorisága a Monarchia társadalmában. **Orv Hetil** 1981 Jun 28;122(26):1593–5
Pollitzer WS: The development of genetics and population studies. **Am J Phys Antropol** 1981 Dec;56(4):483–9
Portugal FH, Cohen JS: A century of DNA: a history of the discovery of the structure and function of the genetic substance. Cambridge, MIT Press, 1977. xiii, 384 p.
Rheinberger HJ: Naudin, Darwin, Nägeli: Bemerkungen zu den Vererbungsvorstellungen des 19. Jahrhunderts. **Medizinhist J** 1983;18(3):198–212
Ríman J: From Mendel to molecular genetics and biotechnologies. **Folia Biol (Praha)** 1983;29(1):1–8
Roberts DF: Dermatoglyphics and human genetics. **Birth Defects** 1979;15(6):475–94
Robson EB: Gene mapping and chromosome 21: history and methodology. **Hum Genet [Supp]** 1981;2:147–53
Romanova NN: E. S. London's contribution to the problem of DNA structure. **Istor Biol Issled** 1983;9:166–75
Romeo G: X come cromosoma. **Kos** 1984 May;1(4):115–21
Root-Bernstein RS: Mendel and methodology. **Hist Sci** 1983 Sep;21(53 pt 3):275–95
Rose H: The social determinants of reproduction science and technology. In Knorr KD, et al, ed: Determinants and controls of scientific development. Dordrecht, Boston, D. Reidel, 1975. (Theory and decision library, v. 10). p. 407–30.
Ruffié J: La signification du polymorphisme humain. **Rev Palais Decouv** 1983;11(107):46–51
Sandler IL: Pierre Louis Moreau de Maupertuis––a precursor of Mendelian genetics?: an inquiry into the biological ideas of Maupertuis, the Mendelian principles of heredity and the nature of the precursor. Ph.D. diss. University of Washington. Seattle, 1979. 265 leaves.
Sapp J: The struggle for authority in the field of heredity, 1900–1932: new perspectives on the rise of genetics. **J Hist Biol** 1983 Fall;16(3):311–42
Schroeder WA: The background of our knowledge of the mutant hemoglobins. **Tex Rep Biol Med** 1980–81;40:137–42
Searle GR: Eugenics and class. In C. Webster, ed: Biology, medicine and society 1840–1940. Cambridge, Cambridge University Press, 1981. p. 217–42.
Serre JL: Mendel's rejection of the concept of blending inheritance. **Fundam Sci** 1981;2(1):55–66
Sinding C: Le concept de gène. Une approche épistémologique. **Arch Fr Pediatr** 1984 Jan;41(1):1–3
Smith TF, Morowitz HJ: Between history and physics. **J Mol Evol** 1982;18(4):265–82
Szabó G: A gén fogalmának fejlödése. **Orv Hetil** 1982 Jan 31;123(5):259–65
Thaler L: La génétique des populations dans la théorie moderne de l'évolution. In Actes du Colloque R.A. Fisher.... Paris, 5–6 déc. 1979. p. 351–79. **Rev Synth (Paris)** 1981;102(103–104)
Valderas JM: Vuelve el lamarckismo? **Folia Hum (Barc)** 1981;19(216):57–65
Vicente R de: La investigación genética, entre la confusión y la esperanza. **Arbor** 1977;98(383):7–23
Wallace B: Changes in the genetic mentality. **Perspect Biol Med** 1984 Summer;27(4):598–610
White BN, Holden JJ: From genetic engineering to biotechnology. **Queens Q** 1982;89(3):538–49
Witkop CJ: History of genetics in dentistry. **Birth Defects** 1980;16(5):13–26
Wolstenholme G: Genetic engineering and public concern. **Clin Radiol** 1979 Nov;30(6):601–5
Yoxen EJ: Constructing genetic diseases. In P. Wright, A. Treacher, ed: The problem of medical knowledge. Examining the social construction of medicine. Edinburgh, Edinburgh University Press, 1982. p. 144–61.
Zalesova ZG: The history of the establishment of the genetic role of DNA. **Istor Biol Issled** 1983;9:66–84

### Austria

Cock AG: Faking and the intent to deceive. **Br Med J** 1980 Nov 1;281(6249):1214–5
Gregor Johann Mendel 1822–1884. In centenary commemoration: **Hereditas** 1984;100(1):2–13
Karp LE: Genetic drift. A question of discovery: Part I. **Am J Med Genet** 1983 Jul;15(3):379–81
Oldroyd D: Gregor Mendel: founding-father of modern genetics? **Endeavour** 1984;8(1):29–31
Pilgrim I: The too-good-to-be-true paradox and Gregor Mendel. **J Hered** 1984 Nov–Dec;75(6):501–2
Sermonti G: Gregor Mendel (1822–1884). **Riv Biol** 1984 Spring;77(1):105–13
Soudek D: Gregor Mendel and the people around him (commemorative of the centennial of Mendel's death). **Am J Hum Genet** 1984 May;36(3):495–8

### Chile

Villarroel H, Lazo B, Campusano C, et al: Consanguinidad y migración en Viña del Mar durante 1888 a 1967. **Rev Med Chil** 1980 May;108(5):407–12

### China

Lo WH, Wu M: Medical genetics in China. **Am J Med Genet**

1981;10(3):257-60
Renkonen KO: Old Chinese observation correlated to ABO groups. **Hum Genet** 1980;55(2):279
Spiess EB: Ching Chun Li, courageous scholar of population on genetics, human genetics, and biostatistics: a living history essay. **Am J Med Genet** 1983 Dec;16(4):603-30

**Czechoslovakia**

Levine HM, Gilderdale S: Genetics and communism. **Colo Q** 1975;24(1):17-24
Matalová A: G. Mendel and the foundation of genetics. **Folia Mendeliana** 1983;18:277-85

**Denmark**

Czeizel E: Tage Kemp, a nagy dán orvos-genetikus, az elsö gentikai tanácsadó megalapítója. **Orv Hetil** 1980 Jun 15;121(24):1460-2

**France**

Borie J: Mythologies de l'hérédité au XIXe siècle. Paris, Editions Galilée, 1981. 215 p.
Bouchard G: Nouvelles perspectives pour les recherches génétiques. Le fichier-réseau de la population du Saguenay. **Ann Demogr Hist (Paris)** 1984;:81-8
Buican D: Histoire de la génétique et de l'évolutionnisme en France. Paris, Presse universitaires de France, 1984. 421 p.
Buican D: La génétique classique en France devant le neo-lamarckisme tardif. **Arch Int Hist Sci (Paris)** 1983 Dec;33(111):300-24
Buican D: Lucien Cuénot et la redécouverte de la génétique. **Pour Sci** 1981;45:21-9
Fischer JL: Yves Delage (1854-1920): l'epigenèse néo-lamarckienne contre la prédétermination weismannienne. **Rev Synth (Paris)** 1979;100(95-6):443-61
Schneider W: Toward the improvement of the human race: the history of eugenics in France. **J Mod Hist** 1982;54(2):268-91

**Germany**

Glass B: A hidden chapter of German eugenics between the two world wars. **Proc Am Philos Soc** 1981;125(5):357-67
Günther M: Die Institutionalisierung der Rassenhygiene an den deutschen Hochschulen vor 1933. Diss., Johannes Gutenberg-Universität, Mainz, 1982. 148 p.
Harwood J: The reception of Morgan's chromosome theory in Germany: inter-war debate over cytoplasmic inheritance. **Medizinhist J** 1984;19(1-2):3-32
Harwood JH: The history of genetics in Germany. **Mendel Newsl** 1984;(24):1-3
Koch G: Inhaltsreiche Jahre eines Humangenetikers: Mein Lebensweg in Bildern und Dokumenten. Erlangen, Perimed Fachbuchgesellschaft, 1982. 472 p.
Lilienthal G: 'Rheinlandbastarde', Rassenhygiene und das Problem der rassenideologischen Kontinuität. Zur Untersuchung von Reiner Pommerin: 'Sterilisierung der Rheinlandbastarde'. **Medizinhist J** 1980;15(4):426-36
Pirchner F: Wilhelm Weinberg's contribution to quantitative genetics. **Folia Mendeliana** 1978;13(63):261-6
Propping P: Genetic disorders presenting as 'schizophrenia'. Karl Bonhoeffer's early view of the psychoses in the light of medical genetics. **Hum Genet** 1983;65(1):1-10
Rissom R: Fritz Lenz und die Rassenhygiene. Husum, Matthiesen, 1983. 143 p. (Abhandlungen zur Geschichte der Medizin und der Naturwissenschaften, 47).
Saha MS: The Carl Correns papers. **Mendel Newsl** 1981 Nov;21:1-6
Seidler E: Johann Friedrich Meckel the Younger (1781-1833). **Am J Med Genet** 1984 Aug;18(4):571-86

**Great Britain**

Amos DB: Peter Alfred Isaac Gorer. In Dictionary of national biography, 1961-1970. Suppl. 8, 1981. p. 443-5.
Anderson NF: The 'marriage with a deceased wife's sister bill' controversy: incest anxiety and the defense of family purity in Victorian England. **J Br Stud** 1982;21(2):67-86
Armytage WH: Issue at stake: the biosocial background. **Hist Educ** 1981;10(3):183-94
Auerbach C: A pilgrim's progress through mutation research. **Perspect Biol Med** 1978 Spring;21(3):319-34
Bateson W: Problems of genetics. Reprint of 1913 ed. Historical introduction by G. E. Hutchinson and S. Rachootin. New Haven and London, Yale University Press, 1979. xxii, 258 p.
Beer CG: Darwin, instinct, and ethology. **J Hist Behav Sci** 1983 Jan;19(1):68-80
Billig M: The origins of race psychology - I. **Patterns Prejudice** 1982;16(3):3-16
Box JF: R. A. Fisher: the life of a scientist. New York, Wiley, 1978. xii, 512 p.
Close HG: A genetic Odyssey. **S Afr Med J** 1982 Jun 26;61(26):1010-2
Conry Y: Organisme et organisation: de Darwin à la génétique des populations. In Actes du Colloques R.A. Fisher.... Paris, 5-6 déc. 1979. p. 291-330. **Rev Synth (Paris)** 1981;102(103-104)
Cornell JF: Analogy and technology in Darwin's vision of nature. **J Hist Biol** 1984 Fall;17(3):303-44
Corney G: Sir Francis Galton, 1822-1911. **Acta Genet Med Gemellol (Roma)** 1984;33(1):13-8
Freeden M: Eugenics and progressive thought: a study in ideological affinity. **Hist J (Gt Brit)** 1979;22(3):645-72
Gilbert SF: Owen's vertebral archetype and evolutionary genetics -- a Platonic appreciation. **Perspect Biol Med** 1980 Spring;23(3):475-88
Gottesman II: James Shields, 1918-1978. **Acta Genet Med Gemellol (Roma)** 1979;28(1):83-90
Lewis D, Hunt DM: Hans Grüneberg: 26 May 1907-23 October 1982. **Biogr Mem Fellows R Soc** 1984;30:227-47
Lowe RA: Eugenicists, doctors and the quest for national efficiency: an educational crusade, 1900-1939. **Hist Educ** 1979;8(4):293-306
Mazumdar PM: The eugenists and the residuum: the problem of the urban poor. **Bull Hist Med** 1980 Summer;54(2):204-15
Norton B: Fisher and the neo-Darwinian synthesis. In Forbes EG, ed: Human implications of scientific advance. Edinburgh, Edinburgh University Press, 1978. p. 481-94.
Rheinberger HJ, McLaughlin P: Darwin's experimental natural history. **J Hist Biol** 1984 Fall;17(3):345-68
Roberts JA: Reginald Ruggles Gates. In Dictionary of national biography, 1961-1970. Suppl. 8, 1981. p. 424-5.
Schall JV: The rarest of all revolutions: G. K. Chesterton on the relation of human life to Christian doctrine. **Am Benedictine Rev** 1981;32(4):304-27
Scott-Moncrieff R: The classical period in chemical genetics; recollections of Muriel Wheldale Onslow, Robert and Gertrude Robinson and J. B. S. Haldane. **Notes Rec R Soc Lond** 1981;36(1):125-54
Shepherd JA: Lawson Tait - disciple of Charles Darwin. **Br Med J [Clin Res]** 1982 May;284(6326):1386-7
Sinohara H: [Archibald Edward Garrod (1857-1936): a biographical assay (author's transl)] (Jpn). **Seikagaku** 1980 Nov;52(11):1155-72
Smith JM: John Burdon Sanderson Haldane. In Dictionary of national biography, 1961-1970. Suppl. 8, 1981. p. 473-5.
Smith MT, Hudson BL: Isonymic relationships in the parish of Fylingdales, North Yorkshire, in 1851. **Ann Hum Biol** 1984 Mar-Apr;11(2):141-8
Woodhouse J: Eugenics and the feeble-minded: the Parliamentary debates of 1912-14. **Hist Educ** 1982;11:127-37
Yates F: Sir Ronald Aylmer Fisher. In Dictionary of national biography, 1961-1970. Suppl. 8, 1981. p. 361-2.

**Hungary**

Czeizel A: A historical evaluation of the doctrine of heredodegeneration. **Orvostort Kozl** 1979;87-88(25 no 1-2):157-79
Kiszely G: Visszaemlékezés a magyar humángenetika elmúlt 50 évére. **Orv Hetil** 1984 Mar 18;125(12):709-12

**Italy**

Lucchetti E: Historical reconstitution of Varaita Valley population 1770-1970. **Acta Anthropogenet** 1981;5(4):255-70
Martucci V: Il discusso fascino di una ipotesi: la pangenesi di Darwin e gli studiosi italiani (1868-1888). **Hist Philos Life Sci** 1981;3(2):243-57
Martucci V: Sviluppo ontogenetico e citologia nell'ologenesi di Daniele Rosa. **Physis** 1980;22(1):73-84

**Netherlands**

Heimans J: Hugo De Vries and the gene theory. In Forbes EG, ed: Human implications of scientific advance. Edinburgh, Edinburgh University Press, 1978. p. 469-80.
Opitz JM: In memoriam: Petrus Johannes Waardenburg, 1886-1979. **Am J Med Genet** 1980;7(1):35-9

**Norway**

Roll-Hansen N: Eugenics before World War II; the case of Norway. **Hist Philos Life Sci** 1980;2(2):269-98

**Poland**

Kasperek S: Przymusowe sterylizacje w rejencji opolskiej 1934-1938. **Przegl Lek** 1980;37(1):33-9
Kinastowski W: Próba analizy założeń weismannowskiej teorii dziedziczenia. Wrocław, Zakład Narodowy im. Ossolińskich, 1977. 42 p.

**Romania**


Popa LM, Repanovici R, Iliescu R: Investigations in the field of recombinant DNA technology performed in the 'Stefan S. Nicolau' Institute of Virology. **Virologie** 1984 Oct–Dec;35(4):315–22


**Sweden**


Hed HM, Rasmuson M: Cohort study of opportunity for selection on two Swedish 19th century parishes with a survey of other estimates. **Hum Hered** 1981;31(2):78–83

Kempe C: Detaljstudier av kromosomer en diagnostisk revolution. **Lakartidningen** 1980 Feb 13;77(7):503–4


**Switzerland**


Kitchener RF: The nature and scope of genetic epistemology. **Philos Sci** 1981;48(3):400–15


**United States**


Allen G: The transformation of a science: T. H. Morgan and the emergence of a new American biology. In Oleson A, Voss J, ed: The organization of knowledge in modern America, 1860–1920. Baltimore and London, Johns Hopkins University Press, 1979. p. 173–210.

Baxter AL: E. B. Wilson's 'Destruction' of the germ-layer theory. **Isis** 1977 Sep;68(243):363–74

Bird RD, Allen G: The J.H.B. Archive report: the papers of Harry Hamilton Laughlin, eugenicist. **J Hist Biol** 1981 Fall;14(2):339–53

Byard PJ: Population history, demography, and genetics of the St. Lawrence Island Eskimos. Ph.D. Diss., University of Kansas. Lawrence, 1981. v, 143 leaves.

Carlson EA: Genes, radiation, and society. The life and work of H. J. Muller. Ithaca, Cornell University Press, 1981. xiv, 457 p.

Carmelli D, Hasstedt S, Andersen S: Demography and genetics of human twinning in the Utah Mormon Genealogy. **Prog Clin Biol Res** 1981;69A:81–93

Caspari EW, Allen GE, et al: Controversial geneticist and creative biologist. [Richard B. Goldschmidt] A critical review on his contributions. **Experientia [Suppl]** 1980;Suppl 35:1–154

Cotterman CW: Relationship and probability in Mendelian populations. **Am J Med Genet** 1983 Nov;16(3):393–440

Cravens H: The triumph of evolution: American scientists and the heredity-environment controversy 1900–1941. [Philadelphia], University of Pennsylvania Press, 1978. xvi, 351 p.

Crow JF: Sewall Wright, the scientist and the man. **Perspect Biol Med** 1982 Winter;25(2):279–94

DelCastillo AR: Sterilization: an overview. In Mora, Magdalena and DelCastillo, Adelaida R., ed. Mexican Women in the United States: Struggles past and present. Los Angeles, U. of California Chicano Studies Res. Center, 1980. p. 65–70.

Eichwald EJ, Silmser CR: H-Y and serendipity. **Hum Genet** 1981;58(1):6–8

Feinleib M: History of the genetic epidemiology of coronary heart disease. **Prog Clin Biol Res** 1984;147:1–7

Fuller MB: Alexander Hollaender Papers (1898– ). **Mendel Newsl** 1984;(24):5–7

Fuller MB: Theodosius Dobzhansky Papers. **Mendel Newsl** 1980 Jun;(18):1–8

Fuller MB: Thomas Hunt Morgan papers at the American Philosophical Society. **Mendel Newsl** 1981 Nov;21:6–8

Gershon ES: The historical context of Franz Kallmann and psychiatric genetics. **Arch Psychiatr Nervenkr** 1981;229(4):273–6

Green HP: The recombinant DNA controversy: a model of public influence. **Bull At Sci** 1978;34(9):12–16

Holstein J: The first fifty years at the Jackson Laboratory. Edited by W. L. Dupuy. [Bar Harbor, Me.], Jackson Laboratory, 1979. xiii, 231 p.

Karp LE: Adrien Bleyer: in the right place at the wrong time. **Am J Med Genet** 1981;10(3):209–11

Karp LE: Genetic drift. A question of discovery: Part II. **Am J Med Genet** 1983 Aug;15(4):533–5

Karp LE: Past perfect: John Humphrey Noyes, stirpiculture, and the Oneida community - part II. **Am J Med Genet** 1982 Jun;12(2):127–30

Keller EF: A feeling for the organism: the life and work of Barbara McClintock. New York, Freeman, 1983. xix, 235 p.

Kelly TE: Clinical genetics on the road: be Oslerian, young man. **Am J Med Genet** 1983 Aug;15(4):561–5

Kimmelman BA: The American Breeders' Association: genetics and eugenics in an agricultural context, 1903–13. **Soc Stud Sci** 1983 May;13(2):163–204

Kopp C: The Edward Lawrie Tatum papers. **Mendel Newsl** 1981 Jul;20:1–2

Kopp C: The J. H. B. Archive report; the Edward Lawrie Tatum papers at the Rockefeller University Archives. **J Hist Biol** 1982 Spring;15(1):153–4

Lear J: Recombinant DNA: the untold story. New York, Crown, 1978. 280 p.

Lederberg J: Edward Lawrie Tatum. **Annu Rev Genet** 1979;13:1–5

Lengeler J: Barbara McClintock und die Entdeckung der beweglichen Gene. **MMW** 1983 Nov 25;125(47):1095–7

McCarty M: Reminiscenses of the early days of transformation. **Annu Rev Genet** 1980;14:1–15

McCoy JJ: The cancer lady: Maud Slye and her heredity studies. Nashville, Nelson, 1977. 191 p.

McDermott W: Colin Munro MacLeod: January 28, 1909–February 11, 1972. **Biogr Mem Natl Acad Sci** 1983;54:183–219

Mehler B: Madge Thurlow Macklin. In: Notable American women. The modern period. Cambridge, Mass., Belknap-Harvard Univ. Press, 1980. 4:451–2

Norrby E: Den medicinska betydelsen av rörliga strukturer i arvsmassan. **Lakartidningen** 1983 Oct 19;80(42):3911–3

On the rôle of Laurence H. Synder in the development of human and medical genetics in the United States; an oral history tape interview: **Am J Med Genet** 1981;8(4):449–68

Opitz JM: Cotterman and combinatorial genetics. **Am J Med Genet** 1983 Nov;16(3):389–92

Opitz JM: Introduction of Sewall Wright on the occasion of receiving the first Meckel medal and prize in mammalian developmental genetics. **Am J Med Genet** 1984 Aug;18(4):587–90

Oppenheimer JM: Walter Landauer and developmental genetics. In Subtelny S, Abbott U, ed: Levels of genetic control in development. New York, Liss, 1981. p. 1–13.

Pfund N, Hofstadter L: Biomedical innovation and the press. **J Commun** 1981;31(2):138–54

Piternick LK: Richard Goldschmidt, controversial geneticist and creative biologist: a critical review of his contribution. Basal, Boston, Birkhäuser, 1980. 153 p.

Ramage JA: Thomas Hunt Morgan: family influences in the making of a great scientist. **Filson Club Hist Q** 1979;53(1):5–25

Ravin AW: Genetics in America: a historical overview. **Perspect Biol Med** 1978 Winter;21(2):214–31

Reed SC: A short history of genetic counseling. Minneapolis, Dight Institute for Human Genetics of the Univ. of Minnesota, 1974. p. 1–10. (Bull. 14).

Reilly P: The Virginia Racial Integrity Act revisited: the Plecker-Laughlin correspondence: 1928–1930. **Am J Med Genet** 1983 Dec;16(4):483–92

Rife DC, et al: Dr. Harold Cummins and dermatoglyphics. **Birth Defects** 1979;15(6):1–797, passim

Ringertz NR: Upptäckt av 'hoppande gener' hos majs gav 81-årig kvinna hela medicinpriset Barbara McClintock--en unik medicinsk nobelpristagare. **Lakartidningen** 1983 Oct 19;80(42):3908–10

Russel ES: A century of mammalian genetics and cancer, 1929–2029, a view at midpassage. **Prog Clin Biol Res** 1981;45:xi–xiv

Schwartz RJ, Weiss KM, Buchanan AV: Looking into the black box: practical approaches to record linkage. **Ann Demogr Hist (Paris)** 1984;:119–28

Skolnick MH, Bean LL, Mineau GP, et al: Etudes génétiques et démographiques et base de données généalogiques de l'Utah. **Ann Demogr Hist (Paris)** 1984;:103–13

Sullivan DJ: Biological engineering. **Thought** 1981;56(221):199–211

Taylor CM: W. E. B. Dubois's challenge to scientific racism. **J Black Stud** 1981;11(4):449–60

Tobach E, Proshansky HM, ed: Genetic destiny: race as a scientific and social controversy. New York, AMS Press, 1976. 163 p. Contributions by A. Edel, R. Cancro, D. Layzer, H. Padfield, A. Chase, E. Drucker, V. W. Sidel, G. Piel, J. C. King, E. A. Mauss.

Vigue CL, Vigue LC: The eugenics movement in America. **Essays Arts Sci** 1982;11:1–12

Weiss KM, Chakraborty R: Genes, populations, and disease, 1930–1980: a problem-oriented review. In F. Spencer, ed: A history of American physical anthropology, 1930–1980. New York, Academic Press, 1982. p. 371–404.


**USSR**


Adams MB: Biology after Stalin: a case study. **Survey** 1977–78;23(1):53–80

Alikhanian SI: Kafedra genetiki Moskovskogo gosudartsvennogo universiteta imeni M. V. Lomonosova--1930–1948 gg. **Genetika (Moskva)** 1981;17(7):1320–7

Astaurov BL: Problemy obshcheĭ biologii i genetiki. Moskva, Nauka, 1979. 292 p.

Baglaĭ EB: [The first attempt to prove the dominant role of the nucleus in heredity.] (Rus). **Istor Biol Issled** 1978;7:156–62

Beliaev DK: Vydaiushchiesia sovetskie genetiki: sbornik biograficheskikh ocherkov. Moskva, Nauka, 1980. 147 p.

Berg RL: The life and research of Boris L. Astaurov. **Q Rev Biol** 1979 Dec;54(4):397–419

Bochkov NP: Vklad s. n. Davidenkova v razrabotku probelmy nasledstvennykh nervynkh i psikhicheskikh zabolevaniĭ. **Zh Nevropatol Psikhiatr** 1982;82(3):1–4

Davidenkova EF: Zanchenie nauchnogo naslediia S. N. Davidenkova v razvitii klinicheskoĭ genetiki (k 100-letiiu so dnai rozhdeniia). **Klin Med (Mosk)** 1981;59(4):112–6

Dogel' LV, Shalagina TL: S. N. Davidenkov v Leningradskom gosudarstvennom institute usovershenstvovaniia vracheĭ. **Zh Nevropatol Psikhiatr** 1982;82(3):107–9

## GENETICS AND HEREDITY

Dubinin NP, ed: Nauchno-teoreticheskaia konferentsiia 'Perspektivy razvitiia genetiki v SSSR v svete soedineniia uspekhov nauchno-tekhnicheskoĭ revoliutsii s preimushchestvami sotsializma', Moscow?, 1976?
Gaissinovitch AE: The origins of Soviet genetics and the struggle with Lamarckism, 1922-1929. **J Hist Biol** 1980 Spring, 13(1):1-51
Golda DM: Iu. A. Filipchenko--osnovopolozhnik otechestvennoĭ genetiki (1882-1930 gg.). **Tsitol Genet** 1982;16(1):73 passim
Golda DM, Berdyshev GD: Prepodavanie genetiki v Kievskom universitete (k 150-letiiu KGU). **Tsitol Genet** 1984 Sep-Oct;18(5):393-4
Kafedre genetiki Moskovskogo gosudarstvennogo universiteta imeni M. V. Lomonosova--50 let: **Genetika (Moskva)** 1981;17(7):1318-20
Kuchenbecker D: Entwicklungstendenzen der sowjetischen Genetik. Frankfurt am Main, Diagnal, 1978. 47 p.
Melnick M: Sakharov and genetic science in the Soviet Union [editorial] **J Craniofac Genet Dev Biol** 1984;4(3):171-2
Nikolai Wladimirovich Timof'eeff-Ressovsky, (1900-1981): **Genetics** 1982 Jan;100(1):1-5

## GERONTOLOGY

See also **Human Development and Growth**

Banziger G: Intergenerational communication in prominent western drama. **Gerontologist** 1979 Oct;19(5 pt 1):471-80
Becker KF: Kirche und Alter in Geschichte Gegenwart. **Z Gerontol** 1984 Jan-Feb;17(1):32-8
Blum L: The youth of geriatrics. **Mt Sinai J Med (NY)** 1983 Nov-Dec;50(6):476-82
Bourlière F: Geschichte der Pflege und Behandlung des alten Menschen. In Sournia JC, Martiny M, Poulet J, ed: Illustrierte Geschichte der Medizin. Salzburg, Andreas, 1980. Vol. 6. p. 2075-101.
Challinor JR: The aged in families: a retrospective view. **Long Term Care Health Serv Adm Q** 1978 Sep;2(3)189-96
Emerson GM, ed: Aging. Stroudsburg, Pa., Dowden, Hutchinson & Ross, 1977. xii, 372 p. (Benchmark Papers in Human Physiology, 11).
Figallo Espinal L: Vejez y envejecimiento (resumen historico). **Rev Soc Venez Hist Med** 1980;29(43-44):39-53
Freeman JT: Aging: its history and literature. New York, Human Sciences Press, 1979. 161 p.
Freeman JT: Collecting books on old age. **Spec Collect** 1982;1(3-4):131-48
Imbault-Huart MJ: La vieillesse: état pathologique ou ultime equilibre de vie? **Asclepio** 1983;35:301-15
Ladendorf H: Der alte Mensch in der Kunst. In Göpfert W, Otten HH, ed: Metavoeite: wandelt euch durch neues Denken. Düsseldorf, Triltsch, 1983. p. 55-68.
Leibowitz JO: Early accounts in geriatric pathology (Leonardo, Harvey, James Keill). **Koroth** 1980 Jun;7(11-12):CCLIII-CCLXIV
Peterson M, Rose Cl: Historical antecedents of normative vs pathologic perspectives in aging. **J Am Geriatr Soc** 1982 Apr;30(4):289-94
Quadagno JS: From poor laws to pensions: the evolution of economic support for the aged in England and America. **Milbank Mem Fund Q** 1984 Summer;62(3):417-46
Spicker SF, Van Tassel DD, Woodward KM, ed: Aging and the elderly; humanistic perspectives in gerontology. Atlantic Highlands, New Jersey, Humanities Press, 1978. viii, 406 p. Historical contributions by D. E. Stannard, H. M. Stahmer, E. E. Whitehead, R. Freedman, S. S. Tamke, G. Berg, S. Gadow, B. G. Rosenkrantz, M. A. Vinovskis, S. R. Smith, D. Luke, W. G. Moss, D. Bronsen, D. S. Smith, T. W. Ganschow, D. Marquis, G. J. Gruman.
Willmuth LR: Medical views of depression in the elderly: historical notes. **J Am Geriatr Soc** 27(11):495-9, Nov 79

**Byzantium**

Eftychiadis AC, Marketos SG: [Geriatrics in Byzantium.] (Gre). **Mater Med Greca** 1981;9:217-20

**Germany**

Altwerden in der Bundesrepublik Deutschland: Geschichte - Situationen - Perspektiven: Berlin, Deutsches Zentrum für Altersfragen, 1982. 3 volumes. (Beiträge zur Gerontologie und Altenarbeit).

**India**

Mahdihassan S: Indian alchemy or Rasayana in the light of asceticism [and] geriatrics. New Delhi, Vikas, 1979. x, 139 p.

**United States**

Cole T: The ideology of old age and death in American history. **Am Q** 1979;31(2):223-31
Demos J: Old age in early New England. In Demos, J, Boocock, SS, ed.: Turning points: historical and sociological essays on the family. Chicago, U. of Chicago Press, 1978. p. 248-87.
Haber C: Beyond sixty-five: the dilemma of old age in America's past. Cambridge, New York, Cambridge University Press, 1983. ix, 181 p.

**Before 500 A.D.**

Kudlien F: Medizinische Aspekte der antiken Unsterblichkeitsvorstellung. **Rheinisches Mus Philol** n.f. 1978;121:218-25

**China**

Lin Qianliang, Liu Zhengcai: [Notions about gerontism, longevity and life span in ancient China.] (Chi). **Chin J Med Hist** 1981;11:84-6

**Greco-Roman**

Hooff AJ van: Oud-zijn in het oude Hellas. **Tijdschr Gerontol Geriatr** 1983 Aug;14(4):141-8
Marinone N: Galeno, De victu attenuante, 79 e 98. **Riv Filol Istruz Classica** 1976;104:328-36

**Greece**

Keil G: Altern und Alter in der Antike. **Aktuel Gerontol** 1983 Mar;13(2):47-52

**1450-1700**

Scheller, EF: Langlebigkeit mit Paracelsus-Arzneien: Versuch einer Geriatrie nach Paracelsus. Heidelberg, Haug, 1977. 150 p.

**Great Britain**

Pelling M: Old people and poverty in early modern towns. **Soc Soc Hist Med Bull (Lond)** 1984 Jun;34:42-7
Smith SR: Age in old England. **Hist Today** 1979;29(3):172-8

**United States**

Boyett GW: Aging in seventeenth-century New England. **N Engl Hist Geneal Regist** 1980 Jul;134:181-93

**1700 to Present**

Austrian R: Pneumonia in the later years. **J Am Geriatr Soc** 1981 Nov;29(11):481-9
Berk SL: Bacterial pneumonia in the elderly: the observations of Sir William Osler in retrospect. **J Am Geriatr Soc** 1984 Sep;32(9):683-5
Davis BA: The gerontological nursing specialty. **J Gerontol Nurs** 1983 Oct;9(10):527-32
Djordjević M: [Surgeon and gerontologist Dr. Adolf L. Vischer: a contribution to Serbo-Swiss relations] (Serbo-Croat). **Srp Arh Celok Lek** 1979;107:1079-92
Fockert JA de: De klinisch geriatrische afdeling in een ziekenhuis: officële erkenning als experiment. **Tijdschr Ziekenverpl** 1982 Sept 21;35(19):621-5
Friedsam HJ: The coming on of years: social science perspectives on aging and death. **Soc Sci Q** 1970;51(1):120-8
Gruman GJ, ed: Roots of modern gerontology and geriatrics. Frederic D. Zeman's 'Medical history of old age' and selected studies by other writers. New York, Arno, 1979. Various paginations.
Gruman GJ, ed: The 'Fixed period' controversy: prelude to modern ageism. New York, Arno Press, 1979. Various paginations. Reprint of passages by George M. Beard, William Osler, and James Crichton-Browne.
Gsell O: Geschichte und Bedeutung der Pneumonie im hohen Alter. **Z Gerontol** 1982 Nov-Dec;15(6):325-31
Haber C: Geriatrics: a specialty in search of specialists. **Z Gerontol** 1984 Jan-Feb;17(1):26-31
Livečka E: Nástin konstituování gerontopedagogiky. **Acta Univ Carol Philos Hist** 1978;(4):41-76
Oesterreich K, Wagner O: Psychopathologie des Alterns und der Voralterung--Historische Entwicklung der Begriffsbildung. **Z Gerontol** 1982 Nov-Dec;15(6):314-20
Pollak O: The shadow of death over aging. **Ann Am Acad Polit Soc Sci** 1980; 447:71-7
Ryant C: Comment: oral history and gerontology. **Gerontologist** 1981 Feb;21(1):104-5
Schulz R, Schulz H, Hartman B: Experimental social gerontology: a social psychological perspective. **J Soc Issues** 1980;36(2):30-46
Smith RM: The structured dependency of the elderly: a twentieth-century creation? **Soc Soc Hist Med Bull (Lond)** 1984 Jun;34:35-41
Stearns PN: Old women: some historical observations. **J Fam Hist** 1980 Spring;5(1):44-57
Stoddard S: The hospice movement. Briarcliff Manor, N. Y., Stein and Day, 1978. xviii, 266 p.
Witkowski JA: Dr. Carrel's immortal cells. **Med Hist** 1980 Apr;24(2):129-42

**Austria**

Amann A, Majce G: A short history of the development of social-scientific research on aging in Austria. **ZFA** 1984 Jan–Feb;39(1):9–15
Hofecker G, Seitelberger F: The state and goals of basic research in gerontology in Austria. **ZFA (Dresden)** 1980;35(2):91–6

**Belgium**

Ter herinnering aan professor dr. jan hellemans: **Tijdschr Gerontol Geriatr** 1982 Oct;13(5):171–8

**Canada**

Holzberg CS: Anthropology, life histories, and the aged: the Toronto Baycrest Centre. **Int J Aging Hum Dev** 1983–84;18(4):255–75

**France**

Eisele FR: Origins of 'gerontocracy'. **Gerontologist** 1979 Aug;19(4):403–7
Huard P: La gérontologie de J. M. Charcot. **Rev Neurol (Paris)** 1982;138(12):989–95
Lamarre C: Vivre de charité à l'hôpital de Dijon au XVIIIe siècle: les secours aux enfants et aux viellards. **Bull Soc Fr Hist Hop** 1981;(42):25–35
Stearns PN: The modernization of old age in France: approaches through history. **Int J Aging Hum Dev** 1981;13(4):297–315
Voldman D: Guérir du cancer et mourir de vieillesse: histoire de l'hospice Paul-Brousse de 1905 à 1975. **Asclepio** 1983;35:317–26

**Germany**

Dieck M: Residential and community provisions for the frail elderly in Germany: current issues and their history. **Gerontologist** 1980 Jun;20(3 Pt 1):260–72
Eitner S: Das gerontologische Engagement von Maxim Zetkin in seinen späten Lebensjahren. **ZFA** 1984 Jan–Feb;39(1):5–8

**Great Britain**

Aoki N: [Aging report: an observation on geriatric care in England. 4. History of geriatric care] (Jpn). **Kangogaku Zasshi** 1982 Apr;46(4):466–8
Charles DC, Charles LA: Charles Dickens' old people. **Int J Aging Hum Dev** 1979–80;10(3):231–7
Florence Nightingale: the original geriatric nurse. **Okla Nurse** 1980 May;25(4):6
Godlove C, Mann A: Thirty years of the welfare state: current issues in British social policy for the aged. **Aged Care Serv Rev** 1980;2(1):1, 3–13
Matthews DA: Dr. Marjory Warren and the origin of British geriatrics. **J Am Geriatr Soc** 1984 Apr;32(4):253–8
Paulshock BZ: When should a physician retire? – William Heberden's view. **Del Med J** 1983;55(6):359–60
Quadagno JS: Aging in early industrial society. Work, family, and social policy in nineteenth-century England. New York, Academic Press, 1982. xvi, 231 p. (Studies in Social Discontinuity).
Richardson R: Old people's attitudes to death in the twentieth century. **Soc Soc Hist Med Bull (Lond)** 1984 Jun;34:48–51
Thane P: The perception and experience of old age 1945–1965. **Soc Soc Hist Med Bull (Lond)** 1984 Jun;34:52–4
Thomson WA: The hospice tradition. **J R Soc Med** 1981 Feb;74(2):90–1
Williamson J: Three views on geriatric medicine: 3. Notes on the historical development of geriatric medicine as a medical specialty. **Age Ageing** 1979 Aug;8(3):144–8

**Hungary**

Vértes L: Elsö gerontológusunk: Rózsay József akadémikus. **Orv Hetil** 1983 Oct 16;124(42):2564–8

**Ireland**

Relethford JH, Lees FC: The effects of aging and secular trend on adult stature in rural western Ireland. **Am J Phys Anthropol** 1981;55(1):81–8

**Netherlands**

Van Proosdij C, Sipsma DH: Dertig jaar vaderlandse geschiedenis. De lijdensweg van de klinische geriatrie in Nederland. **Tijdschr Gerontol Geriatr** 1984 Feb;15(1):3–5

**Scandinavia**

Gray JA: The elderly in Scandinavia: demographic, economic, social and health conditions in 1834. **Scand J Soc Med** 1984;12(2):65–8

**Sweden**

Olsson L: Altern im gesellschaftlichen Wandel--Ein interdisziplinäres Forschungsprojekt über Schweden im 19. und 20. Jahrhundert. **Z Gerontol** 1984 Jan–Feb;17(1):6–12

**United States**

Achenbaum WA: Old age in a new land: the American experience since 1970. Baltimore, Johns Hopkins Univ. Press, 1978. xiii, 237 p.
[Blank MI]: Research on the mental health of the aging 1960–1976. Rockville, Md., National Institute of Mental Health, 1977 (and 1981), xii, 69 p.
Cole TR: The prophecy of Senescence: G. Stanley Hall and the reconstruction of old age in America. **Gerontologist** 1984 Aug;24(4):360–6
Dahlin M: Perspectives on the family life of the elderly in 1900. **Gerontologist** 1980 Feb;20(1):99–107
Davis BA: Nursing care of the aged: past, present, future. **Imprint** 1980 Feb;27(1):38, 65, 72–3
Decker DL: Sociological theory and the social position of the aged. **Int J Contemp Sociol** 1978;15(3–4):303–17
Delprato DJ: The reactional biography concept: early contribution to a perspective for the psychology of aging. **Hum Dev** 1980;23(5):314–22
Dubin JL, Roney JL: The public welfare project on aging. **Public Welf** 1971;29(4):439–46
Freeman JT: Some notes on the history of the National Institute on Aging. **Gerontologist** 1980 Oct;20(5 pt 1):610–4
Hess BB: The politics of aging. **Society** 1978;15(5):22–3
Hickey T, Oriol WE: New directions and societal responses to aging: a symposium in honor of Ollie A. Randall. Introduction. **Gerontologist** 1983 Aug;23(4):397–8
History of the American Geriatrics Society: Malford W. Thewlis, J. Am. Geriatrics Soc. 1: 3, 1953. **J Am Geriatr Soc** 1981 Dec;29(12):544–9
Johnson RA: On the psychology of the aging woman. Mary Baker Eddy as a religious leader. **J Geriatr Psychiatry** 1979;12(1):27–35
Lave JR, Silverman HA: Financing the health care of the aged. **Ann Am Acad Polit Soc Sci** 1983;(468):149–64
Pollard LJ: Aging and slavery: gerontological perspective. **J Negro Hist** 1981 Fall;66:228–34
Rosenwaike I: A note on new estimates of the mortality of the extreme aged. **Demography** 1981 May;18(2):257–66
Siegel JS: On the demography of aging. **Demography** 1980 Nov;17(4):345–64
Silberger J: On the psychology of the aging woman. Mourning and transformation: how Mary Baker Eddy found in middle age a way of making a new life for herself. **J Geriatr Psychiatry** 1979;12(1):9–25
Smith DS: A community-based sample of the older population from the 1880 and 1900 United States manuscript census. **Hist Methods Newsl** 1978;11(2):67–74
Vladeck BC, Firman JP: The aging of the population and health services. **Ann Am Acad Polit Soc Sci** 1983;(468):132–48

**USSR**

Chebotarev DF: Idei A. A. Bogomol'tsa razvitie sovremenno i gerontologii. **Fiziol Zh** 1981 May–Jun;27(3):400–6
Chebotarev DF: 25 let deiatel'nosti Instituta gerontologii AMN SSSR v razvitii nauki o starenii. **Vestn Akad Med Nauk SSSR** 1984;(3):3–9
Duplenko IuK: Istoki sovremennogo razvitiia fiziologii stareniia na Ukraine. **Fiziol Zh** 1984 Jan–Feb;30(1):102–6
Nikitin VN, Perskiĭ EE, Utevskiĭ LA: Molekuliarnye mekhanizmy vozrastnogo razvitiia kollagenovykh struktur i teoriia stareniia A. A. Bogomol'tsa. **Fiziol Zh** 1981 May–Jun;27(3):407–12
Nikitin VN, Perskiĭ EE, Utevskaia LA: Uchenie A. A. Bogomol'tsa o roli soedinitel'noĭ tkani v starenii i sovremennye predstavleniia o mekhanizmakh vozrastnogo razvitiia kollagenovyk struktur. **Patol Fiziol Eksp Ter** 1981 Mar–Apr;(2):30–9

# GYNECOLOGY

See also **Birth Control; Generation and Reproduction; Obstetrics**

Caffaratto TM: Dalle origini. **Minerva Ginecol** 1984 Sep;36(9):541–66
Fergusson IL, Taylor RW, Watson JM, ed: Records and curiosities in obstetrics and gynaecology. London, Baillière Tindall, 1982. x, 115 p.
Fourcroy JL: L'éternel couteau: review of female circumcision. **Urology** 1983 Oct;22(4):458–61
Fox A: Obstetrics and Gynecology in Macbeth. **Shakespeare Stud** 1979;12:127–41
Knibiehler Y, Fouquet C: La femme et les médecins. Analyse historique. [Paris], Hachette, 1983. 333 p.
Kraatz H: Gedanken zur Geschichte der Frauenheilkunde. **Zentralbl Gynakol** 1981;103(11):593–616
Pecker A: Gynäkologie und Geburtshilfe vom Altertum bis zum Anfang des 18. Jahrhunderts. In Sournia JC, Martiny M, Poulet J, ed: Illustrierte Geschichte der Medizin. Salzburg, Andreas, 1980. Vol. 3. p. 1023–73.
Pickering MJ: A history of elderly exercises. **J Fla Med Assoc** 1980 Apr;67(4):398–400
Snyder CC: The beginnings. **Clin Plast Surg** 1980 Apr;7(2):137–9
Thornton JL, Want PC: Antique books in the library of the Royal College

of Obstetricians and Gynaecologists. **Br J Obstet Gynaecol** 1981 Apr;88(4):337–45
Wilbush J: La menespausie---the birth of a syndrome. **Maturitas** 1979;1(3):145–51

**Bulgaria**

Stoimenov G: Istoriia na bŭlgarskoto akusherstvo i ginekologiia. **Akush Ginekol (Sofiia)** 1980;19(5–6):395–401

**Spain**

Botella Llusiá J: La ginecología de Cataluña vista por un madrileño. In Congrés International d'Història de la Medicina Catalana, 2nd, Barcelona, 1975. Llibre d'Actes. Barcelona, Socitra, 1977. p. 163–84.

**United States**

Leavitt JW, ed: Women and health in America: historical readings. Madison, University of Wisconsin Press, 1984. ix, 526 p. (Previously published articles by various authors)

**Before 500 A.D.**

Dumont M: Curieuses observations anciennes d'inversion utérine. **J Med Lyon** 1978;59:503–5
Steinfeld AD, McDuff HC: An ancient report of a dermoid cyst of the vagina. **Surg Gynecol Obstet** 1980 Jan;150(1):95–6

**Egypt**

Diener L: Från antikonception till amning - om tillökning i familjen i det faraoniska Egypten. **Nord Medicinhist Arsbok** 1983;:41–58

**Greco-Roman**

Grensemann H: Eine jüngere Schicht in den gynäkologischen Schriften. In La collection hippocratique et son rôle dans l'histoire de la médecine. Colloque de Strasbourg (23–27 octobre 1972) organisé par le Centre de Recherches sur la Grèce Antique, avec le concours des Facultés de Philosophie et des Langues Classiques. Leiden, E. J. Brill, 1975. p. 151–69.

**Greece**

Bobbio S: Sorano de Efeso. **Femina** 1979;7:791–6
Grensemann H, ed: Hippokratische Gynäkologie. Die gynäkologischen Texte des Autors C nach den pseudohippokratischen Schriften De muliebribus I, II, und De sterilibus. Wiesbaden, Steiner, 1982. 191 p.
Hanson AE: Hippocrates: Diseases of women. 1. **Signs** 1975;1:567–84

**500 A.D.–1450**

Jacquart D: Un jalon dans l'histoire du syndrome hystérique. La 'suffocation de la matrice' dans la tradition médicale médiévale. **Penelope** 1983;(8):7–9
Pinto LB: The folk practice of gynecology and obstetrics in the Middle Ages. **Bull Hist Med** 1973 Sep–Oct;47(5):513–23
Thomasen AL: 'Historia animalium' contra 'Gynaecia' in der Literatur des Mittelalters. **Clio Med** 1980;15(1/2):5–23

**Arabic**

Gewargis AA: Gynäkologisches aus dem Kamil as-Sina a At Tibbiya des Ali ibn Al-Abbas Al-Magusi. Die Abschnitte über Anatomie, Pathologie und konservative Therapie des nichtschwangeren Uterus. Diss. Erlangen-Nürnberg, 1980. 153 p.
Weisser U: Beiträge Ibn Sina's zur Kenntnis der weiblichen Genitalien und zur Embryologie. Eine kritische Betrachtung. In International Congress of the History of Medicine, 27th, Barcelona, 1980. Actas. Barcelona, Acadèmia de Ciències Mèdiques de Catalunya i Balears, 1981. p. 761–5.

**Great Britain**

Medieval woman's guide to health: The first English gynecological handbook. Middle English text, with introduction and Modern English translation by B. Rowland. Kent, Kent State University Press, 1981. xvii, 192 p.

**Italy**

Caffaratto TM: Rilettura e commento dell'opera 'De Mulierum passionibus' di Trotula de Ruggiero, o Trocta Salernitana. **Minerva Med** 1981 Nov 17;72(46):3123–31
Rowland B: Exhuming Trotula, sapiens matrona of Salerno. **Florilegium** 1979;1:42–57

**Spain**

Vázquez de Benito C, Herrera MT: Dos capitulos ginecologicos: arabe y castellano. **Asclepio** 1981;33:183–241

**1450–1700**

**Europe**

Ozment S: The family in Reformation Germany: the bearing and rearing of children. **J Fam Hist** 1983 Summer;8(2):159–76

**Great Britain**

Eccles A: Obstetrics and gynaecology in Tudor and Stuart England. Kent, Kent State University Press, 1982. 145 p.
Huard P, Imbault-Huart MJ: Les étapes du traitement des tumeurs par ischémie, priorité de Harvey. **Hist Sci Med** 1980;14(2):171–5
Porst S: Gynäkologie und Geburtshilfe bei Shakespeare. **Zentralbl Gynakol** 1984;106(12):863–75
Porst S: Gynäkologische, geburtshilfliche, embryologische und teratologische Beschreibungen im Werke Shakespeares. Würzburg, Horst Wellm, 1981. 178 p. (Dissertation, Julius-Maximilians-Universität Würzburg).

**Italy**

Maeder H: Die Frau im 17. Jahrhundert im Spiegel der 'Quaestiones medico-legales' des Paolo Zacchia (1584–1659). Diss. Bern, 1981. 101 p.

**1700 to Present**

Bauer C, Ritt L: 'The little health of ladies.' An anatomy of female invalidism in the nineteenth century. **J Am Med Wom Assoc** 1981 Oct;36(10):300–6
Becker V: Carl Ruge: 100 Jahre Stückchen-Diagnose. **Arch Gynecol** 1979 Sep;227(3):193–204
Blönningen J: Die Osteomalazie als Indikation für eine bilaterale Oophorektomie im späten 19. und frühen 20. Jahrhundert. Ergebnisse und Erklärungsversuche. Diss. Erlangen-Nürnberg, 1980. 113 p.
Burger G: Nerven- und Geisteskrankheiten als Indikationen für eine bilaterale Oophorektomie im späten 19. Jahrhundert. Diss. Erlangen-Nürnberg, 1984. 185 p.
Curtis CH: Autotransfusion in gynecologic hemoperitoneum. **Am J Obstet Gynecol** 1983 Jul 1;146(5):501–4
Danilischina EI, Schneck P: D. O. Ott (1855–1929) und die russisch-deutschen medizinischen Beziehungen. **Z Arztl Fortbild (Jena)** 1981 Oct 1;75(19):924–7
Dieckmann I: Untersuchungen des menschlichen Endometriums durch Hanns Kundrat (1845–1893) und George Julius Engelmann (1847–1903). Diss. Erlangen-Nürnberg, 1980. 73 p.
Fischer-Homberger E: 'Krankheit Frau'. In Imhof AE, ed: Leib und Leben in der Geschichte der Neuzeit. Berlin, Duncker & Humblot, 1983. p. 215–29.
Funk TG: Uterine Fibromyome und Blutungen als Indikation für eine bilaterale Oophorektomie im späten 19. Jahrhundert. Diss. Erlangen-Nürnberg,1984. 158 p.
Higier J: Sto lat sporu o autorstwo (priorytet) operacji pośrodkowego zeszycia pochwy (colpocleisis mediana) 1881–1981. **Ginekol Pol** 1982;53(3)
Holle S: Die Widerlegung des Postulates von der Gleichzeitigkeit der Ovulation und Menstruation bei der Frau. Klinische und histologische Untersuchungen im frühen 20. Jahrhundert. Diss. Erlangen-Nürnberg, 1984. 100 p.
Honegger C: Überlegungen zur Medikalisierung des weiblichen Körpers. In Imhof AE, ed: Leib und Leben in der Geschichte der Neuzeit. Berlin, Duncker & Humblot, 1983. p. 203–13.
Lenzi E: Nota informativa sull'U.P.I.G.O. e sull'U.E.M.S. **Minerva Ginecol** 1981 Feb–Mar;33(2–3):153–5
Mielke HP: Brustgläser, Uringläser und Urinale. Zur Typologie dreier im medizinischen Gebrauch beheimateter Gläser. In Göpfert W, Otten HH, ed: Metavoeite: wandelt euch durch neues Denken. Düsseldorf, Triltsch, 1983. p. 209–12.
Mitchinson W: Gynecological operations on the insane. **Archivaria** 1980 Summer;10:125–44
Muller P: Geschichte der Gynäkologie vom 18. Jahrhundert bis zur Gegenwart. In Sournia JC, Martiny M, Poulet J, ed: Illustrierte Geschichte der Medizin. Salzburg, Andreas, 1980. Vol. 4. p. 1311–57.
Shorter E: Women's diseases before 1900. In M. Albin, R. J. Devlin, G. Heeger, ed: New directions in psychohistory. The Adelphi papers in honor of Erik H. Erikson. Lexington, Toronto, D. C. Heath, 1980. p. 183–208.
Simmer HH: Bilaterale Oophorektomie der Frau im späten 19. Jahrhundert. Zum methodologischen Wert der Kastration für die Entdeckung ovarieller Hormone. **Geburtshilfe Frauenheilkd** 1983 Jun;43 Suppl 1:54–9
Simmer HH: Zur Geschichte der hormonalen Auslösung einer echten

Menstruation. Versuche an menstruierenden Affen und an Frauen in den frühen dreissiger Jahren unseres Jahrhunderts. In Göpfert W, Otten HH, ed: Metavoeite: wandelt euch durch neues Denken. Düsseldorf, Triltsch, 1983. p. 161–71.
Stallworthy J: Progress in gynecologic oncology: a personal retrospective view. **Gynecol Oncol** 1979 Dec;8(3):253–64
Swain G: Les métamorphoses de l'hystérie à la fin du XIX siècle. **Penelope** 1983;(8):13–4

**Australia**

McDonald IA, Cope I, Forster FM: Super Ardua. The Royal College of Obstetricians and Gynaecologists in Australia, 1929–1979. Melbourne, Australian Council RCOG, 1981. iv, 107 p.

**Austria**

Roazen P: The menopause. By Helene Deutsch. **Int J Psychoanal** 1984;65(Pt 1):55–62
Seidenschnur G: Hans Hermann Schmid--Zum 100. Geburtstag. **Zentralbl Gynakol** 1984;106(18):1288–91
Siefert H: Hermann Knaus. **Neue Dtsch Biogr** 1980;12:163–4

**Bulgaria**

Gunev V: Chetvŭrt vek spisanie 'Akusherstvo i ginekologiia'. **Akush Ginekol (Sofiia)** 1983;22(3):242–3

**Canada**

Godfrey CM: Theophilus Mack. In Dictionary of Canadian Biography, 1881–1890. 1982;11:558–9.
Mitchinson W: Causes of disease in women: the case of late 19th century English Canada. In Roland CG, ed: Health, disease and medicine. Toronto, Hannah Institute for the History of Medicine, 1984. p. 381–95.
Mitchinson W: Gynecological operations on insane women: London, Ontario, 1895–1901. **J Soc Hist** 1982;15(3):467–84

**Czechoslovakia**

Balák K: Třicet let výzkumného ústavu MZ CSR. **Cesk Gynekol** 1982 Mar;47(2):81–112
Dopis prof. J. Trapla prof. L. Havláskovi: **Cesk Gynekol** 1983 Feb;48(1):51–5
K 60. narodeninám doc. MUDr. Jána Simku, CSc: **Cesk Gynekol** 1983 Mar;48(2):151–8
Kahle E: Kleinwächter, Ludwig. In Neue Deutsche Biographie 12. 1980. p. 9–10.
Kvíz D: Příspěvek k historiografii moravské gynekologie. **Cesk Gynekol** 1980 Mar;45(2):142–52
Pros JR: Padesát let gynekologické poradny pro sportovkyně. **Cesk Gynekol** 1983 Feb;48(1):55–6
Sebek V: Josef Jerie--jeho život, doba, činnost, zásluhy. **Cesk Gynekol** 1980 Feb;45(1):55–68
Zivotní jubileum prof. MUDr. Františka Gazárka, CSc: **Cesk Gynekol** 1983 Feb;48(1):75–80

**France**

Monroziès M: Au service des femmes. Les services de gynécologie et d'obstétrique de l'hôpital de la Grave à Toulouse, 250 ans d'histoire 1729–1919. Toulouse, Privat, 1980. 88 p.
Wilson LB: Les maladies des femmes: women, charlatanry, and professional medicine in eighteenth–century France. Ph.D. Diss., Stanford University. Palo Alto, 1982. vi, 449 p.

**Germany**

Bayer H: Walter Stoeckel--Leben und Werk. **Zentralbl Gynakol** 1983;105(1):52–5
Danilishina EI: Ernst Bumm (k 125–letiiu so dnia rozhdeniia). **Akush Ginekol (Mosk)** 1984 Jan;(1):69–70
Easton L: Hermann Johannes Pfannenstiel (1862–1909). **Br J Obstet Gynaecol** 1984 Jun;91(6):538–41
Geiger A: Lorenz Heister als Geburtshelfer und gynäkologischer Chirurg. Vergleichende Untersuchung anhand der verschiedenen Auflagen seiner 'Chirurgie'. Zürich, Juris Druck, 1983. 140 p. (Zürcher Medizingeschichtliche Abhandlungen, Neue Reihe, Nr. 162).
Kirchhoff H: 40 Jahre miterlebte wissenschaftliche Forschung auf dem Gebiet der Gynäkologie und Geburtshilfe. **Ther Ggw** 1981 Jul;120(7):654–68
Klausch B, Schwarz R: Die Geschichte der Frauenklinik der Universität Rostock von den Anfängen bis zur Gegenwart. Rostock, Wilhelm–Pieck–Universität, 1980. 31 p.
Kyank H, Möbius W: Zum 100. Geburtstag von Robert Schröder. **Zentralbl Gynakol** 1984;106(15):1092–8
Ober WB: History of the Brenner tumor of the ovary. **Pathol Annu** 1979;14 Pt 2:107–24
Pfister G: The influence of women doctors on the origins of women's sports in Germany. In Borms J, Hebbelinck M, Venerando A, ed: Women and sport. Basel, Karger, 1981. p. 58–65.
Richter K: Die II. Frauenklinik der Universität München und Richard Fikentscher. **MMW** 1983 Sep 23;125(38):827–30
Rihner F: Alfred Hegar--Zum 150. Geburtstag. **Med Welt** 1980 Oct 17;31(42):1522–3
Schneck P: Ernst Bumm (1858–1925) und die Gynäkologie seiner Zeit. Eine bioergographische Skizze anlässlich seines 125. Geburtstages. **Zentralbl Gynakol** 1983;105(10):662–5
Schneck P: Frauenheilkunde und Geburtshilfe in der Zeit des deutschen Faschismus 1933 bis 1945--Zum Schicksal der sozialen Gynäkologie im 'Dritten Reich'. **Z Gesamte Hyg** 1983 Oct;29(10):645–7
Schneck P: Max Hirsch (1877–1948)--der Mitbegründer der sozialgynäkologischen Forschungrichtung. **Zentralbl Gynakol** 1983;105(24):1600–4
Schneck P: Wilhelm Liepmann (1878–1939)--ein Gynäkologenschicksal zwischen Kaiserreich und faschistischer Diktatur. **Zentralbl Gynakol** 1984;106(17):1223–8
Schneck P: Wilhelm Liepmann (1878–1939) und die soziale Gynäkologie im Spiegel der Aktenbestände des Archivs der Humboldt–Universität zu Berlin. **NTM** 1980;17(2):102–20
Schneck P: Zum Wandel ärztlich–ethischer und deontologischer Auffassungen auf dem Gebiete der Frauenheilkunde während des ersten Drittels des 20. Jahrhunderts. **Z Gesamte Hyg** 1984 Apr;30(4):246–8
Semm K, Giese KP: Ernst Gräfenberg, das Leben und Werk des Kieler Facharztes. Zum 100. Geburtstag am 26. September 1981. **Geburtshilfe Frauenheilkd** 1981 Jun;41(6):444–8
Semm K, Giese KP: Ernst Gräfenberg: the life and work of the specialist of Kiel on the hundredth anniversary of his birth on 26 September 1881. **Int J Fertil** 1983;28(3):141–8
Spitzbart H: Hugo Sellheim (1871 – 1936). **Zentralbl Gynakol** 1984;106(10):693–5

**Great Britain**

Classic articles in colonic and rectal surgery: James Young Simpson 1811–1870. **Dis Colon Rectum** 1982 Sep;25(6):611–22
Edwards SS: Femina sexualis: medico–legal control in Victoriana. **Soc Soc Hist Med Bull (Lond)** 1981 Jun;28:17–20
Harrison B: Women's health and the women's movement in Britain: 1840–1940. In C. Webster, ed: Biology, medicine and society 1840–1940. Cambridge, Cambridge University Press, 1981. p. 15–71.
Peel J: Sir Eardley Lancelot Holland. In Dictionary of national biography, 1961–1970. Suppl. 8, 1981. p. 525–7.
Peel J: The lives of the fellows of the Royal College of Obstetricians and Gynaecologists, 1929–1969. London, Heinemann, 1976. xviii, 390 p.
Sheehan E: Victorian clitoridectomy: Isaac Baker Brown and his harmless operative procedure. **Med Anthropol Newsl** 1981;12(4):9–15
Wilbush J: Historical perspective: Tilt, E. J. and the change of life (1857)--the only work on the subject in the English language. **Maturitas** 1980 Dec;2(4):259–67

**Hungary**

Gyöngyössy A: Kovács Ferenc (1890–1974). **Orv Hetil** 1984 Aug 19;125(34):2085–6

**Ireland**

Browne AD: The section of obstetrics and obstetric and gynaecological development over the century. **Ir J Med Sci** 1983 Jan;152(1):26–38

**Japan**

Ono K, Yamada S: [Hygienic supplies for women used from the end of the Meiji era to the early Showa period: accounts by women who grew up in the Meiji period] (Jpn). **Josanpu Zasshi** 1983 Oct;37(10):819–27

**Norway**

Bergsjø P, Ulstein M: Jørgen Løvset 1896–1981. **Acta Obstet Gynecol Scand** 1982;61(3):193–4

**Philippines**

Agris J: Stamps commemorating medicine. 'Honoria Acosta Sison' pioneer gynecologist and obstetrician. **J Dermatol Surg Oncol** 1980 Mar;6(3):178

**Poland**

Heimrath T: Organizacja wrocławskiej kliniki Kobiecej jako wyraz poglądów medycznych epoki (1890 r.). **Arch Hist Med (Warsz)** 1981;44(3/4):381–4
Heimrath T: Położnictwo i genekologia w Akademii Medycznej we Wrocławiu w latach 1945–1980. **Ginekol Pol** 1982 Jul–Aug;53(7–8):563–8

# GYNECOLOGY

Królikowska M: XXXV-lecie ginekologii i położnictwa w Akademii Medycznej w Lodzi. **Ginekol Pol** 1980 Nov;51(11):973–9
Krzyś J, Krzyś Z: Przebieg pierwszych w Polsce wycieć jajników. **Wiad Lek** 1983 Dec 1;36(23):2005–11
Krzyś J, Krzyś Z: Przebieg pierwszych w Polsce wycieć macicy. **Wiad Lek** 1983 Nov 1;36(21):1827–32
Lembrych S: 25-lecie działalności Opolskiego Oddziału Polskiego Towarzystwa Ginekologicznego. **Ginekol Pol** 1984 Jan;55(1):71–3
Malarewicz A: 50 lat cytodiagnostyki ginekologicznej -- George Nicholas Papanicolaou. **Arch Hist Med (Warsz)** 1978;41(4):465–8
Waszyński E: 'Primitiae physico-medicae ...' (1750–1753). Problematyka połozniczo-ginekologiczna. **Arch Hist Med (Warsz)** 1984;47(3):447–61

**Scandinavia**

Asplund J: The Scandinavian Association of Obstetricians and Gynecologists 1933–1983. **Acta Obstet Gynecol Scand [Suppl]** 1984;120:9–26
Borell U: Opening speech at the 50th anniversary congress of the Scandinavian Association of Obstetricians and Gynecologists in Stockholm, January 28–29, 1983. **Acta Obstet Gynecol Scand [Suppl]** 1984;120:5–7
Kjellgren O: The development of gynecological oncology in Scandinavia during the last 50 years. **Acta Obstet Gynecol Scand [Suppl]** 1984;120:27–34

**Singapore**

Ratnam SS, Karim SM, Ng CS, et al: Research and development in obstetrics and gynaecology in the Department of Obstetrics and Gynaecology at the National University of Singapore. **Ann Acad Med Singapore** 1982 Jul;11(3):313–21

**South Africa**

Daubenton F: Professor Cuthbert Crichton--the man and his times. **S Afr Med J** 1979 Dec 15;56(25):1064–75
Sharp RG: Tribute to a great teacher. **S Afr Med J** 1979 Dec 15;56(25):1059–64

**Spain**

Rodríguez García JR: Circulacion mundial de la obstetricia y ginecologia española a traves de Excerpta Medica (1951–71). **Asclepio** 1980;32:401–14
Simón Palmer M del C: Las neurosis femeninas y la educación española. **Asclepio** 1983;35:327–42

**Sweden**

Hagenfeldt K: Dramatiskt minskad mödramortalitet. Framsynta åsikter i abortfrågan. **Lakartidningen** 1983 Nov 9;80(45):4299–302
Kock W: Sven Sköldberg och ovariotomien en pionjärinsats i svensk gynekologi. **Nord Medicinhist Arsbok** 1983;:103–16
Stolt CM, Oberg L: En ovariotomi i Borås 1814. **Sydsven Medicinhist Sallsk Arsskr** 1984;21:109–21

**Switzerland**

Stamm H: 75 Jahre Société de Gynécologie et d'Obstétrique de la Suisse Romande--70 Jahre Gynäkologische Gesellschaft der deutschen Schweiz. **Gesnerus** 1981;38(3/4):313–30

**United States**

Barker-Benfield GJ: A historical perspective on women's health care--female circumcision. **Women Health** 1976 Jan–Feb;1(1):13–15,18–20
Breathnach CS: Biographical sketches no. 36 -- Sims. **Ir Med J** 1984 Jan;77(1):27
Bullough VL: Female physiology, technology and women's liberation. In Trescott, Martha Moore, ed. Dynamos and Virgins revisited: Women and technological change in history. Metuchen, N. J., Scarecrow Pr., 1979. p. 236–51.
Chesley LC: Evolution of the Department of Obstetrics and Gynecology at Downstate, 1860–1980. [New York?, s.n., 1982?] 96 p.
Cohen MR: A tribute to Martin J. Clyman, M.D., 1914–1979. **J Reprod Med** 1983 Apr;28(4):233–4
Dittmer I: James Marion Sims. 1813–1883. **MMW** 1984 Feb 10;126(6):159–60
Djordjević S: Dr. George N. Papanicolaou (13. V 1883--19. II 1962). **Srp Arh Celok Lek** 1983 May;111(5):699–703
Dwork D: Sophia Josephine Kleegman. In: Notable American women. The modern period. Cambridge, Mass., Belknap-Harvard Univ. Press, 1980. 4:398–400.
Fellman AC, Fellman M: Man amuck. **Rev Am Hist** 1976;4(4):558–64
Gordon L: Lena Levine. In: Notable American women. The modern period. Cambridge, Mass., Belknap-Harvard Univ. Press, 1980. 4:419–20.
Grubb JM: The first successful cesarean section and the first oophorectomy in the Americas. **W Va Med J** 1984 Oct;80(10):221–3
Hill EC: The Rubin test. **JAMA** 1983 Nov 4;250(17):2366–8
Kase NG: Gynecologic endocrinology and infertility. A tribute to Martin J. Clyman, M.D. **J Reprod Med** 1983 Apr;28(4):231–2
Keettel WC: A history of the Department of Obstetrics & Gynecology, the University of Iowa, 1848–1980. Iowa City, University of Iowa, 1981. xi, 186 p.
Kelly HA: Pre-1933 history of gynecology in Maryland. Part 1. **Md State Med J** 1980 Mar;29(3):81–5
Kelly HA: Pre-1933 history of gynecology in Maryland. Part 2. **Md State Med J** 1980 Jul;29(7):21–30
Klosky BA: Daring venture: a biography of Anne Austin Young, pioneer woman doctor. Columbia, S.C., Bryan, 1978. xiii, 193 p.
Levin BS: Women and medicine. Metuchen, N. J., London, Scarecrow, 1980. vii, 257 p.
Longo LD: A short history of the Society for Gynecologic Investigation (1953–1983). Los Angeles, Calif., [s.n.], 1983. 70 p.
McDonell KM: Women and medicine in early nineteenth century Indiana. **Indiana Med Hist Q** 1980;6(2):3–23
McIntosh K: Folk obstetrics, gynecology, and pediatrics in Utica, New York. **NY Folkl** 1978;4(1–4):49–59
Masters WH: Half a century of unnecessary sexual myths. **JAMA** 1983 Jul 8;250(2):244
Puchkov IuG, Buslaeva MM, Volodina MN: Georg Papanikolau (k 100-letiiu so dnia rozhdeniia). **Vopr Onkol** 1983;29(12):87–9
Ramsey EM: The story of spiral arteries. **J Reprod Med** 1981 Aug;26(8):393–9
Ranney B: Geschichte, Organisation und Praxis der amerikanischen Gynäkologie und Geburtshilfe. Eine Ubersicht. **Zentralbl Gynakol** 1984;106(9):626–32
Reproductive immunology. A festschrift in honor of Dr. Saul B. Gusberg.: **Mt Sinai J Med (NY)** 1980 Sep–Oct;47(5):i–vii, 427–560
Saffron MH: Isidor Clinton Rubin. In Dictionary of American Biography, Suppl. 6, 1956–1960. p. 554–6, 1980.
Scully D, Bart P: A funny thing happened on the way to the orifice: women in gynecology textbooks. **Am J Sociol** 1973 Jan;78(4):1045–50
Scully D: [A history of] 'Baby catchers and uterus snatchers'. In her: Men who control women's health; the miseducation of obstetrician-gynecologists. Boston, Houghton Mifflin, 1980. p. 25–67.
Stage S: Female complaints: Lydia Pinkham and the business of women's medicine. New York, Norton, 1979. 304 p.
Stevens R: The changing idea of a medical specialty. **Trans Stud Coll Physicians Phila** 1980 Sep;5(2 no 3):159–77
Sugitani A: [First successful case of intentional laparotomy (author's transl)]. (Jpn) **Nippon Geka Hokan** 1980 Jan 1;49(1):1–2
Taylor ES: Commemorative issue: Georgeanna Seegar Jones, Howard W. Jones, Jr. Twenty-five years as editors-in-chief for Gynecology, Obstetrical & Gynecological Survey. **Obstet Gynecol Surv** 1982 Jun;37(6):355–84
Wetzel N: Loyal Davis; Allen Kanavel; surgery, gynecology and obstetrics, and the development of neurosurgery. **Surg Gynecol Obstet** 1983 Aug;157(2):135–9
Wilbush J: Climacteric symptom formation: Donovan's contribution. **Maturitas** 1981 Aug;3(2):99–105

**USSR**

Gerasimovich GT: Belorusskomu Nauchnomu Meditsinskomu obshchestvu Akusherov-Ginekologov 50 let. **Akush Ginekol (Mosk)** 1981 Sep;(9):59–61
Granat NE: 'Skorbnyĭ list' ginekologicheskoĭ bol'noĭ kontsa XIX stoletiia. **Med Sestra** 1979 Dec;38(12):51–5
Manuilova IM, Chervakova TV: Uspekhi otechestvennoĭ akushersko-ginekologicheskoĭ nauki k 60-letiiu obrazovaniia SSSR. **Sov Med** 1982;(12):35–41
Mirskiĭ MB, Verbitskiĭ VM, Khil'chenko MA: K 170-letiiu so dnia rozhdeniia A. A. Kitera. **Akush Ginekol (Mosk)** 1983 Sep;(9):72–3
Sol'skiĭ IP: Razvitie i dostizheniia akushersko-ginekologicheskoĭ sluzhby v USSR. **Akush Ginekol (Mosk)** 1982 Sep;(9):3–5
60 Let deiatel'nosti zhurnala 'Akusherstvio i ginekologiia': **Akush Ginekol (Mosk)** 1982;(12):16–7

**Yugoslavia**

Berić B, Rajković D, Babić-Ilić N: Dr Nikola Hadži-Nikolić (1855–1915) prvi akušer-ginekolog u Srbiji i Njegov značaj za razvoj akušerstva i ginekologije u Srbiji. **Jugosl Ginekol Opstet** 1981 Dec;21(5–6):143–8
Berić BM: Dr Eva Haljecka (18??–1947) prva žena akušer-ginekolog u jugoslovenskim zemljama. **Jugosl Ginekol Opstet** 1983 May–Aug;23(3–4):95–9
Berić BM: Prvi ginekolog-akušer u Vojvodini--dr Aleksander Sosberger (1873–1944). **Jugosl Ginekol Opstet** 1984 May–Aug;24(3–4):71–2
Juvan V: Djelatnost za zdravstvenu zaštitu žena Medicinskog centra u Varaždinu. **Jugosl Ginekol Opstet** 1978;18(5–6):445–53

## HEALTH EDUCATION

See also **Hygiene; Preventive Medicine; Public Health**

Moore PV, Williamson GC: Health promotion. Evolution of a concept. **Nurs Clin North Am** 1984 Jun;19(2):195-206

**Germany**

Rodegra H: Zur Geschichte der Gesundheitserziehung in deutschen Schulen. **Med Welt** 1979 Oct 26;30(43):1615-20

**United States**

Struna NL: Sport and colonial education: a cultural perspective. **Res Q Exerc Sport** 1981 Mar;52(1):117-35

**1700 to Present**

Grosshans OR: Biographical research in health education. **Health Educ (Wash)** 1981 Sep-Oct;12(5):40-1

**Austria**

Gross-Bachmann M: Daniel Sailer, Leben und Wirken eines Idealisten. **Tirol Heimat** 1976;40:163-90

**Belgium**

Velle K: Gezondheidsopvoeding in België in de 19de eeuw. **Spiegel Hist** 1982;17(12):619-25

**China**

Verma A: Birth control and planned parenthood in China. **China Rep (India)** 1971;7(2):41-8

Yip KC: Health and society in China: public health education for the community, 1912-1937. **Soc Sci Med** 1982;16(12):1197-205

**Czechoslovakia**

Ustav zdravotní výchovy: 20 years of health education in the Czech Socialist Republic. Prague, Institute of Health Education, 1973. 31 p.

**Germany**

Alt K: In der Weimarer Zeit war der Rundfunk ein beliebtes Fortbildungs-Instrument. **Zahnarztl Mitt** 1984 Oct 16;74(20):2325-6

Kneist W: Arzte als Gesundheitserzieher von Kindern. **Z Gesamte Hyg** 1982 Apr;28(4):256-9

Ochmann A: Kritische Bemerkungen zur Gesundheitserziehung. **Off Gesundheitswes** 1982 Apr;44(4):230-1

Reis K: Gesundheitserziehung in der DDR - Versuch einer historischen Betrachtung. **Z Gesamte Hyg** 1982 Apr;28(4):253-5

**Great Britain**

Charlton C: The National Health Society Almanack, 1883. **Local Popul Stud (Matlock)** 1984;32:54-7

Fox B, Maddick I: A hundred years of dental health education. **Br Dent J** 1980 Jul 1;149(1):28-32

Towers BA: Health education policy 1916-1926: venereal disease and the prophylaxis dilemma. **Med Hist** 1980 Jan;24(1):70-87

**Hungary**

Antall J: Gesundheitliche Aufklrung und Gesundheitserziehung in Ungarn im 18-19. Jahrhundert. **Orvostort Kozl** 1979;86(24 no 4):25-37

Ferenczy M: Csokonai Vitéz Mihály egészségügyi tanácsai. **Orv Hetil** 1982 Nov 28;123(48):2973-4

**Ireland**

Walsh BM: Health education and the demand for tobacco in Ireland, 1953-76: a note. **Econ Soc Rev (Irel)** 1980;11(2):147-51

**Japan**

Uchibori C: [History of national public health activities in the Gunma Prefecture. 2. Stimulating seminars] (Jpn). **Hokenfu Zasshi** 1982 Feb;38(2):148-50

**Netherlands**

Kerkhoff AH: Het eerste Nederlandstalinge tijdschrift op het terrein van gezondheids- voorlichting in de negentiende eeuw. **Ned Tijdschr Geneeskd** 1981 Nov 21;125(47):1935-40

**United States**

Abish M: A guest's column. **Urology** 1979 Dec;14(6):545-P, 545-V

Brannan JH: A history of health education at the Ohio State University, 1872-1981. Ph.D. Diss., Ohio State University. Columbus, 1981. xi, 579 p.

Contento I: Thinking about nutrition education: what to teach, how to teach it, and what to measure. **Teach Coll Rec** 1980;81(4):421-47

Edwards R: Graham-Kellogg, early American contributors to health education. **J Sch Health** 1981 Nov;51(9):589-91

Gussow JD: Food and nutrition education: a redefinition. **Teach Coll Rec** 1980;81(4):411-6

Gussow JD: Who pays the piper? **Teach Coll Rec** 1980;81(4):448-66

Imber M: Analysis of a curriculum reform movement: the American Social Hygiene Association's campaign for sex education 1900-1930. Ph.D. Diss., Stanford University. Stanford, 1981. v, 173 leaves.

Imber M: The First World War, sex education, and the American Social Hygiene Association's campaign against venereal disease. **J Educ Adm Hist** 1984;16(1):47-56

Neilson EA: Reflections on health promotion through health education historical perspectives: options for the future. **Health Values** 1980 Jul-Aug;4(4):161-7

Notle A, Brannan J: Through the looking glass: health education curriculum. **Health Educ (Wash)** 1979 Nov-Dec;10(6):5-11

Penland L: A decade of dental health education: review of the 1970s. **Dent Hyg (Chic)** 1982 Sep;56(9):16-8, 20-2

Penland LR: Sex education in 1900, 1940 and 1980: an historical sketch. **J Sch Health** 1981 Apr;51(4):305-9

Reed J: Louise Frances Stevens Bryant. In Dictionary of American Biography, Suppl. 6, 1956-1960. p. 80-2, 1980.

Rice CN: The history of the Society of State Directors of Health, physical education, and recreation, 1953-1976. Ed.D. Diss., University of Alabama. University, 1977. v, 199 p.

Selections from The health-education series. New York, Arno, 1977. Various paginations. (Reprint of articles published in Boston between 1906 and 1910).:

Strong B: Ideas of the early sex education movement in America, 1890-1920. **Hist Educ Q** 1972;12(2):129-62

Strong C: Historical research: does it apply to health education? **Health Educ (Wash)** 1981 Jul-Aug;12(4):34-5

Tank RM: Young children, families, and society in America since the 1820s: the evolution of health, education, and child care programs for preschool children. Ph.D. Diss., University of Michigan. Ann Arbor, 1980. v, 471 leaves.

Turner TB: Joseph Earle Moore. In Dictionary of American Biography, Suppl. 6, 1956-1960. p, 460-1, 1980.

Welch JE: Pioneering in health education and services at Amherst College. **J Am Coll Health** 1982 Jun;30(6):289-95

Young JH: Adelle Davis. In: Notable American women. The modern period. Cambridge, Mass., Belknap-Harvard Univ. Press, 1980. 4:179-80.

**USSR**

Iskhakov SI: Razvitie sanitarnogo prosveshcheniia v Tadzhikskoĭ SSR. **Feldsher Akush** 1982;47(11):26-9

Kulak VM, Evdokimov PP: Iz istorii sanitarnogo prosveshcheniia v Simbirskoĭ gubernii i Ul'ianovskoĭ oblasti. **Sov Zdravookhr** 1979;(10):62-4

Kvitnitskiĭ-Ryzhov IuN: Iz istorii populiarizatsii meditsinskikh znaniĭ v Rosii. L.M. Chichagov i ego 'Meditsinskie besedy'. **Sov Zdravookhr** 1984;(8):66-70

## HEALTH OCCUPATIONS AND PROFESSIONS

Novak DE: Dental auxiliary evolution: a historical perspective. **Dent Assist** 1984 Sep-Oct;53(5):17-22

Reiser SJ: Technology, specialization, and the allied health professions. **J Allied Health** 1983 Aug;12(3):177-82

The residents: **MD** 1978 Jul;22(7):89-99

**Belgium**

Daem M: Van baardemaker tot barbier (Gentse chirurgijn-barbiers). Brussel, Aurelia Books, 1976. 170 p. (Aureliae Folklorica, no. 9).

**Canada**

Gelfand T: Who practised medicine in New France?: a collective portrait. In Roland CG, ed: Health, disease and medicine. Toronto, Hannah Institute for the History of Medicine, 1984. p. 16-35.

**Great Britain**

Dobson J: Some associations of St. Thomas's Hospital with the Company of Barber-Surgeons of London. **St Thomas Hosp Gaz** 1981;79:73-8

**Switzerland**

Fehlmann HR: Beziehungen zwischen Arzt und Apotheker im 16. bis 18. Jahrhundert in der Schweiz. **Gesnerus** 1983;40(1-2):67-74

**500 A.D.-1450**

**Great Britain**

Gottfried RS: English medical practitioners, 1340-1530. **Bull Hist Med** 1984 Summer;58(2):164-82

**1450-1700**

**Great Britain**

Pelling M: A survey of East Anglian medical practitioners 1500-1640. **Local Popul Stud (Matlock)** 1980;:(25):54-5
Pelling M: Occupational diversity: barbersurgeons and the trades of Norwich, 1550-1640. **Bull Hist Med** 1982;56(4):484-511

**1700 to Present**

The changing look of dental assisting: **Dent Assist** 1984 Sep-Oct;53(5):23-6
Colón Roure C, Rivera Nieves M: La intervención del terapista ocupacional en el equipo interdisciplinario en el area de la salud mental. **Bol Asoc Med PR** 1984 Jul;76(7):319-22
Heidenheimer AJ: Organized medicine and physician specialization in Scandinavia and West Germany. **West Eur Polit** 1980;3(3):373-87
Levine RE: A historical perspective on professional values. **J Allied Health** 1983 Aug;12(3):183-91
Paciorkiewicz M: Izby lekarskie. Przyczynki do dziejów. **Pol Tyg Lek** 1982 Jul 5;37(21):621-4
Shortt SE: Physicians, science, and status: issues in the professionalization of Anglo-American medicine in the nineteenth century. **Med Hist** 1983 Jan;27(1):51-68
Tornero N: O emprego de auxiliares de saúde em áreas em desenvolvimento: breve histórico. **Rev Saude Publica** 1979 Sep;13(3):254-61
Wattley LA: Male physicians and female health and sexuality in 19th century English and American society. **J Adv Nurs** 1983 Sep;8(5):423-8
Werner R: Medicine men (traditional medical practitioners) in primary health care and the role of traditional medicine towards modern medicine. **Off Gesundheitswes** 1980;42(9):637-56

**Austria**

Wimmer J: Die medizinisch-technische Assistentin in Osterreich: eine entwicklungsgeschichtliche Berufskunde oder eine berufskundliche Entwicklungsgeschichte. Wien, Maudrich, 1983. xii, 79 p.

**Canada**

Bernier J: Les practiciens de la santé à Québec, 1871-1921: quelques données statistiques. **Rech Sociogr** 1979;20(1):41-58
Boase J: Regulation and the paramedical professions: an interest group study. **Can Public Adm** 1982;25(3):332-53
Coburn D, Torrance GM, Kaufert JM: Medical dominance in Canada in historical perspective: the rise and fall of medicine? **Int J Health Serv** 1983;13(3):407-32
Howell CD: Reform and the monopolistic impulse: the professionalization of medicine in the Maritimes. **Acadiensis** 1981;11(1):3-22
Kutcher SP: Toronto's metaphysicians: the social gospel and medical professionalization in Victorian Toronto. **HSTC Bull** 1981;5(1):41-51
Tumbridge JE: Home-workplace separation in Kingston: the legal and medical professions - past, present and future. **Urban Hist Rev** 1982;11(1):11-6

**Chile**

Pérez G: Evolución de los recursos humanos y físicos de salud 1952-1977. **Rev Med Chil** 1977 Oct;105(10):732-8

**China**

Lisowski FP: The emergence and development of the barefoot doctor in China. **East Horiz** 1980;19(4):6-20
Rosenthal MM, Greiner JR: The barefoot doctors of China: from political creation to professionalization. **Hum Organ** 1982;41(4):330-41
Yü Ming: Barefoot doctors in mainland China: a unique medical corps. **Issues Stud** 1978;14(2):53-64

**Colombia**

Mallarino Paz A: Sintesis historica de los programas de personal auxiliar de odontologia en Colombia. **Rev Fac Odontol Univ Nac Colomb** 1980 Jan-Mar;27(132):50-2

**Czechoslovakia**

Remišová M: Národnostná otázka v stavovskom živote lekárov na Slovensku v prvej CSR. **Cesk Zdrav** 1983 Jul;31(6):260-5

**France**

Léonard J: Les médecins au XIXe siècle. **Histoire** 1978;4:15-23
Petrequin J: Un manuel pour le service des malades. **Rev Infirm** 1982 Oct;32(16):17-9

**Germany**

Clasen U: Deutsche und deutschstämmige Arzte in New South Wales und South Australia zwischen 1846 und 1911. Diss., Universität Düsseldorf. Düsseldorf, 1982. 66 p.
Heller R: Johann Christian Reil's training scheme for medical auxiliaries. **Med Hist** 1975 Oct;19(4):321-32
Hinze E: Feldscherer und Feldmedici in deutschen wie fremden Heeren und Flotten. (Biographisches Lexikon deutscher Militärärzte bis 1870) Band I. Hannover, Im Selbstverlag, 1979. 43 p.
Spree R: The impact of the professionalization of physicians on social change in Germany during the late 19th and early 20th century. **Hist Soc Res** 1980;15:24-39

**Great Britain**

Brown PS: Defining the medical profession in mid-nineteenth century Bristol. **Bristol Med Chir J** 1981 Jan-Apr;96(357-358):4-7
Crowther MA: Paupers or patients? Obstacles to professionalization in the Poor Law medical service before 1914. **J Hist Med Allied Sci** 1984 Jan;39(1):33-54
Loudon I: Two thousand medical men in 1847. **Soc Soc Hist Med Bull (Lond)** 1983 Dec;33:4-8
Weir JG: The way they lived then. **Br Med J [Clin Res]** 1982 Dec 18-25;285(6357):1809-10

**Hungary**

Kapronczay K: Orvosi érdekvédelem a múlt század végén. **Orv Hetil** 1982 Sep 19;123(38):2373-5

**Norway**

Hjort EF: Rekruttering av Norges leger på 1800-tallet. **Tidsskr Nor Laegeforen** 1983 May 20;103(14):1149-54

**Poland**

Czeley-Wybieralska M: Nobilitacje lekarzy i aptekarzy w Królestwie Polskim w latach 1817-1861. **Arch Hist Med (Warsz)** 1983;46(2):205-4

**Singapore**

Lee YK: The origins of medical registration in Singapore (Part I). **Singapore Med J** 1983 Oct;24(5):314-22

**Spain**

Marset Campos P, Saturno Hernández PJ: Los sanitarios murcianos de 1750 a 1850. Evolucion numerica, tipos profesionales y procendencia geografica. **Asclepio** 1980;32:255-70
Ortiz Gómez T: El profesional medico en Andalucia: evolucion y distribucion de los medicos en la provincia de Granada (1901-1981). **Dynamis** 1982;2:325-51

**Sweden**

Thomasson J: Arbetsmiljö, förhandlingar, MBL, behörighet och utbildning. En kort berättelse om SHSTFs första fem år. **Vardfacket** 1982 Jan 14;6(1):34-6

**Switzerland**

Wankmüller A: Die Tätigkeit deutscher Apotheker-Gehilfen in der Schweiz im 19. Jahrhundert. **Beitr Gesch Pharm** 1983;31(21):41-3

**United States**

Beardsley EH: Making separate, equal: black physicians and the problems of medical segregation in the pre-World War II South. **Bull Hist Med** 1983 Fall;57(3):382-96
Bosk CL: The doctors. **Wilson Q** 1980;4(2):75-86
Day HG: E. V. McCollum and dietitians in nutrition education. **J Am Diet Assoc** 1980 Feb;76(2):126-7
Drachman VG: Female solidarity and professional success: the dilemma of women doctors in late nineteenth-century America. **J Soc Hist**

1982;15(4):607–19

Duffy J: American perceptions of the medical, legal, and theological professions. **Bull Hist Med** 1984 Spring;58(1):1–15

Falk LA: Black Abolitionist doctors and healers, 1810–1885. **Bull Hist Med** 1980 Summer;54(2):258–72

Grob GN, ed: The medical professions and drug addiction: six studies, 1882–1832. New York, Arno, 1981. various pagings. Reprinted works.

Hamilton WA, Hamilton PR: Sex and the dental practice: a reinterpretation of the history of dental hygienists. **Bull Hist Dent** 1980 Oct;28(2):64–8

King LS: Medicine in the USA: historical vignettes. XXII. Medical practice: making a living. **JAMA** 1984 Apr 13;251(14):1887–92

Mooring PK: Residency training. **MD** 1978 Jul;22(7):23, 27

Morrow CK: Sick doctors: the social construction of professional deviance. **Soc Probl** 1982;30(1):92–108

Powsner R: Women physicians--expanding the domain. **Mich Med** 1983 Aug;82(37):483–4, 502

Sekscenski ES: The health services industry: a decade of expansion. **Mon Labor Rev** 1981;104(5):9–16

Shortt SE: Approaches to the physician's life. **Bull Hist Med** 1981 Spring;55(1):124–7

Summerville J: Formation of a black medical profession in Tennessee, 1880–1920. **J Tenn Med Assoc** 1983 Oct;76(10):644–6

Supply of manpower in selected health occupations: 1950–1990. Hyattsville, U. S. Bureau of Health Professions, 1980. xiii, 62 p:

Vittetoe MC: Development of administrative roles for medical technologists. **Am J Med Technol** 1982 Sept;48(9):727–31

Weiss GN, Weiss EB: The health care profession on the threshold of the eighties: physician and nurse. **J La State Med Soc** 1980 Oct;132(10):151–4

75 years of dental hygiene education.: **Dent Hyg (Chic)** 1980 Mar;54(3):115–7

### USSR

Frieden NM: Russian physicians in an era of reform and revolution, 1856–1905. Princeton, Princeton University Press, 1981. xvii, 378 p.

Furmanchuk VM: Uchastie rabochikh sester i sanitarok v Oktiabr'skoĭ revoliutsii. **Med Sestra** 1982 Apr;41(4):49–51

Gel'fman AA: Fel'dshera-iskrovtsy v revoliutsionnom dvizhenii. **Feldsher Akush** 1984 Apr;49(4):49–50

Hutchinson JF: Society, corporation or Union? Russian physicians and the struggle for professional unity (1890–1913). **Jahrb Gesch Osteur** 1982;30(1):37–53

Ianovskiĭ AG: Fel'dshera i akusherki v revoliutsii 1905–1907 gg. **Feldsher Akush** 1980;45(11):41–4

Il'in AI: Iz istorii sanitarnogo prosveshcheniia vo Vladimirskoĭ gubernii v zemskiĭ period. **Gig Sanit** 1984 Jun;(6):32–5

Ionov IuV, Ionov AIu: Fel'dsher P. K. Beletskiĭ--pisatel', publitsist, étnograf, obshchestvennyĭ deiatel'. **Feldsher Akush** 1982;47(1):55–8

Ionov IuV: Fel'dshera i meditsinskie sestry--sportsmeny. **Feldsher Akush** 1980;45(7):5–7

Khromchenko OM, Sapegina AV: Dvadtsatipiatletniĭ opyt usovershenstvovaniia rukovodiashchikh kadrov sanitarno-épidemiologicheskoĭ sluzhby v Tsentral'nom institute usovershenstvovaniia vracheĭ. **Gig Sanit** 1981 Mar;(3):51–3

Korsunskiĭ MA: Voennyĭ fel'dsher P. E. Lazimir. **Feldsher Akush** 1980;45(12):41–4

Lobanov GP, Zhuravskiĭ VA: Nekotorye voprosy organizatsii spetsial'noĭ podgotovki lichnogo sostava voenno-meditsinskoĭ sluzhby v period Voĭny. **Voen Med Zh** 1980 May;(5):28–33

Miliavskiĭ VM: K istorii prepodavaniia psikhiatrii v fel'dsherskikh shkolakh. **Feldsher Akush** 1982;47(4):53–4

Moskovskomu gorodskomu sovetu sanitarnykh fel'dsherov i laborantov 25 let: **Feldsher Akush** 1980;45(2):57–9

Shabunin AV: P. F. Lesgaft i razvitie fel'dshersko-akusherskogo obrazovaniia v Rossii. **Feldsher Akush** 1981;46(4):57–8

Tsvetkov VL: Srednie meditsinskie rabotniki Orlovskoĭ gubernii v XIX veke. **Med Sestra** 1983 Oct;42(10):49–50

Viduta VK: Tobol'skaia fel'dsherskaia shkola i ee rol' v formirovanii revoliutsionerov. **Sov Zdravookhr** 1984;(8):57–9

### Yugoslavia

Rajkov M: Jedan popis zdravstvenih radnika u velikokikindskom dištriktu 1875. Godine. **Naucni Sastanak Zb Rad Naucno Drus Istor Zdrav Kult Jugosl** 1976;(13):157–62

## HEMATOLOGY

See also **Blood Transfusion; Cardiology and Circulatory System**

Bassis M, Delpech G: Discovery of the red blood cell with notes on priorities and credits of discoveries, past, present and future. **Blood Cells** 1981;7(3):447–80

Bernard J: Le sang et l'histoire. Paris, Buchet/Chastel, 1983. 157 p.

Verso ML: The evolution of haemoglobinometry: and other essays on the history of haematology. Melbourne, Trefusis Publications, 1981. 105 p.

Wintrobe MM: Perspective in hematology. **Pharos** 1983 Winter;46(1):7–12

### France

Bernard J: Hématologie et transfusion sanguine. **Nouv Rev Fr Hematol** 1982;24(5):277–9

### Before 500 A.D.

### Mesopotamia

André-Leicknam B: Les premiers écrits médicaux. Le sang en Mésopotamie. **Nouv Rev Fr Hematol** 1983;25(2):141–4

### Spain

Bernard J, Wintrobe M, Faure E, et al: Le sang d'Altamira ou la naissance de l'hématologie. **Nouv Rev Fr Hematol** 1981;23(4):249–51

### 1700 to Present

Binet JL: Aspect des cellules sanguines au XIXe siècle. **Clio Med** 1982 Dec;17(2–3):133–44

Boić V: Hematologija u prvoj polovici našega stoljeća. **Lijec Vjesn** 1980 Feb;102(2):107–8

Caen JP: A propos du hasard et de la nécessité: la découverte du facteur Fletcher (prékallikréine). **Nouv Rev Fr Hematol** 1981 Dec;23(5):309–10

Cirillo VJ: Nineteenth-century views on blood fluidity. **J Med Soc NJ** 1983 Jul;80(7):535–9

Dacie J: Evolution of ideas on the life-span of the red blood cell. **J R Soc Med** 1979 Jun;72(6):417–52

Golliet P, Binet JL: Deux historiens du sang, ou Réponse de Lucien Lévy-Bruhl et de Wifredo Lam à Jean Bernard. **Nouv Rev Fr Hematol** 1983;25(5):337–41

Gutt RW: The development of hematology. **Hexagon Roche** 1981;9(3):9–16

Haight V: A brief history of hemoglobinometry. **Am J Med Technol** 1983 Feb;49(2):127–8

Owen CA: The revolution of concepts of coagulation. **Ann NY Acad Sci** 1981;370:5–10

Robb-Smith AH: Osler's influence on haematology. **Blood Cells** 1981;7(3):513–36

Schneider WH: Chance and social setting in the application of the discovery of blood groups. **Bull Hist Med** 1983 Winter;57(4):545–62

Wintrobe B: Mrs. Wintrobe writes about her husband. **Med Times** 1979 Nov;107(11):59–64

### Argentina

Pavlovsky S, Dosne Pasqualini C: XXV Aniversario 1956–1981: Instituto de Investigaciones Hematológicas Mariano R. Castex, Academia Nacional de Medicina, Buenos Aires. **Medicina (B Aires)** 1981;41 Suppl:1–4

### Brazil

Costa V: HEMOPE, luta pelo sangue. Recife, Fundação de Ensino Superior de Pernambuco, 1979. 129 p.

### Czechoslovakia

Adamec J: Jan Janský. **Cas Lek Cesk** 1983 Sep 23;122(38):1180–2

Donner L: Ctyřicet let od vydání prvé české klinické hematologie. **Vnitr Lek** 1983 Feb;29(2):184–9

Libánský J: Vývoj hematologie od dob profesora Hynka a její další perspektivy. **Vnitr Lek** 1979 Sep;25(9):915–20

Skala E: Kdo objevil krevní skupiny? **Cas Lek Cesk** 1984 Oct 19;123(42):1292–4

### France

Andral G: Pathological hematology: an essay on the blood in disease. Reprint of the 1844 ed. With a historical introduction by L. A. May. Oceanside, N. Y. Dabor Science Publications, 1977. 129 p.

Bernard J: Evolution de l'hématologie. **Nouv Rev Fr Hematol** 1980 Dec;22(4):453–8

Binet JL: Historical notes on quantitative blood cell measurements. **Blood Cells** 1980 Jun;6(3):507–11

Binet JL: Les premiers clichès du sang. **Nouv Rev Fr Hematol** 1981;23(2):135–7

### Germany

Bast G: Viktor Schilling 1883–1983. Selbstzeugnisse und Erinnerungen an den Altmeister der morphologischen Hämatologie. **Folia Haematol (Leipz)** 1983;110(5):617–29

Neumann-Redlin von Meding E: Ernst Neumann. Zum 150. Geburtstag des Königsberger Pathologen und Hämatologen am 30.1. 1984.

Pathologe 1984 Jan;5(1):53-6
Stahnke J: Häminkristalle--Ludwik Teichmanns Blutnachweis. **Medizinhist J** 1981;16(4):391-413
Stobbe H: Viktor Schilling 1883-1983. Sein hämatologisches Lebenswerk unter Bevorzugung der Tätigkeiten in Berlin. **Folia Haematol (Leipz)** 1983;110(5):630-3

**Great Britain**

Dodd BE: Early work on the Rh factor including the finding of anti-E. **Vox Sang** 1984;47(6):449-51
Qvist G: John Hunter, 1728-1793. London, Heinemann, 1981. xvi, 216 p.

**Italy**

Baserga A, Zavagli G: Ferrata's stem cells: an historical review on hemocytoblasts and hemohistioblasts. **Blood Cells** 1981;7(3):537-45
Baserga A: Una descrizione della forma dei globuli rossi dell'emolisi nella Pavia del settecento. **Haematologica (Pavia)** 1980 Feb;65(1):131-34
Coller BS: Bizzozero and the discovery of the blood platelet. **Lancet** 1984 Apr 7;1(8380):804
Giusti GV: Leone Lattes: Italy's pioneer in forensic serology. **Am J Forensic Med Pathol** 1982 Mar;3(1):79-81

**Japan**

Oguro M: [Late Dr. Satoru Inagaki, a member of the Council of the Japan Society of Clinical Hematology: his life and contributions] (Jpn) **Rinsho Ketsueki** 1979 Nov;20(11):1532-3

**Netherlands**

Hollán SR: An appreciation: J. J. van Loghem. **Haematologia (Budap)** 1980;13(1-4):5-22

**Poland**

Rudowski W: Przemówienie z okazji jubileuszu xxx-lecia działalnośći Instytutu Hematologii. **Acta Haematol Pol** 1982 Jan-Jun;13(1-2):1-4
Rudowski WJ: Instytut Hematologii w Warszawie. Warszawa, Państwowy Zakład Wydawn. Lekarskich, 1976. 90 p.

**Romania**

Gingold N: Data concerning the foundation of the Romanian Society of Hematology. **Med Interne** 1981 Jan-Mar;19(1):99-100

**Spain**

Ralchs A, Rozman C: Veintidós años después. Anotaciones para la historia de la Asociación Española de Hematología y Hemoterapia (AEHH). **Sangre (Barc)** 1982;27(3):377-85

**Switzerland**

Dufek WM: Der Internist Otto Naegeli, 1871-1938. Zürich, Juris Druck, 1983. 76 p. (Zürcher Medizingeschichtliche Abhandlungen, Neue Reihe, Nr. 160).
Hitzig WH: Conrad Gasser 1912-1982. **Schweiz Med Wochenschr** 1982 Oct 16;112(42):1486-7
Späth HU: Der Hämatologe Albert Alder, 1888-1980. Zürich, Juris Druck, 1983. 81 p. (Zürcher Medizingeschichtliche Abhandlungen, Neue Reihe, 164).

**United States**

Benson F: Blood tests showing nonpaternity-conclusive or rebuttable evidence? The Chaplin case revisited. **Am J Forensic Med Pathol** 1981 Sep;2(3):221-3
Blombäck B, Copley AL: Hymie Nossel (11 July 1930-8 October 1983). **Thromb Res** 1984 Apr 1;34(1):1-7
Boggs DR: Experimental hematology and bone marrow transplantation. **Exp Hematol** 1984 Mar;12(3):147-51
Brecher G: A red cell discovery of the 20th century: hemoglobin S. **Blood Cells** 1981;7(3):481-3
Brinkhous KM: W. W. Duke and his bleeding time test. A commentary on platelet function. **JAMA** 1983 Sep 2;250(9):1210-14
Dirckx JH: Armand J. Quick: pioneer and prophet of coagulation research. **Ann Intern Med** 1980 Apr;92(4):553-8
Glueck HI: Twenty years of funding of research by the National Institute of Health grant 02904 entitled 'Determination of Natural Clotting Factors'. **J Am Med Wom Assoc** 1980 Jun;35(6):141-4
Heim LR: Birth and development of a scientific journal, and a society. **Exp Hematol** 1983 Nov;11(10):907-13
Lemon HM: Motivation in cancer education, with an appreciation of Dr. Henry Jackson, Jr., pioneer medical oncologist-hematologist (1892-1968). **Med Pediatr Oncol** 1980;8(4):407-22
McMillan CW: Evolution of modern concepts of hemostasis. A backward glance at the discoveries that made modern practice possible. **Am J Pediatr Hematol Oncol** 1981 Spring;3(1):97-103
Owen CA: H. P. Smith's place in the history of blood coagulation. **Am J Clin Pathol** 1984 Apr;81(4):424-6
Pisciotta AV: Concepts of haemostasis and thrombosis: a study of the coagulation defect in hemophilia and in jaundice (Quick, Stanley-Brown and Bancroft 1935). Armand J. Quick (1894-1978)--a short biography. **Thromb Haemost** 1980 Aug 29;44(1):1-5

**USSR**

Bogomolova LG, Andrianova IG, Selivanov EA: Zaslugi A. N. Filatova v razvitie problemy sozdaniia lechebnykh preparatov krovi i krovezameniteleĭ. **Vestn Khir** 1982 Oct;129(10):9-13
Borob'ev RI: I. A. Kassirskiĭ i razvitie Sovetskoĭ meditsiny. **Ter Arkh** 1982;54(2):148-50
Petrov NS: Idei S. P. Botkina v funktsional'noĭ gematologii i ikh dal'neishee razvitie. **Vestn Akad Med Nauk SSSR** 1983;(3):47-51

**Yugoslavia**

Milić N: Imunoproliferativne bolesti. Uvod. **Lijec Vjesn** 1983 Feb-Mar;105(2-3):105-6
Stručno-znanstveni sastanak u povodu tridesete obljetnice o snutka sekcije za hematologiju i transfuziologiju ZLH (1948-1978): **Lijec Vjesn** 1981;103(3):105-30

# HERBALS

See also **Botany; Printing and Bibliography**

Dence CS: Herbs and spices through the ages. 5. **Herbal Rev** 1979;4(2):4-9
Frey EF: The herbal in the healing arts. In: Congrès international d'histoire de la médecine, XXVe, Québec, 1976. Actes. Québec, 1977. p. 659-79.
Lańcucki J: Współczesne ziołolecznictwo. **Pol Tyg Lek** 1979 Jul 2;34(27):1095-8
Opsomer JE: Problèmes d'identification de plantes dans les 'herbiers' anciens. Erreurs et confusions anciennes et récentes. Fédération des Cercles d'Archéologie et d'Histoire de Belgique. 44e session. Congrès de Huy, 1976. Annales. Tielt, 1978. p. 593-6.
Riddle JM: Dioscorides. In Cranz FE, Kristeller PO, ed: Catalogus translationum et commentariorum: mediaeval and Renaissance Latin translations and commentaries. Annotated lists and guides. Vol. IV. Washington, D.C., Catholic University of America Press, 1980. p. 1-143.

**China**

Griffin RJ: Herbal medicine revisited: science looks anew at ancient Chinese pharmacology. **Am Pharm** 1979 Sep;19(10):16-22
Hyatt R: Chinese herbal medicine. **Herbal Rev** 1979;4(3):9-15

**Hungary**

Fazekas A: A magyar nyelvu herbárium irodalomról. **Orvostort Kozl** 1982;28(1-3):43-64
Oláh A: Zwiebel und Knoblauch in der Volksmedizin; das ungarische Theriak und Mithridaticum früher und heute. **Ethnomedizin** 1981-82;7(1-4):333-48

**Poland**

Dembińska M: Dieetvoedsel en medicijnen voor kinderen in Polen van de 16de tot de 19de eeuw. **Spiegel Hist** 1981;16(11):623-6
Szostak J: Funkcja społeczna pierwszych zielników polskich. **Farm Pol** 1979;4:195-200

**Before 500 A.D.**

**China**

Liu ZZ: Shen Nong's Herbal, the earliest extant treatise on Chinese materia medica. **Chung Yao Tung Pao** 1982 Sep;7(5):43-5
Ma JX: [An investigation on the dosage of herbal drug administration described in the medical works unearthed in Ma Wan Dui tomb of Han Dynasty (author's transl)] (Chi). **Chung Yao Tung Pao** 1982 May;6(3):41-3

**Rome**

Dirckx JH: Virgil and medicine. **JAMA** 1981 Sep 18;246(12):1326-9

**500 A.D.-1450**

Halleux-Opsomer C: Les herbiers comme source pour l'histoire de la pathologie et de la thérapeutique au Moyen Age. In International Congress of the History of Medicine. 26th, Plovdiv, 1978. Actes du

Congress. Sofia, 1981. Volume II. p. 91–3.
Halleux–Opsomer C: Un herbier médicinal du haut moyen âge: l'alfabetum Galieni. **Hist Philos Life Sci** 1982;4(1):65–97
Riddle JM: Pseudo–Dioscorides' Ex herbis femininis and early medieval medical botany. **J Hist Biol** 1981 Spring;14(1):43–81
Stannard J: Albertus Magnus and medieval herbalism. In Weisheipl JA, ed: Albertus Magnus and the sciences. Toronto, Pontifical Institute of Mediaeval Studies, 1980. p. 355–77.
Stannard J: Folkloristic elements in medieval herbalism. In International Congress of the History of Medicine. 26th, Plovdiv, 1978. Actes du Congress. Sofia, 1981. Volume II. p. 203–5.

**Arabic**

Johnstone P: Arab herbals and herbalists. In: Mashriq. Proc. of the Eastern Mediterranean Seminar ... 1977–1978. Manchester, University, 1980. p. 19–24.

**Hungary**

Kadár Z, Vizkelety A: Zu den Pflanzen– und Tierdarstellungen in einem mittelalterlichen deutschen Kodex zu Debrecen (Ungarn). In Hein WH, ed: Pharmaziehistorischer Kongress, Budapest, 1981. Stuttgart, Wissenschaftliche Verlagsgesellschaft, 1983. p. 35–40.

**Spain**

Hussenot C: Sur un Erbier de Me Arnauld de Villeneuve (manuscrit médiéval). Thèse de doctorat, Université René–Descartes. Paris, 1983. 119 leaves. (U. E. R. des Sciences pharm. et biol. de Paris–Luxembourg, 1982–1983, no U 558).

**1450–1700**

Cabello de la Torre P: El herbario medico medieval Macer Floridus en la medicina de la baja edad media. **Asclepio** 1978–79;30–31:157–65
Kuźnicka B: The earliest printed herbals and evolution of pharmacy. **Organon** 1980/81;16–17:255–66
Le Traité de matière médicale de Dioscoride à la Renaissance: Exposition d'exemplaires des XVe et XVIe siecles. Du 11 au 24 février 1984 à Louvain–en–Woluwe à la Bibliothèque de la Faculté de Médecine de l'U.C.L. Louvain, Université Catholique de Louvain, Centre d'Histoire de la Pharmacie et du Médicament, 1984. 40 p.
Müller–Jahncke WD: Die 'Magnarum Medicine partium herbariae et zoographiae imagines' von Georg Ollinger und Samuel Quicchelberg. **Beitr Gesch Pharm** 1982;31(17):129–33

**Belgium**

Dodoens R: Histoire des plantes. Traduction française, suivie du Petit recueil, auquel est contenue la description d'aucunes gommes et liqueurs etc., par Charles de l'Escluse (1557). Fac–similé avec introduction, commentaires et la concordance avec la terminologie scientifique moderne, par J.–E. Opsomer. Bruxelles, Centre National d'Histoire des Sciences, 1978. 78, 584 p. (Publications du Centre National d'Histoire des Sciences, V).

**Europe**

Schienbein G, Schienbein H: 'Der Zähn stincken verbessern'--Zahnheilkunde in einem Kräuterbuch von 1602 (I, II). **Quintessenz** 1980 Jun–Jul;31(6,7):133–40, 165–70

**Germany**

Bernus A von, ed: Alt–Kräuterbüchlein. Nach dem 'New–Kreüterbüchlein' des Leonhart Fuchs. Mit einem Nachwort von E. Mittler. Frankfurt am Main, Insel, 1980. 153 p.
Dilg P: Vom Ansehen der Arzneikunst; historische Reflexionen in Kräuterbüchern des 16. Jahrhunderts. **Sudhoffs Arch** 1978;62(1):64–79
Guédès M: Une variante de la page de titre du De historia stirpium de L. Fuchs (1542). **J Soc Bibliogr Nat Hist** 1974;7(1):81–5
Plowman T: Brunfelsia in ethnomedicine. **Bot Mus Leafl Harv Univ** 1977;25:289–320

**Great Britain**

Best MR: Medical use of a sixteenth–century herbal: Gervase Markham and the Banckes herbal. **Bull Hist Med** 1979 Fall;53(3):449–58
Callery BG: Ancients, moderns and reliable friends: stated sources of some English herbals. **J Soc Bibliogr Nat Hist** 1978;8(4):435–44
Phelps WH: John Gerard, the herbalist. **Library (Lond)** 1980 Mar;2(1):76–85

**Hungary**

Szlatky M: Lippay János Posoni Kertjének orvos–botanikai vonatkozásai (1664–1667). **Orvostort Kozl** 1979;87(25 no 1–2):79–90

**Mexico**

Bárcena A, Barrera A, Ruiz E, et al: Interpretación etnobotánica de la iconografía del Códice de la Cruz–Badiano. **An Soc Mex Hist Cienc Tec** 1979;5:35–48

**Netherlands**

Blankaart S: Den Nederlandschen Herbarius. Facsimile of 1698 ed. Edited by D. A. Wittop Koning. Alphen, Stafleu–Brussel. 621 p.

**Poland**

Szostak J: Scientia de simpliciis w pierwszych zielnikach polskich. **Arch Hist Med (Warsz)** 1980;43(3):265–87

**Romania**

Spielmann J, Spielmann M: L'herbier de Joanus Kájoni. In: Congrès international d'histoire de la médecine, XXVe, Québec, 1976. Actes. Québec, 1977. p. 1301–15.

**1700 to Present**

**Great Britain**

Pickstone JV: Medical botany (self–help medicine in Victorian England). **Mem Proc Manch Lit Philos Soc** 1976–77;119:85–95

# HISTOLOGY

See also **Anatomy**

Reyman TA, Dowd AM: Processing of mummified tissue for histological examination. In A. Cockburn, E. Cockburn, ed: Mummies, disease, and ancient cultures. Cambridge, Cambridge University Press, 1980. p. 258–73.

**Egypt**

Zimmerman MR: The paleopathology of the human remains from Nebwenenef's tomb. Part II: The histologic findings. **Paleopathol Newsl** 1983 Jun;42:6–7

**Before 500 A.D.**

**USSR**

Reyman TA, Goodman M: The histology of ancient mammoth tissue. **Paleopathol Newsl** 1981 Jan;33:13–5

**1450–1700**

**Italy**

Saraf PG, Cockett AT: Marcello Malpighi--a tribute. **Urology** 1984 Jun;23(6):619–23

**1700 to Present**

Bennett HS: A perception of histochemistry. **J Histochem Cytochem** 1983 Jan;31(1A Suppl):127–30
Black SE: Pseudopods and synapses: the amoeboid theories of neuronal mobility and the early formulation of the synapse concept, 1894–1900. **Bull Hist Med** 1981 Spring;55(1):34–58
Bode UK: Frühe histologische Krebsforschung in Deutschland, Frankreich und Oesterreich. Köln, 1979. 208 p. (Kölner medizinhistorische Beiträge. Arbeiten der Forschungsstelle des Instituts für Geschichte der Medizin der Universität zu Köln, Band 12).
Dr. Alexis Carrel and tissue culture: **JAMA** 1984 Jul 6;252(1):44–5
Drury RA: The golden ages of histological technique. **Malays J Pathol** 1979 Aug;2:33–7
Girod C: Die Geschichte der Histologie. In Sournia JC, Martiny M, Poulet J, ed: Illustrierte Geschichte der Medizin. Salzburg, Andreas, 1980. Vol. 5. p. 1877–937.
Kepner GR, ed: Cell membrane permeability and transport. Stroudsburg, Pa., Dowden, Hutchinson & Ross, 1979. xiii, 410 p. (Benchmark Papers in Human Physiology, 12).
Riopelle JL: A la mémoire du Professeur Pierre Masson, Vingt ans après. **Union Med Can** 1979 May;108(5):473–6
Smith RE: Contributions of histochemistry to the development of the proteolytic enzyme detection system in diagnostic medicine. **J Histochem Cytochem** 1983 Jan;31(1A Suppl):199–209
Stoffregen M: Zur Rolle histochemischer Phänomene bei der Erforschung und Systematisierung des chromaffinen Gewebes. **Medizinhist J** 1984;19(3):191–209
Witkowski JA: Dr. Carrel's immortal cells. **Med Hist** 1980

# HISTOLOGY

Apr;24(2):129–42

**Chile**

Costa C: Prehistoria de la cátedra de histología de la Universidad de Chile (1872–1881). Parte I. El affaire Magalhaes. **Rev Med Chil** 1980 Apr;108(4):367–73

Costa C: Prehistoria de la cátedra de histología de la Universidad de Chile (1872–1881) Parte II. Microscopio e histología en Chile antes de 1873. **Rev Med Chil** 1980 May;108(5):463–9

**Czechoslovakia**

Cech S: Milan Dvorzhak (k 50–letiiu so dnia rozhdeniia). **Arkh Anat Gistol Embriol** 1980 Jul;79(7):121–5

**Denmark**

Rasmussen L: En forstander og hans assistent. **Dan Medicinhist Arbog** 1981;:130–40

**Germany**

Kahle E: Koelliker, Albert Ritter v. In Neue Deutsche Biographie 12. 1980. p. 322–3.

Nabielek R: Zu den wichtigsten Veröffentlichungen des polnischen Histologen Henryk Fryderyk Hoyer (1834–1907) in deutschen Fachzeitschriften. **Z Mikrosk Anat Forsch** 1983;97(3):393–408

Teulón AA: La constitucion de la histologia celular: Schwann, Henle y Kölliker. **Asclepio** 1978–79;30–31:7–18

**Great Britain**

Keel O: La pathologie tissulaire de John Hunter. **Gesnerus** 1980;37(1/2):47–61

**Hungary**

Kenéz J: Hugó Richter, an outstanding Hungarian neurohistologist (1887--1945). **Ther Hung** 1979;27(2):99–100

**Italy**

Breathnach CS: Golgi. **Ir Med J** 1983 Jun;76(6):298

Olagüe G: La 'teoria fibrilar' en la obra de Giorgio Baglivi (1668–1707). Introduccion, traduccion de los capitulos I y II del libro I de su specimen Quatuor librorum de fibra motrice et morbosa (Perusa, 1700), y notas. **Morfol Norm Patol** 1979;3:335–56

**Poland**

Loetzke HH: Die wissenschaftlichen Arbeiten des polnischen Histologen Władysław Szymonowicz während seiner Studienaufenthalthe 1895 und 1896 in Berlin. **Arch Hist Med (Warsz)** 1979;42(3):359–64

**Romania**

Diculescu I, Onicescu D: At the hundredth anniversary of the Department of Histology of the Bucharest Faculty of Medicine. **Morphol Embryol (Bucur)** 1980 Jul–Sep;26(3):199–204

Munteanu A, Dobrescu G, Cotuţiu C, et al: The 100th anniversary of the Jassy Faculty of Medicine and an historical approach to the evolution of its department of histology. **Morphol Embryol (Bucur)** 1980 Oct–Dec;26(4):371–3

**Spain**

García del Carrizo San Millán MG: Breve apunte sobre los estudios histologicos en el departamento de anatomia de San Carlos hasta la creacion de la catedra de histologia. **Asclepio** 1978–79;30–31:89–97

Jokisch R: Probleme der spanischen Wissenschaftsentwicklung. Die Institutionalisierung der spanischen Histologie im 19. Jahrhundert als Beispiel. In International Congress of the History of Medicine, 27th, Barcelona, 1980. Actas. Barcelona, Académia de Ciències Médiques de Catalunya i Balears, 1981. p. 522–9.

Valenciano Gayá L: Cajal (recuerdos y reflexiones de uno de sus últimos alumnos). **Arch Neurobiol (Madr)** 1983 Jul–Aug;46(4):272–81

**Switzerland**

Jonecko A: Uwagi o podręczniku histochemii Freya z roku 1870 na tle osiągnięć histochemicznych połowy XIX wieku. **Wiad Lek** 1979 Dec 15;32(24):1811–4

**United States**

Conn HJ: The history of the Stain Commission. III. Birth of the Stain Commission. 1922–3. **Stain Technol** 1981 Jan;56(1):1–17

Conn HJ: The history of the Stain Commission. V. War and its consequences. **Stain Technol** 1981 May;56(3):135–42

Haraway DJ: Ethel Browne Harvey. In: Notable American women. The modern period. Cambridge, Mass., Belknap–Harvard Univ. Press, 1980. 4:319–21.

Hermanek P: 90 Jahre Schnellschnitthistologie. **Pathologe** 1981 Dec;3(1):53–4

Kasten FH: Ralph D. Lillie, 1896–1979. **Stain Technol** 1980 Jul;55(4):201–15

**USSR**

Afanas'ev IuI, Belova TI, Fel'dman NG: Boris Innokent'evich Lavrent'ev (k 90–letiiu so dnia rozhdeniia). **Arkh Anat Gistol Embriol** 1983 Nov;85(11):98–101

Dyskin EA, Klishov AA: O roli Voenno–meditsinskoĭ akademii im. S. M. Kirova v podgotovke vysokokvalifitsirovannykh kadrov anatomov i gistologov SSSR. **Arkh Anat Gistol Embriol** 1983 Mar;84(3):90–6

Klishov AA: Istoriko–gnoseologicheskiĭ analiz poniatiia 'tkan''. **Arkh Anat Gistol Embriol** 1982 Jul;83(7):74–93

Klishov AA: N. M. Iakubovich--pervyĭ russkiĭ professor-gistolog. **Arkh Anat Gistol Embriol** 1981 Oct;81(10):105–15

Klishov AA, Khilova IuK, Pankov EIa, et al: Zhizn' i deiatel'nost' professora V. Ia. Rubashkina. **Arkh Anat Gistol Embriol** 1983 Nov;85(11):94–8

Kvitnitskiĭ–Ryzhov IuN: Iz istorii pervoĭ Kievskoĭ gistologicheskoĭ shkoly. **Arkh Anat Gistol Embriol** 1980 May;78(5):107–11

Kvitnitskiĭ–Ryzhov IuN: Zhizn' i deiatel'nost' ukrainskogo gistologa F. I. Lominskogo (k 125–letiiu so dnia rozhdeniia). **Arkh Anat Gistol Embriol** 1982 Apr;82(4):96–101

Mikhaĭlov VP: Zhurnal Rudneva (poluzabytaia glava v istorii otechestvennoĭ gistologii). **Arkh Anat Gistol Embriol** 1980 Feb;78(2):104–15

**Yugoslavia**

Posinovec J: Histologija i embriologija u djelu dra Ante Schwarza (u povodu 100. obljetnice njegove smrti). **Lijec Vjesn** 1980 Apr;102(4):208–10

# HISTORIOGRAPHY AND HISTORY OF MEDICINE

Albini G: A proposito di studi recenti die storia della salute nel medioevo e nell'età moderna. **Nuova Riv Stor** 1980;64(1–2):143–63

Alvsvåg H: Sykepleiens historie--er den objektiv? **Sykepleien** 1983 Feb 7;70(3):20–1

Anderson JW: The methodology of psychological biography. **J Interdiscip Hist** 1981;11:455–75

Aulizio F: Principi per una rinnovato metodologia nella ricerca e nell' insegnamento della storia della medicina. **Med Secoli** 1980 Jan–Apr;17(1):129–34

Bibliography of the history of medicine, No. 15, 1975–1979: Bethesda, National Library of Medicine, 1981. lxxii, 924 p. (NIH Publication No. 81–1224).

Bibliography of the history of medicine, No. 16, 1980: Bethesda, National Library of Medicine, 1982. xi, 305 p. (NIH Publication No. 82–315).

Bibliography of the history of medicine, No. 17, 1981: Bethesda, National Library of Medicine, 1983. xi, 240 p. (NIH Publication No. 83–315).

Bibliography of the history of medicine, No. 18, 1982: Bethesda, National Library of Medicine, 1983. ix, 305 p. (NIH Publication No. 84–315).

Bulferetti L: Quantification in the historiography of sciences and techniques. **Organon** 1980/81;16–17:19–41

Bustamante ME: La necesidad para los historiadores de saber leer y de poder leer. **Bol Soc Mex Hist Filos Med** 1979 Dec;4(29):141–52

Charbonneau H, Larose A, ed: The great mortalities: methodological studies of demographic crises in the past. Liège, Belgium, Ordina Editions, [1980]. 373 p. Includes contributions by A. Appleby, S. Sogner, J. N. Biraben. Text in English or French.

Comiti VP: Importance des connaissances médico-biologiques actuelles pour une étude critique de pathocénose historique. In Imhof AE, ed: Mensch und Gesundheit in der Geschichte. Husum, Matthiesen, 1980. p. 35–43.

Daumard A: Les généalogies sociales: un des fondements de l'histoire sociale comparative et quantitative. **Ann Demogr Hist (Paris)** 1984;:9–24

Dieckhöfer K: Geistesgeschichtliche Strömungen in der Biographik--ein kulturhistorischer Abriss. **Z Psychosom Med Psychoanal** 1980 Jul–Sep;26(3):275–81

Durbin PT, ed: A guide to the culture of science, technology, and medicine. New York, Free Press, 1980. xl, 723 p. Contributions by A. Thackray, C. W. Pursell, G. H. Brieger, A. C. Michalos, C. Mitcham, H. T. Engelhardt, J. Gaston, L. Aiken, D. Crane.

Esteva J: La historia y el actual debate epistemológico. **Bol Soc Esp Hist Farm** 1980/81 Dec–Mar;31–32(124–5):287–97

Grensemann H, ed: Hippokratische Gynäkologie. Die gynäkologischen Texte des Autors C nach den pseudohippokratischen Schriften De

muliebribus I, II, und De sterilibus. Wiesbaden, Steiner, 1982. 191 p.
Grmek MD: A plea for freeing the history of scientific discoveries from myth. In M. D. Grmek, R. S. Cohen, G. Cimino, ed: On scientific discovery. The Erice Lectures 1977. Dordrecht, D. Reidel, 1981. p. 9–42. (Boston Studies in the Philosophy of Science, v. 34).
Henle M: Why study the history of psychology? In K. Salzinger, ed: Psychology in progress: an interim report. (Annals of the New York Academy of Sciences, vol. 270). New York, New York Academy of Sciences, 1976. p. 14–20.
Hickel E, Schröder G, ed: Neue Beiträge zur Arzneimittelgeschichte. Festschrift für Wolfgang Schneider zum 70. Geburtstag. Stuttgart, Wissenschaftliche Verlagsgesellschaft, 1982. 285 p. (Veröffentlichungen der Internationalen Gesellschaft für Geschichte der Pharmazie e. V., Neue Folge, Band 51).
Hollingsworth TH: A preliminary suggestion for the measurement of mortality crises. In Charbonneau H, Larose A, ed: The great mortalities: methodological studies of demographic crises in the past. Liège, Belgium, Ordina Editions, 1980. p. 21–8.
Jette R, Charbonneau H: Généalogie descendantes et analyse démographique. **Ann Demogr Hist (Paris)** 1984;:45–54
Keil G: Der Medizin-historiker als Terminologe. **MMW** 1979 Dec 7;121(49):1637–8
Keynes M: Medical sense and nonsense in biography. **Br Med J [Clin Res]** 1983 Mar 26;286(6370):1023–6
Kronick DA: Literature of the life sciences: the historical background. **Bull NY Acad Med** 1984 Nov;60(9):857–75
Lenoir T: A history of biology: an essay review. **J Hist Med Allied Sci** 1983 Jul;38(3):348–51
Lloyd GE: Hippocratic problems. **Classical Rev** 1980;30(2):186–9
Lopez Austin A: En defensa de la historia de la medicina. **Bol Soc Mex Hist Filos Med** 1984;7(50):467–75
Losee J: Whewell and Mill on the relation between philosophy of science and history of science. **Stud Hist Philos Sci** 1983 Jun;14(2):113–26
Lynch KA: Local and regional studies in historical demography. **Hist Methods** 1982;15(1):23–9
Maulitz RC, Poses RM, Young MJ: Medical history as an introduction to clinical reasoning. **J Med Educ** 1983 May;58(5):427–9
Merchant C: Isis' consciousness raised. **Isis** 1982 Sep;73(268):398–409
Morain WD: History and plastic surgery: systems of recovering our past. In Romm S, ed: Symposium on historical perspectives of plastic surgery. Philadelphia, Saunders, 1983. p. 595–601.
Ortiz Monasterio J: Reflexiones en torno a los origenes de la historiografia de la medicina. **Bol Soc Mex Hist Filos Med** 1980 Sep–Dec;5(32–33):83–92
Paterson GR, Neilson JB, Roland CG: History of medicine. **Can Med Assoc J** 1982 Nov 15;127(10):948
Puma A: La escuela de Alejandría y nuestro occidente. In International Congress of the History of Medicine, 27th, Barcelona, 1980. Actas. Barcelona, Académia de Ciències Mèdiques de Catalunya i Balears, 1981. p. 610–5.
Putscher M: Die Geschichte der Medizin zwischen normativem und historischem Denken. In International Congress of the History of Medicine. 26th, Plovdiv, 1978. Actes du Congress. Sofia, 1981. Volume II. p. 190–1.
Rothschuh KE: Das Relevanzproblem in der Geschichte der theoretischen Medizin. Zugleich ein Beitrag zur Interpretation der Entwicklungsdynamik in den Wissenschaften von T. S. Kuhn und L. Fleck. In Ganzinger K, Skopec M, Wyklicky H, ed: Festschrift für Erna Lesky zum 70. Geburtstag. Wien, Brüder Hollinek, 1981. p. 75–86.
Runyan WM: Life histories and psychobiography. Explorations in theory and method. New York, Oxford, Oxford University Press, 1982. xiii, 288 p.
Ruse M: The new dualism: 'Res Philosophica' and 'Res Historica.' In M. Ruse, ed: Nature animated. Historical and philosophical case studies in Greek medicine, nineteenth-century and recent biology, psychiatry, and psychoanalysis. Volume II. Dordrecht, D. Reidel, 1983. p. 3–25.
Ruse M, ed: Nature animated. Historical and philosophical case studies in Greek medicine, nineteenth-century and recent biology, psychiatry, and psychoanalysis. Papers deriving from the Third International Conference on the History and Philosophy of Science, Montreal, Canada, 1980. Volume II. Dordrecht, D. Reidel, 1983. xiii, 274 p.
Sanguinetti FA: Reflexiones en torno a la historia de la medicina. **Rev Fac Cien Med Univ Nac Cordoba** 1981 Jan–Dec;39(1–4):81–6
Scarborough J: The Galenic question. **Sudhoffs Arch** 1981;65(1):1–31
Schaefer H: Das Geschichtliche als Prinzip in der Medizin. In Seidler E, Schott H, ed: Bausteine zur Medizingeschichte. Stuttgart, Steiner, 1984. p. 93–9.
Schneider W: Anleitung zum Gebrauch des Systema Pharmaceuticum. (Zur statistischen Auswertung von Quellen zur Arzneimittelgeschichte). Braunschweig, 1978. 67 p. (Veröffentlichungen aus dem Pharmaziegeschichtlichen Seminar der Technischen Universität Braunschweig, 18).
Schoeneman TJ: Criticisms of the psychopathological interpretation of witch hunts: a review. **Am J Psychiatry** 1982 Aug;139(8):1028–32
Siegel IM: History through artifact. **IMJ** 1982 Sep;162(3):202–3, 217
Stein HF: Historical understanding as sense of history: a psychoanalytic inquiry. **Psychoanal Rev** 1983 Winter;70(4):595–619
Swedlund AC: Historical demography as population ecology. **Annu Rev Anthropol** 1978;7:137–73
Teich M: A history of biochemistry. **Hist Sci** 1980;18(1):46–67
Tröhler U: Medizin mit oder ohne Geschichte? **Praxis** 1981 Dec 15;70(51):2295–7
Vuori H: Lääketieteen historian tutkimuksesta. **Duodecim** 1980;96(1):9–17
Weimann KH: Paracelsus-Lexikographie in vier Jahrhunderten. **Medizinhist J** 1981;16(1–2):167–95
Whitteridge G: The Piltdown Hippocrates. **Hist Sci** 1980 Sep;18(41 pt 3):226–30
Wilkie JS: The history of health and medicine: a social history curriculum for secondary schools. D.A. Diss., Carnegie-Mellon University. Pittsburgh, 1982. 261 p.

**Americas**

Super JC: Sources and methods for the study of historical nutrition in Latin America. **Hist Methods** 1981;14(1):22–30

**Hungary**

Antall J: Az orvostörténelem helyzete Magyarországon. **Orv Hetil** 1981 Mar 8;122(10):555–60

**Ireland**

O'Donnell S: Gilding the anemometer: Irish science of the past. **Eire Irel** 1982;17(4):148–51

**Japan**

Maruyama H, et al: [My way of medical history study] (Jpn). **Igakushi Kenkyu** 1978;50:11–48

**Mexico**

Beltrán E: Reflexiones sobre historiografía de la biología en México. **An Soc Mex Hist Cienc Tec** 1979;5:1–19
Somolinos-Palencia J, Risse GB, Price R, et al: Homenaje a la Sociedad Mexicana de Historia y Filosofía de la Medicina. **Gac Med Mex** 1982 Dec;118(12):471–84

**Poland**

Bujałowska B: Recepcja poglądów hipokratesa w polsce na tle dziejów medycyny powszechnej. **Pol Tyg Lek** 1983 Aug 15;38(33–34):1063–6

**Sri Lanka**

Jayawardane KW: A bibliography of the history of medicine in Sri Lanka. **Ceylon Med J** 1979 Sep–Dec;24(3–4):71–8

**Turkey**

Terzioglu A: Zur Avicenna (Ibn Sina) – Forschung in der Türkei. In International Congress of the History of Medicine, 27th, Barcelona, 1980. Actas. Barcelona, Académia de Ciències Mèdiques de Catalunya i Balears, 1981. p. 750–5.

**United States**

Shortt SE: Approaches to the physician's life. **Bull Hist Med** 1981 Spring;55(1):124–7

**USSR**

Shengeliia MS: Izuchenie istorii meditsiny v soiuznykh respublikakh. **Sov Zdravookhr** 1982;(7):53–5

**Yugoslavia**

Supuk A: Sibenski onomastikon nakon kuge od 1649 godine. **Arh Vjesn** 1978–79;21–22:123–79

**Before 500 A.D.**

**Greece**

Kudlien F: A new testimony for Erasistratus? **Clio Med** 1981 Apr;15(3–4):137–42
Lichtenthaeler C: Outé gar iatori èrkoun to proton therapeuontes agnoia. **Hermes** 1979, 1978;107(3):270–86
Poole JC, Holladay AJ: Thucydides and the plague: a footnote. **Classical Q** 1982;32:235–6
Poole JC, Holladay AJ: Thucydides and the plague of Athens. **Classical Q** 1979;29:282–300
Radt SL: Zu Thukydides' Pestbeschreibung. **Mnemosyne** 1978;31:233–45;

1979;32:163

**500 A.D.–1450**

**Byzantium**

Théodoridès J: Quelle était la maladie décrite par l'historien Agathias (VIe siècle A.D.)? **Hist Sci Med** 1981;15(2):153–8

**1450–1700**

Daems WF: Renward Cysat und Paracelsus. **Gesnerus** 1982;39(3–4):469–72
Guerrino AA: Las traducciones médicas hasta el renacimiento. In International Congress of the History of Medicine, 27th, Barcelona, 1980. Actas. Barcelona, Académia de Ciències Médiques de Catalunya i Balears, 1981. p. 249–52.

**France**

Lebel M: Editions, traductions et lexiques hippocratiques. Le docteur Louis Morin, (1635–1715) et son index des mots d'Hippocrate. In: Congrès international d'histoire de la médecine, XXVe, Québec, 1976. Actes. Québec, 1977. p. 848–65.

**Germany**

Kaempfer E: Amoenitatum Exoticarum Politico-physico-medicarum. Fasciculi V, Quibus Continentur Variae Relationes, Observationes and Descriptiones Rerum Persicarum and Ulterioris Asiae (Lemgo: Meyeri, 1712). **J Hist Med Allied Sci** 1978 Jul;33(3):320–43

**Great Britain**

Shapiro B: History and natural history in sixteenth- and seventeenth-century England: an essay on the relationship between humanism and science. In Shapiro, Barbara and Frank, Robert G. Jr., ed: English scientific virtuosi in the 16th and 17th centuries: Los Angeles, William Andrews Clark Memorial Lib., U. of California, 1980. p. 1–55.

**Spain**

Ehlers AP: Medizinisches und Pharmazeutisches in Bernal Diaz del Castillos, 'Historia verdadera de la conquista de la Nueva-España,' Madrid, 1632. Diss. Düsseldorf, 1980. 118 p.

**1700 to Present**

Abir-Am PG: Essay review: how scientists view their heroes: some remarks on the mechanism of myth construction. **J Hist Biol** 1982 Summer;15(2):281–315
Ackerknecht EH: Causes and pseudocauses in the history of diseases. In Stevenson LG, ed: A celebration of medical history. Baltimore, Johns Hopkins University Press, 1982. (The Henry E. Sigerist supplements to the Bulletin of the History of Medicine; new ser., no. 6). p. 19–31. With commentary by C. E. Rosenberg, 'The history of disease: now and in the future,' p. 32–6.
Albin M, Devlin RJ, Heeger G, ed: New directions in psychohistory. The Adelphi papers in honor of Erik H. Erikson. Lexington, Toronto, D. C. Heath, 1980. xx, 217 p. Includes contributions by E. S. Wolf, M. F. Shore, G. M. Platt, H. Feinstein, S. H. Rudolph, L. I. Rudolph.
Albury WR: Going beyond the introduction: Claude Bernard scholarship in the 1970s, an essay review. **Bull Hist Med** 1982 Summer;56(2):271–5
American Academy of Arts and Sciences, American Philosophical Society: Survey of sources for the history of biochemistry and molecular biology. **Surv Sources Newsl** 1975–1981;1(1–10):various pagings
Anderson TH: Becoming sane with psychohistory. **Historian** 1978;41(1):1–20
Anees MA: History of Islamic medicine and pharmacy: contribution of Sami Hamarneh. **Hamdard** 1983 Apr–Jun;26(2):67–75
Ash L, Murray MA, ed: Serial publications containing medical classics. An index to citations in Garrison/Morton (3rd edition, 1970). 2nd ed., revised and enlarged. Bethany, Connecticut, The Antiquarium, 1979, x, 169 p.
Aulizio F: Ideas for a renewed methodology in the research and in teaching the history of medicine. In: International Congress of the History of Medicine, 26th, Plovdiv (Bulgaria), 1978. Actes du Congres, Vol. 1. Sofia, 1980. p. 113–4.
Baader G: Der ärztliche Stand in der Antike. **Jahrb Univ Dusseld** 1977–78;:301–15
Baader G: Zu den Aufgaben der medizinhistorischen Forschung auf dem Gebiet der Geschichte der mittelalterlichen Medizin in der Gegenwart. In: International Congress of the History of Medicine, 26th, Plovdiv (Bulgaria), 1978. Actes du Congres, Vol. 1. Sofia, 1980. p. 85–8.
Babini J: Historia de la ciencia versus historia de la medicina. **Medicina (B Aires)** 1980 Jul–Aug;40(4):486–8
Barnard K: Research designs: the historical method. **MCN** 1981 Nov–Dec;6(6):391
Beatty J: Essay review: life science in the twentieth century. **Ann Sci** 1981;38(2):207–16
Beauperthuy de Benedetti R: Informe sobre la publicacion del señor Cesar Rodriguez Exposito. **Rev Soc Venez Hist Med** 1972–73;20–21(34–35):141–50
Benison S: Celebration and history: the centenary of Robert Koch's discovery of the tubercle bacillus. **Bull Hist Med** 1982 Summer;56(2):157–9
Bizière JM: 'Before and after': essai de psycho-histoire. **Rev Hist Mod Contemp** 1980 Apr–Jun;27:177–207
Bizière JM: Une psycho-histoire, pourquoi faire? **Bull Soc Hist Mod** 1980;79(6):11–5
Blum RH: Psychological processes in preparing contemporary biography. **Biography** 1981;4(4):293–311
Boehm EH, Pope BH, Ensign MS, ed: Historical periodicals directory. Volume 3: Europe: East and Southeast; USSR. Santa Barbara, Oxford, ABC-Clio, 1984. xv, 252 p. (Clio Periodicals Directories).
Bonora F: Compiti e ruoli attuali della storia della medicina. **Med Secoli** 1982;19(3):249–63
Branca P, ed: The medicine show. Patients, physicians and the perplexities of the health revolution in modern society. New York, Science History Publications, 1977. viii, 280 p. (Mostly articles reprinted from Journal of Social History, vol. 10, Summer 1977).
Brieger GH: The history of health and disease for health professionals: the case study approach. With a commentary by G.B. Risse. In J. J. Bylebyl, ed: Teaching the history of medicine at a medical center. Baltimore, London, Johns Hopkins University Press, 1982. (The Henry E. Sigerist supplements to the Bulletin of the History of Medicine; new ser., no. 7). p. 13–30.
Brock WH: Liebigiana: old and new perspectives. **Hist Sci** 1981 Sep;19(45 pt 3):201–18
Brown TE: The mental hospital and its historians. **Bull Hist Med** 1982 Spring;56(1):109–14
Brozek J, Pongratz LJ, ed: Historiography of modern psychology: aims, resources, approaches. Toronto, Hogrefe, 1980. 336 p. Contributions by R. Ardila, M. G. Ash, L. T. Benjamin, W. Bringmann, R. León, B. Ross, M. Sokal, H. Thomae, G. A. Ungerer, R. I. Watson, M. Wertheimer, W. Woodward, L. J. Pongratz.
Bruce NG: Searching the history of the health sciences. **Med Ref Serv Q** 1982 Fall;1(3):13–35
Buchvarova N: Mezhdunaroden Kongres po istoriia na meditsinata. **Istor Pregl** 1978;34(6):148–52
Buess H: Prof. Dr. med. Dr.h.c. Walter Pagel (1898–1983). **Gesnerus** 1984;41(3–4):359–63
Bujosa i Homar F: La afasia y su historiografía. **Dynamis** 1981;1:131–63
Burns CR: Locating sources in the history of medicine and health care: a guide for students and faculty at UTMB. **Bookman** 1984;11(5):3–9
Burns CR: Medical history and medical humanities: some new styles of learning and teaching. With a commentary by T.L. Savitt. In J. J. Bylebyl, ed: Teaching the history of medicine at a medical center. Baltimore, London, Johns Hopkins University Press, 1982. (The Henry E. Sigerist supplements to the Bulletin of the History of Medicine; new ser., no. 7). p. 31–45.
Bylebyl JJ, ed: Teaching the history of medicine at a medical center. Baltimore, London, Johns Hopkins University Press, 1982. 162 p. (The Henry E. Sigerist supplements to the Bulletin of the History of Medicine; new ser., no. 7).
Congrès international d'histoire de la médecine, XXVe, Québec, 1976: Actes. Québec, 1977. 3 vols. 1403 p.
Cooter R: Anticontagionism and history's medical record. In P. Wright, A. Treacher, ed: The problem of medical knowledge. Examining the social construction of medicine. Edinburgh, Edinburgh University Press, 1982. p. 87–108.
Corsi P, Weindling P, ed: Information sources in the history of science and medicine. London, Boston, Butterworth Scientific, 1983. xvi, 531 p. (Butterworth Guides to Information Sources).
Crimmins EM: The completeness of 1900 mortality data collected by registration and enumeration for rural and urban parts of states: estimates using the Chandra Sekar-Deming technique. **Hist Methods** 1980;13(3):163–9
Dätwyler B, Schmidhofer M, L'adrach U: Unterricht in 'Geschichte der Krankenpflege' oder Hilfe zur Selbsthilfe. **Krankenpflege (Bern)** 1983 May;(5):62
Davies C, ed: Rewriting nursing history. London, Croom Helm, and Totowa, New Jersey, Barnes & Noble, 1980. 226 p. Includes contributions by C. Maggs, K. Williams, M. Dean, G. Bolton, M. Carpenter, P. Bellaby, P. Oribabor, M. C. Versluysen, J. Foster, J. Sheppard, C. Kratz.
Degler C: Can a historian or social scientist learn anything from sociobiology? An attempt at an answer. **Hist Methods** 1981;14(4):173–9
Delatte L, Opsomer-Halleux C: Ancient medical recipes and the computer: the Theorema project. **Pharm Hist** 1981;23(2):87–9
Demandt A: Natur- und Geschichtswissenschaft im 19. Jahrhundert. **Ber Wissenschaftsgesch** 1983;6(1–4):59–78
Domandl S, ed: Paracelsus im Blickfeld heutiger wissenschaftsgeschichtlicher Betrachtung (ein Rundgespräch). Wien, 1974. 59 p. (Salzburger Beiträge zur Paracelsusforschung, 12). Contributions by L. Braun, A. W. Gutsch, V. Bazala, K. Goldammer,

H. Goerke, W. Schneider, R. Blaser, KH Weimann, G. Harrer, A. Dyk.

Dostatni P, Cordoliani A: L'histoire de la médecine et la recherche documentaire automatisée. **Hist Sci Med** 1984;18(1):25–32

Durling RJ: Lexicographical notes on Galen's pharmacological writings. **Glotta** 1979;57(3–4):218–24

Ebel H, et al: The psychohistory of history: a symposium. **J Psychohist** 1981 Winter;8(3):259–79

Eckardt G: Einleitung: Bemerkungen zum Anliegen psychologiegeschichtlicher Forschung. In Eckardt G, ed: Zur Geschichte der Psychologie, Berlin, VEB Deutscher Verlag der Wissenschaften, 1970. p. 7–20.

Eissler KR: K. R. Eissler on errors regarding Freud. **Int J Psychoanal** 1981;62(3):371–2

Engelhardt DV, Henkelmann T: Una excursión de história de la medicina con el renacimiento de la toscana. **Folia Hum (Barc)** 1981;19(216):49–56

Ensign MS, ed: Historical periodicals directory. Volume 1: USA and Canada. Santa Barbara, Oxford, ABC–Clio, 1981. xii, 180 p. (Clio Periodicals Directories).

Federn E: On the difficulty of writing history of ideas: a reply. **J Hist Behav Sci** 1980 Jan;16(1):45–9

Fitch NE: Statistical and mathematical methods for historians: an annotated bibliography of selected books and articles. **Hist Methods** 1980;13(4):222–31

Flanagan TE: Problems of psychobiography. **Queens Q** 1982;89(3):596–610

Flinn MW: Plague in Europe and the Mediterranean countries. **J Eur Econ Hist** 1979;8(1):131–48

Frascani P: Il medico nell'ottocento. **Studi Stor** 1982;23(3):617–37

Fredga A: Varför lärdomshistoria? **Nord Medicinhist Arsb** 1980;Suppl 6:22–4

Friedländer S: History and psychoanalysis. An inquiry into the possibilities and limits of psychohistory. New York and London, Holmes & Meier, 1978. 175 p. (Translation of French edition, 1975)

Fye WB: Librarians in the history of the health sciences: challenges and opportunities in the 80's. **Watermark** 1983 Apr;6(4):14–8

Gajda Z: Niektórzy historycy wobec historii medycyny kilka refleksji sceptycznych. **Arch Hist Med (Warsz)** 1984;47(1):1–10

Galdston I: Social and historical foundations of modern medicine. New York, Brunner/Mazel, 1981. xiv, 147 p. (Reprinted articles from various sources)

Ganzinger K, Skopec M, Wyklicky H, ed: Festschrift für Erna Lesky zum 70. Geburtstag. Wien, Brüder Hollinek, 1981. 212 p.

Gaunt D: Historisk demografi eller demografisk historia? En översikt och ett debattinlägg om ett tvärvetenskapligt dilemma. **Hist Tidskr** 1973;93(3):382–405

Georgievskiĭ AS, Tel'iatev IV: Sistemnyĭ podkhod v istoriko–meditsinskikh issledovaniiakh. **Sov Zdravookhr** 1981;(6):52–5

Ghalioungui [: On the necessity of medical–archaeological cooperation. In: Congrès international d'histoire de la médecine, XXVe, Québec, 1976. Actes. Québec, 1977. p. 699–705.

Gilmore WJ: Media resources available for teaching psychohistory. **Group Psychol Hist Newsl** 1975;3(4):15–20

Giustini PA: Museografia e storia del pensiero scientifico. **Med Secoli** 1982;19(3):265–71

Grmek MD, ed: Hippocratica. Actes du Colloque hippocratique de Paris (4–9 septembre 1978). Paris, Editions du Centre National de la Recherche Scientifique, 1980. 486 p. (Colloques Internationaux du C.N.R.S., No. 583). Contributions by A. Anastassiou, J. Benedum, J. Bertier, L. Bourgey, G. Brătescu, S. Byl, G. Cambiano, V. Di Benedetto, J. Ducatillon, M. P. Duminil, L. Garcia–Ballester, D. Gourevitch, H. Grensemann, G. Harig, J. Irigoin, C. Irmer, D. Irmer, R. Joly, J. Jouanna, H. M. Koelbing, V. Langholf, C. Lichtenthaeler, G. Maloney, W. Frohn Villeneuve, J. Mansfeld, P. Manuli, P. Mudry, J. M. Pigeaud, C. Sandulesco, W. D. Smith, A. Thivel, M. Vegetti.

Grosshans OR: Biographical research in health education. **Health Educ (Wash)** 1981 Sep–Oct;12(5):40–1

Guarner V: El conocimiento de la historia de la medicina en la educacion del cirujano. **Bol Soc Mex Hist Filos Med** 1979 Mar;4(26):73–87

Haeger–Aronsen B, Haeger K: Porfyri hos Mary Stuarts efterkommande: en historisk–medicinsk tvistefråga. **Sydsven Medicinhist Sallsk Arsskr** 1984;21:63–75

Hahn R: A bibliography of quantitative studies on science and its history. Berkeley, Office for History of Science, 1980. 84 p. (Berkeley Papers in History of Science, 3).

Haines MR: Recent developments in historical demography: a review of the European fertility project with some comparisons from Japan. **Hist Methods** 1978;11(4):162–73

Hakfoort C: Wetenschapshistorische etiketten en de gevaren van polaire analyses. **Tijdschr Geschied Geneeskd** 1982;5(1):1–5

Hall AR: On Whiggism. **Hist Sci** 1983 Mar;21(51 Pt 1):45–59

Hamarneh S: Sarton (1884–1956) and the Arabic–Islamic legacy. **J Hist Arabic Sci** 1977 Nov;1(2):299–318

Hareven TK: Cycles, courses and cohorts: reflections on theoretical and methodological approaches to the historical study of family development. **J Soc Hist** 1978;12(1):97–109

Harig G: Zu den Aufgaben der medizinhistorischen Forschung auf dem Gebiet der antiken Medizin in der Gegenwart. In International Congress of the History of Medicine. 26th, Plovdiv, 1978. Actes du Congress. Sofia, 1981. Volume II. p. 109–11.

Hart GD, ed: Disease in ancient man. An international symposium held in London, 1979. Toronto, Clarke Irwin, 1983. 297 p. Contributions by D. A. Birkett, F. F. Cartwright, R. Cramp, J. Dobson, A. J. Duggan, N. G. Gejvall, P. S. Gooch, C. J. Hackett, P. D. Horne, P. Janssens, B. Knight, A. K. Knowles, N. B. Millet, V. Møller–Christensen, W. J. Moore, R. Perrot, F. D. Pooley, D. F. Rideout, A. Rook, W. M. Russell, P. Slack, W. E. Swinton, H. A. Waldron.

Hickel E: Pharmaziegeschichte als Wissenschafts– oder Sozialgeschichte? In: Vorträge des Internationalen Pharmaziehistorischen Kongresses Innsbruck 1977. Stuttgart, Wissenschaftliche Verlagsgesellschaft, 1979. p. 23–8.

Hoffer PC: Psychohistory and empirical group affiliation: extraction of personality traits from historical manuscripts. **J Interdiscip Hist** 1978;9(1):131–45

Holmes FL: The history of biochemistry: a review of the literature of the field. **Spec Collect** 1982;1(2):7–15

Hooykaas R: Wissenschaftsgeschichte––eine Brücke zwischen Natur– und Geisteswissenschaften. **Ber Wissenschaftsgesch** 1982;5:153–72

Hügelow M: Original–Lithographien speziell für Pharmazeuten: Historische Apothekergeräte und Heilpflanzen. **Pharm Unserer Zeit** 1984 Jul;13(4):97–101

Hunyady G: Történelem és pszichológia [History and psychology]. **Tortenelmi Sz** 1981;24(1):71–8

Imhof AE: Man and body in the history of the modern age. Reflections on an International Symposium in Berlin, 1–3 December 1981. **Med Hist** 1983 Oct;27(4):394–406

Imhof AE: Ursachen und Folgen der zunehmenden durchschnittlichen Lebenserwartung seit dem 17. Jahrhundert; Bericht über eine interdisziplinäre Tagung an der Ecole des Hautes Etudes en Sciences Sociales, Paris, 24.–26. Oktober 1979. **Ber Wissenschaftsgesch** 1979;3(3–4):212–18

International Congress of the History of Medicine, 26th, Plovdiv [Bulgaria], 20–25 August 1978: Actes du Congres, 2 volumes. Sofia, 1980–81. Articles in Russian, French, English, German.

International Congress of the History of Medicine, 27th, Barcelona, 1980: XXVII Congreso Internacional de Historia de la Medicina, 31 agosto – 6 septiembre 1980: Actas. Barcelona, Acadèmia de Ciències Mèdique de Catalunya i Balears, 1981. 2 Vol., 799 p.

Jacob M: Science and social passion: the case of seventeenth–century England. **J Hist Ideas** 1982 Apr–Jun;43(2):331–9

James JW: Writing and rewriting nursing history: a review essay. **Bull Hist Med** 1984 Winter;58(4):568–84

Joy RJ: Occupying the visual cortex: using slides to teach the history of medicine. In J. J. Bylebyl, ed: Teaching the history of medicine at a medical center. Baltimore, London, Johns Hopkins University Press, 1982. (The Henry E. Sigerist supplements to the Bulletin of the History of Medicine; new ser., no. 7). p. 103–14.

Judson HF: Reflections on the historiography of molecular biology. **Minerva** 1980 Autumn;18(3):369–421

Kaiser W: Wissenschaftsgeschichtliche Kooperation am Beispiel der slowakisch–ungarisch–halleschen Gemeinschaftsforschung zu Leben und Werk von Johann Andreas Segner und Johann Adam Reimann. **Wiss Z Martin Luther Univ (Math)** 1975;24(3):89–98

Kevles DJ: Genetics in the United States and Great Britain, 1890–1930: a review with speculations. **Isis** 1980 Sep;71(258):441–55

King RH: From creeds to therapies: Philip Rieff's work in perspective. **Rev Am Hist** 1976;4(2):291–6

Knodel J: Seasonal variation in infant mortality: an approach with applications. **Ann Demogr Hist (Paris)** 1983;:208–30

Kollesch J: Zum Problem der Medizingeschichtsschreibung in der griechisch–römischen Antike. In International Congress of the History of Medicine. 26th, Plovdiv, 1978. Actes du Congress. Sofia, 1981. Volume II. p. 124–6.

Labisch A: Zur Sozialgeschichte der Medizin. Methodologische Ueberlegungen und Forschungsbericht. **Arch Sozialgesch** 1980;20:431–70

Ladurie E LeRoy: The territory of the historian. Translated from the French by B. and S. Reynolds. Hassocks, Sussex (England), Harvester Press, 1979. viii, 345 p.

Landsberger M: The story of the history of medicine: essay–review. **Trans Stud Coll Physicians Phila** 1980 Dec;5(2 no 4):315–8

Larsen O: Die Krankheitsauffassung und ihre historische Interpretation. Ein Auswertungsmodell aufgrund von norwegischen Medizinalberichten aus dem 19. Jahrhundert. In Imhof AE, ed: Mensch und Gesundheit in der Geschichte. Husum, Matthiesen, 1980. p. 45–58.

Le mouvement historique: Bibliographie internationale d'histoire de la pharmacie et des sciences connexes. **Rev Hist Pharm (Paris)** 1982 Mar;29(252):60–76 (continued regularly)

Ledermann F: Faire de l'histoire de la pharmacie: pourquoi, comment? Quelques éléments historiographiques et théoriques en guise d'apologie. **Pharm Acta Helv** 1984;59(4):118–28

Lehners JP: Schwerpunkte historisch–demographischer Forschung in West– und Mitteleuropa. **Hist Soc Res** 1982;22:3–14

Leont'ev AA: Lichnost' kak istoriko–etnicheskaia kategoriia. **Sov Etnogr** 1981;3:35–44

LeRoy Ladurie E: Pressure of numbers: medical evidence, changing attitudes and historical demography. In his: The territory of the

historian. Hassocks, Sussex, England, Harvester Press, 1979. p. 221–84.
Levere TH, ed: Editing texts in the history of science and medicine. Papers given at the seventeenth annual Conference on Editorial Problems, University of Toronto, 6–7 November 1981. New York, London, Garland, 1982. 190 p. Contributions by S. Drake, L. E. Voigts, B. S. Hall, A. Beaulieu, I. B. Cohen.
Lichtenthaeler C: Chronologische und gedankliche Bezugssysteme in und um 'Ueber die alte Medizin'. XI. Hippokratische Studie. Genève, Droz, 1980. 30 p. (Etudes d'histoire de la médecine, VI).
Lindskog BI: Europeisk musei-konferens. **Sydsven Medicinhist Sallsk Arsskr** 1984;21:11–4
Littman RA: Psychology's histories: some new ones and a bit about their predecessors--an essay review. **J Hist Behav Sci** 1981 Oct;17(4):516–32
Lockridge KA: Historical demography. In Delzell, Charles F., ed.: the future of history: essays in the Vanderbilt University centennial symposium. Nashville, Vanderbilt U., 1977. p. 53–64.
Loewenberg P: The graduate years: what kind of journey? **Group Psychol Hist Newsl** 1975;4(1):2–7
Longrigg J: Superlative achievement and comparative neglect: Alexandrian medical science and modern historical research. **Hist Sci** 1981 Sep;19(45 pt 3):155–200
Loudon I: How it strikes a historian. **Br Med J [Clin Res]** 1984 Jan 14;288(6411):125–6
Löw R: Was hat die Pharmaziegeschichte der Wissenschaftstheorie zu sagen? In: Vorträge des Internationalen Pharmaziehistorischen Kongresses Innsbruck 1977. Stuttgart, Wissenschaftliche Verlagsgesellscaft, 1979. p. 29–38.
Luckin B: Death and survival in the city: approaches to the history of disease. **Urban Hist Yearb** 1980;:53–62
Ludmerer KM: Writing the history of hospitals. An essay review. **Bull Hist Med** 1982 Spring;56(1):106–9
Mack JE: Psychoanalysis and biography: aspects of a developing affinity. **J Am Psychoanal Assoc** 1980;28(3):543–62
McLoughlin Q: History, science and psychohistory. **Psychohist Rev** 1980;8(4):22–31
Manuscripta alchemica der Sammlung Mellon: Bemerkungen zum Katalog: **Sudhoffs Arch** 1981;65(1):79–96
Marshall ME: Biographical genre and biographical archetype: five studies of Gustav Theodor Fechner. **Stor Crit Psicol** 1980;1(2):197–233
Mattmüller M: Medizingeschichte und allgemeine Historie---Dialog und Zusammenarbeit auf dem Gebiet der modernen Sozialgeschichte. **Gesnerus** 1980;37(1/2):62–72
Maulitz RC: Disciplinary perspectives in the history of medicine: a view from the 1980s. With a commentary by R.P. Hudson. In J. J. Bylebyl, ed: Teaching the history of medicine at a medical center. Baltimore, London, Johns Hopkins University Press, 1982. (The Henry E. Sigerist supplements to the Bulletin of the History of Medicine; new ser., no. 7). p. 46–61.
Mazlish B: The next 'next assignment': leader and led, individual and group. **Psychohist Rev** 1981;9(3):214–37
Mazumdar PM: The history of medicine in a medical context. With a commentary by E. C. Atwater. In J. J. Bylebyl, ed: Teaching the history of medicine at a medical center. Baltimore, London, Johns Hopkins University Press, 1982. (The Henry E. Sigerist supplements to the Bulletin of the History of Medicine; new ser., no. 7). p. 91–102.
Medical history without medicine: **J Hist Med Allied Sci** 1980 Jan;35(1):5–7
Merton RK: George Alfred Léon Sarton. In Dictionary of American Biography, Suppl. 6, 1956–1960. p. 564–6, 1980.
Midelfort HC: Madness and civilization in early modern Europe: a reappraisal of Michel Foucault. In Malament, Barbara C., ed. After the Reformation: Essays in honor of J. H. Hexter, Philadelphia; U. of Pennsylvania Press, 1980. p. 247–65.
Miller G: Henry Ernest Sigerist. In Dictionary of American Biography, Suppl. 6, 1956–1960. p. 580–1, 1980.
Mousnier R: Réflexions d'un historien à la lecture d'un manuel de sociologie. **Rev Hist (Paris)** 1980;263(2):395–401
Mulligan L: Puritans and English science: a critique of Webster. **Isis** 1980 Sep;71(258):456–69
Musto DF: Continuity across generations: the Adams Family myth. In M. Albin, R. J. Devlin, G. Heeger, ed: New directions in psychohistory. The Adelphi papers in honor of Erik H. Erikson. Lexington, Toronto, D. C. Heath, 1980. p. 117–29.
Neu J: One hundred fifth critical bibliography of the history of science and its cultural influences (to January 1980). **Isis** 1980;71(260):1–295
Nielsen JS: Den patografiske tradition og metode. **Dan Medicinhist Arbog** 1983;12:91–104
Noland RW: Psychobiography: case history of life history? **Midwest Q** 1978;20(1):7–17
Nye MJ: Scientific decline: is quantitative evaluation enough? **ISIS** 1984 Dec;75(279):697–708
Ostromęcka H: Na marginesie pewnego zebrania. **Arch Hist Med (Warsz)** 1981;44(3/4):385–8
Outhwaite RB: Population change, family structure and the good of counting. **Hist J (Gt Brit)** 1979;22(1):229–37
Paracelsus-Forschung heute: Bericht über den Jubiläumskongress 1976 und die 25 jährige Geschichte der Gesellschaft, mit Beiträgen von K. Goldammer, A. Dyk, S. Domandl. Wien, 1977. 51 p. (Salzburger Beiträge zur Paracelsusforschung, 15).
Parascandola J: Pharmaceutical history for the pharmacy student. With a commentary by J. K. Crellin. In J. J. Bylebyl, ed: Teaching the history of medicine at a medical center. Baltimore, London, Johns Hopkins University Press, 1982. (The Henry E. Sigerist supplements to the Bulletin of the History of Medicine; new ser., no. 7). p. 78–90.
Parascandola J: Reflections on the history of pharmacology. **Pharm Hist** 1980;22(4):131–40
Pastore N: Dr. High on history. **J Hist Behav Sci** 1981 Oct;17(4):486–9
Pereira M: Alchimia medievale: alcuni studi recenti. **Ann Ist Mus Stor Sci Fir** 1984;9(2):89–98
Pfohl G: Das philosophisch-philologische Element in der medizinischen Fakultät. Ein Beitrag der Medizingeschichte, mehr zu formen als zu informieren. I, II. **Med Welt** 1980 Apr 25, May 9;(17,19):644–6,730–3
Płonka-Syroka B, Wieckowska E: Rozwazania o metodyce pisania prac naukowych z zakresu historii medycyny. **Arch Hist Med (Warsz)** 1984;47(1):11–7
Podgórska-Klawe Z: Kilka uwag o warsztacie historyka medycyny. **Arch Hist Med (Warsz)** 1981;44(1):93–6
Porter R: Death and the doctors. **Med Hist** 1982 Jul;26(3):335–41
Premuda L: La storia della medicina nelle facoltà mediche: ruolo e prospettive dell'insegnamento e della ricerca. **Acta Med Hist Patav** 1978–79;25:15–40
Ravitch MM: The uses of medical history. **Pharos** 1983 Fall;46(4):2–6
Recollections & reflections: Lawrence J. Henderson and George Sarton. **Isis** 1984 Mar;75(276):11–32
Regelmann JP: Struktur des Arguments als Struktur der Geschichte?--oder: Paradigm lost! **Medizinhist J** 1982;17(1/2):37–53
Reverte Coma JM: El trabajo de campo en antropología médica. **Asclepio** 1983;35:69–115
Rödel V: Gedanken zur Archivierung medizinischen Schriftguts. **Medizinhist J** 1984;19(3):167–72
Rodin AE, Reece RD: The teaching of medical history by instructors from a variety of disciplines. With a commentary by L.G. Stevenson. In J. J. Bylebyl, ed: Teaching the history of medicine at a medical center. Baltimore, London, Johns Hopkins University Press, 1982. (The Henry E. Sigerist supplements to the Bulletin of the History of Medicine; new ser., no. 7). p. 152–60.
Römer F: Plinius der Aeltere. III. Bericht. **Anz Altertumswiss** 1978;31:129–206
Rose JC, Corn M: Dr. E. and other patients: new lessons from old case reports. **J Hist Med Allied Sci** 1984 Jan;39(1):3–32
Rosenthal N: The psychology of women. **Psychohist Rev** 1980;8(4):32–6
Röthlisberger P: Charles Greene Cumston (1868–1928): Medizinhistoriker in zwei Kontinenten. **Gesnerus** 1984;41(1/2):137–51
Rothschuh KE: Medicina Historica. Zum Selbstverständnis der historischen Medizin. **Janus** 1980;67(1–2–3):7–19
Rousseau GS: Ephebi, Epigoni, and Fornacalia: some meditations on the contemporary historiography of the eighteenth century. **Eighteenth Cent Stud** 1979;20:203–26
Rousseau GS: Literature and medicine: the state of the field. **Isis** 1981 Sep;72(263):406–24
Rousseau GS, Porter R, ed: The ferment of knowledge. Studies in the historiography of eighteenth-century science. Cambridge, Cambridge University Press, 1980. xiii, 500 p. including contributions by R. Harre, S. Schaffer, S. Shapin, H. J. Bos, J. L. Heilbron, E. G. Forbes, D. S. Cardwell.
Ryant C: Comment: oral history and gerontology. **Gerontologist** 1981 Feb;21(1):104–5
Ryant C: Oral history and psychohistory. **J Psychohist** 1981 Winter;8(3):307–18
Salimbeni F: Psicanalisi e storiografia: un problema pluridisciplinare. **Studium** 1981;77(5):565–80
Salov VI: Vtorzhenie psikhoanaliza v burzhuaznuiu istoriografiiu. (Rus). **Nov Noveishaia Istor** 1972;(4):89–105
Scarborough J: Classical antiquity: medicine and allied sciences. **Trends Hist** 1979 Fall-Winter;1(2):3–14
Scarborough J, ed: Society for Ancient Medicine newsletter. No. 1–10 (Apr. 1976–Sept. 1982). Continued periodically.
Schmidt C: Alchemists, critics and psychohistorians. **J Psychohist** 1981 Winter;8(3):337–67
Schoenwald RL: The psychological study of history. In Iggers, GG, Parker HT, ed: International handbook of historical studies: contemporary research and theory. Westport, Conn., Greenwood, 1979. p. 71–85.
Schott H: Traum und Geschichte. Zur Freudschen Geschichtsauffassung im Kontext der Traumdeutung. **Sudhoffs Arch** 1980;64(3):298–312
Schweber SS: Essay review; early Victorian science: science in culture. **J Hist Biol** 1980 Spring;13(1):121–40
Seidler E: Le rôle de la méthode historique dans la médecine actuelle. In Poirier J, Poirier JL, ed: Médecine et philosohie à la fin du XIXe siècle. Paris, Université de Paris XII - Val de Marne, [1980?]. p. 149–55.
Servais P, Roger FH: Les archives médicales hospitalières: organisation et possibilités d'utilisation. **Ann Soc Belg Hist Hop** 1980;18:71–96
Shelestov DK: U istokov istoricheskoi demografii. **Vestn Mosk Univ Ser 8 Istor** 1982;(3):21–33
Shepherd M: The psycho-historians: a psychiatrist's skepticism. **Encounter (Lond)** 1979;52(3):35–42

Shore MF: The psychogenic theory of history. **J Interdiscip Hist** 1979;9(3):517–23
Shortt SE: Cholera: doctors' dilemma, historians' delight. **Queens Q** 1981;88(1):130–4
Shortt SE: Clinical practice and the social history of medicine: a theoretical accord. **Bull Hist Med** 1981 Winter;55(4):533–42
Shortt SE: Medical professionalization: pitfalls and promise in the historiography. **HSTC** 1981 Sep;19(5 no 3):210–9
Siraisi NG: Some recent work on western European medical learning, ca. 1200–ca. 1500. In History of Universities, II, 1982. p. 225–38.
Smith DC: A renaissance for medical history. **J Hist Med Allied Sci** 1984 Oct;39(4):405–7
Stannard DE: Shrinking history. On Freud and the failure of psychohistory. New York, Oxford University Press, 1980. xx, 187 p.
Steneck NH: Greatrakes the stroker: the interpretations of historians. **ISIS** 1982 Jun;73(267):161–77
Stocking GW: Innovation in the Malinowskian mode: an essay review of long-term field research in social anthropology. **J Hist Behav Sci** 1980 Jul;16(3):281–6
Stroppiana L: La moderne méthodologie scientifique dans le domaine de l'histoire de la medécine. In: International Congress of the History of Medicine, 26th, Plovdiv (Bulgaria), 1978. Actes du Congres, Vol. 1. Sofia, 1980. p. 80–1.
Strout C: Psyche, Clio, and the artist. In M. Albin, R. J. Devlin, G. Heeger, ed: New directions in psychohistory. The Adelphi papers in honor of Erik H. Erikson. Lexington, Toronto, D. C. Heath, 1980. p. 97–115.
Strozier CB: A rationale for teaching psychohistory. **Group Psychol Hist Newsl** 1975;4(1):8–10
Strozier CB: Springfield über alles: role playing and the teaching of psychohistory. **Group Psychol Hist Newsl** 1975;4(2):13–24
Swales RJ: Plague, population and ecology in early modern England. **Can J Hist** 1979;14(2):257–66
Syroka A: Pojecie źródeł do historii medycyny i próba ich klasyfikacji. **Arch Hist Med (Warsz)** 1984;47(1):19–24
Taylor DW: Medical libraries and medical history. **NZ Libr** 1976 Apr;39(2):62–7
Taylor LS: Technical accuracy in historical writing. **Health Phys** 1981 May;40(5):595–9
Teigen PM: Medical libraries and history of medicine libraries. **Newsl Libr Hist Health Sci** 1982 Jul;6(1):1–6
Teigen PM, ed: Books, manuscripts, and the history of medicine. Essays on the fiftieth anniversary of the Osler Library. New York, Science History Publications, 1982. 112 p. Contributions by L. G. Stevenson, C. G. Roland, R. J. Durling, E. Brodman, G. T. Tanselle, E. J. Freeman.
Thibodeau D: Indexing medical history: a guide to the literature: an essay review. **Bull Hist Med** 1982 Summer;56(2):276–9
Timofeyev IS: Izmeneniia v ponimanii predmeta istoriko–nauchnykh issledovanii. **Vopr Istor Estestvozn Tekh** 1981;(2):97–102
Tutzke D: Möglichkeiten und Bedeutung quantifizierbarer Aussagen in der medizingeschichtlichen Forschung. In International Congress of the History of Medicine. 26th, Plovdiv, 1978. Actes du Congress. Sofia, 1981. Volume II. p. 209–10.
VanHartesveldt FR: Disease in the Western world: a review essay. **Teach Hist J Methods** 1980;5(1):75–81
Vann RT: The new demographic history. Iggers, Georg G. and Parker, Harold T., ed: International Handbook of Historical Studies: Contemporary Research and Theory. Westport, Conn., Greenwood Press, 1979. p. 29–42.
Vetter T: Essai sur la littérature hippocratique au dix-huitième siècle. In La collection hippocratique et son rôle dans l'histoire de la médecine. Colloque de Strasbourg (23–27 octobre 1972) organisé par le Centre de Recherches sur la Grèce Antique, avec le concours des Facultés de Philosophie et des Langues Classiques. Leiden, E. J. Brill, 1975. p. 347–67.
Viseltear AJ: Antecedents to contemporary health issues: history, politics, and the policy of health. With a commentary by B.G. Rosenkrantz. In J. J. Bylebyl, ed: Teaching the history of medicine at a medical center. Baltimore, London, Johns Hopkins University Press, 1982. (The Henry E. Sigerist supplements to the Bulletin of the History of Medicine; new ser., no. 7). p. 62–77.
Vovelle M: Rediscovery of death since 1960. **Ann Am Acad Polit Soc Sci** 1980;447:89–99
Vovelle M: The history of mankind in the mirror of death. **Proc Annu Meet West Soc Fr Hist** 1978;6:91–109
Wallace ER: Historiography in history and psychoanalysis. **Bull Hist Med** 1983 Summer;57(2):247–66
Waserman M, Clausen C, ed: Bulletin of the History of Medicine. Index to volumes and supplements, 1933–1982. Baltimore, Johns Hopkins University Press, 1983. 195 p.
Watson RI: A methodological note on the research use of the Syntopicon. **J Hist Behav Sci** 1980 Jul;16(3):275–9
Webster C: Medicine as social history: changing ideas on doctors and patients in the age of Shakespeare. With commentary by D. G. Bates, p. 127–34. In Stevenson LG, ed: A celebration of medical history. Baltimore, Johns Hopkins University Press, 1982. (The Henry E. Sigerist supplements to the Bulletin of the History of Medicine;; new ser., no. 6). p. 103–26..
Whitaker MA: Science, scientists and history of science. **Hist Sci** 1984 Dec;22(58 pt 4):421–4
Whitrow M: A classification scheme for the history of science, medicine and technology. In Forbes EG, ed: Human implications of scientific advance. Edinburgh, Edinburgh University Press, 1978. p. 518–30.
Wick DL: Psychomythology: A phenomenological critique of psychohistory. **Dalhousie Rev** 1980;6(2):290–99
Zaretsky E: A note on Marxism and psychoanalysis. **Marx Perspect** 1979;2(2):134–9
Zysk KG: A note on ancient Indian medicine. **Bull Indian Inst Hist Med (Hyderabad)** 1978;8(1–4):14–23
22.500 thèses françaises de médecine publiées de 1796 à 1896: Un monument de l'histoire de la médecine. Genève, Librairie Slatkine, 1982. Various paginations.

#### Americas

Risse GB: Medical history in Latin America. **Clio Med** 1981 Apr;15(3–4):231–45

#### Australia

Home RW: History of science in Australia. **Isis** 1982 Sep;73(268):337–42
Love R: A note on courses taught by Australian psychology departments in the history and philosophy of psychology. **Newsl Australas Assoc Hist Philos Sci** 1975–6;7:28–33a
Verso ML: The history of medical history; with special reference to Australia. **Victorian Hist J** 1979 May;50(2):58–76

#### Austria

Buess H: Der Wiener Sozialmediziner Ludwig Teleky (1872–1957) und seine 'History of factory and mine hygiene'. **Wien Med Wochenschr** 1981 Oct 15;131(19):479–83
Buess H: Der Wiener Sozialmediziner Ludwig Teleky (1872–1957) und seine 'History of Factory and Mine Hygiene'. In Ganzinger K, Skopec M, Wyklicky H, ed: Festschrift für Erna Lesky zum 70. Geburtstag. Wien, Brüder Hollinek, 1981. p. 31–7.
Risse GB: Erna Lesky and the history of medicine. **Bull Hist Med** 1981 Winter;55(4):575–80
Verzeichnis der wissenschaftlichen Arbeiten von Erna Lesky: In Ganzinger K, Skopec M, Wyklicky H, ed: Festschrift für Erna Lesky zum 70. Geburtstag. Wien, Brüder Hollinek, 1981. p. 193–203.
Wyklicky H: Uber einige Aufgaben des medizinhistorischen Unterrichtes. **Wien Klin Wochenschr** 1981 Nov 13;93(21):660–5

#### Belgium

Edsall JT: Marcel Florkin, August 15, 1900--May 3, 1979. **Isis** 1980 Jun;71(257):286–8
Fruton JS: Marcel Florkin, 1900–1979, historian of biochemistry. **Hist Philos Life Sci** 1980;2(1):167–71
Huard P: Marcel Florkin (1900–1979). **Clio Med** 1980 May;14(2):93–5
In memoriam Professor Dr. Marcel Florkin (1900–1979): **Clio Med** 1980 May;14(2):89–90
Mattelaer B: Le Benelux et son apport à l'histoire égyptienne et arabe de la pharmacie. **Bull Pharm** 1979;1–2:1–5
Schoffeniels E: In memoriam Marcel Florkin (Liège, 15 août 1900–3 mai 1979). Les chênes qu'on abat. **Rev Med Liege** 1979 Jun 1;34(11):481–7
Schoffeniels E: Marcel Florkin et les aspects molecularies de la biologie. **Bull Mem Acad R Med Belg** 1979 Nov 24;134(10):604–16
Théodoridès J: Marcel Florkin (1900–1979). **Rev Hist Sci (Paris)** 1980 Jan;33(1):75–6
Théodoridès J: Marcel Florkin (1900–1979). **Hist Sci Med** 1980;14(2):145–50

#### Bulgaria

Kalŭdov I, et al: Prof. Dr. George Pavlov (a centennial of his birth). **Vet Med Nauki** 1981;18(2):3–89
Pavlova V: Istoriografiia meditsinskoĭ nauki v Bolgarii. **Sov Zdravookhr** 1980;(9):41–5
Pŭrvi Natsionalen kongres po istoriia na meditsinata: Shumen, 9–11 oktomvri 1981 god: reziumeta. Bulgaria], Nauch. druzhestvo po istoriia na meditsinata v Bŭlgariia, [1981?]. 146 p.

#### Canada

Bates DG: Teaching medical history to medical students: the McGill experience, 1966–1981. With a commentary by L.G. Stevenson. In J. J. Bylebyl, ed: Teaching the history of medicine at a medical center. Baltimore, London, Johns Hopkins University Press, 1982. (The Henry E. Sigerist supplements to the Bulletin of the History of Medicine; new ser., no. 7). p. 121–38.
LaRose A: Bibliographie courante sur l'histoire de la population canadienne et la démographie historique au Canada, 1977. **Soc Hist (Canada)** 1979;12(23):192–7

Paterson GR: The Hannah Institute: promoting Canadian history of medicine. **Can Med Assoc J** 1983 Jun 1;128(11):1325-8
Roland CG: Dr. Earl Scarlett: melding tradition and beauty in historical writing. **Can Med Assoc J** 1980 Apr 5;122(7):822-6
Sherrington A: Canadian medical periodicals on microfiche. **Can Med Assoc J** 1981 Feb 15;124(4):361-2
Shortt SE: Andrew Macphail: the ideal in nature. In his The search for an ideal: six Canadian intellectuals and their convictions in an age of transition, 1890-1930. Toronto, Buffalo, University of Toronto Press, 1976. p. 12-38.
Smith K: Maude Abbott: pathologist and historian. **Can Med Assoc J** 1982 Oct 15;127(8):774-6

**China**

Bates DG: Teaching and research in the history of medicine in China. **Bull Hist Med** 1979 Spring;53(1):128-39
[Papers on Chinese medicine and on the study of medical history in China.] (Chi): **Chung Hua I Shih Tsa Chih** 1980;10(1):1-64
Ts'ai HC: [Demographic methodology and its application to studies of historical populations] (Chi). **Ssu yu Yen** 1982;20(4):49-56
Wong M: Contributions récentes à l'histoire de la médecine chinoise. **Clio Med** 1981;15:260-2

**Colombia**

Serpa-Flores R: La enseñanza de la historia de la medicina en la formación del médico. **Educ Med Salud** 1983;17(4):423-32

**Czechoslovakia**

Böhm R: Weniger bekannte historische Schriften aus der CSSR. **Hist Med Vet** 1977;2(2):56-7
Müller C, Nikliček L: Der gegenwärtige Zustand und die Aufgaben des Unterrichts in der Geschichte der Medizin an der hygienischen medizinischen Fakultät der Karlsuniversität. In Congr. Hist. Sci., Prague 1981. p. 419-33. **Acta Hist Rerum Nat Tech** 1981;11, special number
Peňáz J: K úmrtí prof. MUDr. Vladislava Kruty, DrSc. **Cesk Fysiol** 1980 Mar;29(2):159-70
Sídlo R: Příspěvek k významu a metodice výuky dějin lékařství a zdravotnictví na lékařské fakultě. **Sb Ved Pr Lek Fak Univ Karlovy** 1979;22(5 Suppl):579-82
Simon F: Latinčinár ako historik medicíny. **Cas Lek Cesk** 1984 Oct 12;123(40-41):1250
Tamáska P: Az orvostörténet oktatásának és müvelésének története Csehországban. **Orv Hetil** 1984 Aug 5;125(32):1963-4

**Denmark**

Jensen VG: Poul Richard Hauberg, 1887-1959. **Theriaca** 1982 Jun;22:xi-xvi
Schaeffer A, Kruse E: Danske farmacihistoriske arbejder efter året 1800. En kortfattet oversigt med bibliografi. 2. ed. København, Dansk Farmacihistorisk Selskab, 1982. 229 p.

**Europe**

Pope BH, ed: Historical periodicals directory. Volume 2: Europe, West, North, Central and South. Santa Barbara, Oxford, ABC-Clio, 1983. xv, 597 p. (Clio Periodicals Directories).

**Finland**

Teir H: Medicinens historia som akademiskt undervisningsämne--erfarenheter från Finland. **Nord Medicinhist Arsb** 1980;Suppl 6:30-4

**France**

Allan NM: Gustave Alexandre Liétard, orientalist and physician. **Med Hist** 1981 Jan;25(1):85-8
Biraben JN: André Armengaud, 1920-1980. **Ann Demogr Hist (Paris)** 1980;:7-10
Bonnemain H: La Société d'Histoire de la Pharmacie; sa création - son développement - ses activités. In: Vorträge des Internationalen Pharmaziehistorischen Kongresses Innsbruck 1977. Stuttgart, Wissenschaftliche Verlagsgesellschaft, 1979. p. 81-90.
Brumpt L: Eloge de Pierre Huard (1901-1983). **Bull Acad Natl Med (Paris)** 1984 Jan-Feb;168(1-2):181-7
Costa O: Storie sommerse di biologia e medicina. **Scientia** 1980;115:215-25
Delaby PA: Le doyen Guillaume Valette (1902-1982). **Hist Sci Med** 1982;16(2):65-79
Delatte L, Halleux R: Recettes médicales anciennes et ordinateur: le projet Theorema. **Rev Hist Pharm (Paris)** 1980 Sep;27(246):155-160
Dulieu L: Le doyen Jean Turchini (Nice, 1894 - Montpellier, 1979) et l'histoire de la médecine. **Hist Sci Med** 1979;13(4):339-41
Dumaître P: Jean Dezeimeris, médecin et historien (1799-1852). In: Congrès National des Sociétés Savantes, 104e, Bordeaux, 1979. Comptes Rendus. Paris, 1979. Section des Sciences, Fasc. IV. p. 69-80.
Fossard J: Un inédit d'un fondateur de la Société française d'histoire de la médecine, le docteur Paul Delaunay. **Hist Sci Med** 1981;15(4):305-6
Gelfand T: The Annales and the history of medicine. **Bull Hist Med** 1981 Winter;55(4):589-93
Halleux R: Marcellin Berthelot, historien de l'alchimie. In: Congrès National des Sociétés Savantes, 104e, Bordeaux, 1979. Comptes Rendus. Paris, 1979. Section des Sciences, Fasc. IV. p. 169-80.
Imbault-Huart MJ, ed: Table ronde consacrée au recteur Pierre Huard (1901-1983). Contributions by J. L. Plessis, P. M. Niaussat, T. H. Nguyen, J. Théodoridès. **Hist Sci Med** 1983;17(4):381-402
Legee G: P. Flourens, historien des sciences: valeur de son histoire de la découverte de la circulation du sang. In: Congrès National des Sociétés Savantes, 107e. Brest, 1982. Comptes Rendus, Paris, 1983. Section des Sciences, Fasc. IV. p. 313-31.
Leuilliot P: Problèmes de méthode: histoire (et archives) de la santé. In Livet G, Schaff G, ed: Médecine et assistance en Alsace, XVIe-XXe siècle. Strasbourg, Istra, 1976. p. 11-17.
Mazars G: Jean Filliozat (1906-1982). **Watermark** 1983 Jan;12:3-7
Mitchell A: Philippe Ariès and the French way of death. **Fr Hist Stud** 1978;10(4):684-95
Pecker A: André Finot (24 mars 1884 - 3 janvier 1980). **Hist Sci Med** 1980;14(1):23-7
Poussou JP: In memoriam: Philippe Aries (1914-1984). **Ann Demogr Hist (Paris)** 1984;:5-6
Sedgwick P: Michel Foucault: the anti-history of psychiatry. **Psychol Med** 1981 May;11(2):235-48
Société française d'histoire des hôpitaux: [1978-79 prizes in hospital history]: **Bull Soc Fr Hist Hop** 1980;(40):4-22
Sournia JC: L'histoire de la médecine en France. **Clio Med** 1980;15(1/2):83-9
Spagnoli PG: Philippe Ariès, historian of the family. **J Fam Hist** 1981 Winter;6(4):434-41
Subba Reddy DV: Prof. Jean Filliozat (1906-1981). **Bull Indian Inst Hist Med Hyderabad** 1982;12(1-4):85-8
Théodoridès J: Pierre Chabbert (1924-1981). **Hist Sci Med** 1981;15(4):287-92
Valentin M, Niaussat PM: Le rôle fondamental d'Amédée Lefèvre, médecin de la Marine (1798-1869), en médecine du travail et en histoire de la médecine. **Hist Sci Med** 1979;13(4):407-17

**Germany**

Bugyi B: Tagung der Deutschen Gesellschaft für Geschichte der Medizin und der Naturwissenschaften im Jahre 1929 zu Budapest. **Orvostort Kozl** 1979;86(24 no 4):65-71
Diehl B: Der Wandel der Historiographie von Medizin und Naturwissenschaften in ihrer gesellschaftlichen Bedingtheit. **Sudhoffs Arch** 1982;66(3):276-300
Dilg, P, et al., ed: Perspektiven der Pharmaziegeschichte: Festschrift für Rudolf Schmitz zum 65. Geburtstag. Bibliography by F. J. Kühlen. Graz, Austria, Akademische Druck- u. Verlagsanstalt, 1983. xviii, 497 p.
Dumont F: Bericht über das Soemmerring-Symposion 1983. **Ber Wissenschaftsgesch** 1984;7(1):58-64
Durling R: Corrigenda and addenda to Diels' Galenica: II. codices miscellanei. **Traditio** 1981;37:373-81
Fichtner G, ed: Index wissenschaftshistorischer Dissertationen (IWD). Verzeichnis abgeschlossener Dissertationen auf dem Gebiet der Geschichte der Medizin, der Pharmazie, der Naturwissenschaften und der Technik. Nr. 1:1970-1980. Tübingen, Institut für Geschichte der Medizin, 1981. 285 p.
Fichtner G, ed: Laufende wissenschaftshistorische Dissertationen (LWD). Verzeichnis in Bearbeitung befindlicher Dissertationen auf dem Gebiet der Geschichte der Medizin, der Pharmazie, der Naturwissenschaften und der Technik. Nr. 1, Tübingen, Institut für Geschichte der Medizin, 1981. 125 p.
Forbes EG: Scientific archives in the Federal Republic of Germany. **Ber Wissenschaftsgesch** 1979;2(3-4):197-201
Fürderer C: Medizin- und geistesgeschichtliche Vorläufer klinisch-psychiatrischer Biographik in der Epoche der Aufklärung und Romantik. Diss. Bonn, 1981. 151 p.
Geuter U, Mattes P: Historiography of psychology in West Germany: approaches from social history. A review of the past ten years. **Stor Crit Psicol** 1984 Jun;5(1):111-26
Göpfert W, Otten HH, ed: Metavoeite: wandelt euch durch neues Denken: Festschrift für Professor Hans Schadewaldt zur Vollendung des 60. Lebensjahres. Düsseldorf, Triltsch, 1983. 226 p.
Gourevitch M: Le musée Adler d'histoire de la médecine à Johannesburg. **Hist Sci Med** 1982;16(1):21-2
Habrich C, Marguth F, Wolf JH, et al: Medizinische Diagnostik in Geschichte und Gegenwart. Festschrift für Heinz Goerke zum sechzigsten Geburtstag. München, Fritsch, 1978. 656 p. Historical contributions by J. Antall, G. Baader, V. Bazala, L. Belloni, G. Bratescu, W. Brendel, L. Burilkova, C. J. Clemedson, K. Goldammer, H. Henne, S. Hofmann, G. Keil, K. P. Killian, W. Klinner, W. Kloppe, M. Knedel, W. Kock, F. Köcher, H. M. Koelbing, K. S. Kolta, E. Kreuzer, V. Krizek, O. Larsen, B. I. Lindskog, N. Mani, V. Møller-Christensen, Y.

Otsuka, G. Preiser, L. Premuda, E. Püschel, H. Röhrich, E. Rosner, G. Rudolph, J. Sájner, H. Schadewaldt, H. Schipperges, H. H. Simmer, J. Spielmann, M. Stürzbecher, A. Terzioglu, R. Winau, N. Plovdiv. (Neue Münchner Beiträge zur Geschichte der Medizin und Naturwissenschaften, Medizinhistorische Reihe, Band 7/8).

Harig G: Bemerkungen zum medizinhistorischen Unterricht in der DDR. **Z Gesamte Hyg** 1980;26(5):383–5

Imhof AE: Mensch und Gesundheit in der Geschichte; Bericht über eine internationale Tagung in Berlin, 20.–23. September 1978. **Ber Wissenschaftsgesch** 1978;1(3–4):235–44

Kahle E, Stupp JA: Hochschulschriften zur Geschichte der Medizin, Pharmazie, und Naturwissenschaften der Friedrich–Alexander–Universität Erlangen–Nürnberg 1885–1975. Erlangen, Verlagsbuchhandlung Hannelore Lüling, 1980. 94 p. (Medizinhistorische Materialien, 2).

Kaiser W: Bericht über die 61. Jahrestagung der Deutschen Gesellschaft für Geschichte der Medizin, Naturwissenschaft und Technik e. V. **Ber Wissenschaftsgesch** 1978;1(3–4):232–4

Keil G: Karl–Sudhoff–Gedächtnissitzung. Sudhoffs Sicht vom deutschen medizinischen Mittelalter. **Nachrichtenbl Dtsch Ges Gesch Med Naturwiss Tech** 1981 Dec;31(3):94–129

Koch HT: Julius Rosenbaum (1807–1874) als Medizinhistoriker. **NTM** 1981;18(1):84–90

Kollesch J: Das Berliner Corpus der antiken Aerzte. **Clio Med** 1981 Sep;16(1):45–7

Krafft F: Forschungsberichte und Spezial–Bibliographien. **Ber Wissenschaftsgesch** 1980;3(3–4):127–88

Kraus I: Hermann Schelenz. In Balde JH, Schmiking W, ed: Festschrift zum 86. Deutschen Ärztetag in Kassel. Kassel, Ärztevereins, 1983 p. 41–9.

Labisch A, Spree R, Weindling P: Conference Report. Social history of nineteenth– and twentieth–century German medicine. **Soc Soc Hist Med Bull (Lond)** 1983;32:40–5

Labisch A: Recent trends in the social history of occupational medicine in the Federal Republic of Germany. **Soc Soc Hist Med Bull (Lond)** 1983 Dec;33:52–7

Lindner H, et al, ed: [Contemporary medical historiography in Germany]. **Nachrichtenbl Dtsch Ges Gesch Med Naturwiss Tech** 1980 Apr;30(1):1–64

Meier P: Paracelsus–Reminiszenzen--Arzt und Medizin im Werk von Reinhold Schneider. **Salzburger Beitr Paracelsusforsch** 1984;23:100–17

Müller–Jahncke WD: In memoriam Walter Pagel (1898–1983). **Ber Wissenschaftsgesch** 1983;6(1–4):165–8

Rödel WG: Mensch und Gesundheit in der Geschichte der Neuzeit. **Medizinhist J** 1984;19(1–2):138–47

Rothschuh KE, Krafft F: Forschungsberichte und Spezial–Bibliographien. **Ber Wissenschaftsgesch** 1978;1(3–4):201–15

Rothschuh KE: Richard Hermann Koch (1882–1949): Arzt, Medizinhistoriker, Medizinphilosoph (Biographisches, Ergographisches). 1. Teil. Zur Biographie. **Medizinhist J** 1980;15(1/2):16–43

Schipperges H: Walther Schönfeld (1888–1977) und seine Verdienste als Medizinhistoriker. **Hautarzt** 1980 Aug;31(8):441–3

Schneider W: Pharmaziegeschichte und ihre Repräsentanten im 20. Jahrhundert. Zum 80. Geburtstag von Prof. Dr. Georg Edmund Dann. **Pharm Ztg** 1978;123:1265–71

Schütt HW: History of science in the Federal Republic of Germany. **Isis** 1980 Sep;71(258):375–80

Schwann H: Zur Gestaltung spezieller Vorlesungen 'Geschichte der Zahnheilkunde' für Stomatologie–Studenten. **Stomatol DDR** 1982 Mar;32(3):229–33

Schwann S: Lekarze polscy w świetle historyczno–medycznego dzieła Grzegorza Matthiasa z XVIII wieku. **Arch Hist Med (Warsz)** 1979;42(2):217–22

Seidler E, Schott H, ed: Bausteine zur Medizingeschichte. Heinrich Schipperges zum 65. Geburtstag. Stuttgart, Steiner, 1984. 154 p. (Sudhoffs Archiv, Beihefte, Heft 24)

Seyda B: O nauczaniu historii medycyny w RFN. **Arch Hist Med (Warsz)** 1982;45(1–4):107–10

Snyder C: Julius Hirschberg, the neglected historian of ophthalmology. **Am J Ophthalmol** 1981 May;91(5):664–76

Strohmaier G: Der arabische Hippokrates. Bemerkungen zu einem Aufsatz von Dieter Irmer. **Sudhoffs Arch** 1980;64(3):234–49

Tutzke D, ed: Zur Entwicklung der Sozialhygiene im 19. und 20. Jahrhundert. Ausgewählte Beiträge vom I. Medizinhistorischen Symposium DDR–UdSSR, Halle (Saale) 1975. Berlin, Akademie für Aerztliche Fortbildung der DDR; Gesellschaft für Geschichte der Medizin in der DDR, 1976, xi, 277 p.

Wankmüller A: Die Bibliothek der Internationalen Gesellschaft für Geschichte der Pharmazie. **Ber Wissenschaftsgesch** 1979;2(3–4):226–8

Wankmüller A: Entstehung des 'Grundriss der Geschichte der deutschen Pharmazie' von Adlung und Urdang. **Pharm Ztg** 1980;125:403–6

Wehler HU: Psychoanalysis and history. **Soc Res (NY)** 1980;47(3):519–36

Winau R: Deutsche Gesellschaft für Geschichte der Medizin, Naturwissenschaft und Tecknik 1901–1976. Wiesbaden, Steiner, 1978. 164 p. (Beiträge zur Geschichte der Wissenschaft und der Technik, 15).

Winkelmann H, Mildner S: Schriftenverzeichnis Hans–Heinz Eulner (19. 4. 1925 - 17. 10. 1980). **Medizinhist J** 1982;17(1/2):148–55

Wittern R: The Robert Bosch Foundation and the establishment of the Institute for the History of Medicine. **Clio Med** 1980;15(1/2):89–91

Wölfel A: Pflanzen in der Volksmedizin. Die volksmedizinischen Studien von Heinrich Marzell. Diss. Erlangen–Nürnberg, 1983. 117 p.

Wussing H: 75 Jahre Karl–Sudhoff–Institut für Geschichte der Medizin und der Naturwissenschaften am Bereich Medizin der Karl–Marx–Universität. **NTM** 1981;18(1):2–3

**Great Britain**

Barry J: Guide to sources and writings on the history of medicine in Bristol, 1600–1900. **Soc Soc Hist Med Bull (Lond)** 1984 Dec;35:48–52

Beloff M: Dr. Darlington's provocative work: the genetic approach to world history. **Encounter (Lond)** 1970;35(4):85–8

Benson B, Wall R: Historical demography in the nineteenth and twentieth centuries in the absence of the civil registers. **Local Popul Stud (Matlock)** 1981 Spring;26:14–28

Carter HE: Who needs veterinary history? **J Small Anim Pract** 1981 Apr;22(4):175–6

Crombie AC: James Sterling Wilkie: 1906–1982. **Br J Hist Sci** 1984 Nov;17(57 pt 3):310–1

Davis AB: Walter Pagel, 14 November 1898–1 April 1983. **ISIS** 1984;75(277):363–5

Debus AG: Walter Pagel (1898–1983). **Bull Hist Med** 1983 Winter;57(4):611–5

Dopson L: The new breed of nurse historian. **Nurs Times** 1984 Sep 19–25;80(38):16–7

Elvin M, et al: The work of Joseph Needham. **Past Present** 1980;87:17–53

Ferguson M: Reflections on teaching a history of nursing. **Nurs Times** 1979 Nov;75(46–47):suppl 29–30:117–20, 121–2

Hartley H: Douglas McKie. In Dictionary of national biography, 1961–1970. Suppl. 8, 1981. p. 695–7.

Jordanova L, ed: Medical records newsletter. (Research Publications of the Wellcome Unit for the History of Medicine, Oxford. No. IV). Oxford, Wellcome Unit for the History of Medicine, 1980. viii, 42 p.

Lock S: A question of confidence. An editor's view. **Br Med J [Clin Res]** 1984 Jan 14;288(6411):123–5

Maggs C: The making of a history man [interview by Jane Salvage]. **Nurs Times** 1983 Aug 17–23;79(33):8–10

Marshall TH, Laslett P: David Glass: an appreciation. **Br J Sociol** 1979;30(1):1–4

Matthews LG: The History of Pharmacy Committee of the Pharmaceutical Society 1952–1967. **Pharm Hist (London)** 1976 Dec;6(3):3–4

Newby MS: Problems of teaching nursing history. 1. **Nurs Times** 1979 Nov 22;75(47):suppl 30:123–4 (continued periodically)

Oakley A: The relevance of the history of medicine to an understanding of current change: some comments from the domain of antenatal care. **Soc Sci Med** 1982;16(6):667–74

Pearson ES, ed: The history of statistics in the 17th and 18th centuries against the changing background of intellectual, scientific and religious thought. Lectures by Karl Pearson given at University College London during the academic sessions 1921–1933. New York, Macmillan, 1978. xix, 744 p.

Poynter N: Douglas James Guthrie, M.D., D. Litt., F.R.C.S.E., F.R.C.P.E., F.R.S.E., 8 September 1885 - 8 June 1975. **Med Hist** 1975 Oct;19(4):400–1

Rowbottom ME: Dr. E. Ashworth Underwood (1899–1980). **Med Hist** 1980 Jul;24(3):349–52

The Scottish society of the history of medicine: report of proceedings, session 1978–79. **Med Hist** 1980 Apr;24(2):209–13

Shepherd MA: Lunacy and labour. **Soc Stud Labour Hist** 1977;(34):61–9

Sheptunova ZI: Dzh R. Partington - vydaiushchiisia istorik khimii. **Vopr Istor Estestvozn Tekh** 1981;3:107–10

Smeaton WA: James Riddick Partington. In Dictionary of national biography, 1961–1970. Suppl. 8, 1981. p. 822–3.

[The need to preserve medical history records]: Evidence presented to the Public Records Committee.: **Soc Soc Hist Med Bull (Lond)** 1979 Dec;25:68–76

**Greece**

Marinéskou–Chýmou M: Ektor saraphídes: iatrós kaí lógis (1872–1950). **Epet Etaireias Stereoelladikon Meleton** 1974–75;5:547–52

Toole HI: Historical studies. Athens, [s.n.], 1984. 608 p. (Greek with English summaries) Includes a collection of the author's previously published essays, mostly on Greek medicine, with a short autobiographical sketch and bibliography.

**Hungary**

Zalai K: Die Geschichte des Universitätsunterrichts der Pharmaziegeschichte in Ungarn. In: Vorträge des Internationalen Pharmaziehistorischen Kongresses Innsbruck 1977. Stuttgart, Wissenschaftliche Verlagsgesellschaft, 1979. p. 197–202.

# HISTORIOGRAPHY AND HISTORY OF

**India**

Broehl WG, McGee VE: Content analysis in psychohistory: a study of three lieutenants in the Indian mutiny, 1857–58. **J Psychohist** 1981 Winter;8(3):281–306
Govinda Reddy C: Recent Indian medical historiography; bibliography for 1973. **Bull Indian Inst Hist Med (Hyderabad)** 1975 Oct;5(4):253–68
Govinda Reddy C: Recent Indian medical historiography: bibliography for 1975. **Bull Indian Inst Hist Med (Hyderabad)** 1978;8(1–4):63–87
Hameed A: A historian of medicine, Major General (Dr) S. L. Bhatia, passes away. **Stud Hist Med** 1981 Sept;5(3):239–41
Hameed HA, Reyaz Ali Parvaz S: Source material of Arab medicine. **Stud Hist Med** 1979 Dec;3(4):225–33
Jopat PD: Abstracts of medico historical articles in Hindi journals. **Bull Indian Inst Hist Med (Hyderabad)** 1978;8(1–4):51–62
Jopat PD: Abstracts of medico historical articles in Hindi journals. **Bull Indian Inst Hist Med (Hyderabad)** 1979;9:128–40
Jopat PD: Abstracts of medico-historical articles in Hindi journals. **Bull Indian Inst Hist Med Hyderabad** 1982;12(1–4):51–65
Jopat PD: Abstracts of select medico-historical articles in Hindi [1974]. **Bull Indian Inst Hist Med (Hyderabad)** 1975 Oct;5(4):249–52
Patterson TJ: Some Indian sources for the study of the history of medicine. **Indian Arch** 1980;29(1):27–30
Subba Reddy DV: Major General S. L. Bhatia (1891–1982). **Bull Indian Inst Hist Med Hyderabad** 1982;12(1–4):88–91
Subba Reddy DV: Prelude to upgraded Department of History of Medicine, Hyderabad. **Bull Indian Inst Hist Med Hyderabad** 1982;12(1–4):92–9
Subba Reddy V: History of Medicine in India. **Bull Indian Inst Hist Med (Hyderabad)** 1980;10(1–4):90–110

**Israel**

Kottek S, Wilk D: Professor Joshua O. Leibowitz; jubilee of his medico-historical activity. **Koroth** 1983 Aug;8(7–8):233–55

**Italy**

Babini J: Para una bibliografía de Aldo Mieli. **Physis** 1979;21(1–4):357–424
Babini VP, Cotti M, Minuz F, et al: La storia della psichiatria nell'Ottocento: i contributi italiani nell'ultimo decennio (1968–1978). **Stor Crit Psicol** 1980;1(2):177–96
L'Istituto di Storia della Medicina dell'Università di Padova: Un triennio di attività (Anni Acc. 1976–77/77–78/78–79). Padova, Tipografia 'La Garangola,' 1979. 23 p.

**Japan**

Nakagawa Y: [Medical history in the medical education] (Jpn). **Igakushi Kenkyu** 1978;50:2–10
Takada M: [Children who do not know Florence Nightingale: teaching of nursing history at a nursing school] (Jpn). **Kango Kyoiku** 1984 Dec;25(12):725–7

**Mexico**

Cárdenas-de la Peña E: La sección de historia de la medicina, de la Academia Nacional de Medicina. Síntesis histórica. **Gac Med Mex** 1980 Feb;116(2):77–91
Flores y Troncoso FA: Historia de la medicina en México desde la época de los indios hasta la presente. Facsimile of 1886 ed. plus new indices. 4 vols. México, Instituto Mexicano del Seguro Social, 1982. Various pagings. Historical and biographical chapters by V. M. Ruiz Naufal, A. G. Medrano, C. Viesca, G. A. Beltrán, J. S. Palencia, J. S. Riquer, B. F. Hernández.
López Hermosa L, ed: Bibliografía historica medica Mexicana 1970–1974. México, Sociedad Mexicana de Historia y Filosofía de la Medicina, (1978?). n.p.
Lozoya X: La herbolaria medicinal en Mexico y el Doctor Del Pozo. **Bol Soc Mex Hist Filos Med** 1980 Mar;5(30):11–6
Mesa de discusion sobre la enseñanza de la historia y filosofia de la medicina en Mexico: **Bol Soc Mex Hist Filos Med** 1984;7(50):439–65
Ortiz Monasterio J: Analisis cuantitativo de la historiografia medica mexicana (1970–1974). **Bol Soc Mex Hist Filos Med** 1983 Mar;6(42):129–36
Sanfilippo J: Bibliografia histórico-odontológica del Dr. Samuel Fastlicht. **Bol Soc Mex Hist Filos Med** 1984 Jun;7(47):317–24
Sanfilippo J: Semblanza del doctor Samuel Fastlicht. **Bol Soc Mex Hist Filos Med** 1984 Jun;7(47):309–15
Somolinos Palencia J: The Mexican Society of History and Philosophy of Medicine – past, present and future. **Clio Med** 1981;15:245–7

**Netherlands**

Ahlrichs EL: Dr. D. A. Wittop Koning 70 jaar. **Pharm Weekbl** 1981 Nov 6;116(45):1365–9
De Moulin D: Gerrit Arie Lindeboom and the history of medicine in the Netherlands. **Janus** 1980;67(1–2–3):1–6
Meininger JV, et al: Geschiednis van Geneeskunde en Gezondheidszorg. Register van publicaties en Lopend Onderzoek. Onderzoek – onderwijs en overige activiteiten gedurende de jaren 1972–1977 in Nederland. Utrecht, Afdeling Maatschappelijke Gezondheidszorg van het Instituut voor Sociale Geneeskunde der Rijksuniversiteit te Utrecht, 1980. 70. p.
Wittop Koning DA: Drei holländische Pharmaziehistoriker. In: Vorträge des Internationalen Pharmaziehistorischen Kongresses Innsbruck 1977. Stuttgart, Wissenschaftliche Verlagsgesellschaft, 1979. p. 129–39.

**Poland**

Barg L, Szpilczynski S: Elements of methodology and searching directions in Polish medical historiography till 1939. In International Congress of the History of Medicine. 26th, Plovdiv, 1978. Actes du Congress. Sofia, 1981. Volume II. p. 72–3.
Bibliografia biezaca: Historii Nauki i Techniki: **Kwart Hist Nauki Tech** 1984;29(Suppl 3–4):1–29
Bojczuk H: Stanisław Konopka (1896–1982), historyk medycyny, bibliotekarz i bibliograf, twórca polskiej bibliografii lekarskiej. **Arch Hist Med (Warsz)** 1983;46(4):439–51
Brzeziński T: Die Entwicklung des medizinhistorischen Unterrichts in Polen. **NTM** 1981;18(2):98–108
Brzeziński T: Problemy nauczania historii medycyny w Polsce. **Arch Hist Med (Warsz)** 1979;42(3):379–82
Dobrzyniecki Z: 'Dzieje Polskie' Jana Długosza jako źródło do dziejów medycyny w Polsce w XIV i XV w. **Arch Hist Med (Warsz)** 1981;44(3/4):265–76
Fijałek J: Dr. N. Med. Jerzy Kasznicki (3.1.1934--20.VII.1979). **Arch Hist Med (Warsz)** 1980;43(2):121–5
Fijałek J: Problemy badań naukowych i kształcenia kadry naukowej w dziedzinie historii medycyny w Polsce. **Arch Hist Med (Warsz)** 1979;42(3):383–8
Gutt RW: Refleksje na temat XXV-lecia Polskiego Towarzystwa Historii Medycyny. **Arch Hist Med (Warsz)** 1982;45(1–4):5–10
Kapronczay K: Az orvostörténelem oktatása a krakkói egyetemen. **Orv Hetil** 1979 Sep 23;120(38):2315–7
Konopka S: Działalność naukowa, redakcyjna i wydawnicza prof. Adama Wrzoska w świetle jego wypowiedzi i listów nie ogłoszonych w druku. **Arch Hist Med (Warsz)** 1982;45(1–4):11–26
Konopka S: O źródłach do dziejów medycyny polskiej i o głównych przeszkodach, utrudniajacych rozwijanie badań naukowych z tej dziedziny. **Arch Hist Med (Warsz)** 1983;46(4):413–37
Konopka S: Relacje profesorów Wydziału lekarskiego Uniwersytetu Jagiellonskiego o dziejach medycyny polskiej. **Arch Hist Med (Warsz)** 1979;42(1):107–24
Majewska-Tronowicz J, Michalczyk B, Kinowskiej M: Zeszyt 35/36 (VII–XII 1979). Dodatek do numeru 2/1980. Kwartalnika Historii Nauki i Techniki. **Kwart Hist Nauki Tech** 1980;25(2):Suppl.1–30
Majewska-Tronowicz J, Michalczyk B, Kinowskiej M: Zeszyt 37 (I–III 1980). Dodatek do numeru 3/1980. Kwartalnika Historii Nauki i Techniki. **Kwart Hist Nauki Tech** 1980;25(3):Suppl 1–28
Meissner RK: In memoriam: Dr med. Edward Stocki (1909--1978), członek honorowy Polskiego Towarzystwa Historii Medycyny. **Arch Hist Med (Warsz)** 1979;42(2):141–55
Michalczyk B, Kinowskiej M: Bibliografia biezaca historii nauki i techniki. **Kwart Hist Nauki Tech** 1984;29(2):Suppl 1–30
Müldner-Nieckowski P: Dr. Jacek Machalski (2.VI.1926--3.X.1979). **Arch Hist Med (Warsz)** 1980;43(2):117–20
Ostrowska T: Dr Aniela Szwejcerowa-Gruszczyńska (1905–1981); Wspomnienie pośmiertne. **Arch Hist Med (Warsz)** 1981;44(3/4):227–35
Ostrowska T: Ksawery Rowiński (1904–1983) i jego działalność w zakresie historii medycyny. **Kwart Hist Nauki Tech** 1984;29(2):445–66
Ostrowska T: Profesor Ksawery Rowiński (1904–1983) i Jego działanść naukowa (Wspomnienie pośmiertne). **Arch Hist Med (Warsz)** 1984;47(3):327–48
Pankiewicz H: Prof. dr hab. Henryk Bukowiecki jako historyk farmacji. **Arch Hist Med (Warsz)** 1984;47(3):389–93
Polska bibliografia biezaca historii medycyny: **Arch Hist Med (Warsz)** 1980;43(2):209–14
Profesor dr med. Stanisław Konopka (1896–1982). Wspomnienie: **Pol Tyg Lek** 1983 Sep 5;38(36):1125–6
Roeske W: Geschichte der Pharmaziehistorik in Polen. In: Vorträge des Internationalen Pharmaziehistorischen Kongresses Innsbruck 1977. Stuttgart, Wissenschaftliche Verlagsgesellschaft, 1979. p. 155–61.
Sieńkowski E: Ekslibris lekarski prof. dr Stanisława Sokoła. **Arch Hist Med (Warsz)** 1978;41(4):473–8
Skład osobowy władz Polskiego Towarzystwa Historii Medycyny i Farmacji: **Arch Hist Med (Warsz)** 1984;47(2):269–85
Sródka A, Wajs S: Bibliografia publikacji w Archiwum Historii Medycyny w latach 1974–1982. **Arch Hist Med (Warsz)** 1984;47(2):287–315
Tadeusz Bilikiewicz (1901–1980)---historyk medycyny i filozof: **Kwart Hist Nauki Tech** 1981;26(2):435–48
Tsouyopoulos N: Auf der Suche nach einer adäquaten Methode für die Geschichte und Theorie der Medizin. Auseinandersetzung mit Ludwik Flecks 'Entstehung und Entwicklung einer wissenschaftlichen Tatsache'.

**Medizinhist J** 1982;17(1/2):20–36
Tyszkiewicz J: Uwagi o historii medycyny w Polsce. **Kwart Hist Kultury Mater** 1975;23(2):245–54
Ziembicki W: Zakład historii Medycyny we Lwowie. Kronika lat 1942–1944. **Arch Hist Med (Warsz)** 1981;44(2):189–215

**Portugal**

Rocchietta S: Le pubblicazioni di storia della farmacia portoghese negli anni '70. **Minerva Med** 1980 Dec 15;71(50):3679–84

**Romania**

Negru I: Istoricul bolilor venerice in studiile clasice ale istoricilor medicinii ramâneşti. **Viata Med [Medii Sanit]** 1981 Dec;29(12):281–5

**Scandinavia**

Lindskog BI, Imhof AE: Mortality in Scandinavia in the 18th century. In: Congrès international d'histoire de la médecine, XXVe, Québec, 1976. Actes. Québec, 1977. p. 205–15.

**South Africa**

Melzer R, Kahn A, Kriel J, ed: Festschrift in honour of Dr. Cyril Adler on the occasion of his 80th birthday.

**Spain**

Balaguer Perigüell E: La historia en la medicina. **Real Acad Med Zaragoza** 1980;34, Curso 1979;:100–16
Ballester R, Bujosa F, Olagüe G: Colección historicomédica de la Facultad de Medicine de Valencia. Valencia, Càtedra e Instituto de Historia de la Medicina, 1976. 54 p. (Cuadernos Valencianos de Historia de la Medicina y de la Ciencia, 18, Serie A (Monografias)).
Beltrán E: Una polémica sobre Francisco Hernández y su obra en 1785. **An Soc Mex Hist Cienc Tec** 1979;5:49–73
Carrillo JL, Paz Torres M: Ibn Al-Baytar y el arabismo español del XVIII. Edicion trilingüe del prologo de su 'Kitab al-chami.' Benalmádena, Ayuntamiento de Benalmádena, 1982. 57 p.
Cornet AM, Sagrera JE de: En memoria de nuestro maestro: José Luis Gómez-Caamaño (1909–1984). **Bol Soc Esp Hist Farm** 1984;35(137):1–22
Folch Jou G, Muñoz Calvo S: Aportación de Olmedilla y Puig al desarrollo de la historiografía farmacéutica en España. **Bol Soc Esp Hist Farm** 1980 Oct;31(123):205–34
Francés C: Manuel Hernández de Gregorio: a Spanish pharmacist dedicated to science and the history of pharmacy. In: Vorträge des Internationalen Pharmaziehistorischen Kongresses Innsbruck 1977. Struttgart, Wissenschaftliche Verlagsgesellschaft, 1979. p. 181–6.
García Ballester L: In memoriam Dr. Vicente Peset Llorca (1914–1981). **Dynamis** 1981;1:221–2
García-Ballester L: Studies on Hippocrates and Galen in modern Spain. **Trans Stud Coll Physicians Phila** 1979 Sep;5(1 No 3):215–29
Gómez Caamaño JL: Historiographie pharmaceutique Catalane-Balear par un groupe universitaire. In: Vorträge des Internationalen Pharmaziehistorischen Kongresses Innsbruck 1977. Stuttgart, Wissenschaftliche Verlagsgesellschaft, 1979. p. 173–8.
Granjel LS: Literatura historico-medica Española de postguerra (1940–1975). Salamanca, 1977. 71 p. (Cuadernos de Historia de la Medicina Española, Monografias, 30).
Holmes JD: A new look at Spanish Louisiana census accounts: the recent historiography of Antonio Acosta. **La Hist** 1980;21(1):77–86
Jimenez Muñoz JM, Riera J: Bibliografía histórica en el siglo médico (1854–1936). Valladolid, Universidad de Valladolid, 1975. 107 p. (Acta Historico-Medica Vallisoletana, Monografias, VI)
López Piñero JM: El estudio histórico de la medicina en la obra de Laín Entralgo. **Dynamis** 1981;1:231–9
Lopez Pinero JM: Los estudios historicos sobre la actividad cientifica en la España de los siglos XVI y XVII. In: Coloquio sobre historia de la ciencia hispano-americana ... 1976. Madrid. 1977. pp. 133–166.
López Piñero JM: The history of science and medicine in Spain. **Clio Med** 1980 Jul;14(3–4):295–9
Marí Balcells VJ: Tres historiadores de la medicina española: Villalba, Hernandez Morejon y Comenge, e influencia del primero en la obra de los otros dos. In: Sociedad Española de Historia de la Medicina. V Congreso Nacional. Madrid, 1977. **Asclepio** 1977;29:167–76
Rof Carballo MC: Le Dr. Jesús Isamat Vila, premier professeur d'histoire de la pharmacie de l'Université de Barcelone. In: Vorträge des Internationalen Pharmaziehistorischen Kongresses Innsbruck 1977. Stuttgart, Wissenschaftliche Verlagsgesellschaft, 1979. p. 189–94.
Sanchez-Moscoso A: José Rodríguez Carracido. **Bol Soc Esp Hist Farm** 1971 Jun;22(86):54–84
Sociedad Española de Historia de la Medicina: V Congreso Nacional. Homenaje al Profesor Pedro Lain Entralgo. Madrid, 29–30 septiembre–1 octubre 1977. **Asclepio** 1977;29:1–358
Tarragó Valentines JF: Un informe sobre el hospital de Santa Maria de Lerida, escrito en el siglo XIX por Marioano Olives. **Asclepio** 1980;32:453–6

**Sweden**

Kock W: Hälsningsanförande. **Nord Medicinhist Arsb** 1980;Suppl 6:12–3
Kock W: Medicinhistorisk krönika. **Nord Medicinhist Arsb** 1981;:5–23
Lindroth S: Medicinens historia som akademiskt undervisningsämne. **Nord Medicinhist Arsb** 1980;Suppl 6:25–9

**Switzerland**

Beer FJ: Le souvenir d'Henri-Ernest Sigerist (1891–1957). **Hist Sci Med** 1982;16(1):49–53
Blaser RH: Paracelsus in Basel. Festschrift für Professor Dr. Robert-Henri Blaser zum 60. Geburtstag. Herausgegeben von der Schweizerischen Paracelsus-Gesellschaft. Biographical introduction by K. Goldammer. Muttenz/Basel, St. Arbogast Verlag, 1979. 210 p. (Reprint of 7 works by Blaser).
Boschung U: Gustav Adolf Wehrli (1888–1949), Gründer der Medizinhistorischen Sammlung der Universität Zürich. **Gesnerus** 1980;37(1/2):91–103
Boschung U, Rüttimann B: Herrn Professor Dr. med. H. M. Koelbing zum 60. Geburtstag. **Gesnerus** 1983;40(1–2):3–13
Buess H: Henry E. Sigerist (1891–1957) und die erste medizinhistorische Konferenz in Pura (Tessin); zur Erinnerung an den 25./26. März 1950. **Gesnerus** 1980;37(1/2):104–12
Ledermann F: L'histoire de la pharmacie dans les 'Pharmaceutica Acta Helvetiae', une bibliographie entre 1926 et 1979. **Pharm Acta Helv** 1981;56(3):93–6
Lichtenthaeler C: [A tribute to Hans Diller.] **Hermes** 1979;109:270–86
Pfohl G: Medizin und Philologie--Allgemeine humanistische Bildung als Anliegen des Schweizer Medizinhistorikers Charles Lichtenthaeler. **Med Welt** 1980 Nov 7;31(45):1651
Walser HH: Der Weg der Schweizer Psychiatrie ins zwanzigste Jahrhundert. **Gesnerus** 1982;39(1):97–108

**United States**

Balog CE: History, medicine, and culture: history for science students. **Indiana Soc Stud Q** 1980–81;33(3):53–62
Barnes J: Aristotle's de Motu Animalium. **Classical Rev** 1980;30(2):222–6
Bean LL, May DL, Skolnick M: The Mormon historical demography project. **Hist Methods Newsl** 1978;11(1):45–53
Beardsley EH: Medical history in South Carolina: the state of the art. **J SC Med Assoc** 1979 Jun;75(6):298–9
Bedini SA: Derek J. de Solla Price (1922–1983). **Technol Cult** 1984 Jul;25(3):701–5
Bedini SA: Derek J. DeSolla Price. **Ann Ist Mus Stor Sci Fir** 1984;9(1):95–115
Bell WJ: George W. Corner (1889–1981): historian. **Bull Hist Med** 1982 Spring;56(1):93–8
Berkowitz ED: The historian as policy analyst: the challenge of HEW. **Public Hist** 1979;1(3):17–25
Blain D, Barton M: The history of American psychiatry: a teaching and research guide. Washington, American Psychiatric Association, 1979. iv, 44 p. Contributions by D. F. Musto, G. Mora, E. T. Carlson.
Bonsett CA: G. W. H. Kemper, M.D. (1839–1927), Indiana medical historian. **J Indiana State Med Assoc** 1980 Jul;73(7):424
Bonsett CA: Medical museum notes: The Indiana Medical History Society. **J Indiana State Med Assoc** 1982 Dec;75(12):839
Brandt AM: James Angus Doull. In Dictionary of American biography, 1961–1965. Suppl. 7, 1981. p. 194–5.
Brieger GH: Fielding H. Garrison: the man and his book. **Trans Stud Coll Physicians Phila** 1981 Mar;3(1):1–21
Brieger GH: The history of medicine and the history of science. **Isis** 1981 Dec;72(264):537–40
Brodman E: Education and attitudes of early medical librarians to their work: a discussion based on the oral history project of the Medical Library Association. **J Libr Hist** 1980;15(2):167–82
Brodman E. Possible uses of MLA's oral history taped interviews. **Bull Med Libr Assoc** 1981 Jan;69(1):34–6
Brozek J, Evans RB, ed: R. I. Watson's selected papers on the history of psychology. Hanover, University of New Hampshire, 1977. xiii, 393 p.
Buchwald H: The scientist-surgeon. **Am J Surg** 1981 Aug;142(2):245–6
Buerki RA, ed: Survey of instructional resources in history of pharmacy undergraduate courses. [Columbus, Ohio], Ohio State University, [1981?]. x, 160 p.
Burnham JC: Will medical history join the American mainstream? **Rev Am Hist** 1978;6(1):43–9
Calcoen R: George Sarton. **Handel Maatsch Geschied Oudheidk Gent** 1980;N.R.,34:181–91
Capps D: Psychohistory in religious studies. **Group Psychol Hist Newsl** 1974;3(2):4–8
Cassedy JH: Highlights in the development of medical history in the United States. (Materials from an exhibit). Bethesda, National Library of Medicine, 1984. 30 p.

# HISTORIOGRAPHY AND HISTORY OF

Christen AG: The oral history interview: a treasurehouse for present and future dental historiographers. **Bull Hist Dent** 1981;29(1):8-14
Christy TE: The need for historical research in nursing. **Res Nurs Health** 1981 Jun;4(2):227-8
Church OM: Preparation in historiography in nursing research. **NLN Publ** 1983;(41-1935):54-6
Churchill FB: In search of the new biology: an epilogue. **J Hist Biol** 1981 Spring;14(1):177-91
Clagett M: Lynn Thorndike. In Dictionary of American biography, 1961-1965. Suppl. 7, 1981. p. 741-2.
Clarke JH: Increased student participation in a dental history course after changing the grading method. **Bull Hist Dent** 1980 Apr;28(1):44-6
Condran GA, Seaman J: Linkage of the 1880-81 Philadelphia death register to the 1880 manuscript census: a comparison of hand and machine-record linkage techniques. **Hist Methods** 1981;14(2):73-84
Corner GW: The seven ages of a medical scientist, an autobiography. Philadelphia, University of Pennsylvania Press, 1981. xi, 411 p.
Cowen DL: New Jersey medical historiography, 1964-1984. **J Med Soc NJ** 1984 Sep;81(9):807-10
Cowen DL: Robert P. Fischelis 1891-1981. **NJ J Pharm** 1982 Feb;55(2):12-4
Cutright PR, Brodhead MJ: Elliott Coues: naturalist and frontier historian. Urbana, University of Illinois Press, 1981. xv, 509 p.
Dann G, Higby G: Bibliography of the publications of George Urdang on his birth centenary. **Pharm Hist** 1982;24(3):106-14
David Shakow, Ph.D., 1901-1981: In Memoriam. **Schizophr Bull** 1981;7(3):383-7
Dekosky RK: The history of science in a history department. **Hist Teacher** 1980;13(3):371-8
Dietrich DJ: Psychohistory: Clio on the couch - or off? **Hist Methods** 1982;15(2):83-90
Donahue EM: Preserving history through oral history reflections. **J Gerontol Nurs** 1982 May;8(5):272-8
Donahue P: Nursing history in the undergraduate curriculum. **NLN Publ** 1983;(41-1935):38-44
Doona ME: The Lucy Lincoln Drown Nursing History Society. **Mass Nurse** 1984 Feb;53(2):6
Ebbert A, et al: [Reminiscences and appreciations of Madeline E. Stanton] Contributions by L. G. Wilson, L. G. Stevenson, T. R. Forbes, S. B. Nuland, F. Gyorgyey, J. Bylebyl, G. L. Geison, W. Le Fanu, G. Robinson. **J Hist Med Allied Sci** 1981 Apr;36(2):129-50
Fedo DA: Liberal arts and pharmacy education: where do we now stand? **Pharm Hist** 1980;22(2):60-8
Fee E, Wallace M: The history and politics of birth control: a review essay. **Feminist Stud** 1979;5(1):201-15
Feinstein HM: Family therapy for the historian?--The case of William James. **Fam Process** 1981 Mar;20(1):97-107
Fox DM: The decline of historicism: the case of compulsory health insurance in the United States. **Bull Hist Med** 1983 Winter;57(4):596-610
Friedman LJ, Shaffer AH: History, politics, and health in early American thought: the case of David Ramsay. **J Am Stud** 1979;13(1):37-56
George Rosen: In Memoriam: With contributions by S. Benison, E. H. Ackerknecht, J. Z. Bowers, L. A. Falk, G. A. Silver, O. H. Wangensteen, A. J. Viseltear, E. H. Thomson. **J Hist Med Allied Sci** 1978 Jul;33(3):244-317
Gifford GE: Medicine and science in early America. Being the collected essays of George Edmund Gifford, Jr., 1930-1981. Edited by Dorothy I. Lansing. Devon, Pa., Published by the friends of George E. Gifford, Jr., 1982. ix, 388 p.
Greene EL: Landmarks of botanical history. Ed., F. N. Egerton, with contributions by R. P. McIntosh and R. McVaugh. 2 vols. Stanford, Stanford University Press, 1983. 1139 p. (Vol. I first published 1909)
Hannaway C: Abraham M. Lilienfeld (1920-1984). **Bull Hist Med** 1984 Winter;58(4):558-9
Has the Republic no need of learning?: **J Hist Med Allied Sci** 1981 Jul;36(3):257-9
Herrmann EK: Strategies for teaching the history of nursing. **NLN Publ** 1983;(41-1935):57-65
Hiebert EN: Report on current activities in the history of science in the United States. **NTM** 1982;19(1):12-5
Hiestand WC: History in graduate teaching. **NLN Publ** 1983;(41-1935):45-8
Hilts VL: History of science at the University of Wisconsin. **Isis** 1984 Mar;75(276):63-94
Hine MK: The status of the teaching of dental history: 1980. **Bull Hist Dent** 1981 Oct;29(2):102-4
Hirsch HN: Clio on the couch. **World Polit** 1980;32(3):406-24
Hornblower H: Henry Furbush Howe. **Mass Hist Soc Proc** 1977,89:184-6
Hughes TP: Convergent themes in the history of science, medicine, and technology. **Technol Cult** 1981 Jul;22(3):550-8
Hutch RA: Explorations in character: Gamaliel Bradford and Henry Murray as psychobiographers. **Biography** 1981;4(4):312-25
Iles JD: Velikovsky: psychiatrist, historian and catastrophist. **Can Med Assoc J** 1981 Sept 1;125(5):496-505
The Indiana Medical History Museum: **Indiana Med Hist Q** 1974;1(1):11-21
Jarcho S: Some experiences with seminars in the history of medicine. In J. J. Bylebyl, ed: Teaching the history of medicine at a medical center. Baltimore, London, Johns Hopkins University Press, 1982. (The Henry E. Sigerist supplements to the Bulletin of the History of Medicine; new ser., no. 7). p. 115-20.
Jones GW: George Edmund Gifford, jr. **Proc Am Antiq Soc** 1981;91(1):22-4
Joy RJ: Starting from scratch: installing a history of medicine program in a new medical school. With a commentary by L.G. Stevenson. In J. J. Bylebyl, ed: Teaching the history of medicine at a medical center. Baltimore, London, Johns Hopkins University Press, 1982. (The Henry E. Sigerist supplements to the Bulletin of the History of Medicine; new ser., no. 7). p. 139-51.
Kaplan E: E.R.N. Grigg, radiologist-historian. **Semin Nucl Med** 1979 Jul;9(3):149-50
Kaufman M: Medicine in America. **Can Rev Am Stud** 1983;14(3):287-96
Keys TE: Chauncey Depew Leake, 1896-1978: an appreciation. **J Hist Med Allied Sci** 1978 Jul;33(3):428-31
Lane AJ: The politics of birth control. **Marx Perspect** 1979;2(3):160-9
LaPenna L: La psychohistory: proposte e studi nella storiografia americana. **Quad Stor** 1981;16(2):574-605
Leavitt JW: Writing public health history: the need for a social scaffolding. **Rev Am Hist** 1976;4(2):150-7
Loewenberg P: Decoding the past: the psychohistorical approach. New York, Knopf, 1983. xiv, 300 p.
Loewenberg P: Psychohistory. In M. Kammen, ed: The Past before us: contemporary historical writing in the United States. Ithaca, Cornell University Press, 1980. p. 408-32.
Mackay A: Derek John de Solla Price: an appreciation. **Soc Stud Sci** 1984 May;14(2):315-20
McLeod DC, Whitney HA: The legacy of Donald E. Francke: DICP--a fifteen-year commitment to clinical pharmacy. **Drug Intell Clin Pharm** 1981 Dec;15(12):990-1
Mandelbaum DR: Women in medicine. **Signs** 1978;4(1):136-45
Mann RJ, Key JD: The Osler Medical Historical Society. Mayo Foundation 'Chapter,' August 28, 1920-July 3, 1925. **Minn Med** 1980 May;63(5):348-54
Miller G: In praise of amateurs: medical history in America before Garrison. **Bull Hist Med** 1973 Nov-Dec;47(6):586-615
Mora G: Gregory Zilboorg. In Dictionary of American Biography, Suppl. 6, 1956-1960. p. 724-5, 1980.
Morison RS: The Foundation interest. In Stevenson LG, ed: A celebration of medical history. Baltimore, Johns Hopkins University Press, 1982. (The Henry E. Sigerist supplements to the Bulletin of the History of Medicine; new ser., no. 6). p. 212-21.
Mrtek RG: Absent the incentive: an example of contemporary history. **Pharm Hist** 1981;23(4):145-51
Navarro V: Medical history as justification rather than explanation: a critique of Starr's The Social Transformation of American Medicine. **Int J Health Serv** 1984;14(4):511-28
Noel NL: Nursing archives - preserving the profession's history. **Deans Notes** 1984 Mar;5(4):1-2
Nojima Y: [Nursing theory by Henderson. 4. Virginia Henderson and the history of nursing theory] (Jpn) **Kango Tenbo** 1979 Oct;4(10):949-57
Norman EM: Who and where are nursing's historians? **Nurs Forum** 1981;20(2):138-52
Nowak JB: Integration of nursing history into the nursing curriculum. **NLN Publ** 1983;(41-1935):49-53
Numbers RL, ed: The education of American physicians: historical essays. [Preface includes biographical tribute to William F. Norwood]. Berkeley, University of California Press, 1980. xiii, 345 p. Contributions by L. G. Stevenson, M. Kaufman, J. B. Blake, J. H. Warner, J. Whorton, D. L. Cowen, R. C. Maulitz, E. C. Atwater, G. H. Brieger, L. D Longo, J. L. Brand, J. W. Leavitt, C R. Burns, G. Miller
Olch PD: Owen H. Wangensteen (1898-1981). **Bull Hist Med** 1981;55:260-2
Oppenheimer JM, Whitfield JB: Biographical Memoirs: George Washington Corner (1889-1981). **Misc Am Philos Soc** 1982?;9 p.
Oral history abstract catalog: Interviews 1969-1978. St. Louis, Archives Section, Washington Univ. School of Medicine Library, 1979. 15 p:
Patzwald GA: Discovering and recording chiropractic history: for a systematic program in the profession. **Chiropr Hist** 1981;1(1):5-9
Pratt-Thomas HR: Joseph I. Waring, M.D.: the man and his times. **J SC Med Assoc** 1981 Dec;77(12):597-601
Radbill SX: Joseph Ioor Waring, 1897-1977. **J Hist Med Allied Sci** 1978 Jul;33(3):427-8
Radbill SX: Remarks on the Kate Hurd Mead lectures. **Trans Stud Coll Physicians Phila** 1977 Apr;44(4):179-81
Raphelson AC: The history course as the capstone of the psychology curriculum. **J Hist Behav Sci** 1982 Jul;18(3):279-85
Reed K, Perakis CR: Medical historiography: its place in osteopathic medicine. Parts I and II. **J Am Osteopath Assoc** 1984 Jun;83(10):738-44
Reverby S, Rosner D: Beyond 'the great doctors.' In their: Health care in America. Philadelphia, Temple University Press, 1979. p. 3-16.
Risse GB: Historia de la medicina en los EE.UU.: nuevos enfoques de investigacion y enseñanza. **Bol Soc Mex Hist Filos Med** 1979 Sep;4(28):113-27
Robert I. Watson and the development of the history of psychology: a symposium: With contributions by E. S. Mills, E. R. Hilgard, B. Ross, J. Popplestone, M. W. McPherson, R. B. Evans, E. S. Goodman, J. Brožek. **J Hist Behav Sci** 1982 Oct;18(4):307-31

Rosenberg C: Science in American society; a generation of historical debate. **Isis** 1983 Sep;74(273):356–67
Ross B: In memoriam: Robert I. Watson, Sr. 1909–1980. **J Hist Behav Sci** 1981 Jan;17(1):1–2
Sahli N: Sexuality in 19th and 20th century America: the sources and their problems. **Radic Hist Rev** 1979;20:89–96
Schnell RL: Contributions to psychohistory: IV. Individual experience in historiography and psychoanalysis: significance of Erik Erikson and Robert Coles. **Psychol Rep** 1980 Apr;46(2):591–612
Schuster CI: Passion and pathology: Richard Selzer's philosophy of doctoring. **Perspect Biol Med** 1984 Autumn;28(1):65–74
Schütt HW: Wissenschaftsgeschichte in Amerika. **Ber Wissenschaftsgesch** 1979;2(3–4):219–23
Shortt SE: History in the medical curriculum. A clinical perspective. **JAMA** 1982 Jul 2;248(1):79–81
Skinner RE: The historical work of William Dosité Postell, Sr. **Watermark** 1983 Fall;7(2):8–10
Skolnick MH, Bean LL, Mineau GP, et al: Etudes génétiques et démographiques et base de données généalogiques de l'Utah. **Ann Demogr Hist (Paris)** 1984;:103–13
Smith DS: The estimates of early American historical demographers: two steps forward, one step back, what steps in the future? **Hist Methods Newsl** 1979;12(1):24–38
Sonnedecker G: The American correspondence between George Urdang and Henry E. Sigerist 1941–1948. In Perspektiven der Pharmaziegeschichte. Festschrift für Rudolf Schmitz zum 65. Geburtstag. Graz, Akademische Druck- u. Verlagsanstalt. p. 343–63.
Stevenson LG: Cushion into launching pad; the fiftieth anniversary of the Institute of the History of Medicine. **Bull Hist Med** 1979 Winter;53(4):487–88
Stevenson LG: The Blake era at HMD. **Bull Hist Med** 1982;56(4):455–9
Stevenson LG: The newest of old journals. **Bull Hist Med** 1980 Spring;54(1):1–3
Stevenson LG, ed: A celebration of medical history. The fiftieth anniversary of The Johns Hopkins Institute of the History of Medicine and The Welch Medical Library. Baltimore and London, Johns Hopkins University Press, 1982. vi, 228 p. (Henry E. Sigerist Supplements to the Bulletin of the History of medicine, new ser., no. 6)
Stowell RE: Esmond R. Long, MD, 1890–1979. **Am J Pathol** 1980 Aug;100(2):321–5
Straight WM: Florida's medical historian––J. Webster Merritt. **J Fla Med Assoc** 1979 Aug;66(8):860–5
Strong C: Historical research: does it apply to health education? **Health Educ (Wash)** 1981 Jul–Aug;12(4):34–5
Susser M: The work of George Rosen: observations on a very small sample. **Int J Health Serv** 1980;10(2):323–8
Swierenga RP: Physicians and abortion reform in the nineteenth century: social control as the new orthodoxy. **Fides Et Hist** 1979;11(2):51–9
Thackray A: The pre-history of an academic discipline: the study of the history of science in the United States, 1891–1941. **Minerva** 1980 Autumn;18(3):448–73
Thibodeau D, ed: A bibliography of the writings of Lloyd G. Stevenson. **Bull Hist Med** 1983 Summer;57(2):267–79
Thomson EH: John Farquhar Fulton. In Dictionary of American Biography, Suppl. 6, 1956–1960. p. 222–4, 1980.
Thomson EH: Madeline Earle Stanton, disciple: the years 1920 to 1941. **J Hist Med Allied Sci** 1981 Apr,36(2):151–67
Weaver B, Britt MC: Dr. Lawrence Reynolds and his medical history collection. **Ala J Med Sci** 1984 Jul;21(3):311–7 contd
Weaver B, Britt MC: Dr. Lawrence Reynolds and his medical history collection. **Ala J Med Sci** 1984 Oct;21(4):441–7
Webster C, ed: Health, medicine and mortality in the sixteenth century. London and New York, Cambridge University Press, 1979. 394 p. In memory of Sanford V. Larkey. Contributions by P. Slack, R. Schofield, E. A. Wrigley, A. B. Appleby, T. R. Forbes, P. Allderidge, M. Pelling, A. Chapman, J. J. Bylebyl.
Weiland S: Historians and psychologists, pluralism and professionalism: a review essay. **Public Hist** 1981;3(2):75–88
Weinstein F: On the social function of intellectuals: a consideration of Erik H. Erikson's contribution to psychoanalysis and psychohistory. In M. Albin, R. J. Devlin, G. Heeger, ed: New directions in psychohistory. The Adelphi papers in honor of Erik H. Erikson. Lexington, Toronto, D. C. Heath, 1980. p. 3–19.
Wilk D: David Israel Macht (1882–1961). **Koroth** 1983 Aug;8(7–8):305–17
Wilson HB: The Medical Annals Committee [interview by B. Taylor]. **Md State Med J** 1981 May;30(5):79–83
Wilson L: Schizophrenia in learned societies: professionalism vs. scholarship. **J Hist Med Allied Sci** 1981 Jan;36(1):5–8
Wilson LG: Dorothy Schullian retires from the Journal. **J Hist Med Allied Sci** 1984 Oct;39(4):457–61
Wilson LG: Madeline Earle Stanton 1898–1980. **Bull Med Libr Assoc** 1981 Jul;69(3):357–8
Wilson LG: Measure in everything: a decade of the journal. **J Hist Med Allied Sci** 1982 Oct;37(4):393–8
[Wilson L]: The education of historians of medicine. **J Hist Med Allied Sci** 1982 Jul;37(3):265–8
Young DM: Eugene H. Conner, M.D., KMA historian. **J Ky Med Assoc** 1982 Apr;80(4):224–6

**Uruguay**

Rial Roade J: Sources for studies of historical demography in Uruguay (1728–1860). **Lat Am Res Rev** 1980;15(2):180–200

**USSR**

Arkhangel'skiĭ GV: L.F. Zmeev-vydaiushchiĭsia otechestvennyĭ istorik meditsiny i bibliograf. **Sov Zdravookhr** 1979;(8):64–7
Bachev VI: K metodike izucheniia memuarno-épistoliarnykh proizvedeniĭ. **Sov Zdravookhr** 1980;(3):60–1
Bachev VI: Klassifikatsiia istoriko-meditsinskikh istochnikov sovetskogo perioda. **Sov Zdravookhr** 1983;9:58–9
Bachev VI: Kompleksnyĭ podkhod k izucheniiu istoriko-meditsinskikh istochnikov sovetskogo perioda. **Sov Zdravookhr** 1984;(7):56–8
Bachev VI: Mestnaia periodicheskaia pechat' kak istoriko-meditsinkiĭ istochnik. **Sov Zdravookhr** 1981;(6):56–8
Bazhan TA: Opyt prepodavaniia kursa istorii meditsiny. **Sov Zdravookhr** 1983;6:46–50
Belov SI: Vrachebnaia étika v kurse istorii meditsiny. **Sov Med** 1981;(6):116–7
Bliakher LI: Ia. A. Borzenkov-istorik biologii. **Vopr Istor Estestvozn Tekh** 1982;1:36–44
Bykov GV, Trifonov DN: Issledovaniia po istorii khimii. **Vopr Istor Estestvozn Tekh** 1981;2:33–8
Duplenko KF, Leonenko NA, Kogan VIa, et al: Organizatsiia istoriko-meditsinskikh isslevaniĭ v Ukrainskoĭ SSR. **Sov Zdravookhr** 1981;(5):57–9
Eleĭnikova VS: Uchebnye plany, programmy i prepodavanie istorii meditsiny. **Sov Zdravookhr** 1984;(1):43–6
Gribanov ED: Rol' Tsentral'nogo instituta usovershenstvovaniia vracheĭ v podgotovke kadrov istorikov meditsiny. **Sov Zdravookhr** 1979;(10):60–1
Grigorian NA: [I. M. Sechenov on science and its history] (Rus). **Istor Biol Issled** 1980;8:173–87
Gritskevich VP: Istoriko-meditsinskoe istochnikovedenie. **Sov Zdravookhr** 1980;(9):56–8
Iarovinskiĭ MIa: K otsenke pammiatnikov istorii meditsiny. **Sov Zdravookhr** 1981;(9):72–4
Iarovinskiĭ MIa: Rol' istorii meditsiny v deontologicheskoĭ podgotovke meditsinskikh rabotnikov. **Sov Zdravookhr** 1982;(4):51–3
Kanep VV: Aktual'nye voprosy muzeevedeniia: iz opyta raboty Muzeia istorii meditsiny im. P. Stradynia : tezisy dokladov. Riga, Ministerstvo zdravookhraneniia Latviĭskoĭ SSR, 1982. 195 p.
Levit MM: Metodologiia i metodika prepodavaniia istorii meditsiny. **Sov Zdravookhr** 1980;(3):54–7
Miliutina IK, Kartasheva LA: K voprosu informatsionnogo obespecheniia i informatsionnoĭ znachimosti istoriko-meditsinskikh issledovanii. **Sov Zdravookhr** 1981;(4):67–9
Petrov BD: Itogi i zadachi istoriko-meditsinskikh issledovaniĭ. **Sov Zdravookhr** 1982;(12):64–7
Petrov BD: O sozdanii polnoĭ istorii gigieny truda v Rossii i SSR. **Gig Tr Prof Zabol** 1980 Jun;(6):1–5
Petrov BD: Zadachi istoriko-meditsinskikh issledovaniĭ v SSSR. **Sov Zdravookhr** 1980;(8):44–7
Piatak OA, Perekhrestenko PM, Sadovskaia AG: Programma issledonvaniĭ po istorii meditsiny i ee znachenie dlia dal'neĭshego razvitiia zdravookhraneniia, meditsinskogo obrazovaniia i meditsinskoĭ nauki v USSR. **Vrach Delo** 1981;(4):7–10
Pomper P: Nečaev, Lenin and Stalin: the psychology of leadership. **Jahrb Gesch Osteur** 1978;26(1):11–30
Pullat R: Istoricheskaia demografiia v SSR (znachenie, mesto, itogi i perspektivy razvitiia). **Probl Istor Demogr SSSR** 1977;8–17
Serebrennikov AB: Dnevniki, memuary, épistoliarnye materialy kak istochniki dlia izucheniia istorii otechestvennoĭ meditsiny. **Sov Zdravookhr** 1981;(7):63–6
Shamin AN: Issledovaniia po istorii biologii. **Vopr Istor Estestvozn Tekh** 1981;2:38–45
Sokolov EI, Suvorova RV, Krechmer MI: M. P. Mul'tanovskiĭ – vidnyĭ sovetskiĭ istorik meditsiny. **Sov Zdravookhr** 1983;(12):46–8
Starchevskiĭ VS, Perfil'ev GN: Ispol'zovanie kraevedcheskikh materialov v prepodavanii istorii meditsiny. **Sov Zdravookhr** 1982;(11):65–6
Suvorova RV, Mikirtichan GL: Metodicheskie voprosy prepodavaniia istorii meditsiny na pediatricheskikh fakul'tetakh. **Sov Zdravookhr** 1982;(1):58–61
Vorob'ev RI: Istoriko-meditsinskie raboty I. A. Kassirskogo. **Feldsher Akush** 1984 Jul;49(7):44–6
Zavalishchenko LI: Podgotovka seriinogo dokumental'nogo izdaniia. **Sov Arkh** 1977;(3):78–81

**Venezuela**

Briceño Romero G: Discurso del doctor Gabriel Briceño Romero al tomar posesion de la presidencia de la Sociedad Venezolana de Historia de la Medicina. **Rev Soc Venez Hist Med** 1972–73;20–21(34–35)79–86
Osuna A: Una biografia del Dr. Ambrosio Perera.

**Rev Soc Venez Hist Med** 1975–76;23(37):71–85
Palabras pronunciadas por el doctor Mario Mazzei Uzcategui, con motivo de la colocacion del retrato del doctor Josa Maria Baptista, en la sede de la Sociedad Venezolana de Historia de la Medicina, en Caracas. Sesion del 8 de febrero de 1972.: **Rev Soc Venez Hist Med** 1972–73;20–21(34–35):41–9
Silva Alvarez A: Juicio critico y discurso de contestacion. **Rev Soc Venez Hist Med** 1977;25(39):93–8
Vélez Boza F: Discurso pronunciado con motivo de la colocacion del retrato del Dr. Jesus Sanabria Bruzual en el salon de sesiones de la Sociedad Venezolana de Historia de la Medicina, el 12 de julio de 1978. **Rev Soc Venez Hist Med** 1980;29(43–44):63–71
Velez Boza F: Homenaje a la memoria del Dr. Jesus A. Yerena. **Rev Soc Venez Hist Med** 1975–76;23(37):91–100

**Yugoslavia**

Tartalja H: Geschichte der Pharmaziehistorik in Jugoslawien bis zum Jahre 1952. In: Vorträge des Internationalen Pharmaziehistorischen Kongresses Innsbruck 1977. Stuttgart, Wissenschaftliche Verlagsgesellschaft, 1979. p. 97–106.

## HOMEOPATHY

Haller JS: Aconite: a case study in doctrinal conflict and the meaning of scientific medicine. **Bull NY Acad Med** 1984 Nov;60(9):888–904
Otten HH: Pedra de mijada, der Pinkelstein. Medizinhistorische Betrachtung zur Lithotherapie. **Med Welt** 1981 May 8;32(19):765–6
Twentyman LR: The nature of homoeopathy. **R Soc Health J** 1982 Oct;102(5):221–5

**Before 500 A.D.**

**Greece**

Müller CW: Die hippokratischen Schriften. In his: Gleiches zu Gleichem. Ein Prinzip frühgriechischen Denkens. Wiesbaden, Harrassowitz, 1965. p. 112–50. (Klassisch-philologische Studien, 31).

**1700 to Present**

Buschauer W: Homöopathie als Vollendung der Hippokratischen Medizin. Heidelberg, Haug, 1982. Historical sections, p. 9–79.
Carlini EA: Homeopatia: ontem, hoje e amanhã. **AMB** 1983 Nov–Dec;29(11–12):210–4
Coulter HL: Homoeopathy and modern medical science. **J Am Inst Homeopath** 1980 Jun;73(2):7–28
Coulter HL: Homoeopathy and modern medical science. **J Am Inst Homeopath** 1980 Sept–Dec;73(3–4):17–38, 23–50
Lecomte J: Sur l'homéopathie. **Rev Med Liege** 1980 May 1;35(9):354–62
Martiny M: Geschichte der Homöopathie. In Sournia JC, Martiny M, Poulet J, ed: Illustrierte Geschichte der Medizin. Salzburg, Andreas, 1980. Vol. 6. p. 2295–317.
Morowitz HJ: Much ado about nothing. **Hosp Pract** 1982 Jul;17(7):215–6
Raj N: The homoeopathic treatment of cholera; a historical study. **Bull Indian Inst Hist Med (Hyderabad)** 1978;8(1–4):39–43
Sananés R: Homéopathie et langage du corps. Paris, Robert Laffont, 1982. 361 p.
Schwanitz HJ: Homöopathie und Brownianismus 1795–1844. Zwei wissenschaftstheoretische Fallstudien aus der praktischen Medizin. Stuttgart Fischer, 1983. 202 p. (Medizin in Geschichte und Kultur, 15).

**Australia**

Gluckman LK: Dr. Carl Fischer MD and the history of homeopathy in Auckland in the 19th century. **NZ Med J** 1979 Jul 25;90(640):66–9

**France**

Haffen M: Structures de l'homéopathie en France: (1919–1982). Paris, Editions médicales internationales, 1982. 158 p.

**Germany**

Cook TM: Samuel Hahnemann. The founder of homoeopathic medicine. Wellingborough, Northamptonshire, Thorsons, 1981. 192 p.
Fritsche H: Samuel Hahnemann: Idee und Wirklichkeit der Homöopathie. Göttingen, Verlag für homöopathische Literatur, 1982. 366 p.
Habacher M: Homöopathische Fernbehandlung durch Samuel Hahnemann. **Medizinhist J** 1980;15(4):385–91
Riet AV: August Bier en de homoeopathie. Eindhoven, Gema, 1978. 320 p. (Diss. Amsterdam).
Schwarz HD: Christian Theodor Lappe (1802–1877). **Pharm Ztg** 1977;122:338
Wittern R: The Robert Bosch Foundation and the establishment of the Institute for the History of Medicine. **Clio Med** 1980;15(1/2):89–91

**Great Britain**

Weeks N: The medical discoveries of Edward Bach, physician. New Canaan, Conn., Keats, 1973. 141 p.

**New Zealand**

Combes RE: J. C. Sharland's pharmacy at Apothecaries' Hall. **J Auckl Waikato Hist Soc** 1979;34:31–4
Gluckman LK: Dr. Carl Frank Fischer M.D.: an early Auckland physician, botanist and viticulturalist. **J Auckl Waikato Hist Soc** 1980;(37):18–20

**Poland**

Lozowski J: Homeopatia (Samuela Hahnemanna). **Pieleg Polozna** 1982;4–5:16–7

**Romania**

Mironţov–Tuculescu V: Homeopatia--specialitate sau metodă? **Rev Med Interna [Neurol Psihiatr]** 1981 Oct–Dec;26(4):247–9

**South Africa**

Bernstein RE: Homeopathic 'firsts' in South Africa. **S Afr Med J** 1981 Jun 27;59(27):968

**Sweden**

Burius A: Lings gymnastik och homeopatien. **Nord Medicinhist Arsb** 1980;:99–123

**United States**

Barlow W, Powell DO: Homeopathy and sexual equality: the controversy over coeducation at Cincinnati's Pulte Medical College, 1873–1879. **Ohio Hist** 1981 Spring;90(2):101–13
Blake JB: Homeopathy in American history; a commentary. **Trans Stud Coll Physicians Phila** 1981 Jun;3(2):83–92
Coulter HL: Divided legacy: the conflict between homoeopathy and the American Medical Association. Science and ethics in American medicine 1800–1914. 2d ed. Richmond, California, North Atlantic Books, 1982. 552 p.
Heindel ND, Foster NI: Medicine, music and 'Money' Munyon. **Pa Folklife** 1982;32(1):44–8
Heindel ND, Foster NI: The Allentown Academy: America's first German medical school. **Pa Folklife** 1980;30(1):2–8
Keeney EB, Lederer SE, Minihan EP: Sectarians and scientists: alternatives to orthodox medicine. In Numbers RL, Leavitt JW, ed: Wisconsin medicine. Historical perspectives. Madison, University of Wisconsin Press, 1981. p. 47–74.
King LS: Medicine in the USA: historical vignettes. III. Medical sects and their influence. **JAMA** 1982 Sep 10;248(10):1221–4
King LS: The 'old code' of medical ethics and some problems it had to face. **JAMA** 1982 Nov 12;248(18):2329–33
Peitzman SJ: 'Thoroughly practical': America's polyclinic medical schools. **Bull Hist Med** 1980 Summer;54(2):166–87
Petrisko TW: Schism and suppression: the elimination of medical protest schools, 1846–1939. **Chiropr Hist** 1982;2(1):35–9
The Robb House: home of the Alachua County Medical Society and Auxiliary: **J Fla Med Assoc** 1982 Aug;69(8):681–2
Rumble W: Homeopathy in the Lehigh Valley, 1881–1920. **Pa Mag Hist Biogr** 1980;104(4):474–90

## HOSPITALS

See also **Hospitals, Psychiatric**

Bravo Peña F: Nociones de historia de la enfermeria. 7a. ed: México, Porrúa, 1980. 191 p.
Caffaratto TM: Le antiche radici della riforma sanitaria. **Minerva Med** 1982 Jun 30;73(27):1905–16
Castro F de: Historia da vida e obras de S. Joao de Deus. Translation and notes by Foão Gameiro, OH. Montemor-O-Novo, Editorial Franciscana, 1982. 166 p.
Chernok NB: Nursing homes--response to a need. **J Long Term Care Adm** 1978 Winter;6(4):41–50
Du Toit DA: Die hospitaal as 'n burokrasie. **Curationis** 1983 Jun;6(2):11–8
Dziob JS: Ten years before 'M A S H'. **RI Med J** 1982 Dec;65(12):499–506
Ellis J: The responsibility of medical schools for teaching hospitals and the provision of clinical services. **Med Educ** 1981 May;15(3):171–83
Filipe NF: S. João de deus um homem que soube amar. 2. edição. Lisboa, Edições Paulistas, [198–?]. 150 p.
Frischauer W: The clinic. London, Frewin, 1976. 200 p.
Gastão M: S. João de Deus: sua vida–sua obra. Lisboa, Centro do Livro Brasileiro, 1982. 733 p.
Gepts–Friedenreich E: Ziekenhuishygiëne vroeger en nu. **FNIB** 1981

Apr;59(2):7-15
Hilario E: Comfort and surroundings in hospitals. **Hosp Eng** 1979 Mar;33(2):20-2, 24-5
Histoire de la médecine aux armées: Tome 1. De l'Antiquité à la Révolution. Paris, Charles Lavauzelle, 1982. 513 p.
Janssen G: L'ingénieur hygiéniste à l'hôpital. **Soins** 1982 Jun;(384):29-30
Jetter D: Klosterhospitäler; St. Gallen, Cluny, Escorial. **Sudhoffs Arch** 1978;62(4):313-38
Kottek SS: The hospital in Jewish History. **Rev Infect Dis** 1981 Jul Aug;3(4):636 9
Murken AH: Das Krankenhaus im Wandel der Zeit ... 19. und 20. Jahrhunderts. **Neue Heimat** 1980;27(11/12):36-45
Murken AH: Geschichte des Hospital- und Krankenhauswesens im deutschsprachigen Raum. In Sournia JC, Martiny M, Poulet J, ed: Illustrierte Geschichte der Medizin. Salzburg, Andreas, 1980. Vol. 5. p. 1595-1653.
Murken AH: Grundzüge des deutschen Krankenhauswesens von 1780 bis 1930 unter Berücksichtigung von Schweizer Vorbildern. **Gesnerus** 1982;39(1):7-45
Shaw S: Seasonal foundations: Santa-the saint who founded hospitals. **Nurs Mirror** 1981 Dec 23-30;153(26):30-1
Smith GH: The excavation of the hospital of St. Mary of Ospringe, commonly called Maison Dieu. **Archaeol Cantiana** 1979,(1980);95:81-184

### Algeria

Friedman EG: Trinitarian hospitals in Algiers: an early example of health care for prisoners of war. **Cathol Hist Rev** 1980;66(4):551-64

### Arabic

Stone C, Lunde P: Early Islamic hospitals: in the hospital bazaar. **Health Soc Serv J** 1981 Dec 17;91(4777):1548-51

### Austria

Jetter D: Die alten Hospitalpläne der Albertina in Wien. **Hist Hosp** 1979-80;13:29-45
Jetter D: Wien von den Anfängen bis um 1900. Wiesbaden, Steiner, 1982. viii, 159 p. (Geschichte des Hospitals, Bd. 5).
Kalzinger W: Das Fürsorgewesen der Stadt Linz bis zu Kaiser Josef II. **Hist Jahrb Stadt Linz** 1978;:11-94
Katzinger W: Das Bürgerspital. **Hist Jahrb Stadt Linz** 1977:11-102

### Belgium

Elaut LJ: Een epos: het Gentse Akademisch Ziekenhuis. Antwerpen, Nederlandsche Boekhandel, 1977. 83 p. (VVA monografie; 3).
Hankart R: L'hôpital Saint-Michel dit des Communs Pauvres-en-Ile à Liège. Histoire de ses origines (XIIe-XVe siècles). **Bull Inst Archeol Liegeois** 1978;90:157-95 Also in Bull Soc R Vieux Liege 1977-79;9:281-7, 385-94
Jacquet-Ladrier F: L'hôpital Saint-Roch et la lutte contre la peste à Namur, aux XVIIe et XVIIIe siècles. **Ann Soc Belg Hist Hop** 1980;18:59-70
Lacroix MT: L'hôpital Saint-Nicolas du Bruille (Saint-André) à Tournai de sa fondation à sa mutation en cloître (ca. 1230-1611). 2 tomes. Louvain, Université Catholique de Louvain, 1977. xxxvi, 892 p. (Publications de l'Institut d'Etudes Médiévales, 2e série, No. 1).
Maurissen AW: De leprozerie van Molenbeek. **Eigen Schoon Brabander** 1979;62:29-40
Pirotte F: Note sur l'évolution de la ladrerie de la Hesse à Tohogne. Du moyen âge à la fin de l'ancien régime. **Ann Inst Archeol Luxemb** 1975-76:106-7:163-81
Servais P, Roger FH: Les archives médicales hospitalières: organisation et possibilités d'utilisation. **Ann Soc Belg Hist Hop** 1980;18:71-96
Spanhove J: De Sieckenhuysen. **Ascania** 1977;20:33-61

### Bolivia

Bravo C: Hospitales de La Paz, datos historicos. **Illimani** 1974;(6):47-63

### Canada

Bernier H: Marie Morin. In Dictionary of Canadian biography, 1701 to 1740. Volume 2, 1969. p. 489-92.
Campeau L: Jeanne-Françoise Juchereau de la Ferté. In Dictionary of Canadian biography, 1701 to 1740. Volume 2, 1969. p. 302-3.
L'Hôtel-Dieu, le premier hôpital de Montréal: **Auxiliaire** 1981 Mar-Apr;:13-5

### Denmark

Brix J: Laegevirke i Sønderjylland før 1864. **Dan Medicinhist Arbog** 1980;:9-10

### France

Amalric P: Dominique Anel et les Quinze Vingts de Paris. **Bull Soc Ophtalmol Fr** 1982 Jan;82(1):87-90
Baillargeat R, et al: Les invalides: trois siècles d'histoire. Paris, Musée de l'armée, 1974. 600 p.
Barré R: Dieppe, l'assistance et la charité au cours des âges. [France? s. n., 1972?]. 20 p.
Bériac F: L'Hôpital Saint-Julien de Bordeaux, XIIIe-XVIe siècle. **Rev Hist Bordeaux Dep Gironde** 1975, 1977,24.47-74
Bernier R: Histoire institutionnelle et sociale de l'hôpital de Tulle sous l'Ancien Régime. Mémoire de fin d'assistanat à l'École Nationale de la Santé Publique de Rennes, 1976, 8 n.p., 114 p.
Bochin A: Et si nous visitions l'Hôpital Saint-Roch de Buzançais? **Bull Soc Fr Hist Hop** 1979;(39):32-49
Burg AM: Les archives hospitalières de Haguenau. In Livet G, Schaff G, ed: Médecine et assistance en Alsace, XVIe-XXe siècle. Strasbourg, Istra, 1976. p. 113-5.
Cheymol J: Hôpitaux des pèlerins de Saint-Jacques-de-Compostelle. IV. Sur la route du Puy: l'hospice de Pradelles. V. L'hôpital de Saint-Géraud et la confrérie des pèlerins d'Aurillac. **Hist Sci Med** 1981;15(1):99-107
Cheymol J: L'hôpital de la Trinité en la rue Saint-Denis à Paris (1201-1790). **Hist Sci Med** 1983;17(2):159-70
Cheymol J: L'hôpital Sainte-Catherine à Paris (1181-1794). **Hist Sci Med** 1982;16(4):239-51
Cotinat L: Vases de l'hôpital Saint-Joseph de Moulins. **Rev Hist Pharm (Paris)** 1980 Mar;27(244):11-14
Coudurier P: Les prix de journée: détermination et contentieux. Nancy, Berger-Levrault, 1978. 225 p.
Curet M, Carre A, Henaff R: Les hôpitaux des ports. **Med Armees** 1980;8(10)spec:795-6
Dinet-Lecomte MC: Les bâtiments hospitaliers de Blois aux XVIIe et XVIIIe siècle (1). **Bull Soc Fr Hist Hop** 1983;46:14-20
Dorche J: Une institution lyonnaise: les religieuses au service des malades dans les hospices civils de Lyon 1500-1950. **Lyon Pharm** 1981 Apr;32(3):155-60
Ferrand F: L'hôpital de Goncelin (Isère) 1658-1793. In Congrès National des Sociétés Savantes, 98e, Saint-Etienne, 1973. Actes. Paris, 1975. Tome II, p. 319-27.
Frenay C: Histoire d'un hôpital: Hôtel-Dieu de Villefranche-sur-Saône. Villefranche-en-Beaujolais, Du Cuvier, 1980. 238 p.
Garnot NS, Simon N: Parigi degli ospedali. **Kos** 1984 May;1(4):95-114
Guillermand J: La tradition hospitalière militaire. **Med Armees** 1980;8(10)spec:817
Helies JC: Aperçu historique sur les hôpitaux de Carcassonne, des origines à la fin du XIXe siècle. Thèse méd., Toulouse, 1977. 94 p.
Ibert M: Contribution à l'étude historique de l'hôpital Ste-Marthe d'Avignon, période 1670-1740. Marseille, Pronto-Offset impr., 1979. 914 p. (Thèse, Marseille, 1979).
Imbert J, Mollat M: Histoire des hôpitaux en France. Toulouse, Privat, 1982. 559 p.
La Salpêtrière: Hier et aujourd'hui. (Numéro spécial hors série, L'Hôpital à Paris, Aout 1982.) 79 p. Contributions by G. Pallez, J. Brunet, R. Poujol, D. Puzin, R. César, F. Greffe, P. Castaigne, R. Brocas, J. Franchi.
Le patrimoine hospitalier en Bourgogne: **Bull Soc Fr Hist Hop** 1979;(39):8-9
Leroy P: L'ancien hôpital de la Charité de Senlis. Senlis, Société d'Histoire et d'Archéologie de Senlis, 1979? 20 p. (Collections Senlisiennes, no. 2).
Malterre-Barthes A: Un service bien particulier: les dispensaires antivénériens. **Soins Gynecol Obstet Pueric** 1981 Sep;(6):37-46
Nguyen-Laissard M: Note sur la pharmacie de l'hôpital de Nuits-Saint Georges. **Rev Hist Pharm (Paris)** 1980 Mar;27(244):15-16
Nguyen-Laissard M: Note sur l'hôpital de Moutiers-Saint-Jean et sa pharmacie. **Rev Hist Pharm (Paris)** 1983 Sep;30(258):233-4
Patrimoine hospitalier de la Bourgogne: [Dijon], Ministère de la Culture et de la Communication; Direction Régionale des Affaires Culturelles de Bourgogne, 1980. 163 p. Contributions by E. Pommier, J. Gaillard, S. Deyts, J. Richard, M. Guillaume, C. Lamarre-Tainturier.
Queyrie G: L'hôpital général de Tulle sous l'Ancien régime: etude économique et sociale (à suivre). **Bull Soc Lett Sci Arts Correze** 1982;85:72-91
Recensement des pharmacies hospitalières: **Bull Soc Fr Hist Hop** 1979;(39):10-18
Roubert J: L'adoption des enfants par des particuliers à Lyon sous l'ancien régime. **Bull Soc Fr Hist Hop** 1978;(36-37):41-67
Simonnet J: L'hospice Saint-Charles d'Amiens. De sa fondation à 1900. Memoire de fin d'assistanant. E.N.S.P. de Rennes, 1977. 155 p.
Société française d'histoire des hôpitaux: [1978-79 prizes in hospital history]: **Bull Soc Fr Hist Hop** 1980;(40):4-22
Zmirou-Lajuzan D: L'hôpital Saint-Jacques de Bordeaux, du XIIe au XVIe siècle. Maîtrise, Univ. de Bordeaux, III, 1977. 309 p.

### Germany

Andrian-Werburg K von: Das Gesundheits- und Medizinalwesen in Sachsen-Coburg und das Coburger Landkrankenhaus.

# HOSPITALS

**Jahrb Coburg Landesstift** 1977;:13–94
Grünberg A: Entwicklungen im Krankenhausbau in Deutschland unter Berücksichtigung funktioneller und hygienischer Aspekte. Diss. Mainz, 1981. 98 p.
Hoffmann H: Urkundenregesten zur Geschichte des Juliusspitals in Würzburg 1576–1849 (Regesta Herbipolensia VI). Würzburg, Kommissionsverlag Ferdinand Schöningh, 1976. xxxi, 434 p. (Quellen und Forschungen zur Geschichte des Bistums und Hochstifts Würzburg, Band 29).
Jetter D: Hospitäler in Salzburg. **Sudhoffs Arch** 1980;64(2):163–86
Jezierska ME: Szpital obozu Buchenwald (na podstawie archiwaliów z okresu 3 IV - 20 VII 1945 r.). **Przegl Lek** 1980;37(1):76–85
Murken AH: Vom Armenhospital zum Grossklinikum. **Waage** 1980;19(1):25–37
Spor E, ed: Das Theresienhospital. Ein Stück Düsseldorfer Stadtgeschichte 1288–1980. Düsseldorf, Triltsch, 1980. 128 p. Contributions by F. L. Greb, M. Antonina, L. Peters.
Stollenwerk M: Die bauliche Entwicklung der Krankenversorgung der Industriestadt Stolberg im Rheinland vor dem Hintergrund der Ursprünge der Messingindustrie. **Hist Hosp** 1979–80;13:164–76

### Great Britain

Barr MB: Looking back: Guy's Hospital. **Lamp** 1980 Aug;37(8):49–51
Barr MB: Looking back. Some London hospitals: St Bartholomew's Hospital. **Lamp** 1980 Jun;37(6):59–61
Barr MB: Looking back: St Thomas's Hospital. **Lamp** 1980 Aug;37(8):51–2
Dainton C: Bart's Hospital, from its refoundation by Henry VIII. **Hist Today** 1978;28(12):810–6
Dainton C: Mustard, vinegar, and hog's grease: a short history of St. Thomas's Hospital. **Br Hist Illus** 1979;6(3):16–26
Dobson J: Some associations of St. Thomas's Hospital with the Company of Barber-Surgeons of London. **St Thomas Hosp Gaz** 1981;79:73–8
Dulake L: Doctors, practices and hospitals through 300 years. A history of general & hospital practice at Reigate & Redhill including Earlswood & Merstham. Redhill, The author, 1977, iv, 154 p.
Jetter D: Hospitäler in London; zur Typologie wohltätiger Einrichtungen im Spannungsfeld politischer Kräfte. **Sudhoffs Arch** 1978;62(3):250–81
Roy I, Porter S: The social and economic structure of an early modern suburb: the Tything at Worcester. **Bull Inst Hist Res** 1980;53:203–17
Winstanley J: St Thomas Hospital a cradle of British ophthalmology. **Trans Ophthalmol Soc UK** 1982;102 (Pt 4):454–60

### Haiti

Barry M, Stansfield SK, Bia FJ: Haiti and the Hôpital Albert Schweitzer. **Ann Intern Med** 1983 Jun;98(6):1018–20

### Hungary

Széll K: Szemelvények a szombathelyi kórház történetéből I. **Orv Hetil** 1979 Dec 16;120(50):3057–60
Szentgyörgyvölgyi G: Szemelvények Debrecen gyógyítástörténeti múltiából. **Orv Hetil** 1982 May 2;123(18):1114–6

### Italy

Bèttica-Giovannini R: Il malgoverno dell'Ospedale di Chivasso dal Cinquecento al Settecento. **Ann Osp Maria Vittoria Torino** 1983 Jan–Jun;26(1–6):183–96
Caffaratto TM: Storia dell'Ospedale Maggiore di Torino della Religione ed Ordine dei SS. Maurizio e Lazzaro--dal secolo XVI al secolo XX. **Ann Osp Maria Vittoria Torino** 1979 Jul–Dec;22(7–12):365–419
Giusberti F: Tra povertà e malattia: il Sant'Orsola a Bologna dal XVII al XVIII secolo. **Ann Fond Luigi Einaudi** 1979;13:117–50
Gnesda L: Gli 'ospizi' nelle Dolomiti. Firenze, Olschki, 1979. 81 p. (Comitato dei Geografi Italiani, 4).

### Japan

Kiikuni K: The development of hospitals and clinics in Japan. In Ogawa T, ed: Public health. Tokyo, Saikon, 1981. p. 1–11.

### Malta

Püschel E: Die Quarantäne auf Malta. Geschichte--Lazarettos und Hospital--Vorschriften. In Göpfert W, Otten HH, ed: Metavoeite: wandelt euch durch neues Denken. Düsseldorf, Triltsch, 1983. p. 95–105.

### Mexico

Alcócer Bernés JM: El Hospital del Divino Salvador. **Salud Publica Mex** 1983 Sep–Oct;25(5):525–30
Morales Meneses J: La congregación y Hospital de San Pedro. **Salud Publica Mex** 1984 Mar–Apr;26(2):190–4
Somolinos Palencia J: Un hospital a raiz de la Conquista. **Bol Soc Mex Hist Filos Med** 1979 Jun;4(27):93–104

### Netherlands

Haneveld GT: Oude medische gebouwen van Nederland. Amsterdam, Meesters, 1976. 218 p.
Van Lieburg MJ: De syfilitische patiënt in de geschiedenis van het Nederlandse ziekenhuiswezen vóór 1900. **Tijdschr Soc Geschied** 1982;8:156–79
Van Malenstein MM: Het Sint-Petersgasthuis te Culemborg een archief-studie vanuit medisch-historisch oogpunt. **Tijdschr Geschied Geneeskd** 1982;5(2):65–77
Van Steijnen C: Van gasthuis tot ziekenhuis; vier eeuwen St. Elisabeth's of Groote Gasthuis te Haarlem. **Ned Tijdschr Geneeskd** 1981 May 9;125(19):761–5

### Norway

Kristiansen K: Hospital services in Oslo. Oslo, Oslo City Hospital Board, 1979. p. 55–70.

### Poland

Krysa-Leszczyńska D: Krótki rys polskiego prawodawstwa szpitalnego w latach 1628–1867. **Wiad Lek** 1983 Aug 15;36(16):1397–401
Maciałek E, Sobocki S, Czyrek G: Pięć wieków szpitalnictwa w Jarosławiu (1462–1977). **Ann Univ Mariae Curie Sklodowska [Med]** 1978;33:341–51
Michalczak W, Lisiewicz J: Z dziejów budynków szpitalnych w Miechowie. **Przegl Lek** 1983;40(9):705
Podgórska-Klawe Z: Szpitale warszawskie, 1388/1945. Warszawa, Państwowe Wydawn. Nauk., 1975. 357 p.

### Portugal

Pina L de: Farmacia ornamental uma historia portuense. **Arch Hist Med Port** 1968–70;3(1–4):117–36

### Puerto Rico

Arana Soto S: El Hospital de Puerto Rico. San Juan de Puerto Rico, [s.n.], 1976. 296 p.
Torres Oliver LJ: Historia del Hospital de la Caridad de Nuestra Señora de la Concepción de San Germán, Puerto Rico. **Cuatricenten San German** 1971;:235–72

### South Africa

Villiers JC de, Keyser AL: Lost hospitals of the Cape. **S Afr Med J** 1983 Jun 29;Spec No:33–9

### Spain

Arnaiz Bonilla A: Las afamadas boticas burgalesas de los hospitales de San Juan y San Julian y San Quirce (Barrantes). Burgos, Exma. Diputacíon Provincial de Burgos, [1981]. 152 p.
Basante Pol RM: La farmacia en los monasterios, hospitales y hospederías del Bierzo. **Bol Soc Esp Hist Farm** 1984 Sep;35(139):165–86
Danon y Bretos J: Visió històrica de l'Hospital General de Santa Creu de Barcelona. Barcelona, Fundació Salvador Vives Casajuana, 1978. 207 p.
Darnés C, Solé A: Influencia de las comunidades religiosas en la enfermería de Cataluña. **Rev Enferm** 1981 Dec–1982 Jan;5(42–43):61–2
Ferrándiz Araujo C: El Hospital de la Caridad de Cartagena. Murcia, Imprenta Provincial, 1981. 286 p.
Garcia Sanchez J: Contribución a la historia de la botica del Hospital de la Pasión, de Ciudad Rodrigo. **Bol Soc Esp Hist Farm** 1980/81 Dec–Mar;31–32(124–5):1–7
Girón Irueste F: En torno al Maristan (hospital arabe) de Granada. **Asclepio** 1978–79;30–31:223–31
Jetter D: Neue Funde zur Geschichte der alten Pilgerherberge in Santiago de Compostela. In Seidler E, Schott H, ed: Bausteine zur Medizingeschichte. Stuttgart, Steiner, 1984. p. 52–64.
Jetter D: Spanien von den Anfängen bis um 1500. Wiesbaden, Steiner, 1980. 239 p. (Geschichte des Hospitals. Band 4).
Juncà i Ramon JM: L'Hospital de Sant Llàtzer: notes històriques. [S.l.]: J. M. Juncà Ramon, 1982. 47 p.
Valverde JL, Pérez Romero JA: La sanidad en Navarra contemplada a través del hospital general de Pamplona en los siglos XVI al XVII. In International Congress of the History of Medicine, 27th, Barcelona, 1980. Actas. Barcelona, Académia de Ciències Médiques de Catalunya i Balears, 1981. p. 636–43.
Velasco B: El hospital de convalescientes de Cuéllar. **Estud Segov** 1973;24(71–72):153–70

### Sri Lanka

Wijesinha SS, Wijesinha CY: Surgery and hospitals: the Sri Lanka tradition. **Ceylon Med J** 1983 Mar;28(1):48–52

**Sweden**

Detlow-Berg AL: Omvårdnad i Vadstena kloster. **Dan Medicinhist Arbog** 1983;12:65-73
Diener L, ed: Röster ur Riksgropen. **Nord Medicinhist Arsb** 1984;:49-61

**Switzerland**

Bächi H: Das Universitätsspital Zürich im Wandel der Zeit 1204-1980. Zürich, Schulthess, 1981. 61 p.
Fehr AM: Geschichte des Winterthurer Spitals. **Gesnerus** 1982;39(1):89-95
Loretan S: Das Antoniusspital in Brig. **Gesnerus** 1982;39(1):109-13

**Tunisia**

Arnoulet F: L'oeuvre hospitalière des Trinitaires et des Capucine dans le Régence de Tunis. **Cah Tunis** 1978;26(3-4):35-48

**Turkey**

Ozbay K: Türk asker hekimligi tarihi ve asker hastaneleri. 3 vols. in 4. Istanbul, Yörük Basimevi, 1976. 686, 349, 576, 493 p.
Said HM: Early hospitals in Turkey. **Med Times** 1981 Nov-Dec;16(11-12):8-14
Terzioglu A: Die Hofspitäler und andere Gesundheitseinrichtungen der osmanischen Palastbauten unter Berücksichtigung der Ursprungsfrage sowie ihre Beziehungen zu den Abendländischen Hofspitälern. München, Rudolf Trofenik, 1979. 303 p. (Beiträge zur Kenntnis Südosteuropas und des Nahen Orients, XXX).

**Uruguay**

Lockhart J: La historia del Hospital Maciel. Montevideo, Editora de Revistas, 1982. 244 p.

**USSR**

Gajeerski SF: Szpitale Zydowskie na Rusi czerwonej w XVI-XVIII w. **Biul Zydowskiego Inst Hist Pol** 1979;(4):25-33

**Before 500 A.D.**

**Asia**

Wijesinha S, Wickremesinghe C: Surgery and hospitals in ancient Sri Lanka and India. **J R Coll Surg Edinb** 1981 Jul;26(4):245-9

**Rome**

Kump WL: The xenodochium of Pammachius. **Minn Med** 1982 Oct;65(10):633

**500 A.D.-1450**

Bonenfant-Feytmans AM: Les organisations hospitalières vues par Jacques de Vitry (1225). **Ann Soc Belg Hist Hop** 1980;18:17-45
Grmek MD: Le médecin au service de l'hôpital médiéval en Europe occidentale. **Hist Philos Life Sci** 1982;4(1):25-64
Jones WR: The clinic in three medieval societies. **Diogenes** 1983;122:86-101

**Arabic**

Atiyeh M: Arab hospitals in history. **King Faisal Spec Hosp Med J** 1982 Apr;2(2):121-6
Sayili A: The emergence of the prototype of the modern hospital in medieval Islam. **Belleten (Turk)** 1980;44:279-86
Valverde JL, Munoz CP, ed: El Formulario de los hospitales De Ibn Abi L-bayan. Introduccion, traduccion espanola y commentarios, con glosarios. Granada, Universidad de Granada, 1981. 256 p. (Cuadernos de historia de la farmacia, 8).
Valverde JL, Peña Muñoz C: El formulario de los hospitales' de Ibn Abi l-Bayan (S. XIII). In International Congress of the History of Medicine, 27th, Barcelona, 1980. Actas. Barcelona, Acadèmia de Ciències Mèdiques de Catalunya i Balears, 1981. p. 346-51.

**Belgium**

De Keyzer W: L'évolution de la léproserie Saint-Ladre de Mons aux XIIIe et XIVe siècles. Fédération des Cercles d'Archéologie et d'Histoire de Belgique. 44e session. Congrès de Huy, 1976. Annales. Tielt, 1978. p. 174-6.
De Spiegeler P: La léproserie de Cornillon et la cité de Liège (XIIe-XVe siècle). **Ann Soc Belg Hist Hop** 1980;18:3-16
Himpens G: Het Sint-Janshospitaal te Brugge en zijn landbouwbedrijf rond 1350. **Biekorf** 1980;80:93-6
Van den Nieuwenhuizen J: Oorkondenboek van het Sint-Elizabeth-ospitaal te Antwerpen (1226-1355). Brussel, Paleis der Academiën, 1976. 414 p. (Koninklijke Commissie voor Geschiedenis).

**Byzantium**

Volk R: Gesundheitswesen und Wohltätigkeit im Spiegel der byzantinischen Klostertypika. München, Institut für Byzantinistik und neugriechische Philologie der Universität München, 1983. lxxx, 326 p. (Miscellanea Byzantina monacensia, Heft 28)

**Denmark**

Jensen KR, Tkocz I: Skeletmaterialet fra udgravningen af St. Jørgensgården i Odense. En foreløbig rapport. **Dan Medicinhist Arbog** 1983;12:52-64
Nielsen E: Udgravningen af Odenses St. Jørgensgård. Foreløbige resultater. **Dan Medicinhist Arbog** 1983;12:39-51

**Europe**

Bannister T, Ireland T: 'Hospitality' in the Middle Ages. **Mich Hosp** 1983 Dec;19(12):31-5

**France**

Assistance et charité: Toulouse, Privat, 1978. 435 p. (Cahiers de Fanjeaux, Collection d'Histoire religieuse du Languedoc au XIIIe et début du XIVe siècles, 13).
Benedetti Y: Les fondations hospitalières pisanes en Corse (XIIIe-XVe siècles). Maîtrise. Univ. d'Aix-en-Provence, 1976, 166 p.
Cheymol J: Hôpitaux et confrérie des pèlerins de Saint-Jacques-de-Compostelle à Paris. **Hist Sci Med** 1980;14(1):29-42
Gonthier N: Les hôpitaux et les pauvres à la fin du moyen âge: l'exemple de Lyon. **Moyen Age** 1978;84:279-308
La Coste-Messelière R de, Jugnot G, Treuille H: Fonda des XVIIe-XVIIIe siècles et sources de l'histoire hospitalière médiévale XIIe-XIVe siècle. Toulouse, E. Privat, 1978. 283-318 p.
La Coste Messelière R de: Sources et illustrations de l'histoire des établissements hospitaliers et du pèlerinage de Saint-Jacques-de-Compostelle. **Bull Soc Hist Sci Deux Sevres** 1977;10:195-269
Le Blevec D: Aux origines des hospitaliers de Saint-Jean de Jérusalem: Gérard dit 'Tenque' et l'établissement de l'Ordre dans le Midi. **Ann Midi** 1977;89:137-51
Neveux F: Un établissement d'assistance en milieu rural au XIVe siècle: l'Hôtel-Dieu de Villers-Bocage. **Ann Normandie** 1977;1:3-17
Peyresblanques J: Histoire de l'Hôpital de Dax au XIIIe siècle. **Bull Soc Borda** 1980;104(377):75-105
Saint-Denis A: Institution hospitalière et société à Laon aux XIIe et XIIIe siècles. **Inf Hist** 1983;45(4):171-9
Touati FO: Une approche de la maladie et du phénomène hospitalier aux XIIe et XIIIe siècles: la léproserie du Grand-Beaulieu à Chartres. **Hist Sci Med** 1980;14:419-24

**Great Britain**

Rawcliffe C: The hospitals of later medieval London. **Soc Soc Hist Med Bull (Lond)** 1983 Jun;32:24-6
Rawcliffe C: The hospitals of later medieval London. **Med Hist** 1984 Jan;28(1):1-21

**Israel**

Dolev E: [A twelfth century hospital in Jerusalem] (Heb). **Harefuah** 1980 Sep:99(5-6):136-7

**Middle East**

Sterns I: Care of the sick brothers by the Crusader Orders in the Holy Land. **Bull Hist Med** 1983;57(1):43-69

**Poland**

Krysa-Leszczyńska D: Polemika wokół daty założenia Szpitala Sw. Ducha w Sandomierzu (w zwiazku z 690 rocznica założenia szpitala). **Wiad Lek** 1984 Feb 1;37(3):237-40

**Spain**

Giron F: Nota sobre un supuesto hospital arabe en Algeciras. **Llull (Spain)** 1978;2:113-5
Imamuddin SM: Maristan (Hospitals) in Medieval Spain. **Islam Stud** 1978;17(1):45-55
Rubio Vela A: Una fundación burguesa en la Valencia medieval: El Hospital de En Clapers (1311). **Dynamis** 1981;1:18-49

# HOSPITALS

## 1450–1700

### Austria

Jäger-Sunstenau H: Auswärtige in einem wiener Totenbuch 1687–1690. **Adler** 1967;7(13–14):205–8

Nowotny E: Die Gründung der Hofspitäler durch Ferdinand I. im 16. Jahrhundert mit besonderer Berücksichtigung des wiener Hofspitals. **Unsere Heimat** 1971;42(2):91–103

### Belgium

Marechal G: Het gebouw van de Brugse Leprozorie in de XVIe eeuw. **Biekorf** 1979;79:316–22

### Canada

Bernier H: Françoise Maumousseau. In Dictionary of Canadian biography, 1701 to 1740. Volume 2, 1969. p. 466–7.

Bernier H: Marie-Madeleine Maufils. In Dictionary of Canadian biography, 1701 to 1740. Volume 2, 1969. p. 466.

Paquin M: Louise Soumande. In Dictionary of Canadian biography, 1701 to 1740. Volume 2, 1969. p. 613.

### Dominican Republic

Marion-Landais G: The first European hospital in the Western Hemisphere. In: Congrès international d'histoire de la médecine, XXVe, Québec, 1976. Actes., Québec, 1977. p. 961–8.

### Europe

Alsop JD: Some notes on seventeenth-century continental hospitals. **Br Libr J** 1981;7(1):70–4

### France

Bériac JP: Le Parlement, la Jurade et l'hôpital Saint-André de Bordeaux face à 'l'effrénée multitude des pauvres' au XVIe siècle et au début du XVIIe. **Rev Hist Bordeaux Dep Gironde** 1977, reçu 1980;26:41–58

Blum A: Les établissements d'assistance en Basse-Alsace au début du XVIIe siècle. In Livet G, Schaff G, ed: Médecine et assistance en Alsace, XVIe-XXe siècle. Strasbourg, Istra, 1976. p. 71–86.

Kneist W: Théophraste Renaudot und die Dispensairebetreuung. **Z Arztl Fortbild (Jena)** 1982 Mar 1;76(5):220–3

Patureau N: L'assistance à Tours au XVIIe siècle; la fondation de l'Hôpital Général de la Charité. In: Congrès National des Sociétés Savantes, 97e, Nantes, 1972. Actes. Paris, 1977. Histoire Moderne et Contemporaine, Tome 1. p. 431–43.

Tessier JF: L'hôpital de Ste-Marguerite de Cadillac et la littérature consacrée à Saint Jean de Dieu et ses disciples en France au XVIIe siècle. **Rev Fr Hist Livre** 1979;23:317–28

Toujas R: La lutte contre la mendicité à la fin du XVIIe siècle: l'établissement d'hôpitaux généraux dans la province ecclśiastique de Toulouse. In: Congrès National des Sociétés Savantes, 97e, Nantes, 1972. Actes. Paris, 1977. Histoire Moderne et Contemporaine, Tome 1. p. 389–401.

Treuille H: L'état des hôpitaux de pèlerins dans le Sud-Ouest de la France dans la seconde moitié du XVIIe siècle. In: Congrès National des Sociétés Savantes, 104e, Bordeaux, 1979. Actes. Paris, 1981. Histoire Moderne et Contemporaine, Tome 2. p. 35–50.

Villard M: Des hôpitaux de Marseille. **Marseille** 1980;122:93–104

Villard M: Des hôpitaux de Marseille. In: Marseille au XVIIème siècle. (Actes du 10ème Colloque de Marseille.) Marseilles Centre Méridional de Rencontres sur le XVIIe siècle. 1980.

### Germany

Fischer H: Zur Entwicklung Bayreuths. Das Hospital und seine Kirche bis zum Ende des 16. Jahrhunderts. **Arch Gesch Oberfranken** 1979;59:41–88

### Great Britain

Kealey EJ: Medieval medicus. A social history of Anglo-Norman medicine. Baltimore, Johns Hopkins University Press, 1981. x, 211 p.

Lynch M: The 'Faithful Brethren' of Edinburgh: the acceptable face of Protestantism. **Bull Inst Hist Res** 1978;51(124):194–9

### Italy

Caffaratto TM: Il Libro Lunghetto, ricettario del '600 dell'Ospedale Mauriziano di Torino. **Minerva Med** 1980 Apr 2;71(13):981–7

Gai L: Interventi rinascimentali nello spedale del Ceppo di Pistoia. Ridefinizione nell'attività pistoiese di Michelozzo architetto. **Boll Stor Pistoiese** 1977;12(1–2):72–155

Ruggiero Pastura MG: Una 'visita' del 1592 all'ospedale dei 'pazzarelli' di Roma. **Rass Arch Stato** 1972;32(1):47–67

### Mexico

Martínez Báez M: La obra hospitalaria del ilustrisismo Señor Don Vasco de Quiroga. **Mem Col Nac (Mex)** 1978;8(4):33–41

Toscano Moreno J: Los hospitales y la 'hospitalidad' de los franciscanos en la Nueva Galicia. **Bol Inst Invest Bibliogr** 1970;4:389–404

### Poland

Karpiński A: Warunkizycia pensjonariuszy szpitali Warszawskich w XVI i w pierwszej połowie XVII wieku. **Kwart Hist Kultury Mater** 1977;25(1):43–62

Skrobacki A: Najstarszy na Warmii Polski regulamin szpitalny. **Komun Mazursko Warm** 1977;(3–4):447–54

### Spain

Bravo Lozano J: La visita del hospital real de San Lázaro de Córdoba (1599–1603). **Hispania** 1979;39(143):639–70

Jordi González R: Inventario incompleto perteneciente a la botica del hospital de Santa Cruz, de Barcelona (21–1–1585). **Circ Farm** 1982 Apr–Jun;40(275):211–21

Marcos Martín A: El sistemo hospitalario de Medina del Campo en el siglo XVI. **Cuad Invest Hist** 1978;2:341–62

Parrilla Hermida M: Un hospital de la Armada en El Ferrol siglo XVI. **Asclepio** 1981;33:407–10

### Switzerland

Waldis V: Hospitalisation und Absonderung in Pestzeiten--die Schweiz im Vergleich zu Oberitalien. **Gesnerus** 1982;39(1):71–8

## 1700 to Present

Apostolov M: D-r Robert Iur'evich Berzin (1887–1950 g.) i bolnitsata na ruskiia Cherven krust v Sofiia. **Khirurgiia (Sofiia)** 1982;35(2):223–7

Beatty WK: Daniel Hale Williams--pioneer surgeon and hospital administrator. **Proc Inst Med Chic** 1979 Jul–Sep;32(7):156

Benedek I: Semmelweis. Budapest, Gondolat, 1980. 269 p.

Elgjo RF: Hospice-bevegelsen. **Tidsskr Nor Laegeforen** 1982 Sep 20;102(26):1352–4

Fockert JA de: De klinisch geriatrische afdeling in een ziekenhuis: officële erkenning als experiment. **Tijdschr Ziekenverpl** 1982 Sept 21;35(19):621–5

Forty A: The modern hospital in England and France: the social and medical uses of architecture. In King, Anthony D., ed. Buildings and society: essays on the social development of the built environment. London, Routledge and Kegan Paul, 1980. p. 61–93.

Foster Z, Wald FS, Wald HJ: The hospice movement: a backward glance at its first two decades. **New Physician** 1978 May;27(5):21–4

Gilbrin E: Le docteur Paul Caujole: l'hôpital français d'Oumiah (septembre 1917 – avril 1918). **Hist Sci Med** 1980;14(2):155–64

Goltz RW: WWII, the 147th General hospital & Harry Arnold. **Hawaii Med J** 1982 Nov;41(11):410

Grellet I, Kruse C: Histoires de la tuberculose. Les fièvres de l'âme 1800–1940. Paris, Ramsay, 1983. 333 p.

Holland MM, Dean L: Mother Joseph: founder, architect, beggar. **Hosp Prog** 1980 Apr;61(4):70–3

Jones PG: 'A man and his hospital'. **Aust Paediatr J** 1981 Mar;17(1):5–14

Knibiehler Y: Les infirmières-visiteuses (1922–1938). **Penelope** 1981;(5):80–4

Kurumada M: ['Introductory notes on lying-in institutions' and problems of management--hospital management and Florence Nightingale] (Jpn). **Sogo Kango** 1983;18(1):107–19

Labisch A: Krankenhauspolitik in der Krankenhausgeschichte. **Hist Hosp** 1979–80;13:217–33

Lejman K: Andrzej Badurski (1740–1789) jako założyciel szpitala akademickiego i inicjator klinicznego nauczania meydycyny. **Przegl Lek** 1981;38(7):567–70

Lorensen M: The contribution of the hospital to health care. **Nurs Times** 1983 Mar 9–15;79(10):42–4

Ludmerer KM: Writing the history of hospitals. An essay review. **Bull Hist Med** 1982 Spring;56(1):106–9

Murken AH: Die Entwicklung des Krankenhauses im 18. und 19. Jahrhundert. **Medita** 1980;10(3):i–xvi (Geschichte der Medizin)

Murken AH: Heilanstalten für Tuberkulöse. Zur Geschichte der Lungensanatorien und ihrer Therpiekonzeption im 19. Jahrhundert. In Göpfert W, Otten HH, ed: Metavoeite: wandelt euch durch neues Denken. Düsseldorf, Triltsch, 1983. p. 107–24.

Murken AH, Rodegra H: Krankenhausrundbauten in Vergangenheit und Gegenwart. Zur historischen Entwicklung von kreisförmigen Bettenhäusern und panoptisch angelegten Krankensälen. **Hist Hosp** 1979–80;13:197–216

Rothman WA: The hospital in literature. **Hosp Health Serv Adm** 1983 Jul–Aug;28(4):85–94

Rüttimann B: Zur Geschichte der Krüppelfürsorge. **Gesnerus**

1980;37(3/4):199-214
Saunders C: Hospice care. **Indian J Cancer** 1979 Sep-Dec;16(3-4):1-4
Schiffczyk D: Vom Therapiekonzept zur Architekturform. Betrachtungen über das Terrassenkrankenhaus. **Hist Hosp** 1979-80;13:177-96
Smith T: Victorian who sent a hospital to war. **Health Soc Serv J** 1983 May 5;93(4845):533-5
Stoddard S: The hospice movement. Briarcliff Manor, N. Y., Stein and Day, 1978. xviii, 266 p.
Terzioglu A, Krebs LM: The development of surgery and of surgical clinics at the turn of the 20th century. Munich, (the authors), 1979. 69 p.
Zambito RF: A history of hospital dental practice. Part I and II. **New Dent** 1979 Oct-Nov;10(2-3):31-3, 35-8

**Africa**

Eddy TP: The evolution of British colonial hospitals in West Africa. **Trans R Soc Trop Med Hyg** 1983;77(4):563-4

**Algeria**

Lefebvre P: L'hôpital Militaire Laveran de Constantine. **Med Trop (Mars)** 1980 Nov-Dec;40(6):645-9

**Americas**

Kalisch PA: Tracadie and Penikese leprosaria: a comparative analysis of societal response to leprosy in New Brunswick, 1844-1880, and Massachusetts, 1904-1921. **Bull Hist Med** 1973 Sep-Oct;47(5):480-512

**Argentina**

Benaim F: Thirty years at the service of the burned in Argentina and South America. **J Trauma** 1981 May;21(5):356-63

**Australia**

A century of health care: **Med J Aust** 1982 Jul 24;2(2):98-9
D'Arbon P: Rehabilitation yesterday and today. **Lamp** 1980 Dec;37(12):16-8
Davidson WS: Havens of refuge. Nedlands, Univ. of Western Australia Press, 1978. xii, 188 p.
Dickey B: St. Vincent's Hospital, Sydney: a note. **J R Aust Hist Soc** 1978;64(2):131-33
Hamilton DG: Hand in hand. Sydney, Ferguson, 1979. 338 p.
Hughes JE: A history of the Royal Adelaide Hospital. Second revised edition. Netley, South Australia, Board of Management of the Royal Adelaide Hospital, 1982. xvii, 240 p.
Lewis M: Hospitalization for childbirth in Sydney, 1870-1939; the modern maternity hospital and the improvement in the health of women. **J R Aust Hist Soc** 1980;66(3):199-205
Loaring K, Wards M: Brief history of Northfield. **Australas Nurses J** 1981 Apr;10(4):5-6, 8
Looking back: the Australian army hospitals: **Lamp** 1980 May;37(5):53-5
Lowe RF: Early Melbourne eye and ear hospital, and Dr. Turnbull's house at 101 (157) Spring Street. **Aust NZ J Surg** 1980 Oct;50(5):546-9
Lowe RF: William R. Wilde, Andrew S. Gray, and two eye and ear hospitals of very similar name. **Aust NZ J Surg** 1981 Dec;51(6):630-6
McLean JA: Direct blood transfusion. Its history, with special reference to the Alfred Hospital, Melbourne. **Med J Aust** 1979 Dec 15;2(12):625-8
Maddox K: Schlink of Prince Alfred. A biography of Sir Herbert Schlink. Sydney, Royal Prince Alfred Hospital, 1978. vii, 283 p.
Neil G: The Scott Memorial Hospital Scone: 90 years of nursing. **Lamp** 1982 Mar-Apr;39(2):19
Pockley JA: An outline of one hundred years' history at St Vincent's Hospital, Sydney, 1872-1972. **Aust J Ophthalmol** 1983 Aug;11(3):221-31
Price L: Sydney Eye Hospital. **Br J Ophthalmol** 1982 Oct;66(10):617-21
Royal Alexandra's century of caring: **Aust Nurses J** 1980 Nov;10(5):20-1
St Vincent's Hospital, Sydney: 1857-1982: **Med J Aust** 1982 Nov 27;2(11):532-3
Smith T: Prince of Wales's Hospital: prince and pauper. **Health Soc Serv J** 1981 Dec 17;91(4777):1552-4
Stubbe JH, Scrymgeour JM, Smith AJ: Medical background; History of Fremantle hospitals and doctors. [Nedlands], Published for the Fremantle Hospital Board by the Univ. of Western Australia Press, 1969. xxvi, 82 p.
Sydney Hospital--a tribute: **Lamp** 1983 Jan-Feb;40(1):14-6
'The Coast' Hospital: remember when?: **Lamp** 1981 May;38(5 Suppl):17-9
(1816) Rum Hospital ... (1844) Infirmary-Dispensary ... (1881) Sydney Hospital ... (1982) ?: **Med J Aust** 1982 Aug 21;2(4):198-200

**Austria**

Ardelt R: Geschichte des Konventes und Krankenhauses der Elisabethinen zu Linz. **Hist Jahrb Stadt Linz** 1978;:95-146
Ebner H: Die Lungenabteilung des Pflegeheimes der Stadt Wien-Lainz im Wandel der Zeit. **Wien Med Wochenschr** 1980 Feb 29;130(4):147-8
Fellner R, Höflechner W: Die Augenheilkunde an der Universität Graz. Graz, Akademische Druck- u. Verlagsanstalt, 1973. ix, 180 p. (Publikationen aus dem Archiv der Universität Graz, Bd. 2).
Holubar K: Ferdinand von Hebra und das Allgemeine Krankenhaus in Wien. Uber die Domizilierung der beiden Hautkliniken um die Mitte des 19. Jahrhunderts und ihr Verhältnis zum II. Hof im Allgemeinen Krankenhaus. **Wien Med Wochenschr** 1982 Sep 30;132(18):423-6
Holubar K: Vienna General Hospital--'Allgemeines Krankenhaus'--bicentennial. **Isr J Med Sci** 1984 Jun;20(6):553-4
Luger A: 70 Jahre Krankenhaus Lainz. **Wien Klin Wochenschr** 1983 Jun 10;95(12):393-6
Mitterstiller S: 100 Jahre chirurgische Klinik in Innsbruck. **Tirol Heimat** 1970;:31-2
Mitterstiller S: 100 Jahre Chirurgische Klinik in Innsbruck. **Tirol Heimat** 1970;34:17-38
Sablik K: Die Finanzierung des Wiener Allgemeinen Krankenhauses (gegründet 1784) durch Kaiser Joseph II. In Schmidtchen V, Jäger E, ed: Wirtschaft, Technik und Geschichte. Beiträge zur Erforschung der Kulturbeziehungen in Deutschland und Osteuropa. Festschrift für Albrecht Timm. Berlin, Verlag Ulrich Camen, 1980. p. 241-50.
Schachter M: Alfred Adler (1870-1937), et sa psycho-pédagogie clinique. **Rev Hist Med Heb** 1981 Dec;139(34 no 4):53-6
Schmalhofer J: Das Werk von Johann Florian Heller mit besonderer Berücksichtigung der Entstehung des ersten pathologisch-chemischen Laboratoriums am Allgemeinen Wiener Krankenhaus und der Ernennung Hellers zum Vorstand des Laboratoriums. Diss. Bonn, 1980. 201 p.
Spängler H, Galle P: 70 Jahre Unfallchirurgie an den Wiener Kliniken. **Wien Klin Wochenschr** 1981 Jun 26;93(13):423-8
Spitzy KH, ed, Lau I, ed: Van Swietens Erbe: die Wiener Medizinische Schule heute in Selbstdarstellungen. Wien, Maudrich, 1982. 400 p.

**Belgium**

Abelshausen M: De Antwerpse Werkhuizen van Liefdadigheid (1802-1870): weldadigheidsinstelling of fabriek? **Ann Soc Belg Hist Hop** 1982;20:61-108
Aernouts R: L'eau de Lourdes est-elle un médicament? **Rev Hist Pharm (Paris)** 1980 Mar;27(244):5-7
Bruneel C: Malades et défunts au Grand Hôpital de Louvain (1767-1796). **Ann Soc Belg Hist Hop** 1978;16:3-33
Dickstein-Bernard C: Genèse del'hôpital universitaire, 1834-1935. **Rev Med Brux** 1984 May;5(5):315-8
Dickstein-Bernard C: La pratique de la chirurgie dans les hôpitaux bruxellois au XIXe siècle. **Ann Soc Belg Hist Hop** 1981;:69-94
Evrard E: Le service de santé militaire hollando-belge à la bataille de Waterloo et dans les hôpitaux de Bruxelles en juin 1815. **Rev Belge Hist Milit** 1983;25(1):61-96
Haesenne-Peremans N: Les asiles pour malades, vieillards et orphelins dans l'arrondissement de Liège au début du XIXe siècle. **Bull Inst Archeol Liegeois** 1979;91:85-157
Haesenne-Peremans N: Les Hospices et Orphelinats de la région Verviétoise au début du XIXe siècle. **Ann Soc Belg Hist Hop** 1978;16:35-56
Joiris A: Le vieux Bavière au XIXe siècle (1830-1895). **Ann Soc Belg Hist Hop** 1982;20:109-44
Jurion F, Parisel F: Le troisième et dernier cimetière de l'hôpital Saint-Jean de Bruxelles (1704-1784). Etude paléopathologique des ossements du cimetière Saint-Jean. **Ann Soc Belg Hist Hop** 1982;20:2-60
Lafosse A: Les hôpitaux temporaires à Verviers durant les épidémies de choléra. **Ann Soc Belg Hist Hop** 1979;17:71-9
Meuwissen E: Les dépôts de mendicité au tribunal de l'histoire. **Ann Soc Belg Hist Hop** 1981;:47-67
Scholliers-van den Eeckhout P: De geschiedenis van de 'Vondelingenbak' te Brussel. Conflicten tussen moraliteit en administratieve zuinigheid. **Ann Soc Belg Hist Hop** 1978;16:57-85
Verheyen H: De zorg voor het gevonden kind te Antwerpen (1830-1870). **Ann Soc Belg Hist Hop** 1978;16:87-109

**Brazil**

Marcondes CH, Colombo MO: Irmandade da Santa Casa de Poços de Caldas. **Enfoque** 1984 Aug;12(1):15-8
Mesgravis L: O primeiro hospital do 'sertão' e a 'corrida do ouro'. **Rev Hist (Brazil)** 1973;46(94):549-62
Nolding Gaffree A: Ana Neri - la première infirmière militaire au Brésil. In: International Congress of the History of Medicine, 26th, Plovdiv (Bulgaria), 1978. Actes du Congres, Vol. 1. Sofia, 1980. p. 114-5.

**Bulgaria**

Beshkov L: Stranitsi ot istoriiata na tolbukhinskata bolnitsa. Tolbukhin, [s.n.], 1967 (Tolbukhin: SPP Kiro Stefanov). 255 p.
Botevgard District Hospital: 90 years (1892-1982). Botevgard, [s.n.], 1982. 25 p.
Nikolaeva I, Vassilev V, Ivanov C, et al: Données statistiques sur l'activité l'hôpital 'Paraskeva Nikolaou' à Varna de 1879 à 1912. In International Congress of the History of Medicine. 26th, Plovdiv, 1978. Actes du Congress. Sofia, 1981. Volume II. p. 68-9.

# HOSPITALS

Zapryanov N: Centennial anniversary of the Plovdiv State Hospital. **Folia Med (Plovdiv)** 1980;22(1):37–9

**Canada**

Andrews MW: St. Luke's Home, Vancouver, 1888–1936: a transitional hospital. **J Can Church Hist Soc** 1982;24(2):90–8
Angus MS: Harriet (Cartwright) Dobbs. In Dictionary of Canadian biography, 1881–1890. 1982;11:265–6.
Audet-Lapointe P, Perrault JL, Deslauriers L, et al: L'Hôpital Notre-Dame de Montréal. **Union Med Can** 1980 Jan;109(1):16–8
Bensley EH: John Poad Drake (1794–1883), the first artist to portray the Hospital. **Montreal Gen Hosp News** 1981;19(1):8–9
Bensley EH: Pages of history. Montreal, [Montreal General Hospital], 1981. 40 p.
Bensley EH: The great remove [1955]. **Montreal Gen Hosp News** 1980;18(2):12–3
Bois P: Le centenaire de l'Hôpital Notre-Dame. **Union Med Can** 1980 Jan;109(1):157–8
Burkinshaw SM: A look at Kingston General Hospital's archives. **Dimens Health Serv** 1982 Nov;59(11):20–1
Ducharme J: Marie-Catherine-Françoise Céloron. In Dictionary of Canadian biography, 1801 to 1820. Volume 5, 1983. p. 174.
Forsey RR: One hundred years ago. A century of hospital administrators. **Montreal Gen Hosp News** 1981;19(1):9
Frost SB: Alexander Skakel, LL.D.: a founder, M.G.H. governor, and a many sided man. **Montreal Gen Hosp News** 1980;18(2):3–5
Gale GL: The changing years. The story of Toronto Hospital and the fight against tuberculosis. Toronto, West Park Hospital, 1979. xvii, 134 p.
Gareau S: L'organisation hospitalière dans le nord-ouest Quebeçois. **Can Cathol Hist Assoc Study Sess** 1982;49:35–58
Historical review (Notre Dame Hospital).: **Nurs Montreal** 1980 Jun;5(1):22–3
Holzberg CS: Anthropology, life histories, and the aged: the Toronto Baycrest Centre. **Int J Aging Hum Dev** 1983–84;18(4):255–75
Johnston AJ: The frères de la charité and the Louisbourg Hôpital du Roi. **Can Cathol Hist Assoc Study Sess** 1981;48:5–25
Knowles V: Leaving with a red rose. A history of the Ottawa Civic Hospital School of Nursing. Ottawa, Ottawa Civic Hospital School of Nursing Alumnae Association, 1981. vi, 218 p.
McGinnis JP: The white plague in Calgary: sanatarium care in southern Alberta. **Alberta Hist** 1980;28(4):1–15
Medovy H: Seven decades of service at the Children's Hospital of Winnipeg. **Can Med Assoc J** 1980 Dec 20;123(12):1259–61
Plamondon L: Marie-Catherine Payen de Noyan. In Dictionary of Canadian biography, 1801 to 1820. Volume 5, 1983. p. 661–2.
Robillard D: L'hôpital Notre-Dame de Montréal célèbre avec dynamisme 100 ans de progrès. **Can Med Assoc J** 1980 Apr 5;122(7):837–9
Ross M: The evolution of hospital care in Alberta. **Dimens Health Serv** 1980 Apr;57(4):A4
Rousseau F: Marie-Geneviève Parent. In Dictionary of Canadian biography, 1801 to 1820. Volume 5, 1983. p. 658–9.
Rousseau F: Marie-Vénérande Melançon. In Dictionary of Canadian biography, 1801 to 1820. Volume 5, 1983. p. 587–8.
Salter RB: Scientific contributions to orthopaedic surgery by the staff of The Hospital for Sick Children, Toronto, 1875 to 1975. In: Congrès international d'histoire de la médecine, XXVe, Québec, 1976. Actes. Québec, 1977. p. 1225–43.
Séguin G: Marie-Angélique Dussaus. In Dictionary of Canadian biography, 1801 to 1820. Volume 5, 1983. p. 293.
Sylvestre PF: Dossier historique: les religieuses infirmières en Ontario français. **Infirm Can** 1983 Nov;25(10):27–9

**Chile**

Chamorro G: El Dr. Hernán Alessandri y el desarrollo de la medicina interna en el Hospital de Salvador. **Rev Med Chil** 1979 May;107(5):438–40
Dooner H: Los ultimos cincuenta años del Hospital San Borja. **Rev Med Chil** 1982 Jul;110(7):698–701
Edwards A, Yerkovic L, Santamaría J: La tuberculosis y el Hospital San José de Santiago. **Rev Med Chil** 1983 Mar;111(3):315–9
Estévez Cordovez R: El Hospital San Francisco de Borja. **Rev Med Chil** 1982 Jul;110(7):694–8
Hervé Lelievre L: La medicina hospitalaria have 50 años. Recuerdos del Hospital San Francisco de Borja. **Rev Med Chil** 1982 Jul;110(7):701–6
Neghme A: Semblanza historica del Hospital San Francisco de Borja. **Rev Med Chil** 1982 Jul;110(7):693–4

**China**

Fox RC, Swazey JP: Critical care at Tianjin's First Central Hospital and the fourth modernization. **Science** 1982 Aug 20;217(4561):700–5
Gilbrin E: Les médecins français au Sseu Tch'ouan au début du XXe siècle; l'hopital de Tch'eng Tou. **Hist Sci Med** 1982;16(3):199–204
Gilbrin E: Les médecins français au Sseu Tch'ouan au début du XXe siècle; l'hôpital de Tch'eng Tou. **Hist Sci Med** 1983;17(1):105–10
Gilbrin E: Les médecins français au Sseu Tch'ouan au début du XXe siècle; l'hôpital de Tch'ong King. **Hist Sci Med** 1982;16(2):125–30

**Cuba**

Torres Medina J: Los barcos hospitales en la campaña de Cuba. **Rev Hist Mil** 1970;14(29):161–86

**Czechoslovakia**

Adamec J: Z historie výuky I. interní kliniky v Praze. **Cas Lek Cesk** 1981;120(49):1475–7
Bolecek O: Protifašistický odboj na zdravotnické frontě. Vzpomínky na ilegální činnost za okupace na Bulovce. **Cas Lek Cesk** 1980 May 9;119(19):538–42
Cerveňanská N: 60 rokov Ortopedickej kliniky University Komenského. **Acta Chir Orthop Traumatol Cech** 1983 Dec;50(6):485–90
Dohnal K: Deset let léčeben pro dlouhodobě nemocné v CSR. **Cas Lek Cesk** 1984 Aug 17;123(33):1027–30
Hlaváčková L: K stému výročí české výuky na I. interní klinice v. Praze. **Cas Lek Cesk** 1981 Nov 26;120(47):1478–82
Hübschmann K: Sambergerovi současníci na klinice Janovského. **Cesk Dermatol** 1980 Oct;55(5):349–53
Krahulec I, Ambrušová L, Dresslerová I, et al: Desat rokov činnosti Foniatrického pracoviska na otolaryngologickej klinike FN v Bratislave. **Cesk Otolaryngol** 1984 Jun;33(3):195–9
Kroupa J: Dvacet pět let výzkumného ústavu traumatologického v brně. **Rozhl Chir** 1979;58(10):675–80
Kroupa J: 50 let od otevření úrazové nemocnice v Brně a 30 let činnosti Výzkumného ústavu traumatologického v Brně. **Rozhl Chir** 1984 Oct;63(10):633–42
Kunc Z: Pěhled cinnosti neurochirurgické kliniky v Praze 1959--1978. **Cas Lek Cesk** 1979 Jul 20;118(29):897–901
Malát L: 85 years of the hospital 'Na tabulovém Vrchu' and 35 years of its change into a faculty hospital. **Acta Univ Palacki Olomuk Fac Med** 1982;103:23–7
Moravec R, Tichý M, Moravcová M, et al: Z dejín chirurgie v Bratislave. Profesor Kostlivý a začiatky chirurgickej•kliniky na LFUK v Bratislava] **Rozhl Chir** 1984 Jul;63(7):526–31
Navrátil M: Padesát let Kojeneckého ústavu v Ostravě. **Cesk Pediatr** 1981 Aug;36(8):475–6
Prokupek J: Pražská psychiatrická klinika před 50 lety. **Cesk Psychiatr** 1982 Apr;78(2):127–36
Rozsívalová E: Příspěvek k vývoji institucionální základny I. interní kliniky v Praze 1881–1938. **Cas Lek Cesk** 1981;120(50):1539–41
Stork A: Sto deset let rozvoje I. interní kliniky v Praze. **Cas Lek Cesk** 1981 Oct 1;120(39):1169–73

**Denmark**

Ehlers H: Bjerrum's Clinic. **Surv Ophthalmol** 1981 Sep–Oct;26(1):101–2
Indretningen af Augustenborg Slot til lazaret i krigen 1848–1850 – en 'chronique scandaleuse'?: **Dan Medicinhist Arbog** 1980;:91–123
Kelly C: Denmark's Rigshospitalet pioneers treatment for torture victims. **Can Med Assoc J** 1983 Jul 15;129(2):178, 180
Ryssing E: Historien om Børnehospitalet i Rigensgade og Dronning Louises Børnehospital. **Dan Medicinhist Arbog** 1981;:58–92
Sell A, Madsen CB: Radiumstationen in Aarhus from 1962 to 1984. **Acta Radiol [Oncol]** 1984;23(2–3):85–90
Sørensen P: Hospitaler og sygehuse i Kolding: er udgivet af Vejle amtsråds sygehusudvalg i anledning af hundredårsdagen for indvielsen af sygehuset i Sct. Jørgensgade i 1880. Kolding, Konrad Jørgensens bogtrykkeri, 1980. 167 p.

**Finland**

Soiva K: Juhlahaastattelu. **Katilolehti** 1980 Dec;85(12):408–11

**France**

Ackerman EB: Use by patients of a French provincial hospital, 1895–1923. **Bull Hist Med** 1980 Summer;54(2):188–203
Ackermann EB: L'Hôpital de Mantes dans la première moitié du XIXe siècle. **Ann Hist Mantois** 1979;6:65–73
Amalric P: La Clinique Ophtalmologique de l'Hôtel Dieu à 100 ans. **Bull Soc Ophtalmol Fr** 1980 Dec;80(12):1177–80
Baradel Y: Quelques aspects de la médecine à Belfort au XVIIIe siècle. In Livet G, Schaff G, ed: Médecine et assistance en Alsace, XVIe–XXe siècle. Strasbourg, Istra, 1976. p. 135–44.
Bergasse JD: Jean Anglade (1698–1764) et la fondation de l'hôpital rural de Cazouls-les-Béziers au XVIIIe siècle. Bergasse (ed.) Hommage à Jacques Fabre de Morlhon. Albi, O.J.S., 1978. p. 133–47.
Bernier R: Les mesures publique d'assistance à la fin de l'Ancien régime dans la généralité de Caen. D.E.S. d'histoire du droit et des faits sociaux, Univ. de Caen, 1972 vii, 89, 56 p.
Bevan-John P: Down memory lane: escape from Alsace. **Nurs Mirror** 1980 Sept 25;151(13):34

Bolzinger R, Beau A: L'hôpital militaire d'instruction de Metz. In: Congrès national des Sociétés Savantes, 103e, Nancy, 1978. Comptes rendus. Paris, Section des Sciences, Fasc. V. p. 11–8.
Bolzinger R, Gilbrin E, Lorrang F: L'hôpital Saint-Nicolas de Metz avant la révolution. Sa fondation laïque, ses singulières prérogatives financières. **Hist Sci Med** 1979;13(4):369–77
Boulle L: La médicalisation des hôpitaux Parisiens dans la première moitié du xixème siècle. **Hist Reflect** 1982;9(1–2):33–44
Buttet H de: Les Invalides en 1709. In: Congrès National des Sociétés Savantes, 97e, Nantes, 1972. Actes. Paris, 1977. Histoire Moderne et Contemporaine, Tome 1. p. 55–65.
Capdebielle A: L'activité médicale à l'Hôtel des Invalides. **Med Armees** 1981;9:631–8
Castaigne P: Centenaire de la Clinique des maladies du système nerveux de la Salpêtrière. Introduction. **Rev Neurol (Paris)** 1982;138(12):879–86
Chambonnet F: Les faiences pharmaceutiques conservées dans les établissements hospitaliers de la région lyonnaise. Le Puy-en-Velay, [s.n.], 1978. 213 p. (Thèse, Lyon).
Cheymol J: Hôpitaux des pèlerins de Saint-Jacques-de-Compostelle. **Hist Sci Med** 1980;14:387–97
Cordoliani A: L'hôpital militaire du Val de Grâce dans la vie sociale parisienne. In Congrès National des Sociétés Savantes, 103e, Nancy-Metz, 1978. Actes. Paris, 1979. Tome I, p. 607–24.
Debré M: Robert Debré, réformateur. **Bull Acad Natl Med (Paris)** 1982 Dec;166(9):1295–303
Delaunay P: Médecins de jadis et d'aujourd'hui; souvenirs des hôpitaux et de la Faculté de Paris de 1895 à 1905. **Hist Sci Med** 1981;15(4):307–20
Devos D, Devos JC: L'hôpital militaire de Barèges (Hautes-Pyrénées) du debut du XVIIIe siècle à la fin du Premier Empire. In: Congrès National des Sociétés Savantes, 97e, Nantes, 1972. Actes. Paris, 1977. Histoire Moderne et Contemporaine, Tome 1. p. 105–13.
Dupré J: Les enfants abandonnés à l'hospice civil et militaire de Châteauroux de 1805 à 1820 inclusivement. **Bull Soc Fr Hist Hop** 1980;(41):9–16
Engrand C: Les abandons d'enfants à Amiens vers la fin de l'Ancien Régime. **Rev Nord** 1982;64(252):73–92
Faure O: A l'hôpital, avant les infirmières: les soeurs hospitalières de Lyon au début du XIXe siècle. **Penelope** 1981;(5):52–5
Faure O: L'hôpital et la médicalisation au début du 19e siècle: l'exemple lyonnais (1800–1830). **Ann Bretagne** 1979;86(3):277–90
Faure O: Médecins, médecine et hôpital à Lyon au début du XIXe siècle. **Bull Soc Fr Hist Hop** 1981;(42):15–24
Ferrières M: Les Donatifs Comtadins: une iconographie hospitalière méconnue. **Bull Soc Fr Hist Hop** 1980;(40):23–8
Fracard ML: L'organisation hospitalière des Frères de Saint-Jean-de-Dieu à Niort (Poitou) dans la seconde moitié du XVIIIe siècle. In: Congrès National des Sociétés Savantes, 97e, Nantes, 1972. Actes. Paris, 1977. Histoire Moderne et Contemporaine, Tome 1. p. 299–327.
Gagnière S, Julien P: Panneaux peints de la pharmacie de l'hôpital de Valréas. **Rev Hist Pharm (Paris)** 1981;28(248):21–4
Garmier JF: Soufflot et Mâcon: La charité, l'Hotel-Dieu. **Cah Rech Archit** 1980;6–7, Suppl:142–51
Gelfand T: Gestation of the clinic. **Med Hist** 1981 Apr;25(2):169–80
Gelfand T: Les caractères originaux d'un hospice parisien à la fin de l'Ancien Régime. In Imhof AE, ed: Mensch und Gesundheit in der Geschichte. Husum, Matthiesen, 1980. p. 339–55.
Gelfand T: The gestation of the clinic. In: Congrès international d'histoire de la médecine, XXVe, Québec, 1976. Actes. Québec, 1977. p. 680–98.
Gelfand T: The hospice of the Paris College of Surgery (1774–1793), 'a unique and invaluable institution.' **Bull Hist Med** 1973 Jul-Aug;47(4):375–93
Gérard A: Quelques aspects du fonctionnement des hospices civils de Lille de 1793 à 1815. **Rev Nord** 1982;64(254–255):803–21
Greenbaum LS: Nurses and doctors in conflict: piety and medicine in the Paris Hôtel-Dieu on the eve of the French Revolution. **Clio Med** 1979 May;13(3–4):247–67
Greenbaum LS: Science, medicine, religion: three views of health care in France on the eve of the French Revolution. **Stud Eighteenth Cent Cult** 1981;10:373–91
Greenbaum LS: Scientists and politicians: hospital reform in Paris on the eve of the French Revolution. **Proc Consort Revolutionary Eur** 1973:168–91
Grivaux M: Soixante-quinzième anniversaire de l'Associaton d'Enseignement médical des Hôpitaux de Paris (1907–1982). **Sem Hop Paris** 1983 Mar 31;59(13):865–7
Guillon J: Un aspect de la population pendant la Révolution. Les entrées à l'Hôtel-Dieu de Paris, ler novembre 1791 - 10 novembre 1799. Maîtrise. Univ. de Paris I, 1976. 104 p.
Harmand L: Une ambulance militaire ouverte par le curé d'une paroisse messine durant les batailles sous Metz (août-décembre 1870). In: Congrès National des Sociétés Savantes, 97e, Nantes, 1972. Actes. Paris, 1977. Histoire Moderne et Contemporaine, Tome 1. p. 121–8.
Jones C: 'Professionalizing modern medicine' in French hospitals. **Med Hist** 1982 Jul;26(3):341–9
Jones C: The French Revolution, hospitals, and the medical profession. **Soc Soc Hist Med Bull (Lond)** 1984 Jun;34:6–9
Jones C, Sonenscher M: The social functions of the hospital in 18th-century France: the case of the Hôtel-Dieu of Nîmes. **Fr Hist Stud** 1983;13:172–214
Keel O: La place et la fonction des modèles étrangers dans la constitution de la problématique hospitalière de l'Ecole de Paris. **Hist Philos Life Sci** 1984;6(1):41–73
La médecine hospitalière française au XVIIIème siècle: Colloque de l'Institut d'Histoire de la Médecine et de la Pharmacie de l'Université René Descartes, Paris, 6 octobre 1977. Strasbourg, Université Louis Pasteur, 1980. 213 p. Travaux d'histoire de la médecine et de la pharmacie, I. Contributions by P. Huard, M. J. Imbault-Huart, M. Baudot, J. Filliozat, P. Niaussat, A. Carré, J. P. Kerneis, V. Comiti
Lamarre C: Vivre de charité à l'hôpital de Dijon au XVIIIe siècle: les secours aux enfants et aux viellards. **Bull Soc Fr Hist Hop** 1981;(42):25–35
Lelu F: La population des 'pauvres malades' de l'Hôtel-Dieu de Provins, de 1762 à 1791. Mém. de maîtrise. Univ. de Paris I, 1976. 13, 204 p.
Leroux-Hugon V: Infirmières des hôpitaux parisiens au début du siècle. **Penelope** 1981;(5):62–7
L'Hôpital Des Enfants-Malades, the world's first children's hospital, founded in Paris in 1802: **Pediatrics** 1981 May;67(5):670
Logeay R: Bonheurs et malheurs de la clinique Tarnier. **Hist Sci Med** 1984;18(3):261–70
Mandrou R: Un problème de diététique à l'Hôtel-Dieu de Paris à la veille de la Révolution. In: Congrès National des Sociétés Savantes, 93e, Tours, 1968. Actes. Paris, 1971. Section d'Histoire Moderne et Contemporaine, Tome 1. p. 125–37.
Manneville P: Le poids des armées à l'hôpital du Havre à l'époque révolutionnaire. In Congrès National des Sociétés Savantes, 103e, Nancy-Metz, 1978. Actes. Paris, 1979. Tome I, p. 593–606.
Medouze RM: Histoire sociale et institutions hospitalières. De la fin de l'Ancient Régime à la veille de la Révolution de 1848. Quelques exemples pris à travers la Société lyonnaise et ses hôpitaus. D.E.S., Univ. des sciences sociales de Grenoble, 1976. 176 p.
Miączyński A: Szpital polski na emigracji w Aix-les-Bains. **Przegl Lek** 1980;37(1):158–62
Monroziès M: Au service des femmes. Les services de gynécologie et d'obstétrique de l'hôpital de la Grave à Toulouse, 250 ans d'histoire 1729–1919. Toulouse, Privat, 1980. 88 p.
Oberlé R: Société et assistance à Mulhouse à la fin du XVIIIe siècle. In Livet G, Schaff G, ed: Médecine et assistance en Alsace, XVIe-XXe siècle. Strasbourg, Istra, 1976. p. 117–34.
Pinel P: The clinical training of doctors. An essay of 1793. Ed. D. B. Weiner. Baltimore, Johns Hopkins University Press, 1980. 102 p. (Henry E. Sigerist suppl. to the Bull. Hist. Med. N.S. no. 3).
Questionnaire aux hôpitaux: **Krankenpflege (Bern)** 1983 May;(5):32–4
Roda JJ: Histoire de la fondation du premier sanatorium populaire français. Ses origines et ses vingt-cinq premières années d'existence (Sanatorium Mangini Hauteville). Thèse. Lyon I, 1976. 85 p.
Roubert J: L'Hôtel-Dieu de Lyon au XVIIIe siècle. **Cah Rech Archit** 1980;6–7:134–41
Sabin LE: The French Revolution: the forgotten era in nursing history. **Nurs Forum** 1981;20(3):225–43
Schwab R: Les relations villes-campagnes: un exemple de mise en place de la zone d'influence d'un service urbain: l'hôpital civil de Strasbourg (1840–1910). **Rev Alsace** 1979;105:151–8
Signoret JL: La création de la chaire de Charcot. **Rev Neurol (Paris)** 1982;138(12):887–92
Simon N: 1979, au musée de l'Assistance publique de Paris. **Bull Soc Fr Hist Hop** 1980;(41):26–8
Thieffry S: Avec Parrot, il y a un siècle, à l'Hospice des Enfants Assistés. **Ann Pediatr (Paris)** 1981 Jan;28(1):63–71
Tijm W: L'évolution de la consommation du fromage dans les hôpitaux de Clermont-Ferrand (1818–1952). **Cah Hist** 1979;24(1):71–8
Tzonis A: Un 'Mémoire sur les hôpitaux' de Condorcet. **Dix-Huit Siecle** 1977;9:109–14
Voldman D: Guérir du cancer et mourir de vieillesse: histoire de l'hospice Paul-Brousse de 1905 à 1975. **Asclepio** 1983;35:317–26
Weiner DB: The role of the doctor in welfare work: the Philanthropic Society of Paris, 1780–1815. **Hist Reflect** 1982;9(1–2):279–304

**Germany**

Abe HR: Die internationale Ausstrahlung der Kehr-Rohdenschen Privatklinik in Halberstadt (1890–1910). Ein Beitrag zur Geschichte der modernen Gallenwegschirurgie. In International Congress of the History of Medicine. 26th, Plovdiv, 1978. Actes du Congress. Sofia, 1981. Volume II. p. 78–80.
Bauer A: Das öffentliche Krankenhaus als wissenschaftliche Bildungs-Anstalt. In Seidler E, Schott, ed: Bausteine zur Medizingeschichte. Stuttgart, Steiner, 1984. p. 9–27.
Baumann J: Das Stadtkrankenhaus Kassel während der Jahre 1942 bis 1965. In Balde JH, Schmiking W, ed: Festschrift zum 86. Deutschen Arztetag in Kassel. Kassel, Arztevereins, 1983. p. 89–98.
Becker J: Die Geschichte des Rheinischen Landeskrankenhauses Düsseldorf-Grafenberg von 1876 bis 1918. Diss. Düsseldorf, 1978. 212 p.
Bethge R, Knöpfler EW: 50 Jahre Orthopädische Klinik der Karl-Marx-Universität Leipzig. **Beitr Orthop Traumatol** 1980

Oct;27(10):545–52
Bijok H: Adolph Carl Gustav Wernher (1809–1883); Sein Leben und Wirken am Giessener Akademischen Hospital. Giessen, Schmitz, 1979. 235 p. (Arbeiten zur Geschichte der Medizin in Giessen, Band 1).
Braun-Falco O: 50 Jahre Dermatologie im Städtischen Krankenhaus Thalkirchnerstrasse - Rückblick und Ausblick. **Hautarzt** 1980 Jan;31(1):37–41
Dietzsch HJ: 50 Jahre Kinderklinik der Medizinischen Akademie 'Carl Gustav Carus' Dresden und ihre Vorgeschichte. **Kinderarztl Prax** 1981 Jun;49(6):318–26
Drabik R: Die Entwicklung des Leistungspotentials der Krankenhausmedizin im 20.Jahrhundert in Deutschland. Diss., Universität Düsseldorf. Düsseldorf, 1982. 98 p.
Eigler J, Müller B: Die Patienten des ersten Jahres (1813–1814) im Allgemeinen Krankenhaus München. **MMW** 1982 Apr 30;124(17):429–33
Engel M: Das Dahlem-Projekt und sein Scheitern. Ein wissenschaftspolitischer Modellfall medizinischer Forschung an der Schwelle zum 20. Jahrhundert - Zur Geschichte des Robert-Koch-Instituts und der Charité. **Fortschr Med** 1982 Jun3;100(21):1009–12
Gabler K: Das Krankenhauswesen der Stadt Krefeld im 19. Jahrhundert. Herzogenrath, Murken-Altrogge, 1983. 405 p. (Studien zur Geschichte des Krankenhauswesens, Band 19)
Gebauer C: Die Lindenburg zu Köln (1848–1965). Beispiel eines grossen Klinikum-Neubaus zu Beginn des 20. Jahrhunderts. Köln, 1979. 340 p. (Kölner medizinhistorische Beiträge, Band 11)
Goerke H: Grandi ospedali in Germania: ieri e oggi. **Acta Med Hist Patav** 1979–80;26:81–93
Hambsch K, Treutler H, Pietruschka WD: Profil und Aufgabenstellung einer medizinischen Universitätspoliklinik in Vergangenheit und Gegenwart am Beispiel des Medizinisch-Poliklinischen Institutes der Karl-Marx-Universität Leipzig. **Z Gesamte Inn Med** 1981 Mar 15;36(6):186–9
Heilwagen W: Das Kasseler Gesundheitswesen der Gegenwart. In Balde JH, Schmiking W, ed: Festschrift zum 86. Deutschen Arztetag in Kassel. Kassel, Arztevereins, 1983. p. 105–12.
Heintel H: Hermann Andreas Reimer und seine 1855 eröffnete 'Heilanstalt für Epileptische' in Görlitz. **Medizinhist J** 1982;17(1/2):156–60
Jungnitz B: Die konfessionellen Krankenhäuser der Stadt Münster im achtzehnten und neunzehnten Jahrhundert. Herzogenrath, Verlag Murken-Altrogge, 1981. 304 p. (Studien zur Geschichte des Krankenhauswesens. 18).
Kaiser W: 100 Jahre Universitätsklinikum Halle. Die Entwicklung der halleschen Universitätskliniken in den ersten Jahrzehnten ihres Bestehens. **Z Gesamte Inn Med** 1982 Jun 15;37(12):354–68
Klausch B, Schwarz R: Die Geschichte der Frauenklinik der Universität Rostock von den Anfängen bis zur Gegenwart. Rostock, Wilhelm-Pieck-Universität, 1980. 31 p.
Kollmeier K: Von der Ueberwasser-Elende zum Militärhospital. Die Entwicklung des militärischen Sanitätswesens in der Provinzhauptstadt Münster/Westfalen. **Hist Hosp** 1979–80;13:96–118
Külz J: 70 Jahre Pädiatrie als Lehrfach an der Universität Rostock. **Kinderarztl Prax** 1981 Feb;49(2):92–100
Labisch A: Das Krankenhaus in der Gesundheitspolitik der deutschen Sozialdemokratie vor dem Ersten Weltkrieg. **Med Soziol** 1981;1:127–51
Labisch A: Das Krankenhaus in der sozialdemokratischen Kommunalpolitik in Berlin um die Jahrhundertwende. **Hist Hosp** 1981–82;14:337–45
Lindemann M: Fürsorge für arme Wöchnerinnen in Hamburg um 1800: die Beschreibung eines 'Entbindungs-Winkels'. **Gesnerus** 1982;39(3–4):395–403
Lipps-Kant B: Das ehemalige Oberamtskrankenhaus in Tettnang. Eine Anlage mit Zentralbau aus dem späten 19. Jahrhundert. **Hist Hosp** 1979–80;13:153–163
Monsées Y: 'Klinisches Ambulatorium' von Andor Dudits, 1890. **Medizinhist J** 1981;16(4):454–8
Müller H: Die Anstalt in Kork (Baden). Von der 'Heil- und Pflegeanstalt für epileptische Kinder' zum 'Epilepsiezentrum Kork'. Freiburg, Schulz, 1979. 190 p. (Freiburger Forschungen zur Medizingeschichte, Neue Folge, 10).
Müller W: Vom Wöchnerinnenasyl zum Universitätsklinikum. Die Geschichte des Städtischen Krankenhauswesens in Essen. Münster, Murken-Altrogge, 1981. 364 p. (Studien zur Geschichte des Krankenhauswesens, 15)
Murken AH: Die bauliche Entwicklung des deutschen Allgemeinen Krankenhauses im 19. Jahrhundert. Göttingen, Vandenhoeck & Ruprecht, 1979. 396 p. (Studien zur Medizingeschichte des neunzehnten Jahrhunderts, Bd. 9).
Murken AH, ed: Kind, Krankheit und Krankenhaus im Bilderbuch von 1900 bis 1982. (Studien zur Medizin-, Kunst- und Literaturgeschichte. Band 5.). Herzogenrath, Verlag Murken-Altrogge, 1982. 238 p.
Neumärker KJ: Zur Geschichte der Abteilung für Kinderneuropsychiatrie an der Berliner Charité. **Acta Paedopsychiatr (Basel)** 1982 Dec;48(6):297–305
Oehler D, Weiner R: Entwicklung und Differenzierung der operativen Therapie urologischer Patienten im Krankenhaus St. Georg, Leipzig, in den letzten 65 Jahren. **Z Urol Nephrol** 1980 Mar;73(3):171–80
Richter K: Die II. Frauenklinik der Universität München und Richard Fikentscher. **MMW** 1983 Sep 23;125(38):827–30
Rodegra H: Johann Carl Georg Fricke (1790–1841): Wegbereiter einer klinischen Chirurgie in Deutschland. Herzogenrath, Murken-Altrogge, 1983. 203 p. (Studien zur Geschichte des Krankenhauswesens, 20)
Seidler E: Die Behinderten in Herten. **Gesnerus** 1982;39(1):133–40
Sendler P: Von der Krüppelheilanstalt zum Universitätsklinikum: die 'Hüfferstiftung' in Münster in Westfalen. Herzogenrath, Murken-Altrogge, 1984. 188 p. (Studien zur Geschichte des Krankenhauswesens, 17)
Skrobacki A, Völker A: Ze starań Profesora Ludwika Bierkowskiego o pozyskanie katedry w berlinie w 1847 r. **Arch Hist Med (Warsz)** 1979;42(3):303–8
Stähler F, ed: Klinik Stähler, Siegen, 1901–1978. Wissenschaftliche Festschrift. Hrsg. zur Eröffnung des Klinik-Neubaus 1978. Siegen, Klinik Stähler, 1978. 104 p.
Stollenwerk M: Der Fakultätsneubau der Medizin in Aachen-Melaten. Versuch einer Deutung. In Göpfert W, Otten HH, ed: Metavoeite: wandelt euch durch neues Denken. Düsseldorf, Triltsch, 1983. p. 125–34.
Thie-Mummenthey G: Vom Säuglingsheim zur Universitätskinderklinik. Die Entwicklung der Kinderklinik der Westfälischen Wilhelms-Universität Münster. Münster, Murken-Altrogge, 1980. 262 p. (Studien zur Geschichte des Krankenhauswesens, 10).
Voss HJ: Beitrag zur Seuchenlage in den Pferdebeständen einer Armee 1940/41 und zur Erfahrung als Leiter eines Seuchenlazarettes für Pferde. **DTW** 1981 Nov 5;88(11):483–6
Weber S: Zur Entstehung der Kieler Universitätskliniken im 19. Jahrhundert. **Hist Hosp** 1979–80;13:46–68
Weiss J: Die Universitätshautklinik Hamburg-Eppendorf im Wandel der Zeit. **Hautarzt** 1981 Jan;32(1):28–32
Westphal J: Das Hospital in Nordkirchen. Ein westfälisches Hospital der Barockzeit von Johann Conrad Schlaun. **Hist Hosp** 1979–80;13:119–34

**Great Britain**

Adler MW: History of the development of a service for the venereal diseases. **J R Soc Med** 1982 Feb;75(2):124–8
Aldis AS: Cardiff Royal Infirmary, 1883–1983. Cardiff, University of Wales Press, 1984. v, 52 p.
Allen DE: Hospital planning: the development of the 1962 hospital plan. London, Pitman Medical, 1979. 191 p.
Allison RS: The second world war 1939–45: an RNVR medical officer's view. **J R Nav Med Serv** 1982;68(2):102–9
Anning ST: A medical case book: Leeds, 1781–84. **Med Hist** 1984 Oct;28(4):420–31
Armstrong D: The Peckham key: ideal project and terrifying dream. **Soc Soc Hist Med Bull (Lond)** 1983 Dec;33:9–10
Arton M: Children first and always. **Nurs Times** 1982 Oct 6–12;78(40):1687–8
Bell M: On the move. **Ulster Med J** 1979;48(1):1–18
Bishop PJ: The history of the Brompton Hospital. **Trans Stud Coll Physicians Phila** 1979 Sep;5(1 No 3):171–82
Bowie DC: Captive surgeon in Hong Kong: the story of the British Military Hospital, Hong Kong 1942–1945. **J Hong Kong Branch R Asiat Soc** 1975;15:150–290
Breakwell J: Birmingham General Hospital and the Birmingham Music Festivals. **Practitioner** 1979 Sep;223(1335):406–10
Broadley ME: Patients come first: nursing at 'The London' between the two World Wars. London, London Hospital Special Trustees, 1980. 282 p.
Bryder L: Papworth Village Settlement--a unique experiment in the treatment and care of the tuberculous? **Med Hist** 1984 Oct;28(4):372–90
Calwell HG: Care of sick children in Belfast in the nineteenth century. **J R Soc Med** 1979 Sep;72(9):706–8
Cherry S: The hospitals and population growth: part 1. The voluntary general hospitals, mortality and local populations in the English provinces in the eighteenth and nineteenth centuries. **Popul Stud** 1980 Mar;34(1):59–75
Cook AL: Liverpool's Northern Hospital, 1834–1978. Liverpool, Liverpool Area Health Authority (Teaching), 1981. v, 141 p.
Cooter R: Open-air therapy and the rise of open-air hospitals. **Soc Soc Hist Med Bull (Lond)** 1984 Dec;35:44–6
Craig P: The 'biographical memoirs' of the Bristol Infirmary. **Soc Soc Hist Med Bull (Lond)** 1984 Dec;35:53–4
Dainton C: The age of specialisation. **Br Herit** 1981;2(2):56–65
Dainton C: The years of reform. **Br Herit** 1981–82;3(1):22–31
Davidson N: Cottage hospital. Just like home. (Meynell Ingram Cottage Hospital, Yoxall, Staffs). **Health Soc Serv J** 1981 Aug 21;:1018–9
Dopson L: From workhouse to workshop. **Nurs Times** 1984 Aug 15–21;80(33):16–7
Dopson L: Hospital history in miniature. **Nurs Times** 1982 Jun 23–29;78(25):1078–9
Dopson L: 100 years of ophthalmic nursing. **Nurs Times** 1981 Jun 11;77(24):1043–4
Eaves Walton PM, et al.: The 250th and 100th anniversaries of the Royal Infirmary of Edinburgh and the 100th anniversary of the Simpson Memorial Maternity Pavilion. Edinburgh, Royal Infirmary of Edinburgh,

1979. 53 p.
Edwards G: William Ernest Henley: early impressions. **Nurs Mirror** 1981 Jun 17;152(25):33-4
Elliott J: The rod and the staff. **Ulster Med J** 1979;48(1):32-42
Evans N: 'The first charity in Wales': Cardiff Infirmary and South Wales Society, 1837-1914. **Welsh Hist Rev** 1979;9(3):n.p.
Evrard E: Chirurgiens militaires britanniques à la bataille de Waterloo et dans les hôpitaux de Bruxelles en juin 1815. **Rev Belge Hist Milit** 1982;24(5):425-64
Forbes TR: Mortality at St. Bartholomew's Hospital, London, 1839-72. **J Hist Med Allied Sci** 1983 Oct;38(4):432-49
Gaffney R: Poor law hospitals 1845-1914. In Checkland O, Lamb M, ed: Health care as social history; the Glasgow case. Aberdeen, Aberdeen University Press, 1982. p. 44-58.
Gelbier S: Frederick Breese and London's first school dental clinic. **Br Dent J** 1981 Nov 3;151(9):309-11
Girdwood RH: The Royal Infirmary of Edinburgh 1729-1979. Its influence on medicine overseas. **Scott Med J** 1979 Apr;24(2):154-8
Glover J: Health and disease in Birmingham, 1770-1830. **Warwickshire Hist** 1978-9;4:40-55
Godber G: The Domesday Book of British hospitals. **Soc Soc Hist Med Bull (Lond)** 1983 Jun;32:4-13
Goldin G: A protohospice at the turn of the century: St. Luke's House, London, from 1893 to 1921. **J Hist Med Allied Sci** 1981 Oct;36(4):383-415
Granshaw LP: St. Thomas's Hospital, London, 1850-1900. Ph.D. Diss., Bryn Mawr College. Bryn Mawr, 1981 v, 564 leaves.
Greene J: Hospital heritage: on the tile trail. **Health Soc Serv J** 1982 Feb 11;92(4783):182-3
Harley JM: The Royal Maternity Hospital, Belfast. Fifty glorious years 1933-1983. **Ulster Med J** 1984;53(1):1-17
Hart H: Some notes on the sponsoring of patients for hospital treatment under the voluntary system. **Med Hist** 1980;24(4):447-60
Hawker R: Rules to control visitors, 1746-1900. **Nurs Times** 1984 Mar 21-27;80(12):48-51
Henderson M: Royal Hospital for Sick Children. A 100-year-old gets a new lease on life. **Health Soc Serv J** 1983 Aug 11;93(4859):966-7
Hovell BC: The Hull Royal Infirmary, 1782-1982. Hull, Hull Health Authority, [1982?]. 75 p.
Hyde A: Still set to serve the needy. **Health Soc Serv J** 1980 Mar 7;90(4683):314-5
Jackson B: The United Hospitals of the Borough. **St Thomas Hosp Gaz** 1981;79:56-61
Kashiwagi T: [Hospice: report on the terminal care in England. 8. St Joseph Hospital. (1): its history and practice] (Jpn) **Kangogaku Zasshi** 1980 Aug;44(8):850-6
Kass EH, Carey AB, Kass AM: Thomas Hodgkin and Benjamin Harrison: crisis and promotion in academia. **Med Hist** 1980 Apr;24(2):197-208
Lenihan J: The history of intensive care. **Nurs Focus** 1979 Oct;1(2):75-6
Lewis J, Brookes B: A reassessment of the work of the Peckham Health Centre, 1926-1951. **Milbank Mem Fund Q** 1983 Spring;61(2):307-50
London PS: Inaugural William Gissane Lecture: man and memorial. **Injury** 1982 Nov;14(3):211-34
Loudon IS: The origins and growth of the dispensary movement in England. **Bull Hist Med** 1981;55(3):322-42
McClure RK: Coram's children, the London Foundling Hospital in the eighteenth century. New Haven, Yale University Press, 1981. xiii, 321 p.
McClure RK: Pediatric practice at the London Foundling Hospital. **Stud Eighteenth Cent Cult** 1981;10:361-71
McGeown MG: Twenty-first birthday of the Renal Unit at the Belfast City Hospital. **Ulster Med J** 1981;50(Suppl 1):2-3
Malmoy CF, ed: The French Protestant Hospital: extracts from the Archives of 'La Providence' relating to inmates and applicants for admission, 1718-1957, and to recipients of and applicants for the Coqueau Charity, 1745-1901. 2 vols. London, Huguenot Society of London, 1977.
Marmoy CF: La Soupe: la Maison de Charité de Spittlefields. **Proc Huguenot Soc Lond** 1979;23:134-47
Marshall RK: Nursing Mirror history of nursing: Scottish hospitals in the 18th century. **Nurs Mirror** 1983 Feb 23;156(8):i-viii
Martin JP: Reminiscenses of Queen Square. **Br Med J [Clin Res]** 1981 Dec 19;283(6307):1640-2
Mayberry JF: The dispensary and the infirmary, Cardiff. **Practitioner** 1980 Jul;224(1345):764-5
Mayberry JF: The Hamadryad Hospital Ship for Seamen, 1866-1905. **Br Med J [Clin Res]** 1980 Dec 20-27;281(6256):1690-2
Mayberry JF: The history of a hospital and its diagnostic index. **Public Health** 1979 Sep;93(5):311-6
Morrant GA: The Eastman reaches its half century. **Br Dent J** 1980 Oct 21;149(8):237-8
Nagasawa Y: [Encounter with Nightingale---a discovery of Nightingale in the field of hospital designs] (Jpn) **Sogo Kango** 1980;15(4):59-69
Nightingale F: [Introductory notes on lying-in institutions (2)] (Jpn). **Sogo Kango** 1983 May 15;18(2):113-30
Nightingale F: [Introductory notes on lying-in institutions. 3] (Jpn). **Sogo Kango** 1983 Aug 15;18(3):89-104
Nightingale F: [Introductory notes on lying-in institutions. 4] (Jpn). **Sogo Kango** 1983 Nov 15;18(4):93-113
Okamura A: [A long road to the hospice movement--life of Mother Mary Aikenhead] (Jpn). **Kango Kyoiku** 1984 Jan;25(1):38-45;25(2):104-11 (continued periodically)
Okamura A: [Let us take a walk in East Side: search of the background of the modern hospice, 3] (Jpn). **Kango Kyoiku** 1982 Oct;23(10):637-43
Peitzman SJ: Bright's disease and Bright's generation--toward exact medicine at Guy's Hospital. **Bull Hist Med** 1981;55(3):307-21
Perry CB: The Bristol Royal Infirmary, 1904-1974. Bristol [Avon], Portishead Press, 1981. 130 p.
Pickstone JV, Butler SV: The politics of medicine in Manchester, 1788-1792: hospital reform and public health services in the early industrial city. **Med Hist** 1984 Jul;28(3):227-49
Powell F: Dean Swift and the Dublin Foundling Hospital. **Studies** 1981;70(278-9):162-70
Prescott LF: The Regional Poisoning Treatment Centre, Edinburgh. In Passmore R, ed: Proceedings of the Royal College of Physicians of Edinburgh Tercentenary Congress, 1981. Edinburgh, Royal College of Physicians of Edinburgh, 1982. p. 211-20.
The preservation of medical and public health records: (Research Publications of the Wellcome Unit for the History of Medicine, Oxford, No. I). Oxford, Wellcome Unit for the History of Medicine, 1979. 52 p. Contributions by C. Webster, P. Barnes, E. Freeman, H. Francis, B. Parry-Jones.
Püchel J: Die Geschichte des German Hospital in London (1845 bis 1948). Münster, Murken-Altrogge, 1980. 207 p. (Studien zur Geschichte des Krankenhauswesens, 14).
Robinson GA: The National Hospitals for Nervous Diseases, 1948-1982. London, The Board of Governors of the National Hospitals for Nervous Diseases, 1982. xvii, 133 p.
Robinson PN: The ANZAC link in the history of Harefield Hospital, Middlesex, England. **NZ Med J** 1983 Oct 26;96(742):807
Rodgers J: Workhouse into hospital: not grim enough for Russia. **Health Soc Serv J** 1982 Feb 11;92(4783):180-1
Sadler C: Hospital report: a tradition for innovation. **Nurs Times** 1983 Sep 7;157(10):26-8
Saunders C: A pioneering approach to the dying [interview by Laurence Dopson] **Nurs Times** 1984 Mar 28-Apr 3;80(13):16-8
Seligman S: The royal maternity charity: the first hundred years. **Med Hist** 1980;24(4):403-18
Smith T: Royal Army Medical Corps. Into battle to save the casualties of war. **Health Soc Serv J** 1983 Aug 18;93(4860):994-5
Spencer EM: Notes on the history of dental dispensaries. **Med Hist** 1982 Jan;26(1):47-66
Spray W: Down memory lane: obituary at Nottingham. **Nurs Mirror** 1980 Mar 27;150(13):27-8
Steiner TJ, Capildeo R, Rose FC: The neurological tradition of Charing Cross Hospital. In Rose FC, Bynum WF, ed: Historical aspects of the neurosciences. New York, Raven, 1982. p. 347-56.
Stetz MD: Charles Dickens and 'The Sanatorium': an unpublished letter and manuscript. **Dickensian** 1980;76(390)22-30
Stevens R: Opening a hospital is easy--isn't it? an account of the commissioning of The William Harvey Hospital. Croydon, South East Thames Regional Health Authority, 1982. 52 p.
Sturrock J: The Edinburgh Royal Maternity and Simpson Memorial Hospital. **J R Coll Surg Edinb** 1980 May;25(3):173-87
Thomson WA: The hospice tradition. **J R Soc Med** 1981 Feb;74(2):90-1
Tröhler U: Britische Spitäler und Polikliniken als Heil- und Forschungsstätten 1720-1820. **Gesnerus** 1982;39(1):115-31
Tröhler U: Towards clinical investigation on a numerical basis: James Lind at Haslar Hospital 1758-1783. In International Congress of the History of Medicine, 27th, Barcelona, 1980. Actas. Barcelona, Académia de Ciències Médiques de Catalunya i Balears, 1981. p. 414-9.
Usui T, Kodama K: [At completion of the translation of the 'Notes on Lying-in Institutions'. A discussion] (Jpn) **Sogo Kango** 1984 Aug 15;19(3):79-91
Vickers HR: Royal Naval Hospital Haslar 1940-44. **J R Nav Med Serv** 1984 Summer;70(2):103-9
Walton E: Royal Infirmary of Edinburgh: preserving a hospital's history. **Nurs Times** 1979 Jul 19;75(29):1239-40
Watkin B: Cottage hospitals: a study in technology and organisation. **Nurs Times** 1979 Jul 5;75(26):suppl 18:73-6
Watkin B: Ivory tower of strength: Hammersmith Hospital. **Health Soc Serv J** 1982 Apr 1;92(4790):394-7
Watkin B: Workhouse into hospital: a house of industry. **Health Soc Serv J** 1982 Mar 4;92(4786):273-5
Watkins D: The man who reformed hospital kitchens (Alexis Benoit Soyer). **Nurs Times** 1981 Nov 18-24;77(47):2029
Weaver JA: A hospital for all seasons. **Ulster Med J** 1984;53(1):18-32
Webster C: The crisis of the hospitals during the Industrial Revolution. In Forbes EG, ed: Human implications of scientific advance. Edinburgh, Edinburgh University Press, 1978. p. 214-23.
Whyler FJ: A history of Orpington Hospital. **Bromley Local Hist** 1979;4:24-31
Willcox RR: The international venereological scene as viewed by Harrison and St Mary's. **Br J Vener Dis** 1982 Apr;58(2):72-85
Worboys M: The development of the sanatorium treatment for consumption in Britain, 1880-1914. **Soc Soc Hist Med Bull (Lond)** 1984

Dec;35:41-3

**Greece**

Slatter EM: Illustrations from the Wellcome Institute Library: the new lazaretto at Siros (Syra), Greece, in 1840. **Med Hist** 1984 Jan;28(1):73-80

**Haiti**

Wallace CE, Marshall FN, Robinson C: A retrospective review of maternal and child health services at the Albert Schweitzer Hospital in rural Haiti. **Bull Pan Am Health Organ** 1982;16(1):7-16

**Hungary**

Balla J: 50 éves a mátraházai gyógyintézet. **Orv Hetil** 1983 Mar 20;124(12):712-3
Bánóczy J, Borós S: A Semmelweis Orvostudományi Egyetem Konzerváló Fogászati Klinika negyedszázados története és munkássága. **Fogorv Sz** 1984 Nov;77(11):321-3
Barzó M: Zur Entwicklung der Dokumentation und Auswertung der stationären Morbidität in Ungarn. **Z Gesamte Hyg** 1980 Apr;26(4):275-80
Biró I: Rekviem a Grósz-iskoláért. **Orv Hetil** 1979 Dec 30;120(52):3183-4
Csillag I: Az elsö magyar orthopédiai intézet. **Orv Hetil** 1982 May 2;123(18):1111-4
Csillag I: Elfelejtett kórházak nyomában. Balassa és Semmelweis a régi zsidó kórházban. **Orv Hetil** 1981 Feb 22;122(8):463-5
Csillag I: L'ancien hôpital juif de Pest. **Rev Hist Med Heb** 1980;33(4):73-4
Dénes J: A Semmelweis Orvostudományi Egyetem Gyermekfogászati és Fogszabályozási Klinikájának negyedszázados története és munkássága. **Fogorv Sz** 1984 Sep;77(9):258-9
Fábián T: A Semmelweis OTE fogpótlástani klinikájának negyedszázados története és munkássága. **Fogorv Sz** 1984 Oct;77(10):289-91
István L: 1945. április 4. Korszakváltás kórházaink történetében. **Orv Hetil** 1983 Apr 3;124(14):803-5
Kapronczay K: A magyar kórházügy elsö reformja a XVIII. században. **Orv Hetil** 1981 May 31;122(22):1337-9
Kemény P: 50 éves a Madarász utcai Gyermekkórház. **Orv Hetil** 1979 Dec 30;120(52):3181-3
Konrády A: A 75 éves Balassa kórház. **Orv Hetil** 1984 Jun 24;125(26):1577-8
Sasvári L: Magyarországi egyházi betegellátó intézetek és testületek a XIX. század második felében. **Orvostort Kozl** 1982;28(1-3):209-18
Sasvári L: Nöi betegápoló rendek szerepe a hazai kórházak munkájában (1867-1918). **Orv Hetil** 1982 Apr 18;123(16):990-2
Széll K: Szemelvények a szombathelyi kórház történetéböl 1946-ig II. **Orv Hetil** 1980 Feb 10;121(6):346-9

**India**

Acworth GW: Acworth Leprosy Hospital, Bombay. **Lepr Rev** 1984 Mar;55(1):77-8
Blatt A: Panchayati raj and the mobilisation of the periphery: the case of the location of a primary health centre. **J Commonw Polit Stud** 1972;10(2):130-48

**Ireland**

Holland D: Corrigan and The House of Industry Hospital. **J Ir Coll Physicians Surg** 1980 Jul;10(1):24-6
O'Dwyer WF: Corrigan and the Charitable Infirmary. **J Ir Coll Physicians Surg** 1980 Jul;10(1):21-3
Okamura A: [Report on 19th century Dublin: the background of the modern hospice movement] (Jpn). **Kango Kyoiku** 1982 Nov;23(11):687-92
Sadler C: Hospital report: mixing the old with the new. **Nurs Mirror** 1984 Mar 21;158(12):23-6

**Israel**

Kohn D, Cohen J, Flatau E: 60 years of medical activities in the Jezreel Valley. From the Archives of Central Emek Hospital in Afula. **Koroth** 1982 Aug;8(3/4):169-75

**Italy**

Bèttica-Giovannini R: Giuseppe Berruti e l'Ospizio Marino Piemontese per ragazzi scrofolosi poveri con una nota su la fondazione dell'Ospedale Maria Vittoria di Torino (1887). **Ann Osp Maria Vittoria Torino** 1977 Jul-Dec;20(7-12):227-340
Bèttica-Giovannini R: Il contributo 1958-1977 degli Annali Dell'Ospedale Maria Vittoria Di Torino alla storia della medicina. **Ann Osp Maria Vittoria Torino** 1980 Jan-Jun;23(1-6):175-223
Caffaratto TM: Storia dell'Ospedale Mauriziano di Lanzo. **Ann Osp Maria Vittoria Torino** 1982 Jan-Jun;25(1-6):97-148
Drey RE: Les vases de pharmacie de l'Hôpital majeur de Novare. **Rev Hist Pharm (Paris)** 1979 Dec;26(243):259-62
Orsini M, Piroli AT, Gaudiosi O: Gli eliporti ospedalieri nell'organizzazione sanitaria militare: l'eliporto dell'ospedale militare di Caserta. **Riv Mil** 1973;29(5):614-26
Vigani P: Per una storia dell'assistenza in Lombardia: la pia casa degli incurabili di Abbiategrasso. **Risorgimento** 1982;34(1):48-64

**Japan**

Ishigaki Y, Uzawa Y: [Historical review of continuing education in Hokkaido University Hospital] (Jpn). **Kango Tenbo** 1984 Nov;9(11):1021-32
Kaneda H: [Development of the concept on open system hospital in Japan] (Jpn). **Igakushi Kenkyu** 1978;50:60-4
Matsuda T: [The Osaka Charity Hospital and private practitioner] (Jpn). **Igakushi Kenkyu** 1977;48:41-5
Okamura A: [Hospice and human rights movement. (2)] (Jpn). **Kango Kyoiku** 1983 May;24(5):294-302
Omiya Sekijui Byoin Yono, Japan: Omiya Sekijuji Byoin yonjunenshi. Yono, Japan, Omiya Sekijuji Byoin, Showa 51 nen, 1976. 173 p.
Showa Byoin Kumiai: Koritsu Showa Byoin gojunen no ayumi. Kodaira, Japan, Showa Byoin Kumiai, Showa 52 nen, 1977. xvii, iii, 384 p.
Tanaka M: [Public health nurses of the Santama area (5). History of public health clinics in the past 40 years since their start: a visit with Ms. Miki Tanaka] (Jpn). **Hokenfu Zasshi** 1982 Aug;38(8):676-83

**Mexico**

Bonequi CC: La huella del Hospital Infantil de México en la pediatría. Cuarenta años de vida institucional. **Bol Med Hosp Infant Mex** 1983 Aug;40 Suppl 2:1-10
Martínez Cortés F: Instituciones médicas de asistencia y de enseñanza. **Salud Publica Mex** 1983 Sep-Oct;25(5):499-503
Robles C: Los hospitales como microsociedades. **Gac Med Mex** 1980 Jan;116(1):1-8

**Nepal**

Dawson P, Uhrig J: Sherpa health and Kunde Hospital. **Can Med Assoc J** 1983 Apr 15;128(8):1010-2

**Netherlands**

Pel JZ: Uit de geschiedenis van het Middleburgse Gasthuis; het ziekenhuispersoneel tijdens de overgangsfase van een 19e-eeuws gasthuis naar een 20e-eeuws ziekenhuis. **Ned Tijdschr Geneeskd** 1982 Sep 18;126(38):1741-5
Stumpel AR: Het Burgerziekenhuis te Amsterdam en de modernisering van de ziekenverpleging in de 19e eeuw. **Tijdschr Ziekenverpl** 1983 Jun 21;36(13):409-15

**New Zealand**

Averill LC: St. George's Hospital, the first fifty years. Christchurch, St. George's Hospital Executive, 1978. 169 p.
Tennant M: Mrs. Grace Neill in the Department of Asylums, Hospitals and Charitable Institutions. **NZ J Hist** 1978 Apr 12;:3-16

**Poland**

Adamczyk A: Ostatnie dni w szpitalu obozu w Litomierzycach. **Przegl Lek** 1980;37(1):184-6
Bergman A: Pobeg V. S. Mitskevicha-Kapsukasa iz suvalkskoi bol'nitsy v 1906 G. **Vopr Istor** 1965;(3):74-6
Borkowski W: Wspomnienia z 'Krankenbau' w Oświecimiu. **Przegl Lek** 1984;41(1):100-8
Bryc S: Thirty five years of activities of the Lublin Medical Centre. **Ann Univ Mariae Curie Sklodowska [Med]** 1979;34:1-5
Ceypek T: Uzupełnienie do artykułu pt. 'Klinika Laryngologii w 30-leciu Slaskiej Akademii Medycznej'. **Otolaryngol Pol** 1979;33(6):671-2
Chojna JW: Warszawskie lazarety wojskowe w czasie powstania listopadowego. **Arch Hist Med (Warsz)** 1981;44(3/4):277-308
Chojna JW: Warszawskie lazarety wojskowe w czasie powstania listopadowego. **Arch Hist Med (Warsz)** 1983;46(1):1-19
Chojna JW: Warszawskie lazarety wojskowe w czasie Powstania Listopadowego. **Arch Hist Med (Warsz)** 1980;43(4):353-75
Chrzanowski A: Instytut Curie w Krakowie, pierwszy zakład leczenia radem w Polsce. **Nowotwory** 1979 Jul-Sep;29(3):239-41
Falkiewiczowa S: Kronika Wrocławskiej Kliniki Neurologicznej. **Neurol Neurochir Pol** 1984 May-Jun;18(3):303-9
Gaertner H: Ordynatorzy oddziału chirurgicznego Krakowskiego Szpitala Braci Miłosiernych (obecnie im. Edmunda Biernackiego). **Nasza Przeslosc** 1979;(51):179-204
Gliński S, Majewska E: Powstanie i działalność szpitala powiatowego w lasinie do roku 1945. **Arch Hist Med (Warsz)** 1984;47(2):249-68
Heimrath T: Organizacja wrocławskiej kliniki Kobiecej jako wyraz poglądów medycznych epoki (1890 r.). **Arch Hist Med (Warsz)** 1981;44(3/4):381-4
Iwankiewicz S, Kossowski S: Klinika Otolaryngologiczna AM we

Wrocławiu (1948-1978). **Otolaryngol Pol** 1980;34(2-3):141-65
Klukowski Z: Szpital w Szczebrzeszynie. **Arch Hist Med (Warsz)** 1981;44(3/4):309-27
Królikowska M: XXXV-lecie ginekologii i położnictwa w Akademii Medycznej w Lodzi. **Ginekol Pol** 1980 Nov;51(11):973-9
Krysa-Leszczyńska D: Przyczynek do powstania szpitala zakaźnego w Sandomierzu. **Wiad Lek** 1979 Jul 15;32(14):1039-42
Lejmbach Z: Myśl pediatryczna wśród pracowników szpitala im. Karola i Marii. **Pediatr Pol** 1984 Sep;59(9):701-3
Losiowski Z: Sanatorium w Zagórzu i jego rola w lecznictwie neurologicznym dzieci. **Pediatr Pol** 1980 Mar;55(3):379-84
Michalowski R: Spital für Geschlechtskranke in Lublin 1832 bis 1982. **Dermatol Monatsschr** 1984;170(4):268-73
Moskwa Z: Założenie kamienia wegielnego pod szpital Dzieciatka Jezus. **Wiad Lek** 1984 Mar 15;37(6):479-80
Opas T: Dawne szpitale województwa Lubelskiego w świetle materiałów lustracyjnych z lat 1790-1791. **Kwart Hist Kultury Mater** 1972;20(2):267-82
Rejmanowski T: Dzieje sióstr miłosierdzia w Szpitalu Powiatowym Sw. Antoniego we Włocławku (1877-1966). **Arch Hist Med (Warsz)** 1984;47(3):433-8
Semczuk B: XXXV-lecie Lubelskiej Kliniki Otolaryngologicznej. **Otolaryngol Pol** 1980;34(1):113-6
Sobolewicz T: Z przeżyć w rewirze oświecimskim. **Przegl Lek** 1984;41(1):108-10
Strzelecka I: Pierwszy szpital obozowy w Brzezince. **Przegl Lek** 1984;41(1):88-93
Strzelecka I: Rozwój szpitali obozowych w Oświecimiu-Brzezince. **Przegl Lek** 1984;41(1):84-8
Stypułkowska J: 25 lat Kliniki Chirurgii Stomatologicznej AM w Krakowie. Historia i kierunki działalności. **Czas Stomatol** 1981 Jan;34(1):51-6
Wunderlich P: Zur Geschichte der Universitäts-Kinderklinik in Breslau unter Adalbert Czerny (1863--1941) von 1894--1910. **Arch Hist Med (Warsz)** 1979;42(3):337-43
Zapaśnik-Kobierska MH: Działalność naukowo-dydaktyczna i społeczna zespołu klinik Państwowego Szpitala Klinicznego Nr 3. **Pediatr Pol** 1984 Sep;59(9):705-12

**Puerto Rico**

Sifontes JE, Valcárcel M: Historical sketch -University Pediatric Hospital-1983. **Bol Asoc Med PR** 1983 Oct;75(10):444-5

**Romania**

Barbu G: Din istoria luptei antiepidemice în România (II). Completări la istoricul spitalului Dudeşti. **Rev Ig [Bacteriol]** 1984 Jul-Sep;29(3):283-7
Bercus CI, ed: Spitalul Coltea: Două sute saptezeci si cinci ani de existentă, 1704-1979. Bucuresti, Spitalul Clinic Coltea, 1979. 582 p.
Costea V: Cîteva date din activitatea primilor trei profesori titulari ai clinicii dermato-venerologice: Gh. Demetriade, E. I. Mironescu şi Gh. Nastase (1901-1962). **Rev Med Chir Soc Med Nat Iasi** 1983 Jan-Mar;87(1):149-55
Cotrău M, Gheorghiţă I: Prescriptii medicale in manuscrisul inedit de la Spitalul Se. Spiridon Iasi, din secolul al XVIII-LEA (IV). **Rev Med Chir Soc Med Nat Iasi** 1983 Apr-Jun;87(2):307-12
Cotrău M, Gheorghiţă I: Prescripţii medicale în manuscrisul inedit de la spitalul SF. Spiridon Iaşi, din secolul al XVIII-lea. **Rev Med Chir Soc Med Nat Iasi** 1983 Jan-Mar;87(1):113-6
Duda R: Spitalul comunal Tutova, Jud. Vaslui 75 ani de activitate. **Rev Med Chir Soc Med Nat Iasi** 1983 Oct-Dec;87(4):667-8
Franche M: Omagiu Profesorului Mihai Ciucă, la 100 ani de la naştere. Profesorul Mihai Ciucă şi spitalul clinic de boli contagioase 'izolarea' Iaşi. **Rev Med Chir Soc Med Nat Iasi** 1983 Oct-Dec;87(4):726-8
Marinescu CG, Vosniuc R: Din istoricul Spitalului din Galaţi filiala epitropiei sf. spiridon. **Rev Med Chir Soc Med Nat Iasi** 1981 Apr-Jun;85(2):399-400
Munteanu M: Inflinţarea clinicii dermato-venerologice din Iaşi şi activitatea desfăşurată în perioada suplinirilor (1882-1901). **Rev Med Chir Soc Med Nat Iasi** 1983 Jan-Mar;87(1):141-8
Negru I: Spitalul de tuberculoză de la 'Filaret' şi doctorul Stefan Irimescu. **Viata Med [Medii Sanit]** 1983 Mar;31(3):68-72
Segal N: 150 de ani de existenţă a Secţiei de oftalmologie Oradea. **Rev Chir [Oftalmol]** 1981 Jan-Mar;25(1):75-9

**Singapore**

Lee YK: Singapore's pauper and Tan Tock Seng Hospitals. **J Malays Branch R Asiatic Soc** 1976;49(2):164-83 1977:50(2):111-35
Singapore General Hospital: Singapore General Hospital 50th anniversary publication, 1926-1976. Singapore, [s. n., 1976?]. 128 p.

**South Africa**

Melzer R: Centenary: Barberton Hospital. **Adler Mus Bull** 1984 Nov;10(3):30-2
Merwe DW van der: Bochum-Blauberg: die ontstaan, stigting en ontwikkeling van die Helene Franz-Hospital, 1895-1935. **Kleio (S Afr)** 1978;10(1-2):2-20

**Spain**

Ferrer D: Dictamen solicitando la erección de los actuales edificios de la Facultad de Medicina y Hospital Clínico de Barcelona. In Congrés International d'Història de la Medicina Catalana, 2nd, Barcelona, 1975. Llibre d'Actes. Barcelona, Socitra, 1977. p. 249-58.
Folch Jou G, Javier Puerto F: Los medicamentos incluidos en los formularios del Hospital General de Madrid (Siglos XVIII y XIX). **Bol Soc Esp Hist Farm** 1982 Mar;33(129):49-76
García Guerra D: El hospital real de Santiago en el siglo XVIII; aspects del ejercicio médico. **Asclepio** 1980;32:211-28, 492-503
García Guerra D: Epidemiologia gallega del siglo XVIII. Su repercusión sobre el Hospital Real de Santiago. In: Sociedad Española de Historia de la Medicina. V Congreso Nacional. Madrid, 1977. **Asclepio** 1977;29:147-65
García Guerra D: La asistencia médica en el Hospital Real de Santiago al final del Antiguo Régimen. **Asclepio** 1983;35:287-300
Jordi R: Bases para un estudio de la evolución del medicamento en el Hospital de la Santa Cruz (1793-1796). Hospital General de Barcelona (1812-1814). Introducción. **Circ Farm** 1981 Jul;12(140):91-7
Jordi R: Notas sobre terapéutica hospitalaria usada en una epidemia en Montblanc. Año 1725. **Circ Farm** 1981 May;12(138):38-73
Kolarov P: Sanitarnata sluzhba na internatsionalnite brigadi v ispaniia (1936-1938). **Izv Inst Istor Bkp** 1967;16:289-312
Morales y Morales A: Francisco Antonio Solano, boticario revalidado. Asentista del Hospital Militar de Santa Cruz de Tenerife (1764-1771). **Bol Soc Esp Hist Farm** 1980 Mar-Jun;3(121-2):109-38
Orozco Acuaviva A: Sabater y el empirismo anatomopatológico en el Hospital de Bellavista del Callao. In International Congress of the History of Medicine, 27th, Barcelona, 1980. Actas. Barcelona, Académia de Ciències Mèdiques de Catalunya i Balears, 1981. p. 401-7.
Pi-Figueras J: Els serveis de cirurgia moderna a l'Hospital de la Santa Creu i Sant Pau. In Congrés International d'Història de la Medicina Catalana, 2nd, Barcelona, 1975. Llibre d'Actes. Barcelona, Socitra, 1977. p. 157-61.
Riera J: Planos de hospitales españoles del siglo XVIII existentes en el Archivo General de Simancas (inventario primero). Valladolid, Ediciones del Seminario de Historia de la Medicine, Universidad de Valladolid, 1975. 18 p., numerous plates. (Acta Historico-Medica Vallisoletana, Monografias, V)
Schadewaldt H: Le lazaret de quarantaine à Mahón (Minorque). In: Congrès National des Sociétés Savantes, 97e, Nantes, 1972. Comptes Rendus. Paris, 1976. Section des Sciences, Tome 1. p. 215-26.
Tarragó Valentines JF: Un informe sobre el hospital de Santa Maria de Lerida, escrito en el siglo XIX por Marioano Olives. **Asclepio** 1980;32:453-6

**Sweden**

Molin C: Karolinska sjukhusets avdelning för tand--och käksjukdomar--en tillbakablick efter fyrtio år. **Nord Medicinhist Arsb** 1981;:183-92
Nyberg A: Södertelge Lazarett--dess tillkomst och första verksamhetsår. **Nord Medicinhist Arsb** 1981;:120-32
Wikström-Haugen I: Patienten im Sahlgren'schen Krankenhaus Göteborg 1782-1822. In Imhof AE, ed: Mensch und Gesundheit in der Geschichte. Husum, Matthiesen, 1980. p. 323-37.

**Switzerland**

Buess H, Portmann ML: Berühmte Schweizer Arzte. **Gesnerus** 1980;37(3/4):289-306
Dr. Guggenbühl's Hospice for cretins on the Abendberg in Switzerland (1840): **Pediatrics** 1983 Mar;71(3):452
L'ecole de soins infirmiers du CHUV: Un cinquantenaire abondamment fêté. **Krankenpflege (Bern)** 1982 Aug;(8):73-4
Mottier G: Histoire de l'Infirmerie de Lausanne et de La Source. **Krankenpflege (Bern)** 1983 Dec;76(12):27-30
Raynier JP de: L'Hôpital de l'Enfance de 1861 à 1979. **Rev Med Suisse Romande** 1980 Jun;100(6):537-65
Rintelen F: Von der Augenheilanstalt zur Universitätsaugenklinik in Basel. **Gesnerus** 1982;39(1):79-83
Rohr A von: Die Medizinische Poliklinik der Universität Zürich 1835 bis 1983. Stuttgart; New York, Thieme, 1983. ix, 418 p.
Sommer P: Die ersten Jahrzehnte des Jenner-Kinderspitals in Bern. **Gesnerus** 1982;39(1):85-8
Steinebrunner WF: Spitalarchitektur und Medizin im Zürich des 19. Jahrhunderts: die Planung des alten Kantonsspitals (1842) und des Burghölzlis (1870), ihre Vorbilder und medizinischen Experten. Zürich, Berichthaus, 1971. 104 p.

**Syria**

Story of the Hosn Hospital: founded by American Hosn Welfare Association, New Kensington, Pennsylvania: New Kensington, Pa., The

Assn., [1971?]. 188 [152] p.

**Tunisia**

L'assistance médicale pendant 50 ans de Protectorat: Dr Mahmoud El Matri: 'La Voie due Tunisien' le 11 mars 1931. **Tunis Med** 1982 Nov-Dec;60(6):378-9

**United States**

Abramson DJ: The surgical residency, the surgical clinic at the Walter Reed Army Medical Center. **Milit Med** 1982 Dec;147(12):1025-8

Ackerman FK: The Geisinger Medical Center. **Natl Forum Hosp Health Aff** 1978;:9-18

Aiken KG: From mission to hospital: the Detroit Florence Crittenton Organization, 1897-1930. **Detroit Perspect** 1982 Spring;6:50-60

Albemarle-Charlottesville Health Department: The history of the Albemarle-Charlottesville Health Department. Charlottesville, Va., Jefferson Printing, 1973. 42 p.

Allen L, Carmichael E: The first sixty-two years: Methodist Hospital, Lubbock, Texas, 1918-1980. Lubbock, Methodist Hospital, 1980. 265 p.

Anderson PG: The spa, the fairgrounds, and the psychiatric hospital: the 21st General Hospital in World War II. **Outlook Mag** 1982 Spring;19(1):2-8

Antler J: Medical women and social reform--a history of the New York Infirmary for Women and Children. **Women Health** 1976 Jul-Aug;1(4):11-15,18

Apffelstaedt G: Militärlazarette während des Bürgerkrieges in den USA anhand von Beispielen aus den Bezirken Washington, District of Columbia, Baltimore, Maryland, Philadelphia, Pennsylvanien und New York. Münster, Murken-Altrogge, 1981. 203 p. (Studien zur Geschichte des Krankenhauswesens, 6)

Aries NR: Abortion clinics and the organization of work: a case study of Charles Circle. **Rev Radic Polit Econ** 1980;12(2):53-62

Aring CD: The Boston City Hospital days with Drs. Merritt and Putnam. **Epilepsia** 1983;24 Suppl 1:S1-3

Barger AC: Some of Carl Walter's contributions to Harvard Medical School and Hospitals. **Am J Surg** 1984 Nov;148(5):578-80

Bass J: Strike at Charleston. **New South** 1969;24(3):35-44

Baylor Medical Center: 75 years old and thriving: **South Hosp** 1978 Nov-Dec;46(6):9-11

Beatty WK: Mary Harris Thompson--pioneer surgeon and hospital founder. **Proc Inst Med Chic** 1981 Jul-Sep;34(3):83-6

Beebe RT: Albany Medical College and Albany Hospital: a history, 1839-1982. Albany, N. Y., New Art Printing, 1983. xxv, 458 p.

Bellush J: A municipal hospital system: myths and realities. **Natl Civ Rev** 1980;69(6):313-20

Bellush J: Indispensable facilities: in defense of municipal hospitals. **NY Aff** 1979;5(4):111-19

Bergstrand CR: Big profit in private hospitals. **Soc Policy** 1982;13(2):50-4

Berk DW: Adventism on the picture post card. **Advent Herit** 1978;5(2):48-53

Berney B: The rise and fall of the UMW Fund. **South Exposure** 6(2):95-102, 1978

Bienia RA, Stein E, Bienia BH: United States Public Health Service hospitals (1798-1981)--the end of an era. **N Engl J Med** 1983 Jan 20;308(3):166-8

Bingham M: Medical education at Hartford Hospital: an historical review. **Conn Med** 1979 Nov;43(11):683-6

Black H: Doctor and teacher, hospital chief. Dr. Samuel Proger and the New England Medical Center. Chester, Connecticut, Globe Pequot Press, 1982. xii, 210 p.

Blanco RL: American army hospitals in Pennsylvania during the Revolutionary War. **Pa Hist** 1981;48(4):347-68

Bonsett CA: Medical museum notes: Indianapolis City Hospital. **J Indiana State Med Assoc** 1983 Oct;76(10):657

Borkenhagen R, Hipskind M, Lewy R: Reminiscences of otorhinolaryngology from Loyola University and Hines Veterans Hospital. **Proc Inst Med Chic** 1982 Apr-Jun;35(2):51-2

Bowman IA, ed: John Sealy Hospital Training School for Nurses. **Bookman** 1982 Oct;9(8):3-11

Boyd DP: Doctor Lahey and his clinic. **Postgrad Med** 1984 Feb 15;75(3):14-6, 18

Boyer S: This is the final issue of The Johns Hopkins Medical Journal [editorial]. **Johns Hopkins Med J** 1982 Dec;151(6):263-82

Brown EG: Notes on the University Hospital: the early decades. **Mich Q Rev** 1964;3(1):8-17

Brown P: National celebrities brought cheer to young patients at Riley Hospital (I. U. Medical Center) in the 1930's. **Indiana Med Hist Q** 1976;2(4):65-9

Brown VK: A cathedral of healing: the story of Wesley Memorial Hospital. Chicago, Northwestern Memorial Hospital, 1981.

Bugbee G: George Bugbee: a first-person profile (Part 2). **Health Serv Res** 1981 Winter;16(4):459-66

Cadmus RR: Intensive care reaches silver anniversary. **Hospitals** 1980 Jan 16;54(2):98-102

Canon BC, Jaros D: The impact of changes in judicial doctrine: the abrogation of charitable immunity. **Law Soc Rev** 1979;13(4):969-86

Castleman B, Sutton SB, Crockett DC: The Massachusetts General Hospital, 1955-1980. Boston, Little, Brown, 1983. xxii, 410 p.

The clinic at Beech Fork--its 57-year history is a mini-history of FNS: **Front Nurs Serv Q Bull** 1984 Summer;60(1):1-10

Connaugton D: Alton Ochsner: not as a legend. **Bull Am Coll Surg** 1981;66(5):27, 31-2

Crawford S: Health science libraries in the United States: III. Hospital health science libraries, 1969-1979. **Bull Med Libr Assoc** 1983 Jan;71(1):30-6

Crombie DH: The founding staff of Hartford Hospital and its legacy. **Conn Med** 1979 Nov;43(11):682-3

Crooks JB: The role of women in volunteerism: a short history. **Volunt Action Leadersh** 1981 Summer;22-8

Cullen JP: Chimborazo Hospital: 'That charnal house of living sufferers.' **Civ War Times Illus** 1981;19(9):36-42

DeMark JL: Chasing the cure--a history of healthseekers to Albuquerque, 1902-1940. **J West** 1982 Jul;21(3):49-58

Derogatis LR, et al: The Hopkins symptom checklist (HSCL): a self-report symptom inventory. **Behav Sci** 1974;19(1):1-15

Dishman M: Coleman Hall. A monument to Indiana medicine. **Indiana Med** 1984 Aug;77(8):622-3

Doona ME: Nursing revisited: the Massachusetts General Hospital, Base Hospital No. 6. **Mass Nurse** 1984 Apr;53(4):9

Doona ME: Nursing revisited: the Worcester State Hospital and nursing. **Mass Nurse** 1984 Jan;53(1):19

Dowling HF: City hospitals. The undercare of the underprivileged. Cambridge, Mass., London, Harvard University Press, 1982. vii, 245 p.

Dr. Harold P. Rusch and the Wisconsin Clinical Cancer Center: **Wis Med J** 1979 Jun;78(6):96-7

Dupont J: At long last 'The TMC Story: premieres'. **EITV** 1984 Mar;16(3):52-4

Durcan J: The Penrose Cancer Hospital. The first thirty-five years, 1941-1976. Colorado Springs, Century One Press, 1976. 120 p.

Dwork D: Elsie Strang L'Esperance. In: Notable American women. The modern period. Cambridge, Mass., Belknap-Harvard Univ. Press, 1980. 4:417-9.

English PC: Pediatrics and the unwanted child in history: foundling homes, disease, and the origins of foster care in New York City, 1860 to 1920. **Pediatrics** 1984 May;73(5):699-711

Farley F: Two generations of women physicians: the New York Infirmary, 1870-1899. **J Am Med Wom Assoc** 1984 Nov-Dec;39(6):189-91

Fath H: A dream come true: the story of St. Jude Children's Research Hospital and ALSAC. Memphis, TN, ALSAC, 1983. 214 p.

Feldman R, Scheffler R: The union impact on hospital wages and fringe benefits. **Ind Labor Relat Rev** 1982;35(2):196-206

Fink L, Greenberg B: Organizing Montefiore: labor militancy meets a progressive health care empire. In Reverby S, Rosner D, ed: Health care in America. Philadelphia, Temple University Press, 1979. p. 226-44.

Finland M: Doting: my early experiences at Boston City Hospital. **Pharos** 1982 Summer;45(3):17-22

Finland M, Castle WB: The Harvard Medical Unit at Boston City Hospital. Boston, Harvard Medical School: Distributed by the University Press of Virginia for The Francis A. Countway Library of Medicine, 1982-83. 2 volumes in 3.

Finlayson G: Osteopathic hospitals and AOHA. United in progress for 50 years. **OH** 1984 Sep;28(8):12-4

Flavin TH: The Clinical Center: twenty-five years of research for people. **Conn Med** 1979 Sep;43(9):563-7

Freymann JG: The origins of disease orientation in American medical education. **Prev Med** 1981 Nov;10(6):663-73

Friedberger M: The decision to institutionalize: families with exceptional children in 1900. **J Fam Hist** 1981 Winter;6(4):396-409

Gault EW, Attwood HD: Medical men in the early history of the Austin Hospital. Five doctors of widely varying ages and backgrounds were associated with the formative years of the Austin Hospital. **Med J Aust** 1981 Dec 12-26;2(12-13):680-3

Gaunt KL: Colorado hospitals of the 1800's. **Denver West Roundup** 1979 Sep-Oct;35:3-19

Gay EW: Atlanta's city hospital had a rough beginning. **J Med Assoc Ga** 1983 Nov;72(11):781-4

Gerhardt RE: The first teaching hospital. **N Engl J Med** 1983 May 19;308(20):1230

Gordon S, ed: All our lives. A centennial history of Michael Reese Hospital and Medical Center, 1881-1981. Chicago, Michael Reese Hospital and Medical Center, 1981. vii, 210 p.

Grace E: House-staff officers: collective bargaining in the health care system. **J Leg Med (Chicago)** 1981 Sep;2(3):415-31

Greisman HC: Wound management and medical organization in the Civil War. **Surg Clin North Am** 1984 Aug;64(4):625-38

Hall D: Ointment of love: Oliver E. Comstock and Tuscon's [sic] tent city. **J Ariz Hist** 19(2):111-30, 1978

Harada M: A brief history of hospital dentistry in the United States. **Bull Hist Dent** 1982 Apr;30(1):46-54

Hartwell SW: From horse and buggy practice to world-renowned medical center. History of the Cleveland Clinic Foundation. **Postgrad Med** 1984

May;75(6):14–6, 21–6

Harvey AM: Clinical investigation of chronic diseases: its successful pursuit in an outpatient setting. **J Chronic Dis** 1980;33(9):529–66

Harvey AM: Henry M. Thomas: Johns Hopkins's first neurologist. **Johns Hopkins Med J** 1982 Jan;150(1):11–21

Harvey AM: Henry Mills Hurd: the first superintendent of the Johns Hopkins Hospital and the first professor of psychiatry. **Johns Hopkins Med J** 1981 Mar;148(3):135–48

Harvey AM: Research and discovery in medicine. Contributions from Johns Hopkins. Baltimore and London, Johns Hopkins University Press, 1981. xiii, 322 p. [Collected historical papers reprinted from various journals].

Harvey AM: Science at the bedside. Clinical research in American medicine, 1905–1945. Baltimore, London, Johns Hopkins University Press, 1981. xix, 554 p.

Harvey KA: Practicing medicine at the Baltimore Almshouse, 1828–1850. **Md Hist Mag** 1979;74(3):223–37

Herman JK: Home of BUMED: a hilltop in Foggy Bottom. Where medical college left off. The U.S. Naval Medical School and Naval Hospital 1902–1917. **US Navy Med** 1983 Jan–Feb;74(1):8–17 contd

Hofmeister LH: The Union Memorial Hospital. Its story...its people. 125 years of caring. Baltimore, Union Memorial Hospital, 1980. xi, 234 p.

Holden C: The hospice movement and its implications. **Ann Am Acad Polit Soc Sci** 1980;447:59–63

Hospital admission tickets: **Profiles Hosp Mark** 1982 3rd Quarter;7:40–1

How the FAH began: **Investor Owned Hosp Rev** 1976 Feb;9(1):43–4

Huff DS, Scrinivasan B: The oldest children's hospital building still in use in the United States? **J Pediatr** 1983 Jan;102(1):165–6

Hunt M: La charité maternelle aux Etats-Unis au 19e siècle: un cas d'étude institutionnelle, un hôpital pédiatrique. **Penelope** 1981;(5):50–1

Hunt M: Women and childsaving: St. Louis Children's Hospital 1879–1979. **Bull Mo Hist Soc** 1980;36(2, pt 1):65–79

Hynes CJ: The regulation of nursing homes: a case study. **Proc Acad Polit Sci** 1980;33(4):126–36

Ivey-Davis EP: Highland Hospital revisited. **NC Med J** 1980 Feb;41(2):85–9

Jacobs SE: 'Our babies shall not die': a community's response to medical neglect. **Hum Organ** 1979;38(2):120–33

Johnson CA, Bond JR: Policy implementation and community linkages: hospital abortion services after Roe V. Wade. **West Polit Q** 1982;35(3):385–405

Kerson TS: Almshouse to municipal hospital: the Baltimore experience. **Bull Hist Med** 1981 Summer;55(2):203–20

Keys TE: The Mayos: a historical vignette. **Adler Mus Bull** 1984 Nov;10(3):16–24

Kingsdale JM: The growth of hospitals: an economic history in Baltimore. Ph.D. Diss., University of Michigan. Ann Arbor, 1981. iv, 527 p.

Kirklin JW: Open-heart surgery at the Mayo Clinic. The 25th anniversary. **Mayo Clin Proc** 1980 May;55(5):339–41

Klein R: Little 'hospital' on the prairie. Roughly the first hundred years of Rochester's Mayo Clinic. **Postgrad Med** 1984 Sep 1;76(3):15–6, 19, 22–4

Korngold S: Memories of the National Jewish Hospital of Denver in 1908. **West States Jew Hist Q** 1980;12(2):161–4

Krell R: At a children's hospital; a folklore survey. **West Folkl** 1980;39(3):223–31

Land LC: Hiran Hitchcock' legacy: the history of the Mary Hitchcock Memorial Hospital School of Nursing. Canaan, N. H., Phoenix Publishing for the Mary Hitchcock Memorial Hospital, 1980. x, 148 p.

Lefemine AA: A recollecton of men and events on the Thoracic Service of the Peter Bent Brigham Hospital: 1958–1966. **Artif Organs** 1980 Aug;4(3):210–8

Leland TM: DaVega's Floating Hospital. **J SC Med Assoc** 1984 Nov;80(11):581

Link EP: The Mayo family: a study in changing social ideas. In: Congrès international d'histoire de la médecine, XXVe, Québec, 1976. Actes. Québec, 1977. p. 895–916.

Loftus MD: St. Vincent Hospital and Health Care Center, Indianapolis, Indiana, 1881–1981. Indianapolis, Litho Press, 1981. xi, 191 p.

Loughry CW: Fifty years of surgical education at Akron City Hospital. **Ohio State Med J** 1982 Oct;78(10):723–6

Ludmerer KM: The rise of the teaching hospital in America. **J Hist Med Allied Sci** 1983 Oct;38(4):389–414

McBryde AM, Pressly JA, Hutchinson F, et al: North Carolina Orthopedic Hospital closes after 58 years of treatment of crippled children. **NC Med J** 1979 Dec;40(12):755–7

McConnell NF, Dore MM: Crittenton services, the first century, 1883–1983. Washington, D.C., National Florence Crittenton Mission, 1983. vi, 95 p.

McConville E: Oliver Harvey: 'Got to take some risks.' **South Exposure** 6(2):24–8, 1978

McDonell KM: The Indianapolis City Hospital, 1833–1866. **Indiana Med Hist Q** 1983 June;9(2):3–23

Mckay DR: A history of the Nordrach Ranch: Colorado's first sanatorium of the open air. **Colo Mag** 1979 Summer-Fall;56:179–96

Martin HE: The history of the Los Angeles County Hospital, 1878–1968. Los Angeles, Univ. of Southern California Press, 1979. xv, 548 p.

Mason LB: Babies hospital, 1920–1978. **NC Med J** 1984 Jan;45(1):53–6

Mayberry WE: The Mayo Clinic in 1984. Preserving the founding values amidst modern diversification. **Postgrad Med** 1984 Sep 1;76(3):13–5

Meier P: Jerome Cornfield and the methodology of clinical trials. **Controlled Clin Trials** 1981 May;1(4):339–45

Miciotto RJ: Anniversary 50: the birth and development of the LSU School of Medicine. The Murmur: LSU Medical Center Yearbook 1981 Fall; 13:34–41, 302–3.

Miller B: The incident. **Lincoln Her** 1980;82(1):342–3

Moldow G: 'For women, by women': women's dispensaries and clinics in Washington, 1882–1900. **Rec Columb Hist Soc** 1980;50:290–308

Mooney EC: The white plague. **Am Heritage** 1979;30(2):54–9

Morantz RM, Zschoche S: Professionalism, feminism, and gender roles: a comparative study of nineteenth-century medical therapeutics. **J Am Hist** 1980 Dec;67(3):568–88

Morgan RF: The Fort McHenry General Hospital for plastic and maxillofacial surgery. **Plast Reconstr Surg** 1983 Aug;72(2):255–9

Morman ET: Clinical pathology in America, 1865–1915: Philadelphia as a test case. **Bull Hist Med** 1984 Summer;58(2):198–214

Mottus JE: New York Nightingales: the emergence of the nursing profession at Bellevue and New York Hospital, 1850–1920. Ann Arbor, Mich., UMI Research Press, 1981. xvii, 277 p. (Ph.D. Diss., New York University, 1980.

Muller SA, Perry HO: The Goeckerman treatment in psoriasis: six decades of experience at the Mayo Clinic. **Cutis** 1984 Sep;34(3):265–8, 270

Mullner R, Byre CS, Kubal JD: Hospital closure in the United States, 1976–1980: a descriptive overview. **Health Serv Res** 1983 Fall;18(3):437–50

Murphy GP: Roswell Park Memorial Institute, Genesis of a cancer center. **Oncology** 1980;37(6):426–8

Musto DF, Ramos MR: Notes on American medical history: a follow-up study of the New Haven morphine maintenance clinic of 1920. **N Engl J Med** 1981 Apr 30;304(18):1071–7

Naisawald LV: Fanny Ricketts, nurse, diarist, devoted wife. **Va Cavalcade** 1972;21(3):14–21

The new Provident Medical Center: **J Natl Med Assoc** 1983 Jul;75(7):727

Nolan E: Children's ward. Lithograph by Robert Riggs, ca. 1940–45. **J Hist Med Allied Sci** 1982 Jul;37(3):322

Okamoto Y: [Nursing home: medical care a nursing practice in the United States. 8. Establishment of the system of nurses' registration and the history of the development of nursing assistants] (Jpn) **Kangogaku Zasshi** 1980 Aug;44(8):858–63

Okamoto Y: [Nursing homes. Status of medical care and nursing in the United States. 5. History of nursing homes]. **Kangogaku Zasshi** 1980 May;44(5):523–7

Orme JG, Stuart P: The Habit Clinics: behavioral social work and prevention in the 1920s. **Soc Serv Rev** 1981;55(2):242–56

Osteopathic hospitals: an historical glimpse: **OH** 1976 Nov–Dec;20(11):12–4

Pearson EF: First hospitals in Southern Illinois. **Proc Inst Med Chic** 1982 Apr–Jun;35(2):43–4

Perry HO: Department of Dermatology, Mayo Clinic. **Cutis** 1984 Sep;34(3):237–8

Perry T: The 48th evacuation hospital. **RI Med J** 1982 Dec;65(12):493

Phipps A: The runaway patient: a legend in oral circulation and the media. **Indiana Folkl** 1980;13(1–2):102–11

Pine Mountain--a clinic with a history: **Front Nurs Serv Q Bull** 1984 Spring;59(4):19–28, 30

Pinsker H, Novick DM, Richman BL: Hospital care at Second Avenue and East 17th Street, New York City, 1894–1984. **Bull NY Acad Med** 1984 Nov;60(9):905–24

Popplestone JA, McPherson MW: Pioneer psychology laboratories in clinical settings. In J. Brozěk, ed: Explorations in the history of psychology in the United States. Lewisburg, Bucknell University Press, 1984. p. 196–272.

Punnett L: Women-controlled medicine--theory and practice in 19th century Boston. **Women Health** 1976 Jul–Aug;1(4)3–11

Rasmussen GL: The history of hospital social work. **Tex Hosp** 1981 Feb;36(9):10–2

Rawlings DM: The history of Hamot Medical Center. **J Erie Stud** 1981 Spring;10:1–16

Redding JS: A historical vignette: intensive care. **Respir Ther** 1979 Jan–Feb;9(1):74–6, 78

Reed J: Who invented the modern hospital and who should tell the story? **Rev Am Hist** 1981;9(1):29–33

Reverby S: The search for the hospital yardstick: nursing and the rationalization of hospital work. In Reverby S, Rosner D, ed: Health care in America. Philadelphia, Temple University Press, 1979. p. 206–35.

Rhoads JE: Development of surgical nutrition at the University of Pennsylvania. **JPEN** 1980 Sep–Oct;4(5):464–6

Risse GB: A letter to Benjamin Rush. **J Hist Med Allied Sci** 1980 Oct;35(4):461

Robbins P: General Grant's calico colonel. **Am Hist Illus** 1979;14(1):4–7, 43–8

Rogers FB: Dr. Edward F. Gleason (1869–1944) of Hyannis, Massachusetts, and the Cape Cod Hospital and Windmill. **J Hist Med Allied Sci** 1980 Oct;35(4):459–60

## HOSPITALS

Rogers JC: Carle: concept and growth. A personal history. Urbana, Carle Foundation, 1978. xix, 228 p.
Rosenberg CE: From almshouse to hospital: the shaping of Philadelphia General Hospital. **Milbank Mem Fund Q** 1982 Winter;60(1):108–54
Rosenberg CE: Inward vision and outward glance: the shaping of the American hospital, 1880–1914. **Bull Hist Med** 1979 Fall;53(3):346–91
Rosenberger HT: Harriet Lane Johnston: pioneer advocate of special care for children with chronic diseases. **J Lanc Cty Hist Soc** 1972;76(1):1–28
Rosner D: A once charitable enterprise: hospitals and health care in Brooklyn and New York, 1885–1915. Cambridge; New York, Cambridge University Press, 1982. ix, 234 p.
Rosner D: Business at the bedside: health care in Brooklyn, 1890–1915. **Health PAC Bull** 1980 Mar–Apr;11(4):23–31
Rosner D: Business at the bedside: health care in Brooklyn, 1890–1915. In Reverby S, Rosner D, ed: Health care in America. Philadelphia, Temple University Press, 1979. p. 117–31.
Rosner D: Gaining control: reform, reimbursement and politics in New York's community hospitals, 1890--1915. **Am J Public Health** 1980 May;70(5):533–42
Rosner D: Social control and social service: the changing use of space in charity hospitals. **Radic Hist Rev** 1979;21:183–97
Roth MA: With mercy toward all. Mercy Hospital, Cedar Rapids, Iowa, 1900–1978. Cedar Rapids, Stamats, 1979. vii, 104 p.
Rumsey TJ: 'The General' -- a history of Hennepin County Medical Center. Part II. **Minn Med** 1980 Feb;63(2):101–6
Sabin TD: The Penikese Hospital: a Massachusetts hospital for the treatment of Hansen's disease. **N Engl J Med** 1981 Jun 25;304(26):1610–2
Sanazaro PJ: Quality assurance in medicine: a brief historical perspective. **World Hosp** 1984 Apr;20(2):16–20
Sayad EG: Alexian Brothers' hospital: unique heritage. **Bull Mo Hist Soc** 1980;36(4):264–7
Schaelchlin P: 'Working for the good of the community': Rest Haven Preventorium for Children. **J San Diego Hist** 1983 Spring;29:96–114
Schlicke CP: Working together. A history of a medical group practice, the Rockwood Clinic, Spokane, Washington. Fairfield, Wash. Ye Galleon Press, 1980. 187 p.
Shane KD: New Mexico: salubrious El Dorado. **NM Hist Rev** 1981;56(4):387–99
Shearer J: History of the Department of Nursing Education at the North Dakota State Hospital. **Prairie Rose** 1984 Oct–Dec;53(4):20–1
Shoemaker P, Jones MV: From infirmaries to intensive care: hospitals in Wisconsin. In Numbers RL, Leavitt JW, ed: Wisconsin medicine. Historical perspectives. Madison, University of Wisconsin Press, 1981. p. 105–31.
Shonick W: Early developments and recent trends in the evolution of the local public hospital. **Annu Rev Public Health** 1984;5:53–81
Skalley M, Skalley R: A medal for Marigold: Seattle's marine medic. Seattle, Superior Pub. Co., 1982. 150 p.
Sloan FA, Steinwald B: Effects of regulation on hospital costs and input use. **J Law Econ** 1980;23(1):81–109
Smith CA: The Children's Hospital of Boston: 'built better than they knew'. Boston, Little, Brown, 1983. ix, 284 p.
Smith DC: The emergence of organized clinical instruction in the nineteenth century American cities of Boston, New York and Philadelphia. Ph.D. Diss. University of Minnesota. Minneapolis, 1979. 357 leaves.
Soth DG: The central processing department: a brief history. **HPN Hosp Purch News** 1983 Mar;7(3):10, 12–3
Southwick HW: The medical center. **Proc Inst Med Chic** 1980 Jul–Sep;33(3):85–7
Staab L: The history of the New Jersey Hospital Association. **J Med Soc NJ** 1984 Sep;81(9):802–4
Stevens R: 'A poor sort of memory': voluntary hospitals and government before the depression. **Milbank Mem Fund Q** 1982 Fall;60(4):551–84
Stevens R: Sweet charity: state aid to hospitals in Pennsylvania, 1870–1910. **Bull Hist Med** 1984 Fall;58(3):287–314
Stevens R: Sweet charity: state aid to hospitals in Pennsylvania, 1870–1910. **Bull Hist Med** 1984 Winter;58(4):474–95
Tasman W: The history of Wills Eye Hospital. Hagerstown, Md., Harper & Row, 1980. ix, 135 p.
Taylor DB: Music in general hospital treatment from 1900 to 1950. **J Music Ther** 1981 Summer;18(2):62–73
Tedeschi CG, Merriam JC, et al: Framingham medical reflections. Framingham, Mass., Tedeschi Library, Framingham Union Hospital, 1975. 120 p.
Thomas RZ: An historical perspective: hospital planning and regulation from 1948 to 1978. **Hosp Health Serv Adm** 1982 Jul–Aug;27(4):66–77
Tilney NL: The original Peter Bent Brigham Hospital surgical staff. **Surg Gynecol Obstet** 1981 Nov;153(5):741–6
Vickers ED: Pensacola's early hospitals. **J Fla Med Assoc** 1981 Aug;68(8):635–43
Vogel MJ: Machine politics and medical care: the city hospital at the turn of the century. In Vogel MJ, Rosenberg CE, ed: The therapeutic revolution. Philadelphia, 1979. p. 159–175.
Vogel MJ: The invention of the modern hospital: Boston 1870–1930. Chicago, University of Chicago Press, 1980. 171 p.
Vogel MJ: The transformation of the American hospital, 1850–1920. In Reverby S, Rosner D, ed: Health care in America. Philadelphia, Temple University Press, 1979. p. 105–16.
Wall HM: Feminism and the New England Hospital, 1949–1961. **Am Q** 1980;32(4):435–52
Wall JH: Westchester County Medical Society and Westchester Division, New York Hospital-Cornell Medical Center; milestones in history. **NY State J Med** 1980 Nov;80(12):1884–5
Walls E: The introduction of prepayment medicine to Arkansas: the Trinity Hospital experience. **Arkansas Hist Q** 1983;42(1):3–26
Wassberg C: The Swedish Hospital Medical Center, Seattle, Washington. **Swed-Am Hist Q** 1983;34(4):312–22
We walk the line: the struggle at preterm.: **Radic Am** 1979;13(2):8–24
Weissmann G: Bellevue: form follows function. **Hosp Pract** 1981 Aug;16(8):18, 21, 24–5
Westerman JH: The Joint Commission on Accreditation of Hospitals: relations with the practicing physician--past, present and future. JCAH and the practicing physician: present issues, current solutions and future considerations 2. **Conn Med** 1982 Feb;46(2):89–92
Westerman MP, Tymorek S: A history of medical research at Mount Sinai Hospital Medical Center of Chicago. **Mt Sinai J Med (NY)** 1984 Apr;51(2):150–6
White WD: The American hospital industry since 1900: a short history. **Adv Health Econ Health Serv Res** 1982;3:143–70
Wilkins EW: Designation or dedication: seven men in the evolution of a trauma center. **Am J Surg** 1982 Apr;143(4):399–403
Wilson JL: 'The daily sanatorium routine was the treatment.' **Am Lung Assoc Bull** 1982 Mar;68(2):7–10
Wilson LB: A women pioneer in a new profession, medical editing. **Mayo Alumnus** 1982 Apr;:20–3
Woosley AI: Fort Burgwin's hospital. **Palacio** 86(1):3–7, 36–9
Wren GR: An historical view of health administration education. **Hosp Health Serv Adm** 1980 Summer;25(3):31–42
Wren GR: The first trained U. S. hospital administrator and his textbook. **Hosp Health Serv Adm** 1981 Winter;26(1):56–9
Wright KW: From poorhouse to medical facility: genesis of Onondaga County Infirmary. **NY State J Med** 1979 Sep;79(10):1612–5
Zainaldin JS, Tyor PL: Asylum and society: an approach to institutional change. **J Soc Hist** 1979;13(1):23–48
Zellweger H, Simpson J, Ionasescu V: Twenty years--Iowa muscle clinic: reminiscences and prospects. **Eur J Pediatr** 1982 Feb;138(1):17–22

### USSR

Artiukhov SA: Sochinskaia gospital'naia baza v gody Velikoĭ Otechestvennoĭ voĭny. **Voen Med Zh** 1981 Mar;(3):70–2
Artiukhov SA: Sochinskaia gospital'naia baza v gody Velikoĭ Otechestvennoĭ voĭny. **Sov Zdravookhr** 1981;(9):66–7
Arzhantsev PZ: Etapy razvitiia spetsializirovannoĭ stomatologicheskoĭ pomoshchi v GVKG imeni N. N. Burdenko. **Voen Med Zh** 1980 Feb;(2):78–80
Baranovskiĭ GIa, Kapitonov GI: Nekotorye voprosy podgotovki i organizatsii raboty sanitarno-transportnykh sudov v period Velikoĭ Otechestvennoĭ voiny. **Voen Med Zh** 1984 May;(5):25–8
Beloborodova NL: Moskovskiĭ vospitatel'nyĭ dom i ego rol' v istorii zdravookhraneniia Rossii. **Sov Zdravookhr** 1984;(7):58–61
Blokhin NN, Trapeznikov NN, Chaklin AV, et al: Vsesoiuznomu onkologicheskomu naushnomu tsentru AMN SSSR 30 let. **Vopr Onkol** 1981;27(12):81–7
Bogdanov EA: 50 Let travmatologicheskomu punktu Moskovskogo raĭona Leningrada. **Ortop Travmatol Protez** 1982 Dec;(12):61–3
Borisov VA: Okruzhnomu voennomu gospitaliu Krasnoznamennogo Zakavkazskogo Boennogo Okruga--175 let. **Voen Med Zh** 1983 Jul;(7):74–5
Burdov VS, Nemchaninov SK, Miziak AN: K istorii okruzhnogo voennogo gospitala Belorusskogo voennogo okruga. **Voen Med Zh** 1984 Aug;(8):71–3
D'iachenko DP: Pervaia bol'nitsa Kamchatskoĭ gubernii (K 75-letiiu Petropavlovsk-Kamchatskoĭ gorodskoĭ bol'nitsy No. 1). **Sov Zdravookhr** 1984;(3):60–2
Dionesov SM: Zhenskie vrachebnye kursy pri Peterburgskom nikolaevskom voennom gospitale. **Sov Med** 1982;(6):117–9
Dzhamadze ShV: Tuberkuleznomu sanatoriiu im. V. I. Lenina v Gul'ripshi - 80 let. **Probl Tuberk** 1983 Feb;(2):73–4
Gorbunov VP: 50 let na strazhe zdorov'ia voĭnov. **Voen Med Zh** 1984 Aug;(8):76–8
Grigorenko GF: K 110-letiiu Vladivostokskogo voenno-morskogo gospitalia. **Vestn Khir** 1983 May;130(5):142–3
Gulida MV: Ialtinskomu protivotuberkuleznomu dispanseru 60 let. **Probl Tuberk** 1984 Mar;(3):71–2
Harmer M: The forgotten hospital: an essay. Chichester, Springwood Books, 1982. 170 p.
Katslan IaD: Iz istorii sozdaniia Glavnogo voennogo klinicheskogo gospitalia im. N. N. Burdenko i razvitiia v nem spetsializirovannoĭ terapevticheskoĭ pomoshchi. **Klin Med (Mosk)** 1983 Jan;61(1):107–10
Khazanov AT: Iz istorii prozektury Obukhovskoĭ bol'nitsy. **Arkh Patol** 1983;45(5):68–73
Komakhidze ME: Ocherki o khirurgicheskoĭ rabote ofitserskogo gospitalia

v period Velikoĭ Otechstvennĭ voĭny (1941–1955 gg.). Tbilisi, Metsniereba, 1977. 102 p.
Kovanov VV: V tylovom gospitale. **Voen Med Zh** 1980 Apr;(4):27–30
Krasnogorskaia ES: V armeĭskom gospitale. **Voen Med Zh** 1980 Mar;(3):69–70
Kravkov IuS: Slavnyĭ jubileĭ. **Med Sestra** 1983 Apr;42(4):50–2
Krylov NL: Stareĭshiĭ meditsinskiĭ tsentr strany (k 275–letiiu Glavnogo voennogo klinicheskogo gospitalia im, Akad. N.N. Burdenko). **Sov Zdravookhr** 1983;(3):65–8
Lukavskiĭ MI, Ugulava SN. Voenno–morskomu Krasnoznamennomu gospitaliu imeni akademika N. I. Pirogova––200 let. **Voen Med ZH** 1983 May;5:71–3
Makhmudov M: Pervaia bol'nitsa v Khorezme. **Sov Zdravookhr** 1984;(1):67–9
Movshovich IA, Kaplan MB: 50 Let so dnia organizatsii travmatologicheskogo otdeleniia v bol'nitse im. S. P. Botkina. **Ortop Travmatol Protez** 1982 Jun;(6):74–5
Nevskiĭ NM: O rabote frontovogo évakopunkta. **Voen Med Zh** 1980 Oct;(10):23–4
Nikulina TD, Ivanov IV: Kuĭbyshevskoĭ oblastnoĭ tuberkuleznoĭ bol'nitse im. Z. P. Solov'eva 125 let. **Probl Tuberk** 1983 Apr;(4):69–71
Okhrimenko NN: Glavnyĭ voennyĭ gospital' i ego rol' v razvitii otechestvennoĭ voennoĭ nevrologii (k 275–letiiu so dnia osnovaniia Glavnogo. **Zh Nevropatol Psikhiatr** 1983;83(7):1069–71
Pavluchkova AV: Pervye sovetskie dispansery po bor'be s tuberkulezom u deteĭ (k Mezhdunarodnomu godu rebenka). **Probl Tuberk** 1979 Dec;(12):11–5
Razvitie nevrologicheskoĭ pomoshchi v Glavnom voennom klinicheskom gospitale imeni N. N. Burdenko (k 275–letiiu osnovaniia gospitalia): **Voen Med Zh** 1982 Jul,(7).71–2
Razvitie otorinolaringologii v Glavnom voennom klinicheskom gospitale imeni N. N. Burdenko (k 275–letiiu osnovaniia gospitalia): **Voen Med Zh** 1982;(9):67–8
Rudakova AIa: Permskaia oblastnaia klinicheskaia bol'nitsa (k 150–letiiu bol'nitsy). **Sov Zdravookhr** 1984;(2):57–8
Ryzhakova GI: Itogi vypolneniia direktiv Dal'kraĭkoma VKP(b) po stroitel'stvu ob'ektov zdravookhraneniia v gody pervykh piatiletok (1928–1937). **Sov Zdravookhr** 1982;(8):55–7
Safarov RN, Shtern MI, Fel'berg MB: K istorii tuberkuleznoĭ bol'nitsy 'Zakhar'ino'. **Probl Tuberk** 1983 Feb;(2):70–3
Salaeva ZM: K istorii kliniki nervnykh bolezně Azerbaĭdzhanskogo orden Trudovogo Krasnogo Znameni gosudarstvennogo meditsinskogo instituta im. N, Narimanova. **Zh Nevropatol Psikhiatr** 1981;81(11):1720–1
Selivanov VI, Tkhostov DR, Selivanov EF: Lechbno– evakuatsionnaia kharakteristika ranenykh i bol'nykh, lechivshikhsia v gospital'noi baze tyla strany. **Voen Med Zh** 1980 Jun;(6):20–3
Selivanov VI: [Organization of rehabilitation of the wounded and sick during World War II in military hospitals]. (Rus) **Voen Med Zh** 1979 Nov;(11):74–5
Senenko AN: Obukhovskaia bol'nitsa (k 200–letiiu so dnia osnovaniia). **Klin Med (Mosk)** 1980 Feb;58(2):111–6
Shereshevskiĭ GM: O stanovlenii i razvitii gospital'nogo dela. **Voen Med Zh** 1983 Oct;10:67–9
Shliapak AE: Partiĭno–politicheskaia rabota v ĕvakogospitaliakh Kavkazskikh Mineral'nykh Vod. **Voen Med Zh** 1981 Nov;(11):69–70
Smorodintsev AA: K istorii izucheniia étiologii i vaktsinoprofilaktiki grippa (nauchnyĭ vklad v étu problemu kliniki M. D. Tushinshinskogo). **Klin Med (Mosk)** 1982 Jan;60(1):108–12
Stahnke J: Skizzen zur Geschichte des russischen Findelhauswesens. Erläutert am St. Petersburger Erziehungshaus. Pattensen (Han.), Wellm, 1983. ix, 628 p. (Würzburger medizinhistorische Forschungen, ix, Bd. 28).
Sukhanov NV: Meditsinakaia i trudovaia reabilitatsiia ranenykh v gospitaliakh Zapadnoĭ Sibiri v period Velikoĭ Otechestvennoĭ voiny. **Voen Med Zh** 1981;(7):72–4
Tambovtsev PD: K istorii organizatsii i razvitiia sanatornoĭ pomoshchi detiam. **Pediatriia** 1983 Sep;:(9):71–3
Tambovtsev PD: K 25–letiiu detskogo pul'monologicheskogo sanatoriia im. M.S. Maslova. **Pediatriia** 1983 Jun;(6):74–5
Telichenas AI, Gritsiutc LA, Skarulis RI, et al: Istoriia razvitiia onkologicheskoĭ sluzhby v Litovskoĭ SSR. **Vopr Onkol** 1982;28(11):8–11
Tkachenko VF: K istorii Smelianskoĭ gorodskoĭ bol'nitsy im. N. A. Semashko. **Med Sestra** 1981 Dec;40(12):5–8
Tsiklik AM: K istorii vozniknoveniia i stanovleniia poliklinicheskoĭ. **Feldsher Akush** 1980;45(10):51–3
Turupanov NL: K istorii organizatsii besplatnoĭ lechebnitsy v Vologde. **Sov Med** 1982;(9):120–2
Vladimirova LB, Gribanov ED: A nagy magyar zeneszerzo, Liszt Ferenc és az ogyesszai gyermekkórház épületének története (orosz nyelven). **Orvostort Kozl** 1982;28(1–3):169–76
Vladimirova LB, Gribanov ED: Emblema meditsiny. **Feldsher Akush** 1981;46(4):58–60
Vlasov AA: Ikh trudom slaven kollektiv. **Voen Med Zh** 1982 Mar;(3):7–10
Volkov MV: Tsentral'nomu institutu travmatologii i ortopedii im. N. N. Priorova––60 let. **Ortop Travmatol Protez** 1981;(4):1–5
Vozchikov-Chernov SP: V polevom podvizhnom gospitale. **Voen Med Zh** 1981 Nov;(11):70

Wunderlich P: Ein Bericht aus dem Jahre 1838 über die Kliniken in Moskau und St. Petersburg. **Z Gesamte Hyg** 1980;26(5):381–2

**Vietnam**

Nguyen TK, Smirnov VS, Mozzhakov VI: Tsentral'nomu voennomu gospitaliu v'et namskoĭ Narodnoĭ armii––30 let. **Voen Med Zh** 1981 Nov;(11):61–2

**Yugoslavia**

Berić B, Miškov D: Pregled istorije bolnice u Novom Sadu (1730–1980). **Med Pregl** 1981;34(5–6):259–65
Djurić L: Vojno–teritorijalna sanitetska služba na baniji u toku nor–a. **Vojnois Glas** 1971;22(3):191–206
Juvan V: Djelatnost za zdravstvenu zaštitu žena Medicinskog centra u Varaždinu. **Jugosl Ginekol Opstet** 1978;18(5–6):445–53
Katan E: Sanitetsko snabdevanje Centralne bolnice Vrhovnog štaba i jedinica Glavne operativne grupe za vreme četvrte i pete ofanzive. **Vojnosanit Pregl** 1980 Nov–Dec;37(6):476–80
Katan E: Ustanove za zbrinjavanje ranjenika NOVJ na području Beograda od 15. oktobra do kraja decembra 1944. godine. **Vojnosanit Pregl** 1980 Mar–Apr;37(2):121–5
Majsec M, Manestar M: Od kupališnog lječilišta do bolnice za reumatske bolesti i rehabilitaciju Krapinske Toplice. **Reumatizam** 1979;26(3):73–6
Mijušković S: Nastojanja kotorske opštine oko osnivanja centralne bolnice za boku sredinom XIX veka. **Istor Zapisi** 1972;25(3–4):443–52
Zorn E: Geschichte und Bedeutung des Marinehospitals von Pola/Jugoslawien. **Hist Hosp** 1979–80;13:135–46

**Zimbabwe**

Morris RM: The Umtali Hospitals. **Rhodesiana** 1979;40:29–33

# HOSPITALS, PSYCHIATRIC

Connor LH: Ships of fools and vessels of the divine: mental hospitals and madness, a case study. **Soc Sci Med** 1982;16(7):783–94
Masters A: Bedlam, London, Michael Joseph, 1977. 206 p.
Porter R: Shutting people up. **Soc Stud Sci** 1982 Aug 3;12(3):467–76
Romano J: Temples, asylums, hospitals ––? **J Natl Assoc Priv Psychiatr Hosp** 1978 Summer;9(4):5–12
Rosenblatt A: Concepts of the asylum in the care of the mentally ill. **Hosp Community Psychiatry** 1984 Mar;35(3):244–50

**Americas**

Viqueira C: Los hospitales para locos e 'inocentes' en hispanoamerica y sus antecedentes españoles. **Rev Esp Antropol Am** 1970;5:341–83

**Canada**

Frankenburg FR: The history of the confinement of the mentally ill in Ontario. **Psychiatr J Univ Ottawa** 1982 Dec;7(4):240–3

**China**

Ng VW: Ch'ing laws governing the insane: an historical survey. **Ch'ing–Shih Wen–t'i** 1980;4(4):55–89

**France**

Alliez J, Cain JR, Thermoz P: L'assistance aux malades mentaux dans le Sud–Est méditerranéen aux XVIIe et XVIIIe siècles: les 'asiles' de Saint–Paul–de–Mausole et de Saint–Pierre–de–Canon, à Saint–Rémy et à Aurons, en Provence. **Ann Med Psychol (Paris)** 1982 Dec;140(10):1122–8
Fourquet F: Histoire de la psychiatrie de secteur. Paris, Recherches, 1980. viii, 338 p.

**Great Britain**

Sumner E: Psychiatry, 1. bordering on bedlam. **Nurs Mirror** 1980 Dec 4;151(23):16–8

**Japan**

Gifu Seishin Byoin: Soritsu gojisshunenshi. Gifu, Japan, Gifu Seishin Byoin, Showa 53 nen, 1978. 283 p.
Kure S, Kashida G: Waga kuni ni okeru seishinbyo ni kansuru saikin no shisetsu. Tokyo, Seishin Igaku Shinkeigaku Koten Kankokai, [1977]. 270 p.

**Poland**

Chrzęściewski L: Pierwsze domy opieki dla dzieci psychicznie chorych w Krakowie. **Psychiatr Pol** 1982 Sep–Dec;16(5–6):437–8

# HOSPITALS, PSYCHIATRIC

**United States**

Jones RE: Moral treatment: the basis of private mental hospital care. **Psychiatr Hosp** 1983 Winter;14(1):5–9

**500 A.D.–1450**

**Spain**

García Ballester L, García-González G: Nota sobre la asistencia a los locos y 'desfallecidos de seso' en la Cordoba medieval: el Hospital de Jesucristo (1419). **Asclepio** 1978–79;30–31:199–207

**1450–1700**

**Canada**

Griffin JD, Greenland C: Institutional care of the mentally disordered in Canada--a 17th century record. **Can J Psychiatry** 1981 Jun;26(4):274–8

**1700 to Present**

Baruk H: L'hôpital psychiatrique d'hier et de demain. **Ann Med Psychol (Paris)** 1980 Jun;138(6):700–7
Brown TE: The mental hospital and its historians. **Bull Hist Med** 1982 Spring;56(1):109–14
Danzinger R, Lyon G: Das Beratungszentrum für psychische und sociale Fragen in Graz. Wien, Osterreichische Akademie der Wissenschaften, 1982. 140 p.
Feinmann J: How a lunatic fared in 1781. **Med News** 1981;13(22):22–3
Goodman LR: Nursing administration in psychiatric hospitals. **J Psychosoc Nurs Ment Health Serv** 1983 Aug;21(8):26–34
Grob GN: Historical origins of deinstitutionalization. **New Dir Ment Health Serv** 1983 Mar;(17):15–29
Janzarik W ed: Psychopathologie als Grundlagenwissenschaft. Stuttgart, Ferdinand Enke, 1979. xi, 202 p. (Klinische Psychologie und Psychopathologie, Bd. 8). Contributions by H. Schipperges, H. D. Middelhoff, R. Avenarius, W. Schmitt, H. Kindt, W. Kretschmer, G. Huber, J. Glatzel, K. P. Kisker, H. Tellenbach, H. Häfner, A. Bader, L. Navratil, W. Baeyer, K. Koehler, O. Dörr-Zegers, B. Kimura.
Jetter D: Grundzüge der Geschichte des Irrenhauses. Darmstadt, Wissenschaftliche Buchgesellschaft, 1981. ix, 244 p.
Jetter D: Zur Typologie des Irrenhauses in Frankreich und Deutschland (1780–1840). Wiesbaden, Steiner, 1971. x, 206 p. (Geschichte des Hospitals, Band 2)
Leighton AH: Caring for mentally ill people. Psychological and social barriers in historical context. Cambridge, Cambridge University Press, 1982. x, 277 p.
Mousnier R: Réflexions d'un historien à la lecture d'un manuel de sociologie. **Rev Hist (Paris)** 1980;263(2):395–401
Risso M: Institution psychiatrique, idéologie médicale et chronification. **Schweiz Arch Neurol Neurochir Psychiatr** 1980;126(2):327–35
Scull A: Humanitarianism or control? Some observations on the historiography of Anglo-American psychiatry. **Rice Univ Stud** 1981;67(1):21–41
Scull A: The domestication of madness. **Med Hist** 1983 Jul;27(3):233–48

**Americas**

Neufeld VH, ed: If we can love: the Mennonite mental health story. Newton, Kan., Faith and Life Press, 1983. xii, 340 p.

**Australia**

McDonald DI: The Newcastle Lunatic Asylum: so human a purpose. **J R Aust Hist Soc** 1980;66(1):20–38
Parkinson JP: The Castle Hill lunatic asylum (1811–1826) and the origins of eclectic pragmatism in Australian psychiatry. **Aust NZ J Psychiatry** 1981 Dec;15(4):319–22

**Austria**

Englisch F: Die Döblinger Privatirrenanstalt. **Wien Geschichtsbl** 1969;24(1):398–406
Jetter D: Wiener Irrenhausprojekte. **Fortschr Neurol Psychiatr** 1981 Feb;49(2):43–52
Skopec M, Wyklicky H: Die Heilpädagogische Abteilung der Universitäts-Kinderklink Wien--die älteste kinderpsychiatrische Forschungs- und Behandlungsstätte. **Erzleh Unterr** 1981 Oct;24:98–105

**Canada**

Goldman DL, Arvanitakis K: D. Ewen Cameron's Day Hospital and the day hospital movement. **Can J Psychiatry** 1981 Aug;26(5):365–8
Greenland C: William George Metcalf. In Dictionary of Canadian biography, 1881–1890. 1982;11:590–1.
Griffin JD, Greenland C: Asylum at lower Fort Garry, 1874–1886. **Beaver** 1980;310(4):18–23
Krasnick CL: 'In charge of the loons': a portrait of the London, Ontario, Asylum for the Insane in the nineteenth century. **Ont Hist** 1982;74(3):138–84
Kroll RE: Confines, wards, and dungeons. **NS Hist Soc Collect** 1980;40:93–107
Mitchinson W: R. M. Bucke: a Victorian asylum superintendent. **Ont Hist** 1981;73(4):239–54
Porter JR: L'Hôpital-Général de Québec et le soin des aliénés (1717–1845). **Can Cathol Hist Assoc Study Sess** 1979;:23–55
Rogers IL: John Mackieson. In Dictionary of Canadian biography, 1881–1890. 1982;11:565–6.
Samuel R: Henry Howard. In Dictionary of Canadian biography, 1881–1890. 1982;11:425–6.
Wallot H: A view on the socio-political history of psychiatric care in French-Canada with particular reference to Quebec asylums. **Soc Sci Med [Med Psychol Med Sociol]** 1980 Dec;14A(6):485–94

**Chile**

Costa-Casaretto C: Ideario psiquiátrico del médico de la Casa de Locos de Santiago en 1862. **Rev Med Chil** 1980 Jun;108(6):559–67

**Czechoslovakia**

Blaták F, Valenčik J: Historické podmínky budování moravakých ústavu pro duševně choré v druhé polovině 19. století. **Cesk Psychiatr** 1981 Oct;77(5):348–51
Dobíšek K: První čtyři primáři Pražského ústavu choromyslných. 2. Josef Pelikan. **Cesk Psychiatr** 1981 Dec;77(6):414–9
Dobíšek K: První čtyři primáři pražského ústavu choromyslných. 3. Karl Damian Schroff, medicinae Doctor et Chirurgae magister. **Cesk Psychiatr** 1982 Feb;78(1):61–6
Dobíšek K: První čtyři primáři pražského ústavu choromyslných. 4. Wenzel Friedrich Rilke, Medicinae et Chirurgiae doctor. **Cesk Psychiatr** 1983 Aug;79(4):275–82
Dobíšek K: První čyři primáři pražského ústavu choromyslných. **Cesk Psychiatr** 1980 Aug;76(4):270–5
Hájek P: 10 let Kroměřížského psychoterapeutického oddělení. **Cesk Psychiatr** 1982 Jun;78(3):196–8
Klik J: Pl Dobřany oslavuje stoleté výročí. **Cesk Psychiatr** 1980 Jun;76(3):204–6
Kunčar K: Olomoucká psychiatrická klinika očima bývalých studentu. **Cesk Psychiatr** 1981 Oct;77(5):346–7
Mečíř J: Dvě instrukce pro zaměstnance prvního ústavu pro choromyslné v Praze. **Cesk Psychiatr** 1984 Aug;80(4):215–9
Mečíř J: Vítězslav Hálek a jeho obec pomatených. **Cesk Psychiatr** 1983 Feb;79(1):60–3
Vencovský E: Jubileum 40 let od založení nemocniční lužkové psychiatrické péče v Plzni. **Cesk Psychiatr** 1982 Dec;78(6):407–8
Vencovský E: Mudr. Josef Cermák a jeho zásluhy o vybudování psychiatrické léčebny v Cernovicích. **Cesk Psychiatr** 1984 Jun;80(3):200–3
Vencovský E: První nemocniční psychiatrické oddělení v Cechách. **Cesk Psychiatr** 1981 Jun;77(3):204–8

**Denmark**

Grodum T: Sindssygehuset i Slesvig. **Dan Medicinhist Arbog** 1983;12:122–43
Jensen E: Et 125-arigt medicinsk bibliotek. **Bogens Verden** 1977;59(5):181–5
Nielsen J: 125 års jubilaeum: fra Jydske asyl 1852 til Psykiatrisk hospital i Arhus 1977: [s. l.: s. n., 1977?]. 139 p.

**Finland**

Salokangas RK: Hospital and outpatient care for psychotic patients during the last three decades. Subsequent hospital and outpatient treatment of psychotic patients hospitalized for the first time in 1949–50, 1959–60 or 1969–70. **Acta Psychiatr Scand** 1980 Jul;62(1):47–62

**France**

Bendiner E: Philippe Pinel: reason for the unreasoning. **Hosp Pract** 1981 Jun;16(6):76E–76P
Cathelin M: Les insensés au XVIIIe siècle: naissance de la solution asilaire. **Bull Soc Fr Hist Hop** 1983;46:21–35
Goldstein J: The hysteria diagnosis and the politics of anticlericalism in late nineteenth-century France. **J Mod Hist** 1982;54(2):209–39
Jones C: The 'new treatment' of the insane in Paris: the formation of the lunatic asylum under the French Revolution. **Hist Today** 1980 Oct;30:5–10
Jones C: The treatment of the insane in eighteenth- and early nineteenth-century Montpellier. A contribution to the prehistory of the lunatic asylum in provincial France. **Med Hist** 1980;24(4):371–90
Quetel C: L'asile d'aliénés en 1900. **Histoire** 1978;7:25–34
Reverzy JF: Petite histoire de la psychiatrie de secteur.

**Soins Psychiatr** 1982 Feb;(16):41
Scherrer P: La débâcle de 1940: recueil des malades mentaux à l'Hôpital Psychiatrique d'Auxerre. **Ann Med Psychol (Paris)** 1984 Feb;142(2):266–70
Telson HW: Une leçon du Docteur Charcot à la Salpêtrière. Lithograph by Eugene Pirodon after a painting (1887) by André Brouillet. **J Hist Med Allied Sci** 1980 Jan;35(1):58

**Germany**

Blasius D: Psychiatrische Versorgung in Preussen, 1880–1910. **Sudhoffs Arch** 1982;66(2):105–28
Cranach M von: Die Münchner Klinik und die psychiatrische Diagnostik. **MMW** 1981 May 8;123(19):777–80
Eichhorn H: Ernst Gottlob Pienitz und die Heil- und Verpflegungsanstalt Sonnenstein. **Psychiatr Neurol Med Psychol (Leipz)** 1982 Jan;34(1):60–3
Hamann P: Peter Willers Jessens ehemaliges Asyl Hornheim in Kiel. Ein Beitrag zur Psychiatriegeschichte Schleswig-Holsteins. **Hist Hosp** 1979–80;13:69–95
Pfeffer R: Professor Franz von Rinecker, 1811–1883. Diss., Bayerische Julius-Maximilians-Universität, Würzburg, 1981. 180 p.
Rodegra H: Philippe Pinels Ideen von der Befreiung der Irren und ihre Verwirklichung im norddeutschen Raum zu Beginn des 19. Jahrhunderts. **Med Welt** 1981 Feb 6;32(6):199–201
Rogoll H, Späte HF: Zur gesellschaftlichen Stellung des psychisch Kranken im Spiegel der Geschichte gesetzlicher Regelungen zur Einweisung in stationäre Einrichtungen. **Z Gesamte Hyg** 1983 Jan;29(1):37–9
Rothkopf A: 'Das Narrenhaus' von W. Kaulbach und die Deutung des Bildes durch J. A. Schilling 1863. **Confin Psychiatr** 1980;23(1):51–64
Rückleben H: Deportation und Tötung von Geisteskranken aus den badischen Anstalten der Inneren Mission Kork und Mosbach. Karlsruhe, Evangelischer Presseverband für Baden, 1981. 104 p. (Veröffentlichungen des Vereins für Kirchengeschichte in der evangelischen Landeskirche in Baden, Band 33).
Schmidt PO: Asylierung oder psychiatrische Familienpflege? Die Diskussionen in den Irrenärzteverbänden um die psychiatrische Versorgungsstruktur im 19. Jahrhundert. **Psychiatr Prax** 1983 Mar;10(2):56–9
Zeller G: Von der Heilanstalt zur Heil- und Pflegeanstalt. Ein Beitrag zur Geschichte des psychiatrischen Krankenhauswesens. **Fortschr Neurol Psychiatr** 1981 Mar;49(3):121–7

**Great Britain**

The Bethlem Royal Hospital and the Maudsley Hospital--a glance at the future...and a look at the past.: **Nurs Times** 1980 Sep 4;76(36):1558–62
Digby A: Changes in the asylum: the case of York, 1777–1815. **Econ Hist Rev** 1983;36:218–39
Digby A: The York Retreat: the growing ascendancy of medicine, 1796–1914. **Pharm Hist (London)** 1984 Jun;14(2):2–3
Fee E: Psychology, sexuality, social control in Victorian England. **Soc Sci Q** 1978;58(4):632–46
McCandless P: 'Build! build!' the controversy over the care of the chronically insane in England, 1855–1870. **Bull Hist Med** 1979 Winter;53(4):553–74
McCandless P: Liberty and lunacy: the Victorians and wrongful confinement. **J Soc Hist** 1978;11(3):366–86
Mellett DJ: The prerogative of asylumdom: social, cultural, and administrative aspects of the institutional treatment of the insane in nineteenth-century Britain. New York, Garland Pub. Co., 1982. 257 p.
Paly D: Portrait of William Norris. Broadside, 1815, with etched portrait (1814) entitled 'William Norris: confined in this manner in Bethlem Hospital'; George Arnald, A.R.A., artist, etcher, and publisher. **Radic Hist Rev** 1979 Spring/Summer;Spec:65
Presly AS: From madhouses to mental hospitals: does history repeat itself? **Scott Med J** 1983 Jan;28(1):71–4
Ray LJ: Models of madness in Victorian asylum practice. **Eur J Sociol** 1981;22(2):229–64
Rollin HR: Changing face of administration of mental hospitals. **J R Soc Med** 1981 Sep;74(9):641–4
Scull A: A convenient place to get rid of inconvenient people: the Victorian lunatic asylum. In King, Anthony D., ed.: Buildings and society: essays on the social development of the built environment. London, Routledge and Kegan Paul, 1980. p. 37–60.
Shepherd MA: Lunacy and labour. **Soc Stud Labour Hist** 1977;(34):61–9
Towers BA: The management and politics of a public exposé: the Prestwich Inquiry 1922. **J Soc Policy** 1984 Jan;13(1):41–61
Walton JK: Lunacy in the Industrial Revolution: a study of asylum admissions in Lancashire, 1848–50. **J Soc Hist** 1979;13(1):1–22
Watkin B: St. Bernard's Hospital: pioneering a humane approach. **Health Soc Serv J** 1981 Dec 3;91(4775):1480–1

**Hungary**

Pisztora F: A schizophrenia és a paranoid kórformák gyógyítási kísérletei a Monarchia korabeli Magyarország különféle psychiátriai intézményeiben. **Orvostort Kozl** 1982;92(4):53–87

**Ireland**

Tumbling walls: The evolution of a community institution over 150 years: 1833, Maryborough District Lunatic Asylum for King's and Queen's Counties, Westmeath and Longford: 1925, Portlaoghise District Mental Hospital: 1983, St. Fintan's Psychiatric Hospital, clinics and community service. Portlaoise, Laois: Midland Health Board at St. Fintan's Hospital, in association with Relay Publications, Tyone, Nenagh, Tipperary, Ireland, 1983. 105 p.

**Italy**

Armocida G: Annotazioni sull'ospedalità privata per malati di mente nella prima metà dell'800: l'esempio di Milano. In International Congress of the History of Medicine, 27th, Barcelona, 1980. Actas. Barcelona, Acadèmia de Ciències Mèdiques de Catalunya i Balears, 1981. p. 23–6.
Armocida G, Ambrosoli C, Finavera L, et al: Gli 'ospizi privati per i pazzi' in Milano nel 1846. **Minerva Psichiatr** 1980 Jan–Mar;21(1):57–62
Ganapini L: Provvedimenti della pietà e della scienza: il frenocomio di Trieste (1908–1914). **Mov Operaio Soc** 1980;3(4):423–39
Lanzavecchia P, Lingua P, Sinigaglia G: La popolazione manicomiale di Alessandria nella seconda metà dell'ottocento. **Mov Operaio Soc** 1980;3(4):405–22
Quaini M: Il modello panoptico nel primo manicomio di Genova. **Mov Operaio Soc** 1980;3(4):395–404
Trabucchi C: Riforma psichiatrica. I vecchi 'manicomi' e la riforma sanitaria. **Minerva Med** 1980 May 7;71(18):1281–5
Villa R: 'Pazzi e criminali': strutture istituzionali e pratica psichiatrica nei manicomi criminali italiani (1876–1915). **Mov Operaio Soc** 1980;3(4):369–93

**Japan**

Okada Y: [The incidence of Kakke-disease (beriberi) in pre-war mental hospitals] (Jpn). **Nihon I-Shigaku Zasshi** 1981;27:95–111
Tokyo Seishin Byoin Kyokai: Tokyo no shiritsu seishin byoin shi. Tokyo, Makino Shuppan, Showa 53 nen, 1978. 378 p.

**Netherlands**

Binneveld JM: Van bewaarplaats tot geneeskundig gesticht. **Spiegel Hist** 1981;16(5):267–73
Van der Esch P: Geschiedenis van het Staatstoezicht op Krankzinningen. 's-Gravenhage, Ministerium van Volksgezondheit en Milieuhygiene, 1975–1980. 3 volumes in 1.

**Norway**

Festy M: Les internements psychiatriques en Norvège. **Population** 1981;36(2):317–36
Haugen A: Sanderud: sykehus i 175 år: psykiatrisk sykehus i 70 år. [s.L.]. Elverum trykk, 1978. 132 p.
Retterstøl N: Gaustad sykehus 125 år (1855–1980). **Tidsskr Nor Laegeforen** 1980 Dec 10;100(34–36):2026–9

**Philippines**

Shegina F: Survey of mental health services of hospitals in the greater Manila area. **Unitas** 1972;45(2):89–113

**Poland**

Jaroszewski Z, Tarmanowska B: Dzieci w Instytucie Higieny Psychicznej (w Warszawie, 1943–1944). **Przegl Lek** 1981;38(1):152–5
Popkowska N: Przeglad problemów diagnostycznych i rehabilitacyjnych dzieci i młodziezy leczonej w Klinice Psychiatrii Akademii Medycznej w Lublinie w latach 1951–1971. **Psychiatr Pol** 1980 May–Jun;14(3):259–64
Sulestrowska H: Zasługi prof. dr. Tadeusza Bilikiewicza dla rozwoju psychiatrii dziecięcej w Polsce. **Psychiatr Pol** 1982;16(4):321–8

**Romania**

Brânzei P: Secvențe din viața spitalului 'Socola' sau despre viitorul psihiatriei. Adaptare – integrare – recuperare. **Rev Med Chir Soc Med Nat Iasi** 1981;85(1):153–7

**Switzerland**

Ernst K: Geisteskrankheit ohne Institution. Eine Feldstudie im Kanton Fribourg aus dem Jahr 1875. **Schweiz Arch Neurol Neurochir Psychiatr** 1983;133(2):239–62
Haenel T: Zur Geschichte der Psychiatrischen Poliklinik Basel. **Schweiz Arch Neurol Neurochir Psychiatr** 1979;124(2):335–50
Müller C: Le Champ-de-l'Air, premier hôpital psychiatrique du Canton

de Vaud. **Gesnerus** 1980;37(1/2):28–33

### United States

Auman C, et al: A state mental hospital and public welfare team up. **Public Welf** 1969;27(1):59–65
Bellows B: 'Insanity is the disease of civilization': the founding of the South Carolina Lunatic Asylum. **SC Hist Mag** 1981;82(3):263–72
Binder G: Penal reform and progressive ideology. **Rev Am Hist** 1981;9(2):224–32
Bower B: St. Elizabeths Museum. **Psychiatr News** 1982 Mar 19;17(6):6–7
Bragg TA: The McLean Hospital archives. **Mass Nurse** 1984 Sep;54(8):3
Bromberg W: Psychiatry between the wars, 1918–1945. A recollection. Westport, London, Greenwood Press, 1982. xxxii, 184 p. (Contributions in Medical History, No. 10).
Cahow CR: People, patients and politics: the history of the North Carolina mental hospitals, 1848–1960. New York, Arno Press, 1980. vii, 254 p (Ph.D. Diss., Duke University, 1967).
Dunkel LM: Moral and humane: patients' libraries in early nineteenth-century American mental hospitals. **Bull Med Libr Assoc** 1983 Jul;71(3):274–81
Dwyer E: Mental health care in early twentieth century Indiana and the limits of reform. **Indiana Med Hist Q** 1983 Mar;9(1):23–7
Emerson RM, Rochford EB, Shaw LL: Economics and enterprise in Board and Care Homes for the mentally ill. **Am Behav Sci** 1981;24(6):771–85
Ewalt DJ: Patients, politics and physicians: the struggle for control of State Lunatic Asylum No. 1, Fulton, Missouri. **Mo Hist Rev** 1983 Jan;77:170–88
Felton BJ, Shinn M: Ideology and practice of deinstitutionalization. **J Soc Issues** 1981;37(3):158–72
Gill D: The dueling doctors of Stockton. **Pac Hist** 1981;25(1):52–8
Golden J, Schneider EC: Custody and control: the Rhode Island Hospital for Mental Diseases, 1870–1970. **RI Hist** 1982;41(4):113–25
Gordon RL: The development of Louisiana's public mental institutions, 1735–1940. 2 vols. in 1. Ph.D. Diss., Louisiana State University. Baton Rouge, 1978, 498 leaves.
Grob GN: Abuse in American mental hospitals in historical perspective: myth and reality. **Int J Law Psychiatry** 1980;3(3):295–310
Grob GN: Rediscovering asylums: the unhistorical history of the mental hospital. In Vogel MJ, Rosenberg CE, ed: The therapeutic revolution. Philadelphia, 1979 p. 135–157.
Grob GN, ed: Public policy and mental illness. Four investigations, 1915–1939. New York, Arno, 1980. Separate paginations.
Haag JE, Jackson LH: The acceptance of chaplains in mental hospitals. **Am Benedictine Rev** 1981;32(4):328–35
Hansen C: Willowbrook: try, try again. **Soc Policy** 1979;10(3):41–5
Hartmann K, Margolin L: The Nebraska Asylum for the Insane, 1870–1886. **Nebr Hist** 1982;63(2):164–83
Hartmann K, Halbert MR, Margolin L: Treatment at the Nebraska asylum for the insane a century ago. **Nebr Med J** 1982 May;67(5):131–3
Hazelrigg C: Central State Hospital. Part 2. **Indiana Med Hist Q** 1981;7(3):3–23
Hendrie HC: Press coverage of Central State Hospital: alarms and excursions. **Indiana Med Hist Q** 1983 Mar;9(1):5–12
Himelhoch MS, Shaffer AH: Elizabeth Packard: nineteenth-century crusader for the rights of mental patients. **J Am Stud** 1979;13(3):343–75
Hollander R: Life at the Washington asylum for the insane, 1871–1880. **Historian** 1982;44(2):229–41
Hollander R: Mental health policy in Washington territory, 1853–1875. **Pac Northwest Q** 1980;71(4):152–61
Jacobs F: Issac Ray and the profession of psychiatry. **RI Hist** 1979;38(4):99–111
Keeney W: Experiences in mental hospitals in World War II. **Mennon Q Rev** 1982;56(1):7–17
Keill SL: Current issues in general hospital psychiatry. Introduction: The evolution of psychiatry in the general hospital. **Gen Hosp Psychiatry** 1981 Dec;3(4):289–91
Kramer ES: The history of art therapy in a large mental hospital. **Am J Art Ther** 1982 Apr;21(3):75–84
Lively CE: Reminiscences of a state mental hospital attendant. **Indiana Med Hist Q** 1983 Mar;9(1):13–22
McFarlane W: Beyond bedlam. **Work Pap Mag** 1982;9(2):10–4
McGovern CM: Doctors or ladies? Women physicians in psychiatric institutions, 1872–1900. **Bull Hist Med** 1981 Spring;55(1):88–107
Mancin S: Days of darkness and hope at the State Hospital: a photographer's perspective. **RI Hist** 1982;41(4):139–41
Massad PM, Sales BD: Guardianship: an acceptable alternative to institutionalization? **Am Behav Sci** 1981;24(6):755–70
Menninger WC: The Menninger Hospitals' Guide to the Order Sheet. **Bull Menninger Clin** 1982 Jan;46(1):1–112
Moore C, Winer JL: Dr. Peterson E. Harrison: pioneer traiblazer for mental health in West Texas. **West Tex Hist Assoc Yearb** 1979;55:49–58
Origins of the State Mental Hospital in America: Reprints of six studies, 1837–1856. New York, Arno Press, 1973. Various pagings.
Pitts JA: The Association of Medical Superintendents of American Institutions for the Insane, 1844–1892: a case study of specialism in American medicine. Ph.F. diss. University of Pennsylvania. Philadelphia, 1979. 267 leaves.
Robison DW: Wisconsin and the mentally ill. A history of the 'Wisconsin Plan' of state and county care 1860–1915. New York, Arno Press, 1980. ix, 322 p. (Historical Issues in Mental Health).
Rochefort DA: Three centuries of care of the mentally disabled in Rhode Island and the nation, 1650–1950. **RI Hist** 1981;40(4):110–32
Rome HP: The troubled world of the psychiatric hospital: the deinstitutionalization problem. **J Natl Assoc Priv Psychiatr Hosp** 1977;9(2):4–13
Rosenkrantz BG: Booby-hatch of booby-trap: a new look at nineteenth-century reform. **Soc Res (NY)** 1972;39(4):733–43
Rosenkrantz BG, Vinovskis MA: Sustaining 'the flickering flame of life': accountability and culpability for death in ante-bellum Massachusetts asylums. In Reverby S, Rosner D, ed: Health care in America. Philadelphia, Temple University Press, p. 155–82.
Rothman DJ: Conscience and convenience. The asylum and its alternatives in progressive America. Boston, Toronto, Little, Brown and Company, 1980. xii, 464 p.
Rothman DJ: The limits of benevolence. **Soc Policy** 1981;12(1):24–8, 37–8
Scull A: A new trade in lunacy: the recommodification of the mental patient. **Am Behav Sci** 1981;24(6):741–54
Scull A: Deinstitutionalization and the rights of the deviant. **J Soc Issues** 1981;37(3):6–20
Sigelman L, Roeder PW, Sigelman CK: Social service innovation in the American states: deinstitutionalization of the mentally retarded. **Soc Sci Q** 1982;62(3):503–15
Smith TG: Detaining the insane: detention hospitals, mental health, and frontier politics in Alaska, 1910–1915. **Pac Northwest Q** 1982;73(3):124–33
Stratton R: The Cherokee National Insane Asylum. **Bull Menninger Clin** 1983 May;47(3):266–8
Tashima N: Asian Americans in psychiatric systems. **Explor Ethnic Stud** 1979;2(1):11–21
Taylor SJ, Bogdan R: Defending illusions: the institution's struggle for survival. **Hum Organ** 1980;39(3):209–18
Ward's Island--a hospital of yesterday: **Psychiatr News** 1979 Mar 16;14(6):4–5
Warren CA: New forms of social control: the myth of deinstitutionalization. **Am Behav Sci** 1981;24(6):724–40
Wells LA: Rural psychiatry on the nineteenth-century frontier: the career of Jacob Bowers. **Perspect Biol Med** 1981 Winter;24(2):270–81
Willis FN, Dean LM, Larsen L: The first mental hospital for American Indians, 1900–1934. **Bull Menninger Clin** 1981 Mar;45(2):149–54
Winkleman M: Institutional retreat. **NY Aff** 1980;6(3):80–3

### USSR

Brown JV: The professionalization of Russian psychiatry: 1857–1911. Ph.D. Diss., Univ. of Pennsylvania. Philadelphia, 1981. 431 p.
Gladkikh PF: Rabota psikhiatricheskikh uchrezhdeniĭ v Leningrade vo vremia blokady. **Zh Nevropatol Psikhiatr** 1980;80(5):760–1
Green D: The Medvedev experience: 1984 and medicine. **Perspect Biol Med** 1976 Autumn;20(1):145–55
Khokhlov LK, Shipov VL: K 200-letiiu Iaroslavskoĭ oblastnoĭ psikhiatricheskoĭ klinicheskoĭ bol'nitsy. **Zh Nevropatol Psikhiatr** 1980;80(9):1393
Popushoĭ EP, Andrievskiĭ VA: Iz istorii sozdaniia Kostiuzhenskoĭ psikhiatricheskoĭ lechebnitsy. **Sov Zdravookhr** 1984;(9):65–6
Reich W: The case of General Grigorenko: a second opinion. **Encounter (Lond)** 1980;54(4):9–24
Saarma IuM: 100-letie kafedry i kliniki psikhiatrii v Tartu. **Zh Nevropatol Psikhiatr** 1981;81(11):1716–20
Sotskov VG: Ot kolonii dlia dushevnobol'nykh k oblastnoĭ psikhiatricheskoĭ bol'nitse (k 100-letiiu Psikhiatricheskoĭ bol'nitsy im. M. P. Litvinova). **Zh Nevropatol Psikhiatr** 1984;84(5):771–3
Tyklina IG, Vol'f MSh: Iz istorii Moskovskoĭ gorodskoĭ klinicheskoĭ psikhiatricheskoĭ bol'nitsy im. P. B. Gannushkina. **Med Sestra** 1984 Jul;43(7):45–6
Vlasova NA, Mokrovskaia AA: 50 let dnevnomu logopedicheskomu polustatsionaru pri detskoĭ psikhiatricheskoĭ bol'nitse No. 6. **Zh Nevropatol Psikhiatr** 1980;80(10):1552–3

### Yugoslavia

Bešlin M: 30 godina neuropsyhijatrijske bolnice 'Dr Slavoljub Bakalović' Vršac. **Med Pregl** 1984;37(1–2):71–4

## HUMAN DEVELOPMENT AND GROWTH

See also **Child Health; Gerontology**

Bastenie PA: Le vieillissement. Vers une nouvelle source de jeunesse. Paris, Flammarion, 1983. 270 p. (De La Science à l'Homme).
Boyd E, Scammon RE: Origins of the study of human growth. Ed. Savara BS, Schilke JF. [Eugene], University of Oregon Health Sciences Center Foundation, 1980. 676 p.
Fox VC, Quitt MH, ed: Loving, parenting and dying: the family cycle in England and America, past and present. New York, Psychohistory

Press, 1980. v, 488 p. Includes original essays by the editors, by M. A. Glendon, and A. Macfarlane. Also includes numerous previously published articles by various other authors.
Grimm H: Zur historischen Vertiefung der Akzelerationsforschung. **Aerztl Jugendkd** 1982;73(3):182–93
Imbault-Huart MJ: La vieillesse: état pathologique ou ultime equilibre de vie? **Asclepio** 1983;35:301–15
Jeggle U: Lebensalter und Körpererleben. In Imhof AE, ed: Leib und Leben in der Geschichte der Neuzeit. Berlin, Duncker & Humblot, 1983. p. 89–102.
Martorell R: Notes on the history of nutritional anthropometry. **Fed Proc** 1981 Sep;40(11):2572–6
Tanner JM: A history of the study of human growth. Cambridge, New York, Cambridge University Press, 1981. 499 p.
Valdiserri RO: Menstruation and medical theory: an historical overview. **J Am Med Wom Assoc** 1983 May–Jun;38(3):66–70
Wilbush J: La menespausie---the birth of a syndrome. **Maturitas** 1979;1(3):145–51

**France**

Flandrin JL: Repression and change in sexual life of young people in medieval and early modern times. In R. Wheaton, T. K. Hareven, ed: Family and sexuality in French history. Philadelphia. University of Pennsylvania Press, 1980. p. 27–48.

**India**

Bhattacharyya NN: Indian puberty rites. Second edition, revised and enlarged. New Delhi, Munshiram Manoharlal, 1980. 124 p.

**Japan**

Inoue N: [Historical view of maxilofacial development] (Jpn). **Nippon Shika Ishikai Zasshi** 1982;35(7):743–8

**Netherlands**

Maat GJ: Boerhaave en zijn tijdgenoten, en de betekenis van hun lichaamslengte (een fysisch-antropologisch onderzoek van begravenen in de Pieterskerk te Leiden). **Ned Tijdschr Geneeskd** 1982 Apr 17;126(16):705–12

### Before 500 A.D.

Bonneau E, Moreau R, Vaillant JM: Notions de craniométrie anthropologique. **Actual Odontostomatol (Paris)** 1983 Jun;142:319–40

**Europe**

Grimm H: Weibliche Figurinen als Zeugnisse vorgeschichtlicher Jugendweihe-Riten? **Aerztl Jugendkd** 1982 Mar;73(1):40–3

**Greco-Roman**

Sandyk R: Brain development and the phylogenesis of writing and drawing direction. **S Afr Med J** 1982 Jul 10;62(2):43–4

**India**

Datta B, Gupta D: The age of menarche in classical India. **Ann Hum Biol** 1981 Jul;8(4):351–9

**Jordan**

Röhrer-Ertl O: Ein Beitrag zur historischen Vertiefung der Akzelerationsforschung: Längenwachstumsänderungen in einer Population vom Tell es Sultan/Jericho aus dem Präkeramischen Neolithikum (ca. 9000–6000 v. Chr.). **Arztl Jugendkd** 1984 Oct,75(5).292–302

### 500 A.D.–1450

Cadden J: The medieval philosophy and biology of growth: Albertus Magnus, Thomas Aquinas, Albert of Saxony and Masilius of Inghen on Book I, Chapter V, of Aristotle's 'De generatione et corruptione.' With translated texts of Albertus Magnus and Thomas Aquinas. Ph. D. Diss. Indiana University. Bloomington, 1971. vii, 267 leaves.

**Hungary**

Pantó E: Wachstum und Reifung der Stadtkinder in Abhängigkeit von soziodemographischen Faktoren. **Anthropol Anz** 1982 Mar;40(1):33–44

### 1450–1700

**Great Britain**

Teigen KH: A note on the origin of the term 'nature and nurture': not Shakespeare and Galton, but Mulcaster. **J Hist Behav Sci** 1984 Oct;20(4):363–4

### 1700 to Present

Beall CM: An historical perspective on studies of human growth and development in extreme environments. In F. Spencer, ed: A history of American physical anthropology, 1930–1980. New York, Academic Press, 1982. p. 447–65.
Cavanaugh JC: Early developmental theories: a brief review of attempts to organize developmental data prior to 1925. **J Hist Behav Sci** 1981 Jan;17(1):38–47
Garn SM: The growth of growth. **Am J Phys Anthropol** 1981 Dec;56(4):521–30
Grimm H: Carl Heinrich Stratz (1858 bis 1924) als Mitbegründer einer ärztlichen Jugendkunde. Zeittafeln zu seinem Leben und seiner Wirksamkeit. **Aerztl Jugendkd** 1979 Jun;70(3):177–92
Lomax EM, Kagan J, Rosenkrantz BG: Science and patterns of child care. San Francisco, W. H. Freeman, 1978. xiv, 247 p.
Meredith HV, Spurgeon JH, Meredith EM: Early seriatim research on human somatic growth. **Growth** 1981 Autumn;45(3):151–67
Stechel RH: Height and per capita income. **Hist Methods** 1983;16(1):1–7

**Australia**

Nicholas S, Shergold PR: The heights of British male convict children transported to Australia, 1825–1840. **Aust Paediatr J** 1982 Jun;18(2):76–83

**Austria**

Roazen P: The menopause. By Helene Deutsch. **Int J Psychoanal** 1984;65(Pt 1):55–62

**Belgium**

Watkins SC, McCarthy J: The female life cycle in a Belgian commune: La Hulpe, 1847–1866. **J Fam Hist** 1980 Summer;5(2):167–79

**Canada**

Siegel LS: Child health and development in English Canada, 1790–1850. In Roland CG, ed: Health, disease and medicine. Toronto, Hannah Institute for the History of Medicine, 1984. p. 360–80.

**France**

Schmid-Kitsikis E: Un certain regard sur l'oeuvre de N. Galifret-Granjon. **Psychiatr Enfant** 1984;27(1):35–48
Shorter E: L'âge des premières règles en France, 1750–1950. **Ann Econ Soc Civilis** 1981;36(3):495–511

**Germany**

Petschauer P: Growing up female in eighteenth-century Germany. **J Psychohist** 1983 Fall;11(2):167–207

**Great Britain**

C[one] TE: Jeremy Bentham's list of data needed to understand the growth and development of children (1797). **Pediatrics** 1981;68:447
Cameron N: The growth of London schoolchildren 1904–1966: an analysis of secular trend and intra-county variation. **Ann Hum Biol** 1979 Nov–Dec;6(6):505–25
Jordan TE: Lancashire lasses and Yorkshire lads: childhood in the early nineteenth century. **R Soc Health J** 1982 Feb,102(1).14–20
Wilbush J: Historical perspective: Tilt, E. J. and the change of life (1857)--the only work on the subject in the English language. **Maturitas** 1980 Dec;2(4):259–67

**Ireland**

Relethford JH, Lees FC: The effects of aging and secular trend on adult stature in rural western Ireland. **Am J Phys Anthropol** 1981;55(1):81–8

**Poland**

Supady J: Wpływ wychowania i nauczania domowego oraz szkolnego na psychofizyczny rozwój młodzieży szlacheckiej w Polsce w XVIII w. **Wiad Lek** 1981 May 1;34(9):789–98

## HUMAN DEVELOPMENT AND GROWTH

**Sweden**

Sandberg LG, Steckel RH: Soldier, soldier, what made you grow so tall? A study of height, health and nutrition in Sweden, 1720–1881. **Econ Hist (Sweden)** 1980;23(2):91–105

**Switzerland**

Staude JR: The adult development of C. G. Jung. Boston, Routledge & Kegan Paul, 1981. xxiv, 134 p.

**Trinidad**

Friedman GC: The heights of slaves in Trinidad. **Soc Sci Hist** 1982;6(4):482–515

**United States**

Chudacoff HP: The life course of women: age and age consciousness, 1865–1915. **J Fam Hist** 1980 Fall;5(3):274–92
Fogel RW, Engerman SL, Trussell J: Exploring the uses of data on height: the analysis of long-term trends in nutrition, labor welfare, and labor productivity. **Soc Sci Hist** 1982;6(4):401–21
Kett JF: Rites of passage. Adolescence in America, 1790 to the present. New York, Basic Books, 1977. ix, 327 p.
Margo RA, Steckel RH: Heights of native-born whites during the antebellum period. **J Econ Hist** 1983;43(1):167–74
Margo RA, Steckel RH: The heights of American slaves: new evidence on slave nutrition and health. **Soc Sci Hist** 1982;6(4):516–38
Powers MN: Menstruation and reproduction: an Oglala case. **Signs** 1980;6(1):54–65
Rhodes SL: Trends in child development research important to day-care policy. **Soc Serv Rev** 1979;53(2):285–94
Sokoloff KL, Villaflor GC: The early achievement of modern stature in America. **Soc Sci Hist** 1982;6(4):453–82
Steckel RH: Slave height profiles from coastwise manifests. **Explor Econ Hist** 1979;16(4):363–80
Wilbush J: Climacteric symptom formation: Donovan's contribution. **Maturitas** 1981 Aug;3(2):99–105

## HYGIENE

See also **Preventive Medicine; Public Health; Sanitation**

Bernard M, Pociello C, Vigarello G: Itinéraire d'un concept. **Esprit** 1975;(5):704–23
Borms J, Hebbelinck M, Venerando A, ed: Women and sport: an historical, biological, physiological and sportsmedical approach. Basel, Karger, 1981. 229 p. (Medicine and sport, Vol. 14)
Engelhardt HT: Philosophical perspectives [of health and disease]. In Reich WT, et al, ed: Encyclopedia of bioethics, v. 2. New York, Free Press, 1978. p. 599–605.
Fan CC: T'i yü ti li shih. **Shih-ta Hsüeh-pao** 1977;22:417–40
Ferenczy M: Izzasztó fürdök és testedzés otthon. **Orv Hetil** 1983 Mar 20;124(12):713–4
Golding PS: The development of the toothbrush. A short history of tooth cleansing. Part 1. **Dent Health (London)** 1982;21(4):25–7
Hoppe B: Arbeit und Gesundheit; historische Aspekte ihrer gegenseitigen Beziehungen. Bericht über eine Tagung der 'International School of History of Biological Sciences' in Ischia/Neapel vom 29. Juni bis 12. Juli 1980. **Ber Wissenschaftsgesch** 1980;3(3–4):214–20
Howell R: Women and sport: an historical overview. In Borms J, Hebbelinck M, Venerando A, ed: Women and sport. Basel, Karger, 1981. p. 11–5.
Imhof AE: Mensch und Gesundheit in Geschichte und Gegenwart. **Jahrb Gesch** 1979;1(3):29–33
Janssen G: L'ingénieur hygiéniste à l'hôpital. **Soins** 1982 Jun;(384):29–30
Kneist W: Rauchen oder Gesundheit. Ein kulturhistorischer Rückblick. **Z Gesamte Hyg** 1981;27(6):477–80
Laín Entralgo P: Being healthy down through history. In Seidler E, Schott H, ed: Bausteine zur Medizingeschichte. Stuttgart, Steiner, 1984. p. 65–72.
Lukas G: Der Beitrag des Sports zur Persönlichkeitsentwicklung unter Berücksichtigung historischer Aspekte. **Wiss Z Martin Luther Univ (Sprachw)** 1975;24(3):29–35
Pickering MJ: A history of elderly exercises. **J Fla Med Assoc** 1980 Apr;67(4):398–400
Rechtman J: De la brosse à dents à la brosse à bouche. **Soc Fr Hist Art Dent** 1979 Mar–Jun;(3–4):23–8
Rechtman J: La brosse à dents et son histoire (1780–1980). **Hist Sci Med** 1980;14(2):221–5
Risse GB: History of the concepts [of health and disease]. In Reich WT, et al, ed: Encyclopedia of bioethics, v. 2. New York, Free Press, 1978. p. 579–85.
Russell HM, Weinberg J, ed: The book of knowledge from the Mishnah Torah of Maimonides. Translated from the Hebrew. Edinburgh, Royal College of Physicians of Edinburgh, 1981. xi, 135 p. (Publication No. 55).
Smith RD: Tribute to Avicenna: one thousand years of the art of preserving health. **J Kans Med Soc** 1981;82:359–60, 372

**China**

Fan Chêng-chih: Chung-kuo t'i-yu ti shih-hsueh Yan-chiu. **Shih-ta Hsueh-pao** 1981;26:117–58
Stiefvater EW, Stiefvater IR: Chinesische Atemlehre und Gymnastik. 2. Auflage. Heidelberg, Haug, 1980. 121 p.

**Egypt**

Badr SM: Women and sports in Egypt: history and problems. In Borms J, Hebbelinck M, Venerando A, ed: Women and sport. Basel, Karger, 1981. p. 45–51.

**France**

Arnaud P: Le Corps en mouvement: précurseurs et pionniers de l'éducation physique. Toulouse, Privat, 1981. 314 p.
Leuilliot P: Problèmes de méthode: histoire (et archives) de la santé. In Livet G, Schaff G, ed: Médecine et assistance en Alsace, XVIe–XXe siècle. Strasbourg, Istra, 1976. p. 11–17.
Vigarello G: L'eau: Un imaginaire pédagogique dans la médecine des enfants aux XVIe–XVIIe et XVIIIe siècles. **Hist Philos Life Sci** 1981;3(2):171–91

**Germany**

Schwarz M: Psychohygienische Verhaltensgebote für schwangere Frauen in medizinischen Ratgebergüchern. Frankfurt am Main, Haag Herchen, 1983. iv, 382 p.

**India**

Rama Rao B: Bath in Ayurveda, Yoga and Dharmashastra. **Bull Indian Inst Hist Med Hyderabad** 1982;12(1–4):13–21
Rama Rao B: Water and usahpana in ayurvedic literature. **Bull Indian Inst Hist Med (Hyderabad)** 1980;10(1–4):1–6
Sitharamiah A: Outline of history of Yoga. **Bull Indian Inst Hist Med (Hyderabad)** 1980;10(1–4):15–22
Tabor DC: Ripe and unripe: concepts of health and sickness in Ayurvedic medicine. **Soc Sci Med** 1981;15B:439–55
Venkat Rao B: Development of naturopathy in Andhra Pradesh. **Bull Indian Inst Hist Med (Hyderabad)** 1979;9:41–5
Venkata Reddy M, Rama Rao B: A note on Kriya Yoga. **Bull Indian Inst Hist Med (Hyderabad)** 1980;10(1–4):69–75

**Italy**

Caffaratto A: Storia della legislazione sanitaria ed igienica in Piemonte da Amedeo VIII all'Unità d'Italia. Parte III. **Minerva Med** 1979 Dec 1;70(54):3729–43

**Japan**

Homma K: On the toothpick. In International Congress of the History of Medicine. 26th, Plovdiv, 1978. Actes du Congress. Sofia, 1981. Volume II. p. 111–4.
Seiwa H: An outline of the history of women and western sport in Japan. In Borms J, Hebbelinck M, Venerando A, ed: Women and sport. Basel, Karger, 1981. p. 52–7.

**Poland**

Kuchowicz Z: Jeszcze o zdrowiu in niezdrowiu magnatów XVII–XVIII W. **Kwart Hist** 1970;77(2):394–403

**United States**

Henderson RW, ed: Early American sport: a checklist of books by American and foreign authors published prior to 1860, including sporting songs. Third edition revised and enlarged. Rutherford, New Jersey, Fairleigh Dickinson University Press, 1977. 309 p.
Kimble C, et al: Health in America. **Wilson Q** 1980 Spring;:60–101
Leavitt JW, ed: Women and health in America: historical readings. Madison, University of Wisconsin Press, 1984. ix, 526 p. (Previously published articles by various authors)
Spears B, Swanson RA: History of sport and physical activity in the United States. Ed. E. T. Smith. Dubuque, Iowa, Wm. C. Brown, 1978. xii, 402 p.
Struna NL: Sport and colonial education: a cultural perspective. **Res Q Exerc Sport** 1981 Mar;52(1):117–35

## Before 500 A.D.

### Egypt

Diener L: Hygieniska förhållanden i det faraoniska Egypten. **Nord Medicinhist Arsb** 1982;:41–55

### Greece

Byl S: Note sur huit recentiores du livre IV Du régime. **Rev Philol (Paris)** 1978;52:37–49
Lämmer M: Women and sport in ancient Greece; a plea for a critical and objective approach. In Borms J, Hebbelinck M, Venerando A, ed: Women and sport. Basel, Karger, 1981. p. 16–23.

## 500 A.D.–1450

Pack RA ed: Pseudo-Aristotelis Epistola ad Alexandrum der regimine sanitatis a quodam Nicolao versificata. **Arch Hist Doctrinale Litt Moyen Age** 1978;53:307–25

### Arabic

Aroua A: L'hygiène et la prevention chez Ibn Sina. **Tunis Med** 1980 Jul–Aug;58(4):556–61
Atabaev ShT, Babakhodzhaev NK, Il'inskiĭ II: Gigiencheskie vzgliady Abu Ali ibn-Siny (k 1000-letiiu so dnia rozhdeniia). **Gig Sanit** 1979 Dec;(12):36–40
Bano M, Ali MI: Cosmetics according to Avicenna. **Bull Indian Inst Hist Med (Hyderabad)** 1981;1–4:110–7
Elkhadem H: Une nouvelle conception de l'hygiène et de la diététique au XIe siècle. **Technologia** 1982;5(3–4):61–73
Moshkov VA: Abu Ali Ibn-Sina (Avitsenna) o fizicheskikh uprazhneniiakh i massazhe. **Vopr Kurortol Fizioter Lech Fiz Kult** 1981 Jan–Feb;(1):66–7
Nassimi MN: The achievements of the Arab Prophet in the field of hygiene and preventive medicine. In: International Symposium for the History of Arabic Science, 1st, University of Aleppo, 1976. Proceedings. Aleppo, Syria, 1976. Papers in European Languages. Vol. II. p. 343–5.
Schipperges H: Grundmuster und Richtlinien arabischer Diätetik. In Dilg P, et al., ed: Perspektiven der Pharmaziegeschichte. Graz, Austria, Akademische Druck- u. Verlagsanstalt, 1983. p. 295–309.

### India

Rama Rao B, Reddy MV: A note on Goraksanātha and his work Yogadipikā. **Bull Indian Inst Hist Med Hyderabad** 1982;12(1–4):34–44

### Iran

Namigohar F, Soltani A: L'hygiène en Iran au temps d'Achemèdes. In International Congress of the History of Medicine. 26th, Plovdiv, 1978. Actes du Congress. Sofia, 1981. Volume II. p. 160–1.

### Italy

Marangon P: Il trattato 'De conservatione sanitatis' di Zanbonino da Gazzo (d. dopo il 1298). **Quad Stor Univ Padova** 1975;8:1–17

### Mexico

Prygova NM: Sanitariia i gigiena v atsteksom obshchestve (k istorii sanitarii i gigieny v Meksike). **Gig Sanit** 1981 Aug;(8):54–6

### Spain

Paniagua Arellano JA, Arnau de Vilanova: El maravilloso regimiento y orden de vivir (una versión castellana del Regimen sanitatis ad regem Aragonum). **Cuad Aragon Hist Med Cienc (B)** 1980;3:1–106

## 1450–1700

English EB: Women and sport during the Renaissance. In Borms J, Hebbelinck M, Venerando A, ed: Women and sport. Basel, Karger, 1981. p. 24–30.

### Europe

Hakulinen E: Hälsoråd till tidigare resenärer. **Nord Med** 1984;99(10):266–7
Schienbein G, Schienbein H: 'Der Zähn stincken verbessern'--Zahnheilkunde in einem Kräuterbuch von 1602 (I, II). **Quintessenz** 1980 Jun–Jul;31(6,7):133–40, 165–70

### Germany

Grasshoff K: Leibesübungen und Gesellschaft im Gemälde 'Melancolia 1558' des Mathias Gerung. **Stadion** 1977;3(1):44–59

### Great Britain

Bowman IA: Thomas Cogan on studying. **Bookman** 1980 Feb;7(2):5–10

### Mexico

Thiemer-Sachse U: Hygiene und Heilkunde bei den Azteca zur Zeit der spanischen Eroberung. **Abh Ber Staatl Mus Voelkerkd Dres** 1978;36:151–213

## 1700 to Present

Als Aerzte den Modeschöpfern ins Handwerk pfuschten: **MMW** 1980 Feb 1;122(5):56–7
Atkinson P: Fitness, feminism and schooling. In Sara Delamont, Lorna Duffin ed: The 19th-century woman: her cultural and physical world. London, Croom Helm, New York, Barnes & Noble, 1978. p. 92–133
Birtalan G: Személyi egeszségvédelem és mentálhygiéne a 18. században. **Orv Hetil** 1982 Mar 7;123(10):607–10
Crellin JK: Internal antisepsis or the dawn of chemotherapy? **J Hist Med Allied Sci** 1981 Jan;36(1):9–18
Eichberg H: Leistung zwischen Wänden--Die sportive Parzellierung der Körper. In Imhof AE, ed: Leib und Leben in der Geschichte der Neuzeit. Berlin, Duncker & Humblot, 1983. p. 119–39.
Emslie RD: A history of oral hygiene measures. **Community Dent Oral Epidemiol** 1980;8(5):225–9
Gold SI: Early origins of hydrogen peroxide use in oral hygiene. A historical note. **J Periodontol** 1983 Apr;54(4):247
Greene VW: Cleanliness and the health revolution. New York, Soap and Detergent Association, 1984. vii, 68 p.
Hannaway C: From private hygiene to public health: a transformation in Western medicine in the eighteenth and nineteenth centuries. In Ogawa T, ed: Public health. Tokyo, Saikon, 1981. p. 108–28.
Heller G: Idéologie et rituels de la propreté aux XIXe et XXe siècles. In Imhof AE, ed: Leib und Leben in der Geschichte der Neuzeit. Berlin, Duncker & Humblot, 1983. p. 193–202.
Helöe LA, Haugejorden O: 'The rise and fall' of dental caries: some global aspects of dental caries epidemiology. **Community Dent Oral Epidemiol** 1981 Dec;9(6):294–9
Jones IH: Menstruation: the history of sanitary protection. **Nurs Times** 1980 Mar 6;76(10):407–8
Jörgensen G: Spiel und Sport aus genetisch-phylogenetischer Sicht. **MMW** 1981 Jun 19;123(25):1039–42
Money J: The genealogical descent of sexual psychoneuroendocrinology from sex and health theory: the eighteenth to the twentieth centuries. **Psychoneuroendocrinology** 1983;8(4):391–400
Pankey LD: Evolution of a philosophy. **Continuum** 1980;:1–9
Rechtman J: De la brosse à dents à la brosse à bouche: deux siècles d'histoire (1780–1977). **Pedod Fr** 1978;12:299–311
Sandler B: An unpalatable but popular gargle. **MIMS Mag** 1981 Jun 15;:59
Schmid R, Barbakow F, Mühlemann H, et al: Amine fluoride and monofluorophosphate: I. Historical review of fluoride dentifrices. **ASDC J Dent Child** 1984 Mar–Apr;51(2):99–103
Seidler E: Die Naturheilkundebewegung, ihre Systeme und Motive. In Dilg P, et al., ed: Perspektiven der Pharmaziegeschichte. Graz, Austria, Akademische Druck- u. Verlagsanstalt, 1983. p. 331–41.
Simri U: Development of women's sport in the 20th century. In Borms J, Hebbelinck M, Venerando A, ed: Women and sport. Basel, Karger, 1981. p. 31–44.
Woodward J: The school medical officer 1880–1914. **Soc Soc Hist Med Bull (Lond)** 1980;27:30–1

### Australia

Anderson DA: Dental health services and the Northern Territory of Australia. A short review of people, places, and programmes to 1981. **Aust Dent J** 1982 Dec;27(6):345–51
Jobling IF: The 'sporty' Australians: women and sport in Australian history. In Borms J, Hebbelinck M, Venerando A, ed: Women and sport. Basel, Karger, 1981. p. 66–72.

### Austria

Wyklicky H: 175 Jahre Hygiene an Oesterreichs Universitäten. **Zentralbl Bakteriol [B]** 1981;172(6):441–53

### Barbados

Phillips GO: Barbados' Battle Creek doctor Charles J. B. Cave 1879–1939. **Advent Herit** 1978;5(2):22–33

### Canada

Fitness for Canadians 1909–1983: **Can J Public Health** 1983 May–Jun;74 Suppl 1:1–45
Gregory CJ: Elfrida K. Berzins: world record holder, olympic athlete, concert soloist, author, and pioneer physical educator.

Can J Hist Sport Phys Educ 1979;10(2):1-14
Lenskyj H: Femininity first, sport and physical education for Ontario girls, 1890-1930. **Can J Hist Sport Phy Educ** 1982;13(2):4-17

**Czechoslovakia**

Horák J, Chrástek J, Novotný V, et al: 30 let práce Ustavu tělovýchovného lékařství fakulty všeobecného lékařství University Karlovy v Praze. **Sb Lek** 1980 Jan;82(1):30-2
Müller C, Niklícek L: Třicet let lékařské fakulty hygienické Univerzity Karlovy. **Cesk Zdrav** 1982 Oct;30(10):402-7

**France**

Fagot A: La philosophie de l'hygiène en 1878. In Poirier J, Poirier JL, ed: Médecine et philosophie à la fin du XIXe siècle. Paris, Université de Paris XII - Val de Marne, [1980?]. p. 61-84.
Guerrand RH: L'âge d'or du bidet. **Histoire** 1983;(57):84-7
Major V: Live in peace and joy. In: Congrès international d'histoire de la médecine, XXVe, Québec, 1976. Actes. Québec, 1977. p. 944-50.
Nye RA: Degeneration, hygiene and sports in fin-de-siècle France. **Proc Annu Meet West Soc Fr Hist** 1980;8:404-12
Quevauviller A: L'hygiène au XVIIIe siècle d'après l'abbé Jacquin. **Rev Hist Pharm (Paris)** 1980 Mar;27(244):24-38
Spivak M: Pour une approche renouvelée de l'histoire de l'éducation physique et du sport. **Hist Educ (France)** 1981;10:21-32
Spivak M: Quelques aperçus de la recherche en histoire de l'éducation physique et des sports en France. **Hist Educ (France)** 1981;10:1-19
Thibault J: Un accouchement laborieux. **Esprit** 1975;(5):696-703
Zabludovskiĭ PE: K 200-letiiu knigi 'Nastavlenie narodu v rassuzhdenii ego zdorov'ia'. **Feldsher Akush** 1982;47(4):52-3

**Germany**

Dietsch H: Die Altershygiene Kants. **Med Welt** 1982 Apr 16;33(15):570-2
Dortmund EK: Daniel Paul Schreber: a case study of private fate as public possibility. **Res Stud** 1978;46(3):141-55
Haase HH: Max von Pettenkofer--einige Gedanken zu Leben, Werk und Hinterlassenschaft. **Z Gesamte Hyg** 1980;26(10):697-9
Haase HH: Uber einige Auswirkungen Robert Kochs und seiner Lehre auf die Entwicklung der Allgemeinen und Kommunalen Hygiene. **Z Gesamte Hyg** 1982 Mar;28(3):154-6
Hiepe T, Odening K, Vater G: Georg Wildführ sen. zum 80. Geburtstag. **Angew Parasitol** 1984 Aug;25(3):117-20
Horn H, Winkler H: 25 Jahre Institut für Allgemeine Hygiene der Medizinischen Akademie Erfurt. **Z Gesamte Hyg** 1984 Sep;30(9):529-30
Kaufmann E: Gustav Jaeger, 1832-1917, Arzt, Zoologe und Hygieniker. Zürich, Juris, 1984. 67 p. (Zürcher Medizingeschichtliche Abhandlungen, Neue Reihe, 171)
Knorr M: 1883-1983. Gedanken zum Jubiläumsband 177. **Zentralbl Bakteriol Mikrobiol Hyg [B]** 1983 Jan;177(1-2):i-iv
Lukas G: Der Neuhumanismus in seiner Stellung zur Körpererziehung. **Wiss Z Martin Luther Univ (Sprachw)** 1978;27(1):47-54
Mader G: Studien zur Gesundheitsbildung und Ordnungslehre bei Sebastian Kneipp: ein Beitrag zur Frage 'machbarer' Gesundheit. Frankfurt am Main, Haag + Herchen, 1984. 198, 49 p.
Nabielek R: Robert Koch und die Begründung des Lehrstuhls für Hygiene an der Berliner Universität. **Z Gesamte Hyg** 1982 Mar;28(3):185-93
Opitz R, Horn H, Heinecke P, et al: Robert Koch. Die Vorgeschichte der Berufung als ersten Ordinarius für Hygiene an die Universität Berlin. **MMW** 1981 Oct 16;123(42):1593-5
Pfister G: The influence of women doctors on the origins of women's sports in Germany. In Borms J, Hebbelinck M, Venerando A, ed: Women and sport. Basel, Karger, 1981. p. 58-65.
Scherrer RM: Friedrich Hoffmanns Anweisung zu gesundem langen Leben, verglichen mit Hufelands Makrobiotik. Zürich, Juris, 1984. 47 p. (Zürcher Medizingeschichtliche Abhandlungen, Neue Reihe, Nr. 170)
Uerckwitz J: Zur Geschichte der Hygiene an der Universität Rostock. **Z Gesamte Hyg** 1981 Jul 7;27(7):501-3

**Great Britain**

Charlton C: The National Health Society Almanack, 1883. **Local Popul Stud (Matlock)** 1984;32:54-7
Cooter R: Open-air therapy and the rise of open-air hospitals. **Soc Soc Hist Med Bull (Lond)** 1984 Dec;35:44-6
Gelbier S, Randall SB: Charles Edward Wallis and London's Toothbrush Clubs: 1909 style. **Dent Health (London)** 1982;21(1):12-5
Haley B: The healthy body and Victorian culture. Cambridge, Massachusetts, Harvard University Press, 1978. 296 p.
Kawakita Y: [Nightingale in the history of medical philosophy--on the meaning of 'health'] (Jpn). **Kango** 1982 Feb;34(2):39-53
Rechtman J: Un précurseur génial de la prévention et de la diététique, du bouche à bouche et du massage cardiaque externe de l'asepsie et parrain de J. P. Marat: Le docteur William Buchan (1729-1805). Diss. Paris VII, 1979. 115 p.
Reichart PA: Toothpastes containing betel nut (Areca catechu L.) from England of the nineteenth century. **J Hist Med Allied Sci** 1984 Jan;39(1):65-79
Smith G: The physiology of air: eighteenth-century fever therapy in the advice literature. **Soc Soc Hist Med Bull (Lond)** 1984 Dec;35:21-3
Thomson I: The origins of physical education in state schools. **Scott Educ Rev** 1978;10(2)
Winter JM: Military fitness and civilian health in Britain during the first World War. **J Contemp Hist** 1980;15(2):211-44

**India**

Ram R, Schultz TW: Life span, health, savings, and productivity. **Econ Dev Cult Change** 1979;27(3):399-421
Rosselli J: The self-image of effeteness: physical education and nationalism in nineteenth-century Bengal. **Past Present** 1980;86:121-48
Rosselli J: The self-image of effeteness: physical education and nationalism in nineteenth-century Bengal. **Past Present** 1980;(86):221-48

**Italy**

Caffaratto TM: Moda e medicina. **Minerva Ginecol** 1980 Sep;32(9):843-6
Cremona GF: Cenni sullo sviluppo della ginnastica educativa e medica in Italia. **Ann Osp Maria Vittoria Torino** 1981 Jan-Jun;24(1-6):210-6

**Japan**

Ono K, Yamada S: [Hygienic supplies for women used from the end of the Meiji era to the early Showa period: accounts by women who grew up in the Meiji period] (Jpn). **Josanpu Zasshi** 1983 Oct;37(10):819-27

**Poland**

Skrobacki A, Völker A: Lekarz olsztyński, Joachim Kornalewskiijego rozprawa o koltunie z 1897 roku. **Komun Mazursko Warm** 1980;(2):155-67

**Portugal**

De Maar FE: The toothpick carvers of Lorvao. **Bull Hist Dent** 1980 Apr;28(1):11-15

**Romania**

Brătescu G: Aerul, soarele şi apa în igiena populară. **Viata Med [Medii Sanit]** 1983 May;31(5):119-20

**Spain**

García Peña de Alexander M del P: Nota biográfica sobre el Doctor Francisco de Asís Pons i Freixa. In Congrés Internacional d'Historie de la Medicina Catalana, 1st, Barcelona-Montpellier, 1970. Barcelona, Editorial Scienta, 1971. v 4, p. 81-6.
Parellada i Feliu D: Comentaris al llibre 'Higiene del alma' del doctor Josep Call i Morros (editat a Barcelona l'any 1888). In Congrés International d'Història de la Medicina Catalana, 2nd, Barcelona, 1975. Llibre d'Actes. Barcelona, Socitra, 1977. p. 263-71.
Park RJ: The 'Enlightenment' in Spain: expressed concern for physical education in Spanish educational thought, 1765-1810. **Can J Hist Sport Phys Educ** 1978;9(2):1-19
Triadan H: Picasso--Pionier der Mundhygiene? **SSO Schweiz Monatsschr Zahnheilkd** 1983 Apr;93(4):250-1

**Sweden**

Burius A: Lings gymnastik och homeopatien. **Nord Medicinhist Arsb** 1980;:99-123
Janzon B: Idrott och ling-gymnastik i populär-medicinsk belysning. **Nord Medicinhist Arsb** 1980;:124-35

**Switzerland**

Burgener L: Pestalozzi et l'education physique. **Paedagog Hist** 1977;17(2):516-18
Godonnèche J: La dégradation de la santé des gens de lettres d'après Tissot. In: Congrès National des Sociétés Savantes, 99e, Besançon, 1974. Comptes Rendus. Paris, 1976. Section des Sciences, Fasc. V. p. 235-41.

**United States**

Berryman JW, Brislin J: The ladies' department of the American Farmer, 1825-1830. A locus for the advocacy of family health and exercise. **J NAL Assoc** 1977;2(2):8-15
Brodkey C, Gaydos JC: United States Army guidelines for troop living space: a historical review. **Milit Med** 1980 Jun;145(6):418-21
Bulger MA: American sportswomen in the 19th century. **J Pop Cult** 1982;16(2):1-16
Burnham JC: Change in the popularization of health in the United States.

**Bull Hist Med** 1984 Summer;58(2):183–97

Cohen S: The mental hygiene movement, the development of personality and the school: the medicalization of American education. **Hist Educ Q** 1983;23(2):123–49

Cutright P, Shorter E: The effects of health on the completed fertility of nonwhite and white U.S. women born from 1867 through 1935. **J Soc Hist** 1979;13(2):191–218

Damsteegt PG: Health reform and the Bible in early Sabbatarian Adventism. **Advent Herit** 1978;5(2):13–21

Dummett CO: Prevention began early: Charles Edwin Bentley, DDS 1859–1929. **J Natl Med Assoc** 1983 Dec;75(12):1235–6

Fox SD: Healing, imagination, and New Mexico. **NM Hist Rev** 1983;58(3):213–37

Fulton MW: Hartley D. Price: his contributions to physical education and gymnastics. Ph.D. Diss., Florida State University. Tallahassee, 1981. xvii, 171 leaves.

Gilbert B: The cry was: go west, young man, and stay healthy. **Smithsonian** 1983;13(12):138–49

Glassberg D: The design of reform: the public bath movement in America. **Am Stud** 1979;20(2):5–21

Kennard JA: The history of physical education. **Signs** 1977;2(4):835–42

Kent MC: A satirical interpretation of the history of selected persons, events and organizations in American physical education. Ed.D. Diss., University of North Carolina. Greensboro, 1981. vi, 266 p.

Langner SR, Innes C: Breathing, holism, and health. **Top Clin Nurs** 1980 Oct;2(3):1–10

McCue RJ: Did the word of wisdom become a commandment in 1851? **Dialogue J Mormon Thought** 1981;14(3):66–77

Michel D: Corps sauvages, corps étranges. **Dix–Huit Siecle** 1977;9:27–38

Millstein CB: W. D. Miller and the beginnings of occupational hygiene in dentistry. **Bull Hist Dent** 1984 Oct;32(2):135–6

Moerchel J: Simon Baruch (1840–1921) und die öffentliche Gesundheitspflege in New York. **Medizinhist J** 1982;17(1/2):138–47

Nightingale TW: A history of physical education, sport, recreation and amusement in Cincinnati, Ohio, in the nineteenth century. Ph.D. Diss., Ohio State University, Columbus, 1979. xi, 279 p.

Nissenbaum S: Sex, diet, and debility in Jacksonian America: Sylvester Graham and health reform. Westport, Connecticut, Greenwood, 1980. 198 p. (Contributions in Medical History, 4).

Park RJ: The research quarterly and its antecedents. **Res Q** 1980 Mar;51(1):1–22

Parry NA: Pioneers of physical education in the 19th century: Alexander Alexander. [1849–1928]. **Bull Hist Educ Soc** 1978;22:21–38

Penland L: A decade of dental health education: review of the 1970s. **Dent Hyg (Chic)** 1982 Sep;56(9):16–8, 20–2

Pennington G: Frederick Rand Rogers: educational provocateur (1894–1972). **Can J Hist Sport Phys Educ** 1981;12(1):24–50

Poirier S: The Weir Mitchell rest cure: doctor and patients. **Womens Stud** 1983;10(1):15–40

Remley ML: Jessie Hubbell Bancroft. In: Notable American women. The modern period. Cambridge, Mass., Belknap–Harvard Univ. Press, 1980. 4:46–7.

Rice CN: The history of the Society of State Directors of Health, physical education, and recreation, 1953–1976. Ed.D. Diss., University of Alabama. University, 1977. v, 199 p.

Ring ME: Oddments in dental history: down with toothbrushes - up with tobacco! **Bull Hist Dent** 1984;32(1):31–2

Rowthorn AW: A history of the evolution and development of therapeutic recreation services for special populations in the United States from 1918 to 1977. Ph.D. Diss. New York University. New York, 1978. 351 leaves.

Schleppi JR: 'It pays': John H. Patterson and industrial recreation at the National Cash Register Company. **J Sport Hist** 1979;6(3):20–8

Stewart TD: Responses of the human skeleton to changes in the quality of life. **J Forensic Sci** 1980 Oct;25(4):912–21

Thomas L: The right track. **Wilson Q** 1980;4(2):87–98

Twin SL: Ethel Perrin. In: Notable American women. The modern period. Cambridge, Mass., Belknap–Harvard Univ. Press, 1980. 4:539–41.

Verbrugge MH: Healthy animals and civic life: Sylvester Graham's physiology of subsistence. **Rev Am Hist** 1981;9(3):359–64

Verbrugge MH: The social meaning of personal health: The Ladies' Physiological Institute of Boston and vicinity in the 1850s. In Reverby S, Rosner D, ed: Health care in America. Philadelphia, Temple University Press, 1979. p. 45–66.

Vertinsky P: Sexual equality and the legacy of Catharine Beecher. **J Sport Hist** 1979;6(1):38–49

Weissman MB: Elizabeth Burchenal. In: Notable American women. The modern period. Cambridge, Mass., Belknap–Harvard Univ. Press, 1980. 4:121–2.

Whorton JC: 'Athlete's heart': the medical debate over athleticism, 1870–1920. **J Sport Hist** 1982;9(1):30–52

Whorton JC: 'Physiologic optimism': Horace Fletcher and hygienic ideology in progressive America. **Bull Hist Med** 1981 Spring;55(1):59–87

Williams MT: New York's public baths: a case study in urban progressive reform. **J Urban Hist** 1981;7(1):49–81

Wosh PJ: Sound minds and unsound bodies: Massachusetts schools and mandatory physical training. **N Engl Q** 1982;55(1):39–60

#### USSR

Belitskaia EIa: O sotsial–gigieniste A. V. Korchake–Chepurkovskom (K 125–letiiu so dnia rozhdeniia). **Sov Zdravookhr** 1982;(6):66–8

Borisenko NF, Slepushkina II, Proklina TL, et al: Stanovlenie i razvitie sanitarnoĭ sluzhby po gigiene deteĭ i podrostkov na Ukraine (1938–1945 gg.). **Gig Sanit** 1984 Aug;(8):44–8

Galin LL: Gotov k trudu i oborone SSSR (k 50–letiiu vvedeniia Vsesouiznogo fizkul'turnogo kompleksa). **Voen Med Zh** 1981 Jun;(6):75–6

Korol'kov AA: Iz istorii pervykh gigienicheskikh kafedr v Rossii. **Zdravookhr Ross Fed** 1980;(5):19–22

Ovsiannikov SI: Dokumenty orazvitii fizicheskoi kul'tury v krasnoi armii (1918–1919 gg). **Sov Arkh** 1977;4:73–8

Petrenko VS: Rozvytok fizychnoi kul'tury na seli USSR v 1951–1968. **Ukr Istor Zh** 1969;9:66–75

Rumiantsev GI, Korostelev NB: Osnovanie kafedry gigieny v Moskovskom universitete (K 100–letiiu kafedry). **Gig Sanit** 1984 Aug;(8):41–4

Shabunin AV: K 150–letiiu izdaniia truda R. S. Chetyrkina 'Opyt voenno–meditsinskoĭ politsii ili pravila k sokhraneniiu zdorov'ia russkikh soldat v sukhoputnoĭ sluzhbe'. **Gig Sanit** 1984 Jun;(6):35–6

Smirnov EI, Garin NS: Znachenie nauchnogo naslediia i deiatel'nosti Ia. L. Okunevskogo dlia sozdaniia dezinfektsionnogo i banno–prachechnogo dela v armii. **Voen Med Zh** 1979 Apr;(4):73–5

V. I. Lenin or razvitii fizicheskoĭ kul'tury i sporta: **Voen Med Zh** 1980 Mar;(3):8–10

## HYPNOSIS

Glowatzki G: Der Mesmerismus––und seine Spuren in der heutigen Medizin. **ZFA (Stuttgart)** 1983 Sep 10,59(25).1360–6

Shelley HS: The Moll Collection on hypnotism at Vanderbilt. **Bull Med Libr Assoc** 1977 Jan;65(1):65–6

Smith DB: The science of medicine and the art of hypnosis. **Pharos** 1980 Winter;43(1):6–9

Spanos NP, Gottlieb J: Demonic possession, mesmerism, and hysteria: a social psychological perspective on their historical interrelations. **J Abnorm Psychol** 88(5):527–46, Oct 79

### Before 500 A.D.

#### Greece

Machovec FJ: The cult of Asklipios. **Am J Clin Hypn** 1979 Oct;22(2):85–90

Stam HJ, Spanos NP: The Asclepian dream healings and hypnosis: a critique. **Int J Clin Exp Hypn** 1982 Jan;30(1):9–22

### 1700 to Present

Chertok L: Hypnosis and suggestion in a century of psychotherapy: an epistemological assessment. **J Am Acad Psychoanal** 1984 Apr;12(2):211–32

Chertok L, De Saussure R: The therapeutic revolution from Mesmer to Freud. New York, Brunner/Mazel, 1979. xiii, 226 p. Translation of French ed., 1973.

Conn JH: Nature of magnetic treatment. **J Am Soc Psychosom Dent Med** 1982;29(2):44–53

Gravitz MA: Bibliographic sources of nineteenth century hypnosis literature. **Am J Clin Hypn** 1981 Jan;23(3):217–9

Gravitz MA, Gerton MI: Freud and hypnosis: report of post–rejection use. **J Hist Behav Sci** 1981 Jan;17(1):68–74

Gravitz MA, Gerton MI: Origins of the term hypnotism prior to Braid. **Am J Clin Hypn** 1984 Oct;27(2):107–10

Hoffeld DR: Mesmer's failure: sex, politics, personality, and the Zeitgeist. **J Hist Behav Sci** 1980 Oct;16(4):377–86

Hypnotherapy––past, present and future: **Med J Aust** 1979 Sep 22;2(6):288

Kornfeld AD: Hypnosis and behavior therapy: historical relationships. **Int J Psychosom** 1984;31(2):22–6

Lesky E: Das Portrait: Franz Joseph Gall 1758–1828. **Med Unserer Zeit** 1980;4(2):57–61

Olness K: Hypnosis in pediatric practice. **Curr Probl Pediatr** 1981 Dec;12(2):1–47

Reis e Almeida FS: Estomatologia sofrologia. **Rev Port Estomatol Cir Maxilofac** 1983 Apr–Jun;24(2):183–97

Ross PJ: The history of hypnosis in dentistry. **Bull Hist Dent** 1981;29(1):24–8

Schott H: Mesmer, Braid und Bernheim: zur Entstehungsgeschichte des Hypnotismus. **Gesnerus** 1984;41(1/2):33–48

Sheehan PW, Perry CW: Methodologies of hypnosis. Hillsdale, N. J., Erlbaum, New York, Halsted Press, 1976. xiii, 329 p.

Simon K: Hypnose––Geschichte und Anwendung heute. **Med Monatsschr Pharm** 1979 Apr;2(4):117–8

#### Austria

Gravitz MA, Gerton MI: Polgar as Freud's hypnotist? contrary evidence. **Am J Clin Hypn** 1982 Apr;24(4):272–6

# HYPNOSIS

**Brazil**

Rezende de Castro Monteiro A: 'Hypnotisme'. Analyse de la thèse présentée à la Faculté de Médecine de Rio de Janeiro par Francisco de Paula Fajardo Junior, en vue d'obtenir le grade de docteur en médecine - Rio de Janeiro, 1888. In: Congrès international d'histoire de la médecine, XXVe, Québec, 1976. Actes. Québec, 1977. p. 980–91.

**Europe**

Klumbies G: Die Entwicklung der Hypnosetherapie in Europa. **Psychiatr Neurol Med Psychol (Leipz)** 1981;28:11–33

**France**

Azouvi F: Irritabilité et magnétisme animal: une lettre inédite de J.-M.-A. Servan. **Dix-huit Siecle** 1982;14:191–7
Barrucand D: Bernheim. Importance historique et actualité de l'Ecole de Nancy. In: Congrès National des Sociétés Savantes, 103e, Nancy, 1978. Comptes Rendus. Paris, 1978. Section des Sciences, Fasc. V. p. 75–86.
Chertok L: On the centenary of Charcot: hysteria, suggestibility and hypnosis. **Br J Med Psychol** 1984 Jun;57(Pt 2):111–20
Josipovici J: Franz Anton Mesmer, magnétiseur, médecin et franc-maçon. Monaco, Editions du Rocher, 1982. 200 p.
Lévy J: Magnétisme animal et médecine à Strasbourg à la fin du XVIIIe siècle. In Livet G, Schaff G, ed: Médecine et assistance en Alsace, XVIe–XXe siècle. Strasbourg, Istra, 1976. p. 201–7.
Mammerickx M: André-Marie Ampère et Claude-Julien Bredin, II. Ampère, Bredin et le magnétisme animal, ou la petite histoire d'une grande découverte. **Hist Med Vet** 1977;2(3):69–75
Pattie FA: A Mesmer-Paradis myth dispelled. **Am J Clin Hypn** 1979 Jul;22(1):29–31
Sandor RS, ed: Bernheim's New studies in hypnotism. New York, International Universities Press, 1980. xix, 407 p. Translation of Hypnotisme, suggestion, psychothérapie: Etudes nouvelles, 1891.
Schott H: Die Mitteilung des Lebensfeuers. Zum therapeutischen Konzept von Franz Anton Mesmer (1734–1815). **Medizinhist J** 1982;17(3):195–214
Sutton G: Electric medicine and mesmerism. **Isis** 1981 Sep;72(263):375–92
Sutton G: The magnetic hands. **Med Instrum** 1984 Jul–Aug;18(4):247
Weitzenhoffer AM: What did he (Bernheim) say? A postscript and an addendum. **Int J Clin Exp Hypn** 1980 July;28(3):252–60
Wilson LB: Les maladies des femmes: women, charlatanry, and professional medicine in eighteenth-century France. Ph.D. Diss., Stanford University. Palo Alto, 1982. vi, 449 p.

**Germany**

Hoff P: Der Einfluss des Mesmerismus auf die Entwicklung der Suggestionstheorie in Deutschland. Diss. Mainz, 1980. 115 p.
Landauer AA: A note on the role of Karl Christian Wolfart (1778–1832) in the study of animal magnetism. **J Hist Behav Sci** 1981;17:206–8

**Great Britain**

Brown PS: Mesmerism, galvanism and quackery. **Bristol Med Chir J** 1983 Apr;98(366):61–4
Miller J: A Gower Street scandal. The Samuel Gee lecture 1982. **J R Coll Physicians Lond** 1983 Oct;17(4):181–5, 188–91
Parssinen TM: Professional deviants and the history of medicine: medical mesmerists in Victorian Britain. **Sociol Rev [Monogr]** 1979;27:103–20

**India**

Pulos L: Mesmerism revisited: the effectiveness of Esdaile's techniques in the production of deep hypnosis and total body hypnoanaesthesia. **Am J Clin Hypn** 1980 Apr;22(4):206–11

**Netherlands**

Verkroost CM: A. W. van Renterghem und Frederik van Eeden, zwei holländische Aerzte als Bahnbrecher auf dem Gebiete der psychischen Therapie. **Janus** 1980;67(1-2-3):191–9

**Sweden**

Luttenberger F: Hypnotisörernas tid. Hypnotismen i svensk medicin 1880–1900. **Lychnos** 1983;:90–119

**United States**

Fuller RC: Mesmerism and the American cure of souls. Philadelphia, University of Pennsylvania Press, 1982. xvi, 227 p.
Gravitz MA: An early case of investigative hypnosis: a brief communication. **Int J Clin Exp Hypn** 1983 Oct;31(4):224–6
Hammond DC: Myths about Erickson and Ericksonian hypnosis. **Am J Clin Hypn** 1984 Apr;26(4):236–45
Laurence JR, Perry C: Forensic hypnosis in the late nineteenth century. **Int J Clin Exp Hypn** 1983 Oct;31(4):266–83
Rosen S: The psychotherapeutic and hypnotherapeutic approaches of Milton H. Erickson, M.D. **Am J Psychoanal** 1984 Summer;44(2):133–45
Triplet RG: The relationship of Clark L. Hull's hypnosis research to his later learning theory: the continuity of his life's work. **J Hist Behav Sci** 1982 Jan;18(1):22–31

# IMMUNOLOGY

Bywaters EG: Historical perspectives in the aetiology of ankylosing spondylitis. **Br J Rheumatol** 1983 Nov;22(4 Suppl 2):1–4
Chase A: Magic shots: a human and scientific account of the long and continuing struggle to eradicate infectious diseases by vaccination. New York, Morrow, 1982. 576 p.
Dodin A: Historique des vaccinations. **Ther Umsch** 1983 Mar;40(3):184–6
Dudgeon JA: Immunization in times ancient and modern. **J R Soc Med** 1980 Aug;73(8):581–6
Henry RL: Paleoserology. In A. Cockburn, E. Cockburn, ed: Mummies, disease, and ancient cultures. Cambridge, Cambridge University Press, 1980. p. 327–34.
Lotzová E: Natural immunity. History, present, and future. **Nat Immun Cell Growth Regul** 1983–84;3(1):1–6
Melnick JL: Toward eradication of poliomyelitis by combined use of killed and liver vaccines. **Cardiovasc Res Cent Bull** 1982 Jan–Mar;20(3):49–60
Paläoimmunologie: **Naturwissenschaften** 1980;67:560
Petrov RV: Immunologiia ot Pastera do nashikh dnei. Moskva, Nauka, 1968. 101 p.
Raymond JF de: Querelle de l'inoculation, ou, Préhistoire de la vaccinaton. Paris, Vrin, 1982. 124 p.
Silverstein AM, Bialasiewicz AA: History of immunology. A history of theories of acquired immunity. **Cell Immunol** 1980 Apr;51(1):151–67
Silverstein AM: History of immunology. Development of the concept of immunologic specificity, I. **Cell Immunol** 1982 Mar 1;67(2):396–409

**China**

Needham J: China and the origins of immunology. **East Horiz** 1980;19(1):6–12

**Before 500 A.D.**

Lowenstein JM: Immunological reactions from fossil material. **Philos Trans R Soc Lond [Biol]** 1981 May 8;292(1057):143–9

**Greece**

Habs H: Immunologische Begriffe bei Thukydides. **Zentralbl Bakteriol Mikrobiol Hyg [A]** 1982 Jun;252(2):143–6

**1450–1700**

Zhu BZ: [History of the vaccination of human pox] (Chi). **Chung Hsi I Chieh Ho Tsa Chi** 1982 Oct;2(4):247–8

**Switzerland**

Guess HA: Bernoulli's cost-benefit analysis of smallpox immunization. **N Engl J Med** 1981 Aug 6;305(6):347

**1700 to Present**

Baggiolini M: Phagozyten und Phagozytose hundert Jahre nach Metschnikoff. Ein aktuelles Bild des neutrophilen Leukozyten. **Schweiz Med Wochenschr** 1982 Oct;112(41):1403–11
Baroian OV: Aspects épidémiologiques de l'immunologie contemporaine. Moscou: [s.n.], 1972 (Cahors: Tardy-Quercy-Auvergne, 1976) 378 p.
Benenson AS: Immunization and military medicine. **Rev Infect Dis** 1984 Jan–Feb;6(1):1–12
Bibel DJ: Sternberg, Metchnikoff, and the phagocytes. **Milit Med** 1982 Jul;147(7):550–3
Billingham RE, Beer AE: Reproductive immunology: past, present, and future. **Perspect Biol Med** 1984;27(2):259–75
Bockemühl J: Die Typhus-Schutzimpfung gestern und heute. **Immun Infekt** 1983 Jan;11(1):16–22
Borek F: Eighty years of Ehrlich's side-chain theory. **J Immunol Methods** 1980;33(4):393
Bornside GH: Waldemar Haffkine's cholera vaccines and the Ferran-Haffkine priority dispute. **J Hist Med Allied Sci** 1982 Oct;37(4):399–422
Bowers JZ: The odyssey of smallpox vaccination. **Bull Hist Med** 1981 Spring;55(1):17–33
Calne RY: The development of immunosuppressive therapy. **Transplant Proc** 1981 Mar;13(1):44–9
Cambier J: De la mort de Louis XV à la vaccination du roi de Rome. **Nouv Presse Med** 1980 Jun 7;9(25):1746
Cazort AG, Gordon VH: History of allergy. University of Arkansas School of Medicine. **J Arkansas Med Soc** 1980 Oct;77(5):197–8

Cooper EL: L'évolution de l'immunité. **Recherche** 1979;103:824–33

Coulanges P: Cinquantenaire du vaccin antipesteux EV (Girard et Robic). **Bull Soc Pathol Exot Filiales** 1983 Mar–Apr;76(2):114–20

Coulanges P: Cinquantenaire du vaccin antipesteux EV (Girard et Robic). **Arch Inst Pasteur Madagascar** 1982;50(1):169–84

Dausset J: The challenge of the early days of human histocompatibility. **Immunogenetics** 1980;10(1):1–5

Dittmann S: Die Welt ist pockenfrei--Durchführung und Erfolg eines grandiosen Programms. **Z Gesamte Inn Med** 1980 Dec 15;35(24):858–63

Dwyer JM: Thirty years of supplying the missing link. History of gamma globulin therapy for immunodeficient states. **Am J Med** 1984 Mar 30;76(3A):46–52

Fenner F: Smallpox and its eradication. In Stanley NF, Joske RA, ed: Changing disease patterns and human behaviour. London, New York, Academic Press, 1980. p. 215–29.

Gordienko SM: Stoletniĭ put' razvitiia teorii fagotsitoza. Sovremennye predstavleniia o roli fagotsitov v nespetsificheskom kletochnom immunitete. **Ter Arkh** 1983;55(8):144–50

Gröschel DH, Hornick RB: Who introduced typhoid vaccination: Almroth Wright or Richard Pfeiffer? **Rev Infect Dis** 1981 Nov–Dec;3(6):1251–4

Hammarsten JF, Tattersall W, Hammarsten JE: Who discovered smallpox vaccination? Edward Jenner or Benjamin Jesty? **Trans Am Clin Climatol Assoc** 1979;90:44–55

Heidelberger M: Recognition of antibodies as labeled globulins. **Ann NY Acad Sci** 1983;420:1–4

Henderson DA: The history of smallpox eradication. In Lilienfeld AM, ed: Times, places, and persons. Baltimore, London, Johns Hopkins Univ. Press, 1980. (Sigerist suppl. to the Bull Hist Med. n.s., no 4) p. 99–108.

Hinman AR: Mass vaccination against polio. **JAMA** 1984 Jun 8;251(22):2994–6

Höring FO: Kritischer Rückblick auf die Entwicklung der Immunitätslehre. **Z Gesamte Inn Med** 1981 Apr 1;36(7):229–35

Johansson SG, Bennich HH: The clinical impact of the discovery of IgE. **Ann Allergy** 1982 Jun;48(6):325–30

Kaul A, Smith GF: Immunobiology of the fetus and newborn--historical perspectives and recent advances. In Smith GF, Smith PN, Vidyasagar D, ed: Historical review and recent advances in neonatal and perinatal medicine. [Chicago?], Mead Johnson Nutritional Division, 1983. Vol. I. p. 197–212.

Keller F, Kirn A: Eradicazione mondiale del vaiolo. Da Sarah Nelmes a Ali Maow Maalin. **Minerva Med** 1980 Oct 20;71(40):2935–40

Klein P: 'Kognitive' Leistungen des Immunsystems. **Medizinhist J** 1983;18(1–2):3–20

Krause RM: The restless tide. The persistent challenge of the microbial world. Washington, D. C., National Foundation for Infectious Diseases, 1981. 152 p.

Kumate J: La immunologia contemporánea. **Mem Col Nac (Mex)** 1978;8(4):11–24

Kumate J: Las herramientas de la inmunología contemporánea: nova et vetera. **Gac Med Mex** 1981 Sep;117(9):382–5

Lindenmann J: Origin of the terms 'antibody' and 'antigen'. **Scand J Immunol** 1984 Apr;19(4):281–5

Lutzker E: Cameron prizewinner: Waldemar M. Haffkine, C.I.E. **Clio Med** 1971 May;13(3–4):269–76

McCracken D: A link with the past. **Br Med J [Clin Res]** 1981 Mar 21;282(6268):964–6

Matsuhashi N: [Introduction to immunology--history] (Jpn). **Shikai Tenbo** 1982 Jan;59(1):169–76

Mazumdar PM: Karl Landsteiner and the problem of species 1838–1968. Ph.D. Diss., Johns Hopkins University. Baltimore, 1976. 725 leaves.

Milhomem AM, Suassuna I: A imunidade na febre tifóide. I. A vacinação anti-tifoídica de Wright, 1896 a 1979. **Mem Inst Oswaldo Cruz** 1982 Jan–Mar;77(1):93–120

Moore DF: The history and development of the BCG. **Practitioner** 1983 Feb;227(1376):i–iii

Moskwa Z: Historia szczepień przeciwgruźliczych i powstanie szczepionki BCG. **Wiad Lek** 1983 Jan 1;36(1):81–5

Moulin AM, Löwi I: La double nature de l'immunologie: histoire de la transplantation rénale. **Fundam Sci** 1983;4(3/4):201–18

O'Brien M: Legal implications of the use of vaccines. **Med Leg J** 1979;47(4):152–9

Possehl I: Impfstoffe, Sera, Diagnostika - Resultate bakteriologischer und immunologischer Forschung. In Hickel E, Schröder G, ed: Neue Beiträge zur Arzneimittelgeschichte. Festschrift für Wolfgang Schneider zum 70. Geburtstag. Stuttgart, Wissenschaftliche Verlagsgesellschaft, 1982. p. 185–203.

Prunet P: Nouvelles technologies et vaccination antirabique. **Arch Inst Pasteur Tunis** 1982 March;59(1):115–20

Ring J: Zur Problematik der Dextran-Unverträglichkeit und ihrer spezifischen Prophylaxe durch Hapten-Hemmung. Ein Stück Geschichte angewandter Immunologie. **Fortschr Med** 1982 Nov 4;100(41):1917–21

Rosenfield RE: Immunobiology of the erythrocyte: perspectives since 1945. **Prog Clin Biol Res** 1980;43:13–7

Rubin LP: Styles in scientific explanations: Paul Ehrlich and Svante Arrhenius on immunochemistry. **J Hist Med Allied Sci** 1980 Oct;35(4):397–425

Sakula A: BCG: who were Calmette and Guérin? **Thorax** 1983 Nov;38(11):806–12

Schneeweiss U: Die Bedeutung der Entdeckung der Tuberkelbakterien für die Immunitäts- und Krankheitslehre. **Padiatr Grenzgeb** 1982;21(2):127–40

Schwaber J: Hybridoma technology. **Science** 1982 May 21;216(4548):798

Sétáló G: Az immunszövettani módszerek fejlődése és jelene. **Morphol Igazsagugyi Orv Sz** 1983 Apr;23(2):85–92

Silverstein AM: Development of the concept of immunologic specificity: III. **Cell Immunol** 1983 May;78(1):174–90

Silverstein AM: Development of the concept of immunologic specificity: IV. **Cell Immunol** 1983 Sep;80(2):416–25

Silverstein AM: History of immunology. Cellular versus humoral immunity: determinants and consequences of an epic 19th century battle. **Cell Immunol** 1979 Nov;48(1):208–21

Silverstein AM: History of immunology: development of the concept of immunologic specificity: II. **Cell Immunol** 1982 Jul 15;71(1):183–95

Sinkovics JG: Early history of specific antibody-producing lymphocyte hybridomas. **Cancer Res** 1981 Mar;41(3):1246–7

Speiser P, Smekal FG: Karl Landsteiner, Entdecker der Blutgruppen und Pionier der Immunologie. Biographie eines Nobelpreisträgers aus der Wiener Medizinischen Schule. 2., vollständig überarb. Aufl. Vienna, Hollinek, 1975. 207 p.

Steege MM: Creating the pneumococcal pneumonia vaccine: a hundred-year story. **Conn Med** 1979 Nov;43(11):717–20

Vorob'ev AA: O tendentsiiakh razvitiia sovremennoĭ immunologii. **Zh Mikrobiol Epidemiol Immunobiol** 1979 Dec;(12):3–9

Wade N: Hybridomas: the making of a revolution [news]. **Science** 1982 Feb 26;215(4536):1073–5

Wyatt HV: Provocation poliomyelitis: neglected clinical observations from 1914 to 1950. **Bull Hist Med** 1981 Winter;55(4):543–57

150e année: La variole et son éradication. Contributions by L. Justin-Besançon, R. Fasquelle, J. Fasquelle, L. Jacques. **J Med Chir Prat** 1979 Sep;17–18:629–708

### Africa

Stewart L: The edge of utility: slaves and smallpox in the early eighteenth century. **Med Hist** 1985 Jan;29(1):54–70

### Australia

Feery B: Impact of immunization on disease patterns in Australia. **Med J Aust** 1981 Aug 22;2(4):172–6

Hamilton DG: Whooping cough immunization. **Med J Aust** 1979 Dec 15;2(12):651

### Austria

Lutzker E, Jochnowitz C: The curious history of Waldemar Haffkine. **Commentary** 1980;69(6):61–4

### Canada

Craig B: Smallpox in Ontario: public and professional perceptions of disease, 1884–1885. In Roland CG, ed: Health, disease and medicine. Toronto, Hannah Institute for the History of Medicine, 1984. p. 215–49.

Spaulding WB: Smallpox control in the Ontario wilderness, 1880–1910. In Roland CG, ed: Health, disease and medicine. Toronto, Hannah Institute for the History of Medicine, 1984. p. 194–214.

Tunis B: Inoculation for smallpox in the Province of Quebec, a re-appraisal. In Roland CG, ed: Health, disease and medicine. Toronto, Hannah Institute for the History of Medicine, 1984. p. 171–93.

### Europe

Emch-Dériaz AS: L'inoculation justifiee–or was it? **Eighteenth Cent Life** 1982;7(2):65–72

### France

Beauchamp C: Les mécomptes d'un bienfait: sur la pratique de la vaccination au XIXe s. l'exemple du Loir-et-Cher. **Asclepio** 1983;35:389–402

Biraben JN: La diffusion de la vaccination en France au 19e siècle. **Ann Bretagne** 1979;86(3):265–76

Cooper EL: Prix D'Immunologie Behring-Metschnikoff. **Dev Comp Immunol** 1982 Summer;6(3):389–90

Danchin A: Une révolution lamarckienne en immunologie. **Recherche** 1981;12(118):84–5

Ferru M: La faillite du BCG. Poitiers, Ferru, 1977. 274 p.

Gilbrin E: Gaston Ramon (1886–1963). Le soixantième anniversaire des anatoxines. **Hist Sci Med** 1984;18(1):53–60

Heifets L: Centennial of Metchnikoff's discovery. **J Reticuloendothel Soc** 1982 May;31(5):381–91

Huard P, Imbault-Huart MJ: Percy, vénéréologue. In: Congrès National des Sociétés Savantes, 99e, Besançon, 1974. Comptes Rendus. Paris, 1976.

Section des Sciences, Fasc. V. p. 259-64.
Kaufmann C: La question de l'inoculation déférée à l'Eglise. **Asclepio** 1983;35:403-11
Kostychev SP: Pasteur: his life and achievements. Annotated translation from the Russian by S. A. Wilde. New Delhi, Oxford & IBH Publishing Co., 1978. 96 p.
Léonard J: Pasteur, un vétérinaire qui ira loin. **Histoire** 1979;12:78-80
Peter JP: Les médecins français face au problème de l'inoculation variolique et de sa diffusion (1750-1790). **Ann Bretagne** 1979;86(3):251-64
Saenz A, Boisvert H: Trois lettres de Louis Pasteur. **Hist Sci Med** 1981;15(4):327-33
Théodoridès J: 'Paris enragé'. **Rev Hist Pharm (Paris)** 1982;29(252):193-8
Wrotnowska D: Lettres inédites de Gilbert Déclat à Louis Pasteur. **Hist Sci Med** 1982;16(2):115-23

**Germany**

Abe HR: Aus der Frühgeschichte der deutschen Impfgesetzgebung. **Z Gesamte Hyg** 1980;26(5):373-4
Bendiner E: Ehrlich: immunologist, chemotherapist, prophet. **Hum Dev** 1980 Nov;15(11):129, 133, 138-9 passim
Beritić T: Carl Prausnitz Giles i saga or reaginima. **Lijec Vjesn** 1981 Jul;103(7):312-4
Blasi A: Der Kochsche Grundversuch und seine gegenwärtigen experimentellen Varianten. **Z Erkr Atmungsorgane** 1983;161(1):51-5
Drössler K: Robert Koch--auch ein Pionier der Immunitätsforschung? **Allerg Immunol (Leipz)** 1982;28(1):13-20
Findeisen DG: Tuberkulose und Allergie. Erkenntnisschritte von der Entdeckung des Mycobacterium tuberculosis durch Robert Koch (24 März 1882). Zu einer umfassenden Immundiagnostik, Immuntherapie und Immunprophylaxe. **Allerg Immunol (Leipz)** 1982;28(1):3-12
Gronski P, Seiler FR: Spezifische Serumtherapie gestern und heute von Antikörper-Präparaten Teil 1: Der Weg zur therapeutischen Anwendung. **Fortschr Med** 1983 Jan 27;101(4):103-6
Kallós P: Immunity and concomitant immunity in infectious diseases. Introduction. **Prog Allergy** 1982;31:IX-XV
Schadewaldt H: Emil von Behring und die Entwicklung der deutschen Immunologie. **Med Welt** 1979;30(48):1795-801
Schneeweiss U: Die Immunitätslehre im Lichte der Vorstellungen von Robert Koch. **Z Erkr Atmungsorgane** 1983;161(1):46-50
Taddey G: Pockenschutz in Hohenlohe. **Medizinhist J** 1983;18(4):313-23
Weingärtner L: Zum Problem der BCG-Impfung. **Wiss Beitr Martin Luther Univ Halle Wittenberg** 1983;5-R80:161-73
Zureck A: 30 Jahre BCG-Impfung in der DDR - 20 Jahre BCG-Impfstoff aus Jena. **Z Erkr Atmungsorgane** 1982;158(1-2)168-84

**Great Britain**

Advances in immunology: a meeting in honor of Sir Peter Medawar: **Cell Immunol** 1981 Aug;62(2):233-310
Amos DB: Peter Alfred Isaac Gorer. In Dictionary of national biography, 1961-1970. Suppl. 8, 1981. p. 443-5.
Baxby D: A death from inoculated smallpox in the English Royal Family. **Med Hist** 1984 Jul;28(3):303-7
Baxby D: Jenner's smallpox vaccine. The riddle of vaccinia virus and its origin. London, Heinemann Educational Books, 1981. xiv, 214 p.
Bendiner E: Jenner: from folklore to scientific triumph. **Hosp Pract [Off]** 1984 Apr;19(4):183-7, 190-1, 196, passim
Bonnabeau RC: Edward Jenner and the advent of vaccination. **Minn Med** 1983 May;66(5):331-3
Charlton C: The fight against vaccination: the Leicester demonstration of 1885. **Local Popul Stud (Matlock)** 1983 Spring;30:60-66
Cordasco F: Laughlin Macleane's Expediency of Inoculation (1756): a checklist of deposit locations. **Am Notes Queries** 1981 Jan-Feb;19(5/6):75
Evans D: Alexander Thomas Glenny. In Dictionary of national biography, 1961-1970. Suppl 8, 1981. p. 434-5.
Guest-Gornall RG: Good servants are scarce. **Br Med J [Clin Res]** 1981 Dec 19;283(6307):1674-5
James DC: HLA-B27 in clinical medicine--historical reflections on the discovery of the disease association. **Br J Rheumatol** 1983 Nov;22(4 Suppl 2):20-4
Kahn A: Highlights of the Adler Museum collections: the Jenner letter. **Adler Mus Bull** 1984 Jun;10(2):15-7
Luckin B: The decline of small pox and the demographic revolution of the eighteenth century. **Soc Hist (Lond)** 1977;(6):793-97
McGregor IA: Thomas Gibson's contribution to immunology. **Plast Reconstr Surg** 1983 Mar;71(3):440
McHenry S: The pox upon her. **Aramco World Mag** 1980, 31(4):13-21
Miller G: Putting Lady Mary in her place: a discussion of historical causation. **Bull Hist Med** 1981 Spring;55(1):2-16
Miller G, ed: Letters of Edward Jenner and other documents concerning the early history of vaccination. From the Henry Barton Jacobs Collection in the William H. Welch Medical Library. Baltimore, London, Johns Hopkins University Press, 1983. xxix, 145 p. (Henry E. Sigerist Supplements to the Bulletin of the History of Medicine, n.s., no. 8).
Perry CB: Edward Jenner. **Ear Nose Throat J** 1984 Dec;63(12):605-17
Peter Brian Medawar: **Cell Immunol** 1981 Aug;62(2):235-42
Razzell P: The conquest of smallpox: the impact of inoculation on smallpox mortality in eighteenth century England. Firle, Sussex, Caliban Books, 1977. x, 190 p.
Saunders P: Edward Jenner. The Cheltenham years 1795-1823. Being a chronicle of the vaccination campaign. Hanover, London, University Press of New England, 1982. xviii, 469 p.
Silverstein AM, Miller G: History of immunology. The royal experiment on immunity: 1721-1722. **Cell Immunol** 1981 Jul 1;61(2):437-47
Tigertt WD: Anthrax. William Smith Greenfield, M.D., F.R.C.P., Professor Superintendent, the Brown Animal Sanatory Institution (1878-81). Concerning the priority due to him for the production of the first vaccine against anthrax. **J Hyg (Lond)** 1980 Dec;85(3):415-20
Wallace EM: The first vaccinator. Benjamin Jesty of Yetminster and Worth Matravers and his family. Wareham and Swanage (England), Anglebury-Bartlett, 1981. 20 p.

**Greece**

Marketos LJ: [Recent data on the inoculation against smallpox in the Ionian Islands] (Gre). **Mater Med Greca** 1981;9:104-9

**Hungary**

Csanak DF: Teleki József Szerepe egy XVIII. századi francia tudományos vitaban. **Szazadok** 1974;108(2):406-22
Gergely J: Az onallosodott immunbiologia: eredmenyek-perspektivak. **Magy Tud** 1981;26(2):93-101
Réthy L: Medico-historical background of the possibility of introducing the compulsory and nation-wide immunization with combined vaccines in Hungary. **Ann Immunol hung** 1984;24:13-38
Schweiger O: A tbc-elleni küzdelem eredményei Magyarországon 100 évvel a mycobacterium felfedezése után. **Orv Hetil** 1983 Jul 10;124(28):1667-70

**India**

Lutzker E: Some unanswered questions in medical history. In: Congrès international d'histoire de la médecine, XXVe, Québec, 1976. Actes. Québec, 1977. p. 917-27.

**Italy**

Imerti AD: Vincenzo Catalani, Neapolitan Jacobin, jurist, reformer (1769-1843), with an appendix containing a translation of his work 'A digression on vaccination.' Lawrence, Kansas, Coronado Press, 1976. 155 p.
Karnovsky ML: Metchnikoff in Messina: a century of studies on phagocytosis. **N Engl J Med** 1981 May 7;304(19):1178-80

**Liechtenstein**

Rheinberger R: Zum 200. Geburtstag von Landesphysikus Gebhard Schaedler. ein Liechtensteinischer Artzt als Pionier der Pockenschutzimpfung. **Jahrb Hist Ver Fuerst Liechtenstein** 1976;76:337-43

**Mexico**

Carrada Bravo T, Gómez Orozco J, Luna Martínez J, et al: La tosferina y la vacunación antitosferinosa. Trabajo para conmemorar el 40 aniversario de la vacunación antitosferinosa en México, Junio 13 de 1940. **Salud Publica Mex** 1982 Jul-Aug;24(4):399-465

**Netherlands**

Janssens U: Matthieu Maty and the adoption of inoculation for smallpox in Holland. **Bull Hist Med** 1981 Summer;55(2):246-56
Steendijk-Kuypers J: De Hoornse Geneeskundige Genootschappen en hun ijver ten aanzien van de vaccinatie in de 19de EEUW. **Tijdschr Geschied Geneeskd** 1982;5(3):105-14

**Poland**

Slopek S: Rozwój immunologii w Polsce w latach 1971-1975. **Nauka Pol** 1976;24(5):41-59
Weissmann G: In quest of Fleck: science from the holocaust. **Hosp Pract** 1980 Oct;15(10):48-9, 52, 54-5 passim

**Puerto Rico**

Ramírez Ronda Ch, Bermúdez RH, Pérez Pabón MJ, et al: Vacunación: principios y práctica 1980. Revisón y conceptos.--Parte I. Desarrollo histórico, efectos secundarios difteria, tétanos y tos ferina, poliomielitis y sarampión. **Bol Asoc Med PR** 1980 Jul;72(7):339-52

**Romania**

Babes V: Opere alese. Vol. I. Bucuresti, Editura Academiei Republicii Socialiste Romania, 1979. 330 p. Biographical contributions by B. Dutescu, N. Marcu, and I. Moraru.

**Spain**

Arce J: De Feijoo a Quintana. Testimonios lingüistico-literarios sobre inoculación y vacuna. **Bol Cent Estud Siglo XVIII** 1978;6:3-18
Bornside GH: Jaime Ferran and preventive inoculation against cholera. **Bull Hist Med** 1981 Winter;55(4):516-32
Dowling J: Smallpox and literature in eighteenth-century Spain. **Stud Eighteenth Cent Cult** 1979;9:59-77

**Sweden**

Grubb R: The discovery of the genetic markers of human immunoglobulins. **Vox Sang** 1983;45(1):89-90
Thulin L: 'Om koppors ympande'--ett vaccinationens förstadium i 1700-talets Sverige. **Nord Medicinhist Arsb** 1981;59-73

**Tunisia**

Eyquem A: L'immuno-pathologie de l'auto-immunisation 1900-1980. **Arch Inst Pasteur Tunis** 1981 Sep-Dec;58(3):281-95

**United States**

Alexander ER: Inactivated poliomyelitis vaccination. Issues reconsidered. **JAMA** 1984 May 25;251(20):2710-2
Alwin M. Pappenheimer, Jr: **Cell Immunol** 1982 Jan 1;66(1):3-8
Benison S: International medical cooperation: Dr. Albert Sabin, live poliovirus vaccine and the Soviets. **Bull Hist Med** 1982;56(4):460-83
Brandt AM: Polio, politics, publicity, and duplicity: ethical aspects in the development of the Salk vaccine. **Conn Med** 1979 Sep;43(9):581-7, 589-90
Brown RW, Henderson JH: The mass production and distribution of HeLa cells at Tuskegee Institute, 1953-55. **J Hist Med Allied Sci** 1983 Oct;38(4):415-31
Carpenter CB: Clinical histocompatibility testing: a brief historical perspective. **Transplant Proc** 1981 Mar;13(1):55-60
Clyde WA, Fernald GW: Mycoplasmas: the pathogens' pathogens. **Cell Immunol** 1983 Nov;82(1):88-97
Cohen IB, ed: The life and scientific and medical career of Benjamin Waterhouse: with some account of the introduction of vaccination in America. 2 vols. New York, Arno Press, 1980. Reprints of various works. Various paginations.
Cohn M: An introduction to 'Le Pap'. **Cell Immunol** 1982 Jan 1;66(1):11-6
Collier RJ: From Pap to ApUp. **Cell Immunol** 1982 Jan 1;66(1):17-23
Dewey FL: Thomas Jefferson's law practice: the Norfolk anti-inoculation riots. **Va Mag Hist Biogr** 1983;91(1):39-53
Festschrift in honor of Robert A. Good on the occasion of his 60th birthday: **Clin Immunol Immunopathol** 1982 May;23(2):155-61
Gara PF de: In celebration of the 75th birthday of 'allergy'. **J Asthma** 1982;19(1):3-4
Green H: Some things that happened on Lew Thomas' floor. **Cell Immunol** 1983 Nov;82(1):98-101
Greenwalt TJ: Rh immunization. The importance of a critical case study. **JAMA** 1984 Mar 9;251(10):1318-20
Heidelberger M: A 'pure' organic chemist's downward path: chapter 3--'retirement'. **Perspect Biol Med** 1981 Summer;24(4):619-36
Immunology and virology--a 25 year retrospective: Proceedings of the Silver Jubilee Symposium sponsored by The Wistar Institute in honor of Hilary Koprowski. **J Cell Physiol [Suppl]** 1982;2:1-147
Kiple KF, Kiple VH: The African connection: slavery, disease and racism. **Phylon** 1980 Fall;41(3):211-22
Kiple KL, Kiple VH: Black yellow fever immunities, innate and acquired, as revealed in the American South. **Soc Sci Hist** 1977;1(4):419-36
Kondratas RA: Biologics Control Act of 1902. In Young JH, ed: The early years of federal food and drug control. Madison, American Institute of the History of Pharmacy, 1982. p. 8-27.
Krause RM: Philadelphia, the Founding Fathers, and systemic lupus erythematosus. **Arthritis Rheum** 1982 Jul;25(7):895-7
Lepow IH: Louis Pillemer, Properdin, and scientific controversy. **J Immunol** 1980 Aug;125(2):471-5
Mascia AV: In memoriam Israel Friedman (1906-1980). **J Asthma** 1982;19(1):59-60
Morris JP: Smallpox inoculation in the American colonies, 1763-1783. **Md Hist** 1977;8:47-58
Moses RJ: Smallpox immunization in Alta California: a story based on José Estrada's 1821 postscript. **South Calif Q** 1979;61(2):125-45
Paterson PY: LT/EAE and the MS quest. Going to the dogs and rats to study the patient. **Cell Immunol** 1983 Nov;82(1):55-74
Raffel S: Fifty years of immunology. **Annu Rev Microbiol** 1982;36:1-26
Reproductive immunology. A festschrift in honor of Dr. Saul B. Gusberg.: **Mt Sinai J Med (NY)** 1980 Sep-Oct;47(5):i-vii, 427-560
Retsinas J: Smallpox vaccination: a leap of faith. **RI Hist** 1979;38(4):113-24
Rubin LP: Gladys Rowena Henry Dick. In: Notable American women. The modern period. Cambridge, Mass., Belknap-Harvard Univ. Press, 1980. 4:191-2.
Silverstein AM: Contributions of A. Edward Maumenee to ocular immunology. **Am J Ophthalmol** 1979 Sep;88(3 Pt 1):302-5
Small WE: Pneumococcal pneumonia vaccine--strange success story. **Am Pharm** 1979 Dec;19(13):39
Spector B: The great Salk vaccine mess. **Antioch Rev** 1980;38(3):291-303
Talmage DW: William Hay Taliaferro: February 10, 1895-December 21, 1973. **Biogr Mem Natl Acad Sci** 1983;54:375-407
Watterson J, ed: Poetic justice; or, an illfated epic by Thomas Burke. **NC Hist Rev** 1978;55(3):339-46
Weissmann G: From Auden to arachidonate: a tribute and a hypothesis. **Cell Immunol** 1983 Nov;82(1):117-26
Wilson CE: The Boston inoculation controversy: a revisionist interpretation. **Journalism Hist** 1980;7(1):16-9, 40

**USSR**

Chebotarev DF, Duplenko IuK: Vklad A. A. Bogomol'tsa v razrabotku aktual'nyk problem medikobiologicheskoĭ nauki (k 100-letiiu so dnia rozhdeniia). **Vrach Delo** 1981 May;(5):6-10
Griffiths J: Doctor Thomas Dimsdale, and smallpox in Russia. The variolation of the Empress Catherine the Great. **Bristol Med Chir J** 1984 Jan;99(369):14-6
Il'chevich NV, Spasokukotskiĭ IuA, Alekseeva IN, et al: Razvitie ideĭ A. A. Bogomol'tsa v oblasti ėksperimental'nogo izucheniia i primeneniia v praktike tsitotoksicheskikh syvorotok. **Fiziol Zh** 1981 May-Jun;27(3):339-46
Koslakov PN: K 100-letniu fagotsitarnoĭ teorii immuniteta I.I. Mechnikova. **Vopr Virusol** 1982 Sep-Oct;27(5):4-9
Kravchenko AT: Razvitie ideĭ prof. I. L. Krichevskogo o priobretennom immuniteta (k 100-letiiu so dnia rozhdeniia I. L. Krichevskogo). **Zh Mikrobiol Epidemiol Immunobiol** 1984 Feb;(2):110-4
Kucharz E, Jabłońska D: Illya Illich Miechnikov -- in seventieth anniversary of being awarded the Nobel Prize. **Mater Med Pol** 1978 Oct-Dec;10(4):342-4
Magazov VS, Morogova VM: 75 let Ufimskomu nauchno-issledovatel'skomu institutu vaktsin i syvorotok im. I. I. Mechnikova. **Zh Mikrobiol Epidemiol Immunobiol** 1981 Jan;(1):110-1
Pinchuk VG: Razvitie ideĭ A. A. Bogomolets v oblasti izucheniia reaktivnosti organizma pri opukholevom protsesse. **Fiziol Zh** 1981 May-Jun;27(3):327-31
Semenov BF: Razvitie ideĭ I.I.Mechnikova v oblasti immunologii. **Zh Mikrobiol Epidemiol Immunobiol** 1984 Jul;(7):50-4
Trubina LM: K 100-letiiu fagotsitarnoĭ teorii I. I. Mechnikova. **Zh Mikrobiol Epidemiol Immunobiol** 1983 Dec;(12):99-101

**Yugoslavia**

Berlot J: Razvitak mikrobiologije i imunologije u Hrvatskoj do 1923. god. In: I simpozij o historiji mikrobiologije i imunologije u Hrvatskoj do 1923. godine. Zagreb, Jugoslavenskoj akademiji, 1973. p. 31-45.
I simpozij o historiji mikrobiologije i imunologije u Hrvatskoj do 1923. godine: Zagreb, Jugoslavenskoj, akademiji, 1973. 126 p.
Kraljević M, Rasuhin-Vekić N, Weisz-Maleček R, et al: O razvoju vakcine i vakcinacije protiv variole (1890-1923). In: I simpozij o historiji mikrobiologije i imunologije u Hrvatskoj do 1923. godine. Zagreb, Jugoslavenskoj akademiji, 1973. p. 63-70.
Topolnik E: Razvoj veterinarske bakteriologije i imunologije u Hrvatskoj do god. In: I simpozij o historiji mikrobiologije i imunologije u Hrvatskoj do 1923. godine. Zagreb, Jugoslavenskoj akademiji, 1973. p. 119-26.

## INSTRUMENTS AND EQUIPMENT

See also **Dentistry; Microscopy; Pharmacy**

Austin RT: Treatment of broken legs before and after the introduction of gypsum. **Injury** 1983 Mar;14(5):389-94
Barnett GH, Hardy RW: Gardner tongs and cervical traction. **Med Instrum** 1982 Nov-Dec;16(6):291-2
Barometer on baromedicine: **MD** 1978 Jun;22(6):53-5, 57
Bean KJ: A history of surgical wound drainage: sump drains and closed wound suction devices. **J Oper Room Res Inst** 1983 Mar;3(3):8-20
Bennion E: Phlebotomy: the art, practice & instruments. **MD** 1981;25(8):43-6
Benzinger TH, ed: Temperature, part 1: arts and concepts. Stroudsburg, Pa., Dowden, Hutchinson & Ross, 1977. viii, 353 p. (Benchmark Papers in Human Physiology, 9).
Berger RL, Clem TR, Harden VA, et al: Historical development and newer means of temperature measurement in biochemistry. **Methods Biochem Anal** 1984;30:269-331
Bernabeo RA, ed: Il ferro chirurgico nella raccolta Vittorio Putti di Bologna. Bologna, Università degli Studi di Bologna, 1981. 14 p. (Catalog of an exhibit Sept.-Nov. 1981).
Beyer C: Temperaturmessung. **Pharm Unserer Zeit** 1983 Jul;12(4):97-110
Black JJ: A stitch in time--1. The history of sutures. **Nurs Times** 1982

Apr 14-20;78(15):619-23
Blum L, Slater S, Reuben D, et al: A consideration of current clinical thermometry. **Bull NY Acad Med** 1982 Oct;58(7)621-7
Bowman IA: History of medical instrumentation. **Bookman** 1982 Dec;9(10):3-8
Buck BA: Ancient technology in contemporary surgery. **West J Med** 1982 Mar;136(3):265-9
Chato JC: Reflections on the history of heat and mass transfer in bioengineering. **J Biomech Eng** 1981 May;103(2):97-101
Conroy BF: The history of faciel prostheses. In Romm S, ed: Symposium on historical perspectives of plastic surgery. Philadelphia, Saunders, 1983. p. 689-707.
Cule J: Catheters: forerunners of Foley. **Nurs Mirror** 1980 Feb 21;150(8):Suppl i-vi
Davis A, Appel T: Bloodletting instruments in the National Museum of History and Technology. Washington, Smithsonian Institution Press, 1979. 103 p.
Davis AB: Medicine and its technology. An introduction to the history of medical instrumentation. Westport, Greenwood Press, 1981. xiii, 285 p. (Contributions in Medical History, 7).
Eisenbud M: Environment, technology, and health: human ecology in historical perspective. New York, New York University Press, 1978. x, 384 p.
Finlay IM: Craniometry and cephalometry: a history prior to the advent of radiography. **Angle Orthod** 1980 Oct;50(4):312-21
Franco Grande A, Martinón JM, Pombo MV, et al: Evolución histórica de la intubación tráqueal. A porpósito de Franz Kuhn en el aniversario de su muerte. **Rev Esp Anestesiol Reanim** 1979 May;26(3):243-54
García-Sainz M: El Sistema Internacional de Unidades en la prática médica. I. **Gac Med Mex** 1981 Dec;117(12):479-83
Halub MA: The catheter--a historical perspective. **AUAA J** 1983 Apr-Jun;3(4):7-9
Harthorne JW: Historic milestones of electrotherapy and cardiac pacing. **Prog Cardiovasc Dis** 1981 May-Jun;23(6):389-92
Hayes B: Ventilation and ventilators. **J Med Eng Technol** 1982 Sep-Oct;6(5):177-92
Heilmann K: Gesundheitstechnologien. [Köln?], Deutscher Instituts-Verlag, 1984. 56 p.
Houston CS: The pressure chamber revisited. A look at the past. **Prog Clin Biol Res** 1983;136:213-20
Hübener KH, Pahl WM: Computertomographische Untersuchungen an altägyptischen Mumien. **ROFO** 1981 Aug;135(2):213-9
Ishiguro T: [History of the abdominal binder. 4. Use of the abdominal binder by pregnant women: views by foreigners and opposition to its use] (Jpn). **Josanpu Zasshi** 1984 Jul;38(7):615-7
Kahn A: Highlights of the Adler Museum collections. **Adler Mus Bull** 1982 Nov;8(2):16-18
Kahn A: Highlights of the Adler Museum collections. **Adler Mus Bull** 1984 Nov;10(3):25-9
Kirkup J: The history and evolution of surgical instruments. III. Handles. **Ann R Coll Surg Engl** 1983 Jul;65(4):269-73
Kirkup JR: The history and evolution of surgical instruments. I. Introduction. **Ann R Coll Surg Engl** 1981 Jul;63(4):279-85
Kirkup JR: The history and evolution of surgical instruments. II Origins: function: carriage: manufacture. **Ann R Coll Surg Engl** 1982 Mar;64(2):125-32
Krukoff S: Utilisation, en craniologie, des vecteurs pour la mise en évidence du degré d'inclinaison du front et de la face chez le chimpanzé, l'homme actuel et fossile. **C R Seances Acad Sci [III]** 1981 May 11;292(17):969-74
Kurzbauer R, Kurzbauer E, Sędzielowski Z: Z historii electrostymulacji. **Pieleg Polozna** 1979;(10):3-4
Lehmann V: Der Gebärstuhl--ein historisches Möbel oder eine sinnvolle Erneuerung. **Z Geburtshife Perinatol** 1983 Mar-Apr;187(2):55-64
Lehmann V: Der Gebärstuhl--ein historisches Möbel oder eine sinnvolle Erneuerung. **Arch Gynecol** 1983;235(1-4):XLVIII-LXIII
McLaury RL: A history of clinical thermometry. **J Okla State Med Assoc** 1983 Dec;76(12):420-6
Mahdihassan S: Alembic and ambix as Sino-Arabic terms with an explanation of Mary's bath. **Stud Hist Med** 1980 Mar;4(1):39-43
Margolin JC: L'histoire des lunettes à nez. **Histoire** 1980;21:14-21
Medical instruments: **MD** 1979 Nov;23(11):71-81
Mitcham C, Grote J: Philosophy of technology [and bioethics]. In Reich WT, et al, ed: Encyclopedia of bioethics, v.4. New York, Free Press, 1978. p. 1638-43.
Molina-Negro P: Le rôle des neurostimulateurs dans le traitement de la douleur chronique rebelle. **Union Med Can** 1980 Jan;109(1):41-54
Mössmer A: Säuglingsflaschen aus Holz. In Göpfert W, Otten HH, ed: Metavoeite: wandelt euch durch neues Denken. Düsseldorf, Triltsch, 1983. p. 201-8.
Olonetzky B, Mez L: Die Sammlung. Darstellung alter Arztinstrumente, Apotheker-Gefässe, Mikroskope, Einnehmelöffel, Terra sigillata, Amulette und anderer interessanter Gegenstände und Kuriositäten. Stuttgart, Thieme, 1980. 3 vol. in one. 123, 114, 127 p.
Orr JF, James WV, Bahrani AS: The history and development of artificial limbs. **Eng Med** 1982 Oct;11(4):155-61
Orr N: Why wear a mask in theatre? **NATNEWS** 1982 Jun;19(6):11-2
Pappas DG: The origin of aural instruments. **Am J Otol** 1979 Oct;1(2):121-4
Perkins WJ: Biomedical engineering--a reappraisal. **J Biomed Eng** 1984 Apr;6(2):157-9
Portele KA: Die Moulagensammlung des Pathologisch-Anatomischen Bundesmuseums in Wien. [Wien, Pathologisch-Anatomisches Bundesmuseum in Wien], 1977. 84 p.
Rádóczy G: Régi gyógyszerészi mértékegységek és kialakulásuk története. **Orvostort Kozl** 1979;87-88(25 no 1-2):229-41
Rall P, Kirchhoff KT, Roberts J: Professional attire at delivery, part I: an historical review. **J Nurse Midwife** 1984 Jul-Aug;29(4):251-6
Raso Rodríguez EJ: La evolucion historica de la profesion de instrumentista. **Asclepio** 1980;32:327-32
Rechtman J: De la brosse à dents à la brosse à bouche. **Soc Fr Hist Art Dent** 1979 Mar-Jun;(3-4):23-8
Reinstein H: Laboratory medicine--then and now. **Am J Med Technol** 1982 Jun;48(6):427-9
Roth N: Life-and-death decisions: electrodiagnosis and premature burial. **Med Instrum** 1980 Nov-Dec;14(6):322
Schmidt J: Individuelle Rettungsmittel für Seenotfälle. In Göpfert W, Otten HH, ed: Metavoeite: wandelt euch durch neues Denken. Düsseldorf, Triltsch, 1983. p. 79-87.
Scott M: 32,000 years of sutures. **NATNEWS** 1983 May;20(5):15-7
Segal A: Les progrès de l'exploration visuelle des organes aux XVIIe et XVIIIe siècles. **Hist Sci Med** 1979;13(4):395-406
Shaw A, Davis PD: The lung ventilator--an engineering appraisal. **Eng Med** 1977 Jul;6(3):85-9
Shehata MA: History of laryngeal intubation. **Middle East J Anaesthesiol** 1981 Feb;6(1):49-53
Simon P, Seifert E: Rollende Hilfsmittel fur Körperbehinderte als Gegenstand in der bildenden Kunst. In KF Schlegel, ed: Der Körperbehinderte in Mythologie und Kunst. Stuttgart, New York, Thieme, 1983. p. 89-125.
Skinner G: The history of surgical instruments. **Nurs Times** 1984 Jul 18-24;80(29):28-30
Stephens SD, Goodwin JC: Non-electric aids to hearing: a short history. **Audiology** 1984;23(2):215-40
Théodoridès J: Considerations on the medical uses of marine invertebrates. In Sears M. Merriman D, ed: Oceanography, the past. New York, Springer, 1980. p. 734-49.
Tucker RA: History of sizing of genitourinary instruments. **Urology** 1982 Sep;20(3):346-9
Turner GL: Antique scientific instruments. Poole, Dorset, Blandford, 1980. 168 p.
Ungethüm M, Kolb W: Elektro-Osteo-Stimulation, Teil 1. Historische Entwicklung und 'Stimulations'-Hypothesen. **Biomed Tech (Berlin)** 1982 Jun;27(6):130-5
Velter A, Lamothe MJ: Les outils du corps. [Paris],? Hier et demain, 1978. 303 p.
Vernon J: The history of masking as applied to tinnitus. **J Laryngol Otol** 1981;4 Suppl:76-9
Wind GG, Rich NM: Historical notes on surgical technique. In their Principles of surgical technique. The art of surgery. Baltimore, Munich, Urban & Schwarzenberg, 1983. p. 9-19.
Zazgornik J, Kallinger W, Graninger W, et al: Uber die Messung der Körpertemperatur. Neue Messgeräte und ihre Bedeutung in der Diagnostik. **Wien Med Wochenschr** 1983 Mar 31;133(6):153-5
Zglinicki F von: Die Wiege: volkskundlich, kulturgeschichtlich, kunstwissenschaftlich, medizinhistorisch. Regensburg, Pustet, 1979. 419 p.

**Asia**

Allan N: The oriental collections in the Wellcome Institute for the History of Medicine, London. **J R Asiat Soc GB Irel** 1981;1:10-25

**Belgium**

Heymans H: Eine Hülse mit Arztinstrumenten aus Maaseik (Belgien). **Archaeol Korrespbl** 1979;9:97-100

**China**

Zheng Jinsheng: [On pulverizing instruments for Chinese herbal drugs and their evolution in ancient China] (Chi). **Chin J Med Hist** 1981;11(1):35-9

**France**

Duchatel F: L'auscultation obstétricale de Philippe Le Goust au monitorage foetal. **Hist Sci Med** 1982;16(1):37-47
Nauroy J: L'équipement technique et le ravitaillement. **Med Armees** 1980;8(10)spec:845-50

**Germany**

Riall CT: Surgical and medical devices and their origins. Chapter XVII. Surgical instrument manufacturers. **J Oper Room Res Inst** 1983 Jan;3(1):33-5, 38-9, 42

**Great Britain**

Ingram A: The country animal doctor. Aylesbury, Bucks, Shire, 1979. 32 p. (Shire album; no. 40).
Lenihan J: Paradox and partnership. The engineer's contribution to medicine. **Scott Med J** 1980 Apr;25(2):107–12

**Poland**

Dutkiewicz M: Z dziejów munduru i symboli służby zdrowia Wojska Polskiego. **Arch Hist Med (Warsz)** 1984;47(1):85–90

**Romania**

Crisan V: Neurochirurgische Beiträge über die Benutzung der keltischen Sägen, sowie die in Galatii Bistritei in Rumanien gefundene Säge. In: International Congress of the History of Medicine, 26th, Plovdiv (Bulgaria), 1978. Actes du Congres, Vol. 1. Sofia, 1980. p. 93–6.

**Before 500 A.D.**

Bliquez LJ: Classical prosthetics. **Archaeology** 1983 Sep–Oct;36(5):25–9

**Egypt**

Narbe S: Egypten: på Ramses tid. **Odontol Foren Tidskr** 1981 Oct;45(4):30–2

**Greco–Roman**

Doederlein G: Arzneiapplikationen in der antiken Chirurgie. **Dtsch Apoth Ztg** 1979 Jun 14;119(24):936–8
Hassel FJ, Künzl E: Ein römisches Arztgrab des 3. Jahrhunderts n. Chr. aus Kleinasien. **Medizinhist J** 1980;15(4):403–21

**Greece**

Pournaropoulos C: The material used for the ancient Greek medical and surgery instruments. In International Congress of the History of Medicine. 26th, Plovdiv, 1978. Actes du Congress. Sofia, 1981. Volume II. p. 188–9.
Pournaropoulos CG: Medical instruments used by ancient Greeks. In International Congress of the History of Medicine. 26th, Plovdiv, 1978. Actes du Congress. Sofia, 1981. Volume II. p. 187–8.

**Rome**

Baxby D: An unauthorized contemporary reprinting of Jenner's paper on the cuckoo. **J Hist Med Allied Sci** 1981 Apr;36(2):218–9
Bliquez LJ: Roman surgical instruments in the Johns Hopkins University Institute of the History of Medicine. **Bull Hist Med** 1982 Summer;56(2):195–217
Cope JC: Roman medical instruments. **Mo Med** 1980 Sep;77(9):574
Engelhardt R, ed: Das römische Aerzte-Instrumentarium. Bingen, Engelhardt, 1974. 47 p. (Binger Annalen, IV) Contributions by C. Palm, K. M. Heidecker, P. Nahm, E. Naujack, A. Engelhardt.
Gilson AG: A group of Roman surgical and medical instruments from Cramond, Scotland. **Medizinhist J** 1983;18(4):384–93

**500 A.D.–1450**

**Arabic**

Hamarneh S: Medical technology in Ibn al-Quff's surgery. In I. El-Sayyad, ed: Papers presented to the First International Conference on Islamic Medicine, celebrating the advent of the fifteenth century hijri. Kuwait, Ministry of Public Health. National Council for Culture, Arts and Letters, 1981. p. 140–7.
Hamarneh SK, Awad EA: Early surgical instruments excavated in old Cairo, Egypt. In: Congrès international d'histoire de la médecine, XXVe, Québec, 1976. Actes. Québec, 1977. p. 761–4.

**China**

Wan Fang: Two questions about the Tian Sheng bronze statue for acupuncture of the Sung dynasty. (Chi). **Chin J Med Hist** 1981;11(1):62–4

**1450–1700**

Kapronczay K: A sebészeti eszközök fejlodése a XV–XVI. században. **Orvostort Kozl** 1982;28(1–3):141–50

**France**

Rudolph G: Les relations entre Denis Papin (1647–1714) et Leibniz (1646–1716). In: Congrès National des Sociétés Savantes, 93e, Tours, 1968. Comptes Rendus. Paris, 1971. Sections des Sciences, Tome II. p. 55–68.

**Germany**

Heintel H: Die Fallhaube: eine Erfindung des 16. Jahrhunderts? **Medizinhist J** 1984;19(3):273–6

**Great Britain**

Krantz JC. An architect designs a needle. **W Va Med J** 1980 Apr,76(4):84–5
Riall CT: Surgical and medical devices and their origins. William Harvey and circulation of the blood. Chapter XVI. **J Oper Room Res Inst** 1982 Nov;2(11):32–6
Robins R: An old Cornish hand. **J Hand Surg [Br]** 1984 Jun;9(2):199–200
Senior JE: Hauksbee's prototypical electrostatic generator. **Med Instrum** 1983 Mar–Apr;17(2):126–7

**Italy**

Oliaro T: Marco Aurelio Severino il perseguitato ricreatore della chirurgia italiana (1580–1656). **Minerva Chir** 1980 Sep 30;35(18 Suppl):32–4

**Netherlands**

Stroup A: Christiaan Huygens & the development of the air pump. **Janus** 1981;68:129–58

**Poland**

Jonecko A. Drzeworyt ukazujacy amputowane i protezowane produdzie w ślaskim poemacie Roździeńskiego 'Officina Ferraria' z roku 1616. **Arch Hist Med (Warsz)** 1984;47(1):107–16

**Switzerland**

Schneider W: Das Lot-Gewicht bei Paracelsus. In Dilg P, et al., ed: Perspektiven der Pharmaziegeschichte. Graz, Austria, Akademische Druck- u. Verlagsanstalt, 1983. p. 325–30.

**1700 to Present**

Amalric P: Ophtalmoscopie et périphérie rétinienne. Quelques aperçus historiques. **Bull Soc Ophtalmol Fr** 1980 Jun–Jul;80(6–7):595–7
Antoszewski Z: Krótki rys historyczny rozwoju pozaustrojowego krażenia krwi i niektórych aparatórych aparatów sztuczne 'płuco-serce'. **Przegl Lek** 1979;36(12):869–72
Arzua Zulaica E de: Historia del fibroscopio. **Rev Esp Enferm Apar Dig** 1980 Jan;57(1):77–80
Baraka A: Evolution of anaesthesia circuits **Middle East J Anaesthesiol** 1979 Jun;5(4):225–7
Belkin NL: Textiles as aseptic barriers: the past, present, and future. **Med Instrum** 1980 Jul–Aug;14(4):233–6
Benison S: Technology the dehumanizer. **Rev Am Hist** 1979;7(4):477–9
Besterman E: Waller before Einthoven in the clinical development of noninvasive ECG. **Am Heart J** 1982 Apr;103(4 pt 1):572
Beynon JH: The history of mass spectrometry and the search for zero. **Biomed Mass Spectrom** 1981 Sep;8(9):380–3
Biadała E: Wiadomości o strzykawkach stosowanych do leczenia chorych z 1820 r. **Wiad Lek** 1980 Nov 15;33(22):1849–50
Bishop PJ: Evolution of the stethoscope. **J R Soc Med** 1980 Jun;73(6):448–56
Bishop PJ: Reception of the stethoscope and Laënnec's book. **Thorax** 1981 Jul;36(7):487–92
Björk VO: The development of the Björk-Shiley artificial heart valve. **Clin Physiol** 1984 Feb;4(1):1–4
Bullough VL: A brief note on rubber technology and contraception: the diaphragm and the condom. **Technol Cult** 1981;22(1):104–11
Bullough VL: Bottle feeding: an amplification. **Bull Hist Med** 1981 Summer;55(2):257–9
Callaghan JC: Early experiences in the study and development of an artificial electrical pacemaker for standstill of the heart: view from 1949. **PACE** 1980 Sep;3(5):618–9
Caraway WT: Major developments in clinical chemical instrumentation. **J Clin Chem Clin Biochem** 1981 Jul;19(7):491–6
Chróścicki A: Osłuchiwanie serca--od stetoskopu do ultradźwi eków. **Pediatr Pol** 1979 Oct;54(10):1095–100
Clark G, White E, White D, et al: Bibliography of biomedical ultrasound from 1 January 1971, No. 20. **Ultrasound Med Biol** 1980;6(1):63–85
Clark LC: Measurement of oxygen tension: a historical perspective. **Crit Care Med** 1981 Oct;9(10):690–2
Coppock JB: Food technology [in the twentieth century]. In Williams TI, ed: A history of technology. Vol. VII. The twentieth century, ca. 1900 to ca. 1950. Part II. Oxford, Clarendon, 1978. p. 1399–445.
Cormack AM: Early two-dimensional reconstruction and recent topics stemming from it. **Science** 1980 Sep 26;209(4464):1482–6
Cormack AM: Recollections of my work with computer assisted tomography. **Mol Cell Biochem** 1980 Sep 15;32(2):59–61

# INSTRUMENTS AND EQUIPMENT

Craggs J: Simple method for auto-ophthalmoscopy. **Br J Ophthalmol** 1983 May;67(5):330-1

Danzin A: Data, evolution and entropy. **Methods Inf Med** 1980 Jan;19(1):2-6

Davis AB: Medical technology [in the twentieth century]. In Williams TI, ed: A history of technology. Vol. VII. The twentieth century, ca. 1900 to ca. 1950, Part II. Oxford, Clarendon Press, 1978. p. 1317-62.

Davis AB: Oscar Otto Rudolf Schwidetzky. In Dictionary of American biography, 1961-1965. Suppl. 7, 1981. p. 678-9.

De Duve C: Le développement de centrifugeuses à haute vitesse et leurs applications au fractionnement cellulaire. Un demi-siècle de collaboration entre la Belgique et l'Institut Rockefeller. **Bull Cl Sci Acad R Belg** 1980;5(66):470-2

Demidova NI: Telefonicheskie issledovaniia v élektrofiziologii. **Zh Vyssh Nerv Deiat** 1982 Jul-Aug;32(4):783-5

Doberneck RC, Kleinman R: The surgical garb. **Surgery** 1984 Jun;95(6):694-8

Doby T: History of cardiovascular catheterization. In: Congrès international d'histoire de la médecine, XXVe, Québec, 1976. Actes. Québec, 1977. p. 596-602.

Dolabjian ZL: The International Congress on Electrocardiography: a brief history. **J Electrocardiol** 1984 Jul;17(3):307-8

Dondelinger R: La tomodensitométrie des années 80. **Bull Soc Sci Med Grand Duche Luxemb** 1980;117(2):23-7

Donovan MG, Barrett DM: Ureteral prostheses. **Semin Urol** 1984 Aug;2(3):158-66

Dunea G: Maintenance dialysis after 20 years. **JAMA** 1980 Jul 4;244(1):67

Edmonson JM: Surgical garb, 1870-1920. Cleveland, Cleveland Health Sciences Library, 1982. 20 p. (Occasional contributions to the history of the health sciences from the Historical Division of the Cleveland Health Sciences Library, no. 1).

Feckenstein KJ: The rheoscopic frog and the study of animal electricity. **Med Instrum** 1983 May-Jun;17(3):235-6

Fleckenstein K: The early ECG in medical practice. **Med Instrum** 1984 May-Jun;18(3):191-2

Fraser I: An historical perspective on mechanical aids in intestinal anastomosis. **Surg Gynecol Obstet** 1982 Oct;155(4):566-74

Fye WB: Coronary arteriography--it took a long time! **Circulation** 1984 Nov;70(5):781-7

García MM: History and design of artifical heart valves. **Bol Asoc Med PR** 1981 Nov;73(11):567-73

Garcia Gamboa MA: Estudio retrospectivo de los forceps de Tarnier 1862-1877. La evolucion de la traccion axial y los forceps curvos tractores sobre su eje sin tractores. 2 vols. 2a. ed. [Rio Piedras, Puerto Rico, Universidad de Puerto Rico, Escuela de Medicina, 1981. 359 leaves.

Gathiram P, Katzeff IE, Edwards H, et al: Dynamic electrocardiography IV. The 'imaginary cardiac vector' hypothesis: the evolution of the vectorcardiographic inverse solution. **Med Hypotheses** 1981 Jul;7(7):825-62

Gersdorff M: Evolution des techniques d'audiométrie objective de 1970 à 1980. **Acta Otorhinolaryngol Belg** 1981;35(3-4):274-80

Giebel G, Rimpler M: Klebungen am Skellettsystem: Klebstoffe, 50 Jahre Hilfsstoffe für den Chirurgen (Teil 1). **Biomed Tech (Berlin)** 1981 Mar;26(3):35-40

Gold RD: Cardiac pacing--from then to now. **Med Instrum** 1984 Jan-Feb;18(1):15-21

Goldwyn RM: The paraffin story. **Plast Reconstr Surg** 1980 Apr;65(4):517-24

Gorham J: A medical triumph: the iron lung. **Respir Ther** 1979 Jan-Feb;9(1):71-3

Gow JG: The evolution of modern endoscopic photography. **Eur Urol** 1984;10(2):133-8

Grenvik A, Eross B, Powner D: Historical survey of mechanical ventilation. **Int Anesthesiol Clin** 1980 Summer;18(2):1-10

Guncheon KF: Diagnostic imaging: an inside look. **Hospitals** 1981 Jan 1;55(1):86-8, 95

Gunnell JG: The technocratic image and the theory of technocracy. **Technol Cult** 1982 Jul;23(3):392-16

Haller JS: Hypodermic medication; early history. **NY State J Med** 1981 Oct;81(11):1671-9

Haugwitz T von: Ophthalmologisch-optische Untersuchungsgeräte. Entwicklung und gegenwärtiger Stand. **Buch Augenarzt** 1981;(85):1-226

Henley KS: History of fiberoptic endoscopy. **Gastroenterology** 1980 May;78(5 Pt 1):1123-4

Herman JR: Old medical instruments. **Urology** 1984 Mar;23(3):301-B, 308-I

Herman JR: Urethral forceps. **Urology** 1983 Jan;21(1):60C

Hicks TP: The history and development of microiontophoresis in experimental neurobiology. **Prog Neurobiol** 1984;22(3):185-240

Huard P, Niaussat P: Calendrier de l'évolution du stéthoscope. In: Congrès National des Sociétés Savantes, 106e, Perpignan, 1981. Comptes Rendus. Paris, Bibliothèque Nationale, 1982. Fasc. IV. p. 105-10.

Huard P, Niaussat P: L'évolution du stéthoscope. In: Congrès National des Sociétés Savantes, 106e, Perpignan, 1981. Comptes Rendus. Paris, Bibliothèque Nationale, 1982. Fasc. IV. p. 91-104.

Il tripode si Sayre: **Chir Organi Mov** 1981;66(2):279-81

Inguaggiato B: Evoluzione tecnologica del pace-maker. **Minerva Med** 1980 Oct 6;71(38):2793-6

Isambert FA: Bio-éthique et techniques biomédicales. **Soc Sci Inf** 1983;22(1):125-37

Jephcott A: The Macintosh laryngoscope. A historical note on its clinical and commercial development. **Anaesthesia** 1984 May;39(5):474-9

Jordanova L: La donna di cera. **Kos** 1984 May;1(4):82-9

Kaleli A, Ansell JS: The artificial bladder: a historical review. **Urology** 1984 Nov;24(5):423-8

Kaltreider S: Tapping the tube. **MCVQ** 1981;16(3):106-12

Kolff WJ: Artificial organs--forty years and beyond. **Trans Am Soc Artif Intern Organs** 1983;29:6-24

Kolff WJ: Past, present, and future of artificial kidneys. **Transplant Proc** 1981 Mar;13(1):35-40

Korepanov VI: Istoriia razvitiia lazernoĭ khirurgii. **Sov Med** 1984;(3):61-5

Lagergren H: Den implanterbara pacemakern 25 år. Utveckling och erfarenheter. **Lakartidningen** 1983 Oct 5;80(40):3688-91

Lavenne F: L'electrocardiographie et vectocardiographie. **Rev Inst Hyg Mines (Hasselt)** 1980;35(3):133-4

Le Tacon J: La pleuroscopie. Rappel historique. **Poumon Coeur** 1981 Jan-Feb;37(1):5-6

Legée G: La notion de temps dans la physiologie neuro-musculaire au XIXe siècle. In: Congrès National des Sociétés Savantes, 99e, Besançon, 1974. Comptes Rendus. Paris, 1976. Section des Sciences, Fasc. V. p. 203-13.

Leme C de A: Desenvolvimento histórico da eletrocardiografia. **Rev Hosp Clin Fac Med Sao Paulo** 1980 Aug;35(4):205-17

Levine JR: The true inventors of the keratoscope and photo-keratoscope. **Br J Hist Sci** 1965;2(8):324-42

Liebenau JM: Medicine and technology. **Perspect Biol Med** 1983 Autumn;27(1):76-92

Lindstedt E, Lundquist SB: Utveckling av den transurethrala kirurgien. **Sydsven Medicinhist Sallsk Arsskr** 1980;:94-111

Lippert GP: Xenogener Ureterersatz in Tierversuch unter besonderer Berücksichtigung der historischen Entwicklung von Ureterbioprothesen. Diss. Mainz, 1979. 43 p.

Lowry LD: Artificial larynges: a review and development of a prototype self-contained intra-oral artificial larynx. **Laryngoscope** 1981 Aug;91(8):1332-55

Lübbers DW: History of transcutaneous PO2 measurement. **Crit Care Med** 1981 Oct;9(10):693

Lux G, Demling L: 100 Jahre Gastroskopie. **Fortschr Med** 1983 Jan 27;101(4):107-12

Mester AF, Stephens SD: Development of the audiometer and audiometry. **Audiology** 1984;23(2):206-14

Meyburg P: Ueber die Entwicklung des Operationstisches im 19. Jahrhundert. Diss. Mainz, 1980. 119 p.

Mielke HP: Brustgläser, Uringläser und Urinale. Zur Typologie dreier im medizinischen Gebrauch beheimateter Gläser. In Göpfert W, Otten HH, ed: Metavoeite: wandelt euch durch neues Denken. Düsseldorf, Triltsch, 1983. p. 209-12.

Morrissey JF: Gastrointestinal endoscopy--20 years of progress. **Gastrointest Endosc** 1983 Feb;29(1):53-6

Murphy RL: Auscultation of the lung: past lessons, future possibilities. **Thorax** 1981 Feb;36(2):99-107

Nice CM: Medical images: past, present, and future. **CRC Crit Rev Diagn Imaging** 1980;14(1):73-109

Nicholson P: Problems encountered by early endoscopists. **Urology** 1982 Jan;19(1):114-9

Pariente L, ed: Les appareils de mesure du pouls et de la pression artérielle. Paris, L. Pariente, 1979. 113 p.

Patev E: Peritonealna dializa--minalo, nastoiashte i budeshte. **Vutr Boles** 1980;19(1):7-11

Peltier LF: A brief historical note on the use of electricity in the treatment of fractures. **Clin Orthop** 1981 Nov-Dec;161:4-7

Picatoste y Patiño J, Martín García B: La cistoscopia (1879-1979) (centenario de un invento trascendental). **Arch Esp Urol** 1980 Jul-Feb;33(1):1-18

Piccolo E: L'elettrocardiografia a una svolta semeiologica. **G Ital Cardiol** 1981;11(1):1-3

Poll M: Die Entwicklung der Gastroskopie. In M. Poll, ed: Gastro-Duodenoskopie. Grundlagen und Hinweise für die Praxis. Weinheim, Edition Medizin, 1982. p. 13-20.

Radner S: Den selektiva angiografins bakgrund och begynnelse. **Sydsven Medicinhist Sallsk Arsskr** 1982;19:109-18

Ravitch MM: Development of intestinal anastomotic devices. **South Med J** 1982 Dec;75(12):1520-4

Ravitch MM, Steichen FM: Staples and staplers. **Adv Surg** 1984;17:241-79

Reiser SJ: Technology and the eclipse of individualism in medicine. **Pharos** 1982 Winter;45(1):10-5

Rendell-Baker L: Nineteenth-century resuscitation apparatus. **Anaesthesia** 1981 Nov;36(11):1058-9

Rendell-Baker L: Principles in design and function of mechanical ventilators. **Respir Ther** 1979 Jan-Feb;9(1):63-4, 66-9

Renggli R: Die Anfänge der Spirometrie im 19. Jahrhundert. **Gesnerus** 1981;38:247-58

Rhoads JE, Vars HM, Dudrick SJ: The development of intravenous hyperalimentation. **Surg Clin North Am** 1981 Jun;61(3):429-35

Riall CT: Surgical and medical devices and their origins. Chapter XIX.

Surgical instrument manufacturers. **J Oper Room Res Inst** 1983 Apr;3(4):36–9
Rijlant P: The coming of age of electrophysiology and electrocardiography. **NTM** 1980;17(1):108–23
Robicsek F: The birth of the surgical stapler. **Surg Gynecol Obstet** 1980 Apr;150(4):579–83
Rodegra H: Die Anfänge der Endoskopie. **Laryngol Rhinol Otol (Stuttg)** 1979 Sep;58(9):723–30
Romm S: Fritz Steinmann and the pin that bears his name. **Plast Reconstr Surg** 1984 Aug;74(2):306–10
Ronchi L, Fronsini R: Sviluppo e applicazioni cliniche dell'elettro-oculografia. Firenze, Baccini and Chiappi, 1975. 84 p.
Roth N: Animal electricity. **Med Instrum** 1980 Jul–Aug;14(4):228
Roth N: Bugs and blasphemy: Andrew Crosse and the Acarus electricus. **Med Instrum** 1979 Nov–Dec;13(6):357
Roth N: Electroresuscitation and the occult. **Med Instrum** 1980 Mar–Apr;14(2):120–1
Rucker CW: A history of the ophthalmoscope. Rochester, Minn., Whiting Printers and Stationers, [1971]. 127 p.
Ruhdorfer UE: Die klinische Blutdruckmessung – rund 100 Jahre alt. **Osterr Arzteztg** 1982;37(4):193
Schechter DC: Flashbacks: containment of tumors through electricity. **PACE** 1979 Jan;2(1):100–14
Schiller F: Neurology: the electrical root. In Rose FC, Bynum WF, ed: Historical aspects of the neurosciences. New York, Raven, 1982. p. 1–11.
Schiller F: Reverend Wesley, Doctor Marat and their electric fire. **Clio Med** 1981 Apr;15(3–4):159–76
Schwan HP: Ultrasound and electromagnetic radiation in hyperthermia--a historical perspective. **Br J Cancer** 1982 Mar;45(5)Suppl:84–92
Seipel L, Breithardt G, Borggrefe M: Die Entwicklung der klinischen Elektrophysiologie. Indikation, Komplikationen und Ergebnisse von 1296 invasiven elektrophysiologischen Untersuchungen 1971 bis 1981 in Düsseldorf. **Z Kardiol** 1984 Apr;73(4):194–8
Serafin D: Microsurgery: past, present, and future. **Plast Reconstr Surg** 1980 Nov;66(5):781–5
Shearing SP: Evolution of the posterior chamber intraocular lens. **J Am Intraocul Implant Soc** 1984 Summer;10(3):343–6
Shehadi WH: X-ray tubes and other historic memorabilia. **Med Radiogr Photogr** 1981;57(2):preceding p 21
Silvay G, Griffin R: The history and development of cardiovascular monitoring during anesthesia. **Mt Sinai J Med (NY)** 1984 Sep;51(5):560–3
Simpson GT, Polanyi TG: History of the carbon dioxide laser in otolaryngologic surgery. **Otolaryngol Clin North Am** 1983 Nov;16(4):739–52
Snellen HA, Dunning AJ, Arntzenius AC, ed: History and perspectives of cardiology. Catheterization, angiography, surgery and concepts of circular control. The Hague, Leiden University Press, 1981. 204 p. Major historical contributions by L. Dexter, H. L. Abrams, H. Swan, A. C. Guyton, J. Sonolet.
Steichen FM, Ravitch MM: History of mechanical devices and instruments for suturing. **Curr Probl Surg** 1982 Jan;19(1):1–52
Steiner W: Fortschritte in der endoskopischen Larynxdiagnostik. **Ther Umsch** 1980 Dec;37(12):1021–8
Stephen RL: Artificial kidneys: past, present and future. **Ann Biomed Eng** 1980;8(4–6):487–502
Stock CR: Laryngoscopy. **Ear Nose Throat J** 1984 Oct;63(10):528–30
Stoecklin WH: Die Erfindung der Magensonde. Ein ethnomedizinischer Beitrag zur Prioritätsfrage. **Gesnerus** 1981;38:237–46
Talyshinskiĭ AM: K istorii éndotrakheal'nykh trukbok s manzhetkami i bronkhoblokatorov. **Anesteziol Reanimatol** 1980 Mar–Apr;(2):68–70
Taylor E: The electrified hand--psychotherapeutic implications. **Med Instrum** 1983 Jul–Aug;17(4):281–2
Timio M: Il rene artificiale: la storia di uno strumento per una vita semiartificiale. **Med Secoli** 1982;19(3):273–301
Van der Star P, ed: Fahrenheit's letters to Leibniz and Boerhaave. Amsterdam, Rodopi, 1983. 195 p. (Nieuwe Nederlandse bijdragen tot de geschiedenis der geneeskunde en der natuurwetenschappen, no. 10).
Walter CW: Use of surgical rubber gloves. **Surgery** 1983 May;93(5):728–9
Watson WF: Development of the PVC endotracheal tube. **Biomaterials** 1980 Jan;1(1):41–6
Wawersik J: Die Geschichte des Narkoseapparates in Grundzügen. **Anaesthesist** 1982 Oct;31(10):541–8
Weerda H, Karl F, Müller-Hermann E: Die Entwicklung der Laryngoskopie. **HNO** 1984 Jul;32(7):307–11
Yechezkel M, Deviri E, Levy MJ: [Prosthetic heart valves--historical review] (Heb). **Harefuah** 1984 May 15;106(10):475–6

**Americas**

Turtle A: Collections of early psychological laboratory apparatus in North America. **Newsl Australas Assoc Hist Philos Sci** 1977–78;9:4–5

**Australia**

Gandevia B: Dr. John Hutchinson: the inventor of the spirometer. **Aust Fam Physician** 1981 Jul;10(7):574–8
Mond HG, Sloman JG, Edwards RH: The first pacemaker. **PACE** 1982 Mar;5(2):278–82

**Austria**

Sakula A: Joseph Skoda 1805–81: a centenary tribute to a pioneer of thoracic medicine. **Thorax** 1981 Jun;36(6):404–11
Zani A: Le origini storiche dell'elettroencefalografia. **Stor Crit Psicol** 1981;2(1):119–84

**Belgium**

Ferkó S: Palfyn Johann (1650–1730) a szülészeti fogó egyik feltalálója halálának 250. évfordulójára. **Orv Hetil** 1980 Mar 17;121(10):585–6
Soeur R: Evocation du passé: le professeur Baron Seutin et sa réaction au bandage plâtré. **Rev Med Brux** 1983 Jun;4(6):447–9

**Brazil**

Leme C de A: História da eletrocardiografia no Brasil. **Rev Hosp Clin Fac Med Sao Paulo** 1981 Aug;36(4):179–83

**Chile**

Costa-Casaretto C: Chile en dueda con el Doctor Francisco Fonck. **Rev Med Chil** 1981 Nov;109(11):1119–25

**Czechoslovakia**

Vlček J, Klánova JV: Akologický kabinet, jeho vznik a osudy. **Rozhl Chir** 1984 Feb;63(2):140–4

**Denmark**

Dragsted PJ: Avendelse af edb i sundhedsvaesenet--det historiske forløb i Danmark. **Nord Med** 1981 Oct;96(10):235–6

**France**

Adler C: René Théophile Hyacinthe Laënnec (1781–1826), inventor of the stethoscope. **Adler Mus Bull** 1981;7(2):3–7
Amalric P: La naissance et les premiers pas de l'ophtalmoscopie binoculaire. **Bull Soc Ophthalmol Fr** 1982 Nov;82(11):1469–71
Bastholm E: Laennec og stetoskopet. **Dan Medicinhist Arbog** 1982;:112–35
Borell M: D'Arsonval's calorimeter: measurement of animal heat, 1877. **Med Instrum** 1982 Nov–Dec;16(6):307–8
Cone TE: The first published report of an incubator for use in the care of the premature infant (1857). **Am J Dis Child** 1981 Jul;135(7):658–60
Delatte L, Halleux R: Recettes médicales anciennes et ordinateur: le projet Theorema. **Rev Hist Pharm (Paris)** 1980 Sep;27(246):155–160
Finot A: Les premiers élèves et collaborateurs (surtout Bretons) de Laennec. In: Congrès National des Sociétés Savantes, 91e, Rennes, 1966. Comptes Rendus. Paris, 1967. Section des Sciences, Tome 1. p. 181–9.
Fleckenstein K: Etienne Marey and the electric torpedo fish. **Med Instrum** 1984 Sep–Oct;18(5):288–9
Fox ER: Mrs. Laennec and the stethoscope. **West J Med** 1981 Jan;134(1):73–4
Gelfand T: Chirurghi dei Lumi. **Kos** 1984 Feb;1(1):51–73
Hanngren A: René Théophile Hyacinthe Laennec (1781–1826). **Nord Medicinhist Arsb** 1981;:106–19
Higier J: J. A. Kergaradec (1787–1877) – zapomniany odkrywca i pionier słuchawki położniczej. **Ginekol Pol** 1982;53(11):817–20
Huard P, Wong M: Ablation d'un polype naso-pharyngien à la Trinité en 1812. In: Congrès National des Sociétés Savantes, 91e, Rennes, 1966. Comptes Rendus. Paris, 1967. Section des Sciences, Tome 1. p. 99–102.
Huard P: Armel-Eugène Gripouilleau (1821–1909) officier de santé à Montlouis (Indre-et-Loire). In: Congrès National des Sociétés Savantes, 93e, Tours, 1968. Comptes Rendus. Paris, 1971. Section des Sciences, Tome II. p. 189–92.
Huard P: Il y a cent ans Constantin Paul présentait à l'Académie de Médecine son stéthoscope autostatique bi-auriculaire. **Bull Acad Natl Med (Paris)** 1981 Nov;165(8):1117–21
Huard P, Chaïa J: La découverte du caoutchouc et ses premières applications médicales en France. In: Congrès National des Sociétés Savantes, 93e, Tours, 1968. Comptes Rendus. Paris, 1971. Section des Sciences, Tome II. p. 69–73.
Huard P, Lefebvre P, Nosny P, et al: La scie ostéotome à chaîne de Bernhard-Franz Heine (1800–1846). **Hist Sci Med** 1983;17(2):147–57
Huard P, Niaussat PM: 'L'arsenal' du service de Santé de la Marine au XIXe siècle. In: Congrès National des Sociétés Savantes, 105e, Caen, 1980. Comptes Rendus, Paris, 1980. Section des Sciences, Fasc. V. p. 85–96.
Huard P, Niaussat PM: L'évolution du stéthoscope de Laennec à nos jours; son influence dans certains domaines des transmissions acoustiques. **Hist Sci Med** 1981;15(2):173–87
Huard P, Imbault-Huart MJ: Travaux de Percy (1754–1825) sur l'hémostase des artères (1790–1810). In: Congrès National des Sociétés Savantes, 99e, Besançon, 1974. Comptes Rendus. Paris, 1976. Section

des Sciences, Fasc. V. p. 251-7.
L'Exposition Universelle de 1889: Recherche des réponses au questionnaire et d'objets. **Bull Soc Fr Hist Hop** 1979;(39):19-21
Maison Nachet: Catalogues de fonds de 1854 à 1910. Facsimile edition. Introduction par G. L'E. Turner. Paris, Brieux, 1979. Various paginations.
Mammerickx M: André-Marie Ampère et Claude-Julien Bredin, II. Ampère, Bredin et le magnétisme animal, ou la petite histoire d'une grande découverte. **Hist Med Vet** 1977;2(3):69-75
Marketos SG: [The concert for Laënnec's stethoscope] (Gre). **Mater Med Greca** 1981;9:125-34
Mercier P: André Bocage et la naissance de la tomographie. **Bull Acad Natl Med (Paris)** 1979;3:188-91
Niaussat P, Huard P: Problèmes acoustiques communs à la médecine, à la marine et aux télécommunications, étudiés par le Docteur Paul Constantin. In: Congrès National des Sociétés Savantes, 106e, Perpignan, 1981. Comptes Rendus. Paris, Bibliothèque Nationale, 1982. Fasc. IV. p. 81-9.
Obermajer J: Endoskopie jako výtvarný motiv. **Cesk Gastroenterol Vyz** 1980 Jan;34(1):51-4
Plessis JL: Un anatomiste militaire mort victime du devoir: Adolphe-Euclide Lacauchie (1806-1853), latiniste distingué et inventeur de l'hydrotomie. **Hist Sci Med** 1982;16(3):151-61
Roth N: Capturing the heart, 1880: Marey's cardiac tongs. **Med Instrum** 1980 Sep-Oct;14(5):285
Sakula A: Acceuil du livre 'De l'auscultation médiate' et du stéthoscope par les médecins de Grande-Bretagne. **Rev Palais Decouv** 1981 Aug;22:280-90
Sakula A: The story of the stethoscope. **Trans Med Soc Lond** 1981-82;98:27-31
Ségal A: Le médecin principal de 1re classe Jean-Pierre Bonnafont (1805-1891); sa place prépondérante dans l'histoire de l'endoscopie aus XIXe siècle. **Hist Sci Med** 1983;17(1):63-70
Snellen HA: E. J. Marey and cardiology: physiologist and pioneer of technology, 1830-1904: selected writings in facsimile with comments and summaries, a brief history of life and work, and a bibliography. 264 p.
Sutton G: Electric medicine and mesmerism. **Isis** 1981 Sep;72(263):375-92
Trautmann M, Trautmann JC: R. T. H. Laennec 1781-1826. Zum 200. Geburtstag des Autors der Auscultation médiate. **MMW** 1981 Nov 6;123(45):1717-20
Turiaf J: Laennec et la pathologie respiratoire. **Bull Acad Natl Med (Paris)** 1981 Feb 17;Spec No:31-6

**Germany**

Bach H: Die Entwicklung der künstlichen Niere aus Hydrodiffusion und Hämodialyse, von J. A. Nollet bis G. Haas. Der Ursprung des ersten Künstlichen inneren Organs. Giessen, Schmitz, 1983. 334 p. (Arbeiten zur Geschichte der Medizin in Giessen, Bd. 7)
Blömer H: 20 Jahre Herzschrittmacher-therapie. **ZFA (Stuttgart)** 1982 Jan 10;58(1):19-25
Engel K: Der Gräfenberg-Ring. Zu seiner Vorgeschichte, Entwicklung, Anwendung und frühen Rezeption. Diss. Erlangen-Nürnberg, 1979. 137 p.
Grapentin F: Veterinärärztliches Gerät im Zweiten Weltkrieg. **DTW** 1981 Nov 5;88(11):473-5
Hollmann W, Valentin H: 50 Jahre Spiroergometrie 1929 bis 1979. **MMW** 1980 Feb 1;122(5):169-74
Howard-Jones N: Cardiac catheterization, a historical note. **Bull Hist Med** 1973 Sep-Oct;47(5):524-6
Jung R, Berger W: Fünfzig Jahre EEG. Hans Bergers Entdeckung des Elektrenkephalogramms und seine ersten Befunde 1924--1931. **Arch Psychiatr Nervenkr** 1979 Dec;227(4):279-300
Koelsch KA: Die Entwicklukng der gastroenterologischen Endoskopie in der DDR während der letzten 10 Jahre, alte und neue Probleme. **Z Arztl Fortbild (Jena)** 1979 Oct 1;73(19-20):981-3
Kugler J: Zur Entwicklung der Deutschen EEG-Gesellschaft. **EEG EMG** 1984 Mar;15(1):1-7
Lopatkin NA, Shchabad AL: Die Zystoskopie und ihre Bedeutung in der Urologie. **Z Urol Nephrol** 1979 Jul;72(12):517-22
Püschel E: Ein hundertjähriger Medizinstudenten-Stock. **Medizinhist J** 1983;18(3):260-5
Rihner F: Alfred Hegar--Zum 150. Geburtstag. **Med Welt** 1980 Oct 17;31(42):1522-3
Schwartz RH: The pneumatic otoscope, a new instrument for the examination of the tympanic membrane--E. Siegle. 1984. **Int J Pediatr Otorhinolaryngol** 1980 Sep;2(3):261-3
Seufert WD: The chain osteotome by Heine. **J Hist Med Allied Sci** 1980 Oct;35(4):454-9
Tautz P, Hein G: Frühformen orthopädischen Denkens und orthopädischer Methoden in den ersten 120 Jahren der Universität Halle (Saale) (III). Heinrich Bass (1690-1754), genannt, 'Bandagen-Bass'. **Beitr Orthop Traumatol** 1979;26(12):705-12
Voswinckel P: Arzt und Auto: das Auto und seine Welt im Spiegel des Deutschen Arztblattes von 1907 bis 1975. Münster, Murken-Altrogge, 1981. iii, 194 p.
Votočková J: 130 let Helmholtzova oftalmoskopu. **Cesk Oftalmol** 1982 Jan;38(1):51-3
Weisser C: Der Ombrédannesche Ather-Inhalator. Ein Beitrag zur Geschichte der Ather-Apparatnarkose. **Anaesthesist** 1983 Feb;32(2):51-4

**Great Britain**

Beneš V, Benešová Z: Horsleyv vosk. **Rozhl Chir** 1982 Feb;61(2):141-3
Chaldecott JA: Wedgwood's ceramic wares for chemical use, production and supply from 1779-1794. **Ambix** 1981 Nov;28(3):184-205
Farr AD: Learn, that you may improve: the history of the Institute of Medical Laboratory Sciences. Sussex, Denley Instruments, 1982. xi, 214 p.
Hounsfield GN: Computed medical imaging. **Med Phys** 1980 Jul-Aug;7(4):283-90
Hunt LB, Buchanan PD: Richard Knight (1768-1844): a forgotten chemist and apparatus designer. **Ambix** 1984 Jul;31(2):57-67
Lawrence C: Alfred Henry Garrod and the indirect measurement of the isometric period of the heart's contraction. **Med Hist** 1980 Jul;24(3):342-6
McLellan I: Nineteenth century resuscitation apparatus. **Anaesthesia** 1981 Mar;36(3):307-11
Ross WM, Day MJ: Mullard 4 MV linear accelerator at Newcastle upon Tyne. **Br J Radiol** 1981 Sep;54(645):819
Sakula A: Laennec's influence on some British physicians in the nineteenth century. **J R Soc Med** 1981 Oct;74(10):759-67
Stephens SD: Centenary of British audiometry. London, Royal National Institute for the Deaf in collaboration with the British Society of Audiology, 1979. 40 p.
Stephens SD: David Edward Hughes and his audiometer. **J Laryngol Otol** 1979 Jan;93(1):1-6
Stephens SD: The British medical profession and the first audimeters. **J Laryngol Otol** 1981 Dec;95(12):1223-35

**Hungary**

Benkö F: A vatta hazai elötörténete. **Orv Hetil** 1984 Nov 25;125(48):2965
A hazai porcragasztás prioritástaról: **Orv Hetil** 1984 Dec 16;125(51):3150
Kempler K: A gyógyszerészeti technológia hazai úttöröje Rozsnyay Mátyás. **Orv Hetil** 1984 Jul 22;125(30):1832-4, 1837
Kempler K: A magyar kereskedelmi tengerjáró hajók kötelezö egészségügyi felszerelése a századfordulón. **Orvostort Kozl** 1981;93-96(27 No 1-4):171-82

**Ireland**

Pinkerton JH: John Creery Ferguson 1802-1865: Physician and fetologist. **Ulster Med J** 1981;50(1):10-20

**Italy**

Azzaroli ML, Lanza B: La Venere scomponibile. **Kos** 1984 May;1(4):65-81
Cremona GF: L'elettroterapia nel XVIII secolo. Ricerche di elettrofisiolgia e di elettroterapia di studiosi piemontesi. **Ann Osp Maria Vittoria Torino** 1981 Jan-Jun;24(1-6):167-77
Dondi RF: Uno strumento chirurgico dimenticato: le forbici del Valtolini. **Ann Osp Maria Vittoria Torino** 1980 Jul-Dec;23(7-12):289-94
Fechner PU, Fechner MU, Reis H: Der Okulist Tadini. Zur Geschichte der künstlichen Augenlinse. **Klin Monatsbl Augenheilkd** 1980 Jun;176(6):1003-11
Fink M: Meduna and the origins of convulsive therapy. **Am J Psychiatry** 1984 Sep;141(9):1034-41
Sakula A: Carlo Forlanini, inventor of artificial pneumothorax for treatment of pulmonary tuberculosis. **Thorax** 1983 May;38(5):326-32

**Japan**

Furukawa T: [Development of neurophysiology in Japan brought by introduction of microelectrodes] (Jpn). **Nippon Seirigaku Zasshi** 1984;46(1):5-7
Nihon Chusha Kigu Kensa Kyokai 15-nenshi: Chusha no rekishi to gyokai no ayumi. Tokyo, Do Kyokai, Showa 51 nen, [1976]. 187 p.

**Netherlands**

Lamas GA, Koller LR, Antman EM, et al: Electrocardiogram by Einthoven 63 years earlier. **Am J Cardiol** 1984 Nov 1;54(8):1163-5
Meijler FL: Vijftig jaar Nederlandse Vereniging voor Cardiologie of, Nederland, debakermat van de elektrocardiografie. **Ned Tijdschr Geneeskd** 1984 Mar 24;128(12):571-3
Van Lieburg MJ: The instrument-collection of Peter Vink, a chapter in the development of the surgical profession in the Netherlands during the 18th century. **Janus** 1980:67(1-2-3):207-19

**Poland**

Rijlant P: Results and perspectives in electrocardiology. **Adv Cardiol** 1981;28:1-8
Wajs S: Obturatory stosowane w leczeniu protetycznym rozszczepów

wrodzonych lub nabytych podniebienia twardego i miękkiego. Czesc III. **Nov Med Tekh** 1979 May–Jun;29(3):211–8
Walewski W, Markowski W, Mosejczuk L, et al: [35 years of service in medical supply to the Polish People's Forces]. (Rus) **Voen Med Zh** 1979 Nov;(11):67–8

**Puerto Rico**

Torres-Gómez JM: Suárez, Ramón M., 1895–19811700 to PresentPuerto Rico **Bol Asoc Med PR** 1983 Nov,75(11).501–2

**Spain**

Herrero P, Frances MC: Influencia de la dosimetria en la farmacia española. **Bol Soc Esp Hist Farm** 1982 Mar;33(130):93–112
Torres Ramírez C, Aguilar Ruíz J, Zuluaga Gómez A, et al: La cristalografía aplicada al análisis de los cálculos urinarios en España. Revisión histórica de la aportacion española al tema. **Arch Esp Urol** 1980 May–Jun;33(3):241–50

**Sweden**

Björk VO: The development of the Björk-Shiley artificial heart valve. **Clin Cardiol** 1984 Jan;7(1):3–5
Elmqvist R: Review of early pacemaker development. **PACE** 1978 Oct;1(4):535–6
Modig M: Raritet från Rörstrand. Från luktvatten till syrgaskuddar-en inhalationshistorik. **Draco Med** 1983;24(7):14–5
Riall CT: Surgical and medical devices and their origins. Chapter XX. The Swedish influence. **J Oper Room Res Inst** 1983 Jun,3(6).18–9, 22, 24

**United States**

Ausman RK, Bellamy D Jr: Problems and resolutions in the development of the flexible plastic blood container (Carl W. Walter). **Am J Surg** 1984 Nov;148(5):559–61
Banta HD, Burns AK, Behney CJ: Policy implications of the diffusion and control of medical technology. **Ann Am Acad Polit Soc Sci** 1983;(468):165–81
Barger AC: New technology for a new century: Walter B. Cannon and the invisible rays. **AJR** 1981 Jan;136(1):187–95
Barrett DM, Donovan MG: Prosthetic bladder augmentation and replacement. **Semin Urol** 1984 Aug;2(3):167–75
Battocletti JH, Halbach RE, Salles-Cunha SX, et al: The NMR blood flowmeter--theory and history. **Med Phys** 1981 Jul–Aug;8(4):435–43
Beatty WK: William T. Bovie. In Dictionary of American Biography, Suppl. 6, 1956–1960. p. 69–70, 1980.
Beatty WK: William T. Bovie, inventor and teacher. **Trans Stud Coll Physicians Phila** 1979 Jun;5(1 no 2):138–44
Bernstein BJ, et al: The artificial heart program. **Cent Mag** 1981;14(3):22–41
Bloomfield DK: Early work on external electrical defibrillation. **N Engl J Med** 1980 Dec 4;303(23):1366–7
Brooks JR: Carl W. Walter, MD: surgeon, inventor, and industrialist. **Am J Surg** 1984 Nov;148(5):555–8
Brumley WC, Sphon JA: Regulatory mass spectrometry. **Biomed Mass Spectrom** 1981 Sep;8(9):390–6
Carlson WB: Innovation in medical technology: Elihu Thomson, General Electric, and X rays in 1896. **Med Instrum** 1982 Jul–Aug;16(4):218
Cole WH: The development of cholecystography. **J Thorac Cardiovasc Surg** 1984 Nov;88(5 Pt 2):827–33
Cormack AM: Early two-dimensional reconstruction and recent topics stemming from it. **Med Phys** 1980 Jul–Aug;7(4):277–82
The cutaneous punch by Edward L. Keyes (J Cutan Genitourin Dis, March 1887): **Arch Dermatol** 1982 Nov;118(11):940–2
Dammann G: Pictorial encyclopedia of Civil War medical instruments and equipment. Missoula, Mont., Pictorial Histories Pub. Co., 1983. iv, 100 p.
Davis AB: Life insurance and the physical examination: a chapter in the rise of American medical technology. **Bull Hist Med** 1981;55(3):392–406
Dobrin L: Origin and evolution of the walkerette. **Mt Sinai J Med (NY)** 1980 Mar–Apr;47(2):172–4
Dupont J: At long last 'The TMC Story: premieres'. **EITV** 1984 Mar;16(3):52–4
Dyer JA: Corneal contact lenses in perspective 1948–1981. **Contact Intraocular Lens Med J** 1982 Jan–Mar;8(1):3–8
Eastman JW: 'Doctors' orders': the American medical profession and the origins of automobile design for crash protection, 1930–1955. **Bull Hist Med** 1981;55(3):407–24
Gorham J: Commercial development of the oxygen tent. **Respir Ther** 1979 Jan–Feb;9(1):48–9
Gotch FA: The evolution of the society. **Trans Am Soc Artif Intern Organs** 1979;25:534–8
Gutman RA: Renal dialysis for kidney failure in North Carolina: history, practice, and lessons. **NC Med J** 1984 Jun;45(6):359–63
Herman JR: Hot water bag for diseased prostate. **Urology** 1979 Dec;14(6):545–V
Hill JD: John H. Gibbon, Jr. Part I. The development of the first successful heart-lung machine. **Ann Thorac Surg** 1982 Sep;34(3):337–41
Holmes JH: Diagnostic ultrasound during the early years of A.I.U.M. **JCU** 1980 Aug;8(4):299–308
Hufnagel CA, Thorn GW: Observations of a colleague (Carl W. Walter). **Am J Surg** 1984 Nov;148(5):581–3
Jones RJ: The NCCLS and medical devices. **JAMA** 1980 May 2;243(17):1748
Kidwell R: Handicapping an innovator. **Reason** 1981;13(4):39–46
Kunitomo T: Development of new artificial kidney systems (Carl W. Walter). **Am J Surg** 1984 Nov;148(5):594–8
Lightdale CJ: Notes on the development of the American Society for Gastrointestinal Endoscopy. **Gastrointest Endosc** 1983 Feb;29(1):51–3
McDonell KM: W. D. Allison: manufacturer of physicians' furniture. **Snakeroot Extr** 1984 Oct;(3):2–3
Miller BJ: The development of heart lung machines. **Surg Gynecol Obstet** 1982 Mar;154(3):403–14
Miller JM: William Stewart Halsted and the use of the surgical rubber glove. **Surgery** 1982 Sep;92(3):541–3
Morgan JP: The first reported case of electrical stimulation of the human brain. **J Hist Med Allied Sci** 1982 Jan;37(1):51–64
Murphy WP: Carl Walter: a pioneer in shaping the medical device industry. **Am J Surg** 1984 Nov;148(5):590–3
Myers WG: The Anger scintillation camera becomes of age. **J Nucl Med** 1979 Jun;20(6):565–7
Olivier A, Bertrand G, Picard C: Discovery of the first human stereotactic instrument. **Appl Neurophysiol** 1983;46(1–4):84–91
Panel on dialysis: **Transplant Proc** 1981 Mar;13(1):67–71
Paquet JB: The gloving of a nurse (Caroline Hampton). **Nurs Success Today** 1984 Summer;1(2):44
Pines M: Modern bioengineers reinvent human anatomy with spare parts. **Smithsonian** 1978;9(8):50–7
Rettig RA: Health care technology. Lessons learned from the end-stage renal disease experience. Santa Monica, Rand Corp., 1976. 36 p.
Rhoads JE: The evolution of intravenous hyperalimentation. **World J Surg** 1982 Jan;6(1):144–8
Riall CT, Hilzinger F: Surgical and medical devices and their origins. Chapter XVIII. Surgical instrument manufacturers. **J Oper Room Res Inst** 1983 Feb;3(2):34–9
Rink E: Technical Americana: a checklist of technical publications printed before 1831. Millwood, N. Y., Kraus International, 1981. 'Medical technology', p. 245–49.
Roth N: Electrotherapy, 19th-century neurasthenia, and the case of Alice James. **Med Instrum** 1981 Mar–Apr;15(2):116
Roth N: Reviving resuscitation: 1900 -- present. **Med Instrum** 1980 May–Jun;14(3):160
Roth N: Tracking by telephone: locating the bullet in President Garfield, 1881. **Med Instrum** 1981 May–Jun;15(3):190
Sammis S, Dummett E: On display: the science and art of healing. **J Med Soc NJ** 1984 Sep;81(9):747–57
Schechter DC: Flashbacks: electrical treatment of aneurysms. **PACE** 1979 Mar;2(2):234–45
Scherlag BJ: The development of the His bundle recording technique. **PACE** 1979 Mar;2(2):230–3
Schwan HP: Biomedical engineering and basic research: historical perspectives. **Med Prog Technol** 1980 Jun;7(2–3):63–7
Shamansky SL, Hamilton WM: Is the public health nurse's bag anachronism? **Nurs Outlook** 1980 Jun;28(6):379–81
Stine JK: Eugene Jules Houdry. In Dictionary of American biography, 1961–1965. Suppl. 7, 1981. p. 367–9.
Studebaker GA: Fifty years of hearing aid research: an evaluation of progress. **Ear Hear** 1980 Mar–Apr;1(2):57–62
Sweeney JK: Earle Ensign Dickson. In Dictionary of American biography, 1961–1965. Suppl. 7, 1981. p. 182–3.
Terreros DA, Grantham JJ: Marshall Barber and the origins of micropipette methods. **Am J Physiol** 1982 Mar;242(3):F293–6
Wolff E: The history and development of surgical tables for large animals. **VM SAC** 1981 Jul;76(7):1033–5

**USSR**

Balikhin LN: 50 let proizvodstva meditsinskikh instrumentov na Mozhaĭskom mediko-instrumental'nom zavode im. P. V. Gusenkova. **Med Tekh** 1981 Sep–Oct;(5):15–7
Demidova NI: [The role of I. M. Sechenov's school in the development of electrophysiology] (Rus). **Istor Biol Issled** 1980;8:156–62
Filatov VI: K stoletiiu otechestvennogo protezirovaniia (1883–1983). **Ortop Travmatol Protez** 1983 March;(3):61–3
Galin LL: Shina Diterikhsa. **Feldsher Akush** 1983 Nov;48(11):46–8
Krasnikov PG: Vydaiushcheesia izobretenie otechestvennogo oftal'mologa (100 let so vremeni sozdaniia applanatsionnogo tonometra Prof. A.N. Maklakova). **Vestn Oftalmol** 1984 Nov–Dec;(6):70–2
Kuz'min MK: V. F. Zelenin i ego rol' v razvitii klinicheskoĭ élektrokardiografii i funktsional'noĭ diagnostike. **Klin Med (Mosk)** 1981 Aug;59(8):115–8
Menshutin AA: 'Krasnogvardeets' v gody Velikoĭ Otechestvennoĭ. **Med Tekh** 1980 May–Jun;(3):3–7

## INSTRUMENTS AND EQUIPMENT

Obrosov AN: Etapy razvitiia metoda impul'snoĭ terapii v SSSR. **Vopr Kurortol Fizioter Lech Fiz Kult** 1980 Mar–Apr;(2):4–10
Roitbak AI: The importance of I. M. Sechenov's electrophysiological research. **Acta Neurobiol Exp (Warsz)** 1980;40(2):451–61
Segall H: N. C. Korotkoff and how he, a surgeon, discovered the sounds for measuring arterial pressure. In: Cóngrès international d'histoire de la médecine, XXVe, Québec, 1976. Actes. Québec, 1977. p. 1253–8.
Voronkov OV: Iz istorii sozdaniia zapasov meditsinskogo imushchestva dlia obespecheniia voĭsk vo vremia voĭny (soobshchenie vtoroe). **Voen Med Zh** 1984 Oct;(10):66–8
Voronkov OV: Obespechenie meditsinskim imushchestvom voĭsk voennogo okruga vo vremia Velikoĭ Otechestvennoĭ voĭny. **Voen Med Zh** 1980 Oct;(10):19–22
Vurgaft MB: The 90th anniversary of Maklakov's applanation tomometer. **Am J Optom Physiol Opt** 1981 Feb;58(2):183–5

**Yugoslavia**

Katan E: Sanitetsko snabdevanje Centralne bolnice Vrhovnog štaba i jedinica Glavne operativne grupe za vreme četvrte i pete ofanzive. **Vojnosanit Pregl** 1980 Nov–Dec;37(6):476–80
Stojan D, Petrović M: Razvoj sanitetske opreme u Ratnom vazduhoplovstvu. **Vojnosanit Pregl** 1981 Jan–Feb;38(1):37–40

## INTERNATIONAL HEALTH

Beer H, Dorolle P, Howard-Jones N: Histoire des institutions médicales internationales. In: Histoire de la médecine, de la pharmacie, de l'art dentaire, et de l'art véterinaire. Tome VIII. Paris, Albin Michel, Laffont, Tchou, 1980. p. 327–41.
Kostrzewski J: Swiat wolny od ospy. **Przegl Epidemiol** 1980;34(4):365–72
Strassburg MA: The global eradication of smallpox. **Am J Infect Control** 1982 May;10(2):53–9

**1700 to Present**

Akpabio SP: World Health Organisation. **Br Dent J** 1983 Feb 5;154(3):83–4
Banta JE: International health: challenges to the basic sciences. **Trans Stud Coll Physicians Phila** 1982 Dec;5(4 no 4):291–303
Beer H, Dorolle P, Howard-Jones N: Geschichte der internationalen Gesundheitsbehörden. In Sournia JC, Martiny M, Poulet J, ed: Illustrierte Geschichte der Medizin. Salzburg, Andreas, 1980. Vol. 8. p. 3109–39.
Belanger M: Une nouvelle branche du droit international: le droit international de la sante. **Etud Int** 1982;13(4):611–32
Bowers JZ, King EE: The conquest of yellow fever: the Rockefeller Foundation. **J Med Soc NJ** 1981 Jul;78(7):539–41
Corning ME: A review of the United States role in international biomedical research and communications: international health and foreign policy. Bethesda, National Library of Medicine, 1980. xxvii, 436 p. (NIH Publication No. 80–1638).
Craig RB, Turner MA: International control of narcotics and dangerous drugs: a synopsis. **Indian Pol Sci Rev** 1977;11(1):33–47
Dittmann S: Die Welt ist pockenfrei--Durchführung und Erfolg eines grandiosen Programms. **Z Gesamte Inn Med** 1980 Dec 15;35(24):858–63
Duffy J, ed: Ventures in world health; the memoirs of Fred Lowe Soper. Washington, Pan American Health Organization, 1977. 365 p. (Scientific Publ. No. 355).
Ermakov VV, Devyatova LN: The experience and the stages of development in USSR of the WHO English International Courses for epidemiology (1969–1978). **Sante Publique (Bucur)** 1980;23(1):3–14
Foster GM: Applied anthropology and international health: retrospect and prospect. **Hum Organ** 1982;41(3):189–97
Friedemann H: Zur Entwicklung der disziplinären Verantwortlichkeit für die Organisation des Gesundheitswesens in einigen internationalen Gesundheitssystemen. **Z Gesamte Hyg** 1980 Apr;26(4):283–90
Glaser S: L'arma batteriologica secondo la convenzione 1971. **Riv Mil** 1975;98(4):56–62
The global eradication of smallpox: Final report of the Global Commission for the certification of smallpox eradication, Geneva, December 1979. Geneva, World Health Organization, 1980. 122 p.
Henderson DA: The deliberate extinction of a species. **Proc Am Philos Soc** 1982 Dec 17;126(6):461–71
The history of the International Epidemiological Association brought up to date: **Int J Epidemiol** 1984 Jun;13(2):139–41
Howard-Jones N: International public health: The organizational problems between the two World Wars (5). **WHO Chron** 1978 Mar;32(3):114–25
Howard-Jones N: The World Health Organization in historical perspective. **Perspect Biol Med** 1981 Spring;24(3):467–82
Kaymakcalan S: Fifty years of international control of dependence-producing drugs. **Natl Inst Drug Abuse Res Monogr Ser** 1979;27:74–6
Keller F, Kirn A: Eradicazione mondiale del vaiolo. Da Sarah Nelmes a Ali Maow Maalin. **Minerva Med** 1980 Oct 20;71(40):2935–40
Moriyama N, Takazoe I: The historical relationship between Japanese dentistry and the Fédération Dentaire Internationale. **Bull Hist Dent** 1984 Oct;32(2):104–8
Morris JP: Gordon Stifler Seagrave. In Dictionary of American biography, 1961–1965. Suppl. 7, 1981. 679–81.
Muller M: The health of nations. A North-South investigation. London, Faber and Faber, 1982. 255 p.
Parnas J: Thorvald Madsen 1870–1957. Leader in international public health. **Dan Med Bull** 1981;28(2):82–6
Petkova M: Seriĭni izdaniia na svetovnata zdravna organizatsiia naukometrichno prouchvane. **Vutr Boles** 1982;21(6):86–91
Raska K: How the smallpox programme began. **World Health Forum** 1981;2:290–1
Rouillon A: The International Union against Tuberculosis. **Tubercle** 1982 Dec;63(4):247–53
Shapiro MF: Medical aid provided by American, Canadian and British Nationals to the Spanish Republic during the Civil War, 1936–1939. **Int J Health Serv** 1983;13(3):443–58
Silver anniversary of the Advisory Committee on Medical Research: **WHO Chron** 1984;38(1):8–16
Smith HH: Life's a pleasant institution: the peregrinations of a Rockefeller doctor. Tucson, The Author, 1978. x, 254 p.
Socknat TP: The Canadian contribution to the China convoy. **Quaker Hist** 1980;69(2):69–90
Sze S: The origins of the World Health Organization: a personal memoir, 1945–1948. Boca Raton, Fla. L.I.S.Z. Publications, [1982]. xiii, 31 p.
Vuori H: The World Health Organization and traditional medicine. **Community Med** 1982 May;4(2):129–37
Ward PS: Antibiotics and international relations at the close of World War II. In J. Parascandola, ed: The history of antibiotics. Madison, American Institute of the History of Pharmacy, 1980. p. 101–12.
Wehrle PF: A reality in our time--certification of the global eradication of smallpox. **J Infect Dis** 1980 Oct;142(4):636–8
Weigold ME: Alice Louise Florence Fitzgerald. In Dictionary of American biography, 1961–1965. Suppl. 7, 1981. p. 247–8.
Wysokiński A: Rola Swiatowej Organizacji Zdrowia w życiu panstw i narodow. **Wiad Lek** 1979 Jul 15;32(14):1031–7
Zaprianov N, Nikolov I: The share of the foreign 'Red Cross' societies in rendering help to the victims of the earthquake in Bulgaria, in the year of 1928. In International Congress of the History of Medicine. 26th, Plovdiv, 1978. Actes du Congress. Sofia, 1981. Volume II. p. 214.
Zhdanov VM, Slepushkin AN: Programma likvidatsii ospy vo vsem mire (istoriia razvitiia i rol' Sovetskogo Soiuza). **Vopr Virusol** 1980 Jul–Aug;(4):395–9

**Americas**

Acuña HR: El Boletín de la Oficina sanitaria panamericana: a los sessenta años. **Bol Of Sanit Panam** 1982 May;92(5):377–8
Boletín panamericano de sanidad de la Oficina sanitaria internacional: **Bol Of Sanit Panam** 1982 May;92(5):429–48
Howard-Jones N: The Pan American Health Organization: origins and evolution (1). **WHO Chron** 1980 Oct;34(10):367–75 (contd)
Howard-Jones N: The Pan American Health Organization: origins and evolution (2). **WHO Chron** 1980 Nov;34(11):419–26 concl.
Neghme A: La organización panamericana de la salud en su 75. aniversario. Tributo al Dr. Abraham B. Horwitz. **Rev Med Chil** 1977 Dec;105(12):950–2
Vaccarezza RF: Devoción a la causa de la salud: Fred Lower Soper. **Medicina (B Aires)** 1981;41(1):101–6

**Chile**

Juricic B: Chile y las organizaciones internacionales de salud. **Rev Med Chil** 1977 Oct;105(10):674–9

**Czechoslovakia**

Slavětínský M: Předchudci československo-sovětských lékařských styku. **Cesk Zdrav** 1982 Sep;30(8–9):381–5

**Europe**

Roscam Abbing HD: International organizations in Europe and the right to health care. Antwerp, Boston, Kluwer-Deventer, 1979. xii, 278 p.

**France**

Lambo TA: Professor Gastaut and his contributions to the World Health Organization programme. **Electroencephalogr Clin Neurophysiol** 1982;35:3–6

**Mexico**

Quijano Narezo M: México en las relaciones internacionales de salud. **Salud Publica Mex** 1983 Sep–Oct;25(5):519–23

**United States**

Kidd CV: The movement of younger scientists into and out of the United States from 1967 to 1980: some aspects of the international movement of scientific knowledge. **Minerva** 1983 Winter;21(4):387–409

## JEWS

See also **Religion and Medicine–Bible and Talmud**

Ackerknecht EH: Jüdische Arzte als Gestalter der Weltmedizin. **Gesnerus** 1981;38:127–33
Barcia Goyanes JJ: Los terminos osteologicos de la Fabrica y la evolucion del lenguaje anatomico hebreo en la Edad Media. **Sefarad** 1982;42:299–326
Baruk H: La médecine et la Torah. **Rev Hist Med Heb** 1981 Oct;34(3):35–9
Baruk H: La médecine hebraïque face à la médecine hippocratique. In La collection hippocratique et son rôle dans l'histoire de la médecine. Colloque de Strasbourg (23–27 octobre 1972) organisé par le Centre de Recherches sur la Grèce Antique, avec le concours des Facultés de Philosophie et des Langues Classiques. Leiden, E. J. Brill, 1975. p. 291–303.
Baruk H: Vers la résurrection de la civilisation hébraïque. La psychiatrie hébraique. **Rev Hist Med Heb** 1983 Jul;36(145):25–7
Cowen DL: The history of pharmacy and the history of the Jews. In H.R. Fehlmann, F. Ledermann, ed: Festschrift für A. Lutz und J. Büchi. Zürich, Juris Druck, 1983. p. 67–83. (Veröffentlichungen der Schweizerischen Gesellschaft für Geschichte der Pharmazie, Bd. 2).
Davis E: [Hebrew medical amulets] (Heb). **Harefuah** 1980 Sept;99(5–6):132–3
Fraikor AL: Fiddling on a drifting roof: genetic implications of Jewish settlement patterns and life style. **Prog Clin Biol Res** 1982;95:535–47
Gachnochi G: La violence de l'antisémitisme. **Ann Med Psychol (Paris)** 1979 Oct;137(8):807–16
The history of science: A collection of manuscripts from the library of the Jewish Theological Seminary. An index to the microfilm collection, reels 1–17. Ann Arbor, University Microfilms, 1980. 79 p. (With Hebrew–English name index).
Jakobovits I: Judaism [and medicine]. In Reich WT, et al, ed: Encyclopedia of bioethics, v. 2. New York, Free Press, 1978. p. 791–802.
Jakobovits I: Medical education––a Jewish perspective. **Isr J Med Sci** 1984 Jan;20(1):2–7
Kass N: Abortion in Jewish law. **Koroth** 1983 Aug;8(7–8):323–31
Kottek SS: The hospital in Jewish History. **Rev Infect Dis** 1981 Jul–Aug;3(4):636–9
Leibowitz JO: The ideal physician as revealed in the Zohar, book of Jewish mysticism. **Koroth** 1982 Aug;8(3/4):111–22
Leibowitz JO: The problem of medical license in Hebrew sources. In International Congress of the History of Medicine. 26th, Plovdiv, 1978. Actes du Congress. Sofia, 1981. Volume II. p. 139–40.
Levin S: Hebrew medical amulets. **Adler Mus Bull** 1981;7(2):8–12
Maeir DM: The physician as a man . . . the man as a physician. A Jewish viewpoint. **NY State J Med** 1983 May;83(6):813–6
Ostow M: Judaism and psychoanalysis. New York, Ktav Publishing House, 1982. 305 p. Includes contributions by J. A. Arlow, R. L. Rubenstein, M. S. Bergmann, L. R. Sillman.
Rosner F: Ancient descriptions of hemophilia and preconception gender selection. **JAMA** 1984 Aug 17;252(7):900
Rosner F, Bleich JD, ed: Jewish bioethics. New York, Sanhedrin Press, 1979. xix, 424 p.
Rothschild H: Diseases of the Jews. In his: Biocultural aspects of disease. New York, Academic Press, 1981. p. 531–55.
Sabin AB: Judaism and medicine. **Perspect Biol Med** 1983 Winter;26(2):188–97
Simon I: Die hebräische Medizin bis zum Mittelalter. In Sournia JC, Martiny M, Poulet J, ed: Illustrierte Geschichte der Medizin. Salzburg, Andreas, 1980. Vol. 3. p. 811–69.
Simon I: La vie et l'oeuvre des médecins juifs d'origine espagnole et portugaise du Moyen Age à la fin du XVIIIe siècle. **Rev Hist Med Heb** 1980 Mar–Apr;33(1):17–20 (continued periodically)
Simon I: L'influence hippocratique sur la médecine hébraique, surtout chez Assaph, Isaac Israèli et Maimonide. In La collection hippocratique et son rôle dans l'histoire de la médecine. Colloque de Strasbourg (23–27 octobre 1972) organisé par le Centre de Recherches sur la Grèce Antique, avec le concours des Facultés de Philosophie et des Langues Classiques. Leiden, E. J. Brill, 1975. 275–89.
Sligmann H: [Some aspects of the physician's law in Jewish traditional sources] (Heb). **Harefuah** 1983 Apr 15;104(8):358–61
Title list for the history of science collection from the Library of the Jewish Theological Seminary of America: Microfilm. 17 reels. Ann Arbor, University Microfilms International, 1980. 46 p.

**France**

Raphaël F: La médecine populaire juive en Alsace. In Livet G, Schaff G, ed: Médecine et assistance en Alsace, XVIe–XXe siècle. Strasbourg, Istra, 1976. p. 287–302.

**Germany**

Zimmermann V: Ein besonderer Eid für die jüdischen Arzte und Wundärzte in Preussen. Ein Beitrag zur Geschichte der jüdischen Arzte in Deutschland. **Medizinhist J** 1982;17(1/2):78–88

**Ireland**

O'Brien E: 'From the waters of Sion to Liffeyside'. The Jewish contribution: medical and cultural. **J Ir Coll Physicians Surg** 1981 Jan;10(3):10 p.

**Malta**

Bercovy D: Quelques Juifs à Malte. **Rev Hist Med Heb** 1984 Jul;37(2):24–5

**Netherlands**

Hes HS: Jewish physicians in the Netherlands 1600–1940. Assen, Van Gorcum, 1980. xxi, 206 p.

**Poland**

Sułowski Z: Les mécanismes de l'expansion démographique des Juifs dans les villes de Pologne aux XVIe–XIXe siècles. **Zesz Nauk KUL** 1978;21:89–100

**USSR**

Gajeerski SF: Szpitale Zydowskie na Rusi czerwonej w XVI–XVIII w. **Biul Zydowskiego Inst Hist Pol** 1979;(4):25–33

**Before 500 A.D.**

Savitz HA: Dreams in the Talmud: the prophets of yore had the noblest dream. **RI Med J** 1981 Sep;64(9):427–30

**Egypt**

Patai R: Maria the Jewess––founding mother of alchemy. **Ambix** 1982 Nov;29(3):177–92

**Greco–Roman**

Robinson PA: The conception of death in Judaism in the Hellenistic and early Roman period. Ph.D. Diss., University of Wisconsin. Madison, 1978. ix, 176 leaves.

**500 A.D.–1450**

Abrahams HJ: A medicine for 'Sickness of the spirit.' **Trans Stud Coll Physicians Phila** 1977 Apr;44(4):202–3
Barber M: Lepers, Jews and Moslems: the plot to overthrow Christendom in 1321. **History** 1981;66:1–17
Kottek S: Medicine in Hebrew poetry: Judah al–Harizi. **Koroth** 1983 Aug;8(7–8):299–304
Kottek SS: The seat of the soul: contribution to the history of Jewish medieval psycho–physiology. **Clio Med** 1979 May;13(3–4):219–46
Leibowitz JO: Jewish translators of medical works in the Middle Ages. In International Congress of the History of Medicine, 27th, Barcelona, 1980. Actas. Barcelona, Académia de Ciències Médiques de Catalunya i Balears, 1981. p. 276–80.
Leibowitz JO: Medical items in the book Torat ha–'Adam of Rabbi Moses ben Nahman (1194–1270). **Koroth** 1983 Aug;8(7–8):257–64
Richler B: Manuscripts of Moses ben Nahman's 'Torat ha–Adam'. **Koroth** 1983 Aug;8(7–8):265–7

**Arabic**

Frank JB: Moses Maimonides: rabbi of medicine. **Yale J Biol Med** 1981 Jan–Feb;54(1):79–88

**Egypt**

Fenton P: The importance of the Cairo Genizah for the history of medicine. **Med Hist** 1980 Jul;24(3):347–8

**France**

Alteras I: Jewish physicians in Southern France during the thirteenth and fourteenth centuries. **Jew Q Rev** 1978 Apr;68–209–23

**Spain**

Kottek S: Eléments de physiologie dans le 'Kusari' de Juda Halevi (Espagne, 12e siècle). In: Congrès international d'histoire de la médecine, XXVe, Québec, 1976. Actes. Québec, 1977. p. 840–7.
Patai R: An unknown Hebrew medicl alchemist: a medieval treatise on the quinta essentia. **Med Hist** 1984 Jul;28(3):308–23

**1450–1700**

Allan N: Illustrations from the Wellcome Institute Library: a Jewish physician in the seventeenth century. **Med Hist** 1984 Jul;28(3):324–8
Kottek S: Aperçu sur l' 'introduction à la pratique médicale', (introitus medici ad praxin) de Zacutus Lusitanus, 1575 - 1642. **Rev Hist Med Heb** 1980 Mar-Apr;33(1):13–16

**France**

Iancu-Agou D: L'inventaire de la bibliothèque et du mobilier d'un médecin juif d'Aix-en-Provence au milieu du XVe siècle. **Rev Etud Juives** 1975;134(1-2):47–80

**Germany**

Kottek S: An oath taken by Jewish community physicians at Frankfort on Main, 1656. **Koroth** 1979 Nov;7(9-10):CCIII-CCVIII(650–7).

**Italy**

Carpi D: R. Yehuda Messer Lion vepe'ulato kerofe. **Michael Hist Jews Diaspora** 1972;1:277–301
Kottek S: Abraham Portaleone (1542-1612): an Italian Jewish physician of the Renaissance period. His life and his will; reflections on early burial. **Koroth** 1983 Aug;8(7–8):269–77
Veronese Ceseracciu E: Ebrei laureati a Padova nel cinquecento. **Quad Stor Univ Padova** 1980;13:151–68

**Netherlands**

Bangs JD: Andries Salomonsz, a converted 'Rabbi and Doctor' in Leiden (1553–1561). **Jew Soc Stud** 1978;40(3–4):271–86
Kerner S: Samuel de Lion Benavente; chirurgien et lithotomiste (1643–1723). **Rev Hist Med Heb** 1981 Jul;34(2):29–30

**Spain**

Gracia D: Chirino en el Retablo de las Maravillas. **Asclepio** 1978–79;30–31:265–76

**1700 to Present**

Aberbach D: Freud's Jewish problem. **Commentary** 1980;69(6):35–9
Blinderman A: Isaac Bashevis Singer; medicinal fiction. **NY State J Med** 1981 Aug;81(9):1382–91
Diamond S: Sigmund Freud, his Jewishness, and scientific method: the seen and the unseen as evidence. **J Hist Ideas** 1982 Oct-Dec;43(4):613–34
Gilman SL: Madness and racial theory in I. J. Singer's The family Carnovsky. **Mod Jud** 1981;1(1):90–100
Kirsch J: Jung's transference on Freud: its Jewish element. **Am Imago** 1984;41:63–84
Klein DB: Jewish origins of the psychoanalytic movement. New York, Praeger, 1981. xvi, 198 p.
Kottek S: Les Juifs et la médecine aux XVIIIe et XIVe siècles (1750–1850). **Rev Hist Med Heb** 1981 Dec;139(34 no 4):57–60
Kottek S, Wilk D: Professor Joshua O. Leibowitz; jubilee of his medico-historical activity. **Koroth** 1983 Aug;8(7–8):233–55
Loker Z: A Franco-Jewish physician--among the pioneers of medicine and science in Central America (Haiti). **Koroth** 1982 Aug;8(3/4):195–7
Miller J: Interpretations of Freud's Jewishness, 1924–1974. **J Hist Behav Sci** 1981;17:357–74
Musatti C: Freud e l'ebraismo. **Belfagor** 1980;35(6):687–96
Nelken LE: Reminiscences of my medical education (1916–1933) before emigrating to Palestine. **Koroth** 1981;8(1–2):51–6
Oring E: The jokes of Sigmund Freud: a study in humor and Jewish identity. Philadelphia, University of Pennsylvania Press, 1984. xiii, 151 p.
Rausky F: Le discours freudien sur l'antisémitisme.
Rosenzweig KA: Dental health service in the Cyprus detention camps, 1946–1948. **Bull Hist Dent** 1982 Oct;30(2):92–5
Schorske CF: Freud: the psycho-archeology of civilizations. **Mass Hist Soc Proc** 1980;92:52–67
Schwartz LL, Isser N: Some involuntary conversion techniques. **Jew Soc Stud** 1981;43(1):1–10
Tal U: On the study of the Holocaust and genocide. **Yad Vashem Stud Eur Jew Catastrophe Resist** 1979;13:7–52

**Austria**

Leitner H: Die jüdischen Arzte in Osterreich und ihr Beitrag zur medizinischen Wissenschaft. In K. Lohrmann, ed: 1000 Jahre Osterreichisches Judentum. Ausstellungskatalog. Eisenstadt, 1982. p. 161–92.

**Canada**

Holzberg CS: Anthropology, life histories, and the aged: the Toronto Baycrest Centre. **Int J Aging Hum Dev** 1983–84;18(4):255–75

**Europe**

Friedländer S: L'extermination des Juifs d'Europe: pour une etude historique globale. **Rev Etud Juives** 1976;135(1–3):113–44
Halpern I: [Rush marriages among Eastern European Jews] (Heb). **Zion** 1962;27(1–2):36–58
Ströder J, Schuster J: Estudio comparativo de la mortalidad infantil entre los niños Judios y no Judios en Europa Central y Oriental a finales del siglo diecinueve y principios del veinte. **Folia Hum (Barc)** 1983;21(240):1–10

**France**

Kottek S: Jacob Rodriguez-Péreire (1715–1780); pionnier de l'éducation des sourds-muets: à l'occasion du 200e anniversaire de sa disparition. **Rev Hist Med Heb** 1981 Mar-Apr;34(1):5–8

**Germany**

Aronsfeld CC: 'Perish Judah': Nazi Extermination Propaganda 1920–1945. **Patterns Prejudice** 1978:12(5):17–26
Bauer Y: Genocide: was it the Nazis' original plan. **Ann Am Acad Polit Soc Sci** 1980;450:35–45
Ebon M: Why did Hitler hate the Jews? **Midstream** 1979;25(8):19–24
Goldhagen E: Nazi sexual demonology. **Midstream** 1981;27(5):7–15
Gumpert M: Hölle im Paradies. Selbstdarstellung eines Arztes. Hildesheim, Gerstenberg, 1983. xxiii, 280 p. (Exilliteratur, Band 17) Reprint of 1939 ed., with new biographical forward by F. Trapp.
Heintel H: Moritz Schiffs gescheiterter Habilitationsversuch an der Universität Göttingen im Jahre 1855. **Medizinhist J** 1980;15(4):378–84
King DF, King LA: Jews in dermatology. **Am J Dermatopathol** 1984 Aug;6(4):415–6
Krebs H: Wie ich aus Deutschland vertrieben wurde: Dokumente mit Kommentaren. **Medizinhist J** 1980;15(4):357–77
Lifton RJ: Medicalized killing in Auschwitz. **Psychiatry** 1982;45(4):283–97
Lowenthal EG: Zur Demographie der Juden im früheren Oberschlesien. **Z Ostforsch** 1979;28(1):81–4
Rosenman S: The late conceptualization of the self in psychoanalysis: the German language and Jewish identity. **J Psychohist** 1983 Summer;11(1):9–42
Rosner F: Julius Preuss. **Med Hist** 1975 Oct;19(4):376–88
Zondek T: Dr. Med. David Viet (1771–1814), eine Gestalt aus der Emanzipationszeit. **Bull Leo Beck Inst** 1976;15(52):49–7

**Great Britain**

Barnett R: Dr. Jacob de Castro Sarmento and Sephardim in medical practice in 18th-century London. **Trans Jew Hist Soc Engl** 1978–80, paru 1982;27:84–114
Guggenheim YK: Jonathan Pereira's contribution to the science of nutrition. **Koroth** 1982 Aug;8(3/4):123–34
Shuttleworth SA: The language of science and psychology in George Eliot's Daniel Deronda. In Paradis J, Postlewait T, ed: Victorian science and Victorian values: literary perspectives. New York, New York Academy of Sciences, 1981. p. 269–98.

**Hungary**

Csillag I: Elfelejtett kórházak nyomában. Balassa és Semmelweis a régi zsidó kórházban. **Orv Hetil** 1981 Feb 22;122(8):463–5
Csillag I: L'ancien hôpital juif de Pest. **Rev Hist Med Heb** 1980;33(4):73–4
Csillag I: Quelques médecins juifs hongrois et les événements viennois de 1848. **Rev Hist Med Heb** 1984;37(1):7–9
Fazekas A: 100 éve volt az eszlári per -nem ölték meg, a tiszának ment Solymosi Eszter-. **Orv Hetil** 1982 Jul 25;123(30):1870–2
Ismét Luzsénszky Talmudja?: **Orv Hetil** 1984 Aug 19;125(34):2086–7
Somogyi E: A tiszaeszlári vérvád a 100. évfordulóra. **Orv Hetil** 1982 Sep 5;123(36):2243–5
Somogyi E: A tiszaeszlári vérvád tanulságai (a budapesti egyetemi tanárok szerepe). **Orv Hetil** 1983 Jan 9;124(2):98–103

**India**

Krishnan P: The historical demography of the Jews in India, 1881–1971. **Ann Demogr Hist (Paris)** 1983;:313–27

**Israel**

Maizels M: Medical literature in Yiddish. **Koroth** 1982 Aug;8(3/4):220–4
Siegel S: [Medical ethics in] contemporary Israel. In Reich ET, et al, ed: Encyclopedia of bioethics, v. 2. New York, Free Press, 1978. p. 895–6.

**Italy**

Giura V: Note sulle caratteristiche demografiche della comunità Ebraica di Napoli nel '700. **Genus** 1979;35(1-2):259-63

**Poland**

Bogusz J: Uwagi lekarza o martyrologii Zydów polskich. **Przegl Lek** 1984;41(1):54-62
Jabłoński C: Wymieralność w getcie w Brzezinach. **Przegl Lek** 1980;37(1):40-3
Lefebvre P: La recherche par le clinicien: une activité inéluctable. **Bull Mem Acad R Med Belg** 1979 Nov 24;134(10):587-96
Zabłotniak R: Towarzystwo opieki nad nerwowo i umysłowo chorymi żydami w Warszawie (1906-1939). **Biul Zydowskiego Inst Hist Pol** 1981;1:37-44

**Portugal**

Lach E: The circumcision of the child on the eighth day...An anonymous engraving after a design by Bernard Picart. **J Hist Med Allied Sci** 1982 Apr;37(2):221

**United States**

Alpert RT: From Jewish science to rabbinical counseling. Philadelphia. [s.n.], 1977. 200 leaves.
Clar R: First Jewish women physician of Los Angeles. **West States Jew Hist Q** 1981;14(1):66-75
DellaPergola S: Patterns of American Jewish fertility. **Demography** 1980 Aug;17(3):261-73
Desnick RJ: Gaucher disease (1882-1982): centennial perspectives on the most prevalent Jewish genetic disease. **Mt Sinai J Med (NY)** 1982 Nov-Dec;49(6):443-55
Dwork D: Health conditions of immigrant Jews on the Lower East Side of New York: 1880-1914. **Med Hist** 1981 Jan;25(1):1-40
Edgar II: A history of early Jewish physicians in the State of Michigan. New York, Philosophical Library, 1982. 249 p.
Edgar II: Dr. Louis Jacob Hirshman. **Mich Jew Hist** 1980;20(2):5-10
Hornbein M: Dr. Charles Spivak of Denver: physician, social worker, Yiddish author. **West States Jew Hist Q** 1979;11(3):195-211
Hornbein M: Dr. John Elsner, a Colorado pioneer. **West States Jew Hist Q** 1981;13(4):291-302
Korngold S: Memories of the National Jewish Hospital of Denver in 1908. **West States Jew Hist Q** 1980;12(2):161-4
The Levy brothers: early San Francisco chiropodists, a picture story: **West States Jew Hist Q** 1981;13(4):317-21
Lindenthal JJ: Health and the eastern European Jewish immigrant. **Am Jew Hist** 1981;70(4):420-41
Watts RK: Jewish fertility trends and differentials: an examination of the evidence from the census of 1970. **Jew Soc Stud** 1980;42(3-4):293-312
Wilk D: David Israel Macht (1882-1961). **Koroth** 1983 Aug;8(7-8):305-17
Wilk D: In memoriam Dr. Leo Kanner, 1894-1981. **Koroth** 1982 Aug;8(3/4):213-20

**USSR**

Dulnik S: Koroteiha shel kehila yehudit bebrit-hamo'atsot. **Yalkut Moreshet Period** 1976;21:89-100
Epstein D: Hayehudi hayehidi (ha'ayarah Libishei bashoah). **Yalkut Moreshet Period** 1975;20:7-34
Gitelman Z: Poriyut hayehudim bivrit hamo'atsot. **Shvut (Israel)** 1977;5:7-20
Radlitzki T: Reshimot mimei hakibush hagermani Be-lvov (Lemberg), 1941-1943. **Yalkut Moreshet Period** 1976;21:7-34
Silber J: Some demographic characteristics of the Jewish population in Russia at the end of the nineteenth century. **Jew Soc Stud** 1980;42(3-4):269-80

## LABORATORIES AND RESEARCH INSTITUTES

See also **Research**

**1450-1700**

**France**

Howard R: Medical politics and the founding of the Jardin des Plantes in Paris. **J Soc Bibliogr Nat Hist** 1980 Apr;9(4):395-402

**Italy**

Bencivenni M: Il Principe dello Studiolo. **Kos** 1984 Jul-Aug;1(6):52-78

**Netherlands**

Beukers H: Het laboratorium van Sylvius. **Tijdschr Geschied Geneeskd** 1980;3(1):28-36

**1700 to Present**

Mercier P: Les instituts Pasteur d'outre-mer: leurs objectifs et moyens d'action. **Bull Acad Natl Med (Paris)** 1981 Apr;165(4):441-8
Rona E: Laboratory contamination in the early period of radiation research. **Health Phys** 1979 Dec;37(6):723-7

**Africa**

Dolman CE: Hideyo Noguchi (1876-1928): his final effort in West Africa. In: Congrès international d'histoire de la médecine, XXVe, Québec, 1976. Actes. Québec, 1977. p. 603-24.

**Americas**

García JC: Historia de las instituciones de investigación en salud en América Latina, 1880-1930. **Educ Med Salud** 1981;15(1):71-90
Turtle A: Collections of early psychological laboratory apparatus in North America. **Newsl Australas Assoc Hist Philos Sci** 1977-78;9:4-5

**Argentina**

Foglia VG: The history of Bernardo A. Houssay's research laboratory, Instituto de Biologia y Medicina Experimental: the first twenty years, 1944-1963. **J Hist Med Allied Sci** 1980 Oct;35(4):380-96
Pavlovsky S, Dosne Pasqualini C: XXV Aniversario 1956-1981: Instituto de Investigaciones Hematológicas Mariano R. Castex, Academia Nacional de Medicina, Buenos Aires. **Medicina (B Aires)** 1981;41 Suppl:1-4

**Australia**

De Vahl Davis V: A history of the Walter and Eliza Hall Institute of Medical Research, 1915-1978. Ph.D. Diss. University of New South Wales. Sydney, 1979.
Lowe TE: The Thomas Baker, Alice Baker and Eleanor Shaw Medical Research Institute. [Melbourne], Trustees of the Institute, [1974?]. xii, 144 p.

**Bulgaria**

Dochev D: Razvitie i segashno sŭstoianie na Katedrata po klinichna laboratoriia. **Vutr Boles** 1981;20(6):15-22

**Burma**

Shi NC: Forensic laboratory work in Burma (with special reference to the Office of the Chemical Examiner, Burma). **Am J Forensic Med Pathol** 1980 Jun;1(2):173-6

**Canada**

Bourassa MG, Goulet C: L'évolution de la recherche à l'Institut de Cardiologie de Montréal. **Union Med Can** 1979 Oct;108(10):1128-38
Cadotte M: Historique du laboratoire de pathologie de l'Hôtel-Dieu de Montréal: de sa création en 1896, à l'arrivée du professeur Pierre Masson en 1928. **Union Med Can** 1979 May;108(5):479-94
Feindel W: The contributions of Wilder Penfield and the Montreal Neurological Institute to Canadian neurosciences. In Roland CG, ed: Health, disease and medicine. Toronto, Hannah Institute for the History of Medicine, 1984. p. 347-58.
Hunt JC: Pourquoi investir dans la recherche biomédicale? **Action Natl** 1980;69(5):372-83

**Czechoslovakia**

Dalák K. Třicet let výzkumného ústavu MZ CSR. **Cesk Gynekol** 1982 Mar;47(2):81-112
Feuereisl R: 30 years of the Research Institute of Tuberculosis and Respiratory Diseases in Prague. **Czech Med** 1983;6(4):193-5
Holub A: Dvacet pět let Výzkumného ústavu veterinárního lékařstvví v Brně. **Vet Med (Praha)** 1982 May;27(5):257-66
Kroupa J: 30 let trvání Výzkumného ústavu traumatologického v Brně. **Cas Lek Cesk** 1984 Jul 20;123(29):904-6
Kyntera F: Přínos vojenské epidemiologie za období 25leté existence Vojenského lékařského výzkumného a doškolovacího ústavu Jana Evangelisty Purkyně v Hradci Králové. **Cesk Epidemiol Mikrobiol Imunol** 1984 Jan;33(1):53-5
Prokupek J: Dvacet roku výzkumného ústavu psychiatrického. **Cesk Psychiatr** 1981 Dec;77(6):361-3

**Denmark**

Rasmussen L, Wheatley DN: The Biological Institute of the Carlsberg foundation: international centre for cell biology for 50 years. **Cell Biol Int Rep** 1983 Dec;7(12):1071–9

**France**

Wrotnowska D: Lettres de Le Dantec, disciple de Pasteur. In: Congrès National des Sociétés Savantes, 107e. Brest, 1982. Comptes Rendus, Paris, 1983. Section des Sciences, Fasc. IV. p. 253–64.

75ème anniversaire de l'Institut de Médecine Tropicale du Service de Santé des Armées (le Pharo Marseille).: **Med Trop (Mars)** 1980 Nov–Dec;40(6):591–604

**Germany**

Benedum J: Vom Giessener pharmakologischen Institut unter Rudolf Buchheim und Karl Gaehtgens (1867–1898). **Medizinhist J** 1980;15(1/2):103–19

Bibergeil H: Vom Diabetikerheim zum Diabetes-Forschungsinstitut--50 jähriges Jubiläum im Zentralinstitut für Diabetes 'Gerhardt Katsch' Karlsburg. **Z Gesamte Inn Med** 1981 Jan 1;36(1):1–3

Breyer H: Max von Pettenkofer: Arzt im Vorfeld der Krankheit. Leipzig, Hirzel, 1980. 234 p.

Bringmann WG, Ungerer GA: The establishment of Wilhelm Wundt's Leipzig laboratory. **Stor Crit Psicol** 1980;1(1):11–28

Deich I: The redistribution of authority in national laboratories in Western Germany. **Minerva** 1979 Autumn;17(3):413–44

Echkardt G: Die Gründung der psychologischen Anstalt in Jena (1923). **Wiss Z Friedrich Schiller Univ (Gesellsch)** 1973;22(4):517–59

Lüst R: Max Planck und die Max-Planck-Gesellschaft. **Gesch Wiss Unterr** 1979;30(9):527–37

Müller-Ruchholtz ER, Haase J, Kaufmann R: Zwanzig Jahre Physiologisches Institut Düsseldorf. Bericht über die Arbeit des Institutes, Verzeichnis der Mitarbeiter und Verzeichnis der Veröffentlichungen 1970–1980. **Jahrb Univ Dusseld** 1977–78;209–47

Schwann H: Richard Kochs Beziehungen zum Karl-Sudhoff-Institut. Archivstudie anlässlich seines 100. Geburtstages. **NTM** 1982;19(1):94–103

**Great Britain**

Farr AD: Learn, that you may improve: the history of the Institute of Medical Laboratory Sciences. Sussex, Denley Instruments, 1982. xi, 214 p.

Hunt LB, Buchanan PD: Richard Knight (1768–1844): a forgotten chemist and apparatus designer. **Ambix** 1984 Jul;31(2):57–67

The Paterson Laboratories, Manchester, England.: **Oncology** 1981;38(1):59–61

**Italy**

Fischer JL: L'aspect social et politique des relations épistolaires entre quelques savants français et la Station zoologique de Naples de 1878 à 1912. **Rev Hist Sci (Paris)** 1980 Jul;33(3):225–51

Groeben C, ed: Guida alla Mostra allestita nella Sala degli Affreschi della Stazione Zoologica nella Villa Comunale (6 luglio – 30 settembre 1982) su Charles Darwin e la Stazione Zoologica di Napoli.

Partsch KJ: Die zoologische Station in Neapel: Modell internationaler Wissenschaftszusammenarbeit. Göttingen, Vandenhoeck & Ruprecht, 1980. 369 p.

Partsch KJ: Die Zoologische Station in Neapel. Modell internationaler Wissenschaftszusammenarbeit. Gottingen, Vandenhoeck & Ruprecht, 1980. 369 p. (Studien zu Naturwissenschaft, Technik und Wirtschaft im Neunzehnten Jahrhundert, Bd. 11).

Sloan JB: The founding of the Naples Table Association for promoting scientific research by women, 1897. **Signs** 1978;4(1):208–16

**Japan**

Hoshasen Igaku Sogo Kenkyusho 20-nenshi Hensan Iinkai: Hoiken nijunenshi. Chiba, Japan, Do Kenkyusho, Showa 52 nen [1977]. 4, 349 p.

Lebedev BI: O nekotorykh parasitologicheskikh uchrezhdeniaikh Iaaponii. **Parazitologiia** 1981 Jul–Aug;15(4):388–91

**Kenya**

Wilson CL, Williams CM: Toward the biological control of insect pests: the rise of the International Center of Insect Physiology and Ecology. **Sci Public Aff Bull At Sci** 1973;29(3):10–16

**Malagasy Republic**

Zeller H, Coulanges P: Les entérovirus à Madagascar. Bilan de vingt ans d'activité du laboratoire de virologie de l'Institut Pasteur de Madagascar. **Arch Inst Pasteur Madagascar** 1980;47(1):121–69

**Malaysia**

Singh RB: Historical development of the laboratory services in Malaysia. **Malays J Pathol** 1982 Aug;5:23–32

**Mali**

Saint André P: The Marchoux Institute. **Lepr Rev** 1980 Mar;51(1):35–42

**Mexico**

Informe de labores con motivo del XXXIV aniversario del Instituto Nacional de la Nutricion: **Rev Invest Clin** 1981 Jan–Mar;33(1):91–108

Izquierdo JJ: Los laboratorios para la investigación, la formación y la especialización del profesorado, en la nueva Facultad de Medicina. In Academia Nacional de Medicina. Libro conmemorativo del primer centenario. México, Comité Editorial de la Comisión Organizadora del Congreso del Centenario, 1964. Tome 2. p. 561–5.

Lomnitz L: Hierarchy and peripherality: the organisation of a Mexican research institute. **Minerva** 1979 Winter;17(4):527–48

Zubirán S: Informe de labores con motivo del XXXIII aniversario del Instituto Nacional de la Nutrición. **Rev Invest Clin** 1980 Jan–Mar;32(1):101–9

40 aniversario del Institute Nacional de Cardiología de México: **Arch Inst Cardiol Mex** 1984 Jul–Aug;54(4):411–26

**Netherlands**

Lindeboom GA: Nederlandse Bijdragen tot de ontwikkeling der moderne fysiologie. Voordracht gehouden op 20 mei 1976 bij de herdenking van het 25-jarig bestaan van het Fysiologisch Laboratorium aan de Vrije Universiteit te Amsterdam. Amsterdam, Laboratorium voor Fysiologie der Vrije Universiteit, 1978. 35 p.

Snelders HA: Het chemisch laboratorium 'de Leeuwenbergh' te Utrecht (1845–1903). **Tijdschr Geschied Geneeskd** 1984;7(3):129–56

Wit JG: Institute of Veterinary Pharmacology, Pharmacy, and Toxicology: its research (1961–1980). **Tijdschr Diergeneeskd** 1981 Oct;106(20):suppl 3:169–75

**Panama**

Chaves-Carballo E: Samuel T. Darling: studies on malaria and the Panama Canal. **Bull Hist Med** 1980 Spring;54(1):95–100

Ocaña G: La misión del 'Smithsonian Tropical Research Institute' (STRI) en Panamá y en el trópico en general. **Rev Med Panama** 1981 Jan;6(1):3–12

**Poland**

Brennan JF, Zieliński K: Science in Poland. The Nencki Institute of Experimental Biology. **Pavlov J Biol Sci** 1981 Apr–Jun;16(2):118–23

Chrzanowski A: Dar Narodowy dla pani Marii Skłodowska-Curie. **Nowotwory** 1980 Jan–Mar;30(1):93–7

Chrzanowski A: Rozwój Instytutu Radowego w Warszawie w okresie 1932–1939. **Nowotwory** 1980 Jul–Sep;30(3):305–9

Kieta M: Instytut higieny SS i Policji w Oświęcimiu. **Przegl Lek** 1980;37(1):172–6

Kołodziejska H: Zarys historii Instytutu Radowego im. Marii Skłodowskiej-Curie. **Nowotwory** 1983 Jan–Mar;33(1):1–5

Koszarowski T: Udział Instytutu Onkologii im. Marii Skłodowskiej-Curie w rozwoju społecznej walki z chorobami nowotworowymi w Polsce w latach 1945–1982. **Nowotwory** 1983 Jan–Mar;33(1):7–12

Luft S: Rys historyczny Instytutu Reumatologicznego. I. Lata 1948–1961. **Reumatologia** 1981;19(2):109–17

Małdyk E: Osiągniecia zakładu anatomii patologicznej IR w zakresie patomorfologii chorób układu ruchu. **Reumatologia** 1981;19(2):123–9

Małdyk E: 25 lat diziałalności Instytutu Rheumatologicznego. **Nauka Pol** 1976;24(9–10):77–83

Małdykowa H: Osiągnięcia Instytutu w zakresie diagnostyki i leczenia układowych chorób tkani łącznej. **Reumatologia** 1981;19(2):119–22

Markiewicz J: Institute of Forensic Research in Cracow (Poland). Its history, organisation and activity. **Acta Med Leg Soc (Liege)** 1979;29(1):85–92

Rudowski WJ: Instytut Hematologii w Warszawie. Warszawa, Państwowy Zakład Wydawn. Lekarskich, 1976. 90 p.

Zieliński K: Sixty years of the Nencki Institute of Experimental Biology. **Rev Pol Acad Sci (Warsz)** 1978;23(4):47–74

50-lecie Zakładu Radiodiagnostyki Instytutu Onkologii im. Marii Skłodowskiej-Curie w Warszawie: **Pol Przegl Radiol (Warszawa)** 1983 Jul–Aug;47(4):261–2

**Portugal**

Sassão solene comemorativa do 75.o aniversário do Instituto de Higiene e Medicina Tropical--14 de Novembro de 1977: **An Inst Hig Med Trop (Lisb)** 1977–1978;5(1–4):21–35

**Puerto Rico**

Busó R: Fundación de Investigaciones Clínicas. (Pro Deus, patriae eus scientia). **Bol Asoc Med PR** 1983 Nov;75(11):500

**Romania**

Babeş VT: Recent research on viral hepatitis performed in the 'Stefan S. Nicolau' Institute of Virology. **Virologie** 1984 Oct-Dec;35(4):251-7

Cajal N: 1949-1984: 35 years devoted to the study of viruses in the 'Stefan S. Nicolau' Institute of Virology. **Virologie** 1984 Oct-Dec;35(4):247-50

Dumitrescu SM: Contribution of the 'Stefan S. Nicolau' Institute of Virology to the electron microscopic study of viruses. **Virologie** 1984 Oct-Dec;35(4):273-80

Eşanu V: Research in the field of antiviral chemotherapy performed in the 'Stefan S. Nicolau' Institute of Virology. **Virologie** 1984 Oct-Dec;35(4):281-93

Negru I: Profesorul Iuliu Moldovan creatorul primului Institut oncologic în România. **Viata Med [Medii Sanit]** 1982 Dec;30(12):281-6

Popa LM, Repanovici R, Iliescu R: Investigations in the field of recombinant DNA technology performed in the 'Stefan S. Nicolau' Institute of Virology. **Virologie** 1984 Oct-Dec;35(4):315-22

Psatta DM: Thirty years of research (II). **Neurol Psychiatr (Bucur)** 1982 Jan-Mar;20(1):3-28

The 'Stefan S. Nicolau': Institute of Virology on its 30th anniversary. **Virologie** 1979 Oct-Dec;30(4):253-5

Sturdza SA: The activity of the Cantacuzino Institute in the field of tuberculosis. A review. **Arch Roum Pathol Exp Microbiol** 1982 Jul-Sep;41(3):195-204

Un secol de activitate de medicină preventivă la Institutul de Medicină şi Farmacie din Iaşi (1882-1982). **Rev Med Chir Soc Med Nat Iasi** 1983 Oct-Dec;87(4):707-25

**South Africa**

Gear JH: Studies of the rickettsial diseases at the South African Institute for Medical Research: epidemic louse-borne typhus fever. **Adler Mus Bull** 1984 Nov;10(3):8-15

Hickman R: The J. S. Marais Surgical Laboratory - 21 years old. **S Afr Med J** 1980 Mar;57(16):677-81

**Spain**

Carrato Ibáñez A: Cajal y su Instituto. **Trab Inst Cajal Invest Biol** 1979;70(3):181-94

**Switzerland**

Picco C: Das Biochemische Institut der Universität Zürich 1931-1981. Aarau, Verlag Sauerländer, 1981. 62 p. (Veröffentlichungen der Schweizerischen Gesellschaft für Geschichte der Medizin und der Naturwissenschaften, 37).

Sulzberger MB: Three lessons learned in Bloch's clinic. **Am J Dermatopathol** 1980 Winter;2(4):321-5

**United States**

Altman SB: A brief history of South Dakota Academy of Ophthalmology and Otorhinolaryngology. **SD J Med** 1981 May;34(5):39

Bayer RA: Q fever as an occupational illness at the National Institutes of Health. **Public Health Rep** 1982 Jan-Feb;97(1):58-60

Benson ES: Laboratory medicine in the United States--the dream and the reality. **Am J Clin Pathol** 1981 Jul;76(1):1-7

Blancher DA: Workshops of the bacteriological revolution: a history of the laboratories of the New York City Department of Health, 1892-1912. Ph.D. Diss., City University of New York. New York, 1979. xiv, 311 leaves.

Brewer NR: Personalities in the early history of laboratory animal science and medicine. **Lab Anim Sci** 1980 Aug;30(4 pt 2):741-58

Clarkson TB: Evolution and history of training and academic programs in laboratory animal medicine. **Lab Anim Sci** 1980 Aug;30(4 pt 2):790-2

Flynn RJ: The founding and early history of the American Association for Laboratory Animal Science. **Lab Anim Sci** 1980 Aug;30(4 pt 2):765-79

Foege WH: Centers for disease control. **J Public Health Policy** 1981 Mar;2(1):8-18

Forrest WR, Christen AG: Recollections of a dental researcher. Fifty years at the U.S. National Bureau of Standards: interviews with George C. Paffenbarger, D.D.S., D.Sc. Part VI. **J Ala Dent Assoc** 1984 Spring;68(2):29-31, 34-7

Foster HL: The history of commercial production of laboratory rodents. **Lab Anim Sci** 1980 Aug;30(4 pt 2):793-8

Freeman JT: Some notes on the history of the National Institute on Aging. **Gerontologist** 1980 Oct;20(5 pt 1):610-4

Glueck HI: Twenty years of funding of research by the National Institute of Health grant 02904 entitled 'Determination of Natural Clotting Factors'. **J Am Med Wom Assoc** 1980 Jun;35(6):141-4

Grafton TS: The founding and early history of the National Society for Medical Research. **Lab Anim Sci** 1980 Aug;30(4 pt 2):759-64

Greenberg JH: Bureau of Laboratories created for protection of public health. **Tex Med** 1980 May;76(5):50

Hill BF: The founding and early history of the Institute of Laboratory Animal Resources. **Lab Anim Sci** 1980 Aug;30(4 pt 2):780-5

Holmes JH: Diagnostic ultrasound during the early years of A.I.U.M. **JCU** 1980 Aug;8(4):299-308

Holstein J: The first fifty years at the Jackson Laboratory. Edited by W. L. Dupuy. [Bar Harbor, Me.], Jackson Laboratory, 1979. xiii, 231 p.

Jones JH: Bad blood: the Tuskegee syphilis experiment. New York, Free Press; London, Collier Macmillan; 1981. xii, 272 p.

Jones RJ: The NCCLS and medical devices. **JAMA** 1980 May 2;243(17):1748

Kanaoka Y: [The chemist in a biomedical environment: personal reflections on a quarter century of research at NIH] (Jpn) **Tanpakushitsu Kakusan Koso** 1979;24(14):1521-30

Kiger JC, ed: Research institutions and learned societies. Westport, Conn., London, Greenwood Press, 1982. xxv, 551 p. (Greenwood Encyclopedia of American Institutions, no. 5).

King LS: Medicine in the USA: Historical vignettes. XVI. Clinical science gets enthroned. Part II. **JAMA** 1983 Oct 14;250(14):1847-50

King LS: XII. Clinical laboratories become important, 1870-1900. **JAMA** 1983 Jun 10;249(22):3025-9

Leake ES: The Henry Phipps Institute: recollections of a foreign research fellow. **Trans Stud Coll Physicians Phila** 1981 Dec;5(3 no 4):256-63

McPherson CW: The origins of laboratory animal science at the National Institutes of Health. **Lab Anim Sci** 1980 Aug;30(4 pt 2):786-9

Martin WR, Isbell H, ed: Drug addiction and the U. S. Public Health Service. Proceedings of symposium commemorating the 40th anniversary of the Addiction Research Center at Lexington, Ky. Rockville, Md., National Institute on Drug Abuse, 1978. xiv, 325 p. Historical contributions by R. H. Felix, C. K. Himmelsbach, J. W. Sloan, C. G. Eades, J. F. Maddux, R. L. DuPont, J. H. Jaffe, E. L. May.

Maulitz RC: 'Physician versus bacteriologist': the ideology of science in clinical medicine. In Vogel MJ, Rosenberg CE, ed: The therapeutic revolution. Philadelphia, 1979. p. 91-107.

Michael JM: The Public Health Service leprosy investigation station on Molokai, Hawaii, 1909-13 -- an opportunity lost. **Public Health Rep** 1980 May-Jun;95(3):203-9

Morman ET: Clinical pathology in America, 1865-1915: Philadelphia as a test case. **Bull Hist Med** 1984 Summer;58(2):198-214

The origins of laboratory animal science and medicine: proceedings of a symposium presented at the 30th annual session of the American Association for Laboratory Animal Science, Atlanta, 16-21 September 1979.: **Lab Anim Sci** 1980 Aug;30(4 pt 2):737-800

Pickett BH: Remarks at the 20th anniversary celebration of the General Clinical Research Center. **Ala J Med Sci** 1984 Apr;21(2 Suppl 2):5-8

Pittman JA: General Clinical Research Center. **Ala J Med Sci** 1984 Apr;21(2 Suppl 2):1-4

Pittman W: Chemical regulation in Mississippi: the State Laboratory (1882- ). **J Miss Hist** 1979;41(2):133-53

Popplestone JA, McPherson MW: Pioneer psychology laboratories in clinical settings. In J. Brozěk, ed: Explorations in the history of psychology in the United States. Lewisburg, Bucknell University Press, 1984. p. 196-272.

Powell MR: H.O. Anger and his work at the Donner Laboratory. **Semin Nucl Med** 1979 Jul;9(3):164-8

Price DE: John Friend Mahoney. In Dictionary of American Biography, Suppl. 6, 1956-1960. p; 423-4, 1980.

Robinton ED: Anna Wessels Williams. In: Notable American women. The modern period. Cambridge, Mass., Belknap-Harvard Univ. Press, 1980. 4:737-9.

Science serving human needs: a history of Battelle Memorial Institute: Columbus, Battelle, 1979. 16 p.

Skinsnes AV, Binford CH: Leprosy research and the Public Health Service -- a brief chronological résumé. **Public Health Rep** 1980 May-Jun;95(3):210-2

Slocum A: Cornelius Packard Rhoads. In Dictionary of American Biography, Suppl. 6, 1956-1960. p. 537-8. 1980.

Ten year progress report of the Center for Population Research: [Bethesda], The Center, 1978. 73 p.

Tilney NL: Carl Walter and the evolution of the Surgical Research Laboratory: 1937 through 1949. **Am J Surg** 1984 Nov;148(5):584-9

Tilney NL: Harvey Cushing and the surgical research laboratory. **Surg Gynecol Obstet** 1980 Aug;151(2):263-70

Trends in biomedical research, 1901-1976: Proceedings of the Second Rockefeller Archive Center Conference, December 10, 1976. North Tarrytown, The Center, 1977. 70 p. Contributions by R. S. Morison, A. M. Harvey, P. H. Mazumdar, S. Benison, M. Heidelberger, M. McCarty, E. H. Ahrens, A. Kappas.

Werdinger J: Embryology at Woods Hole: the emergence of a new American biology. Ph.D. Diss., Indiana University. Bloomington, 1980. xii, 640 leaves.

Wyngaarden JB: Nurturing the scientific enterprise. **J Med Educ** 1984 Mar;59(3):155-61

# LABORATORIES AND RESEARCH

**USSR**

Abramian AIa, Trapeznikova MF: K 50-letiiu urologicheskoĭ MONIKI im. M. F. Vladimirskogo. **Urol Nefrol (Mosk)** 1981 Jul-Aug;(4):64-8
Akademii meditsinskikh nauk SSSR--40 let: **Med Radiol (Mosk)** 1984 Jun;29(6):3-6
Andreeva VN, Kosmachevskaia EA: Ocherk razvitiia fiziologii krovoobrashcheniia v laboratoriiakh Mediko-khirurgicheskoĭ (Voenno-meditsinskoĭ) akademii v XIX veke (K istorii vzaimosviazi teorii i praktiki v issledovatel'skoĭ rabote). **Fiziol Zh SSSR** 1981 Jun;67(6):934-50
Andrianov VL, Veselov NG, Kapitanaki IA: Leningradskiĭ nauchno-issledovatel'skiĭ detskiĭ ortopedicheskiĭ institut im. G.I. Turnera i ego rol' v okhrane zdorov'ia deteĭ (k 50-letiiu so dnia organizatsii). **Pediatriia** 1983 Nov;(11):74-5
Avdeeva TA, Khazenson LB: Osnovnye itogi 60-letnykh issledovaniĭ Leningradskogo instituta épidemiologii i mikrobiologii imeni Pastera po ostrym kishechnym infektsiiam (1923-1983). **Zh Mikrobiol Epidemiol Immunobiol** 1984 Jan;(1):115-9
Bazanov VA: Vsesoiuznyĭ institut éksperimental'noĭ meditsiny im. A. M. Gor'kogo i ego znachenie dlia organizatsii meditsinskoĭ nauki v SSR. **Sov Zdravookhr** 1980;(3):50-4
Bedrin AV, Medvinskaia KG: Sverdlovskomu nauchno-issledovatel'skomu institutu tuberkuleza 50 let. **Probl Tuberk** 1982 May;(5):75-8
Blokhin NN, Trapeznikov NN, Chaklin AV, et al: Vsesoiuznomu onkologicheskomu naushnomu tsentru AMN SSSR 30 let. **Vopr Onkol** 1981;27(12):81-7
Bondar PN: O role uchenykh Kievskogo meditsinskogo instituta v razvitii éndokrinologii. **Vrach Delo** 1981 Aug;(8):124-5
Borisenkova RV, Egorov IuL, Pal'tsev IuP: Vklad Moskovskogo instituta gigieny im. F. F. Érismana v gigienu truda (k 60-letiiu so dnia osnovaniia instituta). **Gig Tr Prof Zabol** 1981 Jul;(7):39-43
Chaĭka NA: Deiatel'nost' Leningradskogo nauchno-issledovatel'skogo instituta épidemiologii i mikrobiologii im. Pastera v gody Velikoĭ Otechestvennoĭ voĭny. **Sov Zdravookhr** 1980;(8):47-51
Chebotarev DF: 25 let deiatel'nosti Instituta gerontologii AMN SSSR v razvitii nauki o starenii. **Vestn Akad Med Nauk SSSR** 1984;(3):3-9
Chernukh AM, Morozov BV, Pogodaev GV: O povyshenii éffektivnosti prioritetnykh issledovaniĭ v nauchnykh uchrezhdeniiakh AMN SSSR. **Vestn Akad Med Nauk SSSR** 1980;(4):22-8
Chissov Vi, Demidov VP, Kapatsinskiĭ EV, et al: Rol' Moskovskogo nauchno-issledovatel'skogo instituta im. P. A. Gertsena Minzdrava RSFSR v razvitii otechestvennoĭ onkologii. **Vopr Onkol** 1983;29(11):3-7
Efremov VV, Shtenberg AI: 50-letnii put' Instituta pitaniia AMN SSSR: ego sozdanie, stanovlenie i razvitie. **Vopr Pitan** 1980 Sept-Oct;(5):4-9
Gusev AV: 150 Jahre Zoologisches Institut der Akademie der Wissenschaften der UdSSR. **Angew Parasitol** 1982 May;23(2):109-11
Institut mikrobiologii i virusologii im. D. K. Zabolotnogo AN USSR--gorodu-iubiliaru: **Mikrobiol Zh** 1982 Mar-Apr;44(2):3-4
Institutu fiziologii imeni A. A. Bogomol'tsa Akademii nauk USSR--50 let: **Neirofiziologiia** 1984;16(3):283-5
Kapatsinskiĭ EV, Kozlova EV: Rol' Moskovskogo nauchno-issledovatel'skogo onkologicheskogo instituta im. P. A. Gertsena v razvitii organizatsionnykh osnov onkologii. **Sov Zdravookhr** 1981;(11):50-2
Kapustin AV, Panfilenko OA: Osnovnye itogia nauchnoĭ deiatel'nosti Nauchno-issledovatel'skogo instituta sudebnoĭ meditsiny za 50 let. **Sud Med Ekspert** 1981 Oct-Dec;24(4):7-10
Kaulen DR: Itogi i perspektivy deiatel'nosti nauchno-issledovatel'skogo instituta épidemiologii i mikrobiologii im. N. F. Gamalei AMN SSSR (k 90-letiiu so dnia osnovaniia). **Zh Mikrobiol Epidemiol Immunobiol** 1982 May;(5):116-20
Konovalov AN, Iartsev VV: 50-letie Nauchno-issledovatel'skogo ordena Trudovogo Krasnogo Znameni instituta neĭrokhirurgii im. akad. N. N. Burdenko AMN SSSR. **Zh Vopr Neirokhir** 1981 Nov-Dec;(6):3-9
Lubegina ZP: K 50-letiiu Sverdlovskogo nauchno-issledovatel'skogo instituta travmatologii i ortopedii. **Ortop Travmatol Protez** 1981 Dec;(12):58-61
Maĭstruk PN, Petrun' AS, Popik SIa, et al: K istorii Kievskogo nauchno-issledovatel'skogo instituta gigieny pitaniia. **Vrach Delo** 1983 Apr;(4):1-5
Medzhidov BF: Istoriia Nauchno-issledovatel'skogo instituta virusologii, mikrobiologii i gigieny imeni G. M. Musabekova. Baku, Azerbaidzhanskoe gos. izd-vo, 1968. 183 p.
Molotkov VN: Rol' Kievskogo ordena Trudovogo Krasnogo Znameni nauchno-issledovatel'skogo instituta tuberkuleza i grudnoĭ khirurgii im. F. G. Ianovskogo v razvitii ftiziatrii i pul'monologii. **Probl Tuberk** 1982 Dec;(12):18-22
Morozova VT: Istoriia kafedry laboratornoĭ klinicheskoĭ diagnostiki Tsentral'nogo instituta usovershenstvovaniia vracheĭ. **Lab Delo** 1981;(6):375-8
Moskovskomu gorodskomu sovetu sanitarnykh fel'dsherov i laborantov 25 let: **Feldsher Akush** 1980;45(2):57-9
Nikitin DP: Nauchno-issledovatel'skaia i proizvodstvennaia deiatel'nost' Moskovskogo nauchno-issledovatel'skogo instituta épidemiologii i mikrobiologii im. G. N. Gabrichevskogo. **Zh Mikrobiol Epidemiol Immunobiol** 1981 Mar;(3):102-5
Ovchinnikov NM, Timchenko GF: Dvadtsatiletniĭ opyt raboty Tsentral'nogo nauchno-issledovatel'skogo kozhnovenerologicheskogo instituta Minzdrava SSR po kontroliu i uluchsheniiu kachestva serologicheskikh laboratorii dermatovenerologicheskikh uchrezhdeniĭ SSSR. **Lab Delo** 1981;(2):120-2
Pozmogov AI, Demin VT, Arendarevskiĭ LF: Kievskomu nauchno-issledovatel'skomu rentgenoradiologicheskomu i onkologicheskomu institutu 60 let. **Vestn Rentgenol Radiol** 1980 May-Jun;(3):78-80
Ptashekas RS: K 25-letiiu patomorfologicheskoĭ laboratorii Litovskogo instituta éksperimental'noĭ i klinicheskoĭ meditsiny. **Arkh Patol** 1983;45(12):76-8
Rakovskaia GG, Khokholia VP: Kievskomu nauchno-issledovatel'skomu institutu klinicheskoĭ i éksperimental'noĭ khirurgii 10 let. **Klin Khir** 1982 May;(5):70-3
Serkov FN, Zadorozhnyĭ AG: Nauchnaia deiatel'nost' Instituta fiziologii im. A. A. Bogomol'tsa AN USSR. K 50-letiiu so dnia osnovaniia. **Fiziol Zh** 1984 May-Jun;30(3):257-66
Shandala MG, Vaĭnrub EM, Kliuzko AS: Edinstvo gigienicheskoĭ nauki i praktiki--osnovnoĭ printsip deiatel'nosti instituta (k 50-letiiu Kievskogo NII obshcheĭ i kommunal'noĭ gigieny im. A. N. Marzeeva). **Gig Sanit** 1981 Oct;(10):45-7
Shandala MG: Ozdorovlenie okruzhaiushcheĭ sredy--put' k obshchestvennomu zdorov'iu (k 50-letiiu Kievskogo NII obshcheĭ i kommunal'noĭ gigieny im. A. N. Marzeeva). **Vrach Delo** 1981 Sep;(9):1-5
Shitskova AP: Moskovskomu ordena Trudovogo Krasnogo Znameni nauchno-issledova-tel'smkou institutu gigieny im. F. F. Erismana--60 let. **Gig Sanit** 1981 Jun;(6):27-31
Shitskova AP: Osnovnye itogi raboty Moskovskogo NII gigieny im. F. F. Erismana v desiatoĭ piatiletke po probleme 'Nauchnye osnovy gigieny pitaniia' (k 60-letiiu so dnia osnovaniia instituta). **Vopr Pitan** 1982 Mar-Apr;(2):64-7
Sidorenko GI: K 50-letiiu Instituta obshcheĭ i kommunal'noĭ gigieny im. A. N. Sysina AMN SSSR. **Gig Sanit** 1981 Oct;(10):41-5
Skripkin IuK, Turanov NM, Mordovtsev VN, et al: Tsentral'nomu nauchno-issledovatel'skomu kozhno-venerologicheskomu institut--60 let. **Vestn Dermatol Venerol** 1981 Dec;(12):4-10
Tkachenko BI, Voronenkova IA, Anoshina AA: 50 let Otdela fiziologii vistseral'nykh sistem imeni akad. K. M. Bykova Instituta éksperimental'nŏ meditsiny AMN SSSR. **Fiziol Zh SSSR** 1981 Aug;67(8):1283-9
Tsentral'nomu institutu tuberkuleza Ministerstva zdravookhraneniia SSSR 60 let: **Probl Tuberk** 1982 May;(5):3-7
Ustinovich AK: 50-letie Belorusskogo nauchno-issledovatel'skogo instituta okhrany materinstva i detstva. **Pediatriia** 1982 Jul;(7):74-6
Vankhanen VD, Grin' NV, Lastkov OA, et al: Aktual'nye problemy gigieny Donbassa (k 50-letiiu so dnia osnovaniia Donetskogo meditsinskogo instituta im. M. Gor'kogo). **Gig Sanit** 1981 Aug;(8):51-3
Volokhov AA, Kolt'tsova MM, Kostandov EA, et al: Institutu vyssheĭ nervnoĭ deiatel'nosti i neĭrofiziologii Adademii nauk 30 let. **Zh Vyssh Nerv Deiat** 1981 Jan-Feb;31(1):202-16
Voloshin PV: 60 let Khar'kovskomu nauchno-issledovatel'skomu institutu nevrologii i psikhiatrii im. V. P. Protopopova. **Zh Nevropatol Psikhiatr** 1983;83(5):780-3

**Yugoslavia**

Fortič B: Sesdeset godina stručnog rada i razvoja Golnika. **Plucne Bolesti Tuberk** 1981 Oct-Dec;33(4):197-215
Sarić M: Institute for Medical Research and Occupational Health in Yugoslavia. Introduction. **Arh Hig Rada Toksikol** 1979;30 Suppl:5-9

# LIBRARIES

See also **Exhibits; Manuscripts; Printing and Bibliography**

Bearman D, Edsall JT, ed: Archival sources for the history of biochemistry and molecular biology. A reference guide and report. Boston, American Academy of Arts and Sciences, Philadelphia, American Philosophical Society, 1980. 338 p. plus microfiche. Contributions by M. Miller, M. Konopka
Fenton P: The importance of the Cairo Genizah for the history of medicine. **Med Hist** 1980 Jul;24(3):347-8
Gibson SS: Scientific societies and exchange: a facet of the history of scientific communication. **J Libr Hist** 1982 Spring;17(2):144-63
Julien P: Le point sur les ex-libris professionnels à l'effigie des saints Côme et Damien. **Rev Hist Pharm (Paris)** 1982;29(252):176-8
Key JD, Keys TE, ed: Classics and other selected readings in medical librarianship. Huntington, N.Y., Krieger, 1980. xvii. 744 p.
Leon L: Cos'è un ex libris. **Kos** 1984 Jun;1(5):112 6
Lorenz B: Il medico bibliofilo. **Kos** 1984 Jun;1(5):101-11
Scholz A: Zur Geschichte der polnischen und deutschen Arzte-Exlibris. **Arch Hist Med (Warsz)** 1979;42(3):365-9
Skolnik H: Historical deveopment of abstracting. **J Chem Inf Comput Sci** 1979 Nov;19(4):215-8
Thornton JL, Want PC: Antique books in the library of the Royal College of Obstetricians and Gynaecologists. **Br J Obstet Gynaecol** 1981 Apr;88(4):337-45

Wells EB: Scientists' libraries: a handlist of printed sources. **Ann Sci** 1983 Jul;40(4):317-89

**Australia**

Gandevia B: The historical role of Australian medical libraries. **Aust Libr J** 1974 Dec;23(11):391-7

**Austria**

Honck K: Die wissenschaftlichen Bibliotheken der Erzdiözese Wien. **Biblos (Vienna)** 1981;30(2):97-102

**Germany**

Broszinski H: Medizinische Handschriften in Kassel. In Balde JH, Schmiking W, ed: Festschrift zum 86. Deutschen Arztetag in Kassel. Kassel, Arztevereins, 1983. p. 5-24.

**Great Britain**

David GR, ed: The manuscript papers of British scientists, 1600-1940. London, H.M.S.O., 1982. 109 p.
Ferguson JP: The College library. In Passmore R, ed: Proceedings of the Royal College of Physicians of Edinburgh Tercentenary Congress, 1981. Edinburgh, Royal College of Physicians of Edinburgh, 1982. p. 103-15.
Lattimore MI: Early naval medical libraries, personal and corporate. **J R Nav Med Serv** 1983 Summer;69(2):107-11

**Hungary**

Grabarits I: A kalocsai érseki könyvtár orvosi könyvritkaságai. **Orv Hetil** 1982 May 30;123(22):1369-70

**Italy**

Sbrana C: Per una ricostruzione dell'antica biblioteca del Giardiono dei Semplici di Pisa. Nuovi Elementi. **Physis** 1982;24(3):423-34

**Mexico**

De Mitcheli A: Libros médicos italianos en la antigua Universidad de México. **Prensa Med Mex** 1979 Jul-Aug;44(7-8):152-6
Micheli A de: Libros médicos italianos en la antigua Universidad de México. **Prensa Med Mex** 1979;44:152-6

**Spain**

Jordi González R: Bibliotecas de boticarios catalanes: aportacion para un estudio. **Circ Farm** 1984;283:127-42
Weiss B: Wissenschaftliche Bibliotheken in Madrid. **Biblos (Vienna)** 1980,29(1):18-26

**Sweden**

Rabo M, Kullberg G: [Swedish Nurses' Association's historical collection: witness to harsh conditions. Nursing departments.] (Swe) **Vardfacket** 1979;3(7):79-82

**United States**

Harris MH, Davis DG: American library history. Austin, Univ. of Texas Press, 1978. xix, 260 p.

**Yugoslavia**

Blažeković T: Entwicklung und Stand der wissenschaftlichen Bibliotheken in Kroatien. **Biblos (Vienna)** 1978;27(1):5-29

**500 A.D.-1450**

**Italy**

Gargan L: [The libraries of Guglielmino de Treviso, Pasquale da Villorba & Niccolo Cesi da Mignagola.] (Ita) In: Cultura et arte nel Veneto al tempo del Petrarca. (Studi sul Petrarca, 5.) Padua, 1978;:101-12, 198-211.
Pesce L: Due inventari di libri del medico umanista trevigiano Nicolò Cesi. **Quad Stor Univ Padova** 1978;11:125-7

**1450-1700**

**Austria**

Kühnel H: Medizinische Bücher im besitz zweier kremser Bürger des 16. Jahrhunderts. **Mitt Krems Stadtarch** 1965;5:123-9

**Czechoslovakia**

Ríhová M: Zamyšlení nad nejstarším lékařským prvotiskem pražské provenience. **Cas Lek Cesk** 1983 Aug 19;122(32-33):1020-2
Spunarová T: Nejstarší katalogy sbírek ve fondech knihovny Narodního Muzea. **Sb Nar Muzea Praze Rada C Lit Hist** 1980;25(1-2):29-40

**Europe**

Gysel G: Renaissance, 'Republique des lettres' et médecine. **Rev Belge Med Dent** 1984 Jun;39(3):99-105

**France**

Iancu-Agou D: L'inventaire de la bibliothèque et du mobilier d'un médecin juif d'Aix-en-Provence au milieu du XVe siècle. **Rev Etud Juives** 1975;134(1-2):47-80

**Germany**

Lorenz B: Notizen zu Privatbibliotheken deutscher Arzte des 15.-17. Jahrhunderts. **Sudhoffs Arch** 1983;67(2):190-8

**Great Britain**

Westfall RS: Alchemy in Newton's library. **Ambix** 1984 Nov;31(3):97-101

**Hungary**

Barlay OS: Boldizsár Batthyány und sein Humanisten-Kreis. Die ersten Jahrzehnten der Güssinger Bibliothek. **Magy Konyvsz** 1979;95(3):231-51

**Italy**

Caroti S: La biblioteca di un medico fiorentino [Simone de Cinozzo di Giovanni Cini]. **Bibliofilia** 1978;80:123-38
Grossi Turchetti ML: La dotazione libraria di un collegio universitario del Quattrocento. **Physis** 1980;22(3-4):463-75

**Poland**

Kamińska-Axer M, Sosińska-Trawińska M: Starodruki medyczne z biblioteki kapitulnez we Wrocławiu XVII w. **Arch Hist Med (Warsz)** 1980;43(2):215-25

**1700 to Present**

American Academy of Arts and Sciences, American Philosophical Society: Survey of sources for the history of biochemistry and molecular biology. **Surv Sources Newsl** 1975-1981;1(1-10):various pagings
Bori PC: Materiale storico-religioso nella biblioteca di Sigmund Freud: alcuni rilievi sul catalogo. **Ann Ist Stor Italo-Ger** 1975;1:281-9
Bruce NG: Searching the history of the health sciences. **Med Ref Serv Q** 1982 Fall;1(3):13-35
Corning ME: A review of the United States role in international biomedical research and communications: international health and foreign policy. Bethesda, National Library of Medicine, 1980. xxvii, 436 p. (NIH Publication No. 80-1638).
Côté RA, Robboy S: Progrès dans la gestion de l'information médicale. La nomenclature systématisée de la médecine (Snomed). **Union Med Can** 1980 Sep;109(9):1243-52
Côté RA, Robboy S: Progress in medical information management. Systematized nomenclature of medicine. **JAMA** 1980 Feb 22-29;243(8):756-62
Dostatni P, Cordoliani A: L'histoire de la médecine et la recherche documentaire automatisée. **Hist Sci Med** 1984;18(1):25-32
Freeman JT: Collecting books on old age. **Spec Collect** 1982;1(3-4):131-48
Fye WB: Librarians in the history of the health sciences: challenges and opportunities in the 80's. **Watermark** 1983 Apr;6(4):14-8
Hodge GP: The preservation of scientific illustrations. **J Biocommun** 1980 Nov;7(3):28-31
Keys TE, Key JD: Osler and Billings: their friendship and contributions to librarianship. **Am Coll Physicians Obs** 1981 Aug;1(8):1, 4-5
Kingsbury M: Book collector, bibliographer, and benefactor of libraries: Sir William Osler. **J Libr Hist** 1981 Winter;16(1):187-98
Kronick DA: The librarian's life, scholarship and librarianship. **Bull Med Libr Assoc** 1980 Oct;68(4):327-35
Mylenki M: Historical collections in psychiatry and psychoanalysis. **Libr Trends** 1982 Spring;:613-29
Peck W, Diethelm O: Review of the Freud library. In International Congress of the History of Medicine, 27th, Barcelona, 1980. Actas. Barcelona, Acadèmia de Ciències Mèdiques de Catalunya i Balears, 1981. p. 130-3.
Richler B: Manuscripts of Avicenna's Kanon in Hebrew translation: a revised and up-to-date list. **Koroth** 1982 Aug;8(3/4):145-68
Rödel V: Gedanken zur Archivierung medizinischen Schriftguts. **Medizinhist J** 1984;19(3):167-72

# LIBRARIES

Taylor DW: Medical libraries and medical history. **NZ Libr** 1976 Apr;39(2):62-7
Teigen PM: Medical libraries and history of medicine libraries. **Newsl Libr Hist Health Sci** 1982 Jul;6(1):1-6
Teigen PM, ed: Books, manuscripts, and the history of medicine. Essays on the fiftieth anniversary of the Osler Library. New York, Science History Publications, 1982. 112 p. Contributions by L. G. Stevenson, C. G. Roland, R. J. Durling, E. Brodman, G. T. Tanselle, E. J. Freeman.
Wojtkowiak S, Stempel A: Z badań nad dziejami szkoleniowych bibliotek medycznych w Polskich Siłach Zbrojnych na Zachodzie w latach II wojny swiatowej. **Arch Hist Med (Warsz)** 1983;46(1):59-65

**Australia**

Lowe RF: The Conjoint Libraries of the Royal Victorian Eye and Ear Hospital and The Royal Australian College of Ophthalmologists. **Aust J Ophthalmol** 1983 May;11(2):127-32
Owen M: The archives of the Royal Australasian College of radiologists: guide to the history collection H706-H765 sundry accessions. **Australas Radiol** 1982 Mar;26(1):30-40
Owen MD: The archives of the Royal Australasian College of Radiologists. **Australas Radiol** 1978 Sep;22(3):222-5
Owen MD: The archives of the Royal Australasian College of Radiologists. **Australas Radiol** 1979 Mar;23(1):15-9
Russell KF, ed: Catalogue of the historical books in the library of the Royal Australasian College of Surgeons. Melbourne, Queensberry Hill Press, 1979. vii, 152 p.

**Austria**

Camerino G, Darbon P, Graber E, et al: I manoscritti medici della Osterreichische Nationalbibliothek di Vienna. **Kos** 1984 Mar;1(2):12-9
Edredge N: I manoscritti medici della Osterreichische Nationalbibliothek di Vienna. (contd). **Kos** 1984 Apr;1(3):7-13

**Belgium**

Servais P, Roger FH: Les archives médicales hospitalières: organisation et possibilités d'utilisation. **Ann Soc Belg Hist Hop** 1980;18:71-96

**Bulgaria**

Apostolov M, Kodov H: The Hilendar medical collection. In International Congress of the History of Medicine. 26th, Plovdiv, 1978. Actes du Congress. Sofia, 1981. Volume II. p. 55-7.

**Canada**

Burkinshaw SM: A look at Kingston General Hospital's archives. **Dimens Health Serv** 1982 Nov;59(11):20-1
Duchesne R: La bibliothèque scientifique de l'Abbé Léon Provancher. **Rev Hist Am Fr** 1981;34(4):535-56
Kalsner J: The unique stress library of Dr. Hans Selye. **Can Med Assoc J** 1983 Aug 1;129(3):288-9
McGill University: The Osler Library. Montreal, McGill University, 1979. 64 p.
McGinnis JP: Records of tuberculosis in Calgary. **Archivaria** 1980;10:173-89
Sherrington A: Canadian medical periodicals on microfiche. **Can Med Assoc J** 1981 Feb 15;124(4):361-2

**Denmark**

Bauer B: Studien zum ersten altdeutschen Pferdearzneibuch des anonymen Kopenhagener Ms. Thott Nr. 202. DMV Diss. Hannover, 1980. 99 p.
Christiansen PA: Bibliotek for Laeger 175 år. **Ugeskr Laeger** 1983 Jun 27;145 Spec No:3-4
Jensen E: Et 125-arigt medicinsk bibliotek. **Bogens Verden** 1977;59(5):181-5

**France**

Burg AM: Les archives hospitalières de Haguenau. In Livet G, Schaff G, ed: Médecine et assistance en Alsace, XVIe-XXe siècle. Strasbourg, Istra, 1976. p. 113-5.
Crosland M: The library of Gay-Lussac. **Ambix** 1981 Nov;28(3):158-70
David-Danel ML: Un ex-libris non professionnel à l'effigie de saint Côme. **Rev Hist Pharm (Paris)** 1982;29(252):171-2
Fontaine-Levent P: Prunelle et la bibliothèque de la Faculté de médecine de Montpellier. **Hist Sci Med** 1980;14(2):241-3
Grmek MD: Vestigia della chirurgia greca: il Codice di Niceta e i suoi discendenti. **Kos** 1984 Jun;1(5):52-60
Hildesheimer F, Robin G, Schenk J, ed: Intendance sanitaire de Marseille. (Répertoire numérique de la sous série 200 E - Archives de la Région Provence-Alpes-Cote d'Azur et du Département des Bouches-du-Rhone). Marseille, Archives Departementales, 1979. 71 p.
Imbault-Huart MJ: La médecine au Moyen Age: à travers les manuscrits de la Bibliothèque Nationale. Paris, Editions de la porte verte: Bibliothèque nationale, 1983. 191 p.
Kernéis JP, Rouzeau L, Cuny J: L'histoire de la médecine navale à l'Université de Nantes. In: Congrès National de Sociétés Savantes, 97e, Nantes, 1972. Comptes Rendus. Paris, 1976. Section des Sciences, Tome 1. p. 149-64.
Leuilliot P: O współczesną historię medyczno-społeczną. **Kwart Hist Kultury Mater** 1975;23(2):255-67
Leuilliot P: Problèmes de méthode: histoire (et archives) de la santé. In Livet G, Schaff G, ed: Médecine et assistance en Alsace, XVIe-XXe siècle. Strasbourg, Istra, 1976. p. 11-17.
Linet J, Hillard D, Lavagne X, ed: Catalogue des ouvrages imprimés au XVIe siècle, Bibliothèque Sainte-Geneviève, Paris: Sciences--Techniques--Médecine. Paris, New York, Saur, 1980. xvi, 493 p.
Roubert J: Les archives médicales en France. **Archivaria** 1980;10:253-8
Schiller J, Rivet R: La bibliographie à la Faculté de Médecine de Paris avant et pendant la Révolution. In: Congrès National des Sociétés Savantes, 91e, Rennes, 1966. Comptes Rendus. Paris, 1967. Section des Sciences, Tome 1. p. 247-54.
Vial F, Merlette B, Roussel CI, et al: Les livres médicaux de la Bibliothèque municipale de Laon. **Hist Sci Med** 1979;13(4):383-93
1879-1979 - centenaire de la bibliothèque de l'Ecole Dentaire de Paris, Centre Français de Documentation Odonto-stomatologique.: **Rev Odontostomatol (Paris)** 1980 Mar-Apr;9(2):13-5

**Germany**

Bircher M: Deutsche Drucke des Barock 1600-1720 in der Herzog August Bibliothek Wolfenbüttel. Abteilung A: Bibliotheca Augusta. Band 2: Arithmetica, Astronomica, Bellica, Geographica, Geometrica, Medica, Oeconomica, Physica. Nendeln, KTO Press, 1979. 408 p.
Forbes EG: Scientific archives in the Federal Republic of Germany. **Ber Wissenschaftsgesch** 1979;2(3-4):197-201
Hoffmann H: Urkundenregesten zur Geschichte des Juliusspitals in Würzburg 1576-1849 (Regesta Herbipolensia VI). Würzburg, Kommissionsverlag Ferdinand Schöningh, 1976. xxxi, 434 p. (Quellen und Forschungen zur Geschichte des Bistums und Hochstifts Würzburg, Band 29).
Saha MS: The Carl Correns papers. **Mendel Newsl** 1981 Nov;21:1-6
Schneck P, Tutzke D: Ueberblick über die Aktenbestände des Staatsarchivs Dresden zur Geschichte der deutsch-polnischen medizinischen Beziehungen im 18. Jahrhundert. **Arch Hist Med (Warsz)** 1979;42(2):205-9
Schumm A: Entwicklung des Medizinalwesens in der Grafschaft Hohenlohe, mit einem Ueberblick über medizingeschichtlich wichtige Bestände des Hohenlohe-Zentralarchivs in Neuenstein. [Tübingen, Präzis], 1964. 109 p.
Wankmüller A: Die Bibliothek der Internationalen Gesellschaft für Geschichte der Pharmazie. **Ber Wissenschaftsgesch** 1979;2(3-4):226-8
Wittern R: The Robert Bosch Foundation and the establishment of the Institute for the History of Medicine. **Clio Med** 1980;15(1/2):89-91
Zachert U, Zeidler U, ed: Herzog August Bibliothek Wolfenbüttel. Verzeichnis medizinischer und naturwissenschaftlicher Drucke, 1472-1830. Band 1-4, Alphabetischer Index. Millwood, New York, Kraus International, 1982. 1857 p.

**Great Britain**

Allan N: Illustrations from the Wellcome Institute Library: a Jewish physician in the seventeenth century. **Med Hist** 1984 Jul;28(3):324-8
Allan N: Some early medical contacts with the Kalmuck tribes of Siberia. **Med Hist** 1983 Jul;27(3):305-9
Allan N: The Wellcome Institute and its Library with special reference to South East Asia. **Southeast Asia Libr Group Newsl** 1980;22:1-4
Appleby JH, Cunningham A: Robert Erskine and Archibald Pitcairne: two Scottish physicians' outstanding libraries. **Bibliotheck** 1982;11:3-16
Benson B, Wall R: Historical demography in the nineteenth and twentieth centuries in the absence of the civil registers. **Local Popul Stud (Matlock)** 1981 Spring;26:14-28
Bird DT: A catalogue of sixteenth-century medical books in Edinburgh libraries. Edinburgh, Royal College of Physicians of Edinburgh, 1982. xxxii, 298 p.
Bridson GD, Phillips VC, Harvey AP, ed: Natural history manuscript resources in the British Isles. London, Mansell; New York, Bowker, 1980. xxxiv, 473 p.
Brody J, Field J, ed: A catalogue of books printed before 1641 in the Science Museum Library. [London], Science Museum, 1979. ii, 43 p. (4 p. supplement to 1981 attached)
Campbell WA: Library resources for the history of science in Newcastle upon Tyne. **Br J Hist Sci** 1982 Nov;15(51 pt 3):281-4
Catton R: The early history of the library of the Royal Veterinary College. **Vet Hist** 1982 Summer;2(3):91-9
Charlton C, Drake M, Gwynne T, et al: The Registrar General's indexes and registers: microfilm copies may be available. **Local Popul Stud (Matlock)** 1984;32:4-11
Clark AJ: Book catalogue of the Library of the Royal Society. University Publication of America, 1982. 5 v.

Comben N: Book values and the book market; some hints for collectors. **Vet Hist** 1982/83;NS2(4):151–60
Dow D: The archives of the Greater Glasgow Health Board. In Checkland O, Lamb M, ed: Health care as social history; the Glasgow case. Aberdeen, Aberdeen University Press, 1982. p. 158–69.
Edsall JT: The papers of W.T. Astbury and J.D. Bernal. **Surv Sources Newsl** 1981 Apr;10:2–6
Elsas M: Archives: the 'memory of man.' **Pharm Hist (London)** 1968 Dec;1(3):1–3
Emmerson JS, ed: Catalogue of the Pybus collection of medical books, letters and engravings, 15th–20th centuries, held in the University Library, Newcastle upon Tyne. Newcastle Upon Tyne, Manchester University Press, for the University Library, 1981. xiv, 270 p.
Foster J, Sheppard J: British archives. A guide to archive resources in the United Kingdom. Surrey, Macmillan, 1982. xxv, 533 p.
Getz FM: Anatomia del medioevo. **Kos** 1984 May;1(4):33–46
Graves V: Graves Medical Audiovisual Library: 1957–82. **Br Med J [Clin Res]** 1982 Dec 4;285(6355):1627–8
Graves V: Twenty-five audiovisual years (the story of GMAL). **J Audiov Media Med** 1983 Jan;6(1):25–7
Gray C: The Wellcome library: reflection of an insatiable collector. **Can Med Assoc J** 1982 Mar 15;126(6):712, 716–20
Hall LA: The Stopes collection in the Contemporary Medical Archives Centre at the Wellcome Institute for the History of Medicine. **Soc Soc Hist Med Bull (Lond)** 1983 Jun;32:50–1
Harrell GT: The Osler-endowed Tudor and Stuart Club. **Pharos** 1984 Summer;47(3):23–6
Hibbott Y: The collection of early printed books in the Medical School Library. **St Thomas Hosp Gaz** 1981;79:64–72
Illustrations from the Wellcome Institute Library: A note on the botanical prints and drawings.
Jordanova L, ed: Medical records newsletter. (Research Publications of the Wellcome Unit for the History of Medicine, Oxford. No. IV). Oxford, Wellcome Unit for the History of Medicine, 1980. viii, 42 p.
Lattimore MI: Early naval medical libraries, personal and corporate. **J R Nav Med Serv** 1983 Winter;69(3):156–60
Muntschick W: Ein Manuskript von Georg Meister, dem Kunst- und Lustgärtner, in der British Library. **Medizinhist J** 1984;19(3):225–32
Newman CE: The history of the College library, 1879–99. **J R Coll Physicians Lond** 1984 Jan;18(1):66–73
Nutton V: Conrad Gesner and the English naturalists. **Med Hist** 1985 Jan;29(1):93–7
Oliver H: The Shore Smith family library: Arthur Hugh Clough and Florence Nightingale. **Book Collect** 1979;28:521–9
Parr LJ: Early libraries for nurses in England, 1860–1914. **J Librariansh** 1980;12(2):102–14
Payne LM, Newman CE: History of the College Library 9: Dr. Munk as Harveian Librarian 2 (1862–1870). **J R Coll Physicians Lond** 1978 Jan;12(2):189–95
Payne LM, Newman CE: The history of the College library: the eighteen-seventies. **J R Coll Physicians Lond** 1984 Jul;18(3):198–202
Pedretti C, Keele K, ed al., ed: Leonardo da Vinci: disegni anatomici dalla Biblioteca Reale di Windsor. Firenze, Barbèra, 1979. 159 p.
Pelling M, ed: Handlist of records of the Society of Medical Officers of Health deposited at the Wellcome Unit for the History of Medicine, Oxford, 4 May 1976, with later deposits and other locations. Oxford, Wellcome Unit for the History of Medicine, 1980 23 p. (Research Publications of the Wellcome Unit for the History of Medicine. Oxford, No. III).
The preservation of medical and public health records: (Research Publications of the Wellcome Unit for the History of Medicine, Oxford, No. I). Oxford, Wellcome Unit for the History of Medicine, 1979. 52 p. Contributions by C. Webster, P. Barnes, E. Freeman, H. Francis, B. Parry-Jones.
Price R: Wellcome Institute for the History of Medicine: American Collections. **Newsl Am Stud Libr Group** 1979;3:13
Price R, ed: An annotated catalogue of medical Americana in the Library of the Wellcome Institute for the History of Medicine. Books and printed documents 1557–1821 from Latin America and the Caribbean Islands and manuscripts from the Americas 1575–1927. London, Wellcome Institute for the History of Medicine, 1983. xix, 319 p.
Sayer K: The ESRC Data Archive. **Soc Soc Hist Med Bull (Lond)** 1984 Dec;35:59–61
Symons H, Nutton V, Schupbach W, et al: [Manuscripts in the Wellcome Library] **Kos** 1984 Jun;1(5):5–26
Tait HP: The McNeil Library and some of its notable volumes. **Univ Edinb J** 1980;29:313–7
Tooley JB: London scientific libraries in the nineteenth century. I: The springs of action. **Libr Hist** 1971;2(4):139–51
Turner H: Henry Wellcome: the man, his collection and his legacy. London, Heinemann for the Wellcome Trust, 1980. 96 p.
Wellcome Institute for the History of Medicine and related Sciences, London: Subject catalogue of the history of medicine and related sciences. 18 vols. München, Kraus-Thomson, 1980.
Whittaker AP: Source-material in the Winchester City Archives 1550-1981. **Pharm Hist (London)** 1981;11(1):5–6
Wood PB, Golinski JV: Library and archive resources in the history of science and medicine at the University of Leeds. **Br J Hist Sci** 1981 Nov;14(3 no 48):263–81

### Hungary

Kapronczay K: Einige alchimistische Werke aus der Raritätensammlung der Semmelweis-Bibliothek für Geschichte der Medizin. In Hein WH, ed: Pharmaziehistorischer Kongress, Budapest, 1981. Stuttgart, Wissenschaftliche Verlagsgesellschaft, 1983. p. 57–72.
Pajorin K: David Verbec könyvtárának töredéke a Semmelweis orvostörténeti könyvtárban. **Magy Konyvsz** 1978;94(3–4):314–21
Sipos G: Egy 1495-re szóló érvágó kalendárium a fővárosi Szabó Ervin könyvtárban. **Magy Konyvsz** 1977;93(1):43–6
Tóth A: Avicenna-kötet a keszthelyi Helikon Könyvtárban. Velencei kiadás, 1564. **Orv Hetil** 1980 Dec 28;121(52):3212–3
Vilmon G: Orvosi közm'úvel'ódésünk – és könyvtáraink – h'óskora. **Orv Hetil** 1983 Feb 6;124(6):341–4

### India

Palanichamy K: Tamil medical manuscripts in Oriental Research Institute, S.V. University, Tirupati. **Bull Inst Hist Med (Hyderabad)** 1973 Oct;3(4):173–81
Patterson TJ: Some Indian sources for the study of the history of medicine. **Indian Arch** 1980;29(1):27–30

### Israel

Maizels M: Medical literature in Yiddish. **Koroth** 1982 Aug;8(3/4):220–4
Ron M: Catalog of the Sidney M. Edelstein Collection of the history of chemistry, dyeing and technology. Jerusalem, The Jewish National and University Library, 1981. 182 p.

### Italy

Adacher S, Bernabò M, Sesti E: I manoscritti medici della Biblioteca Laurenziana di Firenze. **Kos** 1984 Feb;1(1):113–21
Adacher S, Orofino G: I manoscritti medici dell'Archivio dell'Abbazia di Montecassino. **Kos** 1984 Jun;1(5):5–16
Bernabeo RA, ed: Il ferro chirurgico nella raccolta Vittorio Putti di Bologna. Bologna, Università degli Studi di Bologna, 1981. 14 p. (Catalog of an exhibit Sept.-Nov. 1981).
Bernabò M: La 'Rinascenza Macedone' e l'arte dei bendaggi. **Kos** 1984 Jun;1(5):45–51
Libri e manoscritti di Haller, 1777–1977: Nel II centenario della morte di Albrecht von Haller. Milano, Biblioteca Nazionale Braidense, 1977. 69 p.
Sormani E: Il fondo sulla stregoneria della Biblioteca Angelica di Roma. **Mem Riv Stor Donne** 1981;(1):114–5
Tomasi LT: L'isola dei semplici. **Kos** 1984 Jun;1(5):61–84
Torroncelli A, et al: I manoscritti medici della Biblioteca Casanatense di Roma. **Kos** 1984 May;1(4):9–16

### Japan

Akiyoshi T, Takai S, Esaki H: [Old medical books of the Oda family in Kashima, Saga] (Jpn). **Igaku Kenkyu** 1983 Jun;53(3):167–73
Yatsu M: [Miscellaneous records of medico-dental and pharmacological history] (Jpn). **Shikai Tenbo** 1981;57(5):944–5 (continued regularly)

### Lebanon

Haddad FS: Arabic medical manuscripts in the Sami I Haddad Memorial Library. **Clio Med** 1981 Dec;16(2/3):123–7

### Mexico

Alcocer J: El archivo historico de la secretaria de salubridad y asistencia. **Bol Soc Mex Hist Filos Med** 1980 Sep-Dec;5(32–33):103–7
Micheli A de: Libros medicos italianos en la antigua universidad de Mexico. **Bol Soc Mex Hist Filos Med** 1979 Dec;4(29):129–39
Ortiz Monasterio L: La medicina mexicana en el Archivo General de la Nacion. **Bol Soc Mex Hist Filos Med** 1980 Sep-Dec;5(32–33):93–102
Ortiz Monasterio L: La medicina mexicana en el archivo general de la nación. **Prensa Med Mex** 1979 Jul-Aug;44(7–8):157–62

### Netherlands

Catalogus van de Bibliotheek der Nederlandsche Maatschappij tot Bevordering der Geneeskunst, in bruikleen verenigd met de Bibliotheek der Universiteit van Amsterdam: Vol. III. Amsterdam, Rodopi, 1980. 966 columns.
Lindeboom GA: Geschiedenis der geneeskunde: J. N. Ramaer (1817–1887) en zijn bibliotheek. **Ned Tijdschr Geneeskd** 1982 Aug 14;126(33):1504–10

# LIBRARIES

**New Zealand**

Dean DR: The Gideon Mantell collection, New Zealand. **J Soc Bibliogr Nat Hist** 1979 Apr;9(2):121-4
Shearer D: History of the Canterbury Medical Library 1934–1972. **NZ Libr** 1972 Oct;35(5):266-9

**Poland**

Bojczuk H: Stanisław Konopka (1896-1982), historyk medycyny, bibliotekarz i bibliograf, twórca polskiej bibliografii lekarskiej. **Arch Hist Med (Warsz)** 1983;46(4):439-51
Czeley-Wybieralska M: Early medical books in the Jesuits' Library, Małopolska Province, Cracow. **Arch Hist Med (Warsz)** 1980;43:461-3
Czeley-Wybieralska M: Starodruki medyczne w ksiegozbiorze OO. Bonifratrów w Krakowie. **Arch Hist Med (Warsz)** 1982;45(1-4):85-92
Dutkiewicz M, Felchner A, Kuna M: Wystawa czasowa 'Starodruki medyczne w zbiorach łodzkich bibliotek naukowych' zorganizowana w dziesieciolecie Muzeum Polskiej Wojskowej Słuzby Zdrowia WAM. **Arch Hist Med (Warsz)** 1982;45(1-4):93-100
Foltyn W: Biblioteka Towarzystwa Lekarskiego Warszawskiego w latach 1821-1944. **Arch Hist Med (Warsz)** 1983;46(2):151-82
Kaminska-Axer M, Sosińska-Trawinska M: Early medical books in the Capitular Library, Wrocław. **Arch Hist Med (Warsz)** 1981;44:119-26
Kamińska-Axer M, Sosińska-Trawińska M: Starodruki medyczne w Bibliotece Kapitulnej we Wrocławiu. **Arch Hist Med (Warsz)** 1979;42(3):393-402
Kamińska-Axer M: Starodruki medyczne w Bibliotece Seminaryjnej w Warszawie, druki XVII-wieczne (c.d.). **Arch Hist Med (Warsz)** 1978;41(4):483-91
Kaminska-Axer M, Czeley-Wybieralska M: Starodruki medyczne w ksiegozbiorze Biblioteki Seminaryjnej w Tarnowie. **Arch Hist Med (Warsz)** 1979;42(1):125-30
Kamińska-Axer M: Starodruki medyczne z Biblioteki Klasztoru ss Klarysek w Starym Saczu. **Arch Hist Med (Warsz)** 1979;42(3):389-91
Profesor dr med. Stanisław Konopka (1896-1982). Wspomnienie: **Pol Tyg Lek** 1983 Sep 5;38(36):1125-6
Sieńkowski E: Ekslibris lekarski prof. dr Stanisława Sokoła. **Arch Hist Med (Warsz)** 1978;41(4):473-8

**Puerto Rico**

Rivera Villanueva ZE: The collection of the Boletín de la Asociación Médica de Puerto Rico and its preservation (1903-20). **Bol Asoc Med PR** 1984 Sep;76(9):394-6

**Saudi Arabia**

Haddad FS: Arab medical manuscripts in the Sami I. Haddad memorial library. In International Congress of the History of Medicine, 27th, Barcelona, 1980. Actas. Barcelona, Académia de Ciències Médiques de Catalunya i Balears, 1981. p. 253-8.

**Singapore**

Cheng M: The Medical Library in the University of Singapore. **Singapore Libr** 1975;5:50-3

**South Africa**

Cowley J, Adler C, ed: A descriptive catalogue of early medical books in the Adler Museum of the History of Medicine and the University of the Witwatersrand Medical Library. Johannesburg, University of the Witwatersrand Library, 1982. x, 145 p.

**Spain**

Folch Jou G, Muñoz Calvo S: Catalogo de los documentos conservados en el Archivo de la Real Academia de Farmacia. **An R Acad Farm (Madr)** 1978;44(2):199-351
Garcia del Carrizo San Millan MG: Obras de interes medico y cientifico en las bibliotecas universitaria y de Santa Cruz de Valladolid (hasta 1877). Valladolid, Universidad de Valladolid, 1981. 172 p. (Acta Historico-Medica Vallisoletana, Monografias, XI)
Riera J: Planos de hospitales españoles del siglo XVIII existentes en el Archivo General de Simancas (inventario primero). Valladolid, Ediciones del Seminario de Historia de la Medicine, Universidad de Valladolid, 1975. 18 p., numerous plates. (Acta Historico-Medica Vallisoletana, Monografias, V)
Valverde JL, Hidalgo J: Documentos medicofarmaceuticos conservados en archivos de Sevilla. Salamanca, 1971. 120 p. (Cuadernos de Historia de la Medicina Española, Monografias, 17).
Valverde JL, Bautista Mendez MT, De Vinuesa FS: La biblioteca de la Real Botica en 1816. **Bol Soc Esp Hist Farm** 1981 Jun;32(126):65-89
Valverde JL, Bautista T, Montaña MT: Libros de interés histórico-médico-farmaceútico conservados en la Biblioteca de la Real Academia de Medicina de Sevilla. Granada, Universidad de Granada, 1980. 130 p. (Cuadernos de Historia de la Farmacia, 6).

**Sri Lanka**

Uragoda CG, Aloysius DJ, Lionel ND: A history of the Sri Lanka Medical Library. **Ceylon Med J** 1982 Jun;27(2):49-65

**Sweden**

Bahr G von: Upsala Läkareförening 150 år. **Ups J Med Sci [Suppl]** 1982;35:1-33
Modig M: Ex-libris de pharmaciens suédois. **Rev Hist Pharm (Paris)** 1980 Sep;27(246):162-4
Solomon-Bayet C: L'interprétation historique des archives du Comité Nobel de Médecine, 1901-1920. **Soc Sci Inf** 1983;22:487-510

**Switzerland**

Glaus B: Autographen und Manuskripte zur ETH- und zur Wissenschaftsgeschichte. **Gesnerus** 1982;39(3-4):437-42

**Syria**

Kataya S: Les Manuscrits Médicaux et Pharmaceutiques dans Les Bibliothèques publiques d'Alep. Alep, Université d'Alep, Institut du Patrimoine scientifique Arabe, 1976.

**United States**

Adams S: Medical bibliography in an age of discontinuity. Chicago, Medical Library Association, 1981. xviii, 224 p.
Amat N: El médico y el acceso a la información bibliográfica en biomedicina. Guía metodológica para la utilización de fuentes de información. La National Library of Medicine: Index Medicus y Medlars. **Med Clin (Barc)** 1982 Apr 16;78(8):344-50
Appel TA: The archives of the American Physiological Society. **Physiologist** 1984 Jun;27(3):131-2
Apple RD, comp: Illustrated catalogue of the slide archive of historical medical photographs at Stony Brook; Center for Photographic Images of Medicine and Health Care. Westport, Conn., Greenwood, 1984. xi, 442 p.
Archives and manuscripts [in] The Alan Mason Chesney Medical Archives, The Johns Hopkins Medical Institutions: Baltimore, The Johns Hopkins University and The Johns Hopkins Hospital, 1980. 64 p.
ASHP Research and Education Foundation dedicates the Donald E. Francke Memorial Library: **Am J Hosp Pharm** 1982 Jul;39(7):1206-10
Bearman D: A. L. Patterson papers. **Surv Sources Newsl** 1981 Apr;10:9-11
Bearman D: The Alfred Newton Richards papers. **Surv Sources Newsl** 1975 Nov;1(1):9-10
Bell WJ: Private physicians and public collections: medical libraries in the United States before 1900. In Stevenson LG, ed: A celebration of medical history. Baltimore, Johns Hopkins University Press, 1982. (The Henry E. Sigerist supplements to the Bulletin of the History of Medicine; new ser., no. 6). p. 85-102.
Biglow LA: Medical record education: an historical perspective. **J Am Med Rec Assoc** 1982 Aug;53(4):50-8
Bird RD, Allen G: The J.H.B. Archive report: the papers of Harry Hamilton Laughlin, eugenicist. **J Hist Biol** 1981 Fall;14(2):339-53
Blake JB, ed: Centenary of Index Medicus, 1879-1979. Bethesda, National Library of Medicine, 1980. viii, 115 p. (NIH Publication No. 80-2068; Order from U.S. Government Printing Office). Contributions by C. E. Rosenberg, G. Miller, F. B. Rogers, W. B. Bean, E. Wolf, K. G. Huston, S. Jarcho.
Bragg TA: The McLean Hospital archives. **Mass Nurse** 1984 Sep;54(8):3
Braude RM: Medical librarians and the White House Conference: from complacency, to concern, to commitment. **Bull Med Libr Assoc** 1981 Apr;62(2):231-5
Brieger GH: Fielding H. Garrison: the man and his book. **Trans Stud Coll Physicians Phila** 1981 Mar;3(1):1-21
Brodman E: Education and attitudes of early medical librarians to their work: a discussion based on the oral history project of the Medical Library Association. **J Libr Hist** 1980;15(2):167-82
Cain AM, ed: A catalog of the Percival Bailey collection of neurology & psychiatry. Chicago, Library of the Health Sciences, University of Illinois at the Medical Center, Chicago, 1973. viii, 230 p.
Chaff SL: Archives and special collections on women in medicine. **J Am Med Wom Assoc** 1983 May-Jun;38(3):73-4
Cordasco F: Laughlin Macleane's Expediency of Inoculation (1756): a checklist of deposit locations. **Am Notes Queries** 1981 Jan-Feb;19(5/6):75
Corning M: Redes de información biomédica: experiencia de la Biblioteca Nacional de Medicina de los Estados Unidos de América. **Educ Med Salud** 1981;15(4):424-41
Cowen DL: The historical collections of the Pharmacist Institute of New Jersey. **NJ J Pharm** 1980 Oct;53(10):15 and 1982 Jan;55(1):8-9
Crawford S: Health science libraries in the United States: I. Overview of the post-World War II years. **Bull Med Libr Assoc** 1983 Jan;71(1):16-20

Crawford S: Health science libraries in the United States: III. Hospital health science libraries, 1969–1979. **Bull Med Libr Assoc** 1983 Jan;71(1):30–6

Crawford S: Health sciences libraries in the United States: II. Medical school libraries, 1960–1980. **Bull Med Libr Assoc** 1983 Jan;71(1):21–9

Crowe MJ, ed: Witchcraft: catalogue of the witchcraft collection in Cornell University Library. Millwood, N. Y., KTO Press, 1977. xxcviii, 644 p.

Cummings MM: Comments on John Shaw Billings. **J Indiana State Med Assoc** 1981 Oct;74(10):638

Cummings MM: Index Medicus, 1879–1979. **Milit Med** 1979 Dec;144(12):829–30

Davies NE: The health-sciences information struggle: the private information industry versus the National Library of Medicine. **N Engl J Med** 1982 Jul 15;307(3):201–4

Davis NE, Huth EJ: Martin M. Cummings and the National Library of Medicine. **Ann Intern Med** 1983 Dec;99(6):860–1

Donato A: Waring Historical Library, Charleston, South Carolina. **J SC Med Assoc** 1981 Dec;77(12):638

Donato AK: Waring historical library. **South Med J** 1980 Mar;73(3):369–70

Doszkoos TE, Rapp BA, Schoolman HM: Automated information retrieval in science and technology. **Science** 1980 Apr 4;208(4439):25–30

Dunkel LM: Moral and humane: patients' libraries in early nineteenth-century American mental hospitals. **Bull Med Libr Assoc** 1983 Jul;71(3):274–81

Ebbert A, et al: [Reminiscences and appreciations of Madeline E. Stanton] Contributions by L. G. Wilson, L. G. Stevenson, T. R. Forbes, S. B. Nuland, F. Gyorgyey, J. Bylebyl, G. L. Geison, W. Le Fanu, G. Robinson. **J Hist Med Allied Sci** 1981 Apr;36(2):129–50

Evans GT: On-line library networking: a bibliographic essay. **Bull Am Soc Inf Sci** 1979 Jun;5(5):11–4

Everett DE: Dr. Pat Ireland Nixon: letters to and from his book-loving friends. **Friends P. I. Nixon Med Hist Libr** 1974 Oct;3:1–13

Fuller MB: Thomas Hunt Morgan papers at the American Philosophical Society. **Mendel Newsl** 1981 Nov;21:6–8

Gallagher NE: Arabic medical manuscripts at the University of California, Los Angeles. Malibu, Undena Publications, 1983. xix, 24 p. (Aids and Research Tools in Middle East Studies, v. 1).

Garland JE: The centennial history of the Boston Medical Library 1875–1975. Boston, Boston Medical Library, 1975. xiv, 223 p.

Glass B: The preservation of historical materials in genetics. **Bull Hist Med** 1983;57(1):98–105

Haabala SH, Kopper JA, Mann RJ, et al: 'Say please!' A study in library cooperation. **Hosp Libr** 1979 Winter;4(4):26–31

Hamarneh S: Arabic manuscripts of the National Library of Medicine, Washington, D.C. **J Hist Arabic Sci** 1977 May;1(1):72–108

Havighurst W: The mind of John Shaw Billings. In his: Men of old Miami, 1809–1873, a book of portraits. New York, Putnams, 1974. p. 189–207.

Heirs of Hippocrates: The development of medicine in a catalogue of historic books in the Health Sciences Library, The University of Iowa. Compiled by R. Eimas, E. Holtum, D. Curry. Iowa City, Friends of the University of Iowa Libraries, 1980. xiv, 474 p.

Hirsch R, ed: A catalogue of the manuscripts and archives of the Library of the College of Physicians of Philadelphia. Prepared by the Francis Clark Wood Institute for the History of Medicine. Philadelphia, University of Pennsylvania Press, 1983. xx, 259 p.

The history of science: A collection of manuscripts from the library of the Jewish Theological Seminary. An index to the microfilm collection, reels 1–17. Ann Arbor, University Microfilms, 1980. 79 p. (With Hebrew–English name index).

History of the Med–Chi Library: the first decade.: **Md State Med J** 1980 Jun;29(6):38–45

Holden C: Bern Dibner: science bibliophile. **Science** 1980 May 30;208(4447):1012–4

Holland J: A glorious anachronism: the American Philosophical Society. **Wilson Libr Bull** 1982;56(10):740–4

Hoolihan C, Anderson PG: Special collections, Library, Washington University School of Medicine. St. Louis, [Washington University School of Medicine], 1981. iii, 66 p.

Isetts CA: Medical libraries in Cincinnati. **Cinci Hist Soc Bull** 1980 Spring;38(1):51–71

Jensen JE, Weisheit-Smith I: History of the Library of the Medical and Chirurgical Faculty of the State of Maryland. **Md State Med J** 1980 Jun;29(6):35–7

Jones MJ: The Francis E. Fronczak Collection. **Niagara Frontier** 1978;25(4):96–9

Kopp C: The Edward Lawrie Tatum papers. **Mendel Newsl** 1981 Jul;20:1–2

Kopp C: The J. H. B. Archive report; the Edward Lawrie Tatum papers at the Rockefeller University Archives. **J Hist Biol** 1982 Spring;15(1):153–4

Koudelka JB: The genesis of the William H. Welch Medical Library and the Johns Hopkins Institute of the History of Medicine. In Stevenson LG, ed: A celebration of medical history. Baltimore, Johns Hopkins University Press, 1982. (The Henry E. Sigerist supplements to the Bulletin of the History of Medicine; new ser., no. 6). p. 69–76

Kowitz A: You don't have anything, do you? The historical resources of the American Dental Association. **Bull Hist Dent** 1980 Oct;28(2):69–75

Krivatsy P: Medical incunabula and the diffusion of scientific knowledge. Incunabula in the National Library of Medicine. Published in conjunction with an exhibit at the National Library of Medicine, May–Oct. 1984. [Bethesda, National Library of Medicine, 1984.] 14 p.

Kronick DA: Access to the medical journal literature of the 17th and 18th centuries through the Index catalogue. In International Congress of the History of Medicine. 26th, Plovdiv, 1978. Actes du Congress. Sofia, 1981. Volume II. p. 59–62.

Laszlo J: Two long-range clinical data bases are terminated: bang, whimper, or ripple? **J Clin Oncol** 1984 May;2(5):532–3

Lawrence SV: Modern ideas mix with history. **Forum Med** 1978 Nov;1(8):14–9

McCall N, Kanarek H: The Alan Mason Chesney Archives of the Johns Hopkins Medical Institutions. **Bull Hist Med** 1982 Spring;56(1):88–92

Manson Thomas ML, Cooper WC, ed: Catalog of works in the neurological sciences collected by Cyril Brian Courville, M.D., representative of clinical neurology, neuroanatomy and neuropathology, with particular reference to head trauma, and books from historical medicine in the Medical Sciences Library, University of California, Irvine. Irvine, University of California, 1978. 239 p.

Manuscripta alchemica der Sammlung Mellon: Bemerkungen zum Katalog: **Sudhoffs Arch** 1981;65(1):79–96

Mayo Medical Library: selected milestones: **Mayo Alumnus** 1982 Apr;:24–7

Meier RY, ed: The Joseph H. Kiefer catalog of history of urology and medicine. Chicago, Library of the Health Sciences, University of Illinois at the Medical Center, 1981. ix, 207 p. (Special collections catalog).

Miles WD: A history of the National Library of Medicine. The nation's treasury of medical knowledge. Bethesda, National Library of Medicine, 1982. viii, 531 p. (NIH Publication No. 82-1904).

Milner A: The Franklin Institute: as diverse as its namesake. **Wilson Libr Bull** 1982;56(10):735–9

Niles AG: The Dial Access Library for Health Professionals in Wisconsin: an historical account. [Madison,] University of Wisconsin–Extension, 1982. iv, 94 p.

Noore FD: In medicina, veritas; the British and turbulent youth of the faculty of medicine and Harvard College. **N Engl J Med** 1982 Oct 7;307(15):917–25

Ochsenhirt S: The Archives of the History of American Psychology. **Stor Crit Psicol** 1982 Dec;3(2):329–32

Pnina Abir-Am: The I. Fankuchen papers: their relevance to the historian of molecular biology. **Surv Sources Newsl** 1981 Apr;10:6–9

Poland UH: Reflections on the Medical Library Association's international activities. **Bull Med Libr Assoc** 1982 Oct;70(4):359–68

Poppleston JA, McPherson MW: The development of the archives of the history of American psychology. **Manuscripts** 1969;21(3):183–8

Premio Abraham Horwitz. Dr. Martin M. Cummings: **Bol Of Sanit Panam** 1984 Jan;96(1):73–8

Rák K: Korunk orvosi szakirodalma és a klinikai medicina. **Orv Hetil** 1980 Sep 14;121(37):2243–8

Recent acquisitions of the manuscript division: Carl R. Rogers papers. **Q J Libr Congr** 1978;35-258–9

Remembering Maud Mellish Wilson: **Mayo Alumnus** 1982 Apr;:18–20

Robbins C: The collector's legacy. **MD** 1982 May;26(6):193–6, 201

Robert I. Watson and the development of the history of psychology: a symposium: With contributions by E. S. Mills, E. R. Hilgard, B. Ross, J. Popplestone, M. W. McPherson, R. B. Evans, E. S. Goodman, J. Brožek. **J Hist Behav Sci** 1982 Oct;18(4):307–31

Rogers FB: The origins of MEDLARS. In Stevenson LG, ed: A celebration of medical history. Baltimore, Johns Hopkins University Press, 1982. p. 77–84.

Rózsa G: 70 éve halt meg John Shaw Billings. **Orv Hetil** 1983 Sep 4;124(36):2191–2

Schroeder MJ: Manuscript collections: The Jeannette Dean–Throckmorton papers. **Ann Iowa** 1979;44(7):551–4

Scott Adams: A continuing force in the age of discontinuity: **Bull Am Soc Inf Sci** 1982 Dec;9(2):16–8

Shelley HS: The Moll Collection on hypnotism at Vanderbilt. **Bull Med Libr Assoc** 1977 Jan;65(1):65–6

Skinner RE, Marcotte JM: Bibliographic instruction in the health sciences: an historical review. **Med Ref Serv Q** 1982 Summer;1(2):53–76

Skinner RE: The historical work of William Dosité Postell, Sr. **Watermark** 1983 Fall;7(2):8–10

Smith BT: Marcia Crocker Noyes, medical librarian: the shaping of a career. **Bull Med Libr Assoc** 1974 Jul;62(3):314–24

Smith DC: William Budd manuscript at the National Library of Medicine. **J Hist Med Allied Sci** 1980 Jul;35(3):318–19

Sokal MM, ed: A guide to manuscript collections in the history of psychology and related areas. [Wellesley, Mass.], Wellesley College Colloquium on the History of Psychology, 1977. iii, 64 leaves.

Sonnedecker GS: The Richtmann Archive at Auburn University. **Pharm Hist** 1984;26(4):179–81

Stevenson LG: The Blake era at HMD. **Bull Hist Med** 1982;56(4):455–9

Stevenson LG, ed: A celebration of medical history. The fiftieth anniversary of The Johns Hopkins Institute of the History of Medicine and The Welch Medical Library. Baltimore and London, Johns Hopkins University Press, 1982. vi, 228 p. (Henry E. Sigerist Supplements to the Bulletin of the History of medicine, new ser., no. 6)

Stieber MT, Karg AL, Connelly DM, et al: Guide to the botanical records

and papers in the archives of the Hunt Institute. **Huntia** 1981;4(1):3–89
Thomson EH: John Farquhar Fulton. In Dictionary of American Biography, Suppl. 6, 1956–1960. p. 222–4, 1980.
Thomson EH: Madeline Earle Stanton, disciple: the years 1920 to 1941. **J Hist Med Allied Sci** 1981 Apr,36(2):151–67
Tipton R: Continued controversy: the Rutgers Medical School and the Library of Science and Medicine. **J Rutgers Univ Libr** 1983;45(1):1–24
Title list for the history of science collection from the Library of the Jewish Theological Seminary of America: Microfilm. 17 reels. Ann Arbor, University Microfilms International, 1980. 46 p.
Weaver B, Britt MC: Dr. Lawrence Reynolds and his medical history collection. **Ala J Med Sci** 1984 Jul;21(3):311–7 contd
Weaver B, Britt MC: Dr. Lawrence Reynolds and his medical history collection. **Ala J Med Sci** 1984 Oct;21(4):441–7
Webb WM: There's a doctor in the library. The story of John Shaw Billings, M.D. (1838–1913). **J Indiana State Med Assoc** 1981 Jun;74(6):360–6
Williams MR: The scientific library of Charles Babbage. **Ann Hist Comput** 1981;3(3):235–40
Wilson LB: A women pioneer in a new profession, medical editing. **Mayo Alumnus** 1982 Apr;:20–3
Wilson LG: Madeline Earle Stanton 1898–1980. **Bull Med Libr Assoc** 1981 Jul;69(3):357–8
Witten LC, Pachella R, ed: Alchemy and the occult: a catalogue of books and manuscripts from the collection of Paul and Mary Mellon given to Yale University Library. Vols. 3 and 4: Manuscripts 1225–1922. With an introduction by P. Kibre and additional notes by W. McGuire. New Haven, Yale University Library, 1977. 853 p.
Wygant LJ: Archives and manuscripts in the Moody Medical Library. **Bookman** 1983 Sep–Oct;10(5):3–8

**USSR**

Borodyi MK: Arkhivni dzerela z istorii medytsyny na livoberezhnyi ukraini u XVIII st. **Ukr Istor Zh** 1981;(9):137–41
Efimov AE: Neizvestnoe pis'mo N. I. Pirogova. **Sov Zdravookhr** 1983;(8):61–2
Girin VN: Sokrovishchnitsa meditsinskikh znaniĭ (k 50-letiiu Respublikanskoĭ nauchnoĭ meditsinskoĭ biblioteki imeni D. I. Ul'ianova). **Vrach Delo** 1980 Jul;(7):1–4

# LICENSURE AND REGULATION

See also **Ethics, Medical**

Cameron N: Ceremony of presentation of diplomates. **Ann R Coll Surg Engl** 1981 Nov;63(6):447–9
Ell SR: Five hundred years of specialty certification and compulsory continuing medical education. Venice 1300–1801. **JAMA** 1984 Feb 10;251(6):752–3
Emerson RS, Schwartz RM: Professional liability. **NY State J Med** 1983 Jan;83(1):69–74
Leibowitz JO: The problem of medical license in Hebrew sources. In International Congress of the History of Medicine. 26th, Plovdiv, 1978. Actes du Congress. Sofia, 1981. Volume II. p. 139–40.
Sligmann H: [Some aspects of the physician's law in Jewish traditional sources] (Heb). **Harefuah** 1983 Apr 15;104(8):358–61
Wagner HJ: Zur historischen Entwicklung des Begriffs 'Aerztlicher Kunstfehler'. **Z Rechtsmed** 1981;86(4):303–6

**China**

Unschuld PU: Arzneimittelmissbrauch und heterodoxe Heiltätigkeit im kaiserlichen China; ausgewählte Materialien zu Gesetzgebung und Rechtsprechung. **Sudhoffs Arch** 1977;61(4):353–86

**Denmark**

Dübeck I: Jordemødre og jura: en retshistorisk studie. **Tidsskr Rettsvitenskap** 1973;(5):729–57

**Great Britain**

Guy JR: The episcopal licensing of physicians, surgeons and midwives. **Bull Hist Med** 1982;56(4):528–42

**Spain**

Valverde JL, Lopez Andujar G: Las disposiciones legales sobre el certificado de 'Limpieza de sangre' en relación al ejercicio profesional farmacéutico. **Bol Soc Esp Hist Farm** 1980 Oct;31(123):259–71

**United States**

McDonald MO, Utterback N, Wright RA: Medical malpractice and ordinary care in Kentucky. **J Ky Med Assoc** 1983 Jan;81(1):55–7

**500 A.D.–1450**

Amundsen DW: Casuistry and professional obligations: the regulation of physicians by the court of conscience in the late Middle Ages. Part II. **Trans Stud Coll Physicians Phila** 1981 Jun;3(2):93–112

**Great Britain**

Cosman MP: The medieval medical third party: compulsory consultation and malpractice insurance. **Ann Plast Surg** 1982 Feb;8(2):152–62

**1450–1700**

**Great Britain**

Cook HJ: The regulation of medical practice in London under the Stuarts, 1607–1704. Ph.D. Diss., University of Michigan. Ann Arbor, 1981. 438 p.
Cooper DB: The Royal College of Physicians of London during the reign of the House of Stuart (1603–1714). **Trans Stud Coll Physicians Phila** 1983 Sep;5(5 No 3):191–211
Pelling M: Occupational diversity: barbersurgeons and the trades of Norwich, 1550–1640. **Bull Hist Med** 1982;56(4):484–511

**Italy**

Głowacki WW: Ustawy medyczne Królestwa Sycylii z lat 1140–1241. **Arch Hist Med (Warsz)** 1983;46(2):137–47

**Netherlands**

Bangs JD: Andries Salomonsz, a converted 'Rabbi and Doctor' in Leiden (1553–1561). **Jew Soc Stud** 1978;40(3–4):271–86

**Sweden**

Sjövall H: Vem skulle få vårda vad? Fackliga strider i 1600-talets Sverige. **Nord Medicinhist Arsb** 1980;:59–80

**1700 to Present**

Sanitetskollegierne i Slesvig Holsten 1804–1864: **Dan Medicinhist Arbog** 1980;:79–90

**Argentina**

Martín de Codoni E: La politica sanitaria en el primer medio siglo. Mendoza 1810–1860. **Rev Hist Am Argent** 1980;10(19–20):37–52

**Bulgaria**

Kadankov D: Usuvurshenstvuvane na Bulgarskite zubolekari (1890–1930). **Stomatologiia (Sofiia)** 1979 Jul–Aug;61(4):273–5

**Canada**

Howell CD: Reform and the monopolistic impulse: the professionalization of medicine in the Maritimes. **Acadiensis** 1981;11(1):3–22
Tunis B: Medical education and medical licencing in Lower Canada. **Soc Hist (Canada)** 1981;14(27):67–91

**Finland**

Klatt CH: Im 19. Jahrhundert nach Finnland zugezogene und dort zugelassene Tierärzte (Kurzmitteilung). **DTW** 1980 Nov 5;87(11):414

**France**

Dillemann G, Michel ME: La réception des pharmaciens en France de la Révolution à l'application de la loi du 21 germinal an XI (1791–1813). **Rev Hist Pharm (Paris)** 1984;31(260):42–61
Ramsey M: The repression of unauthorized medical practice in eighteenth-century France. **Eighteenth Cent Life** 1982;7(2):118–35
Sigvard J: Cent ans de vie syndicale dans l'industrie pharmaceutique en France, 1880–1980. **Rev Hist Pharm (Paris)** 1982 Jun;29(253):115–23

**Germany**

Weiss C, Specker H, Winckelmann HJ: Die Medizinalgesetzgebung in Württemberg im 19. Jahrhundert. **MMW** 1983 Nov 4;125(44):1005–10

**Great Britain**

Carty MA: The examination of a young surgeon. Hand-colored etching by George Cruikshank, from The Scourge, 1811. **J Hist Med Allied Sci** 1981 Apr;36(2):214
Webster C: General practice under the panel – the last phase.

**Soc Soc Hist Med Bull (Lond)** 1983 Jun;32:20–3
Weeks J: Inverts, perverts, and Mary-Annes. Male prostitution and the regulation of homosexuality in England in the nineteenth and early twentieth centuries. **J Homosex** 1980–81 Fall–Winter;6(1–2):113–34

**Spain**

Carmona-Cornet AM: Actuación de la comisión regia de reforma de los reglamentos de la ciencia de curar (1790–1840). In International Congress of the History of Medicine, 27th, Barcelona, 1980. Actas. Barcelona, Acadèmia de Ciències Mèdiques de Catalunya i Balears, 1981. p. 480–5.

**Switzerland**

Anner E: Gelöbnisse der Medizinalpersonen im Kanton Zürich seit 1798. Zürich, Juris, 1979. 76 p. (Zürcher Medizingeschichtliche Abhandlungen, Neue Reihe Nr. 135).
Kessler N: Die freie Heiltätigkeit im Gesundheitsgesetz des Kantons Appenzell Ausserrhoden. Zürich, Juris, 1981. 51 p. (Züricher medizingeschichtliche Abhandlungen, Neue Reihe Nr. 146).

**United States**

History, information, and examination requirements of the American Board of Prosthodontics. **J Prosthet Dent** 1984 Aug;52(2):281–7
Affeldt JE: Voluntary accreditation. **Proc Acad Polit Sci** 1980;33(4):182–91
Alexander SF: Samuel Alexander, M.D., and the Uniform Medical Practice Act. **J Med Soc NJ** 1984 Sep;81(9):759–62
Baker SL: Physician licensure laws in the United States, 1865–1915. **J Hist Med Allied Sci** 1984 Apr;39(2):173–97
Bugbee G: George Bugbee: a first-person profile (Part 2). **Health Serv Res** 1981 Winter;16(4):459–66
Cirn JT: The birth throes of the Wisconsin Medical Practice Act: the physicians versus the newspaper editors. **Wis Med J** 1980 May;79(5):12–4
Cooper T, Olimpio NA: Medical education. **Proc Acad Polit Sci** 1980;33(4):32–44
Covell RM: The impact of regulation on health care quality. **Proc Acad Polit Sci** 1980;33(4):111–25
Cruft GE, Humphreys JW, Hermann RE, et al: Recertification in surgery, 1980. **Arch Surg** 1981 Aug;116(8):1093–6
Drake DF: The cost of hospital regulation. **Proc Acad Polit Sci** 1980;33(4):45–59
Eckert C: Evarts A. Graham and the American Board of Surgery. **J Thorac Cardiovasc Surg** 1984 Nov;88(5 Pt 2):842–7
Establishment of the American Board of Oral and Maxillofacial Radiology.: **Oral Surg** 1980 Jun;49(6):549–51
Fine DJ, Meyer ER: Quality assurance in historical perspective. **Hosp Health Serv Adm** 1983 Nov–Dec;28(6):94–121
Gilliand E: The legalization of chiropractic in the state of Louisiana. **North La Hist Assoc J** 1981;12(2–3):104–10
Green MW: Epilogue, prologue: from the past comes the future: the first 75 years of the National Association of Boards of Pharmacy. Chicago, National Association of Boards of Pharmacy, 1979. ix, 109 p.
Hall CP: Medical malpractice problem. **Ann Am Acad Polit Soc Sci** 1979;443:82–93
Hamowy R: The early development of medical licensing laws in the United States, 1875–1900. **J Libert Stud** 1979;3(1):73–119
Hanawalt L: The doctors' war in the Michigan legislature, 1835–1861. **Mich Hist** 1979;63(1):29–43
Hayes AH: Science and public policy. **J Assoc Off Anal Chem** 1982 Mar;65(2):202–5
Husing JM: Brief historical background on the certification process in corrective therapy, and a policy statement regarding certification eligibility. **Am Correct Ther J** 1983 Nov–Dec;37(6):153–5
Hynes CJ: The regulation of nursing homes: a case study. **Proc Acad Polit Sci** 1980;33(4):126–36
Isbister JD, McGaw N: Regulation of health care in the United States. **J Health Hum Resour Adm** 1978 Aug;1(1):11–29
Kennedy L: Health planning in an age of austerity. **Policy Stud J** 1980–81;9(2):232–41
Legge D: Peer review in the U.S.A.: an historical perspective. **Med J Aust** 1981 Jun 27;1(13):709–11
Little DM: The founding of the specialty boards. **Anesthesiology** 1981 Sep;55(3):317–21
McCauley HB: The Maryland State Board of Dental Examiners. In the beginning. **J Md State Dent Assoc** 1984 Apr;27(1):22–9
McDonald WH: Then and now. 75 years of Alabama medicine by father and son with comments on the birth of malpractice. **J Med Assoc State Ala** 1979 Jan;48(7):16–8
Numbers RL: Public protection and self-interest: medical societies in Wisconsin. In Numbers RL, Leavitt JW, ed: Wisconsin medicine. Historical perspectives. Madison, University of Wisconsin Press, 1981. p. 75–104.
Pattullo EL: Reconciling risk and regulation. **Society** 1980;18(1):34–8
Regan LJ: Malpractice: 25 years hasn't changed much. **Mich Med** 1981 Oct;80(29):550
Rehm WS: In tribute to a living pioneer: Dr. Lyndon Edmund Lee. **Chiropr Hist** 1981;1(1):47–50
Sanazaro PJ: Quality assurance in medicine: a brief historical perspective. **World Hosp** 1984 Apr;20(2):16–20
Schmidt MS: Why a separate organization for state boards? **Am J Nurs** 1980 Apr;80(4):724–6
Wardwell WI: The cutting edge of chiropractic recognition: prosecution and legislation in Massachusetts. **Chiropr Hist** 1982;2(1):55–65
Westerman JH: The joint commission on accreditation of hospitals: relations with the practicing physician--past, present and future. JCAH and the practicing physician: historical relationships and current issues (First of two parts). **Conn Med** 1982 Jan;46(1):23–6
Westerman JH: The Joint Commission on Accreditation of Hospitals: relations with the practicing physician--past, present and future. JCAH and the practicing physician: present issues, current solutions and future considerations 2. **Conn Med** 1982 Feb;46(2):89–92
Work WP: The American Board of Otolaryngology: 1950–1979. **Ann Otol Rhinol Laryngol [Suppl]** 1982 Mar–Apr;90:1–8

## LITERATURE

Banziger G: Intergenerational communication in prominent western drama. **Gerontologist** 1979 Oct;19(5 pt 1):471–80
Bernard J: Création poétique et création cientifique. **Bull Assoc Guillaume Bude** 1981;3:275–83
Cousins N, ed: The physician in literature. Philadelphia, Saunders, 1982. xxiii, 477 p. Selections from many authors.
Dieckhöfer K: Geistesgeschichtliche Strömungen in der Biographik--ein kulturhistorischer Abriss. **Z Psychosom Med Psychoanal** 1980 Jul–Sep;26(3):275–81
Dubb A: Medical philately: The pen and the scalpel -- the story of medicine and literature. **S Afr Med J** 1979 Nov 17;56(21):847–50
Duff W: An essay on original genius and its various modes of exertion in philosophy and the fine arts, particularly in poetry (1767). Facsimile. Ed. by J. L. Mahoney. Delmar, New York, Scholars' Facsimiles and Reprints, 1978. ix, 296 p.
Erlen J: Medicine in literature: theses; a survey of secondary sources. **Watermark** 1983 Summer;7(1):1–3
Feggetter G: Suicide in opera. **Br J Psychiatry** 1980 Jun;136:552–7
Fox A: Obstetrics and Gynecology in Macbeth. **Shakespeare Stud** 1979;12:127–41
Fox ER: The face of medicine. **West J Med** 1981 Nov;135(5):424–5
Gerevich J: Az elemebeteggé minösítés szépirodalmi modelljei. **Orv Hetil** 1982 Nov 28;123(48):2971–2
Hawkins A: Two pathographies: a study in illness and literature. **J Med Philos** 1984 Aug;9(3):231–52
Horney theory and literature: a symposium: **Am J Psychoanal** 1982 Spring;42(1):3–59
Jones AH: A commentary on 'Two pathographies: a study in illness and literature'. **J Med Philos** 1984 Aug;9(3):257–9
Jones AH, ed: Images of healers. Albany, State University of New York Press, 1983. 160 p. (Literature and medicine, v. 2)
Miller JM: Physicians and prose. **Md State Med J** 1982 Jan;31(1):43–7
Milner M: Freud et l'interprétation de la littérature. Paris, Société d'édition d'enseignement supérieur, 1980. 328 p.
Ober WB: Boswell's clap and other essays. Medical analyses of literary men's afflictions. Carbondale, Southern Illinois University Press; and London, Feffer & Simons, 1979. xiv, 291 p.
Palmer C, Horowitz M, ed: Shaman woman, mainline lady: women's writings on the drug experience. New York, Morrow, 1982. 285 p.
Pascarella F: On 'The physician-writers from the 15th to the 20th century' by Arnaldo Cherubini. Rome, Arti Grafiche E. Cossidente, 1979.
Pastinszky I: A száj müködése: harapás, evés, nevetés, beszéd, ízlelés a klasszikus közmondásokban és idézetekben. **Fogorv Sz** 1984 Jul;77(7):217–8
Pastinszky I: Stomatologia a klasszikus kózmondásokban és idézetekben. **Fogorv Sz** 1984 May;77(5):139–41
Peschel RE, Peschel ER: 'But what if she should die?'--case histories, literary histories: a discussion of maternal death in childbirth. **Pharos** 1981 Winter;44(1):11–8
Peschel RE, Peschel ER: Ritual and the death certificate: case histories, literary histories. **Pharos** 1983 Spring;46(2):11–6
Prioleau E: Leprosy. Reality and metaphor in literature. **Am J Dermatopathol** 1983 Aug;5(4):377–80
Rogers R: Metaphor: a psychoanalytic view. Berkeley, University of California Press, 1979. xi, 148 p.
Rousseau GS: Literature and medicine: the state of the field. **Isis** 1981 Sep;72(263):406–24
Schatzberg W: Relations of literature and science: a bibliography of scholarship, 1978–79. **Clio (US)** 1980;10(1):57–84
Schlegel KF: Der Körperbehinderte in Mythologie und Kunst. Stuttgart; New York, Thieme, 1983. 125 p.
Schlegel KF: Luzifer - ein orthopädischer Patient. In KF Schlegel, ed: Der Körperbehinderte in Mythologie und Kunst. Stuttgart, New York, Thieme, 1983. p. 19–27.
Schlegel KF, ed: Der Körperbehinderte in Mythologie und Kunst. Stuttgart, New York, Georg Thieme Verlag, 1983. 125 p.
Sheerin DJ: A Carolingian cure recovered: Erasmus' citation of Hucbald

of St. Amand's Ecloga de caluis. **Bibl Hum Renaissance** 1980 Jan;42(1):167-71
Shelp EE: The experience of illness: integrating metaphors and the transcendence of illness. **J Med Philos** 1984 Aug;9(3):253-6
Skura MA: The literary use of the psychoanalytic process. New Haven, London, Yale University, 1981. 280 p.
Skvortsov VIa, Skvortsova AI: Obrazy vracheĭ v proizvedeniiakh literatury i iskusstva. **Sov Zdravookhr** 1984;(9):59-62
Smith CU: Don Juan and the vision of Vision. **Perception** 1981;10(4):435-53
Steel D: Plague writing: from Boccaccio to Camus. **J Eur Stud** 1981;11(2):88-110
Thurer S: Disability and monstrosity: a look at literary distortions of handicapping conditions. **Rehabil Lit** 1980 Jan-Feb;41(1-2):12-5
Tissot SA: De la santé des gens de lettres; présentation de F. Azouvi. Genève and Paris, Slatkine, 1981. viii, 246 p. Reprint of Lausanne ed., 1768.
Trautmann J, Pollard C: Literature and medicine. An annotated bibliography. Revised edition. Pittsburgh, University of Pittsburgh Press, 1982. xxi, 228 p. (Contemporary Community Health Series).
Trautmann J: Medical ethics in literature. In Reich WT, et al, ed: Encyclopedia of bioethics, v.3. New York, Free Press, 1978. p. 1008-15.
Trautmann J, ed: Healing arts in dialogue. Medicine and literature. Carbondale, Edwardsville, Southern Illinois University Press, 1981. Contribution by N. C. Andreasen, R. Selzer, J. C. Cowan, I. Lawson, D. Levertov, E. Sewell, H. G. Moss. (Medical Humanities Series).
Wermut W: Rodowody literackie niektórych zespołów klinicznych. **Psychiatr Pol** 1980 Jan-Feb;14(1):69-76

**Austria**

Hochenegg H: Tiroler Aerzte und Pharmazeuten als Künstler und Schriftsteller, Forscher und Volksvertreter. **Tirol Heimat** 1976;40:135-62

**France**

Brann NL: Melancholy and the divine frenzies in the French Pléiade: their conflicting roles in the art of 'beaux exercices spirituels.' **J Mediev Renaiss Stud** 1979;9:81-100
Jackson R: Raynaud and Molière. **Arch Dermatol** 1983 Mar;119(3):263-6

**Germany**

Heidel G: Zur wahrscheinlich ältesten deutschen Ubersetzung des Syphilisgedichtes von Girolamo Fracastoro. **Dermatol Monatsschr** 1983;169(2):130-5

**Great Britain**

Fox D: Henryson's 'Sum Practysis of Medecyne'. **Stud Philol** 1972;69:453-60
Jones GP: The Welsh poet as a medical historian. In J. Cule, ed: Wales and medicine. London, British Society for the History of Medicine, 1975. p. 119-26.
Schuler RM: English magical and scientific poems to 1700: an annotated bibliography. New York, Garland, 1979. xxviii, 120 p.

**Italy**

Dolzani C: Un 'prelievo' di sangue adombrato in una poesia di Giovanni Pascoli? **Acta Med Hist Patav** 1982-83;29:25-8

**Spain**

Rico-Avello C: La enigmatica sexualidad de La Monja-Alferez. **Asclepio** 1980;32:353-60

### Before 500 A.D.

Berle EJ: Legenden om en senantikk bentransplantasjon. **Sydsven Medicinhist Sallsk Arsskr** 1984;21:135-40
Emmerick RE: On the indexation of Sanskrit medical verses and prescriptions. **Sci Orient** 1979;16:3-8
Schadewaldt H: Orthopädische Aspekte der Mythologie. In KF Schlegel, ed: Der Körperbehinderte in Mythologie und Kunst. Stuttgart, New York, Thieme, 1983. p. 1-18.
Sermonti G: Orpheus in Perugia. **Riv Biol** 1981 Winter;74(4):453-8

**Babylon**

Spielmeyer R: The epic of Gilgamesh; resolution of concepts of evil and death in ancient Babylonia. **NY State J Med** 1979 Sep;79(10):1618-21

**Egypt**

Thomas C: First suicide note? **Br Med J** 1980 Jul 26;281(6235):284-5

**Greece**

Anzieu D, Carapanos F, Gillibert J, et al: Psychanalyse et culture grecque. Paris, Société d'Edition 'Les Belles Lettres,' 1980. 243 p.
Geymonat M, ed: Scholia in Nicandri Alexipharmaca, cum glossis. Milan, Cisalpino-Goliardica, 1974. 218 p.
Grmek M: La vita, la morte, la malattia nel mondo di Omero. **Intersezioni** 1983;3:243-64
Hausmann W: Chironica ars-- antike Autoren über Cheiron. **DTW** 1982 Oct 5;89(10):407-11
La Croce E: El concepto de locura en Grecia clásica. **Acta Psiquiatr Psicol Am Lat** 1981 Sep-Nov;27(4-5):285-91
Marketos SG, Ballas CN: Bronchial asthma in the medical literature of Greek antiquity. **J Asthma** 1982;19(4):263-9
Phillips JH: Early Greek medicine and the poetry of Solon. **Clio Med** 1980;15(1/2):1-4
Plaitakis A, Duvoisin RC: Homer's moly identified as Galanthus nivalis L.: physiologic antidote to stramonium poisoning. **Clin Neuropharmacol** 1983 Mar;6(1):1-5
Ruck CA: The wild and the cultivated: wine in Euripides' Bacchae. **J Ethnopharmacol** 1982 May;5(3):231-70

**India**

Hankoff LD, Munver UL: Prenatal experience in Hindu mythology. **NY State J Med** 1980 Dec;80(13):2006-14

**Rome**

Dirckx JH: Virgil and medicine. **JAMA** 1981 Sep 18;246(12):1326-9
Dirckx JH: Virgil on anthrax. **Am J Dermatopathol** 1981 Summer;3(2):191-5
Pearcy LT: Melancholy rhetoricians and melancholy rhetoric: 'black bile' as a rhetorical and medical term in the second century A.D. **J Hist Med Allied Sci** 1984 Oct;39(4):446-56
Richardson WF: Medicine: the art of guessing? **NZ Med J** 1984 Jul 11;97(759):453-5

### 500 A.D.-1450

Gerhardt C: Kröte und Igel in schwankhafter Literatur des späten Mittelalters. **Medizinhist J** 1981;16(4):340-57
Kottek S: Medicine in Hebrew poetry: Judah al-Harizi. **Koroth** 1983 Aug;8(7-8):299-304
Weisser C: Studien zum mittelalterlichen Krankheitslunar. Ein Beitrag zur Geschichte laienastrologischer Fachprosa. Pattensen/Hannover, Horst Wellm, 1982. 468 p. (Würzburger medizinhistorische Forschungen, 21).
Yates D: A fourteenth-century Latin poem on the art of the physician. **Bull Hist Med** 1980 Fall;54(3):447-50

**Germany**

Dirckx JH: The pied piper of Hamelin. A medical-historical interpretation. **Am J Dermatopathol** 1980 Spring;2(1):39-45
Dube WF: Medieval medicine in middle high German epics. Ph.D. Diss. Indiana University. [Bloomington], 1981. 295 leaves.
Farrar WE: Parzival's pericardial puncture. **Ann Intern Med** 1980 May;92(5):640
Grubmüller K: Ein Arzt als Literat: Hans Hartlieb. In Honemann V, Ruh K, et al: Poesie und Gebrauchsliteratur im deutschen Mittelalter. Würzburger Colloquium 1978. Tûbingen, Niemeyer, 1979. p. 14-36.
Keil G: Prosa und gebundene Rede im medizinischen Kurztraktat des Hoch- und Spätmittelalters. In: Poesie und Gebrauchsliteratur im deutschen Mittelalter ... hrsg. von V. Honemann, et al. Würzburger Colloquium, 1978. Tübingen, Max Niemeyer, 1979. p. 76-94.

**Great Britain**

Benson CD: The astrological medicine of Chaucer's physician and Nicholas of Lynn's Kalendarium. **Am Notes Queries** 1984 Jan-Feb;22(5-6):62-6
Hargreaves H: 'De spermate hominis': a Middle English poem on human embryology. [Nat. Libr. Scotland, Advocates' MS. 23.7.11]. **Mediaev Stud** 1977;39:506-10
Mandel SL: Chaucer's vivid medical word pictures (reflections of yore afflictions). **Int J Dermatol** 1983 Jun;22(5):329-31
Mooney LR: A middle English verse compendium of astrological medicine. **Med Hist** 1984 Oct;28(4):406-19
Rowland B: Chaucer's idea of the pardoner. **Chaucer Rev** 1979-80;14(2):138-54
Schmidt PG: Materielle und spirituelle Diät. Ein mittellateinischer Verstraktat des frühen 13. Jahrhunderts aus St. Albans. In Dilg P, et al., ed: Perspektiven der Pharmaziegeschichte. Graz, Austria, Akademische Druck- u. Verlagsanstalt, 1983. p. 311-23.

**Italy**

Bazzi F, Panebianco D: Una lauda di interesse medico poco nota di

Jacopone da Todi. **Minerva Med** 1981 Nov 14;72(45):3039–43

### 1450–1700

Benedek TG: The gout of Desiderius Erasmus and Willibald Pirckheimer: medical autobiography and its literary reflections. **Bull Hist Med** 1983 Winter;57(4):526–44
Blaser RH: Paracelsus und die Dichter. **Salzburger Beitr Paracelsusforsch** 1984;23:9–26
Eden AR, Opland J: Bartolommeo Eustachio's De Auditus Organis and the unique murder plot in Shakespeare's Hamlet. **N Engl J Med** 1982 Jul 22;307(4):259–61
Linden SJ: Alchemy and eschatology in seventeenth-century poetry. **Ambix** 1984 Nov;31(3):102–24
Telle J: Paracelsistische Sinnbildkunst. Bemerkungen zu einer Pseudo-'Tabula smaragdina' des 16. Jahrhunderts. In Seidler E, Schott H, ed: Bausteine zur Medizingeschichte. Stuttgart, Steiner, 1984. p. 129–39.

#### Czechoslovakia

Wondrák E: Der Arzt und Dichter Laurentius Span (1530–1575). **Medizinhist J** 1983;18(3):238–49

#### Europe

Gysel G: Renaissance, 'Republique des lettres' et médecine. **Rev Belge Med Dent** 1984 Jun;39(3):99–105

#### France

Bernoulli R: A propos d'une vieille querelle: Montaigne était-il hypocondriaque? **Hist Sci Med** 1982;16(3):145–9
Duthoit JP: La Marquise de Sévigné et quelques aspects de la thérapeutique médicale au XVIIe siècle. Lille, 1980. 110, 8 p.
Flaumenhaft E: Asian medicinal plants in 17th century French literature. **Econ Bot** 1982;36:147–62
Frey EF: The influence of Rabelais on medicine and its reform. **Clio Med** 1980;15(1/2):25–33
Guyotjeannin C: Un aperçu de la thérapeutique au XVIIe siècle. **Monit Pharm Lab** 1981 Apr–May;1465–6:1677–8, 1680–1, 1845, 1847–8
McBride R: The sceptical view of medicine and the comic vision in Molière. **Studi Francesi** 1979, 23(67):27–42
Swinton WE: Rabelais' coarse humour was therapy for his patients. **Can Med Assoc J** 1981 Feb 15;124(4):500–4

#### Germany

Albert DM: 400th anniversary of Batisch's Der Augendienst. **Arch Ophthalmol** 1983 Dec;101(12):1857

#### Great Britain

Dallett JB: Paracelsus in Moronia. Bischof Joseph Halls satirische Darstellung von 'Bustius Hohenheimius' und dessen Collegium. Wien, 1976. 20 p. (Salzburger Beiträge zur Paracelsusforschung, 14).
Daly RJ: Samuel Pepys and post-traumatic stress disorder. **Br J Psychiatry** 1983 Jul;143:64–8
Davies GC: The Welsh doctor as a poet: Henry Vaughan–Silurist. In J. Cule, ed: Wales and medicine. London, British Society for the History of Medicine, 1975. p. 112–18.
Drew-Bear A: Face-painting scenes in Ben Jonson's plays. **Stud Philol** 1980 Fall;47(4):338–401
Eerie murder in Shakespeare's Hamlet: **N Engl J Med** 1982 Dec 9;307(24):1531
Fleissner RF: Putting Falstaff to rest: 'tabulating' the facts. **Shakespeare Stud** 1983;16:57–74
Harrison DF: Neurochemistry and Sherrington's enchanted loom. **J R Soc Med** 1984 Aug;77(8):706–7
Herring H: The self and madness in Marlowe's 'Edward II' and Webster's 'The Duchess of Malfi'. **J Mediev Renaiss Stud** 1979;9:307–23
Heyd M: Robert Burton's sources on enthusiasm and melancholy: from a medical tradition to religious controversy. **Hist Eur Ideas** 1984;5:17–44
Hill EK: The fierce remedy: a note on The Passion. **Am Notes Queries** 1982 May–Jun;20(9–10):134–5
Junghans RP: Falstaff was drunker than he was fat. **N Engl J Med** 1983 Jun 16;308(24):1483
Kail AC: Medicine in Shakespeare. The bard and the body. 2. Mental illness. **Med J Aust** 1983 Oct 15;2(8):399–405
Kail AC: Medicine in Shakespeare. The bard and the body. 6. Therapeutics. **Med J Aust** 1983 Dec 10–24;2(12):657–62
Kail AC: The bard and the body. 1. Shakespeare' physicians. **Med J Aust** 1983 Oct 1;2(7):338–44
Kail AC: The bard and the body. 3. Venereal disease--'the pox'. **Med J Aust** 1983 Oct 29;2(9):445–9
Kail AC: The bard and the body. 4. Drugs, herbs and poisons. **Med J Aust** 1983 Nov 12;2(10):515–9
Kail AC: The bard and the body. 5. Disease: its causes, diagnosis and cure. **Med J Aust** 1983 Nov 26;2(11):568–77
Keers RY: Richard Morton (1637–98) and his Phthisiologia. **Thorax** 1982 Jan;37(1):26–31
Kolin PC: The Elizabethan stage doctor as a dramatic convention. Salzburg, Institut für englische Sprache und Literatur, Universität Salzburg, 1975. 212 p. (Salzburg studies in English literature; Elizabethan & Renaissance studies, 41).
Kuriyama CB: Hammer or anvil. Psychological patterns in Christopher Marlowe's plays. New Brunswick, Rutgers University Press, 1980. xiv, 240 p.
Lutz LA: Shakespeare on plastic surgery. **Plast Reconstr Surg** 1984 Dec;74(6):841
Madsen V: Medicine in history. Dryden on the doctors and the death of Charles II. **J Dermatol Surg Oncol** 1981 May;7(5):366–9
Miller E: The Browne doublet: 'Religio medici' in the history of English prose style. **Bull Res Humanit** 1979;82:213–21
Muslin HL: Romeo and Juliet: the tragic self in adolescence. **Adolesc Psychiatry** 1982;10:106–17
Mutschmann H: Milton's eyesight and the chronology of his works. New York, Haskell House, 1971. 50 p.
Nelson TG: Death, dung, the devil, and worldly delights: a metaphysical conceit in Harington, Donne, and Herbert. **Stud Philol** 1979 Summer;76(3):272–87
Newman C: Nature of Samuel Pepys's 'wind colic'. **Br Med J [Clin Res]** 1980 Dec 20–27;281(6256):1716–7
Nicholl C: The chemical theatre. London, Boston, Routledge and Kegan Paul, 1980. ix, 292 p.
Ormsby-Lennon H: Radical physicians and conservative poets in Restoration England: Dryden among the doctors. **Stud Eighteenth Cent Cult** 1978;7:389–411
Pady DS: A London medical satire of 1607. **J Hist Med Allied Sci** 1978 Jul;33(3):409–16
Porst S: Gynäkologie und Geburtshilfe bei Shakespeare. **Zentralbl Gynakol** 1984;106(12):863–75
Porst S: Gynäkologische, geburtshilfliche, embryologische und teratologische Beschreibungen im Werke Shakespeares. Würzburg, Horst Wellm, 1981. 178 p. (Dissertation, Julius-Maximilians-Universität Würzburg).
Sawday J: The Leiden Anatomy Theatre as a source for Davenant's 'Cabinet of death' in Gondibert. **Notes Queries** 1983 Oct;30(5):437–9
Webster A: Threefold cord of religion, science, and literature in the character of Sir Thomas Browne. **Br Med J [Clin Res]** 1982 Dec 18–25;285(6357):1801–2
Webster C: Utopian planning and the Puritan revolution. Gabriel Plattes, Samuel Hartlib, and 'Macaria'. Oxford, Wellcome Unit for the History of Medicine, 1979. 89 p. (Research Publications of the Wellcome Unit for the History of Medicine, Oxford, No. II).
Wolfensberger W: Eulogy for a mentally retarded jester. **Ment Retard** 1982 Dec;20(6):269–70
Wooden WW: Childhood and death: a reading of John Skelton's Phillip Sparrow. **J Psychohist** 1980 Spring;7(4):403–14

#### Italy

Graziani R: Fracastoro's 'syphilis' and Priapus. **Clio Med** 1981 Dec;16(2/3):93–9
Schupbach W: Doctor Parma's medicinal macaronic: poem by Bartolotti, pictures by Giorgione and Titian. [Wellcome MS 461]. **J Warburg Courtauld Inst** 1978;41:147–91, 350

#### Netherlands

Moerman AK: Daniël Jonctktys--Dordts dokter en dichter. **Kwartaal Teken** 1979;5(3):5–10
Van Lieburg MJ: De dichter-medicus Daniël Jonctys (1611–1654), zijn strijd tegen het bijgeloof en zijn relatie tot Johan van Beverwijck, William Harvey en Daniël Sennert. **Tijdschr Geschied Geneeskd** 1979;2(4):137–67

#### Poland

Dudziński W: Medicinalia w pierwszej ojczystej gazecie 'Merkuriuszu Polskim'. **Wiad Lek** 1981 Oct 1;34(19):1653–5
Jonecko A: Drzeworyt ukazujący amputowane i protezowane podudzie w śląskim poemacie Roździeńskiego 'Officina ferraria' a roku 1612. **Wiad Lek** 1983 Jun 15;36(12):1025–31
Jonecko A: Drzeworyt ukazujacy amputowane i protezowane produdzie w slaskim poemacie Roździeńskiego 'Officina Ferraria' z roku 1616. **Arch Hist Med (Warsz)** 1984;47(1):107–16

#### Portugal

Reis CS: A 'Doença crua e feia' em 'os lusíadas'. **An Inst Hig Med Trop (Lisb)** 1977–1978;5(1–4):127–69

# LITERATURE

### Spain

Gracia D: Chirino en el Retablo de las Maravillas. **Asclepio** 1978-79;30-31:265-76

Grinberg L, Rodríguez JF: The influence of Cervantes on the future creator of psychoanalysis. **Int J Psychoanal** 1984;65(Pt 2):155-68

### 1700 to Present

Altchek ED: Plus ça change. **Plast Reconstr Surg** 1980 Jun;65(6):849-50

Beer G: Anxiety and interchange: Daniel Deronda and the implications of Darwin's writing. **J Hist Behav Sci** 1983 Jan;19(1):31-44

Blinderman A: Isaac Bashevis Singer; medicinal fiction. **NY State J Med** 1981 Aug;81(9):1382-91

Blumenthal-Barby K: Gedanken zu Sterben und Tod in der Belletristik. **ZFA** 1983 Sep-Oct;38(5):395-8

Bonalumi F: Il medico di Balzac e il curato di Ravizza. **Aevum** 1979;53(3):519-32

Bornstein S, Bitty L: Essai sur folie et roman: un auteur en quête de psychiatres. **Ann Med Psychol (Paris)** 1983 Nov;141(9):957-67

Bower EM, ed: The handicapped in literature. A psychosocial perspective. Denver, Love, 1980. xi, 407 p.

Bowers JZ: Truants from medicine. **Perspect Biol Med** 1979 Autumn;23(1):83-91

Brunclík J: Freud o dostojevském - či naopak. **Cas Lek Cesk** 1982 Aug 13;121(32):1015-6

Caplan RM: The circumstances of the missing biographer or why Watson didn't narrate these four Sherlock Holmes stories. **J Am Acad Dermatol** 1982 Jun;6(6):1112-4

Chabot CB: Freud on Schreber. Psychoanalytic theory and the critical act. Amherst, University of Massachusetts Press, 1982. 171 p.

Crompton R, Gall D: Georgi Markov--death in a pellet. **Med Leg J** 1980;48(2):51-62

Culik H: Mindful of the body: medical allusions in Beckett's Murphy. **Eire-Irel** 1977 Spring;14:84-101

Dellamora R: An essay in sexual liberation, Victorian style: Walter Pater's 'Two early French stories'. **J Homosex** 1983 Spring-Summer;8(3-4):139-50

DuPlessis RB, Friedman SS: 'Woman is perfect': H. D.'s debate with Freud. **Feminist Stud** 1981;7(3):407-30

Engelhardt D von: Das literarische Kunstwerk als Therapeutikum. **Dtsch Apoth Ztg** 1981;33:292-302

Foley GP: A treasury of dentistry. **J Am Coll Dent** 1983 Spring;50(1):42-3

Forschbach G: Tuberculosis and creative man. **Bull Int Union Tuberc** 1984 Mar-Jun;59(1-2):104-7

Frey EF: The physician in nineteenth-century English and American literature. **Bookman** 1981 May-Jun;8(5):3-8

Ginzburg C: Morelli, Freud and Sherlock Holmes: clues and scientific method. **Hist Workshop J** 1980;9:5-36

Graham PW: A mirror for medicine: Richard Selzer, Michael Crichton, and Walker Percy. **Perspect Biol Med** 1981 Winter;24(2):229-39

Grenander ME: Of graver importance than history: psychiatry in fiction. **J Libert Stud** 1978;2(1):29-44

Hall R: Henry James: interpreting an obsessive memory. **J Homosex** 1983 Spring-Summer;8(3-4):83-97

Ham LM: Reflections of nursing: portrait or caricature? **Image (IN)** 1981 Feb;13(1):9-12

Harrington A: After the impossible happened. **Synthesis** 1982;5(2):2-21

Häussermann E: Für den Zahnarzt im Dichter-Schloss nur ein kleines Mansarden-Zimmer. **Zahnarztl Mitt** 1983 Sep 16;73(18):1990, 1993-4

Holland NN: Freud, physics, and literature. **J Am Acad Psychoanal** 1984 Jul;12(3):301-20

Hurst DL, Hurst MJ: Bromide psychosis: a literary case. **Clin Neuropharmacol** 1984;7(3):259-64

Iveson-Iveson J: Vampires: when fantasy meets reality. **Nurs Mirror** 1983 Jan 19;156(3):18-20

Jacoby E: Der Aufstieg ins Bürgertum und sein Preis. Charles Dickens als Beispiel. **Psyche (Stuttg)** 1982 Jul;36(7):609-29

Kaufman P: Burke, Freud, and the Gothic **Stud Burke Time** 1972;13(3):2179-92

Keelan P: Of Pickwick and Ondine. **Ir Med J** 1981 Nov;74(11):339-40

Kramer JC: The metapsychology of opium. **J Psychoactive Drugs** 1981 Jan-Mar;13(1):71-9

Loughman C: Voices of the Wolf Man: the Wolf Man as autobiographer. **Psychoanal Rev** 1984 Sep;71(2):211-25

Macpike L: The social values of childbirth in the nineteenth-century novel. **Int J Womens Stud** 1980;3(2):117-30

Mahler-Schachter E: Svevo, Trieste and the Vienna Circle: Zeno's analyst analysed. **Eur Stud Rev** 1982;12(1):45-66

Mahony P: Freud as a writer. New York, International Universities Press, 1982. xv, 227 p.

Mainetti JA: Leyendo con Freud La peau de chagrin de Balzac. **Asclepio** 1982;34:265-81

Martin E: Mothers, madness, and the middle class in The bell jar and Les mots pour le dire. **Fr Am Rev** 1981;5(1):24-47

Matthews JH: Surrealism, insanity, and poetry. Syracuse, Syracuse University Press, 1982. xii, 154 p.

Meisel P, ed: Freud: a collection of critical essays. Englewood Cliffs, New Jersey, Prentice-Hall, 1981. 240 p. Reprinted works by literary figures.

Montiel L: El psicoanálisis en la Montaña mágica. In International Congress of the History of Medicine, 27th, Barcelona, 1980. Actas. Barcelona, Académia de Ciències Mèdiques de Catalunya i Balears, 1981. p. 116-20.

Montiel L: Freud y el psicoanálisis en dos conferencias de Thomas Mann. In International Congress of the History of Medicine, 27th, Barcelona, 1980. Actas. Barcelona, Académia de Ciències Mèdiques de Catalunya i Balears, 1981. p. 111-5.

Norich I: Kak lechili Toma Soĭera. **Med Sestra** 1984 Feb;43(2):61-3

Ortega Millán A, García Prieto A, Ocio León S: Acercamiento a la vida y obra de Kafka. **Actas Luso Esp Neurol Psiquiatr** 1982 Jul-Aug;10(4):223-7

Reimers D: Die interne Behandlung der Tuberkulose. **Prax Klin Pneumol** 1982 Nov;36(11):475-8

Robert BP: Origines du surréalisme. **Univ Ottawa Q** 1982;52(2):190-205

Rodgers JS: 'Life' in the novel: Tristram Shandy and some aspects of eighteenth-century physiology. **Eighteenth Cent Life** 1980;6(1):1-20

Rothman WA: The hospital in literature. **Hosp Health Serv Adm** 1983 Jul-Aug;28(4):85-94

Sandblom P: Skapande och Sjukdom. Hur lidande påverkar litteratur, konst och musik. Södertälje, Fingraf Tryckeri, 1983. 142 p. (Nordisk Medicinhistorisk Arsbok, Supplementum IX).

Saueressig H: Die Tuberkulose als Paradigma des Lebensgefühls. **Med Welt** 1982 Mar 26;33(12):428-34

Scherg C: Literatur als Lebenshilfe. Am Beispiel Thomas Manns. **Psyche (Stuttg)** 1982 Jul;36(7):630-61

Schings HJ: Melancholie und Aufklärung. Melancholiker und ihre Kritiker in Erfahrungsseelenkunde und Literatur des 18. Jahrhunderts. Stuttgart, Metzler, 1977. x, 476 p.

Schwaber P: Freud and the twenties. **Mass Rev** 1981;22(1):133-51

Sontag S: Illness as metaphor. New York, Farrar, Straus and Giroux, 1978. 87 p.

Spangler GM: Suicide and social criticism: Durkheim, Dreiser, Wharton, and London. **Am Q** 1979;31(4):496-516

Stäuble-Lipman Wulf, M: De Quincey, Baudelaire, e i 'Paradisi artificiali'. **Nuova Antologia** 1972;514(2054):245-54

Strout C: Psyche, Clio, and the artist. In M. Albin, R. J. Devlin, G. Heeger, ed: New directions in psychohistory. The Adelphi papers in honor of Erik H. Erikson. Lexington, Toronto, D. C. Heath, 1980. p. 97-115.

Szállási A: Csehov és Maugham a Nyugat kedvenc írói. **Orv Hetil** 1980 Jan 27;121(4):226-9

Thomas DM: Freud and the 'White Hotel'. **Br Med J [Clin Res]** 1983 Dec 24-31;287(6409):1957-60

Tucker WS: Osler and sleep apnea. **Arch Intern Med** 1984 May;144(5):1085

Vega H: Así sufrieron. Barcelona, Argos Vergara, 1981. 204 p.

Wygant A: Shelley, Hawthorne, and Wells: images of medicine in early science fiction. **Bookman** 1981 Oct;8(8):3-8

Ziegler CR: The image of the physically handicapped in children's literature. New York, Arno, 1980. 156 p. (Also Ed. D. Diss. Philadelphia, Temple University, 1971).

### Austria

Haenel T: Die Suizidproblematik bei Stefan Zweig. **Schweiz Arch Neurol Neurochir Psychiatr** 1981;129(2):297-314

Obermeit W: Die Wirklichkeit des Fiktiven. Literatur und Psychoanalyse. **Psyche (Stuttg)** 1981 Mar;35(3):193-208

Schachter M: L'écrivain-médecin Arthur Schnitzler (1862-1931). **Prov Med** 1979;6/7:347-53

### Brazil

Montenegro TH: A tuberculose na vida e obra de Manuel Bandeira. **Interam Rev Bibliogr** 1969;19(3):278-300

### Canada

Clarke JN: Medicalization and secularization in selected English Canadian fiction. **Soc Sci Med** 1984;18(3):205-10

Moss JB: Pathological images in the Quebec novel. **Am Rev Can Stud** 1980;10(1):39-47

Prescott JF: The extensive medical writings of soldier-poet John McCrae. **Can Med Assoc J** 1980 Jan 12;122(1):110,113-4

### Chile

Casaretto CC: Juan Ignacio Molina (Huaraculén 1740 - Bolonia 1829), fundador de la patografía y de la autopatografía en Chile. **Rev Med Chil** 1979 Nov;107(11):1053-61

Costa-Casaretto C: La descripción de la viruela--su viruela--por el estudiante jesuita Juan Ignacio Molina (1761). **Rev Med Chil** 1979 Dec;107(12):1141-51

Neghme A: La obra literaria de los médicos chilenos. **Rev Med Chil** 1981 Jun;109(6):557-64; Jul;109(7):683-91

Neghme A: Obra literaria de los médicos chilenos. (III, IV). **Rev Med Chil** 1981 Aug-Sep;109(8,9):789-93, 895-900 (continued periodically)

**Czechoslovakia**

Káš S: Básnická tvorba v díle Ceských lékařu. **Cas Lek Cesk** 1983 May 6;122(18):568–70
Káš S: Dramatická tvorba v díle českých lékařu - spisovatelu. **Cas Lek Cesk** 1982 Dec 23;121(51):1592–4
Káš S: Medicínský humor v tvorbě českých lékařu - spisovatelu. **Cas Lek Cesk** 1983 Mar 18;122(11):344–5
Káš S: Románová tvorba českých lékařu--spisovatelu. **Cas Lek Cesk** 1983 Feb 25;122(8):244–6
Mecke G: Der Jäger Gracchus, Kafkas Geheimnis. **Psyche (Stuttg)** 1981 Mar;35(3):209–36
Solana RM: Communication, language and family: a communicational analysis of Kafka's letter to his father. **Psychiatry** 1983 Nov;46(4):387–92
Vilček E: O zdravotnom stave P. O. Hviezdoslava. **Bratisl Lek Listy** 1983;79(1):117–22

**Denmark**

Greenacre P: Hans Christian Andersen and children. **Psychoanal Study Child** 1983;38:617–35

**France**

Balzac et la médecine de son temps: [Paris], Maison de Balzac, [1976?]. [98] p.
Baudry FD: Adolescent love and self-analysis as contributors to Flaubert's creativity. **Psychoanal Study Child** 1980;35:377–416
Bernard J: Lasthénie de Ferjol, Marie de Saint-Vallier, Emilie de Tourville ou le romancier et l'anémie. **Nouv Rev Fr Hematol** 1982;24(1):43–4
Borie J: Mythologies de l'hérédité au XIXe siècle. Paris, Editions Galilée, 1981. 215 p.
Böttiger LE: På spaning i 'På spaning': om homosexualiteten i Prousts verk. **Sydsven Medicinhist Sallsk Arsskr** 1984;21:99–108
Bréhant J: La médecine, dans la vie et l'oeuvre de Voltaire (deuxième partie). **Bull Acad Natl Med (Paris)** 1980 Oct;164(7):675–81
Bréhant J: La médecine dans la vie et l'oeuvre de Voltaire (Première partie). **Bull Acad Natl Med (Paris)** 1980 Oct;164(7):659–64
Bréhant J: Voltaire et la médecine. **Sem Hop Paris** 1982 Dec 23;58(47):2792–801
Bugyi B: G. Flaubert (1821–1880) és az orvosok. **Orv Hetil** 1980 Jun 1;121(22):1339–40
Chasseguet-Smirgel J: De Sade: Der Körper und der Mord an der Realität. **Psyche (Stuttg)** 1981 Mar;35(3):237–52
Cornet A: François Moutier médecin et poète (1881–1961). **Hist Sci Med** 1983;17(2):171–9
Decourt J: Aragon, tendre et fidèle. **Sem Hop Paris** 1983 May 12;59(19):1489–92
Dirckx JH: Voltaire on the pox. **Am J Dermatopathol** 1983 Dec;5(6):581–4
Favre R: La mort dans la littérature et la pensée française au siècle des lumières. Lyon, Presses universitaires de Lyon, 1978. 640 p.
Fouré J: Talma - the dentist who became the greatest French actor of all times. **Bull Hist Dent** 1983 Apr;31(1):3–10
Gastaut H, Gastaut Y, Broughton R: Gustave Flaubert's illness: a case report in evidence against the erroneous notion of psychogenic epilepsy. **Epilepsia** 1984 Oct;25(5):622–37
Gastaut H, Gastaut Y: La maladie de Gustave Flaubert. **Rev Neurol (Paris)** 1982;138(6–7):467–92
Godlewski G: Flaubert l'inassouvi. **Sem Hop Paris** 1980 Dec 18–25;56(47–68):2051–62
Guyotjeannin C: Les médicaments de Marcel Proust. **Monit Pharm** 1983 Sep 10;37(1577):3423, 3425, 3427; 1983 Oct 15;37(1582):3987–8
Halberstadt-Freud HC: Proust and perversion: some clinical and theoretical consideration. **Int J Psychoanal** 1980;61(3):403–10
Hernándex EI: Sindrome de enclaustramiento. **Medicina (B Aires)** 1983;43(1):117–8
Hossard J: Une rencontre inattendue: Flaubert et Dorvault. **Rev Hist Pharm (Paris)** 1980 Jun;27(245):119–22
Hossard J, ed: Flaubert et la médecine. [Catalog of an exhibition July 5–27, 1980.] Rouen, Musée Flaubert, Hôtel Dieu de Rouen, 1980. n. p.
Huard P, Théodoridès J: Jean-Baptiste Pipelet (1759–1823), Constance de Théis (1767–1845), Josef de Salm-Dyck (1773–1861) ou le chirurgien, la poétesse et le botaniste. In: Congrès National des Sociétés Savantes, 93e, Tours, 1968. Comptes Rendus. Paris, 1971. Section des Sciences, Tome II. p. 127–36.
Laurenti H: Une thèse de médecine sur Paul Valéry. **Bull Etud Valeryennes** 1980;(25):5–7
Lemaire JF: Gustave Flaubert, médecin passif. **Nouv Rev Deux Mondes** 1981;9:580–92
Malinas C, Malinas Y: Emile Zola et la génétique. La nevrose des Rougon-Macquart. **J Genet Hum** 1981 Dec;29(5 Suppl):593–602
Matot JP: Filiation problématique roman familial et secret (à propos de Louis Aragon. **Psychiatr Enfant** 1984;27(2):523–38
Mitchell H: Politics, power and psychiatry: a review of L'Ordre psychiatrique: l'age d'or de l'aliénisme by Robert Castel. **Int J Law Psychiatry** 1979;2(2):249–61
Mitzman A: Sartres Flaubert. **Psyche (Stuttg)** 1981 Mar;35(3):268–98
Mitzman A: The unstrung Orpheus: Flaubert's youth and the psycho-social origins of art for art's sake. **Psychohist Rev** 6(1):27–42, Summer 77
Montiel L: La enfermedad como símbolo: la peste en la obra de Albert Camus. **Asclepio** 1983;35:171–6
Potvliege P: Le syndrome 'de Pickwick'. Priorité de sa description par le duc de Saint-Simon (1675–1755). **Nouv Presse Med** 1982 Jul 3;11(31):2360
Robert BP: Profiles de 'La fruite des idées' et surréalisme. **Rev Univ Ottawa** 1977;47(3):345–64
Rocchietta S: Alchimia e medicina nel romanzo 'La rosticceria della regina Pedoca' di Anatole France. **Minerva Med** 1980 Oct 31;71(42):3091–2
Rocchietta S: Medici e speziali in tre romanzi de Voltaire. **Minerva Med** 1982 Feb 11;73(5):219–20
Rocchietta S: Una ricetta contro la gotta trascritta da Stendhal in italiano. **Minerva Med** 1981 Feb 25;72(6):305
Romay Garcia Arias L: La medicina en la obra literaria de Gustave Flaubert. **Galicia Clin** 1978;50:604, 671, 759
Rossier A: L'enfant maudit. **Ann Pediatr (Paris)** 1980 Mar;27(3):195–6
Rossier A: Une jalousie mortelle (Honoré de Balzac). **Ann Pediatr (Paris)** 1981 Apr;28(4):298–300
Roucoules L: Paul Valery et l'art de guérir. **Bull Acad Chir Dent (Paris)** 1981–82;27(27):53–64
Stambolian G, Marks E, ed: Homosexualities and French literature: cultural contexts, critical texts. Ithaca, Cornell University Press, 1979. 387 p. Historical chapters by J. Stockinger, G. H. Storzer, I de Courtivron, P. Schmidt, W. Fowlie, J. E. Rivers, R. Galand, F. P. Bowman, G. H. Bauer, S. Doubrovsky, S. Smith.
Swahn S: Proust och läkarvetenskapen. **Sydsven Medicinhist Sallsk Arsskr** 1984;21:87–98
Théodoridès J: 'Paris enragé'. **Rev Hist Pharm (Paris)** 1982;29(252):193–8
Tytell P: La plume sur le divan. Psychanalyse et littérature en France. Paris, Aubier Montaigne, 1982. 326 p.
Une lettre de Louis Jouvet à la veille d'entreprendre ses études de pharmacie: **Rev Hist Pharm (Paris)** 1981 Jun;28(249):121–4
Viel C: Quelques vers et écrits de jeunesse d'Henri Moissan. **Rev Hist Pharm (Paris)** 1984 Mar;31(260):5–12
Vigliani F, Vigliani MC: La strefopodia nella fantasia e nell'arte di Gustave Flaubert. **Chir Organi Mov** 1980 Jul–Aug;66(4):533–43
Vogt DD, Montagne M: Absinthe: behind the emerald mask. **Int J Addict** 1982 Aug;17(6):1015–29
Wegner PC: Le docteur Gall à Cynthère. **Medizinhist J** 1984;19(3):233–43

**Germany**

Bertaux P: Der Wandel der Auffassungen über Hölderlins Krankheit. War Hölderlin geisteskrank? **Med Welt** 1980 Mar 28;31(13):486–90
Blodi FC: Ophthalmology and philately. **Arch Ophthalmol** 1982 Mar;100(3):425,44 (continuing periodically)
Cremerius J: Robert Musil. Das Dilemma eines Schriftstellers vom Typus 'poeta doctus' nach Freud. **Psyche (Stuttg)** 1979 Aug;33(8):733–72
Dallett JB: Woldemar Nürnbergers Paracelsus-Roman. **Salzburger Beitr Paracelsusforsch** 1984;23:50–60
Dietsch H: Von der Metamorphose zur Homologie. Zum 150. Todestag Goethes. **Med Welt** 1982 Dec 3;33(48):1767–8
Donat K: Goethe aus ärztlicher Sicht. **Fortschr Med** 1982 May 13;100(18):852–8
Drews J: Ein Kratersturz ins Unbewusste. Zur Konstruktion von Traum und Tagtraum [in] Arno Schmidts Roman 'Kaff auch Mare Crisium' (1960). **Psyche (Stuttg)** 1981 Dec;35(12):1103–21
Faber-Castell, K von: Arzt, Krankheit und Tod im erzählerischen Werk Theodor Fontanes. Zürich, Juris Druck, 1983. 97 p. (Zürcher Medizingeschichtliche Abhandlungen, Neue Reihe, Nr. 157).
Hellmich S, Hellmich J: Der Zwischenkieferknochen und Goethes Mephistopheles. **Laryngol Rhinol Otol (Stuttg)** 1982 Oct;61(10):552–6
Hruby K: Goethes Augenleiden. **Klin Monatsbl Augenheilkd** 1984 Jul;185(1):61–3
Ionov IuV: Raboty Fridrikha Shellera kak vracha, ego meditsinskie dissertatsii i bolezn' (k 175-letiiu so dnia smerti). **Klin Med (Mosk)** 1981 Jun;59(6):112–5
Kenéz J: H. Heine betegsége. Egy vita, mely a költ' ó halálának 125. évfordulója után sem zárult le. **Orv Hetil** 1982 May 16;123(20):1246–50
Kleeberg J: Goethe und die 'mal de rosa'. **Z Gastroenterol** 1983 May;21(5):241–3
Klein P: Die Infektionskrankheit im erzählerischen Werk Thomas Manns. **Medizinhist J** 1980;15(1/2):3–15
Kreis R: The history of childhood through German literature: a psychogenic model. **J Psychohist** 1982 Winter;9(3):311–9
Leibowitz JO: The final illness of Gotthold Ephraim Lessing. **Janus** 1980;67(1–2–3):21–30
Montiel L: El escritor y su enfermedad: patobiografía de Thomas Mann. In International Congress of the History of Medicine, 27th, Barcelona, 1980. Actas. Barcelona, Académia de Ciències Médiques de Catalunya i Balears, 1981. p. 586–91.
Montiel L: La 'filosofia de la fisiologia' de Federico Schiller. **Asclepio** 1981;33:163–81

## LITERATURE

Montiel Llorente LE: La ciencia medica en 'La montaña magica' de Thomas Mann. **Asclepio** 1980;32:271–85
Neuhauser W: Goethe sprach nie über die Leiden mit seinen Zähnen. **Zahnarztl Mitt** 1982 Aug 16;72(16):1735–43
Peters UH: Hölderlin: Dichter, Kranker--Simulant? **Nervenarzt** 1981 May;52(5):261–8
Sajner J: Goethuv vztah k přírodním vědám, zvláště k lékařství. **Vnitr Lek** 1982 Jun;28(6):615–6
Schadewaldt H: Das Badewesen in der Goethezeit. **Therapiewoche** 1982;32:4123–33
Théodoridès J: Ernst Jünger ou 'l'oeil vivant'. **Gesnerus** 1983;40(1–2):193–202
Wondrák E: Aerztliches und Arzttum im Werk von Ernst Weiss. In: Bilaterale Germanistenkommission CSSR-DDR. IV. Fachtagung ... 1977. Olomouc, Univerzita Palackého, 1979. pp. 142–54.

**Great Britain**

Aronson ME: Sherlock Holmes, father of forensic pathology. **Trans Stud Coll Physicians Phila** 1978 Jul;45(5):258–61
Austin F, Jones B: The Clifts and the arts. **Ann R Coll Surg Engl** 1984 Jan;66(1):63–70
Bardell EB: Dame Agatha's dispensary. **Pharm Hist** 1984;26(1):13–9
Baudry FD: Problems in the application of psychoanalysis to Mary Shelley's Frankenstein. **Int J Psychoanal Psychother** 1982–83;9:647–56
Beerman H: Sherlock Holmes and medical history. **Trans Stud Coll Physicians Phila** 1978 Jul;45(5):243–8
Bruneteau C: John Arbuthnot (1667–1735) et les idées au début XVIIIe siècle. Univ. de Paris III, 1973. 949 p.
Buchanan WW, Kean WF: Robert Burn's illness revisited. **Scott Med J** 1982 Jan;27(1):75–88
Calcraft LG: Aldous Huxley and the Sheldonian hypothesis. **Ann Sci** 1980 Nov;37(6):657–71
Caplan RM: 'The Lion's Mane'. Concerning the diagnostic acumen of Sherlock Holmes. **Am J Dermatopathol** 1983 Dec;5(6):577–9
Charles DC, Charles LA: Charles Dickens' old people. **Int J Aging Hum Dev** 1979–80;10(3):231–7
Corrigan TJ: Biographia Literaria and the language of science. **J Hist Ideas** 1980 Jul–Sep;41(3):399–419
Crompton L: Don Leon, Byron, and homosexual law reform. **J Homosex** 1983 Spring–Summer;8(3–4):53–71
Curtis FB: William Blake and eighteenth-century medicine. **Blake Stud** 1979;8:187–99
Dauber LG: Dickens and doctors; physicians in fiction of Charles Dickens. **NY State J Med** 1981 Sep;81(10):1522–6
Dervin D: Michael Balint's contributions to the psychoanalysis of literature. **Psychoanal Rev** 1979–80 Winter;66(4):553–70
Dervin D: Rainbow, phoenix, and plumed serpent: D. H. Lawrence's great composite symbols and their vicissitudes. **Psychoanal Rev** 1980 Winter;67(4):515–41
Dirckx JH: Doctor Watson's brothers. **Pharos** 1981 Summer;44(3):24–7
Dirckx JH: Graham Greene's doctors. **Pharos** 1983 Spring;46(2):27–9
Dubovsky H: John Keats (1795–1821)--poet, physician and tuberculosis patient. **S Afr Med J** 1981 Jun 6;59(24):875–8
Edwards G: William Ernest Henley: early impressions. **Nurs Mirror** 1981 Jun 17;152(25):33–4
Fahnestock J: The heroine of irregular features: physiognomy and conventions of heroine description. **Victorian Stud** 1981;24(3):325–50
Fassler B: Theories of homosexuality as sources of Bloomsbury's androgyny. **Signs** 1979;5(2):237–51
Feinstein SC: Why they were afraid of Virginia Woolf: perspectives on juvenile manic-depressive illness. **J Adolesc** 1980 Sep;3(3):187–96
Feinstein SC: Why they were afraid of Virginia Woolf: perspectives on juvenile manic-depressive illness. **Adolesc Psychiatry** 1980;8:332–43
Foster R: United States place names and Sherlock Holmes. **Trans Stud Coll Physicians Phila** 1978 Jul;45(5):249–51
Freeman FW, Law A: Allan Ramsay's first published poem: the poem to the memory of Dr. Archibald Pitcairne. **Bibliotheck** 1979;9:153–60
Fromm H: Virginia Woolf: art and sexuality. **Va Q Rev** 1979;55(3):441–59
Gabriel A: Sir Arthur Conan Doyle: to see and to be seen. **Bull Menninger Clin** 1982 Nov;46(6):530–8
Gittings R: Edward Osler and John Keats. In J. Cule, ed: Wales and medicine. London, British Society for the History of Medicine, 1975. p. 107–11.
Gittings R: Keats and medicine. **Contemp Rev** 1971;219(1268):138–42
Gutierrez D: D. H. Lawrence and modern destructiveness. **Suicide Life Threat Behav** 1980 Winter;10(4):219–29
Haley B: The healthy body and Victorian culture. Cambridge, Massachusetts, Harvard University Press, 1978. 296 p.
Harkness B: Greene's old-fashioned remedy in the heart of the matter. **Am Notes Queries** 1982 Mar–Apr;20(7–8):115–6
Hibberd D: 'Problems A': the solution to Wilfred Owen's 'The Imbecile.' **Notes Queries** 1980 Jun;27(3):232–3
Holbrook DM: John Keats: student at the United Hospitals. **St Thomas Hosp Gaz** 1981;79(1):22–4
Hyman V: The autobiographical present in 'A Sketch of the Past'. **Psychoanal Rev** 1983 Spring;70(1):24–32
Hyman VR: Concealment and disclosure in Sir Leslie Stephen's mausoleum book. **Biography** 1980;3(2):121–31
Johnson JP: Herbert Hoover and David Copperfield: a tale of two childhoods. **J Psychohist** 1980 Spring;7(4):467–75
Kalisch BJ, Kalisch PA: Heroine out of focus: media images of Florence Nightingale. Part I. Popular biographies and stage productions. **Nurs Health Care** 1983 Apr;4(4):181–7
Kittle CF: Sir Arthur Conan Doyle--physician and detective. **Proc Inst Med Chic** 1981 Jan–Mar;34(1):7–11
Knight DM: Chemistry, physiology and materialism in the romantic period. **Durham Univ J** 1972;64(2):139–45
Lasky II: A most benevolent Victorian (Sir Arthur Conan Doyle). **Md State Med J** 1982 Dec;31(12):22–4
Lee RV: The generalist: a jaundiced view. **Am J Med** 1983 Dec;75(6):902–5
Levere TH: Poetry realized in nature. Samuel Taylor Coleridge and early nineteenth-century science. Cambridge, Cambridge University Press, 1981. xiii, 271 p.
MacLaglan D: The ether song, 1850. With an introduction and notes by K. G. Huston. First printed in Edinburgh and now reprinted in Los Angeles, 1982. [12 p.].
Martin RK: Edward Carpenter and the double structure of Maurice. **J Homosex** 1983 Spring–Summer;8(3–4):35–46
Meyer JE, Meyer R: Selbstschilderungen eines Depressiven--Zur Pathobiographie William Cowper's. **Fortschr Neurol Psychiatr** 1984 Apr;52(4):107–12
Miller JM: Poisoning by antimony: a case report (Oliver Goldsmith). **South Med J** 1982 May;75(5):592
Miller WH: The habit of Sherlock Holmes. **Trans Stud Coll Physicians Phila** 1978 Jul;45(5):252–7
Morowitz HJ: The mating poems of D. H. Lawrence. **Hosp Pract [Off]** 1984 May;19(5):233–5, 238
Mulhallen J, Wright DJ: Samuel Johnson: amateur physician. **J R Soc Med** 1983 Mar;76(3):217–22
Murray TJ: The neurology of Alice in Wonderland. **Can J Neurol Sci** 1982 Nov;9(4):453–7
Myers WA: Mary Shelley's Frankenstein: creativity and the psychology of the exception. **Int J Psychoanal Psychother** 1982–83;9:625–45
Nemoianu V: The semantics of Bramble's hypochondria: a connection between illness and style in the eighteenth century. **Clio (US)** 1979;9(1):39–51
Obe JM: Oliver Goldsmith: doctor, poet, writer. **Cent Afr J Med** 1984 Mar;30(3):303–8
Panken S: 'Working through and the novel. **Psychoanal Rev** 1983 Spring;70(1):4–23
Paradis J, Postlewait T, ed: Victorian science and Victorian values: literary perspectives. New York, New York Academy of Sciences, 1981. xiii, 362 p. (Annals of the New York Academy of Sciences, 360).
Perkin GD: Arnold Bennett and medicine: with particular reference to his description of dressing apraxia. **Br Med J [Clin Res]** 1981 Dec 19;283(6307):1666–8
Peters D: The pregnant Pamela: characterizations and popular medical attitudes in the 18th century. **Eighteenth Cent Stud** 1980–81;14:432–51
Poirier S: Tobias Smollett, M.D.--expert on the body--and the bawdy. **Pharos** 1984 Winter;47(1):17–22
Porter R: Le prospettive della 'follia': scienza, medicina, e letteratura nell'Inghilterra dell '700. **Intersezioni** 1982;2:55–76
Powell F: Dean Swift and the Dublin Foundling Hospital. **Studies** 1981;70(278–9):162–70
Riddington Young J: Medicus Magus. **J Hist Med Allied Sci** 1980 Jan;35(1):40–57
Rocchietta S: Due secoli di canzoni inglesi con spunti medico-=farmaceutici. **Minerva Med** 1979 Sep 26;70(41):2839–43
Rodin AE, Key JD: Assessment and significance of Arthur Conan Doyle's medical writings. **South Med J** 1982 Nov;75(11):1392–9
Rogers JS: 'Life' in the novel: Tristram Shandy and some aspects of 18th-century physiology. **Eighteenth Cent Life** 1980;6(1):1–20
Rousseau GS: Six new Hill letters. **Med Hist** 1984 Jul;28(3):293–302
Sakula A: L'histoire du bacille tuberculeux telle qu'il nous la raconte dans 'La Ballade de la Seringue'. **Bull Int Union Tuberc** 1982 Sep–Dec;57(3–4):192–3
Sanders V: 'No ordinary case of a village apothecary': the doctor as hero in Harriet Martineaus's Deerbrook. **Notes Queries** 1983 Aug;30(4):293–4
Schiller F: Thomas de Quincey's lifelong addiction. **Perspect Biol Med** 1976 Autumn;20(1):131–41
Sherman MH: Psychosensory images from Virginia Woolf's 'A Sketch of the Past'. **Psychoanal Rev** 1983 Spring;70(1):33–9
Siegel S: Wilkie Collins: Victorian novelist as psychopharmacologist. **J Hist Med Allied Sci** 1983 Apr;38(2):161–75
Smith FN: Swift and cannabis. **Am Notes Queries** 1983 Nov–Dec;22(3–4):37–9
Smith H: John Keats: poet, patient, physician. **Rev Infect Dis** 1984 May–Jun;6(3):390–404
Smithers DW: Dicken's doctors. Oxford, New York, Pergamon, 1979. xiii, 111 p.
Smithers DW: The Barsetshire doctors. **Br Med J [Clin Res]** 1982 Dec 18–25;285(6357):1806–8
Southgate MT: A summer's reading: Virginia Woolf and her

granddaughters. **Conn Med** 1981 Aug;45(8):483-6
Stetz MD: Charles Dickens and 'The Sanatorium': an unpublished letter and manuscript. **Dickensian** 1980;76(390)22-30
Thomson WA: Rider Haggard and smallpox. **J R Soc Med** 1984 Jun;77(6):506-12
Trombley S: All that summer she was mad: Virginia Woolf and her doctors. **Soc Soc Hist Med Bull (Lond)** 1981 Jun;28:21-5
Trombley S: All that summer she was mad: Virginia Woolf, female victim of male medicine. New York, Continuum, 1982. ix, 338 p.
Waldron HA: Did the Mad Hatter have mercury poisoning? **Br Med J [Clin Res]** 1983 Dec 24-31;287(6409):1961
Walsh W: The Keatsian paradox: the hectic and the healthy. **Ann R Coll Surg Engl** 1984 Mar;66(2):139-44
Weir JG: The way they lived then. **Br Med J [Clin Res]** 1982 Dec 18-25;285(6357):1809-10
Weissman A: The English romantics and modern psychology. **Centerpoint** 1975/76;1(4):9-15
Wendorf R: 'Poor Collins' reconsidered. **Huntington Libr Q** 1979;42(2):91-116

### Hungary

Antall J, Kapronczay K: Toldy Ferenc az orvos. **Orvostort Kozl** 1979;87-88(25 no 1-2):105-22
Bíró I: Babits Mihály szenvedései. **Orv Hetil** 1983 Nov 27;124(48):2937-9
Csorba S: Kölcsey Ferenc hibás szemének kérdéséhez. **Orvostort Kozl** 1982;28(1-3):191-9
Ferenczy M: Csokonai Vitéz Mihály egészségügyi tanácsai. **Orv Hetil** 1982 Nov 28;123(48):2973-4
Gyenes G: Adatok Babits betegségéhez. **Orv Hetil** 1983 Nov 27,124(48).2942-6
Huszár G: Ady Endre fogbántalmairól. **Orv Hetil** 1984 Oct 14;125(42):2575-6
Merényi O: Berzsenyi Dániel (1776-1836) betegségei és halála. **Orvostort Kozl** 1979;87-88(25 no 1-2):243-7
Nagy S: Szépirodalom--orvostörténelem. **Orv Hetil** 1980 Sep 28;121(39):2421
Péter L: Juhász Gyula betegségtudata. **Orv Hetil** 1983 May 15;124(20):1205-7
Péter L: Móra Ferenc betegségei. Halálának 50. évfordulójára. **Orv Hetil** 1984 Feb 5;125(6):341-4
Szállási A: Arany János tanártársa Lengyel Dániel doktor. **Orv Hetil** 1983 Apr 3;124(14):833-4
Szállási A: Babits betegségei. **Orv Hetil** 1983 Nov 27;124(48):2940-2
Szállási A: Babits betegségei a tracheotomia elött. **Orv Hetil** 1981 Sep 6;122(36):2235-9
Szállási A: Diósszilágyi Sámuel, az írók orvosa és az orvosok írója. **Orv Hetil** 1981 Jun 14;122(24):1467-72
Szállási A: Fábián Dániel és József Attila. **Orv Hetil** 1983 Feb 20;124(8):464-6
Szállási A: Orvosok a magyar irodalomban Földi Jánostól napjainkig. **Orv Hetil** 1982 Sep 19;123(38):2367-73

### India

Siddiqi T: Ghalib and Unani medicine. **Stud Hist Med** 1979 Sep;3(3):181-98

### Ireland

Donnelly B: The great famine and the literary imagination. **Studies** 1980;69(275-6):260-72
Lock S: 'O that I were young again': Yeats and the Steinach operation. **Br Med J [Clin Res]** 1983 Dec 24-31;287(6409):1964-8
O'Farrel P: Whose reality?: The Irish famine in history and literature. **Hist Stud** 1982;20(78):1-13
Pruitt VD: Yeats, the Mask, and the poetry of old age. **J Geriatr Psychiatry** 1982;15(1):99-112
Robins AH: Did imprisonment ruin Oscar Wilde? **Practitioner** 1981 May;225(1355):773-5
Shen WW, Soldo JJ: Symbol hunting in James Joyce's 'syphilizations'. **Arch Intern Med** 1981 Apr,141(5).691-2
Spencer FJ: The Gay Nineties: Oscar Wilde reconsidered. **MCVQ** 1981;16(3):67-70
Sullivan E: Ocular history of James Joyce. **Surv Ophthalmol** 1984 Mar-Apr;28(5):412-5
Tashjian LD: Aspects of internalization and individuation: James Joyce's Portrait of the artist as a young man. **Adolesc Psychiatry** 1982;10:75-84

### Italy

Beer M: Suicidio e inettitudine: nota sui romanzi femminili Italiani del ventennio 1880-1890. **Mem Riv Stor Donne** 1981;(2):76-88
Benayahu M: Rabbi Abraham Hacohen of Zante and the Padua group of doctor-poets. **Hasifrut** 1978;26:108-40
Bouissy A: Pirandello, 'psychologue de décadence'. **Rev Etud Ital** 1981;26(2-4):173-94
Giulio L: Un tema ricorrente nello Zibaldone: la memoria. **Stor Crit Psicol** 1982 Jun;3(1):27-40
Pini UA: I medici parmigiani nelle poesie del Frugoni. Il medico dormiglione. **Minerva Med** 1980 Sep 22;71(35):2515
Pini UA: I medici parmigiani nelle poesie del Frugoni. L'Ippocrate dei mori, Medico freddoloso. **Minerva Med** 1980 Sep 19;71(34):2438-9
Pini UA: I medici parmigiani nelle poesie di Carlo Innocenzo Frugoni. **Minerva Med** 1980 Apr 7;71(14):1059-61
Rocchietta S: Canzoni italiane correlate con la medicina e la farmacia. **Minerva Med** 1980 Oct 13;71(39):2861-70
Sansoni J: Considerazioni e riflessioni sul libro 'Lungo Viaggio nel Tunnel della Mallattia' di Gigi Ghirotti. **Prof Inferm** 1980 Jan-March;33(1):3-6
Shneidman ES: The suicidal logic of Cesare Pavese. **J Am Acad Psychoanal** 1982 Oct;10(4):547-63
Smith RD: The cricket and the marionette. **South Med J** 1982 Jan;75(1):59-60

### Japan

Lifton RJ, Kato S, Reich MR: Six lives, six deaths. Portraits from modern Japan. New Haven and London, Yale University Press, 1979. xiii, 305 p.

### Mexico

Cárdenas de la Peña E: Médicos y medicina en la vida de un libro. **Gac Med Mex** 1983 Sep;119(9):370-82
Rodríguez A: Samuel Ramos: influencia de Adler y Jung en su estudio sobre el carácter del Mexicano. **Cuad Hispanoam** 1977;109(326-327):420-30

### Netherlands

Bakker-van der Kooij C: De zoekende zusters. Enige beschouwingen naar aanleiding van de herdruk van de roman 'Zuster Bertha', geschreven door Arnold Aletrino en voor het eerst uitgegeven in 1891. **Tijdschr Ziekenverpl** 1983 Apr 26;36(9):275-8
Dalsimer K: Female adolescent development. A study of the Diary of Anne Frank. **Psychoanal Study Child** 1982;37:487-522
Dieckhöfer K: Der flämische Schriftsteller Hendrik Conscience (1812-1883) und die psychisch Kranken von Geel. **Z Psychosom Med Psychoanal** 1984;30(2):179-90
Visser RP: Arts en geneeskunde in de I83-eeuwse algemene tijdschriften. **Ned Tijdschr Geneeskd** 1981 May 16;125(20):792-4

### Norway

Kierulf H: Farsottenes rolle i dikteren Johan Falkbergets trilogi 'Christianus Sextus' (1720 årene). **Nord Medicinhist Arsb** 1980;Suppl 6:82-9

### Pacific Islands

Austen R: Stoddard's little tricks in South Sea Idyls. **J Homosex** 1983 Spring-Summer;8(3-4):73-81

### Peru

Alarco F: La psicoterápia dinámica y José Carlos Mariátegui. **Rev Neuropsiquiatr** 1979 Sep-Dec;42(3-4):145-64

### Poland

Adelsen CE: The last days of Adam Mickiewicz, poet of freedom. **Mankind** 1976;5(5):16-20, 60-1
Kempa K: Tytus Chałubiński w opiniach współczesnych mu przedstawicieli literatury i sztuki. **Wiad Lek** 1980 Dec;33(23):1931-4
Sieńkowski E: Dr med. Leon Stanisław Szuman (1852-1920), chirurg, społecznik, poeta. **Arch Hist Med (Warsz)** 1984;47(1):133-41

### Portugal

Pina L de, Meneses MO de: Camilo e a historia da medicina. **Arch Hist Med Port** 1968-70;3(1-4):91-116

### Romania

Popushoĭ VP, Spineĭ LV: Viktor Krésesku--vrach, revoliutsioner, pisatel'. **Sov Zdravookhr** 1981;(5):62-4

### South Africa

Cartwright MF: The filthy state of Cape Town in 1858. **Q Bull S Afr Libr** 1978;33(2):53-6
Heyningen EB van: The mysteries of the scarlet phial: spies and plague in Cape Town in 1907. **Q Bull S Afr Libr** 1979;34(2):53-8
Sandler EM: C. Louis Leipoldt--medical student extraordinary. **Adler Mus Bull** 1981 Oct;7(3):8-14

# LITERATURE

**Spain**

Arce J: De Feijoo a Quintana. Testimonios lingüistico-literarios sobre inoculación y vacuna. **Bol Cent Estud Siglo XVIII** 1978;6:3–18
Bouza Brey F: Las enfermedades infantiles de Rosalia de Castro y los ritos de medicina magica en Galicia. **Cuad Estud Gallegos** 1967;22(67):183–97
Corbella Corbella J, Martí Amengual G: Recuerdo de la obra de Pedro Mata y Fontanet (1811–1877) en su centenario. **Asclepio** 1980;32:111–9
Dowling J: Smallpox and literature in eighteenth-century Spain. **Stud Eighteenth Cent Cult** 1979;9:59–77
Gil L, Buño W: La medicina, los médicos y las enfermedades en el epistolario de Manuel Marti. **Med Esp** 1980;79:261–72
Jiménez Herrero F: La medicina y los médicos en el teatro de Casona. **Bol Inst Estud Asturianos** 1968;22(64–65):319–51
Jordi R: Humor colérico. **Circ Farm** 1981 Apr;12(137):61–71
Rubin W: Galdos y la medicina. **Atlantida** 1970;8(43):68–80

**Sweden**

Bergström CO: Den sjuka människan i Hjalmar Bergmans diktning. **Nord Medicinhist Arsb** 1984;:165–73
Briceño-Maaz T: Sobre Axel Munthe y su libro 'La Historia de San Michele'. **Rev Soc Venez Hist Med** 1969–71;17–19(31–33):121–30
Al-Dabbagh F: Aksel Mentah, nafsani Suwidi, wa-mu'allif qissat San Mishel. **Al-Arabi** 1973;179:60–3
Fehrman C: Esaias Tegnér and psychiatry: history of literature from medical view-point. **Sydsven Medicinhist Sallsk Arsskr** 1984;21:47–8

**Switzerland**

Winkler-Trachsel E: Arnold Ott (1840–1910). Arzt und Dichter. Sein ärztliches Wirken. Zürich, Juris Druck, 1983. 83 p. (Zürcher Medizingeschichtliche Abhandlungen, Neue Reihe, Nr. 163).

**Turkey**

Köhbach M: Europäische Aerzte im Osmanischen Reich am Beginn des 18. Jahrhunderts--der Fall Sinasi. **Sudhoffs Arch** 1980;64(1):79–85

**United States**

Allen WR: All the names of death: Walker Percy and Hemingway. **Miss Q** 1982–83;36(1):3–19
Atropine poisoning in Hawthorne's the Scarlet Letter: **N Engl J Med** 1984 Nov 29;311(22):1438–41
Barton M: Painful duties: art, character, and culture in Confederate letters of condolence. **South Q** 1979;17(2):123–34
Beaver H: Parkman's crack-up: a Bostonian on the Oregon Trail. **N Engl Q** 1975;48(1):84–103
Brown CL: Thomas Wolfe: a psychiatric view. **J Med Assoc State Ala** 1981 Oct;51(4):11–5
Burbick J: Emily Dickinson and the revenge of the nerves. **Womens Stud** 1980;7(1–2):95–109
Carson RA: Selzer's surgeon as seer. **Perspect Biol Med** 1981 Winter;24(2):284–9
Coles R: Flannery O'Connor's lupus. A commentary on her collected letters, The habit of being. **JAMA** 1980 Sep 26;244(13):1441–2
Coles R: William Carlos Williams. A writing physician. **JAMA** 1981 Jan 2;245(1):41–2
Conrad B: Genius and intemperance. **Horizon** 1980;23(12):33–40
Crowley JW: Dating Howells' adolescent breakdown. **Old Northwest** 1982;8(1):13–22
Crumpacker L: The art of the healer: women in the fiction of Sarah Orne Jewett. **Colby Libr Q** 1983;19(3):155–66
Dermott R: 'A great black book': East of Eden and Gunn's New family physician. **Am Stud** 1981;22(2):41–57
Duffy S: The origin of speeches: Inherit the Wind, Irving Stone and the Scopes trial. **Am Notes Queries** 1983 Sep-Oct;22(1–2):14–7
Engel BF: Why so doleful? The funereal poetry of the early Midwest. **Old Northwest** 1981;7(2):147–59
Feinstein HM: The use and abuse of illness in the James family circle: a view of neurasthenia as a social phenomenon. **Psychohist Rev** 1979;8(1–2):6–14
Fellman AC, Fellman M: Making sense of self. Medical advice literature in late nineteenth-century America. Philadelphia, University of Pennsylvania Press, 1981. 198 p.
Ferguson RA: Yellow fever and Charles Brockden Brown: the contest of the emerging novelist. **Early Am Lit** 1979–80;14(3):293–305
Francke OC: Tandbehandling för 100 år sedan och Mark Twain som patient. **Nord Medicinhist Arsb** 1984;:137–40
Gardiner JF: Solyman Brown and his epic poem 'Dentologia'. **Bull Hist Dent** 1984;32(1):44–51
Gay EW: Francis O. Ticknor, 19th century physician-poet--Part I and II. **J Med Assoc Ga** 1981;70(7):499–503, (8):561–4
Gilman SL: Madness and racial theory in I. J. Singer's The family Carnovsky. **Mod Jud** 1981;1(1):90–100
Graham TR: William Carlos Williams. In Dictionary of American biography, 1961–1965. Suppl. 7, 1981. p. 788–91.
Jones AH: The healer-patient/family relationship in Vonda N. McIntyre's 'Of mist, and grass, and sand'. **Perspect Biol Med** 1983 Winter;26(2):274–80
Kalisch PA, Kalisch BJ: The image of nurses in novels. **Am J Nurs** 1982 Aug;82(8):1220–4
Kennedy JG: Poe and magazine writing on premature burial. **Stud Am Renaiss** 1977;165–78
Khan JA: Atropine poisoning in Hawthorne's The Scarlet Letter. **N Engl J Med** 1984 Aug 9;311(6):414–6
Kimpel BD, Eaves TC: More on Pound's prison experience. **Am Lit** 1981;53(3):469–76
Kriegel L: The wolf in the pit in the zoo. **Soc Policy** 1982;13(2):16–23
Kurth RT, Kurth DJ: Oliver Wendell Holmes, M.D. (1809–1894); medical and literary knowledge intertwined. **NY State J Med** 1980 Jan;80(1):121–4
Liles DM: William Faulkner's Absalom, Absalom!: an exegesis of the homoerotic configurations in the novel. **J Homosex** 1983 Spring-Summer;8(3–4):99–111
McCann W: (Austin) Merrill Moore. In Dictionary of American Biography, Suppl. 6, 1956–1960. p. 461–2, 1980.
Martin J: Psychic epidemics and American literary history: literature, neurosis, and cultural change. **Amerikastudien** 1983;28(3):265–77
Moore RB: Zane Grey: dentist, novelist, baseball player, outdoors man. **Tic** 1982 Jul;41(7):5–7
Morgan WG: Mark Twain: behaviorist. **J Behav Ther Exp Psychiatry** 1984 Jun;15(2):99
Morowitz HJ: Thoreau as a scientist. **Hosp Pract [Off]** 1984 Nov;19(11):143–6, 151
Muuss RE: Peter Blos' modern psychoanalytic interpretation of adolescence. **J Adolesc** 1980 sep;3(3):229–52
Nelson RB: Occasional notes. Captains of an American credo: Walt and W. O. **N Engl J Med** 1981 Jul 9;305(2):110–2
Nevins MA: Bergen County's poet-physicians. **J Med Soc NJ** 1980 Nov;77(12):831–3
Peschel ER: 'Alchemy of the word'--language and 'the knife' a commentary on Richard Selzer's work. **Pharos** 1979 Winter;42(1):25–32
Prioleau E: The literary epidermists. **Am J Dermatopathol** 1981 Winter;3(4):359–60
Ratzan RM: 'No wreaths please': for William Carlos Williams. **Ann Intern Med** 1982 Dec;97(6):933–7
Reed JF: Samuel Clemens and family: the Hartfold connection and Hartford physicians. **Am J Surg** 1981 Apr;141(4):401–10
Ritchey D: The Baltimore theater and the yellow fever epidemic. **Md Hist Mag** 1972;67(3):298–301
Scarlett C: A tale of ratiocination: the death and burial of Edgar Allan Poe. **Md Hist Mag** 1978;73(4):360–74
Scherlis L: Poetical version of the Rules of the Humane Society for recovering drowned persons. **Crit Care Med** 1981 May;9(5):430–1
Schneck JM: Brain injury, psychiatric sequelae, and surgical intervention in S. Weir Mitchell's Westways. **JAMA** 1983 Dec 9;250(22):3048
Schneck JM: S. Weir Mitchell and Oliver Wendell Holmes. A friendship and poetic tribute. **JAMA** 1981 Aug 28;246(9):974–8
Schneck JM: S. Weir Mitchell, M.D. (1829 to 1914) and D. Hayes Agnew, M.D. (1818 to 1892). Neuropsychiatrist's poetic tribute to a surgeon. **NY State J Med** 1982 Jul;82(8):1264–8
Simberloff D: Entropy, information and life: biophysics in the novels of Thomas Pynchon. **Perspect Biol Med** 1978 Spring;21(3):617–25
Skinner RE: Narcotics, barred windows, and murder: the medical practitioner in the writings of Raymond Chandler. **Perspect Biol Med** 1983 Autumn;27(1):127–34
Spencer S: Delivering the woman artist from the silence of the womb: Otto Rank's influence on Anais Nin. **Psychoanal Rev** 1982 Spring;69(1):111–29
Stoehr T: Hawthorne's mad scientists: Pseudoscience and social science in nineteenth-century life and letters. Hamden, Conn., Shoestring Press, 1978. 313 p.
Stone J: A lifetime of careful listening. A centennial retrospective on the work of William Carlos Williams (1883–1963). **JAMA** 1983 Sep 16;250(11):1421–5
Strout C: Henry James's dream of the Louvre, 'The Jolly Corner,' and psychological interpretation. **Psychohist Rev** 1979 Summer-Fall;8(1–2):47–52
Stupniker S: Suspicious circumstances in Salem. **N Engl J Med** 1983 Nov 10;309(19):1194
Tucker EL: A new letter by Thomas Holley Chivers. **Ga Hist Q** 1971;55(4):582–8
Wand M, Sewall RB: 'Eyes be blind, heart be still': a new perspective on Emily Dickinson's eye problem. **N Engl Q** 1979;52(3):400–6
Warren R: Oliver Wendell Holmes, H.M.S. '36. **Harv Med Alumni Bull** 1982 Spring;56(2):20–6
Watterson J, ed: Poetic justice; or, an illfated epic by Thomas Burke. **NC Hist Rev** 1978;55(3):339–46
White E: The inverted type: homosexuality as a theme in James Merrill's prophetic books. **J Homosex** 1983 Spring-Summer;8(3–4):47–52
White PJ: Medical Leonardo of Boston, Oliver Wendell Holmes, M.D.

(1809–1894): an evaluation of versatility. **Perspect Biol Med** 1981 Spring;24(3):411–21

**USSR**

Arkhangel'skiĭ GV: N. S. Leskov o problemakh zdravookhraneniia (k 150–letiiu so dnia rozhdeniia pisatelia). **Sov Zdravookhr** 1981;(10):63–5

Arkhangel'skiĭ GV: S. P. Botkin i M. E. Saltykov-Shchedrin. **Klin Med (Mosk)** 1982 Oct;60(10):114–8

Arkhangel'skiĭ GV: Vrachebnoe okruzhenie vydaiusnchegosia Russkogo poéta V. A. Zhukovskogo (k 200–letiiu so dnia rozhdeniia). **Klin Med (Mosk)** 1984 May;62(5):139–44

Arkhangel'skiĭ GV: Vrachi meditsina v tvorchestve N. S. Leskova (k 150–letiiu so dnia rozhdeniia pisatelia). **Klin Med (Mosk)** 1981;59(10):114–7

Bugyi B: Csehov, az orvos. **Orv Hetil** 1980 Nov 16;121(46):2834–7

Chokin AR, Kabykenov PS: Voprosy zdorav'ia i meditsiny v trudakh izvestnykh Kazakhskikh prosvetiteleĭ. **Sov Zdravookhr** 1983;6:71–4

Dohnány L: L. N. Tolsztoj az egészségügyröl. **Orv Hetil** 1982 Aug 8;123(32):1985–8

Gaïev A: Suicides d'écrivains sovietiques. **Contrat Soc** 1968;12(4):237–41

Gastaut H: New comments on the epilepsy of Fyodor Dostoevsky. **Epilepsia** 1984 Aug;25(4):408–11

Goscilo H: Lermontov's debt to Lavater and Gall. **Slav East Eur Rev** 1981;59(4):500–15

Gurevich SA: Lev Tolstoĭ i psikhiatriia. **Zh Nevropatol Psikhiatr** 1981;81(9):1386–9

Guyotjeannin C: Les médicaments de Tchékhov. **Monit Pharm** 1983;37(1557):1248–50

Ionov IuV: A. P. Chekhov i meditsina. **Feldsher Akush** 1980;45(6):51–4

Ionov IuV: Meditsinskie temy v proizvedeniiakh V. M. Garshina (k 125–letiiu so dnia rozhdeniia). **Klin Med (Mosk)** 1981 Jan;59(1):110–2

Konovalov II: A. S. Pushkin i M. Iu. Lermontov na Kavkazskikh Mineral'nykh Vodakh (k 200–letiiu Piatigorska). **Vopr Kurortol Fizioter Lech Fiz Kult** 1980 Sep–Oct;(5):68–70

Lieber Z: Is there a relationship between illness and creativity? An analysis of the life and poetry of A. V. Koltsov. **Int J Soc Psychiatry** 1980;26(3):212–7

Melzer R: Chekhov's doctors. **Adler Mus Bull** 1981 Oct;7(3):15–9

Miksanek T: Dostoevsky's The Idiot and psychic disorders in epilepsy. **Perspect Biol Med** 1982 Winter;25(2):231–7

Petrovskiĭ BV: Ranenie na duéli i smert' A. S. Pushkina. **Klin Med (Mosk)** 1983 Apr;61(4):109–17

Retamal P: Consideraciones psicopatológicas sobre el diagnóstico de la enfermedad de Fedor Dostoyevski. **Actas Luso Esp Neurol Psiquiatr** 1983 May–Jun;11(3):231–4

Rice JL: Dostoevsky's medical history: diagnosis and dialectic. **Russ Rev** 1983;42(2):131–61

Schein CJ: The death of Ivan Ilych; an axiomatic hypothesis. **NY State J Med** 1981 Mar;81(3):416

Skvortsov VI, Skvortsova AI: F. M. Dostoevskiĭ i meditsina. **Klin Med (Mosk)** 1982 Feb;60(2):112–6

Smyrniw W: Tolstoy's depiction of death in the context of recent studies of the 'experience of dying.' **Can Slavonic Pap** 1979;21(3):367–79

Uzhanskiĭ IaG: K nauchno–literaturnomu nasledstvu akademika Aleksandra Aleksandrovicha Bogomol'tsa (ob osobennostiakh pis'ma akademika A. A. Bogomol'tsa v nauchnykh trudakh). **Patol Fiziol Eksp Ter** 1981 Mar–Apr;(2):16–20

**Venezuela**

Bonadies A: Manuel Diaz Rodriguez: maestro del estilismo y medico. **Rev Soc Venez Hist Med** 1969–71;17–19(31–33):109–15

**Yugoslavia**

Jakopič B: Slušno in govorno prizadeti in gledališče. **Kronika (Yugosl)** 1978;26(2):100–3

Striković J: Analiza jednog samoubistva u delu Ive Andrića 'Na Drini Cuprija'. **Srp Arh Celok Lek** 1979 Sep;107(9):477–82

## MAGIC AND OCCULT

See also **Folk and Popular Medicine; Witchcraft**

Bardeau F: Les clefs secrètes de la chimie des anciens. Paris, Laffont, 1975. 204 p.

Bernus A von: Alchymie und Heilkunst. Nürnberg, Carl, 1981. 243 p.

Brandenburg D: Medizin und Magie. Heilkunde und Geheimlehre des islamischen Zeitalters. Berlin, Hessling, 1975. 159 p. (Medizingeschichtliche Miniaturen, Band 1).

Deikman AJ: The observing self. Mysticism and psychotherapy. Boston, Beacon Press, 1982. xiii, 194 p.

Gettings F: Dictionary of occult, hermetic and alchemical sigils. London, Routledge & Kegan Paul, 1981. 410 p.

Glowatzki G: Das Magische im menschlichen Denken. Seine Auswirkungen auf die Medizin. **Ther Ggw** 1980 Oct;119(10):1107–28

Grossinger R: Planet medicine. From stone age shamanism to post–industrial healing. Revised edition. Boulder, London, Shambhala, 1982. xviii, 436 p.

Hand WD: Magical medicine: the folkloric component of medicine in the folk belief, custom, and ritual of the peoples of Europe and America: selected essays. Berkeley, University of California Press, 1980. xxvii, 345 p.

Kohnen N: Die Symbolkraft menschlicher Schädel und ihr ritueller Gebrauch. **Med Welt** 1983 May 6;34(18):552–6

Lebrun F: Se soigner autrefois. Médecins saints et sorciers aux 17e et 18e siècles. Paris, Temps Actuels, 1983. 206 p. (La passion de l'histoire).

Leupold–Kirschneck D: Das Handauflegen. Eine ärztliche Urgebärde in Geschichte und Gegenwart. Basel/Stuttgart, Schwabe, 1981. 81 p. (Basler Veröffentlichungen zur Geschichte der Medizin und der Biologie, 33).

Manuscripta alchemica der Sammlung Mellon: Bemerkungen zum Katalog: **Sudhoffs Arch** 1981;65(1):79–96

Mueller–Jahncke WD: Der Höhepunkt der Iatromathematic. **Ber Wissenschaftsgesch** 1981;4(1/2):41–50

Oughourlian JM: Un mime nommé désir. Hystérie, transe, possession, adorcisme. Paris, Bernard Grasset, 1982. 311 p.

Rothschuh KE: Iatromagie, Begriff, Merkmale, Motive, Systematik. Opladen, Westdeutscher Verlag, 1978. 60 p. (Vorträge. Geisteswissenschaften. Rheinisch–Westfälische Akademie der Wissenschaften, G 225).

Schoeneman TJ: Criticisms of the psychopathological interpretation of witch hunts: a review. **Am J Psychiatry** 1982 Aug;139(8):1028–32

Shephard L, ed: Encyclopedia of occultism and parapsychology. A compendium of information on the occult sciences, magic, demonology, superstitions, spiritism, mysticism, metaphysics, psychical science, and parapsychology, with biographical and bibliographical notes and comprehensive indexes. Detroit, Gale, 1978. Two volumes.

Sjöstrand T: Magin i medicinen. **Lakartidningen** 1982 May 26;79(21):2137–40

Witten LC, Pachella R, ed: Alchemy and the occult: a catalogue of books and manuscripts from the collection of Paul and Mary Mellon given to Yale University Library. Vols. 3 and 4: Manuscripts 1225–1922. With an introduction by P. Kibre and additional notes by W. McGuire. New Haven, Yale University Library, 1977. 853 p.

**Americas**

Silverblatt I: The evolution of witchcraft and the meaning of healing in colonial Andean society. **Cult Med Psychiatry** 1983 Dec;7(4):413–27

**Austria**

Hölzl N: Zauberbücher, Vampire und einige vernünftige Köpfe. **Tirol Heimatbl** 1972;47(1–3):35–8

**Bolivia**

Bastien JW: Herbal curing by Qollahuaya Andeans. **J Ethnopharmacol** 1982 Jul;6(1):13–28

**China**

Qiu Renzong: [On the origin of medicine ... from sorcery] (Chi). **Chin J Med Hist** 1981;11(1):6–10

**France**

Léger JM: Incidences de certaines croyances populaires (sorcellerie) sur la pratique médicale courante. **Rev Med Swisse Romande** 1982 Jun;102(6):629–39

**Germany**

Daems WF: Himmel und Erde schaffen den Menschen. Zur Faksimile–Ausgabe eines astromedizinischen Hausbuches (Kodex Schürstab, Zürich, Zentralbibl. Ms. C. 54). **Drei Z Wiss Kunst Soz Leben** 1981;51:177–94

**Great Britain**

Schuler RM: English magical and scientific poems to 1700: an annotated bibliography. New York, Garland, 1979. xxviii, 120 p.

**India**

Sikdar JC: Jaina alchemy. **Indian J Hist Sci** 1980 May;15(1):6–17

Wujastyk D: An alchemical ghost: the Rasaratnâkara by Nâgârjuna. **Ambix** 1984 Jul;31(2):70–83

**Italy**

Coccanari MA: Les plantes et leur action sur le cerveau et sur la psiche:

science et magie. **Med Secoli** 1982 May–Aug;19(2):215–9

**Scandinavia**

Robertson D: Magical medicine in Viking Scandinavia. **Med Hist** 1976 Jul;20(3):317–22

**United States**

Kerr H, Crow CL, ed: The occult in America: new historical perspectives. Urbana, Chicago, University of Illinois Press, 1983. 246 p.
Kuna RR: Hoodoo: the indigenous medicine and psychiatry of the black American. **Ethnomedizin** 1974–75;3(3–4):273–94
Straight WM: Throw downs, fixin, rooting and hexing. **J Fla Med Assoc** 1983 Aug;70(8):635–41

**Before 500 A.D.**

Gregory RL: Gnomenclature of magic mechanisms (2). **Perception** 1982;11(1):1–3
Lewis N: The interpretation of dreams and portents. Toronto, Sarasota, Stevens, 1976. xi, 167 p.

**China**

Unschuld PU: Concepts of illness in ancient China: the case of demonological medicine. **J Med Philos** 1980;5(2):117–32

**France**

Rousselle A: La sage-femme et le thaumaturge dans la Gaule tardive. Les sages-femmes ne font pas de miracles. **Rev Archeol Centre France** 1983;22(Dec):261–71

**Greece**

Lloyd GE: Magic, reason and experience. Studies in the origin and development of Greek science. Cambridge, New York, Cambridge University Press, 1979. xii, 335 p.

**India**

Zimmermann F: Les aspects médicaux du Yavanajataka (traité sankrit d'astrologie). **Sudhoffs Arch** 1981;65(3):299–305

**Peru**

Dobkin de Rios M: Plant hallucinogens, sexuality and shamanism in the ceramic art of ancient Peru. **J Psychoactive Drugs** 1982 Jan–Jun;14(1–2):81–90

**500 A.D.–1450**

Biedermann H: Medicina magica. Metaphysische Heilmethoden in spätantiken und mittelalterlichen Handschriften. 2. Auflage. Graz, Akademische Druck- u. Verlagsanstalt, 1978. 107 p.
Clark CW: The Zodiac man in medieval medical astrology. Ph.D. Diss., University of Colorado. Boulder, 1979. 440 p.
Lemay H: The stars and human sexuality: some medieval scientific views. **Isis** 1980 Mar; 71(256):127–37
Lipton JD: The rational evaluation of astrology in the period of Arabo-Latin translation ca. 1126–1187 AD. Ph.D. Diss., University of California. Los Angeles, 1978. 245 leaves.
Schipperges H: Handschriftliche Funde zu den 'verdrängten Wissenschaften' in der Frühen Neuzeit. **Ber Wissenschaftsgesch** 1981;4(1/2):31–40
Weisser C: Das Krankheitslunar aus medizinhistorischer Sicht. Ein Beitrag zur iatromathematisch-astrologischen Fachliteratur des Mittelalters. **Sudhoffs Arch** 1981;65(4):390–400
Weisser C: Studien zum mittelalterlichen Krankheitslunar. Ein Beitrag zur Geschichte laienastrologischer Fachprosa. Pattensen/Hannover, Horst Wellm, 1982. 468 p. (Würzburger medizinhistorische Forschungen, 21).

**Arabic**

Ullmann M: Die Tadkira des ibn as-Suwaidi, eine wichtige Quelle zur Geschichte der griechisch-arabischen Medicin und Magie. **Islam** 1977;54:33–65

**France**

Charmasson T: L'établissement d'un almanach médical pour l'année 1437. In: Congrès National des Sociétés Savantes, 99e, Besançon, 1974. Comptes Rendus. Paris, 1976. Section des Sciences, Fasc. V. p. 217–34.
Charmasson T: Roland l'Ecrivain, médecin des Ducs de Bourgogne. In: Congrès National des Sociétes Savantes, 101e, Lille, 1976. Comptes Rendus. Paris, 1976. Section des Sciences, Fasc. III. p. 21–32.

**Germany**

Schmitt W: Magie und Mantik bei Hans Hartlieb. Wien, 1966. 25 p. (Salzburger Beiträge zur Paracelsusforschung, 6).

**Great Britain**

Benson CD: The astrological medicine of Chaucer's physician and Nicholas of Lynn's Kalendarium. **Am Notes Queries** 1984 Jan–Feb;22(5–6):62–6
Hill TD: VIII Genitus homo as a nomen sacrum in a twelfth-century Anglo-Latin fever charm. **Notes Queries** 1983 Dec;30(6):487–8
Mooney LR: A middle English verse compendium of astrological medicine. **Med Hist** 1984 Oct;28(4):406–19

**Italy**

Van Egmond W: New light on Paolo dell'Abbaco. **Ann Ist Mus Stor Sci Fir** 1977;2(2):3–21

**1450–1700**

Easlea B: Witch hunting, magic, and the new philosophy: an introduction to debates of the scientific revolution, 1450–1750. Brighton, Sussex, Harvester Press, 1980. xii, 283 p.
Goldammer K: Neues zur Frage der Paracelsischen Spuria. **Sudhoffs Arch** 1984;68(2):235–9
Guinsburg AM: Paracelsian magic and theology; a case study of the Matthew commentaries. **Medizinhist J** 1981;16(1–2):125–39
Hutchison K: What happened to occult qualities in the scientific revolution? **ISIS** 1982 Jun;73(267):233–53
Mixa J: Neues über die Krankheit Wallensteins. **Medizinhist J** 1983;18(3):256–9
Müller-Jahncke WD: Der Höhepunkt der Iatromathematik. **Ber Wissenschaftsgesch** 1981;4(1/2):41–50
Nowotny O: De auro potabili. Wien, 1967. (Salzburger Beiträge zur Paracelsusforschung, 7). p. 13–23.
Rothschuh KE: Der Ausklang der wissenschaftlichen Iatromagie. **Ber Wissenschaftsgesch** 1981;4(1/2):51–60
Van Lieburg MJ: De dichter-medicus Daniël Jonctys (1611–1654), zijn strijd tegen het bijgeloof en zijn relatie tot Johan van Beverwijck, William Harvey en Daniël Sennert. **Tijdschr Geschied Geneeskd** 1979;2(4):137–67
Webster C: From Paracelsus to Newton. Magic and the making of modern science. The Eddington Memorial Lectures delivered at Cambridge University, November 1980. Cambridge, Cambridge University Press, 1982. 107 p.
Wright PW: A study in the legitimisation of knowledge: the 'success' of medicine and the 'failure' of astrology. **Sociol Rev [Monogr]** 1979;27:85–101
Yates FA: The occult philosophy in the Elizabethan age. London, Boston, Routledge & Kegan Paul, 1979. x, 217 p.

**Austria**

Somweber E: Der Zauberer und Hexenmeister Dr. Georg Iserin von Mazo. **Montfort** 1968;20(3):295–325

**Belgium**

Cockx-Indestege E: Cornelis Schuute en de onlangs ontdekte almanak voor 1551. Biekorf, Westvlaams Archief, 1981. 12 p.

**France**

Copenhaver BP: Symphorien Champier and the reception of the occultist tradition in Renaissance France. The Hague, New York, Mouton, 1978. 368 p.
Jiménez-Olivares E: La demonología en el siglo XV. **Prensa Med Mex** 1979 Mar–Apr;44(3–4):72–4
Trevisani F: Un corrispondente di Cartesio: alcune note su Lazare Meyssonnier (1611/12–1673), medico e astrologo lionese e sulla sua Belle Magie (1669). **Hist Philos Life Sci** 1979;1(2):285–308

**Great Britain**

Godwin J: Robert Fludd: hermetic philosopher and surveyor of two worlds. London, Thames and Hudson, 1979. 96 p. An annotated collection of plates from Fludds's works.
MacDonald M: Mystical bedlam: madness, anxiety, and healing in seventeenth-century England. Cambridge, Cambridge University Press, 1981. xvi, 323 p.
Newman W: Thomas Vaughan as an interpreter of Agrippa von Nettesheim. **Ambix** 1982 Nov;29(3):125–40

**Poland**

Gomołka B: On the authorship of an astrologico-medical calendar for 1474.

(Pol) **Biul Bibl Jagiellon** 1978;28(1-2)
Kuchowicz Z, Ojrzyński J: Czy twardowski był niemcem? **Przegl Hist** 1978;69(2):309-15

**1700 to Present**

Duerr HP, ed: Der Wissenschaftler und das Irrationale. Band 1. Beiträge aus Ethnologie und Anthropologie. Frankfurt am Main, Syndikat, 1981. 692 p.
Duerr HP, ed: Der Wissenschaftler und das Irrationale. Band 2. Beiträge aus Philosophie und Psychologie. Frankfurt am Main, Syndikat, 1981. 679 p.
Kaufman P: Burke, Freud, and the Gothic **Stud Burke Time** 1972;13(3):2179-92
Roth N: Electroresuscitation and the occult. **Med Instrum** 1980 Mar-Apr;14(2):120-1

**China**

Sutton D: Pilot surveys of Chinese shamans, 1875-1945: a spatial approach to social history. **J Soc Hist** 1981;15(1):39-50

**France**

Charuty G: La psychiatrisation des croyances: savoir médical et savoirs surnaturels en Languedoc, 1850-1940. **Asclepio** 1983;35:197-215

**Great Britain**

Debus AG: Scientific truth and occult tradition: the medical world of Ebenezer Sibly (1751-1799). **Med Hist** 1982 Jul;26(3):259-77
Myco F: Eighteenth century medicine: of magic and mysticism. **Nurs Mirror** 1982 Sep 8;155(10):50-2

**India**

Wurgaft LD: Another look at Prospero and Caliban: magic and magical thinking in British India. **Psychohist Rev** 6(1):2-26, Summer 77

**Jamaica**

Morrow RC: On obeah, myalism and magical death in Jamaica. **West Indian Med J** 1983 Mar;32(1):4-6

**Japan**

Furukawa F, Bourgeois M: Délires de possession par le renard au Japon (ou délire de Kitsune-Tsuki). **Ann Med Psychol (Paris)** 1984 May;142(5):677-87
Telson H: An explanation of the charm against measles. **J Hist Med Allied Sci** 1978 Jul;33(3):408

**Spain**

Bouza Brey F: Las enfermedades infantiles de Rosalia de Castro y los ritos de medicina magica en Galicia. **Cuad Estud Gallegos** 1967;22(67):183-97

**United States**

Dieffenbach VC: Powwowing among the Pennsylvania Germans. **Pa Folklife** 1975-76;25(2):29-46
Hexham I: Some aspects of religion and spiritual healing in Cultsville, a contemporary North American city. In Sheils WJ, ed: The Church and healing. Papers read at the twentieth summer meeting and the twenty-first winter meeting of the Ecclesiastical History Society. Oxford, Basil Blackwell for the Society, 1982. p. 415-29.
Snow LF: Con men and conjure men: a ghetto image. In Jones AH, ed: Images of healers. Albany, State University of New York Press, 1983. p. 45-78.
Stewart S: Rational powwowing: an examination of choice among medical alternatives in rural York County, Pennsylvania. **Pa Folklife** 1976;26(1):12-7

# MANUSCRIPTS

Adacher S, Bernabò M, Sesti E: I manoscritti medici della Biblioteca Laurenziana di Firenze. **Kos** 1984 Feb;1(1):113-21
Almagro BR: From clay tablets to electronic publications: the history of medical books. **Ariz Med** 1984 Jan;41(1):31-4
Atallah W: L'intérêt des traductions arabes dans l'édition des textes hippocratiques. In La collection hippocratique et son rôle dans l'histoire de la médecine. Colloque de Strasbourg (23-27 octobre 1972) organisé par le Centre de Recherches sur la Grèce Antique, avec le concours des Facultés de Philosophie et des Langues Classiques. Leiden, E. J. Brill, 1975. p. 19-33.
Baader G: Handschrift und Frühdruck als Ueberlieferungsinstrumente der Wissenschaften. **Ber Wissenschaftsgesch** 1980;3(1-2):7-22
Belguedj S: La Collection hippocratique et l'embryologie coranique. In La collection hippocratique et son rôle dans l'histoire de la médecine. Colloque de Strasbourg (23-27 octobre 1972) organisé par le Centre de Recherches sur la Grèce Antique, avec le concours des Facultés de Philosophie et des Langues Classiques. Leiden, E. J. Brill, 1975. p. 321-33.
Boncompagni R: Problemi relativi all'interpretazione e alla composizione del Regime delle malattie acute (Acut.). In La collection hippocratique et son rôle dans l'histoire de la médecine. Colloque de Strasbourg (23-27 octobre 1972) organisé par le Centre de Recherches sur la Grèce Antique, avec le concours des Facultés de Philosophie et des Langues Classiques. Leiden, E. J. Brill, 1975. p. 195-207.
Brătescu G: Eléments archaïques dans la médecine hippocratique. In La collection hippocratique et son rôle dans l'histoire de la médecine. Colloque de Strasbourg (23-27 octobre 1972) organisé par le Centre de Recherches sur la Grèce Antique, avec le concours des Facultés de Philosophie et des Langues Classiques. Leiden, E. J. Brill, 1975. 41-9.
Braun L: Paracelse, commentateur des Aphroismes d'Hippocrate. In La collection hippocratique et son rôle dans l'histoire de la médecine. Colloque de Strasbourg (23-27 octobre 1972) organisé par le Centre de Recherches sur la Grèce Antique, avec le concours des Facultés de Philosophie et des Langues Classiques. Leiden, E. J. Brill, 1975. p. 335-46.
Camerino G, Darbon P, Graber E, et al: I manoscritti medici della Osterreichische Nationalbibliothek di Vienna. **Kos** 1984 Mar;1(2):12-9
Edredge N: I manoscritti medici della Osterreichische Nationalbibliothek di Vienna. (contd). **Kos** 1984 Apr;1(3):7-13
Emmerson JS, ed: Catalogue of the Pybus collection of medical books, letters and engravings, 15th-20th centuries, held in the University Library, Newcastle upon Tyne. Newcastle Upon Tyne, Manchester University Press, for the University Library, 1981. xiv, 270 p.
Fischer KD, Sonderkamp JA: Ein byzantinischer Text zur Altersbestimmung von Pferden; aus Ambrosianus H 2 inf. **Sudhoffs Arch** 1980;64(1):55-68
French RK, Lloyd GE: Greek fragments of the lost books of Galen's Anatomical procedures. **Sudhoffs Arch** 1978;62(3):235-49
Glaus B: Autographen und Manuskripte zur ETH- und zur Wissenschaftsgeschichte. **Gesnerus** 1982;39(3-4):437-42
Grensemann H: Eine jüngere Schicht in den gynäkologischen Schriften. In La collection hippocratique et son rôle dans l'histoire de la médecine. Colloque de Strasbourg (23-27 octobre 1972) organisé par le Centre de Recherches sur la Grèce Antique, avec le concours des Facultés de Philosophie et des Langues Classiques. Leiden, E. J. Brill, 1975. p. 151-69.
The history of science: A collection of manuscripts from the library of the Jewish Theological Seminary. An index to the microfilm collection, reels 1-17. Ann Arbor, University Microfilms, 1980. 79 p. (With Hebrew-English name index).
Hünemörder C: Antike und mittelalterliche Enzyklopädien und die Popularisierung naturkundlichen Wissens. **Sudhoffs Arch** 1981;65(4):339-65
Irigoin J: Tradition manuscrite et histoire du texte. Quelques problèmes relatifs à la collection hippocratique. In La collection hippocratique et son rôle dans l'histoire de la médecine. Colloque de Strasbourg (23-27 octobre 1972) organisé par le Centre de Recherches sur la Grèce Antique, avec le concours des Facultés de Philosophie et des Langues Classiques. Leiden, E. J. Brill, 1975. p. 3-18.
Jouanna J: Le schéma d'exposition des maladies et ses déformations dans les traités dérivés des Sentences cnidiennes. In La collection hippocratique et son rôle dans l'histoire de la médecine. Colloque de Strasbourg (23-27 octobre 1972) organisé par le Centre de Recherches sur la Grèce Antique, avec le concours des Facultés de Philosophie et des Langues Classiques. Leiden, E. J. Brill, 1975. p. 129-50.
Jouanna J: Le traité hippocratique du Régime dans les maladies aiguës: remarques sur la tradition manuscrite et sur le texte. **Rev Hist Textes (Paris)** 1976;6:1-30
Julien P: Une miniature des saints Côme et Damien (fin XVe - début XVIe siècle). **Rev Hist Pharm (Paris)** 1982 Sep;29(254):175-6
Lain-Entralgo P: Quaestiones hippocraticae disputatae tres. In La collection hippocratique et son rôle dans l'histoire de la médecine. Colloque de Strasbourg (23-27 octobre 1972) organisé par le Centre de Recherches sur la Grèce Antique, avec le concours des Facultés de Philosophie et des Langues Classiques. Leiden, E. J. Brill, 1975. p. 305-19.
Manuscripta alchemica der Sammlung Mellon: Bemerkungen zum Katalog: **Sudhoffs Arch** 1981;65(1):79-96
Martiny M: Laënnec et la pensée hippocratique. In La collection hippocratique et son rôle dans l'histoire de la médecine. Colloque de Strasbourg (23-27 octobre 1972) organisé par le Centre de Recherches sur la Grèce Antique, avec le concours des Facultés de Philosophie et des Langues Classiques. Leiden, E. J. Brill, 1975. p. 97-105.
Medizingeschichte wird zum Kassenschlager: Der Faksimile-Boom. **MMW** 1980 Apr 11;122(15):66-7
Nauert CG: Caius Plinius Secundus. In Cranz FE, Kristeller PO, ed: Catalogus translationum et commentariorum: Mediaeval and Renaissance Latin translations and commentaries. Annotated lists and guides. Vol.

IV. Washington, D.C., Catholic University of America Press, 1980. p. 297–422.
Rice EF: Paulus Aegineta. In Cranz FE, Kristeller PO, ed: Catalogus translationum et commentariorum: Mediaeval and Renaissance Latin translations and commentaries. Annotated lists and guides. Vol. IV. Washington, D.C., Catholic University of America Press, 1980. p. 145–91.
Riddle JM: Dioscorides. In Cranz FE, Kristeller PO, ed: Catalogus translationum et commentariorum: mediaeval and Renaissance Latin translations and commentaries. Annotated lists and guides. Vol. IV. Washington, D.C., Catholic University of America Press, 1980. p. 1–143.
Robert E: Les adresses de malades dans les Epidémies II, IV et VI. In La collection hippocratique et son rôle dans l'histoire de la médecine. Colloque de Strasbourg (23–27 octobre 1972) organisé par le Centre de Recherches sur la Grèce Antique, avec le concours des Facultés de Philosophie et des Langues Classiques. Leiden, E. J. Brill, 1975. p. 173–94.
Roselli A: Problemi relativi ai trattati chirurgici De Fracturis e De Articulis. In La collection hippocratique et son rôle dans l'histoire de la médecine. Colloque de Strasbourg (23–27 octobre 1972) organisé par le Centre de Recherches sur la Grèce Antique, avec le concours des Facultés de Philosophie et des Langues Classiques. Leiden, E. J. Brill, 1975. p. 229–34.
Symons H, Nutton V, Schupbach W, et al: [Manuscripts in the Wellcome Library] **Kos** 1984 Jun;1(5):5–26
Teigen PM, ed: Books, manuscripts, and the history of medicine. Essays on the fiftieth anniversary of the Osler Library. New York, Science History Publications, 1982. 112 p. Contributions by L. G. Stevenson, C. G. Roland, R. J. Durling, E. Brodman, G. T. Tanselle, E. J. Freeman.
Telle J: Manuscripta alchemica der Sammlung Mellon. Bemerkungen zum Katalog. **Suddtsch Opt Ztg** 1981;65(1):79–96
Thivel A: Le 'divin' dans la Collection hippocratique. In La collection hippocratique et son rôle dans l'histoire de la médecine. Colloque de Strasbourg (23–27 octobre 1972) organisé par le Centre de Recherches sur la Grèce Antique, avec le concours des Facultés de Philosophie et des Langues Classiques. Leiden, E. J. Brill, 1975. p. 57–76.
Title list for the history of science collection from the Library of the Jewish Theological Seminary of America: Microfilm. 17 reels. Ann Arbor, University Microfilms International, 1980. 46 p.
Witten LC, Pachella R, ed: Alchemy and the occult: a catalogue of books and manuscripts from the collection of Paul and Mary Mellon given to Yale University Library. Vols. 3 and 4: Manuscripts 1225–1922. With an introduction by P. Kibre and additional notes by W. McGuire. New Haven, Yale University Library, 1977. 853 p.

**Americas**

Price R, ed: An annotated catalogue of medical Americana in the Library of the Wellcome Institute for the History of Medicine. Books and printed documents 1557–1821 from Latin America and the Caribbean Islands and manuscripts from the Americas 1575–1927. London, Wellcome Institute for the History of Medicine, 1983. xix, 319 p.

**Arabic**

Gallagher NE: Arabic medical manuscripts at the University of California, Los Angeles. Malibu, Undena Publications, 1983. xix, 24 p. (Aids and Research Tools in Middle East Studies, v. 1).
Haddad FS: Arab medical manuscripts in the Sami I. Haddad memorial library. In International Congress of the History of Medicine, 27th, Barcelona, 1980. Actas. Barcelona, Académia de Ciències Médiques de Catalunya i Balears, 1981. p. 253–8.
Iskandar AZ: An attempted reconstruction of the late Alexandrian medical curriculum. **Med Hist** 1976 Jul;20(3):235–58
Kataya S: Les Manuscrits Médicaux et Pharmaceutiques dans Les Bibliothèques publiques d'Alep. Alep, Université d'Alep, Institut du Patrimoine scientifique Arabe, 1976.

**Armenia**

Vardanian SA: Ancient Armenian translations of the works of Syrian physicians. In International Congress of the History of Medicine, 27th, Barcelona, 1980. Actas. Barcelona, Académia de Ciències Médiques de Catalunya i Balears, 1981. p. 352–7.

**Byzantium**

Kádár Z: Survivals of Greek zoological illuminations in Byzantine manuscripts. Budapest, Akadémiai Kiadó. 1978. 138 p. (With 232 half-tone illustrations and 10 color plates).

**Germany**

Broszinski H: Medizinische Handschriften in Kassel. In Balde JH, Schmiking W, ed: Festschrift zum 86. Deutschen Arztetag in Kassel. Kassel, Arztevereins, 1983. p. 5–24.
Daems WF: Himmel und Erde schaffen den Menschen. Zur Faksimile-Ausgabe eines astromedizinischen Hausbuches (Kodex Schurstab, Zürich, Zentralbibl. Ms. C. 54). **Drei Z Wiss Kunst Soz Leben** 1981;51:177–94

**Great Britain**

David GR, ed: The manuscript papers of British scientists, 1600–1940. London, H.M.S.O., 1982. 109 p.
Schupbach WM: A Venetian 'Plague Miracle' in 1464 and 1576. **Med Hist** 1976 Jul;20(3):312–6

**Hungary**

Grabarits I: A kalocsai érseki könyvtár orvosi könyvritkaságai. **Orv Hetil** 1982 May 30;123(22):1369–70

**India**

Hameed HA, Reyaz Ali Parvaz S: Source material of Arab medicine. **Stud Hist Med** 1979 Dec;3(4):225–33
Palanichamy K: Tamil medical manuscripts in Oriental Research Institute, S.V. University, Tirupati. **Bull Inst Hist Med (Hyderabad)** 1973 Oct;3(4):173–81
Sarma CR, Rama Rao B: A note on the New Edition of Bhela Samhita. **Bull Indian Inst Hist Med (Hyderabad)** 1980;10(1–4):7–14

**Mexico**

De Mitcheli A: Libros médicos italianos en la antigua Universidad de México. **Prensa Med Mex** 1979 Jul–Aug;44(7–8):152–6

**Turkey**

Erdemir-Demirhan A: The evolution and characteristics of important Turkish medical manuscripts by Anatolian Turks. In International Congress of the History of Medicine, 27th, Barcelona, 1980. Actas. Barcelona, Académia de Ciències Médiques de Catalunya i Balears, 1981. p. 238–44.

**USSR**

Shengelia MS: Feudal Georgia translational medical literature (IX–I half of XIX century). In International Congress of the History of Medicine, 27th, Barcelona, 1980. Actas. Barcelona, Académia de Ciències Médiques de Catalunya i Balears, 1981. p. 340–5.

**Before 500 A.D.**

McVaugh MR: The authorship of the Galenic compendium de interioribus, 'Quoniam diversitas...'. **Dynamis** 1981;1:225–9
Ullmann M: Die Schrift des Rufus von Ephesos über die Gelbsucht in arabischer und lateinischer Ubersetzung. Göttingen, Vandenhoeck & Ruprecht, 1983. 87 p. (Abhandlungen der Akademie der Wissenschaften in Göttingen, Philologisch-Historische Klass; Folge 3, No. 138).

**Arabic**

Kruk R: Aristoteles semitico-latinus. The Arabic version of Aristotle's Parts of animals. Book XI–XIV of the Kitab al-Hayawan. A critical edition with introduction and selected glossary. Amsterdam, Oxford, North-Holland Publishing Co., 1979. 96 [107] p.

**China**

Akahori A: Medical manuscripts found in Han Tomb No. 3 at Ma-wang-tui. **Sudhoffs Arch** 1979;63(3):297–300
Bridgman RF: La formation de la théorie médicale en Chine à l'occasion de la récente découverte de manuscrits à Ma Wang Dui. In Mazars G, ed: Les médecines traditionnelles de l'Asie. Strasbourg, Université Louis Pasteur, 1981. p. 5–12.
Chao You Chen: [A study of the ancient medical manuscript 'Tsu-pei-shih-i-mo-chiu-ching' recently found in Ma-wang-t'ui, China.] (Jpn). **Nihon I-Shigaku Zasshi** 1981;27(1):1–5

**Egypt**

Devauchelle D, Pezin M: Un papyrus médical démotique. **Chron Egypte** 1978 Jan;53:57–66
Lipton JS: Oral surgery in Ancient Egypt as reflected in the Edwin Smith Papyrus. **Bull Hist Dent** 1982 Oct;30(2):108–14

**Greco-Roman**

Bourgey L: La relation du médecin au malade dans les écrits de l'Ecole de Cos. In La collection hippocratique et son rôle dans l'histoire de la médecine. Colloque de Strasbourg (23–27 octobre 1972) organisé par le Centre de Recherches sur la Grèce Antique, avec le concours des Facultés de Philosophie et des Langues Classiques. Leiden, E. J. Brill,

1975. p. 209–27.
Chantraine P: Remarques sur la langue et le vocabulaire du Corpus Hippocratique. In La collection hippocratique et son rôle dans l'histoire de la médecine. Colloque de Strasbourg (23–27 octobre 1972) organisé par le Centre de Recherches sur la Grèce Antique, avec le concours des Facultés de Philosophie et des Langues Classiques. Leiden, E. J. Brill, 1975. p. 35–40.
Lactance: L'ouvrage du Dieu créateur. 2 vols. Ed. par M. Perrin. Paris, Editions du Cerf, 1974. 456 p. (Sources Chrétiennes, No. 213, 214).
Riou YF: Un fragment d'un manuscrit disparu d'Oribase, C. L. A. 116 (Vatican, Urb. lat. 293, ff. 95–96, VIIIe siècle). **Scriptorium** 1979,33.235–7
Ullmann M, ed: Rufus von Ephesos Krankenjournale. Wiesbaden, Harrassowitz, 1978. 128 p.

### Greece

Deichgraber K: Die Patienten des Hippokrates. Historisch-prosopographische Beiträge zu den Epidemien des Corpus Hippocraticum. Mainz, Akademie der Wissenschaften und der Literatur, 1982. 41 p. (Abhandlungen der Geistes- und Sozialwissenschaftlichen Klasse, Jahrgang 1982. Nr. 9).
Duffy J: An unnoticed copy of Hippocrates' prognosticon. **Scriptorium** 1982;36(1):89–90
Geymonat M, ed: Scholia in Nicandri Alexipharmaca, cum glossis. Milan, Cisalpino-Goliardica, 1974. 218 p.
Halleux R: Les alchimistes grecs. Tome I. Papyrus de Leyde, Payrus de Stockholm, Fragments de Recettes. Paris. Les Belles Lettres, 1981. xv, 235 p.
Marganne MH: Inventaire analytique des papyrus grecs de médecine. Genève, Droz, 1981. x, 406 p. (Centre des Recherches d'Histoire et de Philologie de la IVe Section de l'Ecole pratique des Hautes Etudes; Hautes Etudes du Monde Gréco-Roman, 12).

### India

Meulenbeld GJ: Observations on the Arkaprakaśa, a medical Sanskrit Text ascribed to Ravana. In Mazars G, ed: Les médecines traditionnelles de l'Asie. Strasbourg, Université Louis Pasteur, 1981. p. 111–39.
Singh RS, Singh AN: On the identity and economico-medicinal uses of hastikarnapalasa (Leea macrophylla Roxb., family: Ampelidaceae) as evinced in the ancient (Sanskrit) texts and traditions. **Indian J Hist Sci** 1981;16(2):219–22

### 500 A.D.–1450

Baraut C: Un manuscrit llatí de medicina de l'Arxiu Capitular de la Seu d'Urgell. In Congrés International d'Història de la Medicina Catalana, 2nd, Barcelona, 1975. Llibre d'Actes. Barcelona, Socitra, 1977. p. 273–94.
Bauer B: Studien zum ersten altdeutschen Pferdearzneibuch des anonymen Kopenhagener Ms. Thott Nr. 202. DMV Diss. Hannover, 1980. 99 p.
Fischer KD: Antike Verse in medizinischen Schriften des Mittelalters. **Gesnerus** 1982;39(3–4):443–50
French RK: An origin for the bone text of the 'five-figure series'. **Sudhoffs Arch** 1984;68(2):143–56
Imbault-Huart MJ: La médecine au Moyen Age: à travers les manuscrits de la Bibliothèque Nationale. Paris, Editions de la porte verte: Bibliothèque nationale, 1983. 191 p.
Koenig GG: Schamane und Schmied, Medicus und Mönch: ein Ueberblick zur Archäologie der merowingerzeitlichen Medizin im südlichen Mitteleuropa. **Helv Archaeol** 1982;13(51–2):75–154
La tradition manuscrite des Quaestiones Nicolai peripatetici. In: J.J.G. Alexander, M.T. Gibson (eds.) Medieval learning and literature: Essays presented to Richard William Hunt. Oxford: Clarendon Pr., 1976. p. 200–219.
Leibowitz JO: Jewish translators of medical works in the Middle Ages. In International Congress of the History of Medicine, 27th, Barcelona, 1980. Actas. Barcelona, Académia de Ciències Médiques de Catalunya i Balears, 1981. p. 276–80.
Leibowitz JO: Medical items in the book Torat ha-'Adam of Rabbi Moses ben Nahman (1194–1270). **Koroth** 1983 Aug;8(7–8):257–64
Marganne MH: A propos du 'Médicinaire liégeois du XIIIe siècle' (manuscrit 815 de Darmstadt). 101. Congrès de Comines, 1, 1980. Actes. p. 348.
Nutton V: Galeno salvato dalle acque. **Kos** 1984 Mar;1(2):33–50
O'Neill YV: An anatomical mystery with global dimensions. In: Congrès international d'histoire de la médecine, XXVe, Québec, 1976. Actes. Québec, 1977. p. 1031–44.
Opsomer-Halleux C: La diététique d'Ibn Butlan dans le manuscrit 887 (1041) de l'Université de Liège. Congrès de Comines, 1, 1980. Actes. p. 350.
Pinto LB: The folk practice of gynecology and obstetrics in the Middle Ages. **Bull Hist Med** 1973 Sep-Oct;47(5):513–23
Rebrikova NL, Mul'diiarov PIa: Elektronno-mikroskopicheskoe izuchenie pergamenta. **Biull Eksp Biol Med** 1982 Dec;94(12):104–7
Richler B: Manuscripts of Moses ben Nahman's 'Torat ha-Adam'. **Koroth** 1983 Aug;8(7–8):265–7
Stuart H: A ninth century account of diets and Dies Aegyptiaci. **Scriptorium** 1979;33(2):237–44
Trynková O: Někteté metody středověkého léčení podle mistra Rhazesa a mistra Salicettiho. I. Rhazesovo a Salicettiho ranná lékařství a jejich vydavatelé. **Sb Lek** 1981;83(11–12):363–7
Wallner B: The Middle English translation of Guy de Chauliac's Treatise on ulcers. Part II. Notes, glossary, marginalia. Book IV of the Great surgery. Edited from Ms. New York Academy of Medicine 12 and related mss. Stockholm, Almqvist & Wiksell International, 1983. 48 p. (Acta Universitatis Lundensis, Sectio I Theologica Juridica Humaniora 44).
Weisser U, ed: Buch über das Geheimnis der Schöpfung und die Darstellung der Natur (Buch der Ursachen), von Pseudo Apollonios von Tyana. Aleppo, Institute for the History of Arabic Science, University of Aleppo, 1979. 66 p. (Sources and Studies in the History of Arabic-Islamic Science, Natural Sciences Series 1).
Zotter H, ed: Antike Medizin. Die medizinische Sammelhandschrift Cod. Vindobonensis 93 in lateinischer und deutscher Sprache. Graz, Akademische Druck- und Verlagsanstalt, xxxii, 380 p.

### Arabic

Haddad FS: Arabic medical manuscripts in the Sami I Haddad Memorial Library. **Clio Med** 1981 Dec;16(2/3):123–7
Hamarneh S: Arabic manuscripts of the National Library of Medicine, Washington, D.C. **J Hist Arabic Sci** 1977 May;1(1):72–108
Hamarneh SK, Hamarneh NT: The physician-surgeon al-Zahrawi and the natural origins and manufacture of drugs. In A. R. El-Gindy, ed: Proceedings of the Second International Conference on Islamic Medicine. No. IV. Kuwait, Islamic Medicine Organization, 1982. (Bulletin of Islamic Medicine, v. 2). p. 375–82, 401–406.
Iskandar AZ: Another fragment from the autograph of Ibn Al-Tilmidh's 'Marginal commentary on Ibn Sina's Canon of medicine'. **Bull Sch Orient Afr Stud** 1981;44:253–61
Jacquart D: Quelques réflexions sur la traduction du Kitab al-Mansuri de Rhazès par Gérard de Crémone. In International Congress of the History of Medicine, 27th, Barcelona, 1980. Actas. Barcelona, Académia de Ciències Médiques de Catalunya i Balears, 1981. p. 264–6.
Kahle E: Der Traktat über das Zusammenwirken der Naturen des Qustā Ibn Lūqā. In Keil G, et al., ed: Fachprosa-Studien. Beiträge zur mittelalterlichen Wissenschafts-und Geistesgeschichte. Berlin, Schmidt, 1982. p. 133–42.
Kahle E: Probleme bei der Ubersetzung mittelalterlicher arabischer pädiatrischer Texte. In International Congress of the History of Medicine, 27th, Barcelona, 1980. Actas. Barcelona, Académia de Ciències Médiques de Catalunya i Balears, 1981. p. 267–70.
Kataya S, ed.: Quelle est la différence (Diagnostics Différentiels) de Abou-Bakr Zakaria Al-Razi (Rhazes). Edition Critique et commentaire de S. Kataya. Alep, Université d'Alep, Institut du Patrimoine Scientifique Arabe, 1978.
Khan MS: An Arabic source for the History of Ancient Indian medicine. **Indian J Hist Sci** 1981, reçu 1982;16(1):47–56
Mendrina GI: Von einer wenig bekannten Ubersetzung aus der 'Augenheilkunde' von Ali Abbas aus dem Latein ins Deutsche, die der russische Arzt gemacht hat. In International Congress of the History of Medicine, 27th, Barcelona, 1980. Actas. Barcelona, Académia de Ciències Médiques de Catalunya i Balears, 1981. p. 316–20.
Rosner F: Moses Maimonides' treatise on asthma. **Thorax** 1981 Apr;36(4):245–51
Valverde JL, Peña Muñoz C: El formulario de los hospitales' de Ibn Abi l-Bayan (S. XIII). In International Congress of the History of Medicine, 27th, Barcelona, 1980. Actas. Barcelona, Académia de Ciències Médiques de Catalunya i Balears, 1981. p. 346–51.
Wilcox J: Problems in the Latin manuscript tradition of De differentia spiritus et animae by the physician Costa ben Luca (9/10 cent.). In International Congress of the History of Medicine, 27th, Barcelona, 1980. Actas. Barcelona, Académia de Ciències Médiques de Catalunya i Balears, 1981. p. 363–5.

### Belgium

Tabanelli M: Gli albori della chirurgia nelle Fiandre. Il libro del maestro Thomas Scellinck. Firenze, Leo S. Olschki, 1974. xxxviii, 284 p. (Biblioteca della 'Rivista di Storia delle Scienze Mediche e Naturali', v. 19).

### Byzantium

Bernabò M: La 'Rinascenza Macedone' e l'arte dei bendaggi. **Kos** 1984 Jun;1(5):45–51
Felici L: L'opera medica die Teofane Nonno in manoscritti inediti. **Acta Med Hist Patav** 1981/82;28:59–74
Grmek MD: Vestigia della chirurgia greca: il Codice di Niceta e i suoi discendenti. **Kos** 1984 Jun;1(5):52–60

### Denmark

Hauberg P: Laegebøger med tilknytning til Henrik Harpestraeng. **Theriaca** 1982 Jun;22:1–362

# MANUSCRIPTS

**Egypt**

Fenton P: L'importance de la guenizah du Caire pour l'histoire de la médecine. **Rev Hist Med Heb** 1980 Mar-Apr;33(1):21-2
Fenton P: The importance of the Cairo Genizah for the history of medicine. **Med Hist** 1980 Jul;24(3):347-8

**France**

Durand J, Hampartzoumian A: Les manuscrits de la faculté de médecine de Montpellier. **Connaiss Pays Occident** 1981;49:26-31
Eastwood BS: The place of medicine in a hierarchy of knowledge: the illustration in Lyon Palais des Arts, ms. 22, f. lr, from the eleventh century. **Sudhoffs Arch** 1982;66(1):20-37
Köpp P: Das Handbuch eines frühmittelalterlichen Arztes in der Stiftsbibliothek St. Gallen. **Helv Archaeol** 1982;13(51-2):163-75
Merlette B, Vial F, Rulliere R: Le Marcellus de Laon: observations paléographiques et critiques. **Hist Sci Med** 1980;14(1):52-60
Vial F, Merlette B, Paris R, et al: Les recettes retenues par les Laonnois: observations médicales. **Hist Sci Med** 1980;14(1):61-9

**Germany**

Bergmann H: Neufunde zum Pesttraktat Jakob Engelins von Ulm. **Sudhoffs Arch** 1978;62(3):282-93
Hirth W: Corpusbildung in der deutschsprachigen medizinischen Fachliteratur des Mittelalters. **Suhoffs Arch** 1982;66(3):239-75
Keil G: Der 'Kodex Kohlhauer'. Ein iatromathematisch-hauswirtschaftliches Arzneibuch aus dem mittelalterlichen Oberfranken. I. Beschreibung der Handschrift. **Sudhoffs Arch** 1980;64(2):130-50
Ott-Voigtländer U: Das St. Georgener Rezeptar. Ein alemannisches Arzneibuch des 14. Jahrhunderts aus dem Karlsruher Kodex St. Georgen 73. Teil I: Text und Wörterverzeichnis. Pattensen/Han., Wellm, 1979. 140 p. (Würzburger medizinhistorische Forschungen, Band 17; also Diss., Würzburg).
Scholle S: Lanfranks 'Chirurgia Parva' in mittelniederfränkischer Ubertragung. Diss. Würzburg, 1978. Pattensen, Horst Wellm Verlag, 1978. 147 p. (Altdeutsche Lanfrank-Ubersetzungen, II, 1).

**Great Britain**

Bitterling K: Zwei bisher unbeachtete Fragmente der mittelenglischen Uebersetzung von Bartholomaeus Anglicus, 'De rerum proprietatibus'. **Neuphilol Mitt** 1977;78:47-56
Bober H, McKinney LC: La prima autopsia. **Kos** 1984 Mar;1(2):51-60
Davies HE, Owen ME: Meddygon Myddfai. In J. Cule, ed: Wales and medicine. London, British Society for the History of Medicine, 1975. p. 156-68.
Getz FM: Anatomia del medioevo. **Kos** 1984 May;1(4):33-46
Hargreaves H: 'De spermate hominis': a Middle English poem on human embryology. [Nat. Libr. Scotland, Advocates' MS. 23.7.11]. **Mediaev Stud** 1977;39:506-10
Harries WG: Bened Feddyg: a Welsh medical practitioner in the late medieval period. In J. Cule, ed: Wales and medicine. London, British Society for the History of Medicine, 1975. p. 169-84.
Medieval woman's guide to health: The first English gynecological handbook. Middle English text, with introduction and Modern English translation by B. Rowland. Kent, Kent State University Press, 1981. xvii, 192 p.
Mooney LR: A middle English verse compendium of astrological medicine. **Med Hist** 1984 Oct;28(4):406-19
Schmidt PG: Materielle und spirituelle Diät. Ein mittellateinischer Verstraktat des frühen 13. Jahrhunderts aus St. Albans. In Dilg P, et al., ed: Perspektiven der Pharmaziegeschichte. Graz, Austria, Akademische Druck- u. Verlagsanstalt, 1983. p. 311-23.
Seymour MC, et al, ed: On the properties of things. John Trevisa's translation of Bartholomaeus Anglicus De proprietatibus rerum. A critical text. 2 vols. Oxford, Oxford University Press, 1975. xix, 1397 p.
Svinhufvud AC: A Late Middle English treatise on horses edited from British Library Ms. Sloane 2584 ff 102-117b. **Acta Univ Stockh** 1978;47:1-281

**India**

Abdul Hai Farooqi: Dafi al-Amrad; an important medical manuscript. **Stud Hist Med** 3(3):199-203, Sep 79
Kausar Chandpuri A: Danish Nama-I Jehan. **Stud Hist Med** 1980 Mar;4(1):53 6

**Israel**

Kottek SS, Metzger M, Metzger T: Manuscrits hebraiques décorés ou illustrés du Canon d'Avicenne. In International Congress of the History of Medicine, 27th, Barcelona, 1980. Actas. Barcelona, Académia de Ciències Médiques de Catalunya i Balears, 1981. p. 739-45.

**Italy**

Billanovich MC: I libri di Benedetto Greco da Salerno, studente a Padova in medicina (1401). **Quad Stor Univ Padova** 1974;7:1-15
Caffaratto TM: Rilettura e commento dell'opera 'De Mulierum passionibus' di Trotula de Ruggiero, o Trocta Salernitana. **Minerva Med** 1981 Nov 17;72(46):3123-31
Jones P: Secreta Salernitana. **Kos** 1984 Feb;1(1):33-50
Müller-Rohlfsen I: Die lateinische Ravennatische Uebersetzung der hippokratischen Aphorismen aus dem 5./6. Jahrhundert n. Chr. Textkonstitution auf der Basis der Uebersetzungscodices. Hamburg, Lüdke, 1980. xlviii, 162 p. (Geistes- und Sozialwissenschaftliche Dissertationen, 55).
Orofino G, Brach CC: Nel nome del bagno. **Kos** 1984 Apr;1(3):33-54
Torroncelli A, et al: I manoscritti medici della Biblioteca Casanatense di Roma. **Kos** 1984 May;1(4):9-16

**Netherlands**

Bauer G: Das 'Haager Aderlassbüchlein'. (Studien zum ärztlichen Vademecum des Spätmittelalters, 1). Pattensen/Hannover, 1978. 198 p. (Würzburger medizinhistorische Forschungen, 14). Also Diss. Würzburg, 1978.
Lindgren A: Das Utrechter Arzneibuch (Ms. 1355,16 degrees, Bibliotheek der Rijksuniversiteit Utrecht). Stockholm, Almqvist & Wiksell, 1977. 199 p. (Acta Universitatis Stockholmiensis, Stockholmer Germanistische Forschungen, 21).

**Poland**

Wysocka F, ed: Głosy i teksty polskie w XV-wiecznym rekopisie lekarskim ze zbiorów Biblioteki Jagiellońskiej nr 132/60 akc. Komitet Jezykoznawstwa Pan. Wydawnictwa Zródłowe. Wrocław, Zakład Narodowy imienia Ossolińskich, 1971. 99 p.

**Spain**

Escudero Mendo A, Sagrera JE de: El Rosario de los filósofos: una copia en castellano del siglo XIII (I). **Bol Soc Esp Hist Farm** 1983;34(136):151-66
Parellada Feliu J: Un text i vuit dibuixos teratològics d'un manuscrit català de l'any 1399. In Congrés International d'Història de la Medicina Catalana, 2nd, Barcelona, 1975. Llibre d'Actes. Barcelona, Socitra, 1977. p. 197-221.

**Switzerland**

Bischoff P, Speiser P: Mittelalterliche Augenheilkunde im Kloster St. Gallen. **Gesnerus** 1982;39(1):47-52
Daems WF: Ermengald Blasius' Tabellen zum 'Antidotarium Nicolai'. **Pharm Acta Helv** 1979;54(4):101-5
Köpp P: Vademecum eines frühmittelalterlichen Arztes. Die gefaltete lateinische Handschrift medizinischen Inhalts im Codex 217 und der Fragmentensammlung 1396 der Stiftsbibliothek in St. Gallen. Aarau, Sauerländer, 1980. 128 p. (Veröffentlichungen der Schweizerischen Gesellschaft für Geschichte der Medizin und der Naturwissenschaften, 34).

**Yugoslavia**

Djordjević SP: Hilandarski medicinski kodeks. **Srp Arh Celok Lek** 1980 Sep;108(9):961-7

**1450–1700**

Alstermark H: Das Arzneibuch des Johan van Segen. Stockholm, Almquist & Wiksell, 1977. 174 p. (Acta Universitatis Stockholmiensis. Stockholmer germanistische Forschungen, 22)
Duka Zólyomi N: Ein ärztliches Vademecum der Aerztefamilie Ruland aus dem 16. Jahrhundert. **Sudhoffs Arch** 1977;61(3):281-97
Hils HP: Die Pestrezepte der Basler Handschrift D II 30. **Sudhoffs Arch** 1983;67(2):210-7
Muntschick W: Ein Manuskript von Georg Meister, dem Kunst- und Lustgärtner, in der British Library. **Medizinhist J** 1984;19(3):225-32
Rohland I, Keil G: Randnotizen zum 'Schüpfheimer Kodex'. Teil I: Allgemeines und Textbestimmung der Traktate. **Gesnerus** 1983;40(3/4):257-74
Schneider W: Ein neuer Textbeleg vom Liber praeparationum. Wien, 1978. 51 p. (Salzburger Beiträge zur Paracelsusforschung, 19).

**Ethiopia**

Pankhurst R: Le piaghe d'Etiopia. **Kos** 1984 Jul-Aug;1(6):33-50

**France**

Husson B, ed: Trois textes alchimiques inédits du XVIIe siècle. L'or potable des anciens; Lettres philosophiques; Le testament d'or. Paris, Librairie de Médicis, 1979. 101 p.

**Germany**

Dilg P: Examen pharmacopoeorum vulgare. Aus einer Handschrift des Laurentius Blumentrost d. A. (1619–1705). In Dilg P, et al., ed: Perspektiven der Pharmaziegeschichte. Graz, Austria, Akademische Druck- u. Verlagsanstalt, 1983. p. 39–64.
Graeser F, Keil G: Die Pestrezepte des Fuldaer Kodex Aa 129 **Z Dtsch Altert Dtsch Lit** 1980;109(1):72–85

**Great Britain**

Boss JM: 'Doctrina de circulatione sanguinis haud immutat antiquam Medendi Methodum': an unpublished manuscript (1662) by Francis Glisson (1597–1677) on the implications of Harvey's physiology. **Physis** 1978;20(1–4):309–35
Guy JR: Doctor's recipe book? **Pharm Hist (London)** 1984;14(1):6–8
Keiser GR: Ms. Rawlinson A.393: another Findern manuscript. **Trans Camb Bibliogr Soc** 1980;7(4):445–8

**Hungary**

Spielmann J: Egy XVII. századi magyar nyelvü orvosi kéziratról. **Orv Hetil** 1982 Jul 11;123(28):1748–51
Szlatky M: Magyar nyelvü, kéziratos orvosló könyvek a 17. századból. **Magy Konyosz** 1980;96(2):131–48

**Italy**

Belloni L: Claudius Aubrius a Francesco M. Fiorentini sull'assunzione di latte da parte del feto nell'utero. **Physis** 1977;19(1–4):378–82
Fehringer WT: Studien zum altitalienischen Pferdearzneibuch des Carlo Bartolomeo Rinaldi (1655). Diss. Hannover, 1978, 247 p.
Jensen JE: More treasures. **Md State Med J** 1982 Nov;31(11):26–9
Peruzzi E: Un trattato inedito di farmacologia di Gerolamo Fracastoro. **Rinascimento** 1978;18:183–228
Tomasi LT: L'isola dei semplici. **Kos** 1984 Jun;1(5):61–84

**Mexico**

Bárcena A, Barrera A, Ruiz E, et al: Interpretación etnobotánica de la iconografía del Códice de la Cruz-Badiano. **An Soc Mex Hist Cienc Tec** 1979;5:35–48

**Netherlands**

Van der Horst K: Inventaire de la correspondance de Caspar Barlaeus (1602–1648). Assen, Van Gorcum, 1978. 214 p.

**Spain**

Garcia-Ballester L: The circulation and use of medical manuscipts in ARabic in 16th century Spain. **J Hist Arabic Sci** 1979;3(2):183–99

**Switzerland**

Funder W: Uber eine bisher unbekannte ophthalmologische Monographie von Jakob Rüff (um 1500–1558). **Klin Monatsbl Augenheilkd** 1981 Oct;179(4):297–8
Koelbing HM: 'De conceptu et generatione hominis'. Die lateinische Fassung von Jakob Rueffs 'Trostbüchle', Zürich 1554. In International Congress of the History of Medicine, 27th, Barcelona, 1980. Actas. Barcelona, Académia de Ciències Médiques de Catalunya i Balears, 1981. p. 271–5.
Schneider-Hiltbrunner V: Wilhelm Fabry von Hilden 1560–1634. Verzeichnis der Werke und des Briefwechsels. Bern, Hans Huber, 1976. 172 p. (Berner Beiträge zur Geschichte der Medizin und der Naturwissenschaften, 8).

**1700 to Present**

Bowman IA: 'My life'; an important Ellis manuscript. **Bookman** 1981 Apr;8(4):3–7
Charles Darwin, 1809–1882; Anton Dohrn, 1840–1909: Correspondence. Napoli, Macchiaroli, 1982. 118 p.
Gysel C: Les relations du jeune Blumenbach avec Camper vieillissant. **Hist Sci Med** 1983;17(2):135–9
Obermajer J: Neznámé dopisy Purkyňova tchána K. A. Rudolphiho J. J. Berzeliovi. **Cas Lek Cesk** 1984 Feb 17;123(7):199–203
Richler B: Manuscripts of Avicenna's Kanon in Hebrew translation: a revised and up-to-date list. **Koroth** 1982 Aug;8(3/4):145–68
Sokal MM, Rafail PA: A guide to manuscript collections in the history of psychology and related areas. Millwood, N.Y., Kraus International, 1982. xi, 212 p.
Van der Star P, ed: Fahrenheit's letters to Leibniz and Boerhaave. Amsterdam, Rodopi, 1983. 195 p. (Nieuwe Nederlandse bijdragen tot de geschiedenis der geneeskunde en der natuurwetenschappen, no. 10).
Vetter T: Essai sur la littérature hippocratique au dix-huitième siècle. In La collection hippocratique et son rôle dans l'histoire de la médecine. Colloque de Strasbourg (23–27 octobre 1972) organisé par le Centre de Recherches sur la Grèce Antique, avec le concours des Facultés de Philosophie et des Langues Classiques. Leiden, E. J. Brill, 1975. p. 347–67.

**Austria**

Dolenc M: 'Nova Gronat-Jabuka'-rokopisne ljudskomedicinske bukve iz 1751. leta. **Cas Zgodovino Narodop** 1980;16(2):311–21

**Canada**

Bethune manuscripts in the Osler Library: **HSTC Bull** 1980;15/16:3

**China**

Saunders JB, Lee FR, ed: The Manchu anatomy and its historical origin. Taipei, Li Ming Cultural Enterprise Co., 1981. 8, 180 p. English and Chinese.

**France**

Boulle L, Grmek MD, Lupovici C, et al: Laennec, Catalogue des manuscrits scientifiques. Paris, Masson, 1982. 316 p.
Vial F, Merlette B, Roussel CI, et al: Les livres médicaux de la Bibliothèque municipale de Laon. **Hist Sci Med** 1979;13(4):383–93

**Germany**

Keil G: Zur Ueberlieferung von Virchows Würzburger Sektionsprotokollen. **Sudhoffs Arch** 1980;64(3):287–97
Schneck P: Die Briefe Paul Ehrlichs an den Moskauer Mikrobiologen Georgij Norbertovič Gabričevskij. **NTM** 1982;19(2):81–7

**Great Britain**

Austin F: The Letters of William Home Clift, 1803–1832. Dorset, Meldon House, 1983. ix, 115 p.
Bridson GD, Phillips VC, Harvey AP, ed: Natural history manuscript resources in the British Isles. London, Mansell; New York, Bowker, 1980. xxxiv, 473 p.
Charlton C, Drake M, Gwynne T, et al: The Registrar General's indexes and registers: microfilm copies may be available. **Local Popul Stud (Matlock)** 1984;32:4–11
Foster J, Sheppard J: British archives. A guide to archive resources in the United Kingdom. Surrey, Macmillan, 1982. xxv, 533 p.
King-Hele D, ed: The letters of Erasmus Darwin. Cambridge, Cambridge University Press, 1981. xxxii, 363 p.
Merrington M, Golden J, ed: A list of the papers and correspondence of Sir Francis Galton (1822–1911) held in the Manuscripts Room, The Library, University College London. London, Galton Laboratory University College London, 1978. 80 p.
Meynell G: Banks papers in the Kent Archives Offices, including notebooks by Joseph Banks and Francis Bauer. **Arch Nat Hist** 1981;10(1):77–88
Rousseau GS: Six new Hill letters. **Med Hist** 1984 Jul;28(3):293–302
Rousseau GS, ed: The letters and papers of Sir John Hill 1714–1775. New York, AMS Press, 1982. li, 208 p.
Sheppard J: Illustrations from the Wellcome Institute Library: the Chain papers. **Med Hist** 1983 Oct;27(4):434–5
Smith DC: William Budd manuscript at the National Library of Medicine. **J Hist Med Allied Sci** 1980 Jul;35(3):318–19
Smith DC, ed: 'On the causes of fevers' (1839) by William Budd. Baltimore and London, Johns Hopkins University Press, 1984. xi, 164 p. (Henry E. Sigerist Supplements to the Bulletin of the History of Medicine, n.s., no. 9)
Sulloway FJ: Further remarks on Darwin's spelling habits and the dating of Beagle voyage manuscripts. **J Hist Biol** 1983 Fall;16(3):361–90
[The need to preserve medical history records]: Evidence presented to the Public Records Committee.: **Soc Soc Hist Med Bull (Lond)** 1979 Dec;25:68–76

**India**

Sidkar JC: Phirangíroga (syphillis) and its management as described in Vaidyaka Samgraka, an old Gujarati manuscript of an unknown author (18th century A.D.). **Indian J Hist Sci** 1982;17(1):132–53

**Italy**

Caracci P: Vicende di una farmacopea di stato della serenissima repubblica di Venezia. **Acta Med Hist Patav** 1981/82;28:29–38
Castellani C: Ricognizione di alcuni inediti spallanzaniani, con particolare riguardo agli studi sui pipistrelli (1793–1794). La Memoria sul volo cieco

dei pipistrelli dedicata al Senebier nelle due versioni: testo e considerazioni. **Physis** 1984;26(3):433–83

Ongaro G, Mazzolini RG: Quasi tradens se totum: i manoscritti morgagnani della Biblioteca Palatina di Parma. **Ann Ist Mus Stor Sci Fir** 1983;8(1):101–5

**Japan**

Yasue M: [On the ancient manuscript named 'A Togoku-ohayashi-ninjin'] (Jpn). **Yakushigaku Zasshi** 1983;18(2):87–94

**Romania**

Cotrău M, Gheorghiţă I: Prescripţii medicale în manuscrisul inedit de la spitalul SF. Spiridon Iaşi, din secolul al XVIII-lea. **Rev Med Chir Soc Med Nat Iasi** 1983 Jan–Mar;87(1):113–6

Cotrău M, Gheorghiţă I: Prescripţii medicale în manuscrisul inedit de la Spitalul Sf. Spiridon Iaşi, din secolul al XVIII-lea (I). **Rev Med Chir Soc Med Nat Iasi** 1982 Jul–Sep;86(3):501–3

Cotrău M, Gheorghiţă I: Prescripţii medicale in manuscrisul inedit de la Spitalul Sf. Spiridon Iaşi, din secolul al XVIII-lea. (II). **Rev Med Chir Soc Med Nat Iasi** 1982 Oct–Dec;86(4):673–6

**Spain**

Basante Pol RM, Castillo Tello MM: La correspondencia dirigida a D. Casimiro Gomez Ortega, desde Valencia en el periodo comprendido entre 1783–1788. **Bol Soc Esp Hist Farm** 1982 Mar;33(130):131–44

Basante Pol RM, Castillo Tello MM: La correspondencia dirigida a D. Casimiro Gómez Ortega por D. Cándido M.a Trigueros. **Bol Soc Esp Hist Farm** 1981 Sep;32(127):137–47

Carrillo JL, Castellanos J, Ramos MD: Enfermedad y sociedad en la Malaga de Comienzos del siglo XIX: el Diálogo de los muertos en la epidemia de Málaga (c. 1803). Introducción y Transcripción. Málaga, Universidad de Málaga, 1980. 41 p.

Parellada Feliu J: Cinc manuscrits catalans escrits entre els anys 1749 i 1835. In Congrés International d'Història de la Medicina Catalana, 2nd, Barcelona, 1975. Llibre d'Actes. Barcelona, Socitra, 1977. p. 235–48.

**Sweden**

Sparre A: Dagboksanteckningar från 1858. **Sydsven Medicinhist Sallsk Arsskr** 1981;:132–50

**Switzerland**

Boschung U: Ein Brief Albrecht Hallers über seinen Aufenthalt in Paris und Strassburg (1728). **Physis** 1977;19(1–4):185–96

Gaberthüel M: Krankengeschichten und Operationsberichte 1784–1811 nach den Aufzeichnungen von Johann Heinrich Steger (1767–1842) und Johann Jakob Steger (1798–1857). Zürich, Juris, 1980. 121 p. (Zürcher Medizingeschichtliche Abhandlungen, Neue Reihe, 140).

Libri e manoscritti di Haller, 1777–1977: Nel II centenario della morte di Albrecht von Haller. Milano, Biblioteca Nazionale Braidense, 1977. 69 p.

**United States**

Archives and manuscripts [in] The Alan Mason Chesney Medical Archives, The Johns Hopkins Medical Institutions: Baltimore, The Johns Hopkins University and The Johns Hopkins Hospital, 1980. 64 p.

Benson KR: 'William Keith Brooks (1848–1908): primary resource material'. **Mendel Newsl** 1983 Nov;23:7–11

Boewe C: Editing Rafinesque's holographs: the case of the short letters. **Filson Club Hist Q** 1980;54(1):37–49

Edsall JT: The William Mansfield Clark papers: a second installment. **Surv Sources Newsl** 1981;10:1

Fuller MB: Theodosius Dobzhansky Papers. **Mendel Newsl** 1980 Jun;(18):1–8

George Sarton's correspondence: **Isis** 1984 Mar;75(276):33–62

Hirsch R, ed: A catalogue of the manuscripts and archives of the Library of the College of Physicians of Philadelphia. Prepared by the Francis Clark Wood Institute for the History of Medicine. Philadelphia, University of Pennsylvania Press, 1983. xx, 259 p.

Jensen JE: Manuscript notes of William Shippen, Jr., MD found in the Faculty Library. **Md State Med J** 1984 Jun;33(6):438–40

Kopp C: The Alfred E. Mirsky papers at the Rockefeller University Archives. **Mendel Newsl** 1983 Nov;23:1–4

Miller G: Edward Jenner letters in Baltimore, Maryland. In International Congress of the History of Medicine. 26th, Plovdiv, 1978. Actes du Congress. Sofia, 1981. Volume II. p. 157–9.

Miller G, ed: Letters of Edward Jenner and other documents concerning the early history of vaccination. From the Henry Barton Jacobs Collection in the William H. Welch Medical Library. Baltimore, London, Johns Hopkins University Press, 1983. xxix, 145 p. (Henry E. Sigerist Supplements to the Bulletin of the History of Medicine, n.s., no. 8).

Rainger R: The Henry Fairfield Osborn Papers at the American Museum of Natural History. **Mendel Newsl** 1980 Jun;(18):8–13

Reingold N, ed: The papers of Joseph Henry. Volume 1. December 1797–October 1832. The Albany years. Washington, Smithsonian Institution Press, 1972. xxxix, 496 p.

Reingold N, ed: The papers of Joseph Henry. Volume 2. November 1832–December 1835. The Princeton Years. Washington, Smithsonian Institution Press, 1975. 524 p.

Sokal MM, ed: A guide to manuscript collections in the history of psychology and related areas. [Wellesley, Mass.], Wellesley College Colloquium on the History of Psychology, 1977. iii, 64 leaves.

Wygant LJ: Archives and manuscripts in the Moody Medical Library. **Bookman** 1983 Sep–Oct;10(5):3–8

**USSR**

Katsnel'bogen AG: Neopublikovannaia rabota N. I. Pirogova. **Sov Zdravookhr** 1982;(11):61–4

Murav'eva EF: Unikal'nyĭ al'bom. **Sov Zdravookhr** 1980;(9):67–72

**500 B.C.–1450**

Adacher S, Orofino G: I manoscritti medici dell'Archivio dell'Abbazia di Montecassino. **Kos** 1984 Jun;1(5):5–16

# MATERNAL HEALTH

Högberg U: Förebyggande mödravård från kinesiska urkunder till moderna MVC. **Lakartidningen** 1983 Dec 21;80(51):5009–12, 5017

Rothman BK: In labor. Women and power in the birthplace. New York, London, W.W. Norton, 1982. 320 p.

Sosa R: Maternal bonding: an overview. In Smith GF, Smith PN, Vidyasagar D, ed: Historical review and recent advances in neonatal and perinatal medicine. [Chicago?], Mead Johnson Nutritional Division, 1983. Vol. I. p. 123–38.

**Great Britain**

Willmott Dobbie BM: An attempt to estimate the true rate of maternal mortality, sixteenth to eighteenth centuries. **Med Hist** 1982 Jan;26(1):79–90

**Before 500 A.D.**

Högberg U: Mödradöd i förhistorisk tid. **Sydsven Medicinhist Sallsk Arsskr** 1983;:103–14

**1700 to Present**

Bardet JP, Lynch KA, Mineau GP, et al: La mortalité maternelle autrefois: une étude comparée (de la France de l'ouest à l'Utah). **Ann Demogr Hist (Paris)** 1981;:31–48

Brickman JP: Mother love – mother death. Maternal and infant care: social class and the role of government. Ph.D. Diss., City University of New York. New York, 1978. vii, 750 leaves. (2 v.).

**Australia**

Lewis MJ: Populate or perish: aspects of infant and maternal health in Sydney, 1870–1939. [S.l.:s.n.], 1976. xx, 365 p.

**Canada**

Buckley S: Efforts to reduce infant maternity mortality in Canada between the two world wars. **Atlantis** 199;2 (2 pt 2):76–84

**Chile**

Kaempffer AM: Evolución de la salud materno infantil en Chile, 1952–1977. **Rev Med Chil** 1977 Oct;105(10):680–6

**Germany**

Cieślawski M: Z przezyć dzieci i matek-robotnic przymusowych na Pomorzu Zachodnim. **Przegl Lek** 1981;38(1):121–4

Lindemann M: Fürsorge für arme Wöchnerinnen in Hamburg um 1800: die Beschreibung eines 'Entbindungs-Winkels'. **Gesnerus** 1982;39(3–4):395–403

Lindemann M. Maternal politics. the principles and practice of maternity care in eighteenth-century Hamburg. **J Fam Hist** 1984 Spring;9(1):44–63

Marcusson H: Zusammenhang zwischen Sozialpolitik und Gesundheitsschutz für Mutter und Kind––Ein Rückblick über 80 Jahre. **Z Gesamte Hyg** 1979 Oct;25(10):775–80

**Ghana**

Ofosu-Amaah S: The maternal and child health services in Ghana (their origins and future). **J Trop Med Hyg** 1981 Dec;84(6):265–9

### Great Britain

Checkland O: Maternal and child welfare. In Checkland O, Lamb M, ed: Health care as social history; the Glasgow case. Aberdeen, Aberdeen University Press, 1982. p. 117-33.
Dyhouse C: Working-class mothers and infant mortality in England, 1895-1914. In C. Webster, ed: Biology, medicine and society 1840-1940. Cambridge, Cambridge University Press, 1981. p. 73-98.
Earwicker R: A study of the BMA-TUC Joint Committee on Medical Questions, 1935-1939. **J Soc Policy** 1979;8:335-56
Gutzke DW: 'The cry of the children': the Edwardian medical campaign against maternal drinking. **Br J Addict** 1984 Mar;79(1):71-84
Harrison B: Women's health and the women's movement in Britain: 1840-1940. In C. Webster, ed: Biology, medicine and society 1840-1940. Cambridge, Cambridge University Press, 1981. p. 15-71.
Lewis J: The politics of motherhood: child and maternal welfare in England, 1900-1939. London, Croom Helm, 1980. 235 p.
Lewis JS: Maternal health in the English aristocracy: myths and realities (1790-1840). **J Soc Hist** 1983;17:97-114
Loudon I: Maternal mortality: an historical audit. **J R Coll Gen Pract** 1984 Nov;34(268):585-6

### Haiti

Wallace CE, Marshall FN, Robinson C: A retrospective review of maternal and child health services at the Albert Schweitzer Hospital in rural Haiti. **Bull Pan Am Health Organ** 1982;16(1):7-16

### Japan

Matsumoto S: [Maternal and child health in Japan during last 80 years (author's transl)] (Jpn). **Nippon Sanka Fujinka Gakkai Zasshi** 1980 Sep;32(9):1171-9

### Mexico

Espinosa de los Reyes V: El doctor Isidro Espinosa de los Reyes y los inicios de la atención materno-infantil en México. **Gac Med Mex** 1981 Feb;117(2):81-7
Frenk S: Historia reciente de la asistencia materno-infantil en México. **Salud Publica Mex** 1983 Sep-Oct;25(5):513-7

### New Zealand

Olssen E: Truby King and the Plunket Society: an analysis of a prescriptive ideology. **NZ J Hist** 1981;15(1):3-23

### Norway

Augensen K, Koller O, Bergsjø P: Mødredødelighet i Norge 1951-1980. **Tidsskr Nor Laegeforen** 1983 Feb 20;103(5):525-30
Maltau JM, Grünfeld B: Mødredødeligheten i Norge 1880-1979. Et medisinsk-historisk tilbakeblikk. **Tidsskr Nor Laegeforen** 1983 Feb 20;103(5):522-5

### Poland

Radiukiewicz S: Opieka nad matką i dzieckiem. **Pieleg Polozna** 1981;(6):1-3

### Romania

Lucaşciuc A: Din istoricul ocrotirii mamei şi copilului în România (II). **Viata Med [Medii Sanit]** 1979 Oct;27(10):235-7
Ploeşteanu I: Aspecte ale activitătii de ocrotire a mamei şi copilului în România, în perioada dintre cele două războaie mondiale. **Viata Med [Medii Sanit]** 1981 Jan;29(1):21-3

### Sweden

Höfberg U: 'Jungfru Mariae nycklar' och mödradödligheten genom två sekler. **Lakartidningen** 1982 Sep 1;79(35):2977-9

### United States

Bullough VL: Female physiology, technology and women's liberation. In Trescott, Martha Moore, ed. Dynamos and Virgins revisited: Women and technological change in history. Metuchen, N. J., Scarecrow Pr., 1979. p. 236-51.
Buss FL: La partera, story of a midwife. Ann Arbor, University of Michigan Press, 1980. viii, 137 p.
Cates W: Abortion attitudes of black women. **Women Health** 1979 Nov-Dec;2(3):3-9
Dye D, Tarpey K: Maternity and infant care services in Chicago--retrospectus: our legacy, our challenge. In Smith GF, Smith PN, Vidyasagar D, ed: Historical review and recent advances in neonatal and perinatal medicine. [Chicago?], Mead Johnson Nutritional Division, 1983. Vol. II. p. 139-58.
Finn WF: Maternal Welfare--Nassau County, New York, 1957-1981. **Obstet Gynecol Surv** 1984 Mar;39(3):127-33
The health of women and children. New York, Arno, 1977. Varius paginations. Five reprinted articles by various authors, 1909-1953.:
Hefner LL: The National Women's Relief Society and the U.S. Sheppard-Towner Act. **Utah Hist Q** 1982;50(3):255-67
Klos SF: Reform initiatives in American maternal health services: 1900-1940. Ed. D. Diss., Harvard University. Cambridge, 1979, vi, 182 p.
Levin BS: Women and medicine. Metuchen, N. J., London, Scarecrow, 1980. vii, 257 p.
McConnell NF, Dore MM: Crittenton services, the first century, 1883-1983. Washington, D.C., National Florence Crittenton Mission, 1983. vi, 95 p.
Robinton ED: Dorothy Reed Mendenhall. In: Notable American women. The modern period. Cambridge, Mass., Belknap-Harvard Univ. Press, 1980. 4:468-70.
Siefert K: An exemplar of primary prevention in social work: the Sheppard-Towner Act of 1921. **Soc Work Health Care** 1983 Fall;9(1):87-103
Wertz DC: What birth has done for doctors: a historical view. **Women Health** 1983 Spring;8(1):7-24

### USSR

Chokin AR, Ibragimov NG: Okhrana materinstva i detstva v Kazakhstane i Bashkirii v pervoe desiatiletie Sovetskoĭ vlasti. **Sov Zdravookhr** 1984;(3):55-9
Danilishina EI, Dzhalalova KM: Materinskaia smertnost' i boriba s neĭ v SSSR v 20-30-e gody. **Sov Zdravookhr** 1983;(8):51-4
Danilishina EI: Razvitie okhrany materinstva i detstva v SSSR. **Sov Zdravookhr** 1983;(1):61-4
Danilishina EI: Rol' Narkomzdrava RSFSR v stanovlenii okhrany zdorov'ia materi i rebenka. **Sov Zdravookhr** 1983;(7):59-63
Dement'ev IuG: V. M. Velichkina (Bonch-Bruevich)--organizator sluzhby okhrany materinstva i detstva. **Pediatriia** 1979 Nov;(11):53-4
Granat NE: K 40-letiiu Ukaza Prezidiuma Verkhovnogo Soveta SSSR ob okhrane materinstva i detstva. **Med Sestra** 1984 Jun;43(6):6-10
Hudzenko PM: Vtilennia ideĭ V. I. Lenina u spravu okhorony zdorov'ia baterynstva i dyttnstva. **Pediatr Akush Ginekol** 1980 Mar-Apr;(2):3-7
Kiriushchenkov AP: Zabota Sovetskogo gosudarstva ob okhrane zdorov'ia materi i rebenka. **Feldsher Akush** 1982;47(8):3-9
Nikonchik OK: Razvitie sistemy okhrany materinstva i detstva v SSSR (1922-1982). **Akush Ginekol (Mosk)** 1982;(7):3-7
Novikova ECh: Okhrana zdorov'ia zhenshchin i deteĭ v strane v 60-iu godovshchinu obrazovaniia Soiuza Sovetskikh Sotsialisticheskikh Respublik. **Pediatriia** 1982 Dec;(12):3-8
Romanenko AE: Okhrana zdorov'ia materi i rebenka v Ukrainskoĭ SSR. **Pediatriia** 1982 Dec;(12):11-4
Shakhmet AV: Deiatel'nost' zhenotdelov Leningrada po okhrane materinstva i detstva (1926--1929). **Sov Zdravookhr** 1980;(4):64-6
Sharmanov TSh: Dostizheniia okhrany materinstva i detstva v Kazakhskoĭ SSR. **Pediatriia** 1982 Dec;(12):18-22
Studenikin MI, Ryleeva RN: Pervyĭ nauchnyĭ tsentr okhrany materinstva idetstva v SSSR. **Pediatriia** 1982 Oct;(10):3-7
Tabolkina NM: Okhrana materinstva i detstva v poslevoennom Leningrade (1945-1948). **Sov Zdravookhr** 1983;(7):67-9
Ustinovich AK: 50-letie Belorusskogo nauchno-issledovatel'skogo instituta okhrany materinstva i detstva. **Pediatriia** 1982 Jul;(7):74-6

### Zambia

Höjeberg P: Mödrovård i Zambia. **Jordemodern** 1982 Jun;95(6):203-7

# MATHEMATICS

Fagot AM: Medicina e probabilità. **Kos** 1984 Feb;1(1):24-31
Smith SB: The great mental calculators: the psychology, methods, and lives of calculating prodigies, past and present. New York, Columbia University Press, 1983. xviii, 374 p.

### Before 500 A.D.

### Greece

Kudlien F: Die Bedeutung des Ungeraden in der hippokratischen Krisenarithmetik. **Hermes** 1980;180:200-5

### 500 A.D.-1450

Weisser C: Das Krankheitslunar aus medizinhistorischer Sicht. Ein Beitrag zur iatromathematisch-astrologischen Fachliteratur des Mittelalters. **Sudhoffs Arch** 1981;65(4):390-400

### 1450-1700

Müller-Jahncke WD: Der Höhepunkt der Iatromathematik.

# MATHEMATICS

**Ber Wissenschaftsgesch** 1981;4(1/2):41–50

**Netherlands**

Beukers H: Mechanistische principes bij Franciscus dele Boë, Sylvius. **Tijdschr Geschied Geneeskd** 1982;5(1):6–15

**1700 to Present**

Brooks GP, Aalto SK: The rise and fall of moral algebra: Frances Hutcheson and the mathematization of psychology. **J Hist Behav Sci** 1981;17:343–56

Luccio R: La percezione della numerosità. **Stor Crit Psicol** 1983 Dec;4(2):215–83

**Czechoslovakia**

Kratochvíl L, Lustig M: K historii tzv. Batemanovy funkce. **Cesk Farm** 1984 Jun;33(5):210–2

**Germany**

Kunze G: Die Anfänge einer biomathematisch – biophysikalischen Denkweise in der Physiologie im Spiegel einiger Arbeiten Leonhard Eulers (1707–1783). Diss., Johannes-Gutenberg-Universität. Mainz, 1981. 182 p.

Leary DE: The historical foundation of Herbart's mathematization of psychology. **J Hist Behav Sci** 1980 Apr;16(2):150–63

Roos A, Boron WF: The buffer value of weak acids and bases: origin of the concept, and first mathematical derivation and application to physico-chemical systems. The work of M. Koppel and K. Spiro (1914). **Respir Physiol** 1980 Apr;40(1):1–32

**Great Britain**

Keller EF: Lewis Carroll: a study of mathematical inhibition. **J Am Psychoanal Assoc** 1980;28(1):133–60

**Italy**

Bèttica-Giovannini R: La sfida di Peano: matematica e paranoia. **Ann Osp Maria Vittoria Torino** 1982 Jul–Dec;25(7–12):241–4

# MEDICAL ILLUSTRATION

See also **Art; Symbolism and Heraldry**

Binet JL: Dessins et traités d'anatomie. Paris, Chêne, 1980. 247 p.

Bowman IA: Anatomical illustrations with superimposed flaps. **Bookman** 1981 Jul–Aug;9(6):3–7

Cohen IB: From Leonardo to Lavoisier 1450–1800. New York, Scribner's, 1980. xiii. 298 p. (Album of Science).

French RK: An origin for the bone text of the 'five-figure series'. **Sudhoffs Arch** 1984;68(2):143–56

Kádár Z, Szlatky M: Orvosi könyvillusztrációk a 15—18. sz'azadban. **Orv Hetil** 1981 Mar 22;122(12):711–4

Lindeboom GA: Cowper's brutale 'plagiaat' van Bidloo's Anatomische Atlas. **Ned Tijdschr Geneeskd** 1982 Oct 9;126(41):1878–82

Medizingeschichte wird zum Kassenschlager: Der Faksimile-Boom. **MMW** 1980 Apr 11;122(15):66–7

Morris AG, Keen EN: Lawrence Herbert Wells and the history of anatomical illustration. **S Afr Med J** 1982 Jan 9;61(2):40–3

Patterson T: La fabbrica dei nasi. **Kos** 1984 Apr;1(3):75–90

Payton BW: An historical survey of illustrations of the medicinal leech. **J Audiov Media Med** 1984 Jul;7(3):105–12

Premuda L, et al: L'illustrazione scientifica: ieri e oggi. **Acta Med Hist Patav** 1980–81;27:9–120

Saban R: Les sinus veineux méningés à travers les traités d'anatomie du XVe au XIXe siècle. In: Congrès National des Sociétés Savantes, 106e, Perpignan, 1981. Comptes Rendus. Paris, Bibliothèque Nationale, 1982. Fasc. IV. p. 119–31.

Thornton JL, Reeves C: Medical book illustration: a short history. Cambridge, New York, Oleander Press, 1983. 142 p.

Tinkelenberg J: On the morphology of creative forms and art. **Acta Morphol Neerl Scand** 1983 Mar;21(1):83–95

Zanca A, Zanca A: Istituti Ospedalieri di Mantova, Mantova, Italy. **Int J Dermatol** 1980 Jan–Feb;19(1):55–8

**China**

Ho J: Medical illustration in the Far East. **J Audiov Media Med** 1981 Apr;4(2):58–61

**500 A.D.–1450**

O'Neill YV: An anatomical mystery with global dimensions. In: Congrès international d'histoire de la médecine, XXVe, Québec, 1976. Actes. Québec, 1977. p. 1031–44.

**Byzantium**

Bernabò M: La 'Rinascenza Macedone' e l'arte dei bendaggi. **Kos** 1984 Jun;1(5):45–51

Grmek MD: Vestigia della chirurgia greca: il Codice di Niceta e i suoi discendenti. **Kos** 1984 Jun;1(5):52–60

**France**

Eastwood BS: The place of medicine in a hierarchy of knowledge: the illustration in Lyon Palais des Arts, ms. 22, f. lr, from the eleventh century. **Sudhoffs Arch** 1982;66(1):20–37

**Great Britain**

Bober H, McKinney LC: La prima autopsia. **Kos** 1984 Mar;1(2):51–60

**1450–1700**

Cavanagh GS: A new view of the Vesalian landscape. **Med Hist** 1983 Jan;27(1):77–9

Eckart WU: Zur Funktion der Abbildung als Medium der Wissenschaftsvermittlung in der medizinischen Literatur des 17. Jahrhunderts. **Ber Wissenschaftsgesch** 1980;3(1–2):35–53

Horowitz M, Collins J: A census of copies of the first edition of Andreas Vesalius' De humani corporis fabrica (1543), with a note on the recently discovered variant issue. **J Hist Med Allied Sci** 1984 Apr;39(2):198–221

Huard P, Imbault-Huart MJ: André Vesale, iconographie anatomique (Fabrica, Epitome, Tabulae sex). Paris, Dacosta, 1980. 255 p.

Putscher M: Ein Totentanz von Tizian. Die 17 grossen Holzschnitte zur Fabrica Vesals (1538–1542). In Göpfert W, Otten HH, ed: Metavoeite: wandelt euch durch neues Denken. Düsseldorf, Triltsch, 1983. p. 23–40.

Roth-Woelfle L: Jan Stephen van Kalkar als Illustrator der Anatomie des Andreas Vesal. **Imprimatur** 1980;8:11

Roth-Wölfle L: Jan Stephan von Kalkar als Illustrator der Anatomie des Andreas Vesal. **Imprimatur** 1980;9:86–100

Sabin JA, Sanmartín Urchaga P: Estudio comparado de las aportaciones iconográficas, en el sistema muscular, en las obras de Leonardo y Vesalio. In International Congress of the History of Medicine, 27th, Barcelona, 1980. Actas. Barcelona, Académia de Ciències Médiques de Catalunya i Balears, 1981. p. 446–53.

**Germany**

Nover A, Kümmel WF: Der Schnitt- und Augenarzt Caspar Stromayr und die ophthalmologischen Illustrationen in seiner 'Practica copiosa' (1559). **Klin Monatsbl Augenheilkd** 1984 Nov;185(5):321–3

**Great Britain**

Godwin J: Robert Fludd: hermetic philosopher and surveyor of two worlds. London, Thames and Hudson, 1979. 96 p. An annotated collection of plates from Fludds's works.

**Italy**

Axdorph S: Den första 'röntgenblicken' – en studie av Leonardo da Vincis anatomiska bilder. **Lakartidningen** 1983 Dec 21;80(51):5005–8

Belloni L: Zur Deutung zweier pathologischer Stellen (eine mit Zeichnung) aus der Anatomie von Leonardo: Lungenechinococcus, Halslymphdrüsenverkalkung. **Gesnerus** 1980;37(1/2):139–44

Duhme L: Die Tabulae anatomicae des Pietro Berrettini da Cortona. Köln, Universität zu Köln, 1980. 185 p. (Kölner medizinhistorische Beiträge, 18) (also Diss.).

Karlan MS: An anatomic plate from Bartolomeo Eustachi. **J Hist Med Allied Sci** 1980 Jul;35(3):316–18

Pedretti C, Keele K, ed al., ed: Leonardo da Vinci: disegni anatomici dalla Biblioteca Reale di Windsor. Firenze, Barbèra, 1979. 159 p.

Roberts KB: Eustachius and his anatomical plates. **Newsl Can Soc Hist** 1979 Apr;:9–13

Todd EM: The neuroanatomy of Leonardo Da Vinci. Ph.D. Diss., University of California, Los Angeles, 1981 xviii, 267 leaves.

Tongiorgi Tomasi L: Inventari della galleria e attivita iconografica dell'orto dei semplici dello studio pisano tra Cinque e Seicento. **Ann Ist Mus Stor Sci Fir** 1979;4(2):21–7

**Switzerland**

Clark H: Foiling the pirates: the preparation and publication of Andreas Vesalius's De humani corporis fabrica. **Libr Q** 1981;51(3):301–11

**1700 to Present**

Dahm S: Frühe Krankenbildnisse: Alibert Esquirol Baumgartner. Köln, 1981. (Kölner medizinhistorische Beiträge; Arbeiten der Forschungsstelle

des Instituts für Geschichte der Medizin der Universität zu Köln, Band 21).
Dumaitre P: Les planches anatomiques d'Antommarchi. **Clio Med** 1981 Sep;16(1):13–23
Gilman SL: Zur Physiognomie des Geisteskranken in Geschichte und Praxis, 1800–1900. **Sudhoffs Arch** 1978;62(3):209–34
Hilloowala R: Illustrations from the Wellcome Institute Library: the origin of the Wellcome anatomical waxes Albinus and the Florentine collection at La Specola. **Med Hist** 1984 Oct;28(4):432–7
Himes JH: An early hand-wrist atlas and its implications for secular change in bone age. **Ann Hum Biol** 1984 Jan–Feb;11(1):71–5
Hodge GP: The preservation of scientific illustrations. **J Biocommun** 1980 Nov;7(3):28–31
Saunders JB, Lee FR, ed: The Manchu anatomy and its historical origin. Taipei, Li Ming Cultural Enterprise Co., 1981. 8, 180 p. English and Chinese.
Thomson LR: Medical illustration: our early years--reminiscing in letters: Harriet Blackstock Thomson to Ranice Crosby. **J Biocommun** 1981 Jul;8(2):13–5

**Australia**

Parkes D, Schachter M: Meige, Brueghel or Blake? **Aust Nurses J** 1981 Feb;10(7):32–5

**Austria**

Portele KA: Die Henning-Moulagen des Pathologisch-anatomischen Bundesmuseums in Wien. **Med Lab (Stuttg)** 1979 Feb;32(2):41–3
Skopec M: Anton Elfinger (1821–1864)--a forgotten medical illustrator. **Int J Dermatol** 1983 May;22(4):256–9

**France**

Endtz LJ: La neurologie et l'illustration photographique du livre médical. **Rev Neurol (Paris)** 1983;139(6–7):439–44
Lach E: The circumcision of the child on the eighth day...An anonymous engraving after a design by Bernard Picart. **J Hist Med Allied Sci** 1982 Apr;37(2):221
Vallat F: Histoire de l'illustration dans l'anatomie vétérinaire française. Bayeux, Bayeusaine, 1973. 157 p.

**Great Britain**

John Hull Grundy, artist and entomologist: **J Audiov Media Med** 1983 Jan;6(1):17–20
Le Fanu W: Natural history drawings collected by John Hunter F.R.S. (1728–1793), at the Royal College of Surgeons of England. **J Soc Bibliogr Nat Hist** 1978;8(4):329–33
Reckert H: Das unbekannte Werk des Pathologen, Robert Carswell (1793–1857). Köln, 1982. 283 p. (Kölner medizinhistorische Beiträge, Band 22)
Van Loghem JJ: Classic illustration (Sir Ronald Fisher). **Eur J Obstet Gynecol Reprod Biol** 1983 Oct;16(2):147–8

**Italy**

Ciardi RP: Fra pelle e ossa. **Kos** 1934 Mar;1(2):93–117

**Netherlands**

Thornton JL: Jan Van Rymsdyk: medical artist of the eighteenth century. Cambridge, New York, Oleander Press, 1982. ix, 111 p.

**United States**

Hodge GP: Medical illustration: our early years. Student days at Johns Hopkins, Evelyn Erickson Sullivan. **J Biocommun** 1982 Mar;9(1):18–22
Hodge GP: The drawings of Raynard N. LeNeil. **J Biocommun** 1983 Mar;10(1):24–9
Wolfe RJ. Jacob Bigelow's American medical botany 1817 1821. An examination of the origin, printing, binding and distribution of America's first color plate book. With special emphasis on the manner of making and printing its colored plates. North Hills, Pennsylvania, and Boston, Bird & Bull Press and Boston Medical Library, 1979. 121 p.

## MEDICINE

Ackerknecht EH: A short history of medicine. Rev. ed. Baltimore and London, Johns Hopkins University Press, 1982. xx, 277 p.
Ackerknecht EH: From barber-surgeon to modern doctor. **Bull Hist Med** 1984 Winter;58(4):545–53
Across the channel: catalogue of an exhibition. London, Royal College of Physicians of London, 1982. iii, 24 p.
Amundsen DW: [History of medical ethics]: ancient Greece and Rome [and] medieval Europe. In Reich WT, et al, ed: Encyclopedia of bioethics, v.3. New York, Free Press, 1978. p. 930–51.
Baran D: Istoriografie. **Rev Med Chir Soc Med Nat Iasi** 1981 Jul–Sep;85(3):468, 472, 510
Bibliography of the history of medicine: no. 14--1978. Bethesda, National Library of Medicine, 1979. 224 p. (NIH Publication No. 80–315).
Bibliography of the history of medicine, No. 15, 1975–1979: Bethesda, National Library of Medicine, 1981. lxxii, 924 p. (NIH Publication No. 81–1224).
Bibliography of the history of medicine, No. 16, 1980: Bethesda, National Library of Medicine, 1982. xi, 305 p. (NIH Publication No. 82–315).
Bibliography of the history of medicine, No. 17, 1981: Bethesda, National Library of Medicine, 1983. xi, 240 p. (NIH Publication No. 83–315).
Bibliography of the history of medicine, No. 18, 1982: Bethesda, National Library of Medicine, 1983. ix, 305 p. (NIH Publication No. 84–315).
Boussel P: Histoire de la médecine et de la chirurgie de la grande peste à nos jours. Paris, Editions de la Porte Verte, 1979. 283 p.
Burrow JG: [History of] organized medicine. In Reich WT, et al, ed: Encyclopedia of bioethics, v.3. New York, Free Press, 1978. p. 1034–42.
Catalogus van de Bibliotheek der Nederlandsche Maatschappij tot Bevordering der Geneeskunst, in bruikleen verenigd met de Bibliotheek der Universiteit van Amsterdam: Vol. III. Amsterdam, Rodopi, 1980. 966 columns.
Cobb WM: Man, the slow learner. **J Natl Med Assoc** 1981 Oct;73(10):973–86
Comaroff J: Medicine: symbol and ideology. In P. Wright, A. Treacher, ed: The problem of medical knowledge. Examining the social construction of medicine. Edinburgh, Edinburgh University Press, 1982. p. 49–68.
Congrès international d'histoire de la médecine, XXVe, Québec, 1976: Actes. Québec, 1977. 3 vols. 1403 p.
Cordera-Pastor A, Corvera-Bernardelli J: A propósito de la deshumanización de la medicina. **Gac Med Mex** 1982 Nov;118(11):431–8
Dolan JP, Holmes GR: Some important epochs in medicine. **South Med J** 1984 Aug;77(8):1022–6
Dumaître P: Médecine et médecins: La longue march de la médecine. Magnard, [1977?]. 174 p.
Durbin PT, ed: A guide to the culture of science, technology, and medicine. New York, Free Press, 1980. xl, 723 p. Contributions by A. Thackray, C. W. Pursell, G. H. Brieger, A. C. Michalos, C. Mitcham, H. T. Engelhardt, J. Gaston, L. Aiken, D. Crane.
Eastwood B: Directory of audio-visual sources. History of science, medicine, and technology. New York, Science History Publications, 1979. 41, [108] p.
Emmerson JS, ed: Catalogue of the Pybus collection of medical books, letters and engravings, 15th–20th centuries, held in the University Library, Newcastle upon Tyne. Newcastle Upon Tyne, Manchester University Press, for the University Library, 1981. xiv, 270 p.
Fearon Z: Patients and doctors. History of their roles and relationships. **Consum Health Perspect** 1982 Oct;9(2):1–3
Fichtner G, ed: Index wissenschaftshistorischer Dissertationen (IWD). Verzeichnis abgeschlossener Dissertationen auf dem Gebiet der Geschichte der Medizin, der Pharmazie, der Naturwissenschaften und der Technik. Nr. 1:1970–1980. Tübingen, Institut für Geschichte der Medizin, 1981. 285 p.
Gabbay J: Asthma attacked? Tactics for the reconstruction of a disease concept. In P. Wright, A. Treacher, ed: The problem of medical knowledge. Examining the social construction of medicine. Edinburgh, Edinburgh University Press, 1982. p. 23–48.
Galdston I: Social and historical foundations of modern medicine. New York, Brunner/Mazel, 1981. xiv, 147 p. (Reprinted articles from various sources)
Ganapathi K: Medicine in social development. **Hindustan Antibiot Bull** 1979 Feb;21(3):102–8
Ganzinger K, Skopec M, Wyklicky H, ed: Festschrift für Erna Lesky zum 70. Geburtstag. Wien, Brüder Hollinek, 1981. 212 p.
García-Ballester L: Studies on Hippocrates and Galen in modern Spain. **Trans Stud Coll Physicians Phila** 1979 Sep;5(1 No 3):215–29
Gass RS: Codes and statements related to medical ethics. In Reich WT, et al, ed: Encyclopedia of bioethics, v.4. New York, Free Press, 1978. p. 1721–1815.
Görtz R: Esculape ou Prométhée: les mutations de la médecine du thaumaturge au démiurge. **Arch Belg Med Soc** 1980 Oct;38(8):479–516
Guarner V, Ortiz-Monasterio F, Somolinos-Palencia J: El enfermo en la historia de la medicina. **Gac Med Mex** 1983 Aug;119(8):301–14
Guerra F: Historia de la medicina. Tomo I. Madrid, Ediciones Norma, 1982. ix, 387 p.
Gutt RW: Rozważania o historii, filozofii i socjologii medycyny, (artykuł dyskusyjny). **Arch Hist Med (Warsz)** 1981;44(1):85–91
Harig G: Mittelalterliche und antike Traditionen in der ärztlichen Ausbildung der Renaissance. **Klio** 1979;61:525–32
Harvey AM: Classics in clinical science. **Am J Med** 1980 Jan;68(1):6–8 (continued periodically)
Henrard G: Histoire et medecine. **Cah Clio** 1981;67:22–31
Imhof AE, ed: Mensch und Gesundheit in der Geschichte. Vorträge eines Internationalen Colloquiums in Berlin vom 20. bis 23. September 1978. Husum, Matthiesen, 1980. viii, 415 p. (Abhandlungen zur Geschichte der Medizin und der Naturwissenschaften, 39).
International Congress of the History of Medicine, 27th, Barcelona, 1980:

# MEDICINE

XXVII Congreso Internacional de Historia de la Medicina, 31 agosto - 6 septiembre 1980: Actas. Barcelona, Acadèmia de Ciències Mèdique de Catalunya i Balears, 1981. 2 Vol., 799 p.

Jinich H, Pérez-Tamayo R, Sepúlveda B, et al: La verdad y el error en medicina. **Gac Med Mex** 1984 Apr;120(4):133-44

Joske RA: The physician and changing patterns of human disease and death. In Stanley NF, Joske RA, ed: Changing disease patterns and human behaviour. London, New York, Academic Press, 1980. p. 551-66.

Kaĭmakchieva R: Belezhiti i iubileĭni dati po istoriia na meditsinata za 1969 godina. Sofiia, Meditsina i fizkultura, 1969. 38 p.

Kaminska-Axer M, Czeley-Wybieralska M: Starodruki medyczne w ksiegozbiorze Biblioteki Seminaryjnej w Tarnowie. **Arch Hist Med (Warsz)** 1979;42(1):125-30

Kapronczay K: Magyar-lengyel orvosi kapcsolatok a XVII-XIX. században. **Orv Hetil** 1981 Jul 12;122(28):1729-31

Klawans HL: The medicine of history. From Paracelsus to Freud. New York, Raven Press, 1982. ix, 238 p.

Klein-Franke F: Die klassische Antike in der Tradition des Islam. Darmstadt, Wissenschaftliche Buchgesellschaft, 1980. ix, 181 p. (Erträge der Forschung, Band 136)

Körtgen A: Die Gesundheit des Fürsten. Diätetische Vorschriften für eine herausgehobene Menschengruppe von der Antike bis zum Anfang des zwanzigsten Jahrhunderts. Diss., Johannes Gutenberg - Universität in Mainz. Frankfurt am Main, Bern, Peter Lang, 1982. 231 p.

Laín Entralgo P: History of the [therapeutic] relationship. In Reich WT, et al, ed: Encyclopedia of bioethics, v.4. New York, Free Press, 1978. p. 1655-63.

Lopez Austin A: En defensa de la historia de la medicina. **Bol Soc Mex Hist Filos Med** 1984;7(50):467-75

López Piñero JM: Medicina, historia, sociedad. Antología de clásicos médicos. 2a ed. Barcelona, Ariel, 1971. 352 p.

Löther R: Geschichte der Medizin und Theorie der Medizin. In International Congress of the History of Medicine. 26th, Plovdiv, 1978. Actes du Congress. Sofia, 1981. Volume II. p. 148-50.

McCullough LB, Jonsen AR, Burns CR, et al: [History of medical ethics in modern Europe and the Americas]. In Reich WT, et al, ed: Encyclopedia of bioethics, v.3. New York, Free Press, 1978. p. 951-75.

Macdonald EM: World-wide conquests of disabilities. The history, development and present functions of the remedial services. London, Baillière Tindall, 1981. 299 p.

Majnoni d'Intignano B, Stephan JC: Hippocrate et les technocrates. Paris, Calmann-Lévy, 1983. 194 p.

Martin HF: Medicine, science and humanism. **RI Med J** 1981 May;64(5):271-4

Médecine et livre médical du XVIème au XIXème siècle: Dunkerque, La Bibliothèque, 1983. 1 v. (various pagings).

Medizinischer Gedenkkalender 1984: **Z Gesamte Hyg** 1984 Jan;30(1):54-9

Mees LF: Blessed by illness. Spring Valley, N.Y., Anthroposophic Press, 1983. Historical section, p. 29-91.

Meier RY, ed: The Joseph H. Kiefer catalog of history of urology and medicine. Chicago, Library of the Health Sciences, University of Illinois at the Medical Center, 1981. ix, 207 p. (Special collections catalog).

Michler M: Zur Toposforschung in der medizinischen Literatur. In Ganzinger K, Skopec M, Wyklicky H, ed: Festschrift für Erna Lesky zum 70. Geburtstag. Wien, Brüder Hollinek, 1981. p. 57-65.

Monod H, Valentin M: Les précurseurs de l'ergonomie. **Ergonomics** 1979 Jun;22(6):673-80

Murphy EA: Skepsis, dogma, and belief. Uses and abuses in medicine. Baltimore, London, Johns Hopkins University Press, 1981. x, 176 p.

Numbers RL: Medicine in the New World: a comparison. In International Congress of the History of Medicine, 27th, Barcelona, 1980. Actas. Barcelona, Acadèmia de Ciències Mèdiques de Catalunya i Balears, 1981. p. 592-5.

Ogawa T, ed: Public health. Proceedings of the 5th International Symposium on the comparative history of medicine--East and West. Division of Medical History, The Taniguchi Foundation. Tokyo, Saikon, 1981. vi, 189 p.

Ohlah A: Changement des relations médecin-malade au cours des millenaires. Méthode socio-psychologique et histoire de la médecine. In International Congress of the History of Medicine. 26th, Plovdiv, 1978. Actes du Congress. Sofia, 1981. Volume II. p. 99-100.

Oliaro T: La medicina attraverso i tempi. Dalla bioritmologia alla cronobiologia. **Minerva Med** 1984 Jan 14;75(1-2):51-2

Ortiz--Monasterio F: La medicina del siglo XX y su proyección futura. II. Los antecedentes. La medicina precientífica. **Gac Med Mex** 1981 Nov;117(11):426-8

Ortiz Monasterio J: Reflexiones en torno a los origenes de la historiografia de la medicina. **Bol Soc Mex Hist Filos Med** 1980 Sep-Dec;5(32-33):83-92

Perkins WJ: Biomedical engineering--a reappraisal. **J Biomed Eng** 1984 Apr;6(2):157-9

Porter R, ed: Liber amicorum. Repertorio biografico di storia della medicina e delle scienze naturali. **Kos Liber Amicorum** 1984;1- (continued regularly)

Premuda L: La storia della medicina nelle facoltà mediche: ruolo e prospettive dell'insegnamento e della ricerca. **Acta Med Hist Patav** 1978-79;25:15-40

Rather LJ: On the source and development of metaphorical language in the history of Western medicine. In Stevenson LG, ed: A celebration of medical history. Baltimore, Johns Hopkins University Press, 1982. (The Henry E. Sigerist supplements to the Bulletin of the History of Medicine; new ser., no. 6). p. 135-53. With commentary by P. H. Niebyl, p. 154-6.

Reier H: Gesundheit, Krankheiten und Arzte bei den Goten. Kiel, 1981. 87 p.

Riad N: L'influence de la médecine pharaonique et arabe sur la médecine européenne et mondiale. In: Congrès international d'histoire de la médecine, XXVe, Québec, 1976. Actes. Québec, 1977. p. 1128-56.

Rice EF: Paulus Aegineta. In Cranz FE, Kristeller PO, ed: Catalogus translationum et commentariorum: Mediaeval and Renaissance Latin translations and commentaries. Annotated lists and guides. Vol. IV. Washington, D.C., Catholic University of America Press, 1980. p. 145-91.

Richardson JP: The surgeon as medical practitioner: an historical appreciation of the role of surgery in the corpus medicum. **Aust NZ J Surg** 1980 Oct;50(5):550-5

Rullière R, Heymans G, Chevalier P: Abrégé d'histoire de la médecine. Paris, Masson, 1981. 376 p.

Ruse M, ed: Nature animated. Historical and philosophical case studies in Greek medicine, nineteenth-century and recent biology, psychiatry, and psychoanalysis. Papers deriving from the Third International Conference on the History and Philosophy of Science, Montreal, Canada, 1980. Volume II. Dordrecht, D. Reidel, 1983. xiii, 274 p.

Russell AW, ed: The town and state physician in Europe from the Middle Ages to the Enlightenment. Wolfenbüttel, Herzog August Bibliothek, 1981. 156 p. (Wolfenbütteler Forschungen, 17).

Said M: Greco-Arabic and modern Western Medicine: conflict or symbiosis? **Stud Philos Med** 1977 Mar;1(1):50-7

Sanguinetti FA: Reflexiones en torno a la historia de la medicina. **Rev Fac Cien Med Univ Nac Cordoba** 1981 Jan-Dec;39(1-4):81-6

Schadewaldt H: Arzt und Gesellschaft im Spannungsfeld der Geschichte. **Therapiewoche** 1983;33:6485-91

Schadewaldt H: Rückblick und Resümee aus der Sicht des Medizinhistorikers. In Rohrmoser G, Lindenlaub E, ed: Fortschritt und Sicherheit Symposium Hotel Schloss Fuschl, Oesterreich, 25-29 Sept. 1979. New York, Schattauer, [u. d.] p. 328-38.

Schadewaldt H: 'Vom Stadtarzt zum öffentlichen Gesundheitsdienst'. **Off Gesundheitswes** 1982 Aug;44(8):512-7

Schipperges H: 'Der Mensch wird geringer'. Verliert die Medizin ihr Humanum? **Scheidewege** 1980;10(1):1-21

Schipperges H: Der Patient als Mensch. **Schleswig Holsteinisches Arztebl** 1979;11:609-14

Schoenberg DG, Schoenberg BS: [Eponyms in medical history] **South Med J** 1979 Dec;72(12):1590-1 (continued periodically)

[Selected gems in medicine.] (Jpn).: **Igaku Sensui** 1974-81 Oct-Dec;1-28: various pagings, issued irregularly

Seyda B: Dzieje medycyny w zarysie. Warszawa, Państwowy Zakład Wydawn. Lekarskich, 1977. 606 p.

Shibaike N, Ogawa S: [A historical study on formation of policy for 'Nambyo' (intractable diseases)] (Jpn). **Igakushi Kenkyu** 1978;50:49-59

Silverman WA: Medicine's millenarianism. **Perspect Biol Med** 1981;24:339-51

Simon I: L'influence hippocratique sur la médecine hébraïque, surtout chez Assaph, Isaac Israëli et Maimonide. In La collection hippocratique et son rôle dans l'histoire de la médecine. Colloque de Strasbourg (23-27 octobre 1972) organisé par le Centre de Recherches sur la Grèce Antique, avec le concours des Facultés de Philosophie et des Langues Classiques. Leiden, E. J. Brill, 1975. 275-89.

Sjöstrand T: Medicinsk vetenskap: Historik, teori och tillämpning. Stockholm, Natur och Kultur, 1979. 183 p.

Smith (Lord of Marlow): Annual oration on some lessons from the history of medicine. **Trans Med Soc Lond** 1977-78;94:86-94

Somolinos Palencia J: El expediente clínico y su importancia en la asistencia y educación médicas. I. El expediente clínico al través de la historia. **Gac Med Mex** 1980 Nov;116(11):477-81

Sournia JC: Histoire et médecine. Paris, Fayard, 1982. 338 p.

Sournia JC, Martiny M, Poulet J, et al., ed: Illustrierte Geschichte der Medizin. Salzburg, Andreas, 1980. 9 vols. (Transl. of Histoire de la médecine de la pharmacie, de l'art dentaire, et de l'art vétérinaire, Paris, 1978).

Stevenson JM: Medicine in a nutshell. **J Indiana State Med Assoc** 1981 Oct;74(10):654-5

Strojnowski J: Stan zdrowotny i medycyna u Słowian według najdawniejszych kronik. **Arch Hist Med (Warsz)** 1979;42(1):93-105

Sugden K: Glimpses of medical history. **Br Dent J** 1981;150(3):75-6

Trevisani F, Moscheo R: Between ancients and moderns: Tommaso Cornelio's medical teaching and an unpublished comment by him on the Galenic Ars parva. **Nouv Repub Lett** 1983;(2):59-73

Tutzke D: Geschichte der Medizin. Berlin, VEB Verlag Volk und Gesundheit, 1983. 248 p.

Tutzke D, ed: Geschichte der Medizin. Berlin, VEB Verlag, 1980. 247 p. Beiträge Von G. Harig, I. Winter.

Vasilenko VKh: Metod Gippokrata. **Klin Med (Mosk)** 1983 Oct;61(10):3-12

Vasilenko VKh: Na grane antichnoĭ i novoĭ meditsiny. **Ter Arkh** 1983;55(1):133-9

Veith I: Changing concepts of health care: an historian's view. **West J Med** 1980 Dec;133(6):532–8

Vengrova IV: Translations of the classics of medicine in the USSR. In International Congress of the History of Medicine, 27th, Barcelona, 1980. Actas. Barcelona, Acadèmia de Ciències Médiques de Catalunya i Balears, 1981. p. 358–62.

Von der Magie zur Medizin. In Becker U: Herders Gesundheitslexikon: Medizin von A biz Z. Freiburg, Herder, 1973. p. 13–36.:

Waserman M, Clausen C, ed: Bulletin of the History of Medicine. Index to volumes and supplements, 1933–1982. Baltimore, Johns Hopkins University Press, 1983. 195 p.

Wellcome Institute for the History of Medicine and related Sciences, London: Subject catalogue of the history of medicine and related sciences. 18 vols. München, Kraus–Thomson, 1980.

Whitrow M: A classification scheme for the history of science, medicine and technology. In Forbes EG, ed: Human implications of scientific advance. Edinburgh, Edinburgh University Press, 1978. p. 518–30.

Who was who in American history – science and technology: (A component of Who's who in American history). Chicago, Marquis, 1976. xiii, 688 p.

Wiench P, ed: Die grossen Arzte. Geschichte der Medizin in Lebensbildern. München, Kindler, 1982. 335 p.

Winder M: Modern and traditional medicine: rivals or friends? Some solutions attempted by India, China, Japan and Tibetans in exile. **Bull Br Assoc Orient** 1979–80,N.Ser;11:35–9

Wright P, Treacher A, ed: The problem of medical knowledge. Examining the social construction of medicine. Edinburgh, Edinburgh University Press, 1982. 232 p.

Yue J: [Ancient Sino–Iraian medical exchanges as seen in Tanksuq–nameh] (Chi). **Chung Hua I Shih Tsa Chih** 1984 Jan;14(1):28–34

Zabludovskiĭ PE: Istoriia meditsiny. Moskva, Meditsnina, 1981. 350 p.

Zachert U, Zeidler U, ed: Herzog August Bibliothek Wolfenbüttel. Verzeichnis medizinischer und naturwissenschaftlicher Drucke, 1472–1830. Band 1–4, Alphabetischer Index. Millwood, New York, Kraus International, 1982. 1857 p.

Znamenatel'nye i iubileĭnye daty istorii meditsiny 1982 g: **Sov Zdravookhr** 1981;(6):68–75

Znamenatel'nye i jubileĭnye daty istorii terapii 1980 g: **Ter Arkh** 1979;51(11):131–3

Zubiri Vidal F: Médicos aragoneses ilustres. Zaragoza, Diputación Provincial, Institución 'Fernando El Católico', [1983]. 395 p.

### Africa

Feierman S, ed: Health and society in Africa: a working bibliography. Waltham, Mass., Crossroads Press, 1979. xii, 210 p.

Janzen JM, Feierman S: The social history of disease and medicine in Africa. I. **Soc Sci Med [Med Anthropol]** 1979 Dec;13B(4):239–43

Ransford O: 'Bid the sickness cease': disease in the history of black Africa. London, John Murray, 1983. x, 235 p.

Waite GM: The indigenous medical system in East-Central African history. Ph.D. Diss., University of California, Los Angeles, 1981. xvi, 277 p.

### Americas

Bowers JZ, Purcell EF, ed: Aspects of the history of medicine in Latin America. [Report of a conference held 10–13 October 1971 in Antigua, Guatemala.] New York, Josiah Macy, Jr. Foundation, 1979. viii, 196 p. Contributions by F. Guerra, F. Cabieses, C. Tejada, E. C. Long, J. M. Gomez, L. C. Santos Filho, D. B. Cooper, A. Seriano Lleras, G. V. Palau, C. R. Boxer, R. Archila.

Guerra F: La evaluacion farmacológica de las fuentes históricas sobre la medicina precolombina. **Guatem Indig** 1978;13(1/2):175–85

Plénot HR: Die präkolumbische Medizin. In Sournia JC, Martiny M, Poulet J, ed: Illustrierte Geschichte der Medizin. Salzburg, Andreas, 1980. Vol. 2. p. 687–729.

Price R, ed: An annotated catalogue of medical Americana in the Library of the Wellcome Institute for the History of Medicine. Books and printed documents 1557–1821 from Latin America and the Caribbean Islands and manuscripts from the Americas 1575–1927. London, Wellcome Institute for the History of Medicine, 1983. xix, 319 p.

Rípodas Ardanaz D: Fuentes inusuales en historia de la medicina hispanoamericana colonial. **Rev Indias** 1980;40(159–62):399–414

Serna Gómez J: Hospitales y beneficencia medicina y métodos curativos en la colonia. **Rev Acad Colomb Hist Ecles** 1973;8(29–30):101–21

### Arabic

Anees MA: History of Islamic medicine and pharmacy: contribution of Sami Hamarneh. **Hamdard** 1983 Apr–Jun;26(2):67–75

Browne EG: Arabian medicine. The FitzPatrick lectures delivered at the College of Physicians in November 1919 and November 1920. Westport, Hyperion, 1983. x, 138 p. Reprint of four lectures.

Bürgel JC: Islam [and Arabic medicine]. In Reich WT, et al, ed: Encyclopedia of bioethics, v. 2. New York, Free Press, 1978. p. 785–9.

Fenton PB: The importance of the Cairo Genizah for the history of medicine. **J Hist Arabic Sci** 1980;4:330–1

Gallagher NE: Arabic medical manuscripts at the University of California, Los Angeles. Malibu, Undena Publications, 1983. xix, 24 p. (Aids and Research Tools in Middle East Studies, v. 1).

Kataya S: Les Manuscrits Médicaux et Pharmaceutiques dans Les Bibliothèques publiques d'Alep. Alep, Université d'Alep, Institut du Patrimoine scientifique Arabe, 1976.

Said HM: al-Tibb al-Islami. Dacca, Islamic Foundation Bangladesh, 1981. 202 p.

Wahab Zuhuri MA: Influence on Ibn Sina on Unani medicine in subsequent ages. **Bull Indian Inst Hist Med (Hyderabad)** 1981;1–4:103–9

### Argentina

Kohn Loncarica AG: Historia de la inmigracion medica en la republica Argentina. Tesis, Universidad de Buenos Aires, 1971–1981. 442 leaves.

Vivas JG: Antecedentes históricos de la medicina en San Luis. In Congreso de Historia de la Medicina Argentina [Transactions], 5th, Mendoza, 1983. p. 197–200.

### Asia

Allan N: The Wellcome Institute and its Library with special reference to South East Asia. **Southeast Asia Libr Group Newsl** 1980;22:1–4

Golden RL: Osler and Oriental medicine: a discursive review. Princeton, Science Press Associates, 1982. iii, 93 p.

Huard P, Bossy J, Mazars G: Les médecines de l'Asie. Paris, Editions du Seuil, 1978. 277 p.

Mazars G, ed: Les médecines traditionnelles de l'Asie. Actes du colloque de Paris 11–12 Juin 1979. Strasbourg, Université Louis Pasteur, 1981. 162 p. (Publication du Séminaire sur les Sciences et les Techniques en Asie).

Said HM: Medieval Chinese, Japanese and Arab medicine: reciprocal impact. In: Congrès international d'histoire de la médecine, XXVe, Québec, 1976. Actes. Québec, 1977. p. 1208–24.

Unschuld PU, Jaggi OP, Kao JJ, et al: [History of medical ethics: South and East Asia]. In Reich WT, et al, ed: Encyclopedia of bioethics, v.3. New York, Free Press, 1978. p. 901–30.

Wasti N: A history of Iran-Pakistan medical relations. (Per) Rawalpindi, Iran Pakistan Institute of Persian Studies, 1974. 199 p.

### Australia

Hagger J: Australian colonial medicine. Adelaide, Rigby, 1979. xii, 219 p.

### Austria

Domandl S: Paracelsus und Paracelsustradition in Salzburg (1524–1976). Ein Beitrag zur Kultur- und Zeitgeschichte. Wien, 1977. (Salzburger Beiträge zur Paracelsusforschung, 17), p. 9–44, 48–59. Includes O. Kostenzer: Das Paracelsusgrabmal in Stams, p. 45–48.

Huter F: Von der medizinischen Versorgung unserer alten Berggemeinden. **Tirol Heimat** 1975;39:5–31

Jetter D: Wien von den Anfängen bis um 1900. Wiesbaden, Steiner, 1982. viii, 159 p. (Geschichte des Hospitals, Bd. 5).

### Belgium

Beerens J: Ombre et lumière sur la médecine. **Cah Biloque** 1980;30:41–53, 81–96

Gerard J: Histoire des médecins belges. [S. l.], Wesmael–Charlier, 1981. 107 p.

Sondervorst FA: Histoire de la medecine belge. Zaventem, Sequoia, 1981. xii, 326 p.

### Bolivia

Bastien JW: Exchange between Andean and Western medicine. **Soc Sci Med** 1982;16(7):795–803

### Brazil

Nóbrega H: As raízes das ciências da saúde na Paraíba: medicina, farmácia, odontologia e enfermagem. Joao Pessoa, Editora Universitária, 1979. 372 p.

Silva LR da: Os Jesuitas e a assistência médica no Brasil colonial. **Rev Inst Hist Georgr Bras** 1978;318:212–32

### Bulgaria

Apostolov M, Kodov H: The Hilendar medical collection. In International Congress of the History of Medicine. 26th, Plovdiv, 1978. Actes du Congress. Sofia, 1981. Volume II. p. 55–7.

Neagu I, Neagu M: Quelques données médico-historiques sur la 'Colonie Bulgare' de Ploiesti. In International Congress of the History of Medicine. 26th, Plovdiv, 1978. Actes du Congress. Sofia, 1981. Volume II. p. 161–3.

# MEDICINE

**Canada**

Jack D: Rogues, rebels, and geniuses. The story of Canadian medicine. Toronto, Garden City, Doubleday, 1981. ix, 662 p.
Macbeth RA: Medicine in French Canada from 1608 to 1763. In: Congrès international d'histoire de la médecine, XXVe, Québec, 1976. Actes. Québec, 1977. p. 931–43.
Poulet J: L'implantation médicale en Nouvelle France. In: Congrès international d'histoire de la médecine, XXVe, Québec, 1976. Actes. Québec, 1977. p. 1081–93.
Roland CG, ed: Health, disease and medicine: essays in Canadian history. Proceedings of the First Hannah Conference on the History of Medicine, McMaster University, June 3-5, 1982. [Toronto?], Hannah Institute for the History of Medicine, 1984. 464 p.
Shortt SE, ed: Medicine in Canadian society: historical perspectives. Montreal, McGill-Queen's University Press, 1981. xiii, 506 p. Reprinted articles by various authors.

**Caribbean**

Halberstein RA, Saunders AB: Traditional medical practices and medicinal plant usage on a Bahamian Island. **Tex Stud Lit Lang** 1978;2:177–203

**China**

Chen Menglai: [Ly Yanshi, life and medical achievements.] (Chi). **Chin J Med Hist** 1981;11:93–4
Chia T: Chung-kuo i hsüeh shih lüeh. Taiyüan, Shan-hsi jen min ch'u pan she, 1979. 4, 316 p.
Dorjee P, Richards E: Cures & concepts of Tibetan medicine. **Tibetan Med** 1981;2:1–83
Elvin M, et al: The work of Joseph Needham. **Past Present** 1980;87:17–53
He Zongyu: [Translation, interpretation and textual research of medical works unearthed in Ma Wang Dui.] (Chi). **Chin J Med Hist** 1981;11:125–7
Hsu HY, Peacher WG: Chen's history of Chinese medical science. Taipei, Modern Drug Publishers, 1977. 148 p.
Jin Shiying: [The influence of 'Pen tsao kang mu' in Japan.] (Chi). **Chin J Med Hist** 1981;11:102–5
Kania I: Médecine tibétaine dans les collections du Musée Ethnographique de Cracovie. In: Proceedings of the Csoma de Körös Memorial Symposium....Matrafüred ... 1976. Budapest: Akad. Kiadó. 1978. pp. 153–160.
Koh TC: Chinese medicine and martial arts. **Am J Chin Med** 1981 Autumn;9(3):181–6
Kong YC: Introduction to basic concepts in Chinese medicine. **Stud Hist Med** 1981 Mar;5(1):1–17
Meyer F: Gso-Ba Rig-Pa. Le système médical tibétain, Paris, Centre National de la Recherche Scientifique, 1981. 237 p.
Meyer F: Médecine tibétaine--l'homme et son milieu. In: Ecologie et géologie de L'Himalaya. (Colloques int. du C.N.R.S., No. 268.) Paris, Centre National de la Recherche Scientifique, 1976. pp. 195–205.
Müller HK: Zur Entwicklung der medizinischen Wissenschaften in China. **Naturwissenschaften** 1980 Feb;67(2):55–60
Pálos, S: Chinesische Heilkunst: Einführung in die Theorie und Praxis der Naturheilkunde der Chinesen--Akupunktur, Moxibustion, Heilmassage, Heilgymnastik, Atemtherapie und Pharmakologie. Bern, Barth, 1984. 286 p.
[Papers on Chinese medicine and on the study of medical history in China.] (Chi): **Chung Hua I Shih Tsa Chih** 1980;10(1):1–64
Porkert M, Ullmann C: Die chinesische Medizin. Düsseldorf, Wien, Econ Verlag, 1982. 416 p.
Rabgay L: The origin and growth of medicine in Tibet. **Tibetan Med** 1981;3:3–31
Thom T: Medicine in China: the continuing revolution - Part II. **J Okla State Med Assoc** 1982 Sep;75(9):308–12
Thom T: Medicine in China: the continuing revolution--part 1. **J Okla State Med Assoc** 1982 Aug;75(8):272–7
Unschuld PU: Die Bedeutung der Ma-wang-tui-Funde für die chinesische Medizin- und Pharmaziegeschichte. In Dilg P, et al., ed: Perspektiven der Pharmaziegeschichte. Graz, Austria, Akademische Druck- u. Verlagsanstalt, 1983. p. 389–416.
Unschuld PU: Medizin in China: eine Ideengeschichte. München, Beck, 1980. 335 p.
Werner R: Offentliches Gesundheitswesen, traditionelle chinesische Medizin, westliche Medizin, Barfussärzte und Heilmittelkunde in der Volksrepublik China. 1. Teil. **Off Gesundheitswes** 1981 Oct;43(10):480–99
Winder M: The buddhist antecedents of Tibetan medicine. **Tibet News Rev** 1981;2(1/2):29–34
Wong M: Die altchinesische Medizin. In Sournia JC, Martiny M, Poulet J, ed: Illustrierte Geschichte der Medizin. Salzburg, Andreas, 1980. Vol. 1. p. 49–89.
Wu Liangzuo: [On the medicine of the Tai Ping Heavenly Kingdom.] (Chi). **Chin J Med Hist** 1981;11:97–100
Xie Z: [On the characteristics and contents of Dian Nan Ben Tsao: an extant work of materia medica featuring traditional medicine of both Chinese (Han) nationality and local minority nationalities] (Chi). **Chung Hua I Shih Tsa Chih** 1984 Jan;14(1):40–5
Yu S: [Talks on the historical materials of medicine in Fujian Province] (Chi). **Chung Hua I Shih Tsa Chih** 1984;14(2):75–7
Zhang W: [Research on the history of medicine and hygiene of Mohe, an ancient Chinese minority nationality] (Chi). **Chung Hua I Shih Tsa Chih** 1984 Jan;14(1):25–7
Zhao PS: [The fine tradition of Chinese medicine in the assimilation of foreign medicine] (Chi). **Chung Hsi I Chieh Ho Tsa Chih** 1982;2(1):55–6

**Czechoslovakia**

Junas J: Z histórie česko-slovenských vztahov v medicíne a zdravotníctve. **Cesk Zdrav** 1983 Mar;31(3):114–8

**Denmark**

Brix J: Laegevirke i Sønderjylland før 1864. **Dan Medicinhist Arbog** 1980;:9–10

**Egypt**

Chirico F: Spunti per un'interpretazione medica del mito egiziano di Horus er Seth. **Acta Med Hist Patav** 1981/82;28:41–57
Ghalioungui P: Medical services throughout Egyptian history. In: Congrès international d'histoire de la médecine, XXVe, Québec, 1976. Actes. Québec, 1977. p. 161–69.
Kolta KS: Neue Erkenntnisse zur Medizin der Kopten. **Sudhoffs Arch** 1984;68(2):157–72

**Europe**

Antall J: Pictorial history of European medicine and pharmaceutics. Budapest, Corvina Kiadó, 1981. 21, [121] p.

**France**

Dulieu L: La médecine à Montpellier. Tome III. L'époque classique. Avignon, Presses Universelles, 1975. 713 p.
Lamare J, ed: Médecine régionale: mystérieuse et pittoresque. Niort [France], Vernaculaires, 1981. 244 p.
Livet G, Schaff G, ed: Médecine et assistance en Alsace, XVIe–XXe siècle. Recherches sur l'histoire de la santé. Strasbourg, Istra, 1976. 368 p. (Publications de la Société Savante d'Alsace et des Régions de l'Est, Tome XI).
Marzocchi J: Essais sur la médecine et la pharmacie à travers l'histoire de la Corse. [S.1], J. P. Marzocchi, [1978?].
Sliosberg R: De la médecine à Saint-Germain en-Laye à travers les siècles. **Bull Soc Amis Vieux St.-Germain** 1978;30:17–33

**Germany**

Andrian-Werburg K von: Das Gesundheits- und Medizinalwesen in Sachsen-Coburg und das Coburger Landkrankenhaus. **Jahrb Coburg Landesstift** 1977;:13–94
Balde JH, Schmiking W, ed: Festschrift zum 86. Deutschen Aerztetag in Kassel. Kassel, Der Arzteverein, 1983. 112 p.
Kaiser W, Träger O: Die Geschichte des Bernburger Gesundheitswesens. Teil I. Von den Anfängen bis zur Mitte des 19. Jahrhunderts. Bernburg, Museum Schloss Bernburg, 1979. 142 p. (Veröffentlichungen zur Heimatgeschichte).
Kaiser W: Ein kurzer Abriss der Medizingeschichte in den Anhaltischen Territorien. **Wiss Z Martin Luther Univ (Math)** 1976;25(4):97–109
Naal W: Arzt und ärztliche Versorgung auf dem Hunsrück seit dem 30jährigen Krieg beispielhaft dargestellt an der Familie Pies. Diss. Düsseldorf, 1979. 198 p.
Rausch U: Das Medizinal- und Apothekenwesen der Landgrafschaft Hessen-Darmstadt und des Grossherzogtums Hessen unter besonderer Berücksichtigung der Provinz Starkenburg. Darmstadt, Marburg, Selbstverlag der Hessischen Historischen Kommission Darmstadt und der Historischen Kommission für Hessen 1978 (Quellen und Forschungen zur Hessischen Geschichte, Bd. 33). 588 p.
Rodegra H: Qualitätssicherung in der Medizin unter medizinhistorischen Aspekten. **Med Welt** 1982 Nov 12;33(45):1607–10
Schumm A: Entwicklung des Medizinalwesens in der Grafschaft Hohenlohe, mit einem Ueberblick über medizingeschichtlich wichtige Bestände des Hohenlohe-Zentralarchivs in Neuenstein. [Tübingen, Präzis], 1964. 109 p.
Stürzbecher M: Quellen zur Geschichte der Medizin und des Gesundheitswesens in und über Berlin. **Baer Berl** 1977;26:113–8

**Ghana**

Twumasi PA: History of pluralistic medical systems: a sociological analysis of the Ghanaian case. **Issue** 1979;9(3):29–34

**Great Britain**

Allan N: Some early medical contacts with the Kalmuck tribes of Siberia.

**Med Hist** 1983 Jul;27(3):305-9
Barry J: Guide to sources and writings on the history of medicine in Bristol, 1600–1900. **Soc Soc Hist Med Bull (Lond)** 1984 Dec;35:48-52
Bayliss JH: The earliest British medical practitioner? **Lancet** 1984 Dec 22;2(8417-18):1458
Blue plaques: London houses of medicohistorical interest: **Br Med J [Clin Res]** 1983 Feb 19;286(6365):641
Collacott RA: Hereditary physicians of the Scottish islands. **Scott Med J** 1983 Oct;28(4):377-81
Cule J: Wales and medicine. A source-list for printed books and papers showing the history of medicine in relation to Wales and Welshmen. [Aberystwyth], National Library of Wales, 1980. xvii, 229 p.
Cule J, ed: Wales and medicine. An historical survey from papers given at the Ninth British Congress on the History of Medicine at Swansea & Cardiff, 4–8th September, 1973. London, British Society for the History of Medicine, 1975. xi, 249 p.
Dulake L: Doctors, practices and hospitals through 300 years. A history of general & hospital practice at Reigate & Redhill including Earlswood & Merstham. Redhill, The author, 1977, iv, 154 p.
Hamilton D: The healers: a history of medicine in Scotland. Edinburgh, Canongate, 1981. xiii, 318 p.
Lobban RD: Edinburgh and the medical revolution. Cambridge, Cambridge University Press, 1980. 48 p.
Pelling M: Medical practice in the early modern period: trade or profession? **Soc Soc Hist Med Bull (Lond)** 1983 Jun;32:27-30
Price R: Wellcome Institute for the History of Medicine: American Collections. **Newsl Am Stud Libr Group** 1979;3:13
Sakula A: Blue plaques: London house of medicohistorical interest. **Br Med J [Clin Res]** 1982 Dec 18-25;285(6357):1799-800
Sandison AT: Glasgow and world medicine. **Pharm Hist (London)** 1971 Dec;2(3):1-2
Schnorrenberg BB: Medical men of Bath. **Stud Eighteenth Cent Cult** 1984;13:189-203
Seki T: [Posthumous manuscripts: medicine and people in Britain] (Jpn). **Igakushi Kenkyu** 1978;51:1-25
Spieckermann ML: Deutsche Uebersetzungen englischer humanmedizinischer Werke 1680-1810. **Medizinhist J** 1984;19(3):280-4
Walton MT: Fifteenth century London medical men in their social context. Ph.D. Diss. The University of Chicago. Chicago, 1979.

**Greece**

Toole HI: Historical studies. Athens, [s.n.], 1984. 608 p. (Greek with English summaries) Includes a collection of the author's previously published essays, mostly on Greek medicine, with a short autobiographical sketch and bibliography.

**Guatemala**

Villacorta Cifuentes JL: Historia de la medicina, cirugia y obstetricia prehispanicas. Guatemala, [s. n.] 1976. 166 p.

**Hungary**

Duka Zolyomi N: Les relations médicales entre la Hongrie et la France jusqu'à la fin du XVIIIe siècle. **Hist Sci Med** 1983;17(2):189-94
Kapronczay K: The history of medicine with special regard to Hungarian studies. **Ther Hung** 1980;28(3):138-42
Réti E: A hazai orvosföldrajz története. **Foldr Kozl** 1979;103(1-3):177-80
Zsebök Z: Famous Hungarian doctors. **New Hung Q** 1982;23(85):131-4

**Iceland**

Steffensen J: Islandske medicinhistoriske kilder, der ikke har påviselige forbilleder i samtidens Europa. **Nord Medicinhist Arsb** 1980;Suppl 6:94-105

**India**

Allan NM: Gustave Alexandre Liétard, orientalist and physician. **Med Hist** 1981 Jan;25(1):85-8
Ammon HP, Kemper FH: Ayurveda: 3000 Jahre indische traditionelle Medizin. **Med Welt** 1982 Jan 29;33(4):148-53
Bagchi AK: The evolution and chronology of ancient Indian medical sciences. **Bull Indian Inst Hist Med (Hyderabad)** 1979;9:21-6
Basham AL: Hinduism [and Hindu medicine]. In Reich WT, et al, ed: Encyclopedia of bioethics, v. 2. New York, Free Press, 1978. p. 661-66.
Devaraj TL: A bird's eye view of history of ayurveda in Karnataka State. **Sachitra Ayurved** 1981 Mar;:185-9
Gaitonde PD: Portuguese pioneers in India: spotlight on medicine. Bombay, Popular Prakashan, 1983. xv, 188 p.
Govinda Reddy C: Recent Indian medical historiography: bibliography for 1975. **Bull Indian Inst Hist Med (Hyderabad)** 1978;8(1-4):63-87
Hausmann W: Medizinhistorische Antiquitäten aus Indien. **Tierarztl Prax** 1981;9(4):421-5
Jee BS: A short history of Aryan medical science. Delhi, New Asian Publishers, 1978. 206 p., x.
Jopat PD: Abstracts of medico historical articles in Hindi journals. **Bull Indian Inst Hist Med (Hyderabad)** 1978;8(1-4):51-62
Jopat PD: Abstracts of medico historical articles in Hindi journals. **Bull Indian Inst Hist Med (Hyderabad)** 1979;9:128-40
Jopat PD: Abstracts of medico-historical articles in Hindi journals. **Bull Indian Inst Hist Med Hyderabad** 1982;12(1-4):51-65
Kakar S: Shamans, mystics, and doctors: a psychological inquiry into India and its healing traditions. New York, Knopf, 1982. x, 306 p.
Kamavisdar SS: Analytical studies in the evidences regarding chemico-culture in the history of Indian medicine in ancient period-allium series. **Indian J Hist Sci** 1980;15(2):210-22
Mazars G: Die klassische indische Medizin. In Sournia JC, Martiny M, Poulet J, ed: Illustrierte Geschichte der Medizin. Salzburg, Andreas, 1980. Vol. 2. p. 631-53.
Mazars G: Jean Filliozat (1906-1982). **Watermark** 1983 Jan;12:3-7
Murthy SR: Vagbhata on medicinal uses of gems. **Indian J Hist Sci** 1979 Nov;14(2):134-8
Ohja J: Chyavanaprasha: a scientific study. Varanasi [India], Tara Publications, 1978. x, 80 p.
Pandya SK: Medicine in Goa--a former Portuguese territory. **J Postgrad Med** 1982 Jul;28(3):123-48
Pandya SK: Medicine in Goa. Bombay, Dr. Ramesh Sanzgiri Foundation, 1980. n. p.
Patterson TJ: Some Indian sources for the study of the history of medicine. **Indian Arch** 1980;29(1):27-30
Patterson TJ: The medical practice of the East India Company. **Soc Soc Hist Med Bull (Lond)** 1980 Jun;26:40-3
Rama Rao B: Contribution of Andhra to ayurveda in Sanskrit. **Bull Indian Inst Hist Med (Hyderabad)** 1978;8(1-4):8-13
Sarma CR, Rama Rao B: Additional material in Astanga sangraha. **Bull Indian Inst Hist Med (Hyderabad)** 1980;10(1-4):23-33
Sarma CR, Rama Rao B: Urine in ancient ayurvedic literature. **Bull Indian Inst Hist Med (Hyderabad)** 1980;10(1-4):48-52
Sastri R: Bharata ke pranacarya: Aśivanikumara, Dhanvantari, Susruta, Atreya Punarvasu, Kaśyapa, Kumara Bhartr Jivaka, Caraka, Nagarjuna, Vagbhata sambandhi ayurvedika, aitihasika sahitya evam puratatva ke gambhira adhyayana, Bharatiya sabhyata, aura Samskrti ka gaveshana-purna paricaya. Dilli [Delhi, India], Atmarama, 1976. xvii, 895 p.
Sharma PV: Dalhana's version of the Suśruta Samhita. **Bull Indian Inst Hist Med (Hyderabad)** 1979;9:27-32
Sharma RK, Dash B, ed: Agniveśa Caraka samhita: text with English translation and critical exposition based on Cakrapani Datta's Ayurveda dipika. Vol I, Sutra Sthana. Varanasi: Chowkhamba Sanskrit Series Office, 1976. xlv, 619 p. (Chowkhamba Sanskrit Studies; 94).
Sharma S, et al: Realms of Ayurveda. Scientific excursions by nineteen scholars. New Delhi, Arnold-Heinemann, 1979. 336 p.
Siddiqi T: Two eminent physicians (of Unani medicine) during Shah Jahan's reign. **Indian J Hist Sci** 1981;16(1):26-30
Siddiqi T: Unani medicine in India during the Delhi Sultanate. **Indian J Hist Sci** 1980 May;15(1):18-24
Siddiqui T: Unani medicine in India. **Indian J Hist Sci** 1981, reçu 1982;16(1):22-5
Subba Reddy DV: Glimpses of health and medicine in Mauryan empire. Hyderabad, Upgraded Dept. of History of Medicine, Osmania Medical College, 1966. 97 p.
Subba Reddy DV: History of Siddha medicine; need for further detailed studies. **Bull Inst Hist Med (Hyderabad)** 1973 Oct;3(4):182-5
Tabor DC: Ripe and unripe: concepts of health and sickness in Ayurvedic medicine. **Soc Sci Med** 1981;15B:439-55
Tripathi RD, Verma KC: Contribution of Kaviraj Gangadhar Ray in the development of ayurvedic education. **Sachitra Ayurved** 1981 Mar;:190-3
Unschuld PU: The Chinese reception of Indian medicine in the first millennium A.D. **Bull Hist Med** 1979 Fall;53(3):329-45
Verma RL: Medical trends in Kashmir during Zain-ul-Abidin's reign. **Indian J Hist Sci** 1980 May;15(1):71-8

**Iran**

Eshraghi R: [History of medical ethics in] Persia. In Reich WT, et al, ed: Encyclopedia of bioethics, v. 2. New York, Free Press, 1978. p. 884-7.
Hampel J: Medizin der Zoroastrier im vorislamischen Iran. Husum, Matthiesen, 1982. 142 p. (Abhandlungen zur Geschichte der Medizin und der Naturwissenschaften, Heft 45).

**Ireland**

Ireland and medicine: **MD** 1979 Mar;23(3):81-93
Woods JO: The history of medicine in Ireland. **Ulster Med J** 1982;51(1):35-45

**Italy**

De Mitcheli A: Libros médicos italianos en la antigua Universidad de México. **Prensa Med Mex** 1979 Jul-Aug;44(7-8):152-6
Fichtner G, Siefert H, ed: Padua. Stuttgart, New York, Schattauer, 1978. 224 p. (Medizinhistorische Reisen, Band 2).

# MEDICINE

Gardner AL: Padua, Italy: the renaissance of medicine. **J Indiana State Med Assoc** 1983 Dec;76(12):842–5

Guarnieri E: La medicina a Firenze durante il governo dei Medici: 1440–1748. **Agressologie** 1981 Dec;22(F):7–9

Micheli A de: Libros medicos italianos en la antigua universidad de Mexico. **Bol Soc Mex Hist Filos Med** 1979 Dec;4(29):129–39

Rosa E: Medicina e salute pubblica a Bologna nel sei e settecento. **Quad Cult Bolognese** 1978 Dec;(2 no 8): 3–60

**Japan**

Bowers JZ: When the twain met. The rise of western medicine in Japan. Baltimore, London, The Johns Hopkins Univ. Press, 1980. xi, 173 p. (Henry E. Sigerist Supplements to the Bulletin of the History of Medicine, n.s., no. 5).

Briot A: Die japanische Medicine. In Sournia JC, Martiny M, Poulet J, ed: Illustrierte Geschichte der Medizin. Salzburg, Andreas, 1980. Vol. 2. p. 655–85.

Fuse S: Ishi no rekishi: sono Nihonteki tokucho. Tokyo, Chuo Koronsha, 1979. ii, 213 p.

Lisowski FP: Development of medicine in Japan. **East Horiz** 1980;19(3):29–34

Lock MM: East Asian medicine in urban Japan: varieties of medical experience. Berkeley, University of California Press, 1980. xiv, 311 p. (Comparative Studies of Health Systems and Medical Care, 4).

Ozaki NT: Conceptual changes in Japanese medicine during the Tokugawa period. Ph.D. Diss., University of California. San Francisco, 1979. viii, 285 leaves.

Schauwecker D: Aspekte der Medizingeschichte Japans im 16.–19. Jhdt. und der Deutschlandaufenthalt des japanischen Schriftstellers und Mediziners Ogai Mori in den Jahren 1884–1888. **Sudhoffs Arch** 1982;66(4):350–89

[Selected gems in medicine.] (Jpn).: **Igaku Sensui** 1974–81 Oct–Dec;1–28: various pagings, issued irregularly

Shimmura T: [Development and alteration of medical system in the Ritsuryo code regimen] (Jpn). **Igakushi Kenkyu** 1978;49:27–30

Shimmura T: [Formation of the medical system in the Ritsyryo code regimen] (Jpn). **Igakushi Kenkyu** 1977;48:25–9

**Korea**

Hall S: With stethoscope in Asia: Korea. McLean, Virginia, MCL Associates, 1978, xiv, 637 p.

Kim T: Han'guk ŭihaksa: chŏn. Seoul, T'amgudang, 1975. xxi, 584 p.

**Mexico**

Alcocer J: El archivo historico de la secretaria de salubridad y asistencia. **Bol Soc Mex Hist Filos Med** 1980 Sep–Dec;5(32–33):103–7

Basich Z, et al: Testimonios sobre medicina de los antiguos mexicanos. México, Instituto Mexicano del Seguro Social, 1980. n. p.

Chavez I: La evolución de la medicina en México. **Cuad Am** 1980;229(2):155–67

Erosa Barbachano A: Historia de la medicina en Yucatan. **Bol Soc Mex Hist Filos Med** 1984 Dec;7(49):399–404

Flores y Troncoso FA: Historia de la medicina en México desde la época de los indios hasta la presente. Facsimile of 1886 ed. plus new indices. 4 vols. México, Instituto Mexicano del Seguro Social, 1982. Various pagings. Historical and biographical chapters by V. M. Ruiz Naufal, A. G. Medrano, C. Viesca, G. A. Beltrán, J. S. Palencia, J. S. Riquer, B. F. Hernández.

López Hermosa L, ed: Bibliografía historica medica Mexicana 1970–1974. México, Sociedad Mexicana de Historia y Filosofía de la Medicina, (1978?). n.p.

Ortiz de Montellano B: Aztec medicine: empirical drug use. **Ethnomedizin** 1974–75;3(3–4):249–71

Ortiz Monasterio L: La medicina mexicana en el Archivo General de la Nacion. **Bol Soc Mex Hist Filos Med** 1980 Sep–Dec;5(32–33):93–102

Somolinos d'Ardois G: Medicina en las culturas mesoamericanas anteriores a la conquista. México, Rendón, for Sociedad Mexicana de Historia y Filosofía de la Medicina, 1978. Capitulos de historia medica Mexicana. I. 97 p.

Torre JM: Historia de la medicina potosina. Cuatro fases de su trayectoria. **Bol Soc Mex Hist Filos Med** 1984 Sep;7(48):351–92

Valverde JL, Martín Martín C: Nuevas aportaciones al estudio del Tribunal del Real Protomedicato en México. In International Congress of the History of Medicine, 27th, Barcelona, 1980. Actas. Barcelona, Académia de Ciències Médiques de Catalunya i Balears, 1981. p. 223–9.

**Netherlands**

Arts en sameleving. Medical history contributions by H. W. Pleket, J. Van Herwaarden, W. Frijhoff, C. Offringa, M. J. Van Lieburg, C. Bakker-Van der Kooij: **Tijdschr Geschied Geneeskd** 1983;96:323–475

Van Lieburg MJ: Het medisch onderwijs te Rotterdam (1467–1967): een kort historisch overzicht. Amsterdam, Rodopi, 1978. 111 p. (Nieuwe Nederlandse Bijdragen tot de Geschiedenis der Geneeskunde, 3).

**Nigeria**

Abdalla IH: Islamic medicine and its influence on traditional Hausa practitioners in northern Nigeria. Ph.D. Diss., University of Wisconsin. Madison, 1981. vii, 240 p.

Osuhor PC: Organisation of health services in Nigeria. **Health Popul Perspect Issues** 1978 Jan–Mar;1(1):1–11

**Poland**

Bujałowska B: Recepcja poglądów hipokratesa w polsce na tle dziejów medycyny powszechnej. **Pol Tyg Lek** 1983 Aug 15;38(33–34):1063–6

Konopka S: O źródłach do dziejów medycyny polskiej i o głównych przeszkodach, utrudniajacych rozwijanie badań naukowych z tej dziedziny. **Arch Hist Med (Warsz)** 1983;46(4):413–37

Lyskanowski M: Medycyna i lekarze dawnej Warszawy. Warszawa, Państwowy Instytut Wydawniczy, 1976. 465 p.

Rudowski W: Polish contribution to the development of biomedical science. **Rev Pol Acad Sci (Warsz)** 1977;22:27–34

Schwann S: Lekarze polscy w świetle historyczno-medycznego dzieła Grzegorza Matthiasa z XVIII wieku. **Arch Hist Med (Warsz)** 1979;42(2):217–22

**Spain**

Albarracín Teulón A, López Piñero JM, Granjel LS, ed: Medicina e historia. Madrid, Editorial de la Universidad Complutense 1980. 387 p. Contributions by P. Laín Entralgo, J. A. Paniagua, E. Balguer Perigüell, R. Ballester Añon, A. Lafuente, J. Riera, A. Carreras Panchón, D. García Guerra, J. L. Peset, M. Luz Terrada, P. Marset.

Alsina i Bofill J: De la medicina d'ahir a la medicina de demà. In Congrés International d'Història de la Medicina Catalana, 2nd, Barcelona, 1975. Llibre d'Actes. Barcelona, Socitra, 1977. p. 139–46.

Comelles JM, Prat Caros J, Pujadas Muñoz JJ: La medicina tradicional en el Estado español y la antropología cultural. In International Congress of the History of Medicine, 27th, Barcelona, 1980. Actas. Barcelona, Académia de Ciències Médiques de Catalunya i Balears, 1981. p. 490–4.

Corbella Corbella J: Notas sobre la historia de la medicina en la comarca del Bagés. **Ascleopio** 1980;32:93–101

Garcia del Carrizo San Millan MG: Obras de interes medico y cientifico en las bibliotecas universitaria y de Santa Cruz de Valladolid (hasta 1877). Valladolid, Universidad de Valladolid, 1981. 172 p. (Acta Historico-Medica Vallisoletana, Monografias, XI)

Granjel LS: La medicina española antigua y medieval. Salamanca, Ediciones Universidad de Salamanca, 1981. 184 p. (Historia general de la medicina española. I.).

Holzinger W: A re-examination of charges of racism in the Converso controversy in the light of Medieval-Renaissance medical lore. **Rev Estud Hisp** 1978;12(3):337–52

López Piñero JM: Medicina moderna y sociedad española (Siglos XVI–XIX). Valencia, Cátedra e Instituto de Historia de la Medicina, 1976. 326 p.

López Piñero JM: Social and economic factors in the translation of medical texts in Spain (16th–19th centuries). In International Congress of the History of Medicine, 27th, Barcelona, 1980. Actas. Barcelona, Académia de Ciències Médiques de Catalunya i Balears, 1981. p. 289–97.

Micheli A de: Los balbuceos de la cardiologia en la medicina islamica. **Bol Soc Mex Hist Filos Med** 1982 Mar;6(38):5–13

Rodríguez Tejerina JM: Historia de la medicina en Mallorca: desde sus orígenes hasta el siglo XVI. Palma de Mallorca, A. Rodríquez Tejerina, 1981. 249 p.

Torres Fontes J: De historia médica murciana. I. Los médicos. Murcia, Academia Alfonso X El Sabio, Biblioteca Murciana de Bolsillo, 1980. 308 p.

**Sweden**

Clemedson CJ: Berömda svenska böcker inom medicin och farmaci. **Nord Medicinhist Arsb** 1980;Suppl 6:35–51

Kock W: Sjuk i Sverige 1578–1978. **Nord Medicinhist Arsb** 1980;Suppl 6:57–66

**Switzerland**

Premuda L: Schweizer Medizinstudenten und Arzte im Gebiet zwischen Padua und Triest. **Gesnerus** 1984;41(3–4):299–321

**Turkey**

Erez S: Ottoman medicine viewed through Western eyes. **Hexagon Roche** 1981;9(3):Suppl I–IV

Said HM: Medicine in Turkey. **Med Times** 1981 Nov–Dec;16(11–12):4–8

**United States**

Barrow MV: Early history of medicine in Alachua County. **J Fla Med Assoc** 1982 Aug;69(8):670–80

Burkhart LL: The good fight: medicine in colonial Pennsylvania, 1681-1765. Ph.D. Diss., Lehigh University. Bethlehem, 1982. 348 p.
Cash P, Christianson EH, Estes JW, ed: Medicine in colonial Massachusetts 1620-1820. A conference held 25 & 26 May 1978 by the Colonial Society of Massachusetts. Boston, Colonial Society of Massachusetts, 1980. xxiii, 425 p. (Publications, Vol. 57) Contributions by R. D. Brown, C. H. Brock, G. B. Warden, W. J. Bell, J. C. Greene, D. L. Jones, W. C. Wigglesworth, J. H. Cassedy, G. E. Gifford.
Estes JW: Medical skills in colonial New England. **N Engl Hist General Regist** 1980 Oct;134:259-75
Gifford GE: A medical tour of Boston. **JAMA** 1981 May 15;245(19):1931-5
Gifford GE: Medicine and science in early America. Being the collected essays of George Edmund Gifford, Jr., 1930-1981. Edited by Dorothy I. Lansing. Devon, Pa., Published by the friends of George E. Gifford, Jr., 1982. ix, 388 p.
Leavitt JW, Numbers RL, ed: Sickness and health in America. Readings in the history of medicine and public health. Madison, University of Wisconsin Press, 1978. ix, 454 p. Reprinted articles by various authors.
Pearson EF: Health care of the French in the Illinois country during the seventeenth and eighteenth centuries. In: Congrès international d'histoire de la médecine, XXVe, Québec, 1976. Actes. Québec, 1977. p. 1063-72.
Saffron MH: A sketch of medicine in New Jersey to 1825. **J Med Soc NJ** 1984 Sep;81(9):709-14
Starr P: The social transformation of American medicine. New York, Basic Books, 1982. xiv, 514 p.
Thomas KB: Some early Welsh contributors to American medicine: the family of Jones. In J. Cule, ed: Wales and medicine. London, British Society for the History of Medicine, 1975. p. 10-22.

**USSR**

Kuzmin MK: [Evolution of medicine in the principality of Moscow] (Rus). **Orvostort Kozl** 1979;87-88(25 no 1-2):91-104
Popushoĭ EP, Ioksa VA: Mediko-geograficheskie opisaniia--vazhnyĭ istochnik izucheniia istorii metitsiny Moldavii. **Sov Zdravookhr** 1983;8:58-61
Shengelia MS: Feudal Georgia translational medical literature (IX-I half of XIX century). In International Congress of the History of Medicine, 27th, Barcelona, 1980. Actas. Barcelona, Académia de Ciències Médiques de Catalunya i Balears, 1981. p. 340-5.
Stahnke J: Synopsis zur neueren Medizingeschichte Russlands. **Medizinhist J** 1980;15(1/2):120-53
U istochnikov mirovoĭ i otechestvennoĭ istorii meditsiny: **Sov Med** 1983;6:107-8
Zguta R: Early Russian medicine: potential sources and directions of research. **J Hist Med Allied Sci** 1980 Apr;35(2):203-14

**Vietnam**

La sagesse de la médecine traditionnelle Sino-Vietnamienne et les maladies de la femme. 2 vols. Paris, Centre de Thuyen d'Europe, 1978. 1260 p.:

**Yugoslavia**

Belicza B: Ranarnici u zdravstvenoj povijesti hrvatske. **Saopcenja** 1973;16(4):213-23
Borisov P: Slovensko-Hrvatske medicinske veze u prošlosti. **Lijec Vjesn** 1981 Oct;103(10):472-4
Dolenc M: Medicinsko bukovništvo na Koroškem, Stajerskem in Prekmurju. **Cas Zgodovino Narodop** 1978;14(1):82-91
Glesinger L: Medicine in old Dubrovnik. In Veteris ragusae medicina et pharmacia. Zagreb, PLIVA, n.d. p. 35-48.
Pertl E: Pregled razvoja zdravstva v Laškem in njegovem okolišu. **Cas Zgodovino Narodop** 1976;12(2):358-91
Tartalja H: [Doctors and biologists in Dubrovník.] (SCC) **Dubrovnik** 1975;18(3-4):5-51

**Before 500 A.D.**

Brandenburg D: Medizinisches bei Herodot. Eine literaturhistorische Studie zur antiken Heilkunde. Berlin, Hessling, 1976. 176 p. (Medizingeschichtliche Miniaturen, Band 2).
Brunet F: Die spätantike und die byzantinische Medizin. In Sournia JC, Martiny M, Poulet J, ed: Illustrierte Geschichte der Medizin. Salzburg, Andreas, 1980. Vol. 2. p. 441-71.
Dastugue J: Les maladies de nos ancétres. **Recherche** 1982;(136):980-8
Ey H: Naissance de la médecine. Paris, New York, Masson, 1981. viii, 230 p.
Filliozat J: Yogaśataka, texte médical attribué à Nagărjuna. Textes sanskrit et tibétain, traduction française, notes, indices. **Publ Inst Fr Indologie** 1979;62:1-206
Harig G: Zu den Aufgaben der medizinhistorischen Forschung auf dem Gebiet der antiken Medizin in der Gegenwart. In International Congress of the History of Medicine. 26th, Plovdiv, 1978. Actes du Congress. Sofia, 1981. Volume II. p. 109-11.
Harrauer H, Sijpesteijn PJ, ed: Medizinische Rezepte und Verwandtes. Wien, Brüder Hollinek, 1981. xv, 56 p. (Mitteilungen aus der Papyrussammlung der Osterreichischen Nationalbibliothek (Papyrus Erzherzog Rainer), Neue Serie, 13. Folge).
Kollesch J: Aerztliche Ausbildung in der Antike. **Klio** 1979;61:507-13
Kollesch J: Antike Heilkunst: ausgewählte Texte aus dem medizinischen Schrifttum der Griechen und Römer. Leipzig, Reclam, 1981. 212 p.
Kollesch J: Das Berliner Corpus der antiken Aerzte. **Clio Med** 1981 Sep;16(1):45-7
Krakovetskaia GA: Gigienicheskie i lechebnye printsipy antichnoĭ meditsiny. **Gig Sanit** 1984 May;(5):37-40
Nickel D: Medizingeschichtliches in den 'Fabulae' des Hyginus. In International Congress of the History of Medicine. 26th, Plovdiv, 1978. Actes du Congress. Sofia, 1981. Volume II. p. 170-3.
Scarborough J, ed: Society for Ancient Medicine newsletter. No. 1-10 (Apr. 1976-Sept. 1982). Continued periodically.
Sorokina TS: Meditsina doklassovogo obshchestva. **Feldsher Akush** 1983;48(1):49-52
Sorokina TS: Meditsina Drevnego Vostoka. **Feldsher Akush** 1983;48(3):50-3
Steiger K: A hippokratészi orvostudomány természetfilozófiai elözményei. **Orvostort Kozl** 1981;93-96(27 No 1-4):17-23
Watermann RA: Mensch und Medizin zwischen Macht und Militär der römischen Kaiserzeit. Frankfurt am Main, Gerhard Michler, 1980. 204 p.
Zotter H, ed: Antike Medizin. Die medizinische Sammelhandschrift Cod. Vindobonensis 93 in lateinischer und deutscher Sprache. Graz, Akademische Druck- und Verlagsanstalt, xxxii, 380 p.

**Arabic**

Khan AJ: A survey of the concepts and measures developed by the Greco-Arab physicians related with the prevention and treatment of the infections and epidemic diseases. **Indian J Hist Sci** 1981;16(2):139-44
Nabielek R: Probleme bei der Edition der nur arabisch überlieferten pseudogalenischen Schrift De sommo et vigilia. **NTM** 1982;19(2):75-80
Valverde JL, Pena Muñoz C: Ibn Al-Haššа Glosario sobre el Mansuri de Razi. **Ars Pharm** 1980;21(4):495-506

**Asia**

Amundsen DW: [Medical ethics in the] ancient Near East. In Reich ET, et al, ed: Encyclopedia of bioethics, v. 2. New York, Free Press, 1978. p. 880-3.
Benedum J: Zur lydischen Arztinschrift IGRR IV 1359. **Z Papyrologie Epigraphik** 1978;29:115-21

**Assyria**

Freydank WF: Zwei medizinische Texte aus Assur. **Schr Gesch Kult Alten Orients** 1977;5:255-8

**China**

Chao You Chen: [A study of the ancient medical manuscript 'Tsu-pei-shih-i-mo-chiu-ching' recently found in Ma-wang-t'ui, China.] (Jpn). **Nihon I-Shigaku Zasshi** 1981;27(1):1-5
Chow Tse-Tsung: The childbirth myth and ancient Chinese medicine: a study of aspects of the 'wu' tradition. In D. T. Roy, T. Tsien, ed: Ancient China. Hong Kong, 1978. p. 43-89.
Dong Renda: [Textual research - on records of ancient Chinese medical history.] (Chi). **Chin J Med Hist** 1981;11:82-3
Duan Yishan: [Examples of special literary problems of ancient medical classics.] (Chi). **Chin J Med Hist** 1981;11:120-3
Emmerick RE: Some lexical items from the rGyud-bźi. In: Proceedings of the Csoma de Körös Memorial Symposium ... Matrafüred ... 1976. Budapest: Akad. Kiadó. 1978. pp.101-108.
Hao B, et al: [My new opinion on the date of writing of the 'Seven Grand Chapters' in Internal Classics of Yellow Emperor: exploration based on the origin and evolution of the historical materials of ancient records on astronomy, classical music and calendar] (Chi). **Chung Hua I Shih Tsa Chih** 1984 Jan;14(1):46-50
Lee FR: The 'silent art' of ancient China; Chung kuo ku tai ssu hsiang: historical analysis of the intellectual and philosophical influences in the earliest medical corpus, Ling shu ching. Taipei, Linking Pub. Co., 1980. ii, 176 p.
Shang ZJ: [Survey of medicin 'Prescription for 52 diseases' (an old medicinal book)] (Chi). **Chung Yao Tung Pao** 1982;7(6):17-20
Wan Fang: [Textual research on some ancient medical figures.] (Chi). **Chin J Med Hist** 1981;11:78-81

**Cyprus**

Papaxenopoulos A: Zypriotische Medizin in der Antike. Diss., Bayerische Julius-Maximilians-Universität. Würzburg, 1981. iii, 104 p.

**Egypt**

Daumas F: Réflexion sur la médecine égyptienne.

# MEDICINE

**Bull Liaison Assoc Amis Mus Pharm Montp** 1978 Dec 10;:23–40
Deines H von, Grapow H, Westendorf W: Grundriss der Medizin der alten Agypter, IX. Ergänzungen: Drogenquanten, Sachgruppen, Nachträge, Bibliographie, Generalregister. Berlin, Akademie Verlag, 1973. 241 p.
Devauchelle D, Pezin M: Un papyrus médical démotique. **Chron Egypte** 1978 Jan;53:57–66
Frey EF: The earliest Egyptian medical texts. **Bookman** 1984 Nov–Dec;11(6):3–7
Ghalioungui P: The last day of Psametik, physician to Pharoah. A tale. **Trans Stud Coll Physicians Phila** 1980 Jun;5(2 no 2):90–111
Ghalioungui [: On the necessity of medical–archaeological cooperation. In: Congrès international d'histoire de la médecine, XXVe, Québec, 1976. Actes. Québec, 1977. p. 699–705.
Kolta KS: Arzt und Hersteller von Heilmitteln im alten Aegypten. **Beitr Gesch Pharm** 1979;31(2):9–12
Kolta KS: Der Arzt und Hersteller von Heilmitteln im alten Agypten. In International Congress of the History of Medicine. 26th, Plovdiv, 1978. Actes du Congress. Sofia, 1981. Volume II. p. 127–8.
Leca AP: Die Medizin im Alten Agypten. In Sournia JC, Martiny M, Poulet J, ed: Illustrierte Geschichte der Medizin. Salzburg, Andreas, 1980. Vol. 1. p. 109–43.
Wu K: [Ancient medical classic – the Papyrus Ebers] (Chi). **Chung Hua I Shih Tsa Chih** 1984;14(2):107–11

**France**

Le Scouëzec G: La médecine en Gaule. Guipavas, Kelenn, 1976, 204 p.
Médecine, villes d'eau, sanctuaires des eaux en Gaule dans l'Antiquité. Ve Partie: La médecine à la fin de l'Antiquité: **Rev Archeol Centre France** 1983;22(Dec):259–82
Rémy B: Répertoire épigraphique des médecins gaulois. **Rev Archeol Centre France** 1983;22(Dec):282

**Greco–Roman**

Amulree L: Pergamum. **Hist Med (Lond)** 1975 Autumn–Winter;6(3–4):15–22
Anastassiou A: Zur hippokratischen Schrift De locis in homine und zum Hippokratesglossar des Galen. **Rheinisches Mus Philol** 1982;125:193–201
Baader G: Der ärztliche Stand in der Antike. **Jahrb Univ Dusseld** 1977–78;:301–15
Baruk H: La médecine hebraïque face à la médecine hippocratique. In La collection hippocratique et son rôle dans l'histoire de la médecine. Colloque de Strasbourg (23–27 octobre 1972) organisé par le Centre de Recherches sur la Grèce Antique, avec le concours des Facultés de Philosophie et des Langues Classiques. Leiden, E. J. Brill, 1975. p. 291–303.
Brătescu G: Eléments archaïques dans la médecine hippocratique. In La collection hippocratique et son rôle dans l'histoire de la médecine. Colloque de Strasbourg (23–27 octobre 1972) organisé par le Centre de Recherches sur la Grèce Antique, avec le concours des Facultés de Philosophie et des Langues Classiques. Leiden, E. J. Brill, 1975. 41–9.
Diller H: Das Selbstverständnis der griechischen Medizin in der Zeit des Hippokrates. In La collection hippocratique et son rôle dans l'histoire de la médecine. Colloque de Strasbourg (23–27 octobre 1972) organisé par le Centre de Recherches sur la Grèce Antique, avec le concours des Facultés de Philosophie et des Langues Classiques. Leiden, E. J. Brill, 1975. p. 77–93.
Durling RJ: Lexicographical notes on Galen's writings. **Glotta** 1981;59:108–16
Harig G, Kollesch J: Galen und Hippokrates. In La collection hippocratique et son rôle dans l'histoire de la médecine. Colloque de Strasbourg (23–27 octobre 1972) organisé par le Centre de Recherches sur la Grèce Antique, avec le concours des Facultés de Philosophie et des Langues Classiques. Leiden, E. J. Brill, 1975. p. 257–74.
Joly R: L'école médicale de Cnide et son évolution. **Antiq Class** 1978;47:528–37
Kollesch J: Zum Problem der Medizingeschichtsschreibung in der griechisch–römischen Antike. In International Congress of the History of Medicine. 26th, Plovdiv, 1978. Actes du Congress. Sofia, 1981. Volume II. p. 124–6.
Kudlien F: Der griechische Arzt im Zeitalter des Hellenismus: seine Stellung in Staat und Gesellschaft. Mainz, Akademie der Wissenschaften und der Literatur; Wiesbaden, Steiner, 1979. 130 p. (Akademie der Wissenschaften und der Literatur. Geists- und sozialwissenschaftlichen Klasse. Abhandlungen, Jahrg. 1979, no. 6)
Lactance: L'ouvrage du Dieu créateur. 2 vols. Ed. par M. Perrin. Paris, Editions du Cerf, 1974. 456 p. (Sources Chrétiennes, No. 213, 214).
Longrigg J: Superlative achievement and comparative neglect: Alexandrian medical science and modern historical research. **Hist Sci** 1981 Sep;19(45 pt 3):155–200
Martiny M: Laënnec et la pensée hippocratique. In La collection hippocratique et son rôle dans l'histoire de la médecine. Colloque de Strasbourg (23–27 octobre 1972) organisé par le Centre de Recherches sur la Grèce Antique, avec le concours des Facultés de Philosophie et des Langues Classiques. Leiden, E. J. Brill, 1975. p. 97–105.
Médioni G: Die griechische Medizin nach Hippokrates. In Sournia JC, Martiny M, Poulet J, ed: Illustrierte Geschichte der Medizin. Salzburg, Andreas, 1980. Vol. 1. p. 351–92.
Moszyński J: Galenus – De victu attenuante. **Arch Hist Med (Warsz)** 1982;45(1–4):61–75
Nutton V: Galen in the eyes of his contemporaries. **Bull Hist Med** 1984 Fall;58(3):315–24
Nutton V, ed: Karl Gottlob Kühn and his edition of the works of Galen. Oxford, Oxford Microform Publications, 1976. 35 p. (First published with the microfiche edition of Kühn's edition of The works of Galen, March 1976).
Palmieri N: Un antico commento a Galeno della scuola medica di Ravenna. **Physis** 1981;23:197–296
Phillips JH: The emergence of the Greek medical profession in the Roman republic. **Trans Stud Coll Physicians Phila** 1980 Dec;5(2 no 4):267–75
Raju TN: Soranus of Ephesus: who was he and what did he do? In Smith GF, Smith PN, Vidyasagar D, ed: Historical review and recent advances in neonatal and perinatal medicine. [Chicago?], Mead Johnson Nutritional Division, 1983. Vol. II. p. 179–86.
Scarborough J: Classical antiquity: medicine and allied sciences. **Trends Hist** 1979 Fall–Winter;1(2):3–14
Scarborough J: The Galenic question. **Sudhoffs Arch** 1981;65(1):1–31

**Greece**

Arts en sameleving. Medical history contributions by H. W. Pleket, J. Van Herwaarden, W. Frijhoff, C. Offringa, M. J. Van Lieburg, C. Bakker–Van der Kooij: **Tijdschr Geschied Geneeskd** 1983;96:323–475
Baissette G: Die Medizin bei den Griechen. In Sournia JC, Martiny M, Poulet J, ed: Illustrierte Geschichte der Medizin. Salzburg, Andreas, 1980. Vol. 1. p. 179–99.
Bonnabeau RC: Hippocratic medicine. **Minn Med** 1984 Jul;67(7):389–91
Bourgey L, Martiny M: Hippokrates und die griechische Medizin des klassischen Zeitalters. In Sournia JC, Martiny M, Poulet J, ed: Illustrierte Geschichte der Medizin. Salzburg, Andreas, 1980. Vol. 1. p. 301–49.
Briceño Maaz T: La isla de Cos y el santuario de esculapio. **Rev Soc Venez Hist Med** 1977;25(39):9–47
Calogirou DK: L'Asclêpieion de Cos, Hippocrate et la maladie des coronaires. **Hist Sci Med** 1979;13(4):427–39
David M: Critical edition of Hippocrates' Aphorisms translated into Hebrew by J.S. Delmedigo (1591–1655), sections IV, V. **Koroth** 1979 Nov;7(9–10):680–709
David M: Critical edition of Hippocrates' Aphorisms, translated into Hebrew by J. S. Delmedigo (1591–1655), sections VI–VIII (cont. and end). **Koroth** 1980 Jun;7(11–12):764–94
Deichgräber K: Der hippokratische Eid. Text griechisch und deutsch – Interpretation – Nachleben. 4., erweiterte Auflage. Stuttgart, Hippokrates Verlag, 1983. 92 p.
Deichgraber K: Die Patienten des Hippokrates. Historisch–prosopographische Beiträge zu den Epidemien des Corpus Hippocraticum. Mainz, Akademie der Wissenschaften und der Literatur, 1982. 41 p. (Abhandlungen der Geistes- und Sozialwissenschaftlichen Klasse, Jahrgang 1982. Nr. 9).
Ducatillon J: Polémiques dans la collection hippocratique. Lille, Atelier de Reproduction des Thèses; Paris, Librairie Honore Champion, 1977. 382 p. (Thèse, Paris, 1976).
Joly R: Hippocrates and the school of Cos. Between myth and skepticism. In M. Ruse, ed: Nature animated. Historical and philosophical case studies in Greek medicine, nineteenth–century and recent biology, psychiatry, and psychoanalysis. Volume II. Dordrecht, D. Reidel, 1983. p. 29–47.
Koelbing HM: The Hippocratic physician at his patient's bedside. **Practitioner** 1980 May;224(1343):551–4
Kudlien F: A new testimony for Erasistratus? **Clio Med** 1981 Apr;15(3–4):137–42
Leebron WM: Reflections on Hippocrates. **Am J Proctol Gastroenterol Colon Rectal Surg** 1982 Jun;33(6):7–8, 24
Lichtenthaeler C: Chronologische und gedankliche Bezugssysteme in und um 'Ueber die alte Medizin'. XI. Hippokratische Studie. Genève, Droz, 1980. 30 p. (Etudes d'histoire de la médecine, VI).
Lloyd GE: Hippocratic problems. **Classical Rev** 1980;30(2):186–9
López Férez JA: El falso Demócrito y los escritos medicos pseudodemocritos. **An Hist Antigua Mediev** 1977–80;20:175–87
Mansfeld J: The historical Hippocrates and the origins of scientific medicine. In M. Ruse, ed: Nature animated. Historical and philosophical case studies in Greek medicine, nineteenth–century and recent biology, psychiatry, and psychoanalysis. Volume II. Dordrecht, D. Reidel, 1983. p. 49–76.
Marganne MH: Inventaire analytique des papyrus grecs de médecine. Genève, Droz, 1981. x, 406 p. (Centre des Recherches d'Histoire et de Philologie de la IVe Section de l'Ecole pratique des Hautes Etudes; Hautes Etudes du Monde Gréco–Roman, 12).
Robert L: Décret pour un médecin de Cos. **Rev Philol (Paris)** 1978;52(2):242–51
Roesch P: Médecins publics dans les cités grecques. **Hist Sci Med** 1984;18(3):279–93
Sakula A: In search of Hippocrates: a visit to Kos. **J R Soc Med** 1984

Aug;77(8):682-8
Sherwin-White SM: The Coan school of medicine. In her: Ancient Cos. An historical study from the Dorian settlement to the Imperial period. Göttingen, Vendenhoeck & Ruprecht, 1978. p. 256-289 (Hypomnemata, 51).
Sorokina TS: Gippokrat i 'Gippokratov sbornik'. **Feldsher Akush** 1984 Mar;49(3):51-5
Sorokina TS: Grecheskaia mifologiia o vrachevanii i vrachevateliakh. **Feldsher Akush** 1983;48(6)::47-54
Thivel A: Cnide et Cos? Essai sur les doctrines médicales dans la collection hippocratique. Paris, Les Belles Lettres, 1981. 135 p. (Publications de la Faculté des Lettres et des Sciences Humaines de Nice, 21).
Warren JV: Hippocrates--man and legend. **Forum Med** 1978 May;1(2):18-9
Wassilew W: Die Medizin im alten Thrazien. In: International Congress of the History of Medicine, 26th, Plovdiv (Bulgaria), 1978. Actes du Congres, Vol. 1. Sofia, 1980. p. 79-80.
Yazdany S, Soltani A: The relationship between ancient Persia and Greece from medical point of view. In International Congress of the History of Medicine. 26th, Plovdiv, 1978. Actes du Congress. Sofia, 1981. Volume II. p. 114-5.

### India

Filliozat J: La doctrine classique de la médecine indienne: ses origines et ses parallèles grecs, Paris, Ecole française d'Extrême-Orient, 1975. vii, 230 p. (also Thèse 1946).
Khan MS: An Arabic source for the History of Ancient Indian medicine. **Indian J Hist Sci** 1981, reçu 1982;16(1):47-56
Lechner-Knecht S: Ayurveda-Wissen vom langen Leben. Eine altindische 'Offenbarungsmedizin'. **Med Klin** 1979 Dec 14;74(50):1938-42
Mazars G: Die Medizin in den Weden. In Sournia JC, Martiny M, Poulet J, ed: Illustrierte Geschichte der Medizin. Salzburg, Andreas, 1980. Vol. 1. p. 145-63.
Meulenbeld GJ: Observations on some medical authors called Madhava and their works. **Sci Orient** 1979;16:59-81
Miltner V: [Ancient Indian concepts of the body and disease] (Cze). **Cas Lek Cesk** 1981 Jun 4;120(22):682-4
Raison A, ed: La Haritasamhita: texte médical sanskrit; avec un index de nomenclature ayurvédique. Pondichéry, Institut français d'indologie, 1974. xlvi, 396 p. (Publications de l'Institut français d'indologie; no. 52).
Sarma CR, Rama Rao B: Additional material in Astanga Sangraha. **Bull Indian Inst Hist Med (Hyderabad)** 1979;9:1-12
Schmidt M: Zur Geschichte der tibetischen Ubersetzungen altindischer medizinischer Werke. In International Congress of the History of Medicine, 27th, Barcelona, 1980. Actas. Barcelona, Académia de Ciències Médiques de Catalunya i Balears, 1981. p. 336-9.
Zysk KG: A note on ancient Indian medicine. **Bull Indian Inst Hist Med (Hyderabad)** 1978;8(1-4):14-23

### Iran

Mazars G: Die altiranische Medizin. In Sournia JC, Martiny M, Poulet J, ed: Illustrierte Geschichte der Medizin. Salzburg, Andreas, 1980. Vol. 1. p. 165-77.

### Israel

Rosner F: Medicine in the Bible and the Talmud. Selections from classical Jewish sources. New York, KTAV Publishing House, Yeshiva University Press, 1977. xiii, 247 p. Includes Muntner S: Medicine in ancient Israel, p. 3-21.

### Mesopotamia

Adamson PB: Medical practice in the ancient Near East, with particular reference to Mesopotamia. **Med Secoli** 1982 May-Aug;19(2):163-73
Ducable G: L'art de guérir en Mésopotamie ancienne. **Hist Sci Med** 1982;16(1):23-7
Zaragoza JR: Die Medizin in Mesopotamien. In Sournia JC, Martiny M, Poulet J, ed: Illustrierte Geschichte der Medizin. Salzburg, Andreas, 1980. Vol. 1. p. 91 107.

### Rome

Engelhardt R, ed: Das römische Aerzte-Instrumentarium. Bingen, Engelhardt, 1974. 47 p. (Binger Annalen, IV) Contributions by C. Palm, K. M. Heidecker, P. Nahm, E. Naujack, A. Engelhardt.
Ma Kanwen: [An introduction to ancient Roman medicine] (Chi). **Chung Hua I Shih Tsa Chih** 1981;11:109-15
Ollero Granados D: New light Celsus' 'De medicina'. **Sudhoffs Arch** 1978;62(4):359-77
Phillips JH: Lucretius on the inefficiency of the medical arts: 6.1179 and 6.1226-38. **Classical Philol** 1982;77:233-5
Puma Fabricatore A: Sobre la medicina romana autoctona. **Rev Soc Venez Hist Med** 1972-73;20-21(34-35):155-60
Riddle JM: Gargilius Martialis as a medical writer. **J Hist Med Allied Sci** 1984 Oct;39(4):408-29
Sorokina TS: Meditsina v Drevnem Rime. **Feldsher Akush** 1983 Dec;48(12):38-43
Villey R: Die Medizin in Rom: Galen. In Sournia JC, Martiny M, Poulet J, ed: Illustrierte Geschichte der Medizin. Salzburg, Andreas, 1980. Vol. 2. p. 411-39.

### Syria

Vardanian SA: Ancient Armenian translations of the works of Syrian physicians. In International Congress of the History of Medicine, 27th, Barcelona, 1980. Actas. Barcelona, Académia de Ciències Médiques de Catalunya i Balears, 1981. p. 352-7.

### 500 A.D.-1450

Agrimi J: Malato, medico, e medicina nel Medioevo. Torino, Loescher Editore, 1980. 301 p.
Alford JA: Medicine in the Middle Ages: the theory of a profession. **Centen Rev** 1979;23(4):377-96
Baader G: Zu den Aufgaben der medizinhistorischen Forschung auf dem Gebiet der Geschichte der mittelalterlichen Medizin in der Gegenwart. In: International Congress of the History of Medicine, 26th, Plovdiv (Bulgaria), 1978. Actes du Congres, Vol. 1. Sofia, 1980. p. 85-8.
Buchet L: Médecine et chirurgie pendant les premiers siècles du Moyen Age. Présentation de quelues vestiges anthropologiques. **Rev Archeol Centre France** 1983;22(Dec):273-81
Cohen W: The blackest hour. **Synthesis** 1980;5(1):2-12
Duffy JM: Stephanus the philosopher: lectures on the Prognosticon of Hippocrates. Critical text and translation. Ph. D. Diss., State University of New York, Buffalo, 1975. xxi, 449 p.
Durling R. Corrigenda and addenda to Diels' Galenica: II. codices miscellanei. **Traditio** 1981;37:373-81
Ell SR: The two medicines: some ecclesiastical concepts of disease and the physician in the high Middle Ages. **Janus** 1981;68:15-25
Gálvez Rodríguez E: Problematica de la medicina en la Baja Edad Media. **Asclepio** 1978-79;30-31:187-97
Imbault-Huart MJ: La médecine au Moyen Age: à travers les manuscrits de la Bibliothèque Nationale. Paris, Editions de la porte verte: Bibliothèque nationale, 1983. 191 p.
Jacquart D: La pratique médicale dans la région du nord au XVe siècle. In: Congrès National des Sociétés Savantes, 101e, Lille, 1976. Comptes Rendus. Paris, 1976. Section des Sciences, Fasc. III. p. 7-19.
Kessel AH: Notes on ps.-Hippocrates De medico. **Mnemosyne** 1978;31:113-33
Kibre P: Arts and medicine in the universities of the later Middle Ages. In Ijsewijn J, Paquet J, ed: The universities in the late Middle Ages. Leuven University Press, 1978. p. 213-27.
Kibre P: Hippocrates latinus: repertorium of Hippocratic writings in the Latin Middle Ages. **Traditio** 1977;33:253-95; 1978;34:193-226
Kibre P: Hippocrates latinus: repertorium of Hippocratic writings in the Latin Middle Ages. (VI). **Traditio** 1980;36:347-72
Kibre P: Hippocrates latinus: repertorium of Hippocratic writings in the Latin Middle Ages (VII). **Zwingliana** 1981;37:267-89
Kibre P: Hippocrates latinus: repertorium of Hippocratic writings in the Latin Middle Ages (VIII). **Traditio** 1982;38:169-71
Koenig GG: Schamane und Schmied, Medicus und Mönch: ein Ueberblick zur Archäologie der merowingerzeitlichen Medizin im südlichen Mitteleuropa. **Helv Archaeol** 1982;13(51-2):75-154
Köpp P: Das Handbuch eines frühmittelalterlichen Arztes in der Stiftsbibliothek St. Gallen. **Helv Archaeol** 1982;13(51-2):163-75
La tradition manuscrite des Quaestiones Nicolai peripatetici. In: J.J.G. Alexander, M.T. Gibson (eds.) Medieval learning and literature: Essays presented to Richard William Hunt. Oxford: Clarendon Pr., 1976. p. 200-219.
Leguay JP: Accidents du travail et maladies professionnelles au Moyen Age. **Inf Hist** 1981;43(5):223-33
Müller RA: Mittelalterliches Konzil und Medizin. **MMW** 1983 Apr 1;125(13):263-4
Pitskhelauri GZ: Meditsina i vydaiushchiesia mediki srednevekovogo Vostoka. Tbilisi, Izd-vo Sabchota Sakartvelo, 1982. 234 p.
Puma FA. Edad media y medicina. **Rev Soc Venez Hist Med** 1975-76;23(37):37-59
Rasheed BM: Avicenna's influence on European medicine. **Bull Indian Inst Hist Med (Hyderabad)** 1981;1-4:99-102
Rofail FF: Why Europe responded to the Muslims' medical achievements in the Middle Ages. **Arabica** 1978;25:292-309
Schipperges H: Das medizinische Denken bei Albertus Magnus. In: Albertus Magnus, Doctor universalis, 1280/1980; hrsg. von G. Meyer, A. Zimmermann. Mainz, Matthias-Grünewald, 1980. p. 279-94.
Schultheisz E: Az Arab medicina assimilatiója a késöközépkori latin orvosi irodalomban. **Demografia** 1976;19(2-3):286-91
Siraisi NG: The medical learning of Albertus Magnus. In Weisheipl JA, ed: Albertus Magnus and the sciences. Toronto, Pontifical Institute of Mediaeval Studies, 1980. p. 379-404.
Trynková O: Některé metody středověkého léčení podle Mistra Rhazesa a Mistra Salicettiho. II. Uspěchy a neúspěchy středověkých léčitelu. **Sb Lek** 1982 Jan;84(1):25-32

# MEDICINE

Uiblein P: Beziehungen der Wiener Medizin zur Universität Padua im Mittelalter. Mit einem Konsilium des Stadtarztes von Udine Jeremias de Simeonibus für Herzog Albrecht VI von Osterreich. **Rom Hist Mitt** 1981;23:271-301

### Arabic

Ammar S: Introduction à l'étude de la médecine arabo-islamique. **Tunis Med** 1980 Jul-Aug;58(4):544-55, 562-77
Arabian medicine in the Middle Ages: **J R Soc Med** 1984 May;77(5):438
Aroua A: Hygiene et prevention médicale chez Ibnou Sina (Avicenne). Alger, S.N.E.D., [1974?]. 106 p.
Arzumetov IuS: Ibn Sina--vrach-éntsiklopedist i nekotorye osnovy ego ucheniia o zdorov'e i bolezni (k 1000-letiiu so dnia rozhdeniia). **Fiziol Zh SSSR** 1980 Sep;66(9):1273-7
El avicenismo: **Med Tradic** 1980;3(10):33-6
Bagchi AK: Indian influences on Arabic and Moorish medicine. **Phronesis** 1978;37:3-12
Baruch JZ: Maimonides as a physician. **Gesnerus** 1982;39(3-4):347-57
Bečka J: Otec lékařu Avicenna v naší vědě a kultuře. Abú Alí ibn Síná (980-1037). **Cas Lek Cesk** 1980 Jan 5;119(1):17-23
Belova LV: Znachenie tvochestva Ibn Sina dlia sovremennoĭ meditsiny. **Med Sestra** 1983 Nov;42(11):46-51
Ben Milad A: Biographie des médécins arabes: Ishaq Ibn Omrane. **Tunis Med** 1979 Nov-Dec;57(6):378-9
Demirhan A: Ibn Sina's canon and some patterns. **Med Bull Istanbul Med Fac** 1979;12:158-62
Durrany KS: Ibn Sinā's concept of man. **Stud Hist Med** 1982 Sep;6(3):161-94
Egri B: Arab triangulum **Orv Hetil** 1981 Jun 28;122(26):1595-600
Egri B: Keleti géniusz. Emlékezés Avicennára, születésének 1000. évfordulóján. **Orv Hetil** 1980 Dec 28;121(52):3207-12
En el milenario de Avicena: **Med Tradic** 1980;2(8):5-9
Ghalioungui P: Hunayn Ibn Ishaq, translator and medical writer. In International Congress of the History of Medicine, 27th, Barcelona, 1980. Actas. Barcelona, Acadêmia de Ciències Médiques de Catalunya i Balears, 1981. p. 245-8.
Haddad FS, Richter-Bernburg L: A hitherto unknown eighth-century commentary on Avicenna's 'Kulliyyat'. **J Hist Arabic Sci** 1980;4:253-8
Hajal F: Galen's ethical psychotherapy: its influence on a medieval Near Eastern physician. **J Hist Med Allied Sci** 1983 Jul;38(3):320-33
Hamarneh SK: Ibn Al-Quff's writings on hygienic regulations and the preservation of health. In A. Hadidi, ed: Studies in the history and archaeology of Jordan. Amman, Department of Antiquities, 1982. p. 373-83.
Hamarneh SK: Introduction to the history and philosophy of Arabic-Islamic medicine and allied sciences. **Stud Hist Med** 1982 Sep;6(3):195-213
Hamarneh SK: Majusi's observations and instructions on medicine and public health. **Hamdard** 1980 Jan-Mar;23(1):3-35
Hau FR: Die Bildung des Arztes im Islamischen Mittelalter. **Clio Med** 1979 May;13(3-4):175-200
Hunayn Ibn Ishak, al-Ibadi: Questions on medicine for scholars. Translated into English, with a preface and historical note, by P. Ghalioungui, M.D., from a critical edition by G. M. Moussa, Ph. D., of the ninth century. Arabic text 'Al Masa'il fi al-Tibb lil Muta'allimin.' Cairo, Al-Ahram Center for Scientific Translations, 1980. xlix, 162 p.
Ibn Masawayh Y: Le livre des axiomes médicaux (aphorismi). Edition du texte arabe et des versions latines avec traduction française et lexique par Danielle Jacquart et Gérard Troupeau. Geneva, Librairie Droz, 1980. iii, 368 p. (Centre de Recherches d'Histoire et de Philologie, II; Hautes Etudes Orientales, 14).
Iqbal Ali M: Contribution of Avicenna to medicine. **Bull Indian Inst Hist Med (Hyderabad)** 1981;1-4:139-45
Isaacs H: European influences in Islamic medicine. In: Mashriq. Proc. of the Eastern Mediterranean Seminar ... 1977-1978. Manchester, University, 1980. p. 25-9.
Iskandar AZ: Another fragment from the autograph of Ibn Al-Tilmidh's 'Marginal commentary on Ibn Sina's Canon of medicine'. **Bull Sch Orient Afr Stud** 1981;44:253-61
Kahle E: Der Traktat über das Zusammenwirken der Naturen des Qustā Ibn Lūqā. In Keil G, et al., ed: Fachprosa-Studien. Beiträge zur mittelalterlichen Wissenschafts-und Geistesgeschichte. Berlin, Schmidt, 1982. p. 133-42.
Kakhorov GK: Gigienicheskie vzgliady Avitsenny. **Feldsher Akush** 1984 Feb;49(2):52
Karmi Ghada: Arabic medicine in the 10th century---a study based on the book Ghina wa Muna by Abu Mansur al-Hasan b. Nuh al-Qumri. In: International Symposium for the History of Arabic Science, 1st, University of Aleppo, 1976. Proceedings. Aleppo, Syria, 1976. Papers in European Languages, Vol. II. p. 326-35.
Klein-Franke F: The Arabic version of Galen's Periethon. **Jerus Stud Arabic Islam** 1979;1:125-50
Kucharz E: Avicenna (Abu Ali Ibn Sina) - życie i działalność Lekarska. **Wiad Lek** 1981 Aug 15;34(16):1405-9
Kunitzsch P: Medizin, Naturwissenschaft und Technik im Mittelalter, Kontinuität und Wandel in Darstellung und Deutung: Die arabisch-islamische Welt. **Medizinhist J** 1982;17(1/2):54-62
Ley H: Ibn Sina (Avicenna, 980-1037): Gründe für 1000 Jahre Rückerinnerung. **Dtsch Z Philos** 1980;28(11):1309-23
Micheau F: La formation des médecins arabes au Proche-Orient (Xe-XIIIe siècle). **Ann Est** 1982;34(1-2):105-25
Milad A ben: Biographie des médécins arabes: Ishaq Ibn Omrane. **Tunis Med** 1979;57:378-9
Muhammad U: Avicenna as a clinician. **Bull Indian Inst Hist Med (Hyderabad)** 1981;1-4:87-90
Pena Munoz C, Girón Irueste F: Aspectos ineditos de la obra medica de Avenzoar: el prologo del 'Kitab al-Taysir'. Edicion, traduccion y comentarios. **Misc Estud Arabes Hebraicos** 1977;26(1):103-16
Peña Muñus C, ed: Indice de sustancias medicinales citadas en el Kitab al-Kulliyyat de Averroes. Granada, Universidad de Granada, 1980. 18 [20] p. (Estudios del Departamento de Historia de la Farmacia y Legislacion Farmaceutica, 5).
Petrov BD: Ibn-Sina--Avitsenna (K 1000-letiiu so dnia rozhdeniia). **Med Sestra** 1980 Aug;39(8):45-51
Petrov BD: Meditsinskoe nasledie Ibn-Siny. **Sov Zdravookhr** 1980;(9):53-6
Petrov BD: Study on the medical heritage of Avicenna (Ibn Sina). In E. Schultheisz, ed: History of physiology. Oxford, Elmsford, New York, Pergamon, 1981. xvi, 208 p. (Advances in Physiological Sciences. Proceedings of the 28th International Congress of Physiological Sciences, Budapest, 1980. Volume 21). p. 49-51.
Pulatov AM: Abuali Ibn-Sina (Avitsenna) i ego nauchno-meditsinskoe nasledie. **Vrach Delo** 1980 Sep;(9):1-6
Rofail Farag F: Why Europe responded to the Muslims' medical achievements in the Middle Ages. **Arabica** 1978;25:292-309
Said HM: Zuviel Erfolg für Avicenna? **Med Welt** 1981 Sep 25;32(39):62-3
Shanks NJ, Al-Kalai D: Arabian medicine in the middle ages. **J R Soc Med** 1984 Jan;77(1):60-5
Smith RD: Avicenna and the Canon of Medicine: a millennial tribute. **West J Med** 1980 Oct;133(4):367-70
Sournia JC: Die arabische Medizin. In Sournia JC, Martiny M, Poulet J, ed: Illustrierte Geschichte der Medizin. Salzburg, Andreas, 1980. Vol. 2. p. 589-629.
Strohmaier G: Aerztliche Ausbildung im islamischen Mittelalter. **Klio** 1979;61:519-24
Vakhidov VV: K 1000-letiiu Avitsenny. **Khirurgiia (Mosk)** 1980 Jul;(7):110-4
Valverde JL, Munoz CP, ed: El Formulario de los hospitales De Ibn Abi L-bayan. Introduccion, traduccion espanola y commentarios, con glosarios. Granada, Universidad de Granada, 1981. 256 p. (Cuadernos de historia de la farmacia, 8).
Vazquez de Benito MC, ed: El libro del 'Amal man tabba li-man habba de Muhammad B. 'Abdallah B. Al-Jatib. Salamanca, Universidad de Salamanca, 1972. liii, 86 p. (Acta Salmanticensia, 66).
Viesca Treviño C: El avicenismo. **Med Tradic** 1980;3(10):33-6
Viesca Trevino C: La medicina de Avicena. **Med Tradic** 1980;3(9):45-52
Weisser U: Ibn Sina und die Medizin des arabisch-islamischen Mittelalters - Alte und neue Urteile und Vorurteile. **Medizinhist J** 1983;18(4):283-305

### Asia

Filliozat J, ed: Yogaśataka. Texte médical attribué à Nagarjuna. Textes sanskrit et tibétain; traduction française. Pondichéry, Institut Français d'Indologie, 1979. xxxviii, 206 p.

### Bulgaria

Kadunkov D: Niakoi danni za meditsinata zubolechenito prez vtoroto bulgarsko tsarstvo i srednovekov neto. **Stomatologiia (Sofiia)** 1979 Jan-Feb;61(1):68-9

### Byzantium

Brunet F: Die spätantike und die byzantinische Medizin. In Sournia JC, Martiny M, Poulet J, ed: Illustrierte Geschichte der Medizin. Salzburg, Andreas, 1980. Vol. 2. p. 441-71.
Felici L: L'opera medica die Teofane Nonno in manoscritti inediti. **Acta Med Hist Patav** 1981/82;28:59-74
Hunger H: 'Zoologie,' 'Botanik,' 'Mineralogie,' 'Alchemie,' and 'Medizin.' In: Die hochsprachliche profane Literatur der Byzantiner. Vol. II. Munich, Beck, 1978 (Part 5, Vol. 2 of the Byzantinisches Handbuch). p. 265-320.
Padis N: The legacy of Byzantine medicine. In: Congrès international d'histoire de la médecine, XXVe, Québec, 1976. Actes. Québec, 1977. p. 1045-51.
Rozos B: The social care during the Eastern Middle Ages according to the sources. In: Congrès international d'histoire de la médecine, XXVe, Québec, 1976. Actes. Québec, 1977. p. 1184-95.
Sorokina TS: Meditsina v Vizantiĭskoĭ imperii. **Feldsher Akush** 1984 May;49(5):49-54

### China

Beckwith CI: The introduction of Greek medicine into Tibet in the seventh

and eighth centuries. **J Am Orient Soc** 1979;99:297–313
Needham J: The social position of scientific men and physicians in mediaeval China. In: International Congress for the History of Science, 14th, Tokyo, Kyoto, 1974. Proceedings. Tokyo, 1975. 4:19–34.

**Denmark**

Hauberg P: Laegebøger med tilknytning til Henrik Harpestraeng. **Theriaca** 1982 Jun;22:1–362

**Europe**

Birtalan G: Avicenna Kánonja és az európai orvostudomány. **Orvostort Kozl** 1980;89–91(26 no 1–3):25–43
Siraisi NG: Some recent work on western European medical learning, ca. 1200–ca. 1500. In History of Universities, II, 1982. p. 225–38.
Werthmann-Haas G: Altdeutsche Ubersetzungen des Prager 'Sendbriefs' ('Missum imperatori') (= Untersuchungen zur mittelalterlichen Pestliteratur, I). Pattensen (Han.), Wellm, 1983. 317 p. (Würzburger medizinhistorische Forschungen, Bd. 27).

**France**

Aron E: Louis XI et ses guérisseurs. Chambray, C. L. D., [1983]. 197 p.
Contreni JJ: The study and practice of medicine in Northern France during the reign of Charles the Bald. **Stud Mediev Cult** 1976;6–7:43–54
Demaitre LE: Doctor Bernard de Gordon: professor and practitioner. Toronto, Pontifical Institute of Mediaeval Studies, 1980. xii, 236 p.
Die französische Medizin im Mittelalter: In Sournia JC, Martiny M, Poulet J, ed: Illustrierte Geschichte der Medizin. Salzburg, Andreas, 1980. Vol. 2. p. 755–65.
Durand J, Hampartzoumian A: Les manuscrits de la faculté de médecine de Montpellier. **Connaiss Pays Occident** 1981;49:26–31
Figarella J: L'art médical au temps du Roi René. **Marseille** 1981;126:10–7
Jacquart D: Le milieu médical en France du XIIe au XVe siècle: en annexe 2e supplément au 'Dictionnaire' d'Ernest Wickersheimer. Genève, Droz; Paris, Champion, 1981. 487 p. (Centre de recherches d'histoire et de philologie de la IVe section de l'Ecole pratique des hautes études. V, Hautes études médiévales et modernes ; 46)
Jacquart D: Le regard d'un médecin sur son temps: Jacques Despars (1380?–1458). **Bibl Ec Chartres** 1980;138:35–86
Janssens PA: Medico-historische gegevens uit de 'Historia Francorum' van Gregorius van Tours. **Hades** 1977;16(30):1–53
Keil G: Randnotizen zu Danielle Jacquarts Wickersheimer-Supplements. **Sudhoffs Arch** 1982;66(2):172–86
Merlette B, Vial F, Rulliere R: Le Marcellus de Laon: observations paléographiques et critiques. **Hist Sci Med** 1980;14(1):52–60
Saint-Blanquat H de: Tableaux de la médecine médiévale. **Sci Avenir** 1984;(445):58–63

**Germany**

Czarnetzki A: Menschen des Frühen Mittelalters im Spiegel der Anthropologie und Medizin: Begleitheft zur Ausstellung. Stuttgart, Würtemmbergisches Landesmuseum Stuttgart, 1982. 103 p.
Dube WF: Medieval medicine in middle high German epics. Ph.D. Diss. Indiana University. [Bloomington], 1981. 295 leaves.
Hildegard von Bingen: Ursachen und Behandlung der Krankheiten (causae et curae). Ubersetzt von H. Schulz. 4. Auflage. Heidelberg, Haug, 1983. 373 p.
Hirth W: Corpusbildung in der deutschsprachigen medizinischen Fachliteratur des Mittelalters. **Suhoffs Arch** 1982;66(3):239–75
Keil G: Der 'Kodex Kohlhauer'. Ein iatromathematisch-hauswirtschaftliches Arzneibuch aus dem mittelalterlichen Oberfranken. I. Beschreibung der Handschrift. **Sudhoffs Arch** 1980;64(2):130–50
Walther H: Ein Magister Ortolf de Bavaria in Paris. **Sudhoffs Arch** 1978;62(3):294–5

**Great Britain**

Davies HE, Owen ME: Meddygon Myddfai. In J. Cule, ed: Wales and medicine. London, British Society for the History of Medicine, 1975. p. 156–68.
Gottfried RS: English medical practitioners, 1340–1530. **Bull Hist Med** 1984 Summer;58(2):164–82
Harries WG: Bened Feddyg: a Welsh medical practitioner in the late medieval period. In J. Cule, ed: Wales and medicine. London, British Society for the History of Medicine, 1975. p. 169–84.
Seymour MC, et al, ed: On the properties of things. John Trevisa's translation of Bartholomaeus Anglicus De proprietatibus rerum. A critical text. 2 vols. Oxford, Oxford University Press, 1975. xix, 1397 p.

**Greece**

Sendrail M: La foi coranique et l'héritage médical grec. **Bull Assoc Guillaume Bude** 1977;:278–99

**Hungary**

Réti E: Early days of medicine in Hungary. **Ther Hung** 1981;29(4):194–6

**India**

Abdul Hai Farooqi: Dafi al-Amrad; an important medical manuscript. **Stud Hist Med** 3(3):199–203, Sep 79
Chauhan DK, Singh RN: Contribution of Medieval India to Ayurvedic Materia Medica. **Indian J Hist Sci** 1982;16(1):17–21
Jaggi OP: Medicine in medieval India. Delhi, Atma Ram, 1977. 244 p.
Mishra SK, Bhatta BR, Bhat PS, et al: Ideas of integration as a process of evolution of Indian system of medicine in the Medieval period. **Indian J Hist Sci** 1981, reçu 1982;16(1):36–40
Muhammad Abad al-Wahab Zahuri: A medical treatise of the time of King Muhammad Tughlaq. **Stud Hist Med** 3(3):173–77, Sep 79
Rahman A, Alvi MA, Khan Ghori SA, et al: Science and technology in Medieval India. A bibliography of source materials in Sanskrit, Arabic and Persian. New Delhi, Indian National Science Academy, 1982. xxxi, 719 p.
Rama Rao B: Medical allusions in some inscriptions of Andhra Pradesh. **Bull Indian Inst Hist Med (Hyderabad)** 1975 Oct, 5(4):198–206
Rama Rao B: References to Ayurveda in the commentaries of Mallinatha. **Bull Indian Inst Hist Med (Hyderabad)** 1979;9:13–20
Sastry VV, Pandey AN: Jajjata. **Bull Indian Inst Hist Med (Hyderabad)** 1975 Jul;5(3):115–22
Siddiqui T: Two eminent physicians (of Unani medicine) during Shah Jahan's reign. **Indian J Hist Sci** 1981, reçu 1982;16(1):26–30
Subba Reddy DV: Glimpses of medicine in Rajatarangini; diseases, drugs, physicians and treatments in medieval Kashmir. **Bull Inst Hist Med (Hyderabad)** 1973 Oct;3(4):189–200

**Iran**

Soltani A: Ancient Jundi-Shahpour and its role in medicine and pharmaceutical progress. In International Congress of the History of Medicine. 26th, Plovdiv, 1978. Actes du Congress. Sofia, 1981. Volume II. p. 196–202.

**Ireland**

Cone TE: Eighth century Irish rules regarding the care of a sick person. **Pediatrics** 1981;67:795

**Italy**

Lucchetta F: La data della morte di Andrea Alpago. **Quad Stor Univ Padova** 1982;15:147–8
Poitras JM: Trotula of Salerno. **Md State Med J** 1980 Apr;29(4):62–4

**Netherlands**

Bauer G: Das 'Haager Aderlassbüchlein'. (Studien zum ärztlichen Vademecum des Spätmittelalters, 1). Pattensen/Hannover, 1978. 198 p. (Würzburger medizinhistorische Forschungen, 14). Also Diss. Würzburg, 1978.

**Poland**

Dobrzyniecki Z: 'Dzieje Polskie' Jana Długosza jako źródło do dziejów medycyny w Polsce w XIV i XV w. **Arch Hist Med (Warsz)** 1981;44(3/4):265–76
Strojnowski J: Nowy obraz polskiej kultury w średniowieczu. **Arch Hist Med (Warsz)** 1983;46(1):21–8
Wysocka F, ed: Głosy i teksty polskie w XV-wiecznym rekopisie lekarskim ze zbiorów Biblioteki Jagiellońskiej nr 132/60 akc. Komitet Jezykoznawstwa Pan. Wydawnictwa Zródłowe. Wrocław, Zakład Narodowy imienia Ossolińskich, 1971. 99 p.

**Rome**

Mudry P: Medicus amicus. Un trait romain dans la médecine antique. **Gesnerus** 1980;37(1/2):17–20

**Spain**

Alvarez de Morales C, Irueste FG: Medicina creencial y medicina racional en la España arabe del siglo IX: el Mujtasar Fi L-tibb (compendio de medicina) de 'Abd al-Malik Ibn Habib al-Ilbiri (c. 790–854). **Asclepio** 1982;34:283–94
Gallent M: Control social de la ciencia medica en Valencia durante el S. XV. **Llull (Spain)** 1978;2:95–105

# MEDICINE

García Ballester L: Evolucion y problematica de las investigaciones sobre historia de la medicina bajomedieval en España. **Asclepio** 1978–79;30–31:121–56
Giran Irueste F: La medicina practica en la España arabe del siglo XII: El 'Kitab al-Yami fi-l-asriba wa-l-Ma ayin de Abu Marwan abd al-Malik ibn Zuhr (Avenzoar). Edicion, traduccion y comentarios. Resumen of Diss. 209. Granada, 1978. 33 p.
Girón Irueste F: Los medicos mozarabes y el proceso de constitucion de la medicina arabe en al-Andalus. Siglos VIII–X. **Asclepio** 1978–79;30–31:209–22
Haven M: La vie et les oeuvres de Maître Arnaud de Villenauve. Genève, Slatkine Reprints, 1972. [192] p.
Kottek SS: Joseph ben Meir ibn Zabara of Barcelona (1140?–?) (his place in the history of medicine). In International Congress of the History of Medicine, 27th, Barcelona, 1980. Actas. Barcelona, Académia de Ciències Médiques de Catalunya i Balears, 1981. p. 181–7.
Paniagua Arellano JA, Arnau de Vilanova: El maravilloso regimiento y orden de vivir (una versión castellana del Regimen sanitatis ad regem Aragonum). **Cuad Aragon Hist Med Cienc (B)** 1980;3:1–106
Sanchez Gozalbo A: Boticarios, medicos y cirujanos en el Castellón del cuatrocientos. **Bol Soc Castell Cult** 1979;55(1):47–80

### Switzerland

Köpp P: Vademecum eines frühmittelalterlichen Arztes. Die gefaltete lateinische Handschrift medizinischen Inhalts im Codex 217 und der Fragmentensammlung 1396 der Stiftsbibliothek in St. Gallen. Aarau, Sauerländer, 1980. 128 p. (Veröffentlichungen der Schweizerischen Gesellschaft für Geschichte der Medizin und der Naturwissenschaften, 34).

### Tunisia

Catahier S: A l'occasion du millénaire de la mort d'Ibnoul-Jazzar (Algizar). **Hist Sci Med** 1984;18(3):247–53

### Venezuela

Kleiss E: Medicine men and conditions of life in pre-Columbian Venezuela. **Arq Anat Antropol** 1978;3(3):83–112

## 1450–1700

Bird DT: A catalogue of sixteenth-century medical books in Edinburgh libraries. Edinburgh, Royal College of Physicians of Edinburgh, 1982. xxxii, 298 p.
Debus AG: The Arabic tradition in the medical chemistry of the scientific revolution. In: International Symposium for the History of Arabic Science, 1st, University of Aleppo, 1976. Proceedings. Aleppo, Syria, 1976. Papers in European Languages, Vol. II. p. 275–90.
Debus AG: The chemical philosophy. Paracelsian science and medicine in the sixteenth and seventeenth centuries. 2 vols. New York, Science History Publications, 1977. xv, 606 p.
Donnellan WL: Medicine and society in the sixteenth and seventeenth centuries: their influence on the life and work of Herman Boerhaave, 1668–1738. Ph.D. Diss., Northwestern University. Evanston, 1981. vii, 483 p.
Durling RJ: Konrad Gessner's Briefwechsel. In: Schmitz R, Krafft F, ed: Humanismus und Naturwissenschaften. Boppard, Boldt, 1979? p. 101–111. (Beiträge zur Humanismusforschung, Band VI).
Eckart W: 'Machiavellus Medicus': eine satirischkritische Schrift zur medizinischen 'Politik' des ausgehenden 17. Jahrhunderts. **Nouv Repub Lett** 1982;(1):97–125
Johannes Adelphus: Ausgewählte Schriften. 3. Band. Das Buch des Lebens. Ed. A. R. Arthur, B. Gotzkowsky. Berlin, New York, De Gruyter, 1980. 413 p.
Kamińska-Axer M, Sosińska-Trawińska M: Starodruki medyczne w Bibliotece Kapitulnej we Wrocławiu. **Arch Hist Med (Warsz)** 1979;42(3):393–402
Kamińska-Axer M: Starodruki medyczne w Bibliotece Seminaryjnej w Warszawie, druki XVII-wieczne (c.d.). **Arch Hist Med (Warsz)** 1978;41(4):483–91
Kapronczay K: Magyar -- lengyel orvosi kapcsolatok a XV–XVI. században. **Orv Hetil** 1981 Feb 22;122(8):465–7
Kottek S: Aperçu sur l'"introduction à la pratique médicale', (introitus medici ad praxin) de Zacutus Lusitanus, 1575 - 1642. **Rev Hist Med Heb** 1980 Jul;33(2):35–8
Maclean I: The Renaissance notion of woman. A study in the fortunes of scholasticism and medical science in European intellectual life. New York, Cambridge University Press, 1980. VIII, 119p.
Mixa J: Neues über die Krankheit Wallensteins. **Medizinhist J** 1983;18(3):256–9
Nutton V: Medicine in the age of Montaigne. In K. Cameron, ed: Montaigne and his age. Univ. of Exeter, 1981. p. 14–25, 163–70.
Paracelsus in der Tradition: Vorträge, Paracelsustag 1978. Wien, Verband der Wissenschaftlichen Gesellschaften Oesterreichs, 1980. 146p. (Salzburger Beiträge zur Paracelsusforschung, Folge 21). Contributions by W. Pagel, F. Baron, H. Rudolph, R. Dilg-Frank, A. Dyk, W. Schneider, A. Miller-Guinsburg, S. Domandl, L. Braun, H. M. Decker-Hauff.
Perret L: René Descartes--drottning Kristinas Cartesius--filosof, matematiker och medicinsk läromästare. **Nord Medicinhist Arsb** 1981;:52–8
Starobinski J: D'Agrippa de Nettesheim à Montaigne: l'embarras de médecins devant l'origine de la semence. **Gesnerus** 1983;40(1–2):175–83
Webster C, ed: Health, medicine and mortality in the sixteenth century. London and New York, Cambridge University Press, 1979. 394 p. In memory of Sanford V. Larkey. Contributions by P. Slack, R. Schofield, E. A. Wrigley, A. B. Appleby, T. R. Forbes, P. Allderidge, M. Pelling, A. Chapman, J. J. Bylebyl.
Wright PW: A study in the legitimisation of knowledge: the 'success' of medicine and the 'failure' of astrology. **Sociol Rev [Monogr]** 1979;27:85–101

### Americas

Ehlers AP: Medizinisches und Pharmazeutisches in Bernal Diaz del Castillos, 'Historia verdadera de la conquista de la Nueva-España,' Madrid, 1632. Diss. Düsseldorf, 1980. 118 p.

### Arabic

Isaacs H: The impact of western medicine on Muslim physicians and their writings in the 17th century. **Bull Br Assoc Orient** 1979–80,N.Ser.;11:52–7
Ullmann M: Die arabische Ueberlieferung der Werke des Rufus von Ephesos. In: International Symposium for the History of Arabic Science, 1st, University of Aleppo, 1976. Proceedings. Aleppo, Syria, 1976. Papers in European Languages, Vol. II. p. 348–57

### Austria

Kostenzer O: Dr. Johannes Cuefner aus Rattenberg (biographische Notizen). **Tirol Heimatbl** 1971;46(1–3):18–20

### Belgium

Jacques E: Médecine et spiritualité: un médecin belge oublié, ami de Port Royal, Philippe Ignace Save (1659–1702). **Rev Hist Eccles** 1980;75(2):322–42
Pagel W: Joan Baptista Van Helmont: reformer of science and medicine. Cambridge, Cambridge University Press, x, 1982. 219 p. (Cambridge monographs on the history of medicine).

### Brazil

Guerra F: Medicine in Dutch Brazil 1624–1654. In: Johan Maurits van Nassau-Siegen 1604–1679 ... Essays on the ... tercentenary of his death. Ed. by E. van den Boogaart et al. The Hague, J. M. van Nassau-Siegen Stichting, 1979. p. 472 ff.

### Bulgaria

Bourilkova L, Israel S: Données sur la médecine et l'hygiène dans les terres bulgares d'après la description du voyageur Ogier Ghiselin de Busbecq (1522–1592). In International Congress of the History of Medicine. 26th, Plovdiv, 1978. Actes du Congress. Sofia, 1981. Volume II. p. 62–3.

### China

Bye Ba Rin Bsrel: Instructions of the great Zur-mkhar Mñam-ñid-rdo-rje on medical treatment comprising the Ma yig, Bu yig, and Kha 'thor collections. (Tib) Reproduced from a print from the Tsharon Sman-dgon blocks. Leh, Ladakh, Tashigangpa, 1974. np (Smanrtsis Shesrig Spendzod, Vol. 58).
Dar-mo Sman-ram Blo-bzan-chos-grags: Dar Mo Bka' Brgya Ma. Man nag zab mo kun gyi snin khu bsdus pa dar-mo sman-rams-pa'i gdams nag bka rgya ma. A collection of profound instructions on the methods and rituals of Tibetan healing transmitted by the physician of the 5th Dalia Lama. Reproduced from a print from the Sde-Dge blocks, 2 vols; and from the Ska-' Bum blocks, 2 vols. Leh, Ladakh, T. S Tashigangpa, 1978. n.p. (Smanrtsis Shesrig Spendzog, Vols. 88–91).
Shi Changyong: [Life and chronology of Xue Lizhai.] (Chi). **Chin J Med Hist** 1981;11:65–9

### Czechoslovakia

Servít Z: Počátky české novověké medicíny a biologie. Jan Marek Marci z Kronlandu (Joannes Marcus Marci, 1595–1667). Stručná biografie. **Cesk Fysiol** 1984;33(5):394–413

### Denmark

Hovesen E: Ole Worm - aegtemand og husfader. **Dan Medicinhist Arbog** 1982;:93–111

Hovesen E: Ole Worm og familien i Arhus. **Dan Medicinhist Arbog** 1981;:9-23

### France

Ackerman RH: Joubert's 'Erreurs populaires'. An insight into some aspects of sixteenth century health care. In: Congrès international d'histoire de la médecine, XXVe, Québec, 1976. Actes. Québec, 1977. p. 455-60.
Brunyate M: Montaigne and medicine. In K. Cameron, ed: Montaigne and his age. Univ. of Exeter, 1981. p. 26-38, 170-71.
Dulieu L: La médecine à Montpellier. Tome II. La Renaissance. Avignon, Presses Universelles, 1979. 481 p.
Heymans G, Vial F, Berti Bock G, et al: Le peuple et la médecine au XVIIe siècle. **Acta Med Hist Patav** 1979-80;26:95-113
Lehoux F: Le cadre de vie des médecins parisiens aux XVIe et XVIIe siècles. Paris, A. & J. Picard, 1976. x, 611 p.
Lingo AK: The rise of medical practitioners in sixteenth-century France: the case of Lyon and Montpellier. Ph.D. diss. University of California. Berkeley, 1980. 318 leaves.
Mistler J: Voyageurs d'autrefois. **Nouv Rev Deux Mondes** 1977;(2):265-75;(3):519-27
Paillard E: Louis Vassé, médecin à Chalôns. **Mem Soc Agric Commer Sci Arts Marne** 1975;90:109-29
Pecker A: Nicolas Venette (1633?-1698) est-il le fils de Guy Patin. **Hist Sci Med** 1982;16(3):167-74
Valverde JL, Arrebola Nacle P: Ayuda sanitaria de Felipe II a Francia. **Bol Soc Esp Hist Farm** 1982 Mar;33(130):123-9

### Germany

Brentini P: Die Institutiones medicinae des Daniel Sennert (1572-1637). Zürich, Juris, 1971. 69 p. (Diss., Zürich).
Häussler S: Johannes Kepler und die Allgemeinmedizin. **ZFA (Stuttgart)** 1982 May 31;58(15):I-1037-8
Senger HG: Thomas Hirschhorn: ein Magdeburger Gelehrter des 15. Jahrhunderts. **Hist Jahrb** 1980;100:217-39
Trüb CL, Eberhard W: Arztliche Berufs- und Standeskunde im 16. und 17. Jahrhundert. **Med Welt** 1982 Oct 2;32(40):1504-9

### Great Britain

Alsop J: A private consultation by Dr. William Harvey in 1642. **Med Hist** 1980 Jan;24(1):93-8
Appleby JH: Ivan the Terrible to Peter the Great: British formative influence on Russia's medico-Apothecary system. **Med Hist** 1983 Jul;27(3):289-304
Bloch H: Francis Bacon (1561-1626), his interest and influence in education, science, and medicine. **NY State J Med** 1981 Jun;81(7):1120-2
Bylebyl JJ, ed: William Harvey and his age: the professional and social context of the discovery of the circulation. Baltimore, Johns Hopkins University Press, 1979. xii, 154 p. (Henry E. Sigerist Supplements to the Bulletin of the History of Medicine, n.s., 2). Includes contributions by S. Jarcho, C. Webster, R. G. Frank.
Cook HJ: The regulation of medical practice in London under the Stuarts, 1607-1704. Ph.D. Diss., University of Michigan. Ann Arbor, 1981. 438 p.
Day RA: Thomas Sydenham (1624-1689). **Friends P. I. Nixon Med Hist Libr** 1977 Oct;6:3-8
Dewhurst K, ed: Willis's Oxford casebook (1650-52). Oxford, Sanford, 1981 xi, 199 p.
Goldstein LM: The life and death of John Lambe. **Guildhall Stud Lond Hist** 1979;4(1):19-32
Kealey EJ: Medieval medicus. A social history of Anglo-Norman medicine. Baltimore, Johns Hopkins University Press, 1981. x, 211 p.
Oakeley HF: The end of my great ... grandfather's second wife, or chest medicine in Lambeth in 1671. **St Thomas Hosp Gaz** 1981;79:50-1
Rawcliffe C: Medicine and medical practice in later medieval London. **Guildhall Stud Lond Hist** 1981;5(1):13-25
Richardson RG: Dr. John Hall, Shakespeare's son-in-law. A vignette of Elizabethan medicine. **Practitioner** 1981 Apr;225(1354):593-5
Webster C: Medicine as social history: changing ideas on doctors and patients in the age of Shakespeare. With commentary by D. G. Bates, p. 127-34. In Stevenson LG, ed: A celebration of medical history. Baltimore, Johns Hopkins University Press, 1982. (The Henry E. Sigerist supplements to the Bulletin of the History of Medicine;; new ser., no. 6). p. 103-26..

### Hungary

Endrei W: Egy korai magyar nyelvü orvoslevél. **Orvostort Kozl** 1980;89-91(26 no 1-3):267-8
Fazekas A: Lencsés György és az elsö magyar nyelvü kéziratos orvosi könyv 1577-böl. **Egeszsegneveles** 1982;23:79-81
Kapronczay K: Magyar-lengyel orvosi kapcsolatok a XVI. században. **Orv Hetil** 1982 Jul 25;123(30):1867-70

### India

Figueiredo JM de: Ayurvedic medicine in Goa according to European sources in the sixteenth and seventeenth centuries. **Bull Hist Med** 1984 Summer;58(2):225-35
Hussain SA: Hakim Nizamuddin Ahmed Geelani; a physician of Qutub Shahi period. **Bull Indian Inst Hist Med (Hyderabad)** 1979;9:67-73
Rama Rao B: Rasapradipika; a Sanskrit medical work attributed to Bharadvaja. **Bull Indian Inst Hist Med (Hyderabad)** 1975 Jul;5(3):123-8
Siddiqi T: Unani medicine in India 1524 to 1605 A.D. **Indian J Hist Sci** 1981;16(1):22-5

### Italy

Busacchi V: Marcello Malpighi (1628-1694), lettore a Bologna, Pisa e Messina, archiatra pontificio. **Strenna Stor Bolognese** 1978;28:81-98
Engelhardt D von, Henkelmann T: Eine medizinhistorische Exkursion in die Renaissance der Toskana. **Wolfenbutteler Renaiss Mitt** 1980;4:87-92
Engelhardt DV, Henkelmann T: Una excursión de história de la medicina con el renacimiento de la toscana. **Folia Hum (Barc)** 1981;19(216):49-56
Głowacki WW: Ustawy medyczne Królestwa Sycylii z lat 1140-1241. **Arch Hist Med (Warsz)** 1983;46(2):137-47
Kapronczay K: Két kevéssé ismert 15. századi orvostörténeti munka. **Orv Hetil** 1983 Jul 10;124(28):1701-5
Matsen HS: Giovanni Garzoni (1419-1505) to Alessandro Achillini (1463-1512): An unpublished letter and defense. In Edward P Mahoney, ed. Philosophy and humanism: Renaissance essays in honor of Paul Oskar Kristeller. New York: Columbia Univ. Press, 1976. p. 518-530.
Olagüe Ros G: Elaboración y difusión de la medicina moderna en la Italia de los siglos XVI y XVII: la peculiaridad del ambiente científico romano (1548-1720). In Albarracin Teulon A, et al, ed: Medicina e Historia. Madrid, Edic. Univ. Comp., 1973. p. 265-90.
Ruggiero G: The status of physicians and surgeons in Renaissance Venice. **J Hist Med Allied Sci** 1981 Apr;36(2):168-84
Saraf PG, Cockett AT: Marcello Malpighi--a tribute. **Urology** 1984 Jun;23(6):619-23
Simili A: Spigolature medicine fra gli inediti aldrovandiani. **Archiginnasio (Italy)** 1968-70;63-65(1):361-488

### Mexico

López Austín A: De las plantas medicinales y de otras cosas medicinales. **Estud Cult Nahuatl** 1971;9:125-230
Micheli A de: Los primeros libros médicos novohispanos. **Arch Inst Cardiol Mex** 1980 Jan-Feb;50(1):107-10
Risse GB: Medicine in New Spain: Institutions and practice 1570-1621. In International Congress of the History of Medicine, 27th, Barcelona, 1980. Actas. Barcelona, Académia de Ciències Médiques de Catalunya i Balears, 1981. p. 207-11.
Sepúlveda MT: Practicas medicas entre los purepecha prehispanicos. **Bol Soc Mex Hist Filos Med** 1980 Sep-Dec;5(32-33):67-81
Somolinos d'Ardois G: El fenomeno de fusion cultural y su trascendencica medica. México, Juan Somolinos Palencia, 1979. (Capitulos de Historia Medica Mexicana, II), p. 99-173.
Somolinos d'Ardois G: Francisco Bravo y su opera medicinalia. **Bol Inst Invest Bibliogr** 1970;4:337-88
Somolinos d'Ardois G: Relacion alfabetica de los profesionistas medicos, o en conexion con la medicina, que practicaron en territorio mexicano (1521-1618). México, Sociedad Mexicana de Historia y Filosofía de la Medicina, [1979?]. (Capitulos de historia medica mexicana, III). p. 175-312.
Somolinos Palencia J: El tiempo medico de Don Vasco de Quiroga. **Bol Soc Mex Hist Filos Med** 1980 Sep-Dec;5(32-33):123-35
Somolinos Palencia J: Vision general de la medicina en la Nueva España durante el siglo XVI. **Bol Soc Mex Hist Filos Med** 1982 Sep;6(40):61-70
Thiemer-Sachse U: Hygiene und Heilkunde bei den Azteca zur Zeit der spanischen Eroberung. **Abh Ber Staatl Mus Voelkerkd Dres** 1978;36:151-213

### Netherlands

Lindeboom GA: De verdiensten van Jan Swammerdam voor de medische wetenschap. **Ned Tijdschr Geneeskd** 1980 Dec 13;124(50):2135-41
Van Lieburg MJ: De genees- en heelkunde in de Noordelijke Nederlanden, gezien vanuit de stedelijke en chirurgijnsgilde-ordonnanties van de 16e eeuw. **Tijdschr Geschied Geneeskd** 1983;6(4):169-84

### Poland

Drygas A: Walka z partactwem aptekarskim i medycznym. **Arch Hist Med (Warsz)** 1981;44(3/4):329-43
Lisiewicz J: Jan Walenty Latos (1539--początek XVII w.) lekarz i astrolog Akademii Krakowskiej. **Wiad Lek** 1982 Dec 15;35(23-24):1589-91
Skulimowski M: Mikołaj Kopernik, wybitny predstawiciel medycyny XVI wieku w Polsce. Kraków, Akademia Medyczna, 1978. 84 p.
Szpilczyński S: Jan Jonston z Szamotuł. Tytaniczny trud barokowego erudyty w świetle wielkiej dydaktyki. **Slaski Kwart Hist Sobotka**

1976;31(2):223–9

**Romania**

Petrescu AD: D. în secolul XVI, un clujean: medic de faimă europeană. **Mag Istor** 1976;10(12):27

**Spain**

Alegría C: Medicos que estimularon a Cristobal Colón en su actividad precursora al descubrimiento de America. **Rev Soc Venez Hist Med** 1969–71;17–19(31–33):199–203

Carreras Panchón A: El ejercicio profesional segun el testimonio de Gaspar Tristan. **Asclepio** 1980;32:87–92

Ferrer D: La sanidad en las 'Leyes de los reinos de las indias'. In International Congress of the History of Medicine, 27th, Barcelona, 1980. Actas. Barcelona, Académia de Ciències Médiques de Catalunya i Balears, 1981. p. 172–6.

Granjel LS: La medicina española del siglo XVII. Salamanca, Ediciones Universidad de Salamanca, 1978. 250 p.

Granjel LS: La medicina española renacentista. Salamanca, Ediciones Universidad de Salamanca, 1980. 289 p. (Historia general de la medicina española, II).

Lopez Piñero JM, Bujosa Homar F: Tradición y renovación de los saberes médicos en la España del siglo XVI. **Med Esp** 1978;77:355–66

López Piñero JM, Bujosa Homar F: Tradicion y renovacion en la medicina española del siglo XVI. **Asclepio** 1978–79;30–31:285–306

Price R: Spanish medicine in the Golden Age. **J R Soc Med** 1979 Nov;72(11):864–74

Riera i Montserrat F: Remeis amatoris, pactes amb el dimoni, encanteris, per a saber de persones absents, cercadors de tresors, remeis per a la salut: bruixes i bruixots davant la inquisició de Mallorca en el segle XVII. Barcelona, Pequña Biblioteca Calamus Scriptorius, 1979. 61 p.

Sayans Castaños M: Importante impulso en el conocimiento cientifico dado por un medico placentino del siglo XVI. In: Sociedad Española de Historia de la Medicina. V Congreso Nacional. Madrid, 1977. **Asclepio** 1977;29:343–50

Somolinos Palencia J: Cristobal Mendez medico y cientifico del siglo XVI. **Bol Soc Mex Hist Filos Med** 1982 Jun;6(39):43–7

Torre E: Las 'Conclusiones' del doctor Estrada de Madrid, contra los 'Avisos particulares' del doctor Hidalgo de Aguero, sevillano. **Asclepio** 1978–79;30–31:389–401

**Sweden**

Hoorn CM van: Willem Lemnius [William Lemnius]. **Spiegel Hist** 1980:15(2):111–4

Perret L: Benedictus Olai: een nyttigh Läkere-Book 1578. Ett 400–årsminne. Några synpunkter på 1500–talets läkekonst. **Nord Medicinhist Arsb** 1980;Suppl 6:118–21

Sjöberg SG: Magister Salomon Rummels libri medici. **Sydsven Medicinhist Sallsk Arsskr** 1982;19:119–36

**Switzerland**

Blaser RH: Paracelsus in Basel. Festschrift für Professor Dr. Robert-Henri Blaser zum 60. Geburtstag. Herausgegeben von der Schweizerischen Paracelsus-Gesellschaft. Biographical introduction by K. Goldammer. Muttenz/Basel, St. Arbogast Verlag, 1979. 210 p. (Reprint of 7 works by Blaser).

Koelbing HM: 'De conceptu et generatione hominis'. Die lateinische Fassung von Jakob Rueffs 'Trostbüchle', Zürich 1554. In International Congress of the History of Medicine, 27th, Barcelona, 1980. Actas. Barcelona, Académia de Ciències Médiques de Catalunya i Balears, 1981. p. 271–5.

Kollautz A: Eine Episode aus der Praxis des Paracelsus. **Carinthia** 1967;157:578–87

Schürmann-Roth J: 'Modus et ratio visendi aegros' des Solothurner Arztes Johann Jakob Scharandaeus (1630–1682). **Gesnerus** 1980;37(1/2):73–82

**United States**

Given FT: Dr. John Pott: maligned early patriot. **Am J Obstet Gynecol** 1983 Sep 15;147(2):115–20

Riker DM: Surgeon Hans Kierstede of New Amsterdam. **Halve Maen** 1983;57(3):11–3, 24

**USSR**

Alekseev GA: Pervye lekari srednego povolzhía. **Sov Zdravookhr** 1983;(4):68–70

Appleby JH: Doctor Christopher Reitinger and a seal of Tsar Boris Godunov. **Oxf Slav Pap** 1979;12:32–9

**Venezuela**

Fortique JR: Hernán Pérez de la Muela, primer médico europeo establecido en Venezuela. **Bol Acad Nac Hist (Caracas)** 1979;62(245):147–58

**1700 to Present**

Achterberg E: Albert Schweitzer: ein Leben in der Zeitenwende. Hameln, Soltsien, 1968. 88 p.

Antall J: Wien und Budapest im Lebenswerk Semmelweis'. In Ganzinger K, Skopec M, Wyklicky H, ed: Festschrift für Erna Lesky zum 70. Geburtstag. Wien, Brüder Hollinek, 1981. p. 13–23.

Appleby JH: 'Rhubarb' Mounsey and the Surinam toad--a Scottish physician--naturalist in Russia. **Arch Nat Hist** 1982 Oct;11(1):137–52

Armstrong D: The doctor-patient relationship: 1930–80. In P. Wright, A. Treacher, ed: The problem of medical knowledge. Examining the social construction of medicine. Edinburgh, Edinburgh University Press, 1982. p. 109–22.

Berliner H: Medical modes of production. In P. Wright, A. Treacher, ed: The problem of medical knowledge. Examining the social construction of medicine. Edinburgh, Edinburgh University Press, 1982. p. 162–73.

Bernard J: L'espérance, ou le nouvel état de la médecine. Paris, Editions Buchet/Chastel, 1978. 255 p.

Bílek V, Niklíček L: K hlavním otázkám historie Ceskoslovensko-sovětských lékãrských styku vletech 1918–1952. **Cesk Zdrav** 1981 Apr;29(4):133–46

Blank RH, Ostheimer JM: Biomedical policy. **Policy Stud Rev** 1982;1(4):789–99

Blantz TE: Thomas Anthony Dooley. In Dictionary of American biography, 1961–1965. Suppl. 7, 1981. p. 190–1.

Bloom SW: Sociohistorical perspectives [on the therapeutic relationship]. In Reich WT, et al, ed: Encyclopedia of bioethics, v.4. New York, Free Press, 1978. p. 1663–68.

Bourget P, Blouin CB: Histoire de la médecine depuis 1940. Plus de progrès en 40 ans qu'en 40 siècles. Paris, Presses de la Cité, 1983. 254 p.

Brady AP: Medical achievements this century--high technology or community health approach. **Ir J Med Sci** 1983 Nov;152(11):413–9

Branca P, ed: The medicine show. Patients, physicians and the perplexities of the health revolution in modern society. New York, Science History Publications, 1977. viii, 280 p. (Mostly articles reprinted from Journal of Social History, vol. 10, Summer 1977).

Brügelmann J: Medikalisierung von Säuglings- und Erwachsenenalter in Deutschland zu Beginn des 19. Jahrhunderts aufgrund von medizinischen Topographien. In Imhof AE, ed.: Leib und Leben in der Geschichte der Neuzeit. Berlin, Duncker & Humblot, 1983. p. 177–92.

Büttner J: Interrelationships between clinical medicine and clinical chemistry, illustrated by the example of the German-speaking countries in the late 19th century. **J Clin Chem Clin Biochem** 1982 Jun;20(6):465–71

Bynum WF: Health, disease and medical care. In G. S. Rousseau, R. Porter, ed. The ferment of knowledge. Studies in the historiography of eighteenth-century science. Cambridge, Cambridge University Press, 1980. p. 211–53.

Cassell EJ: Changing ideas of causality in medicine. **Soc Res (NY)** 1979;46(4):728–43

Català F: Autour d'une consultation par correspondance sous l'Empire. In Congrés International d'Història de la Medicina Catalana, 2nd, Barcelona, 1975. Llibre d'Actes. Barcelona, Socitra, 1977. p. 133–7.

Cockerham WC: The state of medical sociology in the United States, Great Britain, West Germany and Austria: applied vs pure theory. **Soc Sci Med** 1983;17(20):1513–27

Cohen D: The last 100 years, medicine. New York, M. Evans, 1981. 192 p.

Cooter R: Anticontagionism and history's medical record. In P. Wright, A. Treacher, ed: The problem of medical knowledge. Examining the social construction of medicine. Edinburgh, Edinburgh University Press, 1982. p. 87–108.

Corsi P, Weindling P, ed: Information sources in the history of science and medicine. London, Boston, Butterworth Scientific, 1983. xvi, 531 p. (Butterworth Guides to Information Sources).

Crellin JK, Helfand WH: Medical care in the 20th century. Facets of change illustrated by American and British postcards. Durham, Duke University Medical Center, 1982. 106 p. (Readings and Perspectives in Medicine, Booklet Number 3).

Dahlström G: Medicinsk utveckling och grundforskning i historiskt perspektiv. **Nord Medicinhist Arsbok** 1983;:117–25

Fichtner G, ed: Laufende wissenschaftshistorische Dissertationen (LWD). Verzeichnis in Bearbeitung befindlicher Dissertationen auf dem Gebiet der Geschichte der Medizin, der Pharmazie, der Naturwissenschaften und der Technik. Nr. 1, Tübingen, Institut für Geschichte der Medizin, 1981. 125 p.

Forman R: Medical resistance to innovation. **Med Hypotheses** 1981 Aug;7(8):1009–17

Frascani P: Il medico nell'ottocento. **Studi Stor** 1982;23(3):617–37

García JC: Medicina y sociedad. Las corrientes de pensamiento en el campo de la salud. **Educ Med Salud** 1983;17(4):363–97

Gilder SS: Mavericks in medicine. **S Afr Med J** 1984 Aug 18;66(7):252–5

González-Pedrero E: La medicina del siglo XX y su proyección futura. III. Salud, sociedad y política. **Gac Med Mex** 1981 Nov;117(11):428–33

Habrich C: Mediziner und Medizinisches am Hofe des Grafen Casimir zu Sayn-Wittgenstein (1687–1741). **Beitr Gesch Pharm**

1983;31(18/19):138–44
Heirs of Hippocrates: The development of medicine in a catalogue of historic books in the Health Sciences Library, The University of Iowa. Compiled by R. Eimas, E. Holtum, D. Curry. Iowa City, Friends of the University of Iowa Libraries, 1980. xiv, 474 p.
Hoffman W, Shields J: Doctors on the new frontier: breaking through the barriers of modern medicine. New York, Macmillan, 1981. xi, 207 p.
Hordern A: Changing pattern of health care in western countries. In Stanley NF, Joske RA, ed: Changing disease patterns and human behaviour. London, New York, Academic Press, 1980. p. 371–85.
Houtzager HL: A letter from Herman Boerhaave to Johan Philip Burggraaf jr. **Janus** 1980:67(1-2-3):201-5
Imhof AE: Man and body in the history of the modern age. Reflections on an International Symposium in Berlin, 1-3 December 1981. **Med Hist** 1983 Oct;27(4):394-406
Ingelfinger FJ: Medicine. Status and future of applied sciences. **Science** 1980 Jul 4;209(4452):123-6
International Congress of the History of Medicine, 26th, Plovdiv [Bulgaria], 20-25 August 1978: Actes du Congres, 2 volumes. Sofia, 1980-81. Articles in Russian, French, English, German.
Jinich H: La medicina del siglo XX y su proyección futura. IV. Rasgos esenciales de la medicina del siglo XX. **Gac Med Mex** 1981 Nov;117(11):434-8
Kaiser W: Die hallisch-englischen Wissenschaftbeziehungen in der Medizin des 18. Jahrhunderts. **Wiss Z Martin Luther Univ (Math)** 1976;25(5):71-90
Kalisch BJ, Kalisch PA: The Dionne quintuplets legacy: establishing the 'good doctor and his loyal nurse' image in American culture. **Nurs Health Care** 1984 May;5(5):242-51
Kenéz J: 125 éve született Friedrich Kraus (1858-1936). **Orv Hetil** 1984 Oct 28;125(44):2691-3
Koch E: Arzte, die Geschichte machten: Sternkunden der Heilkunde in 30 Lebensbildern. Augsburg, Hofmann, 1981. 195 p.
Kotwas J, Meyer-Wilmes J, Ohlendorf D, ed: Pharmazie und Medizin--Grenzen und Möglichkeiten. Verhandlungsbericht über eine Internationale Tagung der Arbeitsgemeinschaft Deutscher Krankenhausapotheker in Zusammenarbeit mit der Bayerischen Internistenvereinigung München, 18.-19.April 1980. Berlin, Acron, 1981. 152 p. Contributions by R. Winau, D. Ohlendorf, A.G. Hildebrandt, W. Weissauer, R. Quintiliani, D.D. Breimer, R. Preisig, T. Zysset, D. Adam, H. Remmer, G. Dirheimer, K.H. Beyer, H.P.T. Ammon.
Kozlov AM, Kel'ner MS, Losev NI: K. Marks is problemy meditsiny (k 165-letiiu so dnia rozhdeniia K. Marksa). **Patol Fiziol Eksp Ter** 1983 May-Jun;3:3-9
Kunitz SJ: The historical roots and ideological functions of disease concepts in three primary care specialties. **Bull Hist Med** 1983 Fall;57(3):412-32
McCullough LB, Page BB, Blomquist C, et al: [History of medical ethics in contemporary Europe and the Americas]. In Reich WT, et al, ed: Encyclopedia of bioethics, v.3. New York, Free Press, 1978. p. 975-1007.
McKeown T: The role of medicine. Dream, mirage or nemesis? Princeton, Princeton University Press, Oxford, Basil Blackwell, 1979. xvi, 207 p.
Mangel C, Weisse AB: Medicine: the state of the art. New York, Dial Press, 1984. 304 p.
Müller B: Franz Kiwisch, Ritter von Rotterau 1814-1851. Diss. Würzburg, 1980. 111 p.
Nation EF, McGovern JP, ed: Student and chief: the Osler-Camac correspondence. Pasadena, Castle Press, 1980. 131 p.
Nicolle P, Jude A: Réflexions sur les prix Nobel de physiologie ou médecine. **Hist Sci Med** 1980;14(1):83-93
Niklíček L, Müller C: Uloha historie a historické methody v sociálním lékařství. **Cesk Zdrav** 1980 Oct;28(10):416-21
Peter CH: Der Briefwechsel zwischen Paulus Usteri und Melchior Aepli. Zürich, Juris Druck, 1983. 161 p. (Zürcher Medizingeschichtliche Abhandlungen, Neue Reihe, Nr. 155).
Puma FA: Cientificismo (enfermedad de nuestros días). **Rev Soc Venez Hist Med** 1981;30(45-46):57-83
Rose JC, Corn M: Dr. E. and other patients: new lessons from old case reports. **J Hist Med Allied Sci** 1984 Jan;39(1):3-32
Rousseau GS: Ephebi, Epigoni, and Fornacalia: some meditations on the contemporary historiography of the eighteenth century. **Eighteenth Cent Stud** 1979;20:203-26
Schadewaldt H: 100 Jahre deutsch-japanische medizinische Zusammenarbeit. **Dtsch Med Wochenschr** 1980 Oct 17;105(42):1473-7
Schneck P: Iz istorii russko-nemetskikh meditsinskikh sviazeĭ. **Sov Zdravookhr** 1982;(4):61-3
Seidler E: Le rôle de la méthode historique dans la médecine actuelle. In Poirier J, Poirier JL, ed: Médecine et philosohie à la fin du XIXe siècle. Paris, Université de Paris XII - Val de Marne, [1980?]. p. 149-55.
Shortt SE: Clinical practice and the social history of medicine: a theoretical accord. **Bull Hist Med** 1981 Winter;55(4):533-42
Shortt SE: Medical professionalization: pitfalls and promise in the historiography. **HSTC** 1981 Sep;19(5 no 3):210-9
Silló-Seidl G: Arzte ohne Nobelpreis deren Entdeckungen Millionen Menschen geholfen haben. Genf, Ariston, 1978. 256 p.
Spears J, Sydenham D: The evolution of medical practice in two marginal areas of the Western World, 1750-1830. **Hist Reflect** 1982;9(1-2):195-212
Strojnowski J: Orientacja biologiczna a orientacja społeczna w medycynie w ujeciu historycznym. **Arch Hist Med (Warsz)** 1984;47(1):25-37
Szemkeö E: A német orvostudomány szerepe a magyar -- orosz orvosi kapcsolatok XVIII -- XIX. századi történetében. **Orv Hetil** 1981 Jan 11;122(2):104, 107-8
Ten Have HA: Geneeskunde en filosofie, aspecten van een wisselvallige relatie. **Ned Tijdschr Geneeskd** 1982 Apr 10,126(15):668-73
Tsouyopoulos N: Die neue Auffassung der klinischen Medizin als Wissenschaft unter dem Einfluss der Philosophie im frühen 19. Jahrhundert. **Ber Wissenschaftsgesch** 1978;1(1-2):87-100
Vzaimootnosheniia A.I. Gertsena i S. P. Botkina: **Klin Med (Mosk)** 1983 Jun;61(6):108-10
Webb CH: An exciting half century in medicine. **Pharos** 1980 Winter;43(1):14-9
Webster C, ed: Biology, medicine and society 1840-1940. Cambridge, Cambridge University Press, 1981. 344 p. (Past and Present Publications).
Whitby JD: Alcohol in anaesthesia and surgical resuscitation. **Anaesthesia** 1980 May;35(5):502-5
Williams G: The age of miracles. Medicine and surgery in the nineteenth century. London, Constable, 1981. 234 p.
Wunderlich CA: Wien und Paris. Ein Beitrag zur Geschichte und Beurteilung der gegenwärtigen Heilkunde in Deutschland und Frankreich, 1841. Herausgegeben und eingeleitet von H. M. Koelbing. Bern, Huber, 1974. 159 p. (Hubers Klassiker der Medizin und der Naturwissenschaften, Bd. 13).

### Africa

Beck A: Recent changes in attitude toward medicine in East Africa. In: Congrès international d'histoire de la médecine, XXVe, Québec, 1976. Actes. Québec, 1977. p. 493-501.
Domergue D: [French sanitary services on the Ivory Coast.] (Fre). **Rev Fr Hist Outre Mer** 1979;65
Feierman S: History of pluralistic medical systems. Change in African therapeutic systems. **Soc Sci Med [Med Anthropol]** 1979 Dec;13B(4):277-84
Ferguson D: Civilisation for Africa: a study of the impact of modern scientific medicine on Africa. Port Elizabeth, South Africa, E. H. Walton Co., 1981. 160 p.
Gish O: The political economy of primary care and 'health by the people': an historical explanation. **Issue** 1979 Fall;9:6-13
Maier D: Nineteenth-century Asante medical practices. **Comp Stud Soc Hist** 1979;21:63-81
Sabben-Clare EE, Bradley DJ, Kirkwood K, ed: Health in tropical Africa during the colonial period: based on the proceedings of a symposium held at New College, Oxford, 21-23 March 1977. Oxford, Clarendon, 1980. ix, 276 p.
Sai FT: [Medical ethics in modern] sub-Saharan Africa. In Reich WT, et al, ed: Encyclopedia of bioethics, v. 2. New York, Free Press, 1978. p. 897-900.

### Americas

Desrosiers G: Evolution de la médecine et répercussion sur la formation médicale en Amérique du Nord. **Union Med Can** 1981 Sep;110(9):817-20
Plaza Izquierdo F: Medicos presidentes de America. **Rev Soc Venez Hist Med** 1976;24(38):19-36

### Arabic

Abdul-Rauf M: Contemporary Muslim perspective [on medical ethics]. In Reich WT, et al, ed: Encyclopedia of bioethics, v. 2. New York, Free Press, 1978. p. 892-5.
Asper SP, Haddad FS: [History of medical ethics in the] contemporary Arab world. In Reich WT, et al, ed: Encyclopedia of bioethics, v. 2. New York, Free Press, 1978. p. 888-91.
Diaz Garcia A: Three medical recipes in Codex Biblioteca Medicea-Laurenziana Or. 215. **J Hist Arabic Sci** 1980;4:265-86
Kaiser W, Piechocki W: Das hallesche Collegium Orientale und seine Ausstrahlung auf die medizinische Arabistik des 18. Jahrhunderts. **Wiss Z Martin Luther Univ (Math)** 1978;27(5):111-32

### Argentina

Aznárez EP: Juan Bialet Massé, ilustre médico catalán emigrado a la Argentina. In International Congress of the History of Medicine, 27th, Barcelona, 1980. Actas. Barcelona, Académia de Ciències Mèdiques de Catalunya i Balears, 1981. p. 165-7.
Burguéz NA: Los pioneros de la medicina en San Juan de la frontera la institucionalizacion de la medicina en la accíon de los pioneros Sanjuaninos del siglo XIX. In Congreso de Historia de la Medicina Argentina [Transactions], 5th, Mendoza, 1983. p. 183-96.
Kohn Loncarica AG: Contribuciones originales de la medicina argentina a la medicina universal. **Asclepio** 1981;33:411-24
Martín de Codoni EL: Apuntes para un estudio de los pioneros de la medicina en Mendoza en el siglo XIX. In Congreso de Historia de la Medicina Argentina [Transactions], 5th, Mendoza, 1983. p. 145-82.

# MEDICINE

Quiroga MI: Un centro medico en Paris formado por colegas argentinos en 1901. **Bol Acad Nac Med B Aires** 1980;58:611-2

**Asia**

Lucas A: Chinese Medical Modernization. Comparative Policy Continuities, 1930s-1980s. New York, Praeger, 1982. xiii, 188 p.

**Australia**

Clasen U: Deutsche und deutschstämmige Arzte in New South Wales und South Australia zwischen 1846 und 1911. Diss., Universität Düsseldorf. Düsseldorf, 1982. 66 p.
Hicks R: Rum regulation and riches. Sydney, Australian Hospital Association, 1981. vii, 231 p.
Pearn J, O'Carrigan C, ed: Australia's quest for colonial health: some influences on early health and medicine in Australia. Herston, Brisbane, Royal Children's Hospital, 1983. xii, 304 p.
Phillips PJ: Kill or cure? Lotions, potions, characters & quacks of early Australia. Adelaide, Rigby, 1978. 157 p.
Stubbe JH, Scrymgeour JM, Smith AJ: Medical background; History of Fremantle hospitals and doctors. [Nedlands], Published for the Fremantle Hospital Board by the Univ. of Western Australia Press, 1969. xxvi, 82 p.

**Austria**

Gerhartl G: Dr. med. Franz Lorenz (1805-1883). **Mitt Krems Stadtarch** 1971;11:107-14
Leitner H: Die jüdischen Arzte in Osterreich und ihr Beitrag zur medizinischen Wissenschaft. In K. Lohrmann, ed: 1000 Jahre Osterreichisches Judentum. Ausstellungskatalog. Eisenstadt, 1982. p. 161-92.
Lesky E: Heilkunde und Gesundheitswesen unter Maria Theresia. **Osterr Apoth Ztg** 1980 May 17;34(20):357-60
Lesky E: Meilensteine der Wiener Medizin. Grosse Arzte Osterreichs in drei Jahrhunderten. Wien, Wilhelm Maudrich, 1981. 251 p.
Premuda L: The influence of the nineteenth-century Vienna School on Italian medicine: the roles of Padua and Trieste. In Stevenson LG, ed: A celebration of medical history. Baltimore, Johns Hopkins University Press, 1982. (The Henry E. Sigerist supplements to the Bulletin of the History of Medicine; new ser., no. 6). p. 180-99. With commentary by J. J. Bylebyl, p. 200-11.
Wyklicky H: Förderer der Heilkunde. Medizin und Gesundheitswesen Josephs II. In: Was blieb von Joseph II.? Eine Dokumentation; Internationales Symposion Melk, 1980. [Vienna?], Edition Morgen, 1980. p. 66-76.
Wyklicky H: 'Prima inter pares' - Uber die Wiener interne Medizin am Beginn des 20. Jahrhunderts. **Wien Klin Wochenschr** 1983 Sep 16;95(17):601-6

**Belgium**

Darquenne R: Médecine et chirurgie hainuyères au siècle des lumières. **Ann Cerc Archeol Mons** 1976-77;70:139-76
Flameng F: La journée d'un médecin de Bruxelles en 1830. **Folkl Brabancon** 1979 Jun;222:171-214
Kelecom J: Episodes de la médecine liégeoise. Le souvenir de Paracelse au siècle des lumières. **Rev Med Liege** 1981 Sep 1;36(17):638-46
Pasteels JJ: Albert Dalcq, 1893-1973. In Florilège des Sciences en Belgique - II. Bruxelles, Académie Royale de Belgique, 1980. p. 625-39.

**Belize**

Herrmann EK: Health care services in 19th century British Honduras. **Soc Sci Med [Med Psychol Med Sociol]** 1980 Jun;14(4):353-6

**Botswana**

Dennis C: The role of dingaka tsa setswana from the 19th century to the present. **Botsw Notes Rec** 1978;10:53-66

**Brazil**

Costa Filho M: O Erário mineral de Luiz Gomes Ferreira. **Rev Inst Hist Geogr Bras** 1957;235:331-40
De Moulin D: Medizinische und naturwissenschaftliche Aspekte der Regierungszeit des Grafen Johann Moritz von Nassau als Gouverneur in Brasilien (1637-1644). In: Soweit der Erdkreis reicht. J. M. von Nassau-Siegen 1604-1679. Kleve: Städtisches Museum Haus Koekkoek. 1979. pp. 33-46.
Sousa L de C: Miguel Pereira: um cidadão exemplar. **Rev Inst Hist Geogr Bras** 1973;298:306-14

**Bulgaria**

Dulieu L: Les relations entre la Bulgarie et la faculté de médecine de Montpellier (1878-1944). In: International Congress of the History of Medicine, 26th, Plovdiv (Bulgaria), 1978. Actes du Congres, Vol. 1. Sofia, 1980. p. 102-10.
Glavchev P: Pogled vŭrkhu istoriiata na Druzhestvoto na internistite v Bŭlgariia (po sluchaĭ 50 godini ot osnovavaneto mu). **Vutr Boles** 1984;23(2):140-3
Mikhailov C: Etappes dans le développement de l'organisation de l'expertise médicale de la capacité de travail dans la republique populaire de Bulgarie. In International Congress of the History of Medicine. 26th, Plovdiv, 1978. Actes du Congress. Sofia, 1981. Volume II. p. 77-8.
Pavlova V: Istoriografiia meditsinskoĭ nauki v Bolgarii. **Sov Zdravookhr** 1980;(9):41-5
Percebois G: Les Bulgares et la Faculté de Médecine de Nancy à la fin du XIXe siècle et au début du XXe siècle. In International Congress of the History of Medicine. 26th, Plovdiv, 1978. Actes du Congress. Sofia, 1981. Volume II. p. 179-82.
Petkova M: Naukometrichna kharakteristika na publikuvanoto nauchno tvorchestvo na professor Konstantin Chilov. **Vutr Boles** 1984;23(4):102-8
Todorov D: D-r Neno TSarvulvanov. Sofiia, Meditsina i fizkultura, 1981. 113 p.
Vutreshnata meditsina u nas prez poslednoto stoletie: **Vutr Boles** 1979;18(5):1-9
Zaprianov NI, Kazandzhiev NK: D-r Stoian Chomakov. Sofiia, Meditsina i fizkultura, 1979.

**Burma**

Khin Thet Htar: Annotated bibliography of medical literature on Burma, 1866-1976. With supplement up to 1980. New Delhi, World Health Organization, South-East Asia Regional Office, 1981. vii, 484, 35 p. (WHO Regional Publications. South-East Asia series, no. 13).

**Cameroon**

Neumann J: Eingeborenenheilkunde und Europäische Medizin in Kamerun. Arzt und Kranker in der Konfrontation zweier Kulturen. Freiburg, Schulz, 1978. 254 p. (Freiburger Forschungen zur Medizingeschichte, Neue Folge, 7).

**Canada**

Andrews MW: Medical attendance in Vancouver, 1886-1920. **BC Stud** 1978-79(40):32-56
Andrews MW: Medical services in Vancouver, 1886-1920. A study in the interplay of attitudes, medical knowledge, and administrative structures. Ph.D. Diss. The University of British Columbia. Victoria, 1979.
Angus MS: Horatio Yates. In Dictionary of Canadian biography, 1881-1890. 1982;11:940-1.
Angus MS: John Robinson Dickson. In Dictionary of Canadian biography, 1881-1890. 1982;11:263-4.
Aucoin P: Public policy analysis and the Canadian health care system. **Can Public Adm** 1980;23(1):166-74
Bernier J: François Blanchet et le mouvement réformiste en médecine au début du XIXe siècle. **Rev Hist Am Fr** 1980;34(2):223-44
Bernier J: La standardisation des études médicales et la consolidation de la profession dans la deuxième moitié du XIXe siècle. **Rev Hist Am Fr** 1983;37(1):51-65
Bernier J: Le corps médical québecois à la fin du XVIIIe siècle. In Roland CG, ed: Health, disease and medicine. Toronto, Hannah Institute for the History of Medicine, 1984. p. 36-64.
Bernier J: Les practiciens de la santé à Québec, 1871-1921: quelques données statistiques. **Rech Sociogr** 1979;20(1):41-58
Bernier J: L'integration du corps médical Quebeçois à la fin du XIXe siècle. **Hist Reflect** 1983;10(1):91-113
Bernier J: Pierre Beaubien. In Dictionary of Canadian biography, 1881-1890. 1982;11:57-8.
Bredin TF: Henry Septimus Beddome. In Dictionary of Canadian biography, 1881-1890. 1982;11:63-4.
Brown MC: The health care crisis in historical perspective. **Can J Public Health** 1979 Sep-Oct;70(5):300-6
Campbell BJ: Springhill's first doctor. **NS Hist Q** 1979;9(4):297-312
Chi nien Pai Ch'iu-en: in memory of Norman Bethune. Pei-ching, Jen min ch'u pan she, 1979. 285 p.
Coburn D, Torrance GM, Kaufert JM: Medical dominance in Canada in historical perspective: the rise and fall of medicine? **Int J Health Serv** 1983;13(3):407-32
Craig GM: Michael Barrett. In Dictionary of Canadian biography, 1881-1890. 1982;11:53-4.
Desjardins E: Joseph Emery-Coderre. In Dictionary of Canadian biography, 1881-1890. 1982;11:302-3.
Durley MS: Dr. Edmund Bailey O'Callaghan, his early years in medicine, Montreal, 1823-1828. **Study Sess Can Cathol Hist Assoc** 1980;47:23-40
Edwards GT: Bella Coola: Indian and European medicines. **Beaver** 1980;311(3):4-11
Gelfand T: Medicine in New France: les francais look at les canadiens during the seven years' war. In International Congress of the History of Medicine, 27th, Barcelona, 1980. Actas. Barcelona, Académia de

Ciències Mèdiques de Catalunya i Balears, 1981. p. 511-6.
Gidney RD, Millar WP: The origins of organized medicine in Ontario, 1850-1869. In Roland CG, ed: Health, disease and medicine. Toronto, Hannah Institute for the History of Medicine, 1894. p. 65-95.
Godfrey CM: Medicine for Ontario: a history. Belleville, Ont., Mika Pub. Co., 1979. 302 p.
Holling SA: Medicine for heroes: a neglected part of pioneer life. [Mississauga, Ont.], Mississauga South Historical Society in association with the Boston Mills Press, 1981. 93 p.
Lamb WK: William Fraser Tolmie. In Dictionary of Canadian biography, 1881-1890. 1982;11:885-8.
Leblond S: James Douglas. In Dictionary of Canadian biography, 1881-1890. 1982;11:271-2.
Meilicke CA, ed, Storch J, ed: Perspectives on Canadian health and social services policy. Edmonton, Faculty of Medicine, Univ. of Alberta, 1978. xii, 520 p.
Painchaud R: Théogène Fafard. In Dictionary of Canadian biography, 1881-1890. 1982;11:306-7.
Rasporich AW, Getty IA: George Verey. In Dictionary of Canadian biography, 1881-1890. 1982;11:900-1.
Rogers IL: John Mackieson. In Dictionary of Canadian biography, 1881-1890. 1982;11:565-6.
Roland CG: George William Campbell. In Dictionary of Canadian biography, 1881-1890. 1982;11:148-9.
Roland CG: Health and disease among the early Loyalists in Upper Canada. **Can Med Assoc J** 1983 Mar 1;128(5):587-95
Simkin RJ: The inadequacy of health care of women. **Atlantis** 1979;4(2 pt 2):63-70
Tumbridge JE: Separation of [the doctor's] residence from workplace: a Kingston example. **Urban Hist Rev** 1979;(3):23-32

### Chile

Costa-Casaretto C: Don Diego Portales y el Dr. Guillermo C. Blest. **Rev Med Chil** 1984 Jun;112(6):625-31
Costa-Casaretto C: El Dr. D. Jose de Passamán. **Rev Med Chil** 1984 May;112(5):503-8
Costa-Casaretto C: Esomenología (en vez del híbrido futurología) médica. Una visita de médico en 1978, soñada en ... 1878. **Rev Med Chil** 1981 Sep;109(9):901-9
Costa-Casaretto C: Presentación del Dr. Pedro Morán (1771-1840). **Rev Med Chil** 1984 Jul;112(7):729-38
Ionov IuV: Sal'vador Al'ende i ego meditsinskaia deiatel'nost'. **Feldsher Akush** 1981;46(2):39-41
Juricic B: Chile y las organizaciones internacionales de salud. **Rev Med Chil** 1977 Oct;105(10):674-9
Medina E: Bibliografía comentada de la medicina tradicional chilena. **Med Tradic** 1982;3(11):17-26
Medina E: Contribución a la historia de la medicina chilena: 1930-1982. **Rev Med Chil** 1983 Apr;111(4):368-79
Pérez G: Evolución de los recursos humanos y físicos de salud 1952-1977. **Rev Med Chil** 1977 Oct;105(10):732-8
Solar MA: La atención médica en Chile, 1952-1977: una contribución a su estudio. **Rev Med Chil** 1977 Oct;105(10):701-6

### China

Barootes EW: Dr. Norman Bethune: inspiration for a modern China. **Can Med Assoc J** 1980 May 24;122(10):1176-84
Chen KJ: [Historical data of medicine in Qing Dynasty: case records of westerners treated by traditional Chinese medicine] (Chi). **Chung Hsi I Chieh Ho Tsa Chih** 1981;1(2):122
Chu Tinxiang: [A sketch of the life of Lu Liuliang.] (Chi). **Chin J Med Hist** 1981;11:89-90
Gerngross R: Ein bayerischer Arzt in China. **MMW** 1980 Jan 25;122(4):141-2
Hillier SM, Jewell JA: Health care and traditional medicine in China, 1800-1982. London, Routledge & Kegan Paul, 1983, xix, 453 p.
Koo LC: Camminare su due gambe: la medicina nella Cina moderna. **Mondo Cinese** 1974;2(8):100-17
Kunz K: Chinese medicine: a history of revolution. **New Physician** 1979 Jan;28(1):28-30
Lampton DM: Performance and the Chinese political system: a preliminary assessment of education and health policies. **China Q** 1978;(75):509-39
Lisowski FP: The evolution of health care in China (concluded). **East Horiz** 1978;17(4):16-21
Lucas A: Changing medical models in China: organizational options or obstacles? **China Q** 1980;(83):461-89
Shumacker HB: An American surgeon's contribution to Chinese health care. **Am J Surg** 1981 Mar;141(3):311-6
Sun RS: Health services in the People's Republic of China: a blueprint for human and social development. Cambridge, Mass., Schenkman, 1980. xii, 123 p.
Unschuld PU: Das Ch'uan-ya und die Praxis chinesischer Landärzte im 18. Jahrhundert. **Sudhoffs Arch** 1978;62(4):378-407
Wu Y: [An appraisal on Zhang Xichun's thought of amalgamating traditional Chinese medicine with western medicine] (Chi). **Chung Hua I Shih Tsa Chih** 1984 Jan;14(1):16-8

### Colombia

Campo Posada A: Una vida, un médico. Bogota, Colombia, Ediciones Fondo Cultural Cafetero, [1982]. 248 p.
Hernández de Alba G: Una obra postuma cientifica monumental: la bibliografia medica Colombiana (1782-1976). **Bol Cult Bibliogr (Bogota)** 1976;16(7-8):176-9

### Czechoslovakia

Egy történelmi adat pontosításáról és Skoda orvos-beteg kapcsolatáról. **Orv Hetil** 1983 Jan 16;124(3):175-6
Berezowski S: Ceský vědecký přínos v programech sjezdu polských lékařu a přírodovědcu 100. Výročí prvního sjezdu polských lékařu a přírodovědcu. **Cas Lek Cesk** 1979 Nov 23;118(47):1463-5
Bouček K: Problematika zdraví v pracích českých utopistu. **Cas Lek Cesk** 1983 Oct 7;122(40):1217-20
Janeček M: [The father of modern academic medicine (Jan D. Panýrek)] (Cze). **Cas Lek Cesk** 1980;119:1446-8
Kroupa J: Lékařský rod Rincolini v osvíceneckém Brně. **Cas Lek Cesk** 1982 Nov 19;121(46):1429-30
Petrásek J, Adamec J: Prof. MUDr. Emerich Maixner 1847--1920, významná osobnost počátku českého vnitřního lékařství. **Cas Lek Cesk** 1980 Jun 13;119(23-24):684-6
Snajdr J, Thiel L: 30 let obvodního systému v CSSR--vývoj a perspektivy. **Cesk Zdrav** 1984 May;32(5):193-205
Stork A: Sto deset let rozvoje I. interní kliniky v Praze. **Cas Lek Cesk** 1981 Oct 1;120(39):1169-73
Urban F: Historie vzajemných styku ceských a ruských lékařu. **Cas Lek Cesk** 1984 Aug 17;123(33):1037
Vondráček V: Lékař dále vzpromíná (1920-1938). Praha, Avicenum, 1977. 481 p.

### Denmark

Kock W: Nordens första medicinska Nobelpris. **Nord Medicinhist Arsb** 1982;:110-21

### Egypt

Estes JW, Kuhnke L: French observations of disease and drug use in late eighteenth-century Cairo. **J Hist Med Allied Sci** 1984 Apr;39(2):121-52
Sonbol A: The creation of a medical profession in Egypt during the nineteenth century: a study in modernization. Ph.D. Diss., Georgetown University. Washington, D. C., 1981. iv, 296 p.
Sonbol A: The creation of a medical profession in Egypt during the nineteenth century: a study in modernization. Washington, D.C., [s.n.], 1981. iv, 296 p.

### Europe

Claus LM: The development of medical sociology in Europe. **Soc Sci Med** 1983;17(21):1591-7
Giovanni Alessandro Brambilla nella cultura medica del Settecento Europeo: Milano, Istituto Editoriale Cisalpino-La Goliardica, 1980. 371 p.
Lesky E: Die Wiener Medizinische Schule und die Donauländer. In Congress of History, Health, Culture of the Danubian Countries. 1. Novi Sad, 1975. p. 31-6.
Wysokiński A: Analiza rozwoju kadry lekarskiej w Europie w latach 1961-1975. **Wiad Lek** 1979 Nov 1;32(21):1573-7

### Finland

Heikkinen R: Lönnrot Kajaanin piirin ja linnan lääkärinä. **Duodecim** 1983;99(23-24):1726-9

### France

Ackerknecht EH: La médecine française de 1790 à 1850. **Bull Acad Natl Med (Paris)** 1981 Feb 17;Spec No:27-30
Ackerknecht EH: La médecine française de 1790 à 1850. **Bull Acad Natl Med (Paris)** 1981 Feb;165(2):225-8
Albury WR: Heart of darkness: J. N. Corvisart and the medicalization of life. **Hist Reflect** 1982;9(1-2):17-31.
Antoine ME, Waquet J: La médecine civile en France a l'époque napoléonienne et le legs du XVIIIe siècle: étude d'un recrutement professionnel. **Rev Inst Napoleon (Paris)** 1976;(132):67-90
Aron E: Bretonneau et sa légende. **Hist Sci Med** 1980;14(2):187-91
Balzac et la médecine de son temps: [Paris], Maison de Balzac, [1976?]. [98] p.
Bernard J: Laennec et la médecine moderne. **Nouv Rev Deux Mondes** 1981;4:13-9
Bertier de Sauvigny RP: Témoignages américains sur la médecine parisienne (1815-1848). **Hist Sci Med** 1980;14:439-47

# MEDICINE

Bidault R, Ledoux A: La vie médicale bisontine et comtoise à l'aube de l'ère pasteurienne (2ème moitié du XIXe siècle). In: Congrès National des Sociétés Savantes, 99e, Besançon, 1974. Comptes Rendus. Paris, 1976. Section des Sciences, Fasc. V. p. 161–70.
Biserte G: Les grands fondamentalistes médicaux lillois du début du siècle. **Hist Sci Med** 1980;14(1):115–21
Boulle L, Grmek MD, Lupovici C, et al: Laennec, Catalogue des manuscrits scientifiques. Paris, Masson, 1982. 316 p.
Bourgeois P: Laennec et son temps. **Sem Hop Paris** 1981 Dec 18–25;57(47–48):2047–56
Bourget P: Histoire de la médecine depuis 1940: plus de progrès en 40 ans qu'en siècles. [Paris], Presses de la cité, 1983. 254 p.
Bourrus R: Le Docteur Bourrus, professeur et médecin à Mont-de-Marsan (1820–1897). **Bull Soc Borda** 1982;107(386):197–200
Charle C: Histoire professionnelle, histoire sociale? Les médecins de l'ouest au XIXe siècle. **Ann Econ Soc Civilis** 1979;34(4):787–93
Comiti VP: La géographie médicale de la Corse à la fin du XVIIIe siècle. Genève, Droz, 1980. 142 p. (Centre de Recherches d'Histoire et de Philologie de la IVe Section de l'Ecole pratique des Hautes Etudes; Hautes Etudes Médiévales et Modernes, 41).
Commémoration du bicentenaire de la naissance de M.T.H. Laennec 1781–1826: **Bull Acad Natl Med (Paris)** 1981 Feb 17;Spec no.:1–61
Csillag I: David Gruby. **Orvostort Kozl** 1982;28(1–3):177–86
De Vaux de Foletier F: Anoblissements de médecins et chirurgiens de Louis XIV à Louis XVI. **Hist Sci Med** 1982;16(3):163–6
Dulieu L: Prunelle à Montpellier. **Rev Hist Sci (Paris)** 1981 Jan;34(1):59–69
Faure O: Médecins, médecine et hôpital à Lyon au début du XIXe siècle. **Bull Soc Fr Hist Hop** 1981;(42):15–24
Forster R, Ranum O, ed: Medicine and society in France. Selections from the Annales -- Economies, Sociétés, Civilisations. Baltimore and London, Johns Hopkins University Press, 1980. ix, 176 p. Reprinted articles by J. P. Goubert, J. Léonard, M. F. Morel, D. Roche, A. Farge, M. Joerger, M. Laget.
Fossard J: Aperçus médico-politiques en Provence orientale à la Belle Epoque. **Hist Sci Med** 1982;16(4):267–72
Fréor P: Médecins, chirurgiens, épidémies. In: Congrès National des Sociétés Savantes, 97e, Nantes, 1972. Comptes Rendus. Paris, 1976. Section des Sciences, Tome 1. p. 433–44.
Frey EF: Early eighteenth-century French medicine: setting the stage for revolution. **Clio Med** 1982 May;17(1):1–13
Gelfand T: Professionalizing modern medicine: Paris surgeons and medical science and institutions in the 18th century. Westport, Connecticut, Greenwood Press, 1980. xviii, 271 p. (Contributions in medical history, 6)
Gelfand T: Public medicine and medical careers in France during the reign of Louis XV. **Soc Soc Hist Med Bull (Lond)** 1979 Dec;25:48–51
Goubert JP: Die Medikalisierung der französischen Gesellschaft am Ende des Ancien Régime: die Bretagne als Beispiel. **Medizinhist J** 1982;17(1/2):89–114
Goubert JP: La médicalisation de la société française à la fin de l'Ancien Régime. **Francia** 1980, paru 1981;8:245–56
Goubert JP: La médicalisation de la société française, 1770–1830. **Hist Reflect** 1982;9:1–304
Goubert JP: La médicalisation de la société française, 1770–1830. Waterloo, Ont., Historical Reflections Press, 1982. 304 p.
Goubert JP: La pénétration du médecin dans le corps social en France (1770–1850). **Hist Sci Med** 1980;14:435–8
Goubert JP, Lepetit B: Les niveaux de medicalisation des villes Françaises à la fin de l'ancien régime. **Hist Reflect** 1982;9(1–2):45–67
Goubert JP: Réseau médical et médicalisation en France à la fin du 18e siècle. **Ann Bretagne** 1979;86(3):221–9
Goubert JP: The medicalization of French society at the end of the Ancien Régime. With commentary by C. Hannaway, p. 173–9. In Stevenson LG, ed: A celebration of medical history. Baltimore, Johns Hopkins University Press, 1982. (The Henry E. Sigerist supplements to the Bulletin of the History of Medicine; new ser., no. 6). p. 173–9.
Goubert JP: 1770–1830: la premiere croisade medicale. **Hist Reflect** 1982;9(1–2):3–13
Goubert JP: 1789: le corps médical et le changement. **Hist Sci Med** 1982;16(2):99–105
Greenbaum LS: Medicine in revolution: an essay review. **J Hist Med Allied Sci** 1982 Jan;37(1):90–5
Guillaume P: Malades, médecine et médecins à Bordeaux au 19e siècle. **Ann Bretagne** 1979;86(3):291–300
Herzlich C: The evolution of relations between French physicians and the state from 1880 to 1980. **Sociol Health Illn** 1982 Nov;4(3):241–53
Hildreth ML: The foundations of the modern medical system in France: physicians, public health advocates, and the medical legislation of 1892 and 1893. **Proc Annu Meet West Soc Fr Hist** 1980;8:311–27
Huard P, Imbault-Huart MJ: Le professeur Georges Dieulafoy (1839–1911). In: Congrès National des Sociétés Savantes, 96e, Toulouse, 1971. Comptes Rendus. Paris, 1974. Histoire des Sciences, Tome 1. p. 201–5.
Huard P: Les facettes multiples de René Théophile Laennec (1781–1826). **Bull Acad Natl Med (Paris)** 1981 Feb 17;Spec No:51–6
I mutamenti del 'potere medico' in Francia dalla Rivoluzione ad oggi secondo Jean-Paul Aron: **Minerva Med** 1982 Jul 14;73(28–29):2010–2
Jottras PL: Jean Astruc, médecin humaniste. **Hist Sci Med** 1984;18(3):271–7
Laffe F: Médecins et société à Saint-Rémy de Provence au XVIIIe siècle. **Provence Hist** 1983;33(134):461–73
Lecuir J: La médicalisation de la société français dans la deuxième moitié du 18e siècle en France: aux origin premiers traités de médecine légale. **Ann Bretagne** 1979;86(3):231–50
Léonard J: La médecine entre les savoirs et les pouvoirs: histoire intellectuelle et politique de la médecine française au XIXe siècle. Paris, Aubier Montaigne, 1981. 384 p.
Leonard J: La médicalisation de l'Etat: l'exemple des premières décennies de la 3e République. **Ann Bretagne** 1979;86(3):313–20
Léonard J: La restauration et la profession médicale. **Hist Reflect** 1982;9(1–2):69–81
Léonard J: La vie quotidienne du médecin de province au XIXe siècle. Paris, Hachette, 1977. 285 p.
Léonard J: Le corps médical au début de la IIIe République ou l'heureux dénouement d'un malaise professionel. **Third Repub** 1978 Spring;5:94–113
Leonard J: Les médecins de l'Ouest au XIXe siècle. **Ann Demogr Hist (Paris)** 1979;:337–45
Leonard J: Les medecins de l'ouest au XIXème siècle. Lille, Atelier reproduction des thèses, Univ. de Lille III; Paris, Champion, 1978. 3 vols. ccxl, 1570 p. (Thèse, Paris IV, 1976).
Maillé-Virole C: La naissance d'un personnage: le medecin Parisien à la fin de l'ancien régime. **Hist Reflect** 1982;9(1–2):153–79
Marinesco M, Petresco A, Marinesco G: Georges Marinesco et la France. **Hist Sci Med** 1984;18(1):13–8
Mercier P: L'oeuvre scientifique de Robert Debré. **Bull Acad Natl Med (Paris)** 1982 Dec;166(9):1285–94
Merle d'Aubigné R: Paul Broca (1824–1880). **Bull Soc Hist Protestantisme Fr** 1980;126(4):509–24
Mitchell H: Politics in the service of knowledge: the debate over the administration of medicine and welfare in late eighteenth-century France. **Soc Hist (Lond)** 1981;6(2):185–207
Mitchell H: Rationality and control in French eighteenth-century medical views of the peasantry. **Comp Stud Soc Hist** 1979;21(1):82–112
Nocon C: Les médecins à Douai de 1900 à 1939. **Rev Nord** 1979;61(241):439–43
Peter JP: Reparar el desorden del mundo: la medicina ilustrada ante la enfermedad epidemica (Bas-Poitou, 1784–1785). **Asclepio** 1983;35:3–26
Peumery JJ: Une grande figure de la médecine et de la chirurgie française: Pierre-Jean Mauricheau-Beaupré (1778–1857). **Hist Sci Med** 1983;17(1):95–104
Poirier J, Poirier JL, ed: Médecine et philosophie à la fin du XIXe siècle. Paris, Université de Paris XII - Val de Marne, [1980?]. ii, 155 p. (Cahier de l'Institut de recherche universitaire d'histoire de la connaissance, des idées et des mentalités; no. 2).
Pomel ML: La médecine d'autrefois d'après des documents inédits. Le docteur Missoux (1800–1863). Rodez, Editions Subervie, 1979. 162 p.
Ramsey M: Medicina e politica di monopolio professionale nel XIX secolo. **Quad Stor** 1981;16(3):959–1011
Rivet R: Un médecin de Perpignan, professeur à l'Université de Montpellier: Joseph Anglada (1775–1833). In: Congrès National des Sociétés Savantes, 106e, Perpignan, 1981. Comptes Rendus. Paris, Bibliothèque Nationale, 1982. Fasc. IV. p. 111–7.
Rowe C: Jean-Jacques Rousseau: ce qu'il pensait des médecins. **Bull Soc Hist Protestantisme Fr** 1978;124(4):501–17
Sarazin M: Le docteur Fournier de Lempdes (1783–1861). **Bull Hist Sci Auvergne** 1984;92(680):37–47
Shampo MA, Kyle RA: Jacques-Alexandre-César Charles. **JAMA** 1984 May 18;251(19):2547
Vetter T: Témoignages du Strasbourgeois Victor Stoeber sur la médecine parisienne (1824–1825). **Gesnerus** 1983;40(1–2):215–22
Vieuville P: Duhamel et la médecine. **Hist Sci Med** 1980;14(1):71–6
Wrotnowska D: Médecins polonais émigrés en Languedoc et dans les Pyrénées au XIXe siècle. In: Congrès National des Sociétés Savantes, 96e, Toulouse, 1971. Comptes Rendus. Paris, 1974. Histoires des Sciences, Tome 1. p. 175–92.
22.500 thèses françaises de médecine publiées de 1796 à 1896: Un monument de l'histoire de la médecine. Genève, Librairie Slatkine, 1982. Various paginations.

### French Guiana

Chaia J: Vicq d'Azyr, la Société Royale de Médecine et la Guyane. In: Congrès National des Sociétés Savantes, 105e, Caen, 1980. Comptes Rendus, Paris, 1980. Section des Sciences, Fasc. V. p. 9–15.

### Germany

Bach I: Karl Gottlob Springsfeld--Arzt, Gelehrter und Akademiemitglied in der Zeit der Aufklärung. **Z Arztl Fortbild (Jena)** 1984;78(19):829–32
Brücke EW von: Briefe an Emil Du Bois-Reymond. Ed. H. Brücke, W. Hilger, W. Höflechner, W. W. Swoboda. Erster Teil. Graz, Akademische Druck- und Verlagsanstalt, 1978. 308 p. (Publikationen aus dem Archiv der Universität Graz, Band 8/1).
Brügelmann J: Observations on the process of medicalization in Germany, 1770–1830, based on medical topographies. **Hist Reflect**

1982;9(1-2):131-49
Busse H: Christoph Wilhelm Hufeland: der berühmte Arzt der Goethezeit, Leibarzt der Königin Luise. St. Michael, Bläschke, 1982. 334 p.
Curtius F: Richard Siebeck (1883-1965). **Med Welt** 1983 Mar 18;34(11):347-53
Deneke JF: Das Gesundheitswesen der ersten Hälfte des 19.Jahrhunderts im Spiegel der Amts- und Intelligenzpresse. Düsseldorf, Triltsch, 1983. 161 p. (Düsseldorfer Arbeiten zur Geschichte der Medizin, Beiheft IX).
Der dreifache Fluch: Jüdin, Intellektuelle, Sozialistin: Lebenserinnerungen einer Arztin in Deutschland und im Exil: Frankfurt/Main, New York, Campus Verlag, 1981. 320 p.
Drabik R: Die Entwicklung des Leistungspotentials der Krankenhausmedizin im 20.Jahrhundert in Deutschland. Diss., Universität Düsseldorf. Düsseldorf, 1982. 98 p.
Gadacz-Grünefeld G: Die Medizinalentwicklung im Kreise Aurich im 19. und 20. Jahrhundert. Münster, Murken-Altrogge, 1979. 282 p. (Studien zur Geschichte des Krankenhauswesens, 9).
Genschorek W: Christoph Wilhelm Hufeland. Der Arzt, der das Leben verlängern half. Leipzig, Hirzel, 1976. 202 p.
Genschorek W: Christoph Wilhelm Hufeland: der Arzt, der das Leben verlängern half. Leipzig, Hirzel, 1982. 215 p.
Genschorek W: Ernst Ludwig Heim. Das Leben eines Volksarztes. Leipzig, S. Hirzel, 1982. 226 p.
Goerke H, ed: Berliner Aerzte. 2d ed. Berlin, Berlin Verlag, 1984. 328 p.
Gsell O: Hundert Jahre innere Medizin. Eröffnungsreden der Vorsitzenden der Deutschen Gesellschaft für innere Medizin. I. Teil 1882-1932. **Med Welt** 1983 Apr 8;34(14):428-33
Gsell O: Hundert Jahre innere Medizin. Eröffnungsreden der Vorsitzenden der Deutschen Gesellschaft für innere Medizin. II. Teil 1933-1982. **Med Welt** 1983 Apr 15;34(15):462-5
Handrack C: Georg Friedrich Wilhelm Balser (1780-1846). Giessen, Schmitz, 1979. 388 p. (Arbeiten zur Geschichte der Medizin in Giessen, 2).
Hansen E, et al, ed: Seit über einem Jahrhundert ...: Verschüttete Alternativen in der Sozialpolitik. Sozialer Fortschritt, organisierte Dienstleistermacht und nationalsozialistische Machtergreifung: der Fall der Ambulatorien in den Unterweserstädten und Berlin. 100 Jahre kaiserliche Botschaft zur Sozialversicherung: Eine Festschrift. Köln, Bund-Verlag, 1981. 618 p.
Kahle E, Stupp JA: Hochschulschriften zur Geschichte der Medizin, Pharmazie, und Naturwissenschaften der Friedrich-Alexander-Universität Erlangen-Nürnberg 1885-1975. Erlangen, Verlagsbuchhandlung Hannelore Lüling, 1980. 94 p. (Medizinhistorische Materialien, 2).
Kahle E: Hochschulschriften zur Geschichte der Medizin Pharmazie und Naturwissenschaften der Julius-Maximilians-Universität Würzburg, 1885-1970. Medizinhistorische Materialien - 1. Erlangen, Verlagsbuchhandlung, 1979. 48 p.
Kaiser W, Völker A: Das Medizinalwesen von Anhalt-Köthen im Einflussbereich des halleschen Pietismus. **Wiss Z Martin Luther Univ (Math)** 1983;32(2):61-87
Kaiser W, Völker A: Die Aufgaben einer Medizinalbehörde im 19. Jahrhundert am Beispiel von Anhalt-Köthen. **Wiss Z Martin Luther Univ (Math)** 1983;32(2):39-69
Kaiser W: Georg Ernst Stahl (1659-1734)--Zur 250. Wiederkehr seines Todestages am 14. Mai 1984. **Z Gesamte Inn Med** 1984 Aug 1;39(15):371-6
Kaiser W: Johann Reinhold Forster (1729-1798) und Johann Georg Forster (1754-1794) in Halle. Zur 250. Wiederkehr des Geburtstages von Johann Reinhold Forster. **Z Gesamte Inn Med** 1979 Jul 15;34(14):373-81
Kaiser W, Voelker A: Medizingeschichte und Populärwissenschaft bei Johann Heinrich Schulze. **Altertum** 1980;26:243-9
Kater MH: Die 'Gesundheitsführung' des Deutschen Volkes. **Medizinhist J** 1983;18(4):349-75
Klasen EM: Die Diskussion über eine 'Krise' der Medizin in Deutschland zwischen 1925 und 1935. Diss. Mainz, 1984. 169 p.
Kudlien F: Ein Briefwechsel zweier Kieler Professoren aus dem Jahre 1931 und sein zeitgeschichtlicher Hintergrund. **Medizinhist J** 1983;18(4):338-48
Kunze M: Strasse ins Feuer. Vom Leben und Sterben in der Zeit des Hexenwahns. München, Kindler, 1982. 397 p.
Labisch A, Spree R, Weindling P: Conference Report. Social history of nineteenth- and twentieth-century German medicine. **Soc Soc Hist Med Bull (Lond)** 1983;32:40-5
Labisch A, Spree R: Neuere Ergebnisse und Entwicklungen einer Sozialgeschichte der Medizin und des Gesundheitswesens in Deutschland im 19. und 20. Jahrhundert. **Ber Wissenschaftsgesch** 1982;5(3):209-23
Marasanov RA, Mel'nichuk AN: Meditsinskoe obespechenie nemetskogo naseleniia na zavershaiushchem étape Velikoĭ Otechestvennoĭ voĭny i posle ee okonchaniia. **Voen Med Zh** 1981 Jun;(6):16-9
Munk F, ed: Das medizinische Berlin um die Jahrhundertwende. 2d ed. München, Baltimore, Urban & Schwarzenberg, 1979. 182 p.
Ostrowska T: Przedstawiciele medycyny niemieckiej w Towarzystwie Warszawskim Przyjaciół Nauk (1800-1832). **Arch Hist Med (Warsz)** 1979;42(2):257-62
Renker K: Zu einigen Prinzipien der medizinischen Betreuung der Bevölkerung. **Wiss Z Martin Luther Univ (Math)** 1976;25(2):79-89
Rothschuh KE: Das Buch 'Der Arzt' (1906) stammt nicht von Ernst Schweninger! **Medizinhist J** 1983;18(1-2):137-44
Ruff PW: Zum Wandel der gesellschaftlichen Stellung des medizinischen Wissenschaftlers im Deutschland des 19. Jahrhunderts. **Rostocker Wiss Hist Manuskripte** 1981;6:61-7
Rusch T: Detmar Wilhelm Soemmerring, Leben und Werk. Diss. Mainz, 1981. 126 p.
Schattenkirchner M: Rheumatologie. **MMW** 1983 Jul 1;125(26):639-40
Schipperges H: Krankwerden und Gesundsein bei Novalis. **Dtsch Vierteljahresschr Lit Wiss Geistesgesch** 1978;226-42
Schmidt H: Zur Geschichte der Erfurter Kolonne des Arbeiter-Samariter-Bundes. **Beitr Gesch Univ Erfurt** 1979-83;19:283-91
Segebrecht W: Krankheit und Gesellschaft. Zu E.T.A. Hoffmanns Rezeption der Bamberger Medizin. **Dtsch Vierteljahresschr Lit Wiss Geistesgesch** 1978;:267-90
Segebrecht W: Krankheit und Gesellschaft: zu E. T. A. Hoffmanns Rezeption der Bamberger Medizin. In Richard Brinkmann ed: Romantik in Deutschland: ein interdisziplinäres Symposion. Stuttgart, Metzler, 1978.
Speckner W: Carl Friedrich von Heusinger. Sein Leben und sein Wirken in Würzburg (1824-1829). Diss., Bayerische Julius-Maximilians-Universität, Würzburg, 1981. 154 p.
Szwejcerowa A: O Towarzystwie Lekarzy Niemieckich w Paryzu. **Arch Hist Med (Warsz)** 1979;42(3):323-30
Tutzke D: Das sächsische Medizinalwesen um die Wende vom 19. zum 20. Jahrhundert. **Z Gesamte Hyg** 1983 Sep;29(9):556-9
Valentin F: Wandel und Strukturveränderungen im Bereich der Inneren Medizin. **Internist (Berlin)** 1980 Apr;21(4):21-4
Voswinckel P: Arzt und Auto: das Auto und seine Welt im Spiegel des Deutschen Arztblattes von 1907 bis 1975. Münster, Murken-Altrogge, 1981. iii, 194 p.
Weidmann A: Die Arzneiversorgung der Armen zu Beginn der Industrialisierung im deutschen Sprachgebiet, besonders in Hamburg. Braunschweig, 1982. iv, 229 p. (Braunschweiger Veröffentlichungen zur Geschichte der Pharmazie und der Naturwissenschaften, Bd. 25).
Wolf R: Das Leben und Wirken von Carl Friedrich von Marcus (1802-1862). Diss. Würzburg, 1980. 141 p.
Wyklicky H: Arzt und Umwelt im 19. Jahrhundert. **Prakt Arzt** 1982 Feb;36:6-10
Zacher A: Anthropologische Medizin im Wandel. Von Viktor von Weizsäcker zu Dieter Wyss. **Nervenarzt** 1983 Nov;54(11):598-603
Zorn W: Medizinische Volkskunde als sozial-geschichtliche Quelle. Die bayerische Bezirksärzte-Landesbeschreibung von 1860/62. **Vierteljahrsschr Soz Wirtschgesch** 1982;69(2):219-31

### Ghana

Patterson KD: Health in colonial Ghana: disease, medicine, and socio-economic change, 1900-1955. Waltham, Mass., Crossroads Press, 1981. xiii, 187 p.
Twumasi PA: A social history of the Ghanaian pluralistic medical system. **Soc Sci Med [Med Anthropol]** 1979 Dec;13B(4):349-56

### Great Britain

Anning ST: The history of medicine in Leeds. Leeds, Maney, 1980. 218 p.
Appleby JH: Robert Erskine--Scottish pioneer of Russian natural history. **Arch Nat Hist** 1982 Apr;10(3):377-98
Armstrong D: Political anatomy of the body. Medical knowlege in Britain in the twentieth century. Cambridge, Cambridge University Press, 1983. xii, 146 p.
Booth CC: Clinical science in the age of reason. **Perspect Biol Med** 1981 Autumn;25(1):93-114
Bright P: Dr. Richard Bright (1789-1858). London, Bodley Head, 1983. 312 p.
Brown PS: The providers of medical treatment in mid-nineteenth-century Bristol. **Med Hist** 1980 Jul;24(3):297-314
Brown TM: The changing self-concept of the 18th-century London physician. **Eighteenth Cent Life** 1982;7(2):31-40
Bynum WF: Darwin and the doctors: evolution, diathesis, and germs in 19th-century Britain. **Gesnerus** 1983;40(1-2):43-53
Cartwright ML: Sir Edward Foyle Collingwood. In Dictionary of national biography, 1961-1970. Suppl. 8, 1981. p. 232-4.
Checkland O, Lamb M, ed: Health care as social history; the Glasgow case. Aberdeen, Aberdeen University Press, 1982. xix, 285 p.
Chitnis AC: Universities, medicine and science. In his: The Scottish Enlightenment: a social history. 279 pp. London: Croom Helm; Totawa, N.J.: Rowman & Littlefield, 1976. p. 124-94.
Davies NN: Two and a half centuries of medical practice: a Welsh medical dynasty. In J. Cule, ed: Wales and medicine. London, British Society for the History of Medicine, 1975. p. 216-21.
Different letters from the past: Tobias Smollett to William Hunter. **Ann R Coll Surg Engl** 1980 Mar;62(2):146-9
Dobson C., et al: Winchester in the 18th century. **Pharm Hist (London)** 1981 Apr;11(1):4-6

# MEDICINE

Fabian B, Spieckermann ML: Deutsche Uebersetzungen englischer humanmedizinischer Werke 1680–1810. Eine vorläufige Bibliographie. **Medizinhist J** 1980;15(1/2):154–71

Glover J: Health and disease in Birmingham, 1770–1830. **Warwickshire Hist** 1978–9;4:40–55

Gumpert TE: Recollected in tranquillity. Sheffield, [Eng.], Walker and Carson, 1978. 168 p.

Hall IS: John Robert Hume: personal physician to the first Duke of Wellington. **J R Coll Surg Edinb** 1980 Jul;25(4):219–32

Honigsbaum F: The division in British medicine. A history of the separation of general practice from hospital care 1911–1968. London, Kogan Page, 1979. xvi, 445 p.

King-Hele D, ed: The letters of Erasmus Darwin. Cambridge, Cambridge University Press, 1981. xxxii, 363 p.

Kingsley Brown A: 'Mony a mickle...' **Trans Hunter Soc** 1978–80;37–38:7–33

Lane J: The medical practitioners of provincial England in 1783. **Med Hist** 1984 Oct;28(4):353–71

Laundon JR: The date of birth of Sir John Hill (1714–1775). **Arch Nat Hist** 1981 Apr;10(1):65–6

Loudon I: The nature of provincial medical practice in eighteenth-century England. **Med Hist** 1985 Jan;29(1):1–32

Marcovich A: Concerning the continuity between the image of society and the image of the human body - an examination of the work of the English physician, J. C. Lettsom (1746–1815). In P. Wright, A. Treacher, ed: The problem of medical knowledge. Examining the social construction of medicine. Edinburgh, Edinburgh University Press, 1982. p. 69–86.

Murley R: Peace and strife in Hunter's time (part II). **Ann R Coll Surg Engl** 1982 Mar;64(2):81–90

Overmier JA: John Brown's Elementa medicinae: an introductory bibliographical essay. **Bull Med Libr Assoc** 1982 Jul;70(3):310–7

Owen K: John Hunter: a man of his age. **Trans Hunter Soc** 1978–80;37–38:85–97

Porter R: Medicina e illuminismo nell' Inghilterra del settecento. **Quad Stor** 1979;14(1):155–80

Porter R: Medicine and the Enlightenment in Eighteenth century England. **Soc Soc Hist Med Bull (Lond)** 1979 Dec;25:27–40

Porter R: Was there a medical Enlightenment in 18th-century England? **Br J 18th-Cent Stud** 1982;5:49–63

Postlewait T: Bernard Shaw and science: the aesthetics of causality. In Paradis J, Postlewait T, ed: Victorian science and Victorian values: literary perspectives. New York, New York Academy of Sciences, 1981. p. 319–58.

Rook A, Martin L: John Addenbrooke M.D. (1680–1719). **Med Hist** 1982 Apr;26(2):169–78

Rosenberg CE: Medical text and social context: explaining William Buchans's Domestic Medicine. **Bull Hist Med** 1983;57(1):22–42

Rosner LM: Andrew Duncan M.D., F.R.S.E. (1744–1828). Edinburgh, History of Medicine and Science Unit, University of Edinburgh, [1981?]. [12] p.

Sigsworth EM: William Elmhirst 1721–1773: surgeon-apothecary--and medical frontiersman. **Pharm Hist (London)** 1984 Sep;14(3):6–7

Smith R: History of the prison medical services. **Br Med J [Clin Res]** 1983 Dec 10;287(6407):1786–8

Taylor R: Doctors, paupers, and landowners. The evolution of primary medical care in Orkney. **North Scotl** 1981;4(1–2):113–20

Tröhler U: Quantification in British medicine and surgery 1750–1830. Ph.D. Diss., University of London, 1978.

Van Zwanenberg D: The training and careers of those apprenticed to apothecaries in Suffolk. 1815–1858. **Med Hist** 1983 Apr;27(2):139–50

Whitfield AG: Physician to the Prince of Wales. **J R Coll Physicians Lond** 1983 Oct;17(4):231–4

Wilson A: The way it used to be. In Aberdare. **Br Med J** 1981;282:1284–6

**Haiti**

Loker Z: Docteur Michel Lopez de Paz, médecin et savant de Saint-Domingue. **Rev Hist Med Heb** 1980 Oct;134(33 no 3):55–7

**Hungary**

Birtalan G: Dobrudscha in den 60-er Jahren des 19. Jahrhunderts in den Augen eines ungarischen Arztes. In International Congress of the History of Medicine. 26th, Plovdiv, 1978. Actes du Congress. Sofia, 1981. Volume II. p. 103–5.

Bugyi B: Orvosi helyleírásunk történetéhez. **Orvostort Kozl** 1981;93–96(27 No 1–4):219–24

Füves O: Orvosi vonatkozású feljegyzések egy kecskeméti görög naplójában. **Orvostort Kozl** 1979;87–88(25 no 1–2):301–2

Hollán Z: Rusznyák István utca. **Orv Hetil** 1983 Jun 26;124(26):1575–7

Karasszon D: As összehasonlító orvostudomány története hazánkban. **Orv Hetil** 1982 Mar 21;123(12):737–40

Kótay P: István Weszprémi 1723–1799. **Orvostort Kozl** 1980;89–91(26 no 1–3):215–22

Magyar I: Medical trends in interwar Hungary. **Orvostort Kozl** 1980;89–91(26 no 1–3):97–110

Marsovszky P: Herzog Ferenc (1879–1952) emlékezetére. **Orvostort Kozl** 1980;89–91(26 no 1–3):251–6

Pál E: Habent sua fata libelli. Magyar orvosok és gyógyszerészek a nyelvújítás korában. **Orv Hetil** 1981 Feb 22;122(8):467–8

Pisztora F: A bel-, az elme és az ideggyógyászat viszonya hazánkban a századforduló körül. **Orv Hetil** 1982 Jun 27;123(26):1621–9

Serg E: Ethnomedizin und Opfergegenstände auf Wallfahrtsorten in Ungarn. In International Congress of the History of Medicine. 26th, Plovdiv, 1978. Actes du Congress. Sofia, 1981. Volume II. p. 67.

Silló-Seidl G: Die Wahrheit über Semmelweis. Genf, Ariston Verlag, 1978. 214 p.

Simonovits I: Emlékek az 1930–1944. Evi egyetemi diákmozgalomról és orvosmozgalomról. **Parttorteneti Kozl** 1980;26(2):130–41

Somló G: Megemlékezés Diósszilágyi Sámuelröl Makón. **Orv Hetil** 1983 Jul 10;124(28):1705–6

Szállási A: Id. Elischer Gyula élete--a mügyüjtés apológiája. **Orv Hetil** 1984 Oct 14;125(42):2567–9

Szállási A: Ramón y Cajal und die ungarischen Arzte. In International Congress of the History of Medicine, 27th, Barcelona, 1980. Actas. Barcelona, Académia de Ciències Médiques de Catalunya i Balears, 1981. p. 632–5.

**India**

Ata-ur-Rahim M: The contribution of Muslim medical scientists during British period in India -- a bibliography. **JPMA** 1980 Apr;30(4):102–5 contd.

Bigot A: La médecine française à Pondichéry aux XVIIIe et XIXe siècles. In: Congrès National des Sociétés Savantes, 91e, Rennes, 1966. Comptes Rendus. Paris, 1967. Section des Sciences, Tome 1. p. 31–46.

Filliozat J: The expansion of Indian medicine abroad. **Sachitra Ayurved** 1981 Mar;:171–3

Gangadaharan N: The state of Ayurvada in the eighteenth and nineteenth centuries. **Indian J Hist Sci** 1982;17(1):154–63

Garg NK, Nigam SK: Interaction in chemistry and medicine between India and Europe in 18th-19th century. **Indian J Hist Sci** 1981;16(2):145–55

Husain SA: Physicians of Hyderabad during Nizam II & III. **Bull Indian Inst Hist Med (Hyderabad)** 1980;10(1–4):40–7

Jeffery R: Indian medicine and the state. **Bull Br Assoc Orient** 1979–80 N.Ser;11:58–70

Jeffery R: Recognizing India's doctors: the institutionalization of medical dependency, 1918–1939. **Mod Asian Stud** 1979;13(2):301–26

Purushothamacharyulu G: Pandit D. Gopalacharyulu, regenerator of ayurveda. **Sachitra Ayurved** 1981 Mar;:194–200

Rahim MA: The contribution of Muslim medical scientists during the British period in India: a bibliography. **JPMA** 1980 Jan;30(1):17–21

Rama Rao B: Bhishagratna Achanta Lakshmipathi, his dedicated service to Ayurveda. **Bull Indian Inst Hist Med (Hyderabad)** 1980;10(1–4):76–83

Shankara MR, Venkataram BS, Leelavathy S: A 19th century manuscript on traditional medicine. **Bull Indian Inst Hist Med (Hyderabad)** 1979;9:33–7

Shankarashastry V: The eminence of Lakshmipathi. **Bull Indian Inst Hist Med (Hyderabad)** 1980;10(1–4):62–8

Siddiqi T: Hakim Muhammad Akbar Arzani. **Stud Hist Med** 1981 Sep;5(3):167–224

Siddiqi T: Zubdat al-Hukama Allama Hakim Kabiruddin. **Stud Hist Med** 1981 Jun;5(2):87–132

**Iran**

Andreano R: Some personal observations on health policy in Iran, 1973–1978. **Soc Sci Med** 1984;19(1):1–7

**Ireland**

Drury MI: The history of medicine in Dublin. **Q J Med** 1981 Autumn;50(200):485–92

Lyons JB: Letters to an editor. The William Doolin Memorial Lecture. **Ir Med J** 1980 Sep;73(9):323–30

Lyons JB: The section of medicine and medical developments over the century. **Ir J Med Sci** 1983 Jan;152(1):14–24

**Israel**

Margalith D: Physicians, forerunners of modern Israel. Tel-Aviv, Jerusalem Academy of Medicine, 1973. 192, iv, 12 p.

Siegel S: [Medical ethics in] contemporary Israel. In Reich ET, et al, ed: Encyclopedia of bioethics, v. 2. New York, Free Press, 1978. p. 895–6.

**Italy**

Carpinteri F: Sociologia sanitaria a Siracusa ed in altre città della Sicilia: Mali, medici, medicine e terapie: casistiche documentate dal 1728 al 1833. **Cah Int Hist Econ Soc** 1980;12:288–322

Detti T: Medicina, democrazia e socialismo in Italia tra '800 e '900. **Mov Operaio Soc** 1979;2(1):3–49

Frascani P: Medicina e statistica nella formazione del sistema santiario italiano: l'inchiesta del 1885. **Quad Stor** 1980;15(3):942–65

Premuda L: Die Medizin in der Sicht eines italienischen Denkers der Aufklärung. **Gesnerus** 1983;40(3/4):249–56

**Japan**

Bowers JZ: The adoption of German medicine in Japan: the decision and the beginning. **Bull Hist Med** 1979 Spring;53(1):57–80

Johnston WD: [Scientific revolution in 18th century Japanese medicine: intellectual preconditions for the development of the Dutch school of medicine (Rampo).] (Jpn). **Nihon I-Shigaku Zasshi** 1981;27:131–156

Jonston WD: [The scientific revolution in 18th century Japanese medicine – the ideal premise for the development of Dutch learning.] (Jpn). **Nihon I-Shigaku Zasshi** 1981;27(1):6–20

**Kenya**

Beck A: Medicine, tradition, and development in Kenya and Tanzania, 1920–1970. Waltham, Crossroads Press, 1981. viii, 114 p.

Imperato PJ: Early modern medical services at Moyale, Kenya. **East Afr Med J** 1983 Jun;60(6):367–73

**Korea**

Kim DJ: The influence of Western medicine, especially American medicine, on the development of medicine in Korea. **Trans Stud Coll Physicians Phila** 1977 Jan;44(3):131–4

**Mexico**

Córdova Alvelais LT: El surgimiento de la medicina mexicana comtemporánea. **Arch Inst Cardiol Mex** 1981 Jan–Feb;51(1):103–8

Esteyneffer J de: Florilegio medicinal. Edicion, estudio preliminar, notas, glosario e indice analitico by M. del Carmen Anzures y Bolaños. México, Academía Nacional de Medicina, 1978. 2 v. xxiii, 973 p.

Frenk J, Hernández–Llamas H, Alvarez–Klein L: El mercado de trabajo médico. II. Evolución histórica en México. **Gac Med Mex** 1980 Jun;116(6):265–84

Somolinos D'Ardois G, Fernández del Castillo F: Historia de la Academia Nacional de Medicina de México. In Academia Nacional de Medicina. Libro conmemorativo del primer centenario. México, Comité Editorial de la Comisión Organizadora del Congreso del Centenario, 1964. Tome 2. p. 513–21.

Somolinos D'Ardois G: Historia de la fundación de la Academia Nacional de Medicina y su tiempo. In Academia Nacional de Medicina. Libro conmemorativo del primer centenario. México, Comité Editorial de la Comisión Organizadora del Congreso del Centenario, 1964. Tome 2. p. 593–621.

Steimle R: Albert Ehrmann (1821–1871). **Hist Sci Med** 1984;18(3):208–14

Treviño–Zapata N: Valentín Gómez Farías. Patricio, precursor, médico y político. **Gac Med Mex** 1982 Jan;118(1):39–43

Vasconcelos R: La academia y la evolución de la medicina en México desde la Independencia. In Academia Nacional de Medicina. Libro conmemorativo del primer centenario. México, Comité Editorial de la Comisión Organizadora del Congreso del Centenario, 1964. Tome 2. p. 621–9.

**Netherlands**

Lindeboom GA, ed: Boerhaave's correspondence. Part 3. Leiden, Brill, 1979. viii, 281 p. (Part 1 was published 1962, and Part 2 in 1964).

Lindeboom GA, ed: Haller in Holland: het dagboek van Albrecht von Haller van zijn verblijf in Holland (1725–1727). Amsterdam, Rodopi, 1979. 122 p.

Püschel E: 'Dictata' zu den Werken von Johannes de Gorter (1689–1762), professor in Harderwijk: medicinae compendium, praxis medicae systema und chirurgia repurgata. **Janus** 1980;67(1–2–3):41–57

**New Zealand**

Bennett F: A Canterbury tale. The autobiography of Dr. Francis Bennett. Wellington, Oxford University Press, 1980. 249 p.

St. Clair RE: Medical practitioners in early Auckland: part I. **Hist J (NZ)** 1982;40:9–11

Wright-St Clair RE: Early medical practitioners. **NZ Med J** 1980 Mar 12;91(655):190–1

**Nigeria**

Adeloye A: Nigerian pioneers of modern medicine. Selected writings. Ibadan, Nigeria, Ibadan University Press, 1977. xiv. 299 p.

**Pacific Islands**

Howard A: The power to heal in colonial Rotuma. **J Polynesian Soc** 1979;88(3):243–75

Johnston EG: Medical services for the island of Guam until World War Two. **Guam Rec** 1971;1(1):38–46

**Pakistan**

Ata-ur-Rahim M: Medical literature on Pakistan from 1840–1947. **JPMA** 1980 Dec;30(12):281–2 concl

**Philippines**

Guerra F: El medico politico. Estudios biográficos sobre la influencia del médico en la Historia Politica de Hispanoamérica y Filipinas. Madrid, Afrodisio Aguado, 1975. 350 p.

Harvey AM: Johns Hopkins's pioneer venture into international medicine: the commission to the Philippine Islands. **Johns Hopkins Med J** 1980 Jul;147(1):13–27

Kohnen N: Nationalheld und Wissenschaftler; der philippinische Arzt José Rizal. **Dtsch Arztebl** 1983 Apr 22;80(16):102–6

**Poland**

Bayer S: Z dziejów konspiracyjnej służby zdrowia w Warszawie (1939–1944). **Przegl Lek** 1980;37(1):131–7

Berezowski S: Joseph Dietl, a great Polish physician of the 19th century. In International Congress of the History of Medicine. 26th, Plovdiv, 1978. Actes du Congress. Sofia, 1981. Volume II. p. 64–5.

Chojna JW: Pierwsza próba opracowania metodologii historii medycyny w piśmiennictwie polskim. **Arch Hist Med (Warsz)** 1981;44(1):77–84

Dega W: Zapiski do autobiografii moja droga zyciowa do wiedzy i zawodu. **Kwart Hist Nauki Tech** 1984;29(2):259–322

Górski M: Wspomnienia wojenne. **Arch Hist Med (Warsz)** 1983;46(1):91–112

Gutt RW: Historia Recentiorum. (Próba oceny osiągnięć medycyny od zakończenia i Wojny do r. 1950.) **Arch Hist Med (Warsz)** 1981;44(3/4):355–62

Gutt RW: O medycynie w Polsce XVIII–wiecznej. Próba wprowadzenia. **Arch Hist Med (Warsz)** 1979;42(2):211–15

Guzek JW: Profesor Franciszek Venulet (1878–1967) w 15 rocznice śmierci. **Arch Hist Med (Warsz)** 1982;45(1–4):27–38

Kaiser W: Dokumente zur halleschen Promotion polnischer Mediziner in den Jahren 1791 und 1792. **Wiss Z Martin Luther Univ (Math)** 1976;25(6):75–81

Koba S, Koba–Ryszewska T: Sylwetki zasłużonych lekarzy kieleckich z końca XIX i początku XX wieku. **Arch Hist Med (Warsz)** 1980;43(4):429–38

Konopka S: Odrodzenie się niektórych ważnych działów polskiej służby zdrowia w roku 1945. **Pol Tyg Lek** 1981 Sep 7;36(36):1369–75

Kostrzewski JK: Rozwój nauk medycznych w Polsce na tle nauki światowej. **Nauka Pol** 1980;28(5):33–41

Lambert M: Udział niemieckich ośrodków naukowych w kształtowaniu polskiej myśli medycznej w czasach saskich (1697–1763). **Arch Hist Med (Warsz)** 1979;42(2):223–30

Makowiec J: Kaliskie lecznictwo w latach 1874–1914. **Wiad Lek** 1984 Jul 15;37(14):1135–44

Michalczyk B, Kinowskiej M: Bibliografia biezaca historii nauki i techniki. **Kwart Hist Nauki Tech** 1984;29(2):Suppl 1–30

Milik JR: W 20 rocznicę śmierci Bolesława Skarżyńskiego o jego zasługach w rozwoju historii medycyny w Polsce. **Wiad Lek** 1983 Sep 15;36(18):1561–2

Miłosz S, Stański M: O niektórych tendencjach filozoficzno-metodologicznych medycyny w polsce na przełomie XIX i XX w. **Stud Filoz** 1977;11:127–38

Ostrowska T: Dr Karol Sulima Przyborowski (1824–1879), lekarz społecznik w Kamieńcu Podolskim. **Arch Hist Med (Warsz)** 1984;47(1):117–9

Schneck P, Tutzke D: Ueberblick über die Aktenbestände des Staatsarchivs Dresden zur Geschichte der deutsch–polnischen medizinischen Beziehungen im 18. Jahrhundert. **Arch Hist Med (Warsz)** 1979;42(2):205–9

Stecko P: O dalsza poprawe ochrony zdrowia. **Nowe Drogi** 1976;(6):51–62

Stembrowicz W. Lekarze berlińscy pierwszej Połowy XIX wieku w relacjach lekarzy polskich. **Arch Hist Med (Warsz)** 1979;42(3):273–9

Wacek S: Sytuacja zdrowotna Podola w świetle pism dr med Józefa Apolinarego Rollego. **Arch Hist Med (Warsz)** 1981;44(1):99–110

Walter–Janke Z: Z dziejów służby zdrowia okupowanego Śląska. **Przegl Lek** 1980;37(1):104–12

Wieckowska E: Formy opieki zdrowotnej na ziemiach polskich w końcu XIX wieku do lat 30 wieku XX. **Wiad Lek** 1984 Jul 1;37(13):1049–55

**Portugal**

Guerra M: Os primeiros passos na clínica de há 70 anos descritos por Romão Loff. **Acta Med Port** 1983 Jul–Aug;4(7–8):379–80

Pina L de, Meneses MO de: Camilo e a historia da medicina. **Arch Hist Med Port** 1968–70;3(1–4):91–116

**Puerto Rico**

Veray FX: Betances, el médico. **Bol Asoc Med PR** 1983 Mar;75(3):110-3

**Romania**

Bugyi B: Medical geography of Moldavia: historical contribution. **Geogr Med** 1979;9:109-15
Haliţa M: Cinci decenii de la o afirmare a medicinii româneşti. **Rev Med Interna [Med Interna]** 1980 Mar-Apr;32(2):189-92
Kozhokaru I, Maslev S: Novootkriti dokumenti ot i za D-R Petur Beron. **Izv Inst Istor** 1968;20:229-341
Negru I: Din primele realizări sanitare româneşti în Transilvania. **Viata Med [Medii Sanit]** 1980 Dec;28(12):281-4
Negru I: Originile medicinii române sti după dr. N. Vătămanu. **Viata Med [Medii Sanit]** 1980 Jun;28(6):141-4

**Scandinavia**

Oberg L: Sjukdoms--och sjukvårdshistoriens källor. **Nord Medicinhist Arsb** 1980;Suppl 6:90-3

**Singapore**

Seah CS: Medical progress in Singapore--a review of the last three decades, 1951-1980. **Ann Acad Med Singapore** 1982 Jul;11(3):309-12

**South Africa**

Baker TC: Half a century of medical practice in East London. **S Afr Med J** 1983 Jun 29;Spec No:23
Benson RP: Organized medicine in the Eastern Cape. **S Afr Med J** 1981 Oct 17;60(16):631-8
Collins TF: John Max Mehliss, M.D. A Transvaal medical pioneer. **S Afr Med J** 1983 Jun 29;Spec No:14-6
Ferguson D: Civilisation for Africa: a study of the impact of modern scientific medicine on Africa. Port Elizabeth, South Africa, E. H. Walton Co., 1981. 160 p.
Gilder SS: South African medicine in the 1880s. **S Afr Med J** 1984 Aug 18;66(7):247-9
Gilder SS: South African medicine in the 1890s. **S Afr Med J** 1983 Jun 29;Spec No:4-7
Gilder SS: South African patients and their diseases in the 1880s. **S Afr Med J** 1984 Aug 18;66(7):250-2
Kahn A: A-Z in South African medical history. V. The Versveld family. **Adler Mus Bull** 1981;7(2):19-22
Kretzmar N: A half century of medical life in Kimberley. Personal reminiscences. **S Afr Med J** 1981 Aug 22;60(8):331-4
Lucas MB: Diamond jubilee medicine. The medical world of 1897 and 1898 seen in the pages of the South African Medical Journal. **S Afr Med J** 1979 Oct 20;56(17):688-94
Melzer R: William Osler's connection with South Africa. **S Afr Med J** 1983 Jun 29;Spec No.:8-13
Slotow M: Medical Africana. **S Afr Med J** 1983 Jun 29;Spec No:43-6

**Spain**

Campos J, Miguel JM de: Sociologos-de-bata-blanca y medicos-con-barba: relaciones entre las ciencias sociales y la medicina en España. **Rev Esp Invest Sociol** 1981;15:133-41
Carmona-Cornet AM: Actuación de la comisión regia de reforma de los reglamentos de la ciencia de curar (1790-1840). In International Congress of the History of Medicine, 27th, Barcelona, 1980. Actas. Barcelona, Académia de Ciències Médiques de Catalunya i Balears, 1981. p. 480-5.
Cepeda Adán J: Enfermos and enfermedades en el siglo XVII: el marqués y la Marquesa de San Leonardo. **Rev Univ Complut Madr** 1978;27(112):165-84
Corbella Corbella J, Doménech Llabería E: Notas sobre medicos de la comarca del Priorato en el siglo XIX. **Asclepio** 1980;32:103-9
Danon J: Enseñanza de la historia de la medicina en España durante el siglo XIX. In: International Congress of the History of Medicine, 26th, Plovdiv (Bulgaria), 1978. Actes du Congres, Vol. 1. Sofia, 1980. p. 97-100.
Francès Causapè MC, Zubiri García MD: Estudio de la 'revista popular de conocimientos utiles', años 1880-1885, desde el punto de vista sanitario. **Bol Soc Esp Hist Farm** 1983 Sep;135:69-83
Gómez-Santos M: Vida de Gregorio Marañón. Esplugas de Llobregat, Plaza & Janés, 1977. 478 p.
Granjel LS: La medicina española del siglo XVIII. Salamanca, Ediciones Universidad de Salamanca, 1979. 285 p. (Historia general de la medicina española, IV).
Guerra F: La neurosis del exilio en Mariano Batllés, 1827. In International Congress of the History of Medicine, 27th, Barcelona, 1980. Actas. Barcelona, Académia de Ciències Médiques de Catalunya i Balears, 1981. p. 177-80.
Monserrat JT: Medicina y médicos: Mallorca: siglo XIX. Palma de Mallorca, El autor, 1976. 98 p.
Pennini de Vega E, Landáburu AJ, Kohn Loncarica AG, et al: La inmigración médica española en la Argentina. In International Congress of the History of Medicine, 27th, Barcelona, 1980. Actas. Barcelona, Académia de Ciències Médiques de Catalunya i Balears, 1981. p. 188-94.
Riera J: José Masdevall y la medicina española ilustrada (Enseñanza, epidemias y guerra a finales del siglo XVIII). Valladolid, Universidad de Valladolid, 1980. 257 p. (Acta Historico-Medica Vallisoletana, Monografias, X)
Riera J: Medicinas y ciencia en la España ilustrada, epistolario y documentos, I. Valladolid, Universidad de Valladolid, 1981. 159 p. (Acta Historico-Medica Vallisoletana, Monografias, XII)
Riera J: Medicinas y ciencia en la España ilustrada, epistolario y documentos, I. Valladolid, Universidad de Valladolid, 1981. 159 p. (Acta Historico-Medica Vallisoletana, Monografias, XII)
Saturno Hernández PJ: Los medicos de la comarca de la huerta de Murcia. Numero, distribucion espacial, movilidad, grado de especializacion, tipo de ejercicio, edad y años de colegiacion. Evolucion de 1960 a 1974. **Asclepio** 1981;33:23-80
Valverde López JL, Vidal Casero MC: Notas sobre médicos y cirujanos que trabajaron para el Jardín Botánico de Madrid. In International Congress of the History of Medicine, 27th, Barcelona, 1980. Actas. Barcelona, Académia de Ciències Médiques de Catalunya i Balears, 1981. p. 650-5.
Victoria Ortiz M: Vida y obra del doctor Areilza. Bilbao, La Gran Enciclopedia Vasca, 1975. 329 p.

**Sudan**

Gruenbaum ER: Medical anthropology, health policy and the state: a case study of Sudan. **Policy Stud Rev** 1981;1(1):47-65

**Sweden**

Boström H: Internmedicinen - en produkt av vårt eget århundrade. **Lakartidningen** 1983 Nov 16;80(46):4405-7
Brück C: Tidsbilder kring en läkargeneration för 100 år sedan. Efter ett föredrag av Johan Hellström 1935. **Nord Medicinhist Arsb** 1984;:141-52
Höök O: Pehr Dubb -- en medicinsk storman inom västsvensk sjukvård på 1700-talet. **Lakartidningen** 1979 Dec 19;76(51):4710-3
Ober L: Från förspelet till segern över de stora epidemierna. **Hist Foren Arsskr** 1972;:33-45
Oberg L: Malte Ljungdahl 1882-1957. **Sydsven Medicinhist Sallsk Arsskr** 1983;:59-64
Sydow C von: Notiser från Frans von Sydows utrikes studieresor 1861-1886. **Nord Medicinhist Arsb** 1984;:117-28

**Switzerland**

Dr. med. Willy Bircher-Schwarzenbach (1898-1970): s. l., s. n., 1970?. 28 p.
Dufek WM: Der Internist Otto Naegeli, 1871-1938. Zürich, Juris Druck, 1983. 76 p. (Zürcher Medizingeschichtliche Abhandlungen, Neue Reihe, Nr. 160).
Fasol E: Der Internist Hermann Eichhorst, 1849-1921. Zürich, Juris Druck, 1983. 98 P. (Zürcher Medizingeschichtliche Abhandlungen, Neue Reihe, Nr. 159).
Feitknecht-Gallati S: Wandel in der medizinischen Versorgung des Oberwallis in den Jahren 1930-1980. Diss. Bern, 1984. 91 p.
Jéquier MC: Auguste Tissot (1728-1797). **Rev Med Suisse Romande** 1984 May;104(5):337-41
Lamprecht-Naef E: Albert Schweitzer und die Schweiz. Zürich, Juris Druck, 1982. 116 p. (Zürcher Medizingeschichtliche Abhandlungen, Neue Reihe, Nr. 153).
Lichtenthaeler C: Préambule historique au 'baptême' des auditoires. **Rev Med Suisse Romande** 1984 May;104(5):335-6
Meyer-Salzmann M: Michel Schüppach, 1707-1781. Ein Höhepunkt handwerklicher Heilkunst. Bern, Haupt, 1981. 135 p. (Berner Heimatbücher, 126).
Portmann ML: Relations d'Auguste Tissot (1728-1797), médecin à Lausanne, avec le patriciat bernois. **Gesnerus** 1980;37(1/2):21-7
Riva G: Zum 50jährigen Bestehen der Schweizerischen Gesellschaft für Innere Medizin. **Schweiz Med Wochenschr [Suppl]** 1982;13:5-22
Stoffel G: Christian Friedrich Fritzsche, 1851-1938. Erster Glarner Spitalarzt und Beschreiber der Akromealie. Zürich, Juris Druck, 1983. 66 p. (Zürcher Medizingeschichtliche Abhandlungen, Neue Reihe, Nr. 161).

**Thailand**

Matics KI: Medical arts at Wat Phra Chetuphon: various Rishi statues. **J Siam Soc** 1977;65(2):145-52
Smith HE: Doctors and society: a Northern Thailand study. **Soc Sci Med** 1982,16(5):515-26

**Tunisia**

Gallagher NE: Medicine and power in Tunisia, 1780-1900. Cambridge;

New York, Cambridge University Press, 1983. xii, 145 p.

**Turkey**

Becker H: Helmuth von Moltke als Beobachter der hygienischen und medizinischen Situation im osmanischen Kaiserreich (1835-39). In Göpfert W, Otten HH, ed: Metavoeite: wandelt euch durch neues Denken. Düsseldorf, Triltsch, 1983. p. 147-59.
Kapronczay K: Magyar orvosok a török birodalomban a XIX. század közepén. **Orv Hetil** 1980 Mar 17;121(10):581-3
Köhbach M: Europäische Aerzte im Osmanischen Reich am Beginn des 18. Jahrhunderts--der Fall Sinasi. **Sudhoffs Arch** 1980;64(1):79-85

**United States**

Andrews LB, Levin LS: Self-care and the law. **Soc Policy** 1979;9(4):44-9
Baer HA: The organizational rejuvenation of osteopathy: a reflection of the decline of professional dominance in medicine. **Soc Sci Med [A]** 1981 Sep;15(5):701-11
Baird ND: David Wendel Yandell, physician of old Louisville. Lexington: University Press of Kentucky, 1978. x, 116 p.
Banks CS: Two pioneer physicians of San Antonio. **Friends P. I. Nixon Med Hist Libr** 1973 Oct;2:2-17
Barker LF: History of internal medicine. **Md State Med J** 1981 May;30(5):43-4, 47-8, 50, passim
Barlow W, Powell DO: To find a stand: New England physicians on the western and southern frontier, 1790-1840. **Bull Hist Med** 1980 Fall; 54(3):386-401
Bloch H: Guillaume Dupuytren, M.D. (1777-1835). Surgeon of Hôtel Dieu and his American students. **NY State J Med** 1981 Feb;81(2):259-60
Bloch H: William Charles Wells, M.D., F.R.S., 1757-1817. An American physician-scientist America almost forgot. **NY State J Med** 1983 Feb;83(2):248-50
Bluemle LW: John Morgan--the father of American medicine. In Passmore R, ed: Proceedings of the Royal College of Physicians of Edinburgh Tercentenary Congress, 1981. Edinburgh, Royal College of Physicians of Edinburgh, 1982. p. 159-61.
Brainard MD, Plyer CO: Historical perspectives in family practice. **J Fla Med Assoc** 1980 Sep;67(9):812-6
Breeden JO: 'Medicine in the West'--an introduction. **J West** 1982 Jul;21(3):3-4
Bridgforth LR: Heroics and heretics: medical practice in antebellum Mississippi. **J Miss State Med Assoc** 1984 Jan;25(1):8-12
Brodman E: A medical dynasty in New Jersey. **J Med Soc NJ** 1984 Sep;81(9):779-84
Bryant AW: A history of medicine in Atlanta and Fulton County, Georgia. Part I: Terminus to the turn of the century. **J Med Assoc Ga** 1980 Apr;69(4):273-9
Bryant AW: A history of medicine in Atlanta and Fulton County. Part II. **J Med Assoc Ga** 1980 Jul;69(7):589-95 (continued)
Burnham JC: American medicine's golden age: what happened to it? **Science** 1982 Mar 19;215(4539):1474-9
Byrne JJ: Lengthening shadows. **N Engl J Med** 1981 Oct 29;305(18):1051-9
Caplan RL: Pasteurized patients and profits: the changing nature of self-care in American medicine. Ph.D. Diss., University of Massachusetts. Amherst, 1981. xi, 463 p.
Carmichael AG: The Lindsay-Stipp debate. **Indiana Med Hist Q** 1981;7(4):6-19
Carmichael JL: Medical reminiscences. **Ala Med** 1984 Jun;53(12):16-27; July;54(1):13-5, 17
Carroll D: The state of medical knowledge in Maryland, 1870s. **Md State Med J** 1980 Sep;29(9):12-5
Cassedy JH: American medicine and statistical thinking, 1800-1860. Cambridge, Mass., Harvard University Press, 1984. x, 306 p.
Chambers WL: Contributions to American history by physicians. **Am J Surg** 1981 Dec;142(6):640-5
Christianson EH: The emergence of medical communities in Massachusetts, 1700-1794: the demographic factors. **Bull Hist Med** 1980 Spring;54(1):64-77
Clark RB: John L McAlmont, M.D. 1821-1896. **J Arkansas Med Soc** 1984 Apr;80(11):552
Cohen EP, ed: Medicine in transition: the centennial of the University of Illinois College of Medicine: a symposium in Chicago, October 1-2, 1981. [Chicago], University of Illinois College of Medicine, and University of Illinois Press, 1981. 340 p.
Connors DM: Doctors afield in early Wisconsin. **Wis Med J** 1980 Mar;79(3):14-6
Couto R: Property, pinmakers, and physicians: liberal myths and American health care anomalies. **Soundings** 1979;62(3):275-92
Cowen DL: New Jersey medical historiography, 1964-1984. **J Med Soc NJ** 1984 Sep;81(9):807-10
Cranefield PF: Alfred Einstein Cohn. In Dictionary of American Biography, Suppl. 6, 1956-1960. p. 117-18, 1980.
Crellin JK: Medical care in pioneer Illinois. Springfield, Pearson Museum, Southern Illinois University, School of Medicine, 1982. xi, 128 p.
Crutcher JC: A memorial lecture for Dr. Ben Wells. **Ala J Med Sci** 1979 Oct;16(4):346-9
Cushman P: Medicine at turn of century. Perspectives from press. **NY State J Med** 1982 Jan;82(1):81-4
DeFriese GH, Woomert A: The policy implications of self-care. **Soc Policy** 1982;13(2):55-8
Delaney JJ: The doctors Amesse. **Colo Med** 1984 Mar;81(3):77-9
Derrick AA: Old volumes provide links with medicine of today. **J Miss State Med Assoc** 1981 Dec;22(12):331-2
Duffy J: American perceptions of the medical, legal, and theological professions. **Bull Hist Med** 1984 Spring;58(1):1-15
Duffy J: Medicine in the West: an historical overview. **J West** 1982 Jul;21(3):5-14
Eberson F: Early physicians of the West. Forerunners of modern medicine. St. Petersburg, Valkyrie Press, 1979. ix, 140 p.
Eberson FW: Kentucky biographical notebook: Dr. Frederick Ridgely, 1757-1824. **Filson Club Hist Q** 1983;57(2):223-5
Ellison RC, ed: A pioneer Alabama doctor's ledger. **Ala Hist Q** 1981;43(4):315-32
Emmons J: The medical career of Samuel H. Stout. **J Med Assoc Ga** 1980 Nov;69(11):904-10, 1981 Mar;80(3):169-77
Estes JW: Hall Jackson and the purple foxglove: medical practice and research in revolutionary America 1760-1820. Hanover, NH, University Press of New England, 1979. xvi, 291 p.
Estes JW: The practice of medicine in 18th-century Massachusetts: a bicentennial perspective. **N Engl J Med** 1981 Oct 29;305(18):1040-7
Fischoff E: Elizabeth Blackwell: first woman M.D. **Pearson Mus Monogr Ser** 1981;4:1-22
Freymann JG: American health care system: its genesis and trajectory. new ed. Huntington, N. Y., Krieger, 1980. xxiii, 407 p.
Gay EW: The medical profession in Georgia, 1733-1983. Atlanta, Auxiliary to the Medical Association of Georgia, 1983. xvi, 447 p.
Gegenheimer E: Selected letters of Humphrey Hood, Litchfield physician. **J Ill State Hist Soc** 1979;72:193-212, 243-56
Gillett MC: Medicine in the United States in the late eighteenth century. In Medical-Science colloquium. Special edition of Topic: a journal of the liberal arts. Washington, Pennsylvania, Washington and Jefferson College, 1983. p. 13-25.
Gorman BM, McKinzie RD, Wilson TA: From shamans to specialists: a history of medicine and health care in Jackson County, Missouri. Kansas City, Mo., Jackson County Medical Society, 1981. 240 p.
Halas MA: Sexism in women's medical care. **Frontiers** 1979;4(2):11-5
Haller JS: American medicine in transition, 1840-1910. Urbana, University of Illinois Press, 1981. xii, 457 p.
Harstad PT: Frontier medicine in the Territory of Wisconsin. In Numbers RL, Leavitt JW, ed: Wisconsin medicine. Historical perspectives. Madison, University of Wisconsin Press, 1981. p. 13-23.
Harvey AM: Stanhope Bayne-Jones, 1886-1970: the story of a lifetime devoted to country and to medicine. **Johns Hopkins Med J** 1981 Oct;149(4):150-66
Henker FO, Shorey JJ: Dr. P. O. Hooper--father of Arkansas medicine. **J Arkansas Med Soc** 1981 Oct;78(5):189-92
Hess AJ: History of medicine in Harrison County, West Virginia. Clarksburg, Harrison County Medical Society, 1978. xxiii, 662 p.
Holland MR: People, conditions, and activities in the 1880s and 1890s. **Northwest Dent** 1983 Mar-Apr;62(2):45-57
Holley HL: Highlights in history of nineteenth century medicine in Alabama. **Ala J Med Sci** 1983 Jul;20(3):326-33
Holley HL: The history of medicine in Alabama. Birmingham, for University of Alabama School of Medicine, by University of Alabama Press, 1981. xiv, 418 p.
Hollingsworth R: Causes and consequences of the American medical system. **Rev Am Hist** 1983;11(3):326-32
Hood WH: Physicians of Butte County, California, 1850-1900. Chico, Calif., W. H. Hood, 1980. 46 leaves.
Hoyt HF: A frontier doctor. Ed. D. B. Nunis. Chicago, Donnelley -- Lakeside Press, 1979. liii, 518 p.
Hunter WH: South Carolina medicine 110 years ago. **J SC Med Assoc** 1984 Sep;80(9):459-60
Jackson DW: The history of sports medicine. **Am J Sports Med** 1984 Jul-Aug;12(4):255-7
Jirka FJ: One hundred years of American medicine. **J Tenn Med Assoc** 1983 Jul;76(7):450-1
Johnson BH: Doctors, druggists and dentists in the Oklahoma Territory, 1889-1907. **Ariz West** 1977;19:121-34
Johnson RE: Isaac Israel Hayes. In Dictionary of Canadian biography, 1881-1890. 1982;11:393-4.
Johnson TP, Cooper JK: Physician shortage in Kentucky, 1930-1980. **Am J Public Health** 1982 Mar;72(3):257-60
Jones TB: Calvin Jones, M.D.: a case study in the practice of early American medicine. **NC Hist Rev** 1972;49(1):56-71
Judd CS: Some early physicians of Hawaii--1800s. **Hawaii Med J** 1984 Jul;43(7):250
Kampmeier RH: Practice in Nashville--1905 and succeeding years. **J Tenn Med Assoc** 1983 Jan;76(1):9-15
Kampmeier RH: The early history of medicine in Nashville. **J Tenn Med Assoc** 1983 Feb;76(2):89-96
Katsuki B: Medical men who helped to shape Hawaii. **Hawaii Med J** 1981 Oct;40(10):279-82

## MEDICINE

Katz C: The growth of group practice. **Postgrad Med** 1983 Feb;73(2):127–9
Kaufman M: Medicine in America. **Can Rev Am Stud** 1983;14(3):287–96
Kaufman M: Orthodoxy in medicine. In Reich WT, et al, ed: Encyclopedia of bioethics, v.3. New York, Free Press, 1978. p. 1173–6.
Kestigian MC: Early medical care in Deerfield. **Hist J West Mass** 1979;7(2):5–14
King LS: Medicine in the USA: Historical vignettes. X. The changing scene. **JAMA** 1983 Apr 8;249(14):1897–900
King LS: Medicine in the USA: historical vignettes. XXIII. The automobile makes an impact. **JAMA** 1984 May 11;251(18):2352–5
King LS: Medicine in the USA: historical vignettes. XXIV. The continuity of history. **JAMA** 1984 Jun 22–29;251(24):3233–6
King LS: XI. Medicine seeks to be 'scientific'. **JAMA** 1983 May 13;249(18):2475–9
Knox PL, Bohland J, Shumsky NL: The urban transition and the evolution of the medical care delivery system in America. **Soc Sci Med** 1983;17(1):37–43
Koblenzer PJ: Edinburgh's influence on medicine in the new world. In Passmore R, ed: Proceedings of the Royal College of Physicians of Edinburgh Tercentenary Congress, 1981. Edinburgh, Royal College of Physicians of Edinburgh, 1982. p. 143–58.
Kolisch P deR: Paul Revere and medicine. **JAMA** 1984 Jun 22–29;251(24):3224
Krevans JR: Transformation of medicine since 1945. **J Med Educ** 1984 Feb;59(2):75–8
Kunitz SJ: Efficiency and reform in the financing and organization of American medicine in the progressive era. **Bull Hist Med** 1981 Winter;55(4):497–515
Lahiri K: Clara Swain, MD (1834–1910) and her work in India. **Women Health** 1983 Spring;8(1):3–6
Landon SJ: Giants of Paumanok. **York State Tradit** 1972;26(3):24–6, 48–54, 56, 64
Leland TM: Albertus Adair Moore, M.D. 1834–1910. **J SC Med Assoc** 1984 Jul;80(7):358
Lesky E: American medicine as viewed by Viennese physicians, 1893–1912. **Bull Hist Med** 1982 Fall;56(3):368–76
Linder SC: Medicine in Marlboro County 1736 to 1980. Baltimore, Gateway, 1980. 206 p.
Linder SC: Pioneer physicians in Marlboro County, 1760–1824. **SC Hist Mag** 1980 Jul;81:232–44
Linder SG: Pioneer physicians in Marlboro County, 1760–1824. **SC Hist Mag** 1980;81(3):232–44
Lunde AS: Health in the United States. **Ann Am Acad Polit Soc Sci** 1981;453:28–69
Luongo EP: A biography of Wallace Mason Yater, M.D. [S.l., s.n.], 1982. iv, 180 p.
McDonell KM: Dr. William A. Lindsay, innovator, physician, enterpreneur. **Indiana Med Hist Q** 1980;6(1):5–23
McDonell KM: Medicine in antebellum Indiana: conflict, conservatism, and change. Indianapolis, Indiana Historical Society, 1984. 58 p. (Publications in Indiana Medical History, No. 1).
McDonell KM: William A. Lindsay in perspective. **Indiana Hist Soc** 1981 Jun;7(2):3–20
Mason EM: Some insights into the life of a country doctor. **Md State Med J** 1981 Nov;30(11):20–1
Mills GH: Hawaiians and medicine. **Hawaii Med J** 1981 Oct;40(10):272–6
Moes RJ: The elusive Dr. Burrough: Alta California's first physician. **South Calif Q** 1982;64(4):265–80
Murphy RL, Nodyne KR: The healing science in the Mountain State: some notable medical personalities of West Virginia. **W Va Hist** 1981 Spring–Summer;42(3–4):285–306
Nadig P, Wyatt BW: A personal history of Bexar County medicine. **Friends P.I. Nixon Med Hist Libr** 1981;10:6–13
Navarro V: Medical history as justification rather than explanation: a critique of Starr's The Social Transformation of American Medicine. **Int J Health Serv** 1984;14(4):511–28
Nixon PI: Pat Nixon of Texas. Autobiography of a doctor. Ed. by H. H. Lang. College Station, Texas, and London, Texas A & M University Press, 1979. 288 p.
Novotny A, Smith C, ed: Images of healing. A portfolio of American medical & pharmaceutical practice in the 18th, 19th, & early 20th centuries. New York, Macmillan, 1980, 144 p.
Numbers RL, Leavitt JW, ed: Wisconsin medicine. Historical perspectives. Madison, University of Wisconsin Press, 1981. ix, 212 p.
Peitzman SJ: Forgotten reformers: the American Academy of Medicine. **Bull Hist Med** 1984 Winter;58(4):516–28
Pernick MS: A calculus of suffering: pain, anesthesia, and utilitarian professionalism in nineteenth-century American medicine. Ph.D. Diss. Columbia University. New York, 1979.
Pernick MS: [History of] medical professionalism [in the United States]. In Reich WT, et al, ed: Encyclopedia of bioethics, v.3. New York, Free Press, 1978. p. 1028–34.
Petersdorf RG: Managing the revolution in medical care. **J Med Educ** 1984 Feb;59(2):79–90
Pfund N, Hofstadter L: Biomedical innovation and the press. **J Commun** 1981;31(2):138–54
Pickens DR: Medical practice in early Nashville. **J Tenn Med Assoc** 1981 Sep;74(9):637–42
Plummer BL: Document: letters of James Durham to Benjamin Rush. **J Negro Hist** 1980;65(3):261–9
Pollack NS: Medicine nineteenth-century style. **Echoes** 1981 Mar;20:4–5
Quattlebaum JK: Medicine in early Georgia (Savannah). **J Med Assoc Ga** 1983 Dec;72(12):829–32
Rabin PL, Rabin D: Landmark perspective: The care of the patient. Francis Peabody revisited. **JAMA** 1984 Aug 10;252(6):819–20
Raffel MW: The U. S. health system. New York, Wiley, 1980. ix, 639 p.
Reitman N: The history of medicine and medical care in New Brunswick. **J Med Soc NJ** 1984 Sep;81(9):737–9
Reverby S, Rosner D, ed: Health care in America: essays in social history. Philadelphia, Temple University Press, 1979. 275 p.
Reverby S: Stealing the golden eggs: Ernest Amory Codman and the science and management of medicine. **Bull Hist Med** 1981 Summer;55(2):156–71
Revolutionary doctors of Anne Arundel County: **Md Geneal Soc Bull** 1978 Fall;19:303–7
Rice TB: One hundred years medicine: Indianapolis, 1820–1920. **Indiana Med Hist Q** 1976;2(3):40–4
Risse GB: From horse and buggy to automobile and telephone: medical practice in Wisconsin, 1848–1930. In Numbers RL, Leavitt JW, ed: Wisconsin medicine. Historical perspectives. Madison, University of Wisconsin Press, 1981. p. 25–45.
Roland CG: Russell Morse Wilder. In Dictionary of American Biography, Suppl. 6, 1956–1960. p. 697–8, 1980.
Rosales VJ: The medicotrophic syndrome: an acute modern phenomenon. **Unitas** 1970;43(4):30–59
Rundall TG: Environmental selection and physician supply. **AJS** 1982 Mar;87(5):1090–1112
Salazar JG, Espinosa JM: A sociodemographic profile of Hispanic physicians in three United States metropolitan areas. **Aztlan** 1979;10:111–22
Sammis S, Dummett E: On display: the science and art of healing. **J Med Soc NJ** 1984 Sep;81(9):747–57
Schlicke CP: West Coast medicine in 1776. **Pac Northwest** 1976 Winter;20:58–68
Schmitt RC: Health and medical firsts in Hawaii. **Hawaii Med J** 1981 Oct;40(10):284–9
Shimkin MB: Roads to Oz. II. A personal account of some U.S.–USSR medical exchanges and contacts. 1942––1962. **Perspect Biol Med** 1979 Autumn;23(1):118–44
Siddall AC: George Chauncey Jameson, M.D., 1865–1948. From bloodletting to antibiotics. **Northwest Ohio Q** 1980;52(1):168–78
Silver P: From chloroform to CT scans––doctors recall early days of practice. **J Miss State Med Assoc** 1981 Dec;22(12):312–5
Simpson HN: Doctors afield: David Cobb, M.D. **N Engl J Med** 1980 Dec 25;303(26):1517–9
Smith DC: The triumph of scientific medicine in America: an essay review. **J Hist Med Allied Sci** 1982 Apr;37(2):231–5
Sorensen AA, Kunitz SJ: The changing distribution of physicians in Regionville. **Rural Sociol** 1978;43(4):711–25
Stevenson LG: The emergence of American medicine in the nineteenth century. **Cah Hist Mond** 1968;11(3):455–66
Strickland WA: Requiem for a frontier physician: James W. Parker, M.D., doctor to the wagon trains and mountaineers of old Westport. **Mo Med** 1981 Oct;78(10):631–6
Swinton WE: Cadwallader Colden: physician, historian and government official. **Can Med Assoc J** 1981 Mar 15;124(6):805–9
Sydenham DM: Practitioner and patient. The practice of medicine in eighteenth-century South Carolina. Ph.D. Diss. Johns Hopkins University. Baltimore, 1979. vii, 323 leaves.
Thomas L: The youngest science. Notes of medicine-watcher. New York, Viking Press, 1983. xvi, 270 p.
Thompson HE: Early history of the Medical Society of the U. S. and Mexico. **Ariz Med** 1982 Jan;39(1):55–8
Valle RK, Valle AR: La disertacion fisico–médica en la qual se prescribe un método seguro para preservar a los pueblos de viruelas hasta lograr la completa extincion de ellas en todo el reyno, by Dr. Francisco Gil. In International Congress of the History of Medicine, 27th, Barcelona, 1980. Actas. Barcelona, Académia de Ciències Médiques de Catalunya i Balears, 1981. p. 217–22.
Van Voorhis Wendler M: Doctors and diseases on the Ohio frontier. **Ohio Hist** 1980 Spring;89(2):222–40
Vogel MJ, Rosenberg CE, ed: The therapeutic revolution. Essays in the social history of American medicine. Philadelphia, University of Pennsylvania Press, 1979. xiii, 270 p.
Wallerstein RO: ABIM certification revisited–what a difference 30 years make. **Trans Am Clin Climatol Assoc** 1982;94:182–9
Walsh JP, Adelson R: Health care: no time for placebos. **NY Aff** 1978;5(2):151–61
Walton JC: The state of medicine in 1912. **NC Med J** 1984 Feb;45(2):123–4
Weisert JJ: Dr. Anthony Hunn: from storm and stress to tempest and sunshine. **Filson Club Hist Q** 1982;56(2):211–24
Weiss GN, Weiss EB: The health care profession on the threshold of the eighties: physician and nurse. **J La State Med Soc** 1980 Oct;132(10):151–4

Weisse AB: Conversations in medicine. **J Med Soc NJ** 1984 Jul;81(7):576–9
Wilcox HG: The president ails: American medicine in retrospect (George Washington). **Eval Program Plann** 1981 Apr;53(4):201–10
[Willis Dew Gatch. Includes reprints of three of his articles.]: **Indiana Med Hist Q** 1977;3(3):43–60
Workman M: Medical practice in Philadelphia at the time of the yellow fever epidemic, 1793. **Pa Folklife** 1978;27(4):33–9
Wylie MS: Images of sickness and health in American medical thought: 1776–1800 and 1835–1865. Ph.D. Diss. American University. Washington, 1981. 541 p.
Wyman M: Medicine and surgery in 1881. **N Engl J Med** 1981 Oct 29;305(18):1059–62

### USSR

Abdullaev RA: Uspekhi i perspektivy vnutrenneĭ meditsiny v Uzbekskoĭ SSR. **Ter Arkh** 1982;54(12):7–11
Al'bitskiĭ VIu: K 150–letiiu so dnia rozhdeniia Nikolaia Andreevicha Vinogradova - uchenika S. P. Botkina. **Klin Med (Mosk)** 1982 Sep;60(9):121–3
Alekseev GA, Sergeev TS, Galkina ND: N. K. Adrianov--pervyĭ vrach-chuvash. **Sov Zdravookhr** 1981;(11):65–7
Alexander JT: Medical professionals and public health in 'Doldrums' Russia (1725–62). **Can Am Slav Stud** 1978;12(1):116–35
Anisimov VE: Nikolaĭ Andreevich Vinogradov (k 150–letiiu so dnia rozhdeniia). **Klin Med (Mosk)** 1982 Mar;60(3):118–9
Anisimov VE: Professor L. E. Pikulin (1784–1824) (k 200–letiiu so dnia rozhdeniia). **Sov Zdravookhr** 1984;(10):75–6
Anisimov VE: Ucheniki i psoledovateli S. P. Botkina v. Kazani. **Klin Med (Mosk)** 1982 Sep;60(9):113–6
Arkhangel'skiĭ GV: A. I. Gertsen i S. P. Botkin. **Klin Med (Mosk)** 1982 Nov;60(11):118–20
Arkhangel'skiĭ GV: S. P. Botkin i M. E. Saltykov–Shchedrin. **Klin Med (Mosk)** 1982 Oct;60(10):114–8
Arkhangel'skiĭ GV: S. P. Botkin i pisateli-revoliutsionery demokraty. **Sov Zdravookhr** 1983;(2):60
Arkhangel'skiĭ GV: Teoreticheskie vzgliady S. P. Botkina po klinicheskim i obshchepatologicheskim voprosam meditsiny (k 150–letiiu so dnia rozhdeniia). **Klin Med (Mosk)** 1981 Nov;59(11):109–13
Bagdasarian SM: Velikiĭ Russkiĭ klinitsist S. P. Botkin (k 150–letiiu so dnia rozhdeniia). **Klin Med (Mosk)** 1982 Dec;60(12):94–9
Bezkorovainy A: Science and medicine in Imperial Russia. Chicago, (The Author), 1980. 271 p.
Blokhin NN: 60-letie Soiuza Sovetskikh Sotsialisticheskikh Respublik i razvitie Sovetskoĭ meditsinskoĭ nauki. **Vestn Akad Med Nauk SSSR** 1983;6:3–5
Borodiĭ NK: Mediki na Ukraine v XVIII veke. **Sov Zdravookhr** 1980;(9):64–7
Borodiĭ NK: O razvitii meditsiny Ukrainy v XVIII veke. **Sov Zdravookhr** 1981;(11):53–6
Borodulin VI: Vydaiushchiĭsia terapevt V. F. Zelenin i ego rol' v razvitii sovetskoĭ meditsiny. **Feldsher Akush** 1982;47(3):52–4
Borodyi MK: Arkhivni dzerela z istorii medytsyny na livoberezhnyi ukraini u XVIII st. **Ukr Istor Zh** 1981;(9):137–41
Bragin AM: I. M. Sechenov i otechestvennaia meditsina (k 150–letiiu so dnia rozhdeniia. **Klin Med (Mosk)** 1980 Jun;58(6):113–7
Brzheskiĭ VCh: Mestnaia pechat' - o meditsinskikh rabotnikakh. **Sov Zdravookhr** 1983;6:70–1
Burchinskiĭ GI: Razvitie kliniki vnutrennikh bolezneĭ v USSR za 60 let. **Klin Med (Mosk)** 1982 Dec;60(12):22–9
Frieden NM: Russian physicians in an era of reform and revolution, 1856–1905. Princeton, Princeton University Press, 1981. xvii, 378 p.
Frieden NM: The roots of Russian zemstvo medicine. In: Congrès international d'histoire de la médecine, XXVe, Québec, 1976. Actes. Québec, 1977. p. 99–120.
Galiev VZ: Meditsinskaia deiatel'nost' ssyl'nykh revoliutsionerov v Kazakhstane (vtoraia polovina XIX veka). Alma-Ata, Kazakhstan, 1982. 158 p.
Geselvich AM: Letopis' zhizni N.I. Pirogova, 1810–1881. Moskva, Meditsina, 1976. 97 p.
Golovteev VV, Korchagin VP: [Rates and proportions of the development of prophylactic medical care in the USSR] (Rus). **Sov Zdravookhr** 1980;12:9–13
Graham L: Biomedicine and the politics of science in the USSR. **Sov Union** 1981;8(2):147–58
Gritskevich VP: Istoriko-meditsinskoe istochnikovedenie. **Sov Zdravookhr** 1980;(9):56–8
Iuldashev KIu: Vnutrenniaia meditsina Uzbekistana za 60 let. **Klin Med (Mosk)** 1982 Dec;60(12):29–32
Ivaniushkin AIa: Lenin--kul'tura--meditsina. **Farmakol Toksikol** 1980 May–Jun;43(3):261–5
Kaladze NN: Nikolaĭ Fedorovich Golubov (k 125–letiiu so dnia rozhdeniia). **Klin Med (Mosk)** 1982 Nov;60(11):120–3
Kanep VV: Aktual'nye voprosy muzeevedeniia: iz opyta raboty Muzeia istorii meditsiny im. P. Stradynia : tezisy dokladov. Riga, Ministerstvo zdravookhraneniia Latviĭskoĭ SSR, 1982. 195 p.
Katsnel'bogen AG: Dekabrist G. S. Baten'kov. **Sov Zdravookhr** 1982;(8):62–7
Katsnel'bogen AG: Delo o rassmotrenii lektsiĭ I. E. Diad'kovskogo. **Klin Med (Mosk)** 1981;59(4):116–8
Kaveckij RE, Balickij KP: Les sciences médicales. (Rus). In: L'histoire de l'Académie des sciences d'Ukraine. 1919–1979. (Rus). Kiev: Naukova Dumka, 1979, Académie Ukrainienne des Sciences, URSS, 483–490.
Kliachkin LM: Ucheniki S. P. Botkina v. Saratove. **Klin Med (Mosk)** 1982 Sep;60(9):119–21
Knel'ts VF: Deiatel'nost' vracheĭ pervoĭ poloviny XIX veka na territorii sovremennoĭ Udmurtii. **Sov Zdravookhr** 1980;(10):55–7
Komarov FI: S. P. Botkin--vydaiushchiisia deiatel' otechestvennoi meditsiny. **Vestn Akad Med Nauk SSSR** 1983;(3):3–7
Kopelev L: Der heilige Doktor Fjodor Petrowitsch: die Geschichte des Friedrich Joseph Haass, Bad Münstereifel 1780–Moskau 1853. 2. Aufl. Hamburg, Hoffmann und Campe, 1984. 231 p.
Kuzmin MK: [Medicine in the Soviet Union and the impact of the scientific–technical revolution on its development.] (Rus). **Orvostort Kozl** 1981;93–96(27 No 1–4):201–10
Lopatenok AA: M. D. Tushinskiĭ, 1882–1962. Moskva, Meditsina, 1983. 47 p.
Manafov IT: N. Narimanov--vrach, revoliutsioner, partiĭnyi ĭ gosudarstvennyĭ deiatel'. **Sov Zdravookhr** 1982;(4):58–61
Matkovskiĭ NI: Vydaiushchiisia Sovetskiĭ terapevt-infektsionist Nikolaĭ Ivanovich Ragoza (k 100–letiiu so dnia rozhdeniia). **Klin Med (Mosk)** 1983 Oct;61(10):136–8
Müller-Dietz HE: Aerzte im Russland des achtzehnten Jahrhunderts. Esslingen/Neckar, Robugen, 1973. 111 p.
Müller-Dietz HE: Friedrich Joseph Haass, ein deutscher Arzt in Moskau. **Clio Med** 1981 Apr;15(3–4):177–89
Neiman IM: Predvidenie--osnovnaia osobennost' tvorchestva Aleksandra Aleksandrovicha Bogomol'tsa. **Fiziol Zh** 1981 May–Jun;27(3):307–10
Peleshchuk AP, Koliadenko VG, Zhukovskiĭ LI: Ucheniki S. P. Botkina na Ukraine. **Klin Med (Mosk)** 1982 Sep;60(9):110–3
Petrov BD: Izuchenie nauchnogo naslediia S. P. Botkina. **Sov Zdravookhr** 1983;(2):57–9
Petrov NS: Sergeĭ Petrovich Botkin (k 150–letiius so dnia rozhdeniia). **Probl Gematol Pereliv Krovi** 1982 Dec;27(12):49–51
Polenova IV: N. A. Iaroshenko i ucheniki S. P. Botkina. **Klin Med (Mosk)** 1982 Sep;60(9):117–9
Riabov SI, Stavskaia VV: Idei S. P. Botkina v nefrologii. **Klin Med (Mosk)** 1982 Sep;60(9):27–32
Salnikova GP: Zhizn' i deiatel' nost' A.N. Rubakina. **Sov Med** 1981;(2):114–6
Savel'ev VS: N. I. Pirogov -- veljkiĭ russkiĭ khirurg i uchenyĭ. **Sov Med** 1981;(11):116–8
Schtschepin OP, Wladimirova LJ: Die Zusammenarbeit der UdSSR mit den anderen sozialistischen Ländern auf dem Gebiet der medizinischen Wissenschaft und des Gesundheitswesens. **Med Ges** 1979;(6):123–39
Shalaev NF: Terapevt, uchenyĭ i pedagog V.I. Glinchikov. **Klin Med (Mosk)** 1984 Oct;62(10):146–9
Shimkin MB: Roads to Oz. II. A personal account of some U.S.-USSR medical exchanges and contacts. 1942--1962. **Perspect Biol Med** 1979 Autumn;23(1):118–44
Shingarov Gkh: Teoreticheskie nasledie V. I. Lenina i nekotorye metodologicheskie problemy sovremennoĭ meditsiny. **Vestn Akad Med Nauk SSSR** 1980;(4):9–16
Shul'tsev GP: Khronologiia zhizni i deiatel'nosti Sergeia Petrovicha Botkina (k 150–letiiu so dnia rozhdenia). **Klin Med (Mosk)** 1983 Oct;61(10):142–8
Shul'tsev GP: Perechityvaia 'Klinicheskie Lektsii' S. P. Botkina (k 100–letiu so dnia izdaniia). **Klin Med (Mosk)** 1983 Oct;61(10):132–6
Shul'tsev GP: Zhizn' i deiatel'nost' Sergeia Petrovicha Botkina. **Klin Med (Mosk)** 1982 Sep;60(9):12–21
Slavětínský M: Předchudci československo-sovětských lékařských styku. **Cesk Zdrav** 1982 Sep;30(8–9):381–5
Solimonov SL: Mediko-sotsial'nye issledovaniia problemy narodonaseleniia Latviskoi SSR. **Latv PSR Zinat Acad Vestis** 1981;8:75–84
Tareev EM: Sergeĭ Petrovich Botkin i sovremennaia klinika. **Klin Med (Mosk)** 1982 Sep;60(9):4–11
Tsiklik AM: S. M. Vasil'ev i ego klinicheskoe nasledie (K 125–letiiu so dnia rozhdeniia). **Ter Arkh** 1980;52(7):143–6
Uspenskaia EP: Mikhail Vasil'evich Chernorutskiĭ (k 100–letiiu so dnia rozhdeniia). **Ter Arkh** 1984;56(7):151–3

### Venezuela

Beauperthuy de Benedetti R: Au sujet des quatre faits importants de la medecine au Venezuela. In: International Congress of the History of Medicine, 26th, Plovdiv (Bulgaria), 1978. Actes du Congres, Vol. 1. Sofia, 1980. p. 90–2.
Beauperthuy de Benedetti R: Un cirujano y un medico de Montpellier en el siglo pasado en Caracas. **Rev Soc Venez Hist Med** 1979;28(42):29–30
Fébres–Cordero F: Algunos aspectos de la medicina venezolana del siglo XIX y su relación con el período histórico a que corresponde. **Tec Hosp** 1981 Mar–Jun;28(1–2)41–7
Los médicos en la batalla de Carabobo: Caracas, Ministerio de Educación,

Dirección General, Dept. de Publicaciones, 1972. 93 p.
Mazzei Uzcátegui M: Dos figuras medicas venezolanas. **Rev Soc Venez Hist Med** 1969-71;17-19(31-33):163-94
Octavio O: Algunos momentos familiares de Don Lisandro Alvarado. **Bol Acad Nac Hist (Caracas)** 1981;64(254):419-23
Plaza Izquierdo F: Palabras pronunciadas con motivo de su incorporacion como individuo de numero de la Sociedad Venezolana de Historia de la Medicina. **Rev Soc Venez Hist Med** 1981;30(45-46):89-99
Sociedad Venezolana de Historia de la medicina: En homenaje al Dr. Placido Daniel Rodriguez Rivero en el 100e aniversario de su nacimiento. Revista de la Sociedad Venezolana de Historia de la Medicina, 1977; 26(40), p. 11-85. Contributions by M. Rodríguez Navarro, G. Briceño Romero, D. W. Fernándex Pérez, A. Osuna, C. R. Travieso, A. Silva Alvarez, N. Perazo, R. Beauperthuy de Benedetti, M. Granier-Doyaux, R. Caldera.

**Vietnam**

Huard P, Nguyên Trân Huân: La médecine vietnamienne au XVIIIe siècle. In: Congrès National des Sociétés Savantes, 101e, Lille, 1976. Comptes Rendus. Paris, 1976. Section des Sciences, Fasc. III. p. 61-8.
Tran Huan N: Quelques aspects de la médecine et de la pharmacie au Vietnam. **Sci Orient** 1978;13:1-11

**Yugoslavia**

Djordjević SP: Akademik prof. dr Dušan Borić (1. IX 1889-3. IX 1978). **Srp Arh Celok Lek** 1980 May;108(5):541-53
Djordjević SP: General Prof. Dr. Vladimir S. Stanojević (3. III 1886 - 5. VI 1978. **Srp Arh Celok Lek** 1980 Mar;108(3):281-92
Grujić V: Nekolike korespondentne veze ismedju Vladana Djordjevića i Valtazara Bogišića. **Srp Ark Celok Lek** 1981 Jan;109(1):161-8
Jelić R: Zdravstvo u zadru i njegovu podrucju. Zadar, Narodni List, 1978. 383 p.
Pejčić M: Lekari i narodna medicina u Pirotu pre oslobodjenja od Turaka. **Srp Arh Celok Lek** 1981 Dec;108(12):1349-55
Pejčić M: O nekim lekarima, apotekarima, i narodonoj medicini u Nišu za vreme Turaka (XIX vek). **Srp Arh Celok Lek** 1981 Oct;109(10):1405-12
Pertl E: Prvi slovenski zdravniki v Mariboru. **Zb Zgodovino Naravoslovja Teh** 1981;5-6:95-191
Rajkov M: Jedan popis zdravstvenih radnika u velikokikindskom dištriktu 1875. Godine. **Naucni Sastanak Zb Rad Naucno Drus Istor Zdrav Kult Jugosl** 1976;(13):157-62

**Zambia**

Frankenberg R: Man, society and health: towards the definition of the role of sociology in the development of Zambian medicine. **Afr Soc Res** 1969;(8):573-87

**Zimbabwe**

Bergmar M: Stor förändring i nya, självständiga Zimbabwe: en sjukvård som gäller alla - inte går efter hudfärg. **Vardfacket** 1981 Apr 9;5(7):64-6
Roberts RS: A socio-historical view of the struggle for health in Zimbabwe. **Cent Afr J Med** 1979 Oct;25(10):235-6

# MENTAL HEALTH

See also **Psychiatry; Psychology; Psychosomatic Medicine**

Blasius D: Der verwaltete Wahnsinn: eine Sozialgeschichte des Irrenhauses. Frankfurt am Main, Fischer, 1980. 201 p.
Pompey H: Pastoralmedizin--der Beitrag der Seelsorge zur psycho-physischen Gesundheit. Eine bibliographisch-historische Analyse. In Imhof AE, ed: Mensch und Gesundheit in der Geschichte. Husum, Matthiesen, 1980. p. 115-34.
Richardson WJ: Religion and mental health. In Reich WT, et al, ed: Encyclopedia of bioethics, v.3. New York, Free Press, 1978. p. 1064-71.

**Great Britain**

Noble P: Mental health services and legislation--an historical review. **Med Sci Law** 1981 Jan;21(1):16-24

**United States**

Rochefort DA: Three centuries of care of the mentally disabled in Rhode Island and the nation, 1650-1950. **RI Hist** 1981;40(4):110-32

**Before 500 A.D.**

**Rome**

Dieckhöfer K: Psychohygienische Konzepte in der römischen Kaiserzeit. **Ther Ggw** 1981;120(1):80-95

**1700 to Present**

Birtalan G: Személyi egeszségvédelem és mentálhygiéne a 18. században. **Orv Hetil** 1982 Mar 7;123(10):607-10
Colón Roure C, Rivera Nieves M: La intervención del terapista ocupacional en el equipo interdisciplinario en el area de la salud mental. **Bol Asoc Med PR** 1984 Jul;76(7):319-22
Danzinger R, Lyon G: Das Beratungszentrum für psychische und sociale Fragen in Graz. Wien, Osterreichische Akademie der Wissenschaften, 1982. 140 p.
Gibelli A: La guerra laboratorio: eserciti e igiene sociale verso la guerra totale. **Mov Operaio Soc** 1982;5(3):335-49
Leighton AH: Caring for mentally ill people. Psychological and social barriers in historical context. Cambridge, Cambridge University Press, 1982. x, 277 p.
Zax M: History and background of the community mental health movement. In Gibbs M, et. al., ed: Community psychology: theoretical and empirical approaches. New York, Gardner, 1980. p 3-28.

**Africa**

Lambo TA: Changing patterns of mental health needs in Africa. **Contemp Rev** 1973;222(1286):146-54

**Canada**

Frankenburg F: The 1978 Ontario Mental Health Act in historical context. **RSTC** 1982;22(6 No 3):172-7

**Germany**

Kalcher J: Ambrosius war kein Dinosaurier--dem Hansischen Jugendbund nachträglich zum Geburtstag. Versuch einer Deutung. **Prax Kinderpsychol Kinderpsychiatr** 1979 Aug-Sep;28(6):212-24

**Great Britain**

Iveson-Iveson J: The art of observation, 3. Attitudes to mental health. **Nurs Mirror** 1982 Sep 8;155(10):17
Templar M: Historical perspectives. **Nurs Mirror** 1984 Oct 24;159(15):vii-viii
Wilder F: The remarkable world of John Wesley, pioneer in mental health. Hicksville, Exposition Press, 1978. 192 p.

**Nicaragua**

Ahearn FL: Disaster mental health: a pre- and post-earthquake comparison of psychiatric admission rates. **Urban Soc Change Rev** 1981;14(2):22-8

**Poland**

Jaroszewski Z, Tarmanowska B: Dzieci w Instytucie Higieny Psychicznej (w Warszawie, 1943-1944). **Przegl Lek** 1981;38(1):152-5

**Spain**

Parellada i Feliu D: Comentaris al llibre 'Higiene del alma' del doctor Josep Call i Morros (editat a Barcelona l'any 1888). In Congrés International d'Història de la Medicina Catalana, 2nd, Barcelona, 1975. Llibre d'Actes. Barcelona, Socitra, 1977. p. 263-71.

**United States**

Bair B: 'The full light of the dawn': Congressman John Fogarty and the historical cycle of community mental health policy in Rhode Island. **RI Hist** 1982;41(4):127-38
Benson PR: Labeling theory and community care of the mentally ill in California: the relationship of social theory and ideology to public policy. **Hum Organ** 1980;39(2):134-41
[Blank MI]: Research on the mental health of the aging 1960-1976. Rockville, Md., National Institute of Mental Health, 1977 (and 1981), xii, 69 p.
Cohen S: The mental hygiene movement, the development of personality and the school: the medicalization of American education. **Hist Educ Q** 1983;23(2):123-49
Dain N: Clifford W. Beers: advocate for the insane. Pittsburgh, Univ. of Pittsburgh Press, 1980. xxix, 392 p.
Dwyer E: Mental health care in early twentieth century Indiana and the limits of reform. **Indiana Med Hist Q** 1983 Mar;9(1):23-7
Ediger EM: Influences on the origin and development of Mennonite mental health centers. **Mennon Q Rev** 1982;56(1):32-46
Fishbein L: The snake pit (1948): the sexist nature of sanity. **Am Q** 1979;31(5):641-65
Goldman HH: Integrating health and mental health services: historical obstacles and opportunities. **Am J Psychiatry** 1982 May;139(5):616-20
Griffin JD: The amazing careers of Hincks and Beers. **Can J Psychiatry** 1982 Dec;27(8):668-71

Grob GN, ed: Mental hygiene in twentieth century America: four studies, 1921–1924. New York, Arno Press, 1979. Separate paginations.
Grob GN, ed: Public policy and mental illness. Four investigations, 1915–1939. New York, Arno, 1980. Separate paginations.
Grob GN, ed: The beginnings of mental hygiene in America. Three selected essays 1833–1850. New York, Arno, 1973. Various paginations. Includes works by Amariah Brigham (1833); William Sweetser (1850); Samuel B. Woodward (1840).
Hodge MJ: Social forces, ideology, and the domain of mental health services. **Psychiatr Q** 1979 Winter;51(4):280–93
Jackson JS, Chatters LM, Neighbors HW: The mental health status of older black Americans: a national study. **Black Scholar** 1982;13(1):21–35
Levine M: The history and politics of community mental health. New York, Oxford University Press, 1981. 232 p.
Lindy JD, Lindy JG: Planning and delivery of mental health services in disaster: the Cincinnati experience. **Urban Soc Change Rev** 1981;14(2):16–21
Lounsbury JW, Roisum KG, Pokorny L, et al: An analysis of topic areas and topic trends in the Community Mental Health Journal from 1965 through 1977. **Community Ment Health J** 1979 Winter;15(4):267–76
Mennel RM: Ethel Sturges Dummer. In: Notable American women. The modern period. Cambridge, Mass., Belknap–Harvard Univ. Press, 1980. 4:208–10.
Miller B, Chambers EB, Coleman CM: Indo-Chinese refugees: a national mental health need assessment. **Migr Today** 1981;9(2):26–31
Naske CM: Bob Bartlett and the Alaska Mental Health Act. **Pac Northwest Q** 1980;71(1):31–9
Neufeld V: The Mennonite mental health story. **Mennon Q Rev** 1982;56(1):18–31
Nyman GW, Solomon N: Mental hygiene within the state health care delivery system: the Maryland perspective. **Md State Med J** 1980 Jun;29(6):62–6
Robbins T, Anthony D: Deprogramming, brainwashing and the medicalization of diviant religious groups. **Soc Probl** 1982;29(3):283–97
Rosenheck S: Money in the streets. **Work Pap Mag** 1982;9(2):19–23
Salter SS: Toward community mental hygiene. A history of state policy in California, 1939–1969. Doctor of Social Welfare Diss. University of California. Berkeley, 1978. iv, 382 leaves.
Satin DG: Erich Lindemann: the humanist and the era of community mental health. **Proc Am Philos Soc** 1982 Aug;126(4):327–46
Spaulding J, Balch P: A brief history of primary prevention in the twentieth century: 1908 to 1980. **Am J Community Psychol** 1983 Feb;11(1):59–80
Todd DM, Trickett EJ: The 1978 Division 27 award for distinguished contributions to community psychology and community mental health: James G. Kelly. **Am J Community Psychol** 1979 Jun;7(3):239–61
Weisz R: Stress and mental health in a boom town. **Univ Wyo Publ** 1979;43:31–47

## MICROBIOLOGY

See also **Cytology; Histology; Molecular Biology; Pathology**

Belloni L: Leeuwenhoek's Sehversuch am zusammengesetzten Auge und die entsprechende Beobachtung Boll's an der Stäbchenschicht der Netzhaut. **Janus** 1980;67(1-2-3):59–61
Bonsdorff B von: Smittämnenas historia; en översikt. **Nord Medicinhist Arsbok** 1983;:89–101
Cafiso, LM: Storia della teoria sulla generazione spontanea: Redi, Spallanzani, Pasteur. **Cult Sc** 1981;20(80):236–43
Classics of infectious diseases: **Rev Infect Dis** 1981 Mar–Apr;3(2):372–95 (continued regularly)
Demain Al, Solomon NA: Industrial microbiology. **Sci Am** 1981 Sep;245(3):67–75
Eron C: The virus that ate cannibals. New York, Macmillan, 1981. xii, 1983 p.
Greenberg L: Serratia marcescens in human affairs. **Drug Intell Clin Pharm** 1978 Nov;12(11):674–9
Majno G: Inflammation and infection: historic highlights. **Monogr Pathol** 1982;(23):1–17
Marchette NJ, Stiller D: Ecological relationships and evolution of the rickettsiae. Boca Raton, CRC Press, 1982. 2 v.
Micoud M: Die ansteckenden Krankheiten. In Sournia JC, Martiny M, Poulet J, ed: Illustrierte Geschichte der Medizin. Salzburg, Andreas, 1980. Vol. 6. p. 2243–93.
Ogasawara K: [Recollections on microbiological research] (Jpn). **Nippon Saikingaku Zasshi** 1982 Jul;37(4):757–9
Pohle HD, Grossgebauer K: Erreger und Infektion--Begriffe und Wandel ihrer Sinngehalte. **Off Gesundheitswes** 1982 Dec;44(12):767–73
Richmond PA: The germ theory of disease. In Lilienfeld AM, ed: Times, places, and persons. Baltimore, London, Johns Hopkins Univ. Press, 1980. (Sigerist suppl. to the Bull Hist Med, n.s., no 4) p. 84–93.
Riley RL: Airborne contagion. Historical background. **Ann NY Acad Sci** 1980;353:3–9

**Germany**

Koch T: Gedanken zur 100. Wiederkehr des Tages der Entdeckung des Tuberkuloseerregers durch Robert Koch. **Gegenbaurs Morphol Jahrb** 1982;128(1):1–11

**Netherlands**

Luyendijk-Elshout AM: Antoni van Leeuwenhoek (1632–1723) herdacht. **Ned Tijdschr Geneeskd** 1983 Jun 18;127(25):1111–2

**Before 500 A.D.**

Groves D, Dunlop J, Buick R: Les premières traces de vie. **Pour Sci** 1981;50:22–35
Schoental R: A corner of history. Moses and mycotoxins. **Prev Med** 1980 Jan;9(1):159–61

**1450–1700**

Bibel DJ: The discovery of the oral flora--a 300-year retrospective. **J Am Dent Assoc** 1983 Oct;107(4):569–70

**Great Britain**

Selwyn S: The transition from mythology to medical microbiology in 1589. In: Congrès international d'histoire de la médecine, XXVe, Québec, 1976. Actes. Québec, 1977. p. 1262–73.

**Italy**

Gottdenker P: Francesco Redi and the fly experiments. **Bull Hist Med** 1979 Winter;53(4):575–92

**Netherlands**

Bardell D: The roles of the sense of taste and clean teeth in the discovery of bacteria by Antoni van Leeuwenhoek. **Microbiol Rev** 1983 Mar;47(1):121–6
Ford BJ: Cytological examination of Leeuwenhoek's first microbial specimens. **Tissue Cell** 1982;14(2):207–17
López-Ochoterena E: La décima octava carta de Leeuwenhoek. (Delft en Holanda, 9 octubre, 1676). **An Soc Mex Hist Cienc Tec** 1979;5:85–90
Mikx F: Antoni van Leeuwenhoek--300 sodina oralne mikrobiologije. **Acta Stomatol Croat** 1983;17(4):323–5
Mikx FH: Het tandplaque-onderzoek van Antoni van Leeuwenhoek in 1683. **Ned Tijdschr Tandheelkd** 1983 Sep;90(9):421–4

**1700 to Present**

Austrian R: Pneumococcus: the first one hundred years. **Rev Infect Dis** 1981 Mar–Apr;3(2):183–9
Austrian R: Tracking the identity of Lister's pneumococcal groups T and V (Danish types 45 and 46). **Yale J Biol Med** 1982 May–Aug;55(3-4):173–8
Baguenier-Desormeaux L: Henry Drysdale Dakin à Compiègne, en 1915. **Rev Hist Pharm (Paris)** 1981 Jun;28(249):79–88
Baldacci G, Frontali L, Lattanzi A: The debate on spontaneous generation and the birth of microbiology. **Fundam Sci** 1981;2(2):123–36
Barile MF: A brief history of the IOM. **Yale J Biol Med** 1983 Sep–Dec;56(5-6):353–4
Bazanov VA, Schneck P: Robert Koch und die deutsch-russischen Beziehungen auf dem Gebiete der Mikrobiologie. **Z Gesamte Hyg** 1982 Mar;28(3):201–5
Bednarski Z: Sto lat od odkrycia prątka gruźlicy (1882–1982) przez Roberta Kocha: szybka reakcja w polskich czasopismach lekarskich. **Pol Tyg Lek** 1983 Mar 28;38(13):419–21
Beltrán E: Conmemoración del descubrimiento de uno de los gérmenes patogénicos del paludismo. **Gac Med Mex** 1981 May;117(5):195–201
Beltrán E: Notas de historia protozoológica V. el renacimiento de la protozoología. Siete fecundos lustros: 1941–1976. **An Soc Mex Hist Cienc Tec** 1979;5:91–114
Beltrán E: Notas de historia protozoológica VI. la regeneración en los protozoarios. **An Soc Mex Hist Cienc Tec** 1979;5:115–26
Birtalan G: Klinisch-ätiologische Konzeptionen der achtziger Jahre des 19. Jahrhunderts im Spiegel der ungarischen Fachliteratur. **Wiss Beitr Martin Luther Univ Halle Wittenberg** 1983;5–R80:123–7
Burchall JJ: The development of the diaminopyrimidiness. **J Antimicrob Chemother** 1979 Nov;5(B):3–14
Carter KC: Germ theory, hysteria, and Freud's early work in psychopathology. **Med Hist** 1980 Jul;24(3):259–74
Chamberlain RW: Arbovirology--then and now. **Am J Trop Med Hyg** 1982 May;31(3 Pt 1):430–7
Collier LH: Recherches sur les Chlamydia - une vue rétrospective. **Rev Int Trach Pathol Ocul Trop Subtrop Sante Publique** 1982;(2-3):17–23
Crellin JK: Antibiosis in the nineteenth century. In J. Parascandola, ed: The history of antibiotics. Madison, American Institute of the History of Pharmacy, 1980. p. 5–13.
Crellin JK: Internal antisepsis or the dawn of chemotherapy? **J Hist Med Allied Sci** 1981 Jan;36(1):9–18

# MICROBIOLOGY

Downs WG: The Rockefeller Foundation virus program: 1951–1971 with update to 1981. **Annu Rev Med** 1982;33:1–29

Endicott SL: Germ warfare and 'plausible denial': the Korean war, 1952–1953. **Mod China** 1979;5(1):79–104

Fasquelle R, Delaunay A: Geschichte der Mikrobiologie. In Sournia JC, Martiny M, Poulet J, ed: Illustrierte Geschichte der Medizin. Salzburg, Andreas, 1980. Vol. 7. p. 2459–97.

Fraenkel-Conrat H: Portraits of viruses: tobacco mosaic virus. **Intervirology** 1981;15(4):177–89

Freundt EA: Mycoplasma hominis: historical outline and taxonomy. **Sex Transm Dis** 1983 Oct–Dec;10(4 Suppl):226–9

Ginneken J van: Bacteriological warfare. **J Contemp Asia** 1977;7(2):130–52

Girstenbrey W: Robert Koch und sein Erbe. Bedingungen, Konsequenzen und aktuelle Bedeutung einer historischen Leistung für Medizin und Gesundheitspolitik. **Fortschr Med** 1982 Mar 25;100(12):541, 544–6

Glaser S: L'arma batteriologica secondo la convenzione 1971. **Riv Mil** 1975;98(4):56–62

Gottdenker P: Three clerics in pursuit of 'little animals.' **Clio Med** 1980 Jul;14(3–4):213–24

Grange JM: Koch's Tubercle Bacillus - a centenary reappraisal. **Zentralbl Bakteriol Mikrobiol Hyg [A]** 1982 Mar;251(3):297–307

Greenberg SC: The entry of microbiology into clinical medicine. **Conn Med** 1980 Oct;44(10):641–3

Grellet I, Kruse C: Histoires de la tuberculose. Les fièvres de l'âme 1800–1940. Paris, Ramsay, 1983. 333 p.

Hahn FE: Virus chemotherapy: the problem, its development and nature. In Hahn FE, ed: Virus chemotherapy. Basel, New York, Karger, 1980. p. 1–21. (Antibiotics and chemotherapy, v. 27).

Hirsch JG: The greatest success story in the history of medicine. **Med Times** 1980 Sep;108(9):36–43

Hsiung GD: Progress in clinical virology--1960 to 1980: a recollection of twenty years. **Yale J Biol Med** 1980 Jan–Feb;53(1):1–4

Johnson KM, Scribner Cl, McCormick JB: Ecology of ebola virus: a first clue? **J Infect Dis** 1981 May;143(5):749–51

Kaiser W, Hübner H, ed: Robert Koch (1843–1910). **Wiss Beitr Martin Luther Univ Halle Wittenberg** 1983;5–R80:3–321

Kaiser W, Werner K, Rothe J: Sozialmedizinische Konsequenzen aus dem Wirken von Robert Koch unter halleschem Aspekt. **Z Gesamte Hyg** 1982 Mar;28(3):179–84

Kampmeier RH: Establishment of Treponema pallidum as the etiologic agent in general paralysis. **Sex Transm Dis** 1980 Oct–Dec;7(4):197–8

Koehler W, Mochmann H: The development of the staining of bacteria up to the introduction of Gram's method in 1884. **Medicamentum** 1980;54:27–31; 55:29–31

Krause RM: Koch's postulates and the search for the AIDS agent. **Rev Infect Dis** 1984 Mar–Apr;6(2):270–9

Krause RM: The restless tide. The persistent challenge of the microbial world. Washington, D. C., National Foundation for Infectious Diseases, 1981. 152 p.

Lutzker E: Some unanswered questions in medical history. In: Congrès international d'histoire de la médecine, XXVe, Québec, 1976. Actes. Québec, 1977. p. 917–27.

McIntosh K: Sense and nonsense in viral diagnosis--past, present, and future. **Curr Top Microbiol Immunol** 1983;104:1–6

Mathews-Roth MM: Carotenoid pigments and protection against photosensitization: how studies in bacteria suggested a treatment for a human disease. **Perspect Biol Med** 1984 Autumn;28(1):127–39

Mazumdar PM: Karl Landsteiner and the problem of species 1838–1968. Ph.D. Diss., Johns Hopkins University. Baltimore, 1976. 725 leaves.

Mollaret HH: Contribution à la connaissance des relations entre Koch et Pasteur. **NTM** 1983;20(1):57–65

Moseley JE: Travels of Alexandre Yersin: letters of a pastorian in Indochina, 1890–1894. **Perspect Biol Med** 1981 Summer;24(4):607–18

Mucha V, Bobková M: K histórii poznatkov o Pseudomonas aeruginosa. **Bratisl Lek Listy** 1982 Feb;77(2):229–34

Plamenac SD: Pojam antibioze i otkriće penicilina (I–II). **Srp Arh Celok Lek** 1981;108(6):675–87;(7–8):823–33

Plesset IR: Noguchi and his patrons. Rutherford, N.J., Fairleigh Dickinson, 1980. 314 p.

Possehl I: Impfstoffe, Sera, Diagnostika - Resultate bakteriologischer und immunologischer Forschung. In Hickel E, Schröder G, ed: Neue Beiträge zur Arzneimittelgeschichte. Festschrift für Wolfgang Schneider zum 70. Geburtstag. Stuttgart, Wissenschaftliche Verlagsgesellschaft, 1982. p. 185–203.

Prince AM: Detection of the relation between the Australia antigen and hepatitis B virus. **Vox Sang** 1984;47(3):257–60

Ravitch MM, McAuley CE: Airborne contamination of the operative wound. **Surg Gynecol Obstet** 1984 Aug;159(2):177–88

Rothe J, Werner K, Kaiser W: Sozialhygienische Konsequenzen aus der Klärung der Tuberkulose-Atiologie durch Robert Koch. **Z Gesamte Hyg** 1982 Mar;28(3):176–9

Seal SC: Centenary of discovery of cholera vibrio. **Indian J Public Health** 1983 Jan–Mar;27(1):1–5

Seal SC: Centenary of discovery of cholera vibrio. **J Indian Med Assoc** 1983 Dec;81(11–12):210–2

Siqueira LF, de Almeida RG, Belda W: Métodos tintoriais utilizados na identificação do Mycobacterium leprae. Revisão histórica. **Rev Saude Publica** 1984 Jun;18(3):246–58

Snell EE: Lactic acid bacteria and identification of B-vitamins: some historical notes, 1937–1940. **Fed Proc** 1979 Dec;38(13):2690–3

Toellner R: 'Ein Unding vor der Vernunft': Die generatio spontanea im Weltbild der aufgeklärten Naturforschung. In Dilg P, et al., ed: Perspektiven der Pharmaziegeschichte. Graz, Austria, Akademische Druck- u. Verlagsanstalt, 1983. p. 377–88.

Trenckmann U: Das mikrobiologische Modell im theoretischen Denken der Psychiatrie. **Wiss Beitr Martin Luther Univ Halle Wittenberg** 1983;5–R80:301–6

Zhdanov VM: Andre L'vov protiv D. I. Ivanovskogo. **Vopr Virusol** 1982 Jul–Aug;27(4):499–502

Zhdanova LG: K 100–letiiu otkrytiia pnevmokokka. **Zh Mikrobiol Epidemiol Immunobiol** 1981 Dec;(12):3–9

**Austria**

Carter KC: Ignaz Semmelweis, Carl Mayrhofer, and the rise of germ theory. **Med Hist** 1985 Jan;29(1):33–53

Lutzker E, Jochnowitz C: The curious history of Waldemar Haffkine. **Commentary** 1980;69(6):61–4

Majno G, Joris I: Billroth and Penicillium. **Rev Infect Dis** 1979 Sep–Oct;1(5):880–4

**Belgium**

Hennebert GL: Philibert Biourge, microbiologiste et mycologue (1864–1942). Colloque d'histoire des sciences III. Louvain, 1979. p. 61–98.

Welsch M: André Gratia, 1893–1950. In Florilège des Sciences en Belgique - II. Bruxelles, Académie Royale de Belgique, 1980. p. 663–72.

**Canada**

Lortie L: Joseph-Alexandre Crevier. In Dictionary of Canadian biography, 1881–1890. 1982;11:217–8.

**Cuba**

López Sánchez J: Karlos KH. Finlai i teoriia peredachi infektsii. **Vopr Istor Estestvozn Tekh** 1981;(4):29–34

**Czechoslovakia**

Blaškovič D: Twenty-five years of Acta Virologica. **Acta Virol (Praha)** 1982 Sep;26(5):408–16

Dr. Zdeněk Fencl 1922–1981: **Folia Microbiol (Praha)** 1982;27(5):285–94

Patočka F: Počátky české mikrobiologie. **Cesk Epidemiol Mikrobiol Imunol** 1983 May;32(3):121–5

Selected bibliography of Dr. J. Macura: **Folia Microbiol (Praha)** 1980;25(2):81–5

Skovránek V: Naše epidemiologie a mikrobiologie v posledních třiceti letech. **Cesk Epidemiol Mikrobiol Imunol** 1982 May;31(3):132–4

**Denmark**

Jacobson W: Gram's discovery of his staining technique. **J Infect** 1983 Sep;7(2):97–101

Medici TC: Das Gram-Präparat wird hundert Jahre alt. **Schweiz Rundsch Med Prax** 1983 Dec 13;72(50):1587–91

Vogt HH: 100 Jahre Gram-Färbung. Ein Forschungsbeitrag aus den Anfängen dieser Zeitschrift. **Fortschr Med** 1984 Apr;102(16):94–5

**France**

Aharonowitz Y, Cohen G: Les micro-organismes et l'industrie pharmaceutique. **Pour Sci** 1981;49:92–105

Baudin C: Pasteur: un homme, une oeuvre. **Chir Dent Fr** 1983 Jul 7;53(211):23–5

Berndt H: Emile Roux zum 50. Todestag. **Z Arztl Fortbild (Jena)** 1983;77(3):126–7

Brumpt L: L'oeuvre de Laveran en protozoologie et ses conséquences. **Bull Acad Natl Med (Paris)** 1980 Jan;164(1):88–93

Decourt P: Les zymases ou ferments solubles de Béchamp à la lumière des connaissances du XXe siècle. **Hist Sci Med** 1984;18(2):147–51

Delaunay A, ed: Présence de Pasteur. Paris, Fayard, 1973. 225 p. Includes contributions by P. Bidan, A. Gamet, J. Guillaume, L. Léger, J. Piton, J. De Rosnay, R. Scriban, C. Vago.

Dodin A: Albert Calmette. Président de la Société de Pathologie Exotique. **Bull Soc Pathol Exot Filiales** 1983 May–Jun;76(3):211–4

Fasquelle R: Pasteur et l'épopée pasteurienne. **Sem Hop Paris** 1983 Dec 22;59(48):3395–404

Geison GL: Pasteur on vital versus chemical ferments: a previously unpublished paper on the inversion of sugar. **Isis** 1981 Sep;72(263):425–45

Hourlier: 7 juin 1983: Cérémonie d'hommage public à Calmette (Hôpital des Armées de Lorient). **Bull Soc Pathol Exot Filiales** 1983 May–Jun;76(3):312–6

Kler JH: Pasteur. **J Med Soc NJ** 1981 Feb;78(2):121–4

Kostychev SP: Pasteur: his life and achievements. Annotated translation from the Russian by S. A. Wilde. New Delhi, Oxford & IBH Publishing Co., 1978. 96 p.
Mollaret P: La découverte, par Alphonse Laveran de l'agent du paludisme. Constantine, 6 Novembre 1880. **Nouv Presse Med** 1980 Nov 1;9(41):3055-63
Nicolle P: Un événement capital dans la vie passionnée de Charles Nicolle: le Prix Nobel de physiologie ou médecine. Souvenirs évoqués par Pierre Nicolle. **Bull Soc Pathol Exot Filiales** 1981 Jan-Feb;74(1):101-18
Nosny P: Alphonse Laveran et la découverte de l'hématozoaire du paludisme. **Bull Acad Natl Med (Paris)** 1980 Jan;164(1):80-7
Olsson JE, Reichard H: Mannen bakom syndromet: Pierre Ménétrier. Tumörpatolog och mikrobiolog med tidig insikt om precancerösa förändringar. **Lakartidningen** 1984 Oct 10;81(41):3705-6
Saenz A, Boisvert H: Correspondance inédite d'Albert Calmette (1863-1933). **Hist Sci Med** 1983;17(4):419-27
Saenz A, Boisvert H: Trois lettres de Louis Pasteur. **Hist Sci Med** 1981;15(4):327-33
Svarch Scharager N: Obra y vida de Luis Pasteur. **Rev Cubana Med Trop** 1980 Jan-Apr;32(1):79-90
Théodoridès J: Claude Bernard et la microbiologie médicale. In: Congrès international d'histoire de la médecine, XXVe, Québec, 1976. Actes. Québec, 1977. p. 1354-60.
Théodoridès J: La contribution d'A. Laveran à l'étude des Sporozoaires (Hémosporidies exceptées) et des Myxosporidies. **Hist Nat** 1980-81;17-18:77-84
Théodoridès J: Un précurseur girondin de la pathologie infectieuse: Jean Hameau (1779-1851). In: Congrès National des Sociétés Savantes, 104e, Bordeaux, 1979. Comptes Rendus. Paris, 1979. Section des Sciences, Fasc. IV. p. 81-95.
Wrotnowska D: Pasteur. Premières recherches sur les fermentations (1855-1857). **Clio Med** 1981 Apr;15(3-4):191-9

### Germany

Algeorge G: La 100 de ani de la descoperirea de către Robert Koch a agentului etiologic al tuberculozei. **Rev Ig [Pneumoftiziol]** 1982 Jan-Mar;31(1):13-7
Allen BW, Hinkes WF: Koch's cultivation of tubercle bacilli. **Med Lab Sci** 1983 Jan;40(1):85-7
Allen BW, Hinkes WF: La coloration de Koch pour les bacilles de la tuberculose. **Bull Int Union Tuberc** 1982 Sep-Dec;57(3-4):194-6
Ananthanarayan R: Robert Koch's contribution to microbiology. **Indian J Pathol Microbiol** 1982 Apr;25(2):169-71
Anastasatu C: Centenarul descoperirii bacilului Koch. **Rev Ig [Pneumoftiziol]** 1982 Jan-Mar;31(1):1-3
Bednarski Z: Robert Koch (1843-1910). **Wiad Lek** 1983 Mar 1;36(5):425-7
Benison S: Celebration and history: the centenary of Robert Koch's discovery of the tubercle bacillus. **Bull Hist Med** 1982 Summer;56(2):157-9
Bretey J: Robert Koch et son bacille. Un reportage. **Bull Acad Natl Med (Paris)** 1982 Mar;166(3):399-406
Bulla A: Reîntîlnire cu opera ştiinţficǎ a lui Robert Koch. **Rev Ig [Pneumoftiziol]** 1982 Jan-Mar;31(1):5-11
Daniel TM: Robert Koch, tuberculosis, and the subsequent history of medicine. **Am Rev Respir Dis** 1982 Mar;125(3 Pt 2):1-3
Döhner L: Die Kochschen Postulate und die Virologie. **Z Erkr Atmungsorgane** 1983;161(1):21-4
Dubb A: Medical philately: Robert Koch (1843-1910) the man, his germ and history. **Adler Mus Bull** 1984 Mar;10(1):16-22
Dubovsky H: Robert Koch (1843-1910)--the man and his work. **S Afr Med J** 1982 Nov 17;Spec No:3-5
Ferrari Sacco A, Oliaro T: A cent'anni dalla scoperta del micobatterio della tbc. (1822-1982). Robert Koch autore della grande scoperta. **Minerva Med** 1982 Sep 8;73(34):2199-202
Fleck L: Genesis and development of a scientific fact. Edited by T. J. Trenn and R. K. Merton. Chicago, Univ. of Chicago Press, 1979. xxviii, 203 p.
Foreman T, Gordon B, Weese WC: In honor of Robert Koch, M.D. **Ariz Med** 1983 Mar;40(3):149
Freerksen E: Die Atiologie der Tuberkulose--Der Weg dahin und die Folgen. **Prax Klin Pneumol** 1982 Mar;36(3):122-34
Fritzsche K: Erfahrungen bei der Tätigkeit in zwei 'Beweglichen Veterinär-Untersuchungsstellen' an der Ost- und Westfront während des letzten Weltkrieges. **DTW** 1982 Feb 5;89(2):65-70
Genschorek W: Robert Koch. Selbstloser Kampf gegen Seuchen und Infektionskrankheiten. Leipzig, Hirzel, 1981. 224 p. (Hervorragende Arzte im Dienste des Menschen).
Gergely J: Ehrlich 'varázslövedéke' a megvalósulás útján (gyógyszerek irányított célbajuttatása specifikus ellenanyagokkal). **Orv Hetil** 1982 Sep 19;123(38):2331-6
Grange JM, Bishop PJ: 'Uber Tuberkulose'. A tribute to Robert Koch's discovery of the tubercle bacillus, 1882. **Tubercle** 1982 Mar;63(1):3-17
Grujić M: Stogodišnjica otkrića bacila tuberkuloze. Zivot i delo Roberta Kocha. **Plucne Bolesti Tuberk** 1982 Jan-Jun;34(1-2):5-7
Haase HH: Uber einige Auswirkungen Robert Kochs und seiner Lehre auf die Entwicklung der Allgemeinen und Kommunalen Hygiene. **Z Gesamte Hyg** 1982 Mar;28(3):154-6
Henderson AR: A centennial remembrance of Koch's discovery of the tubercle bacillus. **Md State Med J** 1982 May;31(5):47-51
Hidvegi J: Die Resonanz der Kochschen Entdeckung in der medizinischen Fachpresse Ungarns. **Wiss Beitr Martin Luther Univ Halle Wittenberg** 1983;5-R80:87-90
Hoppe B: Die Biologie der Mikroorganismen von F. J. Cohn (1828-1898). **Sudhoffs Arch** 1983;67(2):158-89
Howard-Jones N: Robert Koch and the cholera vibrio: a centenary. **Br Med J [Clin Res]** 1984 Feb 4;288(6414):379-81
Jenschorek N: Robert Koch: Leben, Werk, Zeit. 2. durchgesehene Auflage. Leipzig, Hirzel, 1976. 247 p.
Kaiser W: Vor 100 Jahren beschrieb Robert Koch den Tuberkulose-Erreger. **Z Gesamte Inn Med** 1982 Mar 1;37(5):137-44
Klieneberger-Nobel E: Pionierleistungen für die medizinische Mikrobiologie: Lebenserinnerungen. Stuttgart, New York, Fischer, 1977. x, 144 p.
Knoke M: Viktor van der Reis--Wegbereiter der gastrointestinalen Mikroökologie des Menschen. **Nahrung** 1984;28(6-7):593-8
Knorr M: Das Jahr 1882 - Anfang und Folgen einer neuren medizinischen Methodik um und von Robert Koch. **Zentralbl Bakteriol Mikrobiol Hyg [B]** 1982;176(5-6):413-24
Koch centennial supplement: 100th anniversary of the announcement of the discovery of the tubercle bacillus by Robert Koch, March 24, 1882. **Am Rev Respir Dis** 1982 Mar;125(3 pt 2):1-132
Koch's bacillus: **Tubercle** 1982 Mar;63(1):1-2
Krakówka P: W 100-lecie odkrycia prątka gruźlicy. **Pneumonol Pol** 1982 Nov;50(11):557-8
Kreibich H: Betrachtungen zum 100. Jahrestag der Entdeckung des Mycobacterium tuberculosis durch Robert Koch. **Zentralbl Gynakol** 1982;104(5):258-67
Lammel HU: Virchow contra Koch? Neue Untersuchungen zu einer alten Streitfrage. **Z Gesamte Hyg** 1982 Mar;28(3):206-10
Lock W: Robert Koch. Bemerkungen aus heutiger Sicht. **Prax Klin Pneumol** 1982 Mar;36(3):106-10
Lock W: Robert Koch, Leben und Werk. **Prax Klin Pneumol** 1983 Oct;37 Suppl 1:409-11
Mecklinger L: Robert Koch. **Bull Int Union Tuberc** 1982 Jun;57(2):109-10
Meijer J: De tuberkelbacterie een eeuw bekend; 1882 - 24 Maart - 1982 (Heinrich Hermann Robert Koch). **Ned Tijdschr Geneeskd** 1982 Mar 13;126(11):488-9
Mendoza F: Acerca del descubrimiento del bacilo de Koch. **Rev Med Chil** 1983 May;111(5):539-43
Meve EB: Put' iskaniĭ Roberta Kokha. **Klin Med (Mosk)** 1982 Nov;60(11):111-4
Mochmann H: Biographische und literarische Notizen über Robert Koch aus Anlass des 100. Jahrestages -- 24. März 1982 -- seiner Bekanntgabe der Entdeckung des Tuberkelbazillus. **Padiatr Grenzgeb** 1982;21(2):83-112
Mochmann H, Kohler W: The clarification of the etiology of Asiatic cholera by the German cholera commission under the direction of Robert Koch in the year 1883--1884. **Indian J Public Health** 1983 Jan-Mar;27(1):6-20
Morowitz HJ: How E. coli got its name. **Hosp Pract** 1982 Dec;17(12):58-9
Moskwa Z: W setną rocznic e odkrycia prątka grużlicy. **Wiad Lek** 1983 May 1;36(9):799-802
Oliveira JC de: Em louvor de Koch. A propósito da descoberta do bacilo da tuberculose. **Acta Med Port** 1983 Mar;4(3):195-9
Ovchinnikov NM: K 75-letiiu otkrytiia vozbuditelia sifilisa. **Vestn Dermatol Venerol** 1980 Mar;(3):74-8
Ranasinghe L: Koch and Koch's bacillus: 100 years ago and today. **Ceylon Med J** 1982 Mar;27(1):1-5
Robert Koch: father of bacteriology and infectious diseases: **Ceylon Med J** 1982 Mar;27(1):6-7
Röhrer H: Friedrich Loeffler. Begründer der medizinischen Virusforschung vor 80 Jahren. **Hist Med Vet** 1979;4(2):46-8
Sakula A: Centenary of the discovery of the tubercle bacillus. **Lancet** 1982 Mar 27;1(8274):750
Sakula A: Robert Koch: centenary of the discovery of the tubercle bacillus, 1882. **Thorax** 1982 Apr;37(4):246-51
Sakula A: Robert Koch (1843-1910): founder of the science of bacteriology and discoverer of the tubercle bacillus. A study of his life and work. **Br J Dis Chest** 1979 Oct;73(4):389-94
Schadewaldt H: Anfänge der Medizinischen Mykologie in Deutschland. **Mykosen** 1981 Nov;24(11):654-67
Schadewaldt H: Die Entdeckung des Tuberkuloseerregers durch Robert Koch vor 100 Jahren. **Krankenhausarzt** 1983 Mar 3;56:157-66
Schadewaldt H: L'histoire de la découverte du bacille de Koch. **Hist Sci Med** 1982;16(4):337-41
Schmidt G: O znachenii otkrytiĭ Roberta Kokha dlia razvitiia bakteriologii i épidemiologii. **Zh Mikrobiol Epidemiol Immunobiol** 1983 Mar;(3):106-9
Schmidt G: Zur Bedeutung der Entdeckung Robert Kochs für die Entwicklungen der Bakteriologie. **Z Erkr Atmungsorgane** 1983;161(1):15-20
Schmitt W: Robert Koch, Mensch und Werk. **Zentralbl Chir** 1982;107(5-6):251-9
Steinbrück P: Der Erkenntnisprozess in Robert Koch auf seinem Wege

zum Begründer der Tuberkulosebekämpfung. **Z Erkr Atmungsorgane** 1983;161(1):6–14
Steinbrück P: Robert Koch und sein Werk. Seine Auswirkungen auf die Tuberkulosebekämpfung. **Z Erkr Atmungsorgane** 1982;158(1–2):5–23
Süla L: The 100th anniversary of the discovery of Koch's bacillus, the etiologic agent of tuberculosis. **J Hyg Epidemiol Microbiol Immunol** 1982;26(3):227–9
Szabó I: A Koch bacilus 100 éve. **Orv Hetil** 1982 Jan 24;123(4):227–9
Takeda Y, Zinnaka Y: [Centenary of the discovery of Vibrio cholerae by Robert Koch] (Jpn) **Nippon Saikingaku Zasshi** 1984 Jul;39(4):709–12
Talewski R: Robert Koch 11.XII.1843--27.V.1910. **Pneumonol Pol** 1982 Nov;50(11):553–5
Thom A: Theorie und Empirie in der Entstehungsgeschichte der Bakteriologie - der Beitrag von Edwin Klebs zur Begründung der bakteriologischen Ara.
**Wiss Beitr Martin Luther Univ Halle Wittenberg** 1983;5–R80:71–8
Viswanathan R: Robert Koch's contribution to medical science.
**Indian J Chest Dis Allied Sci** 1982 Apr–Sep;24(2–3):65–7
Wagner G: Robert Koch--Leistungen für die Menschheit.
**Z Arztl Fortbild (Jena)** 1982 Jul 15;75(14):653–5
Weise W: Die Entdeckung des Erregers der Tuberkulose durch Robert Koch vor 100 Jahren. **MMW** 1982 Mar 26;124(12):299–300
Weuffen W: Der Beitrag Robert Koch zur Begründung der Desinfektionslehre und heutige Schwerpunkte der Desinfektionsforschung und -praxis. **Z Gesamte Hyg** 1982 Mar;28(3):167–71
Weuffen W: Der Beitrag Robert Kochs zur Begründung der Desinfektionslehre und heutige Schwerpunkte der Desinfektionsforschung und -praxis. **Z Erkr Atmungsorgane** 1983;161(1):28–35
Wildfuehr G: Robert Koch, Begründer der modernen Mikrobiologie.
**Z Gesamte Hyg** 1982 Mar;28(3):145–8
Znachenie otkrytiia Roberta Kokha dlia razvitiia bakteriologii tuberkuleza: **Probl Tuberk** 1982 Mar;(3):3–7
Zolyomi ND: Die Kochsche Entdeckung in der Pressburger Tagespresse.
**Wiss Beitr Martin Luther Univ Halle Wittenberg** 1983;5–R80:79–84
100 de ani de la descoperirea de către Robert Koch a bacilului tuberculozei: **Rev Ig [Pneumoftiziol]** 1982 Oct–Dec;31(4):289–90

**Great Britain**

Abraham EP: Leonard Colebrook. In Dictionary of national biography, 1961–1970. Suppl. 8, 1981. p. 230–2.
Andrewes CH: Alick Isaacs. In Dictionary of national biography, 1961–1970. Suppl. 8, 1981. p. 569–70.
Burke JF: Ashley A. Miles and the prevention of infection following surgery. **Arch Surg** 1984 Jan;119(1):17–9
Carr JG: Microbes I have known: a study of those associated with fermented products. **J Appl Bacteriol** 1983 Dec;55(3):383–401
Cule J: Griffith Evans (1835–1935) and his trypanosome. **Vet Hist** 1979–80;1(3):94–101
Downie AW: Sir Samuel Phillips Bedson. In Dictionary of national biography, 1961–1970. Suppl. 8, 1981. p. 86–7.
Druett H: David Willis Wilson Henderson. In Dictionary of national biography, 1961–1970. Suppl. 8, 1981. p. 504–6.
Freundt EA: Derrick Graham ffarington Edward: a pioneer in mycoplasmology. **Rev Infect Dis** 1982 May–Jun;(4 Suppl):S3–7
Gale EF: Donald Devereux Woods. In Dictionary of national biography, 1961–1970. Suppl. 8, 1981. p. 1102–3.
Green DM: William John Tulloch. In Dictionary of national biography, 1961–1970. Suppl. 8, 1981. p. 1019–20.
Hamlin C: Edward Frankland's early career as London's official water analyst, 1865–1876: the context of 'previous sewage contamination'.
**Bull Hist Med** 1982 Spring;56(1):56–76
Henderson WM: Wellcome research: virology and the promotion of animal health. **Vet Rec** 1980 Oct 11;107(15):347–50
Howard-Jones N: Fake! **Br Med J [Clin Res]** 1982 Feb 13;284(6314):511
Lowbury EJ: Leonard Colebrook (1883–1967). **Br Med J [Clin Res]** 1983 Dec 24–31;287(6409):1981–3
Smith G: Ogston's Coccus: 102 years and still going strong.
**South Med J** 1982 Dec;75(12):1559–62
Tiburskaia NA, Dukhanina NN: Pamiati P. G. Shute (issledovaniia P. G. Shute shtammov Plasmodium vivax). **Med Parazitol (Mosk)** 1980 Jan–Feb;49(1):87–90
Voyatzakis E, et al: [The research work of Sir Alexander Fleming] (Gre).
**Mater Med Greca** 1981;9:367–76
Weindling PJ: Die Anfänge der Tuberkulose-Fürsorgestellen in Grossbritannien. **Wiss Beitr Martin Luther Univ Halle Wittenberg** 1983;5–R80:243–9
Zikeev PD: Aleksandr Fleming (k 100-letiiu so dnia rozhdeniia).
**Klin Med (Mosk)** 1983 Feb;61(2):110–2

**Hungary**

Kenéz J: József Tomcsik. Life and activity of an outstanding Hungarian microbiologist. **Ther Hung** 1980;28(4):189–90
Kerekes L: Miért vallott kudarcot Balogh Kálmán, a bakteriológia magyar úttöroje? **Orvostort Kozl** 1982;28(1–3):65–85
Wyklicky H, Skopec M: Ignaz Philipp Semmelweis, the prophet of bacteriology. **Infect Control** 1983 Sep–Oct;4(5):367–70

**Italy**

Karnovsky ML: Metchnikoff in Messina: a century of studies on phagocytosis. **N Engl J Med** 1981 May 7;304(19):1178–80
Subba Rao M: Original observations of Filippo Pacini on vibrio cholera.
**Bull Indian Inst Hist Med (Hyderabad)** 1978;8(1–4):32–8
Théodoridès J: Sebastiano Rivolta (1832–1893) parasitologiste et microbiologiste. **Hist Sci Med** 1980;14(2):227–32

**Japan**

Fujita S: Robert Kochs Bedeutung für die japanische Medizin--Tuberkuloseforschung in Japan. **Prax Klin Pneumol** 1983 Oct;37 Suppl 1:423–9
Hayashi T: [Reflection on my research in bacteriology] (Jpn).
**Nippon Saikingaku Zasshi** 1984 Mar;39(2):81–4
Kimura Y: [Reflections on my research] (Jpn).
**Nippon Saikingaku Zasshi** 1984 Jan;39(1):19–23
Masaki T: [Hideyo Noguchi and oral spirochaete]. (Jpn) **Dent Outlook** 1978;51(6):1265
Mitsuhashi S: [Recollection of my research activities in microbiology] (Jpn). **Nippon Saikingaku Zasshi** 1984 Jul;39(4):733–7
Tajima Y: [30 years of research using experimental animals--transition from bacteriology to the study of experimental animals] (Jpn).
**Nippon Saikingaku Zasshi** 1984 Jul;39(4):739–43

**Korea**

Cowdrey AE: 'Germ warfare' and public health in the Korean conflict.
**J Hist Med Allied Sci** 1984 Apr;39(2):153–72

**Malagasy Republic**

Zeller H, Coulanges P: Les entérovirus à Madagascar. Bilan de vingt ans d'activité du laboratoire de virologie de l'Institut Pasteur de Madagascar.
**Arch Inst Pasteur Madagascar** 1980;47(1):121–69

**Mexico**

Beltran E: La protozoología médica en México. In Academia Nacional de Medicina. Libro conmemorativo del primer centenario. México, Comité Editorial de la Comisión Organizadora del Congreso del Centenario, 1964. Tome 1. p. 109–12.
León AP: La brucelosis en México. In Academia Nacional de Medicina. Libro conmemorativo del primer centenario. México, Comité Editorial de la Comisión Organizadora del Congreso del Centenario, 1964. Tome 2. p. 527–32.
Olarte J: La bacteriología intestinal en México. In Academia Nacional de Medicina. Libro conmemorativo del primer centenario. México, Comité Editorial de la Comisión Organizadora del Congreso del Centenario, 1964. Tome 2. p. 521–3.
Ruiloba J: Listeriosis, toxoplasmosis y leptospirosis. In Academia Nacional de Medicina. Libro conmemorativo del primer centenario. México, Comité Editorial de la Comisión Organizadora del Congreso del Centenario, 1964. Tome 2. p. 532–5.

**Netherlands**

de Knecht-van Eekelen A: Abraham Pieter Fokker (1840–1906) en de serumtherapie bij difterie.
**Tijdschr Geschied Geneeskd Natuurwet Wiskd Tech** 1984;7(4):161–71
Haneveld GT: Bij het eeuwfeest van de gonokok: het belang van zijn ontdekking en de ontvangst daarvan in Nederland (Ludwig Sigesmund Albert Neisser). **Ned Tijdschr Geneeskd** 1979 Oct 27;123(43):1875–8

**Norway**

Irgens LM: The discovery of Mycobacterium leprae. A medical achievement in the light of evolving scientific methods.
**Am J Dermatopathol** 1984 Aug;6(4):337–43

**Poland**

Galiński J, Hebanowski M, Lipińska-Namysł E: Serotypy uropatogenne Escherichia coli w materiałach z klinik i przychodni gdańskich w latach 1973–1976. **Przegl Epidemiol** 1980;34(2):155–61
Garfield E: W hołdzie Hilaremu Koprowskiemu: uczonemu, muzykowi i przyjacielowi. **Pol Tyg Lek** 1983 Sep 5;38(36):1119–23
Gruszkiewicz E, Głośnicka R, Kunikowska D: Seroreactions in detecting Yersinia enterocolitica and Yersinia pseudotuberculosis in the Gdánsk region, years 1973–1976. **Bull Inst Marit Trop Med Gdynia** 1980;31(1–2):97–102
Henneberg G: Das Robert Koch-Haus in Wollstein. **Med Welt** 1982 Mar

26;33(12):427

Horbowska-Marzec H, Grodzicka-Królak H, Wielopolska H: Wirusy ECHO-11 u chorych hospitalizowanych w Warszawie w latach 1968-1977. **Pediatr Pol** 1980 Feb;55(2):203-5

Janowiec M, Pichulowa K: Rozwój mikrobiologicznej diagnostyki gruźlicy w Polsce. **Pneumonol Pol** 1982 Nov;50(11):559-62

Kucharz E: Odo Bujwid - the pioneer in microbiology in Poland. In International Congress of the History of Medicine. 26th, Plovdiv, 1978. Actes du Congress. Sofia, 1981. Volume II. p. 128-9.

Marzec M: Ksawery Lewkowicz (1869-1958) wybitny pediatra i bakteriolog. **Wiad Lek** 1982 Aug 15;35(13):845-7

**Romania**

Alexa I: La 100 ani de la naşterea doctorului Mihai Ciucă (1883-1983). **Rev Med Chir Soc Med Nat Iasi** 1983 Oct-Dec;87(4):731-6

Algeorge G, Jemna I: Dezvoltarea micobacteriologici pe plan internaţional şi in ţara noastră. **Rev Ig [Pneumoftiziol]** 1982 Oct-Dec;31(4):291-5

Babes V: Opere alese. Vol. I. Bucuresti, Editura Academiei Republicii Socialiste Romania, 1979. 330 p. Biographical contributions by B. Dutescu, N. Marcu, and I. Moraru.

Babeş VT: Some less well-known priorities of Victor Babeş. **Virologie** 1979 Jul-Sep;30(3):235-6

Cajal N: 1949-1984: 35 years devoted to the study of viruses in the 'Stefan S. Nicolau' Institute of Virology. **Virologie** 1984 Oct-Dec;35(4):247-50

Dumitrescu SM: Contribution of the 'Stefan S. Nicolau' Institute of Virology to the electron microscopic study of viruses. **Virologie** 1984 Oct-Dec;35(4):273-80

Eşanu V: Research in the field of antiviral chemotherapy performed in the 'Stefan S. Nicolau' Institute of Virology. **Virologie** 1984 Oct-Dec;35(4):281-93

Iftimovici R: Constantin Levaditi, a forerunner of the modern research and interpretation of virus multiplication. **Virologie** 1979 Jul-Sep;30(3):237-42

Marcu N: Viaţa si activitatea doctorului Constantin C. Pastia (1883-1926). **Rev Ig [Bacteriol]** 1983 Jan-Mar;28(1):89-95

On the 125th anniversary of Victor Babeş birth: **Virologie** 1979 Jul-Sep;30(3):169-70

On the 35th anniversary of our journal: **Virologie** 1984 Jan-Mar;35(1):3-4

Panaitescu D, Mihalcu F, Neguţ M: Activitatea stiinţifică a prof. Mihai Ciucă. **Rev Iq [Bacteriol]** 1984 Jan-Mar;29(1):80-8

Sefer M, Sefer M: Evocare: Dumitru Combiescu (6 ianuarie 1887 - 25 noiembrie 1961)] (Rom). **Rev Ig [Bacteriol]** 1981 Jul-Sep;26(3):199-204

Sefer M, Sefer M: [10 years after the death of Professor Mihai Ciucă (18 July 1883 - 20 Feb. 1969). Mihai Ciucă and the study of bacteriophage, recorded in his working notebooks.] (Rum) **Rev Ig [Bacteriol]** 1979;24:123-6

The 'Stefan S. Nicolau': Institute of Virology on its 30th anniversary. **Virologie** 1979 Oct-Dec;30(4):253-5

**South Africa**

Bernstein RE: Dr. Harvey Pirie: versatile man of science and pioneer explorer of sub-antarctic regions eighty years ago. **Adler Mus Bull** 1984 Mar;10(1):4-10

Dwork D: Koch and the Colonial Office: 1902-1904; the second South Africa Expedition. **NTM** 1983;20(1):67-74

**Sweden**

Kock W: 80-talet: da å upptäcktes bisköldkörtlarna och då gjorde bakterierna sin entré. **Lakartidningen** 1979 Dec 19;76(51):4697-9

**Switzerland**

Bonifas V: Alexandre Yersin (1863-1943). **Rev Med Suisse Romande** 1984 May;104(5):349-51

Mayer R: Il y a cent ans, à Genève, au 4e Congrès international d'hygiène et de démographie, l''altercation' Pasteur - Koch. **Rev Med Suisse Romande** 1982 Aug;102(8):805-9

**Turkey**

Erk N: Adil Mustafa (Adil-Bey), a pioneer veterinary bacteriologist in Turkey. **Hist Med Vet** 1977;2(4):99-101

**United States**

Dr. Frank M. Schabel Jr. **Cancer** 1984 Sep 15;54(6 Suppl):1132-52

Andrews WH: A perspective review of the development of AOAC microbiological methods. **J Assoc Off Anal Chem** 1984 Jul-Aug;67(4):661-73

Animalcular and cryptogamic theories on the origins of fevers. Reprinted works by John Kearsley Mitchell (1849), John L. Riddell (1836), Josiah Clark Nott (1848). New York, Arno, 1977. Various paginations.:

Arvy L: Clara Louise Maass (1876-1901) et la fièvre jaune. **Clio Med** 1979 May;13(3-4):277-82

Baldwin RS: The fungus fighters: two women scientists and their discovery. Ithaca, Cornell University Press, 1981. 212 p.

Bendiner E: Enders, Weller, and Robbins: the trio that 'fished in troubled waters'. **Hosp Pract** 1982 Jan;17(1):163, 169, 174-5 passim

Blancher DA: Workshops of the bacteriological revolution: a history of the laboratories of the New York City Department of Health, 1892-1912. Ph.D. Diss., City University of New York. New York, 1979. xiv, 311 leaves.

Bovee EC: Theodore Louis Jahn. 1905-1979. In memoriam. **J Protozool** 1979 Nov;26(4):527-9

Brachman PS: Inhalation anthrax. **Ann NY Acad Sci** 1980;353:83-93

The carrier state. New York, Arno, 1977. Various paginations. Four reprinted papers on microbiology by William H. Park and George Soper, 1895-1919.:

Classics in infectious diseases. Letter from Theobald Smith to Edward Krumbhaar: **Rev Infect Dis** 1984 Mar-Apr;6(2):280-1

Conn HJ: The history of the Stain Commission. **Stain Technol** 1980 Sep;55(5):269-79

Conn HJ: The history of the Stain Commission. II. Organization 1921-2. **Stain Technol** 1980 Nov;55(6):327-52

Conn HJ: The history of the Stain Commission IV. Expansion of the work, 1924-39. **Stain Technol** 1981 Mar;56(2):59-66

Corner GW: Louise Pearce. In: Notable American women. The modern period. Cambridge, Mass., Belknap-Harvard Univ. Press, 1980. 4:531-2.

Corner GW: Thomas Milton Rivers. In Dictionary of American biography, 1961-1965. Suppl. 7, 1981. p. 648-9.

Cravens H: Samuel Cate Prescott. In Dictionary of American biography, 1961-1965. Suppl. 7, 1981. p. 629-30.

Dubos R: Hattie Elizabeth Alexander. In: Notable American women. The modern period. Cambridge, Mass., Belknap-Harvard Univ. Press, 1980. 4:10-1.

Garrett CG: Frederick George Novy. In Dictionary of American Biography, Suppl. 6, 1956-1960. p. 481-2, 1980.

Goldhaft TM: Historical note on the origin of the LaSota strain of Newcastle disease virus. **Avian Dis** 1980 Apr-Jun;24(2):297-301

Hungate RE: Evolution of a microbial ecologist. **Annu Rev Microbiol** 1979;33:1-20

King LS: Medicine in the USA: historical vignettes. VIII. Germ theory and its influence. **JAMA** 1983 Feb 11;249(6):794-8

Krause RM: Koch's postulates and the search for the AIDS agent. **Public Health Rep** 1984 May-Jun;99(3):291-9

Kundsin RB: Creative crusader against sepsis (Carl W. Walter). **Am J Surg** 1984 Nov;148(5):573-4

Laufman H: Carl Walter's half century of achievement in asepsis. **Am J Surg** 1984 Nov;148(5):565-70

Lowell JD: The ultraviolet environment in a nutshell (Carl W. Walter). **Am J Surg** 1984 Nov;148(5):575-7

McDermott W: Colin Munro MacLeod: January 28, 1909-February 11, 1972. **Biogr Mem Natl Acad Sci** 1983;54:183-219

Maulitz RC: 'Physician versus bacteriologist': the ideology of science in clinical medicine. In Vogel MJ, Rosenberg CE, ed: The therapeutic revolution. Philadelphia, 1979. p. 91-107.

Maulitz RC: Robert Koch and American medicine. **Ann Intern Med** 1982 Nov;97(5):761-6

Maulitz RC: Robert Koch in the United States of America. **NTM** 1983;20(1):75-84

Millstein CB: W. D. Miller and the beginnings of occupational hygiene in dentistry. **Bull Hist Dent** 1984 Oct;32(2):135-6

Milza P: La guerre froide à Paris: 'Ridgway la peste'. **Histoire** 1980;25:38-47

Niemi SM: D. E. Salmon and the first bacterin. **Mod Vet Pract** 1981 Dec;62(12):913-7

O'Hern EM: Alice Catherine Evans. In: Notable American women. The modern period. Cambridge, Mass., Belknap-Harvard Univ. Press, 1980. 4:219-21.

Riley HD: The history of histoplasmosis. **J Okla State Med Assoc** 1983 Feb;76(2):31-40

Robinton ED: Anna Wessels Williams. In: Notable American women. The modern period. Cambridge, Mass., Belknap-Harvard Univ. Press, 1980. 4:737-9.

Rubin LP: Elizabeth Lee Hazen. In: Notable American women. The modern period. Cambridge, Mass., Belknap-Harvard Univ. Press, 1980. 4:326-8.

Rubin LP: Gladys Rowena Henry Dick. In: Notable American women. The modern period. Cambridge, Mass., Belknap-Harvard Univ. Press, 1980. 4:191-2.

Salk J: The virus of poliomyelitis. From discovery to extinction. **JAMA** 1983 Aug 12;250(6):808-10

Sandusky WR: Frank L. Meleney: pioneer surgeon-bacteriologist. **Arch Surg** 1983 Feb;118(2):151-5

Smithcors JF: Discovery of the arthropod vector of disease. **Mod Vet Pract** 1981 May;62(5):371-4

Talmage DW: William Hay Taliaferro: February 10, 1895-December 21, 1973. **Biogr Mem Natl Acad Sci** 1983;54:375-407

Van Ginneken J: Bacteriological warfare. **J Contemp Asia** 1977;7(2):130-52

Viseltear AJ: Charles-Edward Amory Winslow. In Dictionary of American Biography, Suppl. 6, 1956-1960. p. 701-3, 1980.

# MICROBIOLOGY

Woodruff HB: A soil microbiologist's odyssey. **Annu Rev Microbiol** 1981;35:1–28

**USSR**

Bardell D: An 1898 report by Gamaleya for a lytic agent specific for Bacillus anthracis. **J Hist Med Allied Sci** 1982 Apr;37(2):222–5
Bazanov VA, Schneck P: Nauchnye sviazi Roberta Kokha i ego shkoly s russkimi issledovateliami. **Sov Zdravookhr** 1982;(3)64–7
Bochkov NP: V. D. Timakov (1905--1977). Moskva, Meditsina, 1982. 62 p.
Chaïka NA: Deiatel'nost' Leningradskogo nauchno-issledovatel'skogo instituta épidemiologii i mikrobiologii im. Pastera v gody Velikoï Otechestvennoï voïny. **Sov Zdravookhr** 1980;(8):47–51
Dekhtsunian KM: Nauchnaia deiatel'nost' Armianskogo ordena Trudovogo Krasnogo Znameni NII épidemiologii, virusologii i meditsinskoï parazitologii im. A. B. Aleksaniana (k 60-letiiu so dnia osnovaniia instituta). **Zh Mikrobiol Epidemiol Immunobiol** 1984 Feb;(2):114–7
Diachenko SS: Iz istorii izucheniia semeïstva kishechnykh bakteriï v Ukrainskoï SSR. **Mikrobiol Zh** 1982 Jan-Feb;44(1):95–9
Diachenko SS: Stanovlenie i razvitie meditsinskoï virusologii v Ukraine. **Mikrobiol Zh** 1980 Nov-Dec;42(6):798–802
Diachenko SS: U istochnikov meditsinskoï mikrobiologii v Kieve. **Mikrobiol Zh** 1982 Mar-Apr;44(2):5–10
Elkin II, Frolova VV: Rol' N. I. Pirogova v podgotovke I. I. Mechnikova k nauchnoï deiatel'nosti (k 135-letiiu so dnia rozhdeniia I. I. Mechnikova. **Zh Mikrobiol Epidemiol Immunobiol** 1980 Sep;(9):114–8
Heifets L: Metchnikoff's recollections of Robert Koch. **Tubercle** 1982 Jun;63(2):139–41
Iastrebov VK: Nauchnoe nasledie S. P. Karpova v oblasti prirodno-ochagovykh infektsiï. **Zh Mikrobiol Epidemiol Immunobiol** 1983 Oct;(10):113–5
Institut mikrobiologii i virusologii im. D. K. Zabolotnogo AN USSR--gorodu-iubiliaru: **Mikrobiol Zh** 1982 Mar-Apr;44(2):3–4
Kalina GP: Nekotorye voprosy istorii sanitarnoï mikrobiologii. **Gig Sanit** 1982 Nov;(11):47–50
Kaulen DR: Itogi i perspektivy deiatel'nosti nauchno-issledovatel'skogo instituta épidemiologii i mikrobiologii im. N. F. Gamalei AMN SSSR (k 90-letiiu so dnia osnovaniia). **Zh Mikrobiol Epidemiol Immunobiol** 1982 May;(5):116–20
Kocere V: Latvijas PSR Zinātnu akademijas akademike Rita Kukaine: biobibliogrāfiskais rādītājs. Riga, Zinātne, 1982. 129 p.
Kochemasova ZN, Dykhno MM: 60 let kafedre mikrobiologii i Moskovskogo meditsinskogo instituta im. I. M. Sechenova. **Zh Mikrobiol Epidemiol Immunobiol** 1981 May;(5):113–6
Koroliuk AM: K stoletiiu so dnia rozhdeniia Viacheslava Mikhaïlovicha Aristovskogo. **Zh Mikrobiol Epidemiol Immunobiol** 1983 Mar;(3):109–12
Kravchenko AT: Pamiati professora Glotovoï Eleny Vladimirovny (k 100-letiiu so dnia rozhdeniia). **Zh Mikrobiol Epidemiol Immunobiol** 1983 Mar;(3):112–3
Mazurik EV: Pervye shagi nauchnoï deiatel'nosti D. K. Zabolotnogo. **Zh Mikrobiol Epidemiol Immunobiol** 1983 May;(5):99–101
Nikitin DP: Nauchno-issledovatel'skaia i proizvodstvennaia deiatel'nost' Moskovskogo nauchno-issledovatel'skogo instituta épidemiologii i mikrobiologii im. G. N. Gabrichevskogo. **Zh Mikrobiol Epidemiol Immunobiol** 1981 Mar;(3):102–5
Schneck P: Die Briefe Paul Ehrlichs an den Moskauer Mikrobiologen Georgij Norbertovič Gabričevskij. **NTM** 1982;19(2):81–7
Skobulovich GV: Itogi deiatel'nosti Amursjkogo otdeleniia Nauchnogo obshchestva épidemiologov, mikrobiologov i parazitologov za 25 let (1957–1982). **Zh Mikrobiol Epidemiol Immunobiol** 1984 Feb;(2):117–9
Smirnov VV, Bilaï VI: Zhizn' i deiatel'nost' D. K. Zabolotnogo v Kieve. **Mikrobiol Zh** 1982 May-Jun;44(3):86–90
Sobolev VR: K 50-letiiu kafedry mikrobiologii Tsentral'nogo ordena Lenina instituta usovershenstvovaniia vracheï. **Zh Mikrobiol Epidemiol Immunobiol** 1983 Mar;(3):113–5
Vasil'ev KK: Rol' nauchnykh s'ezdov v nauchnoï meditsinskoï informatsii (iz istorii vserossiïskikh i vsesoiuznykh s'ezdov bakteriologov, épidemiologov i sanitarnykh vracheï, 1918–1928 gg.) **Sov Zdravookhr** 1980;(6):58–60
Vasil'ev KK: Rol' pervykh Vserossiïskikh sezdov bakteriologov i épidemiologov v bor'be s épidemiiami parazitarnykh tifov (k 60-letiiu IV sezda). **Zh Mikrobiol Epidemiol Immunobiol** 1981 Apr;(4):106–9
Vasil'ev KK: 60 let VII Vserossi ïskogo s'ézda bakteriologov, épidemiologov i sanitarnykh vracheï. **Zh Mikrobiol Epidemiol Immunobiol** 1983 Oct;(10):111–3
Ved'mina EA, Tatarinova SD: 50-Letie kafedry mikrobiologii Tsentral'nogo ordena Lenina instituta usovershenstvovaniia vracheï. **Antibiotiki** 1982;27(9):714–5
Zasukhin DN, Alekseev GA: Vydaiushchiï protozoolog A. G. Alekseev (1882–1950). **Parazitologiia** 1982 May-Jun;16(3):262–4
Zavarzin GA: Aleksandr Aleksandrovich Imshenetskiï. Moskva, Nauka, 1967. 82 p.
Zykin LF, Metlin VN: Nauchnaia deiatel'nost' professora V. V. Akimovicha. **Zh Mikrobiol Epidemiol Immunobiol** 1984 Apr;(4):113–4

**Yugoslavia**

Antunović-Mikačič S: O počecima mikrobiološke dijagnostike u Dalmaciji do 1923. g. In: I simpozij o historiji mikrobiologije i imunologije u Hrvatskoj do 1923. godine. Zagreb, Jugoslavenskoj akademiji, 1973. p. 5–15.
Berlot J: Razvitak mikrobiologije i imunologije u Hrvatskoj do 1923. god. In: I simpozij o historiji mikrobiologije i imunologije u Hrvatskoj do 1923. godine. Zagreb, Jugoslavenskoj akademiji, 1973. p. 31–45.
Brudnjak Z: Razvoj virologije u Hrvatskoj do god. 1940. **Lijec Vjesn** 1982 Oct;104(10):448–51
Glesinger L: Uloga stranih liječnika i prirodoslovaca u istraživanju i suzbijanju zaraznih bolesti u Hrvatskoj. In: I simpozij o historiji mikrobiologije i imunologije u Hrvatskoj do 1923. godine. Zagreb, Jugoslavenskoj akademiji, 1973. p. 47–61.
I simpozij o historiji mikrobiologije i imunologije u Hrvatskoj do 1923. godine: Zagreb, Jugoslavenskoj, akademiji, 1973. 126 p.
Rapić S: O zivotu i radu Ferde Kerna. In: I simpozij o historiji mikrobiologije i imunologije u Hrvatskoj do 1923. godine. Zagreb, Jugoslavenskoj akademiji, 1973. p. 85–93.
Skarić J: O osnutku i razvoju bakteriološke stanice u Splitu do 1923. god., s biografijom osnivača dr Josipa Skarića. In: I simpozij o historiji mikrobiologije i imunologije u Hrvatskoj do 1923. godine. Zagreb, Jugoslavenskoj akademiji, 1973. p. 95–105.
Tomič-Karović K: Ljudevit Gutschy. In: I simpozij o historiji mikrobiologije i imunologije u Hrvatskoj do 1923. godine. Zagreb, Jugoslavenskoj akademiji, 1973. p. 107–17.
Topolnik E: Razvoj veterinarske bakteriologije i imunologije u Hrvatskoj do god. In: I simpozij o historiji mikrobiologije i imunologije u Hrvatskoj do 1923. godine. Zagreb, Jugoslavenskoj akademiji, 1973. p. 119–26.

# MICROSCOPY

Archinard M: Nouvelle salle de microscopes au Musée d'histoire des Sciences. **Mus Geneve** 1982;224:7–13
Belloni L: Il Morgagni tra il Malpighi e il Cotugno. **Gesnerus** 1982;39(2):195–213
Ford BJ: Bacteria and cells of human origin on van Leeuwenhoek's sections of 16741,2. **Trans Am Microsc Soc** 1982 Jan;101(1):1–9
Ford BJ: Revelation and the single lens. **Br Med J [Clin Res]** 1982 Dec 18–25;285(6357):1822–4
Kalderon AE: The evolution of microscope design from its invention to the present days. **Am J Surg Pathol** 1983 Jan;7(1):95–102
Lumley JS: Microsurgery. **Practitioner** 1982 Oct;226(1372):1723–6
Riddle JM: A survey of ancient specimens by electron microscopy. In A. Cockburn, E. Cockburn, ed: Mummies, disease, and ancient cultures. Cambridge, Cambridge University Press, 1980. p. 274–86.
Shipman P: Applications of scanning electron microscopy to taphonomic problems. **Ann NY Acad Sci** 1981;376:357–85
Turner GL'E: Essays on the history of the microscope. Oxford, Senecio, 1980. 245 p. (Reprint of the author's journal articles).
Wade NJ: A note on the history of binocular microscopes. **Perception** 1981;10(5):591–2

**Netherlands**

Palm LC, Snelders HA, ed: Antoni van Leeuwenhoek, 1632–1723. Studies on the life and work of the Delft scientist commemorating the 350th anniversary of his birthday. Amsterdam, Rodopi, 1982. 209 p. (Nieuwe Nederlandse Bijdragen tot de Geschiedenis der Geneeskunde en der Natuurwetenschappen, no. 8). Contributions by W. H. van Seters, B. C. Damsteegt, J. van Zuylen, P. Bass, J. E. van Bronswijk, G. A. Lindeboom, P. Smit, K. van Berkel.

**1450–1700**

Kler JH: Along the path of modern medicine. **J Med Soc NJ** 1983 Jul;80(7):552

**Netherlands**

Bendiner E: The man who did not invent the microscope. **Hosp Pract [Off]** 1984 Aug;19(8):139, 144–5, 149 passim
Ford BJ: Correlated optical and electron microscopy of Leeuwenhoek's elder-pith sections. **J Microsc** 1982 Nov;128 Pt 2:211–3
Ford BJ: Found - van Leeuwenhoek's original specimens. **New Sci** 1981;91:301
Ford BJ: Leeuwenhoek's specimens discovered after 307 years [news]. **Nature** 1981 Jul 30;292(5822):407
Ford BJ: The van Leeuwenhoek specimens. **Notes Rec R Soc Lond** 1981;36(1):37–59
Fournier M: Huygens' microscopical researches. **Janus** 1981;68:199–209
Fournier M: Jan Swammerdam en de 17e eeuwse microscopie. **Tijdschr Geschied Geneeskd** 1981;4(2)74–86
Fournier M: 'Ontdeckte onsightbaarheden'. **Spiegel Hist** 1982;17(2):612–8
Houtzager HL: Antonie van Leeuwenhoek. **Eur J Obstet Gynecol Reprod Biol** 1983 Jul;15(3):199–203

Lindeboom GA: Jan Swammerdam als microscopist. **Tijdschr Geschied Geneeskd** 1981;4(2):87-110
Lukács D: Háromszázötven éve született Antony van Leeuwenhoek. **Orv Hetil** 1982 Oct 31;123(44):2732-7
Mikx F: A. van Leeuwenhoek's microscopes: upside down? **Lancet** 1983 Jun 18;1(8338):1387-8
Palm LC: Van Leeuwenhoek en Swammerdam cartesiaanse microscopisten. **Spiegel Hist** 1979;14(4):223-9
Roger J: Two scientific discoveries: their genesis and destiny. In M. D. Grmek, R. S. Cohen, G. Cimino, ed: On scientific discovery. The Erice Lectures 1977. Dordrecht, D. Reidel, 1981. p. 229-37. (Boston Studies in the Philosophy of Science, v. 34).
Ruestow EG: Images and ideas: Leeuwenhoek's perception of the spermatozoa. **J Hist Biol** 1983 Summer;16(2):185-224
Van Zuylen J: The microscopes of Antoni van Leeuwenhoek. **J Microsc** 1981 Mar;121(pt 3):309-28
Zuylen J van: On the microscopes of Antoni van Leeuwenhoek. **Janus** 1981;68:159-98

**1700 to Present**

Barraquer JI: The history of the microscope in ocular surgery. **J Microsurg** 1980 Jan-Feb;1(4):288-99
Cifuentes Delatte L: Historia del estudio microscópico de los cálculos del aparato urinario en el siglo XIX. **Arch Esp Urol** 1981 Sep-Oct;34(5):375-84
Donaghy RM: The history of microsurgery in neurosurgery. **Clin Neurosurg** 1979;26:619-25
Fields K, Kontrovitz M: An invisible art blazes into life under microscope. **Smithsonian** 1980;11(7):109-13
Gelberman RH: Microsurgery and the development of the operating microscope. **Contemp Surg** 1978 Dec;13(6):43-6
Gibson WP: The operating microscope and the development of ear surgery. **J R Soc Med** 1980 Jan;73(1):53-5
Girod C: Die Geschichte der Histologie. In Sournia JC, Martiny M, Poulet J, ed: Illustrierte Geschichte der Medizin. Salzburg, Andreas, 1980. Vol. 5. p. 1877-937.
Lenz F: Theorie und Praxis in der Elektronenoptik. **Mikroskopie** 1982 Dec;39(11-12):359-73
Nuttall RH: Microscopes from the Frank Collection 1800-1860. Illustrating the development of the achromatic instrument. Jersey, Channel Islands, A. Frank, 1979, 64 p.
Porter KR: The cytomatrix: a short history of its study. **J Cell Biol** 1984 Jul;99(1 Pt 2):3s-12s
Ruska E: Die frühe Entwicklung der Elektronenlinsen und der Elektronenmikroskopie. **Acta Hist Leopoldina** 1979;12:7-136
Théodoridès J: Les recherches histologiques sur la rage au 19e siècle. **Clio Med** 1981 Dec;16(2/3):83-92

**Chile**

Costa C: Prehistoria de la cátedra de histología de la Universidad de Chile (1872-1881) Parte II. Microscopio e histología en Chile antes de 1873. **Rev Med Chil** 1980 May;108(5):463-9

**France**

Maison Nachet: Catalogues de fonds de 1854 à 1910. Facsimile edition. Introduction par G. L'E. Turner. Paris, Brieux, 1979. Various paginations.
Stanguennec A: Le scalpel contre le microscope: Auguste Comte et la théorie cellulaire. **Sci Tech Perspect** 1981-82;1:11.1-.12

**Germany**

Afzelius BA: Half a century of electron microscopy: the early years. **Ultrastruct Pathol** 1981 Jul-Sep;2(3):309-11
Hildebrand R: Beitrag der Würzburger Anatomie zur Entwicklung des mikroskopisch-anatomischen Unterrichts (1847 Kölliker--Petersen 1940). **Anat Anz** 1984;155(1-5):115-22
Klermayer O: Werke von Dr. h. c. Hans-Henning Heunert. **Mikroskopie** 1981 Feb;38(1-2):3-12
Ruska E: The early development of electron lenses and electron microscopy. **Microsc Acta** 1980;(Suppl 5):1-140
Schneider HJ, Seiyfarth HH: Die mikroskopische Harnsteinanalyse von den Anfängen 1879 bis zur Gegenwart. Jena, Friedrich-Schiller-Universität, 1980. 81 p.

**Great Britain**

Allen E, Turk JL: Microscopes in the Hunterian Museum. **Ann R Coll Surg Engl** 1982 Nov;64(6):414-8
Barer R: Cosslett's contribution to microscopy (Ellis Cosslett). **J Microsc** 1979 Sep;117(1):5-10
Hirsch PB: Foreword: the Cosslett festschrift (Ellis Cosslett). **J Microsc** 1979 Sep;117(1):1-4
Nuttali RH: An early microscope by John Benjamin Dancer of Manchester. **Microscope** 1980;28(3/4):93-100

**Netherlands**

Beukers H: De beginjaren van de microscopie aan de geneeskundige faculteiten te Utrecht en Leiden. **Tijdschr Geschied Geneeskd** 1983;6(2):65-81
Fournier M: Hoofdlijnen van de microscopie in de negentiende eeuw. **Tijdschr Geschied Geneeskd** 1983;6(2):59-64
Lieburg MJ van: De microscopie in het onderwijs van de klinische scholen in Nederland (1824-1865). **Tijdschr Geschied Geneeskd** 1983;6(2):82-98
Moulin D de: Microscopie en kankerdiagnostiek in de eerste helft van de negentiende eeuw. **Tijdschr Geschied Geneeskd** 1983;6(2):99-107
Mulder WJ: Microscopische preparaten van de praktizerend geneesheer G. J. Luchtmans. **Tijdschr Geschied Geneeskd** 1983;6(2):108-14

**Romania**

Dumitrescu SM: Contribution of the 'Stefan S. Nicolau' Institute of Virology to the electron microscopic study of viruses. **Virologie** 1984 Oct-Dec;35(4):273-80

**Switzerland**

Speiser P: Vogts Lehrbuch und Atlas der Spaltlampenmikroskopie des lebenden Auges. **Gesnerus** 1981:38(3/4):339-45

**United States**

De Duve C, Beaufay H: A short history of tissue fractionation. **J Cell Biol** 1981 Dec;91(3 pt 2):293s-99s
Edgar RK: An annotated bibliography of the American microscopist and diatomist Jacob Whitman Bailey (1811-1857). **Occas Pap Farlow Herb Cryptogam Bot Harv Univ** 1977;11:1-26
Lamping KA, Albert DM, Snyder C, et al: The Harrower collection and its place in the history of ophthalmic pathology. **Surv Ophthalmol** 1983 May-Jun;27(6):374-80
Pease DC, Porter KR: Electron microscopy and ultramicrotomy. **J Cell Biol** 1981 Dec;91(3 pt 2):287s-92s
Prescott GW: American Microscopical Society: the first one-hundred years. Part II. **Trans Am Microsc Soc** 1979 Apr;98(2):165-94
Warner JH: 'Exploring the inner labyrinths of creation': popular microscopy in nineteenth-century America. **J Hist Med Allied Sci** 1982 Jan;37(1):7-33

**USSR**

Magazov VS, Morogova VM: 75 let Ufimskomu nauchno-issledovatel'skomu institutu vaktsin i syvorotok im. I. I. Mechnikova. **Zh Mikrobiol Epidemiol Immunobiol** 1981 Jan;(1):110-1
Rebrikova NL, Mul'diiarov PIa: Elektronno-mikroskopicheskoe izuchenie pergamenta. **Biull Eksp Biol Med** 1982 Dec;94(12):104-7

**Venezuela**

Beauperthuy de Benedetti R: Beauperthuy y su microscopio. **Rev Soc Venez Hist Med** 1978;27(41):59-64
Vélez Boza F: Historia de la microscopia en Venezuela. **Rev Soc Venez Hist Med** 1981;30(45-46):125-97

## MILITARY MEDICINE

See also **Aerospace Medicine; Naval Medicine; Red Cross; Transportation of Patients; War**

Adams DB: Abdominal gunshot wounds in warfare: a historical review. **Milit Med** 1983 Jan;148(1):15-20
Adamson PB: The military surgeon: his place in history. **J R Army Med Corps** 1982 Feb;128(1):43-50
Aker F, Schroeder DC, Baycar RS: Cause and prevention of maxillofacial war wounds: a historical review. **Milit Med** 1983 Dec;148(12):921-7
Cameron N: Ceremony of presentation of diplomates. **Ann R Coll Surg Engl** 1981 Nov;63(6):447-9
Cornand G: Trachome et armées. **Rev Int Trach Pathol Ocul Trop Subtrop** 1979;56(3-4):99-110
Dziob JS: Ten years before 'M A S H'. **RI Med J** 1982 Dec;65(12):499-506
Ellis PS: The origins of the war neuroses. **J R Nav Med Serv** 1984 Winter;70(3):168-77 contd
Engle EK: Medic. New York, Day, [c 1967]. 255 p.
Gestewitz HR, Steiner ER, et al: Historische Entwicklung und Charakteristik der Militärmedizin. In their: Militärmedizin: Hochschullehrbuch für Studenten der Medizin und Stomatologie. 2. Auflage. Berlin, Militärverlag der Deutschen Demokratischen Republik, 1981. p. 13-49.
Guerra F: Three battles that changed military surgery: Avigliana 1536. Moscow 1812. Ebro 1938. In International Congress of the History of Medicine. 26th, Plovdiv, 1978. Actes du Congress. Sofia, 1981. Volume

II. p. 82–3.
Histoire de la médecine aux armées: Tome 1. De l'Antiquité à la Révolution. Paris, Charles Lavauzelle, 1982. 513 p.
Kessler RH: Gunpowder altered the physician's wartime role. Should nuclear weapons change it again? **Arch Intern Med** 1983 Apr;143(4):784–6
Maisel AQ: Miracles of military medicine. Freeport, N.Y., Books for Libraries Press, 1972. xiv, 373 p.
Ragsdale BD: Gunshot wounds: a historical perspective. **Milit Med** 1984 Jun;149(6):301–15
Roberts A: The fifth little horseman. **Nurs Times** 1983 Nov 2–8;79(44):49–53
Watt J: Doctors in the wars. **J R Soc Med** 1984 Apr;77(4):265–7
West CG: A short history of the management of penetrating missile injuries of the head. **Surg Neurol** 1981 Aug;16(2):145–9

**Brazil**

Souza LC: Medicina militar brasileira: nomes marcantes et fatos notáveis. **Rev Inst Hist Geogr Bras** 1975;306:150–63

**China**

Li Yousong: [Exploration of the relationship between defeating Cao Cao in Chibi and schistosomiasis.] (Chi). **Chin J Med Hist** 1981;11:87–8

**Europe**

Wangensteen OH: A few renowned European military surgeons. In Ganzinger K, Skopec M, Wyklicky H, ed: Festschrift für Erna Lesky zum 70. Geburtstag. Wien, Brüder Hollinek, 1981. p. 167–84.

**France**

Baillargeat R, et al: Les invalides: trois siècles d'histoire. Paris, Musée de l'armée, 1974. 600 p.
Fabre A: Les traditions de la médecine de l'avant. **Med Armees** 1980;8(10)spec:781–6
Guillermand J: La tradition hospitalière militaire. **Med Armees** 1980;8(10)spec:817
Lefebvre P: Tradition de l'enseignement dans le Service de santé de l'armée de terre. **Med Armees** 1980;8(10)spec:827–44
Nauroy J: L'équipement technique et le ravitaillement. **Med Armees** 1980;8(10)spec:845–50

**Great Britain**

Crowdy JP: The science of the soldier's food. **Army Q Def J** 1980;110(3):266–79
Ross JA: Men in battle. The factors affecting their lives and well-being. **J R Army Med Corps** 1980 Feb;126(1):4–17
Wickes HL: The Royal Army Dental Corps. **Br Dent J** 1980 Jun 3–17;148(11–12):269–70

**India**

Wilson HH: The art of war and medical & surgical sciences of Hindus. Delhi, Nag Publishers, 1979. 44 p.

**Japan**

Matsuki A: [Prevalence of scurvy among soldiers of the Hirosake feudal clan in Yezo area.] (Jpn). **Nihon I-Shigaku Zasshi** 1981;27(1):56–63

**Poland**

Dutkiewicz M: Z dziejów munduru i symboli służby zdrowia Wojska Polskiego. **Arch Hist Med (Warsz)** 1984;47(1):85–90

**Puerto Rico**

Arana Soto S: El Hospital de Puerto Rico. San Juan de Puerto Rico, [s.n.], 1976. 296 p.

**Switzerland**

Büchi J: Die Arzneiversorgung und der Sanitätsdienst der schweizerischen Truppen vom 15.–18. Jahrhundert. Stuttgart, Wissenschaftliche Verlagsanstalt, 1981. 94 p. (Veröffentlichungen der Internationalen Gesellschaft für Geschichte der Pharmazie, Neue Folge, 49).

**Turkey**

Ozbay K: Türk asker hekimligi tarihi ve asker hastaneleri. 3 vols. in 4. Istanbul, Yörük Basimevi, 1976. 686, 349, 576, 493 p.

**USSR**

Voronkov OV: Iz istorii sozdaniia sapasov meditsinskogo imushchestva dlia obespecheniiavoĭsk na sluchaĭ voĭny (soobshchenie pervoe). **Voen Med Zh** 1984 Feb;(2):72–3

### Before 500 A.D.

Watermann RA: Mensch und Medizin zwischen Macht und Militär der römischen Kaiserzeit. Frankfurt am Main, Gerhard Michler, 1980. 204 p.

**Great Britain**

Wright RP: A Roman veterinary physician from the Thames Valley. **Britannia** 1977;8:279–82

**Greece**

Angulo Arvelo LA: Acerca de la probable causa de la muerte de Alejandro el Grande. **Rev Soc Venez Hist Med** 1981;30(45–46):105–10
Rozos B: Pathological syndromes as mentioned by Xenophon in the march of the ten thousand. In International Congress of the History of Medicine. 26th, Plovdiv, 1978. Actes du Congress. Sofia, 1981. Volume II. p. 163–6.

**Rome**

Wooden AC: Medical services of the Roman army. In International Congress of the History of Medicine. 26th, Plovdiv, 1978. Actes du Congress. Sofia, 1981. Volume II. p. 211–3.

### 500 A.D.–1450

**Arabic**

Wooden AC: Medical care in Islamic armies. In International Congress of the History of Medicine, 27th, Barcelona, 1980. Actas. Barcelona, Acadèmia de Ciències Mèdiques de Catalunya i Balears, 1981. p. 694–8.

**India**

Thakral KK: Techniques for extraction of foreign bodies from war wounds in medieval India. **Indian J Hist Sci** 1981, reçu 1982;16(1):11–6

**Poland**

Dudziński W: Smierć króla Władysława Warneńczvka. **Wiad Lek** 1981 Jun 1;34(11):953–5

### 1450–1700

Krzys J: Problemy medyczne w czasie kampanii wiedeńskiej 1683 roku. **Arch Hist Med (Warsz)** 1981;44(3/4):257–64

**France**

Bendiner E: From barbershop to battlefield--Paré and the renaissance of surgery. **Hosp Pract** 1983 Aug;18(8):193–5, 199, 202 passim
Chaboche R: Le clergé de France et l'assistance aux invalides de guerre au XVIIe siècle. In: Congrès National des Sociétés Savantes, 97e, Nantes, 1972. Actes. Paris, 1977. Histoire Moderne et Contemporaine, Tome 1. p. 31–47.
Prouzet J: Le Service de Santé au cours des guerre de religion dans les pays d'Aude. **Bull Soc Etud Sci Aude** 1979, 1980;79:85–7

**Mexico**

Rico-Avello C: Patologia en la conquista de Mejico. **Asclepio** 1978–79;30–31:377–87

### 1700 to Present

Bartley RL, Kucewicz WP: 'Yellow rain' and the future of arms agreements. **Foreign Aff** 1983;61(4):805–26
Bay A: Chemical warfare: perspectives and potentials. **Strategy Tactics** 1980;81:23–33
Bedwell SF: D'Anville's doom--a neurological vignette from historic Halifax. **Can J Neurol Sci** 1980 Feb;7(1):1–8
Benenson AS: Immunization and military medicine. **Rev Infect Dis** 1984 Jan–Feb;6(1):1–12
Bentham A: Down Memory Lane: as it happened. **Nurs Mirror** 1982 Aug 11;155(6):28–30
Brewer LA: The contributions of the Second Auxiliary Surgical Group to military surgery during World War II with special reference to thoracic surgery. **Ann Surg** 1983 Mar;197(3):318–26
Bruton EM, ed: M A S H: binding up the wounds. An exhibition at the National Museum of American History, Smithsonian Institution,

Washington, D.C. New York, George Fenmore Associates, 1983. 32 p.
Butkus DE: Post-traumatic acute renal failure in combat casualties: a historical review. **Milit Med** 1984 Mar;149(3):117–24
Cullinan J: The roses of no man's land. **Nurs Times** 1980 Oct 16;76(42):1823–5
Curtis DE: Nurses and war. The way it was. **Am J Nurs** 1984 Oct;84(10):1253–4
Dauber LG: Compound X given intravenously. On the history of the nitrogen mustards. **NY State J Med** 1984 Mar;84(3 pt 1):122–4
Davies GR: The invasion of Normandy--D-day. **NATNEWS** 1984 Sep;21(9):24–6
Dobek R, Kolmsee P: Maxim Zetkin--Arzt, Kriegschirurg und Kommunist. **Militaergesch** 1978;17(5):595–603
Dunbar-Miller RA: Alcohol and the fighting man--an historical review. **J R Army Med Corps** 1984 Jun;130(2):117–21
Endicott SL: Germ warfare and 'plausible denial': the Korean war, 1952–1953. **Mod China** 1979;5(1):79–104
Farolfi B: Dall'antropometria militare alla storia del corpo. **Quad Stor** 1979;14(3):1056–91
Gibelli A: La guerra laboratorio: eserciti e igiene sociale verso la guerra totale. **Mov Operaio Soc** 1982;5(3):335–49
Goltz RW: WWII, the 147th General hospital & Harry Arnold. **Hawaii Med J** 1982 Nov;41(11):410
Gray TC: 'Another side of Mars'. **J R Army Med Corps** 1984 Feb;130(1):3–11
Huard P, Imbault-Huart MJ: Geschichte der Militärmedizin. In Sournia JC, Martiny M, Poulet J, ed: Illustrierte Geschichte der Medizin. Salzburg, Andreas, 1980. Vol. 8. p. 2961–97.
Ilnicki S: Pomoc psychiatryczna na polu walki-ewolucja poglądów i metod postępowania. **Psychiatr Pol** 1980 Sep–Oct;14(5):539–46
Juillet P: Aspects évolutifs de la psychiatrie aux armées. In: Congrès National des Sociétés Savantes, 103e, Nancy, 1978. Comptes Rendus. Paris, 1978. Section des Sciences, Fasc. V. p. 99–111.
Karasszon Denes BB: Militärärztliches zur ungarischen Legion im Kampfe der Vereinigung Italiens / Risorgimento/. In International Congress of the History of Medicine. 26th, Plovdiv, 1978. Actes du Congress. Sofia, 1981. Volume II. p. 58–59.
Kuś J: Profesor dr. Tadeusz Rogalski i jego działalność w czasie II wojny światowej (w stulecie jego urodzin). **Przegl Lek** 1982;39(10):683–9
McBryde B: A nurse's war - 2. A trip to Rouen. **Nurs Times** 1979 Jul 5;75(26):1150–2
Price HH: The Falklands: rate of British psychiatric combat casualties compared to recent American wars. **J R Army Med Corps** 1984 Jun;130(2):109–13
Richardson FM: Amateur Palestinian guerrilla. **J R Army Med Corps** 1980 Feb;126(1):48–54
Robinson HS: Anderson Ruffin Abbott, MD, 1837–1913. **J Natl Med Assoc** 1980 Jul;72(7):713–6
Sadler C: Edith Cavell: from Blakeney Point to Brussels. **Nurs Mirror** 1982 Sep 15;155(11):52–4
Sidel'nikov AI: O nekotorykh osobennostiakh raboty otdel'nogo meditsinskogo batal'ona divizii v usloviiakh gorno-pustynnoĭ mestnosti (soobshchenie pervoe). **Voen Med Zh** 1983 Aug;8:20–5
Simeone FA: Studies of trauma and shock in man: William S. Stone's role in the military effort. **J Trauma** 1984 Mar;24(3):181–7
Smith KM: Dr. James Barry: military man--or woman? **Can Med Assoc J** 1982 Apr 1;126(7):854–7
Smith T: Victorian who sent a hospital to war. **Health Soc Serv J** 1983 May 5;93(4845):533–5
Trumpener U: The road to Ypres: the beginnings of gas warfare in World War I. **J Mod Hist** 1975;47(3):460–8
Zemskov MV: Protivoépidemicheskoe obespechenie Iassko-Kisshinevskoĭ operatsii. **Zh Mikrobiol Epidemiol Immunobiol** 1980 May;(5):21–5

**Afghanistan**

Ionov IuV, Ionov AIu: Vrach I. L. Iavorskiĭ - issledovatel' Afganistana. **Sov Zdravookhr** 1983;(12):49–51

**Africa**

Baylon H: L'oeuvre du Service de Santé des Armées en Afrique noire d'expression française. **Bull Acad Natl Med (Paris)** 1981 Apr;165(4):449–60
Brown JS: Of battle and disease: the East African Campaign of 1914–18. **Parameters** 1982;12(2):16–24

**Algeria**

Lefebvre P: L'hôpital Militaire Laveran de Constantine. **Med Trop (Mars)** 1980 Nov–Dec;40(6):645–9

**Argentina**

Agüero AL: La Sanidad Militar Argentina en la guerra con el territorio del Brasil. In Congreso de Historia de la Medicina Argentina [Transactions], 5th, Mendoza, 1983. p. 79–101.
Benencia JA: Los restos del general D. Juan Galo de Lavalle. **Historia (Argentina)** 1965;10(39):84–5
González JL: La medicina militar en la guerra del Paraguay. In Congreso de Historia de la Medicina Argentina [Transactions], 5th, Mendoza, 1983. p. 103–10.
Kohn Loncarica AG: La medicina en las campañas militares del siglo XIX. Las guerras de frontera. In Congreso de Historia de la Medicina Argentina [Transactions], 5th, Mendoza, 1983. p. 111–32.
Loza Colomer JC, Olascoaga ML: La Sanidad del Ejército de los Andes. In Congreso de Historia de la Medicina Argentina [Transactions], 5th, Mendoza, 1983. p. 7–17.
Zarranz A: La Sanidad Militar en las Guerras Civiles Argentinas (Desde el sitio de Buenos Aires a la Revolución del 90). In Congreso de Historia de la Medicina Argentina [Transactions], 5th, Mendoza, 1983. p. 133–40.

**Australia**

Davis E: Irene's diary of nursing in World War I. **Australas Nurses J** 1980 Dec;10(1):16–8
Looking back: the Australian army hospitals: **Lamp** 1980 May;37(5):53–5
O'Carrigan C: Two veteran nurses of World War I days (Sister Mary MacDonald, Sister Mary Vianney). **Med J Aust** 1984 Jun 23;140(13):782–4

**Austria**

Eissler KR: Freud und Wagner-Jauregg vor der Kommission zur Erhebung militärischer Pflichtverletzungen. Wien, Löcker, 1979. 333 p.
Lupinc P: Das zahnärztliche Lehrbuch des Wiener Militärarztes Joseph Georg Pasch 1767. Zürich, Juris Druck, 1984. 80 p. (Zürcher Medizingeschichtliche Abhandlungen, Neue Reihe, Nr. 165).

**Belgium**

Bouckaert A: Le paludisme, maladie professionnelle du soldat belge avant 1900. **Rev Belge Hist Milit** 1980;23:525–8
Evrard E: Le service de santé militaire hollando-belge à la bataille de Waterloo et dans les hôpitaux de Bruxelles en juin 1815. **Rev Belge Hist Milit** 1983;25(1):61–96
Vilain M: Inventaire du fonds d'archives 'Service de santé et Croix-Rouge, 1831–1914'. Bruxelles, Musée royal de l'Armée, 1981. 25 p.

**Brazil**

Nolding Gaffree A: Ana Neri - la première infirmière militaire au Brésil. In: International Congress of the History of Medicine, 26th, Plovdiv (Bulgaria), 1978. Actes du Congres, Vol. 1. Sofia, 1980. p. 114–5.
Souza L de C: A medicina na guerra do Paraguai (Mato-Grosso) V. **Rev Hist (Brazil)** 1971;42(85):129–46
Souza LC: João Moniz Barreto de Aragão-médico militar e pioneiro da veterinária brasileira. **Rev Inst Hist Georgr Bras** 1974;305:51–68

**Bulgaria**

Güdev Kh, Iliev N: Pŭrvi rŭkopisen uchebnik po veterinarana medistina za kusistite ot Voennoto veterinarnofeldshersko uchilishte v Sofiia. **Vet Med Nauki** 1980;17(9–10):84–8
Rusanov GA, Simbirtsev SA, Balanski R: Sto godini ot publikuvaneto na truda na N. I. Pirogov vurkhu opita v meditsinata, pridobit vuv voĭnata za osvobozhdenieto na Bulgariia prez 1877–1878 g. **Khirurgiia (Sofiia)** 1979;32(3):247–53

**Burma**

Whyte D: A trying Chindit. **Br Med J [Clin Res]** 1982 Dec 18–25;285(6357):1776–9

**Canada**

Barr JW: Canadian Forces medicine: 25 years of unified service. **Can Med Assoc J** 1984 Apr 15;130(8):1061–5
Brown T: Shell shock in the Canadian Expeditionary Force, 1914–1918: Canadian psychiatry in the Great War. In Roland CG, ed: Health, disease and medicine. Toronto, Hannah Institute for the History of Medicine, 1984. p. 308–32.
Kernaghan LK: William James Almon. In Dictionary of Canadian biography, 1801 to 1820. Volume 5, 1983. p. 23–4.
Morton D: 'Noblest and best': retaining Canada's war disabled 1915–23. **J Can Stud** 1981;16(3–4):75–85
Pennefather JP: A surgeon with the Alberta Field Force. **Alberta Hist** 1978;26(4):1–14
Pierson RR: The double bind of the double standard: VD control and CWAC in World War II. **Can Hist Rev** 1981;62(1):31–58
Tunis B: George Longmore. In Dictionary of Canadian biography, 1801 to 1820. Volume 5, 1983. p. 501–3.

# MILITARY MEDICINE

**China**

Gong Chun: [Army medical organization of Qing Dynasty after the Opium War] (Chi). **Chin J Med Hist** 1980;10:86-9
Kelkar GS: Kotnis in Kokung. **China Rep (India)** 1979;15(2):97-111
Summers GV: Norman Bethune, Canadian surgeon: his Chinese connection. **Can J Surg** 1983 Jul;26(4):379-82

**Czechoslovakia**

Dohnany L: Der Sanitätsdienst bei den Militär- und Partisaneneinheiten im Slowakischen Nationalaufstand des Jahres 1944. In International Congress of the History of Medicine. 26th, Plovdiv, 1978. Actes du Congress. Sofia, 1981. Volume II. p. 69-71.
Kyntera F: Přínos vojenské epidemiologie za období 25leté existence Vojenského lékařského výzkumného a doškolovacího ústavu Jana Evangelisty Purkyně v Hradci Králové. **Cesk Epidemiol Mikrobiol Imunol** 1984 Jan;33(1):53-5
Pidrman V: Hlavní směry činnosti katedry válečného vnitřního lékřství. K 25. výročí VLVDU JEvP. **Vnitr Lek** 1984 Jan;30(1):86-7
Slezák K: Vývoj oboru 'Organizace a řízení vojenského zdravotnictví' za 25 let existence Vojenského lékařského výzkumného a doškolovacího ústavu J. E. Purkyně v Hradci Králové. **Cesk Zdrav** 1984 Jan;32(1):1-5

**Denmark**

Brix J: Laegevirke i Sønderjylland før 1864. **Dan Medicinhist Arbog** 1980;:9-10
Indretningen af Augustenborg Slot til lazaret i krigen 1848-1850 - en 'chronique scandaleuse'?: **Dan Medicinhist Arbog** 1980;:91-123

**Europe**

Verdoorn JA: Arts en oorlog. Medische en sociale zorg voor oorlogsslachtoffers in de geschiedenis von Europa: inleiding in de medische polemologie. Amsterdam, Lynx, 1972. 2 v.

**Finland**

Teir H: Das Sanitätswesen der finnischen Truppen in Bulgarien sowie die Tätigkeit des finnischen Roten Kreuzes im Kriege von 1877-78 und die positiven Auswirkungen dieser Ereignisse auf die Entwicklung der finnischen Medizin und Krankenpflege. In International Congress of the History of Medicine. 26th, Plovdiv, 1978. Actes du Congress. Sofia, 1981. Volume II. p. 208.

**France**

Amalric P: De l'Hôpital de la Grave à la Grande Armée. L'ophtalmologie de Dominique Larrey. **Bull Soc Ophtalmol Fr** 1979 Feb;79(2):151-4
Baguenier-Desormeaux L: Henry Drysdale Dakin à Compiègne, en 1915. **Rev Hist Pharm (Paris)** 1981 Jun;28(249):79-88
Brullard P: Pierre Christophe (1758-1826), médecin, soldat et humaniste. In: Congrès National des Sociétés Savantes, 103e, Nancy, 1978. Comptes Rendus. Paris, 1978. Section des Sciences, Fasc. V. p. 43-53.
Buttet H de: Les Invalides en 1709. In: Congrès National des Sociétés Savantes, 97e, Nantes, 1972. Actes. Paris, 1977. Histoire Moderne et Contemporaine, Tome 1. p. 55-65.
Cantarel-Besson Y: Les morts exemplaires dans la peinture militaire sous le consulat et l'empire. **Rev Inst Napoleon (Paris)** 1977;(133):97-105
Capdebielle A: L'activité médicale à l'Hôtel des Invalides. **Med Armees** 1981;9:631-8
Chabbert P: Maxence Audouard (1776-1856). In: Congrès National des Sociétés Savantes, 96e, Toulouse, 1971. Comptes Rendus. Paris, 1974. Histoire des Sciences, Tome 1. p. 83-97.
Cordoliani A: L'hôpital militaire du Val de Grâce dans la vie sociale parisienne. In Congrès National des Sociétés Savantes, 103e, Nancy-Metz, 1978. Actes. Paris, 1979. Tome I, p. 607-24.
Courtine JC: L'Armée d'Afrique et l'anesthésie-réanimation: de Baudens (1853) au Corps expéditionnaire française à la Première Armée (1942-1945) et à la guerre d'Algérie. **Hist Sci Med** 1983;17(4):411-17
Courtois D: Naissance de l'Institut de Médecine Tropicale du Service de Santé des Armées. **Med Trop (Mars)** 1980 Nov-Dec;40(6):631-4
Csillag I: Eckstein Ferenc és a hadisebészet a Napóleon elleni háborúban. **Orv Hetil** 1984 Feb 19;125(8):467-70
Delaby PA: Un groupe de brancardiers pendant la bataille de Verdun. **Hist Sci Med** 1980;14:293-303
Demerson P: Le chirurgien Larrey et 'l'invasion française' à l'academie de médecine de Madrid. **Melanges Casa Velasquez** 1973;9:483-501
Des Cilleuls J: L'inspecteur général Jacques de Villemanzy, Sénateur et Pair de France (1751-1830). **Hist Sci Med** 1979;13(4):379-81
Devos D, Devos JC: L'hôpital militaire de Barèges (Hautes-Pyrénées) du debut du XVIIIe siècle à la fin du Premier Empire. In: Congrès National des Sociétés Savantes, 97e, Nantes, 1972. Actes. Paris, 1977. Histoire Moderne et Contemporaine, Tome 1. p. 105-13.
DiGioia JM, Rocko JM, Swan KG: Baron Larrey. Modern military surgeon. **Am Surg** 1983 May;49(5):226-30
Egeblad K: Militaerkirurgen Dominique Jean Larrey: Om pesten i felttoget til Aegypten og Syrien 1798-1801. **Dan Medicinhist Arbog** 1979;132-59
Fabre A, ed: Histoire de la médecine aux armées. Tome 2. De la Révolution française au conflit mondial de 1914. Paris, Charles-Lavazelle, 1984. 491 p.
Gaudiot C: Le Service de Santé dans la bataille de Verdun. **Hist Sci Med** 1980;14(2):193-200
Gerard A, Milot J: Histoire médicale du Camp de Boulogne d'après les papiers du général Vandamme. **Hist Sci Med** 1982;16(1):29-36
Harmand L: Une ambulance militaire ouverte par le curé d'une paroisse messine durant les batailles sous Metz (août-décembre 1870). In: Congrès National des Sociétés Savantes, 97e, Nantes, 1972. Actes. Paris, 1977. Histoire Moderne et Contemporaine, Tome 1. p. 121-8.
Hebbert FJ: Belle-Ile and the secret expedition. **Trans Hunter Soc** 1978-80;37-38:193-210
Hockemeyer H: Die Zeit seiner Schiffsarzttätigkeit in den Memoiren des napoleonischen Chirurgen Dominique-Jean Larrey. Diss., Universität Düsseldorf. Düsseldorf, 1982. 44 p.
Huard P, Lefebvre P, Plessis JL: François-Félix Jacquot (1819-1857). **Hist Sci Med** 1983;17(4):403-10
Jensen JE: Napoleonic medicine. **Md State Med J** 1981 Jul;30(7):66-8
Kalis F: Albert Leulier (1883-1957): a l'occasion du centenaire de sa naissance. Thèse, Univ. Claude-Bernard-Lyon I, U.E.R. de Pharm., 1983. 98 leaves.
Larcan A: Le médecin inspecteur F. C. Maillot. In: Congrès National des Sociétés Savantes, 103e, Nancy, 1978. Comptes Rendus. Paris, 1978. Section des Sciences, Fasc. V. p. 19-30.
Leboutte R: D'Austerlitz à Liège, mourir dans les armées de Bonaparte. **Tijdschr Geschied Geneeskd** 1978;91(3):429-46
Lefebvre P: Il y a deux siècles mourait Germain Pichault de la Martinière (1697-1783). **Chirurgie** 1983;109(10):805-8
Lefebvre P, Godon A: Les cendres du baron Larrey. **Nouv Presse Med** 1982 Jan 30;11(4):235-9
Lefebvre P, Barbas S: L'hystérie de guerre. Etude comparative de ses manifestations au cours des deux derniers conflits mondiaux. **Ann Med Psychol (Paris)** 1984 Feb;142(2):262-6
Lemaire JF: Le chirurgien-baron François Girardot (1773-1831) un oublié de l'histoire. **Hist Sci Med** 1980;14(1):107-14
Manneville P: Le poids des armées à l'hôpital du Havre à l'époque révolutionnaire. In Congrès National des Sociétés Savantes, 103e, Nancy-Metz, 1978. Actes. Paris, 1979. Tome I, p. 593-606.
Mars FL, Théodoridès J: Un savant angevin de l'époque révolutionnaire: Urbain-Philippe Salmon (1768-1805) médecin militaire, géologue et ami de Stendhal. In: Congrès National des Sociétés Savantes, 93e, Tours, 1968. Comptes Rendus. Paris, 1971. Section des Sciences, Tome II. p. 103-25.
Marshall G: A doctor in the Great War--an interview with Sir Geoffrey Marshall. **Br Med J [Clin Res]** 1982 Dec 18-25;285(6357):1780-3
Nauroy J: Les historiographes de la pharmacie militaire française. In: Vorträge des Internationalen Pharmaziehistorischen Kongresses Innsbruck 1977. Stuttgart, Wissenschaftliche Verlagsgesellschaft, 1979. p. 91-6.
Oliver G: Le Service de santé militaire dans les Pyrénées-Orientales pendant la guerre de 1914-1918. In: Congrès National des Sociétés Savantes, 97e, Nantes, 1972. Comptes Rendus. Paris, 1976. Section des Sciences, Tome 1. p. 351-62.
Perçebois G: Jean-Antoine Villemin (1827-1892). In: Congrès National des Sociétés Savantes, 103e, Nancy, 1978. Comptes Rendus. Paris, 1978. Section des Sciences, Fasc. V. p. 31-41.
Peumery JJ: La prodigieuse carrière de Jean-François Coste (1741-1819) médicin-chef des armées. **Hist Sci Med** 1980;14(2):177-86
Plessis JL, Huard P, Lefebvre P, et al: Louis-René Villermé, chirurgien-major à la Grande Armée. **Hist Sci Med** 1982;16(4):305-15
Poulet J: La mort de Junot. **Rev Inst Napoleon (Paris)** 1972;(123):57-62
Richard A: L'évolution de la condition militaire des chirurgiens-dentistes. **Bull Acad Chir Dent (Paris)** 1979-1980;25(25):59-69
Steimle R: Albert Ehrmann (1821-1871). **Hist Sci Med** 1984;18(3):208-14
Tournier-Lasserve C: La Peyronie et la présence des chirurgiens militaires au sein de l'Académie de Chirurgie. **Chirurgie** 1981;107(9):719-22
Tournier-Lasserve C: Le Service de santé des armées et la recherche au fil du temps. **Med Armees** 1980,8(10)spec:851-6
Tournier-Lasserve C: Les chirurgiens militaires et l'Académie de médecine. **Bull Acad Natl Med (Paris)** 1982 May;166(5):601-8
Voelckel J: L'école du Pharo. Tradition-permanence-avenir. **Med Trop (Mars)** 1980 Nov-Dec;40(6):635-8
75ème anniversaire de l'Institut de Médecine Tropicale du Service de Santé des Armées (le Pharo Marseille).: **Med Trop (Mars)** 1980 Nov-Dec;40(6):591-604

**Germany**

Becker H: Helmuth von Moltke als Beobachter der hygienischen und medizinischen Situation im osmanischen Kaiserreich (1835-39). In Göpfert W, Otten HH, ed: Metavoeite: wandelt euch durch neues Denken. Düsseldorf, Triltsch, 1983. p. 147-59.
Enigh K: Als Parasitologe im Veterinärdienst des Heeres. **DTW** 1981 Nov 5;88(11):479-83

FiscHer H: Der deutsche Sanitätsdienst, 1921-1945: Organisation, Dokumente und persönliche Erfahrungen. Band 1. Osnabrück, Biblio, 1982. viii, 289 p.
Frielinghaus E: Initiativen des Veterinär-Inspekteurs der deutschen Wehrmacht auf dem Gebiet der Pferdezucht im Kriege 1939-45. **DTW** 1981 Nov 5;88(11):457-61
Fritzsche K: Erfahrungen bei der Tätigkeit in zwei 'Beweglichen Veterinär-Untersuchungsstellen' an der Ost- und Westfront während des letzten Weltkrieges. **DTW** 1982 Feb 5;89(2):65-70
Grapentin F: Veterinärärztliches Gerät im Zweiten Weltkrieg. **DTW** 1981 Nov 5;88(11):473-5
Hinze E: Feldscherer und Feldmedici in deutschen wie fremden Heeren und Flotten. (Biographisches Lexikon deutscher Militärärzte bis 1870) Band I. Hannover, Im Selbstverlag, 1979. 43 p.
Kaemmerer K: Die Arzneimittel des Veterinärdienstes im Zweiten Weltkrieg. **DTW** 1981 Nov 5;88(11):461-73
Kenéz J: F. Esmarch jelentösége a hadisebészet fejlödésében. **Orv Hetil** 1984 Jul 8;125(28):1708-10
Kłodziński S: Ppłk lek. med. Jan Zielina. **Przegl Lek** 1981;38(1):202-6
Kollmeier K: Von der Ueberwasser-Elende zum Militärhospital. Die Entwicklung des militärischen Sanitätswesens in der Provinzhauptstadt Münster/Westfalen. **Hist Hosp** 1979-80;13:96-118
Machalett G: Ludwig Stromeyer--sein Beitrag zur Entwicklung der Militärmedizin in Deutschland. **Militaergesch** 1975;14(6):694-705
Moskwa Z: Powstańcza søużba zdrowia na Górnym Slasku w latach 1919-1921. **Wiad Lek** 1984 Feb 15;37(4):313-20
Rebentisch E: 100 Jahre Wehrmedizin. Arztliche Erfahrungen zwischen Krieg und Frieden. **Fortschr Med** 1984 Mar 8;102(9):225-31
Schneider J: Beiträge zur Geschichte der Wehrpharmazie von 1935-1945. Düsseldorf, Triltsch Druck, 1982. vi, 160 p. (Düsseldorfer Arbeiten zur Geschichte der Medizin, Beiheft VIII).
Seidler FW: Prostitution, Homosexualität, Selbstverstummelung. Probleme der deutschen Sanitätsführung 1939-1945. Neckargemünd, Vowinkel, 1977. 323 p.
Sons HU: Gesundheitspolitik während der Besatzungszeit: das öffentliche Gesundheitswesen in Nordrhein-Westfalen 1945-1949. Wuppertal, Hammer, 1983. 207 p.
Spann W: Prof. Dr. med. Theo Morell, Hitlers Leibarzt. **MMW** 1983 Jun 17;125(24):534-6
Valentin R: Die Krankenbataillone. Sonderformationen der deutschen Wehrmacht im zweiten Weltkrieg. Düsseldorf, Droste, 1981. 250 p. (Schriftenreihe Erfahrungen des deutschen Sanitätsdienstes im zweiten Weltkrieg, 2).
Vella EE: Belsen: medical aspects of a World War II concentration camp. Paper 1. **J R Army Med Corps** 1984 Feb;130(1):34-59
Voss HJ: Beitrag zur Seuchenlage in den Pferdebeständen einer Armee 1940/41 und zur Erfahrung als Leiter eines Seuchenlazarettes für Pferde. **DTW** 1981 Nov 5;88(11):483-6
Zieger W: Zur 100. Wiederkehr des Geburtstages von Generaloberstabsveterinär Professor Dr. Curt Schulze. **DTW** 1981 Nov 5;88(11):449-52

**Great Britain**

Bird JR: Group approaches and Army health. **J R Army Med Corps** 1980 Oct;126(3):112-9
Boyd J: Sir William Porter MacArthur. In Dictionary of national biography, 1961-1970. Suppl. 8, 1981. p. 688-9.
Craig RP: Military cold injury during the war in the Falkland Islands 1982: an evaluation of possible risk factors. **J R Army Med Corps** 1984 Jun;130(2):89-96
Davis E: Queen Alexandra's Royal Army Nursing Corp. **Australas Nurses J** 1981 Oct;10(10):16-9
De mortuis nil nisi bonum: **J Am Acad Dermatol** 1982 May;6(5):968-76
Devlin R: The VADs nursing in no man's land. **Nurs Mirror** 1980 Oct 23;151(17):8-9
Dopson L: The QA museum. **Nurs Times** 1981 Nov 11-17;77(46):1974
Dopson L: Volunteer nurses. One. VADs at war. **Nurs Times** 1984 Aug 1-7;80(31):36-8
Dunbar-Miller RA: Alcohol and the fighting man--an historical review. **J R Army Med Corps** 1984 Feb;130(1):12-5
Evrard E: Chirurgiens militaires britanniques à la bataille de Waterloo et dans les hôpitaux de Bruxelles en juin 1815. **Rev Belge Hist Milit** 1982;24(5):425-64
Forsythe-Jauch WE: L Cpl Joseph John Farmer, VC, AHC. Centenary of the battle of Majuba 1881. **J R Army Med Corps** 1981 Jun;127(2):100-2
Fraser I: Sir William MacCormac and his times. **Ann R Coll Surg Engl** 1983 Sep;65(5):339-46
Fry J: First David Bruce lecture in the David Bruce tradition. The evolution of general practice in the British Army. **J R Army Med Corps** 1982 Oct;128(3):152-9
Guntrip G: The unknown Edith Cavell. **Nurs Times** 1984 Apr 25-May 1;80(17):63-4
Hardy JH: Royal Army Dental Corps diamond jubilee (1921-1981). **Br Dent J** 1981 Nov 17;151(10):351-2
Harrison JA: Military medicine in the United Kingdom: similarities and differences with respect to the United States and other NATO allies. **Milit Med** 1980 Jun;145(6):388-92
Harrison JA: Military medicine in the United Kingdom: similarities and differences with respect to the United States and other NATO allies. **J R Nav Med Serv** 1980 Winter;66(3):173-9
Howie J: Gonorrhoea--a question of tactics. **Br Med J** 1979 Dec 22-29;2(6205):1631-2
Hunter GM: Pathologist turned general practitioner. Reflections of an ex-Army pathologist. **J R Army Med Corps** 1981 Jun;127(2):93-7
James T: A history of the medical branch of the Royal Air Force: part II aviation medicine. **Adler Mus Bull** 1984 Nov;10(3):2-7
Kaminsky AP: Morality legislation and British troops in late nineteenth century India. **Milit Aff** 1979;43(2):78-83
Lankford ND: The Victorian medical profession and military practice: army doctors and national origins. **Bull Hist Med** 1980 Winter;54(4):511-28
Macfie C: Down Memory Lane: for king and country. **Nurs Mirror** 1982 Jul 21;155(3):41-4
MacKenna RM: Robert M. B. MacKenna. **J Am Acad Dermatol** 1982 Jan;6(1):135-44
Morris M: Normandy 1944. One. D-Day diary. **Nurs Times** 1984;80(23):46-7; (24):44-5
Nuttall P: Miss Florence Nightingale: 'the passionate statistician'. **Nurs J India** 1984 Jun;75(6):128-9
Patton MA: An early case of battle hysteria. **Br J Psychiatry** 1981 Feb 1;138:182-3
Ramsey LJ: Bullet wounds and X-Rays in Britain's little wars. **J Soc Army Hist Res** 1982 Summer;:91-102
Rogers L: Odabrana poglavlja iz ratne kirurgije 8. Britanske armije. **Lijec Vjesn** 1979 Nov;101(11):699-701
Searle CG: A soldier pharmacist. **Pharm Hist (London)** 1974 Jan;4(1):2-3
Smith T: Royal Army Medical Corps. Into battle to save the casualties of war. **Health Soc Serv J** 1983 Aug 18;93(4860):994-5
Spriggs EA: Hector Gavin, MD, FRCSE (1815-1855) - his life, his work for the sanitary movement, and his accidental death in the Crimea. **Med Hist** 1984 Jul;28(3):283-92
Stott R: The Scottish dimension of Enlightenment medicine; the political economy of health. **Soc Soc Hist Med Bull (Lond)** 1979 Dec;25:41-4
Thompson FG: Assistant surgeon William Bradshaw, V.C. **Ir Sword** 1981;14(56):237-9
Vella EE: Brucellosis (the Corps disease). **J R Army Med Corps** 1983 Jun;129(2):97-100
Warren-Farrow D: A perilous night. **Nurs Times** 1982 Jul 14-20;78(28):1203-4
Wickes HL: History of nursing in the Army: behind the lines. **Nurs Mirror** 1981 Jul 8;153(2):23-4
Williams E: Diary of a VAD 1940-49. **Nurs Mirror** 1981 Jul 8;153(2):25-7 (continued regularly)
Winter JM: Military fitness and civilian health in Britain during the first World War. **J Contemp Hist** 1980;15(2):211-44

**Hungary**

Antall J: Organisatorische Reformbestrebungen im militärärztlichen Dienst des ungarischen Freiheitskampfes 1848/49. In: International Congress of the History of Medicine, 26th, Plovdiv (Bulgaria), 1978. Actes du Congres, Vol. 1. Sofia, 1980. p. 83-5.
Kapronczay K, Szemkeö E: A betegápolás szervezése a szabadságharc idején. **Orvostort Kozl** 1981;93-96(27 No 1-4):113-22
Takáts L: A magyarországi utolsó török háború egészségügyi ellátásának megszervezése 1788-89-ben. **Hadtortenelmi Kozl** 1966;13(1):40-63
Takáts L, Fäller J, Leitner F: Katonaegeszségügyi szolgálatunk megalakulása és müködése a felszabadulás évében (1945). **Hadtortenelmi Kozl** 1977;24(1):31-59
Verseghi G: A honvédorvosi kar vázlatos története 1968-1914 között. **Orv Hetil** 1980 Jul 13;121(28):1709-12

**India**

Acharya AM: The first Indian War of Independence and military surgery. **Bull Indian Inst Hist Med (Hyderabad)** 1975 Oct;5(4):225-39
Carré A: Aspects médicaux de la Campagne de l'Inde. **Rev Hist Armees** 1983;(153):50-61
Hameed A: A historian of medicine, Major General (Dr) S. L. Bhatia, passes away. **Stud Hist Med** 1981 Sept;5(3):239-41

**Ireland**

Eakins WA: Thomas Crawford, regimental medical officer in the Crimea, 1855. **Ulster Med J** 1982;51(1):46-51

**Italy**

Miniati M: Lo strumentario di G. A. Brambilla. **Kos** 1984 Feb;1(1):74-6
Orsini M, Piroli AT, Gaudiosi O: Gli eliporti ospedalieri nell'organizzazione sanitaria militare: l'eliporto dell'ospedale militare di Caserta. **Riv Mil** 1973;29(5):614-26

**Japan**

Duncan IL: Life in a Japanese prisoner-of-war camp. **Med J Aust** 1982 Apr 3;1(7):302–6
Fukase Y: [Tezuka Ryosen, army doctor-in-chief of the infantry regiment.] (Jpn). **Nihon I-Shigaku Zasshi** 1981;27(1):21–34
Liebow AA: Encounter with disaster: a medical diary of Hiroshima, 1945. Condensed from the original publication, 1965. **Yale J Biol Med** 1983 Jan–Feb;56(1):23–38

**Korea**

Cowdrey AE: 'Germ warfare' and public health in the Korean conflict. **J Hist Med Allied Sci** 1984 Apr;39(2):153–72
Milza P: La guerre froide à Paris: 'Ridgway la peste'. **Histoire** 1980;25:38–47

**Middle East**

Quin NE: The impact of diseases on military operations in the Persian Gulf. **Milit Med** 1982 Sep;147(9):728–34

**New Guinea**

Hope RB: Dateline--New Guinea 1942. **Forum Med** 1980 Aug;3(8):539–42

**Pacific Islands**

McKinnon DA: Battalion surgeon on Iwo Jima. **Marine Corps Gaz** 1982;66(2):28–37

**Philippines**

Foronda MA: An army doctor in Leyte. **Leyte-Samar Stud** 1980;14(1):1–37

**Poland**

Basinski J: Leczenie rannych i chorych w przebiegu Powstania Wielkopolskiego. Czas od 27.12.1918 do 13.11.1919. **Arch Hist Med (Warsz)** 1979;42(2):189–204
Basiński J: Organizacja i działalność słuzby zdrowia w pierwszym okresie powstania Wielkopolskiego. **Arch Hist Med (Warsz)** 1979;42(1):1–18
Basinski J: Zaplecze i środki sanitarno-medyczne wojsk sanitarnych Powstańczej Armii Wielkopolskiej. Czas od 16.01.1919 do 13.11.1919. **Arch Hist Med (Warsz)** 1979;42(2):161–76
Brzeziński T: Słuzba Zdrowia i Dywizji Piechoty im. T. Kościuszki i jej udział w bitwie pod Lenino. **Arch Hist Med (Warsz)** 1978;41(4):413–22
Chojna JW: Warszawskie lazarety wojskowe w czasie powstania listopadowego. **Arch Hist Med (Warsz)** 1981;44(3/4):277–308
Chojna JW: Warszawskie lazarety wojskowe w czasie powstania listopadowego. **Arch Hist Med (Warsz)** 1983;46(1):1–19
Chojna JW: Warszawskie lazarety wojskowe w czasie Powstania Listopadowego. **Arch Hist Med (Warsz)** 1980;43(4):353–75
Dorsz-Szteke E, Maciejewska-Dorsz K: Pomoc wojskowej służby zdrowia dla ludności cywilnej Pomorza Zachodniego w latach 1945–1946. **Wiad Lek** 1981;34(7):615–8
Dutkiewicz M: Ubiór służby zdrowia Wojska Polskiego w okresie Królestwa Polskiego i wojny 1830–1831 roku. **Arch Hist Med (Warsz)** 1981;44(2):157–62
Felchner A, Pepłowska E: Polski Komitet Pomocy Sanitarnej jednym z prekursorów świeckiego pielegniarstwa w Polsce. **Arch Hist Med (Warsz)** 1984;47(1):91–7
Gerwel T: Słuzba zdrwia w obronie Wybrzeza w r. 1939. **Przegl Lek** 1981;38(1):80–92
Majewski W: Słuzba zdrowia l. armii Wojska Polskiego, 1943–1945. Warszawa, Wydawn. Ministerstwa Obrony Narodowej, 1976. 277 p.
Markowski W, Zychowicz G: Materiały archiwalne dotyczące służby zdrowia w twierdzy Modlin z okresu Powstania Listopadowego. **Arch Hist Med (Warsz)** 1981;44(2):217–24
Markowski W, Szewko S: Sylwetki lekarzy i farmaceutów obrońców modlina w 1939 r. **Arch Hist Med (Warsz)** 1980;43(3):243–63
Odrowaz-Szukiewicz H: Wojskowa słuzba zdrowia na Sadybie podczas Powstania Warszawskiego. **Arch Hist Med (Warsz)** 1978;41(4):447–63
Raiter AW: Wspomnienia z piotrkowskiej partyanckiej słuzby sanitarnej. **Przegl Lek** 1981;38(1):155–9
Rudnicki J: Słuzba zdrowia 1 Polskiej Samodzielnej Brygady Spadochronowej w operacji 'Market-Garden'--relacje uczestników. **Arch Hist Med (Warsz)** 1984;47(1):127–31
Stembrowicz W: Rys historyczny wojskowej służby zdrowia w okresie Powstania Listopadowego. **Arch Hist Med (Warsz)** 1981;44(2):129–41
Terlecki O: Służba zdrowia Drugiego Korpusu Polskiego w bitwie o Monte Cassino. **Przegl Lek** 1980;37(1):92–100
Tkaczewski W: Dwudziestopi ęciolecie Wojskowej Akademii Medycznej im. gen. dyw. prof. Bolesława Szareckiego. **Pol Tyg Lek** 1983 Jul 11–18;38(28–29):857–9
Walewski W, Markowski W, Mosejczuk L, et al: [35 years of service in medical supply to the Polish People's Forces]. (Rus) **Voen Med Zh** 1979 Nov;(11):67–8
Wankiewicz R: Próba oceny działalności słuzby zdrowia w wojnie obronnej 1939 r. **Arch Hist Med (Warsz)** 1984;47(2):183–90
Wankiewicz R: Służba zdrowia Wojska Polskiego w bitwie nad Bzura. **Przegl Lek** 1984;41(1):68–79

**Portugal**

Iria A: Evocação de Júlio Dantas no l. centenário do seu nascimento: duas raridades bibliográficas do médico militar. **An Acad Port Hist** 1979;25:359–84

**Romania**

Cernovodeanu D: Din corespondenta inedită a medicului militar Nicolae Stonescu in timpul Războiului de Independenta. **Rev Istor** 1977;30(6):1051–70
Negru I: Misiuni sanitare române în războiul balcanic din anul 1912. **Viata Med [Medii Sanit]** 1983 Apr;31(4):91–6

**South Africa**

Gear JH: The Anglo-Boer War of 1899–1902:enteric fever and Captain Maxwell Louis Hughes. **Adler Mus Bull** 1981;7(1):10–3
Salter AL: Veterinary life in the Boer War 1899–1902. Correspondence of James William Hall Masheter M.R.C.V.S. **Vet Hist** 1984;3(3):87–92

**Spain**

Broggi M: Progressos assolits en sanitat militar durant la guerra civil espanyola (1936–39). In International Congress of the History of Medicine, 27th, Barcelona, 1980. Actas. Barcelona, Académia de Ciències Médiques de Catalunya i Balears, 1981. p. 168–71.
Gutmann R: Une lettre signée de Larrey, Desgenettes, Coste et Parmentier, à propos d'une épidémie de fièvre jaune en Espagne. **Hist Sci Med** 1980;14:337–41
Kolarov P: Sanitarnata sluzhba na internatsionalnite brigadi v ispaniia (1936–1938). **Izv Inst Istor Bkp** 1967;16:289–312
Matilla Gómez V: Sesión necrológica del Excmo. Sr. D. Manuel Gómez Durán. Día 3 de abril de 1984. **An R Acad Nac Med (Madr)** 1984;101(2):273–88
Morales y Morales A: Francisco Antonio Solano, boticario revalidado. Asentista del Hospital Militar de Santa Cruz de Tenerife (1764–1771). **Bol Soc Esp Hist Farm** 1980 Mar–Jun;3(121–2):109–38
Parrilla Hermida M: La direccion de Sanidad Militar---su primer director. **Asclepio** 1980;32:295–302
Silgo Gamero J: El servicio de sanidad en las guerras Carlistas. **Rev Hist Mil** 1969;13(26):93–103

**Sweden**

Modig M: Karl XII:s siste fältskär. **Sydsven Medicinhist Sallsk Arsskr** 1983;:77–86

**Switzerland**

Nussbaum W: Die Grippe-Epidemie 1918/1919 in der schweizerischen Armee. **Gesnerus** 1982;39(2):243–59
Zanobio B: Je le pansai, Dieu le guérit. Gli aforismi di chirurgia militare di Louis Appia (1818–1898) sulla cura delle ferite d'armi da fuoco. **G Accad Med Torino** 1980;143(Spec No):7–95

**United States**

Agris J: Stamps commemorating medicine. 'Dr. Mary Edwards Walker' (1832–1919). **J Dermatol Surg Oncol** 1982 Nov;8(11)::926
Aldrete JA, Marron GM, Wright AJ: The first administration of anesthesia in military surgery: on occasion of the Mexican-American War. **Anesthesiology** 1984 Nov;61(5):585–8
Anderson DL, Anderson GT: Nostalgia and malingering in the military during the Civil War. **Perspect Biol Med** 1984 Autumn;28(1):156–66
Anderson PG: The spa, the fairgrounds, and the psychiatric hospital: the 21st General Hospital in World War II. **Outlook Mag** 1982 Spring;19(1):2–8
Apffelstaedt G: Militärlazarette während des Bürgerkrieges in den USA anhand von Beispielen aus den Bezirken Washington, District of Columbia, Baltimore, Maryland, Philadelphia, Pennsylvanien und New York. Münster, Murken-Altrogge, 1981. 203 p. (Studien zur Geschichte des Krankenhauswesens, 6)
Appell RA: Medical aspects of the Confederacy (1861--1865). **South Med J** 1980 Jun;73(6):784–6
Armstrong PC, Beary JF: Office of the Assistant Secretary of Defense for Health Affairs: a history. **Milit Med** 1983 Aug;148(8):637–43
Arthurs R: The man who played doctor. **Civ War Times Illus** 1980;19(5):36–8
Arvy L: Clara Louise Maass (1876–1901) et la fièvre jaune. **Clio Med** 1979 May;13(3–4):277–82

Askew M: The health of General Douglas MacArthur. **Practitioner** 1982 Oct;226(1372):1814–5
Baird ND: There is no Sunday in the army: Civil War letters of Lunsford P. Yandell, 1861–62. **Filson Club Hist Q** 1979;53(4):317–27
Beacham EG: Fortieth anniversary of D-Day June 6, 1944, a physician remembers. **Md State Med J** 1984 Jun;33(6):450–3
Bean WB: Walter Reed. A biography. Charlottesville, University Press of Virginia, 1982. 190 p.
Bean WB: Walter Reed and yellow fever. **JAMA** 1983 Aug 5;250(5):659–62
Bell J: Crisis at Gettysburg. **Nurs Times** 1981 Feb 12;77(7):294–5
Blake JB: Medicine and the Revolution. **Milit Med** 1984 Apr;149(4):189–95
Blanco RL: American army hospitals in Pennsylvania during the Revolutionary War. **Pa Hist** 1981;48(4):347–68
Blanco RL: Medicine in the Continental Army, 1775–1781. **Bull NY Acad Med** 1981 Oct;57(8):677–704
Blanco RL: Military medicine in northern New York, 1776–1777. **NY Hist** 1982;63(1):39–58
Blanco RL: Physician of the American revolution, Jonathan Potts. New York, Garland STPM Press, 1979. xv, 276 p.
Bowen TE: William Crawford Gorgas, physician to the world. **Milit Med** 1983 Dec;148(12):917–20
Brady ER: The thread of a concept. **Marine Corps Gaz** 1971;55(5):35–42
Breeden JO: Andersonville--a southern surgeon's story. **Bull Hist Med** 1973 Jul–Aug;47(4):317–43
Breeden JO: 'The case of the miraculous bullet' revisited. **Milit Aff** 1981;45(1):23–6
Brewer LA: A historical account of the 'wet lung of trauma' and the introduction of intermittent positive-pressure oxygen therapy in World War II. **Ann Thorac Surg** 1981 Apr;31(4):386–93
Brodkey C, Gaydos JC: United States Army guidelines for troop living space: a historical review. **Milit Med** 1980 Jun;145(6):418–21
Brown GC, ed: With the ambulance service in France: the wartime letters of William Gorham Rice, jr. **Wis Mag Hist** 1981;64(4):278–93
Brumgardt JR, ed: Civil war nurse. The diary and letters of Hannah Ropes. Knoxville, University of Tennessee Press, 1980. 149 p.
Burch M: 'I don't know only what we hear': the soldiers' view of the 1918 influenza epidemic. **Indiana Med Hist Q** 1983 Dec;9(4):23–7
Caldwell GG, Kelley D, Zack M, et al: Mortality and cancer frequency among military nuclear test (Smoky) participants, 1957 through 1979. **JAMA** 1983 Aug 5;250(5):620–4
Carnegie ME: Nurses and war. Black nurses at the front. **Am J Nurs** 1984 Oct;84(10):1250–2
Cash P: An analysis of the social, political and professional impact of the Revolution upon the Boston medical community. (1759–1789). In: Congrès international d'histoire de la médecine, XXVe, Québec, 1976. Actes. Québec, 1977. p. 546–59.
Chapman JS: Forts and fevers: medicine on the Texas frontier. **Friends P. I. Nixon Med Hist Libr** 1979 Oct;8:1–8
Clary DA, ed: 'I am already quite a Texan': Albert J. Myer's letters from Texas. **Southwest Hist Q** 1978;82(1):25–76
Cox MK: Victory through defeat: a character analysis of Robert E. Lee. **Psychoanal Rev** 1980 Winter;67(4):443–63
Crosby WH: The golden age of the Army Medical Corps: a perspective from 1901. **Milit Med** 1983 Sep;148(9):707–11
Cutright PR, Brodhead MJ: Elliott Coues: naturalist and frontier historian. Urbana, University of Illinois Press, 1981. xv, 509 p.
Dammann G: Pictorial encyclopedia of Civil War medical instruments and equipment. Missoula, Mont., Pictorial Histories Pub. Co., 1983. iv, 100 p.
Dammann GE: Dental care during the Civil War. **Ill Dent J** 1984 Jan–Feb;53(1):12–7
Davis RA: A surgeon at war. **Surg Gynecol Obstet** 1983 Aug;157(2):147–59
Denny FW: Atypical pneumonia and the Armed Forces Epidemiological Board. **J Infect Dis** 1981 Mar;143(3):305–16
Deranian HM: The miracle man of the western front: the story of Dr. Varaztad Kazanjian. **Bull Hist Dent** 1984 Oct;32(2):85–103
Doona ME: Nursing revisited: the Massachusetts General Hospital, Base Hospital No. 6. **Mass Nurse** 1984 Apr;53(4):9
Eckert WG: History of the U.S. Army Graves Registration Service (1917–1950s). **Am J Forensic Med Pathol** 1983 Sep;4(3):231–43
Flynn JP: Maryland physicians in World War II. **Md State Med J** 1984 Jun;33(6):455
Gardner KD: Looking upon the water: in which we return to the Civil War. **Am J Kidney Dis** 1984 Sep;4(2):101–2
Gillett MC: The Army Medical Department 1775–1818. Washington, Center of Military History, U. S. Army, 1981. xiii, 299 p.
Gillett MC: Thomas Lawson, second Surgeon General of the U. S. Army: a character sketch. **Prologue J Nat Arch** 1982 Spring;14(1):15–24
Gladstone W: Early medical photography in America (1839–1883); VI. Civil war medical photography. **NY State J Med** 1981 Jan;81(1):5, 8
Greisman HC: Wound management and medical organization in the Civil War. **Surg Clin North Am** 1984 Aug;64(4):625–38
Hall CA: Doctors afield: John Calef, M.D. **N Engl J Med** 1981 Oct 29;305(18):1048–51
Hammarsten JF, Caylor JA: Physicians and the Lewis and Clark expedition. **Trans Am Clin Climatol Assoc** 1979;91:115–27
Hassler WW: Dr. Hunter Holmes McGuire: surgeon to Stonewall Jackson, the Confederacy, and the Nation. **Va Cavalcade** 1982;32(2):52–61
Havighurst W: The mind of John Shaw Billings. In his: Men of old Miami, 1809–1873, a book of portraits. New York, Putnams, 1974. p. 189–207.
Henderson JV: The importance of operational definitions in design of a combat casualty information system. **J Med Syst** 1983 Oct;7(5):413–26
Henry LJ: Florence Aby Blanchfield. In: Notable American women. The modern period. Cambridge, Mass., Belknap-Harvard Univ. Press, 1980. 4:83–5.
Henry WD: Stonewall Jackson--the soldier eccentric. **Practitioner** 1979 Oct;223(1336):580–7
Hyson JM: William Saunders: the United States Army's first dentist--West Point's forgotten man. **Milit Med** 1984 Aug;149(8):435–41
Irey TR: Soldiering, suffering, and dying in the Mexican War. **J West** 1972;11(2):285–98
Jelenko C, Matthews JB, Matthews JC: Emergency medicine in colonial America: Revolutionary War casualties. **Ann Emerg Med** 1982 Jan;11(1):73–6
Joy RJ: Jonathan Letterman of Jefferson: medical director of the Army of the Potomac. In Medical-Science colloquium. Special edition of Topic: a journal of the liberal arts. Washington, Pennsylvania, Washington and Jefferson College, 1983. p. 26–38.
Kampmeier RH: Venereal disease in the United States Army: 1775–1900. **Sex Transm Dis** 1982 Apr–Jun;9(2):100–3
Keisling P: Old soldiers never die: can we pay for the VA's version of the baby boom? **Wash Mon** 1982;14(1):20–9
Kellen K: War on the mind: a commentary. **Armed Forces Soc** 1980;6(2):313–25
Kennedy JW: The California-Arizona Maneuver Area World War II. Some medical and nonmedical notes about this desert training center--1942–1944. Part I. **Ariz Med** 1983 Jul;40(7):484–7
Kennedy JW: The California-Arizona maneuver area World War II. Some medical and nonmedical notes about this desert training center--1942–1944. Part 2. **Ariz Med** 1983 Aug;40(8):571–5
Kennedy JW: The California-Arizona maneuver area, World War II. Some medical and nonmedical notes about this desert training center--1942–1944. Part 3. **Ariz Med** 1983 Sep;40(9):642–7
Keough G: History and heritage of the Veterans Administration Nursing Service 1930–1980. **League Exch** 1981;(127):i–vi, 1–16
Knudson KG: Walt Disney, dentistry and the armed forces during World War II. **Bull Hist Dent** 1984 Oct;32(2):112–7
Leland TM: Anesthesiology in the Civil War (Dr. Julian John Chisolm). **J SC Med Assoc** 1981 Nov;77(11):524
Leland TM: DaVega's Floating Hospital. **J SC Med Assoc** 1984 Nov;80(11):581
Leland TM: Francis Lejan Parker, M.D. 1836–1913. **J SC Med Assoc** 1983 Feb;79(2):99
Leonard Wood, M.D.: Some Arizona Territory influences. **Ariz Med** 1982 Sep;39(9):593–6
Link K: Potomac fever: the hazards of camp life. **Vt Hist** 1983;51(2):69–88
Loehr WJ: Civil war medicine in North Carolina. **NC Med J** 1982 Feb;43(2):120–1
McLean RB: Leonard D. Heaton--military surgeon. **Milit Med** 1982 Sep;147(9):717–27
McSherry JA: Reiter's syndrome and the American revolutionary war. **Practitioner** 1982 Apr;226(1366):794–5
Miller B: The incident. **Lincoln Her** 1980;82(1):342–3
Musick M, ed: 'Glorious war': the diary of Westwood James, 16th Alabama. **Civ War Times Illus** 1978;17(6)34–42
Naisawald LV: Fanny Ricketts, nurse, diarist, devoted wife. **Va Cavalcade** 1972;21(3):14–21
Olch PD: Medicine in the Indian-fighting army, 1866–1890. **J West** 1982 Jul;21(3):32–41
Parsons ME: Mothers and matrons. **Nurs Outlook** 1983 Sep–Oct;31(5):274–8
Pearlman M: Leonard Wood, William Muldoon and the medical profession: public health and universal military training. **N Engl Q** 1979;52(3):326–44
Perkins JH: Reshaping technology in wartime: the effect of military goals on entomological research and insect-control practices. **Technol Cult** 1978 Apr;19(2):169–86
Perry T: The 48th evacuation hospital. **RI Med J** 1982 Dec;65(12):493
Peyton W: Tender loving care: a study of the doctors, their medicines and medical treatment during the American Civil War era. **Lincoln Her** 1982;84(2):106–13
Pillsbury DM: General Eisenhower's 'melanoma'. **J Am Acad Dermatol** 1981 May;4(5):631–2
Posner RM: Thomas Starr King and the mercy million. **Calif Hist Soc Q** 1964;43(4);291–308
Quilali air strip: **Marine Corps Gaz** 1970;54(11):41–3
Rausch DA, ed: Civil War medicine: a patient's account. **Pa Folklife** 1977;26(5):46–8
A report on the quality of ambulance service as observed in 1862 by S. L. Abbot, Francis Minot. Transactions of the New York State Medical Society, 1863: **NY State J Med** 1982 Mar;82(3):393–4
Rhoades ER: Medicine at Fort Sill, Indian Territory 1975–1880. **J Okla State Med Assoc** 1982 Feb;75(2):36–41
Robbins P: General Grant's calico colonel. **Am Hist Illus** 1979;14(1):4–7, 43–8

## MILITARY MEDICINE

Roberson JW: A view from Oklahoma, 1866–1868: the diary and letters of Dr. James Reagles, Jr., Assistant Surgeon, U. S. Army. **Red River Val Hist Rev** 1978;3(4):19–46

Romm S: Morris Joseph Asch. **Plast Reconstr Surg** 1983 May;71(5):724–8

Rowe WF: Discussion of 'George Armstrong Custer and the Battle of the Little Bighorn: homicide or mass suicide'. **J Forensic Sci** 1984 Jul;29(3):696–9

Rózsa G: 70 éve halt meg John Shaw Billings. **Orv Hetil** 1983 Sep 4;124(36):2191–2

Sandos JA: Prostitution and drugs: the United States Army on the Mexican-American border, 1916–1917. **Pac Hist Rev** 1980;49(4):621–45

Sanford WL: The influenza epidemic of 1918 and its effects on the military. **Indiana Med Hist Q** 1983 Dec;9(4):16–22

Scarchuk JM, ed: The first pharmacopoeia published in the Federated States of America, by William Brown, entitled Pharmacopoeia Simpliciorum et Efficiorum in Usum Nosocomii Militaris, published by Styner Cist. 1778. Coventry, Conn., the Author, 1976. xii, 32 p.

Scheips PJ: Albert James Myer, an army doctor in Texas, 1854–1857. **Southwest Hist Q** 1978;82(1):1–24

Schott TE: Paul Ramsey Hawley. In Dictionary of American biography, 1961–1965. Suppl. 7, 1981. p. 328–9.

Shields EA: A history of the United States Army Nurse Corps (female): 1901–1937. Ed. D. Diss., Columbia University Teachers College. New York, 1980. 232 leaves.

Skinner RE: The making of the air surgeon: the early life and career of David N. W. Grant. **Aviat Space Environ Med** 1983 Jan;54(1):75–82

Smith JD: Kentucky Civil War recruits: a medical profile. **Med Hist** 1980 Apr;24(2):185–96

Smith NB: The women who went to the war: the Union Army nurse in the Civil War. Ph.D. Diss., Northwestern Univ. Evanston, 1981. 183 p.

Smith R: The first American officer wounded in World War I. **JAMA** 1982 Mar 26;247(12):1743

Spring JH: Psychologists and the war: the meaning of intelligene in the alpha and beta tests. **Hist Educ Q** 1972;12(1):3–16

Steiner PE: Medical history of a Civil War regiment: disease in the sixty-fifth United States colored infantry. Clayton, Mo., Institute of Civil War Studies, 1977. xxii, 137 p.

Stephenson LW: Reflections on the military involvement of a medical school. **Surg Gynecol Obstet** 1982 Jun;154(6):888–96

Stewart MJ: Moving the wounded. Litters, cacolets and ambulance wagons, U. S. Army, 1776–1876. Ft. Collins, Colorado, Old Army Press, 1979. 134 p.

Straight WM: Fort Dallas, a most salubrious post. **J Fla Med Assoc** 1982 Aug;69(8):706–12

Tatlock H: Clarification of the cause of Fort Bragg fever (pretibial fever) – January 1982. **Rev Infect Dis** 1982 Jan–Feb;4(1):157–8

Thompson ME: Sixty years of progress: nursing and the times in U. S. A. – and Vermont, 1919. An overview of nursing's accomplishment in World War I – under its chief – Jane A. Delano. **Vt Regist Nurse** 1979 Jul;:6–8

Tilney NL: The marrow of the tragedy (Harvey Cushing). **Surg Gynecol Obstet** 1983 Oct;157(4):380–8

Trice ER: Hugh Mercer: physician-hero of the American Revolution. **Va Med** 1981 Feb;108(2):104–6

Vernon HA: Medical crisis at Fort Niagara, 1779–80. **Niagara Frontier** 1977;24:89–94

Vester JW: The valiant physicians. **Milit Med** 1982 Dec;147(12):1041–7

Webb WM: There's a doctor in the library. The story of John Shaw Billings, M.D. (1838–1913). **J Indiana State Med Assoc** 1981 Jun;74(6):360–6

Weir JA: The army doctor looks at Indian medicine. **Denver West Roundup** 1977 Sep–Oct;33:12–28

Weir JA: The history of Fitzsimons Army Medical Center. **Denver West Roundup** 1980 Jan–Feb;36:3–14

Weir RF: Remarks on the gunshot wounds of the Civil War by Robert F. Weir. New York State Journal of Medicine, April, 1904. **NY State J Med** 1982 Mar;82(3):391–3

Wier JA: 19th century army doctors on the frontier and in Nebraska. **Nebr Hist** 1980;61(2):192–214

Wilbur CK: Revolutionary medicine 1700–1800. Chester, Connecticut, Glove Pequot Press, 1980. 80 p.

Wilkenson F: Spotsylvania: reflections. How men die in battle. **Civ War Times Illus** 1983;22(2):16–8

Williams WH: Norman Thomas Kirk. In Dictionary of American Biography, Suppl. 6, 1956–1960. p. 344–5, 1980.

Wilson JW: Some aspects of medical services in the Trans-Mississippi Department of the Confederate States of America, 1863–1865. **J North LA Hist Assoc** 1981 Fall;12(4):123–46

Woodward TE: The public's debt to military medicine. **Milit Med** 1981 Mar;146(3):168–73

Woosley AI: Fort Burgwin's hospital. **Palacio** 86(1):3–7, 36–9

Zeidenfelt A: Surgeon General William Hammond. **Civ War Times Illus** 1978;17(6):24–32

Zollinger RM: The legacies of William Beaumont, pioneer investigator. **Pharos** 1983 Winter;46(1):20–3

### USSR

Abramov VV: O geroizme meditsinskikh rabotnikov v period oborony Kerchenskikh kamenolomen v 1942 g. **Voen Med Zh** 1982 May;(5):71–3

Aleksanian IV, Kulish IM: Sanitarno-gigienicheskoe i protivoé pidemicheskoe obespechenie voĭsk v gody Velikoĭ Otechestvennoĭ voĭny.

Aleksanian IV: Sovetskaia voennaia meditsina v Velikoĭ Otechestvennoĭ voĭne (k 35-letiiu pobedy nad fashistskoĭ Germanieĭ). **Sov Zdravookhr** 1980;(5):3–6

Aleksanian IV, Knopov MSh: Vidnyĭ sovetskiĭ khirurg V. S. Levit (k 100-letiiu so dnia rozhdeniia). **Klin Khir** 1983 Jun;6:58–60

Andreeva VN, Kosmachevskaia EA: Ocherk razvitiia fiziologii krovoobrashcheniia v laboratoriiakh Mediko-khirurgicheskoĭ (Voenno-meditsinskoĭ) akademii v XIX veke (K istorii vzaimosviazi teorii i praktiki v issledovatel'skoĭ rabote). **Fiziol Zh SSSR** 1981 Jun;67(6):934–50

Artiukhov SA: Sochinskaia gospital'naia baza v gody Velikoĭ Otechestvennoĭ voĭny. **Voen Med Zh** 1981 Mar;(3):70–2

Artiukhov SA: Sochinskaia gospital'naia baza v gody Velikoĭ Otechestvennoĭ voĭny. **Sov Zdravookhr** 1981;(9):66–7

Arzhantsev PZ: Etapy razvitiia spetsializirovannoĭ stomatologicheskoĭ pomoshchi v GVKG imeni N. N. Burdenko. **Voen Med Zh** 1980 Feb;(2):78–80

Babin VP: Iz opyta organizatsii lecheniia legkoranenykh v mediko-sanitarnom batal'one mekhanizirovannogo korpusa v gody Velikoĭ Otechestvennoĭ voĭny. **Voen Med Zh** 1981 Jun;(6):73–4

Babin VP: Mediki 554-go mediko-sanitarnogo batal'ona v bitve za Dnepr. **Voen Med Zh** 1983 Oct;10:63–4

Babin VP: Nekotorye osobennosti raboty mediko-sanitarnogo batal'ona mekhanizirovannogo korpusa v period Velikoĭ Otechestvennoĭ voĭny. **Voen Med Zh** 1982 Feb;(2):74–6

Babushkin A: Razvedka khimicheskikh sredstv protivnika (po opytu v 1944–1945 gg.). **Voen Istor Zh** 1973;(1):85–9

Bagdasar'ian SM: Velikiĭ russkiĭ khirurg N. I. Pirogov (k 100-letiiu so dnia smerti). **Klin Med (Mosk)** 1982 Jul;60(7):111–5

Bagdasar'ian SM: Voennye vrachi--veterany pervoĭ piatiletki. **Voen Med Zh** 1982 Jun;(6):75–6

Bagdasar'ian SM: Vydaiushchiĭsia sovetskiĭ uchenyĭ (k 40-letiiu prisvoeniia zvaniia Geroia Sotsialisticheskogo Truda N. N. Burdenko). **Voen Med Zh** 1983 May;5:64–8

Baranovskiĭ GIa, Kapitonov GI: Nakotorye osobennosti meditsinskoĭ évakuatsii v Stalingradskoĭ bitve. (K 40-letiiu Stalingradskoĭ bitvy). **Voen Med Zh** 1983;(1):71–4

Baranovskiĭ GIa, Kapitonov GI: Ob évakuatsii ranenykh i bol'nykh zheleznodorozhnym transportom vo vremia Velikoĭ Otechestvennoĭ voĭny. **Voen Med Zh** 1981 Mar;(3):9–10

Barsukov MI: Zdravookhranenie v gody Velikoĭ Otechestvennoĭ voĭny 1941–1945. Sbornik dokumentov i materialov. Moskva, Meditsina, 1977. 575 p.

Beloborodova NL: Moskovskoe otdelenie mediko-khirurgicheskoĭ akademii v Otechestvennuiu voinu 1812 goda. **Voen Med Zh** 1982 Nov;(11):66–7

Belozerov VV, Galin LL: Zhurnal dlia ranenykh i bol'nykh krasnoarmeĭtsev. **Voen Med Zh** 1984 Apr;(4):65–9

Berezhniak AP: Polirabotniki meditsinskikh chasteĭ i uchrezhdeniĭ v gody Velikoĭ Otechestvennoĭ voĭny. **Voen Med Zh** 1981 Sep;(9):70–1

Bogatyrev MF: Meditsinskoe obespechenie 25-i Krasnoznamennoĭ gvardeĭskoĭ Sinel'nikovskoĭ strelkovoĭ divizii v Budapeshtskoĭ nastupatel'noĭ operatsii. **Voen Med Zh** 1983 Oct;10:64–6

Borisov EN, Stepanov AA, Voronkov OV, et al: Organizatsiia meditsinskogo snabzheniia Krasnoĭ Armii. **Voen Med Zh** 1980 May;(5):61–4

Borodin VG: Govorit veteran Velikoĭ Otechestvennoĭ. **Voen Med Zh** 1984 May;(5):66–9

Borodin VG: Nekotorye voprosy organizatsii lecheniia i voenno-vrachebnoĭ ékspertizy ranenykh i bol'nykh v évakuatsionnykh gospitaliakh Urala vo vremia Velikŏ Otechestvennoi voiny. **Voen Med Zh** 1983 Mar;(3):71–4

Broshevan VM: Pikluvannia partiinykh, radians'kykh i viis'kovykh orhaniv Krymu pro okhoronu zdorov'ia osobovoho skladu chervonoi armii. **Ukr Istor Zh** 1981;(12):64–8

Buianov MI: Vrach-puteshestvennik A. V. Eliseev. **Klin Med (Mosk)** 1982;60(8):113–4

Bukov VA: Opyt meditsinskogo obespecheniia 13-ĭ armii. Soobshchenie vtoroe. Meditsinskoe obespechnie armii v khode operatsoi. **Voen Med Zh** 1982 Aug;(8):12–7

Bukov VA: Opyt meditsinskogo obespecheniia 13-ĭ armii v bitve pod Kurskom. **Voen Med Zh** 1982;(7):14–9

Burdov VS, Nemchaninov SK, Miziak AN: K istorii okruzhnogo voennogo gospitala Belorusskogo voennogo okruga. **Voen Med Zh** 1984 Aug;(8):71–3

Chirkov AI: Meditsinskoe snabzhenie russkoĭ armii v voĭnakh XVIII veka. **Voen Med Zh** 1981 Aug;(8):74–6

Chirkov AI: Organizatsiia meditsinskogo snabzheniia russkoĭ armii v Otechestvennuiu voĭnu 1812 goda. **Voen Med Zh** 1982 Apr;(4):70–2

Denisenko VZ: 60 Let na strazhe zdorov'ia voennosluzhashchikh. **Voen Med Zh** 1982;(9):78–9

Derbenev NE: Zdravnitsa dlia ranenykh voinov. **Voen Med Zh** 1980 Jul;(7):21-2
Deriabin II, Berkutov AN: Razvitie voenno-polevoĭ khirurgii za 60 let Soiuza SSR. **Vestn Khir** 1983 Feb;2:3-7
Dyskin EA, Klishov AA: O roli Voenno-meditsinskoĭ akademii im. S. M. Kirova v podgotovke vysokokvalifitsirovannykh kadrov anatomov i gistologov SSSR. **Arkh Anat Gistol Embriol** 1983 Mar;84(3):90-6
Elkin II: Voenno-épidemicheskaia doktrina (po opytu protivoépidemicheskoĭ zashchity voĭsk v Velikuiu Otechestvennuiu voinu 1941-1945). **Zh Mikrobiol Epidemiol Immunobiol** 1980 May;(5):11-7
Epifanov NS: Khirurg, uchenyĭ, patriot (k110-letiiu so dnia rozhdeniia V.A. Oppelia). **Khirurgiia (Mosk)** 1982 Nov;(11):101-3
Ermakov MA: Iz istorii organizatsii évakuatsii ranenykh i bol'nykh partizan na Bol'shuiu zemliu. **Med Sestra** 1982 Mar;41(3):43-5
Ermakov ME: Meditsinskiĭ punkt partizanskogo otriada. **Feldsher Akush** 1983;48(5):47-9
Fedotov V: Zabota partii i naroda o ranenykh v gody voiny. **Voen Istor Zh** 1977;6:90-4
Furmanchuk VM: Podvigi meditsinskikh sester v pervyĭ period Velikoĭ Otechestvennoĭ voĭny. **Med Sestra** 1980 Oct;37(10):60-2
Galin LL: Deiatel'nost' voenno-sanitarnoĭ sluzhby v gody Velikoĭ Otechestvennoĭ voĭny (po materialam 'Voenno-meditsinskogo zhurnala'). **Sov Zdravookhr** 1984;(5):58-61
Galin LL: Gotov k trudu i oborone SSSR (k 50-letiiu vvedeniia Vsesouiznogo fizkul'turnogo kompleksa). **Voen Med Zh** 1981 Jun;(6):75-6
Galin LL: Publikatsii N. I. Pirogova na stranitsakh 'Voenno--meditsinskogo zhurnala. **Voen Med Zh** 1980 Nov;(11):69-71
Galin LL: Shina Diterikhsa. **Feldsher Akush** 1983 Nov;48(11):46-8
Galin LL: Vklad P. P. Potiralovskogo v razvitie organizatsionnykh voprosov voennoĭ meditsiny. **Voen Med Zh** 1982 Apr;(4):68-70
Galin LL, Pal'chikov PA: Vklad 'Voenno-Meditsinskogo Zhurnala' v razvitie voennoĭ meditsiny. **Sov Zdravookhr** 1983;(2):63-7
Gembitskiĭ EV: Opyt raboty terapevtov v boevykh usloviiakh i ego znachenie dlia razvitiia voenno-polevoĭ terapii. **Voen Med Zh** 1980 May;(5):46-9
Gembitskiĭ EV: S. P. Botkin kak voennyĭ terapevt. **Klin Med (Mosk)** 1982 Sep;60(9):22-7
Georgievskiĭ AS, Lobanov GP: Meditsinskoe obespechnenie Rzhevsko-Sychevskoĭ nastupatel'noĭ operatsii. **Voen Med Zh** 1982 Oct;(10):62-6
Georgievskiĭ AS: Vklad russkikh voennykh vracheĭ v stanovlenie i razvitie profilakticheskogo napravleniia meditsiny. **Sov Zdravookhr** 1982;(10):66-70
Georgievskiĭ AS: Vklad S. P. Botkina v razvitie otechestvennoĭ voennoĭ meditsiny. **Sov Zdravookhr** 1983;6:62-6
Gladkikh PF, Galin LL: K istorii teoreticheskoi razrabotki sistemy étapnogo lecheniia ranenykh i bol'nykh. **Voen Med Zh** 1984 May;(5):74-5
Gladkikh PF: Meditsinskoe obespechenie 2-ĭ udarnoĭ armii v period proryva blokady Leningrada. **Voen Med Zh** 1981 Feb;(2):71-3
Gladkikh PF: Ob évakuatsii ranenykh i bol'nykh iz gospital'noĭ bazy Leningradskogo fronta v period polnoĭ blokady Leningrada. **Voen Med Zh** 1983 Feb;(2):70-3
Gladkikh PF: Perestroĭka sistemy podgotovki voenno-meditsinskikh kadrov v tridtsatye gody. **Voen Med Zh** 1983 Sep;9:70-2
Gladkikh PF: Zabota M. I. Kutuzova o zdorov'e Russkogo soldata (k 170-letiiu so dnia Borodinskogo srazheniia). **Sov Zdravookhr** 1983;(3):68-70
Golosov BA: Ob organizatsii meditsinskogo obespecheniia voĭsk v bitve pod Kurskom (K 40-letiiu bitvy pod Kurskom). **Voen Med Zh** 1983 Jul;(7):17-21
Gorbunov VP: 50 let na strazhe zdorov'ia voĭnov. **Voen Med Zh** 1984 Aug;(8):76-8
Granat NE: K 35-letiiu pobedy (vospominaniia o sluzhbe v voenno-sanitarnom poezde). **Med Sestra** 1980 May;39(5):7-11
Grebenev AL: S. P. Botkin o N. I. Pirogove. **Klin Med (Mosk)** 1982 Sep;60(9):108-10
Grin' V: Organizatsiia meditsinskogo obespecheniia v oboronitel'nykh operatsiiakh pervogo perioda voiny. **Voen Istor Zh** 1978;3:101-6
Grin' VA: O meditsinskom obespechenii bitvy pod Kurskom. **Voen Med Zh** 1980 Apr;(4):21-6
Gurvich MM, Georgievskiĭ AS: Nekotorye uroki organizatsii meditsinskogo obespecheniia voĭsk Zapadnogo i Kalininskogo frontov v kontrnastuplenii (k 40-letiiu razgroma nemetsko-fashistskikh voĭsk pod Moskvoĭ). **Voen Med Zh** 1982 Jan;(1):14-9
Gvozdev MP, Petrov VA: Iustin Iulianovich Dzhanelidze (K 100-letiiu so dnia rozhdeniia). **Voen Med Zh** 1983 Aug;(8):72-4
Ibragimov NG: Meditsinskaia obshchestvennost' Bashkirii v gody grazhdanskoĭ i Velikoĭ Otechestvennoĭ voĭn. **Feldsher Akush** 1980;45(5):56-9
Iurov IA, Grin' VA: K 40-letiiu bitvy pod Moskvoĭ. **Voen Med Zh** 1981 Dec;(12):9-15
Iurov IA, Grin' VA: K 40-letiiu Stalingradskoĭ bitvy. **Voen Med Zh** 1982 Dec;(12):26-33
Iurov IA, Grin' VA: O meditsinskom obespechenii Belorusskoĭ operatsii. **Voen Med Zh** 1984 Jul;(7):8-16
Ivan'kovich FA: Opyt évakuatsii ranenykh i bol'nykh voenno-sanitarnymi letuchkami vo vremia Stalingradskoĭ bitvy. **Voen Med Zh** 1983 Feb;(2):68-70
Ivanov NG, Georgievskiĭ AS: Sergeĭ Petrovich Botkin i voenno-meditsinskaia akademiia. **Vestn Akad Med Nauk SSSR** 1983;(3):8-14
Ivanov NG: Sovetskoe voennoe zdravookhranenie nakanune i v gody Velikoĭ Otechestvennoĭ voĭny. **Sov Med** 1980;(5):3-10
Ivanov NG: Znachenie opyta Velikoĭ Otechestvennoĭ Voĭny dlia podgotovki voenno-meditsinskikh kadrov. **Voen Med Zh** 1980 May;(5):21-4
Ivashchenko IK: Organizatsiia sanitarno-protivoépidemicheskikh meropriiatiĭ v voĭskakh Sibirskogo voennogo okruga v gody voĭny. **Voen Med Zh** 1981 Mar;(3):11-2
K 40-letiiu organov urpavleniia Tylom Vooruzhennykh Sil SSSR: **Voen Med Zh** 1981 Aug;(8):7-11
Kantorovich MM: Neutomimye truzheniki--geroi Velikoĭ Otechestvennoĭ voĭny. **Med Sestra** 1980 May;39(5):3-7
Katsnel'bogen AG, Stiazhkov AV: Slavnye bol'shevichki--krasnye sestry miloserdiia. **Med Sestra** 1980 Nov;39(11):58-61
Katsnel'bogen AG: Vzgliady P.I. Pestelia na meditsinu. **Klin Med (Mosk)** 1980 Aug;58(8):117-21
Khodorkov LA: Meditsinskaia sluzhba Krasnoĭ Armii v operatsii na reke Khalkin-Gol. **Voen Med Zh** 1979 Aug;(8):76-8
Kishkovskiĭ AN, Tiutin LA: K 50-letiiu kafedry rentgenologii i radiologii VMA imeni S.M. Kirov. **Voen Med Zh** 1980 Sep;(9):76-8
Kolmsee P: Nikolai Iwanowitsch Pirogow - Kriegschirurg und militärmedizinischer Organisator in Russland des 19. Jahrhunderts. **Militaergesch** 1981;20(5):536-45
Kolontaĭ IuIu, Kondrashov AN, Kolod'ko ED: 50 let kafedre travmatologii, ortopedii i voenno-polevoĭ khirurgii Dnepropetrovskogo ordena Trudovogo Krasnogo Znameni meditsinskogo instituta. **Ortop Travmatol Protez** 1980 Mar;(3):76-7
Komarov FI: Vklad voennykh medikov v pobedu nad vragom. **Voen Med Zh** 1980 May;(5):7-13
Koroliuk AM: K stoletiiu so dnia rozhdeniia Viacheslava Mikhaĭlovicha Aristovskogo. **Zh Mikrobiol Epidemiol Immunobiol** 1983 Mar;(3):109-12
Korsunskiĭ MA: Voennyĭ fel'dsher P. E. Lazimir. **Feldsher Akush** 1980;45(12):41-4
Kostrov NI: Opyt sovetskoĭ voennoĭ otorinolaringologii v Velikoĭ Otechestvennoĭ voĭne. **Voen Med Zh** 1980 Aug;(8):17-9
Kotel'nikov VP: V. A. Oppel' i razvitie fiziologicheskoĭ khirurgii. **Klin Med (Mosk)** 1984 May;62(5):145-8
Kovanov VV: V tylovom gospitale. **Voen Med Zh** 1980 Apr;(4):27-30
Kozovenko MN: Rol' N. I. Pirogova v organizatsii truda meditsinskikh sester na voĭne. **Voen Med Zh** 1980 Nov;(11);72-3
Kozubenko ID: Uchastie meditsinskikh rabotnikov Dona v revoliutsionnoĭ bor'be. **Sov Zdravookhr** 1984;(1):47-8
Krasil'shchik SI: Zarubezhnye otzyvy o dostizheniiakh Sovetskoĭ meditsiny v gody Velikoĭ Otechestvennoĭ voĭny. **Voen Med Zh** 1984 May;(5):71-3
Krasnogorskaia ES: V armeĭskom gospitale. **Voen Med Zh** 1980 Mar;(3):69-70
Krasnopeev II: Blokadnyĭ vypusk vracheĭ Voenno-meditsinskoĭ akademii (K 40-letiiu sniatiia blokady Leningrada). **Voen Med Zh** 1984 Jan;(1):69-71
Kurkotkin S: Tyl sovetskikh vooruzhennykh sil v velikoi otechestvennoi voine. **Voen Istor Zn** 1975(5):44-52
Kurpita PN: Osobennosti sanitarno-gigienicheskogo obespecheniia na fronte i v tylu. **Voen Med Zh** 1980 May;(5):54-7
Kuzin M, Antipenko E: Zhizn' otdannaia nauke. **Voen Istor Zh** 1969;11(12):47-50
Kuz'min MK: Muzhestvo i geroizm meditsinskikh rabotnikov. **Voen Med Zh** 1980 May;(5):65-8
Kuz'min MK: Rol' sovetskikh uchenykh-medikov v Velikoĭ Otechestvennoĭ voĭne (k 35-letiiu Pobedy nad fashistskoĭ Germanieĭ). **Sov Med** 1980;(8):118-20
Kuz'min MK: Sovetskaia meditsina v gody Velikoĭ Otechestvennoĭ voĭny ocherki. Moskva, Meditsina, 1979. 237 p.
Kuz'min MK: Velikiĭ Russkiĭ khirurg N. I. Pirogov i sovremennost'. **Sov Med** 1983;(2):117-9
Leonov IT: Bol'sheviki-lenintsy--vospitanniki Voenno-meditsinskoĭ akademii. **Voen Med Zh** 1984 Oct;(10):62-5
Leonov IT: N. I. Pirogov i voennaia meditsina. **Feldsher Akush** 1981;46(11):51-3
Leonov IT: Vydaiushchiĭsia organizator meditsinskoĭ sluzhby i voenno-meditsinskogo obrazovaniia (k 90-letiiu so dnia rozhdeniia B. K. Leonardova). **Sov Zdravookhr** 1982;(9):60-2
Lidov IP: Terapevty v Velikoĭ Otechestvennoĭ voĭne. **Ter Arkh** 1980;52(5):3-5
Lisitsyn KM: Voenno-polevaia khirurgiia vo vremia Velikoĭ Otechestvennoĭ voĭny i perspektivy ee razvitiia. **Voen Med Zh** 1980 May;(5):42-5
Lobanov GP, Zhuravskiĭ VA: Nekotorye voprosy organizatsii spetsial'noĭ podgotovki lichnogo sostava voenno-meditsinskoĭ sluzhby v period Voĭny. **Voen Med Zh** 1980 May;(5):28-33
Lobanov GP: Razvitie i sovershenstvovanie meditsinskoĭ sortirovki v period Velikoĭ Otechestvennoĭ Voĭny. **Voen Med Zh** 1983 May;5:15-20
Lobastov OS: Meditsinskoe obespechenie voĭsk vo frontovykh nastukpatel'nykh operatsiiakh na zavershaiuschchem étape Voĭny.

**Voen Med Zh** 1980 May;(5):25-8
Lomakina NM, Merinov AP, Anoshkin IG: Podvig medikov v Stalingradskoĭ bitve. **Voen Med Zh** 1980 Nov;(11):14-6
Maiat VS: Vladimir Semenovich Levit (K 100-letiiu so dnia rozhdeniia). **Khirurgiia (Mosk)** 1983 Jun;6:111-3
Makovoz AA: D. V. Volchenetskiĭ--vydaiushchiĭsia vrach Rossii. **Feldsher Akush** 1983;48(4):57-8
Marasanov RA, Mel'nichuk AN: Meditsinskoe obespechenie ranenykh i bol'nykh nemetskikh voennoplennykh v gody Velikoĭ Otechestvennoĭi voĭny. **Voen Med Zh** 1981 May;(5):19-22
Marchenko MA: Meditsinskaia sluzhba 4-ĭ Gvardeĭskoĭ Apostolovskoĭ Krasnoznamennoĭ strelkovoĭ divizii v Iassko-Kishinevskoĭ operatsii. **Voen Med Zh** 1984 Aug;(8):15-8
Melkumian GA: Hasarakakan kazmakerputyunneri dere kovkasyan banaki bezheshkakan spasarkmen gortsum arajin hamashkharhayin paterazmi tarinerin. **Patma Banasirakan Handes. Ist Filol Zh** 1977;3:221-34
Milashkin AG: Ispol'zovanie mazi Vishnevskogo v gody Velikoĭ Otechestvennoĭ voĭny. **Voen Med Zh** 1982 Feb;(2):76
Milashkin AG: Nauchno-issledovatel'skaia rabota po voprosam travmaticheskogo shoka v gody Velikoĭ Otechestvennoĭ voĭny. **Voen Med Zh** 1983 Aug;(8):74-5
Mirskiĭ MB: Vydaiushchiĭsia russkiĭ khirurg E. I. Bogdanovskiĭ (k 150-letiiu so dnia rozhdeniia). **Vestn Khir** 1984 Mar;132(3):143-5
Mitrofanov VG: K 90-letiiu so dnia rozhdeniia Mikhaila Semenovicha Lisitsyna. **Vestn Khir** 1983 May;130(5):141-2
Mitsura DI: Vsegda riadom s voinom. **Med Sestra** 1981 Oct;40(10):58-62
Na strazhe Rodiny: **Voen Med Zh** 1980 Feb;(2):3-6
Nagaev IM: Krasnye medsestry na frontakh grazhdanskoĭ voĭny. **Med Sestra** 1980 Dec;39(12):41-2
Nazarov VF: K 60-letiiu organizatsii sanatorno-kurortnogo dela v Vooruzhennykh Silakh SSSR. **Voen Med Zh** 1982 Aug;(8):75-8
Nevskiĭ NM: O rabote frontovogo évakopunkta. **Voen Med Zh** 1980 Oct;(10):23-4
Nikolaĭ Ivanovich Ragoza (K 100-letiiu so dnia rozhdeniia): **Voen Med Zh** 1983 Jul;(7):76
Novikov FG, Tomashuk IP: Iz istorii otechestvennoĭ voenno-polevoĭ khirurgii. **Klin Khir** 1980 May;(5):69-72
Okhrimenko NN: Glavnyĭ voennyĭ gospital' i ego rol' v razvitii otechestvennoĭ voennoĭ nevrologii (k 275-letiiu so dnia osnovaniia Glavnogo. **Zh Nevropatol Psikhiatr** 1983;83(7):1069-71
Pal'chikov PA: Oni zhertvovali soboĭ radi pobedy. **Voen Med Zh** 1983 May;(5):68-70
Petrov BD: I. A. Pribil' (k 200-letiiu so dnia rozhdeniia). **Zh Mikrobiol Epidemiol Immunobiol** 1983 Oct;(10):108-9
Petrov NS, Georgievskiĭ AS, Antonov VB: Sergeĭ Petrovich Botkin i voennaia meditsina (k 150-letiiu so dnia rozhdeniia). **Voen Med Zh** 1982;(9):64-6
Petrov VP, Shamko VI: Oni zashchishchali Odessu. **Med Sestra** 1984 Apr;43(4):55-7
Popov MIa: Ranenie i smert' bagrationa. **Vopr Istor** 1975;(3):211-4
Porter J: Nursing in Imperial Russia. Nurses under siege. **Nurs Mirror** 1980 Oct 16;151(16):24-6
Potulov VM: [V. I. Lenin's concern for the health of the soldiers]. (Rus) **Voen Med Zh** 1979 Dec;(12):7-10
Pozyvaĭ TT: Organizatsiia protivoépidemicheskoĭ zashchity voĭsk na Zapadnom (3-m Belorusskom) fronte. **Voen Med Zh** 1980 Aug;(8):20-1
Pozyvaĭ TT: Protivoépidemicheskaia rabota sredi naseleniia v polose boevykh deĭstvii Zapadnogo (3-go Belorusskogo) fronta. **Zh Mikrobiol Epidemiol Immunobiol** 1980 May;(5):17-21
Ripp GKh, Salamatov EI: Uchastie medikov Zapadnoĭ Sibiri v lechenii ranenykh i bil'nykh voinov. **Voen Med Zh** 1980 Jun;(6):24-6
Rodionov AV: O partiĭno-politicheskoĭ rabote sredi ranenykh i meditsinskogo personala vo vremia Kurskoĭ bitvy. **Voen Med Zh** 1984 Aug;(8):11-5
Rudenko AT: Kafedre cheliustno-litsevoĭ khirurgii so stomatologieĭ VMA imeni S. M. Kirova--50 let. **Voen Med Zh** 1980 Mar;(3):77
Samotokin BA, Nechaĭ AI, Sitenko VM, et al: Vladimir Nikolaevich Shamov (k 100-letiiu so dnia rozhdeniia). **Voen Med Zh** 1982 Jun;(6):73-4
Sanzharov BN: Deiatel'nost' glavnykh épidemiologov frontov v 1941-1945 gg. **Voen Med Zh** 1980;(12):13-4
Sapov IA, Tiurin VI: K 100-letiiu Kronshtadtskoĭ shkoly vodolazov. **Voen Med Zh** 1982 Aug;(8):70-2
Selivanov EF, Pasiukov FV: Pamiatnik medikam Velikoĭ Otechestvennoĭ voĭmy (o Voenno-meditsinskom muzee Ministerstva oborony SSSR). **Feldsher Akush** 1983 Nov;48(11):48-52
Selivanov EF, Kantorovich MM: Relikvii N. I. Pirogova v Noenno-meditsinskom muzee. **Voen Med Zh** 1983 Nov;(11):71-3
Selivanov EF, Pasiukov FV: 40-let Voenno-meditsinskogo muzeia. **Sov Zdravookhr** 1983;(2):67-70
Selivanov VI, Tkhostov DR, Selivanov EF: Lechbno- evakuatsionnaia kharakteristika ranenykh i bol'nykh, lechivshikhsia v gospital'noi baze tyla strany. **Voen Med Zh** 1980 Jun;(6):20-3
Selivanov VI: [Organization of rehabilitation of the wounded and sick during World War II in military hospitals]. (Rus) **Voen Med Zh** 1979 Nov;(11):74-5
Shabunin AV: K 150-letiiu izdaniia truda R. S. Chetyrkina 'Opyt voenno-meditsinskoĭ politsii ili pravila k sokhraneniiu zdorov'ia russkikh soldat v sukhoputnoĭ sluzhbe'. **Gig Sanit** 1984 Jun;(6):35-6
Shabunin AV: Vasiliĭ Ivanovich Priselkov--vidnyĭ deiatel' otechestvennyĭ meditsiny. **Sov Zdravookhr** 1984;(2):62-4
Shalaev NF: Organizatsiia terapevticheskoĭ pomoshchi v Krasnoĭ Armii v gody inostrannoĭ voennoĭ interventsii i grazhdanskoĭ voĭny. **Voen Med Zh** 1982 Jun;(6):68-9
Shalaev NF: Vrach-bol'shevik I. D. Orakhelashvili. **Sov Zdravookhr** 1984;(1):51-3
Shcherbina VP, Liashenko NI: Vsia zhizn'--vdokhnovennyĭ trud. **Voen Med Zh** 1983 Mar;3:70-1
Shliapak AE: Partiĭno-politicheskaia rabota v ěvakogospitaliakh Kavkazskikh Mineral'nykh Vod. **Voen Med Zh** 1981 Nov;(11):69-70
Shulimin VA: Osobennosti meditsinskogo obespecheniia 193-ĭ strelkovoĭ divizii v boiakh za Stalingrad. **Voen Med Zh** 1982 Nov;(11):61-2
Sinitsyn AM: Zabota o ranenykh frontovikakh i invalidakh v gody otechestvennoi voiny. **Istor SSSR** 1973;(1):130-8
Skorogliadov AV: K 50-letiiu so dnia organizatsii kafedry travmatologii, ortopedii i voenno- polevoĭ khirurgii II MOLGMI im. N.I. Pirogova. **Ortop Travmatol Protez** 1983 Dec;(12):60-1
Sluchanko BP: Kerchenskoe meditsinskoe uchilishche im. Geroia Sovetskogo Soiuza glavstarshiny meditsinskoĭ sluzhby G. K. Petrovoĭ. **Med Sestra** 1983 Oct;42(10):56-8
Smirnov EI: Voĭna i voennaia meditsina, 1939-1945. Moskva, Meditsina, 1979. 524 p.
Smirnov EI, Garin NS: Znachenie nauchnogo naslediia i deiatel'nosti Ia. L. Okunevskogo dlia sozdaniia dezinfektsionnogo i banno-prachechnogo dela v armii. **Voen Med Zh** 1979 Apr;(4):73-5
Sovetskaia voenno-polevaia khirurgiia v Velikuiu Otechestvennuiu voinu 1941-1945 gg. i osnovnye napravleniia ee dal'neĭshego razvitiia: **Khirurgiia (Mosk)** 1980 May;(5):3-8
Stegunin SI, Razumov VI: Pomoshch' narodov SSSR ranenym i bol'nym voinam Krasnoĭ Armii (1941-1945). **Sov Zdravookhr** 1982;(8):59-62
Stegunin SI, Razumov VI: Voprosy organizatsii pomoshchi ranenym voinam Krasnoĭ Armii v gody Velikoĭ Otechestvennoĭ voĭny na stranitsakh gazety 'Pravda'. **Sov Zdravookhr** 1984;(6):65-7
Szállási A: Magyar orvosíró és az orosz forradalom. **Orv Hetil** 1984 Mar 18;125(12):712-5
Tiuliandin A, Vlasova-Leshtaeva TF: Muzhestvo i miloserdie meditsinskikh sester. **Med Sestra** 1980 May;39(5):55-60
Tiurin EI, Kovachev VI: Kafedre rentgenologii i radiologii voenno-meditsinskoĭ akademii im. S. M. Kirova. **Vestn Rentgenol Radiol** 1981 Mar-Apr;(2):87-9
Torzhestvo leninskikh ideĭ: **Voen Med Zh** 1980 Apr;(4):3-12
Trubnikov VF: K 60-letiiu osnovanii kafedry ortopedii, travmatologii i voenno-polevoi khirurgii Khar'kovskogo meditsinskogo instituta. **Ortop Travmatol Protez** 1981 Sep;(9):68-70
Tsvang RL: Sovetskaia meditsina v gody Velikoĭ Otechestvennoĭ voĭny. **Feldsher Akush** 1984 May;49(5):3-7
Varlamov VM, Selivanov EF: Voenno-meditsinskomu muzeiu Ministerstva oborony SSSR - 40 let. **Voen Med Zh** 1982 Nov;(11):77-80
Veselkin PN: K 100-letiiu kafedry patologicheskoĭ fiziologii ordena Lenina Krasnoznamennoĭ voenno-meditsinskoĭ akademii im. S. M. Kirova. **Patol Fiziol Eksp Ter** 1980;(4):3-11
Veselov EI, Belevitin AB: A. V. Eliseev--vrach, puteshestvennik, uchenyĭ (k 125-letiiu so dnia rozhdeniia). **Voen Med Zh** 1984 Sep;(9):68-9
Veterany Velikoĭ Otechestvennoĭ voĭny za 'kruglym stolom' redaktsii 'Voenno-medistinskogo zhurnala': **Voen Med Zh** 1980 May;(5):14-20
Vklad sovetskikh voennykh medikov v pobedu nad militaristskoĭ Iaponieĭ.: **Voen Med Zh** 1980 Sep;(9):17-21
Vlasov AA: Ikh trudom slaven kollektiv. **Voen Med Zh** 1982 Mar;(3):7-10
Vodolagin MA: Partiia--organizator pomoshchi ranenym boitsam i komandiram krasnoi armii v gody volikoi otechestvennoi voiny. **Vopr Istor KPSS** 1978;2:64-75
Voĭtenko MF: Organizatsiia meditsinskogo obespecheniia 64-ĭ armii pri vydvizhenii ee iz raĭona Stalingrada v novyĭ raĭon voennykh deĭstviĭ. **Voen Med Zh** 1984 Feb;(2):69-71
Voĭtenko MF: Organizatsiia meditsinskogo obespecheniia 7-ĭ gvardeĭskoĭ armii v Belgorodsko-Kharkovskoĭ nastupatel'noĭ operatsii (K 40-letiiu bitvy pod Kurskom). **Voen Med Zh** 1983 Aug;8:16-20
Voĭtenko MF, Zil'berberg LB: Organizatsiia raboty DMP pri massovom postuplenii ranenykh v period Velikoĭ Otechestvennoĭ voiny. **Voen Med Zh** 1983 Nov;(11):15-8
Volkov VV, Shiliaev VG: Voennaia Oftal'mologiia v period Velikoĭ Otechestvennoĭ Voĭny. **Voen Med Zh** 1980 May;(5):50-3
Voronkov OV: Iz istorii sozdaniia zapasov meditsinskogo imushchestva dlia obespecheniia voĭsk vo vremia voĭny (soobshchenie vtoroe). **Voen Med Zh** 1984 Oct;(10):66-8
Voronkov OV: Obespechenie meditsinskim imushchestvom voĭsk voennogo okruga vo vremia Velikoĭ Otechestvennoĭ voĭny. **Voen Med Zh** 1980 Oct;(10):19-22
Voronkov OV: Remont meditsinskogo imushchestva vo vremia Velikoĭ Otechestvennoĭ voĭny. **Voen Med Zh** 1982 May;(5):73-5
Vozchikov-Chernov SP: V polevom podvizhnom gospitale. **Voen Med Zh** 1981 Nov;(11):70
Zhukova LA: Periodicheskaia pechat' o geroizme sovetskikh medikov v gody Velikoĭ Otechestvennoĭ voĭny. **Voen Med Zh** 1984 Oct;(10):10-2

**Venezuela**

Fernández DW: Manuel Pantoja. **Bol Acad Nac Hist (Caracas)** 1982;65(259):685–8

Jahn F: Los cirujanos del ejercito libertador en la batalla de Carabobo. **Bol Acad Nac Hist (Caracas)** 1972;55(217):134–40

**Vietnam**

Nguyen TK, Smirnov VS, Mozzhakov VI: Tsentral'nomu voennomu gospitaliu v'etnamskoĭ Narodnoĭ armii 30 let. **Voen Med Zh** 1981 Nov;(11):61–2

**Yugoslavia**

Birtašević B: Razvoj naše vojne preventivne medicine. **Vojnosanit Pregl** 1981 Sep–Oct;38(5):308–13

Božović B: Osvrt na nedostatke u dosadašnjem radu našeg vojnog saniteta. **Lijec Vjesn** 1979 Nov;101(11):690–3

Brecilj B: Medicinska doktrina u NOR u Sloveniji. **Vojnosanit Pregl** 1982 Mar–Apr;39(2):121–6

Cetrdeset godina Vojnosanitetskog pregleda: **Vojnosanit Pregl** 1984 Sep–Oct;41(5):315–9

Djordjević SP: Sećanja na rad u vojnom sanitetu Srbije u toku II balkanskog rata 1913. godine. Iz sećanja dr Julija Budisavljevinja i njegovih kolega iz Hirurške klinike u Insbruku. **Srp Arh Celok Lek** 1983 Jun;111(6):853–9

Djurić L: Vojno–teritorijalna sanitetska služba na baniji u toku nor–a. **Vojnois Glas** 1971;22(3):191–206

Dragić D: Drug tito i njegov doprinos razvoju vojnomedicinske misli. **Vojnosanit Pregl** 1980 May;37:54–7

Dragić D: Hronologija znaćajnijih dogadaja za sanitetsku službu u toku NOR–a 1941–1945. **Vojnosanit Pregl** 1981 Nov–Dec;38(6):423–8

Dragić D, Anić N: Nastanak i razvoj sanitetskih jedinca sa hronologijom dogadjaja iz sanitetske službe u narodnooslobodilačkom ratu. **Vojnois Glas** 1981;32(1):181–94

Dragić D: Sanitetska služba u Bosni i Hercegovini u vreme održavanja Prvog kongresa partizanskih lekara. **Vojnosanit Pregl** 1983 Sep–Oct;40(5):386–94

Finderle V: Mobilne kirurške ekipe. **Lijec Vjesn** 1979 Nov;101(11):706

Georgievski M: Zdravstveni radnici--narodni heroji. **Lijec Vjesn** 1983 Feb–Mar;105(2–3):99–104

Harding PM: A Red Cross nurse in Belgrade: Mary Gladwin saw World War I from the inside of a hospital. Her battles were no easier than those of the soldiers. **Am Hist Illus** 1982;17(1):41–7

Jovanovič J: Izvještaj ruskih ljekara o crnogorskim ranjenicima i borbama crnogoraca s turcima 1876. godine. **Istor Zapisi** 1979;32(3):77–88

Južnič M: Razvoj partizanskog saniteta u Sloveniji u toku nardnooslobodilačkog rata (II). **Vojnosanit Pregl** 1982 Mar–Apr;39(2):127–42

Južnič M: Razvoj partizanskog saniteta u Sloveniji za vreme Narodnooslobodilačkog rata. **Vojnosanit Pregl** 1981 Nov–Dec;38(6):412–22

Katan E: Napori za ublažavanje oskudice i očuvanje sanitetskih sredstava u toku bitaka na Neretvi i Sutjesci. **Vojnosanit Pregl** 1984 Jan–Feb;41(1):49–53

Katan E: Sanitetsko snabdevanje Centralne bolnice Vrhovnog štaba i jedinica Glavne operativne grupe za vreme četvrte i pete ofanzive. **Vojnosanit Pregl** 1980 Nov–Dec;37(6):476–80

Katan E: Stručne publikacije sanitetske službe NOVJ izdavane pre Vojnosanitetskog pregleda. **Vojnosanit Pregl** 1984 Sep–Oct;41(5):424–30

Katan E: Ustanove za zbrinjavanje ranjenika NOVJ na području Beograda od 15. oktobra do kraja decembra 1944. godine. **Vojnosanit Pregl** 1980 Mar–Apr;37(2):121–5

Kovačević M: Izrada i proizvodnja lekova u apotekarskoj službi NOVJ (JA). **Vojnosanit Pregl** 1981 Nov–Dec;38(6):404–11

Kralj I: O dostignućima sanitetske službe u NOB na teritoriji Hrvatske do jeseni 1942. godine. **Vojnosanit Pregl** 1983 Sep–Oct;40(5):379–85

Kralj I: Zdravstvo u NOB uoči prvog kongresa liječnika NOF Hrvatske. **Lijec Vjesn** 1979 Nov;101(11):656–62

Kučišec A: Neki aspekti stanja i razvoja kirurgije i kirurške službe u NOB–i Hrvatske od 1941. do 1944. godine. **Lijec Vjesn** 1979 Nov;101(11):669–73

Kulenović H: Cetrdeset godina razvoja sanitetske službe JNA. **Vojnosanit Pregl** 1981 Nov–Dec;38(6):387–98

Kulenović H: Titov doprinos stvaranju i razvoju sanitetske službe--i stalna briga za ljude. **Vojnosanit Pregl** 1980 May;37:46–53

Mićić R: General prof. dr Milan Arsenijević (24. III 1901 – 10. XI 1981). **Srp Arh Celok Lek** 1982 Sep;110(9):1109–13

Milošević P: Organizacija i razvoj partizanske zdravstvene službe u crnoj gori 1941–1942. godine. **Istor Zapisi** 1969;22(4):521–52

Papo I: Izvještaj o četveromjesečnom radu ekipe SOVS–a. **Lijec Vjesn** 1979 Nov;101(11):707–8

Perin J: Depedikulacija u uslovima partizanskog rata. **Lijec Vjesn** 1979 Nov;101(11):716–7

Perin J: Medicinsko–preventivni aspekti zdravstvene službe u narodnooslobodilačkom ratu. **Lijec Vjesn** 1979 Nov;101(11):663–8

Prvi kongres liljećnika Narodnooslobodilačke Fronte Hrvatske: Glina--Topusko--Slunj, 24--27. Veljače 1944. **Lijec Vjesn** 1979 Nov;101(11):686–90

Radović M, Taseski J: Služba za transfuziju krvi i ratovi. **Vojnosanit Pregl** 1979 Sep–Oct;36(5):359–64

Rasuhin J: Epidemiologija i profilaksa zaraznih bolesti u partizanskim prilikama. **Lijec Vjesn** 1979 Nov;101(11):714–6

Sustić V: Naša ratna zdravstvena služba i njezino značenje za zadatke u općenarodnoj obraini. (O nekim pitanjima iz kompenzacije sanitetskih kadrova i korištenja improvizacijama). **Lijec Vjesn** 1979 Nov;101(11):679–81

Vukas A: Organizacija borbe protiv kožnih i spolnih bolesti i dosadašnji nedostaci u tom pogledu. **Lijec Vjesn** 1979 Nov;101(11):718–9

Zarković G: Historijsko značenje prvog kongresa liječnika partizana NOF Hrvatske. **Lijec Vjesn** 1979 Nov;101(11):654–5

Zimolo A: Kongelacije s naročitim osvrtom na preventivne mjere. **Lijec Vjesn** 1979 Nov;101(11):710–3

Zimolo A: Rad i značenje prvog kongresa liječnika Narodnooslobodilačke Fronte Hrvatske 24–27. 2. 1944. **Lijec Vjesn** 1979 Nov;101(11):674–8

# MOLECULAR BIOLOGY

See also **Biology; Cytology; Microbiology**

Bearman D, Edsall JT, ed: Archival sources for the history of biochemistry and molecular biology. A reference guide and report. Boston, American Academy of Arts and Sciences, Philadelphia, American Philosophical Society, 1980. 338 p. plus microfiche. Contributions by M. Miller, M. Konopka

**1700 to Present**

Abir–Am P: Beyond deterministic sociology and apologetic history: reassessing the impact of research policy upon new scientific disciplines (Reply to Fuerst, Bartels, Olby and Yoxen). **Soc Stud Sci** 1984 May;14(2):252–63

Abir–Am P: From biochemistry to molecular biology: DNA and the acculturated journey of the critic of science Erwin Chargaff. **Hist Philos Life Sci** 1980;2(1):3–60

American Academy of Arts and Sciences, American Philosophical Society: Survey of sources for the history of biochemistry and molecular biology. **Surv Sources Newsl** 1975–1981;1(1–10):various pagings

Bartels D: The Rockefeller Foundation's funding policy for molecular biology: success or failure? **Soc Stud Sci** 1984 May;14(2):238–43

Day M, Burton N: Plasmids. **Endeavour** 1982;6(3):108–13

Edsall JT: Essay review; Horace Judson and the molecular biologists. **J Hist Biol** 1980 Spring;13(1):141–58

Fasquelle R, Delaunay A: Geschichte der Mikrobiologie. In Sournia JC, Martiny M, Poulet J, ed: Illustrierte Geschichte der Medizin. Salzburg, Andreas, 1980. Vol. 7. p. 2459–97.

Fuerst JA: The definition of molecular biology and the definition of policy: the role of the Rockefeller Foundation's policy for molecular biology. **Soc Stud Sci** 1984 May;14(2):225–37

Judson HF: Reflections on the historiography of molecular biology. **Minerva** 1980 Autumn;18(3):369–421

Judson HF: The eighth day of creation. New York, Simon and Schuster, 1979. 686 p.

Kendrew G: Some remarks on the history of molecular biology. **Istor Biol Issled** 1983;9:127–34

Kimbrough SO: On the reduction of genetics to molecular biology. **Philos Sci** 1979;46:389–406

Marbach JU: Wilhelm Bernhard, 1920–1978. **Gesnerus** 1979;36(3–4):303–11

Morange M: Schrödinger et la biologie moléculaire. **Fundam Sci** 1983;4(3/4):219–33

Nathans D: The new genetics. **Trans Am Clin Climatol Assoc** 1979;91:75–97

Olby R: The sheriff and the cowboys: or Weaver's support of Astbury and Pauling. **Soc Stud Sci** 1984 May;14(2):244–7

Olby RC: The history of molecular biology. **Hist Philos Life Sci** 1980;2(2):299–310

Olby RC: The significance of the macromolecules in the historiography of molecular biology. **Hist Philos Life Sci** 1979;1(2):185–98

Ota J: [History of biology and the current status of molecular biology] (Jpn). **Kango Gijutsu** 1981 Apr;27(6):700–7

Portugal FH, Cohen JS: A century of DNA: a history of the discovery of the structure and function of the genetic substance. Cambridge, MIT Press, 1977. xiii, 384 p.

Potter VR: Physiological adaptation at the molecular level: the frontier where research on differentiation and malignancy meet. **Perspect Biol Med** 1981 Summer;24(4):525–42

Saget H: L'essor de la biologie moléculaire (1950–1965). Paris, Centre de Documentation Sciences Humaines, CNRS, xi, 1978. 43 p.

Shdanov VM: Molekularbiologie und Okologie der Virusgrippe. **Z Erkr Atmungsorgane** 1983;161(1):74–9

Sibatani A: Two faces of molecular biology: revolution and normal science. **Riv Biol** 1981 Autumn;74(3):279–96

Stent GS: Max Delbrück, 1906–1981. **Genetics** 1982 May;101(1):1–16

Stent GS: To the Stockholm station: makers of the molecular–biological revolution. **Encounter (London)** 1980;54(3):79–85

# MOLECULAR BIOLOGY

Taylor DM: Blutzellmarkierung: Rückblick und Ausblick. **Wien Klin Wochenschr** 1984 Feb 3;96(3):89-92
Thirty years of DNA--and after: **Nature** 1983 Apr 14;302(5909):557-8
Vigue CL, Stanziale WG: Recombinant DNA: history of the controversy. **Am Biol Teach** 1979;41:480-3, 491
Wiewiórkowski M: Chemia a biologia. **Nauka Pol** 1979;27(11):64-74
Yoxen EJ: Scepticism about the centrality of technology transfer in the Rockefeller Foundation programme in molecular biology. **Soc Stud Sci** 1984 May;14(2):248-52

**Belgium**

Brachet J: Esquisse d'une histoire de la biochimie de la biologie cellulaire et de la biologie moléculaire en Belgique. In Florilège des Sciences en Belgique - II. Bruxelles, Académie Royale de Belgique, 1980. p. 289-314.

**Great Britain**

Cornforth J: Portrait of Dorothy Hodgkin, O.M., F.R.S. **Notes Rec R Soc Lond** 1982 Aug;37(1):1-4
Dodson G, Glusker JP, Sayre D, ed: Structural studies on molecules of biological interest. A volume in honour of Professor Dorothy Hodgkin. Oxford, Clarendon, 1981. xviii, 610 p. Historical and biographical chapters by M. F. Perutz, D. Phillips, D. P. Riley, F. Welch, C. H. Carlisle, L. Pauling, T. You-chi, J. H. Robertson, D. F. Steiner, J. G. White, J. D. Dunitz.
Edsall JT: The papers of W.T. Astbury and J.D. Bernal. **Surv Sources Newsl** 1981 Apr;10:2-6
Preston RD: William Thomas Astbury. In Dictionary of national biography, 1961-1970. Suppl. 8, 1981. p. 41-2.

**Poland**

Ostrowski W: Biologia molekularna: rozwój i zadania w nauce polskiej. **Nauka Pol** 1976;24(3):3-13
Szafrański P, Zagórski W, Filipowicz W: Studies on protein biosynthesis at the Institute of Biochemistry and Biophysics, Polish Academy of Sciences, initiated by Professor J. Heller in 1956. **Acta Biochim Pol** 1984;31(1):9-16

**Sweden**

Klein G, Klein E: Torbjörn Caspersson: some personal perspectives. **Cytometry** 1984 Jul;5(4):318
Mayall BH: Torbjörn Oskar Caspersson: curriculum vitae and selected publications. **Cytometry** 1984 Jul;5(4):314-7

**United States**

Abir-Am P: The discourse of physical power and biological knowledge in the 1930s: a reappraisal of the Rockefeller Foundation's 'policy' in molecular biology. **Soc Stud Sci** 1982 Aug 3;12(3):341-82
Bearman D: A. L. Patterson papers. **Surv Sources Newsl** 1981 Apr;10:9-11
Jardetzky O, Wade-Jardetzky NG: Nuclear magnetic resonance as a structural method in molecular biology. **Rice Univ Stud** 1980;66(3):57-79
Lear J: Recombinant DNA: the untold story. New York, Crown, 1978. 280 p.
McDermott W: Colin Munro MacLeod: January 28, 1909-February 11, 1972. **Biogr Mem Natl Acad Sci** 1983;54:183-219
Pnina Abir-Am: The I. Fankuchen papers: their relevance to the historian of molecular biology. **Surv Sources Newsl** 1981 Apr;10:6-9

# MORTUARY PRACTICE

See also **Death**

Ascenzi A, Cockburn A, Kleiss E: Miscellaneous mummies. In A. Cockburn, E. Cockburn, ed: Mummies, disease, and ancient cultures. Cambridge, Cambridge University Press, 1980. p. 224-38.
Cockburn A, Cockburn E, ed: Mummies, disease, and ancient cultures. Cambridge, Cambridge University Press, 1980. x, 340 p.
Croix A: L'homme et son corps dans l'Au-delà. In Imhof AE, ed: Leib und Leben in der Geschichte der Neuzeit. Berlin, Duncker & Humblot, 1983. p. 155-62.
Huntington R, Metcalf P: Celebrations of death: the anthropology of mortuary ritual. Cambridge, New York, Cambridge University Press, 1979. xv, 230 p.
Martinetto P, Riggi G, Valtz A, et al: Microbiological research on specimens (dusts) drawn from the Holy Shroud. **G Batteriol Virol Immunol** 1981 Jul-Dec;74(7-12):202-8
Paleopathology Association: Ninth annual meeting and first Aidan Cockburn memorial symposium: Mummies, disease, and ancient cultures: retrospect and prospect. Toledo, Paleopathology Association, 1982. 16 p.
Roth N: Life-and-death decisions: electrodiagnosis and premature burial. **Med Instrum** 1980 Nov-Dec;14(6):322

**Australia**

Pretty GL, Calder A: Mummification in Australia and Melanesia. In A. Cockburn, E. Cockburn, ed: Mummies, disease, and ancient cultures. Cambridge, Cambridge University Press, 1980. p. 194-210.

**France**

Thibaut-Payen J: Les morts, l'Eglise et l'Etat: recherches d'histoire administrative sur la sépulture et les cimetières dans le ressort du parlement de Paris aux XVIIe et XVIIIe siècles. Paris, Lanore, 1977. (Also Thèse, Paris, 1974). 465 p.

**Great Britain**

Dawes JD, Magilton JR: The cemetery of St Helen-on-the-Walls, Aldwark. London, Council for British Archaeology (for the York Archaeological Trust), 1980. 120 p. (The Archaeology of York. Volume 12: The Medieval Cemeteries).

**Japan**

Sakurai K, Ogata T: Japanese mummies. In A. Cockburn, E. Cockburn, ed: Mummies, disease, and ancient cultures. Cambridge, Cambridge University Press, 1980. p. 211-23.

**Peru**

Riddle JM, Vreeland JM: Identification of insects associated with Peruvian mummy bundles by using scanning electron microscopy. **Paleopathol Newsl** 1982 Sep;39:5-9
Vreeland JM, Cockburn A: Mummies of Peru. In A. Cockburn, E. Cockburn, ed: Mummies, disease, and ancient cultures. Cambridge, Cambridge University Press, 1980. p. 135-74.

**Spain**

López de Guereñu G: Muerte, entierro y funerales in algunos lugares de Alava. **Bol Inst Sancho Sabio** 1978;22:189-242

**United States**

Frayer DW, Bradley LE: A late woodland burial from Platte County, Missouri. **Plains Anthropol** 1979;24(83):21-27
Frisbie CJ: Burial as a disposition mechanism for Navajo jish or medicine bundles. **Am Indian Q** 1978;4(4):347-66
El-Najjar MY, Mulinski TM: Mummies and mummification practices in the southwestern and southern United States. In A. Cockburn, E. Cockburn, ed: Mummies, disease, and ancient cultures. Cambridge, Cambridge University Press, 1980. p. 103-17.
Owsley DW, Bennett SM, Jantz RL: Intercemetery morphological variation in Arikara crania from the Mobridge Site (39WW1). **Am J Phys Anthropol** 1982 Jun;58(2):179-85
Shepardson M: Changes in Navajo mortuary practices and beliefs. **Am Indian Q** 1978;4(4):383-96
Stewart KM: Mortuary practices of the Mojave Indians. **Palacio** 1973;79(4):2-12
Ubelaker DH, Jantz RL: Plains Caddoan relationships: the view from craniometry and mortuary analysis. **Nebr Hist** 1979;60(2):249-59

**USSR**

Kvitnitskiĭ-Ryzhov IuN: Kievskie nekropoli v istoriko-meditsinskom aspekte (k 1500-letiiu Kieva). **Sov Zdravookhr** 1982;(9):65-8

**Zaire**

Kimpianga KM: The religious therapeutic functions of the cemetery for the Kongo of Zaire. **Cah Relig Afr** 1978;12:107-24

**Before 500 A.D.**

Bryce TR: Burial practices in Lycia. **Mankind Q** 1980 Winter;21(2):165-78

**Egypt**

Cockburn A, Peck WH, Barraco RA, et al: A classic mummy: PUM II. In A. Cockburn, E. Cockburn, ed: Mummies, disease, and ancient cultures. Cambridge, Cambridge University Press, 1980. p. 52-70.
Jarcho S: Some historical problems connected with the study of Egyptian mummies. **Bull Inst Egypte (Cairo)** 1981;:58-9, 106-22
Millet NB, Hart GD, Reyman TA, et al: ROM I: mummification for the common people. In A. Cockburn, E. Cockburn, ed: Mummies, disease, and ancient cultures. Cambridge, Cambridge University Press, 1980. p. 71-84.
Peck WH: Mummies of ancient Egypt. In A. Cockburn, E. Cockburn, ed: Mummies, disease, and ancient cultures. Cambridge, Cambridge

University Press, 1980. p. 11–28.
Reyman TA, Peck WH: Egyptian mummification with evisceration per ano. In A. Cockburn, E. Cockburn, ed: Mummies, disease, and ancient cultures. Cambridge, Cambridge University Press, 1980. p. 85–100.
Vahey T, Brown D: Comely Wenuhotep: computed tomography of an Egyptian mummy. **J Comput Assist Tomogr** 1984 Oct;8(5):992–7
Verbov JL: Mummified skin--an exercise in preservation. **Int J Dermatol** 1983 Jan–Feb;22(1):46–60

**Greco–Roman**

Hassel FJ, Künzl E: Ein römisches Arztgrab des 3. Jahrhunderts n. Chr. aus Kleinasien. **Medizinhist J** 1980;15(4):403–21

**500 A.D.–1450**

**Mexico**

Angot J: Un crâne à face décorée de la civilisation mixtèque. **Hist Sci Med** 1984;18(3):255–9

**1450–1700**

**Chile**

Horne PD: The prince of El Plomo. **Paleopathol Newsl** 1982 Dec;40:7–10

**Great Britain**

Lawless DS: On Shakespeare's death, funeral, and burial. **Notes Queries** 1980 Apr;27(2):176–7

**Italy**

Fornaciari G: The mummies of the Abbey of Saint Domenico Maggiore in Naples. **Paleopathol Newsl** 1984 Sep;(47):10–4

**Peru**

Ravines R: Reconocimiento arqueologico en el rio corientes, nororiente del Peru. **Rev Mus Nac** 1978–80;44:111–38

**1700 to Present**

Urbain JD: Les cimetières d'occident: des sociétés de conservation. **Etudes (Fr)** 1982;357(2–3):193–204

**Belgium**

Jurion F, Parisel F: Le troisième et dernier cimetière de l'hôpital Saint-Jean de Bruxelles (1704–1784). Etude paléopathologique des ossements du cimetière Saint-Jean. **Ann Soc Belg Hist Hop** 1982;20:2–60

**Germany**

Spann W: Die Leichenschau bei Feuerbestattung. **Dtsch Med Wochenschr** 1980 Oct 3;105(40):1376–7
Staiger U: Die Auseinandersetzung um die Feuerbestattung in Deutschland im 19. Jahrhundert. Diss. Mainz, 1981. 72 p.

**Great Britain**

Edwards IG: Down memory lane: burial at sea. **Nurs Mirror** 1980 Jul 3;150(21):36–7

**Hungary**

Szerbák E: Halál, temetés és búcsúztatás a XIX. század eleji Magyarországon. **Orvostort Kozl** 1980;89–91(26 no 1–3):175–90

**Netherlands**

Groos KS: Enkele opmerkingen met betrekking tot het graf van Herman Boerhaave in de Pieterskerk te Leiden. **Tijdschr Geschied Geneeskd** 1979;2(4):176–81

**United States**

Barrick ME: Cumberland county death lore. **Pa Folklife** 1979;28(4):37–46
Eckert WG: History of the U.S. Army Graves Registration Service (1917–1950s). **Am J Forensic Med Pathol** 1983 Sep;4(3):231–43
Farrell JJ: The dying of death: the meaning and management of death in America, 1830–1920. Ph.D. diss. University of Illinois, Urbana, Ill., 1980. 329 p.
Jordan TG: 'The roses so red and the lilies so fair': southern folk cemeteries in Texas. **Southwest Hist Q** 1980;83(3):227–58
Lancaster RK: Green Mount: the introduction of the rural cemetry into Baltimore. **Md Hist Mag** 1979;74(1):62–79
Ray DJ: Mortuary art of the Alaskan Eskimos. **Am Indian Art Mag** 1982;7(2):50–7
Salem J: Coon dog graveyard. **South Exposure** 1979;7(3):27–9

## MUSCULOSKELETAL SYSTEM

Etessami S: La contraction musculaire: de l'antiquité jusqu'à nos jours. In: Congrès international d'histoire de la médecine, XXVe, Québec, 1976. Actes. Québec, 1977. p. 644–9.
Finlay IM: Craniometry and cephalometry: a history prior to the advent of radiography. **Angle Orthod** 1980 Oct;50(4):312–21
Skorecki J: What have we learned about walking in twenty four centuries? **Manch Lit Phil Soc Mem Proc** 1977–80;120:56–71

**Ghana**

Macadam PS: A small skeletal sample from northern Ghana. **Paleopathol Newsl** 1981 Jan;33:5–7

**United States**

Gregg JB, Steele JP: Mastoid development in ancient and modern populations. A longitudinal radiological study. **JAMA** 1982 Jul 23;248(4):459–64
Jantz RL, Owsley DW: Temporal changes in limb proportionality among skeletal samples of Arikara Indians. **Ann Hum Biol** 1984 Mar–Apr;11(2):157–63

**Before 500 A.D.**

Rodnan GP, Benedek TG: Synovial fluid in antiquity. **Ann Rheum Dis** 1981 Feb;40(1):103

**Sudan**

Martin DL, Armelagos GJ: Morphometrics of compact bone: an example from Sudanese Nubia. **Am J Phys Anthropol** 1979 Nov;51(4):571–7

**500 A.D.–1450**

**France**

Wackenheim A, Dietemann J, Babin E, et al: Hémi-occipitalisation de l'atlas chez un Mérovingien du bas Moyen Age. **J Radiol** 1981 Oct;62(10):545–7

**Iran**

Usmanova RA: Ibn Sina o Kostnoĭ i myshechnoĭ sisteme. **Arkh Anat Gistol Embriol** 1980 Sep;79(9):112–4

**Peru**

Sawyer DR, Allison MJ, Pezzia A: Elongated styloid process in a pre-Columbian Peruvian. **J Dent Res** 1980 Jan;59(1):79

**1450–1700**

Sabin JA, Sanmartín Urchaga P: Estudio comparado de las aportaciones iconográficas, en el sistema muscular, en las obras de Leonardo y Vesalio. In International Congress of the History of Medicine, 27th, Barcelona, 1980. Actas. Barcelona, Académia de Ciències Médiques de Catalunya i Balears, 1981. p. 446–53.

**Netherlands**

Gysel C: Jan Swammerdam (1637- 1680- 1980), zijn Cartesianisme en de fysiologie van het kauwstelsel (SLOT). **Ned Tijdschr Tandheelkd** 1981 Nov;88(11):414–6

**Sweden**

Sourander P: Drottning Christina och Giovanni Alfonso Borelli till 300-årsminnet av kinesiologins födelse. **Nord Medicinhist Arsb** 1982;:56–65

**1700 to Present**

Armelagos GJ, Carlson DS, Van Gerven DP: The theoretical foundations and development of skeletal biology. In F. Spencer, ed: A history of American physical anthropology, 1930–1980. New York, Academic Press, 1982. p. 305–28.
Banga I: Az izomkutatás eredményei. **Orv Hetil** 1983 Oct 2;124(40):2440–3
Delaporte F: Theories of osteogenesis in the eighteenth century. **J Hist Biol** 1983 Fall;16(3):343–60
Gould SJ: The mismeasure of man. New York, London, W.W., Norton

& Co., 1981. 352 p.
Matthews PB: Evolving views on the internal operation and functional role of the muscle spindle. **J Physiol (Lond)** 1981 Nov;320:1–30
Mommaerts WF: Gondolatok az izomkutatás történetéröl (A. Katschalsky-Katzir professzor emlékezetére). **Orv Hetil** 1983 Oct 2;124(40):2436–40

**United States**

Lovejoy CO, Mensforth RP, Armelagos GJ: Five decades of skeletal biology as reflected in the American Journal of Physical Anthropology. In F. Spencer, ed: A history of American physical anthropology, 1930–1980. New York, Academic Press, 1982. p. 329–36.
Nicolai JP: Earliest free muscle graft? **Br J Plast Surg** 1980 Jul;33(3):350–2
Stewart TD: Responses of the human skeleton to changes in the quality of life. **J Forensic Sci** 1980 Oct;25(4):912–21

# MUSEUMS

See also **Exhibits**

**France**

Huard PO, Imbault-Huart MJ: Le cabinet de l'Académie Royale de Chirurgie. In: Congrès National des Sociétés Savantes, 102e, Limoges, 1977. Comptes Rendus. Paris, 1977. Section des Sciences, Fasc. III. p. 15–20.
Laissus Y: Les voyageurs naturalistes du Jardin du roi et du Muséum d'histoire naturelle: essai de portrait-robot. **Rev Hist Sci (Paris)** 1981 Jul–Oct;34(3–4):259–317

**Germany**

Die Alte Kunst des Apothekers: Wiederentdeckt bei einem Besuch im Deutschen Apotheken-Museum in Heidelberg. Mannheim, Boehringer Mannheim, 1980. 39 p.
Fetzer W: Pharmazie: Historisches aus Museen und Sammlungen der DDR. Leipzig, VEB Deutscher Verlag für Grundstoffindustrie, 1983. 279 p.

**Great Britain**

Bracegirdle B: Displaying the history of medicine: the Wellcome Museum in the Science Museum. **J Audiov Media Med** 1982 Oct;5(4):124–9

**Hungary**

Kelly C, Lage O da: Semmelweis Museum: a reminder of Hungary's 'mothers' saviour'. **Can Med Assoc J** 1983 Jun 15;128(12):1481–2

**Italy**

Aulizio F: Come si estraevano i denti un tempo. Lo strumentario dentistico della Fondazione Putti ... Bologna. **Strenna Stor Bolognese** 1979;29:29–41
Berzi A, Cipriani C, Poggesi M: Florentine scientific museums. **J Soc Bibliogr Nat Hist** 1980 Apr;9(4):413–25

**Poland**

Kania I: Médecine tibétaine dans les collections du Musée Ethnographique de Cracovie. In: Proceedings of the Csoma de Körös Memorial Symposium....Matrafüred ... 1976. Budapest: Akad. Kiadó. 1978. pp. 153–160.

**USSR**

Murav'eva EF: Meditsinskie temy v ékspozitsii Gosudarstvennogo Ermitazha. **Sov Zdravookhr** 1984;(9):62–5
Shengeliia MS: Izuchenie istorii meditsiny v soiuznykh respublikakh. **Sov Zdravookhr** 1982;(7):53–5

**Before 500 A.D.**

**United States**

Bliquez LJ: Roman surgical instruments in the Johns Hopkins University Institute of the History of Medicine. **Bull Hist Med** 1982 Summer;56(2):195–217

**1450–1700**

**Czechoslovakia**

Spunarová T: Nejstarší katalogy sbírek ve fondech knihovny Narodního Muzea. **Sb Nar Muzea Praze Rada C Lit Hist** 1980;25(1–2):29–40

**Netherlands**

Lindeboom GA, ed: Het cabinet van Jan Swammerdam (1637–1680). Facsimile reprinted from 1681 ed., Amsterdam, Rodopi, 1980. xxiv, 16 p.

**1700 to Present**

Geppert W, Hartmann E, Hennis I, et al: Die Entwicklung dentaler Technologien, dargestellt am Bestand einer historischen Sammlung. (II). **Quintessenz Zahntech** 1982 Nov;8(11):1261–70
Giustini PA: Museografia e storia del pensiero scientifico. **Med Secoli** 1982;19(3):265–71
Hamarneh SK, Stieb EW: Pharmacy museums and historical collections on public view in the United States and Canada. Madison, American Institute of the History of Pharmacy in cooperation with the National Museum of American History. Washington, D.C., Smithsonian, 1981. 144 p. (Publication/American Institute of the History of Pharmacy, new series, no. 6).
Hilloowala R: Illustrations from the Wellcome Institute Library: the origin of the Wellcome anatomical waxes Albinus and the Florentine collection at La Specola. **Med Hist** 1984 Oct;28(4):432–7
Koning DA: Grosse Funde in kleinen Museen. Einige Neuentdeckungen auf dem Gebiet der Apotheken-Fayencen. In Dilg P, et al., ed: Perspektiven der Pharmaziegeschichte. Graz, Austria, Akademische Druck- u. Verlagsanstalt, 1983. p. 431–39.
Lindskog BI: Europeisk musei-konferens. **Sydsven Medicinhist Sallsk Arsskr** 1984;21:11–4
Megvinov LS: Izgotovlenie anatomicheskikh muzeĭnykh preparatov s sokhraneniem ikh tsveta i konsistentsii. **Arkh Patol** 1981;43(8):71–2

**Americas**

Turtle A: Collections of early psychological laboratory apparatus in North America. **Newsl Australas Assoc Hist Philos Sci** 1977–78;9:4–5

**Austria**

Heilmittel aus Pflanzen und Tieren: Ausstellung des Oberösterreichischen Landesmuseums im Schlossmuseum zu Linz vom 9. 5. bis 3. 8. 1980. Linz, Landesmuseum, 1980. 359 p. (Katalog des Oberösterr. Landesmuseums, 105). Contributions by W. Kubelka, R. Schmidt, F. Speta, H. Heltmann, B. Kopp, B. Gruber, E. Speta, R. Steinwendtner. K. Rumpler, A. Kump, F. Grims, B. Heinzl.
Portele KA: Die Henning-Moulagen des Pathologisch-anatomischen Bundesmuseums in Wien. **Med Lab (Stuttg)** 1979 Feb;32(2):41–3
Portele KA: Die Moulagensammlung des Pathologisch-Anatomischen Bundesmuseums in Wien. [Wien, Pathologisch-Anatomisches Bundesmuseum in Wien], 1977. 84 p.

**Canada**

Duchesne R: Magasin de curiosités ou musée scientifique? Le musée d'histoire naturelle de Pierre Chasseur à Québec (1824–1854). **HSTC** 1983 May;24(7 No 2):59–79
Rodin AE: Oslerian pathology: an assessment and annotated atlas of museum specimens. Lawrence, Kansas, Coronado, 1981. xviii, 250 p.

**Czechoslovakia**

Rusek V: Historie farmacie na farmaceutické fakultě University Karlovy. **Cas Lek Cesk** 1981 Jan 30;120(3–4):100–3

**Denmark**

Baerentsen K: Gamle Apoteker Krukker. Kobenhavn, Danmarks Apotekerforening, 1980. 65 p.

**Finland**

Aberg S: Tämäkin on yhteinen asiamme. **Katilolehti** 1982 May;87(5):172–3
Ylppö A: Ensimmäinen Gunnar Soininen -luento. **Katilolehti** 1983 Mar;88(3):112–4

**France**

Antoine JP: 'Les horreurs' anatomiques de Florence. **Histoire** 1980;26:96–8
Chambonnet F: Les faiences pharmaceutiques conservées dans les établissements hospitaliers de la région lyonnaise. Le Puy-en-Velay, [s.n.], 1978. 213 p. (Thèse, Lyon).
Delaveau P, Paris RR, Clair G: The Museum of Materia Medica of Paris. **Pharm Hist** 1984;26(3):143–5
Garnot NS, Simon N: Parigi degli ospedali. **Kos** 1984 May;1(4):95–114
Limoges C: The development of the Muséum d'Histoire Naturelle of Paris, c. 1800–1914. In R. Fox, G. Weisz, ed: The organization of science and technology in France 1808–1914. Cambridge, Cambridge University Press, 1980. p. 211–40.

Maire M: L'or du temps. Le musée de la chirurgie dentaire de la faculté d'odontologie de Lyon. **Chir Dent Fr** 1979 May 31;49(22):25–30
Musée de la Pharmacie: Exposition: Montpellier: de l'apothicairerie à la pharmacie. Montpellier, Faculté de Pharmacie, n.d.
Saumande P: Une collection d'instruments scientifiques anciens au Laboratoire de Physique pharmaceutique de la Faculté de Médecine et de Pharmacie de Limoges. **Bull Soc Archeol Hist Limousin** 1981;108:157–8
Solente G: Le Musée de l'Hôpital Saint-Louis. **Am J Dermatopathol** 1983 Oct;5(5):483–9

**Germany**

Alberti H: Die heiligen Kosmas und Damian auf einer Prozessionsfahne im Deutschen Apotheken-Museum. **Dtsch Apoth Ztg** 1979 Jun 14;119(24):948–50 (also in Pharm Ztg 1979 Jun 14;24:1155–7
Engelhardt R, ed: Das römische Aerzte-Instrumentarium. Bingen, Engelhardt, 1974. 47 p. (Binger Annalen, IV) Contributions by C. Palm, K. M. Heidecker, P. Nahm, E. Naujack, A. Engelhardt.
Gerweck U: Die Huf- und Hufeisensammlung des Instituts für Tiermedizin und Tier-hygiene mit Tierklinik der Universität Hohenheim, zugleich ein Rückblick auf die historische Entwicklung des Hufeisens. Diss. Hannover, 1979. 139p.
Gourevitch M: Le musée Adler d'histoire de la médecine à Johannesburg. **Hist Sci Med** 1982;16(1):21–2
Modig M: Deutsches Apotheken-Museum i Heidelberg. **Sydsven Medicinhist Sallsk Arsskr** 1984;21:15–26
Poulet W: Atlas on the history of spectacles. Bonn-Bad Godesberg, Wayenborgh, 1978. xxxv, 396 p. Includes contributions by H. W. Holtmann, H. W. Roth Ulm, W. Pfeiffer.
Querner H: 'Ein Wort über den Einfluss naturwissenschaftlicher Institute auf humane Bildung' (G. A. Goldfuss 1821). In Seidler E, Schott H, ed: Bausteine zur Medizingeschichte. Stuttgart, Steiner, 1984. p. 86–93.
Schneider W: Entwicklung der pharmazeutischen Museologie in Deutschland. **Pharm Ztg** 1980 Jan 10;125(2):68–71
Schuster E: Erbauungsbilder in der Totentanzsammlung (Mensch und Tod) der Universität Düsseldorf. In Göpfert W, Otten HH, ed: Metavoeite: wandelt euch durch neues Denken. Düsseldorf, Triltsch, 1983. p. 41–54.

**Great Britain**

Allan N: The oriental collections in the Wellcome Institute for the History of Medicine, London. **J R Asiat Soc GB Irel** 1981;1:10–25
Allen E, Turk JL: Microscopes in the Hunterian Museum. **Ann R Coll Surg Engl** 1982 Nov;64(6):414–8
Austin F, Jones B: William Home Clift: the first assistant Conservator of the Hunterian Museum. **Ann R Coll Surg Engl** 1980 Jul;62(4):299–303
Bracegirdle B: The Wellcome Museum of the History of Medicine. **J Audiov Media Med** 1980 Apr;3(2):59–63
Brock CH: Dr. Thomas Bond of Philadelphia and his 'Worm'. **Trans Stud Coll Physicians Phila** 1981 Sep;5(3 no 3):209–13
Brock CH: Dr. William Hunter's Museum, Glasgow University. **J Soc Bibliogr Nat Hist** 1980 Apr;9(4):403–12
Cave AJ: A constellation of conservators. **Ann R Coll Surg Engl** 1980 Jan;62(1):66–70
Court WE: The pharmaceutical society's collection of materia medica and herbaria. **Pharm Hist (London)** 1980 Dec;10(3):2–3
Davies J: Cambridge Museum of Technology. **Ind Archaeol** 1980;15(4):335–55
Dopson L: The QA museum. **Nurs Times** 1981 Nov 11–17;77(46):1974
Duggan AJ: A brief history of the Wellcome Museum of Medical Science. **Trans R Soc Trop Med Hyg** 1981;75 Suppl:29–31
Gilson AG: A group of Roman surgical and medical instruments from Cramond, Scotland. **Medizinhist J** 1983;18(4):384–93
Gray C: The remarkable surgical collection of John Hunter. **Can Med Assoc J** 1983 May 15;128(10):1225–8
Gray C: The Wellcome library: reflection of an insatiable collector. **Can Med Assoc J** 1982 Mar 15;126(6):712, 716–20
Lawrence C: Wellcome revisited. **Nurs Times** 1982 Dec 8–14;78(49):2089–90
Le Fanu W: Natural history drawings collected by John Hunter F.R.S. (1728–1793), at the Royal College of Surgeons of England. **J Soc Bibliogr Nat Hist** 1978;8(4):329–33
Nuttall RH: Microscopes from the Frank Collection 1800–1860. Illustrating the development of the achromatic instrument. Jersey, Channel Islands, A. Frank, 1979, 64 p.
A pharmaceutical museum: **Pharm Hist (London)** 1977 Jul;7(2):4–5
Qvist G: John Hunter, 1728–1793. London, Heinemann, 1981. xvi, 216 p.
Salsbury D: Step into the twenties with Jen-Sal's veterinary display. [An early 20th cent. veterinarian's office.] **Found News** 1979 Nov;:12–13
Skinner GM: The Wellcome Museum. **Sydsven Medicinhist Sallsk Arsskr** 1983;:13–22
Tansey V, Mekie DE: Report of the Museum of the Royal College of Surgeons of Edinburgh. **J R Coll Surg Edinb** 1980 Mar;25(2):67–75 contd
Tansey V, Mekie DE: The museum of the Royal College of Surgeons of Edinburgh. **J R Coll Surg Edinb** 1980 Jul;25(4):248–56
Tansey V, Mekie DE: The Museum of the Royal College of Surgeons of Edinburgh. **J R Coll Surg Edinb** 1980 May;25(3):188–93 (continued periodically)
Tansey V, Mekie DE: The Museum of the Royal College of Surgeons of Edinburgh (Part 4). **J R Coll Surg Edinb** 1980 Nov;25(6):481–4
Turner H: Henry Wellcome: the man, his collection and his legacy. London, Heinemann for the Wellcome Trust, 1980. 96 p.
Watts DC: The Wellcome Museum of the History of Medicine. **Biochem Soc Trans** 1982 Jun;10(3):187–8
Winder M: Il Buddha della medicina. **Kos** 1984 Apr;1(3):55–74
Wright D: Moving the Wellcome Collection to the Science Museum. **Vet Hist** 1982 Summer;2(3):100–11

**Hungary**

Kapronczay K: Az állatgyógyászat múltjából Magyarországon (a Semmelweis Orvostörténeti Múzeum új időszakos kiállítása. **Orv Hetil** 1980 Aug 10;121(32):1859–60

**Israel**

Kottek SS: 'Andre Vesale'. Some remarks on a painting by E. J. C. Hamman. **Koroth** 1982 Aug;8(3/4):135–43

**Italy**

Bonilauri F: Museo e città. Le collezioni Spallanzani e chierici a Reggio Emilia. Firenze, Olschki, 1978. 199 p. (Biblioteca della 'Rivista di Storia delle Scienze Mediche e Naturali').
Caffaratto AT: La raccolta di fotografie segnaletiche del Museo di Antropologia Criminale di Torino: la fotografia come documento e testimonianza dell'opera di Cesare Lombroso. **Ann Osp Maria Vittoria Torino** 1980 Jul-Dec;23(7–12):295–332

**Mexico**

Fernández del Castillo F, Castañeda H: El Museo de la Medicina. **Salud Publica Mex** 1982 Sep–Oct;24(5):509–21

**Netherlands**

Apothekerspotten: Apothecary jars. The Hague, Gemeentemuseum, 1979. [59] p.
Haneveld GT: Koning Willem I en de aankoop van anatomische kabinetten. **Spiegel Hist** 1978;13(7–8):488–95
Van der Leun C, ed:: NG 200 – Natuurkundig Gezelschap te Utrecht 1777–1977. Utrecht, Natuurkundig Gezelschap te Utrecht, 1977. 143 p. With contributions by R. Hooykaas, J.G. van Cittert-Eymers, H.A.M. Snelders, N.G. van Kampen, P.H. Kylstra.

**Norway**

Hopstock C: The Norwegian pharmacy museum; a presentation. In: Vorträge des Internationalen Pharmaziehistorischen Kongresses Innsbruck 1977. Stuttgart, Wissenschaftliche Verlagsgesellschaft, 1979. p. 141–5.
Konkoly Thege A: A Bergeni Orvosi Múzeum. **Orv Hetil** 1981 Nov 15;122(46):2858
Norsk Farmasihistorisk Museum. Das Norwegische Pharmaziehistorische Museum (Apothekenmuseum). Le Musée norvégien de la pharmacie. Oslo, Norsk Folkemuseum, 1979, 16 p.:
Svaboe HM: Sykepleiemuseet på Lovisenberg. **Sykepleien** 1983 Apr 21;70(7):12–3
Zirinsky L: The Leprosy Museum of Bergen. **St Mary Hosp Gaz** 1979 Autumn;85:23

**Poland**

Henneberg G: Das Robert Koch-Haus in Wollstein. **Med Welt** 1982 Mar 26;33(12):427
Roeske W: Ceramika apteczna z Proszkowa w Muzeum Farmacji Am w Krakowie. Krakow, 1978. 20 p.
Roeske W: Muzeum Farmacji Akademii medycznej w Krakowie. Krakow, 1977. 22 p.

**Puerto Rico**

Trías de Gómez L, Pagán Ramos IH: Organización del Museo de la Enfermería en Puerto Rico. **Bol Col Prof Enferm PR** 1983 Jun;9(34):24–5

**Romania**

Negru I: Muzeul memorial 'Prof. dr. Gh. Marinescu'. **Viata Med [Medii Sanit]** 1981 Aug;29(8):187–90

# MUSEUMS

**South Africa**

Adler C: Historical perspectives. A corner of history in South Africa: the Adler Museum. **Prev Med** 1984 Mar;13(2):226–30
Adler C: Why a medical historical museum? **Tydskr Tandheelkd Ver S Afr** 1982 Apr;37(4):261–3
Cowley J, Adler C, ed: A descriptive catalogue of early medical books in the Adler Museum of the History of Medicine and the University of the Witwatersrand Medical Library. Johannesburg, University of the Witwatersrand Library, 1982. x, 145 p.
Kahn A: Highlights of the Adler Museum collections. **Adler Mus Bull** 1984 Nov;10(3):25–9
Kahn A: Highlights of the Adler Museum collections: the Jenner letter. **Adler Mus Bull** 1984 Jun;10(2):15–7

**Spain**

Ballester R, Bujosa F, Olagüe G: Colección historicomédica de la Facultad de Medicine de Valencia. Valencia, Càtedra e Instituto de Historia de la Medicina, 1976. 54 p. (Cuadernos Valencianos de Historia de la Medicina y de la Ciencia, 18, Serie A (Monografías)).
Swanson BZ: Spain's private dental museum. **Bull Hist Dent** 1984;32(1):27–30

**Sweden**

Ahlström CG, Ekström P, Persson O: Cartesius' kranium. **Sydsven Medicinhist Sallsk Arsskr** 1983;:23–50
Ahlström CG: Ett gammalt museum berättar; glimtar från patologiska institutionens museum i Lund. **Sydsven Medicinhist Sallsk Arsskr** 1982;:15–31
Brogården in Skaba – the cradle of Swedish veterinary medicine: **Vet Hist** 1982 Summer;2(3):124–7
Francke OC: Svenska Tandläkare-Sällskapets samlingar. **Nord Medicinhist Arsb** 1980;Suppl 6:143–6
Holmertz V: Museet som berättar om m ormors sjukvård. **Vardfacket** 1982 May 13;6(9):8–9
Strandell B: Svenska medicinska medaljer. **Nord Medicinhist Arsb** 1980;Supp 6:52–6

**Switzerland**

Archinard M: Nouvelle salle de microscopes au Musée d'histoire des Sciences. **Mus Geneve** 1982;224:7–13
Boschung U: Gustav Adolf Wehrli (1888–1949), Gründer der Medizinhistorischen Sammlung der Universität Zürich. **Gesnerus** 1980;37(1/2):91–103

**United States**

Anderson RA: Chiropractic in American history: the ins and outs of museums. **Chiropr Hist** 1982;2(1):15–9
Bonsett CA: Medical museum notes: Indianapolis City Hospital. **J Indiana State Med Assoc** 1983 Oct;76(10):657
Bonsett CA: Medical museum notes: The Indiana Medical History Society. **J Indiana State Med Assoc** 1982 Dec;75(12):839
Bonsett CA: Medical museum notes: Thomas B. Harvey. **J Indiana State Med Assoc** 1983 Jun;76(6):371
Bonsett CA: Museum notes [John Shaw Billings' birthplace] **J Indiana State Med Assoc** 1981;74:348
Borowitz HO: A medical tour through The Cleveland Museum of Art. **Cleve Clin Q** 1983 Winter;50(4):417–38
Bower B: St. Elizabeths Museum. **Psychiatr News** 1982 Mar 19;17(6):6–7
Bruton EM, ed: M A S H: binding up the wounds. An exhibition at the National Museum of American History, Smithsonian Institution, Washington, D.C. New York, George Fenmore Associates, 1983. 32 p.
Caplan RM: On the creation of a new medical museum. **J Iowa Med Soc** 1983 Jun;73(6):229
Cohen MS: American civilization in three dimensions: the evolution of the Museum of History and Technology of the Smithsonian Institution. Ph.D. Diss., George Washington University. Washington, D.C., 1980. iv, 349 leaves.
Davis A, Appel T: Bloodletting instruments in the National Museum of History and Technology. Washington, Smithsonian Institution Press, 1979. 103 p.
Fournier GA, Albert DM, Bachrach A, et al: Symbol of Boston's Museum of Science has eye tumor. **N Engl J Med** 1983 Mar 31;308(13):782–3
The healing art: **Am Heritage** 1981;32(4):16–27
The Indiana Medical History Museum: **Indiana Med Hist Q** 1974;1(1):11–21
Lawrence SV: Modern ideas mix with history. **Forum Med** 1978 Nov;1(8):14–9
Liberti L, Coyle G, Der Marderosian A: Historical pharmaceutical exhibits at PCP&S. **Pharm Hist** 1980;22(3):115–18
McIntyre RL: Medical history museum. **J Med Soc NJ** 1982 Dec;79(13):1017
Menczer LF, Mittelmann M, Don RS: Pharmacy in Hartford's Historical Museum of Medicine and Dentistry. **Pharm Hist** 1984;26(3):156–7
Nordstrom WR: How a dental museum – built and staffed by dental students – helps generate interest in dental history. **Bull Hist Dent** 1983 Apr;31(1):18–22
Radbill SX: Josef Hyrtl's Philadelphia connection. **J Hist Med Allied Sci** 1984 Apr;39(2):222–4
Skillman K: The struggle to save a dental shrine. **Ohio Dent J** 1983 May;57(3):44–6
Sognnaes RF: President Washington's most famous dentures stolen from the Smithsonian. **J Am Dent Assoc** 1983 Feb;106(2):216–8
Stadnik J: Why our pharmacy museum is an attraction for old and new customers. **Pharm Times** 1982 Aug;48(8):52–4
Tyson RA, Alcauskas ES, ed: Catalogue of the Hrdlička paleopathology collection. Foreword and glossary by S. L. Rogers. Descriptions by C. F. Merbs. San Diego, San Diego Museum of Man, 1980. xi, 359 p.

**USSR**

Antonovich T: Ima podviga--gumanizm. **Med Sestra** 1981 Dec;40(12):41–4
Bobrik II, Chernyshenko LV: Istoriia anatomicheskikh muzeev na Ukraine i ikh znachenie dlia ateisticheskoĭ propagandy i populiarizatsii dostizheniĭ nauki. **Vrach Delo** 1984 Feb;(2):119–22
Grando AA, Mezhirov LS: Muzeĭ meditsiny Ukrainskoĭ SSR. **Sov Zdravookhr** 1984;(8):59–62
Gribanov ED: Muzeĭ Tsentral'nogo ordena Lenina instituta usovershenstvovaniia vracheĭ. **Sov Zdravookhr** 1982;(8):77–8
Iaremchuk AIâ, et al: [Importance of museums in optimizing the academic process and academic research work of students in a department of surgery.] (Rus). **Klin Khir** 1981;2:47–9
Iarovinskiĭ MIa: K otsenke pammiatnikov istorii meditsiny. **Sov Zdravookhr** 1981;(9):72–4
Idel'chik KhI: Vrachi-bol'sheviki S. I. Mitskevich i S. I. Chernomordik u istokov Tsentral'nogo muzeia revoliutsii SSSR (k 60-letiiu muzeia). **Sov Zdravookhr** 1984;(9):56–9
Kanep VV: Aktual'nye voprosy muzeevedeniia: iz opyta raboty Muzeia istorii meditsiny im. P. Stradynia : tezisy dokladov. Riga, Ministerstvo zdravookhraneniia Latviĭskoĭ SSR, 1982. 195 p.
Khusainova DZh: Muzeĭnaia komnata 'Molodaia gvardiia' v meditsinskom uchilishche. **Med Sestra** 1982 Mar;41(3):56–7
Makovoz AA, Gorskiĭ AN: Muzei istorii meditsiny i zdravookhraneniia Kirovogradskoĭ oblasti. **Feldsher Akush** 1983;48(1):52–4
Murav'ev EV: Ugolok istorii. **Med Sestra** 1980 Oct;37(10):52–4
Nosal' VI: Muzeĭ istorii zdravookhraneniia goroda. **Sov Zdravookhr** 1983;(4):44–5
Pendler MB: Muzeĭ-usad'ba N. I. Pirogova (k 100-letiiu so dnia smerti N. I. Pirogova). **Feldsher Akush** 1981;46(12):40–2
Rudenko AK: Muzeĭ istorii Donetskogo meditsinskogo instituta. **Sov Zdravookhr** 1980;(9):61–4
Selivanov EF: Meditsinskie muzei i vospitanie sovetskogo vracha. **Sov Med** 1982;(7):82–5
Selivanov EF, Pasiukov FV: Pamiatnik medikam Velikoĭ Otechestvennoĭ voĭny (o Voenno-meditsinskom muzee Ministerstva oborony SSSR). **Feldsher Akush** 1983 Nov;48(11):48–52
Selivanov EF, Kantorovich MM: Relikvii N. I. Pirogova v Noenno-meditsinskom muzee. **Voen Med Zh** 1983 Nov;(11):71–3
Selivanov EF, Pasiukov FV: 40-let Voenno-meditsinskogo muzeia. **Sov Zdravookhr** 1983;(2):67–70
Speranskiĭ VS, Burdeĭ GD, Iudin KA: Muzeĭ i biblioteka kafedry anatomii cheloveka Saratovskogo. **Arkh Anat Gistol Embriol** 1980 Jun;78(6):115–9
Tiuliandin AD: Muzeĭ Sovetskogo Krasnogo Kresta. **Zdravookhr Ross Fed** 1980;(5):22–6
Varlamov VM, Selivanov EF: Voenno-meditsinskomu muzeiu Ministerstva oborony SSSR - 40 let. **Voen Med Zh** 1982 Nov;(11):77–80
Zerbino DD: Unikal'nyĭ arkhiv protokolov vskrytiĭ. **Vrach Delo** 1980 Jul;(7):6–9

**Yugoslavia**

Mićić M: Pharmaziegeschichtliche Museen und Sammlungen in Jugoslawien. In: Vorträge des Internationalen Pharmaziehistorischen Kongresses Innsbruck 1977. Stuttgart, Wissenschaftliche Verlagsgesellschaft, 1979. p. 107–25.

# MUSIC

Abbott EC: Composers and tuberculosis: the effects on creativity. **Can Med Assoc J** 1982 Mar 1;126(5):534, 536–8, 543–4
Breuer R: Berufskrankheiten von Instrumentalmusikern aus medizinhistorischer Sicht (vom 15. Jahrhundert bis 1930). Diss., Johannes Gutenberg-Universität. Mainz, 1982. 110 p.
Feggetter G: Suicide in opera. **Br J Psychiatry** 1980 Jun;136:552–7
Graham RM: Music therapy: the state of the field. **J Natl Assoc Priv Psychiatr Hosp** 1979;11(2):32–9
James T: Eunuchs and eunuchism--an historical discourse. **Adler Mus Bull** 1981 Oct;7(3):2–7
Musikterapi förr och nu för barn och vuxna: **Lakartidningen** 1981;78(20):2045–55
Nissen TP: Musiktherapie. Ihre Ursprünge und modernen Formen.

Fortschr Med 1983 Jun 2;101(21):972-8
Perelló J: Los cantantes castrados. **An Otorrinolaringol Ibero Am** 1980;7(1):57-76
Stefani WH: The psycho-physiological effects of volume, pitch, harmony and rhythm in the development of Western art music: implications for a philosophy of music history. M. A. Thesis, Andrews University. Berrien Springs, 1981. 293 leaves.

**France**

Rocchietta S: Musica e litotomia in una composizione di Marin Marais (1656-1728). **Minerva Med** 1983 Nov 16;74(44):2713

**Italy**

Melicow MM: Castrati singers and the lost 'cords'. **Bull NY Acad Med** 1983 Oct;59(8):744-64

**USSR**

Berman IW: Musicogenic epilepsy. **S Afr Med J** 1981 Jan 10;59(2):49-52

### 500 A.D.-1450

**Arabic**

Burgel JC: Musicotherapy in the Islamic Middle Ages as reflected in medical and other sources. **Stud Hist Med** 1980 Mar;4(1):23-8

**France**

Cosman MP: Machaut's medical musical world. In Cosman MP, Chandler B, ed: Machaut's world: science and art in the fourteenth century. New York, New York Academy of Sciences, 1978. (Annals of the New York Academy of Sciences, v. 314). p. 1-36.

**Italy**

Bazzi F, Panebianco D: Una lauda di interesse medico poco nota di Jacopone da Todi. **Minerva Med** 1981 Nov 14;72(45):3039-43

### 1450-1700

Koenigsberger D: Renaissance man and creative thinking. A history of concepts of harmony 1400-1700. Hassocks, Sussex, Harvester Press, 1979. xiii, 282 p.

**Germany**

Stadler F: Paracelsus und die Musik in Salzburg. **Salzburger Beitr Paracelsusforsch** 1984;23:118-25

### 1700 to Present

Aterman K, MacSween HM, Perry PE, et al: Recurrent infections, diarrhea, ascites and phonophobia in a 57-year-old man. **Can Med Assoc J** 1982 Mar 15;126(6):623-8
Böhme G: Medizinische Porträts berühmter Komponisten: Wolfgang Amadeus Mozart, Ludwig van Beethoven, Carl Maria von Weber, Frédéric Chopin, Peter Iljitsch Tschaikowski, Béla Bartók. 2. verbesserte und erweiterte Auflage. Stuttgart, New York, Gustav Fischer Verlag, 1981. xi, 199 p.
Bowers JZ: Truants from medicine. **Perspect Biol Med** 1979 Autumn;23(1):83-91
Czeizel A: Ludwig van Beethoven. **Ther Hung** 1982;30(1):43-7
Forschbach G: Tuberculosis and creative man. **Bull Int Union Tuberc** 1984 Mar-Jun;59(1-2):104-7
Franken FH: Krankheit und Tod grosser Komponisten. Baden-Baden, New York, Witzstrock, 1979. 280 p.
Kerner D: Béla Bartóks Tod in New York. Zu seinem 100. Geburtstag am 25. März 1981. **MMW** 1981 Mar 27;123(13):525-9
Keynes M: Handel's illnesses. **Lancet** 1980 Dec 20-27;2(8208-8209):1354-5
Meyer A: The search for a morphological substrate in the brains of eminent persons including musicians: a historical review. In Critchley M, Henson RA, ed: Music and the brain: studies in the neurology of music. London, Heinemann, 1977. p. 255-81.
Reichsman F: Life experiences and creativity of great composers: a psychosomaticist's view. **Psychosom Med** 1981 Aug;43(4):291-300
Sandblom P: Skapande och Sjukdom. Hur lidande påverkar litteratur, konst och musik. Södertälje, Fingraf Tryckeri, 1983. 142 p. (Nordisk Medicinhistorisk Arsbok, Supplementum IX).
Sieluźycki C: Choroby Fryderyka Chopina, ich patogeneza i leczenie. **Arch Hist Med (Warsz)** 1981;44(3/4):237-56
Suppan W: Biologische und kulturelle Bedingungen des Musikgebrauches. **Universitas (Stuttg)** 1982;37(12):1279-84
Trethowan WH: Ivor Gurney's mental illness. **Music Lett** 1981;62(3-4):300-9
Weir NF: Theodor Billroth and Johannes Brahms--a thirty year friendship. **Hist Med (Lond)** 1975 Autumn-Winter;6(3-4):8-14

**Austria**

Alonso HO: La enfermedad cardíaca de Gustav Mahler. **Medicina (B Aires)** 1981;41(3):373-7
Barthelme E: Sur la fièvre miliaire ardente, a propos de la mort de Mozart. **Hist Sci Med** 1983;17(1):23-8
Blodi FC: Was Mozart cross-eyed? **Arch Ophthalmol** 1981 May;99(5):823
Collins DT: Gustav Mahler's summer of 1910. **Bull Menninger Clin** 1982 May;46(3):255-79
Davies PJ: Mozart's illness and death. **J R Soc Med** 1983 Sep;76(9):776-85
Davies PJ: Mozart's illness & death. **Bol Asoc Med PR** 1984 Aug;76(8):355-61
Franken FH: Mozarts Todeskrankheit. **Fortschr Med** 1980 Mar 6;98(9):301-2
Holinka C: Theodor Billroth: the life of a surgeon in the spirit of music. **Mt Sinai J Med (NY)** 1981 Jan-Feb;48(1):21-41
Kern E: Das chirurgische Erbe. Theodor Billroth und die Musik. **Zentralbl Chir** 1982;107(21):1408-16
Landsberger M: Percussion discovered. **Trans Stud Coll Physicians Phila** 1981 Dec;5(3 no 4):255
Rocchietta S: Alcuni valzer viennesi di interesse medico. **Minerva Med** 1982 Oct 6;73(38):2603-4
Sakula A: 'Amadeus' was Mozart poisoned? **Hist Med (Lond)** 1980 Jan-Feb;8(1):6-9
Schoental R: Mozart's illnesses and death. **J R Soc Med** 1983 Dec;76(12):1079-80
Zagarra MJ: Ludwig van Beethoven: hipótesis sobre su sordera. **CERON** 1979 Dec;4(3):7-9

**Czechoslovakia**

Bořík O, Khel R, Zdichynec B: Několik poznámek k ušnímu onemocnění Bedřicha Smetany. **Cesk Otolaryngol** 1983 Nov;32(6):367-71
Ober WB: The sticky end of Frantisek Koczwara, composer of 'The Battle of Prague'. **Am J Forensic Med Pathol** 1984 Jun;5(2):145-9
Sajner J: Patografická studie o Leoši Janáckovi. **Vnitr Lek** 1982 Aug;28(8):823-7

**France**

Brøndum N: Et kirurgisk indgreb skildret i musik. **Dan Medicinhist Arbog** 1983;12:170-4
Wegner PC: Le docteur Gall à Cynthère. **Medizinhist J** 1984;19(3):233-43

**Germany**

Andre P: Schumann. Les chants de l'ombre. Paris, Jean-Claude Lattes, 1982. 225 p.
Guillemin J: La maladie de Richard Wagner. Pour le centenaire de sa mort à Venise. **Sem Hop Paris** 1983 May 12;59(19):1493-6
Isliker B: Christian Ludwig Bachmanns Dissertation 'Über die Wirkungen der Musik auf den Menschen' (Erlangen 1792). Zürich, Juris Druck, 1982. 76 p. (Zürcher Medizingeschichtliche Abhandlungen, Neue Reihe, Nr. 154).
Kerner D: El último Brahms. **Folia Hum (Barc)** 1981;19:27-34
Rather LJ: The dream of self-destruction. Wagner's Ring and the modern world. Baton Rouge, Louisiana State Univ. Press, 1979. xx, 215 p.
Schein CJ, Koch E: Jenny Lind's concert in Göttingen. Billroth's letter to his mother. **NY State J Med** 1979 Oct;79(11):1786-1891
Shafar J: The Brahms-Billroth friendship. **Br Med J** 1981;282:1775
Vértes L: Georg Händel (Händel apja, a 'hallei chirurgus'). **Orv Hetil** 1980 Apr 6;121(14):851-3
Wurmser L: Idealization and aggression in Beethoven's creativity. **Am Imago** 1979 Winter;36(4):328-44

**Great Britain**

Breakwell J: Birmingham General Hospital and the Birmingham Music Festivals. **Practitioner** 1979 Sep;223(1335):406-10
Rocchietta S: Due secoli di canzoni inglesi con spunti medico-=farmaceutici. **Minerva Med** 1979 Sep 26;70(41):2839-43
Wainapel SF: Frederick Delius; medical assessment. **NY State J Med** 1980 Nov;80(12):1886-7

**Hungary**

Bugyi B: Lichtenthal Péter, egy elfelejtett nagy magyar orvos-zenetudós.
Vladimirova LB, Gribanov ED: A nagy magyar zeneszerzo, Liszt Ferenc és az ogyesszai gyermekkórház épületének története (orosz nyelven). **Orvostort Kozl** 1982;28(1-3):169-76

**Italy**

Blum MH: Toscanini's relation to his orchestra.

# MUSIC

**Hillside J Clin Psychiatry** 1983;5(1):91–127
Kerner D: Bellinis Tod in Paris. **Orchester** 1976;24:712–6
Rocchietta S: Canzoni italiane correlate con la medicina e la farmacia. **Minerva Med** 1980 Oct 13;71(39):2861–70
Rocchietta S: Musica e medicina negli scritti di Felice La Torre (1846–1923). **Minerva Ginecol** 1980 Oct;32(10):949–53
Rocchietta S: Musica e medicina negli scritti di Felice La Torre (1846–1923). **Minerva Med** 1980 Jul;71(27):1949–53
Schoenfeld MR: Nicolo Paganini--musical magician and Marfan mutant? **Med Times** 1980 Nov, 108(11):117–8, 120, 125
Smith RD: Paganini's hand. **Arthritis Rheum** 1982 Nov;25(11):1385–6

**Poland**

Godlewski G: Chopin génie asexué. **Sem Hop Paris** 1979 Dec 18–25;55(43–44):2051–63
Pačes V: Uvahy o nemoci Fryderyka Chopina. **Vnitr Lek** 1980 Oct;26(10):1027–31

**Romania**

Sărmăşanu-Cortez ML, Cortez PP: Un distins psihiatru la confluenta dintre muzică şi medicină: dr. Stefan S. Braşcu (1895–1965). **Rev Med Interna [Neurol Psihiatr]** 1980 Apr–Jun;24(2):143–8

**United States**

Dentistry--for music's sake. I. How dental 'miracles' helped jazz greats with their careers (Buck Clayton): **Tic** 1979 Dec;38(12):1–3
Heindel ND, Foster NI: Medicine, music and 'Money' Munyon. **Pa Folklife** 1982;32(1):44–8
Jensen JE: 166 years ago this month ... William Beanes: the doctor behind 'The Star-Spangled Banner'. **Md State Med J** 1980 Sep;29(9):60–5
Ljunggren B: The case of George Gershwin. **Neurosurgery** 1982 Jun;10(6 Pt 1):733–6
Parrott JR, Harrison DB: Surgically dividing pianists' hands. **J Hand Surg** 1980 Nov;5(6):619
Taylor DB: Music in general hospital treatment from 1900 to 1950. **J Music Ther** 1981 Summer;18(2):62–73

**USSR**

Arkhangel'skii GV: S. P. Botkin i otechestvennye deiateli muzykal'noĭ i khudozhestvennoĭ kul'tury. **Klin Med (Mosk)** 1982 May;60(5):112–7
Evdokimov PP: K istorii bolezni F. I. Shaliapina. **Klin Med (Mosk)** 1983 May;61(5):115–6
Lasky II: Medicine and music. **NY State J Med** 1982 Dec;82(13):1862–4
Shul'tsev GP: Aleksandr Porfir'evich Borodin (k 150-letiiu so dnia rozhdeniia). **Klin Med (Mosk)** 1984 Jul;62(7):144–7

# NAVAL MEDICINE

See also **War**

Carré A: Scorbut marin historique et biologie moderne. In: Congrès National des Sociétés Savantes, 104e, Bordeaux, 1979. Comptes Rendus. Paris, 1979. Section des Sciences, Fasc. IV. p. 219–30.
Haneveld GT: 'De secrete' toiletfacilities in sea-going vessels. In International Congress of the History of Medicine, 27th, Barcelona, 1980. Actas. Barcelona, Académia de Ciències Médiques de Catalunya i Balears, 1981. p. 384–6.
Huard P, Imbault-Huart MJ: A propos du scorbut. In: Congrès National des Sociétés Savantes, 101e, Lille, 1976. Comptes Rendus. Paris, 1976. Section des Sciences, Fasc. III. p. 157–72.
Kernéïs JP: Geschichte der Schiffahrtsmedizin am Beispiel der Schiffschirurgen. In Sournia JC, Martiny M, Poulet J, ed: Illustrierte Geschichte der Medizin. Salzburg, Andreas, 1980. Vol. 8. p. 2999–3023.
Marr JJ: Merchants of death: the role of slave trade in the transmission of disease from Africa to the Americas. **Pharos** 1982 Winter;45(1):31–5
Orozco Acuaviva A: Historia de una enfermedad de los navegantes: el escorbuto. **An R Acad Med Cir Cadiz** 1979;15(1):7–30
Schadewaldt H: A propos de l'histoire de l'hygiène navale. In: Congrès National des Sociétés Savantes, 91e, Rennes, 1966. Comptes Rendus. Paris, 1967. Section des Sciences, Tome 1. p. 47–53.
Schadewaldt H: Das Sargassokraut als Antiskorbutikum. In Dilg P, et al., ed: Perspektiven der Pharmaziegeschichte. Graz, Austria, Akademische Druck- u. Verlagsanstalt, 1983. p. 281–94.
Schadewaldt H: Skorbut. **Zahnarztl Prax** 1980 Jul 11;31(7):297–301
Schmidt J: Individuelle Rettungsmittel für Seenotfälle. In Göpfert W, Otten HH, ed: Metavoeite: wandelt euch durch neues Denken. Düsseldorf, Triltsch, 1983. p. 79–87.
Volbehr K: Gesundheit an Bord. Kleine Geschichte der Hygiene und Arzneimittelversorgung auf Schiffen. Bremerhaven, Ditzen, 1979. 72 p. (Führer des Deutschen Schiffahrtsmuseums, Nr. 11).
Watt J: Nutrition in adverse environments, 1. Forgotten lessons of maritime nutrition. **Hum Nutr Appl Nutr** 1982 Feb;36(1):35–45
Watt J: The burns of seafarers under oars, sail and steam. **Injury** 1980 Jul;12(1):69–81
Watt J: The surgery of sea warfare from the galley to the nuclear age. **Trans Med Soc Lond** 1980–81;97:1–15

**France**

Carré A: La révolution colbertienne et l'assistance aux familles maritimes des origines à 1673. In: Congrès National des Sociétés Savantes, 97e, Nantes, 1972. Comptes Rendus. Paris, 1976. Section des Sciences, Tome 1. p. 227–48.
Carré A: L'évolution du système classes-invalides de 1673 (Edit de Nancy) à 1784 (Réformes de Castries). In: Congrès National des Sociétés Savantes, 97e, Nantes, 1972. Comptes Rendus. Paris, 1976. Section des Sciences, Tome 1. p. 249–67.
Chippaux C: Le Service de Santé des troupes de Marine. **Med Trop (Mars)** 1980 Nov–Dec;40(6):605–30
Curet M, Carre A, Henaff R: Les écoles de chirurgie et de médecine navales. **Med Armees** 1980;8(10)spec:797–800
Curet M, Carre A, Henaff R: Les hôpitaux des ports. **Med Armees** 1980;8(10)spec:795–6
Curet M, Huard P, Carre A, et al: Les traditions de la marine: une médecine de la mer. **Med Armees** 1980;8(10)spec:787–94
Darsel J: L'assistance sociale dans la marine sous l'Ancien Régime en la Province de Bretagne. In: Congrès National des Sociétés Savantes, 97e, Nantes, 1972. Comptes Rendus. Paris, 1976. Section des Sciences, Tome 1. p. 293–309.
Ehrhardt JP: L'Ecole du Service de Santé de la Marine de Bordeaux des origines à nos jours. In Congrès National des Sociétés Savantes, 103e, Nancy-Metz, 1978. Actes. Paris, 1979. Tome I, p. 9–21.
Kernéis JP, Rouzeau L, Cuny J: L'histoire de la médecine navale à l'Université de Nantes. In: Congrès National de Sociétés Savantes, 97e, Nantes, 1972. Comptes Rendus. Paris, 1976. Section des Sciences, Tome 1. p. 149–64.
Lemperier B: Le système d'assistance dans la marine marchande. In: Congrès National des Sociétés Savantes, 97e, Nantes, 1972. Comptes Rendus. Paris, 1976. Section des Sciences, Tome 1. p. 311–7.
Niaussat PM: L'activité scientifique des médecins et pharmaciens de la marine du XVIIe siècle à nos jours. **Med Armees** 1980;8(10)spec:800–6

**Great Britain**

Cannell H: Struck by lightning -- the effects upon the men and the ships of HM Navy. **J R Nav Med Serv** 1979;65(3):165–70
Clark SG: Farewell to the SBA. **J R Nav Med Serv** 1984 Spring;70(1):3–8
Hanson RD: Medical services at Chatham Dockyard 1625–1984. **J R Nav Med Serv** 1984 Spring;70(1):38–40
Lattimore MI: Early naval medical libraries, personal and corporate. **J R Nav Med Serv** 1983 Summer;69(2):107–11

**Spain**

Valverde Lopez JL, Sanchez F, Vinuesa L, et al: La dotacion de medicamentos en los buques de la Armada durante los siglos XVII y XVIII. Granada, Universidad de Granada, 1979. 60 [47] p.

**USSR**

Ivanov EM: Stanovlenie i razvitie otechestvennoĭ voenno-morskoĭ meditsiny. Leningrad, Meditsina, Leningradskoe otd-nie, 1976. 398 p.

**Before 500 A.D.**

**Egypt**

Ghalionungui P: A naval physician in ancient Egypt. In International Congress of the History of Medicine, 27th, Barcelona, 1980. Actas. Barcelona, Académia de Ciències Médiques de Catalunya i Balears, 1981. p. 373–5.

**1450–1700**

Dauber LG: Peter Blood and the Brethren of the Coast. Fictional physicians afield. **NY State J Med** 1982 Jun;82(7):1107–9
Poynter FN: James Yonge. In Dictionary of Canadian biography, 1701 to 1740. Volume 2, 1969. p. 670–2.

**France**

Cadotte M: A propos de la description par Jacques Cartier d'une 'grosse maladie' survenue au cours de son deuxième voyage au Canada. **Union Med Can** 1984 Aug;113(8):651–5

**Great Britain**

Appleby JH: New light on John Woodall, surgeon and adventurer. **Med Hist** 1981 Jul;25(3):251–68
Beaconsfield M, Beaconsfield T: Marine archeology seen from the 'Wasa'

and the 'Mary Rose': a physician's eye-view. **Nord Medicinhist Arsbok** 1983;:65-9
Forbes TR: When did Lionel Wafer die? **J Hist Med Allied Sci** 1981 Jan;36(1)69-70
Harper E: The sailor's surgeon (James Yonge). **J R Nav Med Serv** 1979 Spring;65(1):35-7
Ring ME: Oddments in dental history: what every sea surgeon of around 1600 ought to know concerning treating teeth. **Bull Hist Dent** 1984 Oct;32(2):109-11
Stirland A: The burials from King Henry VIII's ship, the Mary Rose: an interim statement. **Paleopathol Newsl** 1984 Sep;(47):7-10
Watt J: Surgeons of the Mary Rose: the practice of surgery in Tudor England. **Mar Mirror** 1983;69:3-18
Woodall J: The surgions mate. Facsimile of 1617 ed. Ed. J. Kirkup Bath, England, Kingsmead, 1978. xxxiv, 348 p.

**Italy**

Burnett J: The Giustiniani medicine chest. **Med Hist** 1982 Jul;26(3):325-33

**Netherlands**

DeJong CJ: Een verklaring door Anthony van Riebeeck als scheepschirurgijn in 1636. **Historia (S Afr)** 1973;18(4):231-3

**Spain**

Brotóns Picó J: Un medico en el descubrimiento de America. **Rev Gen Mar** 1980 Jul;199:3-11
Parrilla Hermida M: Un hospital de la Armada en El Ferrol siglo XVI. **Asclepio** 1981;33:407-10

**West Indies**

Burg BR: Sodomy and the perception of evil: English sea rovers in the seventeenth-century Caribbean. New York, New York University Press, 1983. xxxiii, 215 p.

**1700 to Present**

Boucher M: The Cape passage: some observations on health hazards aboard Dutch East Indiamen outward-bound. **Historia (S Afr)** 1981;26(1):24-36
Bouchier IA: Some experiences of ships' surgeons during the early days of the sperm whale fishery. **Br Med J [Clin Res]** 1982 Dec 18-25;285(6357):1811-3
Cole BL, Vingrys AJ: A survey and evaluation of lantern tests of color vision. **Am J Optom Physiol Opt** 1982 Apr;59(4):346-74
Fleming AF: HTLV from Africa to Japan. **Lancet** 1984 Feb 4;1(8371):279
Goethe H, Vuksanović P: Bei Seeleuten häufig vorkommende Erkrankungen. In Göpfert W, Otten HH, ed: Metavoeite: wandelt euch durch neues Denken. Düsseldorf, Triltsch, 1983. p. 69-78.
Moretti G, Bosredon J: Le paludisme nautique tropical de la côte d'Afrique, hier et aujourd'hui. In: Congrès National des Sociétés Savantes, 104e, Bordeaux, 1979. Comptes Rendus. Paris, 1979. Section des Sciences, Fasc. IV. p. 309-17.
Pruett CE: Naval medicine and modern sea power. **Nav Rev** 1965;10:238-59
Seidel T: Medizinische Beobachtungen während der Weltumsegelung des Adam Johann von Krusenstern. Diss. Düsseldorf, 1979. 89 p.
Servat A, Servat C: Pierre-Alphonse Doué, médecin de marine, médecin major de 'l'Aigle' à l'inauguration du canal de Suez. **Med Armees** 1981;9:453-68
Watt J: Lettsomian lectures. Medical perspectives of some voyages of discovery. **Trans Med Soc Lond** 1979;95:61-91
Winton R: Food and fitness at sea. **Med J Aust** 1980 Oct 18;2(8):411-2
75 years of caring: **US Navy Med** 1983 May-Jun;74(3):14-7

**Argentina**

López McCabe A: Francisco Javier Villanueva y Godoy: cirujano major de la armada. **Rev Mar** 1981;98(1):72-87

**Australia**

Gurd DP: Australia and around the world. **J R Nav Med Serv** 1982 Winter;68(3):159-66 contd

**Belgium**

Lefevre P: Les voyages de la Marine Royale Belge au Sénégal, en Gambie et en Basse Guinée. Récits des médecins qui accompagnèrent les navires de guerre belges 'Louise-Marie' et 'Duc de Brabant' (1847-1856) dans le cadre de la tentative de colonisation au Rio Nunez. **Rev Belge Hist Milit** 1978-79;22-23:647-68, 39-64, 137-48

**Bulgaria**

Ispirsky N: Medical attendance for seafarers of the Bulgarian Marine from its establishments to present days. In International Congress of the History of Medicine. 26th, Plovdiv, 1978. Actes du Congress. Sofia, 1981. Volume II. p. 215-6.

**Canada**

Bensley EH: James Grant: ship's surgeon on the ill-fated Empress of Ireland. **Can Med Assoc J** 1982 Feb 1;126(3):318-9

**Cuba**

Torres Medina J: Los barcos hospitales en la campaña de Cuba. **Rev Hist Mil** 1970;14(29):161-86

**Denmark**

Winge M: Urban Bruun Aaskow. **Dan Medicinhist Arbog** 1981;:94-127

**France**

Carré A: Essai de synthèse des maladies des gens de mer au XVIIIe siècle et leur évolution au début du XIXe siècle. In: Congrès National des Sociétés Savantes, 91e, Rennes, 1966. Comptes Rendus. Paris, 1967. Section des Sciences, Tome 1. p. 11-29.
Chaïa J: A propos des malheurs de l'escadre du Duc D'Anville (1746). In: Congrès National des Sociétés Savantes, 107e. Brest, 1982. Comptes Rendus, Paris, 1983. Section des Sciences, Fasc. IV. p. 333-9.
Dalat J: Un chirurgien de mer à la fin du XVIIIe siècle. **Rev Hist Pharm (Paris)** 1983 Dec;71(30):275-81
Dejussieu L: Note sur le jardin botanique de la Marine à Rochefort-sur-Mer. In: Congrès National des Sociétés Savantes, 91e, Rennes, 1966. Comptes Rendus. Paris, 1967. Section des Sciences, Tome 1. p. 129-33.
Dulieu L: Pierre Chirac et les maladies des équipages des vaisseaux. **Rev Hist Sci (Paris)** 1984 Jan;37(1):65-70
Dulieu L: Un projet d'Ecole de santé de la Marine à Montpellier. In: Congrès National des Sociétés Savantes, 91e, Rennes, 1966. Comptes Rendus. Paris, 1967. Section des Sciences, Tome 1. p. 103-7.
Ehrhardt JP: Les médecins naturalistes de 'La Coquille' et de 'L'Astrolabe', ex-gabare 'La Coquille'. In: Congrès National des Sociétés Savantes, 104e, Bordeaux, 1979. Comptes Rendus. Paris, 1979. Section des Sciences, Fasc. IV. p. 205-17.
Hockemeyer H: Die Zeit seiner Schiffsarzttätigkeit in den Memoiren des napoleonischen Chirurgen Dominique-Jean Larrey. Diss., Universität Düsseldorf. Düsseldorf, 1982. 44 p.
Huard P, Niaussat PM: Die Medizinisch-Chirurgische Schule der Marine in Brest. **Hist Hosp** 1979-80;13:147-52
Huard P, Imbault-Huart MJ: La stomatologie navale au XVIIIe siècle. In: Congrès National des Sociétés Savantes, 101e, Lille, 1976. Comptes Rendus. Paris, 1976. Section des Sciences, Fasc. III. p. 145-56. (also in 97e Congrès National des Sociétés Savantes, Nantes, 1972, Sciences, Tome I, p. 167-9).
Huard P, Niaussat PM: 'L'arsenal' du service de Santé de la Marine au XIXe siècle. In: Congrès National des Sociétés Savantes, 105e, Caen, 1980. Comptes Rendus, Paris, 1980. Section des Sciences, Fasc. V. p. 85-96.
Huard P: L'oeuvre du Service de Santé de la Marine francaise au XIXe siècle. In: Congrès National des Sociétés Savantes, 91e, Rennes, 1966. Comptes Rendus. Paris, 1967. Section des Sciences, Tome 1. p. 93-8.
Huard P, Lacombe C, Théodoridès J: Marine et botanique aux XVIIIe et XIXe siècles; les jardins botaniques de la Marine. In: Congrès National des Sociétés Savantes, 91e, Rennes, 1966. Comptes Rendus. Paris, 1967. Section des Sciences, Tome 1. p. 109-27.
Léonard J: A propos de l'hygiène navale sur les navires de guerre français dans la première moitié du XIXe siècle. In: Congrès National des Sociétés Savantes, 91e, Rennes, 1966. Comptes Rendus. Paris, 1967. Section des Sciences, Tome 1. p. 55-77.
McKee ME, McKee HS: E. Vieillard et E. Deplanche, deux grands botanistes collecteurs en Nouvelle-Calédonie. **Hist Nat** 1980-81;17-18:49-68
Marc JC: Pharmaciens de la Marine et voyages de découvertes en océanie au XIXe siècle. In: Congrès National des Sociétés Savantes, 104e, Bordeaux, 1979. Comptes Rendus. Paris, 1979. Section des Sciences, Fasc. IV. p. 193-204.
Niaussat P: Les 'coliques sèches' dans la Marine au XIXe siècle: Amédée Lefevre et son combat contre une tenace erreur médicale. In: Congrès National des Sociétés Savantes, 104e, Bordeaux, 1979. Comptes Rendus. Paris, 1979. Section des Sciences, Fasc. IV. p. 183-91.
Niaussat PM: Delioux de Savignac et le traitement des dysenteries. In: Congrès National des Sociétés Savantes, 107e. Brest, 1982. Comptes Rendus, Paris, 1983. Section des Sciences, Fasc. IV. p. 299-309.
Niaussat PM: Sociologie des médecins de marine au XIXe siècle. In Congrès National des Sociétés Savantes, 103e, Nancy-Metz, 1978. Actes. Paris, 1979. Tome I, p. 397-410.
Schadewaldt H: Der Schiffbruch der Méduse im Jahre 1816. In W. Treue, ed: Geschichte der französischen Marine. Herford, Mittler, 1982. p. 107-25.

# NAVAL MEDICINE

Stein R: Mortality in the eighteenth-century French slave trade. **J Afr Hist** 1980, 21(1):35–41
Valentin M, Niaussat PM: Le rôle fondamental d'Amédée Lefèvre, médecin de la Marine (1798–1869), en médecine du travail et en histoire de la médecine. **Hist Sci Med** 1979;13(4):407–17
Voelckel J: Les traditions du service outre-mer. **Med Armees** 1980;8(10)spec:807–12

**Germany**

Goethe H, Rodegra H: The history of nautical medicine in Hamburg at the time of Bernhard Nocht around 1900. In International Congress of the History of Medicine, 27th, Barcelona, 1980. Actas. Barcelona, Académia de Ciències Médiques de Catalunya i Balears, 1981. p. 376–83.
Mit Stücken von Silberteller füllte Zahnarzt kranke Zähne: **Niedersachs Zahnarztebl** 1982 Sep;17(9):403
Püschel E: Die Seenotverbände der Deutschen Luftwaffe und ihr Sanitätsdienst 1939–1945. Düsseldorf, Droste, 1978. 180 p. ((Schriftenreihe Erfahrungen des deutschen Sanitätsdienst im zweiten Weltkrieg, 1).
Schadewaldt H: Le développement de la quarantaine dans les ports allemands. In International Congress of the History of Medicine, 27th, Barcelona, 1980. Actas. Barcelona, Académia de Ciències Médiques de Catalunya i Balears, 1981. p. 408–13.
Schmidt R, Kludas A: Die deutschen Lazarettschiffe im Zweiten Weltkrieg. Stuttgart, Motorbuch, 1978. 174 p.

**Great Britain**

Allison RS: The second world war 1939–45: an RNVR medical officer's view. **J R Nav Med Serv** 1982;68(2):102–9
Barnard EE: Physiological aspects of naval problems. **J R Nav Med Serv** 1980 Spring;66(1):23–5
Cannell H: Struck by lightning--the effects upon the men and the ships of HM Navy. **J R Nav Med Serv** 1980 Summer;66(2):152–6
Cannell H: Struck by lightning -- the effects upon the men and the ships of HM Navy. **J R Nav Med Serv** 1980 Spring;66(1):71–6
Different letters from the past. 4) Horatio, Viscount Nelson to Earl Spencer.: **Ann R Coll Surg Engl** 1980 Sep;62(5):388–9
Donald KW: Submarine escape breathing air. A review and analysis of animal and human experiments by the Royal Navy. **Bull Physiopathol Respir (Nancy)** 1979 Sep–Oct;15(5):739–54
Forbes TR: Coroners' inquisitions on the deaths of prisoners in the hulks at Portsmouth, England, in 1817–27. **J Hist Med Allied Sci** 1978 Jul;33(3):356–66
Goldsworthy BM: The end of an era--the story of mass miniature chest radiography in the Royal Navy. **J R Nav Med Serv** 1981;67(1):32–6
Gurd DP: As it was in the beginning. . . **J R Nav Med Serv** 1980 Summer;66(2):140–6
Gurd DP: Headquarters Queen Anne's Mansions. **J R Nav Med Serv** 1983 Winter;69(3):161–6
Gurd DP: Mediterranean memories. **J R Nav Med Serv** 1981;67(3):169–76 contd.
Harland KM: A short history of Queen Alexandra's Royal Naval Nursing Service. **J R Nav Med Serv** 1984 Summer;70(2):59–65
Iveson-Iveson J: History of the navy nurses: a life on the ocean waves. **Nurs Mirror** 1981 Jul 1;153(1):22–4
Johnson RE: Robert McCormick. In Dictionary of Canadian biography, 1881–1890. 1982;11:543–4.
Lance D: Meals on the mess deck: from canteen messing to professional catering. **Hist Today** 1978;28(7):476–9
Lattimore MI: Early naval medical libraries, personal and corporate. **J R Nav Med Serv** 1983 Winter;69(3):156–60
Lattimore MI: Sir David James Hamilton Dickson, MD (1780–1850). **J R Nav Med Serv** 1981;67(2):92–100
Leach RD: Sir Gilbert Blane, Bart, MD FRS (1749–1832). **Ann R Coll Surg Engl** 1980 May;62(3):232–9
Levien M, ed: Naval surgeon. The voyages of Dr. Edward H. Cree, Royal Navy, as related in his private journals, 1837–1856. New York, E. P. Dutton, 1982. 275 p.
Ljunggren B: The sleepy sea lord who was Churchill's friend. **Surg Neurol** 1982 Nov;18(5):307–19
Lloyd C: Cook and scurvy. **Mar Mirror** 1979 Feb;65:23–8
Mathews M, Harris M: The Royal Naval Medical Air Evacuation Unit. **J R Nav Med Serv** 1980 Summer;66(2):147–51
Mayberry JF: The Hamadryad Hospital Ship for Seamen, 1866–1905. **Br Med J [Clin Res]** 1980 Dec 20–27;281(6256):1690–2
Northrup D: African mortality in the suppression of the slave trade: the case of the bight of Biafra. **J Interdiscip Hist** 1978;9(1):47–64
Oliver TP: 67 years ago--the Journal of the Royal Naval Medical Service, Vol I. **J R Nav Med Serv** 1982 Winter;68(3):167–70
Oliver TP: 67 years ago--the Journal of the Royal Naval Medical Service Vol 1, No. 1. **J R Nav Med Serv** 1982;68(2):98–101
Rice AL, Burstyn HL, Jones AG: G. C. Wallich M.D.---megalomaniac or mis-used oceanographic genius? **J Soc Bibliogr Nat Hist** 1976;7(4):423–50
Taylor B: Health in history. Britain's Admiral Lord Horatio Nelson. **Md State Med J** 1979 Dec;28(12):35–50
Tilghman RC: Captain James Cook (1728–1779). **Trans Am Clin Climatol Assoc** 1980;92:1–15
Tröhler U: Towards clinical investigation on a numerical basis: James Lind at Haslar Hospital 1758–1783. In International Congress of the History of Medicine, 27th, Barcelona, 1980. Actas. Barcelona, Académia de Ciències Médiques de Catalunya i Balears, 1981. p. 414–9.
Vickers HR: Royal Naval Hospital Haslar 1940–44. **J R Nav Med Serv** 1984 Summer;70(2):103–9
Wallace AF: The influence of the Battle of Jutland on plastic surgery. In Romm S, ed: Symposium on historical perspectives of plastic surgery. Philadelphia, Saunders, 1983. p. 657–63.
Wharton M: Sir Gilbert Blane Bt (1749–1834). **Ann R Coll Surg Engl** 1984 Sep;66(5):375–6
Williams E: Diary of a VAD 1940–9: cry havoc... **Nurs Mirror** 1981 Jul 1;153(1):25–8
Winge M: James Lind Grundlaeggeren af den maritime medicin. **Dan Medicinhist Arbog** 1983;12:9–20
Zuckerman A: Scurvy and the ventilation of ships in the Royal Navy: Samuel Sutton's contribution. **Eighteenth Cent Stud** 1976/77;10:222–34

**Guinea**

Sheridan RB: The Guinea surgeons on the middle passage: the provision of medical services in the British slave trade. **Int J Afr Hist Stud** 1981;14(4):601–25

**Hungary**

Kempler K: A magyar kereskedelmi tengerjáró hajók kötelezö egészségügyi felszerelése a századfordulón. **Orvostort Kozl** 1981;93–96(27 No 1–4):171–82
Kempler K: Bonyodalmak a hazai kereskedelmi tengerhajózás egészségügyi ellátásáról szóló rendelet körül a szádfordulón. **Orv Hetil** 1980 Nov 30;121(48):2954–6

**Ireland**

Morton G: Henderson Wightman, R. N., 1810–16. **Ir Sword** 1980;14(54):69–72

**Netherlands**

Haneveld GT: Medische aspecten van de slag bij Doggersbank. **Tijdschr Geschied Geneeskd** 1982;5(2):78–88
Muller CF: 'N blad uit die joernaal van 'n sieketrooster, 1709–1710. **Historia (S Afr)** 1978;23(2):90–8

**Poland**

Brodniewicz A: Józef Jakóbkiewicz M.D., pioneer of maritime and tropical medicine in Poland. **Bull Inst Marit Trop Med Gdynia** 1980;31(1–2):5–13
Gerwel T: Słuzba zdrowia Marynarki Wojennej w konspiracji 1941–1945. **Przegl Lek** 1981;38(1):92–5
Krynicki A: Occurrence of occupational diseases among Polish seamen and fishermen in the years 1969–1977. **Bull Inst Marit Trop Med Gdynia** 1979;30(3–4):245–51

**Polar Regions**

Houston CS: New light on Dr. John Richardson. **Can Med Assoc J** 1984 Sep 15;131(6):653–4, 656–8, 660

**Spain**

Carmona Cornet AM: Ensayo sobre la medicina naval del año 1847. In International Congress of the History of Medicine, 27th, Barcelona, 1980. Actas. Barcelona, Académia de Ciències Médiques de Catalunya i Balears, 1981. p. 369–72.
Gella Iturriaga J: El médico mayor de la escuadra del pacífico: Oliva Muñoz. **Rev Gen Mar** 1980 Aug;199:3–14
Jordi R: Legislación sanitaria marítima española en vigor durante el siglo XIX. **Circ Farm** 1981 Jun;12(139):75–84
Orozco Acuaviva A: Pedro María González y el tratado de las enfermedades de la gente del mar. In International Congress of the History of Medicine, 27th, Barcelona, 1980. Actas. Barcelona, Académia de Ciències Médiques de Catalunya i Balears, 1981. p. 394–8.
Orozco Acuaviva A: Sabater y el empirismo anatomopatológico en el Hospital de Bellavista del Callao. In International Congress of the History of Medicine, 27th, Barcelona, 1980. Actas. Barcelona, Académia de Ciències Médiques de Catalunya i Balears, 1981. p. 401–7.
Orozco Acuaviva, A: El 'Compendio de medicina práctica' de Josef Salvaresa del Real Colegio de Cirugía de Cádiz. In International Congress of the History of Medicine, 27th, Barcelona, 1980. Actas. Barcelona, Académia de Ciències Médiques de Catalunya i Balears, 1981. p. 387–93.
Paredes Salido F: La cartilla de las compañias sanitarias de la armada

en el siglo XIX. **Rev Gen Mar** 1981 Aug;201:137-9
Richter T: Das Sargassokraut in Vicente de Lardizábals Werk 'Consuelo de Navegantes' (Madrid 1772). Diss., Universität Düsseldorf. Düsseldorf, 1982. 111 p.
Valverde JL, Sánchez F, Vinuesa L: Algunas consideraciones sobre la creación del empleo de boticario inspector de medicinas de la Armada. In International Congress of the History of Medicine, 27th, Barcelona, 1980. Actas. Barcelona, Acadèmia de Ciències Mèdiques de Catalunya i Balears, 1981. p. 426-31.
Valverde JL, Bautista Méndez II: Estudio del 'Formulario medicinal de embarco para uso de los cirujanos de la Armada durante la navegación' de 1789. In International Congress of the History of Medicine, 27th, Barcelona, 1980. Actas. Barcelona, Acadèmia de Ciències Mèdiques de Catalunya i Balears, 1981. p. 420-5.
Valverde JL, Sanchez L. De Vinuesa F: Los inspectores de medicinas de la Armada en el siglo XVIII. **Bol Soc Esp Hist Farm** 1980 Oct;31(123):191-203

**Sweden**

Goerke H: Carl von Linné als Marinearzt (1739-1741). In Göpfert W, Otten HH, ed: Metavoeite: wandelt euch durch neues Denken. Düsseldorf, Triltsch, 1983. p. 89-94.
Strandell B: Linné och Stockholm. **Sven Farm Tidskr** 1979;83:677-84

**Turkey**

Gençer AI: Istanbul tersansesinde acilan ilk tib mektebi **Tarih Dergesi (Turkey)** 1977;31:301-16

**United States**

Beatty WK: James Nevins Hyde: pioneer dermatologist and staunch Navy man. **Proc Inst Med Chic** 1982 Oct-Dec;35(4):139-42
Cushman P: Amos Evans, M.D.; surgeon on U.S.S. Constitution in War of 1812. **NY State J Med** 1980 Oct;80(11):1753-6
The Dental Corps of the United States Navy: Washington, Bureau of Medicine and Surgery, Navy Dept. 73 p.
Estes JW: Naval medicine in the age of sail: the voyage of the New York, 1802-1803. **Bull Hist Med** 1982 Summer;56(2):238-53
Foraker AG: A reluctant surgeon at sea. **JAMA** 1981 Jun 12;245(22):2302-3
Fortuine R: Ships' surgeons and naturalists in the early history of Alaska. **Alaska Med** 1984 Apr-Jun;26(2):57-61
Fortuine R: Ships' surgeons and naturalists in the early history of Alaska. Parts 2 and 3. **Alaska Med** 1984 Jul-Sep;26(3):82-6; Oct-Dec;26(4):117-21
Guthorn PJ: William Augustus Newell, M.D., and the Life Saving Service. **J Med Soc NJ** 1984 Sep;81(9):769-72
Herman JK: Home of BUMED, a hilltop in Foggy Bottom. **US Navy Med** 1982 Feb;73(2):9-15 contd.
Herman JK: Home of BUMED: a hilltop in Foggy Bottom. Controversy and transition, 1917-1942. **US Navy Med** 1983 Mar-Apr;74(2):8-17 concl
Herman JK: Home of BUMED: a hilltop in Foggy Bottom. The golden age (part 1). **US Navy Med** 1982 Jun;73(6):11-21
Herman JK: Home of BUMED: a hilltop in Foggy Bottom. Where medical college left off. The U.S. Naval Medical School and Naval Hospital 1902-1917. **US Navy Med** 1983 Jan-Feb;74(1):8-17 contd
Langley HD: Edward Field: a pioneer practitioner of the old Navy. **Conn Med** 1982 Nov;46(11):667-72
Langley HD: Respect for civilian authority: the tragic career of Captain Angus. **Am Neptune** 1980;40(1):23-37
Logue DC: Treating the wounded abroad USS Monitor, 1862. **US Navy Med** 1982 Jan;73(1):4-5
Murphey GT: A Navy dentist's diary: from Okinawa to Viet Nam. (Griffin T. Murphey). **Dent Stud** 1979 Oct;58(2):52-4, 59, 67
Skalley M, Skalley R: A medal for Marigold: Seattle's marine medic. Seattle, Superior Pub. Co., 1982. 150 p.
Stewart WJ: Ross McIntire. In Dictionary of American Biography, Suppl. 6, 1956-1960. p. 413-14, 1980.
Steyn RW: Retrospections: a sketch of nautical psychiatry through World War II. **Milit Med** 1980 Jun;145(6):407-12
Wilbur DA: The inimitable surgeon Pleadwell. **US Navy Med** 1983 May-Jun;74(3):5-10

**USSR**

Baranovskiĭ GIa, Kapitonov GI: Nekotorye voprosy podgotovki i organizatsii raboty sanitarno-transportnykh sudov v period Velikoĭ Otechestvennoĭ voiny. **Voen Med Zh** 1984 May;(5):25-8
Caudill RP: Soviet naval medicine: Military Medical Order of Lenin Medical Academy Imeni S. M. Kirov (VNEA). **US Navy Med** 1980;71(10):16-7
Cherokov VS: Mediki Krasnoznamennoĭ Ladozhskoĭ voennŏi flotilii. **Voen Med Zh** 1980 Jan;(1):66-7
Grigorenko GF: K 110-letiiu Vladivostokskogo voenno-morskogo gospitalia. **Vestn Khir** 1983 May;130(5):142-3
Krymkevich NI: Kniga D.P. Sinopeusa 'Parerga medica'. **Sov Zdravookhr** 1980;(11):66-8
Krymkevich NI: Vklad vracheĭ russkogo voenno-morskogo flota v razvitie gigieny pitaniia v Rossii (II polovina XIX - nachalo XX veka). **Vopr Pitan** 1981 Sep-Oct;(5):72-4
Lukavskiĭ MI, Ugulava SN: Voenno-morskomu Krasnoznamennomu gospitaliu imeni akademika N. I. Pirogova--200 let. **Voen Med ZH** 1983 May;5:71-3
Matusov AL: Iz istorii meditsinskogo obespecheniia russkikh morskikh i poliarnykh ekspeditsiĭ. Leningrad, Gidrometeoizdat, 1972. 118 p.
Nikitin EA: Fel'dsher revoliutsionnogo korablia P. F. Glinkov. **Feldsher Akush** 1982;47(11):36-7
Petrov BD: 'Sposob sokhraneniia zdorov'ia morskikh sluzhiteleĭ'. **Gig Sanit** 1981 Feb;(2):42-3
Potemkin NT, Donchenko GP: Meditsinskoe obespechenie Voenno-Morskogo Flota v gody voĭny. **Voen Med Zh** 1980 May;(5):38-41
Semenov SV: K istorii organizatsii gosudarstvennogo sanitarnogo nadzora na vodnom transporte v RSFSR. **Gig Sanit** 1984 Jan;(1):36-8
Zolotarev V: Zapiska starshego vracha kreisera avrora. **Voen Istor Zh** 1976;(1):51-60

**Yugoslavia**

Popović M: Razvoj Instituta za pomorsku medicinu Ratne mornarice. **Vojnosanit Pregl** 1980 Sep-Oct;37(5):319-26
Zorn E: Geschichte und Bedeutung des Marinehospitals von Pola/Jugoslawien. **Hist Hosp** 1979-80;13:135-46

# NEUROLOGY

See also **Psychiatry; Surgery-Neurological**

Abdullaev MS: Aristotel'i razvitie predstavleniĭ o nervnoĭ sisteme. **Arkh Anat Gistol Embriol** 1984 Sep;87(9):97-103
Angelis E de: Rapporti tra mente e corpo dall'eta' classica al XIX secolo. **Med Secoli** 1982 May-Aug;19(2):193-213
Bell BA: A history of the study of cerebral edema. **Neurosurgery** 1983 Dec;13(6):724-8
Bonica JJ: Pain. **Res Publ Assoc Res Nerv Ment Dis** 1980;58:1-17
Bossy J: Acupuncture et organisation nerveuse periphérique, segmentaire et intersegmentaire. In Mazars G, ed: Les médecines traditionnelles de l'Asie. Strasbourg, Université Louis Pasteur, 1981. p. 41-8.
Brazier MA: A history of neurophysiology in the 17th and 18th centuries: from concept to experiment. New York, Raven Press, 1984. xiii, 230 p.
Brazier MA: Challenges from the philosophers to the neuroscientists. In Brain and mind. Ciba Foundation Symposium 69 (new series). Amsterdam, Oxford, New York, Excerpta Medica, 1979. p. 5-43.
Bruyn GW: The seat of the soul. In Rose FC, Bynum WF, ed: Historical aspects of the neurosciences. New York, Raven, 1982. p. 55-81.
Cain AM, ed: A catalog of the Percival Bailey collection of neurology & psychiatry. Chicago, Library of the Health Sciences, University of Illinois at the Medical Center, Chicago, 1973. viii, 230 p.
Casey AE, Copeland H, Downey-Prince EL, et al: Differential craniometry: (A) Maori 3000 BC--Thera? (B). Ptolemaic Egyptians--New Guinea, America. **Ala J Med Sci** 1979 Oct;16(4):382-9
Castro-Vázquez A: The dawn of neuroendocrinology: conquest and heroes. **Acta Physiol Lat Am** 1981;31(3):151-9
Cilenti V, Milasi G, Jori A: Evoluzione storica del concetto di dolore. **Med Secoli** 1982 May-Aug;19(2):225-30
Drazan JG: The nightmare: a checklist of the world literature to 1976. Palo Alto, R & E Research Associates, 1979.
Dyck P: Lumbar nerve root: the enigmatic eponyms. **Spine** 1984 Jan-Feb;9(1):3-6
Ehni G: Seeking the hidden flaw. **Spine** 1981 Jul-Aug;6(4):369-74
Farina G: Interpretazioni cartesiane. **Med Secoli** 1982 May-Aug;19(2):221-4
Gawel M: The development of concepts concerning cerebral circulation. In Rose FC, Bynum WF, ed: Historical aspects of the neurosciences. New York, Raven, 1982. p. 171-8.
Gibson HB: Pain and its conquest. London, Boston, Peter Owen, 1982. 224 p.
Girard P: Geschichte der Neurologie. In Sournia JC, Martiny M, Poulet J, ed: Illustrierte Geschichte der Medizin. Salzburg, Andreas, 1980. Vol. 3. p. 1125-88.
Hartmann F: Homo patiens. Zur ärztlichen Anthropologie von Leid und Mitleid. In Seidler E, Schott H, ed: Bausteine zur Medizingeschichte. Stuttgart, Steiner, 1984. p. 35-44.
Hufschmidt HJ: Das Rechts-Links-Profil im kulturhistorischen Längsschnitt. Ein Dominanzproblem. **Arch Psychiatr Nervenkr** 1980;229(1):17-43
Kassler JC: Man - a musical instrument: models of the brain and mental functioning before the computer. **Hist Sci** 1984 Mar;22(55 pt 1):59-92
McHenry LC: Neurology and Art. In Rose FC, Bynum WF, ed: Historical aspects of the neurosciences. New York, Raven, 1982. p. 481-519.
Manson Thomas ML, Cooper WC, ed: Catalog of works in the neurological sciences collected by Cyril Brian Courville, M.D., representative of

clinical neurology, neuroanatomy and neuropathology, with particular reference to head trauma, and books from historical medicine in the Medical Sciences Library, University of California, Irvine. Irvine, University of California, 1978. 239 p.
Medvei VC: Some notes on the history of neuroendocrinology. In Rose FC, Bynum WF, ed: Historical aspects of the neurosciences. New York, Raven, 1982. p. 307–15.
Meier RY: 'Sympathy' as a concept in early neurophysiology. Ph.D. Diss. The University of Chicago. Chicago, 1979.
Merskey H: Some features of the history of the idea of pain. **Pain** 1980 Aug;9(1):3–8
Mianet JC: Contribution à l'histoire des nerfs craniens. Diss. Paris V, René Descartes, 1981. 162, xiii leaves.
Michler M: Zur Entstehung des medizinischen Schmerzbegriffes. **Orthop Prax** 1979;15(5):347–50
Milos G, Akert K: Die neurobiologischen Grundlagen der binoculären Raumwahrnehmung. Historische Übersicht über die Entwicklung der Vorstellungen und Erkenntnisse. **Schweiz Arch Neurol Neurochir Psychiatr** 1982;130(1):39–67
Molina-Negro P: Le rôle des neurostimulateurs dans le traitement de la douleur chronique rebelle. **Union Med Can** 1980 Jan;109(1):41–54
Möller HJ: Die Begriffe 'Reizbarkeit' und 'Reiz': Konstanz und Wandel ihres Bedeutungsgehaltes sowie die Problematik ihrer exakten Definition. Stuttgart, Fischer, 1975. viii, 104 p. (Medizin in Geschichte und Kultur, 11).
Nakajima M: [Clinical study of pain]. Continued regularly. (Jpn). **Kangogaku Zasshi** 1984 May;48(5):569–72
Neuburger M: The historical development of experimental brain and spinal cord physiology before Flourens. Edited by E. Clarke. Baltimore and London, Johns Hopkins University Press, 1981. xxiii, 391 p. (Trans. of 1897 ed).
Ochs S: The early history of material transport in nerve. **Physiologist** 1979 Oct;22(5):16–9
Ohry A: On pain. **Koroth** 1982;8(3–4):199–204
O'Neill YV: Speech and speech disorders in Western thought before 1600. Westport, Connecticut, Greenwood, 1980. xii, 246 p. (Contributions in medical history, No. 3).
Ottoson D: Smärta och smärtbehandling genom tiderna. **Sydsven Medicinhist Sallsk Arsskr** 1980;:134–48
Peacock A: The relationship between the soul and the brain. In Rose FC, Bynum WF, ed: Historical aspects of the neurosciences. New York, Raven, 1982. p. 83–98.
Riese W: Selected papers on the history of aphasia. With an introduction by W. Gooddy. Edited with prefatory notes by R. Hoops, Y. Lebrun, E. Buyssens. Amsterdam, Swets and Zeitlinger, 1977. 144 p. (Neurolinguistics, 7).
Salomone G, Lambiase M: Appunti storici sulla teoria del neurone. **Acta Neurol (Napoli)** 1983 Feb;5(1):62–76
Schadewaldt H: Geschichte der Schmerzbehandlung. **Med Welt** 1980 Sep 5;31(36):1277–9
Schiller F: Historical note on sleep and eye movements. **Sleep** 1984;7(3):199–201
Schiller F: Semantics of sleep. **Bull Hist Med** 1982 Fall;56(3):378–97
Seitelberger F: The role of neuropathology in the neurosciences. In Rose FC, Bynum WF, ed: Historical aspects of the neurosciences. New York, Raven, 1982. p. 265–72.
Soriano V: Neurotransmitters. **Int J Neurol** 1979;13(1–4):9–23
Stoessel I: Scheintod und Todesangst. Aeusserungsformen der Angst in ihren geschichtlichen Wandlungen (17.–20. Jahrhundert). Köln, 1983. 247 p. (Kölner medizinhistorische Beiträge, Band 30)
Torack RM: Historical aspects of normal and abnormal brain fluids. **Arch Neurol** 1982 Apr;39(4):197–201; May;39(5):276–9
Velasco-Suárez M: El cerebro humano. Su evolución conceptual. **Gac Med Mex** 1982 Oct;118(10):395–402
Zimmermann M: Electrical stimulation of the human brain. **Hum Neurobiol** 1982;1(4):227–9

**Americas**

Lex BW: Neurological bases of revitalization movements. **Zygon** 1978;13(4):276–312

**Germany**

Brooks CM, Seller H: Early and late contributions to our knowledge of the autonomic nervous system and its control made by German scientists. **J Auton Nerv Syst** 1981 Apr;3(2–4):105–19
Heintel B: Historische Stätten der Neurologie in Baden-Württemberg. Stuttgart; New York, G. Fischer, 1982. [66] p.

**Great Britain**

Harris R: An excursion in serendipity--the conquest of pain. **Ann R Australas Coll Dent Surg** 1979 Nov;6:103–11

**Netherlands**

Schulte BP, Endtz LJ: A short history of neurology in the Netherlands. **Int J Neurol** 1979;13(1–4):62

**Spain**

Campillo D, Turbón D: Cráneo trepanado de la Bauma dels Ossos. In International Congress of the History of Medicine, 27th, Barcelona, 1980. Actas. Barcelona, Académia de Ciències Médiques de Catalunya i Balears, 1981. p. 472–9.

**Before 500 A.D.**

Escobar A, Aruffo C: La paleoneurología y el desarrollo del cerebro en los homínidos. **Gac Med Mex** 1980 Mar;116(3):115–32
Holloway RL: Exploring the dorsal surface of hominoid brain endocasts by stereoplotter and discriminant analysis. **Philos Trans R Soc Lond [Biol]** 1981 May 8;292(1057):155–66
Holloway RL: Volumetric and asymmetry determinations on recent hominid endocasts: Spy I and II, Djebel Ihroud I, and the Sale Homo erectus specimens, with some notes on Neanderthal brain size. **Am J Phys Anthropol** 1981 Jul;55(3):385–93
Swinton WE: Brains of dinosaurs. In Rose FC, Bynum WF, ed: Historical aspects of the neurosciences. New York, Raven, 1982. p. 473–9.

**Denmark**

Halaburt H, Langfeldt B, Rasmussen P: Computerized tomography (CT-scan) of a 2,500-year-old Danish 'Queen'. **Acta Neurochir (Wien)** 1981;56(3–4):153–5

**Greece**

Lokhorst GJ: An ancient Greek theory of hemispheric specialization. **Clio Med** 1982 May;17(1):33–8
Oberhelman SM: The interpretation of prescriptive dreams in ancient Greek medicine. **J Hist Med Allied Sci** 1981 Oct;36(4):416–24

**Tanzania**

Holloway RL: The O.H. 7 (Olduvai Gorge, Tanzania) hominid partial brain endocast revisited. **Am J Phys Anthropol** 1980 Aug;53(2):267–74

**500 A.D.–1450**

Barcia Goyanes JJ: Los nombres medievales del 'infundibulum'. **Med Esp** 1981;80:139–44

**Great Britain**

Rowland B: Bishop Bradwardine on the artificial memory. **J Warburg Courtauld Inst** 1978;41:307–12

**1450–1700**

Faller A: Die Präparation der weissen Substanz des Gehirns bei Stensen, Willis und Vieussens. **Gesnerus** 1982;39(2):171–93
Lokhorst GJ: The oldest printed text on hemispheric specialization. **Neurology** 1982 Jul;32(7):762

**Denmark**

Faller A: Wertschätzung von Stensens 'Discours sur l'anatomie du cerveau' im Verlaufe von drei Jahrhunderten. Aarau, Verlag Sauerländer, 1981. 96 p. (Veröffentlichungen der Schweizerischen Gesellschaft für Geschichte der Medizin und der Naturwissenschaften, 35).

**France**

Amalric P: La naissance de la neuro-ophtalmologie à Montpellier au XVIIme siècle à travers l'oeuvre de Raymond Vieussens et de Guilhem Briggs. **Bull Soc Ophtalmol Fr** 1983 Jan;83(1):83–8

**Great Britain**

Dewhurst K: Thomas Willis and the foundations of British neurology. In Rose FC, Bynum WF, ed: Historical aspects of the neurosciences. New York, Raven, 1982. p. 327–46.
Hughes JT: Spinal cord arteries described by Willis. In Rose FC, Bynum WF, ed: Historical aspects of the neurosciences. New York, Raven, 1982. p. 195–203.
Meier RY: 'Sympathy' in the neurophysiology of Thomas Willis. **Clio Med** 1982 Dec;17(2–3):95–111
Whitteridge G: Harvey and sensory neuropathy. **J R Coll Physicians Lond** 1981 Jan;15(1):61–2

### Italy

Schott GD: Some neurological observations on Leonardo da Vinci's handwriting. **J Neurol Sci** 1979 Aug;42(3):321–9

Todd EM: The neuroanatomy of Leonardo da Vinci. Santa Barbara, Capra Press, 1983. 189 p.

### Netherlands

Brazier MA: The problem of neuromuscular action: two 17th century Dutchmen. In Rose FC, Bynum WF, ed: Historical aspects of the neurosciences. New York, Raven, 1982. p. 13–22.

Pytel' AIa: Bol', prishedshaia iz glubiny vekov (k 375-letiiu so dnia rozhdeniia Rembrandta). **Sov Med** 1980;(12):98–9

### Switzerland

Schiller F: A note on the Pickwickian syndrome and Felix Platter (1536–1614). **J Hist Med Allied Sci** 1985 Jan;40(1):66–7

### 1700 to Present

Arendt A: Die Rolle der Neuropathologie in der Allgemeinen Pathologie und Speziellen Pathologischen Anatomie. **Zentralbl Neurochir** 1983;44(2):113–20

Bakalkin GIa, Taborko MM: Neĭropeptidy: istoriia izucheniia i perspektivy primeneniia v meditsine. **Bol Serv Odontol Saint (Porto Alegre)** 1981;4(2):100–5

Bay E: Neurologie im Wandel. **Jahrb Univ Dusseld** 1977–78;:135–52

Bay E: Sigmund Freud's contribution to the early history of aphasiology. In Rose FC, Bynum WF, ed: Historical aspects of the neurosciences. New York, Raven, 1982. p. 103–7.

Bedwell SF: D'Anville's doom--a neurological vignette from historic Halifax. **Can J Neurol Sci** 1980 Feb;7(1):1–8

Bender MB, Shanzer S: History of binocular movements. In Rose FC, Bynum WF, ed: Historical aspects of the neurosciences. New York, Raven, 1982. p. 45–54.

Black SE: Pseudopods and synapses: the amoeboid theories of neuronal mobility and the early formulation of the synapse concept, 1894–1900. **Bull Hist Med** 1981 Spring;55(1):34–58

Blaschko H: Frederick Hughes Scott and his contribution to the early history of the transmitter concept. **Notes Rec R Soc Lond** 1983 Mar;37(2):235–47

A brief history of the European meetings on electroencephalography and epileptology better known as the 'Colloques de Marseille': **Electroencephalogr Clin Neurophysiol** 1982;(35):VIII–XI

Bucy PC: The pioneers of neurology and neurosurgery in the world and their contributions. A lecture for young Japanese neurosurgeons. **No Shinkei Geka** 1982 May;10(5):490–8

Bull JW: The history of neuroradiology. In Rose FC, Bynum WF, ed: Historical aspects of the neurosciences. New York, Raven, 1982. p. 255–64.

Degleris N: Contribution à l'étude des relations Franco-Helleniques au point de vue de la presse neuro-psychiatrique française (1880–1914); les membres associés grecs de la Société Médico-Psychologique. Mémoire pour le titre d'assistant étranger, Université Paris V, René Descartes, Faculté de Médecine Cochin-Port Royal, Paris, 1984. 96 leaves.

Denny-Brown D: The development of procedures in clinical neurology. **Trans Stud Coll Physicians Phila** 1980 Mar;5(2 no 1):26–30

Ebers GC, Stewart J: In defence of Osler. **J R Soc Med** 1982 Dec;75(12):989

Ecker A: The discovery of human cerebral arterial spasm in angiograms: an autobiographical note.. **Neurosurgery** 1982 Jan;10(1):90

Elliott FA: Biological roots of violence. **Proc Am Philos Soc** 1983 Apr 20;127(2):84–94

Estévez González A: Anotaciones a la historia de la neuropsicoloía. **Arch Neurobiol (Madr)** 1980 Nov–Dec;43(6):401–20

Estévez González A: El cerebro frontal y motor, según Luria. Su patologia, síndromes y afasias. **Arch Neurobiol (Madr)** 1981 Mar–Apr;44(2):75–94

Euler US von: Chemical neurotransmission--yesterday and today. **Ciba Found Symp** 1982;(91):3–12

Feldberg WS: Fifty years on--looking back on some developments in neurohumoral physiology. Liverpool, Liverpool University Press, 1982. xiii, 106 p.

Fullinwider SP: Sigmund Freud, John Hughlings Jackson, and speech. **J Hist Ideas** 1983 Jan–Mar;44(1):151–8

Fulton JF: History of medicine-Arnold Klebs and Harvey Cushing at the 1st International Neurological Congress at Berne in 1931. **Int J Neurol** 1980;14(1):103–15

Galaburda AM: La région de Broca: observations anatomiques faites un siècle après la mort de son découvreur. **Rev Neurol (Paris)** 1980;136(10):609–16

Gallistel CR: Bell, Magendie, and the proposals to restrict the use of animals in neurobehavioral research. **Am Psychol** 1981 Apr;36(4):357–60

Gooddy W: Charles Edward Brown-Séquard. In Rose FC, Bynum WF, ed: Historical aspects of the neurosciences. New York, Raven, 1982. p. 371–8.

Gooddy W: Dr. Brown-Sequard in space and time. **Trans Hunter Soc** 1978–80;37–38:153–9

Hamanaka Y: [Basic neuropsychologic concepts and their origins (conclusion)] (Jpn). **No To Shinkei** 1983 Mar;35(3):310–1

Hamburger V: S. Ramón y Cajal, R. G. Harrison, and the beginnings of neuroembryology. **Perspect Biol Med** 1980;23(4):600–16

Hebb DO: Neuropsychology: retrospect and prospect. **Can J Psychol** 1983 Mar;37(1):4–7

Hécaen H: L'evolution et les perspectives de la neuropsychologie. **Acta Neurol Latinoam** 1980;26(2):75–102

Heywood C: D. H. Lawrence's 'blood consciousness' and the work of Xavier Bichat and Marshall Hall. **Etud Anglaises** 1979;32:397–413

Hicks TP: The history and development of microiontophoresis in experimental neurobiology. **Prog Neurobiol** 1984;22(3):185–240

Hubel DH: Cortical neurobiology: a slanted historical perspective. **Annu Rev Neurosci** 1982;5:363–70

Hubel DH: Evolution of ideas on the primary visual cortex, 1955–1978: a biased historical account. **Biosci Rep** 1982 Jul;2(7):435–69

Hubel DH: Exploration of the primary visual cortex, 1955–78. **Nature** 1982 Oct 7;299(5883):515–24

Illingworth R: Historical concepts of spinal cord pathways subserving pain. In Rose FC, Bynum WF, ed: Historical aspects of the neurosciences. New York, Raven, 1982. p. 209–12.

Jasper HH, Sourkes TL: Nobel laureates in neuroscience: 1904–1981. **Annu Rev Neurosci** 1983;6:1–42

Jokl E: Sherrington, his life and thought: essay-review. **Trans Stud Coll Physicians Phila** 1980 Sep;5(2 no 3):223–35

Joynt RJ: The great confrontation: the meeting between Broca and Jackson in 1868. In Rose FC, Bynum WF, ed: Historical aspects of the neurosciences. New York, Raven, 1982. p. 99–102.

Kleinman LC, McHenry LC: Fragments of neurologic history: phrenology's founders look at the spinal cord. **Neurology** 1984 Apr;34(4):505

Kugler J: Von den Anfängen der Neurophysiologie zur Gegenwart. **MMW** 1981 May 8;123(19):789–90

Lanteri-Laura G: La constitution civile du cerveau. **Rev Int Hist Psychiatr** 1983;1(1):23–45

Lanteri Laura G: L'hystérie. Matrice de la sémiologie neurologique. In Poirier J, Poirier JL, ed: Médecine et philosophie à la fin du XIXe siècle. Paris, Université de Paris XII - Val de Marne, [1980?]. p. 141–8.

Lavie P: Nasal obstructions, sleep, and mental function. **Sleep** 1983;6(3):244–6

Legée G: Evolution de l'histologie du système nerveux au XIXe siècle; l'impulsion donnée par Camillo Golgi (1844–1926). **Clio Med** 1982 May;17(1):15–32

Legée G: La notion de temps dans la physiologie neuro-musculaire au XIXe siècle. In: Congrès National des Sociétés Savantes, 99e, Besançon, 1974. Comptes Rendus. Paris, 1976. Section des Sciences, Fasc. V. p. 203–13.

Lepore FE: Toward a definition of papilledema: a historical review, 1851–1911. **Surg Neurol** 1982 Mar;17(3):178–80

Leys R: Background to the reflex controversy: William Alison and the doctrine of sympathy before Hall. **Stud Hist Biol** 1980;4:1–66

Lissak K: Tvorcheskoe sodruzhestvo vengerskikh i sovetskikh issledovateleĭ mozga. **Zh Vyssh Nerv Deiat** 1982 Nov–Dec;32(6):1183–4

Livingston KE, Hornykiewicz O, ed: Limbic mechanisms. The continuing evolution of the limbic system concept. New York and London, Plenum, 1976. xv, 542 p. Tribute to James W. Papez; biographical contributions by P. D. MacLean, J. B. Angevine, P. I. Yakovlev.

Ljunggren B, Säveland H, Brandt L: Aneurysmal subarachnoid hemorrhage--historical background from a Scandinavian horizon. **Surg Neurol** 1984 Dec;22(6):605–16

Lohff B: Die Entwicklung des Experimentes im Bereich der Nervenphysiologie; Gedanken und Arbeiten zum Begriff der Irritabilität und der Lebenskraft. **Sudhoffs Arch** 1980;64(2):105–29

McGuigan FJ: The historical development of cognitive psychophysiology: theory and measurement. In E. Schultheisz, ed: History of physiology. Oxford, Elmsford, New York, Pergamon, 1981. xvi, 208 p. (Advances in Physiological Sciences. Proceedings of the 28th International Congress of Physiological Sciences, Budapest, 1980. Volume 21). p. 29–47.

McHenry LC: L'idea e la mano. **Kos** 1984 Jul–Aug;1(6):79–90

McMurry JF: Oskar Hirsch and surgery for exophthalmos. In Romm S, ed: Symposium on historical perspectives of plastic surgery. Philadelphia, Saunders, 1983. p. 649–52.

Madrid Arias JL: Evolución histórica de los agentes neurolíticos utilizados para tratamiento del dolor crónico. **Rev Esp Anestesiol Reanim** 1984 Sep–Oct;31(5):197–204

Maiat VS, Kliminskiĭ IV, Maiat KE: K istorii vagotomii. **Klin Med (Mosk)** 1980 Sep;58(9):105–11

Marinesco M, Argemi-Lloveras J: Georges Marinescu (Roumanie) et Santiago Ramon y Cajal; deux représentants du génie latin. In International Congress of the History of Medicine, 27th, Barcelona, 1980. Actas. Barcelona, Acadèmia de Ciències Mèdiques de Catalunya i Balears, 1981. p. 570–4.

Massey EW, Schoenberg B: Foster Kennedy syndrome. **Arch Neurol** 1984 Jun;41(6):658–9

Mattar E: Reminiscênias históricas da endocrinologia. Uma introdução à

neuroendocrinologia e suas fronteiras. **Rev Hosp Clin Fac Med Sao Paulo** 1980 Aug;35(4):218–22
Matthews PB: Evolving views on the internal operation and functional role of the muscle spindle. **J Physiol (Lond)** 1981 Nov;320:1–30
Mecacci L: Le illusioni ottiche nell'Ottocento tra fenomenologia e neurofisiologia. **Stor Crit Psicol** 1983 Dec;4(2):287–9
Meyer A: The search for a morphological substrate in the brains of eminent persons including musicians: a historical review. In Critchley M, Henson RA, ed: Music and the brain: studies in the neurology of music. London, Heinemann, 1977. p. 255–81.
Meyer L: Cristofredo Jakob. A veinticinco años de su muerte. **Acta Psiquiatr Psicol Am Lat** 1981 Mar;27(1):13–4
Money J: The genealogical descent of sexual psychoneuroendocrinology from sex and health theory: the eighteenth to the twentieth centuries. **Psychoneuroendocrinology** 1983;8(4):391–400
Morte PD: Neurologic aspects of human anomalies. **West J Med** 1983 Aug;139(2):250–6
Neu I: Entwicklung und heutiger Stand der klinishen Neurologie. **Fortschr Med** 1980 Oct 2;98(37):1397–9
Nielzén S: Ljudets väg från öra till perception; en sammanställning av biologiska bakgrunder till ljudupplevande bl.a. med utblick mot psykiatrin. **Sydsven Medicinhist Sallsk Arsskr** 1982;19:99–108
Ojemann RG: Biography of C. Miller Fisher, M.D. **Clin Neurosurg** 1983;31:xiii–xxviii
Pallis C: From brain death to brain stem death. **Br Med J [Clin Res]** 1982 Nov 20;285(6353):1487–90
Présentation des grands syndromes cliniques par atteinte focale des hémisphères cérébraux et par lésion du corps calleux. Données historiques: **Rev Med Suisse Romande** 1984 Jul;104(7):477–91
Pretresco A: Dos conmemoraciones. **Rev Neuropsiquiatr** 1980 Jun;43(2):115–23
Reis DJ: The brain and hypertension: reflections on 35 years of inquiry into the neurobiology of the circulation. **Circulation** 1984 Nov;70(5 Pt 2):III31–45
Riabinina MA: K istorii otkrytiia ritmiki élektricheskikh protsessov golovnogo mozga. **Zh Vyssh Nerv Deiat** 1981 Jan–Feb;31(1):192–5
Rokhlin LL, Shereshevskiĭ AM, Tom A: Znamenatel'nye daty 1982 g. **Zh Nevropatol Psikhiatr** 1982;82(1):130–40
Rokhlin LL, Shereshevskiĭ AM, Tom A: Znamenatel'nye i iubileĭnye daty nevropatologii i psikhiatrii 1983 g. **Zh Nevropatol Psikhiatr** 1983;83(1):122–33
Sarnat HB: The discovery, proof and reproof of neurosecretion (Speidel, 1917; Scharrer and Scharrer, 1934). **Can J Neurol Sci** 1983 Aug;10(3):208–12
Schierhorn H: Egas Moniz, Wilhelm Löhr und die cerebrale Angiographie. Ein Streifzug durch die Entdeckungsgeschichte der Hirngefässe. **J Hirnforsch** 1981;22(5):491–515
Schiller F: A Möbius strip. Fin-de-siècle neuropsychiatry and Paul Möbius. Berkeley, University of California Press, 1982. 134 p.
Schiller F: Neurology: the electrical root. In Rose FC, Bynum WF, ed: Historical aspects of the neurosciences. New York, Raven, 1982. p. 1–11.
Schiller F: When is posterior not dorsal but medial? **Neurology** 1984 Apr;34(4):511–4
Schneck JM: Sigmund Freud, Josef Breuer, and Freud's self-observations on meralgia paresthetica. **NY State J Med** 1983 Jun;83(7):968–9
Sicuteri F: The Enrico Greppi International Headache Award. A tribute to the memory of one of medicine's pioneers. **Cephalalgia** 1983 Mar;3(1):11–3
Smith DB, Delgado Escueta AV, Cramer JA, et al: Historical perspective on the choice of antiepileptic drugs for the treatment of seizures in adults. **Neurology** 1983 Mar;33(3 Suppl 1):2–7
Spillane JD: The evolution of the concepts of peripheral paralysis and of sensory ataxia in the 19th century. In Rose FC, Bynum WF, ed: Historical aspects of the neurosciences. New York, Raven, 1982. p. 23–36.
Steiner TJ: Development of the concept of supraspinal control. In Rose FC, Bynum WF, ed: Historical aspects of the neurosciences. New York, Raven, 1982. p. 37–43.
Stoffregen M: Zur Rolle histochemischer Phänomene bei der Erforschung und Systematisierung des chromaffinen Gewebes. **Medizinhist J** 1984;19(3):191–209
Sunderland S: Advances in diagnosis and treatment of root and peripheral nerve injury. **Adv Neurol** 1979;22:271–305
Tammisto T: Kipu muuttuvassa maailmassa. **Duodecim** 1981;97(14):1013–6
Tolosa ES, Klawans HL: Meiges disease: a clinical form of facial convulsion, bilateral and medical. **Arch Neurol** 1979 Oct;36(10):635–7
Torack RM: Historical aspects of normal and abnormal brain fluids. III. Cerebral edema. **Arch Neurol** 1982 Jun;39(6):355–7
Troncale JA: Nineteenth century neurology/psychiatry. **J Med Assoc State Ala** 1982 Aug;52(2):29–30, 32–5
Tyler KL, McHenry LC: Fragments of neurological history: the knee jerk and other tendon reflexes. **Neurosci Behav Physiol** 1983 May;13(5):609–10
Van der Kloot W: Otto Loewi. In Dictionary of American biography, 1961–1965. Suppl. 7, 1981. p. 475–7.
Vidal F: La discontinuité de la douleur chez les physiologistes du XVIIIe siècle. **Inf Dent** 1983 Dec 8;65(43):4243–8
Voogd J: Morphology and clinical neurology. The history and evolution of Wallenberg's syndrome. **Acta Morphol Neerl Scand** 1983 Mar;21(1):27–47
Wilberger JE: Transplantation of central nervous tissue. **Neurosurgery** 1983 Jul;13(1):90–4
Yamakawa T: Wonders in glycolipids--a historical view. **Adv Exp Med Biol** 1984;174:3–13
Zieliński K: Ezras A. Asratyan. **Acta Neurobiol Exp (Warsz)** 1981;41(6):521–42

**Australia**

Eadie MJ: A. W. Campbell: Australia's first neurologist. **Clin Exp Neurol** 1980;17:27–35
Hooper R: Graeme Robertson and the golden age of neurology. **Proc Aust Assoc Neurol** 1978;15:1–10

**Austria**

Henn V: E. Mach on the analysis of motion sensation. **Hum Neurobiol** 1984;3(3):145–8
Zani A: Le origini storiche dell'elettroencefalografia. **Stor Crit Psicol** 1981;2(1):119–84

**Belgium**

Gerebtzoff MA: Recherches sur la structure du système nerveux et ses modifications expérimentales publiées dans les Archives de Biologie de 1880 à 1900. Analyse critique. **Arch Biol (Liege)** 1980;91(2):223–42

**Bulgaria**

Kilimov N: Georgi Uzunov. Sofiia, Izd-vo na Bŭlgarskata akademiia na naukite, 1978. 178 p.

**Canada**

Feindel W: The contributions of Wilder Penfield and the Montreal Neurological Institute to Canadian neurosciences. In Roland CG, ed: Health, disease and medicine. Toronto, Hannah Institute for the History of Medicine, 1984. p. 347–58.
Feindel W: The contributions of Wilder Penfield to the functional anatomy of the human brain. **Hum Neurobiol** 1982;1(4):231–4

**Chile**

Costa-Casaretto C: La cátedra de neuropsiquiatría de la Universidad de Chile desde 1891 hasta 1906. **Rev Med Chil** 1980 Sep;108(9):855–62
Costa-Casaretto C: Sobre el. Dr. Carlos Sazie, primer profesor de neurología y segundo de psiquiatria en la universidad de Chile (1881-1891). **Rev Med Chil** 1980 Aug;108(8):749–56
Pérez-Olea J: Don Augusto Orrego Luco. **Rev Med Chil** 1984 Feb;112(2):193–200

**China**

Hsu K: [Tao Lieh---the pioneer in neurosciences of our country] (Chi). **Sheng Li Ko Hsueh Chin Chan** 1980 Apr;11(4):376–8

**Cuba**

Rivero de la Calle M, Collado Lopez O: Reporte sobre las primeras mediciones craneometricas de tipo comparativo realizadas en Cuba. [H. J. Dumont.]. **Cienc Habana Ser 9** 1976;6:3–27

**Czechoslovakia**

Cernáček J: Počiatky neurológie na Slovensku. **Bratisl Lek Listy** 1982 Sep;78(3):363–9
Grüsser OJ: J.E. Purkyně's contributions to the physiology of the visual, the vestibular and the oculomotor systems. **Hum Neurobiol** 1984;3(3):129–44

**France**

Arquiola E: La antropologia criminal y la 'Societe d'Anthropologie' de Paris. **Asclepio** 1978–79;30–31:63–82
Biographical sketches no. 31--Lasèque: **Ir Med J** 1983 Aug;76(8):367
Brazier MA: The birth of the International Brain Research Organization: a tribute to Henri Gastaut. **Electroencephalogr Clin Neurophysiol** 1982;35:13–4
Broughton R: A brief outline of the career and accomplishments of Henri Gastaut. **Electroencephalogr Clin Neurophysiol** 1982;35:XII–XV
Capildeo R: Charcot in the 80s. In Rose FC, Bynum WF, ed: Historical aspects of the neurosciences. New York, Raven, 1982. p. 383–96.
Castaigne P: Centenaire de la Clinique des maladies du système nerveux de la Salpêtrière. Introduction. **Rev Neurol (Paris)** 1982;138(12):879–86
Castaigne P, Lhermitte F, Signoret JL, et al: Description et étude scannographique du cerveau de Leborgne. La découverte de Broca.

**Rev Neurol (Paris)** 1980;136(10):563–83
Castaigne P: Photographies et tomodensitométrie des deux cerveaux sur lesquels Broca fonda sa conception anatomoclinique de l'"aphémie'. **Bull Acad Natl Med (Paris)** 1979 Oct;163(7):663–7
Charbonnel A: Histoire de l'oto-neuro-ophtalmologie. **Rev Otoneuroophtalmol** 1979 Oct–Dec;51(5):399–416
Cimino G: Claude Bernard sulle 'funzioni del cervello'. **Physis** 1980;22(1):85–119
Clark D: Jules Tinel and Tinel's sign. In Romm S, ed: Symposium on historical perspectives of plastic surgery. Philadelphia, Saunders, 1983. p. 627–8.
Cohn DF: Joseph Babinski and his reflex (1857–1932). **Koroth** 1982 Aug;8(3/4):191–4
Critchley M: Dax's law. **Int J Neurol** 1978;11(4):404–11
Delmas A: Paul Broca et l'anatomie. **Bull Acad Natl Med (Paris)** 1980;164(6):552–6
Dubarry JJ: J. Vincent Laborde et son procédé de réanimation par tractions rythmées de la langue; la survie neuro-musculaire après décapitation. **Hist Sci Med** 1980;14(1):77–82
Ekbom K: Mannen bakom syndromen: Jean-Martin Charcot. Under hans inspirerande ledning skapades den klassiska franska neurologin. **Lakartidningen** 1984 Jun 6;81(23):2363–4
Endtz LJ: La neurologie et l'illustration photographique du livre médical. **Rev Neurol (Paris)** 1983;139(6–7):439–44
Henri Gastaut and the Marseilles school's contribution to the neurosciences: Proceedings of the 25th and final Colloque de Marseille. **Electroencephalogr Clin Neurophysiol** 1982;35:1–447
Houdart R: Paul Broca, précurseur des disciplines neurologiques. **Chirurgie** 1980;106(10):783–6
Huard P, Aaron C, Askienazy S, et al: Le cerveau de Paul Broca (1824–1880). Confrontation anatomo-pathologique et tomo-densitométrique. **J Radiol** 1982 Mar;63(3):175–80
Huard P, Imbault-Huart MJ: Vicq d'Azyr et la nomenclature moderne des nerfs crâniens. In: Congrès National des Sociétés Savantes, 105e, Caen, 1980. Comptes Rendus, Paris, 1980. Section des Sciences, Fasc. V. p. 61–83.
Kenéz J: Joseph Babinski (1857–1932) a francia klinikai neurológia egyik úttörője. **Orv Hetil** 1984 Jan 22;125(4):222–7
Kraetschmer K: Broca's localization theory reconsidered. **Br J Disord Commun** 1980 May;15(1):5–8
Lambo TA: Professor Gastaut and his contributions to the World Health Organization programme. **Electroencephalogr Clin Neurophysiol** 1982;35:3–6
Laporte Y: La sensibilité récurrente des racines rachidiennes antérieures. **Hist Sci Med** 1983;17(4):351–5
Lee DA: Paul Broca and the history of aphasia. **Neurology** 1981 May;31(5):600–2
Legée G: Influence du vitalisme montpelliérain sur la neurophysiologie de Pierre Flourens. **Hist Nat** 1982;21:13–45
Legée G: La place de Magendie dans la physiologie expérimentale du système nerveux. **Hist Sci Med** 1983;17(4):357–66
Legée G: Les concepts de localisation et de coordination dans la neurophysiologie de Maire-Jean-Pierre Flourens (1794–1867). In: Congrès National des Sociétés Savantes, 96e, Toulouse, 1971. Comptes Rendus. Paris, 1974. Histoire des Sciences, Tome 1. p. 123–51.
Legée G: Les relations épistolaires de P. Flourens et de ses collègues de l'Institut de France. In: Congrès National des Sociétés Savantes, 106e, Perpignan, 1981. Comptes Rendus. Paris, Bibliothèque Nationale, 1982. Fasc. IV. p. 171–85.
Lennox MA: Professor Gastaut's contribution to the International League against Epilepsy. **Electroencephalogr Clin Neurophysiol** 1982;35:9–12
Low MD, Purves SJ, Reeves B, et al: Cerebral evoked potentials: a historical review of the marseilles contributions and a preliminary report on a study of the effects of various stimulus parameters on the P90 component of the pattern visual evoked potential. **Electroencephalogr Clin Neurophysiol** 1982;(35):369–79
Lukács D: Pierre Paul Broca, az antropológia és a beszéd agykérgi központjának felfedezője. **Orv Hetil** 1980 Aug 24;121(34):2081–2
Medaer R: Classics in neurology. Etching showing Claude Bernard doing an experiment surrounded by his colleagues. **Neurology** 1982 Oct;32(10):1145
Naquet R: Gastaut and the EEG Federation. **Electroencephalogr Clin Neurophysiol** 1982;35:7–8
Passouant P: Doctor Gelineau (1828–1906): narcolepsy centennial. **Sleep** 1981 Sep;4(3):241–6
Role A: La vie étrange d'un grand savant: le professeur Brown-Sequard, 1817–1894. Paris, Plon, 1977. 219 p.
Satran R: Les débuts de la Société française de neurologie. **Hist Sci Med** 1981;15(2):188–95
Schiller F: Paul Broca, founder of French anthropology, explorer of the brain. Berkeley, University of California Press, 1979. ix, 350 p.
Signoret JL, Castaigne P, Lhermitte F, et al: Rediscovery of Leborgne's brain: anatomical description with CT scan. **Brain Lang** 1984 Jul;22(2):303–19

### Germany

Aumüller G: Benedict Stillings (1810–1879) Untersuchungen über das Rückenmark--ein Wendepunkt in der neuroanatomischen Forschung. **Medizinhist J** 1984;19(1–2):53–69
Duffy RJ, Liles BZ: A translation of Finkelnburg's (1870) lecture on aphasis as 'asymbolia' with commentary. **J Speech Hear Disord** 1979 May;144(2):156–68
Ehrhardt H: 130 Jahre Deutsche Gesellschaft für Psychiatrie und Nervenheilkunde. Wiesbaden, Steiner, 1972. 125 p.
Fischer W: Franz Joseph Gall und Johann Kaspar Spurzheim--Vorläufer einer biologischen Psychiatrie. **Psychiatr Neurol Med Psychol (Leipz)** 1984 Jul;36(7):433–7
Fleischhauer K: In memoriam Philipp Stöhr jr. **Anat Anz** 1981;150(3):239–47
Heintel B, Heintel H: Historische Stätten der Neurologie in Baden-Württemberg. Stuttgart and New York, Fischer, 1982. n.p.
Heintel H: Ein unbekanntes Porträt des Hirnforschers Oskar Vogt (1870–1959). **Medizinhist J** 1984;19(3):277–9
Jung R, Berger W: Fünfzig Jahre EEG. Hans Bergers Entdeckung des Elektrenkephalogramms und seine ersten Befunde 1924--1931. **Arch Psychiatr Nervenkr** 1979 Dec;227(4):279–300
Lauschke HP: Der Epileptologe Herrmann Andreas Reimer in Görlitz. **Psychiatr Neurol Med Psychol (Leipz)** 1982 Dec;34(12):745–8
Loebe FM: Karl Eskuchen--ein fast vergessener Pionier der Liquorforschung. **Psychiatr Neurol Med Psychol (Leipz)** 1983 Sep;35(9):561–5
Meyer A: Paul Flechsig's system of myelogenetic cortical localization in the light of recent research in neuroanatomy and neurophysiology. Part I. **Can J Neurol Sci** 1981 Feb;8(1):1–6
Meyer A: Paul Flechsig's system of myelogenetic cortical localization in the light of recent research in neuroanatomy and neurophysiology part II. **Can J Neurol Sci** 1981 May;8(2):95–104
Neumärker KJ: Zur Geschichte der Abteilung für Kinderneuropsychiatrie an der Berliner Charité. **Acta Paedopsychiatr (Basel)** 1982 Dec;48(6):297–305
Pauly PJ: The political structure of the brain: cerebral localization in Bismarckian Germany. **Int J Neurosci** 1983 Oct;21(1–2):145–9
Rafaelsen OJ: Thudichum: the founder of neurochemistry. In Rose FC, Bynum WF, ed: Historical aspects of the neurosciences. New York, Raven, 1982. p. 293–305.
Ross HE, Bischof K: Wundt's views on sensations of innervation: a reevaluation. **Perception** 1981;10(3):319–29
Sărmăşanu-Cortez ML, Cortez P: Bernhard von Gudden şi drama de la lacul Starnberg (1824–1886). **Rev Med Interna [Neurol Psihiatr]** 1983 Jul–Sep;28(3):233–8
Schaefer H: Some remarks on the history of research on sympathetic nerve action potentials: research at Heidelberg. **J Auton Nerv Syst** 1981 Apr;3(2–4):123–31
Schierhorn H: Die Hirnanatomie im Spiegel der ersten 50 Bände des Anatomischen Anzeigers. **Anat Anz** 1981;150(1–2):77–118
Schierhorn H: Samuel Thomas Soemmerring (1755–1830) als Neuroanatom. **Z Mikrosk Anat Forsch** 1980;94(6):1051–76
Schmutz HK: Rüdingers 'Atlas des peripherischen Nervensystems des menschlichen Körpers' mit Photographien von Joseph Albert; zur Frühgeschichte der medizinischen Photographie. **Gesnerus** 1980;37(1/2):83–90
Schulz M: Dr. John Rittmeister--Nervenarzt und Widerstandskämpfer. **Psychiatr Neurol Med Psychol (Leipz)** 1979 Apr;31(4):213–6
Theopold W: Paul Julius Möbius (1853–1907). **Medizinhist J** 1983;18(1–2):100–17
Thom A: Zur disziplinären Genese der Neurologie im ausgehenden 19. Jahrhundert--aus den Briefen Wilhelm Erbs an Adolf Strümpell. **Z Gesamte Inn Med** 1982 Jun 1;37(11):340–6
Tower DB: Hensing, 1719. An account of the first chemical examination of the brain and the discovery of phosphorus therein, set against the background of Europe in the 17th and early 18th centuries. A source book in the history of neurochemistry. New York, Raven, 1983. xvi, 407 p.
Waldeck-Semadeni EK: Paul Julius Moebius, 1853–1907, Leben und Werk. Diss. Bern, 1980. 222 p.
Westheimer G: Helmholtz on eye movements. **Hum Neurobiol** 1984;3(3):149–52

### Great Britain

Ashworth B: The Bramwells and neurology in Edinburgh. **Scott Med J** 1981 Oct;26(4):364–70
Bacq ZM: Les expériences de W. Feldberg en l'année 1932. **Bull Mem Acad R Med Belg** 1982;137 Suppl:9–30
Behan PO, Behan WM: Sir Robert Carswell: Scotland's pioneer pathologist. In Rose FC, Bynum WF, ed: Historical aspects of the neurosciences. New York, Raven, 1982. p. 273–92.
Bell S: George Henry Lewes: a man of his time. **J Hist Biol** 1981 Fall;14(2):278–98
Bülbring E, Walker JM: Joshua Harold Burn: 6 March 1892–13 July 1981. **Biogr Mem Fellows R Soc** 1984;30:45–89

# NEUROLOGY

Cohen B: Erasmus Darwin's observations on rotation and vertigo. **Hum Neurobiol** 1984;3(3):121–8

Cooper WM, Platt H: John Sebastian Bach Stopford. In Dictionary of national biography, 1961–1970. Suppl. 8, 1981. p. 985–7.

Eccles JC, Gibson WC: Sherrington: his life and thought. Berlin, New York, Springer International, 1979. xv, 269 p.

Fee E: Nineteenth-century craniology: the study of the female skull. **Bull Hist Med** 1979 Fall;53(3):415–33

Gibson WC: Some British contributors to cortical localization. In Rose FC, Bynum WF, ed: Historical aspects of neurosciences. New York, Raven, 1982. p. 109–13.

Gillespie JS: Antagonists of alpha adrenoceptors and adrenergic transmission. **Bull Mem Acad R Med Belg** 1982;137 Suppl:45–55

Gregory RL: Forty years on: Kenneth Craik's The Nature of Explanation (1943). **Perception** 1983;12(3):233–7

Hamanaka Y: [Jackson's theory of stratification of neurological functions--a controversy involving Broca at a symposium (1868) at Norwich] (Jpn). **No To Shinkei** 1982 Oct;34(10):1018–9

Jacyna LS: Principles of general physiology: the comparative dimension to British neuroscience in the 1830s and 1840s. **Stud Hist Biol** 1984;7:47–92

Jacyna LS: The physiology of mind, the unity of nature, and the moral order in Victorian thought. **Br J Hist Sci** 1981 Jul;14(pt 2 no 47):109–32

Lepore FE: Neuro-ophthalmology according to Gordon Holmes. **Neurol Clin** 1983 Nov;1(4):789–805

Lyons JB: The neurology of Robert Bentley Todd. In Rose FC, Bynum WF, ed: Historical aspects of the neurosciences. New York, Raven, 1982. p. 137–50.

McIlwain H: Neurochemistry and Sherrington's enchanted loom. **J R Soc Med** 1984 May;77(5):417–25

Mahta M: The history of the Intractable Pain Society of Great Britain and Ireland. **Pain** 1980 Feb;8(1):121–2

Manuel DE: Marshall Hall, F.R.S. (1790–1857); a conspectus of his life and work. **Notes Rec R Soc Lond** 1980 Dec;35(2):135–66

Martin JP: Reminiscenses of Queen Square. **Br Med J [Clin Res]** 1981 Dec 19;283(6307):1640–2

Merton PA: Neurophysiology on man. **J Neurol Neurosurg Psychiatry** 1981 Oct;44(10):861–70

Moruzzi G: In memoriam Lord Adrian (1889–1977). **Rev Physiol Biochem Pharmacol** 1980;87:1–24

Parsons-Smith BG: Sir Gordon Holmes. In Rose FC, Bynum WF, ed: Historical aspects of the neurosciences. New York, Raven, 1982. p. 357–70.

Paton W: Chemical transmission: exploitation and follow up. **Bull Mem Acad R Med Belg** 1982;137 Suppl:31–44

Penfield W: Sir Gordon Morgan Holmes. In Dictionary of national biography, 1961–1970. Suppl. 8, 1981. p. 534–6.

Picard C, Olivier A, Bertrand G: The first human stereotaxic apparatus. The contribution of Aubrey Mussen to the field of stereotaxis. **J Neurosurg** 1983 Oct;59(4):673–6

Pickering G: Walter Russell Brain. In Dictionary of national biography, 1961–1970. Suppl. 8, 1981. p. 127–9.

Smith CU: Evolution and the problem of mind: part II. John Hughlings Jackson. **J Hist Biol** 1982 Summer;15(2):241–62

Steiner TJ, Capildeo R, Rose FC: The neurological tradition of Charing Cross Hospital. In Rose FC, Bynum WF, ed: Historical aspects of the neurosciences. New York, Raven, 1982. p. 347–56.

### Hungary

Kenéz J: Hugó Richter, an outstanding Hungarian neurohistologist (1887--1945). **Ther Hung** 1979;27(2):99–100

Pisztora F: A bel-, az elme és az ideggyógyászat viszonya hazánkban a századforduló körül. **Orv Hetil** 1982 Jun 27;123(26):1621–9

Szentágothai J: Too 'much' and too 'soon'. A lifetime of inquiry into the functional organization of the nervous system. **Acta Biol Acad Sci Hung** 1982;33(2–3):107–26

### Italy

Armocida G, Ambrosoli C, Majeron MA: Note biografich intorno a Vincenzo Racchetti (1777–1819). Contributo alla storia della neurologia. **Minerva Med** 1980 Apr 21;71(16):1221–6

Arquiola E: La lesión neurologica en 'De sedibus et causis morborum' de Morgagni. In: Congrès international d'histoire de la médecine, XXVe, Québec, 1976. Actes. Québec, 1977. p. 461–8.

Disertori B, Piazza M: Felice Fontana precursore delle moderne neuroscienze. **Ann Osp Maria Vittoria Torino** 1981 Jan–Jun;24(1–6)178–209

Lambertini G: Il pensiero e i trovati di Angelo Ruffini nella sua opera 'Physiogeny'. [Italian and English] Padova, Piccin, 1980. 111 p.

Macchi G: Historia de la neuropatología italiana. Evolución de una problemática. **Arch Neurobiol (Madr)** 1984 Jan–Feb;47(1):45–8

Premuda L, Bonuzzi L: Morgagni e la neuropatologia. **Acta Med Hist Patav** 1982–83;29:75–81

### Japan

Aki M: The history of neurology in Japan, with special reference to its postwar period. In Rose FC, Bynum WF, ed: Historical aspects of the neurosciences. New York, Raven, 1982. p. 451–62.

Fukuyama Y: A quarter-century of the Japanese Society of Child Neurology. **Brain Dev** 1984;6(2):109–18

Fukuyama Y: [Progress of the Japanese Society of Pediatric Neurology in the past quarter of a century] (Jpn). **No To Hattatsu** 1984;16(3):179–88

Furukawa T: [Development of neurophysiology in Japan brought by introduction of microelectrodes] (Jpn). **Nippon Seirigaku Zasshi** 1984;46(1):5–7

Matsuki A: [Current view of the studies on the history of anesthesiology (7)--Tekisai Okubo, a pioneer of the pain clinic in Japan] **Masui** 1980 Feb;29(2):182–4

Tomita T: [Development of neurophysiology following the decrement-nondecrement controversy] (Jpn). **Nippon Seirigaku Zasshi** 1984;46(1):1–4

Tsubaki T: [History of the Japanese Society of Neurology for 20 years (author's transl)]. (Jpn) **Rinsho Shinkeigaku** 1979 Dec;19(12):804–8

### Norway

Refsum S: Some aspects of the history of neurology in Norway. In Rose FC, Bynum WF, ed: Historical aspects of the neurosciences. New York, Raven, 1982. p. 415–33.

### Poland

Falkiewiczowa S: Kronika Wrocławskiej Kliniki Neurologicznej. **Neurol Neurochir Pol** 1984 May–Jun;18(3):303–9

Falkiewiczowa S, Swiątkowski S, Teppa S: Neurologia lwowska. **Neurol Neurochir Pol** 1982 Jan–Jun;16(1–3):85–107

Majdecki T: Powstanie i rozwój w okresie miedzywojennym neurologicznego lecznictwa kolejowej służby zdrowia. **Neurol Neurochir Pol** 1984 Jan–Feb;18(1):87–91

Pacyńska M, Kedzia A, Smereka J: Tematy neurologiczne w pracach doktorskich polaków studiujacych we Wrocławiu w XIX wieku. **Arch Hist Med (Warsz)** 1980;43(2):199–204

Prusiński A: Professor dr hab. nauk med. Eufemiusz Herman - nestor polskiej neurologii (w 90 urodziny). **Neurol Neurochir Pol** 1982;(5–6):306–28

### Romania

Alexandru O: Nicolae Ionescu-Siseşti, neurolog, 1888--1954 (91 ani de la naşterea sa). **Rev Med Interna [Neurol Psihiatr]** 1979 Apr–Jun;24(2):143–6

Marinesco M, Petresco A, Marinesco G: Georges Marinesco et la France. **Hist Sci Med** 1984;18(1):13–8

Marinescu M, Petrescu A: Ecouri contemporane ale operei stiinţifice a lui Gh. Marinescu. **Rev Med Interna [Neurol Psihiatr]** 1980 Oct–Dec;25(4):311–4

Psatta DM: Thirty years of research (II). **Neurol Psychiatr (Bucur)** 1982 Jan–Mar;20(1):3–28

### Spain

Abarracín Teulón A: Santiago Ramón y Cajal, o la pasión de España. Barcelona, Editorial Labor, [1978?] 319 p.

Albarracín A: Ramón y Cajal entre los poderes y los saberes. **Med Hist (Barc)** 1984;4:1–16

Barraquer i Bordás L, Gutiérrez Gómez D: En el centenario de la neurología clínica española. **Arch Neurobiol (Madr)** 1982 Mar–Apr;45(2):157–62

Bustamante M: Nicolás Achúcarro: el hombre y su obra. **Arch Neurobiol (Madr)** 1982 Jan–Feb;45(1):55–72

Carrato Ibáñez A: Cajal y su Instituto. **Trab Inst Cajal Invest Biol** 1979;70(3):181–94

Izquierdo JM: Contribución a la historia de la neuropatología española. **Arch Neurobiol (Madr)** 1983 Sep–Oct;46(5):327–34

Izquierdo Rojo JM: Historia de la neurologia clinica Española (1882–1936). Madrid, Universidad Complutense-Madrid, 1978. 333 p.

Izquierdo Rojo JM: Wenceslao López Albo. **Arch Neurobiol (Madr)** 1983 Mar–Apr;46(2):131–46

Kock W: Santiago Ramón y Cajal och Nobelpriset. **Nord Medicinhist Arsb** 1981;:151–9

Lorenzo Velázquez B: Algunos recuerdos sobre Cajal en el XLVII aniversario de su muerte. **An R Acad Nacl Med (Madr)** 1981;98(4):663–88

Marín Fernández JL: Aspectos bibliometricos de la obra de Roman Alberca Lorente (1903–1967). **Asclepio** 1980;32:229–53

Ricoy JR: In memoriam: J. F. Tello. **Arch Neurobiol (Madr)** 1980 Nov–Dec;43(6):347–52

Simmer HH: Santiago Ramón y Cajal und die Typologie des Wissenschaftlers. **Medizinhist J** 1981;16(4):414–23

Valenciano Gayá L: Cajal (recuerdos y reflexiones de uno de sus últimos alumnos). **Arch Neurobiol (Madr)** 1983 Jul–Aug;46(4):272–81

### Sweden

Gejvall NG: Swedenborg--a man with head enough for two. **Ossa** 1978;5:123-31

Sourander P: Linnaeus and Neurology. **Sven Linnesallskap Arsskr** 1978; Commemorative Volume:88-117

### Switzerland

Aeschlimann J: Rudolf Brun (1885-1969). Leben und Werk des Züricher Neurologen, Psychoanalytikers and Entomologen. Zürich, Juris, 1980. 70p. (Zürcher medizingeschichtliche Abhandlungen. Neue Reihe, Nr. 144).

Tröhler U: Theodor Kocher und die neurotopographische Diagnostik: angewandte Forschung mit grundlegendem Ergebnis um 1900. **Gesnerus** 1983;40(1-2):203-14

### United States

Aring CD: A medical perspective. **Neurology** 1984 Oct;34(10):1357-61

Austin JH: Chase, chance, and creativity: the lucky art of novelty. New York, Columbia Univ. Press, 1978. xvii, 237 p.

Barlow W, Powell DO: The cure of Rachel Baker's 'Devotional Somnium' (Sleep-preaching). **Acad Bookman** 1978;31(1-2):3-10

Bibliography of Dr. E. H. Lambert: **Muscle Nerve** 1982;5(9S):S166-72

Blustein BE: A New York medical man: William Alexander Hammond, M.D. (1828-1900), Neurologist. Ph.D. Diss. University of Pennsylvania. Philadelphia, 1979. 418 leaves.

Bodian D: Normand Louis Hoerr. In Dictionary of American Biography, Suppl. 6, 1956-1960. p. 295-6, 1980.

Brand JL: Evolutionary years of American neurology, 1865-1875. In: Congrès international d'histoire de la médecine, XXVe, Québec, 1976. Actes. Québec, 1977. p. 507-21.

Brandt AM: Herbert Spencer Gasser. In Dictionary of American biography, 1961-1965. Suppl. 7, 1981. p. 279-81.

Brown EM: Neurology and spiritualism in the 1870s. **Bull Hist Med** 1983 Winter;57(4):563-77

Burnham JC: The founding of the Archives of Neurology and Psychiatry; or, what was wrong with the Journal of Nervous and Mental disease? **J Hist Med Allied Sci** 1981 Jul;36(3):310-24

Carlson ET: The history of multiple personality in the United States: Mary Reynolds and her subsequent reputation. **Bull Hist Med** 1984 Spring;58(1):72-82

Cowan WM: Jerzy E. Rose. **J Comp Neurol** 1980 Aug 1;192(3):401-6

Davenport HW: Signs of anxiety, rage, or distress. **Physiologist** 1981 Oct-Nov;24(5):1-5

DeJong RN: A history of American neurology. New York, Raven Press, 1982. 157 p.

Dreifuss JJ: W. L. Gaines, précurseur du concept de réflexe neuroendocrine. **Gesnerus** 1981;38(3/4):331-8

Falk D: Primate neuroanatomy: an evolutionary perspective. In F. Spencer, ed: A history of American physical anthropology, 1930-1980. New York, Academic Press, 1982. 75-103.

Friedman AP: Houston Merritt. In Rose FC, Bynum WF, ed: Historical aspects of the neurosciences. New York, Raven, 1982. p. 379-82.

Fullinwider SP: Technicians of the finite. The rise and decline of the schizophrenic in American thought 1840-1960. Westport, Conn., Greenwood, 1982. ix, 253 p. (Contributions in Medical History, 9).

Gerlach J: Hartwig Kuhlenbeck--60 Jahre vergleichend neuroanatomische Forschung. **J Hirnforsch** 1979;20(2):107-13

Gutiérrez C: The birth and growth of neuroradiology in the USA. **Neuroradiology** 1981;21(4):227-37

Hamburger V: Trophic interactions in neurogenesis: a personal historical account. **Annu Rev Neurosci** 1980;3:269-78

Harvey AM: Henry M. Thomas: Johns Hopkins's first neurologist. **Johns Hopkins Med J** 1982 Jan;150(1):11-21

Holden C: Paul MacLean and the triune brain. **Science** 1979 Jun 8;204(4397):1066-8

Holmes GL: Roberts Bartholow. In search of anatomic localization. **NY State J Med** 1982 Feb;82(2):238-41

Joynt RJ: Landmark perspective: A new look at death. **JAMA** 1984 Aug 3;252(5):680-2

Kandel E: The origins of modern neuroscience. **Annu Rev Neurosci** 1982;5:299-303

Kety SS: The metamorphosis of a psychobiologist. **Annu Rev Neurosci** 1979;2:1-15

Ludmerer KM: Joseph Erlanger. In Dictionary of American biography, 1961-1965. Suppl. 7, 1981. p. 225-7.

Morgan JP: The first reported case of electrical stimulation of the human brain. **J Hist Med Allied Sci** 1982 Jan;37(1):51-64

Morris JP: Walter Timme. In Dictionary of American Biography, Suppl. 6, 1956-1960. p. 634-5, 1980.

Oppenheim RW: Laura Bridgeman's brain: an early consideration of functional adaptations in neural development. **Dev Psychobiol** 1979 Nov;12(6):533-7

Page IH: The discovery of serotonin. **Perspect Biol Med** 1976 Autumn;20(1):1-8

Powell RC: Daniel Joseph McCarthy. In Dictionary of American Biography, Suppl. 6, 1956-1960. p. 402-4, 1980.

Reese WG: 'Don't count the bricks'. Scientific contributions of W. H. Gantt. **Pavlov J Biol Sci** 1982 Jul-Sep;17(3):111-4

Rowland LP: Thirty years of progress and problems in clinical neurology. **Ann Neurol** 1982 Apr;11(4):327-34

Sandelowski M: Pain, pleasure, and American childbirth: from the twilight sleep to the Read Method, 1914-1960. Westport, Conn., Greenwood Press, 1984. xix, 152 p. (Contributions in Medical History, No. 13).

Schneck JM: S. Weir Mitchell, M.D. (1829 to 1914) and D. Hayes Agnew, M.D. (1818 to 1892). Neuropsychiatrist's poetic tribute to a surgeon. **NY State J Med** 1982 Jul;82(8):1264-8

Stumpf DA: The founding of pediatric neurology in America. **Bull NY Acad Med** 1981 Nov;57(9):804-16

Thomson EH: John Farquhar Fulton. In Dictionary of American Biography, Suppl. 6, 1956-1960. p. 222-4, 1980.

Tyler HR, Tyler KL: Charles Edouard Brown-Séquard: professor of physiology and pathology of the nervous system at Harvard Medical School. **Neurology** 1984 Sep;34(9):1231-6

Waites L: American pioneers in the topic of word blindness. In Rose FC, Bynum WF, ed: Historical aspects of the neurosciences. New York, Raven, 1982. p. 115-6.

Wilkerson SY: Mind over body. James Jackson Putnam and the impact of neurology on psychotherapy in late nineteenth-century America. Ph.D. Diss. Duke University. Durham, 1978. v, 377 leaves.

Willison RG: Dr. E. H. Lambert's contributions to electromyography. **Muscle Nerve** 1982;5(9S):S2-5

Windle WF: Recollections of research in spinal cord regeneration. **Exp Neurol** 1981 Jan;71(1):1-5

Wortis J: Johannes Maargaard Nielsen, pioneer. **Biol Psychiatry** 1983 Feb;18(2):135-7

Zeidenfelt A: Surgeon General William Hammond. **Civ War Times Illus** 1978;17(6):24-32

### Uruguay

Speroni Verner J: Vida y obra de José Verocay. Montevideo, Universidad de la Republica, Division Publicaciones y Ediciones, 1980. 51 p.

### USSR

Afanas'ev IuI, Belova TI, Fel'dman NG: Boris Innokent'evich Lavrent'ev (k 90-letiiu so dnia rozhdeniia). **Arkh Anat Gistol Embriol** 1983 Nov;85(11):98-101

Alekseev MA, Person RS: I. M. Sechenov i nekotorye voprosy fiziologii dvizheniĭ. **Usp Fiziol Nauk** 1979 Jul-Sep;10(3):15-25

Arkhangel'skiĭ GV: V. E. Larionov--odin iz osnovopolozhnikov otechestvennoĭ otonevrologii. **Vestn Otorinolaringol** 1984 Mar-Apr;(2):88-93

Arkhangel'skiĭ GV: V. M. Bekhterev--vydaiushchiĭsia deiatel' otechestvennoĭ nauki (k 125-letiiu so dnia rozhdeniia). **Klin Med (Mosk)** 1983 Feb;61(2):106-10

Arkhangel'skiĭ GV: Vklad Akademika G.I. Markelova v teoriiu otechestvennoĭ nevrologii (k 100-letiiu so dnia rozhdeniia). **Klin Med (Mosk)** 1980 Oct;58(10):114-8

Arkhangel'skiĭ GV: Znachenie S. P. Botkina v razvitii otechestvennoĭ nevrologii. **Klin Med (Mosk)** 1983 Apr;61(4):105-9

Asratian EA, Shingarov GKh: Leninskaia teoriia otrazheniia i uchenie I. P. Pavlova o vyssheĭ nervnoĭ deiatel'nosti (k 110-i godovshchine so dnia rozhdeniia V. I. Lenina). **Zh Vyssh Nerv Deiat** 1980 Mar-Apr;30(2):227-34

Bal'dysh G: Bekhterev v Peterburge-Leningrade. Leningrad, Lenizdat, 1979. 318 p.

Bechtereva NP, Bundzen PV, Malyshev VN: [Sechenov's tradition in the development of physiology of mental activity, its origins and perspectives] (Rus). **Istor Biol Issled** 1980;8:163-72

Buzsàki G: Situational conditional reflexes. Physiologic studies of the higher nervous activity of freely moving animals: P. S. Kupalov. **Pavlov J Biol Sci** 1983 Jan-Mar;18(1):13-21

Demidova NI: [The role of I. M. Sechenov's school in the development of electrophysiology] (Rus). **Istor Biol Issled** 1980;8:156-62

Dionesov SM: Stranitsa iz istorii Pervogo s'ezda Russkogo soiuza psikhiatrov i nevropatologov. **Zh Nevropatol Psikhiatr** 1981;(5):744-5

Dogel' LV, Shalagina TL: S. N. Davidenkov v Leningradskom gosudarstvennom institute usovershenstvovaniia vracheĭ. **Zh Nevropatol Psikhiatr** 1982;82(3):107-9

Durinian RA, Dubrov AP: Leninskaia teoriia otrazheniia i metodologicheskie problemy fiziologii i refleksoterapii. **Vestn Akad Med Nauk SSSR** 1981;(4):41-5

Grigori'ian NA: Razvitie ucheniia o vyssheĭ nervnoĭ deiatel'nosti v trudakh L. A. Orbeli. **Zh Vyssh Nerv Deiat** 1982 Nov-Dec;32(6):1011-9

K 80-letiiu zhurnala nevropatologii i psikhiatrii im. S. S. Korsakova: **Zh Nevropatol Psikhiatr** 1981;81(1):3-5

Kabanov MM: Razvitie v deiatel'nosti Leningradskogo nauchno-issledovatel'skogo psikhonevrologicheskogo instituta im. V. M. Bekhtereva ideĭ ego osnovatelia. **Zh Nevropatol Psikhiatr** 1982;82(11):1234-7

## NEUROLOGY

Karamian AI: Ivan Mikhaĭlovich Sechenov i evoliutsionnaia neĭrofiziologiia. Leningrad, Nauka, Leningradskoe otd-nie, 1980. 112 p.
Karamyan AI: The importance of I. M. Sechenov's ideas on formation of human nervous and mental activity for evolutionary neurophysiology. **Hum Physiol** 1979 Nov–Dec;5(5):717–23
Kelemen G: 125 éve született V. M. Bekhterev. **Orv Hetil** 1983 Apr 3;124(14):831–3
Khodos KhG: Epidemicheskiĭ éntsefalit Ekonomo--nereshennaia nevrologicheskaia problema (k 60–letiiu opisaniia éntsefalita Ekonomo sovetskimi nevropatologami). **Zh Nevropatol Psikhiatr** 1981;81(2):124–7
Kokina NN: P. K. Anokhin's concept of systems genesis and its subsequent development. **Neurosci Behav Physiol** 1980 Mar–Apr;10(2):142–6
Kukuev LA: V. M. Bekhterev i znachenie ego trudov dlia sovremennoĭ nevrologii i meditsiny. **Klin Med (Mosk)** 1982 Oct;60(10):118–21
Lisitsyn IuP, Arkhangel'skiĭ GV: S. P. Botkin--nevrolog. **Zh Nevropatol Psikhiatr** 1982;82(10):127–30
Lobzin VS, Pinchuk VK: Pervaia v Rossii kafedra dlia usovershenstvovaniia nevropatologov. **Zh Nevropatol Psikhiatr** 1983;83(8):1240–5
Makarov VA: Razvitie I. M. Sechenovym ucheniia o edinstve organizma i sredy. **Usp Fiziol Nauk** 1979 Jul–Sep;10(3):5–14
Maslov EV: Iz istorii kliniki nervnykh i dushevnykh bolezniĭ Severo–Kavkazskogo meditsinskogo instituta (Rostov–na–Donu). **Zh Nevropatol Psikhiatr** 1983;83(4):601–3
Matiushkin DP: Obzor: uchenie N. E. Vvedenskogo o vozbuzhdenii i tormozhenii v svete sovremennoĭ neĭrofiziologii. **Fiziol Zh SSSR** 1981 Mar;67(3):349–56
Mecacci L: Brain and history. The relationship between neurophysiology and psychology in Soviet research. New York, Brunner/Mazel. 1977. xxiv, 198 p. (Translation of Cervello e storia).
Medvedev VI: I. M. Sechenov's ideas in modern physiology. **Hum Physiol** 1979 May–Jun;5(3):261–8
Molchanov VV, Kulikova TN: K 70–letiiu kafedry nervnykh bolezneĭ Saratovskogo meditsinskogo instituta. **Zh Nevropatol Psikhiatr** 1983;83(9):1399–401
Mozzhukhin AS: [I. M. Sechenov - The founder of the first physiological school in Russia] (Rus). **Istor Biol Issled** 1980;8:124–37
Okhrimenko NN: Glavnyĭ voennyĭ gospital' i ego rol' v razvitii otechestvennoĭ voennoĭ nevrologii (k 275–letiiu so dnia osnovaniia Glavnogo. **Zh Nevropatol Psikhiatr** 1983;83(7):1069–71
Prokhorova MI: E. S. London i funktsional'naia neĭrokhimiia. **Nerv Sist** 1982;23:137–42
Razvitie nevrologicheskoĭ pomoshchi v Glavnom voennom klinicheskom gospitale imeni N. N. Burdenko (k 275–letiiu osnovaniia gospitalia): **Voen Med Zh** 1982 Jul;(7):71–2
Roitbak AI: The importance of I. M. Sechenov's electrophysiological research. **Acta Neurobiol Exp (Warsz)** 1980;40(2):451–61
Rokhlin LL, Shereshevskiĭ AM, Tom A: Znamenatel'nye i iubileĭnye daty nevropatologii i psikhiatrii 1984 g. **Zh Nevropatol Psikhiatr** 1984;84(2):271–80
Salaeva ZM: K istorii kliniki nervnykh bolezně Azerbaĭdzhanskogo orden Trudovogo Krasnogo Znameni gosudarstvennogo meditsinskogo instituta im. N, Narimanova. **Zh Nevropatol Psikhiatr** 1981;81(11):1720–1
Shlykov IP, Dedov II: Anatoliĭ Anatol'evich Voĭtkevich. **Arkh Anat Gistol Embriol** 1979 Dec;77(12):81–4
Simonov PV: Half a century of pursuing the truth. Dedicated to the 80th anniversary of E. A. Asratyan. **Pavlov J Biol Sci** 1983 Apr–Jun;18(2):63–8
Skudarnova ZA: Stanovlenie, razvitie i zadachi nevrologicheskoĭ sluzhby Smolenskoĭ oblasti. **Zh Nevropatol Psikhiatr** 1983;83(11):1732–4
Sokolova LV: Obzor: Problema vzaimodeĭstviia vozbuzhdeniia i tormozheniia pri formirovanii ucheniia A. A. Ukhtomskogo o printsipe dominanty. **Fiziol Zh SSSR** 1981 Jun;67(6):781–6
Sokolova LV: Uchenie A. A. Ukhtomskogo o dominante ka vektore povedeniia. **Nerv Sist** 1982;23:5–13
Tonkikh AV: K mekhanizmu sechenovskogo tormozheniia. **Zh Vyssh Nerv Deiat** 1980 Sep–Oct;30(5):1037–43
Tsybul'kin AG: Vklad Konstantina Monakova v izuchenie anatomii mozga. **Arkh Anat Gistol Embriol** 1979 Nov;77(11):115–7
Viktor Petrovich Babmindra (k 60–letiiu so dnia rozhdeniia): **Arkh Anat Gistol Embriol** 1983 Oct;85(10):102–4
Volokhov AA, Kolt'tsova MM, Kostandov EA, et al: Institutu vyssheĭ nervnoĭ deiatel'nosti i neĭrofiziologii Adademii nauk 30 let. **Zh Vyssh Nerv Deiat** 1981 Jan–Feb;31(1):202–16
Voloshin PV: Razvitie nevrologicheskoĭ nauki na Ukraine za gody Sovetskoĭ vlasti. **Vrach Delo** 1983 Feb;(2):116–20

**Yugoslavia**

Novak Z: 30 godina 'Neuropsyhijatrije' i 'Neurologije'. **Neurologija** 1983;31(1–2):7–9

## NUMISMATICS

Allen CR: A survey of medical numismatics. Medicina in Nummis. **JAMA** 1981 Nov 20;246(20):2347–9
Kottek SS: 'Medicina in Nummis': an exhibition of medical medals in the Hebrew University Hadassah Medical School--Jerusalem (May–June 1979). **Koroth** 1979 Nov;7(9–10):CCXXXI–CCXXXIV(722–3)
Müller–Jahncke WD: Apothekerbildnisse auf Medaillen und Plaketten. 1. Deutschsprachiger Raum. Stuttgart, Wissenschaftliche Verlagsgesellschaft, 1980. 164 p. Veröffentlichungen der Internationalen Gesellschaft für Geschichte der Pharmazie, Neue Folge, 48).
Palmieri TJ: Hands on coins. **Hand** 1982 Oct;14(3):341–2
Schmidt F: Apothekerbildnisse auf Medaillen und Plaketten. **Beitr Gesch Pharm** 1981;31(13):100–1

**Germany**

Wischermann H: Mors meditans: Ein Beitrag zu drei Medaillen auf den Augsburger Arzt Occo III. **Arch Kulturgesch** 1978;58(2):432–3

**Great Britain**

Whittet TD: A survey of apothecaries' tokens including some previously unrecognised specimens. **Pharm J** 1982;228:719–24; 1983;230:133–40; 1983;231:42–5, 641–9; 1984;232:583–5, 790–2

**Hungary**

Huszár L, Varannai G: Medicina in nummis: Hungarian medals relating to medicine. Budapest, Semmelweis Medical Historical Museum, Library, and Archives, 1977. 215 p.
Süle T: Az Erzsébet Tudományegyetem Orvosi Kara, az önálló Pécsi Orvostudományi Egyetem rövid története és numizmatikai emlékei. **Orvostort Kozl** 1982;28(1–3):227–39

**Sweden**

Strandell B: Svenska medicinska medaljer. **Nord Medicinhist Arsb** 1980;Supp 6:52–6

**Before 500 A.D.**

**Greco–Roman**

Chabert JM, Bocquet JP: A propos d'un denier de la république romaine. **Hist Sci Med** 1982;16(2):89–92
Sandyk R: Brain development and the phylogenesis of writing and drawing direction. **S Afr Med J** 1982 Jul 10;62(2):43–4

**Rome**

Klawans HL: The acromegaly of Maximinus I: the possible influence of a pituitary tumor on the life and death of a Roman emperor. In Rose FC, Bynum WF, ed: Historical aspects of the neurosciences. New York, Raven, 1982. 317–26.

**1450–1700**

Kottek S: The humble physician, explanation of and notes on a Renaissance medal. **Koroth** 1980 Jun;7(11–12):747–53

**1700 to Present**

Commemorative coin for Dr. Zamenhof: **Newsl Optom Hist Soc** 1981;12(1):6
Golden RL: Medallic tributes to Sir William Osler and their historical associations. **JAMA** 1979 Dec 28;242(26):2862–7
Julien P: Médailles modernes à sujet pharmaceutique et médical. **Rev Hist Pharm (Paris)** 1980 Mar;27(244):39–47

**France**

Hildebrand R: F. V. Raspail, Begründer der Histochemie und Wegbereiter der Zelltheorie, im Spiegel zeitgenössischer Medaillen. **Anat Anz** 1983;154(4):353–8

**Germany**

Müller–Jahncke WD: Weitere Apothekerbildnisse auf Medaillen und Plaketten des deutschsprachigen Raums. **Beitr Gesch Pharm** 1984;31(24):205–9

**Hungary**

Tóth A: Hévízi érmek. **Orv Hetil** 1982 Jul 11;123(28):1751–3

**Italy**

Tergolina U: Le medaglie fatte coniare dal Nobile Collegio Chimico Farmaceutico di Roma. Nobile Collegio Chimico–Farmaceutico Roma, (Atti e Memorie) 1975 Jan–Mar; 5(1):13–6.

**USSR**

Gribanov ED: Memorial'nye medali N. I. Pirogova (k 100-letiiu so dnia smerti). **Feldsher Akush** 1981;46(12):42-5

# NURSING

See also **Women**

Alvsvåg H: Sykepleiens historie--er den objektiv? **Sykepleien** 1983 Feb 7;70(3):20-1
Anderson NE: The historical development of American nursing education. **JNE** 1981 Jan;20(1):18-36
Bingham S: Ministering angels. Oradell, New Jersey, Medical Economics Company, 1979. 224p.
Bravo Peña F: Nociones de historia de la enfermeria. 7a. ed: México, Porrúa, 1980. 191 p.
Bullough B, Bullough VL, Elcano B: Nursing. A historical bibliography. New York, London, Garland, 1981. xxiv, 408 p. (Garland reference library of social science, v. 66).
Cahall JB: The history of occupational health nursing. **Occup Health Nurs** 1981 Oct;29(10):11-3
Collière MF: Promouvoir la vie. Paris, Inter-Editions, 1982. Historical chapters, p. 23-35, 125-87.
Connell MT: Feminine consciousness and the nature of nursing practice: a historical perspective. **Top Clin Nurs** 1983 Oct;5(3):1-10
Cunningham SG, Mitchell PH: The use of animals in nursing research. **ANS** 1982 Jul;4(4):72-84
Dagsland H, Lysnes M: Sykepleiens historie--forskning og objektivitet. **Sykepleien** 1983 Mar 7;70(5):17-9
Devlin R: A new look at old wives. **Nurs Mirror** 1981 Sep 16;153(12):8-9
Dolan JA: Nursing in society, a historical perspective. 14th ed. Philadelphia, Saunders, 1978. viii, 402 p.
Doona ME: Nursing revisited: nursing at the winter's solstice. **Mass Nurse** 1983 Dec;52(12):1, 3
Duxbury ML: Nursing in neonatology. In Smith GF, Smith PN, Vidyasagar D, ed: Historical review and recent advances in neonatal and perinatal medicine. [Chicago?], Mead Johnson Nutritional Division, 1983. Vol. I. p. 107-22.
Enfermería y sociedad (notas para una historia social de la enfermería): **Rev Enferm** 1981 Feb;4(31):35-44
Fitzpatrick JJ: Suicidology and suicide prevention: historical perspectives from the nursing literature. **J Psychosoc Nurs Ment Health Serv** 1983 May;21(5):20-8
Grobbelaar WC: Die gemeenskapsverpleegkundige in perspektief. **Curationis** 1982 Sep;5(3):44-9
Humphries SV: The place of the nurse in society. **Cent Afr J Med** 1981 Sep;27(9):187-9
Iveson-Iveson J: History of nursing. **Nurs Mirror** 1982 Mar 24;154(12):34-6(continued periodically)
Iveson-Iveson J: St. David's day. **Nurs Mirror** 1984 Feb 29;158(9):16
James JW: Writing and rewriting nursing history: a review essay. **Bull Hist Med** 1984 Winter;58(4):568-84
Kanei H: [The role of women and nursing - a lesson in folk medicine. 3]. **Sogo Kango** 1982;17(1):79-89
Malterre-Barthes A: L'infirmière face aux problèmes de la prostitution. **Infirm Fr** 1981 May;(225):9-12 contd
Mericle BP: The male as psychiatric nurse. **J Psychosoc Nurs Ment Health Serv** 1983 Nov;21(11):28-34
Réflexions sur les soins infirmiers en psychiatrie: L'equipe soignante de Castelluccio. **Soins Psychiatr** 1980 Mar 1;(1):3-8
Seethalakshmi: Nursing education through the ages. **Nurs J India** 1983 Oct;74(10):279-81

**Czechoslovakia**

Tamura S: [History of Czechoslovakia and its system for nursing education] (Jpn). **Kango Kyoiku** 1983 Oct;24(10):605-13

**France**

Dorche J: Une institution lyonnaise: les religieuses au service des malades dans les hospices civils de Lyon 1500-1950. **Lyon Pharm** 1981 Apr;32(3):155-60
Dubrulle C: Soins infirmiers, rétrospective, perspectives. **Soins** 1980 Jul 5-20;25(13-14):67-72
Le Guen Y: Etre infirmier en psychiatrie. **Rev Infirm** 1980 Nov;30(9):19-22

**Germany**

Del Prado S: Einblick in eine Krankenpflegehilfe--Schule (Ausbildung). Der historische Weg zum Selbstverständnis in der Krankenpflegehilfe. **Krankenpflege (Frankfurt)** 1982 Jul-Aug;36(7-8):260-2
Höfert R: Krankenpflege im Spiegel der Zeiten. **Krankenpflege (Frankfurt)** 1983 Jan;37(1):6-8

**Great Britain**

Baly M: Care or cure? **Nurs Mirror** 1982 Sep 22;155(12):43-4
Clark SG: Farewell to the SBA. **J R Nav Med Serv** 1984 Spring;70(1):3-8

**Hungary**

Kapronczay K: A magyar ápolón óképzés kezdetei. **Orv Hetil** 1983 Feb 6;124(6):344-50
Sasvári L. Kiegészítő adatok a női beteg-ápolórendekröl. **Orv Hetil** 1982 Sep 12;123(37)2321-2

**Japan**

Mito M: [Lessons in Oriental medicine: its application in nursing] (Jpn). **Kango** 1981 May;33(6):26-30

**Norway**

Wyller I: Et nytt år med 'gammel-nytt'? **Sykepleien** 1982 Jan 5;69(1):4-7

**Poland**

Mazurkiewicz B: Polskie słownictwo pielęgniarskie. **Pieleg Polozna** 1980;(12):10-2

**Spain**

Darnés C, Solé A: Influencia de las comunidades religiosas en la enfermería de Cataluña. **Rev Enferm** 1981 Dec-1982 Jan;5(42-43):61-2
Domínquez Alcón C: Historia de la enfermería Catalana. **Rev Enferm** 1981 Dec-1982 Jan;5(42-43):57-8

**Sweden**

Rabo M, Kullberg G: [Swedish Nurses' Association's historical collection: witness to harsh conditions. Nursing departments.] (Swe) **Vardfacket** 1979;3(7):79-82

**Turkey**

Akçiçek E: Islâm tibbinda hemşirelik. **Turk Hemsire Derg** 1983;33(3):23-4

**United States**

Doona ME: District nurses celebrate nursing's past. **Mass Nurse** 1983 Nov;52(11):9
Leavitt JW, ed: Women and health in America: historical readings. Madison, University of Wisconsin Press, 1984. ix, 526 p. (Previously published articles by various authors)
Lynch EA: An historical survey of the test services of the National League for Nursing. **NLN Publ** 1980;(17-1777):i-viii, 1-78
Nursing hall of fame: Kansas City, Mo., American Nurses' Association, 1982. 16 p.

**Before 500 A.D.**

**Japan**

Onishi W: [Life among the frontier farmers of Hokkaido: public health nursing in the history of the Showa period. 10.] (Jpn). **Kango** 1982 Feb;34(2):65-71; 97-103

**500 A.D.-1450**

**Great Britain**

Mish IR: Nursing process--medieval style. **Nurs Forum** 1979;18(2):196-203

**1450-1700**

Berriot-Salvadore E: La femme soignante à la Renaissance: de la profession médicale à la vocation charitable. **Penelope** 1981;(5):24-8
Díaz F: Influencia de San Juan de Dios en la enfermería. **Rev Enferm** 1982 Mar;5(45):12-4

**France**

Humm E: Vinzenz von Paul und seine Aktualität. Sein Aufruf zur patientenorientierten Pflege. **Krankenpflege (Frankfurt)** 1982 Jan;36(1):3-4

**Great Britain**

Versluysen MC: A forgotten chapter. **Nurs Times** 1981 Jul 15-21;77(29):1239

# NURSING

## 1700 to Present

Allan P, Jolley M, ed: Nursing, midwifery and health visiting since 1900. London, Faber and Faber, 1982. 316 p. With contributions by R. H. Pyne, B. Watkin, V. H. Darling, M. E. Lee, C. R. Kratz, G. M. Owen, R. Everest, P. D. Birchenall, D. M. Saunders, B. M. Slaney, D. Blenkinsop, M. D. Green, C. M. Chapman, E. A. Bent, J. C. Hayward, S. R. Lelean, A. V. Cowie, S. Quinn, I. S. Palmer, D. H. Rye.
Arcuri EA: Conheça um pouco de sua opção: enfermagem. **Rev Esc Enferm USP** 1982 Aug;16(2):127–36
Arnold O: Charité et maladie dans la 1re moitié du XIXe siècle. **Penelope** 1981;(5):41–4
Barkley S: A nurse who made a difference. **Pulse** 1984 May;20(5):1–2
Barnard K: Research designs: the historical method. **MCN** 1981 Nov–Dec;6(6):391
Bentham A: Down Memory Lane: as it happened. **Nurs Mirror** 1982 Aug 11;155(6):28–30
Bowman IA: The image of the nurse on international postage stamps, 1920–1970. In Jones AH, ed: Images of healers. Albany, State University of New York, Press, 1983. p. 91–100.
Brooks JA, Kleine-Kracht AE: Evolution of a definition of nursing. **ANS** 1983 Jul;5(4):51–85
Carroll MA, Humphrey RH: Moral problems in nursing: case studies. Washington, University Press of America, 1979. Historical chapters, p. 6–28.
Chernetskiĭ OE: Meditsinskie sestry na pochtovykh markakh. **Med Sestra** 1980 Apr;39(4):53–6
Cullinan J: The roses of no man's land. **Nurs Times** 1980 Oct 16;76(42):1823–5
Curtis DE: Nurses and war. The way it was. **Am J Nurs** 1984 Oct;84(10):1253–4
Davies C: Making sense of the census in Britain and the U.S.A.: the changing occupational classification and the position of nurses. **Sociol Rev** 1980;28(3):581–610
Davies GR: The invasion of Normandy--D-day. **NATNEWS** 1984 Sep;21(9):24–6
Davis BA: The gerontological nursing specialty. **J Gerontol Nurs** 1983 Oct;9(10):527–32
Devlin J: Nurses join the stamp set. **Nurs Times** 1984 May 2–8;80(18):40–1
Díaz-Jano-Sov C: Feminism and the evolution of the profession of nursing. **Bol Col Prof Enferm PR** 1981 Jun;7(26):6–12
Dumont-Johnson M: Les infirmières: cols roses? **Nurs Que** 1981 Sep–Oct;1(6):10–9
Fiori L: Les origines du CICIAMS et son évolution pendant 50 ans. **Nouv Com Int Cathol Infirm Assist Med Soc** 1983;(3):41–8
Fitzpatrick ML: Nursing. **Signs** 1977;2(4):818–34
Germain CP: Nursing the dying: implications of Kübler-Ross' staging theory. **Ann Am Acad Polit Soc Sci** 1980;447:46–58
Gibbons LK: La investigación en enfermería: un campo interdisciplinario. **Educ Med Salud** 1980;14(1):76–94
Goodman LR: Nursing administration in psychiatric hospitals. **J Psychosoc Nurs Ment Health Serv** 1983 Aug;21(8):26–34
Ham LM, Chamings PA: Nursing history: our wasted asset. **Nurs Health Care** 1982 Oct;3(8):434–7
Ham LM: Reflections of nursing: portrait or carricature? **Image (IN)** 1981 Feb;13(1):9–12
Heinrich J: Historical perspectives on public health nursing. **Nurs Outlook** 1983 Nov–Dec;31(6):317–20
Henderson V: Nursing--yesterday and tomorrow. **Nurs Times** 1980 May 22;76(21):905–7
Hiestand WC: Nursing, the family, and the 'new' social history. **ANS** 1982 Apr;4(3):1–12
Hutner R: O rozwoju teorii pielęgnowania. **Pieleg Polozna** 1983;(6):8–9
Iveson-Iveson J: Profile: the forgotten heroine. (Mary Seacole). **Nurs Times** 1983 Sep 7;157(10):44–7
Kalisch BJ, Kalisch PA, McHugh M: Content analysis of film stereotypes of nurses. **Int J Womens Stud** 1980;3(6):531–58
Kalisch BJ, Kalisch PA: The Dionne quintuplets legacy: establishing the 'good doctor and his loyal nurse' image in American culture. **Nurs Health Care** 1984 May;5(5):242–51
Kim JS, Pyo YS: [Panel discussion: nurses' status in the community] (Kor). **Taehan Kanho** 1983 Sep 20;22(3):66–73, 41
Knibiehler Y: Les infirmières-visiteuses (1922–1938). **Penelope** 1981;(5):80–4
Lee SH: [Historical review of the nurses' status abroad] (Kor). **Taehan Kanho** 1983 Sep 20;22(3):42–8
McBryde B: A nurse's war - 2. A trip to Rouen. **Nurs Times** 1979 Jul 5;75(26):1150–2
McGinnis S: History of nursing audit: a survey of the literature. **QRB** 1978;Spec No:2–4
Maggs CJ: Oral history and nursing history. **Nurs Times** 1983 Oct 19–25;79(42):55–7
Makabe G: [A visit at Kaiserwerth. (1) (Florence Nightingale)] (Jpn). **Sogo Kango** 1982;16(4):61–74
Makabe G: [Visit to Kaiserwerth (2) (Florence Nightingale)]. (Jpn). **Sogo Kango** 1982;17(1):59–78
Nalepka C: Entry into professional nursing in the United States and in England viewed with a historical and comparative perspective. **Australas Nurses J** 1983 Jan–Feb;11(12):1–7
Netzel Riera C: Dirección de enfermería. Perspectiva histórica y encrucijada actual. **Rev Enferm** 1982 Dec;5(53):11–6
Osorio RA: Reflexión con madurez. Reseña histórica del propósito y origen de la ceremonia del 'capping' (coronamiento). **Bol Col Prof Enferm PR** 1983 Jun;9(34):26–7
Palmer IS: Florence Nightingale and international origins of modern nursing. **Image (IN)** 1981 Jun;13(2):28–31
Sadler C: Edith Cavell: from Blakeney Point to Brussels. **Nurs Mirror** 1982 Sep 15;155(11):52–4
Shimabukuro R: [History of the white nursing uniform. A study on the origin of the white uniform as the symbol of nursing] (Jpn). **Kurinikaru Sutadi** 1984 Jun;5(6):688–94
Smoyak SA, Rouslin S, ed: A collection of classics in psychiatric nursing literature. Thorofare, N. J., Slack, 1982. xi, 295 p.
Thompson JD: [The passionate humanist: from Nightingale to the new nurse] (Jpn). **Sogo Kango** 1981;16(1):60–73
Tokugawa S: [Encounter with history of nursing: on Linda Richards and others] (Jpn). **Kango Kyoiku** 1982 Sep;23(9):539–43
Tsuboi Y, Haga S, Matsuda M, et al: [Relationship between the Nightingale Nursing School and Tokyo Hospital Nursing School] (Jpn). **Sogo Kango** 1981;16(1):36–46
Vaksman IA, Popugaĭlo VM: Zhenshchiny mediki na pochtovykh markakh mira. **Feldsher Akush** 1984 Jul;49(7):38–43
Whitman M: Toward a new psychology for nurses. **Nurs Outlook** 1982 Jan;30(1):48–52
Yan YB, Chang NJ: [Panel discussion: historical review of the nurses' status - educational perspective] (Kor). **Taehan Kanho** 1983 Sep 20;22(3):56–65
Yoshikawa R: [Biography of Nightingale published in the early Meiji era - on 'Self-Help for Women'] (Jpn). **Sogo Kango** 1982;17(1):91–102

### Americas

Sihelvik L: Diamond jubilee of the Vincentian Sisters of Charity. **Jednota Annu Furdek (US)** 1978;17:197–200

### Australia

Adamson J: 75th Anniversary of the Royal Australian Nursing Federation. **Australas Nurses J** 1980 Nov;9(12):3–4
Davis E: Irene's diary of nursing in World War I. **Australas Nurses J** 1980 Dec;10(1):16–8
Fitzgerald M: A 50 years' overview of paediatric nursing practice. **Aust Nurses J** 1982 Aug;12(2):63–4
Hall EM: In the ward next door to Sister Kenny. **Aust Nurses J** 1981 May;10(10):57–8
Hobbs V: But westward look: nursing in Western Australia, 1829–1979. [Perth], University of Western Australia Press, 1980. xvi, 256 p.
Ibell BM: The development of nursing as a profession. In her: Integrated basic theory and practice of nursing. Victoria, Pitmen, 1979. p. 65–75.
Kellett AM: Minor rules and regulations for the nursing staff circa 1930. **Lamp** 1981 May;38(5 Suppl):41–4
Leucah F: Looking back: 'A psychological problem.' **Lamp** 1980 Dec;37(12):41–2
Looking back: the Australian army hospitals: **Lamp** 1980 May;37(5):53–5
Neil G: The Scott Memorial Hospital Scone: 90 years of nursing. **Lamp** 1982 Mar–Apr;39(2):19
O'Carrigan C: Two veteran nurses of World War I days (Sister Mary MacDonald, Sister Mary Vianney). **Med J Aust** 1984 Jun 23;140(13):782–4
Origin of the NSW Nurses' Association: **Lamp** 1981 May;38(5 Suppl):9–10
Parkes D, Schachter M: Meige, Brueghel or Blake? **Aust Nurses J** 1981 Feb;10(7):32–5
Place J: A summary of nurse training at the Royal Women's Hospital, Melbourne. **Aust Nurses J** 1981 Aug;11(2):2–4
Royal Alexandra's century of caring: **Aust Nurses J** 1980 Nov;10(5):20–1
Russell RL: We worked hard, but we enjoyed it! General nurse training in NSW--the first 50 years. **Lamp** 1981 May;38(5 Suppl):57–63
Tracy B: Explorations in industry No. V. The 'ministering angel'. **Lamp** 1981 Dec;38(12):30–4
Vance G: Nursing administration. **Aust Nurses J** 1983 Mar;12(1):12–4
Vance G: Reflections of nurse training. **Australas Nurses J** 1983 Jan–Feb;11(12):26–30

### Austria

Rettig A: 35 Jahre Osterr. Krankenpflegeverband--Permanenz eines Auftrages oder einer Entwicklung. **Osterr Krankenpflegez** 1982;35(3):69–70

### Belgium

In honor of the memory of Ghislaine van Massenhove, international president of CICIAMS: **Nouv Com Int Cathol Infirm Assist Med Soc** 1980;(1):1–24

Quinn S: [Nursing in the European Community; nursing in Belgium]. **Kango** 1982 Mar;34(3):67–79

### Belize

Hermann EK: Belizean nursing education in the 19th century. **Belizean Stud** 1979;7(4):16–24

### Brazil

Carvalho AC de: Escola de Enfermagem da Universidade de São Paulo. Resumo histórico 1942–1980. **Rev Esc Enferm USP** 1980 Aug;14 Suppl:1–271

Nogueira MJ: A pesquisa em enfermagem no Brasil: retrospective histórica. **Rev Esc Enferm USP** 1982 Apr;16(1):17–26

### Canada

Bonin M: Depuis l'Institut Marguerite–d'Youville, 50 ans d'études supérieures au Québec. **Infirm Can** 1984 Oct;26(9):31–4

Glass H: [The Canadian nursing scene] (Jpn). **Kango** 1984 Jul;36(8):11–9

Godfrey CM: Theophilus Mack. In Dictionary of Canadian Biography, 1881–1890. 1982;11:558–9.

The history and future of psychiatric nursing: **Can J Psychiatr Nurs** 1983 Oct–Nov;24(4):6–12

Kerr ME: A capsule history of your journal. **Can Nurse** 1980 Mar;76(3):20–1

Kirkwood L: Hier, aujourd'hui et demain. **Infirm Can** 1983 Oct;25(9):34–6

Knowles V: Leaving with a red rose. A history of the Ottawa Civic Hospital School of Nursing. Ottawa, Ottawa Civic Hospital School of Nursing Alumnae Association, 1981. vi, 218 p.

Le 75e anniversaire de l'association des infirmières et infirmiers du Canada: **Infirm Can** 1983 Oct;25(9):17–38

Michaud A: Evolution du syndicalisme infirmier vis–à–vis les associations professionnelles. **Infirm Can** 1981 Jul–Aug;23(7):24–7

Sylvestre PF: Dossier historique: les religieuses infirmières en Ontario français. **Infirm Can** 1983 Nov;25(10):27–9

Warrington–Türcke K: 75th anniversary. The evolution of accountability in nursing in Canada. **Can Nurse** 1983 Oct;79(9):34–7

Whittaker JA: Distinguishing nurses 'from other types of frauds'. **RNABC News** 1984 Jul–Aug;16(4):20–3

Wood V: Nursing education: the move from hospital schools of nursing––an historical perspective. **Int J Nurs Stud** 1984;21(3):183–92

60 ans déjà ...: **Nurs Que** 1980 Nov–Dec;1(1):12–26

75th anniversary. CNA's twelve member association: Without them where would we be? **Can Nurse** 1983 Oct;79(9):22–34

### Caribbean

Focus on the Bahamas: **Jamaican Nurse** 1982;22(1):19–22

### China

Paung PP: [The memoirs of Judy Chu] (Chi). **Hu Li Tsa Chih** 1980 Jul;27(3):63–71

Suzuki M: [Past and present nursing in China] (Jpn) **Sogo Kango** 1982;17(4):59–74

### Europe

Ikezawa Y, Kono H: [The starting point in nursing––an observation through the history of European ideology] (Jpn). **Kango Tenbo** 1981 Oct;6(10):905–13

Quinn S, ed: Nursing in the European community. London, Croom Helm, 1980. 192 p. With contributions by S. Russell, J. Delaide, K. Stallknecht, C. Allaire, R. Elster, I. Leydon, P. Breccia, D. Schol, M. Van Driel Krol, R. I. Emblin.

### Finland

Fock G: Om sköterskor, havandeskap, förlossning samt barnsäng i Finland på Elias Lönnrots tid. **Katilolehti** 1982 Jan;87(1):11–4

Ohquist M: Hälsosyster i Esbo på 1920–talet. **Hist Litteraturhist Studier (Finl)** 1979;54:201–38

Tallberg M: Sophie Mannerheim: en historisk beskrivning och analys av hennes verksamhet 1904–1928. **Vard Nord Utveckl Forsk** 1983 Spring;3(4):123–30

### France

Collière MF: La profession infirmière en quête de son histoire 1870–1980. **Rev Infirm** 1980 Dec;30(10):13–24

Faure O: A l'hôpital, avant les infirmières: les soeurs hospitalières de Lyon au début du XIXe siècle. **Penelope** 1981;(5):52–5

Greenbaum LS: Nurses and doctors in conflict: piety and medicine in the Paris Hôtel–Dieu on the eve of the French Revolution. **Clio Med** 1979 May;13(3–4):247–67

Jaeger M: La profession d'infirmier psychiatrique: le poids de son passé. **Soins Psychiatr** 1984 Jun–Jul;(44–45):63–4

Joblin J: Monseigneur André Jacques Fougerat; ecclesiastical advisor of CICIAMS (1952–1982). **Nouv Com Int Cathol Infirm Assist Med Soc** 1983;(3):1–8

Leroux–Hugon V: Infirmières des hôpitaux parisiens au début du siècle. **Penelope** 1981;(5):62–7

Loux F: La femme soignante dans les traditions rurales du XIXe siècle. **Penelope** 1981;(5):37–40

Massé G, Petitjean F. L'infirmier en psychiatrie. Loi du 30 juin 1838 –– 2e partie. **Infirm Fr** 1982 Jan;(231):3–4, 36 concl.

Morel MF: Mères et nourrices au XVIIIe siècle: les soins aux jeunes enfants. **Penelope** 1981;(5):29–32

Sabin LE: The French Revolution: the forgotten era in nursing history. **Nurs Forum** 1981;20(3):225–43

### Germany

Elster R: Porträt unserer Zeitschrift. **Krankenpflege (Frankfurt)** 1981 Jan;35(1):7–10

Fricke A: Die thematische Entwicklung unserer Zeitschrift; Rückblick––Gegenwart––Ausblick. **Krankenpflege (Frankfurt)** 1981 Jan;35(1):11–5

Koch F: Geschichte der Krankenpflege von 1930–1950. Bericht über ein Seminar im Bildungszentrum Essen (BZE) des DBfK. **Krankenpflege (Frankfurt)** 1984 Mar;38(3):85–6

Lindemann M: Love for hire: the regulation of the wet–nursing business in eighteenth–century Hamburg. **J Fam Hist** 1981 Winter;6(4):379–95

Lungershausen M: Unsere Rückblende aus dem Jahr 1952. Agnes Karll (25. 3. 1868 12. 2. 1927). **Krankenpflege (Frankfurt)** 1982 Feb;36(2):71–2

Makabe G: [Early nursing textbooks in Germany – 'Establishment of modern nursing' by Anna Sticker. (1)] (Jpn). **Sogo Kango** 1982 May;17(2):103–24

Makabe G: [Early nursing textbooks in Germany––'Establishment of Modern Nursing' by Anna Sticker. (2)] (Jpn). **Sogo Kango** 1982;17(3):59–77

Reimann R: Das Bildungszentrum Essen des DBfK besteht zehn Jahre. **Krankenpflege (Frankfurt)** 1984 Jul–Aug;38(7–8):222–4

Sticker A: Agnes Karll, die Reformerin der deutschen Krankenpflege. Ein Wegweiser für heute zu ihrem 50. Todestag am 12. Februar 1927. Wuppertal, Aussat, 1977. 240 p.

Sticker DA: [Theodor Fliedner and nursing] (Jpn). **Sogo Kango** 1980;15(4):146–55

Torp H: 75 Jahre Fachzeitschrift: Dokumentation von Kontinuität und Wandel in der Krankenpflege. **Krankenpflege (Frankfurt)** 1981 Jun;35(6):235–7

Wolff J, Wolff HP: Die Förderung der Krankenpflege im vollentwickelten Kapitalismus durch Arzte an der Charité. Eine biographische Studies aus Anlass des 150 jährigen Bestehens der Ausbildung von Pflegekräften in Berlin. **Z Arztl Fortbild (Jena)** 1982 Sep 1;76(17):803–7

### Great Britain

Arton M: The development of psychiatric nursing education in England and Wales. **Nurs Times** 1981 Jan 15;77(3):124–7

Baly M: A leading light. **Nurs Mirror** 1982 Nov 10;155(19):49–51

Baly M: A new history of nursing. Three. The nurse élite (Florence Nightingale). **Nurs Times** 1984 Oct 17–23;80(42):55–7

Berentson L: Florence Nightingale: change agent. **RN Id** 1982 Apr–May;6(2):3, 7

Boisvert DJ: Florence Nightingale's cap. **N Engl Galaxy** 1978;20(2):42–51

Bolton G, Dean M: Nursing history: women of good character. **Nurs Mirror** 1980 Nov 20;151(21):24–7

Brimley R: Health visiting as it was. Interview by Shirley Goodwin. **Nurs Mirror** 1981 Jul 22;153(4):22–4

Broadley ME: Patients come first: nursing at 'The London' between the two World Wars. London, London Hospital Special Trustees, 1980. 282 p.

Calton S: Nursing past, present and future: keeping pace with the times. **Nurs Mirror** 1980 Jan 31;150(5):36–7

Carter L: Down memory lane: the bottomless pit. **Nurs Mirror** 1982 Jan 27;154(4):26–7

Clocotici L: Sănătatea este un mod de a exista. **Viata Med [Medii Sanit]** 1981 Nov;29(11):259–60

Cohen IB: Florence Nightingale. **Sci Am** 1984 Mar;250(3):128–37

Collins SM: Nursing––the next 100 years. **J Adv Nurs** 1981 May;6(3):165–71

Connolly MP: Health visiting 1850–1900: a review. **Midwife Health Visit Community Nurse** 1980 Jul;16(7):282–5

Connolly MP: Health visiting 1900–1910: a review. **Midwife Health Visit Community Nurse** 1980 Sep;16(9):375–8

Cowell B, Wainwright D: The battle for status. **Nurs Times** 1981 Jul 15–21;77(29):1237–8

Cruse P: Florence Nightingale. **Surgery** 1980 Sep;88(3):394–9

Davies C: Past and present in nursing education. **Nurs Times** 1980 Sep 25;76(39):1703–7

Davies C: Where next for nursing history? **Nurs Times** 1980 May 22;76(21):920–2

## NURSING


Davies C, ed: Rewriting nursing history. London, Croom Helm, and Totowa, New Jersey, Barnes & Noble, 1980. 226 p. Includes contributions by C. Maggs, K. Williams, M. Dean, G. Bolton, M. Carpenter, P. Bellaby, P. Oribabor, M. C. Versluysen, J. Foster, J. Sheppard, C. Kratz.

Davis E: Queen Alexandra's Royal Army Nursing Corp. **Australas Nurses J** 1981 Oct;10(10):16–9

Dawe AM: A case for community psychiatric nurses. **J Adv Nurs** 1980 Sept;5(5):485–90

Devlin R: The VADs nursing in no man's land. **Nurs Mirror** 1980 Oct 23;151(17):8–9

Dopson L: Celebrating 75 years. **Nurs Times** 1980 May 22;76(21):923–36

Dopson L: The cut-throat world of nursing politics – 18th century-style. **Nurs Times** 1984 Apr 25–May 1;80(17):19–20

Dopson L: The new breed of nurse historian. **Nurs Times** 1984 Sep 19–25;80(38):16–7

Dopson L: The QA museum. **Nurs Times** 1981 Nov 11–17;77(46):1974

Dopson L: Volunteer nurses. One. VADs at war. **Nurs Times** 1984 Aug 1–7;80(31):36–8

Dopson L: 100 years of ophthalmic nursing. **Nurs Times** 1981 Jun 11;77(24):1043–4

Ducrocq F: Des thérapeutes du corps médical. **Penelope** 1981;(5):45–9

Edwards IG: Down memory lane: burial at sea. **Nurs Mirror** 1980 Jul 3;150(21):36–7

Ferguson M: Reflections on teaching a history of nursing. **Nurs Times** 1979 Nov;75(46–47):suppl 29–30:117–20, 121–2

Ferrer M: The Royal College of Midwives 1881 – 1981. **Midwife Health Visit Community Nurse** 1981 Jul;17(7):288–94

Florence Nightingale: the original geriatric nurse. **Okla Nurse** 1980 May;25(4):6

Fraga M, Tenenbaum L: Florence Nightingale--model for today's nurse. **Fla Nurse** 1981 May;29(5):11

French J: Nurses in society: far from home. **Nurs Mirror** 1984 May 23;158(21):32

Gaffney R: Women as doctors and nurses. In Checkland O, Lamb M, ed: Health care as social history; the Glasgow case. Aberdeen, Aberdeen University Press, 1982. p. 134–48.

Glupker DF: The yesteryear of orthopaedic nursing (Agnes Hunt). **Orthop Nurs** 1984 Nov–Dec;3(6):48

Gould ME, Gamlen C: [A woman of parts. Florence Nightingale]. (Jpn) **Sogo Kango** 1980;15(1):95–9

Graham S: Notes on nursing, 1860–1980. Angels of plain speech. **Nurs Times** 1980 Oct 23;76(43):1874

Grant AS: The RCM--the first 100 years: some things never change. **Midwives Chron** 1981 Oct;95(1125):348–50

Greene J: Where now for psychiatric nursing? Steps along the way. **Nurs Mirror** 1980 Jun 26;150(20):suppl iv–vii

Guha M, Wood M: Does health visiting have a history? **Health Visit** 1981 Dec;54(12):540

Guntrip G: The unknown Edith Cavell. **Nurs Times** 1984 Apr 25–May 1;80(17):63–4

Hardy G: William Rathbone and the early history of district nursing. Ormskirk, Hesketh, 1981. 54 p.

Hardy L, Rafferty AM: Nursing and history. **Nurs Times** 1982 Sep 15–21;78(37):1564–5

Harland KM: A short history of Queen Alexandra's Royal Naval Nursing Service. **J R Nav Med Serv** 1984 Summer;70(2):59–65

Hebert RG: Florence Nightingale: saint, reformer or rebel? Malabar, Florida, Robert E. Krieger, 1981. 236 p.

Hepplethwaite A: Nursing in the thirties. **Nurs Times** 1984 Jul 11–17;80(28):40–2

Hill AJ: Nightingale, sainte ou diablesse? **Infirm Can** 1980 Nov;(10):34–6

Hosono K: [The logical structure in the 'Notes on Nursing' (Florence Nightingale)] (Jpn). **Sogo Kango** 1982;16(4):51–60

Iveson-Iveson J: A pin to see a peep show (Mary Seacole, Cicely Saunders). **Nurs Mirror** 1984 Mar 28;158(13):36

Iveson-Iveson J: Diploma of nursing. Part A: development of nursing as a profession. **Nurs Mirror** 1981 Feb 5;152(6):29–30

Iveson-Iveson J: History of nursing in the Air Force: string, sealing wax and individual daring. **Nurs Mirror** 1981 Jul 15;153(3):27–8

Iveson-Iveson J: History of the navy nurses: a life on the ocean waves. **Nurs Mirror** 1981 Jul 1;153(1):22–4

Iveson-Iveson J: Lesson from the past for trauma nursing. **Nurs Mirror** 1982 Jun 16;154(24):10

Iveson-Iveson J: Nurses in society: a legend in the breaking (Florence Nightingale). **Nurs Mirror** 1983 May 11;156(19):26–7

Iżycka J: Międzynarodowa Rada Pielęgniarek. **Pieleg Polozna** 1982;(9):24–6

Jones IH: Wages through the ages. **Nurs Times** 1980 Jul 17;76(29):1279–80

Kalisch BJ, Kalisch PA: Heroine out of focus: media images of Florence Nightingale. Part 1. Popular biographies and stage productions. **Nurs Health Care** 1983 Apr;4(4):181–7

Kanai H: [What Nightingale would have written about summer heat and nursing – a thought in connection with folk remedy] (Jpn). **Kango** 1982 Aug;34(9):4–14

Kaneko M: [An encounter with Nightingale] (Jpn) **Sogo Kango** 1980;15(4):22–8

Kaneko M: [The nature of observation expressed in the 'Observation of the sick' (Florence Nightingale)] (Jpn). **Sogo Kango** 1982;16(4):40–50

Karll A: Florence Nightingale. **Nurs J India** 1983 May;74(5):110

Kawakita Y: [Nightingale in the history of medical philosophy--on the meaning of 'health'] (Jpn). **Kango** 1982 Feb;34(2):39–53

Keeffe D: Development of care for the mentally ill. **Physiotherapy** 1980 Dec;66(12):407–8

Kodama K: [Care and cure defined in the 'Notes on Nursing' (Florence Nightingale)] (Jpn). **Sogo Kango** 1982;16(4):29–39

Kodama K: [From the old notes on Florence Nightingale] (Jpn) **Sogo Kango** 1980;15(4):12–7

Kodama K: [Scenes associated with Florence Nightingale] (Jpn) **Kango** 1980 Nov;32(11):48–59

Koike A: [Hitherto unknown profile of Florence Nightingale]. (Jpn) **Sogo Kango** 1980;15(1):100–8

Konami Y: [Studies on Nightingale: the role of the matron] (Jpn) **Sogo Kango** 1980;15(4):29–36

Livingston RH: They comfort me. The history of nursing in Belfast. **Ulster Med J** 1981;50(1):33–45

McCulloch I: Nursing Mirror mental health forum. 3. From colony to community care. **Nurs Mirror** 1983 Apr 20:156(16):i–ii

Macfie C: Down Memory Lane: for king and country. **Nurs Mirror** 1982 Jul 21;155(3):41–4

McMillan M: Looking back: school nursing in England. **Lamp** 1980 Mar;37(3):69–71

Maggs C: A new history of nursing. Four. **Nurs Times** 1984 Nov 21–27;80(47):49–51

Maggs C: A new history of nursing. One. Changing perspectives. **Nurs Times** 1984 Sep 19–25;80(38):28–31

Maggs C: Control mechanisms and the 'new nurses' 1881–1914. **Nurs Times** 1981 Sep 2–8;77(36)suppl 25:97–100

Maggs C: The making of a history man [interview by Jane Salvage]. **Nurs Times** 1983 Aug 17–23;79(33):8–10

Maggs C: The register of nurses in the Scottish poor law service 1885–1919. **Nurs Times** 1981 Nov 25–Dec 1;77(48):suppl 33:129–32

Makabe G: [Foundation of nursing. Letter collection of Florence Nightingale] (Jpn). **Sogo Kango** 1982;17(4):8–34

Makabe G: [Nightingale's expectation on women--an impression of her writings] (Jpn) **Sogo Kango** 1980;15(4):70–2

Mathews M, Harris M: The Royal Naval Medical Air Evacuation Unit. **J R Nav Med Serv** 1980 Summer;66(2):147–51

Montague L: Ambassadors of the king. **Nurs Times** 1983 Dec 14–20;79(50):57–60

Morris M: Normandy 1944. One. D-Day diary. **Nurs Times** 1984;80(23):46–7; (24):44–5

Nagasawa Y: [Encounter with Nightingale---a discovery of Nightingale in the field of hospital designs] (Jpn) **Sogo Kango** 1980;15(4):59–69

Nauright L: Politics and power: a new look at Florence Nightingale. **Nurs Forum** 1984;21(1):5–7

Newby MS: Problems of teaching nursing history. 1. **Nurs Times** 1979 Nov 22;75(47):suppl 30:123–4 (continued periodically)

Ninan R: The lady with the lamp: a profile. **Nurs J India** 1982 Jun;73(6):154–5

Nishida A: [In preparation of the key words for Nightingale's 'Notes on Nursing'--introduction to a humanistic theory] **Sogo Kango** 1980;15(4):46–58

Nishida A: [Understanding of man in the 'Notes on Nursing' (Florence Nightingale)] (Jpn). **Sogo Kango** 1982;16(4):9–22

Nuttall P: Miss Florence Nightingale: 'the passionate statistician'. **Nurs J India** 1984 Jun;75(6):128–9

Nuttall P: The passionate statistician (Florence Nightingale). **Nurs Times** 1983 Sep 28–Oct 4;79(39):25–7

Okada M: [Notes on 'Cassandra'. 1 (Florence Nightingale)] (Jpn) **Sogo Kango** 1984 Aug 15;19(3):63–78

Okamura A: [A long road to the hospice movement--life of Mother Mary Aikenhead] (Jpn). **Kango Kyoiku** 1984 Jan;25(1):38–45;25(2):104–11 (continued periodically)

Om dårlige arbeidsrutiner. Med hilsen fra Florence Nightingale: **Sykepleien** 1984 Sep 20;71(16):6–8, 30

Ota S: [Florence Nightingale's expectations on modern nursing--thoughts on nursing science] (Jpn). **Sogo Kango** 1984 May 15;19(2):79–88

Palmer IS: Florence Nightingale: the myth and the reality. **Nurs Times** 1983 Aug 3–9;79(31):40–2

Palmer IS: Nightingale revisited. **Nurs Outlook** 1983 Jul–Aug;31(4):229–33

Palmer IS: [Nightingale revisited] (Jpn). **Kango** 1983 Nov;35(12):112–22

Parr LJ: Early libraries for nurses in England, 1860–1914. **J Librariansh** 1980;12(2):102–14

Prince J: Education for a profession: some lessons from history (Florence Nightingale). **Int J Nurs Stud** 1984;21(3):153–63

Quinn S: [Development in nursing practice in the United Kingdom since 1948] (Jpn). **Kango** 1984 Jul;36(8):31–6

Rains AJ: 'The Nightingale touch'. **J R Army Med Corps** 1982 Feb;128(1):4–17

Rogers P: Florence Nightingale: the myth and the reality. **Nurs Focus** 1982 Jul;3(11):10

Rothrock JC: Nursing diagnosis: in the days of Florence Nightingale. **AORN J** 1984 Aug;40(2):189–90

Schmidt V: Hvad fejlede Florence Nightingale? **Sygeplejersken** 1980 Aug 6;80(31):4–10; Oct 5;67(17):16–21

Shannon R: [Re-evaluation of Florence Nightingale: a review of 'Florence Nightingale: Reputation and Power' by F. B. Smith] (Jpn). **Kango Kyoiku** 1982 Nov;23(11):677-85
Slaney B: The development of occupational health nursing. **Nursing (Oxford)** 1984 May;2(25):suppl 1-3
Smith FB: Florence Nightingale. Reputation and power. London, Canberra, Croom Helm, 1982. xii, 216 p.
Smith FT: Florence Nightingale: early feminist. **Am J Nurs** 1981 May;81(5):1021-4
Smith FT: [Florence Nightingale: early feminist] (Jpn). **Kango Kyoiku** 1982 Nov,23(11).671-6
Smith L: The influence of tradition in nursing. **Nurs Times** 1982 Apr 28-May 4;78(17):suppl 12:45-8
Spray W: Down memory lane: obituary at Nottingham. **Nurs Mirror** 1980 Mar 27;150(13):27-8
Swain V: No plaster saint! **Nurs Times** 1983 Mar 16-22;79(11):62-3
Takahashi M: [A tour of the areas related to Florence Nightingale. (1)] (Jpn). **Kango Kyoiku** 1981 Jan;22(1):54-60
Takahashi M: [On participating in the tour of the 'Areas related to Nightingale' (2)] (Jpn). **Kango Kyoiku** 1981 Apr;22(4):262-7
Takeyama M: [Conclusion of the translation of the 'Life of Florence Nightingale'] (Jpn). **Sogo Kango** 1981 Aug;16(3):76-83
Tamura M: [On research on Florence Nightingale -- a future overview] (Jpn). **Sogo Kango** 1980;15(4):18-21
Teramoto M: [Me and the Florence Nightingale letter collection] (Jpn). **Sogo Kango** 1982;17(4):35-8
Thompson JD: The passionate humanist: from Nightingale to the new nurse. **Nurs Outlook** 1980 May;28(5):290-5
Tiffany R: The development of oncology nursing in the United Kingdom. **Prog Clin Biol Res** 1983;132E:435-40
Usui T. [The influence of Nightingale on my nursing activities] (Jpn) **Sogo Kango** 1980;15(4):37-45
Van der Peet R: Florence Nightingale en haar visie op verplegen in relatie tot het leven en werk van Charles Darwin. **Tijdschr Ziekenverpl** 1983 Aug 23;36(17):530-6
Warren-Farrow D: A perilous night. **Nurs Times** 1982 Jul 14-20;78(28):1203-4
Weller B: The spy who nursed me (Edith Cavell). **Nurs Times** 1984 Oct 17-23;80(42):18-9
Wheeler CE: Viewpoint: essay in response to republication of a biography (Florence Nightingale). **ANS** 1984 Jul;6(4):74-9
Wickes HL: History of nursing in the Army: behind the lines. **Nurs Mirror** 1981 Jul 8;153(2):23-4
Wiewiórowska M: Koncepcja piel egniarstwa Florencji Nightingale. **Pieleg Polozna** 1981;(8):7-8
Wiewiórowska M: Koncepcja pielegniarstwa Florencji Nightingale. **Pieleg Polozna** 1981;(5):8
Wiewiórowska M: Koncepcja pielęgniarstwa Florencji Nightingale. **Pieleg Polozna** 1981;(6):10-2 contd
Wiewiórowska M: Koncepcja pielęgniarstwa Florencji Nightingale. **Pieleg Polozna** 1981;(7):9-10, 15
Williams E: Diary of a VAD 1940-49. **Nurs Mirror** 1981 Jul 8;153(2):25-7 (continued regularly)
Williams E: Diary of a VAD 1940-9: cry havoc... **Nurs Mirror** 1981 Jul 1;153(1):25-8
Woodall ME: Ruolo e identita' dell'infermiere: riscoprire il pensiero di Florence Nightingale. **Prof Inferm** 1980 Oct-Dec;33(4):166-9
Yumaki M: [Nightingale's concept of God] (Jpn). **Sogo Kango** 1982;16(4):23-8
Yumaki M: [50 years of the studies on Florence Nightingale] (Jpn). **Sogo Kango** 1980;15(4):7-11

### Hungary

Hogye I: 'Bábai mesterség' a Hegyalján (1711-1849). **Orvostort Kozl** 1982;28(1-3):201-8
Sasvári L: Nöi betegápoló rendek szerepe a hazai kórházak munkájában (1867-1918). **Orv Hetil** 1982 Apr 18;123(16):990-2

### India

Adranvala TK: Vital aspects of nursing: the historical perspective. **Nurs J India** 1982 May;73(5):125-8
Khurana SL: Origin and development of nursing in India. **Nurs J India** 1984 Jan;75(1):9-11
Platinum jubilee almanac: A calendar of developments and activities of TNAI and in the related discipline during last seventy-five years. **Nurs J India** 1983 Nov;74(11):291-7
Sood RK: Vital aspects of nursing: development of education and services. **Nurs J India** 1982 May;73(5):128-32
TNAI in retrospect: The Agra Conference: 1909. **Nurs J India** 1983 Nov;74(11):300-9
Watts EA: Down Memory Lane - a pioneer remembers. **Nurs J India** 1983 Nov;74(11):298-9

### Israel

Bergman R: [Israel nursing--35 years of evolutionary change] (Jpn). **Kango** 1984 Jul;36(8):44-9

### Italy

Morgan K: No boots in Sicily. **Nurs Mirror** 1983 Nov 2;157(18):42

### Jamaica

Dopson L: One hundred years on. **Nurs Times** 1982 May 12-18;78(19):781-2
Marshall-Burnett S: A brief reflection on the life of Mary Seacole 1805-1881. **Jamaican Nurse** 1981 Dec;21(2):14-5
Seivwright M: The Florence Nightingale of Jamaica: Mary Seacole. **Jamaican Nurse** 1981 Dec;21(2):16
Smith JP: Mary Jane Seacole 1805-1881: a black British nurse. **J Adv Nurs** 1984 Sep;9(5):427-8

### Japan

[A meeting to commemorate the 100th anniversary of Ms. Haya Ishibashi, a pioneer in psychiatric nursing] (Jpn): **Kango** 1980 Jun;32(6):88
Besscho C: [Life of Mrs. Seki Hora, the founder of Japanese public health nursing] (Jpn). **Kango** 1980 Jun;32(6):112-20
Bessho C: [Nursing as image. From nurses' point of view: nurses of past and present] (Jpn). **Kango** 1984 Aug;36(9):20-6
Chiyo: [Illustrated history of nursing] (Jpn). **Kango Kyoiku** 1984 Feb;25(2):95-102 contd
Endo E: [Nurse's images in the Taisho period; nurses described in women's magazines] (Jpn). **Igakushi Kenkyu** 1980;54:28-35
Endo E: [Visiting nurse after the World War II] (Jpn). **Igakushi Kenkyu** 1978;49:22-6
Endo E: [Visiting nursing in 1926-1945] (Jpn). **Igakushi Kenkyu** 1977;48:30-8
Hasegawa A: [Social events in the history of nursing after World War II. I. Hospital and nurses on strike] (Jpn). **Kango** 1984 Aug;36(9):126-44
[History of public health nursing activities among frontier farmers in Hokkaido] (Jpn): **Hokenfu Zasshi** 1982 Jan;38(1):10-49
Ishigaki Y, Uzawa Y: [Historical review of continuing education in Hokkaido University Hospital] (Jpn). **Kango Tenbo** 1984 Nov;9(11):1021-32
Kameyama M: Evaluation of the social position of the nurse in the modern history of nursing in Japan. Chapter 1. The Japan Red Cross and nurses (Jpn). **Kango** 1980 Jun;32(6):78-87 (continued periodically)
Kato M, Araki S, Sadahiro U, et al: [History of public health nursing in Hokkaido--through the war, postwar transition, repatriation, and reconstruction periods. A discussion] (Jpn). **Hokenfu Zasshi** 1982 Jan;38(1):58-75
Kawamura Z: [Compilation of the history of public health nursing and observation of its significance] (Jpn). **Hokenfu Zasshi** 1981 Jul;37(7):570-86
Kishi Y, Uzawa Y, Hanashima T: [Postwar transitions in the theories of nursing education: with special reference to the period between 1945 to 1955] (Jpn) **Kango Kyoiku** 1984 Sep;25(9):541-60
Koba F: [History of school health nursing] (Jpn). **Kango** 1984 Jun;36(7):38-46
Lundeen E: [An interview with Miss Elizabeth Lundeen, a former GHQ nursing officer who contributed to the improvement of post-war Japanese nursing and recently visited Japan after 22 years] (Jpn) **Kango** 1982 Nov;34(12):76-7
Nakazato T: [The early days of modern nursing in Japan--the Kyoto School of Nursing] (Jpn). **Kango** 1981 Jan;33(1):70-83
Okuni M: [A chronological table on district nurse (Hokenfu) in after the war. Part I] (Jpn). **Igakushi Kenkyu** 1977;48:39-40
Onishi W: [A life among frontier farmers in Hokkaido: a public health nurse in a segment of history of the Showa era] (Jpn). **Kango** 1981 Aug;33(9):88-91
Onishi W: [Life among farmers of a reclamation project in Hokkaido: a life of a public health nurse in a segment of the history of the Showa period] (Jpn). **Kango** 1981 Dec;33(14):82-7
Onishi W: [Public health nurse working among the farmers in the Hokkaido Reclamation Project: a segment of the history of the Showa period] (Jpn). **Kango** 1981 Apr;33(4):73-9
Onishi W: [Public health nursing at land reclamation project in Hokkaido: a segment of the history of the Showa period] (Jpn). **Kango** 1981 Sep;33(10):98-103, Nov;33(12):81-91
Ryder R: [Nursing reformation in postwar Japan: a reflection on the period of occupation] (Jpn). **Kango Kyoiku** 1981 Oct;22(10):601-11
Shima K: [Endless voyage. The life of Ms. Shin Tanaka. 7. Chapter 2] (Jpn). **Josanpu Zasshi** 1983 Jan;37(1):72-9
Shimoyama K: [Care and nursing given at Koishikawa Clinic] (Jpn). **Kurinikaru Sutadi** 1983 Jul;4(7):837-42
Tagochi T: [Nursing and nursing education in the past 35 years since the end of the Second World War. (1)] (Jpn) **Kango Kyoiku** 1981 Jan;22(1):34-40

Takada M: [Children who do not know Florence Nightingale: teaching of nursing history at a nursing school] (Jpn). **Kango Kyoiku** 1984 Dec;25(12):725–7
Takahashi M: [Illustrated history of nursing - toward teaching of more attractive nursing history (3). The first nursing school in Japan and trained nurses] (Jpn). **Kango Kyoiku** 1983 Sep;24(9):560–3
Takahashi M: [Illustrated history of nursing--towards a more attractive study of nursing history] (Jpn). **Kango Kyoiku** 1984 Jan;25(1):46–9 contd
Takahashi M: [Illustrated nursing history--for teaching of more interesting nursing history (2). The image of midwives described in 'Fujin Juso' and 'Baba Hikken'] (Jpn). **Kango Kyoiku** 1983 Aug;24(8):496–9
Takahashi M: [Illustrated nursing history--teaching of more interesting nursing history (1). Focus on Japanese nursing history] (Jpn). **Kango Kyoiku** 1983 Jul;24(7):432–5
Takahashi M: [Mrs. Fuji Hirano, an early graduate of Jikei Hospital Nursing School] (Jpn). **Kango Kyoiku** 1983 Nov;24(11):686–91
Takahashi M: [Nurses in the history of nursing. (1) Masa Suzuki] (Jpn). **Kango Kyoiku** 1981 Jun;22(6):399–403
Takâhashi M: [Nurses in the history of nursing. (2). Kyo Takano] (Jpn). **Kango Kyoiku** 1981 Jul;22(7):451–6
Takahashi M: [Nurses in the history of nursing. (3). 'Infant Jesus' Mission and its nursing activities] (Jpn). **Kango Kyoiku** 1981 Aug;22(8):513–20
Takahashi M: [Nurses in the history of nursing (6). Mrs. Miki Sawada and a home nurse] (Jpn). **Kango Kyoiku** 1981 Nov;22(11):718–24
Takahashi M: [Personalities in the history of nursing. (4). Ms. Chika Ozeki] (Jpn). **Kango Kyoiku** 1981 Sep;22(9)575–82
Tanaka K, Uzawa Y, Hanashima T: [Further and continuing education of nurses in Japan; historical overview by literature.] (Jpn). **Kango Tenbo** 1983 Nov;8(11):996–1005
Tanaka M: [Public health nurses of the Santama area (5). History of public health clinics in the past 40 years since their start: a visit with Ms. Miki Tanaka] (Jpn). **Hokenfu Zasshi** 1982 Aug;38(8):676–83
Tsubota S: [Public health nurses in the frontier of Hokkaido--a historical background] (Jpn). **Hokenfu Zasshi** 1982 Jan;38(1):50–6
Uchibori C: [Personal record of the government-operated public health nursing activities at Gunma Prefecture. 8. The era of post-war confusion] (Jpn). **Hokenfu Zasshi** 1983 Jan;39(1):38–9
Uchibori C: [Problems faced by public health nurses during World War II] (Jpn). **Hokenfu Zasshi** 1982 Aug;38(8):694–6
Uchibori C: [Public health nursing activities in Gunma Prefecture: a personal history. At the end of World War II] (Jpn). **Hokenfu Zasshi** 1982 Nov;38(11):924–6
Uchibori C: [Reflection on public health nursing retraining seminars immediately after the Second World War] (Jpn). **Hokenfu Zasshi** 1983 Apr;39(4):294–6
Ueda M, Usui K, Kawasaki S, et al: [History of public health nurses associated with Osaka public health clinics: social health of the Meiji, Taisho, and Showa eras and the birth of public health nurses] (Jpn). **Hokenfu Zasshi** 1981 Apr;37(4):250–7
Uzawa Y, Hanajima T: [Modern nursing education observed in nursing text books-from 'Kongo Kokoroe' dated 1877 to those published by the end of World War II] (Jpn). **Kango Kyoiku** 1982 Sep;23(9):544–54
Watanabe K: [History of nursing in the Taisho era.] (Jpn). **Kango Kyoiku** 1982 Jan 25;23(1):60–6 (continued regularly)
Yagi K: [Improvement of teaching/learning method of nursing history.] (Jpn). **Kango Tenbo** 1983 Nov;8(11):1041–50
Yumai M: [Growing pain - a personal history (9)] (Jpn). **Sogo Kango** 1980;15(1):74–81
Yumaki M, Kodama K: [Changes in nursing during the 30 years after the war] (Jpn). **Kango** 1981 Jan;33(1):114–21 (continued periodically)
Yumaki M, Kodama K, Usui H: [Discussion: at the conclusion of 'Growing Pain'] (Jpn) **Sogo Kango** 1980;15(3):90–109
Yumaki M, Kodama K: [Transition in nursing in the 30 years since the end of World War II] (Jpn) **Kango** 1980 Nov;32(11):98–106

**Korea**

Chun SC: [Historical review of the nurses' status in Korea] (Kor). **Taehan Kanho** 1983 Sep 20;22(3):30–41
[The 1st quadrennial convention in commemoration of the diamond jubilee of the KNA] (Kor): **Taehan Kanho** 1983 Sep 20;22(3):15–29

**Malta**

Waterman BB: Memories of Malta 1940–42. **J R Nav Med Serv** 1984 Winter;70(3):182–5

**Mexico**

Bustamente ME: La primera enfermera en la historia de la salud publica, Isabel Cendala y Gómez. **Rev Col Nac Enferm** 1980 Jul, 1981 Feb;27–28(107):7–12
Pérez Loredo Díaz L: Relato de acontecimientos sobresalientes en la enfermería sanitaria y asistencial 1943 a 1983. **Salud Publica Mex** 1983 Sep–Oct;25(5):509–12

**Netherlands**

Knecht, van Eekelen A de: Bakerboekjes in de 19e eeuw: en aanvulling. **Tijdschr Geschied Geneeskd** 1981;4(1):45–7
Kragt VE: De ontwikkeling van het verpleegkundig beroep in Nederland (I). **Tijdschr Ziekenverpl** 1980 Aug 26;33(17):791–8
Kragt VE: De ontwikkeling van het verpleegkundig beroep in Nederland (II). **Tijdschr Ziekenverpl** 1980 Sep 9;33(18):853–60
Lieburg MJ van: De verpleegkundige literatuur in Nederland in de 19e eeuw. **Tijdschr Geschied Geneeskd** 1980;3(3):97–122
Stumpel AR: Het Burgerziekenhuis te Amsterdam en de modernisering van de ziekenverpleging in de 19e eeuw. **Tijdschr Ziekenverpl** 1983 Jun 21;36(13):409–15

**Netherlands Antilles**

Buma S: De ontwikkeling van het verpleegkundig beroep op Curaçao, I--Van de vroegste periode tot 1940. **Tijdschr Ziekenverpl** 1980 Feb 12;33(4):150–6
Buma S: De ontwikkeling van het verpleegkundig beroep op Curaçao. II. Het einde van het Missietijdperk en de introductie van de opleidingen; van 1940 tot heden. **Tijdschr Ziekenverpl** 1980 Feb 26;33(5):210–8

**New Zealand**

Campbell H: Mary Lambie: a biography. Wellington, New Zealand Nursing Education and Research Foundation, 1976. x, 100 p.
Hughes B: 75 years of Kai Tiaki. **NZ Nurs J** 1983 Jan;76(1):4–6
Kinross NJ: Nursing education in New Zealand: a developmental perspective. **Int J Nurs Stud** 1984;21(3):193–9
Pages from the past: **NZ Nurs J** 1983 Jan;76(1):16–25
Shadbolt Y: Nursing education - a major shift. **NZ Nurs J** 1983 Jan;76(1):6–9
Skudder S, Barber LH: The New Zealand nursing team at the Spanish Civil War. **NZ Med J** 1983 May 25;96(732):397–9
Smith MG: Resources for nursing history. **NZ Nurs J** 1983 Jan;76(1):26–7

**Norway**

Aasveien J: A vaere sykepleier for 50 år siden. **Sykepleien** 1984 Aug 20;71(14):14–5, 23
Alvaer I: Sykepleier i 'de gode, gamle dager'. **Sykepleien** 1981 Dec 5;68(21):8–11
Alvsvåg H: Sykepleiens historie og kvinnesynet. **Sykepleien** 1982 Oct 5;69(17):6–10, 29
Bergenheim AL: Jubileumsår i NSF. **Sykepleien** 1982 Apr 5;69(7):5
Fagermoen MS: From apprenticeship to study--the development of nursing education in Norway. **Int J Nurs Stud** 1984;21(3):165–75
Lysnes M: Marie Lysnes: sykepleie var vårt liv. **Sykepleien** 1984 Oct 5;71(17):22–7
Matinsen K: Diakonissene--de første faglaerte sykepleiere. **Sykepleien** 1982 Apr 5;69(7):6–9
Norsk Sykepleierforbund 70–års dag: historisk høytidsstund på Vettre: 'Arhundrets sykepleier' har fått sitt monument. **Sykepleien** 1982 Oct 20;69(18):6–7, 31
Semmelmann E: Sykepleier i de 'gode gamle dager'. **Sykepleien** 1984 Jul 6;71(12):14–7
Svaboe HM: Sykepleiemuseet på Lovisenberg. **Sykepleien** 1983 Apr 21;70(7):12–3
Tofte R: Haukeland Sykepleierhøgskole 75 år: fra 'våkekoner' til moderne sykepleie. **Sykepleien** 1983 Jun 20;70(11):13, 17
Wyller I: Sykepleiens historie og kvinnesynet. **Sykepleien** 1982 Nov 19;69(20):20–1

**Philippines**

Valdez FM: [Perspectives on Philippine nursing] (Jpn). **Kango** 1984 Jul;36(8):50–7

**Poland**

Bogdanow: Wrzesień w Lublinie. **Pieleg Polozna** 1979;(9):26–7
Czapska I: Whołdzie najlepszym (Anita Zofia Brodniewicz). **Pieleg Polozna** 1983;(6):28–9
Czapska I, Kamińska A: Whołdzie najlepszym (Halina Bandurska). **Pieleg Polozna** 1983;(5):27, 31
Dobrowolska-Nowak J: XXV-lecie Studium Nauczycielskiego Szkół Medicznych w Waszawie. **Pieleg Polozna** 1982;(6):19–20
Dwudziestolatka: **Pieleg Polozna** 1982;(3):21
Falkowski W: W Bielsku Podlaskim. **Pieleg Polozna** 1984;(2):26–7
Felchner A, Pepłowska E: Polski Komitet Pomocy Sanitarnej jednym z prekursorów świeckiego pielegniarstwa w Polsce. **Arch Hist Med (Warsz)** 1984;47(1):91–7
Ginalska A: 35 lat mineło. Szkole Pielegniarstwa w Chełmie. **Pieleg Polozna** 1984;(4):26–8
Goszczyńska W: Szkoła im. piel ęgniarek Warszawy. **Pieleg Polozna** 1979;(9):20–2

Jendrysik I: 25 lat Koła PTP w Istebnej. **Pieleg Polozna** 1984;(5):30-1
Konderska Z: Drogi pielegniarstwa polskiego. **Pieleg Polozna** 1984;(7):16-8
Konderska Z: Powstanie Polskiego Towarzystwa Pielęgniarskiego. **Pieleg Polozna** 1982;(10):28-9
Konderska Z: Sprawa rodowodu. **Pieleg Polozna** 1981;(10-11-12):16-7, 27
Konderska Z: 25 lat Polskiego Towarzystwa Pielęgniarskiego. **Pieleg Polozna** 1982;(4-5):26-8, 31
Krzanowska Z: Nauczycielka najbardziej humanistycznego zawodu. **Pieleg Polozna** 1982;4-5:23-4
Leśnikowska M: Wspomnienia z tamtych lat. **Pieleg Polozna** 1980;(1):23-4, 26
Leszczak M: 200 lat. **Pieleg Polozna** 1984;(3):30-1
Lisowski W: Sanitariuszki walczącej Warszawy. **Pieleg Polozna** 1979;(9):23-5
Minęło 25 lat: **Pieleg Polozna** 1983;(11):16-7
Moskwa Z: Pielęgniarstwo polskie w świetle ustawy z 1935 roku. **Wiad Lek** 1982 Sep 15;35(15-16):1017-9
Paciorkiewicz M: Z historii ... **Pieleg Polozna** 1984;(5):21-3
Pszczółkowska-Simiczyjew J: Kształcenie pielegniarek ogólnych na dolnym śląsku w pierwszym xx-leciu Polski Ludowej. **Slaski Kwart Hist Sabotka** 1979;34(4):529-40
Rejmanowski T: Dzieje sióstr miłosierdzia w Szpitalu Powiatowym Sw. Antoniego we Włocławku (1877-1966). **Arch Hist Med (Warsz)** 1984;47(3):433-8
Rodowód przyszłości. 10: Sekcja Pielęgniarek i Położnych ZZPSZ **Pieleg Polozna** 1982;(12):27-9
Rodowód przyszłoścl. 4. Doskonalenie nauczycieli szkół medycznych: **Pieleg Polozna** 1982;(6):22-3
Screbrny jubileusz: **Pieleg Polozna** 1983;(5):28-9
Stanisława Leszczyńska nasza patronka: **Pieleg Polozna** 1984;(3):29
Strzałkowska W: Rodowód przyszłości. 9. Klimat tamtych lat. **Pieleg Polozna** 1982;(11):31-2
Urbanek B: Godzina W na Ochocie. **Pieleg Polozna** 1979;(8):25-6
Urbanek B: Z konspiracyjnej działalności sanitariuszek i pielęgniarek w okupowanej Warszawie. **Przegl Lek** 1980;37(1):137-41
Wadecki Z: Nadgraniczny jubileusz. **Pieleg Polozna** 1984;(2):27
Weber-Pieluszyńska H: PTP w Katowicach. **Pieleg Polozna** 1983;(8-9):32
Witkiewicz H: Jubileusz Warszawskiej Szkoły Pielęgniarstwa. **Pieleg Polozna** 1982;(3):20-1

### Puerto Rico

Cruz Dones A: Escuela de Enfermería de la Clínica Díaz García. **Bol Col Prof Enferm PR** 1982 Sep;8(31):23
Trías de Gómez L, Pagán Ramos IH: Organización del Museo de la Enfermería en Puerto Rico. **Bol Col Prof Enferm PR** 1983 Jun;9(34):24-5
Vilaro de Descartes M: Esbozo de una historía... educación de enfermería en la Universidad Católica de Puerto Rico. **Bol Col Prof Enferm PR** 1979 Sep;5(19):14

### Romania

Clocotici L: Asociația națională a surorilor de ocrotire din românia, cadru de acțiune pentru dezvoltarea și afirmarea profesiei (partea a ii-a). **Viata Med [Medii Sanit]** 1982 Nov;30(11):257-61
Clocotici L: Organiza tii profesionale ale personalului sanitar mediu III. **Viata Med [Medii Sanit]** 1980 Jan;28(1):19-21
Clocotici L: Organizații profesionale ale personalului sanitar mediu (I). **Viata Med [Medii Sanit]** 1979 Jul;27(7):163-6
Clocotici L: Organizații profesionale ale personalului sanitar mediu (II). **Viata Med [Medii Sanit]** 1979 Nov;27(11):261-4
Clocotici L: Sora de ocrotire. **Viata Med [Medii Sanit]** 1982 Sep;30(9):213-6
Negru I: Istoria medicinii: Sora de ocrotire--Teodora Gându. **Viata Med [Medii Sanit]** 1979 Apr;27(4):89-92
Negru I: O școală de surori de ocrotire mai puțin cunoscută-școala din Timișoara (septembrie 1939-februarie 1942). **Viata Med [Medii Sanit]** 1984 Jul;32(7):163-6

### Scandinavia

Stallknecht K: [Development in nursing] (Jpn). **Kango** 1984 Jul;36(8):37-43

### South Africa

Harrison PH: Salute to some nursing pioneers. **Curationis** 1979 Sep;2(2):53-5
Kotze WJ: Verpleegnavorsing in Suid-Afrika in historiese perspektief. **Curationis** 1984 Sep;7(3):11-8
Mellish FM: The birth, growth and development and future dimensions of occupational health nursing. **Curationis** 1980 Sep;3(2):48-53

### Spain

Alberdi RM: La enfermería profesión femenina? **Rev Enferm** 1983 Apr;6(57):21-6
Dominguez Alcon C: Les soins et la profession d'infirmière en Espagne. Une étude de sociologie de la connaissance appliquée. Thèse de doct 3e cycle. Paris, Ecole des hautes études en sciences sociales, 1983. 437 p.

### Sweden

Erikson B: Sjuksköterskeutbildningen i Sverige genom tiderna. **Nord Medicinhist Arsb** 1980;Suppl 6:69-75
Johansson B: 'God bless you, my dear Miss Nightingale.' Letters from Emmy Carolina Rappe to Florence Nightingale 1867-1870. Stockholm, Almqvist & Wiksell International, 1977. 57 p. (Stockholm studies in English, 38).
Kock W: Från Siukwakterska till sjuksköterska. **Nord Medicinhist Arsb** 1984;:129-35
SSF--grande dame på 70--firades med tal och musik: **Vardfacket** 1980 Apr 24;4(8):63-6
Westin M: Så var det då. **Sjukskoterskan** 1984 Apr;:17-20

### Switzerland

Bersch MC: Notre revue a 75 ans. **Krankenpflege (Bern)** 1983 Jan;(1):18-22
Boyer M: Hier et aujourd'hui: l'école d'infirmières de La Source. **Krankenpflege Soins Infirm** 1984 May;77(5):38-43
Jucker-Wannier E: Zum Jubiläumsjahr der Ingenbohler Schwestern. Ein Rückblick auf Festfeiern und Ausstellung an der Schule für allgemeine Krankenpflege des Instituts Ingenbohl am St.-Clara-Spital Basel. **Krankenpflege (Bern)** 1980 Aug;(8):406-7
L'ecole de soins infirmiers du CHUV: Un cinquantenaire abondamment fêté. **Krankenpflege (Bern)** 1982 Aug;(8):73-4
Mordacq C: Ecoles et soignants d'hier à demain, ou les sources du renouvellement d'une institution d'enseignement professionnel **Krankenpflege (Bern)** 1981 Feb;(2):15-9
Pittet-Faessler E: Krankenpflege--Soins infirmiers à 75 ans. **Krankenpflege (Bern)** 1983 Jan;(1):17
Renner M: 'Krankenpflege' stellt sich vor. **Krankenpflege (Bern)** 1981 Dec;(12):58-9
Renner M: 75 Jahre Zeitschrift Krankenpflege. **Krankenpflege (Bern)** 1983 Jan;(1):57-65
75 Jahre Zeitschrift Krankenpflege: Krankenschwestern erinnern sich. **Krankenpflege (Bern)** 1983 Jan;(1):66-9

### Turkey

Conk Z: Cumhuriyet dönemi ve hemşirelik. **Turk Hemsire Derg** 1983;33(4):3-5
Uyer G: Nursing education in Turkey: past and present. **Int J Nurs Stud** 1984;21(3):209-19

### United States

American Nurses' Association. Nursing Hall of Fame. **ANA Publ** 1984 Jun;(G-123):1-21
Abdellah FG: [Nursing in the world: 35 years of development after World War II. Changes affecting nursing in the United States 1949-1984] (Jpn). **Kango** 1984 Jul;36(8):2-10
Allen JC: The history of Cornell University - New York Hospital School of Nursing, 1942-1979. Ed.D. Diss., Columbia University Teachers College. New York, 1982.
American Nurses' Association: A force through history. **Nurs Careers** 1982 May-Jun;3(3):3
ANA's economic and general welfare program: a historical perspective: **ANA Publ** 1981;(EC-143):1-10
Arvy L: Clara Louise Maass (1876-1901) et la fièvre jaune. **Clio Med** 1979 May;13(3-4):277-82
Austin AL: Isabel Maitland Stewart. In: Notable American women. The modern period. Cambridge, Mass., Belknap-Harvard Univ. Press, 1980. 4:660-2.
Baer ED: The conflictive social ideology of American nursing: 1893, a microcosm. Ph.D. Diss , New York University. New York, 1982. vii, 237 p.
Barckley V: The best of times and the worst of times. Historical reflections from an American Cancer Society national nursing consultant. **Oncol Nurs Forum** 1982 Summer;9(3):54-6
Barger J: Origin of flight nursing in the United States Army Air Forces. **Aviat Space Environ Med** 1979 Nov;50(11):1176-8
Bauman M: Intrepid nurses faced the challenges. **Alaska J** 1980;10:36-42
Bell J: Crisis at Gettysburg. **Nurs Times** 1981 Feb 12;77(7):294-5
Benham L: The labor market for registered nurses: a three equation model. **Rev Econ Stat** 1971;53(3):246-52
Benoliel JQ: The historical development of cancer nursing research in the United States. **Cancer Nurs** 1983 Aug;6(4):261-8
Bowman IA, ed: John Sealy Hospital Training School for Nurses. **Bookman** 1982 Oct;9(8):3-11
Bragg TA: The McLean Hospital archives. **Mass Nurse** 1984 Sep;54(8):3
Brodie B: One long step: Virginia nursing moves into the university setting. **Va Nurse** 1983 Winter;51(4):201-4
Brown JM: History of masters education in nursing in the United States,

1945–1969. Ed.D. Diss., Columbia University. New York, 1979. 225 leaves.
Brumgardt JR, ed: Civil war nurse. The diary and letters of Hannah Ropes. Knoxville, University of Tennessee Press, 1980. 149 p.
Buckwalter KC, Church OM: Euphemia Jane Taylor: an uncommon psychiatric nurse. **Perspect Psychiatr Care** 1979 May–Jun;17(3):125–31
Bullough B, Bullough V: Education problems in a woman's profession. **JNE** 1981 Sep;20(7):6–17
Butterworth VE: The girls in white. Independence, Mo., Herald Publishing House, 1979. 176 p.
Carnegie ME: Nurses and war. Black nurses at the front. **Am J Nurs** 1984 Oct;84(10):1250–2
Champagne MT: Innovation in nurse education: a history of the Associate degree program, 1940–1964. Ph.D. Diss., University of Texas. Austin, 1981. xvi, 474 p.
Christy TE: Clinical practice as a function of nursing education: an historical analysis. **Nurs Outlook** 1980 Aug;28(8):493–7
Christy TE: The need for historical research in nursing. **Res Nurs Health** 1981 Jun;4(2):227–8
Church OM, Buckwalter KC: Harriet Bailey---a psychiatric nurse pioneer. **Perspect Psychiatr Care** 1980 Mar–Apr;18(2):62–6
Church OM: Preparation in historiography in nursing research. **NLN Publ** 1983;(41–1935):54–6
The clinic at Beech Fork--its 57-year history is a mini-history of FNS: **Front Nurs Serv Q Bull** 1984 Summer;60(1):1–10
Conrad GB von: The first eighty years: the history of Lutheran Medical Center School of Nursing, 1898–1978. Ph.D. Diss., Saint Louis University. Saint Louis, 1980. 157 p.
Craytor JK: Highlights in education for cancer nursing. **Oncol Nurs Forum** 1982 Fall;9(4):51–9
Crowder EM: Nursing in Texas: a pictorial history. Waco, Texas, Texian Press, 1980, ix, 184 p.
Davis BA: Nursing care of the aged: past, present, future. **Imprint** 1980 Feb;27(1):38, 65, 72–3
Davis CC: The tribulations of Mrs. Turner: an episode after Guilford Court House. **Md Hist Mag** 1981;76(4):376–9
Devine P: Mental retardation: an early subspecialty in psychiatric nursing. **J Psychosoc Nurs Ment Health Serv** 1983 Mar;21(3):21–30
Donahue EM: Preserving history through oral history reflections. **J Gerontol Nurs** 1982 May;8(5):272–8
Donahue MP: Isabel Maitland Stewart's philosophy of education. **Nurs Res** 1983 May–Jun;32(3):140–6
Donahue P: Nursing history in the undergraduate curriculum. **NLN Publ** 1983;(41–1935):38–44
Doona ME: At least as well cared for ... Linda Richards and the mentally ill. **Image J Nurs Sch** 1984 Spring;16(2):51–6
Doona ME: Nursing at Boston College: glimpses of the past. **Mass Nurse** 1983 Dec;52(12):6–7, 20
Doona ME: Nursing revisited: Mary Gerrin and the idea of nursing. **Mass Nurse** 1984 Feb;53(2):5
Doona ME: Nursing revisited: memories - Armistice and suffrage. **Mass Nurse** 1983 Nov;52(11):15
Doona ME: Nursing revisited: the Massachusetts General Hospital, Base Hospital No. 6. **Mass Nurse** 1984 Apr;53(4):9
Doona ME: Nursing revisited: the Worcester State Hospital and nursing. **Mass Nurse** 1984 Jan;53(1):19
Doona ME: Nursing revisited: the 1903 convention. **Mass Nurse** 1984 Jun;54(6):6
Doona ME: The cause is just: Mary E. P. Davis. **Mass Nurse** 1982 Jul;51(7):4–6
Doona ME: The Lucy Lincoln Drown Nursing History Society. **Mass Nurse** 1984 Feb;53(2):6
Doona ME: The Massachusetts Nurses Association eighty years young. **Mass Nurse** 1983 Feb;52(2):8–9
Dye NS: Mary Breckinridge, the Frontier Nursing Service and the introduction of nurse-midwifery in the United States. **Bull Hist Med** 1983 Winter;57(4):485–507
Elmore JA: Frances Elliott Davis. In: Notable American women. The modern period. Cambridge, Mass., Belknap–Harvard Univ. Press, 1980. 4:180–2.
Faust DG: Mary Breckinridge. In: Notable American women. The modern period. Cambridge, Mass., Belknap–Harvard Univ. Press, 1980. 4:103–5.
Fenn D: White slaves. **Wash Mon** 1981;13(9):21–8
Fickeissen JL: A history lesson for today: the creation of the State Board. **NJ Nurse** 1983 Nov–Dec;13(6):20–1
Fickeissen JL: New Jersey State Nurses' Association. **J Med Soc NJ** 1984 Sep;81(9):805–6
Fiedler LA: Images of the nurse in fiction and popular culture. In Jones AH, ed: Images of healers. Albany, State University of New York Press, 1983. p. 79–90.
Fitzpatrick ML: A history of the National Organization for Public Health Nursing, 1912–1952. [New York, N. Y., s. n.], 1973. 3, vi, 451 leaves.
Fitzpatrick ML: Nursing history: route to professional identity. **NLN Publ** 1983;(41–1935):27–38
Flanagan L, ed: One strong voice: the story of the American Nurses' Association. Kansas City, Mo., American Nurses' Assn., 1976. xiii, 692 p.
Fondiller S: Nursing history in undergraduate curriculum: renewal and relevance. **Deans List** 1983 Mar;4(4):1–2
Fondiller SH: The entry dilemma: the National League for Nursing and the higher education movement, 1952–1972, with an epilogue to 1983. New York, N.Y., National League for Nursing, 1983. vii, 136 p.
Friedman A: Nursing revisited: oral history in nursing, Mary A. Maher. **Mass Nurse** 1984 May;53(5):7, 28
Gillies K: Out of the past. Diamond jubilee 1909–1984. **Fla Nurse** 1984 Sep;32(9):4, 12
Gortner SR: The history and philosophy of nursing science and research. **ANS** 1983 Jan;5(2):1–8
Haggerty L: Nursing revisited: Strong public health nurse leader and educator. **Mass Nurse** 1984 Jul–Aug;54(7):7
Hanron J: Nursing revisited: Clarissa Harlow Barton. **Mass Nurse** 1983 Sep;52(9):9, 27
Harmon MD: The evolution of nursing education in the U.S. **Nev Rnformation** 1984 May;:6
Henry LJ: Florence Aby Blanchfield. In: Notable American women. The modern period. Cambridge, Mass., Belknap–Harvard Univ. Press, 1980. 4:83–5.
Herrmann EK: Strategies for teaching the history of nursing. **NLN Publ** 1983;(41–1935):57–65
Hiestand WC: History in graduate teaching. **NLN Publ** 1983;(41–1935):45–8
Hiestand WC: Midwife to nurse-midwife: a history. The development of nurse-midwifery education in the continental United States to 1965. Ed. D. Diss., Columbia University. New York, 1976. 294 p.
Highlights of the Georgia Nurses Association in action 1907–1982: **Ga Nurse** 1982 Dec;42(6):4–15
Hilkemeyer R: A historical perspective in cancer nursing. **Oncol Nurs Forum** 1982 Spring;9(2):47–56
Hine DC: From hospital to college: black nurse leaders and the rise of collegiate nursing schools. **J Negro Educ** 1982 Summer;51:222–37
Hine DC: The Ethel Jones Report: black women in the nursing profession, 1925. **J Negro Hist** 1982 Fall;67:212–28
The history of the National Association of Operating Room Nurses: **Va Nurse** 1982 Summer;50(2):43
Hunter JA, ed: Anna May: eighty-two years in New England. **Northeast Folkl** 1979;20:7–106
Jachimowicz E: Remember the nurses: Michael Reese Hospital School of Nursing, 1890–1981. **Chic Hist** 1981;10(2):96–8
Jackson BS: Nurses at work in America: a history of nursing's economic and general welfare posture. **Nurs Leadersh** 1983 Sep;6(3):93–9
James JW: Isabel Hampton and the professionalization of nursing in the 1890s. In Vogel MJ, Rosenberg CE, ed: The therapeutic revolution. Philadelphia, 1979. p. 201–244.
James JW: Lavinia Lloyd Dock. In: Notable American women. The modern period. Cambridge, Mass., Belknap–Harvard Univ. Press, 1980. 4:195–8.
Johnson JM: The water cure at 'the San.' **NY Folkl Q** 1966;22(3):201–5
Kalisch PA, Kalisch BJ, Scobey M: Images of nurses on television. New York, Springer Pub. Co., 1983. ix, 214 p.
Kalisch PA, Kalisch BJ: The image of nurses in novels. **Am J Nurs** 1982 Aug;82(8):1220–4
Kantrov I, Wittenstein K: Mary Sewall Gardner. In: Notable American women. The modern period. Cambridge, Mass., Belknap–Harvard Univ. Press, 1980. 4:262–4.
Keough G: History and heritage of the Veterans Administration Nursing Service 1930–1980. **League Exch** 1981;(127):i–vi, 1–16
King WH: Caroline Hampton Halsted and her family, revisited. **NC Med J** 1982 Jul;43(7):501–4
Kiser TS: A story of true devotion (Mary Breckinridge). **Front Nurs Serv Q Bull** 1981 Autumn;57(2):16–8
Krampitz SD: Historical development of baccalaureate nursing education in the American university: 1899–1935. **West J Nurs Res** 1983 Fall;5(4):371–80
Lady L: Home visits by FNS nurses. **Front Nurs Serv Q Bull** 1980 Winter;56(3):35–41
Land LC: Hiran Hitchcock' legacy: the history of the Mary Hitchcock Memorial Hospital School of Nursing. Canaan, N. H., Phoenix Publishing for the Mary Hitchcock Memorial Hospital, 1980. x, 148 p.
Levi M: Functional redundancy and the process of professionalization: the case of registered nurses in the United States. **J Health Polit Policy Law** 1980 Summer;5(2):333–53
Litoff JB: Carolyn Conant van Blarcom. In: Notable American women. The modern period. Cambridge, Mass., Belknap–Harvard Univ. Press, 1980. 4:703–4.
Markolf AS: Industrial nursing begins in Vermont. **Vt Regist Nurse** 1980 Jun;:15–7
Matejski MP: Nursing education, professionalism, and autonomy: social constraints and the Goldmark Report. **ANS** 1981;3(3):17–30
Matthies K: Mary Breckinridge and the frontier nursing service. **DAR Mag** 1980;114(5):692–4
Mauksch IG: Nursing is coming of age--the journey from nursing service to nursing as a professional practice. **Fla Nurse** 1982 Nov;30(10):2–9
Melosh B: 'The physician's hand'. Work culture and conflict in American nursing. Philadelphia, Temple University Press, 1982. ix, 260 p.
Milio N: Margaret Gene Arnstein. In: Notable American women. The

modern period. Cambridge, Mass., Belknap-Harvard Univ. Press, 1980. 4:37-8.
Minami H: [American nursing. Outline of the history of the development of studies in the United States. (I)] (Jpn). **Kango** 1982 Apr;34(5):46-54
Moss C, Marchfield F, Hansen H, et al: A treasury of practice history. (Amy Elizabeth Pope). **Calif Nurse** 1983 Sep;79(3):6-7
Mottus JE: New York Nightingales: the emergence of the nursing profession at Bellevue and New York Hospital, 1850-1920. Ann Arbor, Mich., UMI Research Press, 1981. xvii, 277 p. (Ph.D. Diss., New York University, 1980.
Nichols BL: Nurse practitioners: a national perspective. **J Fla Med Assoc** 1982 May;69(5):391-5
NLN's 30th year - leading the way: Renew the spirit! 1952-1982. **Nurs Health Care** 1982 Sep;3(5):398-9
Noel NL: Nursing archives - preserving the profession's history. **Deans Notes** 1984 Mar;5(4):1-2
Nojima Y: [Nursing theory by Henderson. 4. Virginia Henderson and the history of nursing theory] (Jpn) **Kango Tenbo** 1979 Oct;4(10):949-57
Norman EM: Who and where are nursing's historians? **Nurs Forum** 1981;20(2):138-52
Nowak JB: Integration of nursing history into the nursing curriculum. **NLN Publ** 1983;(41-1935):49-53
Nowak JB: The forty-seven hundred. The story of the Mount Sinai Hospital School of Nursing. Canaan, N. H., Phoenix Pub., 1981. xii, 146 p.
Nursing revisited: Mary M. Riddle (1856-1936). **Mass Nurse** 1983 Oct;52(10):4
Nursing revisited: Linda Richards (1841-1930): **Mass Nurse** 1983 Jul;52(7):8
Nursing revisited: Louisa May Alcott: **Mass Nurse** 1983 Jun;52(6):13
Okamoto Y: [Nursing home: medical care a nursing practice in the United States. 8. Establishment of the system of nurses' registration and the history of the development of nursing assistants] (Jpn) **Kangogaku Zasshi** 1980 Aug;44(8):858-63
Paquet JB: The gloving of a nurse (Caroline Hampton). **Nurs Success Today** 1984 Summer;1(2):44
Parsons ME: Mothers and matrons. **Nurs Outlook** 1983 Sep-Oct;31(5):274-8
Pediatric nurse pioneers (Helen Hogan): **Am J Nurs** 1980;80:2084
Peplau HE: Some reflections on earlier days in psychiatric nursing. **J Psychosoc Nurs Ment Health Serv** 1982 Aug;20(8):17-24
Pletsch PK: Mary Breckinridge: a pioneer who made her mark. **Am J Nurs** 1981 Dec;81(12):2188-90
Ponak AM: Unionized professionals and the scope of bargaining: a study of nurses. **Ind Labor Relat Rev** 1981;34(3):396-407
Reed J: Margaret Sanger. In: Notable American women. The modern period. Cambridge, Mass., Belknap-Harvard Univ. Press, 1980. 4:623-7.
Reverby S: The search for the hospital yardstick: nursing and the rationalization of hospital work. In Reverby S, Rosner D, ed: Health care in America. Philadelphia, Temple University Press, 1979. p. 206-35.
Richards EL: 50 years ago--blazing the trail. **Alumni Mag** 1984;84(2):9-12
Richardson L: Breakthrough to nursing: the black nurse's story. **Imprint** 1981 Dec;28(5):27, 60, 73
Rihm A, Montag M, Mock HK: A transition in nursing education. Santa Fe, Research Coordinating Unit, State Dept. of Education, 1967. viii, 114 p.
Robbins P: General Grant's calico colonel. **Am Hist Illus** 1979;14(1):4-7, 43-8
Rooks JB, Fishman SH: American nurse-midwifery practice in 1976-1977: reflections of 50 years of growth and development. **Am J Public Health** 1980 Sep;70(9):990-6
Sanborn A: The seed for a dream: M. Adelaide Nutting. **Alumni Mag** 1984 Jul;84(1):3-5
Sanders RE: History of the Illinois Association of School Nurses: the formative years. Ph.D. Diss., Southern Illinois University, Carbondale, 1979. viii, 175 leaves.
Schmidt MS: Why a separate organization for state boards? **Am J Nurs** 1980 Apr;80(4):724-6
Schor I: The continuing nursing education and adult education movements in the United States. **Nurs Forum** 1981;20(1):87-101
Schwartz D: Reminiscence: those fabulous forties. **Am J Nurs** 1981 Jul;81(7):1414
Selavan IC: Angel in hell-with-the-lid-off. **Am J Nurs** 1980;80:2064-5
Shamansky SL, Hamilton WM: Is the public health nurse's bag anachronism? **Nurs Outlook** 1980 Jun;28(6):379-81
Sharp ES: Nurse-midwifery education: Its successes, failures, and future. **J Nurse Midwife** 1983 Mar-Apr;28(2):17-23
Shearer AW: A commitment to excellence: a history of the School of Nursing, College of Allied Health Sciences, Thomas Jefferson University, 1891-1982. Wynnewood, Pa., Heden-Livingston, 1982. x, 148 p.
Shearer J: History of the Department of Nursing Education at the North Dakota State Hospital. **Prairie Rose** 1984 Oct-Dec;53(4):20-1
Shields EA: A history of the United States Army Nurse Corps (female): 1901-1937. Ed. D. Diss., Columbia University Teachers College. New York, 1980. 232 leaves.
Skinner RE: The roots of flight nursing: Lauretta M. Schimmoler and the Aerial Nurse Corps of America. **Aviat Space Environ Med** 1984 Jan;55(1):72-7
Skinner RE: The U. S. flight nurse: a supplementary bibliography. **Aviat Space Environ Med** 1983 Aug;54(8):735-7
Skinner RE: The U. S. flight nurse: an annotated historical bibliography. **Aviat Space Environ Med** 1981 Nov;52(11 pt 1):707-12
Slavinsky AT, Krauss JB: Mutual withdrawal... or Gwen Tudor revisited. **Perspect Psychiatr Care** 1980 Sep-Oct;18(5):194-203
Smith NB: The women who went to the war: the Union Army nurse in the Civil War. Ph.D. Diss., Northwestern Univ. Evanston, 1981. 183 p.
Smola BK: A study of the development of diploma and baccalaureate degree nursing education programs in Iowa from 1907-1978. Ph.D. Diss., Iowa State University. Ames, 1980. iv, 319 p.
Spiegel AD, Domanowski GF: Beginnings of home health care: a brief history. **Pride Inst J Long Term Home Health Care** 1983 Summer;2(3):28-33
Stewart RF: Nursing education in Texas 1890-1982. Part I. **Tex Nurs** 1982 Jun-Jul;56(6):19-22
Story DK: A study of practical and associate degree nursing education in Iowa from 1918 to 1978. Ph. D. Diss., Iowa State University. Ames, 1980. iii, 308 leaves.
Sullivan AM: Nursing revisited: a tour of nursing history in Massachusetts. **Mass Nurse** 1983 Aug;52(8):9-10
Swenson RS: Associate degree nursing: the gift of thirty years. **NLN Publ** 1983;23-1948:1-9
Talbot DM: Federation of Specialty Nursing Organizations and the American Nurses' Association: a history. **Occup Health Nurs** 1981 Oct;29(10):27-33
Teichmann E: Glimpses into the North Dakota story. **Prairie Rose** 1980 Apr-Jun;59(2):10
This is the National League for Nursing: New York, League, [1977?] 13 p.
Thompson M: Sixty years of progress: nursing and the times in U.S.A.--and in Vermont 1919-1920. **Vt Regist Nurse** 1980 Mar;:9-12
Thompson M: Sixty years of progress. Nursing and the times--in Vermont 1919: past/prospective. **Vt Regist Nurse** 1979 Dec;6-8
Thompson ME: Public health nursing faces challenges in rural health. **Vt Regist Nurse** 1981 May;:7-8, Jul; 3-4
Thompson ME: Sixty years of progress: nursing and the times in U. S. A. - and Vermont, 1919. An overview of nursing's accomplishment in World War I - under its chief - Jane A. Delano. **Vt Regist Nurse** 1979 Jul;:6-8
Thurston HI: An historical perspective of continuing education in Kansas. Part I. **Kans Nurse** 1983 Jan;58(1):5-8
Thurston HI: An historical perspective of continuing education in Kansas. The 70's--voluntary to mandatory. Part II. **Kans Nurse** 1983 Mar;58(3):5-7, 18-9
Tigertt HB, Tigertt WD: Clara Louise Maass: a nurse volunteer for yellow fever inoculations--1901. **Milit Med** 1983 Mar;148(3):252-3
TNA and nursing in Texas: a 75-year perspective: **Tex Nurs** 1982 Jan;56(1):12-3; Feb;56(2):6-7
Tom SA: The evolution of nurse-midwifery: 1900-1960. **J Nurse Midwife** 1982 Jul-Aug;27(4):4-13
Tomes N: Annie Warburton Goodrich. In: Notable American women. The modern period. Cambridge., Mass., Belknap-Harvard Univ. Press, 1980. 4:286-8.
Tomes N: Mary May Roberts. In: Notable American women. The modern period. Cambridge, Mass., Belknap-Harvard Univ. Press, 1980. 4:581-3.
Toppin EA: Alma Cecelia Haupt. In Dictionary of American Biography, Suppl. 6, 1956-1960. p. 283-5, 1980.
Trandel-Korenchuk D, Trandel-Korenchuk K: Entry into nursing practice: does nursing history repeat itself? **Nurse Pract** 1984 Mar;9(3):15-6, 21, 24-5
Trolander JA: Lavinia Lloyd Dock. In Dictionary of American Biography, Suppl. 6, 1956-1960. p. 166-8, 1980.
Vickers ED: F. Elisabeth Cromwell: Pensacola's pioneer nurse. **J Fla Med Assoc** 1983 Aug;70(8):642-6
Visiting Nurse Service of Toledo--eighty-three years of caring: **Caring** 1984 Apr;3(4):57-61
The Visiting Nurses Association of Dayton and Montgomery County: Celebrating 85 years of service. **Caring** 1983 Sep;2(9):18-22
Wagner D: The proletarianization of nursing in the United States. **Int J Health Serv** 1980;10(2):271-90
Weigold ME: Alice Louise Florence Fitzgerald. In Dictionary of American biography, 1961-1965. Suppl. 7, 1981. p. 247-8.
Weiss GN, Weiss EB: The health care profession on the threshold of the eighties: physician and nurse. **J La State Med Soc** 1980 Oct;132(10):151-4
Wilson HS: Research in nursing has a history. **J Nurs Adm** 1984 Dec;14(12):4-5

**USSR**

Antonovich T: Ima podviga--gumanizm. **Med Sestra** 1981 Dec;40(12):41-4
Borich I: O zhurnale 'Meditsinskaia sestra'. **Med Sestra** 1982 Aug;41(8):42-4
Epifanov NS: Nastavnik pervykh russkikh meditsinskikh sester. **Med Sestra** 1983 Mar;42(3):48-50
Ermakov MA: Iz istorii organizatsii évakuatsii ranenykh i bol'nykh partizan na Bol'shuiu zemliu. **Med Sestra** 1982 Mar;41(3):43-5

## NURSING

Furmanchuk VM: Podvigi meditsinskikh sester v pervyĭ period Velikoĭ Otechestvennoĭ voĭny. **Med Sestra** 1980 Oct;37(10):60–2

Furmanchuk VM: Uchastie rabochikh sester i sanitarok v Oktiabr'skoĭ revoliutsii. **Med Sestra** 1982 Apr;41(4):49–51

Granat NE: O 1-ĭ obshchegorodskoĭ nauchno-prakticheskoĭ konferentsii akusherok i meditsinskikh sester akushersko-ginekologicheskikh uchrezhdeniĭ Leningrada (1939 g.). **Med Sestra** 1980 Jun;39(6):40–2

Ibragimov NG: Iz istorii podgotovki meditsinskikh sester v nasheĭ strane. **Med Sestra** 1982 Feb;41(02):55–7

Ionov IuV: Narodovolets Sof'ia Perovskaia i ee meditsinskaia deiatel'nost'. **Feldsher Akush** 1982;47(10):41–2

Kantorovich MM: Neutomimye truzheniki--geroi Velikoĭ Otechestvennoĭ voĭny. **Med Sestra** 1980 May;39(5):3–7

Kantorovich MM: Oni zashchishchali Leningrad (k 40-letiiu sniatiia blokady Leningrada). **Med Sestra** 1984 Jan;43(1):46–9

Katsnel'bogen AG, Stiazhkov AV: Slavnye bol'shevichki--krasnye sestry miloserdiia. **Med Sestra** 1980 Nov;39(11):58–61

Kokhan AI, Miliavskiĭ VM: Sestry miloserdiia v bor'be s épidemieĭ difterii. **Med Sestra** 1983 Oct;42(10):48–9

Korsunskiĭ MA: Voennyĭ fel'dsher P. E. Lazimir. **Feldsher Akush** 1980;45(12):41–4

Kozovenko MN: Rol' N. I. Pirogova v organizatsii truda meditsinskikh sester na voĭne. **Voen Med Zh** 1980 Nov;(11);72–3

Makhrova A: Patrioticheskoe dvizhenie za podgotovku medsester v krasnoi armii i na flote(1938–1940 gg). **Voen Istor Zh** 1974;(3):93–6

Mitsura DI: Vsegda riadom s voinom. **Med Sestra** 1981 Oct;40(10):58–62

Murav'ev EV: Ugolok istorii. **Med Sestra** 1980 Oct;37(10):52–4

Nagaev IM: Krasnye medsestry na frontakh grazhdanskoĭ voĭny. **Med Sestra** 1980 Dec;39(12):41–2

Petrov VP, Shamko VI: Oni zashchishchali Odessu. **Med Sestra** 1984 Apr;43(4):55–7

Porter J: Nursing in Imperial Russia. Nurses under siege. **Nurs Mirror** 1980 Oct 16;151(16):24–6

Tiuliandin A, Vlasova-Leshtaeva TF: Muzhestvo i miloserdie meditsinskikh sester. **Med Sestra** 1980 May;39(5):55–60

Tiuliandin AD: Dasha Sevastopol'skaia--pervaia sestra miloserdiia. **Med Sestra** 1982 Dec;41(12):60–1

Valatkene R: Kaunasskoe meditsinskoe uchilishche im. P. Mazhilisa. **Med Sestra** 1981 Apr;40(4):55–6

Vlasov AA: Ikh trudom slaven kollektiv. **Voen Med Zh** 1982 Mar;(3):7–10

Zabludovskiĭ PE: N. I. Pirogov i meditsinskiĭ trud zhenshchin. **Feldsher Akush** 1981;46(11):53–4

40 let nashemu zhunalu: **Med Sestra** 1982 Aug;41(8):9–12

#### Zambia

Schuster I: Perspectives in development: the problem of nurses and nursing in Zambia. **J Dev Stud** 1981;17(3):77–97

#### Zimbabwe

Tonkin RE: Mother Patrick Cosgrave, O.S.D. 1863–1900. **Zimbabwe Rhod Nurse** 1979;:46–54

## NUTRITION AND DIET

See also **Foods and Food Supply**

Carré A: Scorbut marin historique et biologie moderne. In: Congrès National des Sociétés Savantes, 104e, Bordeaux, 1979. Comptes Rendus. Paris, 1979. Section des Sciences, Fasc. IV. p. 219–30.

Cone TE: History of infant and child feeding: from the earliest years through the development of scientific concepts. In Bond JT, et. al., ed: Infant and child feeding. New York, Academic Press, 1981. p. 3–34.

Covert HH, Kay RF: Dental microwear and diet: implications for determining the feeding behaviors of extinct primates, with a comment on the dietary patterns of Sivapithecus. **Am J Phys Anthropol** 1981 Jul;55(3):331–6

Degen R: The Kitab al-Aghdhiya of Hunayn ibn Ishaq. In: International Symposium for the History of Arabic Science, 1st, University of Aleppo, 1976. Proceedings. Aleppo, Syria, 1976. Papers in European Languages, Vol. II. p. 291–9.

Forster R, Ranum O, ed: Food and drink in history. Selections from the Annales economies, sociétés, civilisations. Volume 5. Baltimore, London, Johns Hopkins University Press, 1979. xiii, 173 p. Reprinted articles by M. Aymard, M. Morineau, J. Revel, JJ. Hémardinquer, W. Frijhoff, JC. Bonnet, R. Barthes, D. Julia, J. Leclant, J.P. Aron, G. Thuillier, J. Soler.

Greenberg MH: Neonatal feeding. In Smith GF, Smith PN, Vidyasagar d, ed: Historical review and recent advances in neonatal and perinatal medicine. [Chicago?], Mead Johnson Nutritional Division, 1983. Vol. I. p. 55–85.

Grivetti LE: Cultural nutrition: anthropological and geographical themes. **Annu Rev Nutr** 1981;1:47–68

Guggenheim KY: Nutrition and nutritional diseases. The evolution of concepts. Lexington, Massachusetts, Toronto, D.C. Heath and Company, 1981. xii, 378 p.

Hirth W: Uberlieferungen der pseudo-aristotelischen 'Secretum-secretorum'-Diätetik mit abweichenden Verfasserangaben. In International Congress of the History of Medicine, 27th, Barcelona, 1980. Actas. Barcelona, Académia de Ciències Médiques de Catalunya i Balears, 1981. p. 259–63.

Huard P, Imbault-Huart MJ: A propos du scorbut. In: Congrès National des Sociétés Savantes, 101e, Lille, 1976. Comptes Rendus. Paris, 1976. Section des Sciences, Fasc. III. p. 157–72.

Kahn A: Highlights of the Adler Museum collections. **Adler Mus Bull** 1984 Nov;10(3):25–9

Körtgen A: Die Gesundheit des Fürsten. Diätetische Vorschriften für eine herausgehobene Menschengruppe von der Antike bis zum Anfang des zwanzigsten Jahrhunderts. Diss., Johannes Gutenberg - Universität in Mainz. Frankfurt am Main, Bern, Peter Lang, 1982. 231 p.

Levenson SM, Hopkins BS, Waldron M, et al: Early history of parenteral nutrition. **Fed Proc** 1984 Apr;43(5):1391–406

Martorell R: Notes on the history of nutritional anthropometry. **Fed Proc** 1981 Sep;40(11):2572–6

Merritt DH, ed: Infant nutrition. Stroudsburg, Pennsylvania, Dowden, Hutchinson & Ross, 1976. xv, 431 p. (Benchmark Papers in Human Physiology, 7).

Moore JG, Krotoszynski BK, O'Neill HJ: Fecal odorgrams. A method for partial reconstruction of ancient and modern diets. **Dig Dis Sci** 1984 Oct;29(10):907–11

Mössmer A: Säuglingsflaschen aus Holz. In Göpfert W, Otten HH, ed: Metavoeite: wandelt euch durch neues Denken. Düsseldorf, Triltsch, 1983. p. 201–8.

Riordan J, Countryman BA: Basics of breastfeeding. Part I: Infant feeding patterns past and present. **JOGN Nurs** 1980 Jul-Aug;9(4):207–10

Schadewaldt H: Skorbut. **Zahnarztl Prax** 1980 Jul 11;31(7):297–301

Schadewaldt H: Zur Entwicklung der wissenschaftlichen Ernährungslehren. **Med Welt** 1982 Jun 4;33(22):799–802

Schönbauer D, Dibold H: Die Diätassistentin. Wien, Göschl, 1978. 223 p.

Senczek D: Zur frühgeschichtlichen Entwicklung der tierärztlichen Nahrungsmittelhygiene aus freiberuflicher Sicht. **Z Ernaehrungswiss** 1980 Mar;19(1):40–6

Sharman IM: Symposium on 'Vitamin A in nutrition and disease.' Historical introduction. **Proc Nutr Soc** 1983 Jan;42(1):1–5

Shimazono N: Eiyogakushi. Tokyo: Asakura Shoten, Showa 53 nen [1978]. viii, 202 p.

Teaford MF, Walker A: Quantitative differences in dental microwear between primate species with different diets and a comment on the presumed diet of Sivapithecus. **Am J Phys Anthropol** 1984 Jun;64(2):191–200

Todhunter EN: Some aspects of the history of nutrition and dietetics. **Ala J Med Sci** 1983 Oct;20(4):460–3

Vanderbilt's history of nutrition collection bookplate: **Nutr Hist Notes** 1979;5:2–7

Walker AR, Richardson BD: What did our forefathers eat? **S Afr Med J** 1981 Jan 3;59(1):3–4

Watt J: Nutrition in adverse environments, 1. Forgotten lessons of maritime nutrition. **Hum Nutr Appl Nutr** 1982 Feb;36(1):35–45

Weyrauch E: Mahl-Zeiten. Beobachtungen zur sozialen Kultur des Essens in der Ständegesellschaft. In Imhof AE, ed: Leib und Leben in der Geschichte der Neuzeit. Berlin, Duncker & Humblot, 1983. p. 103–18.

#### Americas

Richman EA, Ortner DJ, Schulter-Ellis FP: Differences in intracortical bone remodeling in three aboriginal American populations: possible dietary factors. **Calcif Tissue Int** 1979 Nov 6;28(3):209–14

Super JC: Sources and methods for the study of historical nutrition in Latin America. **Hist Methods** 1981;14(1):22–30

#### Asia

Wong M: Contribution à l'histoire des carences en Extrême-Orient: le béribéri. In: Congrès National des Sociétés Savantes, 93e, Tours, 1968. Comptes Rendus. Paris, 1971. Section des Sciences, Tome II. p. 9–15.

#### China

Hou HC: Concerning the study of nutrition in China. **Proc Soc Exp Biol Med** 1982 Oct;171(1):1–6

#### Great Britain

Crowdy JP: The science of the soldier's food. **Army Q Def J** 1980;110(3):266–79

#### Morocco

Rosenberg B: Cultures complémentaires et nourritures de substitution au Maroc (XVe-XVIIIe siècle). **Ann Econ Soc Civilis** 1980;35:477–503

**Panama**

Cooke RG: Los hábitos alimentarios de los indígenas precolombinos de Panamá. **Rev Med Panama** 1981 Jan;6(1):65–89

**Poland**

Dembińska M: Dieetvoedsel en medicijnen voor kinderen in Polen van de 16de tot de 19de eeuw. **Spiegel Hist** 1981;16(11):623–6

Dembińska M: Pożywienie dziecka w polskich żródlach historycznych. **Kwart Hist Kultury Mater** 1980;28(4):481–99

**United States**

Billick G ed.: References for the history of human nutrition in America, 1600 to the present: a selected bibliography. **J NAL Assoc** 1980;5(1–2):45–61

McMahon SF: 'A comfortable subsistence': a history of diet in New England, 1630–1850. Ph.D. Diss., Brandeis University. Waltham, 1982. v, 351 p.

**USSR**

Ashmianskas IuI: Prepodavanie gigieny pitaniia v Vil'niusskom universitete. **Gig Sanit** 1980 Jan;(6):42–3

**Before 500 A.D.**

Brown AB: Assessment of paleonutrition from skeletal remains. **Ann NY Acad Sci** 1981;376:405–16

Dennell RW: Prehistoric diet and nutrition: some food for thought. **World Archaeol** 1979;11:121–35

Dombrowski DA: Vegetarianism and the argument from marginal cases in Porphyry. **J Hist Ideas** 1984 Jan–Mar;45(1):141–3

Grimm H: Was wissen wir über ur- und frühgeschichtliche Kindernahrung? **Aerztl Jugendkd** 1981;72(3):170–3

Puech PF, Prone A, Albertini H: Reproduction expérimentale des processus d'altération de la surface dentaire par friction non abrasive et non adhésive: application à l'étude de l'alimentation de l'homme fossile. **C R Seances Acad Sci [III]** 1981 Nov 9;293(9):497–502

Schoeninger MJ, DeNiro MJ, Tauber H: Stable nitrogen isotope ratios of bone collagen reflect marine and terrestrial components of prehistoric human diet. **Science** 1983 Jun 24;220(4604):1381–3

Schoental R: Mycotoxins and the Bible. **Perspect Biol Med** 1984 Autumn;28(1):117–20

Walker A: Diet and teeth. Dietary hypotheses and human evolution. **Philos Trans R Soc Lond [Biol]** 1981 May 8;292(1057):57–64

**Egypt**

Saffirio L: Razioni e salari in natura nell'antico Egitto. Considerazioni dietetiche e socio economiche. **Aegyptus (Milano)** 1977;57:14–78

**Greece**

Makler PT: New information on nutrition in ancient Greece. **Klio** 1980, reçu 1983;62(2):317–9

**United States**

Blakely RL, Beck LA: Trace elements, nutritional status, and social stratification at Etowah, Georgia. **Ann NY Acad Sci** 1981;376:417–31

**500 A.D.–1450**

Bullough V, Campbell C: Female longevity and diet in the Middle Ages. **Speculum** 1980 Apr;55(2):317–25

Cadden J: Albertus Magnus' universal physiology: the example of nutrition. In Weisheipl JA, ed: Albertus Magnus and the sciences. Toronto, Pontifical Institute of Mediaeval Studies, 1980. 321–39.

Cosman MP: A feast for Aesculapius: historical diets for asthma and sexual pleasure. **Annu Rev Nutr** 1983;3:1–33

Stuart H: A ninth century account of diets and Dies Aegyptiaci. **Scriptorium** 1979;33(2):237–44

**Arabic**

Elkhadem H: Une nouvelle conception de l'hygiène et de la diététique au XIe siècle. **Technologia** 1982;5(3–4):61–73

Kahle E: Das Ammenregimen des Avicenna (Ibn Sina) in seinem Qanun. Erlangen, Verlagsbuchhandlung Hannelore Lüling, 1980. 45, [13] p.

Opsomer-Halleux C: La diététique d'Ibn Butlan dans le manuscrit 887 (1041) de l'Université de Liège. Congrès de Comines, 1, 1980. Actes. p. 350.

Rahman Baig MA: Avicenna's principles of dietetics. **Bull Indian Inst Hist Med (Hyderabad)** 1981;1–4:95–8

Schipperges H: Grundmuster und Richtlinien arabischer Diätetik. In Dilg P, et al., ed: Perspektiven der Pharmaziegeschichte. Graz, Austria, Akademische Druck- u. Verlagsanstalt, 1983. p. 295–309.

**Denmark**

Tauber H: 13C evidence for dietary habits of prehistoric man in Denmark. **Nature** 1981 Jul 23;292(5821):332–3

**Europe**

Hodges R. Diet in the Dark Ages. **Nature** 1984 Aug 30 Sep 5;310(5980):726–7

**France**

Misaki K: Diet in Provence in the late Middle Ages; an analysis according to the Annales School. **Shakai Keizai Shigaku** 1978;44(4):60–80

**Germany**

Schipperges H: Diätetische Lebensführung nach der 'Regula Benedicti' bei Hildegard von Bingen. **Arzt Christ** 1980;2:87–97

**Great Britain**

Schmidt PG: Materielle und spirituelle Diät. Ein mittellateinischer Verstraktat des frühen 13. Jahrhunderts aus St. Albans. In Dilg P, et al., ed: Perspektiven der Pharmaziegeschichte. Graz, Austria, Akademische Druck- u. Verlagsanstalt, 1983. p. 311–23.

**Turkey**

Bowman IA: Ottoman and European diet in the fifteenth century **Bookman** 1981 Mar;8(3):3–9

**1450–1700**

Margolin JC, Sauzet R, ed: Pratiques et discours alimentaires à la Renaissance. Actes du colloque de Tours de mars 1979, Centre d'études supérieures de la Renaissance. Paris, Maisonneuve et Larose, 1982. 305 p. Contributions on medicine and diet by Y. Pélicier, J. Céard, M. de Gandillac, J. Dupèbe, M. M. Fontaine, M. Lazard, J. L. Flandrin, M. Reulos, M. C. Pouchelle-Peter.

**Belgium**

Bruce-Chwatt LJ: Ludovicus Nonnius, M.D., 1553–1645. **Bull NY Acad Med** 1984 Nov;60(9):938–43

**Italy**

Guggenheim YK: Leonardo da Vinci's views on nutrition. **Koroth** 1981;8(1–2):31–9

**Poland**

Wyczanski A: The social structure of nutrition: a case. **Acta Pol Hist** 1968;18:63–74

**United States**

Kupperman KO: Apathy and death in early Jamestown. **J Am Hist** 1979;66(1):24–40

**1700 to Present**

Adams P: Health of the state. New York, N.Y., Praeger, 1982. x, 198 p.

Almquist HJ: Vitamin K; discovery, identification, synthesis, functions. **Fed Proc** 1979 Dec;38(13):2687–9

Aronson N: Social factors in the development of nutrition studies: 1880–1920. **J NAL Assoc** 1980;5(1–2):32–7

Bender AE: Importance of proteins and protein quality. **Bibl Nutr Dieta** 1983;(32):55–66

Berger H: Kurzer historischer Rückblick auf den Beginn der 'Ernährungsprobleme bei frühgeborenen Kindern'. **Padiatr Padol** 1983;18(2):99–103

Guggenheim YK: Forerunners of the vitamin doctrine. **Koroth** 1979 Nov;7(9–10):CLXXXI–CXCIV(634–43)

Howard AN: The historical development, efficacy and safety of very-low-calorie diets. **Int J Obes** 1981;5(3):195–208

Keys A: From Naples to seven countries––a sentimental journey. **Prog Biochem Pharmacol** 1983;19:1–30

Lunden K: Marknadsverdi i forhold til naeringsverdi av poteter og korn 1832–1865. **Hist Tidsskr** 1980;59(4):389–405

Maclean V: A short-title catalogue of household and cookery books published in the English tongue 1701–1800. London, Prospect, 1981. 197

p.
Mayer J: The impact of Elmer Verner McCollum on national and global nutritional problems. **Trans Kans Acad Sci** 1982 Aug;85(3):142–51
Mosek C: Nutrition and fertility: a review essay. **Hist Methods** 1981;14(1):43–6
Reese WJ: After bread, education: nutrition and urban school children, 1890–1920. **Teach Coll Rec** 1980;81(4):496–525
Rhoads JE, Vars HM, Dudrick SJ: The development of intravenous hyperalimentation. **Surg Clin North Am** 1981 Jun;61(3):429–35
Schubert JN: The impact of food aid on world malnutrition. **Int Organ** 1981;35(2):329–54
Shils ME: Historical aspects of minerals and vitamins in parenteral nutrition. **Fed Proc** 1984 Apr;43(5):1412–6
Snell EE: Lactic acid bacteria and identification of B-vitamins: some historical notes, 1937–1940. **Fed Proc** 1979 Dec;38(13):2690–3
Stechel RH: Height and per capita income. **Hist Methods** 1983;16(1):1–7
Van Eys J: Nutritional therapy in childhood malignancies--a historical perspective. In Van Eys J, Seelig MS, Nichols BL, ed: Nutrition and cancer. New York and London, SP, 1979. P. 91–110.
Widdowson EM: The first fifty years. **Curr Concepts Nutr** 1984;13:1–20
Winters RW: An historical review of the development of criteria for intravenous amino acid requirements. **Acta Chir Scand [Suppl]** 1983;517:7–15
Winters RW, Heird WC, Dell RB: History of parenteral nutrition in pediatrics with emphasis on amino acids. **Fed Proc** 1984 Apr;43(5):1407–11
Winton R: Food and fitness at sea. **Med J Aust** 1980 Oct 18;2(8):411–2

**Americas**

Escudero JC: Desnutrición en América Latina, su magnitud (una primera aproximación). **Rev Mex Cienc Polit Soc** 1976;22(84):83–130

**Australia**

Shepherd JJ: Nutrition in the history of Tasmania. **JPEN J Parenter Enteral Nutr** 1980 May–Jun;4(3):312–3

**Belgium**

Masuy-Stroobant G: La surmortalité infantile des Flandres au cours de la deuxième moitié du XIXe siècle: mode d'alimentation ou mode de développement? **Ann Demogr Hist (Paris)** 1983;:231–56
Noirfalise A: Cent ans de bromatologie à l'Université de Liège. **Arch Belg** 1982;40(7–8):365–76

**Brazil**

Ward JO, Sanders JH: Nutritional determinants and migration in the Brazilian northeast: a case study of rural and urban Ceará. **Econ Dev Cult Change** 1980;29(1):141–63

**Canada**

Schurman M: 'Nirkit': good food. **Beaver** 1981;312(2):2–9
Ward WP, Ward PC: Infant birth weight and nutrition in industrializing Montreal. **Am Hist Rev** 1984;89(2):324–45

**Caribbean**

Kiple KF, Kiple VH: Deficiency diseases in the Caribbean. **J Interdiscip Hist** 1980 Autumn;11(2):197–215

**Chile**

Monckeberg F: Lucha contra la desnutrición del niño en Chile, 1952–1977. **Rev Med Chil** 1977 Oct;105(10):687–95

**Cuba**

Handelman H: Cuban food policy and popular nutritional levels. **Cuban Stud** 1981–82;11–12(2–1):127–46

**Czechoslovakia**

Mašek J: Zkoumání výživy dřive a dnes. **Cas Lek Cesk** 1983 May 27;122(21):645–8

**Finland**

Talve I: Piirilläkärit suomen kansan ravinnosta v. 1857–1870. **Kotiseutu** 1972;4–5:196–202

**France**

Aron JP: Le régime des nourrices au début du XIXe siècle à Paris. In: Congrès National des Sociétés Savantes, 93e, Tours, 1968. Actes. Paris, 1971. Section d'Histoire Moderne et Contemporaine, Tome 1. p. 207–15.
Cottet J: Evolution de la consommation du sel en France. **Bull Mem Acad R Med Belg** 1981;136(11):556–65
Desaive JP: L'alimentation populaire d'après les archives de l'Académie de Médecine (1774–1794). In: Congrès National des Sociétés Savantes, 93e, Tours, 1968. Actes. Paris, 1971. Section d'Histoire Moderne et Contemporaine, Tome 1. p. 39–53.
Laissus J: Les conserves alimentaires: Nicolas Appert (1749–1841) bienfaiteur de l'humanité. In: Congrès National des Sociétés Savantes, 93e, Tours, 1968. Comptes Rendus. Paris, 1971. Section des Sciences, Tome II. p. 137–57.
Major V: Live in peace and joy. In: Congrès international d'histoire de la médecine, XXVe, Québec, 1976. Actes. Québec, 1977. p. 944–50.
Mandrou R: Un problème de diététique à l'Hôtel-Dieu de Paris à la veille de la Révolution. In: Congrès National des Sociétés Savantes, 93e, Tours, 1968. Actes. Paris, 1971. Section d'Histoire Moderne et Contemporaine, Tome 1. p. 125–37.

**Germany**

Hoppe B: Adolf Windaus, Heinrich Wieland, Richard Kuhn, Leopold Ružička, Alexander Todd und Adolf Bunenandt. Die Erforschung der Vitamine und der Hormone. In: Die Grossen der Weltgeschichte. Zürich, Kindler, 1978. p. 336–81.
Pfarrwaller-Stieve A: Friedrich von Müller (1858–1941) und seine Stoffwechseluntersuchungen. Zürich, Juris Druck, 1983. 58 p. (Zürcher Medizingeschichtliche Abhandlungen, Neue Reihe, 156).
Teuteberg HJ: Der Verzehr von Nahrungsmitteln in Deutschland pro Kopf und Jahr seit Beginn der Industrialisierung (1850–1975). Versuch einer quantitativen Lang-Zeitanalyse. **Arch Sozialgesch** 1979;19:331–88
Wiegert J: Anfangsprobleme der Nahrungsmittelchemie in Deutschland unter besonderer Berücksichtigung pharmazeutischer Verhältnisse. Braunschweig, 1975. 180 p. (Veröffentlichungen aus dem Pharmaziegeschichtlichen Seminar der Technischen Universität Braunschweig, Band 15).

**Ghana**

Williams CD: Fifty years ago. Archives of Diseases in Childhood 1933. A nutritional disease of childhood associated with a maize diet. **Arch Dis Child** 1983 Jul;58(7):550–60

**Great Britain**

Fildes V: Weaning the Elizabethan child. **Nurs Times** 1980 July–Aug 7;76:31–32:1357–9,1402–3
Guggenheim YK: Jonathan Pereira's contribution to the science of nutrition. **Koroth** 1982 Aug;8(3/4):123–34
Hamilton D: The nineteenth-century surgical revolution--antisepsis or better nutrition? **Bull Hist Med** 1982 Spring;56(1):30–40
Hollingsworth DF: Sir Norman Charles Wright. In Dictionary of national biography, 1961–1970. Suppl. 8, 1981. p. 1115–6.
Hughes RE: James Lind and the cure of scurvy: an experimental approach. **Med Hist** 1975 Oct;19(4):342–51
Jones FA: Presidential address. Lettsom, food and fibre. **Trans Med Soc Lond** 1977–78;94:1–14
Passmore R: Obituary Notice. Wallace Ruddell Aykroyd, CBE, MD, ScD (30 July 1899–7 February 1979). **Br J Nutr** 1980 Mar;43(2):245–50
Passmore R: Reflexions on energy balance. **Proc Nutr Soc** 1982 Jun;41(2):161–5
Pyke M: Alfred Louis Bacharach. In Dictionary of national biography, 1961–1970. Suppl. 8, 1981, p. 59–60.
Rechtman J: Un précurseur génial de la prévention et de la diététique, du bouche à bouche et du massage cardiaque externe de l'asepsie et parrain de J. P. Marat: Le docteur William Buchan (1729–1805). Diss. Paris VII, 1979. 115 p.
Widdowson EM: Adventures in nutrition over half a century. **Proc Nutr Soc** 1980 Sep;39(3):293–306
Yellowlees WW: Ill fares the land. **J R Coll Gen Pract** 1979 Jan;29(198):7–21

**Hungary**

Sergo E: Gyermekágyas asszony étkeztetése Magyarországon. **Orvostort Kozl** 1982;28(1–3):245–50
Spielmann J: Az erdélyi néptáplálkozás kérdései Mátyus István müvében. **Nor Tannlaegeforen Tid** 1982 Jun 13;123(24):1495–8

**India**

Azeez Pasha M: Yusrul Ilaj; a Persian medical manuscript compiled in India by Hakeem Hidaetullah, in 1731 A.D. **Bull Inst Hist Med (Hyderabad)** 1973 Oct;3(4):201–6
Bagley C: Social policy and development: the case of child welfare, health and nutritional services in India. **Plural Soc** 1979;10(1):3–26

### Italy

Bevilacqua P: Emigrazione transoceanica e mutamenti dell'alimentazione contadina calabrese fra otto e novecento. **Quad Stor** 1981;16(2):520–55
Fidanza F, Alberti Fidanza A: Attempts to improve food habits in rapidly changing societies; e.g. Italy. **Bibl Nutr Dieta** 1983;(32):32–9

### Japan

Dwyer JT, Oiso T: Changing food patterns. **Prog Clin Biol Res** 1981;77:509–23

### Mexico

Cross HE: Dieta y nutricion en el medio rural de Zacatecas y San Luis Potosi (siglos XVIII y XIX). **Hist Mex** 1981;31(1):101–16
Gual Castro C: Informe de labores con motivo del XXXV aniversario de la fundación del instituto Nacional de la Nutrición Salvador Zubirán. **Rev Invest Clin** 1982 Jan–Mar;34(1):85–9
Informe de labores con motivo del XXXIV aniversario del Instituto Nacional de la Nutricion: **Rev Invest Clin** 1981 Jan–Mar;33(1):91–108
XXXVI aniversario de la fundación del Instituto nacional de la nutrición Salvador Zubirán. Homenaje al Dr. Salvador Zubirán: **Rev Invest Clin** 1983 Jan–Mar;35(1):85–103
Zubirán S: Informe de labores con motivo del XXXIII aniversario del Instituto Nacional de la Nutrición. **Rev Invest Clin** 1980 Jan–Mar;32(1):101–9

### Netherlands

Hartog AP den: Werklozen en hun voeding in de jaren 1930–1939. **Spiegel Hist** 1982;17(9):445–51

### South Africa

Richardson BD: The historical background of research on diet and dental caries in South Africa. **Tydskr Tandheelkd Ver S Afr** 1982 May;37(5):327–33

### Spain

Grande Covian F: Vitamin deficiencies during the Spanish Civil War in Madrid: a reminiscence. **Acta Vitaminol Enzymol** 1982;4(1–2):99–103
Muñoz Calvo S, Turegano Lopez A: El control de alimentos del Laboratorio Químico Municipal de Madrid en el siglo XIX: contribución a su estudio. **Bol Soc Esp Hist Farm** 1981 Sep;32(127):149–67

### Sweden

Brändström A, Broström G, Persson LA: The impact of feeding patterns on infant mortality in a nineteenth century Swedish parish. **J Trop Pediatr** 1984 Jun;30(3):154–9
Engström A: Reflexioner kring våra matvanor förr och nu. **Nord Medicinhist Arsb** 1984;:83–90
Sandberg LG, Steckel RH: Soldier, soldier, what made you grow so tall? A study of height, health and nutrition in Sweden, 1720–1881. **Econ Hist (Sweden)** 1980;23(2):91–105

### Switzerland

Picard CW: Vitamin B12: an area of darkness. **Br Med J** 1979 Oct 6;2(6194):867

### United States

Ames SR: Karl Ernest Mason (1900–1978): a biographical sketch. **J Nutr** 1984 Mar;114(3):463–6
Aronson N: Nutrition as a social problem: a case study of entrepreneurial strategy in science. **Soc Probl** 1982;29(5):474–87
Bammi V: Nutrition, the historian, and public policy: a case study of U. S. national nutrition policy in the 20th century. **J Soc Hist** 1980;14(4):627–48
Bean WB: Personal reflections on clinical investigations. **Annu Rev Nutr** 1982;2:1–20
Bing FC, Prebluda HJ: E. V. McCollum: pathfinder in nutrition investigations and world agriculture. **Agric Hist** 1980;54(1):157–66
Brandt P: The Howard Bishop Lewis papers. **Surv Sources Newsl** 1976 Dec;4:5–7
Broquist HP, Olson RE: Progress in nutrition research: 1942–1982. **Nutr Rev** 1982 Nov;40(11):343–8
Conable CW: Louise Stanley. In: Notable American women. The modern period. Cambridge, Mass., Belknap–Harvard Univ. Press, 1980. 4:657–9.
Contento I: Thinking about nutrition education: what to teach, how to teach it, and what to measure. **Teach Coll Rec** 1980;81(4):421–47
Darby WJ: The Nutrition Foundation: 1942–1982. **Nutr Rev** 1982 Nov;40(11):348–52
Davis DR: Some legacies of nutrition pioneer E. V. McCollum. **Trans Kans Acad Sci** 1979 Aug;82(3):133–45
Day HG: E. V. McCollum and dietitians in nutrition education. **J Am Diet Assoc** 1980 Feb;76(2):126–7
Day HG, Prebluda HJ: E. V. McCollum: 'lamplighter' in public and professional understanding of nutrition. **Agric Hist** 1980 Jan;54(1):149–56
Day HG: The science of nutrition. **J NAL Assoc** 1980;5(1–2):27–31
Dinning JS: Reflections on Nutrition Reviews from an international nutritionist. **Nutr Rev** 1982 Nov;40(11):328–30
Edwards R: Graham–Kellogg, early American contributors to health education. **J Sch Health** 1981 Nov;51(9):589–91
Egan MC: Public health nutrition services: issues today and tomorrow. **J Am Diet Assoc** 1980 Oct;77(4):423–7
Etheridge EW: Grace Arabell Goldsmith. In: Notable American women. The modern period. Cambridge, Mass., Belknap–Harvard Univ. Press, 1980. 4:283–4.
Fogel RW, Engerman SL, Trussell J: Exploring the uses of data on height: the analysis of long-term trends in nutrition, labor welfare, and labor productivity. **Soc Sci Hist** 1982;6(4):401–21
Gilbert B: The cry was: go west, young man, and stay healthy. **Smithsonian** 1983;13(12):138–49
Gussow JD: Food and nutrition education: a redefinition. **Teach Coll Rec** 1980;81(4):411–6
Gussow JD: Who pays the piper? **Teach Coll Rec** 1980;81(4):448–66
Hadwiger DF: Nutrition, food safety, and farm policy. **Proc Acad Polit Sci** 1982;34(3):79–88
Harper AE: McCollum and directions in the evaluation of protein quality. **J Agric Food Chem** 1981 May–Jun;29(3):429–35
Harper AE: Reflections on Nutrition Reviews from a university professor. **Nutr Rev** 1982 Nov;40(11):330–1
Herriott RM: Life and contributions of Elmer V. McCollum. **Fed Proc** 1980 Aug;39(10):2713–5
Horton LE: The boys in the club. **J Am Diet Assoc** 1982 Jul;81(1):17–25
Ihde AJ: Lydia Jane Roberts. In: Notable American women. The modern period. Cambridge, Mass., Belknap–Harvard Univ. Press, 1980. 4:580–1.
Johnson RE: Carlo Frank Consolazio: March 9, 1913--December 23, 1976. **Prog Food Nutr Sci** 1983;7(1–2):1–10
Jukes TH: Living history: nutritional discoveries of the 1930's: introductory remarks. **Fed Proc** 1979 Dec;38(13):2679–80
Jukes TH: Philip Handler (1917–1981). A biographical sketch. **J Nutr** 1983 Jun;113(6):1086–94
King CG: The isolation of vitamin C from lemon juice. **Fed Proc** 1979 Dec;38(13):2681–3
Kiple KF, King VH: Another dimension to the black diaspora: diet, disease, and racism. Cambridge, Cambridge University Press, 1981. 295 p.
Kiple KF, Kiple VH: Slave child mortality: some nutritional answers to a perennial puzzle. **J Soc Hist** 1977 Mar;10(3):284–309
Klevay LM: Changing patterns of disease: some nutritional remarks. **J Am Coll Nutr** 1984;3(2):149–58
Levenstein H: The New England kitchen and the origins of modern American eating habits. **Am Q** 1980;32(4):369–86
Margo RA, Steckel RH: The heights of American slaves: new evidence on slave nutrition and health. **Soc Sci Hist** 1982;6(4):516–38
Nissenbaum S: Sex, diet, and debility in Jacksonian America: Sylvester Graham and health reform. Westport, Connecticut, Greenwood, 1980. 198 p. (Contributions in Medical History, 4).
Ostenso GL: National Nutrition Monitoring System: a historical perspective. **J Am Diet Assoc** 1984 Oct;84(10):1181–5
Raacke ID: Agnes Fay Morgan. In: Notable American women. The modern period. Cambridge, Mass., Belknap–Harvard Univ. Press, 1980. 4:495–7.
Raacke ID: Herbert Mclean Evans (1882–1971). A biographical sketch. **J Nutr** 1983 May;113(5):929–43
Rhoads JE: Development of surgical nutrition at the University of Pennsylvania. **JPEN** 1980 Sep–Oct;4(5):464–6
Risse GB: A letter to Benjamin Rush. **J Hist Med Allied Sci** 1980 Oct;35(4):461
Sebrell WH: Reflections on Nutrition Reviews from a clinical investigator. **Nutr Rev** 1982 Nov;40(11):326–8
Sokoloff KL, Villaflor GC: The early achievement of modern stature in America. **Soc Sci Hist** 1982;6(4):453–82
Sommer R, Fjeld C: Consumer protection programs in food cooperatives. **Policy Stud Rev** 1983;2(3):455–64
Stare FJ: Forty years of Nutrition Reviews. **Nutr Rev** 1982 Nov;40(11):321–5
Szepesi B: Carp--a nutritional food: preliminary studies on the use of carp in the American diet. **J Nal Assoc** 1981;6(1–4):14–6
Todhunter EN: Reflections on nutrition history. **J Nutr** 1983 Aug;113(8):1681–5
Totter JR, Darby WJ: Paul Louis Day (1899–1980). A biographical sketch. **J Nutr** 1984 Feb;114(2):241–6
Trecker JL: Katharine Blunt. In: Notable American women. The modern period. Cambridge, Mass., Belknap–Harvard Univ. Press, 1980. 4:87–8.
Vanderbilt's influence on world nutrition: **Nutr Hist Notes** 1980;8:2–5; 1980;9:3–8; 1981;10:4–6
Vars HM: Early research in parenteral nutrition. **JPEN** 1980 Sep–Oct;4(5):467–8
Verbrugge MH: Healthy animals and civic life: Sylvester Graham's

physiology of subsistence. **Rev Am Hist** 1981;9(3):359-64
Weigley ES: Sarah Tyson Rorer: first American dietitian? **J Am Diet Assoc** 1980 Jul;77(1):11-5
Welsh SO, Marston RM: Review of trends in food use in the United States, 1909 to 1980. **J Am Diet Assoc** 1982 Aug;81(2):120-8
Whorton JC: Muscular vegetarianism: the debate over diet and athletic performance in the progressive era. **J Sport Hist** 1981;8(2):58-75
Whorton JC: 'Physiologic optimism': Horace Fletcher and hygienic ideology in progressive America. **Bull Hist Med** 1981 Spring;55(1):59-87
Williams HH: Icie Gertrude Macy Hoobler (1892-1984). A biographical sketch. **J Nutr** 1984 Aug;114(8):1351-62
Young JH: Adelle Davis. In: Notable American women. The modern period. Cambridge, Mass., Belknap-Harvard Univ. Press, 1980. 4:179-80.
Young JH, Stitt RS: Nutrition quackery. Upholding the right to criticize. **Food Technol** 1981 Dec;:42-7
Young JH: Nutritional eccentricities. In Neuberger A, Jukes TH, ed: Human nutrition: current issues and controversies. Lancaster, England, MTP Press, 1982. p. 217-32.
Young JH: Nutritional quackery. **Assoc Food Drug Off Q Bull** 1983 Jan;47:3-11
Zikakis JP: Agricultural and food chemistry: accomplishments and perspectives. **J Agric Food Chem** 1983 Jul-Aug;31(4):672-5

**USSR**

Efremov VV, Shtenberg AI: 50-letnii put' Instituta pitaniia AMN SSSR: ego sozdanie, stanovlenie i razvitie. **Vopr Pitan** 1980 Sept-Oct;(5):4-9
Hoch SL: Serf diet in nineteenth-century Russia. **Agric Hist** 1982;56(2):391-414
Krymkevich NI: Vklad vracheĭ russkogo voenno-morskogo flota v razvitie gigieny pitaniia v Rossii (II polovina XIX - nachalo XX veka). **Vopr Pitan** 1981 Sep-Oct;(5):72-4
Levit AZ, Vankhanen NV: V. I. Lenin o sotsial'nykh aspektakh narodnogo pitaniia. **Gig Sanit** 1981 Jan;(1):37-9
Maĭatruk PN, Popik SIa, Petrun' AS, et al: Stanovlenie, puti i perspektivy razvitiia gigieny pitaniia na Ukraine. **Vopr Pitan** 1982 Nov-Dec;(6):15-20
Maĭstruk PN, Petrun' AS, Popik SIa, et al: K istorii Kievskogo nauchno-issledovatel'skogo instituta gigieny pitaniia. **Vrach Delo** 1983 Apr;(4):1-5
Maĭstruk PN, Popik SIa, Petrun' AS, et al: Organizatsiia deiatel'nosti sanitarno-épidemiologicheskoĭ sluzhby v oblasti gigieny pitaniia na Ukraine v period stanovleniia Sovetskoĭi vlasti i v gody pervykh piatiletok. **Gig Sanit** 1982 Apr;(4):54-6
Petrovskiĭ KS: Razvitie nauki o pitanii v SSSR. **Gig Sanit** 1982 Dec;(12):16-9
Samsonov MA: Dostizheniia sovetskoĭ dietologii za piat'desiat let. **Vopr Pitan** 1980 Sep-Oct;(5):15-21
Shaternikov VA, Konyshev VA: 50-ia godovshchina pervogo piatiletnego plana razvitiia narodnogo khoziaĭstva SSSR i nauka o pitanii v nasheĭ strane. **Vopr Pitan** 1979 Sep-Oct;(5):3-7
Shitskova AP: Osnovnye itogi raboty Moskovskogo NII gigieny im. F. F. Erismana v desiatoĭ piatiletke po probleme 'Nauchnye osnovy gigieny pitaniia' (k 60-letiiu so dnia osnovaniia instituta). **Vopr Pitan** 1982 Mar-Apr;(2):64-7
Shmidt AA: Stranitsy vospominanii o blokade goroda Lenina. **Latv PSR Zinat Akad Vestis** 1975;(5):10-7
Shtenberg AI: Osnovnye itogi razvitiia gigieny pitaniia. **Vopr Pitan** 1980 Sep-Oct;(5):9-15

# OBSTETRICS

See also **Gynecology; Maternal Health**

Albert-Puleo M: The obstetrical use in ancient and early modern times of Convolvulus scammonia or Scammony: another non-fugal source of ergot alkaloids? **J Ethnopharmacol** 1979 Apr;1(2):193-5
Baldock D: Early midwifery: one of the oldest professions. **Nurs Mirror** 1981 Jul 15;153(3):40-2
Boschung U: Geburtshilfliche Lehrmodelle. Notizen zur Geschichte des Phantoms und der Hysteroplasmata. **Gesnerus** 1981;38:59-68
Boschung U: Medizinische Lehrmodelle. **Medita** 1980;10(Geschichte der Medizin, 4):xv
Bowler S: Nursing Mirror midwifery forum. 3. Survival test for babies. **Nurs Mirror** 1983 Mar 16;156(11):viii
Bowman IA: Herbal medicines and the midwife. **Bookman** 1982 Jul-Aug;9(6):3-9
Caffaratto TM: Breve storia delle ostetriche. **Minerva Ginecol** 1981 Sep;33(9):867-80
Dommisse J: Gestational age--fact or fallacy? **S Afr Med J** 1980 Sep 13;58(11):449-50
Drury MI: Diabetes in pregnancy--Matthews Duncan revisited. **Ir J Med Sci** 1984 Apr;153(4):144-51
Dunlop JM: Midwifery--ancient and modern. **Hist Med (Lond)** 1975 Autumn-Winter;6(3-4):51-7
Dunstan GR: The moral status of the human embryo: a tradition recalled. **J Med Ethics** 1984 Mar;10(1):38-44
Farkas G: Eclampsia in the course of times. In: Congrès international d'histoire de la médecine, XXVe, Québec, 1976. Actes. Québec, 1977. p. 650-3.
Fergusson IL, Taylor RW, Watson JM, ed: Records and curiosities in obstetrics and gynaecology. London, Baillière Tindall, 1982. x, 115 p.
Fox A: Obstetrics and Gynecology in Macbeth. **Shakespeare Stud** 1979;12:127-41
Gebbie DA: Reproductive anthropology--descent through woman. New York, Wiley, 1981. 371 p.
Harrison MR: Unborn: historical perspective of the fetus as a patient. **Pharos** 1982 Winter;45(1):19-24
Haynes DM: History of placental studies. **Obstet Gynecol Annu** 1983;12:1-14
Heimrath T: Ewolucja doboru pozycji podczas rodzenia. **Wiad Lek** 1984 May 15;37(10):797-9
Högberg U: Förebyggande mödravård från kinesiska urkunder till moderna MVC. **Lakartidningen** 1983 Dec 21;80(51):5009-12, 5017
Houtzager HL: Cesarean section till the end of the 16th century. **Eur J Obstet Gynecol Reprod Biol** 1982 Feb;13(1):57-8
Ishiguro T: [History of the abdominal binder. 4. Use of the abdominal binder by pregnant women: views by foreigners and opposition to its use] (Jpn). **Josanpu Zasshi** 1984 Jul;38(7):615-7
Iveson-Iveson J: Nursing Mirror midwifery forum. 10. Virgins and viragos. **Nurs Mirror** 1983 Nov 30;157(22):viii
Knibiehler Y, Fouquet C: La femme et les médecins. Analyse historique. [Paris], Hachette, 1983. 333 p.
Kogiso M, Ishihara T, Kamata H: [On the history of midwifery. A discussion] (Jpn). **Josanpu Zasshi** 1981 Aug;35(8):562-76
Laget M: La césarienne ou la tentation de l'impossible, 17 et 18e siècle. **Ann Bretagne** 1979;86(3):177-89
Laget M: Naissances: l'accouchement avant l'âge de la clinique. Paris, Seuil, 1982. 346 p.
Lehmann V: Der Gebärstuhl--ein historisches Möbel oder eine sinnvolle Erneuerung. **Z Geburtshife Perinatol** 1983 Mar-Apr;187(2):55-64
Lehmann V: Der Gebärstuhl--ein historisches Möbel oder eine sinnvolle Erneuerung. **Arch Gynecol** 1983;235(1-4):XLVIII-LXIII
Loughlin N: The caesarean section: some historical qualifying perspectives. **Todays OR Nurse** 1981 Feb;2(12):7-10
Marshall R: Nursing Mirror midwifery forum. 10. Birth of a profession. **Nurs Mirror** 1983 Nov 30;157(22):i-vii
Ney D, Hollingsworth DR: Nutritional management of pregnancy complicated by diabetes: historical perspective. **Diabetes Care** 1981 Nov-Dec;4(6):647-55
Pecker A: Gynäkologie und Geburtshilfe vom Altertum bis zum Anfang des 18. Jahrhunderts. In Sournia JC, Martiny M, Poulet J, ed: Illustrierte Geschichte der Medizin. Salzburg, Andreas, 1980. Vol. 3. p. 1023-73.
Peschel RE, Peschel ER: 'But what if she should die?'--case histories, literary histories: a discussion of maternal death in childbirth. **Pharos** 1981 Winter;44(1):11-8
Rall P, Kirchhoff KT, Roberts J: Professional attire at delivery, part I: an historical review. **J Nurse Midwife** 1984 Jul-Aug;29(4):251-6
Rothman BK: In labor. Women and power in the birthplace. New York, London, W.W. Norton, 1982. 320 p.
Russell JG: The rationale of primitive delivery positions. **Br J Obstet Gynaecol** 1982 Sep;89(9):712-5
Smith GF, Smith PN, Vidyasagar D, ed: Historical review and recent advances in neonatal and perinatal medicine. 2 vols. [Chicago?], Mead Johnson Nutritional Division, 1983. xxii, 212 p.; viii, 189 p. Historical contributions by B. F. Andrews, L. Ballowitz, L. J. Butterfield, V. Chernick, T. E. Cone, R. L. Day, M. L. Duxbury, D. Dye, L. M. Gartner, P. J. Goldstein, M. H. Greenberg, L. Johnson, A. Kaul, J. O. Klein, J. Lind, L. O. Lubchenco, N. M. Nelson, K. C. Pringle, T. N. Raju, A. C. Rambar, R. Sosa, M. T. Stahlman, L. Stern, K. Tarpey, A. Zipursky.
Strohmaier G: Der arabische Hippokrates. Bemerkungen zu einem Aufsatz von Dieter Irmer. **Sudhoffs Arch** 1980;64(3):234-49
Thiery M: Het epos van de keizersnede. **Verh K Acad Geneeskd Belg** 1984;46(3):221-30
Thiery M: Historische beschouwingen over obstetrische wanverhouding. **Verh K Acad Geneeskd Belg** 1983;45(6):509-32
Thornton JL, Want PC: Antique books in the library of the Royal College of Obstetricians and Gynaecologists. **Br J Obstet Gynaecol** 1981 Apr;88(4):337-45
The traditional birth attendant in seven countries: Case studies in utilization and training. **Public Health Pap** 1981;75:1-211
Trolle D: The history of Caesarean section. Copenhagen, University Library, 1982. 109 p. (Acta Historica Scientiarum Naturalium Et Medicinalium, v. 33).
Weisner ME: Early modern midwifery: a case study. **Int J Womens Stud** 1983;6(1):26-43
Weisser U: Die hippokratische Lehre von den Siebenmonatskindern bei Galen und Tabit ibn Qurra. **Sudhoffs Arch** 1979;63(3):209-38
Wilken H: Intrauterine und neonatale Infektionen. Geschichtlicher Rückblick. **Zentralbl Gynakol** 1983;105(16):1035-40
York R: The history of induction. **Midwife Health Visit Community Nurse** 1984 Apr;20(4):109-16
Zglinicki F: Geburt, eine Kulturgeschichte in Bildern. Braunschweig, Westermann, 1983. 384 p.

**Americas**

Rosengarten F: A neglected Mayan galactagogue, Ixbut (Euphorbia lancifolia). **Bot Mus Leafl Harv Univ** 1978;26:277-309

**Bulgaria**

Stoimenov G: Istoriia na bŭlgarskoto akusherstvo i ginekologiia. **Akush Ginekol (Sofiia)** 1980;19(5-6):395-401

**Czechoslovakia**

Pontuch A: Pokrokové tradície slovenského pôrodníctva. **Cesk Gynekol** 1981 Jul;46(6):423-6

**Denmark**

Dübeck I: Jordemødre og jura: en retshistorisk studie. **Tidsskr Rettsvitenskap** 1973;(5):729-57
Manniche E: [History of induced abortion in Denmark from 1200 to 1979] (Jpn). **Josanpu Zasshi** 1982 Oct;36(10):842-7

**Europe**

Nissen AJ: Kvinneslektens hemmelige historie. **Samtiden (Norway)** 1979;88(1):99-103

**France**

Bideau A: Accouchement 'Naturel' et accouchement à 'haut risque'. **Ann Demogr Hist (Paris)** 1981;:49 66
Duchatel F: L'auscultation obstétricale de Philippe Le Goust au monitorage foetal. **Hist Sci Med** 1982;16(1):37-47

**Germany**

Böhmer W, Helmbold P: Die reproduktionsbedingte Mortalität während früherer Jahrhunderte. **Zentralbl Gynakol** 1984;106(13):939-46
Schwarz M: Psychohygienische Verhaltensgebote für schwangere Frauen in medizinischen Ratgebergüchern. Frankfurt am Main, Haag Herchen, 1983. iv, 382 p.

**Great Britain**

Dewhurst J: Royal confinements. **Ala J Med Sci** 1982 Oct;19(4):445-52
Dewhurst J: Royal midwives of former times. **Midwife Health Visit Community Nurse** 1983 Oct;19(10):386-92
Dewhurst J: Royal twins. **Br Med J [Clin Res]** 1983 Dec 24-31;287(6409):1937-9
Fraser A: RCM supplement. The modest midwife. **Nurs Times** 1984 Jul 18-24;80(29):suppl 20-1
Guy JR: The episcopal licensing of physicians, surgeons and midwives. **Bull Hist Med** 1982;56(4):528-42
Milne GP: The history of midwifery in Aberdeen. **Aberdeen Univ Rev** 1978;47:293-303
Wilson A: Ignorant midwives - a rejoinder. **Soc Soc Hist Med Bull (Lond)** 1983 Jun;32:46-9

**Guatemala**

Villacorta Cifuentes JL: Historia de la medicina, cirugia y obstetricia prehispanicas. Guatemala, [s. n.] 1976. 166 p.

**Iceland**

Magnussyni SS: Den Isländska obstetrikens historia. **Katilolehti** 1983 Nov;88(11):310-4

**India**

Stork H: La détermination du sexe dans la pédiatrie traditionnelle de l'Inde. In Mazars G, ed: Les médecines traditionnelles de l'Asie. Strasbourg, Université Louis Pasteur, 1981, p. 150-62.

**Ireland**

O'Sullivan JF: Some highlights of obstetrics in Ireland. **Ulster Med J** 1980;49(2):105-11

**Japan**

Ishigoro T: [Historical background of the 'hara-obi' (a piece of cloth wrapped around the abdomen of a pregnant woman) and the origin of its name] (Jpn). **Josanpu Zasshi** 1984;38(4):336-9; (5):437-40; (6):519-23
Kamata H: [The past and present of customs related to childbirth. 7. Ceremonial bathing of the infant] (Jpn). **Josanpu Zasshi** 1982 Jul;36(7):590-3
Obayashi M: [Historical background of the acceptance of induced abortion] (Jpn). **Josanpu Zasshi** 1982 Dec;36(12):1011-6

**Netherlands**

De Bruijn J: Geschiedenis van de abortus in Nederland. Een analyse van opvattingen en discussies, 1600-1979. Amsterdam, Van Gennep, 1979. 330 p.
Houtzager HL: Frederik Ruysch. **Eur J Obstet Gynecol Reprod Biol** 1982 May;13(3):199-201

**Romania**

Farkas G, Farkas G Jr: People's customs related to pregnancy and delivery in former Transylvania. In: Congrès international d'histoire de la médecine, XXVe, Québec, 1976. Actes. Québec, 1977. p. 654-8.

**Sweden**

Högberg U: Allmogens förlossningsställningar. **Jordemodern** 1982 Jun;95(6):199-202

**Switzerland**

Stamm H: Die Entwicklung der Geburtshilfe in Basel. **Gesnerus** 1981;38:23-50

**United States**

Chaney JA: Birthing in early America. **J Nurse Midwife** 1980 Mar-Apr;25(2):5-13
Dye NS: History of childbirth in America. **Signs** 1980;6(1):97-108
Leavitt JW, ed: Women and health in America: historical readings. Madison, University of Wisconsin Press, 1984. ix, 526 p. (Previously published articles by various authors)
Michejda M: Advances in fetal medicine. **J Med Primatol** 1983;12(3):117-23
Robinson SA: A historical development of midwifery in the black community: 1600-1940. **J Nurse Midwife** 1984 Jul-Aug;29(4):247-50

## Before 500 A.D.

**China**

Chow Tse-Tsung: The childbirth myth and ancient Chinese medicine: a study of aspects of the 'wu' tradition. In D. T. Roy, T. Tsien, ed: Ancient China. Hong Kong, 1978. p. 43-89.

**Egypt**

Diener L: Från antikonception till amning - om tillökning i familjen i det faraoniska Egypten. **Nord Medicinhist Arsbok** 1983;:41-58
Ghalioungui P: The persistence and spread of some obstetric concepts held in ancient Egypt. **Ann Serv Antiq Egypte** 1977;62:141-54

**France**

Rousselle A: La sage-femme et le thaumaturge dans la Gaule tardive. Les sages-femmes ne font pas de miracles. **Rev Archeol Centre France** 1983;22(Dec):261-71

**Germany**

Kühl I: Zur Frage nach einer frühen Konzeption in ur- und frühgeschichtlicher Zeit: Beispiel vermutlicher Mutter-Kind-Bestattungen aus der vorrömischen Eisenzeit aus Holstein. **Aerztl Jugendkd** 1983 Jun;74(3):176-87

**Greece**

Benge MO: Midwifery history: How to bring away the after-burden. **Nurs Times** 1984 Oct 10-16;80(41):37
Bobbio S: Sorano de Efeso. **Femina** 1979;7:791-6
Hippokrates: Ueber Nachempfängnis, Geburtshilfe, und Schwangerschaftsleiden. Herausgegeben, übersetzt und erläutert von C. Lienau. Berlin, Akademie Verlag, 1973. 143 p. (Corpus Medicorum Graecorum, I, 2, 2).
Lonie IM: The Hippocratic treatises: 'On Generation', 'On the Nature of the Child', 'Diseases IV'. A commentary. Berlin, New York, Walter de Gruyter, 1981. xxxix, 406 p. (Ars medica. II. Abteilung, Griechisch-lateinische Medizin; Bd. 7, 2).

**India**

Hankoff LD, Munver UL: Prenatal experience in Hindu mythology. **NY State J Med** 1980 Dec;80(13):2006-14
Singhal GD, Guru LV: Anatomical and obstetric considerations in ancient Indian surgery: based on Sarirasthana of Susruta Samhita. Varanasi, India,

Institute of Medical Sciences, Banaras Hindu University, 1973. L, 241 p.

### 500 A.D.-1450

Kerherve J: Un accouchement dramatique à la fin du Moyen Age. **Ann Bretagne** 1982;89(3):391-6
Pinto LB: The folk practice of gynecology and obstetrics in the Middle Ages. **Bull Hist Med** 1973 Sep-Oct;47(5):513-23
Rowland B, Jennings M: Medieval multiple birth. **Neuphilol Mitt** 1980;81:169-73
Salvat M: L'accouchement dans la littérature scientifique médiévale. **Senefiance** 1980;9:87-106

#### Arabic

Asımova MZ, Kuznetsov VK, Piotrovskiĭ SM: Abu Ali Ibn-Sina i znachenie ego nauchnogo naslediia v istorii akusherstva. **Feldsher Akush** 1980;45(5):59-61

#### France

Gélis J: Obstétrique et classes sociales en milieu urbain aux XVIIe et XVIIIe siècles: évolution d'une pratique. **Hist Sci Med** 1980;14:425-33

#### Great Britain

Butler J: Mediaeval midwifery. **Nurs Times** 1981 Oct 7-13;77(41):1762-3
Iveson-Iveson J: A country midwife's tale. **Nurs Mirror** 1984 Apr 4;158(14):34-5
Medieval woman's guide to health: The first English gynecological handbook. Middle English text, with introduction and Modern English translation by B. Rowland. Kent, Kent State University Press, 1981. xvii, 192 p.

#### Italy

Rowland B: Exhuming Trotula, sapiens matrona of Salerno. **Florilegium** 1979;1:42-57

#### Netherlands

Iveson-Iveson J: Joined in parenthood. **Nurs Mirror** 1982 Sep 15;155(11):24

### 1450-1700

Bergamaschi MT, et al: Streghe e raccoglitrici di bambori: al confine tra la medicina colta, empiria e pratiche magiche (XV-XVI secolo). **Mem Riv Stor Donne** 1981;(1):106-13
Darmon P: Le mythe de la procréation a l'âge baroque. [Paris], Pauvert, 1977. 283 p.
Marshall RK: 17th century midwifery: the treatment of miscarriage. **Nurs Mirror** 1982 Dec 15;155(24):31-6

#### Europe

Ozment S: The family in Reformation Germany: the bearing and rearing of children. **J Fam Hist** 1983 Summer;8(2):159-76

#### France

Bernos M: Une 'suscitation' au Buis-les-Baronnies en 1699. Nouvelle contribution à l'étude des sanctuaires 'a répit'. **Ann Midi** 1980;92(146):87-93
Duchatel F: Paul Portal (1630? - ler juillet 1703): un accoucheur méconnu du XVIIe siècle. **Hist Sci Med** 1980;14:407-18
Kalisch PA, Scobey M, Kalisch BJ: Louyse Bourgeois and the emergence of modern midwifery. **J Nurse Midwife** 1981 Jul-Aug;26(4):3-17

#### Germany

Böhmer W: Der Wittenberger Kaiserschnitt von 1610. **Zentralbl Gynakol** 1983;105(19):1265-70
Rösslin E: Der Swangern Frauwen und hebammen Rosengarten. Facsimile of Strasbourg edition of 1513. Einführung von H. M. Koelbing. Dietikon/Zürich, Stocker, 1976. 137 p.
Watanabe N: [On Siegemundine and her 'The most needed training in difficult and abnormal delivery'] (Jpn). **Josanpu Zasshi** 1980 Dec;34(12):812-7

#### Great Britain

Barker AE: The Kelsale wonder. **Local Popul Stud (Matlock)** 1981 Spring;26:43
Crawford P: Attitudes to pregnancy from a woman's spiritual diary, 1687-8. **Local Popul Stud (Matlock)** 1978;21:43-5
Dewhurst J: The alleged miscarriages of Catherine of Aragon and Anne Boleyn. **Med Hist** 1984 Jan;28(1):49-56
Eccles A: Obstetrics and gynaecology in Tudor and Stuart England. Kent, Kent State University Press, 1982. 145 p.
Huard P, Imbault-Huart MJ: Les étapes du traitement des tumeurs par ischémie, priorité de Harvey. **Hist Sci Med** 1980;14(2):171-5
Porst S: Gynäkologie und Geburtshilfe bei Shakespeare. **Zentralbl Gynakol** 1984;106(12):863-75
Porst S: Gynäkologische, geburtshilfliche, embryologische und teratologische Beschreibungen im Werke Shakespeares. Würzburg, Horst Wellm, 1981. 178 p. (Dissertation, Julius-Maximilians-Universität Würzburg).
Versluysen MC: A forgotten chapter. **Nurs Times** 1981 Jul 15-21;77(29):1239

#### Italy

Maeder H: Die Frau im 17. Jahrhundert im Spiegel der 'Quaestiones medico-legales' des Paolo Zacchia (1584-1659). Diss. Bern, 1981. 101 p.

#### Netherlands

Houtzager HL: Medicyns, Vroedwyfs en Chirurgyns. Schets van de gezondheidszorg in Delft en beschrijving van het Theatrum Anatomicum aldaar in de 16e en 17e eeuw. Amsterdam, Rodopi, 1979. 133 p. (Serie-nitgave van het Genootschap Delfia Batavorum, 5).

#### Poland

Krzyś J: Pośmiertne cięcie cesarskie z czasów Zygmunta III. **Wiad Lek** 1980 Sept 1;33(17):1421-5

#### Switzerland

Houtzager HL: Jacob Rueff. **Eur J Obstet Gynecol Reprod Biol** 1982 Mar;13(2):105-7
Koelbing HM: 'De conceptu et generatione hominis' - die lateinische Fassung von Jakob Rueffs 'Trostbüchle', Zürich 1554. **Gesnerus** 1981;38:51-8
Portmann ML: Der Basler Medizinprofessor Johann Jacob Harder (1656-1711) als Geburtshelfer. **Gesnerus** 1983;40(1-2):139-47
Rueff J: Ein schön lustig Trostbüchle von den Empfengknussen und Geburten der Menschen. 2 v. Facsimile of 1554 ed., with Einführung von H. M. Koelbing. Dietikon-Zürich, Verlag Bibliophile Drucke, 1981. 29, cxliii p.

#### Yugoslavia

Sterijev K, Utvić V: Najsariji carski rez u Slavoniji (1694. godine). **Jugosl Ginekol Opstet** 1978 May-Aug;18(3-4):343-7

### 1700 to Present

Allan P, Jolley M, ed: Nursing, midwifery and health visiting since 1900. London, Faber and Faber, 1982. 316 p. With contributions by R. H. Pyne, B. Watkin, V. H. Darling, M. E. Lee, C. R. Kratz, G. M. Owen, R. Everest, P. D. Birchenall, D. M. Saunders, B. M. Slaney, D. Blenkinsop, M. D. Green, C. M. Chapman, E. A. Bent, J. C. Hayward, S. R. Lelean, A. V. Cowie, S. Quinn, I. S. Palmer, D. H. Rye.
Arney WR: Power and the profession of obstetrics. Chicago, London, University of Chicago Press, 1982. xi, 290 p.
Barnhart RJ: Cesarean section: changing indications, 1968-1977. **J Kans Med Soc** 1980 Feb;81(2):57-62, 78
Brickman JP: Mother love - mother death. Maternal and infant care: social class and the role of government. Ph.D. Diss., City University of New York. New York, 1978. vii, 750 leaves. (2 v.).
Curelaru I, Sandu L: Eugen Bogdan Aburel (1899-1975). The pioneer of regional analgesia for pain relief in childbirth. **Anaesthesia** 1982 Jun;37(6):663-9
Fischer-Homberger E: 'Krankheit Frau'. In Imhof AE, ed: Leib und Leben in der Geschichte der Neuzeit. Berlin, Duncker & Humblot, 1983. p. 215-29.
Garcia Gamboa MA: Estudio retrospectivo de los forceps de Tarnier 1862-1877. La evolucion de la traccion axial y los forceps curvos tractores sobre su eje sin tractores. 2 vols. 2a. ed. [Rio Piedras, Puerto Rico, Universidad de Puerto Rico, Escuela de Medicina, 1981. 359 leaves.
Garcia Gamboa MA: La cesarea abdominal: historia y evolucion. [Río Piedras] Universidad de Puerto Rico, Recinto de Ciencias Medicas, Escuela Medicina, 1982. 139 p.
Gélis J: Quand les femmes accouchaient sans médecin. **Histoire** 1981;34:105-12
Gélis J: Regard sur l'Europe médicale des Lumières: la collaboration internationale des acchoucheurs et la formation des sages-femmes au XVIIIe siècle. In Imhof AE, ed: Mensch und Gesundheit in der Geschichte. Husum, Matthiesen, 1980. p. 279-99.
Gillespie SA: Childbirth in the 1980s: what are the options? **Issues Health Care Women** 1981 Mar-Apr;3(2):101-28

Goodlin RC: Why fetal monitoring. **Semin Perinatol** 1981 Apr;5(2):105–7

Hartemann J: Geschichte der Geburtshilfe vom 18. Jahrhundert bis zur Gegenwart. In Sournia JC, Martiny M, Poulet J, ed: Illustrierte Geschichte der Medizin. Salzburg, Andreas, 1980. Vol. 4. p. 1359–427.

Hiestand WC: Nursing, the family, and the 'new' social history. **ANS** 1982 Apr;4(3):1–12

Hirschhorn K: Overview and historical perspective of prenatal diagnosis. **Methods Cell Biol** 1982;26:1–9

Jack DB, Laugher SJ: The earliest demonstration of the placental passage of morphine? **Pharm Hist (London)** 1982 Aug;12(2):7–8

Knight N: Early moral and medical opposition to inhalation anesthesia and childbirth. In The history and sociology of technology: Proceedings of the 24th annual meeting of the Society for the History of Technology. Milwaukee, Milwaukee Public Museum, 1982. p. 29–37.

Kvashenko BK, Konyk IeB: [Obstetrical care in Rovno Province]. (Ukr) **Pediatr Akush Ginekol** 1979;(6):56–8

Lenzi E: Nota informativa sull'U.P.I.G.O. e sull'U.E.M.S. **Minerva Ginecol** 1981 Feb–Mar;33(2–3):153–5

Lomax E: Changing attitudes during the past century as to the hazards of parental alcoholism to the progeny. In International Congress of the History of Medicine. 26th, Plovdiv, 1978. Actes du Congress. Sofia, 1981. Volume II. p. 144–7.

Lundström R: Rubella under graviditet--historik och nomenklatur. **Lakartidningen** 1979 Oct 10;76(41):3512–3

Macpike L: The social values of childbirth in the nineteenth-century novel. **Int J Womens Stud** 1980;3(2):117–30

Malcolm MT: Foetal alcohol syndrome: historical aspects. **Alcohol Alcohol** 1984;19(3):261–2

Matsuki A: [Current findings on the studies of the history of anesthesiology (8) -- Erwin Von Baelz and obstetrical anesthesia] (Jpn). **Masui** 1980 Mar;29(3):287–90

Mellgren A: Grossesse nerveuse--en psykosomatisk sjukdom. **Nord Medicinhist Arsb** 1982;:101–9

Nars PW: Frühgeburten gestern und heute. **Praxis** 1981 Apr 21;70(17):757–62

Potter EL: Yesterday and today. **Pediatr Pathol** 1983 Jan–Mar;1(1):1–3

Roberts J, Mendez-Bauer C: A perspective of maternal position during labor. **J Perinat Med** 1980;8(6):255–64

Sakula A: Augustus Bozzi Granville (1783–1872): London physician-accoucheur and Italian patriot. **J R Soc Med** 1983 Oct;76(10):876–82

Schneck P: Standpunkte russischer und deutscher Geburtshelfer zur Problematik der Eklampsietherapie um die Wende vom 19. zum 20. Jahrhundert. **Z Gesamte Hyg** 1980;26(5):374–6

Stampar-Plasaj B: Razvoj neonatologije. **Lijec Vjesn** 1979 Dec;101(12):737–42

Suitor JJ: Husband's participation in childbirth: a nineteenth-century phenomenon. **J Fam Hist** 1981 Fall;6:278–93

Thacker SB, Banta HD: Benefits and risks of episiotomy: an interpretative review of the English language literature, 1860–1980. **Obstet Gynecol Surv** 1983 Jun;38(6):322–38

This B: La requête des enfants à naître. Paris, Seuil, 1982. 256 p.

Tigertt WD: An annotated life of Egerton Yorrick Davis, M.D., an intimate of Sir William Osler. **J Hist Med Allied Sci** 1983 Jul;38(3):259–97

Zuck D: Early opposition to obstetric anasthesia [letter] **Anaesthesia** 1981 May;36(5):538–42

### Australia

Forster FM: David D. Davis' Obstetric Atlas in Tasmania in 1846. Edmund Bowden's gift to Robert Officer. **Aust NZ J Obstet Gynaecol** 1983 May;23(2):88–92

Lewis M: Hospitalization for childbirth in Sydney, 1870–1939; the modern maternity hospital and the improvement in the health of women. **J R Aust Hist Soc** 1980;66(3):199–205

McDonald IA, Cope I, Forster FM: Super Ardua. The Royal College of Obstetricians and Gynaecologists in Australia, 1929–1979. Melbourne, Australian Council RCOG, 1981. iv, 107 p.

Place J: A summary of nurse training at the Royal Women's Hospital, Melbourne. **Aust Nurses J** 1981 Aug;11(2):2–4

### Austria

Epifanov NS: I. F. Zemmel'veĭs. **Med Sestra** 1983 Aug;42(8):50–1

Frisch H: Die Entwicklung der Neonatologie in Tirol von 1968 bis 1978 und deren Einfluss auf die Morbidität und Mortalität von Früh- und Neugeborenen. **Wien Klin Wochenschr** 1980;92(116):1–58

Lesky E: Theorie und Praxis, aufgezeigt an den Wiener geburtshilflichen Lehrkanzeln 1752–1859. **Gesnerus** 1983;40(1–2):99–107

### Belgium

Ferkó S: Pálfyn Johann (1650–1730) a szülészeti fogó egyik feltalálója halálának 250. évfordulójára. **Orv Hetil** 1980 Mar 17;121(10):585–6

### Brazil

Lobo FB: Duas pioneiras-Madame Dubocher, Rita Lobato. **Rev Inst Hist Geogr Bras** 1980;(328):53–6

### Canada

Hurlburt J: Midwifery in Canada: a capsule history. **Can Nurse** 1981 Feb;77(2):30–1

Kennedy JE: Jane Soley Hamilton, midwife. **NS Hist Rev** 1982;2(1):6–29

Key JD. Osler's baby on the tracks. **Minn Med** 1983 Aug;66(8):515

Lessard R: Alexandre Serres. In Dictionary of Canadian biography, 1801 to 1820. Volume 5, 1983. p. 752.

Mitchinson W: Historical attitudes toward women and childbirth. **Atlantis** 1979;4(2 pt 2):13–34

Richardson G: Letitia Munson. In Dictionary of Canadian biography, 1881–1890. 1982;11:629–30.

Robb-Smith AH: Egerton Y. Davis, M.D., and placentophagy. **Bull NY Acad Med** 1980 Mar;56(2):258–60

### Chile

Costa-Casaretto C: Presentación del Dr. Lorenzo Sazié. **Rev Med Chil** 1983 Dec;111(12):1289–98

### Czechoslovakia

Cernoch A: Třicet pět let československěho porodnictví. **Cesk Gynekol** 1980 Jun;45(5):281–4

Doležal A: Císařský řez na živé v Cechách v roce 1789. **Cesk Gynekol** 1982 Jul;47(6):436–41

Fink A: Historie českého porodnictví, a to nedávná aneb jak je to s českými mezikrajovými semináři. **Cesk Gynekol** 1983 Apr;48(3):230–3

Kahle E: Kleinwächter, Ludwig. In Neue Deutsche Biographie 12. 1980. p. 9–10.

Presl J: K stoletému výročí narození prof. MUDr. Jiřího Trapla--zakladatele československé perinatologie. **Cesk Gynekol** 1980 Sep;45(8):611–3

Subrtová A, Cervený J: About the history of caesarean section and its first performance in Prague in 1792. **Acta Univ Carol [Med] (Praha)** 1983;29(5–6):373–93

Wondrák E: Die Anfänge der chirurgischen und geburtshilflichen Ausbildung in Mähren. In Ganzinger K, Skopec M, Wyklicky H, ed: Festschrift für Erna Lesky zum 70. Geburtstag. Wien, Brüder Hollinek, 1981. p. 185–92.

Zivotní jubileum prof. MUDr. Františka Gazárka, CSc: **Cesk Gynekol** 1983 Feb;48(1):75–80

### Denmark

Dübec I: Jordemødre i retshistorisk belysning. **Historie** 1973;10(3):337–90

### Finland

Aberg S: Tämäkin on yhteinen asiamme. **Katilolehti** 1982 May;87(5):172–3

Fock G: Om sköterskor, havandeskap, förlossning samt barnsäng i Finland på Elias Lönnrots tid. **Katilolehti** 1982 Jan;87(1):11–4

Kölli E: 1920-luvun kätilön työstä. **Katilolehti** 1981 Dec;86(12):392–8

Pakkala K: Kätilönä kolttien parissa. **Katilolehti** 1979 Dec;84(12):473–6

Pöyry M: Mikkelin läänin kätilöyhdistys 80 vuotta. **Katilolehti** 1980 Mar;85(3):97–100

Soiva K: Juhlahaastattelu. **Katilolehti** 1980 Dec;85(12):408–11

Teramo K: Savusaunasta monitoroituun synnytyssaliin. **Duodecim** 1981;97(20):1682–9

### France

Bénard JC: Fille ou garçon à volonté: un aspect du discours médical au XIXe siècle. **Ethnol Fr** 1981;11:63–76

Calot G: Le mouvement journalier des naissances à l'intèrieur de la semaine. **Population** 1981;36(3):477 504

Cone TE: The first published report of an incubator for use in the care of the premature infant (1857). **Am J Dis Child** 1981 Jul;135(7):658–60

Corps de mère, corps d'enfant: Paris, Stock, 1980. 223 p.

Dumont M, Rochefrette J: Un chirurgien-accoucheur au dix-huitième siècle. **J Gynecol Obstet Biol Reprod (Paris)** 1980;9(5):595–9

Gelis J: De la matrone à la sage-femme: les transformations de l'accoucheuse de campagne au XVIIIe siècle. **Penelope** 1981;(5):33–6

Gélis J: La pratique obstétricale dans la France moderne: les carnets du chirurgien accoucheur Pierre Robin (1770–1797). **Ann Bretagne** 1979;86:191–210

Gélis J: L'enquête de 1786 sur les sages-femmes du royaume. **Ann Demogr Hist (Paris)** 1980;:301–43

Houtzager HL: Jean Louis Baudelocque. **Eur J Obstet Gynecol Reprod Biol** 1982 Aug;13(5):323–4

Lamy ML, Leridon H: Les grossesses tardives donnant lieu à amniocentèse: enquête menée dans les trois centres de la région parisienne.

**Population** 1981;36(1):174–82
Logeay R: Bonheurs et malheurs de la clinique Tarnier. **Hist Sci Med** 1984;18(3):261–70
Monroziès M: Au service des femmes. Les services de gynécologie et d'obstétrique de l'hôpital de la Grave à Toulouse, 250 ans d'histoire 1729–1919. Toulouse, Privat, 1980. 88 p.
Riet D: Les déclarations de grossesses dans la région de Dinan à la fin de l'Ancien Régime. **Ann Bretagne** 1981;88(2):181–7
Roux L: 'La sage-femme'. **Ann Demogr Hist (Paris)** 1984;:269–78
Stofft H: Kergaradec à l'écoute du foetus. **J Gynecol Obstet Biol Reprod (Paris)** 1981;10(6):611–22
Stofft H: L'école des sages-femmes de Morlaix à fin du règne de Louis XV et sous le règne de Louis XVI. **Hist Sci Med** 1983;17(1):41–61
Thébaud F: Etre sage-femme entre les deux guerres: une profession en crise. **Penelope** 1981;(5):76–9
Tišer H, Mastný A: O narození Napoleonova syna Orlíka. **Cesk Gynekol** 1982 Jul;47(6):442–4
Tucat D: Les sages-femmes parisiennes à la fin du XIXe siècle. **Penelope** 1981;(5):58–61

**Germany**

Asendorf MI: Die gelehrten Arzte Joseph und Karl Wenzel, ihr Leben und Werk in Mainz und Frankfurt am Main. Diss. Mainz, 1981. 269 p.
Danilishina EI: Ernst Bumm (k 125-letiiu so dnia rozhdeniia). **Akush Ginekol (Mosk)** 1984 Jan;(1):69–70
Duchatel F: Insertion vélamenteuse du cordon ombilical et hémorragie de Benckiser. **Hist Sci Med** 1982;16(3):185–92
Easton L: Hermann Johannes Pfannenstiel (1862–1909). **Br J Obstet Gynaecol** 1984 Jun;91(6):538–41
Geiger A: Lorenz Heister als Geburtshelfer und gynäkologischer Chirurg. Vergleichende Untersuchung anhand der verschiedenen Auflagen seiner 'Chirurgie'. Zürich, Juris Druck, 1983. 140 p. (Zürcher Medizingeschichtliche Abhandlungen, Neue Reihe, Nr. 162).
Hofmann-Meier B: Ein Geburtshelfer und Hebammenlehrer des 18. Jahrhunderts. Leben und Werk des Johann Philipp Hagen (1734–1792), Hebammenlehrer und Professor für Entbindungskunst in Berlin. Diss. Bern, 1982. 75 p.
Kibel MA: Silver nitrate and the eyes of the newborn--a centennial. **S Afr Med J** 1981 Dec 26;60(26):979–80
Kirchhoff H: 40 Jahre miterlebte wissenschaftliche Forschung auf dem Gebiet der Gynäkologie und Geburtshilfe. **Ther Ggw** 1981 Jul;120(7):654–68
Klausch B, Schwarz R: Die Geschichte der Frauenklinik der Universität Rostock von den Anfängen bis zur Gegenwart. Rostock, Wilhelm-Pieck-Universität, 1980. 31 p.
Kraatz H: Zwischen Klinik und Hörsaal. Ein Frauenarzt sieht sich in seiner Zeit. Berlin, Verlag der Nation, 1977. 351 p.
Lindemann M: Fürsorge für arme Wöchnerinnen in Hamburg um 1800: die Beschreibung eines 'Entbindungs-Winkels'. **Gesnerus** 1982;39(3–4):395–403
Makowski HM: Georg Wilhelm Stein und die frühe Geburtshilfe in Bonn. Diss. Bonn, 1979. 110 p.
Müller W: Vom Wöchnerinnenasyl zum Universitätsklinikum. Die Geschichte des Städtischen Krankenhauswesens in Essen. Münster, Murken-Altrogge, 1981. 364 p. (Studien zur Geschichte des Krankenhauswesens, 15)
Schneck P: Frauenheilkunde und Geburtshilfe in der Zeit des deutschen Faschismus 1933 bis 1945--Zum Schicksal der sozialen Gynäkologie im 'Dritten Reich'. **Z Gesamte Hyg** 1983 Oct;29(10):645–7
Schneegans HJ: Die Müttersterblichkeit im 17. bis 19. Jahrhundert. **Zentralbl Gynakol** 1982;104(22):1416–20
Scholz A: Geburtshilfe vor 150 Jahren. **Z Arztl Fortbild (Jena)** 1980 Oct 1;74(19):930–3
Semm K, Giese KP: Ernst Gräfenberg: the life and work of the specialist of Kiel on the hundredth anniversary of his birth on 26 September 1881. **Int J Fertil** 1983;28(3):141–8
Winkelmann H: Entbindungswissenschaft und Entbindungskunst bei Friedrich Benjamin Osiander. **Medizinhist J** 1983;18(4):306–12

**Great Britain**

Ashton RM: The Royal College of Midwives: past, present and future. **Int J Gynaecol Obstet** 1979–80 Sep–Oct;17(2):124–7
Baker M: Midwifery by gaslight. **Nurs Times** 1984 Aug 29–Sep 4;80(35):40–3
Bent EA: From three hours to three days in 101 years. **Midwife Health Visit Community Nurse** 1983 Jul;20(7):267–73
Breathnach CS: Biographical sketches No. 26--W. Hunter. **Ir Med J** 1983 Feb;76(2):59
Classic articles in colonic and rectal surgery: James Young Simpson 1811–1870. **Dis Colon Rectum** 1982 Sep;25(6):611–22
Cowell B, Wainwright D: Behind the blue door: the history of the Royal College of Midwives, 1881–1981. London, Baillière Tindall, 1981. 111 p.
Cowell B: Royal College of Midwives: one hundred years young! **Nurs Mirror** 1981 Jul 15;153(3):18–20
Cowell B, Wainwright D: The battle for status. **Nurs Times** 1981 Jul 15–21;77(29):1237–8
Defalque RJ: The first experiment in obstetrical anesthesia. **Anesth Analg (Cleve)** 1983 Dec;62(12):1136
Eaves Walton PM, et al.: The 250th and 100th anniversaries of the Royal Infirmary of Edinburgh and the 100th anniversary of the Simpson Memorial Maternity Pavilion. Edinburgh, Royal Infirmary of Edinburgh, 1979. 53 p.
Farr AD: Early opposition to obstetric anaesthesia. **Anaesthesia** 1980 Sept;35(9):896–907
Ferrer M: The Royal College of Midwives 1881 - 1981. **Midwife Health Visit Community Nurse** 1981 Jul;17(7):288–94
Harley DN: Ignorant midwives--a persistent stereotype. **Soc Soc Hist Med Bull (Lond)** 1981 Jun;28:6–9
Harley JM: The Royal Maternity Hospital, Belfast. Fifty glorious years 1933–1983. **Ulster Med J** 1984;53(1):1–17
Lewis JS: Manners and medicine. Childbearing in the English aristocracy 1790–1840. Ph.D. Diss., Johns Hopkins University. Baltimore, 1979. vi, 301 leaves.
Loudon I: Maternal mortality: an historical audit. **J R Coll Gen Pract** 1984 Nov;34(268):585–6
The male midwife.: **Bygone Kent** 1980;1(9):532
Maulitz RC: Metropolitan medicine and the man-midwife: the early life and letters of Charles Locock. **Med Hist** 1982 Jan;26(1):25–46
Oakley A: The relevance of the history of medicine to an understanding of current change: some comments from the domain of antenatal care. **Soc Sci Med** 1982;16(6):667–74
Peel J: Sir Eardley Lancelot Holland. In Dictionary of national biography, 1961–1970. Suppl. 8, 1981. p. 525–7.
Peel J: The lives of the fellows of the Royal College of Obstetricians and Gynaecologists, 1929–1969. London, Heinemann, 1976. xviii, 390 p.
Peters D: The pregnant Pamela: characterizations and popular medical attitudes in the 18th century. **Eighteenth Cent Stud** 1980–81;14:432–51
Pinkerton JH: John Creery Ferguson. Friend of William Stokes and pioneer of auscultation of the fetal heart in the British Isles. **Br J Obstet Gynaecol** 1980 Apr;87(4):257–60
Schnorrenberg BB: Is childbirth any place for a woman? The decline of midwifery in eighteenth-century England. **Stud Eighteenth Cent Cult** 1981;10:393–408
Seligman S: The royal maternity charity: the first hundred years. **Med Hist** 1980;24(4):403–18
Sørensen T: James Blundell 27.XII.1790–15.I.1878. Professor i fysiologi og obstetrik ved Guy's Hospital 1823–1834. **Ugeskr Laeger** 1983 Jun 27;145 Spec No:5–49
Stewart J: Women pioneers of medicine. **Midwife Health Visit Community Nurse** 1983 Jun;20(6):240, 242
Sturrock J: The Edinburgh Royal Maternity and Simpson Memorial Hospital. **J R Coll Surg Edinb** 1980 May;25(3):173–87
Thornton JL, Want PC: William Hunter (1718–1783) and his contributions to obstetrics. **Br J Obstet Gynaecol** 1983 Sep;90(9):787–94
Tröhler U: Klinisch-numerische Forschung in der britischen Geburtshilfe 1750–1820. **Gesnerus** 1981;38:69–80
Usui T, Kodama K: [At completion of the translation of the 'Notes on Lying-in Institutions'. A discussion] (Jpn) **Sogo Kango** 1984 Aug 15;19(3):79–91
Ward AR: The passing of the Midwives' Act, 1902. **Midwives Chron** 1981 Jun;94(1121):190–4

**Hungary**

Gyöngyössy A: Kovács Ferenc (1890–1974). **Orv Hetil** 1984 Aug 19;125(34):2085–6
Hogye I: 'Bábai mesterség' a Hegyalján (1711–1849). **Orvostort Kozl** 1982;28(1–3):201–8
Lampé L: Egységes nemzetközi szülészeti adatgyüjtés (Tauffer nyomdokain). **Orv Hetil** 1982 Apr 11;123(15):895–903
Raics J: Tauffer Vilmos mint szülészeti miniszteri biztos. **Orvostort Kozl** 1980;89–91(26 no 1–3):137–55
Sergo E: Gyermekágyas asszony étkeztetése Magyarországon. **Orvostort Kozl** 1982;28(1–3):245–50

**Iceland**

Einarsdóttir ES: Midwifery education in Iceland: yesterday and today. **J Nurse Midwife** 1983 Nov–Dec;28(6):31–2
Snoedal G: Jordenmödrenes arbejde for 100 år siden. **Nord Medicinhist Arsb** 1982;:171–8

**Ireland**

Browne AD: The section of obstetrics and obstetric and gynaecological development over the century. **Ir J Med Sci** 1983 Jan;152(1):26–38
Connolly SJ: Illegitimacy and pre-nuptial pregnancy in Ireland before 1864: the evidence of some Catholic parish registers. **Ir Econ Soc Hist** 1979;6:5–23
Froggatt P: The resignation of Robert Little from the chair of midwifery

at Inst [Academical Institution, Belfast] **Ulster Med J** 1979;48(1):19–31
Pinkerton JH: Evory Kennedy: a master controversial. **Ir Med J** 1984 Mar;77(3):77–81
Pinkerton JH: John Creery Ferguson 1802–1865: Physician and fetologist. **Ulster Med J** 1981;50(1):10–20
Pinkerton JH: Sir James Young Simpson: Irish influences. **Ir Med J** 1982 Jun;75(6):183–7

**Japan**

Matsuki A: [Erwin von Baelz as a pioneer in obstetrical anaesthesia in Japan.] (Jpn). **Nihon I-Shigaku Zasshi** 1981;27(1):47–55
Miyasato K, Ishihara T, Oshima K: [Impression of the Symposium on the History of Obstetrics] (Jpn). **Josanpu Zasshi** 1983 Jul;37(7):566–77
Okamoto K: [Historical significance of midwifery activities--with special reference to the Meiji period] (Jpn). **Josanpu Zasshi** 1981 Aug;35(8):577–99
Seki M, Nonaka R: [55 years of midwifery activities--oral history by Ms. Shin Tanaka]. (Jpn) **Josanpu Zasshi** 1981 Aug;35(8):600–9
Shima K: [Endless voyage. The life of Ms. Shin Tanaka. 5. Chapter 2.] (Jpn). **Josanpu Zasshi** 1982 Nov;36(11):946–53 (continued regularly)
Sugitachi G: [Gen-etsu Kagawa and his obstetric practice] (Jpn). **Josanpu Zasshi** 1983 Jun;37(6):484–9

**Netherlands**

Benedek-Jaszmann LJ: Hendrik van Deventer (1651–1724); the silversmith who became the co-founder of modern obstetrics. **Orvostort Kozl** 1980;89–91(26 no 1–3):241–9
Koning AT: De 'Kweekschool der Vroedkunde', de eerste verloskundige periodiek? **Ned Tijdschr Geneeskd** 1981 Aug 8;125(32):1299–302
Macpherson AI: Blue babies before Fallot. **J R Coll Surg Edinb** 1984 Jul;29(4):199–204
Merriënboer FJ: Eene buitenbaarmoederlijke zwangerschap, waar het foetus na 18 Jaren bij de moeder vertoefd te hebben door de anus is ontlast, beschreven door C.H. van der Looy (1850). **Tijdschr Geschied Geneeskd** 1980;3(1):37–40

**Norway**

Bergsjø P, Ulstein M: Jørgen Løvset 1896–1981. **Acta Obstet Gynecol Scand** 1982;61(3):193–4

**Philippines**

Agris J: Stamps commemorating medicine. 'Honoria Acosta Sison' pioneer gynecologist and obstetrician. **J Dermatol Surg Oncol** 1980 Mar;6(3):178
Kohnen N: Geburtsbräuche bei den Kankanai-Igorot. Ein Beitrag zur 'natürlichen' Geburt. **Dtsch Med Wochenschr** 1983 Jul 29;108(30):1163–7

**Poland**

Heimrath T: Położnictwo i genekologia w Akademii Medycznej we Wrocławiu w latach 1945–1980. **Ginekol Pol** 1982 Jul–Aug;53(7–8):563–8
Królikowska M: XXXV-lecie ginekologii i położnictwa w Akademii Medycznej w Lodzi. **Ginekol Pol** 1980 Nov;51(11):973–9
Krzyś J: Przebieg pierwszych w Polsche cięć cesarskich. **Wiad Lek** 1981 Jan 15;34(2):171–6
Mazurczak T, Wiśniewski L, Wald I, et al: Rozwój i stan obecny diagnostyki prenatalnej w Polsce. **Ginekol Pol** 1983 Mar;54(3):141–5
Moskwa Z: Zawód położnej w świetle rozporządzeń z lat 1928/29. **Wiad Lek** 1983 Jun 1;36(11):941–4
Rodowód przyszłości. 10: Sekcja Pielęgniarek i Położnych ZZPSZ **Pieleg Polozna** 1982;(12):27–9
Rybak J: Tradycje Krakowskiej Szkoły Połżnych. **Pieleg Polozna** 1980;(3):25–7
Słupczyński S, Skrzypczak I: Cięia cesarskie wykonane w szpitalu miejskim w Lukowie w latach 1971–1978. **Ginekol Pol** 1979 Oct;50(10):855–8
Waszyński E: 'Primitiae physico-medicae ...' (1750–1753). Problematyka położniczo-ginekologiczna. **Arch Hist Med (Warsz)** 1984;47(3):447–61
Zrubek H. 35 lat w służbie macierzyństwa na Lubelszczyźnie. **Ginekol Pol** 1980 Dec;51(12):1057–61

**Romania**

Clocotici L: Aspecte din tecutul profesiei de moaşă. **Viata Med [Medii Sanit]** 1983 Nov;31(11):261–4

**Scandinavia**

Asplund J: The Scandinavian Association of Obstetricians and Gynecologists 1933–1983. **Acta Obstet Gynecol Scand [Suppl]** 1984;120:9–26
Borell U: Opening speech at the 50th anniversary congress of the Scandinavian Association of Obstetricians and Gynecologists in Stockholm, January 28–29, 1983. **Acta Obstet Gynecol Scand [Suppl]** 1984;120:5–7

**Singapore**

Ratnam SS, Karim SM, Ng CS, et al: Research and development in obstetrics and gynaecology in the Department of Obstetrics and Gynaecology at the National University of Singapore. **Ann Acad Med Singapore** 1982 Jul;11(3):313–21

**South Africa**

Daubenton F: Professor Cuthbert Crichton--the man and his times. **S Afr Med J** 1979 Dec 15;56(25):1064–75
Lewis JS: Obstetric reminiscences in the course of general practice in Basutoland (over 50 years ago). **S Afr Med J** 1983 Jun 29;Spec No:20–2
Sharp RG: Tribute to a great teacher. **S Afr Med J** 1979 Dec 15;56(25):1059–64

**Spain**

Jordi González R: Dos curiosos impresos, supuestos del siglo XIX. **Circ Farm** 1980 May;12(126):85–9
Rodríguez García JR: Circulacion mundial de la obstetricia y ginecologia española a traves de Excerpta Medica (1951–71). **Asclepio** 1980;32:401–14

**Sweden**

Engel A: Hälsan före födelsen. Prenatal forskning i Sverige. Stockholm, 1981. 128 p. (Nordisk Medicinhistorisk Arsbok, Supplementum, VIII).
Hagenfeldt K: Dramatiskt minskad mödramortalitet. Framsynta åsikter i abortfrågan. **Lakartidningen** 1983 Nov 9;80(45):4299–302
Höfberg U: 'Jungfru Mariae nycklar' och mödradödligheten genom två sekler. **Lakartidningen** 1982 Sep 1;79(35):2977–9
Malmstedt J: Hon förlöste vävarnas barn--barnmorskan Anna Norin. **Jordemodern** 1982 Oct;95(10):341–4
Mattsson V: Ammor och barnafödande i Malmö 1750–1850. **Scandia** 1980;46(2):173–98

**Switzerland**

Buess H, Portmann ML: Berühmte Schweizer Arzte. **Gesnerus** 1980;37(3/4):289–306
Stamm H: 75 Jahre Société de Gynécologie et d'Obstétrique de la Suisse Romande--70 Jahre Gynäkologische Gesellschaft der deutschen Schweiz. **Gesnerus** 1981;38(3/4):313–30
Waszyński E: W dwusetną rocznicę urodzin Franciszka Izaaka Mayora (1779–1855), odkrywcy tonów serca płodu. **Ginekol Pol** 1980 Aug;51(8):765–6

**United States**

Alexander SF, Nevins MA: Home care delivery in Bergen County in the 19th century. **J Med Soc NJ** 1983 Apr;80(4):283–7
Aries NR: Abortion clinics and the organization of work: a case study of Charles Circle. **Rev Radic Polit Econ** 1980;12(2):53–62
Bogdan J: Care or cure? Childbirth practices in 19th-century America. **Feminist Stud** 1978;4(2):92–9
Bond JR, Johnson CA: Implementing a permissive policy: hospital abortion services after Roe V. Wade. **Am J Pol Sci** 1982;26(1):1–24
Bullough VL, Groeger S: Irving W. Potter and internal podalic version: the problems of disciplining a skilled but heretical doctor. **Soc Probl** 1982;30(1):109–16
Burst HV: The influence of consumers on the birthing movement. **Top Clin Nurs** 1983 Oct;5(3):42–54
Buss FL: La partera, story of a midwife. Ann Arbor, University of Michigan Press, 1980. viii, 137 p.
Calmes SH: Virginia Apgar: a woman physician's career in a developing specialty. **J Am Med Wom Assoc** 1984 Nov–Dec;39(6):184–8
Chesley LC: Evolution of the Department of Obstetrics and Gynecology at Downstate, 1860–1980. [New York?, s.n., 1982?] 96 p.
Devitt N: The statistical case for elimination of the midwife: fact versus prejudice, 1890–1935. **Women Health** 1979;4:81–96, 169–86
Devitt N: The statistical case for elimination of the midwife: fact versus prejudice, 1890–1935 (part 2). **Women Health** 1979 Summer;4(2):121–33
Devitt N: The transition from home to hospital birth in the United States, 1930–1960. **Birth Fam J** 1977;4(2):47–58
Dishman M: Coleman Hall. A monument to Indiana medicine. **Indiana Med** 1984 Aug;77(8):622–3
Drachman VG: The Loomis trial: social mores and obstetrics in the mid-nineteenth century. In Reverby S, Rosner D, ed: Health care in America. Philadelphia, Temple University Press, 1979. p. 67–83.
Dwork D: Sophia Josephine Kleegman. In: Notable American women. The modern period. Cambridge, Mass., Belknap-Harvard Univ. Press, 1980. 4:398–400.
Dye NS: Mary Breckinridge, the Frontier Nursing Service and the introduction of nurse-midwifery in the United States. **Bull Hist Med** 1983 Winter;57(4):485–507
Francome C: Abortion politics in the United States. **Polit Stud** 1980;28(4):613–21

# OBSTETRICS

Gibbons RW: Forgotten parameters of general practice: the chiropractic obstetrician. **Chiropr Hist** 1982;2(1):27–33
Graveley A: Midwives celebrate century of professional advancement. **Australas Nurses J** 1981 Mar;10(3):8–9
Grubb JM: The first successful cesarean section and the first oophorectomy in the Americas. **W Va Med J** 1984 Oct;80(10):221–3
Hansen SB: State implementation of supreme court decision: abortion rates since Roe v. Wade. **J Polit** 1980;42(2):372–95
Hiestand WC: Midwife to nurse-midwife: a history. The development of nurse-midwifery education in the continental United States to 1965. Ed. D. Diss., Columbia University. New York, 1976. 294 p.
Higgins PG, Wayland JR: Labour and delivery in North America. **Nurs Times** 1981 Sept 16; Midwifery Suppl:4, 6, 8, 10
Holmes L: Alabama granny midwife. **J Med Soc NJ** 1984 May;81(5):389–91
Huckle P: The womb factor: pregnancy policies and employment of women. **West Polit Q** 1981;34(1):114–26
Ivić J: Povodom 100-te obljetnice rodenja George N. Papanicolaoua 1883–1983. **Jugosl Ginekol Opstet** 1983 May–Aug;23(3–4):53–4
Jones EF: Ways in which childbearing affects women's employment: evidence from the U. S. 1975 national fertility study. **Popul Stud** 1982;36(1):5–14
Keettel WC: A history of the Department of Obstetrics & Gynecology, the University of Iowa, 1848–1980. Iowa City, University of Iowa, 1981. xi, 186 p.
Klos SF: Reform initiatives in American maternal health services: 1900–1940. Ed. D. Diss., Harvard University. Cambridge, 1979, vi, 182 p.
Klosky BA: Daring venture: a biography of Anne Austin Young, pioneer woman doctor. Columbia, S.C., Bryan, 1978. xiii, 193 p.
Labor under ether: Hilo, 1850. **Hawaii Med J** 1981 Oct;40(10):291–2
Lay midwifery--still an 'illegal' profession: **Women Health** 1977 Nov–Dec;2(3):19–26
Leavitt JW: Birthing and anesthesia: the debate over twilight sleep. **Signs** 1980;6(1):147–64
Leavitt JW: 'Science' enters the birthing room: obstetrics in America since the eighteenth century. **J Am Hist** 1983;70(2):281–304
Levin BS: Women and medicine. Metuchen, N. J., London, Scarecrow, 1980. vii, 257 p.
Litoff JB: Carolyn Conant van Blarcom. In: Notable American women. The modern period. Cambridge, Mass., Belknap-Harvard Univ. Press, 1980. 4:703–4.
Longo LD: John Whitridge Williams and academic obstetrics in America. **Trans Stud Coll Physicians Phila** 1981 Dec;5(3 no 4):221–54
McDonell KM: Women and medicine in early nineteenth century Indiana. **Indiana Med Hist Q** 1980;6(2):3–23
McIntosh K: Folk obstetrics, gynecology, and pediatrics in Utica, New York. **NY Folkl** 1978;4(1–4):49–59
Matthies K: Mary Breckinridge and the frontier nursing service. **DAR Mag** 1980;114(5):692–4
Miller LG: Pain, parturition, and the profession: twilight sleep in America. In Reverby S, Rosner D, ed: Health care in America. Philadelphia, Temple University Press, 1979. p. 19–44.
Modern midwives: **MD** 1978 Oct;22(10):53–5
Morantz RM, Zschoche S: Professionalism, feminism, and gender roles: a comparative study of nineteenth-century medical therapeutics. **J Am Hist** 1980 Dec;67(3):568–88
Nipe GM: 'Jessee Bennett decided to operate on his wife at once'. **Va Med** 1979 Dec;106(12):884–5
Pearson CL: 'Nine children were born': a historical problem from the Sugar Creek episode. **Brigham Young Univ Stud** 1981;21(4):441–4
Pebley AR, Westoff CF: Women's sex preferences in the United States: 1970 to 1975. **Demography** 1982 May;19(2):177–89
Perry DS: The early midwives of Missouri. **J Nurse Midwife** 1983 Nov–Dec;28(6):15–23
Pinsker H, Novick DM, Richman BL: Hospital care at Second Avenue and East 17th Street, New York City, 1894–1984. **Bull NY Acad Med** 1984 Nov;60(9):905–24
Ranney B: Geschichte, Organisation und Praxis der amerikanischen Gynäkologie und Geburtshilfe. Eine Ubersicht. **Zentralbl Gynakol** 1984;106(9):626–32
Rooks JB, Fishman SH: American nurse-midwifery practice in 1976–1977: reflections of 50 years of growth and development. **Am J Public Health** 1980 Sep;70(9):990–6
Rothman BK: Midwives in transition: the structure of a clinical revolution. **Soc Probl** 1983;30(3):262–71
Ryan MP: Reproduction in American history. **J Interdiscip Hist** 1979;10(2):319–32
Sablosky AH: The power of the forceps: a comparative analysis of the midwife--historically and today. **Women Health** 1976 Jan–Feb;1(1):10–13
Sandelowski M: Pain, pleasure, and American childbirth: from the twilight sleep to the Read Method, 1914–1960. Westport, Conn., Greenwood Press, 1984. xix, 152 p. (Contributions in Medical History, No. 13).
Scully D: [A history of] 'Baby catchers and uterus snatchers'. In her: Men who control women's health; the miseducation of obstetrician-gynecologists. Boston, Houghton Mifflin, 1980. p. 25–67.
Sharp ES: Nurse-midwifery education: Its successes, failures, and future. **J Nurse Midwife** 1983 Mar–Apr;28(2):17–23
Siddall AC: Bloodletting in American obstetric practice, 1800–1945. **Bull Hist Med** 1980 Spring;54(1):101–10
Strane S: Childbirth – yesterday and today. **J Nurs Care** 1982 Apr;15(4):22–4
Taylor ES: Commemorative issue: Georgeanna Seegar Jones, Howard W. Jones, Jr. Twenty-five years as editors-in-chief for Gynecology, Obstetrical & Gynecological Survey. **Obstet Gynecol Surv** 1982 Jun;37(6):355–84
Thalidomide: 20 years on: **Lancet** 1981 Sep 5;2(8245):510–1
Tom SA: The evolution of nurse-midwifery: 1900–1960. **J Nurse Midwife** 1982 Jul–Aug;27(4):4–13
Tyndall RM: A history of the Bellevue School for midwives 1911–1936. Diss (Ed D), Columbia University. New York, 1978. xi, 260 p.
Wertz DC: What birth has done for doctors: a historical view. **Women Health** 1983 Spring;8(1):7–24

**USSR**

Abramenko VV, Gendel' MG: Rol' A. Ia. Krassovskogo v razvitii operativnogo akusherstva. **Akush Ginekol (Mosk)** 1984 Jan;(1):67–9
Bell JD: Giving birth to the new Soviet man: politics and obstetrics in the USSR. **Slavic Rev** 1981;40(1):1–16
Borodiĭ NK: K biografii N. M. Maksimovicha-Ambodika. **Akush Ginekol (Mosk)** 1982;(8):60–1
D'iachkov VI: Revoliutsionnoe proshloe pervogo meditsinskogo uchebnogo zavedeniia v Sibiri (o Tobol'skoĭ povival'noĭ shkole). **Feldsher Akush** 1984 Mar;49(3):55–6
Dmitriev VG: 'Nauka o babich'em dele' i ee avtor. (N. Maksimovich-Ambodik). **Feldsher Akush** 1984 Feb;49(2):50–1
Dudchenko MA: Aleksandr Mikhaĭlovich Shumlianskiĭ. **Klin Med (Mosk)** 1983 Jan;61(1):114–6
Gerasimovich GT: Belorusskomu Nauchnomu Meditsinskomu obshchestvu Akusherov-Ginekologov 50 let. **Akush Ginekol (Mosk)** 1981 Sep;(9):59–61
Granat NE: Zhurnal 'Akusherka' (po stranitsam starinnogo zhurnala). **Feldsher Akush** 1983;48(4):58–60
Ianovskiĭ AG: Fel'dshera i akusherki v revoliutsii 1905–1907 gg. **Feldsher Akush** 1980;45(11):41–4
Manuilova IM, Chervakova TV: Uspekhi otechestvennoĭ akushersko-ginekologicheskoĭ nauki k 60-letiiu obrazovaniia SSSR. **Sov Med** 1982;(12):35–41
Mirskiĭ MB, Verbitskiĭ VM, Khil'chenko MA: K 170-letiiu so dnia rozhdeniia A. A. Kitera. **Akush Ginekol (Mosk)** 1983 Sep;(9):72–3
Mirskiĭ MB, Verbitskiĭ VM, Khil'chenko MA: Vklad A. Ia. Krassovskiĭ v organizatsiiu rodovspomozheniia v Peterburge. **Sov Zdravookhr** 1984;(3):62–4
Palkin BN, Daniuk GI: Iz istorii akusherstva v Rossii kontsa XVIII-nachala XIX veka. **Feldsher Akush** 1983 Aug;48(8):44–6
Ramer SC: Childbirth and culture: midwifery in the nineteenth-century Russian countryside. In Ransel, David L., ed. The family in Imperial Russia. New lines of historical research. Urbana, U. of Illinois Press, 1978. p. 218–35.
Shabunin AV: P. F. Lesgaft i razvitie fel'dshersko-akusherskogo obrazovaniia v Rossii. **Feldsher Akush** 1981;46(4):57–8
Sol'skiĭ IP: Razvitie i dostizheniia akushersko-ginekologicheskoĭ sluzhby v USSR. **Akush Ginekol (Mosk)** 1982 Sep;(9):3–5
60 Let deiatel'nosti zhurnala 'Akusherstvio i ginekologiia': **Akush Ginekol (Mosk)** 1982;(12):16–7

**Yugoslavia**

Berić B, Babić N: Dr. Antun Lobmayer (1844–1906) pionir savremenog akušerstva i školovanja primalja u Hrvatskoj. **Jugosl Ginekol Opstet** 1979;19(1–2):113–8
Berić B, Rajković D, Babić-Ilić N: Dr Nikola Hadži-Nikolić (1855–1915) prvi akušer-ginekolog u Srbiji i Njegov značaj za razvoj akušerstva i ginekologije u Srbiji. **Jugosl Ginekol Opstet** 1981 Dec;21(5–6):143–8
Berić BM: Dr Eva Haljecka (18??–1947) prva žena akušer-ginekolog u jugoslovenskim zemljama. **Jugosl Ginekol Opstet** 1983 May–Aug;23(3–4):95–9
Berić BM: Prvi ginekolog-akušer u Vojvodini--dr Aleksander Sosberger (1873–1944). **Jugosl Ginekol Opstet** 1984 May–Aug;24(3–4):71–2
Dавić P, Popov K, Popov-Dragin O: Prve babice i razvoj akušerske službe u Somboru u XVIII veku. **Med Pregl** 1982;35(1–2):59–67
Juvan V: Djelatnost za zdravstvenu zaštitu žena Medicinskog centra u Varaždinu. **Jugosl Ginekol Opstet** 1978;18(5–6):445–53
Rosenzweig E: Porodništvo u starom Zagrebu (18. stoljeće). **Lijec Vjesn** 1981 Aug;103(8):363–6

**Zambia**

Höjeberg P: Mödrovård i Zambia. **Jordemodern** 1982 Jun;95(6):203–7

# OCCUPATIONAL MEDICINE

Cahall JB: The history of occupational health nursing. **Occup Health Nurs** 1981 Oct;29(10):11–3

Geerts A, Kornblith BA, Urmson WJ: Compensation for bodily harm. L'indemnisation des lésions corporelles à travers les siècles. Brussels, Fernand Nathan, Labor, 1977. 213 p.

Haeublein HG: Early studies of miners and smelters. **Am J Ind Med** 1982;3(3):357–8

Hoppe B: Arbeit und Gesundheit; historische Aspekte ihrer gegenseitigen Beziehungen. Bericht über eine Tagung der 'International School of History of Biological Sciences' in Ischia/Neapel vom 29. Juni bis 12. Juli 1980. **Ber Wissenschaftsgesch** 1980;3(3–4):214–20

Jenss H: Jugendarbeitsschutz: von den Anfängen der Industrialisierung bis zur Gegenwart. Frankfurt, New York, Campus, 1980. xiv, 260 p.

Karrh BW: The critical balance: the influence of government regulation, past and present. **J Occup Med** 1983 Jan;25(1):21–5

Kilburn KH: Chronic disease in the workplace and the environment. Lung disease: lessons from the past--keys to the future. **Arch Environ Health** 1984 May–Jun;39(3):139–43

Valentin M: Geschichte der Arbeitsmedizin. In Sournia JC, Martiny M, Poulet J, ed: Illustrierte Geschichte der Medizin. Salzburg, Andreas, 1980. Vol. 7. p. 2431–57.

Valentin M: Travail des hommes et savants oubliés: histoire de la médecine du travail, de la sécurité: et l'ergonomie. [Paris], DOCIS, 1978. xi, 329 p.

Zabludovskiĭ PE: Izistorii professional'noĭ patologii i gigieny truda. **Gig Tr Prof Zabol** 1983 Dec;(12):40–2

**Germany**

Müller R: Occupational health statistics in Germany and in the Federal Republic of Germany: a patient in need of care. Some contributions to the history of reporting of industrial pathology. **Soc Soc Hist Med Bull (Lond)** 1983 Dec;33:63–6

Stollenwerk M: Die bauliche Entwicklung der Krankenversorgung der Industriestadt Stolberg im Rheinland vor dem Hintergrund der Ursprünge der Messingindustrie. **Hist Hosp** 1979–80;13:164–76

Wilde J: Historische Aspekte zum Schneeberger Lungenkrebs. **Z Arztl Fortbild (Jena)** 1982 Feb;76(3):118–20

**Great Britain**

Batty Shaw A: Knappers' rot; silicosis in East Anglian flint-knappers. **Med Hist** 1981 Apr;25(2):151–68

Hanson RD: Medical services at Chatham Dockyard 1625–1984. **J R Nav Med Serv** 1984 Spring;70(1):38–40

**USSR**

Beĭlikhis GA: Ob issledovaniiakh po gigienie truda v XVII–XVIII vekakh v Rossii. **Gig Tr Prof Zabol** 1980 Aug;(8):40–2

**Before 500 A.D.**

**Greco–Roman**

Nriagu JO: Occupational exposure to lead in ancient times. **Sci Total Environ** 1983 Nov;31(2):105–16

**1450–1700**

Rosner E: Hohenheims Bergsuchtmonographie. **Medizinhist J** 1981;16(1–2):20–52

**Germany**

Kaiser W: Eisleben und das Mansfelder Land im medizinhistorischen Aspekt. Ein Beitrag zum Lutherjahr 1983. **Z Gesamte Inn Med** 1983 Oct 15;38(20):539–46

**Italy**

Bertelli G, Foà V: Ramazzini, cinquanta anni dopo, su 'la medicina del lavoro'. **Med Lav** 1983 Nov–Dec;74(6):423–5

Parmeggiani L: L'opera di Bernadino Ramazzini nel campo della medicina del lavoro. **Med Lav** 1983 Nov–Dec;74(6):426–32

Pericle di Pietro: Le fonti bibliografiche nella 'De morbis artificum diatriba' di Bernardino Ramazzini. **Hist Philos Life Sci** 1981;3(1):95–114

Premuda L: L'istanza sociale in Ramazzini pre-illuminista. **Med Lav** 1983 Nov–Dec;74(6):433–41

Sakula A: Ramazzini's De Morbis Artificum and occupational lung disease. **Br J Dis Chest** 1983 Oct;77(4):349–61

**1700 to Present**

Bartrip PW, Fenn PT: The administration of safety: the enforcement policy of the early factory inspectorate, 1844–64. **Public Adm** 1980;58(1)

Bazhan TA: K. Marks ob okhrane zdorov'ia rabochego klassa. **Gig Sanit** 1984 Feb;(2):37–40

Black D: The spirit of occupational medicine. **Br Med J** 1979 Dec 22–29;2(6205):1622–6

Burke G, Richardson P: The profits of death: a comparative study of miners' phthisis in Cornwall and the Transvaal, 1876–1918. **J South Afr Stud** 1978;4(2):147–71

Cartwright RA: Historical and modern epidemiological studies on populations exposed to N-substituted aryl compounds. **Environ Health Perspect** 1983 Mar;49:13–9

Felton JS: Classical syndromes in occupational medicine: Phosphorus necrosis--a classical occupational disease. **Am J Ind Med** 1982;3(1):77–120

Figlio K: How does illness mediate social relations? Workmen's compensation and medico-legal practices, 1890–1940. In P. Wright, A. Treacher, ed: The problem of medical knowledge. Examining the social construction of medicine. Edinburgh, Edinburgh University Press, 1982. p. 174–224.

Hunt VR: A brief history of women workers and hazards in the workplace. **Feminist Stud** 1979;5(2):274–85

Izmerov NF, Hoiblain HG: K 10-letiiu mezhdunarodnogo sotrudnichestva mezhdu SSSR i GDR po probleme 'Gigiena truda i profzabolevaniia'. **Gig Tr Prof Zabol** 1982 Jan;(1):3–6

Karbe KH: Die Arbeitsmedizin als Gegenstand historischer Quellenforschung. In International Congress of the History of Medicine. 26th, Plovdiv, 1978. Actes du Congress. Sofia, 1981. Volume II. p. 120–2.

Laurig W: Feiert der Begriff 'Ergonomie' 1982 seinen 125. Geburtstag? **Zentralbl Arbeitsmed Arbeitsschutz Prophyl Ergonomie** 1982 Sep;32(9):341–4

Osborn SB: New regulations for old. **Phys Med Biol** 1984 Feb;29(2):153–6

Parson DO: The male labour force participation decision: health, reported health and economic incentives. **Economica** 1982;49(193):81–91

Rona E: Laboratory contamination in the early period of radiation research. **Health Phys** 1979 Dec;37(6):723–7

The rubber industry: Historical overview. In IARC monographs on the evaluation of the carcinogenic risk of chemicals to humans. (Volume 28: The rubber industry). [Geneva], International Agency for Research on Cancer, 1982. p. 31–46.

Witt M, Early S: The worker as safety inspector. **Work Pap New Soc** 1980;7(5):20–9

**Australia**

Willis E: Sister Elizabeth Kenny and the evolution of the occupational division of labour in health care. **Aust NZ J Sociol** 1979;15(3):30–8

**Austria**

Buess H: Der Wiener Sozialmediziner Ludwig Teleky (1872–1957) und seine 'History of factory and mine hygiene'. **Wien Med Wochenschr** 1981 Oct 15;131(19):479–83

Buess H: Der Wiener Sozialmediziner Ludwig Teleky (1872–1957) und seine 'History of Factory and Mine Hygiene'. In Ganzinger K, Skopec M, Wyklicky H, ed: Festschrift für Erna Lesky zum 70. Geburtstag. Wien, Brüder Hollinek, 1981. p. 31–7.

Popper L: Die Entwicklung der Arbeitsmedizin in Osterreich und die sozialhygienische Tradition. **Arbeitsmed praventive Gesundheitspolitik** 1982;5:41–5

**Belgium**

Abelshausen M: De Antwerpse Werkhuizen van Liefdadigheid (1802–1870): weldadigheidsinstelling of fabriek? **Ann Soc Belg Hist Hop** 1982;20:61–108

Hausman A: Historique et activités du C.C.R. **Rev Inst Hyg Mines (Hasselt)** 1983;38(2):138–9

Lemoine P: L'Organe permanent pour la sécurité et la salubrité dans les mines de houille et les autres industries extractives. **Rev Inst Hyg Mines (Hasselt)** 1983;38(2):140–2

**Brazil**

Berrance de Castro J, Scarano JM, Aissar A: A mortalidade entre os filhos de trabalhadores pretos e brancos estrangeiros numa regiõ cafeeira paulista: 1875–1930. **Rev Hist (Brazil)** 1973;46(94):603–17

**Bulgaria**

Kolarov NI: Iz istoriiata na zhelezopŭtnata meditsinska sluzhba v Bŭlgariia, 1888–1944. Sofiia, Meditsina i fizkultura, 1978. 119 p.

**Canada**

Bercuson DJ: Tragedy at Bellevue: anatomy of a mine disaster. **Labour** 1978;3:221–31

Doern GB: Science and technology in the nuclear regulatory process: the case of Canadian uranium miners. **Can Public Adm** 1978;21(1):51–82

Norris J: The country doctor in British Columbia: 1887–1975. **BC Stud** 1981;(49):15–39

Sauvé R: Legislative developments in Québec. **J Occup Med** 1982

Dec;24(12):981-4

**Czechoslovakia**

Rozsívalová E, Fuchsová V: Zájem lékařu o zdravotní stav dělnictva v druhých dvacetipěti ročnících Casopisu lékařu českých. **Cas Lek Cesk** 1981;120(52):1594-8

**France**

Comiti VP: Les maladies et le travail lors de la révolution industrielle française. **Hist Philos Life Sci** 1980;2(2):215-39
Delmas J: Le travail des enfants dans les manufactures de 1841 à 1914. **Bull Soc Fr Hist Hop** 1980;(41):17-25
Gueniot-Le Minor G: La peste des chiffonniers à Paris en 1920. Diss. Paris, 1980. 83 lv.
Martinon JF, Riou R: Conditions de travail et de santé au XIX siècle: les verriers de Rive-de-Gier. **Cah Hist** 1981;26(1):27-39
Perrot M: De la nourrice à l'employée. Travaux de femmes dans la France du XIXe siècle. **Mouvement Soc** 1978 Oct-Dec;3-10
Tilly LA: Structure de l'emploi, travail des femmes et changements démographiques dans deux villes industrielles, Anzin et Roubaix, 1872-1906.. In: Le mouvement social. Paris, Les éditions ouvrières, 1978; 105:33-58.
Valentin M, Niaussat PM: Le rôle fondamental d'Amédée Lefèvre, médecin de la Marine (1798-1869), en médecine du travail et en histoire de la médecine. **Hist Sci Med** 1979;13(4):407-17

**Germany**

Bury C: Workers' health protection as an issue of industrial hygiene and occupational medical science in the early Kaiserreich (1871-84). **Soc Soc Hist Med Bull (Lond)** 1983 Dec;33:34-6
Dittmann S, Paulenz H, Scheel G, et al: 30 Jahre Staatliche Hygieneinspektion der DDR. **Z Gesamte Hyg** 1983 Oct;29(10):584-8
Hoerger H: Mortalität, Krankheit und Lebenserwartung der Penzberger Bergarbeiterschaft im 19. und beginnenden 20. Jahrhundert. **Z Bayer Landesgesch** 1980;43(1):185-222
Hörger H: Mortalität, Krankheit und Lebenserwartung der Penzberger Bergarbeiterschaft im 19. und beginnenden 20. Jahrhundert. **Z Bayer Landesgesch** 1980:43(1);185-222
Karbe KH: Das Betriebsarztsystem und zum Schicksal der Arbeitsmedizin im faschistischen Deutschland. **Z Gesamte Hyg** 1983 Oct;29(10):640-4
Klein P, Labisch A, Milles D, et al: Zur Entwicklung der Arbeitsmedizin in Deutschland bis zum Ende der Weimarer Republik. **Arbeitsmed praventive Gesundheitspolitik** 1982;5:28-40
Kunze J: Ein geschichtlicher Beitrag zum Arbeitsschutz an der Porzellanmanufaktur zu Meissen um 1820. **Z Arztl Fortbild (Jena)** 1982 May 1;76(9):421-3
Labisch A: Recent trends in the social history of occupational medicine in the Federal Republic of Germany. **Soc Soc Hist Med Bull (Lond)** 1983 Dec;33:52-7
Labisch A: Selbsthilfe zwischen Auflehnung und Anpassung. Arbeiter-Sanitätskommission und Arbeiter-Samariterbund. **Jahrb Krit Med** 1983;77:11-26
Labisch A: The Workingmen's Samaritan Federation (Arbeiter-Samariter-Bund) 1888-1933. **J Contemp Hist** 1978;13:297-322
Machtan L: Workers' insurance versus protection of the workers. Remarks on state social policy in the early Kaiserreich. **Soc Soc Hist Med Bull (Lond)** 1983 Dec;33:33
Milles D: From workers' diseases to occupational diseases: the causality of experts' evidence on liability in the development of social medicine. **Soc Soc Hist Med Bull (Lond)** 1983 Dec;33:58-62
Moschke G: Der Einfluss der Arbeiterklasse auf die Berufskrankheitengesetzgebung und Gewerbehygiene in der Weimarer Republik von 1925-1929. **Z Gesamte Hyg** 1981 Apr;27(4):307-9
Moschke G: Die Stellung der KPD zur Berufskrankheitengesetzgebung in der Weimarer Republik. **Z Exp Chir** 1982 Jul;28(7):471-3
Renker U: Zur Entwicklung des Betriebsgesundheitswesens in der DDR. **Wiss Z Martin Luther Univ (Math)** 1976;25(2):95-8
Robert JS: Drink and industrial work discipline in 19th century Germany. **J Soc Hist** 1981;15(1):25-38
Vetter L, Thiess AM: 100 Jahre Frauenarbeit. Teil 1: Historische Entwicklung, Arbeitsschutz-Gesetzgebung. **Fortschr Med** 1983 Feb 10;101(6):206-10

**Great Britain**

Archibald RM: A short historical note on the Conjoint DIH. **J Soc Occup Med** 1984 Aug;34(3):80
Barnes M, Pratt PK: Women sanitary inspectors. **Hist Workshop J** 1978;6:225
Bartley M: Coronary heart disease: a disease of affluence or a disease of industry? **Soc Soc Hist Med Bull (Lond)** 1983 Dec;33:50-1
Bartrip P: Workmen's compensation in British law, society and politics, 1897-1946. **Soc Soc Hist Med Bull (Lond)** 1983 Dec;33:30-2
Beckett JV: An eighteenth-century case history: Carlisle Spedding 1738. **Med Hist** 1982 Jul;26(3):303-6
Bloor DU: The certifying surgeons. **J R Coll Gen Pract** 1981 Jan;31(222):33-7
Brown RH: The development of methods for the determination of hazardous substances in factory atmospheres: an historical perspective. **Ann Occup Hyg** 1984;28(2):183-8
Bryder L: Tuberculosis, silicosis, and the slate industry in North Wales: Medical examinations of the high tuberculosis death rates in the North Wales slate mining and quarrying districts, 1927-1939. **Soc Soc Hist Med Bull (Lond)** 1983;33:43-6
Burke G: Disease, labour migration and technological change: the case of the Cornish miners. **Soc Soc Hist Med Bull (Lond)** 1983 Dec;33:37-9
Carpenter M: Unity in action. **Nurs Times** 1980 Jul 10;76(28):1204-5
Cunningham W: The control of woolsorter's disease. **Pharm Hist (London)** 1975 May;5(1):4-5
Earwicker R: Miners' medical services before the First World War: the South Wales coalfield. **Llafur J Soc Stud Welsh Labour Hist** 1981;3(2):39-52
Figlio K: What is an accident? **Soc Soc Hist Med Bull (Lond)** 1983 Dec;33:27-9
Greenberg M: Classical syndromes in occupational medicine: the Montague Murray case. **Am J Ind Med** 1982;3(3):351-6
Hall AR: Homo fabricator: a new species. **Hist Philos Life Sci** 1980;2(2):193-14
Harrison B: Women's health and the women's movement in Britain: 1840-1940. In C. Webster, ed: Biology, medicine and society 1840-1940. Cambridge, Cambridge University Press, 1981. p. 15-71.
Hodgson GA: The history of coal miners' skin diseases. In J. Cule, ed: Wales and medicine. London, British Society for the History of Medicine, 1975. p. 54-67.
Houston RA: Colliers with colic? **Local Popul Stud (Matlock)** 1979;22:57-9
Livock R: Science, law and safety standards: a case study of industrial disease. **Br J Law Soc** 1979;6(2):172-99
Luxon SG: A history of industrial hygiene. **Am Ind Hyg Assoc J** 1984 Nov;45(11):731-9
Matsufuji G: [Phosphor-poisoning in match factories and the Salvation Army General Booth] (Jpn). **Igakushi Kenkyu** 1980;54:1-6
Morgan JG: The place of nickel in the history of industrial disease. In J. Cule, ed: Wales and medicine. London, British Society for the History of Medicine, 1975. p. 68-74.
Morris J: The Gertrude Tuckwell collection (Trades Union Congress, Gt. Russell St., London, W.C.l.). **Hist Workshop J** 1978;5:155-62
Posner E: Milestones in the history of mineral dust pneumoconioses. In J. Cule, ed: Wales and medicine. London, British Society for the History of Medicine, 1975. p. 42-53.
Schilling R: Bradford Hill's contribution to occupational health. **Stat Med** 1982 Oct-Dec;1(4):317-24
Schilling RS: Donald Hunter--the first editor of the British Journal of Industrial Medicine. **J Cell Biol** 1979 Aug;36(3):243
Scott J: Taming a revolution - the real achievements of early factory reformers. **Occup Health (Lond)** 1983 Oct;35(10):439-44
Sinclair HM: Sherrington and industrial fatigue. **Notes Rec R Soc Lond** 1984 Sep;39(1):91-104
Slaney B: The development of occupational health nursing. **Nursing (Oxford)** 1984 May;2(25):suppl 1-3
Spiers FW: 40 years of development in radiation protection. **Phys Med Biol** 1984 Feb;29(2):145-51
Sternbach G: C.S. Campbell: Gamekeeper's thumb. **J Emerg Med** 1984;1(4):345-7
Taylor PJ, Burridge J: Trends in death, disablement, and sickness absence in the British Post Office since 1981. **Br J Ind Med** 1982 Feb;39(1):1-10
Thom D, Ineson A: TNT poisoning among women workers in the First World War. **Soc Soc Hist Med Bull (Lond)** 1983 Dec;33:40-2
Williams E: The history of brucellosis in Wales. In J. Cule, ed: Wales and medicine. London, British Society for the History of Medicine, 1975. p. 75-85.
150 years of factory inspectorate: **J R Soc Health** 1983 Dec;103(6):244-5

**Guyana**

Boisanger B de, Cudennec Y, Buffe P: Aperçu sur la médecine de soins et la médecine du travail, dans une plantation de Guyane au XVIIIe siècle. **Hist Sci Med** 1984;18(3):215-21

**Hungary**

Bugyi B: Genersich Antal vasutépítés orvosakénti tevékenységéről. **Orv Hetil** 1983 Jul 24;124(30):1825-6

**Iceland**

Eliasson Orn: Farmer's lung disease: a new historical perspective from Iceland. **J Hist Med Allied Sci** 1982 Oct;37(4):440-4

**India**

Simmons CP: Housing, health and educational facilities in the Indian

coalfields during the colonial era. **South Asia** 1978;1(1):52–62
Vilanilam JV: A historical and socioeconomic analysis of occupational safety and health in India. **Int J Health Serv** 1980;10(2):233–49

**Italy**

Assennato G, Navarro V: Workers' participation and control in Italy: the case of occupational medicine. **Int J Health Serv** 1980;10(2):217–32
Bagnara S, Biocca M, Mazzonis DG: Consiglio Nazionale delle Ricerche, Rome, Italy. **Int J Health Serv** 1981,11(3).431–50
Caffaratto TM: Aspetti medico-sociali delle malattie dei lavoratori piemontesi della terra, nella seconda metà del secolo XIX. **Minerva Med** 1984 Apr;75(14–15):842–51; (17):999–1012; (18):1079–88
Campiglio L: La dinamica degli infortuni sul lavoro nel periodo 1951–1970. **Riv Int Sci Sociali** 1973;81(1–2):134–65
Casula D: I cinquanti'anni della Società Italiana di Medicina del Lavoro e Igiene Industriale. **Med Lav** 1980 Mar–Apr;71(2):115–8
Dodi Osnaghi L: Aspetti della condizione operaia e della nocività attarverso le riviste di medicina del lavoro. **Ann Ist Giangiacomo Feltrinelli** 1979–80;20:231–83
Malamani A: Medicina ottocentesca e medicina del lavoro: l'opera scientifico-sociale di Luigi Devoto a Pavia. **G Ital Med Lav** 1983 Jan;5(1):1–16
Reich MR, Goldman RH: Italian occupational health: concepts, conflicts, implications. **Am J Public Health** 1984 Sep;74(9):1031–41
Willson PR: Industrial health and rationalisation in an Italian light engineering firm: the Magneti Marelli in the Fascist period. **Soc Soc Hist Med Bull (Lond)** 1983 Dec;33:47–9

**Japan**

Matsufuji H: [Chukichi Kubokawa and industrial Hygiene] (Jpn). **Igakushi Kenkyu** 1978;49:14–7

**Norway**

Kierulf H: Farsottenes rolle i dikteren Johan Falkbergets trilogi 'Christianus Sextus' (1720 årene). **Nord Medicinhist Arsb** 1980;Suppl 6:82–9

**Poland**

Bojanowski T: Zdrowotne warunki pracy polaków zatrudnionych w przemyśle łódzkim podczas okupacji hitlerowskiej. **Przegl Lek** 1981;38(12):869–72
Brożek K: Dr med. Karol Zahorski (1879--1970) lekarz-społecznik w Zagłębiu Dąbrowskim (w 100-lecie urodzin). **Pol Tyg Lek** 1979 Jun 25;34(26):1057–9
Brożek K: Społeczne tradycje medycyny w regionie śląsko-dąbrowskim (1901–1950). **Kult Spoleczenstwo** 1979;23(3):67–78
Brzeziński T: Problemy robotnicze w pismach lekarzy Polskich przełomu XIX i XX wieku. **Arch Hist Med (Warsz)** 1984;47(1):75–83
Grzegorczyk L: Uwagi na temat sytuacji epidemiologicznej w zakresie chorób zawodowych skóry w Polsce w latach 1971–1977. **Przegl Dermatol** 1980 Jul–Aug;67(4):455–7
Kieć E, et al: Prof. Dr. Leon Cholewa. **Przegl Lek** 1984;41(7):465–76
Kieć-Swierczyńska M: Uczuleniowy zawodowy wyprysk skóry rozpoznany w Instytucie Medycyny Pracy w Lodzi w latach 1972–1978. **Przegl Dermatol** 1980 Jul–Aug;67(4):449–53
Kowieski L: Działalność Wydziału Higieny Zawodowej i Przemysłu Oddziału Lubelskiego Warszawskiego Towarzystwa Higienicznego w latach 1903–1905. **Arch Hist Med (Warsz)** 1984;47(3):429–31
Krynicki A: Occurrence of occupational diseases among Polish seamen and fishermen in the years 1969–1977. **Bull Inst Marit Trop Med Gdynia** 1979;30(3–4):245–51
Majdecki T: Powstanie i rozwój w okresie miedzywojennym neurologicznego lecznictwa kolejowej służby zdrowia. **Neurol Neurochir Pol** 1984 Jan–Feb;18(1):87–91
Sadowska J: Działalność Inspekcji Pracy w zakresie bezpieczeństwa i higieny w przemyśle łódzkim II Rzeczypospolitej. **Arch Hist Med (Warsz)** 1981;47(3):439–42
Sadowska J: Postulaty zdrowotne klasy robotniczej w rewolucji 1905–1907 roku. **Arch Hist Med (Warsz)** 1980;43(4):377–81
Szymczykiewicz K: XXX lat działalności Instytutu Medycyny Pracy w Sosnowcu. **Med Pr** 1981;32(5):309–15

**Romania**

Crisan E: Aspekte der ärztlichen Betreuung der Eisenbahnarbeiter im XIX. Jahrhundert (Rom) **Acta Mus Napocensis (Cluj)** 1978;15:461–5
Marinescu CG: Concepțiile progresiste ale Doctorului N. Vasiliu. **Rev Med Chir Soc Med Nat Iasi** 1980 Jul–Sep;84(3)578–80

**South Africa**

Brain JB, Brain P: The health of indentured Indian migrants to Natal, 1860–1911. **S Afr Med J** 1982 Nov 6;62(20):739–42
Harington JS, McGlashan ND: Migrant workers and cancer patterns in South Africa. **J South Afr Stud** 1976;3(1):92–101
Mellish FM: The birth, growth and development and future dimensions of occupational health nursing. **Curationis** 1980 Sep;3(2):48–53

**Spain**

Simón Palmer M del C: Las neurosis femeninas y la educación española. **Asclepio** 1983;35:327–42

**Sweden**

Sundin J, Tedebrand LG: Dödlighet och sjuklighet i svenskjärnbruksmiljo, 1750–1875. **Scandia** 1981;47(1):67–108

**Switzerland**

Amstutz P: Für Gesundheitsschutz am Arbeitsplatz: Die Fachkommission der Schweizerischen Gesellschaft für Arbeitsmedizin, Arbeitshygiene und Arbeitssicherheit. **Soz Praventivmed** 1981 Jul;26(3):120–5
Godonnèche J: La dégradation de la santé des gens de lettres d'après Tissot. In: Congrès National des Sociétés Savantes, 99e, Besançon, 1974. Comptes Rendus. Paris, 1976. Section des Sciences, Fasc. V. p. 235–41.
Hansch-Mock B: Arbeitshygiene in schweizerischen Kalendern des 19. Jahrhunderts. **Gesnerus** 1981;38:165–74
Lang K: Kritiker, Ketzer, Kämpfer: das Leben des Arbeiterarztes Fritz Brupbacher. Zürich, Limmat, 1983. 360 p.
Lob M: Aspects de la médecine du travail. **Soz Praventivmed** 1981 Jul;26(3):114–7
Peduzzi R, Piffaretti JC: Ancylostoma duodenale and the Saint Gothard anaemia. **Br Med J [Clin Res]** 1983 Dec 24–31;287(6409):1942–5

**United States**

Aldrich M: Determinants of mortality among New England cotton mill workers during the Progressive era. **J Econ Hist** 1982;42(4):847–63
Aldrich M: Mortality from byssinosis among New England cotton mill workers. 1905–1912. **J Occup Med** 1982 Dec;24(12):977–80
Baetjer AM: The early days of industrial hygiene--their contribution to current problems. **Am Ind Hyg Assoc J** 1980 Nov;41(11):773–7
Baetjer AM: The early days of industrial hygiene – their contribution to current problems. **Am Ind Hyg Assoc J** 1980;41:773–7
Banks A, ed: Monumental stone. Barre, Vermont, 1939 and 1940. In her: First-person America. New York, Knopf, 1980. p. 93–119.
Barclay WR: Landmark perspective: Asbestos. An industrial asset with a health cost. **JAMA** 1984 Jul 6;252(1):96
Bayer RA: Q fever as an occupational illness at the National Institutes of Health. **Public Health Rep** 1982 Jan–Feb;97(1):58–60
Bell C: Implementing safety and health regulations for women in the workplace. **Feminist Stud** 1979;5(2):286–301
Berger LR, Johansson SR: Child health in the workplace: the Supreme Court in Hammer v. Dagenhart (1918). **J Health Polit Policy Law** 1980 Spring;5(1):81–97
Berkowitz M: Occupational safety and health. **Ann Am Acad Polit Soc Sci** 1979;443:41–53
Berman DM: Death on the job. Occupational health and safety struggles in the United States. New York, Monthly Review Press, 1978. xii, 260 p.
Berman DM: Worker's compensation: preventive care for industry. **Health PAC Bull** 1976 Jul–Aug;(71):9–14
Berney B: The rise and fall of the UMW Fund. **South Exposure** 6(2):95–102, 1978
Bing RK: Nationally speaking--living forward, understanding backwards, Part I. **Am J Occup Ther** 1984 Jun;38(6):363–6
C[one] TE: The appalling industrial hazards to which American working children were exposed in 1900. **Pediatrics** 1981;68:378
Cambrosio A: Quand la psychologie fait son entrée à l'usine: sélection et contrôle des ouvriers aux Etats-Unis pendant les années 1910. **Mouvement Soc** 1980;113:37–65
Chavkin W: Occupational hazards to reproduction: a review essay and annotated bibliography. **Feminist Stud** 1979;5(2):310–25
Chelius JR: Economic and demographic aspects of the occupational injury problem. **Q Rev Econ Bus** 1979;19(2):65–70
Cloutier RJ: Florence Kelley and the radium dial painters. **Health Phys** 1980 Nov;39(5):711–6
Corn JK: 'Dark as a dungeon': environment and coal miners' health and safety in nineteenth century America. **Environ Rev** 1983;7(3):257–68
Curran DJ: Symbolic solutions for deadly dilemmas: an analysis of federal coal mine health and safety legislation. **Int J Health Serv** 1984;14(1):5–29
Donnelly PG: The origins of the Occupational Safety and Health Act of 1970. **Soc Probl** 1982 Oct;30:13–25
Eisenbud M: Origins of the standards for control of beryllium disease (1947–1949). **Environ Res** 1982 Feb;27(1):79–88
Felker M: The political economy of sexism in industrial health. **Soc Sci Med** 1982;16(1):3–13
Felton JS: Industrial medicine to occupational health and safety: a 50-year retrospective. **Occup Health Saf** 1982 Sep;51(9):14–22
Fennel ML, Rodin MB, Kantor GK: Problems in the work setting,

drinking, and reasons for drinking. **Soc Forces** 1981;60(1):114–32
Fox DM, Stone JF: Black lung: miners' militancy and medical uncertainty, 1968–1972. **Bull Hist Med** 1980 Spring;54(1):43–63
Freudenberg N: Alice Hamilton 1869–1970. **Women Health** 1976 Sep–Oct;1(5):1–2
Garbelotto N: Teoria e politica nella psicosociologia di E. Mayo. **Stor Crit Psicol** 1980;1(1):61–78
Gersuny C: New England mill casualties: 1890–1910. **N Engl Q** 1979;52(4):467–82
Graebner W: Doing the world's unhealthy work: the fiction of free choice. **Hastings Cent Rep** 1984 Aug;14(4):28–37
Hilaski HJ, Wang CL: How valid are estimates of occupational illness? **Mon Labor Rev** 1982;105(8):27–35
Hornblower H: Henry Furbush Howe. **Mass Hist Soc Proc** 1977,89:184–6
Judkins BM: Occupational health and the developing class consciousness of southern textile workers: the case of the Brown Lung Association. **Md Hist** 1982 Spring–Summer;13:55–71
Kalisch PA: Ordeal of the Oklahoma coal miners: coal mine disasters in the Sooner state, 1886–1945. **Chron Okla** 1979;48(3):331–40
Keiser KR: The new regulation of health and safety. **Polit Sci Q** 1980;95(3):479–91
Kerr LE: The health of workers. **J Public Health Policy** 1981 Mar;2(1):3–7
Kotarba JA: Chronic pain center: A study of voluntary client compliance and entrepreneurship. **Am Behav Sci** 1981;24(6):786–800
Lauer DJ: T. Lyle Hazlett: his role in industrial medicine, 1920–50. **JOM** 1979 Jun;21(6):403–6
Leigh JP: Education, working conditions, and worker's health. **Soc Sci J** 1983;20(2):99–107
Licorish KA: Hypersensitivity pneumonitis--economic and legal aspects. **Clin Rev Allergy** 1983 Dec;1(4):487–96
Lindop PJ, Rotblat J: Radiation pollution of the environment. **Bull At Sci** 1971;27(7):17–24
Liveright T, Stanbury M: An historical prospective study of mortality within a cohort of gas distribution workers. **Am J Ind Med** 1983;4(5):651–7
MacLaury J: The job safety law of 1970: its passage was perilous. **Mon Labor Rev** 1981;104(3):18–24
Markolf AS: Industrial nursing begins in Vermont. **Vt Regist Nurse** 1980 Jun;:15–7
Marshall JR, Dowdall GW: Employment and mental hospitalization: the case of Buffalo, New York, 1914–55. **Soc Forces** 1982;60(3):843–53
Nugent A: Fit for work: the introduction of physical examinations in industry. **Bull Hist Med** 1983 Winter;57(4):578–95
Pappagianis D: Dangerous dust. **Nat Hist** 1983;92(3):36–40
Pettus BE: Osha inspection costs, compliance costs, and other outcomes: the first decade. **Policy Stud Rev** 1982;1(3):596–614
Pochin EE: Sieverts and safety. **Health Phys** 1984 Jun;46(6):1173–9
Rosen G: Urbanization, occupation and disease in the United States 1870–1920. The case of New York City. In Forbes EG, ed: Human implications of scientific advance. Edinburg, Edinburgh University Press, 1978. p. 224–50.
Schleppi JR: 'It pays': John H. Patterson and industrial recreation at the National Cash Register Company. **J Sport Hist** 1979;6(3):20–8
Sicherman B: Alice Hamilton. In: Notable American women. The modern period. Cambridge, Mass., Belknap–Harvard Univ. Press, 1980. 4:303–6.
Smith BE: Black lung: the social production of disease. **Int J Health Serv** 1981;11(3):343–59
Smith HC: Douglas Henry Fryer. In Dictionary of American Biography, Suppl. 6, 1956–1960. p. 222, 1980.
Stacey M: Comment on the paper 'The Political Economy of Sexism in Industrial Health' by Marcia Felker. **Soc Sci Med** 1982;16(1):15–8
Sweeney RE, Castleman B: Asbestos disease and compensation. **Ann NY Acad Sci** 1979;330:273–80
Taylor W, Wasserman D, Behrens V, et al: Effect of the air hammer on the hands of stonecutters. The limestone quarries of Bedford, Indiana, revisited. **Br J Ind Med** 1984 Aug;41(3):289–95
Uselding P: In dispraise of the muckrakers: United States occupational mortality, 1890–1910. **Res Econ Hist** 1976;1:334–71
Ward RD, Rogers WW: Racial inferiority, convict labor, and modern medicine: a note on the Coalburg affair. **Ala Hist Q** 1982;44(3–4):203–10
Wasserman H, Solomon N, Alvarez R, et al: Killing our own: the disaster of America's experience with atomic radiation. New York, Dell, 1982. xiii, 368 p.
Wolkinson BW, Barton D: Arbitration and the rights of mentally handicapped workers. **Mon Labor Rev** 1980;103(4):41–7
Yandle B: A social regulation controversy: the cotton dust standard. **Soc Sci Q** 1982;63(1):58–69

**USSR**

Bazhan TA: Rol' pervykh Sovetov rabochikh deputatov v bor'be za okhranu zdorov'ia trudiashchikhsia na Ukraine v gody pervoĭ russkoĭ revoliutsii (1905–1907). **Gig Sanit** 1983 Nov;:(11):8–12
Bazhan TA: Voprosy okhrany truda i zdorov'ia rabochikh v deiatel'nosti mestnykh komitetov RSDRP iuga Rossi (1898–1917). **Gig Sanit** 1979 Dec;(12):32–6
Bazhan TA: Voprosy okhrany zdorov'ia rabochikh v listovkakh sotsial–demikraticheskikh organizatsiĭ Ukrainy (1896–1904). **Sov Zdravookhr** 1984;(2):53–6
Bogovski P: Historical perspectives of occupational cancer. **J Toxicol Environ Health** 1980 Sep–Nov;6(5–6):921–39
Borisenkova RV, Egorov IuL, Pal'tsev IuP: Vklad Moskovskogo instituta gigieny im. F. F. Erismana v gigienu truda (k 60–letiiu so dnia osnovaniia instituta). **Gig Tr Prof Zabol** 1981 Jul;(7):39–43
Dogle NV: Issledovaniia F. F. Erismana v Moskovskoĭ gubernii i sovremennost'. **Gig Tr Prof Zabol** 1983 Jul;(7):38–41
Ibragimov NG: K istorii okhrany zdorov'ia neftianikov Bashkirii v 30–40–e gody. **Sov Zdravookhr** 1984;(4):65–8
Idel'chik KhI: K istorii izucheniia zdorov'ia rabochikh, zaniatykh v neftianoĭ promyshlennosti Azerbaĭdzhanskoĭ SSR v 20--30–e gody. **Sov Zdravookhr** 1982;(7):55–9
Idel'chik KhI: Nauchno–issledovatel'skie instituty gigieny truda i professional'nykh zabolevaniĭ v SSSR v 20--30–kh godakh (k 60–letiiu organizatsii pervogo instituta). **Gig Tr Prof Zabol** 1984 Sep;(9):30–2
Il'in AI: Iz istorii sanitarno–statisticheskogo issledovaniia Vladimirskoĭ gubernii. **Gig Sanit** 1984 May;(5):35–7
Izmerov NF, Bogolepova LS: Sokhranit' i priumnozhit' nasledie gigieny truda. **Gig Tr Prof Zabol** 1980 Apr;(4):41–2
Izmerov NF: 60 let Nauchno–issledovatel'skomu institutu gigieny truda i professional'nykh zabolevaniĭ AMN SSSR. **Gig Tr Prof Zabol** 1983 Jun;(6):1–5
Kazantsev BN: Okhrana truda v promyshlennosti v 1946–1965 gg. **Istor SSSR** 1971;4:121–32
Klapchuk VV: Razvitie lechebnoĭ fizkul'tury na kurortakh Kryma (k 60–letiiu dekreta 'Ob ispol'zovanii Kryma dlia lechniia trudiahchikhsia'). **Vopr Kurortol Fizioter Lech Fiz Kult** 1981 Mar–Apr;(2):65–7
Letavet AA: K 35–letiiu Velikoĭ Pobedy. **Gig Tr Prof Zabol** 1980 May;(5):1–3
Lotova EI, Idel'chik KhI, Vengrova IV: Mesto i rol' sotsial'no–gigienicheskikh issledovaniĭ v izuchenii zdorov'ia rabochikh v SSSR v 20–30–e gody. **Sov Zdravookhr** 1981;(12):51–4
Mikhaĭlov GN: Voprosy okhrany truda v rabotakh A. N. Sysina. **Gig Tr Prof Zabol** 1982 Oct;(10):41–3
Moikin IuV, Tarasenko NIu, Anan'ev BV: Znachenie naslediia I. M. Sechenova dlia razvitiia otechestvennoĭ fiziologii i gigieny truda. **Gig Tr Prof Zabol** 1980 Mar;(3):1–5
Narimanov ZM: Dostizheniia gigieny truda i profpatologii v Sovetskoĭ Armenii. **Gig Tr Prof Zabol** 1982;(11):1–4
Osipov EO: Kommunisticheskaia Partiia na strazhe zdorov'ia trudiashchikhsia (k 80–letiiu II s'ezda RSDRP). **Sov Med** 1983;8:8–12
Pavlov AS: Epidemiia travmatizma na fabrikakh i zavodakh Peterburga perioda kapitalizma. **Ortop Travmatol Protez** 1979 Jul;(7):64–5
Pavlov AS: Fabrichno–zavodskaia meditsina v Peterburge. **Feldsher Akush** 1981;46(2):41–3
Petrov BD: O sozdanii polnoĭ istorii gigieny truda v Rossii i SSR. **Gig Tr Prof Zabol** 1980 Jun;(6):1–5
Prokhorov AA: Dostizheniia gigieny na zheleznodorozhnom transporte. **Gig Sanit** 1982 Dec;(12):49–52
Retnev VM: 60 let kafedre gigieny truda i professional'nykh bolezneĭ. **Gig Tr Prof Zabol** 1984 May;(5):34–7
Rezanov II: Raboty sanitarnykh vracheĭ v trudakh V. I. Lenina. **Gig Tr Prof Zabol** 1983 Feb;(2):41–3
Roshchin AV, Kozik IV, Arkhangel'skaia LN, et al: Piatidesiatiletie kafedry promyshlennoĭ gigeny Tsentral'nogo ordena Lenina instituta usovershenstvovaniia vracheĭ. **Gig Tr Prof Zabol** 1981 Aug;(8):37–41
Shafranov BV: Iz istorii gigieny promyshlennogo osveshcheniia v SSSR. **Gig Tr Prof Zabol** 1980 Jul;(7):46–7
Shakhgel'diants AE: Okhrana zdorov'ia promyshlennykh rabochikh v SSSR. **Sov Zdravookhr** 1980;(3):8–13
Sheliuzhenko A: Ekonomicheskie posledstviia poteri rabochego vremeni v sviazi s netrudosposobnost'iu po bolezni. **Ekon Sov Ukr** 1972;14(3):63–6
Shitskova AP: Moskovskomu ordena Trudovogo Krasnogo Znameni nauchno–issledova–tel'smkou institutu gigieny im. F. F. Erismana--60 let. **Gig Sanit** 1981 Jun;(6):27–31
Shtrom RS: Meditsinskoe obsluzhivanie shakhterov i metallurgov Donbassa v gody pervoĭ piatiletki (k 50–letiiu pervoĭ piatiletki). **Sov Zdravookhr** 1980;(3):57–9
Sivolob NI: Vklad I.V. Beliaeva v organizatsiiu sanitarnogo dela v Donbasse. **Sov Zdravookhr** 1984;(5):65–7
Stegunin SI, Palagin DA, Veselova AM: Bor'ba Samarskikh bol'shevikov za okhranu zdorov'ia trudiashchikhsia v 1921–1922 gg. **Sov Zdravookhr** 1984;(5):61–4
Tarasenko NIu: Gigiena truda i okhrana zdorov'ia trudiashchikhsia v rabotakh V. I. Lenina. **Gig Tr Prof Zabol** 1982 Apr;(4):1–3
Tarasenko NIu, Moĭkin IuV, Anan'ev BV: Razvitie ideĭ I. M. Sechenova v sovremennykh issledovaniiakh po gigiene i fiziologii truda. **Vestn Akad Med Nauk SSSR** 1981;(1):3–9
Tarasenko NIu: Rol' sanitarno–gigienicheskogo fakul'teta v podgotovke vracheĭ profilakticheskoĭ meditsiny i v razvitii gigieny truda (k 50–letiiu obrazovaniia sanitarno–gigienicheskogo fakul'teta I Moskovskogo meditsinskogo instituta im I. M. Sechenova). **Gig Tr Prof Zabol** 1980 Oct;(10):29–32
Vankhanen VD, Grin' NV, Lastkov OA, et al: Aktual'nye problemy gigieny Donbassa (k 50–letiiu so dnia osnovaniia Donetskogo

meditsinskogo instituta im. M. Gor'kogo). **Gig Sanit** 1981 Aug;(8):51–3

Vasil'ev KK: K istorii zhurnala 'Gigiena i sanitariia'. **Gig Sanit** 1982 Sep;(9):51–2

Vengrova IV: Izuchenie zdorov'ia rabochikh Sibiri. **Sov Zdravookhr** 1982;(11):51–5

Vengrova IV: O deiatel'nosti pervykh Otechestvennykh fabrichnykh inspektorov (k 100–letiiu sozdaniia fabrichnoĭ inspektsii v Rossii). **Sov Zdravookhr** 1983;(3):61–5

Zorina LA, Rashevskaia AM: Postdiplomnoe obuchenie vracheĭ na kafedre profpatologii (k 50–letiiu iubileiu Tsentral'nogo instituta usovershenstvovaniia vracheĭ). **Gig Tr Prof Zabol** 1980 Oct;(10):32–4

**Yugoslavia**

Sarić M: Institute for Medical Research and Occupational Health in Yugoslavia. Introduction. **Arh Hig Rada Toksikol** 1979;30 Suppl:5–9

# OPHTHALMOLOGY

Anis AY: Principles and evolution of intraocular lens implantation. **Int Ophthalmol Clin** 1982 Summer;22(2):1–13

Belloni L: Leeuwenhoek's Sehversuch am zusammengesetzten Auge und die entsprechende Beobachtung Boll's an der Stäbchenschicht der Netzhaut. **Janus** 1980;67(1–2–3):59–61

Blodi FC: Ophthalmology and philately: I. Ophthalmologists on stamps--Ricardo Vertiz. **Arch Ophthalmol** 1979 Sep;97(9):1706 (continued periodically)

Dollfus MA: Geschichte der Augenheilkunde. In Sournia JC, Martiny M, Poulet J, ed: Illustrierte Geschichte der Medizin. Salzburg, Andreas, 1980. Vol. 4. p. 1211–49.

Dyer NA: The artificial eye. **Aust J Ophthalmol** 1980 Nov;8(4):325–7

Eastwood BS: Cosmology and physiology in Galenic visual theory: Hunayn Ibn Ishaq. **Trans Stud Coll Physicians Phila** 1980 Dec;5(2 no 4):276–83

Firoiu I: Istoria ochelarilor. **Rev Chir [Oftalmol]** 1983 Jul–Sep;27(3):231–4

Galand A: Historique de la chirurgie transsclérale. **J Fr Ophtalmol** 1980 Dec;3(12):763–4

Griffin JR: Historical summary of visual fields methods. **J Am Optom Assoc** 1980 Sep;51(9):833–5

Heitz R: Leonardo da Vinci did not invent contact lenses. **CLAO J** 1983 Oct–Dec;9(4):313–6

Hirschberg J: The history of ophthalmology. Translated from the German edition of 1899–1918 by F. C. Blodi. 11 vols. Bonn, Wayenborgh, 1982.

Hughes WL, Castroviejo R, Blaydes JE, et al: The evolution of ophthalmic sutures. **Ann Plast Surg** 1981 Jan;6(1):48–65

Lindberg DC: Theories of vision from Al-Kindi to Kepler. Chicago, London, University of Chicago Press, 1976. xii, 324 p.

Lindberg DC, ed: Opticae thesaurus. Alhazeni Arabis libri septem, nuncprimùm editi. Eiusdem liber De Crepusculis et nubium ascensionibus. Item Vitellonis Thuringopoloni libri X. Reprint of the 1572 ed. New York, Johnson Reprint Corp., 1972. xxxiv, 288, 474 p.

Margolin JC: L'histoire des lunettes à nez. **Histoire** 1980;21:14–21

Martin O, Clodius L: The history of the artificial eye. **Ann Plast Surg** 1979 Aug;3(2):168–71

Milos G, Akert K: Die neurobiologischen Grundlagen der binoculären Raumwahrnehmung. Historische Übersicht über die Entwicklung der Vorstellungen und Erkenntnisse. **Schweiz Arch Neurol Neurochir Psychiatr** 1982;130(1):39–67

Montandon D: History of plastic surgery of the orbital region. In S. J. Aston, et al., ed: Third international symposium of plastic and reconstructive surgery of the eye and adnexa. Baltimore, London, Williams & Wilkins, 1982. p. 2–10.

Muggeridge JF: Progress of optical discovery. **J R Soc Health** 1983 Aug;103(4):150–1

Muggeridge JF: The discovery of spectacles. **R Soc Health J** 1982 Aug;102(4):174

Musiał G: Historia operacji zaćmy. 1. Od czasów starożytnych do X wieku. **Klin Oczna** 1983 Aug–Sep;85(8–9):325–7

Musiał G: Historia operacji zaćmy. 2. Od średniowiecza do XVIII wieku. **Klin Oczna** 1983 Oct;85(10):371–3

Orłowski WJ: Słowo wprowadzające do XI sympozjonu retinologicznego. **Klin Oczna** 1982 Sep;84(9):241–3

Orłowski WJ: Z teki szperacza–bibliografa. **Klin Oczna** 1984 Feb;86(2):90 contd

Pascarella F: Il colore degli occhi: 'teorie' del passato e 'conoscenze' attuali. **Med Secoli** 1979 Jan–Apr;16(1):105–12

Poulet W: Atlas on the history of spectacles. Bonn-Bad Godesberg, Wayenborgh, 1978. xxxv, 396 p. Includes contributions by H. W. Holtmann, H. W. Roth Ulm, W. Pfeiffer.

Poulet W: Atlas on the history of spectacles. Volume Two. The arts and spectacles over five centuries. Bonn-Bad Godesberg, Wayenborgh, 1980. 505 p.

Pritikin RI: History of the development of physical modalities in ophthalmology. In: Congrès international d'histoire de la médecine, XXVe, Québec, 1976. Actes. Québec, 1977. p. 1095–111.

Remy C, Aracil P: Histoire de la chirurgie du strabisme. **J Fr Ophtalmol** 1984;7(6–7):493–8

Rogers BO: History of cosmetic blepharoplasty. In S. J. Aston, et al., ed: Third international symposium of plastic and reconstructive surgery of the eye and adnexa. Baltimore, London, Williams & Wilkins, 1982. p. 276–81.

Schadewaldt H: Kunst und Ophthalmologie. **Ber Zusammenkunft Dtsch Ophthalmol Ges** 1979;76:9–16

Smith AM: Getting the big picture in perspectivist optics. **Isis** 1981 Dec;72(264):568–89

Smith CU: Don Juan and the vision of Vision. **Perception** 1981;10(4):435–53

Trevor–Roper P: The Noysome cataract. **Trans Ophthalmol Soc UK** 1980 Jul:100 (pt 2):299–308

Vipmanis VE, Magil'nitskiĭ SG: Pamiatnye oftal'mologicheskie daty na 1984 g. **Vestn Oftalmol** 1984 Jan–Feb;(1):65–6

**China**

Chen YZ: Ramble in Chinese ophthalmology, past and present. **Chin Med J [Engl]** 1981 Jan;94(1):1–4

Huard P: Un traité chinois d'oculistique. **Rev Hist Sci (Paris)** 1984 Jan;37(1):71–4

**Egypt**

Mawas LJ, Mawas E, Weiss JB: Intérêt en strabologie de la plaquette modifiée de Al Hazen. **Bull Soc Belge Ophtalmol** 1981;196:53–65

**France**

Amalric P: Dominique Anel et les Quinze Vingts de Paris. **Bull Soc Ophtalmol Fr** 1982 Jan;82(1):87–90

Bailliart JP, Royer J, Faure MH, ed: L'ophtalmologie des origines à nos jours. Tome 2. Annoynay, France, Laboratoires H. Faure, 1979. 191 p. Selections by various authors.

**Germany**

Jaeger W: Wege der Forschung auf dem Gebiet der optischen Wahrnehmung. Ein wissenschaftshistorischer Rückblick. **MMW** 1982 Sep 10;124(36):785–8

Jopp R: Einzelheiten zur Geschichte der Augenheilkunde von der Antike bis um 1800 am Beispiel von Köln. Köln, Universität zu Köln, 1980. 225 p. (Kölner medizinhistorische Beiträge, 16), (also Diss.).

Marré E: Zur Geschichte der Augenheilkunde in Dresden. **Wiss Beitr Martin Luther Univ Halle Wittenberg** 1982;52(R77):1–4

Putscher M, ed: Rheinische Splitter und Augenblicke. Köln, Institut für Geschichte der Medizin der Universität zu Köln, 1976. 75 p.

**Great Britain**

Winstanley J: St Thomas Hospital a cradle of British ophthalmology. **Trans Ophthalmol Soc UK** 1982;102 (Pt 4):454–60

**Japan**

Ogawa K: Kohon Nippon gankagaku shi. Kyotol, Shibunkaku, [Showa 46 nen, 1971]. 218 p.

**Sweden**

Bahr G von: Den fysiologiska optikens utveckling i Sverige. **Nord Medicinhist Arsb** 1982;:66–75

**Before 500 A.D.**

Suzuki Y: [Origin of cataract surgery (author's transl)] (Jpn). **Nippon Ganka Gakkai Zasshi** 1980;84(3):183–90

Theisen WR: 'Liber de visu': the Greco–Latin translation of Euclid's 'Optics'. **Mediaev Stud** 1979;41:44–105

**Egypt**

Helbling M: Der altägyptische Augenkranke, sein Arzt und seine Götter. Zürich, Juris, 1980. 78 p. (Zürcher medizingeschichtliche Abhandlungen, Neue Reihe, Nr. 141) Also Diss., Zürich.

Marganne MH: Deux questionnaires d'ophtalmologie: P. Aberdeen 11 et P. Ross. Georg. 1.20. **Chron Egypte** 1978;53:313–20

Youtie LC: [Eye-salves.] **Bull Am Soc Papyrologists** 1979;16:149–51

**Greco–Roman**

Marganne MH: Glaucome ou cataracte? sur l'emploi des dérivés de GLAUKOS en ophtalmologie antique. **Hist Philos Life Sci** 1979;1(2):199–214

# OPHTHALMOLOGY

### Greece

Mansfeld J: Alcmaeon: 'Physikos' or physician? With some remarks on Calcidius' 'On vision' compared to Galen's Plac. Hipp. Plat. VII. In J. Mansfeld, L. M. de Rijk, eds. Kephalaion: Studies in Greek philosophy and its continuation. Assen, Van Gorcum, 1975. p. 26–38.

### 500 A.D.–1450

Akdogan C: Optics in Albert the Great's De sensu et sensato; an edition, English translation, and analysis. Ph.D. Diss., University of Wisconsin. Madison, 1978. iv, 267 leaves.

### Arabic

Eastwood BS: The elements of vision: the micro-cosmology of Galenic visual theory according to Hunayn Ibn Ishaq. Philadelphia, American Philosophical Society, 1982. 59 p. (Transactions of the American Philosophical Society, Vol. 72, pt. 5).

Ismail M, Raheem Rafeeq MA: Anatomy of eye and the mechanism of vision according to Avicenna. **Bull Indian Inst Hist Med (Hyderabad)** 1981;1-4:146-51

Mendrina GI: Von einer wenig bekannten Ubersetzung aus der 'Augenheilkunde' von Ali Abbas aus dem Latein ins Deutsche, die der russische Arzt gemacht hat. In International Congress of the History of Medicine, 27th, Barcelona, 1980. Actas. Barcelona, Académia de Ciències Médiques de Catalunya i Balears, 1981. p. 316–20.

Omar S: Ibn Al-Haytham's theory of knowledge and its significance for later science. **Arab Stud Q** 1979;1(1):67–82

### China

Thomas L: Un manuel d'oculistique chinoise attribué a Sun Si-Miao des tang: le Yin hai jing wei. In Mazars G, ed: Les médecines traditionnelles de l'Asie. Strasbourg, Université Louis Pasteur, 1981. p. 85–92.

### Great Britain

Rhodes M: A pair of late medieval spectacles from the Trig Lane site. **Lond Archaeol** 1980;4:23–5

### Poland

Szpilczyński S: A látás kérdése Witelon (Vitellio) Peri optices (1275) c. munkájában. **Orvostort Kozl** 1979;87–88(25 no 1–2)219–22

Szpilczynski S: La théorie de la vision chez Witelo 'Peri optikes', 1273. In: Congrès international d'histoire de la médecine, XXVe, Québec, 1976. Actes. Québec, 1977. p. 1347–53.

### 1450–1700

Jaeger W: Die Ordnungsprinzipien der Farbsysteme des 17. Jahrhunderts. (Franciscus Aguilonius--Athanasius Kircher--Isaac Newton). **Klin Monatsbl Augenheilkd** 1984 Apr;184(4):321–5

Jaeger W: Sinnesphysiologische Forschungen der Jesuitengelehrten des 17. Jahrhunderts. **Klin Monatsbl Augenheilkd** 1981 Oct;179(4):288–96

Massironi M: Considerazioni psicologiche su alcuni fenomeni della visione descritti nei trattati di prospettiva dei secoli XV–XVII. **Stor Crit Psicol** 1983 Dec;4(2):171–214

### France

Amalric P: La naissance de la neuro-ophtalmologie à Montpellier au XVIIme siècle à travers l'oeuvre de Raymond Vieussens et de Guilhem Briggs. **Bull Soc Ophtalmol Fr** 1983 Jan;83(1):83–8

### Germany

Albert DM: 400th anniversary of Batisch's Der Augendienst. **Arch Ophthalmol** 1983 Dec;101(12):1857

Gregory RL: Two pins and a length of string: Kepler's vision. **Perception** 1983;12(4):371–4

Jaeger W: Symbolische Augendarstellungen in einer Ars Memorandi des 16. Jahrhunderts. **Klin Monatsbl Augenheilkd** 1983 Apr;182(4):337–40

Nover A, Kümmel WF: Der Schnitt- und Augenarzt Caspar Stromayr und die ophthalmologischen Illustrationen in seiner 'Practica copiosa' (1559). **Klin Monatsbl Augenheilkd** 1984 Nov;185(5):321–3

Stefani FH, Riedel K: 400 Jahre Augendienst von George Bartisch (1535–1606). **Klin Monatsbl Augenheilkd** 1984 Jan;184(1):64–5

### Great Britain

Gregory RL: The oldest optical society in the world. **Perception** 1979;8(3):245–6

### Hungary

Bartók I: A magyar szemészet legrégibb emlékei. **Orvostort Kozl** 1981;93–96(27 No 1–4):211–7

### Italy

Bonelli ML, Helden A van: Divini and Campani: a forgotten chapter in the history of the Academia del Cimento. **Ann Ist Mus Stor Sci Fir** 1981;6(1):3–176

Huizink L: Die Abhandlung über das Sehen von Hieronymus Fabricius ab Aquapendente (1537–1619): Ubersetzung von 'De actione oculorum' mit Kommentar. Zürich, Juris Druck, 1984. 58 p. (Zürcher Medizingeschichtliche Abhandlungen, Neue Reihe, Nr. 166).

Kleberger E: Fin Brillenfan des 16. Jahrhunderts. **Klin Monatsbl Augenheilkd** 1982 Sep;181(3):223–6

### Switzerland

Funder W: Uber eine bisher unbekannte ophthalmologische Monographie von Jakob Rüff (um 1500–1558). **Klin Monatsbl Augenheilkd** 1981 Oct;179(4):297–8

### 1700 to Present

Amalric P: Ophtalmoscopie et périphérie rétinienne. Quelques aperçus historiques. **Bull Soc Ophtalmol Fr** 1980 Jun–Jul;80(6–7):595–7

Bailliart JP: Quelques uns des liens privilégiés unissant les ophtalmologies grecque et française. **Bull Soc Ophtalmol Fr** 1980 Oct;80(10):807–9

Barraquer JI: The history of the microscope in ocular surgery. **J Microsurg** 1980 Jan–Feb;1(4):288–99

Berar L: History of ophthalmology in stamps. **Metab Pediatr Syst Ophthalmol** 1982;6(3–4):367–9

Berneaud-Kötz G: Wilhelm Conrad Röntgen: aus den Erinnerungen des Schweizer Ophthalmologen Ernst Wölfflin. **Klin Monatsbl Augenheilkd** 1982 Aug;181(2):138–41

Biró I: A szemészet haladása Helmholtztól napjainkig. **Orv Hetil** 1982 Feb 21;123(8):475–8

Bores LD: Historical review and clinical results of radial keratotomy. **Int Ophthalmol Clin** 1983 Fall;23(3):93–118

Braff SM: Contact lens horizons. **Am J Optom Physiol Opt** 1983 Oct;60(10):851–8

Cole BL, Vingrys AJ: A survey and evaluation of lantern tests of color vision. **Am J Optom Physiol Opt** 1982 Apr;59(4):346–74

Coston TO: A personal sketch of Frank Burton Walsh. **Surv Ophthalmol** 1983 Jul–Aug;28(1):50–4

Craggs J: Simple method for auto-ophthalmoscopy. **Br J Ophthalmol** 1983 May;67(5):330–1

Crookes GP: Communication in ophthalmology. **Trans Ophthalmol Soc UK** 1981;101 (Pt 4):409–21

Dannheim E: Orthoptische Uebungsbehandlung des Binokularsehens. Ein geschichtlicher Ueberblick. **Klin Monatsbl Augenheilkd** 1981 Mar;178(3):212–5

Drews RC: The Barraquer experience with intraocular lenses. 20 years later. **Ophthalmology (Rochester)** 1982 Apr;89(4):386–93

Evens L: History of strabismus treatment. **Bull Soc Belge Ophtalmol** 1981;195:19–52

Feibel RM: Edward J. Curran and the concept of relative pupillary block. **Surv Ophthalmol** 1981 Jan–Feb;25(4):270–8

Feibel RM: Historical error. **Ophthalmology (Rochester)** 1983 Jul;90(7):857

Feibel RM: John Vetch and the Egyptian ophthalmia. **Surv Ophthalmol** 1983 Sep–Oct;28(2):128–34

Gaertner H: Adam Marian Langie. **Klin Oczna** 1982 Apr;84(4):131–4

Goldberg MF: Cocaine: the first local anesthetic and the 'third scourge of humanity'. A centennial melodrama. **Arch Ophthalmol** 1984 Oct;102(10):1443–7

Gutner R, Miller D: Inside the fundus camera. **Ann Ophthalmol** 1983 Jan;15(1):13–6

Haugwitz T von: Ophthalmologisch-optische Untersuchungsgeräte. Entwicklung und gegenwärtiger Stand. **Buch Augenarzt** 1981;(85):1–226

Henkind P: An historical look at the retina, 1880–1980. **Trans Ophthalmol Soc UK** 1980 Apr;100(pt 1):20–4

Hubel DH: Evolution of ideas on the primary visual cortex, 1955–1978: a biased historical account. **Biosci Rep** 1982 Jul;2(7):435–69

Kluxen G: Augenheilkunde deutscher Tropenärzte vor 1918. Düsseldorf, Triltsch Druck, 1980. 50 p. (Düsseldorfer Arbeiten zur Geschichte der Medizin, Beiheft V).

Leonnard P, Rommel J: Lens implantation. Thirty years of progress. **Bull Soc Belge Ophtalmol** 1981;194:1–600

Levine JR: The true inventors of the keratoscope and photo-keratoscope. **Br J Hist Sci** 1965;2(8):324–42

McMurry JF: Oskar Hirsch and surgery for exophthalmos. In Romm S, ed: Symposium on historical perspectives of plastic surgery. Philadelphia, Saunders, 1983. p. 649–52.

Mannis MJ, Krachmer JH: Keratoplasty: a historical perspective. **Surv Ophthalmol** 1981 Mar–Apr;25(5):333–8

Margulis ML: An optometric detective: in search of antique eyewear.

**J Am Optom Assoc** 1979 Dec;50(12):1337–42
Mazzolini RG: The iris in eighteenth-century physiology. Bern, Hans Huber, 1980. 193 p. (Berner Beiträge zur Geschichte der Medizin und der Naturwissenschaften, n. F., Bd. 9).
Mecacci L: Le illusioni ottiche nell'Ottocento tra fenomenologia e neurofisiologia. **Stor Crit Psicol** 1983 Dec;4(2):287–9
Meyer-Schwickerath GR: Biometrical studies of the eye and retinal detachment. **Doc Ophthalmol** 1983 Dec 15;56(1–2):27–34
Musiał G: Historia operacji zaćmy. 3. XIX iXX wiek. **Klin Oczna** 1983 Nov–Dec;85(11–12):439–41
Nussbaum JJ, Pruett RC, Delori FC: Historic perspectives. Macular yellow pigment. The first 200 years. **Retina** 1981;1(4):296–310
Orłowski WJ: Z teki szperacza-bibliografa (VIII). Przed 100 laty. **Klin Oczna** 1981;83(3):193–4
Orłowski WJ: Z teki szperacza-bibliografa (XIII). Przed 75 laty. **Klin Oczna** 1982 Apr;84(4):135–6
Perritt RA: Intraocular lens implantation from Ridley to the present: my 25 years' experience. **Int Ophthalmol Clin** 1979 Fall;19(3):11–31
Ronchi L, Fronsini R: Sviluppo e applicazioni cliniche dell'elettro-oculografia. Firenze, Baccini and Chiappi, 1975. 84 p.
Ross D: Vision and the artist. **Occup Health (Lond)** 1980 Feb;32(2):68–73
Rucker CW: A history of the ophthalmoscope. Rochester, Minn., Whiting Printers and Stationers, [1971]. 127 p.
Rudolph G: Herkunft und Schicksal des Humor aqueus. Physiologische Untersuchungen im Vorfeld der Atiologie des Glaukoms während des ersten Viertels des 20. Jahrhunderts. **Gesnerus** 1983;40(3/4):241–8
Shearing SP: Evolution of the posterior chamber intraocular lens. **J Am Intraocul Implant Soc** 1984 Summer;10(3):343–6
Sherman PD: Colour vision in the nineteenth century: the Young-Helmholtz-Maxwell theory. Bristol, Adam Hilger, 1981. xiii, 233 p.
Sorsby A, Benjamin B, Bennett AG: Steiger on refraction: a reappraisal. **Br J Ophthalmol** 1981 Dec;65(12):805–11
Sugar HS: The filtering operations--past, present, and future. **Int Ophthalmol Clin** 1981 Spring;21(1):1–13
Trevor-Roper P: Then and now--therapy. **Trans Ophthalmol Soc UK** 1980 Apr;100(pt 1):30–3
Villaseñor RA: Introduction to and historical overview of surgical procedures for the correction of refractive errors. **Int Ophthalmol Clin** 1983 Fall;23(3):1–9

**Americas**

Newell FW: Pan-American Association of Ophthalmology--40 years. **Am J Ophthalmol** 1980 Mar;89(3):456–7

**Australia**

Hertzberg R: Ronald Francis Lowe. **Aust J Ophthalmol** 1980 May;8(2):109–15
Hertzberg R: Three great ophthalmologists (E. C. Temple-Smith, Norman Gregg, Arthur D'Ombrain). **Med J Aust** 1979 Dec 15;2(12):649–50
Lowe RF: An outline history of ophthalmology in Australia. **Aust J Ophthalmol** 1984 Feb;12(1):5–14
Lowe RF: Early Melbourne eye and ear hospital, and Dr. Turnbull's house at 101 (157) Spring Street. **Aust NZ J Surg** 1980 Oct;50(5):546–9
Lowe RF: John Box (1863–1934) and William Box (1905–1982). **Aust J Ophthalmol** 1983 Feb;11(1):51–3
Lowe RF: T. Aubrey Bowen, oculist, 1837–93. **Aust J Ophthalmol** 1981 May;9(2):155–62
Lowe RF: T. Aubrey Bowen, oculist, 1837–93. His charitable bequest in Victoria. **Aust NZ J Surg** 1983 Apr;53(2):183–7
Lowe RF: The Conjoint Libraries of the Royal Victorian Eye and Ear Hospital and The Royal Australian College of Ophthalmologists. **Aust J Ophthalmol** 1983 May;11(2):127–32
Lowe RF: The Ophthalmological Society of Melbourne (1899–1913). **Aust J Ophthalmol** 1980 Aug;8(3):257–70
Lowe RF: William R. Wilde, Andrew S. Gray, and two eye and ear hospitals of very similar name. **Aust NZ J Surg** 1981 Dec;51(6):630–6
Pockley JA: An outline of one hundred years' history at St Vincent's Hospital, Sydney, 1872–1972. **Aust J Ophthalmol** 1983 Aug;11(3):221–31
Price L: Sydney Eye Hospital. **Br J Ophthalmol** 1982 Oct;66(10):617–21
Wood RF: Ophthalmology in colonial Queensland. **Aust J Ophthalmol** 1982 May;10(2):141–5

**Austria**

Fellner R, Höflechner W: Die Augenheilkunde an der Universität Graz. Graz, Akademische Druck- u. Verlagsanstalt, 1973. ix, 180 p. (Publikationen aus dem Archiv der Universität Graz, Bd. 2).
Henn V: E. Mach on the analysis of motion sensation. **Hum Neurobiol** 1984;3(3):145–8
Hruby K: Das Auge war meine Welt: ein Leben als Augenarzt. Wien, W. Maudrich, 1983. x, 275 p.
Streiff B: Ernst Fuchs (1851–1930)--Gedächtnisvorlesung Wien 31. 5. 1984. **Klin Monatsbl Augenheilkd** 1984 Nov;185(5):316–20
Sugar HS, Foster CC: Maximilian Salzmann. Ophthalmic pioneer and artist. **Surv Ophthalmol** 1981 Jul–Aug;26(1):28–30

**Canada**

Samuel R: Henry Howard. In Dictionary of Canadian biography, 1881–1890. 1982;11:425–6.

**Chile**

Costa-Casaretto C: Chile en dueda con el Doctor Francisco Fonck. **Rev Med Chil** 1981 Nov;109(11):1119–25

**Costa Rica**

Blodi FC: Ophthalmology and philately: V. The diagnosis and treatment of occular diseases.--Eye banks. **Arch Ophthalmol** 1982 Nov;100(11):1794

**Cuba**

Blodi FC: Ophthalmology and philately: II. Ophthalmologists who became famous in other areas of endeavor--Carlos Finlay (1833–1915). **Arch Ophthalmol** 1980 Oct;98(10):1763

**Czechoslovakia**

Boguszaková J: Třicet let oftalmologické katedry institutu pro další vzdělávání lékařu a farmaceutu v Praze. **Cesk Oftalmol** 1983 May;39(3):145–8
Dienstbier E: Prof. MUDr. Roman Kadlický. Jeho život a dílo. **Cas Lek Cesk** 1980 Aug 22;119(33–34):915–20
Grüsser OJ: J.E. Purkyně's contributions to the physiology of the visual, the vestibular and the oculomotor systems. **Hum Neurobiol** 1984;3(3):129–44
Kadlecová V, Matoušek O: Deník Dr. Med. Josefa A. Ryby. Překlad z Německého Rukopisu Věra Kadleová. **Cesk Oftalmol** 1981 Sep;37(5):383–8
Kadlecová V, Maloušek O, ed: Deník Dr. Med. Josefa Ryby. Překlad z německého rukopisu. **Cesk Oftalmol** 1981 Jul;37(4):293–6
Kadlecová V: Počátky oční kliniky v Praze, Jej í první profesor J.N. Fischer a jeho asistenti. III. První profesor pražské oční kliniky J.N. Fischer: jeho život; Fischer - učitel, operatér, člověk. **Cesk Oftalmol** 1983 Jul;39(4):268–80
Kadlecová V: Počátky oční kliniky v Praze, její první profesor J. N. Fischer a jeho asistenti. **Cesk Oftalmol** 1983 Mar;39(2):131–8
Kadlecová V: Počátky oční kliniky v Praze, její první profesor J. N. Fischer a jeho asistenti. **Cesk Oftalmol** 1983 May;39(3):202–14
Kadlecová V: Počátky oční kliniky v Praze, její první profesor J. N. Fischer a jeho asistenti. IV. Asistenti pražké oční kliniky do r. 1847. **Cesk Oftalmol** 1983 Sep;39(5):357–64
Libicky H: A personal sketch of Professor Anton Elschnig. **Surv Ophthalmol** 1982 Mar–Apr;26(5):266–8
Malec J: 100 let české oční kliniky. **Cas Lek Cesk** 1983 Nov 25;122(47):1466–7
Malec J: 100 let České oční kliniky. **Sb Lek** 1984 Jan;86(1):27–30
Rejchrt B: K počátkum Ceskoslovensko-sovětské spolupráce v oftalmologii. **Cesk Oftalmol** 1981 Sep;37(5):381–2

**Denmark**

Ehlers H: Bjerrum's Clinic. **Surv Ophthalmol** 1981 Sep–Oct;26(1):101–2

**France**

Amalric P: Claude Bernard et l'ophtalmologie. **Bull Soc Ophtalmol Fr** 1979 Nov–Dec;79(11–12):995–7
Amalric P: De l'Hôpital de la Grave à la Grande Armée. L'ophtalmologie de Dominique Larrey. **Bull Soc Ophtalmol Fr** 1979 Feb;79(2):151–4
Amalric P: La Clinique Ophtalmologique de l'Hôtel Dieu à 100 ans. **Bull Soc Ophtalmol Fr** 1980 Dec;80(12):1177–80
Amalric P: La naissance et les premiers pas de l'ophtalmoscopie binoculaire. **Bull Soc Ophtalmol Fr** 1982 Nov;82(11):1469–71
Bacin F, Gibert C: Activité chirurgicale d'un ophthalmologiste clermontois de 1934 à 1938. **Bull Soc Ophtalmol Fr** 1981 Oct;81(10):771–4
Bec P: Le prochain centenaire de la société française d'ophtalmologie (1883–1983). **J Fr Ophtalmol** 1980;3(5):313–4
Bonnaud L: Pierre ophtalmiques en Haut-Limousin. **Bull Soc Archeol Hist Limousin** 1978;105:164–70
Centenaire de la Société Française d'Ophtalmologie: **Bull Mem Soc Fr Ophtalmol** 1983;95:clxxxiii–cxcix
Charbonnel A: Histoire de l'oto-neuro-ophtalmologie. **Rev Otoneuroophtalmol** 1979 Oct–Dec;51(5):399–416
Ciuffreda KJ: Astigmatic amblyopia: George Martin. 1890. Translation. **Am J Optom Physiol Opt** 1978 Feb;55(2):133–6
Crawford WL: On the movements of the iris, and, incidentally, on the essential portion of the organ of vision. **Am J Optom Physiol Opt** 1979 Oct;56(10):658–60
Figarella J: Jacques Daviel à Marseille. **Hist Sci Med** 1979;13(4):347–62

# OPHTHALMOLOGY

Firmin F: Quelques reconstructions palpébrales au XIXe siècle. **Ann Chir Plast** 1981;26(1):77–81

Ourgaud AG: Souvenirs concernant la création de la Sociéte d'ophtalmologie du Midi de la France et du Journal d'Ophtalmologie. **Bull Soc Ophtalmol Fr** 1983 Feb;83(2):309–12

Royer J, Haut J, Amalric P: L'opération de la cataracte de Claude Monet, correspondence inédite du peintre et de G.-Clemenceau au docteur Coutela. **Hist Sci Med** 1984;18(2):109–27

Théodoridès J: Le docteur Basile Scrini (1869–1931) et la thérapeutique oculaire. **Rev Hist Pharm (Paris)** 1982 Jun;29(253):101–6

**Germany**

Bahr G von: Mannen bakom Graefes symtom: dog ung, men ändå ett världsnamn inom oftalmologin. **Lakartidningen** 1984 Mar 21;81(12):1168

Blodi FC: Ophthalmology and philately. **Arch Ophthalmol** 1982 Mar;100(3):425,44 (continuing periodically)

Dodt E: Die erste Beschreibung des Knicks in der Dunkeladaptationskurve durch H. Aubert (1865). **Klin Monatsbl Augenheilkd** 1983 Jan;182(1):107–8

Enoch JM: To woo a Helmholtz. **Am J Optom Physiol Opt** 1982 Oct;59(10):843

Fodor F: 100 de ani de la introducerea procedeului profilactic Credé. **Rev Chir [Oftalmol]** 1981 Jul–Sep;25(3):161–3

Fuhrmeister H: Hallesche Duplikate der Majolikareliefs vom Berliner Albrecht-von-Graefe-Denkmal. **Klin Monatsbl Augenheilkd** 1980 May;176(5):867–9

Goldwyn RM: Carl August Burow. **Plast Reconstr Surg** 1984 Apr;73(4):687–90

Harms H: Zum 100. Geburtstag von Walther Löhlein. **Klin Monatsbl Augenheilkd** 1983 Jun;182(6):585–90

Heitz RF: The invention of contact lenses by August Müller (1887). **CLAO J** 1984 Jan–Mar;10(1):88–95

Hertzberg R: Bielschowsky's sign. Its genesis and other observations by Bielschowsky. **Aust J Ophthalmol** 1982 Nov;10(4):282–4

Hoss J: Albert Mooren: ein Augenarzt im 19. Jahrhundert. Düsseldorf, Triltsch, 1980. 183 p. (Düsseldorfer Arbeiten zur Geschichte der Medizin, 55).

Klauss K: Ein neuentdecktes frühes Dokument zur Geschichte der Erfindung des Augenspiegels durch Hermann v. Helmholtz. **NTM** 1981;18(1):58–61

Klix F: Hermann von Helmholtz' Beitrag zur Theorie der Wahrnehmung--Bleibendes und Vergängliches in einem grossen Lebenswerk. In Eckardt G, ed: Zur Geschichte der Psychologie. Berlin, VEB Deutscher Verlag der Wissenschaften, 1979. p. 45–59.

Lund OE: 125 Jahre Deutsche Ophthalmologische Gesellschaft. **MMW** 1982 Sep 10;124(36):761

Mehlhose F: Der gottesfürchtige Jung-Stilling. Ein Pionier der Star-Extraktion. Düsseldorf, Triltsch, 1983. 63 p. (Düsseldorfer Arbeiten zur Geschichte der Medizin, Beiheft VII).

Münchow W: Albrecht von Graefe (1828–1870) in Memoriam. **Orvostort Kozl** 1979;86(24 no 4):55–64

Nover A: 100 Jahre Augenheilkunde. **Fortschr Med** 1982 Dec 16;100(47–48):2222–7

Perkin GD: Leber's optic atrophy. In Rose FC, Bynum WF, ed: Historical aspects of the neurosciences. New York, Raven, 1982. p. 463–72.

Schadewaldt H: Albert Clemens Mooren als geschichtliche Persönlichkeit. **Jahrb Univ Dusseld** 1977–78;:259–68

Snyder C: Julius Hirschberg, the neglected historian of ophthalmology. **Am J Ophthalmol** 1981 May;91(5):664–76

Théodoridès J: Ernst Jünger ou 'l'oeil vivant'. **Gesnerus** 1983;40(1–2):193–202

Votočková J: 130 let Helmholtzova oftalmoskopu. **Cesk Oftalmol** 1982 Jan;38(1):51–3

Wertheim T: Peripheral visual acuity: Th. Wertheim. **Am J Optom Physiol Opt** 1980 Dec;57(12):915–24

Westheimer G: Helmholtz on eye movements. **Hum Neurobiol** 1984;3(3):149–52

**Great Britain**

Ashton N: Ophthalmological Societies of the United Kingdom. Centenary Meeting, April 1980. **Trans Ophthalmol Soc UK** 1980 Apr;100(pt 1):1–8

Cohen B: Erasmus Darwin's observations on rotation and vertigo. **Hum Neurobiol** 1984;3(3):121–8

Dopson L: 100 years of ophthalmic nursing. **Nurs Times** 1981 Jun 11;77(24):1043–4

Foulds WS: The changing pattern of eye surgery. **Br J Anaesth** 1980 Jul;52(7):643–7

Gregory RL: The 4th dimension of 3-D. **Perception** 1980;9(6):613–6

Hodgkin AL: Some recollections of William Rushton and his contributions to neurophysiology. (1925–52). **Vision Res** 1982;22(6):623–5

Lepore FE: Neuro-ophthalmology according to Gordon Holmes. **Neurol Clin** 1983 Nov;1(4):789–805

Lowe RF: T. Aubrey Bowen, Oculist, 1837–93: his bequests to English charities. **Br J Ophthalmol** 1982 Oct;66(10):622–4

Mitchell M: History of the British Optical Association, 1895–1978: with additional material covering the founding of the British College of Ophthalmic Opticians (Optometrists) and the liquidation of the B.O.A. [London], The Association and the British Optical Association Foundation, [1982]. 304 p.

Newell FW: The Ophthalmological Society of the United Kingdom: its first hundred years. **Am J Ophthalmol** 1980 Apr;89(4):605–7

Obituary William Albert Hugh Rushton F.R.S.: **Vision Res** 1982;22(6):611–21

Ono H: On Wells's (1792) law of visual direction. **Percept Psychophys** 1981 Oct;30(4):403–6

Storey JK: Ultrasound in ophthalmic optics. **Ophthalmic Physiol Opt** 1981;1(3):133–57

**Hungary**

Bak M: Lux Jakab dr. (1822–1876) munkássága mai orvosi szemléletünkben. **Orv Hetil** 1984 Apr 29;125(18):1082–4

Bíró I: Szily Adolf, Szily Aurél. **Orv Hetil** 1983 Aug 21;124(34):2065–6

Radnót M: Ifj. Imre József (1884–1945). **Orv Hetil** 1984 Jun 10;125(24):1453–4

**Ireland**

Pappas DG: Sir William Wilde: a historical review. **Ear Nose Throat J** 1983 Jun;62(6):58, 60–2

**Israel**

Patz A: Retinal neovascularisation: early contributions of Professor Michaelson and recent observations. **Br J Ophthalmol** 1984 Jan;68(1):42–6

**Italy**

Belloni L: Der Beitrag von Francesco Buzzi zur Entdeckung der 'Macula lutea' under 'Fovea centralis' des menschlichen Auges. **Gesnerus** 1983;40(1–2):23–30

Fechner PU, Fechner MU, Reis H: Der Okulist Tadini. Zur Geschichte der künstlichen Augenlinse. **Klin Monatsbl Augenheilkd** 1980 Jun;176(6):1003–11

Fechner PU, Fechner MU: Tadini, the man who invented the artificial lens. **J Am Intraocul Implant Soc** 1979 Jan;5(1):22–3

Pini UA: Cristoforo Matteo Lusardi oculista giramondo. **Arch Stor Prov Parmensi** 1979;31:271–4

**Japan**

Inomata H: Yoshiaki Taniguchi, M.D. **Jpn J Ophthalmol** 1983;27(1):1–8

**Mexico**

Limón E: Homenaje al doctor Antonio Torres Estrada. **Gac Med Mex** 1984 May;120(5):205–12

**Netherlands**

Bardell D: Antoni van Leeuwenhoek's explanation in 1704 of the function of eyelids. **J Hist Med Allied Sci** 1984 Oct;39(4):464–7

Brajkovich HL: Dr. Snellen's 20/20: the development and use of the eye chart. **J Sch Health** 1980 Oct;50(8):472–4

Opitz JM: In memoriam: Petrus Johannes Waardenburg, 1886–1979. **Am J Med Genet** 1980;7(1):35–9

**Poland**

Gaertner H: Kazimierz Karelus, Stefan Pasierbiński, Ignacy Chrzanowski i Czesław Klinowski--ordynatorzy i konsulenci okulistyki krakowskiego szpitala Braci Miłosiernych (obecnie im. E. Biernackiego). **Klin Oczna** 1983 Mar;85(3):129–32

Kałużny J: W 25-lecie redagowania Kliniki Ocznej przez prof. dra Witolda Orowskiego. **Klin Oczna** 1981;83(2):55–8

Orłowski WJ: Polska historiografia okulistyczna. **Klin Oczna** 1980;82(11):553–5

Orłowski WJ: Słowo wprowadzające do IX sympozjonu retinologicznego. **Klin Oczna** 1979 Dec;81(12):645–8

Orłowski WJ: Słowo wprowadzające do XII sympozjonu retinologicznego. **Klin Oczna** 1984 Jan;86(1):1–6

Orłowski WJ: W stulecie polskich zjazdów okulistycznych. **Klin Oczna** 1981 Oct–Dec;83(10–12):465–6

Orłowski WJ: Z teki szperacza-bibliografa (X). Przed 50 laty. **Klin Oczna** 1981;83(9):433–4

Orłowski WJ: Z teki szperacza--bibliografa (XVIII). Przed 50 laty. **Klin Oczna** 1983 Apr;85(4):189–91

Smereka J: Rozprawy doktorskie obronione przez lekarzy polskich we Wrocławskiej Klinice Okulistycznej przed r. 1918. **Klin Oczna** 1979 Nov;81(11):635–6

Sokołowski T: Badanie ostrości wxroku przed 50 latami i dzfiś. **Klin Oczna** 1981;83(9):451

Szwarc B: Spis prac Prof. Tadeusza Krwawicza. **Klin Oczna** 1980 Jan;82(1):1–4
Zygulska-Machowa H, Starzycka M: Professor Bolesław Wicherkiewicz jako współtwórca krakowskiej szkoły okulistycznej. **Klin Oczna** 1982 Sep;84(9):245–9

**Portugal**

Blodi FC: Ophthalmology and philately: I. Ophthalmologist on stamps--M.R. de Gama Pinto (1853–1945). **Arch Ophthalmol** 1980 Jan;98(1):143

**Puerto Rico**

Arana Soto S: La oftalmología en Puerto Rico hasta el 1898. [s.l., s. n.], 1977. 61 p.

**Romania**

Segal N: 150 de ani de existenţă a Secţiei de oftalmologie Oradea. **Rev Chir [Oftalmol]** 1981 Jan–Mar;25(1):75–9

**Sweden**

Palm E: Oftalmologin--perfekt och futurum. **Lakartidningen** 1980 Jun 11;77(24):2258–61

**Switzerland**

Mannen bakom syndromet: Friedrich Horner. Först att införa antiseptisk behandling i ögonsjukvården. **Lakartidningen** 1984 Mar 21;81(12):1165 7
Huber A: W. R. Hess, the ophthalmologist. **Experientia** 1982 Dec 15;38(12):1397–400
Huber A: Walter Rudolf Hess als Ophthalmologe. **Gesnerus** 1982;39(2):287–93
Ott E: Friedrich Horner, 1831–1886, Leben und Werk. Zürich, Juris, 1980. 54 p. (Zürcher Medizingeschichtliche Abhandlungen, Neue Reihe Nr. 136).
Rintelen F: Von der Augenheilanstalt zur Universitätsaugenklinik in Basel. **Gesnerus** 1982;39(1):79–83
Rintelen F: Zum 100. Geburtstag von Alfred Vogt -- Versuch einer Würdigung seines wissenschaftlichen Werkes. **Klin Monatsbl Augenheilkd** 1979 Oct;175(4):439–41
Rintelen F: 75. Jahresversammlung der Schweizerischen ophthalmologischen Gesellschaft; zu ihrer Gründung und ihren Gründen. **Klin Monatsbl Augenheilkd** 1983 May;182(5):348–51
Speiser P: Vogts Lehrbuch und Atlas der Spaltlampenmikroskopie des lebenden Auges. **Gesnerus** 1981:38(3/4):339–45
Winkler-Trachsel E: Arnold Ott (1840–1910). Arzt und Dichter. Sein ärztliches Wirken. Zürich, Juris Druck, 1983. 83 p. (Zürcher Medizingeschichtliche Abhandlungen, Neue Reihe, Nr. 163).

**United States**

Alpern M: Presentation of the Procter Medal for Research in vision and Ophthalmology to Gerald Westheimer. **Invest Ophthalmol Vis Sci** 1979 Sep;18(9):883–92
Altman SB: A brief history of South Dakota Academy of Ophthalmology and Otorhinolaryngology. **SD J Med** 1981 May;34(5):39
Black E: The great contact-lens con. **Wash Mon** 1980;12(7):23–9
Bryan SA: Pioneering specialists: a history of the American Academy of Ophthalmology and Otolaryngology. San Francisco, American Academy of Ophthalmology, Rochester, Minn.: American Academy of Otolaryngology-Head and Neck Surgery, 1982. viii, 305 p.
Coon LJ: Orthokeratology: part I historical perspective. **J Am Optom Assoc** 1982 Mar;53(3):187–95
Delaney JJ: Edward Jackson. **Colo Med** 1983 Apr;80(4):116–7
Dyer JA: Corneal contact lenses in perspective 1948–1981. **Contact Intraocular Lens Med J** 1982 Jan–Mar;8(1):3–8
Enoch JM: Joseph Le Conte. **Am J Optom Physiol Opt** 1983 Dec;60(12):1003
Garber E: Marie Gertrude Rand. In: Notable American women. The modern period. Cambridge, Mass., Belknap-Harvard Univ. Press, 1980. 4:565.
Girard LJ: Contributions to ophthalmology by contact lens research and development. **Contact Intraocular Lens Med J** 1982 Apr–Jun;8(2):77–80
Keeney AH, Keeney VT: Frederick Herman Verhoeff, M. D. **Filson Club Hist Q** 1981;55(2):202–9
Lamping KA, Albert DM, Snyder C, et al: The Harrower collection and its place in the history of ophthalmic pathology. **Surv Ophthalmol** 1983 May–Jun;27(6):374–80
Leeds JP: Review of the Transactions of the American Academy of Optometry, 1922 to 1939. **Am J Optom Physiol Opt** 1982 Sep;59(9):735–7
McDonald PR: Evolution of cataract surgery since the deSchweinitz era. **Ophthalmic Surg** 1979 May;10(5):44–52
McPherson SD: A brief history of ophthalmology in North Carolina. **NC Med J** 1983 Oct;44(10):641–3
Maurizi AR, Moore RL, Shepard L: Competing for professional control: professional mix in the eyeglass industry. **J Law Econ** 1981;24(2):351–64
Morgan MW: The Maddox classification of vergence eye movements. **Am J Optom Physiol Opt** 1980;57:537–9
Newell FW, Blodi FC, Henkind P, et al: In commemoration of 25 years of Survey of Ophthalmology. **Surv Ophthalmol** 1981 May–Jun;25(6):397–403
Newell FW: The first editor--Edward Jackson. **Am J Ophthalmol** 1982 Dec;94(6):809–10
Paton D: The surgery of A. Edward Maumenee. **Am J Ophthalmol** 1979 Sep;88(3 Pt 1):297–302
Patz A: Contributions of A. Edward Maumenee in the field of retinal and choroidal diseases. **Am J Ophthalmol** 1979 Sep;88(3 Pt 1):295–6
Patz A: Jonas S. Friedenwald, man of science. **Invest Ophthalmol Vis Sci** 1980 Oct;19(10):1139–49
Randolph ME: A. Edward Maumenee--an appreciation. **Am J Ophthalmol** 1979 Sep;88(3 Pt 1):289–92
Silverstein AM: Contributions of A. Edward Maumenee to ocular immunology. **Am J Ophthalmol** 1979 Sep;88(3 Pt 1):302–5
Snyder C: A look at George Frick's Treatise on diseases of the eye. In: Congrès international d'histoire de la médecine, XXVe, Québec, 1976. Actes. Québec, 1977. p. 1289–1300.
Stephens LD: Joseph LeConte and the development of the physiology and psychology of vision in the United States. **Ann Sci** 1980 May;37(3):303–21
Sugar HS: In appreciation of the contributions of Harry Searls Gradle. **Surv Ophthalmol** 1981 Nov–Dec;26(3):170–3
Talbott MW: Intraocular lenses and the Food and Drug Administration: regulation amid controversy. **Int Ophthalmol Clin** 1979 Fall;19(3):1–10
Tasman W: The history of Wills Eye Hospital. Hagerstown, Md., Harper & Row, 1980. ix, 135 p.
To honor A. Edward Maumenee: **Am J Ophthalmol** 1979 Sep;88(3 Pt 1):285, 288–316
Waites L: American pioneers in the topic of word blindness. In Rose FC, Bynum WF, ed: Historical aspects of the neurosciences. New York, Raven, 1982. p. 115–6.
Wittenberg S: Brock's research in stereopsis. **Am J Optom Physiol Opt** 1981 Aug;58(8):663–6, 667–70

**USSR**

Belous VI, Mesiats NK: S. M. Ter-Arutiuniants--osnovatel' glaznoĭ sluzhby na Zhitomirshchine. **Oftalmol Zh** 1984;(1):63–4
Bezkorovainy A: Ophthalmologic research in pre-World War I Russia. **Bull Hist Med** 1979 Winter;53(4):593–605
Brzheskiĭ VCh: K istorii pervoĭ v mire kafedry oftal'mologii. **Vestn Oftalmol** 1981 Sep–Oct;(5):69–70
Filimonov AR: Pervyi tom zhurnala 'Vestnik oftal'mologii: (1884 g.). **Vestn Oftalmol** 1984 Jul–Aug;(4):5–7
Filimonov AR: 'Vestnik oftal'mologii' 50 let nazad. **Vestn Oftalmol** 1984 Nov–Dec;(6):6–8
Filimonov AR: 'Vestnik oftal'mologii' 75 let nazad. **Vestn Oftalmol** 1984 Sep–Oct;(5):7–8
Golenkov AK, Zaslavskaia LA: Oftal'mologiia na tselinnoĭ zemle. **Vestn Oftalmol** 1980 Mar–Apr;(2):3–4
Krasnikov PG: L. G. Belliarminov--vydaiushchiĭsia uchenyĭ, obshchestvennyĭ deiatel' i organizator oftal'mologicheskoĭ pomoshchi naseleniiu (k 125-letiiu so dnia rozhdeniia). **Vestn Oftalmol** 1984 Sep–Oct;(5):69–70
Krasnikov PG: Vydaiushcheesia izobretenie otechestvennogo oftal'mologa (100 let so vremeni sozdaniia applanatsionnogo tonometra Prof. A.N. Maklakova). **Vestn Oftalmol** 1984 Nov–Dec;(6):70–2
Krasnov MM: Proshloe v nastoiashchem: Adrian Aleksandrovich Kriukov, redaktor 'Vestnika oftal'mologii' i osnovatel' Moskovskogo oftal'mologicheskogo veshchestva (k 75-letiiu zhurnala). **Vestn Oftalmol** 1984 Nov–Dec;(6):4–6
Leninskie printsipy v rabote oftal'mologov: **Vestn Oftalmol** 1980 May–Jun;(3):3–5
Magil'nitskiĭ SG: Oftal'mologi-revoliutsionery. **Vestn Oftalmol** 1983 Nov–Dec;(6):72–5
Magil'nitskiĭ SG: Pervyĭ opyt otechestvennoĭ oftal'morentgenologii pri travmakh. **Oftalmol Zh** 1983;38(2):119–21
Magil'nitskiĭ SG: Raisa Vasil'evna Putiata--revoliutsionerka-oftal'molog. **Vestn Oftalmol** 1983;3:73–5
Magil'nitskiĭ SG: 'Vestniku oftal'mologii' - 100 let. **Vestn Oftalmol** 1984 May–Jun;(3):3–7
Shul'pina NB, Krasnov ML, Shmeleva VV: Postdiplomnoe usovershenstvovanie oftal'mologov (k 50-letiiu Tsentral'nogo instituta usovershenstvovaniia vracheĭ). **Vestn Oftalmol** 1980 Sep–Oct;(5):7–10
Tret'iak TP, Stetsula TI: Zaslugi N. I. Pirogova v oftal'mologii. **Oftalmol Zh** 1981;36(8):506–8
Volkov VV, Danilichev VF: Professor A.V. Khodin - osnovatel' i pervyĭ redaktor-izdatel' 'Vestnika oftal'mologii' (k 100-letiiu zhurnala). **Vestn Oftalmol** 1984 Nov–Dec;(6):3–4
Volkov VV, Shiliaev VG: Voennaia Oftal'mologiia v period Velikoĭ Otechestvennoĭ Voĭny. **Voen Med Zh** 1980 May;(5):50–3
Vurgaft MB: The 90th anniversary of Maklakov's applanation tomometer.

# OPHTHALMOLOGY

**Am J Optom Physiol Opt** 1981 Feb;58(2):183-5

**Yugoslavia**

Dugački V: Počeci organizirane skrbi za slijepe u Hrvatskoj. Prosvećeno Međunarondoj godini invalida. **Lijec Vjesn** 1981 Nov;103(11):531-3
Dugački V: Povijesni pregled zaštite vida školske djece i omladine u Hrvatskoj. **Lijec Vjesn** 1979 Aug;101(8):503-5
Pavišić Z, Dugački V: Značenje znanstvenog, stručnog i nastavnog rada prof. dr. Alberta Botterija za razvoj oftalmologije u Jugoslaviji. **Lijec Vjesn** 1980 Jan;102(1):43-7
Plamenac SD: Dr. Pavao Popović (30. X 1854 - 17. X 1937), pionir oftalmologije u Srbiji. **Srp Arh Celok Lek** 1980 Feb;108(2):169-80

# ORTHOPEDICS

Allgöwer M: Die Behandlung der Tibiaschaftfraktur im Wandel der Zeit. **Hefte Unfallheilkd** 1982;158:417-21
The classics: **Clin Orthop** 1982 May;(165):6-32 (continued regularly)
Dustmann HO, Ebel V: Darstellungen von Fussdeformierungen und deren Behandlung in der Kunst. In KF Schlegel, ed: Der Körperbehinderte in Mythologie und Kunst. Stuttgart, New York, Thieme, 1983. p. 41-56.
Orr JF, James WV, Bahrani AS: The history and development of artificial limbs. **Eng Med** 1982 Oct;11(4):155-61
Ray JM: The fractured hip: the historical development of fracture management. **Friends P. I. Nixon Med Hist Libr** 1980 Oct;9:1-9
Schlegel KF: Luzifer - ein orthopädischer Patient. In KF Schlegel, ed: Der Körperbehinderte in Mythologie und Kunst. Stuttgart, New York, Thieme, 1983. p. 19-27.
Schlegel KF, ed: Der Körperbehinderte in Mythologie und Kunst. Stuttgart, New York, Georg Thieme Verlag, 1983. 125 p.
Simon P, Seifert E: Rollende Hilfsmittel fur Körperbehinderte als Gegenstand in der bildenden Kunst. In KF Schlegel, ed: Der Körperbehinderte in Mythologie und Kunst. Stuttgart, New York, Thieme, 1983. p. 89-125.
Vander Elst E: Die Geschichte der Orthopädie und der Traumatologie. In Sournia JC, Martiny M, Poulet J, ed: Illustrierte Geschichte der Medizin. Salzburg, Andreas, 1980. Vol. 5. p. 1655-1721.
Verdan C: Evolution historique de la chirurgie des tendons fléchisseurs. **Rev Med Suisse Romande** 1980 Jul;100(7):639-52
Ziller R: Zur Geschichte des künstlichen Gelenkersatzes. **Beitr Orthop Traumatol** 1984 Oct;31(10):526-32

**Denmark**

Fossgreen J: Manuel medicin. Historie og nutid. **Ugeskr Laeger** 1982 May 24;144(21):1545-7

**Germany**

Sollmann AH, Blaurock-Busch E: Manipulative therapy of the spine: the development of 'manual medicine' in Germany and Europe. **Chiropr Hist** 1981;1(1):37-41

**Netherlands**

Haneveld GT: De ledezetters van Jisp. **Spiegel Hist** 1977;12(100):514-17

**Before 500 A.D.**

Beasley AW: The origins of orthopaedics. **J R Soc Med** 1982 Aug;75(8):648-55
Schadewaldt H: Orthopädische Aspekte der Mythologie. In KF Schlegel, ed: Der Körperbehinderte in Mythologie und Kunst. Stuttgart, New York, Thieme, 1983. p. 1-18.

**500 A.D.-1450**

Baumgartner R: Fussprothese aus einem frühmittelalterlichen Grab aus Bonaduz. **Helv Archaeol** 1982;13(51-2):155-62
Beasley AW: Orthopaedic aspects of mediaeval medicine. **J R Soc Med** 1982 Dec;75(12):970-5

**Byzantium**

Bernabò M: La 'Rinascenza Macedone' e l'arte dei bendaggi. **Kos** 1984 Jun;1(5):45-51
Grmek MD: Vestigia della chirurgia greca: il Codice di Niceta e i suoi discendenti. **Kos** 1984 Jun;1(5):52-60

**Mexico**

Alarcon-Segovia D: Descriptions of therapeutic arthrocenthesis and of synovial fluid in a Nahuatl text from prehispanic Mexico. **Ann Rheum Dis** 1980 Jun;39(3):291-3

**1700 to Present**

Bibliography of original works on orthopaedic surgery, traumatology and related sciences, 1872-1972.: Belgrade, Yugoslav Association for Orthopaedic Surgery and Traumatology, 1980. 251 p.
Black J, Sholtes V: Biomaterial aspects of surface replacement arthroplasty of the hip. **Orthop Clin North Am** 1982 Oct;13(4):709-28
Blauth W, Donner K: Zur Geschichte der Arthroplastik. **Z Orthop** 1979 Dec;117(6):997-1006
Charnley J: Evolution of total hip replacement. **Ann Chir Gynaecol** 1982;71(2):103-7
Il tripode si Sayre: **Chir Organi Mov** 1981;66(2):279-81
Livio JJ: L'orthopédie, quelle place dans la société? **Rev Med Suisse Romande**
Romm S: Fritz Steinmann and the pin that bears his name. **Plast Reconstr Surg** 1984 Aug;74(2):306-10
Rüttimann B: Zur Geschichte der Krüppelfürsorge. **Gesnerus** 1980;37(3/4):199-214
Sisk TD: External fixation. Historic review, advantages, disadvantages, complications, and indications. **Clin Orthop** 1983 Nov;(180):15-22
Snook GA: A short history of the anterior cruciate ligament and the treatment of tears. **Clin Orthop** 1983 Jan-Feb;(172):11-3
Soren A, Waugh TR: The historical evolution of arthrodesis of the foot. **Int Orthop** 1980;4(1):3-11
Sprague NF: Operative arthroscopy. **Clin Orthop** 1982 Jul;(167):4-5
Steinberg ME: Evolution and development of surface replacement arthroplasty. **Orthop Clin North Am** 1982 Oct;13(4):661-6
Strubell M, ed: Trueta: surgeon in war and peace. The memoirs of Joep Trueta. London, Gollancz, 1980. 288 p.
Taylor DW: Orthopaedics--a brief historical overview. **Australas Nurses J** 1981 Aug;10(8):24-5
Vidal J: External fixation. Yesterday, today, and tomorrow. **Clin Orthop** 1983 Nov;(180):7-14
Waugh W: Breve storia dell'ortopedia. **Kos** 1984 Jun;1(5):33-44

**Australia**

Clarke J: Dr. Max Herz. Sydney, Alternative Publishing Co-operative, 1976. xv, 184 p.

**Austria**

Peltier LF: The classic. Concerning traumatic malacia of the lunate and its consequences: degeneration and compression fractures. **Clin Orthop** 1980 Jun;149:4-8

**Belgium**

Colard A: Evocation du passé: sur le professeur Baron Seutin et sa méthode amovo-inamovible. **Rev Med Brux** 1983 Jan;4(1):39-44
de Marneffe R: Albin Lambotte, pionnier de l'ostéosynthèse moderne. **Rev Med Brux** 1982 Sep;3(7):493-5

**Canada**

Salter RB: Scientific contributions to orthopaedic surgery by the staff of The Hospital for Sick Children, Toronto, 1875 to 1975. In: Congrès international d'histoire de la médecine, XXVe, Québec, 1976. Actes. Québec, 1977. p. 1225-43.

**Czechoslovakia**

Cerveňanská N: Ian Chervenianskiĭ--osnovopolozhnik chekhoslovatsko-sovetskikh sviazeĭ v ortopedii. **Ortop Travmatol Protez** 1983 Apr;(4):68-71
Cerveňanská N: 60 rokov Ortopedickej kliniky University Komenského. **Acta Chir Orthop Traumatol Cech** 1983 Dec;50(6):485-90
Kubat R, Mřena V: Operatsiia Zagradnicheka pri vrozhdennom vyvikhe bedra segodnia (posviashchaetsia 100-letiiu so dnia rozhdeniia professora Iana Zagradnicheka). **Ortop Travmatol Protez** 1982 Jul;(7):69-71
Rozsívalová E, Adamec J: Podmínky vzniku I. ortopedické kliniky v Praze. **Cas Lek Cesk** 1979 Nov 16;118(46):1429-31

**France**

D'Aubigné RM: Notre orthopédie, hier...et demain. **Rev Chir Orthop** 1980;66 Suppl 2:13-20
D'Aubigné RM: Paul Broca et la chirurgie de l'appareil moteur. **Chirurgie** 1980;106(10):791-3
Evans PE: Cerclage fixation of a fractured humerus in 1775. Fact or fiction? **Clin Orthop** 1983 Apr;(174):138-42
Merle d'Aubigné R: Surfing the wave: fifty years in the growth of French orthopedic surgery. **Clin Orthop** 1982 Nov-Dec;(171):3-23
Mourgues G de: Léopold Ollier, 1830-1900, père de la chirurgie orthopédique. **Rev Chir Orthop** 1979;65(11):2-3
Peltier LF: Guerin versus Malgaigne: a precedent for the free criticism of scientific papers. **J Orthop Res** 1983;1(1):115-8

Peltier LF: The 'back school' of Delpech in Montpellier. **Clin Orthop** 1983 Oct;179:4-9
Peltier LF: The classic. Separations of the epiphyses. By Jean Timothée Emile Foucher. 1867. **Clin Orthop** 1984 Sep;(188):3-9
Ramadier JO: La revue de chirurgie orthopédique et réparatrice de l'appareil moteur--90e anniversaire. **Rev Chir Orthop** 1981;67(3):161-3
Sharrard WJ: 90th anniversary of the Revue de Chirurgie Orthopédique: an outsider's view. **Rev Chir Orthop** 1981;67(3):165-6
Vitoria Ortiz M: Ollier et sa contribution à l'étude de l'appareil locomotor. In International Congress of the History of Medicine, 27th, Barcelona, 1980. Actas. Barcelona, Académia de Ciències Mèdiques de Catalunya i Balears, 1981. p. 680-9.

**Germany**

Abe HR: Zur Biographie von Hans Kehr (1862-1916). **Beitr Gesch Univ Erfurt** 1979-83;19:233-40
Bethge R: Erstes orthopädisches Lehrbuch der Welt für den Gebrauch der Arzte. Zum 200. Geburtstage von Johann Christian Gottfried Jörg. **Beitr Orthop Traumatol** 1979 Sep;26(9):520-4
Bethge R, Knöfler EW: 30 Jahre Gesellschaft für Orthopädie der DDR--Zur Erinnerung an ihren Mitbegründer und ersten Vorsitzenden Friedrich Loeffler. **Beitr Orthop Traumatol** 1983 May;30(5):233-6
Bethge R, Knöpfler EW: 50 Jahre Orthopädische Klinik der Karl-Marx-Universität Leipzig. **Beitr Orthop Traumatol** 1980 Oct;27(10):545-52
Hellinger J, Hornuf H: Zum Einfluss Dresdner Arzte und Wissenschaftler auf die Entwicklung der Orthopädie. **Beitr Orthop Traumatol** 1981 Dec;28(12):637-44
Hipp E: 100 Jahre Orthopädie. **Fortschr Med** 1983 Feb 3;101(5):147-50, 179
Idelberger K: Erlebte Orthopädie (1937-1977). **Jahrb Univ Dusseld** 1977-78;:135-52
Parnitzke C, Schaeper M: Bedeutende Magdeburger antifaschistische Aerzte und die Entwicklung der Orthopädie in Magdeburg. **Z Arztl Fortbild (Jena)** 1980 Aug 15;74(16):781-6
Paul U: Paul Friedrich Scheel zum 100. Geburtstag. **Beitr Orthop Traumatol** 1983 Oct;30(10):505-7
Sendler P: Von der Krüppelheilanstalt zum Universitätsklinikum: die 'Hüfferstiftung' in Münster in Westfalen. Herzogenrath, Murken-Altrogge, 1984. 188 p. (Studien zur Geschichte des Krankenhauswesens, 17)
Staheli LT: A visit with Professor Heinz Wagner: Orthopädische Klinik Wichernhaus Rummelsberg/Nuremberg. **J Pediatr Orthop** 1982 Oct;2(4):448-52
Tautz P, Hein G: Frühformen orthopädischen Denkens und orthopädischer Methoden in den ersten 120 Jahren der Universität Halle (Saale) (III). Heinrich Bass (1690-1754), genannt, 'Bandagen-Bass'. **Beitr Orthop Traumatol** 1979;26(12):705-12

**Great Britain**

Elliott CK: Bonesetters. **Practitioner** 1981 Feb;225(1352):253-5
Glupker DF: The yesteryear of orthopaedic nursing (Agnes Hunt). **Orthop Nurs** 1984 Nov-Dec;3(6):48
Nisbet NW, Woodruff M: John Charnley: 29 August 1911-5 August 1982. **Biogr Mem Fellows R Soc** 1984;30:119-37
Peltier LF: The classic. The growth of bone. Chapter III. Osteogenic power of bone bereft of periosteum. William Macewen, F.R.S. **Clin Orthop** 1983 Apr;(174):5-14
Peltier LF: Ununited fractures in children. James Paget, 1891. **Clin Orthop** 1982 Jun;(166):2-4
Poal-Manresa J: Comentarios sobre la evolución de la prótesis de cadera: a propósito de la muerte de Sir John Charnley. **Med Clin (Barc)** 1983 May 7;80(16):715-6
Ratliff AH: Ernest William Hey Groves and his contributions to orthopaedic surgery. **Bristol Med Chir J** 1983 Jul;98(367):98-103
Taylor RG: G. R. Girdlestone, M.D., F.R.C.S. **Clin Orthop** 1983 Mar;(173):125-9
Thompson U: Liverpool--'the home of orthopaedics'. **Physiotherapy** 1983 Jul 10;69(7):241-2

**Hungary**

Csillag I: Az elsö magyar orthopédiai intézet. **Orv Hetil** 1982 May 2;123(18):1111-4

**Ireland**

Zarzycki D, Zarzycka M: Abraham Colles życie i twórczość. **Chir Narzadow Ruchu Ortop Pol** 1980;45(1):103-4

**Italy**

Paltrinieri M: Cinquant'anni vissuti fra gli splendori dell'ortopedia. **Chir Organi Mov** 1982;67(1):1-6
Riunione straordinaria dei Consigli Comunale e Provinciale in occasione del 1 centenario della morte di Francesco Rizzoli (24-5-1880) e della nascita di Vittorio Putti (1-3-1880): **Chir Organi Mov** 1979 Jul-Aug;65(4):367-98

**Japan**

Takagi K: Arthroscope. Kenji Takagi. J. Jap. Orthop. Assoc., 1939. **Clin Orthop** 1982 Jul;(167):6-8

**Poland**

Dega W: Profesor dr Ireneusz Wierzejewski jako prekursor rehabilitacji. (Z okazji setnej rocznicy jego urodzin). **Chir Narzadow Ruchu Ortop Pol** 1981;46(6):599-602
Dziak A: Zainteresowania ortopedyczne niektórych chirurgów polskich wieku XIX. **Chir Narzadow Ruchu Ortop Pol** 1980;45(1):95-102
Labaziewicz L: Pisarstwo naukowe Ireneusza Wierzejewskiego. **Chir Narzadow Ruchu Ortop Pol** 1981;46(6):595-7
Lempicki A: Ireneusz Wierzejewski (1881-1930). **Chir Narzadow Ruchu Ortop Pol** 1981;46(6):589-93
Marciniak W: Zagadnienia wrodzonego zwichni ęcia biodra w pracach prof. dr Wiktora Degi - z okazji 85 rocznicy urodzin. **Chir Narzadow Ruchu Ortop Pol** 1982;47(3):219-23

**South Africa**

Mackenzie DB: The treatment of recurrent anterior shoulder dislocation by the modified Bristow-Helfet procedure. **S Afr Med J** 1984 Mar 3;65(9):325-30

**Sweden**

Eriksson E: Ivar Palmer, a great name in the history of cruciate ligament surgery. **Clin Orthop** 1983 Jan-Feb;(172):3-10
Goldie I: Progress in Sweden. **Clin Orthop** 1984 Dec;(191):2-3
Husberg K, Räf L: John Charnley efter 30 års arbete med höftledskirurgi: 'intuition och slump hjälpte fram genombrotten men protesens livslängd måste förbättras'. **Lakartidningen** 1982 Jun 9;79(23):2301-3

**Switzerland**

Rüttimann B: Wilhelm Schulthess (1855-1917) und die Schweizer Orthopädie seiner Zeit. Zürich, Schulthess Polygraphischer Verlag, 1983. xv, 272 p.

**United States**

Aufranc OE: Trends in contemporary practice. Prefatory chapter. **Clin Orthop** 1983 May;(175):2-7
Brown JE, Finder JG, Lidge RT: The Clinical Orthopaedic Society, Inc.: an informal history, 1912-1981. Brunswick, Ga., Glover Printing Co., [1982?]. vii, 288 p.
Burd JG: Forty years on the same job (or orthopedic surgery can be fun). **J Tenn Med Assoc** 1979 Jul;72(7):534-6
Clawson DK: The founding of the Association of Orthopaedic Chairmen. **Clin Orthop** 1983 Dec;181:298-303
Dobrin L: Origin and evolution of the walkerette. **Mt Sinai J Med (NY)** 1980 Mar-Apr;47(2):172-4
Elliott J: Orthopedist is pioneer in prosthetic design. **JAMA** 1976 Oct 26;242(17):1831-3, 1837
Fraider CT: Arthroscopic surgery of the knee: history and state of the art. **JAOA** 1981 Aug;80(12):817-22
Harvey AM: Orthopaedic surgery at Johns Hopkins: a heritage of excellence in clinical practice, training and research. **Johns Hopkins Med J** 1982 Jun;150(6):221-45
Heck CV: Fifty years of progress: in recognition of the 50th anniversary of the American Academy of Orthopaedic Surgeons. Chicago, American Academy of Orthopaedic Surgeons, 1983. vi, 361 p.
McBryde AM, Pressly JA, Hutchinson F, et al: North Carolina Orthopedic Hospital closes after 58 years of treatment of crippled children. **NC Med J** 1979 Dec;40(12):755-7
Nolan E: Children's ward. Lithograph by Robert Riggs, ca. 1940-45. **J Hist Med Allied Sci** 1982 Jul;37(3):322
Siegel IM: John B. Murphy - early American orthopaedic surgeon. **Int Surg** 1979 Jan-Feb;64(1):83-5

**USSR**

Andrianov VL, Veselov NG, Kapitanaki IA: Leningradskiĭ nauchno-issledovatel'skiĭ detskiĭ ortopedicheskiĭ institut im. G.I. Turnera i ego rol' v okhrane zdorov'ia deteĭ (k 50-letiiu so dnia organizatsii). **Pediatriia** 1983 Nov;(11):74-5
Andrianov VL: Leningradskomu nauchno-issledovatel'skomu detskomu ortopedicheskomu institutu im. G. I. Turnera 50 let. **Ortop Travmatol Protez** 1983 Mar;(3):56-60
Chaplinskiĭ VV, Iatsekevich IaE: L'vovskomu nauchnomu obshchestvu travmatologov-ortopedov 25 let. **Ortop Travmatol Protez** 1982

Dec;(12):60–1
Dusmuratov MD, Semeniuta AIa: Travmatologiia i ortopediia v Uzbekskoĭ SSR (istoriia, sostoianie i perspektivy razvitiia). **Ortop Travmatol Protez** 1982 Dec;(12):4–7
Kolontaĭ IuIu, Kondrashov AN, Kolod'ko ED: 50 let kafedre travmatologii, ortopedii i voenno-polevoĭ khirurgii Dnepropetrovskogo ordena Trudovogo Krasnogo Znameni meditsinskogo instituta. **Ortop Travmatol Protez** 1980 Mar;(3):76–7
Korzh AA, Simenach BI: Kharkovskiĭ nauchno-issledovatel'skiĭ institut ortopedii i travmatologii im. prof. M.I. Sitenko. **Vestn Khir** 1983 Mar;130(3):23–5
Lubegina ZP: K 50-letiiu Sverdlovskogo nauchno-issledovatel'skogo instituta travmatologii i ortopedii. **Ortop Travmatol Protez** 1981 Dec;(12):58–61
Movshovich IA, Kaplan MB: 50 Let so dnia organizatsii travmatologicheskogo otdeleniia v bol'nitse im. S. P. Botkina. **Ortop Travmatol Protez** 1982 Jun;(6):74–5
Revenko TA, Matiashina OM, Sokolenko OM, et al: Travmatologo-ortopedicheskaia nauka v Donbasse za gody sotsialisticheskogo stroitel'stva. **Ortop Travmatol Protez** 1983 March;(3):47–51
Revenko TA, Matiashina OM, Tsimidanova NB, et al: Travmatologo-ortopedicheskaia sluzhba v Donbasse za 60 let Soiuza SSR. **Vestn Khir** 1983;130(4):10–3
Rusakov AB: Zhiznennyĭ i tvorcheskiĭ put' V. V. Gorinevskoĭ (K 100-letiiu so dnia rozhdeniia). **Ortop Travmatol Protez** 1983 Mar;(3):63–5
Shumada IV, Gorodniaia VN: K istorii Kievskogo obshchestva travmatologov-ortopedov. **Ortop Travmatol Protez** 1984 Aug;(8):69–73
Shumada IV, Gorodniaia VN: Rol' Kievskoĭ shkoly ortopedov v razvitii protezirovaniia i protezostroeniia na Ukraine. **Ortop Travmatol Protez** 1984 Jan;(1):69–70
Skorogliadov AV: K 50-letiiu so dnia organizatsii kafedry travmatologii, ortopedii i voenno- polevoĭ khirurgii II MOLGMI im. N.I. Pirogova. **Ortop Travmatol Protez** 1983 Dec;(12):60–1
Stamatin SI, Marin IM: Rol'kafedry meditsinskogo instituta v razvitii ortopedii i travmatologii v Moldavskoĭ SSR. **Ortop Travmatol Protez** 1982 Jul;(7):64–6
Tkachenko SS, Andrianov VL, Kapitanaki IA: K 125-letiiu so dnia rozhdeniia G. I. Turnera--osnovopolozhnika otechestvennoĭ travmatologii i ortopedii. **Ortop Travmatol Protez** 1984 Jun;(6):68–70
Trubnikov VF: K 60-letiiu osnovanii kafedry ortopedii, travmatologii i voenno-polevoi khirurgii Khar'kovskogo meditsinskogo instituta. **Ortop Travmatol Protez** 1981 Sep;(9):68–70
Volkov MV, Mattis ER: Osnovnye itogi napravleniia razvitiia Sovetskoĭ travmatologii i ortopedii. **Vestn Khir** 1982 Nov;129(11):3–9
Volkov MV: Tsentral'nomu institutu travmatologii i ortopedii im. N. N. Priorova--60 let. **Ortop Travmatol Protez** 1981;(4):1–5

**Yugoslavia**

Bumbaširević Z: Sedamdeset pet godina ortopedske hirurgije u Srbiji. **Srp Arh Celok Lek** 1981 Mar;109(3):425–38
Marinović I: 'Balkanski okvir' (ram) ili 'Balkanska metoda' i njegov tvorac. **Srp Arh Celok Lek** 1984 Jan;112(1):127–36

## OSTEOPATHY

Soutas-Little RW: Louisa Burns memorial lecture: biomechanics and osteopathic manipulative treatment. **J Am Osteopath Assoc** 1983 Sep;83(1):63–5

**1700 to Present**

Gryfe CI: James E. Kadwo Kwegyir Aggrey, D.D., D.O., 1875–1927. **Scalpel Tongs** 1981;25:53–5

**Canada**

Gray C: Osteopathy: is there a place in Canadian medicine? **Can Med Assoc J** 1981 Jul 1;125(1):108–11

**Germany**

Seufert WD: The chain osteotome by Heine. **J Hist Med Allied Sci** 1980 Oct;35(4):454–9

**United States**

Baer HA: The organizational rejuvenation of osteopathy: a reflection of the decline of professional dominance in medicine. **Soc Sci Med [A]** 1981 Sep;15(5):701–11
Finlayson G: Osteopathic hospitals and AOHA. United in progress for 50 years. **OH** 1984 Sep;28(8):12–4
Finlayson G: The birth of a profession: osteopathic medicine. **OH** 1984 Sep;28(8):16–7
Gevitz N: The D.O.'s Osteopathic medicine in America. Baltimore, London, Johns Hopkins University Press, 1982. x, 183 p.
Greenman PE: Osteopathic medicine--origins and outlook. **Postgrad Med** 1980 Nov;68(5):31, 33
Keeney EB, Lederer SE, Minihan EP: Sectarians and scientists: alternatives to orthodox medicine. In Numbers RL, Leavitt JW, ed: Wisconsin medicine. Historical perspectives. Madison, University of Wisconsin Press, 1981. p. 47–74.
Mercer SR: America's minority medical profession. In: Congrès international d'histoire de la médecine, XXVe, Québec, 1976. Actes. Québec, 1977. p. 969–79.
Northup GW: Louisa Burns Memorial Lecture: Re--search. **J Am Osteopath Assoc** 1984 Sep;84(1):67–70
Osteopathic hospitals: an historical glimpse: **OH** 1976 Nov–Dec;20(11):12–4
Reed K, Perakis CR: Medical historiography: its place in osteopathic medicine. Parts I and II. **J Am Osteopath Assoc** 1984 Jun;83(10):738–44
Thompson RL, Chico C: The first 40 years of osteopathic medicine in New Jersey. **J Med Soc NJ** 1984 Sep;81(9):798–801
Wren GR: The history of osteopathic medicine in Georgia. Atlanta, Georgia State University, 1978. iii, 39 p. (Occasional publications of the Institute of Health Administration, Georgia State University, no. 18).

## OTORHINOLARYNGOLOGY

Barbaix M, Clotuche J, Jonckere P de, et al: Naissance et développement de l'Oto-rhino-laryngologie dans l'histoire de la médecine. **Acta Otorhinolaryngol Belg** 1981;35 Suppl 2:1–392
Barbaix M, Clotuche J, De Jonckere P, et al: Naissance et développement de l'oto-rhino-laryngologie dans l'histoire de la médecine. (Suite). **Acta Otorhinolaryngol Belg** 1981;35 Suppl 4:1045–622 contd
Bořík O: Vstřebávací schopnost anatomick ych část i ucha pro léčiva jako jev známý již v historické medicíně. **Cesk Fysiol** 1979;28(5):463–70
Earlam R, Cunha-Melo JR: Benign oesophageal strictures; historical and technical aspects of dilatation. **Br J Surg** 1981 Dec;68(12):829–36
Eisenberg I: A history of rhinoplasty. **S Afr Med J** 1982 Aug 21;62(9):286–92
Guerrier Y, Mounier-Kuhn P: Histoire des maladies de l'oreille, du nez et de la gorge. Les grandes étapes de l'otorhino-laryngologie. Paris, Dacosta. 1980. 492 p.
Hauben DJ: Die Geschichte der Rhinoplastik. **Laryngol Rhinol Otol (Stuttg)** 1983 Feb;62(2):53–5
Hedman D: Medicinhistoriska synpunkter på avhuggna näsor och andra näsdefekter. **Nord Medicinhist Arsb** 1981;:40–51
Lawrence M: Otologic research and the Zeitgeist. **Ear Hear** 1983 Mar–Apr;4(2):73–8
Leden H von: Laryngology: from Galen to Garcia. **Otolaryngol Head Neck Surg** 1982 Mar–Apr;90(2):226–32
Micheli Pellegrini V: Histoire des glandes salivaires. **Acta Otorhinolaryngol Belg** 1981;35(2):351–92
O'Neill YV: Speech and speech disorders in Western thought before 1600. Westport, Connecticut, Greenwood, 1980. xii, 246 p. (Contributions in medical history, No. 3).
Pappas DG: The origin of aural instruments. **Am J Otol** 1979 Oct;1(2):121–4
Pariente L: De la synanche à l'angine. Paris, Pariente, 1982. 250 p.
Patterson T: La fabbrica dei nasi. **Kos** 1984 Apr;1(3):75–90
Pialoux P, Soudant J: Geschichte der Hals-, Nasen- und Ohrenheilkunde. In Sournia JC, Martiny M, Poulet J, ed: Illustrierte Geschichte der Medizin. Salzburg, Andreas, 1980. Vol. 7. p. 2711–47.
Politzer A: History of otology. Volume I. From earliest times to the middle of the nineteenth century. An English translation by S. Milstein, C. Portnoff, A. Coleman from the original German edition (Stuttgart, 1907). Phoenix, Columella Press, 1981. xv, 324 p.
Saban R: Les sinus veineux méningés à travers les traités d'anatomie du XVe au XIXe siècle. In: Congrès National des Sociétés Savantes, 106e, Perpignan, 1981. Comptes Rendus. Paris, Bibliothèque Nationale, 1982. Fasc. IV. p. 119–31.
Shehata MA: History of laryngeal intubation. **Middle East J Anaesthesiol** 1981 Feb;6(1):49–53
Stephens SD: Some historical aspects of ototoxicity. **Br J Audiol** 1982 May;16(2):76–80
Tainmont J: La langue grecque classique et le vocabulaire ORL d'aujourd'hui. **Acta Otorhinolaryngol Belg** 1982;36(6):1039–60
Willemot J: Anatomie et traumatismes du nez. Septorhinoplastie. Nez et esthétique. **Acta Otorhinolaryngol Belg** 1981;35(2):201–350
Willemot J: Naissance et développement de l'oto-rhino-laryngologie dans l'histoire de la médecine. **Acta Otorhinolaryngol Belg** 1981;35(Suppl 3):393–1044
Willemot J: Rhinologie, Pharyngologie. **Acta Otorhinolaryngol Belg** 1981,35(2):11–200
Wilson KS: Mandibular reconstruction: introduction. **Otolaryngol Head Neck Surg** 1982 Sep–Oct;90(5):576
Yonkers AJ: My specialty: otorhinolaryngology and maxillofacial surgery. **Nebr Med J** 1981 Jan;66(1):4–5

**China**

Yang D: [10 kinds of symptom and sign of the pharynx and throat in ancient Chinese historical materials] (Chi).

**Chung Hua I Shih Tsa Chih** 1984 Jan;14(1):4–6

### Before 500 A.D.

#### Spain

Vives E, Campillo D: Otoantritis en un individuo del dolmen del Torrent (Girona). In International Congress of the History of Medicine, 27th, Barcelona, 1980. Actas. Barcelona, Académia de Ciències Mèdiques de Catalunya i Balears, 1981. p. 671–4.

### 500 A.D.–1450

#### Arabic

Iskhaki IuB, Kal'shteĭn LI: Rol' Abu Ali Ibn-Siny v razvitii otorinolaringologii. **Vestn Otorinolaringol** 1980 Nov–Dec;(6):81–5
Lakshmipathi G: Avicenna on ear, nose and throat diseases. **Bull Indian Inst Hist Med (Hyderabad)** 1981;1–4:79–82
Shehata MA: The larynx in Islamic medicine. **Middle East J Anaesthesiol** 1981 Jun;6(2):113–9
Willemot J: Le nez et la gorge dans le poème de la médecine et le premier livre du Canon d'Avicenne. In International Congress of the History of Medicine, 27th, Barcelona, 1980. Actas. Barcelona, Académia de Ciències Mèdiques de Catalunya i Balears, 1981. p. 766–70.

#### Spain

Vives E, Campillo D: Hipertrofia de un cornete nasal en una mujer procedente del cementerio medieval de Sant Marçal en Avinyó (Barcelona). In International Congress of the History of Medicine, 27th, Barcelona, 1980. Actas. Barcelona, Académia de Ciències Mèdiques de Catalunya i Balears, 1981. p. 669–70.

#### United States

Gregg JB, Steele JP, Zimmerman L, et al: Otolaryngic osteopathology in 14th century mid-America. The crow creek massacre. **Ann Otol Rhinol Laryngol** 1981 May–Jun;90(3 pt 1):288–93

### 1450–1700

Eden AR, Opland J: Bartolommeo Eustachio's De Auditus Organis and the unique murder plot in Shakespeare's Hamlet. **N Engl J Med** 1982 Jul 22;307(4):259–61

#### Germany

Pirsig W: Hals-Nasen-Ohrenheilkunde im Werk des Ulmer Stadtarztes Johannes Scultetus (1595–1645). **HNO** 1984 Apr;32(4):149–54

### 1700 to Present

Canalis RF: Laryngeal ventricle. Historical features. **Ann Otol Rhinol Laryngol** 1980 Mar–Apr;89(2 Pt 1):184–7
Catlin FI: Pioneers in stapedectomy. **Am J Otolaryngol** 1983 May–Jun;4(3):217
Diamant H: Robert Bárány och Nobel-priset. **Sydsven Medicinhist Sallsk Arsskr** 1984;21:123–8
Ergetowski R: Akta personalne prof. Antoniego Stanisława Jurasza w Heidelbergu i Karlsruhe. **Arch Hist Med (Warsz)** 1983;46(2):215–35
Fitz-Hugh GS: Anesthesia in otolaryngology: historical overview. **Otolaryngol Clin North Am** 1981 Aug;14(3):467–81
García Ballester L: Factores sociomédicos en el proceso de constitución de las especialidades médicas: el caso de la otología. In Albarracin Teulon A, et al, ed: Medicina e Historia. Madrid, Edic. Univ. Comp., 1973. p. 321–38.
Gersdorff M: Evolution des techniques d'audiométrie objective de 1970 à 1980. **Acta Otorhinolaryngol Belg** 1981;35(3–4):274–80
Gibson WP: The operating microscope and the development of ear surgery. **J R Soc Med** 1980 Jan;73(1):53–5
Goodman WS, Wallace IR: Tympanoplasty--25 years later. **J Otolaryngol** 1980 Apr;9(2):155–64
Hellström S, Stenfors LE: The original description of Shrapnell's membrane reviewed in the light of recent experimental studies. **J Laryngol Otol** 1983 Nov;97(11):985–9
Hickson FS, Newton VE: Sound localization. Part I: a brief history. **J Laryngol Otol** 1981 Jan;95(1):29–40
Hillel AD: History of stapedectomy. **Am J Otolaryngol** 1983 Mar–Apr;4(2):131–40
Jahn AF: Stapes surgery in the nineteenth century. **Am J Otol** 1981 Jul;3(1):74–8
Jephcott A: The Macintosh laryngoscope. A historical note on its clinical and commercial development. **Anaesthesia** 1984 May;39(5):474–9
Lavie P: Nasal obstructions, sleep, and mental function. **Sleep** 1983;6(3):244–6
Lowry LD: Artificial larynges: a review and development of a prototype self-contained intra-oral artificial larynx. **Laryngoscope** 1981 Aug;91(8):1332–55
Michel J: Recherches historiques sur la découverte des maladies des sinus, le XIXe siècle. **J Fr Otorhinolaryngol** 1979 Nov;28(9):577–90
Milstein S: The history of mastoid surgery. **Am J Otol** 1980 Jan;1(3):174–8
Missotten FE: Historical review of pharyngo-oesophageal reconstruction after resection for carcinoma of pharynx and cervical oesophagus. **Clin Otolaryngol** 1983 Oct;8(5):345–62
Pappas DG: Barany's History of Vestibular Physiology. Translation and commentary. **Ann Otol Rhinol Laryngol [Suppl]** 1984 Mar–Apr;110:1–16
Pensak ML, Yanagisawa E: Tympanic membrane photography: historical perspective. **Am J Otol** 1984 Apr;5(4):324–32
Pirsig W: Septumdeviation 1882: Beginn der systematischen submukösen Septumchirurgie. **Laryngol Rhinol Otol (Stuttg)** 1982 Oct;61(10):547–51
Portmann M, Bebear JP, Bagot D'Arc M: L'histoire de l'otosclérose du XIXe siècle à 1952. **Acta Otorhinolaryngol Belg** 1982;36(2):297–305
Pracy R: Recent developments in paediatric otolaryngology. **J Laryngol Otol** 1981 Nov;95(11):1097–108
Rhys Evans PH: Prominent ears and their surgical correction. **J Laryngol Otol** 1981 Sep;95(9):9881–92
Shambaugh GE: Pre and post-antibiotic otology. **Rev Laryngol Otol Rhinol (Bord)** 1980 Nov–Dec;101(11–12):529–36
Shea JJ: Management of the stapes footplate with special reference to otosclerosis. **J Laryngol Otol** 1982 May;96(5):383–403
Simpson GT, Polanyi TG: History of the carbon dioxide laser in otolaryngologic surgery. **Otolaryngol Clin North Am** 1983 Nov;16(4):739–52
Stock CR: Laryngoscopy. **Ear Nose Throat J** 1984 Oct;63(10):528–30
Weerda H, Karl F, Müller-Hermann E: Die Entwicklung der Laryngoskopie. **HNO** 1984 Jul;32(7):307–11
Willemot J: L'endoscopie en oto-rhino-laryngologie de 1850 à 1950. **J Fr Otorhinolaryngol** 1983 Apr;32(4):233–6

#### Australia

Lowe RF: Early Melbourne eye and ear hospital, and Dr. Turnbull's house at 101 (157) Spring Street. **Aust NZ J Surg** 1980 Oct;50(5):546–9
Lowe RF: John Box (1863–1934) and William Box (1905–1982). **Aust J Ophthalmol** 1983 Feb;11(1):51–3
Lowe RF: William R. Wilde, Andrew S. Gray, and two eye and ear hospitals of very similar name. **Aust NZ J Surg** 1981 Dec;51(6):630–6

#### Austria

Majer EH: Zur Geschichte der HNO-Heilkunde in Oesterreich. **Laryngol Rhinol Otol (Stuttg)** 1980 Jul;59(7):406–11
Stool SE: A historical vignette: memoirs of an otologist's European study in 1883. **Am J Otol** 1983 Apr;4(4):346–9

#### Czechoslovakia

Barta T: História otolaryngologickej starostlivosti v Bratislave. **Cesk Otolaryngol** 1984 Jul;33(4):268–71
Barta T, Klačanský I: Tridsat rokov Slovenskej otolaryngologickej spoločnosti. **Cesk Otolaryngol** 1984 Feb;33(1):47–51
Bečer A, Tichý M: Začiatky otolaryngológie na lekárskej fakulte UK v Bratislave. **Bratisl Lek Listy** 1983;79(3):369–74
Klačanský I: Rozvoj detskej otolaryngológie na Slovensku. **Cesk Otolaryngol** 1984 Jun;33(3):193–4
Kontúrová Z: 30 rokov logopédie v zdravotníctve na Slovensku. **Cesk Otolaryngol** 1983 Jun;32(3):188–91
Kuniak B, Strelka J: Vývoj chirurgie strmienka pri otoskleróze na Slovensku. **Bratisl Lek Listy** 1983;79(2):222–6
Novák A: Doc. MUDr. Eva Sedláčková, csc., a československá foniatrie. **Cesk Otolaryngol** 1982 Apr;31(2):68–71
Sedláček K: Sedesáté výročí založení československé foniatrie prof. MUDr. Miloslavem Seemanem, DrSc. **Cesk Otolaryngol** 1982 Apr;31(2):65–8
Síbl O: Katedra otolaryngologie v rámci třicetileté činnosti institutu pro další vzdělávání lékařu a farmaceutu. **Cesk Otolaryngol** 1983 Jun;32(3):171–5

#### France

Chalat NI: Jean Marc Gaspard Itard – 1774–1838. **Laryngoscope** 1982 Jun;92(6 Pt 1):627–9
Charbonnel A: Histoire de l'oto-neuro-ophtalmologie. **Rev Otoneuroophtalmol** 1979 Oct–Dec;51(5):399–416
Cinquantenaire de la Société d'Oto-Rhino-Laryngologie de Lyon et de la Région. Le ler mars 1931: **J Fr Otorhinolaryngol** 1982 Jun;31(6):389–96
Herrera Casado A: Aportación francesa a la amigdalectomiá. **An Otorrinolaringol Ibero Am** 1981;8(6):487–94
Huard P, Wong M: Ablation d'un polype naso-pharyngien à la Trinité en 1812. In: Congrès National des Sociétés Savantes, 91e, Rennes, 1966. Comptes Rendus. Paris, 1967. Section des Sciences, Tome 1. p. 99–102.
Legée G: La découverte des fonctions des canaux semi-circulaires de l'oreille interne. In: Congrès National des Sociétés Savantes, 91e, Rennes, 1966. Comptes Rendus. Paris, 1967. Section des Sciences, Tome 1. p.

291-300.
Lisfranc J: Mémoire sur la rhynoplastie, ou l'art de refaire le nez. **Ann Chir Plast** 1982;27(2):189-93
Morgon A: L'oto-rhino-laryngologie et la communication humaine. **J Fr Otorhinolaryngol** 1982 Jun;31(6):405-8
Pappas DG, Galanos AN: Prosper Ménière: beyond the controversial autopsy report. **South Med J** 1982 Apr;75(4):470-2
Perello J: The Bordeaux School of ENT in the nineteenth century as seen by a Spanish practitioner, Ricardo Botey. **Rev Laryngol Otol Rhinol (Bord)** 1980 Jan-Feb;101(1-2):15-30
Portmann G: The 'Revue de Laryngologie' and the E. N. T. School of Bordeaux are a hundred years old. **Rev Laryngol Otol Rhinol (Bord)** 1980 Jan-Feb;101(1-2):1-14
Un siècle d'oto-rhino-laryngologie: **J Fr Otorhinolaryngol** 1983 Feb;32(2):81-110 contd

**Germany**

Becker KP, Sovák M: Lehrbuch der Logopädie. 2. Auflage. Königstein/Ts., Verlagsgruppe Athenäum, Hain, Scriptor, Hanstein, 1979. Historical section, p. 31-48.
Habermann G: Max Joseph Oertel 1835-1897. **Folia Phoniatr (Basel)** 1983;35(1-2):91
Hauben DJ: Jacques Joseph (1865-1934). **Laryngol Rhinol Otol (Stuttg)** 1983 Feb;62(2):56-7
Hellmich S, Hellmich J: Der Zwischenkieferknochen und Goethes Mephistopheles. **Laryngol Rhinol Otol (Stuttg)** 1982 Oct;61(10):552-6
Jakobi H: Hermann Schwartze. 100 Jahre Ohrchirurgie in Halle/S. **Wiss Z Martin Luther Univ (Math)** 1976;25(2):109-12
Lange G: Die Vereinigung Westdeutscher Hals-, Nasen- und Ohrenärzte besteht im 85-sten Jahr. **HNO** 1982 Mar;30(3):114-5
Schwann H: Anton Jurasz's Bedeutung für die Rhinolaryngologie aus heutiger Sicht. **Arch Hist Med (Warsz)** 1979;42(3):317-21
Schwartz RH: The pneumatic otoscope, a new instrument for the examination of the tympanic membrane--E. Siegle. 1984. **Int J Pediatr Otorhinolaryngol** 1980 Sep;2(3):261-3
Wentges RT: Wilhelm Fliess en de nasale reflexneurose. **Ned Tijdschr Geneeskd** 1981 Feb 14;125(7):278-84
Wullstein HL: Das Schicksal unserer HNO-Zeitschrift bei der Neugründung nach dem Kriege. **HNO** 1980 Jan;28(1):33-4

**Great Britain**

Chalat NI: Sir Morell Mackenzie revisited. **Laryngoscope** 1984 Oct;94(10):1307-10
Fisch L: Development of school screening audiometry. **Br J Audiol** 1981 May;15(2):87-95
Macbeth R: Sir Terence Edward Cawthorne. In Dictionary of national biography, 1961-1970. Suppl. 8, 1981. p. 179-80.
McGovern FH: Sir Astley Cooper and his otological papers. **Ann Otol Rhinol Laryngol** 1984 Nov-Dec;93(6 Pt 1):531-3
McGovern FH: The elusive Henry Jones Shrapnell. **Laryngoscope** 1983 Jul;93(7):903-5
Stephens SD: David Edward Hughes and his audiometer. **J Laryngol Otol** 1979 Jan;93(1):1-6
Whitteridge D, Merton PA: Charles Skinner Hallpike: 19 July 1900-26 September 1979. **Biogr Mem Fellows R Soc** 1984;30:283-95
Wilson TG: Historical vignette. Sir Astley Cooper. **Am J Otol** 1984 Jul;5(5):411-4

**Hungary**

Mester AF: Six great men in Hungarian otorhinolaryngology. **Am J Otolaryngol** 1982 Jan-Feb;3(1):67-72
Torok N: Robert Bárány. **JAMA** 1980 Dec 5;244(22):2520

**Ireland**

Pappas DG: Sir William Wilde: a historical review. **Ear Nose Throat J** 1983 Jun;62(6):58, 60-2

**Italy**

Milstein S: Domenico Cotugno. **Am J Otol** 1982 Jul;4(1):95-7
Phelps PD, Lloyd GA, Windle-Taylor PC, et al: Mondini dysplasia. **Ann Otol Rhinol Laryngol** 1982 Mar-Apr;91(2 Pt 1):254

**Japan**

Ono J: Legacies of Jefferson men to Japanese medicine. **Ann Otol Rhinol Laryngol [Suppl]** 1981 Sep-Oct;90(5 pt 2 Suppl 87):1-10

**Kenya**

Meschig R, Schadewaldt H: Uvulektomie--ein Initiationsritus? **MMW** 1981;123(11):437-40

**Mexico**

del Villar R: La otología en el Hospital Infantil de México; evolución y enseñanza. **Bol Med Hosp Infant Mex** 1983 Aug;40 Suppl 2:22-7

**Mongolia**

Shagdar L: Otorinolaringologiia v Mongol'skoï Narodnoï Respublike. **Vestn Otorinolaringol** 1982 Mar-Apr;(2):59-62

**Poland**

Ceypek T: Uzupełnienie do artykułu pt. 'Klinika Laryngologii w 30-leciu Slaskiej Akademii Medycznej'. **Otolaryngol Pol** 1979;33(6):671-2
Iwankiewicz S, Kossowski S: Klinika Otolaryngologiczna AM we Wrocławiu (1948-1978). **Otolaryngol Pol** 1980;34(2-3):141-65
Semczuk B: XXXV-lecie Lubelskiej Kliniki Otolaryngologicznej. **Otolaryngol Pol** 1980;34(1):113-6
Sienkiewicz H: Wspomnienie pośmiertne o doc. dr. med. Romanie Karwowskim. **Otolaryngol Pol** 1980;34(4):417-9
Waspomnienie pósmiertne o prof. dr med. Tadeuszu Bardadinie.: **Otolaryngol Pol** 1980;34(1):I-VI

**Romania**

Miloşescu P, Bercuş CI: Constituirea otorinolaringologiei ca specialitate medicală în România. **Rev Chir [Otorinolaringol]** 1979 Apr-Jun;24(2):145-8

**Spain**

Botey i Puig A: L'obra del Dr. Ricard Botey i Ducoing. In Congrés Internacional d'Historie de la Medicina Catalana, 1st, Barcelona-Montpellier, 1970. Barcelona, Editorial Scientia, 1971. v 4, p. 20-6.
Perelló J: Historia de la otorrinolaringología en España. **An Otorrinolaringol Ibero Am** 1979;6(6):405-81

**Sweden**

Gejrot T: Frans Vilhelm Törne. **Sydsven Medicinhist Sallsk Arsskr** 1984;21:129-34

**Switzerland**

Terrier G: Louis Secrétan et les débuts de l'enseignement de l'ORL en Suisse Romande. **Acta Otorhinolaryngol Belg** 1982;36(2):306-10

**Thailand**

Varavej P: The history of otorhinolaryngology in Thailand. **Adv Otorhinolaryngol** 1983;29:1-5

**United States**

Altman SB: A brief history of South Dakota Academy of Ophthalmology and Otorhinolaryngology. **SD J Med** 1981 May;34(5):39
Anderson JR: An old medical specialty puts on a new face...and head...and neck. **South Med J** 1980 Aug;73(8):1058-62
Bordley JE: History of research training. **Arch Otolaryngol** 1982 Oct;108(10):612-5
Bordley JE: The American Rhinologic Society: its foundation and its future responsibilities. **Laryngoscope** 1980 May;90(5 Pt 1):876-9
Borkenhagen R, Hipskind M, Lewy R: Reminiscences of otorhinolaryngology from Loyola University and Hines Veterans Hospital. **Proc Inst Med Chic** 1982 Apr-Jun;35(2):51-2
Bryan SA: Pioneering specialists: a history of the American Academy of Ophthalmology and Otolaryngology. San Francisco, American Academy of Ophthalmology, Rochester, Minn.: American Academy of Otolaryngology-Head and Neck Surgery, 1982. viii, 305 p.
Bryant BJ: The Harvard residency program in otolaryngology: an overview. **Am J Otol** 1979 Jul;1(1):60-3
Bryant BJ: The residency program in otolaryngology at Baylor College of Medicine. **Am J Otol** 1979 Oct;1(2):132-4
Bryce DP, Nuis DB, ed: The American Laryngological Association, 1878-1978. Washington, American Laryngological Assn., 1978. xiv, 152 p.
Butler RA: Basic science researcher in otolaryngology at the University of Chicago. **Ann Otol Rhinol Laryngol [Suppl]** 1983 Jan-Feb;102:27-9
Catlin FI: Pulmonary complications of tonsillectomy as originally described by Samuel J. Crowe, M.D. **Laryngoscope** 1981 Jan;91(1):52-61
Fernandez C: Pioneers in research in otolaryngology at the University of Chicago. **Ann Otol Rhinol Laryngol [Suppl]** 1983 Jan-Feb;102:23-6
Fifteen years of the Otological Research Laboratory, Baylor College of Medicine: **Acta Otolaryngol [Suppl] (Stockh)** 1983;393:1-112
Fredrickson JM: Otoneurology. **Ann Otol Rhinol Laryngol [Suppl]** 1983 Jan-Feb;102:17-9

Friedberg SA: The memorable life of Hosmer A. Johnson, early midwestern laryngologist. **Ann Otol Rhinol Laryngol** 1983 Sep–Oct;92(5 Pt 1):470–2
Gay EC, Anderson J, Graham SS: An old medical specialty puts on a new face ... and head ... neck. **J Arkansas Med Soc** 1982 Feb;78(9):359–62
Hanckel RW: A brief history of otolaryngology and head and neck surgery in South Carolina. **J SC Med Assoc** 1984 Aug;80(8):376–7
Kohut RI: The clinical research of John Lindsay. **Ann Otol Rhinol Laryngol [Suppl]** 1983 Jan–Feb;102:20–2
Mhoon EE, Lanzl EF, ed: John Ralston Lindsay, MD, 1898–1981. Contributions by H. F. Schuknecht, J. M. Fredrickson, R. I. Kohut, C. Fernandez, R. A. Butler, R. F. Naunton. (Supplement 102). **Ann Otol Rhinol Laryngol [Suppl]** 1983 Jan–Feb;92(1 Pt.3):1–36
Mounier-Kuhn P: Un siècle d'oto-rhino-laryngologie. **J Fr Otorhinolaryngol** 1983 Jan;32(1):12–30
Naunton RF: Clinical research in otolaryngology at the University of Chicago. **Ann Otol Rhinol Laryngol [Suppl]** 1983 Jan–Feb;102:30–1
Pratt LW: Chiron's contributions. **Arch Otolaryngol** 1980 Nov;106(11):662–7
Publications by John R. Lindsay: **Ann Otol Rhinol Laryngol [Suppl]** 1983 Jan–Feb;102:33–6
Romm S: Morris Joseph Asch. **Plast Reconstr Surg** 1983 May;71(5):724–8
Schuknecht HF: Harvard Medical School and the Massachusetts Eye and Ear Infirmary. **Adv Otorhinolaryngol** 1983;31:1–7
Shambaugh GE: French Keller Hansel and the history of allergy. **Arch Otolaryngol** 1983 Feb;109(2):126–9
Stool SE, Brown SL: Ellen James Patterns, MD. **Arch Otolaryngol** 1983 Jan;109(1):60–1
Stool SE, Kemper M, Kemper B: The compleat otolaryngologist: Burton Alexander Randall. **Laryngoscope** 1984 Jan;94(1):16–9
Watson JA: The residency program in otolaryngology at the Washington University School of Medicine. **Am J Otol** 1980;1:247–9
Wechsler HL: Chevalier Jackson. In Dictionary of American Biography, Suppl. 6, 1956–1960. p. 317–18, 1980.
Work WP: The American Board of Otolaryngology: 1950–1979. **Ann Otol Rhinol Laryngol [Suppl]** 1982 Mar–Apr;90:1–8

### USSR

Arkhangel'skiĭ GV: V. E. Larionov--odin iz osnovopolozhnikov otechestvennoĭ otonevrologii. **Vestn Otorinolaringol** 1984 Mar–Apr;(2):88–93
Gorokhov AA, Gofman VR: K istorii razvitiia spetsializirovannoĭ otorinolaringologicheskoĭ pomoshchi. **Voen Med Zh** 1981 Aug;(8):76–7
Kharshak EM: Nauchnaia deiatel'nost' oblastnykh obshchestv otolaringologov v USSR za period 1957–1978 gg. (po protokolam i godovym otchetam obshchestv, opublikovannym v ZhUNGB s 1959 po 1978 g.). **Zh Ushn Nos Gorl Bolezn** 1980 May–Jun;(3):56–64
Kostrov NI: Opyt sovetskoĭ voennoĭ otorinolaringologii v Velikoĭ Otechestvennoĭ voĭne. **Voen Med Zh** 1980 Aug;(8):17–9
Preobrazhenskiĭ NA, Konstantinova NP: Vsesoiuznoe nauchnoe obshchestvo otorinolaringologov k 60-letiiu obrazovaniia SSSR. **Vestn Otorinolaringol** 1982 Nov–Dec;(6):8–13
Razvitie otorinolaringologii v Glavnom voennom klinicheskom gospitale imeni N. N. Burdenko (k 275-letiiu osnovaniia gospitalia): **Voen Med Zh** 1982;(9):67–8

### Yugoslavia

Djordjević SP: Prvo Otorinolaringološko odeljenje u Srbiji u Opštoj državnoj bolnici u Beogradu, i prvi otorinolaringolog dr Dragoljub Sraga. **Srp Arh Celok Lek** 1982 Oct;110(10):1245–60
Djordjević SP: Stampani radovi i prikazi bolesnika prvog otorhinolaringologa u Beogradu i Srbiji dr Dragoljuba Srage. **Srp Arh Celok Lek** 1982 Oct;110(10):1261–6

## PALEOPATHOLOGY

Ahlström CG: Ett gammalt museum berattar; glimtar från patologiska institutionens museum i Lund. **Sydsven Medicinhist Sallsk Arsskr** 1982;:15–31
Andrik P, Stukovský R: K otázkám terminálnej redukcie chrupu. **Cesk Stomatol** 1980 Jul;80(4):242–5
Angel JL: History and development of paleopathology. **Am J Phys Anthropol** 1981 Dec;56(4):509–15
Angel JL: Physical anthropology: determining sex, age, and individual features. In A. Cockburn, E. Cockburn, ed: Mummies, disease, and ancient cultures. Cambridge, Cambridge University Press, 1980. p. 241–57.
Ascenzi A, Cockburn A, Kleiss E: Miscellaneous mummies. In A. Cockburn, E. Cockburn, ed: Mummies, disease, and ancient cultures. Cambridge, Cambridge University Press, 1980. p. 224–38.
Baker J: Animal diseases in archaeology. London, New York, Academic Press, 1980. ix, 235 p.
Barraco RA: Paleobiochemistry. In A. Cockburn, E. Cockburn, ed: Mummies, disease, and ancient cultures. Cambridge, Cambridge University Press, 1980. p. 312–26.
Benitez JT, Lynn GE: Temporal bone studies. In A. Cockburn, E. Cockburn, ed: Mummies, disease, and ancient cultures. Cambridge, Cambridge University Press, 1980. p. 301–11.
Bliquez LJ: Classical prosthetics. **Archaeology** 1983 Sep–Oct;36(5):25–9
Bromage TG, Horne PD: Stafne defect: a histological approach. **Paleopathol Newsl** 1981 Jan;33:7–9
Buikstra JE, Gordon CC: The study and restudy of human skeletal series: the importance of long term curation. **Ann NY Acad Sci** 1981;376:449–65
Burns PE: Log-linear analysis of dental caries occurrence in four skeletal series. **Am J Phys Anthropol** 1979 Nov;51(4):637–47
Caccialanza E: Il problema delle cranioplastiche dal punto di vista storico ed etio-patogenetico. **Minerva Chir** 1983 Jun 30;38(12):815–8
Campillo D, Viñas R: Contribución a la paleopatología a través del arte rupestre. In International Congress of the History of Medicine, 27th, Barcelona, 1980. Actas. Barcelona, Académia de Ciències Médiques de Catalunya i Balears, 1981. p. 462–71.
Casey AE, Copeland H, Downey-Prince EL, et al: Differential craniometry: (A) Maori 3000 BC--Thera? (B). Ptolemaic Egyptians--New Guinea, America. **Ala J Med Sci** 1979 Oct;16(4):382–9
Chapel A, Mehregan AH, Reyman TA: Histologic findings in mummified skin. **J Am Acad Dermatol** 1981 Jan;4(1):27–30
Cockburn A, Cockburn E, ed: Mummies, disease, and ancient cultures. Cambridge, Cambridge University Press, 1980. x, 340 p.
Cockburn E, Reyman TA: Paleopathology. **JAMA** 1982 Jul 23;248(4):472–3
Colangelo G, Luzi V, Mattioni R: Analisi craniometrica comparativa tra crani etruschi e moderni. **Dent Cadmos** 1982 Jan;50(1):47–51
Corruccini RS, Ciochon RL: Primate facial allometry and interpretations of australopithecine variation. **Nature** 1979 Sep 6;281(5726):62–4
Covert HH, Kay RF: Dental microwear and diet: implications for determining the feeding behaviors of extinct primates, with a comment on the dietary patterns of Sivapithecus. **Am J Phys Anthropol** 1981 Jul;55(3):331–6
Dastugue J: Die Paläopathologie. In Sournia JC, Martiny M, Poulet J, ed: Illustrierte Geschichte der Medizin. Salzburg, Andreas, 1980. Vol. 1. p. 19–47.
Dastugue J: Les maladies de nos ancêtres. **Recherche** 1982;(136):980–8
Doerr W: Evolutionstheorie und pathologische Anatomie. **Verh Dtsch Ges Pathol** 1983;67:663–84
Domen RE: Paleopathological evidence of rheumatoid arthritis. **JAMA** 1981 Oct 23–30;246(17):1899
Földes V, Kósa F, Virágos-Kis E, et al: Atomabsorptions-spektrophotometrische Untersuchung des Gehaltes an anorganischen Substanzen von Skelettbefunden zur Ermittlung der Dauer des Begrabenseins in der Erde. **Arch Kriminol** 1980 Sep–Oct;166(3–4):105–11
Gantt DG: A method of interpreting enamel prism patterns. **Scan Electron Microsc** 1979;(3):491–6
Glazer J: Ancestors. **J Am Dent Assoc** 1984 Jul;109(1):17
Gow CE: The dentitions of the Tritheledontidae (therapsida: cynodontia). **Proc R Soc Lond [Biol]** 1980 Jul 17;208(1173):461–81
Grant PG: A prehistoric case of congenital radioulnar synostosis. **Ossa** 1978;5:13–15
Gürtler LG, Jäger V, Gruber W, et al: Presence of proteins in human bones 200, 1200 and 1500 years of age. **Hum Biol** 1981 Feb;53(1):137–50
Hart GD, ed: Disease in ancient man. An international symposium held in London, 1979. Toronto, Clarke Irwin, 1983. 297 p. Contributions by D. A. Birkett, F. F. Cartwright, R. Cramp, J. Dobson, A. J. Duggan, N. G. Gejvall, P. S. Gooch, C. J. Hackett, P. D. Horne, P. Janssens, B. Knight, A. K. Knowles, N. B. Millet, V. Møller-Christensen, W. J. Moore, R. Perrot, F. D. Pooley, D. F. Rideout, A. Rook, W. M. Russell, P. Slack, W. E. Swinton, H. A. Waldron.
Henry RL: Paleoserology. In A. Cockburn, E. Cockburn, ed: Mummies, disease, and ancient cultures. Cambridge, Cambridge University Press, 1980. p. 327–34.
Hübener KH, Pahl WM: Computertomographische Untersuchungen an altägyptischen Mumien. **ROFO** 1981 Aug;135(2):213–9
Janssens PA: Antropologisch en paleopathologisch onderzoek van de beenderresten uit het centrale graf in de Onze-Lieve-Vrouwe-kerk te Brugge. De identificatie van de hertogin Maria van Bourgondie. **Verh K Acad Geneeskd Belg** 1981;43(4–5):213–70
Kelley MA: Intervertebral osteochondrosis in ancient and modern populations. **Am J Phys Anthropol** 1982 Nov;59(3):271–9
Kristen KT, Reyman TA: Radiographic examination of mummies with autopsy correlation. In A. Cockburn, E. Cockburn, ed: Mummies, disease, and ancient cultures. Cambridge, Cambridge University Press, 1980. p. 287–300.
Krukoff S: Utilisation, en craniologie, des vecteurs pour la mise en évidence du degré d'inclinaison du front et de la face chez le chimpanzé, l'homme actuel et fossile. **C R Seances Acad Sci [III]** 1981 May 11;292(17):969–74
Laitman JT, Heimbuch RC: The basicranium of Plio-Pleistocene hominids as an indicator of their upper respiratory system. **Am J Phys Anthropol** 1982 Nov;59(3):323–43
Lowenstam HA, Margulis L: Evolutionary prerequisites for early Phanerozoic calcareous skeletons. **Biosystems** 1980;12(1–2):27–41
Meir E, Gedalia I, Smith P, et al: Analysis for establishing chronological age of bone. **J Oral Rehabil** 1982 Jan;9(1):53–4

# PALEOPATHOLOGY

Meschig R: Zur Geschichte der Trepanation unter besonderer Berücksichtigung der Schädeloperationen bei den Kisii im Hochland Westkenias. Düsseldorf, Triltsch, 1983. xiii, 166 p. (Düsseldorfer Arbeiten zur Geschichte der Medizin, 57).
Moore JG, Krotoszynski BK, O'Neill HJ: Fecal odorgrams. A method for partial reconstruction of ancient and modern diets. **Dig Dis Sci** 1984 Oct;29(10):907–11
Ortner DJ, Putschar WG: Identification of pathological conditions in human skeletal remains. Washington, Smithsonian Institution Press, 1981. 479 p. (Smithsonian Contributions to Anthropology, 28).
Paleopathology Association: Ninth annual meeting and first Aidan Cockburn memorial symposium: Mummies, disease, and ancient cultures: retrospect and prospect. Toledo, Paleopathology Association, 1982. 16 p.
Papers and exhibits on Paleopathology: presented at the Annual Meeting of the Paleopathology Association. Niagara Falls, New York, 16. April, 1980.
Papers on paleopathology: presented at the Annual Meeting of the Paleopathology Association, 22 April, 1981. [Supplement to Paleopathology Newsletter, No. 34, June 1981] **Paleopathol Newsl** 1981 Jun;34:D1–D6
Papers on Paleopathology presented at the Third European Members Meeting of the Paleopathology Association. 1980, Sept. 26–28. Caen, France.: **Paleopathol Newsl** 1980 Dec;32 Suppl:C1–C18
Passi S, Rothschild-Boros MC, Fasella P, et al: An application of high performance liquid chromatography to analysis of lipids in archaelogical samples. **J Lipid Res** 1981 Jul;22(5):778–84
Pérez PJ, Arsuaga JL de: Estudio paleoepidemiológico y paleodemográfico de la necrópolis de Mirmad (Argin-Sur, Nubia sudanesa). In International Congress of the History of Medicine, 27th, Barcelona, 1980. Actas. Barcelona, Acadèmia de Ciències Mèdiques de Catalunya i Balears, 1981. p. 596–602.
Porter RW: Variations in shape and size of the lumbar spinal canal. **Paleopathol Newsl** 1980 Dec;32:9–11
Resnick D, Greenway G: Distal femoral cortical defects, irregularities, and excavations. **Radiology** 1982 May;143(2):345–54
Reyman TA, Dowd AM: Processing of mummified tissue for histological examination. In A. Cockburn, E. Cockburn, ed: Mummies, disease, and ancient cultures. Cambridge, Cambridge University Press, 1980. p. 258–73.
Riddle JM: A survey of ancient specimens by electron microscopy. In A. Cockburn, E. Cockburn, ed: Mummies, disease, and ancient cultures. Cambridge, Cambridge University Press, 1980. p. 274–86.
Rogers J, Dieppe P: Lessons from paleopathology. **Practitioner** 1983 Jul;227(1381):1191–9
Sellevold BJ: Mandibular torus morphology. **Am J Phys Anthropol** 1980 Nov;53(4):569–72
Shapiro HL: Peking man. London, George Allen & Unwin, 1976. 190 p.
Shipman P: Applications of scanning electron microscopy to taphonomic problems. **Ann NY Acad Sci** 1981;376:357–85
Steinbock RT, ed: Annotated bibliography [of paleopathology] **Paleopathol Newsl** 1984 Sep;(47):15–20
Stenn F: The contributions of paleopathology to modern medicine. An update. **Arch Pathol Lab Med** 1981 Dec;105(12):633–7
Stout SD: Histological structure and its preservation in ancient bone. **Curr Anthropol** 1978;19:601–4
Sullivan CH, Krueger HW: Carbon isotope analysis of separate chemical phases in modern and fossil bone. **Nature** 1981 Jul 23;292(5821):333–5
Teaford MF, Walker A: Quantitative differences in dental microwear between primate species with different diets and a comment on the presumed diet of Sivapithecus. **Am J Phys Anthropol** 1984 Jun;64(2):191–200
Theunissen B: Theorie en praktijk van Cuviers Recherches sur les ossemens fossiles. **Tijdschr Geschied Geneeskd** 1983;6(1):1–17
Tyson RA, Alcauskas ES, ed: Catalogue of the Hrdlička paleopathology collection. Foreword and glossary by S. L. Rogers. Descriptions by C. F. Merbs. San Diego, San Diego Museum of Man, 1980. xi, 359 p.
Van Gerven DP: The contribution of time and local geography to craniofacial variation in Nubia's Batn el Hajar. **Am J Phys Anthropol** 1982 Nov;59(3):307–16
Wells C, Woodhouse N: Paget's disease in an Anglo-Saxon. **Med Hist** 1975 Oct;19(4):396–400
Wolpoff MH, Russell MD: Anterior dental cutting at Laetolil. **Am J Phys Anthropol** 1981 Jun;55(2):223–4
Wong PA: Computed tomography in paleopathology: technique and case study. **Am J Phys Anthropol** 1981 May;55(1):101–10
Zimmerman MR: Annotated bibilography of paleopathology: 1970–1979. Part IV, T–Z and Index. **Trans Stud Coll Physicians Phila** 1980 Dec;5(2 no 4):289–314
Zimmerman MR: Annotated bibliography of paleopathology: 1970–1979. Part I, A–C. **Trans Stud Coll Physicians Phila** 1980 Mar;5(2 no 1):41–66
Zimmerman MR: Annotated bibliography of paleopathology: 1970–1979. Part II, D–J. **Trans Stud Coll Physicians Phila** 1980 Jun;5(2 no 2):112–43
Zimmerman MR: Annotated bibliography of paleopathology: 1970–1979; Part III, K–S. **Trans Stud Coll Physicians Phila** 1980 Sep;5(2 no 3):187–222
Zimmerman M, et al: Annotated bibliography [of Paleopathology]. **Paleopathol Newsl** 1980 Sep;(31):17–20. Continued regularly

**Africa**

Lambrecht FL: Palaeoecology of Tsetse flies and sleeping sickness in Africa. **Proc Am Philos Soc** 1980 Oct 10;124(5):367–85

**Americas**

Anjard R: Mayan dental wonders. **J Oral Implantol** 1981;9(3):423–6
Laughlin WS, Harper AB, ed: The first Americans: origins, affinities, and adaptations. New York and Stuttgart, Fischer, 1979. xi, 340 p.
Perzigian AJ: Allometric analysis of dental variation in a human population. **Am J Phys Anthropol** 1981 Mar;54(3):341–5
Pfeiffer S: Paleopathology in an Iroquoian ossuary, with special reference to tuberculosis. **Am J Phys Anthropol** 1984 Oct;65(2):181–9
Richman EA, Ortner DJ, Schulter-Ellis FP: Differences in intracortical bone remodeling in three aboriginal American populations: possible dietary factors. **Calcif Tissue Int** 1979 Nov 6;28(3):209–14
Ryn L: Los Andes y la medicina. **Actas Luso Esp Neurol Psiquiatr** 1981 May–Jun;9(3):213–30, Jul–Aug;9(4):315–24

**Argentina**

Zimmerman MR: Enterobiasis in precolumbian America. **Paleopathol Newsl** 1983 Jun;42:8

**Australia**

Pretty GL, Calder A: Mummification in Australia and Melanesia. In A. Cockburn, E. Cockburn, ed: Mummies, disease, and ancient cultures. Cambridge, Cambridge University Press, 1980. p. 194–210.

**Barbados**

Corruccini RS, Handler JS, Mutaw RJ, et al: Osteology of a slave burial population from Barbados, West Indies. **Am J Phys Anthropol** 1982 Dec;59(4):443–59

**Brazil**

Ferreira LF, Araújo AJ de, Confalonieri UE: The finding of helminth eggs in a Brazilian mummy. **Trans R Soc Trop Med Hyg** 1983;77(1):65–7
Kliks MM: Parasites in archaeological material from Brazil. **Trans R Soc Trop Med Hyg** 1982;76(5):701
Mascarenhas S, Baffa Filho O, Ikeya M: Electron spin resonance dating of human bones from Brazilian shell-mounds (Sambaquís). **Am J Phys Anthropol** 1982 Dec;59(4):413–7

**Chile**

Horne PD: The prince of El Plomo. **Paleopathol Newsl** 1982 Dec;40:7–10

**Costa Rica**

Weaver DS, Vazquez Leiva R: A survey of the paleopathology of the Vidor site, Guanacaste Province, Costa Rica. **Paleopathol Newsl** 1980 Jun;(30):6–7

**Egypt**

Kolta KS, Rothe R: Ein Bericht über die Röntgen- und Tomographiebefunde bei den Mumien der ägyptischen Staatssammlung in München. In International Congress of the History of Medicine, 27th, Barcelona, 1980. Actas. Barcelona, Acadèmia de Ciències Mèdiques de Catalunya i Balears, 1981. p. 557–9.
Zimmerman MR: The paleopathology of the human remains from Nebwenenef's tomb. Part II: The histologic findings. **Paleopathol Newsl** 1983 Jun;42:6–7

**Germany**

Grimm H: Paläopathologische Befunde an Menschenresten der römischen Kaiserzeit und Völkerwanderungszeit in der DDR. **Ausgrab Funde** 1979;24:267–74
Petsch K, Krekeler G, Otten JE: Pathologische Veränderungen im alveolären Bereich an Funden einer historischen Grablege. **Dtsch Zahnarztl Z** 1982 Apr;37(4):358–60
Seidel K: Vergleichende Untersuchungen über die Häufigkeit des Auftretens degenerativer Wirbelsäulen-veränderungen bei Menschen des Neolitikums, des Mittelalters und der Jetztzeit. **Z Gesamte Inn Med** 1981 Mar;36(5):159–62

**Ghana**

Macadam PS: A small skeletal sample from northern Ghana.

**Paleopathol Newsl** 1981 Jan;33:5-7

**Great Britain**

Dawes JD, Magilton JR: The cemetery of St Helen-on-the-Walls, Aldwark. London, Council for British Archaeology (for the York Archaeological Trust), 1980. 120 p. (The Archaeology of York. Volume 12: The Medieval Cemeteries).
Goose DH: Changes in human face breadth since the Mediaeval period in Britain. **Arch Oral Biol** 1981;26(9):757-8
Rogers J, Watt I, Dieppe P: Arthritis in Saxon and mediaeval skeletons. **Br Med J [Clin Res]** 1981 Dec 19;283(6307)1668-70

**Italy**

D'Amore C, Radice A, Schiano Di Zenise M: Studio radiologico del cranio 1 della necropoli di Madonna delle Grazie a Mirabella Eclano (Avellino). **Radiol Med (Torino)** 1981 Jul-Aug;67(7-8):503-8
Fornaciari G: Natural mummies in central Italy: a preliminary survey. **Paleopathol Newsl** 1982 Dec;40:11-2

**Japan**

Inoue N, Kuo CH, Ito G, et al: [Dental caries in Japanese remains (author's transl)] (Jpn). **Koku Eisei Gakkai Zasshi** 1981 Jul;31(2):90-7
Sakurai K, Ogata T: Japanese mummies. In A. Cockburn, E. Cockburn, ed: Mummies, disease, and ancient cultures. Cambridge, Cambridge University Press, 1980. p. 211-23.
Watanabe S: [Studies on the history of the anthropology of the Ainu skulls.] (Jpn). **Nihon I-Shigaku Zasshi** 1981;27:203-5

**Mexico**

Fastlicht S: Tooth mutilations and dentistry in pre-Columbian Mexico. Berlin, Buch- und Zeitschriften-Verlag 'Die Quintessenz', 1976. 164 p.
Sanfilippo J: The life and accomplishments of Dr. Samuel Fastlicht. **Bull Hist Dent** 1983 Oct;31(2):87-92

**Peru**

Allison MJ: Paleopathology in Peru. **Nat Hist** 1979;88(2):74-82
Cone RO, Danzig L, Resnick D, et al: The bicipital groove: radiographic, anatomic, and pathologic study. **AJR** 1983 Oct;141(4):781-8
Ponec DJ, Resnick D: On the etiology and pathogenesis of porotic hyperostosis of the skull. **Invest Radiol** 1984 Jul-Aug;19(4):313-7
Riddle JM, Vreeland JM: Identification of insects associated with Peruvian mummy bundles by using scanning electron microscopy. **Paleopathol Newsl** 1982 Sep;39:5-9
Sawyer DR, Allison MJ, Pezzia A, et al: Crown dimensions of deciduous teeth from pre-Columbian Peru. **Am J Phys Anthropol** 1982 Dec;59(4):373-6
Vreeland JM, Cockburn A: Mummies of Peru. In A. Cockburn, E. Cockburn, ed: Mummies, disease, and ancient cultures. Cambridge, Cambridge University Press, 1980. p. 135-74.

**Spain**

Campillo D, Turbón D: Cráneo trepanado de la Bauma dels Ossos. In International Congress of the History of Medicine, 27th, Barcelona, 1980. Actas. Barcelona, Académia de Ciències Médiques de Catalunya i Balears, 1981. p. 472-9.
Campillo D: Paleopatologia del craneo en Cataluña, Valencia y Baleares. Barcelona, Editorial Montblanc-Martin, 1977. 630 p.
Pérez PJ, Arsuaga JL, Bermudez de Castro JM: Atypical toothwear in fossil man. **Paleopathol Newsl** 1982 Sep;39:11-3

**Sweden**

Diener L: Osteologi och historia--röntgenologiska aspekter. **Nord Medicinhist Arsb** 1980;Suppl 6:112-7
Diener L, ed: Röster ur Riksgropen. **Nord Medicinhist Arsb** 1984;;49-61
Gejvall NG: Skelettmaterial från utgråvningar som bidrag till medicinhistorisk forkning. **Nord Medicinhist Arsb** 1980;Suppl 6:106-11

**United States**

Aufderheide AC, Neiman FD, Wittmers LE, et al: Lead in bone II: skeletal-lead content as an indicator of lifetime lead ingestion and the social correlates in an archaeological population. **Am J Phys Anthropol** 1981 Jul;55(3):285-91
Costa RL: Periodontal disease in the prehistoric Ipiutak and Tigara skeletal remains from Point Hope, Alaska. **Am J Phys Anthropol** 1982 Sep;59(1):97-110
Devor EJ, Cordell LS: Neural-tube defects in a prehistoric south-western Indian population. **Ann Hum Biol** 1981 Jan-Feb;8(1):65-75
Elting JJ, Starna WA: A possible case of pre-Columbian treponematosis from New York State. **Am J Phys Anthropol** 1984 Nov;65(3):267-73
Frayer DW, Bradley LE: A late woodland burial from Platte County, Missouri. **Plains Anthropol** 1979;24(83):21-27
Fritz G: Analysis of human skeletal remains from the Montgomery farm, Barry County, Missouri. **Arkansas Archeol** 1979;20:69-78
Goodman AH, Armelagos GJ, Rose JC: The chronological distribution of enamel hypoplasias from prehistoric Dickson Mounds populations. **Am J Phys Anthropol** 1984 Nov;65(3):259-66
Gregg JB, Zimmerman LJ, Steele JP, et al: Ante-mortem osteopathology at Crow Creek. **Plains Anthropol** 1981;26(94 pt 1):287-300
Gregg JB, Steele JP: Mastoid development in ancient and modern populations. A longitudinal radiological study. **JAMA** 1982 Jul 23;248(4):459-64
Gregg JB, Steele JP, Bass WM: Unusual osteolytic defects in ancient South Dakota skulls. **Am J Phys Anthropol** 1982 Jul;58(3):243-54
Hinton RJ: Differences in interproximal and occlusal tooth wear among prehistoric Tennessee Indians: implications for masticatory function. **Am J Phys Anthropol** 1982 Jan;57(1):103-15
Hogue H: Analyzing ossurary skeletal remains: techniques and problems. **South Indian Stud (NC)** 1977;29:2-22
Jurmain RD: The pattern of involvement of appendicular degenerative joint disease. **Am J Phys Anthropol** 1980 Jul;53(1):143-50
Morse D: Ancient disease in the Midwest. 2d ed. Springfield, Illinois, Illinois State Museum, 1978. xiii, 181 p. (Illinois State Museum Reports of Investigations, No. 15). Includes contributions by A. A. Dahlberg, D. Ubelaker, D. F. Dickson, J. R. Caldwell, R. C. Dailey, G. M. Comer.
El-Najjar MY, Andrews J, Moore JG, et al: Iron deficiency anemia in two prehistoric American Indian skeletons: a dietary hypothesis. **Plains Anthropol** 1982;27(97):205-9
Ortner DJ: [Case report on paleopathology.] **Paleopathol Newsl** 1983 Jun;42:10
Owsley DW, Bennett SM, Jantz RL: Intercemetery morphological variation in Arikara crania from the Mobridge Site (39WW1). **Am J Phys Anthropol** 1982 Jun;58(2):179-85
Palkovich AM: Demography and disease patterns in a protohistoric plains group: a study of the mobridge site (39WW1). **Plains Anthropol** 1981;26(94 pt 2):71-84
Ruff CB: Age differences in craniofacial dimensions among adults from Indian Knoll, Kentucky. **Am J Phys Anthropol** 1980 Jul;53(1):101-8
Ubelaker DH, Jantz RL: Plains Caddoan relationships: the view from craniometry and mortuary analysis. **Nebr Hist** 1979;60(2):249-59
Von Endt DW, Ortner DJ: Amino acid analysis of bone from a possible case of prehistoric iron deficiency anemia from the American Southwest. **Am J Phys Anthropol** 1982 Dec;59(4):377-85
Zimmerman MR: Aleutian and Alaskan mummies. In A. Cockburn, E. Cockburn, ed: Mummies, disease, and ancient cultures. Cambridge, Cambridge University Press, 1980. p. 118-34.

**USSR**

Derums VIa, Pfafrod GO, Vilks IuK: Dinamika strukturnykh i biomekhanicheskikh izmeneniĭ bedrennoĭ. **Arkh Anat Gistol Embriol** 1980 Aug;79(8):78-84

**Before 500 A.D.**

Brown AB: Assessment of paleonutrition from skeletal remains. **Ann NY Acad Sci** 1981;376:405-16
Campillo D: Los traumatismos en la prehistoria y en los tiempos antiguos. **Med Hist (Barc)** 1984;2:1-16
Campillo D: Neurosurgical pathology in prehistory. **Acta Neurochir (Wien)** 1984;70(3-4):275-90
Chen LB, Hung T: [Scanning electron microscopic view of parasitic worm ova in an ancient corpse (author's transl)] (Chi). **Chung Kuo I Hsueh Ko Hsueh Yuan Hsueh Pao** 1981 Mar;3(1):64-5
Clarke SK: Early childhood morbidity trends in prehistoric populations. **Hum Biol** 1980 Feb;52(1):79-85
Cockburn A, Cockburn E: Autopsies in mummies. **N Engl J Med** 1981 Dec 17;305(25):1534
Conroy GC: Evolutionary significance of cerebral venous patterns in paleoprimatology. **Z Morphol Anthropol** 1980;71(2):125-34
Ericson JE, Coughlin EA: Archaeological toxicology. **Ann NY Acad Sci** 1981;376:393-403
Escobar A, Aruffo C: La paleoneurología y el desarrollo del cerebro en los homínidos. **Gac Med Mex** 1980 Mar;116(3):115-32
Gingerich PD: Dental and cranial adaptations in Eocene Adapidae. **Z Morphol Anthropol** 1980;71(2):135-42
Graham EE: A probable submandibular gland defect in a prehistoric mandible. **Oral Surg** 1980 Aug;50(2):187-9
Grimm M: Frakturen und Frakturheilung in der Ur- und Frühgeschichte. **Beitr Orthop Traumatol** 1982 Feb;29(2):61-70
Hayman J: Mycobacterium ulcerans: an infection from Jurassic time? **Lancet** 1984 Nov 3;2(8410):1015-6
Henke W: Das Calvarium von Binshof (Speyer) im Vergleich mit anderen Jungpaläolithikern. **Z Morphol Anthropol** 1980;70(3):275-94
Holloway RL: Exploring the dorsal surface of hominoid brain endocasts by stereoplotter and discriminant analysis. **Philos Trans R Soc Lond [Biol]** 1981 May 8;292(1057):155-66

# PALEOPATHOLOGY

Holloway RL: Volumetric and asymmetry determinations on recent hominid endocasts: Spy I and II, Djebel Ihroud I, and the Sale Homo erectus specimens, with some notes on Neanderthal brain size. **Am J Phys Anthropol** 1981 Jul;55(3):385-93
Jaworski Z: Abrazja z ebów a zmiany w budowie anatomicznej żuchwy ludzi sprzed 3.000 lat z okolic Tarnobrzega. **Protet Stomatol** 1983 Jan-Feb;33(1):59-66
Jaworski Z, Jaworska M: Morfologia i topografia dna zatoki szczękowej w ciałopalnych szczątkach kostnych prasłowian. **Czas Stomatol** 1982 Apr;35(4):199-210
Kielan-Jaworowska Z: Polska Akademia Nauk, Zaklad Paleobiologii, Warsaw, Poland. **Nature** 1979 Feb 1;277(5695):402-3
Kramar C, Baud CA, Lagier R: Presumed calcified leiomyoma of the uterus. Morphologic and chemical studies of a calcified mass dating from the Neolithic period. **Arch Pathol Lab Med** 1983 Feb;107(2):91-3
Lagier R, Baud CA, Kramar C: Brodie's abscess in a tibia dating from the Neolithic period. **Virchows Arch [A]** 1983;401(2):153-7
Lambert JB, Vlasak SM, Thometz AC, et al: A comparative study of the chemical analysis of ribs and femurs in Woodland populations. **Am J Phys Anthropol** 1982 Nov;59(3):289-94
Lewis OJ: The joints of the evolving foot. Part III. The fossil evidence. **J Anat** 1980 Sep;131(Pt 2):275-98
Lowenstein JM: Immunological reactions from fossil material. **Philos Trans R Soc Lond [Biol]** 1981 May 8;292(1057):143-9
Lowenstein JM: Species-specific proteins in fossils. **Naturwissenschaften** 1980 Jul;67(7):343-6
McHenry HM: Relative cheek-tooth size in Australopithecus. **Am J Phys Anthropol** 1984 Jul;64(3):297-306
Nardoux M, Montarnal: Carie--abrasion--dimension. Dents de la préhistoire. **Ligament (Montp)** 1980;137:88-91
Osborn JW, Hillman J: Enamel structure in some therapsids and mesozoic mammals. **Calcif Tissue Int** 1979 Nov;29(1):47-61
Pontius AA: Icono-diagnosis, a medical-humanistic approach, detecting Crouzon's malformation in Cook Islands' prehistoric art. **Perspect Biol Med** 1983 Autumn;27(1):107-20
Prager EM, Wilson AC, Lowenstein JM, et al: Mammoth albumin. **Science** 1980 Jul 11;209(4453):287-9
Puech PF, Prone A, Albertini H: Reproduction expérimentale des processus d'altération de la surface dentaire par friction non abrasive et non adhésive: application à l'étude de l'alimentation de l'homme fossile. **C R Seances Acad Sci [III]** 1981 Nov 9;293(9):497-502
Puech PF, Prone A: Reproduction expérimentale des processus d'usure dentaire par abrasion: implications paléoécologiques chez l'homme fossile. **C R Acad Sci [D] (Paris)** 1979 Nov 19;289(13):895-8
Putschar WG, Ortner DJ: Zur Paläopathologie der Skelett-Missbildungen und -Dysplasien. **Verh Dtsch Ges Pathol** 1982;66:147-50
Rodnan GP, Benedek TG: Synovial fluid in antiquity. **Ann Rheum Dis** 1981 Feb;40(1):103
Rudney JD, Katz RV, Brand JW: Interobserver reliability of methods for paleopathological diagnosis of dental caries. **Am J Phys Anthropol** 1983 Nov;62(3):243-8
Sakai T: [Morphology of premolar in primitive anthropoidea] (Jpn). **Shikai Tenbo** 1983 Jan;61(1):81-90
Schwartz JH: Dentofacial growth and development in Homo sapiens: evidence from perinatal individuals from Punic Carthage. **Anat Anz** 1982;152(1):1-26
Setoguchi T: [Paleontological view points on the morphological characteristics of human molar teeth. I (author's transl)] (Jpn). **Shikai Tenbo** 1981;(7):31-8
Setoguchi T: [Paleontological view points on the morphological characteristics of human molar teeth. II, III (author's transl)] (Jpn). **Shikai Tenbo** 1981;(8,9):319-25,441-8
Sullivan CH, Krueger HW: Carbon isotope ratios of bone apatite and animal diet reconstruction. **Nature** 1983 Jan 13;301(5896):177-8
Symposium: adaptive grades in the evolution of primates: **Z Morphol Anthropol** 1980;71(2):113-227
Szalay FS: A critique of some recently proposed paleogene primate taxa and suggested relationships. **Folia Primatol (Basel)** 1982;37(3-4):153-62
Szalay FS, Dagosto M: Locomotor adaptations as reflected on the humerus of paleogene primates. **Folia Primatol (Basel)** 1980;34(1-2):1-45
Tattersall I, Schwartz JH: A new genus and species of adapid primate from the middle Eocene of Alsace, and a new genus for 'Adapis' ruetimeyeri Stehlin, 1912. **Folia Primatol (Basel)** 1983;41(3-4):231-9
Thompson DD, Trinkaus E: Age determination of the Shanidar 3 Neanderthal. **Science** 1981 May 1;212(4494):575-7
Walker A, Zimmerman MR, Leakey RE: A possible case of hypervitaminosis A in Homo erectus. **Nature** 1982 Mar 18;296(5854):248-50
Walker A: Diet and teeth. Dietary hypotheses and human evolution. **Philos Trans R Soc Lond [Biol]** 1981 May 8;292(1057):57-64
Williams JA: Fourier analysis and homology of the first molars of the Palaeocene primate family Picrodontidae. **Arch Oral Biol** 1981;26(2):111-6
Yamada M, Horibe H, Fujimori K, et al: Paleobiophysical studies on tooth tisues by microfluorometry and Raman-spectrometry. **Cell Mol Biol** 1979;25(3):167-72
Yinyun Z: Variability and evolutionary trends in tooth size of Gigantopithecus blacki. **Am J Phys Anthropol** 1982 Sep;59(1):21-32
Zakharov BI, Zakharova NP, Beliaskiĭ EA: Proiavleniia mielomnoĭ bolezni v kostiakh drevnikh liudeĭ. **Vopr Onkol** 1983;29(2):86-8

**Africa**

Wood BA, Abbott SA: Analysis of the dental morphology of Plio-pleistocene hominids. I. Mandibular molars: crown area measurements and morphological traits. **J Anat** 1983 Jan;136 (Pt 1):197-219

**Americas**

Allison MJ, Gerszten E, Munizaga J, et al: Metastatic tumor of bone in a Tiahuanaco female. **Bull NY Acad Med** 1980 Jul-Aug;56(6):581-7
Buikstra JE: Prehistoric tuberculosis in the Americas. Evanston, Northwestern University, Archeological Program, 1981. xii, 182 p.
Cook DC: Hereditary enamel hypoplasia in a prehistoric Indian child. **J Dent Res** 1980 Sep;59(9):1522
Fragoso Uribe R: Algunas observaciones que apoyan el origen precolombino de la 'enfermedad de Robles' en América. **SPM** 1979 Nov-Dec;21(6):697-706
Hanson CL, Owsley DW: Frontal sinus size in Eskimo populations. **Am J Phys Anthropol** 1980 Aug;53(2):251-5

**Arabic**

Højgaard K: Dentition on Umm an-Nar (Trucial Oman), 2500 B.C. **Scand J Dent Res** 1980 Oct;88(5):355-64

**Argentina**

Fleagle JG, Bown TM: New primate fossils from late Oligocene (Colhuehuapian) localities of Chubut Province, Argentina. **Folia Primatol (Basel)** 1983;41(3-4):240-66
Hershkovitz P: Comparative anatomy of platyrrhine mandibular cheek teeth dpm4, pm4, ml with particular reference to those of Homunculus (Cebidae), and comments on platyrrhine origins. **Folia Primatol (Basel)** 1981;35(2-3)179-217

**Asia**

Hojgaard K: Dilmun-tidens taender. Umm an-Nar (2500 f.v.t.). Al-Bahrain (2000 f.v.t.). **Tandlaegebladet** 1980 Sep;84(16):548
Rathbun TA: Morphological affinities and demography of metal-age Southwest Asian populations. **Am J Phys Anthropol** 1982 Sep;59(1):47-60

**Australia**

Thorne AG, Wolpoff MH: Regional continuity in Australasian Pleistocene hominid evolution. **Am J Phys Anthropol** 1981 Jul;55(3):337-49

**Austria**

Nicola M, Stiebitz R: Morphologische und pathologische Befunde von Zähnen und Kiefern aus der Mittleren Bronzezeit (Pitten, Niederösterreich). **Anthropol Anz** 1979 Oct;37(3):182-203

**Bahrain**

Højgaard K: Dentition on Bahrain, 2000 B.C. **Scand J Dent Res** 1980 Dec;88(6):467-75

**Brazil**

Araújo AJ, Confalonieri UE, Ferreira LF: Oxyurid infestations in small animals from 9,000 B.P. in Brazil. **Paleopathol Newsl** 1980 Sep;(31):13-14
Ferreira LF, Aráujo AJ de, Confalonieri UE: The finding of eggs and larvae of parasitic helminths in archaeological material from Unai, Minas Gerais, Brazil. **Trans R Soc Trop Med Hyg** 1980;74(6):798-800
Pereira CB, Galvao CA, Evans WG, et al: A cephalometric evaluation of a Brazilian pre-historic man. **Tydskr Tandheelkd Ver S Afr** 1983 Oct;38(10):627-31

**Chile**

Aráujo A, Ferreira LF, Confalonieri UE, et al: Eggs of Diphyllobothrium pacificum in precolumbian human coprolites. **Paleopathol Newsl** 1983 Mar;41:11-3
Ferreira LF, Ribeiro Filho BM, Araújo AJ de, et al: Enterobius vermicularis eggs in preColumbian human coprolites from Chile. **Paleopathol Newsl** 1984;46:4-5
Turner CG, Bird J: Dentition of Chilean paleo-Indians and peopling of the Americas. **Science** 1981 May 29;212(4498):1053-5

### China

Cheng TO: Glimpses of the past from the recently unearthed ancient corpses in China. **Ann Intern Med** 1984 Nov;101(5):714–5

Hu SY: [Study on the parasite eggs in an ancient corpse from Zhangguo Chu Tomb No. 1 in Mashan brick-field of Jiangling County, Hubei] (Chi). **Chi Sheng Chung Hsueh Yu Chi Sheng Chung Ping Tsa Chih** 1984;2(1):8

Pindborg JJ: Nyt om Peking-manden og hans forgaengere. **Tandlaegebladet** 1981 Feb;85(3):82–5

Wei DX, Yang WY, Huang SQ, et al: Parasitological investigation on the ancient corpse of the Western Han Dynasty unearthed from tomb No. 168 on Phoenix Hill in Jianglin county. **Acta Acad Med Wuhan** 1981;1(2):16–23

Wu BM, Wang JH: Female cadaver in the Han Tomb No. 1. X-ray diffraction studies on two kinds of fibrous protein. **Sci Sin** 1980 Jul;23(7):915–22

Yang KL, Qui BS, Zhang YE, et al: Skin changes of 2,100 year old Changsha female corpse. **Chin Med J [Engl]** 1982 Oct;95(10):765–76

Yang WY, Wei DX, Song GF, et al: Parasitologische Untersuchung einer alten Leiche aus der Chu-Dynastie der Streitenden Reiche aus dem Mazhuan-Grab Nr. 1, Kreis Jiangling, Provinz Hubei. **Acta Acad Med Wuhan** 1984;4(1):23–7

Zhang YZ: Dental disease of neolithic age skulls excavated in Shaanxi Province. **Chin Med J [Engl]** 1982 Jun;95(6):391–6

Zheng GZ, Feng WH, Boa YH, et al: Microscopic and submicroscopic studies on the peripheral nerve and the skeletal muscle of the female. Cadaver found in the Han Tomb No. 1. **Sci Sin** 1979 Sep;22(9):1095–8

### Cyprus

Taramides G: Ta dontia ton Kyprios tes neolithikos epoches (5800–3000 P.Ch.). **Odontostomatol Proodos** 1983 Jul–Aug;37(4):213–8

### Denmark

Andersen SR, Geertinger P: Moselig i retsmedicinsk belysning. **Dan Medicinhist Arbog** 1982;:23–42

Fischer C: Bog bodies of Denmark. In A. Cockburn, E. Cockburn, ed: Mummies, disease, and ancient cultures. Cambridge, Cambridge University Press, 1980. p. 177–93.

Halaburt H, Langfeldt B, Rasmussen P: Computerized tomography (CT-scan) of a 2,500-year-old Danish 'Queen'. **Acta Neurochir (Wien)** 1981;56(3–4):153–5

### Egypt

Cockburn A, Peck WH, Barraco RA, et al: A classic mummy: PUM II. In A. Cockburn, E. Cockburn, ed: Mummies, disease, and ancient cultures. Cambridge, Cambridge University Press, 1980. p. 52–70.

Cockburn A: Ancient parasites on the West Bank of the Nile. **Lancet** 1981 Oct 24;2(8252)938

Fodor J, Malott JC, King AY: The radiographic investigation of two Egyptian mummies. **Radiol Technol** 1983 Jul–Aug;54(6):443–8

Harris JE, Wente EF: An X-ray atlas of the royal mummies. Chicago, University of Chicago Press, 1980. xix, 403 p.

Harris JE, Ponitz PV: Dental health in ancient Egypt. In A. Cockburn, E. Cockburn, ed: Mummies, disease, and ancient cultures. Cambridge, Cambridge University Press, 1980. p. 45–51.

Hart GD, Millett N, Scott J: Paleopathology and the autopsy of an Egyptian mummy. In: Congrès international d'histoire de la médecine, XXVe, Québec, 1976. Actes. Québec, 1977. p. 765–70.

Harwood-Nash DC: Computed tomography of ancient Egyptian mummies. **J Comput Assist Tomogr** 1979 Dec;3(6):768–73

Iles JD: Autopsy of an Egyptian mummy (Nakht--ROM I). **Can Med Assoc J** 1980 Mar 8;122(5):512–3

Jarcho S: Some historical problems connected with the study of Egyptian mummies. **Bull Inst Egypte (Cairo)** 1981;:58–9, 106–22

Leek FF: Observations on a collection of crania from the mastabas of the reign of Cheops at Gîza. **J Egypt Archaeol** 1980;66:36–45

Leek FF: Palaeodontology of the Nile Valley. **Paleopathol Newsl** 1981 Jan;33:9–12

Mann P: Taking a look at 3,000-year-old teeth. **Br Dent J** 1980 Jul 15;149(2):57–8

Millet NB, Hart GD, Reyman TA, et al: ROM I: mummification for the common people. In A. Cockburn, E. Cockburn, ed: Mummies, disease, and ancient cultures. Cambridge, Cambridge University Press, 1980. p. 71–84.

Paulshock BZ: Tutankhamun and his brothers. Familial gynecomastia in the Eighteenth Dynasty. **JAMA** 1980 Jul 11;244(2):160–4

Peluso A: Patologia orale in una antica popolazione egiziana. **Dent Cadmos** 1980 Dec;48(12):9–28

Reyman TA, Peck WH: Egyptian mummification with evisceration per ano. In A. Cockburn, E. Cockburn, ed: Mummies, disease, and ancient cultures. Cambridge, Cambridge University Press, 1980. p. 85–100.

Sandison AT: Diseases in ancient Egypt. In A. Cockburn, E. Cockburn, ed: Mummies, disease, and ancient cultures. Cambridge, Cambridge University Press, 1980. p. 29–44.

Turner PJ, Holtom DB: The use of a fabric softener in the reconstitution of mummified tissue prior to paraffin wax sectioning for light microscopical examination. **Stain Technol** 1981 Jan;56(1):35–8

Vahey T, Brown D: Comely Wenuhotep: computed tomography of an Egyptian mummy. **J Comput Assist Tomogr** 1984 Oct;8(5):992–7

Zimmerman MR: The mummies of the tomb of Nebwenenef: paleopathology and archaeology. **J Am Res Cent Egypt** 1977;14:33–6

Zimmerman MR, Zimmerman BH: The paleopathology of the human remains from Nebwenenef's tomb--the 1979 season. **Paleopathol Newsl** 1980 Sep;(31):15–16

Zimmermann MR: A possible histiocytoma in an Egyptian mummy. **Arch Dermatol** 1981 Jun;117(6):364–5

Zuckerman AJ: Palaeontology of smallpox. **Lancet** 1984 Dec 22;2(8417–18):1454

### Ethiopia

Kimbel WH, White TD, Johanson DC: Cranial morphology of Australopithecus afarensis: a comparative study based on a composite reconstruction of the adult skull. **Am J Phys Anthropol** 1984 Aug;64(4):337–88

Pliocene hominid fossils from Hadar, Ethiopia: **Am J Phys Anthropol** 1982 Apr;57(4):373–719

### Europe

Scholz F, Rossiwall B: Taurodontismus: Eine anthropologische Streitfrage und ein Mikrosymptom für genetische Störungen. **Osterr Z Stomatol** 1981 Oct;78(10):373–8

### France

Hammond M: The expulsion of the Neanderthals from human ancestry: Marcellin Boule and the social context of scientific research. **Soc Stud Sci** 1982 Feb;12(1):1–36

Saban R: Le système veineux méningé de l'homme fossile de Biache-Saint-Vaast (Pas-de-Calais), d'après le moulage endocranien. **C R Acad Sci [D] (Paris)** 1979 Dec 10;289(15):1129–32

Tillier AM: Evolution de la région symphysaire chez les homo sapiens juvéniles du paléolithique moyen: pech de l'azé 1, roc de marsal et la chaise 13. **C R Seances Acad Sci [III]** 1981 Nov 9;293(9):493–5

Tillier AM, Genet-Varcin E: La plus ancienne mandibule d'enfant découverte en France dans le gisement de La Chaise de Vouthon (Abri Suard) en Charente. **Z Morphol Anthropol** 1980;71(2):196–214

### Germany

Bräuer G: Die morphologischen Affinitäten des jungpleistozänen Stirnbeines aus dem Elbmündungsgebiet bei Hahnöfersand. **Z Morphol Anthropol** 1980;71(1):1–42

Jaworski Z: Morfologia zębów stałych z dziecięcych grobów ciałopalnych kultury łuzyckiej. **Czas Stomatol** 1981 May;34(5):487–92

Jaworski Z: Przyżyciowe braki zębowe w szczatkach kostnych z grobów ciałopalnych kultury łużyckiej. **Czas Stomatol** 1981 Oct;34(10):969–74

Jaworski Z: Szczątki szczęk i żuchw Prasłowian z grobów ciałopalnych kultury łużychiej. **Czas Stomatol** 1981 Sep;34(9):897–907

Kühl I: Zur Frage nach einer frühen Konzeption in ur- und frühgeschichtlicher Zeit: Beispiel vermutlicher Mutter-Kind-Bestattungen aus der vorrömischen Eisenzeit aus Holstein. **Aerztl Jugendkd** 1983 Jun;74(3):176–87

### Great Britain

Ivanhoe F: Interglovular dentine in first and third molars: relation to hours of sunshine during growth in two archeological populations from England. **Calcif Tissue Int** 1982 Mar;34(2):136–44

Newman HN, Levers BG: Tooth eruption and function in an early Anglo-Saxon population. **J R Soc Med** 1979 May;72(5):341–50

Seddon RP: A cephalometric study of the Romano-British. **Eur J Orthod** 1984 Nov;6(4):303–12

Singer R, Wolff RG, Gladfelter BG, et al: Pleistocene Macaca from Hoxne, Suffolk, England. **Folia Primatol (Basel)** 1982;37(3–4):141–52

Whittaker DK, Parker JH, Jenkins C: Tooth attrition and continuing eruption in a Romano-British population. **Arch Oral Biol** 1982;27(5):405–9

### Greece

Zapfe H: Ein Schädel von Mesopithecus mit Biss-Spuren. **Folia Primatol (Basel)** 1981;35(4):248–58

### Hungary

Kretzoi M: The significance of the Rudabánya prehominid finds in hominization research. **Acta Biol Acad Sci Hung** 1980;31(4):503–6

# PALEOPATHOLOGY

**India**

Lukacs JR: Crown dimensions of deciduous teeth from prehistoric India. **Am J Phys Anthropol** 1981 Jun;55(2):261-6

**Indonesia**

Holloway RL: Indonesian 'Solo' (Ngandong) endocranial reconstructions: some preliminary observations and comparisons with Neandertal and Homo erectus groups. **Am J Phys Anthropol** 1980 Aug;53(2):285-95

**Iraq**

Trinkaus E, Zimmerman MR: Trauma among the Shanidar Neandertals. **Am J Phys Anthropol** 1982 Jan;57(1):61-76

**Italy**

Bucklin R: The Shroud of Turin: a pathologist's viewpoint. **J Miss State Med Assoc** 1983 Apr;24(4):95-8

Gavazzi C: Odontoiatria del passato. I denti umani fossili di Salto (Valle Orco). **Dent Cadmos** 1981 Oct, Nov;49(10,11):59-63 contd, 71-9

Nihlén B: 2 000-åriga skelett med perfekta tänder. **Tandlakartidningen** 1983 Dec 1;75(23):1356-7

**Japan**

Noriyasu S, Higashinakagawa T, Matsushita T, et al: Human skeletal remains of the Yayoi Period excavated from the Tsumayama site, Saga Prefecture, Kyushu, Japan. **Fukuoka Igaku Zasshi** 1982 May;73(5):241-9

Noriyasu S, Isotani S, Akiyoshi T: Human skulls of the Yayoi Period excavated from Himekata site, Saga Prefecture, Kyushu, Japan. **Fukuoka Igaku Zasshi** 1982 May;73(5):232-40

**Jordan**

Ortner DJ: Disease and mortality in the Early Bronze Age people of Bab edh-Dhra, Jordan. **Am J Phys Anthropol** 1979 Nov;51(4):589-97

Röhrer-Ertl O: Ein Beitrag zur historischen Vertiefung der Akzelerationsforschung: Längenwachstumsänderungen in einer Population vom Tell es Sultan/Jericho aus dem Präkeramischen Neolithikum (ca. 9000-6000 v. Chr.). **Arztl Jugendkd** 1984 Oct;75(5):292-302

**Kenya**

McHenry HM, Andrews P, Corruccini RS: Miocene hominoid palatofacial morphology. **Folia Primatol (Basel)** 1980;33(4):241-52

Senut B: Quelques remarques à propos d'un humérus d'homino ide pliocène provenant de Chemeron (bassin du lac Baringo, Kenya). **Folia Primatol (Basel)** 1983;41(3-4):267-76

**Libya**

Boaz NT: A hominoid clavicle from the Mio-Pliocene of Sahabi, Libya. **Am J Phys Anthropol** 1980 Jul;53(1):49-54

**Nigeria**

Fraudet JR: La pression antéro-postérieure des lèvres sur l'arcade dentaire inférieure à l'époque néolithique. **Rev Stomatol Chir Maxillofac** 1984;85(5):438-40

**Norway**

Holck P: Harris' linjer. Røntgenfunn på et prehistorisk skjelett. **Tidsskr Nor Laegeforen** 1984 May 30;104(14):1028-31

**Pakistan**

Pilbeam D: New hominoid skull material from the Miocene of Pakistan. **Nature** 1982 Jan 21-27;295(5846):232-4

**Peru**

Miura F, Soma K, Hatate M: [The orthodontic observation of ancient Peruvian calvaria--orthopedically induced deformity of the skull]. (Jpn) **Kokubyo Gakkai Zasshi** 1979 Sep;46(3):220-7

**Poland**

Biedowa J: Morfologia zębów trzonowych na tle ich tendencji ewolucyjnych. **Czas Stomatol** 1980 Mar;33(3):191-6

**South Africa**

Tobias PV: The natural history of the helicoidal occlusal plane and its evolution in early Homo. **Am J Phys Anthropol** 1980 Aug;53(2):173-87

**Spain**

Campillo D: Estudio etiopatogenico de la lesion encontrada en un craneo procedente del Yacimiento Talayotico de cales coves en Menorca (146, L. P.). **Asclepio** 1980;32:77-85

Campillo D: Malformacion vertebral en un individuo perteneciente a la cultura Talayotica Menorquina (L. P. 147). **Asclepio** 1980;32:65-76

Castro JM de: Etude anthropologique de la denture de la population préhispanique de l'Ile de Grande Canarie. **Bull Group Int Rech Sci Stomatol Odontol** 1984 Jan;27(1):11-29

Vives E, Campillo D: Otoantritis en un individuo del dolmen del Torrent (Girona). In International Congress of the History of Medicine, 27th, Barcelona, 1980. Actas. Barcelona, Académia de Ciències Médiques de Catalunya i Balears, 1981. p. 671-4.

**Sudan**

Bassett EJ, Keith MS, Armelagos GJ, et al: Tetracycline-labeled human bone from ancient Sudanese Nubia (A.D. 350). **Science** 1980 Sep 26;209(4464):1532-4)

Martin DL, Armelagos GJ: Morphometrics of compact bone: an example from Sudanese Nubia. **Am J Phys Anthropol** 1979 Nov;51(4):571-7

**Tanzania**

Holloway RL: The O.H. 7 (Olduvai Gorge, Tanzania) hominid partial brain endocast revisited. **Am J Phys Anthropol** 1980 Aug;53(2):267-74

Rightmire GP: Middle Pleistocene hominids from Olduvai Gorge, northern Tanzania. **Am J Phys Anthropol** 1980 Aug;53(2):225-41

**United States**

Blakely RL, Beck LA: Trace elements, nutritional status, and social stratification at Etowah, Georgia. **Ann NY Acad Sci** 1981;376:417-31

Cook DC, Buikstra JE: Health and differential survival in prehistoric populations: prenatal dental defects. **Am J Phys Anthropol** 1979 Nov;51(4):649-64

Goodman AH, Armelagos GJ, Rose JC: Enamel hypoplasias as indicators of stress in three prehistoric populations from Illinois. **Hum Biol** 1980 Sept;52(3):515-28

Gregg JB, Reed A: Monostotic fibrous dysplasia in the temporal bone: a late prehistoric occurrence. **Am J Phys Anthropol** 1980 May;52(4):587-93

Hinton RJ, Smith MO, Smith FH: Tooth size changes in prehistoric Tennessee Indians. **Hum Biol** 1980 May;52(2):229-45

Lagier R, Baud CA, Arnaud G, et al: Lesions characteristic of infection or malignant tumor in Paleo-Eskimo skulls. An anatomical and radiological study of two specimens. **Virchows Arch [Pathol Anat]** 1982;395(3):237-43

El-Najjar MY, Benitez J, Fry G, et al: Autopsies on two native American Mummies. **Am J Phys Anthropol** 1980 Aug;53(2):197-202

Neiburger EJ: Lesions in a prehistoric bear: differential diagnosis. **Paleopathol Newsl** 1984 Dec;(48):8-11

Streitz JM, Aufderheide AC, El Najjar M, et al: A 1,500-year-old bladder stone. **J Urol** 1981 Oct;126(4):452-3

**USSR**

Barnhart MI, Barmatoski SP, Goodman M, et al: Tissue vestiges of an ancient Magadan mammoth calf. **Scan Electron Microsc** 1980;(pt 2):163-70

Dérums VIa: Rentgenomorfologicheskaia kharakteristika travmaticheskikh povrezhdeniĭ i raneniĭ kosteĭ zhiteleĭ drevneĭ Pribaltiki. **Arkh Patol** 1980;42(2):64-8

Reyman TA, Goodman M: The histology of ancient mammoth tissue. **Paleopathol Newsl** 1981 Jan;33:13-5

**Yugoslavia**

Burleigh R, Zivanovic S: Radiocarbon dating of a Cro-Magnon population from Padina, Yugoslavia, with some general recommendations for dating human skeletons. **Z Morphol Anthropol** 1980;70(3):269-74

**Zimbabwe**

Koritzer RT, St. Hoyme LE: Extensive caries in early man circa 110,000 years before present. **J Am Dent Assoc** 1979 Oct;99(4):642-3

**500 A.D.-1450**

Baumgartner R: Fussprothese aus einem frühmittelalterlichen Grab aus Bonaduz. **Helv Archaeol** 1982;13(51-2):155-62

Larsson E: Malocclusions in a juvenile medieval skull material. **Swed Dent J** 1983;7(5):185-90

Sagne S: The use of the scanning electron microscope with X-ray

equipment for the analysis of elements in medieval bones. **Ossa** 1978;5:85–91
Scheidegger S: Gelenkerkrankungen bei Skelettfunden aus dem Mittelalter. **Aktuel Gerontol** 1980 Nov;10(11):509–10
Steudel K: New estimates of early hominid body size. **Am J Phys Anthropol** 1980 Jan;52(1):52–63

**Americas**

Speck FL, Wheeland RG: Cutaneous histopathology of southwestern American Indian mummies. **Int J Dermatol** 1984 Sep;23(7):487–92

**Austria**

Kloiber A, Glowatzki G, Mullis ML, et al: Zur Identifizierung der mutmasslichen Gebeine des 'letzten Minnesängers', Oswald von Wolkenstein. **Anthropol Anz** 1982;40(4):285–98
Stiebitz R, Teschler-Nicola M: Pathologische Befunde am Kauapparat eines Schädels aus dem 6. Jh. n. Chr., Fundort: Schwechat, Niederösterreich. **Wien Klin Wochenschr** 1981 Nov 27;93(22):703–7

**Chile**

Horne PD, Kawasaki SQ: The Prince of El Plomo: a paleopathological study. **Bull NY Acad Med** 1984 Nov;60(9):925–31

**Denmark**

Helm S, Prydsö U: Assessment of age-at-death from mandibular molar attrition in medieval Danes. **Scand J Dent Res** 1979 Apr;87(2):79–90
Helm S, Prydsö U: Prevalence of malocclusion in medieval and modern Danes contrasted. **Scand J Dent Res** 1979 Apr;87(2):91–7
Jakobsen J, Jorgensen JB, Kreiborg S, et al: Kong Valdemar Atterdag: antropologiske fund under en odontologisk synsvinkel. **Tandlaegebladet** 1981 Jan;85(1):9–16
Jensen KR, Tkocz I: Skeletmaterialet fra udgravningen af St. Jørgensgården i Odense. En foreløbig rapport. **Dan Medicinhist Arbog** 1983;12:52–64
Klafstad J: Odontopathology of a Norwegian medieval population––a pilot study. **Ossa** 1978;5:43–55
Tauber H: 13C evidence for dietary habits of prehistoric man in Denmark. **Nature** 1981 Jul 23;292(5821):332–3
Williams S: En tidlig dansk henrettelse: et kraniefund. **Tandlaegebladet** 1983 Oct;87(18):632–4

**Dominican Republic**

Garcia-Godoy F: Caries dental en cráneos primitivos de la Isla Santo Domingo. **Rev Asoc Odontol Argent** 1978 Jul–Sep;66(3):147–50

**Egypt**

Sheldrick P: 'Skinny bones' from the Dakhleh Oasis. **Paleopathol Newsl** 1980 Jun;(30):7–10

**Europe**

Bergman P, Aue-Hauser G: Methodische Beiträge zu kraniometrischen Studien einiger frühmittelalterlicher Populationen des oberen Donauraumes. I. Die gebräuchlichsten Schädelindices als Grundlage für Populationsvergleiche (graphische und Approximationsverfahren). **Anthropol Anz** 1980 Nov;38(4):251–64

**France**

Gotz I: Untersuchungen an drei Schädeln des 14./15. Jahrhunderts aus einem mittelfränkischen Rittergeschlecht. **ZWR** 1982 Sep;91(9):62–4
Wackenheim A, Dietemann J, Babin E, et al: Hémi-occipitalisation de l'atlas chez un Mérovingien du bas Moyen Age. **J Radiol** 1981 Oct;62(10):515 7

**Germany**

Bergman P, Hauser G: Methodische Beiträge zu kraniometrischen Studien einiger frühmittelalterlicher Populationen des oberen Donauraumes. II. Vergleich der frümittelalterlichen Populationen anhand absoluter Schädelmasse. **Anthropol Anz** 1982 Sep;40(3):173–84
Röhrer-Ertl O: Bemerkungen zur Identifikation des Hl. Emmeram aus St. Emmeram in Regensburg. Ein methodenkritischer Vergleich. **Anthropol Anz** 1981 Sep;39(3):173–88
Schollmayer E: Skelettfunde aus fränkischen Reihengräberfriedhöfen in Eltville und Langenlonsheim. Vergleiche mit anderen merowingerzeitlichen Serien. **Z Morphol Anthropol** 1983;74(2):173–89
Schultz M: Aseptic bone necrosis found in the skeletal material from the Merovingian cemetery of Kleinlangheim, Southern Germany. **Paleopathol Newsl** 1981 Jun;34:7–9

**Great Britain**

Barry PS, Connolly R: Lead concentrations in mediaeval bones. **Int Arch Occup Environ Health** 1981;48(2):173–7

**Hungary**

Kocsis SG, Marcsik A: Zománcképzödmények a VII–VIII. századból származó koponyák fogain. **Fogorv Sz** 1981 Mar;74(3):89–93

**Japan**

Fujimori K, Chikamori K, Matsubara H, et al: Human bones from three burial mounds in Tokushima. **Tokushima J Exp Med** 1979 Dec;26(3–4):73–9

**Malta**

Ramaswamy S, Pace JL: The medieval skeletal remains from St. Gregory's Church at Zejtun (Malta) Part I. Paleopathological studies. **Arch Ital Anat Embriol** 1979 Jan–Mar;84(1):43–53
Ramaswamy S, Pace JL: The medieval skeletal remains from St. Gregory's Church at Zejtun (Malta) Part II. Anthropological studies. **Arch Ital Anat Embriol** 1980;85(1):55–69

**Norway**

Haugen LK: The human upper and middle face. A morphological investigation in a Norwegian medieval population. **Acta Morphol Neerl Scand** 1980 Jun;18(23):93–112,113–23

**Peru**

Canalis RF, Aragon RM, Cabieses F, et al: Fibrous dysplasia: findings in a pre-Columbian skull. **Am J Otolaryngol** 1980 Feb;1(2):131–5
Sawyer DR, Allison MJ, Pezzia A: Elongated styloid process in a pre-Columbian Peruvian. **J Dent Res** 1980 Jan;59(1):79
Sawyer DR, Nwoku AL, Elzay RP, et al: Two probable cases of a depression in the mandible caused by the submandibular salivary gland in Pre-Columbian Peruvians. **J Maxillofac Surg** 1981 Aug;9(3):194–6

**Poland**

Dawidowicz A, Hornowski J: O wieku królowej Jadwigi. **Arch Hist Med (Warsz)** 1978;41(4):423–46
Gładykowska-Rzeczycka J: Dislocation of the hip joint (probably congenital) in the woman from the mediaeval burial ground in Poland. **Folia Morphol (Warsz)** 1980;39(2):211–4

**Sudan**

Hummert JR, Van Gerven DP: Tetracycline-labeled human bone from a medieval population in Nubia'Batn el Hajar (550–1450 A.D.). **Hum Biol** 1982 May;54(2):355–63

**Sweden**

Bergman LE, Hansson T: Hard tissue changes of the temporomandibular joint in an archaeo-osteological material from the 11th century. **Swed Dent J** 1979;3(5):149–55

**Switzerland**

Roulet JF, Ulrich-Bochsler S: Zahnärztliche Untersuchung frühmittelalterlicher Schädel aus Biel-Mett. **SSO Schweiz Monatsschr Zahnheilkd** 1979 Jun;89(6):526–40
Ulrich-Bochsler S, Schäublin E, Zeltner TB, et al: Invalidisierende Wirbelsäulenverkrümmung an einem Skelettfund aus dem Frühmittelalter (7./8. bis Anfang 9. Jh.). Ein Fall einer wahrscheinlichen Spondylitis tuberculosa. **Schweiz Med Wochenschr** 1982 Sep 18;112(38):1318–23
Ulrich-Bochsler S, Glowatzki G: Ossäre Folgezustände einer langzeitig unbehandelten osteomyelitis. Fallbeschreibung an einem mittelalterlichen Skelett. **Anthropol Anz** 1982 Mar;40(1):1–18
Ulrich-Bochsler S, Glowatzki G, Zeltner T: Ossäre Folgezustände einer unbehandelten Osteomyelitis. **Praxis** 1981 Oct;70(43):1913–8
Wiederkehr M, Roulet JF, Ulrich-Bochsler S: Zahnärztliche Untersuchung mittelalterlicher Schädel aus drei Regionen des Kantons Bern. **SSO Schweiz Monatsschr Zahnheilkd** 1982 Feb;92(2):127–36

**United States**

Gregg JB, Steele JP, Zimmerman L, et al: Otolaryngic osteopathology in 14th century mid-America. The crow creek massacre. **Ann Otol Rhinol Laryngol** 1981 May–Jun;90(3 pt 1):288–93
Gregg JB, et al: Possible treponematosis in fourteenth century Dakota territory: a progress report. **Paleopathol Newsl** 1981 Jun;34:5–6

## PALEOPATHOLOGY

Titche LL, Wachter RD, Coulthard SW, et al: Mastoiditis in prehistoric Arizona Indians. **Ariz Med** 1981 Sep;38(9):712–4

Zimmerman LJ, Gregg JB, Gregg PS: Para-mortem osteopathology in the Crow Creek masacre victims. **SD J Med** 1981 Feb;34(2):7–12

**USSR**

Kopshitser IZ: Trepanirovannyĭ cherep iz Dargavskogo nekropolia 'Goroda Mertvykh' v selenii Dargavs Severnoĭ Osetii. **Zh Vopr Neirokhir** 1983 Jul–Aug;4:61–2

**Yugoslavia**

Zivanović S: Povrede i prelomi kostiju u Srpskog srednjovekovnog stanoviništva iz nekropole Vajuga na Dunavu kod Kladova. **Srp Arh Celok Lek** 1982 Mar;110(3):273–89

**1450–1700**

Dierżykray-Rogalski T: Historia Badán szczątków kostnych Jana z Czarnolasu Kochanowskiego. **Kwart Hist Nauki Tech** 1983;28(2):425–35

**Great Britain**

Manchester K: Paleopathology of a royalist garrison. **Ossa** 1978;5:25–33

Stirland A: The burials from King Henry VIII's ship, the Mary Rose: an interim statement. **Paleopathol Newsl** 1984 Sep;(47):7–10

**Italy**

Fornaciari G: The mummies of the Abbey of Saint Domenico Maggiore in Naples. **Paleopathol Newsl** 1984 Sep;(47):10–4

**1700 to Present**

Eckert WG: Identification of the remains of John Paul Jones: a look at early methods. **Am J Forensic Med Pathol** 1982 Jun;3(2):143–52

Lasky II: Autopsy of Admiral John Paul Jones 113 years postmortem; historic and forensic aspects. **NY State J Med** 1982 Jun;82(7):1110–5

**Belgium**

Jurion F, Parisel F: Le troisième et dernier cimetière de l'hôpital Saint-Jean de Bruxelles (1704–1784). Etude paléopathologique des ossements du cimetière Saint-Jean. **Ann Soc Belg Hist Hop** 1982;20:2–60

**United States**

Stewart TD: Essentials of forensic anthropology, especially as developed in the United States. Springfield, Ill, Thomas, 1979. xvii, 300 p.

Stewart TD: J. Lawrence Angel. **Am J Phys Anthropol** 1979 Nov;51(4):509–16

Ubelaker DH: The development of American paleopathology. In F. Spencer, ed: A history of American physical anthropology, 1930–1980. New York, Academic Press, 1982. p. 337–56.

Zimmerman MR, et al: The paleopathology of an Aleutian mummy. **Arch Pathol Lab Med** 1981 Dec;105(12):638–41

## PARASITOLOGY

See also **Microbiology; Tropical Medicine**

Ascuasiati de Alfau C: Efémerides en la historia de la parasitología. [Santo Domingo], Dept. de Microbiología y Parasitología, Universidad Autónoma de Santa Domingo, 1982. 24 p.

Bonsdorff B von: Smittämnenas historia; en översikt. **Nord Medicinhist Arsbok** 1983;:89–101

Busvine JR: The evolution and mutual adaptation of insects, microorganisms and man. In Stanley NF, Joske RA, ed: Changing disease patterns and human behaviour. London, New York, Academic Press, 1980. p. 55–68.

Grundy JH: The evolution and impact of medical entomology. **J R Army Med Corps** 1980 Oct;126(3):140–50

Janssens PG: Parasitism, parasites and disease. **Ann Soc Belg Med Trop** 1982;62(3):183–212

Kean BH, Mott K, Russell AJ: Tropical medicine and parasitology: classic investigations. 2 v. Ithaca, N. Y., Cornell Univ. Press, 1978. xxiii, 677 p.

Théodoridès J: Geschichte der Parasitologie. In Sournia JC, Martiny M, Poulet J, ed: Illustrierte Geschichte der Medizin. Salzburg, Andreas, 1980. Vol. 8. p. 2933–59.

**Africa**

Lambrecht FL: Palaeoecology of Tsetse flies and sleeping sickness in Africa. **Proc Am Philos Soc** 1980 Oct 10;124(5):367–85

**Japan**

HTLV missionaries and parasites: **Lancet** 1984 Oct 20;2(8408):927–8

**Before 500 A.D.**

Chen LB, Hung T: [Scanning electron microscopic view of parasitic worm ova in an ancient corpse (author's transl)] (Chi). **Chung Kuo I Hsueh Ko Hsueh Yuan Hsueh Pao** 1981 Mar;3(1):64–5

**Brazil**

Araújo AJ, Confalonieri UE, Ferreira LF: Oxyurid infestations in small animals from 9,000 B.P. in Brazil. **Paleopathol Newsl** 1980 Sep;(31):13–14

**Chile**

Aráujo A, Ferreira LF, Confalonieri UE, et al: Eggs of Diphyllobothrium pacificum in precolumbian human coprolites. **Paleopathol Newsl** 1983 Mar;41:11–3

Ferreira LF, Ribeiro Filho BM, Araújo AJ de, et al: Enterobius vermicularis eggs in preColumbian human coprolites from Chile. **Paleopathol Newsl** 1984;46:4–5

**China**

Hu SY: [Study on the parasite eggs in an ancient corpse from Zhangguo Chu Tomb No. 1 in Mashan brick-field of Jiangling County, Hubei] (Chi). **Chi Sheng Chung Hsueh Yu Chi Sheng Chung Ping Tsa Chih** 1984;2(1):8

**Egypt**

Cockburn A: Ancient parasites on the West Bank of the Nile. **Lancet** 1981 Oct 24;2(8252)938

**1450–1700**

**Great Britain**

Selwyn S: The transition from mythology to medical microbiology in 1589. In: Congrès international d'histoire de la médecine, XXVe, Québec, 1976. Actes. Québec, 1977. p. 1262–73.

**1700 to Present**

Biocca E: Problemi parassitologici in rapporto ad una politica dell'ambiente. **Parassitologia** 1979;21(1–3):1–9

Chebotarev RS: Ocherki po istorii meditsinskoĭ i veterinarnoĭ parazitologii. Minsk, Nauka i tekhnika, 1977. 308 p.

Chernin E: The curious case of the lateral-spined egg: schistosoma mansoni. **Trans R Soc Trop Med Hyg** 1983;77(6):847–50

Crosskey RW, Post RJ: Which cytospecies of the Simulium damnosum complex did Blacklock incriminate in the transmission of Onchocerca volvulus? **Ann Trop Med Parasitol** 1981 Oct;75(5):569–71

Desowitz RS: New Guinea tapeworms and Jewish grandmothers. Tales of parasites and people. New York, London, W. W. Norton, 1981. 224 p.

Grundy JH: The evolution and impact of medical entomology. In Burgess NR, ed: John Hull Grundy's Arthropods of medical importance. Watch Cottage, Chilbolton, Hampshire, Noble Books, 1981. p. 13–25.

Hartree EF: David Keilin. In Dictionary of national biography, 1961–1970. Suppl. 8, 1981. p. 604–5.

Hesse PG: Współpraca naukowa Schaudinn--Siedlecki w roku 1897. **Przegl Dermatol** 1983 May–Jun;70(3):307–10

Hoogstraal H: Changing patterns of tickborne diseases in modern society. **Annu Rev Entomol** 1981;26:75–99

Laird M: Integrirovannye metody bor'by s perenoschikami i ugroza gemorragicheskoĭ likhoradlki Denge v tropicheskoĭ zone Tikhogo Okeana. **Parazitologiia** 1984 Mar–Apr;18(2):99–105

Rosický B: Razvitie ideĭ akademika E. N. Pavlovskogo v stranakh Tsentral'noĭ Evropy. **Med Parazitol (Mosk)** 1984 Mar–Apr;(2):21–8

Sandbach FR: The history of schistosomiasis research and policy for its control. **Med Hist** 1976 Jul;20(3):259–75

Théodoridès J, Rousset JJ: A propos de la découverte de Trichomonas tenax, Protozaire parasite de l'homme, par O. F. Müller. **Rev Hist Sci (Paris)** 1980 Apr;33(2):163–4

**Africa**

Nicolle P: Alphonase Laveran et Charles Nicolle. **Arch Inst Pasteur Tunis** 1981 Sep–Dec;58(3):265–79

Senft AW: Parasitic disease and exploration: a glimpse of Central Africa in the 1860s. **RI Med J** 1983 Jan;66(1):31–6

# PARASITOLOGY

**Algeria**

Laveran CL: Classics in infectious diseases: A newly discovered parasite in the blood of patients suffering from malaria. Parasitic etiology of attacks of malaria: Charles Louis Alphonse Laveran (1845–1922). **Rev Infect Dis** 1982 Jul–Aug;4(4):908–11

**Australia**

Spratt DM. Dr Ian Murray Mackerras. **Int J Parasitol** 1980 Nov–Dec;10(5–6):329–36

**Brazil**

Lewinsohn R: Carlos Chagas and the discovery of Chagas' disease (American trypanosomiasis). **J R Soc Med** 1981 Jun;74(6):451–5

**Burundi**

Perich P: Les foyers de trypanosomiase humaine africaine à Trypanosoma rhodesiense (vecteur Glossina morsitans) au Burundi. Aspects historiques et actuels. **Med Trop (Mars)** 1982 Jan–Feb;42(1):33–41

**Canada**

Fallis AM: John L. Todd: Canada's first professor of parasitology. **Can Med Assoc J** 1983 Sep 1;129(5):486, 488–90

**Cuba**

Delgado García G: Libros de texto cubanos sobre parasitología y enfermedades tropicales. Comentarios bibliográficos. Primera et segunda parte. **Rev Cubana Med Trop** 1982 Sep–Dec;34(3):327–41

**Czechoslovakia**

Rosický B: Professor Evgenii Nikonorovich Pavlovsky--100 years since his birth. **J Hyg Epidemiol Microbiol Immunol** 1984;28(2):115–8

**Egypt**

Classics in infectious diseases: A contribution to human helminthology: Theodore Bilharz (1825–1862). **Rev Infect Dis** 1982 May–Jun;4(3):727–32

**France**

Brumpt L: L'oeuvre de Laveran en protozoologie et ses conséquences. **Bull Acad Natl Med (Paris)** 1980 Jan;164(1):88–93

Bykhovskaia-Pavlovskaia IE: Istoriia otkrytiia Sharlem Nikollem puti zarazheniia sypnym tifom. **Parassitologia** 1981 Jan–Feb;15(1):87–91

Lamy LH: Sur un point particulier de la contribution de Robert Deschiens à la connaissance des amibes. **Bull Soc Pathol Exot Filiales** 1978;71 Spec No:502–8

Nosny P: Alphonse Laveran et la découverte de l'hématozoaire du paludisme. **Bull Acad Natl Med (Paris)** 1980 Jan;164(1):80–7

Séance du 11 octobre 1978: Séance solennelle à la mémoire du Professeur Robert Deschiens (Professeur et Chef de Service honoraire à l'Institut Pasteur, Membre de l'Académie Nationale de Médecine, Secrétaire Général de la Société de Pathologie Exotique). **Bull Soc Pathol Exot Filiales** 1978;71 Spec No:499–511

Théodoridès J: Claude Bernard et les parasites. (Contribution au centenaire de la mort de Claude Bernard). **Hist Nat** 1979;(14):31–8

**Germany**

Althoff A: Wissenschaftlicher Briefwechsel von und mit Theodor Bilharz. Düsseldorf, Triltsch, 1980. 133 p. (Düsseldorfer Arbeiten zur Geschichte der Medizin, 56; also Diss.) **Dusseld Arb Gesch Med Hefte** 1980;56:1–133

Boray JC: Obituary: Georg Lämmler. **Int J Parasitol** 1981 Oct;11(5):335–40

Eichler W, Jahn I: Fritz Peus 1904--1978. **Angew Parasitol** 1979 Oct;20(3):164–72

Eichler W: Nachruf auf Günter Timmermann (zugleich eine wissenschaftsgeschichtliche Studie zum Disput um die Fahrenholzsche Regel). **Angew Parasitol** 1981 Feb;22(1):53–6

Engelbrecht H, Gräfner G, Müller P, et al: 20 Jahre Parasitologische Gesellschaft der DDR. **Angew Parasitol** 1981 Nov;22(4):185–92

Enigh K: Als Parasitologe im Veterinärdienst des Heeres. **DTW** 1981 Nov 5;88(11):479–83

Enigk K: Abriss der Geschichte der deutschen vet. med. Parasitologie. **Berl Munch Tierarztl Wochenschr** 1982 Oct 1;95(19):374–82

Hesse PG: F. R. Shaudinn i jego dzieło. **Przegl Dermatol** 1983 May–Jun;70(3):303–6

Hiepe T, Odening K, Vater G: Georg Wildführ sen. zum 80. Geburtstag. **Angew Parasitol** 1984 Aug;25(3):117–20

Hiepe T, Odening K: Zur Entwicklung der Parasitologie in der DDR. **Angew Parasitol** 1979 Nov;20(4):177–85

**Great Britain**

Cule J: Griffith Evans (1835–1935) and his trypanosome. **Vet Hist** 1979–80;1(3):94–101

Southgate VR: Obituary. Dr. Christopher A. Wright. **Int J Parasitol** 1984 Jun;14(3):223–7

**India**

Gibson ME: The identification of kala azar and the discovery of Leishmania donovani. **Med Hist** 1983 Apr;27(2):203–13

Naidis M: 'Ants, muskeetoes, flies and stinking chints': the British battle against disease in India. **West Hum Rev** 1964;17(1):39–47

**Italy**

Balbo T: In memoria di Edoardo Perroncito nel centenario di fondazione della prima Cattedra di Parassitologia. **Parassitologia** 1980 Dec;22(3):233–7

De Carneri I: Un secolo di ricerche di parassitologia umana in Italia: riflessioni e prospettive. **Parassitologia** 1981 Dec;23(1–3):1–30

Théodoridès J: Sebastiano Rivolta (1832–1893) parasitologiste et microbiologiste. **Hist Sci Med** 1980;14(2):227–32

**Japan**

Lebedev BI: O nekotorykh parasitologicheskikh uchrezhdeniaikh Iaaponii. **Parazitologiia** 1981 Jul–Aug;15(4):388–91

**Kenya**

Wilson CL, Williams CM: Toward the biological control of insect pests: the rise of the International Center of Insect Physiology and Ecology. **Sci Public Aff Bull At Sci** 1973;29(3):10–16

**Malaysia**

Reid JA: Was Anopheles Donaldi a vector of malaria in Kuala Lumpur, Malaysia, in the past? **Trans R Soc Trop Med Hyg** 1980;74(3):337–9

**Netherlands**

Palm LC: De paalwormepidemie van 1730. **Spiegel Hist** 1980;15(5):266–72

**Poland**

Furmaga S: 30 lat Polskiego Towarzystwa parazytologicznego. **Wiad Parazytol** 1980;26(4–5):293–8

Gundłach JL: Prof. Dr Stefan Furmaga (1924–1983). Wspomnienie pośmiertne. **Wiad Parazytol** 1984;30(3):385–91

Slusarski W: W pięćdziesiątą rocznicę śmierci Konstantego S. Janickiego (1876–1932). **Wiad Parazytol** 1983;28(5–6):507–15

**South Africa**

Findlay GH: South African tick-bite fever (1931–1981). **S Afr Med J** 1981 Dec 26;60(26):998–1000

**Sri Lanka**

Mirando EH: Dr E. M. Wijerama. **Ceylon Med J** 1981 Mar;26(1):5–7

Ranasinghe L: The medical writings of Dr. E. M. Wijerama. **Ceylon Med J** 1981 Mar;26(1):1–4

**United States**

Aldridge WN: Insecticides, past, present and future: practice and the understanding of mechanisms. **Ann Occup Hyg** 1979;22(4):407–9

Govier WM: A helminthic tale. **Perspect Biol Med** 1984 Autumn;28(1):104–6

Jones JE: Parasites in Kentucky: the past seven decades. **J Ky Med Assoc** 1983 Aug;81(8):621–7

Perkins JH: Reshaping technology in wartime: the effect of military goals on entomological research and insect-control practices. **Technol Cult** 1978 Apr;19(2):169–86

Ross RT: Statute and legislative history of the Federal Insecticide, Fungicide, and Rodenticide Act and its impact on agriculture. **J Environ Sci Health [B]** 1980;B15(6):665–76

Sawyer DJ: The lady with the snake in her. **NY Folkl Q** 1969;25(4):299–305

Smithcors JF: Discovery of the arthropod vector of disease. **Mod Vet Pract** 1981 May;62(5):371–4

Talmage DW: William Hay Taliaferro: February 10, 1895–December 21, 1973. **Biogr Mem Natl Acad Sci** 1983;54:375–407

**USSR**

Balashov IuS: Issledovaniia paraziticheskikh chlenistonogikh i perenoschikov v Zoologicheskom institute AN SSSR. **Parazitologiia** 1982 Sep–Oct;16(5):428–31

Burgasov PN: Shest'desiat let SSSR: itogi i perspektivy raboty parazitologov nasheĭ strany. **Med Parazitol (Mosk)** 1982 Nov–Dec;60(6):3–9

Chagin KP: Rol' akademika E. N. Pavlovskogo v izuchenii épidemiologii parazitarnykh i transmissivnykh bolezneĭ (k 100–letiiu so dnia rozhdeniia). **Zh Mikrobiol Epidemiol Immunobiol** 1984 Jun;(6):117–20

Gusev AV: Commemorating the 100th birthday of Valentin Aleksandrovich Dogiel (1882–1955). **J Parasitol** 1982 Dec;68(6):1188–9

Kupriianova ES, Detinova TS, Anufrieva VN, et al: Osnovnye napravleniia rabot V. N. Baklemisheva v oblasti meditsinskoĭ éntomologii i ikh znachenie v épidemiologii i profilaktike transmissivnykh bolezneĭ. **Med Parazitol (Mosk)** 1982 Jan–Feb;51(1):33–9

Oshmarin AP: Gel'mintologicheskie issledovaniia M. M. Zavadovskogo. **Parazitologiia** 1980 May–Jun;14(3):282–7

Oshmarin AP: Razvitie ékologicheskogo napravleniia v otechestvennoĭ gel'mintologii nauchnoĭ shkoloĭ A. A. Soboleva. **Parazitologiia** 1983 Jul–Aug;17(4):324–8

Pervomaĭskiĭ GS, Podolian VIa, Chagin KP, et al: Rol' akademika Evgeniia Nikanorovicha Pavlovskogo v stanovlenii i razvitii parazitologii v SSSR (k 100–letiiu so dnia rozhdeniia). **Parazitologiia** 1984 Mar–Apr;18(2):89–98

Ryzhikov KM, Sonin MD: Biologicheskie problemy gel'mintologii. Kratkaia istoriia razvitiia issledovaniĭ v SSSR i vazhneĭshie dostizheniia. **Parazitologiia** 1982 Nov–Dec;16(6):433–40

Shcherbina VP, Liashenko NI: Akademik Evgeniĭ Nikanorovich Pavlovskiĭ (k 100–letiiu so dnia rozhdeniia). **Voen Med Zh** 1984 Feb;(2):65–8

Shipitsina NK: Vliianie issledovaniĭ V. N. Beklemisheva v oblasti obshcheĭ biologii, parazitologii i épidemiologii transmissivnykh bolezneŭ na razvitie étikh otrasleĭ nauki (k 90–letiiu so dnia rozhdeniia). **Med Parazitol (Mosk)** 1982 Mar–Apr;60(2):86–8

Shusterov AK, Shcherbina VP: Nikolaĭ Aleksandrovich Kholodkovskiĭ (K 125–letiiu so dnia rozhdeniia). **Parazitologiia** 1983 Jul–Aug;17(4):322–4

Skobulovich GV: Itogi deiatel'nosti Amursjkogo otdeleniia Nauchnogo obshchestva épidemiologov, mikrobiologov i parazitologov za 25 let (1957–1982). **Zh Mikrobiol Epidemiol Immunobiol** 1984 Feb;(2):117–9

Smirnova KV: O razvitii ékologicheskoĭ parazitologii v Kazakhstane. **Parazitologiia** 1982 Jan–Feb;16(1):85–7

Soprunov FF: K 90–letiiu so dnia rozhdeniia Petra Grigor'evicha Sergieva (1893–1983). **Med Parazitol (Mosk)** 1983 Nov–Dec;(6):3–6

Tamarina NA, Lange AB: Razvitie ideĭ V. N. Beklemisheva v oblasti sravnitel'noĭ parazitologii. **Med Parazitol (Mosk)** 1982 Jan–Feb;51(1):3–9

**Venezuela**

Iriarte DR: [Public health in Venezuela]. **Rev Soc Venez Hist Med** 1975–76;23(37):107–21

# PATHOLOGY

Ackerknecht EH: Causes and pseudocauses in the history of diseases. In Stevenson LG, ed: A celebration of medical history. Baltimore, Johns Hopkins University Press, 1982. (The Henry E. Sigerist supplements to the Bulletin of the History of Medicine; new ser., no. 6). p. 19–31. With commentary by C. E. Rosenberg, 'The history of disease: now and in the future,' p. 32–6.

Autopsy: necessity or anachronism?: **MD** 1980 Dec;24(12):75–8

Bean WB: Changing patterns of ideas about disease. In Rothschild H, ed: Biocultural aspects of disease. New York, Academic Press, 1981. p. 25–51.

Belloni L: Il Morgagni tra il Malpighi e il Cotugno. **Gesnerus** 1982;39(2):195–213

Bollet AJ: The rise and fall of disease. **Am J Med** 1981 Jan;70(1):12–6

Busvine JR: The evolution and mutual adaptation of insects, microorganisms and man. In Stanley NF, Joske RA, ed: Changing disease patterns and human behaviour. London, New York, Academic Press, 1980. p. 55–68.

Chernukh AM: Ocherki obshcheĭ (teoreticheskoĭ) patologii. **Patol Fiziol Eksp Ter** 1983 May–Jun;3:51–78

Comiti VP: Importance des connaissances médico–biologiques actuelles pour une étude critique de pathocénose historique. In Imhof AE, ed: Mensch und Gesundheit in der Geschichte. Husum, Matthiesen, 1980. p. 35–43.

Doerr W: Evolutionstheorie und pathologische Anatomie. **Verh Dtsch Ges Pathol** 1983;67:663–84

Dustin P: Die pathologische Anatomie. In Sournia JC, Martiny M, Poulet J, ed: Illustrierte Geschichte der Medizin. Salzburg, Andreas, 1980. Vol. 6. p. 2103–47.

Fenner F: Sociocultural change and environmental diseases. In Stanley NF, Joske RA, ed: Changing disease patterns and human behaviour. London, New York, Academic Press, 1980. p. 7–26.

Fitzgerald PJ: Medical anecdotes concerning some diseases of the pancreas. **Monogr Pathol** 1980;21:1–29

Geller SA: Autopsy. **Mt Sinai J Med (NY)** 1984 Jan–Feb;51(1):77–81

Gurevitsh SA: [The pathographic method in the history of medicine.] (Rus). **Orvostort Kozl** 1981;93–96(27 No 1–4):155–69

Hudson RP: Disease and its control. The shaping of modern thought. Westport, London, Greenwood Press, 1983. xvii, 259 p. (Contributions in Medical History, no. 12).

Joske RA: The physician and changing patterns of human disease and death. In Stanley NF, Joske RA, ed: Changing disease patterns and human behaviour. London, New York, Academic Press, 1980. p. 551–66.

Klepinger LL: The evolution of human disease: new findings and problems. **J Biosoc Sci** 1980 Oct;12(4):481–6

Lambrecht M: Die Krankheitsauffassung in der ätiologischen Ara. **Wiss Beitr Martin Luther Univ Halle Wittenberg** 1983;5–R80:63–70

Leibowitz JO: Early accounts in geriatric pathology (Leonardo, Harvey, James Keill). **Koroth** 1980 Jun;7(11–12):CCLIII–CCLXIV

Mims C: The emergence of new infectious diseases. In Stanley NF, Joske RA, ed: Changing disease patterns and human behaviour. London, New York, Academic Press, 1980. p. 231–50.

Nutton V: The seeds of disease: an explanation of contagion and infection from the Greeks to the Renaissance. **Med Hist** 1983 Jan;27(1):1–34

Putscher M: Le malattie nell'iconografia scientifica. **Acta Med Hist Patav** 1980–81:27:43–53

Robins RS: Disease, political events, and populations. In Rothschild H, ed: Biocultural aspects of disease. New York, Academic Press, 1981. p. 153–75.

Rothschild H: Diseases of the Jews. In his: Biocultural aspects of disease. New York, Academic Press, 1981. p. 531–55.

Schadewaldt H: Das Verhältnis zur Krankheit im Wandel der Zeit. **Wien Med Wochenschr** 1980 Nov 15;130(21):673–82

Taylor FK: Disease concepts and the logic of classes. **Br J Med Psychol** 1981 Sep;54(pt 3):277–86

Temkin O: Some moral implications of the concept of disease. In Ganzinger K, Skopec M, Wyklicky H, ed: Festschrift für Erna Lesky zum 70. Geburtstag. Wien, Brüder Hollinek, 1981. p. 153–60.

VanHartesveldt FR: Disease in the Western world: a review essay. **Teach Hist J Methods** 1980;5(1):75–81

Watts ES: The biological race concept and diseases of modern man. In Rothschild H, ed: Biocultural aspects of disease. New York, Academic Press, 1981. p. 3–23.

**Germany**

Kössling FK, Prölss E: Die Pathologie in Bremen. **Verh Dtsch Ges Pathol** 1980;64:XXIX–XXXV

**India**

Krishan Y: The meaning of prajnā–aparādha and karma in Ayurveda. **Bull Indian Inst Hist Med Hyderabad** 1982;12(1–4):28–33

**Italy**

Bucklin R: The Shroud of Turin: a pathologist's viewpoint. **Leg Med** 1982;:33–9

**Spain**

López Piñero JM, Bumosa F, Terrada ML: Clásicos españoles de la anatomía patológica anteriores a Cajal. Spanish classics on pathology before Cajal. Valencia, Cátedra e Instituto de Historia de la Medicina, 1979. 254 p. (Cuadernos Valencianos de Historia de la Medicina y de la Ciencia, 21, Serie B).

López Piñero JM, Bujosa F, Terrada ML, ed: Clásicos españoles de la anatomía patológica anteriores a Cajal. Valencia, Cátedra e Instituto de Historia de la Medicina, 1979. xv, 254 p. (Cuadernos Valencianos de Historia de la Medicina y de la Ciencia, XXI, Serie B (Textos Clasicos)).

**Turkey**

Demirhan A: The development of education of pathology and anatomy in Ottoman Turks. **Stud Hist Med** 1981 Jun;5(2):160–6

**USSR**

Truupyl'd AIu: Patologicheskaia anatomiia v Tartuskom universitete. **Arkh Patol** 1983;45(9):66–72

**Before 500 A.D.**

Kuttner RE: Protohistoric hepatomancy: an oracular form of pathology. **Proc Inst Med Chic** 1982 Jan–Mar;35(1):14

Steinberg A: [Scientific pathology in the books of Talmud.] (Heb). **Harefuah** 1983 Mar 1;104(5):201–2

**Babylon**

Adamson PB: Anatomical and pathological terms in Akkadian. **J R Asiat Soc GB Irel** 1974;102–6: 1979;2–8: 1981;125–32.

**India**

Filliozat J: Sur l'identification des maladies dans l'Ayurveda. In Mazars G, ed: Les médecines traditionnelles de l'Asie. Strasbourg, Université Louis Pasteur, 1981. p. 140–9.
Miltner V: [Ancient Indian concepts of the body and disease] (Cze). **Cas Lek Cesk** 1981 Jun 4;120(22):682–4

**Rome**

Phillips JH: The etiology of disease: a Late Republican view. In International Congress of the History of Medicine, 27th, Barcelona, 1980. Actas. Barcelona, Académia de Ciències Mèdiques de Catalunya i Balears, 1981. p. 327–30.

**500 A.D.–1450**

**Arabic**

Carreras Panchón A: Sobre el concepto de pestilencia (WABA') en el Canon de Avicena. **Asclepio** 1981;33:265–73
Harmarneh SK: Ibn al-Ayn Zarbi and his definitions of diseases and their diagnoses. In: International Symposium for the History of Arabic Science, 1st, University of Aleppo, 1976. Proceedings. Aleppo, Syria, 1976. Papers in European Languages, Vol. II. p. 305–23.

**Great Britain**

Bober H, McKinney LC: La prima autopsia. **Kos** 1984 Mar;1(2):51–60

**1450–1700**

Crellin J: Théophile Bonet (1620–1689). **Am J Pathol** 1980 Jan;98(1):212
Mani N: Neue Konzepte der Pathologie im 17. Jahrhundert. **Gesnerus** 1983;40(1–2):109–17

**Italy**

Belloni L: Zur Deutung zweier pathologischer Stellen (eine mit Zeichnung) aus der Anatomie von Leonardo: Lungenechinococcus, Halslymphdrüsenverkalkung. **Gesnerus** 1980;37(1/2):139–44
Campan L: Le tricentenaire de Morgagni (1682–1721). **Agressologie** 1982;23(7):291–2
Rodriguez-Castellon JA: Selected items from the history of pathology - Girolamo Fracastoro (1478–1553). **Am J Pathol** 1980;101(1):62

**Mexico**

Rico-Avello C: Patologia en la conquista de Mejico. **Asclepio** 1978–79;30–31:377–87

**Netherlands**

Lindeboom GA: Anton de Heide als proefondervindelijk onderzoeker. **Tijdschr Geschied Geneeskd** 1983;6(3):121–34
Veltheer W: Erasmus, in de grond niet so slecht. **Spiegel Hist** 1982;17(4):190–6

**Switzerland**

Trebbin H: Frühe Pathologie. **MMW** 1980 Feb 8;122(6):209–11

**1700 to Present**

Ackerman LV: H. P. Smith Award lecture. Tumor pathologists I have known. **Am J Clin Pathol** 1982 Apr;77(4):385–90
Arendt A: Die Rolle der Neuropathologie in der Allgemeinen Pathologie und Speziellen Pathologischen Anatomie. **Zentralbl Neurochir** 1983;44(2):113–20
Astor G: The disease detectives. Deadly medical mysteries and the people who solved them. New York, Scarborough, Ont., NAL Books, 1983. 216 p.
Belloni L: The discovery of duodenal ancylostoma and of its pathogenic power. In M. D. Grmek, R. S. Cohen, G. Cimino, ed: On scientific discovery. The Erice Lectures 1977. Dordrecht, D. Reidel, 1981. p. 261–79. (Boston Studies in the Philosophy of Science, v. 34).
Bendiner E: Noguchi: many triumphs and a brilliant failure. **Hosp Pract [Off]** 1984 Feb;19(2):222–3, 227, 231 passim
Biraben JN: Histoire des classifications de causes de décès et de maladies aux XVIIIe et XIXe siècles. In Imhof AE, ed: Mensch und Gesundheit in der Geschichte. Husum, Matthiesen, 1980. p. 23–34.
Bleker J: Die historische Pathologie, Nosologie und Epidemiologie im 19. Jahrhundert. **Medizinhist J** 1984;19(1–2):33–52
Brodin MB: William Osler and dermatology, pathology, and dermatopathology. **Am J Dermatopathol** 1981 Fall;3(3):261–4
Cabanne F: Pierre Masson. Précurseur et rénovateur (1880–1959). **Ann Pathol** 1983;3(1):95–7
Carter KC: Semmelweis's possible influence on Karl Mayrhofer and on those who subsequently developed nineteenth century etiological theories. **Orvostort Kozl** 1982;28(1–3):23–31
Cleveland FP: History of environmental pathology. **Am J Forensic Med Pathol** 1983 Dec;4(4):331–6
Comiti VP: Intérêts et apports d'une étude historique des maladies aux XVIIIe et XIXe siècles. **Hist Sci Med** 1980;14(2):201–6
Frable WJ: Fine-needle aspiration biopsy: a review. **Hum Pathol** 1983 Jan;14(1):9–28
Hazard JB: An introduction to the history of surgical pathology. **Am J Clin Pathol** 1981 Mar;75(3 Suppl):444–6
Hill IR: The historical background to aerospace pathology. **Aviat Space Environ Med** 1982 Jan;53(1):1–5
Imhof AE: The analysis of eighteenth-century causes: some methodological considerations. **Hist Methods Newsl** 1978;2(1):3–36
Keel O: La généalogie de l'histopathologie; une révision déchirante. Philippe Pinel, lecteur discret de J.-C. Smyth (1741–1821). Paris, Librairie Philosophique J. Vrin, 1979. ii, 135 p. (Histoire des Sciences: Textes et Etudes).
Keel O: Les conditions de la décomposition 'analytique' de l'organisme: Haller, Hunter, Bichat. **Etud Philos** 1982;:37–62
Michalany I: Masson's contribution to pathology and to histological technique. With special reference to the discovery of argentaffin cells. **Ann Pathol** 1983;3(1):85–93
Miřejovský P, Bednář B, Elleder M, et al: Současné zaměření a metodický základ poznávacího procesu v patologii. **Cas Lek Cesk** 1983 Oct 28;122(43):1317–9
Morgenstern L: The Virchow-Troisier node: a historical note. **Am J Surg** 1979 Nov;138(5):703
Ober WB: Ghon but not forgotten: Anton Ghon and his complex. **Pathol Annu** 1983;18 (pt 2):79–85
Rechtman J: De l'asepsie... ou un siècle avant Semmelweis. **Hist Sci Med** 1980;14(2):165–70
Reverend AP: La enfermedad y los ultimos momentos de Simon Bolivar, libertador de Colombia y del Peru. **Rev Soc Bolivar Venez** 1980;37(128):57–94
Rodin AE: Oslerian pathology: an assessment and annotated atlas of museum specimens. Lawrence, Kansas, Coronado, 1981. xviii, 250 p.
Seemayer TA: The life and legacy of Professor Pierre Masson. **Am J Surg Pathol** 1983 Mar;7(2):179–83
Waitzkin H: The social origins of illness: a neglected history. **Int J Health Serv** 1981;11(1):77–103
Wright RK, Tate LG: Forensic pathology. Last stronghold of the autopsy. **Am J Forensic Med Pathol** 1980 Mar;1(1):57–60

**Australia**

Attwood HD: Patients, pathologists and practice. **Aust NZ J Obstet Gynaecol** 1982 Feb;22(1):11–4
Pounder DJ: Death investigation in early colonial South Australia, 1839–40. **Med Sci Law** 1984 Oct;24(4):273–82
Pridmore S: The history of disease in Tasmania. **Mater Med Pol** 1980;12(4):302–3
Winton R: The nature of things: a history of the Royal College of Pathologists of Australasia. Sydney, The College, 1982. x, 120 p.

**Austria**

Carter KC: Ignaz Semmelweis, Carl Mayrhofer, and the rise of germ theory. **Med Hist** 1985 Jan;29(1):33–53
Miciotto RJ: Carl Rokitansky: nineteenth-century pathologist and leader of the new Vienna school. Ph.D. diss. Johns Hopkins University, 1979. 301 leaves.
Mikuz G: Die Pathologie in Innsbruck. **Verh Dtsch Ges Pathol** 1981;65:XXI–XXVI
Propst A: Bernd Lederer. **Verh Dtsch Ges Pathol** 1982;66:652–7
Schmalhofer J: Das Werk von Johann Florian Heller mit besonderer Berücksichtigung der Entstehung des ersten pathologisch-chemischen Laboratoriums am Allgemeinen Wiener Krankenhaus und der Ernennung Hellers zum Vorstand des Laboratoriums. Diss. Bonn, 1980. 201 p.
Wyklicky H: The role of the Vienna Medical School in the investigation and treatment of infectious diseases. In [The Vienna Medical School]. Produced under a grant from the Squibb Institute for Medical Research, [1983]. p. 6–20.

**Canada**

Bonenfant JL: La pathologie à l'âge des incertitudes. **Union Med Can** 1984 May;113(5):352–4
Cadotte M: Historique du laboratoire de pathologie de l'Hôtel-Dieu de Montréal: de sa création en 1896, à l'arrivée du professeur Pierre Masson en 1928. **Union Med Can** 1979 May;108(5):479–94
Cadotte M: L'héritage scientifique du professeur Pierre Masson. **Union Med Can** 1984 May;113(5):344–5
Michalany J: Masson que j'ai connu: mon maître et mon ami. **Union Med Can** 1984 May;113(5):386–9
Smith K: Maude Abbott: pathologist and historian. **Can Med Assoc J** 1982

Oct 15;127(8):774–6

**Czechoslovakia**

Dobiás J, Marek J: Dr. Václav Treitz (1819–1872). K 110. výročí úmrtí a 125. výročí vybudování patologickoanatomického ústavu v Praze. **Cas Lek Cesk** 1983 Apr 1;122(13):405–7
Dobiáš J, Marek J: Patologická anatomie na pražské univerzitě před rokem 1882. **Cesk Patol** 1984 Feb;20(1):1–10
Fingerland A: Iaroslav Glava--osnovatel' chekhoslovatskoĭ shkoly patologoanatomov. **Arkh Patol** 1981;43(10):62–6
Fingerland A: 100. Výroči rozděleni Karlovy univerzity na českou a německou. Následný vliv na československou patologii. **Cesk Patol** 1983 Aug;19(3):129–32
Wondrák E: Ceský anatom a patolog V. A. Bochdalek--100 let od smrti. **Cas Lek Cesk** 1983 Oct 28;122(43):1334–7

**Europe**

Knapp VJ: Postmortems and the growth of modern medical knowledge in 19th century Europe. **J Okla State Med Assoc** 1983 Mar;76(3):73–6

**France**

Albury WR: French nosologies around 1800 and their relationship with chemistry. In Forbes EG, ed: Human implications of scientific advance. Edinburgh, Edinburgh University Press, 1978. p. 502–17.
Andral G: Pathological hematology: an essay on the blood in disease. Reprint of the 1844 ed. With a historical introduction by L. A. May. Oceanside, N. Y. Dabor Science Publications, 1977. 129 p.
Arquiola E: La enfermedad en la antropologia fisica francesa durante el positivismo. **Asclepio** 1983;35:217–26
Baumann J: Destinée de la méthode anatomo-clinique. **Bull Acad Natl Med (Paris)** 1981 Feb 17;Spec No:45–50
Comiti VP: Evolution de la pathologie française au XXe siècle. **Bull Sect Geogr Com Trav Hist Sci** 1978;83(2):11–28
Denoix P: Paul Broca. L'anatomie pathologique, le cancer, la statistique. **Chirurgie** 1980;106(10):787–90
De Saint-Maur PP: Que pensait Laennec de l'anatomie pathologique? **Ann Pathol** 1981;1(4):249–50
Lazorthes G, Campan L: Jean-Baptiste Morgagni (1682–1771), initiateur de la méthode anatomo-clinique. **Bull Acad Natl Med (Paris)** 1982 Dec;166(9):1317–21
Leroy D: Laennec étudiant en médecine. **Bull Acad Natl Med (Paris)** 1979 Nov 6–27;163(8):849–56
Mann RJ, Mann FD: Laennec as a critical pathologist. **J Hist Med Allied Sci** 1981 Oct;36(4):446–54
Maulitz RC: Channel crossing: the lure of French pathology for English medical students, 1816–36. **Bull Hist Med** 1981 Winter;55(4):475–96
Saint-Maur PP: Que pensait Laennec de l'anatomie pathologique? **Ann Pathol** 1981;1(4):249–50
Théodoridès J: Hippolyte Bernheim et la pathologie infectieuse. In: Congrès National des Sociétés Savantes, 103e, Nancy, 1978. Comptes Rendus. Paris, 1978. Section des Sciences, Fasc. V. p. 87–94.
Théodoridès J: Magendie et la pathologie infectieuse. **Hist Sci Med** 1983;17(4):367–80

**Germany**

Abe HR, Tiedt N: August Friedrich Hecker (1763–1811) und die Anfänge der modernen Pathophysiologie. **Beitr Gesch Univ Erfurt** 1979–83;19:165–85
Bauer A: Rudolf Virchow: der politische Arzt. Berlin, Stapp, 1982. 131 p. (Preussische Köpfe, 6).
Baumberger HR: Carl Liebermeister 1833–1901. Zürich, Juris, 1980. 181 p (Zürcher Medizingeschichtliche Abhandlungen, Neue Reihe, 137).
Bijok H: Adolph Carl Gustav Wernher (1809–1883); Sein Leben und Wirken am Giessener Akademischen Hospital. Giessen, Schmitz, 1979. 235 p. (Arbeiten zur Geschichte der Medizin in Giessen, Band 1).
Büchner F: Der junge Rudolf Virchow. **Verh Dtsch Ges Pathol** 1981;65:458–61
Crump T: Translation of case reports in Ueber die multiplen Fibrome der Haut und ihre Beziehung zu den multiplen Neuromen by F. v. Recklinghausen. **Adv Neurol** 1981;29:259–75
Doerr W: Gestalt theory and morbid anatomy. **Virchows Arch [A]** 1984;403(2):103–15
Eberhard Altenähr (4. 12. 1940 bis 5. 4. 1981): **Verh Dtsch Ges Pathol** 1981;65:561–70
Geiler G: Bedeutungsvolle Leistungen des Pathologischen Instituts Leipzig zur experimentell-theoretischen Pathologie und ätiopathogenetischen Forschung. **Zentralbl Allg Pathol** 1982;126(3–4):237–44
Hans-Jürgen Mohr (1. 11. 1922 bis 7. 6. 1982): **Verh Dtsch Ges Pathol** 1983;67:762–71
Haschen RJ: Entwicklung der Forschung auf dem Gebiet der Pathologischen und Klinischen Biochemie. **Z Med Lab Diagn** 1983;24(7):381–6
Hecht A: Wesen und geistige Wurzeln der Leipziger Pathologischen Anatomie. **Zentralbl Allg Pathol** 1982;126(3–4):229–36
Hollander A: P. G. Unna revisited. **Am J Dermatopathol** 1981 Summer;3(2):187–9
Holle G: Entwicklungslinien der morphologischen Forschung im Spiegel des Greifswalder Lehrstuhls für pathologische Anatomie. **Zentralbl Allg Pathol** 1982;126(5–6):417–23
Hundeiker M: Wilhelm Knoth. **Verh Dtsch Ges Pathol** 1982;66:646–52
Jakob Schoenmackers (26. 5. 1912 bis 22. 11. 1982): **Verh Dtsch Ges Pathol** 1983;67:778–85
Karlferdinand Kloos (17. 8. 1911 bis 29. 12. 1980): **Verh Dtsch Ges Pathol** 1981;65:548–59
Keil G: Zur Ueberlieferung von Virchows Würzburger Sektionsprotokollen. **Sudhoffs Arch** 1980;64(3):287–97
Kohl EW: Virchow in Würzburg. Pattensen/Han., Wellm, 1976. 129 p. (Diss., Würzburg).
Krumholz W: Eugen Woldemar Bostroem (1850–1928), Lehrer der Bathologie und Förderer der Medizin in Giessen. Giessen, Schmitz, 1983. 311 p. (Arbeiten zur Geschichte der Medizin in Giessen, Bd. 8)
Lechtenböhmer S: Die Dissertationen aus dem Institut für Pathologie der Tierärztlichen Hochschule Hannover seit Erteilung des Promotionsrechtes im Jahre 1910 bis Ende 1980. Diss., Tierärzliche Hochschule Hannover. Hannover, 1983. 162 p.
Lie JT: Carl Weigert (1845–1904), a pathfinder in medicine. **Mayo Clin Proc** 1980 Nov;55(11):716–20
Lin JI: Virchow's pathological reports on Frederick III's cancer. **N Engl J Med** 1984 Nov 8;311(19):1261–4
Mahnke PF: Die pathologisch-anatomische Schule Leipzig--ihre Stellung, Bedeutung und Wandlung in der klinischen Pathologie. Ein Beitrag zur Geschichte der Prosektur am Pathologisch-anatomischen Institut der Karl-Marx-Universität Leipzig. **Zentralbl Allg Pathol** 1982;126(3–4):245–52
Mai A: Diagnosestellung niedergelassener Arzte bei der Leichenschau im Vergleich zu den Ergebnissen der gerichtlichen Obduktion. Diss., Johannes Gutenberg - Universität in Mainz. Mainz, 1982. 143 p.
Martha Schmidtmann (4. 8. 1892 bis 28. 4. 1981): **Verh Dtsch Ges Pathol** 1981;65:571–5
Neumann-Redlin von Meding E: Ernst Neumann. Zum 150. Geburtstag des Königsberger Pathologen und Hämatologen am 30.1. 1984. **Pathologe** 1984 Jan;5(1):53–6
Richard Neuhold (17. 10. 1917 bis 14. 8. 1982): **Verh Dtsch Ges Pathol** 1983;67:774–7
Schauer A: Die Pathologie in Göttingen seit 1967. **Verh Dtsch Ges Pathol** 1982;66:XXIII–IX
Schellmann B: Kunst und Pathologie: Joseph Beuys--'zeige deine Wunde'. **Pathologe** 1983 Nov;4(6):325–7
Schubert GE: Christian Jakob Hackmann. **Verh Dtsch Ges Pathol** 1982;66:640–4
Walter Sandritter (7. 7. 1920 bis 12. 11. 1980): **Verh Dtsch Ges Pathol** 1981;65:533–48
Warkany J: Friedrich Daniel von Recklinghausen and his times. **Adv Neurol** 1981;29:251–7
Warzok R: 125 Jahre Lehrstuhl für pathologische Anatomie an der Universität Greifswald. **Zentralbl Allg Pathol** 1982;126(5–6):405–15
Weidenbach H, Massmann J: Der Beitrag des Pathologischen Instituts Leipzig zu den gegenwärtigen Vorstellungen über die Atiopathogenese der Arteriosklerose. **Zentralbl Allg Pathol** 1982;126(3–4):253–9
Willi Busanny-Caspari (8. 4. 1922 bis 7. 7. 1982): **Verh Dtsch Ges Pathol** 1983;67:772–3

**Great Britain**

Aronson ME: Sherlock Holmes, father of forensic pathology. **Trans Stud Coll Physicians Phila** 1978 Jul;45(5):258–61
Barrie HJ: Sir William Boyd: a legacy in print. **Can Med Assoc J** 1982 Feb 15;126(4):421,423–4
Björkholm M: Mannen bakom syndromet: Thomas Hodgkin. Temperamentsfull föregångare inom patologin och kämpe för rättvisa åt förtryckta folk. **Lakartidningen** 1983 Feb 2;80(5):334–5
Cahn LR: Some notes on Sir Jonathan Hutchinson (1828–1913). **Am J Surg Pathol** 1979 Dec;3(6):563–6
Christie AB: Infection in Britain yesterday. **J R Coll Physicians Lond** 1981 Apr;15(2):95–7
Eckert WG: The Whitechapel murders: the case of Jack the Ripper. **Am J Forensic Med Pathol** 1981 Mar;2(1):53–60
Greenwald MW, Greenwald GI: Coroner's inquests. A source of vital statistics: Westminster, 1761–1866. **J Leg Med (Chicago)** 1983 Mar;4(1):51–86
Henkelmann T: Zur Geschichte des pathophysiologischen Denkens. John Brown (1735–1788) und sein System der Medizin. Berlin, New York, Springer, 1981. 104 p.
Hunter GM: Pathologist turned general practitioner. Reflections of an ex-Army pathologist. **J R Army Med Corps** 1981 Jun;127(2):93–7
Keel O: La pathologie tissulaire de John Hunter. **Gesnerus** 1980;37(1/2):47–61
Macfarlane RG: Howard Florey; the making of a great scientist. Oxford and New York, Oxford University Press, 1979. xvi, 396 p.
Macfarlane RG: Howard Walter Florey. In Dictionary of national

biography, 1961–1970. Suppl. 8, 1981. p. 370–4.
Oakley CL: Sir Gordon Roy Cameron. In Dictionary of national biography, 1961–1970. Suppl. 8, 1981. p. 167–9.
Reckert H: Das unbekannte Werk des Pathologen, Robert Carswell (1793–1857). Köln, 1982. 283 p. (Kölner medizinhistorische Beiträge, Band 22)

### Hungary

Bugyi B: Az iskolázottak betegségeiről. **Magy Konyvsz** 1976;92(4):397–401
Frankl J: Entz Béla professzor tudomanyos müködése. **Orvostort Kozl** 1979;86(24 no 4):107–11
Gyenes G: Adatok Babits Mihaly betegségéhez. **Orvostort Kozl** 1981;93–96(27 No 1–4):193–200
Hogye I: Kazinczy Ferenc feljegyzései a betegségekrol. **Orvostort Kozl** 1982;28(1–3):241–3
Lambrecht M: Entz Béla, a klinikai pathológia egyik hazai úttörője. **Orv Hetil** 1984 Oct 28;125(44):2694–5
Lambrecht M: Virchow és Pertik. **Orvostort Kozl** 1980;89–91(26 no 1–3):233–9
Somogyi E: A tiszaeszlári vérvád tanulságai (a budapesti egyetemi tanárok szerepe). **Orv Hetil** 1983 Jan 9;124(2):98–103
Szállási A: Högyes Endre pesti kinevezésének centenáriuma. **Orv Hetil** 1983 Oct 30;124(44):2691–3

### India

Jhala HI: Contribution of Bombay to progress of science of pathology. **Indian J Med Sci** 1980 Apr;34(4):65–71

### Ireland

Dahlin DC: James Watson Kernohan: 1896–1981. **Surg Neurol** 1984 Feb;21(2):107–9
Holland PD: The section of pathology and the development of pathology over the century. **Ir J Med Sci** 1983 Jan;152(1):50–6

### Italy

Arquiola E: La lesión neurologica en 'De sedibus et causis morborum' de Morgagni. In: Congrès international d'histoire de la médecine, XXVe, Québec, 1976. Actes. Québec, 1977. p. 461–8.
Giordano A: Morgagni and the first steps of a European pathology. A brief historical report. **Pathol Res Pract** 1984 Jul;178(6):642–3
Honti J: Morgagni kórbonctana. **Orv Hetil** 1983 Jan;124(4):219–20
Sarkisov DS: Dzh. B. Morgan'i (k 300–letiiu so dnia rozhdeniia). **Klin Med (Mosk)** 1983 Jan;61(1):110–4
Squartini F: L'Instituto di Anatomia Patologica di Perugia dall'anno accademico 1941–42 all'anno accademico 1977–78. **Pathologica** 1983 Nov–Dec;75(1040):763–74
Tavassoli M: Selected items from the history of pathology - Giulio Bizzozero (1846–1901). **Am J Pathol** 1980;101(1):50
Thiene G, Pennelli N: Terzo centenario della nascita di Giovanni Battista Morgagni (1682–1982): c'è ancora bisogno dell'autopsia? **G Ital Cardiol** 1983 Oct;13(10):262–4

### Japan

Ishii T: [Clinical pathology in the past 30 years] (Jpn) **Rinsho Byori** 1984 May;32(5):484–9
Kageyama K, Shimanine T, Ishikawa E: A seventy–year history of the Japanese pathological society. **Acta Pathol Jpn** 1982;32 Suppl 1:1–21

### Netherlands

Haneveld GT: Pathologische Anatomie in Utrecht, circa 1800–1850. Amsterdam, Meesters, 1978. x, 371 p.

### Norway

Larsen O: Hundre år med sykdomsoppfatningen og dens konsekvenser. **Tidsskr Nor Laegeforen** 1981 Jan;101(1):11–4

### Poland

Guzek JW: Professor Karol Klecki 1866–1931. **Przegl Lek** 1981;38(12):873–4
Guzek JW: Two hundred years of the pathologic physiology in Poland--a survey of its past and its present status. **Acta Physiol Pol** 1983 Jan–Feb;34(1):1–4
Kobuszewska–Faryna M: Rok 1978--rokiem ważnych rocznic dla patomorfologów polskich. **Patol Pol** 1979 Apr–Jun;30(2):153–6
Szymańska R: Karol Klecki (1866–1931) - wybitny patofizjolog i profesor Fakultetu Medycznego w Krakowie (w 50 rocznicę śmierci). **Pol Tyg Lek** 1981 Sep 21;36(38):1487–90

### Romania

Achievements in the normal and pathological morphology in Romania: **Morphol Embryol (Bucur)** 1981 Apr–Jun;27(2):105–8
Marcu N: Viața si activitatea doctorului Constantin C. Pastia (1883–1926). **Rev Ig [Bacteriol]** 1983 Jan–Mar;28(1):89–95

### Spain

Izquierdo JM: Contribución a la historia de la neuropatología española. **Arch Neurobiol (Madr)** 1983 Sep–Oct;46(5):327–34

### Sweden

Ahlström CG: Patologisk anatomi i Lund, 1668–1962. Lund, 1983. 155 p. (Sydsvenska Medicinhistoriska Sällskapets Arsskrift, Suppl. 2, 1983).
Falkmer S: Patologi i Umeå. **Nord Medicinhist Arsb** 1980;:147–76
Retzius' stilling i den svenske patologiske anatomi: **Tandlaegebladet** 1979 Oct;83(18):659

### Switzerland

Kis J: Der Knochenpathologe Emil Looser (1877–1936). Zürich, Juris, 1982. 68 p. Zürcher Medizingeschichtliche Abhandlungen, Neue Reihe, 149; also Diss.).

### Tunisia

Eyquem A: L'immuno–pathologie de l'auto–immunisation 1900–1980. **Arch Inst Pasteur Tunis** 1981 Sep–Dec;58(3):281–95

### United States

Ackerman LV: Dr. Evarts Graham and surgical pathology. **J Thorac Cardiovasc Surg** 1984 Nov;88(5 Pt 2):851–3
Alfred A. Angrist: **NY State J Med** 1983 May;83(6):809–11, 872–6
Azar HA: Arthur Purdy Stout (1885–1967). The man and the surgical pathologist. **Am J Surg Pathol** 1984 Apr;8(4):301–7
Beatty WK: Ludvig Hektoen--scientist and counselor. **Proc Inst Med Chic** 1982 Jan–Mar;35(1):7–9
Benson ES: Laboratory medicine in the United States--the dream and the reality. **Am J Clin Pathol** 1981 Jul;76(1):1–7
Brandt AM: Virginia Kneeland Frantz. In: Notable American women. The modern period. Cambridge, Mass., Belknap–Harvard Univ. Press, 1980. 4:247–8.
Coleman FC: A brief look at the sociopolitical and economic history of pathology in the United States. **J Fla Med Assoc** 1980 Feb;67(2):89–96
Corner GW: Leo Loeb. In Dictionary of American Biography, Suppl. 6, 1956–1960. p. 385–7, 1980.
Corner GW: Louise Pearce. In: Notable American women. The modern period. Cambridge, Mass., Belknap–Harvard Univ. Press, 1980. 4:531–2.
Crellin J: Selected items from the history of pathology. **Am J Pathol** 1980 Jan;98(1):60
Dwork D: Elsie Strang L'Esperance. In: Notable American women. The modern period. Cambridge, Mass., Belknap–Harvard Univ. Press, 1980. 4:417–9.
Eckert WG: Dr. Benjamin M. Vance (1886–1962). **Am J Forensic Med Pathol** 1980 Mar;1(1):73–6
Geller SA: Autopsy. **Sci Am** 1983 Mar;248(3):124–9, 132, 135–6
Harvey AM: Amebic dysentery gets its name: the story of William Thomas Councilman. **Johns Hopkins Med J** 1980 May;146(5):185–92, 199–201
Helpern M: History of the methods of detecting murder. **Am J Forensic Med Pathol** 1981 Mar;2(1):61–5
Kissane JM: Founders of Pediatric Pathology. Margaret G. Smith. 1896–1970. **Perspect Pediatr Pathol** 1982;7:v–viii
Lamping KA, Albert DM, Snyder C, et al: The Harrower collection and its place in the history of ophthalmic pathology. **Surv Ophthalmol** 1983 May–Jun;27(6):374–80
Longley JD: Ralph Dougall Lillie. 1896--1979. **J Histochem Cytochem** 1980 Apr;28(4):291–6
Machol L: Dorothy Hansine Andersen. In: Notable American women. The modern period. Cambridge, Mass., Belknap–Harvard Univ. Press, 1980. 4:18–20.
McLendon WW: The Archives of Pathology and Laboratory Medicine. A new beginning. **Arch Pathol Lab Med** 1984 Jan;108(1):13–4
Morman ET: Clinical pathology in America, 1865–1915: Philadelphia as a test case. **Bull Hist Med** 1984 Summer;58(2):198–214
Parascandola J: Maud Caroline Slye. In: Notable American women. The modern period. Cambridge, Mass., Belknap–Harvard Univ. Press, 1980. 4:651–2.
Patterson JN, Moore MJ: Laboratory medicine and pathologists in Florida prior to 1950. **J Fla Med Assoc** 1980 Feb;67(2):97–102
Patz A: Jonas S. Friedenwald, man of science. **Invest Ophthalmol Vis Sci** 1980 Oct;19(10):1139–49
Rothstein WG: Pathology: the evolution of a specialty in American medicine. **Med Care** 1979 Oct;17(10):975–88
Sharpe WD: Autopsies at Newark City Hospital, 1908 to 1911.

**J Med Soc NJ** 1984 Jan;81(1):53–62
Smith DC: Gerhard's distinction between typhoid and typhus and its reception in America, 1833–1860. **Bull Hist Med** 1980 Fall; 54(3):368–85
Spencer F: Samuel George Morton's doctoral thesis on bodily pain: the probable source of Morton's polygenism. **Trans Stud Coll Physicians Phila** 1983 Dec;5(5 no 4):321–38
Stewart HL: Reflections on Colonel James Earle Ash on the occasion of his 100th birthday September 8, 1984. **Lab Invest** 1984 Jan;50(1):1–2
Stowell RE: Esmond R. Long, MD, 1890–1979. **Am J Pathol** 1980 Aug;100(2):321–5
Tedeschi LG: Shields Warren: the legend and the man. **Am J Forensic Med Pathol** 1980 Dec;1(4):297–301
Wegner PN, Wegner KH, Diamond BE: A brief history of pathology in South Dakota. **SD J Med** 1981 May;34(5):65–6
Witkowski JA: Experimental pathology and the origins of tissue culture: Leo Loeb's contribution. **Med Hist** 1983 Jul;27(3):269–88

**USSR**

Abbott WF: The density-pathology hypothesis in comparative perspective: density, status and pathology in prerevolutionary Moscow. **Int J Comp Sociol** 1982;23(1–2):17–33
Akimov GA, Arkhangel'skiĭ AE: K istorii deiatel'nosti Leningradskogo nauchnogo obshchestva nevropatologov i psikhiatrov (pervye gody). **Zh Nevropatol Psikhiatr** 1983;83(7):1067–9
Antonov AM: Kafedre patologicheskoĭ anatomii Saratovskogo ordena Trudovogo Krasnogo Znameni meditsinskogo instituta 70 let (1911–1981). **Arkh Patol** 1981;43(7):80–3
Bobkov AG, Mikhaĭlov VP: Nauchnaia deiatel'nost' V. G. Garshina (1887–1956) i razvitie nauchnykh kontseptsiĭ v rabotakh sovetskikh morfologov. **Arkh Patol** 1983;45(4):77–80
Borisova MA, Bychkovskiĭ AV: Vklad Sergeia Petrovicha Bokina v izuchenie infektsionnykh bolezneĭ (k 150–letiiu so dnia rozhdeniia). **Vrach Delo** 1982 Sep;(9):116–9
Chekareva GA: I. V. Davydovskiĭ, 1887–1968. Moskva, Meditsina, 1980. 79 p.
Dikshteĭn EA, Orlova NL: Kafedre patologicheskoĭ anatomii Donetskogo meditsinskogo instituta 50 let. **Arkh Patol** 1984;46(1):73–4
Dorokhov II: Iz istorii kafedry patologicheskoĭ anatomii Rostovskogo meditsinskogo instituta. **Arkh Patol** 1984;46(1):69–73
Dorokhov II: Sravnitel'nyĭ amaliz sektsionnykh materialov Rostova-na-Donu za dovoennyĭ i poslevoennyĭ periody. **Arkh Patol** 1980;42(8):29–33
Dorosevich AE: Professor Petr L'vovich Poznanin--predstavitel' moskovskoĭ shkoly patologoanatomov. **Arkh Patol** 1983;45(1):79–80
Garmash VIa, Ushmarov AK: Znachenie ucheniia I. P. Pavlova dlia kliniki vnutrennikh bolezneĭ. **Med Sestra** 1981 Feb;40(2):8–10
Garshin VG: Tam, gde smert' pomogaet zhizni. **Arkh Patol** 1984;46(5):83–8
Gorizontov PD: Patologicheskaia fiziologiia v SSSR (k 60–letiiu obrazovaniia SSSR). **Patol Fiziol Eksp Ter** 1983 May–Jun;3:14–22
Ivanovskaia TE: Patologicheskaia anatomiia bolezneĭ detskogo vozrasta na sovremennom étape. **Arkh Patol** 1983;45(10):3–8
Khazanov AT: Iz istorii prozektury Obukhovskoĭ bol'nitsy. **Arkh Patol** 1983;45(5):68–73
Khmel'nitskiĭ OK: Klavdiia Petrovna Ulezko-Stroganova (1856–1943). **Arkh Patol** 1981;43(8):72–4
Natadze TG: Osnovnye dostizheniia gruzinskikh patofiziologov. **Patol Fiziol Eksp Ter** 1983 May–Jun;3:23–4
Onopchenko NA, Gun'ko MA, Eremin VM: Nikolaĭ Fedotovich Mel'nikov-Razvedenkov--zamechatel'nyĭ organizator i vidnyĭ uchenyĭ-patologoanatom. **Arkh Patol** 1983;45(10):78–82
Ordina OM: Professor V. P. Miroliubov (k 110–letiiu so dnia rozhdeniia). **Arkh Patol** 1982;44(7):80–3
Ptashekas RS: K 25–letiiu patomorfologicheskoĭ laboratorii Litovskogo instituta éksperimental'noĭ i klinicheskoĭ meditsiny. **Arkh Patol** 1983;45(12):76–8
Saunders LZ: Veterinary pathology in Russia, 1860–1930. Ithaca, Cornell University Press, 1980. xxi, 327 p.
Serov VV: M. N. Nikiforov i Moskovskaia shkola patologoanatomov (k 125–letiiu so dnia rozhdeniia). **Arkh Patol** 1984;46(2):3–12
Siudikas VP, Kutorga VV, Stalioraĭtite EI, et al: Patologiia i ee prepodavanie v Vil'niusskom universitete (k 400–letiiu Vil'niusskogo universiteta i 200–letiiu meditsinskogo fakul'teta étogo universiteta). **Arkh Patol** 1980;42(9):70–5
Smol'iannikov AV: Kafedre patologicheskoĭ anatomii Tsentral'nogo ordena Lenina instituta usovershenstvovannia vracheĭ 50 let. **Arkh Patol** 1980;42(12):59–61
Smol'iannikov AV, Sarkisov DS, Serebrennikov AB: N. I. Pirogov--velikiĭ uchenyĭ, vrach, grazhdanin. **Arkh Patol** 1982;44(9):3–13
Strukov AI, Smol'iannikov AV, Sarkisov DS: Razrabotka problem patologicheskoĭ anatomii v sisteme Akademii Meditsinskikh Nauk SSSR za 40 let ee sushchestvovaniia (1944–1984). **Arkh Patol** 1984;46(6):3–15
Strukov AI, Puzik VI, Zemskova ZS, et al: V. G. Shtefko i otechestvennaia shkola patologov-ftiziatrov. **Arkh Patol** 1984;46(2):81–5
Vaĭl' SS: M.M.Rudnev--odin iz osnovopolozhnikov otechestvennoĭ patologicheskoĭ anatomii (k 100–letiiu so dnia smerti). **Klin Med (Mosk)** 1979 Jul;57(7):107–10
Veselkin PN: K 100–letiiu kafedry patologicheskoĭ fiziologii ordena Lenina Krasnoznamennoĭ voenno-meditsinskoĭ akademii im. S. M. Kirova. **Patol Fiziol Eksp Ter** 1980;(4):3–11
Zerbino DD: Unikal'nyĭ arkhiv protokolov vskrytiĭ. **Vrach Delo** 1980 Jul;(7):6–9
Zhuravleva TB: Uchenie G. V. Shora o tanatogeneze i rol' ego shkoly v razvitii sovetskoĭ patologicheskoĭ anatomii (k 110–letiiu so dnia rozhdeniia). **Arkh Patol** 1984;46(3):76–80
Zhurnalu 'Patologicheskaia fiziologiia i éksperimental'naia terapiia' 25 let: **Patol Fiziol Eksp Ter** 1982 Jul–Aug;(4):3–10

**Venezuela**

Salfelder K, Novoa Montero D: Patologos alemanes en Venezuela 1936–1981. Merida, Universidad de los Andes, 1982. 131 p.

# PEDIATRICS

See also **Child Health; Human Development and Growth**

Ajuriaguerra J de: L'enfant dans l'histoire---problèmes psychologiques. **Psychiatr Enfant** 1979;22(1):101–26
Aulizio F: Il bambino nel passato e nel presente. **Minerva Pediatr** 1980 Jul 31;32(14):881–5
Demirhan A: Pediatrics and history of medicine. In: Congrès international d'histoire de la médecine, XXVe, Québec, 1976. Actes. Québec, 1977. p. 564–69.
Frenk SF: El raquitismo: un hito en la historia de la pediatria. **Bol Soc Mex Hist Filos Med** 1982 Dec;6(41):89–104
Huard P, Laplane R: Histoire illustrée de la pédiatrie. Tome premier. Paris, Dacosta, 1981. 198 p.
Kloë E, Kindt H: Zur Entstehung und Entwicklung des kindlichen Hysteriebegriffes. **Gesnerus** 1981;38(3/4):281–300
Kotek S: Geschichte der Kinderheilkunde von ihren Anfängen bis zum Ende des 18. Jahrhunderts. In Sournia JC, Martiny M, Poulet J, ed: Illustrierte Geschichte der Medizin. Salzburg, Andreas, 1980. Vol. 7. p. 2499–523.
Oehme J: Kinderkrankheiten und Kinderheikunde. **Klin Padiatr** 1984 Nov–Dec;196(6):325–6
Smith GF, Smith PN, Vidyasagar D, ed: Historical review and recent advances in neonatal and perinatal medicine. 2 vols. [Chicago?], Mead Johnson Nutritional Division, 1983. xxii, 212 p.; viii, 189 p. Historical contributions by B. F. Andrews, L. Ballowitz, L. J. Butterfield, V. Chernick, T. E. Cone, R. L. Day, M. L. Duxbury, D. Dye, L. M. Gartner, P. J. Goldstein, M. H. Greenberg, L. Johnson, A. Kaul, J. O. Klein, J. Lind, L. O. Lubchenco, N. M. Nelson, K. C. Pringle, T. N. Raju, A. C. Rambar, R. Sosa, M. T. Stahlman, L. Stern, K. Tarpey, A. Zipursky.
Spicer RD: Infantile hypertrophic pyloric stenosis: a review. **Br J Surg** 1982 Mar;69(3):128–35
Tait HP: The McNeil Library and some of its notable volumes. **Univ Edinb J** 1980;29:313–7
Teysseire D: Pédiatrie des lumières: maladies et soins des enfants dans l'Encyclopédie et le Dictionnaire de Trévoux. Paris, Vrin, 1982. 255 p.
Wójciak L, Maćkowiak K: Problemy stomatologii wieku rozwojowego w aspekcie rozwoju historycznego. **Czas Stomatol** 1979 Nov;32(11):1063–8

**France**

Gineste T: Naissance de la psychiatrie de l'enfant. De l'idiotie aux psychoses infantiles. **Soins Psychiatr** 1982 Feb;(16):21–6

**India**

Trivedi RP: Glimpses of Ayurvedic contribution to paediatrics & allied subjects. **Sachitra Ayurved** 1981 Aug;:113–7

**Poland**

Dembińska M: Dieetvoedsel en medicijnen voor kinderen in Polen van de 16de tot de 19de eeuw. **Spiegel Hist** 1981;16(11):623–6

**United States**

Cone TE: History of American pediatrics. Historical introduction by S. X. Radbill. Boston, Little, Brown, 1979. xiv, 278 p.

**500 A.D.–1450**

Kottek SS: 'Mater puerorum'. A medieval naming for an enigmatic children's disease. **Eur J Pediatr** 1981 Sep;137(1):75–9

**Arabic**

Kahle E: Probleme bei der Ubersetzung mittelalterlicher arabischer

pädiatrischer Texte. In International Congress of the History of Medicine, 27th, Barcelona, 1980. Actas. Barcelona, Académia de Ciències Médiques de Catalunya i Balears, 1981. p. 267–70.
Shamansurov SS, Madzhidova AT: Ibn-Sina i bolezni detskogo vozrasta. **Pediatriia** 1980 Jul;(7):70–1

### 1450–1700

#### China

Zhi Y: [Research on You Ke Lei Cui (Classified Collections in Pediatrics): a rare edition of pediatrics printed in the Ming dynasty] (Chi). **Chung Hua I Shih Tsa Chih** 1984;14(2):121–2

#### France

Simon de Vallambert on the treatment of diarrhea in infants (1565): **Pediatrics** 1982 Feb;69(2):163

#### Great Britain

Bloch H: Nicholas Culpeper, M.D. (1616 to 1654). Medical maverick in seventeenth-century England. **NY State J Med** 1982 Dec;82(13):1865–7
Cone TE: 'The boke of children' (1544) by Thomas Phaire [Phaer], the first pediatric text published in English. **Pediatrics** 1981;68:182

#### Spain

Ballester R: La utilizacion de los clasicos en la obra pediatrica de Luis Mercado (1525–1611). **Asclepio** 1978–79;30–31:307–18
Carreras Panchón A: Perez Cascales y la clinica del garrotillo. **Asclepio** 1978–79;30–31:319–22

#### Switzerland

Rickham PP: Johannes Fatio: Sein Leben, sein Werk und sein schreckliches Ende. **Z Kinderchir** 1984 Oct;39(5):289–95

### 1700 to Present

Berger H: Kurzer historischer Rückblick auf den Beginn der 'Ernährungsprobleme bei frühgeborenen Kindern'. **Padiatr Padol** 1983;18(2):99–103
Bolzinger A: Jalons pour une histoire de la psychiatrie à travers la Revue de Neuropsychiatrie infantile. **Neuropsychiatr Enfance Adolesc** 1981 Mar;29(3):127–40
Carter KC: Infantile hysteria and infantile sexuality in late nineteenth-century German-language medical literature. **Med Hist** 1983 Apr;27(2):186–96
Chawla PL: Child psychiatry--historical perspective. **Indian J Pediatr** 1984 Mar–Apr;51(409):191–2
Cole RB: Noonan's syndrome: a historical perspective. **Pediatrics** 1980 Sep;66(3):468–9
Cone TE: Is this the first published report on the diagnostic value of the telephone in pediatric practice (1879)? **Pediatrics** 1981;68:321
Cone TE: The first journal devoted exclusively to pediatrics (1834). **Pediatrics** 1981;68:321
Cone TE: The first journal devoted to the diseases of children. **Pediatrics** 1981;67:810
Ekstein R: As I remember her: Anna Freud, 1895–1982. **Adolesc Psychiatry** 1983;11:5–8
Fetterman GH: Maud L. Menten (1879–1960). **Perspect Pediatr Pathol** 1984 Spring;1(1):5–7
Gallagher JR: The origins, development, and goals of adolescent medicine. **J Adolesc Health Care** 1982 Aug;3(1):57–63
Gottschalk E: Quo vadit chirurgia paediatrica? **Beitr Gesch Univ Erfurt** 1979–83;19:361–7
Greenacre P: A historical sketch of the use and disuse of reconstruction. **Psychoanal Study Child** 1980;35:35–40
Hirschberg JC: History of child psychiatry. In H. I. Kaplan, et al, ed: Comprehensive textbook of psychiatry/III. Third edition. Baltimore, London, Williams and Wilkins, 1980. p. 2417–21.
Jones PG: 'A man and his hospital'. **Aust Paediatr J** 1981 Mar;17(1):5–14
Kretchmer N: Science and scholarship in pediatrics. **Pediatr Res** 1980 Oct;14(10):1093–9
McNamara DG: Twenty-five years of progress in the medical treatment of pediatric and congenital heart disease. **J Am Coll Cardiol** 1983 Jan;1(1):264–73
Neimann N, Pierson M: Geschichte der Kinderheilkunde im 19. und 20. Jahrhundert. In Sournia JC, Martiny M, Poulet J, ed: Illustrierte Geschichte der Medizin. Salzburg, Andreas, 1980. Vol. 7. p. 2525–39.
Olness K: Hypnosis in pediatric practice. **Curr Probl Pediatr** 1981 Dec;12(2):1–47
Phillips WR, Rosenberg J, ed: The origins of modern treatment and education of physically handicapped children. Reprint of articles. New York, Arno, 1980. Various pagings. (The physically handicapped in society).
Pirsig W: Historical notes and actual observations on the nasal septal abscess especially in children. **Int J Pediatr Otorhinolaryngol** 1984 Oct;8(1):43–54
Pracy R: Recent developments in paediatric otolaryngology. **J Laryngol Otol** 1981 Nov;95(11):1097–108
Rashkind WJ: Tricuspid atresia: a historical review. **Pediatr Cardiol** 1982;2(1):85–8
Segal H: Klein. Brighton, England, Harvester Press with Fontana Books, 1979. 189 p.
Seidler E: Der 'kleine Patient'– traditionelle Probleme der Kindertherapie. **Monatsschr Kinderheilkd** 1982 Jun;130(6):332–6
Solnit AJ. Anna Freud. December 3, 1895 October 9, 1982. **J Am Acad Child Psychiatry** 1984 Mar;23(2):233–6
Velasco D: La psychiatrie infantile dans les pays en voie de développement. **Ann Med Psychol (Paris)** 1981 Jun;139(6):626–8
Winters RW, Heird WC, Dell RB: History of parenteral nutrition in pediatrics with emphasis on amino acids. **Fed Proc** 1984 Apr;43(5):1407–11
Woodruff M: The master surgeon. **J R Coll Surg Edinb** 1981 Sep;26(5):257–63
Wunderlich P: Zur Vorgeschichte und Geschichte der 'Kinderärztlichen Praxis' 4.: Weitere deutschsprachige Zeitschriften für Kinderheilkunde, die bis 1930 gegründet wurden. **Kinderarztl Prax** 1980 Jun;48(6):312–6

#### Australia

Hall EM: In the ward next door to Sister Kenny. **Aust Nurses J** 1981 May;10(10):57–8
Hamilton DG: Hand in hand. Sydney, Ferguson, 1979. 338 p.
Hamilton DG: 100 years of paediatric surgery in Sydney. **Med J Aust** 1980 Dec 27;2(13):721–6
Royal Alexandra's century of caring: **Aust Nurses J** 1980 Nov;10(5):20–1

#### Austria

Festschrift Otto Thalhammer zum 60. Geburtstag: **Padiatr Padol** 1982;17(2):127–548
In memoriam. Dorothy Burlingham. 1891–1979.: **Psychoanal Study Child** 1980;35:ix–xxii
Rachman AW, Raubolt RR: The pioneers of adolescent group psychotherapy. **Int J Group Psychother** 1984 Jul;34(3):387–413
Skopec M, Wyklicky H: Die Heilpädagogische Abteilung der Universitäts-Kinderklink Wien--die älteste kinderpsychiatrische Forschungs- und Behandlungsstätte. **Erzieh Unterr** 1981 Oct;24:98–105
Swoboda W: 20 Jahre Osterreichische Gesellschaft für Kinderheilkunde. **Padiatr Padol** 1982;17(4):651–6

#### Bulgaria

Christozov C: Histoire de la psychiatrie infantile en Bulgarie. **Acta Paedopsychiatr (Basel)** 1981 Jan;46(4):207–11

#### Canada

De la Broquerie F: Les débuts de la pédiatrie à Québec 1892 à 1929. **Union Med Can** 1983 Jul;112(7):656–63
Ebbs JH: The Canadian Paediatric Society: its early years. **Can Med Assoc J** 1980 Dec 20;123(12):1235–7
Letondal P: Introduction à l'histoire de la pédiatrie au Canada français. In: Congrès international d'histoire de la médecine, XXVe, Québec, 1976. Actes. Québec, 1977. p. 885–94.
Medovy H: Seven decades of service at the Children's Hospital of Winnipeg. **Can Med Assoc J** 1980 Dec 20;123(12):1259–61
Salter RB: Scientific contributions to orthopaedic surgery by the staff of The Hospital for Sick Children, Toronto, 1875 to 1975. In: Congrès international d'histoire de la médecine, XXVe, Québec, 1976. Actes. Québec, 1977. p. 1225–43.
Shandling B: History of the Canadian Association of Paediatric Surgeons. **J Pediatr Surg** 1979 Oct;14(5):509–10
Steinhauer PD: The Canadian Academy of Child Psychiatry. The development of child psychiatry in Canada. **J Am Acad Child Psychiatry** 1982 May;21(3):217–8
Wiglesworth FW: Maude E. Abbott. **Perspect Pediatr Pathol** 1984 Winter;8(4):291–4

#### Chile

Artía A: Centenario de la fundación de la Sociedad Alemana de Pediatría. Influencia de ésta en la pediatría chilena. **Rev Chil Pediatr** 1983 Nov–Dec;54(6):387–9
Reyes H: Cincuentenario de la revista chilena de pediatria. **Rev Med Chil** 1980 Jul;108(7):597–8
Wiederhold Rotter A: La pediatría en la Provincia de Cautín en la década del 20 al 30. **Rev Chil Pediatr** 1981 Jan–Feb;52(1):75–81

# PEDIATRICS

### Czechoslovakia

Březina Z: Sociální pediatrie v Ostravě. **Cesk Zdrav** 1982 Nov;30(11):480–3
Dunovský J: Třicet let katedry pediatrie ILF a její další činnost. **Cesk Pediatr** 1983 Oct;38(10):629–32
Dunovský J: Zur Geschichte der Sozialpädiatrie. **Padiatr Grenzgeb** 1984;23(3):127–31
Houštěk J: Professor MUDr. Ján Birčák šedesátiletý. **Cesk Pediatr** 1983 Feb;38(2):117–9
Houštěk J: Professor MUDr. Otto Hrodek, DrSc., šedesátiletý. **Cesk Pediatr** 1983 Jan;38(1):58–60
Houštěk J: Sto let od narození profesora MUDr. Jiřího Brdlíka, DrSc., vedoucí osobnosti československé pediatrie (24. října 1883--6. července 1965). **Cesk Pediatr** 1983 Nov;38(11):680–1
Hrodek O, Kubát K: Akademik Josef Houštěk sedmdesátiletý. **Cesk Pediatr** 1983 Aug;38(8):496–9
Klačanský I: Rozvoj detskej otolaryngológie na Slovensku. **Cesk Otolaryngol** 1984 Jun;33(3):193–4
Michaličková J: Vývoj a dalšie perspektívy rozvoja pediatrických odborov na lekárskej fakulte Univerzity Komenského v Bratislave. **Cas Lek Cesk** 1979 Dec 21;118(51):1581–3
Svejcar J: Vznik a vývoj Ceskoslovenské spolupráce na poli doškolování pediatru. **Cesk Zdrav** 1983 Oct;31(10):401–7
Tichý M, Volná A: Bratislavské roky profesora Brdlíka. **Cesk Zdrav** 1983 Jul;31(6):250–5
Vendl L: Dvacet let Detské nefrologické léčebny Miramonte v Mariánských Láznich. **Cesk Pediatr** 1982 Jul;37(7):419

### Denmark

Frenckner B: Pionjär för pediatrisk forskning - omtyckt kliniker, mindre värderad föreläsare. **Lakartidningen** 1983 Nov 30;80(48):4664–5
Roed-Petersen K, Madsen CM: Harald Hirschsprung (1830–1916). **Dan Medicinhist Arbog** 1980;:182–99

### Europe

Dunovský J: K istorii razvitiia sotsial'noĭ pediatrii. **Pediatriia** 1982 Jun;(6):4–9
Koller M: Kinderzahnmedizin im 18. und 19. Jahrhundert. **Swiss Dent** 1980 Dec;1(12):32–3
Stutte H: Ueber die Anfänge der 'Europäischen Kinderpsychiatrie'. **Acta Paedopsychiatr (Basel)** 1981 Jan;46(4):189–92

### France

Barner S: Die Entwicklung der Kinderpsychiatrie in Frankreich von den Anfängen bis 1948. Freiburg, Schulz 1980. 300 p. (Freiburger Forschungen zur Medizingeschichte, Neue Folge, 11).
Bernard J: Robert Debré: l'humanisme et les académies. **Bull Acad Natl Med (Paris)** 1982 Dec;166(9):1281–4
Debré M: Robert Debré, réformateur. **Bull Acad Natl Med (Paris)** 1982 Dec;166(9):1295–303
Gineste T: Une histoire de la psychiatrie de l'enfant. Janvier 1800 - novembre 1800: Découverte d'une 'créature très intéressante', l'enfant connu sous le nom de Sauvage de l'Aveyron. Mém. pour le diplôme de psychiatrie. Univ. de Paris XI, 1977. 233 p, 8 n.p.
L'Hôpital Des Enfants-Malades, the world's first children's hospital, founded in Paris in 1802: **Pediatrics** 1981 May;67(5):670
Mande R: Robert Debré et la pédiatrie sociale. **Bull Acad Natl Med (Paris)** 1982 Dec;166(9):1275–9
Marie J: Robert Debré (1882–1978): l'homme, le médecin, le professeur. **Bull Acad Natl Med (Paris)** 1982 Dec;166(9):1257–64
Popescu V: Centenar Robert Debré. **Rev Pediatr Obstet Ginecol [Pediatr]** 1983 Apr–Jun;32(2):97–100
Schmid-Kitsikis E: Un certain regard sur l'oeuvre de N. Galifret-Granjon. **Psychiatr Enfant** 1984;27(1):35–48
Steffen C: Eugène Apert (1868–1940). **Am J Dermatopathol** 1984 Jun;6(3):223–4
Thieffry S: La découverte de la syphilis congénitale par Jules Parrot à l'Hospice des Enfants Assistés il y a un siècle. **Bull Acad Natl Med (Paris)** 1980 Nov;164(8):725–9
Thieffry S: La vie quotidienne avec Robert Debré, pionnier de la pédiatrie: le médecin d'enfants, le chef de service, le chef d'école. **Bull Acad Natl Med (Paris)** 1982 Dec;166(9):1265–77

### Germany

Bescherer J: Krankheitsbilder und Verhaltensweisen bei langfristigen Schülern in Klinik und Körperbehindertenschule--Eindrücke und Erfahrungen eines Sonderschullehrers aus 40 Berufsjahren. Zugleich ein Beitrag zur Geschichte der Pädiatrie und der Sonderpädagogik. **Arztl Jugendkd** 1984 Apr;75(2):88–102
Betke K: 125 Jahre Pädiatrie. **MMW** 1983 Jul 1;125(26):619–20
Butenandt O: Pädiatrie vor 100 Jahren. Aus Berichten des 'Jahrbuches für Kinderheilkunde', Band 18, 1882. **Fortschr Med** 1983 Feb 17;101(7):251–4
Dietzsch HJ: 50 Jahre Kinderklinik der Medizinischen Akademie 'Carl Gustav Carus' Dresden und ihre Vorgeschichte. **Kinderarztl Prax** 1981 Jun;49(6):318–26
Hellbrügge T: Zum 100jährigen Jubiläum der Deutschen Gesellschaft für Kinderheilkunde. **Fortschr Med** 1983 Sep 8;101(34):1513–6
Joppich G: Begegnung mit grossen Pädiatern aus der Frühzeit der deutschen Kinderheilkunde. **Monatsschr Kinderheilkd** 1984 Jun;1132(6):318–24
Külz J: Interessantes und Amüsantes aus dem Nachlass von Karl Stolte. **Kinderarztl Prax** 1981 Nov;49(11):583–90
Külz J: 70 Jahre Pädiatrie als Lehrfach an der Universität Rostock. **Kinderarztl Prax** 1981 Feb;49(2):92–100
Müller H: Die Anstalt in Kork (Baden). Von der 'Heil- und Pflegeanstalt für epileptische Kinder' zum 'Epilepsiezentrum Kork'. Freiburg, Schulz, 1979. 190 p. (Freiburger Forschungen zur Medizingeschichte, Neue Folge, 10).
Murken AH, ed: Kind, Krankheit und Krankenhaus im Bilderbuch von 1900 bis 1982. (Studien zur Medizin-, Kunst- und Literaturgeschichte. Band 5.). Herzogenrath, Verlag Murken-Altrogge, 1982. 238 p.
Ocklitz HW, Landmann H: Robert Koch und die Kindertuberkulose. **Kinderarztl Prax** 1982 Mar;50(3):117–29
Ocklitz HW, Schmitz HH: Unserem Lehrer Karl Stolte zum 100. Geburtstag. **Kinderarztl Prax** 1981 Nov;49(11):591–5
Oehme J: Rückbesinnung zum 100 jährigen Bestehen der Deutschen Gesellschaft für Kinderheilkunde. **Klin Paediatr** 1983 Jan–Feb;195(1):1–3
Pfeffer R: Professor Franz von Rinecker, 1811–1883. Diss., Bayerische Julius-Maximilians-Universität, Würzburg, 1981. 180 p.
Ratzmann GW, Jährig K: Karl Stolte in seiner Zeit und für unsere Zeit. **Kinderarztl Prax** 1981 Dec;49(12):617–27
Schweier P: Lebendige Pädiatrie. München, Marseille, 1983. 302 p.
Seidler E: Carl Gerhardt und seine Rede: 'Die Aufgaben und Ziele der Kinderheilkunde' (1879). **Monatsschr Kinderheilkd** 1983 Sep;131(9):545–8
Stehr S: Zur Geschichte der Münchner Kinderheilkunde (1818 bis 1980, insbesondere die Zeit nach dem Zweiten Weltkrieg). Diss., Technischen Universität München, 1982. 178 p.
Thie-Mummenthey G: Vom Säuglingsheim zur Universitätskinderklinik. Die Entwicklung der Kinderklinik der Westfälischen Wilhelms-Universität Münster. Münster, Murken-Altrogge, 1980. 262 p. (Studien zur Geschichte des Krankenhauswesens, 10).
Wunderlich P: Arthur Schlossmann (1867–1932) als Vorbild für unsere Zeit. **Kinderarztl Prax** 1982 Dec;50(12):589–95

### Ghana

Williams CD: Fifty years ago. Archives of Diseases in Childhood 1933. A nutritional disease of childhood associated with a maize diet. **Arch Dis Child** 1983 Jul;58(7):550–60

### Great Britain

Armstrong D: Child development and medical ontology. **Soc Sci Med [Med Psychol Med Sociol]** 1979 Jan;13(1):9–12
Arton M: Children first and always. **Nurs Times** 1982 Oct 6–12;78(40):1687–8
Buchanan M: The sick child. **Nurs Times** 1983 Feb 23–Mar 1;79(8):66–9
Calwell HG: Care of sick children in Belfast in the nineteenth century. **J R Soc Med** 1979 Sep;72(9):706–8
Cone TE: Overdosing with opium, a serious pediatric problem in England a century and a half ago. **Pediatrics** 1981;68:86
Dobbs R, Robinson R, MacCarthy D, et al: Douglas Gairdner, editor of the Archives 1964–79. **Arch Dis Child** 1979 Nov;54(11):813, 815–21
Dopson L: 'Sick Kids'--100 years on. **Nurs Times** 1983 Mar 30–Apr 5;79(13):8–9
Edgcumbe R: Anna Freud--child analyst. **Int J Psychoanal** 1983;64 (Pt 4):427–33
Feinstein SC: Why they were afraid of Virginia Woolf: perspectives on juvenile manic-depressive illness. **J Adolesc** 1980 Sep;3(3):187–96
Garralda Hualde ME: El modelo inglés de formación en psiquiatría infantil. **Actas Luso Esp Neurol Psiquiatr** 1981 Mar–Apr;9(2):103–12
Hellman I: Work in the Hampstead war nurseries. **Int J Psychoanal** 1983;64 (Pt 4):435–9
Henderson M: Royal Hospital for Sick Children. A 100-year-old gets a new lease on life. **Health Soc Serv J** 1983 Aug 11;93(4859):966–7
Howells JG, Osborn ML: The history of child psychiatry in the United Kingdom. **Acta Paedopsychiatr (Basel)** 1981 Jan;46(4):193–202
Jones IH: Wages through the ages. **Nurs Times** 1980 Jul 17;76(29):1279–80
Lomax E: A mid-nineteenth century British pediatrician's interpretations of the mental peculiarities and disorders of childhood. **Clio Med** 1983 Mar;17(4):223–33
McClure RK: Pediatric practice at the London Foundling Hospital. **Stud Eighteenth Cent Cult** 1981;10:361–71
Paediatrics and psychoanalysis--Miss Anna Freud: **Arch Dis Child** 1983 Jun;58(6):472–3
Sandler J: Discussions with Anna Freud on The Ego and the Mechanisms of Defence: The Ego and the Id at Puberty. **Int J Psychoanal** 1983;64 (Pt 4):401–6
Solnit AJ: Anna Freud's contributions to child and applied analysis.

Int J Psychoanal 1983;64 (Pt 4):379-90
Spray W: Down memory lane: obituary at Nottingham. **Nurs Mirror** 1980 Mar 27;150(13):27-8
Wilkinson AW: Development of modern neonatal surgery. **Trans Hunter Soc** 1978-80;37-38:65-83

**Hungary**

Gegesi Kiss P: Bókay János junior a tanítvány szemével. **Orv Hetil** 1983 May 29;124(22):1329-34
Kemény P: 50 éves a Madarasz utcai Gyermekkórház. **Orv Hetil** 1979 Dec 30;120(52):3181-3
Kiss PG: János Bókay junior as seen by a disciple. **Acta Paediatr Hung** 1984;25(1-2):7-10
Miltényi M: Emlékezés ifjú Bókay Jánosra. **Orv Hetil** 1983 May 29;124(22):1327-9
Miltényi M: Professor János Bókay, Jr. **Acta Paediatr Hung** 1984;25(1-2):3-5

**India**

Hussain SA: Ilajul Atfal: a treatise on pediatrics by Fezl-e-Ali-Shifa-ee Khan. **Bull Indian Inst Hist Med Hyderabad** 1982;12(1-4):45-50

**Israel**

Winter ST, Ginott N: Two pioneer paediatricians in Palestine under the Turks. **Adler Mus Bull** 1983 Nov;Spec issue:58-61

**Italy**

Cheli E: Le decisioni d'interesse pediatrico del Consiglio Superiore di Sanita'. **Minerva Med** 1979 Nov 3;70(48):XVI-XIX

**Japan**

Fukuyama Y: [Progress of the Japanese Society of Pediatric Neurology in the past quarter of a century] (Jpn). **No To Hattatsu** 1984;16(3):179-88
Niigata Daigaku Igakubu Shonikagaku Kyoshitsu shi: [Niigata, Japan], Do Iinkai, Showa 52 nen [1977]. 180 p.

**Mexico**

Bonequi CC: La huella del Hospital Infantil de México en la pediatría. Cuarenta años de vida institucional. **Bol Med Hosp Infant Mex** 1983 Aug;40 Suppl 2:1-10
Carrillo-Rascón J: Escherichia coli: historia de una hipótesis. **Bol Med Hosp Infant Mex** 1983 Aug;40 Suppl 2:28-33
La investigación biomédica en el Hospital Infantil de México: **Bol Med Hosp Infant Mex** 1983 Nov;40 Suppl 3:3-23

**Netherlands**

Koning AT: Vijftig jaar Tijdschrift voor Kindergeneeskunde. **Tijdschr Kindergeneeskd** 1983 Feb;51(1):1-7

**Poland**

Heimrath T, Smereka J: Lekarze polscy wykształceni we wrocławskiej Klinice Kobiecej w latach 1811--1918. **Arch Hist Med (Warsz)** 1979;42(3):345-9
Klein F: Janusz Korczak--Arzt und Erzieher--Ein Symbol gelebter Menschlichkeit für die heutige medizinische und heilpädagogische Praxis. **Off Gesundheitswes** 1984 May;46(5):244-8
Lejmbach Z: Myśl pediatryczna wśród pracowników szpitala im. Karola i Marii. **Pediatr Pol** 1984 Sep;59(9):701-3
Losiowski Z: Sanatorium w Zagórzu i jego rola w lecznictwie neurologicznym dzieci. **Pediatr Pol** 1980 Mar;55(3):379-84
Marzec M: Ksawery Lewkowicz (1869-1958) wybitny pediatra i bakteriolog. **Wiad Lek** 1982 Aug 15;35(13):845-7
Moskwa Z: Założenie kamienia węgielnego pod szpital Dzieciatka Jezus. **Wiad Lek** 1984 Mar 15;37(6):479-80
Ostrowska T: Profesor Ksawery Rowiński (1904-1983) i Jego działanść naukowa (Wspomnienie pośmiertne). **Arch Hist Med (Warsz)** 1984;47(3):327-48
Popkowska N: Przeglad problemów diagnostycznych i rehabilitacyjnych dzieci i młodziezy leczonej w Klinice Psychiatrii Akademii Medycznej w Lublinie w latach 1951-1971. **Psychiatr Pol** 1980 May-Jun;14(3):259-64
Sobień-Kopczyńska S, Gęsicka T, Rybus B, et al: Epidemiologia choroby Wrzodowej u dzieci w latach 1968-1978 w dzielnicy Lódź-Bałuty. **Pediatr Pol** 1980 Apr;55(4):487-93
Staszyc J: Doktór Janusz Korczak -- lekarz, literat i twórca pedagogicznej koncepcji wychowania. **Ann Univ Mariae Curie Sklodowska [Med]** 1978;33:333-9
Tabeński Z: Wkład polskich chirurgów w rozwój leczenia choroby Hirschsprunga u dzieci. **Pediatr Pol** 1981 Jun;56(6):695-7
Wilkoszewski E: Z dziejów polskich czasopism pediatrycznych (lata 1908-1983). **Pediatr Pol** 1983 Aug-Sep;58(8-9):673-84
Wunderlich P: Zur Geschichte der Universitäts-Kinderklinik in Breslau unter Adalbert Czerny (1863--1941) von 1894--1910. **Arch Hist Med (Warsz)** 1979;42(3):337-43
Zapaśnik-Kobierska MH: Działalność naukowo-dydaktyczna i społeczna zespołu klinik Państwowego Szpitala Klinicznego Nr 3. **Pediatr Pol** 1984 Sep;59(9):705-12

**Puerto Rico**

Sifontes JE, Valcárcel M: Historical sketch -University Pediatric Hospital-1983. **Bol Asoc Med PR** 1983 Oct;75(10):444-5

**South Africa**

Louw JH: Leipoldt the paediatrician. **S Afr Med J** 1980 Dec 6;58(23):915-20

**Sweden**

Paborn K: Något om barnavård år 1908. **Omvardaren** 1982;29(4):8-9

**Switzerland**

Raynier JP de: L'Hôpital de l'Enfance de 1861 à 1979. **Rev Med Suisse Romande** 1980 Jun;100(6):557-65
Sommer P: Die ersten Jahrzehnte des Jenner-Kinderspitals in Bern. **Gesnerus** 1982;39(1):85-8
Wall WD: Jean Piaget - 1896-1979. **J Child Psychol Psychiatry** 1982 Apr;23(2):97-104

**United States**

Allen R: The evolution of pediatric surgery. **J Pediatr Surg** 1980 Dec;15(6):711-8
Arena JM: The pediatrician's role in the poison control movement and poison prevention. **Am J Dis Child** 1983 Sep;137(9):870-3
Brent RL: Biography of Josef Warkany. **Teratology** 1982 Apr;25(2):137-51
C[one] TE: Mrs. Nathaniel Hawthorne's invalidism, until her marriage at age 31, was attributed to difficult teething in infancy. **Pediatrics** 1981;67:606
C[one] TE: On the proper treatment of infants according to David Ramsay of South Carolina (1790). **Pediatrics** 1981;68:353
Cone TE: Abraham Jacobi on the establishment of systematic instruction in the diseases of childhood in the United States. **Pediatrics** 1981;67:357
Daeschner CW: Education for primary care of children. A report to Abraham and Mary Jacobi. **Am J Dis Child** 1983 Jun;137(6):566-71
Dubos R: Hattie Elizabeth Alexander. In: Notable American women. The modern period. Cambridge, Mass., Belknap-Harvard Univ. Press, 1980. 4:10-1.
Duncalf D: History of anesthesia for pediatric cardiac surgery. **Int Anesthesiol Clin** 1980 Spring;18(1):1-3
Engle MA: Biographies of great American pediatricians--Helen Brooke Taussig: the mother of pediatric cardiology. **Pediatr Ann** 1982 Jul;11(7):629-31
English PC: Pediatrics and the unwanted child in history: foundling homes, disease, and the origins of foster care in New York City, 1860 to 1920. **Pediatrics** 1984 May;73(5):699-711
Fath H: A dream come true: the story of St. Jude Children's Research Hospital and ALSAC. Memphis, TN, ALSAC, 1983. 214 p.
Festschrift in honor of David W. Smith: **J Pediatr** 1982 Nov;101(5):797-804
Graebner W: The unstable world of Benjamin Spock: social engineering in a democratic culture, 1917-1950. **J Am Hist** 1980 Dec;67(3):612-29
Harrell GT: Pediatrics in an academic health center. **J Fla Med Assoc** 1984 Mar;71(3):163-6
Hayden GF, Saulsbury FT: A review of The Journal of Pediatrics: the first 50 years. **J Pediatr** 1982 Jul;101(1):5-11
Hoekelman RA: Well-child visits revisited. **Am J Dis Child** 1983 Jan;137(1):17-20
Holaday B: Changing views of infant care 1914-1980. **Pediatr Nurs** 1981 Jan-Feb;7(1):21-5
Huff DS, Scrinivasan B: The oldest children's hospital building still in use in the United States? **J Pediatr** 1983 Jan;102(1):165-6
Hunt M: A coming of age with pediatrics: Park Jerauld White, attending physician. **Outlook Mag** 1982 Spring;19(1):18-24
Hunt M: La charité maternelle aux Etats-Unis au 19e siècle: un cas d'étude institutionnelle, un hôpital pédiatrique. **Penelope** 1981;(5):50-1
Hunt M: Women and childsaving: St. Louis Children's Hospital 1879-1979. **Bull Mo Hist Soc** 1980;36(2, pt 1):65-79
Kissane JM: Founders of Pediatric Pathology. Margaret G. Smith. 1896-1970. **Perspect Pediatr Pathol** 1982;7:v-viii
Koop CE: Pediatric surgery: the newest specialty for the youngest patient. **Trans Stud Coll Physicians Phila** 1981 Sep;5(3 no 3):195-208
Krell R: At a children's hospital; a folklore survey. **West Folkl** 1980;39(3):223-31
Leitner J: Leaders in medicine--George H. Garrison, MD.

# PEDIATRICS

**J Okla State Med Assoc** 1981 Sep;74(9):298-304

McBryde AM, Pressly JA, Hutchinson F, et al: North Carolina Orthopedic Hospital closes after 58 years of treatment of crippled children. **NC Med J** 1979 Dec;40(12):755-7

Machol L: Dorothy Hansine Andersen. In: Notable American women. The modern period. Cambridge, Mass., Belknap-Harvard Univ. Press, 1980. 4:18-20.

McIntosh K: Folk obstetrics, gynecology, and pediatrics in Utica, New York. **NY Folkl** 1978;4(1-4):49-59

Mason LB: Babies hospital, 1920-1978. **NC Med J** 1984 Jan;45(1):53-6

Nelson WE: The first 50 years of The Journal of Pediatrics. **J Pediatr** 1982 Jul;101(1):1-4

Nolan E: Children's ward. Lithograph by Robert Riggs, ca. 1940-45. **J Hist Med Allied Sci** 1982 Jul;37(3):322

Pawluch D: Transitions in pediatrics: a segmental analysis. **Soc Probl** 1983;30(4):449-65

Pediatric nurse pioneers (Helen Hogan): **Am J Nurs** 1980;80:2084

Pioneers in pedodontics: influential leaders of the past (John C. Brauer): **Pediatr Dent** 1982 Jun;4(2):143-4

Radbill SX: Arnold Lucius Gesell. In Dictionary of American biography, 1961-1965. Suppl. 7, 1981. p. 283-5.

Radbill SX: Joseph Ioor Waring, 1897-1977. **J Hist Med Allied Sci** 1978 Jul;33(3):427-8

Rosenberger HT: Harriet Lane Johnston: pioneer advocate of special care for children with chronic diseases. **J Lanc Cty Hist Soc** 1972;76(1):1-28

Schaelchlin P: 'Working for the good of the community': Rest Haven Preventorium for Children. **J San Diego Hist** 1983 Spring;29:96-114

Schmidt WM: Ethel Collins Dunham. In: Notable American women. The modern period. Cambridge, Mass., Belknap-Harvard Univ. Press, 1980. 4:212-3.

Slaff B: The history of adolescent psychiatry. **Adolesc Psychiatry** 1981;9:7-21

Smith CA: The Children's Hospital of Boston: 'built better than they knew'. Boston, Little, Brown, 1983. ix, 284 p.

Stanage WF: Pediatrics in South Dakota. **SD J Med** 1981 May;34(5):61-2

Ström J: Männen bakom syndromet: Albert Stevens och Frank Johnson. Först att beskriva 'okänd infektionssjukdom'--allergi utlöst av läkemedel eller infektion. **Lakartidningen** 1983 Mar 16;80(11):1076-7

Stumpf DA: The founding of pediatric neurology in America. **Bull NY Acad Med** 1981 Nov;57(9):804-16

Ternberg JL: Surgical treatment of idiopathic hyperinsulinemic hypoglycemia in children. First successful subtotal pancreatectomy with preservation of spleen reported by Evarts A. Graham (1934). **J Thorac Cardiovasc Surg** 1984 Nov;88(5 Pt 2):898-901

Thompson HC: 20th-century US child health care. Past, present, future. **Am J Dis Child** 1984 Sep;138(9):804-9

Vedder JS: Pediatric respiratory therapy of the 1930s. **Respir Ther** 1979 Jan-Feb;9(1):42, 44

Waserman MJ: The emergence of modern child health care: pediatrics, public health, and the federal government. Ph.D. Diss., The Catholic University of America, Washington, D. C., 1982. v, 232 p.

Wolf ES: Tomorrow's self: Heinz Kohut's contribution to adolescent psychiatry. **Adolesc Psychiatry** 1980;8:41-50

**USSR**

Andrianov VL, Veselov NG, Kapitanaki IA: Leningradskiĭ nauchno-issledovatel'skiĭ detskiĭ ortopedicheskiĭ institut im. G.I. Turnera i ego rol' v okhrane zdorov'ia deteĭ (k 50-letiiu so dnia organizatsii). **Pediatriia** 1983 Nov;(11):74-5

Balasheva II, Zhukova IV: K 90-letiiu kafedry pediatrii Tomskogo meditsinskogo instituta. **Pediatriia** 1982;(9):71-3

Borodiĭ NK: K biografii N. M. Maksimovicha-Ambodika. **Akush Ginekol (Mosk)** 1982;(8):60-1

Garmasheva NL, Konstantinova NN: Osnovnye étapy razvitiia perinatologii v SSSR. **Akush Ginekol (Mosk)** 1982;(7):7-10

Ivanovskaia TE: Patologicheskaia anatomiia bolezneĭ detskogo vozrasta na sovremennom étape. **Arkh Patol** 1983;45(10):3-8

Kliorin AI: N. I. Krasnogorskiĭ (k 100-letiiu so dnia rozhdeniia). **Pediatriia** 1983 May;5:76-8

Kononov VS: Perspektivy i problemy khirurgii detskogo vozrasta v Kirgizii. **Vestn Khir** 1982 Dec;129(12):14-8

Lebedev DD, Kovaleva EV, Semenova VN: Nekotorye voprosy revmatizma, éndokrinnykh i nervnykh zabolevaniĭ u deteĭ v trudakh V.I. Molchanova i ego uchenikov (k 110-letiiu so dnia rozhdeniia). **Pediatriia** 1980 Aug;(8):64-7

Matveev MP, Klaĭshevich GI, Gavriushova LP, et al: Rol' kafedry pediatrii v sisteme poslediplomnogo obucheniia pediatrov (k 50-letiiu Tsentral'nogo ordena V. I. Lenina instituta usovershenstvovaniia vracheĭ. **Pediatriia** 1981 Jul;(7):77-8

Matveev MP: Slovo o Georgii Nestoroviche Speranskom (K 110-letiiu so dnia rozhdeniia). **Pediatriia** 1983 Feb;(2):3-9

Mikirtichan GL: S. P. Botkin i okhrana zdorov'ia deteĭ (k 150-letiiu so dnia rozhdeniia). **Pediatriia** 1982 Oct;(10):62-4

Orlova NV, Pariĭskaia TV, Vorob'ev AS: 20 Let raboty po usovershenstvovaniiu znaniĭ pediatrov v oblasti kardiorevmatologii. **Pediatriia** 1982 Jun;(6):59-61

Pavluchkova AV: Pervye sovetskie dispansery po bor'be s tuberkulezom u deteĭ (k Mezhdunarodnomu godu rebenka). **Probl Tuberk** 1979 Dec;(12):11-5

Ponomareva PA, Kuznetsova AI: K 50-letiiu klinicheskikh pediatricheskikh kafedr II Moskovskogo meditsinskogo instituta im. N. I. Pirogova. **Pediatriia** 1981 Dec;(12):61-3

Sukharev AG, Fokina NS, Telenchi VI: Kafedre Gigieny Deteĭ i Podrostkov Tsentral'nogo Ordena Lenina Instituta Usovershenstvovaniia Vracheĭ 50 let. **Gig Sanit** 1984 Aug;(8):38-40

Tambovtsev PD: K 25-letiiu detskogo pul'monologicheskogo sanatoriia im. M.S. Maslova. **Pediatriia** 1983 Jun;(6):74-5

Tarasov OF: A. F. Tur: 1894-1974. Moskva, Meditsina, 1980. 125 p.

Timofeeva GA, Valenkevich LN: O podgotovke pediatricheskikh kadrov v SSSR. **Pediatriia** 1980;(1):3-5

Usov IN: Belorusskomu nauchnomu obschchestvu detskikh vracheĭ 50 let. **Pediatriia** 1983 Nov;(11):72-4

Vel'tishchev IuE: A. A. Koltypin--uchenyĭ, vrach, obshchestvennyĭ deiatel' (k 100-letiiu so dnia rozhdeniia). **Pediatriia** 1983 Sep;(9):73-4

Vladimirova LB, Gribanov ED: A nagy magyar zeneszerzo, Liszt Ferenc és az ogyesszai gyermekkórház épületének története (orosz nyelven). **Orvostort Kozl** 1982;28(1-3):169-76

Vladimirova LB, Gribanov ED: Emblema meditsiny. **Feldsher Akush** 1981;46(4):58-60

**Venezuela**

Alvarez PJ: Doctor J. M. de los Ríos: precursor de la pediatria en Venezuela. **Rev Sos Venez Hist Med** 1972-73;20-21(34-35):15-20

Caricote N: Formacion odontopediatrica del odontologo general en la UCV. **Acta Odontol Venez** 1980 Jan-Apr;18(1):69-85

**Yugoslavia**

Kolbas V: Marginalije u povodu dvadeset pete godišnjice 'Arhiva za zaštitu majke i djeteta'. **Lijec Vjesn** 1983 Jul-Aug;105(7-8):315-8

Vukadinović S: Razvoj i zadaci pedijatrijske kardiologije. **Lijec Vjesn** 1979 Dec;101(12):733-6

# PERIODICALS

Berry EM: The evolution of scientific and medical journals. **N Engl J Med** 1981;305:400-2

Gibson SS: Scientific societies and exchange: a facet of the history of scientific communication. **J Libr Hist** 1982 Spring;17(2):144-63

Kronick DA: Access to the medical journal literature of the 17th and 18th centuries through the Index catalogue. In International Congress of the History of Medicine. 26th, Plovdiv, 1978. Actes du Congress. Sofia, 1981. Volume II. p. 59-62.

La información documental y su divulgación en medicina: I. Breve reseña de los antecedentes y funciones del periodismo medico Mexicano. **Gac Med Mex** 1981 Apr;117(4):127-41

Maire M: Une mini histoire de la presse dentaire. **Chir Dent Fr** 1979 Dec 13;49(44):53-7

Oliaro T: La funzione storica e didattica della stampa medica. **Minerva Stomatol** 1984 May-Jun;33(3):536-7

Schadewaldt H: Betrachtungen zur Entwicklung des medizinischen Buch- und Zeitschriftenwesens. In:Die Zeitung als Persönlichkeit. Festschrift Bringmann. Düsseldorf, 1982. p. 125-34.

**Great Britain**

Booth CC: Medical communication: the old and new. The development of medical journals in Britain. **Br Med J [Clin Res]** 1982 Jul 10;285(6335):105-8

**1450-1700**

**Great Britain**

Cooke AM: Sir Hans Sloane and the Philosophical Transactions. **J R Coll Physicians Lond** 1984 Jul;18(3):170-1

Hall AR, Boas Hall M: The first human blood transfusion: priority disputes. **Med Hist** 1980;24(4):461-5

**Poland**

Dudziński W: Medicinalia w pierwszej ojczystej gazecie 'Merkuriuszu Polskim'. **Wiad Lek** 1981 Oct 1;34(19):1653-5

**1700 to Present**

Ash L, Murray MA, ed: Serial publications containing medical classics. An index to citations in Garrison/Morton (3rd edition, 1970). 2nd ed., revised and enlarged. Bethany, Connecticut, The Antiquarium, 1979, x, 169 p.

Bednarski Z: Sto lat od odkrycia prątka gruźlicy (1882-1982) przez Roberta Kocha: szybka reakcja w polskich czasopismach lekarskich.

**Pol Tyg Lek** 1983 Mar 28;38(13):419–21
Boehm EH, Pope BH, Ensign MS, ed: Historical periodicals directory. Volume 3: Europe: East and Southeast; USSR. Santa Barbara, Oxford, ABC–Clio, 1984. xv, 252 p. (Clio Periodicals Directories).
Bolzinger A: Jalons pour une histoire de la psychiatrie à travers la Revue de Neuropsychiatrie infantile. **Neuropsychiatr Enfance Adolesc** 1981 Mar;29(3):127–40
Bugyi B: Az orvosi sajtó etikájáról--hetven évvel ezelött. **Orv Hetil** 1979 Dec 30;120(52):3184–6
Cone TE: The first journal devoted exclusively to pediatrics (1834) **Pediatrics** 1981;68:321
Cone TE: The first journal devoted to the diseases of children. **Pediatrics** 1981;67:810
Ensign MS, ed: Historical periodicals directory. Volume 1: USA and Canada. Santa Barbara, Oxford, ABC–Clio, 1981. xii, 180 p. (Clio Periodicals Directories).
The first fifty years 1931–1981: **Dent Assist** 1981 Jan–Feb;50(1):24–6
Fletcher SW, Fletcher RH, Greganti MA: Clinical research trends in general medical journals, 1946–1976. In E. B. Roberts, et al, ed: Biomedical innovation. Cambridge, London, MIT Press, 1981. p. 284–300.
Freshwater MF: Priorities in plastic surgery. **Plast Reconstr Surg** 1984 Jun;73(6):987–90
Gielen JE, Laduron P, Lapière CM: Receptors in classical pharmacology and cell biology. A report of a symposium held on the occasion of the 25th anniversary of the first publication of Biochemical Pharmacology. **Biochem Pharmacol** 1983 Dec 15;32(24):3891–2
In memoriam Professor Dr. Marcel Florkin (1900–1979): **Clio Med** 1980 May;14(2):89–90
Lister J: By the London post. The last post. **N Engl J Med** 1980 Dec 25;303(26):1528–31
Petkova M: Seriĭni izdaniia na svetovnata zdravna organizatsiia naukometrichno prouchvane. **Vutr Boles** 1982;21(6):86–91
Rodríguez García JR: Circulacion mundial de la obstetricia y ginecologia española a traves de Excerpta Medica (1951–71). **Asclepio** 1980;32:401–14
Sammons JH, Miller JD, Hannon TF: The Journal and publication in the other languages and countries. From hesitant beginnings to firm commitment. **JAMA** 1983 Jul 8;250(2):236–41
Schnitzler H, Lieth H: 25 year activities of the International Society of Biometeorology and 25 year publication index. **Int J Biometeorol** 1983 Dec;27(4):287–434
Strbánová S: Biochemical journals and their profile in 1840–1930. **Acta Hist Rerum Nat Tech** 1981;16:149–95
Szállási A: Csehov és Maugham a Nyugat kedvenc írói. **Orv Hetil** 1980 Jan 27;121(4):226–9
Viney W, Michaels T, Ganong A: A note on the history of psychology in magazines. **J Hist Behav Sci** 1981;17:270–2
Wankmüller A: Hinweise zur Literatur für die Pharmaziegeschichte. **Beitr Gesch Pharm** 1982;31(14):110–1
Wedeen RP: 'Punch cures the gout'. **J Med Soc NJ** 1981 Mar;78(3):201–6
Wunderlich P: Zur Vorgeschichte und Geschichte der 'Kinderärztlichen Praxis' 4.: Weitere deutschsprachige Zeitschriften für Kinderheilkunde, die bis 1930 gegründet wurden. **Kinderarztl Prax** 1980 Jun;48(6):312–6

### Americas

Acuña HR: El Boletín de la Oficina sanitaria panamericana: a los sessenta años. **Bol Of Sanit Panam** 1982 May;92(5):377–8
Boletín panamericano de sanidad de la Oficina sanitaria internacional: **Bol Of Sanit Panam** 1982 May;92(5):429–48

### Australia

25th anniversary issue of Australasian Radiology: **Australas Radiol** 1982;Spec. No.:1–162

### Austria

Ganzinger K: Die 'Oesterreichische pharmazeutische Gesellschaft' 1873 bis 1938. **Osterr Apoth Ztg** 1980;34:3–6
Nowotny O: Hans Heger und seine Bedeutung für die Geschichte der Pharmazie in Oesterreich. In: Vorträge des Internationalen Pharmaziehistorischen Kongresses Innsbruck 1977. Stuttgart, Wissenschaftliche Verlagsgesellschaft, 1979. p. 147–52.
Wyklicky H: Vor hundert Jahren. Billroths erste Pylorusresektion, seine diesbezüglichen Publikationen in der 'Wiener Medizinischen Wochenschrift' und ein Rückblick auf seine Zeit. **Wien Med Wochenschr** 1981 Jan 15;131(1):1–13

### Belgium

Fautrez J: Les Archives de Biologie, les fondateurs et les éditeurs de la revue. **Arch Biol (Liege)** 1980;91(2):133–40
Gerebtzoff MA: Recherches sur la structure du système nerveux et ses modifications expérimentales publiées dans les Archives de Biologie de 1880 à 1900. Analyse critique. **Arch Biol (Liege)** 1980;91(2):223–42
Herlant M: Travaux consacrés aux glandes endocrines parus dans les Archives de Biologie entre 1880 et 1931. **Arch Biol (Liege)** 1980;91(2):243–65
Lecomte J, Schoffeniels E: L'oeuvre de Léon Frédéricq et son école (1853–1934) à travers les Archives de Biologie (1880–1904). **Arch Biol (Liege)** 1980;91(2):267–70
Mulnard J: Les vingt premières années des Archives de Biologie. **Arch Biol (Liege)** 1980;91(2):285–95

### Brazil

Knoplich J: Cinqüentenario das Revista Paulista de Medicina. **Rev Paul Med** 1982 Nov–Dec;100(3):3–5
Lemos AA de: Infra–estrutura da literatura biomédica: considerações acerca de um núcleo de revistas brasileiras do setor saúde. **Educ Med Salud** 1981;15(4):406–23

### Bulgaria

Gunev V: Chetvŭrt vek spisanie 'Akusherstvo i ginekologiia'. **Akush Ginekol (Sofiia)** 1983;22(3):242–3

### Canada

Bell SK: Plus ça change, plus c'est la même chose: CPhA 1907–1982. **Can Pharm J** 1982 Oct;115(10):367–8
Gridgeman NT: A semicentennial. The NRCC research journals 1929–1979. **Can J Physiol Pharmacol** 1979 Jul;57(7):i–xiv; Also in Can J Biochem 1979 Jul;57(7):iv–xvi; Also in Can J Zool 1979 Jul; 57(7):i–xiv
Kerr ME: A capsule history of your journal. **Can Nurse** 1980 Mar;76(3):20–1
Roland CG: Canadian medical journalism in the 19th century. **Can Med Assoc J** 1983 Feb 15;128(4):449–51, 454–9, 458–9
Roland CG: John Fulton, In Dictionary of Canadian biography, 1881–1890. 1982;11:328–9.
Roland CG: Ontario medical periodicals as mirrors of change. **Ont Hist** 1980;72:3–15
Sherrington A: Canadian medical periodicals on microfiche. **Can Med Assoc J** 1981 Feb 15;124(4):361–2
Sherrington A: Seventy years of editorial excellence. **Can Med Assoc J** 1981 Jul 1;125(1):85, 88, 91–3

### Chile

Costa–Casaretto C: Recuerdos olvidados de los orígenes de la Sociedad Médica de Santiago y del la 'Revista Médica de Chile'. **Rev Med Chil** 1979 Jul;107(7):663–72
Reyes H: Cincuentenario de la revista chilena de pediatria. **Rev Med Chil** 1980 Jul;108(7):597–8

### Czechoslovakia

Adamec J: Lékařská na stránkách Casopisu lékařu českých v prvním pulstoletí jeho existence. **Cas Lek Cesk** 1981;120(52):1589–93
Blaškovič D: Twenty–five years of Acta Virologica. **Acta Virol (Praha)** 1982 Sep;26(5):408–16
Bunčáková V, Bednárová E, Ivanová A, et al: Vývoj slovenskej lekárskej terminológie od vzniku Bratislavských lekárskych listov a Lekárskej fakulty Univerzity Komenského. **Bratisl Lek Listy** 1983 Aug;80(2):221–35
Cerveňanská N: Príspevok k histórii Slovensko–sovietskych stykov v medicíne. **Bratisl Lek Listy** 1982 Jan;77(1):85–105
Cižmář J: Závodní časopisy Mediky. **Cesk Farm** 1982 Dec;31(10):393–5
Drábek P: Casopis českého lékárnictva a jeho předchudci. **Cesk Farm** 1982 May;31(3–4)85–96
Hanzlíček Z: Ostatní Ceské farmaceutické časopisy. (Příspěvek k dějinám českého farmaceutického periodického tisku). **Cesk Farm** 1982 Dec;31(10):384–92
Hanzlíček Z: Redaktoři Casopisu českého lékárnictva. **Cesk Farm** 1982 May;31(3–4):97–109
Hanzlíček Z: Sto let českých farmaceutických časpisu. **Cesk Farm** 1982 May;31(3–4):83–4
Hlaváčková L: Casopis lékařu českých a Spolek českých lékařu v boji za českou universitu a lékařskou fakultu. **Cas Lek Cesk** 1982 Dec 23;121(51):1569–73
Hlaváčková L: Význam založení Casopisu lékařu českých v rámci rozvoje naší odborné publicistiky. **Cas Lek Cesk** 1981;120(52):1585–8
Hromádková J: Cesko–ruské lékařské vztahy na stránkách prvních dvaceti ročníku Casopisu lékařů českých. **Cas Lek Cesk** 1980 Nov 14;119(46):1259–61
Ondrejička M: 60 Rokov Bratislavských lekárskych listov. **Bratisl Lek Listy** 1982 Jan;77(1):3–5
Potměšilová R: RNDr. Blažena Jirsová zemřela první vedoucí redaktorka oddělení lékařských časopisu 6. 6. 1901--3. 9. 1979. **Cas Lek Cesk** 1979 Dec;118(52)1632
Rozsívalová E, Fuchsová V: Zájem lékařu o zdravotní stav dělnictva v druhých dvacetipěti ročnících Casopisu lékařu českých. **Cas Lek Cesk** 1981;120(52):1594–8
Zadina R: Casopis lékařu českých před sto lety. **Cas Lek Cesk** 1980 Jan

5;119(1):32
Zadina R: Casopis lékařučeských před sto lety. **Cas Lek Cesk** 1984 Jan 6;123(1):32
Zolyomi ND: Die Kochsche Entdeckung in der Pressburger Tagespresse. **Wiss Beitr Martin Luther Univ Halle Wittenberg** 1983;5-R80:79–84

**Denmark**

Vogt HH: 100 Jahre Gram-Färbung. Ein Forschungsbeitrag aus den Anfängen dieser Zeitschrift. **Fortschr Med** 1984 Apr;102(16):94–5

**Dutch Guiana**

Lindeboom GA: Jacob Voegen van Engelen, medisch journalist; 'De Surinaamsche Artz'. **Ned Tijdschr Geneeskd** 1981 Jun 27;125(26):1044–9

**Europe**

Pope BH, ed: Historical periodicals directory. Volume 2: Europe, West, North, Central and South. Santa Barbara, Oxford, ABC-Clio, 1983. xv, 597 p. (Clio Periodicals Directories).

**Finland**

Duodecim: Satavuotisjuhliene satao: **Duodecim** 1982;98(8):623–56
Raivio K: Satavuotias duodecim-seura ja kehittyyä lääketiede. **Duodecim** 1981;97(20):1661–3

**France**

Achard E: 1956--numéro 1 des 'Annales de Chirurgie Plastique'. **Ann Chir Plast** 1980;25(2):191–2
Centenary of a medical journal.: **S Afr Med J** 1979 Sep 8;56(11):419–20
Degleris N: Contribution à l'étude des relations Franco-Helleniques au point de vue de la presse neuro-psychiatrique française (1880–1914); les membres associés grecs de la Société Médico-Psychologique. Mémoire pour le titre d'assistant étranger, Université Paris V, René Descartes, Faculté de Médecine Cochin-Port Royal, Paris, 1984. 96 leaves.
Di Matteo J: Les Archives des maladies du coeur et des vaisseaux. **Arch Mal Coeur** 1980 Jun;73(6):563–84
Lemaire JF: Cent cinquante ans de médecine dans 'La Revue'. **Rev Deux Mondes** 1979 Oct;73–8
Léonard J: Les débuts du 'Concours médical'. **Hist Sci Med** 1980;14:453–8
Portmann G: The 'Revue de Laryngologie' and the E. N. T. School of Bordeaux are a hundred years old. **Rev Laryngol Otol Rhinol (Bord)** 1980 Jan-Feb;101(1-2):1–14
Ramadier JO: La revue de chirurgie orthopédique et réparatrice de l'appareil moteur--90e anniversaire. **Rev Chir Orthop** 1981;67(3):161–3
Rivet R: Un essai de journalisme médical en l'an VII (1799). In: Congrès National des Sociétés Savantes, 105e, Caen, 1980. Comptes Rendus, Paris, 1980. Section des Sciences, Fasc. V. p. 41–7.
Sharrard WJ: 90th anniversary of the Revue de Chirurgie Orthopédique: an outsider's view. **Rev Chir Orthop** 1981;67(3):165–6
Tachon J: La revue 'Médecine Tropical'--retrospective. **Med Trop (Mars)** 1980 Nov-Dec;40(6):639–41
Woehrle R, Touraine JL, Garin JP, et al: Comité de lecture d'une revue régionale. Fonctionnement et résultats. **Bull Soc Sci Med Grand Duche Luxemb** 1979;116(1):137–41

**Germany**

Bayer FW: Der Merck'sche Jahresbericht als Quelle zur Geschichte der Therapie. **Pharm Ind** 1980;42(7):701–6
Butenandt O: Pädiatrie vor 100 Jahren. Aus Berichten des 'Jahrbuches für Kinderheilkunde', Band 18, 1882. **Fortschr Med** 1983 Feb 17;101(7):251–4
Deneke JF: Das Gesundheitswesen der ersten Hälfte des 19.Jahrhunderts im Spiegel der Amts- und Intelligenzpresse. Düsseldorf, Triltsch, 1983. 161 p. (Düsseldorfer Arbeiten zur Geschichte der Medizin, Beiheft IX).
Elster R: Porträt unserer Zeitschrift. **Krankenpflege (Frankfurt)** 1981 Jan;35(1):7–10
Fodor B: 100 Jahre 'Fortschritte der Medizin'--Höhepunkte der Medizin 1882-1982. **Fortschr Med** 1982 Dec 16;100(47-48):2207–13
Fricke A: Die thematische Entwicklung unserer Zeitschrift; Rückblick--Gegenwart--Ausblick. **Krankenpflege (Frankfurt)** 1981 Jan;35(1):11–5
Gieger G: Schwachsinnigenfürsorge und Hilfe für das geistig behinderte Kind. Eine Analyse der 'Zeitschrift für das Idiotenwesen' (1880–1934). Freiburg, Schulz, 1977. 245 p. (Freiburger Forschungen zur Medizingeschichte, Neue Folge, 6).
Hein WH: Historische und kritische Betrachtungen zu den Veröffentlichungen der Gesellschaft. In: Vorträge des Internationalen Pharmaziehistorischen Kongresses Innsbruck 1977. Stuttgart, Wissenschaftliche Verlagsgesellschaft, 1979. p. 15–22.
Hellbrügge T: Anwalt des praktizierenden Arztes: 100 Jahre 'Fortschritte der Medizin'. **Fortschr Med** 1982 Apr 15;100(14):613–4
Knorr M: 1883-1983. Gedanken zum Jubiläumsband 177. **Zentralbl Bakteriol Mikrobiol Hyg [B]** 1983 Jan;177(1-2):i–iv
Linss W: Karl von Bardeleben--der Begründer des 'Anatomischen Anzeigers'. **Anat Anz** 1981;150(1-2):5–10
Lohff B: Johannes Müller, 'Jahresberichte zur Physiologie', in Müllers Archiv der Jahre 1834–1838. **Sudhoffs Arch** 1981;65(1):32–78
Michel D: 100 Jahre 'Fortschritte der Medizin'--100 Jahre Kardiologie. **Fortschr Med** 1982 Dec 16;100(47-48):2191–3
Nabielek R: Zu den wichtigsten Veröffentlichungen des polnischen Histologen Henryk Fryderyk Hoyer (1834–1907) in deutschen Fachzeitschriften. **Z Mikrosk Anat Forsch** 1983;97(3):393–408
Nauels I: Arzt und Medizin in fünf Jahrgängen. Spiegel (1971–1975). Diss. Düsseldorf, 1981. 137 p.
Referent Robert Koch: Der Entdecker des Tuberkulose-Erregers als sachverständiger Referent in der ersten Ausgabe der 'Fortschritte der Medicin'. **Fortschr Med** 1982 Jun 3;100(21):1012–3
Renker K: 25 Jahre Zeitschrift für die gesamte Hygiene. **Z Gesamte Hyg** 1979 Oct;25(10):792
Schierhorn H: Die Hirnanatomie im Spiegel der ersten 50 Bände des Anatomischen Anzeigers. **Anat Anz** 1981;150(1-2):77–118
Schipperges H: Bildung zu gesunder Vernunft. Zu einer wiederentdeckten Magazin der Aufklärung. **Arztebl Baden Wurttemberg** 1981;6
Schneider HG, Witte B: Die Zeitschrift 'Deutsche Stomatologie/Stomatologie der DDR' in den Jahren 1961–1980. Eine Analyse ihrer Beiträge hinsichtlich Inhalt, Form und thematischer Trends. **Stomatol DDR** 1982 Jan;32(1):2–9
Simmer HH: Die Anfänge der hormonalen Kontrazeption und die Münchener Medizinische Wochenschrift. **MMW** 1982 May 21;124(20):499–503
Torp H: 75 Jahre Fachzeitschrift: Dokumentation von Kontinuität und Wandel in der Krankenpflege. **Krankenpflege (Frankfurt)** 1981 Jun;35(6):235–7
Wankmüller A: Hinweise zur Literatur für die Pharmaziegeschichte. 2. Deutschsprachige periodische Veröffentlichungen. **Beitr Gesch Pharm** 1981;31:86
Wimmel B, Geus A, ed: Die tiermedizinischen Zeitschriften des 18. Jahrhunderts. Stuttgart, Hiersemann, 1981. 200 p. (Indices naturwissenschaftlich-medizinischer Periodica bis 1850, 3).
Wullstein HL: Das Schicksal unserer HNO-Zeitschrift bei der Neugründung nach dem Kriege. **HNO** 1980 Jan;28(1):33–4
Zander W: Grussworte zum 25 jährigen Jubiläum der Zeitschrift für Psychosomatische Medizin und Psychoanalyse. **Z Psychosom Med Psychoanal** 1979 Oct-Dec;25(4):301–2

**Great Britain**

Bell C: A hundred years of Lancet language. **Lancet** 1984 Dec 22;2(8417-18):1453
Bliquez LJ: An unidentified Roman surgical instrument in Bingen. **J Hist Med Allied Sci** 1981 Apr;36(2):219–20
Brown PS: The venders of medicines advertised in eighteenth-century Bath newspapers. **Med Hist** 1975 Oct;19(4):352–69
Centenary issue: 1880–1980.: **Br Dent J** 1980 Jul 1;149(1):1–36
Davies C: Where next for nursing history? **Nurs Times** 1980 May 22;76(21):920–2
Dobbs R, Robinson R, MacCarthy D, et al: Douglas Gairdner, editor of the Archives 1964–79. **Arch Dis Child** 1979 Nov;54(11):813, 815–21
Dopson L: Celebrating 75 years. **Nurs Times** 1980 May 22;76(21):923–36
Fee E: Science and the 'woman question', 1860–1920: a study of English scientific periodicals. Ph. D. Diss., Princeton University. Princeton, 1978. v, 351 leaves.
From Gazette to Review: 1904–1979: **Hosp Health Serv Rev** 1980 Jan;76(1):19–22
Graham AN: Contribution of the International Journal of Social Psychiatry. **Int J Soc Psychiatry** 1979;25(4):238–9
Hillson RM: The Lancet 1823. **Lancet** 1983 Dec 24-31;2(8365-66):1507–8
History in the pharmaceutical press: **Pharm Hist (London)** 1971 Mar;2(1):2–8
John Mitchell Bruce (1846–1929): **Practitioner** 1982 Apr;226(1366):800
Leavy BF: Fathering and the British Mother's Magazine, 1845-1864. **Victorian Period Rev** 1980;13(1-2):10–7
O'Brien E: The Lancet maketh the man? Sir Dominic John Corrigan (1802–80). **Lancet** 1980 Dec 20-27;2(8208-8209):1356–7
Oliver TP: 67 years ago--the Journal of the Royal Naval Medical Service, Vol I. **J R Nav Med Serv** 1982 Winter;68(3):167–70
Oliver TP: 67 years ago--the Journal of the Royal Naval Medical Service Vol 1, No. 1. **J R Nav Med Serv** 1982;68(2):98–101
Owen M: The Journal of the Roentgen Society, Number 1, Volume 1: an outline. **Australas Radiol** 1983 Jul;27(2):170–3
Peterson MJ: Specialist journals and professional rivalries in Victorian medicine. **Victorian Period Rev** 1979;12(1):25–32
Roos DA: The 'aims and intentions' of Nature. In Paradis J, Postlewait T, ed. Victorian science and Vicorian values: literary perspectives. New York, New York Academy of Sciences, 1981. p. 159–80.
Schilling RS: Donald Hunter--the first editor of the British Journal of Industrial Medicine. **J Cell Biol** 1979 Aug;36(3):243
Seward M: More than a century of change. **Br Dent J** 1980 Jul 1;149(1):35–6

Sheets-Pyenson S: Darwin's data: his reading of natural history journals, 1837-1842. **J Hist Biol** 1981 Fall;14(2):231-48

Sheets-Pyenson S: From the north to Red Lion Court: the creation and early years of the Annals of Natural History. **Arch Nat Hist** 1981 Oct;10(2):221-49

Zuckerman L: The launching of the Journal of Endocrinology and the founding of the Society for Endocrinology. **J Endocrinol** 1984 Jan;100(1):1-5

**Greece**

Degleris N: [The 19th-century Greek medical journals index: sources of information--results] (Gre). Athens, Athens University Medical Faculty, 1980. 171 p.

Degleris NE, Rozos BP: [Public health, medical education and social care of Ionian Isles in the middle of the 19th century (press documents)] (Gre). **Arch Hyg** 1980;:90-101

**Hungary**

Az Orvosi Hetilap múltjából: **Orv Hetil** 1982 Jan 10;123(2):111

Az Orvosi Hetilap múltjából: **Orv Hetil** 1982 Apr 18;123(16):992-3 (continued periodically)

Az Orvosi Hetilap múltjából: **Orv Hetil** 1982 May 16;123(20):1250-1

Az Orvosi Hetilap 125. évfordulója: **Orv Hetil** 1982 Jan 3;123(1):3-4

Batári G: Az elsö gyógyászati szakfolyóiratok magyarországon. **Magy Konyvsz** 1982;98(1):72-5

Batari G: Az orvosi sajtóreferálás kezdetei Magyarországon. **Orv Hetil** 1982 Oct 17;123(42):2611-3

Batári G: Schmidt Béla és az erdélyi Magyar Népegészségügyi Szemle. **Orv Hetil** 1982 Oct 31;123(44):2737-8

Batári G: Schwartzer Ottó mint az orvosi sajtóreferálás kezdeményezöje. **Orv Hetil** 1979 Jul 1;120(26):1586-7

Fábián T: 75 éves a Fogorvosi Szemle. **Fogorv Sz** 1982 Jan;75(1):1-3

Hidvégi J: Az ifjú Markusovszky világa. **Orv Hetil** 1982 Dec 26;123(52):3207-13

Hidvegi J: Die Resonanz der Kochschen Entdeckung in der medizinischen Fachpresse Ungarns. **Wiss Beitr Martin Luther Univ Halle Wittenberg** 1983;5-R80:87-90

Honti J: A fiziológia az Orvosi Hetilap korai évfolyamaiban. **Orv Hetil** 1981 Aug 9;122(32):1979-80

Kapronczay K: Markusovszky Lajos utolsó levele Fodor Józsefhez. **Orv Hetil** 1982 Dec 26;123(52):3213-4

Littmann I: A 125 éves Orvosi Hetilap és a modern sebészet kialakulása. Merre tart ma a sebészet? **Orv Hetil** 1982 Feb 7;123(6):323-6

Mészárosné Varga M: A Magyar Tanácsköztársaság egészségügye Veszprém megyében - a korabeli sajtó alapján. **Orvostort Kozl** 1982;28(1-3):219-26

Petrányi L: Markusovszky szellemének idézése a 3. évezred küszöbén. **Orv Hetil** 1984 Jun 17;125(25):1487-92

Rixer A: A magyar gyógyszerészi szaksajtó kialakulása és fejlödése a xix. században. **Acta Pharm Hung** 1983 Jul;53(4):183-90

Rixer A: A magyar nyelvü gyógyszerészeti szaksajtó kialakulása és jelenentösége 1831-1872 között. Diss., Budapest, 1976. 193 p.

Szállá A: Arthur Schnitzler és Georges Duhamel a Nyugatban. **Orv Hetil** 1982 Sep 5;123(36):2246-50

Szállási A: A Nyugat, gyógyszerészei'. **Orv Hetil** 1982 Jan 24;123(4):229-32

Szállási A: A salvarsan felfedezésének visszhangja a Nyugat-ban. **Orv Hetil** 1980 Apr 20;121(16):966-7

Szállási A: Donath Gyula és a Klinikai Füzetek. **Orv Hetil** 1984 Apr 15;125(16):960-3

Szállási A: Freud, Ferenczi és a Nyugat. **Orv Hetil** 1980 May 18;121(20):1207-8

Szállási A: Németh Lázzló és a Nyugat. **Orv Hetil** 1981 Jan 25;122(4):226-7

Szállási A: Orvosok és a Nyugat elsö évfolyamai. **Orv Hetil** 1979 Sep 23;120(38):2311-3

Szállási A: Rekviem a 'Gyógyászat'--ért Schachter Miksa szerkesztése ürügyén. **Orv Hetil** 1980 Dec 14;121(50):3073-6

Szállási A: Székey Agoston--a szerkesztöi másodvonalból. **Orv Hetil** 1983 Jan 9;124(2):95-7

Trencséni T: A 125 éves Orvosi Hetilap és szerkesztése az újraindulás óta. **Orv Hetil** 1982 Dec 26;123(52):3179-85

**Indonesia**

Luyendijk-Elshout AM: Het medisch tijdschrift in Nederlands Oost-Indië (1844-1865). **Ned Tijdschr Geneeskd** 1981 Jun 6;125(23):923-6

**Ireland**

Brophy L: Towards a golden jubilee. The Career of 'Caritas' through a half-century. **Caritas** 1983-84;49(49):4-6

**Italy**

Bèttica-Giovannini R: Il contributo 1958-1977 degli Annali Dell'Ospedale Maria Vittoria Di Torino alla storia della medicina. **Ann Osp Maria Vittoria Torino** 1980 Jan-Jun;23(1-6):175-223

Buscaino GA, Guadagnino M: Ulteriore contributo a 'orientamenti teorici e pratici della psichiatria italiana'. Dal 1950 al 1976. **Acta Neurol [Quad]** 1978;37:131-59

Guadagnino M, Buscaino GA: Un secondo contributo a 'orientamenti teorici e pratici della psichiatria italiana dal 1950 al 1970'. **Acta Neurol [Quad]** 1978;37:116-30

Masoni A: Continuita' e novita'. **G Ital Cardiol** 1979;9(1):1-3

Rovelli F: Il 'giornale italiano di cardiologia': 10 anni di storia della cardiologia in italia. **G Ital Cardiol** 1981;11 Suppl 1:1-7

Spirito A: Breve istoria della 'rivista di biologia' con particolare riguardo all'ultimo trentennio. **Riv Biol** 1979 Jan-Jun;72(1-2):3-10

**Japan**

Fukuyama Y: A quarter-century of the Japanese Society of Child Neurology. **Brain Dev** 1984;6(2):109-18

Kikuchi S: [The progress of 'Shigaku' in the past 70 years] (Jpn). **Shigaku** 1982 Jun;70(1):iii-ix

**Luxembourg**

Nahas GG: Bilinguisme médical: vingt cinq ans d'expérience. **Bull Soc Sci Med Grand Duche Luxemb** 1979;116(1):83-7

**Mexico**

Díaz y de Ovando C: Odontología y publicidad en la prensa mexicana del siglo XIX. **Bol Soc Mex Hist Filos Med** 1984 Jun;7(47):325-46

Marcial LD: Las publicaciones oficiales de la Secretaría de Salubridad y Asistencia. **Salud Publica Mex** 1983 Sep-Oct;25(5):489-97

Miguel Torre J: Treinta años de vida de la Sociedad Potosina de Estudios Médicos. Una experiencia interesante. **Gac Med Mex** 1982 Apr;118(4):165-70

**Netherlands**

Beukers H: De tijdschriften van Willem van Ranouw. **Ned Tijdschr Geneeskd** 1981 Oct 3;125(40):1613-7

Jongkees LB: 125 jaar Nederlands Tijdschrift voor Geneeskunde, uit het verleden via het heden naar de toekomst. **Ned Tijdschr Geneeskd** 1982 Jan 2;126(1):1-3

Kerkhoff AH: Het eerste Nederlandstalinge tijdschrift op het terrein van gezondheids- voorlichting in de negentiende eeuw. **Ned Tijdschr Geneeskd** 1981 Nov 21;125(47):1935-40

Koning AT: De 'Kweekschool der Vroedkunde', de eerste verloskundige periodiek? **Ned Tijdschr Geneeskd** 1981 Aug 8;125(32):1299-302

Koning AT: Vijftig jaar Tijdschrift voor Kindergeneeskunde. **Tijdschr Kindergeneeskd** 1983 Feb;51(1):1-7

Moulin D de: Heelkundige onderwerpen in het Nederlandsch Weekblad voor Genesskundigen (1851-1856). **Ned Tijdschr Geneeskd** 1981 Aug 25;125(35):1427-30

Snelders HA: De natuur- en scheikundige wetenschappen in de medische tijdschriften. **Ned Tijdschr Geneeskd** 1981 Apr 25;125(17):668-73

Van der Korst JK: Bataafse geneeskunde in periodiek perspectief; in- en uitwendige historische aspecten van het Geneeskundig Magazijn (1801-1815). **Ned Tijdschr Geneeskd** 1981 Nov 28;125(48):1975-9

Van der Korst JK: Geneeskunde in de eerste internationale geleerdentijdschriften van Nederlandse origine (1680-1709). **Ned Tijdschr Geneeskd** 1981 Feb 28;125(9):355-60

Verslag van de bijzondere wetenschappelijke vergadering ter viering van het honderdvijfentwintigjarig bestaan der Vereniging Nederlands Tijdschrift voor Geneeskunde.: **Ned Tijdschr Geneeskd** 1982 Jan 2;126(1):33-8

Visser RP: Arts en geneeskunde in de I83-eeuwse algemene tijdschriften. **Ned Tijdschr Geneeskd** 1981 May 16;125(20):792-4

Wittop Koning DA: De farmacie en de medische tijdschriften. **Ned Tijdschr Geneeskd** 1981 Dec 5;125(49):2021-4

**New Zealand**

Hughes B: 75 years of Kai Tiaki. **NZ Nurs J** 1983 Jan;76(1):4-6

New Zealand Dental Journal. Seventy-fifth jubilee issue: **NZ Dent J** 1980 Jul;76(345):107-48

Pages from the past: **NZ Nurs J** 1983 Jan;76(1):16-25

Shadbolt Y: Nursing education - a major shift. **NZ Nurs J** 1983 Jan;76(1):6-9

Smith MG: Resources for nursing history. **NZ Nurs J** 1983 Jan;76(1):26-7

**Norway**

Gilder SB: A Norwegian centenary. **Tidsskr Nor Laegeforen** 1981 Jan;101(1):70-1

Johansen O: Klipp fra 'Tidsskriftet' gjennom tidene. **Tidsskr Nor Laegeforen** 1981 Jan;101(1):25-35

# PERIODICALS

**Poland**

Kaiser W: Ernst Jeremias Neifeld (1721-1773), Herausgeber der ersten medizinischen Fachzeitschrift in Polen. **Wiss Z Martin Luther Univ (Math)** 1977;26(3):123-31
Kałużny J: W 25-lecie redagowania Kliniki Ocznej przez prof. dra Witolda Orowskiego. **Klin Oczna** 1981;83(2):55-8
Konopka S: Działalność naukowa, redakcyjna i wydawnicza prof. Adama Wrzoska w świetle jego wypowiedzi i listów nie ogłoszonych w druku. **Arch Hist Med (Warsz)** 1982;45(1-4):11-26
Konopka S: Odrodzenie się niektórych ważnych działów polskiej służby zdrowia w roku 1945. **Pol Tyg Lek** 1981 Sep 7;36(36):1369-75
Michałowski R: Wspomnienie o 'Wiadomościach medycznych' (Warszawa 1934-1939) przez ich Redaktora Naczelnego w latach 1936-1938. **Arch Hist Med (Warsz)** 1981;44(3/4):369-79
Mlosek K: W 50 rocznicę polskiego czasopiśmiennictwa radiologicznego. **Pol Przegl Radiol** 1979 Nov-Dec;43(6):339-43
Sosińska-Trawińska M: Zalecenia lecznicze w chorobach dzieci zawarte w wybranych czasopismach nielekarskich XVIII w w Polsce. **Arch Hist Med (Warsz)** 1983;46(3):285-94
Sródka A, Wajs S: Bibliografia publikacji w Archiwum Historii Medycyny w latach 1974-1982. **Arch Hist Med (Warsz)** 1984;47(2):287-315
Waszyński E: O mechanizmie żucia w 'Primitiae Physico-Medicae...' (1750-1753), pierwszym w Polsce czasopiśmie medycznym. **Czas Stomatol** 1984 Mar;37(3):227-32
Waszyński E: 'Primitiae physico-medicae ...' (1750-1753). Problematyka położniczo-ginekologiczna. **Arch Hist Med (Warsz)** 1984;47(3):447-61
Wilkoszewski E: Z dziejów polskich czasopism pediatrycznych (lata 1908-1983). **Pediatr Pol** 1983 Aug-Sep;58(8-9):673-84

**Puerto Rico**

Rivera Villanueva ZE: The collection of the Boletín de la Asociación Médica de Puerto Rico and its preservation (1903-20). **Bol Asoc Med PR** 1984 Sep;76(9):394-6

**Romania**

Creteanu G, Teodorovici G: Revista Medico-chirurgicală si contributia sa la progresul asistentei medicale. **Rev Med Chir Soc Med Nat Iasi** 1980 Oct-Dec;84(4):625-9
Nepohoda-Seredenciuc I: Our magazine is 25. **Sante Publique (Bucur)** 1983;26(1):3-8
On the 35th anniversary of our journal: **Virologie** 1984 Jan-Mar;35(1):3-4

**South Africa**

Gilder SS: Leipoldt the editor. **S Afr Med J** 1980 Dec 6;58(23):926-32
Lucas MB: Diamond jubilee medicine. The medical world of 1897 and 1898 seen in the pages of the South African Medical Journal. **S Afr Med J** 1979 Oct 20;56(17):688-94

**Spain**

Aragon F: La politica cientifica en la España del s. XVIII a traves de la revista 'Anales de Ciencias Naturales', Madrid, 1799-1804. **Llull (Spain)** 1978;2:19-25
Basas M: La epidemia del cólera morbo de 1854-1855 en Bilbao y otras noticias de este tiempo. **Estud Duesto** 1969;17:135-73
Carreras Panchon A: La obra de Juan de Villarreal y otros estudios historico-medicos. Salamanca, Ediciones Universidad de Salamanca, 1978. 69 p. (Cuadernos de Historia de la Medicina Española, Mongrafias, XXXIII).
Delgado B: La revista de psicologia i pedagogia de Barcelona (1933-1937). **Perspect Pedagog (Barc)** 1982;12(49):47-70
Jimenez Muñoz JM, Riera J: Bibliografia histórica en el siglo médico (1854-1936). Valladolid, Universidad de Valladolid, 1975. 107 p. (Acta Historico-Medica Vallisoletana, Monografias, VI)
Lopez Piñero JM, Terrada ML: Las etapas históricas del periodismo médico en España. Estudio bibliométrico. **Med Esp** 1979:78:95-108
Mendez Alvaro F: Historia del periodismo medico y farmacéutico en España. Ed. J. Riera. Valladolid, Universidad de Valladolid, 1978. 179 p. (Acta Historico-Medica Vallisoletana, Monografias, VIII).
Parra Hidalgo P, Marset Campos P, Ramos García E, et al: Cincuenta años de la Revista de Sanidad e Higiene Pública (1926-1975). Análisis bibliométrico de su producción científica. **Rev Sanid Hig Publica (Madr)** 1983 Sep-Oct;57(9-10):969-1038

**Sri Lanka**

Aloysius DJ, Ranasinghe L: Historical perspective of the Sri Lanka Medical Association. **Ceylon Med J** 1981 Mar;26(1):8-34

**Sweden**

Achté K, Turunen S: Den första psykiatriska artikeln i Finland. **Dan Medicinhist Arbog** 1983;12:74-81
Bahr G von: Upsala Läkareförening 150 år. **Ups J Med Sci [Suppl]** 1982;35:1-33
Engel A: Hälsan före födelsen. Prenatal forskning i Sverige. Stockholm, 1981. 128 p. (Nordisk Medicinhistorisk Arsbok, Supplementum, VIII).

**Switzerland**

Barblan MA: Journalisme médical et échanges intellectuels au tournant du XVIIIe siècle: le cas de la Bibliothèque Britannique. **Arch Sci** 1977;30(3):283-398
Bersch MC: Notre revue a 75 ans. **Krankenpflege (Bern)** 1983 Jan;(1):18-22
Bonard JF: 1980---Année du centenaire de la 'Revue médicale de la Suisse Romande'. **Rev Med Suisse Romande** 1980 Jan;100(1):1-3
Fankhauser R: Dem 125. Bande zum Geleit. **Schweiz Arch Tierheilkd** 1983 Jan;125(1):1-15
Mayer R: Ils étaient trois! Jacques-Louis Reverdin, Jean-Louis Prévost et Constant Picot, fondateurs de la Revue médicale de la Suisse Romande. Evocation de la naissance d'une revue médicale et esquisse biographique de ses premiers rédacteurs. **Rev Med Suisse Romande** 1980 Dec;100(12):1013-41
Pittet-Faessler E: Krankenpflege--Soins infirmiers à 75 ans. **Krankenpflege (Bern)** 1983 Jan;(1):17
Renner M: 'Krankenpflege' stellt sich vor. **Krankenpflege (Bern)** 1981 Dec;(12):58-9
Renner M: 75 Jahre Zeitschrift Krankenpflege. **Krankenpflege (Bern)** 1983 Jan;(1):57-65
75 Jahre Zeitschrift Krankenpflege: Krankenschwestern erinnern sich. **Krankenpflege (Bern)** 1983 Jan;(1):66-9

**United States**

Abelson PH, Kulstad R, et al: Science centennial--3 July 1880 to 4 July 1980. **Science** 1980 Jul 4;209(4452):19-198
Adams DP: The penicillin mystique and the popular press (1935-1950). **Pharm Hist** 1984;26(3):134-42
After seventy-five years, 1890-1965: Baltimore, Waverly Press, William & Wilkins, 1965. 46 p.
Agins TC: Year of the twenty-dollar gold piece. **NY J Dent** 1980 Apr;50(4):123-6
American Academy of Arts and Sciences, American Philosophical Society: Survey of sources for the history of biochemistry and molecular biology. **Surv Sources Newsl** 1975-1981;1(1-10):various pagings
Arndt KA: Archives of Dermatology. Second century. **Arch Dermatol** 1984 Jan;120(1):42-3
Aufricht G: Story of the foundation of the Plastic and Reconstructive Surgery journal and reminiscences of the early formative years of plastic surgery as a specialty. **Plast Reconstr Surg** 1981 Sep;68(3):370-5
Baue AE: 60 years of the Archives of Surgery. July 1920-July 1980. **Arch Surg** 1980 Jul;115(7):809-11
Bean WB: Occasional notes. My sampler of editors: a Fishbein, a Fox, and a Garland. **N Engl J Med** 1980 Jul 24;303(4):229-33
Beawer D de B: The American scientific community, 1800-1860; a statistical-historical study (Doctoral Dissertation, Yale University, 1966). New York, Arno Press, 1980. 379 p.
Berryman JW, Brislin J: The ladies' department of the American Farmer, 1825-1830. A locus for the advocacy of family health and exercise. **J NAL Assoc** 1977;2(2):8-15
Binford Ch: Esmond Ray Long, M.D., Ph. D., 1890-1979, Editor, International Journal of Leprosy, 1964-1968. **Int J Lepr** 1980 Sep;48(3):322-6
Blake JB, ed: Centenary of Index Medicus, 1879-1979. Bethesda, National Library of Medicine, 1980. viii, 115 p. (NIH Publication No. 80-2068; Order from U.S. Government Printing Office). Contributions by C. E. Rosenberg, G. Miller, F. B. Rogers, W. B. Bean, E. Wolf, K. G. Huston, S. Jarcho.
Bonsett CA: Dr. G. W. H. Kemper and his work in indexing the Transactions of the Indiana State Medical Society. **J Indiana State Med Assoc** 1980 Sept;73(9):561
Boyd DP: A half century of publishing. **Chest** 1984 Nov;86(5):654-5
Boyer S: This is the final issue of The Johns Hopkins Medical Journal [editorial]. **Johns Hopkins Med J** 1982 Dec;151(6):263-82
Burnham JC: The founding of the Archives of Neurology and Psychiatry; or, what was wrong with the Journal of Nervous and Mental disease? **J Hist Med Allied Sci** 1981 Jul;36(3):310-24
Carroll D: The state of medical knowledge in Maryland, 1870s. **Md State Med J** 1980 Sep;29(9):12-5
Cassedy JH: The flourishing and character of early American medical journalism, 1797-1860. **J Hist Med Allied Sci** 1983 Apr;38(2):135-50
Castle M, Klimek JJ: From newsletter to journal: a 10-year review. **Am J Infect Control** 1982 Aug;10(3):79-83
Chapman CB: An aspect of medical publication: 1846 and 1982. **N Engl J Med** 1982 Dec 9;307(24):1531
Christianson EH: Wound management advice in antebellum America. In Romm S, ed: Symposium on historical perspectives of plastic surgery. Philadelphia, Saunders, 1983. p. 671-7.
Cirn JT: The birth throes of the Wisconsin Medical Practice Act: the physicians versus the newspaper editors. **Wis Med J** 1980 May;79(5):12-4

# PERIODICALS


Cobb WM: The Black American in medicine. **J Natl Med Assoc** 1981 Dec;73 Suppl:1185–244

Covert C: A view of the press in the twenties. **Journalism Hist** 1975;2(3):66–7, 92–6

Cowen DL: Fifty years of the New Jersey Journal of Pharmacy. **NJ J Pharm** 1977 Oct;50(10):14–17

Dinning JS: Reflections on Nutrition Reviews from an international nutritionist. **Nutr Rev** 1982 Nov;40(11):328–30

Dubos R: Peyton Rous. **J Exp Med** 1979 Oct 1;150(4):735–7

Edsall JT: The Journal of Biological Chemistry after seventy–five years. **J Biol Chem** 1980 Oct 10;255(19):8939–51

Fairbanks RJ: The Journal of Pastoral Care: an historical perspective. **J Pastoral Care** 1975 Sep;29(3):204–6

Felton JS: Industrial medicine to occupational health and safety: a 50–year retrospective. **Occup Health Saf** 1982 Sep;51(9):14–22

Fishman AP: Hail and farewell. **Am J Physiol** 1981 May;240(5):C161–3

Four from '44: the Winslow editorials: **J Public Health Policy** 1980 Mar;1(1):15–24

Garland J: Jerome Van Crowningshield Smith. **N Engl J Med** 1970 Aug 6;283:303–4

Gillies K: Out of the past. Diamond jubilee 1909–1984. **Fla Nurse** 1984 Sep;32(9):4, 12

Goldwyn RM: Transition. **Plast Reconstr Surg** 1980 Jan;65(1):70–1

Greenberg HR, Greenberg RR: 'A bintel brief;' the editor as compleat therapist. **Psychiatr Q** 1980 Fall;52(3):222–30

Gromala T: Broadsides, epigrams, and testimonials: the evolution of chiropractic advertising. **Chiropr Hist** 1984;4(1):41–5

Harper AE: Reflections on Nutrition Reviews from a university professor. **Nutr Rev** 1982 Nov;40(11):330–1

Hayden GF, Saulsbury FT: A review of The Journal of Pediatrics: the first 50 years. **J Pediatr** 1982 Jul;101(1):5–11

Hayden GF: Clinical research in Southern Medical Journal: current trends. **South Med J** 1983 Dec;76(12):1473–6

'Health Physics': 25th anniversary issue commemorating the founding of the Health Physics Society 1955–1980.: **Health Phys** 1980 Jun;38(6):883–1209

Heim LR: Birth and development of a scientific journal, and a society. **Exp Hematol** 1983 Nov;11(10):907–13

Herman BL: Folk medical recipes in nineteenth–century American farm journals. **Pa Folklife** 1976;25(4):16–25

Hidvégi J: A száz éves JAMA–ról. **Orv Hetil** 1984 Jul 8;125(28):1705–7

In the spirit of C.–E. A. Winslow: **J Public Health Policy** 1980 Mar;1(1):3–5

Jackman SW: The tribulations of an editor: Benjamin Silliman and the early days of the American Journal of Science and the Arts. **N Engl Q** 1979;52(1):99–106

Josephson ME: The AJC in March 1959. **Am J Cardiol** 1984 Mar 1;53(6):803–4

The Journal of the American Medical Association: Reproduction of first issue Saturday, July 14, 1883. **JAMA** 1983 Jul 8;250(2):Centennial Issue.

The Journal's 30th anniversary: **J Prosthet Dent** 1980 Jan;43(1):4–8

Kampmeier RH: Seventy–five years of the journal. **J Tenn Med Assoc** 1983 Jul;76(7):431–8

Kennedy JW: Publications of the Arizona Territorial Medical Society. **Ariz Med** 1981 Apr;38(4):290–3 contd

King LS: Medical journalism, 1847–1883. **JAMA** 1983 Aug 12;250(6):744–8

King LS: XIII. The founding of JAMA, 1883. **JAMA** 1983 Jul 8;250(2):177–80

Kinney JR: The first medical journal in Illinois. **J Hist Med Allied Sci** 1983 Apr;38(2):151–60

Knoebel SB: On the occasion of the 25th year of the Journal of the American College of Cardiology. **J Am Coll Cardiol** 1983 Jan;1(1):1–2

Kohlstedt SG: Science: the struggle for survival, 1880 to 1894. **Science** 1980 Jul 4;209(4452):33–42

König S: Arzt und Medizin in der TIME 1971–1975. Diss. Düsseldorf, 1980. 205 p.

Krosnick A: The history of medical journalism in New Jersey. **J Med Soc NJ** 1984 Sep;81(9):723–6

Krosnick A: We are seventy–five. **J Med Soc NJ** 1979 Nov;76(12):809

Lounsbury JW, Roisum KG, Pokorny L, et al: An analysis of topic areas and topic trends in the Community Mental Health Journal from 1965 through 1977. **Community Ment Health J** 1979 Winter;15(4):267–76

Lovejoy CO, Mensforth RP, Armelagos GJ: Five decades of skeletal biology as reflected in the American Journal of Physical Anthropology. In F. Spencer, ed: A history of American physical anthropology, 1930–1980. New York, Academic Press, 1982. p. 329–36.

Lundberg GD: One medical world. **JAMA** 1983 Jul 8;250(2):242–3

McClary A: 'Swat the Fly': popular magazines and the anti–fly campaign. **Prev Med** 1982 May;11(3):373–8

McLendon WW: The Archives of Pathology and Laboratory Medicine. A new beginning. **Arch Pathol Lab Med** 1984 Jan;108(1):13–4

McLeod DC, Whitney HA: The legacy of Donald E. Francke: DICP––a fifteen–year commitment to clinical pharmacy. **Drug Intell Clin Pharm** 1981 Dec;15(12):990–1

Mazur A: The journalists and technology: reporting about Love Canal and Three Mile Island. **Minerva** 1984 Spring;22(1):45–66

Meiling RL: Reflections in a diamond year. **Ohio State Med J** 1980 Aug;76(8):481–3

Method HL: Doctor Loyal Davis––the editor. **Surg Gynecol Obstet** 1983 Aug;157(2):144–6

Nelson WE: The first 50 years of The Journal of Pediatrics. **J Pediatr** 1982 Jul;101(1):1–4

Newell FW, Blodi FC, Henkind P, et al: In commemoration of 25 years of Survey of Ophthalmology. **Surv Ophthalmol** 1981 May–Jun;25(6):397–403

Newell FW: The first editor––Edward Jackson. **Am J Ophthalmol** 1982 Dec;94(6):809–10

Nuland SB: Ingelfinger rule violated in 1846. **N Engl J Med** 1983 Apr 14;308(15):907

The official publication of the American Association of Physical Anthropologists 1930–1980: Jubilee Issue: **Am J Phys Anthropol** 1981 Dec;56(4):327–557

Parish LC: Amerikanische dermatologische Zeitschriften und die New Yorker Dermatologische Gesellschaft. **Hautarzt** 1981 Mar;32(3):136–8

Park RJ: The research quarterly and its antecedents. **Res Q** 1980 Mar;51(1):1–22

Pearson RW: The Archives of Dermatology: the first hundred years. **Arch Dermatol** 1982 Oct;118(10):699–709

Porter KR, Bennett HS: Introduction: recollections on the beginnings of the Journal of Cell Biology. **J Cell Biol** 1981 Dec;91(3 pt 2):IX–XI

Rák K: Korunk orvosi szakirodalma és a klinikai medicina. **Orv Hetil** 1980 Sep 14;121(37):2243–8

Ramsey FB: January 1982: 75th birthday of the ISMA Journal; history and highlights, Indiana State Medical Association and its journal. **J Indiana State Med Assoc** 1982 Jan;75(1):14–9

Riley RW: A century of editors. **JAMA** 1983 Jul 8;250(2):230–5

Robert I. Watson and the development of the history of psychology: a symposium: With contributions by E. S. Mills, E. R. Hilgard, B. Ross, J. Popplestone, M. W. McPherson, R. B. Evans, E. S. Goodman, J. Brožek. **J Hist Behav Sci** 1982 Oct;18(4):307–31

Roberts WC, Warnes CA: The AJC in December 1958. **Am J Cardiol** 1983 Dec 1;52(10):1355

Robinson RG: JAMA at 100. **NZ Med J** 1983 Aug 24;96(738):654

Rogers FB: The origins of MEDLARS. In Stevenson LG, ed: A celebration of medical history. Baltimore, Johns Hopkins University Press, 1982. p. 77–84.

Scheinman MM: The AJC in September 1959. **Am J Cardiol** 1984 Sep 1;54(6):702–3

Sebrell WH: Reflections on Nutrition Reviews from a clinical investigator. **Nutr Rev** 1982 Nov;40(11):326–8

Selections from Public health: reports and papers presented at meetings of the American Public Health Association (1884–1907). New York, Arno, 1977. Various paginations.:

Selections from Public health: reports and papers presented at the meetings of the American Public Health Association (1873–1883). New York, Arno, 1977. Various paginations.:

Selections from the Journal of the Massachusetts Association of Boards of Health (1891–1904). New York, Arno, 1977. Various paginations.:

Shultz SM, Wood MS: Medical journals of Pennsylvania before the Civil War. **Trans Stud Coll Physicians Phila** 1983 Sep;5(5 No 3):244–70

Sokal MM: Science and James McKeen Cattell, 1894 to 1945. **Science** 1980 Jul 4;209(4452):43–52

Spady JG: Dr. W. Montague Cobb: anatomist, physician, physical anthropologist, editor emeritus of the Journal of the National Medical Association, and first black president of NAACP. **J Natl Med Assoc** 1984 Jul;76(7):739–44

Stare FJ: Forty years of Nutrition Reviews. **Nutr Rev** 1982 Nov;40(11):321–5

Stevenson LG: The newest of old journals. **Bull Hist Med** 1980 Spring;54(1):1–3

Taylor ES: Commemorative issue: Georgeanna Seegar Jones, Howard W. Jones, Jr. Twenty–five years as editors–in–chief for Gynecology, Obstetrical & Gynecological Survey. **Obstet Gynecol Surv** 1982 Jun;37(6):355–84

Taylor JS: The Cleveland Clinic Quarterly: the first fifty years. **Cleve Clin Q** 1982 Winter;49(4):149–58

Tomes N: Mary May Roberts. In: Notable American women. The modern period. Cambridge, Mass., Belknap–Harvard Univ. Press, 1980. 4:581–3.

Tuchman LR: The Mount Sinai Journal: past. **Mt Sinai J Med (NY)** 1984 Jan–Feb;51(1):i–iv

Walsh J: Science in transition, 1946 to 1962. **Science** 1980 Jul 4;209(4452):52–7

Waserman M, Clausen C, ed: Bulletin of the History of Medicine. Index to volumes and supplements, 1933–1982. Baltimore, Johns Hopkins University Press, 1983. 195 p.

Watson WG: Dentofacial orthopedics: fifty years of concern. **Am J Orthod** 1981 Nov;80(5):561–3

Watson WG: The journal––a record of professional transition and progress. **Am J Orthod** 1981 Feb;79(2):219–22

Waugh ES, McGoldrick KE: On the history of JAMWA. **J Am Med Wom Assoc** 1980 Jun;35(6):137–9

When 'more doctors smoked Camels': Cigarette advertising in the Journal. **NY State J Med** 1983 Dec;83(13):1347–52

Wilkins RH: Birth of a journal: the origin and early years of Neurosurgery. **Neurosurgery** 1982 Jun;10(6 Pt 2):820–6

## PERIODICALS

Wilson CE: The Boston inoculation controversy: a revisionist interpretation. **Journalism Hist** 1980;7(1):16–9, 40
Wilson LG: Dorothy Schullian retires from the Journal. **J Hist Med Allied Sci** 1984 Oct;39(4):457–61
Wilson LG: Measure in everything: a decade of the journal. **J Hist Med Allied Sci** 1982 Oct;37(4):393–8
Wolfle D: Science: a memoir of the 1960's and 1970's. **Science** 1980 Jul 4;209(4452):57–60

**USSR**

Akopov VI, Akopov AI: Iz istorii otechestvennykh sudebno-meditsinskikh zhurnalov. **Sud Med Ekspert** 1982 Jan–Mar;25(1):53–5
Anokhin VN: K 20-letiiu zhurnala 'Voprosy revmatizma'. **Vopr Revm** 1981 Apr–Jun;(2):3–4
Arkhangel'skiĭ GA: N. A. Belogolovyĭ--obshchestvennyĭ vrach, zhurnalist (k 150-letiiu so dnia rozhdeniia). **Sov Zdravookhr** 1984;(10):67–70
Bachev VI: Mestnaia periodicheskaia pechat' kak istoriko-meditsinkiĭ istochnik. **Sov Zdravookhr** 1981;(6):56–8
Baĭsogolov GD: Rol' zhurnala 'Meditsinskaia Radiologiia' v razvitii luchevoĭ terapii v SSSR. **Med Radiol (Mosk)** 1982 Apr;27(4):3–6
Bazanov VA: Zhurnal 'Vrach' kak istochnik izucheniia Russko-Nemetskikh meditsinskikh sviazeĭ. **Sov Zdravookhr** 1983;(4):60–3
Belozerov VV, Galin LL: Zhurnal dlia ranenykh i bol'nykh krasnoarmeĭtsev. **Voen Med Zh** 1984 Apr;(4):65–9
Borich I: O zhurnale 'Meditsinskaia sestra'. **Med Sestra** 1982 Aug;41(8):42–4
Estrin GB: Voprosy khirurgii i travmatologii v zhurnale 'Vrach' V. A. Manasseina (1880–1901 gg.). **Vestn Khir** 1981 Oct;127(10):142–4
Filimonov AR: Pervyi tom zhurnala 'Vestnik oftal'mologii: (1884 g.). **Vestn Oftalmol** 1984 Jul–Aug;(4):5–7
Filimonov AR: 'Vestnik oftal'mologii' 50 let nazad. **Vestn Oftalmol** 1984 Nov–Dec;(6):6–8
Filimonov AR: 'Vestnik oftal'mologii' 75 let nazad. **Vestn Oftalmol** 1984 Sep–Oct;(5):7–8
Galin LL: Deiatel'nost' voenno-sanitarnoĭ sluzhby v gody Velikoĭ Otechestvennoĭ voĭny (po materialam 'Voenno-meditsinskogo zhurnala'). **Sov Zdravookhr** 1984;(5):58–61
Galin LL: Publikatsii N. I. Pirogova na stranitsakh 'Voenno--meditsinskogo zhurnala. **Voen Med Zh** 1980 Nov;(11):69–71
Galin LL, Pal'chikov PA: Vklad 'Voenno-Meditsinskogo Zhurnala' v razvitie voennoĭ meditsiny. **Sov Zdravookhr** 1983;(2):63–7
Granat NE: Zhurnal 'Akusherka' (po stranitsam starinnogo zhurnala). **Feldsher Akush** 1983;48(4):58–60
Gurevich SA: Aktual'nye problemy psikhiatrii v 'Vestnike klinicheskoĭ i sudebnoĭ psikhiatrii i nevropatologii' (k 100-letiiu osnovaniia otechestvennoĭ psikhiatricheskoĭ periodiki). **Zh Nevropatol Psikhiatr** 1983;83(8):1236–40
Iarmonenko SP: Klinicheskaia radiobiologiia--nauchnaia osnova luchevoĭ terapii opukholeĭ. **Med Radiol (Mosk)** 1982 Mar;27(3):6–9
K 80-letiiu zhurnala nevropatologii i psikhiatrii im. S. S. Korsakova: **Zh Nevropatol Psikhiatr** 1981;81(1):3–5
Kharshak EM: Nauchnaia deiatel'nost' oblastnykh obshchestv otolaringologov v USSR za period 1957–1978 gg. (po protokolam i godovym otchetam obshchestv, opublikovannym v ZhUNGB s 1959 po 1978 g.). **Zh Ushn Nos Gorl Bolezn** 1980 May–Jun;(3):56–64
'Klinicheskoĭ meditsine' 60 let!: **Klin Med (Mosk)** 1980 Aug;58(8):4–6
Krasnov MM: Proshloe v nastoiashchem: Adrian Aleksandrovich Kriukov, redaktor 'Vestnika oftal'mologii' i osnovatel' Moskovskogo oftal'mologicheskogo veshchestva (k 75-letiiu zhurnala). **Vestn Oftalmol** 1984 Nov–Dec;(6):4–6
Lindenbraten LD: Voprosy prepodavaniia i podgotovki kadrov po rentgenologii i radiologii na stranitsakh zhurnala 'Meditsinskaia Radiologiia' (1956–1981). **Med Radiol (Mosk)** 1981;26(10):49–53
Magil'nitskiĭ SG: 'Vestniku oftal'mologii' - 100 let. **Vestn Oftalmol** 1984 May–Jun;(3):3–7
Mikhaĭlov VP: Zhurnal Rudneva (poluzabytaia glava v istorii otechestvennoĭ gistologii). **Arkh Anat Gistol Embriol** 1980 Feb;78(2):104–15
Morogues IM de: N. S. Leskov: premieres polemiques. janvier 1860–mai 1862. **Cah Monde Russe Sovietique** 1982;23(2):243–55
Petrovskiĭ KS, Novikov IV: Zhurnalu 'Gigiena i sanitariia' 60 let. **Gig Sanit** 1982 Aug;(8):4–7
Petrowskij KS, Novikov JV: 60 Jahre 'Gigiena i sanitarija'. **Z Gesamte Hyg** 1983 Sep;29(9):564–5
Piatak OA, Perekhrestenko PM, Semenova NA: 120 let meditsinskoĭ periodicheskoĭ pechati na Ukraine. **Vrach Delo** 1980 Oct;(10):1–5
Shabunin AV: Vklad zhurnala 'Khirurgicheskiĭ vestnik' v razvitie khirurgicheskoĭ mysli v Rossii. **Vestn Khir** 1984 Aug;133(8):146–7
Shalimov AA, Khokholia VP: Zhurnalu 'Klinicheskaia khirurgiia' 60 let. **Klin Khir** 1981 Jun;(6):1–6
Shul'tsev GP: Vnutrennie bolezni v 'Klinicheskoĭ meditsine' za 1970–1979 gg. (obzor materialov.). **Klin Med (Mosk)** 1980 Aug;58(8):112–6
Vasil'ev KK: K istorii zhurnala 'Gigiena i sanitariia'. **Gig Sanit** 1982 Sep;(9):51–2
Veterany Velikoĭ Otechestvennoĭ voĭny za 'kruglym stolom' redaktsii 'Voenno-medistinskogo zhurnala': **Voen Med Zh** 1980 May;(5):14–20
Volkov VV, Danilichev VF: Professor A.V. Khodin - osnovatel' i pervyĭ redaktor-izdatel' 'Vestnika oftal'mologii' (k 100-letiiu zhurnala). **Vestn Oftalmol** 1984 Nov–Dec;(6):3–4
Winter I: Die Zeitschrift 'Russische Medicinische Rundschau' als Mittlerin zwischen deutscher und russischer Medizin. **Z Gesamte Hyg** 1980;26(5):379–80
Zhukova LA: Periodicheskaia pechat' o geroizme sovetskikh medikov v gody Velikoĭ Otechestvennoĭ voĭny. **Voen Med Zh** 1984 Oct;(10):10–2
Zhurnalu 'Antibiotiki' chetvert' veka: **Antibiotiki** 1981;26(8):564–6
Zhurnalu 'Grudnaia khirurgiia' 20 let.: **Grudn Khir** 1980 Jan–Feb;(1):5–6
Zhurnalu 'Patologicheskaia fiziologiia i éksperimental'naia terapiia' 25 let: **Patol Fiziol Eksp Ter** 1982 Jul–Aug;(4):3–10
Zhurnalu 'Uspekhi sovremennoĭ biologii'--50 let:
Zhurnalu 40 let: **Sov Zdravookhr** 1982;(6):3–7
40 let nashemu zhunalu: **Med Sestra** 1982 Aug;41(8):9–12
60 Let deiatel'nosti zhurnala 'Akusherstvio i ginekologiia': **Akush Ginekol (Mosk)** 1982;(12):16–7
[80th anniversary of the 'Zhurnal Nevropatologii i Psikhiatrii im. S. S. Korsakov'] (Rus): **Zh Nevropatol Psikhiatr** 1981;81(1):3–5

**Venezuela**

Canelón JS: Dos artículos odontológicos en la 'Gaceta Cientifica de Venezuela' de 1877. **Acta Odontol Venez** 1980 Jan–Apr;18(1):87–95
Febres-Cordero F: Publicaciones periodicas odontologicas de Venezuela. **Acta Odontol Venez** 1983;21(2):129–47; 21(3):237–59
Saturno Canelón J: Dos articulos odontologicos en la Gaceta Cientifica de Venezuela de 1877. **Acta Odontol Venez** 1980 Jan–Apr;18(1):87–95

**Yugoslavia**

Belicza B: Liječnička udruženja i razvoj medicinske periodike s posebnim osvrtom na 'Liječnički vjesnik' Glasilo Zbora liječnika Hrvatske (1877–1977). **Saopcenja** 1978;21(1–2):133–56
Cetrdeset godina Vojnosanitetskog pregleda: **Vojnosanit Pregl** 1984 Sep–Oct;41(5):315–9
Dragić M: Povodom stogodišnjice osnivanja časopisa 'Zdravlje' dr Milana Jovanović-Batuta. **Srp Arh Celok Lek** 1980 Apr;108(4):391–5
Dugački V: 'Hrvatsko društvo za čuvanje narodnog zdravlja' i njegov časopis 'Zivot i zdravlje'. **Lijec Vjesn** 1982 May;104(5):208–10
Katan E: Stručne publikacije sanitetske službe NOVJ izdavane pre Vojnosanitetskog pregleda. **Vojnosanit Pregl** 1984 Sep–Oct;41(5):424–30
Kolbas V: Marginalije u povodu dvadeset pete godišnjice 'Arhiva za zaštitu majke i djeteta'. **Lijec Vjesn** 1983 Jul–Aug;105(7–8):315–8
Novak Z: 30 godina 'Neuropsyhijatrije' i 'Neurologije'. **Neurologija** 1983;31(1–2):7–9

## PHARMACOLOGY

See also **Chemistry and Biochemistry; Drugs and Chemicals; Pharmacy**

Ackerknecht EH: Zur Geschichte der Krebsbehandlung. **Gesnerus** 1980;37(3/4):189–97
Boussel P, Bonnemain H, Bove FJ: Histoire de la pharmacie et de l'Industrie pharmaceutique. Paris, Editions de la Porte Verte, 1982. 287 p.
Bowman WC: Drugs ancient and modern. **Scott Med J** 1979 Apr;24(2):131–40
Estes JW: Making therapeutic decisions with protopharmacologic evidence. **Trans Stud Coll Physicians Phila** 1979 Jun;5(1 no 2):116–37
Galzigna L, Galzigna M: La produzione del corpo curabile. **Acta Med Hist Patav** 1982–83;29:29–65
Hamel P: Le remède et l'apparence. Plan de la Tour, Editions d'aujourd'hui, 1981. 128 p.
Holmstedt B, Bruhn JG: Ethnopharmacology--a challenge. **J Ethnopharmacol** 1983 Sep;8(3):251–6
Karger-Decker B: Kräuter, Pillen, Präparate: Abenteuer der Arzneimittelforschung. Leipzig, Koehler & Amelang, 1981. 313 p.
Valette G: Auto-expérimentation en pharmacologie. **Bull Ordre Natl Pharm** 1978 Dec;217;1609–30

**China**

Griffin RJ: Herbal medicine revisited: science looks anew at ancient Chinese pharmacology. **Am Pharm** 1979 Sep;19(10):16–22
Porkert M: Sens et non-sens des recherches modernes sur la pharmacopée traditionnelle de la Chine. In Mazars G, ed: Les médecines traditionnelles de l'Asie. Strasbourg, Université Louis Pasteur, 1981. p. 49–56.

**Hungary**

Fleishmann-Bánó M, Zalai K: St. Cosmas and St. Damian relics in Hungary. **Ther Hung** 1981;29(3):142–6

**India**

Nand Raj L: Human experimentation of Drugs. **Bull Indian Inst Hist Med (Hyderabad)** 1980;10(1–4):53–61

**Mexico**

Díaz JL: Ethnopharmacology and taxonomy of Mexican psychodysleptic plants. **J Psychedelic Drugs** 1979 Jan-Jun;11(1-2):71-101

**Spain**

Esplugues J: Tradición farmacológica valenciana: sus momentos estelares. Valencia, Real Academia de Medicina de Valencia, 1975. 71 p.

**Before 500 A.D.**

**Egypt**

Valette S: Die Pharmakologie im alten Agypten. In Sournia JC, Martiny M, Poulet J, ed: Illustrierte Geschichte der Medizin. Salzburg, Andreas, 1980. Vol. 2. p. 479-95.

**Greco-Roman**

Valette G: Die Pharmakologie bei den Griechen und Römern. In Sournia JC, Martiny M, Poulet J, ed: Illustrierte Geschichte der Medizin. Salzburg, Andreas, 1980. Vol. 2. p. 496-521.

**500 A.D.-1450**

**Arabic**

Denisenko PP, Nuraliev IuN: Abu Ali Ibn-Sina i farmakologiia; k 1000 letiiu so dnia rozhdeniia Avitsenny. **Farmakol Toksikol** 1980 Nov-Dec;43(6):753-4

Habib KM: Pharmacology and materiae medicae in the medical formulary of Al-Kindi. **Hamdard** 1981;24(1-2):92-101

**1450-1700**

**Italy**

Peruzzi E: Un trattato inedito di farmacologia di Gerolamo Fracastoro. **Rinascimento** 1978;18:183-228

**1700 to Present**

Ahlquist RP: Historical perspective. Classification of adrenoreceptors. **J Auton Pharmacol** 1980 Nov;1(1):101-6

Alvares AP: Cytochrome P-450s: research highlights of the last two decades. **Drug Metab Rev** 1981;12(2):431-6

Archer S: Historical perspective on the chemistry and development of naltrexone. **Natl Inst Drug Abuse Res Monogr Ser** 1981;28:3-10

Beaver WT: Analgesic development: a brief history and perspective. **J Clin Pharmacol** 1980 Apr;20(4 Pt 2):213-5

Berghaus A: Die Entwicklung der Methoden zur physiologischen Wertbestimmung von Digitalispräparaten. Husum, Matthiesen, 1982. 135 p. (Abhandlungen zur Geschichte der Medizin und der Naturwissenschaften, 42).

Bindra JS, Lednicer D, ed: Chronicles of drug discovery. Volume 1. New York, John Wiley & Sons, 1982. xiii, 283 p.

Boura AL, Green AF: Noradrenergic neurone blocking agents. **J Auton Pharmacol** 1981 Jun;1(3):255-67

Chen KK: Two pharmacological traditions: notes from experience. **Annu Rev Pharmacol Toxicol** 1981;21:1-6

De Meyts P, Rousseau GG: Receptor concepts. A century of evolution. **Circ Res** 1980 Jun;46(6 Pt 2):13-9

Deniker P: Psychopharmacologie et psychiatrie biologique rappel historique. **Soins Psychiatr** 1983 Nov;(37):5-6

Dorkins HR: Suxamethonium--the development of a modern drug from 1906 to the present day. **Med Hist** 1982 Apr;26(2):145-68

Estes JW: The protopharmacological basis of therapeutics. **Pharmacologist** 1984;26(1):25-30

Farnsworth N: Sobre la preparacion de extractos de plantas para su evaluacion farmacologica en animales. **Med Tradic** 1982;3(11):27-33

Fifty years of chemotherapy: **Endeavour** 1982;6(4):145

Garner J: Burroughs and Wellcome: American architects of a British empire. **Can Pharm J** 1980 Dec;:417-9

Gielen JE, Laduron P, Lapière CM: Receptors in classical pharmacology and cell biology. A report of a symposium held on the occasion of the 25th anniversary of the first publication of Biochemical Pharmacology. **Biochem Pharmacol** 1983 Dec 15;32(24):3891-2

Green AF: The discovery of bretylium and bethanidine. **Br J Clin Pharmacol** 1982 Jan;13(1):25-34

Hahn FE: Virus chemotherapy: the problem, its development and nature. In Hahn FE, ed: Virus chemotherapy. Basel, New York, Karger, 1980. p. 1-21. (Antibiotics and chemotherapy, v. 27).

Helfand WH, Cowen DL: Evolution of a revolutionary oral dosage form. **Pharm Int** 1982 Dec;3(12):393-5

Hinshaw HC: The dawn of chemotherapy of tuberculosis. **Indian J Chest Dis Allied Sci** 1982 Apr-Sep;24(2-3):179-83

Isaac O, Kristen G: Alte und neue Wege der Kamillentherapie. Die Kamille als Beispiel für moderne Arzneipflanzenforschung. **Med Welt** 1980 Aug 8;31(31-32):1145-9

Kanai O: [Chemotherapy for tuberculosis--experimental studies over the past 100 years. (1) Development of chemotherapy] (Jpn) **Kekkaku** 1982 Dec;57(12):643-51

Kelwala S, Stanley M, Gershon S: History of antidepressants: successes and failures. **J Clin Psychiatry** 1983 May;44(5 Pt 2):40-8

Kempler K: A kemoterápia haladása napjainkig. **Orv Hetil** 1982 Apr 4;123(14):861-4

Kotwas J, Meyer-Wilmes J, Ohlendorf D, ed: Pharmazie und Medizin--Grenzen und Möglichkeiten. Verhandlungsbericht über eine Internationale Tagung der Arbeitsgemeinschaft Deutscher Krankenhausapotheker in Zusammenarbeit mit der Bayerischen Internistenvereinigung München, 18.-19.April 1980. Berlin, Acron, 1981. 152 p. Contributions by R. Winau, D. Ohlendorf, A.G. Hildebrandt, W. Weissauer, R. Quintiliani, D.D. Breimer, R. Preisig, T. Zysset, D. Adam, H. Remmer, G. Dirheimer, K.H. Beyer, H.P.T. Ammon.

Kramer JC: The opiates: two centuries of scientific study. **J Psychedelic Drugs** 1980 Apr-Jun;12(2):89-103

Maddox VH: The discovery of phencyclidine [proceedings]. **Psychopharmacol Bull** 1980 Oct;16(4):53-4

Marks V: Therapeutic drug monitoring: an historical introduction. **Am J Med Technol** 1983 Aug;49(8):543-8

Maxwell RA: Guanethidine after twenty years: a pharmacologist's perspective. **Br J Clin Pharmacol** 1982 Jan;13(1):35-44

Moriarty KM, Alagna SW, Lake CR: Psychopharmacology. An historical perspective. **Psychiatr Clin North Am** 1984 Sep;7(3):411-33

Oehme P: Entwicklungstendenzen der Arzneimittelforschung. **Z Gesamte Inn Med** 1980 Jul 15;35(14):20-5

Parascandola J: Reflections on the history of pharmacology **Pharm Hist** 1980;22(4):131-40

Parascandola J: The search for the active oxytocic principle of ergot: laboratory science and clinical medicine in conflict. In Hickel E, Schröder G, ed: Neue Beiträge zur Arzneimittelgeschichte. Festschrift für Wolfgang Schneider zum 70. Geburtstag. Stuttgart, Wissenschaftliche Verlagsgesellschaft, 1982. p. 205-27.

Parascandola J, ed: The history of antibiotics. Madison, Wis., 1980. vi, 136 p. (Publication/American Institute of the History of Pharmacy. new series, no. 5)

Płaźnik A, Kostowski W, Puciłowski O: Historia i postepy współczesnej psychofarmakologii. **Pol Tyg Lek** 1983 Dec 19-26;38(51-52):1633-7

Pulewka P: Seit 56 Jahren Arzt und Forscher. **Ther Ggw** 1980;119:216-28

Ruckebusch Y: An historical profile of veterinary pharmacology and therapeutics. **J Vet Pharmacol Ther** 1982 Mar;5(1):1-20

Schicke RK: Sozialpharmakologie, makrosystemische Aspekte. **Fortschr Med** 1982 May 13;100(18):823-4, 845

Sepúlveda B: Nuevas orientaciones de la medicina: los receptores celulares en terapéutica. I. Introducción. **Gac Med Mex** 1981 Dec;117(12):463-5

Smith DB, Delgado Escueta AV, Cramer JA, et al: Historical perspective on the choice of antiepileptic drugs for the treatment of seizures in adults. **Neurology** 1983 Mar;33(3 Suppl 1):2-7

Van der Kloot W: Otto Loewi. In Dictionary of American biography, 1961-1965. Suppl. 7, 1981. p. 475-7.

Van Noordwijk J: Farmacologie, een erkende wetenschap. **Ned Tijdschr Geneeskd** 1983 Jul 9;127(28):1230-2

Wagner JG: History of pharmacokinetics. **Pharmacol Ther** 1981;12(3):537-62

Zubrod CG: The cure of cancer by chemotherapy - reflections on how it happened. (The fifth Myron Karon Memorial Lecture). **Med Pediatr Oncol** 1980;8:107-14

**Austria**

Brandl E, Spitzy KH: Chemotherapie in Osterreich. Geschichte und Ausblick. **Wien Med Wochenschr** 1983;133 Suppl 1:3-10

Schweppe KW, Probst C: Die Versuche zur medikamentösen Karzinomtherapie des Anton Störck (1731 bis 1803). Ein Beitrag zur Geschichte der experimentellen Arzneimittelforschung in der älteren Wiener medizinischen Schule. In Ganzinger K, Skopec M, Wyklicky H, ed. Festschrift für Erna Lesky zum 70. Geburtstag. Wien, Brüder Hollinek, 1981. p. 105-22.

Schweppe KW, Probst C: Die Versuche zur medikamentösen Karzinomtherapie des Anton Störck (1731-1803). Ein Beitrag zur Geschichte der experimentellen Arzneimittelforschung in der älteren Wiener medizinischen Schule. **Wien Med Wochenschr** 1982 Mar 15;132(5):107-17

**Bulgaria**

Furnadzhiev G: Razvitie i segashno sŭstoianie na Katedrata p farmakologiia i fitoterapiia. **Vutr Boles** 1981;20(6):22-6

**Czechoslovakia**

Kratochvíl L, Lustig M: K historii tzv. Batemanovy funkce. **Cesk Farm** 1984 Jun;33(5):210-2

# PHARMACOLOGY

**Finland**

Järnefelt J: P. E. Simola ja sitruunahappokierto. **Duodecim** 1981;97(13):928–30

**France**

Bonnemain H: François Magendie et ses perspectives pharmacologiques. **Hist Sci Med** 1983;17(4):333–43

Colard A: Evocation du passé: propos d'un vieux médecin sur la thérapeutique. **Rev Med Brux** 1983 May;4(5):391–3

Lesch JE: Science and medicine in France: the emergence of experimental physiology, 1790–1855. Cambridge, Mass., Harvard University Press, 1984. viii, 276 p.

Nica-Udangiu S: J. Moreau de Tours (1804–1884). **Rev Med Interna [Neurol Psihiatr]** 1984 Jan–Mar;29(1):77–80

**Germany**

Bäumler E: Paul Ehrlich, Forscher für das Leben. Frankfurt, Societäts-Verlag, 1979. 370 p.

Bendiner E: Ehrlich: immunologist, chemotherapist, prophet. **Hum Dev** 1980 Nov;15(11):129, 133, 138–9 passim

Benedum J: Vom Giessener pharmakologischen Institut unter Rudolf Buchheim und Karl Gaehtgens (1867–1898). **Medizinhist J** 1980;15(1/2):103–19

Burkhardt R, Kienle G: Controlled clinical trials and drug regulations: a report of recent developments in the Federal Republic of Germany. **Controlled Clin Trials** 1980 Sep;1(2):153–66

Kempler K: Az alkaloida-kutatás kezdetei. **Orv Hetil** 1983 Jul 24;124(30):1821–5

Ledermann F: La thérapeutique médicamenteuse et la psychiatrie allemande du XIXe siècle: concordances, oppositions, indifférence? **Gesnerus** 1982;39(3–4):451–67

Mothes K: Pharmakognosie--gestern, heute, morgen. **Pharmazie** 1981 Mar;36(3):174–8

Thorburn AL: Paul Ehrlich: pioneer of chemotherapy and cure by arsenic (1854–1915). **Br J Vener Dis** 1983 Dec;59(6):404–5

Vom Germanin zum Acylureidopenicillin.: Forschung die Geschichte machte. Dokumentation einer wissenschaftlichen Revolution. Leverkusen, Bayer AG, 1980. 77 p.

**Great Britain**

Breathnach CS: Biographical sketches No. 27--Ringer. **Ir Med J** 1983 Mar;76(3):119

Bülbring E, Walker JM: Joshua Harold Burn: 6 March 1892–13 July 1981. **Biogr Mem Fellows R Soc** 1984;30:45–89

Drury VW: Foxglove and chips. **J R Coll Gen Pract** 1984 Mar;34(260):129–39

Feldberg W: Sir Henry Hallett Dale. In Dictionary of national biography, 1961–1970. Suppl. 8, 1981. p. 262–5.

Feldberg W: Sir John Henry Gaddum. In Dictionary of national biography, 1961–1970. Suppl. 8, 1981. p. 412–3.

Fye WB: Sydney Ringer, calcium, and cardiac function. **Circulation** 1984 Apr;69(4):849–53

Johnson AW, Rose FL, Suckling CW: Alfred Spinks: 25 February 1917–11 February 1982. **Biogr Mem Fellows R Soc** 1984;30:567–94

Parascandola J: Chemistry and pharmacology in Britain 1840–1916. **Pharm Hist (London)** 1976 May;6(1):2

Pickford M: Ernest Basil Verney. In Dictionary of national biography, 1961–1970. Suppl. 8, 1981. p. 1035.

Shellard EJ: Some early women research workers in British pharmacy 1886–1912. **Pharm Hist (London)** 1982 Aug;12(2):2–3

Siegel S: Wilkie Collins: Victorian novelist as psychopharmacologist. **J Hist Med Allied Sci** 1983 Apr;38(2):161–75

Vane JR: The Wellcome centenary. Henry S. Wellcome, his research philosophy and current excitements. **Trans Med Soc Lond** 1980–81;97:41–50

West R: An excursion into pharmacology: curare in medicine. **Med Hist** 1984 Oct;28(4):391–405

Young FG: Alastair Campbell Frazer. In Dictionary of national biography, 1961–1970. Suppl. 8, 1981. p. 397–8.

**India**

Ramalingaswami V, Satyavati GV: Sir Ram Nath Chopra. **Indian J Med Res** 1982 Dec;76 Suppl:V–VI

**Italy**

Montorsi W, Pezzuoli G, Guzzon V: Influenza della farmacologia di Emilio Trabucchi nelle discipline chirurgiche e parachirurgiche. **Minerva Med** 1982 May 7;73(19):1255–68

**Mexico**

Sánchez Reséndiz J, et al: Investigaciones mexicans recientés sobre las propriedades medicinalesd del yumel (guatteria gaumeri). **Med Tradic** 1980;3(9):19–27

**Netherlands**

Miert AS van: Van Materia Medica tot rationele farmacotherapie. **Tijdschr Diergeneeskd** 1984 Jan 1;109(1):3–11

Van Ree JM: Nederlandse Farmacologie. I. Bouwstenen van de geneesmiddelentherapie: verantwoording. **Ned Tijdschr Geneeskd** 1983 Jul 9;127(28):1229–30

Wit JG: Institute of Veterinary Pharmacology, Pharmacy, and Toxicology: its research (1961–1980). **Tijdschr Diergeneeskd** 1981 Oct;106(20):suppl 3:169–75

**Poland**

Hołyński J: Wytwórczość przedprzemysłowa chemikaliów i środków leczniczych na przełomie XIX i XX wieku w Lodzi i regionie. **Arch Hist Med (Warsz)** 1983;46(3):273–84

Roeske W: Antonina Leśniewska, 1866–1937. [Warszawa], Zarzad Główny Polskiego Towarzystwa Farmaceutycznego, 1970. 26 p.

**Romania**

Eşanu V: Research in the field of antiviral chemotherapy performed in the 'Stefan S. Nicolau' Institute of Virology. **Virologie** 1984 Oct–Dec;35(4):281–93

Negru I: Prof. dr. Nicolae Gh. Lupu în lumina autobiografică şi a istoriei medicinii româneşti. **Viata Med [Medii Sanit]** 1983 Feb;31(2):45–7

**Singapore**

Teo SK, Chew CH: Tuberculosis chemotherapy--developments in Singapore from 1957–1982. **Ann Acad Med Singapore** 1982 Jul;11(3):366–9

**Sweden**

Ottoson D: Ulf von Euler. Tre milstolpar inom medicinen: substans P, prostaglandin och noradrenalin. **Lakartidningen** 1983 Apr 13;80(15):1579–82

Uvnäs B: From physiologist to pharmacologist--promotion or degradation? Fifty years in retrospect. **Annu Rev Pharmacol Toxicol** 1984;24:1–18

**Switzerland**

Klingler M: A glimpse into Roche research: antiparkinson treatment. **Int J Clin Pharmacol Ther Toxicol** 1982 Apr;20(4):190–3

**Turkey**

Pulewka P: Neunzehn Jahre als Pharmakologe in der Türkei. **Ther Ggw** 1980 Feb;119(2):199–211

**United States**

Bearman D: The Alfred Newton Richards papers. **Surv Sources Newsl** 1975 Nov;1(1):9–10

Becker RA: The John Jacob Abel papers--primary sources for the history of American pharmacology. **Pharm Hist** 1982;24(3):115–6

Farrar GE: Advances in pharmacology--the golden age of therapeutics. **Penn Med** 1983 Dec;86(12):48–9

Govier WM: A helminthic tale. **Perspect Biol Med** 1984 Autumn;28(1):104–6

Gross EG, Long JP: Pharmacology at Iowa 1920–1980. **Life Sci** 1980 Dec 22–29;27(25–26):2423–6

Keys TE: Chauncey Depew Leake, 1896–1978: an appreciation. **J Hist Med Allied Sci** 1978 Jul;33(3):428–31

Krantz JC: Recollections: a medical scientist remembers. Baltimore, Schneidereith, 1978. xvi, 185 p.

Lepow IH: Louis Pillemer, Properdin, and scientific controversy. **J Immunol** 1980 Aug;125(2):471–5

Miller RR: History of clinical pharmacy and clinical pharmacology. **J Clin Pharmacol** 1981 Apr;21(4):195–7

Page IH: The discovery of serotonin. **Perspect Biol Med** 1976 Autumn;20(1):1–8

Parascandola J, Swann J: Development of Pharmacology in American Schools of Pharmacy. **Pharm Hist** 1983;25(3):95–115

Parascandola J: John J. Abel and the early development of pharmacology at the Johns Hopkins University. **Bull Hist Med** 1982;56(4):512–27

Parascandola J: John J. Abel and the founding of ASPET. **Pharmacologist** 1984;26(1):37–40

Parascandola J, Keeney E: Sources in the history of American pharmacology. Madision, American Institute of the History of Pharmacy,

1983. 59 p.

Stork G: Samuel Marion McElvain: December 9, 1897–April 11, 1973. **Biogr Mem Natl Acad Sci** 1983;54:221–48

Swain HH: G & G: the textbook which structured American pharmacology. **Pharmacologist** 1984;26(1):41–4

Tang LC: A personal and scientific biography of Dr. George C. Cotzias. **Neurotoxicology (Park Forest Il)** 1984 Spring;5(1):5–12

Welsh JS: The trial pharmacist. **Am Pharm** 19(5):16–7, 33, May 79

Zubrod CG: Origins and development of chemotherapy research at the National Cancer Institute. **Cancer Treat Rep** 1984 Jan;68(1):9–19

### USSR

Dagurov VG: Razvitie farmakologii v Moskovskom universitete vo vtoroĭ polovine XIX veka. **Farmakol Toksikol** 1983 Jan–Feb;46(1):92–8

Dagurov VG, Miazdrikova AA: Stanovlenie farmakologii v Moskovskom universitete. **Farmakol Toksikol** 1981 Nov–Dec;;44(6):733–7

Fisher JW: The influence of Dorpat on modern pharmacology. **Pharmacologist** 1984;26(1):31–6

Guseĭnov DIa, Guseĭnova ZN: Razvitie farmakologii v Azerbaĭdzhane (k 60–letiiu Azerbaidzhanskoi SSR). **Farmakol Toksikol** 1980 Jul–AUg;43(4):443–5

Ianushkevichus ZI: Razvitie ideĭ i rabot S. P. Botkina i ego shkoly v kardiologii i klinicheskoĭ farmakologii. **Vestn Akad Med Nauk SSSR** 1983;(3):14–7

Jack DB: Dastardly deeds at Dorpat. **Pharm Hist (London)** 1984 Sep;14(3):9–12

Laties VG: I. V. Zavadskii and the beginnings of behavioral pharmacology: an historical note and translation. **J Exp Anal Behav** 1979 Nov;32(3):463–72

Perevodchikova NI, Garin AM: Osnovnye étapy razvitiia klinicheskoĭ khimioterapii opukholeĭ v SSSR. **Vopr Onkol** 1982;28(5):31–8

Vklad farmakologov soiuznykh respublik v razvitie otechestvennoĭ farmakologii: **Farmakol Toksikol** 1982 Nov–Dec;45(6):5–13

Voronov IB, Zeimal EV: Obituary: Professor M. J. Michelson (died 16 August 1978). The contribution of Professor M. J. Michelson to comparative and evolutionary pharmacology. **Comp Biochem Physiol** 1979;62C(1):1–4

Zakusov VV: Farmakologiia v Akademii meditsinskikh nauk SSSR. **Farmakol Toksikol** 1984 Jan–Feb;47(1):5–13

## PHARMACY

See also **Chemistry and Biochemistry; Drugs and Chemicals; Pharmacology**

Adly A, ed: The history of medicinal and aromatic plants. Proceedings of the Second International Congress organised by The Arab Society for the History of Pharmacy in co-operation with The World Union of Societies of the History of Pharmacy, Alexandria - Egypt, December 15th to 19th, 1980. Karachi, Hamdard Foundation Press, 1982. 216 p.

Barcs–Masson ML: Les femmes et la pharmacie. Nice, Belisane, 1977. 149 p.

Bartels K: Apotheker–Dienstbriefe. In Dilg P, et al., ed: Perspektiven der Pharmaziegeschichte. Graz, Austria, Akademische Druck- u. Verlagsanstalt, 1983. p. 1–12.

Berges P: Grenzen sollte man vergessen. [S.l., s.n., 1981?] 32 p.

Berges PH: Mäusedreck für Pfeifer... Der Apotheker und die Substitution. Ein kleines Mosaik. **Dtsch Apoth Ztg** 1981 Jan 8;121(2):53–9

Berges PH, ed: Internationaler Kongress für Geschichte der Pharmazie in Basel/Lausanne, vom 13. bis 19. Juni 1979. [Summary of events plus abstracts of papers] Sonderdruck aus: Deutsche Apotheker Zeitung 119 (1979): 973–976, 1081–1084, 1133–1138, 1170–1173.

Bonnemain H: La Société d'Histoire de la Pharmacie; sa création - son développement - ses activités. In: Vorträge des Internationalen Pharmaziehistorischen Kongresses Innsbruck 1977. Stuttgart, Wissenschaftliche Verlagsgesellschaft, 1979. p. 81–90.

Bosman–Jelgersma HA: 'Gräfinnenpulver'. In Hickel E, Schröder G, ed: Neue Beiträge zur Arzneimittelgeschichte. Festschrift für Wolfgang Schneider zum 70. Geburtstag. Stuttgart, Wissenschaftliche Verlagsgesellschaft, 1982. p. 165–71.

Boussel P, Bonnemain H, Bove FJ: Histoire de la pharmacie et de l'Industrie pharmaceutique. Paris, Editions de la Porte Verte, 1982. 287 p.

Boussel P, Bonnemain H, Bové FJ: History of pharmacy and pharmaceutical industry. Paris, Lausanne, Asklepios, 1983. 285 p.

Bowman IA: Herbal medicines and the midwife. **Bookman** 1982 Jul–Aug;9(6):3–9

Cowen DL: Pharmacy and freedom. **Am J Hosp Pharm** 1984 Mar;41(3):459–67

Cowen DL: The history of pharmacy and the history of the Jews. In H.R. Fehlmann, F. Ledermann, ed: Festschrift für A. Lutz und J. Büchi. Zürich, Juris Druck, 1983. p. 67–83. (Veröffentlichungen der Schweizerischen Gesellschaft für Geschichte der Pharmazie, Bd. 2).

Crellin JK, ed: Plants in medicine: from yesterday to today. Durham, Duke University Medical Center, 1982. 114 p. Readings and Perspectives in Medicine, Booklet Number 2.

Daems WF: Die Apoteca ein 'Stall' und die 'Stall–Apotheke'. **Sudhoffs Arch** 1978;62(1):95–6

Dann G, Higby G: Bibliography of the publications of George Urdang on his birth centenary. **Pharm Hist** 1982;24(3):106–14

Debus AG: History with a purpose: the fate of Paracelsus. **Pharm Hist** 1984;26(2):83–96

Delatte L, Opsomer–Halleux C: Ancient medical recipes and the computer: the Theorema project. **Pharm Hist** 1981;23(2):87–9

Delatte L, Halleux R: Recettes médicales anciennes et ordinateur: le projet Theorema. **Rev Hist Pharm (Paris)** 1980 Sep;27(246):155–160

Delaveau P: Histoire et renouveau des plantes médicinales. Paris, Albin Michel, 1982. 354 p.

de Pasquale A: Pharmacognosy: the oldest modern science. **J Ethnopharmacol** 1984 Jun;11(1):1–16

Dilg, P, et al., ed: Perspektiven der Pharmaziegeschichte: Festschrift für Rudolf Schmitz zum 65. Geburtstag. Bibliography by F. J. Kühlen. Graz, Austria, Akademische Druck- u. Verlagsanstalt, 1983. xviii, 497 p.

Earles MP: Cutting the tapestry. **Pharm Hist (London)** 1972 Sep;2(4):1–4

Ganzinger K, ed: Die Vorträge des Internationalen Pharmaziehistorischen Kongresses Innsbruck 1977. Stuttgart, Wissenschaftliche Verlagsgesellschaft, 1979. 213 p. (Veröffentlichungen der Internationalen Gesellschaft für Geschichte der Pharmazie, Neue Folge, 47).

Gicklhorn R, Göpfert W, Müller I, et al: Bemerkungen zur Geschichte und Ikonographie des Drachenbaumes. **Dtsch Apoth Ztg** 1980 Jul 3;120(27):1260–6

Girre L: La médecine par les plantes, à travers les âges. Rennes, Ouest–France. 1981, 187 p.

Heilmittel aus Pflanzen und Tieren: Ausstellung des Oberösterreichischen Landesmuseums im Schlossmuseum zu Linz vom 9. 5. bis 3. 8. 1980. Linz, Landesmuseum, 1980. 359 p. (Katalog des Oberösterr. Landesmuseums, 105). Contributions by W. Kubelka, R. Schmidt, F. Speta, H. Heltmann, B. Kopp, B. Gruber, E. Speta, R. Steinwendtner. K. Rumpler, A. Kump, F. Grims, B. Heinzl.

Hein WH: Historische und kritische Betrachtungen zu den Veröffentlichungen der Gesellschaft. In: Vorträge des Internationalen Pharmaziehistorischen Kongresses Innsbruck 1977. Stuttgart, Wissenschaftliche Verlagsgesellschaft, 1979. p. 15–22.

Hickel E, Schröder G, ed: Neue Beiträge zur Arzneimittelgeschichte. Festschrift für Wolfgang Schneider zum 70. Geburtstag. Stuttgart, Wissenschaftliche Verlagsgesellschaft, 1982. 285 p. (Veröffentlichungen der Internationalen Gesellschaft für Geschichte der Pharmazie e. V., Neue Folge, Band 51).

Hickel E: Pharmaziegeschichte als Wissenschafts- oder Sozialgeschichte? In: Vorträge des Internationalen Pharmaziehistorischen Kongresses Innsbruck 1977. Stuttgart, Wissenschaftliche Verlagsgesellschaft, 1979. p. 23–8.

Hutton DA: Cordial waters and cordial chests. **Pharm Hist (London)** 1973 Sep;3(2):6–8

Izsák S: Farmacia de–a lungul secolelor. Bucuresti, Editura Stiintifică si Enciclopediă, 1979. 418 p.

Joannis C: Santé et sagesse traditionnelle. Le Puy, France, Bonneton, 1981. 127 p.

Jordi Gonzalez R: Oportunas consideraciones sobre la auto--medicacion. **An Med Cir** 1979 Apr–Jun;(256):99–114

Julien P: Pharmacie et philatélie. **Rev Hist Pharm (Paris)** 1981;28:69–73

Julien P: Une miniature des saints Côme et Damien (fin XVe - début XVIe siècle). **Rev Hist Pharm (Paris)** 1982 Sep;29(254):175–6

Jünemann J: Nachlese zu Rillen und Näpfchen auf sakralen Denkmalen (2). **Beitr Gesch Pharm** 1980;31(7):49–54

Jüttner G: Der Dialog in Pharmazie, Chemie und Botanik. Zum Anteil einer literarischen Gattung in der Darstellung, Vermittlung und im Unterricht der Naturwissenschaften. **Ber Wissenschaftsgesch** 1980;3(1–2):23–34

Kallinich G, Schmidt–Glassner H: Schöne alte Apotheken. 2. Auflage. München, Callwey, 1977. 251 p.

Kuhlen FJ: Zur Geschichte der Schmerz–, Schlaf- und Betäubungsmittel in Mittelalter und früher Neuzeit. Stuttgart, Deutscher Apotheker, 1983. xiv, 445 p. (Quellen und Studien zur Geschichte der Pharmazie, Bd. 19).

Le mouvement historique: Bibliographie internationale d'histoire de la pharmacie et des sciences connexes. **Rev Hist Pharm (Paris)** 1982 Mar;29(252):60–76 (continued regularly)

Leden I: Reumatologisk farmakoterapi ur historiskt/filatelistiskt perspektiv. **Lakartidningen** 1980 Dec 24;77(52):4943–6

Löw R: Was hat die Pharmaziegeschichte der Wissenschaftstheorie zu sagen? In: Vorträge des Internationalen Pharmaziehistorischen Kongresses Innsbruck 1977. Stuttgart, Wissenschaftliche Verlagsgesellscaft, 1979. p. 29–38.

Mattelaer B: Le Benelux et son apport à l'histoire égyptienne et arabe de la pharmacie. **Bull Pharm** 1979;1–2:1–5

Mez–Mangold L: Aus der Geschichte des Medikaments. Basel, Editiones 'Roche', 1980, 175 p.

Miyasita S: Son Shibo no keikenbô. (Sun Ssu–mo's empirical remedies.) **Kampo No Rinsho** 1973;20:544–7

Modig M: The allegory of Christ in a pharmacy. **Pharm Hist** 1984;26(1):44–5

Müller–Jahncke WD: Apothekerbildnisse auf Medaillen und Plaketten. 1. Deutschsprachiger Raum. Stuttgart, Wissenschaftliche

Verlagsgesellschaft, 1980. 164 p. Veröffentlichungen der Internationalen Gesellschaft für Geschichte der Pharmazie, Neue Folge, 48).
Parascandola JL, Bender GA: Historical hobbies for the pharmacist. Symposium on historical hobbies for the pharmacist. Madison, Wis., 1974. iv, 57 p. (Publication/American Institute of the History of Pharmacy. no. 2)
Rádóczy G: Régi gyógyszerészi mértékegységek és kialakulásuk története. **Orvostort Kozl** 1979;87-88(25 no 1-2):229-41
Rocchietta S: Un 'Christ à la pharmacie' ou 'Les Saints Côme et Damien'? **Rev Hist Pharm (Paris)** 1984 Jun;31(261):131-3
Rusek V, Solich J: Vědeckotechnická revoluce ve farmaceutických vědách a výzkumu. **Cesk Farm** 1982 Jun;31(5):145-8
Said HM, ed: Pharmacy and medicine thru' the ages. Karachi, Hamdard Foundation, 1980. 264 p. Contributions by S. K. Hamarneh, Y. Ahmad, I. H. Qureshi, S. S. Ali, K. M. Habib, M. S. Akhtar, V. M. Tirmizi, M. Amin, M. Ashraf, M. K. Bhatty, S. F. Hussain, S. Mahdihassan, U. Schaffer, I. Haq.
Schadewaldt H: Die Nebenwirkungen der Heilmittel aus medizinhistorischer Sicht. **Dtsch Apoth Ztg** 1981 Mar 26;121(13):657-9
Schadewaldt H: Die pharmazeutische Ausbildung aus der Sicht eines Medizinhistorikers. **Dtsch Apoth Ztg** 1981 Oct 15;121(42):2338-41
Schmidt F: Apothekerbildnisse auf Medaillen und Plaketten. **Beitr Gesch Pharm** 1981;31(13):100-1
Schneider W: Anleitung zum Gebrauch des Systema Pharmaceuticum. (Zur statistischen Auswertung von Quellen zur Arzneimittelgeschichte). Braunschweig, 1978. 67 p. (Veröffentlichungen aus dem Pharmaziegeschichtlichen Seminar der Technischen Universität Braunschweig, 18).
Schneider W: Pharmaziegeschichte und ihre Repräsentanten im 20. Jahrhundert. Zum 80. Geburtstag von Prof. Dr. Georg Edmund Dann. **Pharm Ztg** 1978;123:1265-71
Schuster E: Arzt, Apotheker und Tod in den Totentanzdarstellungen. **Apoth J** 1984;7:47-52
Schwaiberger R: Zu einigen Aspekten der Entwicklung der Pharmazie im Rahmen der Aufklärung, beeinflusst durch hallesche Systematiker. **Rostocker Wiss Hist Manuskripte** 1981;6:35-44
Short GR: Postal and pharmaceutical history. **Pharm Hist (London)** 1974 Dec;4(3):5-6
Simco EL: The history of perfumery. **Pharm Hist (London)** 1981;11(1):2-3
Simon G: Kosmetische Präparate vom 16. bis 19. Jahrhundert. Braunschweig, Deutscher Apotheker Verlag, 1983. 396 p. (Braunschweiger Veröffentlichungen zur Geschichte der Pharmazie und der Naturwissenschaften, Bd. 27).
Smollich R: Der Bisamapfel in Kunst und Wissenschaft. Stuttgart, Deutscher Apotheken Verlag, 1983. 342 p. (Quellen und Studien zur Geschichte der Pharmazie, Bd. 21).
Smollich R: Der Bisamapfel in Kunst und Wissenschaft. Stuttgart, Deutscher Apotheker Verlag, 1983. 342 p. (Quellen und Studien zur Geschichte der Pharmazie, Bd. 21).
Soldi A: Agitare prima dell'uso. L'avventurosa storia dei medicamenti. Milano, Ferro, 1979. 176 p.
Sommer J: Dusledky filozofické orientace pro farmacii. **Cesk Farm** 1982 Oct;31(8):297-302
Thiveaud D, Benejeam M: La pharmacopée traditionnelle dans le département du lot. **Quercy Rech** 1982;(49-50):30-9
Vaeth JM: Role of the pharmacist in cancer care throughout history. **Front Radiat Ther Oncol** 1980;15:1-4
Whittaker AP: Source-material in the Winchester City Archives 1550-1981. **Pharm Hist (London)** 1981;11(1):5-6
Wietschoreck H: Aethiops---eine neue Arzneimittelgruppe der Nachchemiatrie---und ihre Bedeutung in Verbindung mit anderen Antimon-Präparaten. (Ein Beispiel für den Einsatz chemischer Untersuchungen bei der Bearbeitung arzneimittelgeschichtlicher Fragen). In: Vorträge des Internationalen Pharmaziehistorischen Kongresses Innsbruck 1977. Stuttgart, Wissenschaftliche Verlagsgesellschaft, 1979. p. 49-55.
Wietschoreck H: Die historische Entwicklung von Tartarusverbindungen in Arzneimitteln unter besonderer Berücksichtigung von Tartarus Chalybeatus und Terra Foliata Tartari in der Nachchemiatrie. In International Congress of the History of Medicine, 27th, Barcelona, 1980. Actas. Barcelona, Académia de Ciències Médiques de Catalunya i Balears, 1981. p. 675-9.
Yazu M: [Medico-dental and pharmacological history--miscellaneous records (1)] **Dent Outlook** 1980 Jan;(1):130-1 (contd. regularly)
Zalai K: Vinum Tokajense passum. In Hickel E, Schröder G, ed: Neue Beiträge zur Arzneimittelgeschichte. Festschrift für Wolfgang Schneider zum 70. Geburtstag. Stuttgart, Wissenschaftliche Verlagsgesellschaft, 1982. p. 41-6.

### Africa

Amakoue A: Médecine et pharmacopée traditionnelle en Afrique. **Dialogue J Mormon Thought** 1978 Nov-Dec;46-70
Elom-Ntouzo'o E: Médecine, pharmacopées traditionelles et développement en Afrique. **Presence Afr** 1978;108:38-49

### Americas

Dominguez XA: Conocimientos médicos de los mayas, aztecas, tarascos y la herbolaria médica mexicana. **Guatem Indig** 1978;13(1/2):220-38
Erichsen-Brown C: Use of plants for the past 500 years. Aurora, Ont., Breezy Creeks Press, 1980, xxii, 512 p.
Guerra F: La evaluacion farmacológica de las fuentes históricas sobre la medicina precolombina. **Guatem Indig** 1978;13(1/2):175-85
Hirschhorn HH: Botanical remedies of South and Central America, and the Caribbean: an archival analysis. Pt. 1. **J Ethnopharmacol** 1981;4:129-58
Schultes RE: Evolution of the identification of the major South American narcotic plants. **J Psychedelic Drugs** 1979 Jan-Jun;11(1-2):119-34
Valverde Lopez JL: La experimentacion farmacologica sobre drogas americanas. (Discurso de ingreso, Academico Correspondiente Electo, 17 de marzo 1981.) Barcelona, Real Academia De Farmacia, 1981. 42 p.

### Arabic

Anees MA: History of Islamic medicine and pharmacy: contribution of Sami Hamarneh. **Hamdard** 1983 Apr-Jun;26(2):67-75
Kataya S: Les Manuscrits Médicaux et Pharmaceutiques dans Les Bibliothèques publiques d'Alep. Alep, Université d'Alep, Institut du Patrimoine scientifique Arabe, 1976.

### Asia

Delaveau P: Les fonds des pharmacopées traditionnelles et l'expérimentation. **Sci Orient** 1977;12:1-16

### Austria

Ganzinger K: Zur Geschichte der Universitätsapotheke. In Dilg P, et al., ed: Perspektiven der Pharmaziegeschichte. Graz, Austria, Akademische Druck- u. Verlagsanstalt, 1983. p. 79-88.
Halmai J: Beiträge zur Geschichte der Pharmazie in Burgenland bis 1918. **Burgenl Heimatbl** 1969;31(4):181-7
Hochenegg H: Tiroler Aerzte und Pharmazeuten als Künstler und Schriftsteller, Forscher und Volksvertreter. **Tirol Heimat** 1976;40:135-62
Huter F: Apothekenwesen und Apothekerstudium in Tirol. **Anz Philol Hist Kl Osterr Akad Wiss** 1979;116:199-221
Huter F: Beiträge zur Geschichte des Apothekenwesens in Tirol [pt. 1]. **Tirol Heimat** 1977;41:5-43
Ryslavy K: Materialien zur Geschichte der Apotheken und Apotheker im Burgenland. Eisenstadt, Amt der Burgenländischen Landesregierung, Landesarchiv, 1979. 285 p. (Burgenländische Forschungen, Heft/68).

### Belgium

Vandewiele LJ: Een vergeten Belgische farmakopee. Het dispensatorium van Triller. **Farm Tijdschr Belg** 1979;56:375-82
Vandewiele LJ: Geschiedenis van de farmacie in België met een inleiding tot de algemene geschiedenis van de farmacie. Beveren, Orion, 1981. 379 p.
Vandewiele LJ: Historiek van de pharmacieopleiding in België. **Sartonia** 1979 Mar;42:6-15

### Canada

Dulong G: Médecine populaire au Canada français. In: Congrès international d'histoire de la médecine, XXVe, Québec, 1976. Actes. Québec, 1977. p. 625-33.

### Caribbean

Halberstein RA, Saunders AB: Traditional medical practices and medicinal plant usage on a Bahamian Island. **Tex Stud Lit Lang** 1978;2:177-203

### China

Chen KJ: Certain progress in the treatment of coronary heart disease with traditional medicinal plants in China. **Am J Chin Med** 1981 Autumn;9(3):193-6
Hu SY: An enumeration of Chinese materia medica. Hong Kong, Chinese University Press, 1980. 287 p.
Hu Naichang: [Textual research on 'Xiao pin (short and miscellaneous) prescriptions'.] (Chi). **Chin J Med Hist** 1981;11:116-9
McCormick JP, Parascandola J: Dragon bones and drugstores: the interaction of pharmacy and paleontology in the search for early man in China. **Pharm Hist** 1981;23(2):55-70
Miyasita S: Honzo no'rui' gainen. (Categorization concepts in Chinese materia medica.) **Tohogaku** 1976;51:104-13
Morimura K: Advancement of the scientific character of Chinese materia medica from Ta-kuan pen-ts'ao to Pen-ts'ao kang-mu. In: International Congress for the History of Science, 14th, Tokyo, Kyoto, 1974. Proceedings. Tokyo, 1975. 3:323-326.

Neumeyer JL, Guan JH: Pharmacy and the pharmaceutical industry, past, present and future, The People's Republic of China. **Am Pharm** 1982 Jan;22(1):14–21
Unschuld PU: Die Bedeutung der Ma-wang-tui-Funde für die chinesische Medizin- und Pharmaziegeschichte. In Dilg P, et al., ed: Perspektiven der Pharmaziegeschichte. Graz, Austria, Akademische Druck- u. Verlagsanstalt, 1983. p. 389–416.
Xie Zongwan: [Present state and prospect of the study and systematization of works on Chinese materia medica written in past dynasties] (Chi). **J Tradit Chin Med** 1981;22(3):64–7
Xu X: [An introduction to the pharmaceutical administration of ancient Chinese feudal dynasties] (Chi). **Chung Hua I Shih Tsa Chih** 1984;14(2):117–20
Zheng Jinsheng: [On pulverizing instruments for Chinese herbal drugs and their evolution in ancient China] (Chi). **Chin J Med Hist** 1981;11(1):35–9

**Czechoslovakia**

Rusek V, Müller D: Příspěvky k dějinám lékáren v Těšíně. **Cesk Farm** 1981 Jun;30(5):171–6

**Denmark**

Kofod H: Danish contributions to the unicorn story. **Beitr Gesch Pharm** 1979;31(2):12–15

**Ethiopia**

Abebe W: Traditional pharmaceutical practice in Gondar region, northwestern Ethiopia. **J Ethnopharmacol** 1984 Jun;11(1):33–47

**Europe**

Antall J: Pictorial history of European medicine and pharmaceutics. Budapest, Corvina Kiadó, 1981. 21, [121] p.

**Finland**

Niemineva K, Haavisto H, Perälä M: Vanhoista Turkulaisia lääkemääräyksistä ja niiden kirjoittajista. **Turun Hist Ark (Finl)** 1979;33:146–63
Peldán K: Huvuddragen i farmaciens historia i Finland. **Sven Farm Tidskr** 1979;83:657–65

**France**

Bonnot I: Du clystère au quinquina. Pour une étude des comptes d'apothicaires aux XVIIe et XVIIIe siècles. **Bull Liaison Assoc Amis Mus Pharm Montp** 1983;:(8):61–75
Chambonnet F: Les faiences pharmaceutiques conservées dans les établissements hospitaliers de la région lyonnaise. Le Puy-en-Velay, [s.n.], 1978. 213 p. (Thèse, Lyon).
Coignerai-Devillers L: Médecine, diététique et santé à la cour de Louis XIV d'après les lettres de la princesse Palatine (1652–1722). **Rev Hist Pharm (Paris)** 1983 Dec;71(30):265–74
De Backer C: De apothekers Van Baudeloo te Gent, 1586–1785. **Farm Tijdschr Belg** 1980;57:351–5
Devaux G: Pharmaciens éponymes des rues de l'agglomération bordelaise. **Rev Hist Pharm (Paris)** 1983 Dec;71(30):299–304
Devaux G: Saint Michel, patron des apothicaires de Bordeaux et d'autres lieux. **Rev Hist Pharm (Paris)** 1982;29(252):151–9
Dillemann G: Die französische Pharmazie vom 3. Jahrhundert bis zur Gegenwart. In Sournia JC, Martiny M, Poulet J, ed: Illustrierte Geschichte der Medizin. Salzburg, Andreas, 1980. Vol. 5. p. 1723–77.
Dillemann G: Les illustres pharmaciens dont les noms ont été donnés aux amphithéatres de la Faculté de Pharmacie de Paris. **Bull Ordre Natl Pharm** 1979 Apr;221:517–41
Dulieu L: La pharmacie à Montpellier de ses origines à nos jours. [Marseilles], Presses Universelles, 1973. 343 p.
Girard P: Toxiques et poisons dans le passé pharmaceutique de la Savoie. **Rev Hist Pharm (Paris)** 1983 Sep;30(258):177–90
Guyotjeannin C: Remèdes d'autrefois aux îles Saint-Pierre-et-Miquelon. **Rev Hist Pharm (Paris)** 1984 Jun;31(261):115–20
Julien P: Deux saints médecins et pharmaciens, Côme et Damien. **Bull Liaison Assoc Amis Mus Pharm Montp** 1982;:(7):13–35
Le Breton D: Apothicaires et moines à Bordeaux à la fin de l'Ancien Régime. Diss., Université de Bordeaux, II, 1983. 131 leaves.
Le Minor JM: Origine et développement des pharmacies de l'arrondissement de Molsheim. **Soc d'Hist d'Archeol Molsheim environs Annu** 1982;:129–44
Marzocchi J: Essais sur la médecine et la pharmacie à travers l'histoire de la Corse. [S.1], J. P. Marzocchi, [1978?].
Musée de la Pharmacie: Exposition: Montpellier: de l'apothicairerie à la pharmacie. Montpellier, Faculté de Pharmacie, n.d.
Nguyen-Laissard M: Note sur la pharmacie de l'hôpital de Nuits-Saint Georges. **Rev Hist Pharm (Paris)** 1980 Mar;27(244):15–16
Nguyen-Laissard M: Note sur l'hôpital de Moutiers-Saint-Jean et sa pharmacie. **Rev Hist Pharm (Paris)** 1983 Sep;30(258):233–4
Niaussat PM: L'activité scientifique des médecins et pharmaciens de la marine du XVIIe siècle à nos jours. **Med Armees** 1980;8(10)spec:800–6
Recensement des pharmacies hospitalières: **Bull Soc Fr Hist Hop** 1979;(39):10–18
Rèche A: Mille ans de médecine et de pharmacie à Bordeaux. Bordeaux, Mollat, 1980. 190 p.
Villeval G: La Pharmacie de N.-D.-de-Lorette, à Alan. **Rev Comminges** 1975;88:307–13

**Germany**

Alberti H: Die heiligen Kosmas und Damian auf einer Prozessionsfahne im Deutschen Apotheken-Museum. **Dtsch Apoth Ztg** 1979 Jun 14;119(24):948–50 (also in Pharm Ztg 1979 Jun 14;24:1155–7
Articus R: Geschichte der alten Husumer Apotheken: ein Beitrag zur Geschichte des Gesundheitswesens in Schleswig-Holstein. Husum, Schwan-Apotheke, 1981. 76 p.
Bartels K: Die ersten Apotheken und Apotheker Coburgs. Ergänzungen zur Geschichte des Coburger Apothekenwesens I. **Pharm Ztg** 1980;125:457–60
Bartels K: Miscellanea civitatis et ducatus Coburgiae pharmaceutica. Ergänzungen zur Coburger Apothekengeschichte II. **Pharm Ztg** 1980;125:1780–4
Becker H: Roter Graben 10: ausgewählte Kapital aus der Pharmaziegeschichte, 1790–1870. Herzogenrath [Germany], Murken-Altrogge, [1982]. 288 p.
Bessler O, Kaiser W: Hallesche und wittenbergische Absolventen in der Frühgeschichte des Pharmakopöewesens. **Wiss Z Martin Luther Univ (Math)** 1973;22(5):139–46
Büsing W: Bedeutende Apotheker aus fünf Jahrhunderten im Weser-Ems-Raum. **Dtsch Apoth Ztg** 1979 Nov 22;119(47):1913–9
Die Alte Kunst des Apothekers: Wiederentdeckt bei einem Besuch im Deutschen Apotheken-Museum in Heidelberg. Mannheim, Boehringer Mannheim, 1980. 39 p.
Dobras W: Cosmas und Damian in oberbayerischen Kirchen. **Pharm Ztg** 1981 Dec 24;126(52-53):2715–6
Drews FH, Guenter M: Die herrschaftliche Apotheke. 400 Jahre Pharmazie in Celle. Celle, Löwen-Apotheke, 1980. 65 p.
Fetzer W: Pharmazie: Historisches aus Museen und Sammlungen der DDR. Leipzig, VEB Deutscher Verlag für Grundstoffindustrie, 1983. 279 p.
Fischer H: Die Apothekenanfänge in Bayreuth bis zum Beginn des 18. Jahrhunderts und die Entwicklung des Apothekenrechts in der Markgrafschaft bis um 1800. **Arch Gesch Oberfranken** 1978;57–58:187–271
Gaude W: Die alte Apotheke. Eine tausendjährige Kulturgeschichte. Stuttgart, Deutscher Apotheker Verlag, 1979. 219 p.
Graepel PH: Die Calwer Apothekerfamilie Gärtner im Bild. **Beitr Gesch Pharm** 1981;31(12):92–5
Hein WH, Wittop Koning AW: Apothekengefässe der Durlacher Fayence-Fabrik. **Pharm Ztg** 1980;125:25–7
Hein WH, Schwarz HD, ed: Deutsche Apotheker-Biographie. Band II, M–Z. Stuttgart, Wissenschaftliche Verlagsgesellschaft, 1978. p. 393–788. (Veröffentlichungen der Internationalen Gesellschaft für Geschichte der Pharmazie, Neue Folge, Band 46).
Höfner C: Geschichte der Apotheke zu Rodach. **Jahrb Coburg Landesstift** 1978;23:1–34
Kohlhaas-Christ C: Zur Geschichte des Apothekenwesens im Hamburg von den Anfängen bis zum Erlass der Medizinalordnung 1818. Stuttgart, Deutscher Apotheker Verlag, 1985. 279 p. (Quellen und Studien zur Geschichte der Pharmazie, Bd. 29)
Meyer v. Froreich H: Zur Geschichte des Apothekenwesens der Grafschaft und des Fürstentums Lippe von den Anfängen bis zum Jahre 1918. Diss. rer. nat. Marburg, 1979. 437 p.
Modig M: Deutsches Apotheken-Museum i Heidelberg. **Sydsven Medicinhist Sallsk Arsskr** 1984;21:15–26
Nordau CG: Grilles du temps jadis. **Monit Pharm Lab** 1980 Dec 6;34(1445):4363, 4365, 4367
Rausch U: Das Medizinal- und Apothekenwesen der Landgrafschaft Hessen-Darmstadt und des Grossherzogtums Hessen unter besonderer Berücksichtigung der Provinz Starkenburg. Darmstadt, Marburg, Selbstverlag der Hessischen Historischen Kommission Darmstadt und der Historischen Kommission für Hessen 1978 (Quellen und Forschungen zur Hessischen Geschichte, Bd. 33). 588 p.
Schaefer M: Zur Geschichte des Gesundheitswesens in der Stadt Leer/Ostfriesland unter besonderer Berücksichtigung der Apotheken von den Anfängen bis zum Jahre 1900. Diss. rer. nat. Marburg, 1980. 272 p.
Schienbein H: Die 'Neu-Vermehrte Heylsame Dreck-Apotheke' (1696/1734) des Hof- und Stadtarztes Christian Frantz Paulini. **Quintessenz** 1981 Sep;32(9):1699–1702
Schneider W: Entwicklung der pharmazeutischen Museologie in Deutschland. **Pharm Ztg** 1980 Jan 10;125(2):68–71
Sommer R: Zur Geschichte des Medizinal- und Apothekenwesens in einem kleinen souveränen Staat (Schaumburg-Lippe). Diss. Braunschweig, 1979. vi, 295 p. (Veröffentlichungen aus dem Pharmaziegeschichtlichen Seminar der Technischen Universität Braunschweig, 19).

# PHARMACY

Sonntag CD: Zur Geschichte der Apothekenprivilegien im Gebiet des Herzogtums Kleve vom Vertrag zu Xanten (1614) bis zur Errichtung der Rheinprovinz (1822). Stuttgart, Deutscher Apotheker Verlag, 1982. v, 268, xviii p. (Quellen und Studien zur Geschichte der Pharmazie, Bd. 18).
Steinkamp U: Zur Geschichte des Apothekenwesens in den Grafschaften und dem späteren Fürstentum Waldeck und Pyrmont von den Anfängen bis zur Gegenwart. Diss. rer. nat. Marburg, 1980. 278 p.
Völksen W: Die Stuckbilder der Berg-Apotheke in Clausthal-Zellerfeld. **Beitr Gesch Pharm** 1984;31(23):197–203
Wankmüller A: Die Bibliothek der Internationalen Gesellschaft für Geschichte der Pharmazie. **Ber Wissenschaftsgesch** 1979;2(3–4):226–8

**Great Britain**

Boorman WH: Local history and the pharmacist. **Pharm Hist (London)** 1968 Mar;1(2):3–6
Burnby J: House and home for apothecaries and druggists. **Pharm Hist (London)** 1978 Dec;8(3):2–3
Burnby JG: Some Derbyshire apothecaries. **Pharm Hist (London)** 1970 Dec;1(6):5–8
Girdwood RH: Doctors, pharmacists and the public. In Passmore R, ed: Proceedings of the Royal College of Physicians of Edinburgh Tercentenary Congress, 1981. Edinburgh, Royal College of Physicians of Edinburgh, 1982. p. 190–8.
Matthews LG: Apothecaries of the Spicers and Kings Lynn, Norfolk. **Pharm Hist (London)** 1971 Dec;2(3):9–10
Matthews LG: The city of York's first spicers, grocers and apothecaries. **Pharm Hist (London)** 1967 Oct;1(1):2–3
A pharmaceutical museum: **Pharm Hist (London)** 1977 Jul;7(2):4–5
Teigen PM: This sea of simples; the materia medica in three early English receipt books. **Pharm Hist** 1980;22(3):104–8
Turner I, Turner TD: Ymarfer Fferylliaeth Meddygon Myddfai (The pharmacy of the physicians of Myddfai. **Pharm Hist (London)** 1983 Jun;13(2):2–5
Whittet TD: A survey of apothecaries' tokens including some previously unrecognised specimens. **Pharm J** 1982;228:719–24; 1983;230:133–40; 1983;231:42–5, 641–9; 1984;232:583–5, 790–2
Whittet TD: Project for a directory of provincial apothecaries. **Pharm Hist (London)** 1970 Mar;1(4):2–3
Whittet TD, White PM: Some midland apothecaries. **Pharm Hist (London)** 1978 Jul;8(2):6–8

**Hungary**

Antall J: Entwicklungstendenzen des Apothekerberufs in Ungarn. **Pharm Ztg** 1981;126:417–23
Antall J: Herausbildung der wissenschaftlichen Pharmazie in Ungarn und die Pester Medizinische Schule. In Hein WH, ed: Pharmaziehistorischer Kongress, Budapest, 1981. Stuttgart, Wissenschaftliche Verlagsgesellschaft, 1983. p. 101–4.
Bano-Fleischmann M, Zalai K: Gegenstände der Erinnerung an Kosma und Damian in Ungarn. **Ther Hung** 1981;29(3):152–6
Benko F: Die Gemälde der Apotheke zum Goldenen Einhorn im Debrecziner Déri Museum. In Hein WH, ed: Pharmaziehistorischer Kongress, Budapest, 1981. Stuttgart, Wissenschaftliche Verlagsgesellschaft, 1983. p. 85–96.
Blázy A: Die Namensgebung der Apotheken in Ungarn in Vergangenheit und Gegenwart. In Hein WH, ed: Pharmaziehistorischer Kongress, Budapest, 1981. Stuttgart, Wissenschaftliche Verlagsgesellschaft, 1983. p. 105–10.
Hegedüs L: Zwei berühmte ungarische Arcana aus dem 14. und 15. Jahrhundert. In Hein WH, ed: Pharmaziehistorischer Kongress, Budapest, 1981. Stuttgart, Wissenschaftliche Verlagsgesellschaft, 1983. p. 41–7.
Hein WH, ed: Pharmaziehistorischer Kongress, Budapest, 1981. I. Vorträge zur ungarischen Pharmaziegeschichte. II. Vorträge in Zusammenfassungen. Stuttgart, Wissenschaftliche Verlagsgesellschaft, 1983. 191 p. (Veröffentlichungen der Internationalen Gesellschaft für Geschichte der Pharmazie e. V., 52).
Zalai K: Die Entwicklungsperioden der wissenschaftlichen Pharmazie in Ungarn. In Hein WH, ed: Pharmaziehistorischer Kongress, Budapest, 1981. Stuttgart, Wissenschaftliche Verlagsgesellschaft, 1983. p. 17–22.

**India**

Filliozat J, Raison A: Problèmes d'identification de la matière médicale indienne. **Sci Orient** 1979;16:41–50
Joshi VK: Evolution of the concept of Astavarga. **Indian J Hist Sci** 1983 May;18(1):9–14
Khan AB, Tariq M, Afaq SH, et al: Poisons and antidotes in Unani system of medicine. **Indian J Hist Sci** 1981, reçu 1982;16(1):57–63
Rama Rao B: Development of dravyaguna in India. **Bull Indian Inst Hist Med (Hyderabad)** 1978;8(1–4):1–7
Sarma CR, Rama Rao B: Urine in ancient ayurvedic literature. **Bull Indian Inst Hist Med (Hyderabad)** 1980;10(1–4):48–52

**Italy**

Celant E: L'empirico dei mali e dei rimedi. Palermo, 'Il Vespro', 1979. 173 p.
Coghi Ruggiero T: L'antica spezieria del monastero di San Giovanni Evangelista in Parma: un libro mastro de 1588 e una controversia del 1722. **Arch Stor Prov Parmensi** 1980;32:231–44
Montanari L, Ponci R: I prezzi delle specialità medicinali in Italia--evoluzione storica della disciplina dei prezzi dei farmaci--attuale metodo per la determinazione dei prezzi delle specialità medicinali. **Farmaco [Prat]** 1982 Nov;37(11):343–64
Olmi G: Farmacopea antica e medicina moderna: la disputa sulla teriaca nel cinquecento Bolognese. **Physis** 1977;19(1–4):197–246
Tergolina U: Le medaglie fatte coniare dal Nobile Collegio Chimico Farmaceutico di Roma. Nobile Collegio Chimico-Farmaceutico Roma, (Atti e Memorie) 1975 Jan–Mar; 5(1):13–6.

**Japan**

Jin Shiying: [The influence of 'Pen tsao kang mu' in Japan.] (Chi). **Chin J Med Hist** 1981;11:102–5
Murakami S, ed: Hokkaido baiyaku shi. [Sapporo, Japan], Hokkaido Haichi Kateiyaku Kyogikai, Showa 52 nen [1977]. 428 p.
Nagasaki-ken Yakuzaishikai, Yakushi Kenkyukai: Nagasaki yakushi. Nagasaki, Nagasaki-ken Yakuzaishikai, Showa 53 nen, 1978. 502 p.

**Mexico**

Ortiz de Montellano B: Aztec medicine: empirical drug use. **Ethnomedizin** 1974–75;3(3–4):249–71

**Morocco**

Venzlaff H: Der marokkanische Drogenhändler und seine Ware. Wiesbaden, Steiner, 1977. 242 p.

**Netherlands**

Bosman-Jelgersma HA: De functie van de hofapotheker. **Pharm Weekbl** 1981 Nov 6;116(45):1373–9
Bosman-Jelgersma HA: Vijf eeuwen delftse apothekers, een bronnenstudie over de geschiedenis van de farmacie in een hollandse stad. Amsterdam, Ronald Meesters, 1979. xx, 446 p. (Thesis, Amsterdam).
Braekman WL: Recepten en pokkentraktaat uit een Middelnederlands handschrift. **Volkskunde** 1977;78:177–98
Wittop Koning DA: Drei holländische Pharmaziehistoriker. In: Vorträge des Internationalen Pharmaziehistorischen Kongresses Innsbruck 1977. Stuttgart, Wissenschaftliche Verlagsgesellschaft, 1979. p. 129–39.

**Norway**

Hopstock C: The Norwegian pharmacy museum; a presentation. In: Vorträge des Internationalen Pharmaziehistorischen Kongresses Innsbruck 1977. Stuttgart, Wissenschaftliche Verlagsgesellschaft, 1979. p. 141–5.
Norsk Farmasihistorisk Museum. Das Norwegische Pharmaziehistorische Museum (Apothekenmuseum). Le Musée norvégien de la pharmacie. Oslo, Norsk Folkemuseum, 1979, 16 p.:

**Poland**

Bukowiecki H, Kuznicka B: The pharmacy in the Warsaw royal castle. A monument of pharmaceutical culture. **Q J Hist Sci Technol (Polish Acad Sci)** 1980;25(4):755–67
Bukowiecki H, Kuźnicka B: The pharmacy in the Warsaw Royal Castle – a monument of pharmaceutical culture. **Kwart Hist Nauki Tech** 1980;25(4):755–67
Kuźnicka B: Kierunki rozwoju farmacji w Polsce epoki Oświecenia. Wrocław; Gdańsk, Zakład Narodowy im. Ossolińskich, Oddz. w Gdańsku, 1982. 172 p.
Roeske W: Freski z dawnych polskich aptek. **Arch Hist Med (Warsz)** 1980;43(2):191–7
Roeske W: Geschichte der Pharmaziehistorik in Polen. In: Vorträge des Internationalen Pharmaziehistorischen Kongresses Innsbruck 1977. Stuttgart, Wissenschaftliche Verlagsgesellschaft, 1979. p. 155–61.
Roeske W: Muzeum Farmacji Akademii medycznej w Krakowie. Krakow, 1977. 22 p.

**Portugal**

Marques Leal A, Silveira C: Hospital pharmacy in Portugal and its future trends. **Drug Intell Clin Pharm** 1983 Nov;17(11):843–6
Pina L de: Farmacia ornamental uma historia portuense. **Arch Hist Med Port** 1968–70;3(1–4):117–36
Rocchietta S: Le pubblicazioni di storia della farmacia portoghese negli anni '70. **Minerva Med** 1980 Dec 15;71(50):3679–84

**Romania**

Neagu I, Neagu M: Vieux médicament utilisé dans la thérapeutique populaire de Roumanie. In: Congrès international d'histoire de la médecine, XXVe, Québec, 1976. Actes. Québec, 1977. p. 1015–25.

**Spain**

Arnaiz Bonilla A: Las afamadas boticas burgalesas de los hospitales de San Juan y San Julian y San Quirce (Barrantes). Burgos, Exma. Diputacíon Provincial de Burgos, [1981]. 152 p.
Basante Pol RM: La farmacia en los monasterios, hospitales y hospederías del Bierzo. **Bol Soc Esp Hist Farm** 1984 Sep;35(139):165–86
Beya Alonso E: La farmacia en la trapa. **Bol Soc Esp Hist Farm** 1983 Sep;135:85–94
Folch Jou G, Muñoz Calvo S: Aportación de Olmedilla y Puig al desarrollo de la historiografía farmacéutica en España. **Bol Soc Esp Hist Farm** 1980 Oct;31(123):205–34
Folch Jou G, Muñoz Calvo S: Catalogo de los documentos conservados en el Archivo de la Real Academia de Farmacia. **An R Acad Farm (Madr)** 1978;44(2):199–351
Folch Jou G, Basante Pol RM, Sanchez-Villacañas CM: La farmacia madrileña de la plaza de Santo Domingo num. 6. **Bol Soc Esp Hist Farm** 1983;34(136):111–37
Folch Jou G, Puerto Sarmiento FJ: Las Cantaridas en Espana. In Hickel E, Schröder G, ed: Neue Beiträge zur Arzneimittelgeschichte. Festschrift für Wolfgang Schneider zum 70. Geburtstag. Stuttgart, Wissenschaftliche Verlagsgesellschaft, 1982. p. 131–47.
Garcia Sanchez J: Contribución a la historia de la botica del Hospital de la Pasión, de Ciudad Rodrigo. **Bol Soc Esp Hist Farm** 1980/81 Dec–Mar;31–32(124–5):1–7
Javier Puerto F: La Farmacia de la Plaza de San Ildefonso (Madrid). **Bol Soc Esp Hist Farm** 1981 Sep;32(127):169–205
Javier Puerto F, Sanz Diaz L: Las ideas cientificas de Felix Palacios. **Bol Soc Esp Hist Farm** 1982 Mar;33(132):237–47
Jordi Gonzàlez FR: Contribució a la genealogia dels farmacèutics catalans; consideracions sobre Narcís Viader i Font. Barcelona, the author, 1981. p. 4–10.
Jordi González R: Bibliotecas de boticarios catalanes: aportacion para un estudio. **Circ Farm** 1984;283:127–42
Rof Carballo MC: Le Dr. Jesús Isamat Vila, premier professeur d'histoire de la pharmacie de l'Université de Barcelone. In: Vorträge des Internationalen Pharmaziehistorischen Kongresses Innsbruck 1977. Stuttgart, Wissenschaftliche Verlagsgesellschaft, 1979. p. 189–94.
Sorní J, Suñé JM: Barcelona. Baja edad media. Especieros o Boticarios? **Bol Soc Esp Hist Farm** 1983;34(136):139–50
Valverde JL, Hidalgo J: Documentos medicofarmaceuticos conservados en archivos de Sevilla. Salamanca, 1971. 120 p. (Cuadernos de Historia de la Medicina Española, Monografías, 17).
Valverde JL, Bautista Mendez T: La evolucion de las formas farmaceuticos a traves de textos españoles. II. Ungüentos. **Ars Pharm** 1980;21:291–315
Valverde JL, Lopez Andujar G: Las disposiciones legales sobre el certificado de 'Limpieza de sangre' en relación al ejercicio profesional farmacéutico. **Bol Soc Esp Hist Farm** 1980 Oct;31(123):259–71
Valverde JL, Bautista T, Montaña MT: Libros de interés histórico–médico–farmaceútico conservados en la Biblioteca de la Real Academia de Medicina de Sevilla. Granada, Universidad de Granada, 1980. 130 p. (Cuadernos de Historia de la Farmacia, 6).
Valverde JL, Vinuesa SL de: Panoramica legal de la introduccion de remedios quimicos en Navarra. **Llull (Spain)** 1978;2:81–94
Valverde Lopez JL, Sanchez F, Vinuesa L, et al: La dotacion de medicamentos en los buques de la Armada durante los siglos XVII y XVIII. Granada, Universidad de Granada, 1979. 60 [47] p.
Vernia P: La farmacopea Valenciana. Villarreal, Seriols–Sichet–Herrero, 1981. 168 p.

**Sweden**

Clemedson CJ: Berömda svenska böcker inom medicin och farmaci. **Nord Medicinhist Arsb** 1980;Suppl 6:35–51
Diener L, ed: Röster ur Riksgropen. **Nord Medicinhist Arsb** 1984;:49–61

**Switzerland**

Büchi J: Die Arzneiversorgung und der Sanitätsdienst der schweizerischen Truppen vom 15.–18. Jahrhundert. Stuttgart, Wissenschaftliche Verlagsanstalt, 1981. 94 p. (Veröffentlichungen der Internationalen Gesellschaft für Geschichte der Pharmazie, Neue Folge, 49).
Fehlmann HR: Beziehungen zwischen Arzt und Apotheker im 16. bis 18. Jahrhundert in der Schweiz. **Gesnerus** 1983;40(1–2):67–74

**United States**

Fitzpatrick TP: The Lenape contribution to New Jersey medicine. **J Med Soc NJ** 1984 Sep;81(9):701–6
Gramling LG: A history of pharmacy in Florida. Gainesville, Ewing Printing, 1973. iv, 225 p.
Liberti L, Coyle G, Der Marderosian A: Historical pharmaceutical exhibits at PCP&S. **Pharm Hist** 1980;22(3):115–18

**USSR**

Fayle R: Introducing the history of Russian pharmacy. **Pharm Hist (London)** 1975 Dec;5(3):1
Natradze AG: Russkie i sovetskie farmakopei. Moskva, Meditsina, 1978. 111 p

**Yugoslavia**

Mićić M: Pharmaziegeschichtliche Museen und Sammlungen in Jugoslawien. In: Vorträge des Internationalen Pharmaziehistorischen Kongresses Innsbruck 1977. Stuttgart, Wissenschaftliche Verlagsgesellschaft, 1979. p. 107–25.
Tartalja H: Pharmacy in old Dubronik. In Veteris ragusae medicina et pharmacia. Zagreb, PLIVA, n.d. p. 49–77.

**Before 500 A.D.**

Emmerick RE: On the indexation of Sanskrit medical verses and prescriptions. **Sci Orient** 1979;16:3–8
Harrauer H, Sijpesteijn PJ, ed: Medizinische Rezepte und Verwandtes. Wien, Brüder Hollinek, 1981. xv, 56 p. (Mitteilungen aus der Papyrussammlung der Osterreichischen Nationalbibliothek (Papyrus Erzherzog Rainer), Neue Serie, 13. Folge).
Jouanna J: Une forme étymologique retrouvée: omelesis dans le Glossaire hippocratique de Galien et dans le traité hippocratique des Maladies II c, 31. **Rev Philol (Paris)** 1979;53:260–63
Youtie LC: Two Michigan medical papyri [1. P. Mich. Inv. 1455; 2. P. Mich. Inv. 488 = P. Coll. Youtie II 87]. **Z Papyrologie Epigraphik** 1977;27:140–46

**Arabic**

Khan AJ: A survey of the concepts and measures developed by the Greco–Arab physicians related with the prevention and treatment of the infections and epidemic diseases. **Indian J Hist Sci** 1981;16(2):139–44

**Asia**

Mulholland J: Soma, an attempt to classify the plant and the drug. **J Asiat Soc** 1976;18(1–3):47–55

**China**

Unschuld PU: Ma-wang-tui materia medica: a comparative analysis of early Chinese pharmaceutical knowledge. **Zinbun** 1982;:(18):11–63

**Egypt**

Kolta KS: Arzt und Hersteller von Heilmitteln im alten Aegypten. **Beitr Gesch Pharm** 1979;31(2):9–12

**Greco–Roman**

Durling RJ: Lexicographical notes on Galen's pharmacological writings. **Glotta** 1979;57(3–4):218–24
Pintaudi R: Frammento di un trattato di materia medica in un Papiro Laurenziano (PL 68). **Z Papyrologie Epigraphik** 1976;23:203–7
Scarborough J: Roman pharmacy and the eastern drug trade. **Pharm Hist** 1982;24(4):135–43
Youtie LC: A medical text (P. Corn. Inv. 47). **Z Papyrologie Epigraphik** 1978;29:279–86

**Greece**

Geymonat M, ed: Scholia in Nicandri Alexipharmaca, cum glossis. Milan, Cisalpino–Goliardica, 1974. 218 p.
Ullmann M: Die Schrift des Rufus von Ephesos über die Gelbsucht in arabischer und lateinischer Ubersetzung. Göttingen, Vandenhoeck & Ruprecht, 1983. 87 p. (Abhandlungen der Akademie der Wissenschaften in Göttingen, Philologisch–Historische Klass; Folge 3, No. 138).

**India**

Emmerick RE: Contributions to the study of the 'Jivaka–pustaka'. **Bull Sch Orient Afr Stud** 1979;42:235–43
Joshi D: Concept of Rasa sala (pharmacy) in ancient India. **Nagarjun** 1978;22:88–90
Sharma PV: Fruits and vegetables in ancient India. Varanasi and Delhi, Chaukhambha Orientalia, 1979. xxvl, 188 p. (Jaikrishnadas Ayurveda Series, No. 28).

# PHARMACY

**Iran**

Yazdany S, Soltani A: The relationship between ancient Persia and Greece from medical point of view. In International Congress of the History of Medicine. 26th, Plovdiv, 1978. Actes du Congress. Sofia, 1981. Volume II. p. 114–5.

**Iraq**

Farber W: Drogerien in Babylonien und Assyrien. **Iraq** 1977;2:223–8

**Mesopotamia**

Valette G: Die pharmazeutische Lehre bei den mesopotamischen Völkern. In Sournia JC, Martiny M, Poulet J, ed: Illustrierte Geschichte der Medizin. Salzburg, Andreas, 1980. Vol. 2. p. 473–8.

**Rome**

Amberger G: Die Mulomedicina Chironis, ein Buch über Pferdeheilkunde aus dem 4. Jahrhundert n. Chr. **Ethnomedizin** 1978–79;5(3–4):233–61
Janiszewski J: Veterinärmedizin Catos des Aelteren. **Hist Med Vet** 1979;4(2):42–5
Stannard J: Medicinal plants and folk remedies in Pliny, Historia Naturalis. **Hist Philos Life Sci** 1982;4(1):3–23
Vidal F: La pharmacologie bucco–dentaire au temps d'Auguste. **Chir Dent Fr** 1983 Mar 10;53(194):21–30

**Sumer**

Meere J: Het eerste receptarium uit Sumer. **Farm Tijdschr Belg** 1979;56:265–6

**500 A.D.–1450**

Beya y Alonso E: Prescripciones medicas y sanitarias en la Regla de San Benito. **Bol Soc Esp Hist Farm** 1984;35(137):61–7
Escudero Mendo A, Sagrera JE de: El Rosario de los filósofos: una copia en castellano del siglo XIII (I). **Bol Soc Esp Hist Farm** 1983;34(136):151–66
Franke H: Materialien zur Arzneimittelgesetzgebung der Yüan–Zeit. **Asiat Forsch** 1980;71:22–9
Jordi González R: Fórmulas medicinales populares y supersticiosas pertenecientes a la primera mitad del siglo XV (1417–1459). **Circ Farm** 1981 Oct–Dec;39(273):469–82
Keil G, et al: Arzneibücher.––Arzneiformen.––Arzneimittelverfälschung. Arzt. In: Lexikon des Mittelalters. Munich. 1977. Bd 1. p. 1091–3.
Stannard J: Bibliographical references in medieval pharmaceutical writings. In: Vorträge des Internationalen Pharmaziehistorischen Kongresses Innsbruck 1977. Stuttgart, Wissenschaftliche Verlagsgesellschaft, 1979. p. 39–46.
Stannard J: '... findet man in den apotecken': Notices concerning the availability of medicamenta in medieval Fachliteratur. In Dilg P, et al., ed: Perspektiven der Pharmaziegeschichte. Graz, Austria, Akademische Druck- u. Verlagsanstalt, 1983. p. 365–76.

**Arabic**

Degen R: The Kitab al–Aghdhiya of Hunayn ibn Ishaq. In: International Symposium for the History of Arabic Science, 1st, University of Aleppo, 1976. Proceedings. Aleppo, Syria, 1976. Papers in European Languages, Vol. II. p. 291–9.
De Marco O, Nebbia G, Pizzoli Mazzacane EM: Ibn Jazla et les connaissances de l'Islam médiéval en sciences naturelles. **Rev Hist Pharm (Paris)** 1979 Dec;26(243):249–58
Folch Jou G: Medicamentos empleados por los árabes y su influencia en la farmacia de occidente en especial española. **Bol Soc Esp Hist Farm** 1979 Dec;30(120):319–35
Hamarneh SK: Al–Biruni, the father of Arabic pharmacy and marine biology as demonstrated in al–Saydanah. In: International Congress held in Pakistan on the occasion of Millenary of Abu Raihan Muhammad ibn Ahmad al–Biruni (973–ca 1051 A.D.) November 26, 1973 thru December 12, 1973. Proceedings. Karachi, Hamdard National Foundation, 1979. p. 479–500.
Hamarneh SK, Hamarneh NT: The physician–surgeon al–Zahrawi and the natural origins and manufacture of drugs. In A. R. El–Gindy, ed: Proceedings of the Second International Conference on Islamic Medicine. No. IV. Kuwait, Islamic Medicine Organization, 1982. (Bulletin of Islamic Medicine, v. 2). p. 375–82, 401–406.
Hein WH: Ein arabisches Apothekeninterieur vom Jahre 1222. **Pharm Ztg** 1979 Jan 4;124(1):3–4
Valverde JL, Munoz CP, ed: El Formulario de los hospitales De Ibn Abi L–bayan. Introduccion, traduccion espanola y commentarios, con glosarios. Granada, Universidad de Granada, 1981. 256 p. (Cuadernos de historia de la farmacia, 8).
Valverde JL, Peña–Muñoz C: Ibn al–Hassa: Glosario sobre el 'Mansuri' de Razi. **Ars Pharm** 1980;21:317–32

**Belgium**

Marganne MH: A propos du 'Médicinaire liégeois du XIIIe siècle' (manuscrit 815 de Darmstadt). 101. Congrès de Comines, 1, 1980. Actes. p. 348.

**Denmark**

Hauberg P: Laegebøger med tilknytning til Henrik Harpestraeng. **Theriaca** 1982 Jun;22:1–362

**France**

Dressendörfer W: Französische Apothekendarstellungen aus dem 13. Jahrhundert. **Beitr Gesch Pharm** 1980;31(8):57–61
Norwood FE, ed: The fourteenth–century medico–botanical glossary of Raimon de Castelnou. Leeds, W. S. Maney for the Leeds Philosophical and Literary Society, 1974. (Proceedings of the Leeds Philosophical and Literary Society, Literary and Historical Section, Vol. XV, Part VI, pp. 135–225).
Opsomer C: Les plantes exotiques du Livre des Simples Medecines de Lille. In: Congrès National des Sociétés Savantes, 101e, Lille, 1976. Comptes Rendus. Paris, 1976. Section des Sciences, Fasc. III. p. 33–44.
Vial F, Merlette B, Paris R, et al: Les recettes retenues par les Laonnois: observations médicales. **Hist Sci Med** 1980;14(1):61–9

**Germany**

Crossgrove W: Ein frühes Zeugnis für Ortolfs Arzneibuch. **Z Dtsch Altert Dtsch Lit** 1979;108:234–9
Daems WF, Keil G: Zum Ansehen des Apothekers im spätmittelalterlichen Deutschland. **Sudhoffs Arch** 1980;64(1):86–9
Dressendörfer W: Spätmittelalterliche Arzneitaxen des Münchner Stadtarztes Sigmund Gotzkircher aus dem Grazer Codex 311. Ein Beitrag zur Frühgeschichte des süddeutschen Apothekenwesens. Pattensen/Hannover, Wellm, 1978. 327 p. (Würzburger medizinhistorische Forschungen, 15). Also Diss. (Pharm) München.
Hils HP: Konrad der Münzmeister oder Konrad der Apotheker? Zur Analyse eines spätmittelalterlichen Pesttraktates. **Sudhoffs Arch** 1984;68(1):105–9
Keil G: Der 'Kodex Kohlhauer'. Ein iatromathematisch–hauswirtschaftliches Arzneibuch aus dem mittelalterlichen Oberfranken. I. Beschreibung der Handschrift. **Sudhoffs Arch** 1980;64(2):130–50
Keil G: Zur Frage der kurativ–konsiliarischen Tätigkeit des mittelalterlichen deutschen Apothekers. In Dilg P, et al., ed: Perspektiven der Pharmaziegeschichte. Graz, Austria, Akademische Druck- u. Verlagsanstalt, 1983. p. 181–96.
Kramer WG: Das vindt man in der Appentegg. . . **Beitr Gesch Pharm** 1980;31(5):38
Mueller I: Krankheit und Heilmittel im Werk Hildegards von Bingen. In: Hildegard von Bingen. Festschrift 1179–1979. [1979] pp. 311–349.
Ott–Voigtländer U: Das St. Georgener Rezeptar. Ein alemannisches Arzneibuch des 14. Jahrhunderts aus dem Karlsruher Kodex St. Georgen 73. Teil I: Text und Wörterverzeichnis. Pattensen/Han., Wellm, 1979. 140 p. (Würzburger medizinhistorische Forschungen, Band 17; also Diss., Würzburg).
Schipperges H: Barmherzigkeit als Heilmittel bei Hildegard von Bingen. In Ganzinger K, Skopec M, Wyklicky H, ed: Festschrift für Erna Lesky zum 70. Geburtstag. Wien, Brüder Hollinek, 1981. p. 97–103.

**Great Britain**

Matthews LG: The pepperers, spicers, and apothecaries of London during the thirteenth and fourteenth centuries. London, The Faculty of the History and Philosophy of Medicine and Pharmacy of the Society of Apothecaries of London, 1980. 64 p.
Voigts LE: British Library, Royal 12 D. XVII, f. 30v. **Old Engl Newsl** 1979 Fall;13(1):12–3

**Hungary**

Kadár Z, Vizkelety A: Zu den Pflanzen– und Tierdarstellungen in einem mittelalterlichen deutschen Kodex zu Debrecen (Ungarn). In Hein WH, ed: Pharmaziehistorischer Kongress, Budapest, 1981. Stuttgart, Wissenschaftliche Verlagsgesellschaft, 1983. p. 35–40.
Vida M: Ursprung und Deutung des Kosmas–Damian–Kultes in Ungarn (11.–14. Jahrhundert). In Hein WH, ed: Pharmaziehistorischer Kongress, Budapest, 1981. Stuttgart, Wissenschaftliche Verlagsgesellschaft, 1983. p. 23–33.
Zalai K: Medizin–pharmazeutische Erwähnungen in einem ungarischen Codex des XII. Jahrhunderts. **Acta Pharm Hung** 1980 Mar;50(2):87–95

**India**

Chauhan DK, Singh RN: Contribution of Medieval India to Ayurvedic Materia Medica. **Indian J Hist Sci** 1982;16(1):17–21

Sharma PV: Contributions of Sarngadhara in the field of materia medica and pharmacy. **Indian J Hist Sci** 1981, reçu 1982;16(1):3–10

Singh BN: Contribution of Madanapala Nighantu to the knowledge of Indian materia medica with particular reference to fig [Anjira] **Indian J Hist Sci** 1981, reçu 1982;16(1):89–94

Singh RS: Contribution of Unani materia medicas to the identification of Vedic plants with special reference to Usana. **Indian J Hist Sci** 1981, reçu 1982;16(1):41–6

**Italy**

Staccini R: L'inventario di una spezieria del Quattrocento. **Stud Mediev** 1981;22:377–420

**Netherlands**

Lindgren A: Das Utrechter Arzneibuch (Ms. 1355,16 degrees, Bibliotheek der Rijksuniversiteit Utrecht). Stockholm, Almqvist & Wiksell, 1977. 199 p. (Acta Universitatis Stockholmiensis, Stockholmer Germanistische Forschungen, 21)

**Portugal**

Sousa Dias JP: Problemas e perspectivas na historia das origens de farmacia em Portugal. **Farm Port** 1983 Jan–Feb;1::23–8

**Spain**

Beya Alonso E: Boticarios de Gerona en el siglo XV. **Bol Soc Esp Hist Farm** 1979 Dec;30(120):337–42

Folch Jou G: Medicamentos empleados por los árabes y su influencia en la farmacia de occidente en especial española. **Bol Soc Esp Hist Farm** 1979 Dec;30(120):319–35

Hussenot C: Sur un Erbier de Me Arnauld de Villeneuve (manuscrit médiéval). Thèse de doctorat, Université René-Descartes. Paris, 1983. 119 leaves. (U. E. R. des Sciences pharm. et biol. de Paris-Luxembourg, 1982–1983, no U 558).

Mendo AE, Sagrera JE de: El rosario de los filosofos: una copia en castellano del siglo XIII (II). **Bol Soc Esp Hist Farm** 1984;35(137):36–59

Sorní J, Suñé JM: La farmacia en Barcelona desde Jaume I a Jaume II (1213–1327). **Bol Soc Esp Hist Farm** 1983 Sep;135:59–68

Valverde JL, Alvarez C, Suñé JM: El primer 'Libro de botica' escrito en la España musulmana. **Bol Soc Esp Hist Farm** 1971 Jun;22(86):49–53

Vazquez C: Sobre la cosmetica (zina) del S. XIV en Al-Andalus. **Bol Soc Esp Hist Farm** 1982 Mar;33(129):9–48

**Switzerland**

Daems WF: Ermengald Blasius' Tabellen zum 'Antidotarium Nicolai'. **Pharm Acta Helv** 1979;54(4):101–5

**USSR**

Salukvadze SS: Starodavnia apteka Vardziï. **Farm Zh** 1979;(6):66–9

**1450–1700**

Alstermark H: Das Arzneibuch des Johan van Segen. Stockholm, Almquist & Wiksell, 1977. 174 p. (Acta Universitatis Stockholmiensis. Stockholmer germanistische Forschungen, 22)

Bosch K: Zur Vorgeschichte chemiatrischer Pharmakopöepräparate im 16./17. Jahrhundert. Braunschweig, 1980. 223 p. (Veröffentlichungen aus dem Pharmaziegeschichtlichen Seminar der Technischen Universität Braunschweig, 21).

Domandl S, ed: Paracelsus im Blickfeld heutiger wissenschaftsgeschichtlicher Betrachtung (ein Rundgespräch). Wien, 1974. 59 p. (Salzburger Beiträge zur Paracelsusforschung, 12). Contributions by L. Braun, A. W. Gutsch, V. Bazala, K. Goldammer, H. Goerke, W. Schneider, R. Blaser, KH Weimann, G. Harrer, A. Dyk.

Duka Zólyomi N: Ein ärztliches Vademecum der Aerztefamilie Ruland aus dem 16. Jahrhundert. **Sudhoffs Arch** 1977;61(3):281–97

Elferink JG: The significance of the pre-Columbian pharmaceutical knowledge for European medicine in the XVIth century. **Pharm Acta Helv** 1979;54(9–10):299–302

Fischer H: Der Streit um das Arzneimittel im Spiegel frühzeitlicher Antimonliteratur. **Beitr Gesch Pharm** 1983;31(18/19):150–4

Hils HP: Die Pestrezepte der Basler Handschrift D II 30. **Sudhoffs Arch** 1983;67(2):210–7

Jordi Gonzáles R: Curiosas formulas de medicina popular pertenecientes al ultimo cuarto del siglo XV. **Offarm** 1982;1(4):239–46

Kuźnicka B: The earliest printed herbals and evolution of pharmacy. **Organon** 1980/81;16–17:255–66

Le Traité de matière médicale de Dioscoride à la Renaissance: Exposition d'exemplaires des XVe et XVIe siecles. Du 11 au 24 février 1984 à Louvain-en-Woluwe à la Bibliothèque de la Faculté de Médecine de l'U.C.L. Louvain, Université Catholique de Louvain, Centre d'Histoire de la Pharmacie et du Médicament, 1984. 40 p.

Scheller, EF: Langlebigkeit mit Paracelsus-Arzneien: Versuch einer Geriatrie nach Paracelsus. Heidelberg, Haug, 1977. 150 p.

Schmitz R: Der Anteil des Renaissance-Humanismus an der Entwicklung von Arzneibüchern und Pharmakopöen. In F. Krafft, D. Wuttke, ed: Das Verhältnis der Humanisten zum Buch. (Deutsche Forschungsgemeinschaft, Kommission für Humanismusforschung, Mitteilung 4.) Boppard: Boldt, 1977.

Schmitz R: Pharmazie und angewandte Naturwissenschaften in ihrer Beziehung zum Renaissance-Humanismus. In: Humanismusforschung seit 1945. Ein Bericht aus interdisziplinärer Sicht. (Deutsche Forschungsgemeinschaft, Kommission für Humanismusforschung, Mitteilung 2.) Boppard, Boldt, 1975. p. 185–91, 215–6.

Schneider W: Arzneirezepte von Paracelsus. **Medizinhist J** 1981;16(1–2):151–66

Schneider W: Ein neuer Textbeleg vom Liber praeparationum. Wien, 1978. 51 p. (Salzburger Beiträge zur Paracelsusforschung, 19).

Vandewiele LJ: Een recept met gezegende distel uit Sint-Truiden anno 1456. **Pharm Weekbl** 1981 Nov 6;116(45):1406–8

**Americas**

Ehlers AP: Medizinisches und Pharmazeutisches in Bernal Diaz del Castillos, 'Historia verdadera de la conquista de la Nueva-España,' Madrid, 1632. Diss. Düsseldorf, 1980. 118 p.

**Asia**

Bowers JZ, Carrubba RW: Exotic antidotes in seventeenth century Asia: two assays from the Amoenitatum Exoticarum of Engelbert Kaempfer. **Clio Med** 1980 May;14(2):129–40

**Austria**

Huter F: Beiträge zur Geschichte des Apothekerwesens in Tirol: I. Kapitel: Die voruniversitäre Periode. **Tirol Heimat** 1978;41:5–43

**Belgium**

Toussaint R: Médicinaire du 17e siècle provenant d'Aywaille. **Enquetes Mus Vie Wallonne** [1980?];13:205–20

**Canada**

Garner J: Louis Hébert: his pharmaceutical skills helped Canada's first permanent settlement to survive. **Can Pharm J** 1982 Oct;115(10):380–1

**Denmark**

Vial G: Studien zum ersten altdeutschen Pferdearzneibuch des dänischen Lehnsmannes Mogens Sehestedt (1598–1657). Diss. Hannover, 1978. 272 p.

**France**

Bono JJ, Schmitt CB: An unknown letter of Jacques Daléchamps to Jean Fernel: local autonomy versus centralized government. **Bull Hist Med** 1979 Spring;53(1):100–27

De Backer C: Gérard d'Attenhoven, apothicaire liégois de la fin du XIVe siècle. **Rev Hist Pharm (Paris)** 1982 Jun;29(253):107–8

Rendinger C de: Un apothicaire du 'Grand Siècle', Claude Bourdelin (1621–1699), de l'Académie des Sciences, sa vie et les événements de son temps. **Bull Ordre Natl Pharm** 1980 Sep;236:1415–24

**Germany**

Dilg P: Examen pharmacopoeorum vulgare. Aus einer Handschrift des Laurentius Blumentrost d. A. (1619–1705). In Dilg P, et al., ed: Perspektiven der Pharmaziegeschichte. Graz, Austria, Akademische Druck- u. Verlagsanstalt, 1983. p. 39–64.

Dilg P: Vom Ansehen der Arzneikunst; historische Reflexionen in Kräuterbüchern des 16. Jahrhunderts. **Sudhoffs Arch** 1978;62(1):64–79

Dilg P: Zur Geschichte des 'alteren deutschen Apothekenwesens', XVI. Die Strassburger Apothekerordnung (um 1500). **Pharm Ztg** 1979;124:2664–70

Dressendörfer W: Drogeneinkaufsmengen einer Münchener Apotheke um die Mitte des 15. Jahrhunderts. Beiträge zur Geschichte des Arzneimittelhandels im Mittelalter. 1. Mitteilung. **Beitr Gesch Pharm** 1982;31(14):105–7

Głowacki WW: Ein verlorenes pharmazeutisches Wörterbuch des siebzehnten Jahrhunderts aus Schlesien. **Pharmazie** 1983 Nov;38(11):759–61

Klutz M: Die Rezepte in Oswald Crolls Basilica Chymica (1609) und ihre Beziehungen zu Paracelsus. Braunschweig, 1974. 124 p. (Veröffentlichungen aus dem Pharmaziegeschichtlichen Seminar der Technischen Universität Braunschweig, 14).

Kraft ES: Andreas Cleyer. In Balde JH, Schmiking W, ed: Festschrift zum 86. Deutschen Arztetag in Kassel. Kassel, Arztevereins, 1983.

p.40.
Lenz HG: Der hessische Paracelsist Johann Thoelde. **Salzburger Beitr Paracelsusforsch** 1984;23:89–99
Morys P: Medizin und Pharmazie in der Kosmologie Leonhard Thurneissers zum Thurn (1531–1596). Husum, Matthiesen, 1982. 179 p. (Abhandlungen zur Geschichte der Medizin und der Naturwissenschaften, 43).
Müller-Jahncke WD: Die 'Magnarum Medicine partium herbariae et zoographiae imagines' von Georg Ollinger und Samuel Quicchelberg. **Beitr Gesch Pharm** 1982;31(17):129–33
Vogel H: Fraunhofer-Wappen auf einem Apothekenmörser aus dem 17. Jahrhundert. **Dtsch Apoth Ztg** 1980;120:2065–7
Zimmermann A: Pharmazeutisches aus dem Nachlassinventar des Octavianus Secundus Fugger (1549-1600). **Beitr Gesch Pharm** 1981;31(12):89–91

**Great Britain**

Bonnabeau RC: The Royal College of Physicians and the apothecaries in the 17th century. A dispute for all seasons. **Minn Med** 1983 Sep;66(9):565–7
Burnby J: Three 17th century London apothecaries; Richard Meynell, Charles Needham, William Booker. **Pharm Hist (London)** 1975 May;5(1):2–3
Cook LG: A 17th century drug account. **Pharm Hist (London)** 1974 Jul;4(2):2–4
Earles MP: The Pharmacopoeia Londinenis 1618. A new look at an old problem. **Pharm Hist (London)** 1982 Aug;12(2):4–5
Guy JR: Doctor's recipe book? **Pharm Hist (London)** 1984;14(1):6–8
Herman JR: The compleat English physician: or, the druggist's shop opened. **Urology** 1983 Mar;21(3):277H, 300D
Jones DA: Nicholas Culpeper and his Pharmacopoeia. **Pharm Hist (London)** 1980 Aug;10(2):9–10
Martin L: John Crane (1571–1652); the Cambridge apothecary and philanthropist. **Med Hist** 1980;24(4):432–46
Monk BE: Thomas Dover, physician and pirate. **J R Coll Physicians Lond** 1982 Jan;16(1):60–1
O'Rourke DT: John Houghton (1645–1705) Journalist, apothecary and F.R.S. **Pharm Hist (London)** 1979 Apr;9(1):2–3
Pelling M: Apothecaries and other medical practitioners in Norwich around 1600. **Pharm Hist (London)** 1983 Jun;13(2):5–8
Rawlings FH: Two 17th century women apothecaries. **Pharm Hist (London)** 1984 Sep;14(3):7
Todd RG: Some drugs of the 17th century. **Pharm Hist (London)** 1980 Aug;10(2):10–12
Whittet TD: John Badger, apothecaryite. **Pharm Hist (London)** 1973 May;3(1):2–4
Whittet TD: Seen in west country. **Pharm Hist (London)** 1975 Aug;5(2):5–6
Whittet TD: Some Oxford apothecaries. **J R Soc Med** 1979 Dec;72(12):940–5

**Hungary**

Grabarits I: Der Arzneischatz des Herbariums von Melius. In Hein WH, ed: Pharmaziehistorischer Kongress, Budapest, 1981. Stuttgart, Wissenschaftliche Verlagsgesellschaft, 1983. p. 49–56.
Grynaeus T, Papp J: Régi magyar (gyógy) növénynevek mutatója, 15–17. század. **Orvostort Kozl** 1979;86(24 no 4):131–7

**Italy**

Caffaratto TM: Il Libro Lunghetto, ricettario del '600 dell'Ospedale Mauriziano di Torino. **Minerva Med** 1980 Apr 2;71(13):981–7
Fehringer WT: Studien zum altitalienischen Pferdearzneibuch des Carlo Bartolomeo Rinaldi (1655). Diss. Hannover, 1978, 247 p.
Hein WH: Sur le frontispice de la Pharmacopée de Milan de 1698. **Rev Hist Pharm (Paris)** 1982 Jun;29(253):87–90
Müller-Jahncke WD: Der 'latheinisch aussgestrichene Matthiolus' Landgraf Wilhelms IV von Hessen-Kassel und sein Schicksal. **Pharm Ztg** 1983 Feb 17;128(7):357–61
Palmer R: The influence of botanical research on pharmacists in sixteenth century Venice. **NTM** 1984;21(2):69–80
Rocchietta S: Le edizioni italiane del ricettario di Madame Fouquet. **Minerva Med** 1981 Jan 21;72(2):111–2
Russo A: Il 'Petitorium' del 1614: prima farmacopea a stampa nel Regno di Napoli. In Hickel E, Schröder G, ed: Neue Beiträge zur Arzneimittelgeschichte. Festschrift für Wolfgang Schneider zum 70. Geburtstag. Stuttgart, Wissenschaftliche Verlagsgesellschaft, 1982. p. 107–10.

**Mexico**

Comas J: Influencia de la farmacopea y terapéutica indígenas de Nueva España en la obra de Juan de Barrios (1607). **An Antropol** 1971;8:125–50

**Netherlands**

Hoppe B: Darstellung der Alchemie in Gemälden von Jan Brueghel d. A. (1568–1625). **Beitr Gesch Pharm** 1983;31(18/19):144–9
Van Lieburg MJ: De 'Materia Chirurgica' in de ordonnanties en examens der Noord-Nederlandse chirurgijnsgilden vóór 1600. **Pharm Weekbl** 1981;116(45):1393–8
Wittop Koning DA: Ein Niederlassungszettel des Chymisten Mattheus Rabs. In Hickel E, Schröder G, ed: Neue Beiträge zur Arzneimittelgeschichte. Festschrift für Wolfgang Schneider zum 70. Geburtstag. Stuttgart, Wissenschaftliche Verlagsgesellschaft, 1982. p. 47–58.

**Poland**

Drygas A: Walka z partactwem aptekarskim i medycznym. **Arch Hist Med (Warsz)** 1981;44(3/4):329–43
Roeske W: Lexicon Synonymorum Mineralo-Chymico-Pharmaceuticorum Trilingue Latino-Germano-Polonicum Collectum et Conscriptum a Johanne Stanko anno MCDLXXII (1472). In Hickel E, Schröder G, ed: Neue Beiträge zur Arzneimittelgeschichte. Festschrift für Wolfgang Schneider zum 70. Geburtstag. Stuttgart, Wissenschaftliche Verlagsgesellschaft, 1982. p. 29–39.
Szostak J: Scientia de simpliciis w pierwszych zielnikach polskich. **Arch Hist Med (Warsz)** 1980;43(3):265–87

**Portugal**

Falcao RF: A proposito do quarto centenario de publicão do 'Tratado de las drogas' de Cristóvão da Costa. **Rev Port Farm** 1980;30:234–44

**Saudi Arabia**

Faust E: Arabien 1680. Olfert Dappers Arabienbuch und seine Quellen, geprüft an Nachrichten über Kaffee, Sesam und Träumen. Köln, Universität zu Köln, 1977, 256 p. (Kölner medizinhistorische Beiträge, 5; also Diss).

**Spain**

Gago R, Olagüe G, Carrillo JL: Aportación al estudio del movimiento novator en España: el Laboratorio Químico del Palacio Real (1694) y la obra del boticario aragonés Juan del Bayle (fl. 1698). **Bol Soc Esp Hist Farm** 1981 Jun;32(126):95–107
Jordi R: Segundas nupcias de Catalina Barbara con Juan Vilarrubia. Inventario y Pacto. (3-10/ 3-11/ 11-11 de 1608). **Circ Farm** 1981 Aug-Sep;12(141-2)57-60, 56–66
Jordi González R: Duedas y cuentas de boticarios: una reivindicación histórica obligada. [Barcelona], Réal Academía de Farmacía de Barcelona, 1985. 63 p.
Jordi González R: Formulas de medicina popular y supersticiosa pertenecientes a la primera mitad del siglo XVI (1504–1568). **Circ Farm** 1983;281:283–309
Jordi González R: Inventario incompleto perteneciente a la botica del hospital de Santa Cruz, de Barcelona (21-1-1585). **Circ Farm** 1982 Apr–Jun;40(275):211–21
Jordi González R: Notas sobre boticarios y drogueros a finales del siglo XVI. Testigos en un pleito 1587–1589. In: Estudis històrics i documents dels arxius de protocols, VIII (1980). Barcelona, Col. Legi Notarial de Barcelona. 1980. p. 171–222.
Pla Dalmáu JM: La farmacia de Llivia. **Prensa Med Mex** 1979 Mar–Apr;44(3–4):75–9
Sanchez-Moscoso Hermida A: Distinción entre alimento y medicamento en un texto médico del siglo XVI. **Bol Soc Esp Hist Farm** 1980 Oct;31(123):151–90
Sánchez-Moscoso Hermida A: La peligrosidad del medicamento a través del 'Discurso Farmacéutico sobre los Cánones de Mesué', de Miguel Martínez de Leache (1652). **Bol Soc Esp Hist Farm** 1984 Jun;35(138):103–23
Sanchez Tellez MC, Guerra F, Valverde JL: La doctrina farmacéutica del Renacimiento en la obra de Francisco Hernández, c. 1515–1587. Granada, Universidad de Granada, Hospital Real, 1979. 140 p. (Estudios del Departamento de Historia de la Farmacia y Legislación Farmacéutica, Universidad de Granada, 6).
Suñé JM, ed: Pharmacopea cathalana sive antidotarium barcinonense. (Edición Facsímil). Barcelona, Catedra de Historia de la Farmacia y Legislacion Farmaceutica, Universidad de Barcelona, 1975. Various paginations.

**Sweden**

Modig M: Pharmacy ruins from 1600's excavated in Stockholm. **Pharm Hist** 1983;25(3):137–41

**Switzerland**

Blaser RH: Paracelsus und die Basler Apotheker. **Pharm Acta Helv**

1979;54(9-10):281-5

Brunner-Wildisen B: Medizinisches aus den Schriften des Renward Cysat, 1545-1614. Zürich, Juris, 1980. 75 p. (Zürcher Medizingeschichtliche Abhandlungen, Neue Reihe, Nr. 138).

Gilly C: Zwischen Erfahrung und Spekulation. Theodor Zwinger und die religiöse und kulturelle Krise seiner Zeit. **Basler Z Gesch Altertumskd** 1977;77:57-137

Goldammer K: Zur philosophischen und religiösen Sinngebung von Heilung und Heilmittel bei Paracelsus. In Dilg P, et al., ed: Perspektiven der Pharmaziegeschichte. Graz, Austria, Akademische Druck- u. Verlagsanstalt, 1983. p. 113-29.

Jaeschke G, Diesbachs A von: Berner 'Arzneibüchlein' in der Erlacher Fassung Daniel von Werdts (1658). Teil I: Text. Pattensen/Han., Wellm, 1978. 180 p. (Würzburger medizinhistorische Forschungen, Band 16).

Rocchietta S: Sulle edizioni degli 'Antidotari' e di altre opere di J.-J. Wecker. **Minerva Med** 1981 Sep 19;72(34):2297

Schneider W: Das Lot-Gewicht bei Paracelsus. In Dilg P, et al., ed: Perspektiven der Pharmaziegeschichte. Graz, Austria, Akademische Druck- u. Verlagsanstalt, 1983. p. 325-30.

**USSR**

Appleby JH: Ivan the Terrible to Peter the Great: British formative influence on Russia's medico-Apothecary system. **Med Hist** 1983 Jul;27(3):289-304

## 1700 to Present

Artiges A: L'institution de la Pharmacopée Européenne: un bilan à l'issue de la première édition. **Inf Pharm** 1980 Apr;(232):506-44

Cowen DL: A note on pharmaceutical literature and the introduction of the new chemical nomenclature. **Beitr Gesch Pharm** 1981;11:84-5

Cowen DL, King LD, Lordi NG: Drug use in the 19th century: a computer analysis. In Hickel E, Schröder G, ed: Neue Beiträge zur Arzneimittelgeschichte. Festschrift für Wolfgang Schneider zum 70. Geburtstag. Stuttgart, Wissenschaftliche Verlagsgesellschaft, 1982. p. 59-67.

Cowen DL: Pharmacy and freedom. **Pharm Hist** 1984;26(2):70-82

Cowen DL: The influence of the Edinburgh Pharmacopoeia and the Edinburgh Dispensatories. **Pharm Hist (London)** 1982;12(3):2-4

Crellin JK, Helfand W: Picture postcards; a resource for social history of pharmacy. **Pharm Hist** 1983;25(3):116-30

Ganzinger K: Zur Geschichte der chemischen Nomenklatur in den amtlichen Arzneibüchern. **Beitr Gesch Pharm** 1980;31(5):33-7

Gheorghiu E: Opinions on old pharmacopeias integration into modern therapy. **Sante Publique (Bucur)** 1984;27(1):83-8

Götz W: Die Briefe Jacques Peschiers aus Genf an Joh. Barth. Trommsdorff, Erfurt, als Beispiel für internationale pharmazeutische Kontakte zu Beginn des 19. Jahrhunderts. **Pharm Acta Helv** 1979;54(9-10):303-7

Götz W: J. B. Trommsdorffs 'Chemische Receptirkunst'. Bisher unbekannte Übersetzungen und Ausgaben. **Beitr Gesch Pharm** 1982;31(14):107-10

Haller JS: Opposition to compressed tablets in 19th and early 20th century medicine. **NY State J Med** 1984 Nov;84(11):554-8

Haller JS: With a spoonful of sugar. The art of prescription writing in the late 19th and early 20th century. **Pharm Hist** 1984;26(4):171-8

Helfand WH, Crellin JK: The pharmacy in comic postcards. **Pharm Hist** 1981;23(3):107-13

Hickel E: 1848 und 1871 als Epochen in der Entwicklung des modernen Arzneimittelbegriffs. In Hickel E, Schröder G, ed: Neue Beiträge zur Arzneimittelgeschichte. Festschrift für Wolfgang Schneider zum 70. Geburtstag. Stuttgart, Wissenschaftliche Verlagsgesellschaft, 1982. p. 281-5.

Jordi R: De los sabios de ayer al 'bichito' de hoy. **Periodico** 1981 Sep 5;4:883

Julien P: Médailles modernes à sujet pharmaceutique et médical. **Rev Hist Pharm (Paris)** 1980 Mar;27(244):39-47

Julien P: Sur le célèbre 'dentiste' ou 'pharmacien' de Pietro Longhi. **Pharm Weekbl** 1981 Nov 6;116(45):1389-92

King LS: The British background for American medicine. **JAMA** 1982 Jul 9;248(2).217-20

Koning A: Die Pharmazie in der holländischen politischen Karikatur. **Pharm Acta Helv** 1979;54(9-10):308-10

Kotwas J, Meyer-Wilmes J, Ohlendorf D, ed: Pharmazie und Medizin--Grenzen und Möglichkeiten. Verhandlungsbericht über eine Internationale Tagung der Arbeitsgemeinschaft Deutscher Krankenhausapotheker in Zusammenarbeit mit der Bayerischen Internistenvereinigung München, 18.-19.April 1980. Berlin, Acron, 1981. 152 p. Contributions by R. Winau, D. Ohlendorf, A.G. Hildebrandt, W. Weissauer, R. Quintiliani, D.D. Breimer, R. Preisig, T. Zysset, D. Adam, H. Remmer, G. Dirheimer, K.H. Beyer, H.P.T. Ammon.

Krafft M: Die anthroposophische Heilmittellehre und ihre geistesgeschichtliche Beziehung zu Heilmittelkonzepten. des 19. Jahrhunderts. Stuttgart, Deutscher Apotheker Verlag, 1984. 210 p. (Quellen und Studien zur Geschichte der Pharmazie, Bd. 27).

Ledermann F: El precio de los medicamentos en el canton de Neuchatel y en Suiza: 1930-1960. **Bol Soc Esp Hist Farm** 1982 Sep;33(131):163-72

Ledermann F: Faire de l'histoire de la pharmacie: pourquoi, comment? Quelques éléments historiographiques et théoriques en guise d'apologie. **Pharm Acta Helv** 1984;59(4):118-28

Ligterink JH: De apotheker en de zelfmedicatie. **Pharm Weekbl** 1981 Nov 6;116(45):1398-1400

Löhr HG: Ein Vierteljahrhundert gemeinsamen Weges von Karl Marx und Friedrich Engels mit ihrem treuen Freund und Kampfgefährten Carl Schorlemmer. **Pharmazie** 1983 Nov;38(11):768-72

Mitteilung zur Tschirch Biographie: **Schweiz Apoth Ztg** 1979;117:558 (continued irregularly here and in Pharm. Ztg, Dtsch Apoth Ztg, and Oesterr. Apoth Ztg)

Niemi SM: Early veterinary biologics. **Mod Vet Pract** 1980 Nov;61(11):926-9

Peeters A: Pharmacopées et médecines traditionnelles: un exemple d'abus de langage. **J Agric Tradit Bot Appl** 1982;29(1):97-100

Pollay RW: Pills, potions and palliatives: some of the social history of drug usage. **Hist Med (Lond)** 1975 Autumn-Winter;6(3-4):58-63

Scarpa A: Pre-scientific medicines: their extent and value. **Soc Sci Med** 1981 May;15A(3):317-26

Schröder G: Die 'Wiedergeburt' der Pharmazie - 1933 bis 1934. In: Naturwissenschaft, Technik und NS-Ideologie. Frankfurt a.M.: Suhrkamp 1980 (stw 303). pp 166-88.

Spiers CH: The drug suppliers of George Washington and other Virginians. **Pharm Hist (London)** 1977 Mar;7(1):2-3

Wade A: 'Martindale'. The International Use of 'Martindale: the Extra Pharmacopoeia'. **Farm Tid** 1979 Dec 1;89(48):1001-4

Wankmüller A: Hinweise zur Literatur für die Pharmaziegeschichte. **Beitr Gesch Pharm** 1982;31(14):110-1

Whorton J: 'Thialion!!!' Anatomy of a pseudo-ethical proprietary. **Pharm Hist** 1981;23(3):114-25

Woods D: Roche: blending independent and commercial research. **Can Med Assoc J** 1983 Oct 1;129(7):743-52

Zuring J: Saint Côme et Saint Damien dans la philatélie. **Rev Hist Pharm (Paris)** 1984 Mar;31(260):69-72

**Africa**

Slotow M: The opening up of Africa. **S Afr Med J** 1981 Oct 3;60(14):557-8

Valverde JL, Arrebola Nacle P: Los servicios farmacéuticos des los presidios menores de Africa. In International Congress of the History of Medicine, 27th, Barcelona, 1980. Actas. Barcelona, Académia de Ciències Médiques de Catalunya i Balears, 1981. p. 644-9.

**Algeria**

Ait Khaled N, Oussedik N, Chaulet P: Evolution du coût des médicaments antituberculeux de 1964 à 1980; son influence dans le choix d'une politique de traitement de la tuberculose en Algérie. **Bull Int Union Tuberc** 1981 Sep-Dec;56(3-4):170-4

**Americas**

Kay MA: The Florilegio Medicinal: source of Southwest ethnomedicine. **Ethnohistory** 1977;24(3):251-9

Rosengarten F: A neglected Mayan galactagogue--ixbut (Euphorbia lancifolia). **J Ethnopharmacol** 1982 Jan;5(1):91-112

Whittet TD: Two restored historical pharmacies. **Pharm Hist (London)** 1974 Jan;4(1):6

Wisswaesser C: Roots and ramifications of medicinal herbs in eighteenth-century North America. **Trans Stud Coll Physicians Phila** 1977 Apr;44(4):194-9

**Argentina**

Muestra en homenaje a los doctores Miguel Puiggari y Miguel Puiggari (h.): **Publ Mus Farm** 1983 Jul-Sep;2(7-9):1-13

**Asia**

Solomon R, Barlow T, Kostal R: The opiate trade of Taiwan and Japan: an historical note. **J Psychoactive Drugs** 1981 Jan-Mar;13(1):35-8

**Australia**

Griffenhagen G: Pharmacy centennials in Australia and New Zealand. **Scalpel Tongs** 1981;25:75

**Austria**

Ganzinger K: Die 'Oesterreichische pharmazeutische Gesellschaft' 1873 bis 1938. **Osterr Apoth Ztg** 1980;34:3-6

Ganzinger K: Naturwissenschaften und Pharmazie unter Maria Theresia und Joseph II. **Osterr Apoth Ztg** 1980;34:361-5

Grabner E: Zwischen Wunderbuch und Rezeptbuchweisheit. Zum Aussagewert eines handschriftlichen burgenländischen Arzneibuches aus der ersten Hälfte des 19. Jahrhunderts. **Ethnomedizin** 1978-79;5(1-2):25-43

# PHARMACY

Nowotny O: Hans Heger und seine Bedeutung für die Geschichte der Pharmazie in Oesterreich. In: Vorträge des Internationalen Pharmaziehistorischen Kongresses Innsbruck 1977. Stuttgart, Wissenschaftliche Verlagsgesellschaft, 1979. p. 147-52.

**Belgium**

Cultures industrielles au pays des collines: plantes médicinales, chicorée, tabac (1890-1914): Ath [Belgium], 1982. 146 p.
Vandewiele LJ: De realisaties van de Belgische apotekers in de 19e eeuw. **Sartonia** 1979 Mar;42:16-44

**Brazil**

Massa F: Alexandre Brethel, pharmacien et planteur au Carangolo: recherche sur sa correspondence brésilienne (1862-1901). Rennes, Université de Haute-Bretagne, Institut Armoricain de recherches économiques et humaines de Rennes, 1977. v, 462 p.

**Bulgaria**

Bakalova L, Draganova T: Stomatologichni retsepti vuv vuzrozhdenski lekarstven spravochnik ot 1870 g. **Stomatologiia (Sofiia)** 1979;(3):203-6

**Canada**

Bell SK: Plus ça change, plus c'est la même chose: CPhA 1907-1982. **Can Pharm J** 1982 Oct;115(10):367-8
Birchall S: A disowned apothecary. **Pharm Hist (London)** 1984 Sep;14(3):8
Desjardins E: Jacques Dénéchaud. In Dictionary of Canadian biography, 1801 to 1820. Volume 5, 1983. p. 248-9.
Hiller JK: John Joseph Dearin. In Dictionary of Canadian biography, 1881-1890. 1982;11:239-40.
Janson G: Charles Blake. In Dictionary of Canadian biography, 1801 to 1820. Volume 5, 1983. p. 88-9.
Kernaghan LK: Duncan Clark. In Dictionary of Canadian biography, 1801 to 1820. Volume 5, 1983. p. 187-8.
Kernaghan LK: William James Almon. In Dictionary of Canadian biography, 1801 to 1820. Volume 5, 1983. p. 23-4.
Larose R: The growth and development of the pharmaceutical industry in Montreal. **Can Pharm J** 1984;117:74-7
Morin J: Liveright Piuze. In Dictionary of Canadian biography, 1801 to 1820. Volume 5, 1983. p. 676.
Stieb EW: Some branches of Canadian pharmacy's family tree--how they sprouted and grew. **Can Pharm J** 1982 Oct;115(10):374-9
Wilson E: How pharmacy developed in the shadow of Parliament Hill. **Can Pharm J** 1982 Oct;115(10):369-73

**Chile**

Presentación de José Vicente Bustillos. Una paradoja?: **Rev Med Chil** 1983 Oct;111(10):1075-84
Valdivieso R: La ley de medicina curativa para empleados y el Formulario Nacional de Medicamentos. **Rev Med Chil** 1977 Oct;105(10):663-7

**China**

Sági E: A kinai gyógyszerészet a századfordulón. Diss., Budapest, 1979. 130 p.
VanderKuijp LW: An index to Tibeto-Mongolian Materia Medica. **Can-Mong Rev** 1975;1(2):15-46

**Czechoslovakia**

Bartunek A, Petrociová O: Vzájomné vztahy medzi levočským a prešovským lekárenstvom v 17. až 19. storočí. **Cesk Farm** 1984 Sep;33(7):308-11
Cižmář J: Botanist Carl Theimer (1823--1870) in the cultural context of Brno during the period of Mendel's research. **Folia Mendeliana** 1979;14:265-70
Cižmář J: Závodní časopisy Mediky. **Cesk Farm** 1982 Dec;31(10):393-5
Drábek P: Casopis českého lékárnictva a jeho předchudci. **Cesk Farm** 1982 May;31(3-4)85-96
Fürst L: O Březnické lékárně a lékárnících. **Cesk Farm** 1979 Mar;28(2):82-7
Hanzlíček Z: Ostatní České farmaceutické časopisy. (Příspěvek k dějinám českého farmaceutického periodického tisku). **Cesk Farm** 1982 Dec;31(10):384-92
Hanzlíček Z: Redaktoři Casopisu českého lékárnictva. **Cesk Farm** 1982 May;31(3-4):97-109
Hanzlíček Z: Sto let českých farmaceutických časpisu. **Cesk Farm** 1982 May;31(3-4):83-4
Hošek E: Dr. phil. PhMr. Ferdinand Daubrawa, světlý zjev mezi lékárníky Moravského venkova v l9. století. **Cesk Farm** 1979 Jun;28(5):223-4
Majtás J: K dialektike zmien profesnej štruktúry vo vývine farmaceutického profesionalizmu. **Cesk Zdrav** 1984 Jan;32(1):18-22
Santavý F: Prof. Dr. chem. PhMr. Martin Ehrmann a jeho pusobení na medicínskochirurgickém učilišti v Olomouci v letech 1836--1866. **Cesk Farm** 1979 Jun;28(5):221-2
Tomiček F, Křepelka J, Beran M: In memoriam Doc. Dr. Ing. M. Semonského, DrSc. **Cesk Farm** 1979 Dec;28(9-10):362-6
Vignati J: Návrh na zřizení farmakologických oddělení u větších nemocnic. **Cas Lek Cesk** 1982 Dec 23;121(51):1590-1
Votavová J: Prof. PhDr. PhMr. O. Tomíček a jeho analytická škola. **Cesk Farm** 1984 Jun;33(5):213-4

**Denmark**

Jensen VG: Poul Richard Hauberg, 1887-1959. **Theriaca** 1982 Jun;22:xi-xvi
Schaeffer A, Kruse E: Danske farmacihistoriske arbejder efter året 1800. En kortfattet oversigt med bibliografi. 2. ed. København, Dansk Farmacihistorisk Selskab, 1982. 229 p.

**Egypt**

Estes JW, Kuhnke L: French observations of disease and drug use in late eighteenth-century Cairo. **J Hist Med Allied Sci** 1984 Apr;39(2):121-52

**El Salvador**

Ferguson AE: Commercial pharmaceutical medicine and medicalization: a case study from El Salvador. **Cult Med Psychiatry** 1981 Jun;5(2):105-34

**Europe**

Wysoki'nski A, Strużak-Wysokińska M: Ocena rozwoju stanu osobowego kadry farmaceutów w Europie w latach 1961-1975. **Wiad Lek** 1980 Mar 1;33(5):409-14

**France**

Aharonowitz Y, Cohen G: Les micro-organismes et l'industrie pharmaceutique. **Pour Sci** 1981;49:92-105
Aiache JM, Dussaud MD: Ordonnancier et préparations magistrales de 1906 à 1960. **Rev Hist Pharm (Paris)** 1984 Jun;31(261):151-7
Bachoffner P: Vulgarisation thérapeutique à travers la 'Materia Medica' de Georges-Henri Behr, médecin strasbourgeois. In Livet G, Schaff G, ed: Médecine et assistance en Alsace, XVIe-XXe siècle. Strasbourg, Istra, 1976. p. 145-53.
Berman A: An unpublished letter from Eugene Soubeiran to Antoine Portal, June 3, 1828. **Pharm Hist** 1982;24(1):32-7
Bonnemain H: Un recueil de recettes 'éprouvées'. **Rev Hist Pharm (Paris)** 1982;29(252):160-4
Bonnemain H: Une famille médico-pharmaceutique: les Augiéras-Bernou. **Rev Hist Pharm (Paris)** 1981;28(248):14-20
Bordes F: Le livre des remèdes de Labadie. Contribution à l'histoire de la médecine populaire landaise au XVIIIe siècle. **Bull Soc Borda** 1982;107(387):399-412
Bouquet A: Note sur la pharmacopée traditionnelle d'une province française. **Rev Hist Pharm (Paris)** 1981 Jun;28(249):100-2
Bouriez J: Lens, trois savants oubliés: Auguste Behal, Amand Valeur, Raymond Delaby. [France], Société de recherches historiques de la région d'Henin-Carvin, [1981] 69 leaves.
Boussel P: Dorvault, sa vie et son oeuvre. Honfleur [France], Editions de la porte verte, 1979. 301 p.
Burke JT: Bref historique de la pharmacovigilance du maléate de perhexiline. **Therapie** 1981 May-Jun;36(3):279-80
Chabbert P: Maxence Audouard (1776-1856). In: Congrès National des Sociétés Savantes, 96e, Toulouse, 1971. Comptes Rendus. Paris, 1974. Histoire des Sciences, Tome 1. p. 83-97.
Chaigneau M: Christophe-Augustin Lamare-Picquot, pharmacien, naturaliste, explorateur. **Rev Hist Pharm (Paris)** 1982 Mar;29(252):5-26
Chalbert P: Une lignée d'apothicaires et de pharmaciens languedociens: les Audouard, d'Agde, Béziers et Castres. **Rev Hist Pharm (Paris)** 1980 Sep;27(246):175-88
Cluchard J: Quelques aspects de la vie sociale des apothicaires bordelais au XVIIIe siècle. Thèse. Bordeaux, 1982. in various pagings.
Cotereau Y: L''Officine' de Dorvault. **Rev Hist Pharm (Paris)** 1980 Jun;27(245):95-107
Courtois JE: Le pharmacien Jacques Personne (1816-1880) pionnier de la chimie analytique. **Rev Hist Pharm (Paris)** 1980 Dec;247(68 no 27):263-71
Darquenne R: Remous autour de la Pharmacopée Montoise (1755). **Mem Publ Soc Sci Arts Lett Hainaut** 1981-82;92:169-201
Delaby PA: Le doyen Guillaume Valette (1902-1982). **Hist Sci Med** 1982;16(2):65-79
Delaby PA: Une 'marmotte' de pâtes et pastilles selon le Codex de 1908 **Rev Hist Pharm (Paris)** 1983 Sep;30(258):191-8
Delaveau P: Sur le 'registre pour l'inscription des poisons' d'un pharmacien tourangeau (1833-1841). **Rev Hist Pharm (Paris)** 1984 Jun;31(261):144-50
Delaveau P, Paris RR, Clair G: The Museum of Materia Medica of Paris. **Pharm Hist** 1984;26(3):143-5
Deutsch Delanoy G: Quelques ephemera des cent ans écoulés. **Rev Hist Pharm (Paris)** 1980 Sep;27(246):189-98
Deutsch-Delanoy G: Un catalogue de la 'Pharmacie Universelle', à Paris,

vers 1900. **Rev Hist Pharm (Paris)** 1982 Mar;29(252):31–6
Dillemann G, Michel ME: La réception des pharmaciens en France de la Révolution à l'application de la loi du 21 germinal an XI (1791–1813). **Rev Hist Pharm (Paris)** 1984;31(260):42–61
Dillemann G: Le Doyen Guillaume Valette (1902–1982). **Rev Hist Pharm (Paris)** 1982 Jun;29(253):83–6
Dillemann G: Les cumuls d'emplois en 1821. **Rev Hist Pharm (Paris)** 1981 Jun;28(249):109–11
Duquénois P: Devenir des plantes médicinales et des médications végétales aux XVIIIe et XIXe siècles sous l'influence de la chimie moderne. In Livet G, Schaff G, ed: Médecine et assistance en Alsace, XVIe–XXe siècle. Strasbourg, Istra, 1976. p. 227–39.
Flahaut S: Le pharmacien Charles-Louis Cadet de Gassicourt, bâtard de Louis XV, et sa famille. **Rev Hist Pharm (Paris)** 1980 Mar;27(244):53–61
Gagnière S, Julien P: Panneaux peints de la pharmacie de l'hôpital de Valréas. **Rev Hist Pharm (Paris)** 1981;28(248):21–4
Gaignault JC: Alfred Houdé. Un bel exemple de fondateur d'une industrie pharmaceutique française au XIXe siècle. **Bull Ordre Natl Pharm** 1980 Dec;239:1816–26
Granger R: Histoire de la chimie organique à la Faculté de Pharmacie de Montpellier. **Trav Soc Pharm Montp** 1978;38:301–8
Grass U: Zu Leben und Werk von Jakob Reinbold Spielmann (1722–1783). Stuttgart, Deutscher Apotheker, 1983. 254 p. (Quellen und Studien zur Geschichte der Pharmazie, Bd. 20).
Griffenhagen G: Drug and underprints from France. [Laboratoire Veyron-Froment, Marseilles.] **Scalpel Tongs** 1981;25:61–3
Guesdon C: Contribution à l'étude de l'évolution de la pharmacie rouennaise: les différents titulaires d'une officine rue du Gros-Horloge. Thèse Dipl. d'Etat Dr. en Pharm., Université Rouen. Rouen, 1982. 65 (13) leaves.
Hossard J: Une rencontre inattendue: Flaubert et Dorvault. **Rev Hist Pharm (Paris)** 1980 Jun;27(245):119–22
Julien P: La France envahie par Hunyadi János. In Hein WH, ed: Pharmaziehistorischer Kongress, Budapest, 1981. Stuttgart, Wissenschaftliche Verlagsgesellschaft, 1983. p. 111–28.
Julien P: Le Dr. Véron et Daumier, ou le fabricant de pâté pectorale en proie à la caricature. In: Congrès international d'histoire de la médecine, XXVe, Québec, 1976. Actes. Québec, 1977. p. 807–21.
Julien P: Le lunch des 12 millions. **Rev Hist Pharm (Paris)** 1980 Jun;27(245):91–3
Julien P: Les apothicaires et autres vendeurs de médicaments de la rue Dauphine, à Paris, dans la seconde moitié du XVIIIe siècle, et l'importation de produits pharmaceutiques. In Dilg P, et al., ed: Perspektiven der Pharmaziegeschichte. Graz, Austria, Akademische Druck- u. Verlagsanstalt, 1983. p. 165–79.
Julien P: Les 'Eléments de pharmacie' de Baumé et la contrefaçon. **Rev Hist Pharm (Paris)** 1981 Jun;28(249):103–6
Julien P: Remarque sur l'édition 1936 de 'l'Officine' de Dorvault. **Rev Hist Pharm (Paris)** 1982 Mar;29(252):37–8
Julien P: Trois expositions. **Rev Hist Pharm (Paris)** 1980 Dec;247(68 no 27):272–6
Julien P: Un empire industriel issu d'une droguerie pharmaceutique. **Rev Hist Pharm (Paris)** 1982 Sep;29(254):180–2
Kalis F: Albert Leulier (1883–1957): a l'occasion du centenaire de sa naissance. Thèse, Univ. Claude-Bernard-Lyon I, U.E.R. de Pharm., 1983. 98 leaves.
Labrude P: Albin Haller 1849–1925 pharmacien et chimiste. **Rev Hist Pharm (Paris)** 1982 Sep;29(254):207–9
Ledermann F: La psychiatrie française et les médicaments: Pomme, Pinel, Esquirol, Morel. **Rev Hist Pharm (Paris)** 1982 Sep;29(254):189–206
Lemoine P: Une entreprise de répartition: l'Office Commercial Pharmaceutique de ses origines (1840) à 1965. **Rev Hist Pharm (Paris)** 1983 Mar;30(256):5–29
Marc JC: Pharmaciens de la Marine et voyages de découvertes en océanie au XIXe siècle. In: Congrès National des Sociétés Savantes, 104e, Bordeaux, 1979. Comptes Rendus. Paris, 1979. Section des Sciences, Fasc. IV. p. 193–204.
Monod T, Hureau JC: Un pharmacien niçois, Antoine Risso (1777–1845), sa vie et son oeuvre. In their: Antoine Risso, 1777–1845. Nice, Editions du Centre d'Etudes Méditerranéennes, 1977. pp. 9–28 (Annales du Muséum d'Histoire Naturelle de Nice, V, 1977).
Mory B: Dorvault et la 'Pharmacie centrale de France.' **Rev Hist Pharm (Paris)** 1980 Jun;27(245):79–90
Nauroy J: Les historiographes de la pharmacie militaire française. In: Vorträge des Internationalen Pharmaziehistorischen Kongresses Innsbruck 1977. Stuttgart, Wissenschaftliche Verlagsgesellschaft, 1979. p. 91–6.
Nauroy J, Bossard E: Louis-Marie Gessard, pharmacien et édile de Saint-Denis. **Rev Hist Pharm (Paris)** 1979 Dec;26(243):235–9
Nauroy J: Une pharmacienne confrontée malgré elle à la conspiration de Malet. **Rev Hist Pharm (Paris)** 1984 Mar;31(260):18–20
Nonclercq M: A. Béchamp, un' ingiustizia nella storia delle scienze. **Empedocle** 1983 Sep–Oct;1(1):39–49
Nonclercq M: Antoine Béchamp 1816–1908: l'homme et le savant originalité et fécondité de son oeuvre. Preface et note documentaire par le Docteur Philippe Decourt. Paris, Maloine, 1982. 249 p.
Pougetoux G: Contribution a l'etude de l'histoire de la pharmacie en correze au XIXème siècle. Thèse. Bordeaux, Unitersité de Bordeaux II, 1984. 226 p.
Ridolphi N: Création des pharmacies en Alsace (1870–1938). Mémoire de diplôme d'Etat de docteur en pharmacie, Université Louis-Pasteur, Strasbourg, 1983. 91 leaves.
Rocchietta S: Medici e speziali in tre romanzi de Voltaire. **Minerva Med** 1982 Feb 11;73(5):219–20
Saumande P: La vie d'un pharmacien limousin à la fin du XIXe siècle d'après les documents d'archives de son officine. **Rev Hist Pharm (Paris)** 1982 Jun;29(253):91–4
Sigvard J: Cent ans de vie syndicale dans l'industrie pharmaceutique en France, 1880–1980. **Rev Hist Pharm (Paris)** 1982 Jun;29(253):115–23
Sigvard J: L'industrie du médicament en France: quelques points d'histoire. **Bull Acad Natl Med (Paris)** 1982 Jun;166(6):829–34
Smeaton WA: Pharmacy in Revolutionary and Napoleonic Paris, 1789–1815. **Pharm Hist (London)** 1979 Apr;9(1):4–5
Thuillier G: Pour une histoire du médicament en Nivernais, au XIXe siècle. **Rev Hist Econ Soc** 1975;53:73–98
Une lettre de Louis Jouvet à la veille d'entreprendre ses études de pharmacie: **Rev Hist Pharm (Paris)** 1981 Jun;28(249):121–4
Valette S: L'histoire de la pharmacie en France au XIXe siécle. In: Vorträge des Internationalen Pharmaziehistorischen Kongresses Innsbruck 1977. Stuttgart, Wissenschaftliche Verlagsgesellschaft, 1979. p. 73–80.
Vidal F: Les drogues tirées du corps de l'homme dans la matière médicale du XVIIIe siècle. **Chir Dent Fr** 1983 Dec 15–22;53(229–230):49–52
Vidal F: Les drogues tirées du corps des animaux dans la matière médicale du XVIIIe siècle. **Chir Dent Fr** 1984 Feb 2;54(235):21–9
Viel C: Quelques vers et écrits de jeunesse d'Henri Moissan. **Rev Hist Pharm (Paris)** 1984 Mar;31(260):5–12

**Germany**

Abe HR: Zum Leben und Werk bedeutender Thüringischer Apotheker. **Pharmazie** 1981 Jun;36(6):435–7
Bartels K: Ein vielseitiger Apotheker der ersten Hälfte des 19. Jahrhunderts: Anselm Franz Strauss. **Beitr Gesch Pharm** 1979;31(4):26–30
Barthel I: Arzneimittelversuche des 19.Jahrhunderts am gesunden Menschen im deutschsprachigen Raum. Diss., Universität Düsseldorf. Düsseldorf, 1982. 105 p.
Bayer FW: Der Merck'sche Jahresbericht als Quelle zur Geschichte der Therapie. **Pharm Ind** 1980;42(7):701–6
Berges PH: Goldene Zwanziger? Not der Krankenkassen und Arzneimittelsubstitution. **Beitr Gesch Pharm** 1983;31(18/19):155–9
Blum W: Der Apotheker und Chemiker Otto A. Ziurek (1821–1886) und die Apothekenreformbewegung von 1848. Braunschweig, 1980. 110 p. (Veröffentlichungen aus dem Pharmaziegeschichtlichen Seminar der Technischen Universität Braunschweig, 22).
Engels W: Zur Geschichte des Verstaatlichungsgedankens im deutschen Apothekenwesen. Stuttgart, Deutscher Apotheker Verlag, 1984. 261 p. (Quellen und Studien zur Geschichte der Pharmazie, Bd. 28).
Fehlmann HR: 'Herrn Adams äusseres Augenmittel.' Eine Frankfurter Merkwürdigkeit aus dem Jahre 1794. **Pharm Ztg** 1980;125:407–8
Friedrich C, Seidlein HJ: Beiträge zur Geschichte der Pharmazeutischen Wissenschaft. **Pharmazie** 1984 May;39(5):340–5
Friedrich C, Seidlein HJ: Beiträge zur Geschichte der Pharmazeutischen Wissenschaft. 11. Mitteilung: Die Bedeutung Johannes (Hans) Valentin für die Entwicklung der Pharmazeutischen Wissenschaft. **Pharmazie** 1984 Apr;39(4):262–9
Friedrich C, Langer H, Seidlein HJ: Beiträge zur Geschichte der Pharmazeutischen Wissenschaft 3. Mitteilung: Christian Ehrenfried von Weigel -- Seine Bedeutung für die Entwicklung der Pharmazeutischen Wissenschaft. Teil 1: Herkunft und Entwicklung. **Pharmazie** 1982 Apr;37(4):290–3
Friedrich C, Langer H, Seidlein HJ: Beiträge zur Geschichte der Pharmazeutischen Wissenschaft. 5. Mitteilung: Christian Ehrenfried von Weigel--Seine Bedeutung für die Entwicklung der pharmazeutischen Wissenschaft. **Pharmazie** 1982 Jul;37(7):514–7
Froböse HH: Beiträge des Apothekers zur Therapieoptimierung--ein Rückblick. **Pharmazie** 1983 Sep;38(9):618–20
Froböse HH: Die Tagung des preussischen Apothekerrates im Jahre 1897--ein Beitrag zur Frage der Zulassung der Frauen zur Pharmazie. **Pharmazie** 1982 Aug;37(8):596–9
Ganzinger K: Der Lippe-Detmoldische Leibarzt Johann Christian Friedrich Scherf (1750–1818) als Medizinalpolitiker und Reformator der Pharmazie. **Beitr Gesch Pharm** 1981;31(10):73–8
Ganzinger K: Johann Peter Frank und die Apothekerordnung für die österreichische Lombardei. **Osterr Apoth Ztg** 1981;35:410–4
Ganzinger K: Johann Peter Frank und die Apothekerordnung für die österreichische Lombardei. In Ganzinger K, Skopec M, Wyklicky H, ed: Festschrift für Erna Lesky zum 70. Geburtstag. Wien, Brüder Hollinek, 1981. p. 39–47.
Gerecke K, Richter J, Koch H: Třicet let Německé demokratické republiky a jejich přínos mezinárodímu vývoji farmacie. **Cesk Farm** 1981 Jun;30(5):142–6
Gericke D: '100 Jahre Dienst am Menschen'. Meilensteine der Pharma-Hoechst. **Fortschr Med** 1984 May 24;102(20):75–7

# PHARMACY

Giebel A: Drei Generationen Constantini als Hofapotheker in Rotenburg a. d. Fulda. **Hess Familienkd** 1977;13:445-8

Habrich C: Therapeutische Grundsätze pietistischer Arzte des 18. Jahrhunderts. **Beitr Gesch Pharm** 1982;31(16):121-3

Höpfinger E: Höchster Anspruch an die Arbeit: Gesundheit bezahlbar machen. Rückblick auf eine langjährige Firmentradition der Boehringer Mannheim GmbH. **Fortschr Med** 1984 Apr 26;102(16):91-2

Kaemmerer K: Die Arzneimittel des Veterinärdienstes im Zweiten Weltkrieg. **DTW** 1981 Nov 5;88(11):461-73

Kahle E, Stupp JA: Hochschulschriften zur Geschichte der Medizin, Pharmazie, und Naturwissenschaften der Friedrich-Alexander-Universität Erlangen-Nürnberg 1885-1975. Erlangen, Verlagsbuchhandlung Hannelore Lüling, 1980. 94 p. (Medizinhistorische Materialien, 2).

Kahle E: Hochschulschriften zur Geschichte der Medizin Pharmazie und Naturwissenschaften der Julius-Maximilians-Universität Würzburg, 1885-1970. Medizinhistorische Materialien - 1. Erlangen, Verlagsbuchhandlung, 1979. 48 p.

Kaiser W: 275 Jahre hallesche Medikamenten-Expedition. Aus der Frühgeschichte der pharmazeutischen Industrie in Deutschland. **Beitr Gesch Pharm** 1984;31(22):1-12

Kaiser W: 275 Jahre hallesche Medikamentenexpedition. **Z Gesamte Inn Med** 1984 Apr 1;39(7):125-33

Korn E: Die Apotheke in Hovestadt. Werl, Dietrich-Coelde-Verlag, 1977. 87 p.

Kraus I: Hermann Schelenz. In Balde JH, Schmiking W, ed: Festschrift zum 86. Deutschen Arztetag in Kassel. Kassel, Arztevereins, 1983. p. 41-9.

Leibecke-Englisch B: Die lokale Wundbehandlung aus pharmakologischer and pharmazeutischer Sicht in der deutschsprachigen medizinischen Literatur von 1800 bis 1867. Diss. Mainz, 1979. 89p.

Müller-Jahncke WD: Weitere Apothekerbildnisse auf Medaillen und Plaketten des deutschsprachigen Raums. **Beitr Gesch Pharm** 1984;31(24):205-9

Oldenburg D: Georg August Bertele (1767-1818) und die Arzneimittellehre der romantischen Naturphilosophie. **Medizinhist J** 1981;16(3):240-56

Oldenburg D: Romantische Naturphilosophie und Arzneimittellehre 1800-1840. Diss. (Doktor der Naturwissenschaften), Braunschweig, 1979. 267 p. (Veröffentlichungen aus dem Pharmaziegeschichtlichen Seminar der Technischen Universität Braunschweig, 20).

Possehl T: Probleme der Arzneipreisgestaltung im 19. Jahrhundert. **Medizinhist J** 1981;16(4):358-90

Rödel W: Die wichtigsten Forderungen der revolutionären deutschen Sozialdemokratie zum Apothekenwesen ausgangs des 19. Jahrhunderts. **Pharmazie** 1983 Nov;38(11):772-4

Rumpf-Lehmann B: Seltene Drogen von 'Dr. Dittrich aus Prag' in der Wigandschen Drogensammlung der Universität Marburg. **Beitr Gesch Pharm** 1982;31(16):123-6

Schneider J: Beiträge zur Geschichte der Wehrpharmazie von 1935-1945. Düsseldorf, Triltsch Druck, 1982. vi, 160 p. (Düsseldorfer Arbeiten zur Geschichte der Medizin, Beiheft VIII).

Schröder G: Die Wiederbelebung der Phytotherapie im Zusammenhang mit den Reformbestrebungen der NS-Pharmazie. In Hickel E, Schröder G, ed: Neue Beiträge zur Arzneimittelgeschichte. Festschrift für Wolfgang Schneider zum 70. Geburtstag. Stuttgart, Wissenschaftliche Verlagsgesellschaft, 1982. p. 111-28.

Schwarz HD: Christian Theodor Lappe (1802-1877). **Pharm Ztg** 1977;122:338

Simmer HH: Organotherapie mit Ovarialpräparaten in der Mitte der neunziger Jahre des 19. Jahrhunderts; Medizinische und pharmazeutische Probleme. In Hickel E, Schröder G, ed: Neue Beiträge zur Arzneimittelgeschichte. Festschrift für Wolfgang Schneider zum 70. Geburtstag. Stuttgart, Wissenschaftliche Verlagsgesellschaft, 1982. p. 229-64.

Telle J: Pharmazie und der gemeine Mann: Hausarznei und Apotheke in deutschen Schriften der frühen Neuzeit: Ausstellung der Herzog August Bibliothek Wolfenbüttel in der Halle des Zeughauses vom 23. August 1982 bis März 1983. Wolfenbüttel, Herzog August Bibliothek, 1982. 144 p.

Wankmüller A: Deutschsprachige Lehrbücher der pharmazeutischen Technologie von 1845 bis 1945. **Dtsch Apoth Ztg** 1982 Oct 6;122(23):1236-9

Wankmüller A: Die Apotheker von Lenzburg im Kanton Aargau. Zum 25 jährigen Bestehen der Schweizerischen Gesellschaft für Geschichte der Pharmazie im Juni 1982. **Pharm Ztg** 1982 Jun 3;127(22):1207-8

Wankmüller A: Die Pharmaziegeschichtsschreibung in Württemberg. In: Vorträge des Internationalen Pharmaziehistorischen Kongresses Innsbruck 1977. Stuttgart, Wissenschaftliche Verlagsgesellschaft, 1979. p. 63-9.

Wankmüller A: Entstehung des 'Grundriss der Geschichte der deutschen Pharmazie' von Adlung und Urdang. **Pharm Ztg** 1980;125:403-6

Wankmüller A: Hinweise zur Literatur für die Pharmaziegeschichte. 2. Deutschsprachige periodische Veröffentlichungen. **Beitr Gesch Pharm** 1981;31:86

Wankmüller A: [Studies in German pharmaceutical history] (Ger). **Beitr Wuerttemb Apothekengesch** 1978;12(2):33-64

Weidmann A: Die Arzneiversorgung der Armen zu Beginn der Industrialisierung im deutschen Sprachgebiet, besonders in Hamburg. Braunschweig, 1982. iv, 229 p. (Braunschweiger Veröffentlichungen zur Geschichte der Pharmazie und der Naturwissenschaften, Bd. 25).

Wiegert J: Anfangsprobleme der Nahrungsmittelchemie in Deutschland unter besonderer Berücksichtigung pharmazeutischer Verhältnisse. Braunschweig, 1975. 180 p. (Veröffentlichungen aus dem Pharmaziegeschichtlichen Seminar der Technischen Universität Braunschweig, Band 15).

Wittop Koning DA, Van Gelder JB: Die Offizin aus der Meteorologia philosophica-politica des Fr. Reinzer. **Beitr Gesch Pharm** 1984;31(24):210

Wölfel A: Pflanzen in der Volksmedizin. Die volksmedizinischen Studien von Heinrich Marzell. Diss. Erlangen-Nürnberg, 1983. 117 p.

**Great Britain**

Anning S: Yorkshire apothecaries. **Pharm Hist (London)** 1980 Dec;10(3):3-4

Bardell EB: Dame Agatha's dispensary. **Pharm Hist** 1984;26(1):13-9

Boden IM: Fifty years of pharmaceutical development. **Practitioner** 1980 May;224(1343):513-5

Burnby J: Some provincial apothecaries. **Pharm Hist (London)** 1978 Mar;8(1):5-6,4

Burnby J: The mortar of Charles Angibaud. **Pharm Hist (London)** 1979 Apr;9(1):6-8

Burnby J: The Raggs of Edmonton Green. **Pharm Hist (London)** 1975 Dec;5(3):2-3

Burnby JG: A study of the English apothecary from 1660 to 1760. London, Wellcome Institute for the History of Medicine, 1983. 128 p. (Medical History, Suppl. no. 3).

Burnby JG: Robert Drane: no ordinary pharmacist. **Pharm Hist (London)** 1984 Dec;14(4):3-6

Cowen DL: The trustees' garden at Savannah. **Ga Pharm Q** 1983 Spring;60(2):5-3

Crellin JK: Pharmacies as general stores in the 19th century. **Pharm Hist (London)** 1979 Apr;9(1):5-6

Drummond CG: Adam Drummond of Megginch, surgeon-apothecary. **Pharm Hist (London)** 1971 Dec;2(3):3-5

Drummond CG: Charles Wilson (1804-1884). In Passmore R, ed: Proceedings of the Royal College of Physicians of Edinburgh Tercentenary Congress, 1981. Edinburgh, Royal College of Physicians of Edinburgh, 1982. p. 199-203.

Ellis R: Pharmacy in Stamford a century ago. **Pharm Hist (London)** 1967 Oct;1(1):4-8

Fletcher G, Harris JI: Pharmacy in Bath during the Regency period. **Pharm Hist (London)** 1970 Jun;1(5):2-4

Ford JM: Apothecaries' roles reassessed. **J R Soc Med** 1983 Aug;76(8):634

Franke NH: James Bell Heyl, Bermuda's pharmacist-photographer. **Pharm Hist** 1982;24(3):117-9

Hanbury J: A reminiscence: pharmacy in the first half of the 20th century. **Pharm Hist (London)** 1978 Jul;8(2):2-4

Hartley F: Pharmacy in the time of John Hunter (1728-1793). **Trans Hunter Soc** 1978-80;37-38:99-107

History in the pharmaceutical press: **Pharm Hist (London)** 1971 Mar;2(1):2-8

Holloway S: Significance of the Apothecaries' Act, 1815. **Pharm Hist (London)** 1970 Jun;1(5):6-9

Hopkinson GD: Alexander Dalmahoy: chemist to Her Majesty. **Pharm Hist (London)** 1984 Dec;14(4):8-11

Jackson WA: Farr's Patent Ampulla. **Pharm Hist (London)** 1977 Dec;7(3):2-3

Jackson WA: Lupton of Levenshulme. **Pharm Hist (London)** 1977 Jul;7(2):2-4

Jackson WA: The Carbolic smoke ball. **Pharm Hist (London)** 1984;14(1):9-10

Livesley CA: 1839 advertisements. **Pharm Hist (London)** 1981 Apr;11(1):10-11

Macdonald G: One hundred years Wellcome, 1880-1980: in pursuit of excellence. London, Wellcome Foundation, Ltd., 1980. 120 p.

McGuckin A: Nineteenth-century pharmacists of Newcastle. **Pharm Hist (London)** 1971 Jul;2(2):4-6

Matthews LG: Apothecaries' apprentices in Wiltshire and Surrey in the eighteenth century. **Pharm Hist (London)** 1971 Jul;2(2):7-8

Myco F: Eighteenth century medicine: of magic and mysticism. **Nurs Mirror** 1982 Sep 8;155(10):50-2

Pharmacist -cum-printer: **Pharm Hist (London)** 1971 Dec;2(3):5-6

Rawlings FH: 18th century Bristol Poll Books; source list of apothecaries and chemists and druggists. **Pharm Hist (London)** 1973 May;3(1):5

Robinson WJ: Physick in Bolton in 1779. **Pharm Hist (London)** 1981 Apr;11(1):6-7

Rocchietta S: Due secoli di canzoni inglesi con spunti medico-=farmaceutici. **Minerva Med** 1979 Sep 26;70(41):2839-43

Searle CG: A soldier pharmacist. **Pharm Hist (London)** 1974 Jan;4(1):2-3

Selleck AD: William Cookworthy, an 18th century polymath. **Pharm Hist (London)** 1979 Dec;9(3):8-12

Short AL: Portraits, paintings and caricatures. **Pharm Hist (London)** 1970 Jun;1(5):10-11

Sigsworth EM, Swan P: An eighteenth-century surgeon and apothecary: William Elmhirst (1721-1773). **Med Hist** 1982 Apr;26(2):191-8

Sigsworth EM: William Elmhirst 1721-1773: surgeon-apothecary--and medical frontiersman. **Pharm Hist (London)** 1984 Sep;14(3):6-7
Thomas PH: Professor Theophilus Redwood (1806-92). **Pharm Hist (London)** 1983 Jun;13(2):9-12
Tring FC: Thomas Holloway and his patent pills. **Pharm Hist (London)** 1977 Dec;7(3):4-5
Turner H: Henry Wellcome: the man, his collection and his legacy. London, Heinemann for the Wellcome Trust, 1980. 96 p.
Vane JR: The research heritage of Henry Wellcome. **Pharm Hist (London)** 1980 Aug;10(2):2-8
Van Zwanenberg D: The training and careers of those apprenticed to apothecaries in Suffolk. 1815-1858. **Med Hist** 1983 Apr;27(2):139-50
Wright A: Some Yorkshire proprietaries. **Pharm Hist (London)** 1980 Dec;10(3):6-8
Yaffe G: Wigan Dispensary. **Pharm Hist (London)** 1981;11(2):6

### Hungary

Antall J: Der Einfluss der Apotheker auf das öffentliche Leben Ungarns im 19. Jahrhundert. **Pharm Acta Helv** 1979;54(9-10):295-8
Duka Zólyomi N: A magyarországi gyógyszertári vizsgálatok alapveto reformjai a 18. szádban. **Orvostort Kozl** 1982;28(1-3):151-4
Grabarits I: Die Klassifizierung des ungarischen Arzneischatzes im 18. Jahrhundert. In Hickel E, Schröder G, ed: Neue Beiträge zur Arzneimittelgeschichte. Festschrift für Wolfgang Schneider zum 70. Geburtstag. Stuttgart, Wissenschaftliche Verlagsgesellschaft, 1982. p. 87-105.
Kapronczay K: Personalstand und territoriale Verteilung der ungarischen Apotheken am Ende des 18. Jahrhunderts. In Hein WH, ed: Pharmaziehistorischer Kongress, Budapest, 1981. Stuttgart, Wissenschaftliche Verlagsgesellschaft, 1983. p. 81-4.
Kempler K: A gyógyszerészeti technológia hazai úttörője Rozsnyay Mátyás. **Orv Hetil** 1984 Jul 22;125(30):1832-4, 1837
Kempler K: Lex Szapáryana. **Acta Pharm Hung** 1980 Jul;50(4):166-72
Kempler K: Száz éves az elsö magyar gyógyszerkönyv kommentárja. Tallózás évszázados gyógyszerkincsünkben. **Orv Hetil** 1979 Dec 16;120(50):3055-7
Pál E: Habent sua fata libelli. Magyar orvosok és gyógyszerészek a nyelvújítás korában. **Orv Hetil** 1981 Feb 22;122(8):467-8
Rádóczy G: A Magyarországon Hivatalos gyógyszernormatívumok. **Orvostort Kozl** 1981;93-96(27 No 1-4):123-53
Rádóczy G: Norma Pauperum: Amtliche Standardrezeptsammlungen neben dem Arzneibuch in Ungarn. In Hickel E, Schröder G, ed: Neue Beiträge zur Arzneimittelgeschichte. Festschrift für Wolfgang Schneider zum 70. Geburtstag. Stuttgart, Wissenschaftliche Verlagsgesellschaft, 1982. p. 71-80.
Rixer A: A magyar gyógyszerészi szaksajtó kialakulása és fejlödése a xix. században. **Acta Pharm Hung** 1983 Jul;53(4):183-90
Rixer A: A magyar nyelvü gyógyszerészeti szaksajtó kialakulása és jelenentösége 1831-1872 között. Diss., Budapest, 1976. 193 p.
Soproni L: Nógrád megye gyógyszerészetének kialakualása és története 1701-1918-ig. Diss., Budapest, 1979. 133 p.
Sugár I: Az 'Egri Víz' története. **Orvostort Kozl** 1980;89-91(26 no 1-3):191-207
Szállási A: A Nyugat, gyógyszerészei'. **Orv Hetil** 1982 Jan 24;123(4):229-32
Szemkeö E: Die Teilnahme des ungarischen Landesrates für Gesundheitswesen an der Zusammenstellung eines internationalen Arzneibuches zur Zeit der Jahrhundertwende. In Hein WH, ed: Pharmaziehistorischer Kongress, Budapest, 1981. Stuttgart, Wissenschaftliche Verlagsgesellschaft, 1983. p. 129-33.
Szentgyörgyvölgyi G: Egy régi hajdúszoboszlói gyógyszerész: Trocsányi Imre és köre. **Orv Hetil** 1982 Nov 28;123(48):2972-3
Szigetváry F: Die Apotheke der Jesuiten von Köszeg. In Hein WH, ed: Pharmaziehistorischer Kongress, Budapest, 1981. Stuttgart, Wissenschaftliche Verlagsgesellschaft, 1983. p. 73-80.
Varga P: Bacsó Bálint debreceni orvos-gyógyszerész élete és munkássága. **Orvostort Kozl** 1982;28(1-3):155-67
Zalai K: A gyógyszerészi szemlélet és gondolkodás változása századunkban Magyarországon. **Acta Pharm Hung** 1983 Jul;53(4):145-9
Zalai K: A gyógyszerügyi szervezéstudomány, a társadalmogyógyszerészet hazai és külföldi fejlödése. **Acta Pharm Hung** 1984 Jan;54(1):1-14

### Iceland

Bödvarsdóttir I: Apoteks oprettelse og de første apotekere i Island. **Nord Medicinhist Arsb** 1982;:157-61

### Italy

Caracci P: Vicende di una farmacopea di stato della serenissima repubblica di Venezia. **Acta Med Hist Patav** 1981/82;28:29-38
Drey RE: Les vases de pharmacie de l'Hôpital majeur de Novare. **Rev Hist Pharm (Paris)** 1979 Dec;26(243):259-62
Rocchietta S: Canzoni italiane correlate con la medicina e la farmacia. **Minerva Med** 1980 Oct 13;71(39):2861-70
Talenti M: Cenni storici su la Farmacopea Ufficiale Italiana. **Nuovi Ann Ig Microbiol** 1982 Jul-Dec;33(4-6):889-99

### Malta

Cassar P: Impact of British pharmacy in Malta. **Pharm Hist (London)** 1978 Mar;8(1):2-4

### Mexico

Cervantes V: 'Ensayo a la materia medica vegetal de Mexico' (Introduccion). **Med Tradic** 1982;3(11):34-6
Gereffi G: Drug firms and dependency in Mexico: the case of the steroid hormones industry. **Int Organ** 1978;32:237-86

### Netherlands

Ahlrichs EL: Dr. D. A. Wittop Koning 70 jaar. **Pharm Weekbl** 1981 Nov 6;116(45):1365-9
Jüttner G: Ein 'Pharmacopoeus spagyricus': Johann Conrad Barkhausen (1666-1723) und die Pharmazie. In Dilg P, et al., ed: Perspektiven der Pharmaziegeschichte. Graz, Austria, Akademische Druck- u. Verlagsanstalt, 1983. p. 147-64.
Snelders HA: Nederlandse apothekers en het acceptatieproces van Lavoisiers nieuwe scheikunde. **Pharm Weekbl** 1981 Nov 6;116(45):1401-6
Wittop Koning DA: De farmacie en de medische tijdschriften. **Ned Tijdschr Geneeskd** 1981 Dec 5;125(49):2021-4

### New Zealand

Combes RE: J. C. Sharland's pharmacy at Apothecaries' Hall. **J Auckl Waikato Hist Soc** 1979;34:31-4

### Nigeria

Carlson DG: Drug supply systems in West Africa; a historical overview with particular reference to Nigeria. **Pharm Hist** 1982;24(2):73-82

### Norway

Kringlen E: Legemidler for behov eller profitt. **Samtiden (Norway)** 1970;79(9):546-63

### Philippines

Sánchez Téllez MC: Remedios filipinos descritos por Fr. Antonio Mozo (1763). **Bol Soc Esp Hist Farm** 1983 Sep;135:95-100

### Poland

Czeley-Wybieralska M: Nobilitacje lekarzy i aptekarzy w Królestwie Polskim w latach 1817-1861. **Arch Hist Med (Warsz)** 1983;46(2):205-4
Jeśman C: Organizacja niemieckiej Izby Aptekarskiej i gospodarka lekami w tzw. Generalnym Gubernatorstwie w latach 1939-1945. **Arch Hist Med (Warsz)** 1984;47(3):403-15
Krówczyński L: Dorobek naukowy katedry i Zakładu Farmacji Stosowanej AM w Krakowie. **Folia Med Cracov** 1979;21(1):133-9
Ostrowska T: Rozprawy składane Towarzystwu Warszawskiemu Przyjaciół Nauk (1800--1832) przez jego członków -- lekarzy i farmaceutów. **Arch Hist Med (Warsz)** 1979;42(1):61-81
Pabis-Braunstein M: Aptekarstwo w Bieczu. Dzieje rodziny Fusków. **Arch Hist Med (Warsz)** 1984;47(2):191-206
Pabis-Braunstein M: Ponad stuletnie tradycje farmaceutycznej rodziny Nitribittów. **Arch Hist Med (Warsz)** 1983;46(3):295-313
Pankiewicz H: Prof. dr hab. Henryk Bukowiecki jako historyk farmacji. **Arch Hist Med (Warsz)** 1984;47(3):389-93
Skład osobowy władz Polskiego Towarzystwa Historii Medycyny i Farmacji: **Arch Hist Med (Warsz)** 1984;47(2):269-85
Sosińska-Trawińska M: Zalecenia lecznicze w chorobach dzieci zawarte w wybranych czasopismach nielekarskich XVIII w w Polsce. **Arch Hist Med (Warsz)** 1983;46(3):285-94
Szwarczyński W: Rozwój badań w dziedzinie oryginalnego polskiego leku syntetycznego. **Arch Hist Med (Warsz)** 1984;47(3):443-6

### Portugal

Mosch E: Der Apotheker Pedro José da Silva, ein unbekannter Lebenslauf. **Beitr Gesch Pharm** 1980;31(9):65-71

### Romania

Centenarul Institutului de Medicină şi Farmacie din Iaši (1879-1979): **Rev Med Chir Soc Med Nat Iasi** 1979 Oct-Dec;83(4):727-32
Cotrău M, Gheorghiță I: Prescriptii medicale in manuscrisul inedit de la Spitalul Se. Spiridon Iasi, din secolul al XVIII-LEA (IV). **Rev Med Chir Soc Med Nat Iasi** 1983 Apr-Jun;87(2):307-12
Cotrău M, Gheorghiță I: Prescripții medicale în manuscrisul inedit de la spitalul SF. Spiridon Iaşi, din secolul al XVIII-lea. **Rev Med Chir Soc Med Nat Iasi** 1983 Jan-Mar;87(1):113-6
Cotrău M, Gheorghiță I: Prescripții medicale în manuscrisul inedit de la

Spitalul Sf. Spiridon Iaşi, din secolul al XVIII-lea (I). **Rev Med Chir Soc Med Nat Iasi** 1982 Jul-Sep;86(3):501-3

Cotrău M, Gheorghiţă I: Prescripţii medicale in manuscrisul inedit de la Spitalul Sf. Spiridon Iaşi, din secolul al XVIII-lea. (II). **Rev Med Chir Soc Med Nat Iasi** 1982 Oct-Dec;86(4):673-6

Năstasă V: Activitatea ştiinţifică a farmaciştilor în cadrul 'societăţii de medici şi naturalişti' din iaşi. **Rev Med Chir Soc Med Nat Iasi** 1981;85(1):158-60

Pincu P: Din istoricul unei farmacii bicentenare 'spiţeria mănăstirii neamţ'. **Rev Med Chir Soc Med Nat Iasi** 1980 Jan-Mar;84(1):137-9

Samborschi E, Baicu G, Suliman M, et al: Die Tradition der Spezialitätenherstellung in Apotheken Rumäniens. In Hickel E, Schröder G, ed: Neue Beiträge zur Arzneimittelgeschichte. Festschrift für Wolfgang Schneider zum 70. Geburtstag. Stuttgart, Wissenschaftliche Verlagsgesellschaft, 1982. p. 81-5.

Scripcaru G: Un secol de învătămînt medical universitar la Iaşi. **Rev Med Chir Soc Med Nat Iasi** 1979 Oct-Dec;83(4):557-63

Un secol de activitate de medicină preventivă la Institutul de Medicină şi Farmacie din Iaşi (1882-1982): **Rev Med Chir Soc Med Nat Iasi** 1983 Oct-Dec;87(4):707-25

**South Africa**

Steenkamp WF: The pharmaceutical industry in South Africa. **S Afr J Econ** 1979;47:75-89

**Spain**

Alegre Pérez E, González García M: Estudio de la vida y obra científica de D. Manuel Jiménez Murillo. **Bol Soc Esp Hist Farm** 1983;34(136):185-201

Alegre Perez E, Andres Turrion L de: La altea en las prescripciones hechas a la Real familia durante el reinado de Carlos IV (1788-1808). In Hickel E, Schröder G, ed: Neue Beiträge zur Arzneimittelgeschichte. Festschrift für Wolfgang Schneider zum 70. Geburtstag. Stuttgart, Wissenschaftliche Verlagsgesellschaft, 1982. p. 159-63.

Alegre Pérez E: La asistencia social en la Real Botica durante el último cuarto del siglo XVIII. **Bol Soc Esp Hist Farm** 1984 Sep;35(139):199-210

Alegre Perez E, Caraballo Ortega T: Utilización de las aguas de 'El Molar' por las reales personas durante los años 1841, 42, 43 y 1851. **Bol Soc Esp Hist Farm** 1981 Sep;32(127):115-36

Alegre Perez ME, Santonja R: Delito o previsión de futuro? **Bol Soc Esp Hist Farm** 1980 Mar-Jun;31(121-2):31-7

Alegre Perez ME, Fuente Souviron E: Noticias sobre los farmaceuticos habilitados para atender por cuenta de la Real Hacienda a los individuos del Real Servicio y personas agraciadas por los Reyes (Reinado de Fernando VII). **Bol Soc Esp Hist Farm** 1982 Mar;33(130):113-22

Alegre Perez ME, Andres Turrion ML de: Polémica surgida con motivo de la convocatoria a oposiciones para la Real Botica, en el año 1816. **Bol Soc Esp Hist Farm** 1980/81 Dec-Mar;31-32(124-5):35-45

Andrés Turrión ML de: Normativa sobre la confección de recetas en la Real Botica durante el siglo XIX. **Bol Soc Esp Hist Farm** 1984 Jun;35(138):89-102

Arques J, Suñe JM: Razones que motivaron la individualizacion de la Catedra de Historia de la Farmacia de la Universidad Central, en 1896. **Bol Soc Esp Hist Farm** 1983 Mar-Jun;34(133-134):3-10

Basante Pol RM, Garcia Ada R: La botica del Colegio Imperial de Madrid. **Bol Soc Esp Hist Farm** 1982 Mar;33(132):219-36

Basante Pol RM, Castillo Tello MM: La correspondencia dirigida a D. Casimiro Gómez Ortega por D. Cándido M.a Trigueros. **Bol Soc Esp Hist Farm** 1981 Sep;32(127):137-47

Basante Pol RM: La real oficina de farmacia en las postrimerias del reinado de Isabel II (1843-1868). **Bol Soc Esp Hist Farm** 1983 Mar-Jun;34(133-134):11-23

Basante Pol RM: Notas sobre algunos de los boticarios madrileños de los primeros años de siglo XVIII. **Bol Soc Esp Hist Farm** 1980 Oct;31(123):235-58

Bel E, María Suñé J: La 'Farmacopea Matritense en Castellano' y la 'Farmacopea en Castellano o colección de las fórmulas más usuales y acreditadas de la matritense y española'. **Bol Soc Esp Hist Farm** 1984 Jun;35(138):69-87

Beya Alonso E: Un comentario sobre los 'Elementos de Farmacia', de Carbonell. **Bol Soc Esp Hist Farm** 1980/81 Dec-Mar;31-32(124-5):315-22

Cabal Gonzalez M: Historia de los boticarios de Oviedo en el siglo XIX. Oviedo, Instituto de Estudios Asturianos, 1979. 107 p.

Donoso V: La industria farmacéutica en España. Oligopolio y colonización. **Rev Fom Soc** 1978;129:79-90;130:187-201;131:287-302

Esteva de Sagrera J: La farmacia española frente al cambio político. Barcelona, Ketres, 1978. 102 p.

Folch Jou G: L'influence de Dorvault en Espagne. **Rev Hist Pharm (Paris)** 1980 Jun;27(245):109-18

Folch Jou G, Javier Puerto F: Los medicamentos incluidos en los formularios del Hospital General de Madrid (Siglos XVIII y XIX). **Bol Soc Esp Hist Farm** 1982 Mar;33(129):49-76

Folch Jou G, Sanz Diaz L, Puerto Sarmiento FJ: Los proyectos de socialización de la farmacia durante la Segunda República española. **Pharm Acta Helv** 1979;54(9-10):286-94

Folch Jou G, Nuñez Varela V: Un examen de farmaceutico por comisionados del protomedicato en la Andalucia del siglo XIX. **Bol Soc Esp Hist Farm** 1982 Sep;33(131):193-8

Francés C: Manuel Hernández de Gregorio: a Spanish pharmacist dedicated to science and the history of pharmacy. In: Vorträge des Internationalen Pharmaziehistorischen Kongresses Innsbruck 1977. Stuttgart, Wissenschaftliche Verlagsgesellschaft, 1979. p. 181-6.

Frances M del C: Problemática sobre la botica de Villaluenga de la Sagra a fines del siglo XVIII. **Bol Soc Esp Hist Farm** 1980/81 Dec-Mar;31-32(124-5):283-5

Frances MC: Contrata suscrita entre José Terraza y el partido de Beteta en el siglo XIX. **Bol Soc Esp Hist Farm** 1981 Sep;32(127):207-16

Frances MC: Noticias de farmacéuticos que ejercieron en Buendía (Cuenca) en el siglo XVIII. **Bol Soc Esp Hist Farm** 1980 Mar-Jun;3(121-2):139-46

Gomez Caamaño JL, Rof Carballo MC: Los boticarios catalanes de la ilustración. **Bol Soc Esp Hist Farm** 1980 Mar-Jun;3(121-2):39-50

Herrero P, Frances MC: Influencia de la dosimetria en la farmacia española. **Bol Soc Esp Hist Farm** 1982 Mar;33(130):93-112

History of Pharmacy at the University of Granada: **Pharm Hist** 1983;25(2):74-9

Javier Puerto F: Pedro Calvo Asensio (1821-1863): farmaceutico liberal. **Bol Soc Esp Hist Farm** 1983;34(136):203-28

Jordi FR: Un capítulo de la propaganda farmacéutica: troquelados. **Circ Farm** 1981;12(134-5):58-61,68-72

Jordi R: Antonio Sala, un boticario barcelon/B//es aficionado a la botánica. **Farm Univers** 1980;13(1,2):10-7,78-82

Jordi R: Bases para un estudio de la evolución del medicamento en el Hospital de la Santa Cruz (1793-1796). Hospital General de Barcelona (1812-1814). Introducción. **Circ Farm** 1981 Jul;12(140):91-7

Jordi R: Notas sobre terapéutica hospitalaria usada en una epidemia en Montblanc. Año 1725. **Circ Farm** 1981 May;12(138):38-73

Jordi González FR: Recetas en circulación en Barcelona durante la Guerra Civil de 1936-1939. **Circ Farm** 1979 Nov;11(120):40-5

Jordi González FR: Recuerdos para un Montepío. **Circ Farm** 1980 Dec;12(133):75-84

Jordi González R: Anotaciones a los discursos botánicos del boticario barcelonés Antonio Sala Domènech. **An Med Cir** 1982;60(261):24-45

Jordi Gonzalez R: Cien año de vida farmacéutica barcelonesa (1830-1939). Barcelona, Circular Farmaceutica. [1982]. 615 p.

Jordi González R: Contribución para el estudio sociológico de la farmacia barcelonesa durante la guerra civil, a través de la prensa política. **Circ Farm** 1984;282:55-62

Jordi González R: Contribución para el estudio sociológico de la Farmacia barcelonesa durante la guerra civil, a través de la prensa política. (pt. I-VI). **Circ Farm** 1981-82 Dec, Jan, Feb, Mar, Jun, Sep;12-13:145-52

Jordi González R: Criterios del boticario y academico barcelones Jose Ignacio Mollar sobre la tinta de escribir. **Offarm** 1982;1(9):453-67

Jordi González R: Dos curiosos impresos, supuestos del siglo XIX. **Circ Farm** 1980 May;12(126):85-9

Jordi González R: Notas dispersas sobre la Facultad de Farmacia de Barcelona. **Circ Farm** 1980 Apr;12(125):91-8

Jordi González R: Notas sobre la clausura de una farmacia cooperativa, después del 6 de octubre de 1934. **Circ Farm** 1980 Feb;12(123):70-3

Jordi González R: Notas sobre la economía de una farmacia barcelonesa colectivizada durante la guerra civil española. **Circ Farm** 1980;12(122):51-67

Jordi Gonzalez R: Reflexiones sobre el inventario de una botica barcelonesa del siglo XVIII. **Circ Farm** 1981;12(143):83-95

Lavaque RJ: Botica publica de la capital de Don Felipe Vicente Reynoso. **Bol Soc Esp Hist Farm** 1983 Mar-Jun;34(133-134):35-7

Lorenzo Velázquez B: Presentación de dos formularios: 'Formulario de Terapéutica Clínica' (XV edición) y 'Formulario de Urgénica' (XVII edición). **An R Acad Nac Med (Madr)** 1981;98(2):211-26

Morales y Morales A: Francisco Antonio Solano, boticario revalidado. Asentista del Hospital Militar de Santa Cruz de Tenerife (1764-1771). **Bol Soc Esp Hist Farm** 1980 Mar-Jun;3(121-2):109-38

Muñoz Calvo S: Notas para elaboracion de una sociologia farmaceutica en el sexenio revolucionario (1868-1874). **Bol Soc Esp Hist Farm** 1982 Sep;33(131):173-84

Orozco Acuaviva A: El inventario de la botica del Convento-Hospital de San Juan de Dios de Cadiz, de 1822. **Bol Soc Esp Hist Farm** 1981 Dec;32(128):223-33

Paredes Salido F: La cartilla de las compañias sanitarias de la armada en el siglo XIX. **Rev Gen Mar** 1981 Aug;201:137-9

Puerto Sarmiento FJ: Andrés Alcón (1782-1850), farmacéutico, político y profesor de Química. **Bol Soc Esp Hist Farm** 1984 Sep;35(139):143-64

Puerto Sarmiento FJ, Cobo Cobo J: La evolucion de la quimica farmaceutica durante el siglo XVIII. **Bol Soc Esp Hist Farm** 1983 Mar-Jun;34(133-134):25-33

Puerto Sarmiento FJ: Las luchas en torno al monopolio farmacéutico, vistas desde el Colegio de Farmacéuticos de Madrid, durante el periodo de la Junta Superior Gubernativa de Farmacia (1800-1839). **Bol Soc Esp Hist Farm** 1980 Mar-Jun;3(121-2):69-96

Rof Carballo MC: Biografía y labor docente de Francisco Carbonell y Bravo. Diss. Barcelona, Facultad de Farmacia, Universidad de Barcelona, 1975. 189 p. (Publicaciones del Seminario de Historia de la Farmacia).

Sanchez-Moscoso A: José Rodríguez Carracido. **Bol Soc Esp Hist Farm** 1971 Jun;22(86):54–84
Sorní J, Suñé JM: Marcofilia farmacéutica española. III. **Bol Soc Esp Hist Farm** 1984 Sep;35(139):211–6
Valverde JL, Sánchez Tellez MC: Dos boticarios reales de origen frances del siglo XVII. **Ars Pharm** 1979;20:309–27
Valverde JL, Sanchez Tellez MC: Inventario de todos los efectos de la Botica del Monasterio de la Cartuja del Paular (1811). **Bol Soc Esp Hist Farm** 1980 Mar–Jun;3(121–2):51–67
Valverde JL, Bautista Mendez MT, De Vinuesa FS: La biblioteca de la Real Botica en 1816. **Bol Soc Esp Hist Farm** 1981 Jun;32(126):63–89
Valverde JL, Perez Romero JA: Remedios secretos: expedientes de autorización en España en el siglo XVIII. **Bol Soc Esp Hist Farm** 1980 Mar–Jun;31(121–2):7–20
Vidal Casero MC: Aportacion a la historia del Jardin de Aclimatacion de San Lucard de Barrameda. **Bol Soc Esp Hist Farm** 1981 Dec;32(128):235–49

**Sweden**

Bruun NW, Baerentsen K, Jensen VG: Anders Jahan Retzius: 'Fragmentum historiae pharmaceutices veterum'. Med dansk oversaettelse, biografiske noter og kommentarer. **Theriaca** 1981;20:5–151
Erichsen SW: Dronning Caroline Mathildes reiseapotek og litt om Stadsfysikus Johan Gotfried Erichsen. **Aust Agder Arv** 1977–78;:55–69
Ericsson R: Mineralvatten på svenska apotek--en svunnen epok. **Nord Medicinhist Arsb** 1980;Suppl 6:129–38
Goerke H: Linné und die Pharmacopoea Svecica (1775). In Dilg, P, et al., ed: Perspektiven der Pharmaziegeschichte. Graz, Austria, Akademische Druck- u. Verlagsanstalt, 1983. p. 89–96.
Modig M: Ex-libris de pharmaciens suédois. **Rev Hist Pharm (Paris)** 1980 Sep;27(246):162–4
Modig M: Kungliga hus--och reseapotek. **Livrustkammaren** 1980;15(1):1–16
Retzius AJ: Fragmentum historiae pharmaceutices veterum. Med dansk oversaettelse, biografiske noter og kommentarer, ved N. W. Bruun, K. Baerentsen, V. G. Jensen. København, Dansk Farmacihistorisk Selskab, 1981. 152 p. (Theriaca, 20).
Söderström N: Infusum amarum alkalinum militare; en arabesk kring ett gammalt amarum. **Sydsven Medicinhist Sallsk Arsskr** 1982;19:137–43
Strandell B: Linné och Stockholm. **Sven Farm Tidskr** 1979;83:677–84

**Switzerland**

Büchi J: Das Dispensatorium Medicum seu Pharmacopoea Noșocomii Thuricensis 1757. **Pharm Acta Helv** 1981;56(4–5):101–5
Büchi J: Die wiederaufgefundene 'Pharmacia contracta' des Johann Jakob Scheuchzer (1672–1733). **Gesnerus** 1982;39(2):145–69
Fehlmann HR: Bearbeitung des pharmazeutischen Reiseführers Schweiz. In: Vorträge des Internationalen Pharmaziehistorischen Kongresses Innsbruck 1977. Stuttgart, Wissenschaftliche Verlagsgesellschaft, 1979. p. 165–70.
Keller O: Apotheken und Apotheker der Stadt Schaffhausen. **Schaffhauser Beitr Vaterl Gesch** 1979;56:29–142
Ledermann F: La dispensation des médicaments dans le canton de Neuchâtel (Suisse) 1930–1960. - S.l.n.n., 1978, in-4., 336 p., multigraphié. (Thèse doct. Univ., Pharm., Univ. René-Descartes, U.E.R. Sciences pharm. et biol. Paris-Luxembourg, 1978).
Ledermann F: L'histoire de la pharmacie dans les 'Pharmaceutica Acta Helvetiae', une bibliographie entre 1926 et 1979. **Pharm Acta Helv** 1981;56(3):93–6
Wankmüller A: Die Tätigkeit deutscher Apotheker-Gehilfen in der Schweiz im 19. Jahrhundert. **Beitr Gesch Pharm** 1983;31(21):41–3

**United States**

Barrow MV: Self-treatment practices in North Florida. **J Fla Med Assoc** 1979 Aug;66(8):840–4
Bender GA: Henry Hurd Rusby: scientific explorer, societal crusader, scholastic innovator. **Pharm Hist** 1981;23(2):71–85
Bender GA: Nineteenth century pharmaceutical research into plants of the southwestern deserts. **Pharm Hist** 1980;22(2):49–59
Berman A: The eclectic 'concentrations' and American pharmacy (1847–1861). **Pharm Hist** 1980;22(3):91–103
Bogard MO: Facts about artifacts; drugstore perfumes in the 1890s. **Pharm Hist** 1983;25(2):80–2
Bogard MO: Peoria's pioneer druggists, the Farrells, and Farrell's Arabian liniment. **Pharm Hist** 1982;24(3):99–105
Bowers RA: Frederick B. Kilmer: a notable New Jersey pharmacist. **J Med Soc NJ** 1984 Sep;81(9):765–8
Conn HJ: The history of the Stain Commission. V. War and its consequences. **Stain Technol** 1981 May;56(3):135–42
Corgan JX: Richard Owen Currey, a little known intellectual figure of antebellum Tennessee. **East Tenn Hist Soc Publ** 1978;50:58–70
Cowen DL: A century of American pharmacy. **Carol J Pharm** 1980 May;60(5):5,7,9–10. Also in: Md Pharm 1981;57(1–3):8–9 and 58(4):8–9. Ala Pharm 1981 Aug–Oct;13(2–4). LA Pharm 1982 Jan–Feb;41(1–2)
Cowen DL: A century of American pharmacy. In Alabama Pharmaceutical Association: Centennial celebration, 1881–1981. (Birmingham?), Alabama Pharmaceutical Association, 1981. 11 p.
Cowen DL: Fifty years of the New Jersey Journal of Pharmacy. **NJ J Pharm** 1977 Oct;50(10):14–17
Cowen DL, King LD, Lordi NG: Nineteenth century drug therapy: computer analysis of the 1854 prescription file of a Burlington pharmacy. **J Med Soc NJ** 1981 Oct;78(11):758–61
Cowen DL: Robert P. Fischelis 1891–1981. **NJ J Pharm** 1982 Feb;55(2):12–4
Cowen DL: The nineteenth century German immigrant and American pharmacy. In Dilg P, et al., ed: Perspektiven der Pharmaziegeschichte. Graz, Austria, Akademische Druck- u. Verlagsanstalt, 1983. p. 13–28.
Cowen DL, Helfand WH: The progressive movement and its impact on pharmacy. **Pharm Acta Helv** 1979;54(11):317–23
Cowen DL, Helfand WH: The Progressive Movement and its impact on pharmacy. **Pharm Acta Helv** 1979;(11):1–6
Cowen DL: Tying the knot - secundum artem. **NJ J Pharm** 1983;56(3):6
Crellin J: 'The past recaptured'...five North Carolina pharmacies. **Pharm Hist** 1980;22(2):77–8
Friedman BL: Productivity gains in the drugstore industry, 1958–79. **Mon Labor Rev** 1980;103(11):18–22
Haller JS: The United States Pharmacopoeia: its origin and revision in the 19th century. **Bull NY Acad Med** 1982 Jun;58(5):480–92
Hanzlícěk Z: První česká lékárna v Chicagu. **Cesk Farm** 1981 May;30(3–4):125–30
Hayles AB, Key JD: Adventures of two prairie pioneers. **Minn Med** 1981 Oct;64(10):629–32
Helfand WH, Cowen DL: American pharmaceutical posters. In W.H. Hein, G. Schramm, ed: Die Vorträge des Internationalen Pharmazihistorischen Kongresses Basel 1979. Stuttgart, Wissenschaftliche Verlagsgesellschaft, 1981. (Veröffentlichungen der Internationalen Gesellschaft für Geschichte der Pharmazie e.V., Neue Folge, Bd. 50).
Heller WM: Dispensing in 1982. **Drug Intell Clin Pharm** 1983 Jul–Aug;17(7–8):570–3
Higby GJ: Practical Pharmacy by Mohr, Redwood, and Procter: an international pharmacy textbook. **Pharm Hist** 1984;26(2):97–102
Holcombe HW: Patent medicine tax stamps. A history of the firms using United States private die proprietary medicine tax stamps. Ed. G. B. Griffenhagen. Lawrence, Quarterman, 1979. xxv, 604 p. Reprinted articles from various journals.
Ingells DT: Miss Cora Dow. **Cinci Hist Soc Bull** 1982;40(3):151–66
Johnson BH: Doctors, druggists and dentists in the Oklahoma Territory, 1889–1907. **Ariz West** 1977;19:121–34
Johnson VB: Drug product selection through the decades. **Am Pharm** 1980 Oct;20(10):20–4
Lewis ER: Prairie state pharmacy. [Chicago?], Illinois Pharmacists Association, 1980. vi, 163 p.
Lewis ER: The anatomy of a pharmacist. **Pharm Hist** 1982;24(2):87–9
Liebenau JM: Medical science and medical industry, 1890–1929: a study of pharmaceutical manufacturing in Philadelphia. Ph. D. Diss., University of Pennsylvania. Philadelphia, 1981. vii, 489 p.
Loudon B: Pioneer pharmacist J. Walter Moyer's notes on Crawford and Fort Robinson in the 1890's. **Nebr Hist** 1977;58(1):89–117
Marion JF: The fine old house. Philadelphia, Smith Kline Corp., 1980. 251 p.
Menczer LF, Mittelmann M, Don RS: Pharmacy in Hartford's Historical Museum of Medicine and Dentistry. **Pharm Hist** 1984;26(3):156–7
Miller RR: History of clinical pharmacy and clinical pharmacology. **J Clin Pharmacol** 1981 Apr;21(4):195–7
Morgan GR: 'Sugar bowls' (Clematis hirsutissima): a horse restorative of the Nez Perces. **J Ethnopharmacol** 1981 Jul;4(1):117–20
Mrtek RG: Absent the incentive: an example of contemporary history. **Pharm Hist** 1981;23(4):145–51
Novotny A, Smith C, ed: Images of healing. A portfolio of American medical & pharmaceutical practice in the 18th, 19th, & early 20th centuries. New York, Macmillan, 1980, 144 p.
Scarchuk JM, ed: The first pharmacopoeia published in the Federated States of America, by William Brown, entitled Pharmacopoeia Simpliciorum et Efficiorum in Usum Nosocomii Militaris, published by Styner Cist. 1778. Coventry, Conn., the Author, 1976. xii, 32 p.
Shirkey HC: Clinical pharmacy--past, present & future. **Drug Intell Clin Pharm** 1977 Nov;(11):674–7
Sonnedecker G: The American correspondence between George Urdang and Henry E. Sigerist 1941–1948. In Perspektiven der Pharmaziegeschichte. Festschrift für Rudolf Schmitz zum 65. Geburtstag. Graz, Akademische Druck- u. Verlagsanstalt. p. 343–63.
Sonnedecker GS: The Richtmann Archive at Auburn University. **Pharm Hist** 1984;26(4):179–81
Stadnik J: Why our pharmacy museum is an attraction for old and new customers. **Pharm Times** 1982 Aug;48(8):52–4
Stage S: Female complaints: Lydia Pinkham and the business of women's medicine. New York, Norton, 1979. 304 p.
Strickland WA: Quinine pills, manufactured on the Missouri frontier (1832–1862). **Pharm Hist** 1983;25(2):61–8
Stuart RB, ed: Memoirs of a Council Bluffs druggist. **Palimpsest**

1980;61(3):66–79
Swiderski RM: Chinese-American patent medicines. **Ethnomedizin** 1978–79;5(1–2):97–126
Thomas SJ: Nostrum advertising and the image of woman as invalid in late Victorian America. **J Am Cult** 1982 Fall;5(3):104–12
Tyler VE: Damiana – history of a herbal hoax. **Pharm Hist** 1983;25(2):55–60
Tyler VE: Three proprietaries and their claim as American 'Indian' remedies. **Pharm Hist** 1984;26(3):146–9
Wallace DJ: Thomsonians: the people's doctors. **Clio Med** 1980 Jul;14(3–4):169–86
Wankmüller A, Cowen D, ed: A visitor's view of American pharmacy, 1851. **Pharm Hist** 1981;23(2):101–3
White JS: The Hedden's Store handbook of proprietary medicines. Portland, Durham & Downey, 1974. 94 p.
Whitney HA: Let us now praise famous men... **Drug Intell Clin Pharm** 1983 Jan;17(1):45–7
Young JH: George Wilhelm Merck. In Dictionary of American Biography, Suppl. 6, 1956–1960. p. 447–8, 1980.
Young JH: Public policy and drug innovation. **Pharm Hist** 1982;24(1):3–31
Zopf LC: Iowa pharmacy, a century of service: a chronology of the Iowa Pharmacists Association, 1880–1980. West Des Moines, Rob Lee Hill Pub. Co., 1980. xv, 408 p.

**USSR**

Bastenchuk AZ, Vladova MI, Siur HA, et al: Dosiahnennia aptechnoiï sluzhby Zaporiz'koï oblasti z chasu pryïniattia dekretu pro natsionalizatsiiu aptek na Ukraïni. **Farm Zh** 1979;(6):9–11
Borodiï MK: Do istoriï aptechnoï spravy na Ukraïni u druhii polovyni XVIII storichchia. **Farm Zh** 1980;(2):76–9
Borodiï MK: Do istoriï aptechnoï spravy na Ukraïni v pershiï polovyni XVIII storichchia. **Farm Zh** 1980;(1):77–9
Guyotjeannin C: Les médicaments de Tchékhov. **Monit Pharm** 1983;37(1557):1248–50
Jack DB: Dastardly deeds at Dorpat. **Pharm Hist (London)** 1984 Sep;14(3):9–12
Kaiser W: Vertreter der Ars pharmaceutica im petrinischen und nachpetrinischen Russland. **Wiss Z Martin Luther Univ (Math)** 1973;22(5):147–52
Kokoska U: Johann Georg Noël Dragendorff (20.4.1836 - 7.4.1898): Sein Beitrag zur Gerichtsmedizin, Pharmakologie und Pharmazie an der Universität Dorpat. Diss. Berlin, 1983. 234 p.
Shishkin NA, Orlova RV: Stanovlenie aptechnoï sistemy v Iaroslavskoi oblasti. **Farmatsiia** 1980 Mar–Apr;29(2):52–5
Tashmukhamedov IR, Dzhuraev IN: 60 let aptechnoï sistemy v Uzbekistane. **Farmatsiia** 1980 Mar–Apr;29(2):49–51
Tolmachov VF: Rozvytok aptechnoï spravy na Donechchyni za roky Radians'koï vlady. **Farm Zh** 1980;(1):9–12
Zolotnitskiï IaI: O knige O. Kalinskogo 'Retseptura ili nastavlenie sochiniat' pravil'nye retsepty dlia studentov imperatorskoï mediko-khirurgicheskoï akademii'. **Klin Med (Mosk)** 1984 Apr;62(4):151

**Vietnam**

Tran Huan N: Quelques aspects de la médecine et de la pharmacie au Vietnam. **Sci Orient** 1978;13:1–11

**Yugoslavia**

Kovačević M: Izrada i proizvodnja lekova u apotekarskoj službi NOVJ (JA). **Vojnosanit Pregl** 1981 Nov–Dec;38(6):404–11
Pejčić M: O nekim lekarima, apotekarima, i narodonoj medicini u Nišu za vreme Turaka (XIX vek). **Srp Arh Celok Lek** 1981 Oct;109(10):1405–12
Tartalja H: Geschichte der Pharmaziehistorik in Jugoslawien bis zum Jahre 1952. In: Vorträge des Internationalen Pharmaziehistorischen Kongresses Innsbruck 1977. Stuttgart, Wissenschaftliche Verlagsgesellschaft, 1979. p. 97–106.
Tartalja H: Mouvement social des pharmaciens en Croatie. **Orvostort Kozl** 1982;28(1–3):187–90

## EDUCATION

**Austria**

Huter F: Beiträge zur Geschichte des Apothekerwesens in Tirol (II). Von der Errichtung der Universität Innsbruck (1669) bis zu ihrer ersten Aufhebung (1782). **Tirol Heimat** 1978;42:5–51

**France**

Dillemann G: Histoire de l'enseignement pharmaceutique en France. **Pharm Acta Helv** 1979;54(9–10):269–72

**Hungary**

Zalai K: Die Geschichte des Universitätsunterrichts der Pharmaziegeschichte in Ungarn. In: Vorträge des Internationalen Pharmaziehistorischen Kongresses Innsbruck 1977. Stuttgart, Wissenschaftliche Verlagsgesellschaft, 1979. p. 197–202.

**Netherlands**

Grendel E: Het had een excursie van de Kring kunnen zijn. **Pharm Weekbl** 1981 Nov 6;116(45):1383–6

**Spain**

Gómez Caamaño JL: Historiographie pharmaceutique Catalane–Balear par un groupe universitaire. In: Vorträge des Internationalen Pharmaziehistorischen Kongresses Innsbruck 1977. Stuttgart, Wissenschaftliche Verlagsgesellschaft, 1979. p. 173–8.
Valverde López JL: Estudio sobre los fueros y privilegios del Antiguo Colegio de Apotecarios de Valencia. [Granada], Universidad de Granada, 1979. 90 p.

**1450–1700**

**Spain**

Jordi González R: La tarifa del Colegio de Boticarios de Barcelona año 1588. **Circ Farm** 1982 Jul–Sep;40(276):313–25

**1700 to Present**

Parascandola J: Pharmaceutical history for the pharmacy student. With a commentary by J. K. Crellin. In J. J. Bylebyl, ed: Teaching the history of medicine at a medical center. Baltimore, London, Johns Hopkins University Press, 1982. (The Henry E. Sigerist supplements to the Bulletin of the History of Medicine; new ser., no. 7). p. 78–90.

**Brazil**

Madeira AA, Rosa JE: O curso de odontologia da Faculdade de Farmacia e Odontologia de Santa Catarina. **Rev Catarinense Odontol** 1979 Jul–Dec;6(2):9–20
Rosa JE, Madeira AA: A fundação da faculdade de farmácia e odontologia de Santa Catarina antecedentes e funcionamento. **Rev Catarinense Odontol** 1979 Jan–Jun;6(1):7–20

**Canada**

Hughes FN: The Faculty of Pharmacy--a retrospective look. **Contin Pract** 1980;7(3):3–8
Stieb EW: A century of formal pharmaceutical education in Ontario. **Can Pharm J** 1983;116(3):104–7; 116(4):153–7

**Czechoslovakia**

Chlumský J: Třicet let Institutu pro další vzdělávání lékařu a farmaceutu. **Cesk Gastroenterol Vyz** 1983 Nov;37(6–7):361–3
Heinl E: Třicet let výchovně vzdělávací činnosti Institut pro další vzdělávání lékařu a farmaceutu. **Cas Lek Cesk** 1983 Oct 21;122(42):1286–90
Jirouš J: Třicetiletá bilance a perspektivy Katedry sociálního lékařství a organizace zdravotnictví Institutu pro další vzdělávání lékařu a farmaceutu Praha. **Cesk Zdrav** 1983 Sep;31(8–9):360–7
Macúch P: K 30. výročí činnosti Institutu pro další vzdělávání lékařu a farmaceutu v Praze. **Cesk Zdrav** 1983 Sep;31(8–9):337–45
Macúch P: Třicet let činnosti Institutu pro další vzdělávání lékařu a farmaceutu v Praze--integrální součást vývoje socialistického zdravotnictví v Ceskoslovensku. **Cas Lek Cesk** 1983 Oct 21;122(42):1281–4
Makovický E: Desat rokov Katedry metodiky a plánovania dalšieho vzdelávania Inštitútu pre dalšie vzdelávanie lekárov a farmaceutov Praha. **Cesk Zdrav** 1983 Sep;31(8–9):346–9
Mandák M: K jubileu farmaceutického štúdia. **Cesk Farm** 1982 Jul;31(6):201–2
Melichar B, Rusek V: Příspěvek farmaceutické fakulty brněnské univerzity k vývoji farmaceutických věd. **Cesk Farm** 1983 Jul;32(6):201–4
Rusek V: Historie farmacie na farmaceutické fakultě University Karlovy. **Cas Lek Cesk** 1981 Jan 30;120(3–4):100–3
Rybová J: Vývoj ideově výchovné práce Institutu pro další vzdělávání lékařu a farmaceutu. **Cas Lek Cesk** 1983 Oct 21;122(42):1291–4
Solich J: Prvních deset let farmaceutické fakulty University Karlovy. **Cesk Farm** 1980 Sep;29(7):217–25

**France**

Biserte G: L'Histoire de la Faculté Mixte de Médecine et de Pharmacie de Lille. (2 vols). Vol I. Lille, l'Association Corporative des Etudiants en Médecine de Lille, 1975. 169 p.
Bonnemain H: La Faculté de Pharmacie de Paris depuis cent ans Avenue de de l'Observatoire. **Rev Hist Pharm (Paris)** 1982 Mar;29(252):39–48

Dillemann G: La difficile conquête des prérogatives universitaires par les pharmaciens. **Rev Hist Pharm (Paris)** 1982 Sep;29(254):155-63
Dillemann G: Les dénominations successives des établissements autonomes d'enseignement pharmaceutique.
**Bull Liaison Assoc Amis Mus Pharm Montp** 1983;:(8):77-82
Dolique R: Sur les projets de masse pour l'Ecole de Pharmacie de Montpellier (en 1809) et la Faculté de Pharmacie (en 1966).
**Bull Liaison Assoc Amis Mus Pharm Montp** 1979;4:1-6
Michel ME: Bibliographie internationale d'histoire de la pharmacie et des sciences connexes. **Rev Hist Pharm (Paris)** 1982 Sep;29(254):214-6
Sordet D: Un homme, une famille. Le médecin principal Pierre Spillmann, professeur agrégé du Val-de-Grâce, professeur à l'Ecole préparatoire de Médecine et de Pharmacie d'Alger (1833-1883). Lyon, Association corporative des Etudiants en Médecine de Lyon, 1978. 40 p. (Thèse, Lyon).
Wankmüllert A: Studierende der Pharmazie an der Universität Strassburg vom Jahre 1872 an. **Pharm Ztg** 1982 Sep 9;127(36):1905-8

**Germany**

Friedrich C, Langer H, Seidlein HJ: Beiträge zur Geschichte der Pharmazeutischen Wissenschaft. 4. Mitteilung: Christian Ehrenfried von Weigel--Seine Bedeutung für die Entwicklung der Pharmazeutischen Wissenschaft. Teil 2: Christian Ehrenfried von Weigel als Hochschullehrer. **Pharmazie** 1982 Jun;37(6):446-50
Friedrich C, Seidlein HJ: Otto Anselmino--Seine Bedeutung für die Entwicklung der Pharmazeutischen Wissenschaft, insbesondere an der Universität Greifswald. **Pharmazie** 1981 Dec;36(12):846-52
Hellmuth H: Heinrich Wilhelm Ferdinand Wackenroder 8. März 1798--14. September 1854. **Pharmazie** 1980;34(5-6):321-3
Hermann A, Wankmüller A: Physik, Physiologische Chemie und Pharmazie an der Universität Tübingen. Tübingen, J.C.B. Mohr, 1980. 181 p. (Contubernium, Bd. 21).
Poethke W: Einige Bemerkungen zum Pharmaziestudium an der Universität Leipzig. **Pharmazie** 1980;35(10):641-2
Renner I: Zur Entwicklungsgeschichte der Pharmakognosie als selbständiges Hochschulfach an der Ludwig-Maximilians-Universität Ingolstadt - Landshut - München. Stuttgart, Deutscher Apotheker Verlag, 1982. 377 p. (Quellen und Studien zur Geschichte der Pharmazie, Bd. 17).
Wankmüller A: Anfänge des Chemie- und Pharmaziestudiums in Stuttgart unter Professor Hermann Fehling. **Dtsch Apoth Ztg** 1982 Sep 9;122(36):1805-6
Wankmüller A: Die deutschen Lehrbücher von Ira Remsen.
**Dtsch Apoth Ztg** 1979 Aug 30;119(35):1381-2
Wankmüller A: Pharmaziestudenten in den Universitäts-Matrikeln.
**Dtsch Apoth Ztg** 1979 Jun 14;119(24):945-7
Wankmüller A: Schlickums Lehrbuch für den Apothekerlehrling.
**Dtsch Apoth Ztg** 1981 Sep 3;121(36):1921-3

**Great Britain**

Education of a provincial apothecary: **Pharm Hist (London)** 1978 Jul;8(2):5-6

**Hungary**

Kempler K: Hugo Issekutz, der Begründer der ersten ungarischen Universitätsapotheke. In Hein WH, ed: Pharmaziehistorischer Kongress, Budapest, 1981. Stuttgart, Wissenschaftliche Verlagsgesellschaft, 1983. p. 135-9.
Tóth Z: Az orvosdoktori értekezések jelentösége a gyógyszerészeti tudomanyok hazai kialakulásában és fejlödésében 1770-1848. Diss., Budapest, 1976. 131 p.
Zalai K: 'Systema Artis Pharmaceuticae'. La première dissertation à la Faculté Hongroise de médecine, présentée par Maritius Fabi.
**Beitr Gesch Pharm** 1983;31(20):25-7

**Italy**

Colapinto L: Il Nobile Collegio Chimico Farmaceutico Romano. Cenni storici. Roma, Stomygen, 1979, 30 p.

**Japan**

Koyama T: [A history of pharmaceutical education in Okayama (I). Private Okayama pharmaceutical school (primary)] (Jpn). **Yakushigaku Zasshi** 1983;18(2):95-100

**Lebanon**

Zablotniak R: Polscy studenci medycyny i farmcji w uniwersytetach bejruckich (1941-1945). **Przegl Lek** 1981;38(1):124-5

**Netherlands**

Ahlrichs EL: Van leerjongen tot meester-apotheker (VII).
**Pharm Weekbl** 1981 Nov 6;116(45):1369-73
Van Ree JM: Nederlandse Farmacologie. I. Bouwstenen van de geneesmiddelentherapie: verantwoording. **Ned Tijdschr Geneeskd** 1983 Jul 9;127(28):1229-30

**Poland**

Dawidowicz A: Tajne nauczanie medycyny i farmacji w latach 1939-1945. Warszawa, Państwówy Zakład Wydawn. Lekarskich, 1977. 398 p.

**Spain**

Carmona Cornet AM, Gómez Caamaño JL: Historia de la Cátedra de técnica física aplicada a la Farmacia y análisis químico y en particular de los alimentos, medicamentos y venenos de la Facultad de Farmacia de la Universidad de Barcelona (1886-1936). **Bol Soc Esp Hist Farm** 1984 Jun;35(138):125-37
Jordi González R: Activitat del col.legi de Farmacèutics de Barcelona durant la Renaixença. **Figueres** 1981 (Separata: Ciència Renaixença Catalana)
Jordi Gonzalez R: Criterios basicos para una modificacion de los colegios de farmaceuticos catalanes. **Monit Farm Ter** 1980-81;2116-8:var. pagings
Puerto Sarmiento FJ: Las luchas en torno al monopolio farmacéutico vistas desde el Colegio de Farmacéuticos de Madrid (1839-1855).
**Bol Soc Esp Hist Farm** 1980/81 Dec-Mar;31-32(124-5):9-33
Sánchez-Moscoso Hermida A, Alfonso Galán MT: Estudio histórico de una tesis de farmacia juzgada hace 100 años: 'Las divisiones de la naturaleza y de la ciencia', de Francisco Fernández Iparraguirre.
**Bol Soc Esp Hist Farm** 1983;34(136):167-84

**Switzerland**

Ledermann F: Formation du pharmacien. Règlements, tendances, opinions.
**Schweiz Apoth Ztg** 1979 Dec 13;117(24):664-8; 1980 Jan 10;118(1):11-15
Meyer-Salzmann M: Aus der medizinischen Vergangenheit in Langenthal.
**Gesnerus** 1983;40(1-2):129-37
Wankmüller A: Die Schweizer Apotheker-Examen von 1874 bis 1880.
**Pharm Ztg** 1979 Jun 14;124(24):1161-4

**United States**

Allen B: David Stewart: first professor of pharmacy in America.
**Md Pharm** 1982 Feb;:4-8
Allen BF: Maryland College of Pharmacy and the doctor of pharmacy degree. **Md Pharm** 1982 Mar;:12-4
Autian J, Wood G: The role of toxicology in the pharmacy curriculum.
**Am J Pharm Educ** 1976 Nov,;40(4):378-82
Bardell EB: America's only school of pharmacy for women.
**Pharm Hist** 1984;26(3):127-33
Buerki RA, ed: Survey of instructional resources in history of pharmacy undergraduate courses. [Columbus, Ohio], Ohio State University, [1981?]. x, 160 p.
Fedo DA: Liberal arts and pharmacy education: where do we now stand?
**Pharm Hist** 1980;22(2):60-8
Parascandola J, Swann J: Development of Pharmacology in American Schools of Pharmacy. **Pharm Hist** 1983;25(3):95-115
Rodowskas CA Jr: A matter of degrees. **Drug Intell Clin Pharm** 1982 Jul-Aug;16(7-8):607-12
Russell JC: Werrett Wallace Charters, Sr. (1875-1952): his life, career and influence upon pharmaceutical education. Ph.D. Diss., Loyola University. Chicago, 1981. vii, 259 leaves.
Swintosky JV: Maturing of pharmaceutical education.
**Drug Intell Clin Pharm** 1976 Mar;10(3):153-60
Swinyard EA: Research and graduate education in pharmacy: looking back--looking forward. **Am J Pharm Educ** 1977 Nov;41(4):409-14

**USSR**

Dagurov VG: Razvitie farmakologii v Moskovskom universitete vo vtoroĭ polovine XIX veka. **Farmakol Toksikol** 1983 Jan-Feb;46(1):92-8
Elinov NP: 60 let Leningradskomu khimiko-farmatsevticheskomu institutu.
**Farmatsiia** 1979 Nov-Dec;28(6):49-56
Zabłotniak R: Polacy studiujący medycynę i farmację w Kownie (1940-1944). **Przegl Lek** 1980;37(1):101-4

**EQUIPMENT**

Apothekerspotten: Apothecary jars. The Hague, Gemeentemuseum, 1979. [59] p.
Baerentsen K: Gamle Apoteker Krukker. Kobenhavn, Danmarks Apotekerforening, 1980. 65 p.
Drey RE: Drug jars from hospitals and from royal pharmacies.
**Pharm Hist (London)** 1971 Dec;2(3):11-12
Fredgant D: Antique pharmacy bottles: sources and pricing.
**Pharm Hist** 1984;26(1):46-9
Habrich C: Die Ausstattung von Haus- und Reise-apotheken in ihrer pharmazie- und medizinhistorischen Bedeutung. **Pharm Ztg** 1979 Jun

14;124(24):1151–5
Hamarneh SK, Stieb EW: Pharmacy museums and historical collections on public view in the United States and Canada. Madison, American Institute of the History of Pharmacy in cooperation with the National Museum of American History. Washington, D.C., Smithsonian, 1981. 144 p. (Publication/American Institute of the History of Pharmacy, new series, no. 6).
Hömberg W: Bronzemörser für Apotheken Herstellung–Stilmerkmale–Fälschungen. **Beitr Gesch Pharm** 1983;31(21):33–40
Koning DA: Grosse Funde in kleinen Museen. Einige Neuentdeckungen auf dem Gebiet der Apotheken-Fayencen. In Dilg P, et al., ed: Perspektiven der Pharmaziegeschichte. Graz, Austria, Akademische Druck- u. Verlagsanstalt, 1983. p. 431–39.

**France**

Cotinat L: Les vases de pharmacie à l'exposition de faïences françaises du Grand-Palais (juin–août 1980). **Rev Hist Pharm (Paris)** 1981;28(248):49–53
Cotinat L: Vases de l'hôpital Saint-Joseph de Moulins. **Rev Hist Pharm (Paris)** 1980 Mar;27(244):11–14
Fourest HP, Sainte-Fare-Garnot PN: Les pots de pharmacie: Paris et l'Ile-de-France. Paris, Dacosta, 1981. 229 p.
Saumande P: Une collection d'instruments scientifiques anciens au Laboratoire de Physique pharmaceutique de la Faculté de Médecine et de Pharmacie de Limoges. **Bull Soc Archeol Hist Limousin** 1981;108:157–8

**Great Britain**

Lothian A, Short GR: Angel design drug jars. **Pharm Hist (London)** 1977 Mar;7(1):1
Matthews LG: Apothecaries' memorials. **Pharm Hist (London)** 1968 Mar;1(2):2

**Israel**

Drey RE: Drug jars from the Convent of St. Saviour of Jerusalem. **Pharm Hist (London)** 1984;14(1):11–2

**Yugoslavia**

Herkov Z: Srpska apotekarska funta. **Glas Srp Akad Nauka Umet** 1982;328(22):87–95

**Before 500 A.D.**

Haneveld GT: De antieke reisapotheek. **Arts Auto** 1981;47:896–9

**500 A.D.–1450**

**Arabic**

Bernus-Taylor M, Kalus L: Musée du Louvre, département des Antiquités orientales. Un vase d'apothicaire islamique. **Rev Louvre Mus Fr** 1980;30(2):95–101

**Great Britain**

Hutton DA: York bellfounders and their mortars. **Pharm Hist (London)** 1984 Sep;14(3):2–5

**1450–1700**

**Great Britain**

Burnby J: The Thomas Fautrart pill tile. **Pharm Hist (London)** 1977 Dec;7(3):6
Drey RE: A dated slipware drug jar. **Pharm Hist (London)** 1975 May;5(1):1

**Italy**

Burnett J: The Giustiniani medicine chest. **Med Hist** 1982 Jul;26(3):325–33
Drey RE: Trois familles nobles de Florence et leur vases de pharmacie. **Rev Hist Pharm (Paris)** 1982 Sep;29(254):177–9
Lise G: Ceramica del '600 e farmacia / Giorgio Lise. Milano, Giuliani, 1974. 113 p.

**1700 to Present**

Bogard MO, Higby GJ: A look at covered mortars and pestles. **Pharm Hist** 1984;26(2):106–8
Bogard MO: Colored glass in pharmacy. **Pharm Hist** 1984;26(1):20–7
Bogard MO: Eighteenth-century poison phials. **Pharm Hist** 1984;26(4):183–4
Bogard MO: Vials and bottles for peppermint and other essences. **Pharm Hist** 1983;25(3):142–6
Jackson WA: Aether rounds. **Pharm Hist (London)** 1976 Aug;6(2):4
Jacobs D: Israel health stamps [on medicine bottles] **Scalpel Tongs** 1981;25:68–9
Sheldon PB: Mortar and pestle. **J Med Soc NJ** 1983 Feb;80(2):134

**Caribbean**

Watters DR: A Turlington balsam phial from Montserrat, West Indies: genuine or counterfeit? **Hist Archaeol** 1981;15(1):105–8

**Germany**

Hein WH: Fälschungen deutscher Apothekengläser. **Beitr Gesch Pharm** 1982;31(15):113–16
Hügelow M: Original-Lithographien speziell für Pharmazeuten: Historische Apothekergeräte und Heilpflanzen. **Pharm Unserer Zeit** 1984 Jul;13(4):97–101

**Great Britain**

Jackson WA: Antiques of Mander, Weaver and Co., Wolverhampton. **Pharm Hist (London)** 1978 Dec;8(3):4–6

**Poland**

Roeske W: Ceramika apteczna z Proszkowa w Muzeum Farmacji Am w Krakowie. Krakow, 1978. 20 p.

**Spain**

Carmona Cornet AM, Bofill Pellicer C: Instruments i operacions farmacéutiques del segle XIX a Catalunya: creació d'un aparell destl.latori de vapor per a ús farmacéutic. **Bol Soc Esp Hist Farm** 1980/81 Dec–Mar;31–32(124–5):275–82

**United States**

Levy B: Pharmacy graduates in use from 1880 to 1920. **Pharm Hist** 1984;26(3):150–4
Sheldon PB: Wooden medicine chest. **J Med Soc NJ** 1983 May;80(5):383

## GOVERNMENT REGULATION

Goldberg A: A Committee on Safety of Medicines. **Health Bull (Edinb)** 1981 Nov;39(6):393–7
Penn RG: The state control of medicines: the first 3000 years. **Br J Clin Pharmacol** 1979 Oct;8(4):293–305

**Great Britain**

Penn RG: Veterinary drugs: the beginnings of legislative control in the U.K. **Vet Res Commun** 1983 Dec;7(1–4):377–81

**Hungary**

Zolyomi ND: Ein Beitrag zur Entwicklung der Apothekenvisitationen in Ungarn des 17. und 18. Jahrhunderts. Von den Theriakvorführungen zur wissenschaftlich fundierten Apothekenvisitation. **Pharm Acta Helv** 1979;54(4):114–6

**1450–1700**

**France**

Bachoffner P: Le premier règlement des apothicaires de Strasbourg (vers 1500). **Rev Hist Pharm (Paris)** 1981;28(248):35–8

**Poland**

Drygas A: Uprawnienia rektorów Uniwersytetu Krakowskiego w zakresie kontroli aptek krakowskich w XV i XVI wieku w świetle źródeł i prezekazów pośrednich. **Arch Hist Med (Warsz)** 1983;46(2):183–203

**Switzerland**

Dilg P: Die 'Reformation der Apotecken' (1536) des Berner Stadtarztes Otto Brunfels. **Gesnerus** 1979;36(3–4):181–205

**1700 to Present**

Craig RB, Turner MA: International control of narcotics and dangerous drugs: a synopsis. **Indian Pol Sci Rev** 1977;11(1):33–47
Frey EF: The regulations of patent medicines in the United States and France. **Bookman** 1983 Jan–Feb;10(1):3–6
Kaymakcalan S: Fifty years of international control of dependence-producing drugs. **Natl Inst Drug Abuse Res Monogr Ser**

1979;27:74-6
Scheerer S: The new Dutch and German drug laws: social and political conditions for criminalization and decriminalization. **Law Soc Rev** 1978;12(4):585-606

### Asia

Solomon R: The rise and fall of the Laotian and Vietnamese opiate trades. **J Psychedelic Drugs** 1979 Jul-Sep;11(3):159-71

### Canada

Stieb EW: Three centennials: a retrospective view of Canada's pure food and drug legislation. In: Congrès international d'histoire de la médecine, XXVe, Québec, 1976. Actes. Québec, 1977. p. 1327-40.

### Cuba

Valverde JL, Martin C: Situacion de los boticarios cubanos en sus relaciones con el Tribunal del Protomedicato S. XVIII. **Bol Soc Esp Hist Farm** 1982 Mar;33(129):3-7

### Czechoslovakia

Drábek P: Dějiny Státního ústavu pro kontrolu léčiv (1918-1983). II. Vývoj Státního ústavu pro kontrolu léčiv (1952-1983). **Cesk Farm** 1984 Jun;33(5):201-9
Hanzlíček Z: Dějiny Státního ústavu pro kontrolu léčiv (1918-1983). Dějiny ustavu pro zkoumáni léčiv (1918-1952). **Cesk Farm** 1984 Mar;33(2):83-91

### France

Dillemann G: Le monopole pharmaceutique et le décret du 2 mars 1791. **Rev Hist Pharm (Paris)** 1980 Dec;247(68 no 27):235-8
Ramsey M: Traditional medicine and medical enlightenment: the regulation of secret remedies in the ancien regime. **Hist Reflect** 1982;9(1-2):215-32

### Germany

Burkhardt R, Kienle G: Controlled clinical trials and drug regulations: a report of recent developments in the Federal Republic of Germany. **Controlled Clin Trials** 1980 Sep;1(2):153-66
Posseh1 I: Die Arzneitaxe--auch im 19. Jahrhundert ein Problem. **Beitr Gesch Pharm** 1980;8:61-3

### Great Britain

Campbell WA: Oxalic acid, epsom salt and the poison bottle. **Hum Toxicol** 1982 Mar;1(2):187-93
Goldberg A: Ten years of The Medicines Act. **Br J Clin Pharmacol** 1981 Oct;12(4):447-8

### Mexico

Craig RB: Human rights and Mexico's antidrug campaign. **Soc Sci Q** 1980;60(4):691-701

### Spain

Alvarez de Abajo M, Frances Causape MC: La inspeccion de boticas en el Obispado de Malaga entre 1824 y 1830. **Bol Soc Esp Hist Farm** 1981 Dec;32(128):251-63
Folch Jou G, Muñoz Calvo S: El concepto de 'Legislacion Farmaceutica' a traves de la Historiografia Universitaria de la Facultad de Farmacia de Madrid (1884-1965). **Bol Soc Esp Hist Farm** 1982 Mar;33(131):145-61
Folch Jou G, Muñoz Calvo S: Un intento de reforma legislativa en la Farmacia Española del siglo XIX: J. Guerrero Fernández y su 'Proyecto de Servicio Farmacéutico'. **Bol Soc Esp Hist Farm** 1980/81 Dec-Mar;31-32(124 5):299 314
Jordi González R: Visita de boticas en Cataluña a principios del siglo XVIII (16-3-1710/10-4-1710). **Circ Farm** 1982 Jan-Mar;40(274):111-39
Lobo F: Perspectivas de la autorización de medicamentos en España. **Rev Sanid Hig Publica (Madr)** 1983 May-Jun;57(5-6):509-15
Muñoz Calvo S: Notas para un estudio historiográfico de la legislación farmacéutica en España. **Bol Soc Esp Hist Farm** 1979 Dec;30(120):305-17

### United States

Ballentine C: Taste of raspberries, taste of death: the 1937 elixir sulfanilamide incident. **FDA Consum** 1981 Jun;15(5):18-21
Cowen DL: Louisiana--pioneer in the regulation of pharmacy. **La Pharm** 1982 Apr;41(4):4-9
Goedde AG: Internal diversification and US regulatory controls in the pharmaceutical industry. **Q Rev Econ Bus** 1982;22(1):101-10
Goyan JE: Dr. Harvey Wiley's brainchild, 75 years later. **J Assoc Off Anal Chem** 1981 Mar;64(2):256-9
Grabowski HG, Vernon JM, Thomas LG: Estimating the effects of regulation on innovation: an international comparative analysis of the pharmaceutical industry. **J Law Econ** 1978;21(1):133-63
Hammer SN, ed: Symposium for the 75th Anniversary of the Food, Drug & Cosmetic Act, Meat Inspection Act, 1906-1981. Monday, June 8, 1981. Washington, D.C. **Food Drug Cosmet Law J** 1982 Jan;37(1):3-149
Harvey W. Wiley and the Pure Food and Drug Act: **Nutr Hist Notes** 1981;11:2-4
Hayes AH: Food and drug regulation after 75 years. **JAMA** 1981 Sep 11;246(11):1223-6
History of FDA patient package insert requirements.: **Am J Hosp Pharm** 1980 Dec;37(12):1660-1
Hutt PB: About fairness in applying the law. **FDA Consum** 1981 Jun;15(5):23-5
Hutt PB: Food and drug law: a strong and continuing tradition. In Hammer SN, ed: Symposium for the 75th Anniversary of the Food, Drug & Cosmetic Act, Meat Inspection Act, 1906-1981. Monday, June 8, 1981. Washington, D.C. **Food Drug Cosmet Law J** 1982 Jan;37(1):123-37
Hutt PB: Investigations and reports respecting FDA regulation of new drugs (Part I). **Clin Pharmacol Ther** 1983 Apr;33(4):537-48
Jackson CO: A difficult pill to swallow. **Rev Am Hist** 1981;9(4):516-20
Janssen WF: FDLI's unforgettable character: Charles Wesley Dunn. **Food Drug Cosmet Law J** 1982 Oct;37(4):446-56
Janssen WF: Food and Drug Administration celebrates 75 years of consumer protection -- an album from the archives. **Public Health Rep** 1981 Nov-Dec;96(6):487-94
Janssen WF: Pharmacy .. and the Food and Drug Law. **Am Pharm** 1981 Apr;21(4):28-36
Janssen WF: The story of the laws behind the labels. **FDA Consum** 1981 Jun;15(5):32-45
Johnson DR: The history of the 1906 Pure Food and Drugs Act and the Meat Inspection Act. In Hammer SN, ed: Symposium for the 75th Anniversary of the Food, Drug & Cosmetic Act, Meat Inspection Act, 1906-1981. Monday, June 8, 1981. Washington, D.C. **Food Drug Cosmet Law J** 1982 Jan;37(1):5-9
Lambert EI: The United States labeling regulations for vegetable proteins: an historical perspective. **J Am Oil Chem Soc** 1979 Mar;56(3):234-7
Laubach GD: Federal regulation and pharmaceutical innovation. **Proc Acad Polit Sci** 1980;33(4):60-80
Litman RC, Litman DS: Protection of the American consumer: the congressional battle for the enactment of the First Federal Food and Drug Law in the United States. **Food Drug Cosmet Law J** 1982 Jul;37(3):310-29
Markle GE, Petersen JC, ed: Politics, science, and cancer: the laetrile phenomenon. Boulder, Westview Press, for the American Association for the Advancement of Science, 1980. xiii, 190 p. (AAAS Selected Symposium, v. 46). Contributions by JH Young, RD Smith, RF Rich, GP Monaco, Al Caplan, D Nelkin.
Miller HD: Patent license restrictions in the prescription drug industry. **Va Law Rev** 1967;53(6):1283-313
Monson MC: The dirty little secret behind our drug laws. **Reason** 1980;12(7):48-52
Priebe PM, Kauffman GB: Making governmental policy under conditions of scientific uncertainty: a century of controversy about saccharin in Congress and the laboratory. **Minerva** 1980 Winter;18(4):556-74
Rothschild L: FDA's changing role in food safety. **FDA Consum** 1981 Jun;15(5):28-31
Shapiro LJ, Angorn RA, McCormick WC: Look-alike prescription drugs. A historical perspective of the legal issues. **Am Pharm** 1982 Aug;22(8):26-30
Silverman M, Lee PR, Lydecker M: Pills and the public purse: the routes to national drug insurance. Berkeley, University of California Press, 1981. xviii, 232 p.
Small WE: FDA: today's strengths built on turbulent past. **Am Pharm** 1980 Jan;20(1):25-7
Steele H: The fortunes of economic reform legislation: the case of the Drug Amendments Act of 1962. **Am J Econ Sociol** 1966;25(1):39-52
Stewart D: Unapproved generics. A generation of confusion. **Am Pharm** 1980 Nov;20(11):12-7
Talbott MW: Intraocular lenses and the Food and Drug Administration: regulation amid controversy. **Int Ophthalmol Clin** 1979 Fall;19(3):1 10
Taylor MR: History of cosmetic color additive regulation: creative maneuvering by FDA bodes well for the future. **Food Drug Cosmet Law J** 1982 Apr;37(2):152-62
Temin P: Regulation and the choice of prescription drugs. **Am Econ Rev** 1980;70(2):301-5
Temin P: Taking your medicine. Drug regulation in the United States. Cambridge, Massachusetts, and London, Harvard Univ. Press, 1980. 274 p.
Temin P: The origin of compulsory drug prescriptions. **J Law Econ** 1979;22(1):91-106
Tocus EC, Nelson RC, Vocci FJ: Regulatory perspectives and the benzodiazepines. **J Psychoactive Drugs** 1983 Jan-Jun;15(1-2):151-7
Wiggins SN: The impact of regulation on pharmaceutical research expenditures: a dynamic approach. **Econ Inq** 1983;21(1):115-28
Wolfe MR: Lucius Polk Brown and progressive food and drug control. Tennessee and New York City 1908-1920. Lawrence, Regents Press of

Kansas, 1978. 194 p.
Young JH: Laetrile in historical perspective. **Conn Med** 1979 Aug;43(8):497-500
Young JH: Laetrile in historical perspective. In Markle GE, Petersen JC, ed: Politics, science and cancer: the laetrile phenomenon. Boulder, CO. Westview Press, for American Association for the Advancement of Science, Washington, D. C., 1980. p. 11-60.
Young JH: Nutritional eccentricities. In Neuberger A, Jukes TH, ed: Human nutrition: current issues and controversies. Lancaster, England, MTP Press, 1982. p. 217-32.
Young JH: Self-dosage medicine in America, 1906 and 1981. **South Atl Q** 1981 Autumn;80(4):379-90
Young JH: The early years of federal food and drug control. Madison, Wis., 1982. 60 p. (Publication/American Institute of the History of Pharmacy. new series, no. 7)
Young JH: The long struggle for the 1906 law. **FDA Consum** 1981 Jun;15(5):12-7
Young JH: The regulation of health quackery. **Pharm Hist** 1984;26(1):3-12
Young JH: 'This greasy counterfeit': butter versus oleomargarine in the United States Congress, 1886 (the Fielding H. Garrison Lecture). **Bull Hist Med** 1979 Fall;53(3):392-414
Young JH: Three southern food and drug cases. **J South Hist** 1983:49(1):3-36

### SOCIETIES

**France**

Bournique CP: La S.H.P. a Douai, Seclin et Lille. **Rev Hist Pharm (Paris)** 1981;28(248):5-13

**Great Britain**

Whittet TD: The octocentenary of the Pepperers' Gild. **Pharm Hist** 1980;22(3):111-13

#### 1450-1700

**Italy**

Rocchietta S: Von der Apothekergilde während des 15. Jahrhunderts gestiftete Glasfenster im Dom von Mailand. **Beitr Gesch Pharm** 1981;31(13):97-100

**Spain**

Jordi González R: Control de substancias medicinales por el colegio de boticarios de Barcelona en el siglo XVI (1531-1574). Federacion Farmaceutica, Sociedad Cooperative, Seccion Cienfica, 28th, Barcelona, April 7, 1983. 12 p.

#### 1700 to Present

**Australia**

Sekuless P: The first fifty years: an historical review of the Pharmacy Guild of Australia 1928-78. Canberra, Pharmacy Guild of Australia, 1978. 45 p.

**France**

Dehillerin B, Goubert JP: A la conquete du monopole pharmaceutique: le College de Pharmacie de Paris (1777-96). **Hist Reflect** 1982;9(1-2):233-48
Dehillerin B: Le Collège de Pharmacie de Paris: du régime des corporations au régime de germinal ou de l'étonnante vitalité du modèle parisien. Th. doct. 3e cycle. Paris, Univ. Paris I, 1981. 346 leaves.
Dehillerin B: Les maîtres apothicaires de Paris au XVIIIe siècle: le Collège de Pharmacie. Mém. de maîtrise. Paris, Univ. Paris I, 1976. 333 leaves.
Poillot J: Pharmaciens de la Côte-d'Or: Cent ans de vie syndicale, 1880-1980. Dijon, Chambre Syndicale des Pharmaciens de la Côte-d'Or, 1981. 235 p.
Procès-verbaux des délibérations du Collège de Pharmacie de Paris: **Rev Hist Pharm (Paris)** 1981;28(248):45-8 (continued regularly)
Procès-Verbaux des délibérations du Collège de Pharmacie, puis Société libre des Pharmaciens de Paris: **Rev Hist Pharm (Paris)** 1982 Jun;29(253):109-14
Procès-verbaux des délibérations du Collège de Pharmacie, puis Société libre des Pharmaciens de Paris: **Rev Hist Pharm (Paris)** 1984 Mar;31(260):73-6
Procès-verbaux des délibérations du Collège de Pharmacie, puis Société libre des Pharmaciens de Paris: **Rev Hist Pharm (Paris)** 1984 Jun;31(261):171-6

**Germany**

Wankmüller A: Die Anfänge der Pharmazeutischen Gesellschaft Tübingen. **Dtsch Apoth Ztg** 1980 Jul 31;120(31):1460-2

**Great Britain**

Court WE: The pharmaceutical society's collection of materia medica and herbaria. **Pharm Hist (London)** 1980 Dec;10(3):2-3
Matthews LG: The History of Pharmacy Committee of the Pharmaceutical Society 1952-1967. **Pharm Hist (London)** 1976 Dec;6(3):3-4
Neild FG: Lieutenant Colonel C. T. Samman, OStJ, MRCS, LSA, DPH, Master of the Society of Apothecaries, 1928-31. **J R Army Med Corps** 1983 Oct;129(3):184-5
Whittet TD: The Crown & Anchor and the arts and sciences. **Pharm Hist (London)** 1983 Sept;13(3-4):2-6, 5-8

**Hungary**

Zalai K: A Magyar Gyógyszerészeti Társaság ötven éve (1924-1974). Budapest, Magyar Gyógyszerészeti Társaság, 1974. 75 p.

**Spain**

Folch Jou G, Muñoz Calvo S: Datos para la historia del Colegio de Boticarios de Madrid. Actos con motivo de la preparacion de la Triaca en el siglo XVIII. **An R Acad Farm (Madr)** 1979;45(4):599-606
Jordi González FR: Un desconocido anteproyecto de confederación de farmacias nacido en Barcelona durante la guerra civil de 1936-1939. **Circ Farm** 1979 Dec;11(121):54-8

**United States**

Allen BF: Formation of the Maryland State Pharmaceutical Association. **Med Pharm (Tokyo)** 1982 Apr;:4-7
The American Institute of Pharmacy: 50th anniversary: **Am Pharm** 1984 Aug;NS24(8):suppl 1-16
ASHP Research and Education Foundation dedicates the Donald E. Francke Memorial Library: **Am J Hosp Pharm** 1982 Jul;39(7):1206-10
Cowen DL: The historical collections of the Pharmacist Institute of New Jersey. **NJ J Pharm** 1980 Oct;53(10):15 and 1982 Jan;55(1):8-9
Green MW: Epilogue, prologue: from the past comes the future: the first 75 years of the National Association of Boards of Pharmacy. Chicago, National Association of Boards of Pharmacy, 1979. ix, 109 p.
Magalian P: Florida Society of Hospital Pharmacists, Inc.: thirty-five years, 1947-1982. [Miami?], The Society, 1983. iii, 15 p.
Sonnedecker G: The records of the American Association of Colleges of Pharmacy. **Pharm Hist** 1980;22(3):113-14

## PHILATELY

Blodi FC: Ophthalmology and philately: I. Ophthalmologists on stamps--Ricardo Vertiz. **Arch Ophthalmol** 1979 Sep;97(9):1706 (continued periodically)
Drinnan AJ: Odontophilately. **NY State Dent J** 1980 Apr;46(4):173
Dubb A: Medical philately. Doctors in politics. **S Afr Med J** 1980 Aug 23;58(8):326-9
Dubb A: Medical philately: The pen and the scalpel -- the story of medicine and literature. **S Afr Med J** 1979 Nov 17;56(21):847-50
Geschichte der Tuberkulose - philatelistisch illustriert: **MMW** 1982 Apr 23;124(16):92-3
Kler JH: Medicine and religion. **J Med Soc NJ** 1983 May;80(5):382
Kyle RA, Shampo MA: [Historical aspects of medicine and philately]. **JAMA** 1982 Feb 12;247(6):796 (continued regularly)
Kyle RA, Shampo MA, ed: Medicine and stamps. Vol. 2. Huntington, New York, Krieger, 1980. xv, 209 p. (Reprinted articles from Journal of the American Medical Association).
Leden I: Reumatologisk farmakoterapi ur historiskt/filatelistiskt perspektiv. **Lakartidningen** 1980 Dec 24;77(52):4943-6
Light TR: Hands on stamps. **J Hand Surg** 1982 Jan;7(1):20
Loevy HT, Kowitz A: Dentistry on stamps. **J Am Dent Assoc** 1980 Jun;100(6):917, 924
Loevy HT, Kowitz A: Dentistry on stamps. **J Am Dent Assoc** 1981 Jul;103(1):143
Loevy HT, Kowitz A: Dentistry on stamps. **J Am Dent Assoc** 1983 Oct;107(4):618 (continued periodically)
Loevy HT, Kowitz A: Health science on stamps. **J Am Dent Assoc** 1980 Jan;100(1):86
Loevy HT, Kowitz A: Health science on stamps. **J Am Dent Assoc** 1980 Jul;101(1):156
Shampo MA, Kyle RA: [Contributions to the history of medical philately]. **JAMA** 1981 Dec 4;246(22):2572 (continued periodically)
Short GR: Postal and pharmaceutical history. **Pharm Hist (London)** 1974 Dec;4(3):5-6
Ullman AH: Analytical chemists on postage stamps. **Anal Chem** 1982 Jun;54(7):780A-785A
Vaksman IA, Popugaĭlo VM: Istoriia anesteziologii i reanimatsii v filatelii. **Anesteziol Reanimatol** 1984 Mar-Apr;(2):75-7
Verveen G: Chirurgia: the handicraft of medicine. Philatelically illustrated historic survey of surgery. **Am J Surg** 1982 May;143(5):640-8

Verveen G: Venerologie auf Briefmarken; Philatelistisch illustrierte Geschichte der Venerologie. **Z Hautkr** 1981 Feb 15;56(4):227-33

**Australia**

Pearn J: Medical philately of Australia. Sydney, [s.n.], 1978. 32 p.

**Germany**

Loevy HT, Kowitz A: Dentistry on stamps. **J Am Dent Assoc** 1982 Jun;104(6):890

**Syria**

Drinnan AJ: Odontophilately (Abul Kasim). **NY State Dent J** 1979 Aug-Sep;45(7):332

**United States**

Brewer AF: U.S. philately in medicine. **J Fla Med Assoc** 1979 Aug;66(8):866-70

**1450-1700**

Kler JH: Along the path of modern medicine. **J Med Soc NJ** 1983 Jul;80(7):552
Light TR: Hands on stamps. **J Hand Surg** 1981 Sep;6(5):441

**1700 to Present**

Agris J: Stamps commemorating medicine: Emily Bissell. **J Dermatol Surg Oncol** 1980;6(9):705
Agris J: Stamps commemorating medicine: 'Indian folk art: the medicine man'. **J Dermatol Surg Oncol** 1981;7(1):82
Berar L: History of ophthalmology in stamps. **Metab Pediatr Syst Ophthalmol** 1982;6(3-4):367-9
Bläsig W: Die Sondermarken zum Internationalen Jahr der Behinderten - geordnet nach Gesichtspunkten der Rehabilitation. **Rehabilitation (Stuttg)** 1983 Nov;22(4):162-5
Bluefarb SM: Dermatologists on postage stamps (Hulusi Behçet, Ruzar Briffa). **Int J Dermatol** 1982 Jan-Feb;21(1):54
Bowman IA: The image of the nurse on international postage stamps, 1920-1970. In Jones AH, ed: Images of healers. Albany, State University of New York, Press, 1983. p. 91-100.
Bowman IA, ed: Child health on postage stamps. **Bookman** 1982 Feb;9(2):3-7
Chernetskiĭ OE: Meditsinskie sestry na pochtovykh markakh. **Med Sestra** 1980 Apr;39(4):53-6
Devlin J: Nurses join the stamp set. **Nurs Times** 1984 May 2-8;80(18):40-1
Dubb A: Medical philately: Robert Koch (1843-1910) the man, his germ and history. **Adler Mus Bull** 1984 Mar;10(1):16-22
Dubb A: Medical philately: sport and medicine. **S Afr Med J** 1981 Jul 25;60(4):144-6
Durnin E: Cancels unite world against malaria. **Scalpel Tongs** 1981;25:49
Evans M: Medicine and stamps. **Hist Med (Lond)** 1981;9(1):21-2
Griffenhagen G: Drug and underprints from France. [Laboratoire Veyron-Froment, Marseilles.] **Scalpel Tongs** 1981;25:61-3
Harsch OM: Philatelistisch-Odontologises Panopticum. **Zahnarztl Mitt** 1983 Jul 1;73(13):1470-1 contd
Julien P: Pharmacie et philatélie. **Rev Hist Pharm (Paris)** 1981;28:69-73
Kler JH: Medical philately. Missionary medicine. **J Med Soc NJ** 1983 Apr;80(4):302
Kler JH: Medical pioneers. **J Med Soc NJ** 1982 Dec;79(13):1025
Martin MW: Stamping out dentistry. **Tic** 1979;38(7):11;(9):5
Palmieri TJ: Scientists' hands on stamps. **J Hand Surg** 1983 Jan;8(1):3
Red Cross in philately: **Scalpel Tongs** 1981;25:39-43
Spina MB: '... Nothing beats stamp collecting ...' **Tic** 1979;38(8):12-5
Vaksman IA, Popugaĭlo VM: Zhenshchiny mediki na pochtovykh markakh mira. **Feldsher Akush** 1984 Jul;49(7):38-43
Zuring J: Saint Côme et Saint Damien dans la philatélie. **Rev Hist Pharm (Paris)** 1984 Mar;31(260):69-72

**Costa Rica**

Blodi FC: Ophthalmology and philately: V. The diagnosis and treatment of occular diseases.--Eye banks. **Arch Ophthalmol** 1982 Nov;100(11):1794

**Cuba**

Blodi FC: Ophthalmology and philately: II. Ophthalmologists who became famous in other areas of endeavor--Carlos Finlay (1833-1915). **Arch Ophthalmol** 1980 Oct;98(10):1763

**France**

Shampo MA, Kyle RA: Jacques-Alexandre-César Charles. **JAMA** 1984 May 18;251(19):2547

**Germany**

Bäsig W: Die Philatelie im Dienste der Rehabilitation. **Rehabilitation (Stuttg)** 1981 May;20(2):86-9
Blodi FC: Ophthalmology and philately. **Arch Ophthalmol** 1982 Mar;100(3):425,44 (continuing periodically)
Drinnan AJ: Odontophilately. **NY State Dent J** 1980 Feb;46(2):73
Rehder K, Shampo MA, Kyle RA: Physician's personal in-flight medical kit. **JAMA** 1982 Feb 19;247(7):1011

**Israel**

Jacobs D: Israel health stamps [on medicine bottles] **Scalpel Tongs** 1981;25:68-9

**Mauritius**

Sir Thomas Lewis centenary stamp: **Lancet** 1981;ii:378

**New Zealand**

Griffenhagen G: Pharmacy centennials in Australia and New Zealand. **Scalpel Tongs** 1981;25:75

**Philippines**

Agris J: Stamps commemorating medicine. 'Honoria Acosta Sison' pioneer gynecologist and obstetrician. **J Dermatol Surg Oncol** 1980 Mar;6(3):178

**Portugal**

Blodi FC: Ophthalmology and philately: I. Ophthalmologist on stamps--M.R. de Gama Pinto (1853-1945). **Arch Ophthalmol** 1980 Jan;98(1):143

**Spain**

Sorní J, Suñé JM: Marcofilia farmacéutica española. III. **Bol Soc Esp Hist Farm** 1984 Sep;35(139):211-6

**Sweden**

Loevy HT, Kowitz A: Dentistry on stamps (Dr. Kerstin Palm). **J Am Dent Assoc** 1984 Nov;109(5):755

**United States**

Agris J: 'Henry Dearborn'. Physician, soldier, civil servant, diplomat. **J Dermatol Surg Oncol** 1979 Sep;9(5):677
Agris J: 'Jane Addams'. Medical student, social worker and activist, humanitarian. **J Dermatol Surg Oncol** 1979 Dec;5(12):936
Agris J: 'John McLoughlin' physician, pioneer, fur trader, settler. **J Dermatol Surg Oncol** 1979 Oct;5(10):760
Agris J: Stamps commemorating medicine. 'American Red Cross'. **J Dermatol Surg Oncol** 1981 Sep;7(9):697
Agris J: Stamps commemorating medicine. 'Dr. Charles R. Drew'. **J Dermatol Surg Oncol** 1982 Feb;8(2):96
Agris J: Stamps commemorating medicine. 'Dr. Crawford Williamson Long' the father of anesthesia. **J Dermatol Surg Oncol** 1980 May;6(5):415
Agris J: Stamps commemorating medicine. 'Dr. Mary Edwards Walker' (1832-1919). **J Dermatol Surg Oncol** 1982 Nov;8(11)::926
Agris J: Stamps commemorating medicine: 'Ephraim McDowell' (1771-1830). **J Dermatol Surg Oncol** 1980 Aug;6(8):621
Agris J: Stamps commemorating medicine. 'The Doctors William James and Charles Horace Mayo'. **J Dermatol Surg Oncol** 1980 Jul;6(7):523
Chakravorty RC: Charles Richard Drew (1904-1950). **Scalpel Tongs** 1981;25:69-70
Drew GR: The Dr. Charles R. Drew stamp. **J Afro-Am Hist Geneol Soc** 1981;2(4):139-42
Holcombe HW: Patent medicine tax stamps. A history of the firms using United States private die proprietary medicine tax stamps. Ed. G. D. Griffenhagen. Lawrence, Quarterman, 1979. xxv, 604 p. Reprinted articles from various journals.
Yancey AG: US postage stamp issued in honor of Charles R. Drew, MD, MDSc. **J Natl Med Assoc** 1982 Jun;74(6):561-5

# PHILOSOPHY

Baumann HU: Ueber Mehrfachentdeckungen. Eine Darstellung des allgemeinen Problems mit Beispielen aus drei Teilgebieten der theoretischen Medizin. Diss. Münster, 1972. 133 p.
Bean WB: Changing patterns of ideas about disease. In Rothschild H, ed: Biocultural aspects of disease. New York, Academic Press, 1981. p. 25-51.
Beering SC: 'The spark within.' **J Indiana State Med Assoc** 1982 Jan;75(1):22-4
Bouchet A, Masson JL: Les localisations anatomiques de l'âme au cours

des siècles. **Hist Sci Med** 1980;14(1):95–106

Brazier MA: Challenges from the philosophers to the neuroscientists. In Brain and mind. Ciba Foundation Symposium 69 (new series). Amsterdam, Oxford, New York, Excerpta Medica, 1979. p. 5–43.

Brody H: Placebos and the philosophy of medicine: clinical, conceptual and ethical issues. Chicago and London, University of Chicago Press, 1980. vii, 164 p.

Buschauer W: Homöopathie als Vollendung der Hippokratischen Medizin. Heidelberg, Haug, 1982. Historical sections, p. 9–79.

Cilenti V, Milasi G, Jori A: Evoluzione storica del concetto di dolore. **Med Secoli** 1982 May–Aug;19(2):225–30

Costa O: Storie sommerse di biologia e medicina. **Scientia** 1980;115:215–25

D'Arcy E: [History of the theory of] natural law [in bioethics]. In Reich WT, et al, ed: Encyclopedia of bioethics, v.3. New York, Free Press, 1978. p. 1131–7.

Duminil MP: La recherche hippocratique aujourd'hui. **Hist Philos Life Sci** 1979;1(1):153–81

Eastwood BS: Cosmology and physiology in Galenic visual theory: Hunayn Ibn Ishaq. **Trans Stud Coll Physicians Phila** 1980 Dec;5(2 no 4):276–83

Engelhardt D von: Medizin und Philosophie - Positionen und Gegenstand in der Entwicklung der Neuzeit. **MMG** 1980;5:94–100

Engelhardt HT: Philosophical perspectives [of health and disease]. In Reich WT, et al, ed: Encyclopedia of bioethics, v. 2. New York, Free Press, 1978. p. 599–605.

Engelhardt HT, Erde EL: [Philosophy of medicine]. In Reich WT, et al, ed: Encyclopedia of bioethics, v.3. New York, Free Press, 1978. p. 1049–54.

Epistemologia, metodologia clinica e storia della scienza medica, 1: Roma, Cossidente, 1977. xliii, 225 p. (Collana di Studi Epistemologici). Introduction by D. Antiseri. Contributions by D. Antiseri, G. Giunchi, M. Baldini, O. Todisco, M. D. Grmek, P. Potestà, V. Scalera.

Epistemologia, metodologia clinica e storia della scienza medica, 2: Roma, Cossidente, 1978. 172 p. (Collana di Studi Epistemologici). Introduction by D. Antiseri. Contributions by V. Mathieu, V. Tomini, E. Urbani, V. Somenzi, G. Federspil, C. Scandellari, M. Austoni, M. Di Giandomenico, E. Riverso, E. Garulli.

Galzigna L, Galzigna M: La produzione del corpo curabile. **Acta Med Hist Patav** 1982–83;29:29–65

Goldstein-Préaud T: Albert le Grand et les questions du XIIIe siècle sur le De animalibus d'Aristote. **Hist Philos Life Sci** 1981;3(1):61–71

Görtz R: Esculape ou Prométhée: les mutations de la médecine du thaumaturge au démiurge. **Arch Belg Med Soc** 1980 Oct;38(8):479–516

Grmek MD: La légende et la réalité de la nocivité des fèves. **Hist Philos Life Sci** 1980;2(1):61–121

Grmek MD, Cohen RS, Cimino G, ed: On scientific discovery. The Erice Lectures 1977. Dordrecht, D. Reidel, 1981. 333 p. (Boston Studies in the Philosophy of Science, v. 34).

Guerra F: The historical cycles in traditional medicine. **Stud Hist Med** 1980 Mar;4(1):57–63

Hahn U: Die Entwicklung des Tierschutzgedankens in Religion und Geistesgeschichte. DMV Diss. Hannover, 1980. 192 p.

Hakfoort C: Wetenschapshistorische etiketten en de gevaren van polaire analyses. **Tijdschr Geschied Geneeskd** 1982;5(1):1–5

Haller JS: Aconite: a case study in doctrinal conflict and the meaning of scientific medicine. **Bull NY Acad Med** 1984 Nov;60(9):888–904

Hartmann F: Homo patiens. Zur ärztlichen Anthropologie von Leid und Mitleid. In Seidler E, Schott H, ed: Bausteine zur Medizingeschichte. Stuttgart, Steiner, 1984. p. 35–44.

Hasler L, ed: Schelling: seine Bedeutung für eine Philosophie der Natur und der Geschichte. Referate und Kolloquien der Internationalen Schelling-Tagung Zürich 1979. Stuttgart-Bad Cannstaff, Frommann-Holzboog, 1981. 319 p. Includes contributions by H. Krings, D. von Engelhardt, R. Löw, N. Tsouyopoulos, R. Toellner, H. Poser, H. Querner, K. E. Rothschuh, F. Moiso, S. Dietzch, D. v. Uslar, W. Bonsiepen.

Herrmann B: Zur Entstehung und Wirkung ästhetischer Prinzipien in der menschlichen Rassenkunde. In Imhof AE, ed: Leib und Leben in der Geschichte der Neuzeit. Berlin, Duncker & Humblot, 1983. p. 165–75.

Herzog H: Wirklichkeit und Wahrheit--Weg und Ziel ärztlichen Wirkens. **Praxis** 1982 Aug 10;71(32):1254–61

Jackson SW: Melancholia and the waning of the humoral theory. **J Hist Med Allied Sci** 1978 Jul;33(3):367–76

Jinich H, Pérez-Tamayo R, Sepúlveda B, et al: La verdad y el error en medicina. **Gac Med Mex** 1984 Apr;120(4):133–44

Kampmeier RH: Medicine as an art: the history and physical examination. **South Med J** 1982 Feb;75(2):203–10

King LS: Medical logic. **J Hist Med Allied Sci** 1978 Jul;33(3):377–85

King LS: Medical thinking, a historical preface. Princeton, Princeton University Press, 1982. vii, 336 p.

Klein-Franke F: Die klassische Antike in der Tradition des Islam. Darmstadt, Wissenschaftliche Buchgesellschaft, 1980. ix, 181 p. (Erträge der Forschung, Band 136)

Kohnen N: Arzt und Philosoph. Das Verhältnis von Medizin und Philosophie in seinem geschichtlichen Wandel. **Med Welt** 1981 Oct 16;32(42):1586–92

Labhart A: Diskursives Denken und Intuition in der medizinischen Forschung. **Helv Chir Acta** 1981 Feb;47(6):859–72

Laín Entralgo P: Being healthy down through history. In Seidler E, Schott H, ed: Bausteine zur Medizingeschichte. Stuttgart, Steiner, 1984. p. 65–72.

Laudan L: Progress and its problems. Toward a theory of scientific growth. Berkeley, Univ. of California Press, 1977. x, 257 p.

Lenihan J: Descartes versus Hippocrates--a conflict resolved? **Br J Radiol** 1984 Oct;57(682):861–5

Lichtenthaeler C: Humanismus und Aufklärung aus der Sicht der allgemeinen Medizingeschichte. In: Aufklärung und Humanismus; hrsg. von R. Toellner. Heidelberg, Lambert Schneider, 1980. p. 235–49.

Lock MM: L'homme machine et l'homme-microcosme: l'approche occidentale et l'approche japonaise des soins médicaux. **Ann Econ Soc Civilis** 1980;35:1116–36

Lonie IM: Hippocrates the iatromechanist. **Med Hist** 1981 Apr;25(2):113–50

Lorenz K, ed, Wuketits FM, ed: Die Evolution des Denkens. München, Piper, 1983. 393 p. Contributions by G. Vollmer, R. Kaspar, R. Riedl, F. Seitelberger, G. P. Wagner, W. Leinfellner, E. Oeser, H. Mohr, R. Löw.

Löw R: Was hat die Pharmaziegeschichte der Wissenschaftstheorie zu sagen? In: Vorträge des Internationalen Pharmaziehistorischen Kongresses Innsbruck 1977. Stuttgart, Wissenschaftliche Verlagsgesellscaft, 1979. p. 29–38.

Lu Gwei-djen, Needham J: Celestial lancets: a history and rationale of acupuncture and moxa. Cambridge, Cambridge University Press, 1980. xxi, 427 p.

McCullough LB: Thought-styles, diagnosis, and concepts of disease: commentary on Ludwig Fleck. **J Med Philos** 1981 Aug;6(3):257–61

Martiny M: Laënnec et la pensée hippocratique. In La collection hippocratique et son rôle dans l'histoire de la médecine. Colloque de Strasbourg (23–27 octobre 1972) organisé par le Centre de Recherches sur la Grèce Antique, avec le concours des Facultés de Philosophie et des Langues Classiques. Leiden, E. J. Brill, 1975. p. 97–105.

Massey RU: Reflections from the Dean's office. The cheerful physicians. **Conn Med** 1979 Nov;43(11):747

Merskey H: Some features of the history of the idea of pain. **Pain** 1980 Aug;9(1):3–8

Morison RS: Is there a biological person? **Milbank Mem Fund Q** 1983 Winter;61(1):3–18

Murphy EA: Skepsis, dogma, and belief. Uses and abuses in medicine. Baltimore, London, Johns Hopkins University Press, 1981. x, 176 p.

Oide S: Der Einfluss der galenischen Pneumatheorie auf die cusanische Spiritustheorie. Eine Anmerkung zu 'De quaerendo deum'. **Mitt Forschungsbeitr Cusanus Ges** 1978;13:198–207

Pfohl G: Das philosophisch-philologische Element in der medizinischen Fakultät. Ein Beitrag der Medizingeschichte, mehr zu formen als zu informieren. I, II. **Med Welt** 1980 Apr 25, May 9;(17,19):644–6,730–3

Pigeaud J: La maladie de l'ame: étude sur la relation de l'âme et du corps dans la tradition médico-philosophique antique.

Pouchelle-Peter MC: La enfermedad y sus representaciones: una ojeada sobre la persistencia. **Asclepio** 1983;35:117–28

Rather LJ: On the source and development of metaphorical language in the history of Western medicine. In Stevenson LG, ed: A celebration of medical history. Baltimore, Johns Hopkins University Press, 1982. (The Henry E. Sigerist supplements to the Bulletin of the History of Medicine; new ser., no. 6). p. 135–53. With commentary by P. H. Niebyl, p. 154–6.

Risse GB: Epidemics and medicine: the influence of disease on medical thought and practice. **Bull Hist Med** 1979 Winter;53(4):505–19

Risse GB: History of the concepts [of health and disease]. In Reich WT, et al, ed: Encyclopedia of bioethics, v. 2. New York, Free Press, 1978. p. 579–85.

Rosenbaum M, ed: Ethics and values in psychotherapy: a guidebook. New York, Free Press; London, Collier Macmillan; 1982. xvi, 464 p. Historical chapter by J. F. Drane.

Rosoff L: Roger Bacon, William of Occam and Lord Houghton: guides for the perplexed physician. **Am J Surg** 1981 Jan;141(1):2–9

Rothschuh KE: Aus der Geschichte der Naturheilbewegung (III). 'Vorläufer' des Rousseauschen Naturismus in der römischen Kaiserzeit. Die Philosophie der Stoa und die Methodische Medizin. **ZFA (Stuttgart)** 1981 May 31;57(15):1172–9

Rothschuh KE: Die Konzeptualisierung der Medizin in Geschichte und Gegenwart. **Acta Hist Leopoldina** 1980;13:27–38

Ruse M: Ought philosophers consider scientific discovery? A Darwinian case-study. In T. Nickles, ed: Scientific discovery: case studies. Dordrecht, D. Reidel, 1980. (Boston Studies in the Philosophy of Science, v. 60). p. 131–49.

Ruse M. The new dualism: 'Res Philosophica' and 'Res Historica.' In M. Ruse, ed: Nature animated. Historical and philosophical case studies in Greek medicine, nineteenth-century and recent biology, psychiatry, and psychoanalysis. Volume II. Dordrecht, D. Reidel, 1983. p. 3–25.

Sadegh-Zadeh K: World 5 and medical knowledge. **J Med Philos** 1981 Aug;6(3):263–70

Salemme MA, Celani AM: La valeur de la logique dans l'ancienne et la moderne science. In International Congress of the History of Medicine. 26th, Plovdiv, 1978. Actes du Congress. Sofia, 1981. Volume II. p. 94–6.

Santambrogio M: Minima methodica: una rubrica che affronta problemi di metodo e di concetto, e intende stimolare nella cultura medica una riflessione 'di fondo'. (continued regularly). **Kos** 1984 Feb;1(1):16–8
Schaefer H: Das Geschichtliche als Prinzip in der Medizin. In Seidler E, Schott H, ed: Bausteine zur Medizingeschichte. Stuttgart, Steiner, 1984. p. 93–9.
Schaffner KF: Discovery in the biomedical sciences: logic or irrational intuition? In T. Nickles, ed: Scientific discovery: case studies. Dordrecht, D. Reidel, 1980. (Boston Studies in the Philosophy of Science, v. 60). p. 171–212. With commentary by N. L. Maull.
Schiller F: Stepmother nature: a medico-historical scan. **Clio Med** 1979 May;13(3–4):201–18
Schipperges H: Vindication of the doctor's decisions. **Hexagon Roche** 1981;9(3):1–8
Sharkey PW, ed: Philosophy, religion and psychotherapy. Essays in the philosophical foundations of psychotherapy. Washington, University Press of America, 1982. xiii, 227 p. Contributions by R. Macklin, J. E. Morris, R. N. Sollod, J. Needleman, C. E. Scott, M. Friedman, J. F. Rychlak, E. Weisskopf-Joelson, T. S. Szasz, R. J. Sullivan.
Siniak KM, Davidenko OS: Materialisticheskoe ponimanie razvitiia épidemiologii. **Zh Mikrobiol Epidemiol Immunobiol** 1980 Sep;(9):12–7
Sjöstrand T: Medicinsk vetenskap: Historik, teori och tillämpning. Stockholm, Natur och Kultur, 1979. 183 p.
Smith CU: Don Juan and the vision of Vision. **Perception** 1981;10(4):435–53
Sommer J: Dusledky filozofické orientace pro farmacii. **Cesk Farm** 1982 Oct;31(8):297–302
Spicker SF, ed: Organism, medicine, and metaphysics. Essays in honor of Hans Jonas on his 75th birthday May 10, 1978. Dordrecht and Boston, Reidel, 1978. xxvii, 330 p. Contributions by A. Lowe, M. Landmann, P. O. Kristeller, O. E. Guttentag, E. J. Cassell, L. R. Kass, M. Grene, C. Hartshorne, S. Donnelley, B. S. Currie, R. Kennington, W. Magnus, M. Greene, R. M. Zaner, J. N. Mohanty, H. Arendt.
Tatoń J: Filozoficzna koncepcja człowieka a medycyna. **Pol Tyg Lek** 1983 Aug 15;38(33–34):1015–8
Temkin O, Frankena WK, Kadish SH: Respect for life in medicine, philosophy, and the law. (Thalheimer lectures, 1975). Baltimore: Johns Hopkins Univ. Press, 1977. ix, 107 p.
Trenn TJ: Ludwik Fleck's 'On the question of the foundations of medical knowledge'. **J Med Philos** 1981 Aug;6(3):237–56
Tubesing DA: Whole person health care: an idea in evolution. Hinsdale, Il., Wholistic Health Centers, Inc.: distributed by Society for Wholistic Medicine, 1977. 52 p.
Vahiduddin S: Body and soul. **Stud Philos Med** 1977 Mar;1(1):22–30
Vuori H, Rimpela M: The development and impact of the medical model. **Perspect Biol Med** 1981 Winter;24(2):217–28
Wayman A: The human body as microcosm in India, Greek cosmology, and sixteenth-century Europe. **Hist Relig** 1982;22(2):172–90
Wuketits FM: Wissenschaftsgeschichte und gegenwärtige Theoriendiskussion in der Biologie. **Nat Mus** 1980;110:175–81
Wuttke-Groneberg W: 'Parasitäre Glücksgefrässigkeit'. Irrationalismus in der Medizin. **Bl Dtsch Int Polit** 1980;25:572–83
Wyschogrod E: Empathy and sympathy as tactile encounter. **J Med Philos** 1981 Feb;6(1):25–43

### Afghanistan

Penkala D: 'Hot' and 'cold' in the traditional medicine of Afghanistan. **Ethnomedizin** 1980;6(1–4):201–28

### Arabic

Gran P: Medical pluralism in Arab and Egyptian history: an overview of class structures and philosophies of the main phases. **Soc Sci Med [Med Anthropol]** 1979 Dec;13B(4):339–48
Mansursov KhKh: Vrachebnoe nasledie Ibn-Siny i sovremennaia klinicheskaia meditsina. **Ter Arkh** 1980;52(11):149–51

### Asia

Mahdihassan S: An analytical and comparative study of Indian and Chinese cosmologies. **Bull Indian Inst Hist Med Hyderabad** 1982;12(1–4):1–12
Mahdihassan S: Indian and Chinese cosmic elements. **Am J Chin Med** 1979 Winter;7(4):316–23

### China

Finckh E: Tibetan medicine, theory and practice. In: Tibetan studies in honor of H. E. Richardson. Warminster, Aris and Phillips, 1980. p. 103–10.
Koh TC: Chinese medicine and martial arts. **Am J Chin Med** 1981 Autumn;9(3):181–6
Li Q: [Discussion on the time of formation of the theoretical system of Ziwuliuzhu (Selection of acupoint for treatment varied with the circadian changes of vital energy and blood flow in the channels and collaterals relevant to heavenly stem and earthly branches)] (Chi). **Chung Hua I Shih Tsa Chih** 1984;14(2):85–9
Mahdihassan S: Interpreting Chinese cosmology and its association with the dualistic doctrine of Yin-Yang. **Stud Hist Med** 1982 Sep;6(3):214–24
Pálos, S: Chinesische Heilkunst: Einführung in die Theorie und Praxis der Naturheilkunde der Chinesen--Akupunktur, Moxibustion, Heilmassage, Heilgymnastik, Atemtherapie und Pharmakologie. Bern, Barth, 1984. 286 p.
Schiffeler JW: An essay on some of the fundamental philosophical tenets found in traditional Chinese medicine. **Chin Cult** 1976;17(4):141–7
Unschuld PU: Medizin in China: eine Ideengeschichte. München, Beck, 1980. 335 p.

### Egypt

Gran P: Medical pluralism in Arab and Egyptian history: an overview of class structures and philosophies of the main phases. **Soc Sci Med [Med Anthropol]** 1979 Dec;13B(4):339–48

### Europe

Myíri JK: Philosophy and suicide--statistics in Austria-Hungary. **East Cent Eur** 1978;5(1):69–89

### France

Gysel C: Cartesianisme en tandheelkunde bij Henricus Regius (1598--1679--1979). **Rev Belge Med Dent** 1979;34(2):213–22

### Great Britain

Brown T: The mechanical philosophy and the 'animal oeconomy'. New York, Arno Press, 1981. viii, 419 p.

### Hungary

Oláh A: Althergebrachte Tierheilpraktiken im Komitat Békés, Ungarn. **Ethnomedizin** 1978–79;5(3–4):301–18

### India

Krishan Y: The doctrine of Karma and Ayurveda. **Bull Indian Inst Hist Med (Hyderabad)** 1980;10(1–4):34–9
Krishan Y: The meaning of prajnā-aparādha and karma in Ayurveda. **Bull Indian Inst Hist Med Hyderabad** 1982;12(1–4):28–33
Mahdihassan S: A comparative study of the early system of Indian cosmology and the tridosa humoral doctrine. **Indian J Hist Sci** 1980;15:223–9
Mahdihassan S: Indian alchemy or Rasayana in the light of asceticism [and] geriatrics. New Delhi, Vikas, 1979. x, 139 p.
Tabor DC: Ripe and unripe: concepts of health and sickness in Ayurvedic medicine. **Soc Sci Med** 1981;15B:439–55

### Japan

Manaka Y: [The concept of Oriental medicine] (Jpn). **Kango** 1981 May;33(6):19–25
Mito M: [Lessons in Oriental medicine: its application in nursing] (Jpn). **Kango** 1981 May;33(6):26–30
Otsuka Y: [History of logic of Oriental medicine] (Jpn). **Kango** 1981 May;33(6):4–18
Ozaki NT: Conceptual changes in Japanese medicine during the Tokugawa period. Ph.D. Diss., University of California. San Francisco, 1979. viii, 285 leaves.

### Mexico

Lopez Austin A: Almas y experiencia entre los antiguos nahuas. **Bol Soc Mex Hist Filos Med** 1983;6(45):223–33

### United States

Puckrein GA: Humoralism and social development in Colonial America. **JAMA** 1981 May 1;245(17):1755–7

### Before 500 A.D.

Israili AH: Humoral theory of Unani Tibb. **Indian J Hist Sci** 1981, reçu 1982;16(1):95–9
Kudlien F: Medizinische Aspekte der antiken Unsterblichkeitsvorstellung. **Rheinisches Mus Philol** n.f. 1978;121:218–25
Manuli P, Vegetti M: Cuore, sangue e cervello. Biologia e antropologia nel pensiero antico. Milano, Episteme, 1977. 241 p.
Sermonti G: Orpheus in Perugia. **Riv Biol** 1981 Winter;74(4):453–8
Vickers DW: The naive empiricism of an ancient medicine. **Apeiron** 1979;13(1):1–8

### China

Bridgman RF: La formation de la théorie médicale en Chine à l'occasion de la récente découverte de manuscrits à Ma Wang Dui. In Mazars G, ed: Les médecines traditionnelles de l'Asie. Strasbourg, Université Louis Pasteur, 1981. p. 5–12.

**Greco–Roman**

De Lacy PH: Galen's concept of continuity. **Greek Roman Byz Stud (Cambridge, Mass.)** 1979;20:355–69
Dierauer U: Tier und Mensch im Denken der Antike: Studien zur Tierpsychologie, Anthropologie, und Ethik. Amsterdam, Grüner, 1977. xvii, 320 p. (Studien zur antiken Philosophie, 6.).
Hameed A: Attemperament in medicine. **Stud Philos Med** 1977 Mar;1(1):31–9
Joly R: Le système cnidien des humeurs. In La collection hippocratique et son rôle dans l'histoire de la médecine. Colloque de Strasbourg (23–27 octobre 1972) organisé par le Centre de Recherches sur la Grèce Antique, avec le concours des Facultés de Philosophie et des Langues Classiques. Leiden, E. J. Brill, 1975. p. 107–27.
Jouanna J: Le schéma d'exposition des maladies et ses déformations dans les traités dérivés des Sentences cnidiennes. In La collection hippocratique et son rôle dans l'histoire de la médecine. Colloque de Strasbourg (23–27 octobre 1972) organisé par le Centre de Recherches sur la Grèce Antique, avec le concours des Facultés de Philosophie et des Langues Classiques. Leiden, E. J. Brill, 1975. p. 129–50.
Kollesch J: Galen als Vertreter der zweiten Sophistik. **Orvostort Kozl** 1981;93–96(27 No 1–4):47–54
Maróth M: Apodeiksis und Endeiksis bei Galen. **Orvostort Kozl** 1981;93–96(27 No 1–4):55–62
Pearcy LT: Galen and Stoic rhetoric. **Greek Roman Byz Stud** 1983;24:259–72
Rabel RJ: Diseases of soul in Stoic psychology. **Greek Roman Byz Stud (Cambridge, Mass.)** 1981;22:385–93
Siclari A: L'antropologia di Nemesio di Emesa. Padova, La Garangola, 1974. 318 p. (Filosofia e religione; 9).
Smith WD: Galen on Coans versus Cnidians. **Bull Hist Med** 1973 Nov–Dec;47(6):569–85

**Greece**

Abdullaev MS: Anatomiia v trudakh Aristotelia. **Arkh Anat Gistol Embriol** 1984 Mar;86(3):95–9
Azeez Pasha M: Biography of the Unani physician Arestu. **Bull Indian Inst Hist Med (Hyderabad)** 1978;8(1–4):26–31
Boylan M: The Galenic and Hippocratic challenges to Aristotle's conception theory. **J Hist Biol** 1984 Spring;17(1):83–112
Daglio P: L'epistemologia medica: nuova filosofia della medicina. **Minerva Med** 1982 Dec 8;73(47):3359–67
Dieckhöfer K: Zur Rolle einer Psychohygiene im Griechenland des 5. vorchristlichen Jahrhunderts bis zur Zeitenwende. **Clio Med** 1982 Dec;17(2–3):81–94
Galen: On the doctrines of Hippocrates and Plato. Edition, translation and commentary by P De Lacy. Second Part: Books VI–IX. Berlin, Akademie Verlag, 1980. p. 361–609. (Corpus Medicorum Graecorum, V, 4, 1, 2).
Gracia D: The structure of medical knowledge in Aristotle's philosophy. **Sudhoffs Arch** 1978;62(1):1–36
Hoffmann WF: Socrates revisited: his relevance today. **J Fam Pract** 1982 Jan;14(1):179–80
Joly R: Hippocrates and the school of Cos. Between myth and skepticism. In M. Ruse, ed: Nature animated. Historical and philosophical case studies in Greek medicine, nineteenth–century and recent biology, psychiatry, and psychoanalysis. Volume II. Dordrecht, D. Reidel, 1983. p. 29–47.
Kibre P: Hippocrates latinus: repertorium of Hippocratic writings in the Latin Middle Ages (VIII). **Traditio** 1982;38:169–71
Kozlov AM, Kozlov IA: Filosofskie vzgliady Gippokrata. **Klin Med (Mosk)** 1983 May;61(5):111–5
Kullmann W: Wesen und Bedeutung der 'Zweckursache' bei Aristoteles. **Ber Wissenschaftsgesch** 1982;5:25–39
Laín Entralgo P: Relieves hipocráticos. **Med Hist (Barc)** 1984;1:1–16
Leikola A: Alkmaion - den vetenskapliga medicinens pionjär. **Nord Medicinhist Arsbok** 1983;:59–63
Lennox J: Teleology, chance, and Aristotle's theory of spontaneous generation. **J Hist Philos** 1981;19:219–38
Lloyd GE: Magic, reason and experience. Studies in the origin and development of Greek science. Cambridge, New York, Cambridge University Press, 1979. xii, 335 p.
Lohr CH: Renaissance Latin Aristotle Commentaries: authors N–Ph. **Renaiss Q** 1979 Winter;32(4):529–80 (continued periodically)
Lohr CH: Renaissance Latin Aristotle commentaries: authors So–Z. **Renaiss Q** 1982 Summer;35(2):164–256
Müller CW: Die hippokratischen Schriften. In his: Gleiches zu Gleichem. Ein Prinzip frühgriechischen Denkens. Wiesbaden, Harrassowitz, 1965. p. 112–50. (Klassisch–philologische Studien, 31).
Müller–Rohlfsen I: Die lateinische Ravennatische Uebersetzung der hippokratischen Aphorismen aus dem 5./6. Jahrhundert n. Chr. Textkonstitution auf der Basis der Uebersetzungscodices. Hamburg, Lüdke, 1980. xlviii, 162 p. (Geistes– und Sozialwissenschaftliche Dissertationen, 55).
Nussbaum MC, ed: Aristotle's De motu animalium. Text with translation, commentary, and interpretive essays. Princeton, Princeton University Press, 1978. xxiii, 430 p.
Pfohl G: Humanitas Hippocratica. **ZFA (Stuttgart)** 1983 Dec 20;59(35–36):1943–54
Plass P: A Greek alchemical formula. **Ambix** 1982 Jul;29(2):69–73
Pomeroy SB: Plato and the female physician ('Republic', 454d 2). **Am J Philol** 1978;99:496–500
Robert F: Hippocrate, Platon, Aristote et les notions de genre et d'espèce. **Hist Philos Life Sci** 1982;4(2):173–201
Romilly J de: Théorie politique et théorie médicale dans la Grèce antique. **Actual Odontostomatol (Paris)** 1982;138:157–70
Ruck CA: Mushrooms and philosophers. **J Ethnopharmacol** 1981 Sep;4(2):179–205
Staden H von: Hairesis and heresy: the case of the haireseis iatrikai. In B. F. Meyer, E. P. Sanders, ed: Jewish and Christian self–definition. Volume three. Self–definition in the Graeco–Roman world. London, SCM Press, 1982. p. 76–100, 199–206.
Thivel A: Cnide et Cos? Essai sur les doctrines médicales dans la collection hippocratique. Paris, Les Belles Lettres, 1981. 435 p. (Publications de la Faculté des Lettres et des Sciences Humaines de Nice, 21).

**India**

Filliozat J: La doctrine classique de la médecine indienne: ses origines et ses parallèles grecs, Paris, Ecole française d'Extrême–Orient, 1975. vii, 230 p. (also Thèse 1946).

**Rome**

Dieckhöfer K: Aspekte einer rudimentären Psychologie, Psychopathologie und Psychotherapie bei Seneca. In: Congrès international d'histoire de la médecine, XXVe, Québec, 1976. Actes. Québec, 1977. p. 579–95.
Harig G: Die philosophischen Grundlagen des medizinischen Systems des Asklepiades von Bithynien. **Philologus** 1983;127:43–60
Richardson WF: Medicine: the art of guessing? **NZ Med J** 1984 Jul 11;97(759):453–5

**500 A.D.–1450**

Burchardt J: List Witelona do Ludwika we Lwowku Slaskim. Problematyka teoriopoznawcza, kosmologiczna i medyczna. Wroclaw, Polish Academy of Sciences, 1979. 225 p. (Studia Copernicana, 19).
Cadden J: A matter of life and death: water in the natural philosophy of Albertus Magnus. **Hist Philos Life Sci** 1980;2(2):241–52
Escudero Mendo A, Sagrera JE de: El Rosario de los filósofos: una copia en castellano del siglo XIII (I). **Bol Soc Esp Hist Farm** 1983;34(136):151–66
Gracia D: En torno al averroismo medico latino. **Asclepio** 1978–79;30–31:233–64
Hajal F: Galen's ethical psychotherapy: its influence on a medieval Near Eastern physician. **J Hist Med Allied Sci** 1983 Jul;38(3):320–33
Livesey SJ: Metabasis: the interrelationship of the sciences in antiquity and the Middle Ages. Ph.D. Diss., University of California. Los Angeles, 1982. x, 742 p.

**Arabic**

Arnaldez R: The theory and practice of science according to Ibn Sina and al–Biruni. **Stud Philos Med** 1977 Mar;1(1):58–69
Eastwood BS: The elements of vision: the micro–cosmology of Galenic visual theory according to Hunayn Ibn Ishaq. Philadelphia, American Philosophical Society, 1982. 59 p. (Transactions of the American Philosophical Society, Vol. 72, pt. 5).
Frank JB: Moses Maimonides: rabbi of medicine. **Yale J Biol Med** 1981 Jan–Feb;54(1):79–88
Gracia D, Vidal JL: Avicena, sobre la definición de la medicina. In International Congress of the History of Medicine, 27th, Barcelona, 1980. Actas. Barcelona, Académia de Ciències Médiques de Catalunya i Balears, 1981. p. 723–30.
Hamarneh SK: Introduction to the history and philosophy of Arabic–Islamic medicine and allied sciences. **Stud Hist Med** 1982 Sep;6(3):195–213
Kataya S, ed.: Quelle est la différence (Diagnostics Différentiels) de Abou–Bakr Zakaria Al–Razi (Rhazes). Edition Critique et commentaire de S. Kataya. Alep, Université d'Alep, Institut du Patrimoine Scientifique Arabe, 1978.
Lauer HH: Ethik und ärztliches Denken im arabischen Mittelalter. In Seidler E, Schott H, ed: Bausteine zur Medizingeschichte. Stuttgart, Steiner, 1984. p. 72–86.
Maĭmonid kak estestvoispytatel' i vrach: **Ter Arkh** 1982;54(10):137–9
Rahman F: Essence and existence in Ibn Sina: the myth and the reality. **Hamdard** 1981;4(1):3–14
Van Riet S, ed: Avicenna Latinus. Liber de philosophia prima sive scientia divina, I–IV. Louvain, Peeters; Leiden, Brill, 1977. 225 p.

Wilcox J: Problems in the Latin manuscript tradition of De differentia spiritus et animae by the physician Costa ben Luca (9/10 cent.). In International Congress of the History of Medicine, 27th, Barcelona, 1980. Actas. Barcelona, Académia de Ciències Médiques de Catalunya i Balears, 1981. p. 363–5.
Zedler BH: The prince of physicians on the nature of man. **Mod Schoolman** 1978;55(2):165–77

**France**

Eastwood BS: The place of medicine in a hierarchy of knowledge: the illustration in Lyon Palais des Arts, ms. 22, f. lr, from the eleventh century. **Sudhoffs Arch** 1982;66(1):20–37

**Great Britain**

Bitterling K: Zwei bisher unbeachtete Fragmente der mittelenglischen Uebersetzung von Bartholomaeus Anglicus, 'De rerum proprietatibus'. **Neuphilol Mitt** 1977;78:47–56

**India**

Bala P: The Ayurvedic system of medicine: its fate in medieval India. **Bull Indian Inst Hist Med Hyderabad** 1982;12(1–4):22–7

**Italy**

Siraisi NG: Taddeo Alderotti and his pupils. Two generations of Italian medical learning. Princeton, Princeton University Press, 1981. xxiii, 461 p

**Spain**

Esteva de Sagrera J: Alquimia seudoluliana y medicina. In Congrés International d'Història de la Medicina Catalana, 2nd, Barcelona, 1975. Llibre d'Actes. Barcelona, Socitra, 1977. p. 301–3.
Esteva de Sagrera J: Aplicación del 'Ars' luliana a la medicina. In Congrés International d'Història de la Medicina Catalana, 2nd, Barcelona, 1975. Llibre d'Actes. Barcelona, Socitra, 1977. p. 295–300.
Esteva de Sagrera J: Influencia decisiva de la biografía y la filosofía de Ramón Llull en su obra médica. In Congrés International d'Historia de la Medicina Catalana, 2nd, Barcelona, 1975. Llibre d'Actes. Barcelona, Socitra, 1977. p. 305–7.
Kottek S: Eléments de physiologie dans le 'Kusari' de Juda Halevi (Espagne, 12e siècle). In: Congrès international d'histoire de la médecine, XXVe, Québec, 1976. Actes. Québec, 1977. p. 840–7.
Rodríguez-Tejerina JM: El pensamiento medico de Ramon Llull en la epoca de Miramar. **Asclepio** 1978–79,30–31:277–82

**1450–1700**

Boss J: The methodus medendi as an index of change in the philosophy of medical science in the sixteenth and seventeenth centuries. **Hist Philos Life Sci** 1979;1(1):13–42
Braun L: Nature et philosophie. **Medizinhist J** 1981;16(1–2):140–50
Braun L: Paracelsus und die Philosophiegeschichte. Eine systematische Betrachtung. Wien, 1965. 26 p. (Salzburger Beiträge zur Paracelsusforschung, 5).
Cohen LJ: Bayesianism versus Baconianism in the evaluation of medical diagnoses. **Br J Philos Sci** 1980;31(1):45–62
Domandl S: Erziehung und Menschenbild bei Paracelsus. Anfänge einer verantwortungsbewussten Pädagogik. Wien, Notring, 1970. 144 p. (Salzburger Beiträge zur Paracelsusforschung, 9).
Glesinger L: Der Humanist Andreas Dudith im Kreise der Antiparacelsisten. Wien, 1967. (Salzburger Beiträge zur Paracelsusforschung, 7). p. 3–12.
Gysel C: Jan Swammerdam (1637–1680–1980), zijn Cartesianism en de fysiologie van het kauwstelsel (I). **Ned Tijdschr Tandheelkd** 1981 Jun;88(6):238–41
Gysel C: Jan Swammerdam (1637–1680–1980), zijn Cartesianisme en de fysiologie van het kauwstelsel (II). **Ned Tijdschr Tandheelkd** 1981 Jul–Aug;88(7–8):274–7
Gysel C: Odontologie et cartesianisme naissant (1637--1650). **Rev Belge Med Dent** 1979;34(2):223–30
Koch CH: Petrus Severinus, Francis Bacon og Naturiagttagelsen. **Dan Medicinhist Arbog** 1979;161–72
Koenigsberger D: Renaissance man and creative thinking. A history of concepts of harmony 1400–1700. Hassocks, Sussex, Harvester Press, 1979. xiii, 282 p.
Kraemer S: A note on Spinoza's contribution to systemic therapy. **Fam Process** 1982 Sep;21(3):353–7
Lindeboom GA: Descartes and medicine. Amsterdam, Rodopi, 1979. 134 p. (Nieuwe Nederlandse Bijdragen tot de Geschiedenis der Geneeskunde, No. 1).
Linden SJ: Alchemy and eschatology in seventeenth-century poetry. **Ambix** 1984 Nov;31(3):102–24
Maclean I: The Renaissance notion of woman. A study in the fortunes of scholasticism and medical science in European intellectual life. New York, Cambridge University Press, 1980. VIII, 119p.
Maria CI: La disputa sulle scienze e la medicina come venne affrontata nel corso del XV secolo da Platonismo e Aristotelismo. **Med Secoli** 1982;19(3):323–8
Nutton V: John Caius und Johannes Lange: medizinischer Humanismus zur Zeit Vesals. **NTM** 1984;21(2):81–7
Pagel W: Mother nature and the scientific revolution. **Hist Sci** 1981 Jun:19(44 pt 2):148–53
Rudolph H: Schriftauslegung und Schriftverständnis bei Paracelsus. **Medizinhist J** 1981;16(1–2):101–24
Schipperges H: Kranksein und Heilung bei Paracelsus. Wien, Verband der wissenschaftlichen Gesellschaften Oesterreichs, 1978. 32 p. (Salzburger Beiträge zur Paracelsusforschung, 18).
Toellner R: Logical and psychological aspects of the discovery of the circulation of the blood. In M. D. Grmek, R. S. Cohen, G. Cimino, ed: On scientific discovery. The Erice Lectures 1977. Dordrecht, D. Reidel, 1981. p. 239–59. (Boston Studies in the Philosophy of Science, v. 34).
Tomaselli S: The first person: Descartes, Locke and mind-body dualism. **Hist Sci** 1984;22(pt 2):185–205

**Belgium**

Gysel C: Helmontianisme en odontologie (I). **Rev Belge Med Dent** 1979;34(3):295–312
Pagel W: Joan Baptista Van Helmont: reformer of science and medicine. Cambridge, Cambridge University Press, x, 1982. 219 p. (Cambridge monographs on the history of medicine).

**Denmark**

Skov H, Bastholm E, ed: Petrus Severinus og hans Idea medicinae philosophicae. En dansk paracelsist. Copenhagen, Odense Universitetsforlag, 1979. 299 p. (Acta Historica Scientiarum et Medicinalium, 32).

**Europe**

Gysel C: Renaissance, filosofie en geneeskunde. **Rev Belge Med Dent** 1983 Jan;38(1):16–20

**France**

Arbini R: Did Descartes have a philosophical theory of sense perception? **J Hist Philos** 1983;21:317–37
Carter RB: Descartes' medical philosophy. The organic solution to the mind-body problem. Baltimore, London, Johns Hopkins University Press, 1983. xi, 301 p.
Gysel C: Odontoiatria e cartesianesimo nascente (1637–1650). **Dent Cadmos** 1980 Mar;48(3):53–5
Limbrick E: Franciscus Sanchez 'Scepticus': un médecin philosophe précurseur de Descartes (1550–1623). **Renaiss Reformation** 1982;18:264–72
Locke D: Mind, matter, and the 'Meditations'. **Mind** 1981;90:343–66
Trevisani F: Un corrispondente di Cartesio: alcune note su Lazare Meyssonnier (1611/12–1673), medico e astrologo lionese e sulla sua Belle Magie (1669). **Hist Philos Life Sci** 1979;1(2):285–308

**Germany**

Baader G: Medizinisches Reformdenken und Arabismus im Deutschland des 16. Jahrhunderts. **Sudhoffs Arch** 1979;63(3):261–96
Morys P: Medizin und Pharmazie in der Kosmologie Leonhard Thurneissers zum Thurn (1531–1596). Husum, Matthiesen, 1982. 179 p. (Abhandlungen zur Geschichte der Medizin und der Naturwissenschaften, 43).

**Great Britain**

Boss J: The relation of clinical to non-clinical medicine according to Thomas Sydenham (1624–1689). In E. Schultheisz, ed: History of physiology. Oxford, Elmsford, New York, Pergamon, 1981. xvi, 208 p. (Advances in Physiological Sciences. Proceedings of the 28th International Congress of Physiological Sciences, Budapest, 1980. Volume 21). p. 9–21.
Bylebyl JJ: Boyle and Harvey on the valves in the veins. **Bull Hist Med** 1982 Fall;56(3):351–67
Dirckx JH: Sir Thomas Browne (1605–1682). A model for medical humanists. **JAMA** 1982 Oct 15;248(15):1845–7
Godwin J: Robert Fludd: hermetic philosopher and surveyor of two worlds. London, Thames and Hudson, 1979. 96 p. An annotated collection of plates from Fludds's works.
Oldroyd DR: Some 'philosophical scribbles' attributed to Robert Hooke. **Notes Rec R Soc Lond** 1980 Jul;35(1):17–32
Romanell P: The scientific and medical genealogy of Locke's 'historical, plain method'. **Trans Stud Coll Physicians Phila** 1983 Dec;5(5 no

4):339–52

Stewart MA: The authenticity of Robert Boyle's anonymous writings on reason. **Bodleian Libr Rec** 1981 Aug;10(5):280–9

Taylor FK: Sydenham's disease entities. **Psychol Med** 1982 May;12(2):243–50

**India**

Venkata Reddy M: Hatharatnavali of Srinivasabhatta, a late medieval treatise on yoga and tantra. **Bull Indian Inst Hist Med (Hyderabad)** 1979;9:74–81

**Italy**

Mugnai Carrara D: Una polemica umanistico-scolastica circa l'interpretazione delle tre dottrine ordinate di Galeno. **Ann Ist Mus Stor Sci Fir** 1983;8(1):31–57

Premuda L: L'istanza sociale in Ramazzini pre-illuminista. **Med Lav** 1983 Nov–Dec;74(6):433–41

**Netherlands**

Farina P: Il corpuscolarismo di Henricus Regius: materialismo e medicina in un cartesiano olandese del Seicento. In: Ricerche sull'atomismo del Seicento. Florence: La Nuova Italia, 1977. p. 119–78.

**Poland**

Miller JM: Copernicus, medicine, and the heliocentric concept. **South Med J** 1983 Sep;76(9):1167–8

Szpilczyński S: Das traditionelle und progressive Gesicht der Medizin in der Renaissance-Epoche im Lichte der Polemik zwischen S. Simonius und N. Buccella nach dem Tode des Königs Stefan Batory. **Organon** 1979;15:229–37

**Spain**

Cappelletti AJ: Servet, teologo, filosofo y medico. **Rev Soc Venez Hist Med** 1975–76;23(37):147–61

Corsano A: Medicina e teologia nel pensiero rinascimentale. La fisiologia di Michele Serveto. **G Crit Filos Ital** 1975;6(1):84–8

Trueta J: Els orígens del 'Welfare State' i de les lleis socials: Lluí Vives. In Congrés International d'Història de la Medicina Catalana, 2nd, Barcelona, 1975. Llibre d'Actes. Barcelona, Socitra, 1977. p. 39–47.

**Sweden**

Eriksson G: Om ingenting. Olof Rudbeck föreläsningsprogram 1679. **Lychnos** 1979–80;:79–108

**Switzerland**

Braun L: Vom Wesen des Grundes bei Paracelsus. **Salzburger Beitr Paracelsusforsch** 1984;23:27–35

Braun L, et al: Paracelse. Paris, Albin Michel, 1980. 280 p. (Cahiers de l'Hermétisme).

Domandi S: Hohenheims De natura rerum. Eine Einführung in die geistige Welt des Paracelsus. **Salzburger Beitr Paracelsusforsch** 1984;23:61–88

Goldammer K: Zur philosophischen und religiösen Sinngebung von Heilung und Heilmittel bei Paracelsus. In Dilg P, et al., ed: Perspektiven der Pharmaziegeschichte. Graz, Austria, Akademische Druck- u. Verlagsanstalt, 1983. p. 113–29.

Pagel W: Paracelsus. An introduction to philosophical medicine in the era of the Renaissance, 2nd, revised edition. Basel, Karger, 1982. xii, 399 p.

Schipperges H: Paracelsus. Das Abenteuer einer sokratischen Existenz. Freiburg im Breisgau, Aurum Verlag, 1983. 108 p. (Reihe: Sokratische Weisheit, Bd. 3).

**1700 to Present**

Abbott P, Wertheimer R: Philosophers and the abortion question. **Polit Theory** 1978;6(3):313–44

Albarello B, Collorio C: Analisi dei collegamenti tra l'opera freudiana e il positivismo ottocentesco. **Acta Med Hist Patav** 1982–83;29:9–18

Antiseri D: Metaphysical ideas and the development of science. **Riv Biol** 1981 Winter;74(4):529–42

Bechtel W: The evolution of our understanding of the cell: a study in the dynamics of scientific progress. **Stud Hist Philos Sci** 1984 Dec;15(4):309–56

Bednarczyk A: Antymechanicyzm w osiemnastowiecznej filozofii medycyny: Georg Ernst Stahl (1659–1734) i animizm. **Arch Hist Med (Warsz)** 1981;44(2):163–87

Benedetti G: Die neurotische Lebensproblematik Nietzsches als eine Wirkkraft und eine Grenze seiner Philosophie. **Gesnerus** 1984;41(1/2):111–32

Carter KC: Semmelweis's possible influence on Karl Mayrhofer and on those who subsequently developed nineteenth century etiological theories. **Orvostort Kozl** 1982;28(1–3):23–31

Chambers RW, Durkin JT, ed: Papers of the Alexis Carrel centennial conference, Georgetown University June 28, 1973. Washington, Georgetown University, 1973. 107 p. Contributions by C. A. Lindbergh, A. Gros, S. Maggio, L. G. Walker, C. A. Hufnagel, T. I. Malinin.

Cohen RS, Laudan L, ed: Physics, philosophy and psychoanalysis. Essays in honor of Adolf Grünbaum. Dordrecht, D. Reidel, 1983. xviii, 339 p. (Boston Studies in the Philosophy of Science, v. 76).

Cowen DL: Pharmacy and freedom. **Pharm Hist** 1984;26(2):70–82

Duerr HP, ed: Der Wissenschaftler und das Irrationale. Band 2. Beiträge aus Philosophie und Psychologie. Frankfurt am Main, Syndikat, 1981. 679 p.

Ellacuría I: Seguridad social y solidaridad humana: aproximacion filosofica al fenomeno de la seguridad social. **Estud Cent Am** 1969;24(253):357–66

Engelhardt D von, Schipperges H: Die inneren Verbindungen zwischen Philosophie und Medizin im 20. Jahrhundert. Darmstadt, Wissenschaftliche Buchgesellschaft, 1980. vii, 190 p.

Greene JC: Science, ideology, and world view: essays in the history of evolutionary ideas. Berkeley/Los Angeles, Univ. of California Press, 1981. x, 202 p.

Gunnell JG: The technocratic image and the theory of technocracy. **Technol Cult** 1982 Jul;23(3):392–16

Habacher M: Auf der suche nach dem 'Od'; Karl Ludwig Freiherr von Reichenbach (1788–1869) und Karl Wilhelm Mayrhofer (1806–1853), zwei Verbündete contra Justus von Liebig. **Clio Med** 1980 May;14(2):105–18

Haffter C: Die Entstehung des Begriffs der Zivilisationskrankheiten. **Gesnerus** 1979;36(3–4):228–37

Hassani AM: The appearance of scientific naturalism in Syria and Egypt. **J Hist Arabic Sci** 1977 Nov;1(2):284–98

Hoffmann P: La théorie de l'âme dans la pensée médicale vers 1778. **Dix-Huit Siecle** 1979;11:201–12

Knežević S: Iličijada i 'nakon' Ivana Ilića. **Lijec Vjesn** 1983 Sep;105(9):337–42

Krafft M: Die anthroposophische Heilmittellehre und ihre geistesgeschichtliche Beziehung zu Heilmittelkonzepten. des 19. Jahrhunderts. Stuttgart, Deutscher Apotheker Verlag, 1984. 210 p. (Quellen und Studien zur Geschichte der Pharmazie, Bd. 27).

Lohff B: Zur Geschichte der Lehre von der Lebenskraft. **Clio Med** 1981 Dec;16(2/3):101–12

Löther R, ed: Philosophische Schriften von Marx, Engels und Lenin und ihre Bedeutung für die Medizin heute. Jena, Fischer, 1979. 127 p. Contributions by U. Körner, I. Löther, P. W. Ruff, R. Stach, G. Straass.

Luyendijk-Elshout AM: Samuel Musgrave's attack upon Stahl's and Boerhaave's doctrines in 1763. **Janus** 1980;67(1–2–3):141–56

Macpike L: The social values of childbirth in the nineteenth-century novel. **Int J Womens Stud** 1980;3(2):117–30

Manier E: History, philosophy and sociology of biology: a family romance. **Stud Hist Philos Sci** 1980 Mar;11(1):1–24

Mann G: Gunter Mann: Neovitalismus. **Medizinhist J** 1983;18(4):376–83

May R: The discovery of being. Writings in existential psychology. New York, London, W.W. Norton, 1983. 192 p.

Mazet P: Points de vue théoriques en psychosomatique. Historique et actualité. **Sem Hop Paris** 1984 Mar 22;60(13):887–93

Morrison LR: 'Nearer to the brute creation': the scientific defense of American slavery before 1830. **South Stud** 1980;19(3):228–42

Nierhaus G: Ludwig von Bertalanffy 1901–1972. **Sudhoffs Arch** 1981;65(2):144–72

Nyiri JK: Philosophy and suicide--statistics in Austria-Hungary. **East Cent Eur** 1978;5(1):69–89

Ojeda Figueroa C: Karl Jaspers: filosofía y psicoterapia. **Acta Luso Esp Neurol Psiquiatr** 1983 Mar–Apr;11(2):181–8

Oppitz R: Freiherr von Ehrenfels (1859–1932) und die Entwicklung des 'Neuen Menschen' zu Beginn des 20. Jahrhunderts. Diss. Mainz, 1980. 256 p.

Pansera MT: Per un'antropologia filosofica freudiana: il valore della negazione. **Physis** 1982;24(1):76–108

Proffitt E: Science and Romanticism. **Ga Rev** 1980;34(1):55–80

Puma A: Medicinas pretécnicas? In International Congress of the History of Medicine, 27th, Barcelona, 1980. Actas. Barcelona, Académia de Ciències Mèdiques de Catalunya i Balears, 1981. p. 616–20.

Querner H: La cuestion metodologica en la biologia del siglo XIX. **Folia Hum (Barc)** 1981;19(225):595–611

Rawlinson MC: Psychiatric discourse and the feminine voice. **J Med Philos** 1982 May;7(2):153–77

Reiser SJ: Technology and the eclipse of individualism in medicine. **Pharos** 1982 Winter;45(1):10–5

Rissmann W: Ernst Freiherr von Feuchtersleben (1806–1849). Sein Beitrag zur medizinischen Anthropologie und Psychopathologie. Freiburg im Breisgau, Schulz, 1980. 243 p. (Freiburger Forschungen zur Medizingeschichte, Neue Folge, Band 12).

Risso M: Institution psychiatrique, idéologie médicale et chronification. **Schweiz Arch Neurol Neurochir Psychiatr** 1980;126(2):327–35

Rothschuh KE: Aus der Geschichte der Naturheilbewegung (I). Ueber den 'Naturismus' als die weltanschauliche Grundlage der Naturheilbewegung. **ZFA (Stuttgart)** 1981 May 10;57(13):1011–8

Sandler IL: Pierre Louis Moreau de Maupertuis--a precursor of Mendelian genetics?: an inquiry into the biological ideas of Maupertuis, the Mendelian principles of heredity and the nature of the precursor. Ph.D. diss. University of Washington. Seattle, 1979. 265 leaves.
Schmitz R: Der Beginn der organischen Chemie und der Neo-Vitalismus von heute. In Seidler E, Schott H, ed: Bausteine zur Medizingeschichte. Stuttgart, Steiner, 1984. p. 105-11.
Schwanitz HJ: Homöopathie und Brownianismus 1795-1844. Zwei wissenschaftstheoretische Fallstudien aus der praktischen Medizin. Stuttgart Fischer, 1983. 202 p. (Medizin in Geschichte und Kultur, 15).
Seidler E: Die Naturheilkundebewegung, ihre Systeme und Motive. In Dilg P, et al., ed: Perspektiven der Pharmaziegeschichte. Graz, Austria, Akademische Druck- u. Verlagsanstalt, 1983. p. 331-41.
Smith LD: Psychology and philosophy: towards a realignment, 1905-1935. **J Hist Behav Sci** 1981 Jan;17(1):28-37
Sródka A: Racjonalistyczne i empiryczne podstawy rozwoju medycyny na przełomie XVIII i XIX wieku. Krótki przegląd doktryn filozoficznych i teorii przyrodniczych. **Arch Hist Med (Warsz)** 1983;46(3):333-45
Stephenson W: Micheal Polanyi, science and belief. **Ethics Sci Med** 1980;7(2):97-110
Stevenson LG: Exemplary disease: the typhoid pattern. **J Hist Med Allied Sci** 1982 Apr;37(2):159-81
Stratone N: Filosofia în secolul 'luminilor'. **Rev Med Chir Soc Med Nat Iasi** 1983 Jul-Sep;87(3):509-11
Ten Have HA: Geneeskunde en filosofie, aspecten van een wisselvallige relatie. **Ned Tijdschr Geneeskd** 1982 Apr 10,126(15):668-73
Toellner R: Die Bedeutung des physico-theologischen Gottesbeweises für die nachcartesianische Physiologie im 18. Jahrhundert. **Ber Wissenschaftsgesch** 1982;5:75-82
Toellner R: 'Ein Unding vor der Vernunft': Die generatio spontanea im Weltbild der aufgeklärten Naturforschung. In Dilg P, et al., ed: Perspektiven der Pharmaziegeschichte. Graz, Austria, Akademische Druck- u. Verlagsanstalt, 1983. p. 377-88.
Torrance TF: The place of Michael Polanyi in the modern philosophy of science. **Ethics Sci Med** 1980;7(2):57-95
Tsouyopoulos N: Andreas Röschlaub und die Romantische Medizin. Die philosophischen Grundlagen der modernen Medizin. **Med Gesch Kult** 1982;14:1-259
Tsouyopoulos N: Auf der Suche nach einer adäquaten Methode für die Geschichte und Theorie der Medizin. Auseinandersetzung mit Ludwik Flecks 'Entstehung und Entwicklung einer wissenschaftlichen Tatsache'. **Medizinhist J** 1982;17(1/2):20-36
Tsouyopoulos N: Die neue Auffassung der klinischen Medizin als Wissenschaft unter dem Einfluss der Philosophie im frühen 19. Jahrhundert. **Ber Wissenschaftsgesch** 1978;1(1-2):87-100
van Hoorn W: Psychoanalysis, romanticism and biology. **Stor Crit Psicol** 1982 Jun;3(1):5-25
Weissmann G: Against Aequanimitas. **Hosp Pract [Off]** 1984 Jun;19(6):159-69

**Austria**

Broda E: Ludwig Boltzmann als evolutionistischer Philosoph. **Ber Wissenschaftsgesch** 1983;6(1-4):103-14
Premuda L: The influence of the nineteenth-century Vienna School on Italian medicine: the roles of Padua and Trieste. In Stevenson LG, ed: A celebration of medical history. Baltimore, Johns Hopkins University Press, 1982. (The Henry E. Sigerist supplements to the Bulletin of the History of Medicine; new ser., no. 6). p. 180-99. With commentary by J. J. Bylebyl, p. 200-11.

**Belgium**

Havelange C: Pléthore et art de guérir. Le malaise des médecins liégeois au XIXe siècle. **Rev Med Liege** 1984 Oct 1;39(19):676-95

**Canada**

Shortt SE: Andrew Macphail: the ideal in nature. In his The search for an ideal: six Canadian intellectuals and their convictions in an age of transition, 1890-1930. Toronto, Buffalo, University of Toronto Press, 1976. p. 12-38.

**Czechoslovakia**

Daněk K: Bernard Bolzano v historii medicíny. **Cas Lek Cesk** 1981 Sep 24;120(38)1160-3

**Europe**

Ikezawa Y, Kono H: [The starting point in nursing--an observation through the history of European ideology] (Jpn). **Kango Tenbo** 1981 Oct;6(10):905-13

**France**

Albury WR: Heart of darkness: J. N. Corvisart and the medicalization of life. **Hist Reflect** 1982;9(1-2):17-31.
Arquiola E: Anatomia y antropologia en el positivismo frances. **Asclepio** 1978-79;30-31:19-32
Arquiola E: La enfermedad en la antropología física francesa durante el positivismo. **Asclepio** 1983;35:217-26
Atwood GE: The pursuit of being in the life and thought of Jean-Paul Sartre. **Psychoanal Rev** 1983 Summer;70(2):143-62
Cappelletti AJ: Lamettrie medico y filosofo del hombre. **Rev Soc Venez Hist Med** 1972-73;20-21(34-35):211-27
Cappelletti V: Bernard, oltre meccanicismo e vitalismo. **Med Secoli** 1979 Jan-Apr;16(1):5-11
Cappelletti V: Claude Bernard between history and the 'principles' of science. **Riv Biol** 1980 Spring;73(1):21-33
Cid F: Broussais, su concepto de irritación en el cuadro de la locura durante el siglo XIX. **Med Hist (Barc)** 1984;(5):3-7
Favre R: La mort dans la littérature et la pensée française au siècle des lumières. Lyon, Presses universitaires de Lyon, 1978. 640 p.
Frey EF: Voltaire's relation to the discipline of medicine. **Bookman** 1982 May-Jun;9(5):3-7
Gregory RL: French without fears: Denis Diderot. **Perception** 1983;12(5):509-12
Gusdorf G: Médecine romantique. A la mémoire du Pr Marc Klein. **Etud Philos** 1981;(1):11-23
Lagoutte J: Claude Bernard, un physiologiste, un philosophe. Lyon, Centre régional de documentation pédagogique, 1978. 40 p.
Legée G: Influence du vitalisme montpelliérain sur la neurophysiologie de Pierre Flourens. **Hist Nat** 1982;21:13-45
McManners J: Death and the Enlightenment. Changing attitudes to death among Christians and unbelievers in eighteenth-century France. Oxford, Clarendon Press; New York, Oxford University Press; 1981. vii, 619 p.
Matsuda K: L'enseignement des sourds-muets et les philosophes au siècle de Lumières. **Zinbun** 1979;15:141-74
Poirier J, Poirier JL, ed: Médecine et philosophie à la fin du XIXe siècle. Paris, Université de Paris XII - Val de Marne, [1980?]. ii, 155 p. (Cahier de l'Institut de recherche universitaire d'histoire de la connaissance, des idées et des mentalités; no. 2).
Rauch A: Le souci du corps chez Condillac. **Stadion** 1977;3(1):60-89
Schneiderman L: Henri Saint-Simon: his ideology and personality. **Am J Psychoanal** 1980 Winter;40(4):349-64
Sloan AW: Claude Bernard's philosophy of medical science. **S Afr Med J** 1984 May 19;65(20):817-9
Staum MS: Cabanis. Enlightenment and medical philosophy in the French Revolution. Princeton, Princeton University Press, 1980. xi, 430 p.
Stratone M: Metoda analizei la E.B. Condillac. **Rev Med Chir Soc Med Nat Iasi** 1979 Jan-Mar;83(1):163-6

**Germany**

Arndal S: Krop, sjael og ånd Georg Ernst Stahls og Christian Friedrich Richters medicinske antropologi. **Dan Medicinhist Arbog** 1980;:126-66
Bleker J: Die Naturhistorische Schule 1825-1845. Ein Beitrag zur Geschichte der klinischen Medizin in Deutschland. Stuttgart, New York, Fischer, 1981. ix, 174 p.
Brister L: J. G. Zimmermanns Essay 'Von der Erfahrung in der Arzneikunst': Ein Beitrag zur rationalen Medizin. **Schweiz Med Wochenschr** 1980 Apr 19;110(16):615-9
Dieckhöfer K: Menschliches, Allzumenschliches---zur verstehenden Psychologie bei Nietzsche. **Z Klin Psychol Psychother** 1980;28(2):101-5
Doerr W: Gestalt theory and morbid anatomy. **Virchows Arch [A]** 1984;403(2):103-15
Duchesneau F: G. E. Stahl: Antimécanisme et physiologie. **Arch Int Hist Sci (Paris)** 1976;26:3-26
Engelhardt D von: Historisches Bewusstein in der Medizin der Romantik. In Seidler E, Schott H, ed: Bausteine zur Medizingeschichte. Stuttgart, Steiner, 1984. p. 26-34.
Engelhardt D von: Polemik und Kontroversen um Haeckel. **Medizinhist J** 1980;15(3):284-304
Gilman SL: The Nietzsche murder case. **New Lit Hist** 1983;14(2):359-72
Goldammer K: Paracelsus in der deutschen Romantik. Eine Untersuchung zur Geschichte der Paracelsus-Rezeption und zu geistesgeschichtlichen Hintergründen der Romantik. Mit einem Anhang über die Entstehung und Entwicklung der Elementargeister-Vorstellungen seit dem Mittelalter. Wien, 1980. 212 p. (Salzburger Beiträge zur Paracelsusforschung, 20).
Gusdorf G: Médecine romantique. **Etud Philos** 1983;:11-23
Hayman R: Nietzsche's madness. **Partisan Rev** 1980;47(1):29-44
Henkelmann T: Die Struktur des Lebendigen. Die Fragmente zur Physiologie von Novalis. In Seidler E, Schott H, ed: Bausteine zur Medizingeschichte. Stuttgart, Steiner, 1984. p. 45-52.
Kaiser W: Georg Ernst Stahl (1659-1734)--Zur 250. Wiederkehr seines Todestages am 14. Mai 1984. **Z Gesamte Inn Med** 1984 Aug 1;39(15):371-6
Kovel J: Marx and Freud. In M. Albin, R. J. Devlin, G. Heeger, ed: New directions in psychohistory. The Adelphi papers in honor of Erik H. Erikson. Lexington, Toronto, D. C. Heath, 1980. p. 21-6.
Legée G: Schopenhauer (1788-1860) et les sciences de la nature.

**Hist Nat** 1979;(14):39-62
Lenoir T: Kant, Blumenbach, and vital materialism in German biology. **Isis** 1980 Mar;71(256):77-108
Lenoir T: The strategy of life: teleology and mechanics in nineteenth century German biology. Dordrecht, Holland; Boston, Reidel, 1982. xii, 314 p.
Löther I, Löther R: Engels' 'Ludwig Feuerbach und der Ausgang der klassischen deutschen Philosophie', die Grundrichtungen des philosophischen Denkens und die Medizin. **Med Ges** 1979;(5):79-91
Mann G, ed: Naturwissen und Erkenntnis im 19. Jahrhundert: Emil Du Bois-Reymond. Hildesheim, Gerstenberg, 1981. 243 p. Contributions by K. E. Rothschuh, H. Hensel, R. Malter, C. von Campenhausen, B. Lohff, H. Lübbe, D. von Engelhardt, W. F. Gutmann, K. Bonink, C. Andree
Mück H: Die rechtliche Entwicklung des Arzt-Patient-Verhältnisses in der DDR; vom Dienstvertrag zum medizinischen Betreuungsverhältnis. Köln, 1982. 322 p. (Kölner medizinhistorische Beiträge, Band 24)
Oldenburg D: Georg August Bertele (1767-1818) und die Arzneimittellehre der romantischen Naturphilosophie. **Medizinhist J** 1981;16(3):240-56
Oldenburg D: Romantische Naturphilosophie und Arzneimittellehre 1800-1840. Diss. (Doktor der Naturwissenschaften), Braunschweig, 1979. 267 p. (Veröffentlichungen aus dem Pharmaziegeschichtlichen Seminar der Technischen Universität Braunschweig, 20).
Ortmann F: Dietrich Georg Kieser (1779-1862)--nur ein romantischer **Z Gesamte Inn Med** 1979 Sep 1;34(17):486-9
Pfohl G: Das philosophisch-philologische Element in der medizinischen Fakultät. **Med Welt** 1980 May 16;31(20):775-8
Rather LJ: The dream of self-destruction. Wagner's Ring and the modern world. Baton Rouge, Louisiana State Univ. Press, 1979. xx, 215 p.
Rehder K, Shampo MA, Kyle RA: Physician's personal in-flight medical kit. **JAMA** 1982 Feb 19;247(7):1011
Rothschuh KE: Naturphilosophische Konzepte der Medizin aus der Zeit der deutschen Romantik.
**Dtsch Vierteljahresschr Lit Wiss Geistesgesch** 1978;:243-66
Rothschuh KE: Richard Hermann Koch (1882-1949). **Medizinhist J** 1980;15(3):223-43
Rothschuh KE: Richard Hermann Koch (1882-1949): Arzt, Medizinhistoriker, Medizinphilosoph (Biographisches, Ergographisches). 1. Teil. Zur Biographie. **Medizinhist J** 1980;15(1/2):16-43
Rothschuh KE: Therapia rationalis systematica bei Friedrich Hoffmann (1660-1742). In Dilg P, et al., ed: Perspektiven der Pharmaziegeschichte. Graz, Austria, Akademische Druck- u. Verlagsanstalt, 1983. p. 269-80.
Schleiffer R: Zur Methodologie von Psychopathologie und Historik. **Nervenarzt** 1980 Jan;51(1):17-21
Schott H: Der versteckte Poet in uns; zur Sprachtheorie in der naturphilosophischen Seelenlehre von Gotthilf Heinrich von Schubert (1780-1860). **Sudhoffs Arch** 1981;65(3):226-50
Sohni H: Die Medizin der Frühromantik. Novalis' Bedeutung für den versuch einer Umwertung der 'Romantischen Medizin.' Freiburg, Schulz, 1973. 270 p. (Freiburger Forschungen zur Medizingeschichte, Neue Folge, 2).
Sprung L: Immanuel Kant in der Geschichte der Psychologie--Aspekte seines Beitrages in der Entwicklung zur Einzelwissenschaft. In Eckardt G, ed: Zur Geschichte der Psychologie. Berlin, VEB Deutscher Verlag der Wissenschaften, 1979. p. 33-42.
Tellenbach H: Martin Bubers Einfluss auf die anthropologische Wende in der Medizin. **Nervenarzt** 1980 May;51(5):302-6
Tsouyopoulos N: Andreas Röschlaub und die Romantische Medizin. Stuttgart, Fischer, 1982. 258 p. (Medizin in Geschichte und Kultur, 14).
Weinberger C: Wissenschaftstheoretische Anmerkungen zu Konrad Lorenz' 'Vergleichende Verhaltensforschung'.
**Z Allg Wissenschaftstheorie** 1980;10(1):147-61

**Great Britain**

Ball T: Platonism and penology: James Mill's attempted synthesis. **J Hist Behav Sci** 1982 Jul;18(3):222-9
Boss J: An early eighteenth-century criticism of clinical medicine as experimental philosophy. **Koroth** 1980 Jun;7(11-12):CCLXV-CCLXXV
Brink A: Love and conflict in Bertrand Russell's letters. **Queens Q** 1979;86(1):1-15
Colp R: Dr. Erasmus Darwin consults with another physician. **Radic Hist Rev** 1979 Spring/Summer;Spec:66-71
Corrigan TJ: Biographia Literaria and the language of science. **J Hist Ideas** 1980 Jul-Sep;41(3):399-419
Daněk K: Incitabilita, stenie a astenie. K 200. výročí Brownových Základu medicíny. **Cas Lek Cesk** 1980 Jul 11;119(27-28):774-6
Douglas A: Promises to keep. **Thorax** 1984 Jul;39(7):481-6
Gaustad ES: George Berkeley in America. New Haven, Yale University Press, 1979. xi, 225 p.
Gilbert SF: Owen's vertebral archetype and evolutionary genetics -- a Platonic appreciation. **Perspect Biol Med** 1980 Spring;23(3):475-88
Henkelmann T: Zur Geschichte des pathophysiologischen Denkens. John Brown (1735-1788) und sein System der Medizin. Berlin, New York, Springer, 1981. 104 p.
Jacyna LS: Immanence or transcendence; theories of life and organization in Britain, 1790-1835. **Isis** 1983 Sep;74(273):311-29
Jacyna LS: The physiology of mind, the unity of nature, and the moral order in Victorian thought. **Br J Hist Sci** 1981 Jul;14(pt 2 no 47):109-32
Kawakita Y: [Nightingale in the history of medical philosophy--on the meaning of 'health'] (Jpn). **Kango** 1982 Feb;34(2):39-53
Kinch MP: Geographical distribution and the origin of life: the development of early nineteenth-century British explanations. **J Hist Biol** 1980 Spring;13(1):91-119
Kowalewski D: Politics and emotion in the thought of John Stuart Mill. **J Psychohist** 1980 Spring;7(4):455-66
Lenoir T: The Göttingen School and the development of transcendental Naturphilosophie in the Romantic Era. **Stud Hist Biol** 1981;5:111-205
McEvoy JG: Joseph Priestley, scientist, philosopher and divine. **Proc Am Philos Soc** 1984 Sep;128(3):193-9
Paradis JG: T. H. Huxley, Man's place in nature. Lincoln, University of Nebraska Press, 1978. xi, 226 p.
Porter R: Medicina e illuminismo nell' Inghilterra del settecento. **Quad Stor** 1979;14(1):155-80
Porter R: Was there a medical Enlightenment in 18th-century England? **Br J 18th-Cent Stud** 1982;5:49-63
Smith CU: Evolution and the problem of mind: part I. Herbert Spencer. **J Hist Biol** 1982 Spring;15(1):55-88
Smith DC: William Budd manuscript at the National Library of Medicine. **J Hist Med Allied Sci** 1980 Jul;35(3):318-19
Trotter WR: John Brown, and the nonspecific component of human sickness. **Perspect Biol Med** 1978 Winter;21(2):258-64

**Greece**

Stavros T: Erokles basiades o teleytaios iatrophilosophos. **Epeirotike Hestia** 1975;24(279-280):419-32

**Hungary**

Réti E: Idées d'avant-garde dans les thèses hongroises séculaires. **Orvostort Kozl** 1979;86(24 no 4):73-9

**Italy**

Doise W: Dalla filosofia alla psicologia sociale. Una 'lettura' di Carlo Cattaneo. **Stor Crit Psicol** 1983;4(1):117-29
Renaldo JJ: A note on the history of medicine and a debate on Parnassus. **Bull Hist Med** 1979 Winter;53(4):606-13

**Netherlands**

Luyendijk-Elshout AM: Mechanicisme contra vitalisme de school van Herman Boerhaave en de beginselen van het leven. **Tijdschr Geschied Geneeskd** 1982;5(1):16-26

**Poland**

Chrześciewski L: Filozofia medycyny Władysława Szumowskiego (1875-1954). **Wiad Lek** 1984 Apr 15;37(8):653-4
Chrześciewski L: Filozofia medycyny Wøadysøawa Szumowskiego (1875-1954). **Wiad Lek** 1984 Feb 15;37(4):321-2
Jakubik A: Antoni Kępiński -- Twórca psychiatrii aksjologicznej. **Psychiatr Pol** 1980 Jul-Aug;14(4):403-7
Jakubik A: Psychiatria fenomenologiczna w ujęciu Antoniego Kępińskiego. **Psychiatr Pol** 1980 Jul-Aug;14(4):395-401
Miłosz S, Stański M: O niektórych tendencjach filozoficzno-metodologicznych medycyny w polsce na przełomie XIX i XX w. **Stud Filoz** 1977;11:127-38
Podgórska-Klawe Z: Kierunki rozwoju Polskiej medycyny w dobie pozytywizmu. **Arch Hist Med (Warsz)** 1984;47(1):121-6
Porus VN: Ludwick Flecks's epistemological conception and contemporary discussion on the nature and dynamics of scientific knowledge. **Kwart Hist Nauki Tech** 1983;28(3-4):545-60
Tadeusz Bilikiewicz (1901-1980)---historyk medycyny i filozof: **Kwart Hist Nauki Tech** 1981;26(2):435-48

**Romania**

Stratone N, Stratone A: Probleme de gnoseologie în lucrările doctorului Grigore T. Popa. **Rev Med Chir Soc Med Nat Iasi** 1979 Oct-Dec;83(4):713-6
Stratone N: Spațiul si timpul in concepția lui Vasile Conta (1845-1882). **Rev Med Chir Soc Med Nat Iasi** 1982 Jul-Sep;86(3):513-5

**Spain**

Albarracín A: Gaspar Casal y el concepto moderno de especie morbosa. **Asclepio** 1983;35:189-95
Albarracín Teulón A: Cajal y el problema del conocimiento científico. **Asclepio** 1980;32:7-17
Arquiola E: Anatomia y antropologia fisica en el positivismo español. **Asclepio** 1981;33:3-22
Carreras i Roca M: La introducció del positivisme mèdic a Catalunya. In Congrés International d'Història de la Medicina Catalana, 2nd,

Barcelona, 1975. Llibre d'Actes. Barcelona, Socitra, 1977. p. 7–18.
Montiel L: La influencia de la ideologia en la clinica medica del S. XIX español. La obra de Tomas Santero y Moreno (1817–1888). **Asclepio** 1981;33:127–42
Riera J: [Dr. Matias Nieto y Serrano and Romantic medicine in Spain.] (Spa) **Cuad Invest Hist** 1979;:3
Riera J: Matías Nieto y Serrano (1813–1902) y la medicina romántica. **Cuad Invest Hist** 1979;3:275–306
Riera J: Matias Nieto y Serrano (1813–1902) y la medicina romantica. **Asclepio** 1980;32:367 81

**Sweden**

Gejrot T: Medikofilosofisk examen; om medikofilare och medikofilen. **Sydsven Medicinhist Sallsk Arsskr** 1982;19:45–53

**Switzerland**

Marx J: Charles Bonnet contre les Lumières. 2 v. Oxford, Voltaire Foundation at the Taylor Institution, 1976. 782 p.
Modgil S, Modgil C, ed: Jean Piaget. Consensus and controversy. New York, Praeger, 1982. 446 p.
Roe SA, ed: The natural philosophy of Albrecht von Haller. New York, Arno, 1981. Various pagings. Reprint of works published 1750–1936.

**United States**

Andrews LB, Levin LS: Self-care and the law. **Soc Policy** 1979;9(4):44–9
Animalcular and cryptogamic theories on the origins of fevers. Reprinted works by John Kearsley Mitchell (1849), John L. Riddell (1836), Josiah Clark Nott (1848). New York, Arno, 1977. Various paginations.:
Blight JG: Jonathan Edwards's theory of the mind: its applications and implications. In J. Brozĕk, ed: Explorations in the history of psychology in the United States. Lewisburg, Bucknell University Press, 1984. p. 61–120.
Carlson ET: Benjamin Rush and his friends on human nature. **Psychiatr Q** 1979 Winter;51(4):300–6
Carlson RJ: Holism and reductionism as perspectives in medicine and patient care. **West J Med** 1979 Dec;131(6):466–70
Coulter HL: Divided legacy: the conflict between homoeopathy and the American Medical Association. Science and ethics in American medicine 1800–1914. 2d ed. Richmond, California, North Atlantic Books, 1982. 552 p.
Couto R: Property, pinmakers, and physicians: liberal myths and American health care anomalies. **Soundings** 1979;62(3):275–92
Crawford R: Individual responsibility and health politics in the 1970s. In Reverby S, Rosner D, ed: Health care in America. Philadelphia, Temple University PRess, 1979. p. 247–68.
Davis L: The philosophy of a neurosurgeon. **J Kans Med Soc** 1980 May;81(5):252–5
Gavin WJ: Vagueness and empathy: a Jamesian view. **J Med Philos** 1981 Feb;6(1):45–65
Greenstone JD: Dorothea Dix and Jane Addams: from transcendentalism to pragmatism in American social reform. **Soc Serv Rev** 1979;53(4):527–59
Maulitz RC: 'Physician versus bacteriologist': the ideology of science in clinical medicine. In Vogel MJ, Rosenberg CE, ed: The therapeutic revolution. Philadelphia, 1979. p. 91–107.
Michel D: Corps sauvages, corps étranges. **Dix-Huit Siecle** 1977;9:27–38
Palmer BB: The philosophy of dental health service: its relation to the changing social order. Advice from 1934. **J Am Coll Dent** 1981 Fall;48(3):179–92
Rabin PL, Rabin D: Landmark perspective: The care of the patient. Francis Peabody revisited. **JAMA** 1984 Aug 10;252(6):819–20
Romanell P: Medical history in the religious psychology of William James. In: Congrès international d'histoire de la médecine, XXVe, Québec, 1976. Actes. Québec, 1977. p. 1171–83.
Schuster CI: Passion and pathology: Richard Selzer's philosophy of doctoring. **Perspect Biol Med** 1984 Autumn;28(1):65–74
Warner MH: Vindicating the minister's medical role: Cotton Mather's concept of the nishmath-chajim and the spiritualization of medicine. **J Hist Med Allied Sci** 1981 Jul;36(3):278–95
Whorton JC: 'Antibiotic abandon': the resurgence of therapeutic rationalism. In Parascandola J, ed: The history of antibiotics. Madison, American Institute of the History of Pharmacy, 1980. p. 125–136.
Wylie MS: Images of sickness and health in American medical thought: 1776–1800 and 1835–1865. Ph.D. Diss. American University. Washington, 1981. 541 p.

**USSR**

Cherkasov SV: Leninskoe uchenie ob istine i problema kriteriia praktiki v diagnostike. **Klin Khir** 1980 Jun;(6):1–6
Katsnel'bogen AG: Idei Russkogo Prosveshcheniia i formirovanie obshchestvenno-meditsinskoĭ mysli vo vtoroĭ polovine XVIII veka. **Klin Med (Mosk)** 1984 Jan;62(1):146–51
Löther R: Lenins 'Zur Frage der Dialektik' und die Bedeutung dialektischen Denkens in der Medizin. **Med Ges** 1979;(5):106–12
Nichik VM: Filosofskie vzgliady A. A. Bogomol'tsa. **Patol Fiziol Eksp Ter** 1981 Mar-Apr;(2):20–30, also in Fiziol Zh 1981 May-Jun;27(3):302–6

# PHOTOGRAPHY

See also **Art; Medical Illustration**

Hammond JH: Camera, camera, camera. **J Audiov Media Med** 1984 Jan;7(1):19–20
Mayoz de la Vega R: La fotografía en medicina. Habana, Instituto del Libro Cubano, 1970. Historical sections, p. 271–304.
Miller VD, Pellicori SF: Ultraviolet fluorescence photography of the Shroud of Turin. **J Biol Photogr** 1981 Jul;49(3):71–85

**1700 to Present**

Bogdan R, Biklen D, Shapiro A, et al: The disabled: media's monster. **Soc Policy** 1982;13(2):32–5
Crellin JK, Helfand WH: Medical care in the 20th century. Facets of change illustrated by American and British postcards. Durham, Duke University Medical Center, 1982. 106 p. (Readings and Perspectives in Medicine, Booklet Number 3).
Crellin JK, Helfand W: Picture postcards; a resource for social history of pharmacy. **Pharm Hist** 1983;25(3):116–30
Engelman E: Berggasse 19, Sigmund Freud's home and offices, Vienna, 1938: the photographs of Edmund Engelman. Chicago, University of Chicago Press, 1981. 153 p.
Gilman SL: Zur Physiognomie des Geisteskranken in Geschichte und Praxis, 1800–1900. **Sudhoffs Arch** 1978;62(3):209–34
Gow JG: The evolution of modern endoscopic photography. **Eur Urol** 1984;10(2):133–8
Joy RJ: Occupying the visual cortex: using slides to teach the history of medicine. In J. J. Bylebyl, ed: Teaching the history of medicine at a medical center. Baltimore, London, Johns Hopkins University Press, 1982. (The Henry E. Sigerist supplements to the Bulletin of the History of Medicine; new ser., no. 7). p. 103–14.
Lithner K: Bilden i ögat. **Sydsven Medicinhist Sallsk Arsskr** 1983;:51–8
Lugli T: Hand diseases in early photographs. **Hand** 1980 Feb;12(1):97–104
Pensak ML, Yanagisawa E: Tympanic membrane photography: historical perspective. **Am J Otol** 1984 Apr;5(4):324–32
Stannard T: The history of medical photography. **Soc Soc Hist Med Bull (Lond)** 1980;27:33–43
Taureck R: Die Bedeutung der Photographie für die medizinische Abbildung im 19. Jahrh, Köln, 1980, 258 p. (Kölner medizinhistorische Beiträge, 15).
Terry JS, Herskovitz A, Fox DM: Photographs tell more than meets the eye. **J Biol Photogr** 1980 Jul;48(3):111–5
Verso ML: Doctors and daguerrotypes. Contributions of medical men to the history of photography. **Victorian Hist Mag** 1969 Feb–May;40(155/6 No 1/2):3–24
Veylon R: La photographie. Petit essai de 'psychopathologie'. **Nouv Presse Med** 1980 Jul 12–26;9(30):2073–5
Williams AR: Victorian clinical photography. **J Audiov Media Med** 1982 Jul;5(3):100–3

**France**

Aterman K, Grimaud JA: The brothers Lumière. Pioneers in medical photography. **Am J Dermatopathol** 1983 Oct;5(5):479–81
Binet JL: Les premiers clichès du sang. **Nouv Rev Fr Hematol** 1981;23(2):135–7
Dupuis M: Etienne-Jules Marey, le photographe du mouvement. **Sci Avenir** 1980;400:95–100
Esman AH: Henri Dagonet. Pioneer of psychiatric photography. **NY State J Med** 1984 Feb;84(2):79–81

**Germany**

Aulas JJ: La folie dans le cinéma allemand (1913–1933). **Ann Med Psychol (Paris)** 1980;138(8):925–38
Kiermayer O: Werke von Dr. h. c. Hans-Henning Heunert. **Mikroskopie** 1981 Feb;38(1–2):3–12
Schmutz HK: Rüdingers 'Atlas des peripherischen Nervensystems des menschlichen Körpers' mit Photographien von Joseph Albert; zur Frühgeschichte der medizinischen Photographie. **Gesnerus** 1980;37(1/2):83–90

**Great Britain**

Burrows A, Schumacher I: Doktor Diamonds Bildnisse von Geisteskranken. Transl. of Doctor Diamond's portraits of the insane. Frankfurt am Main, Syndikat, 1979. 159 p.
Hansell P: A backward glance — 2. **J Audiov Media Med** 1979 Jul;2(3):107–11

# PHOTOGRAPHY

**Italy**

Caffaratto AT: La raccolta di fotografie segnaletiche del Museo di Antropologia Criminale di Torino: la fotografia come documento e testimonianza dell'opera di Cesare Lombroso.
**Ann Osp Maria Vittoria Torino** 1980 Jul-Dec;23(7-12):295-332

**United States**

Apple RD, comp: Illustrated catalogue of the slide archive of historical medical photographs at Stony Brook; Center for Photographic Images of Medicine and Health Care. Westport, Conn., Greenwood, 1984. xi, 442 p.
Boatner EB: Captioned films of the deaf. **Am Ann Deaf** 1981 Aug;126(5):520-5
Bonsett CA: Mystery photo: why was it shown to med students?
**J Indiana State Med Assoc** 1980 Mar;73(3):123
Burns SB: Early medical photography in America (1839-1883).
**NY State J Med** 1980 Aug;80(9):1444-69 (continued regularly)
Burns SB: Early medical photography in America (1839--1883); IV. Early wet-plate era. **NY State J Med** 1979 Nov;79(12):1931-8
Burns SB: Early medical photography in America (1839-1883) V. Beginnings of psychiatric photography. **NY State J Med** 1980 Feb;80(2):270-82
Burns SB: Early medical photography in America (1839-1883). VII. American medical publications with photographs. **NY State J Med** 1981 Jul;81(8):1126-64
Dean JB: A retrospective look through the camera of Fred A. Hitchcock. **Physiologist** 1984 Jun;27(3):128-30
Fishbein L: The snake pit (1948): the sexist nature of sanity. **Am Q** 1979;31(5):641-65
Gibson HL: The Biological Photographic Association, its half century. The era of maturation, 1965-1980. **J Biol Photogr** 1980 Apr;48(2):41-86
Gladstone W: Early medical photography in America (1839-1883); VI. Civil war medical photography. **NY State J Med** 1981 Jan;81(1):5, 8
Johnson CS: Anesthesia and photography. **Harv Mag** 1980 Jul-Aug;82(6):57
Kalisch PA, Kalisch BJ, Scobey M: Images of nurses on television. New York, Springer Pub. Co., 1983. ix, 214 p.
Knudson KG: Walt Disney, dentistry and the armed forces during World War II. **Bull Hist Dent** 1984 Oct;32(2):112-7
Layne GS: The Kirkbride-Langenheim collaboration: early use of photography in psychiatric treatment in Philadelphia.
**Pa Mag Hist Biogr** 1981;105(2):182-202
Mancin S: Days of darkness and hope at the State Hospital: a photographer's perspective. **RI Hist** 1982;41(4):139-41
Palmquist PE: Photography in medicine. **J West** 1982 Jul;21(3):59-64
Quart L, Auster A: The wounded vet in postwar film. **Soc Policy** 1982;13(2):24-31
Skinner RE: Photography, advertising, and the history of medicine: notes on the medico-historical art of Lejaren a Hiller. **Watermark** 1983 Jan;6(2-3):11-2

# PHYSICAL MEDICINE AND REHABILITATION

See also **Balneology, Hydrotherapy, and Health Resorts; Radiology; Sports Medicine**

Daněk K: Skiing in and through the history of medicine.
**Nord Medicinhist Arsb** 1982;:86-100
Fletcher GF: The history of exercise in the practice of medicine.
**J Med Assoc Ga** 1983 Jan;72(1):35-40
Harris P, Ross JC, et al: [Ludwig Guttmann - special issue].
**Paraplegia** 1979 May;17(1): passim
Hindermeyer J: Geschichte der physikalischen Therapie und der Rehabilitation. In Sournia JC, Martiny M, Poulet J, ed: Illustrierte Geschichte der Medizin. Salzburg, Andreas, 1980. Vol. 7. p. 2649-79.
Macdonald EM: World-wide conquests of disabilities. The history, development and present functions of the remedial services. London, Baillière Tindall, 1981. 299 p.
Macdonald EM: World-wide conquests of disabilities. The history, development and present functions of the remedial services. London, Baillière Tindall, 1981. 299 p.
Merikas G: The philosophy of exercise. **Curr Probl Clin Biochem** 1982;11:13-23
Ohry A: Historical perspectives of medical rehabilitation. **Koroth** 1981;8(1-2):57-60
Orr JF, James WV, Bahrani AS: The history and development of artificial limbs. **Eng Med** 1982 Oct;11(4):155-61
Smith WC: Brief history of the treatment of disabled citizens--since the beginning of written history. **Am Correct Ther J** 1980 Nov-Dec;34(6):182-3
Stensman R: The paraplegic Viking and the one-armed pianist--some well known persons with locomotor disability.
**Scand J Rehabil Med [Suppl]** 1983;9:82-7
Verdan C: Geschichte der plastischen und wiederherstellenden Chirurgie. In Sournia JC, Martiny M, Poulet J, ed: Illustrierte Geschichte der Medizin. Salzburg, Andreas, 1980. Vol. 8. p. 2911-31.
Wilken U: Zur geschichtlichen Entwicklung der Körperbehinderten-Selbsthilfe-Vereinigungen. **Rehabilitation (Stuttg)** 1983 May;22(2):65-8
Zhuo O: Chinese traditional medicine: its contribution to physical rehabilitation. **Arch Phys Med Rehabil** 1982 Oct;63(10):499-500

**China**

Zhou DH: The contribution of traditional Chinese medicine to rehabilitation medicine. **Chin Med J [Engl]** 1981 Sep;94(9):593-6

**Germany**

Wilken U: Zur Geschichte von Einstellungsdeterminanten gegen über Körperbehinderten. **Rehabilitation (Stuttg)** 1984 May;23(2):81-3

**United States**

Obermann CE: A history of vocational rehabilitation in America. New York, Arno Press, 1980. 389 p.

**USSR**

Kunichev LA: Iz istorii lechebnogo massazha. **Feldsher Akush** 1981;46(2):43-5

**500 A.D.-1450**

**Arabic**

Estestvennye i preformirovannye fizicheskie faktory vo vrachebnoĭ deiatel'nosti Abu-Ali Ibn-Siny (k 1000-letiiu so dnia rozhdneiia):
**Vopr Kurortol Fizioter Lech Fiz Kult** 1981 Jan-Feb;(1):64-6

**1700 to Present**

Barker JT: Women as leaders in the field of rehabilitation. **J Rehabil** 1982 Jan-Mar;48(1):9-18, 68-70
Bläsig W: Die Sondermarken zum Internationalen Jahr der Behinderten - geordnet nach Gesichtspunkten der Rehabilitation.
**Rehabilitation (Stuttg)** 1983 Nov;22(4):162-5
Dyer L: Rock or sand? **Physiotherapy** 1982 Jun;68(6):177-81
Geddes LA: A short history of the electrical stimulation of excitable tissue. Including electrotherapeutic applications. **Physiologist** 1984 Feb;27(1 Suppl):S1-47
Herbison GJ: Research: ends, setting, environment, activities, resources, creativity, health. **Arch Phys Med Rehabil** 1984 Mar;65(3):112-4
Kersley GD: The scope of rheumatology. **Ann Rheum Dis** 1981 Dec;40(6):631-2
Leyendecker CH: Erfahrung und Theorie in der Sonderpädagogik Körperbehinderter--ein Diskurs zum Theorie-Praxis-Bezug.
**Rehabilitation (Stuttg)** 1983 Aug;22(3):100-9
McGuiness-Scott J: Benesh movement notation. An introduction to recording clinical data. Part 12: an historical perspective and clinical uses. **Physiotherapy** 1982 Jun;68(6):182-4
Peltier LF: A brief historical note on the use of electricity in the treatment of fractures. **Clin Orthop** 1981 Nov-Dec;161:4-7
Phillips WR, Rosenberg J, ed: The origins of modern treatment and education of physically handicapped children. Reprint of articles. New York, Arno, 1980. Various pagings. (The physically handicapped in society).
Sheon RP: Transcutaneous electrical nerve stimulation. From electric eels to electrodes. **Postgrad Med** 1984 Apr;75(5):71-4

**Australia**

D'Arbon P: Rehabilitation yesterday and today. **Lamp** 1980 Dec;37(12):16-8

**Canada**

Martin D: Dr. Robert Tait McKenzie: Canada's renaissance man.
**Can Med Assoc J** 1984 Sep 1;131(5):493-6
Morton D: 'Noblest and best': retaining Canada's war disabled 1915-23. **J Can Stud** 1981;16(3-4):75-85

**Chile**

Paolinelli L: Acciones de rehabilitación médica en Chile, 1952-1977.
**Rev Med Chil** 1977 Oct;105(10):707-13

**France**

Colas des Francs G: L'oeuvre de Jules Amar entre 1914 et 1918. Thèse,

Université René-Descartes, Faculté Cochin-Port-Royal. Paris, 1984. 21, 29, 7, 70 p.
Huard P: Armel-Eugène Gripouilleau (1821-1909) officier de santé à Montlouis (Indre-et-Loire). In: Congrès National des Sociétés Savantes, 93e, Tours, 1968. Comptes Rendus. Paris, 1971. Section des Sciences, Tome II. p. 189-92.
Monod H: Evocation de d'Arsonval. **J Belge Med Phys Rehabil** 1981;4(3):103-15
Montès F: La réinsertion professionnelle et sociale des handicapés. **Etudes (Fr)** 1981;354(4):467-83
Swain Gladys: Une logique de l'inclusion: les infirmes du signe. **Esprit** 1982;5:61-75

**Germany**

Asdonk J: Die Physikalische Lymphdrainage- und Odemtherapie der Feldbergklinik. Eine historische Übersicht über den derzeitigen Stand der physikalisch-lymphologischen Medizin. **Z Lymphol** 1983 Jul;7(1):40-6
Bäsig W: Die Philatelie im Dienste der Rehabilitation. **Rehabilitation (Stuttg)** 1981 May;20(2):86-9
Becker KP: 30 Jahre Lehre, Forschung und Wissenschaftsentwicklung im Dienste der Bildung, Erziehung und Rehabilitation Geschädigter. **Wiss Z Humboldt Univ Berl [Gesellschaftswiss Sprachwiss Reihe]** 1979;28(2):157-64
Klessen D, Albrecht U, Grützmacher KH, et al: Stand und weitere Aufgaben der physikalischen Therapie in Berlin--Hauptstadt der DDR. **Sante Publique (Bucur)** 1981;24(4):347-57
Seidler E: Die Entwicklung des Rehabilitations-Verständnisses. **Krankenpflege (Frankfurt)** 1980 Oct;34(10):338-41
Trettin H: Der Weg der Manuellen Lymphdrainage nach Vodder zur Therapeutischen Lymphdrainage nach Kuhnke/Asdonk--ein halbes Jahrhundert geschichtlicher Entwicklung der Odemtherapie. **Z Lymphol** 1983 Jul;7(1):47-9
Volkert G: Die Entwicklung der Körperbehindertenfürsorge. **ZFA (Stuttgart)** 1980 Apr 10;56(10):725-30

**Great Britain**

Compton A: Developments of skills in physiotherapy over the last 60 years. **Midwife Health Visit Community Nurse** 1980 Oct;16(10):412-4
Myers-Levin A: Cerebral palsy: the early years of occupational therapy in Scotland. Edingburgh, Scottish Council for Spastics, 1978. xv, 131 p.

**Hungary**

Balóné Fleischmann M: A rehabilitáció hazai úttörõje Gárdi Jenö dr. (1886-1944). **Orv Hetil** 1984 Feb 19;125(8):470-2

**India**

Nimbkar KV: A new life for the handicapped: a history of rehabilitation and occupational therapy in India. Bombay, Nimbkar Rehabilitation Trust, 1980. xviii, 374 p.

**Mexico**

Ibarra LG: Rehabilitationsdienste in territorialen Gesundheitseinrichtungen. **Z Gesamte Hyg** 1981;27(2):111-3

**United States**

Balasalle NM: A history of public policy for the education of handicapped children in Massachusetts. Ed.D. Dissertation, Harvard University. Cambridge, 1980. viii, 273 p.
Berkowitz ED: Rehabilitation: the federal government's response to disability, 1935-1954. New York, Arno, 1980. xv, 339 p. (The Physically Handicapped in Society.) Also Ph.D. Diss., Northwestern University. Evanston, 1976.
Berkowitz ED: The federal government and the emergence of rehabilitation medicine. **Historian** 1981;43(4):530-45
Christie J: Mary Elizabeth Switzer. In: Notable American women. The modern period. Cambridge, Mass., Belknap-Harvard Univ. Press, 1980. 4:669-70.
Husing JM: Brief historical background on the certification process in corrective therapy, and a policy statement regarding certification eligibility. **Am Correct Ther J** 1983 Nov-Dec;37(6):153-5
Kidwell R: Handicapping an innovator. **Reason** 1981;13(4):39-46
Lehmann JF: Rehabilitation medicine: past, present and future. **Arch Phys Med Rehabil** 1982 Jul;63(7):291-7
Murphy EF: Reflections on automotive adaptive equipment--an essay. **Bull Prosthet Res** 1979 Fall;16(2):191-207
Ostrow PC: The historical precedents for quality assurance in health care. **Am J Occup Ther** 1983 Jan;37(1):23-6
Pittenger JC, Kuriloff P: Educating the handicapped: reforming a radical law. **Public Interest** 1982;66:72-96
Stillwell GK: Whence our academy? **Arch Phys Med Rehabil** 1983 Mar;64(3):97-100
Yanes-Hoffman N: Howard Rusk, MD: an equal chance. **JAMA** 1981 Oct 2;246(14):1503-5, 1509-10

**USSR**

Bogoliubov VM, Sokolova NF: [Department of Physiotherapy of the Order of Lenin Central Institute of Physician Advanced Training in preparing medical personnel] (Rus). **Vopr Kurortoi Fizioter Lech Fiz Kult** 1980;6:62-3
Orzheshkovskiĭ VV, Chopchik DI: 20-letie Ukrainskogo respublikanskogo nauchnogo obshchestva fizioterapevtov i kurortologov. **Vopr Kurortol Fizioter Lech Fiz Kult** 1979 Sep-Oct;(5):69-70
Shukurov AK, Pulatov RP: [Development of health resort science and physiotherapy in Uzbekistan]. (Rus) **Vopr Kurortol Fizioter Lech Fiz Kult** 1979 Nov-Dec;(6):7-11
Sukhanov NV: Meditsinakaia i trudovaia reabilitatsiia ranenykh v gospitaliakh Zapadnoĭ Sibiri v period Velikoĭ Otechestvennoĭ voiny. **Voen Med Zh** 1981;(7):72-4

# PHYSIOGNOMY

**Before 500 A.D.**

**Greco-Roman**

Evans EC: Physiognomics in the ancient world. Philadelphia, American Philosophical Society, 1969. 101 p. (Transactions of the American Philosophical Society, n. s., Vol. 59, Part 5).

**500 A.D.-1450**

**France**

Charmasson T: Roland l'Ecrivain, médecin des Ducs de Bourgogne. In: Congrès National des Sociétes Savantes, 101e, Lille, 1976. Comptes Rendus. Paris, 1976. Section des Sciences, Fasc. III. p. 21-32.

**1450-1700**

Müller-Jahncke WD: Kleiner Beitrag zum Prioritätenstreit um die Metoposkopie: Hájek contra Cardano. **Sudhoffs Arch** 1982;66(1):79-84
Pack RA: Magister Iodocus: 'Regule phisonomie'. **Mediaev Stud** 1980;42:212-37

**Germany**

Dotz W: Albrecht Dürer. Depictions of facies as expressions of personality. **Am J Dermatopathol** 1981 Spring;3(1):59-65

**Italy**

Baur O, Bott B, Braunfels-Esche S, et al: Leonardo da Vinci Anatomie, Physiognomik, Proportion und Bewegung. Köln, 1984. 343 p. (Kölner medizinhistorische Beiträge: Arbeiten der Forschungsstelle des Instituts für Geschichte der Medizin der Universität zu Köln, Band 23/1)

**1700 to Present**

Gilman SL: Zur Physiognomie des Geisteskranken in Geschichte und Praxis, 1800-1900. **Sudhoffs Arch** 1978;62(3):209-34

**France**

Wechsler J: A human comedy. Physiognomy and caricature in 19th century Paris. Chicago, University of Chicago Press, 1982. 208 p.

**Germany**

Glandien O: Franz Xaver Messerschmidt (1736-1783) - Ausdrucksstudien und Charakterköpfe, Köln: 1981. 205 p. (Kölner medizinhistorische Beiträge: Arbeiten der Forschungsstelle des Instituts für Geschichte der Medizin der Universität zu Köln, Band 20).

**Great Britain**

Fahnestock J: The heroine of irregular features: physiognomy and conventions of heroine description. **Victorian Stud** 1981;24(3):325-50

**Italy**

Bazzi F, Bèttica-Giovannini R: L'atlante fisiognomonico e frenologico del sig. Ysabeau tra quelli di Lavater e di Fall e quello di Lombroso. **Ann Osp Maria Vittoria Torino** 1980 Jul-Dec;23(7-12):343-416

## PHYSIOGNOMY

**United States**

Mainwaring M: 'Phys/phren': why not to take each other at face value. **Smithsonian** 1980;11(8):193–212

**USSR**

Goscilo H: Lermontov's debt to Lavater and Gall. **Slav East Eur Rev** 1981;59(4):500–15

## PHYSIOLOGY

Angelis E de: Rapporti tra mente e corpo dall'eta' classica al XIX secolo. **Med Secoli** 1982 May–Aug;19(2):193–213
Baumann HU: Ueber Mehrfachentdeckungen. Eine Darstellung des allgemeinen Problems mit Beispielen aus drei Teilgebieten der theoretischen Medizin. Diss. Münster, 1972. 133 p.
Bell BA: A history of the study of the cerebral circulation and the measurement of cerebral blood flow. **Neurosurgery** 1984 Feb;14(2):238–46
Belloni L: Il Morgagni tra il Malpighi e il Cotugno. **Gesnerus** 1982;39(2):195–213
Benzinger TH, ed: Temperature, part 1: arts and concepts. Stroudsburg, Pa., Dowden, Hutchinson & Ross, 1977. viii, 353 p. (Benchmark Papers in Human Physiology, 9).
Bouvenot G, Delboy C: Geschichte der grossen physiologischen Konzepte. In Sournia JC, Martiny M, Poulet J, ed: Illustrierte Geschichte der Medizin. Salzburg, Andreas, 1980. Vol. 8. p. 2881–909.
Brazier MA: A history of neurophysiology in the 17th and 18th centuries: from concept to experiment. New York, Raven Press, 1984. xiii, 230 p.
Brooks CM: An event in the history of physiology. Transfer of Aristotelian corpus of science and the Hippocratic–Galenic corpus of medicine to the Islamic world by the Nestorians. In E. Schultheisz, ed: History of physiology. Oxford, Elmsford, New York, Pergamon, 1981. xvi, 208 p. (Advances in Physiological Sciences. Proceedings of the 28th International Congress of Physiological Sciences, Budapest, 1980. Volume 21). p. ix–xvi.
Brooks CM: Origin, essence and survival of physiology: queen of sciences. **Isr J Med Sci** 1982 Jan;18(1):3–7
Copley AL: The endo–endothelial fibrin lining. A historical account. **Thromb Res [Suppl]** 1983;5:1–26
Crosby WH: An historical sketch of splenic function and splenectomy. **Lymphology** 1983 Jun;16(2):52–5
Duchesneau F: De Boerhaaave et Baglivi à Haller: vers un concept 'analytique' de la structure organique. **Arch Int Hist Idees** 1982;95:103–40
Duchesneau F: De l'épigenèse au vitalisme (C. F. Wolff et Blumenbach). **Arch Int Hist Idees** 1982:95:312–60
Duchesneau F: La physiologie des lumières. Empirisme, modèles et théories. The Hague, Martinus Nijhoff, 1982. xxi, 611 p. (International Archives of the History of Ideas, no. 95).
Etessami S: La contraction musculaire: de l'antiquité jusqu'à nos jours. In: Congrès international d'histoire de la médecine, XXVe, Québec, 1976. Actes. Québec, 1977. p. 644–9.
Fontaine M: From the physiology of marine organisms to oceanographic physiology or physiological oceanography. In Sears M, Merriman D, ed: Oceanography, the past. New York, Springer, 1980. p. 353–59.
Fontaine M: The history of comparative physiology. In E. Schultheisz, ed: History of physiology. Oxford, Elmsford, New York, Pergamon, 1981. xvi, 208 p. (Advances in Physiological Sciences. Proceedings of the 28th International Congress of Physiological Sciences, Budapest, 1980. Volume 21). p. 23–28.
Glass E: Chemistry and physiology in their historical and philosophical relations. Delft, Delft University Press, 1979. xiii, 199 p.
Hall DL: Why do animals breathe? New York, Arno Press, 1981. xviii, 296 p.
Hoffmann P: Modèle mécaniste et modèle animiste. De quelques aspects de la représentation du vivant chez Descartes, Borelli et Stahl. **Rev Sci Hum** 1982–3;186–7:199–211
Imhof AE: Leib und Leben unserer Vorfahren: eine rhythmisierte Welt. In Imhof AE, ed: Leib und Leben in der Geschichte der Neuzeit. Berlin, Duncker & Humblot, 1983. p. 21–38.
Knell AJ: Liver function and failure: the evolution of liver physiology. **J R Coll Physicians Lond** 1980 Jul;14(3):205–8
Kurzbauer R, Kurzbauer E, Sędzielowski Z: Z historii electrostymulacji. **Pieleg Polozna** 1979;(10):3–4
Macdonald AA: Studies on the anatomy and physiology of the pig fetus and placenta: an historical review. In E. Schultheisz, ed: History of physiology. Oxford, Elmsford, New York, Pergamon, 1981. xvi, 208 p. (Advances in Physiological Sciences. Proceedings of the 28th International Congress of Physiological Sciences, Budapest, 1980. Volume 21). p. 53–60.
Möller HJ: Die Begriffe 'Reizbarkeit' und 'Reiz': Konstanz und Wandel ihres Bedeutungsgehaltes sowie die Problematik ihrer exakten Definition. Stuttgart, Fischer, 1975. viii, 104 p. (Medizin in Geschichte und Kultur, 11).
Neuhausen T: Das Cholesterin. Vorstellungen über seine Rolle im Körper. Köln, Universität zu Köln, 1977. 187 p. (Kölner medizinhistorische Beiträge, 6).
Schiller J: Physiology and classification: historical relations. Paris, Maloine, 1980. xiii, 194 p.
Schultheisz E: The beginning of quantification in physiology. **Clio Med** 1983 Mar;17(4):193–7
Schultheisz E, ed.: History of physiology. Oxford, Elmsford, New York, Pergamon, 1981. xvi, 208 p. (Advances in Physiological Sciences. Proceedings of the 28th International Congress of Physiological Sciences, Budapest, 1980. Volume 21).
Starobinski J: Breve storia della coscienza del corpo. **Intersezioni** 1981;1(1):27–43

**China**

Dakpa N: La Sphygnologie tibétaine. In Mazars G, ed: Les médecines traditionnelles de l'Asie. Strasbourg, Université Louis Pasteur, 1981. p. 23–9.

**France**

Buffat M: Diderot, le corps le la machine. **Rev Sci Hum** 1982–3;186–7:185–97

**Germany**

Witschel H: Die Physiologie zu Erlangen von der Gründung der Universität bis zum Ausklang der Romantik. Erlangen, 1964. 141 p.

**Great Britain**

Brown T: The mechanical philosophy and the 'animal oeconomy'. New York, Arno Press, 1981. viii, 419 p.

**India**

Sinha A: Physiological concepts in ancient and medieval India. In E. Schultheisz, ed: History of physiology. Oxford, Elmsford, New York, Pergamon, 1981. xvi, 208 p. (Advances in Physiological Sciences. Proceedings of the 28th International Congress of Physiological Sciences, Budapest, 1980. Volume 21). p. 61–75.

**Netherlands**

Ruestow EG: The rise of the doctrine of vascular secretion in the Netherlands. **J Hist Med Allied Sci** 1980 Jul;35(3):265–87

**USSR**

Ocherki istorii fiziologicheskikh nauk v SSSR: Istoki i osobennosti razvitiia: materialy Pervoĭ Vsesoiuznoĭ konferentsii po istorii fiziologicheskikh nauk, Tartu, 1981. Leningrad, Nauka, Leningradskoe otd–nie, 1984. 287 p.

**Vietnam**

Nguyen–Tran–Huan: La sphygmologie dans la médecine vietnamienne traditionnelle. Contribution à l'étude du traité 'Bin hú mài xué' de Lĭ Shí Zhen. In Mazars G, ed: Les médecines traditionnelles de l'Asie. Strasbourg, Université Louis Pasteur, 1981. p. 13–22.

**Before 500 A.D.**

**China**

Bridgman RF: Les fonctions physiologiques chez l'homme dans la Chine antique. **Hist Philos Life Sci** 1981;3(1):3–17

**Greco–Roman**

Cheng Zhifan: [Galen's thought, physiology and anatomy as taught by him] (Chi). **Chin J Med Hist** 1980;10:92–5

**Greece**

Bugaj R: Koncepcje elementów ognia i powietrza u Arystotelesa i ich rola w procesach spalania i oddychania. **Kwart Hist Nauki Tech** 1980;25(1):89–103
Kullmann W: Aristoteles' Grundgedanken zu Aufbau und Funktion der Körpergewebe. **Sudhoffs Arch** 1982;66(3):209–38
Kung J: Aristotle's De motu animalium and the separability of the sciences. **J Hist Philos** 1982;20:65–76
Pigeaud JM: Du rhythme dans le corps. Quelques notes sur l'interprétation du pouls par le médecin Hérophile. **Bull Assoc Guillaume Bude** 1978;3:258–67
Roselli A: Aristotele e il sistema della sensazione. **Physis** 1980;22(2):157–73
Smith WD: Erasistratus's dietetic medicine. **Bull Hist Med** 1982 Fall;56(3):398–409

### 500 A.D.–1450

Cadden J: A matter of life and death: water in the natural philosophy of Albertus Magnus. **Hist Philos Life Sci** 1980;2(2):241–52
Henkel N: Studien zum Physiologus im Mittelalter. Tübingen, Max Niemeyer, 1976. xi, 227 p. (Hermaea Germanistische Forschungen, N. F. xi, Bd. 38).
Leibowitz JO: R. Simon ben Zemah Duran (1361–1444) and his conception of metabolism in Magen Avot. **Koroth** 1979 Nov;7(9–10):CLXIX–XXIX(626–33)

#### Arabic

Rahman SA: Avicenna on digestion of food. **Bull Indian Inst Hist Med (Hyderabad)** 1981;1–4:59–63
Sankaran JR: Avicenna's thoughts and concepts of the pulse (sphygmology). **Bull Indian Inst Hist Med (Hyderabad)** 1981;1–4:64–74
Shetty PS: A critical analysis of Avicenna's contribution to physiology. **Bull Indian Inst Hist Med (Hyderabad)** 1981;1–4:152–60

#### Germany

Schultheisz E: Beginning of quantification in physiology. **Orvostort Kozl** 1980;89–91(26 no 1–3):209–13

#### Spain

Kottek S: Eléments de physiologie dans le 'Kusari' de Juda Halevi (Espagne, 12e siècle). In: Congrès international d'histoire de la médecine, XXVe, Québec, 1976. Actes. Québec, 1977. p. 840–7.

### 1450–1700

Boss J: Helmont, Glisson, and the doctrine of the common reservoir in the seventeenth-century revolution in physiology. **Br J Hist Sci** 1983 Nov;16(54 Pt 3):261–72
Lindeboom GA: Descartes and medicine. Amsterdam, Rodopi, 1979. 134 p. (Nieuwe Nederlandse Bijdragen tot de Geschiedenis der Geneeskunde, No. 1).
Nakamura T: T. Willis' and Lower's physiology with special reference to the theory of heart movement. **Jpn Stud Hist Sci** 1977;16:23–41
Trevisani F: 'Ratio' und 'Experimentum': Johannes Bohn (1640–1718) und die italienische Experimentalphysiologie. **Clio Med** 1983 Mar;17(4):199–206

#### France

Pflug G: Descartes und das mechanistische Menschenbild. **Medizinhist J** 1982;17(1/2):3–19
Vetter T: Louis de la Forge (1632–1667?) angevin et fidèle adepte de la physiologie cartésienne. In: Congrès National des Sociétés Savantes, 93e, Tours, 1968. Comptes Rendus. Paris, 1971. Section des Sciences, Tome II. p. 31–50.

#### Great Britain

Bonnabeau RC, Bonnabeau MM: William Harvey revisited 1578–1978. **Minn Med** 1981 Jan;64(1):28–33
Frank RG: Harvey and the Oxford physiologists: scientific ideas and social interaction. Berkeley, University of California Press, 1980. xviii, 368 p.
Knobil E: William Harvey and the physiology of reproduction. **Physiologist** 1981 Feb;24(1):3–7
Nikolov G: Uiliam Kharveĭ, otkrivateliat na krŭvoobrashtenieto. Sofiia, Meditsina i fizkultura, 1981. 74 p.
Schadewaldt H: 'Le génie, c'est une longue patience'. (Teil 1). **Arztl Fortbild** 1982;32(11):12–23
Schadewaldt H: 'Le génie, c'est une longue patience'. (Teil 2). **Arztl Fortbild** 1982;32(12):16–8
Schadewaldt H: 'Le génie, c'est une longue patience'. (Teil 3). **Arztl Fortbild** 1982;32(13):32–40
Whitteridge G: Of the local movement of animals. **Proc R Soc Lond [Biol]** 1979 Nov 30;206(1162):1–13

#### Italy

Baur O, Bott B, Braunfels-Esche S, et al: Leonardo da Vinci Anatomie, Physiognomik, Proportion und Bewegung. Köln, 1984. 343 p. (Kölner medizinhistorische Beiträge: Arbeiten der Forschungsstelle des Instituts für Geschichte der Medizin der Universität zu Köln, Band 23/1)

#### Netherlands

Lindeboom GA: Anton de Heide als proefondervindelijk onderzoeker. **Tijdschr Geschied Geneeskd** 1983;6(3):121–34

#### Spain

Corsano A: Medicina e teologia nel pensiero rinascimentale. La fisiologia di Michele Serveto. **G Crit Filos Ital** 1975;6(1):84–8

#### Sweden

Sourander P: Drottning Christina och Giovanni Alfonso Borelli till 300–årsminnet av kinesiologins födelse. **Nord Medicinhist Arsb** 1982;:56–65

### 1700 to Present

Almoyna JM, Almoyna CM: Continencia anal. Antecedentes históricos. **Rev Esp Enferm Apar Dig** 1983 Dec;64(6):549–55
Altschule MD: Invalidity of using so-called Starling curves in clinical medicine. **Perspect Biol Med** 1983 Winter;26(2):171–87
Brazier MA: Pioneers in the discovery of evoked potentials. **Electroencephalogr Clin Neurophysiol** 1984 Feb;59(1):2–8
Chang S: In memory of our visiting professor: Walter B. Cannon at Peking. **Physiologist** 1980 Jun;23(3):39–40
Cirillo VJ: Nineteenth-century views on blood fluidity. **J Med Soc NJ** 1983 Jul;80(7):535–9
Clark LC: Measurement of oxygen tension: a historical perspective. **Crit Care Med** 1981 Oct;9(10):690–2
Demidova NI: Telefonicheskie issledovaniia v élektrofiziologii. **Zh Vyssh Nerv Deiat** 1982 Jul–Aug;32(4):783–5
Duchesneau F: Monades, molécules organiques et ordre physiologique: de Maupertuis et Buffon à Haller. **Arch Int Hist Idees** 1982;95:235–311
Duchesneau F: Sensibilité et structure organique: l'alternative Whytt–Haller. **Arch Int Hist Idees** 1982;95:171–234
Erickson RP: Ohrwall, Henning and von Skramlik; the foundations of the four primary positions in taste. **Neurosci Biobehav Rev** 1984 Spring;8(1):105–27
Franzini C: La evoluzione del concetto di stress in fisiologia. **Arch Sci Biol (Bologna)** 1978 Jan–Dec;62(1–4):131–7
Gago R, Carrillo JL: La obra fisiológica de Ignacio María Ruiz de Luzuriaga (1763–1822) y su plagio del científico británico Adair Crawford (1748–1795). **Dynamis** 1981;1:87–100
Glas E: Chemistry and physiology in their historical and philosophical relations. Delft, Delft University Press, 1979. 199 p.
Günther B: Génesis del de homeostasis: de Claude Bernard a Walter Cannon. **Rev Med Chil** 1981 May;109(5):484–5
Harrison G, Collins K: In memoriam Joseph Sydney Weiner (1915–1982). **Ann Hum Biol** 1982 Nov–Dec;9(6):583–92
Hoppe B: Chemophysiologie zwischen vitalistischer und mechanistischer Biologie im 19. Jahrhundert. **Medizinhist J** 1983;18(3):163–83
Hubel DH: Exploration of the primary visual cortex, 1955–78. **Nature** 1982 Oct 7;299(5883):515–24
Huf EG: Echoes of the past. Reflections on the early history of the concept of 'active transport'. **Physiologist** 1979 Dec;22(6):18–24
Imhof AE, ed: Leib und Leben in der Geschichte der Neuzeit: Vorträge eines internationalen Colloquiums. Berlin, Duncker & Humblot, 1983. 266 p. Text in German and French. (Berliner Historische Studien, Bd. 9. Einzelstudien 2).
Jones IH: Menstruation: the history of sanitary protection. **Nurs Times** 1980 Mar 6;76(10):407–8
Kaiser W: Ernst Mach und das Mechanismusproblem in der Biologie. **Medizinhist J** 1982;17(3):179–94
Keel O: John Hunter et Xavier Bichat: les rapports de leurs travaux en pathologie tissulaire. In International Congress of the History of Medicine, 27th, Barcelona, 1980. Actas. Barcelona, Académia de Ciències Médiques de Catalunya i Balears, 1981. p. 535–49.
Kempner W: The Durham connection to Germany. **NC Med J** 1984 Jan;45(1):25–6
Leach DH, Dagg AI: Evolution of equine locomotion research. **Equine Vet J** 1983 Apr;15(2):87–92
Lohff B: Zur Geschichte der Lehre von der Lebenskraft. **Clio Med** 1981 Dec;16(2/3):101–12
Lübbers DW: History of transcutaneous PO2 measurement. **Crit Care Med** 1981 Oct;9(10):693
Mani N: Physiologische und medizinische Chemie zwischen 1800 und 1850. **Pharm Acta Helv** 1979;54(9–10):273–80
Miller MJ: Tissue oxygenation in clinical medicine: an historical review. **Anesth Analg (Cleve)** 1982 Jun;61(6):527–35
Nicolle P, Jude A: Réflexions sur les prix Nobel de physiologie ou médecine. **Hist Sci Med** 1980;14(1):83–93
Paál A: Az aero-ionizáció orvos-biológiai felhasználásának lehetöségei a XVIII–XIX-ik században és mai idöszerüségük. **Orv Hetil** 1984 Mar 4;125(10):595–6, 599
Pakovich BI: To commemorate the 80th year since discovery of conditional reflexes. **Pavlov J Biol Sci** 1983 Oct–Dec;18(4):175–80
Pavel I: Aperçu historique de l'existence du rôle du shunt disse-canalicule biliaire dans la sécrétion biliaire et dans la pathogénie de certains ictères. **Med Interne** 1981 Oct–Dec;19(4):389–96
Potter VR: Physiological adaptation at the molecular level: the frontier where research on differentiation and malignancy meet.

# PHYSIOLOGY

**Perspect Biol Med** 1981 Summer;24(4):525-42

Rijlant P: The coming of age of electrophysiology and electrocardiography. **NTM** 1980;17(1):108-23

Robin ED, ed: Claude Bernard and the internal environment: a memorial symposium. New York, Dekker, 1979. xvi, 299 p. Historical contributions by J. Bernard, M. Bertrand, J. S. Fruton, R. H. Unger, J. P. Changeux, A. Cournand, F. Morel, R. Guillemin, H. Rahn, S. S. Cohen.

Rodgers JS: 'Life' in the novel: Tristram Shandy and some aspects of eighteenth-century physiology. **Eighteenth Cent Life** 1980;6(1):1-20

Roth N: Animal electricity. **Med Instrum** 1980 Jul-Aug;14(4):228

Rothschuh KE: Ursprünge und Wandlungen der physiologischen Denkweisen im 19. Jahrhundert. **Forschungsunternehm Fritz Thyssen Stift Stud Naturwiss Tech Wirtsch Neunzehn Jahrhundert** 1976;2:135-60

Rudolph G: Herkunft und Schicksal des Humor aqueus. Physiologische Untersuchungen im Vorfeld der Atiologie des Glaukoms während des ersten Viertels des 20. Jahrhunderts. **Gesnerus** 1983;40(3/4):241-8

Sechzer JA: The ethical dilemma of some classical animal experiments. **Ann NY Acad Sci** 1983;406:5-12

Stoffregen M: Zur historischen Entwicklung der experimentellen Physiologie der Nebennierenrindensuffizienz. **Sudhoffs Arch** 1981;65(3):266-98

Stremel RW: Historical development of the anaerobic threshold concept. **Physiologist** 1984 Aug;27(4):295-8

[The history of physiology:] essay review: **Ann Sci** 1981;38(3):343-52

Van der Kloot W: Otto Loewi. In Dictionary of American biography, 1961-1965. Suppl. 7, 1981. p. 475-7.

Vengrova IV, Egorysheva IV, Rabinovich RS, et al: Znamenatel'nye i iubileĭnye daty istorii fiziologii 1980 g. **Fiziol Zh SSSR** 65(9):1396-9, Sep 79

Vidal F: L'inflammation chez les physiologistes du XVIIIe siècle. **Chir Dent Fr** 1983 Oct 27;53(222):43-6

West JB: Man at extreme altitude. **J Appl Physiol** 1982 Jun;52(6):1393-9

West JB, ed: Translations in respiratory physiology. Stroudsburg, Pennsylvania, Dowden, Hutchinson & Ross, 1975. 772 p. (Translations of 19th-20th century articles by various authors).

Zieliński K: Ezras A. Asratyan. **Acta Neurobiol Exp (Warsz)** 1981;41(6):521-42

### Belgium

Florkin M, Théodoridès J: Henri de Lacaze-Duthiers et Léon Fredericq: correspondance (1876-1900). **Arch Int Physiol Biochim** 1982 Jul;90(2):Suppl 1-94

Florkin M: L'Ecole Liégeoise de Physiologie et son Maître Léon Fredericq (1851-1935), pionnier de la zoologie chimique. Liège, Vaillant-Carmanne, 1979. 211 p. (Publication des Archives Internationales de Physiologie et de Biochimie, Médecine et Médicins au Pays de Liège, IV).

Lecomte J, Schoffeniels E: L'oeuvre de Léon Frédéricq et son école (1853-1934) à travers les Archives de Biologie (1880-1904). **Arch Biol (Liege)** 1980;91(2):267-70

Lecomte J, Bacq ZM: Physiologie animale et humaine. In Florilège des Sciences en Belgique - II. Bruxelles Académie Royale de Belgique, 1980. p. 273-86.

### Canada

Roland CG: John Fulton, In Dictionary of Canadian biography, 1881-1890. 1982;11:328-9.

### Chile

Croxatto H: Homenaje al Dr. Teodoro Muhm (1869-1939). **Rev Med Chil** 1984 Jan;112(1):81-8

Dill DB: International high altitude expedition to Chile, 1935. **Prog Clin Biol Res** 1983;136:201-4

### China

Tang PS: [An unfinished project--recollections of fifty years of physiological research] (Chi). **Sheng Li Ko Hsueh Chin Chan** 1984 Jul;15(3):193-7

Tsai C: [Retrospect of a physiologist engaged in scientific research and education for 60 years] (Chi). **Sheng Li Ko Hsueh Chin Chan** 1982 Jul;13(3):193-200

### Czechoslovakia

Drahota Z: Třicet let Fyziologického ústavu CSAV. **Cesk Fysiol** 1984;33(4):289-92

Kruta V: Jiří Procháska. Professor anatomie a fysiologie 1778-1786. K dějinám fysiologie v Praze. **Cesk Fysiol** 1980;29(1):84-9

Obermajer J: Neznámé dopisy Purkyňova tchána K. A. Rudolphiho J. J. Berzeliovi. **Cas Lek Cesk** 1984 Feb 17;123(7):199-203

Peňáz J: K úmrtí prof. MUDr. Vladislava Kruty, DrSc. **Cesk Fysiol** 1980 Mar;29(2):159-70

První české přednášky na Pražské lékařské fakultě - Kuřákovy přednášky z fysiologie: **Cesk Fysiol** 1983;32(5):467-8

Trojan S, Trávníčkova E: Přednášky Vladimíra Tomsy. **Cesk Fysiol** 1979;80(5):471-2

### Denmark

Schmidt-Nielsen B: August and Marie Krogh and respiratory physiology. **J Appl Physiol** 1984 Aug;57(2):293-303

### France

Albury WR: Going beyond the introduction: Claude Bernard scholarship in the 1970s, an essay review. **Bull Hist Med** 1982 Summer;56(2):271-5

Azouvi F: Irritabilité et magnétisme animal: une lettre inédite de J.-M.-A. Servan. **Dix-huit Siecle** 1982;14:191-7

Bacq ZM: Le centenaire de la mort de Claude Bernard. **Rev Med Liege** 1979 Jun 1;34(11):525-8

Baron JB: Etienne-Jules Marey. **Acta Belg Med Phys** 1983 Oct-Dec;6(4):187-97

Bert P: La pression barométrique. Recherches de physiologie expérimentale. Facsimile of 1878 edition. Biographical introduction by P. Dejour. Paris, Editions du Centre National de la Recherche Scientifique, 1979. viii, 1183 p.

Borell M: D'Arsonval's calorimeter: measurement of animal heat, 1877. **Med Instrum** 1982 Nov-Dec;16(6):307-8

Bourguignon A: Certains problèmes épistemologiques évoqués par Claude Bernard. In Poirier J, Poirier JL, ed: Médecine et philosophie à la fin du XIXe siècle. Paris, Université de Paris XII - Val de Marne, [1980?]. p. 85-100.

Cappelletti V: Bernard, oltre meccanicismo e vitalismo. **Med Secoli** 1979 Jan-Apr;16(1):5-11

Cappelletti V: Claude Bernard between history and the 'principles' of science. **Riv Biol** 1980 Spring;73(1):21-33

Claude Bernard fut-il un médecin praticien?: Entretiens de Bichat, Faculté de médecine, Pitié-Salpêtrière, Paris, 29 septembre-8 Octobre 1978. [France], Expansion scientifique, 1978 printing. [32] p.

Czeisler CA, Guilleminault C: 250 years ago: tribute to a new discipline (1729--1979). **Sleep** 1979;2(2):155-60

De Neve M: E. J. Marey, inventieve registrator van de fysiologische fenomenen. **Acta Belg Med Phys** 1983 Oct-Dec;6(4):153-5

Dillemann G: L'éloge de Magendie par Claude Bernard. **Hist Sci Med** 1983;17(4):345-9

Dreyfus G: Médecine scientifique et art médical. Une controverse à propos de Claude Bernard. **Sem Hop Paris** 1983 May 19;59(20):1569-71

Duchesneau F: Vers une théorie analytique de l'organisme (Bichat). **Arch Int Hist Idees** 1982;95:431-76

Dupuis M: Etienne-Jules Marey, le photographe du mouvement. **Sci Avenir** 1980;400:95-100

Fleckenstein K: Etienne Marey and the electric torpedo fish. **Med Instrum** 1984 Sep-Oct;18(5):288-9

Kayser C: Note historique sur l'évolution de la chaire de physiologie de la Faculté de Médecine. In Livet G, Schaff G, ed: Médecine et assistance en Alsace, XVIe-XXe siècle. Strasbourg, Istra, 1976. p. 303-19.

Kenéz J: Forradalmi átalakulás a medicinában a XIX. század elején. **Orv Hetil** 1984 May 27;125(22):1330-3

Knaus WA: Claude Bernard fut-il l'inventeur de l'indice de gravité? **Presse Med** 1983 Jul 2;12(28):1755-6

La Vergata A: Claude Bernard, 'punti di vista fisiologici', ed economia della natura. **Riv Filos** 1982;73:361-95

Lagoutte J: Claude Bernard, un physiologiste, un philosophe. Lyon, Centre régional de documentation pédagogique, 1978. 40 p.

Lazorthes G, Campan L: François Magendie (1783-1855). **Bull Acad Natl Med (Paris)** 1984 Jan-Feb;168(1-2):105-11

Lecomte J: Apologie de Zénon Bacq 1903-1983. **Rev Med Liege** 1983 Sep 1;38(17):627-30

Légée G: A. Vulpien (1826-1887), physiologiste élève de P. Flourens (1794-1867). In: Congrès international d'histoire de la médecine, XXVe, Québec, 1976. Actes. Québec, 1977. p. 873-80.

Legée G: Henri Ducrotay de Blainville (1777-1850) et la physiologie. In: Congrès National des Sociétés Savantes, 105e, Caen, 1980. Comptes Rendus, Paris, 1980. Section des Sciences, Fasc. V. p. 49-59.

Legée G: L'activité parisienne d'un physiologiste languedocien Marie-Jean-Pierre Flourens (1794-1867). In: Congrès National des Sociétés Savantes, 96e, Toulouse, 1971. Comptes Rendus. Paris, 1974. Histoire des Sciences, Tome 1. p. 107-22.

Legée G: L'influence de la Société d'Auteuil sur les travaux des physiologistes. In: Congrès National des Sociétés Savantes, 100e, Paris, 1975. Actes. Paris, 1976. Histoire Moderne et Contemporaine et Histoire des Sciences. p. 229-42.

Legée G: Physiologie et phrenologie au temps du physiologiste Pierre Flourens (1794-1867). In International Congress of the History of Medicine, 27th, Barcelona, 1980. Actas. Barcelona, Académia de Ciències Médiques de Catalunya i Balears, 1981. p. 91-7.

Lesch JE: Science and medicine in France: the emergence of experimental physiology, 1790-1855. Cambridge, Mass., Harvard University Press, 1984. viii, 276 p.

Lichtenthaeler C: Die sechs Leitgedanken von Magendies medizinischer Revolution. **Z Arztl Fortbild (Jena)** 1983;77(18):785-8
Mayer J: Quand Diderot corrige Diderot: l'élaboration des Eléments de physiologie. In J. Proust, ed: Recherches nouvelles sur quelques écrivains des lumières (II). Montpellier, Univ. Paul Valéry, 1979. p. 73-129.
Pickstone JV: Bureaucracy, liberalism and the body in post-revolutionary France: Bichat's physiology and the Paris school of medicine. **Hist Sci** 1981 Jun;19(44 pt 2):115-42
Pozo EC del: La medicina como ciencia en Claudio Bernard. Homenaje en el primer centenario de su muerte. **Gac Med Mex** 1979 Jun;115(6):245-56
Premuda L: Claude Bernard e gli indirizzi della fisiologia e della medicina nel secolo XIX. **Minerva Med** 1982 Feb 25;73(7):329-35
Schiller J: Henri Dutrochet et la terminologie scientifique. In: Congrès National des Sociétés Savantes, 97e, Nantes, 1972. Comptes Rendus. Paris, 1976. Section des Sciences, Tome 1. p. 83-9.
Snellen HA: E. J. Marey and cardiology: physiologist and pioneer of technology, 1830-1904: selected writings in facsimile with comments and summaries, a brief history of life and work, and a bibliography. 264 p.
Sutton G: The physical and chemical path to vitalism: Xavier Bichat's Physiological Researches on Life and Death. **Bull Hist Med** 1984 Spring;58(1):53-71
Vartanian A: Le frère de Maupertuis et l'homme machine. **Dix-huit Siecle** 1982;14:305-23
Vial F, Rullière R: François Magendie. **Hist Sci Med** 1983;17(4):323-32

### Germany

Abe HR, Tiedt N: August Friedrich Hecker (1763-1811) und die Anfänge der modernen Pathophysiologie. **Beitr Gesch Univ Erfurt** 1979-83;19:165-85
Belloni L: Hermann Helmholtz und Franz Boll. **Medizinhist J** 1982;17(1/2):129-37
Coleman W: Bergmann's rule: animal heat as a biological phenomenon. **Stud Hist Biol** 1979;3:67-88
Cranefield PF, ed: Two great scientists of the nineteenth century. Correspondence of Emil Du Bois-Reymond and Carl Ludwig. Collected by Estelle Du Bois-Reymond. Foreword, notes, and indexes by Paul Diepgen. Translation of 1927 German ed. Baltimore, London, Johns Hopkins Univ. Press, 1982. xix, 183 p.
Duchesneau F: G. E. Stahl: antimécanisme et concept d'organisme. **Arch Int Hist Idees** 1982;95:1-31
Duchesneau F: G. E. Stahl: Antimécanisme et physiologie. **Arch Int Hist Sci (Paris)** 1976;26:3-26
Duchesneau F: Le système mécaniste de Friedrich Hoffmann. **Arch Int Hist Idees** 1982;95:32-64
Eulner HH, Hoepke H, ed: Der Briefwechsel zwischen Rudolph Wagner und Jacob Henle 1838-1862. Göttingen, Vandenhoeck & Ruprecht, 1979. 115 p. (Arbeiten aus der Niedersächsischen Staats- und Universitätsbibliothek Göttingen, Band 16).
Hall VM: The role of force or power in Liebig's physiological chemistry. **Med Hist** 1980 Jan;24(1):20-59
Heintel H: Moritz Schiffs gescheiterter Habilitationsversuch an der Universität Göttingen im Jahre 1855. **Medizinhist J** 1980;15(4):378-84
Henkelmann T: Die Struktur des Lebendigen. Die Fragmente zur Physiologie von Novalis. In Seidler E, Schott H, ed: Bausteine zur Medizingeschichte. Stuttgart, Steiner, 1984. p. 45-52.
Jung R: Walter R. Hess (1881-1973). **Rev Physiol Biochem Pharmacol** 1981;88:1-21
Kaiser W, Völker A: Der Arbeitskreis um den halleschen Physiologen Julius Bernstein (1839-1917) und seine Bedeutung für die klinische Medizin. **Wiss Z Martin Luther Univ (Math)** 1982;31(6):75-100
Klix F: Hermann von Helmholtz' Beitrag zur Theorie der Wahrnehmung--Bleibendes und Vergängliches in einem grossen Lebenswerk. In Eckardt G, ed: Zur Geschichte der Psychologie. Berlin, VEB Deutscher Verlag der Wissenschaften, 1979. p. 45-59.
Kunze G: Die Anfänge einer biomathematisch - biophysikalischen Denkweise in der Physiologie im Spiegel einiger Arbeiten Leonhard Eulers (1707-1783). Diss., Johannes-Gutenberg-Universität, Mainz, 1981. 182 p.
Lindemann M, Cesnokova S: Wissenschaftliche Schulen in Deutschland im XIX. Jahrhundert und ihre Rolle für die Entwicklung der Physiologie in der Welt. In International Congress of the History of Medicine. 26th, Plovdiv, 1978. Actes du Congress. Sofia, 1981. Volume II. p. 140-3.
Lohff B: Johannes Müller, 'Jahresberichte zur Physiologie', in Müllers Archiv der Jahre 1834-1838. **Sudhoffs Arch** 1981;65(1):32-78
Mann G, ed: Naturwissen und Erkenntnis im 19. Jahrhundert: Emil Du Bois-Reymond. Hildesheim, Gerstenberg, 1981. 243 p. Contributions by K. E. Rothschuh, H. Hensel, R. Malter, C. von Campenhausen, B. Lohff, H. Lübbe, D. von Engelhardt, W. F. Gutmann, K. Bonink, C. Andree
Mayer JR von: Die Mechanik der Wärme: sämtliche Schriften. In Zusammenarbeit mit dem Stadtarchiv Heilbronn herausgegeben von Hans Peter Münzenmayer. Heilbronn, Stadtarchiv, 1978. 457 p. (Veröffentlichungen des Archivs der Stadt Heilbronn; 22).
Montiel L: La 'filosofia de la fisiologia' de Federico Schiller. **Asclepio** 1981;33:163-81
Moschner H: Wissenschaftliche Arbeit und Lehre des Bonner Physiologen Eduard Friedrich Wilhelm Pflüger auf dem Gebiet des tierischen Stoffwechsels. Diss. Bonn, 1981. 233 p.
Müller-Ruchholtz ER, Haase J, Kaufmann R: Zwanzig Jahre Physiologisches Institut Düsseldorf. Bericht über die Arbeit des Institutes, Verzeichnis der Mitarbeiter und Verzeichnis der Veröffentlichungen 1970-1980. **Jahrb Univ Dusseld** 1977-78;209-47
Pfarrwaller-Stieve A: Friedrich von Müller (1858-1941) und seine Stoffwechseluntersuchungen. Zürich, Juris Druck, 1983. 58 p. (Zürcher Medizingeschichtliche Abhandlungen, Neue Reihe, 156)
Reale E: Wissenschaftliche Arbeiten von H. von Mayersbach. **Mikroskopie** 1981;38(3-4):67-77
Rudolph G: Das Mechanismusproblem in der Physiologie des 19. Jahrhunderts. **Ber Wissenschaftsgesch** 1983;6(1-4):7-28
Sandführ K: Das Verständnis vom Leben und vom Organismus im Werk von Johannes Müller (1801-1858). Die Eigenart des Lebendigen und die Methode seiner Erforschung. Diss, Bonn, 1979. 153 p.
Seller H: Physiology at Heidelberg. **J Auton Nerv Syst** 1981 Apr;3(2-4):121-2
Simmer HH: Experimentelle Prüfungen der pflügerschen Reflexhypothese der Menstruation im späten 19. Jahrhundert. **Clio Med** 1980 Jul;14(3-4):235-54
Yamaguchi C: [Betrachtungen über die frühesten physiologischen Arbeiten Hermann von Helmholtz, die zu seiner Entdeckung des Gesetzes von der Erhaltung der Energie führen] (Jpn). **Kagakushi Kenkyu** 1984;23(151):169-76

### Great Britain

Bacq ZM: Les expériences de W. Feldberg en l'année 1932. **Bull Mem Acad R Med Belg** 1982;137 Suppl:9-30
Barnard EE: Physiological aspects of naval problems. **J R Nav Med Serv** 1980 Spring;66(1):23-5
Butler SV: From physician to scientist: changing styles of thought in late Victorian physiology. **Soc Soc Hist Med Bull (Lond)** 1980 Jun;26:7-10
Capper WM, Johnson D, ed: The faith of a surgeon. Belief and experience in the life of Arthur Rendle Short. Exeter, England, Paternoster Press, 1976. 156 p.
Cross SJ: John Hunter, the animal oeconomy, and late eighteenth-century physiological discourse. **Stud Hist Biol** 1981;5:1-110
Cunningham DJ: Claude Gordon Douglas. In Dictionary of national biography, 1961-1970. Suppl. 8, 1981. p. 303-4.
Eccles JC, Gibson WC: Sherrington: his life and thought. Berlin, New York, Springer International, 1979. xv, 269 p.
Evans C: Thomas Graham Brown. In Dictionary of national biography, 1961-1970. Suppl. 8, 1981. p. 151-2.
Feldberg W: Sir Henry Hallett Dale. In Dictionary of national biography, 1961-1970. Suppl. 8, 1981. p. 262-5.
Gregory RL: Forty years on: Kenneth Craik's The Nature of Explanation (1943). **Perception** 1983;12(3):233-7
Henkelmann T: Zur Geschichte des pathophysiologischen Denkens. John Brown (1735-1788) und sein System der Medizin. Berlin, New York, Springer, 1981. 104 p.
Himsworth H: Thomas Renton Elliott. In Dictionary of national biography, 1961-1970. Suppl. 8, 1981. p. 329-30.
Jacyna LS: Principles of general physiology: the comparative dimension to British neuroscience in the 1830s and 1840s. **Stud Hist Biol** 1984;7:47-92
Jacyna LS: The romantic programme and the reception of cell theory in Britain. **J Hist Biol** 1984 Spring;17(1):13-48
Knight DM: Chemistry, physiology and materialism in the romantic period. **Durham Univ J** 1972;64(2):139-45
Manuel DE: Marshall Hall, F.R.S. (1790-1857); a conspectus of his life and work. **Notes Rec R Soc Lond** 1980 Dec;35(2):135-66
Mazumdar PM: Anatomical physiology and the reform of medical education: London, 1825-1835. **Bull Hist Med** 1983 Summer;57(2):230-46
Miller M: A. V. Hill papers. **Surv Sources Newsl** 1978 Oct;8:8-10
Nayler WG: Sydney Ringer--physician and scientist. **J Mol Cell Cardiol** 1984 Feb;16(2):113-6
Pickford M: Ernest Basil Verney. In Dictionary of national biography, 1961-1970. Suppl. 8, 1981. p. 1035.
Rogers JS: 'Life' in the novel: Tristram Shandy and some aspects of 18th-century physiology. **Eighteenth Cent Life** 1980;6(1):1-20
Short RV: The scientific contributions of Professor Emmanuel Ciprian Amoroso, CBE, TC, FRS. **J Reprod Fertil [Suppl]** 1982 Nov;31:1-8
Sinclair HM: Sherrington and industrial fatigue. **Notes Rec R Soc Lond** 1984 Sep;39(1):91-104
Smyth DH: Sir Charles Arthur Lovatt Evans. In Dictionary of national biography, 1961-1970. Suppl. 8, 1981. p. 334-6.
Sørensen T: James Blundell 27.XII.1790-15.I.1878. Professor i fysiologi og obstetrik ved Guy's Hospital 1823-1834. **Ugeskr Laeger** 1983 Jun 27;145 Spec No:5-49
Warner JH: Physiological theory and therapeutic explanation in the 1860s: the British debate on the medical use of alcohol. **Bull Hist Med** 1980 Summer;54(2):235-57
West JB: Stephen Hales: neglected respiratory physiologist. **J Appl Physiol** 1984 Sep;57(3):635-9

# PHYSIOLOGY

**Hungary**

Antall J, Kapronczay K: Jan Nepomuk Czermak in Hungary. In E. Schultheisz, ed: History of physiology. Oxford, Elmsford, New York, Pergamon, 1981. xvi, 208 p. (Advances in Physiological Sciences. Proceedings of the 28th International Congress of Physiological Sciences, Budapest, 1980. Volume 21). p. 77–84.
Banga I: A Magyar Elettani Társaság 50 éves jubileuma. **Orv Hetil** 1981 Dec 13;122(50):3093–6
Honti J: A fiziológia az Orvosi Hetilap korai évfolyamaiban. **Orv Hetil** 1981 Aug 9;122(32):1979–80
Kovách AG, Schultheisz E: A physiologianak rövid sommája - a short summation of physiology. The first book of physiology in Hungarian. In E. Schultheisz, ed: History of physiology. Oxford, Elmsford, New York, Pergamon, 1981. xvi, 208 p. (Advances in Physiological Sciences. Proceedings of the 28th International Congress of Physiological Sciences, Budapest, 1980. Volume 21). p. 85–87.
Néhány F: Farkas Géza professzorról a tanítványai. **Orv Hetil** 1984 Nov 11;125(46):2817
Racz S: Selected paragraphs from the 1789 edition of Samuel Rácz's textbook of physiology. With corresponding English translation by E. Kovács and C. Szabó. In E. Schultheisz, ed: History of physiology. Oxford, Elmsford, New York, Pergamon, 1981. xvi, 208 p. (Advances in Physiological Sciences. Proceedings of the 28th International Congress of Physiological Sciences, Budapest, 1980. Volume 21). p. 89–203.
Varga E: Megemlékezés Went Istvánról. **Orv Hetil** 1983 Sep 18;124(38):2319–20

**Italy**

Bonuzzi L: Alberto Brighenti nella storia della fisiologia. **Acta Med Hist Patav** 1981/82;28:21–8
Cremona GF: L'elettroterapia nel XVIII secolo. Ricerche di elettrofisiolgia e di elettroterapia di studiosi piemontesi. **Ann Osp Maria Vittoria Torino** 1981 Jan–Jun;24(1–6):167–77
Fadiga E: Giulio Cesare Pupilli. Milano, 5–10–1893–Pescia (PT), 17–8–1973. **Arch Fisiol** 1979 Jun 30;71(1–4):3–22
Pinotti O: Giulio Stella 1899–1978. **Arch Sci Biol (Bologna)** 1978 Jan–Dec;62(1–4):i–xiv

**Mexico**

Guzmán-Flores C: El Doctor Efrén C. Del Pozo, Fisiólogo y Maestro. **Bol Estud Med Biol** 1980 Jul–Oct;31(3–4):116–26

**Nepal**

Hornbein TF: Everest without oxygen. **Prog Clin Biol Res** 1983;136:409–14
Pugh LG, Sutton JR: Everest then and now. **Prog Clin Biol Res** 1983;136:415–30

**Netherlands**

Lindeboom GA: Nederlandse Bijdragen tot de ontwikkeling der moderne fysiologie. Voordracht gehouden op 20 mei 1976 bij de herdenking van het 25-jarig bestaan van het Fysiologisch Laboratorium aan de Vrije Universiteit te Amsterdam. Amsterdam, Laboratorium voor Fysiologie der Vrije Universiteit, 1978. 35 p.
Luyendijk-Elshout AM: Mechanicisme contra vitalisme de school van Herman Boerhaave en de beginselen van het leven. **Tijdschr Geschied Geneeskd** 1982;5(1):16–26

**Norway**

Svebak S: Helga Eng: a Norwegian precursor to Darrow and Lacey. **Psychophysiology** 1983 Sep;20(5):600–1

**Poland**

Demel M: Wysoko jak król Zygmunt. Zycie i dzieło dra Stanisława Markiewicza. Warszawa, Państwowy Zakład Wydawn. Lekarskich, 1977. 102 p.
Guzek JW: Two hundred years of the pathologic physiology in Poland--a survey of its past and its present status. **Acta Physiol Pol** 1983 Jan–Feb;34(1):1–4
Zefirova GS, Lebedev VV: Oskar Minkovskiĭ. **Klin Med (Mosk)** 1983 Apr;61(4):119–20

**South Africa**

Sloan AW: Highlights of physiological research at the University of Cape Town, 1912–1978. **S Afr Med J** 1979 Nov 24;56(22):974–6

**Spain**

Kock W: Santiago Ramón y Cajal and the Nobel prize. In International Congress of the History of Medicine, 27th, Barcelona, 1980. Actas. Barcelona, Acadèmia de Ciències Mèdiques de Catalunya i Balears, 1981. p. 550–6.
Puche J, Folch i Pi A: El Doctor August Pi Sunyer. **Xaloc** 1980;16(105):10–2

**Sweden**

Gutt RW: Jöns Jacob Berzelius (1779–1848) i poczatki chemii fizjologicznej). **Arch Hist Med (Warsz)** 1979;42(1):83–92
Marks LS, Maxwell MH: Tigerstedt and the discovery of renin. An historical note. **Hypertension** 1979 Jul–Aug;1(4):384–8
Nunn JB, Holmdahl MH: Henrik Enghoff and the volumen inefficax. **Ups J Med Sci** 1979;84(2):105–8
Uvnäs B: From physiologist to pharmacologist--promotion or degradation? Fifty years in retrospect. **Annu Rev Pharmacol Toxicol** 1984;24:1–18

**Switzerland**

Albrecht von Haller, 1708–1777: Zehn Vorträge gehalten am Berner Haller-Symposion vom 6. bis 8. Oktober 1977. Basel, Birkhäuser, 1978. x, 182 p. With contributions by M. Stettler, K. S. Guthke, U. Im Hof, N. Mani, L. Premuda, H. Zoller, R. Toellner, A. Lindt, W. Zimmerli, W. Killy.
Duchesneau F: La théorie physiologique de Haller: irritabilité et sensibilité. **Arch Int Hist Idees** 1982;95:141–70
Jung R: W. R. Hess und das Ordnungsprinzip in der Physiologie. **Schweiz Arch Neurol Neurochir Psychiatr** 1983;132(2):277–308
Muralt A von: A life with several facets. **Annu Rev Physiol** 1984;46:1–13
Roe SA, ed: The natural philosophy of Albrecht von Haller. New York, Arno, 1981. Various pagings. Reprint of works published 1750–1936.

**United States**

Adolph EF: Growing up in the American Physiological Society. **Physiologist** 1979 Oct;22(5):11–5
Alexander RS: History of the Cardiovascular Section. **Physiologist** 1984 Apr;27(2):67–8
Alexander RS: Pitts and urine acidification. **Physiologist** 1983 Dec;26(6):364–6
Annegers JH: Department of Physiology Northwestern University Medical School. **Physiologist** 1983 Jun;26(3):120–1
Appel TA: The archives of the American Physiological Society. **Physiologist** 1984 Jun;27(3):131–2
Appel TA: The 1941–42 search for an APS emblem. **Physiologist** 1984 Apr;27(2):69–70
Bacq ZM: Marcel Florkin. Harvard et Californie 1929–1930. **Rev Med Liege** 1983 Apr 1;38(7):257–60
Barger AC: The meteoric rise and fall of William Townsend Porter, one of Carl J. Wigger's 'Old Guard'. **Physiologist** 1982 Oct;25(5):407–13
Beatty W: Cecil Kent Drinker. In Dictionary of American Biography, Suppl. 6, 1956–1960. p. 174–5, 1980.
Beatty WK: Sarah Hackett Stevenson--concerned practitioner and social activist. **Proc Inst Med Chic** 1982 Jul–Sep;35(3):99–101
Benison S, Barger AC, Wolfe EL: Changing of the guard. **Harv Med Alumni Bull** 1982 Spring;56(2):34–41
Bibliography of Dr. E. H. Lambert: **Muscle Nerve** 1982;5(9S):S166–72
Bishop DW: H. Burr Steinbach: Prosit! **Soc Gen Physiol Ser** 1981;36:xi–xiv
Bowditch HP: The life and writings of Henry Pickering Bowditch. 2 vols. New York, Arno Press, 1980. Various paginations.
Brandt AM: Herbert Spencer Gasser. In Dictionary of American biography, 1961–1965. Suppl. 7, 1981. p. 279–81.
Brinkhous KM: Judith Graham Pool. In: Notable American women. The modern period. Cambridge, Mass., Belknap-Harvard Univ. Press, 1980. 4:553–4.
Brooks CM: Walter Joseph Meek: August 15, 1878–February 15, 1963. **Biogr Mem Natl Acad Sci** 1983;54:251–68
Burchell HB: The investigator as volunteer subject. **Mayo Clin Proc** 1982 Jul;57 Suppl:28–33
Cannon B: Walter Bradford Cannon, M. D.: Reflections on the physician, the man, and his contributions. **Gastrointest Radiol** 1982;7(1):1–6
Chasis H: History of collaboration by Department of Physiology at New York University School of Medicine. **Physiologist** 1983 Apr;26(2):64–70
Cohen IB, ed: The career of William Beaumont and the reception of his discovery. New York, Arno Press, 1980. Various pagings. Reprint of G. Miller: William Beaumont's formative years: two early notebooks 1811–1821 (1946); G. Rosen: The reception of William Beaumont's discovery in Europe (1942); G. Rosen: Notes on the reception and influence of William Beaumont's discovery (1943). (Three centuries of Science in America).
Davenport HW: Carbonic anhydrase, or, the strange case of the disappearing scientist. **Physiologist** 1980 Apr;23(2):11–5
Davenport HW: Physiology, 1850–1923. The view from Michigan. **Physiologist** 1982 Feb;24(1 Suppl):1–96
Davis AB: Winthrop John Vanleuven Osterhout. In Dictionary of American biography, 1961–1965. Suppl. 7, 1981. p. 592–3.
Dean JB: A retrospective look through the camera of Fred A. Hitchcock.

**Physiologist** 1984 Jun;27(3):128-30
Dustan A, ed: In memoriam Wallace O. Fenn 1893-1971. [S.l., s.n.] 1979? [127] p.
Elizondo RS, Jacobs N, Moore WW: Physiology at Indiana University-Bloomington. A history. **Physiologist** 1984 Oct;27(5):319-24
Fee E: William Henry Howell: physiologist and philosopher of health. **Am J Epidemiol** 1984 Mar;119(3):293-300
Fishman AP: Hail and farewell. **Am J Physiol** 1981 May;240(5):C161-3
Fye WB: S. Weir Mitchell, Philadelphia's 'lost' physiologist. **Bull Hist Med** 1983 Summer;57(2):188-202
Fye WB: Why a physiologist?--the case of Henry P. Bowditch. **Bull Hist Med** 1982 Spring;56(1):19-29
Gantt WH: E. Cowles Andrus (1896--1978), eighth president of the Pavlovian Society. **Pavlov J Biol Sci** 1979 Jan-Mar;14(1):74-5
Garrett CG: Anton Julius Carlson. In Dictionary of American Biography, Suppl. 6, 1956-1960. p. 99-100, 1980.
Geison GL: Divided we stand: physiologists and clinicians in the American context. In Vogel MJ, Rosenberg CE, ed: The therapeutic revolution. Philadelphia, 1979. p. 67-90.
Handbook of Physiology 1959-1978.: **Physiologist** 1980 Oct;23(5):14-6
Hansel W, Leonard EP, Dukes HH: A backward look from far above Cayuga's waters. **Physiologist** 1982 Dec;25(6):469-74
Johnson EE: Ida Henrietta Hyde: early experiments. **Physiologist** 1981 Dec;24(6):10-1
Kline DL: Department of Physiology, University of Cincinnati, College of Medicine. **Physiologist** 1983 Dec;26(6):366-8
Kopp C: The Alfred E. Mirsky papers at the Rockefeller University Archives. **Mendel Newsl** 1983 Nov;23:1-4
Landor JH: Lester Reynold Dragstedt--physiologist-surgeon. **Gastroenterology** 1981 Apr;80(4):846-53
Loew ER: Departmental history. Department of Physiology. Boston University School of Medicine (1873-1948). **Physiologist** 1984 Feb;27(1):4-12
Ludmerer KM: Joseph Erlanger. In Dictionary of American biography, 1961-1965. Suppl. 7, 1981. p. 225-7.
McMillan CW: Evolution of modern concepts of hemostasis. A backward glance at the discoveries that made modern practice possible. **Am J Pediatr Hematol Oncol** 1981 Spring;3(1):97-103
Marshall LH: More on Burt Green Wilder at Cornell. **Physiologist** 1983 Dec;26(6):361-3
Myer JS: William Beaumont: a pioneer American physiologist. New ed. of his: Life and letters of Dr. William Beaumont. With historical introductions by E. Brodman and R. E. Shank. Includes reprint of 1833 ed. of Beaumont's Experiments and observations on the gastric juice and the physiology of digestion. St. Louis, Mosby, 1981. xi, 394 p.
Numbers RL, Orr WJ: William Beaumont's reception at home and abroad. **Isis** 1981 Dec;72(264):590-612
Owen CA: H. P. Smith's place in the history of blood coagulation. **Am J Clin Pathol** 1984 Apr;81(4):424-6
Ransom JF: The origins of chiropractic physiological therapeutics: Howard, Forester and Schulze. **Chiropr Hist** 1984;4(1):47-52
Reese WG: 'Don't count the bricks'. Scientific contributions of W. H. Gantt. **Pavlov J Biol Sci** 1982 Jul-Sep;17(3):111-4
Riley HD: Homer William Smith. In Dictionary of American biography, 1961-1965. Suppl. 7, 1981. p. 699-700.
Rosenfeld LM: Physiology at Jefferson Medical College (1842-1982). **Physiologist** 1984 Jun;27(3):113-27
Schmidt-Nielsen B: A history of renal physiology at the Mount Desert Island Biological Laboratory. **Physiologist** 1983 Oct;26(5):260-6
Selkurt EE: Physiology at Indiana University School of Medicine-Indianapolis. **Physiologist** 1984 Oct;27(5):325-9
Spencer F: Samuel George Morton's doctoral thesis on bodily pain: the probable source of Morton's polygenism. **Trans Stud Coll Physicians Phila** 1983 Dec;5(5 no 4):321-38
Starr I: Concerning Dr. Grayson Prevost McCouch with recollections of the earlier days of physiology in Philadelphia. **Neurol Res** 1983;5(1):1-17
Stinson JM: Department of Physiology, Meharry Medical College, Nashville, Tennessee. **Physiologist** 1983 Jun;26(3):119-20
Symposium on capillary permeability and mechanism of transport, American Physiological Society, New Orleans, 1979. A salute to Professor Hyman S. Mayerson.: **Physiologist** 1980 Feb;23(1):34-93
Taylor AE: Dr. Mayerson, the scientist. **Physiologist** 1980 Feb;23(1):38-40
Terreros DA, Grantham JJ: Marshall Barber and the origins of micropipette methods. **Am J Physiol** 1982 Mar;242(3):F293-6
Tucker GS: Ida Henrietta Hyde: the first woman member of the society. **Physiologist** 1981 Dec;24(6):1-9
Verbrugge MH: The social meaning of personal health: The Ladies' Physiological Institute of Boston and vicinity in the 1850s. In Reverby S, Rosner D, ed: Health care in America. Philadelphia, Temple University Press, 1979. p. 45-66.
Weissmann G: Loeb and a Gloria. **Hosp Pract [Off]** 1984 Oct;19(10):65-74
Wilber JA: The founding of Georgia and the discovery of blood pressure. **J Med Assoc Ga** 1981 May;70(5):333
Wood EH: Four decades of physiology, musing, and what now. **Physiologist** 1982 Feb;25(1):19-32
Zollinger RM: The legacies of William Beaumont, pioneer investigator. **Pharos** 1983 Winter;46(1):20-3

**USSR**

Batuev AS: Fiziologicheskaia nauchnaia shkola Leningradskogo universiteta. **Fiziol Zh SSSR** 1984 Oct;70(10):1353-60
Berezovskiĭ VA: Ivan Mikhaĭlovich Sechenov. Kiev, Nauk. dumka, 1981. 173 p.
Berezovskiĭ VA, Nazarenko AI: Krupnyĭ vklad v gepatologiiu. **Fiziol Zh** 1980 Mar-Apr;26(2):244-9
Berezovskiĭ VA: Ritmy biologicheskikh protsessov kak proiavlenie individual'noĭ reaktivnosti i konstitutsii individa. **Patol Fiziol Eksp Ter** 1981 May-Jun;(3):3-7
Brestkin AP: Iz vospominanii ob akademike L. A. Orbeli: vstrechi i besedy v sviazi s issledovaniiami po fiziologii vodolaznogo truda. **Vopr Istor Estestvozn Tekh** 1982;2:27-37
Buzsàki G: Situational conditional reflexes. Physiologic studies of the higher nervous activity of freely moving animals: P. S. Kupalov. **Pavlov J Biol Sci** 1983 Jan-Mar;18(1):13-21
Chernov AZ: Aleksandr Filippovich Samoĭlov. **Klin Med (Mosk)** 1983 Jan;61(1):116-20
Fiziologiia v SSSR: **Fiziol Zh SSSR** 1982 Dec;68(12):1593-630
Gorizontov PD: K 130-letiiu so dnia rozhdeniia I. P. Pavlova (vstupitel'noe slovo k Pervym Pavlovskim chteniiam). **Zh Vyssh Nerv Deiat** 1980 May-Jun;30(3):627-30
Gorizontov PD: Patologicheskaia fiziologiia v SSSR (k 60-letiiu obrazovaniia SSSR). **Patol Fiziol Eksp Ter** 1983 May-Jun;3:14-22
Govyrin VA, Grigor'ian RA: Akademik L. A. Orbeli: étapy zhizni i nauchnoĭ deiatel'nosti (k 100-letiiu so dnia rozhdeniia). **Usp Fiziol Nauk** 1982 Jun-Sep;13(3):3-8
Iaroshevskiĭ MG: Genezis issledovatel'skoĭ programmy I. P. Pavlova (istoricheskoe znachenie madridskoĭ rechi I. P. Pavlova). **Zh Vyssh Nerv Deiat** 1984 Jan-Feb;34(1):3-13
IAroshevskiĭ MG: Uolter Kennon (1871-1945). Moskva, Nauka, 1976. 374 p.
Institutu fiziologii imeni A. A. Bogomol'tsa Akademii nauk USSR--50 let: **Neirofiziologiia** 1984;16(3):283-5
K 100-letiiu so dnia rozhdeniia akademika A. A. Bogomol'tsa: **Fiziol Zh** 1981 May-Jun;27(3):291-443
Karamian AI: Ivan Mikhaĭlovich Sechenov i evoliutsionnaia neĭrofiziologiia. Leningrad, Nauka, Leningradskoe otd-nie, 1980. 112 p.
Kol'tsova MM: Mekhanizmy integratsii uslovnykh refleksov v trudakh E. A. Asratiana. **Zh Vyssh Nerv Deiat** 1983 Mar-Apr;33(2):216-20
Kotel'nikov VP: V. A. Oppel' i razvitie fiziologicheskoĭ khirurgii. **Klin Med (Mosk)** 1984 May;62(5):145-8
Lebedev KV: Iz istorii Kazanskoĭ fiziologicheskoĭ shkoly. Kazan', Izd-vo Kazanskogo universiteta, 1978. 246 p.
Leĭbson LG: L. A. Orbeli i nekotorye aspekty évoliutsionnoĭ fiziologii. **Zh Evol Biokhim Fiziol** 1983 Jul-Aug;19(4):322-32
Makarov VA: [I. M. Sechenov and the development of physiology in the Moscow University] (Rus). **Istor Biol Issled** 1980;8:138-55
Makarov VA: Uspekhi fiziologii v SSSR i perspektivy ee razvitiia (k 60-letiiu obrazovaniia Soiuza Sovetskikh Sotsialisticheskikh respublik). **Usp Fiziol Nauk** 1982 Oct-Dec;13(4):3-26
Makarov VA: 50 let kafecre normal'noĭ fiziologii 1-go Moskovskogo meditsinskogo instituta im. I. M. Sechenova (1930-1980). **Fiziol Zh SSSR** 1980 Dec;66(12):1860-4
Merkulov VL: I. P. Pavlov--organizator nauchnykh issledovaniĭ. Moskva, Nauka, Glav. red. vostochnoĭ lit-ry, 1971. 8 p.
Moikin IuV, Tarasenko NIu, Anan'ev BV: Znachenie naslediia I. M. Sechenova dlia razvitiia otechestvennoĭ fiziologii i gigieny truda. **Gig Tr Prof Zabol** 1980 Mar;(3):1-5
Mozzhukhin AS: [I. M. Sechenov - The founder of the first physiological school in Russia] (Rus). **Istor Biol Issled** 1980;8:124-37
Mozzhukhin AS: Rol' L. A. Orbeli v stanovlenii i razrabotke fiziologicheskikh problem radiobiologii. **Fiziol Zh SSSR** 1982 Jul;68(7):914-7
Natadze TG: O prioritete V. V. Voronina v nekotorykh oblastakh meditsiny i biologii (k 110-letiiu so dnia rozhdeniia V. V. Voronina). **Patol Fiziol Eksp Ter** 1981 May-Jun;(3):53-7
Natadze TG: Osnovnye dostizheniia gruzinskikh patofiziologov. **Patol Fiziol Eksp Ter** 1983 May-Jun;3:23-4
Nikitin VN: Vedushchie problemy sovremennykh vozrastnykh fiziologii, biokhimii i biofiziki i isledovaniia shkoly A. V. Nagornogo. **Usp Sovrem Biol** 1982 Nov-Dec;94(3):421-32
Panchenko DI, Vilenskiĭ IuG: Leon Abgarovich Orbeli v Kieve (k 100-letiiu so dnia rozhdeniia). **Vrach Delo** 1982 Sep;(9):119-22
Pappenheimer JR: Pavlov's contributions to physiology before 1900. **J Hist Behav Sci** 1981;17:239-41
Podachin VP: Cherty nauchnogo tvorchestva. E. A. Asratiana (k 80-letiiu so dnia rozhdeniia). **Usp Fiziol Nauk** 1983 Jul-Sep;14(3):3-13
Pressman IaM: E. A. Asratian i nauchnoe sodruzhestvo neĭrofiziologiov sotsialisticheskikh stran. **Zh Vyssh Nerv Deiat** 1983 Mar-Apr;33(2):211-5
Rosliakova NA: Contribution of academician P. K. Anokhin to physiology. **Agressologie** 1982;23(5):165-6
Serkov FN: Fiziologicheskaia nauka v USSR za 60 let. **Fiziol Zh** 1982 Nov-Dec;28(6):643-52

## PHYSIOLOGY

Serkov FN, Zadorozhnyĭ AG: Nauchnaia deiatel'nost' Instituta fiziologii im. A. A. Bogomol'tsa AN USSR. K 50-letiiu so dnia osnovaniia. **Fiziol Zh** 1984 May-Jun;30(3):257-66
Serkov FN: Problemy normal'noĭ fiziologii v issledovaniiakh A. A. Bogomolets. **Fiziol Zh** 1981 May-Jun;27(3):438-43
Severin SE: V. V. Parin. Zhizn' i deiatel'nost'. **Vestn Akad Med Nauk SSSR** 1984;(4):3-7
Shik LL: Akademik V. V. Parin kak fiziolog. **Vestn Akad Med Nauk SSSR** 1984;(4):12-5
Shingarov GKh: Filosofskie voprosy ucheniia o vyssheĭ nervnoĭ deiatel'nosti v tvorchestve E. A. Asratiana. **Zh Vyssh Nerv Deiat** 1983 Mar-Apr;33(2):204-10
Shingarov GKh: Gordost' russkoĭ nauki (k 150-letiiu so dnia rozhdeniia I. M. Sechenova). **Patol Fiziol Eksp Ter** 1979 Nov-Dec;(6):3-8
Simonov PV: Polveka neotstupnykh iskaniĭ istiny (k 80-letiiu so dnia rozhdeniia E. A. Asratiana). **Zh Vyssh Nerv Deiat** 1983 Mar-Apr;33(2):197-203
Sokolova LV: Uchenie A. A. Ukhtomskogo o dominante ka vektore povedeniia. **Nerv Sist** 1982;23:5-13
Suvorov NF, Lange KA: Sovětská fysiologie-hlavní etapy a tendence vývoje. **Cesk Fysiol** 1983;32(3):193-6
Svetaĭlo EN: Vydaiuschiĭsia uchenyĭ sovremennosti (k 100-letiiu so dnia rozhdeniia L. A. Orbeli). **Fiziol Zh SSSR** 1983 Feb;69(2):281-3
Tkachenko BI, Voronenkova IA, Anoshina AA: 50 let Otdela fiziologii vistseral'nykh sistem imeni akad. K. M. Bykova Instituta éksperimental'nŏ meditsiny AMN SSSR. **Fiziol Zh SSSR** 1981 Aug;67(8):1283-9
Uzhanskiĭ IaG: K mekhanizmu stimuliatsii funksiĭ i regeneratsii kletok i tkaneĭ po A. A. Bogomol'tsa. **Fiziol Zh** 1981 May-Jun;27(3):322-6
Uzhanskiĭ IaG: K nauchno-literaturnomu nasledstvu akademika Aleksandra Aleksandrovicha Bogomol'tsa (ob osobennostiakh pis'ma akademika A. A. Bogomol'tsa v nauchnykh trudakh). **Patol Fiziol Eksp Ter** 1981 Mar-Apr;(2):16-20
Vasilevskiĭ NN: D. A. Biriukov, 1904-1969. Moskva, Meditsina, 1981 95 p.
Viktor Petrovich Babmindra (k 60-letiiu so dnia rozhdeniia): **Arkh Anat Gistol Embriol** 1983 Oct;85(10):102-4
Vorob'ev AI: Ivan Mikhaĭlovich Sechenov. **Klin Med (Mosk)** 1980;58(11):105-8
Windholz G: Pavlov's position toward American behaviorism. **J Hist Behav Sci** 1983 Oct;19(4):394-407
Zaĭchik ASh: Teoreticheskoe i prakticheskoe znachenie ucheniia o tsitotoksinakh. **Patol Fiziol Eksp Ter** 1981 Mar-Apr;(2):46-55
Zaiko NN: A. A. Bogomolets, zhizn i deiatel nost. K 100-letiiu so dnia rozhdeniia. **Fiziol Zh** 1981 May-Jun;27(3):291-301
Zhurnalu 'Patologicheskaia fiziologiia i éksperimental'naia terapiia' 25 let: **Patol Fiziol Eksp Ter** 1982 Jul-Aug;(4):3-10
Zimkin NV: 60 let kafedre fiziologii Leningradskogo instituta fizicheskoĭ kul'tury imeni P. F. Lesgafta. **Fiziol Zh SSSR** 1979 Dec;65(12):1854-6

## PODIATRY

Dustmann HO, Ebel V: Darstellungen von Fussdeformierungen und deren Behandlung in der Kunst. In KF Schlegel, ed: Der Körperbehinderte in Mythologie und Kunst. Stuttgart, New York, Thieme, 1983. p. 41-56.
Rossi WA: High heels. The agony and the ecstasy. **J Am Podiatry Assoc** 1981 Dec;71(12):698-9

**China**

Veith I: The history of medicine dolls and foot-binding in China. **Clio Med** 1980 Jul;14(3-4):255-67

**1700 to Present**

Block P: Podiatric medicine in Britain and the United States: contrasts in development. **Milit Med** 1981 Mar;146(3):205-10

**France**

Laforest NL: L'art de soigner les pieds. Fac-simile de l'édition de 1782. Ed. R. Habert. Bruxelles, Caducea, 1979. 257 p.

**United States**

The Levy brothers: early San Francisco chiropodists, a picture story: **West States Jew Hist Q** 1981;13(4):317-21
Skipper JK, Hughes JE: Podiatry: a medical care specialty in quest of full professional status and recognition. **Soc Sci Med** 1983;17(20):1541-8

## POLITICS

See also **State Medicine**

Bolton C, Leasure JW: Evolution politique et baisse de la fécondité en occident. **Population** 1979;34(4-5):825-43
Chorover SL: From genesis to genocide. The meaning of human nature and the power of behavior control. Cambridge, Mass., MIT Press, 1979. xiii, 238 p.
Dubb A: Medical philately. Doctors in politics. **S Afr Med J** 1980 Aug 23;58(8):326-9
Eckart W: 'Medicus Politicus' oder 'Machiavellus Medicus'? Wechselwirkungen von Ideal und Realität des Arzttypus im 17. Jahrhundert. **Medizinhist J** 1984;19(3):210-24
Ezrahi Y: Utopian and pragmatic rationalism: the political context of scientific advice. **Minerva** 1980 Spring;18(1):111-31
Fischer-Homberger E: Aerztliche Ethik und ärztliche Standespolitik--ein Aspekt der Geschichte der ärztlichen Ethik. **Bull Schweiz Akad Med Wiss** 1980 Nov;36(4-6):395-410
Luckin B: States and epidemic threats. **Soc Soc Hist Med Bull (Lond)** 1984 Jun;34:25-7
Ness DE: C'est fini. . . .le pouls ne bat plus! Drawn by Paul Bernay, for Le Charivari, in 1872. **J Hist Med Allied Sci** 1980 Jul;35(3):312
Plaza Izquierdo F: Enfermedad final de Francisco Franco, a proposito de los que mueren en el poder. **Rev Soc Venez Hist Med** 1980;29(43-44):95-124
Robins RS: Disease, political events, and populations. In Rothschild H, ed: Biocultural aspects of disease. New York, Academic Press, 1981. p. 153-75.
Trevor-Roper H: Medicine in politics. **Am Scholar** 1981-82;51(1):23-41

**Austria**

Hochenegg H: Tiroler Aerzte und Pharmazeuten als Künstler und Schriftsteller, Forscher und Volksvertreter. **Tirol Heimat** 1976;40:135-62

**Germany**

Jezierska ME: Szpital obozu Buchenwald (na podstawie archiwaliów z okresu 3 IV - 20 VII 1945 r.). **Przegl Lek** 1980;37(1):76-85

**Great Britain**

Carlton C: Three British revolutions and the personality of kingship. In Pocock, JG. ed: Three British revolutions: 1641, 1688, 1776. Princeton, N.J., Princeton U. Press, 1980. p. 165-207.
Jetter D: Hospitäler in London; zur Typologie wohltätiger Einrichtungen im Spannungsfeld politischer Kräfte. **Sudhoffs Arch** 1978;62(3):250-81

**Switzerland**

Fehlmann HR: Beziehungen zwischen Arzt und Apotheker im 16. bis 18. Jahrhundert in der Schweiz. **Gesnerus** 1983;40(1-2):67-74

**Before 500 A.D.**

Kuttner RE: Protohistoric hepatomancy: an oracular form of pathology. **Proc Inst Med Chic** 1982 Jan-Mar;35(1):14

**Greece**

Coulomb J: La mort d'Alexandre Le Grand. **Hist Sci Med** 1984;18(2):137-45
Hughes JD: The dreams of Alexander the Great. **J Psychohist** 1984 Fall;12(2):168-92
Romilly J de: Théorie politique et théorie médicale dans la Grèce antique. **Actual Odontostomatol (Paris)** 1982;138:157-70

**Rome**

Klawans HL: The acromegaly of Maximinus I: the possible influence of a pituitary tumor on the life and death of a Roman emperor. In Rose FC, Bynum WF, ed: Historical aspects of the neurosciences. New York, Raven, 1982. 317-26.

**500 A.D.-1450**

Barber M: Lepers, Jews and Moslems: the plot to overthrow Christendom in 1321. **History** 1981;66:1-17

**Great Britain**

Sass LJ: Religion, medicine, politics and spices. **Appetite** 1981 Mar;2(1):7-13

**1450-1700**

**Austria**

Beck-Mannagetta P: Zum 300. Todestag des Johann Wilhelm Ritter von Mannagetta und seinem Wirken in Niederösterreich. **Unsere Heimat** 1966;37(4-6):125-9

### France

Howard R: Medical politics and the founding of the Jardin des Plantes in Paris. **J Soc Bibliogr Nat Hist** 1980 Apr;9(4):395–402
Vally G: Ludovic cel stăruitor si misterioasa sa moarte. **Mag Istor** 1976;10(10):52–4

### Germany

Baader G: Medizinisches Reformdenken und Arabismus im Deutschland des 16. Jahrhunderts. **Sudhoffs Arch** 1979;63(3):261–96

### Great Britain

Birken WJ: The Royal College of Physicians of London and its support of the parliamentary cause in the English civil war. **J Br Stud** 1983;23(1):47–62
Bruce-Chwatt LJ: George Bate--Cromwell's devious physician. **J R Coll Physicians Lond** 1983 Apr;17(2):144–6
Bruce-Chwatt LJ: Myth of quartan malaria. **Trans R Soc Trop Med Hyg** 1982;76(1):133–4
Carlton C: Towards a psychobiography of Charles I. **J Psychohist** 1984 Spring;11(4):513–31
Cook HJ: The regulation of medical practice in London under the Stuarts, 1607–1704. Ph.D. Diss., University of Michigan. Ann Arbor, 1981. 438 p.
Dewhurst J: The alleged miscarriages of Catherine of Aragon and Anne Boleyn. **Med Hist** 1984 Jan;28(1):49–56
Rattansi PM: Medicine and the Puritan Revolution. **Soc Soc Hist Med Bull (Lond)** 1984 Jun;34:4–5

### Italy

Davico R: La morte barocca: popolazione, quartieri e campagne Messina nella rivolta del 1674–1678. La rivolta di Messina e il mondo Mediterraneo nella seconda metà del seicento, Cosenza, Pelligrini, 1979, p. 359–394.

### Netherlands

Pollitt R: The wounding and treatment of William of Orange in 1582. **J Hist Med Allied Sci** 1982 Apr;37(2):135–58

### Romania

Milin M, Popescu A: Sfîrsitul Lui Serban Cantacuzino. **Mag Istor** 1980;14(9):53–8
Vătămanu N: Contribution à l'étude de la vie et de l'oeuvre di Giovanni Mascellini, médecin et secrétaire princier. **Rev Etud Sud Est Eur** 1978;16(2):269–87

### 1700 to Present

Adelman H: Hitler and Gandhi: the will as spirit and as flesh. **Psychoanal Rev** 1980 Winter;67(4):543–61
Ash MG: Disziplinentwicklung und Wissenschaftstransfer--Deutschsprachige Psychologen in der Emigration. **Ber Wissenschaftsgesch** 1984;7(4):207–26
Bazhan TA: K. Marks ob okhrane zdorov'ia rabochego klassa. **Gig Sanit** 1984 Feb;(2):37–40
Berlan JP: The world food problem: Malthus, Marx and their epigones. **Mon Rev** 1980;31(10):20–32
Cameron S, Falk LA: Some black medical history: Dr. Martin R. Delany's Canadian years as medical practitioner and abolitionist (1856–1864). In: Congrès international d'histoire de la médecine, XXVe, Québec, 1976. Actes. Québec, 1977. p. 537–45.
Concepcion R: Medical ethics in connection with torture of prisoners and other persons under some form of detention. **Unitas** 1976;49(4):542–92
Cowen DL: Pharmacy and freedom. **Pharm Hist** 1984;26(2):70–82
Davidson WD, Montville JV: Foreign policy according to Freud. **Foreign Policy** 1981–82;45:145–57
Dobek R, Kolmsee P: Maxim Zetkin--Arzt, Kriegschirurg und Kommunist. **Militaergesch** 1978;17(5):595–603
Dwudziesty drugi zeszył poświęcony zagadnieniom lekarskim okresu hitlerowskiej okupacji: **Przegl Lek** 1982;39(1–3):1–267
Dynamite doctors: **Practitioner** 1980 Feb;224(1340):119–20
Foerster I, Kirschke S: Soziobiologie oder Biosoziologie? **Wiss Z Martin Luther Univ (Math)** 1984;33(4):51–67
Gish O: The political economy of primary care and 'health by the people': an historical exploration. **Soc Sci Med** 1979 Dec;13C(4):203–11
Heidenheimer AJ: Organized medicine and physician specialization in Scandinavia and West Germany. **West Eur Polit** 1980;3(3):373–87
Hoffman LE: War, revolution, and psychoanalysis: Freudian thought begins to grapple with social reality. **J Hist Behav Sci** 1981;17:251–69
Jarrell RA: Colonialism and the truncation of science in Ireland and French Canada during the nineteenth century. **HSTC** 1981 May;18(5 no 2):140–57
Jordanova LJ: Towards the light? Science, politics and the enlightenment. **Eur Stud Rev** 1982;12(4):479–88
Koning A: Die Pharmazie in der holländischen politischen Karikatur. **Pharm Acta Helv** 1979;54(9–10):308–10
Kornfeld H: Nuclear weapons and civil defense. The influence of the medical profession in 1955 and 1983. **West J Med** 1983 Feb;138(2):207–12
Kozlov AM, Kel'ner MS, Losev NI: K. Marks is problemy meditsiny (k 165-letiiu so dnia rozhdeniia K. Marksa). **Patol Fiziol Eksp Ter** 1983 May–Jun;3:3–9
Labisch A: Krankenhauspolitik in der Krankenhausgeschichte. **Hist Hosp** 1979–80;13:217–33
L'Etang H: Fit to lead? London, Heinemann, 1980. 211 p.
Löhr HG: Ein Vierteljahrhundert gemeinsamen Weges von Karl Marx und Friedrich Engels mit ihrem treuen Freund und Kampfgefährten Carl Schorlemmer. **Pharmazie** 1983 Nov;38(11):768–72
Luther E: Humanismus und gesellschaftliche Verantwortung. **Wiss Z Martin Luther Univ (Math)** 1984;33(2):122–7
Magner LN: Women and the scientific idiom: textual episodes from Wollstonecraft, Fuller, Gilman, and Firestone. **Signs** 1978;4(1):61–80
Mullaney MM: Gender and revolution: Rosa Luxemburg and the female revolutionary personality. **J Psychohist** 1984 Spring;11(4):463–76
Nilius B: Heuristische Aspekte im Verhältnis zwischen Philosophie und Einzelwissenschaft. **Wiss Z Martin Luther Univ (Math)** 1984;33(2):134–42
Odajnyk VW: Jung and politics. The political and social ideas of C. G. Jung. New York, New York University Press, 1976. xv, 190 p.
Orlov DA, Galakhov EV, Zhiliaeva EP: Uchastie mirovoĭ meditsinskoĭ obshchestvennosti v bor'be za mir i razoruzhenie. **Sov Zdravookhr** 1980;(10):38–44
Paul D: Eugenics and the Left. **J Hist Ideas** 1984 Oct–Dec;45(4):567–90
Pharmacology of leadership: **Practitioner** 1980 Feb;224(1340):119
Renshon SA: Life history and character development: some reflections on political leadership. In M. Albin, R. J. Devlin, G. Heeger, ed: New directions in psychohistory. The Adelphi papers in honor of Erik H. Erikson. Lexington, Toronto, D. C. Heath, 1980. p. 57–68.
Schullian DM: Notes on William Gladston, Karl Marx, Charles Darwin, Kliment Timiriazev, and the 'Eastern question' of 1876–78. **J Hist Med Allied Sci** 1983 Apr;38(2):178–85
Sheiman I: Kapitalizm i problemy zdravo-okhraneniia. **Mirovaia Ekon Mezhdunar Otnosheniia** 1979;12:116–23
Smirnov EI, Garin NS: Agressivnaia sushchnost' amerikanskogo imperializma i vozmozhnye posledstviia primeneniia iadernogo oruzhiia. **Zh Mikrobiol Epidemiol Immunobiol** 1982 May;(5):3–11
Stewart R: Bethune. 2nd ed. Hamden, Connecticut, Archon, 1979. 210 p.
Studer KE, Chubin DE: The cancer mission. Social contexts of biomedical research. Beverly Hills, London, Sage, 1980. 319 p. (Sage Library of Social Research, V. 103).
Szymanski A: On the uses of disinformation to legitimize the revival of the cold war: health in the U.S.S.R. **Sci Soc** 1981–82;45(4):453–74
Tal U: On the study of the Holocaust and genocide. **Yad Vashem Stud Eur Jew Catastrophe Resist** 1979;13:7–52
Tesh S: Political ideology and public health in the nineteenth century. **Int J Health Serv** 1982;12(2):321–42
Thiel C: Folgen der Emigration deutscher und österreichischer Wissenschaftstheoretiker und Logiker zwischen 1933 und 1945. **Ber Wissenschaftsgesch** 1984;7(4):227–56
Ward PS: Antibiotics and international relations at the close of World War II. In J. Parascandola, ed: The history of antibiotics. Madison, American Institute of the History of Pharmacy, 1980. p. 101–12.
Wright PW: The radical sociology of medicine. **Soc Stud Sci** 1980;10(1):103–20
Zaretsky E: A note on Marxism and psychoanalysis. **Marx Perspect** 1979;2(2):134–9

### Africa

Sabben-Clare EE, Bradley DJ, Kirkwood K, ed: Health in tropical Africa during the colonial period: based on the proceedings of a symposium held at New College, Oxford, 21–23 March 1977. Oxford, Clarendon, 1980. ix, 276 p.

### Americas

Figueroa Marroquin H: De qué murió Simon Bolivar? **Bol Soc Mex Hist Filos Med** 1981 Dec;5(37):217–47
Guerra F: El medico politico. Estudios biográficos sobre la influencia del médico en la Historia Politica de Hispanoamérica y Filipinas. Madrid, Afrodisio Aguado, 1975. 350 p.
Mérida F: Las enfermedades odontologicas y dermatologicas del Libertador. **Rev Soc Venez Hist Med** 1981;30(47):81–7
Mérida F: Semblanzas de Alejandro Prospero Révérend, primicias para calificar su actuacion frente a la ultima enfermedad del Libertador. **Rev Soc Venez Hist Med** 1981;30(47):71–80
Randall M: La penetración imperialista y sus consecuencias para la mujer Latinoamericana. **Santiago (Cuba)** 1974;(15):227–47
Weaver JL: The politics of Latin American family-planning policy. **J Dev Areas** 1978;12(4):415–37

# POLITICS

**Argentina**

Martín de Codoni E: La politica sanitaria en el primer medio siglo. Mendoza 1810–1860. **Rev Hist Am Argent** 1980;10(19–20):37–52
Zarranz A: La Sanidad Militar en las Guerras Civiles Argentinas (Desde el sitio de Buenos Aires a la Revolución del 90). In Congreso de Historia de la Medicina Argentina [Transactions], 5th, Mendoza, 1983. p. 133–40.

**Australia**

Hunter T: Medical politics: decline in the hegemony of the Australian Medical Association? **Soc Sci Med** 1984;18(11):973–80
Hunter T: Pressure groups and the Australian political process: the case of the Australian Medical Association. **J Commonw Comp Polit** 1980;18(2):190–206

**Austria**

Hubenstorf M: Osterreichische Arzteemigration 1934–1945--Zwischen neuem Tätigkeitsgebiet und organisierten Rückkehrplänen. **Ber Wissenschaftsgesch** 1984;7(2):85–107
Huter F: Ein tiroler Student erlebt den Beginn der Wiener Märzrevolution. **Tirol Heimat** 1972;36:131–9
Pisźtora F: Tipikus társadalmi konfliktusok és reaktív neurosisok-psychosisok a Monarchia idöszakában hazánkban. **Orv Hetil** 1980 Aug 10;121(32):1956–9
Spiro HM: Eppinger of Vienna: scientist and villain? **J Clin Gastroenterol** 1984 Dec;6(6):493–7
Wyklicky H: Maria Theresia und Joseph II. als Reformatoren des Gesundheitswesens in Oesterreich. **Wien Tierarztl Monatsschr** 1981;68(1):3–7

**Bulgaria**

Micheva Z: Shesta sesiia na Bulgaro-Polskata Komisiia na istoritsite. **Istor Pregl** 1978;34(5):162–4
Nicolov IC: Doctors, participants in the national liberation movement of the Bulgarian people in Macedonia. In International Congress of the History of Medicine. 26th, Plovdiv, 1978. Actes du Congress. Sofia, 1981. Volume II. p. 167–8.

**Canada**

Audet LP: Louis Giard. In Dictionary of Canadian biography, 1881–1890. 1982;11:345–6.
Beck JM: George Murray. In Dictionary of Canadian biography, 1881–1890. 1982;11:633–4.
Bilas I: Pierre-Etienne Fortin. In Dictionary of Canadian biography, 1881–1890. 1982;11:320–1.
Boudreau F: The Quebec psychiatric system in transition: a case study in psychopolitics. **Can Rev Sociol Anthropol** 1980;17(2):122–37
Caissie F: Joseph-Godric Blanchet. In Dictionary of Canadian biography, 1881–1890. 1982;11:85–6.
Guerra F: Les médecins patriotes. In: Congres international d'histoire de la médecine, XXVe, Québec, 1976. Actes. Québec, 1977. p. 746–54.
Hiller JK: John Joseph Dearin. In Dictionary of Canadian biography, 1881–1890. 1982;11:239–40.
MacDougall H: Public health in Toronto's municipal politics: the Canniff years, 1883–1890. **Bull Hist Med** 1981 Summer;55(2):186–202
McGahan EW: Sylvester Zobieski Earle. In Dictionary of Canadian biography, 1881–1890. 1982;11:295–6.
Swainson D: William Henry Brouse. In Dictionary of Canadian biography, 1881–1890. 1982;11:114.
Teece WK: John Ash. In Dictionary of Canadian biography, 1881–1890. 1982;11:32–3.
Whalen JM: Edwin Arnold Vail. In Dictionary of Canadian biography, 1881–1890. 1982;11:896–7.
Wier RA: Federalism, interest groups, and parliamentary government: the Canadian Medical Association. **J Commonw Polit Stud** 1973;11(2):159–75

**Chile**

Costa-Casaretto C: Don Diego Portales y el Dr. Guillermo C. Blest. **Rev Med Chil** 1984 Jun;112(6):625–31

**China**

Buck P: American science and modern China, 1876–1936. Cambridge, Cambridge University Press, 1980. viii, 283 p.
Chi nien Pai Ch'iu-en: in memory of Norman Bethune. Pei-ching, Jen min ch'u pan she, 1979. 285 p.
Dodds WR: From medicine to president [Sun Yat Sen]. **Practitioner** 1981 Sep;225(1359):1342–3
Garfield R, Salmon JW: Struggles over health care in the People's Republic of China. **J Contemp Asia** 1981;11(1):91–103
Kelkar GS: Kotnis in Kokung. **China Rep (India)** 1979;15(2):97–111
Lampton DM: The roots of interprovincial inequality in education and health services in China since 1949. **Am Pol Sci Rev** 1979,73(2):459–77
Lucas A: Chinese Medical Modernization. Comparative Policy Continuities, 1930s–1980s. New York, Praeger, 1982. xiii, 188 p.

**Costa Rica**

Rosenberg MB: Reforma social y conflicto político: La huelga médica como preludio a la guerra civil costarricense de 1948. **Rev Hist (Costa Rica)** 1977 Jul-Dec;3:149–70

**Cuba**

Expósito CR: Dr. Félix Figueredo y Diaz (Un hombre del 68 y de la Protesta de Baraguá). Habana, Organismos, 1973. 417 p. (Cuadernos de Historia de la Salud Pública, 55).
Fernandez-Conde A: One Cuban physician's odyssey. **J Fla Med Assoc** 1979 Aug;66(8):845–52
Figueredo Díaz F: La guerra de Cuba en 1878 (La protesta de Baragua). Habana, Organismos, 1973. 338 p. (Cuadernos de Historia de la Salud Pública, 56).

**Czechoslovakia**

Bolecek O: Protifašistický odboj na zdravotnické frontě. Vzpomínky na ilegální činnost za okupace na Bulovce. **Cas Lek Cesk** 1980 May 9;119(19):538–42
Remišová M: Slovenské národné povstanie a nový prístup k organizovaniu odborného spolkového života lekárov. **Bratisl Lek Listy** 1979 Aug;72(2):141–6
Winters SB: The health of Edvard Beneš: an unpublished letter from 1948. **East Cent Eur** 1977;4:60–6

**Ethiopia**

Rosenfeld CP: The medical history of Menilek II, Emperor of Ethiopia (1844–1913): a case of medical diplomacy. **Munger Afr Libr Notes** 1978(45–46):3–43

**France**

Besombes A: Odonto-stomatologie et diplomatie de l'Impératrice Eugénie à Clemenceau. **Hist Sci Med** 1983;17(1):13–22
Biéder J: L'odyssée d'Ulysse Trélat (1795–1879). **Ann Med Psychol (Paris)** 1984 Jan;142(1):128–41
Bourquelot L: Le congrès médical de France: défense d'und profession libérale sous la Monarchie de Juillet. **Ann Bretagne** 1979,86(3):301–12
Bulhan HA: Frantz Fanon: the revolutionary psychiatrist. **Race Cl** 1980 Winter;21:251–72
Dillemann G, Michel ME: La réception des pharmaciens en France de la Révolution à l'application de la loi du 21 germinal an XI (1791–1813). **Rev Hist Pharm (Paris)** 1984;31(260):42–61
Dillemann G: Le monopole pharmaceutique et le décret du 2 mars 1791. **Rev Hist Pharm (Paris)** 1980 Dec;247(68 no 27):235–8
Fouré J: A French woman dentist who gave her life as a freedom fighter against the Nazis. **Bull Hist Dent** 1984 Oct;32(2):133–4
Gerard A: Chronique médico-chirurgicale Lilloise sous la Révolution et l'Empire. **Lille Med** 1979 Dec;24(10):774–83
Godlewski G: Le Docteur Clemenceau. **Sem Hop Paris** 1981 Dec 18–25;57(47–48):2057–71
Godlewski G: Le docteur Combes, pourfendeur de l'Eglise. **Sem Hop Paris** 1982 Dec 23;58(47):2802–13
Goubert JP: Réseau médical et médicalisation en France à la fin du 18e siècle. **Ann Bretagne** 1979;86(3):221–9
Goubert JP: 1789: le corps médical et le changement. **Hist Sci Med** 1982;16(2):99–105
Greenbaum LS: Medicine in revolution: an essay review. **J Hist Med Allied Sci** 1982 Jan;37(1):90–5
Greenbaum LS: Scientists and politicians: hospital reform in Paris on the eve of the French Revolution. **Proc Consort Revolutionary Eur** 1973:168–91
Guillon J: Un aspect de la population pendant la Révolution. Les entrées à l'Hôtel-Dieu de Paris, ler novembre 1791 - 10 novembre 1799. Maîtrise. Univ. de Paris I, 1976. 104 p.
Haeberle EJ: Human rights and sexual rights. The legacy of René Guyon. **Med Law** 1983;2(2):159–72
Houdaille J: Mortalité des députés élus de 1789 à 1794. **Population** 1979;34(3):714–7
Jones C: The French Revolution, hospitals, and the medical profession. **Soc Soc Hist Med Bull (Lond)** 1984 Jun;34:6–9
Kreiser BR: Miracles, convulsions, and ecclesiastical politics in early eighteenth-century Paris. Princeton, Princeton University Press, 1978. xvii, 485 p.
Leonard J: La médicalisation de l'Etat: l'exemple des premières décennies de la 3e République. **Ann Bretagne** 1979;86(3):313–20
Léonard J: La restauration et la profession médicale. **Hist Reflect** 1982;9(1–2):69–81
Leonard J: Le corps médical au début de la IIIe République, ou l'heureux

dénouement d'un malaise professionnel. In Poirier J, Poirier JL, ed: Médecine et philosophie à la fin du XIXe siècle. Paris, Université de Paris XII - Val de Marne, [1980?]. p. 9-21.
Levin A: Venel, Lavoisier, Fourcroy, Cabanis and the idea of scientific revolution: the French political context and the general patterns of conceptualization of scientific change. **Hist Sci** 1984 Sep;22(57 pt 3):303-20
Lorillot D: 1789: les medecins ont la parole. **Hist Reflect** 1982;9(1-2):103-129
Makarenko EM: Molodoi Lafarg. **Vopr Istor** 1981;(6):115-22
Martiny M: Projet de loi présenté le 31 janvier 1923 par le député Edouard Grinda sur les assurances sociales. **Hist Sci Med** 1979;13(4):363-7
Mitchell H: Politics in the service of knowledge: the debate over the administration of medicine and welfare in late eighteenth-century France. **Soc Hist (Lond)** 1981;6(2):185-207
Mitchell H: Politics, power and psychiatry: a review of L'Ordre psychiatrique: l'age d'or de l'aliénisme by Robert Castel. **Int J Law Psychiatry** 1979;2(2):249-61
Musset J: L'intervention de l'administration en matière d'épidémie au XVIIIe siècle: l'élection de Saint-Lô en 1785. **Ann Normandie** 1978 Dec;28:344-6
Nauroy J: Une pharmacienne confrontée malgré elle à la conspiration de Malet. **Rev Hist Pharm (Paris)** 1984 Mar;31(260):18-20
Oguse, D: 'Socialisme et néo-malthusianisme', la Revue Socialiste, t. XLVI, juillet-décembre 1907, p. 27-124. **Ann Demogr Hist (Paris)** 1983;:371-89
Outram D: Politics and vocation: French science, 1793-1830. **Br J Hist Sci** 1980 Mar;13(43 pt 1):27-43
Outram D: The ordeal of vocation: the Paris Academy of Sciences and the Terror, 1793-95. **Hist Sci** 1983 Sep;21(53 pt 3):251-73
Peset JL: La sociedad enferma: algunas reflexiones sobre la muerte del presidente Carnot (1894). **Asclepio** 1983;35:177-88
Pickstone JV: Bureaucracy, liberalism and the body in post-revolutionary France: Bichat's physiology and the Paris school of medicine. **Hist Sci** 1981 Jun;19(44 pt 2):115-42
Ramsey M: Medicina e politica di monopolio professionale nel XIX secolo. **Quad Stor** 1981;16(3):959-1011
Raspail S: Raspail, savant et militant. **Histoire** 1978 Dec;7:89-91
Redlich FC: Medical ethics under National Socialism. In Reich WT, et al, ed: Encyclopedia of bioethics, v.3. New York, Free Press, 1978. p. 1015-20.
Ronsin F: La classe ouvrière et le néo-Malthusianisme: l'exemple français avant 1914. **Mouvement Soc** 1979;106:85-117
Rullière R: Les morts subites à la Cour de Louis XIV de 1690 à 1709, d'après Pierre Dionis. **Hist Sci Med** 1984;18(1):19-24
Shulim JI: The birth of a revolutionary: Robespierre in Artois. **Consortium Revolut Eur 1750-1850 Proc** 1977;:22-33
Smeaton WA: Pharmacy in Revolutionary and Napoleonic Paris, 1789-1815. **Pharm Hist (London)** 1979 Apr;9(1):4-5
Staum MS: Cabanis. Enlightenment and medical philosophy in the French Revolution. Princeton, Princeton University Press, 1980. xi, 430 p.
Szaluta J: Apotheosis to ignominy: the martyrdom of Marshal Pétain. **J Psychohist** 1980 Spring;7(4):415-53
Weiner DB: Les handicapés et la révolution française: aspects de médecine sociale. In: Congrès international d'histoire de la médecine, XXVe, Québec, 1976. Actes. Québec, 1977. p. 333-70.

### Germany

Arendt HJ: Eine demokratische Massenbewegung unter Führung der KPD im Frühjahr 1931. **Z Geschichtswiss** 1971;19(2):212-23
Baader G: Politisch motivierte Emigration deutscher Arzte. **Ber Wissenschaftsgesch** 1984;7(2):67-84
Bayertz K: Naturwissenschaft und Sozialismus: Tendenzen der Naturwissenschafts-Rezeption in der deutschen Arbeiterbewegung des 19. Jahrhunderts. **Soc Stud Sci** 1983 Aug;13(3):355-94
Benjamin H: Georg Benjamin: eine Biographie. 2d ed. Leipzig, S. Hirzel, 1982. 363 p.
Bogusz J: Wpływ norymberskiego procesu lekarzy hitlerowskich na kształtowanie się pojeć o dokonywaniu badań na ludziach. **Przegl Lek** 1981;38(1):72-9
Boozer JS: Children of Hippocrates: doctors in Nazi Germany. **Ann Am Acad Polit Soc Sci** 1980;450:83-97
Born GV: The effect of the scientific environment in Britain on refugee scientists from Germany and their effects on science in Britain. **Ber Wissenschaftsgesch** 1984;7(3):129-43
Brainin E, Kaminer IJ: Psychoanalyse und Nationalsozialismus. **Psyche (Stuttg)** 1982 Nov;36(11):989-1012
Broszat M: Hitler und die Genesis der 'Endlösung.' Aus Anlass der Thesen von David Irving. **Vierteljahrsh Zeitgesch** 1977;25(4):739-75
Büttner L, Meyer B: Karl Marx und die Begründung der Gesundheitspolitik der revolutionären Arbeiterbewegung I. Vormarxistische Kritik der bürgerlichen Gesundheitspolitik. **Z Arztl Fortbild (Jena)** 1983;77(17):743-8
Büttner L, Meyer B: Karl Marx und die Begründung der Gesundheitspolitik der revolutionären Arbeiterbewegung. II. Marx' Aufdeckung des Klasseninhalts der bürgerlichen Gesundheitspolitik. **Z Arztl Fortbild (Jena)** 1983;77(19):819-23
Büttner L, Meyer B: Zur Herausbildung und Entwicklung der Gesundheitspolitik der SED nach 1945. **Wiss Z Martin Luther Univ (Math)** 1975;24(3):5-14
Cieślawski M: Z przeżyć dzieci i matek-robotnic przymusowych na Pomorzu Zachodnim. **Przegl Lek** 1981;38(1):121-4
Cocks GC: Psychoanalyse, Psychotherapie und Nationalsozialismus. **Psyche (Stuttg)** 1983 Dec;37(12):1057-106
Cohen CB: 'Quality of life' and the analogy with the Nazis. **J Med Philos** 1983 May;8(2):113-35
Dahmer H: 'Psychoanalyse unter Hitler'--Rückblick auf eine Kontroverse. **Psyche (Stuttg)** 1984 Oct;38(10):927-42
Dortmund EK: Daniel Paul Schreber: a case study of private fate as public possibility. **Res Stud** 1978;46(3):141-55
Dulnik S: Koroteiha shel kehila yehudit bebrit-hamo'atsot. **Yalkut Moreshet Period** 1976;21:89-100
Engel M: Das Dahlem-Projekt und sein Scheitern. Ein wissenschaftspolitischer Modellfall medizinischer Forschung an der Schwelle zum 20. Jahrhundert - Zur Geschichte des Robert-Koch-Instituts und der Charité. **Fortschr Med** 1982 Jun3;100(21):1009-12
Epstein D: Hayehudi hayehidi (ha'ayarah Libishei bashoah). **Yalkut Moreshet Period** 1975;20:7-34
Figlio K, Weindling P: Was social medicine revolutionary? Rudolf Virchow and the revolutions of 1848. **Soc Soc Hist Med Bull (Lond)** 1984 Jun;34:10-8
Flehr H: Geschichte des Arztlichen Vereins in Frankfurt am Main und sein standespolitisches Wirken. Diss. Mainz, 1982. 144 p.
Friedländer S: L'extermination des Juifs d'Europe: pour une etude historique globale. **Rev Etud Juives** 1976;135(1-3):113-44
Ganzinger K: Der Lippe-Detmoldische Leibarzt Johann Christian Friedrich Scherf (1750-1818) als Medizinalpolitiker und Reformator der Pharmazie. **Beitr Gesch Pharm** 1981;31(10):73-8
Gebhardt O, Kubik G: Zur Bündnispolitik der Arbeiterklasse und ihrer marxistisch-leninistischen Partei mit der medizinischen Intelligenz. **Med Ges** 1978;(3):28-47
Gehrke H, Dückert M: Gesundheitspolitik der deutschen Arbeiterklasse und ihre Unterstützung durch die fortschrittlichsten Vertreter der medizinischen Intelligenz. **Z Arztl Fortbild (Jena)** 1983;77(12):530-4
Geuter U: Die Professionalisierung der deutschen Psychologie im Nationalsozialismus. Frankfurt am Main, Suhrkamp, 1984. 592 p.
Glass B: A hidden chapter of German eugenics between the two world wars. **Proc Am Philos Soc** 1981;125(5):357-67
Gotovitch J: Quelques données relatives à l'extermination des Tsiganes de Belgique. **Cah Hist Seconde Guerre Mond** 1976;4:161-80
Gumpert M: Hölle im Paradies. Selbstdarstellung eines Arztes. Hildesheim, Gerstenberg, 1983. xxiii, 280 p. (Exilliteratur, Band 17) Reprint of 1939 ed., with new biographical forward by F. Trapp.
Güse HG, Schmacke N: Psychiatrie zwischen bürgerlicher Revolution und Faschismus. Kronberg, Ger., Athenäum Verlag, 1976.
Güse HG, Schmacke N: Psychiatry and the origins of Nazism. **Int J Health Serv** 1980;10(2):177-96
Haeberle EJ: 'Stigmata of degeneration'. Prisoner markings in Nazi concentration camps. **J Homosex** 1980-81 Fall-Winter;6(1-2):135-9
Hahn S: Positionen der Kommunistischen Partei Deutschlands zur lebensbewahrenden Aufgabe der Medizin in der Zeit der Weimarer Republik. **Z Exp Chir** 1982 Jul;28(7):468-71
Heston LL, Heston R: The medical casebook of Adolf Hitler: his illnesses, doctors, and drugs. New York, Stein and Day, 1980. 184 p.
Hieronimi S: Nationalsozialistische Vernichtungsaktionen an geistig Kranken im Spiegel psychiatrie-historischer Publikationen des Nachkriegsdeutschlands. Eine Auseinandersetzung mit psychiatrischen Positionen zur Geschichte der deutschen Psychiatrie 1933-1945. Diss. Mainz, 1981. 75 p.
Hoffmann-Axthelm W: Wilhelm Dieck--Lehrer, Forscher und Standespolitiker. **Quintessenz** 1984 Feb;35(2):365-9
Hollander A: Geschichtliches aus vergangener Zeit: Politische Bekämpfung der Geschlechtskrankheiten? **Fortschr Med** 1981 Jun 25;99(24):927-8
Jagoda Z, Kłodziński S, Masłowski J: Stosunek ofiar Oświecimia-Brzezinki do prześladowców. **Przegl Lek** 1981;38(1):37-62
Kaiser W: Medizinhistorische Impressionen zum Karl-Marx-Jahr 1983. **Z Gesamte Inn Med** 1983 Dec 15;38(24):669-72
Karbe KH: Das Betriebsarztsystem und zum Schicksal der Arbeitsmedizin im faschistischen Deutschland. **Z Gesamte Hyg** 1983 Oct;29(10):640-4
Kater MH: Die 'Gesundheitsführung' des Deutschen Volkes. **Medizinhist J** 1983;18(4):349-75
Katz O: Der 'Führer' behandelte sich selbst. Aus jetzt verfügbaren Aufzeichnungen des Leibarztes Theo Morell werden realistische Konturen der geheimnisvollen Krankheiten Adolf Hitlers erkennbar (I). **Fortschr Med** 1984 Oct 4;102(37):70-1
Katz O: Prof. Dr. Med. Theo Morell: Hitlers Leibarzt. Bayreuth, Hestia, 1983. 397 p.
Klasen EM: Die Diskussion über eine 'Krise' der Medizin in Deutschland zwischen 1925 und 1935. Diss. Mainz, 1984. 169 p.
Klee E: 'Euthanasie' im NS-Staat: die 'Vernichtung lebensunwerten Lebens'. Frankfurt am Main, S. Fischer, 1983. 502 p.
Kłodzinski S: Uwagi o sytuacji zdrwotnej robotników przymusowych w Niemczech hitlerowskich. **Przegl Lek** 1981;38(1):62-72

# POLITICS

Kober R: Abteilung Gesundheits- und Sozialwesen des Rates des Bezirkes Gera. **Z Arztl Fortbild (Jena)** 1979 Oct 1;73(19-20):983-6

Kozlov AM: Genial'nyĭ myslitel', plamennyĭ revoliutsioner i velikiĭ chelovek (k 165-letiiu so dnia rozhdeniia i 100-letiiu so dnia smerti Karla Marksa). **Feldsher Akush** 1983;48(5):3-4

Krebs H: Wie ich aus Deutschland vertrieben wurde: Dokumente mit Kommentaren. **Medizinhist J** 1980;15(4):357-77

Krüger M: Uber progressive Traditionen in der haltung bürgerlicher deutscher ärzte der 20er Jahre gegenüber der Sowjetunion und ihrer Medizin am Beispiel des Hämatologen Viktor Schilling. **Wiss Z Univ Rostock** 1971;20(5):329-32

Kudlien F, Andree C: Sauerbruch und der Nationalsozialismus. **Medizinhist J** 1980;15(3):201-222

Labisch A: Das Krankenhaus in der Gesundheitspolitik der deutschen Sozialdemokratie vor dem Ersten Weltkrieg. **Med Soziol** 1981;1:127-51

Labisch A: Das Krankenhaus in der sozialdemokratischen Kommunalpolitik in Berlin um die Jahrhundertwende. **Hist Hosp** 1981-82;14:337-45

Labisch A: Neue Quellen zum gesundheitspolitischen Programm der MSPD von 1920/22. **Int Wiss Korresp Gesch Dtsch Arb-bew** 1980 June;16(2):231-47

Labisch A: Selbsthilfe zwischen Auflehnung und Anpassung. Arbeiter-Sanitätskommission und Arbeiter-Samariterbund. **Jahrb Krit Med** 1983;77:11-26

Labisch A: The Workingmen's Samaritan Federation (Arbeiter-Samariter-Bund) 1888-1933. **J Contemp Hist** 1978;13:297-322

Lautmann R: The pink triangle. The persecution of homosexual males in concentration camps in Nazi Germany. **J Homosex** 1980-81 Fall-Winter;6(1-2):141-60

Lekisch K: Drugs and politics. **Scalpel Tongs** 1981;25:93-4

Lifton RJ: Medicalized killing in Auschwitz. **Psychiatry** 1982;45(4):283-97

Lilienthal G: 'Rheinlandbastarde', Rassenhygiene und das Problem der rassenideologischen Kontinuität. Zur Untersuchung von Reiner Pommerin: 'Sterilisierung der Rheinlandbastarde'. **Medizinhist J** 1980;15(4):426-36

Lohmann HM, Rosenkötter L: Psychoanalyse in Hitlerdeutschland. Wie war es wirklich? **Psyche (Stuttg)** 1982 Nov;36(11):961-88

Lohmann HM, Rosenkötter L: Psychoanalyse in Hitlerdeutschland. Wie war es wirklich? Ein Nachtrag. **Psyche (Stuttg)** 1983 Dec;37(12):1107-15

Löther I: Probleme der Wissenschaftlich-technischen Revolution und einige Aufgaben des sozialistischen Gesundheitsschutzes. **Med Ges** 1978;(3):69-78

McKale D: Purging Nazis: the postwar trials of female German doctors and nurses. **Proc SC Hist Assoc** 1981;:156-70

Moe K: Should the Nazi research data be cited? **Hastings Cent Rep** 1984 Dec;14(6):5-7

Moschke G: Die Stellung der KPD zur Berufskrankheitengesetzgebung in der Weimarer Republik. **Z Exp Chir** 1982 Jul;28(7):471-3

Moschke G: Samaritianskiĭ soiuz rabochikh Germanii--primer tvorcheskoĭ deiatel'nosti nemetskogo rabochego klassa v 1909-1930 gg. v bor'be protiv burzhuaznoĭ politiki zdravookhraneniia. **Sov Zdravookhr** 1981;(2):52-6

Moskwa Z: Powstańcza søużba zdrowia na Górnym Slasku w latach 1919-1921. **Wiad Lek** 1984 Feb 15;37(4):313-20

Parnitzke C, Schaeper M: Bedeutende Magdeburger antifaschistische Aerzte und die Entwicklung der Orthopädie in Magdeburg. **Z Arztl Fortbild (Jena)** 1980 Aug 15;74(16):781-6

Paton A: Mission to Belsen 1945. **Br Med J [Clin Res]** 1981 Dec 19;283(6307):1656-9

Perl G: I was a doctor in Auschwitz. New York, Arno Press, 1979. 189 p.

Pommerin R: The fate of mixed blood children. **Ger Stud Rev** 1982;5(3):315-23

Przyboś A: Smierć wieźnia Stefana Przybosia w Mauthausen. **Przegl Lek** 1984;41(1):97-9

Przychodzki M: Lekarze Poznanscy w latach hitlerowskiej okupacji 1939-1945. **Przegl Zachod** 1977;33(1):106-39

Rödel W: Die wichtigsten Forderungen der revolutionären deutschen Sozialdemokratie zum Apothekenwesen ausgangs des 19. Jahrhunderts. **Pharmazie** 1983 Nov;38(11):772-4

Schachter M: La personnalité de Frédéric II Le Grand, Roi de Prusse (1712-1786). Essai de psychologie adlérienne. **Hist Sci Med** 1984;18(2):181-7

Scharfetter C: Ein Anliegen der Menschheitserziehung: Delegierte Destruktivität. Massenmord an Psychiatriepatienten in Hitler-Deutschland. **Schweiz Arch Neurol Neurochir Psychiatr** 1984;134(2):279-93

Schmidt H: Zur Kostenfreiheit ärztlicher Hilfeleistung; eine Betrachtung aus Anlass des 90. Jahrestages des Erfurter Programms der SPD. **Beitr Gesch Univ Erfurt** 1979-83;19:265-70

Schneck P: Frauenheilkunde und Geburtshilfe in der Zeit des deutschen Faschismus 1933 bis 1945--Zum Schicksal der sozialen Gynäkologie im 'Dritten Reich'. **Z Gesamte Hyg** 1983 Oct;29(10):645-7

Schneck P: Wilhelm Liepmann (1878-1939)--ein Gynäkologenschicksal zwischen Kaiserreich und faschistischer Diktatur. **Zentralbl Gynakol** 1984;106(17):1223-8

Schneck P: Wilhelm Liepmann (1878-1939) und die soziale Gynäkologie im Spiegel der Aktenbestände des Archivs der Humboldt-Universität zu Berlin. **NTM** 1980;17(2):102-20

Schwann H, Wilke J: 'Erbliche Taubheit' im Faschismus. **Z Gesamte Hyg** 1984 Apr;30(4):232-4

Seidler E: Die Freiburger Gobineau-Vereinigung und die Verbreitung des Arier-Gedankens in Deutschland. In Seidler E, Schott H, ed: Bausteine zur Medizingeschichte. Stuttgart, Steiner, 1984. p. 121-9.

Späte HF, Thom A: Psychiatrie im Faschismus--Bilanz der historischen Analyse. **Z Gesamte Hyg** 1980;26(8):553-60

Stahlschmidt S: Professor Dr. med. habil. Fritz Gietzelt--Arzt, Wissenschaftler, Kommunist: ein Lebensbild. Berlin, Humboldt-Universität zu Berlin, 1982. 64 p.

Szemraj-Lochynska A, Kempisty C: Stan adaptacji do zycia na emeryturze nauczycieli akademickich represjonowanych przez hitleryzm. **Przegl Lek** 1981;38(1):33-6

Ungerer GA: Wilhelm Wundt als Psychologe und Politiker: Anmerkungen zur Biographie. **Psychol Rundschau** 1980;31:99-110

Vella EE: Belsen: medical aspects of a World War II concentration camp. Paper 1. **J R Army Med Corps** 1984 Feb;130(1):34-59

Weindling P: Theories of the cell state in Imperial Germany. In C. Webster, ed: Biology, medicine and society 1840-1940. Cambridge, Cambridge University Press, 1981. p. 99-155.

Winkle S: Johann Friedrich Struensee: Arzt, Aufklärer und Staatsmann: Beitrag zur Kultur-, Medizin- und Seuchengeschichte der Aufklärungszeit. Stuttgart, Fischer, 1983. 654 p.

Wolfensberger W: The extermination of handicapped people in World War II Germany. **Ment Retard** 1981 Feb;19(1):1-7

**Ghana**

Twumasi PA: Colonialism and international health: a study in social change in Ghana. **Soc Sci Med [Med Anthropol]** 1981 Apr;15B(2):147-51

**Great Britain**

Ashby E: The politics of clean air. Oxford, Clarendon Press, 1981. viii, 178 p.

Brayshay M, Pointon VF: Local politics and public health in mid-nineteenth-century Plymouth. **Med Hist** 1983 Apr;27(2):162-78

Cooke AM: Queen Victoria's medical household. **Med Hist** 1982 Jul;26(3):307-20

Deacon R: The PSI factor. An examination of the medical and psychological aspects of intelligence work. **Practitioner** 1982 Jan;226(1363):97-102

Dopson L: The cut-throat world of nursing politics - 18th century-style. **Nurs Times** 1984 Apr 25-May 1;80(17):19-20

Dupâquier J, Fauve-Chamoux A, Grebenik E, ed: Malthus past and present. London; New York, Academic Press, 1983. xix, 416 p. Contributions by A. Béjin, Y. Breton, Y. Charbit, L. Devance, A. Digby, M. W. Flinn, R. E. Frisch, M. Godelier, L. Gordon, P. Guillaume, G. Heinsohn, T. H. Hollingsworth, P. A. Jewell, N. Keyfitz, R. Keynes, H. Le Bras, M. Perrot, F. Rausky, M. Rebérioux, R. Remond, F. Ronsin, G. R. Searle, B. Stapleton, O. Steiger, P. Vallin, E. Van de Walle, A. Waterman, J. Wolff, E. A. Wrigley, V. Wynne-Edwards.

Earwicker R: The emergence of a medical strategy in the Labour Movement 1906-1919. **Soc Soc Hist Med Bull (Lond)** 1981 Dec;29:6-9

Eder NR: National health insurance, social politics and medical practice in Britain, 1913-1939. Ph.D. diss. University of Illinois. Chicago, 1980. 375 leaves.

Freeden M: Eugenics and progressive thought: a study in ideological affinity. **Hist J (Gt Brit)** 1979;22(3):645-72

Greenblatt RB: The humiliating demise of Lord Randolph Churchill, 1849-1895. **Postgrad Med** 1984 Jan;75(1):129-31, 134

Hamilton M: Opposition to the Contagious Diseases Act, 1864-1886. **Albion** 1978;10:14-27

Hansen B: The historical construction of homosexuality. **Radic Hist Rev** 1979;20:66-73

Harrison B: Women's health and the women's movement in Britain: 1840-1940. In C. Webster, ed: Biology, medicine and society 1840-1940. Cambridge, Cambridge University Press, 1981. p. 15-71.

Honigsbaum F: Medical politics and the state: the part played by the medical profession in the development of the National Health Service. **Soc Soc Hist Med Bull (Lond)** 1981 Dec;29:20-1

Ingle ST: Parliament and health policy: the role of MPs, 1970-75. Farnborough, Gower, 1981 vi, 171 p.

Levere TH: Dr. Thomas Beddoes (1750-1808): science and medicine in politics and society. **Br J Hist Sci** 1984 Jul;17(56 pt 2):187-204

Lewis J: The ideology and politics of birth control in inter-war Britain. **Womens Stud** 1979;2(l)

Livock R: Science, law and safety standards: a case study of industrial disease. **Br J Law Soc** 1979;6(2):172-99

McHugh PF: The campaign against the Contagious Diseases Act: Some organizational aspects, 1869-1886. Ph.D thesis, Oxford Univ, 1976.

Morgan KO: Dr. Christopher Addison and social reform. **Soc Soc Hist Med Bull (Lond)** 1981 Dec;29:21-5

Nauright L: Politics and power: a new look at Florence Nightingale. **Nurs Forum** 1984;21(1):5-7

Navarro V: Class struggle, the state and medicine. An historical and contemporary analysis of the medical sector in Great Britain. New York, Prodist, 1978. xviii, 156 p.
Ofcansky TP: British colonial administration in the Fiji Islands during the 1875 measles epidemic. **Adler Mus Bull** 1984 Mar;10(1):23-7
Pickstone JV: Ferriar's fever to Kay's cholera: disease and social structure in cottonopolis. **Hist Sci** 1984 Dec;22(58 pt 4):401-19
Pickstone JV, Butler SV: The politics of medicine in Manchester, 1788-1792: hospital reform and public health services in the early industrial city. **Med Hist** 1984 Jul;28(3):227-49
Porter R: The rage of party: a glorious revolution in English psychiatry? **Med Hist** 1983 Jan;27(1):35-50
Santurri EN: Theodicy and social policy in Malthus' thought. **J Hist Ideas** 1982 Apr-Jun;43(2):315-30
Towers BA: The management and politics of a public exposé: the Prestwich Inquiry 1922. **J Soc Policy** 1984 Jan;13(1):41-61
Weindling P: Science and sedition: how effective were the acts licensing lectures and meetings, 1795-1819? **Br J Hist Sci** 1980 Jul;13(44 no 2):139-53
Werskey G: The visible college. London, Allen Lane, 1978. 376 p.
Whitfield AG: Disraeli's doctors. **J R Coll Physicians Lond** 1980 Jul;14(3):202-4
Woodhouse J: Eugenics and the feeble-minded: the Parliamentary debates of 1912-14. **Hist Educ** 1982;11:127-37
Wurgaft LD: Another look at Prospero and Caliban: magic and magical thinking in British India. **Psychohist Rev** 6(1):2-26, Summer 77

### Greece

Degleris NE, Rozos BP: [Public health, medical education and social care of Ionian Isles in the middle of the 19th century (press documents)] (Gre). **Arch Hyg** 1980;:90-101

### Hungary

Csillag I: Quelques médecins juifs hongrois et les événements viennois de 1848. **Rev Hist Med Heb** 1984;37(1):7-9
Csorba S: Kölcsey Ferenc hibás szemének kérdéséhez. **Orvostort Kozl** 1982;28(1-3):191-9
Harmat P: Psychoanalyse und Marxismus in Ungarn (1900-1980). **Psyche (Stuttg)** 1984 Mar;38(3):254-69
Honti J: A magyar progresszió egészségpolitikai törekvései és a Nagy Októberi Szocialista Forradalom hatása. **Orvostort Kozl** 85(24 No 3):85-90, 1978
Tóth A: Orvosok Széchenyi naplójában. **Orv Hetil** 1981 May 31;122(22):1329-37

### India

Chandpuri K: Hakim Aziz al-Din; foreign minister of the Sikh kingdom. **Stud Hist Med** 1979 Sep;3(3):178-80
Rosselli J: The self-image of effeteness: physical education and nationalism in nineteenth-century Bengal. **Past Present** 1980;86:121-48

### Ireland

Smith BA: Irish prison doctors--men in the middle, 1865-90. **Med Hist** 1982 Oct;26(4):371-94

### Israel

Falk A: Moshe Dyan: the infantile roots of political action. **J Psychohist** 1983 Fall;11(2):271-88
Margalith D: Physicians, forerunners of modern Israel. Tel-Aviv, Jerusalem Academy of Medicine, 1973. 192, iv, 12 p.
Sherman ED: David Ben-Gurion (1886-1973). **J Am Geriatr Soc** 1983 Aug;31(8):501-5

### Italy

Detragiache D: Un aspect de la politique demographique de l'Italie fasciste: la repression de l'avortement. **Melanges Archeol Hist Ec Fr Rome** 1980;92(2):691-735
Detti T: Medicina, democrazia e socialismo in Italia tra '800 e '900. **Mov Operaio Soc** 1979;2(1):3-49
Imerti AD: Vincenzo Catalani, Neapolitan Jacobin, jurist, reformer (1769-1843), with an appendix containing a translation of his work 'A digression on vaccination.' Lawrence, Kansas, Coronado Press, 1976. 155 p.
Weber-Unger S: Wahnsinn und Politik: zur neuen Psychiatrie in Italien. Frankfurt; New York, Campus Verlag, 1984. 181 p.

### Kenya

Mburu FM: Socio-political imperatives in the history of health development in Kenya. **Soc Sci Med [A]** 1981 Sep;15(5):521-7

### Mexico

Fernández del Castillo F: El expediente médico de Valentín Gómez Farias. **Bol Inst Invest Bibliogr** 1970;(4):125-9

### Netherlands

Juffermans P: Economic crisis and health policy in the Netherlands. **Int J Health Serv** 1984;14(1):147-58

### New Zealand

Henderson J: Muldoon and Rowling: a preliminary analysis of contrasting personalities. **Pol Sci** 1980;32(1):26-46

### Nigeria

Pearce TO: Political and economic changes in Nigeria and the organization of medical care. **Soc Sci Med [Med Anthropol]** 1980 May;14(2):91-8

### Norway

Nilsen KH: Det Norske Arbeiderparti og befolkningsspørsmålet i mellomkrigstida. **Hist Tidsskr** 1979;58(3):287-304

### Pacific Islands

Boyd M: Coping with Samoan restistance after the 1918 influenza epidemic: Colonel Tate's problems and perplexities. **J Pac Hist** 1980;15(3):155-74

### Philippines

Barón Fernández J: La faceta medica del gran patriota Filipino Jose Rizal. **Asclepio** 1980;32:47-52
Pearlman M: Emotional factors in America's Western Pacific policy: Wood and Stimson in the Philippines. **J Psychohist** 1983 Fall;11(2):243-69

### Poland

Adamczyk A: Ostatnie dni w szpitalu obozu w Litomierzycach. **Przegl Lek** 1980;37(1):184-6
Bendiner E: Korczak: pediatrician on the road to hell. **Hosp Pract** 1981 Jul;16(7):125-8, 132-4, 138-9 passim
Dwudziesty trzeci zeszyt poświęcony zagadnieniom lekarskim okresu Hitlerowskiej okupacji: **Przegl Lek** 1983;40(1):1-247
Fijałek J, Machalski J: Publiczna opieka zdrowotna u poczatków Polski Niepodległej. **Arch Hist Med (Warsz)** 1978;41(4):393-404
Jabłoński C: Wymieralność w getcie w Brzezinach. **Przegl Lek** 1980;37(1):40-3
Jagoda Z, Kłodziński S, Masłowski J: Agresja i agresywność w obozie oświęcimskim. **Przegl Lek** 1980;37(1):43-75
Jakóbczyk W: Karol Marcinkowski, 1800-1846. Warszawa; Poznań, Państwowe Wydawn. Nauk., Oddz. w Poznaniu, 1981. 189 p.
Kaiser W, Skrobacki A: Resonanz des polnischen Novemberaufstandes (1831) an der Königsberger Universität. **Arch Hist Med (Warsz)** 1979;42(3):281-4
Kasperek S: Przymusowe sterylizacje w rejencji opolskiej 1934-1938. **Przegl Lek** 1980;37(1):33-9
Kieta M: Instytut higieny SS i Policji w Oświęcimiu. **Przegl Lek** 1980;37(1):172-6
Kłodziński S, Masłowski J: Patologia pracy w Oświecimiu-Brzezince. **Przegl Lek** 1984;41(1):37-54
Lefebvre P: La recherche par le clinicien: une activité inéluctable. **Bull Mem Acad R Med Belg** 1979 Nov 24;134(10):587-96
Maisel W: Plany Hitlerowskie w odniesieniu do chorych na gruźlicę Polaków w Wartegau. **Przegl Zachod** 1981;37(3-4):99-106
Masłowski J: Okupacyjna tematyka lekarska w polskich publikacjach z roku 1979. **Przegl Lek** 1980;37(1):213-28
Meclewski E: Der faschistische völkermord in polen. **Dtsch Aussenpolit** 1967;12(2):169-76
Ryn Z, Kłodziński S: Głód w obozie koncentracyjnym. **Przegl Lek** 1984;41(1):21-37
Ryn Z: Zakopiańskie placówki słyzby zdrowia podczas okupacji hitlerowskiej. **Przegl Lek** 1981;38(1):114-21
Sadowska J: Postulaty zdrowotne klasy robotniczej w rewolucji 1905-1907 roku. **Arch Hist Med (Warsz)** 1980;43(4):377-81
Strzelecka I: Pierwszy szpital obozowy w Brzezince. **Przegl Lek** 1984;41(1):88-93
Strzelecki A: O postawach więźniów konspiratorów w Oświecimiu. **Przegl Lek** 1984;41(1):93-6
Treść poprzednich zeszytów 'Przegladu lekarskiego' poświeconych zagadnieniom lekarskim okupacji hitlerowskiej: **Przegl Lek** 1984;41(1):178-202
Urban A: Konspiracyjna działalnść dydaktyczna profesor Janiny Kowalczykowej w okresie okupacji 1939-1944. **Patol Pol** 1980 Apr-Jun;31(2):161-9
Wrotnowska D: Médecins polonais émigrés en Languedoc et dans les

Pyrénées au XIXe siècle. In: Congrès National des Sociétés Savantes, 96e, Toulouse, 1971. Comptes Rendus. Paris, 1974. Histoires des Sciences, Tome 1. p. 175–92.
Zajusz K, Ornowski J: Rudolf Virchow a problemy niepodległościowe i społeczne narodu polskiego. **Arch Hist Med (Warsz)** 1979;42(3):285–9

**Puerto Rico**

Figueroa L: Betances, el irreductible. **Atenea (Puerto Rico)** 1972;9(3–4):29–39

**Romania**

Barbu G: Medici sub steagul revoluției în tara românească. **Rev Arhiv** 1973;35 suppl:153–69
Cernovodeanu D: Din corespondenta inedită a medicului militar Nicolae Stonescu in timpul Războiului de Independenta. **Rev Istor** 1977;30(6):1051–70
Marinescu CG: Concepţiile social-politice ale Profesorului Dr. E. I. Mironescu (II). **Rev Med Chir Soc Med Nat Iasi** 1979 Jan–Mar;83(1):159–62
Marinescu CG, Stratone M, Teodorovici G: Contributia unor medici la lupta pentru făurirea statului national unitar român. **Rev Med Chir Soc Med Nat Iasi** 1979 Jan–Mar;83(1):155–8
Marinescu CG, Stratone N: Contributii ale unor medici ieseni la promovarea gîndirii democratice si progresiste în perioada interbelică. **Rev Med Chir Soc Med Nat Iasi** 1979 Apr–Jun;83(2):341–5
Popushoĭ EP, Ioksa VA: N. P. Zubku-Kodrianu--progressivnyĭ vrach, vidnyĭ uchastnik revoliutsionno-demokraticheskogo dvizheniia. **Sov Zdravookhr** 1979;(3):59–63
Popushoĭ VP, Spineĭ LV: Viktor Krésesku--vrach, revoliutsioner, pisatel'. **Sov Zdravookhr** 1981;(5):62–4
Tudor C: Răscoala de la 1888. **Rev Arhiv** 1978;40(3):348–9

**South Africa**

Appelgryn MS: Die siektetoestand en laaste dae van president T. F. Burgers. **Kleio (S Afr)** 1980;12(1–2):18–31
Gutsche T: There was a man. The life and times of Sir Arnold Theiler K.C.M.G. of Onderstepoort. Cape Town, Timmins, 1979. 487 p.
Marks S, Andersson N: Epidemics and social control in twentieth-century South Africa. **Soc Soc Hist Med Bull (Lond)** 1984 Jun;34:32–4
Retief FP: President J. H. Brand en sy siekte-geskiedenis. **S Afr Med J** 1981 Mar 14;59(11):384–6

**Spain**

Aragon F: La politica cientifica en la España del s. XVIII a traves de la revista 'Anales de Ciencias Naturales', Madrid, 1799–1804. **Llull (Spain)** 1978;2:19–25
Espinosa Iborra J: El enfermo mental al final del Antiguo Régimen. **Asclepio** 1983;35:277–85
Esteva de Sagrera J: La farmacia española frente al cambio político. Barcelona, Ketres, 1978. 102 p.
García Guerra D: La asistencia médica en el Hospital Real de Santiago al final del Antiguo Régimen. **Asclepio** 1983;35:287–300
Javier Puerto F: Pedro Calvo Asensio (1821–1863): farmaceutico liberal. **Bol Soc Esp Hist Farm** 1983;34(136):203–28
Jordi González FR: Notas legislativas sobre los estatutos de autonomia catalanes 1932/1979. **Circ Farm** 1979 Oct;11(119):19–27
Jordi González R: Contribución para el estudio sociológico de la farmacia barcelonesa durante la guerra civil, a través de la prensa política. **Circ Farm** 1984;282:55–62
Jordi González R: Contribución para el estudio sociológico de la Farmacia barcelonesa durante la guerra civil, a través de la prensa política. (pt. I–VI). **Circ Farm** 1981–82 Dec, Jan, Feb, Mar, Jun, Sep;12–13:145–52
Mas i Perera P: Tribut al Doctor Domènec Martí i Julià. **Xaloc** 1972;56:182–5
Puerto Sarmiento FJ: Andrés Alcón (1782–1850), farmacéutico, político y profesor de Química. **Bol Soc Esp Hist Farm** 1984 Sep;35(139):143–64
Shapiro MF: Medical aid to the Spanish Republic during the Civil War (1936–1939). **Ann Intern Med** 1982 Jul;97(1):119–24
Strubell M, ed: Trueta: surgeon in war and peace. The memoirs of Joep Trueta. London, Gollancz, 1980. 288 p.

**Switzerland**

Buess H, Portmann ML: Berühmte Schweizer Arzte. **Gesnerus** 1980;37(3/4):289–306
Gautier A: Heurs et malheurs politiques d'une loi fédérale sur les épidémies. **Rev Med Suisse Romande** 1980 Dec;100(12):1061–2
Lang K: Kritiker, Ketzer, Kämpfer: das Leben des Arbeiterarztes Fritz Brupbacher. Zürich, Limmat, 1983. 360 p.
Müller C: Historische Vignette. August Forel und der Nationalsozialismus. **Nervenarzt** 1984 Sep;55(9):504–5
Scalabrin HR: Heinrich Ludwig Attenhofer, 1783–1856. Arzt und Politiker. Zürich, Juris Druck, 1983. 67 p. (Zürcher Medizingeschichtliche Abhhandlungen, Neue Reihe, Nr. 158).

**Tunisia**

Gallagher NE: Medicine and power in Tunisia, 1780–1900. Cambridge; New York, Cambridge University Press, 1983. xii, 145 p.

**United States**

Adler S: The operation on President McKinley. In Plesur M, ed.: An American Historian: essays to honor Selig Adler (Buffalo: State U. of N.Y., 1980): 37–49.
Altenstetter C, Bjorkman JW: Federal-state health policies and impacts: the politics of implementation. Washington, University Press of America, 1978. xi, 116 p.
Arseneau JC, Thigpen JT: The new quack--pseudoscience, public relations and politics. **J Miss State Med Assoc** 1981 Aug;22(8):202–7
Baird ND: Luke Pryor Blackburn: physician, governor, reformer. Lexington, University Press of Kentucky, 1979. viii, 127 p.
Bakan D: Politics and American psychology. In R. W. Rieber, K. Salzinger, ed: Psychology: theoretical-historical perspectives. New York, Academic Press, 1980. p. 125–44.
Banta HD, Burns AK, Behney CJ: Policy implications of the diffusion and control of medical technology. **Ann Am Acad Polit Soc Sci** 1983;(468):165–81
Barber D: Secret operation on US president. **Probe (Lond)** 1982 May;23(11):415–6
Beatty WK: Charles Volney Dyer: physician, promoter, and abolitionist. **Proc Inst Med Chic** 1982 Apr–Jun;35(2):45–8
Beatty WK: Levi Day Boone--Physician and politician. **Proc Inst Med Chic** 1980 Oct–Dec;33(4):139–41
Behn RD, Sperduto K: Medical Schools and the 'entitlement ethic'. **Public Interest** 1979;57:48–68
Benison S: Ideology über alles: an essay review. **J Hist Med Allied Sci** 1982 Jan;37(1)83–90
Bennett DH: Francis Everett Townsend. In Dictionary of American Biography, Suppl. 6, 1956–1960. p. 645–7, 1980.
Berkowitz E, McQuaid K: Welfare reform in the 1950s. **Soc Serv Rev** 1980 Mar;54(1):45–58
Berkowitz ED: The historian as policy analyst: the challenge of HEW. **Public Hist** 1979;1(3):17–25
Berkowitz ED: The politics of mental retardation during the Kennedy Administration. **Soc Sci Q** 1980;61(1):128–43
Bernstein BJ: The swine flu vaccination campaign of 1976: politics, science, and the public. **Congr Pres J Cap Stud** 1983;10(1):95–103
Blake JB: Medicine and the Revolution. **Milit Med** 1984 Apr;149(4):189–95
Blakeley PR: Francis Green: 'a suffering loyalist and friend to the British government. **NS Hist Q** 1979;9(1):1–14
Bollet AJ: Wounded presidents: 1981 almost repeats the events of 1881. **Med Times** 1981 Jul;109(7):19–23
Boor M: Effects of United States presidential elections on suicide and other causes of death. **Am Sociol Rev** 1981;46(5):616–8
Bradley JP: Shaping administrative policy with the aid of congressional oversight: the Senate Finance Committee and Medicare. **West Polit Q** 1980;33(4):492–501
Brandt AM: Polio, politics, publicity, and duplicity: ethical aspects in the development of the Salk vaccine. **Conn Med** 1979 Sep;43(9):581–7, 589–90
Brooks JJ, Enterline HT, Aponte GE: The final diagnosis of President Cleveland's lesion. **Trans Stud Coll Physicians Phila** 1980 Mar;(2 no 1):1–25
Brown ER: Rockefeller medicine men. Medicine and capitalism in America. Berkeley, University of California Press, 1979. xii, 283 p.
Brown LD: Competition and health care policy: experience and expectations. **Ann Am Acad Polit Soc Sci** 1983;(468):48–59
Cahow CR: People, patients and politics: the history of the North Carolina mental hospitals, 1848–1960. New York, Arno Press, 1980. vii, 254 p (Ph.D. Diss., Duke University, 1967).
Caravati CM: President Andrew Jackson: despite infirmities, a strong leader. **Va Med** 1983 Mar;110(3):194–5
Carson SL: Presidential children: abandonment, hysteria and suicide. **J Psychohist** 1984 Spring;11(4):533–44
Cash P: An analysis of the social, political and professional impact of the Revolution upon the Boston medical community. (1759–1789). In: Congrès international d'histoire de la médecine, XXVe, Québec, 1976. Actes. Québec, 1977. p. 546–59.
Cash P: Pride, prejudice and politics. **Harv Med Alumni Bull** 1980 Dec;54(6):20–5
Cavanaugh G: The corruptions of science. **Dissent** 1981;28(2):195–202
A chronology of health legislation in the U.S., 1798–1983: **Conn Med** 1984 Apr;48(4):251–7
Clarke JW: American assassins: an alternative typology. **Br J Polit Sci** 1981;11(1):81–104
Corning ME: A review of the United States role in international biomedical research and communications: international health and foreign policy. Bethesda, National Library of Medicine, 1980. xxvii, 436 p. (NIH Publication No. 80–1638).
Coulter HL: Divided legacy: the conflict between homoeopathy and the

American Medical Association. Science and ethics in American medicine 1800–1914. 2d ed. Richmond, California, North Atlantic Books, 1982. 552 p.
Cowen DL, Helfand WH: The Progressive Movement and its impact on pharmacy. **Pharm Acta Helv** 1979;(11):1–6
Cowen DL, Helfand WH: The progressive movement and its impact on pharmacy. **Pharm Acta Helv** 1979;54(11):317–23
Crawford R: Individual responsibility and health politics in the 1970s. In Reverby S, Rosner D, ed: Health care in America. Philadelphia, Temple University PRess, 1979. p. 247–68.
Cross W, Moses J: 'My God, sir, I think the president is doomed!' [Grover Cleveland's cancer surgery] **Am Hist Illus** 1982 Nov;17:40–5
Curran DJ: Symbolic solutions for deadly dilemmas: an analysis of federal coal mine health and safety legislation. **Int J Health Serv** 1984;14(1):5–29
Davis C: Hazardous waste politics and policy. **Policy Stud J** 1983;12(1):171–4
Delaney JJ: Hubert Work. **Colo Med** 1983 Oct;80(10):285–6
deMause L: The making of a fearful leader: 'Where's the rest of me?' **J Psychohist** 1984 Summer;12(1):5–21
Downing PB: Bargaining in pollution control. **Policy Stud J** 1983;11(4):577–86
Duffy S: The origin of speeches: Inherit the Wind, Irving Stone and the Scopes trial. **Am Notes Queries** 1983 Sep–Oct;22(1–2):14–7
Dupree AH: The rise and fall of the American establishment. **Minerva** 1984 Spring;22(1):116–24
Dusseau JL: Tertium Quid: a third something in a muddied puzzle. **Perspect Biol Med** 1982 Winter;25(2):238–53
Ewalt DJ: Patients, politics and physicians: the struggle for control of State Lunatic Asylum No. 1, Fulton, Missouri. **Mo Hist Rev** 1983 Jan;77:170–88
Fink L, Greenberg B: Organizing Montefiore: labor militancy meets a progressive health care empire. In Reverby S, Rosner D, ed: Health care in America. Philadelphia, Temple University Press, 1979. p. 226–44.
Fox DM, Stone JF: Black lung: miners' militancy and medical uncertainty, 1968–1972. **Bull Hist Med** 1980 Spring;54(1):43–63
Francome C: Abortion politics in the United States. **Polit Stud** 1980;28(4):613–21
Freud S, Bullitt WC: Thomas Woodrow Wilson, twenty-eighth President of the United States: a psychological study. Boston, Houghton Mifflin; and Cambridge, Riverside, 1967. 307 p.
Fries SD: The ideology of science during the Nixon years: 1970–76. **Soc Stud Sci** 1984 Aug;14(3):323–41
Galishoff S: Germs know no color line: black health and public policy in Atlanta, 1900–1918. **J Hist Med Allied Sci** 1985 Jan;40(1):22–41
Gallagher HG: FDR: handicapped American. **Public Welf** 1984 Spring;42(2):6–18
Gambill J: Potential problems of detecting and treating psychosis in the White House. Potential psychosis in the White House. **Int J Soc Psychiatry** 1980;26(4):255–62
Garbelotto N: Teoria e politica nella psicosociologia di E. Mayo. **Stor Crit Psicol** 1980;1(1):61–78
Giglio JN: Voluntarism and public policy between World War I and the New Deal: Herbert Hoover and the American Child Health Association. **Pres Stud Q** 1983;13(3):430–52
Green E: U. S. population policies, development, and the rural poor of Africa. **J Mod Afr Stud** 1982;20(1):45–67
Green HP: The recombinant DNA controversy: a model of public influence. **Bull At Sci** 1978;34(9):12–16
Grob GN, ed: Narcotic addiction and American foreign policy: seven studies, 1924–1938. New York, Arno Press, 1981. 276 p. in various pagings. (Reprinted works).
Has the Republic no need of learning?: **J Hist Med Allied Sci** 1981 Jul;36(3):257–9
Hasson GS: The medical activities of the Freedmen's Bureau in Reconstruction Alabama, 1865–1868. Ph.D. Diss, University of Alabama, University, 1982. 252 p.
Henderson P: Psychohistorical perspectives on the presidency. **Mich J Polit Sci** 1981;1(1):1–11
Hershkowitz L: Powdered tin and rose petals: Myer Myers, Goldsmith, and Peter Middleton, physician. **Am Jew Hist** 1981;70(4):462–7
Hess BB: The politics of aging. **Society** 1978;15(5):22–3
Hill D: The politics of schizophrenia: psychiatric oppression in the United States. Lanham, MD, University Press of America, 1983. xii, 577 p.
Hine WC: Dr. Benjamin A. Boseman, Jr.: Charleston's black physician-politician. In Rabinowitz HN, ed: Southern Black leaders of the reconstruction era. Urbana, University of Illinois Press, 1982. p. 335–62.
Hirsch HN: Clio on the couch. **World Polit** 1980;32(3):406–24
Huch RK: 'Typhoid' Truelsen, water and politics in Duluth, 1896–1900. **Minn Hist** 1981;47(5):189–99
Isacsson A: A study of Louis J. Weichmann. **Lincoln Her** 1978;80(1):25–38
Jameson MG: Physicians and American political leadership. **JAMA** 1983 Feb 18;249(7):929–30
Johnson JP: Herbert Hoover: the orphan as children's friend. **Prologue J Nat Arch** 1980;12(4):193–206
Jones DP: American chemists and the Geneva protocol. **Isis** 1980 Sep;71(258):426–40
Katsnel'bogen AG: Dekabristy i peredovaia meditsinskaia obshchestvennost' Rossii. **Sov Zdravookhr** 1980;(10):51–5
Keigher SM: Reagan's 'New' federalism and the 1971 California Medi-cal reforms. **Urban Soc Change Rev** 1983;16(2):3–8
Kopp C: The origins of the American Scientific debate over fallout hazards. **Soc Stud Sci** 1979;9(4):403–22
Landon SJ: Giants of Paumanok. **York State Tradit** 1972;26(3):24–6, 48–54, 56, 64
Leavitt JW: Politics and public health: small pox in Milwaukee, 1894–1895. In Reverby S, Rosner D, ed: Health care in America. Philadephia, Temple University Press, 1979. p. 84–101.
Leavitt JW: The healthiest city: Milwaukee and the politics of health reform. Princeton, Princeton University Press, 1982. xvii, 294 p.
Lee PR, Estes CL: New federalism and health policy. **Ann Am Acad Polit Soc Sci** 1983;(468):88–102
Lester JP, Franke JL, Bowman AO, et al: Hazardous wastes, politics, and public policy: a comparative state analysis. **West Polit Q** 1983;36(2):257–85
Litman RC, Litman DS: Protection of the American consumer: the congressional battle for the enactment of the First Federal Food and Drug Law in the United States. **Food Drug Cosmet Law J** 1982 Jul;37(3):310–29
Maddox RF: The politics of World War II science: Senator Harley M. Kilgore and the legislative origins of the National Science Foundation. **W Va Hist** 1979;41(1):20–39
Marcus AI: Professional revolution and reform in the Progressive era: Cincinnati physicians and the city elections of 1897 and 1900. **J Urban Hist** 1979;5(2):183–208
Marcus AI: The strange career of municipal health initiatives: Cincinnati and city government in the early nineteenth century. **J Urban Hist** 1980;7(1):3–29
Margolis M, Neary K: Pressure politics revisited: the anti-abortion campaign. **Policy Stud J** 1980;8(5):698–716
Markle GE, Petersen JC, ed: Politics, science, and cancer: the laetrile phenomenon. Boulder, Westview Press, for the American Association for the Advancement of Science, 1980. xiii, 190 p. (AAAS Selected Symposium, v. 46). Contributions by JH Young, RD Smith, RF Rich, GP Monaco, Al Caplan, D Nelkin.
Markowitz GE, Rosner D: Doctors in crisis: medical education and medical reform during the Progressive era, 1895–1915. In Reverby S, Rosner D, ed: Health care in America. Philadelphia, Temple University Press, 1979. p. 185–205.
Massey EW: Dr. Samuel Mudd: justice at last. **South Med J** 1980 Oct;73(10):1375–6
Mevers FC, ed: The papers of Josiah Bartlett, Hanover, University Press of New England, for the New Hampshire Historical Society, 1979. xxxvii, 477 p.
Miller JM, Sakowski RA: Doctors and the Declaration of Independence. **Surg Gynecol Obstet** 1980 Jun;150(6):903–5
Morgan AH: Is there a doctor in the house? or for the house? **Rev Am Hist** 1980;8(1):129–33
Naske CM: Bob Bartlett and the Alaska Mental Health Act. **Pac Northwest Q** 1980;71(1):31–9
Navarro P: The politics of air pollution. **Public Interest** 1980;59:36–44
Olson GD: Dr. David Ramsay and Lt. Colonel Thomas Brown: patriot historian and loyalist critic. **SC Hist Mag** 1976;77:256–67
Peroff K, Podolak-Warren M: Does spending on defence cut spending on health? A time-series analysis of the U. S. economy 1929–74. **Br J Polit Sci** 1979;9(1):21–39
Petersen JC, Markle GE: Politics and science in the laetrile controversy. **Soc Stud Sci** 1979;9(2):139–66
Poen MM: Harry S. Truman versus the medical lobby. The genesis of Medicare. Columbia, London, University of Missouri Press, 1979. xii, 260 p.
Pond MA: Block grants for health: a brief history of presidential initiatives. **Health Policy Q** 1982 Fall-Winter;2(3–4):180–98
Pond MA: Presidential initiatives in organizing health affairs: from Harding to Roosevelt. **Pres Stud Q** 1983;13(3):417–29
Putney DT: Fighting the scourge: American Indian morbidity and federal policy, 1897–1928. Ph.D. Diss., Marquette University. Milwaukee, 1980. 355 leaves.
Robins RS, Rothschild H: Hidden health disabilities and the presidency: medical management and political consideration. **Perspect Biol Med** 1981 Winter;24(2):240–53
Rodgers BL: The great depression, 1929-1940: an era of reform. **Va Nurse** 1984 Spring;52(1):12–3
Rogers FA: The American Medical Association: yesterday, today and tomorrow. **J La State Med Soc** 1981 Sep;133(9):129–35
Rosner D: Gaining control: reform, reimbursement and politics in New York's community hospitals, 1890--1915. **Am J Public Health** 1980 May;70(5):533–42
Ruscio KP: A new regime in the republic of science. **Policy Stud Rev** 1983;2(4):790–4
Saffron MH: James Peter Warbasse. In Dictionary of American Biography, Suppl. 6, 1956–1960. p. 663–5, 1980.
Savitt TL: Politics in medicine: the Georgia Freedmen's Bureau and the organization of health care, 1865–1866. **Civ War Hist** 1982;28(1):45–64

# POLITICS


Scalettar R: Presidential candidate disability. **JAMA** 1984 Jun 1;251(21):2811

Spady JG: Dr. W. Montague Cobb: anatomist, physician, physical anthropologist, editor emeritus of the Journal of the National Medical Association, and first black president of NAACP. **J Natl Med Assoc** 1984 Jul;76(7):739–44

Starr P, Esping-Anderson G: Passive intervention. **Work Pap New Soc** 1979;7(2):15–25

Strauss MJ: The political history of the artificial heart. **N Engl J Med** 1984 Feb 2;310(5):332–6

Taylor RC: The politics of prevention. **Soc Policy** 1982;13(1):32–41

Vogel MJ: Machine politics and medical care: the city hospital at the turn of the century. In Vogel MJ, Rosenberg CE, ed: The therapeutic revolution. Philadelphia, 1979. p. 159–175.

Walker FA: Americanism versus Sovietism: a study of the reaction to the committee on the costs of medical care. **Bull Hist Med** 1979 Winter;53(4):489–504

Wasserman H, Solomon N, Alvarez R, et al: Killing our own: the disaster of America's experience with atomic radiation. New York, Dell, 1982. xiii, 368 p.

Weinstein EA: Woodrow Wilson: a medical and psychological biography. Princeton, Princeton University Press, 1981. xi, 399 p.

Whittet TD: Botanic garden of the trustees of the Georgia colony at Savannah. **Pharm J** 1983;231:770–1

Yankauer A: Refugees, immigrants, and the public health. **Am J Public Health** 1982 Jan;72(1):12–4

Young JH: Laetrile in historical perspective. In Markle GE, Petersen JC, ed: Politics, science and cancer: the laetrile phenomenon. Boulder, CO. Westview Press, for American Association for the Advancement of Science, Washington, D. C., 1980. p. 11–60.

Young JH: Public policy and drug innovation. **Pharm Hist** 1982;24(1):3–31

Young JH: 'This greasy counterfeit': butter versus oleomargarine in the United States Congress, 1886 (the Fielding H. Garrison Lecture). **Bull Hist Med** 1979 Fall;53(3):392–414


## USSR


Adams MB: Biology after Stalin: a case study. **Survey** 1977–78;23(1):53–80

Alekseev GA, Butsevitskiĭ VS, Galkina ND: Revoliutsionnaia deiatel'nost' vracha A.A. Buĭnovskogo. **Sov Zdravookhr** 1979;(8):54–5

Aleksentsev AI: Otchet o deiatel'nosti prodovol'stvennoi armii za pervyi god ee sushchestvovaniia. **Sov Arkh** 1981;5:33–8

Asratian EA, Shingarov GKh: Leninskaia teoriia otrazheniia i uchenie I. P. Pavlova o vyssheĭ nervnoĭ deiatel'nosti (k 110–i godovshchine so dnia rozhdeniia V. I. Lenina). **Zh Vyssh Nerv Deiat** 1980 Mar–Apr;30(2):227–34

Bazhan TA: Voprosy okhrany truda i zdorov'ia rabochikh v deiatel'nosti mestnykh komitetov RSDRP iuga Rossi (1898–1917). **Gig Sanit** 1979 Dec;(12):32–6

Berezhniak AP: Polirabotniki meditsinskikh chasteĭ i uchrezhdeniĭ v gody Velikoĭ Otechestvennoĭ voĭny. **Voen Med Zh** 1981 Sep;(9):70–1

Bergman A: Pobeg V. S. Mitskevicha-Kapsukasa iz suvalkskoi bol'nitsy v 1906 G. **Vopr Istor** 1965;(3):74–6

Brzheskiĭ VCh, Evdokimov PP: K istorii bolezni V.G. Belinskogo. **Klin Med (Mosk)** 1984 Aug;62(8):150–2

Cherkasov SV: Leninskoe uchenie ob istine i probleme kriterii praktiki v diagnostike. **Ter Arkh** 1980;52(7):146–40

Chokin AR, Ibragimov NG: Obshchestvenno-politicheskaia deiatel'nost' progressivnykh medikov dorevoliutsionnogo Kazakhstana i Bashkirii. **Sov Zdravookhr** 1981;(7):59–62

Ciucura TB: Dissent, law and psychiatry in the Soviet Union. **Can Slavonic Pap** 1979;21(1):98–108

Conquest R: Forced labour statistics: some comments. **Sov Stud** 1982;34(3):434–9

Elkin II: Leninskiĭ étap v razvitii épidemiologii. **Zh Mikrobiol Epidemiol Immunobiol** 1981 Jan;(1):3–8

Emeksuzian VS: A. P. Golubkov v sibirskoĭ ssylke. **Sov Zdravookhr** 1981;(11):59–62

Engel BA: Women medical students in Russia, 1872–1882: reformers or rebels? **J Soc Hist** 1979;12(3):394–415

Epifanov NS: I. K. Spizharnyĭ v Viatskoĭ ssylke (materialy biografii). **Sov Zdravookhr** 1983;(2):70–1

Evdokimov PP: Lechashchie vrachi sem'i I.N. Ul'ianova. **Sov Zdravookhr** 1980;(11):64–5

Evdokimov PP: Mediki, privlekaemye i sudimye po 'Delu 193–kh'. **Sov Zdravookhr** 1980;(6):61–3

Evdokimov PP: Uchastie studentov-medikov Kazani v revoliutsionnom dvizhenii 1870–1880 gg. **Sov Zdravookhr** 1981;(1):60–2

Fel' II, Truman GL: A. M. Aliev--vydaiushchiĭsia pertiĭnyĭ, gosudarstvennyĭ deiatel', organizator zdravookhraneniia i meditsinskoĭ nauki v Sovetskom Azerbaĭdzhane. **Sov Zdravookhr** 1982;(8):57–9

Frieden NM: Russian physicians in an era of reform and revolution, 1856-1905. Princeton, Princeton University Press, 1981. xvii, 378 p.

Furmanchuk VM: Uchastie rabochikh sester i sanitarok v Oktiabr'skoĭ revoliutsii. **Med Sestra** 1982 Apr;41(4):49–51

Gavrilov OK: Meditsinskaia nauka k 60–ĭ godoshchine obrazovaniia Soiuza Sovetskikh Sotsialisticheskikh Respublik. **Sov Zdravookhr** 1982;(8):3–8

Gel'fman AA: Fel'dshera–iskrovtsy v revoliutsionnom dvizhenii. **Feldsher Akush** 1984 Apr;49(4):49–50

Grando AA, Kogan Via: Rol' Narkomzdrava RSFSR v stanovlenii zdravookhraneniia Sovetskoĭ Ukrainy. **Sov Zdravookhr** 1983;9:55–7

Green D: The Medvedev experience: 1984 and medicine. **Perspect Biol Med** 1976 Autumn;20(1):145–55

Gurvich KI: Uchastiie meditsinskikh rabotnikov v revoliutsionnom dvizhenii v Rossii XIX- nachala XX veka. **Vopr Istor** 1972;4:203–6

Hutchinson JF: Science, politics, and the alcohol problem in post-1905 Russia. **Slav East Eur Rev** 1980;58(2):232–54

Ianovskiĭ AG: Fel'dshera i akusherki v revoliutsii 1905-1907 gg. **Feldsher Akush** 1980;45(11):41–4

Ibragimov NG: Sanitarnyĭ aktiv Bashkirii v pervye desiatiletiia Sovetskoĭ vlasti. **Sov Zdravookhr** 1980;(7):56–60

Idel'chik KhI: Vrachi–bol'sheviki S. I. Mitskevich i S. I. Chernomordik u istokov Tsentral'nogo muzeia revoliutsii SSSR (k 60–letiiu muzeia). **Sov Zdravookhr** 1984;(9):56–9

Jack DB: Dastardly deeds at Dorpat. **Pharm Hist (London)** 1984 Sep;14(3):9–12

Johanson C: Autocratic politics, public opinion, and women's medical education during the reign of Alexander II, 1855–1881. **Slavic Rev** 1979;38(3):426–43

Katsnel'bogen AG: Dekabristy i obshcestvennaia meditsina. **Sov Zdravookhr** 1979;(12):47–51

Katsnel'bogen AG: Doktor N. V. Maĭer i dekabristy. **Sov Zdravookhr** 1980;(8):59–62

Katsnel'bogen AG: M. Ia. Mudrov i voprosy vrachebnoĭ étiki. **Sov Zdravookhr** 1983;(10):58–61

Katsnel'bogen AG: Meditsinskaia zapiska dekabrista A. O. Kornilovicha. **Sov Zdravookhr** 1981;(11):62–4

Katsnel'bogen AG: Neizuchennyĭ dokument dekabristov. **Sov Zdravookhr** 1980;(7):60–1

Katsnel'bogen AG: Obshchestvenno–politicheskaia deiatel'nost' vracha–dekabrista F. B. Vol'fa. **Sov Zdravookhr** 1981;(1):66–70

Katsnel'bogen AG: Vrachi–dekabristy. **Klin Med (Mosk)** 1980 Apr;58(4):107–10

Knel'ts VF: Revoliutsionnaia deiatel'nost' medikov Udmurtii v 1905–1907 gg. **Feldsher Akush** 1982;47(11):32–3

Knel'ts VF: Uchastie zemskikh vracheĭ Udmurtii v revoliutsionnom dvizhenii 1905–1907 gg. **Sov Zdravookhr** 1982;(6):64–6

Kokhan AI: Mediki–uzniki Petropavlovskoĭ kreposti. **Sov Zdravookhr** 1979;(12):52–5

Kozubenko ID: Partĭnye organizatsii Dona vo glave razvitiia zdravookhraneniia v 1923–1924 gg. **Sov Zdravookhr** 1982;(6):56–9

Krasil'shchikov MI, Kulish EA, Rumer LZ, et al: Tsentral'naia pechat' v propagande meditsinskikh i gigienicheskikh znaniĭ (1921–1932). **Sov Zdravookhr** 1983;(10):53–5

Leninskie printsipy v rabote oftal'mologov: **Vestn Oftalmol** 1980 May–Jun;(3):3–5

Leonov IT: Bol'sheviki–lenintsy--vospitanniki Voenno–meditsinskoĭ akademii. **Voen Med Zh** 1984 Oct;(10):62–5

Levitin MN: Stoĭkiĭ bol'shevik–leninets A. P. Golubkov. **Feldsher Akush** 1980;45(11):44–6

Malozemova AI: Revoliutsionery–mediki Pribylevy. **Sov Zdravookhr** 1984;(8):62–5

Malozemova AI: Uchastie meditsinskikh rabotnikov v 'Politicheskom Krasnom Kreste 'Nardonoĭ voli'. **Sov Zdravookhr** 1984;(4):59–63

Malozemova AI: Zhenshchiny–mediki v politicheskikh protsessakh 1881 g. (k 100–letiiu protsessov). **Sov Zdravookhr** 1981;(7):54–9

Manafov IT: N. Narimanov--vrach, revoliutsioner, partiĭnyi ĭ gosudarstvennyĭ deiatel'. **Sov Zdravookhr** 1982;(4):58–61

Merman MM: Za kommunisticheskoe otnoshenie k zdorov'iu i trudu. **Feldsher Akush** 1983 Oct;48(10):3–8

Morogues IM de: N. S. Leskov: premieres polemiques. janvier 1860–mai 1862. **Cah Monde Russe Sovietique** 1982;23(2):243–55

Osipov EO: Kommunisticheskaia Partiia na strazhe zdorov'ia trudiashchikhsia (k 80–letiiu II s'ezda RSDRP). **Sov Med** 1983;8:8–12

Paul DB: A war on two fronts: J. B. S. Haldane and the response to lysenkoism in Britain. **J Hist Biol** 1983 Spring;16(1):1–37

Podolyan VY: Development of medico–geographical ideas in the epoch of the developed socialism and scientific and technological progress. **Geogr Med** 1984;14:284–93

Popushoĭ EP, Ioksa VA: Progressivnaia rol' vracha–revoliutsionera P. P. Tutyshkina v razvitii nauchnoĭ mysli v Moldavii. **Sov Zdravookhr** 1984;(4):69–71

Potulov BM: Leninskie zavety meditsinskim rabotnikam. **Voen Med Zh** 1980 Jan;(1):11–4

Potulov BM: V. I. Lenin o sotsial'noĭ obuslovlennosti zdorov'ia i zdravookhraneniia. **Sov Zdravookhr** 1984;(4):3–10

Potulov BM: Voprosy bor'by s épidemiiami v trudakh V. I. Lenina. **Zh Mikrobiol Epidemiol Immunobiol** 1980 Apr;(4):3–9

Potulov BM: Vrach–bol'shevik (k 110–ĭ godovshchine so dnia rozhdeniia D.I. Ul'ianova). **Voen Med Zh** 1984 Aug;(8):69–70

Prokop M: Pro vorkutu, holod ta problemy samooborony narodu. **Sucasnist** 1980;(3):48–56

Reich W: The case of General Grigorenko: a psychiatric reexamination of a Soviet dissident. **Psychiatry** 1980 Nov;43(4):303–23

Reich W: The case of General Grigorenko: a second opinion. **Encounter (Lond)** 1980;54(4):9-24
Rodionov AV: O partiĭno-politicheskoĭ rabote sredi ranenykh i meditsinskogo personala vo vremia Kurskoĭ bitvy. **Voen Med Zh** 1984 Aug;(8):11-5
Ryzhakova GI: Itogi vypolneniia direktiv Dal'kraĭkoma VKP(b) po stroitel'stvu ob'ektov zdravookhraneniia v gody pervykh piatiletok (1928-1937). **Sov Zdravookhr** 1982;(8):55-7
Schtschepin OP, Wladimirova LJ: Die Zusammenarbeit der UdSSR mit den anderen sozialistischen Ländern auf dem Gebiet der medizinischen Wissenschaft und des Gesundheitswesens. **Med Ges** 1979;(6):123-39
Shalaev NF: Uchastie studentov Voenno-meditsinskoĭ akademii v revoliutsii 1905-1907 gg. **Sov Zdravookhr** 1980;(8):53-6
Shaternikov VA, Konyshev VA: 50-ia godovshchina pervogo piatiletnego plana razvitiia narodnogo khoziaĭstva SSSR i nauka o pitanii v nasheĭ strane. **Vopr Pitan** 1979 Sep-Oct;(5):3-7
Shengeliia MS: Georgievskiĭ traktat i istoriia russko-gruzinskikh vzaimootnosheniĭ v oblasti meditsiny. **Sov Zdravookhr** 1984;(3):54-5
Shliapak AE: Partiĭno-politicheskaia rabota v ĕvakogospitaliakh Kavkazskikh Mineral'nykh Vod. **Voen Med Zh** 1981 Nov;(11):69-70
Skachilov VA: S. Ia. Elpat'evskiĭ v Ufimskoĭ ssylke. **Sov Zdravookhr** 1980;(8):56-9
Stegunin SI, Palagin DA, Veselova AM: Bor'ba Samarskikh bol'shevikov za okhranu zdorov'ia trudiashchikhsia v 1921-1922 gg. **Sov Zdravookhr** 1984;(5):61-4
Tepun PD: Deiatel'nost' partiĭnykh organizatsiĭ i naseleniia Severnogo Kavkaza po okazaniiu pomoshchi ranenym v gody Velikoĭ Otechestvennoĭ voĭny. **Sov Zdravookhr** 1980;(5):61-3
Tikotin MA: Peterburgskiĭ zhenskiĭ meditsinskiĭ institut v revoliutsionnom dvizhenii. **Sov Zdravookhr** 1981;(7):51-4
Tiukina AP: S. A. Nikonov--vrach-revoliutsioner. **Sov Zdravookhr** 1984;(10):64-7
Todes DP: Biological psychology and the Tsarist censor: the dilemma of scientific development. **Bull Hist Med** 1984 Winter;58(4):529-44
Tsaregorodtsev GI, Anokhin AM: V. I Lenin i problemy okhrany zdorov'ia cheloveka v razvitom sotsialisticheskom obshchestve. **Ter Arkh** 1980;52(4):3-7
Vasil'ev KG, Vasil'ev KK: Vrach-revoliutsioner V. L. Elin. **Sov Zdravookhr** 1983;(8):57-8
Viduta VK: Studenty-mediki v Tartuskom (Iur'evskom) Marksistskom kruzhke. **Sov Zdravookhr** 1983;(10):55-7
Viduta VK: Tobol'skaia fel'dsherskaia shkola i ee rol' v formirovanii revoliutsionerov. **Sov Zdravookhr** 1984;(8):57-9
Vovk IG: Meropriiatiia KPSS po razvitiiu nardonogo zdravookhraneniia v predvoennye gody. **Voen Med Zh** 1980 Jun;(6):18-20
Weiner DR: Community ecology in Stalin's Russia: 'socialist' and 'bourgeois' science. **ISIS** 1984 Dec;75(279):684-96
Weinrib A: Zikhronot shel rofe migetto Vilna. **Yalkut Moreshet Period** 1979;(27):7-60
Wheatcroft SG: Doctors and the Revolution in Russia. **Soc Soc Hist Med Bull (Lond)** 1984 Jun;34:19-24
Wyziembło M: Losy polaków ... **Zesz Hist** 1974;(30):16-23
Yaremovich AJ: Collectivization through famine. **Ukr Q** 1978;34(4):349-62

#### Venezuela

Alegría C: Dos medicos en la aurora de la gesta emancipadora de Venezuela. **Rev Soc Venez Hist Med** 1969-71;17-19(31-33):29-48
Grisanti A: La medicina, libertada por el libertador. **Rev Soc Venez Hist Med** 1972-73;20-21(34-35):203-5
Silva Alvarez A: Ensayo patobiografico sobre el Dr. Juan Pablo Rojas Paúl. **Bol Acad Nac Hist (Caracas)** 1981;64(256):859-68

#### Yugoslavia

Tartalja H: Mouvement social des pharmaciens en Croatie. **Orvostort Kozl** 1982;28(1-3):187-90

## PORTRAITS

Glowatzki G: Der Mesmerismus--und seine Spuren in der heutigen Medizin. **ZFA (Stuttgart)** 1983 Sep 10;59(25):1360-6
Lipscomb JM: New light on some Harvey portraits, in memoriam Sir Geoffrey Keynes. **Med Hist** 1983 Apr;27(2):197-202

#### Germany

Benedum J, Giese C: Die Professoren der Medizin in der giessener Gemäldegalerie. Giessen, Schmitz, 1983. 230 p. (Arbeiten zur Geschichte der Medizin in Giessen, Bd. 5)
Graepel PH: Die Calwer Apothekerfamilie Gärtner im Bild. **Beitr Gesch Pharm** 1981;31(12):92-5

#### Great Britain

Gibson T: The Royal College of Physicians and Surgeons of Glasgow: a short history based on the portraits and other memorabilia. Edinburgh, Macdonald Publishers, 1983. 301 p.
Sakula A: The Betchworth Portraits: members of the family of William Harvey. **Med Hist** 1980 Jul;24(3):333-41

### Before 500 A.D.

#### Rome

Klawans HL: The acromegaly of Maximinus I: the possible influence of a pituitary tumor on the life and death of a Roman emperor. In Rose FC, Bynum WF, ed: Historical aspects of the neurosciences. New York, Raven, 1982. 317-26.

### 500 A.D.-1450

#### Arabic

Brandenburg D: Das Portrait des Ibn Sînâ (Avicenna). **Med Welt** 1983 Jun 10;34(23):682-4

### 1450-1700

#### Czechoslovakia

Wondrák E: Drei Bilder eines Arztes des 16. Jahrhunderts. **Medizinhist J** 1983;18(3):250-55

#### France

Rudolph G: Iconographie de La Mettrie (1709-1751) à propos de la découverte d'un portrait inconnu du médecin et philosophe breton. In: Congrès National des Sociétés Savantes, 91e, Rennes, 1966. Comptes Rendus. Paris, 1967. Section des Sciences. Tome 1, p. 171-9.
Schiller N: L'iconographie de Claude Perrault (1613-1688). In: Congrès National des Sociétés Savantes, 91e, Rennes, 1966. Comptes Rendus. Paris, 1967. Section des Sciences, Tome 1. p. 217-34.

#### Germany

Schnelbögl F: Auerbacher Lebensbilder. Zum 500. Geburtsjahr Heinrich Stromers, genannt Auerbach. **Altnurnb Landsch** 1976;25(Sonderh. 1):1-26

#### Great Britain

Morris GC: A portrait of Thomas Hollier, Pepy's surgeon. **Ann R Coll Surg Engl** 1979 May;61(3):224-9

### 1700 to Present

Böhme G: Medizinische Porträts berühmter Komponisten: Wolfgang Amadeus Mozart, Ludwig van Beethoven, Carl Maria von Weber, Frédéric Chopin, Peter Iljitsch Tschaikowski, Béla Bartók. 2. verbesserte und erweiterte Auflage. Stuttgart, New York, Gustav Fischer Verlag, 1981. xi, 199 p.
Chen KK: Two pharmacological traditions: notes from experience. **Annu Rev Pharmacol Toxicol** 1981;21:1-6
Kottek SS: 'Andre Vesale'. Some remarks on a painting by E. J. C. Hamman. **Koroth** 1982 Aug;8(3/4):135-43

#### France

Schiller N: Henri Dutrochet contributions biographiques et iconographiques. In: Congrès National des Sociétés Savantes, 97e, Nantes, 1972. Comptes Rendus. Paris, 1976. Section des Sciences, Tome 1. p. 71-82.

#### Germany

Heintel H: Ein unbekanntes Porträt des Hirnforschers Oskar Vogt (1870-1959). **Medizinhist J** 1984;19(3):277-9
Rosler HP: Samuel Thomas von Soemmerring (1755-1830), Aquarell, gemalt 1794 von seiner Frau Margarethe Elisabeth, geb. Grunelius (1768-1802), Grösse des Bildovals 12,8 cm (Höhe): 11,5 cm (Breite) (Privatbesitz). **Medizinhist J** 1980;15(4):422-5
Schulze W: Conrad Felixmüller 1897 - 1977--ein Maler der Tierärzte. **Hist Med Vet** 1977;2(2):51-5
Winau R, Vaubel E: Chirurgen in Berlin. 100 Porträts. Berlin, New York, Walter de Gruyter, 1983. 106 p.

#### Great Britain

Cornforth J: Portrait of Dorothy Hodgkin, O.M., F.R.S. **Notes Rec R Soc Lond** 1982 Aug;37(1):1-4
[Pigalle's bust of Dr. Maloët acquired by Fitzwilliam Museum, Cambridge, 1979.]: **Burlington Mag** 1980 Jan;122:83
Sakula A: Baroness Burdett-Coutts' garden party: the International Medical Congress, London, 1881. **Med Hist** 1982 Apr;26(2):183-90

## PORTRAITS

Swain VA: Some portraits of Sir Thomas Spencer Wells (1818–1897). **Ann R Coll Surg Engl** 1983 May;65(3):201–2

**Italy**

Gamba A: Un ritratto inedito di Giambattista Morgagni. **Acta Med Hist Patav** 1982–83;29:67–74

**United States**

Bonsett CA: Medical museum notes. **J Indiana State Med Assoc** 1981 Dec;74(12):770

**Venezuela**

Vélez Boza F: Discurso pronunciado con motivo de la colocacion del retrato del Dr. Jesus Sanabria Bruzual en el salon de sesiones de la Sociedad Venezolana de Historia de la Medicina, el 12 de julio de 1978. **Rev Soc Venez Hist Med** 1980;29(43–44):63–71

## PREVENTIVE MEDICINE

See also **Immunology; Public Health; Health Education; Hygiene; Sanitation**

Reverzy JF: La biocratie. Esquisse d'une histoire de la notion de prévention en médecine et en psychiatrie en Occident. **Soins Psychiatr** 1982 Feb;(16):27–35

**Africa**

Gelfand M: African customs in relation to preventive medicine. **Cent Afr J Med** 1981 Jan;27(1):1–8

**France**

Malterre-Barthes A: Un service bien particulier: les dispensaires antivénériens. **Soins Gynecol Obstet Pueric** 1981 Sep;(6):37–46

**Before 500 A.D.**

Häusermann R, Koelbing H, Biener K: Präventivmedizin in den alten Religionen. **Soz Praventivmed** 1984;29(2):72–7

**500 A.D.–1450**

**Arabic**

Aroua A: L'hygiène et la prevention chez Ibn Sina. **Tunis Med** 1980 Jul–Aug;58(4):556–61

**1700 to Present**

Forum: the place of prevention in medical education: past, present, and future: **Prev Med** 1981 Nov;10(6):661–740

Howard-Jones N: Prelude to modern preventive medicine. In Stanley NF, Joske RA, ed: Changing disease patterns and human behaviour. London, New York, Academic Press, 1980. p. 69–80.

Hunstadbråten K: Fluor in der Kariesprophylaxe der Jahrhundertwende. **Quintessenz J** 1984 Feb;14(2):147–51

Krister CJ: Safety evaluation ... it ain't all science. **Vet Hum Toxicol** 1980 Jun;22(3):156–9

**Canada**

Gaucher D: La formation des hygiénistes à l'Université de Montréal, 1910–1975: de la santé publique à la médecine préventive. **Rech Sociogr** 1979;20(1):59–85

Reid D: De la médecine traditionnelle à la médecine préventive: analyse des réformes de santé au Québec. **Union Med Can** 1980 May;109(5):774–7

**Czechoslovakia**

Kukura J: Preventívne disciplíny na lekárskej fakulte Univerzity Komenského v Bratislave za roky 1919–1979. **Cas Lek Cesk** 1979 Dec 21;118(51):1588–92

**France**

Hommage au professeur Armand Delachaux à l'occasion de son 70e anniversaire: **Soz Praventivmed** 1982 May;27(2–3):59–67

**Germany**

Dittmann S, Paulenz H, Scheel G, et al: 30 Jahre Staatliche Hygieneinspektion der DDR. **Z Gesamte Hyg** 1983 Oct;29(10):584–8

Kaiser W, Völker A: Hygiene, Präventiv, und Unfallmedizin in den Schriften des halleschen Ordinarius Johann Heinrich Schulze (1687–1744). **Z Gesamte Hyg** 1981 Oct;27(10):779–84

**Great Britain**

Extracts from the last century: Dental preventive medicine. **Br Dent J** 1981 Jul 7;151(1):23

Levere TH: Dr. Thomas Beddoes: the interaction of pneumatic and preventive medicine with chemistry. **Interdiscip Sci Rev** 1982;7:137–47

Ott PW: A corner of history. John Wesley and the non-naturals. **Prev Med** 1980 Jul;9(4):578–84

Taylor: The natural history of preventive medicine, or breaking the chains of causation. **Br Med J** 1980 Sep 27;281(6244):849–53

Yellowlees WW: Ill fares the land. **J R Coll Gen Pract** 1979 Jan;29(198):7–21

**Hungary**

Bánóczy J, Borós S: A Semmelweis Orvostudományi Egyetem Konzerváló Fogászati Klinika negyedszázados története és munkássága. **Fogorv Sz** 1984 Nov;77(11):321–3

**Ireland**

Doll R: Back to Methuselah? Opportunities for preventive medicine. **Ir J Med Sci** 1983 Jan;152(1):64–8

**Mexico**

Bustamante ME: La medicina preventiva. In Academia Nacional de Medicina. Libro conmemorativo del primer centenario. México, Comité Editorial de la Comisión Organizadora del Congreso del Centenario, 1964. Tome 2. p. 640–2.

**Romania**

Alexa I: La 100 ani de la naşterea doctorului Mihai Ciucă (1883–1983). **Rev Med Chir Soc Med Nat Iasi** 1983 Oct–Dec;87(4):731–6

Arion R: Prof. C. Ionescu-Mihăieşti, o personalitate de însemnătate fundamentală în istoria medicinii preventive din România. **Rev Ig [Bacteriol]** 1984 Jan–Mar;29(1):89–95

Un secol de activitate de medicină preventivă la Institutul de Medicină şi Farmacie din Iaşi (1882–1982): **Rev Med Chir Soc Med Nat Iasi** 1983 Oct–Dec;87(4):707–25

**United States**

Barker WH, Jonas S: The teaching of preventive medicine in American medical schools, 1940–1980. **Prev Med** 1981 Nov;10(6):674–88

Christen AG: Charles C. Bass, M.D.--1875–1975: that cantankerous genius of preventive dentistry. **Bull Hist Dent** 1982 Apr;30(1):8–18

Eastman JW: 'Doctors' orders': the American medical profession and the origins of automobile design for crash protection, 1930–1955. **Bull Hist Med** 1981;55(3):407–24

Evans RD: Inception of standards for internal emitters, radon and radium. **Health Phys** 1981 Sep;41(3):437–48

Kathren RL: Elda Emma Anderson. In: Notable American women. The modern period. Cambridge, Mass., Belknap-Harvard Univ. Press, 1980. 4:20–1.

Litoff JB: Carolyn Conant van Blarcom. In: Notable American women. The modern period. Cambridge, Mass., Belknap-Harvard Univ. Press, 1980. 4:703–4.

McClary A: 'Swat the Fly': popular magazines and the anti-fly campaign. **Prev Med** 1982 May;11(3):373–8

Parker HM: Invited paper delivered at the 25th Annual Meeting of the Health Physics Society. Protection programs of the Plutonium Project. **Health Phys** 1981 Oct;41(4):571–6

Steneck NH, Cook HJ, Vander AJ, et al: The origins of U.S. safety standards for microwave radiation. **Science** 1980 Jun 13;208(4449):1230–7

Taylor RC: The politics of prevention. **Soc Policy** 1982;13(1):32–41

Terris M: The primacy of prevention. **Prev Med** 1981 Nov;10(6):689–99

Viseltear AJ: John R. Paul and the definition of preventive medicine. **Yale J Biol Med** 1982 May–Aug;55(3–4):167–72

**USSR**

Georgievskiĭ AS: Vklad russkikh voennykh vracheĭ v stanovlenie i razvitie profilakticheskogo napravleniia meditsiny. **Sov Zdravookhr** 1982;(10):66–70

Kucheruk VV: Itogi i rabot sovetskikh uchenykh po izucheniiu i profilaktike prirodno-ochagovykh bolezneĭ (soobshchenie 1). **Med Parazitol (Mosk)** 1982 Nov–Dec;60(6):9–17

Kuz'min MK, Rumiantsev GI: Razvitie osnovnykh napravleniĭ profilakticheskoĭ meditsiny na sanitarno-gigienicheskom fakul'tete (1930–1980). **Sov Med** 1981;(5):115–9

Shishkin AP: Voprosy profilaktiki v deiatel'nosti Gosudarstvennogo Instituta Sotsial'noĭ Gigieny Narkomzdrava RSFSR (k 65-letiiu obrazovaniia N rodnogo Komissariata Zdravookhraneniia RSFSR).

**Sov Zdravookhr** 1983;6:55–8
Tarasenko NIu: Rol' sanitarno-gigienicheskogo fakul'teta v podgotovke vracheĭ profilakticheskoĭ meditsiny i v razvitii gigieny truda (k 50-letiiu obrazovaniiu sanitarno-gigienicheskogo fakul'teta I Moskovskogo meditsinskogo instituta im I. M. Sechenova). **Gig Tr Prof Zabol** 1980 Oct;(10):29–32
Vorontsova EI, Moĭkin IuV: V. I Lenin o profilakticheskom napravlenii sovetskogo zdravookhraneniia (k 110-ĭ godovshchine so dnia rozhdeniia Vladimira Il'icha Lenina). **Gig Tr Prof Zabol** 1980 Apr;(4):1–4

**Yugoslavia**

Birtašević B: Razvoj naše vojne preventivne medicine. **Vojnosanit Pregl** 1981 Sep–Oct;38(5):308–13
Perin J: Medicinsko-preventivni aspekti zdravstvene službe u narodnooslobodilačkom ratu. **Lijec Vjesn** 1979 Nov;101(11):663–8

## PRIMITIVE MEDICINE

See also **Folk and Popular Medicine; Religion and Medicine; Magic and Occult; Witchcraft**

Cook DC: Koniag Eskimo tooth ablation: was Hrdlička right after all? **Curr Anthropol** 1981;22(2):159–63
Grossinger R: Planet medicine. From stone age shamanism to post-industrial healing. Revised edition. Boulder, London, Shambhala, 1982. xviii, 436 p.
La Barre W: Shamanic origins of religion and medicine. **J Psychedelic Drugs** 1979 Jan–Jun;11(1–2):7–11
Newman LF: [Medical ethics in] primitive societies. In Reich WT, et al, ed: Encyclopedia of bioethics, v. 2. New York, Free Press, 1978. p. 877–9.
Rogers SL: The shaman's healing way. Ramona, California, Acoma Books, 1976. 40 p.
Shemluck M: Medicinal and other uses of the Compositae by Indians in the United States and Canada. **J Ethnopharmacol** 1982 May;5(3):303–58
Wassén SH: On concepts of disease among Amerindian tribal groups. **J Ethnopharmacol** 1979 Oct;1(3):285–93

**Africa**

Amakoue A: Médecine et pharmacopée traditionnelle en Afrique. **Dialogue J Mormon Thought** 1978 Nov–Dec;46–70
Tella A: The practice of traditional medicine in Africa. **Niger Med J** 1979 May–Jun;9(5–6):607–12

**Americas**

Dominguez XA: Conocimientos médicos de los mayas, aztecas, tarascos y la herbolaria médica mexicana. **Guatem Indig** 1978;13(1/2):220–38
Lex BW: Neurological bases of revitalization movements. **Zygon** 1978;13(4):276–312
Mora X: La medicina pre y post Colombina aplicada en la herborística. In Ureña Morales, Gabriel, ed. Memoria del Congreso Sobre el Mundo Centroamericano de su Tiempo: V. Centenario de Gonzalo Fernández de Oviedo. Nicoya, Costa Rica, Comisión Nac. Organizadora, 1980. p. 433–9.
Naranjo P: Medicina indigena y popular de América Latina y medicina contemporánea. **Guatem Indig** 1978;13(1/2):186–219

**Australia**

Cowlishaw G: Infanticide in aboriginal Australia. **Oceania** 1978;48:262–83

**Bolivia**

Bastien JW: Herbal curing by Qollahuaya Andeans. **J Ethnopharmacol** 1982 Jul;6(1):13–28

**Canada**

Edwards GT: Bella Coola: Indian and European medicines. **Beaver** 1980;311(3):4–11
Stewart WB: Indian medicine in New Brunswick. In: Congrès international d'histoire de la médecine, XXVe, Québec, 1976. Actes. Québec, 1977. p. 1320–6.

**Mexico**

Davidson JR, Ortiz de Montellano BR: The antibacterial properties of an Aztec wound remedy. **J Ethnopharmacol** 1983 Aug;8(2):149–61
Díaz JL: Ethnopharmacology and taxonomy of Mexican psychodysleptic plants. **J Psychedelic Drugs** 1979 Jan–Jun;11(1–2):71–101
Lopez Austin A: Almas y experiencia entre los antiguos nahuas. **Bol Soc Mex Hist Filos Med** 1983;6(45):223–33
McGuire TM: Ancient Maya mushroom connections: a transcendental interaction model. **J Psychoactive Drugs** 1982 Jul–Sep;14(3):221–38

**Pacific Islands**

Clarke MC: Some medical customs of the Cocos-Keeling Islanders. **Aust Nurses J** 1979 Oct;9(4):42–4, 50

**Panama**

Reverte Coma JM: El chamanismo en Panama. **Asclepio** 1980;32:341–52

**Peru**

Ryn L: Medicina popular andina. **Actas Luso Esp Neurol Psiquiatr** 1982 Jan–Feb;10(1):33–42

**United States**

Agris J: Stamps commemorating medicine: 'Indian folk art: the medicine man'. **J Dermatol Surg Oncol** 1981;7(1):82
Cox WW, Evans RJ: Health practices in Collier County: a study in diversity and contrast. **J Fla Med Assoc** 1982 Aug;69(8):695–701
Fitzpatrick TP: The Lenape contribution to New Jersey medicine. **J Med Soc NJ** 1984 Sep;81(9):701–6
Frisbie CJ: Burial as a disposition mechanism for Navajo jish or medicine bundles. **Am Indian Q** 1978;4(4):347–66
Hanson JR: Structure and complexity of medicine bundle systems of selected Plains Indian tribes. **Plains Anthropol** 1980;25(89):199–216
Laird C: Chemehuevi shamanism, sorcery, and charms. **J Calif Great Basin Anthropol** 1980;2(1):80–7
Langenwalter RE: A possible shamans's cache from CA-RIV-102, Hemet, California. **J Calif Great Basin Anthropol** 1980;2(2):233–44
Martin M: Native American medicine. Thoughts for posttraditional healers. **JAMA** 1981 Jan 9;245(2):141–3
Mathes VS: Native American women in medicine and the military. **J West** 1982;21(2):41–8
Milling CJ: Indian medicine. **SC Hist Illus** 1970;1(4):31–5
Shepardson M: Changes in Navajo mortuary practices and beliefs. **Am Indian Q** 1978;4(4):383–96
Snyderman GS: Witches, witchcraft, and Allegany Seneca medicine. **Proc Am Philos Soc** 1983;127(4):263–77

**Before 500 A.D.**

Schadewaldt H: Orthopädische Aspekte der Mythologie. In KF Schlegel, ed: Der Körperbehinderte in Mythologie und Kunst. Stuttgart, New York, Thieme, 1983. p. 1–18.

**1450–1700**

**Canada**

Griffin JD, Greenland C: Manifestations of madness in New France. In: Congrès international d'histoire de la médecine, XXVe, Québec, 1976. Actes. Québec, 1977. p. 727–45.

**Mexico**

López Austin A: Textos acerca de las partes del cuerpo humano y de las enfermedades y medicinas en los primeros memoriales de Sahagún. **Estud Cult Nahuatl** 1972;10:129–53
Wasserman M: Aztec psychotherapy: a study of help-giving in ancient Mexico. **Int J Soc Psychiatry** 1982 Spring;28(1):54–9

**1700 to Present**

Scarpa A: Pre-scientific medicines: their extent and value. **Soc Sci Med** 1981 May;15A(3):317–26

**Africa**

Janzen JM: Ideologies and institutions in the precolonial history of equatorial African therapeutic systems. **Soc Sci Med [Med Anthropol]** 1979 Dec;13B(4):317–26

**Brazil**

Williams PV: Primitive religion and healing. A study of folk medicine in North-East Brazil. Cambridge, England, and Totowa, New Jersey, D. S. Brewer and Rowman and Littlefield, 1979. xi, 212 p.

**Canada**

Robb-Smith AH: Egerton Y. Davis, M.D., and placentophagy. **Bull NY Acad Med** 1980 Mar;56(2):258–60
Romaniuk A: Increase in natural fertility during the early stages of modernization: Canadian Indians case study. **Demography** 1981 May;18(2):157–72

# PRIMITIVE MEDICINE

**United States**

Albanese CL: The poetics of healing: root metaphors and rituals in nineteenth-century America. **Soundings** 1980;63(4):381–406
Allen VR: Medical practices and health in the Choctaw Nation. 1831–1885. **Chron Okla** 1970;48(1):60–73
Blackwood L: Alaska native fertility trends, 1950–1978. **Demography** 1981 May;18(2):173–9
Blanchard D: Who or what's a witch: Iroquois persons of power. **Am Indian Q** 1982;6(3–4):218–37
Documents in Hopi Indian sexuality: Imperialism, culture and resistance. **Radic Hist Rev** 1979 Spring/Summer;Spec:99–130
Fenton WN: The 'Great Good Medicine.' **NY State J Med** 1979 Sep;79(10):1603–9
Fortuine R: Traditional surgery of the Alaska natives. **Alaska Med** 1984 Jan–Mar;26(1):22–5
Grant RE: Tuuhikya: the Hopi healer. **Am Indian Q** 1982;6(3–4):291–304
Hart JA: The ethnobotany of the Northern Cheyenne Indians of Montana. **J Ethnopharmacol** 1981 Jul;4(1):1–55
Jaskoski H: 'My heart will go out': healing songs of native American women. **Int J Womens Stud** 1981;4(2):118–34
Lewis TH: The changing practice of the Oglala medicine man. **Plains Anthropol** 1980;25(89):265–7
Mooney J: Cherokee theory and practice of medicine. **J Cherokee Stud** 1982;7(1):25–9
Powers MN: Menstruation and reproduction: an Oglala case. **Signs** 1980;6(1):54–65
Thornton R: Demographic antecedents of a revitalization movement: population change, population size, and the 1890 Ghost Dance. **Am Sociol Rev** 1981;46(1):88–96
Tyler VE: Three proprietaries and their claim as American 'Indian' remedies. **Pharm Hist** 1984;26(3):146–9
Weir JA: The army doctor looks at Indian medicine. **Denver West Roundup** 1977 Sep–Oct;33:12–28

**Zambia**

Prins G: Disease at the crossroads: towards a history of therapeutics in Bulozi since 1876 [1]. **Soc Sci Med [Med Anthropol]** 1979 Dec;13B(4):285–315

# PRINTING AND BIBLIOGRAPHY

See also **Exhibits; Herbals; Libraries; Manuscripts; Periodicals**

Almagro BR: From clay tablets to electronic publications: the history of medical books. **Ariz Med** 1984 Jan;41(1):31–4
Baader G: Handschrift und Frühdruck als Ueberlieferungsinstrumente der Wissenschaften. **Ber Wissenschaftsgesch** 1980;3(1–2):7–22
Bruneel C: Répertoire des thèses imprimées de l'Université de Louvain (1425–1797). Louvain, Université Catholique de Louvain, 1977. xxv, 113 p. (Catalogues, inventaires et répertoires de la Bibliothèque Centrale. III.).
Kronick DA: Literature of the life sciences: the historical background. **Bull NY Acad Med** 1984 Nov;60(9):857–75
Lebel M: Editions, traductions et lexiques hippocratiques. Le docteur Louis Morin, (1635–1715) et son index des mots d'Hippocrate. In: Congrès international d'histoire de la médecine, XXVe, Québec, 1976. Actes. Québec, 1977. p. 848–65.
Maire M: Une mini histoire de la presse dentaire. **Chir Dent Fr** 1979 Dec 13;49(44):53–7
Nauert CG: Caius Plinius Secundus. In Cranz FE, Kristeller PO, ed: Catalogus translationum et commentariorum: Mediaeval and Renaissance Latin translations and commentaries. Annotated lists and guides. Vol. IV. Washington, D.C., Catholic University of America Press, 1980. p. 297–422.
Oliaro T: La funzione storica e didattica della Stampa Medica. **Minerva Med** 1983 Dec 15;74(47–48):2801–2
Oliaro T: La funzione storica e didattica della stampa medica. **Minerva Stomatol** 1984 May–Jun;33(3):536–7
Rice EF: Paulus Aegineta. In Cranz FE, Kristeller PO, ed: Catalogus translationum et commentariorum: Mediaeval and Renaissance Latin translations and commentaries. Annotated lists and guides. Vol. IV. Washington, D.C., Catholic University of America Press, 1980. p. 145–91.
Riddle JM: Dioscorides. In Cranz FE, Kristeller PO, ed: Catalogus translationum et commentariorum: mediaeval and Renaissance Latin translations and commentaries. Annotated lists and guides. Vol. IV. Washington, D.C., Catholic University of America Press, 1980. p. 1–143.
Scarborough J, ed: Society for Ancient Medicine newsletter. No. 1–10 (Apr. 1976–Sept. 1982). Continued periodically.
Schadewaldt H: Betrachtungen zur Entwicklung des medizinischen Buch- und Zeitschriftenwesens. In:Die Zeitung als Persönlichkeit. Festschrift Bringmann. Düsseldorf, 1982. p. 125–34.
Stafleu FA, Cowan RS: Taxonomic literature. A selective guide to botanical publications and collections with dates, commentaries and types. Second edition. Utrecht; Bohn, Scheltema and Holkema; The Hague, Junk; Vol. II, 1979, 991 p; Vol. III, 1981, xii, 980 p.

**Americas**

Price R, ed: An annotated catalogue of medical Americana in the Library of the Wellcome Institute for the History of Medicine. Books and printed documents 1557–1821 from Latin America and the Caribbean Islands and manuscripts from the Americas 1575–1927. London, Wellcome Institute for the History of Medicine, 1983. xix, 319 p.

**China**

Schmidt M: Zur Geschichte der tibetischen Ubersetzungen altindischer medizinischer Werke. In International Congress of the History of Medicine, 27th, Barcelona, 1980. Actas. Barcelona, Académia de Ciències Médiques de Catalunya i Balears, 1981. p. 336–9.

**Europe**

Meadows AJ, ed: Development of science publishing in Europe. Amsterdam, Elsevier Science, 1980. ix, 269 p.

**Germany**

Spieckermann ML: Deutsche Uebersetzungen englischer humanmedizinischer Werke 1680–1810. **Medizinhist J** 1984;19(3):280–4

**Great Britain**

Barry J: Guide to sources and writings on the history of medicine in Bristol, 1600–1900. **Soc Soc Hist Med Bull (Lond)** 1984 Dec;35:48–52
Getz FM: Gilbertus Anglicus anglicized. **Med Hist** 1982 Oct;26(4):436–42

**Hungary**

Buzinkay G: Az egyetemi nyomda és orvosi-természettudományos szakirodalmunk kialakulása. **Magy Konyvsz** 1977;93(1):25–37

**India**

Hameed HA, Reyaz Ali Parvaz S: Source material of Arab medicine. **Stud Hist Med** 1979 Dec;3(4):225–33

**Italy**

Micheli A de: Libros médicos italianos en la antigua Universidad de México. **Prensa Med Mex** 1979;44:152–6

**Netherlands**

Witkam HJ: Catalogues of all the chiefest rarities in the Publick Anatomie Hall of the University of Leyden. Leiden, Witkam, 1980. xv, 86 leaves.

**Spain**

López Piñero JM: Social and economic factors in the translation of medical texts in Spain (16th–19th centuries). In International Congress of the History of Medicine, 27th, Barcelona, 1980. Actas. Barcelona, Académia de Ciències Médiques de Catalunya i Balears, 1981. p. 289–97.

**1450–1700**

Bird DT: A catalogue of sixteenth-century medical books in Edinburgh libraries. Edinburgh, Royal College of Physicians of Edinburgh, 1982. xxxii, 298 p.
Eamon W: Arcana disclosed: the advent of printing, the books of secrets tradition and the development of experimental science in the sixteenth century. **Hist Sci** 1984;22(pt 2):111–50
Guerrino AA: Las traducciones médicas hasta el renacimiento. In International Congress of the History of Medicine, 27th, Barcelona, 1980. Actas. Barcelona, Académia de Ciències Médiques de Catalunya i Balears, 1981. p. 249–52.
Horowitz M, Collins J: A census of copies of the first edition of Andreas Vesalius' De humani corporis fabrica (1543), with a note on the recently discovered variant issue. **J Hist Med Allied Sci** 1984 Apr;39(2):198–221
Krivatsy P: Medical incunabula and the diffusion of scientific knowledge. Incunabula in the National Library of Medicine. Published in conjunction with an exhibit at the National Library of Medicine, May–Oct. 1984. [Bethesda, National Library of Medicine, 1984.] 14 p.
Linet J, Hillard D, Lavagne X, ed: Catalogue des ouvrages imprimés au XVIe siècle, Bibliothèque Sainte-Geneviève, Paris: Sciences--Techniques--Médecine. Paris, New York, Saur, 1980. xvi, 493 p.
Lohr CH: Renaissance Latin Aristotle Commentaries: authors N–Ph. **Renaiss Q** 1979 Winter;32(4):529–80 (continued periodically)
Lohr CH: Renaissance Latin Aristotle commentaries: authors So–Z. **Renaiss Q** 1982 Summer;35(2):164–256
Schneider W: Ueber den Liber praeparationum des Paracelsus. **Sudhoffs Arch** 1980;64(1):69–78

**China**

Zhi Y: [Research on You Ke Lei Cui (Classified Collections in Pediatrics): a rare edition of pediatrics printed in the Ming dynasty] (Chi). **Chung Hua I Shih Tsa Chih** 1984;14(2):121-2

**Europe**

Eisenstein EL: The printing press as an agent of change. Communications and cultural transformations in early-modern Europe. 2 vols. Cambridge, Cambridge University Press, 1979. xxi, 794 p.

**France**

Desgraves L, ed: Répertoire bibliographique des livres imprimés en France au XVIIe siècle. Tome VI. Baden-Baden, Koerner, 1982. 248 p. (Bibliotheca Bibliographica Aureliana, XCI).

Rulliere R, Heymans G, Vial F: La version en langue française (1679) du Tractatus de Corde (1669) de Richard Lower. In International Congress of the History of Medicine, 27th, Barcelona, 1980. Actas. Barcelona, Acadèmia de Ciències Mèdiques de Catalunya i Balears, 1981. p. 331-5.

**Germany**

Amelung P: Dinckmuts Drucke des Regimen sanitatis. **Gutenberg Jahrb** 1979;:58-71

Bircher M: Deutsche Drucke des Barock 1600-1720 in der Herzog August Bibliothek Wolfenbüttel. Abteilung A: Bibliotheca Augusta. Band 2: Arithmetica, Astronomica, Bellica, Geographica, Geometrica, Medica, Oeconomica, Physica. Nendeln, KTO Press, 1979. 408 p.

Guédès M: Une variante de la page de titre du De historia stirpium de L. Fuchs (1542). **J Soc Bibliogr Nat Hist** 1974;7(1):81-5

Junkte F: Ueber Leonhard Thurneisser zum Thurn und seine deutschen Kalendar 1572-1584. **Arch Gesch Buchwes** 1978;19:1349-400

**Great Britain**

Cule J: Medical translations in sixteenth century Wales. In International Congress of the History of Medicine, 27th, Barcelona, 1980. Actas. Barcelona, Acadèmia de Ciències Mèdiques de Catalunya i Balears, 1981. p. 233-7.

**Italy**

Jarcho S: Some early Italian epidemiological maps. **Imago Mundi** 1983;35:9-19

**Mexico**

Micheli A de: Los primeros libros médicos novohispanos. **Prensa Med Mex** 1979 Jan-Feb;43(1-2):25-30

**Spain**

Balaguer i Perigüell E, Ballester i Añón R, Bujosa i Homar F, et al: Els impresos clientífics a Catalunya en els segles XV i XVI. In Congrés International d'Història de la Medicina Catalana, 2nd, Barcelona, 1975. Llibre d'Actes. Barcelona, Socitra, 1977. p. 185-96.

Sanchez Granjel Santander L, Sanchez Granjel Santander M: El libro medico español renacentista. Salamanca, Universidad de Salamanca, 1980. 41 p. (Trabajos de la Catedra de Historia de la Medicina, 5).

**Switzerland**

Clark H: Foiling the pirates: the preparation and publication of Andreas Vesalius's De humani corporis fabrica. **Libr Q** 1981;51(3):301-11

Rocchietta S: Sulle edizioni degli 'Antidotari' e di altre opere di J.-J. Wecker. **Minerva Med** 1981 Sep 19;72(34):2297

**1700 to Present**

Burns CR: Locating sources in the history of medicine and health care: a guide for students and faculty at UTMB. **Bookman** 1984;11(5):3-9

Faulkner TC: Computer applications for an edition of Robert Burton's The anatomy of melancholy: a system for scholarly publishing. **Comput Hum** 1981 Nov;15(3):163-82

Götz W: J. B. Trommsdorffs 'Chemische Receptirkunst'. Bisher unbekannte Ubersetzungen und Ausgaben. **Beitr Gesch Pharm** 1982;31(14):107-10

Hügelow M: Original-Lithographien speziell für Pharmazeuten: Historische Apothekergeräte und Heilpflanzen. **Pharm Unserer Zeit** 1984 Jul;13(4):97-101

Karger T: A short history of the Karger Publishing firm. **Bull Med Libr Assoc** 1981 Apr;69(2):254-7

Lampert RH: Osler and his publishers. **Trans Stud Coll Physicians Phila** 1983 Sep;5(5 No 3):177-90

Levere TH, ed: Editing texts in the history of science and medicine. Papers given at the seventeenth annual Conference on Editorial Problems, University of Toronto, 6-7 November 1981. New York, London, Garland, 1982. 190 p. Contributions by S. Drake, L. E. Voigts, B. S. Hall, A. Beaulieu, I. B. Cohen.

Maclean V: A short-title catalogue of household and cookery books published in the English tongue 1701-1800. London, Prospect, 1981. 197 p.

Matthews WB: Osler Oration. **J R Soc Med** 1982 May;75(5):307-14

Schiller J: Les traductions en français des ouvrages scientifiques de Haller. In: Congrès National des Sociétés Savantes, 91e, Rennes, 1966. Comptes Rendus. Paris, 1967. Section des Sciences, Tome 1. p. 241-5.

Teigen PM, ed: Books, manuscripts, and the history of medicine. Essays on the fiftieth anniversary of the Osler Library. New York, Science History Publications, 1982. 112 p. Contributions by L. G. Stevenson, C. G. Roland, R. J. Durling, E. Brodman, G. T. Tanselle, E. J. Freeman.

Thibodeau D: Indexing medical history: a guide to the literature: an essay review. **Bull Hist Med** 1982 Summer;56(2):276-9

**Asia**

Golden RL: Osler and Oriental medicine: a discursive review. Princeton, Science Press Associates, 1982. iii, 93 p.

**Colombia**

Hernández de Alba G: Una obra postuma cientifica monumental: la bibliografia medica Colombiana (1782-1976). **Bol Cult Bibliogr (Bogota)** 1976;16(7-8):176-9

**France**

Julien P: Les 'Eléments de pharmacie' de Baumé et la contrefaçon. **Rev Hist Pharm (Paris)** 1981 Jun;28(249):103-6

Sournia JC: Littré l'Académie de Médecine. **Bull Acad Natl Med (Paris)** 1981 Oct;165(7):941-7

**Germany**

Deneke JF: Das Gesundheitswesen der ersten Hälfte des 19.Jahrhunderts im Spiegel der Amts- und Intelligenzpresse. Düsseldorf, Triltsch, 1983. 161 p. (Düsseldorfer Arbeiten zur Geschichte der Medizin, Beiheft IX).

Fabian B, Spieckermann ML: Deutsche Uebersetzungen englischer humanmedizinischer Werke 1680-1810. Eine vorläufige Bibliographie. **Medizinhist J** 1980;15(1/2):154-71

Gumpert M: Hölle im Paradies. Selbstdarstellung eines Arztes. Hildesheim, Gerstenberg, 1983. xxiii, 280 p. (Exilliteratur, Band 17) Reprint of 1939 ed., with new biographical forward by F. Trapp.

Kollesch J: Das Berliner Corpus der antiken Aerzte. **Clio Med** 1981 Sep;16(1):45-7

Nutton V, ed: Karl Gottlob Kühn and his edition of the works of Galen. Oxford, Oxford Microform Publications, 1976. 35 p. (First published with the microfiche edition of Kühn's edition of The works of Galen, March 1976).

**Hungary**

Friedrich I: 18. századi magyar nyelvu orvosi könyvek az 'ügyefogyott szegények' szolgálatában. **Magy Konyvsz** 1978;94(2):158-67

Rixer A: A magyar nyelvü gyógyszerészeti szaksajtó kialakulása és jelenentösége 1831-1872 között. Diss., Budapest, 1976. 193 p.

Szállási A: Aki szerkesztönek született, az orvostudomány sem menti meg. **Orv Hetil** 1981 Apr 5;122(14):837-9

**Italy**

Kligfield PD: A survey of variant title page vignettes in Lancisi's De subitaneis mortibus. **J Hist Med Allied Sci** 1983 Jul;38(3):336-9

Rocchietta S: Libri di interesse medico stampati da Giambattista Bodoni (1740-1813). **Minerva Med** 1983 Oct 13;74(39):2327-8

**Spain**

Beltrán E: Una polémica sobre Francisco Hernández y su obra en 1785. **An Soc Mex Hist Cienc Tec** 1979;5:49-73

Granjel LS: El libro medico en España (1808-1936). Salamanca, 1975. 111 p (Cuadernos de Historia de la Medicina Española, Monografias, 28).

**United States**

Adams S: Medical bibliography in an age of discontinuity. Chicago, Medical Library Association, 1981. xviii, 224 p.

After seventy-five years, 1890-1965: Baltimore, Waverly Press, William & Wilkins, 1965. 46 p.

Blake JB, ed: Centenary of Index Medicus, 1879-1979. Bethesda, National Library of Medicine, 1980. viii, 115 p. (NIH Publication No. 80-2068; Order from U.S. Government Printing Office). Contributions by C. E. Rosenberg, G. Miller, F. B. Rogers, W. B. Bean, E. Wolf, K. G. Huston,

S. Jarcho.
Clagett M: Lynn Thorndike. In Dictionary of American biography, 1961-1965. Suppl. 7, 1981. p. 741-2.
Girard DE: The history of Osler's Principles and practice of medicine. **Med Times** 1981 Jul;109(7):1s-4s, 13s
Hodgson MN: The University of North Carolina Press may be a rare bargain. **NC Med J** 1983 May;44(5):315-6
Jekel JF: The 'Rainbow Reviews': publications of the National Center for Health Statistics. **J Chronic Dis** 1984;37(9-10):681-8
Kohlstedt SG: Science: the struggle for survival, 1880 to 1894. **Science** 1980 Jul 4;209(4452):33-42
Rogers FB: The origins of MEDLARS. In Stevenson LG, ed: A celebration of medical history. Baltimore, Johns Hopkins University Press, 1982. p. 77-84.
Sokal MM: Science and James McKeen Cattell, 1894 to 1945. **Science** 1980 Jul 4;209(4452):43-52
Swain HH: G & G: the textbook which structured American pharmacology. **Pharmacologist** 1984;26(1):41-4
Wilson LB: A women pioneer in a new profession, medical editing. **Mayo Alumnus** 1982 Apr;:20-3
Wolfe RJ: Jacob Bigelow's American medical botany 1817-1821. An examination of the origin, printing, binding and distribution of America's first color plate book. With special emphasis on the manner of making and printing its colored plates. North Hills, Pennsylvania, and Boston, Bird & Bull Press and Boston Medical Library, 1979. 121 p.

### USSR

Bawden CR: W. A. Unkrig's correspondence with the British and Foreign Bible Society. A contribution to ... printing in Mongolian. **Zentralasiat Stud** 1980;14(1):65-108
Idel'chik KhI: K isotorii izdatel'stva 'Meditsina'. **Sov Zdravookhr** 1979;(10):54-9
Vengrova IV: Translations of the classics of medicine in the USSR. In International Congress of the History of Medicine, 27th, Barcelona, 1980. Actas. Barcelona, Académia de Ciències Mèdiques de Catalunya i Balears, 1981. p. 358-62.

## PSYCHIATRY

See also **Hospitals, Psychiatric; Hypnosis; Mental Health; Neurology; Psychology; Psychosomatic Medicine; Sex Behavior; Witchcraft**

Aaron PG, Clouse RG: Freud's psychohistory of Leonardo de Vinci: A matter of being right or left. **J Interdiscip Hist** 1982;13(1):1-16
Ballbé R: El psiquiatra y el hombre contemporáneo. **Actas Luso Esp Neurol Psiquiatr** 1981 Mar-Apr;9(2):89-102
Baruk H: Quelques réflexions sur l'histoire de la psychiatrie. **Hist Sci Med** 1984;18(3):205-7
Bernard H: L'histoire de la psychiatrie selon Ey (sa forme et son sens, le mythe). **Rev Int Hist Psychiatr** 1983;1(1):59-77
Braceland FJ: Psychiatry, medicine's erring sibling, returns: a history and a prophecy. **Trans Stud Coll Physicians Phila** 1981 Sep;5(3 no 3):181-94
Brennan JF: History and systems of psychology. Englewood Cliffs, Prentice-Hall, 1982. x, 374 p.
Buckley P, Galanter M: Altered states of consciousness during psychotherapy: a historical and cultural perspective. **Int J Soc Psychiatry** 1979 Summer;25(2):118-24
Cain AM, ed: A catalog of the Percival Bailey collection of neurology & psychiatry. Chicago, Library of the Health Sciences, University of Illinois at the Medical Center, Chicago, 1973. viii, 230 p.
Castorina JA, Lerner BD: Comentarios sobre la investigación clínica en Freud y Piaget. **Acta Psiquiatr Psicol Am Lat** 1983 Jun;29(2):85-95
Cervera S: La influencia de los acontecimientos de la vida en los trastornos psiquiátricos: planteamiento del problema. **Rev Med Univ Navarra** 1982 Sep;26(3):147-9
Davis B, Shanley E: The history of psychiatry. **Nursing (Oxford)** 1982 Jul;2(3):59-62
De Fréminville B: La raison du plus fort. Paris, Editions du Seuil, 1977. 189 p.
Doerner K: Madmen and the bourgeoisie. A social history of insanity and psychiatry. (First published in German as Bürger und Irre, 1969.) Oxford, Basil Blackwell, 1981 vi, 361 p.
Fernandez G: The social structure of the medical model of madness and the physician's role. **Psychiatry** 1981 Aug;44(3):241-52
Fischer-Homberger E: On the medical history of the doctrine of imagination. **Psychol Med** 1979 Nov;9(4):619-28
Fitzpatrick JJ: Suicidology and suicide prevention: historical perspectives from the nursing literature. **J Psychosoc Nurs Ment Health Serv** 1983 May;21(5):20-8
Giuseppe Capailla D: El psiquiatra frente a los derechos del hombre. **An R Acad Nac Med (Madr)** 1981;98(3):463-72
Graham RM: Music therapy: the state of the field. **J Natl Assoc Priv Psychiatr Hosp** 1979;11(2):32-9
Hajal F: Galen's ethical psychotherapy: its influence on a medieval Near Eastern physician. **J Hist Med Allied Sci** 1983 Jul;38(3):320-33
Hare E: Great books in psychiatry. **Br J Psychiatry** 1981 Mar;138:261-3
Hoffman LE: From instinct to identity: implications of changing psychoanalytic concepts of social life from Freud to Erikson. **J Hist Behav Sci** 1982 Apr;18(2):130-46
Howells JG, Osborn ML: A reference companion to the history of abnormal psychology. Westport, Conn., Greenwood Press, 1984. 2 v. xviii, 1141 p.
Jackson BS: Historical aspects of legal drafting in the light of modern theories of cognitive development. **Int J Law Psychiatry** 1980;3(4):349-69
Jones WL: Ministering to minds diseases: a history of psychiatric treatment. London, W. Heinemann Medical Books, 1983. x, 157 p.
Kalinowsky LB: The discoveries of somatic treatments in psychiatry: facts and myths. **Compr Psychiatry** 1980 Nov-Dec;21(6):428-35
Lanteri-Laura G: Lecture des perversions: histoire de leur appropriation médicale. Paris, New York, Masson, 1979. 160 p.
Maeder C: Zur Geschichte der Psychiatrie. Umgang mit psychisch Kranken--gestern und heute. **Krankenpflege (Frankfurt)** 1984 Apr;38(4):115-6, 121-2 contd
Mark B: From 'lunatic' to 'client': 300 years of psychiatric patienthood. **J Psychiatr Nurs** 1980 Mar;18(3):32-6
Menninger WW: A psychiatric perspective of medical history. **J Okla State Med Assoc** 1980 Nov;73(11):386-90
Merani AL: Freud y el Talmud: seguido de crítica de los fundamentos de la psicopatología. México, Grijalbo, 1974. 159 p.
Mylenki M: Historical collections in psychiatry and psychoanalysis. **Libr Trends** 1982 Spring;:613-29
Oberhelman S: Popular dream-interpretation in ancient Greece and Freudian psychoanalysis. **J Pop Cult** 1978;11:682-95
Pethö B: A psychiatria mint történeti rendszer. **Orvostort Kozl** 1982;92(4):23-52
Pigeaud J: La maladie de l'ame: étude sur la relation de l'âme et du corps dans la tradition médico-philosophique antique.
Pivnicki D: On psychopathology of exile. An essay. **Confin Psychiatr** 1980;23(2):109-17
Postel J, Quétel C, ed: Nouvelle histoire de la psychiatrie. Toulouse, Privat, 1983. 774 p. Contributions by J. Bancaud, P. Berner, F. Bing.
The process of child therapy: **Publ Group Adv Psychiatry** 1982;11(111):3-220
Quen JM: Forensic psychiatry. **JAMA** 1980 Jan 4;243(1):30
Réflexions sur les soins infirmiers en psychiatrie: L'equipe soignante de Castelluccio. **Soins Psychiatr** 1980 Mar 1;(1):3-8
Reverzy JF: La biocratie. Esquisse d'une histoire de la notion de prévention en médecine et en psychiatrie en Occident. **Soins Psychiatr** 1982 Feb;(16):27-35
Rieber RW, Green M, ed: Milestones in the history of forensic psychology and psychiatry; a book of readings. New York, Da Capo, 1981. xi, 271 p.
Rosenbaum M, ed: Ethics and values in psychotherapy: a guidebook. New York, Free Press; London, Collier Macmillan; 1982. xvi, 464 p. Historical chapter by J. F. Drane.
Sahakian WS, ed: History of psychology. A source book in systematic psychology. Revised edition. Itasca, Illinois, F. E. Peacock, 1981. xvi, 497 p.
Sedgwick P: Psycho politics: Laing, Foucault, Goffman, Szasz, and the future of mass psychiatry. New York, Harper & Row, 1982. 292 p.
Sharkey PW, ed: Philosophy, religion and psychotherapy. Essays in the philosophical foundations of psychotherapy. Washington, University Press of America, 1982. xiii, 227 p. Contributions by R. Macklin, J. E. Morris, R. N. Sollod, J. Needleman, C. E. Scott, M. Friedman, J. F. Rychlak, E. Weisskopf-Joelson, T. S. Szasz, R. J. Sullivan.
Sjöstrand T: Magin i medicinen. **Lakartidningen** 1982 May 26;79(21):2137-40
Smith JC, Weisstub DN: The evolution of Western legal consciousness. **Int J Law Psychiatry** 1979;2(2):215-34
Stein HF: Historical understanding as sense of history: a psychoanalytic inquiry. **Psychoanal Rev** 1983 Winter;70(4):595-619
Tellenbach H, ed: Psychiatrische Therapie heute. Antike Diaita und moderne Therapeutik. Ein Symposium in Salzburg 1979. Stuttgart, Ferdinand Enke, 1982. 135 p. Contributions by P. L. Entralgo, D. Gracia-Guillen, H. Schipperges, W. Schmitt, K. P. Kisker, D. Wyss, W. Blankenburg.
Verdiglione A: Fondations de la psychanalyse: la peste. Paris, Galilée/Spirali, 1981. 282 p.
Vié J: Die grossen klassischen Traditionen von Hippokrates bis Pinel. In Sournia JC, Martiny M, Poulet J, ed: Illustrierte Geschichte der Medizin. Salzburg, Andreas, 1980. Vol. 6. p. 2008-33.
Vié J, Baruk H: Geschichte der Psychiatrie. In Sournia JC, Martiny M, Poulet J, ed: Illustrierte Geschichte der Medizin. Salzburg, Andreas, 1980. Vol. 6. p. 2003-7.
Wajeman G: Le Maître et l'hystérique. Paris, Navarin Editeur, 1982. 286 p. (Bibliothèque des Analytica).
Weiss L: The resurgence of biological psychiatry: new promise or false hope for a troubled profession. **Perspect Biol Med** 1977 Summer;20(4):573-85
Wolf SG: Psychosocial and neural mechanisms in health and disease; historical perspectives. **J Okla State Med Assoc** 1982 Mar;75(3):53-61

**Africa**

Moersch E: Psychiatrie in Afrika zwischen Tradition und Moderne. **Psyche (Stuttg)** 1984 Aug;38(8):673–95

**Austria**

Berner P: Zur Geschichte der Psychiatrie in Wien: eine Bilddokumentation. Wien, C. Brandstätter, 1983. 143 p.

**Brazil**

Seibel SD, Coura SH, Alho Filho JL: Evolution de la politique brésilienne d'assistance psychiatrique et de santé mentale. **Ann Med Psychol (Paris)** 1979 Dec;137(10):1001–7

**China**

Clifford T: Tibetan Buddhist medicine and psychiatry: the diamond healing. Introduction by Lokesh Chandra. York Beach, Me., S. Weiser, 1983. xx, 268 p.
Collins JL: Psychiatry in China. **J Natl Med Assoc** 1982 Oct;74(10):993–8
Liu X: Psychiatry in traditional Chinese medicine. **Br J Psychiatry** 1981 May;138:429–33

**France**

Gineste T: Naissance de la psychiatrie de l'enfant. De l'idiotie aux psychoses infantiles. **Soins Psychiatr** 1982 Feb;(16):21–6
Jaeger M: Le d'esordre psychiatrique: des politiques de la santé mentale en France. Paris, Payot, 1981. 262 p.
Kurz C: De l'enfermement au secteur. **Soins Psychiatr** 1982 Feb;(16):2
Le Guen Y: Etre infirmier en psychiatrie. **Rev Infirm** 1980 Nov;30(9):19–22
Tisseron S: Une préhistoire de la psychiatrie? Plutôt quelques économies différentes de la folie. **Soins Psychiatr** 1982 Feb;(16):5–8

**Germany**

Heinemeyer W, Pünder T: 450 Jahre Psychiatrie in Hessen. Marburg, Elwert (Kommissionsverlag), 1983. x, 461 p.

**Great Britain**

Eigen JP: Historical developments in psychiatric forensic evidence: the British experience. **Int J Law Psychiatry** 1983;6(3–4):423–9
Okamura A: [Abnormal psychology and England from 1660 to 1760] (Jpn). **Kango Kyoiku** 1983 Jun;24(6):360–7

**Italy**

Loré C, Piva I: Pensiero e pratica psichiatrici in Toscana da chiarugi a livi. In International Congress of the History of Medicine, 27th, Barcelona, 1980. Actas. Barcelona, Académia de Ciències Médiques de Catalunya i Balears, 1981. p. 103–10.

**Japan**

Kato N: [Psychiatric treatment at Iwakura-Mura and in Kyoto] (Jpn). **Seishin Shinkeigaku Zasshi** 1982;84(11):889–94
Kure S, Kashida G: Waga kuni ni okeru seishinbyo ni kansuru saikin no shisetsu. Tokyo, Seishin Igaku Shinkeigaku Koten Kankokai, [1977]. 270 p.
Makita K, Kamiide H: Jido seishin igaku sosetsu. Tokyo, Yasuda Seimei Shakai Jigyodan, [1977]. 146 p.

**Spain**

Contreras Mas A: Notas para la historia de la psiquiatría Bajomedieval en Mallorca. In International Congress of the History of Medicine, 27th, Barcelona, 1980. Actas. Barcelona, Académia de Ciències Médiques de Catalunya i Balears, 1981. p. 56–63.
Dieckhöfer K: El desarrollo de la psiquiatría en España. Aspectos historicos y culturales. **Actas Luso Esp Neurol Psiquiatr** 1983 Nov–Dec;11(6):487–96
Dieckhöfer K: II. El desarrollo de la psiquiatría en España. Aspectos históricos y culturales. **Actas Luso Esp Neurol Psiquiatr** 1983 Sep–Oct;11(5):407–22

**Sweden**

Seeman K, Lauren K: Psychotherapy in Sweden: historical background, current status, and future projections. **Am J Psychother** 1984 Jan;38(1):97–110

**United States**

Kuna RR: Hoodoo: the indigenous medicine and psychiatry of the black American. **Ethnomedizin** 1974–75;3(3–4):273–94

**Before 500 A.D.**

**Greco-Roman**

Gourevitch D, Gourevitch M: Chronique anachronique III. Simulation. **Evol Psychiatr (Paris)** 1981;46(1):205–9

**Greece**

Anzieu D, Carapanos F, Gillibert J, et al: Psychanalyse et culture grecque. Paris, Société d'Edition 'Les Belles Lettres,' 1980. 243 p.
Chessick RD: Socrates: first psychotherapist. **Am J Psychoanal** 1982 Spring;42(1):71–83
La Croce E: El concepto de locura en Grecia clásica. **Acta Psiquiatr Psicol Am Lat** 1981 Sep–Nov;27(4–5):285–91
Mann L: The wax block metaphor: Plato's views on learning disabilities. **J Learn Disabil** 1980 Oct;13(8):420–4

**India**

Weiss MG: Critical study of Unmada in the early sanskrit medical literature. An analysis of ayurvedic psychiatry with reference to present-day diagnostic concepts. Ph.D. Diss., University of Pennsylvania. Philadelphia, 1977. 353 leaves.

**Rome**

Dieckhöfer K: Aspekte einer rudimentären Psychologie, Psychopathologie und Psychotherapie bei Seneca. In: Congrès international d'histoire de la médecine, XXVe, Québec, 1976. Actes. Québec, 1977. p. 579–95.

**500 A.D.–1450**

Stephanos S: Zur Problematik des omnipotenten Objekts – eine psychoanalytische Studie über Psoriasis. Ein Fall aus dem Jahre 802. **Krankenpfl J** 1984 Mar 1;22(3):20–3
Williman JP, Kvarnes RG: A medieval example of psychotherapy. **Psychiatry** 1984 Feb;47(1):93–5

**Arabic**

Moussaoui D, Touhami M, Msefer W: Psychiatrie et psychosomatique dans la médecine arabe. **Ann Med Psychol (Paris)** 1980;138(8):967–74

**1450–1700**

Fischer-Homberger E: The medicalization of demonology--the contribution of forensic medicine to early modern psychiatry. In International Congress of the History of Medicine, 27th, Barcelona, 1980. Actas. Barcelona, Académia de Ciències Médiques de Catalunya i Balears, 1981. p. 69–73.
Midelfort HC: The anthropological roots of Paracelsus' psychiatry. **Medizinhist J** 1981;16(1–2):67–77

**Americas**

Alvarado JM: El primer episodio psiquiátrico de la conquista hispana. **Acta Psiquiatr Psicol Am Lat** 1979 Sep;25(3):225–8

**France**

Jiménez-Olivares E: La demonología en el siglo XV. **Prensa Med Mex** 1979 Mar–Apr;44(3–4):72–4

**Spain**

Dieckhöfer K: Juan Huarte de San Juan, precursor de la psicología diferencial. In International Congress of the History of Medicine, 27th, Barcelona, 1980. Actas. Barcelona, Académia de Ciències Médiques de Catalunya i Balears, 1981. p. 64–8.

**1700 to Present**

Aberbach D: Freud's Jewish problem. **Commentary** 1980;69(6):35–9
Ackerknecht EH: Wilhelm Reich (1897–1957). In Ganzinger K, Skopec M, Wyklicky H, ed: Festschrift für Erna Lesky zum 70. Geburtstag. Wien, Brüder Hollinek, 1981. p. 5–12.
Ader R, Schmale AH: George Libman Engel: on the occasion of his retirement. **Psychosom Med** 1980;42(1 Suppl):79–101
Albarello B, Collorio C: Analisi dei collegamenti tra l'opera freudiana e il positivismo ottocentesco. **Acta Med Hist Patav** 1982–83;29:9–18
Albarello B: Il concetto di regressione in Freud. **Minerva Psichiatr** 1984 Jan–Mar;25(1):23–36
Albin M, Devlin RJ, Heeger G, ed: New directions in psychohistory. The Adelphi papers in honor of Erik H. Erikson. Lexington, Toronto, D.

C. Heath, 1980. xx, 217 p. Includes contributions by E. S. Wolf, M. F. Shore, G. M. Platt, H. Feinstein, S. H. Rudolph, L. I. Rudolph.
Angelini A: Wilhelm Reich nel dibattito psicoanalitico degli anni Trenta. **Stor Crit Psicol** 1984;5(2):373–88
Antón Fructuoso P: Las ideas biológicas en la psiquiatría de ayer. **Rev Med Univ Navarra** 1981 Sep;25(3):59–62
Bakan D: Freud e la tradizione mistica ebraica: psicoanalisi e cabala. **Comunita** 1976;39(176):206–44
Balmary M: Psychoanalyzing psychoanalysis--Freud and the hidden fault of the father. Baltimore, Johns Hopkins University Press, 1982. xxiii, 184 p.
Barahona Fernándes H: O sentido actual de obra de K. Kleist e as repercusões nos países Ibero-Americanos. **Actas Luso Esp Neurol Psiquiatr** 1979 Nov–Dec;7(6):341–52
Baruk H: Die französische und europäische Psychiatrie von Pinel bis heute. In Sournia JC, Martiny M, Poulet J, ed: Illustrierte Geschichte der Medizin. Salzburg, Andreas, 1980. Vol. 6. p. 2034–43.
Baruk H: Moïse, Freud et le veau d'or. **Rev Hist Med Heb** 1984 Jul;37(2):19–23
Baruk H: Vers la résurrection de la civilisation hébraïque. La psychiatrie hébraique. **Rev Hist Med Heb** 1983 Jul;36(145):25–7
Basch MF: Selfobject disorders and psychoanalytic theory: a historical perspective. **J Am Psychoanal Assoc** 1981;29(2):337–51
Baumer G, Greulich G: Otto Rank. In J. Rattner, ed: Wandlungen der Psychoanalyse. Wien, Europaverlag, 1980. p. 31–52.
Beierlein C: Zum Leben und Schaffen von Sigmund Freud (1856–1939) im Umfeld seiner Zeit. **Wiss Z Martin Luther Univ (Math)** 1984;33(2):101–12
Benedetti G: Die neurotische Lebensproblematik Nietzsches als eine Wirkkraft und eine Grenze seiner Philosophie. **Gesnerus** 1984;41(1/2):111–32
Berlin JB: Richard Beer-Hofmann and Theodor Reik: a letter in exile. **Psychoanal Rev** 1981–82 Winter;68(4):479–86
Berliner AK: Psychoanalysis and society. The social thought of Sigmund Freud. Washington, D.C., University Press of America, 1983. x, 205 p.
Berrios GE: Descriptive psychopathology: conceptual and historical aspects. **Psychol Med** 1984 May;14(2):303–13
Biniek EM: Psychotherapie mit gestalterischen Mitteln. Eine Einführung in die Gestaltungstherapie. (Die Medizin) Darmstadt, Wissenschaftliche Buchgesellschaft, 1982. 169 p.
Biondani P, Frazzingaro S: Evoluzione storica del concetto di aggressività in psicoanalisi ed etologia. **Acta Med Hist Patav** 1981/82;28:9–20
Bocock R: Freud and modern society. An outline and analysis of Freud's sociology. New York, Holmes & Meier, 1978. xv, 200 p.
Bocock R: Sigmund Freud. Chichester, Horwood; London; New York, Tavistock, 1983. 145 p.
Bolzinger A: Jalons pour une histoire de la psychiatrie à travers la Revue de Neuropsychiatrie infantile. **Neuropsychiatr Enfance Adolesc** 1981 Mar;29(3):127–40
Bori PC: Materiale storico-religioso nella biblioteca di Sigmund Freud: alcuni rilievi sul catalogo. **Ann Ist Stor Italo-Ger** 1975;1:281–9
Boss M: Entwicklung der Psychotherapie im 20. Jahrhundert. **Universitas (Stuttg)** 1981;6:
Boss M: Exposé sur le développement de la psychothérapie au XXe siècle. **Schweiz Arch Neurol Neurochir Psychiatr** 1981;128(2):183–96
Boulanger JB: Dissidences, sécessions et défections dans l'histoire du mouvement psychanalytique. **Union Med Can** 1983 Aug;112(8):744–6
Bourguignon A: Geschichte der Psychoanalyse. In Sournia JC, Martiny M, Poulet J, ed: Illustrierte Geschichte der Medizin. Salzburg, Andreas, 1980. Vol. 7. p. 2403–29.
Boyer LB: Die Psychoanalyse in der Ethnologie. Ein Literaturbericht. **Psyche (Stuttg)** 1980 Aug;34(8):694–715
Brill H: Notes on the history of social psychiatry. **Compr Psychiatry** 1980 Nov–Dec;21(6):492–9
Brun D: Les sources infantiles de la théorie chez Freud. Une scène d'enfance dans l'après-coup. **Rev Fr Psychanal** 1982;46(3):583–99
Brunclík J: Freud o dostojevském - či naopak. **Cas Lek Cesk** 1982 Aug 13;121(32):1015–6
Buckley NL: Women psychoanalysts and the theory of feminine development: a study of Karen Horney, Helene Deutsch, and Marie Bonaparte. Ph.D. Diss., University of California. Los Angeles, 1982. 178 p.
Burnham JC, McGuire W: Jelliffe: American psychoanalyst and physician & his correspondence with Sigmund Freud and C. G. Jung. Chicago, University of Chicago Press, 1983. xx, 324 p. With contributions by A. R. D'Amore and J. E. Sauer.
Burnham JC: The acceptance of psychoanalysis in Western cultures: an afterword on its comparative history. **Comp Stud Soc Hist** 1982;24(4):603–10
Bynum WF: Alcoholism and degeneration in 19th century European medicine and psychiatry. **Br J Addict** 1984 Mar;79(1):59–70
Cade JF: Mending the mind. A short history of twentieth-century psychiatry. Melbourne, Sun Books, 1979. 108 p.
Caire JB: A holographic model of a psychosomatic pattern: Freud's specimen dream re-interpreted. **Psychother Psychosom** 1981;36(2):132–42
Campbell RJ: Flashbacks: scenes from psychiatry's revolutions. **Bull NY Acad Med** 1984 Jun;60(5):479–93
Camus CH: La psychoanalyse, avènement d'une connaissance originale (Sigmund Freud). **Soins Psychiatr** 1980 Dec;(6):3–8
Carotenuto A: A secret symmetry: Sabina Spielrein between Jung and Freud. New York, Pantheon Books, 1982. xix, 250 p.
Carr V: The concept of clinical state in psychiatry: a review. **Compr Psychiatry** 1983 Jul–Aug;24(4):370–91
Carrillo Broatch A: Aspectos del linde de la psiquiatría y la terapéutica biológica. **Rev Neuropsiquiatr** 1980 Jun;43(2):87–96
Carter KC: Germ theory, hysteria, and Freud's early work in psychopathology. **Med Hist** 1980 Jul;24(3):259–74
Chabot CB: Freud on Schreber. Psychoanalytic theory and the critical act. Amherst, University of Massachusetts Press, 1982. 171 p.
Chawla PL: Child psychiatry--historical perspective. **Indian J Pediatr** 1984 Mar–Apr;51(409):191–2
Chazaud J: Les contestations actuelles de la psychanalyse. Toulouse, Privat, 1974. 227 p.
Chemin A, Ganry C: Approche systémique et thérapie familiale. Place et histoire du mouvement systémique. **Soins Psychiatr** 1983 Dec;(38):3–7
Chertok L: Hypnosis and suggestion in a century of psychotherapy: an epistemological assessment. **J Am Acad Psychoanal** 1984 Apr;12(2):211–32
Chertok L, De Saussure R: The therapeutic revolution from Mesmer to Freud. New York, Brunner/Mazel, 1979. xiii, 226 p. Translation of French ed., 1973.
Chessick RD: Freud teaches psychotherapy. Indianapolis, Cambridge, Hackett, 1980. viii, 342 p.
Chromý K: Masturbace a historie psychiatrie. **Cesk Psychiatr** 1984 Jun;80(3):180–3
Clark RW: Freud: the man the cause. New York, Random House, 1980. 652 p.
Clark RW: Sigmund Freud's sortie to America. **Am Heritage** 1980;3(3):34–43
Cohen RS, Laudan L, ed: Physics, philosophy and psychoanalysis. Essays in honor of Adolf Grünbaum. Dordrecht, D. Reidel, 1983. xviii, 339 p. (Boston Studies in the Philosophy of Science, v. 76).
Cole DR: Helping: origins and development of the major psychotherapies. Toronto, Butterworths, 1982. xv, 390 p.
Cooper AM: Psychoanalysis at one hundred: beginnings of maturity. **J Am Psychoanal Assoc** 1984;32(2):245–67
Cournut J: L'innocence de la Marquise ou spécificités et vicissitudes de l'après-coup dans la théorie freudienne et la pratique analytique. **Rev Fr Psychanal** 1982;46(3):535–57
Cremerius J: Die ödipal verkleidete präödipale Liebe oder Feydeaus professionelles Missverständnis. **Psyche (Stuttg)** 1981;35:253–67
Cremerius J: Freuds Sterben--Die Identität von Denken, Leben und Sterben. **Psychother Psychosom Med Psychol** 1983 Sep;33(5):163–6
Csiky K, Csiky CE, Grecu G: Electroşocul în psihiatrie. **Rev Med Interna [Neurol Psihiatr]** 1981 Oct–Dec;26(4):259–66
Danzinger R, Lyon G: Das Beratungszentrum für psychische und sociale Fragen in Graz. Wien, Osterreichische Akademie der Wissenschaften, 1982. 140 p.
Dauven J: La genèse de la psychanalyse (Freud, Wagner, et la Walkyrie Materna). Paris, Nouvelles Editions latines, 1979. 163 p.
Decker HS: Freud and Dora: constraints on medical progress. **J Soc Hist** 1981;14(3):445–64
Decker HS: The choice of a name: 'Dora' and Freud's relationship with Breuer. **J Am Psychoanal Assoc** 1982;30(1):113–36
Degleris N: Contribution à l'étude des relations Franco-Helleniques au point de vue de la presse neuro-psychiatrique française (1880–1914); les membres associés grecs de la Société Médico-Psychologique. Mémoire pour le titre d'assistant étranger, Université Paris V, René Descartes, Faculté de Médecine Cochin-Port Royal, Paris, 1984. 96 leaves.
Deniker P: Psychopharmacologie et psychiatrie biologique rappel historique. **Soins Psychiatr** 1983 Nov;(37):5–6
Dews PB: Pavlov and psychiatry. **J Hist Behav Sci** 1981;17:246–50
Diamond S: Sigmund Freud, his Jewishness, and scientific method: the seen and the unseen as evidence. **J Hist Ideas** 1982 Oct–Dec;43(4):613–34
Dieckhöfer K: Frühe Formen der Antipsychiatrie und die Reaktion der Psychiatrie. **Medizinhist J** 1984;19(1–2):101–11
Dilman I: Freud and human nature. Oxford, Basil Blackwell, 1983. 207 p.
DuPlessis RB, Friedman SS: 'Woman is perfect': H. D.'s debate with Freud. **Feminist Stud** 1981;7(3):407–30
Eagle MN: The epistemological status of recent developments in psychoanalytic theory. In R.S. Cohen, L. Laudan, ed: Physics, philosophy and psychoanalysis. Dordrecht, D. Reidel, 1983. p. 31–55.
Eissler KR: K. R. Eissler on errors regarding Freud. **Int J Psychoanal** 1981;62(3):371–2
Eissler KR: Victor Tausk's suicide. New York, International Universities Press, 1983. 322 p.
Ekstein R: As I remember her: Anna Freud, 1895–1982. **Adolesc Psychiatry** 1983;11:5–8
Ellenberger H: Le secret pathogène et son traitement. **Rev Int Hist Psychiatr** 1983;1(1):5–22
Engelman E: Berggasse 19, Sigmund Freud's home and offices, Vienna, 1938: the photographs of Edmund Engelman. Chicago, University of Chicago Press, 1981. 153 p.

Fähndrich E, Helmchen H, Hippius H: The history of the AMDP-System. **Mod Probl Pharmacopsychiatry** 1983;20:1-9

Federn E: On the difficulty of writing history of ideas: a reply. **J Hist Behav Sci** 1980 Jan;16(1):45-9

Fenichel O: Psychoanalyse und Gesellschaftswissenschaften (1938). **Psyche (Stuttg)** 1981 Nov;35(11):1055-71

Fischer-Homberger E: Psychiatrie im Wandel der Zeit. **Schweiz Spital** 1980;44(2):24-7

Fischle-Carl H, ed: Theorie und Praxis der Psychoanalyse. Fellbach, Bonz, 1979. Historical contributions p. 7-132, by H. Thomä, J. Cremerius, A. Dührssen, P. Kutter, W. Bräutigam, G. Benedetti.

Fisher S, Greenberg RP, ed: The scientific evaluation of Freud's theories and therapy; a book of readings. New York, Basic Books, 1978. xv, 446 p. (Reprinted articles of various authors).

Flegenheimer WV: Techniques of brief pschotherapy. New York, London, Jason Aronson, 1982. xiii, 206 p.

Forrester J: Language and the origins of psychoanalysis. London, Macmillan, 1980. xvi, 285 p.

Frances A, Cooper AM: Descriptive and dynamic psychiatry: a perspective on DSM-III. **Am J Psychiatry** 1981 Sep;138(9):1198-202

Freeman L, Strean HS: Freud and women. New York, Frederick Ungar, 1981. xiii, 238 p.

Frey-Rohn L: Von Freud zu Jung. Eine vergleichende Studie zur Psychologie des Unbewussten. (2. überarbeitete Ausgabe) Zürich, Daimon Verlag, 1980?. 456 p.

Fullinwider SP: Sigmund Freud, John Hughlings Jackson, and speech. **J Hist Ideas** 1983 Jan-Mar;44(1):151-8

Gautier J: Freud a menti. Périgny-sur-Yerres, Mandres-les-Roses, Edition de 'La vie claire, 1977. vii, 566 p.

Gershenowitz H: The influence of Lamarckism on the development of Freud's psychoanalytic theory. **Indian J Hist Sci** 1979 Nov;14(2):105-13

Gilman SL: Den Geisteskranken sehen: Mackenzie, Kleist, William James. **Confin Psychiatr** 1979;22(3):127-44

Ginzburg C: Morelli, Freud and Sherlock Holmes: clues and scientific method. **Hist Workshop J** 1980;9:5-36

Glymour C: The theory of your dreams. In R.S. Cohen, L. Laudan, ed: Physics, philosophy and psychoanalysis. Dordrecht, D. Reidel, 1983. p. 57-71.

Gmelin OF: Anti-Freud: von der Psychoanalyse zur Medienwissenschaft. Mit einem Beitrag von Helene Saussure. Frankfurt am Main, Haag and Herchen, 1979. 175 p.

Goering JD: Sigmund Freud, Carl Jung and religion. **Mennon Q Rev** 1982;56(1):47-56

Goldberg A, ed: The future of psychoanalysis. Essays in honor of Heinz Kohut. New York, International Universities Press, 1983. xx, 514 p. Contributions by A. M. Cooper, R. S. Wallerstein, W. W. Meissner, R. D. Stolorow, G. E. Atwood, A. H. Modell, R. Michels, L. Friedman, J. S. Grotstein, J. D. Lichtenberg, M. Kanzer, P. Tolpin, E. Schwaber, E. S. Wolf, B. Brandchaft, M. Tolpin, A. Ornstein, B. E. Litowitz, N. S. Litowitz, M. F. Basch, P. H. Knapp, N. J. London, C. B. Strozier.

Goldstein RL: Sigmund Freud: forensic psychiatrist. **Bull Am Acad Psychiatry Law** 1983;11(3):273-7

Goldwert M: Toynbee and Jung: the historian and analytical psychology--a brief comment. **J Anal Psychol** 1983 Oct;28(4):363-6

Gómez EA: El problema del liderazgo en psicoanalisis. **Rev Neuropsiquiatr** 1978 Sep-Dec;41(3-4):92-100

Goodheart WB: C. G. Jung's first 'patient': on the seminal emergence of Jung's thought. **J Anal Psychol** 1984 Jan;29(1):1-34

Gras VW: Myth and the reconciliation of opposites: Jung and Lévi-Strauss. **J Hist Ideas** 1981 Jul-Sep;42(3):471-88

Gravitz MA, Gerton MI: Freud and hypnosis: report of post-rejection use. **J Hist Behav Sci** 1981 Jan;17(1):68-74

Grayson RS: Collection of psychoanalytic classics. **J Am Psychoanal Assoc** 1979;27(4):913-20

Greenacre P: A historical sketch of the use and disuse of reconstruction. **Psychoanal Study Child** 1980;35:35-40

Greisman HC: Social structure, psychoanalysis, and collective aggression. **Hist Eur Ideas** 1981;2(1):35-48

Grenander ME: Of graver importance than history: psychiatry in fiction. **J Libert Stud** 1978;2(1):29-44

Grinberg L, Rodríguez JF: The influence of Cervantes on the future creator of psychoanalysis. **Int J Psychoanal** 1984;65(Pt 2):155-68

Grinstein A: Sigmund Freud's dreams. New York, International Universities Press, 1980. 486 p.

Grotjahn M: Remembering Theodor Reik and the third ear. **Psychoanal Rev** 1981-82 Winter;68(4):473-6

Grubrich-Simitis I: Siegfried Bernfeld: Historiker der Psychoanalyse und Freud-Biograph. **Psyche (Stuttg)** 1981 May;35(5):397-434

Guerrero AC: The superego concept. Part I: historical review; object relations approach. **Psychoanal Rev** 1981 Fall;68(3):321-42

Gunter PA: Bergson and Jung. **J Hist Ideas** 1982 Oct-Dec;43(4):635-52

Gutmann A: Freud versus feminism. **Dissent** 1979;26(2):204-12

Hamanaka Y: [Basic neuropsychologic concepts and their origins (conclusion)] (Jpn). **No To Shinkei** 1983 Mar;35(3):310-1

Hausmann J: Die Syndrome 'Manie' und 'Melancholie' an der Wende zum 18. Jahrhundert. Dargestellt an zwei zeitgenössischen Dissertationen. Diss., Rheinische Friedrich-Wilhelms-Universität. Bonn, 1982. 148 p.

Havens LL: Twentieth-century psychiatry: a view from the sea. **Am J Psychiatry** 1981 Oct;138(10):1279-87

Heimann H: De Kraepelin au sytème AMDP. **Acta Psychiatr Belg** 1983 Mar-Apr;83(2):147-54

Herren R: Freud und die Kriminologie: Einführung in die psychoanalytische Kriminologie. Stuttgart, Enke, 1973. x, 281 p.

Hirschberg JC: History of child psychiatry. In H. I. Kaplan, et al, ed: Comprehensive textbook of psychiatry/III. Third edition. Baltimore, London, Williams and Wilkins, 1980. p. 2417-21.

Hoff SG: Frieda Fromm-Reichmann. In Dictionary of American Biography, Suppl. 6, 1956-1960. p. 219-20, 1980.

Hoffman LE: War, revolution, and psychoanalysis: Freudian thought begins to grapple with social reality. **J Hist Behav Sci** 1981;17:251-69

Hogenson GB: Jung's struggle with Freud. Notre Dame, London, University of Notre Dame Press, 1983. xi, 180 p.

Ilnicki S: Pomoc psychiatryczna na polu walki-ewolucja poglądów i metod postępowania. **Psychiatr Pol** 1980 Sep-Oct;14(5):539-46

Ingleby D: The social construction of mental illness. In P. Wright, A. Treacher, ed: The problem of medical knowledge. Examining the social construction of medicine. Edinburgh, Edinburgh University Press, 1982. p. 123-43.

Jaccard R: Histoire de la psychanalyse. [France], Hachette, 1982. 2 v.

Jarrick A: Freud och historien. **Scandia** 1982;48(1):107-48

Juillet P: Aspects évolutifs de la psychiatrie aux armées. In: Congrès National des Sociétés Savantes, 103e, Nancy, 1978. Comptes Rendus. Paris, 1978. Section des Sciences, Fasc. V. p. 99-111.

Kanzer M, Glenn J, ed., et al: Freud and his patients. New York and London, Aronson, 1980. 452 p.

Kanzer M, Glenn J, ed: Freud and his self-analysis. New York and London, Aronson, 1979. x, 308 p. (Downstate Psychoanalytic Institute, Twenty-Fifth Anniversary Series, Vol. I). Includes reprinted papers by various authors.

Kanzer M: Freud, Theodor Lipps, and 'scientific psychology'. **Psychoanal Q** 1981;50(3):393-410

Kaplan AH: From discovery to validation: a basic challenge to psychoanalysis. **J Am Psychoanal Assoc** 1981;29(1):3-26

Kardiner A: My analysis with Freud. New York, Norton, 1977. 123 p.

Karl Menninger: a literary self-portrait: A celebration issue for his 90th birthday. **Bull Menninger Clin** 1983 Jul;47(4):293-400

Kätzel S: Individuum contra Gesellschaft? Ein Beitrag zur Kritik der Gesellschaftsauffassung von Sigmund Freud. **Wiss Z Karl Marx Univ Math Natur Wiss Reihe** 1973;22(5):467-82

Kazdin AE: History of behavior modification. Baltimore, University Park Press, 1978. xi, 468 p.

Kennedy H: Anna Freud, 1895-1982. **Psychoanal Q** 1983 Oct;52(4):501-6

Kern S: The prehistory of Freud's dream theory: Freud's masterpiece anticipated. **Hist Med (Lond)** 1975 Autumn-Winter;6(3-4):83-92

Kernberg OF: The contributions of Edith Jacobson: an overview. **J Am Psychoanal Assoc** 1979;27(4):793-819

Kirsch J: Jung's transference on Freud: its Jewish element. **Am Imago** 1984;41:63-84

Klein DB: Jewish origins of the psychoanalytic movement. New York, Praeger, 1981. xvi, 198 p.

Knobel P: Relations entre la psychiatrie francaise et le Brésil. **Ann Med Psychol (Paris)** 1984 Apr;142(4):499-503

Knoepfmacher H: Sigmund Freud in high school. **Am Imago** 1979 Fall;36(3):287-300

Kobarg I: Das Leben und Werk von Sandor Rado. Diss. Mainz, 1979. 73 p.

Koehler KG: The Schreber case and affective illness: a research diagnostic re-assessment. **Psychol Med** 1981 Nov;11(4):689-96

Kottayarikil C: Sigmund Freud on religion and morality: a challenge to Christianity. Innsbruck, Resch, 1977. xx, 399 p.

Kovel J: Marx and Freud. In M. Albin, R. J. Devlin, G. Heeger, ed: New directions in psychohistory. The Adelphi papers in honor of Erik H. Erikson. Lexington, Toronto, D. C. Heath, 1980. p. 21-6.

Kraus A, ed: Leib. Geist. Geschichte. Brennpunkte anthropologischer Psychiatrie. Festschrift zum 60. Geburtstag von Hubertus Tellenbach. With contributions by W. Baeyer, W. Blankenburg, H. G. Gadamer, W. Jacob, B. Kimura, H. Lang, A. Leder, G. Marcel, A Métraux, B. Pauleikhoff, H. Schipperges. Heidelberg, Hüthig, 1978. (Medizin im Wandel).

Kringlen E: Personlighet og psykiatrisk teori. **Tidsskr Samfunnsforskning** 1980;21(2):179-85

Krüll M: Freud und sein Vater. München, Beck, 1979. 344 p.

Lacorre B: Role des savoirs constitués dans la justification de la notion d'inconscient psychique. In Poirier J, Poirier JL, ed: Médicine et philosophie à la fin du XIXe siècle. Paris, Université de Paris XII - Val de Marne, [1980?]. p. 127-40.

Langer D: Paul Ferdinand Schilder, Leben und Werk. Diss. Mainz, 1979. 259 p.

Langer M: Memoria, historia y diálogo psicoanalítico. With Jaime del Palacio and Enrique Guinsberg. Mexico City. Folios Ediciones S. A., 1981. 240 p.

Langs R: The psychotherapeutic conspiracy. New York, Aronson, 1982. xiii, 338 p.

Langs R, ed: Classics in psychoanalytic technique. New York, London,

Jason Aronson, 1981. xii, 523 p. Contains 44 papers from various authors.

Langsley DG: Community psychiatry. In H. I. Kaplan, et al, ed: Comprehensive textbook of psychiatry/III. Third edition. Baltimore, London, Williams and Wilkins, 1980. p. 2836–54.

Lanteri-Laura G: La constitution civile du cerveau. **Rev Int Hist Psychiatr** 1983;1(1):23–45

Lebzeltern G: S. Freud und das Kokain. **Wien Klin Wochenschr** 1983 Nov 11;95(21):765–9

Lerner EA: Franz Gabriel Alexander. In Dictionary of American Biography, 1961–1965. Suppl. 7, 1981. p. 5–7.

Lerner L: Esther Menaker. **Psychoanal Rev** 1984 Spring;71(1):iii–viii

Leupold-Löwenthal H: Zur Geschichte der 'Frage der Laienanalyse'. **Psyche (Stuttg)** 1984 Feb;38(2):97–120

Lipton SD: An addendum to 'The advantages of Freud's technique, as shown in his analysis of the Rat Man'. **Int J Psychoanal** 1979;60(pt2):215–6

Lohmann HM, ed: Die Psychoanalyse auf der Couch. Frankfurt am Main, Qumran, 1984. 330 p. Historical contributions by E. Federn, J. Cremerius, K. Brede, A. Lorenzer, M. Pohlen.

Lomax EM, Kagan J, Rosenkrantz BG: Science and patterns of child care. San Francisco, W. H. Freeman, 1978. xiv, 247 p.

Lothane Z: Listening with the Third Ear as an instrument in psychoanalysis: the contributions of Reik and Isakower. **Psychoanal Rev** 1981–82 Winter;68(4):487–503

McCarthy T: Freud and the problem of sexuality. **J Hist Behav Sci** 1981;17:332–9

McGuinness BF: Freud e Wittgenstein. **Ann Sc Norm Super Pisa** 1979;9(1):409–24

Maeder C: Zur Geschichte der Psychiatrie. Umgang mit psychisch Kranken--gestern und heute. **Krankenpflege (Frankfurt)** 1984;38(5):155–8;(6):197–200

Mahler-Schachter E: Svevo, Trieste and the Vienna Circle: Zeno's analyst analysed. **Eur Stud Rev** 1982;12(1):45–66

Mahony P: Freud as a writer. New York, International Universities Press, 1982. xv, 227 p.

Mainetti JA: Leyendo con Freud La peau de chagrin de Balzac. **Asclepio** 1982;34:265–81

Mann WE, Hoffman E: The man who dreamed of tomorrow. A conceptual biography of Wilhelm Reich. Los Angeles, Tarcher, 1980. 295 p.

Manus A, Bourguignon A: Réflexions sur les limites de la psychiatrie. **Nouv Presse Med** 1979 Oct 8;8(38):3051–3

Marchais P: Vers la fin de l'ère Kraepelinienne? **Ann Med Psychol (Paris)** 1980 Nov;138(9):1061–78

May R: Freud and the phallic defense. **Psychiatry** 1979;42(2):147–56

Meisel P, ed: Freud: a collection of critical essays. Englewood Cliffs, New Jersey, Prentice-Hall, 1981. 240 p. Reprinted works by literary figures.

Menaker E: Otto Rank: a rediscovered legacy. New York, Columbia University Press, 1982. xvii, 166 p.

Meyer L: Cristofredo Jakob. A veinticinco años de su muerte. **Acta Psiquiatr Psicol Am Lat** 1981 Mar;27(1):13–4

Meynell GG: Freud translated: an historical and bibliographical note. **J R Soc Med** 1981 Apr;74(4):306–9

Midelfort HC: Madness and civilization in early modern Europe: a reappraisal of Michel Foucault. In Malament, Barbara C., ed. After the Reformation: Essays in honor of J. H. Hexter, Philadelphia; U. of Pennsylvania Press, 1980. p. 247–65.

Miller J: Interpretations of Freud's Jewishness, 1924–1974. **J Hist Behav Sci** 1981;17:357–74

Milner M: Freud et l'interprétation de la littérature. Paris, Société d'édition d'enseignement supérieur, 1980. 328 p.

Mindham RH: My father knew Adolf Meyer. The currency of Meyer's ideas in British psychiatry. **Br J Psychiatry** 1984 Mar;144:323–5

Mitscherlich A: Probleme und Standort der Psychoanalyse. **Universitas (Stuttg)** 1982;37(6):575–80

Montiel L: El psicoanálisis en la Montaña mágica. In International Congress of the History of Medicine, 27th, Barcelona, 1980. Actas. Barcelona, Acadèmia de Ciències Mèdiques de Catalunya i Balears, 1981. p. 116–20.

Montiel L: Freud y el psicoanálisis en dos conferencias de Thomas Mann. In International Congress of the History of Medicine, 27th, Barcelona, 1980. Actas. Barcelona, Acadèmia de Ciències Mèdiques de Catalunya i Balears, 1981. p. 111–5.

Mora G: 1979 anniversaries. **Am J Psychiatry** 1980 Jan;137(1):56–60

Mora Merida JA: Freud: De la libido al eros. La coherencia del discurso freudiano. Malaga, Universidad de Malaga, 1979. 284 p.

Mormont C, Bobon D, Frenckell R von, et al: Introduction aux Journées AMDP d'hommage à Jean Bobon. **Acta Psychiatr Belg** 1982 Jul–Aug;82(4):367–70

Muldworf B: Freud. Paris, Les Editeurs français réunis, 1976. 349 p.

Muñoz PE: Psiquiatría social: un punto de vista sobre el enfermar. **Actas Loso Esp Neurol Psiquiatr** 1983 Mar–Apr;11(2):163–80

Musatti C: Freud e l'ebraismo. **Belfagor** 1980;35(6):687–96

Neill JR, Ludwig AM: Psychiatry and psychotherapy: past and future. **Am J Psychother** 1980 Jan;34(1):39–50

Neubauer PB: Anna Freud's legacy. **Psychoanal Q** 1983 Oct;52(4):507–13

Nica-Udangiu S: Karl Jaspers (1883–1969). **Rev Med Interna [Neurol Psihiatr]** 1983 Oct–Dec;28(4):311–6

Obholzer K: The Wolf-man. Conversations with Freud's patient--sixty years later. New York, Continuum, 1982. 250 p.

Odajnyk VW: Jung and politics. The political and social ideas of C. G. Jung. New York, New York University Press, 1976. xv, 190 p.

Pagel G: Narziss und Prometheus: die Theorie der Phantasie bei Freud und Gehlen. Würzburg, Königshausen & Neumann, 1984. 195 p. (Studien zur Anthropologie, Band 8).

Pansera MT: Per un'antropologia filosofica freudiana: il valore della negazione. **Physis** 1982;24(1):76–108

Parry-Jones WL: The development of the psychotherapies: a brief historical overview. In M. Weller, ed: The scientific basis of psychiatry. London, Baillière Tindall, 1983. p. 391–401.

Parson T: The articulation of the personality and the social-action system: Sigmund Freud and Max Weber. In M. Albin, R. J. Devlin, G. Heeger, ed: New directions in psychohistory. The Adelphi papers in honor of Erik H. Erikson. Lexington, Toronto, D. C. Heath, 1980. p. 27–35.

Pauleikhoff B: Das Menschenbild im Wandel der Zeit: Ideengeschichte der Psychiatrie und der klinischen Psychologie. Hürtgenwald, Pressler, 1983. 2 vol. 416 p., 439 p.

Peck W, Diethelm O: Review of the Freud library. In International Congress of the History of Medicine, 27th, Barcelona, 1980. Actas. Barcelona, Acadèmia de Ciències Mèdiques de Catalunya i Balears, 1981. p. 130–3.

Peters UH, ed: Psychiatrie. Weinheim, Beltz, 1983. 2 v. 588, 581 p. (Kindlers 'Psychologie des 20. Jahrhunderts'). Historical contributions by R. Tölle, H. Kindler, W. Schmitt, D. von Zerssen, Y. Fried, P. Berner.

Petot JM: Mélanie Klein: le moi et le bon objet, 1932–1960. [Paris], Dunod, 1982. xvi, 303 p.

Phillilps S: Psychoanalysis and childhood education: a historical review. **Paedagog Hist** 1977;17(2):378–85

Pichot P: Historical introduction to psychiatry. In M. Weller, ed: The scientific basis of psychiatry. London, Baillière Tindall, 1983. p. 34–46.

Pichot P: Un siècle de psychiatrie. Neuilly-sur-Seine [France], Roche, [1983] 189 p.

Pletsch C: Freud's case studies. **Partisan Rev** 1982;49(1):101–18

Pohlen M, Wittmann L: 'Die Unterwelt bewegen.' Versuch über Wahrnehmung und Phantasie in der Psychoanalyse. Frankfurt am Main, Syndikat, 1980. 112 p.

Porter R: Was there a moral therapy in eighteenth century psychiatry? **Lychnos** 1981–82;:12–26

Powell RC: Manfred Joshua Sakel. In Dictionary of American Biography, Suppl. 6, 1956–1960. p. 563–4, 1980.

Raditsa L: Some sense about Wilhelm Reich. New York, Philosophical Library, 1978. 126 p.

Ramas M: Freud's Dora, Dora's hysteria: the negation of a woman's rebellion. **Feminist Stud** 1980;6(3):472–510

Rangell L: The Anna Freud experience. **Psychoanal Study Child** 1984;39:29–43

Rattner J, ed: Wandlungen der Psychoanalyse. Wien, Europaverlag, 1980. 373 p.

Rausky F: Le discours freudien sur l'antisémitisme.

Rawlinson MC: Psychiatric discourse and the feminine voice. **J Med Philos** 1982 May;7(2):153–77

Rawn ML: Some reflections on the work of Theodor Reik. **Psychoanal Rev** 1981–82 Winter;68(4):477–8

Reich W: Psychiatry's second coming: the way we analyse now. **Encounter (Lond)** 1981;57(2):66–72

Reverzy JF: Introduction au secteur psychiatrique, définitions et historique. **Soins Psychiatr** 1980 Oct;(5):3–8

Reverzy JF: Pour une compréhension historique de la psychiatrie. **Soins Psychiatr** 1982 Feb;(16):3

Rice JL: Russian stereotypes in the Freud-Jung correspondence. **Slavic Rev** 1982 Spring;41(1):19–34

Rissmann W: Ernst Freiherr von Feuchtersleben (1806–1849). Sein Beitrag zur medizinischen Anthropologie und Psychopathologie. Freiburg im Breisgau, Schulz, 1980. 243 p. (Freiburger Forschungen zur Medizingeschichte, Neue Folge, Band 12).

Roazen P: Paul Roazen on errors regarding Freud. **Int J Psychoanal** 1982;63(pt 2):260–1

Robert BP: Origines du surréalisme. **Univ Ottawa Q** 1982;52(2):190–205

Rodero Vicente B: Psiquiatría comunitaria: reforma psiquiátrica. **Rev Sanid Hig Publica (Madr)** 1982 Sep–Oct;56(9–10):941–51

Rogers FB: Analytical psychology: Carl Jung and his circle. **Trans Stud Coll Physicians Phila** 1980 Dec;5(2 no 4):284–8

Rogers FB: The legacy of Carl Jung. **Trans Stud Coll Physicians Phila** 1979 Sep;5(1 No 3):211–14

Rokhlin LL, Shereshevskiĭ AM, Tom A: Znamenatel'nye daty 1982 g. **Zh Nevropatol Psikhiatr** 1982;82(1):130–40

Rokhlin LL, Shereshevskiĭ AM, Tom A: Znamenatel'nye i iubileĭnye daty nevropatologii i psikhiatrii 1983 g. **Zh Nevropatol Psikhiatr** 1983;83(1):122–33

Roustang F: Dire mastery. Discipleship from Freud to Lacan. Translated by Ned Lukacher. Baltimore, London, Johns Hopkins University Press, 1982. (Translation of: Un destin si funeste).

Rubinstein BB: Freud's early theories of hysteria. In R.S. Cohen, L. Laudan, ed: Physics, philosophy and psychoanalysis. Dordrecht, D. Reidel, 1983. p. 169–90.

Ruse M: Medicine as social science: the case of Freud on homosexuality.

**J Med Philos** 1981 Nov;6(4):361–86

Ruse M, ed: Nature animated. Historical and philosophical case studies in Greek medicine, nineteenth-century and recent biology, psychiatry, and psychoanalysis. Papers deriving from the Third International Conference on the History and Philosophy of Science, Montreal, Canada, 1980. Volume II. Dordrecht, D. Reidel, 1983. xiii, 274 p.

Rychlak JF: Freud's confrontation with the telic mind. **J Hist Behav Sci** 1981;17:176–83

Salimbeni F: Psicanalisi e storiografia: un problema pluridisciplinare. **Studium** 1981;77(5):565–80

Salvetti ME: Gefässpsychopathologie bei Richard von Krafft-Ebing (1840–1902). Bern, Huber, 1984. 125 p. (Berner Beiträge zur Geschichte der Medizin und der Naturwissenschaften, Neue Folge, Band 10)

Sander FM: Individual and family therapy: toward an integration. New York Aronson, 1979. Historical chapters, p. 1–42, 89–109.

Sandler J: On the psychoanalytic theory of affects. A historical and developmental review. **Isr J Psychiatry Relat Sci** 1983;20(1-2):81–94

Sarro R: Razon y sinrazon de las heterodoxias psicoanaliticas. **Asclepio** 1980;32:421–32

Sartorius N: La classification: une optique internationale. **Acta Psychiatr Belg** 1983 Mar–Apr;83(2):88–103

Satin DG: Erich Lindemann as humanist, scientist, and change agent. **Am J Community Psychol** 1984 Oct;12(5):519–27

Schachter M: Le professeur Erich Stern (1889–1959) psychiatre et psychologue. **Rev Hist Med Heb** 1980 Oct;134(33 no 3):53–4)

Schiller F: A Möbius strip. Fin-de-siècle neuropsychiatry and Paul Möbius. Berkeley, University of California Press, 1982. 134 p.

Schmitt W: Das Modell der Naturwissenschaft in der Psychiatrie im Ubergang vom 19. zum 20. Jahrhundert. **Ber Wissenschaftsgesch** 1983;6(1–4):89–101

Schöpf A: Sigmund Freud. München, Beck, 1982. 244 p.

Schorr A: Die Verhaltens-Therapie: ihre Geschichte von den Anfängen bis zur Gegenwart. Weinheim, Beltz, 1984. 364 p.

Schott H: Freuds Selbstanalyse (Freud und Fliess). In International Congress of the History of Medicine, 27th, Barcelona, 1980. Actas. Barcelona, Académia de Ciències Mèdiques de Catalunya i Balears, 1981. p. 145–8.

Schott H: Traum und Geschichte. Zur Freudschen Geschichtsauffassung im Kontext der Traumdeutung. **Sudhoffs Arch** 1980;64(3):298–312

Schott HG: Elemente der Selbstanalyse in den 'Studien über Hysterie'. **Gesnerus** 1980;37(3/4):235–56

Schou M: Lithium perspectives. **Neuropsychobiology** 1983;10(1):7–12

Schwaber P: Freud and the twenties. **Mass Rev** 1981;22(1):133–51

Schwaber P: Scientific art: the interpretation of dreams. **Colby Libr Q** 1977;13(1):5–18

Scull A, ed: Madhouses, mad-doctors, and madmen. The social history of psychiatry in the Victorian era. Philadelphia, University of Pennsylvania Press, 1981. xv, 384 p. Contributions by W. F. Bynum, R. Cooter, N. J. Tomes, J. Walton, W. L. Parry-Jones, B. Sicherman, B. E. Blustein, M. J. Clark, E. Showalter, P. McCandless, R. Smith.

Sebald H: Freud: instinctivist or behaviorist? The mirages of American sociology. **J Hist Sociol** 1982;4(2):64–89

Segal H: Klein. Brighton, England, Harvester Press with Fontana Books, 1979. 189 p.

Seidler E, Kindt H, Schaub N: Jaspers und Freud. **Sudhoffs Arch** 1978;62(1):37–63

Selective bibliography of Selma Fraiberg (1945–1982): **Psychoanal Q** 1982;51(4):636–41

Sharaf M: Fury on Earth. A biography of Wilhelm Reich. New York, St. Martin's Press/Marek, 1983. xiii, 550 p.

Sherman MH: The paradox of Theodor Reik. **Psychoanal Rev** 1981–82 Winter;68(4):467–72

Sifneos PE: Short-term dynamic psychotherapy: its history, its impact and its future. **Psychother Psychosom** 1981;35(4):224–9

Sirkin M, Fleming M: Freud's 'Project' and its relationship to psychoanalytic theory. **J Hist Behav Sci** 1982 Jul;18(3):230–41

Sirota M: On the Freud-Jung correspondence. **Mod Stud** 1977;2(3):45–8

Slochower H: The permanence of our Freudian heritage. **Mod Stud** 1977;2(3):13–18

Smoyak SA, Rouslin S, ed: A collection of classics in psychiatric nursing literature. Thorofare, N. J., Slack, 1982. xi, 295 p.

Socarides CW: Homosexuality. New York, Aronson, 1978. Historical chapters, p. 7–61.

Solnit AJ: Anna Freud. December 3, 1895–October 9, 1982. **J Am Acad Child Psychiatry** 1984 Mar;23(2):233–6

Spence DP: Narrative truth and historical truth: meaning and interpretation in psychoanalysis. New York, W. W. Norton, 1982. 320 p.

Stainback S, Stainback W: Historical development of treatments for maladaptive behavior. In their: Educating children with severe maladaptive behaviors. New York, Grune & Stratton, 1980. p. 36–60.

Steele RS, Swinney SV: Freud and Jung: conflicts of interpretation. London, Boston, Routledge and Kegan Paul, 1982. x, 390 p.

Steiner H: Freud against himself. **Perspect Biol Med** 1977 Summer;20(4):510–27

Stolorow RD, Atwood GE: Faces in a cloud: subjectivity in personality theory. New York, Aronson, 1979. 217 p.

Sulloway FJ: Freud as psychobiologist: a study in scientific revolution and revolutionary ideology. Ph.D. Diss. Harvard University. Cambridge, Mass., 1979.

Sulloway FJ: Freud, biologist of the mind: beyond the psychoanalytic legend. New York, Basic Books, 1979. xxvi, 612 p.

Szasz TS: The lying truths of psychiatry. **J Libert Stud** 1979;3(2):121–39

Tedeschi G: Jung-Freud: un dilemma inattuale. Roma, Astrolabio, 1979. 88 p.

Tengwall R: A note on the influence of F. M. Alexander on the development of Gestalt therapy. **J Hist Behav Sci** 1981 Jan;17(1):126–30

Thomas DM: Freud and the 'White Hotel'. **Br Med J [Clin Res]** 1983 Dec 24–31;287(6409):1957–60

Thornton EM: Freud and cocaine: the Freudian fallacy. London, Blond & Briggs, 1983. 340 p.

Trenckmann U: Das mikrobiologische Modell im theoretischen Denken der Psychiatrie. **Wiss Beitr Martin Luther Univ Halle Wittenberg** 1983;5–R80:301–6

Trenckmann U, Ortmann F: Das psychodynamische Krankheitskonzept der Romantik--Testfall für die Anwendung des Kuhnschen Paradigmabegriffs in einer Humanwissenschaft. **Z Psychol** 1980;188(3):331–9

Trenckmann U: Vergleich der psychiatrischen Versorgungssysteme in Polen und Sachsen im 18. und 19. Jahrhundert. **Arch Hist Med (Warsz)** 1979;42(2):241–4

Troncale JA: Nineteenth century neurology/psychiatry. **J Med Assoc State Ala** 1982 Aug;52(2):29–30, 32–5

Ujhely GB: Jungian approach to clinical practice. **ANA Publ** (NP-59):319–32, 1979

Vagniluca G: Epistemologia e psichiatria (II). **Sapienza** 1981;34(3):310–27

Valdivia Ponce O: Bases dinámicas de la psicoterapia tradicional. **Rev Neuropsiquiatr** 1979 Mar;42(1):31–46

Valenstein AF: Insight as an embedded concept in the early historical phase of psychoanalysis. **Psychoanal Study Child** 1981;36:307–15

Vallaud D: Infanticide et folie au XIX siècle. **Penelope** 1983;(8):51–3

van Hoorn W: Psychoanalysis, romanticism and biology. **Stor Crit Psicol** 1982 Jun;3(1):5–25

Velasco D: La psychiatrie infantile dans les pays en voie de développement. **Ann Med Psychol (Paris)** 1981 Jun;139(6):626–8

Ventura P: Freud e la giuridicità della coesistenza. Per un ritorno filosofico alla psicologia del profondo. Vol. I. La psicoanalisi individuale. Milano, Giuffrè, 1979. xvi, 420 p.

Vikár G: Emlékezés Anna Freudra. **Orv Hetil** 1983 Nov 13;124(46):2819–20

Wachinger L: Buber und Freud. **Stimmen Zeit** 1978;196(11):754–62

Wallace ER: A commentary on the Freud-Jung letters. **Psychoanal Rev** 1980 Spring;67(1):112–37

Wallace ER, Pressley LC, ed: Essays in the history of psychiatry: a tenth anniversary supplementary volume to the Psychiatric Forum. Columbia, Wm. S. Hall Psychiatric Institute, 1980. xviii, 205 p. Contributions by E. Ackerknecht, R. Bosnak, E. T. Carlson, H. Decker, C. Fox, J. Gach, G. Gifford, M. Gildea, S. Jackson, O. Marx, W. McGuire, G. Mora, R. C. Powell, P. Stepansky.

Wallace ER: Freud and anthropology. A history and reappraisal. New York, International Universities Press, 1983. xi, 306 p. (Psychological Issues, Monograph 55).

Wallace ER: Historiography in history and psychoanalysis. **Bull Hist Med** 1983 Summer;57(2):247–66

Wallace ER: The primal parricide. **Bull Hist Med** 1980 Summer;54(2):153–65

Walser HH: Adolf Meyer--student of the Zurich psychiatric school. **Gesnerus** 1984;41(1/2):49–52

Walser HH: Geschichtliche Anmerkungen zum Problem der Aggressivität in der klinischen Psychiatrie. **Schweiz Arch Neurol Neurochir Psychiatr** 1981;129(1):83–91

Weber M: Kerners 'Kleksographien' und Rorschachs 'Psychodiagnostik'. **Gesnerus** 1984;41(1/2):101–9

Whitehead CC: Technical implications of the post-metapsychological era: toward a developmental psychoanalysis. **Int J Psychoanal Psychother** 1984–85;10:437–56

Widlocher D: L'hystérie, cent ans après. **Rev Neurol (Paris)** 1982;138(12):1053–60

Wilmer HA: Defining and understanding the therapeutic community. **Hosp Community Psychiatry** 1981 Feb;32(2):95–9

Wilson C: The quest for Wilhelm Reich. Garden City, N.Y., Anchor, 1981. xv, 272 p.

Woodman RG: Freud and Jung: the parting of the ways. **Queens Q** 1978;85(1):93–108

Wyss D: Die tiefenpsychologischen Schulen von den Anfängen bis zur Gegenwart. Entwicklung, Probleme, Krisen. Göttingen, Vandenhoeck & Ruprecht, 1977. xxxii, 562 p.

Yorke C: Anna Freud, CBE (1895–1982). **J Child Psychol Psychiatry** 1983 Jul;24(3):333–8

Zaretsky E: A note on Marxism and psychoanalysis. **Marx Perspect** 1979;2(2):134–9

Zaretsky E: Evolutionary biology and psychoanalysis: a review essay on Frank J. Sulloway's Freud: biologist of the mind. **Psychohist Rev** 1981;10(2):109–22

Zottl A: Otto Rank: das Lebenswerk eines Dissidenten der Psychoanalyse. München, Kindler, 1982. 316 p.

# PSYCHIATRY

**Africa**

Sow I: Psychiatrie dynamique africaine. Paris, Payot, 1977. 280 p.
Zempléni A: Henri Collomb (1913–1979) et l'équipe de Fann. **Soc Sci Med [Med Anthropol]** 1980 May;14(2):85–90

**Argentina**

Lardies González J: Panorama historico de la psiquiatria argentina. **Asclepio** 1981;33:251–64

**Australia**

Dax EC: Crimes, follies and misfortunes in the history of australasian psychiatry. **Aust NZ J Psychiatry** 1981 Sep;15(3):257–63
Edwards GA, Hall W: The case of William Chidley: a study in psychiatry, morality and lunacy law. **Aust NZ J Psychiatry** 1980 Jun;14(2):133–9

**Austria**

Ansbacher HL: 'To love and to work'. Adlerian thoughts on an anecdote about Freud. **Bull Menninger Clin** 1981 Sep;45(5):439–41
Baruk H: Viktor Frankl et la psychanalyse. **Ann Med Psychol (Paris)** 1982 Apr;140(4):438–42
Bernfeld S: Freuds früheste Theorien und die Helmholtz-Schule (1944). **Psyche (Stuttg)** 1981 May;35(5):435–55
Dacquino G: Psicoanalisi e ipnosi nella dottrina e nella pratica clinica. **Minerva Med** 1982 Nov 24;73(45):3207–12
Delion P: Freud, l'hystérique et la psychanalyse. **Soins Psychiatr** 1983 Jan;(27):7–10
Doering D: Die Logotherapie Viktor Emil Frankls. Köln, 1981, 272 p. (Kölner medizinhistorische Beiträge; Arbeiten der Forschungsstelle des Instituts für Geschichte der Medizin der Universität zu Köln, Band 19).
Drell MJ: Hermine Hug-Hellmuth, a pioneer in child analysis. **Bull Menninger Clin** 1982 Mar;46(2):139–50
Eissler KR: Freud und Wagner-Jauregg vor der Kommission zur Erhebung militärischer Pflichtverletzungen. Wien, Löcker, 1979. 333 p.
Erdheim M: Freuds Grössenphantasien, sein Konzept des Unbewussten und die Wiener Décadence. **Psyche (Stuttg)** 1981 Oct;35(10):857–74;Nov;35(11):1006–33
Federn E: Psychoanalyse und Sozialarbeit in Osterreich. **Zeitgesch** 1980;7(5):141–9
Glenn J: 'The open-air closet'. **Am J Psychoanal** 1980 Summer;40(2):165–8
Huber W: Psychoanalytische Pädagogik in der Zeit des Ständestaates. **Zeitgesch** 1979;6(11–12):386–400
In memoriam. Dorothy Burlingham. 1891–1979.: **Psychoanal Study Child** 1980;35:ix–xxii
Kästle O: Zwei wiederentdeckte Rezensionen Sigmund Freuds von 1895. Wissenschaftlicher Kontext und biographischer Hintergrund. **Psyche (Stuttg)** 1983 Sep;37(9):805–27
Katzenstein A, Thom A: Die historische Leistung und die Grenzen des Werkes von Sigmund Freud (1856–1939). **Psychiatr Neurol Med Psychol (Leipz)** 1982 Feb;34(2):68–78
Kuper A, Stone AA: The dream of Irma's injection: a structural analysis. **Am J Psychiatry** 1982 Oct;139(10):1225–34
Laor N: Szasz, Feuchtersleben, and the history of psychiatry. **Psychiatry** 1982;45(4):316–24
Laor N: The myth of mental illness: the Feuchtersleben version. **Gesnerus** 1984;41(1/2):3–32
Lebzeltern G: Ein vielsagender Irrtum S. Freuds. **Z Klin Psychol Psychother** 1982;30(1):25–30
Lebzeltern G: Eine interessante Fehlleistung S. Freuds. **Z Klin Psychol Psychother** 1980;28(1):14–20
Lesky E, ed: Franz Joseph Gall, 1758–1828, Naturforscher und Anthropologe. Wien, Huber, 1979. (Hubers Klassiker der Medizin und der Naturwissenschaften, Band 15) 217 p.
Pappenheim E: More on the case of Anna O. **Am J Psychiatry** 1980 Dec;137(12):1625–6
Pilleri G: Josef Breuer, 1842–1925. Waldau-Bern (Schweiz), Verlag des Hiranatomischen Institutes, 1983. 81 p.
Rachman AW, Raubolt RR: The pioneers of adolescent group psychotherapy. **Int J Group Psychother** 1984 Jul;34(3):387–413
Rattner J: Alfred Adler. New York, Frederick Ungar, 1983. 226 p.
Roazen P: A note on the Vienna Psychoanalytic Society: Felix Deutsch's letters, 1923 and 1935. **J Hist Behav Sci** 1984 Oct;20(4):359–62
Schachter M: Alfred Adler (1870–1937), et sa psycho-pédagogie clinique. **Rev Hist Med Heb** 1981 Dec;139(34 no 4):53–6
Segal H: Melanie Klein. New York, Viking, 1980. vii, 194 p.
Sherman MH, ed: Psychoanalysis and old Vienna: Freud, Reik, Schnitzler, Kraus. New York, Human Sciences Press, 1978. 192 p.
Strotzka H: Laudatio auf Anna Freud. **Wien Klin Wochenschr** 1983 Jan 21;95(2):35–7
Székács I: Freud és pszichoanalízis természettudományos alapjai. **Orv Hetil** 1982 Dec 12;123(50):3091–9
Wyklicky H: Economo als Psychiater. **Osterr Arzteztg** 1982;37(8):533
Zur Geschichte der Psychiatrie in Wien: Psychiatry in Vienna. Eine Bilddokumentation. An illustrated documentation. With contributions by P. Berner, W. Spiel, H. Strotzka, H. Wyklicky. Wien, Brandstätter, 1983. 144 p.

**Belgium**

Dor J: Jean Bobon et la psychopathologie du langage. **Acta Psychiatr Belg** 1983 May–Jun;83(3):197–206

**Bulgaria**

Christozov C: Histoire de la psychiatrie infantile en Bulgarie. **Acta Paedopsychiatr (Basel)** 1981 Jan;46(4):207–11
Christozov C: Histoire de la psychiatrie infantile en Bulgarie. In International Congress of the History of Medicine. 26th, Plovdiv, 1978. Actes du Congress. Sofia, 1981. Volume II. p. 65–6.
Kilimov N: Georgi Uzunov. Sofiia, Izd-vo na Bŭlgarskata akademiia na naukite, 1978. 178 p.

**Canada**

Boudreau F: The Quebec psychiatric system in transition: a case study in psychopolitics. **Can Rev Sociol Anthropol** 1980;17(2):122–37
Brown T: Shell shock in the Canadian Expeditionary Force, 1914–1918: Canadian psychiatry in the Great War. In Roland CG, ed: Health, disease and medicine. Toronto, Hannah Institute for the History of Medicine, 1984. p. 308–32.
Cleghorn RA: The emergence of psychiatry at McGill. **Can J Psychiatry** 1984 Nov;29(7):551–6
Delage J: Cinquante ans de pédopsychiatrie à Quebec. De l'Ecole La Jemmerais à la Chaire de Psychiatrie infantile et juvénile (Hôtel-Dieu du Sacré-Coeur). **Neuropsychiatr Enfance Adolesc** 1980 Jun;28(6):239–41
Dickson I: Early history of CPA. The Canadian Psychiatric Association. **Can J Psychiatry** 1980 Feb;25(1):86–97
Greben SE: CPA--yesterday and today. **Can J Psychiatry** 1980 Feb;25(1):27–9
Roberts CA: Perspectives on 25 years of Canadian psychiatric research. **Psychiatr J Univ Ottawa** 1984 Sep;9(3):95–101
Shortt SE: R. M. Bucke: vital force, evolution and somatic psychiatry, 1862–1902. In International Congress of the History of Medicine, 27th, Barcelona, 1980. Actas. Barcelona, Académia de Ciències Médiques de Catalunya i Balears, 1981. p. 149–53.
Steinhauer PD: The Canadian Academy of Child Psychiatry. The development of child psychiatry in Canada. **J Am Acad Child Psychiatry** 1982 May;21(3):217–8
Weisstub DN, ed: Law and psychiatry in the Canadian context. New York, Pergamon Press, 1980. xlvi, 911 p.

**Chile**

Costa-Casaretto C: Condiciones de la asistencia psiquiátrica en Chile durante el último cuarto del siglo XIX. **Rev Med Chil** 1980 Jul;108(7):657–65
Costa-Casaretto C: La cátedra de neuropsiquiatría de la Universidad de Chile desde 1891 hasta 1906. **Rev Med Chil** 1980 Sep;108(9):855–62
Costa-Casaretto C: Sobre el. Dr. Carlos Sazie, primer profesor de neurología y segundo de psiquiatria en la universidad de Chile (1881–1891). **Rev Med Chil** 1980 Aug;108(8):749–56

**China**

Lu YC: The collective approach to psychiatric practice in the People's Republic of China. **Soc Probl** 1978;26(1):2–14
Xia ZY, Zhang MY: History and present status of modern psychiatry in China. **Chin Med J [Engl]** 1981 May;94(5):277–82

**Czechoslovakia**

Ambrus O: Historie a přehled lázeňské péče v psychiatrii v Ceskoslovensku. **Fysiatr Reumatol Vestn** 1982 Apr;60(2):105–7
Baudiš P: Franz Köstl a jeho práce s epidemiologickým zaměřením. **Cesk Psychiatr** 1979 Apr;75(2):144–7
Hájek P: 10 let Kroměřížského psychoterapeutického oddělení. **Cesk Psychiatr** 1982 Jun;78(3):196–8
Junas J: K starším dejinám psychiatrie na Slovensku. **Bratisl Lek Listy** 1981;76(3):383–7
Medvecký J, Medvecká E: K histórii psychiatrického ústavníctva vo Východoslovenskom krji. **Cesk Psychiatr** 1981 Jun;77(3):209–12
Prokupek J: Dvacet roku výzkumného ústavu psychiatrického. **Cesk Psychiatr** 1981 Dec;77(6):361–3
Richterová L: Příspěvek k historii psychiatrie z doby před 'velkou přeměnou'. **Cesk Psychiatr** 1980 Apr;76(2):134–8

**Denmark**

Smith JH, ed: Kierkegaard's truth: the disclosure of the self. New Haven, London, Yale University, 1981. xvii, 438 p. (Psychiatry and the Humanities. Volume 5.) With contributions by P. L. Holmer, P. B.

Armstrong, J. Collins, H. A. Durfee, W. Kerrigan, B. H. Kirmmse, L. H. Mackey, V. A. McCarthy, W. W. Meissner, P. Ricoeur, M. C. Taylor, M Theunissen.

Wang AG: Establishment of a local psychiatric service. **Acta Psychiatr Scand** 1981 Aug;64(2):150–7

### Europe

Decker HS: Psychoanalysis and the Europeans. In J. M. Quen, E. T. Carlson, ed: American psychoanalysis: origins and development. The Adolf Meyer seminars. New York, Brunner/Mazel, 1978. p. 1–19.

Stutte H: Ueber die Anfänge der 'Europäischen Kinderpsychiatrie'. **Acta Paedopsychiatr (Basel)** 1981 Jan;46(4):189–92

### Finland

Achté K, Turunen S: Den första psykiatriska artikeln i Finland. **Dan Medicinhist Arbog** 1983;12:74–81

### France

Alliez J: Jean-Baptiste Lautard et la 'maison des fous' de Marseille. **Marseille** 1981;127:44–9

Alliez J, Huber JP: L'assistance aux malades mentaux en Provence au XVIIIe siècle. **Ann Med Psychol (Paris)** 1984 Mar;142(3):321–42

Atwood GE: The pursuit of being in the life and thought of Jean-Paul Sartre. **Psychoanal Rev** 1983 Summer;70(2):143–62

Barner S: Die Entwicklung der Kinderpsychiatrie in Frankreich von den Anfängen bis 1948. Freiburg, Schulz 1980. 300 p. (Freiburger Forschungen zur Medizingeschichte, Neue Folge, 11)

Baruk H: Actualité du traitement moral et de la nosographie de Pinel. **Ann Med Psychol (Paris)** 1982 Apr;140(4):442–7

Baruk H: L'Ecole de Nancy et la découverte de la psychothérapie. La régression psychanalytique à l'ancienne hystérie. In: Congrès National des Sociétés Savantes, 103e, Nancy, 1978. Comptes Rendus. Paris, 1978. Section des Sciences, Fasc. V. P. 71–4.

Biéder J: L'odyssée d'Ulysse Trélat (1795–1879). **Ann Med Psychol (Paris)** 1984 Jan;142(1):128–41

Biéder J: Un aliéniste du XIXe siècle: Louis-Antoine Evrat (1797–1876). **Ann Med Psychol (Paris)** 1983 Jan;141(1):122–33

Biéder J: Un président de la Société Médico-Psychologique: Prosper Lucas (1808–1885). **Ann Med Psychol (Paris)** 1983 Sep–Oct;141(8):908–15

Bourgeois M: Jules Cotard et son syndrome cent ans après. **Ann Med Psychol (Paris)** 1980 Dec;138(10);1165–80

Bulhan HA: Frantz Fanon: the revolutionary psychiatrist. **Race Cl** 1980 Winter;21:251–72

Butts HF: Frantz Fanon's contribution to psychiatry: the psychology of racism and colonialism. **J Natl Med Assoc** 1979 Oct;71(10):1015–8

Capildeo R: Charcot in the 80s. In Rose FC, Bynum WF, ed: Historical aspects of the neurosciences. New York, Raven, 1982. p. 383–96.

Castel R: L'ordre psychiatrique: l'âge d'or de l'aliénisme. Paris, Editions de Minuit, 1976. 334 p.

Chabbert P, Mangin P: Les premières publications de Philippe Pinel consacrées à la médecine mentale. In International Congress of the History of Medicine, 27th, Barcelona, 1980. Actas. Barcelona, Acadèmia de Ciències Mèdiques de Catalunya i Balears, 1981. p. 42–7.

Charuty G: La psychiatrisation des croyances: savoir médical et savoirs surnaturels en Languedoc, 1850–1940. **Asclepio** 1983;35:197–215

Colmin J: L'aventure du quartier ney. Paris, Editions du Scarabée, 1980. 167 p.

Dahm S: Frühe Krankenbildnisse: Alibert Esquirol Baumgartner. Köln, 1981. (Kölner medizinhistorische Beiträge; Arbeiten der Forschungsstelle des Instituts für Geschichte der Medizin der Universität zu Köln, Band 21).

Ducommun C: Paul Dubois (1848–1918). Sa place dans l'histoire de la psychothérapie. **Gesnerus** 1984;41(1/2):61–99

Elmore R: View from the Rive Gauche: a comment on Annales Historiography. **Psychohist Rev** 1978;7(2):30–5

Esman AH: Henri Dagonet. Pioneer of psychiatric photography. **NY State J Med** 1984 Feb;84(2):79–81

Fisher DJ: Lacans's ambiguous impact on French psychoanalysis. **Contemp Fr Civiliz** 1981–82;6(1–2):89–114

Forrester J: Michel Foucault and the history of psychoanalysis. **Hist Sci** 1980 Dec;18(42 pt 4):286–303

Gineste T, Postel J: J. M. G. Itard et l'enfant connu sous le nom de 'sauvage de l'Aveyron'. **Psychiatr Enfant** 1980;23(1):251–307

Gineste T: Une histoire de la psychiatrie de l'enfant. Janvier 1800 – novembre 1800: Découverte d'une 'créature très intéressante', l'enfant connu sous le nom de Sauvage de l'Aveyron. Mém. pour le diplôme de psychiatrie. Univ. de Paris XI, 1977. 233 p, 8 n.p.

Gorney JE: The clinical application of Lacan in the psychoanalytic situation. **Psychoanal Rev** 1982 Summer;69(2):241–8

Gourevitch M: Coup d'oeil sur la naissance de la psychiatrie à Paris. **Soins Psychiatr** 1982 Feb;(16):9–11

Gourevitch M: Esquirol et la medicalisation de la psychiatrie: théorie médicale et pratique clinique. In International Congress of the History of Medicine, 27th, Barcelona, 1980. Actas. Barcelona, Acadèmia de Ciències Mèdiques de Catalunya i Balears, 1981. p. 74–7.

Heinrichs HJ: Bibliographie der Schriften von Jacques Lacan. **Psyche (Stuttg)** 1980 Oct;34(10):958–73

Hooton A, Hooton C: A critical analysis of French psychiatric nosology. **Can J Psychiatry** 1981 Mar;26(2):120–5

Jaeger M: La profession d'infirmier psychiatrique: le poids de son passé. **Soins Psychiatr** 1984 Jun–Jul;(44–45):63–4

Julien P: Un psychanalyste, Jacques Lacan. **Etudes (Fr)** 1982;357(4):333–46

Khuton A, Khuton K: Kriticheskiĭ analiz frantsuzskoĭ psikhiatricheskoĭ nozologii. **Zh Nevropatol Psikhiatr** 1982;82(4):121–3

Lebovici S: Jacques Lacan and French psychiatry. **Psychol Med** 1983 Feb;13(1):9–13

Ledermann F: La psychiatrie française et les médicaments: Pomme, Pinel, Esquirol, Morel. **Rev Hist Pharm (Paris)** 1982 Sep;29(254):189–206

Legée G: Evolution de l'étude clinique, sociale et juridique de l'aliénation mentale, sous l'impulsion de Jean-Etienne-Dominique Esquirol (1772–1840), médecin aliéniste d'origine Toulousaine. In: Congrès National des Sociétés Savantes, 96e, Toulouse, 1971. Comptes Rendus. Paris, 1974. Histoire des Sciences, Tome 1. p. 63–81.

Legée G: P. Flourens (1794–1867) et la psychiatrie de son temps. In: Congrès National des Sociétés Savantes, 103e, Nancy, 1978. Comptes Rendus. Paris, 1978. Section des Sciences, Fasc. V. p. 113–23.

Lemaire A: Jacques Lacan. London and Boston, Rutledge and Kegan Paul, 1977. xxiv, 266 p.

Lieberman LM: Itard: the great problem solver. **J Learn Disabil** 1982 Nov;15(9):566–8

Mai FM: Pierre Briquet: 19th century savant with 20th century ideas. **Can J Psychiatry** 1983 Oct;28(6):418–21

Massé G, Petitjean F: L'infirmier en psychiatrie. Loi du 30 juin 1838 -- 2e partie. **Infirm Fr** 1982 Jan;(231):3–4, 36 concl.

Mitchell H: Politics, power and psychiatry: a review of L'Ordre psychiatrique: l'age d'or de l'aliénisme by Robert Castel. **Int J Law Psychiatry** 1979;2(2):249–61

Mordier JP: Les débuts de la psychanalyse en France 1895–1926. Paris, Francois Maspero, 1981. 275 p.

Nica-Udangiu S: Henri Ey (1900–1977). **Rev Med Interna [Neurol Psihiatr]** 1984 Apr–Jun;29(2):151–6

Nica-Udangiu S: J. Moreau de Tours (1804–1884). **Rev Med Interna [Neurol Psihiatr]** 1984 Jan–Mar;29(1):77–80

Petitjean F, Bonnefoy JP, Caroli F, et al: Le secteur et la loi du 30 juin 1838. **Ann Med Psychol (Paris)** 1982;140(3):301–19

Pichot P: La recherche psychiatrique en France. **Ann Med Psychol (Paris)** 1981 Jun;139(6):640–3

Pichot PJ: The French approach to psychiatric classification. **Br J Psychiatry** 1984 Feb;144:113–8

Pinell P, Zafiropoulos M: Un siècle d'échecs scolaires (1882–1982). Paris, Les Editions Ouvrières, 1983. (Collection Politique Sociale).

Pontalis JB: Regards sur la psychanalyse en France. Paris, Gallimard, 1979. 301 p.

Postel J: Les premières expériences psychiatriques de Philippe Pinel à la Maison de santé Belhomme. **Can J Psychiatry** 1983 Nov;28(7):571–6

Postel J: Un manuscrit inédit de Philippe Pinel sur 'Les guérisons opérées dans le 7ème emploi' de Bicêtre, en 1794. **Rev Int Hist Psychiatr** 1983;1(1):79–82

Rappard P: La folie et l'Etat: aliénation mentale et aliénation sociale. Toulouse, Privat, 1981. 261 p.

Roudinesco E: La bataille de cent ans. Histoire de la psychanalyse en France. Volume I. 1885–1939. Paris, Ramsay, 1982. 498 p.

Russ, J: Histoire de la folie [de] Michel Foucault: analyse critique. Paris, Hatier, 1979. 79 p.

Sandor RS, ed: Bernheim's New studies in hypnotism. New York, International Universities Press, 1980. xix, 407 p. Translation of Hypnotisme, suggestion, psychothérapie: Etudes nouvelles, 1891.

Schepisi MA: Il bilancio e le prospettive della psicoanalisi francese nella riflessione critica di alcuni protagonisti (1970–1980). **Stor Crit Psicol** 1984;5(2):345–71

Schmid-Kitsikis E: Un certain regard sur l'oeuvre de N. Galifret-Granjon. **Psychiatr Enfant** 1984;27(1):35–48

Schneiderman S: Jacques Lacan, the death of an intellectual hero. Cambridge, Harvard University Press, 1983. vii, 182 p.

Sedgwick P: Michel Foucault: the anti-history of psychiatry. **Psychol Med** 1981 May;11(2):235–48

Sedler MJ: Falret's discovery: the origin of the concept of bipolar affective illness. Translated by M. J. Sedler and Eric C. Dessain. **Am J Psychiatry** 1983 Sep;140(9):1127–33

Sutter J: Aperçu historique de la psychopathologie française. **Acta Psychiatr Belg** 1983 Mar–Apr;83(2):104–14

Swain G: Le sujet de la folie. Naissance de la psychiatrie. Toulouse, Edouard Privat, 1977. 174 p.

Thiry U: Le professeur Joseph Guislain (1797–1860), apôtre des aliénés. **Cah Biloque** 1980;30:35–40

Turkle S: 'Mon oncle de Marienbad: sociobiology comes to the land of the structuralists. **Contemp Fr Civiliz** 1981–82;6(1–2):67–87

Turkle S: Psychoanalytic politics: Freud's French Revolution. Cambridge, MIT Press, 1981, c1978. x, 278 p.

Tytell P: La plume sur le divan. Psychanalyse et littérature en France. Paris, Aubier Montaigne, 1982. 326 p.

# PSYCHIATRY

Valla JP: L'oeuvre psychothérapeutique de Déjerine. **Inf Psychiatr** 1978 Feb;54(2):171–8

Weiner DB: Trois moments-clefs dans la vie de Ph. Pinel. In International Congress of the History of Medicine, 27th, Barcelona, 1980. Actas. Barcelona, Acadèmia de Ciències Mèdiques de Catalunya i Balears, 1981. p. 154–61.

Yáñez Cortés RJ: La intervención de conceptos psicoanalíticos en el pensamiento epistemológico de Gastón Bachelard. **Acta Psiquiatr Psicol Am Lat** 1979 Jun;25(2):135–41

**Gabon**

Vencovský E: Ceskoslovenský psychiatr spolupracovníkem profesora dr. Alberta Schweitzera v Lambarène. **Cesk Psychiatr** 1984 Apr;80(2):125–8

**Germany**

Alexander Mitscherlich: Aus der Analyse eines Gummi-Fetischisten. **Psyche (Stuttg)** 1983 Oct;37(10):867–904

Alexander Mitscherlich: Zur Dynamik des Wechsels von Depression und organischem Symptom. **Psyche (Stuttg)** 1983 Oct;37(10):905–20

Amitai M, Cremerius J: Dr. med. Arthur Muthmann. Ein Beitrag zur Frühgeschichte der Psychoanalyse. **Psyche (Stuttg)** 1984 Aug;38(8):738–53

Aus dem Archiv der Psychoanalyse: Carl Müller-Braunschweig: Psychoanalyse und Weltanschauung. **Psyche (Stuttg)** 1983 Dec;37(12):1136–45

Aus dem Archiv der Psychoanalyse. John F. Rittmeister: Voraussetzungen und Konsequenzen der Jungschen Archetypenlehre: **Psyche (Stuttg)** 1982 Nov;36(11):1032–44

Baeyer WR von, Pongratz LJ, ed: Psychiatrie in Selbstdarstellungen. Bern, Huber, 1977. 516 p.

Bergener M: Gestalt-wandel in der Psychiatrie. **MMW** 1980 Jan 11;122(2):41–2

Blankenburg W: Unausgeschöpftes in der Psychopathologie von Karl Jaspers. **Nervenarzt** 1984 Sep;55(9):447–60

Brainin E, Kaminer IJ: Psychoanalyse und Nationalsozialismus. **Psyche (Stuttg)** 1982 Nov;36(11):989–1012

Bräutigam W: Rückblick auf das Jahr 1942. Betrachtungen eines psychoanalytischen Ausbildungskandidaten des Berliner Instituts der Kriegsjahre. **Psyche (Stuttg)** 1984 Oct;38(10):905–14

Brede K, Irion U, Lohmann HM, et al: Mitscherlich, Alexander, 1908–19821700 to PresentGermany **Psyche (Stuttg)** 1984 Nov;38(11):1023–52

Cocks GC: Psychoanalyse, Psychotherapie und Nationalsozialismus. **Psyche (Stuttg)** 1983 Dec;37(12):1057–106

Cremerius J: Die Reszeption der Psychoanalyse in der Soziologie, Psychologie und Theologie im deutschsprachigen Raum bis 1940. Frankfurt am Main, Suhrkamp, 1981. 339 p.

Cremerius J: Robert Musil. Das Dilemma eines Schriftstellers vom Typus 'poeta doctus' nach Freud. **Psyche (Stuttg)** 1979 Aug;33(8):733–72

Dahmer H, Rosenkötter L: Jasager und Weisswäscher. **Psyche (Stuttg)** 1983 Dec;37(12):1146–53

Dahmer H: Kapitulation vor der 'Weltanschauung'. Zu einem Aufsatz von Carl Müller-Braunschweig aus dem Herbst 1933. **Psyche (Stuttg)** 1983 Dec;37(12):1116–35

Dahmer H: 'Psychoanalyse unter Hitler'--Rückblick auf eine Kontroverse. **Psyche (Stuttg)** 1984 Oct;38(10):927–42

Decker HS: The reception of psychoanalysis in Germany. **Comp Stud Soc Hist** 1982 Oct;24(4):589–602

Eggert GH: Wernicke's works on aphasia. The Hague, New York, Mouton, 1977. xiii, 307 p.

Ehrhardt H: 130 Jahre Deutsche Gesellschaft für Psychiatrie und Nervenheilkunde. Wiesbaden, Steiner, 1972. 125 p.

Fetscher I: Alexander Mitscherlich--zur Pathologie der bundesdeutschen Gesellschaft. **Psyche (Stuttg)** 1983 Apr;37(4):298–310

Fichtner G: Psychiatrie zur Zeit Hölderlins: Ausstellung anlässlich der 63. Jahrestagung der Deutschen Gesellschaft für Geschichte der Medizin, der Naturwissenschaften und Technik in Tübingen, Universitätsbibliothek Tübingen, Bonatzbau 27. September bis 30. Oktober 1980. Tübingen, Universitätsbibliothek, 1980. 99 p.

Finck J: Thomas Mann et la psychanalyse. Précédé de Thomas Mann et l' irrationnel par J-M Palmier. Paris, Société d'Edition 'Les Belles Lettres', 1982. 216 p. (Confluents Psychanalytiques).

Fischer W: Der Psychiater Heinroth--eine kritische Betrachtung. **Psychiatr Neurol Med Psychol (Leipz)** 1983 Oct;35(10):623–8

Fischer W: Die Psychiatrie des Mediziners J.C. Reil--eine kritische Betrachtung. **Psychiatr Neurol Med Psychol (Leipz)** 1984 Apr;36(4):229–35

Fischer W: Franz Joseph Gall und Johann Kaspar Spurzheim--Vorläufer einer biologischen Psychiatrie. **Psychiatr Neurol Med Psychol (Leipz)** 1984 Jul;36(7):433–7

Fritsche C: Wandlungen in Struktur und Funktion der Psychotherapie ab 1933. **Z Gesamte Hyg** 1984 Feb;30(2):115–7

Fürderer C: Medizin- und geistesgeschichtliche Vorläufer klinisch-psychiatrischer Biographik in der Epoche der Aufklärung und Romantik. Diss. Bonn, 1981. 151 p.

Garrison D: Karen Horney and feminism. **Signs** 1981;6(4):672–91

Gercke H, Jarchov I, ed: Die Prinzhorn-Sammlung. Bilder, Skulpturen, Texte aus psychiatrischen Anstalten (ca. 1890–1920). Königstein/Taunus, Athenäum Verlag, 1980. 312 p.

Glandien O: Franz Xaver Messerschmidt (1736–1783) - Ausdrucksstudien und Charakterköpfe, Köln: 1981. 205 p. (Kölner medizinhistorische Beiträge: Arbeiten der Forschungsstelle des Instituts für Geschichte der Medizin der Universität zu Köln, Band 20).

Glatzel J: Die Psychopathologie Karl Jaspers' in der Kritik. **Nervenarzt** 1984 Jan;55(1):10–7

Grunert J: Zur Geschichte der Psychoanalyse in München. **Psyche (Stuttg)** 1984 Oct;38(10):865–904

Güse HG, Schmacke N: Psychiatrie zwischen bürgerlicher Revolution und Faschismus. Kronberg, Ger., Athenäum Verlag, 1976.

Güse HG, Schmacke N: Psychiatry and the origins of Nazism. **Int J Health Serv** 1980;10(2):177–96

Heinrichs HJ: Harold Linckes Versuch einer Vermittlung von Natur- und Geisteswissenschaften. **Psyche (Stuttg)** 1980 Feb;34(2):152–67

Hermanns LM: John F. Rittmeister und C. G. Jung. **Psyche (Stuttg)** 1982 Nov;36(11):1022–31

Hieronimi S: Nationalsozialistische Vernichtungsaktionen an geistig Kranken im Spiegel psychiatrie-historischer Publikationen des Nachkriegsdeutschlands. Eine Auseinandersetzung mit psychiatrischen Positionen zur Geschichte der deutschen Psychiatrie 1933–1945. Diss. Mainz, 1981. 75 p.

Hippius H: Ziele und Wege der psychiatrischen Forschung. **MMW** 1981 May 8;123(19):770–1

Hoenig J: Kurt Schneider and Anglophone psychiatry. **Compr Psychiatry** 1982 Sep–Oct;23(5):391–400

Homenaje al Doctor Erich Fromm: **Gac Med Mex** 1980 Oct;116(10):431–45

Huber G: Die Bedeutung von Karl Jaspers für die Psychiatrie der Gegenwart. **Nervenarzt** 1984 Jan;55(1):1–9

Huber G: Erich Sternberg 1903–1980. **Arch Psychiatr Nervenkr** 1981;230(1):1–3

Janzarik W: Der schizoaffektive Zwischenbereich und die Lehre von den primären und sekundären Seelenstörungen. **Nervenarzt** 1980 May;51(5):272–9

Janzarik W: Jaspers, Kurt Schneider und die Heidelberger Psychopathologie. **Nervenarzt** 1984 Jan;55(1):18–24

Kahle E: Laehr, Heinrich. In Neue Deutsche Biographie 13. 1982. p. 396–7.

Kaiser W, Trenckmann U: Christian Friedrich Nasse (1778–1851). **Wiss Z Martin Luther Univ (Math)** 1980;29(2):65–89

Kaiser W: Moritz O. Fränkel (1814–1902) als Mitarbeiter der 'Allgemeinen Zeitschrift für Psychiatrie'. **Wiss Z Martin Luther Univ (Math)** 1983;32(2):89–94

Kick H: Antipsychiatrie um 1900: Zur Tradition des Konfliktes zwischen Psychiatrie und Presseberichterstattung. **Nervenarzt** 1982 May;53(5):299–300

Kick H: Der Forschungsansatz Kraepelins aus der Sicht seiner klinischen Praxis. **Fortschr Neurol Psychiatr** 1981 Jul;49(7):259–64

König R: Alexander Mitscherlich: Psychoanalyse und Zeitkritik (1969). **Psyche (Stuttg)** 1983 Oct;37(10):921–60

Krauss P: 'Mediale' Psychotherapie einer depressiven Krise. Ein Kuriosum aus den Jahren 1833/34. **Psyche (Stuttg)** 1981 Oct;35(10):963–71

Kröber HL: K. Schneiders Psychopathiebegriff als Hemmnis psychosomatischen Denkens. **Nervenarzt** 1984 Jan;55(1):25–9

Kugler J: Zur Entwicklung der Deutschen EEG-Gesellschaft. **EEG EMG** 1984 Mar;15(1):1–7

Kulessa C, Böhme K: Ursprung und Entwicklung der Selbstmordverhütung in der deutschsprachigen Psychiatrie. **Fortschr Neurol Psychiatr** 1980 Dec;48(12):629–42

Lacan J: The neurotic's individual myth. **Psychoanal Q** 1979 Jul;48(3):405–25

Lange E: Die Rodewischer Thesen 1963--Vermächtnis und Verpflichtung, Bekenntnis und Verwirklichung. **Psychiatr Neurol Med Psychol (Leipz)** 1979 Jul;31(7):385–92

Ledermann F: La thérapeutique médicamenteuse et la psychiatrie allemande du XIXe siècle: concordances, oppositions, indifférence? **Gesnerus** 1982;39(3–4):451–67

Leonhard K: Psychiatrische Behandlungsmethodik von Kraepelin nach seinen Lebenserinnerungen. **Psychiatr Neurol Med Psychol (Leipz)** 1984 Jul;36(7):395–405

Loch W: Alexander Mitscherlich und die Wiedergeburt der Psychoanalyse in Deutschland. **Psyche (Stuttg)** 1983 Apr;37(4):336–45

Lohmann HM, Rosenkötter L: Psychoanalyse in Hitlerdeutschland. Wie war es wirklich? **Psyche (Stuttg)** 1982 Nov;36(11):961–88

Lohmann HM, Rosenkötter L: Psychoanalyse in Hitlerdeutschland. Wie war es wirklich? Ein Nachtrag. **Psyche (Stuttg)** 1983 Dec;37(12):1107–15

Lohmann HM: Scheiden tut weh. **Psyche (Stuttg)** 1984 Oct;38(10):943–8

López Ibor JJ: Karl Jaspers en su centenario. **Actas Luso Esp Neurol Psiquiatr** 1982 Nov–Dec;10(6):321–30

Maeder C: Zur Geschichte der Psychiatrie. Umgang mit psychisch Kranken--gestern und heute. 3. **Krankenpflege (Frankfurt)** 1984 Jul–Aug;38(7–8):247–50

Müller M: Erinnerungen, erlebte Psychiatriegeschichte, 1920–1960. Berlin; New York, Springer-Verlag, 1982. 504 p.

Neiss R: Alfred Lorenzer. In J. Rattner, ed: Wandlungen der

Psychoanalyse. Wien, Europaverlage, 1980. p. 233-56.
Neumann H: Leben, wissenschaftliche Studien, Krankheiten und Tod Alfred Döblins. St. Michael [Austria], Bläschke, 1982. 110 p.
Neumärker KJ: Zur Geschichte der Abteilung für Kinderneuropsychiatrie an der Berliner Charité. **Acta Paedopsychiatr (Basel)** 1982 Dec;48(6):297-305
Parin P: Psychoanalyse als Gesellschaftskritik im Werk von Alexander Mitscherlich. **Psyche (Stuttg)** 1983 Apr;37(4):364-73
Pivnicki D: Paradoxes of psychotherapy. In honor and memory of Ludwig Binswanger. **Confin Psychiatr** 1979;22(4):197-203
Rattner J: Alexander Mitscherlich. In J. Rattner, ed: Wandlungen der Psychoanalyse. Wien, Europaverlag, 1980. p. 211-32.
Rattner J: Fritz Künkel. In J. Rattner, ed: Wandlungen der Psychoanalyse. Wien, Europaverlag, 1980. p. 141-63.
Rattner J: Karl Abraham. In J. Rattner, ed: Wandlungen der Psychoanalyse. Wien, Europaverlag, 1980. p. 9-29.
Rattner J: Victor Emil von Gebsattel. In J. Rattner, ed: Wandlungen der Psychoanalyse. Wien, Europaverlag, 1980. p. 257-79.
Rodegra H: Philippe Pinels Ideen von der Befreiung der Irren und ihre Verwirklichung im norddeutschen Raum zu Beginn des 19. Jahrhunderts. In International Congress of the History of Medicine, 27th, Barcelona, 1980. Actas. Barcelona, Académia de Ciències Médiques de Catalunya i Balears, 1981. p. 140-4.
Rosenkötter L: Alexander Mitscherlich als Chef und Lehrer. **Psyche (Stuttg)** 1983 Apr;37(4):346-51
Roth JK: Verleihung des Ehrendoktors der Johann-Wolfgang-Goethe-Universität an Anna Freud. **Psyche (Stuttg)** 1982 Oct;36(10):951-3
Sărmăşanu-Cortez ML, Cortez P: Bernhard von Gudden şi drama de la lacul Starnberg (1824-1886). **Rev Med Interna [Neurol Psihiatr]** 1983 Jul-Sep;28(3):233-8
Schleiffer R: Zur Methodologie von Psychopathologie und Historik. **Nervenarzt** 1980 Jan;51(1):17-21
Schmitt W: Grundlinien psychiatrischer Praxis bei Karl Jaspers. In Seidler E, Schott H, ed: Bausteine zur Medizingeschichte. Stuttgart, Steiner, 1984. p. 99-104.
Schröder C, König W: Die Integration der Psychotherapie in die klinische Medizin in Deutschland--der Beitrag von J. H. Schultz. **Psychiatr Neurol Med Psychol (Leipz)** 1984 Oct;36(10):586-90
Schulze HA: Karl Bonhoeffer, seine Persönlichkeit, sein Werk, seine Wirkung. **Psychiatr Neurol Med Psychol (Leipz)** 1981 Jun;33(6):321-6
Schweighofer F: Der Fall Schreber. **Psychother Psychosom Med Psychol** 1982 Jan;32(1):4-8
Seletskiĭ AI: Gegel' o patologii psikhiki--psikhoze i slaboumii. **Zh Nevropatol Psikhiatr** 1982;82(6):102-5
Siefert H: Emil Kraepelin. **Neue Dtsch Biogr** 1980;12:639-40
Siemen HL: Das Grauen ist vorprogrammiert: Psychiatrie zwischen Fashismus und Atomkrieg. Giessen, Focus, 1982. 248 p.
Späte HF, Thom A: Psychiatrie im Faschismus--Bilanz der historischen Analyse. **Z Gesamte Hyg** 1980;26(8):553-60
Thom A: Zur Geschichte der Psychiatrie im 19. Jahrhundert. Berlin, Volk und Gesundheit, 1984. 168 p.
Thomä H: Von der Psychosomatischen Medizin zur Psychoanalyse--Heidelberg 1949-1967. **Psyche (Stuttg)** 1983 Apr;37(4):322-35
Trenckmann U: Der Wandel der Epidemiologie in der Psychiatrie in der mikrobiologisch-antibiotischen Ara und seine Konsequenzen für das psychiatrische Denken im 19. und 20. Jahrhundert. **Z Gesamte Hyg** 1982 Mar;28(3):211-3
Unseld S: Versuch, die Welt besser zu bestehen. **Psyche (Stuttg)** 1983 Apr;37(4):311-21
Vojáček M: Cíle a úkoly psychoterapie v díle Ernsta Kretschmera. **Cesk Psychiatr** 1979 Feb;75(1):69-72
Waldeck-Semadeni EK: Paul Julius Moebius, 1853-1907, Leben und Werk. Diss. Bern, 1980. 222 p.
Wehler HU: Psychoanalysis and history. **Soc Res (NY)** 1980;47(3):519-36
Will H: Die Geburt der Psychosomatik: Georg Groddeck, der Mensch und Wissenschaftler. München, Baltimore, Urban & Schwarzenberg, 1984. vi, 231 p.
Wunderlich G: Die psychodynamische Theorie von Ideler (1835). **Z Psychosom Med Psychoanal** 1983;29(3):286-92
Wunderlich G: Kranheits- und Therapiekonzepte am Anfang der deutschen Psychiatrie (Haindorf, Heinroth, Ideler). Husum, Matthiesen, 1981. 132 p. (Abhandlungen zur Geschichte der Medizin und der Naturwissenschaften, 41).
Wyatt F: Erinnerungen vom ersten psychoanalytischen Kongress in Wiesbaden 1932. **Psyche (Stuttg)** 1984 Apr;38(4):360-7
Zander E: Was hat Schultz-Hencke uns heute noch zu sagen? **Z Psychosom Med Psychoanal** 1982;28(2):231-8
Zander W: Grusswort zum 25 jährigen Jubiläum der Zeitschrift für Psychosomatische Medizin und Psychoanalyse. **Z Psychosom Med Psychoanal** 1979 Oct-Dec;25(4):301-2

**Great Britain**

Arton M: The development of psychiatric nursing education in England and Wales. **Nurs Times** 1981 Jan 15;77(3):124-7
Bean P: The Mental Health Act 1959: rethinking an old problem. **Br J Law Soc** 1979;6(1):99-108
Bird JR: Group approaches and Army health. **J R Army Med Corps** 1980 Oct;126(3):112-9
Brome V: Ernest Jones, Freud's alter ego. London, Caliban Books, 1982. 250 p.
Bynum WF: Themes in British psychiatry, J. C. Prichard (1786-1848) to Henry Maudsley (1835-1918). With comments by S. Poggi. In M. Ruse, ed: Nature animated. Historical and philosophical case studies in Greek medicine, nineteenth-century and recent biology, psychiatry, and psychoanalysis. Volume II. Dordrecht, D. Reidel, 1983. p. 225-66.
Bynum WF: Theory and practice in British psychiatry from J. C. Prichard (1785-1848) to Henry Maudsley (1835-1918). **Nihon I-Shigaku Zasshi** 1981;27(1):94-73
Clark MJ: 'A plastic power ministering to organisation': interpretations of the mind-body relation in late nineteenth-century British psychiatry. **Psychol Med** 1983 Aug;13(3):487-97
Dawe AM: A case for community psychiatric nurses. **J Adv Nurs** 1980 Sept;5(5):485-90
Edgcumbe R: Anna Freud--child analyst. **Int J Psychoanal** 1983;64 (Pt 4):427-33
Etchegoyen RH: Fifty years after the mutative interpretation. **Int J Psychoanal** 1983;64 ( Pt 4):445-59
Fordham M: Analytical psychology in England. **J Anal Psychol** 1979 Oct;24(4):279-97
Freeman T: Anna Freud--psychiatrist. **Int J Psychoanal** 1983;64 (Pt 4):441-4
Garralda Hualde ME: El modelo inglés de formación en psiquiatría infantil. **Actas Luso Esp Neurol Psiquiatr** 1981 Mar-Apr;9(2):103-12
Goldstein J: Anna Freud in law. **Psychoanal Study Child** 1984;39:3-13
Graham AN: Contribution of the International Journal of Social Psychiatry. **Int J Soc Psychiatry** 1979;25(4):238-9
Greene J: Where now for psychiatric nursing? Steps along the way. **Nurs Mirror** 1980 Jun 26;150(20):suppl iv-vii
Hellman I: Work in the Hampstead war nurseries. **Int J Psychoanal** 1983;64 (Pt 4):435-9
Herzka HS, Otti L: Geschichte der Kindheit--zum Belspiel: Industrialisierung. **Acta Paedopsychiatr (Basel)** 1984 May;50(1):5-6
Hill D: The changing role of psychiatry in medicine and society. **Br J Med Psychol** 1983 Mar;56(Pt 1):27-38
Howells JG, Osborn ML: The history of child psychiatry in the United Kingdom. **Acta Paedopsychiatr (Basel)** 1981 Jan;46(4):193-202
Jacyna LS: Somatic theories of mind and the interests of medicine in Britain. **Med Hist** 1982 Jul;26(3):233-58
Jones K: Robert Gardiner Hill and the non-restraint movement. **Can J Psychiatry** 1984 Mar;29(2):121-4
Keeffe D: Development of care for the mentally ill. **Physiotherapy** 1980 Dec;66(12):407-8
King P: The contributions of Ernest Jones to the British Psycho-Analytical Society. **Int J Psychoanal** 1979;60(Pt 3):280-4
King PH: The life and work of Melanie Klein in the British Psycho-Analytical Society. **Int J Psychoanal** 1983;64 (Pt 3):251-60
Kris AO: The analyst's conceptual freedom in the method of free association. **Int J Psychoanal** 1983;64 (Pt 4):407-11
Langley GE: Sir John Charles Bucknill 1817-1897: our founder. **Br J Psychiatry** 1980;137:105-10
Lebovici S: L'oeuvre D'Anna Freud (1895-1982). **Psychiatr Enfant** 1984;27(1):5-34
Limentani A: Anna Freud's contribution to the work of the International Psychoanalytical Association. **Int J Psychoanal** 1983;64 (Pt 4):375-7
Lipton MA: A letter from Anna Freud. **Am J Psychiatry** 1983 Dec;140(12):1583-4
Marley E: Sir Aubrey Lewis: the golden age of a career. **J Psychiatr Res** 1982-83;17(1):93-9
Maudsley H: The pathology of mind: a study of its distempers, deformities and disorders. Reprint of 1895 ed. Biographical introduction by A. Lewis. London, Friedmann, 1979. 571 p.
Mellett DJ: Bureaucracy and mental illness: the Commissioner in Lunacy 1845-90. **Med Hist** 1981 Jul;25(3):221-50
Netzer C: Annals of psychoanalysis: Ella Freeman Sharpe. **Psychoanal Rev** 1982 Summer;69(2):207-19
Newcombe N, Lerner JC: Britain between the wars: the historical context of Bowlby's theory of attachment. **Psychiatry** 1982 Feb;45(1):1-12
Paediatrics and psychoanalysis--Miss Anna Freud: **Arch Dis Child** 1983 Jun;58(6):472-3
Porter R: The rage of party: a glorious revolution in English psychiatry? **Med Hist** 1983 Jan;27(1):35-50
Ray LJ: Models of madness in Victorian asylum practice. **Eur J Sociol** 1981;22(2):229-64
Reid DD: The historical background to wartime research in psychology and psychiatry in the Royal Air Force. In Dearnaley EJ, Warr PB, ed: Aircrew stress in wartime operations. London, New York, Academic Press, 1979. p. 1-8.
Rice F: Care and treatment of the mentally ill. In Checkland O, Lamb M, ed: Health care as social history; the Glasgow case. Aberdeen, Aberdeen University Press, 1982. p. 59-73.
Sandler J: Discussions with Anna Freud on The Ego and the Mechanisms

of Defence: The Ego and the Id at Puberty. **Int J Psychoanal** 1983;64 (Pt 4):401–6
Sandler J, Sandler AM: The 'second censorship', the 'three box model' and some technical implications. **Int J Psychoanal** 1983;64 (Pt 4):413–25
Savage GH: Psychiatry in the 1880s. **Psychol Med** 1984 Aug;14(3):723–4
Sclare AB: John Carswell: a pioneer in Scottish psychiatry. **Scott Med J** 1981 Jul;26(3):265–70
Scull A: A brilliant career? John Conolly and Victorian psychiatry. **Victorian Stud** 1984;27:203–35
Shepherd M: From social medicine to social psychiatry: the achievement of Sir Aubrey Lewis. **Psychol Med** 1980 May;10(2):211–8
Shepherd M: Social psychiatry and epidemiology. **Practitioner** 1983 Jan;227(1375):148–50
Slater E: Psychiatry in the thirties. **Contemp Rev** 1975;226(1309):70–5
Smith R: Criminal insanity: from a historical point of view. **Bull Am Acad Psychiatry Law** 1983;11(1):27–34
Solnit AJ, Newman LM: Anna Freud: the child expert. **Psychoanal Study Child** 1984;39:45–63
Solnit AJ: Anna Freud 1895–1982. **Am J Psychiatry** 1983 Dec;140(12):1632–3
Solnit AJ: Anna Freud's contributions to child and applied analysis. **Int J Psychoanal** 1983;64 (Pt 4):379–90
Swan M: Fitness to plead. **Br J Hosp Med** 1981 Nov;26(5):503, 505–9
Taylor FK: Sir Aubrey Lewis: Inquiries in Psychiatry; The State of Psychiatry; The Later Papers of Sir Aubrey Lewis. **Br J Psychiatry** 1983 Jul;143:89–93
Two jubilees in psychotherapy: **Br Med J** 1980 Jul 26;281(6235):256–7
Wallerstein RS: Anna Freud: radical innovator and staunch conservative. **Psychoanal Study Child** 1984;39:65–80
Watt DC: Social psychiatry. **J R Soc Med** 1981 Feb;74(2):88–90
Yorke C: Anna Freud and the psychoanalytic study and treatment of adults. **Int J Psychoanal** 1983;64 (Pt 4):391–400

**Hungary**

Antal G: Freud in Hungary. An interview with Imre Hermann, the psychoanalyst. **New Hung Q** 1982;23(85):88–95
Cremerius J: 'Die Sprache der Zärtlichkeit und der Leidenschaft'. Reflexionen zu Sándor Ferenczis Wiesbadener Vortrag von 1932. **Psyche (Stuttg)** 1983 Nov;37(11):988–1015
Füredi J, Buda B: A pszichiátria önállósodásának problémája Magyarországon. **Orv Hetil** 1980 May 11;121(19):1115–20
Hárdi I: Ferenczi Sándor jelentősége a mai orvostudomány számára. **Orv Hetil** 1983 Aug 21;124(34):2067–70
Hárdi I: Hollós István (születésének 110–ik évfordulójára). **Orv Hetil** 1982 Dec 12;123(50):3099–100
Harmat P, Hebenstreit G: Freud, Ferenczi und die Psychoanalyse in Ungarn. **Wien Med Wochenschr** 1982 Feb 15;132(3):63–6
Harmat P: Psychoanalyse und Marxismus in Ungarn (1900–1980). **Psyche (Stuttg)** 1984 Mar;38(3):254–69
Harmat P, Hebenstreit G: Sándor Ferenczis theoretisches Werk. **Wien Med Wochenschr** 1984 Jan 31;134(2):49–53
Hörcsik E, Pisztora F: Ritkuló és halványuló babonás hiedelmek valamint széles körben elterjedt technikai ismeretek napjaink pszichiátriai kórképeiben. **Orvostort Kozl** 1982;92(4):93–9
Pisztora F: A bel–, az elme és az ideggyógyászat viszonya hazánkban a századforduló körül. **Orv Hetil** 1982 Jun 27;123(26):1621–9
Stucke W: Balintgruppen-Arbeit. **Med Monatsschr Pharm** 1982 Jun;5(6):176–82
Szállási A: Freud, Ferenczi és a Nyugat. **Orv Hetil** 1980 May 18;121(20):1207–8
Szentgyörgyvölgyi G: Csáth Géza--Dr. Brenner József (1887–1919). **Orv Hetil** 1984 Sep 30;125(40):2446–8
Walter H: Sándor Ferenczi. In J. Rattner, ed: Wandlungen der Psychoanalyse. Wien, Europaverlag, 1980. p. 53–86.

**Israel**

Alex W: The significance of Erich Neuman in Jungian psychology. **Isr Ann Psychiatry** 1979 Dec;17(4):263–8
Edelston H: A psychiatrist in Youth Aliah (1956–57). **Midstream** 1981;27(9):42–5
Fifty years of psychoanalysis in Israel: past, present and future: **Isr J Psychiatry Relat Sci** 1983;20(1–2):1–203
Hertz DG: Pioneers and psychoanalysis: beginnings of the psychoanalytic movement in Eretz Israel. **Isr J Psychiatry Relat Sci** 1983;20(1–2):5–12

**Italy**

Babini VP, Cotti M, Minuz F, et al: La storia della psichiatria nell'Ottocento: i contributi italiani nell'ultimo decennio (1968–1978). **Stor Crit Psicol** 1980;1(2):177–96
Babini VP, Cotti M, Minuz F, et al: Tra sapere e potere. La psichiatria italiana nella seconda metà dell'Ottocento. Bologna, Società Editrice il Mulino, 1982. 272 p. (Studi e Ricerche, CLV).
Babini VP: Tra sapere e potere: la psichitria italiana nella seconda metà dell'Ottocento. Bologna, Società editrice il mulino, 1982. 272 p.
Buscaino GA, Guadagnino M: Ulteriore contributo a 'orientamenti teorici e pratici della psichiatria italiana'. Dal 1950 al 1976. **Acta Neurol [Quad]** 1978;37:131–59
Fink M: Meduna and the origins of convulsive therapy. **Am J Psychiatry** 1984 Sep;141(9):1034–41
Guadagnino M, Buscaino GA: Un secondo contributo a 'orientamenti teorici e pratici della psichiatria italiana dal 1950 al 1970'. **Acta Neurol [Quad]** 1978;37:116–30
Schorske CF: Freud: the psycho-archeology of civilizations. **Mass Hist Soc Proc** 1980;92:52–67
Weber-Unger S: Wahnsinn und Politik: zur neuen Psychiatrie in Italien. Frankfurt; New York, Campus Verlag, 1984. 181 p.

**Japan**

[A meeting to commemorate the 100th anniversary of Ms. Haya Ishibashi, a pioneer in psychiatric nursing] (Jpn): **Kango** 1980 Jun;32(6):88
Matsuda H: [Psychiatry in the early 19th century Japan] (Jpn). **Igakushi Kenkyu** 1978;49:18–21

**Kenya**

Ndetei DM: Psychiatry in Kenya: yesterday, today and tomorrow. An overview. **Acta Psychiatr Scand** 1980 Sep;62(3):201–11

**Lebanon**

Katchadourian H: The historical background of psychiatry in Lebanon. **Bull Hist Med** 1980 Winter;54(4):544–53

**Mexico**

Parrés R: Las corrientes psiquiátricas contemporáneas. In Academia Nacional de Medicina. Libro conmemorativo del primer centenario. México, Comité Editorial de la Comisión Organizadora del Congreso del Centenario, 1964. Tome 2. p. 486–9.
Rodríguez A: Samuel Ramos: influencia de Adler y Jung en su estudio sobre el carácter del Mexicano. **Cuad Hispanoam** 1977;109(326–327):420–30

**Netherlands**

Bakker-van der Kooij C: Honderd jaar krankzinnigheid. **Tijdschr Ziekenverpl** 1984 Aug 21;37(17):545–8
Bulhof IN: From psychotherapy to psychoanalysis: Frederik van Eeden and Albert Willem van Renterghem. **J Hist Behav Sci** 1981;17:209–21
Bulhof IN: Psychoanalysis in the Netherlands. **Comp Stud Soc Hist** 1982;24(4):572–88
Lindeboom GA: Geschiedenis der geneeskunde: J. N. Ramaer (1817–1887) en zijn bibliotheek. **Ned Tijdschr Geneeskd** 1982 Aug 14;126(33):1504–10
Verkroost CM: A. W. van Renterghem und Frederik van Eeden, zwei holländische Aerzte als Bahnbrecher auf dem Gebiete der psychischen Therapie. **Janus** 1980;67(1–2–3):191–9

**Nigeria**

Akighir A: Traditional and modern psychiatry: a survey of opinions and beliefs amongst people in plateau state, Nigeria. **Int J Soc Psychiatry** 1982 Autumn;28(3):203–9

**Norway**

Lysnes M: Marie Lysnes: sykepleie var vårt liv. **Sykepleien** 1984 Oct 5;71(17):22–7
Odegård O: Perspektiver efter 55 års psykiatrisk virksomhet. **Nord Med** 1982 Dec;97(12):310–3
Svebak S: Helga Eng: a Norwegian precursor to Darrow and Lacey. **Psychophysiology** 1983 Sep;20(5):600–1

**Peru**

Alarco F: La psicoterápia dinámica y José Carlos Mariátegui. **Rev Neuropsiquiatr** 1979 Sep–Dec;42(3–4):145–64
Mariátegui J: Hermilio Valdizán, la psiquiatría comparativa y la medicina folklórica. **Acta Psiquiatr Psicol Am Lat** 1980 Jun;26(2):96–106
Mariátegui J: Hermilio Valdizán y la psiquiatriá peruana. **Rev Neuropsiquiatr** 1980 Mar;43(1):1–22
Saavedra A: Honorio Delgado y la psiquiatría Peruana. **Rev Neuropsiquiatr** 1980 Jun;43(2):67–86

**Poland**

Aleksandrowicz JW, Bomba J, Broszkiewicz E, et al: Kępiński jako klinicysta. **Przegl Lek** 1983;40(12):843–8
Bilikiewicz A: Problematyka psychiatryczna w polskiej epileptologii ostatniego 35-lecia. **Psychiatr Pol** 1981 Mar–Apr;15(2):189–93
Drozdowski P, Fortuna D, Nieniewska M, et al: Dr med. Małgorzata

Dominik (1941–1979). **Psychiatr Pol** 1980 Sep–Oct;14(5):549–54

Drozdowski P, Kokoszka A: Psychoterapia według Antoniego Kępińskiego. **Przegl Lek** 1983;40(12):877–80

Fortuna D, Nieniewska M, Szymusik A: Kępiński jako nauczyciel i wychowawca. **Przegl Lek** 1983;40(12):837–41

Jakubik A: Antoni Kepiński: człowiek i dzieło. Warszawa, Państwowy Zakład Wydawn. Lekarskich, 1981. 426 p.

Jakubik A: Antoni Kępiński -- Twórca psychiatrii aksjologicznej. **Psychiatr Pol** 1980 Jul–Aug;14(4):403–7

Jakubik A: Psychiatria fenomenologiczna w ujęciu Antoniego Kępińskiego. **Psychiatr Pol** 1980 Jul–Aug;14(4):395–401

Maćkowiak Z: Uwagi o życiu i działalności Witolda Chodźki (1875–1954). **Przegl Lek** 1980;37(4):437–40

Masłowski J: Reakcje na twórczość Antoniego Kępińskiego. **Przegl Lek** 1983;40(12):861–4

Ostrowska T: Dr Franciska Minkowska (1882–1950), psychiatra i psychoannalityk, twórca pojęcia gliskroidii. W 100–lecie urodzin. **Arch Hist Med (Warsz)** 1983;46(1):39–44

Ryn Z: Antoni Kępiński we wspomnieniach. **Przegl Lek** 1983;40(12):881–4

Struzik T: Metabolizm informacyjny Kępińskiego w świetle teorii informacji. **Przegl Lek** 1983;40(12):865–71

Sulestrowska H: Zasługi prof. dr. Tadeusza Bilikiewicza dla rozwoju psychiatrii dziecięcej w Polsce. **Psychiatr Pol** 1982;16(4):321–8

Uszkiewiczowa L: Działalność profesora Stanisława Batawii w dziedzinie psychiatrii sądowej. **Psychiatr Pol** 1979 Sep–Oct;13(5):441–3

Wardaszko–Lyskowska H, Piotrowski A, Włosińska I: Ewolucja celów, treści i form w programie dydaktycznym Kliniki Psychiatrycznej Akademii Medycznej w Warszawie. **Psychiatr Pol** 1982 Jan–Apr;16(1–2):73–6

Zadecki J: O Kępińskiego 'Schizofrenii'. **Przegl Lek** 1983;40(12):873–6

### Romania

Bour P: L'apport de Jacob Lévy Moréno. **Ann Med Psychol (Paris)** 1983 Dec;141(10):1079–87

Cortez P, Sărmăşeanu–Cortez ML: Un psihiatru în căutarea propriului său destin. Dr. Anastse Andrei Periclis Dosis (1900–1974). **Rev Med Interna [Neurol Psihiatr]** 1980 Jul–Sep;25(3):231–7

Sărmąsanu–Cortez ML, Cortez P: A great forerunner of the modern sanitary organization, Prof. Dr. Alexandru Obregia (1860–1937). **Sante Publique (Bucar)** 1979;22(4):387–93

Sărmăşanu–Cortez ML, Cortez P: Dr. Ioan I. Popescu–Sibiu, promotor al psihanalizei şi neobosit animator al vieţii culturale din Romąnia (1901–1974). **Rev Med Interna [Neurol Psihiatr]** 1982 Oct–Dec;27(4):313–8

Sărmăşanu–Cortez ML, Cortez PP: Un distins psihiatru la confluenta dintre muzică şi medicină: dr. Stefan S. Braşcu (1895–1965). **Rev Med Interna [Neurol Psihiatr]** 1980 Apr–Jun;24(2):143–8

Sărmăşanu–Cortez ML, Cortez P: Un luptător neobosit pentru progresul psihiatriei româneşti: dr. Mircea Bruteanu (1882--1957). **Rev Med Interna [Neurol Psihiatr]** 1979 Apr–Jun;24(2):137–42

### Spain

Barcia D: La significacion de la antropologia medica de Lain Entralgo para la psiquiatria actual. **Asclepio** 1980;32:19–45

Comelles JM: El tratamiento moral en Catalunya (I): el 'Proyecto médico razonado' de Emili Pi i Molist (1860). In International Congress of the History of Medicine, 27th, Barcelona, 1980. Actas. Barcelona, Académia de Ciències Médiques de Catalunya i Balears, 1981. p. 48–55.

Dieckhöfer K: El desarrollo de la psiquiatría en España. Aspectos históricos y culturales. **Actas Luso Esp Neurol Psiquiatr** 1983 Jul–Aug;11(4):333–42

Doménech Llabería E: Las ideas de Pedro Mata en el campo de la psicologia de su tiempo. **Asclepio** 1980;32:137–50

Germain J, Solís J: José Miguel Sacristán (1887–1956). **Arch Neurobiol (Madr)** 1982 Jul–Aug;45(4):299–319

Glick TF: The naked science: psychoanalysis in Spain. **Comp Stud Soc Hist** 1982;24(4):533–71

Linares Maza A: La psiquiatría andaluza en la primera mitad de nuestro siglo. Personalidades destacadas. I. Miguel Prados Such (Málaga). **Arch Neurobiol (Madr)** 1983 Jan–Feb;46(1):39–66

López Ibor JJ: Egas Moniz, en su centenario. **Actas Luso Esp Neurol Psiquiatr** 1980 Jul–Aug;8(4):239–46

Lopez–Ibor Alino JJ: Les développements récents de la politique psychiatrique en Espagne. **Ann Med Psychol (Paris)** 1980 Jun;138(6):716–21

Marín Fernández JL: Aspectos bibliometricos de la obra de Roman Alberca Lorente (1903–1967). **Asclepio** 1980;32:229–53

Mas i Perera P: Tribut al Doctor Domènec Martí i Julià. **Xaloc** 1972;56:182–5

Nieto D: José Sanchís Banús. **Arch Neurobiol (Madr)** 1982 Sep–Oct;45(5):407–16

Pigem Serra JM: Emilio Mira y López y su entorno. **Arch Neurobiol (Madr)** 1982 Mar–Apr;45(2):135–56

### Sweden

Essen–Möller E: The psychology and psychiatry of Henrik Sjöbring (1879–1956). **Psychol Med** 1980 May;10(2):201–10

Fehrman C: Esaias Tegnér and psychiatry: history of literature from medical view-point. **Sydsven Medicinhist Sallsk Arsskr** 1984;21:47–8

Johansson–Saleby E: I brottmål: Elsa Johansson–Saleby mot Svenska psykiaterkåren. Stockholm, Johansson–Salebys förlag, 1973. 101 p.

Nielzén S: Sjöbrings tankemodeller för personlighet och psykisk sjukdom. **Sydsven Medicinhist Sallsk Arsskr** 1980;:124–33

### Switzerland

Aeschlimann J: Rudolf Brun (1885–1969). Leben und Werk des Zürcher Neurologen, Psychoanalytikers and Entomologen. Zürich, Juris, 1980. 70p. (Zürcher medizingeschichtliche Abhandlungen. Neue Reihe, Nr. 144).

Bleuler M, ed: Beiträge zur Schizophrenielehre der Zürcher Psychiatrischen Universitätsklinik Burghölzli (1902–1971). Einleitende Uebersicht und gekürzter Nachdruck von Veröffentlichungen. Darmstadt, Wissenschaftliche Buchgesellschaft, 1979. vii, 358 p.

Evans RI: Dialogue with C. G. Jung. New York, Praeger, 1981. xi, 241 p.

Haenel T: Jakob Klaesi--Schlafkur und Antieidodiathese. **Gesnerus** 1979;36(3–4):246–65

Haenel T: Zur Geschichte der Psychiatrie: Gedanken zur allgemeinen und Basler Psychiatriegeschichte. Basel; Boston, Birkhäuser Verlag, 1982. 249 p.

Iijima E: [Records of hallucination: my attraction to Jung's world of hallucination]. (Jpn) **Kango Kyoiku** 1980 Feb;21(2):74–8

Jaffe A: Aufsätze zur Psychologie C. G. Jungs. Zürich, Daimon, 1982. 160 p.

Jung CG: Erinnerungen, Träume, Gedanken. Olten, Walter–Verlag, 1984. 419 p.

Jung CG: The essential Jung. Princeton, Princeton University Press, 1983. 447 p.

Jung–Merker L, Ruf E, ed: C. G. Jung: Bibliographie. Olten [Switzerland], Walter–Verlag, 1983. 295 p. (C. G. Jung gesammelte Werke, 19)

Kaiser W: Leben und Werk des Basler Psychiaters und Psychoanalytikers Hans Christoffel (1888–1959. Zürich, Juris Druck, 1982. 267 p. (Zürcher Medizingeschichtliche Abhandlungen, Neue Reihe, Nr. 152.)

Miéville C: Fortbildungskurs der Schweizerischen Gesellschaft für Psychiatrie. Biologische Aspekte der Psychiatrie. Eröffnung. **Schweiz Arch Neurol Neurochir Psychiatr** 1979;125(2):187–91

Müller C: Historische Vignette. August Forel und der Nationalsozialismus. **Nervenarzt** 1984 Sep;55(9):504–5

Müller C: Un drame dans la famille d'Albrecht de Haller. **Gesnerus** 1984;41(1/2):133–6

Nica–Udangiu S: Hermann Rorschach (1884–1922). **Rev Med Interna [Neurol Psihiatr]** 1984 Jul–Sep;29(3):235–40

Rattner J: Medard Boss. In J. Rattner, ed: Wandlungen der Psychoanalyse. Wien, Europaverlag, 1980. p. 281–308.

Rihner F: Professor Dr. Manfred Bleuler zum 80. Geburtstag. Zürich, Woodtli, 1982. 43 p.

Rogers FB: Psychology in practice: a jungian perspective. **Del Med J** 1982 Mar;54(3):179–81

Smythies JR: A visit to Dr. Jung. **Ala J Med Sci** 1981 Jan;18(1):93–4

Van der Post L: Jung and the story of our time. New York, Vintage Books, 1977. 276 p.

Walser HH: Der Weg der Schweizer Psychiatrie ins zwanzigste Jahrhundert. **Gesnerus** 1982;39(1):97–108

Wilson C: Lord of the underworld: Jung and the twentieth century. Wellingborough, Northamptonshire, Aquarian Press, 1984. 160 p.

Witzig JS: Theodore Flournoy–a friend indeed. **J Anal Psychol** 1982 Apr;27(2):131–48

Zinsstag: Memories of what mother told about her cousin Carl Gustav Jung. **J Am Soc Psychosom Dent Med** 1980;27(2):42–6

### United States

Abbott A: Religion, psychiatry, and problems of everyday life. **Sociol Anal** 1980;41(2):164–71

Abend SM: Charles Brenner. An appreciation. **Psychoanal Q** 1984 Jan;53(1):1–12

Alexander LB: Social work's Freudian deluge: myth or reality? **Soc Serv Rev** 1972;46(4):517–38

Bayer R, Spitzer RL: Edited correspondence on the status of homosexuality in DSM–III. **J Hist Behav Sci** 1982 Jan;18(1):32–52

Bean DW, Fuller WC: Development of the South Dakota Psychiatric Association. **SD J Med** 1981 May;34(5):53–5

Bettelheim B: Reflections: Freud and the Soul [as perceived in America]. **New Yorker** 1982;68(2):52–93

Blain D, Barton M: The history of American psychiatry: a teaching and research guide. Washington, American Psychiatric Association, 1979. iv, 44 p. Contributions by D. F. Musto, G. Mora, E. T. Carlson.

Blain D: Twentieth century psychiatry--living history in the life of

Kenneth E. Appel, M.D., 1896–1979.
**Trans Stud Coll Physicians Phila** 1980 Jun;5(2 no 2):144–54
Bromberg W: Psychiatry between the wars, 1918–1945. A recollection. Westport, London, Greenwood Press, 1982. xxxii, 184 p. (Contributions in Medical History, No. 10).
Brown CL: Fifty years of psychiatry. **J Med Assoc State Ala** 1981 Aug;51(2):40–3
Brown CL: The Four Horsemen of amateur psychiatry, class of '46 [interview by William H McDonald] **J Med Assoc State Ala** 1980 Nov;50(5):8–10, 15
Bruch H: Personal reminiscences of Frieda Fromm-Reichmann. **Psychiatry** 1982;45(2):98–104
Buckwalter KC, Church OM: Euphemia Jane Taylor: an uncommon psychiatric nurse. **Perspect Psychiatr Care** 1979 May–Jun;17(3):125–31
Burnham JC: The founding of the Archives of Neurology and Psychiatry; or, what was wrong with the Journal of Nervous and Mental disease? **J Hist Med Allied Sci** 1981 Jul;36(3):310–24
Burns CR: Richard Cabot and 'The American type' of psychotherapy. In International Congress of the History of Medicine, 27th, Barcelona, 1980. Actas. Barcelona, Académia de Ciències Mèdiques de Catalunya i Balears, 1981. p. 39–41.
Burns SB: Early medical photography in America (1839–1883) V. Beginnings of psychiatric photography. **NY State J Med** 1980 Feb;80(2):270–82
Callan CM: A leader in psychiatry--Carol Nadelson, M.D. **Conn Med** 1981 Aug;45(8):491–2
Carlson ET, Quen JM: American psychoanalysis: origins and development. New York, Brunner/Mazel, 1978.
Carlson ET, Wollock JL, Noel PS, ed: Benjamin Rush's Lectures on the mind. Philadelphia, American Philosophical Society, 1981. xix, 735 p. (Memoirs of the American Philosophical Society, 144).
Castel F, Castel R, Lovell A: La société psychiatrique avancée. Paris, Grasset, 1979. 365 p.
Castel R, Castel F, Lovell A: The psychiatric society. La société psychiatrique avancée. New York, Columbia University Press, 1982. xxiii, 358 p.
Chapman AH, Vieira e Silva D: Base para uma psiquiatria científica: os conceitos de Harry Stack Sullivan. **Arq Neuropsiquiatr** 1980 Mar;38(1):76–80
Chase A: Jerome Frank and American psychoanalytic jurisprudence. **Int J Law Psychiatry** 1979;2(1):29–54
Chatelaine KL: Harry Stack Sullivan, the formative years. Washington, D.C., University Press of America, 1981. xxiv, 553 p.
Church OM, Buckwalter KC: Harriet Bailey---a psychiatric nurse pioneer. **Perspect Psychiatr Care** 1980 Mar–Apr;18(2):62–6
Cohen RA: Notes on the life and work of Frieda Fromm-Reichmann. **Psychiatry** 1982;45(2):90–8
Crowley RM: Frieda Fromm-Reichmann: recollections of a student. **Psychiatry** 1982;45(2):105–7
Crowley RM: Harry Stack Sullivan as social critic. **J Am Acad Psychoanal** 1981 Apr;9(2):211–26
Crowley RM: William V. Silverberg as teacher and colleague. **J Am Acad Psychoanal** 1981 Oct;9(4):493–500
D'Amore AR: Ernest Jones: founder of the American Psychoanalytic Association. **Int J Psychoanal** 1979;60(Pt 3)287–90
D'Amore AR: Psychoanalysis in America: 1930–1939. **Psychoanal Q** 1981;50(4):570–86
Diamond BL: The psychiatrist as expert witness. **Psychiatr Clin North Am** 1983 Dec;6(4):597–609
Doona ME: At least as well cared for ... Linda Richards and the mentally ill. **Image J Nurs Sch** 1984 Spring;16(2):51–6
Evans RI: Dialogue with Erik Erikson. New York, London, Harper & Row, 1967. xvi, 142 p.
Evans RI: Dialogue with R. D. Laing. New York, Praeger, 1981. lxxv, 170 p. (Reprint of 1976 ed; with new introduction).
Feinstein HM: Family therapy for the historian?--The case of William James. **Fam Process** 1981 Mar;20(1):97–107
Field MH: Social casework practice during the 'psychiatric deluge'. **Soc Serv Rev** 1980;54(4):482–507
Fishbein L: Freud and the radicals: the sexual revolution comes to Greenwich Village. **Can Rev Am Stud** 1981;12(2):173–89
Frieda Fromm-Reichmann: A seminar in the history of psychiatry. **Psychiatry** 1982 May;45(2):89–136
Frieda Fromm-Reichmann discusses the 'Rose garden' case: **Psychiatry** 1982 May;45(2):128–36
Frommknecht M: Frieda Fromm-Reichmann. In J. Rattner, ed: Wandlungen der Psychoanalyse. Wien, Europaverlag, 1980. p. 115–39.
Fullinwider SP: Technicians of the finite. The rise and decline of the schizophrenic in American thought 1840–1960. Westport, Conn., Greenwood, 1982. ix, 253 p. (Contributions in Medical History, 9).
Garfield SL: Psychotherapy. A 40-year-appraisal. **Am Psychol** 1981 Feb;36(2):174–83
Gershon ES: The historical context of Franz Kallmann and psychiatric genetics. **Arch Psychiatr Nervenkr** 1981;229(4):273–6
Gilgen AR: American psychology since World War II. A profile of the discipline. Westport, Connecticut, London, Greenwood Press, 1982. xiii, 272 p.
Gill D: Quest, the life of Elisabeth Kübler-Ross. New York, Harper & Row, 1980. xiv, 329 p.
Gill MM: David Rapaport. In Dictionary of American Biography, Suppl. 6, 1956–1960. p. 526–8, 1980.
Gödde G: Theodor Reik. In J. Rattner, ed: Wandlungen der Psychoanalyse. Wien, Europaverlag, 1980. p. 87–113.
Gordon L: Lena Levine. In: Notable American women. The modern period. Cambridge, Mass., Belknap-Harvard Univ. Press, 1980. 4:419–20.
Grayson VS: Mary Cromwell Jarrett. In: Notable American women. The modern period. Cambridge, Mass., Belknap-Harvard Univ. Press, 1980. 4:377–9.
Green M, Rieber RW: The assimilation of psychoanalysis in America. In R. W. Rieber, K. Salzinger, ed: Psychology: theoretical-historical perspectives. New York, Academic Press, 1980. p. 263–304.
Grenander ME: Psychiatry's sacred cow. **Reason** 1979;10(11):30–1, 34
Grinker RR: Fifty years in psychiatry. Springfield, Ill., Thomas, 1979. xiii, 263 p.
Grob GN: Mental illness and American society, 1875–1940. Princeton, Princeton University Press, 1983. xiii, 428 p.
Grob GN, ed: The beginnings of American psychiatric thought and practice. Five accounts, 1811–1830. New York, Arno, 1973. Various paginations. Includes Account of the rise and progress of the Asylum . . . near Philadelphia (1814), and works by Theodric Romeyn Beck (1811); Thomas Eddy (1815); George Parkman (1814); and Rufus Wyman (1830).
Gunst VK: Memoirs-Professional and personal: a decade with Frieda Fromm-Reichmann. **Psychiatry** 1982;45(2):107–15
Hancock V: Women in Arizona medicine: Mary Lawson Neff, M.D. **Ariz Med** 1984 Nov;41(11):750–4; Dec;41(12):819–21
Harper R: A psychoanalytic geronimo. **Queen Q** 1981;88(2):256–63
Harvey AM: Henry Mills Hurd: the first superintendent of the Johns Hopkins Hospital and the first professor of psychiatry. **Johns Hopkins Med J** 1981 Mar;148(3):135–48
Hesselnberg M: Les thérapies familiales et leur histoire. **Soins Psychiatr** 1982 Jan;(15):41–4
Hill D: The politics of schizophrenia: psychiatric oppression in the United States. Lanham, MD, University Press of America, 1983. xii, 577 p.
Iles JD: Velikovsky: psychiatrist, historian and catastrophist. **Can Med Assoc J** 1981 Sept 1;125(5):496–505
Jahoda M: La scuola psicoanalitica dalla Germania agli Stati Uniti. **Comunita** 1971;25(165):189–213
Jones E: Social class and psychotherapy: a critical review of research. **Psychiatry** 1974;37(4):307–20
Jones GW: George Edmund Gifford, jr. **Proc Am Antiq Soc** 1981;91(1):22–4
Kessler RC, McRae JA: Trends in the relationship between sex and psychological distress: 1957–1976. **Am Sociol Rev** 1981;46(4):443–52
Kucharski A: History of frontal lobotomy in the United States, 1935–1955. **Neurosurgery** 1984 Jun;14(6):765–72
Kushner HI: Americanization of the ego. **Can Rev Am Stud** 1979;10(1):95–101
Kushner HI: The suicide of Meriwether Lewis: a psychoanalytic inquiry. **William Mary Q** 1981;38(3):464–81
Laor N: Old whig psychiatry: the Szaszian variant. **Isr J Psychiatr Relat Sci** 1982;19(3):215–27
Layne GS: The Kirkbride-Langenheim collaboration: early use of photography in psychiatric treatment in Philadelphia. **Pa Mag Hist Biogr** 1981;105(2):182–202
Leys R: Meyer's dealings with Jones: a chapter in the history of the American response to psychoanalysis. **J Hist Behav Sci** 1981 Oct;17(4):445–65
Lindemann E: Beyond grief: studies in crisis intervention. Ed. by E. B. Lindemann. Biographical introduction by B. S. Brown. New York and London, Aronson, 1979. 274 p.
Lipowski ZJ: Holistic-medical foundations of American psychiatry: a bicentennial. **Am J Psychiatry** 1981 Jul;138(7):888–95
McCann W: (Austin) Merrill Moore. In Dictionary of American Biography, Suppl. 6, 1956–1960. p. 461–2, 1980.
McGovern CM: Doctors or ladies? Women physicians in psychiatric institutions, 1872–1900. **Bull Hist Med** 1981 Spring;55(1):88–107
Maultsby MC: A historical view of Blacks' distrust of psychiatry. In Turner SM, Jones RT, ed: Behavior modification in Black populations; psychosocial issues and empirical findings. New York, Plenum, 1982. p. 39–55.
Modlin HC: Contributions of the Menninger School of Psychiatry to psychiatric education. **Bull Menninger Clin** 1983 May;47(3):253–61
Mora G: Gregory Zilboorg. In Dictionary of American Biography, Suppl. 6, 1956–1960. p. 724–5, 1980.
Morrissey JP, Goldman HH: Cycles of reform in the care of the chronically mentally ill. **Hosp Community Psychiatry** 1984 Aug;35(8):785–93
Neill JR: Adolf Meyer and American psychiatry today. **Am J Psychiatry** 1980 Apr;137(4):460–4
Payne H, Luthe R: Isaac Ray and forensic psychiatry in the United States. **Forensic Sci Int** 1980 Mar–Apr;15(2):115–27
Perry HS: Clara Mabel Thompson. In: Notable American women. The modern period. Cambridge, Mass., Belknap-Harvard Univ. Press, 1980. 4:680–3.
Perry HS: Psychiatrist of America. The life of Harry Stack Sullivan.

Cambridge, Belknap Press, 1982. 462 p.
Peset JL: Cesare Lombroso y la psiquiatría de su tiempo: el caso U.S.A. In International Congress of the History of Medicine, 27th, Barcelona, 1980. Actas. Barcelona, Acadèmia de Ciències Mèdiques de Catalunya i Balears, 1981. p. 134–9.
Pillard E: Nevada's treatment of the mentally ill, 1882–1961. **Nev Hist Soc Q** 1979;22(2):83–99
Pillard RC: Psychotherapeutic treatment for the invisible minority. **Am Behav Sci** 1982;25(4):407–22
Pines M: The Foundations' Fund for Research in Psychiatry and the growth of research in psychiatry. **Am J Psychiatry** 1983 Jan;140(1):1–10
Powell RC: Anton Theophilus Boisen. In Dictionary of American biography, 1961–1965. Suppl. 7, 1981. p. 63–5.
Powell RC: Daniel Joseph McCarthy. In Dictionary of American Biography, Suppl. 6, 1956–1960. p. 402–4, 1980.
Powell RC, Hoff SG: Frieda Fromm-Reichmann. In: Notable American women. The modern period. Cambridge, Mass., Belknap-Harvard Univ. Press, 1980. 4:252–5.
Powell RC: (Helen) Flanders Dunbar. In Dictionary of American Biography, Suppl. 6, 1956–1960. p. 180–1, 1980.
Quen JM: Isaac Ray and the development of American psychiatry and the law. **Psychiatr Clin North Am** 1983 Dec;6(4):527–37
Quen JM: Remarks on Doctor Isaac Ray (1807–1881). **RI Med J** 1980 Jun;63(6):217–9
Radochoński M: Ewolucja idei terapii rodszinnej w USA. **Psychiatr Pol** 1982;16(3):187–94
Rattner J: Rollo May. In J. Rattner, ed: Wandlungen der Psychoanalyse. Wien, Europaverlag, 1980. p. 309–32.
Reese WG: Academic psychiatry in Arkansas. **J Arkansas Med Soc** 1981 Nov;78(6):220–33
Restak RM: Psychiatry in America. **Wilson Q** 1983;7(4):94–125
Rioch MJ: In memoriam: Abe Fortas. **Psychiatry** 1983;46(1):83–6
Roazen P: Anorexia nervosa: Helene Deutsch, M.D. **Bull Menninger Clin** 1981 Nov;45(6):499–501
Roazen P: Freud and America. **Soc Res (NY)** 1972;39(4):720–32
Rosen S: The psychotherapeutic and hypnotherapeutic approaches of Milton H. Erickson, M.D. **Am J Psychoanal** 1984 Summer;44(2):133–45
Ross JM, Slap JW, Gehrie MJ, et al: George Klein's 'Psychoanalytic theory' in perspective. **Psychoanal Rev** 1980 Summer;67(2):161–216
Rubins JL: Karen Danielson Horney. In: Notable American women. The modern period. Cambridge, Mass., Belknap-Harvard Univ. Press, 1980. 4:351–4.
Saklad SM: Psychiatry in Rhode Island: 1725–1980. **RI Med J** 1980 Jun;63(6):207–16
Satin DG: Erich Lindemann: the humanist and the era of community mental health. **Proc Am Philos Soc** 1982 Aug;126(4):327–46
Schimel JL: Ralph M. Crowley: psychoanalytic pioneer. **J Am Acad Psychoanal** 1981 Oct;9(4):489–91
Schneck JM: S. Weir Mitchell, M.D. (1829 to 1914) and D. Hayes Agnew, M.D. (1818 to 1892). Neuropsychiatrist's poetic tribute to a surgeon. **NY State J Med** 1982 Jul;82(8):1264–8
Schneck JM: S. Weir Mitchell, psychopathology, and 'The Waters of Oblivion'. **Am J Psychiatry** 1984 Jan;141(1):150–1
Schnell RL: Contributions to psychohistory: IV. Individual experience in historiography and psychoanalysis: significance of Erik Erikson and Robert Coles. **Psychol Rep** 1980 Apr;46(2):591–612
Shepherd M: La découverte de la nature de la pellagre. Leçons d'une recherche épidémiologique et psychiatrique remarquable. **Acta Psychiatr Belg** 1983 May–Jun;83(3):295–303
Sifneos PE: A historical account of preventive psychiatry in the greater Boston area, 1942–1979. **Bibl Psychiatr** 1981;(160):1–6
Singerman B: DSM-III: historical antecedents and present significance. **J Clin Psychiatry** 1981 Nov;42(11):409–10
Slaff B: The history of adolescent psychiatry. **Adolesc Psychiatry** 1981;9:7–21
Slavinsky AT, Krauss JB: Mutual withdrawal... or Gwen Tudor revisited. **Perspect Psychiatr Care** 1980 Sep–Oct;18(5):194–203
Snodgrass J: William Healy (1869–1963): pioneer child psychiatrist and criminologist. **J Hist Behav Sci** 1984 Oct;20(4):332–9
Sollod RN: Goodwin Watson's 1940 conference. **Am Psychol** 1981 Dec;36(12):1546–7
Spencer S: Delivering the woman artist from the silence of the womb: Otto Rank's influence on Anais Nin. **Psychoanal Rev** 1982 Spring;69(1):111–29
Stam I, Lahmann F: Carl R. Rogers. In J. Rattner, ed: Wandlungen der Psychoanalyse. Wien, Europaverlag, 1980. p. 165–86.
Stanton AH: Frieda Fromm-Reichmann, MD: her impact on American psychiatry. **Psychiatry** 1982;45(2):121–7
Stokes GA: Helen Flanders Dunbar. In: Notable American women. The modern period. Cambridge, Mass., Belknap-Harvard Univ. Press, 1980. 4:210–2.
Sulman AM: Victor Vance Anderson. In Dictionary of American Biography, Suppl. 6, 1956–1960. p. 16–17, 1980.
Taylor E: Louville Eugene Emerson: psychotherapy, Harvard, and the early Boston scene. **Harv Med Alumni Bull** 1982 Spring;56(2):42–8
Tucker EB: James Jackson Putnam: an American perspective on the social uses of psychoanalysis, 1895–1918. **N Engl Q** 1978;51(4):527–46
Weinberg J: 'Roy R. Grinker, Sr.' Some biographical notes. **J Am Acad Psychoanal** 1980;8:441–9
Weinstein F: On the social function of intellectuals: a consideration of Erik H. Erikson's contribution to psychoanalysis and psychohistory. In M. Albin, R. J. Devlin, G. Heeger, ed: New directions in psychohistory. The Adelphi papers in honor of Erik H. Erikson. Lexington, Toronto, D. C. Heath, 1980. p. 3–19.
Wiegand R: Thomas S. Szasz. In J. Rattner, ed: Wandlungen der Psychoanalyse. Wien, Europaverlag, 1980. p. 333–68.
Wilk D: In memoriam Dr. Leo Kanner, 1894–1981. **Koroth** 1982 Aug;8(3/4):213–20
Wilkerson SY: Mind over body. James Jackson Putnam and the impact of neurology on psychotherapy in late nineteenth-century America. Ph.D. Diss. Duke University. Durham, 1978. v, 377 leaves.
Wolf ES: Tomorrow's self: Heinz Kohut's contribution to adolescent psychiatry. **Adolesc Psychiatry** 1980;8:41–50
Women in psychiatry--a quiet revolution: **Psychiatr News** 1980 Jul 18;15(14):7, 20–1
Wortis J: How shock treatment came to America: what history teaches. **Biol Psychiatry** 1982 Nov;17(11):1203–5
Zahn WM: Erik H. Erikson. In J. Rattner, ed: Wandlungen der Psychoanalyse. Wien, Europaverlag, 1980. p. 187–210.

**USSR**

Akimov GA, Arkhangel'skiĭ AE: K istorii deiatel'nosti Leningradskogo nauchnogo obshchestva nevropatologov i psikhiatrov (pervye gody). **Zh Nevropatol Psikhiatr** 1983;83(7):1067–9
Bal'dysh G: Bekhterev v Peterburge-Leningrade. Leningrad, Lenizdat, 1979. 318 p.
Brown JV: The professionalization of Russian psychiatry: 1857–1911. Ph.D. Diss., Univ. of Pennsylvania. Philadelphia, 1981. 431 p.
Ciucura TB: Dissent, law and psychiatry in the Soviet Union. **Can Slavonic Pap** 1979;21(1):98–108
Dionesov SM: Stranitsa iz istorii Pervogo s'ezda Russkogo soiuza psikhiatrov i nevropatologov. **Zh Nevropatol Psikhiatr** 1981;(5):744–5
Gataullin MM: Razvitie psikhiatrii v Bashkirii (k 425-letiiu dobrovol'nogo prisoedineniia Bashkirii k ruskomu gosudarstvu (1557–1982 gg.). **Zh Nevropatol Psikhiatr** 1982;82(12):99–102
Gerish AG: P. P. Kashchenko: 1859–1920. Moskva, Meditsina, 1980. 77 p.
Gurevich SA: Aktual'nye problemy psikhiatrii v 'Vestnike klinicheskoĭ i sudebnoĭ psikhiatrii i nevropatologii' (k 100-letiiu osnovaniia otechestvennoĭ psikhiatricheskoĭ periodiki). **Zh Nevropatol Psikhiatr** 1983;83(8):1236–40
Gurevich SA: Lev Tolstoĭ i psikhiatriia. **Zh Nevropatol Psikhiatr** 1981;81(9):1386–9
Gurevich SA: Problemy épileptologii v otechestvennoĭ psikhiatrii XIX veka (po materialam pervykh psikhiatricheskikh zhurnalov). **Zh Nevropatol Psikhiatr** 1983;83(6):914–7
K 80-letiiu zhurnala nevropatologii i psikhiatrii im. S. S. Korsakova: **Zh Nevropatol Psikhiatr** 1981;81(1):3–5
Kabanov MM: Razvitie v deiatel'nosti Leningradskogo nauchno-issledovatel'skogo psikhonevrologicheskogo instituta im. V. M. Bekhtereva ideĭ ego osnovatelia. **Zh Nevropatol Psikhiatr** 1982;82(11):1234–7
Kelemen G: V. H. Kandinszkij (1849–1889) a pszichopatológia nagy orosz úttörője. **Orv Hetil** 1984 Nov 25;125(48):2943–4, 2947
Koupernik C: Serbsky and czarist dissidents. **Arch Gen Psychiatry** 1983 Jun;40(6):697–8
Krasik ED, Minevich VB, Potapov AI: Istoriia psikhiatricheskoi pomoshchi v Tomskoĭ oblasti. **Zh Nevropatol Psikhiatr** 1981;81(9):1393–9
Kretschmer W: Psychiatrie in der Sowjetunion. **Osteuropa** 1978;28(4):317–20
Lakosina ND: Idei nevroticheskogo razvitiia v trudakh P. B. Gannushkina. **Zh Nevropatol Psikhiatr** 1982;82(11):127–9
Maslov EV: Iz istorii kliniki nervnykh i dushevnykh bolezní Severo-Kavkazskogo meditsinskogo instituta (Rostov-na-Donu). **Zh Nevropatol Psikhiatr** 1983;83(4):601–3
Mečíř J: Z počátku sovětské dětské psychiatrie. **Cesk Psychiatr** 1979 Dec;75(6):402–7
Miliavskiĭ VM: K istorii prepodavaniia psikhiatrii v fel'dsherskikh shkolakh. **Feldsher Akush** 1982;47(4):53–4
Nicolino F: Trotskij e la psicoanalisi. **Nuova Riv Stor** 1978;62(5–6):605–25
Popushoĭ EP, Ioksa VA: Progressivnaia rol' vracha-revoliutsionera P. P. Tutyshkina v razvitii nauchnoĭ mysli v Moldavii. **Sov Zdravookhr** 1984;(4):69–71
Roĭtel'man AG: Iz istorii razvitiia nezemskoĭ psikhiatricheskoĭ pomoshchi v Rossii vo vtoroĭ polovine XIX veka. **Zh Nevropatol Psikhiatr** 1981;81(9):1390–3
Rokhlin LL, Shereshevskiĭ AM: Znamenatel'nye daty istorii psikhiatrii 1981 g. **Zh Nevropatol Psikhiatr** 1981;81(1):122–7
Rokhlin LL, Shereshevskiĭ AM, Tom A: Znamenatel'nye i iubileĭnye daty nevropatologii i psikhiatrii 1984 g. **Zh Nevropatol Psikhiatr** 1984;84(2):271–80
Shereshevskiĭ AM: Organizatsiia usovershenstvovaniia vracheĭ-psikhiatrov v Rossii. **Zh Nevropatol Psikhiatr** 1980;80(8):1230–4

## PSYCHIATRY

Voloshin PV: 60 let Khar'kovskomu nauchno-issledovatel'skomu institutu nevrologii i psikhiatrii im. V. P. Protopopova. **Zh Nevropatol Psikhiatr** 1983;83(5):780-3
[80th anniversary of the 'Zhurnal Nevropatologii i Psikhiatrii im. S. S. Korsakov'] (Rus): **Zh Nevropatol Psikhiatr** 1981;81(1):3-5

**Yugoslavia**

Jan Z: Biografija Bogomira Magajne. **Goriski Letnik** 1979;6:491-502
Novak Z: 30 godina 'Neuropsyhijatrije' i 'Neurologije'. **Neurologija** 1983;31(1-2):7-9

## PSYCHOLOGY

See also **Neurology; Psychiatry**

Ajuriaguerra J de: L'enfant dans l'histoire---problèmes psychologiques. **Psychiatr Enfant** 1979;22(1):101-26
Anderson JW: The methodology of psychological biography. **J Interdiscip Hist** 1981;11:455-75
Berger M: The 'scientific approach' to intelligence: an overview of its history with special reference to mental speed. In H. J. Eysenck, ed: A model for intelligence. Berlin, Springer-Verlag, 1982. p. 13-43.
Bizière JM: Psychohistory and histoire des mentalités. **J Psychohist** 1983 Summer;11(1):89-109
Brennan JF: History and systems of psychology. Englewood Cliffs, Prentice-Hall, 1982. x, 374 p.
Brink TL: History and depth psychology: some reconsiderations. **Historian** 1979;41(4):738-53
Broughton JM: Psychology and the history of the self: from substance to function. In R. W. Rieber, K. Salzinger, ed: Psychology: theoretical-historical perspectives. New York, Academic Press, 1980. p. 81-99.
Brozek J, Evans RB, ed: R. I. Watson's selected papers on the history of psychology. Hanover, University of New Hampshire, 1977. xiii, 393 p.
Brulin F, Doual A, Gysel C: Evolution des rapports de la psychologie et de l'odontologie. **Orthod Fr** 1980;51:197-202
Calhoun D: On the psychohistory of childhood. **Hist Educ Q** 1974;14(3):371-7
Campillo-Sainz C, Xirau R, Armendares S, et al: La indentidad del hombre. **Gac Med Mex** 1982 Sep;118(9):366-78
Chaplin, JP, Krawiec TS: Systems and theories of psychology. New York, Holt, Rinehart and Winston, 1979. viii, 651 p.
Chorover SL: From genesis to genocide. The meaning of human nature and the power of behavior control. Cambridge, Mass., MIT Press, 1979. xiii, 238 p.
Cofer CN: The history of the concept of motivation. **J Hist Behav Sci** 1981 Jan;17(1):48-53
Coleman SR: Historical context and systematic functions of the concept of the operant. **Behaviorism** 1981;9:207-26
Day WF: The historical antecedents of contemporary behaviorism. In R. W. Rieber, K. Salzinger, ed: Psychology: theoretical-historical perspectives. New York, Academic Press, 1980. p. 203-62.
Deikman AJ: The observing self. Mysticism and psychotherapy. Boston, Beacon Press, 1982. xiii, 194 p.
Devereux G: The family: historical function, dysfunction, lack of function, and schizophrenia. **J Psychohist** 1980;8:183-93
Dieckhöfer K: Geistesgeschichtliche Strömungen in der Biographik--ein kulturhistorischer Abriss. **Z Psychosom Med Psychoanal** 1980 Jul-Sep;26(3):275-81
Earl JW: The role of the men's hall in the development of the Anglo-Saxon superego. **Psychiatry** 1983 May;46(2):139-60
Ebel H, et al: The psychohistory of history: a symposium. **J Psychohist** 1981 Winter;8(3):259-79
Eckardt G, ed: Zur Geschichte der Psychologie. Berlin, VEB, 1979. 128 p.
Eng E: Locke's Tabula Rasa and Freud's 'Mystic writing pad.' **J Hist Ideas** 1980 Jan-Mar;41(1):133-40
Fishman S: The history of childhood sexuality. **J Contemp Hist** 1982;17(2):269-83
Franz ML von: Alchemy: an introduction to the symbolism and the psychology. Toronto, Inner City Books, 1980. 280 p. (Studies in Jungian Psychology, 5).
Friedländer S: History and psychoanalysis. An inquiry into the possibilities and limits of psychohistory. New York and London, Holmes & Meier, 1978. 175 p. (Translation of French edition, 1975)
Gachnochi G: La violence de l'antisémitisme. **Ann Med Psychol (Paris)** 1979 Oct;137(8):807-16
Gilmore WJ: Media resources available for teaching psychohistory. **Group Psychol Hist Newsl** 1975;3(4):15-20
Gregory RL: Mind in science. A history of explanations in psychology and physics. Cambridge, New York, Cambridge University Press, 1981. xi, 641 p.
Grossinger R: Planet medicine. From stone age shamanism to post-industrial healing. Revised edition. Boulder, London, Shambhala, 1982. xviii, 436 p.
Henle M: Why study the history of psychology? In K. Salzinger, ed: Psychology in progress: an interim report. (Annals of the New York Academy of Sciences, vol. 270). New York, New York Academy of Sciences, 1976. p. 14-20.
Hoffer PC: Psychohistory and empirical group affiliation: extraction of personality traits from historical manuscripts. **J Interdiscip Hist** 1978;9(1):131-45
Hogenson GB: Depth psychology, death and the hermeneutic of empathy. **J Med Philos** 1981 Feb;6(1):67-89
Homans P: A personal struggle with religion: significant fact in the lives and work of the first psychologists. **J Relig** 1982;62:128-44
Horney theory and literature: a symposium: **Am J Psychoanal** 1982 Spring;42(1):3-59
Hothersall D: History of psychology. Philadelphia, Temple University Press, 1984. xx, 456 p.
Huguet M: Expérience mystique, pathologie mentale et condition féminine. **Penelope** 1983;(8):25-8
Informazioni bibliografiche: **Stor Crit Psicol** 1981;2(1):187-98
King RH: From creeds to therapies: Philip Rieff's work in perspective. **Rev Am Hist** 1976;4(2):291-6
Laman CA: A prolegomenon to the history of perspectives in personality theory. Ph.D. Diss., Rice University. Houston, 1978. iv, 210 leaves.
Lawry JD: Guide to the history of psychology. Totowa, N. J., Littlefield, Adams, 1981. xi, 114 p.
Leahey TH: A history of psychology: main currents in psychological thought. Englewood Cliffs, Prentice-Hall, 1980. xii, 431 p.
Lerner RM, ed: Developmental psychology: historical and philosophical perspectives. Hillsdale, N. J., London, Lawrence Erlbaum, 1983. xii, 274 p. Contributions by J. Kagan, S. H. White, P. B. Baltes, R. A. Dixon, J. R. Nesselroade. U. Bronfenbrenner, B. Kaplan.
Levin MJ: Psychology. A biographical approach. New York, McGraw-Hill, 1978. 662 p.
Littman RA: Psychology's histories: some new ones and a bit about their predecessors--an essay review. **J Hist Behav Sci** 1981 Oct;17(4):516-32
Loewenberg P: Decoding the past: the psychohistorical approach. New York, Knopf, 1983. xiv, 300 p.
Lôo P: Plaidoyer pour la violence. **Ann Med Psychol (Paris)** 1979 Oct;137(8):836-9
Lorenz K, ed, Wuketits FM, ed: Die Evolution des Denkens. München, Piper, 1983. 393 p. Contributions by G. Vollmer, R. Kaspar, R. Riedl, F. Seitelberger, G. P. Wagner, W. Leinfellner, E. Oeser, H. Mohr, R. Löw.
Lowry RJ: The evolution of psychological theory: a critical history of concepts and presuppositions. New York, Aldine Pub. Co., 1982. x, 246 p.
McReynolds P: The clock metaphor in the history of psychology. In T. Nickles, ed: Scientific discovery: case studies. Dordrecht, D. Reidel, 1980. (Boston Studies in the Philosophy of Science, v. 60). p. 97-112.
Menzen KH: Entwürfe subjektiver Totalität. Frankfurt am Main, Lang, 1980. 546 p.
Menzen KH: Zum Verhältnis von ästhetischer Theorie und ästhetischer Psychologie. **Ber Wissenschaftsgesch** 1981;4:143-8
Merani AL: Historia crítica de la psicología. Barcelona, Grijalbo, 1976. 671 p.
Noland RW: Psychobiography: case history of life history? **Midwest Q** 1978;20(1):7-17
O'Neil WM: The beginnings of modern psychology. Brighton, Harvester Press; Atlantic Highlands, N.J., Humanities Press, 1982. x, 145 p.
Ostow M: Judaism and psychoanalysis. New York, Ktav Publishing House, 1982. 305 p. Includes contributions by J. A. Arlow, R. L. Rubenstein, M. S. Bergmann, L. R. Sillman.
Oughourlian JM: Un mime nommé désir. Hystérie, transe, possession, adorcisme. Paris, Bernard Grasset, 1982. 311 p.
Ouvrard J: Perception de l'angoisse et de l'anxiété par quelques artistes à travers les siècles. **Actual Odontostomatol (Paris)** 1983 Dec;144:593-622
Palmer C, Horowitz M, ed: Shaman woman, mainline lady: women's writings on the drug experience. New York, Morrow, 1982. 285 p.
Pârvu E, Russo G: Une approche psychosociologique de lat tentative de suicide. **Sante Publique (Bucur)** 1981;24(1):61-5
Putscher M: Climbing Jacob's Ladder: on dreams. In: Congrèss international d'histoire de la médecine, XXVe, Québec, 1976. Actes. Québec, 1977. p. 1112-9.
Rieber RW, Green M, ed: Milestones in the history of forensic psychology and psychiatry; a book of readings. New York, Da Capo, 1981. xi, 271 p.
Robinson DN: System of modern psychology. New York, Columbia Univ. Press, 1979. xii, 333 p.
Robinson DN: The mind unfolded. Essays on psychology's historic texts. Washington, D. C., University Publications of America, 1978. xi, 539 p.
Rogers R: Metaphor: a psychoanalytic view. Berkeley, University of California Press, 1979. xi, 148 p.
Ross E: Rethinking 'the family'. **Radic Hist Rev** 1979 Spring/Summer;Spec:76-84
Rousselle R: Comparative psychohistory: snake-handling in Hellenistic Greece and the American South. **J Psychohist** 1984 Spring;11(4):477-89
Runyan WM: Life histories and psychobiography. Explorations in theory

and method. New York, Oxford, Oxford University Press, 1982. xiii, 288 p.
Sahakian WS: Systematic social psychology. New York, Chandler, 1974. xiii, 589 p.
Sahakian WS, ed: History of psychology. A source book in systematic psychology. Revised edition. Itasca, Illinois, F. E. Peacock, 1981. xvi, 497 p.
Sáry G: A megértés müvészete. **Orv Hetil** 1984 May 13;125(20):1210–1
Schiller F: Coenesthesis. **Bull Hist Med** 1984 Winter;58(4):496–515
Schmidt C: Alchemists, critics and psychohistorians. **J Psychohist** 1981 Winter;8(3):337–67
Schoeneman TJ: Criticisms of the psychopathological interpretation of witch hunts: a review. **Am J Psychiatry** 1982 Aug;139(8):1028–32
Schoenwald RL: The psychological study of history. In Iggers, GG, Parker HT, ed: International handbook of historical studies: contemporary research and theory. Westport, Conn., Greenwood, 1979. p. 71–85.
Schott H: Die 'Suggestion' und ihre medizinhistorische Bedeutung. In Seidler E, Schott H, ed: Bausteine zur Medizingeschichte. Stuttgart, Steiner, 1984. p. 111–21.
Shephard L, ed: Encyclopedia of occultism and parapsychology. A compendium of information on the occult sciences, magic, demonology, superstitions, spiritism, mysticism, metaphysics, psychical science, and parapsychology, with biographical and bibliographical notes and comprehensive indexes. Detroit, Gale, 1978. Two volumes.
Shepherd M: The psycho-historians: a psychiatrist's skepticism. **Encounter (Lond)** 1979;52(3):35–42
Shields SA: The variability hypothesis: the history of a biological model of sex differences in intelligence. **Signs** 1982;7:769–97
Skura MA: The literary use of the psychoanalytic process. New Haven, London, Yale University, 1981. 280 p.
Smith SB: The great mental calculators: the psychology, methods, and lives of calculating prodigies, past and present. New York, Columbia University Press, 1983. xviii, 374 p.
Sosa R: Maternal bonding: an overview. In Smith GF, Smith PN, Vidyasagar D, ed: Historical review and recent advances in neonatal and perinatal medicine. [Chicago?], Mead Johnson Nutritional Division, 1983. Vol. I. p. 123–38.
Ushida N: Etude comparative de la psychologie d'Aristote, d'Avicenne et de St. Thomas d'Aquin. Tokyo, Keio Institute of Cultural and Linguistic Studies, 1968. vi, 231 p. (Studies in the humanities and social relations; v. 11.).
Watson RI: A methodological note on the research use of the Syntopicon. **J Hist Behav Sci** 1980 Jul;16(3):275–9
Watson RI: Basic writings in the history of psychology. New York, Oxford Univ. Press, 1979. xviii, 420 p.
Weckowicz TE, Liebel-Weckowicz H: Typologies of the theory of behaviorism since Descartes. **Sudhoffs Arch** 1982;66(2):129–51
Zimmermann RE: The structure of mythos: on the cultural stability of alchemy. **Ambix** 1984 Nov;31(3):125–37

### Americas

Wendorf de Sejas M, Sejas García R: Medicina y psicologia tradicional de la region andina: bibliografía comentada. **Nuevos Libros** 1980;23–24:1–23

### China

Veith I: Psychologische Dimensionen der fernöstlichen Persönlichkeit. **Jahrb Univ Dusseld** 1977–78;:317–25

### France

Vigarello G: L'eau: Un imaginaire pédagogique dans la médecine des enfants aux XVIe–XVIIe et XVIIIe siècles. **Hist Philos Life Sci** 1981;3(2):171–91

### Germany

Belke I: Die Begründung der Völkerpsychologie in Deutschland: Eine Alternative zur etablierten Geschichtswissenschaft? **Riv Filos** 1982;73:192–233
Schwarz M: Psychohygienische Verhaltensgebote für schwangere Frauen in medizinischen Ratgebergüchern. Frankfurt am Main, Haag Herchen, 1983. iv, 382 p.

### Great Britain

Carlton C: Three British revolutions and the personality of kingship. In Pocock, JG. ed: Three British revolutions: 1641, 1688, 1776. Princeton, N.J., Princeton U. Press, 1980. p. 165–207.
McDonald M: Religion, social change, and psychological healing in England, 1600–1800. In Sheils WJ, ed: The Church and healing. Papers read at the twentieth summer meeting and the twenty-first winter meeting of the Ecclesiastical History Society. Oxford, Basil Blackwell for the Society, 1982. p. 101–25.

### India

Kakar S: Shamans, mystics, and doctors: a psychological inquiry into India and its healing traditions. New York, Knopf, 1982. x, 306 p.
Krishan Y: The meaning of prajnā-aparādha and karma in Ayurveda. **Bull Indian Inst Hist Med Hyderabad** 1982;12(1–4):28–33
Roşu A: Les conceptions psychologiques dans les textes médicaux indiens. Paris, Institut de civilisation indienne, 1978. xv, 287 p. (Publications de l'Institut de civilisation indienne. Série in-8; fasc. 43).

### Mexico

Díaz JL: Ethnopharmacology and taxonomy of Mexican psychodysleptic plants. **J Psychedelic Drugs** 1979 Jan–Jun;11(1–2):71–101
Jiménez-Olivares E: La interpretación de los sueños en el México prehispánico. In International Congress of the History of Medicine, 27th, Barcelona, 1980. Actas. Barcelona, Acadèmia de Ciències Mèdiques de Catalunya i Balears, 1981. p. 78–80.
Lopez Austin A: Almas y experiencia entre los antiguos nahuas. **Bol Soc Mex Hist Filos Med** 1983;6(45):223–33
Salinas Quiroga G: Psicologia de los pueblos y del mexicano. **Humanitas** 1981;22:213–8

### United States

Brozěk J, ed: Explorations in the history of psychology in the United States. Lewisburg, [Pa.], Bucknell University Press, 1984. 333 p. Contributions by R. B. Evans, J. G. Blight, W. R. Woodward, J. A. Popplestone, M. W. McPherson, M. M. Sokal.
Davis G: Childhood and history in America. New York, Psychohistory Press, 1976. 281 p.
Murphey MG: The psychodynamics of Puritan conversion. **Am Q** 1979;31(2):135–47
Pontius AA: Face representation linked with literacy level in colonial American tombstone engravings and Third World preliterates' drawings. Toward a cultural-evolutional neurology. **Experientia** 1982 May 15;38(5):577–81
Smith WD, et al: Reflections on black psychology. Washington, University Press of America, 1979. ix, 528 p.

### Before 500 A.D.

Berger J: New views on the Biblical Joseph. **Am J Psychoanal** 1981 Fall;41(3):277–82
Lewis N: The interpretation of dreams and portents. Toronto, Sarasota, Stevens, 1976. xi, 167 p.
Savitz HA: Dreams in the Talmud: the prophets of yore had the noblest dream. **RI Med J** 1981 Sep;64(9):427–30

### Babylon

Spielmeyer R: The epic of Gilgamesh; resolution of concepts of evil and death in ancient Babylonia. **NY State J Med** 1979 Sep;79(10):1618–21

### Greco-Roman

Sandyk R: Brain development and the phylogenesis of writing and drawing direction. **S Afr Med J** 1982 Jul 10;62(2):43–4
Siclari A: L'antropologia di Nemesio di Emesa. Padova, La Garangola, 1974. 318 p. (Filosofia e religione; 9).

### Greece

Cappelletti AJ: El sentido del gusto, segun Aristoteles. **Rev Soc Venez Hist Med** 1978;27(41):41–57
Cappelletti AJ: El sentido del olfato, segun Aristoteles. **Rev Soc Venez Hist Med** 1978;27(41):9–40
Dieckhöfer K: Zur Rolle einer Psychohygiene im Griechenland des 5. vorchristlichen Jahrhunderts bis zur Zeitenwende. **Clio Med** 1982 Dec;17(2–3):81–94
Gaukroger S: Aristotle on the function of sense perception. **Stud Hist Philos Sci** 1981 Mar;12(1):75–89
Hughes JD: The dreams of Alexander the Great. **J Psychohist** 1984 Fall;12(2):168–92
Lefèvre C: Sur l'évolution d'Aristote en psychologie. Louvain, Editions de l'Institut supérieur de philosophie, 1972. ix, 345 p.
Longrigg J: Two notes on Theophrastus 'De sensibus.' **Philologus** 1975;119:163–9
Osborne C: Aristotle's De anima 3.2: how do we perceive that we see and hear? **Classical Q** 1983;33:401–11
Roselli A: Aristotele e il sistema della sensazione. **Physis** 1980;22(2):157–73
Smith NW: Illusions and counter-illusions or aesthetic effects in Greek temples? **Stor Crit Psicol** 1983 Dec;4(2):157–70
Stam HJ, Spanos NP: The Asclepian dream healings and hypnosis: a critique. **Int J Clin Exp Hypn** 1982 Jan;30(1):9–22

# PSYCHOLOGY

### Rome

Eastwood BS: Galen on the elements of olfactory sensation. **Rheinisches Mus Philol** 1981;124:268-90

### 500 A.D.-1450

Dewan L: St. Albert, the sensibles, and spiritual being. In Weisheipl JA, ed: Albertus Magnus and the sciences. Toronto, Pontifical Institute of Mediaeval Studies. p. 291-320.

Kottek SS: The seat of the soul: contribution to the history of Jewish medieval psycho-physiology. **Clio Med** 1979 May;13(3-4):219-46

Kroll J, Bachrach B: Medieval visions and contemporary hallucinations. **Psychol Med** 1982 Nov;12(4):709-21

Park K: Albert's influence on late medieval psychology. In Weisheipl JA, ed: Albertus Magnus and the sciences. Toronto, Pontifical Institute of Mediaeval Studies, 1980. p. 501-35.

Steneck NH: Albert on the psychology of sense perception. In Weisheipl JA, ed: Albertus Magnus and the sciences. Toronto, Pontifical Institute of Mediaeval Studies, 1980. p. 263-90.

Sutto C, ed: Le sentiment de la mort au Moyen Age. Etudes présentées au Cinquième colloque de l'Institut d'études médiévales de l'Université de Montréal. Quebec, L'Aurore, 1979. Contributions by M. Hébert, R. Lavoie, B. Saint-Pierre, C. Dolan-Leclerc, B. Roy, R. M. Kully, A. Chené-Williams, P. Boglioni, G. H. Allard, E. Schulze-Busacker, D. Smoje.

### Arabic

Bel-Haj Mahmoud N: La psychologie des animaux chez les arabes, notamment à travers le kitab al-hayawan de Djahiz. Paris, Klincksieck, 1977. xxiii, 231 p. (Etudes arabes et islamiques, Série 3; Etudes et documents, 8).

### France

Jung R: Sinnesphysiologische Bemerkungen zu Thomas von Aquinos Maxime der Sinneserkenntnis. **Sudhoffs Arch** 1980;64(4):371-84

### 1450-1700

Jaeger W: Die Ordnungsprinzipien der Farbsysteme des 17. Jahrhunderts. (Franciscus Aguilonius--Athanasius Kircher--Isaac Newton). **Klin Monatsbl Augenheilkd** 1984 Apr;184(4):321-5

Kierulf H: L'ergotisme chez Bosch et Grünewald. In International Congress of the History of Medicine, 27th, Barcelona, 1980. Actas. Barcelona, Acadèmia de Ciències Mèdiques de Catalunya i Balears, 1981. p. 81-90.

Legrenzi P, Sonino M: Fisica ingenua a teoria cartesiana degli urti. **Stor Crit Psicol** 1984;5(2):213-28

Martinez Conesa JA: Sobre 'De somniis' de Augerius Ferrerius. **Helmantica** 1975;26:341-55

Massironi M: Considerazioni psicologiche su alcuni fenomeni della visione descritti nei trattati di prospettiva dei secoli XV-XVII. **Stor Crit Psicol** 1983 Dec;4(2):171-214

Starobinski J: Panorama succinct des sciences psychologiques entre 1575 et 1625. **Gesnerus** 1980;37(1/2):3-16

Toellner R: Logical and psychological aspects of the discovery of the circulation of the blood. In M. D. Grmek, R. S. Cohen, G. Cimino, ed: On scientific discovery. The Erice Lectures 1977. Dordrecht, D. Reidel, 1981. p. 239-59. (Boston Studies in the Philosophy of Science, v. 34).

Tomaselli S: The first person: Descartes, Locke and mind-body dualism. **Hist Sci** 1984;22(pt 2):185-205

Waswo R: The reaction of Juan Luis Vives to Valla's philosophy of language. **Bibl Hum Renaissance** 1980 Sep;42(3):595-609

Watkins RN: The Renaissance pater familias - 'Be ye perfect'. **Psychohist Rev** 1980;9:91-110

### France

Arbini R: Did Descartes have a philosophical theory of sense perception? **J Hist Philos** 1983;21:317-37

Blom JJ, ed: Descartes, his moral philosophy and psychology. Hassocks, Sussex, Harvester Press, 1978. xxi, 288 p.

Joubert L: Treatise on laughter. Translated and annotated by G. D. de Rocher. University, Alabama, University of Alabama Press, 1980. xv, 155 p.

Locke D: Mind, matter, and the 'Meditations'. **Mind** 1981;90:343-66

Reed ES: Descartes' corporeal ideas hypothesis and the origin of scientific psychology. **Rev Metaphys** 1982;35:731-52

Stone MH: Modern concepts of emotion as prefigured in Descartes' 'Passions of the Soul'. **J Am Acad Psychoanal** 1980;8:473-95

Wilson C: Sensation and explanation: the problem of consciousness in Descartes. **Nat Syst** 1982;4:151-65

Yolton JW: Perceptual cognition with Descartes. **Stud Cartesiana** 1981;2:63-83

### Germany

Becke U: Eine hinterlassene psychiatrische Studie Paul Johann Reiters über Luther. **Z Kirchengesch** 1979;90(1):85-95

Tschassovnikarov D, Markov G: Personologische Untersuchungen über einige Urbilder im Schaffen von Hieronymus Bosch. **Psychiatr Neurol Med Psychol (Leipz)** 1980 Oct;32(10):623-30

### Great Britain

Carlton C: Towards a psychobiography of Charles I. **J Psychohist** 1984 Spring;11(4):513-31

Cohen A: Prophecy and madness: women visionaries during the Puritan Revolution. **J Psychohist** 1984 Winter;11(3):411-30

Elton GR: The real Thomas More? **Psychol Med** 1980 Nov;10(4):611-7

Heyd D: The place of laughter in Hobbes's theory of emotions. **J Hist Ideas** 1982 Apr-Jun;43(2):285-95

Kuriyama CB: Hammer or anvil. Psychological patterns in Christopher Marlowe's plays. New Brunswick, Rutgers University Press, 1980. xiv, 240 p.

Muslin HL: Romeo and Juliet: the tragic self in adolescence. **Adolesc Psychiatry** 1982;10:106-17

Petryszak NG: Tabula rasa--its origins and implications. **J Hist Behav Sci** 1981 Jan;17(1):15-27

Reynolds E: A treatise of the passions and faculties of the soule of man (1640). Facsimile, with introduction by M. L. Wiley. Gainesville, Florida, Scholars' Facsimiles & Reprints, 1971. 585 p. in various pagings.

Teigen KH: A note on the origin of the term 'nature and nurture': not Shakespeare and Galton, but Mulcaster. **J Hist Behav Sci** 1984 Oct;20(4):363-4

Wooden WW: Childhood and death: a reading of John Skelton's Phillip Sparrow. **J Psychohist** 1980 Spring;7(4):403-14

### Italy

Kraye J: Francesco Filelfo on emotions, virtues and vices: a re-examination of his sources. **Bibl Hum Renaissance** 1981;43(1):129-40

Liebert RS: Michelangelo: a psychoanalytic study of his life and images. New Haven, Yale University Press, 1983. xxii, 447 p.

### Mexico

Gruzinski S: La mère dévorante: alcoolisme, sexualité et déculturation chez les mexicas (1500-1550). **Cah Am Lat** 1979;20:5-36

### Netherlands

Pagel W: The smiling spleen. In H. Lloyd-Jones, et al., ed: History and imagination: essays in honor of H. R. Trevor-Roper. New York, Holmes & Meier, 1982. p. 81-7.

### Spain

Hirsch EF: Michael Servetus and the neoplatonic tradition: God, Christ and Man. **Bibl Hum Renaissance** 1980 Sep;42(3):561-75

Noreña CG: Juan Luis Vives. The Hague, Nijhoff, 1970. xiii, 327 p.

### United States

Demos JP: Entertaining Satan. Witchcraft and the culture of early New England. New York, Oxford, Oxford University Press, 1982. xiv, 543 p.

Green SA: Salem witchcraft: a biopsychosocial analysis. **Pharos** 1982 Summer;45(3):9-13

Spanos NP: Ergotism and the Salem witch panic: a critical analysis and an alternative conceptualization. **J Hist Behav Sci** 1983 Oct;19(4):358-69

### 1700 to Present

Adelman H: Hitler and Gandhi: the will as spirit and as flesh. **Psychoanal Rev** 1980 Winter;67(4):543-61

Albin M, Devlin RJ, Heeger G, ed: New directions in psychohistory. The Adelphi papers in honor of Erik H. Erikson. Lexington, Toronto, D. C. Heath, 1980. xx, 217 p. Includes contributions by E. S. Wolf, M. F. Shore, G. M. Platt, H. Feinstein, S. H. Rudolph, L. I. Rudolph.

Amundson R: E. C. Tolman and the intervening variable: a study in the epistemological history of psychology. **Philos Sci** 1983;50:268-82

Anderson TH: Becoming sane with psychohistory. **Historian** 1978;41(1):1-20

Ansbacher HL: Psychology: a way of living. **J Individ Psychol** 1981 Nov;37(2):153-95

Ardila R: La Psicologia contemporanea. Buenos Aires, Paidos, 1972. 212 p.

Armstrong D: The invention of the normal child. **Soc Soc Hist Med Bull (Lond)** 1980;27:32

Ash MG: Disziplinentwicklung und Wissenschaftstransfer--Deutschsprachige Psychologen in der

Emigration. **Ber Wissenschaftsgesch** 1984;7(4):207–26
Babini VP: La 'Riforma' di Maine de Biran e i dibattiti sulla folia e il sogno all'Académie Impériale de Médecine. **Atti Accad Sci Ist Bologna** 1979, reçu 1980;67(1):199–222
Barz H: Psychologische Probleme des Unbewussten: C.G. Jung und sein Lebenswerk für die moderne Psychologie. **Universitas (Stuttg)** 1980;35(3):275–82
Beach FA: Historical origins of modern research on hormones and behavior. **Horm Behav** 1981 Dec;15(4):325–76
Beeck M: Merkmale epileptischer Bildnerei: mit Pathographie Van Gogh. Bern, Huber, 1982. 134 p.
Beer G: Anxiety and interchange: Daniel Deronda and the implications of Darwin's writing. **J Hist Behav Sci** 1983 Jan;19(1):31–44
Ben-Zeev A: J. J. Gibson and the ecological approach to perception. **Stud Hist Philos Sci** 1981 Jun;12(2):107–39
Bizière JM: 'Before and after': essai de psycho-histoire. **Rev Hist Mod Contemp** 1980 Apr–Jun;27:177–207
Bizière JM: Une psycho-histoire, pourquoi faire? **Bull Soc Hist Mod** 1980;79(6):11–5
Bower EM, ed: The handicapped in literature. A psychosocial perspective. Denver, Love, 1980. xi, 407 p.
Brooks GP, Aalto SK: The rise and fall of moral algebra: Frances Hutcheson and the mathematization of psychology. **J Hist Behav Sci** 1981;17:343–56
Broughton JM, Leadbeater B, Amsel E, ed: Reflections on Piaget: proceedings of the Jean Piaget Memorial Conference. **Teach Coll Rec** 1981;83(2):151–217
Brozek J, Pongratz LJ, ed: Historiography of modern psychology: aims, resources, approaches. Toronto, Hogrefe, 1980. 336 p. Contributions by R. Ardila, M. G. Ash, L. T. Benjamin, W. Bringmann, R. León, B. Ross, M. Sokal, H. Thomae, G. A. Ungerer, R. I. Watson, M. Wertheimer, W. Woodward, L. J. Pongratz.
Bujosa i Homar F: Reconsiderations on the history of aphasia. In International Congress of the History of Medicine, 27th, Barcelona, 1980. Actas. Barcelona, Acadèmia de Ciències Mèdiques de Catalunya i Balears, 1981. p. 27–38.
Burg BR: The sick and the dead: the development of psychological theory on necrophilia from Krafft-Ebing to the present. **J Hist Behav Sci** 1982 Jul;18(3):242–54
Campbell DT: On the conflicts between biological and social evolution and between psychology and moral tradition. **Zygon** 1976;11:167–208
Capps D: Psychohistory in religious studies. **Group Psychol Hist Newsl** 1974;3(2):4–8
Cavanaugh JC: Early developmental theories: a brief review of attempts to organize developmental data prior to 1925. **J Hist Behav Sci** 1981 Jan;17(1):38–47
Cina C: Social science for whom? A structural history of social psychology. Ph.D. Diss., State University of New York. Stony Brook, 1981. xiii, 417 leaves.
Coon DJ: Eponymy, obscurity, Twitmyer, and Pavlov. **J Hist Behav Sci** 1982 Jul;18(3):255–62
Cordeschi R: Dal comportamentismo alla simulazione del comportamento. **Stor Crit Psicol** 1983;4(1):87–113
Danzinger K: The history of introspection reconsidered. **J Hist Behav Sci** 1980 Jul;16(3):241–62
Davidson WD, Montville JV: Foreign policy according to Freud. **Foreign Policy** 1981–82;45:145–57
Dean MC: The evolution of experimental operant psychology: a quantitative analysis of 'progress' in behavioral science. Ph.D. Diss., Syracuse University. Syracuse, 1981. v, 249 leaves.
Diamond S: Buckle, Wundt, and psychology's use of history. **Isis** 1984 Mar;75(276):143–52
DiCori P: Come controllare i sentimenti: tra scienza delle emozioni e identita di genere all'inizio del '900. **Mem Riv Stor Donne** 1981;(1):26–32
Duerr HP, ed: Der Wissenschaftler und das Irrationale. Band 2. Beiträge aus Philosophie und Psychologie. Frankfurt am Main, Syndikat, 1981. 679 p.
Duncan CP: A note on the 1929 International Congress of Psychology. **J Hist Behav Sci** 1980 Jan;16(1):1–5
Ebel H: Notes toward a psychohistory of the movies. **Psychoanal Rev** 1983 Spring;70(1):121–4
Erickson RP: Ohrwall, Henning and von Skramlik; the foundations of the four primary positions in taste. **Neurosci Biobehav Rev** 1984 Spring;8(1):105–27
Erös F: Cooperation, legitimation and some aspects of the history of social psychology. **Stor Crit Psicol** 1981;2(1):87–96
Estévez González A: Anotaciones a la historia de la neuropsicoloía. **Arch Neurobiol (Madr)** 1980 Nov–Dec;43(6):401–20
Evans B, Waites B: IQ and mental testing. An unnatural science and its social history. London, Macmillan, 1981. x, 228 p. (Critical social studies).
Feinstein HM: The sins of the fathers. **Psychoanal Rev** 1983 Spring;70(1):95–100
Feinstein HM: The therapeutic fantasy of psychohistorian. **Psychoanal Rev** 1982 Summer;69(2):221–8
Fischer-Homberger E: Herr und Weib: Zur Geschichte der Beziehung zwischen ordnendem Geist und anderen Impulsen. In Fischer-Homberger E: Krankheit Frau. Zur Geschichte der Einbildungen. Darmstadt, Sammlung Luchterhand, 1984. p. 92–121.
Flanagan OJ: Psychology, progress and the problem of reflexivity: a study in the epistemological foundations of psychology. **J Hist Behav Sci** 1981;17:375–86
Flanagan TE: Problems of psychobiography. **Queens Q** 1982;89(3):596–610
Frey-Rohn L: Von Freud zu Jung. Eine vergleichende Studie zur Psychologie des Unbewussten. (2. überarbeitete Ausgabe) Zürich, Daimon Verlag, 1980?. 456 p.
Galati D: Lacan: un ritorno a Freud? **Stor Crit Psicol** 1980;1(1):79–91
Gladstein GA: The historical roots of contemporary empathy research. **J Hist Behav Sci** 1984 Jan;20(1):38–59
Goldberg H: An early psychologist of the unconscious. **J Hist Ideas** 1982 Apr–Jun;43(2):269–84
Goldberg A, ed: The future of psychoanalysis. Essays in honor of Heinz Kohut. New York, International Universities Press, 1983. xx, 514 p. Contributions by A. M. Cooper, R. S. Wallerstein, W. W. Meissner, R. D. Stolorow, G. E. Atwood, A. H. Modell, R. Michels, L. Friedman, J. S. Grotstein, J. D. Lichtenberg, M. Kanzer, P. Tolpin, E. Schwaber, E. S. Wolf, B. Brandchaft, M. Tolpin, A. Ornstein, B. E. Litowitz, N. S. Litowitz, M. F. Basch, P. H. Knapp, N. J. London, C. B. Strozier.
Gorman M: Pre-war conformity research in social psychology: the approaches of Floyd H. Allport and Muzafer Sherif. **J Hist Behav Sci** 1981 Jan;17(1):3–14
Green BF: Three decades of quantitative methods in psychology. **Am Behav Sci** 1980;23(6):811–34
Gross G: Medizin zwischen Wissenschaft und Spekulation. Die Phrenologie des Dr. Johann Kaspar Spurzheim aus Longwich. **Kurtrier Jahrb** 1977;17:35–52
Gruber HE: Cognitive psychology, scientific creativity, and the case study method. In M. D. Grmek, R. S. Cohen, G. Cimino, ed: On scientific discovery. The Erice Lectures 1977. Dordrecht, D. Reidel, 1981. p. 295–322. (Boston Studies in the Philosophy of Science, v. 34).
Hale M: Psychology and social order: an intellectual biography of Hugo Münsterberg. Ph.D. Diss. University of Maryland. College Park, 1977. ix, 444 leaves.
Hammett JY: A second drink at the well: theological and philosophical context of CPE origins. **J Pastoral Care** 1975 Jun;29(2):86–9
Hartl P: Vývoj pedagogické psychologie a její význam pro oblast výchovy a vzdělávání dospělých. **Acta Univ Carol [Hist] (Praha)** 1977;5:25–52
Harwood J: The IQ in history. **Soc Stud Sci** 1983 Aug;13(3):465–77
Hearst E, ed: The first century of experimental psychology. Hillsdale, N.J., Erlbaum, 1979. xxiii, 693 p. Contributions by R. A. Littman, J. Hochberg, G. Gottlieb, H. M. Jenkins, J. S. Brown, G. Mandler, C. N. Cofer, M. I. Posner, G. L. Shulman, R. F. Thompson, D. N. Robinson, R. B. Cairns, P. A. Ornstein, I. D. Steiner, B. A. Maher, W. B. Maher, W. K. Estes.
Hebb DO: Neuropsychology: retrospect and prospect. **Can J Psychol** 1983 Mar;37(1):4–7
Hécaen H: L'evolution et les perspectives de la neuropsychologie. **Acta Neurol Latinoam** 1980;26(2):75–102
Hetzer H: 100 Jahre kinderpsychologische Forschung. **Fortschr Med** 1983 Feb 17;101(7):255–8
High RP: Shadworth Hodgson and William James's formulation of space perception: phenomenology and perceptual realism. **J Hist Behav Sci** 1981 Oct;17(4):466–85
Hilgard ER: The trilogy of mind: cognition, affection, and conation. **J Hist Behav Sci** 1980 Apr;16(2):107–17
Hilts VL: Obeying the laws of hereditary descent: phrenological views on inheritance and eugenics. **J Hist Behav Sci** 1982 Jan;18(1):62–77
Hunyady G: Történelem és pszichológia [History and psychology]. **Tortenelmi Sz** 1981;24(1):71–8
Inhelder B: Genetic epistemology and developmental psychology. In R. W. Rieber, K. Salzinger, ed: Psychology: theoretical–historical perspectives. New York, Academic Press, 1980. p. 315–27.
Jacoby E: Der Aufstieg ins Bürgertum und sein Preis. Charles Dickens als Beispiel. **Psyche (Stuttg)** 1982 Jul;36(7):609–29
Jacoby R: Social amnesia: a critique of conformist psychology from Adler to Laing. Boston, Beacon, 1975. xxiii, 191 p.
Jaffe NC: A second opinion on delusions and dreams. A reading of Freud's interpretation of Jensen. In Jones AH, ed: Images of healers. Albany, State University of New York Press, 1983. p. 101–7.
Janzarik W ed: Psychopathologie als Grundlagenwissenschaft. Stuttgart, Ferdinand Enke, 1979. xi, 202 p. (Klinische Psychologie und Psychopathologie, Bd. 8). Contributions by H. Schipperges, H. D. Middelhoff, R. Avenarius, W. Schmitt, H. Kindt, W. Kretschmer, G. Huber, J. Glatzel, K. P. Kisker, H. Tellenbach, H. Häfner, A. Bader, L. Navratil, W. Baeyer, K. Koehler, O. Dörr-Zegers, B. Kimura.
Job R, Tabossi P: Umana o artificiale, purché sia intelligenza. **Stor Crit Psicol** 1984 Jun;5(1):69–89
Johnson JP: Herbert Hoover and David Copperfield: a tale of two childhoods. **J Psychohist** 1980 Spring;7(4):467–75
Kalat JW: Evolutionary thinking in the history of the comparative psychology of learning. **Neurosci Biobehav Rev** 1983 Fall;7(3):309–14
Kasschau RA, Cofer CN, ed: Psychology's second century: enduring issues. New York, Praeger, 1981. 303 p. Historical contributions by G. W. Albee, R. Brown, K. H. Pribram, J. F. Rychlak, S. Toulmin.
Katori H: [A special edition on 'the subject and the object'. Commentary: the history of objective conceptualization in psychology] (Jpn).

# PSYCHOLOGY

**Kango Kenkyu** 1983 Summer;16(3):182–5
Kaufman P: Burke, Freud, and the Gothic **Stud Burke Time** 1972;13(3):2179–92
Kenyon J: Brain stimulation and affective behavior: a note on an early demonstration of a 'reward center'. **J Hist Behav Sci** 1981;17:174–5
Kern SR: Freud and the emergence of child psychology. [New York, s. n.], 1973. 3, vii, 415 leaves.
Kleinman LC, McHenry LC: Fragments of neurologic history: phrenology's founders look at the spinal cord. **Neurology** 1984 Apr;34(4):505
Køppe S: The psychology of the neuron: Freud, Cajal and Golgi. **Scand J Psychol** 1983;24(1):1–12
Kramer JC: The metapsychology of opium. **J Psychoactive Drugs** 1981 Jan–Mar;13(1):71–9
Krauss P: Leiden und Hoffnung in der Sicht der Medizin. **Universitas (Stuttg)** 1980;35(3):511–8
Krippner S: Parapsychological research: a century of inquiry. **J Am Soc Psychosom Dent Med** 1982;29(4):121–7
Kurtz E: Why A.A. works; the intellectual significance of Alcoholics Anonymous. **J Stud Alcohol** 1982 Jan;43(1):38–80
Leahey TH: The mistaken mirror: on Wundt's and Titchener's psychologies. **J Hist Behav Sci** 1981;17:273–82
Lehmann HE: De Binet et Wundt aux mesures neuropsychologiques et aux échelles de comportement. **Acta Psychiatr Belg** 1983 Mar–Apr;83(2):135–46
Leont'ev AA: Lichnost' kak istoriko-etnicheskaia kategoriia. **Sov Etnogr** 1981;3:35–44
Levi F: La cecita nella cultura. **Belfagor** 1982;37(5):569–80
Lifton RJ: On the consciousness of holocaust. **Psychohist Rev** 1980;9(1):3–22
Lifton RJ: Psychohistory. In H. I. Kaplan, et al, ed: Comprehensive textbook of psychiatry/III. Third edition. Baltimore, London, Williams & Wilkins, 1980. p. 3104–12.
Lifton RJ: The concept of the survivor. In Dimsdale, Joel E., ed: Survivors, victims, and perpetrators. Essays on the Nazi Holocaust. Washington, Hemisphere Publ., 1980. p. 113–26.
Lloyd-Bostock SM: Psychology and the law: a critical review of research and practice. **Br J Law Soc** 1981;8(1):1–28
Loewenberg P: The graduate years: what kind of journey? **Group Psychol Hist Newsl** 1975;4(1):2–7
Loughman C: Voices of the Wolf Man: the Wolf Man as autobiographer. **Psychoanal Rev** 1984 Sep;71(2):211–25
Luccio R: La percezione della numerosità. **Stor Crit Psicol** 1983 Dec;4(2):215–83
McDermott WV: Endorphins, I presume. **Lancet** 1980 Dec 20–27;2(8208–8209):1353
McGuigan FJ: The historical development of cognitive psychophysiology: theory and measurement. In E. Schultheisz, ed: History of physiology. Oxford, Elmsford, New York, Pergamon, 1981. xvi, 208 p. (Advances in Physiological Sciences. Proceedings of the 28th International Congress of Physiological Sciences, Budapest, 1980. Volume 21). p. 29–47.
Mack JE: Psychoanalysis and biography: aspects of a developing affinity. **J Am Psychoanal Assoc** 1980;28(3):543–62
McLeish J: The development of modern behavioural psychology. Calgary, Detselig Enterprises, 1981. 228 p.
McLoughlin Q: History, science and psychohistory. **Psychohist Rev** 1980;8(4):22–31
Macmillan MB: Freud and Lindner on pleasure sucking. **Stor Crit Psicol** 1980;1(1):111–43
Malinovich MM: On Herbert Marcuse and the concept of psychological freedom. **Soc Res (NY)** 1982;49(1):158–80
May R: The discovery of being. Writings in existential psychology. New York, London, W.W. Norton, 1983. 192 p.
Mazlish B: The next 'next assignment': leader and led, individual and group. **Psychohist Rev** 1981;9(3):214–37
Meares R: Body feeling in human relations: the possible examples of Brancusi and Giacometti. **Psychiatry** 1980 May;43(2):160–7
Mecacci L: Le illusioni ottiche nell'Ottocento tra fenomenologia e neurofisiologia. **Stor Crit Psicol** 1983 Dec;4(2):287–9
Meerwein P: Der Krebspatient und sein Arzt im 19. Jahrhundert. Ursprünge der Psychoonkologie? Zürich, Juris, 1980. 97 p. (Zürcher Medizingeschichtliche Abhandlungen, Neue Reihe, 139).
Mitchell H: The passions according to Adam Smith and Pierre-Jean-Georges-Cabanis. Two sciences of man(1). **Soc Soc Hist Med Bull (Lond)** 1979 Dec;25:20–7
Mowrer OH: Enuresis: the beginning work--what really happened. **J Hist Behav Sci** 1980 Jan;16(1):25–30
Mullaney MM: Gender and revolution: Rosa Luxemburg and the female revolutionary personality. **J Psychohist** 1984 Spring;11(4):463–76
Musto DF: Continuity across generations: the Adams Family myth. In M. Albin, R. J. Devlin, G. Heeger, ed: New directions in psychohistory. The Adelphi papers in honor of Erik H. Erikson. Lexington, Toronto, D. C. Heath, 1980. p. 117–29.
Nielsen JS: Den patografiske tradition og metode. **Dan Medicinhist Arbog** 1983;12:91–104
Nielzén S: Ljudets väg från öra till perception; en sammanställning av biologiska bakgrunder till ljudupplevande bl.a. med utblick mot psykiatrin. **Sydsven Medicinhist Sallsk Arsskr** 1982;19:99–108
Norton B: Psychologists and class. In C. Webster, ed: Biology, medicine and society 1840–1940. Cambridge, Cambridge University Press, 1981. p. 289–314.
O'Connell AN, Russo NF, ed: Models of achievement. Reflections of eminent women in psychology. New York, Columbia University Press, 1983. xiii, 338 p.
Oei TI: Over depressie (I). Enkele ontwikkelingen omtrent de depressie. **Tijdschr Ziekenverpl** 1983 Feb 15;36(4):105–8
Oesterreich K, Wagner O: Psychopathologie des Alterns und der Voralterung--Historische Entwicklung der Begriffsbildung. **Z Gerontol** 1982 Nov–Dec;15(6):314–20
Ojeda Figueroa C: Karl Jaspers: filosofia y psicoterapia. **Acta Luso Esp Neurol Psiquiatr** 1983 Mar–Apr;11(2):181–8
Ono Y: [Human science. Religion (1). Religion as a psychological phenomenon--progress in religious psychology] (Jpn). **Kango Tenbo** 1981 Apr;6(4):350–6
Oring E: The jokes of Sigmund Freud: a study in humor and Jewish identity. Philadelphia, University of Pennsylvania Press, 1984. xiii, 151 p.
Parson T: The articulation of the personality and the social-action system: Sigmund Freud and Max Weber. In M. Albin, R. J. Devlin, G. Heeger, ed: New directions in psychohistory. The Adelphi papers in honor of Erik H. Erikson. Lexington, Toronto, D. C. Heath, 1980. p. 27–35.
Paskaukas RA: Sigmund Freud and Arthur Schopenhauer reexamined. In International Congress of the History of Medicine, 27th, Barcelona, 1980. Actas. Barcelona, Académia de Ciències Médiques de Catalunya i Balears, 1981. p. 125–9.
Pastore N: Dr. High on history. **J Hist Behav Sci** 1981 Oct;17(4):486–9
Pauleikhoff B: Das Menschenbild im Wandel der Zeit: Ideengeschichte der Psychiatrie und der klinischen Psychologie. Hürtgenwald, Pressler, 1983. 2 vol. 416 p., 439 p.
Peters UH: Anna Freud. Ein Leben für das Kind. München, Kindler, 1979. 309 p.
Pinkham JR: The dentist and child-patient encounter: an Adlerian analysis. **ASDC J Dent Child** 1982 Jul–Aug;49(4):266–72
Proffitt E: Science and Romanticism. **Ga Rev** 1980;34(1):55–80
Raphelson AC: The history course as the capstone of the psychology curriculum. **J Hist Behav Sci** 1982 Jul;18(3):279–85
Raubolt RR: The history and development of adolescent group psychotherapy. Ph.D. Diss., The Fielding Institute, 1979. 172 leaves.
Renshon SA: Life history and character development: some reflections on political leadership. In M. Albin, R. J. Devlin, G. Heeger, ed: New directions in psychohistory. The Adelphi papers in honor of Erik H. Erikson. Lexington, Toronto, D. C. Heath, 1980. p. 57–68.
Rieber RW, Salzinger K, ed: Psychology; theoretical-historical perspectives. New York, Academic Press, 1980. xiv, 364 p.
Robinson DN, ed: Significant contributions to the history of psychology 1750–1920. Series A. Orientations. Volume I: E. Condillac, T. Brown. Washington, D. C., University Publications of America, 1977. Various pagings.
Rogers FB: Carl Jung and self-realization. **Penn Med** 1983 Oct;86(10):30, 32
Roland CG: Sir William Osler's dreams and nightmares. **Bull Hist Med** 1980 Fall;54(3):418–46
Romanyshyn RD: Psychological life, from science to metaphor. Austin, University of Texas Press, 1982. xvii, 209 p.
Rosenthal N: The psychology of women. **Psychohist Rev** 1980;8(4):32–6
Rossi L: Il concetto di adattamento nella psicologia evoluzionistica di K. Lorenz e nell'epistemologia genetica di J. Piaget. **Stor Crit Psicol** 1984;5(2):301–17
Rousseau GS: Psychology. In G. S. Rousseau, R. Porter, ed: The ferment of knowledge. Studies in the historiography of eighteenth-century science. Cambridge, Cambridge University Press, 1980. p. 143–210.
Ruel-Kellermann M: Repères historiques de l'évolution du recours de l'odonto-stomatologie à la psychologie. **Inf Dent** 1981 Oct 1;63(33):3071–83
Russell A: Late effects--influence on the children of the concentration camp survivor. In Dimsdale, Joel E., ed: Survivors, victims, and perpetrators: Essays on the Nazi holocaust. Washington, Hemisphere Publ., 1980. p. 175–204.
Ryant C: Oral history and psychohistory. **J Psychohist** 1981 Winter;8(3):307–18
Salmon P: Psychosociologie du collectionneur. **Rev Inst Sociol** 1977;2:271–87
Salov VI: Vtorzhenie psikhoanaliza v burzhuaznuiu istoriografiiu. (Rus). **Nov Noveishaia Istor** 1972;(4):89–105
Scheidhauer M: Un problème épineux entre Freud et Jung: le rêve. **Rev Hist Philos Relig** 1981;61(4):413–25
Scherg C: Literatur als Lebenshilfe. Am Beispiel Thomas Manns. **Psyche (Stuttg)** 1982 Jul;36(7):630–61
Schneider R: Gibt es eine 'Problemkinderkurve' im HAWIK? Zur Geschichte von Intelligenztestergebnissen. **Prax Kinderpsychol Kinderpsychiatr** 1982 Nov–Dec;31(8):286–90
Schott H: Mesmer, Braid und Bernheim: zur Entstehungsgeschichte des Hypnotismus. **Gesnerus** 1984;41(1/2):33–48
Schulz R, Schulz H, Hartman B: Experimental social gerontology: a social

psychological perspective. **J Soc Issues** 1980;36(2):30–46
Schurig V: Die Eingliederung des Begriffs 'Ethologie' in das System der Biowissenschaften im 19. Jahrhundert. **Sudhoffs Arch** 1984;68(1):94–104
Schwartz LL, Isser N: Some involuntary conversion techniques. **Jew Soc Stud** 1981;43(1):1–10
Seaman JD: On phi-phenomena. **J Hist Behav Sci** 1984 Jan;20(1):3–8
Seron X, Feyereisen P: Cent ans de psychologie scientifique. **Rev Nouv** 1981;73(3):283–93
Shore MF: The psychogenic theory of history. **J Interdiscip Hist** 1979;9(3):517–23
Shorter E: Women's diseases before 1900. In M. Albin, R. J. Devlin, G. Heeger, ed: New directions in psychohistory. The Adelphi papers in honor of Erik H. Erikson. Lexington, Toronto, D. C. Heath, 1980. p. 183–208.
Simon HA: The behavioral and social sciences. **Science** 1980 Jul 4;209(4452):72–8
Sizer SS: New spirit, new flesh: the poetics of nineteenth-century mind-cures. **Soundings** 1980;63(4):407–22
Smith LD: Psychology and philosophy: towards a realignment, 1905–1935. **J Hist Behav Sci** 1981 Jan;17(1):28–37
Sokal MM, Rafail PA: A guide to manuscript collections in the history of psychology and related areas. Millwood, N.Y., Kraus International, 1982. xi, 212 p.
Sokal MM, ed: A guide to manuscript collections in the history of psychology and related areas. [Wellesley, Mass.], Wellesley College Colloquium on the History of Psychology, 1977. iii, 64 leaves.
Sokal MM, ed: An education in psychology: James McKeen Cattell's journal and letters from Germany and England. 1880–1888. Cambridge, Mass., MIT Press, 1981, xxvii, 372 p.
Sparvieri F: Teorie freudiane e psicologia aeronautica. **Riv Med Aeronaut Spaz** 1980 Jan–Jun;43(1–2):81–103
Stannard DE: Shrinking history. On Freud and the failure of psychohistory. New York, Oxford University Press, 1980. xx, 187 p.
Stein HF: Implicit ideology in the psychoanalytic study of culture. **Psychohist Rev** 1981;10(2):91–108
Stocking GW: Innovation in the Malinowskian mode: an essay review of long-term field research in social anthropology. **J Hist Behav Sci** 1980 Jul;16(3):281–6
Strout C: Psyche, Clio, and the artist. In M. Albin, R. J. Devlin, G. Heeger, ed: New directions in psychohistory. The Adelphi papers in honor of Erik H. Erikson. Lexington, Toronto, D. C. Heath, 1980. p. 97–115.
Strozier CB: A rationale for teaching psychohistory. **Group Psychol Hist Newsl** 1975;4(1):8–10
Strozier CB: Heinz Kohut and the historical imagination. **Psychohist Rev** 1978;7(2):36–9
Strozier CB: Springfield über alles: role playing and the teaching of psychohistory. **Group Psychol Hist Newsl** 1975;4(2):13–24
Suransky VP: A tyranny of experts. **Wilson Q** 1982;6(4):53–60
Tobach E: The relationship between Preyer's concept of psychogenesis and his views of Darwin's theory of evolution. **Z Psychol** 1983;191(4):388–95
Treher W: Jean-Jacques Rousseau oder die Anatomie eines Pulverfasses mit Betrachtungen über Georg Wilhelm Friedrich Hegel und Adolf Hitler verbunden zu einer Vergleichenden Psychopathologie der Funktionsschizophrenie. Emmendigen, W. Treher, 1982. 208 p.
Tucker RC: A case of mistaken identity: djugashvili-Stalin. **Biography** 1982;5(1):17–24
Vande Kemp H: The dream in periodical literature: 1860–1910. **J Hist Behav Sci** 1981 Jan;17(1):88–113
Varga A: Eksperimental'noe issledovanie faktorov testa Sondi. **Ann Univ Sci Budap Rolando Eotvos Nominatae** 1979;6:171–83
Vermorel H: Un trouble de mémoire sur l'Acropole, 1936–1904. **Rev Fr Psychanal** 1982;46(3):513–26
Veylon R: La photographie. Petit essai de 'psychopathologie'. **Nouv Presse Med** 1980 Jul 12–26;9(30):2073–5
Vidal F, Buscaglia M, Vonèche JJ: Darwinism and developmental psychology. **J Hist Behav Sci** 1983 Jan;19(1):81–94
Viney W, Michaels T, Ganong A: A note on the history of psychology in magazines. **J Hist Behav Sci** 1981;17:270–2
Voronin LG: Vysshaia nervnaia deiatel'nost' i psikhologiia. **Zh Vyssh Nerv Deiat** 1983 Jul–Aug;33(4):611–8
Wallerström A: Johann Friedrich Struensee--en psykologisk gåta. **Nord Medicinhist Arsb** 1981;:74–87
Wegner PC: Le docteur Gall à Cynthère. **Medizinhist J** 1984;19(3):233–43
Weiner PS: The study of childhood language disorders in the nineteenth century. **ASHA** 1984 Apr;26(4):35–8
Wellmann J: Culture and character: some perspectives from psychological anthropology for psychohistorians. **Group Psychol Hist Newsl** 1975;4(3):12–30
Whiteley JM, ed: The history of counseling psychology. Monterey, California, Brooks/Cole, 1980. xiii, 209 p. [Mostly reprinted articles by various authors]
Wick DL: Psychomythology: A phenomenological critique of psychohistory. **Dalhousie Rev** 1980;6(2):290–99
Windholz G: Pavlov vs. Köhler. Pavlov's little-known primate research. **Pavlov J Biol Sci** 1984 Jan–Mar;19(1):23–31
Wolf S: The psyche and the stomach. A historical vignette. **Gastroenterology** 1981 Mar;80(3):605–14
Woodward AM: The problematic science: psychology in nineteenth-century thought. New York, Praeger, 1982. xvii, 384 p.
Woodward WR: 'Visible colleges' and archives in Europe: first impressions. **J Hist Behav Sci** 1981;17:387–98
Zaretsky E: A note on Marxism and psychoanalysis. **Marx Perspect** 1979;2(2):134–9
Zimmerman J: Transcendent psychology: Erik H. Erikson, Erich Fromm, Karen Horney, Abraham H. Maslow, and Harry Stack Sullivan and the quest for a healthy humanity. Ph.D. Diss., Northwestern University, Evanston, 1982. vi, 498 p.

#### Africa

Ross R: Oppression, sexuality and slavery at the Cape of Good Hope. **Hist Reflect** 1979;6(2):421–33

#### Americas

Torres M: La nueva perspectiva psicologica de Bolivar. **Bol Hist Antiq (Bogota)** 1980;67(728):69–85
Turtle A: Collections of early psychological laboratory apparatus in North America. **Newsl Australas Assoc Hist Philos Sci** 1977–78;9:4–5

#### Australia

Gillespie RR: The early development of the scientific movement in Australian education - child study. **Anzhes J** 1982;11(2):1–14
Love R: A note on courses taught by Australian psychology departments in the history and philosophy of psychology. **Newsl Australas Assoc Hist Philos Sci** 1975–6;7:28–33a
Richard J: Psychohistory: an Australian perspective. **Hist Today** 1981 May;31:10–3

#### Austria

Beckh-Widmannstetter HA: Zur Geschichte der Individualpsychologie: Julius Wagner-Jauregg über Alfred Adler. **Unsere Heimat** 1965;36(10–12):182–8
Gilman SL: Freud and the prostitute: male stereotypes of female sexuality in fin-de-siècle Vienna. **J Am Acad Psychoanal** 1981 Jul;9(3):337–60
Hahoda M: Aus den Anfängen der sozialwissenschaftlichen Forschung in Osterreich. **Zeitgesch** 1981;8(4):133–41
Hetzer H: Kinder- und jugendpsychologische Forschung im Wiener Psychologischen Institut von 1922 bis 1938. **Z Entwicklungspsychol Padagog Psychol** 1982;14(3):175–224
Holck P: Galls frenologi. **Tidsskr Nor Laegeforen** 1983 Sep 20;103(26):1805–7
Legrenzi P: L'uomo senza facoltà: modelli del comportamento in Musil. **Stor Crit Psicol** 1982 Dec;3(2):301–13
Lesky E: Der angeklagte Gall. **Gesnerus** 1981;38(3/4):301–11
Lesky E, ed: Franz Joseph Gall, 1758–1828, Naturforscher und Anthropologe. Wien, Huber, 1979. (Hubers Klassiker der Medizin und der Naturwissenschaften, Band 15) 217 p.
Obermeit W: Die Wirklichkeit des Fiktiven. Literatur und Psychoanalyse. **Psyche (Stuttg)** 1981 Mar;35(3):193–208
Roazen P: The menopause. By Helene Deutsch. **Int J Psychoanal** 1984;65(Pt 1):55–62

#### Bulgaria

Marinow W: Uber einige irrationale psychotherapeutische Heilmittel der Volksmedizin. In International Congress of the History of Medicine. 26th, Plovdiv, 1978. Actes du Congress. Sofia, 1981. Volume II. p. 80–1.

#### Canada

Ames EW: The status of women in Canadian psychology: a case study of women in science. **Int J Womens Stud** 1981;4(4):431–40
Ballstadt C, Peterman M, Hopkins E: 'A glorious madness': Susanna Moodie and the spiritualist movement. **J Can Stud** 1982–83;17(4):88–100
Wright MJ: History of academic psychology in Canada. Toronto, Hogrefe, 1982. x, 260 p.

#### Colombia

Sanz de Santamaría MC de, Salas Sánchez M, Sabogal F: Aspectos psicosociales del aborto (mesa redonda). **Cuad Filos Let** 1980;3(2):85–105

#### Cuba

López Segrera F: Psicoanálisis de una generación. **Rev Bibl Nac Jose Marti** 1970;12(1,2):93-125, 101-52

#### Cyprus

Volkan VD: Cyprus--war and adaptation: a psychoanalytic history of two ethnic groups in conflict. Charlottesville, University Press of Virginia, 1979. xxviii, 192 p.

**Czechoslovakia**

Mecke G: Der Jäger Gracchus, Kafkas Geheimnis. **Psyche (Stuttg)** 1981 Mar;35(3):209–36
Solana RM: Communication, language and family: a communicational analysis of Kafka's letter to his father. **Psychiatry** 1983 Nov;46(4):387–92
Stefánek B: Zur Psychologie des slowakischen politischen Realismus. **Bohemia Jahrb Coll Caroninum (Ger)** 1979;20:82–96

**Denmark**

Greenacre P: Hans Christian Andersen and children. **Psychoanal Study Child** 1983;38:617–35

**Europe**

Gay P: On the bourgeoisie: a psychological interpretation. In Merriman, John M., ed: Consciousness and class experience in nineteenth-century Europe. New York, Holmes and Meier, 1979. p. 187–203.
Mann G: Franz Joseph Galls kranioskopische Reise durch Europa (1805–1807). Fundierung und Rechtfertigung neuer Wissenschaft. **Nachrichtenbl Dtsch Ges Gesch Med Naturwiss Tech** 1984;34(3):86–114

**France**

Baudry FD: Adolescent love and self-analysis as contributors to Flaubert's creativity. **Psychoanal Study Child** 1980;35:377–416
Cavallo C, Cei A: Pinel e il magnetismo animale. **Stor Crit Psicol** 1984 Jun;5(1):91–109
Chasseguet-Smirgel J: De Sade: Der Körper und der Mord an der Realität. **Psyche (Stuttg)** 1981 Mar;35(3):237–52
Chertok L: 30 ans après. La petite histoire de la découverte des neuroleptiques. **Ann Med Psychol (Paris)** 1982 Nov;140(9):971–6
Clément PP: Quelques aspects de la vie et de l'oeuvre de Jean-Jacques Rousseau: s'oublier--se surveiller--fixer par l'écriture. **Univ Ottawa Q** 1979;49(3–4):292–9
Elmore R: View from the Rive Gauche: a comment on Annales Historiography. **Psychohist Rev** 1978;7(2):30–5
Fusswerk-Fursay J: A propos d'un inédit de Pierre Janet sur les croyances. **Ann Med Psychol (Paris)** 1984 May;142(5):703–10
Girard R: Force et tension psychologique selon Pierre Janet. **Schweiz Arch Neurol Neurochir Psychiatr** 1981;128(1):33–51
Gregory RL: French without fears: Denis Diderot. **Perception** 1983;12(5):509–12
Halberstadt-Freud HC: Proust and perversion: some clinical and theoretical consideration. **Int J Psychoanal** 1980;61(3):403–10
Hawkins MJ: Reason and sense perception in Comte's theory of mind. **Hist Eur Ideas** 1984;5:149–63
Ito J: [In search of educational humanity (5). Understanding of man in education (2): 'Emile' by Jean Jacques Rousseau] (Jpn). **Kango Kyoiku** 1983 May;24(5):310–4
Leary DE: Nature, art, and imitation: the Wild Boy of Aveyeron as a pivotal case in the history of psychology. **Stud Eighteenth Cult** 1984;13:155–72
Legée G: Physiologie et phrenologie au temps du physiologiste Pierre Flourens (1794–1867). In International Congress of the History of Medicine, 27th, Barcelona, 1980. Actas. Barcelona, Acadèmia de Ciències Mèdiques de Catalunya i Balears, 1981. p. 91–7.
Léon A: Psychopédagogie scientifique et humanisme dans l'oeuvre d'Henri Wallon (1879–1962). **Paedagog Hist** 1979;19(1):132–45
McLaren A: A prehistory of the social sciences: phrenology in France. **Comp Stud Soc Hist** 1981;23(1):3–22
Matot JP: Filiation problématique roman familial et secret (à propos de Louis Aragon. **Psychiatr Enfant** 1984;27(2):523–38
Mitzman A: Sartres Flaubert. **Psyche (Stuttg)** 1981 Mar;35(3):268–98
Mitzman A: The unstrung Orpheus: Flaubert's youth and the psycho-social origins of art for art's sake. **Psychohist Rev** 6(1):27–42, Summer 77
Moravia S: The capture of the invisible. For a (pre)history of psychology in eighteenth-century France. **J Hist Behav Sci** 1983 Oct;19(4):370–8
Muller JP: Ego and subject in Lacan. **Psychoanal Rev** 1982 Summer;69(2):234–40
Rauch A: Le souci du corps chez Condillac. **Stadion** 1977;3(1):60–89
Richardson WJ: Lacan's view of language and being. **Psychoanal Rev** 1982 Summer;69(2):229–33
Robert BP: Profiles de 'La fruite des idées' et surréalisme. **Rev Univ Ottawa** 1977;47(3):345–64
Ryan S: Reflections on the psychohistory of France, 1919–1940. **J Psychohist** 1983 Fall;11(2):225–41
Schneiderman L: Henri Saint-Simon: his ideology and personality. **Am J Psychoanal** 1980 Winter;40(4):349–64
Shulim JI: The birth of a revolutionary: Robespierre in Artois. **Consortium Revolut Eur 1750–1850 Proc** 1977;:22–33
Szaluta J: Apotheosis to ignominy: the martyrdom of Marshal Pétain. **J Psychohist** 1980 Spring;7(4):415–53
Vartanian A: Le frère de Maupertuis et l'homme machine. **Dix-huit Siecle** 1982;14:305–23

**Germany**

Andre P: Schumann. Les chants de l'ombre. Paris, Jean-Claude Lattes, 1982. 225 p.
Ash MG: Academic politics in the history of science: experimental psychology in Germany, 1879–1941. **Cent Eur Hist** 1980;13(3):255–86
Ash MG: The emergence of Gestalt theory: experimental psychology in Germany 1890–1920. Ph.D. Diss., Harvard University. Cambridge, 1982. xlii, 613 p.
Becker KH, Schmidt HD: Uber eine bisher unerschlossene Quelle der Preyer-Forschung. **Z Psychol** 1984;192(2):182–91
Bellinazzi P: Panpsichismo e psicologia nel pensiero di Ernst H. Haeckel. **Stor Crit Psicol** 1982 Dec;3(2):281–99
Blumenthal AL: Wundt - revisions and reappraisals. In K. Salzinger, ed: Psychology in progress: an interim report. (Annals of the New York Academy of Sciences, vol. 270). New York, New York Academy of Sciences, 1976. p. 21–9.
Bosshardt HG: Hans Hörmann (1924–1983). **Arch Psychol (Frankf)** 1983;135(3):163–73
Bringmann WG, Ungerer GA: The establishment of Wilhelm Wundt's Leipzig laboratory. **Stor Crit Psicol** 1980;1(1):11–28
Bringmann WG, Balk MM: Wilhelm Wundt's publication record: a re-examination. **Stor Crit Psicol** 1983;4(1):61–86
Day RH, Knuth H: The contributions of F C Müller-Lyer. **Perception** 1981;10(2):126–46
Dieckhöfer K: Menschliches, Allzumenschliches---zur verstehenden Psychologie bei Nietzsche. **Z Klin Psychol Psychother** 1980;28(2):101–5
Drews J: Ein Kratersturz ins Unbewusste. Zur Konstruktion von Traum und Tagtraum [in] Arno Schmidts Roman 'Kaff auch Mare Crisium' (1960). **Psyche (Stuttg)** 1981 Dec;35(12):1103–21
Echkardt G: Die Gründung der psychologischen Anstalt in Jena (1923). **Wiss Z Friedrich Schiller Univ (Gesellsch)** 1973;22(4):517–59
Eckhardt G, ed: Zur Geschichte der Psychologie. Berlin, VEB Deutscher Verlag der Wissenschaften, 1979. 128p. Mit Beiträgen von H. Hiebsch, F. Klix, W. Schreier, und L. Sprung.
Geuter U: Die Professionalisierung der deutschen Psychologie im Nationalsozialismus. Frankfurt am Main, Suhrkamp, 1984. 592 p.
Geuter U, Mattes P: Historiography of psychology in West Germany: approaches from social history. A review of the past ten years. **Stor Crit Psicol** 1984 Jun;5(1):111–26
Habermas J: Bemerkungen zu Alexander Mitscherlichs analytischer Socialpsychologie. **Psyche (Stuttg)** 1983 Apr;37(4):352–63
Hardesty FP: Louis William Stern: a new view of the Hamburg years. In K. Salzinger, ed: Psychology in progress: an interim report. (Annals of the New York Academy of Sciences, 1976. p. 31–44.
Jagoda Z, Kłodzinski S, Masłowski J: Stosunek ofiar Oświecimia-Brzezinki do prześladowców. **Przegl Lek** 1981;38(1):37–62
Klix F: Hermann Ebbinghaus---Ursprünge und Anfang psychologischer Forschungen an der Berliner Universität. In Eckardt G, ed: Zur Geschichte der Psychologie. Berlin, VEB Deutscher Verlag der Wissenschaften, 1979. p. 85–109.
Kreis R: The history of childhood through German literature: a psychogenic model. **J Psychohist** 1982 Winter;9(3):311–9
Leary DE: German idealism and the development of psychology in the nineteenth century. **J Hist Philos** 1980;18(3):299–317
Leary DE: The historical foundation of Herbart's mathematization of psychology. **J Hist Behav Sci** 1980 Apr;16(2):150–63
Leary DE: The psychology of Jakob Friedrich Fries (1773–1843): its context, nature, and historical significance. **Stor Crit Psicol** 1982 Dec;3(2):217–48
Marion P: La polemica tra Henning e Bühler. **Stor Crit Psicol** 1980;1(2):297–310
Marion P: La psicologia del pensiero dalla polemica di Wundt alla Entwicklungspsychologie di Bühler. **Stor Crit Psicol** 1982 Dec;3(2):249–79
Marshall ME: Biographical genre and biographical archetype: five studies of Gustav Theodor Fechner. **Stor Crit Psicol** 1980;1(2):197–233
Meiers J: Joseph Meiers' autobiography 1894--an Adlerian physician's mostly non-medical life story. **J Individ Psychol** 1981 Nov;37(2):205–26
Petschauer P: Growing up female in eighteenth-century Germany. **J Psychohist** 1983 Fall;11(2):167–207
Poggi I: Wundt e il linguaggio dei gesti. **Stor Crit Psicol** 1981;2(2):297–314
Rather LJ: The dream of self-destruction. Wagner's Ring and the modern world. Baton Rouge, Louisiana State Univ. Press, 1979. xx, 215 p.
Reiter A: Ernst L. Kirchner--Psychoanalytische Perspektiven der Psychoökonomie seines künstlerischen Schaffens. **Confin Psychiatr** 1980;23(2):118–28
Richards RJ: Christian Wolff's prolegomena to empirical and rational psychology: translation and commentary. **Proc Am Philos Soc** 1980 Jun;124(3):227–39
Rieber RW, ed: Wilhelm Wundt and the making of a scientific psychology. New York, Plenum, 1980. xii, 252 p. Includes contributions by S. Diamond, K. Danziger, A. L. Blumenthal, W. James, S. Feldman, H. K. Haebertin.

Rosenkötter L: Die Idealbildung in der Generationenfolge. **Psyche (Stuttg)** 1981 Jul;35(7):593–9
Rosenman S: The late conceptualization of the self in psychoanalysis: the German language and Jewish identity. **J Psychohist** 1983 Summer;11(1):9–42
Ross HE, Bischof K: Wundt's views on sensations of innervation: a reevaluation. **Perception** 1981;10(3):319–29
Schachter M: La personnalité de Frédéric II Le Grand, Roi de Prusse (1712–1786). Essai de psychologie adlérienne. **Hist Sci Med** 1984;18(2):181–7
Schipperges H: Bildung zu gesunder Vernunft. Zu einer wiederentdeckten Magazin der Aufklärung. **Arztebl Baden Wurttemberg** 1981;6
Schöllgen G: Das Problem einer Hitler-Biographie. **Neue Polit Lit** 1978;23(4):421–34
Schott H: Der versteckte Poet in uns; zur Sprachtheorie in der naturphilosophischen Seelenlehre von Gotthilf Heinrich von Schubert (1780–1860). **Sudhoffs Arch** 1981;65(3):226–50
Smith R: Wilhelm Wundt resurrected. **Br J Hist Sci** 1982 Nov;15(51 pt 3):285–91
Sprung H, Sprung L: William Thkerry Preyer (1841–1897) als Methodologe und Methodiker. **Z Psychol** 1984;192(2):170–81
Szemraj-Lochynska A, Kempisty C: Stan adaptacji do zycia na emeryturze nauczycieli akademickich represjonowanych przez hitleryzm. **Przegl Lek** 1981;38(1):33–6
Ungerer GA: Wilhelm Wundt als Psychologe und Politiker: Anmerkungen zur Biographie. **Psychol Rundschau** 1980;31:99–110
Van Ijzendoorn MH, Van der Veer R: Holzkamp's critical psychology and the functional-historical method: a critical appraisal. **Stor Crit Psicol** 1983;4(1):5–26
Waite RG: The psychopathic god – Adolf Hitler. New York, Basic Books, 1977. xx, 482 p.
Wegner PC: Phrenologische Schnupftabakdosen; ein Beitrag zur Wirkung Franz Joseph Galls bei seiner Ankunft in Paris. **Medizinhist J** 1983;18(1–2):69–99
Wurmser L: Idealization and aggression in Beethoven's creativity. **Am Imago** 1979 Winter;36(4):328–44
Wyss D, Zacher A: W. J. Revers' Bedeutung für die moderne Psychologie. Ein Uberblick. **Z Klin Psychol Psychother** 1983;31(2):137–48
Zacher A: Anthropologische Medizin im Wandel. Von Viktor von Weizsäcker zu Dieter Wyss. **Nervenarzt** 1983 Nov;54(11):598–603


**Great Britain**


Ball T: Platonism and penology: James Mill's attempted synthesis. **J Hist Behav Sci** 1982 Jul;18(3):222–9
Baudry FD: Problems in the application of psychoanalysis to Mary Shelley's Frankenstein. **Int J Psychoanal Psychother** 1982–83;9:647–56
Bell S: George Henry Lewes: a man of his time. **J Hist Biol** 1981 Fall;14(2):278–98
Bernard CA: Dickens and Victorian dream theory. In Paradis J, Postlewait T, ed: Victorian science and Victorian values: literary perspectives. New York, New York Academy of Sciences, 1981. p. 197–216.
Bowman IA: 'My life'; an important Ellis manuscript. **Bookman** 1981 Apr;8(4):3–7
Brink A: Love and conflict in Bertrand Russell's letters. **Queens Q** 1979;86(1):1–15
Broadbent DE: Sir Frederic Charles Bartlett. In Dictionary of national biography, 1961–1970. Suppl. 8, 1981. p. 77–9.
Calcraft LG: Aldous Huxley and the Sheldonian hypothesis. **Ann Sci** 1980 Nov;37(6):657–71
Clarke AM: Psychology and education. **Br J Educ Stud** 1982;30(1):43–56
Continenza B: Darwin e la psicologia. **Stor Crit Psicol** 1981;2(1):99–105
Cooter R: The politics of brain: phrenology in Birmingham. **Soc Soc Hist Med Bull (Lond)** 1983 Jun;32:34–6
Cordeschi R: Craik e la psicologia meccanicistica. **Stor Crit Psicol** 1984 Jun;5(1):161–75
Deacon R: The PSI factor. An examination of the medical and psychological aspects of intelligence work. **Practitioner** 1982 Jan;226(1363):97–102
Dervin D: Michael Balint's contributions to the psychoanalysis of literature. **Psychoanal Rev** 1979–80 Winter;66(4):553–70
Dervin D: Rainbow, phoenix, and plumed serpent: D. H. Lawrence's great composite symbols and their vicissitudes. **Psychoanal Rev** 1980 Winter;67(4):515–41
Duff W: An essay on original genius and its various modes of exertion in philosophy and the fine arts, particularly in poetry (1767). Facsimile. Ed. by J. L. Mahoney. Delmar, New York, Scholars' Facsimiles and Reprints, 1978. ix, 296 p.
Fancher RE: Francis Galton's African ethnography and its role in the development of his psychology. **Br J Hist Sci** 1983 Mar;16(12 No. 1):67–79
Fee E: Nineteenth-century craniology: the study of the female skull. **Bull Hist Med** 1979 Fall;53(3):415–33
Fee E: Psychology, sexuality, social control in Victorian England. **Soc Sci Q** 1978;58(4):632–46
Giannattasio ME, Nencini R: Il mito jacksoniano. **Stor Crit Psicol** 1982 Dec;3(2):315–27
Grosskurth P: Havelock Ellis: biography. New York, Knopf, 1980. xvi, 492 p.
Gruber HE: Darwin on man: a psychological study of scientific creativity. 2d. ed. Chicago, University of Chicago Press, 1981. xxvii, 310 p.
Gruber HE: Darwin on psychology and its relation to evolutionary thought. In R. W. Rieber, K. Salzinger, ed: Psychology: theoretical-historical perspectives. New York, Academic Press, 1980. p. 145–74.
Haynes R: The Society for Psychical Research, 1882–1982: a history. London, Macdonald, 1982. xv, 240 p.
Hearnshaw LS: Cyril Burt, psychologist. Ithaca, Cornell University Press, 1979. xi, 370 p.
Henry WD: The case of Captain Colthurst. **Practitioner** 1981;225:418–20
Hyman V: The autobiographical present in 'A Sketch of the Past'. **Psychoanal Rev** 1983 Spring;70(1):24–32
Jacyna LS: The physiology of mind, the unity of nature, and the moral order in Victorian thought. **Br J Hist Sci** 1981 Jul;14(pt 2 no 47):109–32
Karier C: In praise of great men. **Hist Educ Q** 1980;20(4):473–86
Keegan RT, Gruber HE: Love, death, and continuity in Darwin's thinking. **J Hist Behav Sci** 1983 Jan;19(1):15–30
Keller EF: Lewis Carroll: a study of mathematical inhibition. **J Am Psychoanal Assoc** 1980;28(1):133–60
Kirsop W: W. R. Greg and Charles Darwin in Edinburgh and after: an antipodean gloss. **Trans Camb Bibliogr Soc** 1979;7(3):376–90
Kowalewski D: Politics and emotion in the thought of John Stuart Mill. **J Psychohist** 1980 Spring;7(4):455–66
Kris K: A 70-year follow-up of a childhood learning disability. The case of Fanny Burney. **Psychoanal Study Child** 1983;38:637–52
Myers WA: Mary Shelley's Frankenstein: creativity and the psychology of the exception. **Int J Psychoanal Psychother** 1982–83;9:625–45
Panken S: 'Working through and the novel. **Psychoanal Rev** 1983 Spring;70(1):4–23
Ravin JG: Sir Arthur Conan Doyle and his mystical Ohio tour. **Ohio State Med J** 1983 Jun;79(6):425–7, 431–2
Reid DD: The historical background to wartime research in psychology and psychiatry in the Royal Air Force. In Dearnaley EJ, Warr PB, ed: Aircrew stress in wartime operations. London, New York, Academic Press, 1979. p. 1–8.
Richards RJ: Instinct and intelligence in British natural theology: some contributions to Darwin's theory of the evolution of behavior. **J Hist Biol** 1981 Fall;14(2):193–230
Shaw JA: The postadolescent crisis of John Stuart Mill. **Adolesc Psychiatry** 1982;10:85–98
Sherman MH: Psychosensory images from Virginia Woolf's 'A Sketch of the Past'. **Psychoanal Rev** 1983 Spring;70(1):33–9
Shuttleworth SA: The language of science and psychology in George Eliot's Daniel Deronda. In Paradis J, Postlewait T, ed: Victorian science and Victorian values: literary perspectives. New York, New York Academy of Sciences, 1981. p. 269–98.
Siegel S: Wilkie Collins: Victorian novelist as psychopharmacologist. **J Hist Med Allied Sci** 1983 Apr;38(2):161–75
Smith CU: Evolution and the problem of mind: part II. John Hughlings Jackson. **J Hist Biol** 1982 Summer;15(2):241–62
Soffer RN: Ethics and society in England: the revolution in the social sciences, 1870–1914. Berkeley, University of California Press, 1978. ix, 325 p.
Stewart-Robertson JC: The well-principled savage, or the child of the Scottish enlightenment. **J Hist Ideas** 1981;42:503–25
Sutherland G: Measuring intelligence: English local education authorities and mental testing 1919–1939. In C. Webster, ed: Biology, medicine and society 1840–1940. Cambridge, Cambridge University Press, 1981. p. 315–35.
Sutherland G, Sharp S: 'The fust official psychologist in the wurrld': aspects of the professionalization of psychology in early twentieth century Britain. **Hist Sci** 1980 Sep;18(41 pt 3):181–208
Sutherland JD: The British object relations theorists: Balint, Winnicott, Fairbairn, Guntrip. **J Am Psychoanal Assoc** 1980;28(4):829–60
Tweney RD: Isaac Newton's two uses of hypothetical reasoning: dual influences on the history of psychology. **Stor Crit Psicol** 1980;1(2):235–59
Webb ME: A reexamination of the inception, development, and 'Newtonianism' of David Hartley's 'Observations on man.' Ph.D. Diss., University of Oklahoma, 1981. ix, 310 p.
Weissman A: The English romantics and modern psychology. **Centerpoint** 1975/76;1(4):9–15


**Guyana**


Baechler J: Mourir à Jonestown. **Eur J Sociol** 1979;20(2):173–210
Johnson DP: Dilemmas of charismatic leadership: the case of the People's Temple. **Sociol Anal** 1979;40(4):315–23


**Hungary**


Farkas J, Pisztora F, Martos G: Történeti szocio-kulturpsychiátriai vizsgálatok egy zárt faluközösségre, a mezökövesdi matyó populációra vonatkozóan 1895 és 1945 között. **Orvostort Kozl** 1982;92(4):127–31
Juhász F: Die Anfänge und spezifischen Züge der

Persönlichkeitspädagogik im Ungarn der Jahrhundertwende. **Ann Univ Sci Budap Rolando Eotvos Nominatae** 1972;3:41–54

Martos G, Farkas J, Pisztora F: Szocio-kulturális tényezök hatása a mezökövesdi matyók pszichés sajátosságaira és megbetegedéseire a XVIII. és XIX. században. **Orvostort Kozl** 1982;92(4):119–26

Putnoky J: The development of psychology in Hungary between 1945 and 1970. **Ann Univ Sci Budap Rolando Eotvos Nominatae** 1972;(3):95–102

**India**

Broehl WG, McGee VE: Content analysis in psychohistory: a study of three lieutenants in the Indian mutiny, 1857–58. **J Psychohist** 1981 Winter;8(3):281–306

Fellman G: Leaf in a storm: Jayaprakash Narayan as politician and as saint. **Psychohist Rev** 1981;9(3):183–213

Wurgaft LD: Another look at Prospero and Caliban: magic and magical thinking in British India. **Psychohist Rev** 6(1):2–26, Summer 77

**Ireland**

Robins AH: Did imprisonment ruin Oscar Wilde? **Practitioner** 1981 May;225(1355):773–5

**Israel**

Falk A: Moshe Dyan: the infantile roots of political action. **J Psychohist** 1983 Fall;11(2):271–88

**Italy**

Bazzi F, Bèttica-Giovannini R: L'atlante fisiognomonico e frenologico del sig. Ysabeau tra quelli di Lavater e di Fall e quello di Lombroso. **Ann Osp Maria Vittoria Torino** 1980 Jul-Dec;23(7–12):343–416

Bouissy A: Pirandello, 'psychologue de décadence'. **Rev Etud Ital** 1981;26(2–4):173–94

Caffaratto AT: La raccolta di fotografie segnaletiche del Museo di Antropologia Criminale di Torino: la fotografia come documento e testimonianza dell'opera di Cesare Lombroso. **Ann Osp Maria Vittoria Torino** 1980 Jul-Dec;23(7–12):295–332

Doise W: Dalla filosofia alla psicologia sociale. Una 'lettura' di Carlo Cattaneo. **Stor Crit Psicol** 1983;4(1):117–29

Giulio L: Un tema ricorrente nello Zibaldone: la memoria. **Stor Crit Psicol** 1982 Jun;3(1):27–40

Luccio R: De Sanctis e la psicologia italiana. **Stor Crit Psicol** 1981;2(2):317–68

Masin SC: Note on Eugenio Rignano as a forerunner of the 'New Look' theory of visual perception. **J Hist Behav Sci** 1980 Oct;16(4):313–6

Sansoni J: Considerazioni e riflessioni sul libro 'Lungo Viaggio nel Tunnel della Mallattia' di Gigi Ghirotti. **Prof Inferm** 1980 Jan-March;33(1):3–6

**Mexico**

Colotla VA, Jurado S: Contributions to the history of psychology: XXXIV. Enrique O. Aragon, a pioneer in Mexican psychology. **Percept Mot Skills** 1983 Dec;57(3 Pt 1):1013–4

**Netherlands**

Dalsimer K: Female adolescent development. A study of the Diary of Anne Frank. **Psychoanal Study Child** 1982;37:487–522

Runyan WM: Why did Van Gogh cut off his ear? The problem of alternative explanations in psychobiography. **J Pers Soc Psychol** 1981 Jun;40(6):1070–7

**New Zealand**

Henderson J: Muldoon and Rowling: a preliminary analysis of contrasting personalities. **Pol Sci** 1980;32(1):26–46

**Norway**

Eitinger L: The concentration camp syndrome and its late sequelae. In Dimsdale, Joel E., ed: Survivors, victims and perpetrators: Essays on the Nazi holocaust. Washington, Hemisphere Publ., 1980. p. 127–62.

Fagerheim E: Lars Levi Laestadius' teologiske studier. **Nor Teol Tidsskr** 1972;73(1):35–50

Warick LH, Warick ER: Transitional process and creativity in the life and art of Edvard Munch. **J Am Acad Psychoanal** 1984 Jul;12(3):413–24

**Poland**

Chylińska M: W kregu reakcji obronnych. **Przegl Lek** 1984;41(1):121–6

Jagoda Z, Kłodziński S, Masłowski J: Agresja i agresywność w obozie oświęcimskim. **Przegl Lek** 1980;37(1):43–75

Klein F: Janusz Korczak--Arzt und Erzieher--Ein Symbol gelebter Menschlichkeit für die heutige medizinische und heilpädagogische Praxis. **Off Gesundheitswes** 1984 May;46(5):244–8

Later-Chodyłowa E: Psychospołeczne podstawy więzi polonii z krajem pochodzenia. **Przegl Zachod** 1980;36(3):38–70

Leśniak E, Leśniak R, Ryn Z: Nurt oświecimski w twórczości Antoniego Kępińskiego. **Przegl Lek** 1983;40(12):849–54

Tischner J: Refleksje nad dziełem Antoniego Kępińskiego. **Przegl Lek** 1983;40(12):855–9

**Romania**

Vulcanescu R: Les chevaux fantastiques et la psychothérapie populaire. In International Congress of the History of Medicine. 26th, Plovdiv, 1978. Actes du Congress. Sofia, 1981. Volume II. p. 83–5.

**South Africa**

Shore MF: Cecil Rhodes and the ego ideal. **J Interdiscip Hist** 1979;10(2):249–65

**Spain**

Delgado B: La revista de psicologia i pedagogia de Barcelona (1933–1937). **Perspect Pedagog (Barc)** 1982;12(49):47–70

Siguan M: La psicologia a Catalunya. Barcelona, Edicions 62, 1981. 268 p.

**Sweden**

Al-Dabbagh F: Aksel Mentah, nafsani Suwidi, wa-mu'allif qissat San Mishel. **Al-Arabi** 1973;179:60–3

**Switzerland**

Boden MA: Jean Piaget. New York, Viking, 1979. xii, 176 p.

Caramelli N: Introduzione a Piaget. **Stor Crit Psicol** 1981;2(1):5–85

Eckstaedt A: 'Mimi überreicht Madam Grenouillet einen Blumenstrauss'. Eine psychoanalytische Studie über den Weg der Phantasie des vierjährigen Paul Klee anhand einer Kinderzeichnung. **Psyche (Stuttg)** 1980 Dec:34(12):1123–44

Evans RI: Dialogue with Jean Piaget. New York, Praeger, 1981. lxi, 189 p. (Dialogues in Contemporary Psychology Series).

Hug H, ed: Friedrich Liebling, 1893–1982, zum Gedenken: Gedenkfeier vom 28. März 1982. Zürich, Verlag Psychologische Menschenkenntnis, 1983. 140 p.

Iselin HK: Zur Entstehung von C. G. Jungs 'Psychologischen Typen.' Der Briefwechsel zwischen C. G. Jung und Hans Schmid-Guisan im Lichte ihrer Freundschaft. Aarau, Sauerländer, 1982. 152 p. (Veröffentlichungen der Schweizerischen Gesellschaft für Geschichte der Medizin und der Naturwissenschaften, Bd. 38).

Kitchener RF: Genetic epistemology, normative epistemology and psychologism. **Synthese** 1980;45(2):257–80

Meier-Seethaler C: The child: Erich Neumann's contribution to the psychopathology of child development. **J Anal Psychol** 1982 Oct;27(4):357–79

Modgil S, Modgil C, ed: Jean Piaget. Consensus and controversy. New York, Praeger, 1982. 446 p.

Pulaski MS: Understanding Piaget. Revised and expanded ed. New York, Harper & Row, 1980. xvii, 248 p.

Staude JR: The adult development of C. G. Jung. Boston, Routledge & Kegan Paul, 1981. xxiv, 134 p.

Sullivan EV: The career and legacy of Jean Piaget. **Queens Q** 1981;88(2):341–52

[Understanding of man in education: (3). 'Dusk of a Hermit' by Pestalozzi] (Jpn).

Varma VP, Williams P, ed: Piaget, psychology and education; papers in honour of Jean Piaget. Itasca, Illinois, Peacock, 1976. xiv, 233 p. Biographical chapters by E. A. Lunzer, p. xi–xiv, 3–14.

Wall WD: Jean Piaget – 1896–1979. **J Child Psychol Psychiatry** 1982 Apr;23(2):97–104

**United States**

Adler HE: Vicissitudes of Fechnerian psychophysics in America. In R. W. Rieber, K. Salzinger, ed: Psychology: theoretical–historical perspectives. New York, Academic Press, 1980. p. 11–23.

Adler KA: A personal autobiography. **J Individ Psychol** 1981 Nov;37(2):196–204

Allen M: Charlotte Bertha Bühler. In: Notable American women. The modern period. Cambridge, Mass., Belknap-Harvard Univ. Press, 1980. 4.119–21.

Alper TG: Psychology in New England: a retrospective look -- a woman's point of view. **J Hist Behav Sci** 1980 Jul;16(3):220–4

Anderson JW: In search of Mary James. **Psychohist Rev** 8(1–2):63–70, Summer-Fall 79

Anderson JW: 'The worst kind of melancholy': William James in 1869. **Harv Libr Bull** 1982 Oct;30(4):369–86

Asquith GH: Anton T. Boisen and the study of 'living human documents.' **J Presbyt Hist** 1982;60(3):244–65

Averill LA: Recollections of Clark's G. Stanley Hall. **J Hist Behav Sci** 1982 Oct;18(4):341-6
Axinn J: Jessie Taft. In: Notable American women. The modern period. Cambridge, Mass., Belknap-Harvard Univ. Press, 1980. 4:673-5.
Bakan D: Politics and American psychology. In R. W. Rieber, K. Salzinger, ed: Psychology: theoretical-historical perspectives. New York, Academic Press, 1980. p. 125-44.
Bell MJ: The relation of mentality to race: William Wells Newell and the Celtic hypothesis. **J Am Folkl** 1979;92(363):25-43
Benjamin LT, Jones MR: From motivational theory to social cognitive development: twenty-five years of the Nebraska Symposium. **Nebr Symp Motiv** 1978;26:ix-xix
Bernard J: Authority, autonomy, and radical commitment: Stephen and Abby Kelley Foster. **Proc Am Antiq Soc** 1980:90(2):347-86
Bixler RH: The Psychology Department at the University of Louisville, 1907-1953. **Filson Club Hist Q** 1983;57(3):253-69
Bjork DW: The compromised scientist: William James in the development of American psychology. New York, Columbia University Press, 1983. xiv, 221 p.
Blumenthal AL: Wilhelm Wundt and early American psychology: a clash of cultures. In R. W. Rieber, K. Salzinger, ed: Psychology: theoretical-historical perspectives. New York, Academic Press, 1980. p. 25-42.
Brown CL: Thomas Wolfe: a psychiatric view. **J Med Assoc State Ala** 1981 Oct;51(4):11-5
Brudnoy D: An untarnished youth in the gilded age: Theodore Schroeder of Wisconsin and Dakota territory. **ND Hist** 1972;39(4):17-25, 34
Buckley KW: Behaviorism and the professionalization of American psychology: a study of John Broadus Watson, 1878-1958. Ph.D. Diss., University of Massachusetts. Amherst, 1982. vii, 313 p.
Buckley KW: The selling of a psychologist: John Broadus Watson and the application of behavioral techniques to advertising. **J Hist Behav Sci** 1982 Jul;18(3):207-21
Burlingame VS: The family therapy tapestry: a multi-disciplinary history of the family therapy movement in the United States from 1900 to 1957. Ph.D. Diss., Northwestern University. Evanston, 1982. vii, 608 p.
Burnham JC: Augusta Fox Bronner. In: Notable American women. The modern period. Cambridge, Mass., Belknap-Harvard Univ. Press, 1980. 4:108-10.
Burnham JC: John Broadus Watson. In Dictionary of American Biography, Suppl. 6, 1956-1960. p. 670-3, 1980.
Cambrosio A: Quand la psychologie fait son entrée à l'usine: sélection et contrôle des ouvriers aux Etats-Unis pendant les années 1910. **Mouvement Soc** 1980;113:37-65
Carlson ET: The history of multiple personality in the United States: Mary Reynolds and her subsequent reputation. **Bull Hist Med** 1984 Spring;58(1):72-82
Carson SL: Presidential children: abandonment, hysteria and suicide. **J Psychohist** 1984 Spring;11(4):533-44
Cavallo D: Sexual politics and social reform: Jane Addams, from childhood to Hull House. In: Albin, Mel, ed. New Directions in Psychohistory: The Adelphi Papers in Honor of Erik H. Erikson. Lexingon, Mass., Health, 1980: 161-82.
Chapman PD: Schools as sorters: testing and tracking in California, 1910-1925. **J Soc Hist** 1981;14(4):701-17
Clarke JW: American assassins: an alternative typology. **Br J Polit Sci** 1981;11(1):81-104
Cohen D: J. B. Watson, the founder of behaviourism: a biography. London, Routledge and Kegan Paul, 1979. vi, 297 p.
Cole RA, Rudnicky AI: What's new in speech perception? The research and ideas of William Chandler Bagley, 1874-1946. **Psychol Rev** 1983 Jan;90(1):94-101
Cole TR: The prophecy of Senescence: G. Stanley Hall and the reconstruction of old age in America. **Gerontologist** 1984 Aug;24(4):360-6
Continenza B: L'effetto Baldwin. **Stor Crit Psicol** 1982 Dec;3(2):335-42
The Council at midcentury--: the reach for growth and status 1934-1950. **Except Child** 1981 Jan;47(4):286-96
Covert C: A view of the press in the twenties. **Journalism Hist** 1975;2(3):66-7, 92-6
Cowan RS: Lillian Evelyn Moller Gilbreth. In: Notable American women. The modern period. Cambridge, Mass., Belknap-Harvard Univ. Press, 1980. 4:271-3.
Cox MK: Victory through defeat: a character analysis of Robert E. Lee. **Psychoanal Rev** 1980 Winter;67(4):443-63
Cravens H: Robert Mearns Yerkes. In Dictionary of American Biography, Suppl. 6, 1956-1960. p. 717-19, 1980.
Cravens H: The triumph of evolution: American scientists and the heredity-environment controversy 1900-1941. [Philadelphia], University of Pennsylvania Press, 1978. xvi, 351 p.
Davison GC: Politics, ethics, and therapy for homosexuality. **Am Behav Sci** 1982;25(4):423-34
Dazzi N, Ferruzzi F: Wundt, Titchener e la psicologia americana. **Stor Crit Psicol** 1980;1(1):29-52
Delprato DJ: The reactional biography concept: early contribution to a perspective for the psychology of aging. **Hum Dev** 1980;23(5):314-22
DeMause L: Foundations of psychohistory. New York, Creative Roots, 1982. v, 336 p.
deMause L: The making of a fearful leader: 'Where's the rest of me?' **J Psychohist** 1984 Summer;12(1):5-21
Dennis PM: The Edison questionnaire. **J Hist Behav Sci** 1984 Jan;20(1):23-37
Diamond S: Francis Galton and American psychology. In R. W. Rieber, K. Salzinger, ed: Psychology: theoretical-historical perspectives. New York, Academic Press, 1980. p. 43-55.
Dietrich DJ: Psychohistory: Clio on the couch - or off? **Hist Methods** 1982;15(2):83-90
Distinguished contribution for applications in psychology award for 1978 (Alphonse Chapanis).: **Am Psychol** 1979 Jan;34(1):48-55
Distinguished contribution to psychology in the public interest.: **Am Psychol** 1979 Jan;34(1):65-8
Distinguished Professional Contribution Award for 1978: (Arthur L. Benton). **Am Psychol** 1979 Jan;34(1):56-64
Distinguished scientific contribution awards for 1978 (Julian Hochberg, Philip Teitelbaum, Robert B. Zajonc).: **Am Psychol** 1979 Jan;34(1):35-47
Dorsey JM: University Professor John M. Dorsey. Detroit, Wayne State University Press, 1980. 282 p.
Erdt T: Jonathan Edwards: art and the sense of heart. Amherst, University of Massachusetts Press, 1980. xiv, 123 p.
Esman AH: The study of lives: discussion of Tashjian and Shaw. **Adolesc Psychiatry** 1982;10:99-105
Evans RB, MacLeod RB: Foreword to Systematic psychology: Prolegomena by Edward Bradford Titchener. Ithaca, London, Cornell University Press, 1972. v-xvi.
Evans RI: B. F. Skinner, the man and his ideas: dialogue with B. F. Skinner. New York, Praeger, 1981. xiv, 140 p.
Evans RI: Dialogue with Carl Rogers. New York, Praeger, 1981. lxxxviii, 195 p.
Evans RI: Dialogue with Gordon Allport. New York, Praeger, 1981. xxv, 157 p.
Farrah MA: Andrew Carnegie: a psychohistorical sketch. D. A. Diss. Carnegie-Mellon University. Pittsburgh, 1982. ix. 183 p.
Fehrenbacher DE: In quest of the psychohistorical Lincoln. **Rev Am Hist** 1983;11(1):12-9
Feinstein HM: The 'crisis' of William James: a revisionist view. **Psychohist Rev** 1981;10(2):71-80
Feinstein HM: The use and abuse of illness in the James family circle: a view of neurasthenia as a social phenomenon. **Psychohist Rev** 1979;8(1-2):6-14
Fontaine O: Introduction aux thérapies comportementales (behavior therapies). Historique, bases théoriques, pratique. Bruxelles, Mardaga, 1978. 299 p. (Psychologie et sciences humaines).
Freud S, Bullitt WC: Thomas Woodrow Wilson, twenty-eighth President of the United States: a psychological study. Boston, Houghton Mifflin; and Cambridge, Riverside, 1967. 307 p.
Fuller RC: Mesmerism and the American cure of souls. Philadelphia, University of Pennsylvania Press, 1982. xvi, 227 p.
Gantt WH: E. Cowles Andrus (1896--1978), eighth president of the Pavlovian Society. **Pavlov J Biol Sci** 1979 Jan-Mar;14(1):74-5
Gantt WH: Review of the shaping of a behaviorism (B.F. Skinner). **Pavlov J Biol Sci** 1980 Jan-Mar;15(1):42-4
Garbelotto N: Teoria e politica nella psicosociologia di E. Mayo. **Stor Crit Psicol** 1980;1(1):61-78
Gatz M, Gease EI, Tyler FB, et al: Psychosocial competence characteristics of black and white women: the constraining effects of 'triple jeopardy'. **Black Scholar** 1982;13(1):5-12
Gavin WJ: Vagueness and empathy: a Jamesian view. **J Med Philos** 1981 Feb;6(1):45-65
Geldard FA: The Southern Society for Philosophy and Psychology at midstream. **J Hist Behav Sci** 1984 Jan;20(1):60-2
Gilgen AR: American psychology since World War II. A profile of the discipline. Westport, Connecticut, London, Greenwood Press, 1982. xiii, 272 p.
Girden E: Conditioning decorticate canines in Culler's laboratory: some reflexions and second thoughts. **Am J Psychol** 1983 Summer;96(2):243-52
Glenn ND, Weaver CN: Education's effects on psychological well-being. **Public Opin Q** 1981;45(1):22-39
Golbeck AL: Quantification in ethnology and its appearance in regional culture trait distribution studies (1888 to 1939). **J Hist Behav Sci** 1980 Jul;16(3):225-7
Gordon EW, Rubain TJ: Bias and alternatives in psychological testing. **J Negro Educ** 1980;49(3):350-60
Gordon MD: How socially distinctive is cognitive deviance in an emergent science? The case of parapsychology. **Soc Stud Sci** 1982 Feb;12(1):151-65
Hale M: Human science and social order: Hugo Münsterberg and the origins of applied psychology. Philadelphia, Temple University Press, 1980. xii, 239 p.
Hammett HB: The historical context of the origins of CPE. **J Pastoral Care** 1975 Jun;29(2):76-85
Haraway D: The biological enterprise: sex, mind, and profit from human engineering to sociobiology. **Radic Hist Rev** 1979 Spring/Summer;Spec:206-37
Henderson P: Psychohistorical perspectives on the presidency. **Mich J Polit Sci** 1981;1(1):1-11
Henle M: Robert M. Ogden and Gestalt psychology in America.

**J Hist Behav Sci** 1984 Jan;20(1):9-19
Henle M: The influence of Gestalt psychology in America. In R. W. Rieber, K. Salzinger, ed: Psychology: theoretical-historical perspectives. New York, Academic Press, 1980. p. 177-90.
Herrnstein RJ: Karl Spencer Lashley. In Dictionary of American Biography, Suppl. 6, 1956-1960. p. 367-8, 1980.
High RP, Woodward WR: William James and Gordon Allport: parallels in their maturing conceptions of self and personality. In R. W. Rieber, K. Salzinger, ed: Psychology: theoretical-historical perspectives. New York, Academic Press, 1980. p. 57-79.
Hilgard ER: Edward Chace Tolman. In Dictionary of American Biography, Suppl. 6, 1956-1960. p. 639-41, 1980.
Hilgard E, ed: American psychology in historical perspective: addresses of the presidents of the American Psychological Association, 1892-1977. Washington, D.C., The Association, 1978. viii, 558 p.
Hiltner S: Fifty years of CPE. **J Pastoral Care** 1975 Jun;29(2):90-8
Hirsch HN: Clio on the couch. **World Polit** 1980;32(3):406-24
Hoopes J: Jonathan Edwards's religious psychology. **J Am Hist** 1983;69(4):849-65
Hunt JM: Toward equalizing the developmental opportunities of infants and preschool children. **J Soc Issues** 1982;38(4):163-91
Hutch RA: Explorations in character: Gamaliel Bradford and Henry Murray as psychobiographers. **Biography** 1981;4(4):312-25
Hyman HH: Samuel Andrew Stouffer. In Dictionary of American Biography, Suppl. 6, 1956-1960. p. 604-6, 1980.
Irwin LN: Fulfillment and frustration: the confessions of a behavioral biochemist. **Perspect Biol Med** 1978 Spring;21(3):476-91
Jackson DJ: Contributions to the history of psychology: XXXV. Dorothy Burlingham. **Psychol Rep** 1984 Jun;54(3):855-63
Jacobs DW: Mark Schwartz and the Biofeedback Certification Institute of America: an appreciation. **Biofeedback Self Regul** 1983 Jun;8(2):279-80
James W: The principles of psychology. Edited and annotated by FH Burkhardt, F. Bowers and I. K. Skrupskelis. 3 vols. Cambridge, Mass. and London, Harvard University Press, 1981. lxviii, 1740 p. (The Works of William James) Introductory historical and biographical essays by G. E. Myers and R. B. Evans.
Johnson RA: On the psychology of the aging woman. Mary Baker Eddy as a religious leader. **J Geriatr Psychiatry** 1979;12(1):27-35
Joseph A: Intelligence, IQ, and race: When, how, and why they became associated. San Francisco, R & E Research Associates, 1977. vii, 142 p.
Karnani C: William James and I. A. Richards. **Indian J Am Stud** 1980;10(1):78-82
Kellen K: War on the mind: a commentary. **Armed Forces Soc** 1980;6(2):313-25
Kuo P: Lu-mu-ssu ti ch'e-ti ching-yen lun. **Bull Coll Lib Arts (Taiwan)** 1981;30:207-28
LaPenna L: La psychohistory: proposte e studi nella storiografia americana. **Quad Stor** 1981;16(2):574-605
Lawton H: The myth of altruism: a psychohistory of public agency social work. **J Psychohist** 1982 Winter;9(3):265-308
Lehrer PM: How to relax and how not to relax: a re-evaluation of the work of Edmund Jacobson--I. **Behav Res Ther** 1982;20(5):417-28
Linton SJ: The man and the mind: Carl Emil Seashore, a pioneer on two frontiers. **Swed Pioneer Hist Q** 1980;31(2):122-8
Loewenberg P: Psychohistory. In M. Kammen, ed: The Past before us: contemporary historical writing in the United States. Ithaca, Cornell University Press, 1980. p. 408-32.
Logan RD: Charles Lindbergh and the 'right stuff'. **Aviat Space Environ Med** 1982 Jul;53(7):708-11
Lyles MR, Carter JH: Myth and strengths of the black family: a historical and sociological contribution to family therapy. **J Natl Med Assoc** 1982 Nov;74(11):1119-23
Lyon TJ: John Muir's enlightenment. **Pac Hist** 1981;25(2):50-7
McHugh C: Phrenology: getting your head together in ante-bellum America. **Midwest Q** 1981;23(1):65-77
Mackenzie L: William James and the problem of interests. **J Hist Behav Sci** 1980 Apr;16(2):175-85
Mainwaring M: 'Phys/phren': why not to take each other at face value. **Smithsonian** 1980;11(8):193-212
Mauskopf SH, Seymour H, McVaugh MR: The elusive science: origins of experimental psychical research. Baltimore: Johns Hopkins University Press. 1980. xvi, 368 p.
Mills JG, Jones DR: The adaptability rating for military aeronautics: an historical perspective of a continuing problem. **Aviat Space Environ Med** 1984 Jun;55(6):558-62
Minot WS: Millay's 'Ungrafted tree'; the problem of the artist as woman. **New Engl Q** 1975;48(2):260-69
Morgan WG: Màrk Twain: behaviorist. **J Behav Ther Exp Psychiatry** 1984 Jun;15(2):99
Muuss RE: Peter Blos' modern psychoanalytic interpretation of adolescence. **J Adolesc** 1980 sep;3(3):229-52
Napoli DS: Architects of adjustment: the history of the psychological profession in the United States. Port Washington, N. Y., Kennikat Press, 1981. 176 p.
Ochsenhirt S: The Archives of the History of American Psychology. **Stor Crit Psicol** 1982 Dec;3(2):329-32
Orme JG, Stuart P: The Habit Clinics: behavioral social work and prevention in the 1920s. **Soc Serv Rev** 1981;55(2):242-56
Over R: The durability of scientific reputation. **J Hist Behav Sci** 1982 Jan;18(1):53-61
Palermo DS: The history of the Boyd R. McCandless Young Scientist Awards: the first recipients. **Adv Child Dev Behav** 1982;16:1-6
Parker GT: How to win friends and influence people: Dale Carnegie and the problem of sincerity. **Am Q** 1977;29(5):506-18
Pauly PJ: The Loeb-Jennings debate and the science of animal behavior. **J Hist Behav Sci** 1981 Oct;17(4):504-15
Pearlman M: Emotional factors in America's Western Pacific policy: Wood and Stimson in the Philippines. **J Psychohist** 1983 Fall;11(2):243-69
Poppleston JA, McPherson MW: The development of the archives of the history of American psychology. **Manuscripts** 1969;21(3):183-8
Post DL: Floyd H. Allport and the launching of modern social psychology. **J Hist Behav Sci** 1980 Oct;16(4):369-76
Pozovich GJ: Functional psychology and its influence upon the emergence of the mental measurement movement, 1870-1910. Ph.D. Diss. Southern Illinois University. Carbondale, 1978. vii, 221 leaves.
Pruyser PW: Religio medici: Karl A. Menninger, Calvinism and the Presbyterian Church. **J Presbyt Hist** 1981;59(1):59-72
Radbill SX: Arnold Lucius Gesell. In Dictionary of American biography, 1961-1965. Suppl. 7, 1981. p. 283-5.
Rambo LR: Ethics, evolution, and the psychology of William James. **J Hist Behav Sci** 1980 Jan;16(1):50-7
Raphelson AC: Psychology at Michigan: the Pillsbury years, 1897-1947. **J Hist Behav Sci** 1980 Oct;16(4):301-12
Recent acquisitions of the manuscript division: Carl R. Rogers papers. **Q J Libr Congr** 1978;35-258-9
Rhodes SL: Trends in child development research important to day-care policy. **Soc Serv Rev** 1979;53(2):285-94
Richards RJ: The personal equation in science: William James's psychological and moral uses of Darwinian theory. **Harv Libr Bull** 1982 Oct;30(4):387-425
Rieber RW: The Americanization of psychology before William James. In R. W. Rieber, K. Salzinger, ed: Psychology: theoretical-historical perspectives. New York, Academic Press, 1980. p. 103-23.
Rieber RW, Salzinger K, ed: The roots of American psychology: historical influences and implications for the future. (Conference on the roots of American psychology). New York, New York Academy of Sciences, 1977. 394 p.
Roazen P: Erik H. Erikson's America: the political implications of ego psychology. **J Hist Behav Sci** 1980 Oct;16(4):333-41
Robert I. Watson and the development of the history of psychology: a symposium: With contributions by E. S. Mills, E. R. Hilgard, B. Ross, J. Popplestone, M. W. McPherson, R. B. Evans, E. S. Goodman, J. Brožek. **J Hist Behav Sci** 1982 Oct;18(4):307-31
Romanell P: Medical history in the religious psychology of William James. In: Congrès international d'histoire de la médecine, XXVe, Québec, 1976. Actes. Québec, 1977. p. 1171-83.
Ross B: Edwin Ray Guthrie, Jr. In Dictionary of American Biography, Suppl. 6, 1956-1960. p. 261-3, 1980.
Ross B: In memoriam: Robert I. Watson, Sr. 1909-1980. **J Hist Behav Sci** 1981 Jan;17(1):1-2
Ross D: The development of the social sciences. In Oleson A, Voss J, ed: The organization of knowledge in modern America, 1860-1920. Baltimore and London, Johns Hopkins University Press, 1979. p. 107-38.
Ross D: Woodrow Wilson and the case for psychohistory. **J Am Hist** 1982;69(3):659-68
Rubin W: Pollock as Jungian illustrator: the limits of psychological criticism. **Art Am** 1979;67(7):104-23, (8):72-91
Ryan TA: Psychology at Cornell after Titchener: Madison Bentley to Robert Macleod, 1928-1948. **J Hist Behav Sci** 1982 Oct;18(4):347-69
Samelson F: A note on an unpublished article by John B. Watson. **J Hist Behav Sci** 1982 Jan;18(1):20-1
Sarason SB: Psychology misdirected. New York, Free Press, 1981. xiii, 193 p.
Schmidt CG: The group-fantasy origins of AIDS. **J Psychohist** 1984 Summer;12(1):37-78
Schwehn MR: Making the world: William James and the life of the mind. **Harv Libr Bull** 1982 Oct;30(4):426-54
Schwehn MR, ed: A William James renaissance: four essays by young scholars. **Harv Libr Bull** 1982 Oct;30(4):367-480
Sears RR: Lewis Madison Terman. In Dictionary of American Biography, Suppl. 6, 1956-1960. p. 626-7, 1980.
Siegel AW, White SH: The child study movement: early growth and development of the symbolized child. **Adv Child Dev Behav** 1982;17:233-85
Silberger J: On the psychology of the aging woman. Mourning and transformation: how Mary Baker Eddy found in middle age a way of making a new life for herself. **J Geriatr Psychiatry** 1979;12(1):9-25
Skinner BF: Notebooks. Edited with an introduction by R. Epstein. Englewood Cliffs, Prentice-Hall, 1980. xiii, 386 p.
Skinner BF: Pavlov's influence on psychology in America. **J Hist Behav Sci** 1981;17:242-5
Skinner BF: The experimental analysis of operant behavior: a history. In R. W. Rieber, K. Salzinger, ed: Psychology: theoretical-historical

perspectives. New York, Academic Press, 1980. p. 191–202.
Skinner BF: The shaping of a behaviorist. New York, Knopf, 1979. 373 p.
Smith HC: Arthur Sinton Otis. In Dictionary of American biography, 1961–1965. Suppl. 7, 1981. p. 594–5.
Smith HC: Douglas Henry Fryer. In Dictionary of American Biography, Suppl. 6, 1956–1960. p. 222, 1980.
Smith MB: Else Frenkel-Brunswik. In: Notable American women. The modern period. Cambridge, Mass., Belknap-Harvard Univ. Press, 1980. 4:250–2.
Sokal MM: The origins of the psychological corporation. **J Hist Behav Sci** 1981 Jan;17(1):54–67
Spring JH: Psychologists and the war: the meaning of intelligene in the alpha and beta tests. **Hist Educ Q** 1972;12(1):3–16
Stein HF: Sittin' tight and bustin' loose: contradiction and conflict in midwestern masculinity and the psychohistory of America. **J Psychohist** 1984 Spring;11(4):501–12
Stephens LD: Joseph LeConte and the development of the physiology and psychology of vision in the United States. **Ann Sci** 1980 May;37(3):303–21
Stern MB: Margaret Fuller and the phrenologist-publishers. **Stud Am Renaiss** 1980;229:37
Stern MB, comp: A phrenological dictionary of nineteenth-century Americans. Westport, Conn., Greenwood Press, 1982. xx, 430 p.
Strout C: Henry James's dream of the Louvre, 'The Jolly Corner,' and psychological interpretation. **Psychohist Rev** 1979 Summer–Fall;8(1–2):47–52
Stryker S: Social psychology: trends, assessment, and prognosis. **Am Behav Sci** 1981;24(3):386–406
Sullivan OR: Who's testing black children and youth in the public schools? **Freedomways** 1981;21(2):114–8
Susskind JL: Kathryn McHale. In Dictionary of American Biography, Suppl. 6, 1956–1960. p. 412–13, 1980.
Taylor CM: W. E. B. Dubois's challenge to scientific racism. **J Black Stud** 1981;11(4):449–60
Taylor E: William James on psychopathology: the 1896 Lowell lectures on 'Exceptional mental states'. **Harv Libr Bull** 1982 Oct;30(4):455–79
Teahan JF: Warren Felt Evans and mental healing: romantic idealism and practical mysticism in nineteenth-century America. **Church Hist** 1979 Mar;48(1):63–80
Tipton DA, Mohler SR: The Wright brothers: a personality profile. **Aviat Space Environ Med** 1983 Jun;54(6):560–2
Tobach E: A brief history of the Psychology Section of The New York Academy of Sciences. In K. Salzinger, ed: Psychology in progress: an interim report. (Annals of the New York Academy of Sciences, vol. 270). New York, New York Academy of Sciences, 1976. p. 6–13.
Tobach E, Proshansky HM, ed: Genetic destiny: race as a scientific and social controversy. New York, AMS Press, 1976. 163 p. Contributions by A. Edel, R. Cancro, D. Layzer, H. Padfield, A. Chase, E. Drucker, V. W. Sidel, G. Piel, J. C. King, E. A. Mauss.
Tong BR: The ghetto of the mind: notes on the historical psychology of Chinese America. **Amerasia J** 1971;1(3):1–31
Tyor PL: Henry Herbert Goddard. In Dictionary of American Biography, Suppl. 6, 1956–1960. p. 240–1, 1980.
Underwood BJ: Studies in learning and memory: selected papers. New York, Praeger, 1982. x, 331 p.
Van Buren J: Louisa May Alcott: a study in persona and idealization. **Psychohist Rev** 1981;9(4):282–99
van Ijzendoorn MH, Goossens FA, van der Veer R: Klaus F. Riegel and dialectical psychology: in search for the changing individual in a changing society. **Stor Crit Psicol** 1984 Jun;5(1):5–28
Voyat G: In tribute to Piaget: a look at his scientific impact in the United States. In R. W. Rieber, K. Salzinger, ed: Psychology: theoretical-historical perspectives. New York, Academic Press, 1980. p. 305–14.
Ward JF: Arthur F. Bentley and the foundations of behavioral science. **J Hist Behav Sci** 1981;17:222–31
Weiland S: Historians and psychologists, pluralism and professionalism: a review essay. **Public Hist** 1981;3(2):75–88
Weinstein EA: Woodrow Wilson: a medical and psychological biography. Princeton, Princeton University Press, 1981. xi, 399 p.
Weinstein F: On the social function of intellectuals: a consideration of Erik H. Erikson's contribution to psychoanalysis and psychohistory. In M. Albin, R. J. Devlin, G. Heeger, ed: New directions in psychohistory. The Adelphi papers in honor of Erik H. Erikson. Lexington, Toronto, D. C. Heath, 1980. p. 3–19.
Williams DE: Wendell Andrew Leroy Johnson. In Dictionary of American biography, 1961–1965. Suppl. 7, 1981. p. 395–6.
Williams DR: Horses, pigeons, and the therapy of conversion: a psychological reading of Jonathan Edwards's theology. **Harv Theol Rev** 1981;74(4):337–52
Windholz G: Pavlov's position toward American behaviorism. **J Hist Behav Sci** 1983 Oct;19(4):394–407
Wolf TH: Florence Laura Goodenough. In: Notable American women. The modern period. Cambridge, Mass., Belknap-Harvard Univ. Press, 1980. 4:284–6.
Zabarskas J: Psychometric intelligence pattern of the native-born children of Lithuanian immigrants. **Lituanus** 1980;26(1):39–54
Zwelling S: Spiritualist perspectives on antebellum experience. **J Psychohist** 1982 Summer;10(1):3–25

### USSR

Arkhangel'skiĭ GV: V. M. Bekhterev--vydaiushchiĭsia deiatel' otechestvennoĭ nauki (k 125–letiiu so dnia rozhdeniia). **Klin Med (Mosk)** 1983 Feb;61(2):106–10
Barkóczi I: On outstanding achievements of Soviet general psychology. **Ann Univ Sci Budap Rolando Eotvos Nominatae** 1979;6:61–9
Chertok L: La riabilitazione dell'inconscio in Unione Sovietica: il Convegno internazionale di Tbilisi. **Stor Crit Psicol** 1982 Jun;3(1):41–62
Goscilo H: Lermontov's debt to Lavater and Gall. **Slav East Eur Rev** 1981;59(4):500–15
Gray JA: Ivan Pavlov. New York, Viking Press, 1979. vii, 153 p.
Gubko AT: Le rôle de l'Académie de Kiev dans la naissance de la science psychologique en Ukraine. (Rus) **Vopr Psikhol** 1980;(1):82–93
Iaroshevski MG, Gurgenidze GS: L. S. Vygotski o prirode psikhiki. **Vopr Filos** 1981;(1):142–54
Kol'tsova MM: Mekhanizmy integratsii uslovnykh refleksov v trudakh E. A. Asratiana. **Zh Vyssh Nerv Deiat** 1983 Mar–Apr;33(2):216–20
Kozulin A: Peter Blonsky and Russian progressivism: the early years. **Stud Sov Thought** 1982;24(1):11–21
Kozulin A: The influence of the personality of the scientist on his theorizing: I. P. Pavlov and the concept of human signal systems. **Stud Sov Thought** 1981;22(4):249–56
Luria AR: The making of mind. A personal account of Soviet psychology. Edited by M. Cole and S. Cole. Cambridge, London, Harvard University Press, 1979. 234 p.
McGuigan FJ, Szegal B: Covert behavior and mental processes in Russian psychology. **Pavlov J Biol Sci** 1980 Jan–Mar;15(1):35–41
Mecacci L: Brain and history. The relationship between neurophysiology and psychology in Soviet research. New York, Brunner/Mazel. 1977. xxiv, 198 p. (Translation of Cervello e storia).
Mecacci L: Il manifesto della scuola storico-culturale. **Stor Crit Psicol** 1980;1(2):263–95
Mecacci L: Koffka e la psicologia sovietica. **Stor Crit Psicol** 1980;1(1):95–109
Misiti R: Ladygina-Kots and Soviet comparative psychology. **Stor Crit Psicol** 1982 Jun;3(1):109–12
Moiseeva NI: The role of I M. Sechenov's ideas in development of modern views on time perception. **Hum Physiol** 1979 Nov–Dec;5(5):723–7
Natadse R: Die Rolle der Universität Tbilisi bei der entwicklung der Psychologie in Georgien. **Wiss Z Friedrich Schiller Univ (Gesellsch)** 1973;22(3):497–509
Platonov KK: K istorii otechestvennoĭ aviatsionnoĭ psikhologii: dokumenty i materialy. Moskva, Meditsina, 1981. 316 p.
Pomper P: Nečaev, Lenin and Stalin: the psychology of leadership. **Jahrb Gesch Osteur** 1978;26(1):11–30
Pressman IaM: E. A. Asratian i nauchnoe sodruzhestvo neĭrofiziologiov sotsialisticheskikh stran. **Zh Vyssh Nerv Deiat** 1983 Mar–Apr;33(2):211–5
Salamon J: The basic concept of psychical development in Soviet psychology and several of its variants. **Ann Univ Sci Budap Rolando Eotvos Nominatae** 1979;6:89–101
Shingarov GKh: Filosofskie voprosy ucheniia o vyssheĭ nervnoĭ deiatel'nosti v tvorchestve E. A. Asratiana. **Zh Vyssh Nerv Deiat** 1983 Mar–Apr;33(2):204–10
Simonov PV: Podkrepliaiushchaia funktsiia émotsiĭ (k 80–letiiu so dnia rozhdeniia Ezrasa Asratovicha Asratiana). **Fiziol Zh SSSR** 1983 May;69(5):577–86
Simonov PV: Polveka neotstupnykh iskaniĭ istiny (k 80–letiiu so dnia rozhdeniia E. A. Asratiana). **Zh Vyssh Nerv Deiat** 1983 Mar–Apr;33(2):197–203
Todes DP: Biological psychology and the Tsarist censor: the dilemma of scientific development. **Bull Hist Med** 1984 Winter;58(4):529–44
Todes DP: From radicalism to scientific convention: biological psychology in Russia from Sechenov to Pavlov. Ph.D. Diss., University of Pennsylvania. Philadelphia, 1981. v, 557 leaves.
Vacola G, Gayda M, Pélicier Y: Philocalie d'une prière orthodoxe, aspects psycho-physiologiques. **Ann Med Psychol (Paris)** 1984 Mar;142(3):416–22
Vdovin AI, Drobizhev VZ: Sotsial'naia psikhologiia i nekotorye voprosy istorii sovetskogo obshchesta. **Istor SSSR** 1971;5:23–43
Wertsch JV: Trends in Soviet cognitive psychology. **Stor Crit Psicol** 1981;2(2):219–95
Wortman R: Power and responsibility in the upbringing of the nineteenth-century tsars. **Group Psychol Hist Newsl** 1976;4(4):18–27

## PSYCHOSOMATIC MEDICINE

Ackerknecht EH: The history of psychosomatic medicine. **Psychol Med** 1982 Feb;12(1):17–24
Etziony M: History of psychosomatic medicine: semantic and philosophic bird's eye view. **Koroth** 1979 Nov;7(9–10):CCIX–CCX(658–66)
Ikemi Y, Ikemi A: Psychosomatic medicine: a meeting ground of Eastern and Western medicine. **J Am Soc Psychosom Dent Med** 1983;30(1):3–16
Lipowski ZJ: What does the word 'psychosomatic' really mean? A

historical and semantic inquiry. **Psychosom Med** 1984 Mar–Apr;46(2):153–71
Perret L: Kropp, själ och ande i historisk belysning. **Nord Medicinhist Arsb** 1980;:53–8
Zigmond D: A psychosomatic approach. **Practitioner** 1982 Apr;226(1366):699, 701–2, 704 passim

**Before 500 A.D.**

**Greece**

Siefert H: Inkubation, Imagination und Kommunikation im antiken Asklepioskult. In Leuner H, ed: Katathymes Bilderleben. Ergebnisse in Theorie und Praxis. Bern, Stuttgart, Wien, Huber, 1980. p. 324–45.

**500 A.D.–1450**

**Arabic**

Hajal F: Psychological treatment of anorexia: a case from the ninth century. **J Hist Med Allied Sci** 1982 Jul;37(3):325–8
Mora G: Mind-body concepts in the Middle Ages: part II. The Moslem influence, the great theological systems, and cultural attitudes toward the mentally ill in the late Middle Ages. **J Hist Behav Sci** 1980 Jan;16(1):58–72
Moussaoui D, Touhami M, Msefer W: Psychiatrie et psychosomatique dans la médecine arabe. **Ann Med Psychol (Paris)** 1980;138(8):967–74
Schultheisz E: Avicenna és a psychosomatika gyökerei. **Orv Hetil** 1980 Dec 28;121(52):3171–3

**1450–1700**

**Great Britain**

Oldroyd DR: Some 'philosophical scribbles' attributed to Robert Hooke. **Notes Rec R Soc Lond** 1980 Jul;35(1):17–32

**1700 to Present**

Ader R, Schmale AH: George Libman Engel: on the occasion of his retirement. **Psychosom Med** 1980;42(1 Suppl):79–101
Caire JB: A holographic model of a psychosomatic pattern: Freud's specimen dream re-interpreted. **Psychother Psychosom** 1981;36(2):132–42
Gay P: Victorian sexuality: old texts and new insights. **Am Scholar** 1980;49(3):372–8
McMahon CE, Oberg D: Functional illness and the status of psychosomatic concepts in nineteenth century medicine. **J Am Soc Psychosom Dent Med** 1983;30(4):156–61
McMahon CE, Hastrup JL: The role of imagination in the disease process: post-Cartesian history. **J Behav Med** 1980 Jun;3(2):205–17
Mazet P: Points de vue théoriques en psychosomatique. Historique et actualité. **Sem Hop Paris** 1984 Mar 22;60(13):887–93
Mellgren A: Grossesse nerveuse--en psykosomatisk sjukdom. **Nord Medicinhist Arsb** 1982;:101–9
Siefert H: Sigmund Freud, Georg Groddeck und die psychosomatische Medizin. **Prax Psychother Psychosom** 1979;24:63–78

**Canada**

Minde K: The scientific analyst -- a student's perspective. **Can J Psychiatry** 1979 Aug;24(5):498

**France**

Gastaut H, Gastaut Y, Broughton R: Gustave Flaubert's illness: a case report in evidence against the erroneous notion of psychogenic epilepsy. **Epilepsia** 1984 Oct;25(5):622–37

**Germany**

Arndal S: Krop, sjael og ånd Georg Ernst Stahls og Christian Friedrich Richters medicinske antropologi. **Dan Medicinhist Arbog** 1980;:126–66
Brede K, Irion U, Lohmann HM, et al: Mitscherlich, Alexander, 1908–19821700 to PresentGermany **Psyche (Stuttg)** 1984 Nov;38(11):1023–52
Schröder C, König W: Die Integration der Psychotherapie in die klinische Medizin in Deutschland--der Beitrag von J. H. Schultz. **Psychiatr Neurol Med Psychol (Leipz)** 1984 Oct;36(10):586–90
Thomä H: Von der Psychosomatischen Medizin zur Psychoanalyse--Heidelberg 1949–1967. **Psyche (Stuttg)** 1983 Apr;37(4):322–35
Zander W: Grussworte zum 25 jährigen Jubiläum der Zeitschrift für Psychosomatische Medizin und Psychoanalyse. **Z Psychosom Med Psychoanal** 1979 Oct–Dec;25(4):301–2

**United States**

Ackerman SH: Herbert Weiner 'at home'. **Psychosom Med** 1982 Mar;44(1):5–17
Katz JL: Three studies in psychosomatic medicine revisited: a tribute to the psychobiological perspective of Herbert Weiner. **Psychosom Med** 1982 Mar;44(1):29–42
Powell RC: (Helen) Flanders Dunbar. In Dictionary of American Biography, Suppl. 6, 1956–1960. p. 180–1, 1980.
Stokes GA: Helen Flanders Dunbar. In: Notable American women. The modern period. Cambridge, Mass., Belknap-Harvard Univ. Press, 1980. 4:210–2.

**USSR**

Mendelson G, Mendelson D: Psychological aspects of bronchial asthma in the writings of Isaac Babel. **Isr J Psychiatr Relat Sci** 1981;18(1):31–9

# PUBLIC HEALTH

See also **Child Health; Communicable Disease Control; Economics, Medical; Epidemiology; Foods and Food Supply; Health Education; Hygiene; Immunology; Maternal Health; Mental Health; Occupational Medicine; Preventive Medicine; Rural Health; Sanitation; Social Medicine; State Medicine; Statistics and Demography**

Caffaratto A: Storia della legislazione sanitaria ed igienica in Piemonte da Amedeo VIII all'Unità d'Italia. Parte II, III. **Minerva Med** 1979;70(51,54):3511–23, 3729–34 (continued)
Dake WJ: Het medische werk van de zending in Nederlands-Indië. Kampen, Kok, 1972. 235 p.
Ellencweig AY, Yoshpe RB: Definition of public health. **Public Health Rev** 1984;12(1):65–78
Espinosa y León VM: Reseña histórica de los roedores domésticos. **Salud Publica Mex** 1984 Jan–Feb;26(1):77–81
Fruchtbaum H: [History of] public health. In Reich WT, et al, ed: Encyclopedia of bioethics, v.3. New York, Free Press, 1978. p. 1392–99.
Jordanova LJ: Medical police and public health: problems of practice and ideology. **Soc Soc Hist Med Bull (Lond)** 1980;27:15–19
Mani N: Zur Geschichte der Hygiene. Kontinuität und Wandel hygienischer Vorstellungen von der Antike zum 19. Jahrhundert. **ZFA (Stuttgart)** 1981 Nov 20;57(32):2183–92
Means RK: Historical perspectives on school health. Thorofare, New Jersey, Slack, 1975. 253 p.
Radovi sa Medunarodnog simpozija u povodu sestote obljetnice Dubrovacke karantene: Dubrovnik, 29. i 30. rujna 1977. Zagreb, Jugoslavenska Akademija Znanosti i Umjetnosti, 1980. 173 p.
Russell AW, ed: The town and state physician in Europe from the Middle Ages to the Enlightenment. Wolfenbüttel, Herzog August Bibliothek, 1981. 156 p. (Wolfenbütteler Forschungen, 17).
Sournia JC: Die Sozialmedizin. In Sournia JC, Martiny M, Poulet J, ed: Illustrierte Geschichte der Medizin. Salzburg, Andreas, 1980. Vol. 6. p. 2149–93.
Steele JH: International and world developments in veterinary public health with a comment on historical developments. **Int J Zoonoses** 1979 Jun;6(1):1–32
Tracy GD: Evolution of responsibilities in the care of health. **Med J Aust** 1980 Nov 29;2(11):591–6
Weinstein MS: Health in the city. Environmental and behavioral influences. New York, Pergamon, 1980. xvii, 92 p.

**Africa**

Feierman S, ed: Health and society in Africa: a working bibliography. Waltham, Mass., Crossroads Press, 1979. xii, 210 p.

**Belgium**

Vandenbroeke C: De medische konsumptie sinds de 16e eeuw. **Handel Maatsch Geschied Oudheidk Gent** 1980;34:143–65

**Bolivia**

Flores D: Historia de la sanidad publica de Bolivia, durante los primeros años de la republica. **Illimani** 1974;(5):22–38

**Canada**

Canada's amazing health history: let's murder the medical officer: **Can J Public Health** 1984 Sep–Oct;75(5):344–7
Desrosiers G: Histoire de la santé publique au Québec. **Can J Public Health** 1984 Sep–Oct;75(5):359–63

**China**

Werner R: Offentliches Gesundheitswesen, traditionelle chinesische Medizin, westliche Medizin, Barfussärzte und Heilmittelkunde in der

Volksrepublik China. 1. Teil. **Off Gesundheitswes** 1981 Oct;43(10):480–99

**Colombia**

Chandler DL: Health and slavery in colonial Colombia. New York, Arno Press, 1981. iv, 307 p. (Ph.D. Diss., Tulane 1972).

**Denmark**

Brix J: Laegevirke i Sønderjylland før 1864. **Dan Medicinhist Arbog** 1980;:9–10
Fysikatsdistrikter i det sønderjyske område indtil 1864: **Dan Medicinhist Arbog** 1980;:66–78

**Finland**

Strandberg H: Sanitary regulations in calendars in public use to indicate the attitude to the preventive health care in Finland in the 17th and 18th centuries. In International Congress of the History of Medicine, 27th, Barcelona, 1980. Actas. Barcelona, Académia de Ciències Médiques de Catalunya i Balears, 1981. p. 621–5.

**France**

Hildesheimer F, Robin G, Schenk J, ed: Intendance sanitaire de Marseille. (Répertoire numérique de la sous série 200 E – Archives de la Région Provence-Alpes-Cote d'Azur et du Département des Bouches-du-Rhone). Marseille, Archives Departementales, 1979. 71 p.
Hildesheimer F: Le Bureau de la Santé de Marseille sous l'Ancien Régime. Le renfermement de la contagion. Marseille, Fédération historique de Provence, 1980. 256 p.
Leuilliot P: O współczesną historię medyczno-społeczną. **Kwart Hist Kultury Mater** 1975;23(2):255–67
Marzocchi J: Essais sur la médecine et la pharmacie à travers l'histoire de la Corse. [S.1], J. P. Marzocchi, [1978?].
Muchembled R: Le corps, la culture populaire et la culture des élites en France (XVe–XVIIIe siècle). In Imhof AE, ed: Leib und Leben in der Geschichte der Neuzeit. Berlin, Duncker & Humblot, 1983. p. 141–53.

**Germany**

Kaiser W, Völker A: Universität und Physikat in der Frühgeschichte des Amtsarztwesens. Halle, Martin-Luther-Universität, 1980. 95 p. (Beiträge zur Universitätsgeschichte: Wissenschaftliche Beiträge der Martin-Luther-Universität Halle-Wittenberg, 1980/53, T 39).
Labisch A: Entwicklungslinien des öffentlichen Gesundheitsdienstes in Deutschland. Vorüberlegungen zur historischen Soziologie öffentlicher Gesundheitsvorsorge. **Off Gesundheitswes** 1982 Nov;44(11):745–61
Schipperges H: Vom Physikus zum Arzt für Gesundheit. Verwurzelung, Entwicklung und Chancen des öffentlichen Gesundheitsdienstes. **Off Gesundheitswes** 1983 Jun;45(6):290–8
Stürzbecher M: Quellen zur Geschichte der Medizin und des Gesundheitswesens in und über Berlin. **Baer Berl** 1977;26:113–8

**India**

Tindall G: Bombay: City of gold. **Hist Today** 1982 May;32:15–21

**Italy**

Caffaratto A: Storia della legislazione sanitaria ed igienica in Piemonte da Amedeo VIII all'Unità d'Italia. Parte I. **Minerva Med** 1979 Nov 3;70(48):3315–21 (contd)
Giusberti F: Tra povertà e malattia: il Sant'Orsola a Bologna dal XVII al XVIII secolo. **Ann Fond Luigi Einaudi** 1979;13:117–50
Menini C: Rapporto tra storia della medicina e medicina pratica: un contributo paradigmatico in tema di talassemia e favismo nella popolazione ferrarese. **Acta Med Hist Patav** 1978–79;25:40–54
Rosa E: Medicina e salute pubblica a Bologna nel sei e settecento. **Quad Cult Bolognese** 1978 Dec;(2 no 8): 3–60

**Luxembourg**

Goergen A: L'art de guérir et la santé publique dans le grand-duché de Luxembourg. Luxembourg, Cour Victor Buck, 1916. [5], 383 p.

**Spain**

Pérez Moreda V: Las crisis de mortalidad en la España interior (siglos XVI–XIX). Madrid, Siglo XXI de España Editores, 1980. 526 p.
Saiz Moreno L: Antiguas vías de circulación del ganado. La trashumancia del ganado merino en España y las epizootias. **Rev Sanid Hig Publica (Madr)** 1983 Nov–Dec;57(11–12):1229–53

**United States**

Cassedy JH: Church record-keeping and public health in early New England. In: Medicine in Colonial Massachusetts 1620–1820. (Publications of the Colonial Society of Massachusetts, vol. 57), 1980. p. 249–62.
Leavitt JW: Writing public health history: the need for a social scaffolding. **Rev Am Hist** 1976;4(2):150–7

**Before 500 A.D.**

**Greco-Roman**

Callmer C: Ur arkiater-titelns historia. **Sydsven Medicinhist Sallsk Arsskr** 1980;:40–80

**Greece**

Roesch P: Médecins publics dans les cités grecques. **Hist Sci Med** 1984;18(3):279–93

**India**

Sugita K: Public health of ancient India. In Ogawa T, ed: Public health. Tokyo, Saikon, 1981. p. 75–81.

**Japan**

Onishi W: [Life among the frontier farmers of Hokkaido: public health nursing in the history of the Showa period. 10.] (Jpn). **Kango** 1982 Feb;34(2):65–71; 97–103

**Rome**

Scarborough J: Roman medicine and public health. In Ogawa T, ed: Public health. Tokyo, Saikon, 1981. p. 33–74.

**500 A.D.–1450**

**Arabic**

Hamarneh SK: Majusi's observations and instructions on medicine and public health. **Hamdard** 1980 Jan–Mar;23(1):3–35
Petrov BD: Voprosy okhrany zdorov'ia v 'Kanone' Ibn-Siny (k 1000-letiiu so dnia rozhdeniia). **Gig Sanit** 1980 May;(5):22–5

**Bulgaria**

Stamova N, Kurtev V: Khigiennite znaniia i navitsi u bulgarite ot vremeto na pokrustvaneto im. **Probl Khig** 1983;8:155–60

**Ireland**

Moylan TK: Poverty, pigs and pestilence in medieval Dublin. **Dublin Hist Rec** 1978;31(4)

**Italy**

Powell JM: Greco-Arabic influences on the public health legislation in the constitutions of Melfi. **Arch Stor Pugliese** 1978;31:77–96

**Poland**

Tyszkiewicz J, Widy-Tyszkiewicz E: Czynniki kształtujace zdrowie Polsce XIII–XV w. **Kwart Hist Kultury Mater** 1976;24(2):205–15
Tyszkiewicz J, Widy-Tyszkiewicz E: Zdrowie i choroby w Polsce XIII–XV w. **Kwart Hist Kultury Mater** 1976;24(1):55–73

**1450–1700**

Hiller I: Betrachtungen zu medizinischen Aspekten des Umweltschutzes im 17. Jahrhundert. **Z Gesamte Hyg** 1983 Sep;29(9):560–3

**Americas**

Ferrer D: La sanidad en las 'Leyes de los reinos de las indias'. In International Congress of the History of Medicine, 27th, Barcelona, 1980. Actas. Barcelona, Académia de Ciències Médiques de Catalunya i Balears, 1981. p. 172–6.

**Germany**

Böhmer W, Kirsten F: Reformatorische Ausstrahlungen Martin Luthers auf das Gesundheitswesen seiner Zeit. **Z Gesamte Inn Med** 1983 Oct 15;38(20):546–51
Mäder M: Ludwig von Hoernigk: Arzt, Jurist und Bücherkommissar im 17. Jahrhundert. Diss. Bern, 1984. 77 p.

# PUBLIC HEALTH

**Italy**

Cipolla CM: Cristofano e la peste. Bologna, Il Mulino, 1976. 157 p.

**Mexico**

Harvey HR: Public health in Aztec society. **Bull NY Acad Med** 1981 Mar;57(2):157–65

**Spain**

Valverde JL, Sánchez F, Vinuesa L: Controversias jurisdiccionales del Protomedicato castellano. **Asclepio** 1978–79;30–31:403–23
Viana S: El diario de una parroquia: Legrán. **Bol Inst Sancho Sabio** 1971;15:269–76

**USSR**

Alekseev GA: Zarozhdenie organizatsii okhrany zdorov'ia v Srednem Povolzh'e (XVII vek). **Sov Zdravookhr** 1984;(9):49–52

**Yugoslavia**

Rudelić I: Glagolijski grafiti kao svjedočanstva socijalnih i zdravstvenih prilka u Istri. **Lijec Vjesn** 1984 Jun;106(6):261–4

**1700 to Present**

Adams P: Health of the state. New York, N.Y., Praeger, 1982. x, 198 p.
Aleksandrovskiĭ BN, Shchetova GA: K istorii russko-nemetskikh nauchnykh sviazeĭ v oblasti épidemiologii i gigieny. **Sov Zdravookhr** 1982;(1):61–5
Allan P, Jolley M, ed: Nursing, midwifery and health visiting since 1900. London, Faber and Faber, 1982. 316 p. With contributions by R. H. Pyne, B. Watkin, V. H. Darling, M. E. Lee, C. R. Kratz, G. M. Owen, R. Everest, P. D. Birchenall, D. M. Saunders, B. M. Slaney, D. Blenkinsop, M. D. Green, C. M. Chapman, E. A. Bent, J. C. Hayward, S. R. Lelean, A. V. Cowie, S. Quinn, I. S. Palmer, D. H. Rye.
Boden RT: Public health and physical planning--a time to reconsider? **S Afr Med J** 1981 Oct 10;60(15):582–8
Brandt AM: James Angus Doull. In Dictionary of American biography, 1961-1965. Suppl. 7, 1981. p. 194–5.
Brügelmann J: Medikalisierung von Säuglings- und Erwachsenenalter in Deutschland zu Beginn des 19. Jahrhunderts aufgrund von medizinischen Topographien. In Imhof AE, ed.: Leib und Leben in der Geschichte der Neuzeit. Berlin, Duncker & Humblot, 1983. p. 177–92.
Coppock JB: Food technology [in the twentieth century]. In Williams TI, ed: A history of technology. Vol. VII. The twentieth century, ca. 1900 to ca. 1950. Part II. Oxford, Clarendon, 1978. p. 1399–445.
Eberson F: Apostles and prophets. Medicine for society's ills. Hicksville, Exposition Press, 1977. xi, 106 p.
Frankl J: Somogy megyei adatok az abszolutizmus orvostörténelméhez. **Orv Hetil** 1982 Aug 22;123(34):2117–20
Greene VW: Cleanliness and the health revolution. New York, Soap and Detergent Association, 1984. vii, 68 p.
Hackett CJ: McLetchie on mass campaigns. **Trop Doct** 1982 Jan;12(1):35–8
Hannaway C: From private hygiene to public health: a transformation in Western medicine in the eighteenth and nineteenth centuries. In Ogawa T, ed: Public health. Tokyo, Saikon, 1981. p. 108–28.
Hiestand WC: Nursing, the family, and the 'new' social history. **ANS** 1982 Apr;4(3):1–12
Hunstadbråten K: Fluor i kariesprofylaksen omkring århundriskiftet. **Nor Tannlaegeforen Tid** 1981 May;91(7):227–31
Imhof AE, ed: Leib und Leben in der Geschichte der Neuzeit: Vorträge eines internationalen Colloquiums. Berlin, Duncker & Humblot, 1983. 266 p. Text in German and French. (Berliner Historische Studien, Bd. 9. Einzelstudien 2).
Kaiser W, Werner K, Rothe J: Sozialmedizinische Konsequenzen aus dem Wirken von Robert Koch unter halleschem Aspekt. **Z Gesamte Hyg** 1982 Mar;28(3):179–84
Lee SS: Health policy, A social contract: a comparison of the United States and Canada. **J Public Health Policy** 1982 Sep;3(3):293–301
Lilienfeld AM: Epidemiology and health policy: some historical highlights. **Public Health Rep** 1984 May–Jun;99(3):237–41
O'Brien ME: Pragmatic survivalism: behavior patterns affecting low-level wellness among minority group members. **ANS** 1982 Apr;4(3):13–26
Parnas J: Thorvald Madsen 1870–1957. Leader in international public health. **Dan Med Bull** 1981;28(2):82–6
Recht P: La mesure de la santé. **Arch Belg** 1984;42(7–8):418–34
Rothe J, Werner K, Kaiser W: Sozialhygienische Konsequenzen aus der Klärung der Tuberkulose-Ätiologie durch Robert Koch. **Z Gesamte Hyg** 1982 Mar;28(3):176–9
Sheiman I: Kapitalizm i problemy zdravo-okhraneniia. **Mirovaia Ekon Mezhdunar Otnosheniia** 1979;12:116–23
Shishkin AP: Gosudarstvennyĭ institut sotsial'noĭ gigieny Narkomzdrava RSFSR i ego rol' v razvitii teorii i organizatsii sovetskogo. **Sov Zdravookhr** 1982;(6):59–62
Spaar H: Die Begründung der Vorzüge des Gesundheitsschutzes im Sozialismus und seiner gesetzmässigen Schranken im Kapitalismus im Lichte der Lehre von Karl Marx. **Z Gesamte Hyg** 1983 Oct;29(10):573–6
Tesh S: Political ideology and public health in the nineteenth century. **Int J Health Serv** 1982;12(2):321–42
Wagner D: Einige Aspekte von den Anfängen der experimentellen Desinfektionslehre. **Z Gesamte Hyg** 1982 Mar;28(3):172–6
Waitzkin H: The social origins of illness: a neglected history. **Int J Health Serv** 1981;11(1):77–103
Webster C: Healthy or hungry thirties? **Soc Soc Hist Med Bull** 1980;27:22–4
Wilkinson A: Disease in the 19th century urban economy: the medical officer of health and the community. **Soc Soc Hist Med Bull (Lond)** 1980;27:24–6

**Afghanistan**

Ionov IuV, Ionov AIu: Vrach I. L. Iavorskiĭ - issledovatel' Afganistana. **Sov Zdravookhr** 1983;(12):49–51

**Africa**

Gale TS: Segregation in British West Africa. **Cah Etud Afr** 1980;20(4):495–507

**Americas**

Acuña HR: El Boletín de la Oficina sanitaria panamericana: a los sessenta años. **Bol Of Sanit Panam** 1982 May;92(5):377–8
Boletín panamericano de sanidad de la Oficina sanitaria internacional: **Bol Of Sanit Panam** 1982 May;92(5):429–48
Garcia JC: The laziness disease. **Hist Philos Life Sci** 1981;3(1):31–59
González AD: La mision de Carlos M. Ramirez al Brasil y el convenio sanitario de 1887. **Bol Acad Nac Hist (Argentina)** 1964;35:327–53
Vaccarezza RF: Devoción a la causa de la salud: Fred Lower Soper. **Medicina (B Aires)** 1981;41(1):101–6
Zschock DK: Health care financing in Central America and the Andean Region: a workshop report. **Lat Am Res Rev** 1980;15(3):149–68

**Argentina**

Burguéz NA: Los pioneros de la medicina en San Juan de la frontera la institucionalizacion de la medicina en la accíon de los pioneros Sanjuaninos del siglo XIX. In Congreso de Historia de la Medicina Argentina [Transactions], 5th, Mendoza, 1983. p. 183–96.
Martín de Codoni E: La politica sanitaria en el primer medio siglo. Mendoza 1810–1860. **Rev Hist Am Argent** 1980;10(19–20):37–52
Veronelli JC: Medicina, gobierno y sociedad: evolución de las instituciones de atención de la salud en Argentina. Buenos Aires, El Coloquio, [1975]. 227 p.

**Asia**

Iarovinskiĭ MIa, Goncharova SG: Vklad medikov Moskvy v zdravookhranenie sredneaziatskikh respublik. **Sov Zdravookhr** 1983;(1):64–7

**Australia**

Cummins CJ: A history of medical administration in New South Wales 1788–1973. Sydney, Health Commission of New South Wales, 1979. 223 p.
Dickey B: The sick poor in New South Wales, 1840–1880: colonial practice in an amateur age. **J R Aust Hist Soc** 1973;59(1):16–28
Duckett SJ: Structual interests and Australian health policy. **Soc Sci Med** 1984;18(11):959–66
Fisher S: The pastoral interest and Sydney's public health. **Hist Stud** 1982;20(78):73–89
Fisher SH: An accumulation of misery? **Labour Hist** 1981;40:16–28
Lewis M: Milk, mothers, and infant welfare. In J. Roe, ed: Twentieth century Sydney: studies in urban and social history. Sydney, Hale & Iremonger for the Sydney Hist. Group, 1980. p. 193–207.
Mayne AJ: Fever, squalor and vice: sanitation and social policy in Victorian Sydney. St. Lucia, New York, University of Queensland Press, 1982. xviii, 263 p.
Najman JM, Western JS: A comparative analysis of Australian health policy in the 1970s. **Soc Sci Med** 1984;18(11):949–58
Pearn J, O'Carrigan C, ed: Australia's quest for colonial health: some influences on early health and medicine in Australia. Herston, Brisbane, Royal Children's Hospital, 1983. xii, 304 p.
Pryor RJ: Morbidity and minerals: health and mortality in Victoria in the 1850s. Canberra, Department of Demography, Australian National University, 1977. 26 leaves. (Working paper in demography, 5).
Snow D: The progress of public health in Western Australia, 1829–1977. Perth, Public Health Department; Beaverton, Or., International Scholarly Book Services, 1981. xvi, 185 p.

### Austria

Popper L: Die Entwicklung der Arbeitsmedizin in Osterreich und die sozialhygienische Tradition. **Arbeitsmed praventive Gesundheitspolitik** 1982;5:41–5

Skopec M: The development of hygiene in Austria. In Ogawa T, ed: Public health. Tokyo, Saikon, 1981. p. 129–44.

### Belgium

Bruneel C: Un problème de gouvernement: le pouvoir face à l'epidémie de fièvre putride à Bruxelles en 1772–1773. In Imhof AE, ed: Mensch und Gesundheit in der Geschichte. Husum, Matthiesen, 1980. p. 199–221.

Dhoore L, Halter S: Secretaris-generaal van het Ministerie van Volksgezondheid en van het Gezin, Prof. Dr. S. Halter. **Arch Belg Med Soc** 1981 Jul;39(7)Suppl:1–64

Gadeyne G: De plaatselijke commissies van geneeskundkig toevoorzicht in Oost-Vlaanderen (1818–1830). **Handel Maatsch Geschied Oudheidk Gent** 1979;33:175–220

Leboutte R: Conditions d'hygiène et salubrité publique au siècle dernier. Neuf cents ans de vie autour de Saint Remacle au Pont, Liège, Soledi, 1979, p. 177–223.

Prof. Dr S. Halter (1916–1981): **Arch Belg** 1984;42(7–8):349–89

Vilain M: Inventaire du fonds d'archives 'Service de santé et Croix-Rouge, 1831–1914'. Bruxelles, Musée royal de l'Armée, 1981. 25 p.

### Brazil

Alameida BC: Underdevelopment in a 'developing' nation: a quantitative study of health and medicine in Brazil, 1950–1975. Ph. D. Diss., University of California. Los Angeles, 1980. 338 leaves.

Alves M: Dr. Arthur Neiva. **Rev Inst Hist Geogr Bras** 1979;325:123–31

Dr. Marcolino Gomes Candau (30.05.1911--23.01.1983): **Rev Bras Malariol Doencas Trop** 1982;34:119–22

Fraga C: Vida e obra de Osvaldo Cruz. Rio de Janeiro, Livraria José Olympio Editôra em convênio com o Instituto Nacional do Livro, [1972]. 186 p.

Freitas CA de: A memória de Oswaldo Cruz. **Rev Bras Malariol Doencas Trop** 1978;30:129–33

Vasconcellos I de: Francisco de Paula Candido et son 'Rapport sur des mesures d'assainissement réclamées par cité de Rio de Janeiro et sur la fièvre jaune en particulier' - Typographie Nationale - Rio de Janeiro, 1854. In: Congrès international d'histoire de la médecine, XXVe, Québec, 1976. Actes. Québec, 1977. p. 1382–4.

### Bulgaria

Bugyi B: Medical topography of Bulgaria and Serbia in the third quarter of the 19th century. **Geogr Med** 1981;11:158–61

Georgieva K, Dačev B: 100 godini obstesyveno zdraveopazvane. **Stomatologiia (Sofiia)** 1979 Nov–Dec;61(6):337–41

Hadjioloff A, Valtchev A: Problèmes de la médecine et de la santé publique bulgare dans les rapports des semaines médicales balkaniques / 1962–1977. In International Congress of the History of Medicine. 26th, Plovdiv, 1978. Actes du Congress. Sofia, 1981. Volume II. p. 105–6.

Kadunkov D: Purvite obstestveni zubolekarski kabineti v Bulgarija (1907–1971). **Stomatologiia (Sofiia)** 1979 Nov–Dec;61(6):405–8

Nikolaeva I: Istoriia na zdraveopazvaneto vŭv Varna ot drevnostta do sotsialisticheskata revoliutsiia ot 9.IX.1944 g. Sofiia, Meditsina i fizkultura, 1980. 153 p.

Vutov M, Krumova E: Razvitie na stomatologicnata pomost i obrazovanie v bulgariia. **Stomatologiia (Sofiia)** 1979 Mar–Apr;61(2):133–6

### Canada

Baker M: The development of the office of a permanent medical health officer for St. John's, Newfoundland, 1826–1905. **HSTC** 1983 May;24(7 No 2):98–105

Baker M: Thomas Howley. In Dictionary of Canadian biography, 1881–1890. 1982;11:429–30.

Bator PA. Saving lives on the wholesale plan: public health reform in the city of Toronto, 1900–1930. Ph. D. Diss. University of Toronto. Toronto, 1979.

Bator PA: 'The struggle to raise the lower classes': public health reform and the problem of poverty in Toronto, 1910 to 1921. **J Can Stud** 1979;14(1):43–9

Bilson G: A darkened house: cholera in nineteenth century Canada. Toronto, Buffalo, University of Toronto Press, 1980. 222 p.

Bilson G: Cholera and public health in Canada. **Can J Public Health** 1984 Sep–Oct;75(5):352–5

Bilson G: 'Muscles and health': health and the Canadian immigrant, 1867–1906. In Roland CG, ed: Health, disease and medicine. Toronto, Hannah Institute for the History of Medicine, 1984. p. 398–411.

Buckley S, McGinnis JD: Venereal disease and public health reform in Canada. **Can Hist Rev** 1982;63(3):337–54

Farley M, Keel O, Limoges C: Les commencements de l'administration montréalaise de la santé publique (1865–1885). **HSTC** 1982 May;21(6 no 2):85–109

Farley M, Keel O, Limoges C: Les commencements de l'administration montrèalaise de la santé publique (1865–1885)--I. **HSTC** 1982 Jan;20(6 no 1):24–46

Gaucher D: La formation des hygiénistes à l'Université de Montréal, 1910–1975: de la santé publique à la médecine préventive. **Rech Sociogr** 1979;20(1):59–85

Keystone J: The physical health of the Indochinese refugees. In Adelman, Howard, ed: The Indochinese Refugee Movement: The Canadian Experience (Toronto: Operation Lifeline, 1980): 163–5.

Liston A: To cure the sick and protect the healthy. In: Congrès international d'histoire de la médecine, XXVe, Québec, 1976. Actes. Québec, 1977. p. 217–28.

Lloyd S: The Ottawa typhoid epidemics of 1911 and 1912: a case study of disease as a catalyst for urban reform. **Urban Hist Rev** 1979;8(1):66–89

McCombie F, Gray AS: Dental public health in British Columbia. **Can J Public Health** 1984 Sep–Oct;75(5):368–9

MacDougall H: 'Enlightening the public': the views and values of the Association of Executive Health Officers of Ontario, 1886–1903. In Roland CG, ed: Health, disease and medicine. Toronto, Hannah Institute for the History of Medicine, 1984. p. 436–64.

MacDougall H: Public health in Toronto's municipal politics: the Canniff years, 1883–1890. **Bull Hist Med** 1981 Summer;55(2):186–202

MacDougall HA: The genesis of public health reform in Toronto, 1869–1890. **Urban Hist Rev** 1982;10(3):1–9

McGahan EW: John Thomson. In Dictionary of Canadian biography, 1881–1890. 1982;11:878–9.

McLeod K: Hallmarks of reform: social change and the new education in Canada. **Hist Educ Q** 1980;20(3):369–75

Mishler W, Campbell DB: The healthy state. Legislative responsiveness to public health care needs in Canada, 1920–1970. **Comp Pol** 1978 Jul;10:479–97

Oberlander HP: Aspects of public health in Toronto, in the 19th and early 20th centuries. **Can J Public Health** 1984 Sep–Oct;75(5):364–5

Paddon A: Public health in Sub-Arctic Labrador 1912–1978. **Can J Public Health** 1984 Sep–Oct;75(5):356–8

Pierre-Deschênes C: Santé publique et organisation de la profession médicale au Quebec, 1870–1918. **Rev Hist Am Fr** 1981;35(3):355–75

Powell M: Public health litigation in Ontario, 1884–1920. In Roland CG, ed: Health, disease and medicine. Toronto, Hannah Institute for the History of Medicine, 1984. p. 412–35.

Predy GN: A brief history of public health in Alberta. **Can J Public Health** 1984 Sep–Oct;75(5):366–7

Tétreault M: Les maladies de la misère: aspects de la santé publique à Montréal, 1880–1914. **Rev Hist Am Fr** 1983;36(4):507–26

Trent B: Grosse Ile: island of the dead. **Can Med Assoc J** 1984 Oct 15;131(8):960–8

Trépanier P: Victor Barbeau et Albiny Paquette. **Action Natl** 1978;68(4):324–30

Young TK: Indian health services in Canada: a sociohistorical perspective. **Soc Sci Med** 1984;18(3):257–64

### Chile

Medina E: Evolución de la salud pública en Chile en los últimos 25 años. **Rev Med Chil** 1977 Oct;105(10):739–45

Neghme A: La medicina chilena esta de duelo. **Rev Med Chil** 1980 May;108(5):399–406

### China

Brown ER: Exporting medical education: professionalism, modernization and imperialism. **Soc Sci Med [Med Psychol Med Sociol]** 1979 Nov;13A(6):585–95

Bullock MB: An American transplant: the Rockefeller Foundation and Peking Union Medical College. Berkeley, University of California Press, 1980. xxvii, 280 p.

Garfield R, Salmon JW: Struggles over health care in the People's Republic of China. **J Contemp Asia** 1981;11(1):91–103

Hillier SM, Jewell JA: Health care and traditional medicine in China, 1800–1982. London, Routledge & Kegan Paul, 1983, xix, 453 p.

Lisowski FP: The evaluation of health care in China. **East Horiz** 1978;17(3):5–11

Minden K: The development of early Chinese Communist health policy: health care in the border region, 1936–1949. **Am J Chin Med** 1979 Winter;7(4):299–315

### Cuba

Díaz-Briquets S: The health revolution in Cuba. Austin, University of Texas Press, 1983. xvii, 227 p.

Gordon G, Bishop B: Community control, Cuban style. **Freedomways** 1981;21(3):194–200

Richmond JB: A conversation with Fidel Castro about health services. **N Engl J Med** 1984 Apr 12;310(15):994–5

# PUBLIC HEALTH

**Czechoslovakia**

Daněk K: Sto let zdravotnických obvodu na Moravě. Z historie československćh priorit ve zdravotnictví. **Cas Lek Cesk** 1984 Feb 3;123(5):133–6

Fröml F: Pod dohledem městského fyzika. **Cas Lek Cesk** 1982 Jan 15;121(2):58–60

Fröml F: Poslední léta městských chirurgu v Prostějově. **Cas Lek Cesk** 1981;120(51):1573–4

Niklíček L, Manová L: Ceská hygiena a česká společnost na přelomu 19. a 20. století. **Cesk Zdrav** 1981 Apr;29(4):156–64

Skovránek V: Thirty years of the Czechoslovak sanitary and epidemiological service--1952–1982. **J Hyg Epidemiol Microbiol Immunol** 1982;26(4):329–33

Slosarová V, Tomanová M: 100 let školího lékařství v Praze. **Cesk Pediatr** 1984 Jul;39(7):420–4

**Denmark**

Dragsted PJ: Avendelse af edb i sundhedsvaesenet--det historiske forløb i Danmark. **Nord Med** 1981 Oct;96(10):235–6

Madsen KE: Dansk sundhedspolitik 1901–21. **Historie** 1982;14(2):239–71

**Egypt**

Estes JW, Kuhnke L: French observations of disease and drug use in late eighteenth-century Cairo. **J Hist Med Allied Sci** 1984 Apr;39(2):121–52

**Ethiopia**

Stommes E, Sisaye S: The development and distribution of health care services in Ethiopia: a preliminary review. **Can J Afr Stud** 1980;13(3):487–95

**Finland**

Ohquist M: Hälsosyster i Esbo på 1920-talet. **Hist Litteraturhist Studier (Finl)** 1979;54:201–38

**France**

Beauchamp C: Les mécomptes d'un bienfait: sur la pratique de la vaccination au XIXe s. l'exemple du Loir-et-Cher. **Asclepio** 1983;35:389–402

Coleman W: Death is a social disease. Public health and political economy in early industrial France. Madison, University of Wisconsin Press, 1982. xxi, 322 p. (Wisconsin Publications in the History of Science and Medicine, 1).

Coleman W: L'hygiène et l'état selon Montyon. **Dix-Huit Siecle** 1977;9:101–8

Comiti VP: La géographie médicale de la Corse à la fin du XVIIIe siècle. Genève, Droz, 1980. 142 p. (Centre de Recherches d'Histoire et de Philologie de la IVe Section de l'Ecole pratique des Hautes Etudes; Hautes Etudes Médiévales et Modernes, 41).

Fagot A: La philosophie de l'hygiène en 1878. In Poirier J, Poirier JL, ed: Médecine et philosophie à la fin du XIXe siècle. Paris, Université de Paris XII - Val de Marne, [1980?]. p. 61–84.

Guyotjeannin C, Lehuenen J: Contribution à l'étude de la pathologie aux îles Saint-Pierre-et-Miquelon (XIXe siècle - début du XXe siècle). **Hist Sci Med** 1984;18(1):61–5

Jordanova L: Urban health in the French Enlightenment. **Soc Soc Hist Med Bull (Lond)** 1983 Jun;32:31–3

Jordanova LJ: Policing public health in France 1780–1815. In Ogawa T, ed: Public health. Tokyo, Saikon, 1981. p. 12–32.

La Berge AF: The early nineteenth-century French public health movement: the disciplinary development and institutionalization of hygiène publique. **Bull Hist Med** 1984 Fall;58(3):363–79

Lebrun F: L'intervention des autorités face aux crises de mortalité dans la France d'ancien régime. In Imhof AE, ed: Leib und Leben in der Geschichte der Neuzeit. Berlin, Duncker & Humblot, 1983. p. 39–52.

Musset J: L'intervention de l'administration en matière d'épidémie, en milieu rural au XVIIIe siècle: l'élection de Saint-Lô (Généralité de Caen) en 1785. **Bull Soc Fr Hist Hop** 1979;(39):23–31

Pringle JK, Saba SJ: Langage médical et politique locale: l'urbanisme et la santé à Marseille à la fin de l'Ancien Régime. **Ann Midi** 1981;93(154):397–417

Rivet R: Quelques aspects sanitaires de la Bretagne vus à travers les thèses des Facultés de médecine de Paris et de Strasbourg de l'an VII (1798) à 1870. In: Congrès National des Sociétés Savantes, 107e, Brest, 1982. Comptes Rendus, Paris, 1983. Section des Sciences, Fasc. IV. p. 241–52.

Shapiro AL: Private rights, public interest, and professional jurisdiction: the French public health law of 1902. **Bull Hist Med** 1980 Spring;54(1):4–22

Shapiro AL: Working class housing and public health in Paris, 1850–1902. Ph.D. Diss., Brown University. Providence, 1980. 338 leaves.

Stofft H: Bouestard, médecin des épidémies à Morlaix. **Hist Sci Med** 1984;18(3):223–45

**Germany**

Abe HR: Zur medizinhistorischen Topographie und ihrer Bedeutung für die Pflege fortschrittlicher Traditionen auf dem Gebiet des Gesundheitswesens. **Z Gesamte Hyg** 1984 May;30(5):298–301

Bleker J: Die Stadt als Krankheitsfaktor; eine Analyse ärztlicher Auffassungen im 19. Jahrhundert. **Medizinhist J** 1983;18(1–2):118–36

Breustedt A: 30 Jahre DDR--30 Jahre Mitarbeit der stomatologisch-wissenschaftlichen Gesellschaften bei der Gestaltung des sozialistischen Gesundheitswesens in der DDR. **Stomatol DDR** 1979;29(10):729–34

Breyer H: Johann Peter Frank. 'Fürst unter den Arzten Europas.' Leipzig, S. Hirzel, 1983. 184 p.

Dahm I, Schorr R, Niehoff JU: Zum 50. Todestag von Alfred Grotjahn. **Z Arztl Fortbild (Jena)** 1981 Sep 15;75(16):878–81

Dieck M: Residential and community provisions for the frail elderly in Germany: current issues and their history. **Gerontologist** 1980 Jun;20(3 Pt 1):260–72

Eisenberg L: Rudolf Ludwig Karl Virchow, where are you now that we need you? **Am J Med** 1984 Sep;77(3):524–32

Ewert G: Auffassungen der Sozialhygiene zum Organisationsaspekt im Gesundheitswesen. **Z Gesamte Hyg** 1980 Apr;26(4):280–3

FiscHer H: Der deutsche Sanitätsdienst, 1921–1945: Organisation, Dokumente und persönliche Erfahrungen. Band 1. Osnabrück, Biblio, 1982. viii, 289 p.

Haase HH: Uber einige Auswirkungen Robert Kochs und seiner Lehre auf die Entwicklung der Allgemeinen und Kommunalen Hygiene. **Z Gesamte Hyg** 1982 Mar;28(3):154–6

Hagen W: Auftrag und Wirklichkeit: Sozialarzt im 20. Jahrhundert. München-Gräfelfing, Werk-Verlag, 1978. 253 p.

Hahn S: Positionen der Kommunistischen Partei Deutschlands zur lebensbewahrenden Aufgabe der Medizin in der Zeit der Weimarer Republik. **Z Exp Chir** 1982 Jul;28(7):468–71

Hartung K: Einhundert Jahre schulärztlicher Dienst--ein beinahe vergessenes Jubiläum. **Off Gesundheitswes** 1983 Dec;45(12):615–7

Heilwagen W: Das Kasseler Gesundheitswesen der Gegenwart. In Balde JH, Schmiking W, ed: Festschrift zum 86. Deutschen Arztetag in Kassel. Kassel, Arztevereins, 1983. p. 105–12.

Helm D: Die Cholera in Lübeck. Epidemieprophylaxe und -bekämpfung im 19. Jahrhundert. Neumünster, Wachholtz, 1979. 81 p. (Kieler Beiträge zur Geschichte der Medizin und Pharmazie, 16).

Hiller I: Ludwig Formeys 'Versuch einer medicinischen Topographie von Berlin' und kommunale Umweltproblematik im 18. Jahrhundert. **Z Exp Chir** 1982 Jul;28(7):474–6

Jenner H: Organisation des Gesundheitswesens in Schleswig-Holstein in der ersten Hälfte des 19. Jahrhunderts. **Z Ges Schleswig Holstein Gesch** 1982;107:67–112

Kaiser W, Völker A: Die Aufgaben einer Medizinalbehörde im 19. Jahrhundert am Beispiel von Anhalt-Köthen. **Wiss Z Martin Luther Univ (Math)** 1983;32(2):39–69

Kaiser W, Völker A: Hygiene, Präventiv, und Unfallmedizin in den Schriften des halleschen Ordinarius Johann Heinrich Schulze (1687–1744). **Z Gesamte Hyg** 1981 Oct;27(10):779–84

Kaiser W: Johann Friedrich Gottlieb Goldhagen (1742–1788) aus Nordhausen, Stadtphysikus und Ordinarius in Halle. **Beitr Heimatkd Stadt Kreis Nordhausen** 1978;(2–3):58–70

Klein P, Labisch A, Milles D, et al: Zur Entwicklung der Arbeitsmedizin in Deutschland bis zum Ende der Weimarer Republik. **Arbeitsmed praventive Gesundheitspolitik** 1982;5:28–40

Kłodzinski S: Uwagi o sytuacji zdrwotnej robotników przymusowych w Niemczech hitlerowskich. **Przegl Lek** 1981;38(1):62–72

Künzel W: 20 Jahre Trinkwasserfluoridierung in der Deutschen Demokratischen Republik. **Stomatol DDR** 1979;29(10):743–52

Labisch A: Selbsthilfe zwischen Auflehnung und Anpassung. Arbeiter-Sanitätskommission und Arbeiter-Samariterbund. **Jahrb Krit Med** 1983;77:11–26

Labisch A, Tennstedt F: 50 Jahre Gesetz über Vereinheitlichung des Gesundheitswesens. Dr. med. Arthur Gütt und die Gründung des öffentlichen Gesundheitsdienstes. **Off Gesundheitswes** 1984 Jul;46(7):291–8

Lindemann M: Love for hire: the regulation of the wet-nursing business in eighteenth-century Hamburg. **J Fam Hist** 1981 Winter;6(4):379–95

Lindemann ME: Producing policed man: poor relief, population policies and medical care in Hamburg, 1750–1806. Ph. D. Diss., University of Cincinnati. Cincinnati, 1980. vii, 386 p.

Loewenstein G: Kommunale Gesundheitsfürsorge und sozialistische Arztepolitik zwischen Kaiserreich und Nationalsozialismus. Bremen, Universität Bremen, 1980. v, 374 p.

Moschke G: Die Rolle des Sanitäts- und Hilfsdienstes bei der Gestaltung des Systems der medizinischen Versorgung in Leipzig von 1945–1948. **Z Gesamte Hyg** 1979;25(11):845–7

Moschke G: Samaritianskiĭ soiuz rabochikh Germanii--primer tvorcheskoĭ deiatel'nosti nemetskogo rabochego klassa v 1909–1930 gg. v bor'be protiv burzhuaznoĭ politiki zdravookhraneniia. **Sov Zdravookhr** 1981;(2):52–6

Moskwa Z: Powstańcza søużba zdrowia na Górnym Slasku w latach 1919–1921. **Wiad Lek** 1984 Feb 15;37(4):313–20

Nagel A, Nagel R: Von Arzten und Beamten. Ein Collegium Sanitatis für Kleve (1726). **Med Welt** 1983 Sep 16;34(37):1019–20
Opitz R, Horn H, Heinecke P, et al: Robert Koch. Die Vorgeschichte der Berufung als ersten Ordinarius für Hygiene an die Universität Berlin. **MMW** 1981 Oct 16;123(42):1593–5
Piechocki W: Die Gesundheitsverhältnisse in der Stadt Halle im ausgehenden 19. Jahrhundert. **Wiss Beitr Martin Luther Univ Halle Wittenberg** 1983;5-R80:211–23
Reis K: Gesundheitserziehung in der DDR – Versuch einer historischen Betrachtung. **Z Gesamte Hyg** 1982 Apr;28(4):253–5
Renker K. 25 Jahre Zeitschrift für die gesamte Hygiene. **Z Gesamte Hyg** 1979 Oct;25(10):792
Renker K: 30 Jahre Sozialhygiene an der Universität Halle. **Z Gesamte Hyg** 1980;26(2):116–21
Rodegra H: Das Gesundheitswesen der Stadt Hamburg im 19. Jahrhundert, unter Berücksichtigung der Medizinalgesetzgebung (1586–1818–1900). Wiesbaden, Steiner, 1979. 217 p. (Sudhoffs Archiv, Beihefte, Heft 21)
Sanden B: Gesundheitsfürsorge einst und jetzt. **ZFA (Stuttgart)** 1980 Mar;56(8):567–72
Schipperges H: Struktur und Funktion eines Instituts für Gesundheitsbildung. In R. Wittern, ed: Jahrbuch des Instituts für Geschichte der Medizin der Robert Bosch Stiftung. Stuttgart, Hippokrates Verlag, 1984. Bd. 1. p. 42–69.
Sons HU: Gesundheitspolitik während der Besatzungszeit: das öffentliche Gesundheitswesen in Nordrhein-Westfalen 1945–1949. Wuppertal, Hammer, 1983. 207 p.
Sons HU: Lebensbedingungen in Nordrhein-Westfalen nach dem Zweiten Weltkrieg. Teil 1: Die Situation. **Fortschr Med** 1984 Apr 5;102(13):93–5 (cont)
Sons HU: Offentliches Gesundheitswesen und kommunale Selbstverwaltung in Nordrhein-Westfalen (britisches Besatzungsgebiet) 1945–1949. -- Die Kommunalisierung der Gesundheitsämter. **Off Gesundheitswes** 1983 Jul;45(7):343–8
Steinbrück P: 30 Jahre DDR -- 30 Jahre erfolgreicher Kampf um die Gesundheit unserer Bürger. **Z Erkr Atmungsorgane** 1979 Apr;153(11):3–4
Stürzbecher M: Franz Schrakamp (1860–1920) Stadt- und Kreisarzt in Düsseldorf. **Clin Notes Respir Dis** 1980 May;42(5):289–92
Teubel S: Schulhygiene in der Zeit von 1870 bis 1900. Diss. Bonn, 1981. 149 p.
Thomann KD: Wissenschaftliche Sozialhygiene und gesellschaftliche Praxis im Deutschen Reich. **Sudhoffs Arch** 1984;68(1):61–76
Troschke J von: Möglichkeiten und Grenzen ärztlicher Gesundheitsberatung. Freiburg, Gesomed, 1981. 373 p.
Weispfenning I: Pettenkofers Gesundheitswirtschaftslehre. Ein meilenstein in der Entwicklung des öffentlichen Gesundheitswesens. In Seidler E, Schott H, ed: Bausteine zur Medizingeschichte. Stuttgart, Steiner, 1984. p. 146–54.
Wildfuehr G: 100 Jahre Hygiene in Leipzig. **Wiss Z Karl Marx Univ Math Natur Wiss Reihe** 1979;28:9–23
Winter K: Das Gesundheitswesen in der Deutschen Demokratischen Republik. Bilanz nach 30 Jahren. Berlin, Volk und Gesundheit, 1980. 223 p.
Winter K, ed: Das Gesundheitswesen in der Deutschen Demokratischen Republik. Berlin, Verlag Volk und Gesundheit, 1974. 209 p.

**Ghana**

Patterson KD: Health in colonial Ghana: disease, medicine, and socio-economic change, 1900–1955. Waltham, Mass., Crossroads Press, 1981. xiii, 187 p.
Patterson KD: Health in urban Ghana: the case of Accra 1900–1940 [1]. **Soc Sci Med [Med Anthropol]** 1979 Dec;13B(4):251–68

**Great Britain**

Barlow K: The pioneer health centre at Peckham. **Soc Soc Hist Med Bull (Lond)** 1984 Dec;35:47
Barnet MC: Life in 19th century York. **Pharm Hist (London)** 1984 Jun;14(2):3–5
Benjamin B: Changes in public health in London in the past fifty years. **R Soc Health J** 1981 Dec;101(6):245–60
Berridge V: Drugs and social policy: the establishment of drug control in Britain 1900–30. **Br J Addict** 1984 Mar;79(1):17–29
Berridge V, Edwards G: Opium and the people. Opiate use in nineteenth-century England. London and New York; Allen Lane and St. Martin's Press; 1981. 369 p.
Blackden SM: The development of public health administration in Glasgow, 1842–1872. Ph.D. thesis, Univ. of Edinburgh, 1976.
Brayshay M, Pointon VF: Local politics and public health in mid-nineteenth-century Plymouth. **Med Hist** 1983 Apr;27(2):162–78
Brimley R: Health visiting as it was. Interview by Shirley Goodwin. **Nurs Mirror** 1981 Jul 22;153(4):22–4
Brotherston JH: James Macalister Mackintosh. In Dictionary of national biography, 1961–1970. Suppl. 8, 1981. p. 698–9.
Budnick LD: The spirit of Chadwick. **NY State J Med** 1983 Dec;83(13):1345–6
Cardwell D, Mottram J: Fresh light on John Dalton. **Notes Rec R Soc Lond** 1984 Sep;39(1):29–40
Carpenter M: William Farr: a pioneer of public health. **Nurs Times** 1983 Jun 15–21;79(24):9–11
Chave SP: Duncan of Liverpool--and some lessons for today. **Community Med** 1984 Feb;6(1):61–71
Chave SP: The rise and fall of the medical officer of health. **Community Med** 1980 Feb;2(1):36–45
Checkland O, Lamb M, ed: Health care as social history; the Glasgow case. Aberdeen, Aberdeen University Press, 1982. xix, 285 p.
Checkland S: British urban health in general and in a single city. In Checkland O, Lamb M, ed: Health care as social history; the Glasgow case. Aberdeen, Aberdeen University Press, 1982. p. 170–90.
Connolly MP: Health visiting 1850–1900: a review. **Midwife Health Visit Community Nurse** 1980 Jul;16(7):282–5
Connolly MP: Health visiting 1900–1910: a review. **Midwife Health Visit Community Nurse** 1980 Sep;16(9):375–8
Dow D: The archives of the Greater Glasgow Health Board. In Checkland O, Lamb M, ed: Health care as social history; the Glasgow case. Aberdeen, Aberdeen University Press, 1982. p. 158–69.
Elcock H: Regional government in action: the members of two regional health authorities. **Public Adm** 1978 Winter;56:379–97
Elliott A, Freeling P, Owen J: District nurse training. **J R Coll Gen Pract** 1980 Feb;30(211):69–74
Godber GE: Sir Arthur Salusbury MacNalty. In Dictionary of national biography, 1961–1970. Suppl. 8, 1981. p. 706–7.
Guest-Gornall RG: Good servants are scarce. **Br Med J [Clin Res]** 1981 Dec 19;283(6307):1674–5
Guha M, Wood M: Does health visiting have a history? **Health Visit** 1981 Dec;54(12):540
Hardy A: Water and the search for public health in London in the eighteenth and nineteenth centuries. **Med Hist** 1984 Jul;28(3):250–82
Hardy G: William Rathbone and the early history of district nursing. Ormskirk, Hesketh, 1981. 54 p.
Hirst JD: A failure 'without parallel': the School Medical Service and the London County Council 1907–12. **Med Hist** 1981 Jul;25(3):281–300
James DC: Dr. Henry James Paine: medical officer of health for Cardiff 1853–1889. **Public Health** 1981 Jul;95(4):215–21
James PM: One hundred years of dental public health. **Br Dent J** 1981 Jul 7;151(1):20–3
Jones IG: Merthyr Tydfil: the politics of survival. **Llafur J Soc Stud Welsh Labour Hist** 1976;2(1):18–31
Kearns G: Cholera and public health reform in nineteenth-century England and Wales: interpreting the geographical patterns. **Soc Soc Hist Med Bull (Lond)** 1984 Dec;35:30–2
Lawrence C: Sanitary reformers and the medical profession in Victorian England. In Ogawa T, ed: Public health. Tokyo, Saikon, 1981. p. 145–68.
Levere TH: Dr. Thomas Beddoes (1750–1808): science and medicine in politics and society. **Br J Hist Sci** 1984 Jul;17(56 pt 2):187–204
Lewis J, Brookes B: The Peckham Health Centre, 'Pep', and the concept of General practice during the 1930s and 1940s. **Med Hist** 1983 Apr;27(2):151–61
Lilienfeld AM, Lilienfeld DE: Epidemiology and the public health movement: a historical perspective. **J Public Health Policy** 1982 Jun;3(2):140–9
Macrae AD: Laboratory diagnosis of smallpox: role of the Virus Reference Laboratory, Colindale, 1947–70. **J Hyg (Lond)** 1982 Dec;89(3):399–407
Novak SJ: Professionalism and bureaucracy: English doctors and Victorian public health administration. **J Soc Hist** 1973;6(4):440–62
Parfit J: The Oxford Board of Health 1831–1833. **Public Health** 1982 Jan;96(1):25–30
Pelling M, ed: Handlist of records of the Society of Medical Officers of Health deposited at the Wellcome Unit for the History of Medicine, Oxford, 4 May 1976, with later deposits and other locations. Oxford, Wellcome Unit for the History of Medicine, 1980 23 p. (Research Publications of the Wellcome Unit for the History of Medicine. Oxford, No. III).
Pickstone JV: Ferriar's fever to Kay's cholera: disease and social structure in cottonopolis. **Hist Sci** 1984 Dec;22(58 pt 4):401–19
Pickstone JV, Butler SV: The politics of medicine in Manchester, 1788–1792: hospital reform and public health services in the early industrial city. **Med Hist** 1984 Jul;28(3):227–49
The preservation of medical and public health records: (Research Publications of the Wellcome Unit for the History of Medicine, Oxford, No. I). Oxford, Wellcome Unit for the History of Medicine, 1979. 52 p. Contributions by C. Webster, P. Barnes, E. Freeman, H. Francis, B. Parry-Jones.
Radford P: Gilbert White: medical and social aspects of his letters. **Bristol Med Chir J** 1984 Apr;99(370):46–7
Savage R: Croydon's local Board of Health in the early 1850s. **Proc Croydon Nat Hist Sci Soc** 1974;14(13)
Smith FB: Ethics and disease in the later nineteenth century: the Contagious Diseases Acts. **Hist Stud** 1971;15(57):118–35
Spriggs EA: Hector Gavin, MD, FRCSE (1815–1855) – his life, his work for the sanitary movement, and his accidental death in the Crimea. **Med Hist** 1984 Jul;28(3):283–92
Stevens P: The health of Hampshire towns in an age of revolutions. **Pharm Hist (London)** 1981;11(2):4–5

# PUBLIC HEALTH

Stewart AB: Sir William Allen Daley. In Dictionary of national biography, 1961–1970. Suppl. 8, 1981. p. 265–6.
Stewart L: The edge of utility: slaves and smallpox in the early eighteenth century. **Med Hist** 1985 Jan;29(1):54–70
Tait HP: The College and community health. In Passmore R, ed: Proceedings of the Royal College of Physicians of Edinburgh Tercentenary Congress, 1981. Edinburgh, Royal College of Physicians of Edinburgh, 1982. p. 162–78.
Takei Y: [Administrative reform in 19th-century England, a result of the public health problem] (Jpn). **Shakai Keizai Shigaku** 1976;42(3):1–21
Takei Y: [The public health problem in Great Britain at the time of the Industrial Revolution] (Jpn). **Shakai Keizai Shigaku** 1974;40(4):1–24
Templar M: Historical perspectives. **Nurs Mirror** 1984 Oct 24;159(15):vii–viii
Thomas EG: Chelmsford and the Board of Health Report of 1849. **Essex J** 1979;14(1):
Thomas M, ed: Urban and rural social conditions in industrial Britain; series 2. The reports [of the medical officers of health] to the Local Government Board 1869–1908. A complete listing and guide to the Harvester microfiche collection. Brighton, England, Harvester Press Microform Publications, 1979. 251 p.
Thomson I: The origins of physical education in state schools. **Scott Educ Rev** 1978;10(2)
Webster C: Healthy or hungry thirties? **Hist Workshop J** 1982;13:110–29
White B: Public health and civic administration in nineteenth-century Glasgow. **Soc Soc Hist Med Bull (Lond)** 1983 Jun;32:37–9
White BM: Medical police. Politics and police: the fate of John Roberton. **Med Hist** 1983 Oct;27(4):407–22
Williams H: Public health and local history. **Local Hist** 1980;14(4):202–10
Wilson TS: The National Health Service 1948–1980. In Checkland O, Lamb M, ed: Health care as social history; the Glasgow case. Aberdeen, Aberdeen University Press, 1982. p. 149–57.
Winter JM: Infant mortality, maternal mortality and public health in Britain in the 1930's. **J Eur Econ Hist** 1979;13(2):439–62

**Greece**

Degleris NE, Rozos BP: [Public health, medical education and social care of Ionian Isles in the middle of the 19th century (press documents)] (Gre). **Arch Hyg** 1980;:90–101

**Hungary**

Bacsa S: Morfinszármazékok adásának veszélye pancreatitisben. **Orv Hetil** 1982 May 30;123(22):1387–8
Bak M: Lux Jakab dr. (1822–1876) munkássága mai orvosi szemléletünkben. **Orv Hetil** 1984 Apr 29;125(18):1082–4
Batári G: Schmidt Béla és az erdélyi Magyar Népegészségügyi Szemle. **Orv Hetil** 1982 Oct 31;123(44):2737–8
Birtalan G: Adatok a két világháború között Magyarországon végzett szervezett egészségvédelmi munkáról, különös tekintettel az Oki tevékenységére. **Orvostort Kozl** 1979;87–88(25 no 1–2):181–218
Bugyi B: Akit indokolatlanul elfelejtettek: Schnirch Emil (1822–1884). **Orv Hetil** 1982 Oct 17;123(42):2613–4
Fazekas A: Jósa András 150 éve született (1834. nov. 30.–1918. szept. 6.). **Orv Hetil** 1984 Sep 30;125(40):2444–6
Frankl J: Faber Tamás dr., Somogy els ó megyei orvosa. **Orv Hetil** 1983 Feb 20;124(8):466–7
Gyárfás A: Gálfalvi Domby Sámuel, Borsod vármegye föorvosa (1729–1807)]. **Orv Hetil** 1982 Aug 22;123(34):2123–5
Hahn G: Zwanzig Jahre des Ungarischen Gesundheitswesens. Budapest: Ministerium für Gesundheitswesen, 1965. 116 p.
Hidvégi J: Az ifjú Markusovszky világa. **Orv Hetil** 1982 Dec 26;123(52):3207–13
Honti J: A magyar progresszió egészségpolitikai törekvései és a Nagy Októberi Szocialista Forradalom hatása. **Orvostort Kozl** 85(24 No 3):85–90, 1978
Kálmán G: Mészáros Kálmán emlékezete. **Orv Hetil** 1983 Apr;124(16):962–7
Kapronczay K: Az 1848/49-es magyar szabadságharc egészségügyének szervezete. **Orv Hetil** 1984 Jun 10;125(24):1454–6
Kapronczay K: Markusovszky Lajos utolsó levele Fodor Józsefhez. **Orv Hetil** 1982 Dec 26;123(52):3213–4
Kerekes L: In memoriam Halász Géza (1816–1888). **Orvostort Kozl** 1979;86(24 no 4):113–22
Leblancné Kelemen M: Adalékok a reformkori Nógrád megye egészségügyi helyzetéröl Baintner Ferenc megyei föorvos jelentései alapján. **Orvostort Kozl** 1979;87–88(25 no 1–2):269–75
Menner O: Menner Adolf dr. (1824–1901). **Orv Hetil** 1983 Jun 12;124(24):1451–3
Mészárosné Varga M: A Magyar Tanácsköztársaság egészségügye Veszprém megyében – a korabeli sajtó alapján. **Orvostort Kozl** 1982;28(1–3):219–26
Nikodemusz I: Közlekedésünk egészségügye a múltban. **Orv Hetil** 1984 Apr 29;125(18):1084–5
Somogyi E: Korányi Frigyes közéleti munkássága. **Orv Hetil** 1984 Apr 29;125(18):1079–82
Spielmann J: Nyulas Ferenc emlékezete. **Orv Hetil** 1984 Jun 24;125(26):1578–81
Szállási A: [Gusztáv Rigler: prominent figure in Hungarian public health (1868–1930)] (Hun). **Orv Hetil** 1980;121:2209–11
Szállási A: Szociálhigiéne, szociográfia, szépirodalom. **Orv Hetil** 1981 May 17;122(20)1199–202
Szilvágyi I: Fejér megye közegészségügyének története 1865–1903 között. **Orvostort Kozl** 1979;87–88(25 no 1–2):277–90

**India**

All India Institute of Hygiene & Public Health golden jubilee, 1932–1982: [New Delhi], Ministry of Health & Family Welfare, Government of India; Calcutta, The Institute, 1982. 25, 4 p.
Blatt A: Panchayati raj and the mobilisation of the periphery: the case of the location of a primary health centre. **J Commonw Polit Stud** 1972;10(2):130–48
Caldwell JC, Reddy PH, Caldwell P: The social component of mortality decline: an investigation in South India employing alternative methodologies. **Popul Stud** 1983 Jul;37(2):185–205
Deodhar NS: Primary health care in India. **J Public Health Policy** 1982 Mar;3(1):76–99
Naidis M: 'Ants, muskeetoes, flies and stinking chints': the British battle against disease in India. **West Hum Rev** 1964;17(1):39–47
Sastry VV: Health habits of South Indians as recorded by Abbe J. A. Dubois. **Bull Indian Inst Hist Med (Hyderabad)** 1980;10(1–4):84–9
Simmons CP: Housing, health and educational facilities in the Indian coalfields during the colonial era. **South Asia** 1978;1(1):52–62

**Iran**

Andreano R: Some personal observations on health policy in Iran, 1973–1978. **Soc Sci Med** 1984;19(1):1–7

**Ireland**

Elwood JH: Thomas Carnwath. **Ulster Med J** 1982;51(2):98–109
Niven Mackay IM: The relationship between human and animal health in nineteenth century Dublin. **Vet Hist** 1984;3(3):110–4

**Italy**

Balzani A: Primi interventi di bonifica dello stato unitario nella campagna romana. **Studi Romani** 1980;28(1):47–67
Coppola G: Condizioni materiali e problemi sociali in Lombardi tra '700 e '800. **Ann Ist Stor Italo-Ger** 1976;2:553–61
Della Peruta F: Fonti a stampa relative alla storia della sanità in Lombardia, 1816–1859. **Soc Stor** 1978;:369–92
Della Peruta F: Sanità pubblica e legislazione sanitaria dall'unità a Crispi. **Studi Stor** 1980;21(4):713–59
Pontuale L: L'urbanistica 'risanatrice' a Napoli: meglio il colera? **Comunita** 1975;29(174):128–65
Sorcinelli P: Miseria e malattie nel XIX secolo. I ceti popolari nell'Italia centrale fra tifo petecchiale e pellagra. Milano, Franco Angeli, 1979. 285 p.
Trabucchi C: Riforma psichiatrica. I vecchi 'manicomi' e la riforma sanitaria. **Minerva Med** 1980 May 7;71(18):1281–5

**Ivory Coast**

Domergue D: Les vingt premières années de l'action sanitaire en Côte d'Ivoire. **Rev Fr Hist Outre Mer** 1978;65(1):40–63

**Japan**

Besscho C: [Life of Mrs. Seki Hora, the founder of Japanese public health nursing] (Jpn). **Kango** 1980 Jun;32(6):112–20
Endo E: [Visiting nurse after the World War II] (Jpn). **Igakushi Kenkyu** 1978;49:22–6
Endo E: [Visiting nursing in 1926–1945] (Jpn). **Igakushi Kenkyu** 1977;48:30–8
[History of public health nursing activities among frontier farmers in Hokkaido] (Jpn): **Hokenfu Zasshi** 1982 Jan;38(1):10–49
Kato M, Araki S, Sadahiro U, et al: [History of public health nursing in Hokkaido--through the war, postwar transition, repatriation, and reconstruction periods. A discussion] (Jpn). **Hokenfu Zasshi** 1982 Jan;38(1):58–75
Kawamura Z: [Compilation of the history of public health nursing and observation of its significance] (Jpn). **Hokenfu Zasshi** 1981 Jul;37(7):570–86
Komatsu N: [A study on Shimpei Goto/Part II & III. His basic idea on central and rural health organization] (Jpn). **Igakushi Kenkyu** 1980;53:10–21
Marui E: Public health and 'Koshu-Eisei'. Speciality and universality of the modern Japanese public health. In Ogawa T, ed: Public health. Tokyo, Saikon, 1981. p. 99–107.
Okuni M: [A chronological table on district nurse (Hokenfu) in after the

war. Part I] (Jpn). **Igakushi Kenkyu** 1977;48:39–40

Onishi W: [A life among frontier farmers in Hokkaido: a public health nurse in a segment of history of the Showa era] (Jpn). **Kango** 1981 Aug;33(9):88–91

Onishi W: [Public health nurse working among the farmers in the Hokkaido Reclamation Project: a segment of the history of the Showa period] (Jpn). **Kango** 1981 Apr;33(4):73–9

Onishi W: [Public health nursing at land reclamation project in Hokkaido: a segment of the history of the Showa period] (Jpn). **Kango** 1981 Sep;33(10):98–103, Nov;33(12):81–91

Suzuki S: Kenko hoken kumiai hattatsu shi. Tokyo, Kitamura Shakai Hoken Shuppan, Showa 51 nen [1976]. 15, 362 p.

Tatara K: [Interim report on the future provision on medical and allied services, 1920 (I)] (Jpn). **Igakushi Kenkyu** 1978;51:42–51

Tsubota S: [Public health nurses in the frontier of Hokkaido--a historical background] (Jpn). **Hokenfu Zasshi** 1982 Jan;38(1):50–6

Uchibori C: [History of national public health activities in the Gunma Prefecture. 2. Stimulating seminars] (Jpn). **Hokenfu Zasshi** 1982 Feb;38(2):148–50

Ueda M, Usui K, Kawasaki S, et al: [History of public health nurses associated with Osaka public health clinics: social health of the Meiji, Taisho, and Showa eras and the birth of public health nurses] (Jpn). **Hokenfu Zasshi** 1981 Apr;37(4):250–7

### Kenya

Koinange K: Some reflections on development of health services in Kenya. **East Afr Med J** 1983 Sep;60(9):599–602

Mburu FM: Socio-political imperatives in the history of health development in Kenya. **Soc Sci Med [A]** 1981 Sep;15(5):521–7

Wilson CL, Williams CM: Toward the biological control of insect pests. the rise of the International Center of Insect Physiology and Ecology. **Sci Public Aff Bull At Sci** 1973;29(3):10–16

### Korea

Cowdrey AE: 'Germ warfare' and public health in the Korean conflict. **J Hist Med Allied Sci** 1984 Apr;39(2):153–72

### Libya

Abu-Shwairb 'Abd al-Karim: Mushahadati haul al-tib al-sha'bi fi Fazan (tarjamah wa-taqdim limushahadat tabib Turki). **Majallat al-Puhuth al-Tarikhiya (Lybia)** 1979;1(2):37–50

### Liechtenstein

Rheinberger R: Zum 200. Geburtstag von Landesphysikus Gebhard Schaedler. ein Liechtensteinischer Artzt als Pionier der Pockenschutzimpfung. **Jahrb Hist Ver Fuerst Liechtenstein** 1976;76:337–43

### Mexico

Alvarez Amézquita J: Influencia de la salud pública en el desarrollo social. In Academia Nacional de Medicina. Libro conmemorativo del primer centenario. México, Comité Editorial de la Comisión Organizadora del Congreso del Centenario, 1964. Tome 2. p. 630–40.

Bustamante ME: Hechos sobresalientes en la historia de la Secretaría de Salubridad y Asistencia. **Salud Publica Mex** 1983 Sep–Oct;25(5):465–82

Bustamante ME: Historia de la Secretaría de Salubridad y Asistencia. **Salud Publica Mex** 1983 Sep–Oct;25(5):461–4

Bustamante ME: La coordinación de los servicios sanitarios federales y locales como factor de progreso higiénico en México. Su evolución y desarrollo de 1934 a 1964. In Academia Nacional de Medicina. Libro conmemorativo del primer centenario. México, Comité Editorial de la Comisión Organizadora del Congreso del Centenario, 1964. Tome 2. p. 652–64.

Bustamente ME: La primera enfermera en la historia de la salud pública, Isabel Cendala y Gómez. **Rev Col Nac Enferm** 1980 Jul, 1981 Feb;27 28(107):7 12

González-Polo I: La ciudad de México a fines del siglo XVIII-disquisiciones sobre un manuscrito anónimo. **Hist Mex** 1976;26(1):29–47

Marcial LD: Las publicaciones oficiales de la Secretaría de Salubridad y Asistencia. **Salud Publica Mex** 1983 Sep–Oct;25(5):489–97

Price R: Estado, iglesia, caridad y viruela: una crisis epidémica en la Ciudad de México 1797–98. **Bol Soc Mex Hist Filos Med** 1984 Mar;7(46):269–87

Quijano Narezo M: México en las relaciones internacionales de salud. **Salud Publica Mex** 1983 Sep–Oct;25(5):519–23

Rodríguez Domínguez J: La Escuela de Salud Pública de México. **Salud Publica Mex** 1983 Sep–Oct;25(5):505–8

Sepúlveda B: La medicina en la seguridad social. In Academia Nacional de Medicina. Libro conmemorativo del primer centenario. México, Comité Editorial de la Comisión Organizadora del Congreso del Centenario, 1964. Tome 2. p. 678–83.

Soberón G, Sepúlveda B: El Consejo de Salubridad General. **Salud Pubica Mex** 1983 Sep–Oct;25(5):483–7

### Mongolia

Radnabazar Zh: Razvitie zdravookhraneniia v Mongol'skoĭ Narodnoi Respublike. **Sov Zdravookhr** 1983;(4):50–2

### Netherlands

Stemvers FA: Geslachtsziektenbestrijding 1850–1880. **Tijdschr Geschied Geneeskd** 1981;4(1):1–24

### New Zealand

Bryder L: 'Lessons' of the 1918 influenza epidemic in Auckland. **NZ J Hist** 1982;16(2):97–121

New Zealand Dept. of Health: Health expenditures in New Zealand -- trends and growth patterns. Wellington, Management Services and Research Unit, Department of Health, 1979. 62 p.

### Norway

Elstad JI: Helsetilstand og dødelighet i Sogn og Fjordane og Finnmark i sosiologisk perspektiv. **Tidsskr Samfunnsforskning** 1982;23(1):49–70

Lerche C: The National Institute of Public Health--fifty years of activity and development in retrospect. **NIPH Ann** 1979 Dec;2(2):3–10

### Pacific Islands

Johnson G: Micronesia: America's strategic trust. **Bull At Sci** 1979;35(2):10–15

Ofcansky TP: British colonial administration in the Fiji Islands during the 1875 measles epidemic. **Adler Mus Bull** 1984 Mar;10(1):23–7

### Papua New Guinea

Kettle E: That they might live. Sydney, F.P. Leonard, 1979. viii, 368 p.

### Philippines

Tiglao T, Cruz WL: Seven decades of public health in the Philippines (1898–1972). Tokyo, SEAMIC, 1975. xv, 310 p.

### Poland

Dorsz-Szteke E, Maciejewska-Dorsz K: Pomoc wojskowej służby zdrowia dla ludności cywilnej Pomorza Zachodniego w latach 1945–1946. **Wiad Lek** 1981;34(7):615–8

Kasperek J: Zarys organizacji służby zdrowia w Lublinie w okresie okupacji hitlerowskiej. **Przegl Lek** 1980;37(1):149–57

Korczak CW: Jubileusz 80-lecia Polskiego Towarzystwa Higienicznego. **Pol Tyg Lek** 1979 Nov 12;34(46):1813–5

Korczak CW: 80-letie Pol'skogo Gigienicheskogo Obshchestva (1898–1978). **Gig Sanit** 1980 Mar;(3):58–9

Kostrzewski JK: Stan zdrowia ludności Polski--dotychczasowe wyniki i dalsze kierunki badań. **Nauka Pol** 1979;27(4):3–18

Kowieski L: Działalność Wydziału Higieny Zawodowej i Przemysłu Oddziału Lubelskiego Warszawskiego Towarzystwa Higienicznego w latach 1903–1905. **Arch Hist Med (Warsz)** 1984;47(3):429–31

Makowiec J: Kaliskie lecznictwo w latach 1874–1914. **Wiad Lek** 1984 Jul 15;37(14):1135–44

Moskwa Z: Publiczna służba zdrowia w świetle ustawy z 1939 roku. **Wiad Lek** 1983 Nov 1;36(21):1833–4

Sobalski F: Uwagi o pracownikach służby zdrowia w Czestochowie w XIX wieku. **Arch Hist Med (Warsz)** 1984;47(3):375–82

Stembrowicz W: Miscellanea prasy warszawskiej o służbie zdrowia w okresie Powstania Listopadowego. **Arch Hist Med (Warsz)** 1980;43(4):415–21

Trzydziestolecie słuzby zdrowia Ministerstwa Spraw Wewnetrznych w Olsztyńskiem, 1945–1975: materiały sesji naukowej, Olsztyn, 7 pazdziernika 1975. Olsztyn, Wydano na zlecenie Tarchomińskich Zakładów Farmaceutycznych 'Polfa,' 1976. 106 p.

Wieckowska E: Formy opieki zdrowotnej na ziemiach polskich w końcu XIX wieku do lat 30 wieku XX. **Wiad Lek** 1984 Jul 1;37(13):1049–55

### Puerto Rico

Rigau Pérez JG: El Dr. Francisco Oller y el inicio de la salud pública moderna en Puerto Rico, 1790–1831. In International Congress of the History of Medicine, 27th, Barcelona, 1980. Actas. Barcelona, Académia de Ciències Médiques de Catalunya i Balears, 1981. p. 199–202.

### Romania

Brătescu G: Charles Davila et l'organisation sanitaire moderne de la Roumanie. **Sante Publique (Bucur)** 1982;25(1):33–43

Negru I: Concepţia profesorului Victor Babeş asupra instruirii şi formării

agentului sanitar. **Viata Med [Medii Sanit]** 1983 Sep;31(9):211–4
Negru I: O şcoală de surori de ocrotire mai puţin cunoscută–şcoala din Timişoara (septembrie 1939–februarie 1942). **Viata Med [Medii Sanit]** 1984 Jul;32(7):163–6
Nepohoda–Seredenciuc I: Our magazine is 25. **Sante Publique (Bucur)** 1983;26(1):3–8
Ploesteanu I: Pozitia P.C.R. şi a celorlalte forţe democratice din România privind sănătatea publică, în perioada dintre cele două războaie mondiale (I). **Viata Med [Medii Sanit]** 1979 Aug;27(8):189–91
Sărmąsanu–Cortez ML, Cortez P: A great forerunner of the modern sanitary organization, Prof. Dr. Alexandru Obregia (1860–1937). **Sante Publique (Bucar)** 1979;22(4):387–93

**South Africa**

Adler C: Dr. Charles Porter. **Adler Mus Bull** 1984 Jun;10(2):9–14
Applegryn MS: Die ontstaan van die eerste gesondheitskomitee van Johannesburg. **Kleio (S Afr)** 1971;3(2):1–7

**South-East Asia**

A decade of health development in South-East Asia, 1968–1977: New Delhi, NHO Regional Office for South-East Asia, 1978. xx, 418 p.

**Spain**

Arjona Castro A: La poblacion de Córdoba en el siglo XIX. Sanidad y crisis demográfica en la Córdoba decimonónica. Córdoba, Instituto de Historia de Andalucia, Universidad de Córdoba, 1979. 184 p.
Jordi R: Legislación sanitaria marítima española en vigor durante el siglo XIX. **Circ Farm** 1981 Jun;12(139):75–84
Jordi González FR: Notas legislativas sobre los estatutos de autonomia catalanes 1932/1979. **Circ Farm** 1979 Oct;11(119):19–27
Jordi González R: Contribución para el estudio sociológico de la farmacia barcelonesa durante la guerra civil, a través de la prensa política. **Circ Farm** 1984;282:55–62
Jordi González R: Nota sobre higiene ciudadana en la Barcelona de finales del siglo XVIII. **Circ Farm** 1980;12(124):61–4
Miguel JM de: Siete tesis erróneas sobre la política sanitaria española y una alternativa sociológica crítica. **Rev Esp Invest Sociol** 1980;(9):53–80
Parra Hidalgo P, Marset Campos P, Ramos García E, et al: Cincuenta años de la Revista de Sanidad e Higiene Pública (1926–1975). Análisis bibliométrico de su producción científica. **Rev Sanid Hig Publica (Madr)** 1983 Sep–Oct;57(9–10):969–1038
Riera J, Jiménez Muñoz JM: Dos 'ordenanzas' sanitarias de Fernando VI. **Asclepio** 1980;32:389–99
Ruiz–Falcó López F: Escuela Nacional de Sanidad. Problemática pasada, actual y futura. **Rev Sanid Hig Publica (Madr)** 1983 Mar–Apr;57(3–4):359–72
Saiz Moreno L: La Sociedad Española de Higiene (un siglo al servicio de la Salud Pública). **Rev Sanid Hig Publica (Madr)** 1981 Sep–Oct;55(9–10):1073–100

**Switzerland**

Gautier A: Heurs et malheurs politiques d'une loi fédérale sur les épidémies. **Rev Med Suisse Romande** 1980 Dec;100(12):1061–2
Luzi von Scheid C: Ueber die Entwicklung der Sanitätsgesetzgebung in Graubünden. Zürich, Bischofberger, 1970. 48 p. (Diss., Zürich).
Ort–Wädensweiler L: Johann Melchior Aepli: zur Verbesserung des Medizinalwesens in der Schweiz (1783/88). Zürich, Juris Druck, 1984. 70 p. (Zürcher Medizingeschichtliche Abhandlungen, Neue Reihe, Nr. 167).
Poletti R: Il y a 75 ans naissait Le Bon Secours... 1905–1980. **Krankenpflege (Bern)** 1980 Nov;(11):567–9
Scalabrin HR: Heinrich Ludwig Attenhofer, 1783–1856. Arzt und Politiker. Zürich, Juris Druck, 1983. 67 p. (Zürcher Medizingeschichtliche Abhhandlungen, Neue Reihe, Nr. 158).

**Syria**

Drysdale A: The regional equalization of health care and education in Syria since the Ba'thi revolution. **Int J Middle East Stud** 1981;13(1):93–111

**Tanzania**

Beck A: Medicine, tradition, and development in Kenya and Tanzania, 1920–1970. Waltham, Crossroads Press, 1981. viii, 114 p.

**Tunisia**

Ben Yedder W: Enseignement para-médical en Tunisie. L'école professionnelle de la santé publique de Tunis 'Avicenne'. **Tunis Med** 1981 Jan–Feb;59(1):874–5
Gallagher NE: Medicine and power in Tunisia, 1780–1900. Cambridge; New York, Cambridge University Press, 1983. xii, 145 p.

**Turkey**

Becker H: Helmuth von Moltke als Beobachter der hygienischen und medizinischen Situation im osmanischen Kaiserreich (1835–39). In Göpfert W, Otten HH, ed: Metavoeite: wandelt euch durch neues Denken. Düsseldorf, Triltsch, 1983. p. 147–59.

**United States**

History and use of Public Health Service Commissioned Corps: hearing before the Subcommittee on Health and the Environment of the Committee on Energy and Commerce, House of Representatives, Ninety-seventh Congress, session, June 14, 1982. Washington, GPO, 1982. iii, 141 p.
Absher RR: The history of the Indiana State Board of Health from 1922 to 1954. Diss. Indiana University. [Bloomington], 1978. 323 leaves.
Albemarle–Charlottesville Health Department: The history of the Albemarle–Charlottesville Health Department. Charlottesville, Va., Jefferson Printing, 1973. 42 p.
Aldridge WN: Insecticides, past, present and future: practice and the understanding of mechanisms. **Ann Occup Hyg** 1979;22(4):407–9
Alewitz S: Ezra Mundy Hunt--physician, writer, humanitarian. **J Med Soc NJ** 1981 May;78(5):381–5
Alewitz S: Sanitation and public health: Philadelphia, 1870–1900. Ph.D. Diss., Case Western Reserve University. Cleveland, 1981. vii, 421 p.
Alewitz S: The life and times of Camden. **J Med Soc NJ** 1984 Sep;81(9):740–6
Angevine E: History of the National Consumers League, 1899–1979. Washington, The League, 1979. 69 leaves.
Baird ND: A Kentucky physician examines Memphis. **Tenn Hist Q** 1978;37(2):190–202
Barr HH, Barrie FH: Edward G. McGavran: guardian of the body politic. Chapel Hill, School of Public Health, Univ. of North Carolina at Chapel Hill, 1979. xii, 177 p.
Bath CR: Health and environmental problems: the role of the border in El Paso–Ciudad Juarez coordination. **J Interam Stud World Aff** 1982;24(3):375–92
Bernstein NR: The first one hundred years. Essays on the history of the American Public Health Association. Washington, American Public Health Assn., 1972. 97 p.
Bienia RA, Stein E, Bienia BH: United States Public Health Service hospitals (1798–1981)--the end of an era. **N Engl J Med** 1983 Jan 20;308(3):166–8
Blancher DA: Workshops of the bacteriological revolution: a history of the laboratories of the New York City Department of Health, 1892–1912. Ph.D. Diss., City University of New York. New York, 1979. xiv, 311 leaves.
Bowman IA: Prostitution and the medical profession in the nineteenth century. **Bookman** 1982 Jan;9(1):3–9
Brumley WC, Sphon JA: Regulatory mass spectrometry. **Biomed Mass Spectrom** 1981 Sep;8(9):390–6
Buchanan R: Fighting the ubiquitous monarch, disease: the 1866 report on the Sanitary Relations of Kansas. **J Hist Med Allied Sci** 1983 Jan;38(1):78–83
Cannon JE: Rhode Island's health: yesterday, today, tomorrow. **RI Med J** 1979 Aug;62(8):297–307
The carrier state. New York, Arno, 1977. Various paginations. Four reprinted papers on microbiology by William H. Park and George Soper, 1895–1919.:
Cassedy JH: Charles V. Chapin re-visited: an appreciation. **RI Med J** 1983 Jan;66(1):41–4
Chernin E: Two physicians, a landscape architect, and malaria. **Bull NY Acad Med** 1984 Nov;60(9):932–7
Children's Bureau studies: Introduction by W. M. Schmidt. New York, Arno, 1974. Reprinted works by various authors.
Christie J: Mary Elizabeth Switzer. In: Notable American women. The modern period. Cambridge, Mass., Belknap–Harvard Univ. Press, 1980. 4:669–70.
Cobb AB, Riecken WE: Public health in Mississippi. **J Miss State Med Assoc** 1981 Dec;22(12):319–24
Cohen D: Social medicine: amputating the wrong leg. **Work Pap Mag** 1981;8(6):17–20
Cohen S: The mental hygiene movement, the development of personality and the school: the medicalization of American education. **Hist Educ Q** 1983;23(2):123–49
Collingridge D, Douglas J: Three models of policymaking: expert advice in the control of environmental lead. **Soc Stud Sci** 1984 Aug;14(3):343–70
Corgan JX: Richard Owen Currey, a little known intellectual figure of antebellum Tennessee. **East Tenn Hist Soc Publ** 1978;50:58–70
Corn JK: 'Dark as a dungeon': environment and coal miners' health and safety in nineteenth century America. **Environ Rev** 1983;7(3):257–68
Cortes KF: Democracy in the American Public Health Association: a historical analysis. [New York?, s.n.], 1976. 362 leaves.
Curran JA: Founders of the Harvard School of Public Health, with biographical notes, 1909–1946. New York, Josiah Macy, Jr. Foundation, 1970. xviii, 294 p.
Darby WJ: A perspective on food legislation. **Nutr Rev** 1981

Nov;39(11):413-6

Duffy J: Haven Emerson. In Dictionary of American Biography, Suppl. 6, 1956-1960. p. 192-3, 1980.

Duffy J: School vaccination: the precursor to school medical inspection. **J Hist Med Allied Sci** 1978 Jul;33(3):344-55

Duffy J: The American medical profession and public health: from support to ambivalence. **Bull Hist Med** 1979 Spring;53(1):1-22

Dunlap TR: DDT: scientists, citizens, and public policy. Princeton, Princeton University Press, 1981. 318 p.

Dwork D: Health conditions of immigrant Jews on the Lower East Side of New York: 1880-1914. **Med Hist** 1981 Jan;25(1):1-40

Dye D, Tarpey K: Maternity and infant care services in Chicago--retrospectus: our legacy, our challenge. In Smith GF, Smith PN, Vidyasagar D, ed: Historical review and recent advances in neonatal and perinatal medicine. [Chicago?], Mead Johnson Nutritional Division, 1983. Vol. II. p. 139-58.

Eberson F: Eradication of hookworm disease in Florida. **J Fla Med Assoc** 1980 Aug;67(8):736-42

Egan MC: Public health nutrition services: issues today and tomorrow. **J Am Diet Assoc** 1980 Oct;77(4):423-7

Ellis JH: Business leadership in Memphis public health reform, 1880-1900. **West Tenn Hist Soc Pap** 1965;19:94-104

Elmore JA: Frances Elliott Davis. In: Notable American women. The modern period. Cambridge, Mass., Belknap-Harvard Univ. Press, 1980. 4:180-2.

Enarson HL: Perspectives on college health in the 80's: a president's view. **J Am Coll Health Assoc** 1981 Aug;30(1):11-3

Ensley PC: Indiana and the influenza pandemic of 1918. **Indiana Med Hist Q** 1983 Dec;9(4):3-15

Etheridge EW: Grace Arabell Goldsmith. In: Notable American women. The modern period. Cambridge, Mass., Belknap-Harvard Univ. Press, 1980. 4:283-4.

Ettling J: The germ of laziness. Rockefeller philanthropy and public health in the new South. Cambridge, Harvard, 1981. x, 263 p.

Fee E: Competition for the first school of hygiene and public health. **Bull Hist Med** 1983 Fall;57(3):339-63

The first American Medical Association reports on public hygiene in American cities. Twelve reports reprinted from the Transactions of the American Medical Association, Vol. II, 1849. New York, Arno, 197. P. 431-634.:

Fitzpatrick ML: A history of the National Organization for Public Health Nursing, 1912-1952. [New York, N. Y., s. n.], 1973. 3, vi, 451 leaves.

Fitzpatrick SA: Only the poor in a gilded age: public health care for the poor in St. Louis, 1890-1900. Ph.D. diss. Saint Louis University. St. Louis, 1979. 157 leaves.

Flavin TH: The Clinical Center: twenty-five years of research for people. **Conn Med** 1979 Sep;43(9):563-7

Four from '44: the Winslow editorials: **J Public Health Policy** 1980 Mar;1(1):15-24

Fox DM: The decline of historicism: the case of compulsory health insurance in the United States. **Bull Hist Med** 1983 Winter;57(4):596-610

Frank N: From criminal to civil penalties in the history of health and safety laws. **Soc Probl** 1983;30(5):532-44

Freymann JG: The origins of disease orientation in American medical education. **Prev Med** 1981 Nov;10(6):663-73

Galishoff S: Germs know no color line: black health and public policy in Atlanta, 1900-1918. **J Hist Med Allied Sci** 1985 Jan;40(1):22-41

George O: Eskimo medicine man. [Portland], Oregon Historical Society, 1978. xi, 278 p.

Glassberg D: The design of reform: the public bath movement in America. **Am Stud** 1979;20(2):5-21

Goldman HH: Integrating health and mental health services: historical obstacles and opportunities. **Am J Psychiatry** 1982 May;139(5):616-20

Goyan JE: Dr. Harvey Wiley's brainchild, 75 years later. **J Assoc Off Anal Chem** 1981 Mar;64(2):256-9

Goyan JE: FDA at 75--failure, symbiosis, convergence. In Young JH, ed: The early years of federal food and drug control. Madison, American Institute of the History of Pharmacy, 1982. p. 53-60.

Grayson VS: Mary Cromwell Jarrett. In: Notable American women. The modern period. Cambridge, Mass., Belknap-Harvard Univ. Press, 1980. 4:377-9.

Greenberg JH: Bureau of Laboratories created for protection of public health. **Tex Med** 1980 May;76(5):50

Grob GN, ed: Public policy and the problem of addiction: four studies, 1914-1924. New York, Arno Press, 1981. 1 v. (various pagings).

Haggerty L: Nursing revisited: Strong public health nurse leader and educator. **Mass Nurse** 1984 Jul-Aug;54(7):7

Haywood A: The National Health Survey--in the beginning. **Public Health Rep** 1981 May-Jun;96(3):195-9

Health in the southern United States: New York, Arno, 1977. Various paginations. Facsimiles of works by David Ramsay (1790 and 1796), Josiah C. Nott (1847), Edward H. Barton (1851), Wickliffe Rose (1910), Joseph Goldberger (1916).

Heller SA: A Public Health Service wife. Rockville, Printex, 1978. [144] leaves.

Hellman LM: A history and reminiscence of the office of the Deputy Assistant Secretary for Population Affairs, Department of Health, Education and Welfare, 1969-1977. **Bull Hist Med** 1982 Spring;56(1):77-87

Herrick JM: Health care: the dilemma of delivery. **Aztlan** 1979;10:123-7

Higgs R: Edward Franklin Meeker (1943-1980). **Explor Econ Hist** 1981;18(2):209-10

Hildreth PB: Early Red Cross: the Howard Association of New Orleans, 1837-1878. **La Hist** 1979;20(1):77-92

History of the rising costs of the Medicare and Medicaid programs and attempts to control these costs: Washington, U. S. General Accounting Office, 1976. iii, 126 p.

History of the South Dakota State Department of Health (1891-1950): **SD J Med** 1981 May;34(5):67-8

Hornbrook MC: Medicinal drugs: risks and regulations. **Curr Hist** 1980;78(457):201-5, 223-6

Ihde AJ: Food controls under the 1906 act. In Young JH, ed: The early years of federal food and drug control. Madison, American Institute of the History of Pharmacy, 1982. p. 40-50.

In the spirit of C.-E. A. Winslow: **J Public Health Policy** 1980 Mar;1(1):3-5

Jaffe A: Addiction reform in the progressive age: scientific and social responses to drug dependence in the United States, 1870-1930. New York, Arno, 1981. vii, 358 p.

Janssen WF: Food and Drug Administration celebrates 75 years of consumer protection -- an album from the archives. **Public Health Rep** 1981 Nov-Dec;96(6):487-94

Janssen WF: Pharmacy .. and the Food and Drug Law. **Am Pharm** 1981 Apr;21(4):28-36

Janssen WF: The story of the laws behind the labels. **FDA Consum** 1981 Jun;15(5):32-45

Jekel JF: The 'Rainbow Reviews': publications of the National Center for Health Statistics. **J Chronic Dis** 1984;37(9-10):681-8

Jones RL: A note on public health in early Galveston. **Bookman** 1982;9(9):3-7

Kantrov I, Wittenstein K: Mary Sewall Gardner. In: Notable American women. The modern period. Cambridge, Mass., Belknap-Harvard Univ. Press, 1980. 4:262-4.

Katsnel'bogen AG: Dekabristy i peredovaia meditsinskaia obshchestvennost' Rossii. **Sov Zdravookhr** 1980;(10):51-5

Kondratas RA: Biologics Control Act of 1902. In Young JH, ed: The early years of federal food and drug control. Madison, American Institute of the History of Pharmacy, 1982. p. 8-27.

Koplin AN: Anti-smoking legislation: the New Jersey experience. **J Public Health Policy** 1981;2(3):247-55

Kunitz SJ: Underdevelopment, demographic change, and health care on the Navajo Indian Reservation. **Soc Sci Med [Med Psychol Med Sociol]** 1981 Mar;15A(2):175-92

Lady L: Home visits by FNS nurses. **Front Nurs Serv Q Bull** 1980 Winter;56(3):35-41

Leahy PJ, Mazur A: The rise and fall of public opposition in specific social movements. **Soc Stud Sci** 1980 Aug 3;10(3):259-84

Leavitt JW: Health in urban Wisconsin: from bad to better. In Numbers RL, Leavitt JW, ed: Wisconsin medicine. Historical perspectives. Madison, University of Wisconsin Press, 1981. p. 155-75.

Leavitt JW: Politics and public health: small pox in Milwaukee, 1894-1895. In Reverby S, Rosner D, ed: Health care in America. Philadephia, Temple University Press, 1979. p. 84-101.

Leavitt JW: Public Health in Milwaukee 1867-1910. Ph.D. Diss., University of Chicago. Chicago, 1975. 363 leaves.

Leavitt JW: The healthiest city: Milwaukee and the politics of health reform. Princeton, Princeton University Press, 1982. xvii, 294 p.

Lee PR: Health policy and the health of the public. A two hundred year perspective. **Mobius** 1984 Jul;4(3):95-113

Lilienfeld AM: Wade Hampton Frost: contributions to epidemiology and public health. **Am J Epidemiol** 1983 Apr;117(4):379-83

Lohr W: An historical view of the research on the behavioral and organizational factors related to the utilization of health services. [s.l.: s.n.], 1972. 67, 16 leaves.

McClary A: 'Swat the Fly': popular magazines and the anti-fly campaign. **Prev Med** 1982 May;11(3):373-8

Marcus AI: In sickness and in health: the marriage of the municipal corporation to the public interest and the problem of public health, 1820-1870. The case of Cincinnati. Ph.D. diss. University of Cincinnati. Cincinnati, 1979. 379 leaves.

Marcus AI: National history through local social evils and the origin of municipal services in Cincinnati. **Am Stud** 1981;22(2):23-39

Marcus AI: Professional revolution and reform in the Progressive era: Cincinnati physicians and the city elections of 1897 and 1900. **J Urban Hist** 1979;5(2):183-208

Marcus AI: The strange career of municipal health initiatives: Cincinnati and city government in the early nineteenth century. **J Urban Hist** 1980;7(1):3-29

Martin WR, Isbell H, ed: Drug addiction and the U. S. Public Health Service. Proceedings of symposium commemorating the 40th anniversary of the Addiction Research Center at Lexington, Ky. Rockville, Md., National Institute on Drug Abuse, 1978. xiv, 325 p. Historical contributions by R. H. Felix, C. K. Himmelsbach, J. W. Sloan, C. G. Eades, J. F. Maddux, R. L. DuPont, J. H. Jaffe, E. L. May.

Mazur A: The journalists and technology: reporting about Love Canal

and Three Mile Island. **Minerva** 1984 Spring;22(1):45–66
Meeker E: The improving health of the United States, 1850–1915. **Explor Econ Hist** 1972;9(4):353–73
Michael JM, Bender TR: Fighting smallpox on the Texas border: an episode from PHS's proud past. **Public Health Rep** 1984 Nov–Dec;99(6):579–82
Michael JM: The Public Health Service leprosy investigation station on Molokai, Hawaii, 1909–13 -- an opportunity lost. **Public Health Rep** 1980 May–Jun;95(3):203–9
Michigan Department of Public Health: The first 100 years. [Lansing, The Department, 1973?] 116 p.
Milio N: Margaret Gene Arnstein. In: Notable American women. The modern period. Cambridge, Mass., Belknap-Harvard Univ. Press, 1980. 4:37–8.
Miller G, Warriner CK: Professional power and social change at the community level: the case of three prepaid health care programs. **Soc Sci J** 1980;17(3):1–19
Mitchell VL: Louisiana health and the Civil Works Administration. **Red River Val Hist Rev** 1982;7(1):22–32
Models for action: **J Public Health Policy** 1980;1(2):103–9
Moerchel J: Simon Baruch (1840–1921) und die öffentliche Gesundheitspflege in New York. **Medizinhist J** 1982;17(1/2):138–47
Ostenso GL: National Nutrition Monitoring System: a historical perspective. **J Am Diet Assoc** 1984 Oct;84(10):1181–5
Palmer BB: The philosophy of dental health service: its relation to the changing social order. Advice from 1934. **J Am Coll Dent** 1981 Fall;48(3):179–92
Palmer CA: Public health in the South. **Rev Am Hist** 1982;10(2):229–33
Pearlman M: Leonard Wood, William Muldoon and the medical profession: public health and universal military training. **N Engl Q** 1979;52(3):326–44
Pearson EF, Miles W: Disinfection of mail in the United States. **Bull Hist Med** 1980 Spring;54(1):111–24
Peroff K, Podolak-Warren M: Does spending on defence cut spending on health? A time-series analysis of the U. S. economy 1929–74. **Br J Polit Sci** 1979;9(1):21–39
Perry S: Special report. The brief life of the National Center for Health Care Technology. **N Engl J Med** 1982 Oct 21;307(17):1095–100
Phaneuf MM: Sanitation and cholera: Springfield and the 1866 epidemic. **Hist J West Mass** 1980;8(1):26–36
Pivar DJ: Cleansing the nation: the war on prostitution, 1917–21. **Prologue J Nat Arch** 1980;12(1):29–40
Plaut EA, Rubenstein S: State care for the mentally ill: a brief history. **State Gov** 1977;50(4):192–7
Pollard MR: Fostering competition in health care. **Proc Acad Polit Sci** 1980;33(4):158–67
Price DE: John Friend Mahoney. In Dictionary of American Biography, Suppl. 6, 1956–1960. p; 423–4, 1980.
Ptalis P, Porfilio RL: The evolution of a State Department of Health: an example of the shift of the responsibility of health care from the private to the public sector. **Long Term Care Health Serv Adm Q** 1977 Summer;1(2):124–36
Raffel MW: The U. S. health system. New York, Wiley, 1980. ix, 639 p.
Reid JD, Jedlicka D, Lee ES, et al: Trends in black health. **Phylon** 1977;38(2):105–16
Rice DP: Health statistics: past and present. **N Engl J Med** 1981 Jul 23;305(4):219–20
Riley RH: Historical data, Maryland State Department of Health, 1899–1932. **Md State Med J** 1980 Nov;29(11):92–7
Rodgers BL: The great depression, 1929–1940: an era of reform. **Va Nurse** 1984 Spring;52(1):12–3
Rooks JB, Fishman SH: American nurse-midwifery practice in 1976–1977: reflections of 50 years of growth and development. **Am J Public Health** 1980 Sep;70(9):990–6
Rothschild L: FDA's changing role in food safety. **FDA Consum** 1981 Jun;15(5):28–31
Rowthorn AW: A history of the evolution and development of therapeutic recreation services for special populations in the United States from 1918 to 1977. Ph.D. Diss. New York University. New York, 1978. 351 leaves.
Sardell A: Neighborhood health centers and community-based care: federal policy from 1965 to 1982. **J Public Health Policy** 1983 Dec;4(4):484–503
Savitt TL: Politics in medicine: the Georgia Freedmen's Bureau and the organization of health care, 1865–1866. **Civ War Hist** 1982;28(1):45–64
Schwartz JI: Public health: case studies on the origins of government responsibility for health services in the United States. Ithaca, N.Y., Environmental Health Planning Training Program, Dept. of City and Regional Planning, and the Program in Urban and Regional Studies, Cornell University, 1977, 1980 printing. vi, 208 p.
Selections from Public health: reports and papers presented at meetings of the American Public Health Association (1884–1907). New York, Arno, 1977. Various paginations.:
Selections from Public health: reports and papers presented at the meetings of the American Public Health Association (1873–1883). New York, Arno, 1977. Various paginations.:
Selections from the Journal of the Massachusetts Association of Boards of Health (1891–1904). New York, Arno, 1977. Various paginations.:
Shamansky SL, Hamilton WM: Is the public health nurse's bag anachronism? **Nurs Outlook** 1980 Jun;28(6):379–81
Skinsnes AV, Binford CH: Leprosy research and the Public Health Service -- a brief chronological résumé. **Public Health Rep** 1980 May–Jun;95(3):210–2
Small WE: FDA: today's strengths built on turbulent past. **Am Pharm** 1980 Jan;20(1):25–7
Sonnedecker G: Drug standards become official. In Young JH, ed: The early years of federal food and drug control. Madison, American Institute of the History of Pharmacy, 1982. p. 28–39.
Spector B: The great Salk vaccine mess. **Antioch Rev** 1980;38(3):291–303
Speer JB: Pestilence and progress: health reform in Galveston and Houston during the nineteenth century. **Houston Rev** 1980 Fall;2:120–32
The state and public welfare in nineteenth-century America: Five investigations, 1833–1877. New York, Arno, 1976. Various pagings. Reprint of state documents. (Social Problems and Social Policy: The American Experience).
Susser M: The work of George Rosen: observations on a very small sample. **Int J Health Serv** 1980;10(2):323–8
Terris M: The complex tasks of the second epidemiologic revolution. **J Public Health Policy** 1983 Mar;4(1):8–24
Thompson ME: Public health nursing faces challenges in rural health. **Vt Regist Nurse** 1981 May;:7–8, Jul; 3–4
Tokuhata GK, Smith MW: History of health studies around nuclear facilities: a methodological consideration. **Environ Res** 1981 Jun;25(1):75–85
Toppin EA: Alma Cecelia Haupt. In Dictionary of American Biography, Suppl. 6, 1956–1960. p. 283–5, 1980.
Treleven DE: One hundred years of health and healing in rural Wisconsin. In Numbers RL, Leavitt JW, ed: Wisconsin medicine. Historical perspectives. Madison, University of Wisconsin Press, 1981. p. 133–53.
Tunell DN: A regional history of Southern Branch, American Public Health Association. Ed.D. Diss., University of Alabama. University, Alabama, 1977. xv, 694 leaves.
U. S. Bureau of Radiological Health: Legislative history of Radiation control for health and safety act of 1968. Bureau of Radiological Health; Washington: for sale by the Supt. of Docs., U. S. Govt. Print. Off., 1975. 2 v. (ix, 1494 p.).
Viseltear AJ: 'C.-E.A. Winslow and the early years of public health at Yale, 1915–1925'. **Yale J Biol Med** 1982 Mar–Apr;55(2):137–51
Viseltear AJ: Charles-Edward Amory Winslow. In Dictionary of American Biography, Suppl. 6, 1956–1960. p. 701–3, 1980.
Viseltear AJ: John R. Paul and the definition of preventive medicine. **Yale J Biol Med** 1982 May–Aug;55(3–4):167–72
Visiting Nurse Service of Toledo--eighty-three years of caring: **Caring** 1984 Apr;3(4):57–61
Ward RD, Rogers WW: Racial inferiority, convict labor, and modern medicine: a note on the Coalburg affair. **Ala Hist Q** 1982;44(3–4):203–10
Waserman MJ: The emergence of modern child health care: pediatrics, public health, and the federal government. Ph.D. Diss., The Catholic University of America, Washington, D. C., 1982. v, 232 p.
Weingast BR: Consumer product safety. **Curr Hist** 1980;78(457):206–9, 228
Williams MT: New York's public baths: a case study in urban progressive reform. **J Urban Hist** 1981;7(1):49–81
Williams WE: The school physician's notebook: a cameo of William Carlos Williams. In Jones AH, ed: Images of healers. Albany, State University of New York Press, 1983. p. 3–8.
Winslow CE: Health in the twentieth century. New York, Arno, 1977. Reprint of Winslow's The evolution and significance of the modern public health campaign (New Haven, 1923); and Winslow's A city set on a hill: The significance of the health demonstration at Syracuse, New York (Garden City, N. Y., 1934). Various paginations.
The Winslow tradition: **J Public Health Policy** 1984 Sep;5(3):320–6
Wolfe MR: Lucius Polk Brown and progressive food and drug control. Tennessee and New York City 1908–1920. Lawrence, Regents Press of Kansas, 1978. 194 p.
Worth D, Beck AM: Multiple ownership of animals in New York City. **Trans Stud Coll Physicians Phila** 1981 Dec;5(3 no 4):280–300
Yankauer A: Deregulation and the right to life. **Am J Public Health** 1981 Aug;71(8):797–8
Yankauer A: Refugees, immigrants, and the public health. **Am J Public Health** 1982 Jan;72(1):12–4
Yew E: Medical inspection of immigrants at Ellis Island, 1891–1924. **Bull NY Acad Med** 1980 Jun;56(5):488–510
Young JH: Nutritional eccentricities. In Neuberger A, Jukes TH, ed: Human nutrition: current issues and controversies. Lancaster, England, MTP Press, 1982. p. 217–32.
Young JH: The long struggle for the 1906 law. **FDA Consum** 1981 Jun;15(5):12–7
Young JH: 'This greasy counterfeit': butter versus oleomargarine in the United States Congress, 1886 (the Fielding H. Garrison Lecture). **Bull Hist Med** 1979 Fall;53(3):392–414

**USSR**

Akhapkin IA, ed: Leninskie dekrety po zdravookhraneniiu. Moskva, Meditsina, 1980. 510 p.

Akulov KI, Korol'kov AA: Pervaia piateletka strany Sovetov i stanovlenie gosudarstvennogo sanitarnogo nadzora. **Gig Sanit** 1982 Sep;(9):45-8
Aleksandrovskiĭ BN, Shchepetova GA: P. H. Sokolov--vidnyĭ organizator zdravookhraneniia Saratova. **Sov Zdravookhr** 1979;(11):55-9
Alekseev GA, Alekseev VA, Gunin GP: Razvitie sovetskogo zdravookhraneniia v Chuvashii za 60 let avtonomii. **Sov Zdravookhr** 1980;(7):52-4
Alekseev GA, Butsevitskiĭ VS, Galkina ND: Revoliutsionnaia deiatel'nost' vracha A.A. Buĭnovskogo. **Sov Zdravookhr** 1979;(8):54-5
Alekseeva LP: Z. G. Frenkel'. Moskva, Meditsina, 1971. 126 p.
Alexander JT: Bubonic plague in early modern Russia; public health & urban disaster. Baltimore and London, Johns Hopkins University Press, 1980. xviii, 385 p.
Alexander JT: Catherine the great and public health. **J Hist Med Allied Sci** 1981 Apr;36(2):185-204
Alexander JT: Medical professionals and public health in 'Doldrums' Russia (1725-62). **Can Am Slav Stud** 1978;12(1):116-35
Altynbekov MA: Zdravookhranenie Chimkentskoĭ oblasti v dorevoliutsionnyĭ period. **Sov Zdravookhr** 1981;(8):63-5
Altynbekov MA: Zdravookhranenie Chimkentskoĭ oblasti v gody Velikoĭ Otechestvennoĭ voĭny. **Sov Zdravookhr** 1980;(8):51-3
Altynbekov MA: Zdravookhranenie Chimkentskoĭ oblasti v poslevoennyĭ period. **Sov Zdravookhr** 1981;(3):57-9
Arkhangel'skiĭ GV: N. S. Leskov o problemakh zdravookhraneniia (k 150-letiiu so dnia rozhdeniia pisatelia). **Sov Zdravookhr** 1981;(10):63-5
Barsukov MI: Zdravookhranenie v gody Velikoĭ Otechestvennoĭ voĭny 1941-1945. Sbornik dokumentov i materialov. Moskva, Meditsina, 1977. 575 p.
Bazanov VA: Deiatel'nost' Uchenogo meditsinskogo soveta Narodnogo komissariata zdravookhraneniia SSSR v 1937-1941 gg. **Sov Zdravookhr** 1980;(12):57-60
Bazanov VA: Narkomzdrav i organizatsiia meditsinskoĭ nauki. **Sov Zdravookhr** 1983;(7):56-9
Beliatskiĭ DP: K istorii razvitiia zdravookhraneniia BSSR na osnove printsipov leninskoĭ natsional'noĭ politiki KPSS. **Sov Zdravookhr** 1982;(11):57-60
Belitskaia EIa: Gigienicheskie i sotsial'no-gigienicheskie vzgliady S. P. Botkina (k 150-letiiu so dnia rozhdeniia). **Gig Sanit** 1982 Jul;(7):34-8
Belitskaia EIa, Zhuravleva KI: K 60-letiiu Kafedry sotsial'noĭ gigieny i organizatsii zdravookhraneniia Leningradskogo sanitarno-gigienicheskogo meditsinskogo instituta. **Sov Zdravookhr** 1982;(7):61-3
Beloborodova NL: Moskovskiĭ vospitatel'nyĭ dom i ego rol' v istorii zdravookhraneniia Rossii. **Sov Zdravookhr** 1984;(7):58-61
Bokeriia LA: Leninskie dekrety v oblasti zdravookhraneniia. **Anesteziol Reanimatol** 1980 Mar-Apr;(2):3-5
Borisenko NF, Gabovich RD, Goncharuk EI, et al: Osnovnye itogi deiatel'nosti sanitarno-gigienicheskogo fakul'teta Kievskogo meditsinskogo instituta (k 140-letiiu osnovaniia instituta i 50-letiiu osnovaniia fakul'teta. **Gig Sanit** 1982 Oct;(10):48-51
Borisenko NF, Slepushkina II, Proklina TL, et al: Stanovlenie i razvitie sanitarnoĭ sluzhby po gigiene deteĭ i podrostkov na Ukraine (1938-1945 gg.). **Gig Sanit** 1984 Aug;(8):44-8
Borodiĭ NK: A.F. Maslovskiĭ--vydaiushchiĭsia Ukrainskiĭ vrach XVIII v. **Sov Zdravookhr** 1984;(5):70-2
Boziian KA: Razvitie zdravookhraneniia v Nagorno-Karabakhskoĭ Avtonomnoĭ oblasti. **Sov Zdravookhr** 1983;7:69-71
Burenkov SP: Torzhestvo leninskikh ideĭ v zdrakhookhranenii. **Sov Zdravookhr** 1980;(11):3-8
Burenkov SP: 60-letie obrazovaniia SSSR i zadachi Sovetskogo zdravookhraneniia. **Vestn Akad Med Nauk SSSR** 1983;6:5-13
Chechenkina OI: Progress zdravookhraneniia c respublikakh Sredneĭ Azii i Kazakhstane - rezul'tat Leninskoĭ natsional'noĭ politiki. **Sov Zdravookhr** 1982;(11):49-51
Chernov PA: Sanitarno-épidemiologicheskaia sluzhba Kirgizskoĭ SSR. **Gig Sanit** 1982 Dec;(12):43-5
Chikin SIa: Leninskie printsipy okhrany narodnogo zdorov'ia. **Vestn Akad Med Nauk SSSR** 1980;(4):3-9
Chikin SIa: Razvitie zdravookhraneniia SSSR v period mezhdu XXI i XXVI s'ezdami KPSS. **Med Sestra** 1981 Feb;40(2):3-7
Chikin SIa: Sotsial'no-gigienicheskie ideĭ K. Marksa (k 100-letiiu so dnia smerti). **Sov Med** 1983;(3):75-8
Chikin SIa: 60-letie obrazovaniia SSSR i uspekhi razvitiia sovetskogo zdravookhraneniia. **Sov Med** 1982;(12):3-10
Chokin AR, Kabykenov PS: Voprosy zdorav'ia i meditsiny v trudakh izvestnykh Kazakhskikh prosvetiteleĭ. **Sov Zdravookhr** 1983;6:71-4
Dohnány L: L. N. Tolsztoj az egészségügyről. **Orv Hetil** 1982 Aug 8;123(32):1985-8
Dushmanov SKh, Dushmanova TB: Zdravookhranenie Ural'skoĭ oblasti. **Sov Zdravookhr** 1983;6:66-9
Ermolaev MM: Vklad A. N. Marzeeva v stanovlenie i razvitie sanitarnogo prosveshcheniia na Ukraine. **Vrach Delo** 1983 Jan;(1):118-21
Gassiev VI: Iz istorii zdravookhraneniia Iuzhnoĭ Osetii. **Sov Zdravookhr** 1983;(2):61-3
Gassiev VI: Zdravookhranenie Iuzhnoĭ Osetii v gody Velikoĭ Otechestvennoĭ voĭny. **Sov Zdravookhr** 1983;5:55-8
Gavrilov OK: Meditsinskaia nauka k 60-ĭ godoshchine obrazovaniia Soiuza Sovetskikh Sotsialisticheskikh Respublik. **Sov Zdravookhr** 1982;(8):3-8
Gormakh SIa: Razvitie zdravookhraneniia Rovenskoĭ oblasti za gody Sovetskoĭ vlasti. **Vrach Delo** 1979 Nov;(11):1-5
Grando AA, Makarenko IM, Polianskiĭ AA: Kafedre sotsial'noĭ gigieny i organizatsii zdravookhraneniia Kievskogo meditsinskogo instituta--60 let. **Sov Zdravookhr** 1984;(3):52-3
Grando AA, Kogan Via: Rol' Narkomzdrava RSFSR v stanovlenii zdravookhraneniia Sovetskoĭ Ukrainy. **Sov Zdravookhr** 1983;9:55-7
Ianushkevichus ZI, Krikshtopaĭtis MI: O razvitii zdravookhraneniia Litovskoĭ SSR. **Klin Med (Mosk)** 1982 Dec;60(12):38-41
Iarovinskiĭ MI: Zdravookhranenie Moskvy v gody Velikoĭ Otechestvennoĭ voĭny. **Sov Zdravookhr** 1983;(7):63-7
Iarovinskiĭ MIa: 100 let sanitarnoĭ organizatsii goroda Moskvy. **Sov Zdravookhr** 1984;(9):45-9
Ibragimov NG: Rol' obshchestvennosti v deiatel'nosti Ufimskogo gorodskogo Soveta po okhrane zdorov'ia naseleniia v pervye desiatiletiia Sovetskoĭ vlasti. **Sov Zdravookhr** 1981;(2):67-71
Idel'chik KI: A. P. Golubkov: 1880-1945. Moskva, Meditsina, 1980. 78 p.
Il'in AI: S. I. Sychugov--osnovopolozhnik sanitarnoĭ organizatsii Vladimirskoĭ gubernii. **Gig Sanit** 1983 Nov;:(11):53-5
Izmerov NF: 60 let Nauchno-issledovatel'skomu institutu gigieny truda i professional'nykh zabolevaniĭ AMN SSSR. **Gig Tr Prof Zabol** 1983 Jun;(6):1-5
Kadyrov AA: N. A. Semashko v Uzbekistane. **Sov Zdravookhr** 1984;(1):49-50
Kamalov Mkh: Zdravookhranenie Bashkirskoĭ ASSR. **Med Sestra** 1982 Dec;41(12):14-8
Kanep VV: Osnovnye tendentsii razvitiia meditsinskoi nauki i zdravo-okhraneniia latviiskoi SSR. **Latv PSR Zinat Acad Vestis** 1981;3:9-22
Kanep VV: Uspekhi v razvitii zdravookhraneniia Latviĭskoĭ SSR. **Klin Med (Mosk)** 1982 Dec;60(12):33-7
Kaneps V: Padomju latvijas veselibas aizsardzibai 25 gadi. Riga, Izdevnieciba Zvaigzne, 1965. 157 p.
Kas'ianenko AM: Sanitarno-épidemiologicheskaia sluzhba Sovetskoĭ Ukrainy. **Vrach Delo** 1983 Jan;(1):1-6
Kas'ianenko AM: Sanitarno-épidemiologicheskaia sluzhba Ukrainskoĭ SSR. **Gig Sanit** 1982 Dec;(12):22-5
Kasumov TA: Dostizheniia zdravookhraneniia Azerbaĭdzhana za 60 let i perspektivy ego razvitiia. **Sov Zdravookhr** 1980;(4):14-8
Katsnel'bogen AG: Idei Russkogo Prosveshcheniia i formirovanie obshchestvenno-meditsinskoĭ mysli vo vtoroĭ polovine XVIII veka. **Klin Med (Mosk)** 1984 Jan;62(1):146-51
Katsnel'bogen AG: Neizuchennyĭ dokument dekabristov. **Sov Zdravookhr** 1980;(7):60-1
Katsnel'bogen AG: Programmy zdravookhraneniia dekabristov (ot 'Zelenoĭ knigi' do 'Russkoĭ pravdy'). **Klin Med (Mosk)** 1979 Dec;57(12):97-101
Katsnel'bogen AG: Vzgliady P.I. Pestelia na meditsinu. **Klin Med (Mosk)** 1980 Aug;58(8):117-21
Khromchenko OM, Sapegina AV: Dvadtsatipiatletniĭ opyt usovershenstvovaniia rukovodiashchikh kadrov sanitarno-épidemiologicheskoĭ sluzhby v Tsentral'nom institute usovershenstvovaniia vracheĭ. **Gig Sanit** 1981 Mar;(3):51-3
Klantsa OP: Zdravookhranenie na Podolii v period ustanovleniia Sovetskoĭ vlasti. **Sov Zdravookhr** 1983;(3):57-8
Klebanov IaA, Goncharov NP, Chokin AR: Sanitarno-ěpidemiologicheskaia sluzhba Kazakhskoĭ SSR. **Gig Sanit** 1982 Dec;(12):34-7
Knel'ts VF: Pervyĭ s'ezd zemskikh vracheĭ i ego rol' v razvitii zdravookhraneniia Udmurtii. **Sov Zdravookhr** 1981;(7):62-3
Kogan VI, Petrova LF, Tarasenko IV: Slavnaia stranitsa iz istorii sanitarnoĭ organizatsii Ukrainskoĭ SSR (k 60-letiiu sozyva I sessii Sanitarnogo soveta). **Gig Sanit** 1982 Jul;(7):32-4
Kogan VIa: II sessiia Vseukrainskogo tsentral'nogo komiteta i ee znachenie dlia razvitiia zdravookhraneniia Ukrainskoĭ SSR. **Sov Zdravookhr** 1984;(10):51-3
Koroleva LN: Znachenie bratskogo sotrudnichestva Sovetskikh narodov v podgotovke meditsinskikh kradov dlia zdravookhraneniia Kazakhstana (1928-1940). **Sov Zdravookhr** 1983;6:58-62
Korostelev NB: Osnovanie pervykh gigienicheskikh kafedr v Rossii. **Gig Sanit** 1984 Feb;(2):40-4
Kovshilo VE: K 60-letiiu so dnia priniatiia dekreta o sanitarnykh organakh RSFSR. **Gig Sanit** 1982 Sep;(9):4-6
Kozliuk VM, Leonenko NA, Stefanovskaia NV: O razvitii lechebno-profilakticheskoĭ pomoshchi naseleniiu USSR v 1917-1940 gg. **Vrach Delo** 1982 Apr;(4):3-7
Kozubenko ID: Partiĭnye organizatsii Dona vo glave razvitiia zdravookhraneniia v 1923-1924 gg. **Sov Zdravookhr** 1982;(6):56-9
Krotkov FG, Golikov VIa: Gigienicheskaia nauka i klinicheskie distsipliny. **Klin Med (Mosk)** 1982 Dec;60(12):8-15
Krotkov FG: Lenin i sovetskoe zdravookhranenie. **Gig Sanit** 1980 Apr;(4):3-5
Krotkov FG, Golikov VIa: Profilakticheskaia meditsina i gigiena. **Gig Sanit** 1983 Feb;(2):24-8
Kulagin AI: Razvitie zdravookhraneniia Mordovskoĭ ASSR.

Med Sestra 1982 Dec;41(12):18–23
Kusevich GV: Razvitie zadrvookhraneniia v g. Smele. **Med Sestra** 1981 Dec;40(12):3–5
Kuz'min MK: Sovetskaia meditsina na razlichnykh étapakh sotsialisticheskogo stroitel'stva. **Sov Med** 1982;(12):10–6
Kuznetsov DN, Tikhonov AF: V. I. Lenin i sovetskaia meditsina. **Vestn Khir** 1980 Apr;124(4):3–8
Leninskaia zabota o blage naroda: **Vopr Onkol** 1980;26(4):3–9
Levitin MN: Stoĭkiĭ bol'shevik-leninets A. P. Golubkov. **Feldsher Akush** 1980;45(11):44–6
Likhachev AG: Dostizheniia sovetskogo zdravookhraneniia. **Vestn Otorinolaringol** 1982 Nov–Dec;(6):3–8
Lisitsyn IuP: V. I. Lenin i sovremennye voprosy sotsial'noĭ gigieny. **Zdravookhr Ross Fed** 1980;(4):3–9
Lotova EI, Egorysheva IV: Gigienist i obshchestvennyĭ deiatel' I. V. Bertenson (k 150–letiiu so dnia rozhdeniia). **Sov Zdravookhr** 1984;(1):57–60
Maĭboroda VS: Sanitarno–épidemiologicheskaia sluzhba Tadzhikskoĭ SSR. **Gig Sanit** 1982 Sep;(9):15–6
Makovoz AA, Gorskiĭ AN: Muzei istorii meditsiny i zdravookhraneniia Kirovogradskoĭ oblasti. **Feldsher Akush** 1983;48(1):52–4
Makovoz AA: O. A. Iunevich - vidnyĭ zemskiĭ vrach. **Sov Zdravookhr** 1984;(1):64–7
Malozemova AI: Revoliutsionery–mediki Pribylevy. **Sov Zdravookhr** 1984;(8):62–5
Manafov IT: Rol' Narkomzdrava Azerbaĭdzhanskoĭ SSR v stanovlenii Sovetskogo zdravookhraneniia v respublike. **Sov Zdravookhr** 1984;(5):67–70
Mareĭ AN: 50 Let pervogo vypuska sanitarnykh vracheĭ. **Gig Sanit** 1982 Jul;(7):38–40
Medzhidov BF: Istoriia Nauchno–issledovatel'skogo instituta virusologii, mikrobiologii i gigieny imeni G. M. Musabekova. Baku, Azerbaidzhanskoe gos. izd–vo, 1968. 183 p.
Mikirtichan GL: Iu. A. Mendeleva––vidnyĭ organizator sovetskogo zdravookhraneniia (1883–1959). **Sov Zdravookhr** 1983;(11):59–62
Miliavskiĭ VM: Obshchestvo poltavskikh vracheĭ i 'Trudy post oiannoĭ meditsinskoĭ komissii pri Poltavskoĭ gubernnskoĭ zemskoĭ uprave'. **Sov Zdravookhr** 1981;(4):69–71
Miliavskiĭ VM: Znachenie 'Trudov postoiannoĭ meditsinskoĭ komissii pri Poltavskoĭ gubernskoĭ zemskoĭ uprave' dlia razvitiia zemskoĭ meditsiny v Rossii. **Sov Zdravookhr** 1984;(4):63–5
Mozhaev VP: Sanitarnye biulleteni o V. V. Maiakovskom. **Feldsher Akush** 1983 Dec;48(12):36–8
Nosal' VI: Muzeĭ istorii zdravookhraneniia goroda. **Sov Zdravookhr** 1983;(4):44–5
Novoselov VI: Razvitie zakonodatel'stva o narodnom zdravookhranenii. **Sov Zdravookhr** 1980;(6):3–7
Ordabekov S: Zdravookhranenie Dzhambulskoĭ oblasti v dorevoliutsionnyĭ period. **Sov Zdravookhr** 1982;(4):64–5
Ovchinnikov NM, Timchenko GF: Dvadtsatiletniĭ opyt raboty Tsentral'nogo nauchno–issledovatel'skogo kozhnovenerologicheskogo instituta Minzdrava SSR po kontroliu i uluchsheniiu kachestva serologicheskikh laboratorii dermatovenerologicheskikh uchrezhdeniĭ SSSR. **Lab Delo** 1981;(2):120–2
Palkin BN: Gubernskaia reforma 1775 g. i organizatsiia grazhdanskoĭ meditsiny v Rossii. **Sov Zdravookhr** 1983;9:66–70
Palkin BN: Reformy v oblasti organizatsii meditsinskogo dela v Rossii kontsa XVII veka. **Sov Zdravookhr** 1981;(3):67–70
Palkin BN: S. S. Andreevskiĭ v Astrakhani. **Sov Zdravookhr** 1981;(6):66–8
Palkin BN: V. N. Tatishchev i zdravookhranenie Astrakhanskoĭ gubernii. **Sov Zdravookhr** 1982;(4):65–8
Panzer D: Zur historischen Entwicklung des Objektverständnisses der Sozialhygiene während der Entstehung der sozialistischen Gesellschaft am Beispiel der UdSSR. **Z Gesamte Hyg** 1983 Oct;29(10):581–4
Penishkevich IF, Svitun VD: Razvitie zdravookhraneniia za gody Sovetskoĭ vlasti na Bukovine. **Vrach Delo** 1983 Mar;(3):1–4
Perfil'ev GN: Zemskaia meditsina v Krymu. **Sov Zdravookhr** 1981;(1):63–6
Petrovskiĭ BV: 60 let sovetskogo zdravookshraneiia. Moskva, Meditsina, 1977. 414 p.
Petrovskiĭ KS, Novikov IV: Zhurnalu 'Gigiena i sanitariia' 60 let. **Gig Sanit** 1982 Aug;(8):4–7
Petrowskij KS, Novikov JV: 60 Jahre 'Gigiena i sanitarija'. **Z Gesamte Hyg** 1983 Sep;29(9):564–5
Piatak OA, Perekhrestenko PM, Sadovskaia AG: Programma issledonvaniĭ po istorii meditsiny i ee znachenie dlia dal'neĭshego razvitiia zdravookhraneniia, meditsinskogo obrazovaniia i meditsinskoĭ nauki v USSR. **Vrach Delo** 1981;(4):7–10
Pivchenko AG: Sanitarno–épidemiologicheskaia sluzhba Belorusskoĭ SSR. **Gig Sanit** 1982 Dec;(12):29 31
Podolyan VY: Development of medico–geographical ideas in the epoch of the developed socialism and scientific and technological progress. **Geogr Med** 1984;14:284–93
Pogosian UG: Sanitarno–ĕpidemiologicheskaia sluzhbar Armianskoĭ SSR. **Gig Sanit** 1982 Dec;(12):37–40
Poliak VE: Voprosy okhrany zdorov'ia naroda v trudakh V. I. Lenina. **Feldsher Akush** 1980;45(4):5–7
Popushoĭ EP, Ioksa VA: N. A. Doroshevskiĭ - peredovoĭ vrach, uchastnik revoliutsionne–demokraticheskogo dvizheniia. **Sov Zdravookhr** 1982;(11):55–7
Popushoĭ EP, Ioksa VA: Vklad nauchnykh meditsinskikh obshchestv Moldavskoĭ SSR v razvitie narodnogo zdravookhraneniia. **Sov Zdravookhr** 1984;(8):54–7
Portulov BM: Torzhestvo ideĭ V. I. Lenina v meditsine. **Sov Med** 1980;(4):3–9
Potulov BM: Leninskaia zabota o zdorov'e naroda. **Sov Zdravookhr** 1980;(3):3–8
Potulov BM: Leninskie zavety meditsinskim rabotnikam. **Voen Med Zh** 1980 Jan;(1):11–4
Potulov BM: V. I. Lenin and public health. **Sante Publique (Bucur)** 1981;24(1):3–12
Potulov BM: V. I. Lenin o sotsial'noĭ obuslovlennosti zdorov'ia i zdravookhraneniia. **Sov Zdravookhr** 1984;(4):3–10
Potulov BM: Vrach–bol'shevik (k 110–ĭ godovshchine so dnia rozhdeniia D.I. Ul'ianova). **Voen Med Zh** 1984 Aug;(8):69–70
Potulov BM: Vydaiushchiĭsia teoretik i organizator sovetskogo zdravookhraneniia (k 110–ĭ godovshchine so dnia rozhdeniia N. A. Semashko). **Voen Med Zh** 1984 Sep;(9):65–8
Raskin BV: Razrabotka V. I. Leninym programmnykh zadach partii v oblasti zdravookhraneniia. **Zdravookhr Ross Fed** 1980;(4):9–13
Riatsen VI: Uspekhi zdravookhraneniia Estonii. **Sov Zdravookhr** 1982;(11):12–5
Rinchindorzh TS, Tuméngur Z: Pomoshch' Sovetskogo Soiuza v razvitii zdravookhraneniia Mongol'skoĭ Narodnoĭ Respubliki. **Sov Zdravookhr** 1981;(8):59–62
Romanenko AE: V.I. Lenin i zdravookhranenie Sovetskoĭ Ukrainy. **Vrach Delo** 1980 Mar;(3):1–7
Roshchin AV: 100–letie Ustava Moskovskogo gigienicheskogo obshchestva. **Gig Sanit** 1982;(5):48–9
Rumiantsev GI, Korostelev NB: Osnovanie kafedry gigieny v Moskovskom universitete (K 100–letiiu kafedry). **Gig Sanit** 1984 Aug;(8):41–4
Rusiaev AP: Znachenie dekreta o sanitarnykh organakh respubliki dlia razvitiia sanitarno–épidemiologicheskoĭ sluzhby v Belorusskoĭ SSR. **Gig Sanit** 1982 Sep;(9):12–4
Ryzhakova GI: Itogi vypolneniia direktiv Dal'kraĭkoma VKP(b) po stroitel'stvu ob'ektov zdravookhraneniia v gody pervykh piatiletok (1928–1937). **Sov Zdravookhr** 1982;(8):55–7
Savchenko NE: Druzhba narodov i zdravookhranenie Belorussii. **Sov Zdravookhr** 1982;(12):19–22
Savel'ev VN: Zdravookhranenie Udmurtii za 60 let Sovetskoĭ vlasti. **Med Sestra** 1982 Dec;41(12):23–30
Savel'ev VN: 60 let zdravookhraneniia avtonomii Udmurtii. **Sov Zdravookhr** 1981;(4):53–9
Serdiuk AM: Leninskim putem k novym sversheniiam. **Vrach Delo** 1980 Apr;(4):1–7
Serenko AF, Ermakov VV: S. V. Kurashov––vydaiushchiĭsia deiatel' sovetskogo zdravookhraneniia. **Sov Zdravookhr** 1980;(10):45–8
Sergeev VM, Levin AB: Sovetskoe zdravookhranenie v kanun 60–letiia obrazovaniia SSSR. **Grudn Khir** 1982 Nov–Dec;(6):5–8
Shandala MG, Vaĭnrub EM, Kliuzko AS: Edinstvo gigienicheskoĭ nauki i praktiki––osnovnoĭ printsip deiatel'nosti instituta (k 50–letiiu Kievskogo NII obshcheĭ i kommunal'noĭ gigieny im. A. N. Marzeeva). **Gig Sanit** 1981 Oct;(10):45–7
Shandala MG, Kogan VIa: Ot zemskogo sanitarnogo vracha do akademika (k 100–letiiu so dnia rozhdeniia A. N. Marzeeva). **Gig Sanit** 1983 Oct;(10):43–5
Shandala MG: Ozdorovlenie okruzhaiushcheĭ sredy––put' k obshchestvennomu zdorov'iu (k 50–letiiu Kievskogo NII obshcheĭ i kommunal'noĭ gigieny im. A. N. Marzeeva). **Vrach Delo** 1981 Sep;(9):1–5
Sharipov MK: Opyt raboty i dostizheniia sanitarno–épidemiologicheskoĭ sluzhby Uzbekskoĭ SSR. **Gig Sanit** 1982 Dec;(12):31–3
Shishkin AP: Bor'ba s detskoĭ smertnost'iu v pervye gody Sovetskoĭ vlasti. **Sov Zdravookhr** 1981;(12):46–50
Shishkin AP: Organizatsiia Narodnykh komissariatov zdravookhraneniia RSFSR i drugikh soiuznykh respublik (1918–1922) (K 65–letiiu sozdaniia Narodnogo komissariata zdravookhraneniia RSFSR). **Sov Zdravookhr** 1983;(8):47–51
Shishkin AP: Pervyĭ piatiletniĭ plan razvitiia zdravookhraneniia strany Sovetov. **Sov Zdravookhr** 1980;(9):46–9
Shishkin AP: Vazhnyĭ étap v stanovlenii sovetskogo zdravookhraneniia. **Sov Zdravookhr** 1983;(1):57–61
Shishkin AP: Voprosy profilaktiki v deiatel'nosti Gosudarstvennogo Instituta Sotsial'noĭ Gigieny Narkomzdrava RSFSR (k 65–letiiu obrazovaniia N rodnogo Komissariata Zdravookhraneniia RSFSR). **Sov Zdravookhr** 1983;6:55–8
Shitskova AP, Novikov IV, Borisenkova RV, et al: Stanovlenie sanitarnoĭ sluzhby RSFSR. **Gig Sanit** 1982 Sep;(9):6–11
Sidorenko GI: Dostizheniia i perspektivy razvitiia sovetskoĭ gigienicheskoĭ nauki. **Gig Sanit** 1982 Dec;(12):4–9
Sidorenko GI: K 50–letiiu Instituta obshcheĭ i kommunal'noĭ gigieny im. A. N. Sysina AMN SSSR. **Gig Sanit** 1981 Oct;(10):41–5
Sidorenko GI: Razvitie obshcheĭ i kommunal'noĭ gigieny v SSSR za 60 let. **Gig Sanit** 1982 Sep;(9):17–21
Sivolob NI: Rol' A. N. Marzeeva v razvitii otechestvennoĭ gigieny (k 100–letiiu so dnia rozhdeniia). **Sov Zdravookhr** 1983;(8):54–6

Solov'eva VA, ed: Zhizn' deiatel'nost' Z. P. Solov'eva. Moskva, Meditsina, 1980. 205 p.
Strukov AI, Paukov VS, Kazantseva IA: Druzhba i edinstvo narodov SSSR - zalog uspekhov narodnogo zdravookhraneniia. **Arkh Patol** 1982;44(11):3-16
Szymanski A: On the uses of disinformation to legitimize the revival of the cold war: health in the U.S.S.R. **Sci Soc** 1981-82;45(4):453-74
Ternovoĭ KS: V. I. Lenin i okhrana zdorov'ia naroda. **Klin Khir** 1980 Apr;(4):1-7
Tesler DB: Dostizheniia sanitarnoi sluzhby Turkmenistana. **Gig Sanit** 1982 Nov;(11):45-7
Tesler DB: Razvitie i dal'neĭshee sovershenstvovanie sanitarno-épidemiologicheskoĭ sluzhby Turkmenskoĭ SSR. **Gig Sanit** 1982 Dec;(12):40-3
Tikotin MA: Voprosy obshchestvennoĭ gigieny na s'ezdakh russkikh estestvoispytateleĭ i vracheĭ. **Gig Sanit** 1981 Oct;(10):55-8
Treĭman VV: F. G. Mukhamed'iarov--organizator Sovetskogo zdravookhraneniia v Tatarii. **Sov Zdravookhr** 1983;(7):71-2
Tsaregorodtsev GI, Anokhin AM: V. I Lenin i problemy okhrany zdorov'ia cheloveka v razvitom sotsialisticheskom obshchestve. **Ter Arkh** 1980;52(4):3-7
Tumendemberel T: The present situation and the experiment of the primary medical assistance development in the Mongolian People's Republic. **Sante Publique (Bucar)** 1979;22(1):3-13
Vasil'ev KG, Vasil'ev KK: Vrach-revoliutsioner V. L. Elin. **Sov Zdravookhr** 1983;(8):57-8
Vasil'ev KK: K istorii zhurnala 'Gigiena i sanitariia'. **Gig Sanit** 1982 Sep;(9):51-2
Vasil'ev KK: Rol' A. N. Sysina v organizatsii i provendenii vserossiĭskikh (vsesoiuznykh) s'ezdov bakteriologov, epidemiologov i sanitarynykh vracheĭ. **Gig Sanit** 1980 Apr;(4):31-3
Vasil'ev KK: Rol' nauchnykh s'ezdov v nauchnoĭ meditsinskoĭ informatsii (iz istorii vserossiĭskikh i vsesoiuznykh s'ezdov bakteriologov, épidemiologov i sanitarnykh vracheĭ, 1918-1928 gg.) **Sov Zdravookhr** 1980;(6):58-60
Vasil'ev KK: U istokov sanitarno-épidemiologicheskoĭ sluzhby sovetskogo zdravookhraneniia. **Med Sestra** 1983 Mar;42(3):46-8
Vavilin PA: A. P. Dobroslavin--ego obshchestvennaia i prakticheskaia deiatel'nost' (k 140-letiiu so dnia rozdeniia). **Gig Sanit** 1982 Sep;(9):53-6
Vavilin PA: Gigienicheskie prognozy v trudakh A. P. Dobroslavina. **Gig Sanit** 1980 May;(5):25-9
Vavilin PA: Rol' A. P. Dobroslavina v stanovlenii otechestvennoĭ gigienicheskoĭ nauki (k 90-letiiu so dnia smerti). **Gig Sanit** 1980 Mar;(3):45-7
Viduta VK: Tobol'skaia fel'dsherskaia shkola i ee rol' v formirovanii revoliutsionerov. **Sov Zdravookhr** 1984;(8):57-9
Vladimirova LB: Sotsial'nye problemy meditsiny i gigieny na VII s'ezde russkikh estestvoispytateleĭ i vracheĭ. **Sov Zdravookhr** 1984;(1):54-7
Vovk IG: Meropriiatiia KPSS po razvitiiu nardonogo zdravookhraneniia v predvoennye gody. **Voen Med Zh** 1980 Jun;(6):18-20
Vovk IG: Sovetskoe zdravookhranenie v gody pervykh piatiletok. **Voen Med Zh** 1981 Oct;(10):10-2
Zakharov FG, Medik VA: Razvitie zdravookhraneniia v Novgorodskoĭ gubernii v 1864-1917 gg. **Sov Zdravookhr** 1982;(7):59-61
Zakharov FG, Medik VA, Bazylev AE: Stanovlenie zdravookhraneniia Novgorodskoĭ gubernii (1917-1927). **Sov Zdravookhr** 1983;(1):68-71
Zakharov FG, Medik VA, Bazylev AE: Zdravookhranenie Novgorodskoĭ oblasti v poslevoennyĭ period. **Sov Zdravookhr** 1983;(4):53-5
Zavalishchenko LI: Podgotovka seriinogo dokumental'nogo izdaniia. **Sov Arkh** 1977;(3):78-81
Zhukova LA: Narkomzdrav RSFSR v bor'be s detskoĭ besprizornost'iu (1917--1935). **Sov Zdravookhr** 1980;(4):61-3
Zhurnalu 40 let: **Sov Zdravookhr** 1982;(6):3-7
Zuev AI, Sergienko VI: V. I. Lenin--organizator sovetskogo zdravookhraneniia. **Zh Ushn Nos Gorl Bolezn** 1980 Jan-Feb;1:1-6

**Venezuela**

Iriarte DR: [Public health in Venezuela]. **Rev Soc Venez Hist Med** 1975-76;23(37):107-21

**Yugoslavia**

Berber S: Istorija zdravstvene kulture u Somboru. Sombor, Dispanzer za kardiovaskularne bolesti, 1980. 95 p.
Djuretić V: Socijalno-zdravstvena i kulturno-prosvjetna aktivnost organa vlasti u bosñi i hercegovini izmedju drugog i trećeg zasjedanja zavnobih-a. **God Drus Istor Bosne Herceg** 1976;21-27:239-67
Dragić M: Dr. Vladan Djordjević i zakon o zaštiti narodnog zdravlja u Srbiji iz 1881. godine. **Srp Arh Celok Lek** 1982 Jun;110(6):791-8
Dragić M: Zdravstvene prilike u Beogradu za vreme okupacije u prvom svetskom ratu i spanski grip 1918-1919. godine. **Srp Arh Celok Lek** 1980 Sep;108(9):969-74
Dyck RG: Health care planning in Slovenia. **Pap Slov Stud** 1977;105-23
Krajinović S: Povodom stogodišnjice jednog izveštaja dr Vladana Djordjevića objavljenog y 'Srpskom Arhivu' 1883. godine. **Srp Arh Celok Lek** 1983 Jul;111(7):1005-8
Lukić D: O narodnom zdravlju u delima Svetozara markovića. **Srp Arh Celok Lek** 1981 Apr;109(4):579-86
Marjanović V: Zdravstvena kultura Kragujevca u XIX veku. Kragujevac, Farmacija, 1979. 301 p.
Milošević P: Organizacija i razvoj partizanske zdravstvene službe u crnoj gori 1941-1942. godine. **Istor Zapisi** 1969;22(4):521-52
Rakić L: Prilog proučuvanju zdravstvenih prilika u Backoj posle revolucije 1848-1849. **Naucni Sastanak Zb Rad Naucno Drus Istor Zdrav Kult Jugosl** 1980;21:149-52
Stahan J, Jurković P: Materijalni položaj zdravstvene djelatnosti u Zagrebu u razdoblju od godine 1968-1980. **Ekon Pregl** 1982;33(3-4):137-53

**Zaire**

Janssens PG: The colonial legacy: health and medicine in the Belgian Congo. **Trop Doct** 1981 Jul;11(3):132-40

# QUACKERY

See also **Folk and Popular Medicine; Magic and Occult; Therapeutic Cults**

Berges PH: Mäusedreck für Pfeifer... Der Apotheker und die Substitution. Ein kleines Mosaik. **Dtsch Apoth Ztg** 1981 Jan 8;121(2):53-9
Caballero O: De milagros, medicina onírica y curanderos. **Rev Enferm** 1982 Sep;5(50):64-6
Jago JD: Early dental charlatans and quacks. **Bull Hist Dent** 1984 Oct;32(2):118-25
Rolls R: Bark, blisters and the bathe: some problems of pain relief in former times. **J R Soc Med** 1982 Oct;75(10):812-9

**Belgium**

Homblé AG: Het keisnijden. Kwakzalverij of werkelijkheid? **Oostvlaam Zanten** 1980;55:105-14

**Great Britain**

Matthews LG: Italian charlatans in England. **Pharm Hist (London)** 1979 Apr;9(1):2-4

**Before 500 A.D.**

**Greco-Roman**

Kudlien F: Schaustellerei und Heilmittelvertrieb in der Antike. **Gesnerus** 1983;40(1-2):91-8

**500 A.D.-1450**

**France**

Aron E: Louis XI et ses guérisseurs. Chambray, C. L. D., [1983]. 197 p.

**1450-1700**

**Great Britain**

McConchie RW: Additions to OED from John Cotta's Ignorant Practisers of Physicke, 1612. **Notes Queries** 1981 Dec;28(6):490-3
McCray Beier L: The creation of the medical fringe 1500-1700. **Soc Soc Hist Med Bull (Lond)** 1981 Dec;29:29-31
Proust J: Francis Anthonie, charlatan elisabéthain. In: Devins et charlatans au temps de la Renaissance. ed. M.T. Jones-Davies. Paris, Université, Centre de Recherches sur la Renaissance, 1979. p. 101-11.
Walton MT: Thomas Forestier and the 'False Lechys' of London. **J Hist Med Allied Sci** 1982 Jan;37(1):71-3

**Ireland**

Arnold LJ: Valentine Greatrakes, a seventeenth-century 'touch-doctor'. **Eire Irel** 1976;11:3-12

**1700 to Present**

Herman JR: Rejuvenation: Brown-Sequard to Brinkley: monkey glands to goat glands. **NY State J Med** 1982 Nov;82(12):1731-9
Hoffman JH: Dentistry is quack-less. **CAL** 1982 Apr;45(10):18-21
Keene BE: Portrait of a man protected against cholera. **J Hist Med Allied Sci** 1982 Oct;37(4):439
Mertz DP: 100 Jahre Gicht: Von Scharlatanerie und Hypotheses zur gezielten Therapie. **Fortschr Med** 1982 Apr 15;100(14):636-44
Whorton J: 'Thialion!!!' Anatomy of a pseudo-ethical proprietary. **Pharm Hist** 1981;23(3):114-25

# QUACKERY

**Australia**

Forster FM: B. Fawcett, a nineteenth-century Australian quack doctor. **J R Aust Hist Soc** 1981;67(3):272-82
Forster FM: Benjamin Fawcett, a 19th century Australian quack-doctor. In: International Congress of the History of Medicine, 26th, Plovdiv (Bulgaria), 1978. Actes du Congres, Vol. 1. Sofia, 1980. p. 111-2.
Phillips PJ: Kill or cure? Lotions, potions, characters & quacks of early Australia. Adelaide, Rigby, 1978. 157 p.

**Belgium**

Havelange C: Médecine traditionnelle ou exercice illégal de l'art de guérir? Les empiriques liégeois au dix-neuvième siècle. **Rev Med Liege** 1983 Nov 15;38(22):860-8

**France**

Ramsey M: Sous le régime de la législation de 1803: trois enquêtes sur les charlatans au XIVe siècle. **Rev Hist Mod Contemp** 1980 Jul-Sept;27:485-500

**Great Britain**

Brown PS: Mesmerism, galvanism and quackery. **Bristol Med Chir J** 1983 Apr;98(366):61-4
Hambridge RA: 'Empiricomany, or an infatuation in favour of Empiricism or Quackery': the socio-economics of eighteenth-century quackery. In S. Soupel, R. A. Hambridge: Literature and science and medicine. Los Angeles, William Andrews Clark Memorial Library, UCLA, 1982. p. 45-102.

**Ireland**

Cassidy M, Jacobs A, Bresnihan B: The use of unproven remedies for rheumatoid arthritis in Ireland. **Ir Med J** 1983 Nov;76(11):464-5

**United States**

Arata LA: Nostalgia: the medicine show. **J Indiana State Med Assoc** 1980 Jun;73(6):353
Arseneau JC, Thigpen JT: The new quack--pseudoscience, public relations and politics. **J Miss State Med Assoc** 1981 Aug;22(8):202-7
Baker HC: Patent medicine in Pennsylvania before 1906: a history through advertising. **Pa Folklife** 1977-78;27(2):20-33
Boatman BE: On American nostrum making and quackery. **J Okla State Med Assoc** 1982 Jan;75(1):3-7
Ferry AP, Ferry MK: Dr. Isaac Thompson and his celebrated eye water. **Ophthalmology** 1984 May;91(5):528-37
Heindel ND, Foster NI: Medicine, music and 'Money' Munyon. **Pa Folklife** 1982;32(1):44-8
Herman JR: Operating furniture. 'Medical briefs'. **Urology** 1981 Sep;18(3):295 H
Janssen WF: Cancer quackery: past and present. **FDA Consum** 1977 Jul-Aug;11(6):27-32
Janssen WF: The gadget quacks. **FDA Consum** 1977 Feb;11(1):4-11
Japp PM: Pioneer medicines: doctors, nostrums, and folk cures. **J West** 1982 Jul;21(3):15-22
Kardinal CG: Laetrile in historical perspective. **Mo Med** 1980 Sep;77(9):564-9
Kaufman M: 'Step right up, ladies and gentlemen...': Patent medicines in 19th-century America. **Am Hist Illus** 1981;16(5):38-45
Keeney EB, Lederer SE, Minihan EP: Sectarians and scientists: alternatives to orthodox medicine. In Numbers RL, Leavitt JW, ed: Wisconsin medicine. Historical perspectives. Madison, University of Wisconsin Press, 1981. p. 47-74.
Lerner IJ: The whys of cancer quackery. **Cancer** 1984 Feb 1;53(3 Suppl):815-9
Massie LB: Celebrated celery city quacks. **Mich Hist** 1982;66(5):16-23
Miller NJ, Howard-Ruben J: Unproven methods of cancer management part I: background and historical perspectives. **Oncol Nurs Forum** 1983 Fall;10(4):46-52
Pollack CV: Electronic therapeutics of Albert Abrams, M.D. **Pharm Hist** 1984;26(2):109-13
Snow LF: Con men and conjure men: a ghetto image. In Jones AH, ed: Images of healers. Albany, State University of New York Press, 1983. p. 45-78.
Stage S: Female complaints: Lydia Pinkham and the business of women's medicine. New York, Norton, 1979. 304 p.
Stoehr T: Hawthorne's mad scientists: Pseudoscience and social science in nineteenth-century life and letters. Hamden, Conn., Shoestring Press, 1978. 313 p.
Thomas SJ: Nostrum advertising and the image of woman as invalid in late Victorian America. **J Am Cult** 1982 Fall;5(3):104-12
Tyler VE: Damiana - history of a herbal hoax. **Pharm Hist** 1983;25(2):55-60
Tyler VE: Three proprietaries and their claim as American 'Indian' remedies. **Pharm Hist** 1984;26(3):146-9
White JS: The Hedden's Store handbook of proprietary medicines. Portland, Durham & Downey, 1974. 94 p.
Young JH: American health quackery: an historical view. **Ga J Sci** [1979?];38:33-40
Young JH: Laetrile in historical perspective. In Markle GE, Petersen JC, ed: Politics, science and cancer: the laetrile phenomenon. Boulder, CO. Westview Press, for American Association for the Advancement of Science, Washington, D. C., 1980. p. 11-60.
Young JH, Stitt RS: Nutrition quackery. Upholding the right to criticize. **Food Technol** 1981 Dec;:42-7
Young JH: Nutritional eccentricities. In Neuberger A, Jukes TH, ed: Human nutrition: current issues and controversies. Lancaster, England, MTP Press, 1982. p. 217-32.
Young JH: Nutritional quackery. **Assoc Food Drug Off Q Bull** 1983 Jan;47:3-11
Young JH: Self-dosage medicine in America, 1906 and 1981. **South Atl Q** 1981 Autumn;80(4):379-90
Young JH: 'The foolmaster who fooled them'. **Yale J Biol Med** 1980 Nov-Dec;53(6):555-66
Young JH: The regulation of health quackery. **Pharm Hist** 1984;26(1):3-12
Zorgniotti AW: The Civiale Remedial Agency. Urologic quackery in the gay nineties. **Urology** 1981 Jan;17(1):109-12

# RACE

See also **Genetics and Heredity; Jews; Blacks**

Bernard J: Le sang et l'histoire. Paris, Buchet/Chastel, 1983. 157 p.
Gould SJ: The mismeasure of man. New York, London, W.W., Norton & Co., 1981. 352 p.
Herrmann B: Zur Entstehung und Wirkung ästhetischer Prinzipien in der menschlichen Rassenkunde. In Imhof AE, ed: Leib und Leben in der Geschichte der Neuzeit. Berlin, Duncker & Humblot, 1983. p. 165-75.
Hinton RJ: Relationships between mandibular joint size and craniofacial size in human groups. **Arch Oral Biol** 1983 Jan;28(1):37-43
Johnston FE, Selby H: Anthropology: the biocultural view. Dubuque, Iowa, Brown, 1978. Historical sections, p. 73-80, 125-213, 270-275.
Rassengeschichte der Menscheit: 7 vols. Vol. 1 ed. by K. Saller; Vols. 2-7 ed. by I. Schwidetzky. München und Wien, R. Oldenbourg Verlag, 1968-1979. Continuing.
Reyment RA: Moors and Christians: an example of multivariate analysis applied to human blood-groups. **Ann Hum Biol** 1983 Nov-Dec;10(6):505-21
Vora E: Evolution of race: a synthesis of social and biological concepts. **J Black Stud** 1981;12(2):182-91
Watts ES: The biological race concept and diseases of modern man. In Rothschild H, ed: Biocultural aspects of disease. New York, Academic Press, 1981. p. 3-23.

**Americas**

Milner GR: Epidemic disease in the postcontact southeast: a reappraisal. **Midcont J Archaeol** 1980;5(1):39-56

**Canada**

Larocque R: Les maladies chez les Iroquoiens pré-historique. **Rech Amerindiennes Que Bull Inf** 1980;10(3):165-80

**France**

Guy Y: Sur les origines possibles de la ségrégation des Cagots. **Hist Sci Med** 1983;17(1):85-93

**United States**

Cooper R: A note on the biologic concept of race and its application in epidemiologic research. **Am Heart J** 1984 Sep;108(3 Pt 2):715-22
Houck PW: A vanishing tribe: the Monacan Indians of Virginia. **Va Med** 1983 May;110(5):332-4
Mathes VS: Native American women in medicine and the military. **J West** 1982;21(2):41-8

**500 A.D.-1450**

Friedman JB: The monstrous races in medieval art and thought. Cambridge, London, Harvard University Press, 1981. xiii, 268 p.

**1450-1700**

**Peru**

Cook ND: Population data for Indian Peru: sixteenth and seventeenth centuries. **Hisp Am Hist Rev** 1982;62(1):73-120

### 1700 to Present

Anderson CM: Measles mortality and ethnic groups. **S Afr Med J** 1982 Jul 17;62(3):86–8
Chase A: The legacy of Malthus: the social costs of the new scientific racism. Urbana, University of Illinois Press, 1980. xxix, 686, xviii p.
Cooney RS, Min K: Demographic characteristics affecting living arrangements among young currently unmarried Puerto Rican, non-Spanish black, and non-Spanish white mothers. **Ethnicity** 1981,8(2).107–20
Dworkin AG, Stephen RC: Mexican-American adolescent inhalant abuse: a proposed Model. **Youth Soc** 1980;11(4):493–506
Freedman BJ: For debate ... Caucasian. **Br Med J [Clin Res]** 1984 Mar 3;288(6418):696–8
Keystone J: The physical health of the Indochinese refugees. In Adelman, Howard, ed: The Indochinese Refugee Movement: The Canadian Experience (Toronto: Operation Lifeline, 1980): 163–5.
Muthiah A, Jones GW: Fertility trends among overseas Indian populations. **Popul Stud** 1983 Jul;37(2):273–99
O'Brien ME: Pragmatic survivalism: behavior patterns affecting low-level wellness among minority group members. **ANS** 1982 Apr;4(3):13–26
Oppitz R: Freiherr von Ehrenfels (1859–1932) und die Entwicklung des 'Neuen Menschen' zu Beginn des 20. Jahrhunderts. Diss. Mainz, 1980. 256 p.
Schneider WH: Chance and social setting in the application of the discovery of blood groups. **Bull Hist Med** 1983 Winter;57(4):545–62
Yonemoto S: [Progress in life science and humanity--historical changes in the ideological background and the present status of life science] (Jpn). **Kango Gijutsu** 1981 Apr;27(6):739–44

### Africa

Fancher RE: Francis Galton's African ethnography and its role in the development of his psychology. **Br J Hist Sci** 1983 Mar;16(12 No. 1):67–79
Gale TS: Segregation in British West Africa. **Cah Etud Afr** 1980;20(4):495–507

### Canada

Hidgson C: The social and political implications of tuberculosis among native Canadians. **Can Rev Sociol Anthropol** 1982;19(4):502–12
Young TK: Indian health services in Canada: a sociohistorical perspective. **Soc Sci Med** 1984;18(3):257–64

### France

Blanckaert C: Médecine et histoire naturelle de l'homme: l'anthropologie française dans la seconde moitié du XIXe siècle. In Poirier J, Poirier JL, ed: Médecine et philosophie à la fin du XIXe siècle. Paris, Université de Paris XII - Val de Marne, [1980?]. p. 101–16

### Germany

Günther M: Die Institutionalisierung der Rassenhygiene an den deutschen Hochschulen vor 1933. Diss., Johannes Gutenberg-Universität, Mainz, 1982. 148 p.
Heinrich WL: Richard Walther Darré und der Hegehofgedanke. Diss. Mainz, 1980. 161 p.
Lilienthal G: 'Rheinlandbastarde', Rassenhygiene und das Problem der rassenideologischen Kontinuität. Zur Untersuchung von Reiner Pommerin: 'Sterilisierung der Rheinlandbastarde'. **Medizinhist J** 1980;15(4):426–36
Pommerin R: The fate of mixed blood children. **Ger Stud Rev** 1982;5(3):315–23
Rissom R: Fritz Lenz und die Rassenhygiene. Husum, Matthiesen, 1983. 143 p. (Abhandlungen zur Geschichte der Medizin und der Naturwissenschaften, 47).
Seidler E: Die Freiburger Gobineau-Vereinigung und die Verbreitung des Arier-Gedankens in Deutschland. In Seidler E, Schott H, ed. Baustein zur Medizingeschichte. Stuttgart, Steiner, 1984. p. 121–9.
Winau R: Ernst Haeckels Vorstellungen von Wert und Werden menschlicher Rassen und Kulturen. **Medizinhist J** 1981;16(3):270–79

### Mexico

Alba F: La fecundidad entre los mexicano-norteamericanos en relacion a los cambiantes patrones reproductivos en Mexico y los Estados Unidos. **Demogr Econ** 1982;16(2):236–49
Jackson RH: Epidemic disease and population decline in the Baja California Missions, 1697–1834. **South Calif Q** 1981;63(4):308–46

### Norway

Roll-Hansen N: Eugenics before World War II; the case of Norway. **Hist Philos Life Sci** 1980;2(2):269–98

### South Africa

Brain JB, Brain P: Nostalgia and alligator bite--morbidity and mortality among Indian migrants to Natal, 1884–1911. **S Afr Med J** 1984 Jan 21;65(3):98–102

### United States

Arceneaux MG: Acadian to Cajun: population, family, and wealth in southwest Louisiana, 1765–1854. Ph.D. Diss., Brigham Young University, Provo, 1982. xii, 436 p.
Bean FD, Swicegood G: Generation, female education and Mexican-American fertility. **Soc Sci Q** 1982;63(1):131–44
Bell MJ: The relation of mentality to race: William Wells Newell and the Celtic hypothesis. **J Am Folkl** 1979;92(363):25–43
Bieder RE: Scientific attitudes toward Indian mixed-bloods in early nineteenth century America. **J Ethn Stud** 1980;8(2):17–30
Brace CL: The roots of the race concept in American physical anthropology. In F. Spencer, ed: A history of American physical anthropology, 1930–1980. New York, Academic Press, 1982. p. 11–29.
Brod RL, May PA, Stewart TJ: Recruitment and retention of federal physicians on the Navajo Reservation. **Soc Sci J** 1982;19(4):47–66
Byard PJ: Population history, demography, and genetics of the St. Lawrence Island Eskimos. Ph.D. Diss., University of Kansas. Lawrence, 1981. v, 143 leaves.
Cooney RS, Rogler LH, Schroder E: Puerto Rican fertility: an examination of social characteristics, assimilation and minority status variables. **Soc Forces** 1981;59(4):1094–1113
Crozier WL: A people apart: a census analysis of the Polish community of Winona, Minnesota, 1880–1905. **Pol Am Stud** 1981;38(1):5–22
DelCastillo AR: Sterilization: an overview. In Mora, Magdalena and DelCastillo, Adelaida R., ed. Mexican Women in the United States: Struggles past and present. Los Angeles, U. of California Chicano Studies Res. Center, 1980. p. 65–70.
Eberstein IW, Pol LG: Mexican-American ethnicity, socioeconomic status, and infant mortality: a county-level analysis. **Soc Sci J** 1982;19(2):61–71
Gilman SC: Degeneracy and race in the nineteenth century: the impact of clinical medicine. **J Ethn Stud** 1983;10(4):27–50
Gordon EW, Rubain TJ: Bias and alternatives in psychological testing. **J Negro Educ** 1980;49(3):350–60
Guest AM: Fertility variation among the U.S. foreign stock population in 1900. **Int Migr Rev** 1982;16(3):577–94
Harbison SF, Weishaar ME: Samoan migrant fertility: adaptation and selection. **Hum Organ** 1981;40(3):268–73
Hedderson J, Daudistel HC: Infant mortality of the Spanish surname population. **Soc Sci J** 1982;19(4):67–78
Hirschhorn HH: Ethnomedical acculturation of Florida Seminole Indians 1919–1952. **Ethnomedizin** 1981–82;7(1–4):127–47
Joseph A: Intelligence, IQ, and race: When, how, and why they became associated. San Francisco, R & E Research Associates, 1977. vii, 142 p.
Lee ES, Roberts RE: Ethnic fertility differentials in the Southwest: the case of Mexican Americans reexamined. **Sociol Soc Res** 1981;65(2):194–210
McBride DC, Page JB: Adolescent Indian substance abuse: ecological and sociocultural factors. **Youth Soc** 1980;11(4):475–92
Mathes VS: Susan La Flesche Picotte: Indian physician. **Masterkey Ind Lore Hist** 1983;57(1):10–4
Mathes VS: Susan La Flesche Picotte: Nebraska's Indian physician, 1865–1915. **Nebr Hist** 1982;63(4):502–30
Miller B, Chambers EB, Coleman CM: Indo-Chinese refugees: a national mental health need assessment. **Migr Today** 1981;9(2):26–31
Nalven J: Health research on undocumented Mexicans. **Soc Sci J** 1982;19(2):73–88
Nalven J: Who benefits from knowledge about the health of undocumented Mexicans? **Policy Stud J** 1982;10(3):556–80
Pao-Min C: Health and crime among Chinese-Americans: recent trends. **Phylon** 1981;42(4):356–68
Pao-Min C: The age and sex composition of Chinese-Americans: recent trends. **Asian Profile** 1980,8(5).409–20
Putney DT: Fighting the scourge: American Indian morbidity and federal policy, 1897–1928. Ph.D. Diss., Marquette University. Milwaukee, 1980. 355 leaves.
Reilly P: The Virginia Racial Integrity Act revisited: the Plecker-Laughlin correspondence: 1928–1930. **Am J Med Genet** 1983 Dec;16(4):483–92
Roeder BA: Health care beliefs and practices among Mexican Americans: a review of the literature. **Aztlan** 1982;13(1–2):223–56
Sabagh G, Lopez D: Religiosity and fertility: the case of Chicanas. **Soc Forces** 1980;59(2):431–9
St. John C: Race differences in age at first birth and the pace of subsequent fertility: implications for the minority group status hypothesis. **Demography** 1982 Aug;19(3):301–14
Salazar JG, Espinosa JM: A sociodemographic profile of Hispanic physicians in three United States metropolitan areas. **Aztlan** 1979;10:111–22
Schaeffer CE: Plains Kutenai: an ethnological evaluation. **Alberta Hist** 1982;30(4):1–9

## RACE

Schoen R, Nelson VE: Mortality by cause among Spanish surnamed Californians, 1969–71. **Soc Sci Q** 1981;62(2):259–74
Shipek FE: A native American adaptation to drought: the Kumeyaay as seen in the San Diego Mission records, 1770–1798. **Ethnohistory** 1981;28(4):295–312
Spencer F: Samuel George Morton's doctoral thesis on bodily pain: the probable source of Morton's polygenism.
**Trans Stud Coll Physicians Phila** 1983 Dec;5(5 no 4):321–38
Spencer F, ed: A history of American physical anthropology, 1930–1980. New York, Academic Press, 1982. xvi, 495 p.
Tobach E, Proshansky HM, ed: Genetic destiny: race as a scientific and social controversy. New York, AMS Press, 1976. 163 p. Contributions by A. Edel, R. Cancro, D. Layzer, H. Padfield, A. Chase, E. Drucker, V. W. Sidel, G. Piel, J. C. King, E. A. Mauss.
Velez-I CG: Se me acabó la canción: an ethnography of non-consenting sterilizations among Mexican women in Los Angeles. Mora, Magdalena and Del Castillo, Adelaida R., ed. Mexican Women in the United States: Struggles past and present. Los Angeles, U. of California Chicano Studies Res. Center, 1980 p. 71–91.
Westfall LG: Immigrants in society. **Americas (Engl)** 1982;34(4):41–5
Winfree LT, Theis HE, Griffiths CT: Drug use in rural America: a cross-cultural examination of complementary social deviance theories. **Youth Soc** 1981;12(4):465–89
Wong EF: Learned helplessness: the need for self-determination among the Chinese American elderly. **J Ethn Stud** 1980;8(2):45–62
Wright A: An ethnography of the Navajo reproductive cycle.
**Am Indian Q** 1982;6(1–2):52–70
Zimmermann G, Liljeblad S, Frank A, et al: The Indians have many terms for it: stuttering among the Bannock-Shoshoni. **J Speech Hear Res** 1983 Jun;26(2):315–8

## RADIOLOGY

Kristen KT, Reyman TA: Radiographic examination of mummies with autopsy correlation. In A. Cockburn, E. Cockburn, ed: Mummies, disease, and ancient cultures. Cambridge, Cambridge University Press, 1980. p. 287–300.

### Before 500 A.D.

#### Denmark

Halaburt H, Langfeldt B, Rasmussen P: Computerized tomography (CT-scan) of a 2,500-year-old Danish 'Queen'.
**Acta Neurochir (Wien)** 1981;56(3–4):153–5

#### Egypt

Fodor J, Malott JC, King AY: The radiographic investigation of two Egyptian mummies. **Radiol Technol** 1983 Jul–Aug;54(6):443–8

#### Spain

Fernández PL, Quindós LS, Soto J, et al: Radiation exposure levels in Altamira Cave. **Health Phys** 1984 Feb;46(2):445–7

### 1700 to Present

Anger P, Wenz W: Aus der Pionierzeit der Arteriographie. **Radiologe** 1981 Feb;21(2):65–71
Beeching BW: Historical background to radiation safety of dental x-ray sets in the English speaking countries. **Dentomaxillofac Radiol** 1981;10(2):85–92
Berk RN: Gallstones: diagnostic imaging in historical perspective.
**Pharos** 1983 Winter;46(1):30–4
Bird PD: The development of dental radiology. The realisation of a scientific dream. **Br Dent J** 1981 Jul 7;151(1):28–30
Bull JW: The history of neuroradiology. In Rose FC, Bynum WF, ed: Historical aspects of the neurosciences. New York, Raven, 1982. p. 255–64.
Buttermann G: Lungenszintigraphie. Entwicklung, gegenwärtiger Stand und Zukunftsperspektiven. **Fortschr Med** 1983 Mar 17;101(10):403–8
Carr N: The fascinating story of X-rays. **Br Dent Surg Assist** 1980 Sept–Oct;39(5):92–3
Cormack AM: Early two-dimensional reconstruction (CT scanning) and recent topics stemming from it. **J Comput Assist Tomogr** 1980 Oct;4(5):658–64
Darius J: Radiography of the living brain. **Nature** 1984 Mar 15–21;308(5956):225
Donizetti P: I cacciatori d'ombre: storia della radiologia. Milano, Mondadori. 1978. 275 p.
Eckert WG, Garland N: The history of the forensic applications in radiology. **Am J Forensic Med Pathol** 1984 Mar;5(1):53–6
English PC, Grossman H: Radiology and the history of child abuse.
**Pediatr Ann** 1983 Dec;12(12):870–4
Franke OC: Wilhelm Conrad Roentgen and other X-ray pioneers.
**Bull Hist Dent** 1983 Apr;31(1):11–7
Fye WB: Coronary arteriography--it took a long time! **Circulation** 1984 Nov;70(5):781–7
Grainger RG: Intravascular contrast media--the past, the present and the future. **Br J Radiol** 1982 Jan;55(649):1–18
Gyenes G: Klinische, physikalische und biologische Grundlagen der modernen Strahlentherapie. **Radiobiol Radiother (Berl)** 1980;21(3):208–17
Hall EJ: Particles in radiation therapy--Part III.
**Int J Radiat Oncol Biol Phys** 1982 Dec;8(12):2041–4
Hall EJ: The contribution of the physical sciences to the development of radiation therapy. **J Surg Oncol** 1983 Dec;24(4):248–57
Hammer B: Die Geschichte der Computertomographie (anlässlich von 10 Jahren klinischer Computertomographie). **Computertomographie** 1982 Jun;2(2):59–61
Heckmann K: Die Entwicklung der Schlitzaufnahmen. **Rontgenblatter** 1984 Jan;37(1):29–39
Hevesy GC de: Marie Curie and her contemporaries. **J Nucl Med** 1984 Jan;25(1):116–31
Hounsfield GN: Computed medical imaging. **J Comput Assist Tomogr** 1980 Oct;4(5):665–74
Jantsch M: Zur Geschichte der Röntgendiagnostik in der Urologie.
**Wien Klin Wochenschr** 1984 Sep 14;96(17):637–42
Jeanmart L: Le radiodiagnostic de Roentgen à Hounsfield. **Flash Inf** 1983 May–Jun;:3–7
Jennings WA: When did you last see your röntgen?--The SI units and their use. **Phys Med Biol** 1984 Feb;29(2):131–7
Jung T: X-rays in dentistry. **J Am Dent Assoc** 1982 Apr;104(4):438
Klickstein HS: Wilhelm Conrad Röntgen: on a new kind of rays; a bibliographical study. [Philadelphia?], 1966. xvi, 129 p. (Mallinckrodt Classics of Radiology, v. 1).
Kolta KS, Rothe R: Ein Bericht über die Röntgen- und Tomographiebefunde bei den Mumien der ägyptischen Staatssammlung in München. In International Congress of the History of Medicine, 27th, Barcelona, 1980. Actas. Barcelona, Acadèmia de Ciències Mèdiques de Catalunya i Balears, 1981. p. 557–9.
Körbler J: Strahlen, Heilmittel und Gefahr. Wien, Ranner, 1977. 162 p.
Kornfeld H: Nuclear weapons and civil defense. The influence of the medical profession in 1955 and 1983. **West J Med** 1983 Feb;138(2):207–12
Lalanne C, Coussement A: Geschichte der Radiodiagnostik. In Sournia JC, Martiny M, Poulet J, ed: Illustrierte Geschichte der Medizin. Salzburg, Andreas, 1980. Vol. 6. p. 2195–221.
Laughlin JS: AAPM and RAMPS--antecedents and perspectives.
**Med Phys** 1983 Jul–Aug;10(4):387–94
Lederman M: The early history of radiotherapy: 1895–1939.
**Int J Radiat Oncol Biol Phys** 1981 May;7(5):639–48
Maurer HJ, Weber W: Die Entdeckung der Röntgenstrahlen in der Trivialliteratur und der Fachpresse von 1896–1901. **Technikgeschichte** 1977;44:324–39
O'Rahilly R: Plain words on planes and sections. **Radiol Technol** 1981 May–Jun;52(6):615–7
Osborn SB: New regulations for old. **Phys Med Biol** 1984 Feb;29(2):153–6
Pressman D: The development and use of radiolabeled antitumor antibodies. **Cancer Res** 1980 Aug;40(8 Pt 2):2960–4
Proux C: Geschichte der Radiotherapie. In Sournia JC, Martiny M, Poulet J, ed: Illustrierte Geschichte der Medizin. Salzburg, Andreas, 1980. Vol. 6. p. 2223–41.
A review of dental radiography: **J Am Dent Assoc** 1984 Apr;108(4):552–3
Roentgenology 1902.: **AJR** 1981 Mar;136(3):630–1
Rona E: Laboratory contamination in the early period of radiation research.
**Health Phys** 1979 Dec;37(6):723–7
Rosen PP: Specimen radiography and the diagnosis of clinically occult mammary carcinoma. A brief historical review. **Pathol Annu** 1980;15(pt 1):225–37
Róziewicz J: Zwiazki Marii Skłodowskiej-Curie z nauka rosyjska i radziecka. **Kwart Hist Nauki Tech** 1984;29(3–4):535–55
Ryan MT, Fair MF: The radiation warning symbol. **Health Phys** 1981 Aug;41(2):416–7
Schadewaldt H: Anfänge der Röntgentherapie.
**Schriftenr Dtsch Rontgenmus** 1983 Aug;5
Schuur KH: Radiological visualization of the portal venous system. A historical review. **Diagn Imag Clin Med** 1984;53(4):173–6
Sewerin I: Fra katoderør til computer-tomografi. **Tandlaegebladet** 1983 Jun;87(11):383–8
Shehadi WH: X-ray tubes and other historic memorabilia.
**Med Radiogr Photogr** 1981;57(2):preceding p 21
Smirnov EI, Garin NS: Agressivnaia sushchnost' amerikanskogo imperializma i vozmozhnye posledstviia primeneniia iadernogo oruzhiia.
**Zh Mikrobiol Epidemiol Immunobiol** 1982 May;(5):3–11
Süsskind C: The 'story' of nonionizing radiation research.
**Bull NY Acad Med** 1979 Dec;55(11):1152–63
Taylor LS: Organization for radiation protection: the operations of the ICRP and NCRP, 1928–1974. [Washington], U. S. Dept. of Energy. 1979. 2082 p. in various pagings.
Vaeth JM: Historical aspects of tylectomy and radiation therapy in the treatment of cancer of the breast. **Front Radiat Ther Oncol** 1983;17:1–10
Zherbin EA: Rol' radiobiologii v razvitii luchevoĭ terapii.
**Med Radiol (Mosk)** 1982 May;27(5):48–56

### Australia

Hamersley H: Radiation science and Australian medicine, 1896–1914. **Hist Rec Aust Sci** 1982;5(3):41–63
Owen M: The archives of the Royal Australasian College of radiologists: guide to the history collection H706–H765 sundry accessions. **Australas Radiol** 1982 Mar;26(1):30–40
Owen MD: The archives of the Royal Australasian College of Radiologists. **Australas Radiol** 1978 Sep;22(3):222–5
Owen MD: The archives of the Royal Australasian College of Radiologists. **Australas Radiol** 1979 Mar;23(1):15–9
Sutherland SK: Useless X-rays. **Med J Aust** 1983 Aug 20;2(4):165
Transcript of the amorial bearings of the Royal Australasian College of Radiologists in the letters patent: **Australas Radiol** 1982;Spec. No.:3–4
25th anniversary issue of Australasian Radiology: **Australas Radiol** 1982;Spec. No.:1–162

### Austria

Wyklicky H: Zur Geschichte der Strahlentherapie in Oesterreich. **Wien Klin Wochenschr** 1980 Feb 29;92(5 Suppl 110):165–71

### Canada

Aldrich JE: Nova Scotia's pioneers in radiology. **Can Med Assoc J** 1984 Aug 15;131(4):376–80
Becker A: Radiological pioneers in Saskatoon. **Sask Hist** 1983;36(1):31–7
Lipinski JK: Some observations on early diagnostic radiology in Canada. **Can Med Assoc J** 1983 Oct 1;129(7):766–8

### Chile

Costa-Casaretto C: Ochenta y cinco años de radiología chilena. Su partida de nacimiento y su fe de beautismo. **Rev Med Chil** 1981 Jul;109(7):669–78

### Czechoslovakia

Dienstbier Z: 25 years of the Czechoslovak Society for Nuclear Medicine and Radiation Hygiene. **Czech Med** 1981;4(3):97–106
Kutarňa A, Sajter V: Subtrakcia a harmonizácia kontrastu röntgenového obrazu v diele prof. MUDr. Vojtecha Alexandra (1857–1916). **Bratisl Lek Listy** 1983 Dec;80(6):717–24
Vilček E: O prvom röntgenológovi z Moravy. **Cesk Radiol** 1980 Mar;34(2):138–43
Vilček E: O prvopočiatkoch rádiodiagnostiky a rádioterapie na Slovensku. **Bratisl Lek Listy** 1981;76(1):107–21

### Denmark

Rasmussen PG: The history of veterinary roentgenology in Denmark 1895 - 1975. **Hist Med Vet** 1977;2(3):65–8
Sell A, Madsen CB: Radiumstationen in Aarhus from 1962 to 1984. **Acta Radiol [Oncol]** 1984;23(2–3):85–90

### Finland

Pataky L: Az orthopantomográfia kialakulása Paatero munkásságának tükrében. **Fogory Sz** 1979 Sep;72(9):279–80

### France

Arnulf G: A propos de la naissance de la radiologie en France. L'oeuvre d'Etienne Destot à Lyon. **Bull Acad Natl Med (Paris)** 1981 Oct;165(7):955–9
Bendiner E: The Curies: pioneers and victims of the atomic era. **Hosp Pract** 1981 Dec;16(12):80, 82–4 passim
Del Regato JA: Jean Frederic Joliot. **Int J Radiat Oncol Biol Phys** 1980 May;6(5):621–40
Hurwic J: Nieznany list Marii Skłodowskiej-Curie. **Kwart Hist Nauki Tech** 1984;29(3–4):557–8
Mercier P: André Bocage et la naissance de la tomographie. **Bull Acad Natl Med (Paris)** 1979;3:188–91
Ratti A: Antoinette Béclère e il Centro per le Relazioni internazionali in Radiologia. **Radiol Med (Torino)** 1982 Nov;68(11):785–7
Sztanyik BL: Curie és az orvostudomány. **Orv Hetil** 1981 Apr 19;;122(16):961–4
Theil P: Les premières radiographies faites en France, retrouvées à l'Académie Nationale de Médecine. **Bull Acad Natl Med (Paris)** 1980 Nov;164(8):752–6

### Germany

Dörffel EW, Held F, Oelssner W: Zum 30. Jahrestag der Gründung der Deutschen Demokratischen Republik. Die Bedeutung Fritz Gietzelts für die Radiologie und Geschwulst-bekämpfung. **Radiobiol Radiother (Berl)** 1979 Oct;20(5):621–6
Drinnan AJ: Odontophilately. **NY State Dent J** 1980 Feb;46(2):73
Fischmann E: Retracing Röntgen's discovery. **Diagn Imaging** 1979;48(5):294–303
Huttmann A: Nichtärzte als erste Röntgenologen. **ROFO** 1982 Jan;136(1):85–8
Kalok L: Wilhelm Conrad Röntgen in Giessen, 1879–1888: Ausstellung in der Universitätsbibliothek Giessen vom 28. Juni–27. Juli 1979 aus Anlass der Berufung Röntgens nach Giessen vor 100 Jahren: Katalog. Giessen, Universitätsbibliothek, 1979. 34 p.
Kraft E, Finby N: Beginning of radiology in 1896; first newspaper report of discovery of x-ray. **NY State J Med** 1981 Apr;81(5):805–6
Kraft E, Finby N: Röntgen's discovery of X-ray and Lenard's priority claim; award of first Nobel Prize in physics in 1901. **NY State J Med** 1980 Sep;80(10):1623–5
Maurer HJ: Die Entdeckung einer 'neuen Form von Strahlen' durch W. C. Röntgen im Spiegel der Presse. **Med Welt** 1982 Apr 8;33(14):520–4
Ratti A: I 75 anni della Deutsche Röntgengesellschaft. **Radiol Med (Torino)** 1980 Jul–Aug;66(7–8):481–4
Stahlschmidt S: Professor Dr. med. habil. Fritz Gietzelt--Arzt, Wissenschaftler, Kommunist: ein Lebensbild. Berlin, Humboldt-Universität zu Berlin, 1982. 64 p.

### Great Britain

Boag JW: Silvanus Phillips Thompson--some studies in the 'prehistory' of X rays. **Br J Radiol** 1984 Jan;57(673):1–15
Coombs WH: Recollections of a veteran [interview by Peter Center]. **Radiography** 1983 Oct;49(586):235–8
Goldsworthy BM: The end of an era--the story of mass miniature chest radiography in the Royal Navy. **J R Nav Med Serv** 1981;67(1):32–6
Kinloch J: The Society and College of Radiographers--60 years on. **Radiography** 1980 Dec;46(552):271–87
Landes RR, Hall S: A letter from Joseph Lister to Dr. David Walsh. **JAMA** 1984 Jun 15;251(23):3101–3
Loutit JF: Louis Harold Gray. In Dictionary of national biography, 1961–1970. Suppl. 8, 1981. p. 453–5.
Owen M: The Journal of the Roentgen Society, Number 1, Volume 1: an outline. **Australas Radiol** 1983 Jul;27(2):170–3
Ramsey LJ: Bullet wounds and X-Rays in Britain's little wars. **J Soc Army Hist Res** 1982 Summer;:91–102
Ramsey LJ: Some notable early contributors to radiography--Thompson, Jackson and Campbell Swinton. **Radiography** 1980 Dec;46(552):289–97
Ross WM: The Institute: yesterday and tomorrow. **Br J Radiol** 1980 Feb;53(626):55–62
Smith C: Medical radiology: its practical application 1895–1914. In Checkland O, Lamb M, ed: Health care as social history; the Glasgow case. Aberdeen, Aberdeen University Press, 1982. p. 100–116.
Spiers FW: 40 years of development in radiation protection. **Phys Med Biol** 1984 Feb;29(2):145–51

### Hungary

Gyenes G: 65 éves az elsö magyar röntgen tankönyv. **Orv Hetil** 1983 Jul 24;124(30):1829–30
Kárpáti E: Emlékezés Hamburger Jenöre (1883–1936). **Orv Hetil** 1983 Dec 11;124(50):3063–6
Laczay A: Történelmi tévedések a röntgendiagnosztikában és a tévedés etikája. **Orv Hetil** 1983 Dec 4;124(49):2999–3002
Sztanyik BL: A sugárbiológia negyedszázada. **Orv Hetil** 1983 Sep 11;124(37):2223–32

### Italy

Lenarduzzi G, Pescarini L, Miotto D: Un precursore dell'esame radiologico del tubo digerente: il prof. G. Vicentini. **Radiol Med (Torino)** 1980 Apr;66(4):263–4
Toti A: Augusto Righi precursore della xeroradiografia. **Radiol Med (Torino)** 1979 Sep;65(9):615–6

### Japan

Errera M, Einstein A: Effets à court terme d'explosions nucléaires. **Bull Mem Acad R Med Belg** 1982;137(8–9):560–8
Hoshasen Igaku Sogo Kenkyusho 20-nenshi Hensan Iinkai: Hoiken nijunenshi. Chiba, Japan, Do Kenkyusho, Showa 52 nen [1977]. 4, 349 p.
Liebow AA: Encounter with disaster: a medical diary of Hiroshima, 1945. Condensed from the original publication, 1965. **Yale J Biol Med** 1983 Jan–Feb;56(1):23–38
Omuro A: X-sen igakukai no senkusha Miyahara Tatsutaro. Ichihara, Japan. Ichihara-shi Kyoiku Iinkai, Showa 50 nen [1975] 88 p.
Tubiana M: Effets à long terme observés chez les survivants des explosions d'Hiroshima et Nagasaki. Implications pour l'évaluation des risques d'un guerre atomique. **Bull Mem Acad R Med Belg** 1982;137(8–9):533–41

### Poland

Chrzanowski A: Dar Narodowy dla pani Marii Skłodowska-Curie.

Nowotwory 1980 Jan–Mar;30(1):93–7
Chrzanowski A: Instytut Curie w Krakowie, pierwszy zakład leczenia radem w Polsce. **Nowotwory** 1979 Jul–Sep;29(3):239–41
Chrzanowski A: Rozwój Instytutu Radowego w Warszawie w okresie 1932–1939. **Nowotwory** 1980 Jul–Sep;30(3):305–9
Kołodziejska H: Zarys historii Instytutu Radowego im. Marii Skłodowskiej-Curie. **Nowotwory** 1983 Jan–Mar;33(1):1–5
Meissner R: Swiatowy priorytet Karola Mayera w dziedzinie radiodiagnostyki--przyczynek do dziejów tomografii. **Kwart Hist Nauki Tech** 1982;27(1):125–37
Mlosek K: W 50 rocznicę polskiego czasopiśmiennictwa radiologicznego. **Pol Przegl Radiol** 1979 Nov–Dec;43(6):339–43
50-lecie Zakładu Radiodiagnostyki Instytutu Onkologii im. Marii Skłodowskiej-Curie w Warszawie: **Pol Przegl Radiol (Warszawa)** 1983 Jul–Aug;47(4):261–2

**Portugal**

Veiga-Pires JA, Grainger RG: Pioneers in angiography: The Portuguese School of Angiography. Lancaster, Boston, MTP Press, 1982. 131 p.

**Singapore**

Khoo FY, Chow KW: The development of diagnostic radiology in Singapore. **Ann Acad Med Singapore** 1982 Jul;11(3):444–6

**Spain**

Piquer y Jover JJ: Panorama històric de la radiologia a Catalunya. Barcelona, Asociación de Radiología y Electrología, 1971. 160 p.

**Sweden**

Nicou G, Kock W, ed: Från Gösta Forssells och den Svenska röntgenologiens ungdomstid. Södertälje, Sweden, Fingraf Tryckeri, 1984. 84 p. (Nordisk Medicinhistorisk Arsbok, Supplementum X, 1984)

**Switzerland**

Hobi F: Zahnärztliche Röntgenologie von den Anfängen bis zum Jahre 1914: ihre Entwicklung in der Schweiz unter Berücksichtigung der im Ausland geschaffenen Voraussetzungen im Rahmen der Zahnheilkunde jener Zeit. Zürich, Juris, 1981. 126 p. (Zürcher medizingeschichtliche Abhandlungen, Neue Reihe, 145).
Stamm H: 50 Jahre medizinische Forschung in Waldenburg. **Gesnerus** 1983;40(3/4):281–90

**United States**

The American Radium Society: **Am J Clin Oncol** 1982 Apr;5(2):99–100
Annas GJ: The case of Karen Silkwood. **Am J Public Health** 1984 May;74(5):516–8
Barger AC: New technology for a new century: Walter B. Cannon and the invisible rays. **AJR** 1981 Jan;136(1):187–95
Black EF, Libby LM: Commercial food irradiation. **Bull At Sci** 1983;39(6):48–50
Bowers JZ: Yale and the Atomic Bomb Casualty Commission. **Yale J Biol Med** 1983 Jan–Feb;56(1):39–45
Breit DH, Wunder JF: The history of radiology in South Dakota. **SD J Med** 1981 May;34(5):56–8
Caldwell GG, Kelley D, Zack M, et al: Mortality and cancer frequency among military nuclear test (Smoky) participants, 1957 through 1979. **JAMA** 1983 Aug 5;250(5):620–4
Carlson EA: Genes, radiation, and society. The life and work of H. J. Muller. Ithaca, Cornell University Press, 1981. xiv, 457 p.
Carlson WB: Innovation in medical technology: Elihu Thomson, General Electric, and X rays in 1896. **Med Instrum** 1982 Jul–Aug;16(4):218
Carr JD: The great radiology debate: the letters of C. Edmund Kells and Howard R. Raper. **Bull Hist Dent** 1981 Oct;29(2):69–73
Chapman EM: History of the discovery and early use of radioactive iodine. **JAMA** 1983 Oct 21;250(15):2042–4
Cook HJ, Steneck NH, Vander AJ, et al: Early research on the biological effects of microwave radiation: 1940–1960. **Ann Sci** 1980 May;37(3):323–51
del Regato JA: Isadore Lampe. **Int J Radiat Oncol Biol Phys** 1984 Feb;10(2):173–83
Del Regato JA: The tracks of the Compton effect. **Med Phys** 1981 Nov–Dec;8(6):761–5
Detlefsen EG: George Edward Pfahler. In Dictionary of American Biography, Suppl. 6, 1956–1960. p. 505–6, 1980.
Donner MW: Der Weg der amerikanischen Radiologie zu ihrer jetzigen Stellung. **Radiologe** 1982 Jan;22(1):1–6
Elkind MM: Radiobiology in radiotherapy: a personal history. **Int J Radiat Oncol Biol Phys** 1984 Jul;10(7):1143–8
Establishment of the American Board of Oral and Maxillofacial Radiology.: **Oral Surg** 1980 Jun;49(6):549–51
Evans JA: Landmark perspective: Roentgenography of the urinary tract. **JAMA** 1983 Nov 25;250(20):2854–5
Fuller MB: Alexander Hollaender Papers (1898– ). **Mendel Newsl** 1984;(24):5–7
Gutiérrez C: The birth and growth of neuroradiology in the USA. **Neuroradiology** 1981;21(4):227–37
Jacobson HG, Stern WZ: Landmark perspective: The Graham-Cole 'test' revisited. The oral cholecystogram today. **JAMA** 1983 Dec 2;250(21):2977–82
Jacobson LO: From atom to eve. **Perspect Biol Med** 1981 Winter;24(2):195–216
Kaplan E: E.R.N. Grigg, radiologist-historian. **Semin Nucl Med** 1979 Jul;9(3):149–50
Kaufman JA: Francis H. Williams and the shadows of disease. **Conn Med** 1980 Apr;44(4):229–32
Leopold LA: Radiology at the University of Pennsylvania 1890–1975. Philadelphia, University of Pennsylvania Press, 1981. xvi, 163 p.
Moldenhauer W: Aufbau der Röntgendiagnostik an der Wilhelm-Pieck-Universität Rostock in den letzten 30 Jahren. **Wiss Z Univ Rostock** 1979;28(1–2):25–7
Moler CL: The certification of radiological equipment specialists: a historical review. **Radiol Manage** 1980 Spring;2(4):9–13
Ochsner SF: Perspectives in radiology--1922 to 1982. **South Med J** 1983 Dec;76(12):1549–53
Regato JA del: Albert Soiland and the early development of therapeutic radiology in the United States. **Int J Radiat Oncol Biol Phys** 1983 Feb;9(2):243–53
Regato JA del: Francis Henry Williams. **Int J Radiat Oncol Biol Phys** 1983 May;9(5):739–49
Sunshine I: Dr. Alexander O. Gettler's documentation of a radiation hazard. **Am J Forensic Med Pathol** 1983 Dec;4(4):307–9
Wasserman H, Solomon N, Alvarez R, et al: Killing our own: the disaster of America's experience with atomic radiation. New York, Dell, 1982. xiii, 368 p.

**USSR**

Abdurasulov DM: Osnoynye étapy razvitiia i nauchnye dostizheniia meditsinskoĭ radiologii i rentgenologii v Uzbekskoĭ SSR za 60 let. **Med Radiol (Mosk)** 1982 Dec;27(12):21–6
Abramov ShI: Iubileĭ pervoĭ kafedry. **Vestn Rentgenol Radiol** 1980 Jan–Feb;(1):89–91
Baĭsogolov GD: Rol' zhurnala 'Meditsinskaia Radiologiia' v razvitii luchevoĭ terapii v SSSR. **Med Radiol (Mosk)** 1982 Apr;27(4):3–6
Bakhshiev BA, Beĭbutov ShM, Aleskerov DSh, et al: Istoriia razvitiia radiologii v Azerbaĭdzhane. **Med Radiol (Mosk)** 1982 Dec;27(12):18–21
Barrett HH, Hawkins WG, Joy ML: Historical note on computed tomography. **Radiology** 1983 Apr;147(1):172
Iarmonenko SP: Klinicheskaia radiobiologiia--nauchnaia osnova luchevoĭ terapii opukholeĭ. **Med Radiol (Mosk)** 1982 Mar;27(3):6–9
Kindzel'skiĭ LP, Sivachenko TP: Razvitie meditsinskoĭ radiologii v Ukrainskoĭ SSR. **Med Radiol (Mosk)** 1982 Dec;27(12):13–8
Kishkovskiĭ AN, Tiutin LA: K 50-letiiu kafedry rentgenologii i radiologii VMA imeni S.M. Kirov. **Voen Med Zh** 1980 Sep;(9):76–8
Lindenbraten LD: Voprosy prepodavaniia i podgotovki kadrov po rentgenologii i radiologii na stranitsakh zhurnala 'Meditsinskaia Radiologiia' (1956–1981). **Med Radiol (Mosk)** 1981;26(10):49–53
Mikhaĭlov AN: Razvitie rentgenologii i radiologii v Belorusskoĭ SSR. **Vestn Rentgenol Radiol** 1982 Nov–Dec;(6):83–4
Mkrtchian LN: Osnovnye étapy razvitiia onkologii i rentgenologii v Armianskoĭ SSR. **Vopr Onkol** 1982;28(12):20–4
Pozmogov AI, Demin VT, Arendarevskiĭ LF: Kievskomu nauchno-issledovatel'skomu rentgenoradiologicheskomu i onkologicheskomu institutu 60 let. **Vestn Rentgenol Radiol** 1980 May–Jun;(3):78–80
Purévzhav T: Razvitie rentgenoradiologicheskoĭ sluzhby v Mongol'skoĭ Narodnoĭ Respublike. **Vestn Rentgenol Radiol** 1981;(3):74–6
Ragumov RN, Aleskerov DSh: Razvitie i dostizheniia rentgenologii i radiologii v Azerbaĭdzhane. **Vestn Rentgenol Radiol** 1982 Nov–Dec;(6):81–3
Rits IA: O razvitii rentgenologii v Sibiri. **Vestn Rentgenol Radiol** 1982 May–Jun;(3):90–2
Sipukhin IaM: Razvitie rentgenologii na Dal'nem Vostoke. **Vestn Rentgenol Radiol** 1982 Jan–Feb;(1):89–91
Sipukhin IaM: Vladimir Semenovich Kravchenko. K istorii otechestvennoĭ rentgenologii. **Vestn Rentgenol Radiol** 1983 May–Jun;(3):91–2
Sokolov IuN, Rozenshtraukh LS: Kafedre rentgenologii Tsentral'nogo instituta usovershenstvovaniia vrachei 50 let (kratkiĭ istoricheskiĭ ocherk). **Vestn Rentgenol Radiol** 1980 May–Jun;(3):75–8
Tiurin EI, Kovachev VI: Kafedre rentgenologii i radiologii voenno-meditsinskoĭ akademii im. S. M. Kirova. **Vestn Rentgenol Radiol** 1981 Mar–Apr;(2):87–9
Tsyb AF: Nauchno-issledovatel'skomu institutu meditsinskoĭ radiologii AMN SSSR-20 let. **Med Radiol (Mosk)** 1982 Sep;27(9):3–12
Vorob'ev IuI, Veretennikova VP: 25 let kafedry rentgenologii i radiologii Moskovskogo meditsinskogo stomatologicheskogo instituta im. N. A. Semashko. **Vestn Rentgenol Radiol** 1980 Sep–Oct;(5):88–9

**Yugoslavia**

Gavrilović VS: Doprinos Mihajla Pupina svetskoj medicinskoj nauci. **Srp Arh Celok Lek** 1981 Feb;109(2):293-302

# RED CROSS

See also **Nursing; Emergency Medical Services**

**1700 to Present**

Apostolov M: D-r Robert Iur'evich Berzin (1887-1950 g.) i bolnitsata na ruskiia Cherven krust v Sofiia. **Khirurgiia (Sofiia)** 1982;35(2):223-7
Muerant J: La Comité International de la Croix-Rouge et la protection des civils. **Rev Hist Deuxieme Guerre Mond** 1981;31(121):129-38
Red Cross in philately: **Scalpel Tongs** 1981;25:39-43
Sandoz Y: Le droit d'initiative du Comité International de la Croix-Rouge. **Ger Yearb Int Law** 1979;22:352-73
Tiuliandin AD: Sotrudnichestvo obshchestv Krasnogo Kresta SSSR i Bolgarii. **Sov Zdravookhr** 1982;(6):53-5

**Africa**

Clerc B, Hanne M: La Croix-Rouge et l'Afrique: essai bibliographique. **Geneva Afr** 1970;9(1):94-101

**Australia**

Verso ML: Fifty years of the Red Cross Blood Transfusion Service in Victoria. **Victorian Hist J** 1980;51(4):218-36

**Bulgaria**

Dikova S: The Bulgarian Red Cross and the development of blood donation in Bulgaria. In International Congress of the History of Medicine. 26th, Plovdiv, 1978. Actes du Congress. Sofia, 1981. Volume II. p. 220.
Zaprianov N, Nikolov I: The share of the foreign 'Red Cross' societies in rendering help to the victims of the earthquake in Bulgaria, in the year of 1928. In International Congress of the History of Medicine. 26th, Plovdiv, 1978. Actes du Congress. Sofia, 1981. Volume II. p. 214.

**Germany**

Blos D: 100 Jahre Rotes Kreuz. **Fortschr Med** 1983 Mar 31;101(12):524-6
Schlögel A: Neuaufbau des Deutschen Roten Kreuzes nach dem II. Weltkrieg: Geschichte des DRK 1945-1950. Bonn, Das Deutsche Rote Kreuz, 1983. 120 p.

**Great Britain**

Walker J: The British Red Cross in the Bromley area 1910-1919. **Bromley Local Hist** 1979;4:17-23

**Hungary**

Kapronczay K: A Magyar Vöröskereszt centenáriumára. **Orv Hetil** 1981 May 17;122(20):1197-9
Kapronczay K: A Magyar Vöröskereszt száz éve--időszaki kiállítás a Semmelweis Orvostörténeti Múzeumban. **Orv Hetil** 1981 Nov 1;122(44):2732-3

**Japan**

Kameyama M: Evaluation of the social position of the nurse in the modern history of nursing in Japan. Chapter 1. The Japan Red Cross and nurses (Jpn). **Kango** 1980 Jun;32(6):78-87 (continued periodically)

**Poland**

Babecki JW: Ze wspomnień czerwonokrzyskich na emigracji podczas II wojny światowej. **Arch Hist Med (Warsz)** 1980;43(3):317-22

**Romania**

Neagu I, Maracineanu G, Neagu M: Contribution de la Société 'La Jeune Croix Rouge Américaine' au developpement de l'assistance médicale et sociale en Roumanie. In: Congrès international d'histoire de la médecine, XXVe, Québec, 1976. Actes. Québec, 1977. p. 1009-14.

**Spain**

Soteras Elía B: Centenario de la batalla de Oroquieta: primera actuacion de los camilleros de la Cruz Roja. **Pregon** 1972;(111):n p

**Sweden**

Johansson B: 'God bless you, my dear Miss Nightingale.' Letters from Emmy Carolina Rappe to Florence Nightingale 1867-1870. Stockholm, Almqvist & Wiksell International, 1977. 57 p. (Stockholm studies in English, 38).
Lagnelius C: Svenska röda korset som piojärorganisation. **Omvardaren** 1982;29(2):10-1
Stroh O: Svenska röda korset i totalförsvaret. **K Krigsvetensk Akad Handl Tidskr** 1965;169:183-92

**Switzerland**

Hässig A: 40 Jahre Blutspendedienst des Schweizerischen Roten Kreuzes. **Ther Umsch** 1984 Aug;41(8):533-5
Morgenstern S: Henri Dunant and the Red Cross. **Bull NY Acad Med** 1979 Nov;55(10):949-56
Morgenstern S: Henri Dunant and the Red Cross. **Bull NY Acad Med** 1981 May;57(4):311-26

**United States**

Agris J: Stamps commemorating medicine. 'American Red Cross'. **J Dermatol Surg Oncol** 1981 Sep;7(9):697
American Red Cross celebrates 100th anniversary: **Am Nurse** 1981;13(5):15, 17
Bertini RC: The American Red Cross-- a centennial year. **RI Med J** 1981 Apr;64(4):183-4
A bulwark against mighty woes: The hundredth anniversary of the American Red Cross. **Am Heritage** 1981;32(2):81-91
Gilbo PF: Candid 'cranky' Clara Barton gave us the Red Cross. **Smithsonian** 1981;12(2):126-42
Gilbo PF: The American Red Cross. The first century. New York, Harper & Row, 1981 ix, 246 p.
Hanron J: Nursing revisited: Clarissa Harlow Barton. **Mass Nurse** 1983 Sep;52(9):9, 27
Harding PM: A Red Cross nurse in Belgrade: Mary Gladwin saw World War I from the inside of a hospital. Her battles were no easier than those of the soldiers. **Am Hist Illus** 1982;17(1):41-7
Hughes RE, Scott LD: The founding of San Diego's Red Cross. **J San Diego Hist** 1981;27(2):115-28
Levine P: Historical perspectives before 1945--updated. **Prog Clin Biol Res** 1980;43:3-11
The Red Cross: the first hundred years: **MD** 1981 May;25(5):43-7
Rinn WA: A medical anniversary. **Md State Med J** 1981 Dec;30(12):38
Stewart S: Sharing more than marble palaces. **DAR Mag** 1981;115(3):188-91
Woodruff NE: The failure of relief during the Arkansas drought of 1930-1931. **Arkansas Hist Q** 1980;39(4):301-13

**USSR**

Antonovich T: Ima podviga--gumanizm. **Med Sestra** 1981 Dec;40(12):41-4
Egorysheva IV: Novye dannye iz istorii Krasnogo Kresta v dorevoliutsionnoĭ Rossii. **Sov Zdravookhr** 1981;(2):57-60
Ibragimov NG: Sanitarnyĭ aktiv Bashkirii v pervye desiatiletiia Sovetskoĭ vlasti. **Sov Zdravookhr** 1980;(7):56-60
Kirsanov NA, Razumov VI: Iz istorii organizatsii massovogo donorskogo dvizheniia v gody velikoi otechestvennoi voiny. **Vestn Mosk Univ Ser 8 Istor** 1980;(5):32-41
Kokhan AI, Miliavskiĭ VM: Sestry miloserdiia v bor'be s épidemieĭ difterii. **Med Sestra** 1983 Oct;42(10):48-9
Koval' MV: Tovarsystvo chervonoho khresta i chervonoho pivmisiatsia ursr-frontu i tylu (1941-1945). **Ukr Istor Zh** 1975;(4):78-87
Malozemova AI: Uchastie meditsinskikh rabotnikov v 'Politicheskom Krasnom Kreste 'Nardonoĭ voli'. **Sov Zdravookhr** 1984;(4):59-63
Melkumian GA: Hasarakakan kazmakerputyunneri dere kovkasyan banaki bezheshkakan spasarkmen gortsum arajin hamashkharhayin paterazmi tarinerin. **Patma Banasirakan Handes. Ist Filol Zh** 1977;3:221-34
Tiuliandin AD: Muzeĭ Sovetskogo Krasnogo Kresta. **Zdravookhr Ross Fed** 1980;(5):22-6
Tovbin MM: Obshchestvo krasnogo kresta v SSSR (pervoe desiatiletie). **Vopr Istor** 1978;(4):204-10

# RELIGION AND MEDICINE

See also **Primitive Medicine; Magic and Occult; Folk and Popular Medicine**

Baruk H: Moïse, Freud et le veau d'or. **Rev Hist Med Heb** 1984 Jul;37(2):19-23
Becker KF: Kirche und Alter in Geschichte Gegenwart. **Z Gerontol** 1984 Jan-Feb;17(1):32-8
Bleich JD, Harakas SS, Hehir JB, et al: Population ethics: religious traditions. In Reich WT, et al, ed: Encyclopedia of bioethics, v.3. New York, Free Press, 1978. p. 1250-73.
Brandenburg D: Medizin und Magie. Heilkunde und Geheimlehre des islamischen Zeitalters. Berlin, Hessling, 1975. 159 p. (Medizingeschichtliche Miniaturen, Band 1).
Briceño-Maaz T: Sobre Axel Munthe y su libro 'La Historia de San Michele'. **Rev Soc Venez Hist Med** 1969-71;17-19(31-33):121-30

## RELIGION AND MEDICINE

Caffaratto TM: Fantasia e realtà nella storia della medicina. Il diavolo, la strega, il medico. **Minerva Med** 1981 Oct 32;72(42):2837-5
Cook DC: Koniag Eskimo tooth ablation: was Hrdlička right after all? **Curr Anthropol** 1981;22(2):159-63
Croix A: L'homme et son corps dans l'Au-delà. In Imhof AE, ed: Leib und Leben in der Geschichte der Neuzeit. Berlin, Duncker & Humblot, 1983. p. 155-62.
Curran CE: Roman Catholicism [and the history of bioethics]. In Reich WT, et al, ed: Encyclopedia of bioethics, v.4. New York, Free Press, 1978. p. 1522-34.
Davis E: [Hebrew medical amulets] (Heb). **Harefuah** 1980 Sept;99(5-6):132-3
Declaración sobre el aborto provocado: Sagrada Congregación para la Doctrina de la Fe **Rev Med Univ Navarra** 1982 Dec;26(4):255-60
deWachter MA: Is death and dying merely an ethical issue? **Ann Am Acad Polit Soc Sci** 1980;447:78-88
Duncombe DC: [History of the ministry in medicine]. In Reich WT, et al, ed: Encyclopedia of bioethics, v.3. New York, Free Press, 1978. p. 1189-94.
Dunstan GR: The moral status of the human embryo: a tradition recalled. **J Med Ethics** 1984 Mar;10(1):38-44
Fenner ET: Rasayana Siddhi: medicine and alchemy in the Buddhist tantras. Ph.D. diss. University of Wisconsin. Madison, 1979. 272 leaves.
Fichtner G: Christus als Arzt: Ursprünge und Wirkungen eines Motivs. **Fruhmittelalt Stud** 1982;16:1-18
Geller SA: Autopsy. **Mt Sinai J Med (NY)** 1984 Jan-Feb;51(1):77-81
Greenberg DF, Bystryn MH: Christian intolerance of homosexuality. **AJS** 1982 Nov;88(3):515-48
Hackett E: The foreskin saga. **Med J Aust** 1984 Aug 4;141(3):187-9
Hahn U: Die Entwicklung des Tierschutzgedankens in Religion und Geistesgeschichte. DMV Diss. Hannover, 1980. 192 p.
Hartmann F: Homo patiens. Zur ärztlichen Anthropologie von Leid und Mitleid. In Seidler E, Schott H, ed: Bausteine zur Medizingeschichte. Stuttgart, Steiner, 1984. p. 35-44.
Hausmann W: Christliche Votivtäfelchen aus Metall. **Tierarztl Prax** 1981;9(1):3-8
Hausmann W: Weibliche Fruchtbarkeitssymbole der Quanchen und Tarasken. **Tierarztl Prax** 1983;11(3):417-20
Heggelbacher O: Geisteskrankheit und kirchenrechtliche Verantwortlichkeit. **Osterr Arch Kirchenr** 1967;18(1):3-16
Herzog H: Wirklichkeit und Wahrheit--Weg und Ziel ärztlichen Wirkens. **Praxis** 1982 Aug 10;71(32):1254-61
The history of science: A collection of manuscripts from the library of the Jewish Theological Seminary. An index to the microfilm collection, reels 1-17. Ann Arbor, University Microfilms, 1980. 79 p. (With Hebrew-English name index).
Homans P: A personal struggle with religion: significant fact in the lives and work of the first psychologists. **J Relig** 1982;62:128-44
Jaki SL: The road of science and the ways to God. Chicago, London, Univ. of Chicago Press, 1978 vii, 478 p.
Jakobovits I: Judaism [and medicine]. In Reich WT, et al, ed: Encyclopedia of bioethics, v. 2. New York, Free Press, 1978. p. 791-802.
James EO: Cultural and religious taboos related to food. **Prog Food Nutr Sci** 1979;3(3):67-77
Jetter D: Klosterhospitäler; St. Gallen, Cluny, Escorial. **Sudhoffs Arch** 1978;62(4):313-38
Johnson JT: History of Protestant medical ethics. In Reich WT, et al, ed: Encyclopedia of bioethics, v.3. New York, Free Press, 1978. p. 1364-73.
Kierulf H: L'ergotisme chez Bosch et Grünewald. **Nouv Presse Med** 1982 Oct 2;11(38):2803-9
Kler JH: Medicine and religion. **J Med Soc NJ** 1983 May;80(5):382
La Barre W: Shamanic origins of religion and medicine. **J Psychedelic Drugs** 1979 Jan-Jun;11(1-2):7-11
Leibowitz JO: The ideal physician as revealed in the Zohar, book of Jewish mysticism. **Koroth** 1982 Aug;8(3/4):111-22
Maida AJ: The new code of canon law: some historical perspectives. **Hosp Prog** 1982 Dec;63(12):10, 14
Martinetto P, Riggi G, Valtz A, et al: Microbiological research on specimens (dusts) drawn from the Holy Shroud. **G Batteriol Virol Immunol** 1981 Jul-Dec;74(7-12):202-8
Marty ME: Health/medicine and the faith traditions: an inquiry into religion and medicine. Philadelphia, Fortress Press, 1982. xii, 350 p.
Miller VD, Pellicori SF: Ultraviolet fluorescence photography of the Shroud of Turin. **J Biol Photogr** 1981 Jul;49(3):71-85
Modig M: The allegory of Christ in a pharmacy. **Pharm Hist** 1984;26(1):44-5
Musallam BF: Why Islam permitted birth control. **Arab Stud Q** 1981;3(2):181-97
Ostow M: Judaism and psychoanalysis. New York, Ktav Publishing House, 1982. 305 p. Includes contributions by J. A. Arlow, R. L. Rubenstein, M. S. Bergmann, L. R. Sillman.
Pompey H: Pastoralmedizin--der Beitrag der Seelsorge zur psycho-physischen Gesundheit. Eine bibliographisch-historische Analyse. In Imhof AE, ed: Mensch und Gesundheit in der Geschichte. Husum, Matthiesen, 1980. p. 115-34.
Rahman F: Islam and medicine: a general overview. **Perspect Biol Med** 1984 Summer;27(4):585-97
Ranger T: The Church and healing: introduction. In Sheils WJ, ed: The Church and healing. Papers read at the twentieth summer meeting and the twenty-first winter meeting of the Ecclesiastical History Society. Oxford, Basil Blackwell for the Society, 1982. p. xi-xxiv.
Richardson WJ: Religion and mental health. In Reich WT, et al, ed: Encyclopedia of bioethics, v.3. New York, Free Press, 1978. p. 1064-71.
Rosner F: Ancient descriptions of hemophilia and preconception gender selection. **JAMA** 1984 Aug 17;252(7):900
Russell HM, Weinberg J, ed: The book of knowledge from the Mishnah Torah of Maimonides. Translated from the Hebrew. Edinburgh, Royal College of Physicians of Edinburgh, 1981. xi, 135 p. (Publication No. 55).
Schuster E: Erbauungsbilder in der Totentanzsammlung (Mensch und Tod) der Universität Düsseldorf. In Göpfert W, Otten HH, ed: Metavoeite: wandelt euch durch neues Denken. Düsseldorf, Triltsch, 1983. p. 41-54.
Schwabe CW: Cattle, priests, and progress in medicine. Minneapolis, University of Minnesota Press, 1978. xiii, 277 p.
Schweiger K: Medizinisches im Werk des Kirchenvaters Origenes. Diss., Universität Düsseldorf. Düsseldorf, 1983. 96 p.
Sharkey PW, ed: Philosophy, religion and psychotherapy. Essays in the philosophical foundations of psychotherapy. Washington, University Press of America, 1982. xiii, 227 p. Contributions by R. Macklin, J. E. Morris, R. N. Sollod, J. Needleman, C. E. Scott, M. Friedman, J. F. Rychlak, E. Weisskopf-Joelson, T. S. Szasz, R. J. Sullivan.
Sheils WJ, ed: The Church and healing. Papers read at the twentieth summer meeting and the twenty-first winter meeting of the Ecclesiastical History Society. Oxford, Basil Blackwell for the Society, 1982. xxiv, 440 p. (Studies in Church History, v. 19).
Sugimoto S: [An interpretation of a syndrome depicted in Buddhist cannon [sic] through Susruta Samhita] (Jpn). **Igakushi Kenkyu** 1980;54:12-7
Theopold W: Das Kind in der Votivmalerei. Munich, Karl Thiemig, 1981.
Thivel A: Le 'divin' dans la Collection hippocratique. In La collection hippocratique et son rôle dans l'histoire de la médecine. Colloque de Strasbourg (23-27 octobre 1972) organisé par le Centre de Recherches sur la Grèce Antique, avec le concours des Facultés de Philosophie et des Langues Classiques. Leiden, E. J. Brill, 1975. p. 57-76.
Trüb CL: Heilige und Krankheit. Stuttgart, Klett-Cotta, 1978. 307 p.
Vanderpool HY: Dominant health concerns in Protestantism. In Reich WT, et al, ed: Encyclopedia of bioethics, v.3. New York, Free Press, 1978. p. 1373-8.
Vanderpool HY: Miracle and faith healing. In Reich WT, et al, ed: Encyclopedia of bioethics, v.3. New York, Free Press, 1978. p. 1120-5.
Vega Diaz F: El corazón en la simbología y en la iconografía profana y religiosa. In Academia Nacional de Medicina. Libro conmemorativo del primer centenario. México, Comité Editorial de la Comisión Organizadora del Congreso del Centenario, 1964. Tome 2. p. 78-82.
Wayman A: The human body as microcosm in India, Greek cosmology, and sixteenth-century Europe. **Hist Relig** 1982;22(2):172-90

### Americas

Emboden WA: The mushroom and the water lily: literary and pictorial evidence for Nymphaea as a ritual psychotogen in Mesoamerica. **J Ethnopharmacol** 1982 Mar;5(2):139-48
Lex BW: Neurological bases of revitalization movements. **Zygon** 1978;13(4):276-312
Robicsek F: The smoking gods; tobacco in Maya art, history, and religion. Norman, Oklahoma, Univ. of Oklahoma Press, 1978. xxv, 233 p.
Signorini I: Transvestism and institutionalized homosexuality in North America. In: Congresso Intern. degli Americanisti, 40th, Italy, 1972. Atti. Vol. 2. p. 153-63.
Sihelvik L: Diamond jubilee of the Vincentian Sisters of Charity. **Jednota Annu Furdek (US)** 1978;17:197-200
Wasson RG: The wondrous mushroom. Mycolatry in Mesoamerica. New York, McGraw-Hill, 1980. xxvi, 248 p.
Weiss P: La Trepanacion ritual suprainiana--rasgo de culturas peruanas, encontrado también en México y Guatemala. **Bol Soc Mex Hist Filos Med** 1981 Sep;5(36):193-211

### Arabic

Belguedj S: La Collection hippocratique et l'embryologie coranique. In La collection hippocratique et son rôle dans l'histoire de la médecine. Colloque de Strasbourg (23-27 octobre 1972) organisé par le Centre de Recherches sur la Grèce Antique, avec le concours des Facultés de Philosophie et des Langues Classiques. Leiden, E. J. Brill, 1975. p. 321-33.
Bürgel JC: Islam [and Arabic medicine]. In Reich WT, et al, ed: Encyclopedia of bioethics, v. 2. New York, Free Press, 1978. p. 785-9.
Hameed A: Medical ethics in Islam. **Stud Hist Med** 1981 Jun;5(2):133-59
Nahas GG: Hashish in Islam 9th to 18th century. **Bull NY Acad Med** 1982 Dec;58(9):814-31

### Asia

Touw M: The religious and medicinal uses of Cannabis in China, India and Tibet. **J Psychoactive Drugs** 1981 Jan–Mar;13(1):23–34

**Belgium**

Lacroix MT: L'hôpital Saint-Nicolas du Bruille (Saint-André) à Tournai de sa fondation à sa mutation en cloître (ca. 1230–1611). 2 tomes. Louvain, Université Catholique de Louvain, 1977. xxxvi, 892 p. (Publications de l'Institut d'Etudes Médiévales, 2e série, No. 1).
Villa R: Le famiglie di Gheel: utopia, tradizione e storia nel trattamento della follia. **Studi Stor** 1980;21(3):503–26

**Brazil**

Ribeiro da Silva L: Os Jesuitas e a assistencia medica no Brasil colonial. **Rev Inst Hist Geogr Bras** 1978 Jan–Mar;318:212–32

**China**

Clifford T: Tibetan Buddhist medicine and psychiatry: the diamond healing. Introduction by Lokesh Chandra. York Beach, Me., S. Weiser, 1983. xx, 268 p.
Girardot NJ: Taoism [and the history of Chinese medicine]. In Reich WT, et al, ed: Encyclopedia of bioethics, v.4. New York, Free Press, 1978. p. 1631–8.
Liu Chi-Wan: [The rite of a pestilence god in southern Taiwan] (Chi). **Bull Inst Ethnol Acad Sin** 1979;47:73–169
Unschuld PU: The Chinese reception of Indian medicine in the first millennium A.D. **Bull Hist Med** 1979 Fall;53(3):329–45
Winder M: Il Buddha della medicina. **Kos** 1984 Apr;1(3):55–74
Winder M. The buddhist antecedents of Tibetan medicine. **Tibet News Rev** 1981;2(1/2):29–34

**Colombia**

Chandler DL: Health and slavery in colonial Colombia. New York, Arno Press, 1981. iv, 307 p. (Ph.D. Diss., Tulane 1972).

**Denmark**

Gøtzsche I: Andelig omsorg/7. Kristendommens indflydelse på sundhedsvaesenet. **Sygeplejersken** 1983 Mar 9;83(10):12–6

**Ethiopia**

Pankhurst R: Le piaghe d'Etiopia. **Kos** 1984 Jul–Aug;1(6):33–50

**Europe**

Andreski S: The syphilitic shock: puritanism, capitalism, and a medical factor. **Encounter (Lond)** 1980;55(4):76–81
Boswell J: Christianity, social tolerance, and homosexuality: gay people in Western Europe from the beginning of the Christian era to the fourteenth century. Chicago and London, University of Chicago Press, 1980. xviii, 424 p.
Czigány LG: The use of hallucinogens and the shamanistic tradition of the Finno-Ugrian people. **Slav East Eur Rev** 1980;58(2):212–7
Hörger H: Krankheit und religiöses Tabu--die Lepra in der mittelalterlich-frühneuzeitlichen Gesellschaft Europas. **Gesnerus** 1982;39(1):53–70
Palmer R: The Church, leprosy and plague in medieval and early modern Europe. In Sheils WJ, ed: The Church and healing. Papers read at the twentieth summer meeting and the twenty-first winter meeting of the Ecclesiastical History Society. Oxford, Basil Blackwell for the Society, 1982. p. 79–99.

**Finland**

Achté K: Döden i den fornfinska kulturen. Tron påsjälens odödlighet. **Dan Medicinhist Arbog** 1983;12:82–90

**France**

Brann NL: Melancholy and the divine frenzies in the French Pléiade: their conflicting roles in the art of 'beaux exercices spirituels.' **J Mediev Renaiss Stud** 1979;9:81–100
Dinet D: Mourir en religion aux dix-septième et dix-huitième siècles; la mort dans quelques couvents des dioceses d'Auxerre, Langres et Dijon. **Rev Hist (Paris)** 1978;259(3):29–54
Gélis J: La Pierre et le saint: recours populaires pour la guérison des petits enfants (XVIIe–XIXe siècles). **Asclepio** 1983;35:129–58
Gélis J: Miracle et medecine aux siècles classiques: le corps medical et le retour temporaire a la vie des mort-nes. **Hist Reflect** 1982;9(1–2):85–101
Le Breton D: Apothicaires et moines à Bordeaux à la fin de l'Ancien Régime. Diss., Université de Bordeaux, II, 1983. 131 leaves.

**Great Britain**

Harley D: Religious and professional interests in northern spa literature, 1625–1775. **Soc Soc Hist Med Bull (Lond)** 1984 Dec;35:14–6
Larner C: Enemies of God: the witch-hunt in Scotland. Baltimore, Johns Hopkins Univ. Press, 1981. x, 244 p.
McDonald M: Religion, social change, and psychological healing in England, 1600–1800. In Sheils WJ, ed: The Church and healing. Papers read at the twentieth summer meeting and the twenty-first winter meeting of the Ecclesiastical History Society. Oxford, Basil Blackwell for the Society, 1982. p. 101–25.

**Hungary**

Sasvári L: Emlékek és adatok az ingyenorvosok tiszteletére a magyarországi ortodoxok és görög katolikusok köréből. **Orvostort Kozl** 1979;87–88(25 no 1–2):65–78

**India**

Basham AL: Hinduism [and Hindu medicine]. In Reich WT, et al, ed: Encyclopedia of bioethics, v. 2. New York, Free Press, 1978. p. 661–66.
Kakar S: Shamans, mystics, and doctors: a psychological inquiry into India and its healing traditions. New York, Knopf, 1982. x, 306 p.
Neelavathi A: A brief introduction of Siddha system of medicine. **Bull Indian Inst Hist Med (Hyderabad)** 1979;9:38–40
Nicholas RW: The goddess Sitala and epidemic smallpox in Bengal. **J Asian Stud** 1981;41(1):21–45
Pisztora F: Evezredes-évszázados vallások és a religiózus megélés szélsőségei, valamint elmeкóros formái a mai Indiában. **Orv Hetil** 1983 Mar 6;124(10):591–7
Rama Rao B: Bath in Ayurveda, Yoga and Dharmashastra. **Bull Indian Inst Hist Med Hyderabad** 1982;12(1–4):13–21

**Iran**

Hampel J: Medizin der Zoroastrier im vorislamischen Iran. Husum, Matthiesen, 1982. 142 p. (Abhandlungen zur Geschichte der Medizin und der Naturwissenschaften, Heft 45).

**Italy**

Accati L: Lo spirito della fornicazione: virtù dell'anima e virtù del corpo in Friuli, fra '600 e '700. **Quad Stor** 1979;14(2):644–72
Bucklin R: The Shroud of Turin: a pathologist's viewpoint. **Leg Med** 1982;:33–9
Gnesda L: Gli 'ospizi' nelle Dolomiti. Firenze, Olschki, 1979. 81 p. (Comitato dei Geografi Italiani, 4).

**Japan**

Nakazawa O: The faith in Buddha of medicine in Japan. In: Congrès international d'histoire de la médecine, XXVe, Québec, 1976. Actes. Québec, 1977. p. 1002–8.

**Mexico**

Micheli A de: La inquisicion y los medicos en la Nueva España. **Bol Soc Mex Hist Filos Med** 1982 Sep;6(40):71–81
Morales Meneses J: La congregación y Hospital de San Pedro. **Salud Publica Mex** 1984 Mar–Apr;26(2):190–4

**Nigeria**

Abdalla IH: Islamic medicine and its influence on traditional Hausa practitioners in northern Nigeria. Ph.D. Diss., University of Wisconsin. Madison, 1981. vii, 240 p.

**Peru**

Dobkin de Rios M, Cardenas M: Plant hallucinogens, shamanism and Nazca ceramics. **J Ethnopharmacol** 1980 Sept;2(3):233–46

**Romania**

Barbu G: Din istoria combaterii epidemiilor în ţara noastră. (I). Frăţiile milosteniei. **Rev Ig [Bacteriol]** 1984 Apr–Jun;29(2):189–92

**Spain**

Basante Pol RM: La farmacia en los monasterios, hospitales y hospederías del Bierzo. **Bol Soc Esp Hist Farm** 1984 Sep;35(139):165–86
Darnés C, Solé A: Influencia de las comunidades religiosas en la enfermería de Cataluña. **Rev Enferm** 1981 Dec–1982 Jan;5(42–43):61–2
Esteva de Sagrera J, Espinosa Ramos E: El proceso inquisitorial de Proust y el protagonismo cultural de Feijoo en el panorama cientifico de la ilustracion española. **Bol Soc Esp Hist Farm** 1982 Mar;33(129):77–92

# RELIGION AND MEDICINE

Jetter D: Neue Funde zur Geschichte der alten Pilgerherberge in Santiago de Compostela. In Seidler E, Schott H, ed: Bausteine zur Medizingeschichte. Stuttgart, Steiner, 1984. p. 52–64.

**Sweden**

Pontén J: Gudar, präster och läkekonst. Södertälje, Axlings, 1980. 79 p. (Nordisk Medicinhistorisk Arsbok, Supplementum, VII).

**Switzerland**

Monter EW: Sodomy and heresy in early modern Switzerland. **J Homosex** 1980–81 Fall–Winter;6(1–2):41–55

**United States**

Carmelli D, Andersen S: A longevity study of twins in the Mormon genealogy. **Prog Clin Biol Res** 1981;69 pt C:187–200

Cassedy JH: Church record-keeping and public health in early New England. In: Medicine in Colonial Massachusetts 1620–1820. (Publications of the Colonial Society of Massachusetts, vol. 57), 1980. p. 249–62.

Christensen HT: Mormon sexuality in cross-cultural perspective. **Dialogue** 1976;10(2):62–75

King JO: The iron of melancholy: structures of spiritual conversion in America from the Puritan conscience to Victorian neurosis. Middletown, Conn., Wesleyan University Press, 1983. ix, 456 p.

Murphey MG: The psychodynamics of Puritan conversion. **Am Q** 1979;31(2):135–47

**USSR**

Zguta R: The one-day votive church: a religious response to the black death in early Russia. **Slavic Rev** 1981;40(3):423–32

**Zaire**

Kimpianga KM: The religious therapeutic functions of the cemetery for the Kongo of Zaire. **Cah Relig Afr** 1978;12:107–24

**Before 500 A.D.**

Amundsen DW: Medicine and faith in early Christianity. **Bull Hist Med** 1982 Fall;56(3):326–50

Barton NJ: Hand markings of the Shroud of Turin. **Hand** 1980;12:323

Davidson M: Ancient references to dentistry and 'Biblical bites'. **Bull Hist Dent** 1983 Apr;31(1):30–1

Häusermann R, Koelbing H, Biener K: Präventivmedizin in den alten Religionen. **Soz Praventivmed** 1984;29(2):72–7

Hausmann W: Der Stier als Fruchtbarkeitssymbol. Ein Bericht über Funde aus mehreren Ländern. **DTW** 1982 Feb 5:89(2):86–8

Kádár Z: Gyógyító istenségek tisztelete Pannóniában topográfiai adatok tükrében. **Orvostort Kozl** 1981;93–96(27 No 1–4):63–78

Kuttner RE: Protohistoric hepatomancy: an oracular form of pathology. **Proc Inst Med Chic** 1982 Jan–Mar;35(1):14

Noorda S: Illness and sin, forgiving and healing. The connection of medical treatment and religious beliefs in Ben Sira 38, 1–15. In: Studies in Hellenistic Religions; ed. by M. J. Vermaseren. Leiden, Brill, 1979. pp.215–224.

Savitz HA: Dreams in the Talmud: the prophets of yore had the noblest dream. **RI Med J** 1981 Sep;64(9):427–30

Sorokina TS: Meditsina Drevnego Vostoka. **Feldsher Akush** 1983;48(3):50–3

**Asia**

Hausmann W: Der Becher des Gudea. **Tierarztl Prax** 1979;7(2):141–3

**China**

Unschuld PU: Concepts of illness in ancient China: the case of demonological medicine. **J Med Philos** 1980;5(2):117–32

**Egypt**

Briceño Maaz T: Im-Hotep: dios egipcio de la medicina. **Rev Soc Venez Hist Med** 1969–71;17–19(31–33):75–82

Emboden WA: Transcultural use of narcotic water lilies in ancient Egyptian and Maya drug ritual. **J Ethnopharmacol** 1981 Jan;3(1):39–83

Helbling M: Der altägyptische Augenkranke, sein Arzt und seine Götter. Zürich, Juris, 1980. 78 p. (Zürcher medizingeschichtliche Abhandlungen, Neue Reihe, Nr. 141) Also Diss., Zürich.

Patai R: Maria the Jewess--founding mother of alchemy. **Ambix** 1982 Nov;29(3):177–92

**Greco–Roman**

Kerényi K: Der göttliche Arzt. Studien über Asklepios und seine Kultstätten. Darmstadt, Wissenschaftliche Buchgesellschaft, 1975, 3rd ed. xxi, 113 p.

Oberhelman SM: Galen, On Diagnosis from Dreams. **J Hist Med Allied Sci** 1983 Jan;38(1):36–47

Siclari A: L'antropologia di Nemesio di Emesa. Padova, La Garangola, 1974. 318 p. (Filosofia e religione; 9).

Vidal F: Medecine sacerdotale dans le monde antique. **Chir Dent Fr** 1983 Jun 2;53(206):37–5

**Greece**

Briceño Maaz T: Santuario de Esculapio en Epidauro. **Rev Soc Venez Hist Med** 1972–73;20–21(34–35):51–65

Calogirou DK: L'Asclêpieion de Cos, Hippocrate et la maladie des coronaires. **Hist Sci Med** 1979;13(4):427–39

Castner CJ: Epicurean Hetainai as dedicants to healing deities? **Greek Roman Byz Stud (Cambridge, Mass.)** 1982;23:51–7

Oberhelman SM: The interpretation of prescriptive dreams in ancient Greek medicine. **J Hist Med Allied Sci** 1981 Oct;36(4):416–24

Ruck CA: Mushrooms and philosophers. **J Ethnopharmacol** 1981 Sep;4(2):179–205

Siefert H: Inkubation, Imagination und Kommunikation im antiken Asklepioskult. In Leuner H, ed: Katathymes Bilderleben. Ergebnisse in Theorie und Praxis. Bern, Stuttgart, Wien, Huber, 1980. p. 324–45.

Stam HJ, Spanos NP: The Asclepian dream healings and hypnosis: a critique. **Int J Clin Exp Hypn** 1982 Jan;30(1):9–22

Vincelet L: Asklépios, dieu grec de la médecine ou simple praticien grec mortel? **Arch Med Normandie** 1978 Oct, Dec;9(8,10):427–9, 543–4

**India**

Bergemann H: Drachenzähne und Opfergaben. **Zahnarztl Mitt** 1980 May 16;70(10):655–7

Corcos AF: Reproduction and heredity beliefs of the Hindus based on their sacred books. **J Hered** 1984 Mar–Apr;75(2):152–4

Filliozat J: Sur l'identification des maladies dans l'Ayurveda. In Mazars G, ed: Les médecines traditionnelles de l'Asie. Strasbourg, Université Louis Pasteur, 1981. p. 140–9.

Mazars G: Die Medizin in den Weden. In Sournia JC, Martiny M, Poulet J, ed: Illustrierte Geschichte der Medizin. Salzburg, Andreas, 1980. Vol. 1. p. 145–63.

Ranade HG: A note on 'Pata in Atharvaveda 2.27'. **Stud Hist Med** 1981 Sep;5(3):225–7

**Italy**

Bucklin R: The Shroud of Turin: a pathologist's viewpoint. **J Miss State Med Assoc** 1983 Apr;24(4):95–8

Massey EW: An interpretation of the hand and arm markings of the shroud of Turin. **Hand** 1980 Feb;12(1):75–80

**Mesopotamia**

André-Leicknam B: Les premiers écrits médicaux. Le sang en Mésopotamie. **Nouv Rev Fr Hematol** 1983;25(2):141–4

**Peru**

Dobkin de Rios M: Plant hallucinogens, sexuality and shamanism in the ceramic art of ancient Peru. **J Psychoactive Drugs** 1982 Jan–Jun;14(1–2):81–90

**Rome**

Andre JM: La notion de Pestilentia à Rome: du tabou religieux à l'interprétation pré-scientifique. **Latomus** 1980;39:2–16

Richardson WF: Medicine: the art of guessing? **NZ Med J** 1984 Jul 11;97(759):453–5

**500 A.D.–1450**

Abrahams HJ: A medicine for 'Sickness of the spirit.' **Trans Stud Coll Physicians Phila** 1977 Apr;44(4):202–3

Agrimi J: Malato, medico, e medicina nel Medioevo. Torino, Loescher Editore, 1980. 301 p.

Amundsen DW: Casuistry and professional obligations: the regulation of physicians by the court of conscience in the late Middle Ages. Part II. **Trans Stud Coll Physicians Phila** 1981 Jun;3(2):93–112

Brossollet J: Quelques aspects religieux de la grande peste du XIVe siècle. **Rev Hist Philos Relig** 1984 Jan–Mar;64(1):53–66

Dirckx JH: Peter Juliani, physician and pope. **Pharos** 1980 Fall;43(4):8–13

Ell SR: The two medicines: some ecclesiastical concepts of disease and the physician in the high Middle Ages. **Janus** 1981;68:15–25

Jackson SW: Acedia the sin and its relationship to sorrow and melancholia

in medieval times. **Bull Hist Med** 1981 Summer;55(2):172–85
Jenkins M: Medicine and spices, with special reference to medieval monastic accounts. **Gard Hist** 1976;4:47–9
Kroll J, Bachrach B: Visions and psychopathology in the Middle Ages. **J Nerv Ment Dis** 1982 Jan;170(1):41–9
Leibowitz JO: Medical items in the book Torat ha-'Adam of Rabbi Moses ben Nahman (1194–1270). **Koroth** 1983 Aug;8(7–8):257–64
Müller RA: Mittelalterliches Konzil und Medizin. **MMW** 1983 Apr 1;125(13):263–4
Weisheipl JA, ed: Albertus Magnus and the sciences: commenmorative essays 1980. Toronto, Pontifical Institute of Mediaeval Studies, 1980. xiv, 657 p.
Wood CT: The doctors' dilemma: sin, salvation, and the menstrual cycle in medieval thought. **Speculum** 1981;56(4):710–27

#### Americas

Naranjo P: Social function of coca in pre-Columbian America. **J Ethnopharmacol** 1981 Mar–May;3(2–3):161–72

#### Arabic

Abdul Ali: Contribution of Islam to the development of medical science. **Stud Hist Med** 1980 Mar;4(1):44–52
Klein-Franke F: Vorlesungen über die Medizin im Islam. **Sudhoffs Arch Beih** 1982;23:1–146
Leiser G: Medical education in Islamic lands from the seventh to the fourteenth century. **J Hist Med Allied Sci** 1983 Jan;38(1):48–75
Sendrail M: La foi coranique et l'héritage médical grec. **Bull Assoc Guillaume Bude** 1977;:278–99
Wooden AC: Medical care in Islamic armies. In International Congress of the History of Medicine, 27th, Barcelona, 1980. Actas. Barcelona, Académia de Ciències Mèdiques de Catalunya i Balears, 1981. p. 694–8.

#### Byzantium

Volk R: Gesundheitswesen und Wohltätigkeit im Spiegel der byzantinischen Klostertypika. München, Institut für Byzantinistik und neugriechische Philologie der Universität München, 1983. lxxx, 326 p. (Miscellanea Byzantina monacensia, Heft 28)

#### Europe

Ferrari Sacco A: Benedetto da Norcia e la medicina conventuale in Europa (nel 1500th anniversario della nascita). **Minerva Med** 1981 Mar 10;72(9):585–7
Kroll J, Bachrach B: Sin and mental illness in the Middle Ages. **Psychol Med** 1984 Aug;14(3):507–14

#### France

Assistance et charité: Toulouse, Privat, 1978. 435 p. (Cahiers de Fanjeaux, Collection d'Histoire religieuse du Languedoc au XIIIe et début du XIVe siècles, 13).
Cheymol J: Hôpitaux et confrérie des pèlerins de Saint-Jacques-de-Compostelle à Paris. **Hist Sci Med** 1980;14(1):29–42
Eastwood BS: The place of medicine in a hierarchy of knowledge: the illustration in Lyon Palais des Arts, ms. 22, f. lr, from the eleventh century. **Sudhoffs Arch** 1982;66(1):20–37
Karnofsky ES: The vision of Tainard, miraculum de quodam canonico Guatenensi per Sanctum Donatianum curato. In Sheils WJ, ed: The Church and healing. Papers read at the twentieth summer meeting and the twenty-first winter meeting of the Ecclesiastical History Society. Oxford, Basil Blackwell for the Society, 1982. p. 15–24.
La Coste Messelière R de: Sources et illustrations de l'histoire des établissements hospitaliers et du pèlerinage de Saint-Jacques-de-Compostelle. **Bull Soc Hist Sci Deux Sevres** 1977;10:195–269
Wakefield WL: Heretics as physicians in the thirteenth century. **Speculum** 1982 Apr;57(2):328–31

#### Germany

John Paul II Pope: Discurso de Juan Pablo II a los profesores y estudiantes universitarios en la catedral de Colonia (Aalemania), 15.XI.1980. **Rev Med Univ Navarra** 1981 Jun;25(2):61–4
Valentin P: Mit Brevier und Skalpell. Legendäre Bauchoperation Kaiser Heinrichs II. **Med Welt** 1982 Feb 19;33(7):260–2

#### Great Britain

Cohen VL: Bleeding monks. **Lancet** 1981 Jul 18;2(8238):158
Foley GP: A treasury of dentistry. The dental attraction of the Wells Cathedral. **J Am Coll Dent** 1983 Fall;50(3):16–7
Gardner R: Miracles of healing in Anglo-Celtic Northumbria as recorded by the venerable Bede and his contemporaries: a reappraisal in the light of twentieth century experience. **Br Med J [Clin Res]** 1983 Dec 24–31;287(6409):1927–33
Mason E: 'Rocamadour in Quercy above all other churches': the healing of Henry II. In Sheils WJ, ed: The Church and healing. Papers read at the twentieth summer meeting and the twenty-first winter meeting of the Ecclesiastical History Society. Oxford, Basil Blackwell for the Society, 1982. p. 39–54.
Sass LJ: Religion, medicine, politics and spices. **Appetite** 1981 Mar;2(1):7–13
Schmidt PG: Materielle und spirituelle Diät. Ein mittellateinischer Verstraktat des frühen 13. Jahrhunderts aus St. Albans. In Dilg P, et al., ed: Perspektiven der Pharmaziegeschichte. Graz, Austria, Akademische Druck- u. Verlagsanstalt, 1983. p. 311–23.

#### India

Gurjar GK, Anand RM: Apurva Vaidya of Vagbhata. **Bull Indian Inst Hist Med (Hyderabad)** 1975 Oct;5(4):207–10
Rama Rao B, Reddy MV: A note on Goraksanātha and his work Yogadipikā. **Bull Indian Inst Hist Med Hyderabad** 1982;12(1–4):34–44

#### Italy

Bazzi F, Panebianco D: Una lauda di interesse medico poco nota di Jacopone da Todi. **Minerva Med** 1981 Nov 14;72(45):3039–43
Bruce-Chwatt LJ: Jacopone da Todi's mystical pathology. **Br Med J [Clin Res]** 1982 Dec 18–25;285(6357):1803–4
Orofino G, Brach CC: Nel nome del bagno. **Kos** 1984 Apr;1(3):33–54

#### Mexico

Angot J: Un crâne à face décorée de la civilisation mixtèque. **Hist Sci Med** 1984;18(3):255–9

#### Portugal

Reis CS, Jans GJ: Sessão comemorativa do 7.o centenário de Pedro Hispano -- 20 de Maio de 1977. **An Inst Hig Med Trop (Lisb)** 1977–1978;5(1–4):3–19

#### Scandinavia

Steffensen J: Fra hedenskab til katolicisme, de medicinsk-historiske konsekvenser i Norden. **Nord Medicinhist Arsb** 1982;:149–56

#### Spain

Gyug R: The effects and extent of the Black Death of 1348: new evidence for clerical mortality in Barcelona. **Mediaev Stud** 1983;45:385–98
Rodrigo Lizondo M: La protesta de Valencia de 1318 y otros documentos inéditos referentes a Arnau de Vilanova. **Dynamis** 1981;1:241–73

#### Switzerland

Bischoff P, Speiser P: Mittelalterliche Augenheilkunde im Kloster St. Gallen. **Gesnerus** 1982;39(1):47–52

### 1450–1700

Rudolph H: Schriftauslegung und Schriftverständnis bei Paracelsus. **Medizinhist J** 1981;16(1–2):101–24
Secret F: Palingenesis, alchemy and metempsychosis in Renaissance medicine. **Ambix** 1979 Jul;26(2):81–92

#### Belgium

Bloch H: Jan Baptiste Van Helmont, M.D. (1579–1644); religion, mysticism, and science in a century of change. **NY State J Med** 1980 Sep;80(10):1631–3

#### Denmark

Bierbaum M, Faller A: Niels Stensen. Anatom, Geologe und Bischof, 1638–1686. 2d ed. Münster, Aschendorff, 1979. xi, 203 p. Includes Thomasen AL, Der Wandel des Stensenbildes.

#### Europe

Gysel C: Renaissance, filosofie en geneeskunde. **Rev Belge Med Dent** 1983 Jan;38(1):16–20
Niccoli O: 'Menstruum quasi monstruum': parti mostruosi e tabù mestruale nel '500. **Quad Stor** 1980;15(2):402–8

#### France

Bèttica-Giovannini R: La preghiera di Blaise Pascal per il buon uso delle malattie. **Ann Osp Maria Vittoria Torino** 1979 Jul–Dec;22(7–12):420–5
Chaboche R: Le clergé de France et l'assistance aux invalides de guerre

au XVIIe siècle. In: Congrès National des Sociétés Savantes, 97e, Nantes, 1972. Actes. Paris, 1977. Histoire Moderne et Contemporaine, Tome 1. p. 31–47.
Humm E: Vinzenz von Paul und seine Aktualität. Sein Aufruf zur patientenorientierten Pflege. **Krankenpflege (Frankfurt)** 1982 Jan;36(1):3–4
Robert G: La révocation de l'édit de Nantes et les professions de Santé. **Hist Sci Med** 1983;17(2):181–7
Treuille H: L'état des hôpitaux de pèlerins dans le Sud-Ouest de la France dans la seconde moitié du XVIIe siècle. In: Congrès National des Sociétés Savantes, 104e, Bordeaux, 1979. Actes. Paris, 1981. Histoire Moderne et Contemporaine, Tome 2. p. 35–50.
Valverde JL, Arrebola Nacle P: Ayuda sanitaria de Felipe II a Francia. **Bol Soc Esp Hist Farm** 1982 Mar;33(130):123–9

**Germany**

Becke U: Eine hinterlassene psychiatrische Studie Paul Johann Reiters über Luther. **Z Kirchengesch** 1979;90(1):85–95
Böhmer W, Kirsten F: Reformatorische Ausstrahlungen Martin Luthers auf das Gesundheitswesen seiner Zeit. **Z Gesamte Inn Med** 1983 Oct 15;38(20):546–51
Hahn S: Martin Luther--was sagt er uns Arzten heute? **Z Gesamte Inn Med** 1983 Oct 15;38(20):551–4
Imhof A: Les sermons funèbres comme source de la démographie historique pour la période de 1500 à 1650. **Ann Demogr Hist (Paris)** 1980;:79–86
Kaiser W: Eisleben und das Mansfelder Land im medizinhistorischen Aspekt. Ein Beitrag zum Lutherjahr 1983. **Z Gesamte Inn Med** 1983 Oct 15;38(20):539–46
Kapronczay K: Magyar medikusok a wittenbergi egyetemen Luther és Melanchton korában. **Orv Hetil** 1984 Apr 15;125(16):958–60
Ozment S: Luther and the family. **Harv Libr Bull** 1984 Winter;32(1):36–53
Völker A: Martin Luther und seine Arzte. Ein Beitrag zum Lutherjahr 1983. **Z Gesamte Inn Med** 1983 Oct 15;38(20):533–9

**Great Britain**

Ardolino F: The saving hand of God: the significance of the emblematic frontispiece of the Religio medici. **Engl Lang Notes** 1977;15:19–23
Birken W: Dr. John King (1614–1681) and Dr. Assuerus Regemorter (1615–1650). Brethren in the Dutch Church and in the Royal College of Physicians of London, with added references to other 'Dutch' congregants in the Royal College, Dr. Baldwin Hamey and Dr. George Ent. **Med Hist** 1976 Jul;20(3):276–95
Elton GR: The real Thomas More? **Psychol Med** 1980 Nov;10(4):611–7
Force JE: Hume and the relation of science to religion among certain members of the Royal Society. **J Hist Ideas** 1984 Oct–Dec;45(4):517–36
Heyd M: Robert Burton's sources on enthusiasm and melancholy: from a medical tradition to religious controversy. **Hist Eur Ideas** 1984;5:17–44
Huntley FL: 'Well Sir Thomas?': oration to commemorate the tercentenary of the death of Sir Thomas Browne. **Br Med J [Clin Res]** 1982 Jul 3;285(6334):43–7
Kaplan BB: Greatrakes the stroker: the interpretations of his contemporaries. **ISIS** 1982 Jun;73(267):178–85
Lynch M: The 'Faithful Brethren' of Edinburgh: the acceptable face of Protestantism. **Bull Inst Hist Res** 1978;51(124):194–9
MacDonald M: Mystical bedlam: madness, anxiety, and healing in seventeenth-century England. Cambridge, Cambridge University Press, 1981. xvi, 323 p.
Miller E: The Browne doublet: 'Religio medici' in the history of English prose style. **Bull Res Humanit** 1979;82:213–21
Mulligan L: Puritans and English science: a critique of Webster. **Isis** 1980 Sep;71(258):456–69
Neibyl KH: Science, medicine and the Puritan society. **J Eur Econ Hist** 1979;8(1):149–56
Nelson TG: Death, dung, the devil, and worldly delights: a metaphysical conceit in Harington, Donne, and Herbert. **Stud Philol** 1979 Summer;76(3):272–87
Niebyl KH: Science, medicine and the Puritan society. **J Eur Econ Hist** 1979;8(1):
Pineas R: William Turner's Spirituall physik. **Sixteenth Cent J** 1983;14:387–98
Rattansi PM: Medicine and the Puritan Revolution. **Soc Soc Hist Med Bull (Lond)** 1984 Jun;34:4–5
Steneck NH: Greatrakes the stroker: the interpretations of historians. **ISIS** 1982 Jun;73(267):161–77
Webster A: Threefold cord of religion, science, and literature in the character of Sir Thomas Browne. **Br Med J [Clin Res]** 1982 Dec 18–25;285(6357):1801–2

**Italy**

David A: A medical sermon of R. Gedalya ibn Yahya. **Koroth** 1982;8(3–4):187–9
Ruggiero Pastura MG: Una 'visita' del 1592 all'ospedale dei 'pazzarelli' di Roma. **Rass Arch Stato** 1972;32(1):47–67

**Japan**

Hino S, Konoshita K, Kitamura T: HTLV and the propagation of Christianity in Nagasaki. **Lancet** 1984 Sep 8;2(8402):572–3

**Mexico**

Micheli A de: La inquisición y los médicos en la Nueva España. **Prensa Med Mex** 1979 Nov–Dec;44(11–12):273–7

**Netherlands**

Schupbach W: The paradox of Rembrandt's 'Anatomy of Dr. Tulp'. London, Wellcome Institute for the History of Medicine, 1982. 110 p. (Medical History, Suppl. No. 2).

**Portugal**

Pereira I da R: Processos de feitiçaria e de bruxaria na Inquisiçao de Portugal. **An Acad Port Hist** 1977;24(2):83–178

**Spain**

Cappelletti AJ: Servet, teologo, filosofo y medico. **Rev Soc Venez Hist Med** 1975–76;23(37):147–61
Dedieu H: Notes sur les pertes humaines subies par les communautés religieuses de Séville durant l'epidémie de 1649. **Arch Franciscanum Hist** 1978;71(3–4):462–68
Hirsch EF: Michael Servetus and the neoplatonic tradition: God, Christ and Man. **Bibl Hum Renaissance** 1980 Sep;42(3):561–75

**Switzerland**

Bouwsma WJ: John Calvin's anxiety. **Proc Am Philos Soc** 1984 Sep;128(3):252–6
Gilly C: Zwischen Erfahrung und Spekulation. Theodor Zwinger und die religiöse und kulturelle Krise seiner Zeit. **Basler Z Gesch Altertumskd** 1977;77:57–137
Goldammer K: Zur philosophischen und religiösen Sinngebung von Heilung und Heilmittel bei Paracelsus. In Dilg P, et al., ed: Perspektiven der Pharmaziegeschichte. Graz, Austria, Akademische Druck- u. Verlagsanstalt, 1983. p. 113–29.

**1700 to Present**

Bakan D: Freud e la tradizione mistica ebraica: psicoanalisi e cabala. **Comunita** 1976;39(176):206–44
Beckmann P, Kirchhoff HW: Heilkunst und Heilkunde am Beispiel des Pfarrers Sebastian Kneipp. **Ther Ggw** 1980 Aug;119(8):945–53
Bori PC: Materiale storico–religioso nella biblioteca di Sigmund Freud: alcuni rilievi sul catalogo. **Ann Ist Stor Italo–Ger** 1975;1:281–9
Capps D: Psychohistory in religious studies. **Group Psychol Hist Newsl** 1974;3(2):4–8
Clarke JM: Surgery in Jehovah's witnesses. **Br J Hosp Med** 1982 May;27(5):497–500
Farr AD: Religious opposition to obstetric anaesthesia: a myth? **Ann Sci** 1983 Mar;40(2):159–77
Genné WH: Sex, marriage and family: an update from Amsterdam. **J Ecumenical Stud** 1979;16(1):154–60
Goering JD: Sigmund Freud, Carl Jung and religion. **Mennon Q Rev** 1982;56(1):47–56
Gottdenker P: Three clerics in pursuit of 'little animals.' **Clio Med** 1980 Jul;14(3–4):213–24
Hammett JY: A second drink at the well: theological and philosophical context of CPE origins. **J Pastoral Care** 1975 Jun;29(2):86–9
Kottayarikil C: Sigmund Freud on religion and morality: a challenge to Christianity. Innsbruck, Resch, 1977. xx, 399 p.
McCall N: The statue of the Christus Consolator at the Johns Hopkins Hospital: its acquisition and historic origins. **Johns Hopkins Med J** 1982 Jul;151(1):11–9
Money J: The genealogical descent of sexual psychoneuroendocrinology from sex and health theory: the eighteenth to the twentieth centuries. **Psychoneuroendocrinology** 1983;8(4):391–400
Odontoiatria del passato: Dei campanelli de Loreto. **Dent Cadmos** 1981 Jul;49(7):59–60
Ono Y: [Human science. Religion (1). Religion as a psychological phenomenon--progress in religious psychology] (Jpn). **Kango Tenbo** 1981 Apr;6(4):350–6
Pototschnig F: Entwicklungstendenzen im kanonischen Ehe- und Eheprozessrecht. **Osterr Arch Kirchenr** 1978;29(1–2):52–81
Prayer composed during cholera epidemic outbreak 1831 and 1847?: by R. Abraham Bing of Würzburg. **Koroth** 1979 Nov;7(9–10):719–20
Sandler IL: Pierre Louis Moreau de Maupertuis--a precursor of Mendelian genetics?: an inquiry into the biological ideas of Maupertuis, the Mendelian principles of heredity and the nature of the precursor. Ph.D. diss. University of Washington. Seattle, 1979. 265 leaves.
Socknat TP: The Canadian contribution to the China convoy.

Quaker Hist 1980;69(2):69–90
Vader JP: August Forel defends the persecuted Persian Baha'is, 1925–27. **Gesnerus** 1984;41(1/2):53–60
Weinstein MA, Weinstein D: Freud's encounter with religion: a study in bad faith. **Thought** 1981;56:463–76

### Africa

Kiernan J: Saltwater and ashes: instruments of curing among some Zulu zionists. **J Relig Afr** 1978;9:27–32
Ranger T: Medical science and pentecost: the dilemma of anglicanism in Africa. In Sheils WJ, ed: The Church and healing. Papers read at the twentieth summer meeting and the twenty-first winter meeting of the Ecclesiastical History Society. Oxford, Basil Blackwell for the Society, 1982. p. 333–65.
Stöcklin WH: Sakpata, ein Beitrag Afrikanischer Medizinmänner zur Pockeneradikation. **Gesnerus** 1982;39(3–4):405–15

### Americas

Kay MA: The Florilegio Medicinal: source of Southwest ethnomedicine. **Ethnohistory** 1977;24(3):251–9
Neufeld VH, ed: If we can love: the Mennonite mental health story. Newton, Kan., Faith and Life Press, 1983. xii, 340 p.

### Arabic

Abdul-Rauf M: Contemporary Muslim perspective [on medical ethics]. In Reich WT, et al, ed: Encyclopedia of bioethics, v. 2. New York, Free Press, 1978. p. 892–5.

### Australia

Burke JA: The Dominican nun's school for the deaf and dumb in New South Wales. **J R Aust Hist Soc** 1973;59(4):270–85

### Barbados

Phillips GO: Barbados' Battle Creek doctor Charles J. B. Cave 1879–1939. **Advent Herit** 1978;5(2):22–33

### Belgium

Aernouts R: L'eau de Lourdes est-elle un médicament? **Rev Hist Pharm (Paris)** 1980 Mar;27(244):5–7

### Brazil

Williams PV: Primitive religion and healing. A study of folk medicine in North-East Brazil. Cambridge, England, and Totowa, New Jersey, D. S. Brewer and Rowman and Littlefield, 1979. xi, 212 p.

### Canada

Ballstadt C, Peterman M, Hopkins E: 'A glorious madness': Susanna Moodie and the spiritualist movement. **J Can Stud** 1982–83;17(4):88–100
Berger C: Science, God, and nature in Victorian Canada. Toronto; Buffalo, University of Toronto Press, 1983. xiv, 92 p.
DeValk A: Understandable but mistaken: law, morality and the Canadian Catholic Church 1966–1969. **Can Cathol Hist Assoc Study Sess** 1982;49:87–109
Gareau S: L'organisation hospitalière dans le nord-ouest Quebeçois. **Can Cathol Hist Assoc Study Sess** 1982;49:35–58
Janson G: Pierre-Joseph Compain. In Dictionary of Canadian biography, 1801 to 1820. Volume 5, 1983. p. 201–202.
Kutcher SP: Toronto's metaphysicians: the social gospel and medical professionalization in Victorian Toronto. **HSTC Bull** 1981;5(1):41–51
Sylvain P: Jean-Etienne Landry. In Dictionary of Canadian biography, 1881–1890. 1982;11:483–6.

### China

Buck P: American science and modern China, 1876–1936. Cambridge, Cambridge University Press, 1980. viii, 283 p.

### Europe

Lesthaeghe R, Wilson C: Les modes de production, la laïcisation et le rythme de la baisse de la fécondité en Europe de l'Ouest de 1870 à 1930. **Population** 1982;37(3):623–45

### Finland

Pesonen N: Rovasti Wegelius ja hänen lääkärikirjansa. **Duodecim** 1984;100(2):72–9

### France

Billioud J: Les Saints de la Peste. Une grande page de solidarité. **Marseille** 1983;(132–133):56–63
Charuty G: La psychiatrisation des croyances: savoir médical et savoirs surnaturels en Languedoc, 1850–1940. **Asclepio** 1983;35:197–215
Fusswerk-Fursay J: A propos d'un inédit de Pierre Janet sur les croyances. **Ann Med Psychol (Paris)** 1984 May;142(5):703–10
Greenbaum LS: Nurses and doctors in conflict: piety and medicine in the Paris Hôtel-Dieu on the eve of the French Revolution. **Clio Med** 1979 May;13(3–4):247–67
Greenbaum LS: Science, medicine, religion: three views of health care in France on the eve of the French Revolution. **Stud Eighteenth Cent Cult** 1981;10:373–91
Kaufmann C: La question de l'inoculation déférée à l'Eglise. **Asclepio** 1983;35:403–11
Kreiser BR: Miracles, convulsions, and ecclesiastical politics in early eighteenth-century Paris. Princeton, Princeton University Press, 1978. xvii, 485 p.
Léonard J: Les guérisseurs en France au XIXe siècle. **Rev Hist Mod Contemp** 1980 Jul–Sep;27:501–16
McManners J: Death and the Enlightenment. Changing attitudes to death among Christians and unbelievers in eighteenth-century France. Oxford, Clarendon Press; New York, Oxford University Press; 1981. vii, 619 p.
Mammerickx M: André-Marie Ampère et Claude-Julien Bredin, I. Ampère, Bredin et la philosophie, ou la belle histoire d'une amitié. **Hist Med Vet** 1977;2(1):11–19
Muller-Rensmann R: Les trois grands pôles du miracle en France au 19e siècle, la médaille miraculeuse, Lourdes et Thérèse de Lisieux. **Penelope** 1981;(5):56–7
Religion et médecine populaires: **Lemouzi** 1979;71:235–367

### Germany

Arendt HJ: Eine demokratische Massenbewegung unter Führung der KPD im Frühjahr 1931. **Z Geschichtswiss** 1971;19(2):212–23
Arndal S: Krop, sjael og ånd Georg Ernst Stahls og Christian Friedrich Richters medicinske antropologi. **Dan Medicinhist Arbog** 1980;:126–66
Habrich C: Therapeutische Grundsätze pietistischer Arzte des 18. Jahrhunderts. **Beitr Gesch Pharm** 1982;31(16):121–3
Jungnitz B: Die konfessionellen Krankenhäuser der Stadt Münster im achtzehnten und neunzehnten Jahrhundert. Herzogenrath, Verlag Murken-Altrogge, 1981. 304 p. (Studien zur Geschichte des Krankenhauswesens. 18).
Volk L: Episkopat und Kirchenkampf im Zweiten Weltkrieg. Lebensvernichtung und Klostersturm 1939–1941. **Stimmen Zeit** 1980;198(9):597–611

### Ghana

Breidenbach PS: 'Sunsum edwuma': the limits of classification and the significance of an event. **Soc Res (NY)** 1979;46(1):63–87

### Great Britain

Altholz JL: The Huxley-Wilberforce debate revisited. **J Hist Med Allied Sci** 1980 Jul;35(3):313–16
Annear MW: Some healing and holy wells of Wales. In J. Cule, ed: Wales and medicine. London, British Society for the History of Medicine, 1975. p. 185–89.
Aspinwall B: Social Catholicism and health: Dr. and Mrs. Thomas Low Nichols in Britain. In Sheils WJ, ed: The Church and healing. Papers read at the twentieth summer meeting and the twenty-first winter meeting of the Ecclesiastical History Society. Oxford, Basil Blackwell for the Society, 1982. p. 249–70.
Barrow L: Anti-establishment healing: spiritualism in Britain. In Sheils WJ, ed: The Church and healing. Papers read at the twentieth summer meeting and the twenty-first winter meeting of the Ecclesiastical History Society. Oxford, Basil Blackwell for the Society, 1982. p. 225–47.
Barrow L: Deviants in death? Plebeian secularists and spiritualists c. 1860–1910. **Soc Soc Hist Med Bull (Lond)** 1980 Jun;26:22–4
Bolander V: A preliminary examination of John Wesley's 'Primitive physick'. **Bookman** 1983 Jul–Aug;10(4):3–10
Capper WM, Johnson D, ed: The faith of a surgeon. Belief and experience in the life of Arthur Rendle Short. Exeter, England, Paternoster Press, 1976. 156 p.
Champ JF: Bishop Milner, Holywell, and the cure tradition. In Sheils WJ, ed: The Church and healing. Papers read at the twentieth summer meeting and the twenty-first winter meeting of the Ecclesiastical History Society. Oxford, Basil Blackwell for the Society, 1982. p. 153–64.
Connolly GP: Little brother be at peace: the priest as holy man in the nineteenth-century ghetto. In Sheils WJ, ed: The Church and healing. Papers read at the twentieth summer meeting and the twenty-first winter meeting of the Ecclesiastical History Society. Oxford, Basil Blackwell for the Society, 1982. p. 191–206.
Dupâquier J, Fauve-Chamoux A, Grebenik E, ed: Malthus past and

present. London; New York, Academic Press, 1983. xix, 416 p. Contributions by A. Béjin, Y. Breton, Y. Charbit, L. Devance, A. Digby, M. W. Flinn, R. E. Frisch, M. Godelier, L. Gordon, P. Guillaume, G. Heinsohn, T. H. Hollingsworth, P. A. Jewell, N. Keyfitz, R. Keynes, H. Le Bras, M. Perrot, F. Rausky, M. Rebérioux, R. Remond, F. Ronsin, G. R. Searle, B. Stapleton, O. Steiger, P. Vallin, E. Van de Walle, A. Waterman, J. Wolff, E. A. Wrigley, V. Wynne-Edwards.

Gaustad ES: George Berkeley in America. New Haven, Yale University Press, 1979. xi, 225 p.

Guy JR: Archbishop Secker as a physician. In Sheils WJ, ed: The Church and healing. Papers read at the twentieth summer meeting and the twenty-first winter meeting of the Ecclesiastical History Society. Oxford, Basil Blackwell for the Society, 1982. p. 127-35.

Janet RJ: Providence, prayer and cholera: the English general fast of 1832. **Hist Mag Protest Episc Church** 1982;51(3):297-317

Lineham PJ: Restoring man's creative power: the theosophy of the Bible Christians of Salford. In Sheils WJ, ed: The Church and healing. Papers read at the twentieth summer meeting and the twenty-first winter meeting of the Ecclesiastical History Society. Oxford, Basil Blackwell for the Society, 1982. p. 207-23.

Lucas JR: Wilberforce and Huxley: a legendary encounter. **Hist J (Gt Brit)** 1979;22(2):313-30

Malmoy CF, ed: The French Protestant Hospital: extracts from the Archives of 'La Providence' relating to inmates and applicants for admission, 1718-1957, and to recipients of and applicants for the Coqueau Charity, 1745-1901. 2 vols. London, Huguenot Society of London, 1977.

Mews S: The revival of spiritual healing in the Church of England 1920-26. In Sheils WJ, ed: The Church and healing. Papers read at the twentieth summer meeting and the twenty-first winter meeting of the Ecclesiastical History Society. Oxford, Basil Blackwell for the Society, 1982. p. 299-331.

Ospovat D: God and natural selection: the Darwinian idea of design. **J Hist Biol** 1980 Fall;13(2):169-94

Ott PW: A corner of history. John Wesley and the non-naturals. **Prev Med** 1980 Jul;9(4):578-84

Ott PW: John Wesley on health: a word for sensible regimen. **Methodist Hist** 1980;18(3):193-204

Phillips M: Yorkshire, cradle of medical friends. **Pharm Hist (London)** 1984 Jun;14(2):6-9

Pickstone JV: Establishment and dissent in nineteenth-century medicine: an exploration of some correspondence and connections between religious and medical belief-systems in early industrial England. In Sheils WJ, ed: The Church and healing. Papers read at the twentieth summer meeting and the twenty-first winter meeting of the Ecclesiastical History Society. Oxford, Basil Blackwell for the Society, 1982. p. 165-89.

Rack HD: Doctors, demons and early Methodist healing. In Sheils WJ, ed: The Church and healing. Papers read at the twentieth summer meeting and the twenty-first winter meeting of the Ecclesiastical History Society. Oxford, Basil Blackwell for the Society, 1982. p. 137-52.

Richards RJ: Instinct and intelligence in British natural theology: some contributions to Darwin's theory of the evolution of behavior. **J Hist Biol** 1981 Fall;14(2):193-230

Royle SA: Clergymen's return to the 1831 census. **Local Hist** 1980;14(2):79-90

Santurri EN: Theodicy and social policy in Malthus' thought. **J Hist Ideas** 1982 Apr-Jun;43(2):315-30

Wenneker M: Huxley's ethical system: an alternative to evolutionary ethics. **Synthesis** 1980;5(1):13-44

Wilder F: The remarkable world of John Wesley, pioneer in mental health. Hicksville, Exposition Press, 1978. 192 p.

Williams CP: Healing and evangelism: the place of medicine in later Victorian Protestant missionary thinking. In Sheils WJ, ed: The Church and healing. Papers read at the twentieth summer meeting and the twenty-first winter meeting of the Ecclesiastical History Society. Oxford, Basil Blackwell for the Society, 1982. p. 271-85.

Yumaki M: [Nightingale's concept of God] (Jpn). **Sogo Kango** 1982;16(4):23-8

**Guyana**

Baechler J: Mourir à Jonestown. **Eur J Sociol** 1979;20(2):173-210

Johnson DP: Dilemmas of charismatic leadership: the case of the People's Temple. **Sociol Anal** 1979;40(4):315-23

**Hungary**

Bolyki J: Komáromi Csipkés György: Pestis pestise (1664). **Orvostort Kozl** 1979;86(24 no 4):81-9

Sasvári L: Magyarországi egyházi betegellátó intézetek és testületek a XIX. század második felében. **Orvostort Kozl** 1982;28(1-3):209-18

**India**

Rosselli J: The self-image of effeteness: physical education and nationalism in nineteenth-century Bengal. **Past Present** 1980;(86):221-48

**Ireland**

Coward J: Recent characteristics of Roman Catholic fertility in Northern and Southern Ireland. **Popul Stud** 1980 Mar;34(1):31-44

**Israel**

Schmelz UO: [Demography of Moslems and Christians in Jerusalem] (Heb). **Hamizrah Hehadash** 1979;28(1-2):40-73

**Ivory Coast**

Handloff R: Prayers, amulets and charms: health and social control. **Afr Stud Rev** 1982;25(2-3):185-94

Walker SS: Witchcraft and healing in an African church. **J Relig Afr** 1979;10(2):127-138

**Lebanon**

Katchadourian H: The historical background of psychiatry in Lebanon. **Bull Hist Med** 1980 Winter;54(4):544-53

**Mexico**

Esteyneffer J de: Florilegio medicinal. Edicion, estudio preliminar, notas, glosario e indice analitico by M. del Carmen Anzures y Bolaños. México, Academía Nacional de Medicina, 1978. 2 v. xxiii, 973 p.

Price R: State church charity and smallpox: an epidemic crisis in the City of Mexico 1797-98. **J R Soc Med** 1982 May;75(5):356-7

**Nigeria**

Amadi GI: Healing in 'The Brotherhood of the Cross and Star'. In Sheils WJ, ed: The Church and healing. Papers read at the twentieth summer meeting and the twenty-first winter meeting of the Ecclesiastical History Society. Oxford, Basil Blackwell for the Society, 1982. p. 367-83.

Hackett R: Recent developments in the healing concepts and activities of the Aladura churches. **Afr Notes** 1981;8(2):55-8

**Norway**

Fagerheim E: Lars Levi Laestadius' teologiske studier. **Nor Teol Tidsskr** 1972;73(1):35-50

Matinsen K: Diakonissene--de første faglaerte sykepleiere. **Sykepleien** 1982 Apr 5;69(7):6-9

**Pacific Islands**

Stocking GW: Contradicting the doctor: Billy Hancock and the problem of baloma. **Hist Anthropol Newsl** 1977;4(1):4-7

**Poland**

Czeley-Wybieralska M: Early medical books in the Jesuits' Library, Małopolska Province, Cracow. **Arch Hist Med (Warsz)** 1980;43:461-3

**Portugal**

Lach E: The circumcision of the child on the eighth day...An anonymous engraving after a design by Bernard Picart. **J Hist Med Allied Sci** 1982 Apr;37(2):221

**Romania**

Pincu P: Din istoricul unei farmacii bicentenare 'spiţeria mănăstirii neamţ'. **Rev Med Chir Soc Med Nat Iasi** 1980 Jan-Mar;84(1):137-9

**South Africa**

Torrington M, Botha JL, Pilcher GJ, et al: Association between familial hypercholesterolaemia and church affiliation. Is this the result of sociocultural isolation of migrant farmers in 19th-century South Africa? **S Afr Med J** 1984 May 12;65(19):762-7

**Spain**

Carrillo JL: La dialectica ciencia--creencia y su manifestacion en la Malaga de 1803: el conflicto del cierre de los templos. **Jabega (Malaga)** 1979;26(2):3-8

Carrillo JL, García Ballester L: Repercusiones sociales de la epidemia de fiebre amarilla de Malaga (1803-1804): posturas tradicionales e ilustradas en el estamento eclesiastico. In: Sociedad Española de Historia de la Medicina. V Congreso Nacional. Madrid, 1977. **Asclepio** 1977;29:73-99

**Sri Lanka**

Stirrat RL: Shrines, pilgrimage and miraculous powers in Roman Catholic

Sri Lanka. In Sheils WJ, ed: The Church and healing. Papers read at the twentieth summer meeting and the twenty-first winter meeting of the Ecclesiastical History Society. Oxford, Basil Blackwell for the Society, 1982. p. 385–413.

**Sweden**

Lindroth S: The two faces of Linnaeus. In Frängsmyr T, ed: Linnaeus, the man and his work. Berkeley, University of California Press, 1983. p. 1–62.

**Thailand**

Matics KI: Medical arts at Wat Phra Chetuphon: various Rishi statues. **J Siam Soc** 1977;65(2):145–52

**United States**

Abbott A: Religion, psychiatry, and problems of everyday life. **Sociol Anal** 1980;41(2):164–71

Abraham HJ: Religion, medicine, and the state: reflections on some contemporary issues. **J Church State** 1980;22(3):423–36

Alexander TG: The word of wisdom: from principle to requirement. **Dialogue J Mormon Thought** 1981;14(3):78–88

Alpert RT: From Jewish science to rabbinical counseling. Philadelphia. [s.n.], 1977. 200 leaves.

Asquith GH: Anton T. Boisen and the study of 'living human documents.' **J Presbyt Hist** 1982;60(3):244–65

Baer HA: Prophets and advisors in black spiritual churches: therapy, palliative, or opiate? **Cult Med Psychiatry** 1981 Jun;5(2):145–70

Baker AL: The San Francisco evolution debates: June 13–14, 1925. **Advent Herit** 1975;2(2):23–32

Barlow W, Powell DO: The cure of Rachel Baker's 'Devotional Somnium' (Sleep-preaching). **Acad Bookman** 1978;31(1-2):3–10

Bean LL, May DL, Skolnick M: The Mormon historical demography project. **Hist Methods Newsl** 1978;11(1):45–53

Berk DW: Adventism on the picture post card. **Advent Herit** 1978;5(2):48–53

Bishop MG: The celestial family: early Mormon thought on life and death, 1830–1846. Ph.D. Diss., Southern Illinois University. Carbondale, 1981. viii, 165 leaves.

Blight JG: Jonathan Edwards's theory of the mind: its applications and implications. In J. Brozěk, ed: Explorations in the history of psychology in the United States. Lewisburg, Bucknell University Press, 1984. p. 61–120.

Breitwieser MR: Cotton Mather's pharmacy. **Early Am Lit** 1981;16(1):42–9

Brown EM: Neurology and spiritualism in the 1870s. **Bull Hist Med** 1983 Winter;57(4):563–77

Browning DS: Homosexuality, theology, the social sciences and the church. **Encounter (Lond)** 1979;40(3):223–43

Bullock A: Francis Schlatter: a fool for God. **Palacio** 1975;83(1):38–45

Bush LE: Mormon 'physiology' 1850–1875. **Bull Hist Med** 1982 Summer;56(2):218–37

Bush LE: The word of wisdom in early nineteenth-century perspective. **Dialogue J Mormon Thought** 1981;14(3):46–65

Cahill LS: Within shouting distance: Paul Ramsey and Richard McCormick on method. **J Med Philos** 1979 Dec;4(4):398–417

Carmelli D, Hasstedt S, Andersen S: Demography and genetics of human twinning in the Utah Mormon Genealogy. **Prog Clin Biol Res** 1981;69A:81–93

Cassedy JH: An American clerical crisis: ministers' sore throat 1830–1860 (the Fielding H. Garrison Lecture). **Bull Hist Med** 1979 Spring;53(1):23–38

Colbert L: Amish attitudes and treatment of illness. **Pa Folklife** 1980;30(1):9–15

Cunningham RJ: James Moore Hickson and spiritual healing in the American Episcopal church. **Hist Mag Protest Episc Church** 1970;39(1):2–16

Currie R, Driedger L, Linden R: Abstinence and moderation: mixing Mennonite drinking norms. **Mennon Q Rev** 1979;53(4):263–81

Damsteegt PG: Health reform and the Bible in early Sabbatarian Adventism. **Advent Herit** 1978;5(2):13–21

D'Antonio WV, Stack S: Religion, ideal family size, and abortion: extending Renzi's hypothesis. **J Sci Stud Relig** 1980;19(4):397–408

Davis JH: Two martyrs of the yellow fever epidemic of 1878. **West Tenn Hist Soc Pap** 1972;26:20–39

Divett RT: His chastening rod: cholera epidemics and the Mormons. **Dialogue J Mormon Thought** 1979;12(3):6–15

Divett RT: Medicine and the Mormons. An introduction to the history of Latter-Day Saint health care. Bountiful, Utah, Horizon, 1981. 222 p.

Ediger EM: Influences on the origin and development of Mennonite mental health centers. **Mennon Q Rev** 1982;56(1):32–46

Erdt T: Jonathan Edwards: art and the sense of heart. Amherst, University of Massachusetts Press, 1980. xiv, 123 p.

Flowers RB: Freedom of religion versus civil authority in matters of health. **Ann Am Acad Polit Soc Sci** 1979;446:149–61

Haag JE, Jackson LH: The acceptance of chaplains in mental hospitals. **Am Benedictine Rev** 1981;32(4):328–35

Hammett HB: The historical context of the origins of CPE. **J Pastoral Care** 1975 Jun;29(2):76–85

Hansen KJ: Mormon sexuality and American culture. **Dialogue** 1976;10(2):45–56

Hart AW: Religion and education: the Scopes controversy in Utah. **Utah Hist Q** 1983;5(2):183–98

Herring R: Southern Baptist convention resolutions on the family. **Baptist Hist Heritage** 1982;17(1):36–45, 64

Hexham I: Some aspects of religion and spiritual healing in Cultsville, a contemporary North American city. In Sheils WJ, ed: The Church and healing. Papers read at the twentieth summer meeting and the twenty-first winter meeting of the Ecclesiastical History Society. Oxford, Basil Blackwell for the Society, 1982. p. 415–29.

Hiltner S: Fifty years of CPE. **J Pastoral Care** 1975 Jun;29(2):90–8

Hoopes J: Jonathan Edwards's religious psychology. **J Am Hist** 1983;69(4):849–65

Johnson NE: Religious differentials in reproduction: the effects of sectarian education. **Demography** 1982 Nov;19(4):495–509

Johnson RA: On the psychology of the aging woman. Mary Baker Eddy as a religious leader. **J Geriatr Psychiatry** 1979;12(1):27–35

Keeney W: Experiences in mental hospitals in World War II. **Mennon Q Rev** 1982;56(1):7–17

Kenyon FE: Mary Baker Eddy, founder of Christian Science; the sublime hysteric. **Hist Med (Lond)** 1975 Autumn-Winter;6(3-4):29–46

Laur WE: Christian science visited. **South Med J** 1980 Jan;73(1):71–4

Lewis TH: The changing practice of the Oglala medicine man. **Plains Anthropol** 1980;25(89):265–7

McCue RJ: Did the word of wisdom become a commandment in 1851? **Dialogue J Mormon Thought** 1981;14(3):66–77

McLaughlin L: The pill, John Rock, and the church: the biography of a revolution. Boston, Little, Brown, 1982. 243 p.

Mandelker IL: Religion, sex, and utopia in nineteenth-century America. **Soc Res (NY)** 1982;49(3):730–51

Massey EW, Brannon WL, Riley TL: The 'jerks': mass hysteria or epilepsy? **South Med J** 1981 May;74(5):607–9

Massey JM, Massey EW: Ergot, the 'jerks,' and revivals. **Clin Neuropharmacol** 1984;7(1):99–105

Mauss AL: Shall the youth of Zion falter? Mormon youth and sex: a two-city comparison. **Dialogue** 1976;10(2):82–4

Miller L: The role of a Braucher-chiropractor in an Amish community. **Mennon Q Rev** 1981;55(2):157–71

Mineau GP, Anderton DL, Bean LL, et al: Evolution différentielle de la fécondité et groupes sociaux religieux: l'exemple de l'Utah au XIXe siècle. **Ann Demogr Hist (Paris)** 1984;:219–36

Neuerburg N: An early California document. **Masterkey Ind Lore Hist** 1983;57(3):113–6

Neufeld V: The Mennonite mental health story. **Mennon Q Rev** 1982;56(1):18–31

Norwood WF: The CME School of Medicine: its struggle for recognition and status, 1905–1915. **Advent Herit** 1979;6(2):15–24

Patrick JW: Personal faith and the fear of death among divergent religious populations. **J Sci Stud Relig** 1979;18(3):298–305

Powell RC: Anton Theophilus Boisen. In Dictionary of American biography, 1961–1965. Suppl. 7, 1981. p. 63–5.

Powell RC: Mrs. Ethel Phelps Stockes Hoyt (1877–1952) and the Joint Committee on Religion and Medicine (1923–1936): a brief sketch. **J Pastoral Care** 1975 Jun;29(2):99–105

Pruyser PW: Religio medici: Karl A. Menninger, Calvinism and the Presbyterian Church. **J Presbyt Hist** 1981;59(1):59–72

Reynolds KJ: Early days of Loma Linda.....and even before. **Advent Herit** 1975;2(1):42–50

Robbins T, Anthony D: Deprogramming, brainwashing and the medicalization of diviant religious groups. **Soc Probl** 1982;29(3):283–97

Russett CE: Declaring the glory of God. **Hist Educ Q** 1980;20(2):217–21

Shapiro HD: Getting back---and down---to basics. **Rev Am Hist** 1977;5(2):242–48

Skolnick MH, Bean LL, Mineau GP, et al: Etudes génétiques et démographiques et base de données généalogiques de l'Utah **Ann Demogr Hist (Paris)** 1984;:103–13

Smith WE: Mormon sex standards on college campuses: or deal us out of the sexual revolution! **Dialogue** 1976;10(2):76–81

Stack S: The effect of the decline in institutionalized religion on suicide, 1954–1978. **J Sci Stud Relig** 1983;22(3):239–52

Steele TJ: The death cart: it's place among the Santos of New Mexico. **Colo Mag** 1978;55(1):1–14

Studer GC: Powwowing: folk medicine or white magic? **Pa Mennon Heritage** 1980;3(3):17–23

Swan R: Faith healing, Christian Science, and the medical care of children. **N Engl J Med** 1983 Dec 29;309(26):1639–41

Szasz FM: Francis Schlatter: the healer of the southwest. **NM Hist Rev** 1979;54(2):89–104

Teahan JF: Warren Felt Evans and mental healing: romantic idealism and practical mysticism in nineteenth-century America. **Church Hist** 1979 Mar;48(1):63–80

Treolo J: Seeing fingers: the ministry of the Christian Record Braille

Foundation. **Advent Herit** 1982;7(2):28–37
Unger CW: The old Goschenhoppen Lutheran burial register: 1752–1772. **Pa Folklife** 1967–68;17(2):32–5
Wahlquist WL: Population growth in the Mormon core area: 1847–1890. Jackson, Richard H., ed. The Mormon role in the settlement of the West. 1978. Reprint ed., Provo, Utah, Brigham Young U. Pr., 1980. p. 107–34.
Walden DM: Rebels among dissenters: a local history of chiropractic in Provo, Utah. **Chiropr Hist** 1984;4(1):55–61
Warner MH: Vindicating the minister's medical role: Cotton Mather's concept of the nishmath-chajim and the spiritualization of medicine. **J Hist Med Allied Sci** 1981 Jul;36(3):278–95
Yoder D, ed: Advertisements of urban healers. **Pa Folklife** 1978;27(3):44–8
Zwelling S: Spiritualist perspectives on antebellum experience. **J Psychohist** 1982 Summer;10(1):3–25

**USSR**

Bawden CR: W. A. Unkrig's correspondence with the British and Foreign Bible Society. A contribution to ... printing in Mongolian. **Zentralasiat Stud** 1980;14(1):65–108
Vacola G, Gayda M, Pélicier Y: Philocalie d'une prière orthodoxe, aspects psycho-physiologiques. **Ann Med Psychol (Paris)** 1984 Mar;142(3):416–22

**Venezuela**

Alegría C: Dos medicos en la aurora de la gesta emancipadora de Venezuela. **Rev Soc Venez Hist Med** 1969–71;17–19(31–33):29–48

### BIBLE AND TALMUD

Baruk H: La médecine et la Torah. **Rev Hist Med Heb** 1981 Jul;34(2):19–22
Baruk H: La médecine et la Torah. **Rev Hist Med Heb** 1981 Oct;34(3):35–9
Baruk H: La médecine hebraïque face à la médecine hippocratique. In La collection hippocratique et son rôle dans l'histoire de la médecine. Colloque de Strasbourg (23–27 octobre 1972) organisé par le Centre de Recherches sur la Grèce Antique, avec le concours des Facultés de Philosophie et des Langues Classiques. Leiden, E. J. Brill, 1975. p. 291–303.
Davis E: Biblical inscriptions on Hebrew medical amulets. **Adler Mus Bull** 1982 Nov;8(2):19–20
Kass N: Abortion in Jewish law. **Koroth** 1983 Aug;8(7–8):323–31
Kleeberg J: A medical study of the story of Samson and Delilah. **Koroth** 1979 Nov;7(9–10):CXCV–CCII(644–9)
Kottek SS: Embryology in Talmudic and Midrashic literature. **J Hist Biol** 1981 Fall;14(2):299–315
Merani AL: Freud y el Talmud: seguido de crítica de los fundamentos de la psicopatología. México, Grijalbo, 1974. 159 p.
Miller JM: Physicians and prose. **Md State Med J** 1982 Jan;31(1):43–7
Ober WB: Reuben's mandrakes: infertility in the Bible. **Int J Gynecol Pathol** 1984;3(3):299–317
Reier H: Gesundheit, Krankheiten und Arzte bei den Goten. Kiel, 1981. 87 p.
Rosner F: Medicine in the Bible and the Talmud. Selections from classical Jewish sources. New York, KTAV Publishing House, Yeshiva University Press, 1977. xiii, 247 p. Includes Muntner S: Medicine in ancient Israel, p. 3–21.
Simon I: Les notions de cardiologie bibliques et talmudiques. **Rev Hist Med Heb** 1984;37(1):3–6
Simon I: Les notions de cardiologie bibliques et talmudiques. **Rev Hist Med Heb** 1984 Jul;37(2):26–30
Tratner E: A new Talmudic source on the history of diabetes (late onset). **Koroth** 1982 Aug;8(3/4):205–12
Tratner E: 1. Tracheotomy in the Hebrew translation of Ibn-Sina. 2. Intubation mentioned in the Talmud and by Jacob Ben Asher (14th Century). **Koroth** 1983 Aug;8(7–8):333–8

**Hungary**

Egri B: Talmud-tradiciók magyarul. **Orv Hetil** 1984 May 27;125(22):1333–5

**Before 500 A.D.**

Berger J: New views on the Biblical Joseph. **Am J Psychoanal** 1981 Fall;41(3):277–82
Bron B: Depression und Glaube bei Hiob. **Schweiz Arch Neurol Neurochir Psychiatr** 1983;133(1):159–74
Bron B: Zur Psychopathologie und Verkündigung des Propheten Ezechiel. Zum Phänomen der prophetischen Ekstase. **Schweiz Arch Neurol Neurochir Psychiatr** 1981;128(1):21–31
Bubis M: Petroleum in Talmudic sources. **Koroth** 1981;8(1–2):41–4
David, Goliath, et al.: **N Engl J Med** 1984 Mar 22;310(12):790
Dirckx JH: Scientific and medical terms and references in the writings of St. Luke. **Am J Dermatopathol** 1983 Oct;5(5):491–9
Forrai G: Noah or the legend of albinism. **Ther Hung** 1980;28(2):87–9
Freilich AR: Tzaraat--'biblical leprosy'. **J Am Acad Dermatol** 1982 Jan;6(1):131–4
Kaplan AS, Garfinkel PE: Bulimia in the Talmud. **Am J Psychiatry** 1984 May;141(5):721
Kass N: Sex determination--medically and in the Talmud. **Koroth** 1980 Jun;7(11–12):CCLXLIII–CCCI
Koch HA: Zum Nachweis einiger mikrobiologischer Probleme im Buch Leviticus (3. Buch Mose) des Alten Testamentes. **Mykosen** 1983 Mar;26(3):159–62
Kokaska CJ, Woodward S, Tyler L: Disabled people in the Bible. **Rehabil Lit** 1984 Jan–Feb;45(1–2):20–1
Kook H: Introduction to the history of urology in the Bible and Talmud. **Koroth** 1979 Nov;7(9–10):CCXIX–CCXX(710–15)
Kottek SS, Seligman H: Ecology in Talmudic sources. In H. Shuval, ed: Developments in arid zone ecology and environment quality. Philadelphia, Balaban ISS, 1981. p. 119–26.
Littmann SK: King Saul: persecutor or persecuted? **Can J Psychiatry** 1981 Nov;26(7):464–7
Medlen LM: Health care in the Bible and the Talmud. **Curationis** 1980 Sep;3(2):28–31
Neuhauser W: Zur Zeit der Bibel war der Zahn so viel wert wie das Leben selbst. **Zahnarztl Mitt** 1984 Apr 1;74(7):729–33
Rosner F: Earliest description of gout. **Arthritis Rheum** 1983 Feb;26(2):236
Rosner F: Mandrakes and other aphrodisiacs in the Bible & Talmud. **Koroth** 1980 Jun;7(11–12):CCLXXVII–CCLXXXIV
Schoental R: A corner of history. Moses and mycotoxins. **Prev Med** 1980 Jan;9(1):159–61
Schoental R: Mycotoxins and the Bible. **Perspect Biol Med** 1984 Autumn;28(1):117–20
Steinberg A: [Scientific pathology in the books of Talmud.] (Heb). **Harefuah** 1983 Mar 1;104(5):201–2
Steinfeld AD, McDuff HC: An ancient report of a dermoid cyst of the vagina. **Surg Gynecol Obstet** 1980 Jan;150(1):95–6
Unna PG: An exemplary instance of faulty scholarship. **Am J Dermatopathol** 1983 Dec;5(6):569–75
Van der Horst PW: Aelius Aristides and the New Testament. Leiden, E. J. Brill, 1980. ix, 115 p. (Studia ad Corpus Hellenisticum Novi Testamenti. Volumen Sextum.)

**Egypt**

Jacoby MG: The Fifth Plague of Egypt. **JAMA** 1983 May 27;249(20):2779–80

**Israel**

Brian VA: Infant welfare in the Bible. **Nurs Times** 1980 Dec 18–25;76(51):2230–1

**1450–1700**

Guinsburg AM: Paracelsian magic and theology; a case study of the Matthew commentaries. **Medizinhist J** 1981;16(1–2):125–39

**1700 to Present**

**Germany**

Levinger IM, ed: 'Medizinisch-schwierige Talmudstellen' [by Karl Preis]. **Udim** 1977–78;7–8:95–107

**Hungary**

Ismét Luzsénszky Talmudja?: **Orv Hetil** 1984 Aug 19;125(34):2086–7

**Switzerland**

Beerli UP: Medizinisches in Scheuchzers Physica sacra oder Kupferbibel. Zürich, Juris, 1980. 89p. (Zürcher medizingeschichtliche Abhandlungen, Neue Reihe, Nr. 143).

### MISSIONS AND MISSIONARIES

**Japan**

HTLV missionaries and parasites: **Lancet** 1984 Oct 20;2(8408):927–8

**1700 to Present**

Browne SG: The contribution of medical missionaries to tropical medicine. **Trans R Soc Trop Med Hyg** 1979;73(4):357–60
Chesterman C: The medical missionary. **Trans R Soc Trop Med Hyg** 1979;73(4):360–1
Holland MM, Dean L: Mother Joseph: founder, architect, beggar. **Hosp Prog** 1980 Apr;61(4):70–3
Kler JH: Medical philately. Missionary medicine. **J Med Soc NJ** 1983 Apr;80(4):302
Morris JP: Gordon Stifler Seagrave. In Dictionary of American biography, 1961–1965. Suppl. 7, 1981. 679–81.
Scheel M: Mision medica en la transformacion del tiempo.

**Folia Hum (Barc)** 1982;20(233):413–24
Trevor-Roper PD: Sir Henry Tristram Holland. In Dictionary of national biography, 1961–1970. Suppl. 8, 1981. p. 528–9.

**Africa**

Clendennen GW: Livingstone's second book. **Bibliotheck** 1980;10(1):10–9
Jorden PJ: Surgeon on safari. New York, Hawthorn, 1976. xiv, 173 p.
Pierhal J: Albert Schweitzer. München, Kindler, 1979. 363 p.

**Canada**

Cook CS: Clark Bentom. In Dictionary of Canadian biography, 1801 to 1820. Volume 5, 1983. p. 68–9.
Jones F: John Clinch. In Dictionary of Canadian biography, 1801 to 1820. Volume 5, 1983. p. 189–190.

**France**

Gilbrin E: Les médecins français au Sseu Tch'ouan au début du XXe siècle; l'hopital de Tch'eng Tou. **Hist Sci Med** 1982;16(3):199–204
Gilbrin E: Les médecins français au Sseu Tch'ouan au début du XXe siècle; l'hôpital de Tch'eng Tou. **Hist Sci Med** 1983;17(1):105–10
Gilbrin E: Les médecins français au Sseu Tch'ouan au début du XXe siècle; l'hôpital de Tch'ong King. **Hist Sci Med** 1982;16(2):125–30

**Gabon**

Vencovský E: Ceskoslovenský psychiatr spolupracovníkem profesora dr. Alberta Schweitzera v Lambarène. **Cesk Psychiatr** 1984 Apr;80(2):125–8

**Great Britain**

Schram R: Britain's contribution to health and medicine in tropical countries through medical missions. **Trans R Soc Trop Med Hyg** 1981;75 Suppl:56–8
Walls AF: 'The heavy artillery of the missionary army': the domestic importance of the nineteenth-century medical missionary. In Sheils WJ, ed: The Church and healing. Papers read at the twentieth summer meeting and the twenty-first winter meeting of the Ecclesiastical History Society. Oxford, Basil Blackwell for the Society, 1982. p. 287–97.

**India**

Rabe V: Ida Sophia Scudder. In: Notable American women. The modern period. Cambridge, Mass., Belknap-Harvard Univ. Press, 1980. 4:634–6.
Sastry VV: Health habits of South Indians as recorded by Abbe J. A. Dubois. **Bull Indian Inst Hist Med (Hyderabad)** 1980;10(1–4):84–9

**Japan**

Takahashi M: [Nurses in the history of nursing. (3). 'Infant Jesus' Mission and its nursing activities] (Jpn). **Kango Kyoiku** 1981 Aug;22(8):513–20

**Korea**

Phillips CJ: Rosetta Sherwood Hall. In: Notable American women. The modern period. Cambridge, Mass., Belknap-Harvard Univ. Press, 1980. 4:299–301.

**Nepal**

Gross HP: Medical mission to Nepal. **SD J Med** 1983 Jan;36(1):5–7

**Nigeria**

du Toit ML: A mission doctor's experiences in West Africa. **S Afr Med J** 1984 Nov 17;66(20):775–8

**Pacific Islands**

Crawford RJ: Missionary accounts of fofo mo'omo'o. **J Polynesian Soc** 1977;86(4):531–4
Leenhardt RH: Un tournant de l'histoire de la nouvelle caledonie: Maurice Leenhardt (1878–1954). **Rev Fr Hist Outre Mer** 1978;65(2):236–52

**South Africa**

Barker A: A Zulu contribution. **Trans R Soc Trop Med Hyg** 1979;73(4):364–5
Merwe DW van der: Bochum-Blauberg: die ontstaan, stigting en ontwikkeling van die Helene Franz-Hospital, 1895–1935. **Kleio (S Afr)** 1978;10(1–2):2–20

**Tanzania**

Ranger TO: Godly medicine: the ambiguities of medical mission in southeast Tanzania, 1900–1945. **Soc Sci Med [B]** 1981 Jul;15(3):261–77

**Uganda**

Foster WD: The Church Missionary Society and modern medicine in Uganda. The life of Sir Albert Cook, K.C.M.G., 1870–1951. Newhaven, Sussex, [The author], 1978. 234 p.
Ofcansky TP: The life and times of Sir Albert Ruskin Cook. **J Hist Med Allied Sci** 1982 Apr;37(2):225–8

**United States**

Kaiser RM, Chaff SL, Peitzman SJ: A Philadelphia medical student of the 1890's: the diary of Mary Theodora McGavran. **Pa Mag Hist Biogr** 1984 Apr;108(2):217–36
Kim DJ: The influence of Western medicine, especially American medicine, on the development of medicine in Korea. **Trans Stud Coll Physicians Phila** 1977 Jan;44(3):131–4
Valle RK, Valle AR: Medicine and health among the Alta California mission Indians (1769–1834). In: Congrès international d'histoire de la médecine, XXVe, Québec, 1976. Actes. Québec, 1977., p. 1374–81.

## RELIGIOUS ORDERS

Castro F de: Historia da vida e obras de S. Joao de Deus. Translation and notes by Foâo Gameiro, OH. Montemor-O-Novo, Editorial Franciscana, 1982. 166 p.
Filipe NF: S. João de deus um homem que soube amar. 2. edição. Lisboa, Edições Paulistas, [198–?]. 150 p.
Gastão M: S. João de Deus: sua vida-sua obra. Lisboa, Centro do Livro Brasileiro, 1982. 733 p.

**Algeria**

Friedman EG: Trinitarian hospitals in Algiers: an early example of health care for prisoners of war. **Cathol Hist Rev** 1980;66(4):551–64

**Asia**

Schipperges H: Sorge um den Kranken und Dienste am Kranken: ein Beitrag der Benediktiner zur Medizin des Abendlandes. **Arzt Christ** 1980;3:125–34

**Brazil**

Silva LR da: Os Jesuitas e a assistência médica no Brasil colonial. **Rev Inst Hist Georgr Bras** 1978;318:212–32

**Canada**

Bernier H: Charlotte Gallard. In Dictionary of Canadian biography, 1701 to 1740. Volume 2, 1969. p. 235–6.
Bernier H: Marie Morin. In Dictionary of Canadian biography, 1701 to 1740. Volume 2, 1969. p. 489–92.
Campeau L: Jeanne-Françoise Juchereau de la Ferté. In Dictionary of Canadian biography, 1701 to 1740. Volume 2, 1969. p. 302–3.

**France**

Arnoulet F: L'oeuvre hospitalière des Trinitaires et des Capucine dans le Régence de Tunis. **Cah Tunis** 1978;26(3–4):35–48
Cheymol J: L'hôpital Sainte-Catherine à Paris (1181–1794). **Hist Sci Med** 1982;16(4):239–51
Dorche J: Une institution lyonnaise: les religieuses au service des malades dans les hospices civils de Lyon 1500–1950. **Lyon Pharm** 1981 Apr;32(3):155–60
LeBras H, Dinet D: Mortalité des laïcs et mortalité des religieux: les Bénédictins de Saint-Maur aux XVIIe et XVIIIe siècles. **Population** 1980;35(2):347–83

**Germany**

Spor E, ed: Das Theresienhospital. Ein Stück Düsseldorfer Stadtgeschichte 1288–1980. Düsseldorf, Triltsch, 1980. 128 p. Contributions by F. L. Greb, M. Antonina, L. Peters.

**Hungary**

Sasvári L: Kiegészítö adatok a nöi beteg-ápolórendekröl. **Orv Hetil** 1982 Sep 12;123(37)2321–2

**Italy**

Caffaratto TM: Storia dell'Ospedale Maggiore di Torino della Religione ed Ordine dei SS. Maurizio e Lazzaro—dal secolo XVI al secolo XX. **Ann Osp Maria Vittoria Torino** 1979 Jul-Dec;22(7–12):365–419

## RELIGION AND MEDICINE

**Spain**

Beya Alonso E: La dietetica en los cartujos. **Bol Soc Esp Hist Farm** 1982 Sep;33(131):185–92
Beya Alonso E: La farmacia en la trapa. **Bol Soc Esp Hist Farm** 1983 Sep;135:85–94

**Sweden**

Detlow-Berg AL: Omvårdnad i Vadstena kloster. **Dan Medicinhist Arbog** 1983;12:65–73

**500 A.D.–1450**

Biller P: Curate infirmos: the medieval waldensian practice of medicine. In Sheils WJ, ed: The Church and healing. Papers read at the twentieth summer meeting and the twenty-first winter meeting of the Ecclesiastical History Society. Oxford, Basil Blackwell for the Society, 1982. p. 55–57.

**Great Britain**

Dawtry AF: The modus medendi and the Benedictine order in Anglo-Norman England. In Sheils WJ, ed: The Church and healing. Papers read at the twentieth summer meeting and the twenty-first winter meeting of the Ecclesiastical History Society. Oxford, Basil Blackwell for the Society, 1982. p. 25–38.

**Middle East**

Sterns I: Care of the sick brothers by the Crusader Orders in the Holy Land. **Bull Hist Med** 1983;57(1):43–69

**1450–1700**

Jaeger W: Sinnesphysiologische Forschungen der Jesuitengelehrten des 17. Jahrhunderts. **Klin Monatsbl Augenheilkd** 1981 Oct;179(4):288–96

**Belgium**

Toussaint R: Médicinaire du 17e siècle provenant d'Aywaille. **Enquetes Mus Vie Wallonne** [1980?];13:205–20

**Canada**

Bernier H: Françoise Maumousseau. In Dictionary of Canadian biography, 1701 to 1740. Volume 2, 1969. p. 466–7.
Bernier H: Marie-Madeleine Maufils. In Dictionary of Canadian biography, 1701 to 1740. Volume 2, 1969. p. 466.
Paquin M: Louise Soumande. In Dictionary of Canadian biography, 1701 to 1740. Volume 2, 1969. p. 613.
Voisine N: Marguerite Bourdon. In Dictionary of Canadian biography, 1701 to 1740. Volume 2, 1969. p. 92–3.

**Italy**

Salvini S: La mortalità dei gesuiti in Italia nei secoli XVI e XVII. **Quad Depart Stat Univ Studi Fir** 1979;3:1–25

**Mexico**

Toscano Moreno J: Los hospitales y la 'hospitalidad' de los franciscanos en la Nueva Galicia. **Bol Inst Invest Bibliogr** 1970;4:389–404

**Spain**

Bravo Lozano J: La visita del hospital real de San Lázaro de Córdoba (1599–1603). **Hispania** 1979;39(143):639–70

**1700 to Present**

**Austria**

Ardelt R: Geschichte des Konventes und Krankenhauses der Elisabethinen zu Linz. **Hist Jahrb Stadt Linz** 1978;:95–146

**Canada**

Ducharme J: Marie-Catherine-Françoise Céloron. In Dictionary of Canadian biography, 1801 to 1820. Volume 5, 1983. p. 174.
Johnston AJ: The frères de la charité and the Louisbourg Hôpital du Roi. **Can Cathol Hist Assoc Study Sess** 1981;48:5–25
Kennedy E: Immigrants, cholera and the Saint John Sisters of Charity, 1854–64. **Can Cathol Hist Assoc Study Sess** 1977;44:25–44
Plamondon L: Marie-Catherine Payen de Noyan. In Dictionary of Canadian biography, 1801 to 1820. Volume 5, 1983. p. 661–2.
Rousseau F: Marie-Geneviève Parent. In Dictionary of Canadian biography, 1801 to 1820. Volume 5, 1983. p. 658–9.
Rousseau F: Marie-Vénérande Melançon. In Dictionary of Canadian biography, 1801 to 1820. Volume 5, 1983. p. 587–8.
Séguin G: Marie-Angélique Dussaus. In Dictionary of Canadian biography, 1801 to 1820. Volume 5, 1983. p. 293.
Sylvestre PF: Dossier historique: les religieuses infirmières en Ontario français. **Infirm Can** 1983 Nov;25(10):27–9

**France**

Fracard ML: L'organisation hospitalière des Frères de Saint-Jean-de-Dieu à Niort (Poitou) dans la seconde moitié du XVIIIe siècle. In: Congrès National des Sociétés Savantes, 97e, Nantes, 1972. Actes. Paris, 1977. Histoire Moderne et Contemporaine, Tome 1. p. 299–327.

**Germany**

Seidler E: Die Behinderten in Herten. **Gesnerus** 1982;39(1):133–40

**Hungary**

Sasvári L: Nöi betegápoló rendek szerepe a hazai kórházak munkájában (1867–1918). **Orv Hetil** 1982 Apr 18;123(16):990–2
Szigetváry F: Die Apotheke der Jesuiten von Köszeg. In Hein WH, ed: Pharmaziehistorischer Kongress, Budapest, 1981. Stuttgart, Wissenschaftliche Verlagsgesellschaft, 1983. p. 73–80.

**Mexico**

Bustamante ME: Supervivencia y muerte de los Jesuitas de la Provincia de Mexico entre 1767 y 1820. **Bol Soc Mex Hist Filos Med** 1983;6(45):235–63

**Poland**

Rejmanowski T: Dzieje sióstr miłosierdzia w Szpitalu Powiatowym Sw. Antoniego we Włocławku (1877–1966). **Arch Hist Med (Warsz)** 1984;47(3):433–8

**Spain**

Valverde JL, Sanchez Tellez MC: Inventario de todos los efectos de la Botica del Monasterio de la Cartuja del Paular (1811). **Bol Soc Esp Hist Farm** 1980 Mar–Jun;3(121–2):51–67

**United States**

Roth MA: With mercy toward all. Mercy Hospital, Cedar Rapids, Iowa, 1900–1978. Cedar Rapids, Stamats, 1979. vii, 104 p.
Sayad EG: Alexian Brothers' hospital: unique heritage. **Bull Mo Hist Soc** 1980;36(4):264–7
Weiss RE: Mother Joseph: the legendary nun who broke ground for women and men health administrators in the West. **Hosp Forum** 1981 Jan–Feb;24(1):17–8

### SAINTS

Alberti H: Die heiligen Kosmas und Damian auf einer Prozessionsfahne im Deutschen Apotheken-Museum. **Dtsch Apoth Ztg** 1979 Jun 14;119(24):948–50 (also in Pharm Ztg 1979 Jun 14;24:1155–7
Frey EF: Saints in medical history. **Clio Med** 1979 Jul;14(1):35–70
Iveson-Iveson J: St. David's day. **Nurs Mirror** 1984 Feb 29;158(9):16
Julien P: Le point sur les ex-libris professionnels à l'effigie des saints Côme et Damien. **Rev Hist Pharm (Paris)** 1982;29(252):176–8
Lebrun F: Se soigner autrefois. Médecins saints et sorciers aux 17e et 18e siècles. Paris, Temps Actuels, 1983. 206 p. (La passion de l'histoire).
Orłowski WJ: Patronka cierpiacych na oczy. **Klin Oczna** 1984 May;86(5):231–5
Rocchietta S: Un 'Christ à la pharmacie' ou 'Les Saints Côme et Damien'? **Rev Hist Pharm (Paris)** 1984 Jun;31(261):131–3
Schadewaldt H: Heilige in der Medizin. **Dtsch Arztebl** 1980 Apr 3;77(14):922–4
Shaw S: Seasonal foundations: Santa-the saint who founded hospitals. **Nurs Mirror** 1981 Dec 23–30;153(26):30–1
Théodoridès J: Saints in medical history (a complement). **Clio Med** 1980 Jul;14(3–4):269–70
Zuring J: Saint Côme et Saint Damien dans la philatélie. **Rev Hist Pharm (Paris)** 1984 Mar;31(260):69–72

**Byzantium**

Horden P: Saints and doctors in the early Byzantine Empire: the case of Theodore of Sykeon. In Sheils WJ, ed: The Church and healing. Papers read at the twentieth summer meeting and the twenty-first winter meeting of the Ecclesiastical History Society. Oxford, Basil Blackwell for the Society, 1982. p. 1–13.

**France**

David-Danel ML: Un ex-libris non professionnel à l'effigie de saint Côme. **Rev Hist Pharm (Paris)** 1982;29(252):171-2

Devaux G: Saint Michel, patron des apothicaires de Bordeaux et d'autres lieux. **Rev Hist Pharm (Paris)** 1982;29(252):151-9

Julien P: Culte et iconographie des saints médecins Come et Damien dans une province française. In International Congress of the History of Medicine, 27th, Barcelona, 1980. Actas. Barcelona, Académia de Ciències Médiques de Catalunya i Balears, 1981. p. 530-4.

Julien P. Deux saints médecins et pharmaciens, Côme et Damien. **Bull Liaison Assoc Amis Mus Pharm Montp** 1982;:(7):13-35

Schmitt JC: The holy greyhound: Guinefort, healer of children since the thirteenth century. Cambridge, Cambridge University Press; Paris, Editions de la Maison des Sciences de l'Homme, 1983. 215 p. Translation of Le saint lévrier: Guinefort, guérisseur d'enfants depuis le XIIIe siècle, Paris, 1979.

**Germany**

Dobras W: Cosmas und Damian in oberbayerischen Kirchen. **Pharm Ztg** 1981 Dec 24;126(52-53):2715-6

**Hungary**

Bano-Fleischmann M, Zalai K: Gegenstände der Erinnerung an Kosma und Damian in Ungarn. **Ther Hung** 1981;29(3):152-6

Fleishmann-Bánó M, Zalai K: St. Cosmas and St. Damian relics in Hungary. **Ther Hung** 1981;29(3):142-6

Vida M: A Kozma- és Damján-tisztelet írásos és tárgyi emlékei Magyarországon. **Orvostort Kozl** 1980,89-91(26 no 1-3).257-65

**Italy**

Rocchietta S: Iconografia statuaria e pittorica di Santa Apollonia nel Duomo di Milano. **Minerva Med** 1981 Jan 14;72(1):45-9

**Before 500 A.D.**

Berle EJ: Legenden om en senantikk bentransplantasjon. **Sydsven Medicinhist Sallsk Arsskr** 1984;21:135-40

Deutsch-Kasimir M: Die Heilige Apollonia. **Quintessenz J** 1982 Nov;12(11):1025-6

Marí VJ: El martirio de Santa Agatha, un precedente de la mastectomia. Représentacion artistica con especial referencia a una coleccion de tallas. In International Congress of the History of Medicine. 26th, Plovdiv, 1978. Actes du Congress. Sofia, 1981. Volume II. p. 150-7.

**Denmark**

Sct Apollonia og dansk odontologi: **Tandlaegebladet** 1984 Jan;88(1):5-8

**Egypt**

Tronnberg G: S:ta Apollonia av Alexandra--tandlakarnas skyddshelgon. **Odontol Foren Tidskr** 1980 Dec;44(5):22-8

**500 A.D.-1450**

Hofmann B: Kranker und Krankheit um 1500. Die Darstellung des Kranken im Zusammenhang mit den spätgotischen Bildnissen der Heiligen Elisabeth. Herzogenrath, Verlag Murken-Altrogge, 1983. 226 p. (Studien zur Medizin-, Kunst- und Literaturgeschichte, Bd. 3).

Lacey JH: Anorexia nervosa and a bearded female saint. **Br Med J [Clin Res]** 1982 Dec 18-25;285(6357):1816-7

Shahar S: Infants, infant care, and attitudes toward infancy in the medieval Lives of Saints. **J Psychohist** 1983 Winter;10(3):281-309

**Germany**

Baader G: Naturwissenschaft und Medizin im 12. Jahrhundert und Hildegard von Bingen. **Arch Mittelrheinischen Kirchengesch** 1979;31:33-54

Hertzka G: Das Wunder der Hildegard-Medizin. Stein am Rhein, Christiana-Verlag, 1984. 236 p.

Hildegard von Bingen: Ursachen und Behandlung der Krankheiten (causae et curae). Ubersetzt von H. Schulz. 4. Auflage. Heidelberg, Haug, 1983. 373 p.

Mueller I: Krankheit und Heilmittel im Werk Hildegards von Bingen. In: Hildegard von Bingen. Festschrift 1179-1979. [1979] pp. 311-349.

Müller I: Die pflanzlichen Heilmittel bei Hildegard von Bingen. Salzburg, D. Müller, 1982. 215 p.

Pereira M: Maternità e sessualità femminile nell' opera di Ildegarda di Bingen. Una proposta di lettura. **Quad Stor** 1980;2

Röhrer-Ertl O: Bemerkungen zur Identifikation des Hl. Emmeram aus St. Emmeram in Regensburg. Ein methodenkritischer Vergleich. **Anthropol Anz** 1981 Sep;39(3):173-88

Schipperges H: Barmherzigkeit als Heilmittel bei Hildegard von Bingen. In Ganzinger K, Skopec M, Wyklicky H, ed: Festschrift für Erna Lesky zum 70. Geburtstag. Wien, Brüder Hollinek, 1981. p. 97-103.

Schipperges H: Der Mensch und seine Welt bei Hildegard von Bingen. **Arzt Christ** 1978-79;1:2-7

Schipperges H: Diätetische Lebensführung nach der 'Regula Benedicti' bei Hildegard von Bingen. **Arzt Christ** 1980;2:87-97

Schipperges H: Die Kardinaltugenden im Weltbild der Hildegard von Bingen. **Grenzgeb Wiss** 1980;29(1):19-34

Van der May-de Leur AP: Moderne pelgrimage: Sint Elisabeth-expositie Marburg 1981. **Tijdschr Ziekenverpl** 1982 Feb 2;35(3):83-6

**Hungary**

Vida M: Az orvosi gyakorlat és a gyógyítószentek ikonográfiája a XIII-XIV. századi magyarországi falfestészetben. **Orvostort Kozl** 1979;87-88(25 no 1-2):13-63

Vida M: Ursprung und Deutung der Verehrung der Heiligen Kosmas und Damian in Ungarn (11-14. Jahrhundert). **Orvostort Kozl** 1980;89-91(26 no 1-3):45-95

Vida M: Ursprung und Deutung des Kosmas-Damian-Kultes in Ungarn (11.-14. Jahrhundert). In Hein WH, ed: Pharmaziehistorischer Kongress, Budapest, 1981. Stuttgart, Wissenschaftliche Verlagsgesellschaft, 1983. p. 23-33.

**Italy**

Casanovas J: La enfermedad ocular de Francisco de Asís. **Klin Oczna** 1980 May;82(5):243-4

Daglio P: San Benedetto da Norcia patrono d'Europa, nella medicina e nella storia. **Minerva Med** 1982 Sep 8;73(34):2193-8

Eramo S: L'odontoiatria nell'arte. Su un affresco raffigurante S. Apollonia nella Basilica di Santa Maria di Collemaggio a l'Aquila. **Dent Cadmos** 1984 Apr;52(4):135-7

Touati FO: François d'Assise et la diffusion d'un modèle thérapeutique a XIIIe siècle. **Hist Sci Med** 1982;16(3):175-84

**1450-1700**

Díaz F: Influencia de San Juan de Dios en la enfermería. **Rev Enferm** 1982 Mar;5(45):12-4

**Austria**

Grossmann T: Die hl. Ottilie, Patronin der Augenkranken. Eine ungewöhnliche Abbildung am Gnadenstuhlaltar von Bad Aussee mit Krebsscherenattribut. **Klin Monatsbl Augenheilkd** 1981 Jun;178(6):480-1

**France**

Peyresblanques J: Monsieur Vincent, ses maladies, ses médecins. **Hist Sci Med** 1982;16(4):253-61

Tessier JF: L'hôpital de Ste-Marguerite de Cadillac et la littérature consacrée à Saint Jean de Dieu et ses disciples en France au XVIIe siècle. **Rev Fr Hist Livre** 1979;23:317-28

**Great Britain**

Theilmann JM: The miracles of King Henri VI of England. **Historian** 1980;42(3):456-71

**Italy**

Manzi L: I santi protettori degli artisti dello studio bolognese... Santi Cosma e Damiano. **Strenna Stor Bolognese** 1977;27:179-93

Rocchietta S: Von der Apothekergilde während des 15. Jahrhunderts gestiftete Glasfenster im Dom von Mailand. **Beitr Gesch Pharm** 1981;31(13):97-100

Verellen T: Cosmas and Damian in the New Sacristy [Medici Chapel of San Lorenzo, Florence]. **J Warburg Courtauld Inst** 1979;42:274-7

**Spain**

Huguet M: Expérience mystique, pathologie mentale et condition féminine. **Penelope** 1983;(8):25-8

**1700 to Present**

**Italy**

Papàsogli G: Giuseppe Moscati, 1880-1927: Leben eines heiligen Arztes. Stein am Rhein [Schweiz], Christiana-Verlag, 1982. 109 p.

## RESEARCH

See also **Laboratories and Research Institutes**

Brewer NR, et al: The origins of laboratory animal science and medicine: proceedings of a symposium ... American Association for Laboratory Animal Science ... 1979. **Lab Anim Sci** 1980;30:737-800
Brieger GH: History [of human experimentation]. In Reich WT, et al, ed: Encyclopedia of bioethics, v. 2. New York, Free Press, 1978. p. 684-90.
Cunningham SG, Mitchell PH: The use of animals in nursing research. **ANS** 1982 Jul;4(4):72-84
Grmek MD: Planung und Zufall in der Forschung-eine historische Betrachtung. In R. Wittern, ed: Jahrbuch des Instituts für Geschichte der Medizin der Robert Bosch Stiftung. Stuttgart, Hippokrates Verlag, 1984. Bd. 1. p. 9-27.
Gustafsson RA: Omvårdnadsforskning. Forskningen startade på läkarnas villkor. **Vardfacket** 1981 Aug 27;5(15):6-10
Howard-Jones N: Expérimentation humaine et déontologie: une interprétation historique. In: Médicine et expérimentation. Québec, Les Presses de l'Université Laval, 1982. p. 39-65. (Cahiers de Bioethique, 4).
Labhart A: Diskursives Denken und Intuition in der medizinischen Forschung. **Helv Chir Acta** 1981 Feb;47(6):859-72
Lemaine G: Perspectives on the emergence of scientific disciplines. Chicago, Aldine, 1976. xi, 281 p.
McKeown T: The direction of medical research. **Lancet** 1979 Dec 15;2(8155):1281-4
Miké V: Clinical studies in cancer: a historical perspective. In V. Miké, K. E. Stanley, ed: Statistics in medical research. Methods and issues, with applications in cancer research. New York, John Wiley & Sons, 1982. p. 111-55.
Rosinga WM: Clinical trial under trial. **Pharm Weekbl [Sci]** 1983 Feb 25;5(1):1-8
Sambursky S: Einheit und Einfachheit der Natur als Leitmotiv der Forschung. **Biomed Tech (Berlin)** 1979 Oct;24(10):230-6
Warren JV: The evolution of the clinical investigator. **J Lab Clin Med** 1983 Mar;101(3):335-50

**Germany**

Jaeger W: Wege der Forschung auf dem Gebiet der optischen Wahrnehmung. Ein wissenschaftshistorischer Rückblick. **MMW** 1982 Sep 10;124(36):785-8

**Greco-Roman**

Ferngren GB: A Roman declamation on vivisection. **Trans Stud Coll Physicians Phila** 1982 Dec;5(4 no 4):272-90

**Turkey**

Sehsuvaroglu BN: Science and experimentation in Anatolian Turkey. In: Congrès international d'histoire de la médecine, XXVe, Québec, 1976. Actes. Québec, 1977. p. 1259-61.

**1450-1700**

Mani N: Biomedical thought in Glisson's hepatology and in Wepfer's work on apoplexy. With commentary by R. G. Frank, p. 84-8. In Stevenson LG, ed: A celebration of medical history. Baltimore, Johns Hopkins University Press, 1982. (The Henry E. Sigerist supplements to the Bulletin of the History of Medicine; new ser., no. 6). p. 37-63.

**Germany**

Bonn G: Der wissenschaftliche Nachlass des lippischen Forschungsreisenden Engelbert Kaempfer im Britischen Museum. **Lipp Mitt Gesch Landeskd** 1979;48:69-116

**Great Britain**

Hunter M: Early problems in professionalizing scientific research: Nehemiah Grew (1641-1712) and the Royal Society with an unpublished letter to Henry Oldenburg. **Notes Rec R Soc Lond** 1982 Feb;36(2):189-209
Klein J: Sir Francis Bacon's 'Valerius Terminus' (1603). **Sudhoffs Arch** 1982;66(1):38-69

**Italy**

Bacchi W: Su alcune note sperimentali inedite di Francesco Redi. **Ann Ist Mus Stor Sci Fir** 1982;7(1):35-56

**1700 to Present**

Burnet M: Biomedical research: changes and opportunities. **Perspect Biol Med** 1981;24:511-24
Chambers RW, Durkin JT, ed: Papers of the Alexis Carrel centennial conference, Georgetown University June 28, 1973. Washington, Georgetown University, 1973. 107 p. Contributions by C. A. Lindbergh, A. Gros, S. Maggio, L. G. Walker, C. A. Hufnagel, T. I. Malinin.
Chayen Y, Bitensky L: Modern cytological techniques in biological and medical research. **Acta Med Pol** 1982;23(3-4):127-39
Cock AG: Chauvinism and internationalism in science: The International Research Council, 1919-1926. **Notes Rec R Soc Lond** 1983 Mar;37(2):249-88
Comroe JH: Roast pig and scientific discovery. Part II. **Am Rev Respir Dis** 1977 Jun;115(6):1035-44
Corning ME: A review of the United States role in international biomedical research and communications: international health and foreign policy. Bethesda, National Library of Medicine, 1980. xxvii, 436 p. (NIH Publication No. 80-1638).
Ewald BH, Gregg DA: Animal research for animals. **Ann NY Acad Sci** 1983;406:48-58
Fletcher SW, Fletcher RH, Greganti MA: Clinical research trends in general medical journals, 1946-1976. In E. B. Roberts, et al, ed: Biomedical innovation. Cambridge, London, MIT Press, 1981. p. 284-300.
Gibson WC: The cost of not doing medical research. **JAMA** 1980 Oct 17;244(16):1817-9
Hemminki E: Quality of clinical trials--a concern of three decades. **Methods Inf Med** 1982 Apr;21(2):81-5
Herbison GJ: Research: ends, setting, environment, activities, resources, creativity, health. **Arch Phys Med Rehabil** 1984 Mar;65(3):112-4
Howard-Jones N: Human experimentation in historical and ethical perspectives. **Soc Sci Med** 1982;16(15):1429-48
Hubbard WN: The role of controlled therapeutic investigations. **Prog Clin Biol Res** 1980;38:275-80
Jonas AM: The mouse in biomedical research. **Physiologist** 1984 Oct;27(5):330-46
Key JD, Rodin AE: William Osler and Arthur Conan Doyle versus the antivivisectionists: some lessons from history for today. **Mayo Clin Proc** 1984 Mar;59(3):189-96
Kohn A: Errors, fallacies, or deception? **Perspect Biol Med** 1978 Spring;21(3):420-30
Lemaire A: Les aléas de la découverte en thérapeutique ou l'aventure du médicament. **Bull Acad Natl Med (Paris)** 1981 Dec;165(9):1215-27
Levine RJ: [History of biomedical research]. In Reich WT, et al, ed: Encyclopedia of bioethics, v.4. New York, Free Press, 1978. p. 1481-92.
Lilienfeld AM: Ceteris Paribus: the evolution of the clinical trial. (The Fielding H. Garrison Lecture). **Bull Hist Med** 1982 Spring;56(1):1-18
Meagher LR: The influence of Darwinian theory upon biological research of the late nineteenth century. Ph.D. Diss., Duke University. Durham, 1979. xii, 329 leaves.
Peller S: Cancer research since 1900. New York, Philosophical Library, 1979. xv, 394 p.
Reiser SJ: Observer variance and error in clinical medicine. In: Congrès international d'histoire de la médecine, XXVe, Québec, 1976. Actes. Québec, 1977. p. 1120-7
Schaffner KF: Clinical trials: the validation of theory and therapy. In R.S. Cohen, L. Laudan, ed: Physics, philosophy and psychoanalysis. Dordrecht, D. Reidel, 1983. p. 191-208.
Shimamura K: [Chronological review of TB research - from a clinical viewpoint.] (Jpn). **Kekkaku** 1980;55:383-8
Silver anniversary of the Advisory Committee on Medical Research: **WHO Chron** 1984;38(1):8-16
Studer KE, Chubin DE: The cancer mission. Social contexts of biomedical research. Beverly Hills, London, Sage, 1980. 319 p. (Sage Library of Social Research, V. 103).
Szilagyi DE: The elusive target: truth in scientific reporting. Comments on error, self-delusion, deceit, and fraud. **J Vasc Surg** 1984 Mar;1(2):243-53
Wade N: The Nobel duel. Two scientists' 21-year race to win the world's most coveted research prize. Garden City, Anchor Press/Doubleday, 1981. 321 p.
Wondrák E: Lékaři hanby. **Cas Lek Cesk** 1984 Aug 3;123(31):969-72
Yamaguchi Y: [Life science. 5. Progress in medical research] (Jpn) **Kango Tenbo** 1980 Aug;5(8):722-9

**Argentina**

Pasqualini RQ: Houssay y el serendipismo. **Medicina (B Aires)** 1981;41(6):827-30
Taquini AC: XX aniversario de la Fundación de la Sociedad Argentina de Investigación Clínica. **Medicina (B Aires)** 1979 Nov-Dec;39(6):703-5

**Austria**

Spiro HM: Eppinger of Vienna: scientist and villain? **J Clin Gastroenterol** 1984 Dec;6(6):493-7

**Bulgaria**

Georgiev I: Development and scientific research activity achievements in the higher medical institute 'I. P. Pavlov' - Plovdiv. **Folia Med (Plovdiv)** 1981;23(3-4):5-23

**Canada**

Naylor D: Osler's first medical publications. **Can Med Assoc J** 1984 Oct 1;131(7):800–5

Rafter GW: Banting and Best and the sources of useful knowledge. **Perspect Biol Med** 1983 Winter;26(2):281–6

**Chile**

Neghme A: Significado de la investigación biomédica en el desarrollo académico de una escuela de medicina. Remembranzas de un pasado no tan remoto. **Rev Med Chil** 1981 Sep;109(9):878–84

**France**

Albury WR: Going beyond the introduction: Claude Bernard scholarship in the 1970s, an essay review. **Bull Hist Med** 1982 Summer;56(2):271–5

Berman A: An unpublished letter from Eugene Soubeiran to Antoine Portal, June 3, 1828. **Pharm Hist** 1982;24(1):32–7

Bourguignon A: Certains problèmes épistemologiques évoqués par Claude Bernard. In Poirier J, Poirier JL, ed: Médecine et philosophie à la fin du XIXe siècle. Paris, Université de Paris XII - Val de Marne, [1980?]. p. 85–100.

Crosland M: From prizes to grants in the support of scientific research in France in the nineteenth century: the Montyon legacy. **Minerva** 1979 Autumn;17(3):355–80

Grmek MD, Fantini B: Le rôle du hasard dans la naissance du modèle de l'opéron. **Rev Hist Sci (Paris)** 1982 Jul;35(3):193–215

Heron JR: Louis Pasteur: the nature of his illness. In Passmore R, ed: Proceedings of the Royal College of Physicians of Edinburgh Tercentenary Congress, 1981. Edinburgh, Royal College of Physicians of Edinburgh, 1982. p. 116–27.

Miles A: Reports by Louis Pasteur and Claude Bernard on the organization of scientific teaching and research. **Notes Rec R Soc Lond** 1982 Aug;37(1):101–18

Poggi S: Ricerca della verità e metodo sperimentale in Claude Bernard. **Intersezioni** 1981;1:361–79

Théodoridès J: Claude Bernard et les parasites. (Contribution au centenaire de la mort de Claude Bernard). **Hist Nat** 1979;(14):31–8

Tournier–Lasserve C: Le Service de santé des armées et la recherche au fil du temps. **Med Armees** 1980,8(10)spec:851–6

**Germany**

Bogusz J: Wpływ norymberskiego procesu lekarzy hitlerowskich na kształtowanie sie pojeć o dokonywaniu badań na ludziach. **Przegl Lek** 1981;38(1):72–9

Engel M: Das Dahlem–Projekt und sein Scheitern. Ein wissenschaftspolitischer Modellfall medizinischer Forschung an der Schwelle zum 20. Jahrhundert - Zur Geschichte des Robert–Koch–Instituts und der Charité. **Fortschr Med** 1982 Jun3;100(21):1009–12

Friedrich C, Langer H, Seidlein HJ: Beiträge zur Geschichte der Pharmazeutischen Wissenschaft. 5. Mitteilung: Christian Ehrenfried von Weigel--Seine Bedeutung für die Entwicklung der pharmazeutischen Wissenschaft. **Pharmazie** 1982 Jul;37(7):514–7

Jungnickel C: The Royal Saxon Society of Sciences: a study of nineteenth century German science. Ph.D. Diss., Johns Hopkins University. Baltimore, 1978. v, 222 leaves.

Moe K: Should the Nazi research data be cited? **Hastings Cent Rep** 1984 Dec;14(6):5–7

Sass HM: Reichsrundschreiben 1931: Pre–Nuremberg German regulations concerning new therapy and human experimentation. **J Med Philos** 1983 May;8(2):99–111

**Great Britain**

Aitken R: A historical dispute. **Clin Sci** 1981 Sep;61(3):360–2

Boss J: An early eighteenth–century criticism of clinical medicine as experimental philosophy. **Koroth** 1980 Jun;7(11–12):CCLXV–CCLXXV

Doll R: The controlled trial. **Postgrad Med J** 1984 Nov;60(709):719–24

Hare R: The scientific activities of Alexander Fleming, other than the discovery of penicillin. **Med Hist** 1983 Oct;27(4):347–72

Himsworth H: Thomas Lewis and the development of support for clinical research. **Pharos** 1982 Spring;45(2):15–9

Hoffenberg R: Fiftieth anniversary. Medical Research Society. **Clin Sci** 1981 Sep;61(3):355–6

Kempler K: Tervszerü kutatás, vagy véletlen? Gondolatok Fleming születésének centenáriumán. **Orv Hetil** 1981 Nov 29;122(48):2967–9

Krebs H: Reminiscenses and reflections. In collaboration with Anne Martin. Oxford, Clarendon Press, 1981. x, 298 p.

Pochin EE: Early days of the Medical Research Society. **Clin Sci** 1981 Sep;61(3):357–60

Rodin AE: Autoexperimentation with a drug by Arthur Conan Doyle. **J Hist Med Allied Sci** 1980 Oct;35(4):426–30

Vane JR: The Wellcome centenary. Henry S. Wellcome, his research philosophy and current excitements. **Trans Med Soc Lond** 1980–81;97:41–50

Voyatzakis E, et al: [The research work of Sir Alexander Fleming] (Gre). **Mater Med Greca** 1981;9:367–76

Wilkinson L: 'The other' John Hunter, M.D., F.R.S. (1754–1809): his contributions to the medical literature, and to the introduction of animal experiments into infectious disease research. **Notes Rec R Soc Lond** 1982 Feb;36(2):227–41

**Italy**

Azzone GF: L'opinione di studiosi sulla vivisezione. **Minerva Med** 1980 May 7;71(18):1334–5

**Mexico**

La investigación biomédica en el Hospital Infantil de México: **Bol Med Hosp Infant Mex** 1983 Nov;40 Suppl 3:3–23

**Netherlands**

Elzinga A: Christiaan Huygens' theory of research. **Janus** 1980;67:281–300

Hackmann WD: Early societies popularize scientific research. **Med Instrum** 1983 Sep–Oct;17(5):338

**Poland**

Lefebvre P: La recherche par le clinicien: une activité inéluctable. **Bull Mem Acad R Med Belg** 1979 Nov 24;134(10):587–96

**Spain**

Peltier LF: The classic: qualities of intellectual order which the investigator should possess. Santiago Ramón y Cajal. **Clin Orthop** 1981;(160):2–13

**Sweden**

Engel A: Hälsan före födelsen. Prenatal forskning i Sverige. Stockholm, 1981. 128 p. (Nordisk Medicinhistorisk Arsbok, Supplementum, VIII).

**Tanzania**

Beck A: Priorities in biological research at Amani, 1902–1914. **Tanzan Notes Rec** 1981;(86–87):13–6

**United States**

Abir–Am P: The discourse of physical power and biological knowledge in the 1930s: a reappraisal of the Rockefeller Foundation's 'policy' in molecular biology. **Soc Stud Sci** 1982 Aug 3;12(3):341–82

Austin JH: Chase, chance, and creativity: the lucky art of novelty. New York, Columbia Univ. Press, 1978. xvii, 237 p.

Bordley JE: History of research training. **Arch Otolaryngol** 1982 Oct;108(10):612–5

Brieger GH: Florence Rena Sabin. In: Notable American women. The modern period. Cambridge, Mass., Belknap–Harvard Univ. Press, 1980. 4:614–7.

Brown RW, Henderson JH: The mass production and distribution of HeLa cells at Tuskegee Institute, 1953–55. **J Hist Med Allied Sci** 1983 Oct;38(4):415–31

Bulmer M: The early institutional establishment of social science research: the local community research committee at the University of Chicago, 1923–30. **Minerva** 1980 Spring;18(1):51–110

Carmen IH: The constitution in the laboratory: recombinant DNA research as 'free expression.' **J Polit** 1981;43(3):737–62

Chalmers TC: The clinical trial. **Milbank Mem Fund Q** 1981 Summer;59(3):324–39

Dishong A: Highlights of twenty years' research at the University of Florida College of Medicine. **J Fla Med Assoc** 1980 Mar;67(3):288–93

Dubos R: Peyton Rous. **J Exp Med** 1979 Oct 1;150(4):735–7

Eckenhoff EA, Harasymiw SJ: Contributors to research literature: 1948–1973. **Hosp Health Serv Adm** 1979 Summer;24(3):11–20

Eichwald EJ, Silmser CR: H-Y and serendipity. **Hum Genet** 1981;58(1):6–8

Fath H: A dream come true: the story of St. Jude Children's Research Hospital and ALSAC. Memphis, TN, ALSAC, 1983. 214 p.

Fernandez C: Pioneers in research in otolaryngology at the University of Chicago. **Ann Otol Rhinol Laryngol [Suppl]** 1983 Jan–Feb;102:23–6

Flavin TH: The Clinical Center: twenty–five years of research for people. **Conn Med** 1979 Sep;43(9):563–7

Forrest WR, Christen AG: Recollections of a dental researcher. Fifty years at the U. S. Bureau of Standards: Interviews with George C. Paffenbarger. Part I. **J Ala Dent Assoc** 1982 Summer;66(3):24–8

Fredrickson DS: Biomedical research in the 1980s. **N Engl J Med** 1981 Feb 26;304(9):509–17

Frei E: Intramural therapeutic research at the National Cancer Institute, Department of Medicine: 1955–1965. **Cancer Treat Rep** 1984 Jan;68(1):21–30

Haraway D: The biological enterprise: sex, mind, and profit from human

engineering to sociobiology. **Radic Hist Rev** 1979 Spring/Summer;Spec:206–37
Harvey AM: Clinical investigation of chronic diseases: its successful pursuit in an outpatient setting. **J Chronic Dis** 1980;33(9):529–66
Harvey AM: Francis Weld Peabody: the blending of general internal medicine and clinical science. **Pharos** 1981 Summer;44(3):6–8
Harvey AM: Joseph Charles Aub: applying the tools of the basic sciences to clinical investigation. **Am J Med** 1981 Jul;71(1):13–5
Harvey AM: Louis Harry Newburgh: compleat clinical investigator with a passion for measurement. **Am J Med** 1981 Apr;70(4):759–61
Harvey AM: Research and discovery in medicine. Contributions from Johns Hopkins. Baltimore and London, Johns Hopkins University Press, 1981. xiii, 322 p. [Collected historical papers reprinted from various journals].
Harvey AM: Samuel J. Meltzer: pioneer catalyst in the evolution of clinical science in America. **Perspect Biol Med** 1978 Spring;21(3):431–40
Harvey AM: Science at the bedside: the story of Warfield Theobald Longcope. **Trans Stud Coll Physicians Phila** 1981 Sep;5(3 no 3):161–73
Hayden GF: Clinical research in Southern Medical Journal: current trends. **South Med J** 1983 Dec;76(12):1473–6
Jones JH: Bad blood: the Tuskegee syphilis experiment. New York, Free Press; London, Collier Macmillan; 1981. xii, 272 p.
Kelley WN: Clinical investigation and the clinical investigator: the past, present, and future. **J Clin Invest** 1984 Sep;74(3):1117–22
King LS: Medicine in the USA: Historical vignettes. XVI. Clinical science gets enthroned. Part II. **JAMA** 1983 Oct 14;250(14):1847–50
Laszlo J: Two long-range clinical data bases are terminated: bang, whimper, or ripple? **J Clin Oncol** 1984 May;2(5):532–3
Lederer SE: 'The right and wrong of making experiments on human beings': Udo J. Wile and syphilis. **Bull Hist Med** 1984 Fall;58(3):380–97
Loew FM: Animal experimentation. **Bull Hist Med** 1982 Spring;56(1):123–6
McCarthy CR: [History of biomedical research policy]. In Reich WT, et al, ed: Encyclopedia of bioethics, v.4. New York, Free Press, 1978. p. 1492–8.
Maddox RF: The politics of World War II science: Senator Harley M. Kilgore and the legislative origins of the National Science Foundation. **W Va Hist** 1979;41(1):20–39
Miller M: The Simon Flexner papers. **Surv Sources Newsl** 1979 Apr;9:2–4
Miller M: The Walter Bradford Cannon Papers. **Surv Sources Newsl** 1977 May;5:8–9
National Institute of General Medical Sciences. Office of Research Reports: Nobel prize laureates. [Bethesda, Md.], National Institutes of Health, Dept. of Health, Education, and Welfare. [1978]. 24 p.
Naunton RF: Clinical research in otolaryngology at the University of Chicago. **Ann Otol Rhinol Laryngol [Suppl]** 1983 Jan–Feb;102:30–1
Pattullo EL: Reconciling risk and regulation. **Society** 1980;18(1):34–8
Reingold N: The scientist as troubled American. **Am Ind Hyg Assoc J** 1979 Dec;40(12):1107–13
Salsburg D, Heath A: When science progresses and bureaucracies lag: the case of cancer research. **Public Interest** 1981;65:30–9
Savit TL: The use of blacks for medical experimentation and demonstration in the old South. **J South Hist** 1982;48(3):331–48
Savitt TL: The use of Blacks for medical experimentation and demonstration in the Old South. **J South Hist** 1982 Aug;48(3):331–48
Schwan HP: Biomedical engineering and basic research: historical perspectives. **Med Prog Technol** 1980 Jun;7(2–3):63–7
Sechzer JA: Historical issues concerning animal experimentation in the United States. **Soc Sci Med [F]** 1981 Mar;15F(1):13–7
Sechzer JA: The use of animals for experimentation in the United States. **Psychopharmacol Bull** 1981 Apr;17(2):88–91
Smith T: Document: [letter to Dr. Edward B. Krumbhaar]. **Trans Stud Coll Physicians Phila** 1981 Sep;5(3 no 3):214–5
Stetten D: High-powered research and the microscopic viewpoint. **J Med Educ** 1981 Jan;56(1):3–7
Trends in biomedical research, 1901–1976: Proceedings of the Second Rockefeller Archive Center Conference, December 10, 1976. North Tarrytown, The Center, 1977. 70 p. Contributions by R. S. Morison, A. M. Harvey, P. H. Mazumdar, S. Benison, M. Heidelberger, M. McCarty, E. H. Ahrens, A. Kappas.
Ward PS: 'Who will bell the cat?' Andrew C. Ivy and krebiozen. **Bull Hist Med** 1984 Spring;58(1):28–52
Warkany J: Laissez-faire in research. **J Am Coll Nutr** 1984;3(2):177–81
Westerman MP, Tymorek S: A history of medical research at Mount Sinai Hospital Medical Center of Chicago. **Mt Sinai J Med (NY)** 1984 Apr;51(2):150–6
Yalow R: Science and technology: problems and perceptions. In Cohen EP, ed: Medicine in transition. [Chicago], University of Illinois College of Medicine, 1981. p. 53–63.
Zubrod CG: Origins and development of chemotherapy research at the National Cancer Institute. **Cancer Treat Rep** 1984 Jan;68(1):9–19

**USSR**

Avdeeva TA, Khazenson LB: Osnovnye itogi 60-letnykh issledovaniĭ Leningradskogo instituta épidemiologii i mikrobiologii imeni Pastera po ostrym kishechnym infektsiiam (1923–1983). **Zh Mikrobiol Epidemiol Immunobiol** 1984 Jan;(1):115–9
Bazanov VA: Upravlenie meditsinskimi nauchnymi issledovaniiami v gody Velikoĭ Otechestvennoĭ voĭny (1941–1945). **Sov Zdravookhr** 1983;5:52–5
Bramberga VM: Stanovlenie, sovremennoe sostoianie i perspektivy razvitiia onkologii v Latviĭskoĭ SSR. **Vopr Onkol** 1982;28(10):8–13
Frolov VA: K 40-letiiu sozdaniia Akademii meditsinskikh nauk USSR. **Patol Fiziol Eksp Ter** 1984 Jul–Aug;(4):3–9
Kucheruk VV: Itogi i rabot sovetskikh uchenykh po izucheniiu i profilaktike prirodno-ochagovykh bolezneĭ (soobshchenie 1). **Med Parazitol (Mosk)** 1982 Nov–Dec;60(6):9–17

**Yugoslavia**

Fortič B: Sesdeset godina stručnog rada i razvoja Golnika. **Plucne Bolesti Tuberk** 1981 Oct–Dec;33(4):197–215

# RESPIRATORY SYSTEM

See also **Otorhinolaryngology; Resuscitation; Surgery–Thoracic**

Bollinelli R, Carles P: Geschichte der Lungenheilkunde. In Sournia JC, Martiny M, Poulet J, ed: Illustrierte Geschichte der Medizin. Salzburg, Andreas, 1980. Vol. 8. p. 2795–825.
Bunnell JB: Respiratory assistance: a review of techniques, rationale, and problems with a glimpse at the future. **Ann Biomed Eng** 1982;9(5–6):645–67
Hall DL: Why do animals breathe? New York, Arno Press, 1981. xviii, 296 p.
Houston CS: The pressure chamber revisited. A look at the past. **Prog Clin Biol Res** 1983;136:213–20
Otis AB: A perspective of respiratory mechanics. **J Appl Physiol** 1983 May;54(5):1183–7

**China**

Stiefvater EW, Stiefvater IR: Chinesische Atemlehre und Gymnastik. 2. Auflage. Heidelberg, Haug, 1980. 121 p.

**Before 500 A.D.**

**Greece**

Bugaj R: Koncepcje elementów ognia i powietrza u Arystotelesa i ich rola w procesach spalania i oddychania. **Kwart Hist Nauki Tech** 1980;25(1):89–103

**500 A.D.–1450**

**Peru**

Canalis RF, Cabieses F, Hemenway WG, et al: Prehistoric trephination of the frontal sinus. **Ann Otol Phinol Laryngol** 1981 Mar–Apr;90(2 pt 1):186–9

**1700 to Present**

Bendixen HH: Respirators and respiratory care. **Acta Anaesthesiol Scand** 1982 Jun;26(3):279–86
Cartwright FF: Pneumatic medicine. **Pharm Hist (London)** 1970 Jun;1(5):4–6
Grenvik A, Eross B, Powner D: Historical survey of mechanical ventilation. **Int Anesthesiol Clin** 1980 Summer;18(2):1–10
Raskin SP: The pulmonary acinus: historical notes. **Radiology** 1982 Jul;144(1):31–4
Rendell-Baker L: Principles in design and function of mechanical ventilators. **Respir Ther** 1979 Jan–Feb;9(1):63–4, 66–9
Renggli R: Die Anfänge der Spirometrie im 19. Jahrhundert. **Gesnerus** 1981;38:247–58
Saklad M: Revolutionary ideas versus progress--in respiratory care. **Respir Care** 1977 Nov;22(11):1212–9
Stremel RW: Historical development of the anaerobic threshold concept. **Physiologist** 1984 Aug;27(4):295–8
West JB, ed: Translations in respiratory physiology. Stroudsburg, Pennsylvania, Dowden, Hutchinson & Ross, 1975. 772 p. (Translations of 19th–20th century articles by various authors).

**Australia**

Gandevia B: Dr. John Hutchinson: the inventor of the spirometer. **Aust Fam Physician** 1981 Jul;10(7):574–8

**Denmark**

Schmidt-Nielsen B: August and Marie Krogh and respiratory physiology. **J Appl Physiol** 1984 Aug;57(2):293–303

**France**

Hanngren A: R. T. H. Laënnec, lungmedicinens fader, 1781–1826. **Kvartalsskr Sven Hjart Lungsjukdomor** 1981;76:73–82
Turiaf J: Laennec et la pathologie respiratoire. **Bull Acad Natl Med (Paris)** 1981 Feb 17;Spec No:31–6

**Germany**

Hollmann W, Valentin H: 50 Jahre Spiroergometrie 1929 bis 1979. **MMW** 1980 Feb 1;122(5):169–74

**Great Britain**

West JB: Stephen Hales: neglected respiratory physiologist. **J Appl Physiol** 1984 Sep;57(3):635–9

**Hungary**

Kenéz J: A fizikális mellkasvizsgálat és hazai úttöröi. **Orv Hetil** 1982 Oct 3;123(40):2483–7

**Sweden**

Nunn JB, Holmdahl MH: Henrik Enghoff and the volumen inefficax. **Ups J Med Sci** 1979;84(2):105–8

**United States**

Ebert RV: The First Aspen Conference in retrospect. **Chest** 1984 Jun;85(6 Suppl):2S–3S
Levine ER: Fifty years of respiratory therapy. **Respir Ther** 1979 Jan–Feb;9(1):57, 59–60
Onsager LW: That curious book 'The breath of life' by George Catlin. **Int J Oral Myol** 1980 Oct;6(4):7–10
Petty TL: 25 years of Aspen Lung Conferences. **Chest** 1984 Jun;85(6 Suppl):1S
Snider GL: Thirty years of mechanical ventilation. Changing implications. **Arch Intern Med** 1983 Apr;143(4):745–9
Soroka M: Fifty years of progress in respiratory care. **Respir Ther** 1979 Jan–Feb;9(1):21, 24–9, 92–3
Temby KL: Tracheobronchial hygieng circa 1900. **Respir Care** 1977 Aug;22(8):876
Vedder JS: Pediatric respiratory therapy of the 1930s. **Respir Ther** 1979 Jan–Feb;9(1):42, 44
White LW: Adapting commercial oxygen for medical use. **Respir Ther** 1979 Jan–Feb;9(1):30–2
White LW: Education of oxygen-treatment personnel, 1928–1948. **Respir Ther** 1979 Jan–Feb;9(1):35, 38–9

## RESUSCITATION

Barometer on baromedicine: **MD** 1978 Jun;22(6):53–5, 57
DeBard ML: The history of cardiopulmonary resuscitation. **Ann Emerg Med** 1980 May;9(5):273–5
Delaby PA: Appareillages de réanimation. **Hist Sci Med** 1980;14(2):153–4
Hayes B: Ventilation and ventilators. **J Med Eng Technol** 1982 Sep–Oct;6(5):177–92
Shaw A, Davis PD: The lung ventilator--an engineering appraisal. **Eng Med** 1977 Jul;6(3):85–9
Vaksman IA, Popugaĭlo VM: Istoriia anesteziologii i reanimatsii v filatelii. **Anesteziol Reanimatol** 1984 Mar–Apr;(2):75–7

**France**

Gélis J: Miracle et medecine aux siècles classiques: le corps medical et le retour temporaire a la vie des mort-nes. **Hist Reflect** 1982;9(1–2):85–101

**500 A.D.–1450**

**Arabic**

Jasser MT: Anaesthesia and resuscitation in the history of Arabic medicine. In: International Symposium for the History of Arabic Science, 1st, University of Aleppo, 1976. Proceedings. Aleppo, Syria, 1976. Papers in European Languages, Vol. II. p. 324–5.

**1450–1700**

**France**

Bernos M: Une 'suscitation' au Buis-les-Baronnies en 1699. Nouvelle contribution à l'étude des sanctuaires 'a répit'. **Ann Midi** 1980;92(146):87–93

**Great Britain**

Hughes JT: Miraculous deliverance of Anne Green: an Oxford case of resuscitation in the seventeenth century. **Br Med J [Clin Res]** 1982 Dec 18–25;285(6357):1792–3

**1700 to Present**

Bartecchi CE: Cardiopulmonary resuscitation--an element of sophistication in the 18th century. **Am Heart J** 1980 Oct;100(4):580–1
Dünschel D: Berichte von Wiederbelebungsmassnahmen im 18. und 19. Jahrhundert. In: Congrès international d'histoire de la médecine, XXVe, Québec, 1976. Actes. Québec, 1977. p. 634–43.
Elliott LS: A pictorial history of mechanical respiration devices. **Respir Ther** 1979 Jan–Feb;9(1):52–4
Gorham J: A medical triumph: the iron lung. **Respir Ther** 1979 Jan–Feb;9(1):71–3
Rapin M, Lemaire F: La ventilation artificielle prolongée. 1954–1979. **Nouv Presse Med** 1979 Jan 13;8(2):89–92
Rendell-Baker L: Nineteenth-century resuscitation apparatus. **Anaesthesia** 1981 Nov;36(11):1058–9
Roth N: Electroresuscitation and the occult. **Med Instrum** 1980 Mar–Apr;14(2):120–1

**France**

Courtine JC: L'Armée d'Afrique et l'anesthésie-réanimation: de Baudens (1853) au Corps expéditionnaire française à la Première Armée (1942–1945) et à la guerre d'Algérie. **Hist Sci Med** 1983;17(4):411–17
Laget M: Note sur la réanimation des nouveau-nés (XVIIIe–XIXe siècles). **Ann Demogr Hist (Paris)** 1983;:65–72

**Germany**

Biadała E: Sztuczne oddychanie metodą usta-usta i pobudzanie prądem elektrycznym akcji serca opisane przed 200 laty. **Wiad Lek** 1981 Sep 1;34(17):1471–7

**Great Britain**

Fothergill J: Observations on the recovery of a man dead in appearance by distending the lungs with air. Facsimile of London 1745 edition, with biographical note by K. G. Huston. Van Nuys, California, Hoffman, 1980. 13 p.
McLellan I: Nineteenth century resuscitation apparatus. **Anaesthesia** 1981 Mar;36(3):307–11
Rechtman J: Un précurseur génial de la prévention et de la diététique, du bouche à bouche et du massage cardiaque externe de l'asepsie et parrain de J. P. Marat: Le docteur William Buchan (1729–1805). Diss. Paris VII, 1979. 115 p.

**Italy**

Bellucci G: Storia della Società Italiana di Anestesia ed Analgesia, Società Italiana di Anestesiologia, Società Italiana di Anestesia e Rianimazione, Società Italiana di Anestesiologia, Analgesia, Rianimazione e Terapia Intensiva. **Minerva Anestesiol** 1980 Jul;46(7):733–56

**United States**

Cornwell JB, Davis HN: Historical perspective, current applications: the chest cuirass. **Respir Ther** 1979 Jan–Feb;9(1):87–9, 90
Criley JM, Niemann JT, Rosborough JP: Cardiopulmonary resuscitation research 1960–1984: discoveries and advances. **Ann Emerg Med** 1984 Sep;13(9 Pt 2):756–8
Dill DB, Gordon AS: Background on manual artificial respiration and mouth-to-mouth resuscitation. Addendum: Background on cardiopulmonary resuscitation. **Physiologist** 1980 Jun;23(3):33–7
Glover DW: Model No. 110 Kreiselman Resuscitator. **Respir Care** 1977 Feb;22(2):203
Gorham J: Commercial development of the oxygen tent. **Respir Ther** 1979 Jan–Feb;9(1):48–9
Roth N: Reviving resuscitation: 1900 -- present. **Med Instrum** 1980 May–Jun;14(3):160
Scherlis L: Poetical version of the Rules of the Humane Society for recovering drowned persons. **Crit Care Med** 1981 May;9(5):430–1
Sladen A: Landmark perspective: Closed-chest massage, Kouwenhoven, Jude, Knickerbocker. **JAMA** 1984 Jun 15;251(23):3137–40
Stephenson HE: Charles Claude Guthrie's contribution to cardiac resuscitation. **Crit Care Med** 1981 May;9(5):428–9

## RURAL HEALTH

See also **Public Health**

Larsen O: Leben auf dem Lande: dem Körper nicht nur förderlich. In Imhof AE, ed: Leib und Leben in der Geschichte der Neuzeit. Berlin,

Duncker & Humblot, 1983. p. 53-62.

**Bolivia**

Bastien JW: Exchange between Andean and Western medicine. **Soc Sci Med** 1982;16(7):795-803

**China**

Werner R: Offentliches Gesundheitswesen, traditionelle chinesische Medizin, westliche Medizin, Barfussärzte und Heilmittelkunde in der Volksrepublik China. 1. Teil. **Off Gesundheitswes** 1981 Oct;43(10):480-99

**Great Britain**

Tricks N: Man and medicine on Mendip. **Bristol Med Chir J** 1984 Apr;99(370):40-4

**Poland**

Piontek J, Henneberg M: Mortality changes in a Polish rural community (1350-1972) and estimation of their evolutionary significance. **Am J Phys Anthropol** 1981 Jan;54(1):129-38

**Sweden**

Högberg U: Allmogens förlossningsställningar. **Jordemodern** 1982 Jun;95(6):199-202

**Switzerland**

Meyer-Salzmann M: Die Spitalversorgung im Emmental. **Gesnerus** 1980;37(3/4):307-13

**United States**

Cox WW, Evans RJ: Health practices in Collier County: a study in diversity and contrast. **J Fla Med Assoc** 1982 Aug;69(8):695-701

**Before 500 A.D.**

**Japan**

Onishi W: [Life among the frontier farmers of Hokkaido: public health nursing in the history of the Showa period. 10.] (Jpn). **Kango** 1982 Feb;34(2):65-71; 97-103

**1450-1700**

**Australia**

Roberts R: Pioneering, medicine and mind. **Australas Nurses J** 1982 Jun;11(5):16-23

**Great Britain**

Doolittle IG: The effects of the Plague on a provincial town in the sixteenth and seventeenth centuries. **Med Hist** 1975 Oct;19(4):333-41

Sawyer RC: Ordinary medicine for ordinary people: illness and its treatment in the East Midlands, 1600-1630. **Soc Soc Hist Med Bull (Lond)** 1983 Dec;33:20-3

**1700 to Present**

Judd CS: Plantation health. **Hawaii Med J** 1982 Apr;41(4):116, 118

O'Brien ME: Pragmatic survivalism: behavior patterns affecting low-level wellness among minority group members. **ANS** 1982 Apr;4(3):13-26

**Africa**

Green E: U. S. population policies, development, and the rural poor of Africa. **J Mod Afr Stud** 1982;20(1):45-67

**Australia**

Daley EA: The Royal Flying Doctor Service of Australia. **Victorian Hist Mag** 1970;41(3-4):375-95

**Belgium**

Abeele R van den: Jan Albert Roselt, plattelandschirurgijn te Machelen (1714-1785). **Jaarb Kunst Oudheidk Kring Deinze** 1978;:83-117

**Canada**

Norris J: The country doctor in British Columbia: 1887-1975. **BC Stud** 1981;(49):15-39

Weller GR: The delivery of health services in the Canadian north. **J Can Stud** 1981;16(2):69-80

**China**

Lucas A: Chinese Medical Modernization. Comparative Policy Continuities, 1930s-1980s. New York, Praeger, 1982. xiii, 188 p.

**Czechoslovakia**

Fröml F: Venkovský lékař a ranhojič na konci 19. století. **Cas Lek Cesk** 1979 May 25;118(21):662-4

Sípek Z: Norbert Mrštík. (1867-1905) Ze života venkovského lékaře na začátku 20. století. **Cas Lek Cesk** 1982 Jul 30;121(30):955-6

**France**

Bergasse JD: Jean Anglade (1698-1764) et la fondation de l'hôpital rural de Cazouls-les-Béziers au XVIIIe siècle. Bergasse (ed.) Hommage à Jacques Fabre de Morlhon. Albi, O.J.S., 1978. p. 133-47.

Gelis J: De la matrone à la sage-femme: les transformations de l'accoucheuse de campagne au XVIIIe siècle. **Penelope** 1981;(5):33-6

Loux F: La femme soignante dans les traditions rurales du XIXe siècle. **Penelope** 1981;(5):37-40

Morel MF: Health and illness in traditional rural France in the 18th and 19th centuries: the example of wet-nurses. **Soc Soc Hist Med Bull (Lond)** 1983 Dec;33:24-6

**Germany**

Lüth P: Tagebuch eines Landarztes. Stuttgart, Deutsche Verlags-Anstalt, 1983. 303 p.

**Ghana**

Aidoo TA: Rural health under colonialism and neocolonialism: a survey of the Ghanaian experience. **Int J Health Serv** 1982;12(4):637-57

**Haiti**

Wallace CE, Marshall FN, Robinson C: A retrospective review of maternal and child health services at the Albert Schweitzer Hospital in rural Haiti. **Bull Pan Am Health Organ** 1982;16(1):7-16

**Hungary**

Farkas J, Pisztora F, Martos G: Történeti szocio-kulturpsychiátriai vizsgálatok egy zárt faluközösségre, a mezökövesdi matyó populációra vonatkozóan 1895 és 1945 között. **Orvostort Kozl** 1982;92(4):127-31

Kapronczay K: A vidéki orvosok társasága. **Orv Hetil** 1979 Jul 15;120(28):1703-5

Martos G, Farkas J, Pisztora F: Szocio-kulturális tényezök hatása a mezökövesdi matyók pszichés sajátosságaira és megbetegedéseire a XVIII. és XIX. században. **Orvostort Kozl** 1982;92(4):119-26

Menner O: Menner Adolf dr. (1824-1901). **Orv Hetil** 1983 Jun 12;124(24):1451-3

**India**

Simmons GB, Smucker C, Bernstein S, et al: Post-neonatal mortality in rural India: implications of an economic model. **Demography** 1982 Aug;19(3):371-89

**Italy**

Caffaratto TM: Aspetti medico-sociali delle malattie dei lavoratori piemontesi della terra, nella seconda metà del secolo XIX. **Minerva Med** 1984 Apr;75(14-15):842-51; (17):999-1012; (18):1079-88

**Japan**

[History of public health nursing activities among frontier farmers in Hokkaido] (Jpn): **Hokenfu Zasshi** 1982 Jan;38(1):10-49

Kato M, Araki S, Sadahiro U, et al: [History of public health nursing in Hokkaido--through the war, postwar transition, repatriation, and reconstruction periods. A discussion] (Jpn). **Hokenfu Zasshi** 1982 Jan;38(1):58-75

Onishi W: [Life among farmers of a reclamation project in Hokkaido: a life of a public health nurse in a segment of the history of the Showa period] (Jpn). **Kango** 1981 Dec;33(14):82-7

Tsubota S: [Public health nurses in the frontier of Hokkaido--a historical background] (Jpn). **Hokenfu Zasshi** 1982 Jan;38(1):50-6

**Mexico**

Canales Muñoz JL, Almada Bay I, Narro Robles J: La mortalidad en una población rural de México y su relación con el uso de los servicios

médicos antes de la muerte. **Salud Publica Mex** 1984 Jul–Aug;26(4):404–14
Ramírez Almanza MA: La formación de los médicos y su utilización en el área rural. **Salud Publica Mex** 1983 Sep–Oct;25(5):533–9

**Thailand**

Frenzen PD, Hogan DP: The impact of class, education, and health care on infant mortality in a developing society: the case of rural Thailand. **Demography** 1982 Aug;19(3):391–408

**United States**

Ackerman EB: The activities of a country doctor in New York State: Dr. Elias Cornelius of Somers, 1794–1803. **Hist Reflect** 1982 Spring–Summer;9:181–93
Baird WD, ed: Years of discontent. Doctor Frank L. James in Arkansas, 1877–1878. Memphis, Memphis State University Press, 1977. xxviii, 84 p.
Brod RL, May PA, Stewart TJ: Recruitment and retention of federal physicians on the Navajo Reservation. **Soc Sci J** 1982;19(4):47–66
Brown DC: Health of farm children in the South, 1900–1950. **Agric Hist** 1979;53(1):170–87
Downey-Anderson C: The 'Coggins Affair': desegregation and Southern mores in Madison County, Florida. **Fla Hist Q** 1981 Apr;59:464–72
Dye NS: Mary Breckinridge, the Frontier Nursing Service and the introduction of nurse-midwifery in the United States. **Bull Hist Med** 1983 Winter;57(4):485–507
Harstad PT: Frontier medicine in the Territory of Wisconsin. In Numbers RL, Leavitt JW, ed: Wisconsin medicine. Historical perspectives. Madison, University of Wisconsin Press, 1981. p. 13–23.
Hasson GS: The medical activities of the Freedmen's Bureau in Reconstruction Alabama, 1865–1868. Ph.D. Diss, University of Alabama, University, 1982. 252 p.
Herman BL: Folk medical recipes in nineteenth-century American farm journals. **Pa Folklife** 1976;25(4):16–25
Houser HR: Wilderness doctor: the life and times of Dr. John Hole. [Centerville, Ohio], Centerville Historical Society, 1980. 32 p.
Peacock EG: Early Idaho panhandle doctor reached patients on horseback, boats and rails. **Pac Northwest** 1979;23(1):1–15
Pletsch PK: Mary Breckinridge: a pioneer who made her mark. **Am J Nurs** 1981 Dec;81(12):2188–90
Reid RA, Bartlett EE, Kozoll R: The checkerboard area health system: delivering comprehensive care in a remote region of New Mexico. **Hum Organ** 1982;41(2):147–55
Savitt TL: Patient letters to an early nineteenth century Virginia physician. **J Fla Med Assoc** 1982 Aug;69(8):688–94
Scott MH: Say, 'Ah,' the story of a hundred years of medicine in Richland County, Wisconsin, 1840–1940. Richland Center, Wis., Richland County Pub., 1981. 262 p.
Stewart S: Rational powwowing: an examination of choice among medical alternatives in rural York County, Pennsylvania. **Pa Folklife** 1976;26(1):12–7
Stuart R, Stuart W: John Marsh. **Pac Hist** 1980;24(3):369–75
Thompson ME: Public health nursing faces challenges in rural health. **Vt Regist Nurse** 1981 May;:7–8, Jul; 3–4
Treleven DE: One hundred years of health and healing in rural Wisconsin. In Numbers RL, Leavitt JW, ed: Wisconsin medicine. Historical perspectives. Madison, University of Wisconsin Press, 1981. p. 133–53.
Van Riper C: My father, Doctor Van. Marquette, Mich., John M. Longyear Research Library, 1982. ix, 74 p.
Wells LA: Rural psychiatry on the nineteenth-century frontier: the career of Jacob Bowers. **Perspect Biol Med** 1981 Winter;24(2):270–81
Wendler M van Voorhis: Doctors and diseases on the Ohio frontier. **Ohio Hist** 1980;89(2):222–42
Winfree LT, Theis HE, Griffiths CT: Drug use in rural America: a cross-cultural examination of complementary social deviance theories. **Youth Soc** 1981;12(4):465–89

**USSR**

Kamalov MKh, Golubev LV, Petrov ME, et al: K 60-letiiu iubileiu Bashkirskoĭ ASSR: sel'skoe zdravookhranenie Bashkirii i puti dal'neĭshego ego razvitiia. **Sov Med** 1980;(4):101–3
Kozliuk VM, Leonenko NA, Stefanovskaia NV: O razvitii lechebno-profilakticheskoĭ pomoshchi naseleniiu USSR v 1917–1940 gg. **Vrach Delo** 1982 Apr;(4):3–7
Rakov PP: Razvitie zdravookhraneniia Ul'ianovskoĭ oblasti za gody Sovetskoĭ vlasti. **Sov Med** 1980;(4):94–8
Shandala MG: Aleksandr Nikitich Marzeev (k 100-letiiu so dnia rozhdeniia). **Vrach Delo** 1983 May;5:119–21
Shtern MI, Karinskaia GS: Zemskiĭ vrach A. V. Ivanov. **Sov Zdravookhr** 1983;(8):64–7

# SANITATION

See also **Ecology; Hygiene; Public Health**

Eisenbud M: Environment, technology, and health: human ecology in historical perspective. New York, New York University Press, 1978. x, 384 p.
Fitchen JF: The problem of ventilation through the ages. **Technol Cult** 1981 Jul;22(3):485–511
Haneveld GT: 'De secrete' toiletfacilities in sea-going vessels. In International Congress of the History of Medicine, 27th, Barcelona, 1980. Actas. Barcelona, Acadèmia de Ciències Mèdiques de Catalunya i Balears, 1981. p. 384–6.
Pelling M: Social history of medicine and the geographers--a bibliography. **Soc Soc Hist Med Bull (Lond)** 1984 Dec;35:55–8
Schadewaldt H: 'Schulmedizin--Aussenseitermethoden'; eine Betrachtung aus historischer Sicht. **Rheinisches Arztebl** 1980;8:225–30
Schadewaldt H: Von der Cloaca maxima bis zur modernen Kläranlage – historische Aspekte zur Abfallbeseitigung. **Zentralbl Bakteriol Mikrobiol Hyg [B]** 1983 Sep;178(1–2):68–80
Schadewaldt H: Wasser--Hygienische Gefahren früher und heute. **Zentralbl Bakteriol [B]** 1980;172(1–3):275–97
Weinstein MS: Health in the city. Environmental and behavioral influences. New York, Pergamon, 1980. xvii, 92 p.
Wijbenga A, Hutzinger O: Chemicals, man and the environment: a historic perspective of pollution and related topics. **Naturwissenschaften** 1984 May;71(5):239–46

**Belgium**

Leboutte R: Les métaux et l'hygiène alimentaire: la vaisselle en zinc de l'abbé Dony. **Bull Soc R Vieux Liege** 1977–79;9:311–3

**France**

Amiot M, Béguinot P: L'alimentation en eau potable de la ville de Dijon et son assainnissement. **Mem Acad Sci Arts B-Lett Dijon** 1977;122:551–602
Hildesheimer F, Robin G, Schenk J, ed: Intendance sanitaire de Marseille. (Répertoire numérique de la sous série 200 E – Archives de la Région Provence-Alpes-Cote d'Azur et du Département des Bouches-du-Rhone). Marseille, Archives Departementales, 1979. 71 p.

**Great Britain**

Rennison RW: The supply of water to Newcastle upon Tyne and Gateshead, 1680–1837. **Archaeol Aeliana** 1977;5:5

**Italy**

Caffaratto A: Storia della legislazione sanitaria ed igienica in Piemonte da Amedeo VIII all'Unità d'Italia. Parte I. **Minerva Med** 1979 Nov 3;70(48):3315–21 (contd)
Caffaratto A: Storia della legislazione sanitaria ed igienica in Piemonte da Amedeo VIII all'Unità d'Italia. Parte III. **Minerva Med** 1979 Dec 1;70(54):3729–43

**United States**

Capper J, Power G, Shivers FR: Chesapeake waters. Pollution, public health, and public opinion, 1607–1972. Centreville, Maryland, Tidewater Publishers, 1983. xii, 201 p.
Hoy SM, Robinson MC, ed: Public works history in the United States: a guide to the literature. Nashville, American Association for State and Local History, 1982. Sections on water supply and waste disposal, p. 165–215.

**Before 500 A.D.**

Sorokina TS: O drevneĭshikh sanitarno-tekhnicheskikh sooruzheniiakh. **Gig Sanit** 1980 Jul;(7):41–4

**Rome**

Duka Zólyomi N: Sanitäre Beziehungen in privatrechtlichen Bestimmungen des römischen Corpus juris civilis. **Orvostort Kozl** 1981;93–96(27 No 1–4):83–91

**500 A.D.–1450**

**Ireland**

Moylan TK: Poverty, pigs and pestilence in medieval Dublin. **Dublin Hist Rec** 1978;31(4)

**Mexico**

Prygova NM: Sanitariia i gigiena v atsteksom obshchestve (k istorii sanitarii i gigieny v Meksike). **Gig Sanit** 1981 Aug;(8):54–6

# SANITATION

**1450–1700**

Hiller I: Betrachtungen zu medizinischen Aspekten des Umweltschutzes im 17. Jahrhundert. **Z Gesamte Hyg** 1983 Sep;29(9):560–3

**Austria**

Budernik A: Die zweite Türkenbelagerung Wiens, mit besonderer Berücksichtigung der sanitären Verhältnisse vor und während dieser Zeit. **Wien Klin Wochenschr** 1983 Oct 14;95(19):688–92

**Brazil**

Ferreira França M: Panorama medico dos seculos XVI e XVII. **Rev Inst Hist Geogr Bras** 1970;288:255–74

**Germany**

Hiller I: Betrachtungen zu medizinischen Aspekten des Umweltschutzes im 17. Jahrhundert. **Z Gesamte Hyg** 1983 Sep;29(9):560–3

**Great Britain**

Nelson TG: Death, dung, the devil, and worldly delights: a metaphysical conceit in Harington, Donne, and Herbert. **Stud Philol** 1979 Summer;76(3):272–87

Walton MT: Stinking air, corrupt water, and the English Sweat: a footnote to the quality of life in fifteenth-century London. **J Hist Med Allied Sci** 1981 Jan;36(1):67–8

**1700 to Present**

Bruce FE: Water supply and waste disposal [in the twentieth century]. In Williams TI, ed: A history of technology. Vol. VII. The twentieth century, ca. 1900 to ca. 1950, Part II. Oxford, Clarendon, 1978. p. 1363–98.

Budnikowski A, Rusiński M: O skutkach ekonomicznych przeciwdziałani zanieczyszczeniu środowiska w krajach kapitalistycznych. **Ekonomista** 1974;(2):401–14

Fitzgerald GF: Le Canada et le développement du droit international: la contribution de l'affaire de la fonderie de Trail à le formation du nouveau droit de la pollution atmosphérique transfrontière. **Etud Int** 1980;11(3):393–420

Greene VW: Cleanliness and the health revolution. New York, Soap and Detergent Association, 1984. vii, 68 p.

Makliarski B: Bor'ba s zagriaznenniem biosfery: ekonomicheskii i sotsial'nyi aspekt. **Mirovaia Ekon Mezhdunar Otnosheniia** 1974;(5):63–75

Simson JV: Die Flussverunreinigungsfrage im 19. Jahrhundert. **Vierteljahrsschr Soz Wirtschgesch** 1978;65(3):370–90

Tarr JA, Yosie T, McCurley J: Disputes over water quality policy: professional cultures in conflict, 1900–1917. **Am J Public Health** 1980 Apr;70(4):427–35

Templeton WL: Artificial radionuclides in the oceans. In Sears M, Merriman D, ed: Oceanography, the past. New York, Springer, 1980. p. 420–37.

**Americas**

Cain LP: An economic history of urban location and sanitation. **Res Econ Hist** 1977;2:337–89

**Australia**

Dawson B: Sanitary condition of Melbourne, 1888–1891: a study. **Anu Hist J** 1979–80;14:37–49

Mayne A: City back-slums in the land of promise: some aspects of the 1876 report on overcrowding in Sydney. **Labour Hist** 1980;38:26–39

Mayne AJ: Fever, squalor and vice: sanitation and social policy in Victorian Sydney. St. Lucia, New York, University of Queensland Press, 1982. xviii, 263 p.

**Austria**

Wens HM: Zur Geschichte der Tierkörperbeseitigung in Ober- und Nieder-österreich. **Zentralbl Bakteriol [B]** 1980 Mar;170(3–4):211–6

**Brazil**

Greenfield GM: The development of the underdeveloped city: public sanitation in São Paulo, Brazil, 1885–1913. **Luso-Braz Rev** 1980;17(1):107–18

**Canada**

Farley M, Keel O, Limoges C: Les commencements de l'administration montréalaise de la santé publique (1865–1885). **HSTC** 1982 May;21(6 no 2):85–109

Taylor JH: Disease, fire and water in the nineteenth century city: a bibliography. **Urban Hist Rev** 1979;8(1):113–5

Taylor JH: Fire, disease and water in Ottawa: an introduction. **Urban Hist Rev** 1979;8(1):7–37

**Chile**

Unda F: Acciones de saneamiento ambiental del Servicio Nacional de Salud, 1952–1957. **Rev Med Chil** 1977 Oct;105(10):714–23

**Czechoslovakia**

Dohnany L: Der Sanitätsdienst bei den Militär- und Partisaneneinheiten im Slowakischen Nationalaufstand des Jahres 1944. In International Congress of the History of Medicine. 26th, Plovdiv, 1978. Actes du Congress. Sofia, 1981. Volume II. p. 69–71.

**Europe**

Yturriaga Barberán JA de: La Comunidad Económica Europea y la protección del medio acuático contra la contaminación. **Rev Inst Eur** 1976;3(3):691–99

**France**

Abrahams HJ: Lavoisier and his contemporaries debate the supply of water for Paris. **Bull NY Acad Med** 1981 Jun;57(5):355–69

Darquenne R: Controverses sur la nocivité du charbon de terre (18e–19e siècles). **Ann Soc Belg Hist Hop** 1981;:33–45

Goubert JP: A 'quiet revolution': the coming of pure water to contemporary France. **Soc Soc Hist Med Bull (Lond)** 1984 Dec;35:28–9

Goubert JP: L'hygiène de l'eau dans la France contemporaine d'après le thèses de doctorat de la Faculté de Médecine de Paris (1830–1940). In Imhof AE, ed: Mensch und Gesundheit in der Geschichte. Husum, Matthiesen, 1980. p. 59–78.

Goubert JP: Ordre et désordre: l'origine aquatique de la fièvre typhoïde. **Asclepio** 1983;35:161–70

Guerrand RH: L'âge d'or du bidet. **Histoire** 1983;(57):84–7

Guerrand RH: Petite histoire du quotidien: l'avènement de la chasse d'eau. **Histoire** 1982;43:96–9

Guillerme A: Medical topography and the rebuilding of Le Mans. **Soc Soc Hist Med Bull (Lond)** 1984 Dec;35:26–7

Hildesheimer F: La protection sanitaire des côtes françaises au XVIIIe siècle. **Rev Hist Mod Contemp** 1980 Jul–Sep;27:443–67

Jacquemet G: Urbanisme parisien: la bataille du tout-/AF/a-l'égout a la fin du XIXe siècle. **Rev Hist Mod Contemp** 1979;26(Oct–Dec):505–48

Shapiro AL: Working class housing and public health in Paris, 1850–1902. Ph.D. Diss., Brown University. Providence, 1980. 338 leaves.

**Germany**

Breyer H: Max von Pettenkofer: Arzt im Vorfeld der Krankheit. Leipzig, Hirzel, 1980. 234 p.

Cieply J: Warunki sanitarne w zastepcym wiezieniu policyjnym w Mysłowicach. **Przegl Lek** 1981;38(1):95–107

Haase HH: Max von Pettenkofer--einige Gedanken zu Leben, Werk und Hinterlassenschaft. **Z Gesamte Hyg** 1980;26(10):697–9

Kaiser W, Werner K: Das Trinkwasser in der halleschen populärmedizinischen Aufklärungsliteratur des frühen 18. Jahrhunderts. **Z Gesamte Hyg** 1981;27(5):365–71

Schulze B: Probleme der Umwelthygiene im Erfurt des 19. Jahrhunderts. **Z Arztl Fortbild (Jena)** 1980;74(2):89–92

**Great Britain**

Ashby E: The politics of clean air. Oxford, Clarendon Press, 1981. viii, 178 p.

Barnes M, Pratt PK: Women sanitary inspectors. **Hist Workshop J** 1978;6:225

Blamire RV: Meat hygiene: the changing years. **J R Soc Health** 1984 Oct;104(5):180–5

Brown RH: The development of methods for the determination of hazardous substances in factory atmospheres: an historical perspective. **Ann Occup Hyg** 1984;28(2):183–8

Carter JT: Vitiated air: a Victorian villain? **J R Soc Med** 1981 Dec;74(12):914–9

Craig P: Medical topography. **Soc Soc Hist Med Bull (Lond)** 1984 Dec;35:33–4

Davies J: Cambridge Museum of Technology. **Ind Archaeol** 1980;15(4):335–55

Dingle AE: 'The monster nuisance of all': landowners, alkali manufacturers, and air pollution, 1828–64. **Econ Hist Rev** 1982;35(4):529–48

Eyler JM: The conversion of Angus Smith: the changing role of chemistry and biology in sanitary science, 1850–1880. **Bull Hist Med** 1980 Summer;54(2):216–34

Flick C: The movement for smoke abatement in 19th-century Britain. **Technol Cult** 1980 Jan;21(1):29–50

Gorham E: Robert Angus Smith, F.R.S., and 'Chemical climatology'. **Notes Rec R Soc Lond** 1982 Feb;36(2):267–72

Gould MH: The administrative units used for water supply purposes in Northern Ireland from 1828. **R Soc Health J** 1981 Jun;101(3):119–22

Hamlin C: Edward Frankland's early career as London's official water analyst, 1865–1876: the context of 'previous sewage contamination'. **Bull Hist Med** 1982 Spring;56(1):56–76

Hamlin CS: What becomes of pollution? Adversary science and the controversy of self-purification of rivers in Britain, 1850–1900. Ph.D. Diss., University of Wisconsin. Madison, 1982. vi, 618 p.

Hardy A: Water and the search for public health in London in the eighteenth and nineteenth centuries. **Med Hist** 1984 Jul;28(3):250–82

Haugh MC: The Doulton story (Henry Doulton). **Nurs Times** 1979 Jul 19;75(29):1207–8

Herzka HS, Otti L: Geschichte der Kindheit--zum Belspiel: Industrialisierung. **Acta Paedopsychiatr (Basel)** 1984 May;50(1):5–6

Hinton BT: Thomas Crapper (1837–1910). **Invest Urol** 1980 May;17(6):534–5

James DC: The genesis of sanitary reform in Cardiff, 1774–1850. **Welsh Hist Rev** 1982;11(1):50–66

Kerr B: Henry Moule and cholera in Dorset: nineteenth-century sanitary reform. **Hist Today** 1978;28(10):672–80

Knapp MR: Economics of scale in sewage purification and disposal. **J Ind Econ** 1978 Dec;27:163–83

McLaren D: Disease and dirty water in West Somerset in the late nineteenth century. **Soc Soc Hist Med Bull (Lond)** 1974 Dec;35:35–6

Porter R: Cleaning up the Great Wen: public health and eighteenth-century London. **Soc Soc Hist Med Bull (Lond)** 1984 Dec;35:24–5

Ranlett J: The Smoke Abatement Exhibition of 1881. **Hist Today** 1981 Nov;31:10–3

Spavold J: The sanitary pottery industries of South Derbyshire, 1840–1914. **Ind Archaeol Rev** 1981;5(2):143–54

Warner F: Control of pollution. **Proc R Inst GB** 1979;51:95–119

Watterson P: Environmental factors in infant and early childhood mortality decline in England and Wales, 1895 to 1910. **Soc Soc Hist Med Bull (Lond)** 1984 Dec;35:37–40

White BM: Medical police. Politics and police: the fate of John Roberton. **Med Hist** 1983 Oct;27(4):407–22

**India**

Klein I: Cholera: theory and treatment in nineteenth century India. **J Indian Hist** 1980;58(1–3):35–51

Naidis M: 'Ants, muskeetoes, flies and stinking chints': the British battle against disease in India. **West Hum Rev** 1964;17(1):39–47

**Italy**

Sorcinelli P: Miseria e malattie nel XIX secolo. I ceti popolari nell'Italia centrale fra tifo petecchiale e pellagra. Milano, Franco Angeli, 1979. 285 p.

Whiteside T: The pendulum and the toxic cloud. The course of dioxin contamination. New Haven, London, Yale University Press, 1979. 205 p.

**Japan**

Nomiyama K: 'Kogai', environmental pollution and the related public nuisance. In Ogawa T, ed: Public health. Tokyo, Saikon, 1981. p. 82–98.

**Mexico**

Bath CR: Health and environmental problems: the role of the border in El Paso–Ciudad Juarez coordination. **J Interam Stud World Aff** 1982;24(3):375–92

**Netherlands**

Graaff MG: Milieuvervuiling: een oud probleem. **Spiegel Hist** 1982;17(2):86–96

**Romania**

Năstasă V, Sîrghie E, Cuciureanu R, et al: Date istorice privind alimentarea cu apă potabilă a municipiului Iaşi, precum şi variaţiile cantitative şi calitative ale acesteia. **Rev Med Chir Soc Med Nat Iasi** 1982 Jul–Sep;86(3):449–52

Negru I: Aprovizionarea Bucureştilor cu apă prină in pragul secolului al XX-lea. **Viata Med [Medii Sanit]** 1983 Aug;31(8):185–90

Peiu N: Din istoricul alimentării cu apă a oraşului Iaşi în secolele XVIII şi XIX. **Rev Med Chir Soc Med Nat Iasi** 1983 Oct–Dec;87(4):657–9

**South Africa**

Cartwright MF: The filthy state of Cape Town in 1858. **Q Bull S Afr Libr** 1978;33(2):53–6

**Spain**

Rodriguez Ocaña E: Higiene y terapeutica anticolericas en la primera epidemia de colera en España, 1833–1835. **Asclepio** 1982;34:71–100

Sanz Sanjosé MG, Merino Navarro JP: Saneamiento y limpieza en Madrid, siglo XVIII. **An Inst Estud Madrilenos** 1976;(12):119–32

**United States**

Alewitz S: Sanitation and public health: Philadelphia, 1870–1900. Ph.D. Diss., Case Western Reserve University. Cleveland, 1981. vii, 421 p.

Bonte FJ: The notorius decontamination caper. **Semin Nucl Med** 1979 Jul;9(3):218–9

Bowers JZ: Shields Warren's exemplary sanitary survey. **Am J Forensic Med Pathol** 1980 Dec;1(4):365–6

Brown AS: Caroline Bartlett Crane and urban reform. **Mich Hist** 1972;56(4):287–301

Burns LS: Noise. **Horizon** 1977;20(1):66–9

Cain LP: Sanitation strategy for a lakefront metropolis. The case of Chicago. DeKalb, Northern Illinois University Press, 1978. xv, 173 p.

Cain LP: The creation of Chicago's sanitary district and construction of the Sanitary and Ship Canal. **Chic Hist** 1979;8(2):98–110

Clean water and the health of the cities: New York, Arno, 1977. Various paginations. Facsimile reprints of works by William T. Sedgwick (1893), George C. Whipple (1907), and J. Scott MacNutt (1910).

Collingridge D, Douglas J: Three models of policymaking: expert advice in the control of environmental lead. **Soc Stud Sci** 1984 Aug;14(3):343–70

Cox JS: Die Entwicklung der amerikanischen Tierkörperverwertungs-industrie. **Zentralbl Bakteriol [B]** 1980 Mar;170(3–4):217–21

Davis C: Hazardous waste politics and policy. **Policy Stud J** 1983;12(1):171–4

Downing PB: Bargaining in pollution control. **Policy Stud J** 1983;11(4):577–86

Ettling J: The germ of laziness. Rockefeller philanthropy and public health in the new South. Cambridge, Harvard, 1981. x, 263 p.

Galishoff S: The Passaic Valley trunk sewer. **NJ Hist** 1970;88(4):197–214

Greenberg M, O'Neill TF: Solid waste: the end of the bottomless pit. **NY Aff** 1978;5(2):114–29

Hamilton HD, Lander BG: Public policy analysis: water and sewers for McElrath Park. **Phylon** 1979;40(1)41–51

House RV: A brief history of hookworm disease in North Carolina. **NC Med J** 1982 Nov;43(11):765–8

Jacobs M, Stevenson G: Health and housing: a historical examination of alternative perspectives. **Int J Health Serv** 1981;11(1):105–22

Kiefer WE: The Gratiot County landfill: one of Michigan's foremost toxic waste sites. **Mich Acad** 1983;15(3):311–31

Leavitt JW: The wasteland: garbage and sanitary reform in the nineteenth-century American city. **J Hist Med Allied Sci** 1980 Oct;35(4):431–52

Lester JP, Franke JL, Bowman AO, et al: Hazardous wastes, politics, and public policy: a comparative state analysis. **West Polit Q** 1983;36(2):257–85

Lindop PJ, Rotblat J: Radiation pollution of the environment. **Bull At Sci** 1971;27(7):17–24

Liu B: The costs of air quality deterioration and benefits of air pollution control: estimates of mortality costs for two pollutants in 40 U.S. metropolitan areas. **Am J Econ Sociol** 1979;38(2):187–95

McMahon M: Fairmount. **Am Heritage** 1979;30(3):100–7

Maloney MT, McCormick RE: A positive theory of environmental quality regulation. **J Law Econ** 1982;25(1):99–123

Mazur A: The journalists and technology: reporting about Love Canal and Three Mile Island. **Minerva** 1984 Spring;22(1):45–66

Melosi MV: Battling pollution in the Progressive era. **Landscape** 1982;26(3):35–41

Melosi MV: Garbage in the cities. Refuse, reform, and the environment, 1880–1980. College Station, Texas A & M University Press, 1981. xvi, 268 p. (Environmental History Series, no. 4).

Melosi MV: Urban pollution: historical perspective needed. **Environ Rev** 1980;3(3):37–44

Melosi MV, ed: Pollution and reform in American cities, 1870–1930. Austin, Univ. of Texas Press, 1980. xii, 212 p. Contributions by S. Galishoff, J. A. Tarr, J. McCurley, T. F. Yosie, R. D. Grinder, R. W. Smilor, S. K. Schultz, C. McShane, S. M. Hoy.

Morandi M, Eisenbud M: Carbon monoxide exposure in New York City: a historical overview. **Bull NY Acad Med** 1980 Nov–Dec;56(9):817–28

Navarro P: The politics of air pollution. **Public Interest** 1980;59:36–44

Peterson JA: The impact of sanitary reform upon American urban planning, 1840–1890. **J Soc Hist** 1979;13(1):83–103

Polikoff A: The Interlake affair. **Wash Mon** 1971;3(1):7–17

Reid L: Pollution: not a new problem for Missourians. **Gateway Herit** 1980;1(2):18–22

Remes NR: The rural cemetery. **Nineteenth Century Fict** 1979;5(4):52–5

Rhoades ER: Medicine at Fort Sill, Indian Territory 1975–1880. **J Okla State Med Assoc** 1982 Feb;75(2):36–41

Sewering the cities. New York, Arno, 1977. Various paginations. Five reprinted articles by various authors, 1881–1914.:

## SANITATION

Sloyan PJ: The day they shut down Birmingham. **Wash Mon** 1972;4(3):41–50
Stakem KA: Hans Froelicher, Jr.: civic educator. **Md Hist Mag** 1982;77(2):193–201
Stern AC: History of air pollution legislation in the United States. **J Air Pollut Control Assoc** 1982 Jan;32(1):44–61
Stone MN: The plumbing paradox: American attitudes toward late nineteenth-century domestic sanitary arrangements. **Winterthur Portf** 1979;14(3):283–309
Sturgis KR: The driftwood case: pioneering antipollution in Pennsylvania. **Trans Stud Coll Physicians Phila** 1982 Dec;5(4 no 4):259–71
Tarr JA, Lamperes BC: Changing fuel use behavior ... the Pittsburgh smoke control movement, 1940–1950. **J Soc Hist** 1981;14:561–88
Tarr JA: The separate vs. combined sewer problem: a case study in urban technology design choice. **J Urban Hist** 1979;5(3):308–39
Tarr JA, et al: Water and wastes: a retrospective assessment of wastewater technology in the United States, 1800–1932. **Technol Cult** 1984 Apr;25(2):226–63
Thompson K: The notion of air purity in early California. **South Calif Q** 1972;54(3):203–10
Warfe C: The search for pure water in Ottawa: 1910–1915. **Urban Hist Rev** 1979;8(1):90–112
Zimmerman BK: An overview of regulatory responsibilities. **Basic Life Sci** 1982;21:439–60

**USSR**

Akulov KI, Shlepnina TG: Nauchnoe obosnovanie standartizatsii kachestva pit'evoĭ vody v trudakh prof. S. N. Cherkinskogo. **Gig Sanit** 1982 Aug;(8):50–3
Aleksanian IV, Kulish IM: Sanitarno-gigienicheskoe i protivoé pidemicheskoe obespechenie voĭsk v gody Velikoĭ Otechestvennoĭ voĭny.
Galin LL: Deiatel'nost' voenno-sanitarnoĭ sluzhby v gody Velikoĭ Otechestvennoĭ voĭny (po materialam 'Voenno-meditsinskogo zhurnala'). **Sov Zdravookhr** 1984;(5):58–61
Iarovinskiĭ MIa: 100 let sanitarnoĭ organizatsii goroda Moskvy. **Sov Zdravookhr** 1984;(9):45–9
Kalina GP: Nekotorye voprosy istorii sanitarnoĭ mikrobiologii. **Gig Sanit** 1982 Nov;(11):47–50
Kogan VIa, Petrova LF: Sanitarnye s'ezdy USSR i ikh sotsial'no-gigienicheskaia napravlennost'. **Sov Zdravookhr** 1983;(3):58–61
Lubomudrov S: Environmental politics in the Soviet Union: the Baikal controversy. **Can Slavonic Pap** 1978;20(4):529–43
Semenov SV: K istorii organizatsii gosudarstvennogo sanitarnogo nadzora na vodnom transporte v RSFSR. **Gig Sanit** 1984 Jan;(1):36–8
Shirokov IuG, Lebedeva NV, Koliadich MN: Uchastie L. K. Khotsianova v rabote s'ezdov gigienistov i sanitarnykh vracheĭ. **Gig Sanit** 1983 Feb;(2):31–5
Sivolob NI: Vklad I.V. Beliaeva v organizatsiiu sanitarnogo dela v Donbasse. **Sov Zdravookhr** 1984;(5):65–7

**Yugoslavia**

Dragić M: Higijenske prilike u Beogradskoj tvrdjavi i Beogradu 1829. godine (prema putopisu Ota Dubislava Pirha). **Srp Arh Celok Lek** 1982 Jul–Aug;110(7–8):951–7

## SCIENCE

See also **Research; Laboratories and Research Institutes**

Arkhangel'skiĭ GV: Primenenie naukovedcheskikh metodov vi istorii meditsiny. **Sov Zdravookhr** 1981;(3):70–3
Asimov I: Asimov's biographical encyclopedia of science and technology. The lives and achievements of 1510 great scientists from ancient times to the present chronologically arranged. Second revised edition. Garden City, New York, Doubleday, 1982. xxxv, 941 p.
Bibliografia biezaca: Historii Nauki i Techniki: **Kwart Hist Nauki Tech** 1984;29(Suppl 3–4):1–29
Blair GW: The history of rheology. **Biorheology** 1982;19(1/2):231–5
Bulferetti L: Quantification in the historiography of sciences and techniques. **Organon** 1980/81;16–17:19–41
Bunge M: The limits on science. **Physiologist** 1980 Feb;23(1):7–13
Bynum WF, Browne EJ, Porter R, ed: Dictionary of the history of science. Princeton, Princeton University Press, 1981. [xxxiv], 494 p.
Campbell WA: Library resources for the history of science in Newcastle upon Tyne. **Br J Hist Sci** 1982 Nov;15(51 pt 3):281–4
Cohen IB: From Leonardo to Lavoisier 1450–1800. New York, Scribner's, 1980. xiii. 298 p. (Album of Science).
Debus AG: History with a purpose: the fate of Paracelsus. **Pharm Hist** 1984;26(2):83–96
Downs RB: Landmarks in science, Hippocrates to Carson. Littleton, Colo., Libraries Unlimited, 1982. 305 p.
Durbin PT, ed: A guide to the culture of science, technology, and medicine. New York, Free Press, 1980. xl, 723 p. Contributions by A. Thackray, C. W. Pursell, G. H. Brieger, A. C. Michalos, C. Mitcham, H. T. Engelhardt, J. Gaston, L. Aiken, D. Crane.
Eastwood B: Directory of audio-visual sources. History of science, medicine, and technology. New York, Science History Publications, 1979. 41, [108] p.
Edel A: Science: ethical implications. In Reich WT, et al, ed: Encyclopedia of bioethics, v.4. New York, Free Press, 1978. p. 1535–41.
Elkana Y: The discovery of the conservation of energy. Cambridge, Mass., Harvard University Press, 1974. xiv, 213 p.
Epistemologia, metodologia clinica e storia della scienza medica, 1: Roma, Cossidente, 1977. xliii, 225 p. (Collana di Studi Epistemologici). Introduction by D. Antiseri. Contributions by D. Antiseri, G. Giunchi, M. Baldini, O. Todisco, M. D. Grmek, P. Potestà, V. Scalera.
Epistemologia, metodologia clinica e storia della scienza medica, 2: Roma, Cossidente, 1978. 172 p. (Collana di Studi Epistemologici). Introduction by D. Antiseri. Contributions by V. Mathieu, V. Tomini, E. Urbani, V. Somenzi, G. Federspil, C. Scandellari, M. Austoni, M. Di Giandomenico, E. Riverso, E. Garulli.
Ezrahi Y: Utopian and pragmatic rationalism: the political context of scientific advice. **Minerva** 1980 Spring;18(1):111–31
Forbes EG, ed: Human implications of scientific advance. Proceedings of the XVth International Congress of the History of Science, Edinburgh 10–15 August 1977. Edinburgh, Edinburgh University Press, 1978. 596 p. (This volume includes papers delivered at ten special symposia)
Fredga A: Varför lärdomshistoria? **Nord Medicinhist Arsb** 1980;Suppl 6:22–4
Gibson SS: Scientific societies and exchange: a facet of the history of scientific communication. **J Libr Hist** 1982 Spring;17(2):144–63
Gregory RL: Mind in science. A history of explanations in psychology and physics. Cambridge, New York, Cambridge University Press, 1981. xi, 641 p.
Grmek MD: A plea for freeing the history of scientific discoveries from myth. In M. D. Grmek, R. S. Cohen, G. Cimino, ed: On scientific discovery. The Erice Lectures 1977. Dordrecht, D. Reidel, 1981. p. 9–42. (Boston Studies in the Philosophy of Science, v. 34).
Grmek MD, Cohen RS, Cimino G, ed: On scientific discovery. The Erice Lectures 1977. Dordrecht, D. Reidel, 1981. 333 p. (Boston Studies in the Philosophy of Science, v. 34).
Guerlac H: Essays and papers in the history of modern science. Baltimore, London, Johns Hopkins University Press, 1977. xix, 540 p.
Hahn R: A bibliography of quantitative studies on science and its history. Berkeley, Office for History of Science, 1980. 84 p. (Berkeley Papers in History of Science, 3).
Hakfoort C: Wetenschapshistorische etiketten en de gevaren van polaire analyses. **Tijdschr Geschied Geneeskd** 1982;5(1):1–5
Haller JS: Aconite: a case study in doctrinal conflict and the meaning of scientific medicine. **Bull NY Acad Med** 1984 Nov;60(9):888–904
The history of science: A collection of manuscripts from the library of the Jewish Theological Seminary. An index to the microfilm collection, reels 1–17. Ann Arbor, University Microfilms, 1980. 79 p. (With Hebrew–English name index).
Honek K: Die wissenschaftlichen Bibliotheken der Erzdiözese Wien. **Biblos (Vienna)** 1981;30(2):97–102
Hooykaas R: Wissenschaftsgeschichte––eine Brücke zwischen Natur- und Geisteswissenschaften. **Ber Wissenschaftsgesch** 1982;5:153–72
Hünemörder C: Antike und mittelalterliche Enzyklopädien und die Popularisierung naturkundlichen Wissens. **Sudhoffs Arch** 1981;65(4):339–65
Jaki SL: The road of science and the ways to God. Chicago, London, Univ. of Chicago Press, 1978 vii, 478 p.
Jinich H, Pérez-Tamayo R, Sepúlveda B, et al: La verdad y el error en medicina. **Gac Med Mex** 1984 Apr;120(4):133–44
Laudan L: Progress and its problems. Toward a theory of scientific growth. Berkeley, Univ. of California Press, 1977. x, 257 p.
Lemaine G: Perspectives on the emergence of scientific disciplines. Chicago, Aldine, 1976. xi, 281 p.
Losee J: Whewell and Mill on the relation between philosophy of science and history of science. **Stud Hist Philos Sci** 1983 Jun;14(2):113–26
Magner LN: A history of the life sciences. New York, Dekker, 1979. xi, 489 p.
Martin HF: Medicine, science and humanism. **RI Med J** 1981 May;64(5):271–4
Masters J, Lambert D, Paterson H: Scientific prejudice, reproductive isolation, and apartheid. **Perspect Biol Med** 1984 Autumn;28(1):107–16
Medawar P: Pluto's republic. Incorporating The art of the soluble and Induction and intuition in scientific thought. Oxford, New York, Oxford University Press, 1982. x, 351 p.
Merchant C: Isis' consciousness raised. **Isis** 1982 Sep;73(268):398–409
Merton RK: George Alfred Léon Sarton. In Dictionary of American Biography, Suppl. 6, 1956–1960. p. 564–6, 1980.
Nauert CG: Caius Plinius Secundus. In Cranz FE, Kristeller PO, ed: Catalogus translationum et commentariorum: Mediaeval and Renaissance Latin translations and commentaries. Annotated lists and guides. Vol. IV. Washington, D.C., Catholic University of America Press, 1980. p. 297–422.
Neu J: One hundred fifth critical bibliography of the history of science and its cultural influences (to January 1980). **Isis** 1980;71(260):1–295
Pelletier PA, ed: Prominent scientists. An index to collective biographies. New York, Neal-Schuman, 1980. xxviii, 311 p.

Porter R: Dictionaries and the history of science. **Hist Sci** 1980;18(2):148–50
Porter R, ed: Liber amicorum. Repertorio biografico di storia della medicina e delle scienze naturali. **Kos Liber Amicorum** 1984;1– (continued regularly)
Reif AE: Hippocrates and the biomedical scientist: the problems of controlling the dangers of science. **Minerva** 1980 Spring;18(1):29–50
Salemme MA, Celani AM: La valeur de la logique dans l'ancienne et la moderne science. In International Congress of the History of Medicine. 26th, Plovdiv, 1978. Actes du Congress. Sofia, 1981. Volume II, p. 94–6.
Santambrogio M: Minima methodica: una rubrica che affronta problemi di metodo e di concetto, e intende stimolare nella cultura medica una riflessione 'di fondo'. (continued regularly). **Kos** 1984 Feb;1(1):16–8
Sauvy A: Science médicale et science économique. **Ann Med Interne (Paris)** 1982;133(3):216–21
Schaffner KF: Discovery in the biomedical sciences: logic or irrational intuition? In T. Nickles, ed: Scientific discovery: case studies. Dordrecht, D. Reidel, 1980. (Boston Studies in the Philosophy of Science, v. 60). p. 171–212. With commentary by N. L. Maull.
Scheuermann A: Die wissenschaftliche Gesellschaft als Medium des Fortschritts. **Tierarztl Prax** 1981:9(2):161–6
Sjöstrand T: Medicinsk vetenskap: Historik, teori och tillämpning. Stockholm, Natur och Kultur, 1979. 183 p.
Solberg WU: Cotton Mather's indebtedness to Marcello Malpighi. **J Hist Med Allied Sci** 1981 Jul;36(3):326–31
Stuhlhofer F: Unser Wissen verdoppelt sich alle 100 Jahre. **Ber Wissenschaftsgesch** 1983;6(1–4):169–93
Timofeyev IS: Izmeneniia v ponimanii predmeta istoriko-nauchnykh issledovanii. **Vopr Istor Estestvozn Tekh** 1981;(2):97–102
Wallace WA: Prelude to Galileo. Essays on medieval and sixteenth-century sources of Galileo's thought. Dordrecht, D. Reidel, 1981. xvi, 369 p. (Boston Studies in the Philosophy of Science, v. 62).
Walsh J: New niche for science on reference shelf. **Science** 1981 Jan 16;211(4479):263–4
Webster C: From Paracelsus to Newton. Magic and the making of modern science. The Eddington Memorial Lectures delivered at Cambridge University, November 1980. Cambridge, Cambridge University Press, 1982. 107 p.
Wells EB: Scientists' libraries: a handlist of printed sources. **Ann Sci** 1983 Jul;40(4):317–89
Whitaker MA: Science, scientists and history of science. **Hist Sci** 1984 Dec;22(58 pt 4):421–4
Who was who in American history – science and technology: (A component of Who's who in American history). Chicago, Marquis, 1976. xiii, 688 p.
Williams TI, Withers S, ed: A biographical dictionary of scientists. 3rd ed. London, A. & C. Black, 1982. xiv, 674 p.
Williams TI, ed, Withers S, ed: A biographical dictionary of scientists. New York, Wiley, [1974]. 641 p.
Zachert U, Zeidler U, ed: Herzog August Bibliothek Wolfenbüttel. Verzeichnis medizinischer und naturwissenschaftlicher Drucke, 1472–1830. Band 1–4, Alphabetischer Index. Millwood, New York, Kraus International, 1982. 1857 p.

### Arabic

Hamarneh S: Sarton (1884–1956) and the Arabic-Islamic legacy. **J Hist Arabic Sci** 1977 Nov;1(2):299–318

### Austria

Hochenegg H: Tiroler Aerzte und Pharmazeuten als Künstler und Schriftsteller, Forscher und Volksvertreter. **Tirol Heimat** 1976;40:135–62

### Belgium

Danckaert L, De Smet A, ed: Notes bibliographiques [on the history of science in Belgium], 89. [Brussels], Comité belge d'histoire des sciences, 1979. 24 p.

### China

Elvin M, et al: The work of Joseph Needham. **Past Present** 1980;87:17–53
Kim YS: Natural knowledge in a traditional culture: problems in the study of the history of Chinese science. **Minerva** 1982 Spring–Summer;30(1–2):83–104
Needham J: Science in traditional China. A comparative perspective. Cambridge, Harvard University Press; Hong Kong, The Chinese University Press, 1981. x, 134 p.

### Europe

Meadows AJ, ed: Development of science publishing in Europe. Amsterdam, Elsevier Science, 1980. ix, 269 p.

### France

Laissus Y: Les voyageurs naturalistes du Jardin du roi et du Muséum d'histoire naturelle: essai de portrait-robot. **Rev Hist Sci (Paris)** 1981 Jul–Oct;34(3–4):259–317

### Germany

Kohlhauer CE: Mediziner und Naturwissenschaftler im Fürstentum Ansbach. [Ansbach, s. n., 1964]. 30 p.

### Great Britain

David GR, ed: The manuscript papers of British scientists, 1600–1940. London, H.M.S.O., 1982. 109 p.
Matthews LG: Medical men as mapmakers. **Pharm Hist (London)** 1975 Aug;5(2):2–4
Morrell JT: Gentlemen of science: early years of the British Association for the Advancement of Science. Oxford, Clarendon Press; New York, Oxford University Press, 1981. xxiii, 592 p.
Schuler RM: English magical and scientific poems to 1700: an annotated bibliography. New York, Garland, 1979. xxviii, 120 p.

### Hungary

Duka Zólyomi N: Az Academia Leopoldina és a magyarországi tudományosság fejl/ABodése a 18. század végéig. **Orv Hetil** 1982 Nov 28;123(48):2969–71
Duka Zólyomi N: Die Leopoldinische Akademie und die ungarländische Medizin und Naturwissenschaft bis zum Ende des 18. Jahrhunderts. **Acta Hist Leopoldina** 1980;13:51–101

### Ireland

O'Donnell S: Gilding the anemometer: Irish science of the past. **Eire Irel** 1982;17(4):148–51

### Italy

Lolli G: La tradizione scientifica italiana. **Scientia** 1980;115(9–12):713–23

### Poland

Majewska-Tronowicz J, Michalczyk B, Kinowskiej M: Zeszyt 35/36 (VII–XII 1979). Dodatek do numeru 2/1980. Kwartalnika Historii Nauki i Techniki. **Kwart Hist Nauki Tech** 1980;25(2):Suppl.1–30
Majewska-Tronowicz J, Michalczyk B, Kinowskiej M: Zeszyt 37 (I–III 1980). Dodatek do numeru 3/1980. Kwartalnika Historii Nauki i Techniki. **Kwart Hist Nauki Tech** 1980;25(3):Suppl 1–28

### Spain

Beddall BG: Essay review: Spanish science and the New World. **J Hist Biol** 1983 Fall;16(3):433–40
Esteva de Sagrera J, Espinosa Ramos E: El proceso inquisitorial de Proust y el protagonismo cultural de Feijoo en el panorama cientifico de la ilustracion española. **Bol Soc Esp Hist Farm** 1982 Mar;33(129):77–92
Garcia del Carrizo San Millan MG: Obras de interes medico y cientifico en las bibliotecas universitaria y de Santa Cruz de Valladolid (hasta 1877). Valladolid, Universidad de Valladolid, 1981. 172 p. (Acta Historico-Medica Vallisoletana, Monografias, XI)
Gónzalez Blasco P, Jiménez Blanco J, López Piñero JM: Historia y sociología de la ciencia en España. Madrid, Alianza, 1979. 195 p.
López Piñero JM: Diccionario histórico de la ciencia moderna en España. Barcelona, Peninsula, 1983. 2 v.
Vernet Gines J: Historia de la ciencia española. Madrid, Instituto de España, Cátedra Alfonso X el Sabio, 1975. 312 p.
Weiss B: Wissenschaftliche Bibliotheken in Madrid. **Biblos (Vienna)** 1980,29(1):18–26

### Switzerland

Balmer H: Walliser Naturforscher. **Gesnerus** 1979;36(1/2):35–49

### United States

Black GW: American science and technology; a bicentennial bibliography. Carbondale, Ill., Southern Illinois University Press, 1979. xi, 170 p.
Gifford GE: Medicine and science in early America. Being the collected essays of George Edmund Gifford, Jr., 1930–1981. Edited by Dorothy I. Lansing. Devon, Pa., Published by the friends of George E. Gifford, Jr., 1982. ix, 388 p.

### Venezuela

Yépez Tamayo G: Ensayo sobre la historia de las ciencias en Venezuela. **Bol Acad Nac Hist (Caracas)** 1975;58(231):573–95

# SCIENCE

### Before 500 A.D.

**Greece**

Lloyd GE: Magic, reason and experience. Studies in the origin and development of Greek science. Cambridge, New York, Cambridge University Press, 1979. xii, 335 p.

Maloney G: Les particules dans trois traités d'Hippocrate. In: Mélanges d'études anciennes offerts à Maurice Lebel. St-Jean-Chrysostôme, Québec, 1980. p. 125–34.

Pitskhelauri GZ: Aristotle's knowledge in the field of natural and medical sciences (on celebrating 2300 years since his death). **Sante Publique (Bucur)** 1980;23(4):375–9

Sow M: Des couleurs dans quelques traités de la collection hippocratique. Univ. de Strasbourg, Thèse de 3e cycle, 1979. lxiv, 402 p.

### 500 A.D.–1450

Burchardt J: List Witelona do Ludwika we Lwowku Slaskim. Problematyka teoriopoznawcza, kosmologiczna i medyczna. Wroclaw, Polish Academy of Sciences, 1979. 225 p. (Studia Copernicana, 19).

Kollesch J: Papyri mit medizinischen, naturwissenschaftlichen und Mathematischen Texten. **Arch Papyrusforsch** 1978;26:141–8

Livesey SJ: Metabasis: the interrelationship of the sciences in antiquity and the Middle Ages. Ph.D. Diss., University of California. Los Angeles, 1982. x, 742 p.

Stoll C: Nikolaus von Kues (1401–1464) und seine Bedeutung für die Naturwissenschaft. **Pharm Acta Helv** 1979;54(9–10):311–6

Weisheipl JA, ed: Albertus Magnus and the sciences: commenmorative essays 1980. Toronto, Pontifical Institute of Mediaeval Studies, 1980. xiv, 657 p.

Weisser U, ed: Buch über das Geheimnis der Schöpfung und die Darstellung der Natur (Buch der Ursachen), von Pseudo-Apollonios von Tyana. Aleppo, Institute for the History of Arabic Science, University of Aleppo, 1979. 66 p. (Sources and Studies in the History of Arabic-Islamic Science, Natural Sciences Series 1).

**Arabic**

Burnett CS: The impact of Arabic science on western civilisation in the Middle Ages. **Bull Br Assoc Orient** 1979–80 N.Ser;11:40–51

Klein-Franke F: Die klassische Antike in der Tradition des Islam. Darmstadt, Wissenschaftliche Buchgesellschaft, 1980. ix, 181 p. (Erträge der Forschung, Band 136)

Kunitzsch P: Medizin, Naturwissenschaft und Technik im Mittelalter, Kontinuität und Wandel in Darstellung und Deutung: Die arabisch-islamische Welt. **Medizinhist J** 1982;17(1/2):54–62

Marmura ME: Avicenna on the division of the sciences in the 'Isagoge' of his 'Shifa'. **J Hist Arabic Sci** 1980;4:239–51

Tirmizi SM: Ibn Sina as a scientist. **Stud Hist Med** 1981 Sep;5(3):233–8

**Byzantium**

Hunger H: 'Zoologie,' 'Botanik,' 'Mineralogie,' 'Alchemie,' and 'Medizin.' In: Die hochsprachliche profane Literatur der Byzantiner. Vol. II. Munich, Beck, 1978 (Part 5, Vol. 2 of the Byzantinisches Handbuch). p. 265–320.

**China**

Needham J: The social position of scientific men and physicians in mediaeval China. In: International Congress for the History of Science, 14th, Tokyo, Kyoto, 1974. Proceedings. Tokyo, 1975. 4:19–34.

**Germany**

Baader G: Naturwissenschaft und Medizin im 12. Jahrhundert und Hildegard von Bingen. **Arch Mittelrheinischen Kirchengesch** 1979;31:33–54

John Paul II Pope: Discurso de Juan Pablo II a los profesores y estudiantes universitarios en la catedral de Colonia (Aalemania), 15.XI.1980. **Rev Med Univ Navarra** 1981 Jun;25(2):61–4

Kohnen N: Nicolai de Cusa. Liber quasi medicinalis: De staticis experimentis. In Göpfert W, Otten HH, ed: Metavoeite: wandelt euch durch Denken. Düsseldorf, Triltsch, 1983. p. 135–45.

**Great Britain**

McEvoy J: The chronology of Robert Grosseteste's writings on nature and natural philosophy. **Speculum** 1983 July;58(3):614–55

**India**

Rahman A, Alvi MA, Khan Ghori SA, et al: Science and technology in Medieval India. A bibliography of source materials in Sanskrit, Arabic and Persian. New Delhi, Indian National Science Academy, 1982. xxxi, 719 p.

**Iran**

Schöffler HH: Die Akademie von Gondischapur. Aristoteles auf dem Wege in den Orient. Stuttgart, Freies Geistesleben, 1979. 154 p.

**Italy**

Clagett M: The life and works of Giovanni Fontana. **Ann Ist Mus Stor Sci Fir** 1976;1(1):5–28

Jones P: Secreta Salernitana. **Kos** 1984 Feb;1(1):33–50

Olmi G: Osservazione della natura e raffiguarazione in Ulisse Aldrovandi (1522–1605). **Ann Ist Stor Italo-Ger** 1977;3:105–81

### 1450–1700

Boas Hall M: Renaissance science and professionalisation. **Ann Ist Mus Stor Sci Fir** 1982;7(2):53–64

Brody J, Field J, ed: A catalogue of books printed before 1641 in the Science Museum Library. [London], Science Museum, 1979. ii, 43 p. (4 p. supplement to 1981 attached)

Crombie AC: Science and the arts in the Renaissance: the search for truth and certainty, old and new. **Hist Sci** 1980 Dec;18(42 pt 4):233–46

Eamon W: Arcana disclosed: the advent of printing, the books of secrets tradition and the development of experimental science in the sixteenth century. **Hist Sci** 1984;22(pt 2):111–50

Faller A: Elemente einer Wissenschaftslehre und einer Wissenschaftskritik in den Schriften von Niels Stensen (1638–1686). **Gesnerus** 1980;37(3/4):169–88

Hutchison K: What happened to occult qualities in the scientific revolution? **ISIS** 1982 Jun;73(267):233–53

Kirsch I: Demonology and science during the scientific revolution. **J Hist Behav Sci** 1980 Oct;16(4):359–68

Koch CH: Petrus Severinus, Francis Bacon og Naturiagttagelsen. **Dan Medicinhist Arbog** 1979;161–72

Linet J, Hillard D, Lavagne X, ed: Catalogue des ouvrages imprimés au XVIe siècle, Bibliothèque Sainte-Geneviève, Paris: Sciences--Techniques--Médecine. Paris, New York, Saur, 1980. xvi, 493 p.

Maria CI: La disputa sulle scienze e la medicina come venne affrontata nel corso del XV secolo da Platonismo e Aristotelismo. **Med Secoli** 1982;19(3):323–8

Nauert CG: The author of a Renaissance commentary on Pliny: Rivius, Trithemius or Aquaeus. **J Warburg Courtauld Inst** 1979;42:282–6

Pagel W: Mother nature and the scientific revolution. **Hist Sci** 1981 Jun:19(44 pt 2):148–53

Roger J: Two scientific discoveries: their genesis and destiny. In M. D. Grmek, R. S. Cohen, G. Cimino, ed: On scientific discovery. The Erice Lectures 1977. Dordrecht, D. Reidel, 1981. p. 229–37. (Boston Studies in the Philosophy of Science, v. 34).

Sjöstrand T: Medicinen i vetenskapshistorien. **Sydsven Medicinhist Sallsk Arsskr** 1980;:149–58

Slaughter MM: Universal languages and scientific taxonomy in the seventeenth century. Cambridge, Cambridge University Press, 1982. x, 277 p.

Snelders HA: Science in the Low Countries during the sixteenth century. A survey. **Janus** 1983;70(3–4):213–27

Vasoli C: The contribution of humanism to the birth of modern science. **Renaiss Reformation** 1979;3(1):1–15

**Americas**

Cardenas J de: Primera parte de los problemas y secretos maravillosos de las Indias. Edicion, estudio preliminar y notas para X. Lozoya. Mexico, Academia Nacional de Medicina, 1980. 320 p.

**Austria**

Burmeister KH: Achilles Gasser als Stadtarzt von Feldkirch. **Montfort** 1968;20(3):326–42

**Belgium**

Bloch H: Jan Baptiste Van Helmont, M.D. (1579–1644); religion, mysticism, and science in a century of change. **NY State J Med** 1980 Sep;80(10):1631–3

Gysel C: Helmontianisme en odontologie (I). **Rev Belge Med Dent** 1979;34(3):295–312

**Czechoslovakia**

Spunarová T: Nejstarší katalogy sbírek ve fondech knihovny Narodního Muzea. **Sb Nar Muzea Praze Rada C Lit Hist** 1980;25(1–2):29–40

**Denmark**

Bierbaum M, Faller A: Niels Stensen. Anatom, Geologe und Bischof, 1638–1686. 2d ed. Münster, Aschendorff, 1979. xi, 203 p. Includes

Thomasen AL, Der Wandel des Stensenbildes.
Greisman HC: Tycho Brahe: astronomer of renaissance Denmark. In Romm S, ed: Symposium on historical perspectives of plastic surgery. Philadelphia, Saunders, 1983. p. 629–33.

**Europe**

Eisenstein EL: The printing press as an agent of change. Communications and cultural transformations in early-modern Europe. 2 vols. Cambridge, Cambridge University Press, 1979. xxi, 794 p.

**France**

Chabbert P: Problèmes scientifiques évoqués à l'Académie de Castres (1648–1670). In: Congrès National des Sociétés Savantes, 100e, Paris, 1975. Actes. Paris, 1976. Histoire Moderne et Contemporaine et Histoire des Sciences. p. 21–9.
Sutton GV: A science for a polite society: Cartesian natural philosophy in Paris during the reigns of Louis XIII and XIV. Ph.D. Diss., Princeton University. Princeton, 1982. xi, 481 leaves.

**Germany**

Gregory RL: Two pins and a length of string: Kepler's vision. **Perception** 1983;12(4):371–4
Kaiser W: Athanasius Kircher (1602–1680) und die medizinisch-naturwissenschaftlichen Konzeptionen seiner Zeit. **Z Gesamte Inn Med** 1981 Jul 15;36(14):494–9

**Great Britain**

Cooke AM: Sir Hans Sloane and the Philosophical Transactions. **J R Coll Physicians Lond** 1984 Jul;18(3):170–1
Force JE: Hume and the relation of science to religion among certain members of the Royal Society. **J Hist Ideas** 1984 Oct–Dec;45(4):517–36
Frank RG: Harvey and the Oxford physiologists: scientific ideas and social interaction. Berkeley, University of California Press, 1980. xviii, 368 p.
Frank RG: The physician as virtuoso in seventeenth-century England. In Shapiro, Barbara and Frank, Robert G., Jr. ed: English scientific virtuosi in the 16th and 17th centuries. Los Angeles, William Andrews Clark Memorial Lib., U. of California, 1980. p. 57–114.
Godwin J: Robert Fludd: hermetic philosopher and surveyor of two worlds. London, Thames and Hudson, 1979. 96 p. An annotated collection of plates from Fludds's works.
Hunter M: Reconstructing restoration science: problems and pitfalls in institutional history. **Soc Stud Sci** 1982 Aug 3;12(3):451–66
Jacob M: Science and social passion: the case of seventeenth-century England. **J Hist Ideas** 1982 Apr–Jun;43(2):331–9
Jobe TH: The devil in Restoration science: the Glanvill-Webster witchcraft debate. **Isis** 1981 Sep;72(263):343–56
Mulligan L: Puritans and English science: a critique of Webster. **Isis** 1980 Sep;71(258):456–69
Neibyl KH: Science, medicine and the Puritan society. **J Eur Econ Hist** 1979;8(1):149–56
Niebyl KH: Science, medicine and the Puritan society. **J Eur Econ Hist** 1979;8(1):
Niebyl PH: Science and metaphor in the medicine of Restoration England. **Bull Hist Med** 1973 Jul–Aug;47(4):356–74
Nutton V: Conrad Gesner and the English naturalists. **Med Hist** 1985 Jan;29(1):93–7
Sasaki C: Scientific studies at Oxford and Cambridge in the seventeenth century - a research review. **Hist Sci** 1981;(20):57–75
Shapiro B, Frank RG: English scientific virtuosi in the 16th and 17th centuries. Los Angeles, Clark Memorial Library, University of California, 1979, vii, 123 p.
Shapiro B: History and natural history in sixteenth- and seventeenth-century England: an essay on the relationship between humanism and science. In Shapiro, Barbara and Frank, Robert G. Jr., ed: English scientific virtuosi in the 16th and 17th centuries: Los Angeles, William Andrews Clark Memorial Lib., U. of California, 1980. p. 1–55.
Simpson AD: Sir Robert Sibbald--the founder of the College. In Passmore R, ed: Proceedings of the Royal College of Physicians of Edinburgh Tercentenary Congress, 1981. Edinburgh, Royal College of Physicians of Edinburgh, 1982. p. 59–91.
Steneck NH: Greatrakes the stroker: the interpretations of historians. **ISIS** 1982 Jun;73(267):161–77
Walker W: Harvey's contemporaries--science and society. **Scott Med J** 1981 Oct;26(4):356–63

**Italy**

Bencivenni M: Il Principe dello Studiolo. **Kos** 1984 Jul–Aug;1(6):52–78
Fierz M: Girolamo Cardano (1501–1576): Arzt, Naturphilosoph, Mathematiker, Astronom, und Traumdeuter. Basel, Birkhäuser, 1977. 138 p.
Ladendorf H: Leonardo da Vinci und die Wissenschaften: eine Literaturübersicht. Köln, 1984. 190 p. (Kölner medizinhistorische Beiträge: Arbeiten der Forschungsstelle des Instituts für Geschichte der Medizin der Universität zu Köln, Band 23/2)
Middleton WE: Some unpublished correspondence of Giovanni Alfonso Borelli. **Ann Ist Mus Stor Sci Fir** 1984;9(2):99–132
Ubrizsy in Savoia A: I rapport fra Carolus Clusius ed i naturalisti italiani del suo tempo. **Physis** 1978;20(1–4):49–68

**Japan**

Yoshida T: [History of Dutch learning in Tokugawa Japan] (Jpn). **Kagakushi Kenkyu** 1984;23(150):73–80

**Netherlands**

Luyendijk-Elshout AM: Christiaan Huygens en de geneeskunde. **Spiegel Hist** 1979;14(4):230–33
Struik DJ: The land of Stevin and Huygens. A sketch of science and technology in the Dutch Republic during the Golden Century. Dordrecht, D. Reidel, 1981. xx, 162 p. (Studies in the History of Modern Science, v. 7).
Visser RP: Theorie en praktijk van Swammerdams wetenschappelijke methode in zijn entomologie. **Tijdschr Geschied Geneeskd** 1981;4(2):63–72

**Spain**

Balaguer i Perigüell E, Ballester i Añón R, Bujosa i Homar F, et al: Els impresos cientifics a Catalunya en els segles XV i XVI. In Congrés International d'Història de la Medicina Catalana, 2nd, Barcelona, 1975. Llibre d'Actes. Barcelona, Socitra, 1977. p. 185–96.
López Piñero JM: Ciencia y técnica en la sociedad española de los siglos XVI y XVII. Barcelona, Labor, 1979. 511 p.
López Piñero JM: La ciencia en la España de los siglos XVI y XVII. In Tuñón de Lara M, ed.: Historia de España. Tomo V. La frustración de un imperio (1476–1714). Barcelona, Labor, 1982. p. 355–423.
Lopez Pinero JM: Los estudios historicos sobre la actividad cientifica en la España de los siglos XVI y XVII. In: Coloquio sobre historia de la ciencia hispano-americana ... 1976. Madrid. 1977. pp. 133–166.

**1700 to Present**

Abir-Am PG: Essay review: how scientists view their heroes: some remarks on the mechanism of myth construction. **J Hist Biol** 1982 Summer;15(2):281–315
Antiseri D: Metaphysical ideas and the development of science. **Riv Biol** 1981 Winter;74(4):529–42
Babini J: Historia de la ciencia versus historia de la medicina. **Medicina (B Aires)** 1980 Jul–Aug;40(4):486–8
Balan B: L'ordre et le temps. L'anatomie comparée et l'histoire des vivants au XIXe siècle. Paris, Vrin, 1979. 610 p.
Bayertz K: Naturwissenschaft und Sozialismus: Tendenzen der Naturwissenschafts-Rezeption in der deutschen Arbeiterbewegung des 19. Jahrhunderts. **Soc Stud Sci** 1983 Aug;13(3):355–94
Cambrosio A, Keating P: The disciplinary stake: the case of chronobiology. **Soc Stud Sci** 1983 Aug;13(3):323–53
Chappert A: L' autobiographical sketch de Thomas Young. **Rev Hist Sci (Paris)** 1981 Apr;34(2):137–8
Cohen LK: Dentistry and the behavioral/social sciences: an historical overview. **J Behav Med** 1981 Sep;4(3):247–56
Cohen RS, Laudan L, ed: Physics, philosophy and psychoanalysis. Essays in honor of Adolf Grünbaum. Dordrecht, D. Reidel, 1983. xviii, 339 p. (Boston Studies in the Philosophy of Science, v. 76).
Collins HM: The place of the 'core-set' in modern science: social contingency with methodological propriety in science. **Hist Sci** 1981;19:6–19
Corsi P, Weindling P, ed: Information sources in the history of science and medicine. London, Boston, Butterworth Scientific, 1983. xvi, 531 p. (Butterworth Guides to Information Sources).
Coulter HL: Homoeopathy and modern medical science. **J Am Inst Homeopath** 1980 Jun;73(2):7–28
Crane D: Invisible colleges: diffusion of knowledge in scientific communities. Chicago, University of Chicago Press, 1972. x, 213 p.
Duerr HP, ed: Der Wissenschaftler und das Irrationale. Band 1. Beiträge aus Ethnologie und Anthropologie. Frankfurt am Main, Syndikat, 1981. 692 p.
Duerr HP, ed: Der Wissenschaftler und das Irrationale. Band 2. Beiträge aus Philosophie und Psychologie. Frankfurt am Main, Syndikat, 1981. 679 p.
Fourastié J: Réflexions sur la science d'aujourd'hui. **Chirurgie** 1981;107(1):23–5
Geison GL: Scientific change, emerging specialties, and research schools. **Hist Sci** 1981;19(1):20–40
George Sarton's correspondence: **Isis** 1984 Mar;75(276):33–62
Gilbert GN, Mulkay M: Warranting scientific belief. **Soc Stud Sci** 1982 Aug 3;12(3):383–408
Giustini PA: Museografia e storia del pensiero scientifico. **Med Secoli** 1982;19(3):265–71
Gould SJ: Ever since Darwin. Reflections in natural history. New York,

W. W. Norton, 1977. 285 p.
Graham LR: Between science and values. New York, Columbia University Press, 1981. x, 449 p.
Greene JC: Science, ideology, and world view: essays in the history of evolutionary ideas. Berkeley/Los Angeles, Univ. of California Press, 1981. x, 202 p.
Gruber HE: The evolving systems approach to creative scientific work: Charles Darwin's early thought. In T. Nickles, ed: Scientific discovery: case studies. Dordrecht, D. Reidel, 1980. (Boston Studies in the Philosophy of Science, v. 60). p. 113–30.
Gunnell JG: The technocratic image and the theory of technocracy. **Technol Cult** 1982 Jul;23(3):392–16
Harrington A: After the impossible happened. **Synthesis** 1982;5(2):2–21
Hassani AM: The appearance of scientific naturalism in Syria and Egypt. **J Hist Arabic Sci** 1977 Nov;1(2):284–98
Hiebsch H: Ein Jahrhundert wissenschaftliche Psychologie. In Eckardt G, ed: Zur Geschichte der Psychologie. Berlin, VEB Deutscher Verlag der Wissenschaften, 1979. p. 21–31.
Holmes FL: The fine structure of scientific creativity. **Hist Sci** 1981;19(1):60–70
Jarrell RA: Colonialism and the truncation of science in Ireland and French Canada during the nineteenth century. **HSTC** 1981 May;18(5 no 2):140–57
Jordanova LJ: Towards the light? Science, politics and the enlightenment. **Eur Stud Rev** 1982;12(4):479–88
Kaiser W: Wissenschaftsgeschichtliche Kooperation am Beispiel der slowakisch–ungarisch–halleschen Gemeinschaftsforschung zu Leben und Werk von Johann Andreas Segner und Johann Adam Reimann. **Wiss Z Martin Luther Univ (Math)** 1975;24(3):89–98
Krause RM: The restless tide. The persistent challenge of the microbial world. Washington, D. C., National Foundation for Infectious Diseases, 1981. 152 p.
Lemay JA, Rousseau GS: The Renaissance man in the eighteenth century. Papers read at a Clark Library seminar, 9 October 1976. Los Angeles, William Andrews Clark Memorial Library, UCLA, 1978. xi, 139 p.
Levere TH: Poetry realized in nature. Samuel Taylor Coleridge and early nineteenth–century science. Cambridge, Cambridge University Press, 1981. xiii, 271 p.
Levere TH, ed: Editing texts in the history of science and medicine. Papers given at the seventeenth annual Conference on Editorial Problems, University of Toronto, 6–7 November 1981. New York, London, Garland, 1982. 190 p. Contributions by S. Drake, L. E. Voigts, B. S. Hall, A. Beaulieu, I. B. Cohen.
Magner LN: Women and the scientific idiom: textual episodes from Wollstonecraft, Fuller, Gilman, and Firestone. **Signs** 1978;4(1):61–80
Miller M: The Max Bergmann papers. **Surv Sources Newsl** 1976Dec;4:7–8
Moravia S: The Enlightenment and the sciences of man. **Hist Sci** 1980 Dec;18(42 pt 4):247–68
Morrison LR: 'Nearer to the brute creation': the scientific defense of American slavery before 1830. **South Stud** 1980;19(3):228–42
Moseley R: From avocation to job: the changing nature of scientific practice. **Soc Stud Sci** 1979;9(4):511–22
Nye MJ: Scientific decline: is quantitative evaluation enough? **ISIS** 1984 Dec;75(279):697–708
Petit A: L'esprit de la science anglaise et les Français au XIXème siècle. **Br J Hist Sci** 1984 Nov;17(57 pt 3):273–93
Recollections & reflections: Lawrence J. Henderson and George Sarton. **Isis** 1984 Mar;75(276):11–32
Roe W: 'Science' in the practice of medicine: its limitations and dangers as exemplified by a study of the natural history of acute bronchial asthma in children. **Perspect Biol Med** 1984 Spring;27(3):386–400
Rousseau GS, Porter R, ed: The ferment of knowledge. Studies in the historiography of eighteenth–century science. Cambridge, Cambridge University Press, 1980. xiii, 500 p. including contributions by R. Harre, S. Schaffer, S. Shapin, H. J. Bos, J. L. Heilbron, E. G. Forbes, D. S. Cardwell.
Róziewicz J: Zwiazki Marii Skłodowskiej-Curie z nauka rosyjska i radziecka. **Kwart Hist Nauki Tech** 1984;29(3–4):535–55
Rupke NA: The study of fossils in the Romantic philosophy of history and nature. **Hist Sci** 1983 Dec;21(54 Pt 4):389–413
Russell CA: Science and social change in Britain and Europe, 1700–1900. New York, St. Martin's Press, 1983. xvii, 307 p.
Schaffer S: Natural philosophy and public spectacle in the eighteenth century. **Hist Sci** 1983 Mar;21(51 Pt 1):1–43
Shortt SE: Physicians, science, and status: issues in the professionalization of Anglo–American medicine in the nineteenth century. **Med Hist** 1983 Jan;27(1):51–68
Stephenson W: Micheal Polanyi, science and belief. **Ethics Sci Med** 1980;7(2):97–110
Stroppina L, Salemme MA: Le nouveau visage de la science et du savant au XXe siècle, après Einstein et Freud. In International Congress of the History of Medicine, 27th, Barcelona, 1980. Actas. Barcelona, Acadèmia de Ciències Mèdiques de Catalunya i Balears, 1981. p. 626–31.
Thiel C: Folgen der Emigration deutscher und österreichischer Wissenschaftstheoretiker und Logiker zwischen 1933 und 1945. **Ber Wissenschaftsgesch** 1984;7(4):227–56
Toellner R: 'Ein Unding vor der Vernunft': Die generatio spontanea im Weltbild der aufgeklärten Naturforschung. In Dilg P, et al., ed: Perspektiven der Pharmaziegeschichte. Graz, Austria, Akademische Druck- u. Verlagsanstalt, 1983. p. 377–88.
Torrance TF: The place of Michael Polanyi in the modern philosophy of science. **Ethics Sci Med** 1980;7(2):57–95
Trompiz G: Dogmas que se derrumban. **Rev Soc Venez Hist Med** 1981;30(45–46):101–3
Wallace ER: Freud and anthropology. A history and reappraisal. New York, International Universities Press, 1983. xi, 306 p. (Psychological Issues, Monograph 55).
Williams LP: Album of science: the nineteenth century. New York, Scribner's, 1978. xiv, 413 p.

**Australia**

Home RW: History of science in Australia. **Isis** 1982 Sep;73(268):337–42

**Austria**

Lesky E, ed: Franz Joseph Gall, 1758–1828, Naturforscher und Anthropologe. Wien, Huber, 1979. (Hubers Klassiker der Medizin und der Naturwissenschaften, Band 15) 217 p.

**Belgium**

Poll M, Herlant-Meewis H: Esquisse de l'histoire de la zoologie et de la biologie animale en Belgique depuis 1920. In Florilège des Sciences en Belgique - II. Bruxelles, Académie Royale de Belgique, 1980. p. 249–69.

**Brazil**

De Moulin D: Medizinische und naturwissenschaftliche Aspekte der Regierungszeit des Grafen Johann Moritz von Nassau als Gouverneur in Brasilien (1637–1644). In: Soweit der Erdkreis reicht. J. M. von Nassau–Siegen 1604–1679. Kleve: Städtisches Museum Haus Koekkoek. 1979. pp. 33–46.

**Canada**

Berger C: Science, God, and nature in Victorian Canada. Toronto; Buffalo, University of Toronto Press, 1983. xiv, 92 p.
Chapman ID, Farina C: Accountability and the science research board. **J Can Stud** 1982–83;17(4):3–9
Duchesne R: Science et société coloniale: les naturalistes du Canada français et leurs correspondants scientifiques (1860–1900). **HSTC Bull** 1981;5:99–139
Frost SB: Science education in the 19th century: The Natural History Society of Montreal, 1827–1925. **McGill J Educ** 1982;17(1):31–48
Gridgeman NT: A semicentennial. The NRCC research journals 1929–1979. **Can J Physiol Pharmacol** 1979 Jul;57(7):i–xiv; Also in Can J Biochem 1979 Jul;57(7):iv–xvi; Also in Can J Zool 1979 Jul; 57(7):i–xiv
Howell CD: Elite doctors and the development of scientific medicine: the Halifax medical establishment and 19th century medical professionalism. In Roland CG, ed: Health, disease and medicine. Toronto, Hannah Institute for the History of Medicine, 1984. p. 105–22.
Labreche J: NRC: where science fiction often comes true. **Can Geogr** 1980;100(4):24–33
Lithwick NH: Science policy in Canada. **J Can Stud** 1968;3(3):29–38
Lortie L: Joseph–Alexandre Crevier. In Dictionary of Canadian biography, 1881–1890. 1982;11:217–8.
Rasporich AW: John Jeremiah Bigsby. In Dictionary of Canadian biography, 1881–1890. 1982;11:72–3.

**China**

Ho PY: Chinese scientific terminology. **Pap Far East Hist** 1974;(9):1–14
Kühner H: Between autonomy and planning: the Chinese Academy of Sciences in transition. **Minerva** 1984 Spring;22(1):13–44
Schneider LA: The Rockefeller Foundation, the China Foundation, and the development of modern science in China. **Soc Sci Med** 1982;16(12):1217–21

**Czechoslovakia**

Petrášek J: Třicet let Slovenské akademie věd. **Cas Lek Cesk** 1983 Dec 16;122(50):1568
Slavětínský M: Naši lékaři–archeologové. **Vnitr Lek** 1980 Mar;26(3):415–6

**France**

Arquiola E: Topinard: medico y antropologo fisico. **Asclepio** 1978–79;30–31:41–61
Blanckaert C: Médecine et histoire naturelle de l'homme: l'anthropologie française dans la seconde moitié du XIXe siècle. In Poirier J, Poirier JL, ed: Médecine et philosophie à la fin du XIXe siècle. Paris, Université de Paris XII - Val de Marne, [1980?]. p. 101–16
Borie J: Les dents de la mer: Notes sur le rôle du médecin dans l'idéologie

scientifique au 19e siècle. **Stanford Fr Rev** 1978 Fall;2:159–92

Chaïa J: Sur une correspondance, entre 1739 et 1749, de Duhamel du Monceau avec J.-F. Artur, médecin du roy a Cayenne. In: Congrès National des Sociétés Savantes, 102e, Limoges, 1977. Comptes Rendus. Paris, 1977. Section des Sciences, Fasc. III. p. 21–6.

Crosland M: From prizes to grants in the support of scientific research in France in the nineteenth century: the Montyon legacy. **Minerva** 1979 Autumn;17(3):355–80

Dillemann G: Les cumuls d'emplois en 1821. **Rev Hist Pharm (Paris)** 1981 Jun;28(249):109–11

Di Trocchio F: Paul-Joseph Barthez e l' 'Encyclopédie'. **Physis** 1980;22(3–4):379–92

Dulieu L: La Société Royale des Sciences de Montpellier (1706–1792). In: Congrès National des Sociétés Savantes, 100e, Paris, 1975. Actes. Paris, 1976. Histoire Moderne et Contemporaine et Histoire des Sciences. p. 43–8.

Ehrhardt JP: Les médecins naturalistes de 'La Coquille' et de 'L'Astrolabe', ex-gabare 'La Coquille'. In: Congrès National des Sociétés Savantes, 104e, Bordeaux, 1979. Comptes Rendus. Paris, 1979. Section des Sciences, Fasc. IV. p. 205–17.

Fox R, Weisz G: The institutional basis of French science in the nineteenth century. In R. Fox, G. Weisz, ed: The organization of science and technology in France 1808–1914. Cambridge, Cambridge University Press, 1980. p. 1–28.

Fox R: The organization of science and technology in France, 1808–1914. Cambridge, New York, Cambridge University Press, 1980. x, 355 p.

Greenbaum LS: Science, medicine, religion: three views of health care in France on the eve of the French Revolution. **Stud Eighteenth Cent Cult** 1981;10:373–91

Gutina VN: Pasteur's views on the science. **Istor Biol Issled** 1983;9:134–44

Jordanova LJ: Romantic science? Michelet, morals, and nature. **Br J Hist Sci** 1980 Mar;13(43 pt 1):44–50

Laissus Y: Les papiers du docteur J.-B. Mougeot (1776–1858): un fonds important pour l'histoire des sciences naturelles en Lorraine. In: Congrés National des Sociétés Savantes, 103e, Nancy, 1978. Comptes Rendus. Paris, 1978. Section des Sciences, Fasc. V. p. 233–40.

Lanchou G, Veron C: Un évadé de la médecine: Jean-Baptiste Charcot (1867–1936). **Hist Sci Med** 1980;14(1):43–50

Le Grand HE: Chemistry in a provincial context: the Montpellier Société Royale des Sciences in the eighteenth century. **Ambix** 1982 Jul;29(2):88–105

Levin A: Venel, Lavoisier, Fourcroy, Cabanis and the idea of scientific revolution: the French political context and the general patterns of conceptualization of scientific change. **Hist Sci** 1984 Sep;22(57 pt 3):303–20

McClellan JE: The Académie Royale des Sciences, 1699–1793: a statistical portrait. **Isis** 1981 Dec;72(264):541–67

Martínez Báez M: Pasteur, maestro. **Mem Col Nac (Mex)** 1967–68;6(2–3):115–31

Nonclercq M: Un chapitre ignoré de l'histoire des sciences: l'oeuvre de Béchamp. In: Congrés National des Sociétés Savantes, 103e, Nancy, 1978. Comptes Rendus. Paris, 1978. Section des Sciences, Fasc. V. p. 157–69.

Outram D: Politics and vocation: French science, 1793–1830. **Br J Hist Sci** 1980 Mar;13(43 pt 1):27–43

Outram D: The ordeal of vocation: the Paris Academy of Sciences and the Terror, 1793–95. **Hist Sci** 1983 Sep;21(53 pt 3):251–73

Pace D: Claude Lévi-Strauss, the bearer of ashes. Boston, Routledge & Kegan Paul, 1983. x, 263 p.

Paul CB: Science and immortality. The eloges of the Paris Academy of Sciences (1699–1791). Berkeley, University of California Press, 1980. x, 202 p.

Pigeaud J: Cabanis et les rapports du physique et du moral. **Sci Tech Persp** 1981–82;1:8.1–.13

Pineau H: Paul Broca et l'anthropologie. **Bull Acad Natl Med (Paris)** 1980;164(6):557–62

Portal C, Rideau M, Viel C: Quelques aspects de l'oeuvre de Duhamel de Monceau dans le domaine des sciences naturelles et des sciences physiques. In: Congrès National des Sociétés Savantes, 107e. Brest, 1982. Comptes Rendus, Paris, 1982. Section des Sciences, Fasc. IV. p. 341–50.

Pozo EC del. La medicina como ciencia en Claudio Bernard. Homenaje en el primer centenario de su muerte. **Gac Med Mex** 1979 Jun;115(6):245–56

Sebastiani F: Jean-Paul Marat, l'ami de la nature. **Physis** 1984;26(3):325–59

Todericiu D: Balthasar-Georges Sage (1740–1824) chimiste et minéralogiste français, fondateur de la première Ecole des Mines (1783). **Rev Hist Sci (Paris)** 1984 Jan;37(1):29–46

Wrotnowska D: Pasteur, membre du Comice agricole de l'arrondissement de Lille. In: Congrès National des Sociétés Savantes, 101e, Lille, 1976. Comptes Rendus. Paris, 1976. Section des Sciences, Fasc. III. p. 133–44.

Zelbstein MU: Mauduyt de La Varenne (1733–1792) un médecin au siècle des 'Lumières'. **Hist Sci Med** 1984;18(3):295–306

**Germany**

Bleker J: Die Naturhistorische Schule 1825–1845. Ein Beitrag zur Geschichte der klinischen Medizin in Deutschland. Stuttgart, New York, Fischer, 1981. ix, 174 p.

Brücke EW von: Briefe an Emil Du Bois-Reymond. Ed. H. Brücke, W. Hilger, W. Höflechner, W. W. Swoboda. Erster Teil. Graz, Akademische Druck- und Verlagsanstalt, 1978. 308 p. (Publikationen aus dem Archiv der Universität Graz, Band 8/1).

Cranefield PF, ed: Two great scientists of the nineteenth century. Correspondence of Emil Du Bois-Reymond and Carl Ludwig. Collected by Estelle Du Bois-Reymond. Foreword, notes, and indexes by Paul Diepgen. Translation of 1927 German ed. Baltimore, London, Johns Hopkins Univ. Press, 1982. xix, 183 p.

Deich I. The redistribution of authority in national laboratories in Western Germany. **Minerva** 1979 Autumn;17(3):413–44

Engelhardt DV: Virchow et Haeckel et la liberté de la science. In Poirier J, Poirier JL, ed: Médecine et philosophie à la fin du XIXe siècle. Paris, Université de Paris XII - Val de Marne, [1980?]. p. 117–25.

Forbes EG: Scientific archives in the Federal Republic of Germany. **Ber Wissenschaftsgesch** 1979;2(3–4):197–201

Jungnickel C: The Royal Saxon Society of Sciences: a study of nineteenth century German science. Ph.D. Diss., Johns Hopkins University. Baltimore, 1978. v, 222 leaves.

Kahle E, Stupp JA: Hochschulschriften zur Geschichte der Medizin, Pharmazie, und Naturwissenschaften der Friedrich-Alexander-Universität Erlangen-Nürnberg 1885–1975. Erlangen, Verlagsbuchhandlung Hannelore Lüling, 1980. 94 p. (Medizinhistorische Materialien, 2).

Kelley DR: The science of anthropology: an essay on the very old Marx. **J Hist Ideas** 1984 Apr–Jun;45(2):245–62

Krafft F: Der 'Historische Erfahrungsraum' der Entdeckung der Kernspaltung. In Dilg P, et al., ed: Perspektiven der Pharmaziegeschichte. Graz, Austria, Akademische Druck- u. Verlagsanstalt, 1983. p. 209–24.

Krafft F: Forschungsberichte und Spezial-Bibliographien. **Ber Wissenschaftsgesch** 1980;3(3–4):127–88

Larson JL: An alternative science, Linnaean natural history in Germany, 1770–1790. **Janus** 1979;66(4):267–83

Löther I: Probleme der Wissenschaftlich-technischen Revolution und einige Aufgaben des sozialistischen Gesundheitsschutzes. **Med Ges** 1978;(3):69–78

Mann G: Geschichte als Wissenschaft und Wissenschaftsgeschichte bei Du Bois-Reymond. **Hist Z** 1980;231:75–100

Mann G, ed: Naturwissen und Erkenntnis im 19. Jahrhundert: Emil Du Bois-Reymond. Hildesheim, Gerstenberg, 1981. 243 p. Contributions by K. E. Rothschuh, H. Hensel, R. Malter, C. von Campenhausen, B. Lohff, H. Lübbe, D. von Engelhardt, W. F. Gutmann, K. Bonink, C. Andree

Matthes T: Die medizinisch-wissenschaftlichen Gesellschaften der DDR: Geschichte, Funktion, Aufgaben. Berlin, Volk und Gesundheit, 1981. 239 p., 371 p.

Querner H: 'Ein Wort über den Einfluss naturwissenschaftlicher Institute auf humane Bildung' (G. A. Goldfuss 1821). In Seidler E, Schott H, ed: Bausteine zur Medizingeschichte. Stuttgart, Steiner, 1984. p. 86–93.

Rothschuh KE: Ernst Schweninger (1850–1924). Zu seinem Leben und Wirken. Ergänzungen, Korrekturen. **Medizinhist J** 1984;19(3):250–8

Schipperges H: Einheitsbestrebungen und Normbegriff auf der Naturforscherversammlung im 19. Jahrhundert. **Sudhoffs Arch** 1977;61(4):313–30

Schütt HW: History of science in the Federal Republic of Germany. **Isis** 1980 Sep;71(258):375–80

Sucker U: On the history of problems of scientific studies in the beginning of the XXth century in Germany. **Istor Biol Issled** 1983;9:191–200

Winau R: Deutsche Gesellschaft für Geschichte der Medizin, Naturwissenschaft und Tecknik 1901–1976. Wiesbaden, Steiner, 1978. 164 p. (Beiträge zur Geschichte der Wissenschaft und der Technik, 15).

**Great Britain**

Altholz JL: The Huxley-Wilberforce debate revisited. **J Hist Med Allied Sci** 1980 Jul;35(3):313–16

Bayliss RA, Ellis CW: Neil Arnott, F.R.S., reformer, innovator and popularizer of science, 1788–1874. **Notes Rec R Soc Lond** 1981;36(1):103–24

Bernstein RE: Dr Harvey Pirie and the Scottish National Antartic Expedition (1902–4). Scottish science and medicine in the Falklands and Antarctica. **Scott Med J** 1983 Jan;28(1):75–9

Born GV: The effect of the scientific environment in Britain on refugee scientists from Germany and their effects on science in Britain. **Ber Wissenschaftsgesch** 1984;7(3):129–43

Brockway LH: Science and colonial expansion. The role of the British Royal Botanic Gardens. New York, Academic Press, 1979. 215 p. (Studies in Social Discontinuity).

Cannon SF: Science in culture: the early Victorian period. Kent, Eng., Dawson; New York, Science History Publications, 1978. xii, 296 p.

Cardwell D, Mottram J: Fresh light on John Dalton. **Notes Rec R Soc Lond** 1984 Sep;39(1):29–40

Chitnis AC: Universities, medicine and science. In his: The Scottish Enlightenment: a social history. 279 pp. London: Croom Helm; Totawa, N.J.: Rowman & Littlefield, 1976. p. 124–94.

Corrigan TJ: Biographia Literaria and the language of science.

# SCIENCE

J Hist Ideas 1980 Jul-Sep;41(3):399-419
Crosland M: Explicit qualifications as a criterion for membership of the Royal Society: a historical review. **Notes Rec R Soc Lond** 1983 Mar;37(2):167-87
Dean DR: The Gideon Mantell collection, New Zealand. **J Soc Bibliogr Nat Hist** 1979 Apr;9(2):121-4
Edwards PI: Robert Brown (1773-1858) and the natural history of Matthew Flinders' voyage in H.M.S. Investigator, 1801-1805. **J Soc Bibliogr Nat Hist** 1976;7(4):385-407
Fee E: Science and the 'woman question', 1860-1920: a study of English scientific periodicals. Ph. D. Diss., Princeton University. Princeton, 1978. v, 351 leaves.
Flinn D: John Macculloch, M.D., F.R.S., and his geological map of Scotland: his years in the Ordnance. 1795-1826. **Notes Rec R Soc Lond** 1981;36(1):83-101
Gregory RL: Bacon's last egg?--the Exploratory. **Perception** 1982;11(4):371-5
Gruber HE: Darwin on man: a psychological study of scientific creativity. 2d. ed. Chicago, University of Chicago Press, 1981. xxvii, 310 p.
Hartley H: Douglas McKie. In Dictionary of national biography, 1961-1970. Suppl. 8, 1981. p. 695-7.
Inkster I, Morrell J: Metropolis and province; science in British culture, 1780-1850. Philadelphia, University of Pennsylvania Press, 1983. 288 p.
Inkster I: Scientific culture and education in Nottingham, 1800-1843. **Trans Thoroton Soc** 1979;82
Kark RM, Moore DT: The life, work, and geological collections of Richard Bright, M.D. (1789-1858); with a note on the collections of other members of the family. **Arch Nat Hist** 1981 Apr;10(1):119-51
Kitteringham G: Science in provincial society: the case of Liverpool in the early nineteenth century. **Ann Sci** 1982;39:329-48
Lenoir T: The Göttingen School and the development of transcendental Naturphilosophie in the Romantic Era. **Stud Hist Biol** 1981;5:111-205
Levere TH: Dr. Thomas Beddoes (1750-1808): science and medicine in politics and society. **Br J Hist Sci** 1984 Jul;17(56 pt 2):187-204
McEvoy JG: Joseph Priestley, scientist, philosopher and divine. **Proc Am Philos Soc** 1984 Sep;128(3):193-9
MacLeod R, Moseley R: Fathers and daughters: reflections on women, science, and Victorian Cambridge. **Hist Educ** 1979;8:321-33
MacLeod RM, Collins P: The parliament of science: the British Association for the Advancement of Science 1831-1981. London, Science Reviews, 1981. vi, 308 p.
Miller DP: The Royal Society of London 1800-1835: a study in the cultural politics of scientific organization. Ph. D. Diss., University of Pennsylvania, Philadelphia, 1981. vii, 422 leaves.
Paradis J, Postlewait T, ed: Victorian science and Victorian values: literary perspectives. New York, New York Academy of Sciences, 1981. xiii, 362 p. (Annals of the New York Academy of Sciences, 360).
Paradis JG: T. H. Huxley, Man's place in nature. Lincoln, University of Nebraska Press, 1978. xi, 226 p.
Paul DB: A war on two fronts: J. B. S. Haldane and the response to lysenkoism in Britain. **J Hist Biol** 1983 Spring;16(1):1-37
Porter R: Le prospettive della 'follia': scienza, medicina, e letteratura nell'Inghilterra dell '700. **Intersezioni** 1982;2:55-76
Rice AL, Burstyn HL, Jones AG: G. C. Wallich M.D.---megalomaniac or mis-used oceanographic genius? **J Soc Bibliogr Nat Hist** 1976;7(4):423-50
Ross DA: Neglected bibliographical aspects of the works of Thomas Henry Huxley. **J Soc Bibliogr Nat Hist** 1978;8(4):401-20
Ruse M: Darwin's theory: an exercise in science. **New Sci** 1981;90:828-30
Schweber SS: Essay review; early Victorian science: science in culture. **J Hist Biol** 1980 Spring;13(1):121-40
Sheets-Pyenson S: From the north to Red Lion Court: the creation and early years of the Annals of Natural History. **Arch Nat Hist** 1981 Oct;10(2):221-49
Thackray JC: James Parkinson's Organic remains of a former world (1804-1811). **J Soc Bibliogr Nat Hist** 1976;7(4):45-66
Van Keuren DK: Human science in Victorian Britain: anthropology in institutional and disciplinary formation, 1863-1908. Ph.D. Diss., University of Pennsylvania. Philadelphia, 1982. vi, 329 p.
Weindling P: Science and sedition: how effective were the acts licensing lectures and meetings, 1795-1819? **Br J Hist Sci** 1980 Jul;13(44 no 2):139-53
Werskey G: The visible college. London, Allen Lane, 1978. 376 p.
Wright D: Moving the Wellcome Collection to the Science Museum. **Vet Hist** 1982 Summer;2(3):100-11

### Hungary

Páal A: Orvostörténeti adatok a 'Magyar Faust', Hatvani istván professzor (1718-1786 ig) tanulmányairól és munkásságáról. **Orv Hetil** 1984 Aug 5;125(32):1957-8, 1961-2

### India

Gorman M: Sir William Brooke O'Shaughnessy, F.R.S. (1809-1889), Anglo-Indian forensic chemist. **Notes Rec R Soc Lond** 1984 Sep;39(1):51-64
Kumar D: Patterns of colonial science in India. **Indian J Hist Sci** 1980 May;15(1):105-13
Shiva V, Bandyopadhyay J: The large and fragile community of scientists in India. **Minerva** 1980 Winter;18(4):575-94

### Italy

Arrigoni T: Fra la curiosità e la scienza. **Kos** 1984 May;1(4):47-64
Bonilauri F: Museo e città. Le collezioni Spallanzani e chierici a Reggio Emilia. Firenze, Olschki, 1978. 199 p. (Biblioteca della 'Rivista di Storia delle Scienze Mediche e Naturali').
Castellani C: Ricognizione di alcuni inediti spallanzaniani, con particolare riguardo agli studi sui pipistrelli (1793-1794). La Memoria sul volo cieco dei pipistrelli dedicata al Senebier nelle due versioni: testo e considerazioni. **Physis** 1984;26(3):433-83
Cavazza M: Bologna and the Royal Society in the seventeenth century. **Notes Rec R Soc Lond** 1980 Dec;35(2):105-23

### Netherlands

Smit P: Jan Ingen-Housz (1730-1799): some new evidence about his life and work. **Janus** 1980;67(1-2-3):125-39
Snelders HA: De natuur- en scheikundige wetenschappen in de medische tijdschriften. **Ned Tijdschr Geneeskd** 1981 Apr 25;125(17):668-73
Snelders HA: Het fysisch-chemisch werk van de Rotterdamse arts Hendrik Willem Rouppe (1765-1816). **Tijdschr Geschied Geneeskd** 1981;4(1):25-44
Van der Korst JK: Geneeskunde in de eerste internationale geleerdentijdschriften van Nederlandse origine (1680-1709). **Ned Tijdschr Geneeskd** 1981 Feb 28;125(9):355-60
Van der Leun C, ed:: NG 200 - Natuurkundig Gezelschap te Utrecht 1777-1977. Utrecht, Natuurkundig Gezelschap te Utrecht, 1977. 143 p. With contributions by R. Hooykaas, J.G. van Cittert-Eymers, H.A.M. Snelders, N.G. van Kampen, P.H. Kylstra.

### Poland

Labuda G, Rodzik I: Scientists and scholars of Polish origin and Polish men of learning active abroad: their share in the development of science. **Rev Pol Acad Sci (Warsz)** 1980;25(1-2):105-23
Ostrowska T: Rozprawy składane Towarzystwu Warszawskiemu Przyjaciół Nauk (1800--1832) przez jego członków -- lekarzy i farmaceutów. **Arch Hist Med (Warsz)** 1979;42(1):61-81
Ostrowski W: The work of the Committee on Biochemistry and Biophysics during twenty five years of the Polish Academy of Sciences. **Rev Pol Acad Sci (Warsz)** 1978;23(2):101-12
Schnelle T: Ludwik Fleck - a classical scholar of the sociology of science and of epistemology. **Kwart Hist Nauki Tech** 1983;28(3-4):525-43
Sródka A, Sosińska-Trawińska M: O utworzeniu Wydziałow Lekarskich w polskich instytucjach naukowych. II. Towarzystwo Naukowe Warszawskie (TNW). **Arch Hist Med (Warsz)** 1982;45(1-4):81-4
Suchodolski B, Chmielewska-Szlajfer M: Developmental tendencies of Polish 19th- and 20th century science against the background of world science. **Rev Pol Acad Sci (Warsz)** 1980;25(1-2):81-90

### Spain

Albarracín Teulón A: Cajal y el problema del conocimiento cientifico. **Asclepio** 1980;32:7-17
Aragon F: La politica cientifica en la España del s. XVIII a traves de la revista 'Anales de Ciencias Naturales', Madrid, 1799-1804. **Llull (Spain)** 1978;2:19-25
d'Ors A: Cuatro precursores de la ciencia española de nuestro tiempo. **Rev Med Univ Navarra** 1980 Dec;24(4):55-60
Fernández González M, Gago Bohórquez R: La medicina en la obra cientifica de Francisco de Paula Montells y Nadal (1813-1893). **Asclepio** 1980;32:151-9
Puig-Samper Mulero MA: El Doctor Pedro Gonzalez de Velasco y la antropologia española en el siglo XIX. **Asclepio** 1982;34:327-37
Riera J: Medicinas y ciencia en la España ilustrada, epistolario y documentos, I. Valladolid, Universidad de Valladolid, 1981. 159 p. (Acta Historico-Medica Vallisoletana, Monografias, XII)
Riera J: Medicinas y ciencia en la España ilustrada, epistolario y documentos, I. Valladolid, Universidad de Valladolid, 1981. 159 p. (Acta Historico-Medica Vallisoletana, Monografias, XII)
Sala Catalá J: Cambio de paradigma y polemica cientifica entre los biologos españoles (1860-1922). **Asclepio** 1982;34:239-63
Sánchez-Moscoso Hermida A, Alfonso Galán MT: Estudio histórico de una tesis de farmacia juzgada hace 100 años: 'Las divisiones de la naturaleza y de la ciencia', de Francisco Fernández Iparraguirre. **Bol Soc Esp Hist Farm** 1983;34(136):167-84
Simmer HH: Santiago Ramón y Cajal und die Typologie des Wissenschaftlers. **Medizinhist J** 1981;16(4):414-23

### Sweden

Frängsmyr T, ed: Linnaeus. The man and his work. Berkeley, University of California Press, 1983. xii, 203 p. With contributions by S. Lindroth,

G. Eriksson, G. Broberg.

Johannisson K: Naturvetenskap på reträtt. En diskussion om naturvetenskapens status under svenskt 1700-tal. **Lychnos** 1979–80;:109–54

Lindroth S: The two faces of Linnaeus. In Frängsmyr T, ed: Linnaeus, the man and his work. Berkeley, University of California Press, 1983. p. 1–62.

**Switzerland**

Boschung U: Johannes von Muralt, 1645–1733: Arzt, Chirurg, Anatom, Naturforscher, Philosoph. Zürich, Rohr, 1983. 105 p.

Hansen JR: Scientific fellowship in a Swiss community enlightenment: a history of Zurich's Physical Society, 1746–1798. Ph.D. Diss., Ohio State University. Columbus, 1981. viii, 264 leaves.

Schmutz HK: Die Gründung des Zürcher Lehrstuhles für Anthropologie. **Gesnerus** 1983;40(1–2):167–73

Sieber CF: Johann Georg Amstein 'der Jüngere' (1819–1892): ein gelehrter Bündner Arzt und Naturforscher des 19. Jahrhunderts. Zürich, Juris Druck, 1984. 72 p. (Zürcher Medizingeschichtliche Abhandlungen, Neue Rheihe, Nr. 168).

Toellner R: Decora Merenti. Glory, merit and science. Haller spellbound by the Newtonian star. **Janus** 1980;67(1-2-3):171–85

**United States**

Abelson PH, Kulstad R, et al: Science centennial--3 July 1880 to 4 July 1980. **Science** 1980 Jul 4;209(4452):19–198

Baker TS, Eveleth PB: The effects of funding patterns on the development of physical anthropology. In F. Spencer, ed: A history of American physical anthropology, 1930–1980. New York, Academic Press, 1982. p. 31–48.

Bearman D: The Alfred Newton Richards papers. **Surv Sources Newsl** 1975 Nov;1(1):9–10

Beawer D de B: The American scientific community, 1800–1860; a statistical-historical study (Doctoral Dissertation, Yale University, 1966). New York, Arno Press, 1980. 379 p.

Boaz NT: American research on Australopithecines and early Homo, 1925-1980. In F. Spencer, ed: A history of American physical anthropology, 1930-1980. New York, Academic Press, 1982. p. 239–60.

Brieger GH: The history of medicine and the history of science. **Isis** 1981 Dec;72(264):537–40

Buck P: American science and modern China, 1876–1936. Cambridge, Cambridge University Press, 1980. viii, 283 p.

Cavanaugh G: The corruptions of science. **Dissent** 1981;28(2):195–202

Christianson EH: The conditions for science in the academic department of Transylvania University, 1799–1857. **Regist Ky Hist Soc** 1981;79(4):305–25

Clagett M: Lynn Thorndike. In Dictionary of American biography, 1961–1965. Suppl. 7, 1981. p. 741–2.

Cochrane RC: The National Academy of Sciences: the first hundred years, 1863-1963. Washington, D.C., National Academy of Sciences, 1978. xv, 694 p.

Cohen EP, ed: Medicine in transition: the centennial of the University of Illinois College of Medicine: a symposium in Chicago, October 1–2, 1981. [Chicago], University of Illinois College of Medicine, and University of Illinois Press, 1981. 340 p.

Cohen IB, ed: Thomas Jefferson and the sciences. New York, Arno Press, 1980. Reprints of various works. Various paginations. (Three Centuries of Science in America).

Collins R, Restivo S: Development, diversity, and conflict in the sociology of science. **Sociol Q** 1983;24(2):185–200

Cutright PR, Brodhead MJ: Elliott Coues: naturalist and frontier historian. Urbana, University of Illinois Press, 1981. xv, 509 p.

Dekosky RK: The history of science in a history department. **Hist Teacher** 1980;13(3):371–8

Dupree AH: The rise and fall of the American establishment. **Minerva** 1984 Spring;22(1):116–24

Edwards S: Science and secular idealism. **Midwest Q** 1980;22(1):21–31

Elliott CA: Models of the American scientist: a look at collective biography. **Isis** 1982 Mar;73(266):77–93

Erickson P: The anthropology of Charles Caldwell, M.D. **ISIS** 1981 Jun;72(262):252–6

Etzkowitz H: Entrepreneurial scientists and entrepreneurial universities in American academic science. **Minerva** 1983 Summer–Autumn;21(2–3):198–233

Fisher D: The role of philanthropic foundations in the reproduction and production of hegemony: Rockefeller foundations and the social sciences. **Sociology** 1983;17(2):206–33

Fortuine R: Ships' surgeons and naturalists in the early history of Alaska. **Alaska Med** 1984 Apr–Jun;26(2):57–61

Fortuine R: Ships' surgeons and naturalists in the early history of Alaska. Parts 2 and 3. **Alaska Med** 1984 Jul–Sep;26(3):82–6; Oct–Dec;26(4):117–21

Freymann JG: The origins of disease orientation in American medical education. **Prev Med** 1981 Nov;10(6):663–73

Fries SD: The ideology of science during the Nixon years: 1970–76. **Soc Stud Sci** 1984 Aug;14(3):323–41

Gifford GE: James de Berty Trudeau: physician-naturalist. **Bull Hist Med** 1980 Spring;54(1):78–94

Greene JC: American science in the age of Jefferson. Ames, Iowa State University Press, 1984. xiv, 484 p.

Hale DK: Cyrus N. Ray: the Abilene man. **West Tex Hist Assoc Yearb** 1979;55:17-36

Haskins CP: The changing environments of science. **Daedalus** 1965;94(3):682–712

Hayes AH: Science and public policy. **J Assoc Off Anal Chem** 1982 Mar;65(2):202–5

Hiebert EN: Report on current activities in the history of science in the United States. **NTM** 1982;19(1):12–5

Hilts VL: History of science at the University of Wisconsin. **Isis** 1984 Mar;75(276):63–94

Holden C: Bern Dibner: science bibliophile. **Science** 1980 May 30;208(4447):1012–4

Holland J: A glorious anachronism: the American Philosophical Society. **Wilson Libr Bull** 1982;56(10):740–4

Hoobler IG: Boundless horizons. Portrait of a pioneer woman scientist. Smithtown, N. Y., Exposition Press, 1982. 197 p.

Jackman SW: The tribulations of an editor: Benjamin Silliman and the early days of the American Journal of Science and the Arts. **N Engl Q** 1979;52(1):99–106

Kevles DJ, Sturchio JL, Carroll PT: The sciences in America, circa 1880. **Science** 1980 Jul 4;209(4452):26–32

Kidd CV: The movement of younger scientists into and out of the United States from 1967 to 1980: some aspects of the international movement of scientific knowledge. **Minerva** 1983 Winter;21(4):387–409

King LS: XI. Medicine seeks to be 'scientific'. **JAMA** 1983 May 13;249(18):2475–9

Kohlstedt SG: In from the periphery: American women in science, 1830–1880. **Signs** 1978;4(1):81–96

Kohlstedt SG: Science: the struggle for survival, 1880 to 1894. **Science** 1980 Jul 4;209(4452):33–42

Kuritz H: The popularization of science in nineteenth-century America. **Hist Educ Q** 1981;21(3):259–74

Leonard DC: Harvard's first science professor: a sketch of Isaac Greenwood's life and work. **Harv Libr Bull** 1981 Apr;29(2):135–68

Lester JF: John Fiske's philosophy of science: the union of science and religion through the principle of evolution. Ph.D. Diss., Oregon State University, Corvallis, 1979. 275 leaves.

Liebenau J: Charles Albert Browne (1870–1947). **Surv Sources Newsl** 1977 May;5:10–1

Maddox RF: The politics of World War II science: Senator Harley M. Kilgore and the legislative origins of the National Science Foundation. **W Va Hist** 1979;41(1):20–39

Miller M: Hans Thacher Clarke Papers. **Surv Sources Newsl** 1977 May;5:12–3

Milner A: The Franklin Institute: as diverse as its namesake. **Wilson Libr Bull** 1982;56(10):735–9

Morowitz HJ: Thoreau as a scientist. **Hosp Pract [Off]** 1984 Nov;19(11):143–6, 151

Noble I: Contemporary women scientists in America. New York, Messner, 1979. 158 p.

O'Donnell S: Irish-American scientists. **Eire Irel** 1979;14(2):106–9

The official publication of the American Association of Physical Anthropologists 1930-1980: Jubilee Issue: **Am J Phys Anthropol** 1981 Dec;56(4):327–557

Oleson A, Voss J, ed: The organization of knowledge in modern America, 1860–1920. Baltimore and London, Johns Hopkins University Press, 1979. xxi, 478 p.

Reingold N, Reingold IH, ed: Science in America. A documentary history, 1900–1939. Chicago, London, Univ. of Chicago Press, 1981. xii, 490 p. (The Chicago history of science and medicine).

Reingold N, ed: The papers of Joseph Henry. Volume 1. December 1797–October 1832. The Albany years. Washington, Smithsonian Institution Press, 1972. xxxix, 496 p.

Reingold N, ed: The papers of Joseph Henry. Volume 2. November 1832 December 1835. The Princeton Years. Washington, Smithsonian Institution Press, 1975. 524 p.

Reverby S: Stealing the golden eggs: Ernest Amory Codman and the science and management of medicine. **Bull Hist Med** 1981 Summer;55(2):156–71

Rosenberg C: Science in American society; a generation of historical debate. **Isis** 1983 Sep;74(273):356–67

Rossiter MW: The history and philosophy of science program at the National Science Foundation. **Isis** 1984 Mar;75(276):95–104

Rossiter MW: Women scientists in America. Struggles and strategies to 1940. Baltimore, London, Johns Hopkins University Press, 1982. xviii, 439 p.

Rossiter MW: 'Women's work' in science, 1880-1910. **Isis** 1980 Sep;71(258):381–98

Ruscio KP: A new regime in the republic of science. **Policy Stud Rev** 1983;2(4):790–4

Russett CE: Declaring the glory of God. **Hist Educ Q** 1980;20(2):217–21

Schütt HW: Wissenschaftsgeschichte in Amerika.

## SCIENCE

**Ber Wissenschaftsgesch** 1979;2(3-4):219-23
Sloan D: Science in New York City, 1867 - 1907. **Isis** 1980 Mar;71(256):35-76
Sokal MM: Science and James McKeen Cattell, 1894 to 1945. **Science** 1980 Jul 4;209(4452):43-52
Spencer F, Erickson GE: Charter members of the American Association of Physical Anthropologists. **Am J Phys Antropol** 1981 Dec;56(4):531-5
Spencer F, ed: A history of American physical anthropology, 1930-1980. New York, Academic Press, 1982. xvi, 495 p.
Stapleton DH, Carter EC: 'I have the itch of botany, of chemistry, of mathematics ... strong upon me': the science of Benjamin Henry Latrobe. **Proc Am Philos Soc** 1984 Sep;128(3):173-92
Stoehr T: Hawthorne's mad scientists: Pseudoscience and social science in nineteenth-century life and letters. Hamden, Conn., Shoestring Press, 1978. 313 p.
Thackray A: The pre-history of an academic discipline: the study of the history of science in the United States, 1891-1941. **Minerva** 1980 Autumn;18(3):448-73
Trinkaus E: A history of Homo erectus and Homo sapiens paleontology in America. In F. Spencer, ed: A history of American physical anthropology, 1930-1980. New York, Academic Press, 1982. p. 261-80.
Walsh J: Science in transition, 1946 to 1962. **Science** 1980 Jul 4;209(4452):52-7
Williams LP: The history of science at Cornell University. **Hist Teacher** 1980;13(3):379-83
Wilson LG, ed: Benjamin Silliman and his circle: Studies on the influence of Benjamin Silliman on science in America. Prepared in honor of Elizabeth H. Thomson. New York, Science History Publications, 1979. x, 227 p. Contributions by S. D Beckham, J. C. Greene, L. I. Kuslan, G. Robinson, M. W. Rossiter.
Wolfle D: Science: a memoir of the 1960's and 1970's. **Science** 1980 Jul 4;209(4452):57-60
Wyngaarden JB: Nurturing the scientific enterprise. **J Med Educ** 1984 Mar;59(3):155-61
Yalow R: Science and technology: problems and perceptions. In Cohen EP, ed: Medicine in transition. [Chicago], University of Illinois College of Medicine, 1981. p. 53-63.

**USSR**

Alumäe N: Eesti NSV teaduste akadeemia aastail 1965-1972. [toimetuskolleegium N. Alumäe ... et al.]. Tallinn, The Academy, 1973. 274 p.
Appleby JH: 'Rhubarb' Mounsey and the Surinam toad--a Scottish physician--naturalist in Russia. **Arch Nat Hist** 1982 Oct;11(1):137-52
Appleby JH: Robert Erskine--Scottish pioneer of Russian natural history. **Arch Nat Hist** 1982 Apr;10(3):377-98
Frolov VA: K razvitiiu nauki v SSSR. **Med Sestra** 1982 Dec;41(12):7-9
Grigorian NA: I. M. Sechenov i razvitie nauki v Rossii (k 150-letiiu so dnia rozhdeniia). **Sov Zdravookhr** 1979;(10):50-4
Grigorian NA: [I. M. Sechenov on science and its history] (Rus). **Istor Biol Issled** 1980;8:173-87
Grigor'ian NA: I. P. Pavlov o nauke i sotsial'noĭ otvetvennosti uchenogo. **Sov Zdravookhr** 1984;(2):58-61
Ionov IuV, Ionov AIu: Vklad russkikh vracheĭ v issledovanie Kamchatki i Dal'nego Vostoka v XIX veke. **Sov Zdravookhr** 1981;(10):59-62
Issledovaniia po istorii estestvoznaniia i tekhniki v desiatoi piatiletke: **Vopr Istor Estestvozn Tekh** 1981;1:3-12
Komkov GD, Levsĭn BV, Semenov LK: Geschichte der Akademie der Wissenschaften der UdSSR. Ed. C. Grau. Berlin, Akademie Verlag, 1981. 745 p. (Translation from the Russian edition of 1977)
Lebedkina ED: International contacts of Soviet scientists during 1917-1924. **Sov Stud Hist** 1971-72;10(3):267-86
Serebrovskaja KB: The role of scientific school in the formation of the new field of natural science. **Istor Biol Issled** 1983;9:145-58
Tarasov O: Science in Soviet Moldavia. In Science and Technology: humanism and progress. Moscow, Social Science Today, 1981. Vol. 2, p. 53-66. (Problems of the Contemporary World, no. 96).
Tarasov OI: Iz istorii nauki v Moldavskoi SSR. **Vopr Istor Estestvozn Tekh** 1981;1:85-94

**Venezuela**

Arechabaleta G de: Historia de la antropología física en Venezuela. Caracas, Universidad Central de Venezuela, Facultad de Ciencias Económicas y Sociales, División de Publicaciones, 1973. 30 p.
Mercedes Gomez J: La ciencia es la iniciacion del hombre en el conocimiento de la obra de dios. **Rev Soc Venez Hist Med** 1975-76;23(37):135-46
Osuna A: Ambrosio Perera dos historieta relacionadas con su persona la disyuntiva 'Ciencia pura y aplicada'. **Rev Soc Venez Hist Med** 1972-73;20-21(34-35):229-41

## SEX BEHAVIOR

See also **Birth Control; Generation and Reproduction**

Abramson HA: The historical and cultural spectra of homosexuality and their relationship to the fear of being a lesbian. **J Asthma Res** 1980 Jul;17(4):177-88
Ackner D: The crime of incest. **Med Leg J** 1980;48(pt 3):79-91
Bloch RH: Untangling the roots of modern sex roles: a survey of four centuries of change. **Signs** 1978;4(2)
Bullough VL: Homosexuality: a history. New York, New American Library, 1979. ix, 196 p.
Bullough VL, Bullough B: Prostitution--an illustrated social history. New York, Crown Publishers, 1978. xii, 336 p.
Bullough VL, Bullough B: Sin, sickness and sanity. New York, Garland, 1977. ix, 276 p.
Crompton L: The myth of lesbian impunity: capital laws from 1270 to 1791. **J Homosex** 1980-81 Fall-Winter;6(1-2):11-25
Farley MA: [History of] sexual ethics. In Reich WT, et al, ed: Encyclopedia of bioethics, v.4. New York, Free Press, 1978. p. 1575-89.
Fishman S: The history of childhood sexuality. **J Contemp Hist** 1982;17(2):269-83
Foucault MJ: The history of sexuality. Histoire de la sexualité. La volonté de savoir. v. 1. London, Lane, 1978. 168 p.
Greenberg DF, Bystryn MH: Christian intolerance of homosexuality. **AJS** 1982 Nov;88(3):515-48
Greydanus DE, Geller B: Masturbation; historic perspective. **NY State J Med** 1980 Nov;80(12):1892-6
Heath G: The illusory freedom. London, Heinemann, 1978. 131 p.
James T: Eunuchs and eunuchism--an historical discourse. **Adler Mus Bull** 1981 Oct;7(3):2-7
James T: Eunuchs and eunuchism - an historical discourse. Part II - Civil law. **Adler Mus Bull** 1982 Nov;8(2):3-7
Janda LH, Klenke-Hamel KE: Human sexuality. New York, Van Nostrand, 1980. xv, 475 p.
Lanteri-Laura G: Lecture des perversions: histoire de leur appropriation médicale. Paris, New York, Masson, 1979. 160 p.
Laslett P, Oosterveen K, Smith RM, ed: Bastardy and its comparative history. Cambridge, Mass., Harvard University Press, 1980. xv, 431 p. Contributions by Y. Blayo, D. Gaunt, S. Hartley, A. Hayami, S. Hochstadt, A. S. Kälvemark, J. Knodel, D. Levine, A. Newman, A. Macfarlane, M. R. Matovic, J. Meyer, D. S. Smith, C. Smout, S. Stewart, E. van de Walle, R. V. Wells, K. Wrightson.
Licata SJ, Peterson RP ed: Historical perspectives on homosexuality. **J Homosex** 1980-81 Fall-Winter;6(1-2):3-210
Licata SJ: Historical perspectives on homosexuality. New York, Haworth, 1981. 224 p.
London P: [History of] sexual behavior. In Reich WT, et al, ed: Encyclopedia of bioethics, v.4. New York, Free Press, 1978. p. 1560-9.
Maier-Bode S: Die Stellung der lesbischen Frau in der heutigen Gesellschaft und in früheren Jahrhunderten. Diss., Rheinische Friedrich-Wilhelms-Universität. Bonn, 1983. 101 p.
Malterre-Barthes A: L'infirmière face aux problèmes de la prostitution. **Infirm Fr** 1981 May;(225):9-12 contd
Mittwoch U: Whistling maids and crowing hens--hermaphroditism in folklore and biology. **Perspect Biol Med** 1981 Summer;24(4):595-606
Padgug RA: Sexual matters: on conceptualizing sexuality in history. **Radic Hist Rev** 1979;20:3-24
Parker W: Homosexuality in history; an annotated bibliography. **J Homosex** 1980-81 Fall-Winter;6(1-2):191-210
Roberts A: The pox and the people: a history of venereal diseases and sexual attitudes. **Nurs Times** 1982 Jul 14-20;78(28):1177-85
Rosen IL: Aphrodisiacs in the kitchen. **J La State Med Soc** 1980 Oct;132(10):155-9
Rousselle R: Comparative psychohistory: snake-handling in Hellenistic Greece and the American South. **J Psychohist** 1984 Spring;11(4):477-89
Sauri JJ: Nacimiento del concepto de perversión. **Rev Neuropsiquiatr** 1979 Jun;42(2):71-85
Steiner BW: From Sappho to Stand: historical perspective on crossdressing and cross gender. **Can J Psychiatry** 1981 Nov;26(7):502-6

**Americas**

Signorini I: Transvestism and institutionalized homosexuality in North America. In: Congresso Intern. degli Americanisti, 40th, Italy, 1972. Atti. Vol. 2. p. 153-63.

**Belgium**

Vandenbroeke C: Seksualiteit en huwelijksbeleving in Vlaanderen. **Spiegel Hist** 1979;14(7-8):425-33

**Europe**

Boswell J: Christianity, social tolerance, and homosexuality: gay people in Western Europe from the beginning of the Christian era to the fourteenth century. Chicago and London, University of Chicago Press, 1980. xviii, 424 p.

**France**

Flandrin JL: Repression and change in sexual life of young people in medieval and early modern times. In R. Wheaton, T. K. Hareven, ed: Family and sexuality in French history. Philadelphia. University of Pennsylvania Press, 1980. p. 27–48.
Wheaton R: Family and sexuality in French history. Philadelphia, University of Pennsylvania Press, 1980. ix, 274 p.

**Great Britain**

Thompson EP: Happy families. **Radic Hist Rev** 1979 Spring/Summer;Spec:42–50

**Italy**

Accati L: Lo spirito della fornicazione: virtù dell'anima e virtù del corpo in Friuli, fra '600 e '700. **Quad Stor** 1979;14(2):644–72
Pavan E: Police des moeurs, sociètè et politique à Venise à la fin du Moyen Age. **Rev Hist (Paris)** 1980;264(2):241–88

**Netherlands**

Salden MJ: Van doodstraft to straffeloosheid. **Spiegel Hist** 1982;17(11):559–65
Schenk J: Homoseksualiteit in de Nederlandse beeldende kunst voor 1800. **Spiegel Hist** 1982;17(11):576–83

**Peru**

Doig FK: Sexualverhalten im alten Peru. Lima, Kompaktos, 1979. 189 p.
Kauffmann Doig F: Comportamiento sexual en el antiguo Perú. Lima, Kompaktos G. S., [1978]. 189 p.

**Spain**

Rico-Avello C: La enigmatica sexualidad de La Monja-Alferez. **Asclepio** 1980;32:353–60

**Switzerland**

Monter EW: Sodomy and heresy in early modern Switzerland. **J Homosex** 1980–81 Fall-Winter;6(1–2):41–55

**United States**

Gladwin LA: Tobacco and sex: some factors affecting nonmarital sexual behavior in colonial Virginia. **J Soc Hist** 1978;12(1):57–75

**Before 500 A.D.**

Rousselle A: Porneia. De la maitrise du corps à la privation sensorielle. IIe–IVe siècles de l'ère chrétienne. Paris, Presses Universitaires de France, 1983. 254 p. (Les chemins de l'Histoire).

**Greco-Roman**

Hallett JP: Something in excess? Priapea 50, 2. **Mnemosyne** 1978;31:203–6
Krenkel WA: Masturbation in der Antike. **Wiss Z Univ Rostock** 1979;28(3):159–78
Verstraete BC: Homosexuality in ancient Greek and Roman civilization: a critical bibliography with supplement. Toronto, Canadian Gay Archives, 1982. 14 p.

**Greece**

Hoffman RJ: Some cultural aspects of Greek male homosexuality. **J Homosex** 1980 Spring;5(3):217–26

**Rome**

Verstraete BC: Slavery and the social dynamics of male homosexual relations in ancient Rome. **J Homosex** 1980 Spring;5(3):227–36
Veyne P: La vie sexuelle dans l'Empire Romain. **Sci Avenir** 1977;365:698–703

**500 A.D.–1450**

Bullough VL: Transvestites in the middle ages. **Am J Sociol** 1974 May;79(6):1381–94
Cosman MP: A feast for Aesculapius: historical diets for asthma and sexual pleasure. **Annu Rev Nutr** 1983;3:1–33
Gerhardt C: Kröte und Igel in schwankhafter Literatur des späten Mittelalters. **Medizinhist J** 1981;16(4):340–57
Jacquart D, Thomasset C: Albert le Grand et les problèmes de la sexualité. **Hist Philos Life Sci** 1981;3(1):73–93
Lemay H: The stars and human sexuality: some medieval scientific views. **Isis** 1980 Mar; 71(256):127–37
Radcliff-Umstead D, ed: Human sexuality in the Middle Ages and Renaissance. Pittsburgh, University of Pittsburgh Center for Medieval and Renaissance Studies, 1978. viii, 193 p. (University of Pittsburgh publications on the Middle Ages and the Renaissance, 4). Contributions by B. D. Palmer, J. Spisak, D. S. McCoy, T. G. Benedek, J. Schwartz, M. J. Thorssen, M. Novy, H. E. Faletti.
Wood CT: The doctors' dilemma: sin, salvation, and the menstrual cycle in medieval thought. **Speculum** 1981;56(4):710–27

**Germany**

Pereira M: Maternità e sessualità femminile nell' opera di Ildegarda di Bingen. Una proposta di lettura. **Quad Stor** 1980;2

**Italy**

Rowland B: Exhuming Trotula, sapiens matrona of Salerno. **Florilegium** 1979;1:42–57

**Spain**

García Iglesias L: La edad difícil y la sexualidad adolescente en la España visigoda. **Hisp Antiq** 1976;6:79–96

**1450–1700**

**Great Britain**

Burg BR: Ho hum, another work of the devil. Buggery and sodomy in early Stuart England. **J Homosex** 1980–81 Fall–Winter;6(1–2):69–78

**Netherlands**

Matheron A: Spinoza et la sexualité. **G Crit Filos Ital** 1977;56:436–57

**United States**

Oaks BF: 'Things fearful to name': sodomy and buggery in seventeenth-century New England. **J Soc Hist** 1978;12(2):268–81
Oaks RF: Defining sodomy in seventeenth-century Massachusetts. **J Homosex** 1980–81 Fall–Winter;6(1–2):79–83

**West Indies**

Burg BR: Sodomy and the perception of evil: English sea rovers in the seventeenth-century Caribbean. New York, New York University Press, 1983. xxxiii, 215 p.

**1700 to Present**

Ackerknecht EH: Wilhelm Reich (1897–1957). In Ganzinger K, Skopec M, Wyklicky H, ed: Festschrift für Erna Lesky zum 70. Geburtstag. Wien, Brüder Hollinek, 1981. p. 5–12.
Burg BR: The sick and the dead: the development of psychological theory on necrophilia from Krafft-Ebing to the present. **J Hist Behav Sci** 1982 Jul;18(3):242–54
Chromý K: Masturbace a historie psychiatrie. **Cesk Psychiatr** 1984 Jun;80(3):180–3
Dellamora R: An essay in sexual liberation, Victorian style: Walter Pater's 'Two early French stories'. **J Homosex** 1983 Spring–Summer;8(3–4):139–50
Farley J: Gametes & spores. Ideas about sexual reproduction, 1750–1914. Baltimore, London, Johns Hopkins University Press, 1982. x, 299 p.
Fischer-Homberger E: Herr und Weib: Zur Geschichte der Beziehung zwischen ordnendem Geist und anderen Impulsen. In Fischer-Homberger E: Krankheit Frau. Zur Geschichte der Einbildungen. Darmstadt, Sammlung Luchterhand, 1984. p. 92–121.
Gay P: Victorian sexuality: old texts and new insights. **Am Scholar** 1980;49(3):372–8
Genné WH: Sex, marriage and family: an update from Amsterdam. **J Ecumenical Stud** 1979;16(1):154–60
Gilbert AN: Conceptions of homosexuality and sodomy in Western history. **J Homosex** 1980–81 Fall–Winter;6(1–2):57–68
Gmelin OF: Anti-Freud: von der Psychoanalyse zur Medienwissenschaft. Mit einem Beitrag von Helene Saussure. Frankfurt am Main, Haag and Herchen, 1979. 175 p.
Hall R: Henry James: interpreting an obsessive memory. **J Homosex** 1983 Spring–Summer;8(3–4):83–97
Hekma G: Homoseksualiteit: van zonde tot geaardheid. **Spiegel Hist** 1980;15(9):484–91
Israelstam S, Lambert S: Homosexuality as a cause of alcoholism: a historical review. **Int J Addict** 1983 Dec;18(8):1085–107
McCarthy T: Freud and the problem of sexuality. **J Hist Behav Sci** 1981;17:332–9
Macmillan MB: Freud and Lindner on pleasure sucking.

**Stor Crit Psicol** 1980;1(1):111–43
May R: Freud and the phallic defense. **Psychiatry** 1979;42(2):147–56
Money J: The genealogical descent of sexual psychoneuroendocrinology from sex and health theory: the eighteenth to the twentieth centuries. **Psychoneuroendocrinology** 1983;8(4):391–400
Mullaney MM: Gender and revolution: Rosa Luxemburg and the female revolutionary personality. **J Psychohist** 1984 Spring;11(4):463–76
Raboch J: Historický vývoj lékařské sexuologie. **Cesk Psychiatr** 1982 Oct;78(5):353–7
Ruse M: Medicine as social science: the case of Freud on homosexuality. **J Med Philos** 1981 Nov;6(4):361–86
Smith KM: Dr. James Barry: military man--or woman? **Can Med Assoc J** 1982 Apr 1;126(7):854–7
Socarides CW: Homosexuality. New York, Aronson, 1978. Historical chapters, p. 7-61.
Wattley LA: Male physicians and female health and sexuality in 19th century English and American society. **J Adv Nurs** 1983 Sep;8(5):423–8

**Africa**

Ross R: Oppression, sexuality and slavery at the Cape of Good Hope. **Hist Reflect** 1979;6(2):421–33

**Australia**

Finnane M: The popular defence of Chidley. **Labour Hist** 1981;41:57–73

**Austria**

Biliński Z: Przyczynek do poznania zjawiska szerzenia się chorób wenerycznych-w oparciu o problem występowania prostytucji w Jarosławiu w okresie zaboru austriackiego (1895–1916). **Przegl Dermatol** 1982 Jan–Apr;69(1–2):113–5
Gilman SL: Freud and the prostitute: male stereotypes of female sexuality in fin-de-siècle Vienna. **J Am Acad Psychoanal** 1981 Jul;9(3):337–60

**Canada**

Bedford J: Prostitution in Calgary 1905–1914. **Alberta Hist** 1981;29(2):1–11

**Europe**

Calmy C: La sexualité au XIXe siècle: entretien avec Alain Corbin. **Histoire** 1979;12:80–2

**France**

Aldrich R: Homosexuality in France. **Contemp Fr Civiliz** 1982;7(1):1–10
Böttiger LE: På spaning i 'På spaning': om homosexualiteten i Prousts verk. **Sydsven Medicinhist Sallsk Arsskr** 1984;21:99–108
Bullough VL, Elcano BW, Legg WD, et al: An annotated bibliography of homosexuality. 2 vols. Vol. I. New York, Garland, 1976. xxxvii, 405 p.
Coward DA: Attitudes to homosexuality in eighteenth century France. **J Eur Stud** 1980;10(4):231–55
Fernandez D: Francois Carlier, La Prostitution antiphysique (1857). Précédé de La Pederastie (1887) par Ambroise Tardieu. Paris, Le Sycomore, 1981. ix, 250 p.
Haeberle EJ: Human rights and sexual rights. The legacy of René Guyon. **Med Law** 1983;2(2):159–72
Halberstadt-Freud HC: Proust and perversion: some clinical and theoretical consideration. **Int J Psychoanal** 1980;61(3):403–10
Litchfield RB, Gordon D: Closing the 'tour': a close look at the marriage market, unwed mothers, and abandoned children in mid-nineteenth century Amiens. **J Soc Hist** 1980;13(3):458–72
Stambolian G, Marks E, ed: Homosexualities and French literature: cultural contexts, critical texts. Ithaca, Cornell University Press, 1979. 387 p. Historical chapters by J. Stockinger, G. H. Storzer, I de Courtivron, P. Schmidt, W. Fowlie, J. E. Rivers, R. Galand, F. P. Bowman, G. H. Bauer, S. Doubrovsky, S. Smith.

**Germany**

Adam J, Fikentscher E, Liebner K: Untersuchungen zur sexuellen Entwicklung. **Wiss Z Martin Luther Univ (Math)** 1976;25(3):81–91
Eriksson B: A lesbian execution in Germany, 1721: the trial records. **J Homosex** 1980–81 Fall–Winter;6(1–2):27–40
Goldhagen E: Nazi sexual demonology. **Midstream** 1981;27(5):7–15
Haeberle EJ: 'Stigmata of degeneration'. Prisoner markings in Nazi concentration camps. **J Homosex** 1980–81 Fall–Winter;6(1–2):135–9
Kennedy HC: The 'Third sex' theory of Karl Heinrich Ulrichs. **J Homosex** 1980–81 Fall–Winter;6(1–2):103–11
Lautmann R: The pink triangle. The persecution of homosexual males in concentration camps in Nazi Germany. **J Homosex** 1980–81 Fall–Winter;6(1–2):141–60
Seidler FW: Prostitution, Homosexualität, Selbstverstümmelung. Probleme der deutschen Sanitätsführung 1939–1945. Neckargemünd, Vowinkel, 1977. 323 p.

**Great Britain**

Anderson NF: The 'marriage with a deceased wife's sister bill' controversy: incest anxiety and the defense of family purity in Victorian England. **J Br Stud** 1982;21(2):67–86
Bowman IA: 'My life'; an important Ellis manuscript. **Bookman** 1981 Apr;8(4):3–7
Brome V: Havelock Ellis, philospher of sex: a biography. London, Boston, Routledge & Kegan Paul, 1979. xiv, 271 p.
Coleman W: The Queen's women. **Bull Hist Med** 1981 Winter;55(4):580–9
Cott NF: Passionlessness: an interpretation of Victorian sexual ideology, 1790–1850. **Signs** 1978;4(2):219–36
Crompton L: Don Leon, Byron, and homosexual law reform. **J Homosex** 1983 Spring–Summer;8(3–4):53–71
Edwards SS: Femina sexualis: medico-legal control in Victoriana. **Soc Soc Hist Med Bull (Lond)** 1981 Jun;28:17–20
Fassler B: Theories of homosexuality as sources of Bloomsbury's androgyny. **Signs** 1979;5(2):237–51
Fee E: Psychology, sexuality, social control in Victorian England. **Soc Sci Q** 1978;58(4):632–46
Fromm H: Virginia Woolf: art and sexuality. **Va Q Rev** 1979;55(3):441–59
Gabriel A: Sir Arthur Conan Doyle: to see and to be seen. **Bull Menninger Clin** 1982 Nov;46(6):530–8
Gilbert AN: Masturbation and insanity: Henry Maudsley and the ideology of sexual repression. **Albion** 1980;12(3):268–82
Gilbert AN: Sodomy and the law in eighteenth- and early nineteenth-century Britain. **Societas** 1978;8(3):225–41
Hall LA: The Stopes collection in the Contemporary Medical Archives Centre at the Wellcome Institute for the History of Medicine. **Soc Soc Hist Med Bull (Lond)** 1983 Jun;32:50–1
Hansen B: The historical construction of homosexuality. **Radic Hist Rev** 1979;20:66–73
Hansen B: The historical construction of homosexuality. **Radic Hist Rev** 1979 Spring/Summer;Spec:66–73
Harrison F: The dark angel: aspects of Victorian sexuality. New York, Universe, 1977. 288 p.
Harvey AD: Prosecutions for sodomy in England at the beginning of the nineteenth century. **Hist J (Gt Brit)** 1978;21(4):939–48
Hilliard D: Unenglish and unmanly: Anglo-Catholicism and homosexuality. **Victorian Stud** 1982;25(2):181–210
Holtzman EM: Marriage, sexuality, and contraception in the British middle class, 1918–1939: the correspondence of Marie Stopes. Ph.D. Diss., Rutgers University, The State Univ. of New Jersey. New Brunswick, 1982. v, 170 p.
McHugh P: Prostitution and Victorian social reform. New York, St. Martin's Press, 1980. 306 p.
Martin RK: Edward Carpenter and the double structure of Maurice. **J Homosex** 1983 Spring–Summer;8(3–4):35–46
Morowitz HJ: The mating poems of D. H. Lawrence. **Hosp Pract [Off]** 1984 May;19(5):233–5, 238
Spencer FJ: The Gay Nineties: Oscar Wilde reconsidered. **MCVQ** 1981;16(3):67–70
Walkowitz JR: Prostitution and Victorian society. Women, class, and the state. Cambridge, New York, Cambridge University Press, 1980. ix, 347 p.
Weeks J: Inverts, perverts, and Mary-Annes. Male prostitution and the regulation of homosexuality in England in the nineteenth and early twentieth centuries. **J Homosex** 1980–81 Fall–Winter;6(1–2):113–34
Weeks J: Movements of affirmation: sexual meanings and homosexual identities. **Radic Hist Rev** 1979;20:164–79

**Italy**

Cotti C: Il femminismo come caso letterario: un'inchiesta di inizio '900 su amore e sessualita. **Mem Riv Stor Donne** 1981;(2):112–8
DeGiorgio M: Primi sintomi di un carattere appassionato: dal collegio. **Mem Riv Stor Donne** 1981;(1):94–102

**Netherlands**

Boon LJ: 'Utrechtenaren': de sodomieprocessen in Utrecht, 1730–1732. **Spiegel Hist** 1982;17(11):553–8
Kooij CG van der: Rudolf de Mepsche en de Faanse processen. **Spiegel Hist** 1979;14(6):358–64
Tielman RA: De emancipatie van homoseksuelen in Nederland. **Spiegel Hist** 1982;17(11):572–5

**Norway**

Dyrvik S: Marriage and social norms: a study of Etne, 1715–1801. **Tidsskr Samfunnsforskning** 1970;11(4):285–300

**Pacific Islands**

Austen R: Stoddard's little tricks in South Sea Idyls. **J Homosex** 1983

Spring–Summer;8(3–4):73–81

**Singapore**

Lee YK: Prostitution and venereal disease in early Singapore (1819–1889). **Singapore Med J** 1980;21:720–31

**United States**

Armstrong L: The cradle of sexual politics. **Frontiers** 1981;6(1–2):19–25
Barker-Benfield GJ: A historical perspective on women's health care--female circumcision. **Women Health** 1976 Jan–Feb;1(1):13–15,18–20
Bayer R, Spitzer RL: Edited correspondence on the status of homosexuality in DSM-III. **J Hist Behav Sci** 1982 Jan;18(1):32–52
Bowman IA: Prostitution and the medical profession in the nineteenth century. **Bookman** 1982 Jan;9(1):3–9
Brown SE: Sexuality and the slave community. **Phylon** 1981;42(1):1–10
Browning DS: Homosexuality, theology, the social sciences and the church. **Encounter (Lond)** 1979;40(3):223–43
Bush LE: Mormon 'physiology' 1850–1875. **Bull Hist Med** 1982 Summer;56(2):218–37
Christensen HT: Mormon sexuality in cross-cultural perspective. **Dialogue** 1976;10(2):62–75
Christenson CV: Alfred Charles Kinsey. In Dictionary of American Biography, Suppl. 6, 1956–1960. p. 342–4, 1980.
Cook BW: The historical denial of lesbianism. **Radic Hist Rev** 1979 Spring/Summer;Spec:60–5
Davison GC: Politics, ethics, and therapy for homosexuality. **Am Behav Sci** 1982;25(4):423–34
Documents in Hopi Indian sexuality: Imperialism, culture and resistance. **Radic Hist Rev** 1979 Spring/Summer;Spec:99–130
Duberman MB: 'Writhing bedfellows': 1826. Two young men from antebellum South Carolina's ruling elite share 'extravagant delight'. **J Homosex** 1980–81 Fall–Winter;6(1–2):85–101
Fellman AC, Fellman M: Making sense of self. Medical advice literature in late nineteenth-century America. Philadelphia, University of Pennsylvania Press, 1981. 198 p.
Fellman AC, Fellman M: Man amuck. **Rev Am Hist** 1976;4(4):558–64
Fishbein L: Freud and the radicals: the sexual revolution comes to Greenwich Village. **Can Rev Am Stud** 1981;12(2):173–89
Fogarty RS, Grant HR: Free love in Ohio: Jacob Beilhardt and the Spirit Fruit Colony. **Ohio Hist** 1980;89(2):206–21
Gilchrist LD, Schinke SP: Teenage pregnancy and public policy. **Soc Serv Rev** 1983;57(2):307–22
Gordon L: The long struggle for reproductive rights. **Radic Am** 1981;15(1–2):75–88
Gove WR, Hughes M: Beliefs vs. data: more on the illness behavior of men and women. **Am Sociol Rev** 1981;46(1):123–8
Gove WR, Hughes M: Possible causes of the apparent sex differences in physical health: an empirical investigation. **Am Sociol Rev** 1979;44(1):126–46
Hamowy R: Medicine and the crimination of sin: 'self-abuse' in the 19th century America. **J Libert Stud** 1977;1(3):229–70
Hansen KJ: Mormon sexuality and American culture. **Dialogue** 1976;10(2):45–56
Haraway D: The biological enterprise: sex, mind, and profit from human engineering to sociobiology. **Radic Hist Rev** 1979 Spring/Summer;Spec:206–37
Jacob KA: The Mosher report. **Am Heritage** 1981;32(4):56–64
Kampmeier RH: Venereal disease in the United States Army: 1775–1900. **Sex Transm Dis** 1982 Apr–Jun;9(2):100–3
Kern LJ: Ideology and reality: sexuality and women's status in the Oneida community. **Radic Hist Rev** 1979 Spring/Summer;Spec:180–204
Kessler RC, McRae JA: Trends in the relationship between sex and psychological distress: 1957–1976. **Am Sociol Rev** 1981;46(4):443–52
Kitsuse JI: Coming out all over: deviants and the politics of social problems. **Soc Probl** 1980;28(1):1–13
Liles DM: William Faulkner's Absalom, Absalom!: an exegesis of the homoerotic configurations in the novel. **J Homosex** 1983 Spring–Summer;8(3–4):99–111
Mandelker IL: Religion, sex, and utopia in nineteenth-century America. **Soc Res (NY)** 1982;49(3):730–51
Marcus AC, Seeman TE: Sex differences in health status: a reexamination of the nurturant role hypothesis. **Am Sociol Rev** 1981;46(1):119–23
Masters WH: Half a century of unnecessary sexual myths. **JAMA** 1983 Jul 8;250(2):244
Mauss AL: Shall the youth of Zion falter? Mormon youth and sex: a two-city comparison. **Dialogue** 1976;10(2):82–4
May ET: Sex in utopia: a review essay. **NY Hist** 1981;62(4):462–7
Nissenbaum S: Sex, diet, and debility in Jacksonian America: Sylvester Graham and health reform. Westport, Connecticut, Greenwood, 1980. 198 p. (Contributions in Medical History, 4).
Oaks R: Perceptions of homosexuality by justices of the peace in colonial Virginia. **J Homosex** 1979–80 Fall–Winter;5(1–2):35–41
Penland LR: Sex education in 1900, 1940 and 1980: an historical sketch. **J Sch Health** 1981 Apr;51(4):305–9
Pillard RC: Psychotherapeutic treatment for the invisible minority. **Am Behav Sci** 1982;25(4):407–22
Pomerantz MB, Marr JS, Goldman WD: Amebiasis in New York City 1958--1978: identification of the male homosexual high risk population. **Bull NY Acad Med** 1980 Mar;56(2):232–44
Ross E: 'The love crisis': couples advice books of the late 1970s. **Signs** 1980;6(1):109–22
Sahli N: Sexuality in 19th and 20th century America: the sources and their problems. **Radic Hist Rev** 1979;20:89–96
Sandos JA: Prostitution and drugs: the United States Army on the Mexican-American border, 1916–1917. **Pac Hist Rev** 1980;49(4):621–45
Schwarz J: Yellow clover: Katharine Lee Bates and Katharine Coman. **Frontiers** 1979;4(1):59–67
Scully D, Bart P: A funny thing happened on the way to the orifice: women in gynecology textbooks. **Am J Sociol** 1973 Jan;78(4):1045–50
Smith WE: Mormon sex standards on college campuses: or deal us out of the sexual revolution! **Dialogue** 1976;10(2):76–81
Smith-Rosenberg C: Sex as symbol in Victorian purity: an ethnohistorical analysis of Jacksonian America. In Demos, John and Boocock, Sarane Spence, ed: Turning points: historical and sociological essays on the family. Chicago, U. of Chicago Press, 1978. p. 212–47.
Stein HF: Sittin' tight and bustin' loose: contradiction and conflict in midwestern masculinity and the psychohistory of America. **J Psychohist** 1984 Spring;11(4):501–12
Strong B: Ideas of the early sex education movement in America, 1890–1920. **Hist Educ Q** 1972;12(2):129–62
Verbrugge MH: Healthy animals and civic life: Sylvester Graham's physiology of subsistence. **Rev Am Hist** 1981;9(3):359–64
Wangensteen OH: Mandated celibacy in the academic arena. **Surg Gynecol Obstet** 1980 May;150(5):739–45
Weinberg MS, Swensson RG, Hammersmith SK: Sexual autonomy and the status of women: models of female sexuality in U. S. sex manuals from 1950 to 1980. **Soc Probl** 1983;30(3):312–24
White E: The inverted type: homosexuality as a theme in James Merrill's prophetic books. **J Homosex** 1983 Spring–Summer;8(3–4):47–52

**USSR**

Kon IS: O sotsiologicheskoi interpretatsii seksual'nogo povedeniia. **Sotsiol Issled** 1982;(2):113–22

# SOCIAL MEDICINE

See also **Public Health; State Medicine**

Del Nero CR: De polícia médica à medicina social: uma análise genética. **AMB** 1980 Jul;26(7):255–6
McCullough LB: Justice and health care: historical perspectives and precedents. In E. E. Shelp, ed: Justice and health care. Dordrecht, Reidel, 1981. (Philosophy and medicine, Vol. 8), p. 51–71.
Mani N: Zur Geschichte der Hygiene. Kontinuität und Wandel hygienischer Vorstellungen von der Antike zum 19. Jahrhundert. **ZFA (Stuttgart)** 1981 Nov 20;57(32):2183–92
Sournia JC: Die Sozialmedizin. In Sournia JC, Martiny M, Poulet J, ed: Illustrierte Geschichte der Medizin. Salzburg, Andreas, 1980. Vol. 6. p. 2149–93.

**Africa**

Gaye P: La médecine sociale en Afrique de l'ouest (historique, situation actuelle et perspective d'avenir). In: Congrès international d'histoire de la médecine, XXVe, Québec, 1976. Actes. Québec, 1977. p. 121–40.

**Belgium**

Sondervost FA, Wery Ph: Quelques aspects de l'histoire des organisations d'entraide et la médecine sociale en Belgique. In: Congrès international d'histoire de la médecine XXVe, Québec, 1976. Actes. Québec, 1977. p. 371–99.

**Italy**

Stroppiana L: Histoire et perspectives de la médecine sociale en Italie. In: Congrès international d'histoire de la médecine, XXVe, Québec, 1976. Actes. Québec, 1977. p. 321–31.

**Sweden**

Lindgren G: History and perspectives of social medicine. In: Congrès international d'histoire de la médecine, XXVe, Québec, 1976. Actes. Québec, 1977. p. 193–203.

**1700 to Present**

Bílek V, Niklíček L: Dílo Alfreda Grotjahna a jeho vliv na vývoj sociálního lékařství v Cechách. Cást I. **Cesk Zdrav** 1982 Apr;30(4):145–56
Czehák J: November 7: Gondolatok az egészségügy és a társadalom

kapcsolatáról. **Orv Hetil** 1983 Nov 6;124(45):2723–4
Eberson F: Profiles, giants in social medicine. St. Petersburg, Valkyrie Press, 1980. 103 p.
Foucault M: El nacimiento de la medicina social. **Med Tradic** 1982;3(11):3–16
Numbers RL, ed: Compulsory health insurance. The continuing American debate. Westport, Connecticut, London, Greenwood Press, 1982. xv, 172 p. With contributions by A. J. Viseltear, G. Land, T. R. Marmor, M. M. Poen, P. Starr, R. Lubove, W. J. Cohen. (Contributions in medical history, no. 11).
Rodríguez Ocaña E: Aproximacion al concepto y practica de la medicina social en Ludwig Teleky (1872–1957). **Dynamis (Spain)** 1982;2:299–323
Sournia JC: Remarques sur l'évolution de la protection sociale et sanitaire dans les pays en voie de développement. In: Congrès international d'histoire de la médecine, XXVe, Québec, 1976. Actes. Québec, 1977. p. 297–317.
Spaar H: Die Begründung der Vorzüge des Gesundheitsschutzes im Sozialismus und seiner gesetzmässigen Schranken im Kapitalismus im Lichte der Lehre von Karl Marx. **Z Gesamte Hyg** 1983 Oct;29(10):573–6
Thom A: Die spezifische Funktion sozialer und ideologischer Bedingungen in der Erkenntnisentwicklung der Medizin – methodologische Vorbestimmungen und Resultate bisheriger Forschungen. In International Congress of the History of Medicine. 26th, Plovdiv, 1978. Actes du Congress. Sofia, 1981. Volume II. p. 74–6.
Trüb CL: Die Terminologie und Definition Sozialmedizin und Sozialhygiene in den literarischen Sekundärquellen der Jahre 1900 bis 1960. Opladen, Westdeutscher Verlag, 1978. 87 p.
Tutzke D, ed: Zur Entwicklung der Sozialhygiene im 19. und 20. Jahrhundert. Ausgewählte Beiträge vom I. Medizinhistorischen Symposium DDR–UdSSR, Halle (Saale) 1975. Berlin, Akademie für Aerztliche Fortbildung der DDR; Gesellschaft für Geschichte der Medizin in der DDR, 1976, xi, 277 p.
Vengrova IV: K. Marks i razvitie sotsial'noĭ gigieny. **Sov Zdravookhr** 1983;6:3–8

**Australia**

Holton S: Social medicine in nineteenth century South Australia. **Community Health Stud** 1983;7(2):121–35

**Brazil**

Freitas DG de: La médecine sociale dans la plus grande et plus populeuse ville du Brésil: Sao Paulo. In: Congrès international d'histoire de la médecine, XXVe, Québec, 1976. Actes. Québec, 1977. p. 77–97.

**Canada**

Gilbert R: La nouvelle morale sociale et l'état surveillant. In: Congrès international d'histoire de la médecine, XXVe, Québec, 1976. Actes. Québec, 1977. p. 171–92.

**Czechoslovakia**

Filip M: 25 rokov katedry sociálneho lekárstva Lekárskej fakulty UPJS v Košiciach. **Cesk Zdrav** 1980 Oct;28(10):397–402
Junas J: K rozvíjaniu sociálnolekárskych hl'adísk na Slovensku v 19. storočí. **Cesk Zdrav** 1983 Feb;31(2):65–70
Müller C, Niklíček L: K postavení sociálního lékařství v historii systému výuky a výchovy lékařu na Univerzitě Karlově. **Cesk Zdrav** 1982 Jan;30(1):22–33
Porubčinová Z: Pokrokové tradice katedry sociálního lékařstvílékařské faculty UJEP v Brně. **Cesk Zdrav** 1983 Feb;31(2):71–6
Významné životné jubileum prof. MUDr. Adolfa Zácka: **Cesk Zdrav** 1982 Dec;30(12):530–6

**Europe**

Dunovský J: K istorii razvitiia sotsial'noĭ pediatrii. **Pediatriia** 1982 Jun;(6):4–9

**France**

Weiner DB: Les handicapés et la révolution française: aspects de médecine sociale. In: Congrès international d'histoire de la médecine, XXVe, Québec, 1976. Actes. Québec, 1977. p. 333–70.

**Germany**

Dittmann S, Paulenz H, Scheel G, et al: 30 Jahre Staatliche Hygieneinspektion der DDR. **Z Gesamte Hyg** 1983 Oct;29(10):584–8
Ewert G, Rothe J: K vývoji sociální hygieny v Německé Demokratické Republice. **Cesk Zdrav** 1979 Oct;27(10):391–8
Ewert G: Kratkiĭ obzor o razvitii sotsial'noĭ gigieny v GDR. **Sov Zdravookhr** 1980;(3):45–9
Figlio K, Weindling P: Was social medicine revolutionary? Rudolf Virchow and the revolutions of 1848. **Soc Soc Hist Med Bull (Lond)** 1984 Jun;34:10–8
Gehrke H, Dückert M: Gesundheitspolitik der deutschen Arbeiterklasse und ihre Unterstützung durch die fortschrittlichsten Vertreter der medizinischen Intelligenz. **Z Arztl Fortbild (Jena)** 1983;77(12):530–4
Hahn S: Positionen der Kommunistischen Partei Deutschlands zur lebensbewahrenden Aufgabe der Medizin in der Zeit der Weimarer Republik. **Z Exp Chir** 1982 Jul;28(7):468–71
Kaiser W: Medizinhistorische Impressionen zum Karl-Marx-Jahr 1983. **Z Gesamte Inn Med** 1983 Dec 15;38(24):669–72
Karbe KH: Die 'Woche der Sowjet-Medizin' zu Berlin (28. November bis 2. Dezember 1932). **Z Gesamte Hyg** 1981 Oct;27(10):784–8
Karbe KH: Ein Leben für die soziale Medizin––Salomon Neumann zu seinem 75. Todestag. **Z Gesamte Hyg** 1983 Nov;29(11):696–8
Labisch A: Alfred Grotjahn (1869–1931) und das gesundheitspolitische Programm der Mehrheitssozialdemokraten von 1922. **MMG** 1983;8:192–7
Milles D: From workers' diseases to occupational diseases: the causality of experts' evidence on liability in the development of social medicine. **Soc Soc Hist Med Bull (Lond)** 1983 Dec;33:58–62
Moerchel J: Soziale Bedingtheit von Gesundheit und Krankheit in Vergangenheit und Gegenwart. **Off Gesundheitswes** 1980 Nov;42(11):893–901
Moschke G: Die Stellung der KPD zur Berufskrankheitengesetzgebung in der Weimarer Republik. **Z Exp Chir** 1982 Jul;28(7):471–3
Moschke G: Zur Bedeutung des SMAD-Befehls Nr. 234 für die Entwicklung der Lehre über Sozialhygiene an der Leipziger Universität in den Jahren 1948 bis 1952. **Z Gesamte Hyg** 1983 Oct;29(10):620–3
Reis K: Gesundheitserziehung in der DDR – Versuch einer historischen Betrachtung. **Z Gesamte Hyg** 1982 Apr;28(4):253–5
Rothe J, Ewert G: Od pracovního společenství sociálních hygienikuke společnosti sociální hygieny NDR. **Cesk Zdrav** 1981 Jan;29(1):5–9
Schadewaldt H: L'histoire de la médecine sociale et ses perspectives pendant l'Empire et la République Allemande et dans la République Fédérale Allemande. In: Congrès international d'histoire de la médecine, XXVe, Québec, 1976. Actes. Québec, 1977. p. 277–94.
Schneck P: Max Hirsch (1877–1948)––der Mitbegründer der sozialgynäkologischen Forschungrichtung. **Zentralbl Gynakol** 1983;105(24):1600–4
Werner K: Sozialhygienische Aspekte in der frühen Ara der Tuberkulose-Therapie. **Wiss Beitr Martin Luther Univ Halle Wittenberg** 1983;5–R80:273–7

**Great Britain**

Davies J: David Lloyd George and the National Insurance Act of 1911. In J. Cule, ed: Wales and medicine. London, British Society for the History of Medicine, 1975. p. 1–9.

**Italy**

Cherubini A: Medicina e lotte sociali (1900–1920). Roma, Il Pensiero Scientifico, 1980. 358 p.
Malamani A: Medicina ottocentesca e medicina del lavoro: l'opera scientifico-sociale di Luigi Devoto a Pavia. **G Ital Med Lav** 1983 Jan;5(1):1–16

**Poland**

Jacquel R: Trois Alsaciens et les débuts––modestes––de la médecine sociale en Pologne pendant l'époque des lumières (troisième tiers du XVIIIe siècle). Les médecins strasbourgeois Jacques Reinbold Spielmann (1722–1783) et Jean Boecler (1737–1808) et le savant mulhousien Jean-Henri Lambert (1728–1777). In Livet G, Schaff G, ed: Médecine et assistance en Alsace, XVIe–XXe siècle. Strasbourg, Istra, 1976. p. 155–200.
Kirschner H: Geneza i zadania medycyny społecznej. **Pol Arch Med Wewn** 1984 Jul–Aug;72(1–2):1–7

**Romania**

Negru I: Primele anchete medico-sociale ale şcolii clujene de igienă. **Viata Med [Medii Sanit]** 1983 Jul;31(7):165–8

**United States**

Cimini TA, Wong A: The historical development of federal involvement in health care. **Am Arch Rehabil Ther** 1979 Spring;27(1):4–6
Cohen D: Social medicine: amputating the wrong leg. **Work Pap Mag** 1981;8(6):17–20
Coleman FC: The legislative history of Medicare. **Pathologist** 1981 Feb;35(2):97–9
Coleman FC: The legislative history of Medicare: Part II. **Pathologist** 1981 Mar;35(3):156–8
Engquist-Seidenberg G: The States' role in health care cost containment. **Policy Stud Rev** 1981;1(2):275–87
Falk IS: Some lessons from the fifty years since the CCMC final report, 1932. **J Public Health Policy** 1983 Jun;4(2):135–61
Medicaid: an historical perspective up to 1966: **Mich Hosp** 1978

Oct;14(10):2-3
Robison DW: Wisconsin and the mentally ill. A history of the 'Wisconsin Plan' of state and county care 1860-1915. New York, Arno Press, 1980. ix, 322 p. (Historical Issues in Mental Health).
Rosen G: Social medicine in the United States: The role of non-medical individuals and movements in its developments. In: Congrès international d'histoire de la médecine, XXVe, Québec, 1976. Actes. Québec, 1977. p. 247-74.
Uphoff MJ, Uphoff WH, Lewis RK: Group Health: an American success story in prepaid health care. Minneapolis, Dillon Press, 1980. xvii, 173 p.

**USSR**

Arkhangel'skiĭ GA: N. A. Belogolovyĭ--obshchestvennyĭ vrach, zhurnalist (k 150-letiiu so dnia rozhdeniia). **Sov Zdravookhr** 1984;(10):67-70
Bazanov VA: E. A. Osipov--odin iz osnovopolozhnikov obshchestvennoĭ meditsiny i sanitarnoĭ statistiki v dorevoliutsionnoĭ Rossii. **Feldsher Akush** 1980;45(9):40-4
Belitskaia EIa: Gigienicheskie i sotsial'no-gigienicheskie vzgliady S. P. Botkina (k 150-letiiu so dnia rozhdeniia). **Gig Sanit** 1982 Jul;(7):34-8
Grando AA, Makarenko IM, Polianskiĭ AA: Kafedre sotsial'noĭ gigieny i organizatsii zdravookhraneniia Kievskogo meditsinskogo instituta--60 let. **Sov Zdravookhr** 1984;(3):52-3
Grigorian NA: Rol' uchenykh Kazanskogo universiteta v razvitii obshchestvennoĭ meditsiny. **Sov Zdravookhr** 1981;(7):48-51
Ibragimov NG: Stanovlenie i razvitie sotsial'nogo strakhovaniia v Bashkirii. **Sov Zdravookhr** 1983;5:58-61
Katsnel'bogen AG: Dekabristy i obshcestvennaia meditsina. **Sov Zdravookhr** 1979;(12):47-51
Katsnel'bogen AG: Dekabristy i obshchestvenno-meditsinskaia mysl' v Rossii. **Klin Med (Mosk)** 1981 Mar;59(3):115-8
Panzer D: Zur historischen Entwicklung des Objektverständnisses der Sozialhygiene während der Entstehung der sozialistischen Gesellschaft am Beispiel der UdSSR. **Z Gesamte Hyg** 1983 Oct;29(10):581-4
Popushoĭ EP, Spineĭ LV: A.D. Kotsovskiĭ--vidnyĭ predstavitel' obshchestvennoĭ meditsiny Moldavii. **Sov Zdravookhr** 1980;(9):58-61
Shishkin AP: Sozdanie seti institutov zdravookhraneniia i sotsial'noĭ gigieny v SSSR v 20-x--nachale 30-x godov. **Sov Zdravookhr** 1982;(10):57-61
Shishkin AP: Voprosy profilaktiki v deiatel'nosti Gosudarstvennogo Instituta Sotsial'noĭ Gigieny Narkomzdrava RSFSR (k 65-letiiu obrazovaniia N rodnogo Komissariata Zdravookhraneniia RSFSR). **Sov Zdravookhr** 1983;6:55-8
Vengrova IV: Sotsial'no-gigienicheskie issledovaniia 20-kh godov, posviashchennye sel'skomu pereselencheskomu naseleniiu Sibiri. **Sov Zdravookhr** 1981;(7):45-8

**Venezuela**

Risquez-Iribarren R: Some aspects of social medicine in Venezuela. In: Congrès international d'histoire de la médecine, XXVe, Québec, 1976. Actes. Quebec, 1977. p. 237-45.

**Yugoslavia**

Dragić M: Razvoj i pioniri socijalno-medicinskih ideja u Srbiji. **Srp Arh Celok Lek** 1982 Nov;109(11):1543-53

# SOCIAL WELFARE

See also **Child Health; Economics, Medical; Public Health; State Medicine**

Cain LP: Child abuse: historical precedent and legal ramifications. **Health Soc Work** 1980 Aug;5(3):61-7
Karbowski J: Tecza nad Solferino. Warszawa, Państwony Zakład Wydawn. Lekarskich, 1973. 211 p.
Quadagno JS: From poor laws to pensions: the evolution of economic support for the aged in England and America. **Milbank Mem Fund Q** 1984 Summer;62(3):417-46
Robin M: Sheltering arms: the roots of child protection. In E. H. Newberger, ed: Child abuse. Boston, Little, Brown and Company, 1982. p. 1-21.
Sournia JC: Die Sozialmedizin. In Sournia JC, Martiny M, Poulet J, ed: Illustrierte Geschichte der Medizin. Salzburg, Andreas, 1980. Vol. 6. p. 2149-93.
Stiker HJ: Corps infirmes et sociétés. Paris, Aubier Montaigne, 1982. 250 p.

**Austria**

Kalzinger W: Das Fürsorgewesen der Stadt Linz bis zu Kaiser Josef II. **Hist Jahrb Stadt Linz** 1978;:11-94

**France**

Carré A: La révolution colbertienne et l'assistance aux familles maritimes des origines à 1673. In: Congrès National des Sociétés Savantes, 97e, Nantes, 1972. Comptes Rendus. Paris, 1976. Section des Sciences, Tome 1. p. 227-48.
Muchembled R: Le corps, la culture populaire et la culture des élites en France (XVe-XVIIIe siècle). In Imhof AE, ed: Leib und Leben in der Geschichte der Neuzeit. Berlin, Duncker & Humblot, 1983. p. 141-53.
Norberg K: Educating the poor: charity schools and charitable attitudes, Grenoble, 1600-1789. **Proc Annu Meet West Soc Fr Hist** 1980;8:181-90
Roubert J: L'adoption des enfants par des particuliers à Lyon sous l'ancien régime. **Bull Soc Fr Hist Hop** 1978;(36-37):41-67

**Great Britain**

Baker-Jones DL: 'To supply the sick poor'. **Carmarthensh Hist** 1978;:15

**Netherlands**

Alberts WJ: Armen- en ziekenzorg in Gelre en Limburg, 15de - 19de eeuw. **Spiegel Hist** 1982;17(5):278-84

**Romania**

Barbu G: Din istoria combaterii epidemiilor în ţara noastră. (I). Frăţiile milosteniei. **Rev Ig [Bacteriol]** 1984 Apr-Jun;29(2):189-92

**United States**

Breul FR, Diner SJ, ed: Compassion and responsibility. Readings in the history of social welfare policy in the United States. Chicago, London, University of Chicago Press, 1980. 372 p. Contributions by R. F. Pumphrey, C. A. Chambers, M. W. Jernegan, E. Wisner, D. M. Schneider, E. Parkhurst, B. J. Klebaner, M. B. Treudley, N. K. Teeters, W. I. Trattner, S. W. Manning, J. H. Franklin, R. H. Bremner, A. F. Davis, G. C. White, M. H. Leff, J. L. Castrovinci, J. L. Kreader, L. Gordon, B. McArthur.
Lender ME: Dictionary of American temperance biography: from temperance reform to alcohol research, the 1600s to the 1980s. Westport, Conn., Greenwood Press, 1984. xiv, 572 p.

**500 A.D.-1450**

**Belgium**

De Messemaeker-De Wilde G: De parochiale armenzorg te Gent in de late middeleeuwen. **Ann Soc Belg Hist Hop** 1980;18:47-58

**Byzantium**

Volk R: Gesundheitswesen und Wohltätigkeit im Spiegel der byzantinischen Klostertypika. München, Institut für Byzantinistik und neugriechische Philologie der Universität München, 1983. lxxx, 326 p. (Miscellanea Byzantina monacensia, Heft 28)

**France**

Assistance et charité: Toulouse, Privat, 1978. 435 p. (Cahiers de Fanjeaux, Collection d'Histoire religieuse du Languedoc au XIIIe et début du XIVe siècles, 13).
Gonthier N: Les hôpitaux et les pauvres à la fin du moyen âge: l'exemple de Lyon. **Moyen Age** 1978;84:279-308

**Germany**

Van der May-de Leur AP: Moderne pelgrimage: Sint Elisabeth-expositie Marburg 1981. **Tijdschr Ziekenverpl** 1982 Feb 2;35(3):83-6

**Venezuela**

Kleiss E: Medicine men and conditions of life in pre-Columbian Venezuela. **Arq Anat Antropol** 1978;3(3):83-112

**1450-1700**

**Belgium**

Vocht AM de: Het gentse antwoord op de armoede: de sociale instellingen van wevers en volders te Gent in de late middeleeuwen. **Ann Soc Belg Hist Hop** 1981;:3-32

**Canada**

Voisine N: Marguerite Bourdon. In Dictionary of Canadian biography, 1701 to 1740. Volume 2, 1969. p. 92-3.

**Denmark**

Dahlerup T: Den sociale forsorg og reformationen i Danmark. **Historie** 1979;13(1-2):194-207

# SOCIAL WELFARE

**France**

Blum A: Les établissements d'assistance en Basse-Alsace au début du XVIIe siècle. In Livet G, Schaff G, ed: Médecine et assistance en Alsace, XVIe–XXe siècle. Strasbourg, Istra, 1976. p. 71–86.

Patureau N: L'assistance à Tours au XVIIe siècle; la fondation de l'Hôpital Général de la Charité. In: Congrès National des Sociétés Savantes, 97e, Nantes, 1972. Actes. Paris, 1977. Histoire Moderne et Contemporaine, Tome 1. p. 431–43.

Toujas R: La lutte contre la mendicité à la fin du XVIIe siècle: l'établissement d'hôpitaux généraux dans la province ecclśiastique de Toulouse. In: Congrès National des Sociétés Savantes, 97e, Nantes, 1972. Actes. Paris, 1977. Histoire Moderne et Contemporaine, Tome 1. p. 389–401.

**Great Britain**

Evans N: Charitable bequests and their recipients. **Local Hist** 1982;15(4):225–6

Herlan RW: Relief of the poor in Bristol from late Elizabethan times until the Restoration era. **Proc Am Philos Soc** 1982 Jun 8;126(3):212–28

Kent JR: Population mobility and alms: poor migrants in the Midlands during the early seventeenth century. **Local Popul Stud (Matlock)** 1981;27:35–51

Lynch M: The 'Faithful Brethren' of Edinburgh: the acceptable face of Protestantism. **Bull Inst Hist Res** 1978;51(124):194–9

Martin L: John Crane (1571–1652); the Cambridge apothecary and philanthropist. **Med Hist** 1980;24(4):432–46

**Poland**

Karpiński A: Warunkizycia pensjonariuszy szpitali Warszawskich w XVI i w pierwszej połowie XVII wieku. **Kwart Hist Kultury Mater** 1977;25(1):43–62

**Spain**

Carreras Panchon A: El problema del niño exposito en la España ilustrada. Salamanca, 1977. 94 p. (Cuadernos de Historia de la Medicina Española, Monografías, 32).

Trueta J: Els orígens del 'Welfare State' i de les lleis socials: Lluí Vives. In Congrés International d'Història de la Medicina Catalana, 2nd, Barcelona, 1975. Llibre d'Actes. Barcelona, Socitra, 1977. p. 39–47.

**1700 to Present**

Arnold O: Charité et maladie dans la 1re moitié du XIXe siècle. **Penelope** 1981;(5):41–4

Ellacuría I: Seguridad social y solidaridad humana: aproximacion filosofica al fenomeno de la seguridad social. **Estud Cent Am** 1969;24(253):357–66

Miringoff ML: The impact of population policy upon social welfare. **Soc Serv Rev** 1980;54(3):301–16

Reinders RC: Toynbee Hall and the American settlement movement. **Soc Serv Rev** 1982;56(1):39–54

Thoire V de: L'Ordre Souverain de Malte au secours des lépreux. Vingt-cinq ans d'activité du CIOMAL 1958–1983. **Acta Leprol (Geneve)** 1983 Oct–Dec;(93):191–203

Vader JP: August Forel defends the persecuted Persian Baha'is, 1925–27. **Gesnerus** 1984;41(1/2):53–60

Zimbalist SE: Historic themes and landmarks in social welfare research. New York, Harper & Row, 1977. xii, 432 p. (Harper Series in Social Work).

**Africa**

Green E: U. S. population policies, development, and the rural poor of Africa. **J Mod Afr Stud** 1982;20(1):45–67

**Australia**

Dickey B: Care for the aged poor in Australia, 1788–1914. **Community Health Stud** 1983 Oct;7(3):247–55

Dickey B: No charity there: a short history of social welfare in Australia. Melbourne, Nelson, 1980. xix, 252 p.

Dickey B: The sick poor in New South Wales, 1840–1880: colonial practice in an amateur age. **J R Aust Hist Soc** 1973;59(1):16–28

Mendelsohn R: The condition of the people: social welfare in Australia, 1900–1975. Sydney, Allen and Unwin, 1979. 407 p.

Rodgers GF: A question of policy: is provision of special schools for defectives to be undertaken by this department? **Anzhes J** 1980;9(2):42–54

**Austria**

Federn E: Psychoanalyse und Sozialarbeit in Osterreich. **Zeitgesch** 1980;7(5):141–9

Sablik K: Julius Tandler: Mediziner und Sozialreformer: eine Biographie. Wien, A. Schendl, 1983. 389 p.

Wyklicky H: Uber die Fürsorge Josephs II. für elternlose und kranke Kinder. **Padiatr Padol** 1982;17(2):437–40

**Belgium**

Abelshausen M: De Antwerpse Werkhuizen van Liefdadigheid (1802–1870): weldadigheidsinstelling of fabriek? **Ann Soc Belg Hist Hop** 1982;20:61–108

Meuwissen E: Les dépôts de mendicité au tribunal de l'histoire. **Ann Soc Belg Hist Hop** 1981;:47–67

**Canada**

Angus MS: Harriet (Cartwright) Dobbs. In Dictionary of Canadian biography, 1881–1890. 1982;11:265–6.

Bator PA: 'The struggle to raise the lower classes': public health reform and the problem of poverty in Toronto, 1910 to 1921. **J Can Stud** 1979;14(1):43–9

Bilson G: 'Muscles and health': health and the Canadian immigrant, 1867–1906. In Roland CG, ed: Health, disease and medicine. Toronto, Hannah Institute for the History of Medicine, 1984. p. 398–411.

Meilicke CA, ed, Storch J, ed: Perspectives on Canadian health and social services policy. Edmonton, Faculty of Medicine, Univ. of Alberta, 1978. xii, 520 p.

Roland CG: War amputations in Upper Canada. **Archivaria** 1980 Summer;10:73–84

**Czechoslovakia**

Dunovský J: Zur Geschichte der Sozialpädiatrie. **Padiatr Grenzgeb** 1984;23(3):127–31

**France**

Bernier R: Les mesures publique d'assistance à la fin de l'Ancien régime dans la généralité de Caen. D.E.S. d'histoire du droit et des faits sociaux, Univ. de Caen, 1972 vii, 89, 56 p.

Beyt JP: La médecine de bienfaisance et d'assistance dans le Pas-de-Calais, 1856–1914. **Rev Nord** 1983;65(259):683–9

Constantin-Lhuillery A: Les enfants du bureau des pauvres de Chartres (1693–1715). Mém. de maîtrise. Univ. de Tours, 1976, 213 p

Ferrières M: Les Donatifs Comtadins: une iconographie hospitalière méconnue. **Bull Soc Fr Hist Hop** 1980;(40):23–8

Forget M: La fondation Roguet à Clichy. **Bull Soc Fr Hist Hop** 1978;(36–37):31–9

Huard P, Rousseau A, Wong M: Les bagnes et la médecine aux XVIIIe et XIXe siècles. In: Congrès National des Sociétés Savantes, 91e, Rennes, 1966. Comptes Rendus. Paris, 1967. Section des Sciences, Tome 1. p. 79–85.

Imbert J: L'assistance publique à Paris: le poids de l'histoire. **Rev Trav Acad Sci Morales Polit** 1978;131(2):675–89

Lamarre C: Vivre de charité à l'hôpital de Dijon au XVIIIe siècle: les secours aux enfants et aux viellards. **Bull Soc Fr Hist Hop** 1981;(42):25–35

Lamarre-Tainturier C: Les secours aux malades pauvres des campagnes dans la généralité de Bourgogne au XVIIIe siècle. In: Congrès National des Sociétés Savantes, 97e, Nantes, 1972. Actes. Paris, 1977. Histoire Moderne et Contemporaine, Tome 1. p. 499–511.

Lecomte MC: Les enfants trouvés d'après les archives du bureau des pauvres de Chartres, de 1780 à 1792. Mém. de Maîtrise, Univ. de Tours, 1976. vii, 195 p.

Lelu F: La population des 'pauvres malades' de l'Hôtel-Dieu de Provins, de 1762 à 1791. Mém. de maîtrise. Univ. de Paris I, 1976. 13, 204 p.

Oberlé R: Société et assistance à Mulhouse à la fin du XVIIIe siècle. In Livet G, Schaff G, ed: Médecine et assistance en Alsace, XVIe–XXe siècle. Strasbourg, Istra, 1976. p. 117–34.

Pihet C: Les enfants abandonnés à Poitiers dans la seconde moitié du XVIIIe siècle (1755–1789). Maîtrise, Univ. de Poitiers, 1976, XII, 222 p.

Swain Gladys: Une logique de l'inclusion: les infirmes du signe. **Esprit** 1982;5:61–75

Thieffry S: Avec Parrot, il y a un siècle, à l'Hospice des Enfants Assistés. **Ann Pediatr (Paris)** 1981 Jan;28(1):63–71

Tschill Y: Le bureau de bienfaisance de Mulhouse (1798–1848). In Livet G, Schaff G, ed: Médecine et assistance en Alsace, XVIe–XXe siècle. Strasbourg, Istra, 1976. p. 241–64.

Voldman D: Guérir du cancer et mourir de vieillesse: histoire de l'hospice Paul-Brousse de 1905 à 1975. **Asclepio** 1983;35:317–26

Weiner DB: The role of the doctor in welfare work: the Philanthropic Society of Paris, 1780–1815. **Hist Reflect** 1982;9(1–2):279–304

**Germany**

Lindemann ME: Producing policed man: poor relief, population policies and medical care in Hamburg, 1750–1806. Ph. D. Diss., University of Cincinnati. Cincinnati, 1980. vii, 386 p.

**Great Britain**

Behlmer GK: Child abuse and moral reform in England, 1870–1908. Stanford, Stanford University Press, 1982. viii, 320 p.
Berridge V, Edwards G: Opium and the people. Opiate use in nineteenth-century England. London and New York; Allen Lane and St. Martin's Press; 1981. 369 p.
Björkholm M: Mannen bakom syndromet: Thomas Hodgkin. Temperamentsfull föregångare inom patologin och kämpe för rättvisa åt förtryckta folk. **Lakartidningen** 1983 Feb 2;80(5):334–5
Blackden S: The Poor Law and wealth: a survey of parochial medical aid in Glasgow, 1845–1900. In: The search for wealth and stability. Ed. by T. C. Smout. London, Macmillan, 1979.
Bloor DU: The certifying surgeons. **J R Coll Gen Pract** 1981 Jan;31(222):33–7
Brewer C, Lait J: Can social work survive? London, Temple Smith, 1980. Historical chapters, p. 11–85.
Crowther MA: Family responsibility and state responsibility in Britain before the welfare state. **Hist J (Gt Brit)** 1982;25(1):131–45
Crowther MA: Paupers or patients? Obstacles to professionalization in the Poor Law medical service before 1914. **J Hist Med Allied Sci** 1984 Jan;39(1):33–54
Earwicker R: Miners' medical services before the First World War: the South Wales coalfield. **Llafur J Soc Stud Welsh Labour Hist** 1981;3(2):39–52
Evans N: 'The first charity in Wales': Cardiff Infirmary and South Wales Society, 1837–1914. **Welsh Hist Rev** 1979;9(3):n.p.
Gaffney R: Poor law hospitals 1845–1914. In Checkland O, Lamb M, ed: Health care as social history; the Glasgow case. Aberdeen, Aberdeen University Press, 1982. p. 44–58.
Gibson R: Little grains of sand. **Br Med J [Clin Res]** 1981 Dec 19;283(6307):1647–50
Godlove C, Mann A: Thirty years of the welfare state: current issues in British social policy for the aged. **Aged Care Serv Rev** 1980;2(1):1, 3–13
Gould F, Roweth B: Public spending and social policy: the United Kingdom 1950–1977. **J Soc Policy** 1980 Jul;9(3):337–57
Hart H: Some notes on the sponsoring of patients for hospital treatment under the voluntary system. **Med Hist** 1980;24(4):447–60
Huzel JP: The demographic impact of the old poor law: more reflexions on Malthus. **Econ Hist Rev** 1980;33:367–81
Lane J: The provincial practitioner and his services to the poor, 1750–1800. **Soc Soc Hist Med Bull (Lond)** 1981 Jun;28:10–4
Levere TH: Dr. Thomas Beddoes (1750–1808): science and medicine in politics and society. **Br J Hist Sci** 1984 Jul;17(56 pt 2):187–204
Lodge M: How we ran the welfare. **Health Visit** 1983 Jul;56(7):244–6
Loudon IS: The origins and growth of the dispensary movement in England. **Bull Hist Med** 1981;55(3):322–42
McClure RK: Coram's children, the London Foundling Hospital in the eighteenth century. New Haven, Yale University Press, 1981. xiii, 321 p.
Maggs C: The register of nurses in the Scottish poor law service 1885–1919. **Nurs Times** 1981 Nov 25–Dec 1;77(48):suppl 33:129–32
Malmoy CF, ed: The French Protestant Hospital: extracts from the Archives of 'La Providence' relating to inmates and applicants for admission, 1718–1957, and to recipients of and applicants for the Coqueau Charity, 1745–1901. 2 vols. London, Huguenot Society of London, 1977.
Marx R: Angleterre: la legende noire des 'Asiles pour pauvres'. **Histoire** 1982;46:50–9
Mazumdar PM: The eugenists and the residuum: the problem of the urban poor. **Bull Hist Med** 1980 Summer;54(2):204–15
Moore MJ: Social work and social welfare: the organization of philanthropic resources in Britain 1900–1914. **J Br Stud** 1977;16:85–104
Navarro V: Class struggle, the state and medicine. An historical and contemporary analysis of the medical sector in Great Britain. New York, Prodist, 1978. xviii, 156 p.
Neild FG: James Neild (1744–1814) and prison reform. **J R Soc Med** 1981 Nov;74(11):834–40
Pickstone JV: Ferriar's fever to Kay's cholera: disease and social structure in cottonopolis. **Hist Sci** 1984 Dec;22(58 pt 4):401–19
Pickstone JV, Butler SV: The politics of medicine in Manchester, 1788–1792: hospital reform and public health services in the early industrial city. **Med Hist** 1984 Jul;28(3):227–49
Seed P: The expansion of social work in Britain. London and Boston, Routledge and Kegan Paul, 1973. xi, 116 p.
Seligman S: The royal maternity charity: the first hundred years. **Med Hist** 1980;24(4):403–18
Spencer EM: Notes on the history of dental dispensaries. **Med Hist** 1982 Jan;26(1):47–66
Taylor R: Doctors, paupers, and landowners. The evolution of primary medical care in Orkney. **North Scotl** 1981;4(1–2):113–20
Thomas EG: The old Poor Law and medicine. **Med Hist** 1980 Jan;24(1):2–19
Walkowitz JR: Prostitution and Victorian society. Women, class, and the state. Cambridge, New York, Cambridge University Press, 1980. ix, 347 p.
Walters V: Class inequality and health care. London, Croom Helm, 1980. 175 p.
Walton RG: Women in social work. London, Boston, Routledge and Kegan Paul, 1975. xvi, 308 p.

**Greece**

Ballas C: Greek co-operatives of the 18th century and social welfare in Ampelakia of Thessaly. In: International Congress of the History of Medicine, 26th, Plovdiv (Bulgaria), 1978. Actes du Congres, Vol. 1. Sofia, 1980. p. 88–90.

**Hungary**

Friedrich I: 18. századi magyar nyelvu orvosi könyvek az 'ügyefogyott szegények' szolgálatában. **Magy Konyvsz** 1978;94(2):158–67

**Ireland**

Smith BA: Irish prison doctors--men in the middle, 1865–90. **Med Hist** 1982 Oct;26(4):371–94

**Italy**

Caprioli MP: Il patrimonio del povero. L'inchiesta sulle Opere Pie del 1861. **Quad Stor** 1980;15(3):918–41
Vigani P: Per una storia dell'assistenza in Lombardia: la pia casa degli incurabili di Abbiategrasso. **Risorgimento** 1982;34(1):48–64

**Mexico**

Malvido E: El abandono de los hijos--una forma de control del tamaño la familia y del trabajo indígena--Tula (1683–1730). **Hist Mex** 1980;29:521–61
Price R: State church charity and smallpox: an epidemic crisis in the City of Mexico 1797–98. **J R Soc Med** 1982 May;75(5):356–7
Sepúlveda B: La medicina en la seguridad social. In Academia Nacional de Medicina. Libro conmemorativo del primer centenario. México, Comité Editorial de la Comisión Organizadora del Congreso del Centenario, 1964. Tome 2. p. 678–83.
Zuckermann C: Realizaciónes en medicina asistencial. In Academia Nacional de Medicina. Libro conmemorativo del primer centenario. México, Comité Editorial de la Comisión Organizadora del Congreso del Centenario, 1964. Tome 2. p. 642–6.

**Netherlands**

Hart PD: Berustten de armen in Nederland omstreeks 1800 eerbiedig in hun lot? **Spiegel Hist** 1982;17(3):148–55
Hart PD: Waren de armen in Nederland omstreeks 1800 zorgeloze klaplopers? **Spiegel Hist** 1982;17(2):62–8
Hartog AP den: Werklozen en hun voeding in de jaren 1930–1939. **Spiegel Hist** 1982;17(9):445–51

**Poland**

Sieńkowski E: Dr med. Leon Stanisław Szuman (1852–1920), chirurg, społecznik, poeta. **Arch Hist Med (Warsz)** 1984;47(1):133–41

**Scandinavia**

Gray JA: The elderly in Scandinavia: demographic, economic, social and health conditions in 1834. **Scand J Soc Med** 1984;12(2):65–8

**Singapore**

Lee YK: Singapore's pauper and Tan Tock Seng Hospitals. . **J Malays Branch R Asiatic Soc** 1976;49(2):164–83 1977:50(2):111–35

**Spain**

Alegre Perez E: La asistencia social en la Real Botica durante el último cuarto del siglo XVIII. **Bol Soc Esp Hist Farm** 1984 Sep;35(139):199–210
Fernández Picón L: Concepcion Arenal en la historia de la medicina. Ideas medicas de Concepcion Arenal. **Asclepio** 1980;32:161–70
García Guerra D: La asistencia médica en el Hospital Real de Santiago al final del Antiguo Régimen. **Asclepio** 1983;35:287–300
Jordi González FR: Recuerdos para un Montepío. **Circ Farm** 1980 Dec;12(133):75–84

**United States**

Agris J: 'Jane Addams'. Medical student, social worker and activist, humanitarian. **J Dermatol Surg Oncol** 1979 Dec;5(12):936
Altman D: Health care for the poor. **Ann Am Acad Polit Soc Sci** 1983;(468):103–21
ANA's economic and general welfare program: a historical perspective: **ANA Publ** 1981;(EC–143):1–10
Apple RD: Lillie Rosa Minoka-Hill. In: Notable American women. The

modern period. Cambridge, Mass., Belknap-Harvard Univ. Press, 1980. 4:481-3.
Ashcraft ML, Berki SE: Health maintenance organizations as Medicaid providers. **Ann Am Acad Polit Soc Sci** 1983;(468):122-31
Auman C, et al: A state mental hospital and public welfare team up. **Public Welf** 1969;27(1):59-65
Axinn J: Jessie Taft. In: Notable American women. The modern period. Cambridge, Mass., Belknap-Harvard Univ. Press, 1980. 4:673-5.
Balasalle NM: A history of public policy for the education of handicapped children in Massachusetts. Ed.D. Dissertation, Harvard University. Cambridge, 1980. viii, 273 p.
Berkowitz E, McQuaid K: Welfare reform in the 1950s. **Soc Serv Rev** 1980 Mar;54(1):45-58
Berkowitz ED: Rehabilitation: the federal government's response to disability, 1935-1954. New York, Arno, 1980. xv, 339 p. (The Physically Handicapped in Society.) Also Ph.D. Diss., Northwestern University. Evanston, 1976.
Canon BC, Jaros D: The impact of changes in judicial doctrine: the abrogation of charitable immunity. **Law Soc Rev** 1979;13(4):969-86
Cavallo D: Sexual politics and social reform: Jane Addams, from childhood to Hull House. In: Albin, Mel, ed. New Directions in Psychohistory: The Adelphi Papers in Honor of Erik H. Erikson. Lexingon, Mass., Health, 1980: 161-82.
Chambers CA, Romanofsky P, ed: Social service organizations. 2 v. Westport, Conn., Greenwood Press, 1978. xxxiii, 843 p.
Clarke SS: Hyman J Weiner's use of systems and population approaches: their relevance to social work practice in health care today. **Soc Work Health Care** 1983 Winter;9(2):5-14
David SI: To lift a heavy burden: the story of the Medicare and Medicaid law. Ph.D. Diss., City University of New York. New York, 1982. viii, 312 p.
Davoren E: The profession of social work and the protection of children. In E. H. Newberger, ed: Child abuse. Boston, Little, Brown and Company, 1982. p. 257-73.
Dowling HF: City hospitals. The undercare of the underprivileged. Cambridge, Mass., London, Harvard University Press, 1982. vii, 245 p.
Driver WJ: Forty-fifth anniversary of social security. **Soc Secur Bull** 1980;43(8):3-5
English PC: Pediatrics and the unwanted child in history: foundling homes, disease, and the origins of foster care in New York City, 1860 to 1920. **Pediatrics** 1984 May;73(5):699-711
Field MH: Social casework practice during the 'psychiatric deluge'. **Soc Serv Rev** 1980;54(4):482-507
Fink L, Greenberg B: Organizing Montefiore: labor militancy meets a progressive health care empire. In Reverby S, Rosner D, ed: Health care in America. Philadelphia, Temple University Press, 1979. p. 226-44.
Fitzpatrick SA: Only the poor in a gilded age: public health care for the poor in St. Louis, 1890-1900. Ph.D. diss. Saint Louis University. St. Louis, 1979. 157 leaves.
Foster GM: The limitations of federal health care for freed men, 1862-1868. **J South Hist** 1982;48(3):349-72
Galishoff S: Germs know no color line: black health and public policy in Atlanta, 1900-1918. **J Hist Med Allied Sci** 1985 Jan;40(1):22-41
Graebner W: Doing the world's unhealthy work: the fiction of free choice. **Hastings Cent Rep** 1984 Aug;14(4):28-37
Grayson VS: Mary Cromwell Jarrett. In: Notable American women. The modern period. Cambridge, Mass., Belknap-Harvard Univ. Press, 1980. 4:377-9.
Greenstone JD: Dorothea Dix and Jane Addams: from transcendentalism to pragmatism in American social reform. **Soc Serv Rev** 1979;53(4):527-59
Grob GN, ed: Public policy and mental illness. Four investigations, 1915-1939. New York, Arno, 1980. Separate paginations.
Guillory F: Family planning in Louisiana. **New South** 1971;26(4):29-34
Hahn H: Paternalism and public policy. **Society** 1983;20(3):36-46
Hall D: Ointment of love: Oliver E. Comstock and Tuscon's [sic] tent city. **J Ariz Hist** 19(2):111-30, 1978
Harmon SD: Florence Kelley in Illinois. **J Ill State Hist Soc** 1981;74(3):162-78
Harvey KA: Practicing medicine at the Baltimore Almshouse, 1828-1850. **Md Hist Mag** 1979;74(3):223-37
Hasson GS: Health and welfare of freedmen in reconstruction Alabama. **Ala Rev** 1982;35(2):94-110
Herrick JM: Health care: the dilemma of delivery. **Aztlan** 1979;10:123-7
Hessler RK, Beavert CS: Citizen participation in neighborhood health centers for the poor: the politics of reform organizational change, 1965-77. **Hum Organ** 1982;41(3):245-55
History of the provisions of the old-age, survivors, disability, and health insurance program: **Soc Secur Bull** 1980;Suppl:19-40
History of the provisions of the Supplemental Security Income program for the aged, blind, and disabled: **Soc Secur Bull** 1980;Suppl:43-6
Hunt M: La charité maternelle aux Etats-Unis au 19e siècle: un cas d'étude institutionnelle, un hôpital pédiatrique. **Penelope** 1981;(5):50-1
Jacobs F: Issac Ray and the profession of psychiatry. **RI Hist** 1979;38(4):99-111
James JW: Lavinia Lloyd Dock. In: Notable American women. The modern period. Cambridge, Mass., Belknap-Harvard Univ. Press, 1980. 4:195-8.
Jones E: Social class and psychotherapy: a critical review of research. **Psychiatry** 1974;37(4):307-20
Karl BD, Katz SN: The American private philanthropic foundation and the public sphere 1890-1930. **Minerva** 1981 Summer;19(2):236-70
Katz MB: Poorhouses and the origins of the public old age home. **Milbank Mem Fund Q** 1984 Winter;62(1):110-40
Keefe DE: Governor Reagan, welfare reform and AFDC fertility. **Soc Serv Rev** 1983;57(2):234-53
Kendall KA: A sixty-year perspective of social work. **Soc Casework** 1982 Sep;63(7):424-8
Kerson TS: Medical social work. New York, Irvington Publishers, 1980. 320 p.
Lave JR, Silverman HA: Financing the health care of the aged. **Ann Am Acad Polit Soc Sci** 1983;(468):149-64
Lawton H: The myth of altruism: a psychohistory of public agency social work. **J Psychohist** 1982 Winter;9(3):265-308
Leiby J: A history of social welfare and social work in the United States. New York, Columbia University Press, 1978. 426 p.
Levin H: Conservatism of social work. **Soc Serv Rev** 1982;56(4):605-15
Marsh JC: Help seeking among addicted and nonaddicted women of low socioeconomic status. **Soc Serv Rev** 1980;54(2):239-48
Mennel RM: Ethel Sturges Dummer. In: Notable American women. The modern period. Cambridge, Mass., Belknap-Harvard Univ. Press, 1980. 4:208-10.
Morehead J: Government involvement in programs for the handicapped. **Ser Libr** 1982;7(2):7-16
Murray AE: Bright delusion: Presbyterians and African colonization. **J Presbyt Hist** 1980;58(3):224-37
Parker JK, Carpenter EM: Julia Lathrop and the Children's Bureau: the emergence of an institution. **Soc Serv Rev** 1981;55(1):60-77
Romanofsky P: Ellen Culver Potter. In Dictionary of American Biography, Suppl. 6, 1956-1960. p. 515-16, 1980.
Rosenberg CE: From almshouse to hospital: the shaping of Philadelphia General Hospital. **Milbank Mem Fund Q** 1982 Winter;60(1):108-54
Rosenkrantz BG: Booby-hatch of booby-trap: a new look at nineteenth-century reform. **Soc Res (NY)** 1972;39(4):733-43
Rosner D: Health care for the 'truly needy': nineteenth-century origins of the concept. **Milbank Mem Fund Q** 1982 Summer;60(3):355-85
Rosner D: Social control and social service: the changing use of space in charity hospitals. **Radic Hist Rev** 1979;21:183-97
Sexton PC: The life of the homeless. **Dissent** 1983;30(1):79-84
Sicherman B: Alice Hamilton. In: Notable American women. The modern period. Cambridge, Mass., Belknap-Harvard Univ. Press, 1980. 4:303-6.
Siefert K: An exemplar of primary prevention in social work: the Sheppard-Towner Act of 1921. **Soc Work Health Care** 1983 Fall;9(1):87-103
The state and public welfare in nineteenth-century America: Five investigations, 1833-1877. New York, Arno, 1976. Various pagings. Reprint of state documents. (Social Problems and Social Policy: The American Experience).
Stevens R: Sweet charity: state aid to hospitals in Pennsylvania, 1870-1910. **Bull Hist Med** 1984 Fall;58(3):287-314
Stevens R: Sweet charity: state aid to hospitals in Pennsylvania, 1870-1910. **Bull Hist Med** 1984 Winter;58(4):474-95
Stickle DF: Death and class in Baltimore: the yellow fever epidemic of 1800. **Md Hist Mag** 1979;74(3):282-99
Trattner WI: Homer Folks. In Dictionary of American biography, 1961-1965. Suppl. 7, 1981. p. 250-2.
Vogel MJ: Ida Maud Canon. In Dictionary of American Biography, Suppl. 6, 1956-1960. p. 97-8, 1980.
Woodruff NE: The failure of relief during the Arkansas drought of 1930-1931. **Arkansas Hist Q** 1980;39(4):301-13
Zainaldin JS, Tyor PL: Asylum and society: an approach to institutional change. **J Soc Hist** 1979;13(1):23-48

**USSR**

Beloborodova NL: Moskovskiĭ vospitatel'nyĭ dom i ego rol' v istorii zdravookhraneniia Rossii. **Sov Zdravookhr** 1984;(7):58-61
Chepik IK: Moral'nyi zakon nashei zhizni (obzor dokumentov Moskovskoi oblastnoi Partiinoi organizatsii vtorogo perioda velikoi otechestvennoi voiny o pomoshchi sem'iam zashchitnikov rodiny i invalidam voiny). **Sov Arkh** 1975;(6):75-80

**Yugoslavia**

Djuretić V: Socijalno-zdravstvena i kulturno-prosvjetna aktivnost organa vlasti u bosni i hercegovini izmedju drugog i trećeg zasjedanja zavnobih-a. **God Drus Istor Bosne Herceg** 1976;21-27:239-67

## SOCIETIES, ACADEMIES AND FOUNDATIONS

See also **Dentistry; Pharmacy**

Ackerknecht EH: Great doctors and scientists as freemasons. **Clio Med** 1982 Dec;17(2-3):145-56
Coing H: Remarks on the history of foundations and their role in the

promotion of learning. **Minerva** 1981 Summer;19(2):271–81

Gibson SS: Scientific societies and exchange: a facet of the history of scientific communication. **J Libr Hist** 1982 Spring;17(2):144–63

Hall MB: The Royal Society and Italy 1667–1795. **Notes Rec R Soc Lond** 1982 Aug;37(1):63–81

Kaiser W, Völker A: Zur Geschichte der ärztlichen Fortbildung auf der Ebene regionaler Vereine und Gesellschaften. **Z Gesamte Inn Med** 1983 Jul 1;38(13):348–58

Sersiron G: La croix à double barre, symbole de l'UICT. Quelques informations sur ses origines. **Bull Int Union Tuberc** 1982 Sep–Dec;57(3–4):196–9

### France

Huard PO, Imbault-Huart MJ: Le cabinet de l'Académie Royale de Chirurgie. In: Congrès National des Sociétés Savantes, 102e, Limoges, 1977. Comptes Rendus. Paris, 1977. Section des Sciences, Fasc. III. p. 15–20.

Les sociétés savantes: leur histoire: actes du 100e Congrès national des sociétés savantes, Paris, 1975, Section d'histoire moderne et contemporaine et Commission d'histoire des sciences et des techniques: Paris, Bibliothèque nationale, 1976. 386 p.

### Germany

Duka Zólyomi N: Die Leopoldinische Akademie und die ungarländische Medizin und Naturwissenschaft bis zum Ende des 18. Jahrhunderts. **Acta Hist Leopoldina** 1980;13:51–101

### Great Britain

Appleby JH: Ginseng and the Royal Society. **Notes Rec R Soc Lond** 1983 Mar;37(2):121–45

Booth CC: Medical communication: the old and new. The development of medical journals in Britain. **Br Med J [Clin Res]** 1982 Jul 10;285(6335):105–8

Dobson J, Walker RM: Barbers and barber-surgeons of London: a history of the barbers' and barber-surgeons' companies. Oxford, Blackwell Scientific Publications for the Worshipful Company of Barbers, 1979. xix, 171 p.

Ferguson JP: The College library. In Passmore R, ed: Proceedings of the Royal College of Physicians of Edinburgh Tercentenary Congress, 1981. Edinburgh, Royal College of Physicians of Edinburgh, 1982. p. 103–15.

Gibson T: The Royal College of Physicians and Surgeons of Glasgow: a short history based on the portraits and other memorabilia. Edinburgh, Macdonald Publishers, 1983. 301 p.

Girdwood RH: Three hundred years of the Royal College of Physicians of Edinburgh. **Br Med J [Clin Res]** 1981 Sep 5;283(6292):651–4

McWilliam CE: The college buildings and their architects. In Passmore R, ed: Proceedings of the Royal College of Physicians of Edinburgh Tercentenary Congress, 1981. Edinburgh, Royal College of Physicians of Edinburgh, 1982. p. 92–102.

Morrell JT: Gentlemen of science: early years of the British Association for the Advancement of Science. Oxford, Clarendon Press; New York, Oxford University Press, 1981. xxiii, 592 p.

Passmore R, ed: Proceedings of the Royal College of Physicians of Edinburgh Tercentenary Congress, 1981. Edinburgh, Royal College of Physicians of Edinburgh, 1982. xvi, 416 p. (Publication No. 56)

Robinson JO: The barber-surgeons of London. **Arch Surg** 1984 Oct;119(10):1171–5

### Hungary

Duka Zólyomi N: Az Academia Leopoldina és a magyarországi tudományosság fejl/ABodése a 18. század végéig. **Orv Hetil** 1982 Nov 28;123(48):2969–71

Kaiser W, Völker A: Zur Mitgliedschaft ungarländischer Wissenschaftler in der Academia Naturae Curiosorum (17. und 18. Jahrhundert). **Orvostort Kozl** 1981;93–96(27 No 1–4):93–111

### Japan

Neyagawa-shi Ishikai no ayumi: Neyagawa, Japan, Neyagawa-shi, [1977]. xxviii, 466 p.

Yanai Ishikai shi: [Yanai, Japan], Yanai Ishikai, [1977]. 301 p.

### Mexico

Somolinos-Palencia J, Risse GB, Price R, et al: Homenaje a la Sociedad Mexicana de Historia y Filosofía de la Medicina. **Gac Med Mex** 1982 Dec;118(12):471–84

Treviño-García Manzo N, Kumate J, Alarcón-Segovia D, et al: La Academia Nacional de Medicina en las actividades de investigación y enseñanza del país. **Gac Med Mex** 1983 Jul;119(7):274–88

### Netherlands

Veltheer W: Het chirurgijnsgilde van Amersfoort. **Tijdschr Geschied Geneeskd** 1979;2(3):101–9

### Poland

Pankiewicz Z: Cech chirurgów toruńskich w XVI, XVII i XVIII wieku. **Czas Stomatol** 1979;32(10):989–92

Sobocki S, Maciałek E: Rys historyczny towarzystw lekarskich w Jarosławiu. **Ann Univ Mariae Curie Sklodowska [Med]** 1978;33:353–9

Zajusz K: Z dziejów spółek Brackich. **Arch Hist Med (Warsz)** 1979;42(1):33–43

### Spain

Massons JM: El gobierno de las Hermandades de San Cosme y San Damián. In International Congress of the History of Medicine, 27th, Barcelona, 1980. Actas. Barcelona, Académia de Ciències Médiques de Catalunya i Balears, 1981. p. 580–5.

Matilla y Gómez V: Avance de un trabajo sobre la historia de la Academia. **An R Acad Nac Med (Madr)** 1983;100(3):497–513

### United States

Lynch EA: An historical survey of the test services of the National League for Nursing. **NLN Publ** 1980;(17–1777):i–viii, 1–78

Numbers RL: Together but not equal: amateurs and professionals in early American scientific societies. **Rev Am Hist** 1976;4(4):497–503

## 500 A.D.–1450

### Iran

Schöffler HH: Die Akademie von Gondischapur. Aristoteles auf dem Wege in den Orient. Stuttgart, Freies Geistesleben, 1979. 154 p.

## 1450–1700

### France

Chabbert P: Problèmes scientifiques évoqués à l'Académie de Castres (1648–1670). In: Congrès National des Sociétés Savantes, 100e, Paris, 1975. Actes. Paris, 1976. Histoire Moderne et Contemporaine et Histoire des Sciences. p. 21–9.

### Great Britain

Birken WJ: The Royal College of Physicians of London and its support of the parliamentary cause in the English civil war. **J Br Stud** 1983;23(1):47–62

Bonnabeau RC: The Royal College of Physicians and the apothecaries in the 17th century. A dispute for all seasons. **Minn Med** 1983 Sep;66(9):565–7

Cooke AM: Sir Hans Sloane and the Philosophical Transactions. **J R Coll Physicians Lond** 1984 Jul;18(3):170–1

Cooper DB: The Royal College of Physicians of London during the reign of the House of Stuart (1603–1714). **Trans Stud Coll Physicians Phila** 1983 Sep;5(5 No 3):191–211

Farr AD: The first human blood transfusion. **Med Hist** 1980 Apr;24(2):143–62

Force JE: Hume and the relation of science to religion among certain members of the Royal Society. **J Hist Ideas** 1984 Oct–Dec;45(4):517–36

Gregory RL: The oldest optical society in the world. **Perception** 1979;8(3):245–6

Hall AR, Boas Hall M: The first human blood transfusion: priority disputes. **Med Hist** 1980;24(4):461–5

Hunter M: Early problems in professionalizing scientific research: Nehemiah Grew (1641–1712) and the Royal Society with an unpublished letter to Henry Oldenburg. **Notes Rec R Soc Lond** 1982 Feb;36(2):189–209

Hunter M: Reconstructing restoration science: problems and pitfalls in institutional history. **Soc Stud Sci** 1982 Aug 3;12(3):451–66

McHarg JF: Dr. Johne Makluire and the 1630 attempt to establish the College. In Passmore R, ed: Proceedings of the Royal College of Physicians of Edinburgh Tercentenary Congress, 1981. Edinburgh, Royal College of Physicians of Edinburgh, 1982. p. 44–58.

Mulligan L, Mulligan G: Reconstructing restoration science: styles of leadership and social composition of the early Royal Society. **Soc Stud Sci** 1981;11(3):327–64

Simpson AD: Sir Robert Sibbald--the founder of the College. In Passmore R, ed: Proceedings of the Royal College of Physicians of Edinburgh Tercentenary Congress, 1981. Edinburgh, Royal College of Physicians of Edinburgh, 1982. p. 59–91.

Walker W: Harvey's contemporaries--science and society. **Scott Med J** 1981 Oct;26(4):356–63

Whitfield AG: Roger Marbeck--first Registrar. **J R Coll Physicians Lond** 1981 Jan;15(1):59–60

Wyman AL: John Nowell, an Elizabethan Fellow of the College of Physicians. **J R Coll Physicians Lond** 1984 Jul;18(3):166–9

**Netherlands**

Van Lieburg MJ: De 'Materia Chirurgica' in de ordonnanties en examens der Noord-Nederlandse chirurgijnsgilden vóór 1600. **Pharm Weekbl** 1981;116(45):1393–8

**1700 to Present**

Aleksandrowicz R: From the history of the Polish Anatomical Society and the International Federation of Anatomical Societies. **Folia Morphol (Warsz)** 1980;39(4):393–5
Barile MF: A brief history of the IOM. **Yale J Biol Med** 1983 Sep–Dec;56(5–6):353–4
Barone R: L'Association Mondiale des Anatomistes Vétérinaires: 1955–1980. **Anat Histol Embryol** 1980;9(3):280–8
Batári G: Az Erdélyi Orvosok Egyesülete (1833–1836). **Orv Hetil** 1981 Jul 12;122(28):1732
Bowers JZ, King EE: The conquest of yellow fever: the Rockefeller Foundation. **J Med Soc NJ** 1981 Jul;78(7):539–41
Cavazza M: Bologna and the Royal Society in the seventeenth century. **Notes Rec R Soc Lond** 1980 Dec;35(2):105–23
Cochrane RG: Notes concerning the formation of the International Leprosy Association. **Int J Lepr** 1981 Mar;49(1):67–71
Crane D: Invisible colleges: diffusion of knowledge in scientific communities. Chicago, University of Chicago Press, 1972. x, 213 p.
Curtis JB, Miller D, Simpson D: The Neurosurgical society of Australasia: the first forty years. **Aust NZ J Surg** 1980 Aug;50(4):434–7
Downs WG: The Rockefeller Foundation virus program: 1951–1971 with update to 1981. **Annu Rev Med** 1982;33:1–29
Fiori L: Les origines du CICIAMS et son évolution pendant 50 ans. **Nouv Com Int Cathol Infirm Assist Med Soc** 1983;(3):41–8
Frank SB: International Society of Tropical Dermatology in perspective. **Int J Dermatol** 1981 Jan–Feb;20(1):69–71
Helliwell PJ: The Association of Anaesthetists of Great Britain and Ireland. **Anaesthesia** 1982 Sep;37(9):913–23
The history of the International Epidemiological Association brought up to date: **Int J Epidemiol** 1984 Jun;13(2):139–41
Howard-Jones N: International public health: The organizational problems between the two World Wars (5). **WHO Chron** 1978 Mar;32(3):114–25
Howard-Jones N: The World Health Organization in historical perspective. **Perspect Biol Med** 1981 Spring;24(3):467–82
The International Federation of Surgical Colleges: 1958–1980. **Ann R Coll Surg Engl** 1981;63:290–2
Laughlin JS: AAPM and RAMPS--antecedents and perspectives. **Med Phys** 1983 Jul–Aug;10(4):387–94
Leatherman GH: 80 Jahre FDI--eine Chronik moderner Gesundheitspolitik. **Zahnarztliche Mitteilungen** 1980 Sep 1;70(17):1070–9
Leatherman GH: 80 Jahre FDI-- 'Erntejahre' 1962–1980. **Zahnarztliche Mitteilungen** 1980 Nov 1;70(21):1392–7 concl
Leatherman GH: 80 Jahre FDI--1900–1980. Aktivitäten der Kommissionen 1962–1979. **Zahnarztliche Mitteilungen** 1980 Oct 16;70(2):1313–7 contd
Leatherman GH: 80 Jahre FDI--1900–1980. Die Zeit des Wiederaufbaus und der Reformen. **Zahnarztliche Mitteilungen** 1980 Sep 16;70(18):1172–8 contd
Lechat MF: The International Leprosy Association at 50 years. **Int J Lepr** 1981 Mar;49(1):60–4
Lenzi E: Nota informativa sull'U.P.I.G.O. e sull'U.E.M.S. **Minerva Ginecol** 1981 Feb–Mar;33(2–3):153–5
Lochmann EH: Das 16. Internationale Symposion der Welt-Gesellschaft für Geschichte der Veterinärmedizin, 21.–24. Mai 1980 in Bärau, Schweiz. **Ber Wissenschaftsgesch** 1980;3(3–4):207–13
Perelló J: The history of the International Association of Logopedics and Phoniatrics. Barcelona, Augusta, 1976. 73 p.
Recollections & reflections: Lawrence J. Henderson and George Sarton. **Isis** 1984 Mar;75(276):11–32
Sanitetskollegierne i Slesvig Holsten 1804–1864: **Dan Medicinhist Arbog** 1980;:79–90
Schnitzler H, Lieth H: 25 year activities of the International Society of Biometeorology and 25 year publication index. **Int J Biometeorol** 1983 Dec;27(4):287–434
Silver anniversary of the Advisory Committee on Medical Research: **WHO Chron** 1984;38(1):8–16
Stephenson GW: Martin and Mayo plant the seeds: a history of the international program. **Bull Am Coll Surg** 1980 Jul;65(7):22–8
Sulzberger MB: My companions on the International Committee of Dermatology. **J Am Acad Dermatol** 1982 Feb;6(2):179–94
Thoire V de: L'Ordre Souverain de Malte au secours des lépreux. Vingt-cinq ans d'activité du CIOMAL 1958–1983. **Acta Leprol (Geneve)** 1983 Oct–Dec;(93):191–203
Willenegger H, Bandi W: Werdegang und Aufgabe der AO-International. Teil 2. **Unfallchirurgie** 1984 Jun;10(3):107–9

**Americas**

Garcia JC: The laziness disease. **Hist Philos Life Sci** 1981;3(1):31–59
Howard-Jones N: The Pan American Health Organization: origins and evolution (1). **WHO Chron** 1980 Oct;34(10):367–75 (contd)
Howard-Jones N: The Pan American Health Organization: origins and evolution (2). **WHO Chron** 1980 Nov;34(11):419–26 concl.
Jilek-Aall L: Acculturation, alcoholism and Indian-style Alcoholics Anonymous. **J Stud Alcohol [Suppl]** 1981 Jan;9:143–58
Neghme A: La organización panamericana de la salud en su 75. aniversario. Tributo al Dr. Abraham B. Horwitz. **Rev Med Chil** 1977 Dec;105(12):950–2
Newell FW: Pan-American Association of Ophthalmology--40 years. **Am J Ophthalmol** 1980 Mar;89(3):456–7

**Argentina**

Taquini AC: XX aniversario de la Fundación de la Sociedad Argentina de Investigación Clínica. **Medicina (B Aires)** 1979 Nov–Dec;39(6):703–5

**Australia**

Adamson J: 75th Anniversary of the Royal Australian Nursing Federation. **Australas Nurses J** 1980 Nov;9(12):3–4
Hunter T: Medical politics: decline in the hegemony of the Australian Medical Association? **Soc Sci Med** 1984;18(11):973–80
Hunter T: Pressure groups and the Australian political process: the case of the Australian Medical Association. **J Commonw Comp Polit** 1980;18(2):190–206
Kenny PJ, Miller ID: The founders of the College. New South Wales. **Aust NZ J Surg** 1981 Jun;51(3):319–25
Lowe RF: The Ophthalmological Society of Melbourne (1899–1913). **Aust J Ophthalmol** 1980 Aug;8(3):257–70
McEachern AC: The founders of the College. **Aust NZ J Surg** 1981 Aug;51(4):400–5
Origin of the NSW Nurses' Association: **Lamp** 1981 May;38(5 Suppl):9–10
Owen M: The archives of the Royal Australasian College of radiologists: guide to the history collection H706–H765 sundry accessions. **Australas Radiol** 1982 Mar;26(1):30–40
Owen MD: The archives of the Royal Australasian College of Radiologists. **Australas Radiol** 1979 Mar;23(1):15–9
Parkes D, Schachter M: Meige, Brueghel or Blake? **Aust Nurses J** 1981 Feb;10(7):32–5
Royal Australian College of General Practitioners: The Royal Australian College of General Practioners, 1958–1978. [Sydney?] The College, [1979?] 130 p.
Transcript of the amorial bearings of the Royal Australasian College of Radiologists in the letters patent: **Australas Radiol** 1982;Spec. No.:3–4
Weedon D: Conception, birth, and growth of the Australian Dermatopathology Society. **Am J Dermatopathol** 1984 Apr;6(2):159–60
Winton R: The nature of things: a history of the Royal College of Pathologists of Australasia. Sydney, The College, 1982. x, 120 p.
25th anniversary issue of Australasian Radiology: **Australas Radiol** 1982;Spec. No.:1–162

**Austria**

Holubar K: Die Dermatologie in Wien und die Deutsche Dermatologische Gesellschaft (DDG). Eine historische Perspektive. **Hautarzt** 1983;34(Suppl 6):xvii–xviii
Kerl H, Konrad K, Holubar K: The Austrian Society of Dermatopathology. **Am J Dermatopathol** 1984 Jun;6(3):221–2
Kolb A: Sebastian Kneipp und Vorarlberg. **Montfort** 1971;23(2):158–62
Paracelsus-Forschung heute: Bericht über den Jubiläumskongress 1976 und die 25 jährige Geschichte der Gesellschaft, mit Beiträgen von K. Goldammer, A. Dyk, S. Domandl. Wien, 1977. 51 p. (Salzburger Beiträge zur Paracelsusforschung, 15).
Rettig A: 35 Jahre Osterr. Krankenpflegeverband--Permanenz eines Auftrages oder einer Entwicklung. **Osterr Krankenpflegez** 1982;35(3):69–70
Roazen P: A note on the Vienna Psychoanalytic Society: Felix Deutsch's letters, 1923 and 1935. **J Hist Behav Sci** 1984 Oct;20(4):359–62
Swoboda W: 20 Jahre Osterreichische Gesellschaft für Kinderheilkunde. **Padiatr Padol** 1982;17(4):651–6

**Belgium**

In honor of the memory of Ghislaine van Massenhove, international president of CICIAMS: **Nouv Com Int Cathol Infirm Assist Med Soc** 1980;(1):1–24
Quintyn JB: Jozef Frans Kluyskens (1771–1843), eerste voorman van het Vlaams-Belgisch doktersgild. **Sartonia** 1980 Dec;49:1–37
Thielemans MR: Les sociétés scientifiques. **Rev Univ Brux** 1981;1–2:217–31

**Brazil**

Fernandes R: Jose Martins da Cruz Jobim, um fundador da Academia

Nacional de Medicina. **Rev Inst Hist Geogr Bras** 1980;327:247–68

**Bulgaria**

Glavchev P: Pogled vŭrkhu istoriiata na Druzhestvoto na internistite v Bŭlgariia (po sluchaĭ 50 godini ot osnovavaneto mu). **Vutr Boles** 1984;23(2):140–3

**Canada**

Anglin B: Twenty-five years of growing together. A history of the Ontario Association for the Mentally Retarded, 1978. 92, x p.
Angus MS: Harriet (Cartwright) Dobbs. In Dictionary of Canadian biography, 1881–1890. 1982;11:265–6.
Bernier J: Vers un nouvel ordre médical: les origines de la Corporation des Médecins et Chirurgiens du Quebec. **Rech Sociogr** 1981;22(3):307–30
Dickson I: Early history of CPA. The Canadian Psychiatric Association. **Can J Psychiatry** 1980 Feb;25(1):86–97
Ebbs JH: The Canadian Paediatric Society: its early years. **Can Med Assoc J** 1980 Dec 20;123(12):1235–7
Entin MA: Med-Chi is 140 years old: a historical sketch of the Montreal Medical Chirurgical Society. **Can J Surg** 1983 Nov;26(6):563–5
Frost SB: Science education in the 19th century: The Natural History Society of Montreal, 1827–1925. **McGill J Educ** 1982;17(1):31–48
Greben SE: CPA--yesterday and today. **Can J Psychiatry** 1980 Feb;25(1):27–9
Gridgeman NT: A semicentennial. The NRCC research journals 1929–1979. **Can J Physiol Pharmacol** 1979 Jul;57(7):i–xiv; Also in Can J Biochem 1979 Jul;57(7):iv–xvi; Also in Can J Zool 1979 Jul; 57(7):i–xiv
Labreche J: NRC: where science fiction often comes true. **Can Geogr** 1980;100(4):24–33
McCaughey D: Professional militancy: the Medical Defence Association vs. the College of Physicians & Surgeons of Ontario, 1891–1902. In Roland CG, ed: Health, disease and medicine. Toronto, Hannah Institute for the History of Medicine, 1984. p. 96–104.
McCuaig K: 'From social reform to social service': the changing role of volunteers: the anti-tuberculosis campaign, 1900–30. **Can Hist Rev** 1980;61(4):480–501
MacDougall H: 'Enlightening the public': the views and values of the Association of Executive Health Officers of Ontario, 1886–1903. In Roland CG, ed: Health, disease and medicine. Toronto, Hannah Institute for the History of Medicine, 1984. p. 436–64.
Michaud A: Evolution du syndicalisme infirmier vis-à-vis les associations professionnelles. **Infirm Can** 1981 Jul–Aug;23(7):24–7
Naylor CD: The CMA's first code of ethics: medical morality or borrowed ideology? **J Can Stud** 1982–83;17(4):20–32
Paterson GR: The Hannah Institute: promoting Canadian history of medicine. **Can Med Assoc J** 1983 Jun 1;128(11):1325–8
Shandling B: History of the Canadian Association of Paediatric Surgeons. **J Pediatr Surg** 1979 Oct;14(5):509–10
Steinhauer PD: The Canadian Academy of Child Psychiatry. The development of child psychiatry in Canada. **J Am Acad Child Psychiatry** 1982 May;21(3):217–8
Stewart B: CMA's Dr. T. Clarence Routley: 34 years of devoted service. **Can Med Assoc J** 1983 Sep 15;129(6):642–3, 645
Wier RA: Federalism, interest groups, and parliamentary government: the Canadian Medical Association. **J Commonw Polit Stud** 1973;11(2):159–75

**Chile**

Costa-Casaretto C: Recuerdos olvidados de los orígenes de la Sociedad Médica de Santiago y del la 'Revista Médica de Chile'. **Rev Med Chil** 1979 Jul;107(7):663–72

**China**

Brown ER: Exporting medical education: professionalism, modernization and imperialism. **Soc Sci Med [Med Psychol Med Sociol]** 1979 Nov;13A(6):585–95
Kühner H: Between autonomy and planning: the Chinese Academy of Sciences in transition. **Minerva** 1984 Spring;22(1):13–44
Schneider LA: The Rockefeller Foundation, the China Foundation, and the development of modern science in China. **Soc Sci Med** 1982;16(12):1217–21

**Cuba**

Bustamante O'Leary J: La Academia de Ciencias Médicas, Físicas y Naturales de la Habana. **Conf Estud Hist Organ Cienc** 1979;11:1–19
Fernandez-Conde A: One Cuban physician's odyssey. **J Fla Med Assoc** 1979 Aug;66(8):845–52

**Czechoslovakia**

Barta T, Klačanský I: Tridsat rokov Slovenskej otolaryngologickej spoločnosti. **Cesk Otolaryngol** 1984 Feb;33(1):47–51
Dienstbier Z: 25 let Ceskoslovenské společnosti nukleární medicíny a radiační hygieny. **Cas Lek Cesk** 1981 Aug 13;120(31–32):963–7
Dienstbier Z: 25 years of the Czechoslovak Society for Nuclear Medicine and Radiation Hygiene. **Czech Med** 1981;4(3):97–106
Drahota Z: Třicet let Fyziologického ústavu CSAV. **Cesk Fysiol** 1984;33(4):289–92
Hlaváčková L: Casopis lékařu českých a Spolek českých lékařu v boji za českou universitu a lékařskou fakultu. **Cas Lek Cesk** 1982 Dec 23;121(51):1569–73
Homolka J: Třicet let Ceskoslovenské lékařské společnosti J.E. Purkyně. **Cas Lek Cesk** 1979 Dec 14;118(50):1541–7
Homolka J: Ze začátku historie Společnosti klinické biochemie. **Cas Lek Cesk** 1981 Jun 11;120(23):713–5
Hromádková J: Medici v boji za Ceskou Univerzitu a Lékařskou Fakultu. II. Spolek českých mediku a jeho úloha v boji za českou lékařskou fakultu. **Sb Lek** 1984 Apr;86(4):119–28
Janisch R: 60 let Ceskoslovenské biologické společnosti při CSAV v Brně. **Cas Lek Cesk** 1982 Nov;121(47):1467–8
Niederland TR: Desat rokov Slovenskej lekárskej spoločnosti a tridsat rokov Ceskoslovenskej lekárskej spoločnosti Jana E. Purkyne. **Cas Lek Cesk** 1979 Dec 14;118(50):1548–51
Petrášek J: Třicet let Slovenské akademie věd. **Cas Lek Cesk** 1983 Dec 16;122(50):1568
Reiniš Z: Padesát let Ceskoslovenské kardiologické společnosti. **Cas Lek Cesk** 1979 Nov 9;118(45):1404–7
Reiniš Z: Přehled 50 leté činnosti Cs. kardiologické spolčnosti. **Vnitr Lek** 1980 Apr;26(4):306–9
Reiniš Z, Gvozdják J, Widimský J, et al: The fiftieth anniversary of the Czechoslovak Society of Cardiology. **Cor Vasa** 1979;21(6):445–9
Remišová M: Slovenské národné povstanie a nový prístup k organizovaniu odborného spolkového života lekárov. **Bratisl Lek Listy** 1979 Aug;72(2):141–6
Tesař J: Sto let českeho ústavu pro soudní lékařství v Praze. **Soud Lek** 1984 Aug;29(3):33–9
Válek A: Ceskoslovenské nefrologické spolecnosti je dvacet let. **Cas Lek Cesk** 1982 May 7;121(18):568–71
Zadina R: První sjezd českých lékařu a přírodozpytcu v Praze roku 1880. **Cas Lek Cesk** 1980 Jan 11;119(2):64

**Denmark**

[1857–1982 – the National Danish Medical Society: 125th anniversary]: **Ugeskr Laeger** 1982 Aug 30;144(35):2549–616

**Europe**

Brihaye J: Celebration of the 10th anniversary of the European Association of Neurosurgical Societies. **Acta Neurochir (Wien)** 1982;60(1–2):1–6
Brihaye J: History of the European Association of Neurosurgical Societies. **Neurosurgery** 1984 Aug;15(2):262–4
Lindskog BI: Europeisk musei-konferens. **Sydsven Medicinhist Sallsk Arsskr** 1984;21:11–4
Olesińska-Serafin A: Europejskie Stowarzyszenie Kształcenia Medycznego i jego wpływ na rozwój dydaktyki medycznej. **Pol Tyg Lek** 1984 Mar 26;39(13):453–5
Roscam Abbing HD: International organizations in Europe and the right to health care. Antwerp, Boston, Kluwer-Deventer, 1979. xii, 278 p.
Skreb N, McKenzie J: The early days of European Developmental Biology Organisation (E.D.B.O.). **Anat Anz** 1981;150(4):443–8
Snellen HA: Birth and growth of the European Society of Cardiology. **Eur Heart J** 1980 Feb;1(1):5–7

**Finland**

Pöyry M: Mikkelin läänin kätilöyhdistys 80 vuotta. **Katilolehti** 1980 Mar;85(3):97–100
Raivio K: Satavuotias duodecim-seura ja kehittyyä lääketiede. **Duodecim** 1981;97(20):1661–3

**France**

Arquiola E: Darwinism in the Société d'Anthropologie de Paris. **Clio Med** 1980 May;14(2):119–28
Arquiola E: La antropologia criminal y la 'Societe d'Anthropologie' de Paris. **Asclepio** 1978–79;30–31:63–82
Bec P: Le prochain centenaire de la société française d'ophtalmologie (1883–1983). **J Fr Ophtalmol** 1980;3(5):313–4
Bellet P: Les membres résidents de la Société, puis Académie de Pharmacie. **Rev Hist Pharm (Paris)** 1981 Jun;28(249):118–20
Bernard J: Robert Debré: l'humanisme et les académies. **Bull Acad Natl Med (Paris)** 1982 Dec;166(9):1281–4
Biéder J: Un président de la Société Médico-Psychologique: Prosper Lucas (1808–1885). **Ann Med Psychol (Paris)** 1983 Sep–Oct;141(8):908–15
Bonnemain H: La Société d'Histoire de la Pharmacie; sa création – son développement – ses activités. In: Vorträge des Internationalen Pharmaziehistorischen Kongresses Innsbruck 1977. Stuttgart, Wissenschaftliche Verlagsgesellschaft, 1979. p. 81–90.
Brazier MA: The birth of the International Brain Research Organization:

a tribute to Henri Gastaut. **Electroencephalogr Clin Neurophysiol** 1982;35:13–4

Brégeat P: Antoine Portal, fondateur de l'Académie de médecine. **Bull Acad Natl Med (Paris)** 1982 Dec;166(9):1304–16

Centenaire de la Société Française d'Ophtalmologie: **Bull Mem Soc Fr Ophtalmol** 1983;95:clxxxiii–cxcix

Chaia J: Vicq d'Azyr, la Société Royale de Médecine et la Guyane. In: Congrès National des Sociétés Savantes, 105e, Caen, 1980. Comptes Rendus, Paris, 1980. Section des Sciences, Fasc. V. p. 9–15.

Cinquantenaire de la Société d'Oto-Rhino-Laryngologie de Lyon et de la Région. Le ler mars 1931: **J Fr Otorhinolaryngol** 1982 Jun;31(6):389–96

Cosma-Muller P: Entre science et commerce: les eaux minerales en France a la fin de l'ancien regime. **Hist Reflect** 1982;9(1–2):249–62

Crosland M: From prizes to grants in the support of scientific research in France in the nineteenth century: the Montyon legacy. **Minerva** 1979 Autumn;17(3):355–80

Degleris N: Contribution à l'étude des relations Franco-Helleniques au point de vue de la presse neuro-psychiatrique française (1880–1914); les membres associés grecs de la Société Médico-Psychologique. Mémoire pour le titre d'assistant étranger, Université Paris V, René Descartes, Faculté de Médecine Cochin-Port Royal, Paris, 1984. 96 leaves.

Desaive JP: L'alimentation populaire d'après les archives de l'Académie de Médecine (1774–1794). In: Congrès National des Sociétés Savantes, 93e, Tours, 1968. Actes. Paris, 1971. Section d'Histoire Moderne et Contemporaine, Tome 1. p. 39–53.

Dodin A: Albert Calmette. Président de la Société de Pathologie Exotique. **Bull Soc Pathol Exot Filiales** 1983 May–Jun;76(3):211–4

Dulieu L: La Société Royale des Sciences de Montpellier (1706–1792). In: Congrès National des Sociétés Savantes, 100e, Paris, 1975. Actes. Paris, 1976. Histoire Moderne et Contemporaine et Histoire des Sciences. p. 43–8.

Forget M: La fondation Roguet à Clichy. **Bull Soc Fr Hist Hop** 1978;(36–37):31–9

Godlewski G: De l'Académie de médecine à l'Académie française. **Bull Acad Natl Med (Paris)** 1982 Mar;166(3):407–13

Grivaux M: Soixante-quinzième anniversaire de l'Associaton d'Enseignement médical des Hôpitaux de Paris (1907–1982). **Sem Hop Paris** 1983 Mar 31;59(13):865–7

Guillermand J: Un anniversaire et une tradition: l'Académie Royale de Chirurgie. **Med Armees** 1981;9:807–11

Hillemand P, Gilbrin E: Le Père Elisée, premier chirurgien de Louis XVIII et la création de l'Académie de Médecine. **Bull Acad Natl Med (Paris)** 1981 Jan;165(1):23–6

Huard P, Imbault-Huart MJ: L'Académie royale de chirurgie après le 8 aout 1793. In: Congrès National des Sociétés Savantes, 100e, Paris, 1975. Actes. Paris, 1976. Histoire Moderne et Contemporaine et Histoire des Sciences. p. 297–308.

Huard P, Imbault-Huart MJ: Le concept d'Académie en France au XVIIIe siècle; son évolution face à la médecine et à la chirurgie. In: Congrés National des Sociétés Savantes, 100e, Paris, 1975. Actes. Paris, 1976. Histoire Moderne et Contemporaine et Histoire des Sciences. p. 289–96.

Huard P, Imbault-Huart MJ: Les papiers d'Antoine Louis (1723–1792). In: Congrès National des Sociétés Savantes, 102e, Limoges, 1977. Comptes Rendus. Paris, 1977. Section des Sciences, Fasc. III. p. 7–14.

Joblin J: Monseigneur André Jacques Fougerat; ecclesiastical advisor of CICIAMS (1952–1982). **Nouv Com Int Cathol Infirm Assist Med Soc** 1983;(3):1–8

Le Grand HE: Chemistry in a provincial context: the Montpellier Société Royale des Sciences in the eighteenth century. **Ambix** 1982 Jul;29(2):88–105

Legée G: L'influence de la Société d'Auteuil sur les travaux des physiologistes. In: Congrès National des Sociétés Savantes, 100e, Paris, 1975. Actes. Paris, 1976. Histoire Moderne et Contemporaine et Histoire des Sciences. p. 229–42.

Lennox MA: Professor Gastaut's contribution to the International League against Epilepsy. **Electroencephalogr Clin Neurophysiol** 1982;35:9–12

McClellan JE: The Académie Royale des Sciences, 1699–1793: a statistical portrait. **Isis** 1981 Dec;72(264):541–67

Naquet R: Gastaut and the EEG Federation. **Electroencephalogr Clin Neurophysiol** 1982;35:7–8

Ourgaud AG: Souvenirs concernant la création de la Sociéte d'ophtalmologie du Midi de la France et du Journal d'Ophtalmologie. **Bull Soc Ophtalmol Fr** 1983 Feb;83(2):309–12

Paul CB: Science and immortality. The eloges of the Paris Academy of Sciences (1699–1791). Berkeley, University of California Press, 1980. x, 202 p.

Péquignot H: Société Médicale des Hôpitaux de Paris. **Ann Med Interne (Paris)** 1980;131(2):125–8

Ramsey M: Traditional medicine and medical enlightenment: the regulation of secret remedies in the ancien regime. **Hist Reflect** 1982;9(1–2):215–32

Rigault J: Les membres de l'Académie des Sciences Arts et Belles-lettres de Dijon de 1798 à 1914. In: Congrès National des Sociétés Savantes, 100e, Paris, 1975. Actes. Paris, 1976. Histoire Moderne et Contemporaine et Histoire des Sciences. p. 145–50.

Satran R: Les débuts de la Société française de neurologie. **Hist Sci Med** 1981;15(2):188–95

Sicard A: Allocution de André Sicard Président de L'Académie nationale de médecine. **Bull Acad Natl Med (Paris)** 1982 Dec;166(9):1243–9

Sicard A: Historique de l'Académie de Chirurgie. **Chirurgie** 1981;107(9):713–8

Sicard A: Hommage rendu au cimetière Saint-Pierre de Montmartre par l'Académie nationale de médecine au baron Antoine Portal, son fondateur, à l'occasion du 150e anniversaire de sa mort. **Hist Sci Med** 1983;17(2):195–8

Société française d'histoire des hôpitaux: [1978–79 prizes in hospital history]: **Bull Soc Fr Hist Hop** 1980;(40):4–22

Sournia JC: Littré l'Académie de Médecine. **Bull Acad Natl Med (Paris)** 1981 Oct;165(7):941–7

Szállási A: 1925-ben alakult meg a Párizsi Magyar Egyesület. **Orv Hetil** 1980 Sept 21;121(38):2339–40

Szwejcerowa A: O Towarzystwie Lekarzy Niemieckich w Paryzu. **Arch Hist Med (Warsz)** 1979;42(3):323–30

Theil P: Brève histoire de l'Ordre des Médecins. **Bull Acad Natl Med (Paris)** 1981 Jun;165(6):739–45

Théodoridès J: Un correspondant breton de la Société Royale de Médecine: Claude-Marie Robin de Keriavalle (1743–1785). In: Congrès National des Sociétés Savantes, 107e. Brest, 1982. Comptes Rendus, Paris, 1983. Section des Sciences, Fasc. IV. p. 225–39.

Tournier-Lasserve C: La Peyronie et la présence des chirurgiens militaires au sein de l'Académie de Chirurgie. **Chirurgie** 1981;107(9):719–22

Tournier-Lasserve C: Les chirurgiens militaires et l'Académie de médecine. **Bull Acad Natl Med (Paris)** 1982 May;166(5):601–8

Valette G: Allocution du Président de l'Académie Nationale de Médecine. **Bull Acad Natl Med (Paris)** 1980 Dec;164(9):801–4

Weiner DB: The role of the doctor in welfare work: the Philanthropic Society of Paris, 1780–1815. **Hist Reflect** 1982;9(1–2):279–304

Witczak W: Towarzystwo Paryskie Lekarzy Polskich (w 125 rocznice powstania). **Przegl Lek** 1984;41(4):325–7

### Germany

Artía A: Centenario de la fundación de la Sociedad Alemana de Pediatría. Influencia de ésta en la pediatría chilena. **Rev Chil Pediatr** 1983 Nov–Dec;54(6):387–9

Bethge R, Knöfler EW: 30 Jahre Gesellschaft für Orthopädie der DDR--Zur Erinnerung an ihren Mitbegründer und ersten Vorsitzenden Friedrich Loeffler. **Beitr Orthop Traumatol** 1983 May;30(5):233–6

Biermann KR: Alexander von Humboldt in seinem Verhältnis zur Leopoldina und zu anderen Akademien. **Acta Hist Leopoldina** 1980;13:39–49

Bugyi B: Tagung der Deutschen Gesellschaft für Geschichte der Medizin und der Naturwissenschaften im Jahre 1929 zu Budapest. **Orvostort Kozl** 1979;86(24 no 4):65–71

Diercksen G, et al: Aus der Chronik der Aerzteschaft Karlsruhe, 1715–1977: nach alten Aufzeichnungen, aktuellen Berichten, Biographien und Presseveröffentlichungen. Karlsruhe, Aerzteschaft Karlsruhe, 1978. 519, 8 p.

Efkes F: Entstehung und Entwicklung der studentischen Korporationen an der Tierärztlichen Hochschule Hannover im 19. Jahrhundert. Diss. Hannover, 1978. 227 p.

Ehrhardt H: 130 Jahre Deutsche Gesellschaft für Psychiatrie und Nervenheilkunde. Wiesbaden, Steiner, 1972. 125 p.

Engelbrecht H, Gräfner G, Müller P, et al: 20 Jahre Parasitologische Gesellschaft der DDR. **Angew Parasitol** 1981 Nov;22(4):185–92

Flehr H: Geschichte des Arztlichen Vereins in Frankfurt am Main und sein standespolitisches Wirken. Diss. Mainz, 1982. 144 p.

Ganguin HG: Beitrag der medizinisch-wissenschaftlichen Gesselschaft für Bronchopneumonologie der DDR und ihrer Sektionen zur Entwicklung des Fachgebietes Bronchopneumonologie. **Z Erkr Atmungsorgane** 1979 Apr;153(11):5–13

Garnerus K: Die Versammlungen Deutscher Narturforscher und Arzte--Medaillen berichten. **Naturwissenschaften** 1982 Apr;69(4):158–61

Goerke H: 150 Jahre Arztlicher Verein München. Rückschau auf Gründung, Aufgaben und Leistungen. **MMW** 1983 Oct 14;125(41):906–10

Greeff K: Zur 48. Jahrestagung der Deutschen Gesellschaft für Herz- und Kreislaufforschung. Eröffnungsansprache. **Verh Dtsch Ges Herz Kreislaufforsch** 1982;48:XI–XX

Gsell O: Hundert Jahre innere Medizin. Eröffnungsreden der Vorsitzenden der Deutschen Gesellschaft für innere Medizin. I. Teil 1882–1932. **Med Welt** 1983 Apr 8;34(14):428–33

Hamelmann H: Zur Geschichte der Vereinigung Nordwestdeutscher Chirurgen: zur 125. Tagung 12.-14. Juni 1980. Lübeck, Wullenwever, 1980?. 103 p.

Hein WH: Historische und kritische Betrachtungen zu den Veröffentlichungen der Gesellschaft. In: Vorträge des Internationalen Pharmaziehistorischen Kongresses Innsbruck 1977. Stuttgart, Wissenschaftliche Verlagsgesellschaft, 1979. p. 15–22.

Hesse A: Aerztliche Vereine und Standesorganisationen in Freiburg i. Br. Entwicklung und Struktur. Freiburg, Schulz, 1978. 321 p. (Freiburger Forschungen zur Medizingeschichte, Neue Folge, 8).

Jungnickel C: The Royal Saxon Society of Sciences: a study of nineteenth century German science. Ph.D. Diss., Johns Hopkins University. Baltimore, 1978. v, 222 leaves.

Kalcher J: Ambrosius war kein Dinosaurier--dem Hansischen Jugendbund nachträglich zum Geburtstag. Versuch einer Deutung. **Prax Kinderpsychol Kinderpsychiatr** 1979 Aug-Sep;28(6):212-24

Kohlhausen K: 30 Jahre Bundesverband der Vertrauensärzte (jetzt: Bundesverband der Vertrauens- und Rentenversicherungsärzte e.V.). **Off Gesundheitswes** 1982 Apr;44(4):205-8

Kugler J: Zur Entwicklung der Deutschen EEG-Gesellschaft. **EEG EMG** 1984 Mar;15(1):1-7

Labisch A: Neue Quellen zum gesundheitspolitischen Programm der MSPD von 1920/22. **Int Wiss Korresp Gesch Dtsch Arb-bew** 1980 June;16(2):231-47

Labisch A: Selbsthilfe zwischen Auflehnung und Anpassung. Arbeiter-Sanitätskommission und Arbeiter-Samariterbund. **Jahrb Krit Med** 1983;77:11-26

Labisch A: The Workingmen's Samaritan Federation (Arbeiter-Samariter-Bund) 1888-1933. **J Contemp Hist** 1978;13:297-322

Lange G: Die Vereinigung Westdeutscher Hals-, Nasen- und Ohrenärzte besteht im 85-sten Jahr. **HNO** 1982 Mar;30(3):114-5

Lindner H, et al, ed: [Contemporary medical historiography in Germany]. **Nachrichtenbl Dtsch Ges Gesch Med Naturwiss Tech** 1980 Apr;30(1):1-64

Lund OE: 125 Jahre Deutsche Ophthalmologische Gesellschaft. **MMW** 1982 Sep 10;124(36):761

Matthes T: Die medizinisch-wissenschaftlichen Gesellschaften der DDR: Geschichte, Funktion, Aufgaben. Berlin, Volk und Gesundheit, 1981. 239 p., 371 p.

Oehme J: Rückbesinnung zum 100 jährigen Bestehen der Deutschen Gesellschaft für Kinderheilkunde. **Klin Paediatr** 1983 Jan-Feb;195(1):1-3

Querner H: 'Ein Wort über den Einfluss naturwissenschaftlicher Institute auf humane Bildung' (G. A. Goldfuss 1821). In Seidler E, Schott H, ed: Bausteine zur Medizingeschichte. Stuttgart, Steiner, 1984. p. 86-93.

Ratti A: I 75 anni della Deutsche Röntgengesellschaft. **Radiol Med (Torino)** 1980 Jul-Aug;66(7-8):481-4

Rothe J, Ewert G: Od pracovního společenství sociálních hygienikuke společnosti sociální hygieny NDR. **Cesk Zdrav** 1981 Jan;29(1):5-9

Rothschuh KE, Krafft F: Forschungsberichte und Spezial-Bibliographien. **Ber Wissenschaftsgesch** 1978;1(3-4):201-15

Scharkoff H: 25 Jahre Gesellschaft für Bronchopneumonologie und Tuberkulose der DDR. **Z Erkr Atmungsorgane** 1983;160(3):199-200

Scheuch DW, Hoffmann H: 20 Jahre Gesellschaft für Klinische Chemie und Laboratoriumsdiagnostik der DDR. **Z Med Lab Diagn** 1983;24(7):371-80

Schierhorn H: Die Multinationalität der Anatomischen Gesellschaft und die Mehrsprachigkeit ihrer Versammlungen. **Anat Anz** 1980;148(2):168-206

Schober KL: Gedächtnisvorlesung zum 150. Geburtstag von Richard von Volkmann, dem Mit-Gründer der Deutschen Gesellschaft für Chirurgie. **Langenbecks Arch Chir** 1981;355:597-606

Seidler E: Die Freiburger Gobineau-Vereinigung und die Verbreitung des Arier-Gedankens in Deutschland. In Seidler E, Schott H, ed: Bausteine zur Medizingeschichte. Stuttgart, Steiner, 1984. p. 121-9.

Wankmüller A: Die Bibliothek der Internationalen Gesellschaft für Geschichte der Pharmazie. **Ber Wissenschaftsgesch** 1979;2(3-4):226-8

Winau R: Deutsche Gesellschaft für Geschichte der Medizin, Naturwissenschaft und Tecknik 1901-1976. Wiesbaden, Steiner, 1978. 164 p. (Beiträge zur Geschichte der Wissenschaft und der Technik, 15).

Zopff G: Erinnerungen an die Anfänge des Berufsverbandes. **Chirurg** 1980 Aug;51(8):128-9

### Great Britain

Allen DE: James Edward Smith and the Natural History Society of Edinburgh. **J Soc Bibliogr Nat Hist** 1978;8(4):483-93

Ashton N: Ophthalmological Societies of the United Kingdom. Centenary Meeting, April 1980. **Trans Ophthalmol Soc UK** 1980 Apr;100(pt 1):1-8

Ashton RM: The Royal College of Midwives: past, present and future. **Int J Gynaecol Obstet** 1979-80 Sep-Oct;17(2):124-7

Bayliss RA: The Round Table Club, Edinburgh. **Practitioner** 1980 Apr;224(1342):438-40

Bliquez LJ: An unidentified Roman surgical instrument in Bingen. **J Hist Med Allied Sci** 1981 Apr;36(2):219-20

Bloor DU: Club practice. **J R Coll Gen Pract** 1982 May;32(238):310 5

Bradburne P, Williams PO: The Wellcome Trust story. **Grants Mag** 1978 Sep;1(3):196-205

Brown A: COHSE: pioneers from the past. **Nurs Mirror** 1980 Jul 10;151(2):8

Campbell N, Smellie RM: The Royal Society of Edinburgh (1783-1983). The first two hundred years. Edinburgh, The Society, 1983. xvi, 186 p.

Cardwell D, Mottram J: Fresh light on John Dalton. **Notes Rec R Soc Lond** 1984 Sep;39(1):29-40

Charlton C: The National Health Society Almanack, 1883. **Local Popul Stud (Matlock)** 1984;32:54-7

Cockshott WP: Old medical societies. **N Engl J Med** 1980 Dec 4;303(23):1371

Cowell B, Wainwright D: Behind the blue door: the history of the Royal College of Midwives, 1881-1981. London, Baillière Tindall, 1981. 111 p.

Cowell B: Royal College of Midwives: one hundred years young! **Nurs Mirror** 1981 Jul 15;153(3):18-20

Cowell B, Wainwright D: The battle for status. **Nurs Times** 1981 Jul 15-21;77(29):1237-8

Craig P: The first B.M.A. meeting in Bristol. **Bristol Med Chir J** 1983 Jul;98(367):104-8

Crosland M: Explicit qualifications as a criterion for membership of the Royal Society: a historical review. **Notes Rec R Soc Lond** 1983 Mar;37(2):167-87

Douglas A: Promises to keep. **Thorax** 1984 Jul;39(7):481-6

Duncan A: The Royal Counties Veterinary Association 1883-1983. **Vet Rec** 1983 Dec 10;113(24):552-3

Earwicker R: A study of the BMA-TUC Joint Committee on Medical Questions, 1935-1939. **J Soc Policy** 1979;8:335-56

Emerson RL: The Philosophical Society of Edinburgh 1748-1768. **Br J Hist Sci** 1981 Jul;14(pt 2 no 47):133-76

Evans N: 'The first charity in Wales': Cardiff Infirmary and South Wales Society, 1837-1914. **Welsh Hist Rev** 1979;9(3):n.p.

Ferrer M: The Royal College of Midwives 1881 - 1981. **Midwife Health Visit Community Nurse** 1981 Jul;17(7):288-94

Foster WD: The Church Missionary Society and modern medicine in Uganda. The life of Sir Albert Cook, K.C.M.G., 1870-1951. Newhaven, Sussex, [The author], 1978. 234 p.

Fry J, Hunt JH, Pisent RJ, ed: A history of the Royal College of General Practitioners. The first 25 years. Lancaster, Boston, MTP Press, 1983. xiii, 270 p.

Fry J, Hunt JH, Pinsent RJ: The Royal College of General Practitioners: the first 25 years.

Gleason ML: The Royal Society of London: years of reform, 1827-1847. Ph.D. Diss. Harvard University. Cambridge, Mass. 1979.

Grabham AH: Precepts and practice: Charles Hastings's vision and reality. **Br Med J [Clin Res]** 1982 Dec 18-25;285(6357):1789-92

Grant AS: The RCM--the first 100 years: some things never change. **Midwives Chron** 1981 Oct;95(1125):348-50

Hall MB: The Royal Society in Thomas Henry Huxley's time. **Notes Rec R Soc Lond** 1984;38(2):153-8

Hankins TL: Prosopography of the British Association: an essay review. **J Hist Med Allied Sci** 1982 Oct;37(4):451-4

Henderson WM: Wellcome research: virology and the promotion of animal health. **Vet Rec** 1980 Oct 11;107(15):347-50

Hoffenberg R: Fiftieth anniversary. Medical Research Society. **Clin Sci** 1981 Sep;61(3):355-6

Horder J: The origin of the Royal College of General Practitioners. **Soc Soc Hist Med Bull (Lond)** 1983 Dec;33:13-4

Innes J: The Harveians of Edinburgh--their first two hundred years. **Scott Med J** 1983 Jul;28(3):285-9

Jones GR: The King Edward VII Welsh National Memorial Association, 1912-1948. In J. Cule, ed: Wales and medicine. London, British Society for the History of Medicine, 1975. p. 30-41.

Joynt RJ: The great confrontation: the meeting between Broca and Jackson in 1868. In Rose FC, Bynum WF, ed: Historical aspects of the neurosciences. New York, Raven, 1982. p. 99-102.

King P: The contributions of Ernest Jones to the British Psycho-Analytical Society. **Int J Psychoanal** 1979;60(Pt 3):280-4

King PH: The life and work of Melanie Klein in the British Psycho-Analytical Society. **Int J Psychoanal** 1983;64 (Pt 3):251-60

Kinloch J: The Society and College of Radiographers--60 years on. **Radiography** 1980 Dec;46(552):271-87

Landes RR, Hall S: A letter from Joseph Lister to Dr. David Walsh. **JAMA** 1984 Jun 15;251(23):3101-3

Levere TH: Dr. Thomas Beddoes (1750-1808): science and medicine in politics and society. **Br J Hist Sci** 1984 Jul;17(56 pt 2):187-204

Limentani A: Anna Freud's contribution to the work of the International Psychoanalytical Association. **Int J Psychoanal** 1983;64 (Pt 4):375-7

Lyte C: Sir Joseph Banks, 18th century explorer, botanist and entrepreneur. London, David & Charles, 1980. 248 p.

MacLeod RM, Collins P: The parliament of science: the British Association for the Advancement of Science 1831-1981. London, Science Reviews, 1981. vi, 308 p.

Mahta M: The history of the Intractable Pain Society of Great Britain and Ireland. **Pain** 1980 Feb;8(1):121 2

Manson-Bahr PE, Willmott S: Dermatology and the Royal Society of Tropical Medicine and Hygiene. **Int J Dermatol** 1981 Jul-Aug;20(6):429-30

Marks J: The Conference of Local Medical Committees and its executive: an historical review. [London?], Trustees of the General Medical Services Defence Trust, 1979. 32 p.

Matsufuji G: [Phosphor-poisoning in match factories and the Salvation Army General Booth] (Jpn). **Igakushi Kenkyu** 1980;54:1-6

Maxwell VB: The first 2 years--a brief history of the British Association of Aviation Medical Examiners. **Aviat Space Environ Med** 1983 May;54(5):xiii-xiv

Miller DP: The Royal Society of London 1800-1835: a study in the cultural politics of scientific organization. Ph. D. Diss., University of Pennsylvania, Philadelphia, 1981. vii, 422 leaves.

Mitchell M: History of the British Optical Association, 1895-1978: with additional material covering the founding of the British College of

Ophthalmic Opticians (Optometrists) and the liquidation of the B.O.A. [London], The Association and the British Optical Association Foundation, [1982]. 304 p.
Newell FW: The Ophthalmological Society of the United Kingdom: its first hundred years. **Am J Ophthalmol** 1980 Apr;89(4):605–7
Newman CE: The history of the College library, 1879–99. **J R Coll Physicians Lond** 1984 Jan;18(1):66–73
Payne LM, Newman CE: The history of the College library: the eighteen-seventies. **J R Coll Physicians Lond** 1984 Jul;18(3):198–202
Peel J: The lives of the fellows of the Royal College of Obstetricians and Gynaecologists, 1929–1969. London, Heinemann, 1976. xviii, 390 p.
Peel J, Robinson J: The Oxford and Cambridge graduates' medical clubs. **Br Med J [Clin Res]** 1983 Dec 24–31;287(6409):1979–81
Pelling M, ed: Handlist of records of the Society of Medical Officers of Health deposited at the Wellcome Unit for the History of Medicine, Oxford, 4 May 1976, with later deposits and other locations. Oxford, Wellcome Unit for the History of Medicine, 1980 23 p. (Research Publications of the Wellcome Unit for the History of Medicine. Oxford, No. III).
Platt H: The foundation of the Association of Surgeons of Great Britain and Ireland. **Br J Surg** 1982 Oct;69(10):561–3
Pochin EE: Early days of the Medical Research Society. **Clin Sci** 1981 Sep;61(3):357–60
Price R: St. Albans Medical Club. **J Int Wine Food Soc** 1979;6(1):7–12
Proudfit WL: The Fleece Medical Society. **Br Heart J** 1981 Dec;46(6):589–94
Ratcliffe DS: The evolution of medical societies in Britain---have they a future? **Bristol Med Chir J** 1979 Jan–Apr;94(349–350):3–10, 13–4
Ross JP, LeFanu WR, ed: Lives of the Fellows of the Royal College of Surgeons of England 1965–1973. London, Pitman Medical, 1981. 405 p.
Ross WM: Carcinoma of the breast in the section of radiology. **J R Soc Med** 1980 Oct;73(10):734–8
Ross WM: The Institute: yesterday and tomorrow. **Br J Radiol** 1980 Feb;53(626):55–62
Sakula A: Founding of the Athenaeum and Fellows of the Royal College of Physicians. **J R Coll Physicians Lond** 1983 Jul;17(3):206–7
Scadding JG: The Thoracic Society: a retrospect. **Thorax** 1983 Feb;38(2):88–92
The Scottish society of the history of medicine: report of proceedings, session 1978–79. **Med Hist** 1980 Apr;24(2):209–13
Snodgrass N: BVA Centenary. The British Veterinary Association: an historical note. **Vet Rec** 1982 Mar 20;110(12):279–88
Stephens SD: Centenary of British audiometry. London, Royal National Institute for the Deaf in collaboration with the British Society of Audiology, 1979. 40 p.
Tait HP: The College and community health. In Passmore R, ed: Proceedings of the Royal College of Physicians of Edinburgh Tercentenary Congress, 1981. Edinburgh, Royal College of Physicians of Edinburgh, 1982. p. 162–78.
Tansey V, Mekie DE: The Museum of the Royal College of Surgeons of Edinburgh. **J R Coll Surg Edinb** 1980 May;25(3):188–93 (continued periodically)
Tansey V, Mekie DE: The Museum of the Royal College of Surgeons of Edinburgh (Part 4). **J R Coll Surg Edinb** 1980 Nov;25(6):481–4
Taylor S: Surgical Research Society, 1954--79. **Lancet** 1979 Dec 8;2(8154):1234
[The need to preserve medical history records]: Evidence presented to the Public Records Committee.: **Soc Soc Hist Med Bull (Lond)** 1979 Dec;25:68–76
Turner-Warwick M: The British Thoracic Society. **Thorax** 1982 May;37(5):321–3
West GP, Ware F: A history of the overseas veterinary services. London, British Veterinary Assn., 1961–1973. 2 v.
Zuckerman L: The launching of the Journal of Endocrinology and the founding of the Society for Endocrinology. **J Endocrinol** 1984 Jan;100(1):1–5

**Hungary**

Banga I: A Magyar Elettani Társaság 50 éves jubileuma. **Orv Hetil** 1981 Dec 13;122(50):3093–6
Duka Zólyomi N: Orvosi tudós társaságok alapítási kisérletei a 18. századi Magyarországon. **Orv Hetil** 1983 Mar 20;124(12):711–2
Kapronczay K, Szemkeö E: A magyar orvostársaságok kialakulása és fejlödése a 19–20. században. **Orvostort Kozl** 1979;87–88(25 no 1–2):141–55
Kapronczay K: A vidéki orvosok társasága. **Orv Hetil** 1979 Jul 15;120(28):1703–5
Vilmon G: Orvosi közm'úvel'ódésünk – és könyvtáraink – h'óskora. **Orv Hetil** 1983 Feb 6;124(6):341–4

**India**

Garg MG: IMA: its origin, role and prospects. **J Indian Med Assoc** 1983 Oct;81(7–8):142–7

**Ireland**

Breathnach CS: John William Moore. **Ir J Med Sci** 1983 Jan;152(1):69–71
Browne AD: The section of obstetrics and obstetric and gynaecological development over the century. **Ir J Med Sci** 1983 Jan;152(1):26–38
Holland PD: The section of pathology and the development of pathology over the century. **Ir J Med Sci** 1983 Jan;152(1):50–6
Hughes ES, Dooley B: The Royal College of Surgeons in Ireland 1784–1984. **Aust NZ J Surg** 1984 Dec;54(6):502
Kinnear N: The surgical section and surgical developments over the century. **Ir J Med Sci** 1983 Jan;152(1):44–8
Lyons JB: The section of medicine and medical developments over the century. **Ir J Med Sci** 1983 Jan;152(1):14–24
O'Brien E: The bicentenary of the Royal College of Surgeons in Ireland, 1784–1984. **Br Med J [Clin Res]** 1983 Dec 24–31;287(6409):1988–90
Plaisted J: A short history of the Irish Medical Association. **Ir Med J** 1983 May;76(5):221–5
Powell M: The Royal Academy of Medicine in Ireland: the first hundred years. **Ir J Med Sci** 1983 Jan;152(1):3–12
Widdess JD: The Royal College of Surgeons in Ireland and its medical school, 1784–1984. Third edition. Dublin, Royal College of Surgeons in Ireland, 1984. x, 194 p.

**Israel**

Glazer I: A brief history of the Israel Society of Aerospace Medicine--a 1981 affiliate of the Aerospace Medical Association. **Aviat Space Environ Med** 1983 Apr;54(4):371–2

**Italy**

Belloni L: Un circolo bernardiano in Italia: la Società delle Scienze Biologiche in Torino. Luigi Vella de la curaroterapia del tetano. **Physis** 1981;23(3):301–10
Bellucci G: Storia della Società Italiana di Anestesia ed Analgesia, Società Italiana di Anestesiologia, Società Italiana di Anestesia e Rianimazione, Società Italiana di Anestesiologia, Analgesia, Rianimazione e Terapia Intensiva. **Minerva Anestesiol** 1980 Jul;46(7):733–56
Borsarelli F: Storia della Associazione Italiana Donne Medico--A.I.D.M. Affiliata alla Medical Women's International Association--M.W.I.A. Torino, Edizioni Minerva Medica, 1977. 55 p.
Casula D: I cinquanti'anni della Società Italiana di Medicina del Lavoro e Igiene Industriale. **Med Lav** 1980 Mar–Apr;71(2):115–8

**Jamaica**

Vernon C: The early beginnings of the Association of Nurses. **Jamaican Nurse** 1981;21(1):9–10

**Japan**

Aki-gun Ishikaishi Hensan Iinkai: Aki-gun Ishikai shi. Kaida-machi, Japan, Aki-gun Ishikai, Showa 52 nen, 1977. 769 p.
Atomic Bomb Casualty Commission: The Atomic Bomb Casualty Commission, 1947–1975. [Hiroshima?] The Commission, [1978?] vi, 240 p.
[Brief history of the Japan Society of Medical Electronics and Biological Engineering] (Jpn): **Iyodenshi To Seitai Kogaku** 1982 Dec;20(7):486–98
Fukuyama Y: [Progress of the Japanese Society of Pediatric Neurology in the past quarter of a century] (Jpn). **No To Hattatsu** 1984;16(3):179–88
Gotenba-shi I: Gotenba-shi Ishikai shi. [Gotenba, Japan], Do Ishikai, Showa 53 nen, [1978]. 680, [35] p.
Ichinomiya-shi Ishikaishi Henshu Iinkai: Ichinomiya-shi Ishikai shi. Ichinomiya, Japan, Ichinomiya-shi Ishikai, Showa 52 nen, 1977. 21, 1013 p.
Kageyama K, Shimanine T, Ishikawa E: A seventy-year history of the Japanese pathological society. **Acta Pathol Jpn** 1982;32 Suppl 1:1–21
Kagoshima-shi Ishikai: Kagoshima-shi Ishikai sanjunenshi. [Thirty years' history of the Kagoshima City Medical Association]. (Jpn) Kagoshima, Japan, Ishikai, Showa 53 nen [1978]. 537 p.
Kanagawa-ken I: Kanagawa-ken Ishikai shi. Yokohama: Do Ishikai, Showa 52. 1977-. v.
Kumanoto-shi Ishikai, Kaishi Henshu Iinkai: Kumamoto-shi Ishikai shi. Kumamoto, Japan, Do Ishikai, Showa 52 nen, 1977. 10, 465, 7 p.
Matsunaga F: [80 years of the Japanese Society of Gastroenterology] (Jpn). **Nippon Shokakibyo Gakkai Zasshi** 1983 Jul;80(7):1395–409
Okita S, ed: Miyoshi-gun Ishikai shi. Ikeda-cho, Japan, Miyoshi-gun Ishikai, Showa 53 nen. [1978]. 568 p.
Osaka-fu Ishikai: Osaka-fu Ishikai shi nenpyo/G. Osaka: Do Ishikai, Showa 52 nen [1977]. 194, 18 p.
Oshima Ishikai: Oshima Ishikai shi. Kamiiso-cho, Japan, Do Ishikai, Showa 52 nen, 1977. 360 p.
Sakai-shi Ishikai, Kaishi Hensan Iinkai: Nijugoshunen kinen Sakai-shi Ishikai shi. Sakai, Do Ishikai, Showa 52 nen, 1977. 822 p.
Shizuoka-ken I: Shizuoka-ken Ishikai nijunenshi. Shizuoka, Japan Do Ishikai, Showa 50 nen 1975. 13, 999 p.
Suzuki S: Kenko hoken kumiai hattatsu shi. Tokyo, Kitamura Shakai Hoken

Shuppan, Showa 51 nen [1976]. 15, 362 p.
Tsubaki T: [History of the Japanese Society of Neurology for 20 years (author's transl)]. (Jpn) **Rinsho Shinkeigaku** 1979 Dec;19(12):804–8
Yumai M: [Growing pain - a personal history (9)] (Jpn). **Sogo Kango** 1980;15(1):74–81

### Mexico

Academia Nacional de Medicina: Libro conmemorativo del primer centenario. México, Comité Editorial de la Comisión Organizadora del Congreso del Centenario, 1964. 2 v. (xxxii, 454 p.; xxxix, 719 p.)
Bandera B: La Academia Nacional de Medicina y la evolución de la anestesia en México. In Academia Nacional de Medicina. Libro conmemorativo del primer centenario. México, Comité Editorial de la Comisión Organizadora del Congreso del Centenario, 1964. Tome 2. p. 546–52.
Gual Castro C: Informe de labores con motivo del XXXV aniversario de la fundación del instituto Nacional de la Nutrición Salvador Zubirán. **Rev Invest Clin** 1982 Jan–Mar;34(1):85–9
Miguel Torre J: Treinta años de vida de la Sociedad Potosina de Estudios Médicos. Una experiencia interesante. **Gac Med Mex** 1982 Apr;118(4):165–70
Ramos P: Crónica. La Asociación Mexicana de Gastroenterología. **Rev Gastroenterol Mex** 1981 Apr–Jun;46(2):71–3 contd.
Somolinas Palencia J, Campillo Sainz C, Kumate J: Conmemoración del sesquicentenario de la fundación del Establecimiento de Ciencias Médicas. **Gac Med Mex** 1983 Nov;119(11):471–4
Somolinos D'Ardois G, Fernández del Castillo F: Historia de la Academia Nacional de Medicina de México. In Academia Nacional de Medicina. Libro conmemorativo del primer centenario. México, Comité Editorial de la Comisión Organizadora del Congreso del Centenario, 1964. Tome 2. p. 513–21.
Somolinos D'Ardois G: Historia de la fundación de la Academia Nacional de Medicina y su tiempo. In Academia Nacional de Medicina. Libro conmemorativo del primer centenario. México, Comité Editorial de la Comisión Organizadora del Congreso del Centenario, 1964. Tome 2. p. 593–621.
Somolinos Palencia J: The Mexican Society of History and Philosophy of Medicine - past, present and future. **Clio Med** 1981;15:245–7
Thompson HE: Early history of the Medical Society of the U. S. and Mexico. **Ariz Med** 1982 Jan;39(1):55–8
Vasconcelos R: La academia y la evolución de la medicina en México desde la Independencia. In Academia Nacional de Medicina. Libro conmemorativo del primer centenario. México, Comité Editorial de la Comisión Organizadora del Congreso del Centenario, 1964. Tome 2. p. 621–9.
XXXVI aniversario de la fundación del Instituto nacional de la nutrición Salvador Zubirán. Homenaje al Dr. Salvador Zubirán: **Rev Invest Clin** 1983 Jan–Mar;35(1):85–103

### Netherlands

Hackmann WD: Early societies popularize scientific research. **Med Instrum** 1983 Sep–Oct;17(5):338
Karthaus PP, Brongersma LD: H. R. G. J. Brongersma en de Nederlandse Vereniging voor Urologie. **Ned Tijdschr Geneeskd** 1983 Sep 3;127(36):1642–3
Meijler FL: Vijftig jaar Nederlandse Vereniging voor Cardiologie of, Nederland, debakermat van de elektrocardiografie. **Ned Tijdschr Geneeskd** 1984 Mar 24;128(12):571–3
Praag P van: Het nieuw-malthusianisme in Vlaanderen en Holland. **Spiegel Hist** 1978;13(11):662–8
Snelders HA: Het fysisch-chemisch werk van de Rotterdamse arts Hendrik Willem Rouppe (1765–1816). **Tijdschr Geschied Geneeskd** 1981;4(1):25–44
Snelders HA: Het Gezelschap der Hollandsche Scheikundigen. Amsterdamse chemici uit het einde van de achttiende eeuw. Amsterdam, Rodopi, 1980. 111 p. (Nieuwe Nederlandse Bijdragen tot de Geschiedenis der Geneeskunde en der Natuurwetenschappen, no. 4).
Van der Leun C, ed:: NG 200 - Natuurkundig Gezelschap te Utrecht 1777–1977. Utrecht, Natuurkundig Gezelschap te Utrecht, 1977. 143 p. With contributions by R. Hooykaas, J.G. van Cittert-Eymers, H.A.M. Snelders, N.G. van Kampen, P.H. Kylstra.
Verslag van de bijzondere wetenschappelijke vergadering ter viering van het honderdvijfentwintigjarig bestaan der Vereniging Nederlands Tijdschrift voor Geneeskunde.: **Ned Tijdschr Geneeskd** 1982 Jan 2;126(1):33–8
Woerdeman MW: The pre-constitutional years of the Dutch anatomical society. **Acta Morphol Neerl Scand** 1983 Mar;21(1):7–8

### New Zealand

Gluckman LK: Aspects of early medical organisation in Auckland, New Zealand. **NZ Med J** 1980 Mar 26;91(656):224–6
Kenny PJ: The founders of the College. **Aust NZ J Surg** 1981 Feb;51(1):95–101

### Norway

Bergenheim AL: Jubileumsår i NSF. **Sykepleien** 1982 Apr 5;69(7):5
Norsk Sykepleierforbund 70-års dag: historisk høytidsstund på Vettre: 'Arhundrets sykepleier' har fått sitt monument. **Sykepleien** 1982 Oct 20;69(18):6–7, 31

### Poland

Brożek K: Ruch naukowy towarzystw medycznych w regionie śląsko-dąbrowskim. **Wiad Lek** 1980 Aug 1;33(15):1265–9
Dobrowolska J: Wspomnienia z pracy w Warszawskim Towarzystwie Lekarskim. **Wiad Lek** 1980 Jun 1;33(11):927–30
Foltyn W: Biblioteka Towarzystwa Lekarskiego Warszawskiego w latach 1821–1944. **Arch Hist Med (Warsz)** 1983;46(2):151–82
Furmaga S: 30 lat Polskiego Towarzystwa parazytologicznego. **Wiad Parazytol** 1980;26(4–5):293–8
Gutt RW: Refleksje na temat XXV-lecia Polskiego Towarzystwa Historii Medycyny. **Arch Hist Med (Warsz)** 1982;45(1–4):5–10
Hornowski J: O obecnej siebzibie zarządu głownego Polskiego Towarzystwa Lekarskiego i Klubie Lekarza w Warszawie, Aleje Ujazdowskie nr. 24. **Wiad Lek** 1983 Jul 1;36(13):1127–35
Jendrysik I: 25 lat Koła PTP w Istebnej. **Pieleg Polozna** 1984;(5):30–1
Kobuszewska-Faryna M: Rok 1978--rokiem ważnych rocznic dla patomorfologów polskich. **Patol Pol** 1979 Apr–Jun;30(2):153–6
Konderska Z: 25 lat Polskiego Towarzystwa Pielęgniarskiego. **Pieleg Polozna** 1982;(4–5):26–8, 31
Korczak CW: Jubileusz 80-lecia Polskiego Towarzystwa Higienicznego. **Pol Tyg Lek** 1979 Nov 12;34(46):1813–5
Korczak CW: 80-letie Pol'skogo Gigienicheskogo Obshchestva (1898–1978). **Gig Sanit** 1980 Mar;(3):58–9
Kowalczyk S: Lubelskie Towarzystwo Lekarskie w Polsce Ludowej (1945–1951). **Ann Univ Mariae Curie Sklodowska [Med]** 1981;36:283–92
Kowieski L: Działalność Wydziału Higieny Zawodowej i Przemysłu Oddziału Lubelskiego Warszawskiego Towarzystwa Higienicznego w latach 1903–1905. **Arch Hist Med (Warsz)** 1984;47(3):429–31
Kuźnicke L: The Section of Biological Science of the Polish Academy of Sciences over the last 25 years. **Rev Pol Acad Sci (Warsz)** 1978;23:21–35
Kuźnicki L, Radziwiłł M: The section of biological science of the Polish Academy of Sciences over the last 25 years. **Rev Pol Acad Sci (Warsz)** 1978;23(1):21–35
Lembrych S: 25-lecie działalności Opolskiego Oddziału Polskiego Towarzystwa Ginekologicznego. **Ginekol Pol** 1984 Jan;55(1):71–3
Miętkiewskiego E: XXX lat Pomorskiej Akademii Medycznej w Szczecinie. **Ann Acad Med Stetin** 1979;(Suppl 17):1–549
Milik JR: W XXX rocznicę śmierci Wacława Lilpopa i założenia polskiego towarzystwa urologicznego. **Wiad Lek** 1979 Nov 1;32(21):1569–71
Moskwa Z: Izby lekarskie--wczoraj i dziś. **Wiad Lek** 1984 Jul 1;37(13):1064–8
Niziński J: Z historii Towarzystwa Lekarskiego Zagłębia Dąbrowskiego. **Wiad Lek** 1980 Nov 15;33(22):1851–5
Orłowski WJ: W stulecie polskich zjazdów okulistycznych. **Klin Oczna** 1981 Oct–Dec;83(10–12):465–6
Ostrowska T: Przedstawiciele medycyny niemieckiej w Towarzystwie Warszawskim Przyjaciół Nauk (1800–1832). **Arch Hist Med (Warsz)** 1979;42(2):257–62
Ostrowska T: Przedstawiciele nauk medycznych i ich działalność naukowa w Towarzystwie Warszawskim Przyjaciół Nauk (1800–1832). **Arch Hist Med (Warsz)** 1982;45(1–4):77–9
Ostrowska T: Rozprawy składane Towarzystwu Warszawskiemu Przyjaciół Nauk (1800--1832) przez jego członków -- lekarzy i farmaceutów. **Arch Hist Med (Warsz)** 1979;42(1):61–81
Ostrowski W: The work of the Committee on Biochemistry and Biophysics during twenty five years of the Polish Academy of Sciences. **Rev Pol Acad Sci (Warsz)** 1978;23(2):101–12
Rozwadowska-Dowzenko M, Afek-Kamińska M: Rys historyczny Towarzystawa Lekarskiego Warszawskiego w 160-lecie jego powstania. **Pol Tyg Lek** 1982 Apr 19;37(7):211–4
Rudowski W: Przemówienie z okazji jubileuszu xxx-lecia działalności Instytutu Hematologii. **Acta Haematol Pol** 1982 Jan–Jun;13(1–2):1–4
Rudowski W, Kostrzewski J, Mossakowski M: The twenty-fifth anniversary of the Polish Academy of Sciences and the twentieth anniversary of its medical science section. **Rev Pol Acad Sci (Warsz)** 1978;23(2):23–48
Skład osobowy władz Polskiego Towarzystwa Historii Medycyny i Farmacji: **Arch Hist Med (Warsz)** 1984;47(2):269–85
Sosińska-Trawińska M, Sródka A: O utworzeniu Wydziałów Lekarskich W polskich instytucjach naukowych. I. Polska Akademia Umiejętności (PAU). **Arch Hist Med (Warsz)** 1981;44(3/4):363–7
Sródka A, Sosińska-Trawińska M: O utworzeniu Wydziałow Lekarskich w polskich instytucjach naukowych. II. Towarzystwo Naukowe Warszawskie (TNW). **Arch Hist Med (Warsz)** 1982;45(1–4):81–4
Sródka A, Sosińska-Trawińska M: O utworzeniu wydziałów lekarskich w polskich instytucjach naukowych. III. Polska Akademia Nauk (PAN). **Arch Hist Med (Warsz)** 1983;46(1):51–7
Supady J: Powstanie i działalność stowarzyszenia 'Polski Instytut

Przeciwrakowy' we Lwowie (1929–1939). **Wiad Lek** 1982 Nov 1;35(19–20):1301–3
Szwejcerowa A: Siedziby Towarzystwa Lekarskiego Warszawskiego w latach 1820--1944. **Arch Hist Med (Warsz)** 1980;43(2):127–46
Towpik E: Benjaminowskie Towarzystwo Lekarskie (1917–1918). **Arch Hist Med (Warsz)** 1982;45(1–4):101–5
Wilczyńska M: Działalność Warszawskiej Podsekcji Ortodontycznej w latach 1956–78. **Czas Stomatol** 1980 May;33(5):475–8
Zabłotniak R: Polskie Towarzystwo Pomocy Ofiarom Wojny w Rosji (1914–1919). **Arch Hist Med (Warsz)** 1981;44(3/4):345–54

### Romania

Bădărău GH, Ciurea D, Pirozynski T, et al: Societatea de Medici si Naturalisti din Iasi la a 150–a aniversare (1830–1980). **Rev Med Chir Soc Med Nat Iasi** 1980 Oct–Dec;84(4):601–11
Bădărău Gh: Sesiunea stiintifică jubiliară Medicina progresului si umanismul medical. La 150 de ani de activitate a Societatii de Medici si Naturalisti (1830–1980) Iasi, 4 Octombrie 1980. **Rev Med Chir Soc Med Nat Iasi** 1980 Oct–Dec;84(4):613–24
Ciulei SG: Robert Koch (1843–1910), membru de onoare al Societății de Medici şi Naturalişti din Iaşi. **Rev Med Chir Soc Med Nat Iasi** 1983 Jul–Sep;87(3):503–4
Ciurea D: Societatea de Medici şi Naturalişti din Iaşi (1830–1980). **Rev Med Chir Soc Med Nat Iasi** 1980 Jul–Sep;84(3):587–92
Clocotici L: Organiza tii profesionale ale personalului sanitar mediu III. **Viata Med [Medii Sanit]** 1980 Jan;28(1):19–21
Clocotici L: Organizații profesionale ale personalului sanitar mediu (I). **Viata Med [Medii Sanit]** 1979 Jul;27(7):163–6
Gingold N: Data concerning the foundation of the Romanian Society of Hematology. **Med Interne** 1981 Jan–Mar;19(1):99–100
Jitariu P: Societatea de Medici si Naturalisti si dezvoltarea stiintelor biologicie. **Rev Med Chir Soc Med Nat Iasi** 1980 Oct–Dec;84(4):636–42
Manoliu V: History of medical societies in Romania. In: Congrès international d'histoire de la médecine, XXVe, Québec, 1976. Actes. Québec, 1977. p. 957–60.
Năstasă V: Activitatea ştiinţifică a farmaciştilor în cadrul 'societăţii de medici şi naturalişti' din iaşi. **Rev Med Chir Soc Med Nat Iasi** 1981;85(1):158–60
Negru I: 'Secolul copilului' in discuţia congreselor medicale din România (1919 şi 1925). **Viata Med [Medii Sanit]** 1982 Feb;30(2):45–7
Scripcaru G: Traditia si actualitatea relatiei dintre învătămîntul medical si Societatea de Medici si Naturalisti. **Rev Med Chir Soc Med Nat Iasi** 1980 Oct–Dec;84(4):629–35

### Scandinavia

Asplund J: The Scandinavian Association of Obstetricians and Gynecologists 1933–1983. **Acta Obstet Gynecol Scand [Suppl]** 1984;120:9–26
Borell U: Opening speech at the 50th anniversary congress of the Scandinavian Association of Obstetricians and Gynecologists in Stockholm, January 28–29, 1983. **Acta Obstet Gynecol Scand [Suppl]** 1984;120:5–7

### South Africa

Grey–Turner E: The British Medical Association and its South African branches. **S Afr Med J** 1983 Jun 29;Spec No:2–3
James T: Dr. Alfred Cox and the South African Medical Association. **S Afr Med J** 1980 Mar 15;57(11):416–21
Vaughan VH, Vaughan L: Fifty years of service: The S. A. National Council for the Blind, 1929–1979. The story of the South African National Council for the Blind. Pretoria. S. A. National Council for the Blind, 1979. xii, 468 p.

### Spain

Demerson P: Le chirurgien Larrey et 'l'invasion française' à l'academie de médecine de Madrid. **Melanges Casa Velasquez** 1973;9:483–501
García Alfonso C, Pérez García JM: Académicos veterinarios en la Real Academia Nacional de Medicina. **An R Acad Nac Med (Madr)** 1982;99(4):671–704
Matilla V: Cuatro secretarios perpetuos ejemplares de la Real Academia Nacional de Medicina. **An R Acad Nac Med (Madr)** 1981;98(1):31–68
Matilla Gómez V: Presentación del libro 'Galería de Presidentes'. **An R Acad Nac Med (Madr)** 1982;99(1):31–40
Miguel Martínez J, Cabarrocas Gafarot E: Bodas de plata de la associació catalana d'anestesiologia i reanimació (1953–1978). **Rev Esp Anestesiol Reanim** 1981 Mar;28(2):51–110
Palafóx Marqués S: Glosa al libro 'Galería de Presidentes.' **An R Acad Nac Med (Madr)** 1982;99(2):147–65
Quinta de Salud la Alianza, Barcelona: 75 aniversari (1904–1979), editat per la 'Quinta de Salud la Alianza; dirigit y realitzat pel Servei Tecnic de Relacions Publiques de la Comission de Foment. Barcelona, Printer Industria Grafica S. A., 1979. 93 p.
Ralchs A, Rozman C: Veintidós años después. Anotaciones para la historia de la Asociación Española de Hematología y Hemoterapia (AEHH). **Sangre (Barc)** 1982;27(3):377–85

### Sri Lanka

Aloysius DJ, Ranasinghe L: Historical perspective of the Sri Lanka Medical Association. **Ceylon Med J** 1981 Mar;26(1):8–34

### Sweden

Bahr G von: Upsala Läkare Klubb (ULK)--ur en gammal protokollsbok. **Nord Medicinhist Arsb** 1981;:172–5
Bahr G von: Upsala Läkareförening 150 år. **Ups J Med Sci [Suppl]** 1982;35:1–33
Boström H: Internmedicinen – en produkt av vårt eget århundrade. **Lakartidningen** 1983 Nov 16;80(46):4405–7
Kock W: Märkesdagar och märkesmän i svenska läkaresällskapet. **Lakartidningen** 1983 Nov 30;80(48):4667–70
Lindgren S: Ur svenska kirurgförbundets historia. **Nord Medicinhist Arsb** 1981;:160–71
Osterberg S: Svenska läkaresällskapet firar 175–årsjubileum. **Lakartidningen** 1983 Oct 5;80(40):3671–4
SSF--grande dame på 70--firades med tal och musik: **Vardfacket** 1980 Apr 24;4(8):63–6
Thomasson J: Arbetsmiljö, förhandlingar, MBL, behörighet och utbildning. En kort berättelse om SHSTFs första fem år. **Vardfacket** 1982 Jan 14;6(1):34–6

### Switzerland

Amstutz P: Für Gesundheitsschutz am Arbeitsplatz: Die Fachkommission der Schweizerischen Gesellschaft für Arbeitsmedizin, Arbeitshygiene und Arbeitssicherheit. **Soz Praventivmed** 1981 Jul;26(3):120–5
Bernische Liga gegen die Tuberkulose 1930–1980: Festschrift zum 50jährigen Jubiläum 20. Juni 1980 in Bern. Bern, 1980? 72 p. Contributions by S. Weiss, E. R. Mordasini, E. Arnold, R. Keller.
Brühlmann–Jecklin E: Zehn Jahre Gesellschaft für Muskelkrankheiten. Fachleute und Betroffene am gleichen Strick. **Krankenpflege Soins Infirm** 1984 Jun;77(6):34–6
Hansen JR: Scientific fellowship in a Swiss community enlightenment: a history of Zurich's Physical Society, 1746–1798. Ph.D. Diss., Ohio State University. Columbus, 1981. viii, 264 leaves.
Renner M: 'Krankenpflege' stellt sich vor. **Krankenpflege (Bern)** 1981 Dec;(12):58–9
Rintelen F: 75. Jahresversammlung der Schweizerischen ophthalmologischen Gesellschaft; zu ihrer Gründung und ihren Gründen. **Klin Monatsbl Augenheilkd** 1983 May;182(5):348–51
Riva G: Zum 50jährigen Bestehen der Schweizerischen Gesellschaft für Innere Medizin. **Schweiz Med Wochenschr [Suppl]** 1982;13:5–22
Stamm H: 75 Jahre Société de Gynécologie et d'Obstétrique de la Suisse Romande--70 Jahre Gynäkologische Gesellschaft der deutschen Schweiz. **Gesnerus** 1981;38(3/4):313–30

### Syria

Story of the Hosn Hospital: founded by American Hosn Welfare Association, New Kensington, Pennsylvania: New Kensington, Pa., The Assn., [1971?]. 188 [152] p.

### United States

American Nurses' Association. Nursing Hall of Fame. **ANA Publ** 1984 Jun;(G–123):1–21
Abir–Am P: Beyond deterministic sociology and apologetic history: reassessing the impact of research policy upon new scientific disciplines (Reply to Fuerst, Bartels, Olby and Yoxen). **Soc Stud Sci** 1984 May;14(2):252–63
Adolph EF: Growing up in the American Physiological Society. **Physiologist** 1979 Oct;22(5):11–5
Alexander RS: History of the Cardiovascular Section. **Physiologist** 1984 Apr;27(2):67–8
American Dental Association 1859–1880: **J Am Dent Assoc** 1984 Apr;108(4):479–89, 492
American Dental Association 1881–1917: **J Am Dent Assoc** 1984 Apr;108(4):497–510
American Dental Association 1918–1928: **J Am Dent Assoc** 1984 Apr;108(4):515–9, 522
American Dental Association 1929–1945: **J Am Dent Assoc** 1984 Apr;108(4):527–33, 535–6
American Dental Association 1946–1962: **J Am Dent Assoc** 1984 Apr;108(4):541–51, 554–6
American Dental Association 1963–1984: **J Am Dent Assoc** 1984 Apr;108(4):561–71, 574–9
The American Radium Society: **Am J Clin Oncol** 1982 Apr;5(2):99–100
ANA's economic and general welfare program: a historical perspective: **ANA Publ** 1981;(EC–143):1–10
Andrews WH: A perspective review of the development of AOAC

microbiological methods. **J Assoc Off Anal Chem** 1984 Jul-Aug;67(4):661-73
Angevine E: History of the National Consumers League, 1899-1979. Washington, The League, 1979. 69 leaves.
Appel TA: The archives of the American Physiological Society. **Physiologist** 1984 Jun;27(3):131-2
Appel TA: The 1941-42 search for an APS emblem. **Physiologist** 1984 Apr;27(2):69-70
Ashcraft ML, Berki SE: Health maintenance organizations as Medicaid providers. **Ann Am Acad Polit Soc Sci** 1983;(468):122-31
Austin D, Hunnicutt BK: National Therapeutic Recreation Society: the first twelve years. **Ther Recreation J** 1978 3d Quarter;12(3):4-14
Ayvasian LF: American Thoracic Society: the fifty-five Trudeau medalists (1926-1980): a seventy-fifty anniversary review. **Am Rev Respir Dis** 1980 Apr;121(4):753-75
Barckley V: The best of times and the worst of times. Historical reflections from an American Cancer Society national nursing consultant. **Oncol Nurs Forum** 1982 Summer;9(3):54-6
Bartels D: The Rockefeller Foundation's funding policy for molecular biology: success or failure? **Soc Stud Sci** 1984 May;14(2):238-43
Bartlett RM: Meditation on the subject of holes in the head. **Pharos** 1980 Spring;43(2):19
Batchelor AJ: AMWA's founder--the 'red headed dynamo'. **J Am Med Wom Assoc** 1984 Jul-Aug;39(4):123, 139
Bean DW, Fuller WC: Development of the South Dakota Psychiatric Association. **SD J Med** 1981 May;34(5):53-5
Bearn AG, James DG: Dr. William Harvey (1578-1657) and the Harvey Society of New York. **Perspect Biol Med** 1978 Spring;21(3):524-35
Bearn AG: The Harvey Society of New York. **Harvey Lect** 1979;73:1-18
Benison S: Ideology über alles: an essay review. **J Hist Med Allied Sci** 1982 Jan;37(1)83-90
Benson ES: Laboratory medicine in the United States--the dream and the reality. **Am J Clin Pathol** 1981 Jul;76(1):1-7
Berney B: The rise and fall of the UMW Fund. **South Exposure** 6(2):95-102, 1978
Bing RK: Nationally speaking--living forward, understanding backwards, Part I. **Am J Occup Ther** 1984 Jun;38(6):363-6
Blumberg LU: The significance of the alcohol prohibitionists for the Washington temperance societies; with special reference to Paterson and Newark, New Jersey. **J Stud Alcohol** 1980 Jan;41(1):37-77
Blustein BE: The Philadelphia Biological Society, 1857-61: a failed experiment? **J Hist Med Allied Sci** 1980 Apr;35(2):188-202
Bond GR, et al: Mended hearts: a self-help case study. **Soc Policy** 1979;9(4):50-7
Bonsett CA: Medical museum notes: Thomas B. Harvey. **J Indiana State Med Assoc** 1983 Jun;76(6):371
Bordley JE: The American Rhinologic Society: its foundation and its future responsibilities. **Laryngoscope** 1980 May;90(5 Pt 1):876-9
Bricker EM: Evarts A. Graham and the American College of Surgeons. **J Thorac Cardiovasc Surg** 1984 Nov;88(5 Pt 2):834-41
Brown ER: He who pays the piper: foundations, the medical profession, and medical education. In Reverby S, Rosner D, ed: Health care in America. Philadelphia, Temple University Press, 1979. p. 132-54.
Brown ER: Rockefeller medicine men. Medicine and capitalism in America. Berkeley, University of California Press, 1979. xii, 283 p.
Brown JE, Finder JG, Lidge RT: The Clinical Orthopaedic Society, Inc.: an informal history, 1912-1981. Brunswick, Ga., Glover Printing Co., [1982?]. vii, 288 p.
Bryan SA: Pioneering specialists: a history of the American Academy of Ophthalmology and Otolaryngology. San Francisco, American Academy of Ophthalmology, Rochester, Minn.: American Academy of Otolaryngology-Head and Neck Surgery, 1982. viii, 305 p.
Bryce DP, Nuis DB, ed: The American Laryngological Association, 1878-1978. Washington, American Laryngological Assn., 1978. xiv, 152 p.
Buchanan DJ: Huron District Medical Society (No. 5). **SD J Med** 1981 May;34(5):15-7
Bullock MB: An American transplant: the Rockefeller Foundation and Peking Union Medical College. Berkeley, University of California Press, 1980. xxvii, 280 p.
Burstein SS: Prepaid health care in the United States. **IMJ** 1981 Aug;160(2):83-5
Byrne R: Keynote address--50th anniversary BPA meeting, Boston, Massachusetts. **J Biol Photogr** 1981 Apr;49(2):39-44
Cahn JD: A doctor's legacy: Dr. John E. T. Camper and the MeDeSo. **J Natl Med Assoc** 1980 Mar;72(3):283-7
Cameron JE: The Tallapoosa County Medical Society. **J Med Assoc State Ala** 1982 Jul;52(1):20-3
Carson RB: Fifty years of history: Southeastern Section, American Urological Association, 1931-1981. The Section, 1981. 119 p.
Cash P: The phoenix and the eagle: The founding of the Boston and Massachusetts Medical Societies in 1780 and 1781. **N Engl J Med** 1981 Oct 29;305(18):1033-9
Centennial edition: The South Dakota State Medical Association: **SD J Med** 1981 May;34(5):1-80
Chambers CA, Romanofsky P, ed: Social service organizations. 2 v. Westport, Conn., Greenwood Press, 1978. xxxiii, 843 p.
Chase MW: Irreverent recollections from Cooke and Coca, 1928-1978. **J Allergy Clin Immunol** 1979 Nov;64(5):306-20
Clawson DK: The founding of the Association of Orthopaedic Chairmen. **Clin Orthop** 1983 Dec;181:298-303
Cobb WM: The Black American in medicine. **J Natl Med Assoc** 1981 Dec;73 Suppl:1185-244
Cochrane RC: The National Academy of Sciences: the first hundred years, 1863-1963. Washington, D.C., National Academy of Sciences, 1978. xv, 694 p.
Colonel Leverett Hubbard's address to the Society at their meeting Feby 2d 1784: **Conn Med** 1984 Sep;48(9):557
Conn HJ: The history of the Stain Commission. II. Organization 1921-2. **Stain Technol** 1980 Nov;55(6):327-52
Conn HJ: The history of the Stain Commission. III. Birth of the Stain Commission. 1922-3. **Stain Technol** 1981 Jan;56(1):1-17
Conn HJ: The history of the Stain Commission IV. Expansion of the work, 1924-39. **Stain Technol** 1981 Mar;56(2):59-66
Conn HJ: The history of the Stain Commission. V. War and its consequences. **Stain Technol** 1981 May;56(3):135-42
Corgan JX: A preliminary catalog of the scientific and technical societies of Antebellum East Tennessee. **East Tenn Hist Soc Publ** 1976(issued Feb 80);48:21-8
Cortes KF: Democracy in the American Public Health Association: a historical analysis. [New York?, s.n.], 1976. 362 leaves.
Coulter HL: Divided legacy: the conflict between homoeopathy and the American Medical Association. Science and ethics in American medicine 1800-1914. 2d ed. Richmond, California, North Atlantic Books, 1982. 552 p.
The Council at midcentury--: the reach for growth and status 1934-1950. **Except Child** 1981 Jan;47(4):286-96
D'Amato NA: Nathaniel Chapman: first president of the American Medical Association. **Va Med** 1984 Nov;111(11):708-10
D'Amore AR: Ernest Jones: founder of the American Psychoanalytic Association. **Int J Psychoanal** 1979;60(Pt 3)287-90
Darby WJ: The Nutrition Foundation: 1942-1982. **Nutr Rev** 1982 Nov;40(11):348-52
Dean JB: A retrospective look through the camera of Fred A. Hitchcock. **Physiologist** 1984 Jun;27(3):128-30
Dekosky RK: The history of science in a history department. **Hist Teacher** 1980;13(3):371-8
Doona ME: The Lucy Lincoln Drown Nursing History Society. **Mass Nurse** 1984 Feb;53(2):6
Dreiling DA: The first fifty years--a history of evolution of the American College of Gastroenterology as a Society for Clinical Gastroenterology. **Am J Gastroenterol** 1983 Mar;78(3):138-9
Dunphy JE: Look back for tomorrow. **Bull Am Coll Surg** 1975 Dec;60(12):9-14
Ellison RG: Paul C. Samson, M.D., 1905-1982. Part I. His contributions to the Society of Thoracic Surgeons. **Ann Thorac Surg** 1983 Nov;36(5):500-1
Ellison RG: The Society of Thoracic Surgeons: the first twenty years. **Ann Thorac Surg** 1984 Jan;37(1):1-8
Ellman MH: William Crawford Gorgas and the American Medical Association. **JAMA** 1980 Feb 15;243(7):659-60
Ettling J: The germ of laziness. Rockefeller philanthropy and public health in the new South. Cambridge, Harvard, 1981. x, 263 p.
Evans RB, Talmadge P: Dial access: a history of the Southern Medical Association's newest contribution to continuing medical education. **South Med J** 1980 Apr;73(4):489-96
Fath H: A dream come true: the story of St. Jude Children's Research Hospital and ALSAC. Memphis, TN, ALSAC, 1983. 214 p.
Faust DG: Mary Breckinridge. In: Notable American women. The modern period. Cambridge, Mass., Belknap-Harvard Univ. Press, 1980. 4:103-5.
Fickeissen JL: New Jersey State Nurses' Association. **J Med Soc NJ** 1984 Sep;81(9):805-6
Fiftieth anniversary: American College of Gastroenterology. Reprints. The American Journal of Gastroenterology celebrates the Golden Anniversary of the College. **Am J Gastroenterol** 1982 Oct;77(10):701-832
Finlayson G: Osteopathic hospitals and AOHA. United in progress for 50 years. **OH** 1984 Sep;28(8):12-4
The first American Medical Association reports on public hygiene in American cities. Twelve reports reprinted from the Transactions of the American Medical Association, Vol. II, 1849. New York, Arno, 197. P. 431-634.:
Fisher D: The role of philanthropic foundations in the reproduction and production of hegemony: Rockefeller foundations and the social sciences. **Sociology** 1983;17(2):206-33
Fisher DA: The Endocrine Society: past and present. **J Clin Endocrinol Metab** 1984 Dec;59(6):1229-33
Fitzpatrick ML: A history of the National Organization for Public Health Nursing, 1912-1952. [New York, N. Y., s. n.], 1973. 3, vi, 451 leaves.
Flanagan L, ed: One strong voice: the story of the American Nurses' Association. Kansas City, Mo., American Nurses' Assn., 1976. xiii, 692 p.
Flynn RJ: The founding and early history of the American Association for Laboratory Animal Science. **Lab Anim Sci** 1980 Aug;30(4 pt 2):765-79
Fondiller SH: The entry dilemma: the National League for Nursing and

the higher education movement, 1952-1972, with an epilogue to 1983. New York, N.Y., National League for Nursing, 1983. vii, 136 p.
Fox DM: Abraham Flexner's unpublished report: foundations and medical education, 1909-1928. **Bull Hist Med** 1980 Winter;54(4):475-96
Freeman RG: History of the American Society of Dermatopathology. **Am J Dermatopathol** 1984 Feb;6(1):25-33
Fuerst JA: The definition of molecular biology and the definition of policy: the role of the Rockefeller Foundation's policy for molecular biology. **Soc Stud Sci** 1984 May;14(2):225-37
Gantt WH: E. Cowles Andrus (1896--1978), eighth president of the Pavlovian Society. **Pavlov J Biol Sci** 1979 Jan-Mar;14(1):74-5
Gibson HL: The Biological Photographic Association, its half century. The era of maturation, 1965-1980. **J Biol Photogr** 1980 Apr;48(2):41-86
Giglio JN: Voluntarism and public policy between World War I and the New Deal: Herbert Hoover and the American Child Health Association. **Pres Stud Q** 1983;13(3):430-52
Gilliland M: The FMA Auxilliary--a half century of progress and accomplishment. **J Fla Med Assoc** 1981 Mar;68(3):166-8
Gotch FA: The evolution of the society. **Trans Am Soc Artif Intern Organs** 1979;25:534-8
Grafton TS: The founding and early history of the National Society for Medical Research. **Lab Anim Sci** 1980 Aug;30(4 pt 2):759-64
Graham FE, Wright RJ: The American College of Medical Group Administrators: twenty-five years in brief perspective. **Med Group Manage** 1981 Sep-Oct;28(5):60-2, 64, 66
Guthorn PJ: William Augustus Newell, M.D., and the Life Saving Service. **J Med Soc NJ** 1984 Sep;81(9):769-72
Hammond EA: Dr. Newton D. Phillips, Florida Medical Association's eleventh president. **J Fla Med Assoc** 1982 Aug;69(8):683-7
Hamowy R: The early development of medical licensing laws in the United States, 1875-1900. **J Libert Stud** 1979;3(1):73-119
Hanlon CR: The surgical presidency. **Ann Surg** 1982 Sep;196(3):233-8
Harvey AM: Science at the bedside. Clinical research in American medicine, 1905-1945. Baltimore, London, Johns Hopkins University Press, 1981. xix, 554 p.
Harvey AM: The Interurban Clinical Club (1905-1976): a record of achievement in clinical science. [s.l.], Interurban Clinical Club, 1978. xiii, 573 p.
'Health Physics': 25th anniversary issue commemorating the founding of the Health Physics Society 1955-1980.: **Health Phys** 1980 Jun;38(6):883-1209
Heck CV: Fifty years of progress: in recognition of the 50th anniversary of the American Academy of Orthopaedic Surgeons. Chicago, American Academy of Orthopaedic Surgeons, 1983. vi, 361 p.
Heim LR: Birth and development of a scientific journal, and a society. **Exp Hematol** 1983 Nov;11(10):907-13
Hildreth PB: Early Red Cross: the Howard Association of New Orleans, 1837-1878. **La Hist** 1979;20(1):77-92
A history of South Dakota Blue Shield: **SD J Med** 1981 May;34(5):69
History of South Dakota Society of Internal Medicine: **SD J Med** 1981 May;34(5):63-4
History of the American Geriatrics Society: Malford W. Thewlis, J. Am. Geriatrics Soc. 1: 3, 1953. **J Am Geriatr Soc** 1981 Dec;29(12):544-9
The history of the National Association of Operating Room Nurses: **Va Nurse** 1982 Summer;50(2):43
Holland J: A glorious anachronism: the American Philosophical Society. **Wilson Libr Bull** 1982;56(10):740-4
Horton LE: The boys in the club. **J Am Diet Assoc** 1982 Jul;81(1):17-25
Hovland M: Aberdeen District Medical Society (No. 1), 1957-1981. **SD J Med** 1981 May;34(5):8-9
Hutner G: MSNJ: America's first and oldest medical society. **J Med Soc NJ** 1984 Sep;81(9):718-21
Ikard RW: The Nashville Academy of Medicine 'Yankee Gunboat' Gavel. **J Tenn Med Assoc** 1982 Aug;75(8):530-2
Imber M: The First World War, sex education, and the American Social Hygiene Association's campaign against venereal disease. **J Educ Adm Hist** 1984;16(1):47-56
ISMS organization: History of founding and expansion. **IMJ** 1981 Nov;160(5):297
Jaques DA: The fraternity of strangers. **Am J Surg** 1984 Oct;148(4):426-7
Jensen JE: A Med-Chi physician's travelog 1860-62 (Dr. H. Willis Baxley). **Md State Med J** 1984 Feb;33(2):90-2
Johnson EA, Bell G: Whetstone Valley District Medical Society (No. 12). **SD J Med** 1981 May;34(5):32-4
Jones JH: Alan Gregg. In Dictionary of American Biography, Suppl. 6, 1956-1960. p. 252-3, 1980.
Jones RJ: The NCCLS and medical devices. **JAMA** 1980 May 2;243(17):1748
Kampmeier RH: A century of the Tennessee Medical Association. **J Tenn Med Assoc** 1980 Mar;73(3):169-81
Kampmeier RH: History of the American Venereal Disease Association. **Sex Transm Dis** 1984 Jul-Sep;11(3 Suppl):185-265
Kampmeier RH: Seventy-five years of the journal. **J Tenn Med Assoc** 1983 Jul;76(7):431-8
Kampmeier RH: The Asklepion Club of Nashville. **J Tenn Med Assoc** 1982 Feb;75(2):93-9
Kaplan MM: Three decades of collaboration with Hilary Koprowski. **J Cell Physiol [Suppl]** 1982;2:1-6
Karl BD, Katz SN: The American private philanthropic foundation and the public sphere 1890-1930. **Minerva** 1981 Summer;19(2):236-70
Kelley WN: Clinical investigation and the clinical investigator: the past, present, and future. **J Clin Invest** 1984 Sep;74(3):1117-22
Kennedy JW: Publications of the Arizona Territorial Medical Society. **Ariz Med** 1981 Apr;38(4):290-3 contd
Keys TE, Key JD: An overlooked tribute for Dr. William Worrall Mayo. **Minn Med** 1984 Jul;67(7):375-8
Kiger JC, ed: Research institutions and learned societies. Westport, Conn., London, Greenwood Press, 1982. xxv, 551 p. (Greenwood Encyclopedia of American Institutions, no. 5).
King LS: IX. The AMA gets a new code of ethics. **JAMA** 1983 Mar 11;249(10):1338-42
King LS: Medicine in the USA: historical vignettes. IV. The founding of the American Medical Association. **JAMA** 1982 Oct 8;248(14):1749-52
Kohlstedt SG: Science: the struggle for survival, 1880 to 1894. **Science** 1980 Jul 4;209(4452):33-42
Kritchevsky D: Hilary Koprowski and The Wistar Institute. **J Cell Physiol [Suppl]** 1982;2:vi-viii
Lam CR: The Central Surgical Association turns forty. Some highlights of the first twenty years. **Henry Ford Hosp Med J** 1982;30(2):77-80
Leeds JP: Review of the Transactions of the American Academy of Optometry, 1922 to 1939. **Am J Optom Physiol Opt** 1982 Sep;59(9):735-7
Leland TM: James Rufus Bratton 1821-1897. **J SC Med Assoc** 1984 Feb;80(2):84
Lewis BE: A tradition of exceptional women. **J Am Med Wom Assoc** 1983 May-Jun;38(3):75-6, 82
Lightdale CJ: Notes on the development of the American Society for Gastrointestinal Endoscopy. **Gastrointest Endosc** 1983 Feb;29(1):51-3
Linde LM: History of Northwest District Medical Association (No. 11). **SD J Med** 1981 May;34(5):31
Livingood CS: History of the American Board of Dermatology, Inc. (1932-1982). **J Am Acad Dermatol** 1982 Dec;7(6):821-50
Longo LD: A short history of the Society for Gynecologic Investigation (1953-1983). Los Angeles, Calif., [s.n.], 1983. 70 p.
McCarty DJ: The American Rheumatism Association and the Arthritis Foundation: commentary on 14 years of a happy union. **Arthritis Rheum** 1979 Dec;22(12):1394-5
McConville E: Oliver Harvey: 'Got to take some risks.' **South Exposure** 6(2):24-8, 1978
McDonald CJ: Seventh District Medical Society (Sioux Falls). **SD J Med** 1981 May;34(5):19-20
Maddox RF: The politics of World War II science: Senator Harley M. Kilgore and the legislative origins of the National Science Foundation. **W Va Hist** 1979;41(1):20-39
Mann RJ, Key JD: The Osler Medical Historical Society. Mayo Foundation 'Chapter,' August 28, 1920-July 3, 1925. **Minn Med** 1980 May;63(5):348-54
Marino H: Reminiscences of the American Society of Plastic and Reconstructive Surgeons, Inc., and some of its members. **Plast Reconstr Surg** 1981 Sep;68(3):376-80
Marrett CB: Influences on the rise of new organizations: the formation of women's medical societies. **Adm Sci Q** 1980 Jun;25(2):185-99
Marrett CB: On the evolution of women's medical societies. **Bull Hist Med** 1979 Fall;53(3):434-48
Mathews CL: History of the Mississippi State Medical Association. **J Miss State Med Assoc** 1981 Dec;22(12):299-302
Mathews CL: The component society--a 'sine qua non' to membership. **J Miss State Med Assoc** 1981 Dec;22(12):303-5
Mathewson C: Historical review of the San Francisco Surgical Society. **Am J Surg** 1982 Feb;143(2):246-51
Matthews J: Twenty five years of Asha. **ASHA** 1984 Sep;26(9):39-40
Matthies K: Mary Breckinridge and the frontier nursing service. **DAR Mag** 1980;114(5):692-4
Medical highlights in South Dakota--the first 100 years of the South Dakota State Medical Association: **SD J Med** 1981 May;34(5):75-8
Morison RS: The Foundation interest. In Stevenson LG, ed: A celebration of medical history. Baltimore, Johns Hopkins University Press, 1982. (The Henry E. Sigerist supplements to the Bulletin of the History of Medicine; new ser., no. 6). p. 212-21.
Neagu I, Maracineanu G, Neagu M: Contribution de la Société 'La Jeune Croix Rouge Américaine' au developpement de l'assistance médicale et sociale en Roumanie. In: Congrès international d'histoire de la médecine, XXVe, Québec, 1976. Actes. Québec, 1977. p. 1009-14.
NLN's 30th year - leading the way: Renew the spirit! 1952-1982. **Nurs Health Care** 1982 Sep;3(5):398-9
Nuland SB: 'A matter of great importance to mankind': the origins of the New Haven County Medical Association. **Conn Med** 1984 Sep;48(9):559-61
Numbers RL: Public protection and self-interest: medical societies in Wisconsin. In Numbers RL, Leavitt JW, ed: Wisconsin medicine. Historical perspectives. Madison, University of Wisconsin Press, 1981. p. 75-104.
Ochsner A: To our founder [Franklin H. Martin], with reflections. **Bull Am Coll Surg** 1981;66(5):26-30
The official publication of the American Association of Physical

Anthropologists 1930–1980: Jubilee Issue: **Am J Phys Anthropol** 1981 Dec;56(4):327–557
Olby R: The sheriff and the cowboys: or Weaver's support of Astbury and Pauling. **Soc Stud Sci** 1984 May;14(2):244–7
Oleson A, Voss J, ed: The organization of knowledge in modern America, 1860–1920. Baltimore and London, Johns Hopkins University Press, 1979. xxi, 478 p.
Olsen AM: ACCP International--'The world is our classroom'. **Chest** 1984 Nov;86(5):655–6
Page IH: A history of the Council for High Blood Pressure research. Past imperfect, present indicative, and future perfect. **Hypertension** 1984 Mar–Apr;6(2 pt 2):208–10
Paletta FX: History of the American Society of Plastic and Reconstructive Surgeons, Inc., 1931–1981: its growth, change, unity. **Plast Reconstr Surg** 1981 Sep;68(3):292–369
Parascandola J: John J. Abel and the founding of ASPET. **Pharmacologist** 1984;26(1):37–40
Parish LC: Amerikanische dermatologische Zeitschriften und die New Yorker Dermatologische Gesellschaft. **Hautarzt** 1981 Mar;32(3):136–8
Peitzman SJ: Forgotten reformers: the American Academy of Medicine. **Bull Hist Med** 1984 Winter;58(4):516–28
Pines M: The Foundations' Fund for Research in Psychiatry and the growth of research in psychiatry. **Am J Psychiatry** 1983 Jan;140(1):1–10
Pitts JA: The Association of Medical Superintendents of American Institutions for the Insane, 1844–1892: a case study of specialism in American medicine. Ph.F. diss. University of Pennsylvania. Philadelphia, 1979. 267 leaves.
Poland UH: Reflections on the Medical Library Association's international activities. **Bull Med Libr Assoc** 1982 Oct;70(4):359–68
Popper H: History of the American Association for the Study of Liver Diseases. **Hepatology** 1982 Nov–Dec;2(6):874–8
Posner RM: Thomas Starr King and the mercy million. **Calif Hist Soc Q** 1964;43(4);291–308
Prescott GW: American Microscopical Society: the first one-hundred years. Part II. **Trans Am Microsc Soc** 1979 Apr;98(2):165–94
Proceedings of the State Medical Convention, held in Raleigh, April, 1849, and Constitution and Medical Ethics of the Medical Society of the State of North Carolina, then adopted: **NC Med J** 1982 Mar;43(3):212–21
Ramsey FB: January 1982: 75th birthday of the ISMA Journal; history and highlights, Indiana State Medical Association and its journal. **J Indiana State Med Assoc** 1982 Jan;75(1):14–9
Ravitch MM: A century of surgery. The history of the American Surgical Association. 2 vols. Philadelphia and Toronto, Lippincott, 1981.
Ravitch MM: The American Surgical Association. The peaks of excitement. **Ann Surg** 1980 Sep;192(3):282–7
Reding MM: History of the South Dakota State Medical Association Auxiliary 1910–1981. **SD J Med** 1981 May;34(5):72–3
Reed J: Katharine Dexter McCormick. In: Notable American women. The modern period. Cambridge, Mass., Belknap–Harvard Univ. Press, 1980. 4:440–2.
Reese WG: Early history of the Pavlovian Society. Twentyfive plus twentyfive. (W. Horsley Gantt). **Pavlov J Biol Sci** 1982 Oct–Dec;17(4):171–7
Relman AS: Two hundred years young. **N Engl J Med** 1981 Oct 29;305(18):1088–9
Resnik SS: The making of dermatologic surgeons. The first decade of the American Society for Dermatologic Surgery. **J Dermatol Surg Oncol** 1980 Dec;6(12):993–5
Rhodes JS: The Raleigh Academy of Medicine. **NC Med J** 1981 Apr;42(4):263–4
Rice CN: The history of the Society of State Directors of Health, physical education, and recreation, 1953–1976. Ed.D. Diss., University of Alabama. University, 1977. v, 199 p.
The Robb House: home of the Alachua County Medical Society and Auxiliary: **J Fla Med Assoc** 1982 Aug;69(8):681–2
Robert I. Watson and the development of the history of psychology: a symposium: With contributions by E. S. Mills, E. R. Hilgard, B. Ross, J. Popplestone, M. W. McPherson, R. B. Evans, E. S. Goodman, J. Brožek. **J Hist Behav Sci** 1982 Oct;18(4):307–31
Roberts NJ: Presidents's remarks. **Bull NY Acad Med** 1981 Oct;57(8):659–63
Rogers FA: The American Medical Association: yesterday, today and tomorrow. **J La State Med Soc** 1981 Sep;133(9):129–35
Saffron MH: New Jersey or Massachusetts? **JAMA** 1981 May 22–29;245(20):2031–2
Saffron MH: The Academy of Medicine of New Jersey: a brief history. **J Med Soc NJ** 1984 Sep;81(9):785–8
Sanger G, ed: The Charaka Club, 1898–1978. A history. New York, Charles C. Morchand, 1978. 260 p.
Scarborough J, ed: Society for Ancient Medicine newsletter. No. 1–10 (Apr. 1976–Sept. 1982). Continued periodically.
Scherlis L: Poetical version of the Rules of the Humane Society for recovering drowned persons. **Crit Care Med** 1981 May;9(5):430–1
Selections from Public health: reports and papers presented at meetings of the American Public Health Association (1884–1907). New York, Arno, 1977. Various paginations.:
Selections from Public health: reports and papers presented at the meetings of the American Public Health Association (1873–1883). New York, Arno, 1977. Various paginations.:
Selections from the Journal of the Massachusetts Association of Boards of Health (1891–1904). New York, Arno, 1977. Various paginations.:
Sherrard ML: History of the Baltimore County Medical Association. **Md State Med J** 1983 May;32(5):332
Silver P: Auxiliary history is record of service. **J Miss State Med Assoc** 1981 Dec;22(12):316–8
Silver P: MSMA leadership is family tradition. **J Miss State Med Assoc** 1981 Dec;22(12):306–9
Sloan W, Stevens HA: A century of concern: a history of the American Association on Mental Deficiency 1876–1976. Washington, American Association on Mental Deficiency, 1976, viii, 310p.
Smith EK: History of the Pacific Northwest Section, AACC 1961–1981. **Clin Chem** 1981 May;27(5):762–4
Smith HH: Life's a pleasant institution: the peregrinations of a Rockefeller doctor. Tucson, The Author, 1978. x, 254 p.
Smith KC: History of American Society for Photobiology (ASP). The first 10 years, and before. **Photochem Photobiol** 1982 May;35(5):597–614
Spencer ER: A society of physicians. An account of the activities of the members of the Massachusetts Medical Society 1923–1981. Boston, Massachusetts Medical Society, 1981. 410 p.
Spencer ER: The Massachusetts Medical Society bicentennial celebration. **N Engl J Med** 1981 Oct 15;305(16):953–4
Spencer F, Erickson GE: Charter members of the American Association of Physical Anthropologists. **Am J Phys Antropol** 1981 Dec;56(4):531–5
Staab L: The history of the New Jersey Hospital Association. **J Med Soc NJ** 1984 Sep;81(9):802–4
Stanage WF: Yankton District Medical Society (No. 8). **SD J Med** 1981 May;34(5):26
Stephenson GW: A history of the Committee on Pre- and Postoperative Care. **Bull Am Coll Surg** 1981 Nov;66(11):21–2, 24, 26
Stephenson GW: The College's role in hospital standardization. **Bull Am Coll Surg** 1981 Feb;66(2):17–29
Stephenson GW: The Commission on Cancer: an historical review. **Bull Am Coll Surg** 1979 Sep;64(9):7–13
Stephenson GW: The Committee on Trauma: its men and its mission. **Bull Am Coll Surg** 1979 Oct;64(10):17–8, 22–6
Stevens EB: The history of the Medical Group Management Association, 1926–1976. Denver, Medical Group Management Assn, 1976? ix, 135 p.
Stillwell GK: Whence our academy? **Arch Phys Med Rehabil** 1983 Mar;64(3):97–100
Stoltz CR, Stoltz V: Watertown District Medical Society (No. 2). **SD J Med** 1981 May;34(5):10–11
Stone LG: Medical society of the county of Monroe; sesquicentennial–1971. **NY State J Med** 1980 Jun;80(7 Pt 1):1155–7
Summerville J: Formation of a black medical profession in Tennessee, 1880–1920. **J Tenn Med Assoc** 1983 Oct;76(10):644–6
Talbot DM: Federation of Specialty Nursing Organizations and the American Nurses' Association: a history. **Occup Health Nurs** 1981 Oct;29(10):27–33
Tank MC: Synopsis of the Brookings–Madison District medical community (No. 3). **SD J Med** 1981 May;34(5):12–3
Tedeschi LG: The Massachusetts Medico–Legal Society. The early years. **Am J Forensic Med Pathol** 1981 Sep;2(3):257–60
This is the National League for Nursing: New York, League, [1977?] 13 p.
Thomson EH: Esther Pohl Lovejoy. In: Notable American women. The modern period. Cambridge, Mass., Belknap–Harvard Univ. Press, 1980. 4:424–6.
TNA and nursing in Texas: a 75-year perspective: **Tex Nurs** 1982 Jan;56(1):12–3; Feb;56(2):6–7
Tobach E: A brief history of the Psychology Section of The New York Academy of Sciences. In K. Salzinger, ed: Psychology in progress: an interim report. (Annals of the New York Academy of Sciences, vol. 270). New York, New York Academy of Sciences, 1976. p. 6–13.
Touloukian RJ: The legacy of Connecticut surgery: case histories revisited. **Conn Med** 1981 Apr;45(4):241–4
Trout GM: The American Dairy Science Association: the third twenty-five years, 1957–1981. **J Dairy Sci** 1981 Jun;64(6):876–99
Tucker GS: Ida Henrietta Hyde: the first woman member of the society. **Physiologist** 1981 Dec;24(6):1–9
Tunell DN: A regional history of Southern Branch, American Public Health Association. Ed.D. Diss., University of Alabama. University, Alabama, 1977. xv, 694 leaves.
Van Riper C: An early history of ASHA. **ASHA** 1981 Nov;23(11):855–8
Verbrugge MH: The social meaning of personal health: The Ladies' Physiological Institute of Boston and vicinity in the 1850s. In Reverby S, Rosner D, ed: Health care in America. Philadelphia, Temple University Press, 1979. p. 45–66.
Wagner FB: The founding fathers and centennial history of the Philadelphia Academy of Surgery. **Ann Surg** 1980 Jul;192(1):1–8
Wall JH: Westchester County Medical Society and Westchester Division, New York Hospital–Cornell Medical Center; milestones in history. **NY State J Med** 1980 Nov;80(12):1884–5
Walsh J: Science in transition, 1946 to 1962. **Science** 1980 Jul

4;209(4452):52–7

Warren WD: Not for the profession ... for the people. **Ann Surg** 1983 Sep;198(3):241–50

Watne Al, Bartholomew S: Giants in the hills: a brief history of the West Virginia Chapter, American College of Surgeons. **W Va Med J** 1982 Jul;78(7):168–71

Waugh ES, McGoldrick KE: On the history of JAMWA. **J Am Med Wom Assoc** 1980 Jun;35(6):137–9

Webb A: A definitive history of the Raleigh Academy of Medicine. **NC Med J** 1981 Apr;42(4):260–2

Weiner AL: The Noah Worcester Dermatological Society. **Int J Dermatol** 1980 Jun;19(5):288–90

Weinhouse S: Prometheus and Pandora--cancer research on our Diamond Anniversary: American Association for Cancer Research. **Cancer Res** 1982 Sep;42(9):3471–4

Williams JE, Johns RB, Evans P: The Gold-Headed Cane award of the Taylor-Jones County Medical Society. **Tex Med** 1981 Nov;77(11):50–1

Williston CL: 1954–1984 with TMA: a look at 30 years of growth and change. **Tex Med** 1984 Jul;80(7):57–9

Wilson JL: American Thoracic Society--five great teachers in the field of tuberculosis. **Am Rev Respir Dis** 1981 May;123(5):571–5

Wilson L: Schizophrenia in learned societies: professionalism vs. scholarship. **J Hist Med Allied Sci** 1981 Jan;36(1):5–8

Winsten S, Sideman L: History of the Philadelphia Section, American Association for Clinical Chemistry. **Clin Chem** 1981 Jan;27(1):192–4

Wolfle D: Science: a memoir of the 1960's and 1970's. **Science** 1980 Jul 4;209(4452):57–60

Woolverton DK: Taking stock: Med-Chi and its women members. **Md State Med J** 1983 Oct;32(10):787–91

Yoxen EJ: Scepticism about the centrality of technology transfer in the Rockefeller Foundation programme in molecular biology. **Soc Stud Sci** 1984 May;14(2):248–52

75 years of dedication and progress: American Dairy Science Association: **J Dairy Sci** 1981 Jun;64(6):875–1526

**USSR**

Akademii Meditsinskikh Nauk SSSR--40 let. **Biull Eksp Biol Med** 1984 Jul;97(7):3–4

Akimov GA, Arkhangel'skiĭ AE: K istorii deiatel'nosti Leningradskogo nauchnogo obshchestva nevropatologov i psikhiatrov (pervye gody). **Zh Nevropatol Psikhiatr** 1983;83(7):1067–9

Alumäe N: Eesti NSV teaduste akadeemia aastail 1965–1972. [toimetuskolleegium N. Alumäe ... et al.]. Tallinn, The Academy, 1973. 274 p.

Astapenko VG: Belorusskoe Nauchnoe Meditsinskoe Obshchestvo Khirurgov (k 50–letiiu obrazovaniia obshchestva). **Khirurgiia (Mosk)** 1980;1:113–4

Bazanov VA: K istorii sozdaniia Akademii meditsinskikh nauk SSSR. **Sov Zdravookhr** 1981;(1):56–9

Bazanov VA: 35 let Akademii meditsinskikh nauk SSSR. **Feldsher Akush** 1980;45(1):3–6

Chaplinskiĭ VV, Iatsekevich IaE: L'vovskomu nauchnomu obshchestvu travmatologov-ortopedov 25 let. **Ortop Travmatol Protez** 1982 Dec;(12):60–1

Dionesov SM: Vrachebnoe obshchestvo v Derpte. **Sov Zdravookhr** 1983;5:62–3

Dunaev PV, Solov'ev GS, Agarkov VA: Rol' Nauchnogo obshchestva anatomov, gistologov i émbriologov v optimizatsii uchebnogo protsessa na morfologicheskikh kafedrakh i sovershenstvovanii muzeĭnogo dela. **Arkh Anat Gistol Embriol** 1984 Feb;86(2):93–5

Frolov VA: K 40–letiiu sozdaniia Akademii meditsinskikh nauk USSR. **Patol Fiziol Eksp Ter** 1984 Jul–Aug;(4):3–9

Gerasimovich GT: Belorusskomu Nauchnomu Meditsinskomu obshchestvu Akusherov-Ginekologov 50 let. **Akush Ginekol (Mosk)** 1981 Sep;(9):59–61

Gubko AT: Le rôle de l'Académie de Kiev dans la naissance de la science psychologique en Ukraine. (Rus) **Vopr Psikhol** 1980;(1):82–93

K 40–letiiu Akademii meditsinskikh nauk SSSR: **Arkh Anat Gistol Embriol** 1984 Jun;86(6):5–10

Kharshak EM: Nauchnaia deiatel'nost' oblastnykh obshchestv otolaringologov v USSR za period 1957–1978 gg. (po protokolam i godovym otchetam obshchestv, opublikovannym v ZhUNGB s 1959 po 1978 g.). **Zh Ushn Nos Gorl Bolezn** 1980 May–Jun;(3):56–64

Kolesov VI: Khirurgicheskomu obshchestvu Pirogova--100 let. **Vestn Khir** 1982 May;128(5):127–36

Koliadiuk IV, Mamontov AS, Kovaleva NS, et al: Stranitsy nasheĭ istorii. **Sov Med** 1983;(12):111–3

Komkov GD, Levšin BV, Semenov LK: Geschichte der Akademie der Wissenschaften der UdSSR. Ed. C. Grau. Berlin, Akademie Verlag, 1981. 745 p. (Translation from the Russian edition of 1977)

Korol' GG, Denisova TP, Naumenko AM: Iz istorii instituta im. N. V. Sklifosovskogo. **Sov Zdravookhr** 1984;(10):53–5

Kovalev MM, Roĭ VP, Burka AA, et al: Deviat'sot zasedaniĭ nauchnogo obshchestva khirurgov Kieva i Kievskoĭ oblasti. **Klin Khir** 1984 Apr;(4):58–61

Krasnov MM: Proshloe v nastoiashchem: Adrian Aleksandrovich Kriukov, redaktor 'Vestnika oftal'mologii' i osnovatel' Moskovskogo oftal'mologicheskogo veshchestva (k 75–letiiu zhurnala). **Vestn Oftalmol** 1984 Nov–Dec;(6):4–6

Lukash AA: 30 let deiatel'nosti Estonskogo otdeleniia Vsesouiznogo nauchnogo obshchestva sudebnykh medikov. **Sud Med Ekspert** 1982 Apr–Jun;25(2):57–9

Mazurik EV: O pedagogicheskoĭ deiatel'nosti N. I. Pirogova v Kamenets--Polol'ske i o ego sviaziakh s Obshchestvom polol'skikh vracheĭ (k 100–letiiu so dnia smerti N. I. Pirogova). **Sov Zdravookhr** 1981;(8):66–8

Miliavskiĭ VM: Obshchestvo poltavskikh vracheĭ i 'Trudy post oiannoĭ meditsinskoĭ komissii pri Poltavskoĭ gubernnskoĭ zemskoĭ uprave'. **Sov Zdravookhr** 1981;(4):69–71

Orzheshkovskiĭ VV, Chopchik DI: 20–letie Ukrainskogo respublikanskogo nauchnogo obshchestva fizioterapevtov i kurortologov. **Vopr Kurortol Fizioter Lech Fiz Kult** 1979 Sep–Oct;(5):69–70

Petrov BD: Akademii meditsinskikh nauk SSSR - 40 let. **Vestn Akad Med Nauk SSSR** 1984;(6):3–13

Popushoi EP: Rol' meditsinskikh obvshchestv Moldavii v razvitii meditsinskoĭ mysli vo vtoroi polovine XIX--nachale XX veka. **Sov Zdravookhr** 1982;(1):65–8

Popushoĭ EP, Ioksa VA: Vklad nauchnykh meditsinskikh obshchestv Moldavskoĭ SSR v razvitie narodnogo zdravookhraneniia. **Sov Zdravookhr** 1984;(8):54–7

Preobrazhenskiĭ NA, Konstantinova NP: Vsesoiuznoe nauchnoe obshchestvo otorinolaringologov k 60–letiiu obrazovaniia SSSR. **Vestn Otorinolaringol** 1982 Nov–Dec;(6):8–13

Revutskiĭ EL: 50 let Respublikanskogo nauchnogo obshchestva terapevtov USSR. **Vrach Delo** 1981 Oct;(10):120–1

Roshchin AV: 100–letie Ustava Moskovskogo gigienicheskogo obshchestva. **Gig Sanit** 1982;(5):48–9

Sakharov MI, Sorokin EIu: Sverdlovskoe oblastnoe nauchnoe obshchestvo khirurgov (k 50–letiiu so dnia obrazovaniia). **Vestn Khir** 1982 May;128(5):136–7

Shabunin AV: Uchastie N.I. Pirogova v Obshchestve S.-Peterburgskikh prakticheskikh vracheĭ. **Sov Zdravookhr** 1983;(4):63–5

Shumada IV, Gorodniaia VN: K istorii Kievskogo obshchestva travmatologov-ortopedov. **Ortop Travmatol Protez** 1984 Aug;(8):69–73

Skobulovich GV: Itogi deiatel'nosti Amursjkogo otdeleniia Nauchnogo obshchestva épidemiologov, mikrobiologov i parazitologov za 25 let (1957–1982). **Zh Mikrobiol Epidemiol Immunobiol** 1984 Feb;(2):117–9

Stepanskiĭ GA, Fomenko VN: Sovetskaia toksikologicheskaia nauka i deiatel'nost' moskovskikh toksikologov (k 15-letiiu toksikologicheskoĭ sektsii Moskovskogo nauchnogo obshchestva farmakologov). **Farmakol Toksikol** 1980 Nov–Dec;43(6):747–50

Strukov AI, Smol'iannikov AV, Sarkisov DS: Razrabotka problem patologicheskoĭ anatomii v sisteme Akademii Meditsinskikh Nauk SSSR za 40 let ee sushchestvovaniia (1944–1984). **Arkh Patol** 1984;46(6):3–15

Usov IN: Belorusskomu nauchnomu obschchestvu detskikh vracheĭ 50 let. **Pediatriia** 1983 Nov;(11):72–4

Vasil'ev KK: K istorii meditsinskikh obshchestv v Rossii. **Sov Zdravookhr** 1983;(1):71–3

Verenkina TN: Vrachebnye obshchestva v dorevoliutsionnom Sevastopole. **Sov Zdravookhr** 1982;(6):68–71

Zikeev PD: Chrezvychaĭnyĭ kholernyĭ s'ezd Obshchestva russkikh vracheĭ v pamiat' N. I. Pirogova. **Sov Zdravookhr** 1981;(11):56–9

**Venezuela**

Briceño Romero G: Discurso del doctor Gabriel Briceño Romero al tomar posesion de la presidencia de la Sociedad Venezolana de Historia de la Medicina. **Rev Soc Venez Hist Med** 1972–73;20–21(34–35)79–86

**Yugoslavia**

Belicza B: Liječnička udruženja i razvoj medicinske periodike s posebnim osvrtom na 'Liječnički vjesnik' Glasilo Zbora liječnika Hrvatske (1877–1977). **Saopcenja** 1978;21(1–2):133–56

Belicza B: U povodu stote obljetnice Zbora Liječnika Hrvatske (1874–1974). **Saopcenja** 1974;17(1):55–74

Berić BM, Berić ML: Društvo lekara iz Vojvodine (1919–1929). **Med Pregl** 1983;36(5–6):253–7

Dugački V: 'Hrvatsko društvo za čuvanje narodnog zdravlja' i njegov časopis 'Zivot i zdravlje'. **Lijec Vjesn** 1982 May;104(5):208–10

Pavlović BB: Pismo Rista Jeremića povodom osnivanja sekcije za istoriju medicine i farmacije Srpskog lekarskog društva u Beogradu 12. II 1950 godine. **Srp Arh Celok Lek** 1981 Jul;109(7):955–8

Straser P, Protić M: Pečat karlovačkog hiruško-berberskog esnafa iz XVIII veka. **Med Pregl** 1982;35(11–12):493

Stručno-znanstveni sastanak u povodu tridesete obljetnice o snutka sekcije za hematologiju i transfuziologiju ZLH (1948–1978): **Lijec Vjesn** 1981;103(3):105–30

## SPECIALIZATION

Bevan PG: Generalism and specialisation in surgery. **Ann R Coll Surg Engl** 1981 Nov;63(6):383–5

Küss R: Chirurgie générale ou chirurgie spécialisée. Une dualité dépassée? **Nouv Presse Med** 1980 Oct 11;9(37):2757-8
Ritter L: Die Spezialgebiete der Medizin und ihre Geschichte. Darmstadt, Bläschke, 1978. 262 p.
Swenson O: Specialization: What it holds for the future of medicine. **Can J Surg** 1980 Mar;23(2):154-6

**1700 to Present**

García Ballester L: Factores sociomédicos en el proceso de constitución de las especialidades médicas: el caso de la otología. In Albarracin Teulon A, et al, ed: Medicina e Historia. Madrid, Edic. Univ. Comp., 1973. p. 321-38.
Geison GL: Scientific change, emerging specialties, and research schools. **Hist Sci** 1981;19(1):20-40
Haber C: Geriatrics: a specialty in search of specialists. **Z Gerontol** 1984 Jan-Feb;17(1):26-31
Heidenheimer AJ: Organized medicine and physician specialization in Scandinavia and West Germany. **West Eur Polit** 1980;3(3):373-87
Kunitz SJ: The historical roots and ideological functions of disease concepts in three primary care specialties. **Bull Hist Med** 1983 Fall;57(3):412-32
Lenzi E: Nota informativa sull'U.P.I.G.O. e sull'U.E.M.S. **Minerva Ginecol** 1981 Feb-Mar;33(2-3):153-5

**Great Britain**

Dainton C: The age of specialisation. **Br Herit** 1981;2(2):56-65

**United States**

History, information, and examination requirements of the American Board of Prosthodontics. **J Prosthet Dent** 1984 Aug;52(2):281-7
Cone TE: Abraham Jacobi on medical specialization, as viewed in 1880. **Pediatrics** 1981;67:481
Daly WJ: A personal testament--reflections on the Tower of Babel. **J Lab Clin Med** 1982 Jan;99(1):10-4
King LS: Medicine in the USA: historical vignettes. XXI. Medical practice: specialization. **JAMA** 1984 Mar 9;251(10):1333-8
Little DM: The founding of the specialty boards. **Anesthesiology** 1981 Sep;55(3):317-21
Pitts JA: The Association of Medical Superintendents of American Institutions for the Insane, 1844-1892: a case study of specialism in American medicine. Ph.F. diss. University of Pennsylvania. Philadelphia, 1979. 267 leaves.
Ritchey FJ: Medical rationalization, cultural lag, and the malpractice crisis. **Hum Organ** 1981;40(2):97-112
Stevens R: The changing idea of a medical specialty. **Trans Stud Coll Physicians Phila** 1980 Sep;5(2 no 3):159-77
Talbot DM: Federation of Specialty Nursing Organizations and the American Nurses' Association: a history. **Occup Health Nurs** 1981 Oct;29(10):27-33

## SPORTS MEDICINE

Arndt KH, Arndt C: Die Medizin bei Olympia. **Z Arztl Fortbild (Jena)** 1980 Apr 15;74(8):389-92
Borms J, Hebbelinck M, Venerando A, ed: Women and sport: an historical, biological, physiological and sportsmedical approach. Basel, Karger, 1981. 229 p. (Medicine and sport, Vol. 14)
Daněk K: Skiing in and through the history of medicine. **Nord Medicinhist Arsb** 1982;:86-100
Jokl E: Medicine, science and sport. **Trans Stud Coll Physicians Phila** 1980 Jun;5(2 no 2):81-9
Percy EC: Sports medicine: its past, present and future. **Ariz Med** 1983 Nov;40(11):789-92
Snook GA: The history of sports medicine. **Am J Sports Med** 1984 Jul-Aug;12(4):252-4
Stricevic MV, Patel MR, Okazaki T, et al: Karate: historical perspective and injuries sustained in national and international tournament competitions. **Am J Sports Med** 1983 Sep-Oct;11(5):320-4

**Before 500 A.D.**

**Greece**

Retsas S: Medicine and the Olympic games of antiquity. **Hist Med (Lond)** 1981;9(1):4-7
Vandewiele LJ: Herodikos, de eerste sportarts. **Farm Tijdschr Belg** 1978;55:13-4

**Rome**

Wacke A: Unfälle bei Sport und Spiel nach römischem und geltendem Recht. **Stadion** 1977;3(1):4-43

**1700 to Present**

Dubb A: Medical philately: sport and medicine. **S Afr Med J** 1981 Jul 25;60(4):144-6
Hollmann W: 100 Jahre Sportmedizin. **Fortschr Med** 1983 Oct 6;101(37):1660-3
Maud PJ, Pollock ML, Foster C, et al: Fifty years of training and competition in the marathon: Wally Hayward, age 70--a physiological profile. **S Afr Med J** 1981 Jan 31;59(5):153-7

**Chile**

Dill DB: International high altitude expedition to Chile, 1935. **Prog Clin Biol Res** 1983;136:201-4

**Czechoslovakia**

Daněk K: Lyžování v dějinách lékařství. K 90. vtoči začátku lyžování na Vysŏ cině. **Cas Lek Cesk** 1982 Apr 9;121(14):437-40
Pros JR: Padesát let gynekologické poradny pro sportovkyně. **Cesk Gynekol** 1983 Feb;48(1):55-6

**Denmark**

Thorseth K: Idraetsmedicin. **Ugeskr Laeger** 1981;143(34):2189-90

**Italy**

Brieger GH: The diseases of runners: a view from the eighteenth century--a commentary. **Pharos** 1980 Fall;43(4):29-32

**Nepal**

Hornbein TF: Everest without oxygen. **Prog Clin Biol Res** 1983;136:409-14
Pugh LG, Sutton JR: Everest then and now. **Prog Clin Biol Res** 1983;136:415-30

**Spain**

Balius R: Hitos de la historia de la educacion fisica española. **Apuntes Med Deportiva** 1975;12:215-20

**United States**

Brady GM: Lou Gehrig: the iron man. **Manuscripts** 1980;32(2):84-9
Emerson RS: Olympics and sports medicine. **NY State J Med** 1980 May;80(6):992-4
Haycock CE: The female athlete and sportsmedicine in the 70's. **J Fla Med Assoc** 1980 Apr;67(4):411-4
Jackson DW: The history of sports medicine. **Am J Sports Med** 1984 Jul-Aug;12(4):255-7
Morris AF: Sports medicine today. **J Sports Med Phys Fitness** 1982 Jun;22(2):259-73
Novich MM: Early developments in sports medicine. **J Med Soc NJ** 1982 Apr;79(4):309-13
Rowthorn AW: A history of the evolution and development of therapeutic recreation services for special populations in the United States from 1918 to 1977. Ph.D. Diss. New York University. New York, 1978. 351 leaves.
Whorton JC: 'Athlete's heart': the medical debate over athleticism, 1870-1920. **J Sport Hist** 1982;9(1):30-52

**USSR**

Zimkin NV: 60 let kafedre fiziologii Leningradskogo instituta fizicheskoĭ kul'tury imeni P. F. Lesgafta. **Fiziol Zh SSSR** 1979 Dec;65(12):1854-6

## STATE MEDICINE

See also **Economics, Medical; Politics; Public Health; Social Welfare**

Nutton V: Continuity or rediscovery? The city physician in classical antiquity and mediaeval Italy. In Russell AW, ed: The town and state physician in Europe from the Middle Ages to the Enlightenment. Wolfenbüttel, Herzog August Bibliothek, 1981. p. 9-46 (Wolfenbütteler Forschungen, 17).

**Germany**

Stürzbecher M: The physician in German-speaking countries from the Middle-Ages to the Enlightenment. In Russell AW, ed: The town and state physician in Europe from the Middle Ages to the Enlightenment. Wolfenbüttel, Herzog August Bibliothek, 1981. p. 123-29 (Wolfenbütteler Forschungen, 17).

**Hungary**

Zólyomi ND: The development of the district medical officer in Hungary from the Middle-Ages to the 18th century. In Russell AW, ed: The town and state physician in Europe from the Middle Ages to the Enlightenment. Wolfenbüttel, Herzog August Bibliothek, 1981. p. 131–40 (Wolfenbütteler Forschungen, 17).

**Switzerland**

Koelbing HM: Town and state physicians in Switzerland (16th–18th centuries). In Russell AW, ed: The town and state physician in Europe from the Middle Ages to the Enlightenment. Wolfenbüttel, Herzog August Bibliothek, 1981. p. 141–55 (Wolfenbütteler Forschungen, 17).

**500 A.D.–1450**

**Arabic**

Karmi G: State control of the physician in the Middle Ages: an Islamic model. In Russell AW, ed: The town and state physician in Europe from the Middle Ages to the Enlightenment. Wolfenbüttel, Herzog August Bibliothek, 1981. p. 63–84 (Wolfenbütteler Forschungen, 17).

**Italy**

Palmer R: Physicians and the state in post-mediaeval Italy. In Russell AW, ed: The town and state physician in Europe from the Middle Ages to the Enlightenment. Wolfenbüttel, Herzog August Bibliothek, 1981. p. 47–61 (Wolfenbütteler Forschungen, 17).

**Mexico**

Prygova NM: O roli gosudarstva v meditsinskom dele atstekov (k voprosu ob izuchenii metsiny rabovladel'cheskikh obshchestv). **Sov Zdravookhr** 1981;(8):68–71

**1450–1700**

**Spain**

López-Piñero JM: The medical profession in 16th century Spain. In Russell AW, ed: The town and state physician in Europe from the Middle Ages to the Enlightenment. Wolfenbüttel, Herzog August Bibliothek, 1981. p. 85–98 (Wolfenbütteler Forschungen, 17).

**1700 to Present**

Godber G: The NHS in an international setting. **Health Bull (Edinb)** 1982 Mar;40(2):67–76

Shishkin AP: Gosudarstvennyĭ institut sotsial'noĭ gigieny Narkomzdrava RSFSR i ego rol' v razvitii teorii i organizatsii sovetskogo. **Sov Zdravookhr** 1982;(6):59–62

**Bulgaria**

Todorow A: Die Entwicklung des Gesundheitswesens in der Volksrepublik Bulgarien. **Med Ges** 1979;(6):35–46

Vasilev D: Borbata na BKP v pomosht na gladuvashtite v Suvestska Rusiia. **Izv Inst Istor BKP** 1968;18:339–65

**Canada**

Black E: Dealing with the doctors: the Canadian experience. **Mon Rev** 1981;33(4):27–35

Collins LD, Higgins D, ed: The politics of abortion: trends in Canadian fertility policy. **Atlantis** 1982;7(2):2–20

Heeney B: Opposition to state medicine and state education: an historical analogy. **Queens Q** 1968;75(1):72–89

LaBerge R: Medicare is not the health charter for Canadians. **Can Labour** 1969;14(9):14–9

Morton D: 'Noblest and best': retaining Canada's war disabled 1915–23. **J Can Stud** 1981;16(3–4):75–85

Shipley M, Agass M, Bell A, et al: The Quebec Medicare Programme. **R Soc Health J** 1982 Feb;102(1):37–8, 43

Soderstrom L: The Canadian experience. **Proc Acad Polit Sci** 1980;33(4):224–38

Summers JL: A century of health protection. **Can J Hosp Pharm** 1975 Sep–Oct;28(5):143

Walters V: State, capital, and labour: the introduction of Federal-Provincial insurance for physician care in Canada. **Can Rev Sociol Anthropol** 1982;19(2):157–72

**Chile**

Mardones J: Origen del Servicio Nacional de Salud. **Rev Med Chil** 1977 Oct;105(10):654–8

Neghme A: La educación médica y el Servicio Nacional de Salud. **Rev Med Chil** 1977 Oct;105(10):668–73

Unda F: Acciones de saneamiento ambiental del Servicio Nacional de Salud, 1952–1957. **Rev Med Chil** 1977 Oct;105(10):714–23

Urzúa Merion H: Estructuración inicial del Servicio Nacional de Salud. **Rev Med Chil** 1977 Oct;105(10):659–62

**China**

Lucas A: Chinese Medical Modernization. Comparative Policy Continuities, 1930s–1980s. New York, Praeger, 1982. xiii, 188 p.

**Cuba**

Gordon G, Bishop B: Community control, Cuban style. **Freedomways** 1981;21(3):194–200

Ochoa FR: Die Entwicklung des Gesundheitswesens in der Republik Kuba (1959–1973). **Med Ges** 1979;(6):84–98

Parra Hidalgo P: 'Marco téorico y conceptual de la atención médica primaria en Cuba'. **Rev Sanid Hig Publica (Madr)** 1980 Sep–Oct;54(9–10):959–1008

Richmond JB: A conversation with Fidel Castro about health services. **N Engl J Med** 1984 Apr 12;310(15):994–5

**Czechoslovakia**

Prokopec J: Die Entwicklung des Gesundheitswesens in der CSSR. **Med Ges** 1979;(6):110–22

Slavětínský M: Připomínka prukopníka zestátněnú veřejného zdravotnictví z Moravy na sklonku minulého století. **Cesk Zdrav** 1980 May;28(5):219–20

**Europe**

Blanpain J, Delesie L, Nys H: National health insurance and health resources. Cambridge, Harvard Univ. Press, 1978. xiv, 294 p.

**France**

Gelfand T: Public medicine and medical careers in France during the reign of Louis XV. In Russell AW, ed: The town and state physician in Europe from the Middle Ages to the Enlightenment. Wolfenbüttel, Herzog August Bibliothek, 1981. p. 99–122 (Wolfenbütteler Forschungen, 17).

Milliez P: La médecine socialisée. **Acquis Med Recent** 1978;:189–91

**Germany**

Büttner L, Meyer B: Karl Marx und die Begründung der Gesundheitspolitik der revolutionären Arbeiterbewegung. II. Marx' Aufdeckung des Klasseninhalts der bürgerlichen Gesundheitspolitik. **Z Arztl Fortbild (Jena)** 1983;77(19):819–23

Engels W: Zur Geschichte des Verstaatlichungsgedankens im deutschen Apothekenwesen. Stuttgart, Deutscher Apotheker Verlag, 1984. 261 p. (Quellen und Studien zur Geschichte der Pharmazie, Bd. 28).

Kober R: Abteilung Gesundheits- und Sozialwesen des Rates des Bezirkes Gera. **Z Arztl Fortbild (Jena)** 1979 Oct 1;73(19–20):983–6

Nemitz K: Die Bemühungen zur Schaffung eines Reichsgesundheitsministeriums in der ersten Phase der Weimarer Republik 1918–1922. **Medizinhist J** 1981;16(4):424–45

Schmidt H: Zur Kostenfreiheit ärztlicher Hilfeleistung; eine Betrachtung aus Anlass des 90. Jahrestages des Erfurter Programms der SPD. **Beitr Gesch Univ Erfurt** 1979–83;19:265–70

Schüler H: Die Entwicklung des Gesundheitswesens in der Deutschen Demokratischen Republik. **Med Ges** 1979;(6):69–83

**Great Britain**

Bowles G: National Health Dental Services 1948–1955. **Soc Soc Hist Med Bull (Lond)** 1981 Dec;29:1–6

Brown A: COHSE: pioneers from the past. **Nurs Mirror** 1980 Jul 10;151(2):8

Coventry JB: The dental estimates board. Thirty-three years at Eastbourne. **Br Dent J** 1981 Jul 7;151(1):33–4

Earwicker R: The emergence of a medical strategy in the Labour Movement 1906–1919. **Soc Soc Hist Med Bull (Lond)** 1981 Dec;29:6–9

Eder NR: National health insurance, social politics and medical practice in Britain, 1913–1939. Ph.D. diss. University of Illinois. Chicago, 1980. 375 leaves.

Francis H: The reorganisation of the National Health Service in 1974. **Soc Soc Hist Med Bull (Lond)** 1981 Dec;29:9–20

Godber G: Looking back on the NHS. **Hosp Health Serv Rev** 1979 Jan;75(1):23–4

Godber G: The British health system: achievements and limitations. **Isr J Med Sci** 1982 Mar;18(3):365–73

Hamilton D: The early history of the Highlands and Islands Medical Scheme. **Scott Med J** 1979 Jan;24(1):64–8

Harris J: William Beveridge. A biography. Oxford, Clarendon Press, 1977. 488 p.

Health care and its costs: The development of the National Health Service in England. London, H. M. S. O., 1983. 51 p.

Himsworth H: On the integration of expert knowledge into the machinery

of government. **Br Med J** 1980 Nov 1;281(6249):1197–9
Hindley-Smith D: The General Dental Council. Twenty-five years on. **Probe (Lond)** 1981 Jul;23(1):29–30, 32
Honigsbaum F: Medical politics and the state: the part played by the medical profession in the development of the National Health Service. **Soc Soc Hist Med Bull (Lond)** 1981 Dec;29:20–1
Honigsbaum F: The BMA–TUC alliance and the Beveridge report. **Soc Soc Hist Med Bull (Lond)** 1983 Jun;32:19
Ingle ST: Parliament and health policy: the role of MPs, 1970–75. Farnborough, Gower, 1981 vi, 171 p.
Lindsay CM, Seldon A, Feigenbaum B: National health issues. [s.l.], Roche Laboratories, 1980. viii, 130 p.
Marks J: The Conference of Local Medical Committees and its executive: an historical review. [London?], Trustees of the General Medical Services Defence Trust, 1979. 32 p.
Morgan KO: Dr. Christopher Addison and social reform. **Soc Soc Hist Med Bull (Lond)** 1981 Dec;29:21–5
Navarro V: Class struggle, the state and medicine. An historical and contemporary analysis of the medical sector in Great Britain. New York, Prodist, 1978. xviii, 156 p.
Pinsent R: The birth of an NHS practice. **Soc Soc Hist Med Bull (Lond)** 1983 Dec;33:11–2
Stephens SD: The role of the state in hearing health care. **Br J Audiol** 1982 Nov;16(4):255–63
Walters V: Class inequality and health care. London, Croom Helm, 1980. 175 p.
Watkin B: The National Health Service: the first phase, 1948–1974 and after. London, Boston, Allen and Unwin, 1978. 170 p.
Whitehouse WL: The British National Health Service. **Zentralbl Gynakol** 1984;106(14):1028–32
Whiteside N: Central control and the approved societies: access to social support under the interwar health insurance scheme. **Soc Soc Hist Med Bull (Lond)** 1983 Jun;32:14–8
Wilson TS: The National Health Service 1948–1980. In Checkland O, Lamb M, ed: Health care as social history; the Glasgow case. Aberdeen, Aberdeen University Press, 1982. p. 149–57.

### Hungary

The development of social insurance in Hungary over three decades. [Budapest?], The Administration, [1975?]. 114 p.:
Lukázs J, Keresztes L, Hal G, et al: Die Entwicklung des Gesundheitswesens in der Ungarischen Volksrepublik. **Med Ges** 1979;(6):47–68
Mervo Z: A Hajdu-Bihar megyei tanács és Debrecen város egészségügyi szolgálatának ágazati felépítése, hataśköre 1950–1956 között. **Leveltari Sz** 1973;23(2):189–209
Orsós S: A megyei 'fogász-föorvostól' a stomatologus felügyelö szakföorvosig. **Fogorv Sz** 1984 Jun;77(6):165–9

### India

Deodhar NS: Primary health care in India. **J Public Health Policy** 1982 Mar;3(1):76–99

### Italy

Piva I: Su taluni 'momenti di passaggio' dal sistema mutualistico al Servizio Sanitario Nazionale. **Minerva Med** 1981 Sep 26;72(36):2415–21

### Malawi

Baker C: The Government Medical Service in Malawi: an administrative history, 1891–1974. **Med Hist** 1976 Jul;20(3):296–311

### Mexico

Correa Vázquez ME: Capital monopolista, estado e instituciones estatales de salud en Mexico, 1940–1978. **Invest Econ** 1981;40(158):57–83

### Netherlands

Van der Esch P: Geschiedenis van het Staatstoezicht op Krankzinningen. 's-Gravenhage, Ministerium van Volksgezondheit en Milieuhygiene, 1975-1980. 3 volumes in 1.

### Poland

Fijałek J: Kasa Chorych--pierwowzór społecznego, samorzadowego lecznictwa pracowniczego w Polsce. **Arch Hist Med (Warsz)** 1984;47(1):99–106
Leowski J: Die Entwicklung des Gesundheitswesens in der VR Polen. **Med Ges** 1979;(6):99–109

### Spain

Folch Jou G, Sanz Diaz L, Puerto Sarmiento FJ: Los proyectos de socialización de la farmacia durante la Segunda República española. **Pharm Acta Helv** 1979;54(9–10):286–94
Parrilla Hermida M: Apuntes historicos sobre la subdelegacion del promedicato en Cataluña. **Asclepio** 1981;33:391–405

### Sweden

Sandblom P: The tragic development of socialized medicine in Sweden. **Bull Am Coll Surg** 1976 Feb;61(2):13–5
Thulin KE: Infektionernas förändrade sjukdomspanorama under 40 år. **Sydsven Medicinhist Sallsk Arsskr** 1981;.151–69

### United States

History and use of Public Health Service Commissioned Corps: hearing before the Subcommittee on Health and the Environment of the Committee on Energy and Commerce, House of Representatives, Ninety-seventh Congress, session, June 14, 1982. Washington, GPO, 1982. iii, 141 p.
Altenstetter C, Bjorkman JW: Federal-state health policies and impacts: the politics of implementation. Washington, University Press of America, 1978. xi, 116 p.
Altman D: Health care for the poor. **Ann Am Acad Polit Soc Sci** 1983;(468):103–21
Ashcraft ML, Berki SE: Health maintenance organizations as Medicaid providers. **Ann Am Acad Polit Soc Sci** 1983;(468):122–31
Keisling P: Old soldiers never die: can we pay for the VA's version of the baby boom? **Wash Mon** 1982;14(1):20–9
Lave JR, Silverman HA: Financing the health care of the aged. **Ann Am Acad Polit Soc Sci** 1983;(468):149–64
Miller EB: Petition for a Federal Veterinary Sanitary Bureau. **J Am Vet Med Assoc** 1984 May 15;184(10):1224–5
Morgan AH: Is there a doctor in the house? or for the house? **Rev Am Hist** 1980;8(1):129–33
Numbers RL: Compulsory health insurance: the continuing American debate. Westport, Greenwood Press, 1982. xv, 172 p.
Pond MA: Presidential initiatives in organizing health affairs: from Harding to Roosevelt. **Pres Stud Q** 1983;13(3):417–29
Stalheim OH: Contributions of the Bureau of Animal Industry to the veterinary profession. **J Am Vet Med Assoc** 1984 May 15;184(10):1222–4
Starr P: Transformation of defeat: the changing objectives of national health insurance, 1915–1980. **Am J Public Health** 1982 Jan;72(1):78–88
Underhill D: Government health insurance: an analysis of division. **Mich J Polit Sci** 1981;1(1):26–38

### USSR

Bastenchuk AZ, Vladova MI, Siur HA, et al: Dosiahnennia aptechnoiï sluzhby Zaporiz'koï oblasti z chasu pryïniattia dekretu pro natsionalizatsiiu aptek na Ukraïni. **Farm Zh** 1979;(6):9–11
Bazanov VA: Pervaia piatiletka i planirovanie meditsinskoĭ nauki. **Sov Zdravookhr** 1980;(2):68–71
Beliatskiĭ DP: K istorii razvitiia zdravookhraneniia BSSR na osnove printsipov leninskoĭ natsional'noĭ politiki KPSS. **Sov Zdravookhr** 1982;(11):57–60
Belitskaia EIa, Zhuravleva KI: K 60-letiiu Kafedry sotsial'noĭ gigieny i organizatsii zdravookhraneniia Leningradskogo sanitarno-gigienicheskogo meditsinskogo instituta. **Sov Zdravookhr** 1982;(7):61–3
Blokhin NN, Napalkov NP: Razvitie onkologii v SSSR. **Vopr Onkol** 1982;28(12):3–9
Chechenkina OI: Progress zdravookhraneniia c respublikakh Sredneĭ Azii i Kazakhstane - rezul'tat Leninskoĭ natsional'noĭ politiki. **Sov Zdravookhr** 1982;(11):49–51
Chemerisski IA: Kommunisticheskaia partiia: organizator bor'by s golodom (1921–1922 gg). **Vopr Istor KPSS** 1971;11:42–53
Chernobrov IV: Vrach-revoliutsioner N. A. Alekseev. **Sov Zdravookhr** 1983;(11):57–9
Davydov MI: Zabota o detiakh iz istorii deiatel'-nosti Soveta zashchity detei v 1918–1920 godakh. **Istor SSSR** 1979;5:163–71
Drobizhev VZ. Stanovlenie politiki sovetskogo gosudarstva v oblasti estestvennogo dvizheniia naseleniia. **Vestn Mosk Univ Ser 8 Istor** 1981;1:17–26
Edmondson CM: The politics of hunger: the Soviet response to famine. **Sov Stud** 1977;29(4):506–18
Fedotov V: Zabota partii i naroda o ranenykh v gody voiny. **Voen Istor Zh** 1977;6:90–4
Fel' II, Truman GL: A. M. Aliev--vydaiushchiĭsia pertiĭnyĭ, gosudarstvennyĭ deiatel', organizator zdravookhraneniia i meditsinskoĭ nauki v Sovetskom Azerbaĭdzhane. **Sov Zdravookhr** 1982;(8):57–9
Gavrilov OK: Meditsinskaia nauka k 60-ĭ godoshchine obrazovaniia Soiuza Sovetskikh Sotsialisticheskikh Respublik. **Sov Zdravookhr** 1982;(8):3–8
Klessen D: Zur Entwicklung der Beziehungen zwischen Sozialhygiene und Organisation des Gesundheitswesens in der Sowjetunion. **Z Gesamte Hyg** 1980 Apr;26(4):290–4
Korotkikh RV, Gorelova LE, Shtil'man NL: M. Tsetkin (k 100-letiiu so dnia rozhdeniia). **Sov Zdravookhr** 1983;(11):63–6

## STATE MEDICINE

Kozliuk VM, Leonenko NA, Stefanovskaia NV: O razvitii lechebno-profilakticheskoĭ pomoshchi naseleniiu USSR v 1917-1940 gg. **Vrach Delo** 1982 Apr;(4):3-7
Kuz'min MK: Sovetskaia meditsina na razlichnykh étapakh sotsialisticheskogo stroitel'stva. **Sov Med** 1982;(12):10-6
Kuz'min MS: Mezhnarodnye sviazi Narkomzdrava RSFSR v pervye gody Sovetskoĭ vlasti. **Sov Zdravookhr** 1984;(5):53-7
Landa LM: Pomoshch' trudiashchikhsia turkestana golodaiushchemu naseleniiu RSFSR v 1921-1922 gg. **Istor SSSR** 1971;2:136-40
Likhachev AG: Dostizheniia sovetskogo zdravookhraneniia. **Vestn Otorinolaringol** 1982 Nov-Dec;(6):3-8
Maĭstruk PN, Popik SIa, Petrun' AS, et al: Organizatsiia deiatel'nosti sanitarno-épidemiologicheskoĭ sluzhby v oblasti gigieny pitaniia na Ukraine v period stanovleniia Sovetskoŏi vlasti i v gody pervykh piatiletok. **Gig Sanit** 1982 Apr;(4):54-6
Mkrtchian LN: Osnovnye étapy razvitiia onkologii i rentgenologii v Armianskoĭ SSR. **Vopr Onkol** 1982;28(12):20-4
Potulov BM: V. I. Lenin and public health. **Sante Publique (Bucur)** 1981;24(1):3-12
Réti E: Lenin, a modern egészségpolitika úttörője. **Orvostort Kozl** 85(24 No 3):77-84, 1978
Ryzhakova GI: Itogi vypolneniia direktiv Dal'kraĭkoma VKP(b) po stroitel'stvu ob'ektov zdravookhraneniia v gody pervykh piatiletok (1928-1937). **Sov Zdravookhr** 1982;(8):55-7
Savchenko NE, Shitikov BD: Ob uspekhakh i tendentsiiakh razvitiia onkologicheskoĭ sluzhby v Belorusskoĭ SSR. **Vopr Onkol** 1982;28(12):13-20
Skishkin AP: Vazhnyĭ étap v razvitii planirovaniia sovetskoge zdravookhranenia. **Sov Zdravookhr** 1982;(3):61-4
Tschikin SJ: Die Entwicklung des Gesundheitswesens in der UdSSR. **Med Ges** 1979;(6):11-34
Verenkina TN, Davidiuk VG: Zdravookhranenie Sebastopolia v pervye gody Sovetskoĭ vlasti (1920-1923). **Sov Zdravookhr** 1983;(11):54-7
Vodolagin MA: Partiia--organizator pomoshchi ranenym boitsam i komandiram krasnoi armii v gody volikoi otechestvennoi voiny. **Vopr Istor KPSS** 1978;2:64-75
Zhamba G, Gorin OZ, Avilov EN, et al: Itogi bor'by s infektsionnymi zabolevaniiami v Mongol'skoĭ Narodnoĭ Respublike za 60 let narodnoĭ vlasti. **Zh Mikrobiol Epidemiol Immunobiol** 1982 Jun;(6):23-6
Zhukova LA: Deiatel'nost' gosudarstvennykh i obshchestvennykh organizatsiĭ po likvidatsii detskoĭ besprizornosti v SSSR (1917-1932). **Sov Zdravookhr** 1982;(10):62-6

**Yugoslavia**

Farcnik F, Vrbic V: Stomatološka klinika včeraj, danes, jutri. **Zobozdrav Vestn** 1981 Summer;36(3-4):81-7
Health care planning in urban areas: Zagreb: **World Hosp** 1978 May;14(2):123-9

## STATISTICS AND DEMOGRAPHY

See also **Birth Control; Mathematics; Public Health**

Adams RE: Social structural consequences of population growth. **J Biosoc Sci** 1981 Jan;13(1):107-22
Bastenie PA: Le vieillissement. Vers une nouvelle source de jeunesse. Paris, Flammarion, 1983. 270 p. (De La Science à l'Homme).
Bideau A, Poulain M: De la généalogie à la démographie historique: généalogie ascendante et analyse démographique. **Ann Demogr Hist (Paris)** 1984;:55-68
Bideau A: Présentation. **Ann Demogr Hist (Paris)** 1981;:23-30
Bideau A, et al: Démographie historique et génétique des populations: la concentration géographique d'une maladie héréditaire rare. **Ann Econ Soc Civilis** 1979;34:85-105
Biraben JN: Essai sur l'évolution du nombre des hommes. **Population** 1979;34(1):13-24
Black FL: Modern isolated pre-agricultural populations as a source of information on prehistoric epidemic patterns. In Stanley NF, Joske RA, ed: Changing disease patterns and human behaviour. London, New York, Academic Press, 1980. p. 37-54.
Bleich JD, Harakas SS, Hehir JB, et al: Population ethics: religious traditions. In Reich WT, et al, ed: Encyclopedia of bioethics, v.3. New York, Free Press, 1978. p. 1250-73.
Bolton C, Leasure JW: Evolution politique et baisse de la fécondité en occident. **Population** 1979;34(4-5):825-43
Boyd E, Scammon RE: Origins of the study of human growth. Ed. Savara BS, Schilke JF. [Eugene], University of Oregon Health Sciences Center Foundation, 1980. 676 p.
Caldwell JC: The mechanisms of demographic change in historical perspective. **Popul Stud** 1981 Mar;35(1):5-27
Charbonneau H, Larose A, ed: The great mortalities: methodological studies of demographic crises in the past. Liège, Belgium, Ordina Editions, [1980]. 373 p. Includes contributions by A. Appleby, S. Sogner, J. N. Biraben. Text in English or French.
Cohen YA: Shrinking households. **Society** 1981;18(2):48-52
Cohn RL, Jensen RA: The determinants of slave mortality rates on the middle passage. **Explor Econ Hist** 1982;19(3):269-82
Daumard A: Les généalogies sociales: un des fondements de l'histoire sociale comparative et quantitative. **Ann Demogr Hist (Paris)** 1984;:9-24
Dupâquier J, Hollingsworth TH, Köllmann W: Bibliographie internationale sur les crises de mortalité. In Charbonneau H, Larose A, ed: The great mortalities: methodological studies of demographic crises in the past. Liège, Belgium, Ordina Editions, 1980. 257-70.
Dupaquier J: L'analyse statistique des crises de mortalite. In Charbonneau H, Larose A, ed: The great mortalities: methodological studies of demographic crises in the past. Liège, Belgium, Ordina Editions, 1980. p. 83-112.
Fagot AM: Medicina e probabilità. **Kos** 1984 Feb;1(1):24-31
Fox VC, Quitt MH, ed: Loving, parenting and dying: the family cycle in England and America, past and present. New York, Psychohistory Press, 1980. v, 488 p. Includes original essays by the editors, by M. A. Glendon, and A. Macfarlane. Also includes numerous previously published articles by various other authors.
Gaunt D: Historisk demografi eller demografisk historia? En översikt och ett debattinlägg om ett tvärvetenskapligt dilemma. **Hist Tidskr** 1973;93(3):382-405
Groh F: Zu einigen Aspekten der Mortalitäts- und Todesursachenstatistik. **Wiss Z Martin Luther Univ (Math)** 1978;27(6):121-32
Gupta AD: Catastrophes and their population symptoms. In Charbonneau H, Larose A, ed: The great mortalities: methodological studies of demographic crises in the past. Liège, Belgium, Ordina Editions, 1980. p. 61-8.
Haan H de: Fertiliteit in pre-industriële samenlevingen. **Spiegel Hist** 1980;15(10):554-60
Harper AB: Istoriia Aleutskoi populiatsii. **Sov Etnogr** 1980;(6):50-60
Hélin E, Lebrun M, Grégoire-Reiters M: Bibliographie internationale de démographie historique, 1981. **Ann Demogr Hist (Paris)** 1981;:v-cxii
Hélin E, Lebrun M, Grégoire-Reiters M: International bibliography of historical demography, 1980. **Ann Demogr Hist (Paris)** 1980;:I-CXI
Imhof AE: Leib und Leben unserer Vorfahren: eine rhythmisierte Welt. In Imhof AE, ed: Leib und Leben in der Geschichte der Neuzeit. Berlin, Duncker & Humblot, 1983. p. 21-38.
Imhof AE: Ursachen und Folgen der zunehmenden durchschnittlichen Lebenserwartung seit dem 17. Jahrhundert; Bericht über eine interdisziplinäre Tagung an der Ecole des Hautes Etudes en Sciences Sociales, Paris, 24.-26. Oktober 1979. **Ber Wissenschaftsgesch** 1979;3(3-4):212-18
Imhof AE: Von der unsicheren zur sicheren Lebenszeit. Ein folgenschwerer Wandel im Verlaufe der Neuzeit. **Vierteljahrsschr Soz Wirtschgesch** 1984;71(2):175-98
Jette R, Charbonneau H: Généalogie descendantes et analyse démographique. **Ann Demogr Hist (Paris)** 1984;:45-54
Joske RA: The physician and changing patterns of human disease and death. In Stanley NF, Joske RA, ed: Changing disease patterns and human behaviour. London, New York, Academic Press, 1980. p. 551-66.
Knodel J, Van de Walle E: Lessons from the past: policy implications of historical fertility studies. **Popul Dev Rev** 1979;5:217-45
Larsen O: Fårlig a vaere barneår og livesjanser. [Dangers of childhood--life prospects] (Nor). **Forskningsnytt (Norway)** 1979;24(4):14-9
Larsen O: Leben auf dem Lande: dem Körper nicht nur förderlich. In Imhof AE, ed: Leib und Leben in der Geschichte der Neuzeit. Berlin, Duncker & Humblot, 1983. p. 53-62.
Laslett P, Oosterveen K, Smith RM, ed: Bastardy and its comparative history. Cambridge, Mass., Harvard University Press, 1980. xv, 431 p. Contributions by Y. Blayo, D. Gaunt, S. Hartley, A. Hayami, S. Hochstadt, A. S. Kälvemark, J. Knodel, D. Levine, A. Newman, A. Macfarlane, M. R. Matovic, J. Meyer, D. S. Smith, C. Smout, S. Stewart, E. van de Walle, R. V. Wells, K. Wrightson.
Laughlin WS, Harper AB, Thompson DD: New approaches to the pre- and post-contact history of Arctic peoples. **Am J Phys Anthropol** 1979 Nov;51(4):579-87
Lee RD: Econometric studies of topics in demographic history. New York, Arno Press, 1978. 272 (12) p. (Ph.D. Diss, Harvard University, 1970).
LeRoy Ladurie E: Pressure of numbers: medical evidence, changing attitudes and historical demography. In his: The territory of the historian. Hassocks, Sussex, England, Harvester Press, 1979. p. 221-84.
Llewelyn DE, Anderson J: The historical development of the concepts of diagnosis and prognosis and their relationship to probabilistic inference. **Med Inf (Lond)** 1980 Oct-Dec;5(4):267-80
Lockridge KA: Historical demography. In Delzell, Charles F., ed.: the future of history: essays in the Vanderbilt University centennial symposium. Nashville, Vanderbilt U., 1977. p. 53-64.
Lynch KA: Local and regional studies in historical demography. **Hist Methods** 1982;15(1):23-9
McNeill WH: Historical patterns of migration. **Curr Anthropol** 1979;20(1):94-8
McNeill WH: Migration patterns and infection in traditional societies. In Stanley NF, Joske RA, ed: Changing disease patterns and human behaviour. London, New York, Academic Press, 1980. p. 27-36.
Miké V: Clinical studies in cancer: a historical perspective. In V. Miké, K. E. Stanley, ed: Statistics in medical research. Methods and issues, with applications in cancer research. New York, John Wiley & Sons,

1982. p. 111–55.
Ober WB: Reuben's mandrakes: infertility in the Bible. **Int J Gynecol Pathol** 1984;3(3):299–317
Overbeek J, ed: The evolution of population theory: a documentary sourcebook. Westport, Conn., Greenwood Press, 1977. x, 277 p.
Pahl KP: Life expectancy in ancient and modern man. **Acta Anthropogenet** 1981;5(2):119–28
Panzac D: La population de l'empire Ottoman et de ses marges du XVe au XIX siècle: bibliographie (1941–1980) et bilan provisoire. **Rev Occident Musulman Mediterr** 1981;31(1):119–37
Pearson ES, ed: The history of statistics in the 17th and 18th centuries against the changing background of intellectual, scientific and religious thought. Lectures by Karl Pearson given at University College London during the academic sessions 1921–1933. New York, Macmillan, 1978. xix, 744 p.
Pedlow GW: Marriage, family size, and inheritance among Hessian nobles, 1650–1900. **J Fam Hist** 1982 Winter;7(4):333–52
Peterson W: History of population theories. In Reich WT, et al, ed: Encyclopedia of bioethics, v.3. New York, Free Press, 1978. p. 1225–32.
Rassengeschichte der Menscheit: 7 vols. Vol. 1 ed. by K. Saller; Vols. 2–7 ed. by I. Schwidetzky. München und Wien, R. Oldenbourg Verlag, 1968–1979. Continuing.
Risse GB: La ecología de la enfermedad: tema de estudio médico-histórico. **Bol Soc Mex Hist Filos Med** 1984 Mar;7(46):289–304
Robins RS: Disease, political events, and populations. In Rothschild H, ed: Biocultural aspects of disease. New York, Academic Press, 1981. p. 153–75.
Schofield R: Microdemography and epidemic mortality: two case studies. In: Time, space and man, essays on microdemography. Uppsala, Almquist & Wiksell, 1979, p. 53–67.
Schultheisz E: On the beginnings of quantitative thinking in medicine. (Nicholas of Cusa and the Idiot). In E. Schultheisz, ed: History of physiology. Oxford, Elmsford, New York, Pergamon, 1981. xvi, 208 p. (Advances in Physiological Sciences. Proceedings of the 28th International Congress of Physiological Sciences, Budapest, 1980. Volume 21). p. 1–7.
Segalen M: Quelques réflexions pour l'étude de la condition féminine. **Ann Demogr Hist (Paris)** 1981;:11–22
Shelestov DK: U istokov istoricheskoi demografii. **Vestn Mosk Univ Ser 8 Istor** 1982;(3):21–33
Sheynin OB: On the history of medical statistics. **Arch Hist Exact Sci** 1982;26(3):241–86
Sheynin OB: On the history of the statistical method in biology. **Arch Hist Exact Sci** 1980;22(4):323–71
Somolinos Palencia J: El expediente clínico y su importancia en la asistencia y educación médicas. I. El expediente clínico al través de la historia. **Gac Med Mex** 1980 Nov;116(11):477–81
Spengler JJ: History of population policies. In Reich WT, et al, ed: Encyclopedia of bioethics, v.3. New York, Free Press, 1978. p. 1232–6.
Swedlund AC: Historical demography as population ecology. **Annu Rev Anthropol** 1978;7:137–73
Tanner JM: A history of the study of human growth. Cambridge, New York, Cambridge University Press, 1981. 499 p.
Teitelbaum MS: The population problem in demographic perspective. In Reich WT, et al, ed: Encyclopedia of bioethics, v.3. New York, Free Press, 1978. p. 1218–25.
Vann RT: The new demographic history. Iggers, Georg G. and Parker, Harold T., ed: International Handbook of Historical Studies: Contemporary Research and Theory. Westport, Conn., Greenwood Press, 1979. p. 29–42.
Wall R: Inferring differential neglect of females from mortality data. **Ann Demogr Hist (Paris)** 1981;:119–40
Watts ES: The biological race concept and diseases of modern man. In Rothschild H, ed: Biocultural aspects of disease. New York, Academic Press, 1981. p. 3–23.

### Americas

Dobyns HF: Their number become thinned: native American population dynamics in eastern North America. Knoxville, University of Tennessee Press, 1983. 378 p.
Fogel RW, et al: The economics of mortality in North America, 1650–1910: a description of a research project. **Hist Methods Newsl** 1978;11(2):75–108
Harper AB, Laughlin WS: Inquiries into the peopling of the new world: development of ideas and recent advances. In F. Spencer, ed: A history of American physical anthropology, 1930–1980. New York, Academic Press, 1982. p. 281–304.
Situación actual de la población indigena.: **Am Indig** 1979;39:211–418
Viel B: Fertility policies in the Latin American continent. **Proc Annu Symp Eugen Soc** 1981;16:15–22

### Argentina

Comadrán Ruiz J: Evolución demográfica argentina durante el périodo hispano, 1535–1810. Buenos Aires, Editorial Universitaria de Buenos Aires, 1969. xi, 120 p.

### Belgium

Bougard JP: La fécondité au Borinage au XVIIe et au début du XIXe siècle. **Popul Famille** 1979;:109–46
Bruneel C: La mortalité dans les campagnes: Le Duché de Brabant aux XVIIe et XVIIIe siècles. Louvain, Bureau du Recueil, Bibliothèque de l'Université, et Editions Nauwelaerts, 1977. lxiv, 777 p. and atlas, 97 p. (Université de Louvain, Recueil de Travaux d'Histoire et de Philologie, 6e série, Fasc. 10).
Gutmann MR, Wyrick R: Adapting methods to needs: studying fertility and nuptiality in seventeenth- and eighteenth-century Belgium. **Hist Methods** 1981;14(4):163–71
Marechal G: De leprozen in de kwartieren Brugge en het Brugse Vrije. Nieuwe cijfers. **Ann Soc Emulation Bruges** 1979;116:147–62
Vandenbroeke C: Zuigelingensterfte, bevallingsstoornissen en kraambedsterfte (17–19de eeuw). **Bijdr Geschied Geneeskd** 1977;60:133–63

### Brazil

Marcilio ML: Dos registros parroquiais a demografia historica no Brasil. **An Hist** 1970;2:81–100

### Bulgaria

Grozdanova E: Za demografskoto sustoianie na karnobatsko i aitosko prez 17 i 18 vek. **Istor Pregl** 1976;32(6):81–8

### Canada

Goudreault L: Naissance de la statistique alieniste au Canada jusqu'en 1867. In: Congrès international d'histoire de la médecine, XXVe, Québec, 1976. Actes. Québec, 1977. p. 706–26.
Houdaille J: Quelques aspects de la démographie ancienne de l'Acadie. **Population** 1980;35(3):581–602

### Chile

Romero H: Población y planificación de familia. **Rev Med Chil** 1977 Dec;105(12):946–50

### China

Cartier M: Quand la Chine avait cent millions d'habitants. **Histoire** 1980;24:87–9
Lee J: Food supply and population growth in southwest China, 1250–1850. **J Asian Stud** 1982;41(4):711–46
Ts'ai HC: [Demographic methodology and its application to studies of historical populations] (Chi). **Ssu yu Yen** 1982;20(4):49–56
Wülker G: Das grösste Volk der Erde: Bevölkerungsprobleme und Bevölkerungspolitik der Volksrepublik China. **Eur Arch** 1972;27(8):285–94

### Colombia

Chandler DL: Health and slavery in colonial Colombia. New York, Arno Press, 1981. iv, 307 p. (Ph.D. Diss., Tulane 1972).

### Czechoslovakia

Cáňová E: Vývoj úmrtnosti od poloviny 17. do poloviny 19. století. **Arch Cas** 1977;27(4):222–5

### Denmark

Lassen A: Befolkningsudviklingen i Danmark 1660–1769. **Jyske Saml** 1960;5(2):173–97

### Europe

Bach A, Simon K: Sterblichkeit des Menschen im historischen Verlauf unter besonderer Berücksichtigung ihrer Geschlechtsspezifik. **Alt-Thueringen** 1978;15:7–17
Flinn MW: The European demographic system, 1500–1820. Baltimore, Johns Hopkins Univ. Press, 1981. 175 p.
Imhof AE: Från ett osäkert till ett säkert liv. **Sydsven Medicinhist Sallsk Arsskr** 1983;:115–40
Imhof AE: Säuglingssterblichkeit im europäischen Kontext, 17.–20 Jahrhundert. Ueberlegungen zu einem Buch von Anders Brändström. Umeå, Umeå University, 1984. 73 p. (Demographic Data Base, Newsletter No. 2)

### France

Angers D: La vicomté de Bayeux au bas Moyen-Age: esquisse d'histoire démographique. **Francia** 1979;7:141–72
Bideau A: Accouchement 'Naturel' et accouchement à 'haut risque'.

**Ann Demogr Hist (Paris)** 1981;:49–66

Dayras M: La population d'Aubusson (Creuse) du XVIIe au XIXe siècle. In: Congrès National des Sociétés Savantes, 92e, Strasbourg et Colmar, 1967. Actes. Paris, 1970. Section d'Histoire Moderne et Contemporaine, Tome 1. p. 289–295.

Dupâquier J: De l'animal à l'homme: le mécanisme autorégulateur des populations traditionnelles. **Rev Inst Sociol** 1972;2:177–211

Durr M: Contribution à l'étude démographique d'une paroisse de l'ancien Tournugeois: Préty-Lacrost-La Truchère, 1678–1752 (3e partie). **Soc Amis Arts Sci Tournus** 1978;77:92–112

Gélis J: Miracle et medecine aux siècles classiques: le corps medical et le retour temporaire a la vie des mort-nes. **Hist Reflect** 1982;9(1–2):85–101

Grenier JY: Quelques éléments pour une étude des liens entre conjoncture économique et conjoncture démographique aux XVIIe et XVIIIe siècles. **Ann Demogr Hist (Paris)** 1984;:175–99

Houdaille J: Mortalité dans divers groupes de notables du XVIIe au XIXe siècles. **Population** 1980;35(4–5):966–8

LeBras H, Dinet D: Mortalité des laïcs et mortalité des religieux: les Bénédictins de Saint-Maur aux XVIIe et XVIIIe siècles. **Population** 1980;35(2):347–83

Lebrun F: Les crises démographiques en France aux XVIIe et XVIIIe siècles. **Ann Econ Soc Civilis** 1980;35(2):205–34

Poussou JP: In memoriam: Philippe Aries (1914–1984). **Ann Demogr Hist (Paris)** 1984;:5–6

Rebaudo D: Le mouvement annuel de la population française rurale de 1670 à 1740. **Population** 1979;34(3):589–606

**Germany**

Böhmer W, Helmbold P: Die reproduktionsbedingte Mortalität während früherer Jahrhunderte. **Zentralbl Gynakol** 1984;106(13):939–46

Burg P: Demographie und Geschichte. **Rheinische Vierteljahrsbl** 1978;(42):298–383

Houdaille J: La fécondité en Allemagne avant 1850. **Population** 1979;34(3):695–705

**Great Britain**

Barker DJ: Geographical variations in disease in Britain. **Br Med J** 1981;283:398–400

Bradley L: Review essay: The population history of England 1541–1871: a reconstruction. **Local Popul Stud (Matlock)** 1981;27:53–64

Cowgill UM: Marriage and its progeny in the city of York, 1538-1751. **Kroeber Antropol Soc Pap** 1970;(42):47–87

Finlay R: Differential child mortality in pre-industrial England: the example of Cartmel, Cumbria, 1600–1750. **Ann Demogr Hist (Paris)** 1981;:67–80

Finlay R: Distance to church and registration experience. **Local Popul Stud (Matlock)** 1980 Spring;24:26–40

Forbes TR: Births and deaths in a London parish: the record from the registers, 1654–1693 and 1729–1743. **Bull Hist Med** 1981;55(3):371–91

Fryer JG, et al: Comparing the early mortality rates of the local authorities of England and Wales. **J R Stat Soc** 1979;142(2)

Gottfried RS: Bury St. Edmunds and the populations of late medieval English towns, 1270–1530. **J Br Stud** 1980;20(1):1–31

Levine D: Siamese twins in the Parish Registers of Shepshed, Leicestershire. **Local Popul Stud (Matlock)** 1981 Spring;26:44–5

McCallum DM: A demographic study of the parishes of Bruton and Pitcombe in the County of Somerset. **Proc Somerset Archaeol Nat Hist Soc** 1977;121:77–87

Margan V: A case study of population change over two centuries: Blaris, Lisburn 1661–1848. **Ir Econ Soc Hist** 1976;3:5–16

Matossian MK: Mold poisoning: an unrecognized English health problem, 1550–1800. **Med Hist** 1981 Jan;25(1):73–84

Morrow RB: Family limitation in pre-industrial England: a reappraisal. **Econ Hist Rev** 1978;31(3):419–28

Outhwaite RB: Population change, family structure and the good of counting. **Hist J (Gt Brit)** 1979;22(1):229–37

Reynolds G: Infant mortality and sex ratios at baptism ... Willingham ... Cambridgeshire [1559–1812]. **Local Popul Stud (Matlock)** 1979;22:31–7

Skinner J: 'Crisis mortality' in Buckinghamshire 1600–1750. **Local Popul Stud (Matlock)** 1982 Spring;28:67–72

Smith RM: Fertility, economy, and household formation in England over three centuries. **Popul Dev Rev** 1981;7(4):595–622

Swales RJ: Plague, population and ecology in early modern England. **Can J Hist** 1979;14(2):257–66

Weir DR: Rather never than late: celibacy and age at marriage in English cohort fertility, 1541–1871. **J Fam Hist** 1984 Winter;9(4):340–54

Willmott Dobbie BM: An attempt to estimate the true rate of maternal mortality, sixteenth to eighteenth centuries. **Med Hist** 1982 Jan;26(1):79–90

Wrigley EA, Schofield RS: English population history from family reconstitution: summary results 1600–1799. **Popul Stud** 1983 Jul;37(2):157–84

Wrigley EA, Schofield RS: The population history of England, 1541-1871; a reconstruction. Cambridge, Mass., Harvard University Press, 1981. xv, 779 p.

**Ireland**

Relethford JH: Genetic structure and population history of Ireland: a comparison of blood group and anthropometric analyses. **Ann Hum Biol** 1983 Jul–Aug;10(4):321–33

**Italy**

Bellettini A, Samoggia A: Evolution différentielle et mouvement saisonnier de la mortalité infantile et enfantine dans la banlieue de Bologne (XVIIe–XIXe siècles). **Ann Demogr Hist (Paris)** 1983;:195–207

Del Panta L, Livi-Bacci M: Chronology, intensity and diffusion of mortality in Italy, 1600–1850. In Charbonneau H, Larose A, ed: The great mortalities: methodological studies of demographic crises in the past. Liège, Belgium, Ordina Editions, 1980. p. 69–81.

Frassetto F: Le cose son numeri. **Riv Biol** 1981 Autumn;74(3):402–8

Rossi F: Crisi di mortalità ad Adria nel contesto socio-ambientale dei secoli XVII–XIX. **Genus** 1977;33(3–4):83–118

**Japan**

Hanley SB, Yamamura K: Economic and demographic change in preindustrial Japan, 1600–1868. Princeton, N. J., Princeton University Press, 1977. xiii, 409 p.

Mosk C: The evolution of the pre-modern demographic regime in Japan. **Popul Stud** 1981 Mar;35(1):28–52

Okada Y: [Background of Rintaro Mori's debates on statistics] (Jpn). **Igakushi Kenkyu** 1978;49:1–13

**Mexico**

Gurría Lacroix J: La población de la provincia de Tabasco durante el virreinato. **Estud Hist Novohisp** 1978;6:65–88

**Netherlands**

Maat GJ: Boerhaave en zijn tijdgenoten, en de betekenis van hun lichaamslengte (een fysisch-antropologisch onderzoek van begravenen in de Pieterskerk te Leiden). **Ned Tijdschr Geneeskd** 1982 Apr 17;126(16):705–12

Schuurman AJ: De bevolking van Duiven, 1665–1795. Een historisch-demografische studie. **AAG Bijdr** 1979;22:138–89

Van der Woude AM: Population developments in the Northern Netherlands (1500–1800) and the validity of the 'urban graveyard' effect. **Ann Demogr Hist (Paris)** 1982;:55–75

**Norway**

Aaraas O: Demografishe kriser i Norge: hunger eller sykdom? **Socialmed Tidsskr** 1979;56

Rokkan S: National primary socio-economic data structures: Norway. **Int Soc Sci J** 1978;30(3):621–52

**Pacific Islands**

McArthur N: And, behold, the plague was begun among the people. The Changing Pacific: Essays in honour of H. E. Maude. Melbourne, Oxford University Press, 1978. p. 273–84.

**Poland**

Kuchowicz Z: Jeszcze o zdrowiu in niezdrowiu magnatów XVII–XVIII W. **Kwart Hist** 1970;77(2):394–403

Piontek J, Henneberg M: Mortality changes in a Polish rural community (1350–1972) and estimation of their evolutionary significance. **Am J Phys Anthropol** 1981 Jan;54(1):129–38

Sułowski Z: Les mécanismes de l'expansion démographique des Juifs dans les villes de Pologne aux XVIe–XIXe siècles. **Zesz Nauk KUL** 1978;21:89–100

**Scandinavia**

Hansen HO: Some age structural consequences of mortality variations in pre-transitional Iceland and Sweden. In: Charbonneau H., La Rose A., ed.: The great mortalities: methodological studies of demographic crises in the past. Liège, Ordina, 1979, p. 113–32.

**Spain**

García Sanz A, Pérez Moreda V: Análisis histórico de una crisis demográfica: Villacastín de 1466 a 1800. **Estud Segov** 1972;(70):119–46

Marset Campos P, Chacón Jiménez F, Lemeunier G, et al: La sociedad murciana y cartagenera y las epidemias durante los siglos XVII, XVIII y XIX. In: Sociedad Española de Historia de la Medicina. V Congreso Nacional. Madrid, 1977. **Asclepio** 1977;29:177–208

Moreda VP: The intensity of the mortality crises in Spain: an outline of their regional differences over time. In Charbonneau H, Larose A, ed: The great mortalities: methodological studies of demographic crises in the past. Liège, Belgium, Ordina Editions, 1980. p. 179–98.
Pérez Moreda V: Las crisis de mortalidad en la España interior (siglos XVI–XIX). Madrid, Siglo XXI de España Editores, 1980. 526 p.
Pérez Moreda V: Un estudio evolutivo de la mortalidad: el ejemplo de otero de herreros a traves de sus registros parroquiales. **Estud Segov** 1973–74;25(73):37–52

**Sweden**

Hed H: Opportunity for selection during the 17th–19th centuries in the diocese of Linköping as estimated with Crow's index in a population of clergymen's wives. **Hum Hered** 1984;34(6):378–87

**Switzerland**

Perrenoud A: Contribution à l'histoire cyclique des maladies. Deux cents ans de variole à Genève (1580–1810). In Imhof AE, ed: Mensch und Gesundheit in der Geschichte. Husum, Matthiesen, 1980. p. 175–98.
Perrenoud A: Surmortalité féminine et condition de la femme (XVIIe–XIXe siècles). Une vérification empirique. **Ann Demogr Hist (Paris)** 1981;:89–104
Ruesch H: Die Demographie der Alpen zwischen 1650 und 1850: Bericht über den heutigen Wissensstand und Fragen an die künftige Forschung. **Schweiz Z Gesch** 1979;29(1):159–80

**United States**

Byers E: Fertility transition in a New England commercial center: Nantucket, Massachusetts, 1680–1840. **J Interdiscip Hist** 1982;13(1):17–40
Carmelli D, Andersen S: A longevity study of twins in the Mormon genealogy. **Prog Clin Biol Res** 1981;69 pt C:187–200
Cassedy JH: Church record-keeping and public health in early New England. In: Medicine in Colonial Massachusetts 1620–1820. (Publications of the Colonial Society of Massachusetts, vol. 57), 1980. p. 249–62.
Cates GL: 'The seasoning': disease and death among the first colonists of Georgia. **Ga Hist Q** 1980;64(2):146–58
Crosby AW: God... would destroy them, and give their country to another people. **Am Heritage** 1978;29(6):38–43
Demos J: Old age in early New England. In Demos, J, Boocock, SS, ed.: Turning points: historical and sociological essays on the family. Chicago, U. of Chicago Press, 1978. p. 248–87.
Earle CV: Environment, disease, and mortality in early Virginia. In Tate, TW, Ammerman, DL, ed. The Chesapeake in the seventeenth century: essays on Anglo-American society (Chapel Hill, U. of North Carolina Press for the Institute of Early American History and Culture, 1979):96–125.
Gallman JM: Determinants of age at marriage in colonial Perquimans County, North Carolina. **William Mary Q** 1982;39(1):176–91
Gallman JM: Mortality among white males: colonial North Carolina. **Soc Sci Hist** 1980;4(3):295–316
Gladwin LA: Tobacco and sex: some factors affecting nonmarital sexual behavior in colonial Virginia. **J Soc Hist** 1978;12(1):57–75
Hogue H: Analyzing ossurary skeletal remains: techniques and problems. **South Indian Stud (NC)** 1977;29:2–22
Kantrow L: Philadelphia gentry: fertility and family limitation among an American aristocracy. **Popul Stud** 1980 Mar;34(1):21–30
Kenney AP: The rhythm of life among the Hudson Valley Dutch in the eighteenth century. **Trans Stud Coll Physicians Phila** 1978 Apr;45(4):217–23
Kunitz SJ: Mortality change in America, 1620–1920. **Hum Biol** 1984 Sep;56(3):559–82
Palkovich AM: Demography and disease patterns in a protohistoric plains group: a study of the mobridge site (39WW1). **Plains Anthropol** 1981;26(94 pt 2):71–84
Rutman DB, Wetherell C, Rutman AH: Rhythms of life: black and white seasonality in the early Chesapeake. **J Interdiscip Hist** 1980;11(1):29–53
Sharpless J: Population redistribution in the American past: empirical generalizations and theoretical perspectives. **Soc Sci Q** 1980;61(3–4):401–17
Smith DS: The demographic history of colonial New England. **J Econ Hist** 1972;32(1):165–83
Smith DS: The estimates of early American historical demographers: two steps forward, one step back, what steps in the future? **Hist Methods Newsl** 1979;12(1):24–38
Vinovskis MA, ed: Studies in American historical demography. New York, Academic Press, 1979. 530 p. Reprinted articles by various authors.

**USSR**

Pullat R: Istoricheskaia demografiia v SSR (znachenie, mesto, itogi i perspektivy razvitiia). **Probl Istor Demogr SSSR** 1977;8–17
Ransel DL: Recent Soviet studies in demographic history. **Russ Rev** 1981;40(2):143–57

**West Indies**

Mayer FM, Lavoie Y: Généalogie, démographie et génétique; étude d'un cas: Saint-Barthélemy. **Ann Demogr Hist (Paris)** 1984;:89–102

**Yugoslavia**

Supuk A: Sibenski onomastikon nakon kuge od 1649 godine. **Arh Vjesn** 1978–79;21–22:123–79

**Before 500 A.D.**

Clarke SK: Early childhood morbidity trends in prehistoric populations. **Hum Biol** 1980 Feb;52(1):79–85
Scharf JH: Die Sapienten-Populationen im Neolithicum Zentral- und Nordeuropas--Hypothesen, Model und Realität. **Gegenbaurs Morphol Jahrb** 1980;126(4):449–77

**Asia**

Rathbun TA: Morphological affinities and demography of metal-age Southwest Asian populations. **Am J Phys Anthropol** 1982 Sep;59(1):47–60

**Greco-Roman**

Engels D: The problem of female infanticide in the Greco-Roman world. **Classical Philol** 1980;75:112–20

**Spain**

Castillo A: Algunas anotaciones demograficas sobre Cádiz en los primeros siglos del Imperio romano. **Hispania** 1978 Jul–Aug;38:235–57

**500 A.D.–1450**

Bullough V, Campbell C: Female longevity and diet in the Middle Ages. **Speculum** 1980 Apr;55(2):317–25
Bulst N: Der Schwarze Tod. Demographische, wirtschafts- und kulturgeschichtliche Aspekte der Pestkatastrophe von 1347–1352. Bilanz der neueren Forschung. **Saeculum (Freiburg)** 1979;30(1):45–67
Verlinden C: Ist mittelalterliche Sklaverei ein bedeutsamer demographischer Faktor gewesen? **Vierteljahrsschr Soz Wirtschgesch** 1979;66:153–73

**France**

Biget JL, Tricard J: Livres de raison et démographie familiale en Limousin au XVe siècle. **Ann Demogr Hist (Paris)** 1981;:321–63
Higounet-Nadal A: Périgueux aux XIVe et XVe siècles: étude de démographie historique. Bordeaux, Fédération historique du Sud-Ouest, 1978. 458 p.
Riché P: Les 'Gouvernants' et les problèmes de population dans le Haut Moyen-Age (Ve–IXe siècles). **Ann Demogr Hist (Paris)** 1979;:301–9

**Germany**

Schultheisz E: Beginning of quantification in physiology. **Orvostort Kozl** 1980;89–91(26 no 1–3):209–13

**Great Britain**

Ackerman C: The rural demography of medieval England. **Ethnohistory** 1976 Spring;23:105–15
Nash AE: Mortality pattern of the Wiltshire lords of the manor, 1242–1377. **South Hist** 1979;2
Pam DO: The hungry years: the struggle for survival in Edmonton and Enfield before 1400. Enfield, Edmonton Hundred Historical Society, 1980. 31 p. (Occasional paper no. 42.)
Poos LR: Plague mortality and demographic depression in later medieval England. **Yale J Biol Med** 1981 May–Jun;54(3):227–34
Razi Z: Life, marriage and death in a medieval parish: economy, society and demography in Healesowen, 1270–1400. Cambridge, Cambridge University Press, 1980. xi, 162 p.

**Hungary**

Pantó E: Wachstum und Reifung der Stadtkinder in Abhängigkeit von soziodemographischen Faktoren. **Anthropol Anz** 1982 Mar;40(1):33–44

**Poland**

Tyszkiewicz J, Widy-Tyszkiewicz E: Zdrowie i choroby w Polsce XIII–XV w. **Kwart Hist Kultury Mater** 1976;24(1):55–73

**1450–1700**

Cabourdin G: Introduction aux problèmes de la démographie de la période

1500–1670. **Ann Demogr Hist (Paris)** 1980;:13–8

Dobson MJ: Environments of disease and mortality in the New World and the Old World. **Soc Soc Hist Med Bull (Lond)** 1984 Dec;35:7–10

Fenaroli G, Garibaldi U, Penco MA: Giochi, scommesse sulla vita, tabelle di mortalità, nascita del calcolo probabilistico, statistica e teoria delle popolazioni. **Arch Hist Exact Sci** 1981;25(4):329–41

Fenaroli G, Penco MA: Le prime analisi di problemi di mortalità in termini probabilistici. **Physis** 1981;23(1):115–34

Neugebauer R: Application of a capture-recapture method (the Bernoulli census) to historical epidemiology. **Am J Epidemiol** 1984 Oct;120(4):626–34

Webster C, ed: Health, medicine and mortality in the sixteenth century. London and New York, Cambridge University Press, 1979. 394 p. In memory of Sanford V. Larkey. Contributions by P. Slack, R. Schofield, E. A. Wrigley, A. B. Appleby, T. R. Forbes, P. Allderidge, M. Pelling, A. Chapman, J. J. Bylebyl.

**Austria**

Jäger-Sunstenau H: Auswärtige in einem wiener Totenbuch 1687–1690. **Adler** 1967;7(13–14):205–8

Spreitzer H: Pestjahre in Mistelbach. **Unsere Heimat** 1970;41(3):132–6

**Belgium**

Helin E: A la recherche d'une mesure de la léthalité des épidémies: les désignations de tuteurs pour les orphelins servent-elles d'indicateur? **Ann Demogr Hist (Paris)** 1980;:67–78

**China**

Shu-Yuen Yim: Famine relief statistics as a guide to the population of sixteenth-century China: a case-study of Honan province. **Ch'ing-Shih Wen-t'i** 1978;3(9):1–30

Yim SY: Famine relief statistics as a guide to the population of sixteenth century China: a case study of Honan Province. **Ch'ing-Shih Wen-t'i** 1978 Nov;3:1–30

**Finland**

Tamminen S: Varhainen väestökirjanpitokaava Maalahdella ja Sulvassa 1600-luvulla. **Hist Aikak** 1978;76(3):241–50

**France**

Moriceau JM: Les crises démographiques dans le sud de la région parisienne de 1560 à 1670 **Ann Demogr Hist (Paris)** 1980;:105–23

**Germany**

Imhof A: Les sermons funèbres comme source de la démographie historique pour la période de 1500 à 1650. **Ann Demogr Hist (Paris)** 1980;:79–86

Ozment S: Luther and the family. **Harv Libr Bull** 1984 Winter;32(1):36–53

**Great Britain**

Dymond D: The famine of 1527 in Essex. **Local Popul Stud (Matlock)** 1981 Spring;26: 29–40

Finlay R: Health and mortality in London 1580–1650. **Soc Soc Hist Med Bull (Lond)** 1981 Jun;28:1–5

Finlay R: Population and metropolis. The demography of London, 1580–1650. Cambridge, New York, Cambridge University Press, 1981. xii, 188 p.

Herlan RW: Age at baptism in the London Parish of St. Olave, Old Jewry, 1645–1667. **Local Popul Stud (Matlock)** 1980 Spring;24:42–8

Herlan RW: Aspects of population history in the London parish of St. Olave, Old Jewry, 1645–1667. **Guildhall Stud Lond Hist** 1980;4(3):133–40

Kent JR: Population mobility and alms: poor migrants in the Midlands during the early seventeenth century. **Local Popul Stud (Matlock)** 1981;27:35–51

Martin JM: A Warwickshire market town in adversity: Stratford-upon-Avon in the sixteenth and seventeenth centuries. **Midl Hist** 1982;7:26–41

Pelling M: A survey of East Anglian medical practitioners 1500–1640. **Local Popul Stud (Matlock)** 1980;:(25):54–5

Pelling M: Old people and poverty in early modern towns. **Soc Soc Hist Med Bull (Lond)** 1984 Jun;34:42–7

Turner D: A lost seventeenth century demographic crisis? The evidence of two counties. **Local Popul Stud (Matlock)** 1978;(21):11–18

Wrigley EA: Marital fertility in seventeenth century Colyton. **Econ Hist Rev** 1978;31(3):429–36

**Ireland**

Barnard TC: Sir William Petty: his Irish estates and Irish population. **Ir Econ Soc Hist** 1979;6

**Italy**

Bobbioni MT: Strutture demografiche e strutture sociali in una comunità rurale tra '500 e '600: il caso di s. secondo (prime indagini). **Genus** 1979;35(1–2):237–43

Davico R: La morte barocca: popolazione, quartieri e campagne Messina nella rivolta del 1674–1678. La rivolta di Messina e il mondo Mediterraneo nella seconda metà del seicento, Cosenza, Pelligrini, 1979, p. 359–394.

Salvini S: La mortalità dei gesuiti in Italia nei secoli XVI e XVII. **Quad Depart Stat Univ Studi Fir** 1979;3:1–25

**Mexico**

Berthe JP: Les epidémies au Mexique au XVIe siècle. **Asclepio** 1983;35:257–63

Lange FW: Una reevalución de la población del norte de Yucatán en el tiempo del contacto Español: 1528. **Am Indig** 1971;31(1):117–39

**Morocco**

Rosenberger B, Triki H: Famines et épidémies au Maroc aux XVIe et XVIIe siècles. **Hesperis Tamuda** 1973;14:109–75

**Netherlands**

Alter G: Plague and the Amsterdam annuitant: a new look at life annuities as a source for historical demography. **Popul Stud** 1983 Mar;37(1):23–41

Schneider I: Christiaan Huygens's contribution to the development of a calculus of probabilities. **Janus** 1980;67(4):269–79

**Peru**

Cook ND: Population data for Indian Peru: sixteenth and seventeenth centuries. **Hisp Am Hist Rev** 1982;62(1):73–120

Visita de Acarí (1593): **Hist Cult (Peru)** 1973;7:129–209

**Spain**

Cabrillana N: Repoblación y despoblación en Almería (1572–1599). **Rev Arch Bibl Mus** 1977;80(4):703–29

Johansen AH: Zur demographischen Entwicklung Kastiliens im 16. Jahrhundert. **Gesammelte Aufs Kulturgesch Spaniens** 1978;29:538–80

Maza Zorilla E: [Population and plague of Vallalón 16–17 centuries.] (Spa) **Cuad Invest Hist** 1978;2

Maza Zorrilla E: Régimen demográfico de una villa castellana. La natalidad en Villalón de Campos durante los siglos XVI y XVII. **Invest Hist** 1979;1:69–97

Rodríguez Sánchez A: La natalidad ilegítima en Cáceres en el siglo XVI. **Rev Estud Extremenos** 1979;35(1):123–64

**Sweden**

Akerman S: En befolkning före den demografiska revolutionen. **Karolinska Forb Arsb** 1977;66–113

**Switzerland**

Mattmüller M: Die Pest in Liestal. Notizen zu den demographischen Implikationen der frühneuzeitlichen Epidemien. **Gesnerus** 1983;40(1–2):119–28

Perrenoud A, Zumkeller D: Caractères originaux de la démographie genevoise du XVIe siècle: structure ou conjoncture. **Ann Demogr Hist (Paris)** 1980;:125–41

**United States**

Earle C: Environment, disease and mortality in early Virginia. **J Hist Geogr** 1979;5(4):365–90

Rutman DB, Rutman AH: More true and perfect lists: the reconstruction of censuses for Middlesex County, Virginia, 1668–1704. **Va Mag Hist Biogr** 1980;88(1):37–74

Walsh LS: 'Till death us do part': marriage and family in seventeenth-century Maryland. In Tate, TW, Ammerman, DL., ed. The Chesapeake in the seventeenth century: essays on Anglo-American society (Chapel Hill, U. of North Carolina Press for the Institute of Early American Hist. and Culture, 1979): 126–52.

**West Indies**

Moya Pons F: Datos para el estudio de la demografía aborigen en Santo Domingo. **Jahrb Gesch Staat Wirtsch Ges Lateinam** 1979;16:1–11

**1700 to Present**

Anderson CM: Measles mortality and ethnic groups. **S Afr Med J** 1982 Jul 17;62(3):86–8

# STATISTICS AND DEMOGRAPHY


Appleyard RT: Economic demography of the twentieth century. In Stanley NF, Joske RA, ed: Changing disease patterns and human behaviour. London, New York, Academic Press, 1980. p. 389–401.

Baker PT: Human population biology: a viable transdisciplinary science. **Hum Biol** 1982 May;54(2):203–20

Barber CL: Some implications of declining birth rates in developed countries. **Trans R Soc Can** 1979;17:174–85

Bardet JP, Lynch KA, Mineau GP, et al: La mortalité maternelle autrefois: une étude comparée (de la France de l'ouest à l'Utah). **Ann Demogr Hist (Paris)** 1981;:31–48

Berlan JP: The world food problem: Malthus, Marx and their epigones. **Mon Rev** 1980;31(10):20–32

Black LT: Volcanism as a factor in human ecology: the Aleutian case. **Ethnohistory** 1981;28(4):313–40

Brügelmann J: Medikalisierung von Säuglings- und Erwachsenenalter in Deutschland zu Beginn des 19. Jahrhunderts aufgrund von medizinischen Topographien. In Imhof AE, ed.: Leib und Leben in der Geschichte der Neuzeit. Berlin, Duncker & Humblot, 1983. p. 177–92.

Calot G: Données comparées sur l'évolution de la fécondité selon le rang de naissance en Allemagne Fédérale et en France (1950–1977). **Population** 1979;34(Special):1291–347

Calot G: L'observation de la fécondité à court et moyen terme. **Population** 1981;36(1):9–40

Chesnais JC: La baisse de la natalite et ses consequences pour la planification sectorielle dans les pays capitalistes developpes. **Population** 1982;37(6):1133–58

Chesnais JC: La notion de cycle en démographié: la fécondité post-transitionnelle est-elle cyclique? **Population** 1983;38(2):361–90

Collins JJ: The contribution of medical measures to the decline of mortality from respiratory tuberculosis: an age period cohort model. **Demography** 1982 Aug;19(3):409–27

Cooney RS, Min K: Demographic characteristics affecting living arrangements among young currently unmarried Puerto Rican, non-Spanish black, and non-Spanish white mothers. **Ethnicity** 1981;8(2):107–20

Crimmins EM: The completeness of 1900 mortality data collected by registration and enumeration for rural and urban parts of states: estimates using the Chandra Sekar-Deming technique. **Hist Methods** 1980;13(3):163–9

Davies C: Making sense of the census in Britain and the U.S.A.: the changing occupational classification and the position of nurses. **Sociol Rev** 1980;28(3):581–610

Dean MC: The evolution of experimental operant psychology: a quantitative analysis of 'progress' in behavioral science. Ph.D. Diss., Syracuse University. Syracuse, 1981. v, 249 leaves.

Farolfi B: Dall'antropometria militare alla storia del corpo. **Quad Stor** 1979;14(3):1056–91

Fegersten S: Crude death rate and infant mortality (1840–1900) in Norway, Sweden, Denmark, England and Wales with particular attention to the relationship between mortality and population density-urbanisation. **Scand Popul Stud** 1979;5:83–97

Ferrone V: Il dibattito su probabilità e scienze sociali nel secolo XVIII. **Physis** 1980;22(1):27–71

Festy P: La fécondité des pays occidentaux de 1870 à 1970. Paris, I.N.E.D., Presses Universitaires de France, 1979. 390 p. (Travaux et documents, cahier no 85).

Fitch NE: Statistical and mathematical methods for historians: an annotated bibliography of selected books and articles. **Hist Methods** 1980;13(4):222–31

Flegg AT: Inequality of income, illiteracy and medical care as determinants of infant mortality in underdeveloped countries. **Popul Stud** 1982 Nov;36(3):441–58

Franz MM, Chiba M: Abortion, contraception, and motherhood in post-war Japan and the United States. **Int J Womens Stud** 1980;3(1):66–75

Greene VW: Cleanliness and the health revolution. New York, Soap and Detergent Association, 1984. vii, 68 p.

Grigg D: Modern population growth in historical perspective. **Geography** 1982;67(2):97–108

Haines MR: Recent developments in historical demography: a review of the European fertility project with some comparisons from Japan. **Hist Methods** 1978;11(4):162–73

Hareven TK: Cycles, courses and cohorts: reflections on theoretical and methodological approaches to the historical study of family development. **J Soc Hist** 1978;12(1):97–109

Hayashi J: [History of graphs and the basic rules in drawing] (Jpn). **Josanpu Zasshi** 1983 Dec;37(12):1035–9

Imhof AE: The analysis of eighteenth-century causes: some methodological considerations. **Hist Methods Newsl** 1978;2(1):3–36

Imhof AE, ed: Leib und Leben in der Geschichte der Neuzeit: Vorträge eines internationalen Colloquiums. Berlin, Duncker & Humblot, 1983. 266 p. Text in German and French. (Berliner Historische Studien, Bd. 9. Einzelstudien 2).

Isambert FA: Bio-éthique et techniques biomédicales. **Soc Sci Inf** 1983;22(1):125–37

Jeffery T: Mass-observation. **Soc Soc Hist Med Bull** 1980;27:8–14

Juhasz L: Den selvregulerende mekanisme hos befolninger i eldre tid. **Heimen** 1974;16(5):255–8

Kevles DJ: Genetics in the United States and Great Britain, 1890–1930: a review with speculations. **Isis** 1980 Sep;71(258):441–55

Krótki KJ: Some demographic, particularly fertility, correlates of female status in Eastern Europe and the Republics of the Soviet Union. In Yedlin, Tova, ed: Women in Eastern Europe and the Soviet Union, New York, Praeger, 1980. 239–69.

Langford CM: Fertility change in Sri Lanka since the war: an analysis of the experience of different districts. **Popul Stud** 1981 Jul;35(2):285–306

Larsen O: Die Krankheitsauffassung und ihre historische Interpretation. Ein Auswertungsmodell aufgrund von norwegischen Medizinalberichten aus dem 19. Jahrhundert. In Imhof AE, ed: Mensch und Gesundheit in der Geschichte. Husum, Matthiesen, 1980. p. 45–58.

Larsen O: Eighteenth century diseases. Diagnostical trends and mortality. **Scand Popul Stud** 1979;5

Lehners JP: Schwerpunkte historisch-demographischer Forschung in West- und Mitteleuropa. **Hist Soc Res** 1982;22:3–14

Lévy C: La mortalité par accident des enfants et des adolescents dans huit pays développés. **Population** 1980;35(2):291–319

Lithell UB: Breast-feeding habits and their relation to infant mortality and marital fertility. **J Fam Hist** 1981;6:182–94

Littlefield DC: Plantations, paternalism, and profitability: factors affecting African demography in the old British Empire. **J South Hist** 1981;47(2):167–82

Loraine JA: Future patterns of disease: maladies of development. **Contemp Rev** 1983;242(1409):298–302

Loraine JA: The economics of fertility. **Midwife Health Visit Community Nurse** 1982 Jan;18(1):6–8

McIntosh CA: Demographic trends and policies in developed countries. **Int J Polit** 1982;12(3):3–26

McKeown T: The role of medicine. Dream, mirage or nemesis? Princeton, Princeton University Press, Oxford, Basil Blackwell, 1979. xvi, 207 p.

Mazur DP: Procreation and new definitions in the role of women in a Soviet bloc country: the case of Poland. Yedlin Tova, ed. Women in Eastern Europe and the Soviet Union. New York, Praeger, 1980. p. 226–38.

Meindl RS: Components of longevity: developmental and genetic responses to differential childhood mortality. **Soc Sci Med** 1982;16(2):165–74

Merton RK, Sills DL, Stigler SM: The Kelvin dictum and social science: an excursion into the history of an idea. **J Hist Behav Sci** 1984 Oct;20(4):319–31

Miringoff ML: The impact of population policy upon social welfare. **Soc Serv Rev** 1980;54(3):301–16

Mosk C: Patriarchy and fertility: Japan and Sweden, 1880–1960. New York, Academic Press, 1983. xxii, 320 p.

Mosk C: Rural-urban fertility differences and the fertility transition. **Popul Stud** 1980;34(1):77–90

Muñoz-Perez F: L'évolution de la fécondité dans les pays industrialisés depuis 1971. **Population** 1982;37(3):483–512

Muthiah A, Jones GW: Fertility trends among overseas Indian populations. **Popul Stud** 1983 Jul;37(2):273–99

O'Connell M, Rogers CC: Assessing cohort birth expectations data from the current population survey, 1971-1981. **Demography** 1983 Aug;20(3):369–84

Onuigbo WI: Historical notes on cancer in married couples. **Neth J Surg** 1984 Aug;36(4):112–5

Ortmeyer LE: Female's natural advantage? Or, the unhealthy environment of males? The status of sex mortality differentials. **Women Health** 1979 Summer;4(2):121–33

Plews JH: Charles Darwin and Hawaiian sex ratios, or, genius is a capacity for making compensating errors. **Hawaii J Hist** 1980;14:24–49

Pollitzer WS: The development of genetics and population studies. **Am J Phys Antropol** 1981 Dec;56(4):483–9

Porter TM: The calculus of liberalism: the development of statistical thinking in the social and natural sciences of the nineteenth century. Ph.D. Diss., Princeton University. Princeton, 1981. iv, 365 leaves.

Riley JC: Mortality on long-distance voyages in the eighteenth century. **J Econ Hist** 1981;41(3):651–6

Rollet C: Variole et mortalité des enfants au XVIIIe siècle. **Cah Hist** 1978;23(4):417–36

Rosales VJ: The medicotrophic syndrome: an acute modern phenomenon. **Unitas** 1970;43(4):30–59

Rutkowska I: Ludność świata i jej wyżywienie-kierunki zmian po kryzysie żywnościowym lat siedemdziesłątych. **Ekonomista** 1979;(2):445–63

Schultz TP: Fertility and child mortalilty over the llfe cycle: aggregate and additional evidence. **Am Econ Rev** 1978;68(2):208–15

Seidel-Aprin H: Zum Selbstmordgeschehen in der Bundesrepublik und den sozialistischen Staaten Osteuropas. Diss. Bonn, 1980. 94 p.

Sindelar JL: Differential use of medical care by sex. **J Polit Econ** 1982;90(5):1003–19

Sloan DG: The extent of contraceptive use and the social paradigm of modern demography. **Sociology** 1983;17(3):380–7

Stein R: Mortality in the eighteenth-century French slave trade. **J Afr Hist** 1980, 21(1):35–41

Stephan GE, McMullin DR, Stephan KH: Statistical and historical analyses of nations which deviate from the size-density law. **Demography** 1982 Nov;19(4):567–76

Tal U: On the study of the Holocaust and genocide.

# STATISTICS AND DEMOGRAPHY

**Yad Vashem Stud Eur Jew Catastrophe Resist** 1979;13:7–52
Trussell J, Olsen R: Evaluation of the Olsen technique for estimating the fertility response to child mortality. **Demography** 1983 Aug;20(3):391–405
Vandenbroeke C, Van Poppel F, Van Der Woude AM: Le développement séculaire de la mortalité aux jeunes âges dans le territoire du Bénélux. **Ann Demogr Hist (Paris)** 1983;:257–89
Van Dijk JP: Doodsoorzakenclassificaties van 1750 tot 1900. **Tijdschr Geschied Geneeskd** 1982;5(4):145–57
Westing AH: Research communication: war as a human endeavor: the high-fatality wars of the twentieth century. **J Peace Res** 1982;19(3):261–70

**Africa**

Abate Y: Population growth and urbanization in Africa. **Curr Hist** 1980;78(455):102–6, 132–3
Chauleur P: Développement et problèmes démographiques Africains. **Etudes (Fr)** 1981;354(4):437–49
Green E: U. S. population policies, development, and the rural poor of Africa. **J Mod Afr Stud** 1982;20(1):45–67
Gregory JW, Piché V: African population: reproduction for whom? **Daedalus** 1982 Spring;:179–209
Hartwig GW: Demographic considerations in East Africa during the nineteenth century. **Int J Afr Hist Stud** 1979;12(4):653–72
Kocher JE: Socio-economic development and fertility change in rural Africa. **Food Res Inst Stud** 1977;16(2):63–76
Northrup D: African mortality in the suppression of the slave trade: the case of the bight of Biafra. **J Interdiscip Hist** 1978;9(1):47–64
Perova M: V poiskakh resheniia demograficheskikh problem. **Aziia Afr Segodnia** 1981;5:31–3

**Albania**

Misja V, Vejsiu Y: Aspekte të zhvillimit të popullsisë në rps të shqipërisë. **Studime Hist** 1981;35(3):33–54

**Americas**

Festy P: La fécondité en Amérique du nord: vingt années de baisse. **Population** 1979;34(4–5):767–99
Fogel RW, Engerman SL: Recent findings in the study of slave demography and family structure. **Sociol Soc Res** 1979;63(3):566–89
Harrison GA: The past fifty years of human population biology in North America: an outsider's view. In F. Spencer, ed: A history of American physical anthropology, 1930–1980. New York, Academic Press, 1982. p. 467–72.
Johansen HC: Slave demography of the Danish West Indian Islands. **Scand Econ Hist Rev** 1981;29(1):1–20
Palloni A: Mortality in Latin America: emerging patterns. **Popul Dev Rev** 1981;7(4):623–49
Stycos JM: Recent trends in Latin American fertility. **Popul Stud** 1978;31(3):407–26

**Argentina**

Johnson LL, Seibert S: Estimaciones de la población de Buenos Aires en 1744, 1778 y 1810. **Desarrollo Econ** 1979;19(73):107–19

**Asia**

Cho LJ, Kobayashi K, ed: Fertility transition of the East Asian populations. Honolulu, University Press of Hawaii, 1979. vi, 300 p. (Monographs of the Center for Southeast Asian Studies, Kyoto University). Contributions by A. J. Coale, S. B. Hanley, Y. Tsubouchi, H. Y. Lee, P. E. Perry, T. H. Sun, Y. L. Soong, P. K. Liu, B. Mok, V. T. Palan, Y. J. Takeshita, C. T. Chang, C. Tuan, R. Freeman.
Gurevich NM: Dinamika rosta naseleniia zarubezhnoi Azii v nashei ere. **Nar Azii Afriki** 1975;(4):69–80
Loraine JA: Population perspectives in Asia. **Contemp Rev** 1979;235(1363):66–9
Ruzicka LT, Hansluwka H: Mortality transition in South and East Asia: technology confronts poverty. **Popul Dev Rev** 1982;8(3):567–88
Véron J: La mortalité en Asie Méridionale et Orientale. **Population** 1980;35(1):137–65

**Australia**

Gandevia B: Childhood mortality in Australia from 1788. In International Congress of the History of Medicine. 26th, Plovdiv, 1978. Actes du Congress. Sofia, 1981. Volume II. p. 100–3.
Pryor RJ: Morbidity and minerals: health and mortality in Victoria in the 1850s. Canberra, Department of Demography, Australian National University, 1977. 26 leaves. (Working paper in demography, 5).
Yusuf F, Rockett I: Immigrant family patterns and differentials in Australia, 1971–76. **Popul Stud** 1981;35(3):413–24

**Austria**

Auer EM: 80 Geburtsbriefe aus den Büchern des Vizedomamtes in Oesterreich unter der Enns. **Jahrb Landeskd Niederoesterr** 1961–63;35:50–105
Feurstein G: Vorarleberg: das familienfreundlichste Bundesland Oesterreichs. **Montfort** 1979;31(2–3):135–41
Riz R: Geburtenrückgang in Südtirol. **Eur Ethn** 1980;37(1):14–9

**Belgium**

Abelshausen M: De Antwerpse Werkhuizen van Liefdadigheid (1802–1870): weldadigheidsinstelling of fabriek? **Ann Soc Belg Hist Hop** 1982;20:61–108
André R: Etude régionale de la natalité et de la fécondité des populations belge et étrangère. **Rev Inst Sociol** 1969;3:569–86
André R: La mortalité de la population de nationalité belge. **Rev Inst Sociol** 1969;2:305–24
André R, Gyselings R: Variation saisonnière de la mortalité infantile en Belgique. **Rev Inst Sociol** 1970;3:587–97
Bruneel C: Malades et défunts au Grand Hôpital de Louvain (1767–1796). **Ann Soc Belg Hist Hop** 1978;16:3–33
Bruneel C: Un problème de gouvernement: le pouvoir face à l'epidémie de fièvre putride à Bruxelles en 1772–1773. In Imhof AE, ed: Mensch und Gesundheit in der Geschichte. Husum, Matthiesen, 1980. p. 199–221.
Gadeyne G: Oostvlaamse medici en parochiepriesters, slachtoffers van de tyfusepidemie, 1847–48: een episode uit de sociale geschiedenis. **Handel Maatsch Geschied Oudheidk Gent** 1980;34:167–79
Gotovitch J: Quelques données relatives à l'extermination des Tsiganes de Belgique. **Cah Hist Seconde Guerre Mond** 1976;4:161–80
Gutmann MP, Walle E van de: New sources for social and demographic history: the Belgian population registers. **Soc Sci Hist** 1978;2(2):121–43
Haesenne-Peremans N: Les Hospices et Orphelinats de la région Verviétoise au début du XIXe siècle. **Ann Soc Belg Hist Hop** 1978;16:35–56
Houdaille J: La baisse de la fécondité en Belgique au XIXe siècle. **Population** 1980;35(2):450–56
Joiris A: Le vieux Bavière au XIXe siècle (1830–1895). **Ann Soc Belg Hist Hop** 1982;20:109–44
Masuy-Stroobant G: La surmortalité infantile des Flandres au cours de la deuxième moitié du XIXe siècle: mode d'alimentation ou mode de développement? **Ann Demogr Hist (Paris)** 1983;:231–56
Poulain M, Tabutin D: La surmortalité des petites filles en Belgique au XIXe et au début du XXe siècle. [Brussels], Département démographique U.C.L., 1979, 17 p.
Poulain M, Tabutin D: La surmortalité des petites filles en Belgique au XIXe et début du XXe siècle. **Ann Demogr Hist (Paris)** 1981;:105–18
Van Buyten L: Drie 'doopregisters' van de Leuvense vondelingen (1745–1797). **Ann Soc Belg Hist Hop** 1979;17:31–69
Watkins SC, McCarthy J: The female life cycle in a Belgian commune: La Hulpe, 1847–1866. **J Fam Hist** 1980 Summer;5(2):167–79

**Bolivia**

Grieshaber EP: Survival of Indian communities in nineteenth-century Bolivia: a regional comparison. **J Lat Am Stud** 1980;12(2):223–69

**Brazil**

Alameida BC: Underdevelopment in a 'developing' nation: a quantitative study of health and medicine in Brazil, 1950–1975. Ph. D. Diss., University of California. Los Angeles, 1980. 338 leaves.
Berrance de Castro J, Scarano JM, Aissar A: A mortalidade entre os filhos de trabalhadores pretos e brancos estrangeiros numa regiõ cafeeira paulista: 1875–1930. **Rev Hist (Brazil)** 1973;46(94):603–17
Goldberg HI, Rodrigues W, Thome AM, et al: Infant mortality and breast-feeding in North-Eastern Brazil. **Popul Stud** 1984 Mar;38(1):105–15
Lisanti L: Urbanisation et folie São Paulo, 1852–1929. **Jahrb Gesch Staat Wirtsch Ges Lateinam** 1980;17:297–315
Wood CH: Infant mortality trends and capitalist development in Brazil: the case of Sao Paulo and Belo Horizonte. **Lat Am Perspect** 1977:4(4):56–65

**Bulgaria**

McIntyre RJ: The Bulgarian anomaly: demographic transition and current fertility. **Southeast Eur** 1980;7(2):147–70
Nikolaeva I, Vassilev V, Ivanov C, et al: Données statistiques sur l'activité l'hôpital 'Paraskeva Nikolaou' à Varna de 1879 à 1912. In International Congress of the History of Medicine. 26th, Plovdiv, 1978. Actes du Congress. Sofia, 1981. Volume II. p. 68–9.
Stefanov I: A népesedéspolitika jelenlegi problémái Bulgáriában. **Demografia** 1972;15(2):227–34

### Canada

Bilson G: 'Muscles and health': health and the Canadian immigrant, 1867–1906. In Roland CG, ed: Health, disease and medicine. Toronto, Hannah Institute for the History of Medicine, 1984. p. 398–411.
Bouchard G: Démographie et société rurale au Saguenay, 1851–1935. **Rech Sociogr** 1978;19(1):7–31
Bouchard G, Brard P: Le programme de reconstitution automatique des familles saguenayennes: données de base et resultats provisoires. **Soc Hist (Canada)** 1979;12(23):170–83
Bourbeau R, Légaré J: Evolution de la mortalité au Canada et au Québec, 1831–1931. Essai de mesure par génération. Montreal, Les Presses de l'Universite de Montreal, 1982. 140 p.
Chadney JG: Sikh family patterns and ethnic adaptation in Vancouver. **Amerasia J** 1980;7(1):31–50
Collins LD, Higgins D, ed: The politics of abortion: trends in Canadian fertility policy. **Atlantis** 1982;7(2):2–20
Cumming E, Lazer C: Kinship structure and suicide: a theoretical link. **Can Rev Sociol Anthropol** 1981;18(3):271–82
Dufour D, Péron Y: Vingt ans de mortalité au Québec: les causes de décés, 1951–1971. Montréal, Presses de l'Université de Montréal, 1979. 204 p. (Collection 'Démographie canadienne, 4). 204 p.
Ewart WB: Causes of mortality in a subarctic settlement (York Factory, Man.), 1714–1946. **Can Med Assoc J** 1983 Sep 15;129(6):571–4
Igartua JE: Le comportement démographique des marchands de Montréal vers 1760. **Rev Hist Am Fr** 1979;33(3):427–45
Kyriazis N: A parity-specific analysis of completed fertility in Canada. **Can Rev Sociol Anthropol** 1982;19(1):29–43
Kyriazis N, Henripin J: Women's employment and fertility in Québec. **Popul Stud** 1982 Nov;36(3):431–40
LaRose A: Bibliographie courante sur l'histoire de la population canadienne et la démographie historique au Canada, 1977. **Soc Hist (Canada)** 1979;12(23):192–7
Mathieu J, Cyr C, Dinel G, et al: Les alliances matrimoniales exogames dans le gouvernement de Québec 1700–1760. **Rev Hist Am Fr** 1981;35(1):3–32
Norris J: Typhoid in the Rockies: epidemiology in a constrained habitat, 1883–1939. In Roland CG, ed: Health, disease and medicine. Toronto, Hannah Institute for the History of Medicine, 1984. p. 276–95.
Romaniuk A: Increase in natural fertility during the early stages of modernization: Canadian Indians case study. **Demography** 1981 May;18(2):157–72
Trovato F, Grindstaff CF: Decomposing the urban-rural fertility differential: Canada, 1971. **Rural Sociol** 1980;45(3):448–68

### Caribbean

Lamur HE: Demographic performance of two slave populations of the Dutch speaking Caribbean. **Bol Estud Latinoam Caribe** 1981;(30):87–102
Leridon H, Charbit Y: Patterns of marital unions and fertility in Guadeloupe and Martinique. **Popul Stud** 1981;35(2):235–46

### Chile

Villarroel H, Lazo B, Campusano C, et al: Consanguinidad y migración en Viña del Mar durante 1888 a 1967. **Rev Med Chil** 1980 May;108(5):407–12

### China

Barrett RE: Short-term trends in bastardy in Taiwan. **J Fam Hist** 1980 Fall;5(3):293–312
Bianco L: Birth control in China: local data and their reliability. **China Q** 1981;(85):119–37
Bianco L: Voyage en Chine. **Esprit** 1973; (4):595–604
Chan H: [A description of demographic cognition during the Ch'ing Dynasty] (Chi). **Ssu yu Yen** 1973;10(6):425–31
Conger DJ, Luan DC: Dynamic properties of Taiwanese fertility, 1950–1972. **Stud Comp Int Dev** 1979 Summer;14:54–74
Freedman R, Chang MC, Sun TH: Household composition, extended kinship and reproduction in Taiwan: 1973–1980. **Popul Stud** 1982 Nov;36(3):395–411
Lavely WR: The rural Chinese fertility transition: a report from Shifang Xian, Sichuan. **Popul Stud** 1984 Nov;38(3):365–84
Loraine JA: Population and birth control in China. **Contemp Rev** 1981;239(1388):126–130
Maloney JM: Recent developments in China's population planning: notes and comments. **Pac Aff** 1981;54(1):100–14
Molodtsova LI: O chislennosti naseleniia knr. **Nar Azii Afriki** 1975;(4):81–91
Pressat R: Evolution des naissances en Chine. **Population** 1980;35(4–5):968–72
Schultz TP: Explanations of birth rate changes over space and time: a study of Taiwan. **J Polit Econ** 1973;81(2 pt 2):238–74
Yuan Tien H: Induced fertility transition: impact of population planning and socio-economic change in the People's Republic of China. **Popul Stud** 1984 Nov;38(3):385–400

### Costa Rica

Stycos JM: The decline of fertility in Costa Rica: literacy, modernization and family planning. **Popul Stud** 1982 Mar;36(1):15–30
Tjarks GO, Espinoza Guadamuz JC, Paniagua Vargas C: Un procedimiento estadístico para resolver muescas de población: el caso de Heredia. **Rev Hist (Costa Rica)** 1978;3(6):111–27

### Cuba

Díaz-Briquets S, Pérez L: Fertility decline in Cuba: a socioeconomic interpretation. **Popul Dev Rev** 1982;8(3):513–37
Iglesias F: Características de la población cubana en 1862. **Rev Bibl Nac Jose Marti** 1980;22(3):89–110
Losada J, Mayor J: Esclavitud y psicología: una investigación interdisciplinaria. **Rev Bibl Nac Jose Marti** 1980;22(3):133–43

### Czechoslovakia

Matejček J: K populačnímu vývoji severní Moravy a Slezska 1910–1921. **Slezsky Sb** 1978;76(1):43–63
Pitronová B: Hlavní rysy vývoje obyvatelstva severočeské hnědouhelné oblasti v období kapitalismu (do roku 1939). **Slezsky Sb** 1176–77;4:251–78
Sípek Z: Na co umírali lidé v Morašicích na okrese znojemském v letech 1904–1949. **Cas Lek Cesk** 1984 Mar 16;123(11):331
Subrtová A: Antonín Bohác—statistik a demograf: život a dílo. **Sb Nar Muzea Praze Rada A Hist** 1977;32(1–3):1–198

### Denmark

Andersen O: The development in Danish mortality 1735–1850. **Scand Popul Stud** 1979;5:9–21
Hoem JM, Finnäs F: Traek af fertilitetsfaldet i Danmark siden slutningen af tresserne. **Nationalocon Tidsskr** 1980;118(2):171–83
Jensen OM, Larsen A: Blaerecancer i Danmark 1943–1977. Kraeftstatistik 4. **Ugeskr Laeger** 1982 Nov 15;144(46):3458–60
Lamblin-Robert J, Lecomte D, Lathrop M, et al: Epidemies virales et rapport de masculinité des naissances: des données divergentes. **Population** 1983;38(1):162–5
Manniche E: Age at menarche: Nicolai Edvard Ravn's data on 3385 women in mid-19th century Denmark. **Ann Hum Biol** 1983 Jan–Feb;10(1):79–82

### El Salvador

Karush G: Tierra, población y pobreza: las raíces de la crisis demográfica en El Salvador. **Estud Cent Am** 1977;32(350):893–910

### Europe

Berntsen B: Fra Malthus til befolkningsåret 1974. **Samtiden (Norway)** 1973;82(4):232–9
Bourgeois-Pichat J: Recent demographic change in Western Europe: an assessment. **Popul Dev Rev** 1981;7(1):19–42
Calot G, Blayo C: Recent course of fertility in Western Europe. **Popul Stud** 1982 Nov;36(3):349–72
Chaunu P, Dupâquier J, Chesnais JC: La dénatalité. Analyse historique du présent: la dénatalité. 'La vie c'est bon.' Les retournements de l'avenir. **Histoire** 1978;(3,6):62–6, 62–5
Egon S: Az európai országok termékenységét közvetlenül, vagy közvetve befolyásoló törvények. **Demografia** 1973;16(1):114–8
Friedländer S: L'extermination des Juifs d'Europe: pour une etude historique globale. **Rev Etud Juives** 1976;135(1–3):113–44
Girard A, Roussel L: Ideal family size, fertility, and population policy in Western Europe. **Popul Dev Rev** 1982;8(2):323–45
Girard A: Le nouveau régime démographique et la crise des valeurs. **Etudes (Fr)** 1979;350(1):7–23
Halpern I: [Rush marriages among Eastern European Jews] (Heb). **Zion** 1962;27(1–2):36–58
Imhof AE: Recherches macroregionales sur la mortalité en Europe septentrionale sous l'ancien regime. In Charbonneau H, Larose A, ed. The great mortalities: methodological studies of demographic crises in the past. Liège, Belgium, Ordina Editions, 1980. p. 139–56.
Lebrun F: Quand un enfant sur deux mourait. **Histoire** 1982;42:78–81
Lesthaeghe R, Wilson C: Les modes de production, la laïcisation et le rythme de la baisse de la fécondité en Europe de l'Ouest de 1870 à 1930. **Population** 1982;37(3):623–45
Madai L: Les crises de mortalité en Europe dans la deuxième moitie cu XIXe siècle. In Charbonneau H, Larose A, ed: The great mortalities: methodological studies of demographic crises in the past. Liège, Belgium, Ordina Editions, 1980. p. 157–78.
Mitterauer M, Kagan A: Russian and Central European family structures: a comparative view. **J Fam Hist** 1982 Spring;7(1):103–31
Pressat R: Mesures natalistes et relèvement de la fécondité en Europe de l'est. **Population** 1979;34(3):533–48
Ströder J, Schuster J: Estudio comparativo de la mortalidad infantil entre los niños Judios y no Judios en Europa Central y Oriental a finales del siglo diecinueve y principios del veinte. **Folia Hum (Barc)**

# STATISTICS AND DEMOGRAPHY

1983;21(240):1-10

### Finland

Jutikkala E: Finnish mortality in the eighteenth century: the sources and the reality **Scand Econ Hist Rev** 1978;26(2):168-9
Lindgren S: Utomäktenskaplig fertilitet i Helsingfors under 1800-talets senare del. **Hist Arkisto (Finl)** 1981;76:301-20
Lithell UB: Infant mortality rate and standards of living in the past. **Scand J Hist** 1981;6(4):297-315
Mereste U, Pullat R: Tallinna elanikkonna kujune misest 18. sajandil ja aegridade rekonstrueerimis est ajaloolises demograafias (meetrikaraamatute andmeil). **Eesti NSV Tead Akad Toim** 1979;28(4):285-303
Näyhä S: Short and medium-term variations in mortality in Finland. A study on cyclic variations, annual and weekly periods and certain irregular changes in mortality in Finland during period 1868-1972. **Scand J Soc Med [Suppl]** 1981;(21):1-101
Pitkänen K: The changing features of mortality in Finland in the 18th and 19th centuries. The Fifth Scandinavian Demographic Symposium, 13-16 June 1979 at Hurdalssjen, Norway. **Scand Popul Stud** 1979;5:74-82
Turpeinen O: Die Sterblichkeit an Pocken, Masern und Keuchhusten in Finnland in den Jahren 1751 bis 1865. In Imhof AE, ed: Mensch und Gesundheit in der Geschichte. Husum, Matthiesen, 1980. p. 135-61.
Turpeinen O: Infant mortality in Finland 1749-1865. **Scand Econ Hist Rev** 1979;27(1):1-21,67
Turpeinen O: Les causes des fluctuations annuelles du taux de mortalité finlandais entre 1750 et 1806. **Ann Demogr Hist (Paris)** 1980;:287-96
Turpeinen O: Monthly mortality in Finland in 1751-1806. **Yearb Popul Res Finl** 1979;17:59-73
Turpeinen O: Mortalitetskrisen i Finland åren 1788--1791. **Hist Tidskr Finl** 1981;66(1):14-34

### France

Ackerman EB: Use by patients of a French provincial hospital, 1895-1923. **Bull Hist Med** 1980 Summer;54(2):188-203
Adams P: Mortality crises in nineteenth century France. In: Les Grandes mortalités: étude méthodologique des crises démographiques du passé. H. Charbonneau et A. LaRose, ed. Liège, U.I.E.S.P., 1979, p. 29-31.
Arquiola E: La enfermedad en la antropología física francesa durante el positivismo. **Asclepio** 1983;35:217-26
Azemar R: Les causes de décès à La Roque-Sainte-Marguerite, en sud-Rouergue, de 1721 à 1742. **Ann Demogr Hist (Paris)** 1984;:239-58
Barbier F: Les caractères généraux de la démographie de Valenciennes au XIXe siècle. **Rev Nord** 1983;65(258):567-79
Beauquier JP: Quelques aspects de la démographie et de la santé à Marseille pendant la seconde guerre mondiale. **Provence Hist** 1983;33(134):439-47
Bideau A: A demographic and social analysis of widowhood and remarriage: the example of the castellany of Thoissey-en-Dombes, 1670-1840. **J Fam Hist** 1980 Spring;5(1):28-43
Bideau A: Variables familiales de la mortalité infantile. In Imhof AE, ed: Mensch und Gesundheit in der Geschichte. Husum, Matthiesen, 1980. p. 223-50.
Biraben JN: André Armengaud, 1920-1980. **Ann Demogr Hist (Paris)** 1980;:7-10
Blanchet D: Evolution de la fécondite des régions françaises depuis 1960. **Population** 1981;36(4-5):817-44
Bouchard G: Nouvelles perspectives pour les recherches génétiques. Le fichier-réseau de la population du Saguenay. **Ann Demogr Hist (Paris)** 1984;:81-8
Bougard JP: La formation de la classe ouvrière dans le borinage au XVIIIème et au début du XIXème siècle. La cas de Wasmes et de Warquignies. **Rev Nord** 1981;63:248:157-68
Brunet G: Un bourg rural de la Dombes au XVIIIe et XIXe siècles: Saint-Trivier-sur-Moignans. Démographie, société et mentalités, 2 volumes. Lyon II. Thèse de doct de 3e cycle 1979. 128 p.
Calot G: Le mouvement journalier des naissances à l'intèrieur de la semaine. **Population** 1981;36(3):477-504
Cibois P: La natalisme national. **Esprit** 1982;10:76-96
Coleman W: Death is a social disease. Public health and political economy in early industrial France. Madison, University of Wisconsin Press, 1982. xxi, 322 p. (Wisconsin Publications in the History of Science and Medicine, 1).
Coleman W: Medicine against Malthus: François Mélier on the relation between subsistence and mortality (1843). **Bull Hist Med** 1980 Spring;54(1):23-42
Comiti VP: La géographie médicale de la Corse à la fin du XVIIIe siècle. Genève, Droz, 1980. 142 p. (Centre de Recherches d'Histoire et de Philologie de la IVe Section de l'Ecole pratique des Hautes Etudes; Hautes Etudes Médiévales et Modernes, 41).
Denis MN: Un problème de moeurs dans l'Alsace rurale traditionnelle: naissances illégitimes et conceptions prénuptiales à Bosselshausen (Bas-Rhin) de 1738 à 1838. In Congrès National des Sociétés Savantes, 103e, Nancy-Metz, 1978. Actes. Paris, 1979. Tome II, p. 57-69.
Denoix P: Paul Broca. L'anatomie pathologique, le cancer, la statistique. **Chirurgie** 1980;106(10):787-90
Derouet B: Une démographie sociale différentielle: clés pour un système auto-régulateur des populations rurales d'Ancien Régime. **Ann Econ Soc Civilis** 1980;35(1):3-41
Deville JC: Analyse harmonique dul calendrier de constitution des familles en France. Disparités sociales et évolution de 1920 à 1960. **Population** 1977;32(1):17-63
Dumazet A: 'Au pays des nourrices'. **Ann Demogr Hist (Paris)** 1984;:279-84
Dumont GF, Legrand J: Evolution récente du nombre des décès déclarés dus à l'avortement. **Population** 1981;36(2):410-14
Dupâquier J, Lachiver M: Du contresens à l'illusion technique, suivi d'une réponse de John Knodel à Jacques Dupâquier. **Ann Econ Soc Civilis** 1981;36(3):489-92
Dupâquier J: Etude comparative des données sur la fécondité dans 25 monographies concernant le bassin parisien à la fin du XVIIe siècle et au début du XVIIIe siècle. In Leridon H, Menken J, ed: Féconditè naturelle, U. T. E. S. P., 1979, p. 409-39.
Dupaquier M: La famille Bertillon et la naissance d'une nouvelle science sociale: la démographie. **Ann Demogr Hist (Paris)** 1983;:293-310
Feldenkirchen W: Aspekte der Bevölkerungs- und Sozialstruktur der Stadt Köln in der französischen Zeit (1794-1814). **Rheinische Vierteljahrsbl** 1979;43:182-227
Festy P, Rallu JL: Constitution et reconstitution des familles françaises: état civil et recensements de 1968 et 1975. **Population** 1981;36(1):63-92
Fine-Souriac A: La limitation des naissances dans le sud-ouest de la France: fécondité, allaitement et contraception au pays de Sault du milieu du XVIIIe siècle à 1914. **Ann Midi** 1978;90(2):155-88
Gani L: Jules Guesde, Paul Lafargue et les problèmes de population. **Population** 1979;34(4):1023-1044
Ganiage J: La population du Beauvaisis: transformations économiques et mutations démographiques (1790-1975). **Ann Geogr** 1980;89(491):1-36
Gélis J: L'enquête de 1786 sur les sages-femmes du royaume. **Ann Demogr Hist (Paris)** 1980;:301-43
Goubert JP: Die Medikalisierung der französischen Gesellschaft am Ende des Ancien Régime: die Bretagne als Beispiel. **Medizinhist J** 1982;17(1/2):89-114
Gutierrez H: Evolution de la population totale et qualité des previsions démographiques à court terme, par dpartements de la région Midipyrenées, 1821-1976. **Population** 1981;36(1):182-7
Houdaille J: La Réunion, des origines à 1766: étude démographique. **Ann Demogr Hist (Paris)** 1980;:213-37
Houdaille J: Mortalité des députés élus de 1789 à 1794. **Population** 1979;34(3):714-7
Houdaille J: Mouvement saisonnier des conceptions en France de 1740 à 1829. **Population** 1979;34(2):452-57
Huron R: La statistique medicale en France à l'époque romantique. **Mem Acad Sci Insc B-Lett Toulouse** 1976;138:121-39
Knodel J: Espacement des naissances et planification familiale: une critique de la méthode Dupâquier-Lachiver. **Ann Econ Soc Civilis** 1981;36(3):473-88
Le Goff A: La paroisse de Saint-Hélier de Rennes et sa démographie de 1711 à 1790. In Congrès National des Sociétés Savantes, 97e, Nantes, 1972. Actes. Paris, 1977. Tome II, p. 153-63.
Leboutte R: D'Austerlitz à Liège, mourir dans les armées de Bonaparte. **Tijdschr Geschied Geneeskd** 1978;91(3):429-46
Lebrun F: L'intervention des autorités face aux crises de mortalité dans la France d'ancien régime. In Imhof AE, ed: Leib und Leben in der Geschichte der Neuzeit. Berlin, Duncker & Humblot, 1983. p. 39-52.
Lehning JR: The decline of marital fertility: evidence from a French department, la Loire (1851-1891). **Ann Demogr Hist (Paris)** 1984;:201-17
LeRoy Ladurie E: Demographie et 'funestes secrets': le Languedoc (fin XVIIIe-debut XIXe siècle). **Ann Hist Revolut Fr** 1965;37(4):385-400
Lescarret JP: Démographie et société dans le Haute-Lande depuis le XVIIIe siècle, Saugnac-le-Muret, 2 volumes. Univ. de Boredaux III. Thèse de doct. 1979. 642 p.
Levy C: Essai d'estimation de la population handicapée en France. (Handicap sevère). **Population** 1983;38(1):178-84
Lilienfeld DE, Lilienfeld AM: The French influence on the development of epidemiology. In Lilienfeld AM, ed: Times, places, and persons. Baltimore, London, Johns Hopkins Univ. Press, 1980. (Sigerist suppl. to the Bull Hist Med, n.s., no 4) p. 28-38.
McLaren A: Sexuality and social order: the debate over the fertility of women and workers in France, 1770-1920. New York, Holmes & Meier, 1982.
McManners J: Death and the Enlightenment. Changing attitudes to death among Christians and unbelievers in eighteenth-century France. Oxford, Clarendon Press; New York, Oxford University Press; 1981. vii, 619 p.
McQuillan K: Modes of production and demographic patterns in nineteenth-century France. **AJS** 1984;89(6):1324-46
Maillé-Virole C: La naissance d'un personnage: le medecin Parisien à la fin de l'ancien régime. **Hist Reflect** 1982;9(1-2):153-79
Mérigot JG: Le problème des naissances en France. **Def Natl** 1975;31(7):95-104
Moch LP: Marriage, migration, and urban demographic structure: a case from France in the Belle Epoque. **J Fam Hist** 1981 Spring;6(1):70-88
Murphy TD: Medical knowledge and statistical methods in early nineteenth-century France. **Med Hist** 1981 Jul;25(3):301-19

Naranjo B, Estienne P: La mutation des comportements démographiques de la proche banlieue clermontoise: le rôle des étrangers. **Rev Auvergne** 1981;95(1):3-11
Nizard A, Vallin J: Les causes de décès en France. II. couplage des 7e et 8e révisions de la classification internationale. Application à la période 1958-1974. **Population** 1980;35(6):1057-99
Offen K: Depopulation, nationalism, and feminism in fin-de-siècle France. **Am Hist Rev** 1984;89(3):648-76
Oguse, D: 'Socialisme et néo-malthusianisme', la Revue Socialiste, t. XLVI, juillet-décembre 1907, p. 27-124. **Ann Demogr Hist (Paris)** 1983;:371-89
Phillips R: Family breakdown in late eighteenth-century France. Divorces in Rouen 1792-1803. Oxford and New York, clarendon Press, 1980. x, 244 p.
Plessix R: La mortalité à Mamers de Louis XIV à Napoléon III. **Ann Bretagne** 1983;90(3):467-82
Pollet M: Naissances illégitimes, filles-mères et enfants trouvés à Grasse au XVIIIe siècle, 1751-1789. **Bull Inf Soc Demogr Hist** 1979;:5-21
Poussou JP: Les crises démographiques en milieu urbain: l'example de Bordeaux (fin XVIIe-fin XVIIIe siècle). **Ann Econ Soc Civilis** 1980;35(2):235-52
Rallu JL: Evolution du nombre et de la composition des familles françaises entre 1975 et 1979. **Population** 1981;36(3):629-34
Richards T: Weather, nutrition, and the economy: short-run fluctuations in births, deaths, and marriages, France 1740-1909. **Demography** 1983 May;20(2):197-212
Spagnoli PG: High fertility in mid-nineteenth century France: a multivariate analysis of fertility patterns in the arrondissement of Lille. **Res Econ Hist** 1977;2:281-336
Spagnoli PG: Industrialization, proletarianization, and marriage: a reconsideration. **J Fam Hist** 1983 Fall;8(3):230-47
Spagnoli PG: Philippe Ariès, historian of the family. **J Fam Hist** 1981 Winter;6(4):434-41
Sussman GD: The end of the wet-nursing business in France, 1874-1914. In R. Wheaton, T. K. Hareven, ed: Family and sexuality in French history. Philadelphia, University of Pennsylvania Press, 1980. p. 224-52.
Tilly LA: Structure de l'emploi, travail des femmes et changements démographiques dans deux villes industrielles, Anzin et Roubaix, 1872-1906.. In: Le mouvement social. Paris, Les éditions ouvrières, 1978; 105:33-58.
Traer JF: Marriage and the family in eighteenth-century France. Ithaca, Cornell University Press, 1980. 208 p.
Vallin J: Tendances récentes de la mortalité française. **Population** 1983;38(1):77-105
Van de Walle E: Motivation and technology in the decline of French fertility. In R. Wheaton, T. K. Hareven, ed: Family and sexuality in French history. Philadelphia, University of Pennsylvania Press, 1980. p. 135-78.
Weir DR: Fertility transition in rural France, 1740-1829. Ph.D. Diss., Stanford University. Palo Alto, 1983. xiv, 366 p.

**French Guiana**

Henry L, Hurault J: Mortalité de la population européenne de Guyane Française au début du XVIIIe siècle. **Population** 1979;34(6):1087-1100

**Gambia**

Weil PM: The staff of life: food and female fertility in a West African society. **Africa (Gt Brit)** 1976;46(2):182-95

**Germany**

Aronsfeld CC: 'Perish Judah': Nazi Extermination Propaganda 1920-1945. **Patterns Prejudice** 1978:12(5):17-26
Bauer Y: Genocide: was it the Nazis' original plan. **Ann Am Acad Polit Soc Sci** 1980;450:35-45
Becker K: 100 Jahre gesetzliche Krankenversicherung. Entwicklung, Krise, Lösungsansätze in der Krankenversicherung der Rentner. (Mit einem Beitrag von Jens Jessen, Programmierter Kollaps der GKV?) Mainz, MPS, 1980. 74 p.
Bleker J: Die Stadt als Krankheitsfaktor, eine Analyse ärztlicher Auffassungen im 19. Jahrhundert. **Medizinhist J** 1983;18(1-2):118-36
Blohmke M: Stadt-Land-Unterschiede im Gesundheitszustand historischer und heutiger Bevölkerungen. In Imhof AE, ed: Leib und Leben in der Geschichte der Neuzeit. Berlin, Duncker & Humblot, 1983. p. 63-75.
Broszat M: Hitler und die Genesis der 'Endlösung.' Aus Anlass der Thesen von David Irving. **Vierteljahrsh Zeitgesch** 1977;25(4):739-75
Drabik R: Die Entwicklung des Leistungspotentials der Krankenhausmedizin im 20.Jahrhundert in Deutschland. Diss., Universität Düsseldorf. Düsseldorf, 1982. 98 p.
Eigler J, Müller B: Die Patienten des ersten Jahres (1813-1814) im Allgemeinen Krankenhaus München. **MMW** 1982 Apr 30;124(17):429-33
Hecht J: Johann Peter Sussmilch, point alpha ou omega de la science démographique naïve? **Ann Demogr Hist (Paris)** 1979;:101-34
Hohorst G: The decline of fertility once again: a critical note on John Knodel's book and standardized demographic indexes. **Hist Soc Res** 1982;22:50-62
Hörger H: Mortalität, Krankheit und Lebenserwartung der Penzberger Bergarbeiterschaft im 19. und beginnenden 20. Jahrhundert. **Z Bayer Landesgesch** 1980:43(1);185-222
Imhof AE: Die Uebersterblichkeit verheirateter Frauen im fruchtbaren Alter. Eine Illustration der 'condition féminine' im 19. Jahrhundert. **Z Bevoelkerungswiss** 1979;4:487-510
Imhof AE: La surmortalité des femmes mariées en age de procréation: un indice de la condition féminine au XIXe siècle. **Ann Demogr Hist (Paris)** 1981;:81-7
Khalatbari P, Müllen K, Strohbach E: Népesedéspolitikai problémák a német demokratikus koztársasagban. **Demografia** 1972;15(2):184-94
Knodel J, Hermalin AI: Effects of birth rank, maternal age, birth interval, and sibship size on infant and child mortality: evidence from 18th and 19th century reproductive histories. **Am J Public Health** 1984 Oct;74(10):1098-106
Knodel J: From natural fertility to family limitation: the onset of fertility transition in a sample of German villages. **Demography** 1979 Nov;16(4):493-521
Knodel J, De Vos S: Preferences for the sex of offspring and demographic behavior in eighteenth and nineteenth-century Germany: an examination of evidence from village genealogies. **J Fam Hist** 1980 Summer;5(2):145-66
Knodel J: Seasonal variation in infant mortality: an approach with applications. **Ann Demogr Hist (Paris)** 1983;:208-30
Knodel J, Wilson C: The secular increase in fecundity in German village populations: an analysis of reproductive histories of couples married 1750-1899. **Popul Stud** 1981 Mar;35(1):53-84
Landmann H: Die Entwicklung der Tuberkulose in den letzten 100 Jahren unter besonderer Berücksichtigung der epidemiologischen Situation in der Deutschen Demokratischen Republik.
Lee RW: Medicalisation and mortality trends in South Germany in the early 19th century. In Imhof AE, ed: Mensch und Gesundheit in der Geschichte. Husum, Matthiesen, 1980. p. 79-113.
Lee WR: The mechanism of mortality change in Germany, 1750-1850. **Medizinhist J** 1980;15(3):244-68
Lengsfeld W: La population allemande depuis un siècle. **Documents** 1979;34(3):61-70
Lengsfeld W: Un phénomène complexe: la fécondité. **Documents** 1979;34(3):79-85
Lowenthal EG: Zur Demographie der Juden im früheren Oberschlesien. **Z Ostforsch** 1979;28(1):81-4
Mai A: Diagnosestellung niedergelassener Arzte bei der Leichenschau im Vergleich zu den Ergebnissen der gerichtlichen Obduktion. Diss., Johannes Gutenberg - Universität in Mainz. Mainz, 1982. 143 p.
Miura T, Richter J: Changes in the seasonal distribution of births in Görlitz, Germany, during the period between 1657 and 1816. **Hum Biol** 1981 Feb;53(1):15-22
Müller C: Zur Bevölkerungsentwicklung in Westberlin. **Wiss Z Humboldt Univ Berl [Gesellschaftswiss Sprachwiss Reihe]** 1979;28(1):105-13
Rein DB: En République Démocratique d'Allemagne: population et politique. **Documents** 1979;34(4):131-7
Rein DB: Une attitude allemande face à l'évolution démographique. **Population** 1982;37(1):113-30
Rodegra H: Kindestötung und Verheimlichung der Schwangerschaft: eine sozialgeschichtliche und medizinsoziologische Untersuchung mit Einzelfallanalysen. Herzogenrath [Germany], Murken-Altrogge, 1981. 68 p.
Schneegans HJ: Die Müttersterblichkeit im 17. bis 19. Jahrhundert. **Zentralbl Gynakol** 1982;104(22):1416-20
Spree R: Die Entwicklung der differentiellen Säuglingssterblichkeit in Deutschland seit der Mitte des 19. Jahrhunderts. (Ein Versuch zur Mentalitäts-Geschichte). In Imhof AE, ed: Mensch und Gesundheit in der Geschichte. Husum, Matthiesen, 1980. p. 251-78.
Spree R: The German petite bourgeoisie and the decline of fertility: some statistical evidence from the late 19th and early 20th centuries. **Hist Soc Res** 1982;22:15-49
Stephan P: Geburtlichkeit und Kindersterblichkeit in einem Dorf im 17. und 18. Jahrhundert. **Arztl Jugendkd** 1984 Jun;75(3):178-89

**Ghana**

Patterson KD: Health in colonial Ghana: disease, medicine, and socio-economic change, 1900-1955. Waltham, Mass., Crossroads Press, 1981. xiii, 187 p.

**Great Britain**

Anderson O: Did suicide increase with industrialization in Victorian England? **Past Present** 1980;86:149-73
Anning ST: A medical case book: Leeds, 1781-84. **Med Hist** 1984 Oct;28(4):420-31
Armstrong WA: The trend of mortality in Carlisle between the 1780s and the 1840s: a demographic contribution to the standard of living debate. **Econ Hist Rev** 1981;34(1):91-114
Austin Bradford Hill: **Stat Med** 1982 Oct-Dec;1(4):305-9
Banks JA: Victorian values: secularism and the size of families. London,

Boston, Routledge & Kegan Paul, 1981. ix, 203 p.
Benson B, Wall R: Historical demography in the nineteenth and twentieth centuries in the absence of the civil registers. **Local Popul Stud (Matlock)** 1981 Spring;26:14-28
Bibliography: Publications (in English) of Sir Austin Bradford Hill. **Stat Med** 1982 Oct-Dec;1(4):369-75
Box JF: R. A. Fisher: the life of a scientist. New York, Wiley, 1978. xii, 512 p.
Brown HP: Sir Alexander Carr-Saunders. In Dictionary of national biography, 1961-1970. Suppl. 8, 1981. p. 175-6.
Brown PS: The providers of medical treatment in mid-nineteenth-century Bristol. **Med Hist** 1980 Jul;24(3):297-314
Browne J: Darwin's botanical arithmetic and the 'principle of divergence,' 1854-1858. **J Hist Biol** 1980 Spring;13(1):53-89
Buck P: People who counted: political arithmetic in the eighteenth century. **Isis** 1982 Mar;73(266):28-45
Bulber M: The slow and uneven growth of sociology in Great Britain. **Minerva** 1983 Summer-Autumn;21(2-3):338-47
Charlton C, Drake M, Gwynne T, et al: The Registrar General's indexes and registers: microfilm copies may be available. **Local Popul Stud (Matlock)** 1984;32:4-11
Cherry S: The hospitals and population growth: part 1. The voluntary general hospitals, mortality and local populations in the English provinces in the eighteenth and nineteenth centuries. **Popul Stud** 1980 Mar;34(1):59-75
Crafts NF: Illegitimacy in England and Wales in 1911. **Popul Stud** 1982 Jul;36(2):327-31
Doll R: Clinical trials: retrospect and prospect. **Stat Med** 1982 Oct-Dec;1(4):337-44
Doll R: The route back to Methusaleh. **Trans Hunter Soc** 1978-80;37-38:161-74
Dupâquier J: Avez-vous lu Malthus? **Population** 1980;35(2):279-90
Dupâquier J, Fauve-Chamoux A, Grebenik E, ed: Malthus past and present. London; New York, Academic Press, 1983. xix, 416 p. Contributions by A. Béjin, Y. Breton, Y. Charbit, L. Devance, A. Digby, M. W. Flinn, R. E. Frisch, M. Godelier, L. Gordon, P. Guillaume, G. Heinsohn, T. H. Hollingsworth, P. A. Jewell, N. Keyfitz, R. Keynes, H. Le Bras, M. Perrot, F. Rausky, M. Rebérioux, R. Remond, F. Ronsin, G. R. Searle, B. Stapleton, O. Steiger, P. Vallin, E. Van de Walle, A. Waterman, J. Wolff, E. A. Wrigley, V. Wynne-Edwards.
Dyhouse C: Working-class mothers and infant mortality in England, 1895-1914. **J Soc Hist** 1978;12(2):248-67
Eyler JM: The conceptual origins of William Farr's epidemiology: numerical methods and social thought in the 1830s. In Lilienfeld AM, ed: Times, plaes, and persons. Baltimore, London, Johns Hopkins Univ. Press, 1980. (Sigerist suppl. to the Bull Hist Med, n.s., no 4) p. 1-21.
Fildes V: Neonatal feeding practices and infant mortality during the 18th century. **J Biosoc Sci** 1980 Jul;12(3):313-24
Fleiss JL: Multicentre clinical trials: Bradford Hill's contributions and some subsequent developments. **Stat Med** 1982 Oct-Dec;1(4):353-9
Forbes TR: Mortality at St. Bartholomew's Hospital, London, 1839-72. **J Hist Med Allied Sci** 1983 Oct;38(4):432-49
Greenwald MW, Greenwald GI: Coroner's inquests. A source of vital statistics: Westminster, 1761-1866. **J Leg Med (Chicago)** 1983 Mar;4(1):51-86
Haines MR: Age specific and differential fertility in Durham and Easington registration districts, England, 1851 and 1861. **Soc Sci Hist** 1977;2(1):23-52
Hall AR: Homo fabricator: a new species. **Hist Philos Life Sci** 1980;2(2):193-14
Hamilton D: The nineteenth-century surgical revolution--antisepsis or better nutrition? **Bull Hist Med** 1982 Spring;56(1):30-40
Hansen E: 'Overlaying' in 19th-century England: infant mortality in infanticide? **Hum Ecol** 1979;7:333-52
Hardy A: Smallpox in London: factors in the decline of the disease in the nineteenth century. **Med Hist** 1983 Apr;27(2):111-38
Hare EH, Moran PA, Macfarlane A: The changing seasonality of infant deaths in England and Wales 1912-78 and its relation to seasonal temperature. **J Epidemiol Community Health** 1981 Jun;35(2):77-82
Hilts VL: Epidemiology and the statistical movement. In Lilienfeld AM, ed: Times, places, and persons. Baltimore, London, Johns Hopkins Univ. Press, 1980. (Sigerist suppl. to the Bull Hist Med, n.s., no 4) p. 43-55.
Hilts VL: Statist and statistician. New York, Arno, 1981. (Reprint of Ph.D. Diss., Harvard University, 1967). 647 p.
Himsworth H: Bradford Hill and statistics in medicine. **Stat Med** 1982 Oct-Dec;1(4):301-3
Holland WW, Breeze E, Swan AV: Clinical trials: some reflections. **Stat Med** 1982 Oct-Dec;1(4):361-8
Hunnisett RF, ed: Wiltshire coroners' bills, 1752-1796. Devizes, Wiltshire Record Society, 1981. liv, 239 p. (Wiltshire Record Society, v. 36).
Huzel JP: The demographic impact of the old poor law: more reflexions on Malthus. **Econ Hist Rev** 1980;33:367-81
James DC: Disease, debility and death in a Welsh Town: Cardiff 1845-65. **Public Health** 1984 May;98(3):157-62
James P: Population Malthus, his life and times. London, Routledge and Kegan Paul, 1979. xv, 524 p.
Kabir M: Regional variations in nuptiality in England and Wales during the demographic transition. **Genus** 1980;36(3-4):171-87
Knox PL: Convergence and divergence in regional patterns of infant mortality in the United Kingdom from 1949-51 to 1970-72. **Soc Sci Med** 1981;15(3):323-8
Lane J: The medical practitioners of provincial England in 1783. **Med Hist** 1984 Oct;28(4):353-71
Langton J, Laxton P: Parish registers and urban structure: the example of late-eighteenth century Liverpool. **Urban Hist Yearb** 1978:74-84
Laslett P: The centrality of demographic experience. **Proc Annu Symp Eugen Soc** 1981;16:23-40
Lee R, Lam D: Age distribution adjustments for English censuses, 1821-1931. **Popul Stud** 1983 Nov;37(3):445-64
Leneman L: The study of illegitimacy from kirk session records: two eighteenth-century Perthshire parishes. **Local Popul Stud** 1983 Autumn;31:29-33
Levine D: Illiteracy and family life during the first industrial revolution. **J Soc Hist** 1980;14(1):25-44
Lewis JS: Manners and medicine. Childbearing in the English aristocracy 1790-1840. Ph.D. Diss., Johns Hopkins University. Baltimore, 1979. vi, 301 leaves.
Lilienfeld AM: Bradford Hill's influence on epidemiology. **Stat Med** 1982 Oct-Dec;1(4):325-8
Logan WP: Cancer mortality by occupation and social class 1851-1971. **IARC Sci Publ** 1982;(36):1-253
Luckin B: The decline of small pox and the demographic revolution of the eighteenth century. **Soc Hist (Lond)** 1977;(6):793-97
MacKenzie DA: Statistics in Britain, 1865-1930: the social construction of scientific knowledge. Edinburgh, Edinburgh University Press, 1981. viii, 306 p.
McNeil M: Medical theory and demographic concerns in early industrial England. **Soc Soc Hist Med Bull (Lond)** 1979 Dec;25:12-20
Marshall TH, Laslett P: David Glass: an appreciation. **Br J Sociol** 1979;30(1):1-4
Martin JM: The rich, the poor and the migrant in eighteenth century Stratford-on-Avon. **Local Popul Stud (Matlock)** 1978;(20):38-48
Nuttall P: Miss Florence Nightingale: 'the passionate statistician'. **Nurs J India** 1984 Jun;75(6):128-9
Peel J: Changing patterns of contraception. **Proc Annu Symp Eugen Soc** 1981;16:41-8
Petersen W: Malthus. Cambridge, Mass. Harvard University Press, 1979. vi, 302 p.
Peterson MJ: Gentlemen and medical men: the problem of professional recruitment. **Bull Hist Med** 1984 Winter;58(4):457-73
Pharoah PO, Alberman ED: Mortality of low birthweight infants in England and Wales 1953 to 1979. **Arch Dis Child** 1981 Feb;56(2):86-9
Preston B: Further statistics of inequality. **Sociol Rev** 1979;27(2):343-50
Riley D: 'The free mothers': pronatalism and working women in industry at the end of the last war in Britain. **Hist Workshop J** 1981;11:59-118
Royle SA: Clergymen's return to the 1831 census. **Local Hist** 1980;14(2):79-90
Santurri EN: Theodicy and social policy in Malthus' thought. **J Hist Ideas** 1982 Apr-Jun;43(2):315-30
Schoolman HM: The clinician and the statistician. **Stat Med** 1982 Oct-Dec;1(4):311-6
Sigsworth EM, Swan P: Para-medical provision in the West Riding. **Soc Soc Hist Med Bull (Lond)** 1981 Dec;29:37-9
Smith MT, Hudson BL: Isonymic relationships in the parish of Fylingdales, North Yorkshire, in 1851. **Ann Hum Biol** 1984 Mar-Apr;11(2):141-8
Stern J: The relationship between unemployment, morbidity and mortality in Britain. **Popul Stud** 1983 Mar;37(1):61-74
Stewart F: Life and death in an Oxfordshire churchyard. **Local Hist** 1978;13(3):149-62
Tait I: History of our records. **Br Med J [Clin Res]** 1981 Feb 28;282(6265):702-4
Talmor E, ed: Malthus our contemporary. Contributions by K. W. Back, A. J. Field, L. Murard, P. Zylberman. **Hist Eur Ideas** 1983;4:121-214
Tranter NL: The demographic impact of economic growth and decline: Portpatrick, 1820-1891. **Scott Hist Rev** 1978 Apr;57:87-105
Tröhler U: Britische Spitäler und Polikliniken als Heil- und Forschungsstätten 1720-1820. **Gesnerus** 1982;39(1):115-31
Tröhler U: Quantification in British medicine and surgery 1750-1830. Ph.D. Diss., University of London, 1978.
Watterson P: Environmental factors in infant and early childhood mortality decline in England and Wales, 1895 to 1910. **Soc Soc Hist Med Bull (Lond)** 1984 Dec;35:37-40
Watts S: Demographic facts as experienced by a group of families in eighteenth-century Shifnal, Shropshire. **Local Popul Stud (Matlock)** 1984;32:34-43
Webster C: Healthy or hungry thirties? **Hist Workshop J** 1982;13:110-29
Williamson JG: British mortality and the value of life, 1781-1931. **Popul Stud** 1984 Mar;38(1):157-72
Winter JM: Aspects of the impact of the first world war on infant mortality in Britain. **J Eur Econ Hist** 1982;11(3):713-38
Winter JM: Infant mortality, maternal mortality and public health in Britain in the 1930's. **J Eur Econ Hist** 1979;13(2):439-62
Woods R, Smith CW: The decline of marital fertility in the late nineteenth century: the case of England and Wales. **Popul Stud** 1983 Jul;37(2):207-25

Wrigley EA: English mortality in the Industrial Revolution period. In Forbes EG, ed: Human implications of scientific advance. Edinburgh, Edinburgh University Press, 1978. p. 203–13.

**Hungary**

Andorka R: A család és háztartás nagysága és összetétele 1800 körül két déldunántúli faluban (Alsónyéken és Kölkeden). Kisérlet P. Laslett elemzési módszerének felhasználására. **Tort Stat Tanulm** 1977;3:215–36

Barzó M: Zur Entwicklung der Dokumentation und Auswertung der stationären Morbidität in Ungarn. **Z Gesamte Hyg** 1980 Apr;26(4):275–80

Böszörményi E: Hódmezövásárhelyi öngyilkosságok. **Tort Stat Tanulm** 1977;3:237–304

Cook MS, Repetto R: The relevance of the developing countries to demographic transition theory: further lessons from the Hungarian experience. **Popul Stud** 1982 Mar;36(1):105–28

Dányi D: AZ 1964–1976. Evi termékenység elemzése kísírlet II. **Demografia** 1978;21(4):452–66

Dezsö D: Az 1964–1976, évi termékenység elemzése, kísérlet i. **Demografia** 1978;21(2–3):221–43

Dezsö D: Népességi nézetek és népesedéspolitika Magyarországon a kapitalizmus korában. **Demografia** 1962;5(2):143–64

Gizella M: Termékenységi vizsgálat három generáción keresztül a Mezökövesdi népességben. **Demografia** 1980;23(4):370–96

Horváth M: Cigánycsecsmök halálozása Baranya megyében 1973–1977 között, városok és járások szerint. **Demografia** 1978;21(2–3):366–70

Katus L: A demográfiai átmenet kérdései magyarországon a 19. században. **Tortenelmi Sz** 1980;23(2):270–288

Kiss IN: 'A kortól megtört, beteg, nyomorult személyek' összeírása Bártfa városában 1708–ban. **Orvostort Kozl** 1979;87–88(25 no 1–2):299–300

Kováts Z: A XVIII századi népesség fejlödés kérdéséhez. **Agrartort Sz** 1969;11(1–2):218–27

Lampé L: Egységes nemzetközi szülészeti adatgyüjtés (Tauffer nyomdokain). **Orv Hetil** 1982 Apr 11;123(15):895–903

Madai L: Le premier enregistrement statistique des malades cancereux dans l'annee 1904, en hongrie. **Genus** 1981;37(3–4):227–40

Martos G: Termékenységi vizsgálat három generáción keresztül a mezökövesdi népességben. **Demografia** 1980;23(4):370–96

Mikolás M: Gesztációs folyamatokra vonatkozó matematikai statisztikai vizsgálatok (Magyarország, 1931–1978). **Demografia** 1980;23(2–3):163–207

Preston SH: A halandóság és a gazdásági fejlettség szintje közötti változó kapcsolat. **Demografia** 1976;19(2–3):228–55

Reti E: L'évolution des vues en démographie et en planification familiale. In: Congrès international d'histoire de la médecine, XXVe, Québec, 1976. Actes. Québec, 1977. p. 229–35.

Szabady E: Crises of mortality in Hungary in the 19th century. In Charbonneau H, Larose A, ed: The great mortalities: methodological studies of demographic crises in the past. Liège, Belgium, Ordina Editions, 1980. p. 199–205.

Valenti R: Ongyilkosságok Budapesten 1881–82–ben. Egykorú boncjegyzökönyvek összehasonlító vizsgálata. **Morphol Igazsagugyi Orv Sz** 1982 Jan;22(1):67–70

Zadneprovski IA, Podol'ski AG: Borisz Cezarevics Urlanisz (1906–1981). **Demografia** 1981;24(4):553–5

**Iceland**

Hansen HO: A comparison of empirical life tables for Iceland 1785–1860 with selected model life tables. **Scand Popul Stud** 1979;5:22–37

Hansen HO: Some age structural consequences of mortality variations in pre-transitional Iceland and Sweden. In Charbonneau H, Larose A, ed: The great mortalities: methodological studies of demographic crises in the past. Liège, Belgium, Ordina Editions, 1980. p. 113–32.

**India**

Caldwell JC, Reddy PH, Caldwell P: The social component of mortality decline: an investigation in South India employing alternative methodologies. **Popul Stud** 1983 Jul;37(2):185–205

Firebaugh G: Population density and fertility in 22 Indian villages. **Demography** 1982 Nov;19(4):481–94

Jain AK, Adlakha AL: Preliminary estimates of fertility decline in India during the 1970's. **Popul Dev Rev** 1982;8(3):589–606

Krishnan P: The historical demography of the Jews in India, 1881–1971. **Ann Demogr Hist (Paris)** 1983;:313–27

Lardinois R: Une conjoncture de crise démographique en Indé du Sud au XIXe siècle: la famine de 1876–1878. **Population** 1982;37(2):371–404

Ram R, Schultz TW: Life span, health, savings, and productivity. **Econ Dev Cult Change** 1979;27(3):399–421

Simmons GB, Smucker C, Bernstein S, et al: Post-neonatal mortality in rural India: implications of an economic model. **Demography** 1982 Aug;19(3):371–89

**Indonesia**

Bracher MD, Santow G: Breast-feeding in Central Java. **Popul Stud** 1982 Nov;36(3):413–29

Poffenberger M: Toward a new understanding of population change in Bali. **Popul Stud** 1983 Mar;37(1):43–59

**Iran**

Farahani EM: Abridged life tables of Iran, 1956–1966. **Genus** 1978;34(1–2):215–26

**Ireland**

Connolly SJ: Illegitimacy and pre-nuptial pregnancy in Ireland before 1864: the evidence of some Catholic parish registers. **Ir Econ Soc Hist** 1979;6:5–23

Coward J: Birth under-registration in the Republic of Ireland during the twentieth century. **Econ Soc Rev (Irel)** 1982;14(1):1–27

Coward J: Recent characteristics of Roman Catholic fertility in Northern and Southern Ireland. **Popul Stud** 1980 Mar;34(1):31–44

Gráda CO: The population of Ireland 1700–1900: a survey. **Ann Demogr Hist (Paris)** 1979;:281–99

McKenna EE: Marriage and fertility in postfamine Ireland: a multivariate analysis. **Am J Sociol** 1974 Nov;80(3):688–705

Relethford JH: Isonymy and population structure of Irish isolates during the 1890s. **J Biosoc Sci** 1982 Apr;14(2):241–7

**Israel**

Schmelz UO: [Demography of Moslems and Christians in Jerusalem] (Heb). **Hamizrah Hehadash** 1979;28(1–2):40–73

Schmelz UO: Hamivneh hademografi shel ha'Aravim v'Hadruzim b'Yisrael. **Hamizrah Hehadash** 1979;28(3–4):244–54

**Italy**

Canetta R: Mortalità ed epidemie nello stato di Milano durante l'ultimo terzo del Settecento nelle valutazioni dei pubblici amministratori. **Econ Stor** 1978 Jan–Mar;25:52–64

Caprioli MP: Il patrimonio del povero. L'inchiesta sulle Opere Pie del 1861. **Quad Stor** 1980;15(3):918–41

Colombo B: La tradizione italiana negli studi biodemografici. **Genus** 1979;35(3–4):7–22

Dossetti M: La demografia delle valli Valdesi dal 1686 al 1800. **Boll Stori Bibliogr Subalpino** 1981;79(2):535–602

Frascani P: Medicina e statistica nella formazione del sistema santiario italiano: l'inchiesta del 1885. **Quad Stor** 1980;15(3):942–65

Giura V: Note sulle caratteristiche demografiche della comunità Ebraica di Napoli nel '700. **Genus** 1979;35(1–2):259–63

Isenburg T: Il dibattito su Malthus e sulla popolazione nell'Italia di fine '800. **Studi Stor** 1977;18(3):41–67

Kármán T: A nemzetközi összehasonlító népesedésstatisztika fejlödese a XIX. század utolsó negyedében (Luigi Bodio). **Demografia** 1978;21(4):493–504

Lanzavecchia P, Lingua P, Sinigaglia G: La popolazione manicomiale di Alessandria nella seconda metà dell'ottocento. **Mov Operaio Soc** 1980;3(4):405–22

Mattioli E: Una prima analisi della struttura della mortalita' nelle province Italiane al 1960–62 ed al 1970–72. **Genus** 1980;36(1–2):23–57

Pomata G: Madri illegittime tra Ottocento e Novecento: storie cliniche e storie di vita. **Quad Stor** 1980;2

Rallu JL: Permanence des disparités régionales de la fécondité en Italie? **Population** 1983;38(1):29–59

Saraceno C: Trent' anni di storia della famiglia Italiana. **Studi Stor** 1979;20(4):833–56

Schiaffino A: Fecondita e vita conjugale a Bologna nell'ultimo secolo: analisi longitudinale delle discendenze. **Inst Stat Q** 1979;3:199–275

Schiaffino A: Il declino della fecondità in ambiente urbano: Reggio Emilia fra otto e novecento. **Inst Stat Q** 1979;3:7–275

Smith RM: The people of Tuscany and their families in the fifteenth century: Medieval or Mediterranean? **J Fam Hist** 1981 Spring;6(1):107–28

Sorcinelli P: Miseria e malattie nel XIX secolo. I ceti popolari nell'Italia centrale fra tifo petecchiale e pellagra. Milano, Franco Angeli, 1979. 285 p.

**Jamaica**

Hum D, Basilevsky A: Economic activity and cyclical variations in birthrates: some new evidence for Jamaica. **Soc Econ Stud** 1978;27(2):197–203

**Japan**

Mosk C: Fertility and occupation: mining districts in prewar Japan. **Soc Sci Hist** 1981;5(3):293–316

**Korea**

Donaldson PJ, Nichols DJ: The changing tempo of fertility in Korea.

**Popul Stud** 1978;32(2):231–50
Park CB: Preference for sons, family size, and sex ratio: an empirical study in Korea. **Demography** 1983 Aug;20(3):333–52

**Liberia**

Kory WB: Liberia's population figures. **Liberian Stud J** 1970–71;3(1):53–61

**Malaysia**

Davanzo J, Haaga J: Anatomy of a fertility decline: Peninsular Malaysia, 1950–1976. **Popul Stud** 1982 Nov;36(3):373–93
Dodge NN: Population estimates for the Malay Peninsula in the nineteenth century, with special reference to the East Coast States. **Popul Stud** 1980;34(3):437–75

**Mexico**

Brading DA, Wu C: Population growth and crisis: León, 1720–1860. **J Lat Am Stud** 1973;5(1):1–36
Bustamante ME: Supervivencia y muerte de los Jesuitas de la Provincia de Mexico entre 1767 y 1820. **Bol Soc Mex Hist Filos Med** 1983;6(45):235–63
Canales Muñoz JL, Almada Bay I, Narro Robles J: La mortalidad en una población rural de México y su relación con el uso de los servicios médicos antes de la muerte. **Salud Publica Mex** 1984 Jul–Aug;26(4):404–14
Coatsworth JH: Anotaciones sobre la producción de alimentos durante el Porfiriato. **Hist Mex** 1976;26(2):167–87
Houdaille J, Gutierrez H: Exploitation sommaire du recensement de Mexico en 1811. **Population** 1981;36(4–5):933–8
Jackson RH: Epidemic disease and population decline in the Baja California Missions, 1697–1834. **South Calif Q** 1981;63(4):308–46
Laurell AC, et al: Enfermedad y desarrollo: análisis sociológico de la morbilidad en dos pueblos mexicanos. **Rev Mex Cienc Polit Soc** 1976;22(84):131–58
Mina VA: Estimaciones de los niveles, tendencias y diferenciales de la mortalidad infantil y en los primeros años de vida en México, 1940–77. **Demogr Econ** 1981;15(1):85–142
Mota Hernández F: La implantación del expediente clínico organizado por problemas. **Bol Med Hosp Infant Mex** 1981 Jul–Aug;38(4):567–70
Valdés LM: Ensayo sobre política de población 1970–1980 (planificación familiar). **Demogr Econ** 1980;14(4):467–80
Zambrano L, Jorge H: Fecundidad y escolaridad en la ciudad de Mexico. **Demogr Econ** 1979;13(4):405–48
Zavala de Cosio ME: Problèmes de population au Mexique. **Cah Am Lat** 1978;17:89–11

**Middle East**

Allman J: The demographic transition in the Middle East and North Africa. **Int J Middle East Stud** 1980;12(3):277–301

**Morocco**

Sabagh G, Kim SB: The relationship between migration and fertility in an historical context: the case of Morocco in the 1960s. **Int Migr Rev** 1980;14(4):525–38

**Netherlands**

Jansen PC: Demografie in Nederland. **Kleio (Netherl)** 1979;20(8):353–7
Swierenga RP: Dutch immigrant demography, 1820–1880. **J Fam Hist** 1980 Winter;5(4):390–405

**Nigeria**

Onyemacke Ogum GE: Fertility differentials in Nigeria. **Genus** 1980;36(3–4):203–13
Uche C: The contexts of mortality in Nigeria. **Genus** 1981;37(1–2):123–35

**Norway**

Augensen K, Koller O, Bergsjø P: Mødredødelighet i Norge 1951–1980. **Tidsskr Nor Laegeforen** 1983 Feb 20;103(5):525–30
Dyrvik S: Marriage and social norms: a study of Etne, 1715–1801. **Tidsskr Samfunnsforskning** 1970;11(4):285–300
Festy M: Les internements psychiatriques en Norvège. **Population** 1981;36(2):317–36
Grünfeld B, Maltau JM: Et helsepolitisk perspektiv på fruktbarhetsutviklingen i Norge 1880–2000. **Tidsskr Nor Laegeforen** 1983 Mar 20;103(8–9):795–9
Maltau JM, Grünfeld B: Mødredødeligheten i Norge 1880–1979. Et medisinsk-historisk tilbakeblikk. **Tidsskr Nor Laegeforen** 1983 Feb 20;103(5):522–5
Nilsen KH: Det Norske Arbeiderparti og befolkningsspørsmålet i mellomkrigstida. **Hist Tidsskr** 1979;58(3):287–304
Ramsøy NR: Den norske folketellingsdatabanken: forskningspotensial belyst med eksempler. **Tidsskr Samfunnsforskning** 1981;22(4):287–308
Rønnike F: Arstidsfordeling for menneskets undfangelse i landene omkring Norskehavet--med specielt henblik på Nord-Norge. **Tidsskr Nor Laegeforen** 1981 Jan 20;101(2):151–5

**Pacific Islands**

Les maladies des Européens à Tahiti, en 1880. **Bull Soc Etud Oceaniennes** 1983;19(225):1433–1440
Lange R: Plagues and pestilence in Polynesia: the nineteenth-century Cook Islands experience. **Bull Hist Med** 1984 Fall;58(3):325–46
Leenhardt RH: Un tournant de l'histoire de la nouvelle caledonie: Maurice Leenhardt (1878–1954). **Rev Fr Hist Outre Mer** 1978;65(2):236–52
Nelson HE: Disease, demography, and the evolution of social structure in Highland New Guinea. **J Polynesian Soc** 1971;80(2):204–16
Rallu JL: La dépopulation des archipels du Pacifique: l'exemple de quatre villages de l'île Malekula. **Population** 1981;36(3):519–40
Rallu JL: Situation démographique de la Polynésie Française. **Population** 1980;35(2):385–416
Refshauge WF, Walsh RJ: Pitcairn Island: fertility and population growth, 1790–1856. **Ann Hum Biol** 1981 Jul;8(4):303–12

**Pakistan**

Retherford RD, Mirza GM: Evidence of age exaggeration in demographic estimates for Pakistan. **Popul Stud** 1982 Jul;36(2):257–70

**Philippines**

Smith PC: Crisis mortality in the nineteenth century Philippines: data from parish records. **J Asian Stud** 1978;38(1):51–76
Smith PC, Shui-Meng NG: The components of population change in nineteenth-century South-east Asia: village data from the Philippines. **Popul Stud** 1982 Jul;36(2):237–55

**Poland**

Jabłoński C: Wymieralność w getcie w Brzezinach. **Przegl Lek** 1980;37(1):40–3
Jarosz M: Le suicide en Pologne. **Rev Etud Comp Est Ouest** 1978;9(4):65–101
Jastrzebowski Z: Epidemie a rozwój ludności Królestwa Polskiego w latach 1815–1870. **Arch Hist Med (Warsz)** 1984;47(3):355–74
Klonowicz S: Excessive mortality of men. **Sante Publique (Bucur)** 1981;24(2–3):259–73
Mularczyk-Bal MU, Kopzyński J: Smiertelność noworodków z niskim urodzeniowym ciężarem w latach 1970--1974 w szpitalach w Warszawie. **Pediatr Pol** 1980 Aug;55(8):957–63
Piasecki E: Umieralność niemowląt w parafii bejskiej. **Przeszlosc Demograf Pol** 1979;11:23–67
Rosset E: Demographic factors concerning the re-polonization of western and northern territories. **Pol West Aff** 1970;11(1):67–88
Stapiński A: Powojenny wyż demograficzny a zapadalność na kiłę i rzeżączkę w Polsce. **Przegl Dermatol** 1979 Nov–Dec;66(6):667–72
Supady J: Ankieta statystyczna z 1931 r. na temat występowania nowotworów złośliwych w populacji II Rzeczypospolitej. **Wiad Lek** 1981 Feb 15;34(4):351–5

**Portugal**

André R, Pereira-Roque J: La mortalité infantile au Portugal. **Rev Inst Sociol** 1972;3:573–91

**Puerto Rico**

Mosher WD: The theory of change and response: an application to Puerto Rico, 1940 to 1970. **Popul Stud** 1980 Mar;34(1):45–58
Schultz TP: An economic model of family planning and fertility. **J Polit Econ** 1969;77(2):153–80

**Romania**

Marinescu I, Cicu N, Mesaros E: Románia népesedéspolitikájának néhány kérdése. **Demografia** 1972;15(2):195–201
Moskoff W: Pronatalist policies in Romania. **Econ Dev Cult Change** 1980;28(3):597–614
Vasile R: L'évolution démographique en Roumanie au cours des trois dernières décennies du XIXe siècle (II). **Rev Roum Hist** 1981;20(1):65–89

**Scandinavia**

Lindskog BI, Imhof AE: Mortality in Scandinavia in the 18th century. In: Congrès international d'histoire de la médecine, XXVe, Québec, 1976. Actes. Québec, 1977. p. 205–15.

**Senegal**

Becker C, Martin V: Les premiers recensements au Sénégal; le Sénégal centre-ouest et son évolution démographique. **Ann Demogr Hist (Paris)** 1981;:367–86
Bouche D: Dakar pendant la deuxième guerre mondiale: problèmes de surpeuplement. **Rev Fr Hist Outre Mer** 1978;65(3):423–48

**Singapore**

Neville W: The birth rate in Singapore. **Popul Stud** 1978;32(1):113–4

**South Africa**

Brain JB, Brain P: Nostalgia and alligator bite--morbidity and mortality among Indian migrants to Natal, 1884–1911. **S Afr Med J** 1984 Jan 21;65(3):98–102
Kuparinen E: 'Enligt uppgift död i Sydafrika' - suomalaisten siirtolaisten terveydellinen ympäristö vuosisadan vaihteen etelä-Afrikassa. **Turun Hist Ark (Finl)** 1980;34:174–95
Torrington M, Botha JL, Pilcher GJ, et al: Association between familial hypercholesterolaemia and church affiliation. Is this the result of sociocultural isolation of migrant farmers in 19th-century South Africa? **S Afr Med J** 1984 May 12;65(19):762–7

**Spain**

Agüero I, Rey AO: La evolución reciente de la fecundidad en España. **Rev Esp Invest Sociol** 1980;(10):121–50
Arjona Castro A: La poblacion de Córdoba en el siglo XIX. Sanidad y crisis demográfica en la Córdoba decimonónica. Córdoba, Instituto de Historia de Andalucia, Universidad de Córdoba, 1979. 184 p.
Cachinero Sánchez B: El modelo europeo de matrimonio, evolucion, determinantes y consecuencias. **Rev Esp Invest Sociol** 1981;15:33–58
Jiménez MR: La epidemia de colera de 1834 en Zaragoza y su provincia. **Asclepio** 1982;34:3–31
Llombart V: Anotaciones a la introducción del 'ensayo sobre la población de Malthus en España. **Moneda Credito** 1973;126:79–86
Marset Campos P, Saturno Hernández PJ: Los sanitarios murcianos de 1750 a 1850. Evolucion numerica, tipos profesionales y procendencia geografica. **Asclepio** 1980;32:255–70
Miguel A de: La poblacion en Madrid en los primeros años del siglo. **Rev Esp Invest Sociol** 1982;(19):55–71
Rodríguez Galdo MX: Hambre, epidemia y crisis demográfica en la Galicia litoral a mediados del siglo XIX. **Asclepio** 1983;35:53–68
Saez A: La fécondité en Espagne depuis le début du siècle. **Population** 1979;34(6):1007–21
Saturno Hernández PJ: Los medicos de la comarca de la huerta de Murcia. Numero, distribucion espacial, movilidad, grado de especializacion, tipo de ejercicio, edad y años de colegiacion. Evolucion de 1960 a 1974. **Asclepio** 1981;33:23–80
Saturno Hernández PJ: Los veterinarios de la comarca de la huerta de Murcia. Numero, distribucion espacial, movilidad, tipo de ejercicio, edad y años de colegiacion. Evolucion de 1960 a 1975. **Asclepio** 1980;32:433–52

**Sri Lanka**

Langford C: Fertility in Sri Lanka since the war: an analysis of the experience of different districts. **Popul Stud** 1981;35(2):285–306

**Sudan**

El-Bushra ES: Some demographic indicators for Khartoum Conurbation, Sudan. **Middle East Stud** 1979;15(3):295–309

**Sweden**

Brändström A, Broström G, Persson LA: The impact of feeding patterns on infant mortality in a nineteenth century Swedish parish. **J Trop Pediatr** 1984 Jun;30(3):154–9
Hansen HO: Some age structural consequences of mortality variations in pre-transitional Iceland and Sweden. In Charbonneau H, Larose A, ed: The great mortalities: methodological studies of demographic crises in the past. Liège, Belgium, Ordina Editions, 1980. p. 113–32.
Hed HM, Rasmuson M: Cohort study of opportunity for selection on two Swedish 19th century parishes with a survey of other estimates. **Hum Hered** 1981;31(2):78–83
Hofsten E, Lundström H: Swedish population history. Main trends from 1750 to 1970. Stockholm, National Central Bureau of Statistics, 1976. 186 p. (Urval skriftserie utgiven av statistiska centralbyrån. Nummer 8).
Kälvemark AS: Att vänta barn när man gifter sig. Föräktenskapliga förbindelser och giftermålsmönster i 800-talets Sverige. **Hist Tidskr** 1977;(2):181–99
Kälvemark AS: The country that kept track of its population: methodological aspects of Swedish population records. **Scand J Hist** 1977;2(3):211–30
Lindskog BI: Mortalitätsanalyse einer südschwedischen Bevölkerung 1749–1818. In Imhof AE, ed: Mensch und Gesundheit in der Geschichte. Husum, Matthiesen, 1980. p. 163–73.
Mattsson V: Ammor och barnafödande i Malmö 1750–1850. **Scandia** 1980;46(2):173–98
Modrzewska K, Böök JA: Sulla mortalita in un isolato della Svezia del nord, 1875–1975. **Genus** 1981;37(3–4):221–6
Mosher WD: Demographic responses and demographic transitions: a case study of Sweden. **Demography** 1980 Nov;17(4):395–412
Sandberg LG, Steckel RH: Soldier, soldier, what made you grow so tall? A study of height, health and nutrition in Sweden, 1720–1881. **Econ Hist (Sweden)** 1980;23(2):91–105
Sundin J, Tedebrand LG: Dödlighet och sjuklighet i svenskjärnbruksmiljo, 1750–1875. **Scandia** 1981;47(1):67–108

**Switzerland**

Blanc O: La natalité vaudoise: deux cents ans d'histoire. **Schweiz Z Gesch** 1981;31(2):144–73
Gubéran E: Tendances de la mortalité en Suisse. 2. Maladies infectieuses 1876–1977. **Schweiz Med Wochenschr** 1980 Apr 12;110(15):574–83
Suratteau JR: Contribution à l'étude des mouvements de population dans le canton et la ville de Berne à la fin du XVIIIe siècle. In: Congrès National des Sociétés Savantes, 92e, Strasbourg et Colmar, 1967. Actes. Paris, 1970. Section d'Histoire Moderne et Contemporaine, Tome 1. p. 177–272.

**Thailand**

Frenzen PD, Hogan DP: The impact of class, education, and health care on infant mortality in a developing society: the case of rural Thailand. **Demography** 1982 Aug;19(3):391–408
Goldstein S, Goldstein A: The impact of migration on fertility: an 'own children' analysis for Thailand. **Popul Stud** 1981;35(2):265–84

**Uganda**

Miltényi K: Uganda népesedésének néhány jellegzetessége. **Demografia** 1979;(2–3):228–36

**United States**

Alba F: La fecundidad entre los mexicano-norteamericanos en relacion a los cambiantes patrones reproductivos en Mexico y los Estados Unidos. **Demogr Econ** 1982;16(2):236–49
Aldrich M: Determinants of mortality among New England cotton mill workers during the Progressive era. **J Econ Hist** 1982;42(4):847–63
Aldrich M: Progressive economics, and scientific racism: Walter Willcox and black Americans, 1895–1910. **Phylon** 1979;40(1):1–14
Arceneaux MG: Acadian to Cajun: population, family, and wealth in southwest Louisiana, 1765–1854. Ph.D. Diss., Brigham Young University, Provo, 1982. xii, 436 p.
Bean FD, Swicegood G: Generation, female education and Mexican-American fertility. **Soc Sci Q** 1982;63(1):131–44
Bean LL, May DL, Skolnick M: The Mormon historical demography project. **Hist Methods Newsl** 1978;11(1):45–53
Beawer D de B: The American scientific community, 1800–1860; a statistical-historical study (Doctoral Dissertation, Yale University, 1966). New York, Arno Press, 1980. 379 p.
Benham L: The labor market for registered nurses: a three equation model. **Rev Econ Stat** 1971;53(3):246–52
Blackwood L: Alaska native fertility trends, 1950–1978. **Demography** 1981 May;18(2):173–9
Bloom DE: What's happening to the age at first birth in the United States? A study of recent cohorts. **Demography** 1982 Aug;19(3):351–70
Bohme FG, ed: Twenty censuses: population and housing questions 1790–1980. Washington, Bureau of the Census, 1979. 91 p.
Bollen KA: Temporal variations in mortality: a comparison of U. S. suicides and motor vehicle fatalities, 1972–1976. **Demography** 1983 Feb;20(1):45–59
Boor M: Effects of United States presidential elections on suicide and other causes of death. **Am Sociol Rev** 1981;46(5):616–8
Bosk CL: The doctors. **Wilson Q** 1980;4(2):75–86
Buchanan AV, Weiss KM, Schwartz RJ, et al: Reconstruction of genealogies from vital records: the Laredo Epidemiology Project. **Comput Biomed Res** 1984 Aug;17(4):326–51
Bulmer M: Quantification and Chicago social science in the 1920s: a neglected tradition. **J Hist Behav Sci** 1981;17:312–31
Bush LE: Mormon 'physiology' 1850–1875. **Bull Hist Med** 1982 Summer;56(2):218–37
Byard PJ: Population history, demography, and genetics of the St. Lawrence Island Eskimos. Ph.D. Diss., University of Kansas. Lawrence, 1981. v, 143 leaves.
Carmelli D, Hasstedt S, Andersen S: Demography and genetics of human twinning in the Utah Mormon Genealogy. **Prog Clin Biol Res** 1981;69A:81–93
Cassedy JH: American medicine and statistical thinking, 1800–1860. Cambridge, Mass., Harvard University Press, 1984. x, 306 p.

## STATISTICS AND DEMOGRAPHY


Cherlin AJ: Explaining the postwar baby boom. **Soc Sci Res Counc Items** 1981;35(4):57–63

Chernomas R: A comparative view of the relationship between the business cycle and mortality, 1871–1900. **Int J Health Serv** 1984;14(1):127–46

Christianson EH: The emergence of medical communities in Massachusetts, 1700–1794: the demographic factors. **Bull Hist Med** 1980 Spring;54(1):64–77

Chudacoff HP: The life course of women: age and age consciousness, 1865–1915. **J Fam Hist** 1980 Fall;5(3):274–92

Clarke SS: Hyman J Weiner's use of systems and population approaches: their relevance to social work practice in health care today. **Soc Work Health Care** 1983 Winter;9(2):5–14

Cody CA: Slave demography and family formation: a community study of the Ball Family plantations, 1720–1896. Ph.D. Diss., University of Minnesota. Minneapolis, 1982. xiv, 429 p.

Cohen PC: A calculating people. The spread of numeracy in early America. Chicago, London, Univ. of Chicago Press, 1982. ix, 271 p.

Condran GA, Crimmins E: A description and evaluation of mortality data in the federal census: 1850–1900. **Hist Methods Newsl** 1979;12(1):1–23

Condran GA: An evaluation of estimates of undernumeration in the census and the age pattern of mortality, Philadelphia, 1880. **Demography** 1984 Feb 1;21(1):53–69

Condran GA, Seaman J: Linkage of the 1880–81 Philadelphia death register to the 1880 manuscript census: a comparison of hand and machine-record linkage techniques. **Hist Methods** 1981;14(2):73–84

Condran GA, Crimmins E: Mortality differentials between rural and urban areas of states in the Northeastern United States 1890–1900. **J Hist Geogr** 1980;6(2):179–202

Condran GA, Cheney RA: Mortality trends in Philadelphia: age- and cause--specific death rates 1870–1930. **Demography** 1982 Feb;19(1):97–123

Cooney RS, Rogler LH, Schroder E: Puerto Rican fertility: an examination of social characteristics, assimilation and minority status variables. **Soc Forces** 1981;59(4):1094–1113

Crimmins EM, Condran GA: Mortality variation in U.S. cities in 1900: a two-level explanation by cause of death and underlying factors. **Soc Sci Hist** 1983;7(1):31–60

Crimmins EM: The changing pattern of American mortality decline, 1940–1977, and its implications for the future. **Popul Dev Rev** 1981;7(2):229–54

Crowley JE, Shapiro D: Aspirations and expectations of youth in the United States: part I. Education and fertility. **Youth Soc** 1982;13(4):391–422

Crozier WL: A people apart: a census analysis of the Polish community of Winona, Minnesota, 1880–1905. **Pol Am Stud** 1981;38(1):5–22

Cutright P, Shorter E: The effects of health on the completed fertility of nonwhite and white U.S. women born from 1867 through 1935. **J Soc Hist** 1979;13(2):191–218

DeFronzo J: Female labor force participation and fertility in 48 states: cross-sectional and change analyses for the 1960–1970 decade. **Sociol Soc Res** 1980;64(2):263–78

DellaPergola S: Patterns of American Jewish fertility. **Demography** 1980 Aug;17(3):261–73

Devitt N: The statistical case for elimination of the midwife: fact versus prejudice, 1890–1935. **Women Health** 1979;4:81–96, 169–86

Devitt N: The statistical case for elimination of the midwife: fact versus prejudice, 1890–1935 (part 2). **Women Health** 1979 Summer;4(2):121–33

Doerner WG: Why does Johnny Reb die when shot? The impact of medical resources upon lethality. **Sociol Inq** 1983;53(1):1–15

Doll R: Smoking and death rates. **JAMA** 1984 Jun 1;251(21):2854–7

Dwork D: Health conditions of immigrant Jews on the Lower East Side of New York: 1880–1914. **Med Hist** 1981 Jan;25(1):1–40

Easterlin RA: Population issues in American economic history: a survey and critique. **Res Econ Hist** 1977;(supplement 1):131–58

Eberstein IW, Pol LG: Mexican-American ethnicity, socioeconomic status, and infant mortality: a county-level analysis. **Soc Sci J** 1982;19(2):61–71

Ederer F: Jerome Cornfield's contributions to the conduct of clinical trials. **Biometrics** 1982 Mar;38 Suppl:25–32

Elder GH: Scarcity and prosperity in postwar childbearing: explorations from a life course perspective. **J Fam Hist** 1981 Winter;6(4):410–31

Elliott CA: Models of the American scientist: a look at collective biography. **Isis** 1982 Mar;73(266):77–93

Engerman SL: Changes in black fertility, 1880–1940. In T. K. Hareven and M. A. Vinovskis, ed: Family and population in nineteenth-century America. Princeton, Princeton University Press, 1978. p. 126–53.

Estes JW: Naval medicine in the age of sail: the voyage of the New York, 1802–1803. **Bull Hist Med** 1982 Summer;56(2):238–53

Faber JF: Life tables for the United States: 1900–2050. Actuarial Study No. 87. Washington, D.C., Social Security Administration, 1982. ii, 86 p. (SSA Pub. No. 11-11534).

Farnham TJ: New Haven, 1784. **Conn Med** 1984 Sep;48(9):563–5

Figa'Talamanca I, Galmacci G: Infant mortality and economic stability. An analysis of the last century. **Nuovi Ann Ig Microbiol** 1979 Mar–Apr;30(2):107–26

Freedman R, Freedman DS, Thornton AD: Changes in fertility expectations and preferences between 1962 and 1977: their relation to final parity. **Demography** 1980 Nov;17(4):365–78

Gardner B: Economic aspects of the fertility of rural-farm and urban women. **South Econ J** 1972;38(4):518–24

Ginzberg E: How many physicians are enough? **Ann Am Acad Polit Soc Sci** 1983;(468)::205–15

Glenn ND, Weaver CN: Education's effects on psychological well-being. **Public Opin Q** 1981;45(1):22–39

Greenberg MR: A note on the changing geography of cancer mortality within metropolitan regions of the United States. **Demography** 1981 Aug;18(3):411–20

Greenhouse SW: Jerome Cornfield's contributions to epidemiology. **Biometrics** 1982 Mar;38 Suppl:33–45

Guest AM: Fertility variation among the U.S. foreign stock population in 1900. **Int Migr Rev** 1982;16(3):577–94

Guest AM: Social structure and U. S. inter-state fertility differentials in 1900. **Demography** 1981 Nov;18(4):465–86

Haines MR: Fertility and marriage in a nineteenth-century industrial city: Philadelphia, 1850–1880. **J Econ Hist** 1980;40(1):151–8

Haines MR, Avery RC: The American life table of 1830–1860: an evaluation. **J Interdiscip Hist** 1980;11(1):73–95

Hammel EA, Johansson SR, Ginsberg CA: The value of children during industrialization: sex ratios in childhood in nineteenth-century America. **J Fam Hist** 1983 Winter;8(4):346–66

Hansen SB: State implementation of supreme court decision: abortion rates since Roe v. Wade. **J Polit** 1980;42(2):372–95

Harbison SF, Weishaar ME: Samoan migrant fertility: adaptation and selection. **Hum Organ** 1981;40(3):268–73

Hareven TK, Vinovskis MA: Patterns of childbearing in late nineteenth-century America: the determinants of marital fertility in five Massachusetts towns in 1880. In their: Family and population in nineteenth-century America. Princeton, Princeton University Press, 1978. p. 85–125.

Harper JP: Be fruitful and multiply: origins of legal restrictions on planned parenthood in nineteenth-century America. In Berkin, C. R., Norton, M. B. ed: Women of America: a history. Boston, Houghton Mifflin, 1979: 245–69.

Hauptman LM: Smallpox and American Indian; depopulation in colonial New York. **NY State J Med** 1979 Nov;79(12):1945–9

Healthy people: The Minnesota experience. Minnesota Center for Health Statistics, 1982. [xix], 168 p.

Hellman LM: A history and reminiscence of the office of the Deputy Assistant Secretary for Population Affairs, Department of Health, Education and Welfare, 1969–1977. **Bull Hist Med** 1982 Spring;56(1):77–87

Henson PM: Harold Fred Dorn. In Dictionary of American biography, 1961–1965. Suppl. 7, 1981. p. 191–3.

Higgs R: Cycles and trends of mortality in 18 large American cities, 1871–1900. **Explor Econ Hist** 1979;16(4):381–408

Higgs R: Edward Franklin Meeker (1943–1980). **Explor Econ Hist** 1981;18(2):209–10

Higgs R, Booth D: Mortality differentials within large American cities in 1890. **Hum Ecol** 1979;7:353–70

Hilaski HJ, Wang CL: How valid are estimates of occupational illness? **Mon Labor Rev** 1982;105(8):27–35

Holmes JD: A new look at Spanish Louisiana census accounts: the recent historiography of Antonio Acosta. **La Hist** 1980;21(1):77–86

Huber J: Will U. S. fertility decline toward zero? **Sociol Q** 1980;21(4):481–92

Hyman HH: Samuel Andrew Stouffer. In Dictionary of American Biography, Suppl. 6, 1956–1960. p. 604–6, 1980.

Jackson JJ: Death rates of aged blacks and whites, United States, 1964–1978. **Black Scholar** 1982;13(1):36–48

Jackson RH: The last Jesuit censuses of the Pimeria Alta Missions, 1761 and 1766. **Kiva** 1981;46(4):243–72

Jacobs SE: 'Our babies shall not die': a community's response to medical neglect. **Hum Organ** 1979;38(2):120–33

Jekel JF: The 'Rainbow Reviews': publications of the National Center for Health Statistics. **J Chronic Dis** 1984;37(9–10):681–8

Jerome Cornfield's publications: contributions to the literature as they appeared from 1941 through 1980: **Biometrics** 1982 Mar;38 Suppl:47–52

Johansson SR, Preston SH: Tribal demography: the Hopi and Navaho population as seen through manuscripts from the 1900 U.S. census. **Soc Sci Hist** 1978;3(1):1–33

Johnson MP: Smothered slave infants; were slave mothers at fault? **J South Hist** 1981;47(4):493–520

Johnson NE: Minority-group status and the fertility of black Americans, 1970: a new look. **Am J Sociol** 1979;84(6):1386–1400

Johnson NE: Religious differentials in reproduction: the effects of sectarian education. **Demography** 1982 Nov;19(4):495–509

Johnson TP, Cooper JK: Physician shortage in Kentucky, 1930–1980. **Am J Public Health** 1982 Mar;72(3):257–60

Jones EF: The impact of women's employment on marital fertility in the U. S. 1970–1975. **Popul Stud** 1981;35(2):161–74

Jones EF: Ways in which childbearing affects women's employment: evidence from the U. S. 1975 national fertility study. **Popul Stud** 1982;36(1):5–14

Kan SH, Kim Y: Cause-structure of post-transitional mortality decline: the case of Utah. **Soc Sci J** 1982;19(1):63–71

Katz MB, Stern MJ: Fertility, class, and industrial capitalism: Erie County, New York, 1855-1915. **Am Q** 1981;33(1):63-92

Katz MB, Stern MJ: History and the limits of population policy. **Polit Soc** 1981;10(2):225-45

Keisling P: Old soldiers never die: can we pay for the VA's version of the baby boom? **Wash Mon** 1982;14(1):20-9

Keyfitz N: Irene Barnes Taeuber. In: Notable American women. The modern period. Cambridge, Mass., Belknap-Harvard Univ. Press, 1980. 4:672-3.

Kingsland S: Raymond Pearl: on the frontier in the 1920's. Raymond Pearl memorial lecture, 1983. **Hum Biol** 1984 Feb;56(1):1-18

Kiple KF, King VH: Another dimension to the black diaspora: diet, disease, and racism. Cambridge, Cambridge University Press, 1981. 295 p.

Kitagawa EM: New life-styles: marriage patterns, living arrangements, and fertility outside of marriage. **Ann Am Acad Polit Soc Sci** 1981;453:1-27

Laidig GL, et al: Agricultural variation and human fertility in antebellum Pennsylvania. **J Fam Hist** 1981;6:195-204

Leasure JW: La baisse de la fécondité aux Etats-Unis de 1800 à 1860. **Population** 1982;37(3):607-22

Lee AS, Lee ES: The health of slaves and the health of freedmen: a Savannah study. **Phylon** 1977;38(2):170-80

Lee ES, Roberts RE: Ethnic fertility differentials in the Southwest: the case of Mexican Americans reexamined. **Sociol Soc Res** 1981;65(2):194-210

Levison CH, Hastings DW, Harrison JN: The epidemiologic transition in a frontier town--Manti, Utah, 1849-1977. **Am J Phys Anthropol** 1981 Sep;56(1):83-93

Liu B: The costs of air quality deterioration and benefits of air pollution control: estimates of mortality costs for two pollutants in 40 U.S. metropolitan areas. **Am J Econ Sociol** 1979;38(2):187-95

McCoy DR: Jefferson and Madison on Malthus: population growth in Jeffersonian political economy. **Va Mag Hist Biogr** 1980;88(3):259-76

McFalls JA, Masnick GS: Birth control and the fertility of the U. S. Black population, 1880 to 1980. **J Fam Hist** 1981 Spring;6(1):89-106

Mantel N: Jerome Cornfield and statistical applications to laboratory research: a personal reminiscence. **Biometrics** 1982 Mar;38 Suppl:17-23

Manton KG: Temporal trends in U. S. multiple cause of death mortality data: 1968 to 1977. **Demography** 1982 Nov,19(4):527-47

Marcum JP: Explaining fertility differences among U. S. protestants. **Soc Forces** 1981;60(2):532-43

Marcum JP, Radosh M: Religious affiliation, labor force participation and fertility. **Sociol Anal** 1981;42(4):353-62

Margo RA, Steckel RH: Heights of native-born whites during the antebellum period. **J Econ Hist** 1983;43(1):167-74

Marshall JR: Political integration and the effect of war on suicide: United States, 1933-76. **Soc Forces** 1981;59(3):771-85

Matter DE: Biographical factors associated with longevity in male Kansas pioneers. **Psychol Rep** 1979 Dec;45(3):843-52

Meeker E: The improving health of the United States, 1850-1915. **Explor Econ Hist** 1972;9(4):353-73

Meier P: Jerome Cornfield and the methodology of clinical trials. **Controlled Clin Trials** 1981 May;1(4):339-45

Miller MK, Voth DE, Danforth DM: The medical care system and community malady: rural, urban, and suburban variations in impact. **Rural Sociol** 1982;47(4):634-54

Mineau GP: A specification of marital fertility by parents' age, age at marriage and marital duration. **Demography** 1982 Aug;19(3):335-49

Mineau GP, Anderton DL, Bean LL, et al: Evolution différentielle de la fécondité et groupes sociaux religieux: l'exemple de l'Utah au XIXe siècle. **Ann Demogr Hist (Paris)** 1984;:219-36

Miranda GE: Gente de Razón marriage patterns in Spanish and Mexican California: a case study of Santa Barbara and Los Angeles. **South Calif Q** 1981;63(1):1-21

Modell J: An ecology of family decisions: suburbanization, schooling, and fertility in Philadelphia, 1880-1920. **J Urban Hist** 1980;6(4):397-417

Morantz RM, Zschoche S: Professionalism, feminism, and gender roles: a comparative study of nineteenth-century medical therapeutics. **J Am Hist** 1980 Dec;67(3):568-88

Morgan SP: Parity-specific fertility intentions and uncertainty: the United States, 1970 to 1976. **Demography** 1982 Aug;19(3):315-34

Neuerburg N: An early California document. **Masterkey Ind Lore Hist** 1983;57(3):113-6

Normandeau L, Légaré J: La mortalité infantile des Inuit du Nouveau-Quebec. **Can Rev Sociol Anthropol** 1979;16(3):260-74

Notestein FW: Demography in the United States: a partial account of the development of the field. **Popul Dev Rev** 1982;8(4):651-87

Pao-Min C: The age and sex composition of Chinese-Americans: recent trends. **Asian Profile** 1980;8(5):409-20

Pearle KM: Arzteemigration nach 1933 in die USA: der Fall New York. **Medizinhist J** 1984;19(1-2):112-37

Pebley AR, Westoff CF: Women's sex preferences in the United States: 1970 to 1975. **Demography** 1982 May;19(2):177-89

Pyle GF, Rees PH: Modeling patterns of death and disease in Chicago. **Econ Geogr** 1971;47(4):475-88

Ram B: Regional-sub-cultural explanations of black fertility in the United States. **Popul Stud** 1976;30(3):553ff

Reid JD, Jedlicka D, Lee ES, et al: Trends in black health. **Phylon** 1977;38(2):105-16

Rice DP: Health statistics: past and present. **N Engl J Med** 1981 Jul 23;305(4):219-20

Rindfuss RR: Changing patterns of fertility in the South: a social-demographic examination. **Soc Forces** 1978;57(2):621-35

Rosenkrantz BG, Vinovskis MA: Sustaining 'the flickering flame of life': accountability and culpability for death in ante-bellum Massachusetts asylums. In Reverby S, Rosner D, ed: Health care in America. Philadelphia, Temple University Press, p. 155-82.

Rosenwaike I: A note on new estimates of the mortality of the extreme aged. **Demography** 1981 May;18(2):257-66

Ruffin CB: Records of the Sellers Funeral Home, Chambersburg, Pennsylvania, relating to the black families of Franklin County, 1866-1933. **J Afro-Am Hist Geneal Soc** 1982;3(4):165-82; 1983;4(1):32-4

Rundall TG: Environmental selection and physician supply. **AJS** 1982 Mar;87(5):1090-1112

Ryder NB: The future of American fertility. **Soc Probl** 1979;26(3):359-70

Sabagh G, Lopez D: Religiosity and fertility: the case of Chicanas. **Soc Forces** 1980;59(2):431-9

St. John C: Race differences in age at first birth and the pace of subsequent fertility: implications for the minority group status hypothesis. **Demography** 1982 Aug;19(3):301-14

Salazar JG, Espinosa JM: A sociodemographic profile of Hispanic physicians in three United States metropolitan areas. **Aztlan** 1979;10:111-22

Sanderson WC: Quantitative aspects of marriage, fertility and family limitation in nineteenth century America: another application of the Coale specifications. **Demography** 1979 Aug;16(3):339-58

Schapiro MO: Land availability and fertility in the United States, 1760-1870. **J Econ Hist** 1982;42(3):577-600

Schneiderman MA: Trends in cancer mortality and incidence in the United States: is the future clear or clouded? In V. Miké, K. E. Stanley, ed: Statistics in medical research. Methods and issues, with applications in cancer research. New York, John Wiley & Sons, 1982. p. 71-107.

Schoen R, Nelson VE: Mortality by cause among Spanish surnamed Californians, 1969-71. **Soc Sci Q** 1981;62(2):259-74

Schwartz RJ, Weiss KM, Buchanan AV: Looking into the black box: practical approaches to record linkage. **Ann Demogr Hist (Paris)** 1984;:119-28

Shipek FE: A native American adaptation to drought: the Kumeyaay as seen in the San Diego Mission records, 1770-1798. **Ethnohistory** 1981;28(4):295-312

Siegel JS: On the demography of aging. **Demography** 1980 Nov;17(4):345-64

Skolnick MH, Bean LL, Mineau GP, et al: Etudes génétiques et démographiques et base de données généalogiques de l'Utah. **Ann Demogr Hist (Paris)** 1984;:103-13

Sloane DM: Sex of privious children and intentions for further birth in the United States, 1965-1976. **Demography** 1983 Aug;20(3):353-67

Smith DP: A reconsideration of Easterlin cycles. **Popul Stud** 1981 Jul;35(2):247-64

Smith DS: A community-based sample of the older population from the 1880 and 1900 United States manuscript census. **Hist Methods Newsl** 1978;11(2):67-74

Smith HC: Arthur Sinton Otis. In Dictionary of American biography, 1961-1965. Suppl. 7, 1981. p. 594-5.

Spanier GB, Glick PC: The life cycle of American families: an expanded analysis. **J Fam Hist** 1980 Spring;5(1):97-111

Steckel RH: Antebellum southern white fertility: a demographic and economic analysis. **J Econ Hist** 1980;40(2):331-50

Steckel RH: Slave height profiles from coastwise manifests. **Explor Econ Hist** 1979;16(4):363-80

Steckel RH: Slave marriage and the family. **J Fam Hist** 1980 Winter;5(4):406-21

Steckel RH: The fertility of American slaves. **Res Econ Hist** 1982;7:239-86

Stewart JB: The political economy of black male suicides. **J Black Stud** 1980;11(2):249-61

Supply of manpower in selected health occupations: 1950-1990. Hyattsville, U. S. Bureau of Health Professions, 1980. xiii, 62 p:

Temkin-Greener H, Swedlund AC: A test of the child replacement hypothesis: nineteenth century Massachusetts. **Soc Biol** 1983 Summer;30(2):218-27

Thornton R: Demographic antecedents of a revitalization movement: population change, population size, and the 1890 Ghost Dance. **Am Sociol Rev** 1981;46(1):88-96

Tickamyer AR: Women's roles and fertility intentions. **Pac Sociol Rev** 1979;22(2):167-84

Tolnay SE, Guest AM: American family building strategies in 1900: stopping or spacing. **Demography** 1984 Feb 1;21(1):9-18

Tolnay SE: Black fertility in decline: urban differentials in 1900. **Soc Biol** 1980 Winter;27(4):249-60

Tolnay SE: Fertility of southern black farmers in 1900: evidence and speculation. **J Fam Hist** 1983 Winter;8(4):314-32

Tolnay SE, Graham SN, Guest AM: Own-child estimates of U. S. white fertility, 1886-1899. **Hist Methods** 1982;15(3):127-38

Tolnay SE: Trends in total and marital fertility for black Americans,

1886–1899. **Demography** 1981 Nov;18(4):443–63
Uhlenberg P: Death and the family. **J Fam Hist** 1980 Fall;5(3):313–20
Unger CW: The old Goschenhoppen Lutheran burial register: 1752–1772. **Pa Folklife** 1967–68;17(2):32–5
Uselding P: In dispraise of the muckrakers: United States occupational mortality, 1890–1910. **Res Econ Hist** 1976;1:334–71
Van Horn SH: Women's roles: work and fertility for American women between 1900 and 1980. Ph.D. Diss., Carnegie-Mellon University. Pittsburgh, 1980. 344 leaves.
Vinovskis MA: Fertility in Massachusetts from the Revolution to the Civil War. New York, Academic Press, 1981. xii, 253 p.
Vinovskis MA: Mortality rates and trends in Massachusetts before 1860. **J Econ Hist** 1972;32(1):184–213
Vinovskis MA: The Jacobson life table of 1850: a critical reexamination from a Massachusetts perspective. **J Interdiscip Hist** 1978;8(4):703–24
Vinovskis MA: The 1789 life table of Edward Wigglesworth. **J Econ Hist** 1971;31(3):570–90
Vladeck BC, Firman JP: The aging of the population and health services. **Ann Am Acad Polit Soc Sci** 1983;(468):132–48
Wahlquist WL: Population growth in the Mormon core area: 1847–1890. Jackson, Richard H., ed. The Mormon role in the settlement of the West. 1978. Reprint ed., Provo, Utah, Brigham Young U. Pr., 1980. p. 107–34.
Walker JD, Scott JS: Location of mortality schedules of the United States decennial censuses, 1850–1900. **J Afro-Am Hist Geneal Soc** 1981;2(1):1–7
Watts RK: Jewish fertility trends and differentials: an examination of the evidence from the census of 1970. **Jew Soc Stud** 1980;42(3-4):293–312
Wells RV: Women's lives transformed: demographic and family patterns in America, 1600–1970. In Berkin, CR, Norton MB, ed: Women of America: a history. Boston, Houghton Mifflin, 1979. p. 16–33.
Wilcox J, Golden HH: Prolific immigrants and dwindling natives?: fertility patterns in western Massachusetts, 1850 and 1880. **J Fam Hist** 1982 Fall;7(3):265–88
Yankauer A: Refugees, immigrants, and the public health. **Am J Public Health** 1982 Jan;72(1):12–4
Zelen M: The contributions of Jerome Cornfield to the theory of statistics. **Biometrics** 1982 Mar;38 Suppl:11–5

**Upper Volta**

Armagnac C, Retel-Laurentin A: Relations between fertility, birth intervals, foetal mortality and maternal health in Upper Volta. **Popul Stud** 1981 Jul;35(2):217–34

**Uruguay**

Rial Roade J: Sources for studies of historical demography in Uruguay (1728–1860). **Lat Am Res Rev** 1980;15(2):180–200

**USSR**

Abbott WF: The density-pathology hypothesis in comparative perspective: density, status and pathology in prerevolutionary Moscow. **Int J Comp Sociol** 1982;23(1-2):17–33
Afanas'eva GM: Demograficheskaia kharakteristika Avamskikh Nganasan po istochnikam XVIII–XIX. **Sov Etnogr** 1980;2:25–34
Aumont B: La situation démographique en USSR. **Contrat Soc** 1968;12(4):219–22
Azhenov MS: Razvitie sotsial'noi struktury Kazakhstana v usloviiakh sotsializma. **Vopr Filos** 1980;8:44–51
Bazanov VA: E. A. Osipov--odin iz osnovopolozhnikov obshchestvennoĭ meditsiny i sanitarnoĭ statistiki v dorevoliutsionnoĭ Rossii. **Feldsher Akush** 1980;45(9):40–4
Belitskaia EIa: V. I. Lenin on voprosakh narodnonaseleniia. **Sov Zdravookhr** 1980;(4):8–10
Belitskaia EIa: V. V. Paevskiĭ i ego kniga 'Elementy statistiki' (k 50-letiiu opublikovaniia). **Sov Zdravookhr** 1981;(6):64–6
Berelowitch W: L'évolution de la fécondité légitime à Saint-Petersbourg-Petrograd-Leningrad (1869–1926). **Ann Demogr Hist (Paris)** 1982;:243–65
Brambe R: Rigas pilsetas iedzìvotàju skaita dinamika no 1787. lidz 1860. gadam. **Latv PSR Zinat Akad Vestis** 1972;8:55–66
Cesnys G: Lietuvos didžiosios kunigaikštystes demografiniai rodikliai 1790m. gyventoju surašymo duomenimis. **Liet Istor Metrast** 1980:5–16
Chesnais JC: La hausse de la mortalité infantile en Union Sovietique. **Population** 1981;36(6):1176–80
Coale AJ, Anderson BA, Härm E: Human fertility in Russia since the nineteenth century. Princeton, N. J., Princeton Univ. Press, 1979. xxiii, 285 p.
Conquest R: Forced labour statistics: some comments. **Sov Stud** 1982;34(3):434–9
Cooper R: Rising death rates in the Soviet Union. The impact of coronary heart disease [1960–77]. **N Engl J Med** 1981;304:1259–65
Danilishina EI, Dzhalalova KM: Materinskaia smertnost' i boriba s neĭ v SSSR v 20–30-e gody. **Sov Zdravookhr** 1983;(8):51–4
Davis C, Feshbach M: Rising infant mortality in the USSR in the 1970's. Washington, U. S. Dept. of Commerce, Bureau of the Census, 1980. 33 p. (International population reports. Series P–95, no. 74).
Drobizhev VZ: Organizatsiia ucheta estestvennogo dvizheniia naseleniia SSSR v 1917–1926 gg. **Vestn Mosk Univ Ser 8 Istor** 1978;3:27–33
Drobizhev VZ: Stanovlenie politiki sovetskogo gosudarstva v oblasti estestvennogo dvizheniia naseleniia. **Vestn Mosk Univ Ser 8 Istor** 1981;1:17–26
Dulnik S: Koroteiha shel kehila yehudit bebrit-hamo'atsot. **Yalkut Moreshet Period** 1976;21:89–100
Dutton JC: Causes of Soviet adult mortality increases. **Sov Stud** 1981;33(4):548–59
Epstein D: Hayehudi hayehidi (ha'ayarah Libishei bashoah). **Yalkut Moreshet Period** 1975;20:7–34
Gitelman Z: Poriyut hayehudim bivrit hamo'atsot. **Shvut (Israel)** 1977;5:7–20
Il'in AI: Iz istorii sanitarno-statisticheskogo issledovaniia Vladimirskoĭ gubernii. **Gig Sanit** 1984 May;(5):35–7
Mironov BN: Traditsionnoye Demograficheskoye povedeniye krest'yan v XIX - nachale XX V. Brachnost', Rozhdayemost', Smertnost', v Rossii i v sssr, (Vishnevskiy, A. G. ed.), Moskva, 1977, p. 83–104.
Perkovskiy AL: Krizis demograficheskogo vosproizvodstva krepostnogo krest'yanstva rossii v pervoy polovine XIX stoletiya. Brachnost', Rozhdayemost', Smertnost' v Rossii i v sssr, Moskva, Statistika, 1977, p. 167–190.
Poliakov IA, Kiselev IN: Chislennost' i natsional'-nyi sostav naseleniia Rossii v 1917 godu. **Vopr Istor** 1980;6:39–49
Pressat R: Pertes subies par la population de l'U.R.S.S. 1918–1958. **Population** 1979;34(6):1147–52
Pressat R: Situation démographique de l'U.R.S.S. à la veille de son cinquième recensement. **Population** 1979;34(4–5):845–68
Radlitzki T: Reshimot mimei hakibush hagermani Be-lvov (Lemberg), 1941–1943. **Yalkut Moreshet Period** 1976;21:7–34
Shishkin AP: Bor'ba s detskoĭ smertnost'iu v pervye gody Sovetskoĭ vlasti. **Sov Zdravookhr** 1981;(12):46–50
Silber J: Some demographic characteristics of the Jewish population in Russia at the end of the nineteenth century. **Jew Soc Stud** 1980;42(3–4):269–80
Szymanski A: On the uses of disinformation to legitimize the revival of the cold war: health in the U.S.S.R. **Sci Soc** 1981–82;45(4):453–74
Veispak T: Rakvere elanikkonna suurus ja sotsiaalnestruktuur 17. sajandi lõpust 1780. Aastateni. **Eesti NSV Tead Akad Toim** 1981;30(2):169–78
Wheatcroft SG: Famine and epidemic crises in Russia, 1918–1922: the case of Saratov. **Ann Demogr Hist (Paris)** 1983;:329–52

**Venezuela**

Pinto-Cisternas J, Castelli MC, Pineda L: La consanguinidad en la parroquia de Los Teques, Venezuela desde 1790 a 1869. **Acta Cient Venez** 1981;32(3):262–8
Vélez Boza F: Estudio epidemiologico de la mortalidad por malformaciones congenitas letales en Venezuela, de 1950 a 1974. **Rev Soc Venez Hist Med** 1980;29(43–44):73–80

**Vietnam**

Monnier A: Données récentes sur la population du Vietnam. **Population** 1981;36(3):610–19

**Yugoslavia**

Hadjivuković S, Cobanović K: Prirodno kretanje stanovništva jugoslavije, socijalističkih republika i autonomnih pokrajina u posleratnom periodu. **Zb Drus Nauke** 1978;(65):107–22
Harmsen H: Demografische Verluste Kroatien 1941 bis 1946. **Donauraum** 1978;23(4):154–7
Jovin S: Uticaj zdravstvenih prilika na išćeznuce srpskog živla u selu Gložanu. **Naucni Sastanak Zb Rad Naucno Drus Iator Zdrav Kult Jugosl** 1977;15:161–66
Rendulić M: Demografska kretanja u hrvatskoj. **Ekon Pregl** 1971;22(7–8):340–51

**Zaire**

Romaniuk A: Increase in natural fertility during the early stages of modernization: evidence from an African case study, Zaire. **Popul Stud** 1980;34(2):293–310

**Zimbabwe**

Cockcroft IG: They did not leave the valley. **Nada** 1969;10(1):50–3

# SURGERY

See also **Anesthesiology; Dentistry; Gynecology; Obstetrics; Ophthalmology; Orthopedics; Otorhinolaryngology; Urology**

Ackerknecht EH: From barber-surgeon to modern doctor. **Bull Hist Med** 1984 Winter;58(4):545–53

Acuña HR: La medicina y el estado. Recuento histórico y problemas acutales de la cirugía. **Bol Of Sanit Panam** 1981 Oct;91(4):283-8
Adamson PB: The military surgeon: his place in history. **J R Army Med Corps** 1982 Feb;128(1):43-50
Adamson PB: The relationship between medical and veterinary surgeons from Sumer to the present. **Vet Hist** 1983 Summer;3(1):16-24
Andersson L, Kinn AC: Njursten och blåssten--en medicinhistorisk översikt. **Nord Medicinhist Arsb** 1982;:76-85
Arianoff AA: Historique de la chirurgie biliaire. A propos du centenaire de la première cholécystectomie. **Acta Chir Belg** 1983 Jul-Aug;(4):241-52
Babé J: Amigdalectomía extracapsular con reconstrucción de la celda amigdalina. **An Otorrinolaringol Ibero Am** 1983;10(1):19-50
Ballantyne GH: Review of sigmoid volvulus: history and results of treatment. **Dis Colon Rectum** 1982 Jul-Aug;25(5):494-501
Barnett GH, Hardy RW: Gardner tongs and cervical traction. **Med Instrum** 1982 Nov-Dec;16(6):291-2
Bean KJ: A history of surgical wound drainage: sump drains and closed wound suction devices. **J Oper Room Res Inst** 1983 Mar;3(3):8-20
Berk JB: Antiquarian antisepsis. **Contemp Surg** 1980 Jun;16(6):62-3
Bernabeo RA, ed: Il ferro chirurgico nella raccolta Vittorio Putti di Bologna. Bologna, Università degli Studi di Bologna, 1981. 14 p. (Catalog of an exhibit Sept.-Nov. 1981).
Bevan PG: Generalism and specialisation in surgery. **Ann R Coll Surg Engl** 1981 Nov;63(6):383-5
Black JJ: A stitch in time--1. The history of sutures. **Nurs Times** 1982 Apr 14-20;78(15):619-23
Buck BA: Ancient technology in contemporary surgery. **West J Med** 1982 Mar;136(3):265-9
Carstensen G: Die Chirurgie in der Kunst. Düsseldorf, Econ, 1983. 206 p.
Crul JF: [History of anesthesiology]. (Ita) **Minerva Anestesiol** 1979 Sep;45(9):721-9
Cuthbertson DP: Symposium on 'surgery and nutrition'. Historical approach. **Proc Nutr Soc** 1980 May;39(2):101-5
Egorysheva IV, Rabinovich RS, Serdiuk GV, et al: Zhamenatel'nye iubileĭnye daty istorii khirurgii 1983 g. **Khirurgiia (Mosk)** 1982 Nov;(11):103-5
Febres-Cordero F: Cirujanos y odontologos proceden de los barberos medievales? **Acta Odontol Venez** 1981 Sep-Dec;19(3):283-304
Forgue E, Bouchet A: Die Chirurgie bis zum Ende des 18. Jahrhunderts. In Sournia JC, Martiny M, Poulet J, ed: Illustrierte Geschichte der Medizin. Salzburg, Andreas, 1980. Vol. 3. p. 931-1021.
Glenn WW: The lymphatic system. Some surgical considerations. **Arch Surg** 1981 Aug;116(8):989-95
Goldwyn RM: 'Surgeon'. **Plast Reconstr Surg** 1983 Aug;72(2):229-30
Guerra F: Three battles that changed military surgery: Avigliana 1536. Moscow 1812. Ebro 1938. In International Congress of the History of Medicine. 26th, Plovdiv, 1978. Actes du Congress. Sofia, 1981. Volume II. p. 82-3.
Harper RG, Kenigsberg K, Sia CG, et al: Xiphopagus conjoined twins: a 300-year review of the obstetric, morphopathologic, neonatal, and surgical parameters. **Am J Obstet Gynecol** 1980 Jul 1;137(5):617-29
Higgins GA: Chirurgeon generalis--an endangered species. **Am Surg** 1984 Jan;50(1):1-5
Histoire de la médecine aux armées: Tome 1. De l'Antiquité à la Révolution. Paris, Charles Lavauzelle, 1982. 513 p.
Jenkins MT: History of sequestered edema associated with surgical operations and trauma. **Contemp Anesth Pract** 1983;6:1-31
Kernéïs JP: Geschichte der Schiffahrtsmedizin am Beispiel der Schiffschirurgen. In Sournia JC, Martiny M, Poulet J, ed: Illustrierte Geschichte der Medizin. Salzburg, Andreas, 1980. Vol. 8. p. 2999-3023.
Kirby NG: How fertile the blood of warriors. **J R Coll Surg Edinb** 1981 Jan;26(1):1-11
Kirkup J: The history and evolution of surgical instruments. III. Handles. **Ann R Coll Surg Engl** 1983 Jul;65(4):269-73
Kirkup JR: The history and evolution of surgical instruments. I. Introduction. **Ann R Coll Surg Engl** 1981 Jul;63(4):279-85
Kirkup JR: The history and evolution of surgical instruments. II Origins: function: carriage: manufacture. **Ann R Coll Surg Engl** 1982 Mar;64(2):125-32
Küss R: Chirurgie générale ou chirurgie spécialisée. Une dualité dépassée? **Nouv Presse Med** 1980 Oct 11;9(37):2757-8
Levy M: Intraperitoneal drainage. **Am J Surg** 1984 Mar;147(3):309-14
Longmire WP: Historic landmarks in biliary surgery. **South Med J** 1982 Dec;75(12):1548-50, 1552
Lumley JS: Microsurgery. **Practitioner** 1982 Oct;226(1372):1723-6
McCullagh KG, Silver IA: The actual cautery -- myth and reality in the art of firing. **Equine Vet J** 1981 Apr;13(2):81-4
Moss JP: Historical and current perspectives on surgical drainage. **Surg Gynecol Obstet** 1981 Apr;152(4):517-27
Oncel O: Asepsis and antisepsis in the past and today. In International Congress of the History of Medicine. 26th, Plovdiv, 1978. Actes du Congress. Sofia, 1981. Volume II. p. 175-8.
Orr N: Why wear a mask in theatre? **NATNEWS** 1982 Jun;19(6):11-2
Pechter EA, Sherman RA: Maggot therapy: the surgical metamorphosis. **Plast Reconstr Surg** 1983 Oct;72(4):567-70
Peltier LF: A capite ad calcem--a parable for our time. **J Trauma** 1981 Feb;21(2):96-8
Portele KA: Die Moulagensammlung des Pathologisch-Anatomischen Bundesmuseums in Wien. [Wien, Pathologisch-Anatomisches Bundesmuseum in Wien], 1977. 84 p.
Raso Rodríguez EJ: Hitos cumbres en la historia de la cirugia. **Asclepio** 1980;32:333-9
Raso Rodríguez EJ: La evolucion historica de la profesion de instrumentista. **Asclepio** 1980;32:327-32
Richardson JP: Surgeons, physicians, and cardiology. **Aust NZ J Surg** 1980 Dec;50(6):668-71
Richardson JP: The surgeon as medical practitioner: an historical appreciation of the role of surgery in the corpus medicum. **Aust NZ J Surg** 1980 Oct;50(5):550-5
Rosoff L: Roger Bacon, William of Occam and Lord Houghton: guides for the perplexed physician. **Am J Surg** 1981 Jan;141(1):2-9
Rüster D: Alte Chirurgie: Legende und Wirklichkeit. Berlin, VEB Verlag Volk und Gesundheit, 1984. 255 p.
Schmauss AK: Zur Geschichte der chirurgischen Eingriffe am Magen. **Z Arztl Fortbild (Jena)** 1983;77(10):445-8
Schmitt W: Das chirurgische Erbe. Zur Geschichte der modernen Chirurgie; ein Abriss. Teil I. **Zentralbl Chir** 1982;107(12):727-36
Scott M: 32,000 years of sutures. **NATNEWS** 1983 May;20(5):15-7
Shepherd J, Dawber RP: The historical and scientific basis of cryosurgery. **Clin Exp Dermatol** 1982 May;7(3):321-8
Sherman R: Perspectives in management of trauma to the spleen. **J Trauma** 1980 Jan;20(1):1-13
Skinner G: The history of surgical instruments. **Nurs Times** 1984 Jul 18-24;80(29):28-30
Sparacia A: Dal cerusico all'intensivoterapeuta (rassegna storica dell'emostasi). **Minerva Anestesiol** 1980 Jul;46(7):759-71
Stahnke J: Geschichte der Kropfchirurgie. **MMW** 1981 Feb 20;123(8):315-6
Swenson O: Specialization: What it holds for the future of medicine. **Can J Surg** 1980 Mar;23(2):154-6
Tratner E: 1. Tracheotomy in the Hebrew translation of Ibn-Sina. 2. Intubation mentioned in the Talmud and by Jacob Ben Asher (14th Century). **Koroth** 1983 Aug;8(7-8):333-8
Trolle D: The history of Caesarean section. Copenhagen, University Library, 1982. 109 p. (Acta Historica Scientiarum Naturalium Et Medicinalium, v. 33).
Verdan C: Histoire de la chirurgie de la main. **Ann Chir** 1980 Nov;34(9):647-54
Verveen G: Chirurgia: the handicraft of medicine. Philatelically illustrated historic survey of surgery. **Am J Surg** 1982 May;143(5):640-8
Wangensteen OH: Teaching and learning: retrospect and prospect. **Proc Inst Med Chic** 1980 Apr-Jun;33(2):46-53
Watt J: The surgery of sea warfare from the galley to the nuclear age. **Trans Med Soc Lond** 1980-81;97:1-15
Wilson KS: Mandibular reconstruction: introduction. **Otolaryngol Head Neck Surg** 1982 Sep-Oct;90(5):576
Wind GG, Rich NM: Historical notes on surgical technique. In their Principles of surgical technique. The art of surgery. Baltimore, Munich, Urban & Schwarzenberg, 1983. p. 9-19.
Wolner E: Die Chirurgie als Handwerk, Kunst und Wissenschaft. **Wien Klin Wochenschr** 1982 Mar 19;94(6):140-5
Zigiotti GL, Messerotti GF, Cavaliere F: La chirurgia della palatoschisi dalle origini ai giorni nostri. **Minerva Med** 1983 Jan 14;74(1-2):59-68

**Argentina**

Cassone E: Historia de la Cirugia en Mendoza. In Congreso de Historia de la Medicina Argentina [Transactions], 5th, Mendoza, 1983. p. 69-78.
Hernández HH: Historia de la Cirugia en Buenos Aires y Rosario. In Congreso de Historia de la Medicina Argentina [Transactions], 5th, Mendoza, 1983. p. 33-68.

**Belgium**

Daem M: Van baardemaker tot barbier (Gentse chirurgijn-barbiers). Brussel, Aurelia Books, 1976. 170 p. (Aureliae Folklorica, no. 9).
Homble AG: Jan Albert Roselt, plattelandschirurgijn te Machelen. **Ons Heem** 1979;33:1-70

**Bulgaria**

Lukanov A, Altŭnkov P: Khirurgiiata v Bŭlgariia prez vekovete. **Khirurgiia (Sofiia)** 1982;35(1):100-7

**Canada**

Boissonnault CM: Antoine Forestier. In Dictionary of Canadian biography, 1701 to 1740. Volume 2, 1969. p. 226.
Rousseau J: Michel Sarrazin. In Dictionary of Canadian biography, 1701 to 1740. Volume 2, 1969. p. 593-600.

# SURGERY

### Europe

Wangensteen OH: A few renowned European military surgeons. In Ganzinger K, Skopec M, Wyklicky H, ed: Festschrift für Erna Lesky zum 70. Geburtstag. Wien, Brüder Hollinek, 1981. p. 167–84.

### Finland

Lindholm RV: Küntscher bone nailing in Finland. Oulu, Finland, Univ. of Oulu, 1979. 35 p..

### France

Bodemer CW: France, the fundament, and the rise of surgery. **Dis Colon Rectum** 1983 Nov;26(11):743–50

Curet M, Carre A, Henaff R: Les écoles de chirurgie et de médecine navales. **Med Armees** 1980;8(10)spec:797–800

Huard PO, Imbault-Huart MJ: Le cabinet de l'Académie Royale de Chirurgie. In: Congrès National des Sociétés Savantes, 102e, Limoges, 1977. Comptes Rendus. Paris, 1977. Section des Sciences, Fasc. III. p. 15–20.

Rocchietta S: Musica e litotomia in una composizione di Marin Marais (1656–1728). **Minerva Med** 1983 Nov 16;74(44):2713

Vidal F: Odontoiatria del passato. L'"Edit Royal' del maggio 1699. L'"Editto' del 1699 y quello del 1768. **Dent Cadmos** 1982 Jan, Feb;50(1,2):57–63, 67–74

### Germany

Killian H: Meister der Chirurgie und die Chirurgenschulen im gesamten deutschen Sprachraum. 2., neubearbeitete Auflage. Stuttgart, Thieme, 1980. xii, 492 p.

Riall CT: Surgical and medical devices and their origins. Chapter XVII. Surgical instrument manufacturers. **J Oper Room Res Inst** 1983 Jan;3(1):33–5, 38–9, 42

### Great Britain

Dobson J, Walker RM: Barbers and barber-surgeons of London: a history of the barbers' and barber-surgeons' companies. Oxford, Blackwell Scientific Publications for the Worshipful Company of Barbers, 1979. xix, 171 p.

Dobson J: Some associations of St. Thomas's Hospital with the Company of Barber-Surgeons of London. **St Thomas Hosp Gaz** 1981;79:73–8

Guy JR: The episcopal licensing of physicians, surgeons and midwives. **Bull Hist Med** 1982;56(4):528–42

Robinson JO: The barber-surgeons of London. **Arch Surg** 1984 Oct;119(10):1171–5

Wyman AL: The surgeoness: the female practitioner of surgery 1400–1800. **Med Hist** 1984 Jan;28(1):22–41

### Guatemala

Villacorta Cifuentes JL: Historia de la medicina, cirugia y obstetricia prehispanicas. Guatemala, [s. n.] 1976. 166 p.

### Hungary

Petri G: Sebészet és tudomány. **Orv Hetil** 1982 Jan 3;123(1):5–11

### Italy

Fabbi A: La scuola chirurgica di Preci. Preci [s.n.], 1974. 213 p.

### Mexico

Alcocer Andalón A: La cirugia potosina de 1592 a 1911. **Bol Soc Mex Hist Filos Med** 1981 Jun;5(35):171–88

### Netherlands

Veltheer W: Het chirurgijnsgilde van Amersfoort. **Tijdschr Geschied Geneeskd** 1979;2(3):101–9

### Poland

Kobylińska-Szymańska M, Froch W: Poczatki sztuki chirurgicznej w Lublinie i kształcenie jej adeptów (wiek XVI - XVIII). **Arch Hist Med (Warsz)** 1980;43(2):163–78

Pankiewicz Z: Cech chirurgów toruńskich w XVI, XVII i XVIII wieku. **Czas Stomatol** 1979;32(10):989–92

### Spain

Guerra F: La cirurgía catalana y contemporánea y la cirugía castellana del Renacimiento. In Congrés International d'Història de la Medicina Catalana, 2nd, Barcelona, 1975. Llibre d'Actes. Barcelona, Socitra, 1977. p. 49–58.

Guerra F: Las heridas de guerra. Contribución de los cirujanos Españoles en la evolución de su tratamiento. Santander, Catedra de Historia de la Medicina, Universidad de Santander, 1981. XVI, 237 p.

Massons JM: Los cirujanos madrileños del siglo XVIII ante el servicio militar. In International Congress of the History of Medicine, 27th, Barcelona, 1980. Actas. Barcelona, Académia de Ciències Médiques de Catalunya i Balears, 1981. p. 575–9.

### Sri Lanka

Wijesinha SS, Wijesinha CY: Surgery and hospitals: the Sri Lanka tradition. **Ceylon Med J** 1983 Mar;28(1):48–52

### United States

Hightower F: Surgeons of early North Carolina. **Ann Surg** 1981 May;193(5):525–38

### USSR

Bratus' VD: Khirurgiia v Kieve (K 1500-letiiu goroda). **Klin Khir** 1982 May;(5):1–7

Khokholia VP, Stebliak AG: Stranitsy iz istorii razvitiia khirurgii v Kieve. **Klin Khir** 1982 May;(5):65–7

### Venezuela

Travieso CR: Historia de la cirugia en Venezuela. **Rev Soc Venez Hist Med** 1975–76;23(37):21–35

## Before 500 A.D.

### Asia

Wijesinha S, Wickremesinghe C: Surgery and hospitals in ancient Sri Lanka and India. **J R Coll Surg Edinb** 1981 Jul;26(4):245–9

### Egypt

Narbe S: Egypten: på Ramses tid. **Odontol Foren Tidskr** 1981 Oct;45(4):30–2

### Greco-Roman

Roselli A: Problemi relativi ai trattati chirurgici De Fracturis e De Articulis. In La collection hippocratique et son rôle dans l'histoire de la médecine. Colloque de Strasbourg (23–27 octobre 1972) organisé par le Centre de Recherches sur la Grèce Antique, avec le concours des Facultés de Philosophie et des Langues Classiques. Leiden, E. J. Brill, 1975. p. 229–34.

### India

Chakravorty RC: Management of clean wounds and abscesses as described in the Sushrutasamhita. In: Congrès internationale d'histoire de la médecine, XXVe, Québec, 1976. Actes. Québec, 1977. p. 560–3.

Das S: Shusruta of India: pioneer in vesicolithotomy. **Urology** 1984 Mar;23(3):317–9

Das S: Shusruta of India, the pioneer in the treatment of urethral stricture. **Surg Gynecol Obstet** 1983 Dec;157(6):581–2

Pagella P: Il Susruta Samhita: un capitolo originale della chirurgia o una interdipendenza di valori nella storia della medicina? **Ann Osp Maria Vittoria Torino** 1977 Jul–Dec;20(7–12):354–63

Singhal GD, Guru LV: Anatomical and obstetric considerations in ancient Indian surgery: based on Sarirasthana of Susruta Samhita. Varanasi, India, Institute of Medical Sciences, Banaras Hindu University, 1973. L, 241 p.

Singhal GD, Singh RH, Shukla KP: Non-operative considerations in ancient Indian surgery: (based on Susruta Samhita, Cikitsa-Sthana, chapters 24–40). Varanasi, India, Institute of Medical Sciences, Banaras Hindu University, 1971. xlii, 396 p.

### Rome

Baxby D: An unauthorized contemporary reprinting of Jenner's paper on the cuckoo. **J Hist Med Allied Sci** 1981 Apr;36(2):218–9

Bliquez LJ: Roman surgical instruments in the Johns Hopkins University Institute of the History of Medicine. **Bull Hist Med** 1982 Summer;56(2):195–217

Cope JC: Roman medical instruments. **Mo Med** 1980 Sep;77(9):574

Piotrowski E: Chirurgia starożytnego rzymu z okresu zagłady Pompei. **Wiad Lek** 1980 Jul 15;33(14):1175–8

## 500 A.D.–1450

Mirskiĭ MB: Khirurgi v épokhu srednevekov'ia. **Klin Med (Mosk)** 1984

Feb;62(2):144–7
Scholle S: Lanfranks 'Chirurgia Parva' in mittelniederfränkischer Ubertragung. Diss. Würzburg, 1978. Pattensen, Horst Wellm Verlag, 1978. 147 p. (Altdeutsche Lanfrank-Ubersetzungen, II, 1).
Södergård O: La chirurgie de l'Abbé Poutrel. Texte picard de 1300 environ. **Acta Univ Lund** 1980;34:1–94
Trynková O: Některé metody středověkého léčení podle mistra Rhazesa a mistra Salicettiho. I. Rhazesovo a Salicettiho ranná lékařství a jejich vydavatelé. **Sb Lek** 1981;83(11–12):363–7

**Arabic**

Beg MH: Muslim contribution to surgery. **JPMA** 1984 Jul;34(7):218–21
Buniiatov ZM, Kagramanov KM: O 30-m traktate Abu-l-kasima Khalafa Ibn Abbasa Az-Zakhravi. **Vestn Akad Med Nauk SSSR** 1980;9:75–8
Hamarneh S: Medical technology in Ibn al-Quff's surgery. In I. El-Sayyad, ed: Papers presented to the First International Conference on Islamic Medicine, celebrating the advent of the fifteenth century hijri. Kuwait, Ministry of Public Health. National Council for Culture, Arts and Letters, 1981. p. 140–7.
Hamarneh SK, Awad EA: Early surgical instruments excavated in old Cairo, Egypt. In: Congrès international d'histoire de la médecine, XXVe, Québec, 1976. Actes. Québec, 1977. p. 761–4.
Kataye S: L'amygdalectomie dans la médecine arabe. **Hist Sci Med** 1979;13(4):419–25
Mihic DN: Die erste orotracheale Intubation. **Anaesthesist** 1983 Sep;32(9):450–1
Nabri IA: El Zahrawi (936–1013 AD), the father of operative surgery. **Ann R Coll Surg Engl** 1983 Mar;65(2):132–4
Omirov RIu, Mardanov LM: Nekotorye voprosy khirurgii v trudakh Abu Ali Ibn Siny (k 1000-letiiu so dnia rozhdeniia). **Klin Khir** 1980 Mar;(3):66–8
Wijesinha SS: El Zahrawi (936–1013 AD), the father of operative surgery. **Ann R Coll Surg Engl** 1983 Nov;65(6):423

**Belgium**

Tabanelli M: Gli albori della chirurgia nelle Fiandre. Il libro del maestro Thomas Scellinck. Firenze, Leo S. Olschki, 1974. xxxviii, 284 p. (Biblioteca della 'Rivista di Storia delle Scienze Mediche e Naturali', v. 19).

**Byzantium**

Pentogalos GE, Lascaratos JG: A surgical operation performed on Siamese twins during the tenth century in Byzantium. **Bull Hist Med** 1984 Spring;58(1):99–102

**Great Britain**

Cosman MP: The medieval medical third party: compulsory consultation and malpractice insurance. **Ann Plast Surg** 1982 Feb;8(2):152–62

**Italy**

Berg A, ed: Lanfranks 'Chirurgia parva' in der Abschrift Konrad Schrecks von Aschaffenburg. Diss. Würzburg 1975, 145 S. (Altdeutsche Lanfrank-Uebersetzungen III).

**Spain**

Hussenot C: Sur un Erbier de Me Arnauld de Villeneuve (manuscrit médiéval). Thèse de doctorat, Université René-Descartes. Paris, 1983. 119 leaves. (U. E. R. des Sciences pharm. et biol. de Paris-Luxembourg, 1982–1983, no U 558).

**1450–1700**

Kapronczay K: A sebészeti eszközök fejlodése a XV–XVI. században. **Orvostort Kozl** 1982;28(1–3):141–50
Riall CT: Surgical and medical devices and their origins. Chapter XIV. Beginnings of modern surgery (Andreas Vesalius). **J Oper Room Res Inst** 1982 Sep;2(9):30–3
Simeone FA: Andreas Vesalius: anatomist, surgeon, count palatine, and pilgrim. **Am J Surg** 1984 Apr;147(4):432–40

**Canada**

Biron H: Antoine Chaudillon. In Dictionary of Canadian biography, 1701 to 1740. Volume 2, 1969. p. 140–1.
Cormier C: Jacques Bourgeois. In Dictionary of Canadian biography, 1701 to 1740. Volume 2, 1969. p. 94.

**France**

Amalric P: L'influence de Guy de Chauliac à Toulouse au XVIIe siècle. A propos d'un petit livre inédit. **Bull Soc Ophtalmol Fr** 1980 Jun–Jul;80(6–7):617–8
Ayer E, Montandon D: Pierre Franco (1506–1580) and the treatment of a cheek ulcer. **Chir Plast** 1980;5(4):289–93
Bagwell CE: Ambröise Paré and the renaissance of surgery. **Surg Gynecol Obstet** 1981 Mar;152(3):350–4
Bendiner E: From barbershop to battlefield--Paré and the renaissance of surgery. **Hosp Pract** 1983 Aug;18(8):193–5, 199, 202 passim
Colard A: En chirurgie, Ambroise Paré n'a pas innové la ligature vasculaire. **Rev Med Brux** 1980; NS 1;687–9
Colard A: Evocation du passé en chirugie. Ambroise Paré n'a pas innové la ligature vasculaire. **Rev Med Brux** 1980 Dec;1(10):687–9
Pédron F: Histoire d'Ambroise, chirurgien du roi. Paris, Orban, 1980. 468 p.
Touati B: Ambroise paré. **Rev Odontostomatol (Paris)** 1983 Mar–Apr;12(2):85

**French Guiana**

Chaïa J: Contrat d'un chirurgien d'une plantation de Cayenne au XVIIe siècle. In: Congrès National des Sociétés Savantes, 93e, Tours, 1968. Comptes Rendus. Paris, 1971. Section des Sciences, Tome II. p. 51–4.

**Germany**

Böhmer W: Der Wittenberger Kaiserschnitt von 1610. **Zentralbl Gynakol** 1983;105(19):1265–70

**Great Britain**

Appleby JH: New light on John Woodall, surgeon and adventurer. **Med Hist** 1981 Jul;25(3):251–68
Cohen B: A tale of two paintings. **Ann R Coll Surg Engl** 1982 Jan;64(1):4–12
Harper E: The sailor's surgeon (James Yonge). **J R Nav Med Serv** 1979 Spring;65(1):35–7
Morris GC: A portrait of Thomas Hollier, Pepy's surgeon. **Ann R Coll Surg Engl** 1979 May;61(3):224–9
Pelling M: Barbers and barber-surgeons: an occupational group in an English provincial town, 1550–1640. **Soc Soc Hist Med Bull (Lond)** 1981 Jun;28:14–6
Riall CT: Surgical and medical devices and their origins. William Harvey and circulation of the blood. Chapter XVI. **J Oper Room Res Inst** 1982 Nov;2(11):32–6
Robb-Smith AH: The quatercentenary of the Lumleian Lecture. **J R Coll Physicians Lond** 1983 Jan;17(1):74–8
Robins R: An old Cornish hand. **J Hand Surg [Br]** 1984 Jun;9(2):199–200
Watt J: Surgeons of the Mary Rose: the practice of surgery in Tudor England. **Mar Mirror** 1983;69:3–18

**Italy**

Oliaro T: Marco Aurelio Severino il perseguitato ricreatore della chirurgia italiana (1580–1656). **Minerva Chir** 1980 Sep 30;35(18 Suppl):32–4
Pesenti Marañgon T: 'Professores chirurgie', 'medici ciroici' e 'barbitonsores' a Padova nell' età di Leonardo Buffi da Bertipaglia (dopo il 1448). Quad. Stor Univ. Padova, 1978;11:1–38.

**Mexico**

López de Hinojosos A: Suma y recopilación de cirugía con un arte para sangrar muy útil y provechosa. Mexico, Academia Nacional de Medicina, 1977. xxiv, 227 p.

**Netherlands**

Houtzager HL: Medicyns, Vroedwyfs en Chirurgyns. Schets van de gezondheidszorg in Delft en beschrijving van het Theatrum Anatomicum aldaar in de 16e en 17e eeuw. Amsterdam, Rodopi, 1979. 133 p. (Serie-nitgave van het Genootschap Delfia Batavorum, 5).
Kerner S: Samuel de Lion Benavente; chirurgien et lithotomiste (1643–1723). **Rev Hist Med Heb** 1981 Jul;34(2):29–30
Pollitt R: The wounding and treatment of William of Orange in 1582. **J Hist Med Allied Sci** 1982 Apr;37(2):135–58
Pytel' AIa: Nicolaus Van Tul'p - vydaiushchiĭsia anatom i khirurg (k 340-letiiu opublikovania ego znamenitoĭ knigi 'Meditsinskie nabliudeniia'). **Khirurgiia (Mosk)** 1980 Aug;(8):117–9
Van Lieburg MJ: De genees- en heelkunde in de Noordelijke Nederlanden, gezien vanuit de stedelijke en chirurgijnsgilde-ordonnanties van de 16e eeuw. **Tijdschr Geschied Geneeskd** 1983;6(4):169–84
Van Lieburg MJ: De 'Materia Chirurgica' in de ordonnanties en examens der Noord-Nederlandse chirurgijnsgilden vóór 1600. **Pharm Weekbl** 1981;116(45):1393–8

**Spain**

Guerra F: La tradicion medieval en la cirugia española del siglo XVI. **Asclepio** 1978–79;30–31:359–63
Jiménez Muñoz JM: Salarios de medicos y cirujanos (I) (II). (Nóminas

de Corte 1538–1629). **Asclepio** 1981;33:315–47

**Switzerland**

Kuemmel WF: Chirurgie vor 400 Jahren: die Bilderhandschrift des Caspar Stromayr. **Medita** 1980;10, Suppl. (Geschichte der Medizin, f.6:16)
Rickham PP: Johannes Fatio: Sein Leben, sein Werk und sein schreckliches Ende. **Z Kinderchir** 1984 Oct;39(5):289–95
Rintelen F: Der Basler Chirurg und Rebell Johannes Fatio 1649–1691. **Gesnerus** 1983;40(1–2):149–58

**1700 to Present**

Absolon KB: The surgeon's surgeon. Theodor Billroth 1829–1894. Vol. I. Lawrence, Kansas, Coronado Press, 1979. xxi, 282 p.
Absolon KB: The surgeon's surgeon. Theodor Billroth 1829–1894. Volume II. Lawrence, Kansas, Coronado Press, 1981. 232 p.
Aellen HP: Dr. Med. Armin Emil Elsaesser (1875–1952), Schueler von Theodor Kocher: sein Werden und Wirken in der Schweiz und in den Vereinigten Staaten von Amerika. Bern, [s.n.], 1982. x, 187 p.
Altemeier WA: Sepsis in surgery. **Arch Surg** 1982 Feb;117(2):107–12
Balogh J, Sükösd L: Manninger Vilmos akadémiai pályadíjának 80 éves évfordulójára. **Orv Hetil** 1983 Oct 30;124(44):2693–5
Beatty WK: Daniel Hale Williams--pioneer surgeon and hospital administrator. **Proc Inst Med Chic** 1979 Jul–Sep;32(7):156
Belkin NL: Textiles as aseptic barriers: the past, present, and future. **Med Instrum** 1980 Jul–Aug;14(4):233–6
Ben-Hur N, Converse JM: The impact of plastic surgery on transplantation from skin graft to microsurgery. **Transplant Proc** 1980 Dec;12(4):616–20
Bibliography of original works on orthopaedic surgery, traumatology and related sciences, 1872–1972.: Belgrade, Yugoslav Association for Orthopaedic Surgery and Traumatology, 1980. 251 p.
Boschung U: Chirurgiemechanik im 18. Jahrhundert. **Medita** 1980;10:14
Bouchet A: Geschichte der Chirurgie vom Ende des 18. Jahrhunderts bis zur Gegenwart. In Sournia JC, Martiny M, Poulet J, ed: Illustrierte Geschichte der Medizin. Salzburg, Andreas, 1980. Vol. 7. p. 2541–607.
Breen RE, Garnjobst W: Surgical procedures for carcinoma of the rectum. A historical review. **Dis Colon Rectum** 1983 Oct;26(10):680–5
Cady B, Sedgwick CE: History of thyroid and parathyroid surgery. **Major Probl Clin Surg** 1980;15:1–5
Chambers RW, Durkin JT, ed: Papers of the Alexis Carrel centennial conference, Georgetown University June 28, 1973. Washington, Georgetown University, 1973. 107 p. Contributions by C. A. Lindbergh, A. Gros, S. Maggio, L. G. Walker, C. A. Hufnagel, T. I. Malinin.
Charnley J: Evolution of total hip replacement. **Ann Chir Gynaecol** 1982;71(2):103–7
Clarke JM: Surgery in Jehovah's witnesses. **Br J Hosp Med** 1982 May;27(5):497–500
Condon AG: John Caleff. In Dictionary of Canadian biography, 1801 to 1820. Volume 5, 1983. p. 134–5.
De Moulin D: On the early history of antisepsis. **Arch Chir Neerl** 1979;31(4):197–201
Dobek R, Kolmsee P: Maxim Zetkin--Arzt, Kriegschirurg und Kommunist. **Militaergesch** 1978;17(5):595–603
Doberneck RC, Kleinman R: The surgical garb. **Surgery** 1984 Jun;95(6):694–8
Drake CG: Aneurysm surgery: past, present, and future. **Int Anesthesiol Clin** 1982 Summer;20(2):1–9
Edmonson JM: Surgical garb, 1870–1920. Cleveland, Cleveland Health Sciences Library, 1982. 20 p. (Occasional contributions to the history of the health sciences from the Historical Division of the Cleveland Health Sciences Library, no. 1).
Elmslie R: The colonial career of James Patrick Murray. **Aust NZ J Surg** 1979 Feb;49(1):154–62
Fraser I: An historical perspective on mechanical aids in intestinal anastomosis. **Surg Gynecol Obstet** 1982 Oct;155(4):566–74
Fulton JF: History of medicine–Arnold Klebs and Harvey Cushing at the 1st International Neurological Congress at Berne in 1931. **Int J Neurol** 1980;14(1):103–15
Gelberman RH: Microsurgery and the development of the operating microscope. **Contemp Surg** 1978 Dec;13(6):43–6
Gottschalk E: Quo vadit chirurgia paediatrica? **Beitr Gesch Univ Erfurt** 1979–83;19:361–7
Greene NM: Anesthesia and the development of surgery (1846–1896). **Middle East J Anaesthesiol** 1979 Oct;5(5):309–23
Guarner V: El conocimiento de la historia de la medicina en la educacion del cirujano. **Bol Soc Mex Hist Filos Med** 1979 Mar;4(26):73–87
Hazard JB: An introduction to the history of surgical pathology. **Am J Clin Pathol** 1981 Mar;75(3 Suppl):444–6
Higier J: Sto lat sporu o autorstwo (priorytet) operacji pośrodkowego zeszycia pochwy (colpocleisis mediana) 1881–1981. **Ginekol Pol** 1982;53(3)
Hillel AD: History of stapedectomy. **Am J Otolaryngol** 1983 Mar–Apr;4(2):131–40
Höcht B: Operative Behandlung des Hodenhochstandes. Ein Rückblick auf die historische Entwicklung. **MMW** 1983 May 6;125(18):381–4
Illingworth C: The sanguine mystery. 'This bloody and butcherly department of the healing art.' [London], Nuffield Provincial Hospitals Trust, 1970. 72 p.
The International Federation of Surgical Colleges: 1958–1980. **Ann R Coll Surg Engl** 1981;63:290–2
Jain KM, Swan KG, Casey KF: Nobel Prize winner in surgery. Part 2. **Am Surg** 1982 May;48(5):191–6
Jain KM, Swan KG, Casey KF: Nobel prize winners in surgery. Part 3. (Frederick Grant Banting, Walter Rudolph Hess). **Am Surg** 1982 Jul;48(7):287–90
Johnson G: Vistas in the management of bleeding esophageal varices. **NC Med J** 1982 May;43(5):353–7
Kaiser W, Skrobacki A: Królewieckie listy Jana Mukulicza de Fryderyka Althoffa. **Komun Mazursko Warm** 1975;4(130):455–65
Korepanov VI: Istoriia razvitiia lazernoĭ khirurgii. **Sov Med** 1984;(3):61–5
Lawrence W Jr: The scope of surgical oncology. **Aust NZ J Surg** 1982 Aug;52(4):325–30
Les pansements à la ouate de M. Alphonse Guérin: **Union Med Can** 1981 May;110(5):464
Lindholm RV: Küntscher bone nailing – forecast and actuality. **Ann Chir Gynaecol** 1980;69(3):85–91
Littmann I: Theodor Billroth (1829–1894). **Orvostort Kozl** 1979;87–88(25 no 1–2):123–39
Ljunggren B: Harvey Cushing and Sven Hedin. **Surg Neurol** 1982 Mar;17(3):165–71
MacLean LD, Rhode BM: The history of surgery for morbid obesity. **Can J Surg** 1984 Mar;27(2):126–7
Meissner K, Meiser G: Primary open wound management after emergency laparotomies for conditions associated with bacterial contamination. Reappraisal of a historical tradition. **Am J Surg** 1984 Nov;148(5):613–7
Meyburg P: Ueber die Entwicklung des Operationstisches im 19. Jahrhundert. Diss. Mainz, 1980. 119 p.
Mirskiĭ MB: Teodor Bil'rot i ego vklad v khirurgiiu (k 150-letiiu so dnia rozhdeniia). **Klin Med (Mosk)** 1980 Sep;58(9):112–4
Missotten FE: Historical review of pharyngo-oesophageal reconstruction after resection for carcinoma of pharynx and cervical oesophagus. **Clin Otolaryngol** 1983 Oct;8(5):345–62
Moerchel J: Sauerbruch und die Mayos. **Dtsch Med Wochenschr** 1980 May 9;105(19):697–9
O'Connor TW: A historical review of reversed gastric tube esophagoplasty. **Surg Gynecol Obstet** 1983 Mar;156(3):371–4
Oliaro A: La chirurgia cento anni or sono. L'Anatomia Chirurgica del dott. **Minerva Chir** 1982 Dec 15–31;37(23–24):2159–79
Pernick MS: The calculus of suffering in nineteenth-century surgery. **Hastings Cent Rep** 1983 Apr;13(2):26–36
Premuda L: Arthur Menzel (1844–1878), einer der liebsten und tüchtigsten Schüler und der treuesten Freunde Billroths, Primarchirung in Triest. **Gesnerus** 1981;38:191–205
Pringle KC: Neonatal surgery: historical perspectives and a glimpse of the future. In Smith GF, Smith PN, Vidyasagar D, ed: Historical review and recent advances in neonatal and perinatal medicine. [Chicago?], Mead Johnson Nutritional Division, 1983. Vol. II. p. 85–105.
Ravitch MM, McAuley CE: Airborne contamination of the operative wound. **Surg Gynecol Obstet** 1984 Aug;159(2):177–88
Ravitch MM, Steichen FM: Staples and staplers. **Adv Surg** 1984;17:241–79
Ravitch MM: The danger of stating an opinion or the hazards of going on record. **Surg Gynecol Obstet** 1980 Dec;151(6):810–6
Ravitch MM: The reception of new operations. **Ann Surg** 1984 Sep;200(3):231–46
Read RD: Marcy's priority in the development of inguinal herniorrphaphy. **Surgery** 1980 Nov;88(5):682–5
Riall CT: Surgical and medical devices and their origins. Chapter XIX. Surgical instrument manufacturers. **J Oper Room Res Inst** 1983 Apr;3(4):36–9
Robicsek F: The birth of the surgical stapler. **Surg Gynecol Obstet** 1980 Apr;150(4):579–83
Rutkow IM: The letters of William Halsted and Anton von Eiselsberg: a very special friendship. **Arch Surg** 1980 Aug;115(8):993–1001
Saegesser F: César Roux (1857–1934) et son époque. **Rev Med Suisse Romande** 1984 Jun;104(6):403–64
Schober KL: Vor etwa hundert Jahren. **Zentralbl Chir** 1980;105(6):401–3 (continued regularly)
Schoefer G: Die chirurgische Behandlung der Lungentuberkulose. **Zentralbl Chir** 1982;107(5–6):285–94
Serafin D: Microsurgery: past, present, and future. **Plast Reconstr Surg** 1980 Nov;66(5):781–5
Silló-Seidl G: Arzte ohne Nobelpreis deren Entdeckungen Millionen Menschen geholfen haben. Genf, Ariston, 1978. 256 p.
Simpson GT, Polanyi TG: History of the carbon dioxide laser in otolaryngologic surgery. **Otolaryngol Clin North Am** 1983 Nov;16(4):739–52
Starzl TE, Porter KA, Francavilla A: The Eck fistula in animals and humans. **Curr Probl Surg** 1983 Nov;20(11):687–752
Steichen FM, Ravitch MM: History of mechanical devices and instruments for suturing. **Curr Probl Surg** 1982 Jan;19(1):1–52
Stephenson GW: Martin and Mayo plant the seeds: a history of the international program. **Bull Am Coll Surg** 1980 Jul;65(7):22–8
Taylor S: Thomas Richardson Colledge FRCS, 1796–1879.

## SURGERY

**Ann R Coll Surg Engl** 1982 Jul;64(4):266-7

Terzioglu A, Krebs LM: The development of surgery and of surgical clinics at the turn of the 20th century. Munich, (the authors), 1979. 69 p.

Tilney NL: Harvey Cushing and the Oxford connection. **Surg Gynecol Obstet** 1982 Jul;155(1):89-94

Török B: Langenbuch és Halpert Béla. Az elsö cholecytektómia centenáriumára. **Orv Hetil** 1983 Jun 26;124(26):1577-81

Walter CW: Use of surgical rubber gloves. **Surgery** 1983 May;93(5):728-9

Wangensteen OH: The University of Glasgow and the Johns Hopkins schools of surgery. **Am J Surg** 1980 Jun;139(6):870-5

Whitby JD. Alcohol in anaesthesia and surgical resuscitation. **Anaesthesia** 1980 May;35(5):502-5

White FM: Nosocomial infection control: scope and implications for health care--historical view. **Am J Infect Control** 1981 Aug;9(3):61-9

Wondrak E: Johann Nepomuk Rust (1775-1840): der Lebensweg des Chirurgen und Förderers des jungen J.E. Purkyne. **Acta Univ Palacki Olomuc Fac Med** 1977;83:169-76

Woodruff M: The master surgeon. **J R Coll Surg Edinb** 1981 Sep;26(5):257-63

### Asia

Bowie DC: Captive surgeon in Hong Kong: the story of the British Military Hospital, Hong Kong 1942-1945. **J Hong Kong Branch R Asiat Soc** 1975;15:150-290

### Australia

Fleming DW: The founders of the college: Western Australia. **Aust NZ J Surg** 1981 Dec;51(6):623-4

Hamilton DG. 100 years of paediatric surgery in Sydney. **Med J Aust** 1980 Dec 27;2(13):721-6

Howard RN: The founders of the College Victoria. **Aust NZ J Surg** 1981 Apr;51(2):227-38

Leggett CA: The founders of the College. **Aust NZ J Surg** 1981 Oct;51(5):508-12

McEachern AC: The founders of the College. **Aust NZ J Surg** 1981 Aug;51(4):400-5

Nicks R: Australian surgeons and society. **Aust NZ J Surg** 1980 Dec;50(6):659-67

Rank BK: George Grey Turner, F.R.A.C.S. (Hon). **Aust NZ J Surg** 1981 Dec;51(6):627-30

### Austria

Berezowski S: Jan Dolliner--chirurg bocheński (przyczynek do historii zdobywania doktoratów chirurgii w Uniwersytecie Jagiellońskim). **Pol Tyg Lek** 1979 Aug 27;34(35):1403-5

Frick K: Michael Ferdinand Wittmann (1755-1826) Magister und Doktor der Chirurgie, der erste graduierte Chirurg in Kärnten. **Carinthia** 1968;158:643-62

Galle P: Fortschritte in der operativen Behandlung hüftgelenksnaher Frakturen seit W. Denk. **Wien Klin Wochenschr** 1982 Apr 2;94(7):185-9

Holinka C: Theodor Billroth: the life of a surgeon in the spirit of music. **Mt Sinai J Med (NY)** 1981 Jan-Feb;48(1):21-41

Kern E: Das chirurgische Erbe. Theodor Billroth und die Musik. **Zentralbl Chir** 1982;107(21):1408-16

Mitterstiller S: 100 Jahre chirurgische Klinik in Innsbruck. **Tirol Heimat** 1970;:31-2

Mitterstiller S: 100 Jahre Chirurgische Klinik in Innsbruck. **Tirol Heimat** 1970;34:17-38

Paul U: Das chirurgische Erbe. Anton von Eiselsberg. **Zentralbl Chir** 1982;107(7):418-21

Paul U: Das chirurgische Erbe. Eduard Albert. **Zentralbl Chir** 1982;107(23):1535-7

Paul U: Das chirurgische Erbe: Johann von Mikulicz-Radecki. **Zentralbl Chir** 1981;106(7):469-72

Rüden AD von: Medicina Graecensis. Das medizinisch-chirurgische Studium in Graz (1782-1862). Diss. Technischen Universität München, 1978. 195 p.

Spängler H, Galle P: 70 Jahre Unfallchirurgie an den Wiener Kliniken. **Wien Klin Wochenschr** 1981 Jun 26;93(13):423-8

### Belgium

Abeele R van den: Jan Albert Roselt, plattelandschirurgijn te Machelen (1714-1785). **Jaarb Kunst Oudheidk Kring Deinze** 1978;:83-117

Darquenne R: Médecine et chirurgie hainuyères au siècle des lumières. **Ann Cerc Archeol Mons** 1976-77;70:139-76

Dickstein-Bernard C: La pratique de la chirurgie dans les hôpitaux bruxellois au XIXe siècle. **Ann Soc Belg Hist Hop** 1981;:69-94

### Brazil

Sattamini Duarte O: Dr. José Maurício Nunes Garcia. **Rev Inst Hist Geogr Bras** 1971;291:92-103

### Bulgaria

Altŭnkov P: D-r Vladimir Petrov Glavchev (1878-1915 g.). **Khirurgiia (Sofiia)** 1982;35(6):632

Apostolov MA: Pervaia Bolgarskaia khirurgicheskaia shkola. **Klin Med (Mosk)** 1984 Oct;62(10):149-51

### Canada

Beamish RE: Dr. Albert Clifford Abbott: a pioneer surgeon of western Canada. **Can Med Assoc J** 1983 Apr 1;128(7):862-4

Bernier J: Philippe-Louis-François Badelard. In Dictionary of Canadian biography, 1801 to 1820. Volume 5, 1983. p. 46-7.

Boissonnault CM: Michel Bertier. In Dictionary of Canadian biography, 1701 to 1740. Volume 2, 1969. p. 60.

Cook CS: Clark Bentom. In Dictionary of Canadian biography, 1801 to 1820. Volume 5, 1983. p. 68-9.

Desjardins E: Jacques Dénéchaud. In Dictionary of Canadian biography, 1801 to 1820. Volume 5, 1983. p. 248-9.

Entin MA: Med-Chi is 140 years old: a historical sketch of the Montreal Medical Chirurgical Society. **Can J Surg** 1983 Nov;26(6):563-5

The evolution of the O. R.: **Hosp Adm Can** 1978 Apr;20(4):38-9

Fahrni GS: Prairie surgeon. Winnipeg, Queenston House, 1976. vi, 138 p.

Harrison RC, Mills F: Canadian contributions toward the comprehension of hyperinsulinism: the first successful excision of an insulinoma. **Can J Surg** 1980 Jul;23(4):401-3

Janson G: Charles Blake. In Dictionary of Canadian biography, 1801 to 1820. Volume 5, 1983. p. 88-9.

Kernaghan LK: Duncan Clark. In Dictionary of Canadian biography, 1801 to 1820. Volume 5, 1983. p. 187-8.

Lessard R: Alexandre Serres. In Dictionary of Canadian biography, 1801 to 1820. Volume 5, 1983. p. 752.

Lessard R: François-Michel Suzor. In Dictionary of Canadian biography, 1801 to 1820. Volume 5, 1983. p. 788-9.

Moogk PN: Simon Soupiran. In Dictionary of Canadian biography, 1701 to 1740. Volume 2, 1969. p. 613-4.

Morin J: Liveright Piuze. In Dictionary of Canadian biography, 1801 to 1820. Volume 5, 1983. p. 676.

Shandling B: History of the Canadian Association of Paediatric Surgeons. **J Pediatr Surg** 1979 Oct;14(5):509-10

Stewart R: The mind of Norman Bethune. Toronto, Fitzhenry and Whiteside, 1977. ix, 150 p.

Walt AJ: The world's best-known surgeon. **Surgery** 1983 Oct;94(4):582-90

### Chile

Costa-Casaretto C: Presentación del Dr. Lorenzo Sazié. **Rev Med Chil** 1983 Dec;111(12):1289-98

### China

Lee S, Li SJ: Clinical and experimental microsurgery in China: an historical note. **J Microsurg** 1982 Spring;3(3):180-3

Stewart R: Bethune. 2nd ed. Hamden, Connecticut, Archon, 1979. 210 p.

Summers GV: Norman Bethune, Canadian surgeon: his Chinese connection. **Can J Surg** 1983 Jul;26(4):379-82

### Czechoslovakia

Balaš V: I. chirurgická klinika a její vliv na rozvoj chirurgie v Ceskoslovensku. **Rozhl Chir** 1983 Apr;62(4):289-307

Balaš V: 100 years of Czech surgery. **Sb Lek** 1983 Apr;85(4):97-104

Duda M, Serý Z: Historie a současnost chirurgie hiátových hernií a refluxní nemoci jícnu. **Cesk Gastroenterol Vyz** 1979 Sep;33(6):332-41

Fröml F: Poslední léta městských chirurgu v Prostějově. **Cas Lek Cesk** 1981;120(51):1573-4

Knobloch J: Hrst vzpomínek na I. chirurgickou kliniku v době Jiráskově. **Cas Lek Cesk** 1983 Jul 15;122(28):871-5

Kraus B: MUDr. Jaroslav Mathon - chirurg, umelecky a pamatkový praukopník. **Cas Lek Cesk** 1983 Sep 30;122(39):1214-5

Kubat R, Mřena V: Operatsiia Zagradnicheka pri vrozhdennom vyvikhe bedra segodnia (posviashchaetsia 100-letiiu so dnia rozhdeniia professora Iana Zagradnicheka). **Ortop Travmatol Protez** 1982 Jul;(7):69-71

Kuniak B, Strelka J: Vývoj chirurgie strmienka pri otoskleróze na Slovensku. **Bratisl Lek Listy** 1983;79(2):222-6

Moravec R, Tichý M, Moravcová M, et al: Z dejín chirurgie v Bratislave. Profesor Kostlivý a začiatky chirurgickej kliniky na LFUK v Bratislava] **Rozhl Chir** 1984 Jul;63(7):526-31

Subrtová A: Johann Bapt. Michael Sagar (1732-1813). **Cas Nar Muz** 1981;150(3-4):153-90

Vlček J, Klánova JV: Akologický kabinet, jeho vznik a osudy. **Rozhl Chir** 1984 Feb;63(2):140-4

Vlček J: K historii stoletého trvání I. české chirurgické kliniky v Praze. **Cas Lek Cesk** 1983 Jul 15;122(28):865-70

Vojtíšek V: Historie chirurgické kliniky lékařské fakulty hygienické

Univerzity Karlovy v Praze. **Rozhl Chir** 1983 Jul;62(7):533-8
Wondrák E: Die Anfänge der chirurgischen und geburtshilflichen Ausbildung in Mähren. In Ganzinger K, Skopec M, Wyklicky H, ed: Festschrift für Erna Lesky zum 70. Geburtstag. Wien, Brüder Hollinek, 1981. p. 185-92.
Zvara V: O vývoji a ďalších perspektívach rozvoja chirurgických disciplín na lekárskej fakulte Univerzity Komenského v Bratislave. **Cas Lek Cesk** 1979 Dec 21;118(51):1583-5

**Egypt**

Jagailloux S: L'évolution de la chirurgie en Egypte au XIXe siècle. **Hist Sci Med** 1984;18(1):69-73

**Europe**

Vainio K: History of surgery of rheumatoid arthritis in Europe. **Scand J Rheumatol** 1983;12(2):65-8

**Finland**

Mäntylä I, Ylikahri R: Mitä jokaisen välskärinkisällin tulee tietää? Lääketieteellinen kuulustelu vuonna 1751. **Duodecim** 1984;100(14):863-9

**France**

Angot JL: Pierre Fauchard (1677?-1761). Expert pour les dents, et maître chirurgien de Saint-Côme de Paris. **Clio Med** 1983 Mar;17(4):207-21
Baguenier-Desormeaux L: Henry Drysdale Dakin à Compiègne, en 1915. **Rev Hist Pharm (Paris)** 1981 Jun;28(249):79-88
Bloch H: Guillaume Dupuytren, M.D. (1777-1835). Surgeon of Hôtel Dieu and his American students. **NY State J Med** 1981 Feb;81(2):259-60
Bodemer CW: Baron Dominique Jean Larrey, Napoleon's surgeon. **Bull Am Coll Surg** 1982 Jul;67(7):18-21
Brahma B, Singh M: The man behind the name: Eugene Louis Doyen 1859-1916. **NATNEWS** 1981 Dec;18(12):14
Charpin J: Goyrand, d'Aix, un académicien de province au XIX siècle (1803-1866). **Bull Acad Natl Med (Paris)** 1982 Jun;166(6):787-90
Converse JM: Alexis Carrel: the man, the unknown. **Plast Reconstr Surg** 1981 Oct;68(4):629-39
Csillag I: Eckstein Ferenc és a hadisebészet a Napóleon elleni háborúban. **Orv Hetil** 1984 Feb 19;125(8):467-70
Dalat J: Un chirurgien de mer à la fin du XVIIIe siècle. **Rev Hist Pharm (Paris)** 1983 Dec;71(30):275-81
Darracq PJ: Les chirurgiens à Bordeaux au XVIIIe siècle. **Hist Sci Med** 1981;15(4):299-303
Decaux A: Napoléon III et la chirurgie. **Chirurgie** 1984;110(1):23-8
De Vaux de Foletier F: Anoblissements de médecins et chirurgiens de Louis XIV à Louis XVI. **Hist Sci Med** 1982;16(3):163-6
Didier C: Aperçu sur les médecins et chirurgiens à Colmar au XVIIIe siècle. In Livet G, Schaff G, ed: Médecine et assistance en Alsace, XVIe-XXe siècle. Strasbourg, Istra, 1976. p. 87-111.
DiGioia JM, Rocko JM, Swan KG: Baron Larrey. Modern military surgeon. **Am Surg** 1983 May;49(5):226-30
Figarella J: Jacques Daviel, chirurgien marseillais. **Marseille** 1978;113:42-56
Gelfand T: Chirurghi dei Lumi. **Kos** 1984 Feb;1(1):51-73
Gelfand T: Demystification and surgical power in the French Enlightenment. **Bull Hist Med** 1983 Summer;57(2):203-17
Gelfand T: Deux cultures, une profession: les chirurgiens français au XVIIIe siècle. **Rev Hist Mod Contemp** 1980 July-Sep;27:468-84
Gelfand T: Professionalizing modern medicine: Paris surgeons and medical science and institutions in the 18th century. Westport, Connecticut, Greenwood Press, 1980. xviii, 271 p. (Contributions in medical history, 6)
Gelfand T: Two cultures, one profession: the surgeons of France in the eighteenth century. In the consortium on Revolutionary Europe: Proceedings, 1978, 1980. p. 171-87. French language version, Rev Hist Mod Contemp 1980 Jul-Sep; 27:468-84.
Gerard A: Chronique médico-chirurgicale Lilloise sous la Révolution et l'Empire. **Lille Med** 1979 Dec;24(10):774-83
Guarner V: Louis-Hubert Farabeuf (1841-1910). **Gac Med Mex** 1982 Dec;118(12):505-8
Guillermand J: Un anniversaire et une tradition: l'Académie Royale de Chirurgie. **Med Armees** 1981;9:807-11
Gutmann RA: Une lettre de Marjolin sur ses rapports avec Dupuytren. **Hist Sci Med** 1981;15(2):123-7
Haller alla 'Charité' con Ledran: **Dent Cadmos** 1979 Feb 2;47(2):54-6
Hau T: The surgical practice of Dominique Jean Larrey. **Surg Gynecol Obstet** 1982 Jan;154(1):89-94
Hauben DJ: Das chirurgische Erbe. Guillaume Dupuytren (1777-1835). **Zentralbl Chir** 1984;109(11):765-6
Hepp J: Un grand chirurgien du début de ce siècle. **Sem Hop Paris** 1981 Jun 8-15;57(21-24):1049-54
Hillemand P, Gilbrin E: Le Père Elisée, premier chirurgien de Louis XVIII et la création de l'Académie de Médecine. **Bull Acad Natl Med (Paris)** 1981 Jan;165(1):23-6
Hillemand P, Gilbrin E: Le père Elisée (1753-1817); premier chirurgien de Louis XVIII. **Hist Sci Med** 1980;14(2):233-40
Hockemeyer H: Die Zeit seiner Schiffsarzttätigkeit in den Memoiren des napoleonischen Chirurgen Dominique-Jean Larrey. Diss., Universität Düsseldorf. Düsseldorf, 1982. 44 p.
Huard P: Claude Bernard et la chirurgie. In: Congrès National des Sociétés Savantes, 107e. Brest, 1982. Comptes Rendus, Paris, 1983. Section des Sciences, Fasc. IV. p. 267-71.
Huard P: Jacques Delpech (1777-1832). In: Congrès National des Sociétés Savantes, 96e, Toulouse, 1971. Comptes Rendus. Paris, 1974. Histoire des Sciences, Tome 1. p. 99-105.
Huard P, Théodoridès J: Jean-Baptiste Pipelet (1759-1823), Constance de Théis (1767-1845), Josef de Salm-Dyck (1773-1861) ou le chirurgien, la poétesse et le botaniste. In: Congrès National des Sociétés Savantes, 93e, Tours, 1968. Comptes Rendus. Paris, 1971. Section des Sciences, Tome II. p. 127-36.
Huard P, Lefebvre P, Nosny P, et al: La scie ostéotome à chaîne de Bernhard-Franz Heine (1800-1846). **Hist Sci Med** 1983;17(2):147-57
Huard P, Imbault-Huart MJ: L'Académie royale de chirurgie après le 8 aout 1793. In: Congrès National des Sociétés Savantes, 100e, Paris, 1975. Actes. Paris, 1976. Histoire Moderne et Contemporaine et Histoire des Sciences. p. 297-308.
Huard P, Niaussat PM: 'L'arsenal' du service de Santé de la Marine au XIXe siècle. In: Congrès National des Sociétés Savantes, 105e, Caen, 1980. Comptes Rendus, Paris, 1980. Section des Sciences, Fasc. V. p. 85-96.
Huard P, Imbault-Huart MJ: Le concept d'Académie en France au XVIIIe siècle; son évolution face à la médecine et à la chirurgie. In: Congrés National des Sociétés Savantes, 100e, Paris, 1975. Actes. Paris, 1976. Histoire Moderne et Contemporaine et Histoire des Sciences. p. 289-96.
Huard P, Imbault-Huart MJ: Les papiers d'Antoine Louis (1723-1792). In: Congrès National des Sociétés Savantes, 102e, Limoges, 1977. Comptes Rendus. Paris, 1977. Section des Sciences, Fasc. III. p. 7-14.
Imbault-Huart MJ: Les chirurgiens et l'esprit chirurgical en France au XVIIIème siècle. **Clio Med** 1981 Apr;15(3-4):143-57
Lefebvre P: Il y a deux siècles mourait Germain Pichault de la Martinière (1697-1783). **Chirurgie** 1983;109(10):805-8
Leger L: Allocution. **Chirurgie** 1980 Jan;106(1):3-10
Lemaire JF: Le chirurgien-baron François Girardot (1773-1831) un oublié de l'histoire. **Hist Sci Med** 1980;14(1):107-14
Lugnegård H: Mannen bakom dupuytrens kontraktur: 'vilddjuret vid Seine' - sin tids mest namnkunnige kirurg. **Lakartidningen** 1983 Dec 28;80(52):5068-9
Malinin TI: Surgery and life: the extraordinary career of Alexis Carrel. New York, Harcourt Brace Jovanovich, 1979. xiii, 242 p.
Monod-Broca P: Anselme Schwartz 1872-1957. **Chirurgie** 1984;110(1):11-21
Monod-Broca P: Henri Redon, 1899-1974. **Chirurgie** 1983;109(1):15-22
Monod-Broca P: Henry Delagenière, 1858-1930. **Chirurgie** 1982;108(1):17-25
Monod-Broca P: Jacques Leveuf (1885-1948). **Chirurgie** 1980 Jan;106(1):18-25
Monod-Broca P: Louis Michon, 1892-1973. **Chirurgie** 1981;107(1):13-22
Monod-Broca P: Paul Broca (1824-1880). Le chirurgien, l'homme. **Bull Acad Natl Med (Paris)** 1980;164(6):536-44
Najafi H: Landmark perspective: Dr. Alexis Carrel and tissue culture. **JAMA** 1983 Aug 26;250(8):1086-9
Paul U: Das chirurgische Erbe. René Leriche. **Zentralbl Chir** 1983;108(18):1177-80
Pecker J: Thierry de Martel, 1875-1940. **Surg Neurol** 1980;13:401-3
Peltier LF: The 'back school' of Delpech in Montpellier. **Clin Orthop** 1983 Oct;179:4-9
Plessis JL, Huard P, Lefebvre P, et al: Louis-René Villermé, chirurgien-major à la Grande Armée. **Hist Sci Med** 1982;16(4):305-15
Sagaert LLC: Un grand chirurgien français: le docteur Achille-Cléophas Flaubert. **Hist Sci Med** 1980;14:449-52
Schmitt W: Das chirurgische Erbe. Alexis Carrel (1873-1944). **Zentralbl Chir** 1983;108(8):495-503
Sicard A: Historique de l'Académie de Chirurgie. **Chirurgie** 1981;107(9):713-8
Tournier-Lasserve C: La Peyronie et la présence des chirurgiens militaires au sein de l'Académie de Chirurgie. **Chirurgie** 1981;107(9):719-22
Tournier-Lasserve C: Les chirurgiens militaires et l'Académie de médecine. **Bull Acad Natl Med (Paris)** 1982 May;166(5):601-8
Vidal F: Les maîtrises en chirurgie au XVIIIe siècle. **Inf Dent** 1980 Jul 10;62(27):2345-54

**Germany**

Abe HR: Zur Biographie von Hans Kehr (1862-1916). **Beitr Gesch Univ Erfurt** 1979-83;19:233-40
Abe HR: Zur Sicherstellung des Nachlasses von Prof. Dr. Hans Kehr. **Beitr Gesch Univ Erfurt** 1979-83;19:259-64
Absolon KB: Ein einmaliger Brief - Der zwanzigjährige Billroth beschreibt seine Reise durch Thüringen im Jahre 1849. **Pommern** 1982;4:18-27
Allgöwer M, Tröhler U: Biographical note on Theodor Billroth. **Br J Surg** 1981 Oct;68(10):678-9

Asendorf MI: Die gelehrten Arzte Joseph und Karl Wenzel, ihr Leben und Werk in Mainz und Frankfurt am Main. Diss. Mainz, 1981. 269 p.

Bauer KH: Die Deutschen Chirurgenkongresse seit der 50. Tagung aus der Sicht ihrer Vorsitzenden. Berlin, New York, Springer-Verlag, 1983. ix, 262 p.

Becker T: Das chirurgische Erbe. Erwin Payr zum Gedenken. **Zentralbl Chir** 1981;106(23):1563-8

Bienengräber A: Wilhelm Busch und die Medizin. **Zentralbl Chir** 1980;105(24):1644-52

Boschung U: Iatromechanik and Chirurgie bei Lorenz Heister. **Gesnerus** 1983;40(1-2):31-41

Burmeister KJ, Lange-Pfautsch R: Maxim Zetkin--Kommunist und Arzt (1883-1965). **Z Arztl Fortbild (Jena)** 1983;77(16):695-7

Faller A: Welchen Platz nimmt Stensens anatomische Forschung in Lorenz Heisters Chirurgie und Anatomie ein? **Gesnerus** 1983;40(1-2):55-66

Geiger A: Lorenz Heister als Geburtshelfer und gynäkologischer Chirurg. Vergleichende Untersuchung anhand der verschiedenen Auflagen seiner 'Chirurgie'. Zürich, Juris Druck, 1983. 140 p. (Zürcher Medizingeschichtliche Abhandlungen, Neue Reihe, Nr. 162).

Genschorek W: Wegbereiter der Chirurgis: Johann Friedrich Dieffenbach, Theodor Billroth. Leipzig, Hirzel, Teubner, 1983. 252 p.

Gütgemann A: In Memoriam Freiherr von Redwitz. Bonn, Hanstein, 1966. 40 p.

Hamelmann H: Zur Geschichte der Vereinigung Nordwestdeutscher Chirurgen: zur 125. Tagung 12.-14. Juni 1980. Lübeck, Wullenwever, 1980?. 103 p.

Hauben DJ: Das chirurgische Erbe. Bernhard Rudolf Conrad Langenbeck (1810-1887). **Zentralbl Chir** 1984;109(20):1338-9

Hesekiel T, ed: Ein deutscher Chirurg und seine Frau in Japan vor 100 Jahren. Briefe von Dr. Wilhelm Schultze und seiner Frau Emma geb. Wegscheider an die Eltern Dr. Wegscheider in Berlin aus Japan 1878-1881. Lübeck, (the author), 1980. 316 p.

Kahle E: Klinkosch, Joseph Thaddäus. In Neue Deutsche Biographie 12. 1980. p. 101-2.

Kenéz J: F. Esmarch jelentösége a hadisebészet fejlödésében. **Orv Hetil** 1984 Jul 8;125(28):1708-10

Kern E: 100 Jahre Chirurgie. **Fortschr Med** 1982 Dec 16;100(47-48):2199-206

Kudlien F, Andree C: Sauerbruch und der Nationalsozialismus. **Medizinhist J** 1980;15(3):201-222

Leibecke-Englisch B: Die lokale Wundbehandlung aus pharmakologischer and pharmazeutischer Sicht in der deutschsprachigen medizinischen Literatur von 1800 bis 1867. Diss. Mainz, 1979. 89p.

Linde E: Ernst von Bergmann. Rückblick auf das Leben anlässlich der Einweihung der Sanitätsakademie in München. **MMW** 1981 May 1;123(18):751-2

Moll J: Das chirurgische Erbe. Ludwik Rydygier (1850-1920). **Zentralbl Chir** 1983;108(23):1532-5

Neumann A, Heinrich P: Die Bedeutung des Magdeburger Chirurgen Werner Hagedorn (1831 bis 1894) für die Einführung der Antiseptik auf dem europäischen Kontinent. **Zentralbl Chir** 1982;107(11):617-20

Paul U: Das chirurgische Erbe. Albert Hoffa. **Zentralbl Chir** 1981;106(13):901-3

Paul U: Das chirurgische Erbe. Franz König (1832-1910)--Weg und Wandel der Chirurgie seiner Zeit. **Zentralbl Chir** 1983;108(22):1451-6

Pies E: Ich bin der Doktor Eisenbarth. Arzt der Landstrasse. Eine Bildbiographie über das Leben und Wirken des volkstümlichen und berümten Chirurgen Johann Andreas Eisenbarth (1663-1727). Genf, Ariston, 1977. 306 p.

Probst J: Lorenz Heister, 1683-1758 Praeceptor Chirurgiae. **Unfallchirurgie** 1984 Feb;10(1):1-8

Rocchietta S: Vita avventurosa di Johann Andreas Eisenbarth (1663-1727), chirurgo e medico girovago. **Minerva Med** 1981 Jan 28;72(3):173-4

Rodegra H: Johann Carl Georg Fricke (1790-1841): Wegbereiter einer klinischen Chirurgie in Deutschland. Herzogenrath, Murken-Altrogge, 1983. 203 p. (Studien zur Geschichte des Krankenhauswesens, 20)

Romm S: Johann Friedrich August von Esmarch. **Plast Reconstr Surg** 1983 Feb;71(2):271-3

Romm S: The person behind the name: Martin Kirschner. **Plast Reconstr Surg** 1983 Jul;72(1):104-7

Schmauss AK: Das chirurgische Erbe. Johann Friedrich August von Esmarch--Leben und Werk (9. 1. 1823-23. 2. 1908). **Zentralbl Chir** 1983;108(24):1577-83

Schober KL: Das chirurgische Erbe. Richard von Volkmann zum 150. Geburtstag am 17. 8. 1980. **Zentralbl Chir** 1980;105(24):1635-43

Schober KL: Das chirurgische Erbe. Theodor Billroth und seine norddeutsche Heimat. **Zentralbl Chir** 1982;107(20):1317-23

Schober KL: Das chirurgische Erbe: Tragische Chirurgenschicksale. 1882: Die Tragödie des Dr. Block. **Zentralbl Chir** 1984;109(5):366-73

Schober KL: Gedächtnisvorlesung zum 150. Geburtstag von Richard von Volkmann, dem Mit-Gründer der Deutschen Gesellschaft für Chirurgie. **Langenbecks Arch Chir** 1981;355:597-606

Schober KL: Teodor Bil'rot i sovremennaia khirurgiia. **Khirurgiia (Mosk)** 1981 Feb;(2):116-7

Schober KL: Vor etwa hundert Jahren (31). **Zentralbl Chir** 1981;106(11):753-6 (continued periodically)

Schreiber HW: Chirurgie im Wandel der Zeit 1945-1983. Berlin, New York, Springer-Verlag, 1983. xviii, 419 p.

Taubert E: Das chirurgische Erbe. Das Wirken Georg Axhausens an der Chirurgischen Klinik der Charité--Berlin. **Zentralbl Chir** 1983;108(14):913-7

Waas G: Die Berufung von August Bier (1861-1949) an die Berliner Universität im Jahre 1907. **Z Arztl Fortbild (Jena)** 1980 Oct 15;74(20):982-7

Weiss C, Specker H, Winckelmann HJ: Die Medizinalgesetzgebung in Württemberg im 19. Jahrhundert. **MMW** 1983 Nov 4;125(44):1005-10

Winau R, Vaubel E: Chirurgen in Berlin. 100 Porträts. Berlin, New York, Walter de Gruyter, 1983. 106 p.

Winkelmann O: Werner Körte. **Neue Dtsch Biogr** 1980;12:395-6

Winkler EA: Ernst Unger: a pioneer in modern surgery. **J Hist Med Allied Sci** 1982 Jul;37(3):269-86

Wirth M: Das Leben und Wirken des Chirurgen Cajetan von Textor. Diss. Würzburg, 1980. 107 p.

Wolff H: Billroth in Berlin. **Zentralbl Chir** 1982;107(20):1324-6

Zenker R: Die Chirurgie Martin Kirschners in unserer Zeit. **MMW** 1980 Feb 29;122(9):318-9

### Great Britain

Anning ST: William Hey, F.R.S.: the father of Leeds surgery. **Proc Leeds Philos Lit Soc (Lit Hist Sect)** 1980;17(5):101-11

Atkins H: Memoirs of a surgeon. London, Springwood, 1977. xiv, 265 p.

Austin F: The Letters of William Home Clift, 1803-1832. Dorset, Meldon House, 1983. ix, 115 p.

Beneš V, Benešová Z: Horsleyv vosk. **Rozhl Chir** 1982 Feb;61(2):141-3

Brahma B, Singh M: The man behind the name: Ernest William Hey Groves 1872-1944. **NATNEWS** 1982 Jun;19(6):26

Brahma B, Singh M: What lies behind a name? (Sir Thomas Spencer Wells 1818-1897). **NATNEWS** 1981 Jul;18(7):15

Burke JF: Ashley A. Miles and the prevention of infection following surgery. **Arch Surg** 1984 Jan;119(1):17-9

Capper WM, Johnson D, ed: The faith of a surgeon. Belief and experience in the life of Arthur Rendle Short. Exeter, England, Paternoster Press, 1976. 156 p.

Carter L: Snatching the thyroid. **Nurs Times** 1984 Mar 7-13;80(10):38

Carty MA: The examination of a young surgeon. Hand-colored etching by George Cruikshank, from The Scourge, 1811. **J Hist Med Allied Sci** 1981 Apr;36(2):214

Cohen B: John Hunter's application of science to surgery. **Ann R Coll Surg Engl** 1984 Jan;66(1):59-62

Collis JL: The history of British oesophageal surgery. **Thorax** 1982 Nov;37(11):795-802

Douglas DM: Sir James Rögnvald Learmonth. In Dictionary of national biography, 1961-1970. Suppl. 8, 1981. p. 638-40.

Drummond CG: Adam Drummond of Megginch, surgeon-apothecary. **Pharm Hist (London)** 1971 Dec;2(3):3-5

Estévez R: Sir James Paget. **Rev Med Chil** 1984 Jul;112(7):740-3

Fraser I: Sir William MacCormac and his times. **Ann R Coll Surg Engl** 1983 Sep;65(5):339-46

Gelfand M: Joseph Lister. **Cent Afr J Med** 1981 Feb;27(2):31-4

Goldstein HB: Sir James Paget. **Am J Dermatopathol** 1980 Spring;2(1):27-31

Gray C: The remarkable surgical collection of John Hunter. **Can Med Assoc J** 1983 May 15;128(10):1225-8

Greenwood RD: Surgical treatment for facial hemangioma, 1834. **Ala Med** 1984 Sep;54(3):27

Guy JR: Surgeons and surgery in Victorian Yeovil. **Bristol Med Chir J** 1984 Apr;99(370):48-50

Hamilton D, Lamb M: Surgeons and surgery. In Checkland O, Lamb M, ed: Health care as social history; the Glasgow case. Aberdeen, Aberdeen University Press, 1982. p. 74-85.

Hamilton D: The nineteenth-century surgical revolution--antisepsis or better nutrition? **Bull Hist Med** 1982 Spring;56(1):30-40

Harrison SH: Accident surgery--the life and times of William Gissane. **Injury** 1984 Nov;16(3):145-54

Keynes G: The gates of memory. Oxford, Clarendon, 1981. xi, 428 p.

Moore AM: Sir Hugh Lett. In Dictionary of national biography, 1961-1970. Suppl. 8, 1981. p. 650-1.

Moran HM: Looking back: Lister. **Lamp** 1981 Mar;38(3):57-60

Murley R: Peace and strife in Hunter's time. (Part I). **Ann R Coll Surg Engl** 1982 Jan;64(1):20-8

Pattison I: The Veterinary Surgeons Act, 1881. **Vet Rec** 1981 Feb 21;108(8):157-60

Peltier LF: The classic. The growth of bone. Chapter III. Osteogenic power of bone bereft of periosteum. William Macewen, F.R.S. **Clin Orthop** 1983 Apr;(174):5-14

Rains AJ: The continuing message. **Ann R Coll Surg Engl** 1984 May;66(3):151-8

Ratliff AH: Ernest William Hey Groves and his contributions to orthopaedic surgery. **Ann R Coll Surg Engl** 1983 May;65(3):203-6

Ravitch MM: Sir Astley Paston Cooper. **Bull Am Coll Surg** 1977 Feb;62(2):17-20

Reed K, Grage TB: Our surgical heritage. The Paget tradition revisited. **Am J Surg** 1982 Nov;144(5):498-503
Rogers L: Odabrana poglavlja iz ratne kirurgije 8. Britanske armije. **Lijec Vjesn** 1979 Nov;101(11):699-701
Ross JP, LeFanu WR, ed: Lives of the Fellows of the Royal College of Surgeons of England 1965-1973. London, Pitman Medical, 1981. 405 p.
Sellors TH: Sir Henry Sessions Souttar. In Dictionary of national biography, 1961-1970. Suppl. 8, 1981. p. 969-70.
Shenoy BV, Scheithauer BW: Sir James Paget, F.R.S. **Mayo Clin Proc** 1983 Jan;58(1):51-5
Shepherd JA: Lawson Tait, the rebellious surgeon (1845-1899). Lawrence, Kansas, Coronado Press, xv, 249 p.
Sigsworth EM, Swan P: An eighteenth-century surgeon and apothecary: William Elmhirst (1721-1773). **Med Hist** 1982 Apr;26(2):191-8
Sigsworth EM: William Elmhirst 1721-1773: surgeon-apothecary--and medical frontiersman. **Pharm Hist (London)** 1984 Sep;14(3):6-7
Smith AN: Pringle's maneuver. **Curr Surg** 1982 Jan-Feb;39(1):12-7
Tansey V, Mekie DE: Report of the Museum of the Royal College of Surgeons of Edinburgh. **J R Coll Surg Edinb** 1980 Mar;25(2):67-75 contd
Tansey V, Mekie DE: The museum of the Royal College of Surgeons of Edinburgh. **J R Coll Surg Edinb** 1980 Jul;25(4):248-56
Tansey V, Mekie DE: The Museum of the Royal College of Surgeons of Edinburgh. **J R Coll Surg Edinb** 1980 May;25(3):188-93 (continued periodically)
Tansey V, Mekie DE: The Museum of the Royal College of Surgeons of Edinburgh (Part 4). **J R Coll Surg Edinb** 1980 Nov;25(6):481-4
Taylor S: Surgical Research Society, 1954--79. **Lancet** 1979 Dec 8;2(8154):1234
Tröhler U: Quantification in British medicine and surgery 1750-1830. Ph.D. Diss., University of London, 1978.
Walker JB: Charles John Bond of Leicester (1856-1939). **J R Soc Med** 1984 Apr;77(4):316-24
Watkins AH: James Scott, the famous surgeon of Bromley, 1770-1848. **Bromley Local Hist** 1979;4:41-7
Wharton M: Sir Benjamin Brodie, Bt. (1783-1862). **Ann R Coll Surg Engl** 1983 Nov;65(6):418-9
Wilkinson AW: Development of modern neonatal surgery. **Trans Hunter Soc** 1978-80;37-38:65-83

### Hungary

Back F, Ritter L: Adatok a magyar proctológia történetéhez (1700-1847). **Orv Hetil** 1983 Jun 26;124(26):1581-82
Benkö F: A vatta hazai elötörténete. **Orv Hetil** 1984 Nov 25;125(48):2965
A hazai porcragasztás prioritástaról: **Orv Hetil** 1984 Dec 16;125(51):3150
Littmann I: A 125 éves Orvosi Hetilap és a modern sebészet kialakulása. Merre tart ma a sebészet? **Orv Hetil** 1982 Feb 7;123(6):323-6
Péterffy I: Híradás két felvilágosodás kori jeles orvosról. **Orv Hetil** 1983 Jul 31;124(31):1895-6
Robicsek F, Littmann L: The first reported case of external heart massage (János Balassa). **Clin Cardiol** 1983 Nov;6(11):569, 571
Szállási A: Rekviem a 'Gyógyászat'--ért Schachter Miksa szerkesztése ürügyén. **Orv Hetil** 1980 Dec 14;121(50):3073-6
Szeleczky G: Hüttl Tivadar centenáriumára. **Orv Hetil** 1984 Aug 19;125(34):2081-2
Zallár A: Huszonöt éve hunyt el jáki Gyula professzor. **Orv Hetil** 1983 Sep 18;124(38):2321-2

### India

Acharya AM: The first Indian War of Independence and military surgery. **Bull Indian Inst Hist Med (Hyderabad)** 1975 Oct;5(4):225-39
Thatte DG, Tiwari SP, Tiwari GP: Techniques of venupuncture (śiravedha) in India in 18th century. **Indian J Hist Sci** 1981;16(2):181-8

### Ireland

Hughes ES, Dooley B: The Royal College of Surgeons in Ireland 1784-1984. **Aust NZ J Surg** 1984 Dec;54(6):502
Kinnear N: The surgical section and surgical developments over the century. **Ir J Med Sci** 1983 Jan;152(1):44-8
O'Brien E: The bicentenary of the Royal College of Surgeons in Ireland, 1784-1984. **Br Med J [Clin Res]** 1983 Dec 24-31;287(6409):1988-90
Platt H: The foundation of the Association of Surgeons of Great Britain and Ireland. **Br J Surg** 1982 Oct;69(10):561-3
Walsh J: Who was William Doolin? **Ir Med J** 1983 Oct;76(10):436-7
Widdess JD: The Royal College of Surgeons in Ireland and its medical school, 1784-1984. Third edition. Dublin, Royal College of Surgeons in Ireland, 1984. x, 194 p.

### Italy

Dondi RF: Uno strumento chirurgico dimenticato: le forbici del Valtolini. **Ann Osp Maria Vittoria Torino** 1980 Jul-Dec;23(7-12):289-94
Miniati M: Lo strumentario di G. A. Brambilla. **Kos** 1984 Feb;1(1):74-6
Montorsi W, Pezzuoli G, Guzzon V: Influenza della farmacologia di Emilio Trabucchi nelle discipline chirurgiche e parachirurgiche. **Minerva Med** 1982 May 7;73(19):1255-68
Pini UA: Medici e chirurghi parmigiani dell'ottocento. Notizie sulla vita e sulle opere. **Minerva Med** 1980 May 12;71(19-20):1393-8, 1461-6
Riunione straordinaria dei Consigli Comunale e Provinciale in occasione del 1 centenario della morte di Francesco Rizzoli (24-5-1880) e della nascita di Vittorio Putti (1-3-1880): **Chir Organi Mov** 1979 Jul-Aug;65(4):367-98

### Netherlands

Mees LF: Kennis en wijsheid, herinneringen aan leermeesters. **Ned Tijdschr Geneeskd** 1980 Aug 9;124(32):1354-6
Moulin D de: Heelkundige onderwerpen in het Nederlandsch Weekblad voor Genesskundigen (1851-1856). **Ned Tijdschr Geneeskd** 1981 Aug 25;125(35):1427-30
Van Lieburg MJ: The instrument-collection of Peter Vink, a chapter in the development of the surgical profession in the Netherlands during the 18th century. **Janus** 1980:67(1-2-3):207-19

### New Zealand

Bell FG: Surgeon's saga. Wellington, Reed, [1968] 216 p.
Dudley HA: From Edinburgh, an academic surgeon. **Aust NZ J Surg** 1981 Jun;51(3):247-50
Kenny PJ: The founders of the College. **Aust NZ J Surg** 1981 Feb;51(1):95-101
Lambert G: Peter Wilson: colonial surgeon. Palmerston North, N.Z., Dunmore Press, 1981. 213 p.
Wright-St Clair RE: Robert Hall Bakewell, letter writer. **NZ Med J** 1982 Nov 24;95(720):820-2

### Norway

Hjort EF: Vis medicatrix naturae og kirurgiens gjennombrudd i Norge. **Tidsskr Nor Laegeforen** 1981 Apr;101(11):641-5

### Poland

Gaertner H: Ordynatorzy oddziału chirurgicznego Krakowskiego Szpitala Braci Miłosiernych (obecnie im. Edmunda Biernackiego). **Nasza Przeslosc** 1979;(51):179-204
Kłodziński S: Lek. Zbigniew Sobieszczański. **Przegl Lek** 1984;41(1):131-6
Marczyński A: Dr Tadeusz Boczoń. **Przegl Lek** 1984;41(1):127-31
Piotrowski E: Jan Mikulicz Radecki we Wrocławiu. **Arch Hist Med (Warsz)** 1979;42(3):351-7
Sieńkowski E: Dr med. Leon Stanisław Szuman (1852-1920), chirurg, społecznik, poeta. **Arch Hist Med (Warsz)** 1984;47(1):133-41
Skrobacki A, Völker A: Ze starań Profesora Ludwika Bierkowskiego o pozyskanie katedry w berlinie w 1847 r. **Arch Hist Med (Warsz)** 1979;42(3):303-8

### South Africa

Hickman R: The J. S. Marais Surgical Laboratory - 21 years old. **S Afr Med J** 1980 Mar;57(16):677-81
Nel CJ: Die departement chirurgie, universiteit van die oranje-vrystaat--die eerste tien jaar. **S Afr J Surg** 1980 Sep;19(3):81-6

### Spain

Balaguer Perigüell E, Ballester Añon R: El colegio di cirugía de Zaragoza, intento de renovación de las instituciones médicas aragonesas. 2. Jornadas sobre el estado actual de los Estudios sobre Aragón, diciembre de 1979, Esp. 1980: 713-8.
Ferrer D: Representación para el establecimiento de un Colegio de Ciruxia en Barcelona a la manera del de Cádiz (1759). In Congrés International d'Història de la Medicina Catalana, 2nd, Barcelona, 1975. Llibre d'Actes. Barcelona, Socitra, 1977. p. 259-61.
Garcia Gonzalez R, Prieto Cantero A: Licenciados en medicina y cirugia graduados en la Universidad de Valladolid (1871-1936). Vallodolid, Universidad de Valladolid, 1979. 383 p. (Acta Historico-Medica Vallisoletana, Monografias, IX)
Herrera Casado A: Vida y obra del doctor D. Juan Creus y Manso (1828-1897). **An Otorrinolaringol Ibero Am** 1980;7(2):109-32
Kagan RL: From trade to profession: surgical education in eighteenth-century Spain. **Hist Educ Q** 1978;18(2):195-200
Matilla Gómez V: Sesión necrológica del Excmo. Sr. D. Manuel Gómez Durán. Día 3 de abril de 1984. **An R Acad Nac Med (Madr)** 1984;101(2):273-88
Parellada Feliu J: Cinc manuscrits catalans escrits entre els anys 1749 i 1835. In Congrés International d'Història de la Medicina Catalana, 2nd, Barcelona, 1975. Llibre d'Actes. Barcelona, Socitra, 1977. p. 235-48.
Peña Páez I de la, Viesca Treviño C, Casales Ortiz G: Presencia de la cirugía española en México en el siglo XVIII. (Real Colegio de Cirugía). In International Congress of the History of Medicine, 27th, Barcelona, 1980. Actas. Barcelona, Acadèmia de Ciències Mèdiques de Catalunya

i Balears, 1981. p. 195–8.

Pi-Figueras J: Els serveis de cirurgia moderna a l'Hospital de la Santa Creu i Sant Pau. In Congrés International d'Història de la Medicina Catalana, 2nd, Barcelona, 1975. Llibre d'Actes. Barcelona, Socitra, 1977. p. 157–61.

Pi-Figueras J: La cirugía moderna a Catalunya: de Cardenal al 1936. In Congrés Internacional d'Història de la Medicina Catalana, 1st, Barcelona-Montpellier, 1970. Llibr d'actes. Barcelona, Editorial Scientia, 1971. v 2, p. 193–212.

Riera J: Cirurgía española ilustrada y su comunicación con Europa (Estudio y documentos de un influjo cultural). Valladolid, Universidad de Vallodolid, 1976. 332 p. (Acta Historico-Medica Vallisoletana, Monografias, VII)

Uranga E: Un ilustre anatónomo y cirujano con ideas necrofílicas del siglo XIX en Zaragoza. **Bol Real Soc Vascongada Amigos Pais** 1973;29(1–3):375–91

### Sweden

Arenander E: Kirurgi under föranestetisk tid--ur anteckningar efter Anders Johan Hagströms Operations Collegium. **Nord Medicinhist Arsb** 1981;:88–105

Bauer G: Sven Johanssons betydelse för höftfrakturernas behandling. **Sydsven Medicinhist Sallsk Arsskr** 1981;:12–29

Husberg K, Räf L: John Charnley efter 30 års arbete med höftledskirurgi: 'intuition och slump hjälpte fram genombrotten men protesens livslängd måste förbättras'. **Lakartidningen** 1982 Jun 9;79(23):2301–3

Kock W: Sven Sköldberg och ovariotomien en pionjärinsats i svensk gynekologi. **Nord Medicinhist Arsbok** 1983;:103–16

Larsson J: Hermann Boerhaave och 1700-talets Lund. **Sydsven Medicinhist Sallsk Arsskr** 1981;:53–64

Larsson J: Kirurgi och medicinsk teori vid Lunds Universitet under 1700-talet. En medicinhistorisk studie. (Supplementum nr 1). **Sydsven Medicinhist Sallsk Arsskr** 1982;Suppl V:1–262

Lindgren S: Ur svenska kirurgförbundets historia. **Nord Medicinhist Arsb** 1981;:160–71

Lindskog BI: Otto Löfberg 1881–1954. **Sydsven Medicinhist Sallsk Arsskr** 1983;:65–76

Modig M: Karl XII:s siste fältskär. **Sydsven Medicinhist Sallsk Arsskr** 1983;:77–86

Riall CT: Surgical and medical devices and their origins. Chapter XX. The Swedish influence. **J Oper Room Res Inst** 1983 Jun;3(6):18–9, 22, 24

Thorén L: K. G. Lennander och kirurgien i Uppsala kring sekelskiftet. **Nord Medicinhist Arsb** 1984;:153–64

### Switzerland

Biaudet JC: Mathias Mayor (1775–1847). **Rev Med Suisse Romande** 1984 May;104(5):343–7

Buess H, Portmann ML: Berühmte Schweizer Arzte. **Gesnerus** 1980;37(3/4):289–306

Fraser I: Steinach operation. **Br Med J [Clin Res]** 1984 Jan 21;288(6412):242

Gaberthüel M: Krankengeschichten und Operationsberichte 1784–1811 nach den Aufzeichnungen von Johann Heinrich Steger (1767–1842) und Johann Jakob Steger (1798–1857). Zürich, Juris, 1980. 121 p. (Zürcher Medizingeschichtliche Abhandlungen, Neue Reihe, 140).

Kis J: Der Knochenpathologe Emil Looser (1877–1936). Zürich, Juris, 1982. 68 p. Zürcher Medizingeschichtliche Abhandlungen, Neue Reihe, 149; also Diss.).

Meyer-Salzmann M: Aus der medizinischen Vergangenheit in Langenthal. **Gesnerus** 1983;40(1–2):129–37

Morscher E: Entwicklungen in der Chirurgie: das Department Chirurgie der Universität Basel 1967–1983. Basel, Schwabe, 1983. 192 p.

Schneider S: Commentaires sur l'article de Jacques-Louis Reverdin: 'des opérations modernes de cure radicale des hernies'. **Rev Med Suisse Romande** 1980 Dec;100(12):1097–101

Stamm H: 50 Jahre medizinische Forschung in Waldenburg. **Gesnerus** 1983;40(3/4):281–90

Subrtová A: Jean de Carro (1770–1857) - příspěvek k biografi. **Cas Nar Muz** 1980;149(1–2):45–61

Verdan C: Historische Entwicklung der Beugesehnen-Chirurgie. **Handchirurgie** 1981;13(3–4):181–5

Zanobio B: Je le pansai, Dieu le guérit. Gli aforismi di chirurgia militare di Louis Appia (1818–1898) sulla cura delle ferite d'armi da fuoco. **G Accad Med Torino** 1980;143(Spec No):7–95

### United States

Abramson DJ: The surgical residency, the surgical clinic at the Walter Reed Army Medical Center. **Milit Med** 1982 Dec;147(12):1025–8

Ackerman LV: Dr. Evarts Graham and surgical pathology. **J Thorac Cardiovasc Surg** 1984 Nov;88(5 Pt 2):851–3

Adler S: The operation on President McKinley. In Plesur M, ed.: An American Historian: essays to honor Selig Adler (Buffalo: State U. of N.Y., 1980): 37–49.

Aldrete JA, Marron GM, Wright AJ: The first administration of anesthesia in military surgery: on occasion of the Mexican-American War. **Anesthesiology** 1984 Nov;61(5):585–8

Allen R: The evolution of pediatric surgery. **J Pediatr Surg** 1980 Dec;15(6):711–8

Allen TD: Lest we forget. **South Med J** 1983 Jun;76(6):699–700

Allison HM: Doctor Amos Twitchell: pioneer surgeon. **Hist NH** 1978;33(2):167–79

Altemeier WA: Perspectives in surgical infections. **Surg Clin North Am** 1980 Feb;60(1):5–13

Baker HW: The general surgeon and cancer. **Am J Surg** 1980 May;139(5):606–7

Barger AC: Some of Carl Walter's contributions to Harvard Medical School and Hospitals. **Am J Surg** 1984 Nov;148(5):578–80

Baue AE: 60 years of the Archives of Surgery. July 1920–July 1980. **Arch Surg** 1980 Jul;115(7):809–11

Beahrs OH: Surgery of the head and neck--1896–1982. **Surg Gynecol Obstet** 1983 Aug;157(2):180–4

Beatty WK: Mary Harris Thompson--pioneer surgeon and hospital founder. **Proc Inst Med Chic** 1981 Jul-Sep;34(3):83–6

Beatty WK: Nicholas Senn -- surgeon and traveler. **Proc Inst Med Chic** 1980 Jan-Mar;33(1):8–9

Bing RJ: Carrel: a personal reminiscence. **JAMA** 1983 Dec 23–30;250(24):3297–8

Boyd DP: Doctor Lahey and his clinic. **Postgrad Med** 1984 Feb 15;75(3):14–6, 18

Brandt AM: Virginia Kneeland Frantz. In: Notable American women. The modern period. Cambridge, Mass., Belknap-Harvard Univ. Press, 1980. 4:247–8.

Bricker EM: Evarts A. Graham and the American College of Surgeons. **J Thorac Cardiovasc Surg** 1984 Nov;88(5 Pt 2):834–41

Brooks JR: Carl W. Walter, MD: surgeon, inventor, and industrialist. **Am J Surg** 1984 Nov;148(5):555–8

Brown HM: Reminiscences of Dr. Senn. **Milw Hist** 1981;4(3–4):87–94

Buchwald H: The scientist-surgeon. **Am J Surg** 1981 Aug;142(2):245–6

Buell FD: Nineteenth century surgeon: Dr. Alden March, founder, Albany Medical College, 1795–1869. Albany, Albany Medical College, 1981. 12 p.

Buess H: Nikolaus Senn (1844–1908), ein schweizerischer Pionier der Chirurgie in den USA. **Gesnerus** 1979;36(3–4):238–45

Bush RB: Max Thorek. In Dictionary of American Biography, Suppl. 6, 1956–1960. p. 631–2, 1980.

Butcher HR: Evarts Graham and surgical residency education. **J Thorac Cardiovasc Surg** 1984 Nov;88(5 Pt 2):848–50

Butcher HR: What's past is prologue. **Arch Surg** 1980 Apr;115(4):371–6

Cangi EC: Abraham Flexner's philanthrophy: the full-time system in the department of surgery at the University of Cincinnati College of Medicine, 1910–1930. **Bull Hist Med** 1982 Summer;56(2):160–74

Carmichael JL: Dr. James Monroe Mason, Jr. and his era in medicine. **J Med Assoc State Ala** 1982 May;51(11):30–7

Carmichael AG, ed: [John S. Bobbs]. **Indiana Med Hist Q** 1982;8(2):3–24

Carson RA: Selzer's surgeon as seer. **Perspect Biol Med** 1981 Winter;24(2):284–9

Clark D, Hyde GL: A brief history of the University of Kentucky Department of Surgery. **J Ky Med Assoc** 1984 Jul;82(7):343–7

Classic articles in colonic and rectal surgery. Robert Fulton Weir 1838–1927: An improved method of treating high-seated cancers of the rectum. **Dis Colon Rectum** 1982 Jul-Aug;25(5):503–7

Colp R Jr: Notes on Dr. William S. Halsted. **Bull NY Acad Med** 1984 Nov;60(9):876–87

Cowell HR: Osteomyelitis revisited: a 19th century case report. **Del Med J** 1982 May;54(5):263–5

Crellin JK: The surgical teaching of Philip Syng Physick. Durham, Medical History Program and the Trent Collection, Duke University Medical Center, 1981 vi, 101 p.

Cruft GE, Humphreys JW, Hermann RE, et al: Recertification in surgery, 1980. **Arch Surg** 1981 Aug;116(8):1093–6

Cushman P: Amos Evans, M.D.; surgeon on U.S.S. Constitution in War of 1812. **NY State J Med** 1980 Oct;80(11):1753–6

Delaney JJ: Leonard Freeman. **Colo Med** 1983 Aug;80(8):219–20

Duffy J: Rudolph Matas. In Dictionary of American Biography, Suppl. 6, 1956–1960. p. 434–5, 1980.

Dugan DJ: Aequanimitas revisited. **Am J Surg** 1982 Jul;144(1):3–7

Dunphy JE: Look back for tomorrow. **Bull Am Coll Surg** 1975 Dec;60(12):9–14

Eckert C: Evarts A. Graham and the American Board of Surgery. **J Thorac Cardiovasc Surg** 1984 Nov;88(5 Pt 2):842–7

Edlich RF: Reflections on Wangensteen's academic village. **Am J Surg** 1981 May;141(5):601–4

English PC: Shock, physiological surgery, and George Washington Crile. Medical innovation in the Progressive era. Westport, Connecticut, and London, Greenwood, 1980. xi, 271 p. (Contributions in medical history, 5)

The evolution of Mohs' surgery: **J Dermatol Surg Oncol** 1982 Aug;8(8):650–4

Festschrift to Dr. Samuel R. Powers, Jr. September 25, 1919 - March 27, 1980: **Arch Surg** 1981 Oct;116(10):1241–1356

Foraker AG: A reluctant surgeon at sea. **JAMA** 1981 Jun 12;245(22):2302–3

## SURGERY

Fortuine R: Traditional surgery of the Alaska natives. **Alaska Med** 1984 Jan–Mar;26(1):22–5
Geist DC: William Williams Keen, M.D. (1837–1932), surgeon and author. **Trans Stud Coll Physicians Phila** 1977 Apr;44(4):182–93
Gold SI: Robert Neumann: a pioneer in periodontal flap surgery. **J Periodontol** 1982 Jul;53(7):456–9
Graner JL, Frederick W: William Halsted's cocaine habit. **Arch Ophthalmol** 1984 Dec;102(12):1746
Greenwood RD: 19th century medicine in Indiana. An 1869 clinical report by J. S. Bobbs. **Indiana Med** 1984 Jun;77(6):476
Hamlin H: Oskar Hirsch. **Surg Neurol** 1981 Dec;16(6):391–3
Hanlon CR: The surgical presidency. **Ann Surg** 1982 Sep;196(3):233–8
Harvey AM: Alfred Blalock. In Dictionary of American biography, 1961–1965. Suppl. 7, 1981. p. 59.
Harvey AM: Orthopaedic surgery at Johns Hopkins: a heritage of excellence in clinical practice, training and research. **Johns Hopkins Med J** 1982 Jun;150(6):221–45
Harvey AM: The influence of William Stewart Halsted's concepts of surgical training. **Johns Hopkins Med J** 1981 May;148(5):215–36
Hassler WW: Dr. Hunter Holmes McGuire: surgeon to Stonewall Jackson, the Confederacy, and the Nation. **Va Cavalcade** 1982;32(2):52–61
Hayles AB, Key JD: Adventures of two prairie pioneers. **Minn Med** 1981 Oct;64(10):629–32
Heck CV: Fifty years of progress: in recognition of the 50th anniversary of the American Academy of Orthopaedic Surgeons. Chicago, American Academy of Orthopaedic Surgeons, 1983. vi, 361 p.
Herman JR: Operating furniture. 'Medical briefs'. **Urology** 1981 Sep;18(3):295 H
Hufnagel CA, Thorn GW: Observations of a colleague (Carl W. Walter). **Am J Surg** 1984 Nov;148(5):581–3
Jain KM, Swan KG, Casey KF: Nobel prize winners in surgery. **Am Surg** 1982 Oct;48(10):495–500
Johnson CS: Anesthesia and photography. **Harv Mag** 1980 Jul–Aug;82(6):57
Johnston GA: Tribute to a Chicago surgeon: Ulysses Grant Dailey. **IMJ** 1983 Jan;163(1):35–6
Jones OP: A peripatetic surgery in Valhalla (Frank Hastings Hamilton). **Am J Surg** 1982 Mar;143(3):370–3
Key JD, Callahan JA, Nelson CW: William J. Mayo--centennial notes. **Minn Med** 1982 Oct;65(10):636–8
King WH: Caroline Hampton Halsted and her family, revisited. **NC Med J** 1982 Jul;43(7):501–4
Koop CE: Pediatric surgery: the newest specialty for the youngest patient. **Trans Stud Coll Physicians Phila** 1981 Sep;5(3 no 3):195–208
Kukral AJ: The Southwestern surgical story. **Am J Surg** 1982 Dec;144(6):600–4
Kundsin RB: Creative crusader against sepsis (Carl W. Walter). **Am J Surg** 1984 Nov;148(5):573–4
Lam CR: The Central Surgical Association turns forty. Some highlights of the first twenty years. **Henry Ford Hosp Med J** 1982;30(2):77–80
Landor JH: Lester Reynold Dragstedt--physiologist-surgeon. **Gastroenterology** 1981 Apr;80(4):846–53
Laufman H: Carl Walter's half century of achievement in asepsis. **Am J Surg** 1984 Nov;148(5):565–70
Laufman H: Loyal Davis and the young surgeon. **Surg Gynecol Obstet** 1983 Aug;157(2):123–8
Leonard AS: A tribute to Dr. Owen H. Wangensteen, 'the Chief'. **Surgery** 1981;89:402–6
Letton AH: Pyramids or Parthenons? **J Surg Oncol** 1983 Jun;23(2):63–9
Lillehei RC: The Wangensteen tradition: what it is and how can we perpetuate it? **Minn Med** 1981 Oct;64(10):626–8
Longmire WP: Changing patterns of surgical training and practice. **Am J Surg** 1981 Jun;141(6):632–7
Longmire WP: Loyal Davis' personal qualities and their influence on American surgery. **Surg Gynecol Obstet** 1983 Aug;157(2):114–7
Longmire WP: Surgical upbringing in America. **Bull Am Coll Surg** 1978 Sep;63(9):6–11
Longmire WP: Two great American surgeons, each with four aces. **Pharos** 1983 Summer;46(3):9–14
Loughry CW: Fifty years of surgical education at Akron City Hospital. **Ohio State Med J** 1982 Oct;78(10):723–6
Lowell JD: The ultraviolet environment in a nutshell (Carl W. Walter). **Am J Surg** 1984 Nov;148(5):575–7
McDonald JC: Louisiana's place in American surgery. **J La State Med Soc** 1984 Jan;136(1):3–8
McDonell KM: Surgery in early nineteenth century Indiana. **Indiana Med Hist Q** 1980;6(4):3–23
MacDougall JD: Joseph Eastman, M.D., LL.D; citizen, soldier, surgeon and medical educator. **Indiana Med Hist Q** 1974;1(2):26–30
MacKay W: Salesman surgeon. New York, McGraw-Hill, 1978. xii, 187 p.
McLean RB: Leonard D. Heaton--military surgeon. **Milit Med** 1982 Sep;147(9):717–27
Mathewson C: Historical review of the San Francisco Surgical Society. **Am J Surg** 1982 Feb;143(2):246–51
Melick DW: Surgical therapy of pulmonary tuberculosis--a rare necessity of the 1980's. An historical review. **Ariz Med** 1983 Mar;40(3):158–9
Miller JM: William Stewart Halsted and the use of the surgical rubber glove. **Surgery** 1982 Sep;92(3):541–3
Moore FD: The changing mission and status of surgery 1780 to 1980. **Arch Surg** 1983 Sep;118(9):1013–8
Moore FD: Zabdiel Boylston and colonial surgery. American surgery and public health in the early 18th century. **Bull Am Coll Surg** 1983 May;68(5):13–7
Murray JE, Zollinger RM: Carl Walter Appreciation Day: April 28, 1984. **Am J Surg** 1984 Nov;148(5):552–3
Ochsner A: To our founder [Franklin H. Martin], with reflections. **Bull Am Coll Surg** 1981;66(5):26–30
Olch PD: Evarts Ambrose Graham. In Dictionary of American Biography, Suppl. 6, 1956–1960. p. 245–7, 1980.
Olch PD: Owen H. Wangensteen (1898–1981). **Bull Hist Med** 1981;55:260–2
Olch PD: Robert Elman. In Dictionary of American Biography, Suppl. 6, 1956–1960. p. 189–90, 1980.
Paquet JB: The gloving of a nurse (Caroline Hampton). **Nurs Success Today** 1984 Summer;1(2):44
Parrott JR, Harrison DB: Surgically dividing pianists' hands. **J Hand Surg** 1980 Nov;5(6):619
Peschel ER: 'Alchemy of the word'--language and 'the knife' a commentary on Richard Selzer's work. **Pharos** 1979 Winter;42(1):25–32
Rainer JK: Cervical disc surgery--a historical review. **J Tenn Med Assoc** 1984 Jan;77(1):12–6
Ravitch MM: A century of surgery. The history of the American Surgical Association. 2 vols. Philadelphia and Toronto, Lippincott, 1981.
Ravitch MM: The American Surgical Association. The peaks of excitement. **Ann Surg** 1980 Sep;192(3):282–7
Rhoads JE: Development of surgical nutrition at the University of Pennsylvania. **JPEN** 1980 Sep–Oct;4(5):464–6
Rhoads JE: The evolution of intravenous hyperalimentation. **World J Surg** 1982 Jan;6(1):144–8
Riall CT, Hilzinger F: Surgical and medical devices and their origins. Chapter XVIII. Surgical instrument manufacturers. **J Oper Room Res Inst** 1983 Feb;3(2):34–9
Romm S: Maurice Howe Richardson. **Plast Reconstr Surg** 1983 Mar;71(3):432–4
Rutkow IM: The letters of William Halsted and Alexis Carrel. **Surg Gynecol Obstet** 1980 Nov;151(5):676–88
Rutkow IM: William Halsted and Rudolph Matas: their unique alliance. **Surgery** 1980 May;87(5):524–38
Sabiston DC: Deryl Hart: leader in the development of the Duke University Medical Center. **NC Med J** 1983 Jul;44(7):441–2
Saffron MH: James Peter Warbasse. In Dictionary of American Biography, Suppl. 6, 1956–1960. p. 663–5, 1980.
Saffron MH: Russell Story Fowler. In Dictionary of American Biography, Suppl. 6, 1956–1960. p. 214–15, 1980.
Sandusky WR: Frank L. Meleney: pioneer surgeon-bacteriologist. **Arch Surg** 1983 Feb;118(2):151–5
Scannell JG: A sidelight of cholecystography. **Pharos** 1983 Summer;46(3):42
Schmitt W: Das chirurgische Erbe. Zur Geschichte der modernen Chirurgie: ein Abriss. Teil II. **Zentralbl Chir** 1982;107(13):798–808
Schneck JM: S. Weir Mitchell, M.D. (1829 to 1914) and D. Hayes Agnew, M.D. (1818 to 1892). Neuropsychiatrist's poetic tribute to a surgeon. **NY State J Med** 1982 Jul;82(8):1264–8
Shell DH, Sparkman RS: John Allan Wyeth, MD. Surgeon, soldier, author and founder of postgraduate medical education in America. **Am J Surg** 1980 Sep;140(3):447–56
Shields RT: He helped shape Virginia: Dr. Wiliam Fleming, 1728–1795. **Va Med** 1982 Jul;109(7):441–5
Shires GT: The fourth surgical renaissance? **Ann Surg** 1980 Sep;192(3):269–81
Stephenson GW: A history of the Committee on Pre- and Postoperative Care. **Bull Am Coll Surg** 1981 Nov;66(11):21–2, 24, 26
Stephenson GW: The College's role in hospital standardization. **Bull Am Coll Surg** 1981 Feb;66(2):17–29
Sterling Bunnell; 1882–1957: **J Hand Surg** 1982 May;7(3):217–20
Thomson EH: Harvey Cushing, surgeon, author, artist. New York, Neale Watson Academic Publications, 1981, xvii, 347 p.
Tilney NL: Carl Walter and the evolution of the Surgical Research Laboratory: 1937 through 1949. **Am J Surg** 1984 Nov;148(5):584–9
Tilney NL: Harvey Cushing and the surgical research laboratory. **Surg Gynecol Obstet** 1980 Aug;151(2):263–70
Tilney NL: The marrow of the tragedy (Harvey Cushing). **Surg Gynecol Obstet** 1983 Oct;157(4):380–8
Tilney NL: The original Peter Bent Brigham Hospital surgical staff. **Surg Gynecol Obstet** 1981 Nov;153(5):741–6
Touloukian RJ: The legacy of Connecticut surgery: case histories revisited. **Conn Med** 1981 Apr;45(4):241–4
Trice ER: Philip Syng Physick, father of American surgery. **Va Med** 1981 Jul;108(7):456–9
Vandam LD: Robert Hinckley's 'The First operation with ether'. **Anesthesiology** 1980 Jan;52(1):62–70
Wagner FB: Revisit of Samuel D. Gross, M.D. **Surg Gynecol Obstet** 1981 May;152(5):663–74

Wagner FB: The founding fathers and centennial history of the Philadelphia Academy of Surgery. **Ann Surg** 1980 Jul;192(1):1–8
Wangensteen OH: Great opportunity: a binding summons to achieve. Musings upon surgical history. **Am J Surg** 1981 Nov;142(5):605–14
Wangensteen OH: Mandated celibacy in the academic arena. **Surg Gynecol Obstet** 1980 May;150(5):739–45
Wangensteen OH: Surgery's reawakening. **Minn Med** 1979 Dec;62(12):879–82
Warren WD: Not for the profession ... for the people. **Ann Surg** 1983 Sep;198(3):241–50
Watne AI, Bartholomew S: Giants in the hills: a brief history of the West Virginia Chapter, American College of Surgeons. **W Va Med J** 1982 Jul;78(7):168–71
Wilbur DA: The inimitable surgeon Pleadwell. **US Navy Med** 1983 May–Jun;74(3):5–10
Williams WH: Norman Thomas Kirk. In Dictionary of American Biography, Suppl. 6, 1956–1960. p. 344–5, 1980.
Wirthlin LS: Joseph Smith's boyhood operation: an 1813 surgical success. **Brigham Young Univ Stud** 1981;21(2):131–54
Wolff E: The history and development of surgical tables for large animals. **VM SAC** 1981 Jul;76(7):1033–5
Wu YK: Reminiscence of personal association with American thoracic and cardiovascular surgery. **Am J Surg** 1980 Jun;139(6):765–70
Yancey AG: US postage stamp issued in honor of Charles R. Drew, MD, MDSc. **J Natl Med Assoc** 1982 Jun;74(6):561–5

**Uruguay**

Praderi RC, Bergalli L: Notas para una historia de la cirugia Uruguaya desde la independencia hasta principios de este siglo. Montevideo, (The authors?), 1981. 44 p.

**USSR**

Aĭrapetova RA, Kiazimov RA, ed: M. A. Topchibashev. Baku, Izd-vo Akademii nauk Azerbaĭdzhanskoĭ SSR, 1965. 66 p.
Aleksanian IV, Knopov MSh: Akhutinskoe dvizhenie. **Voen Med Zh** 1981;(7):74–5
Aleksanian IV, Knopov MSh: K 125-letiiu so dnia rozhdeniia G. I. Turnera. **Khirurgiia (Mosk)** 1984 Jan;(1):154–5
Aleksanian IV, Knopov MSh: Vidnyĭ sovetskiĭ khirurg V. S. Levit (k 100-letiiu so dnia rozhdeniia). **Klin Khir** 1983 Jun;6:58–60
Aleksanian IV, Knopov MSh: Vladimir Semenovich Levit (k 100-letiiu so dnia rozhdeniia). **Voen Med Zh** 1983 Jun;6:72–3
Aliev MA, Ioffe LTs, Chekurov PR, et al: Razvitie nekotorykh vidov spetsializirovannoĭ khirurgicheskoĭ pomoschi v Kazakhstane. **Vestn Khir** 1983 Mar;130(3):17–23
Altschuller GI, Keenan WA: History of the development of painless surgery in Russia. **Bull NY Acad Med** 1982 Jun;58(5):493–502
Aminev AM: 125 let so dnia rozhdeniia Vasiliia Ivanovicha Razumovskogo. **Vestn Khir** 1983 May;130(5):137–9
Astapenko VG: Belorusskoe Nauchnoe Meditsinskoe Obshchestvo Khirurgov (k 50-letiiu obrazovaniia obshchestva). **Khirurgiia (Mosk)** 1980;1:113–4
Bagdasar'ian SM: Velikiĭ russkiĭ khirurg N. I. Pirogov (k 100-letiiu so dnia smerti). **Klin Med (Mosk)** 1982 Jul;60(7):111–5
Bagdasar'ian SM: Vydaiushchiĭsia sovetskiĭ uchenyĭ (k 40-letiiu prisvoeniia zvaniia Geroia Sotsialisticheskogo Truda N. N. Burdenko). **Voen Med Zh** 1983 May;5:64–8
Beloborodova NL: Moskovskoe otdelenie mediko-khirurgicheskoĭ akademii v Otechestvennuiu voinu 1812 goda. **Voen Med Zh** 1982 Nov;(11):66–7
Berkutov AN: Das chirurgische Erbe. N.I. Pirogov und die gegenwärtige Chirurgie. **Zentralbl Chir** 1984;109(17):1149–52
Berkutov AN: Zavety N. I. Pirogova i sovremennaia khirurgiia. **Vestn Khir** 1982 May;128(5):125–7
Bogush LK: Razvitie i dostizheniia khirurgii tuberkuleza legkikh v SSSR. **Probl Tuberk** 1983 Oct;10:3–7
Bregadze IL: Novoe v pokazaniiakh k khirurgicheskim vmeshatel'stvam pri vnutrennikh zabolevaniiakh (k 40-letiiu so dnia smerti M. P. Konchalovskogo). **Klin Med (Mosk)** 1981;59(10):78–9
Brzheskiĭ VCh: Imena khirurgov v pamiati sovetskogo naroda. **Klin Khir** 1979 Nov;(11):64–70
Deriabin II, Berkutov AN: Razvitie voenno-polevoĭ khirurgii za 60 let Soiuza SSR. **Vestn Khir** 1983 Feb;2:3–7
Epifanov NS: I. K. Spizharnyĭ v Viatskoĭ ssylke (materialy biografii). **Sov Zdravookhr** 1983;(2):70–1
Epifanov NS: Khirurg, uchenyĭ, patriot (k110-letiiu so dnia rozhdeniia V.A. Oppelia). **Khirurgiia (Mosk)** 1982 Nov;(11):101–3
Epifanov NS: Vasiliĭ Ivanovich Razumovskiĭ (k 125-letiiu so dnia rozhdeniia). **Feldsher Akush** 1982;47(7):42–3
Estrin GB: Voprosy khirurgii i travmatologii v zhurnale 'Vrach' V. A. Manasseina (1880–1901 gg.). **Vestn Khir** 1981 Oct;127(10):142–4
Fel'berg MV: S. S. Iudin v 'Zakhar'ine'. **Sov Zdravookhr** 1983;(3):71–3
Filatov VI: K stoletiiu otechestvennogo protezirovaniia (1883–1983). **Ortop Travmatol Protez** 1983 March;(3):61–3
Galin LL: Publikatsii N. I. Pirogova na stranitsakh 'Voenno--meditsinskogo zhurnala. **Voen Med Zh** 1980 Nov;(11):69–71
Gol'braĭkh VR: Velikiĭ khirurg N. I. Pirogov--osnovopolozhnik khirurgii cheliustno-litsevoĭ oblasti (k 100-letiiu so dnia smerti). **Stomatologiia (Mosk)** 1982 Jul–Aug;61(4):66–7
Golovin GV, Depp ME, Dutkevich IG: Vydaiushchiĭsia sovetskiĭ khirurg i transfuziolog (k 80-letiiu so dnia rozhdeniia A. N. Filatova). **Vestn Khir** 1982 Oct;129(10):3–8
Gordeev VI, Gogun KV, Gandziuk VM: Vydaiushchiesia vrachi-khirurgi Khersonshchiny. **Klin Khir** 1983 Jun;(6):56–8
Gvozdev MP, Petrov VA: Iustin Iulianovich Dzhanelidze (K 100-letiiu so dnia rozhdeniia). **Voen Med Zh** 1983 Aug;(8):72–4
Iaremchuk AIâ, et al: [Importance of museums in optimizing the academic process and academic research work of students in a department of surgery.] (Rus). **Klin Khir** 1981;2:47–9
Iurikhin AP: K 140-letiiu so dnia rozhdeniia Sergeia Petrovicha Kolomnina (1842–1886). **Klin Khir** 1982 Dec;(12):61–3
Iurikhin AP: N. I. Pirogov, ego ucheniki i posledovateli. **Klin Khir** 1984 May;(5):62–4
Kapitanenko AM: Talantlivyĭ organizator, iskusnyĭ khirurg (k 100-letiiu so dnia rozhdeniia P. V. Mandryki). **Sov Zdravookhr** 1984;(10):58–60
Katsnel'bogen AG: N. I. Pirogov i brat'ia Pushchiny. **Sov Zdravookhr** 1983;(9):62–5
Katsnel'bogen AG: Obshchestvenno-meditsinskaia deiatel'nost' Kh. I. Lodera. **Klin Med (Mosk)** 1982 Jun;60(6):117–20
Khokholia VP: Nikolaĭ Markiianovich Volkovich (k 125-letiiu so dnia rozhdeniia). **Klin Khir** 1983 Dec;(12):55–6
Kolesov VI: Khirurgicheskomu obshchestvu Pirogova--100 let. **Vestn Khir** 1982 May;128(5):127–36
Kolmsee P: Nikolai Iwanowitsch Pirogow – Kriegschirurg und militärmedizinischer Organisator in Russland des 19. Jahrhunderts. **Militaergesch** 1981;20(5):536–45
Kolomiĭchenko MI: Materialy X plenuma Nauchnogo obshchestva khirurgov USSR. Kiev, Zdorov'ia, 1967. 157 p.
Komakhidze ME: Ocherki o khirurgicheskoĭ rabote ofitserskogo gospitalia v period Velikoĭ Otechstvenniĭ voĭny (1941–1955 gg.). Tbilisi, Metsniereba, 1977. 102 p.
Kononov VS: Perspektivy i problemy khirurgii detskogo vozrasta v Kirgizii. **Vestn Khir** 1982 Dec;129(12):14–8
Korzh AA, Bondarenko NS: Pamiati N. I. Pirogova (k 100-latiiu so dnia smerti). **Ortop Travmatol Protez** 1982 Apr;(4):56–9
Kotel'nikov VP: V. A. Oppel' i razvitie fiziologicheskoĭ khirurgii. **Klin Med (Mosk)** 1984 May;62(5):145–8
Kotel'nikov VP: Znachenie nauchnogo naslediia S. P. Botkina v khirurgii. **Klin Med (Mosk)** 1983 Jul;61(7):140–2
Kovalev MM, Roĭ VP, Burka AA, et al: Deviat'sot zasedaniĭ nauchnogo obshchestva khirurgov Kieva i Kievskoĭ oblasti. **Klin Khir** 1984 Apr;(4):58–61
Kozlov VA, Iarchuk NI, Kotov GA: Razvitie cheliustno-litsevoĭ khirurgii c SSSR. **Vestn Khir** 1982 Nov;129(11):9–12
Kul'chitskiĭ KI, Klantsa PA, Sobchuk GS: Chestvovanie N.I. Pirogova na ego 50-letnem iubilee. **Vrach Delo** 1981;(6):1–5
Kul'chitskiĭ KI: N. I. Pirogov v usad'be Vishnia. Kiev, Zdorov'ia, 1981. 99 p.
Kul'chitskiĭ KI, Romenskiĭ OIu, Sobchuk GS, et al: Nikolaĭ Ivanovich Pirogov v usad'be 'Vishnia'. **Arkh Anat Gistol Embriol** 1980 Aug;79(8):110–7
Kuz'min MK: Velikiĭ Russkiĭ khirurg N. I. Pirogov i sovremennost'. **Sov Med** 1983;(2):117–9
Lisitsyn KM: Voenno-polevaia khirurgiia vo vremia Velikoĭ Otechestvennoĭ voĭny i perspektivy ee razvitiia. **Voen Med Zh** 1980 May;(5):42–5
Maiat VS: Vladimir Semenovich Levit (K 100-letiiu so dnia rozhdeniia). **Khirurgiia (Mosk)** 1983 Jun;6:111–3
Makovoz AA: D. V. Volchenetskiĭ--vydaiushchiĭsia vrach Rossii. **Feldsher Akush** 1983;48(4):57–8
Makovoz AA: O. A. Iunevich – vidnyĭ zemskiĭ vrach. **Sov Zdravookhr** 1984;(1):64–7
Mirskiĭ MB: N. I. Pirogov--krupneĭshiĭ khirurg XIX veka. **Feldsher Akush** 1981;46(12):37–40
Mirskiĭ MB: Novye dokumenty o zhizni i nauchnoĭ deiatel'nosti I. I. Grekova (1867–1941). **Sov Zdravookhr** 1981;(5):64–7
Mirskiĭ MB, Khil'chenko MA: Professor A. A. Kiter--pervyĭ uchenik Pirogova (k 170-letiiu so dnia rozhdeniia A. A. Kitera). **Sov Zhdravookhr** 1983;(11):68–71
Mirskiĭ MB: V. I. Razumovskiĭ kak istorik khirurgii (k 125-letiiu so dnia rozhdeniia). **Sov Zdravookhr** 1983;5:66–70
Mirskiĭ MB: Vydaiushchiĭsia russkiĭ khirurg E. I. Bogdanovskiĭ (k 150-letiiu so dnia rozhdeniia). **Vestn Khir** 1984 Mar;132(3):143–5
Mitrofanov VG: K 90-letiiu so dnia rozhdeniia Mikhaila Semenovicha Lisitsyna. **Vestn Khir** 1983 May;130(5):141–2
Napalkov PN, Shafer II: Professor Vasiliĭ Mikhaĭlovich Nazarov (k 100-letiiu so dnia rozhdeniia). **Vestn Khir** 1983 Mar;130(3):129–30
Napalkov PN, Vigdorchuk IV, Labazanov MM: Razvitie khirurgii v soiuznykh respublikakh za 60 let Soiuza SSR. **Vestn Khir** 1983;130(4):3–9
Nechaĭ AI, Sitenko VM: Vladimir Nikolaevich Shamov (k 100-letiiu so dnia rozhdeniia). **Klin Khir** 1982 May;(5):62–4
Nechiporuk VM, Boliukh BA: Iz istorii s'ézdov khirurgov USSR.

Klin Khir 1979 Nov;(11):61-4
Novakova LIa: Publikatsii o N. I. Pirogove v khirurgicheskom zhurnale Ukrainy. Klin Khir 1982 Feb;(2):49-50
Novikov FG, Tomashuk IP: Iz istorii otechestvennoĭ voenno-polevoĭ khirurgii. Klin Khir 1980 May;(5):69-72
Permiakov NK: B. A. Petrov. Moskva, Meditsina, 1982. 170 p.
Petrov IN: P.G. Kornev i ego shkola. Probl Tuberk 1984 Jul;(7):73-5
Petrova TA: Razvitie khirurgii v dorevoliutsionnoĭ Karelii. Sov Zdravookhr 1981;(12):58-60
Petrovskiĭ BV: Petr Aleksandrovich Gertsen (k 80-letiiu Moskovskogo nauchno-issledovatel'skogo onkologicheskogo instituta im P. A. Gertsena). Khirurgiia (Mosk) 1983 Nov;(11):3-7
Petrovskiĭ BV: Sovetskaia khirurgiia za 60 let. Klin Med (Mosk) 1982 Dec;60(12):15-22
Pokrovskiĭ GA: Razvitie nauchnykh issledovaniĭ vNII Proktologii za poslednie 10 let. Khirurgiia (Mosk) 1983 Mar;(3):40-5
Pytel' AIa: Velikiĭ russkiĭ khirurg Nikolaĭ Ivanovich Pirogov (k 100-letiiu so dnia smerti). Urol Nefrol (Mosk) 1981 Jan-Feb;(1):3-8
Rakovskaia GG, Khokholia VP: Kievskomu nauchno-issledovatel'skomu institutu klinicheskoĭ i ėksperimental'noĭ khirurgii 10 let. Klin Khir 1982 May;(5):70-3
Sakharov MI, Sorokin EIu: Sverdlovskoe oblastnoe nauchnoe obshchestvo khirurgov (k 50-letiiu so dnia obrazovaniia). Vestn Khir 1982 May;128(5):136-7
Schober K: Das chirurgische Erbe: Vor etwa 100 Jahren (9). Zentralbl Chir 1979;104(12):798-9
Serebrennikov AB: Khirurg L. A. Bekkers - uchenik N. I. Pirogova. Klin Med (Mosk) 1983 Mar;61(3):113-5
Shabunin AV: Kalinkinskiĭ khirurgicheskiĭ institut (k 200-letiiu so dnia osnovaniia). Sov Zdravookhr 1983;(11):66-7
Shabunin AV: Uchastie N.I. Pirogova v Obshchestve S.-Peterburgskikh prakticheskikh vracheĭ. Sov Zdravookhr 1983;(4):63-5
Shabunin AV: Vklad zhurnala 'Khirurgicheskiĭ vestnik' v razvitie khirurgicheskoĭ mysli v Rossii. Vestn Khir 1984 Aug;133(8):146-7
Shalimov AA, Kovalev MM, Sakharchuk IM: Leninskaia druzhba narodov SSSR-reshaiushchee uslovie vosstanovleniia khirurgicheskikh kadrov Ukrainy posle ee osvobozhdeniia ot nemetsko-fashistskikh zakhvatchikov. Klin Khir 1982 Dec;(12):7-11
Shalimov AA, Khokholia VP: Zhurnalu 'Klinicheskaia khirurgiia' 60 let. Klin Khir 1981 Jun;(6):1-6
Skopakov Kh: N. I. Pirogov--genialen khirug i osnovopolozhnik na topografskata anatomiia. Khirurgiia (Sofiia) 1982;35(1):99-100
Smol'iannikov AV, Sarkisov DS, Serebrennikov AB: N. I. Pirogov--velikiĭ uchenyĭ, vrach, grazhdanin. Arkh Patol 1982;44(9):3-13
Sovetskaia khirurgiia k 62-ĭ: godovshchine Velikoĭ Oktiabr'skoĭ sotsialisticheskoĭ revoliutsii. Vestn Khir 1979 Nov;123(11):3-8
Sovetskaia voenno-polevaia khirurgiia v Velikuiu Otechestvennuiu voinu 1941-1945 gg. i osnovnye napravleniia ee dal'neĭshego razvitiia: Khirurgiia (Mosk) 1980 May;(5):3-8
Struchkov VI: Ivan Gur'evich Rufanov (k 100-letiiu so dnia rozhdeniia). Sov Med 1984;(7):114-5
Ternovoĭ KS: Dostizheniia sovetskoĭ khirurgii (k 60-letiiu obrazovaniia SSSR). Klin Khir 1982 Dec;(12):1-7
Ternovoĭ KS, Shalimov AA: Vydaiushchiĭsia sovetskiĭ khirurg I. I. Dzhanelidze (k 100-letiiu so dnia rozhdeniia). Klin Khir 1983 Jul;(8):76-9
Trubnikov VF: K 60-letiiu osnovanii kafedry ortopedii, travmatologii i voenno-polevoi khirurgii Khar'kovskogo meditsinskogo instituta. Ortop Travmatol Protez 1981 Sep;(9):68-70
Uglov FG, Afanas'eva AV: Iustin Iulianovich Dzhanelidze (k 100-letiiu so dnia rozhdeniia). Vestn Khir 1983 Aug;131(8):131-4
Uglov FG, Golovin GV, Dutkevich IG: Sovetskaia khirurgiia za 60 let Soiuza Sovetskikh Sotsialisticheskikh Respublik. Vestn Khir 1982 Dec;129(12):3-10
Vytrishchak VIa: Vklad N. I. Pirogova v razvitie cheliustno-litsevoĭ khirurgii. Voen Med Zh 1982 Nov;(11):64-5
Zabludovskiĭ PE: Trudy nauchnykh uchrezhdeniĭ Ukrainskoĭ SSR k Pirogovskoĭ godovshchine. Vrach Delo 1983 Feb;(2):121-2
Zadorozhnyĭ AA, Saks FF, Dolgikh VP, et al: Erast Gavrilovich Salishchev (k 130-letiiu so dnia rozhdeniia). Vestn Khir 1982 Jul;129(7):140-3
Zinevich VP: Razvitie ideĭ A. N. Filatova po probleme parenteral'nogo pitaniia v khirurgii. Vestn Khir 1982 Oct;129(10):16-20
Zivković K: Dr Nikolaj S. Korotkov (13. II. 1874-1920). Srp Arh Celok Lek 1983 Jan;111(1):97-9

**Yugoslavia**

Borisov P: Od ranocelnistva do zacetkov znanstvene kirurgije na Slovenskem. Ljubljana, Slovenska akademija znanosti in umetnosti, 1977. 339 p.
Bumbaširević Z: Sedamdeset pet godina ortopedske hirurgije u Srbiji. Srp Arh Celok Lek 1981 Mar;109(3):425-38
Djordjević SP: Prof. dr Julije Budisavljević (2. III 1882--5. V 1981). Srp Arh Celok Lek 1983 Jun;111(6):861-4
Djordjević SP: Sećanja na rad u vojnom sanitetu Srbije u toku II balkanskog rata 1913. godine. Iz sećanja dr Julija Budisavljevinja i njegovih kolega iz Hirurške klinike u Insbruku. Srp Arh Celok Lek 1983 Jun;111(6):853-9
Finderle V: Mobilne kirurške ekipe. Lijec Vjesn 1979 Nov;101(11):706
Glesinger L: Povijest kirurgije u Hrvatskoj do sredine XIX stoljeća. Acta Chir Iugosl 1967;14:121-35
Kučišec A: Neki aspekti stanja i razvoja kirurgije i kirurške službe u NOB-i Hrvatske od 1941. do 1944. godine. Lijec Vjesn 1979 Nov;101(11):669-73
Papo I: Izvještaj o četveromjesečnom radu ekipe SOVS-a. Lijec Vjesn 1979 Nov;101(11):707-8
Straser P, Protić M: Pečat karlovačkog hirurško-berberskog esnafa iz XVIII veka. Med Pregl 1982;35(11-12):493

**Zimbabwe**

Gann LH, Gelfand M: Huggins of Rhodesia. London, Allen & Unwin [1964]. 285 p.

## ABDOMINAL

Adams DB: Abdominal gunshot wounds in warfare: a historical review. Milit Med 1983 Jan;148(1):15-20
Crosby WH: An historical sketch of splenic function and splenectomy. Lymphology 1983 Jun;16(2):52-5
Read RC: The development of inguinal herniorrhaphy. Surg Clin North Am 1984 Apr;64(2):185-96
Schmauss AK: Die Geschichte der Gastrotomie zur Entfernung von Fremdkörpern. Zentralbl Chir 1982;107(22):1481-5

**Czechoslovakia**

Duda M, Serý Z: Geschichte und Stand der Chirurgie der Hiatushernien und der Refluxkrankheit des Osophagus. Dtsch Z Verdau Stoffwechselkr 1980;40(5):177-83

**500 A.D.-1450**

Classic articles in colonic and rectal surgery: John Arderne 1307-1380 (?). Dis Colon Rectum 1982 Nov-Dec;25(8):832-40

**1700 to Present**

Baker JW: A historical overview of surgical decompression in advanced intestinal obstruction. Surg Gynecol Obstet 1984 Jun;158(6):593-8
Blalock JB: History and evolution of peptic ulcer surgery. Am J Surg 1981 Mar;141(3):317-22
Browne HJ: A century of changing fashions in peptic ulcer surgery. Ir Med J 1979 Nov 30;72(11):458-69
Helmer F: Das chirurgische Erbe. Der Einfluss Theodor Billroths auf die heutige Abdominalchirurgie. Zentralbl Chir 1982;107(22):1469-80
Hughes ES: The development of a restorative operation for carcinoma of the rectum. Aust NZ J Surg 1981;51:117-9
Miguel J de: Anotaciones al desenvolvimiento histórico de la cirugía de la úlcera péptica con especial referencia a la úlcera duodenal en los últimos 50 años. Rev Esp Enferm Apar Dig 1983 Jul;64(1):60-5
Nöske HD: Lithotomia vesicae. München, Zuckschwerdt, 1982. v, 74 p.
Ravitch MM: Development of intestinal anastomotic devices. South Med J 1982 Dec;75(12):1520-4
Sparkman RS: 100th anniversary of the first cholecystectomy. Arch Surg 1982 Dec;117(12):1525
Wyklicky H: 100 Jahre Magenresektion. In H. Brunner, ed: Pathophysiologie und Pharmakotherapie des peptischen Geschwürs. München, Urban & Schwarzenberg, 1982. p. 123-32.

**Austria**

Schreiber HW: Wo steht die Carcinom-Chirurgie des Magens 100 Jahre nach der ersten erfolgreichen Magenresektion durch Theodor Billroth? Langenbecks Arch Chir 1982;358:53-5

**France**

Morer G: La découverte de Charles Krafft. Hist Sci Med 1984;18(1):33-40
Sanderson ER: Henri Hartmann and the Hartmann operation. Arch Surg 1980 Jun;115(6):792-3

**Germany**

Abe HR: Der soziale Aspekt im ärztlichen Wirken des grossen deutschen Gallenchirurgen Dr. Hans Kehr. Beitr Gesch Univ Erfurt 1979-83;19:241-58
Abe HR: Die internationale Ausstrahlung der Kehr-Rohdenschen Privatklinik in Halberstadt (1890-1910). Ein Beitrag zur Geschichte der modernen Gallenwegschirurgie. In International Congress of the History of Medicine. 26th, Plovdiv, 1978. Actes du Congress. Sofia, 1981. Volume II. p. 78-80.
Casal MA: Hace cien años: 1882-1982. 'Carl Langenbuch, la primera colecistectomía y breve historia de una polémia famosa. Acta Gastroenterol Latinoam 1982;12(2):181-4

Rains AJ: A thought for Carl Langenbuch (1846–1901): a centenary. **Ann R Coll Surg Engl** 1982 Jul;64(4):268–9
Schlosser GA, Hrynyschyn K, Zornig C, et al: Die Geschichte der Bauchdeckenschnitte. Historisches und Entwicklungstendenzen (I). **Med Welt** 1981 Oct 30;32(44):1672–6

**Great Britain**

McWhinnie DL, Hamilton DN: The rise and fall of surgery for the 'floating' kidney. **Br Med J [Clin Res]** 1984 Mar 17;288(6420):845–7

**Hungary**

Gyenes G: Adatok a splenectomia történetéhez Magyarországon. **Orv Hetil** 1980 Apr 6;121(14):853–4

**New Zealand**

Wright-St Clair RE: The development of abdominal surgery in New Zealand. **NZ Med J** 1981 Apr;93(682):270–3

**Poland**

Krzyś J, Krzyś Z: Przebieg pierwszych w Polsce wycieć macicy. **Wiad Lek** 1983 Nov 1;36(21):1827–32

**Switzerland**

Jost A: Commentaires sur les articles de Gustave Julliard. Fistule pyo-stercorale--laparotomie et suture de l'intestin--guérison par premiere intention. Hernio-laparotomie--resection de dix-huit centimètres d'intestin--guérison. **Rev Med Suisse Romande** 1980 Dec;100(12):1089–96

**United States**

Bernhard CM: Dr. Ephraim McDowell: father of abdominal surgery. **Am Surg** 1980 Jan;46(1):1–5
Christianson EH: The colonial surgeon's rise to prominence: Dr. Silvester Gardiner (1707–1786) and the practice of lithotomy in New England. **N Engl Hist Geneal Regist** 1982 Apr;136:104–14
Criado FJ, Wilson TH: Posterior transsphincteric approach for surgery of the rectum: the Bevan operation. **Dis Colon Rectum** 1981;24:145–50
Fraser ID, Condon RE: Sutureless bowel anastomosis -- an historical perspective. **Wis Med J** 1980 May;79(5):16–8
Hanley PH: Colon and rectal surgery. Our heritage. **Dis Colon Rectum** 1983 Feb;26(2):81–4
Mumey N: Ephraim McDowell, 1771–1830: a frontiersman who advanced the art of surgery. **Denver West Roundup** 1979 Jul–Aug;35:3–20
Walker LG: L. L. Staton, M.D., and the first successful gastrostomy in America. **Surg Gynecol Obstet** 1984 Apr;158(4):387–8

**USSR**

Pytel' AIa: O pervykh kholetsistektomiiakh v Rossii. **Khirurgiia (Mosk)** 1981 Jan;(1):116–8

### AMPUTATION

Dustmann HO: Das Bildnis des Amputierten in der Kunst. In KF Schlegel, ed: Der Körperbehinderte in Mythologie und Kunst. Stuttgart, New York, Thieme, 1983. p. 57–87.
Murdoch G: Amputation revisited. **Prosthet Orthot Int** 1984 Apr;8(1):8–15

**1450–1700**

**Poland**

Jonecko A: Drzeworyt ukazujący amputowane i protezowane podudzie w śląskim poemacie Roździeńskiego 'Officina ferraria' a roku 1612. **Wiad Lek** 1983 Jun 15;36(12):1025–31
Jonecko A: Drzeworyt ukazujacy amputowane i protezowane produdzie w ślaskim poemacie Roździeńskiego 'Officina Ferraria' z roku 1616. **Arch Hist Med (Warsz)** 1984;47(1):107–16

**1700 to Present**

Liston SL: Traumatic amputation of the external ear: the War of Jenkins' Ear and George Washington. **Am J Surg** 1984 Nov;148(5):599–601

**Canada**

Roland CG: War amputations in Upper Canada. **Archivaria** 1980 Summer;10:73–84

**France**

Firmin F: De la réunion immédiate de quelques doigts amputés. **Ann Chir Plast** 1980;25(2):187–90
Huard P: Armel-Eugène Gripouilleau (1821–1909) officier de santé à Montlouis (Indre-et-Loire). In: Congrès National des Sociétés Savantes, 93e, Tours, 1968. Comptes Rendus. Paris, 1971. Section des Sciences, Tome II. p. 189–92.
Huard P, Plessis JL: L'amputation de jambe à la bordelaise. In: Congrès National des Sociétés Savantes, 104e, Bordeaux, 1979. Comptes Rendus. Paris, 1979. Section des Sciences, Fasc. IV. p 243–57.
Plessis JL: Un anatomiste militaire mort victime du devoir: Adolphe-Euclide Lacauchie (1806–1853), latiniste distingué et inventeur de l'hydrotomie. **Hist Sci Med** 1982;16(3):151–61

**Germany**

Ertl JW von: Die Versorgung von Amputationsstümpfen durch Osteo-Myoplastik nach v. Ertl. **Z Plast Chir** 1981 Sep;5(3):184–9
Schober KL: Vor etwa 100 Jahren (8). Amputatio talo-calcanea von Dr. E. Blasius Geh. Medicinalrath und Professor in Halle. **Zentralbl Chir** 1979;104(11):739–41
Watermann RA: Figures for bone-amputations, introduced by Zur Verth and regarding artificial limbs. In: Congrès international d'histoire de la médecine, XXVe, Québec, 1976. Actes. Québec, 1977. p. 1386–95.

**Great Britain**

Agnew LR: An 18th century amputation (Lady Anne Dawson). **Lancet** 1983 Nov 5;2(8358):1074–5
Beckett JV: Illness and amputation in the eighteenth century: the case of Sir James Lowther (1673–1755). **Med Hist** 1980 Jan;24(1):88–92
Rüttimann B: Nelsons Oberarm-Amputation. **Z Orthop** 1982 Feb;120(1):86–8

**United States**

Brieger GH: Early ambulation. A study in the history of surgery. **Ann Surg** 1983 Apr;197(4):443–9

### BREAST

Dufourmentel C: Reconstruction du sein après mastectomie. Historique, état actuel, perspectives d'avenir. **Bull Acad Natl Med (Paris)** 1981 Jan;165(1):103–8
Raven RW: The surgeon and oncology. **Clin Oncol** 1984 Dec;10(4):311–8

**Netherlands**

Moulin D de: Historical notes on breast cancer, with emphasis on The Netherlands. II. Pathophysiological concepts, diagnosis and therapy in the 18th century. **Neth J Surg** 1981 Oct;33(4):206–16

**Before 500 A.D.**

Marí VJ: El martirio de Santa Agatha, un precedente de la mastectomia. Représentacion artistica con especial referencia a una coleccion de tallas. In International Congress of the History of Medicine. 26th, Plovdiv, 1978. Actes du Congress. Sofia, 1981. Volume II. p. 150–7.

**1450–1700**

**Netherlands**

De Moulin D: Historical notes on breast cancer, with emphasis on the Netherlands. I. Pathological and therapeutic concepts in the seventeenth century. **Neth J Surg** 1980;32(4):129–34

**1700 to Present**

Babayan R: Reduktionsplastik der Mamma. **Med Welt** 1980 Nov 28 and Dec 19;31(48, 51–52):1873–6, 1767–9
Mendelson BC: The evolution of breast reconstruction. **Med J Aust** 1982 Jan 9;1(1):7–8
Vaeth JM: Historical aspects of tylectomy and radiation therapy in the treatment of cancer of the breast. **Front Radiat Ther Oncol** 1983;17:1–10
Vázquez Albaladejo G, Sospedra Ferrer R: Evolución de las técnicas quirúrgicas en el cáncer de mama. **Rev Esp Oncol** 1981;28(1):83–94

**France**

Pérel L: Conception pathogénique et traitement du cancer du sein au 18ème siècle. In: Congrès international d'histoire de la médecine, XXVe, Québec, 1976. Actes. Québec, 1977. p. 1073–80.

# SURGERY

**Germany**

Meyer KK, Beck WC: Mastectomy performed by Lawrence Heister in the eighteenth century. **Surg Gynecol Obstet** 1984 Oct;159(4):391–4

**Great Britain**

Fletcher C: Mastectomy in the 1880s. **Br Med J [Clin Res]** 1983 Mar 19;286(6369):966–7

**Netherlands**

Moulin D de: Historical notes on breast cancer, with emphasis on The Netherlands; III. The growth of scientific surgery in the 19th century. **Neth J Surg** 1982 Dec;34(5):193–200

**United States**

Bland CS: The Halsted mastectomy: present illness and past history. **West J Med** 1981 Jun;134(6):549–55
Crile G: Breast cancer. A personal perspective. **Surg Clin North Am** 1984 Dec;64(6):1145–9

### CARDIOVASCULAR

Borst HG, Hetzer R: Die Rolle des Experiments in der Kardiovaskularchirurgie. **Fortschr Med** 1982 Nov 4;100(41):1889–92
Brewer LA: Open heart surgery and myocardial revascularization. Historical notes. **Am J Surg** 1981 Jun;141(6):618–31
Donovan AJ: Surgical treatment of portal hypertension: a historical perspective. **World J Surg** 1984 Oct;8(5):626–45
McGoon DC: Cardiac surgery. Prologue: From Whence? **Cardiovasc Clin** 1981;12(3):1–8
al-Naaman YD, Wada J: The history of thoracic and cardiovascular surgery. **J Fac Med Baghdad** 1977;19(suppl):1–24
Ouvry PA, Davy A: De la vanité des incisions multiples dans la chirurgie des varices. **Phlebologie** 1982 Oct–Dec;35(4):851–5
Rashkind WJ: Historical aspects of surgery for congenital heart disease. **J Thorac Cardiovasc Surg** 1982 Oct;84(4):619–25
Vecht RJ, Besterman EM, Bromley LL, et al: Acute aortic dissection: historical perspective and current management. **Am Heart J** 1981 Dec;102(6 pt 1):1087–9
Wertenbaker L: To mend the heart. New York, Viking Press, 1980. xiv, 344 p.

**1700 to Present**

Austen WG: Cardiovascular surgery: past, present, and future. **Cardiovasc Res Cent Bull** 1979 Jan–Mar;17(3):56–65
Björk VO: The development of the Björk-Shiley artificial heart valve. **Clin Physiol** 1984 Feb;4(1):1–4
Burchell HB: Contributions of the basic sciences to successful clinical application of cardiopulmonary bypass. **Mayo Clin Proc** 1980 Dec;55(12):754–7
Carney AL: Vertebral artery surgery: historical development, basic concepts of brain hemodynamics, and clinical experience of 102 cases. **Adv Neurol** 1981;30:249–82
English TA: Heart transplantation---1979. **Trans Hunter Soc** 1978–80;37–38:143–51
Faller A: Die 'Tetralogie von Fallot'; zur geschichtlichen Entwicklung von Diagnose und Therapie eines kongenitalen Herzsyndroms von Niels Stensen bis zur modernen Herzchirurgie. **Gesnerus** 1982;39(3–4):321–46
Gott VL: Extracorporeal circulation: 1970–1982. **Trans Am Soc Artif Intern Organs** 1982;28:17–9
Harrison DC: Coronary bypass: the first 10 years. **Hosp Pract** 1981 Jun;16(6):49–56
John S: Mitral valvotomy. Past and present. **Indian J Chest Dis Allied Sci** 1979 Oct–Dec;21(4):163–5
Just Viera JO: Mitral valve commissurotomy by John Alexander: repeat surgery 28 years later. **Bol Asoc Med PR** 1981 Feb;73(2):56–8
Keown KK: A brief history of anesthesia and surgery of the heart and great vessels. **Can Anaesth Soc J** 1982 Jul;29(4):325–9
Kirienko AI, Garibdzhanian LL: Embolektomiia iz legochnoĭ arterii. **Grudn Khir** 1983 Mar–Apr;(2):64–71
Lee S, Frank DH, Choi SY: Historical review of small and microvascular vessel surgery. **Ann Plast Surg** 1983 Jul;11(1):53–62
Lillehei CW: A personalized history of extracorporeal circulation. **Trans Am Soc Artif Intern Organs** 1982;28:5–16
Ljunggren B, Säveland H: Hjärnpulsåderbråckens medicinska historia – ett långtifrån avslutat kapitel. **Sydsven Medicinhist Sallsk Arsskr** 1982;19:63–98
McGoon DC: The dimensions of surgical progress in cardiac surgery. **Bol Asoc Med PR** 1983 Feb;75(2):80–2
Mayer T: Early history of heart surgery. **Pediatrics** 1980 May;65(5):1054
Mulch J, Scheld HH, Köstering B, et al: 20 Jahre Herzklappenchirurgie. (1). Entwicklung der künstlichen Herzklappenventile. **ZFA (Stuttgart)** 1981 Mar 31;57(9):639–44
Nolen WA: A short history of heart surgery. **Am Heritage** 1983;34(5):101–5
Paiement B, Boulanger M, Taillefer J, et al: Anesthésie et cardiopathie: évolution des concepts et perspectives. **Union Med Can** 1979 Oct;108(10):1158–66
Parker EF: Eventful events in the history of cardiovascular surgery. **J SC Med Assoc** 1982 Aug;78(8):441–5
Quijano-Pitman F: Desarrollo y estado actual de la cirugía del corazón. **Arch Inst Cardiol Mex** 1979 Sep–Oct;49(5):984–1002
Rich NM, Clagett GP, Salander JM, et al: Surgical treatment of arterial and venous injuries. **Acta Chir Belg** 1982 Sep–Oct;(5):473–84
Rich NM, Clagett GP, Salander JM, et al: The Matas/Soubbotitch connection. **Surgery** 1983 Jan;93(1 Pt 1):17–9
Robicsek F: An epitaph for cavopulmonary anastomosis. **Ann Thorac Surg** 1982 Aug;34(2):208–20
Rothlin M: Koronarchirurgie vor 25 Jahren und heute. **Praxis** 1980 Dec 9;69(49):1839–43
Rutkow IM, Rutkow BG, Ernst CB: Letters of William Halsted and René Leriche: 'Our friendship seems so deep'. **Surgery** 1980 Dec;88(6):806–25
Scheld HH, Mulch J, Walter P, et al: 20 Jahre Herzklappenchirurgie. (2) Klinische Ergebnisse. **ZFA (Stuttgart)** 1981 Mar 31;57(9):645–51
Shumacker HB: Better early than late. **Am J Surg** 1982 Aug;144(2):170–9
Shumacker HB: Extraperitoneal approach for vascular operations: retrospective review. **South Med J** 1982 Dec;75(12):1499–507, 1516
Warren WD: Reflections on the early development of portacaval shunts. **Ann Surg** 1980 May;191(5):519–27
Weinberg SL: The patient with heart diseases and the cardiovascular physician and surgeon: 1958–1983. **J Am Coll Cardiol** 1983 Jan;1(1):6–12

**Australia**

Maddern GJ, Craddock D, Leppard PI, et al: Twelve years of coronary artery surgery in South Australia. **Med J Aust** 1984 Feb 4;140(3):136–40
Sutherland HD: The metamorphosis of cardiac surgery in Australia. **J Thorac Cardiovasc Surg** 1980;80:808–23

**Austria**

Absolon KB: Theodor Billroth and cardiac surgery. **J Thorac Cardiovasc Surg** 1983 Sep;86(3):451–2

**France**

d'Allaines C: Alexis Carrel (1873–1944), visionnaire de la chirurgie cardio-vasculaire. **Arch Mal Coeur** 1984 Sep;77(9):1074–7
Dubost C: First successful resection of an aneurysm of the abdominal aorta with restoration of the continuity by a human arterial graft. **World J Surg** 1982 Mar;6(2):256–7
Huard P, Imbault-Huart MJ: Travaux de Percy (1754–1825) sur l'hémostase des artères (1790–1810). In: Congrès National des Sociétés Savantes, 99e, Besançon, 1974. Comptes Rendus. Paris, 1976. Section des Sciences, Fasc. V. p. 251–7.
Natali J: Paul Broca, chirurgien vasculaire. **Chirurgie** 1980;106(10):777–82

**Germany**

Neugebauer J, Metz L: 15 Jahre Gefässchirurgie am Städtischen Krankenhaus im Friedrichshain Berlin. **Z Arztl Fortbild (Jena)** 1979 Nov 1;73(21):1032–4
Sabiston DC: Trendelenburg's classic work on the operative treatment of pulmonary embolism. **Ann Thorac Surg** 1983 May;35(5):570–4
Schober KL: The quotation about the heart. Comments on Theodor Billroth's attitude towards cardiac surgery. **Thorac Cardiovasc Surg** 1981 Jun;29(3):131–7
Zenker R, Borst HG, Reichart B: 100 Jahre Herzchirurgie. **Fortschr Med** 1983 Dec 1;101(45):2094–100

**Great Britain**

Black MM, Drury PJ, Tindale WB: Twenty-five years of heart valve substitutes: a review. **J R Soc Med** 1983 Aug;76(8):667–80
Cleland WP: The evolution of cardiac surgery in the United Kingdom. **Thorax** 1983 Dec;38(12):887–96
Lasky II: John Hunter, the Shakespeare of medicine. **Surg Gynecol Obstet** 1983 Apr;156(4):511–8
Murley R: John Hunter, velvet and vascular surgery. **Ann R Coll Surg Engl** 1984 May;66(3):214–8
Shinebourne EA: Ethics of innovative cardiac surgery. **Br Heart J** 1984 Dec;52(6):597–601

**Hungary**

Vas G, Hidvégi J: Balassa érsebészeti munkásságáról. **Orv Hetil** 1983 Mar 20;124(12):709–10

**Jamaica**

A decade of open heart surgery at the University Hospital of the West

Indies, Kingston, Jamaica, 1968–1978: **West Indian Med J** 1980 Dec;29 Suppl:299–345

### Poland

Juszczyński M: 15 lat transplantacji serca. **Pieleg Polozna** 1984;(2):16–7

### Sweden

Björk VO: The development of the Björk–Shiley artificial heart valve. **Clin Cardiol** 1984 Jan,7(1).3–5

### United States

Bland EF: The first ductus revisited. **N Engl J Med** 1984 Jun 28;310(26):1749
Dobell AR: John H. Gibbon, Jr. Part II. Personal reminiscenses. **Ann Thorac Surg** 1982 Sep;34(3):342–4
Duncalf D: History of anesthesia for pediatric cardiac surgery. **Int Anesthesiol Clin** 1980 Spring;18(1):1–3
Edmunds LH: A historical review of shunts for cyanotic heart disease. In B. L. Tucker, G. G. Lindesmith, ed: First clinical conference on congenital heart disease. New York, Grune & Stratton, 1979. p. 207–17.
Fyler DC: The history of treatment of patent ductus arteriosus. In B. L. Tucker, G. G. Lindesmith, ed: First clinical conference on congenital heart disease. New York, Grune & Stratton, 1979. p. 3–11.
Glenn WW: Some account of the early years of cardiac surgery. **Conn Med** 1980 Jun;44(6):338–44
Greenwood RD: Operation for Aneurism of the Axillae'––1834, a historical notation. **J Med Assoc State Ala** 1982 May;51(11):57
Gupta BL: Surgery in angina. **Indian Heart J** 1980,(9).415–24
Hammond GL, Laks H, Geha AS: Development of aortic valve prostheses. **Conn Med** 1980 Jun;44(6):348–52
Hill JD: John H. Gibbon, Jr. Part I. The development of the first successful heart-lung machine. **Ann Thorac Surg** 1982 Sep;34(3):337–41
Kirklin JW: Open-heart surgery at the Mayo Clinic. The 25th anniversary. **Mayo Clin Proc** 1980 May;55(5):339–41
Lam CR: Heart valve surgery at Henry Ford Hospital from a perspective of thirty-two years. **Henry Ford Hosp Med J** 1982;30(3):170–1
Lefemine AA: A recollecton of men and events on the Thoracic Service of the Peter Bent Brigham Hospital: 1958–1966. **Artif Organs** 1980 Aug;4(3):210–8
McNamara DG: Landmark perspective: the Blalock–Taussig operation and subsequent progress in surgical treatment of cardiovascular diseases. **JAMA** 1984 Apr 27;251(16):2139–41
Mills NL: Valvular heart surgery––1984. **J La State Med Soc** 1984 Apr;136(4):43–6
Scott HW: A tribute to Barney Brooks, Alfred Blalock, and the Vanderbilt Surgical Staff (1925 to 1982). **South Med J** 1982 Dec;75(12):1439–52
Sealy WC: The case of the fisherman with the fast pulse and the beginning of arrhythmia surgery. **NC Med J** 1983 Aug;44(8):489–90
Shumacker HB: A history of modern treatment of aortic aneurysms. **World J Surg** 1980 Sep;4(5):503–9
Tilney NL: Cushing, Cutler and the mitral valve. **Surg Gynecol Obstet** 1981 Jan;152(1):91–6
Tomlinson WK, Perret JJ: Rudolph Matas father of cardiovascular surgery. In International Congress of the History of Medicine, 27th, Barcelona, 1980. Actas. Barcelona, Académia de Ciències Médiques de Catalunya i Balears, 1981. p. 212–6.
Valentine Mott: **Surgery** 1979 Dec;86(6):906–7
Wylie EJ: Vascular surgery––reflections of the past three decades. **Surgery** 1980 Dec;88(6):743–7

### USSR

Brzheskiĭ VC: Neskol'ko slov o zabytom prioritete. **Grudn Khir** 1983 May–Jun;3:82–3
Dzhoshibaev SD: Razvitie serdechnoĭ khirurgii v Kirgizii. **Zdravookhr Kirg** 1980 Mar–Apr;2:7–11
Kovalev MM, Suslov VS: Antonin Nikolaevich Filatov, ego rol' v razvitii sovremennoĭ khirurgii. **Klin Khir** 1983 Mar;(3):58 60
Laher M, O'Brien E: In search of Korotkoff. **Br Med J [Clin Res]** 1982 Dec 18–25;285(6357):1796–8
Pokrovskii AV, et al: Sosudistyi zamenitel'iz veny pupochnogo kanatika novorozhdennogo. **Latv PSR Zinat Acad Vestis** 1981;12:80–7
Shalybkova OP: Rol' gipotermii v razvitii khirurgii serdtsa i sosudov. **Med Sestra** 1981 Jan;40(1):6–9
Toporov GN: Khirurgiia krovenosnykh sosudov v trudakh N. I. Pirogova (K stoletiiu vykhoda v svet piatogo izdaniia knigi N. I. Pirogova 'Khirurgicheskaia anatomiia arterial'nykh stvolov i fastsiĭ'. CPB, 1881–1882). **Klin Khir** 1982 Nov;(11):71–3

## NEUROLOGICAL

Bakay L: The ancient fear of trephining through the cranial sutures. **Orvostort Kozl** 1982;28(1–3):15–22
Bakay L: The danger of trephining through the cranial sutures. **Surg Neurol** 1982 Oct;18(4):284–5
Ballantine HT: 'Sciatica' and the neurosurgeon: historical perspectives and personal reminiscenses. **Clin Neurosurg** 1980;27:541–52
Caccialanza E: Il problema delle cranioplastiche dal punto di vista storico ed etio–patogenetico. **Minerva Chir** 1983 Jun 30;38(12):815–8
Flamm ES: The decline of osteology and the rise of surgical neurology in the management of head injuries. In Rose FC, Bynum WF, ed: Historical aspects of the neurosciences. New York, Raven, 1982. p. 243–53.
Harris P, Ross JC, et al: [Ludwig Guttmann - special issue]. **Paraplegia** 1979 May;17(1): passim
Meschig R: Zur Geschichte der Trepanation unter besonderer Berücksichtigung der Schädeloperationen bei den Kisii im Hochland Westkenias. Düsseldorf, Triltsch, 1983. xiii, 166 p. (Düsseldorfer Arbeiten zur Geschichte der Medizin, 57).
Rix A: Oklahoma's neurosurgical heritage. **J Okla State Med Assoc** 1980 Apr;73(4):112–8
West CG: A short history of the management of penetrating missile injuries of the head. **Surg Neurol** 1981 Aug;16(2):145–9

### Africa

Meschig R, Schadewaldt H: Skull trepanation in Eastern Africa. **Hexagon Roche** 1981;9(3):17–24

### Americas

Weiss P: La Trepanacion ritual suprainiana––rasgo de culturas peruanas, encontrado también en México y Guatemala. **Bol Soc Mex Hist Filos Med** 1981 Sep;5(36):193–211

### Italy

Guidetti B, Giuffrè R, Valente V: Italian contribution to the origin of neurosurgery. **Surg Neurol** 1983 Oct;20(4):335–46

### Kenya

Meschig R, Schadewaldt H: Schädeloperationen in Kenia. **Dtsch Med Wochenschr** 1981;106:157

### Romania

Crisan V: Neurochirurgische Beiträge über die Benutzung der keltischen Sägen, sowie die in Galatii Bistritei in Rumanien gefundene Säge. In: International Congress of the History of Medicine, 26th, Plovdiv (Bulgaria), 1978. Actes du Congres, Vol. 1. Sofia, 1980. p. 93–6.

### Syria

Bakdash H: Perspectives in international neurosurgery: neurosurgery in Syria. **Neurosurgery** 1979 Dec;5(6):759–60

### Before 500 A.D.

Campillo D: Neurosurgical pathology in prehistory. **Acta Neurochir (Wien)** 1984;70(3–4):275–90

### USSR

Derums VJ: Extensive trepanation of the skull in ancient Latvia. **Bull Hist Med** 1979 Fall;53(3):459–64

### 500 A.D.–1450

### Peru

Canalis RF, Cabieses F, Hemenway WG, et al: Prehistoric trephination of the frontal sinus. **Ann Otol Phinol Laryngol** 1981 Mar–Apr;90(2 pt 1):186–9

### 1700 to Present

Black DW: Psychosurgery. **South Med J** 1982 Apr;75(4):453–7
Bucy PC: The pioneers of neurology and neurosurgery in the world and their contributions. A lecture for young Japanese neurosurgeons. **No Shinkei Geka** 1982 May;10(5):490–8
Curtis JB, Miller D, Simpson D: The Neurosurgical society of Australasia: the first forty years. **Aust NZ J Surg** 1980 Aug;50(4):434–7
Donaghy RM: The history of microsurgery in neurosurgery. **Clin Neurosurg** 1979;26:619–25
Gillingham FJ: The influence of Harvey Cushing on British and European neurosurgery. **Surg Neurol** 1982 May;17(5):344–9
Goldhahn WE: Die interdisziplinären Verbindungen der Neurochirurgie in Vergangenheit, Gegenwart und Zukunft. **Zentralbl Neurochir** 1983;44(4):295–301
Hart BL: Neurosurgery for behavioral problems. A curiosity or the new

wave? **Vet Clin North Am [Small Anim Pract]** 1982 Nov;12(4):707–14
Laine E: Histoire de la chirurgie des anévrysmes cérébraux. **Bull Mem Acad R Med Belg** 1983;138(12):576–86
Ljunggren B: Cushing och Sven Hedin. **Lakartidningen** 1982 Aug 11;79(32–33):2790–2
Luyendijk W: The arteries of the spinal cord. The history of a paradigmal shift. **Acta Neurochir (Wien)** 1982;61(1–3):25–41
Nakazawa S: [Recent advances in neurological surgery (Jpn). **Nippon Ika Daigaku Zasshi** 1981 Dec;48(6):711
Niculescu SI: Pe marginea corespondenţei dintre Harvey Cushing şi Dumitru Bagdasar. **Rev Med Interna [Neurol Psihiatr]** 1981 Jul–Sep;26(3):229–33
Penzholz H: Development and present state of cerebellopontine angle surgery from the neuro- and otosurgical point of view. **Arch Otorhinolaryngol** 1984;240(2):167–74
Petrescu A: Lumini în marele întuneric din istoria neurochirurgiei. **Rev Med Interna [Neurol Psihiatr]** 1981 Oct–Dec;26(4):311–4
Pothe H: Zur geschichtlichen Entwicklung der operativen Zugangswege zur Sella turcica. **Zentralbl Neurochir** 1983;44(2):151–4
Satoh O: [Transsphenoidal surgery for pituitary tumors: historical review and present trends] (Jpn). **No Shinkei Geka** 1984 Jan;12(1):7–26
Teichman SL, Aldea PA: Pioneers in pituitary physiology: Harvey Cushing and Nicolas Paulescu. **J Hist Med Allied Sci** 1985 Jan;40(1):68–72
Wertheimer P, David M, Sindou M, et al: Naissance et croissance de la neurochirurgie. **Neurochirurgie** 1979;25(5–6):247–63
Wilson CB: A decade of pituitary microsurgery. **J Neurosurg** 1984 Nov;61(5):814–33
Zülch KJ: Reflections on the surgery of the pineal gland (a glimpse into the past). Gleanings from medical history. **Neurosurg Rev** 1981;4(3):159–63

**Asia**

Kariev Mkh: Istoriia i sostoianie neĭrokhirurgicheskoĭ sluzhby v respublikakh Sredneĭ Azii. **Zh Vopr Neirokhir** 1983 Sep–Oct;5:56–8

**Austria**

Diemath HE: Perspectives in international neurosurgery: neurosurgery in Austria. **Neurosurgery** 1981 Nov;9(5):604–5

**Brazil**

Marino R: Perspectives in international neurosurgery: neurosurgery in Brazil. **Neurosurgery** 1982 Sep;11(3):454–6

**Bulgaria**

Petrov P, Bussarsky VA: Perspectives in international neurosurgery: neurosurgery in Bulgaria. **Neurosurgery** 1981 Dec;9(6):758

**Canada**

Botterell EH: Kenneth George McKenzie, M.D., F.R.C.S., 1923–1963. **Surg Neurol** 1982 Feb;17(2):81–9

**China**

Chen BH: Neurosurgery in China. (A report presented in the Italian Cities of Turin, Padua and Florence in October, 1981). **J Neurosurg Sci** 1982 Oct–Dec;26(4):273–7
Shih CJ: Perspectives in international neurosurgery: neurosurgery in Taiwan. **Neurosurgery** 1979 Nov;5(5):637–40
Wu WQ: Neurosurgery in Tibet. **Surg Neurol** 1981 Jun;15(6):419–21
Yu-chuan S: Perspectives in neurosurgery: neurosurgery in the People's Republic of China. **Neurosurgery** 1981 Apr;8(4):497–500

**Czechoslovakia**

Kunc Z: Pěhled cinnosti neurochirurgické kliniky v Praze 1959--1978. **Cas Lek Cesk** 1979 Jul 20;118(29):897–901

**Denmark**

Broager B: Perspectives in international neurosurgery: neurosurgery in Denmark. **Neurosurgery** 1980 Nov;7(5):529–30

**Europe**

Brihaye J: Celebration of the 10th anniversary of the European Association of Neurosurgical Societies. **Acta Neurochir (Wien)** 1982;60(1–2):1–6
Brihaye J: History of the European Association of Neurosurgical Societies. **Neurosurgery** 1984 Aug;15(2):262–4

**Finland**

Törmä T: Perspectives in international neurosurgery: neurosurgery in Finland. **Neurosurgery** 1981 Oct;9(4):479–81

**Germany**

Alexander E, Alexander E (3d): German influences on the work of Harvey Cushing, the pioneer of neurosurgery in America. **Neurosurgery** 1981 Nov;9(5):501–5
Geiger I: Das Leben und Werk von Wilhelm Tönnis unter besonderer Berücksichtigung seiner Würzburger Zeit. Diss. Würzburg, 1981. 109 p.
Gerlach J: Perspectives in international neurosurgery: neurosurgery in West Germany. **Neurosurgery** 1982 Jun;10(6 Pt 1):785–7
Pothoff PC, Schwarz R: Traugott Riechert. **Surg Neurol** 1983 May;19(5):403–5

**Great Britain**

Black SP: Wilfred Trotter. **Surg Neurol** 1983 Mar;19(3):199–204
Cooper IS: Sir Victor Horsley: father of modern neurological surgery. In Rose FC, Bynum WF, ed: Historical aspects of the neurosciences. New York, Raven, 1982. p. 235–8.
Himsworth H: Sir Geoffrey Jefferson. In Dictionary of national biography, 1961–1970. Suppl. 8, 1981. p. 580–1.
Hunter AR: Anaesthesia for intracranial surgery: an autobiographical view. **Ann R Coll Surg Engl** 1981;63:316–21
Hunter AR: Zebulon Mennell. A pioneer of neurosurgical anaesthesia. **Anaesthesia** 1983 Dec;38(12):1214–6
Jefferson A: Geoffrey Jefferson 1886–1961. **Surg Neurol** 1984 Jul;22(1):1–4
Kirkpatrick DB: The first primary brain-tumor operation. **J Neurosurg** 1984 Nov;61(5):809–13
Pattison FL: The Pattison-Miller quarrel. **Scott Med J** 1980 Jul;25(3):234–40

**Honduras**

Diaz CM: Perspectives in international neurosurgery: neurosurgery in Honduras. **Neurosurgery** 1982 Feb;10(2):277–8

**Hungary**

Hullay J: Perspectives in international neurosurgery: neurosurgery in Hungary. **Neurosurgery** 1981 May;8(5):627–8

**Ireland**

Byrnes DP: Perspectives in international neurosurgery: neurosurgery in Ireland. **Neurosurgery** 1983 May;12(5):585–8

**Italy**

Giuffré R: Successful radical removal of an intracranial meningioma in 1835 by Professor Pecchioli of Siena. **J Neurosurg** 1984 Jan;60(1):47–51
Guidetti B: Francesco Durante. June 29, 1844 to October 2, 1934. **Surg Neurol** 1983 Jul;20(1):1–3
Rossi GF: Perspectives in international neurosurgery: neurosurgery in Italy. **Neurosurgery** 1981 Jan;8(1):132–3

**Japan**

Bucy PC: 'Ancora imparo'--'I continue to learn'. **Neurol Med Chir (Tokyo)** 1981 Jul;21(7):629–34
Sano K: Perspectives in international neurosurgery: neurosurgery in Japan. **Neurosurgery** 1980 Mar;6(3):337–9

**Netherlands**

Vet AC de: Perspectives in international neurosurgery: neurosurgery in the Netherlands. **Neurosurgery** 1981 Jul;9(1):92–4

**New Zealand**

MacDonald GM: Perspectives in international neurosurgery: the development of neurosurgical services in New Zealand. **Neurosurgery** 1980 Apr;6(4):466–7

**Norway**

Kristiansen K: Perspectives in neurosurgery: neurosurgery in Norway. **Neurosurgery** 1981 Jun;8(6):750–2

**Portugal**

Guerra M: Corino Andrade na história da medicina Portuguesa. **Acta Med Port** 1983 Apr–May;4(4–5):239–43
Sancho Trabulo AA: Perspectives in international neurosurgery: neurosurgery in Portugal. **Neurosurgery** 1982 Mar;10(3):409–10

**Romania**

Arseni C, Ciurea AV: The history of Romanian neurosurgery. Bucharest, Medical Publishing House, 1981. 21 p.

**South Africa**

De Villiers JC: Perspectives in international neurosurgery: neurosurgery in South Africa. **Neurosurgery** 1983 Nov;13(5):609–10

**Spain**

Zabalogoitia GB: Perspectives in international neurosurgery: neurosurgery in Spain. **Neurosurgery** 1984 Jan;14(1):111–2

**Sweden**

Crişan V: Herbert Olivecrona (1891–1980). **Rev Med Interna [Neurol Psihiatr]** 1981 Oct–Dec;26(4):307–10
Ljunggren B: Reflexioner kring en hjärnsvulst hos 'En förnäm herre af 30 år'. **Sydsven Medicinhist Sallsk Arsskr** 1983;:87–102

**Switzerland**

Richter HR: Perspectives in international neurosurgery: neurosurgery in Switzerland. **Neurosurgery** 1980 Dec;7(6):632–5

**Turkey**

Berkay F: Perspectives in international neurosurgery: neurosurgery in Turkey. **Neurosurgery** 1980 Oct;7(4):419–22

**United States**

Alexander E: Archaeology: the big neurosurgical dig. **Clin Neurosurg** 1981;28:323–73
Beatty WK: William T. Bovie, inventor and teacher. **Trans Stud Coll Physicians Phila** 1979 Jun;5(1 no 2):138–44
Davis L: The philosophy of a neurosurgeon. **J Kans Med Soc** 1980 May;81(5):252–5
Handa H: [Percival Bailey (author's transl)] (Jpn). **No Shinkei Geka** 1981 Mar;9(4):538–41
Horrax G: Some of Harvey's Cushing's contributions to neurological surgery. **J Neurosurg** 1981 Apr;54(4):436–47
Jacobson HG: A revisit with Leo M. Davidoff, M.D.—a titan of his time: some personal notes (1898–1975). **Neurosurgery** 1983 Nov;13(5):601–6
James Garber Galbraith, M.D.: **Clin Neurosurg** 1982;29:xiii–xix
Kelly DL: Eben Alexander, Jr., M.D.: a biographical sketch. **Clin Neurosurg** 1981;28:xiii–xx
Kenéz J: Harvey Williams Cushing (1869–1939) und die moderne Hirnchirurgie. **Med Welt** 1980 Sep 5;31(36):1295–7
Key JD: Winchell McKendree Craig. In Dictionary of American Biography, Suppl. 6, 1956–1960. p. 130–31, 1980.
Kucharski A: History of frontal lobotomy in the United States, 1935–1955. **Neurosurgery** 1984 Jun;14(6):765–72
Ljunggren B: Pionjärer inom hjärnkirurgi. **Lakartidningen** 1982 Apr 7;79(14):1377–8
Ljunggren B: The case of General Wood. **J Neurosurg** 1982 Apr;56(4):471–4
McGrath MH: Scalping: the savage and the surgeon. In Romm S, ed: Symposium on historical perspectives of plastic surgery. Philadelphia, Saunders, 1983. p. 679–88.
Molino-Negro P: Jules Hardy M.D. **Surg Neurol** 1984 Aug;22(2):109–12
Perret GE: Doctor Loyal Davis—the neurosurgeon. **Surg Gynecol Obstet** 1983 Aug;157(2):140–3
Pinkus RL: Innovation in neurosurgery: Walter Dandy in his day. **Neurosurgery** 1984 May;14(5):623–31
Ray BS: The development of neurosurgery in New York City. **Bull NY Acad Med** 1979 Nov;55(10):916–38
Rosegay H: Cushing's legacy to transsphenoidal surgery. **J Neurosurg** 1981 Apr;54(4):448–54
Sano K: [Harvey Williams Cushing] (Jpn). **No Shinkei Geka** 1981 Jan;9(1):32–5
Schneck JM: Brain injury, psychiatric sequelae, and surgical intervention in S. Weir Mitchell's Westways. **JAMA** 1983 Dec 9;250(22):3048
Shutts D: Lobotomy, resort to the knife. New York, Van Nostrand Reinhold, 1982. xxi, 284 p.
Wetzel N: Loyal Davis; Allen Kanavel; surgery, gynecology and obstetrics, and the development of neurosurgery. **Surg Gynecol Obstet** 1983 Aug;157(2):135–9
Wilkins RH: Birth of a journal: the origin and early years of Neurosurgery. **Neurosurgery** 1982 Jun;10(6 Pt 2):820–6
Woodhall B: Walter Dandy, M.D.: personal reminiscences. **Neurosurgery** 1979 Jan;4(1):3–6
Yaksh TL: Obituary for Dr. Frederick W. L. Kerr. **Pain** 1984 Mar;18(3):217–20

**USSR**

Konovalov AN, Iartsev VV: Istoriia i perspektivy razvitiia sovetskoĭ neĭrokhirurgii. **Zh Vopr Neirokhir** 1982 Sep–Oct;(5):3–8
Konovalov AN, Iartsev VV: 50-letie Nauchno-issledovatel'skogo ordena Trudovogo Krasnogo Znameni instituta neĭrokhirurgii im. akad. N. N. Burdenko AMN SSSR. **Zh Vopr Neirokhir** 1981 Nov–Dec;(6):3–9
Panchenko PM, Shereshevskiĭ AM: V. M. Bekhterev i neĭrokhirurgiia (k 125-letiiu so dnia rozhdeniia). **Zh Vopr Neirokhir** 1982 Sep–Oct;(5):59–61
Rachkov BM, Potanina MN: Razvitie neĭrokhirurgii v Rossiĭskoĭ Federatsii. **Zh Vopr Neirokhir** 1982 Nov–Dec;(6):3–7
Romodanov AP: Neirokhirurgiia Sovetskoĭ Ukrainy. **Zh Vopr Neirokhir** 1982 Sep–Oct;(5):9–11
Victorovich YV, Rachmanovna DO: Perspectives in international neurosurgery: neurosurgery in the Union of Soviet Socialist Republics. **Neurosurgery** 1981 Feb;8(2):283–4
Zlotnik EN: Razvitie neĭrokhirurgii v Belorusskoĭ SSR. **Zh Vopr Neirokhir** 1982 Nov–Dec;(6):7–9

**Yugoslavia**

Konjhodžić F, Simunović V: Prve operacije na glavi i mozgu u akufskoj bolnici u Sarajeve. **Med Arh** 1978 Sep–Oct;32(5):325–8

**Zaire**

Djhnga S: Perspectives in international neurosurgery: neurosurgery in Zaire. **Neurosurgery** 1983 Jul;13(1):95–7

**PLASTIC**

Bennett JP: Aspects of the history of plastic surgery since the 16th century. **J R Soc Med** 1983 Feb;76(2):152–6
Busse H, Hollwich F, Jünemann G: Plastische und rekonstruktive Chirururie der Tränenwege. **Ber Zusammenkunft Dtsch Ophthalmol Ges** 1979;(77):111–21
Eisenberg I: A history of rhinoplasty. **S Afr Med J** 1982 Aug 21;62(9):286–92
Hauben DJ: Die Geschichte der Rhinoplastik. **Laryngol Rhinol Otol (Stuttg)** 1983 Feb;62(2):53–5
Hauben DJ, Baruchin A, Mahler A: On the history of the free skin graft. **Ann Plast Surg** 1982 Sep;9(3):242–5
Hauben DJ: Plastic surgery - historical aspects. **Koroth** 1981;8(1-2):71–7
Hauben DJ, Sonneveld GJ: The influence of war on the development of plastic surgery. **Ann Plast Surg** 1983 Jan;10(1):65–9
Kastenbauer ER: Zur Geschichte der Plastischen und Wiederherstellungschirurgie im Kopf- und Halsbereich. **Laryngol Rhinol Otol (Stuttg)** 1981 May;60(5):245–50
Mazzola RF, Lupo G: Evolving concepts in lip reconstruction. **Clin Plast Surg** 1984 Oct;11(4):583–617
Montandon D: History of plastic surgery of the orbital region. In S. J. Aston, et al., ed: Third international symposium of plastic and reconstructive surgery of the eye and adnexa. Baltimore, London, Williams & Wilkins, 1982. p. 2–10.
Patterson T: La fabbrica dei nasi. **Kos** 1984 Apr;1(3):75–90
Rodegra H, Pirsig W: Zur Geschichte der Versorgung von Mittelgesichtsverletzungen. **Laryngol Rhinol Otol (Stuttg)** 1980 Jul;59(7):412–7
Rogers BO: History of cosmetic blepharoplasty. In S. J. Aston, et al., ed: Third international symposium of plastic and reconstructive surgery of the eye and adnexa. Baltimore, London, Williams & Wilkins, 1982. p. 276–81.
Romm S: On the beauty of lips. **Clin Plast Surg** 1984 Oct;11(4):571–81
Romm S, ed: Symposium on historical perspectives of plastic surgery. Philadelphia, Saunders, 1983. p. 593–716. (Clinics in plastic surgery, Oct. 1983, vol. 10, no. 4) Contributions by E. H. Christianson, D. Clark, B. F. Conroy, W. B. Davis, H. C. Greisman, E. A. Luce, M. H. McGrath, J. F. McMurry, W. O. Morain, A. D. Morani, R. F. Morgan, L. S. Nichter, M. A. Nichter, R. L. Ruberg, L. A. Sargent, J. Scarborough, R. R. Shah, C. N. Verheyden, A. F. Wallace, J. B. Zacher.
Verdan C: Geschichte der plastischen und wiederherstellenden Chirurgie. In Sournia JC, Martiny M, Poulet J, ed: Illustrierte Geschichte der Medizin. Salzburg, Andreas, 1980. Vol. 8. p. 2911–31.

**India**

Nichter LS, Morgan RF, Nichter MA: The impact of Indian methods for total nasal reconstruction. In Romm S, ed: Symposium on historical perspectives of plastic surgery. Philadelphia, Saunders, 1983. p. 635–47.

**Before 500 A.D.**

**Egypt**

Goldwyn RM: Is there plastic surgery in the Edwin Smith Papyrus? **Plast Reconstr Surg** 1982 Aug;70(2):263–4

# SURGERY

**India**

Hauben DJ: Sushruta Samhita (Sushruta's Collection) (800–600 B.C.?). Pioneers of plastic surgery. **Acta Chir Plast (Prague)** 1984;26(2):65–8

**Rome**

Hauben DJ: Aulus (Aurelius) Cornelius Celsus (25 v.u.Z.–50 n.u.Z.) – Vater der plastischen Chirurgie. **Zentralbl Chir** 1984;109(6):441–3

Marmelzat Wl: Medicine in history. Celsus (Ad 25), plastic surgeon: on the repair of defects of the ears, lips, and nose. **J Dermatol Surg Oncol** 1982 Dec;8(12):1012–4

**1450–1700**

Hauben DJ: Das chirurgische Erbe. Pioniere der plastischen Chirurgie der Renaissance (1). **Zentralbl Chir** 1984;109(9):631–7

**Belgium**

Vrebos J: Jehan Yperman, medieval cleft lip surgeon. **Plast Reconstr Surg** 1982 Dec;70(6):762–5

**Great Britain**

Lutz LA: Shakespeare on plastic surgery. **Plast Reconstr Surg** 1984 Dec;74(6):841

**1700 to Present**

Bodenham DC: In quest of perfection: training in plastic surgery. (McIndoe Memorial Lecture, 1980). **Ann R Coll Surg Engl** 1981;63:233–8

Chase RA: The development of tissue transfer in hand surgery. **J Hand Surg [Am]** 1984 Jul;9(4):463–77

Converse JM: Experimental human skin allografts, the hla complex, and a Nobel prize. **Plast Reconstr Surg** 1982 Aug;70(2):255–62

Cremone JC, Beddings A: Aesthetic reconstruction [letter]. **Plast Reconstr Surg** 1983 Mar;71(3):440–2

Cremone JC: Thinking before incising. **Plast Reconstr Surg** 1984 Mar;73(3):500

Freshwater MF: Priorities in plastic surgery. **Plast Reconstr Surg** 1984 Jun;73(6):987–90

Goldwyn RM: The paraffin story. **Plast Reconstr Surg** 1980 Apr;65(4):517–24

Hakme F: Abdominoplasty: peri- and supra-umbilical lipectomy. **Aesthetic Plast Surg** 1983;7(4):213–20

Heritier J: Le martyre des nez coupés: les débuts de la chirurgie esthétique. **Histoire** 1983;(57):68–71

Klasen HJ: History of free skin grafting--knowledge or empiricism? Berlin, New York, Springer, 1981. 190 p.

Krag C, Kirkby B: The deltopectoral flap: a historical review with comments on its role in neurovascular reconstruction. **Scand J Plast Reconstr Surg** 1980:14(2):145–50

McCraw JB: The recent history of myocutaneous flaps. **Clin Plast Surg** 1980 Jan;7(1):3–7

Mazzola RF, Marcus S: History of total nasal reconstruction with particular emphasis on the folded forehead flap technique. **Plast Reconstr Surg** 1983 Sep;72(3):408–14

Moermans JP, Bovy A, De Mey A: Aspects historiques des lambeaux libres. **Acta Chir Belg** 1982 May–Jun;82(3):213–8

Nicolai JP: Facial paralysis -- 100 years of treatment. **Arch Chir Neerl** 1979;31(3):159–69

Pirsig W: Septumdeviation 1882: Beginn der systematischen submukösen Septumchirurgie. **Laryngol Rhinol Otol (Stuttg)** 1982 Oct;61(10):547–51

Rhys Evans PH: Prominent ears and their surgical correction. **J Laryngol Otol** 1981 Sep;95(9):9881–92

Rogers BO: Julius von Szymanowski (1829--1868). His life and contributions to plastic surgery. **Plast Reconstr Surg** 1979 Oct;64(4):465–78

Romm S, Zacher J: Anna Coleman Ladd: maker of masks for the facially mutilated. **Plast Reconstr Surg** 1982 Jul;70(1):104–11

Rudert H: Von der sujbmukösen Septumresektion Killians über Cottles Septumplastik zur modernen plastischen Septumkorrektur und funktionellen Septo-Rhinoplastik. **HNO** 1984 Jun;32(6):230–3

Wallace AF: The progress of plastic surgery: an introductory history. Oxford, W. A. Meeuws, 1982. xii, 184 p.

Wallace AF: The surgery of beauty. **Trans Med Soc Lond** 1981–82;98:17–23

Zeis E, Patterson TJ, ed: The Zeis index and history of plastic surgery. Baltimore, Williams and Wilkins, 1977. xxix, 315 p.

**Canada**

Williams HB: The McGill University plastic surgery program. **Ann Plast Surg** 1984 Nov;13(5):362–5

**China**

Lu M: History of plastic surgery in China. **Plast Reconstr Surg** 1982 Aug;70(2):273–4

**Colombia**

Orticochea M: History of the discovery of the musculocutaneous flap method as a substitute for the delay method. **Ann Plast Surg** 1983 Jul;11(1):63–8

**France**

Achard E: 1956--numéro 1 des 'Annales de Chirurgie Plastique'. **Ann Chir Plast** 1980;25(2):191–2

Firmin F: Cancer de la joue et autoplastie en l'an 1838. Opération de génioplastie pratiquée par M. Roux de Brignolles. **Ann Chir Plast** 1982;27(1):91–3

Lisfranc J: Mémoire sur la rhynoplastie, ou l'art de refaire le nez. **Ann Chir Plast** 1982;27(2):189–93

Marchac D: Julien Bourguet. The pioneer in aesthetic surgery of the neck. **Clin Plast Surg** 1983 Jul;10(3):363–5

Ortiz-Monasterio F: Labat and the three-lobed forehead flap. **Plast Reconstr Surg** 1984 Apr;73(4):705

Pons J, Davoust B, Pons ML: Qui êtes-vous Monsieur Camille Bernard? **Ann Chir Plast Esthet** 1983;28(2):199–200

Rogers BO: Hippolyte Morestin (1869–1919). Part I: A brief biography. **Aesthetic Plast Surg** 1982;6(3):141–7

Teimourian B, Adham MN: Louis Ombredanne and the origin of muscle flap use for immediate breast mound reconstruction. **Plast Reconstr Surg** 1983 Dec;72(6):905–10

Yarington CT: The evolution of reconstructive facial surgery. **Otolaryngol Clin North Am** 1983 May;16(2):305–8

**Germany**

Goldwyn RM: Carl August Burow. **Plast Reconstr Surg** 1984 Apr;73(4):687–90

Hauben DJ: Carl Ferdinand von Graefe (1787–1840). **Zentralbl Chir** 1984;109(14):950–1

Hauben DJ: Ernst Blasius's contributions to plastic surgery. **Plast Reconstr Surg** 1984 Oct;74(4):561–70

Hauben DJ: Jacques Joseph (1865–1934). **Laryngol Rhinol Otol (Stuttg)** 1983 Feb;62(2):56–7

Natvig P: Jacques Joseph, surgical sculptor. Philadelphia, Saunders, 1982. xiii, 264 p.

Schmidt-Tintemann U: Plastische Chirurgie. Entwicklung in Deutschland. **MMW** 1983 Jul 1;125(26):566–8

**Great Britain**

As I remember. T. P. Kilner.: **Ann Plast Surg** 1980 Apr;4(4):328–36

Bennett JP: Sir William Fergusson and the Indian Rhinoplasty. **Ann R Coll Surg Engl** 1984 Nov;66(6):444–8

Hauben DJ: Robert Liston's life and work in the renaissance of plastic surgery. **Ann Plast Surg** 1983 Jun;10(6):502–9

Muir IF: The development of plastic surgery in the United Kingdom. **Ann Plast Surg** 1981 May;6(5):411–5

**Italy**

Maxwell GP: Iginio Tansini and the origin of the latissimus dorsi musculocutaneous flap. **Plast Reconstr Surg** 1980 May;65(5):686–92

Zanobio B: Contributi di Scuola Pavese allo sviluppo della chirurgia plastica. **Minerva Chir** 1983 Mar 31;38(6):297–302

**New Zealand**

Beattie D: Plastic surgery in New Zealand (Sir Harold Gillies). **Ann Plast Surg** 1982 Nov;9(5):358–60

**United States**

As I remember: Clarence R. Straatsma: **Ann Plast Surg** 1981 Oct;7(4):327–32

As I remember Earl C. Padgett: **Ann Plast Surg** 1981 Feb;6(2):142–57

Aufricht G: Story of the foundation of the Plastic and Reconstructive Surgery journal and reminiscences of the early formative years of plastic surgery as a specialty. **Plast Reconstr Surg** 1981 Sep;68(3):370–5

Cannon B: External esophageal construction remembered. **Plast Reconstr Surg** 1983 Apr;71(4):540–2

Converse JM: The extraordinary career of Doctor Varaztad Hovhannes Kazanjian. **Plast Reconstr Surg** 1983 Jan;71(1):138–43

Deranian HM: The miracle man of the western front: the story of Dr. Varaztad Kazanjian. **Bull Hist Dent** 1984 Oct;32(2):85–103

Fisher GT, Fisher JB, Stark RB: Origin of the use of subcuticular sutures. **Ann Plast Surg** 1980 Feb;4(2):144–8

Frileck SP: More on Robert Abbe's contributions to the field of plastic surgery. **Ann Plast Surg** 1979 Oct;3(4):357–60
Goldwyn RM: Transition. **Plast Reconstr Surg** 1980 Jan;65(1):70–1
Hamm WG: The development of plastic surgery during the past sixty years. **Ann Plast Surg** 1984 Feb;12(2):102–4
Ketchum LD: An historical account of the development of the calibrated dermatome. **Ann Plast Surg** 1978 Nov;1(6):608–11
Marino H: Reminiscences of the American Society of Plastic and Reconstructive Surgeons, Inc., and some of its members. **Plast Reconstr Surg** 1981 Sep;68(3):376–80
Meals RA, Brody GS: Gatewood and the first thenar pedicle. **Plast Reconstr Surg** 1984 Feb;73(2):315–9
Morgan RF: The Fort McHenry General Hospital for plastic and maxillofacial surgery. **Plast Reconstr Surg** 1983 Aug;72(2):255–9
Murray JE: An interview with Joseph E. Murray, M.D. conducted by Joel M. Noe, M.D. **Ann Plast Surg** 1984 Jan;12(1):84–9
Orenstein HH: How excellent a showman: Joseph Eastman Sheehan, 1885–1951. **Bull NY Acad Med** 1983 Apr;59(3):327–30
Paletta FX: History of the American Society of Plastic and Reconstructive Surgeons, Inc., 1931–1981: its growth, change, unity. **Plast Reconstr Surg** 1981 Sep;68(3):292–369
Romm S: Morris Joseph Asch. **Plast Reconstr Surg** 1983 May;71(5):724–8
Romm S: The persons behind the name: Charles Bingham Penrose. **Plast Reconstr Surg** 1982 Sep;70(3):397–9
Shell DH: John Bingham Roberts: Philadelphia plastic surgeon. **Plast Reconstr Surg** 1982 Jan;69(1):145–54
Spira M, Hardy SB: The history of Baylor College of Medicine affiliated residency in plastic surgery. **Ann Plast Surg** 1983 Oct;11(4):268–72
Yavenditti MJ: The Hiroshima maidens and American benevolence in the 1950's. **Mid-Am** 1982;64(2):21–39

**USSR**

Balon LR: N. I. Pirogov--osnovopolozhnik otechestvennoĭ vosstanovitel'noĭ khirurgii. **Vestn Khir** 1983 Jun;130(6):93–7

### THORACIC

Bahnson HT: Classics in thoracic surgery. **Ann Thorac Surg** 1982 Jan;33(1):96–8 (continued regularly)
Brewer LA: Historical notes on lung cancer before and after Graham's successful pneumonectomy in 1933. **Am J Surg** 1982 Jun;143(6):650–9
Stahnke J: Geschichte der Lungenchirurgie. **MMW** 1980 Oct 24;122(43):1517–8

**1700 to Present**

Bendixen HH: Respirators and respiratory care. **Acta Anaesthesiol Scand** 1982 Jun;26(3):279–86
Bogdan TT: Poluvekovoĭ opyt khirurgii raka legkogo. **Vestn Khir** 1984 Apr;132(4):69–71
Brewer LA: The contributions of the Second Auxiliary Surgical Group to military surgery during World War II with special reference to thoracic surgery. **Ann Surg** 1983 Mar;197(3):318–26
Edwards WS: Alexis Carrel's contributions to thoracic surgery. **Ann Thorac Surg** 1983 Jan;35(1):111–4
Spencer FC: Intellectual creativity in thoracic surgeons. **J Thorac Cardiovasc Surg** 1983 Aug;86(2):163–79
White JJ: 'Classics' and total pneumonectomy. **Ann Thorac Surg** 1981 Aug;32(2):216

**China**

Shumacker HB: An American surgeon's contribution to Chinese health care. **Am J Surg** 1981 Mar;141(3):311–6

**Czechoslovakia**

Procházka J: Poznámky k rozvoji československé plicní chirurgie. **Cas Lek Cesk** 1984 Jan 27;123(4):85–8

**Denmark**

Husfeldt E: Traek af thoraxkirurgiens historie i Danmark. **Dan Medicinhist Arbog** 1982;:9–21

**Germany**

Abe HR, Kaiser L: Ferdinand Sauerbruch und Erfurt. **Beitr Gesch Univ Erfurt** 1979–83;19:271–81
Bertram E, Wengenmayer M: Ein Dezennium Lungenchirurgie. Operative Therapie am Krankengut der Jahre 1958 bis 1967. **Prax Klin Pneumol** 1980 May;34(5):282–94
Hägermark O: Beläst, försynt invärtesmedicinare – piojär även inom lumbalpunktionsteknik och lungkirurgi. **Lakartidningen** 1983 Nov 16;80(46):4429–30

**Great Britain**

Scadding JG: The Thoracic Society: a retrospect. **Thorax** 1983 Feb;38(2):88–92
Smith RA: Development of lung surgery in the United Kingdom. **Thorax** 1982 Mar;37(3):161–8
Turner-Warwick M: The British Thoracic Society. **Thorax** 1982 May;37(5):321–3

**Romania**

Lazăr C, Ionescu C: Istoricul chirurgiei toraco-pulmonare din Moldova. **Rev Med Chir Soc Med Nat Iasi** 1980 Jul-Sept;84(3):575–7

**Switzerland**

Tanner-Weder C: Alfred Brunner und die Entwicklung der Thoraxchirurgie. Zürich, Juris, 1980. 37p. (Zürcher Medizingeschichtliche Abhandlungen, Neue Reihe, Nr. 142).

**United States**

Baue AE: Landmark perspective: Evarts A. Graham and the first pneumonectomy. **JAMA** 1984 Jan 13;251(2):260–4
Breathnach CS: Biographical sketches no. 28 -- Graham. **Ir Med J** 1983 Apr;76(4):167
Brewer LA: The first pneumonectomy. Historical notes. **J Thorac Cardiovasc Surg** 1984 Nov;88(5 Pt 2):810–26
Ellison RG: Paul C. Samson, M.D., 1905–1982. Part I. His contributions to the Society of Thoracic Surgeons. **Ann Thorac Surg** 1983 Nov;36(5):500–1
Ellison RG: The Society of Thoracic Surgeons: the first twenty years. **Ann Thorac Surg** 1984 Jan;37(1):1–8
Ferguson TB: Evarts A. Graham--the man. **J Thorac Cardiovasc Surg** 1984 Nov;88(5 Pt 2):803–9
Meyer BW: An overview of thirty years of thoracic surgery. **J Thorac Cardiovasc Surg** 1982 Feb;83(2):163–7
Moerchel J: The introduction of thoracic surgery into America. **Clio Med** 1980;15(1/2):67–73
Olivier AF: In proper perspective: Daniel Hale Williams, M.D. **Ann Thorac Surg** 1984 Jan;37(1):96–7
Ravitch MM: Progress in resection of the chest wall for tumor with reminiscences of Dr. Blalock. **Johns Hopkins Med J** 1982 Aug;151(2):43–53
Scannell JG: Some thoracic surgeons of Boston--before the cardiac balloon went up. **Pharos** 1984 Fall;47(4):26–30
Shumacker HB: Leo Eloesser, M.D.: eulogy for a free spirit. New York, Philosophical Library, 1982. 483 p.
Sloan H: Let us now praise famous men. **J Thorac Cardiovasc Surg** 1980 Aug;80(2):159–70
Urschel HC: 'Life is short and the art long, the occasion instant, the experiment perilous, the decision difficult'. **Ann Thorac Surg** 1984 Jul;38(1):1–14

**USSR**

Kariev TM: Razvitie khirurgicheskikh metodov lecheniia tuberkuleza legkikh v Uzbekskoĭ SSR. **Probl Tuberk** 1984 Jun;(6):69–71
Miliavskiĭ VM, Ikonnikov MV: K stoletiiu pervoĭ pnevmotomii v Rossii. **Klin Khir** 1983 Oct;:(10):73–4
Molotkov VN: Rol' Kievskogo ordena Trudovogo Krasnogo Znameni nauchno-issledovatel'skogo instituta tuberkuleza i grudnoĭ khirurgii im. F. G. Ianovskogo v razvitii ftiziatrii i pul'monologii. **Probl Tuberk** 1982 Dec;(12):18–22
Zhurnalu 'Grudnaia khirurgiia' 20 let.: **Grudn Khir** 1980 Jan–Feb;(1):5–6

### TRACHEAL

Brewer LA: History of surgery of the esophagus. **Am J Surg** 1980 Jun;139(6):730–43
Franco Grande A, Martinon JM, Pombo MV, et al: Evolucion historica de la intubación tráqueal. A porpósito de Franz Kuhn en el aniversario de su muerte. **Rev Esp Anestesiol Reanim** 1979 May;26(3):243–54
Klippe HJ, Löhr J, Kroeger C: Historische Aspekte zur Entwicklung der endotrachealen Intubation. **Prax Klin Pneumol** 1981 Sep;35(9):413–20

**1700 to Present**

Langston HT: The first successful total repair of congenital atresia of the esophagus with tracheoesophageal fistula. **Ann Thorac Surg** 1984 Jul;38(1):72–4
Talyshinskiĭ AM: K istorii éndotrakheal'nykh trukbok s manzhetkami i bronkhoblokatorov. **Anesteziol Reanimatol** 1980 Mar–Apr;(2):68–70

**Denmark**

Agård S: Mandlernes historie 1953–1983. **Sygeplejersken** 1984 Mar

21;84(12):23-4

**United States**

Brantigan CO, Grow JB: Cricothyroidotomy revisited again. **Ear Nose Throat J** 1980 Jul;59(7):289-95

**TRANSPLANT**

Dymarskiĭ LIu: K istorii razvitiia khirurgicheskogo lecheniia raka molochnoĭ zhelezy, nachinaia s drevnego Egipta i do nashikh dneĭ. **Khirurgiia (Mosk)** 1981 Apr;(4):111-6

**Before 500 A.D.**

Berle EJ: Legenden om en senantikk bentransplantasjon. **Sydsven Medicinhist Sallsk Arsskr** 1984;21:135-40

**1700 to Present**

Balner H, Marquet RL: Transplantation biology--past and present: reappraisal of 'breakthroughs' since 1955. **Transplant Proc** 1981 Mar;13(1 pt 1):13-8
Black J, Sholtes V: Biomaterial aspects of surface replacement arthroplasty of the hip. **Orthop Clin North Am** 1982 Oct;13(4):709-28
Calne RY: The development of immunosuppressive therapy. **Transplant Proc** 1981 Mar;13(1):44-9
Chase RA: The development of tissue transfer in hand surgery. **J Hand Surg [Am]** 1984 Jul;9(4):463-77
Donovan MG, Barrett DM: Ureteral prostheses. **Semin Urol** 1984 Aug;2(3):158-66
Downing R: Historical review of pancreatic islet transplantation. **World J Surg** 1984 Apr;8(2):137-42
English TA: Heart transplantation---1979. **Trans Hunter Soc** 1978-80;37-38:143-51
Hall BM, Sheil AG: Transplantation in Australia and New Zealand. **Transplant Proc** 1984 Aug;16(4):925-6
Hardy JD: Landmark perspective. Transplantation of blood vessels, organs, and limbs. **JAMA** 1983 Aug 19;250(7):954-7
Johnson FL: Marrow transplantation in the treatment of acute childhood leukemia. Historical development and current approaches. **Am J Pediatr Hematol Oncol** 1981 Winter;3(4):389-95
Juszczyński M: Ostatnie osi ągni ęcia transplantacji serca i płuc. **Kardiol Pol** 1983;26(10):733-9
Juszczyński M: Piętnaście lat transplantacji serca. **Pol Tyg Lek** 1983 May 9;38(19):615-8
Kolff WJ: Past, present, and future of artificial kidneys. **Transplant Proc** 1981 Mar;13(1):35-40
McKee GK: Total hip replacement--past, present and future. **Biomaterials** 1982 Jul;3(3):130-5
Merrill JP: A historical perspective of renal trasplantation. **Proc Clin Dial Transplant Forum** 1979;9:221-5
Merrill JP: Early days of the artificial kidney and transplantation. **Transplant Proc** 1981 Mar;13(1):4-8
Mirskiĭ MB: Vklad Revedena v transplantologiiu i khirurgiiu. **Khirurgiia (Mosk)** 1980 Jun;(6):109-10
Moore FD: Transplantation--a perspective. **Transplant Proc** 1980 Dec;12(4):539-50
Moulin AM, Löwi I: La double nature de l'immunologie: histoire de la transplantation rénale. **Fundam Sci** 1983;4(3/4):201-18
Rapaport FT: Perspectives in transplantation. **Transplant Proc** 1981 Mar;13(1 pt 1):6-9
Schreiner GE: Past, present, and future of transplantation. **Kidney Int [Suppl]** 1983 May;(14):S-4-9
Shumway NE: Heart transplantation. **J Arkansas Med Soc** 1982 Dec;79(7):221-7
Smith HL: [Development of] heart transplantation. In Reich WT, et al, ed: Encyclopedia of bioethics, v. 2. New York, Free Press, 1978. p. 654-60.
Starzl TE: The succession from kidney to liver transplantation. **Transplant Proc** 1981 Mar;13(1):50-4
Steinberg ME: Evolution and development of surface replacement arthroplasty. **Orthop Clin North Am** 1982 Oct;13(4):661-6
Timio M: Il rene artificiale: la storia di uno strumento per una vita semiartificiale. **Med Secoli** 1982;19(3):273-301
Válek A, Wing AJ: Development of dialysis and transplant activity in the world during the seventies of the 20th century. **Z Exp Chir Transplant Kunstliche Organe** 1984;17(2):69-78
Wilberger JE: Transplantation of central nervous tissue. **Neurosurgery** 1983 Jul;13(1):90-4

**France**

Hamburger J: Note préliminaire sur les greffes rénales. **Nephrologie** 1982;3(1):2-5
Mirskiĭ MB: L. Oll'e i ego rol' v razvitii khirurgii i transplantologii (k 150-letiiu so dnia rozhdeniia). **Ortop Travmatol Protez** 1981 Oct;(10):75-6
Shaw R, Stubenbord WT: Alexis Carrel, M.D.; contribution to kidney transplantation and preservation. **NY State J Med** 1980 Aug;80(9):1438-42

**Netherlands**

Hamburger J: Past, present, and future of transplantation. **Transplant Proc** 1981 Mar;13(1):41-3

**Poland**

Juszczyński M: 15 lat transplantacji serca. **Pieleg Polozna** 1984;(2):16-7

**Scandinavia**

Groth CG: Kidney transplantations in the Nordic countries 1956-1980. **Scand J Urol Nephrol** 1981;64:12-5

**United States**

Barrett DM, Donovan MG: Prosthetic bladder augmentation and replacement. **Semin Urol** 1984 Aug;2(3):167-75
Carpenter CB: Clinical histocompatibility testing: a brief historical perspective. **Transplant Proc** 1981 Mar;13(1):55-60
Dammin GJ: Transplantation, 1950s. **Transplant Proc** 1981 Mar;13(1):16-23
Goodwin WE: Recollections: early experiences in kidney transplantation. **Transplant Proc** 1981 Mar;13(1):29-31
Murray JE: Reflections on the first successful kidney transplantation. **World J Surg** 1982 May;6(3):372-6
Murray JE: Remembrances of the early days of renal transplantation. **Transplant Proc** 1981 Mar;13(1):9-15
Nicolai JP: Earliest free muscle graft? **Br J Plast Surg** 1980 Jul;33(3):350-2
Pines M: Modern bioengineers reinvent human anatomy with spare parts. **Smithsonian** 1978;9(8):50-7
Santos GW: History of bone marrow transplantation. **Clin Haematol** 1983 Oct;12(3):611-39
Starzl TE: Loyal Davis, surgery of the liver and transplantation of the kidney. **Surg Gynecol Obstet** 1983 Aug;157(2):160-3
Starzl TE: The landmark identical twin case. **JAMA** 1984 May 18;251(19):2572-3
Thorn GW: A 50th anniversary celebration. **Transplant Proc** 1981 Mar;13(1):24-8
Vandam LD: Impressions of anesthetics past. **Transplant Proc** 1981 Mar;13(1):61-4

**USSR**

Hamilton DN, Reid WA: Yu. Yu. Voronoy and the first human kidney allograft. **Surg Gynecol Obstet** 1984 Sep;159(3):289-94
Keĭsevich LV: K piatidesiatiletiiu pervoĭ v mire klinicheskoĭ allotransplantatsii zhiznenno vashnogo organa. **Klin Khir** 1983 Mar;(3):53-5
Mirski MB: [The history of the problem of kidney transplantation in Soviet medicine (Rus). **Orvostort Kozl** 1980;89-91(26 no 1-3):125-36
Mirskiĭ MB: Dostizheniia sovetskoĭ transplantologii: nauchnyĭ obzor. Moskva, Vses. nauchno-issl. int med. i mediko-tekhn. informatsii, 1979. 96 p.
Mirskiĭ MB: Iu. K. Shimanovskiĭ i ego rol' v razvitii otechestvennoĭ khirurgii i transplantologii (k 150-letiiu so dnia rozhdeniia). **Klin Khir** 1980 Mar;(3):68-71
Mirskiĭ MB: Pamiatnaia vekha v razvitii sovetskoĭ transplantologii (k 25-letiiu I Vsesoiuznoĭ konferentsii po probleme tkanevoĭ nesovmestimosti i transplantatsii organov i tkaneĭ. **Sov Zdravookhr** 1982;(10):70-2
Mirskiĭ MB: Pervaia peresadka pochki v klinike (k 50-letiiu operatsii sovetskogo khirurga Iu. Iu. Voronogo). **Klin Med (Mosk)** 1983 Nov;61(11):147-9

# SYMBOLISM AND HERALDRY

See also **Art**

Baruk H: Moïse, Freud et le veau d'or. **Rev Hist Med Heb** 1984 Jul;37(2):19-23
Brinkman AA: Chemie in de Kunst. Amsterdam, Rodopi, 1975. 69 p.
Franz ML von: Alchemy: an introduction to the symbolism and the psychology. Toronto, Inner City Books, 1980. 280 p. (Studies in Jungian Psychology, 5).
Furukawa A: [The rod of Asklepios and Hygieia's cup--medico-dental and pharmacological symbols] (Jpn). **Shikai Tenbo** 1981 Nov;58(5):977-86
Gettings F: Dictionary of occult, hermetic and alchemical sigils. London, Routledge & Kegan Paul, 1981. 410 p.
Gribanov ED: Emblemy meditsiny. Tbilisi, Sabchota Sakartvelo, 1979. 111 p.
Hausmann W: Weibliche Fruchtbarkeitssymbole der Quanchen und Tarasken. **Tierarztl Prax** 1983;11(3):417-20
Hovesen E: Slangen i laegekunsten. **Dan Medicinhist Arbog** 1983;12:105-21

Leon L: Cos'è un ex libris. **Kos** 1984 Jun;1(5):112–6
Levin S: Eshmun, healing of God of Sidon. **Adler Mus Bull** 1983 Nov;Spec issue:39–42
Levin S: Hebrew medical amulets. **Adler Mus Bull** 1981;7(2):8–12
Lorenz B: Il medico bibliofilo. **Kos** 1984 Jun;1(5):101–11
Nechiporenko PI: Meditsinskaia émblema i ee istoriia. **Med Sestra** 1980 Feb;39(2):50–3
Radbill SX: The cock as a symbol of medicine. **Adler Mus Bull** 1981;7(1):7–9
Rosen J: Of serpents and symbols. **J Am Dent Assoc** 1984 Apr,108(4).534
Rousselle R: Comparative psychohistory: snake-handling in Hellenistic Greece and the American South. **J Psychohist** 1984 Spring;11(4):477–89
Sersiron G: La croix à double barre, symbole de l'UICT. Quelques informations sur ses origines. **Bull Int Union Tuberc** 1982 Sep–Dec;57(3–4):196–9
Stöber O: Drudenfuss-Monographie. Linz, Stadt-Verlag Neydharting, 1981. 460 p.
Vega Diaz F: El corazón en la simbología y en la iconografía profana y religiosa. In Academia Nacional de Medicina. Libro conmemorativo del primer centenario. México, Comité Editorial de la Comisión Organizadora del Congreso del Centenario, 1964. Tome 2. p. 78–82.
Wayman A: The human body as microcosm in India, Greek cosmology, and sixteenth-century Europe. **Hist Relig** 1982;22(2):172–90
Zimmermann RE: The structure of mythos: on the cultural stability of alchemy. **Ambix** 1984 Nov;31(3):125–37

**Denmark**

Kofod H: Danish contributions to the unicorn story. **Beitr Gesch Pharm** 1979,31(2).12–15

**Germany**

Benedum J, Michler M: Das Siegel der Medizinischen Fakultät Giessen. Giessen, Universitätsbibliothek, 1982. 47 p., [18 leaves]. (Berichte und Arbeiten aus der Universitätsbibliothek Giessen, no. 35).

**Poland**

Dutkiewicz M: Z dziejów munduru i symboli służby zdrowia Wojska Polskiego. **Arch Hist Med (Warsz)** 1984;47(1):85–90

**Before 500 A.D.**

Hausmann W: Der Stier als Fruchtbarkeitssymbol. Ein Bericht über Funde aus mehreren Ländern. **DTW** 1982 Feb 5:89(2):86–8
Muñoz P: Origins of the caduceus. **Md State Med J** 1981 Oct;30(10):35–40

**Asia**

Hausmann W: Der Becher des Gudea. **Tierarztl Prax** 1979;7(2):141–3

**Great Britain**

Hart G: A medical caduceus from Roman London. **Trans Med Soc Lond** 1979;95:99–105

**Greece**

Bettermann A: Das Attribut des Asklepios. Versuch über das Zeichen des ärztlichen Standes. **ZFA (Stuttgart)** 1982 Dec 20;58(35–36):1903–7

**1450–1700**

Corbett M: The emblematic title-page to Stirpium Adversaria nova by Petro Pena and Mathias de L'Obel (1570). **Arch Nat Hist** 1981 Apr;10(1):111–7
Telle J: Paracelsistische Sinnbildkunst. Bemerkungen zu einer Pseudo-'Tabula smaragdina' des 16. Jahrhunderts. In Seidler E, Schott II, ed. Bausteine zur Medizingeschichte. Stuttgart, Steiner, 1984. p. 129–39.

**Great Britain**

Ardolino F: The saving hand of God: the significance of the emblematic frontispiece of the Religio medici. **Engl Lang Notes** 1977;15:19–23

**Netherlands**

Schupbach W: The paradox of Rembrandt's 'Anatomy of Dr. Tulp'. London, Wellcome Institute for the History of Medicine, 1982. 110 p. (Medical History, Suppl. No. 2).

**1700 to Present**

Osorio RA: Reflexión con madurez. Reseña histórica del propósito y origen de la ceremonia del 'capping' (coronamiento). **Bol Col Prof Enferm PR** 1983 Jun;9(34):26–7
Ryan MT, Fair MF: The radiation warning symbol. **Health Phys** 1981 Aug;41(2):416–7
Shimabukuro R: [History of the white nursing uniform. A study on the origin of the white uniform as the symbol of nursing] (Jpn). **Kurinikaru Sutadi** 1984 Jun;5(6):688–94

**France**

Montiel L. La enfermedad como símbolo: la peste en la obra de Albert Camus. **Asclepio** 1983;35:171–6

**Germany**

Haeberle EJ: 'Stigmata of degeneration'. Prisoner markings in Nazi concentration camps. **J Homosex** 1980–81 Fall–Winter;6(1–2):135–9
Hein WH: Die ephesische Diana als Natursymbol bei Alexander von Humboldt. In Dilg P, et al., ed: Perspektiven der Pharmaziegeschichte. Graz, Austria, Akademische Druck- u. Verlagsanstalt, 1983. p. 131–46.

**Great Britain**

Dervin D: Rainbow, phoenix, and plumed serpent: D. H. Lawrence's great composite symbols and their vicissitudes. **Psychoanal Rev** 1980 Winter;67(4):515–41

**Ireland**

Shen WW, Soldo JJ: Symbol hunting in James Joyce's 'syphilizations'. **Arch Intern Med** 1981 Apr;141(5):691–2

**United States**

Appel TA: The 1941–42 search for an APS emblem. **Physiologist** 1984 Apr;27(2):69–70

**Yugoslavia**

Straser P, Protić M: Pečat karlovačkog hirurško-berberskog esnafa iz XVIII veka. **Med Pregl** 1982;35(11–12):493

# TERMINOLOGY AND NOMENCLATURE

Ackerknecht EH: Diathesis: the word and the concept in medical history. **Bull Hist Med** 1982 Fall;56(3):317–25
Bagchi AK: Sanskrit and modern medical vocabulary. A comparative study. Calcutta, RDDHI-India, 1978. 119 p.
Ballantyne GH: The meaning of ileus. Its changing definition over three millennia. **Am J Surg** 1984 Aug;148(2):252–6
Barcia Goyanes JJ: Los albores del lenguaje anatómico en las lenguas neolatinos. La traduccion del inventarium de Guy de Chauliac por Bernat de Casaldovol. **Med Esp** 1980;79:235–49
Barcia Goyanes JJ: Onomatologia anatomica nova: historia del lenguaje anatomico. Tomo VI. Nares–Profundus. Valencia, Universidad de Valencia, 1983. 467 p.
Barcia Goyanes JJ: Onomatologia anatomica nova; historia del lenguaje anatómico. Tomos I–III. Valencia, Universidad de Valencia, 1978.
Barcia Goyanes JJ: Un extraño nombre del apendice xifoides: 'malum punicum'; a strange name of the xiphoid process: 'malum punicum'. **Med Esp** 1981;80:105–11
Barthelmé E: Histoire de la notion du cancer. **Hist Sci Med** 1981;15(2):167–72
Bernard J, Druon M: La langue française et la médecine dans le monde. **Rev Deux Mondes** 1979;:45–51
Bynum WF, Browne EJ, Porter R, ed: Dictionary of the history of science. Princeton, Princeton University Press, 1981. [xxxiv], 494 p.
Comiti VP: La fièvre et les fièvres. **Doc Hist Vocab Sci** 1983;(5):91–5
Contreras Poza L: La Torre de Babel del léxico sanitario. **Rev Sanid Hig Publica (Madr)** 1982 Mar–Apr;56(3–4):311–40
Daems WF: Die Apoteca ein 'Stall' und die 'Stall-Apotheke'. **Sudhoffs Arch** 1978;62(1):95–6
Delmas A: L'anatomiste devant les problèmes du langage. **Bull Assoc Anat (Nancy)** 1980;64:313–47
Dirckx JH: New meanings for old words. A gentle introduction to semantics. **Am J Dermatopathol** 1983 Jun;5(3):249–54
Dudziński W: Epigramaty i sentencje łacińskie na tematy medyczne. **Pol Tyg Lek** 1980 Dec 1;35(48):1883–6
Dyck P: Lumbar nerve root: the enigmatic eponyms. **Spine** 1984 Jan–Feb;9(1):3–6
Ellencweig AY, Yoshpe RB: Definition of public health. **Public Health Rev** 1984;12(1):65–78
Febres-Cordero F: Incorrecciones en el lenguaje de medicos y odontologos. Trabajo presentado en el X Congreso Venezolano de Ciencias Medicas. Caracas, 8 de marzo de 1983. 19 p.
Fischer KD: 'Three lexicographical notes.' **Glotta** 1979;57:224–6
Fischer KD: Wege zum Verständnis antiker Tierkrankheitsnamen. **Hist Med Vet** 1977;2(4):106–11

# TERMINOLOGY AND NOMENCLATURE


Gravenstein JS: A perspective on science. The language and history of anesthesia. **Ala J Med Sci** 1984 Jul;21(3):304–10

Grmek MD: La légende et la réalité de la nocivité des fèves. **Hist Philos Life Sci** 1980;2(1):61–121

Hakfoort C: Wetenschapshistorische etiketten en de gevaren van polaire analyses. **Tijdschr Geschied Geneeskd** 1982;5(1):1–5

Halpert BP: Development of the term 'senility' as a medical diagnosis. **Minn Med** 1983 Jul;66(7):421–4

Hartree EF: Ethics for authors: a case history of acrosin. **Perspect Biol Med** 1976 Autumn;20(1):82–91

Hirth W: Uberlieferungen der pseudo-aristotelischen 'Secretum-secretorum'-Diätetik mit abweichenden Verfasserangaben. In International Congress of the History of Medicine, 27th, Barcelona, 1980. Actas. Barcelona, Académia de Ciències Médiques de Catalunya i Balears, 1981. p. 259–63.

Hünemörder C: Aims and intentions of botanical and zoological classification in the Middle Ages and Renaissance. **Hist Philos Life Sci** 1983;5(1):53–67

Jackson R: Historical outine of attempts to classify skin diseases. In: Congrès international d'histoire de la médecine, XXVe, Québec, 1976. Actes. Québec, 1977. p. 798–806.

Johansson BW: Hjärtinfarkt--gammal sjukdom med nytt namn. **Sydsven Medicinhist Sallsk Arsskr** 1980;:57–79

Keil G: Der Medizin-historiker als Terminologe. **MMW** 1979 Dec 7;121(49):1637–8

Lipowski ZJ: What does the word 'psychosomatic' really mean? A historical and semantic inquiry. **Psychosom Med** 1984 Mar–Apr;46(2):153–71

Mahdihassan S: Alembic and ambix as Sino-Arabic terms with an explanation of Mary's bath. **Stud Hist Med** 1980 Mar;4(1):39–43

Mianet JC: Contribution à l'histoire des nerfs craniens. Diss. Paris V, René Descartes, 1981. 162, xiii leaves.

Möller HJ: Die Begriffe 'Reizbarkeit' und 'Reiz': Konstanz und Wandel ihres Bedeutungsgehaltes sowie die Problematik ihrer exakten Definition. Stuttgart, Fischer, 1975. viii, 104 p. (Medizin in Geschichte und Kultur, 11).

Pinckers AJ: Leber's congenital amaurosis as conceived by Leber. **Ophthalmologica** 1979;179(1):48–51

Pouchelle-Peter MC: La enfermedad y sus representaciones: una ojeada sobre la persistencia. **Asclepio** 1983;35:117–28

Rather LJ: On the source and development of metaphorical language in the history of Western medicine. In Stevenson LG, ed: A celebration of medical history. Baltimore, Johns Hopkins University Press, 1982. (The Henry E. Sigerist supplements to the Bulletin of the History of Medicine; new ser., no. 6). p. 135–53. With commentary by P. H. Niebyl, p. 154–6.

Reiser SJ: Words as scalpels: transmitting evidence in the clinical dialogue. **Ann Intern Med** 1980 Jun;92(6):837–42

Richter W: Der Anteil des Griechischen an den vorklinischen Nomenklaturen und die didaktischen Konsequenzen für die fachsprachliche Ausbildung von Medizinstudenten. **Wiss Z Univ Rostock** 1979;28(3):145–50

Schiller F: Semantics of sleep. **Bull Hist Med** 1982 Fall;56(3):378–97

Schiller J: Physiology and classification: historical relations. Paris, Maloine, 1980. xiii, 194 p.

Schoenberg DG, Schoenberg BS: [Eponyms in medical history] **South Med J** 1979 Dec;72(12):1590–1 (continued periodically)

Schönfeld J: Zum Ursprung der Krankheitsbezeichnung 'Syphylis'. **Off Gesundheitswes** 1984 Feb;46(2):104–5

Schütter R: Die Namen der Metalle. Herkunt und Bedeutung. **Zahnarzt** 1984 Sep;28(9):726–30

Sheehan DV, Sheehan KH: The classification of anxiety and hysterical states. Part I. Historical review and empirical delineation. **J Clin Psychopharmacol** 1982 Aug;2(4):235–44

Simić V: About correct and incorrect terminology in veterinary medicine. **Hist Med Vet** 1979;4(1):1–7

Sournia JC, Manuila A: Geschichte der medizinischen Fachsprache. In Sournia JC, Martiny M, Poulet J, ed: Illustrierte Geschichte der Medizin. Salzburg, Andreas, 1980. Vol. 8. p. 3093–107.

Tainmont J: La langue grecque classique et le vocabulaire ORL d'aujourd'hui. **Acta Otorhinolaryngol Belg** 1982;36(6):1039–60

Taylor FK: Disease concepts and the logic of classes. **Br J Med Psychol** 1981 Sep;54(pt 3):277–86

The two manias: **Br J Psychiatry** 1981 Sep;139:258–61

Weimann KH: Paracelsus-Lexikographie in vier Jahrhunderten. **Medizinhist J** 1981;16(1-2):167–95

Winau R: Bemerkungen zur 'Sprache' der Medizin. **Ber Wissenschaftsgesch** 1980;3(1–2):95–102


**Americas**


Foster GM, et al: El legado hipocratico latinoamericano: 'caliente' y 'frio' en la medicina popular contemporanea. **Med Tradic** 1979;2(6):5–24


**China**


Hu SY: An enumeration of Chinese materia medica. Hong Kong, Chinese University Press, 1980. 287 p.


**France**


Dillemann G: Les illustres pharmaciens dont les noms ont été donnés aux amphithéatres de la Faculté de Pharmacie de Paris. **Bull Ordre Natl Pharm** 1979 Apr;221:517–41


**Hungary**


Büky B: Rejtett orvosi vonatkozások régi szavainkban. **Orvostort Kozl** 1979;87–88(25 no 1–2):223–8

Fazekas A: A magyar nyelvu herbárium irodalomról. **Orvostort Kozl** 1982;28(1–3):43–64


**India**


Krishan Y: The meaning of prajnā-aparādha and karma in Ayurveda. **Bull Indian Inst Hist Med Hyderabad** 1982;12(1–4):28–33

Singh AN, Pathak SK, Singh RS: Non-plant Vedic epithets in the Sanskrit nomenclature of Indian economic plants. **Stud Hist Med** 1982 Sep;6(3):225–30

Singh RS, Vyas VD: The identity and critical appraisal of the basis of nomenclature and ancient socio-cultural and geographico-historical reflections evinced with the Paninian perfume-plant/plant-part 'Kisara' (Panini IV. IV. 53). **Indian J Hist Sci** 1983 Nov;18(2):166–71


**Poland**


Mazurkiewicz B: Polskie słownictwo pielęgniarskie. **Pieleg Polozna** 1980;(12):10–2


**Spain**


Sorní J, Suñé JM: Barcelona. Baja edad media. Especieros o Boticarios? **Bol Soc Esp Hist Farm** 1983;34(136):139–50


**Before 500 A.D.**


Jouanna J: Une forme étymologique retrouvée: omelesis dans le Glossaire hippocratique de Galien et dans le traité hippocratique des Maladies II c, 31. **Rev Philol (Paris)** 1979;53:260–63

McVaugh MR: The authorship of the Galenic compendium de interioribus, 'Quoniam diversitas...'. **Dynamis** 1981;1:225–9

Pélicier Y: Beständigheit im Sinngehalt des lateinischen Vokabulars für 'La folie' (Verrücktheit). **Z Klin Psychol Psychother** 1982;30(1):68–76

Ramsey WO: Hermetic sealing of root canals--the Greeks had a name for it. **J Endod** 1982 Mar;8(3):100


**Arabic**


Valverde JL, Pena Muñoz C: Ibn Al-Haššа Glosario sobre el Mansuri de Razi. **Ars Pharm** 1980;21(4):495–506


**Babylon**


Adamson PB: Anatomical and pathological terms in Akkadian. **J R Asiat Soc GB Irel** 1974;102–6: 1979;2–8: 1981;125–32.


**China**


Emmerick RE: Some lexical items from the rGyud-bźi. In: Proceedings of the Csoma de Körös Memorial Symposium ... Matrafüred ... 1976. Budapest: Akad. Kiadó. 1978. pp.101–108.

Mahdihassan S: Chinese origin of the word alcohol. **Am J Chin Med** 1980 Autumn;8(3):239–44

Tode I: [Significance of the letter 'u' in ancient Chinese. Did it mean caries or tooth?] (Jpn). **Shikai Tenbo** 1983 Nov;62(5):975–81


**Greco-Roman**


Callmer C: Ur arkiater-titelns historia. **Sydsven Medicinhist Sallsk Arsskr** 1980;:40–80

Daly LW: Miltiades. Aratus and compound fractures. **Am J Philol** 1980;101:59–60

Durling RJ: Lexicographical notes on Galen's pharmacological writings. **Glotta** 1979;57(3–4):218–24

Durling RJ: Lexicographical notes on Galen's writings (part II). **Glotta** 1980;58(3–4):260–5

Fischer KD: The first Latin treatise on horse medicine and its author Pelagonius Saloninus. **Medizinhist J** 1981;16(3):215–26

Fischer KD: Two notes on the Hippiatrica. **Greek Roman Byz Stud (Cambridge, Mass.)** 1979;20:371–9

Grmek MD: La réalité nosologique au temps d'Hippocrate. In La collection hippocratique et son rôle dans l'histoire de la médecine. Colloque de Strasbourg (23-27 octobre 1972) organisé par le Centre de Recherches sur la Grèce Antique, avec le concours des Facultés de Philosophie et

des Langues Classiques. Leiden, E. J. Brill, 1975. p. 239–55.
Marganne MH: Glaucome ou cataracte? sur l'emploi des dérivés de GLAUKOS en ophtalmologie antique. **Hist Philos Life Sci** 1979;1(2):199–214

**Greece**

Anzieu D, Carapanos F, Gillibert J, et al: Psychanalyse et culture grecque. Paris, Société d'Edition 'Les Belles Lettres,' 1980. 243 p.
Lebel M: Editions, traductions et lexiques hippocratiques. Le docteur Louis Morin, (1635–1715) et son index des mots d'Hippocrate. In: Congrès international d'histoire de la médecine, XXVe, Québec, 1976. Actes. Québec, 1977. p. 848–65.
Lichtenthaeler C: Outé gar iatori èrkoun to proton therapeuontes agnoia. **Hermes** 1979, 1978;107(3):270–86
Oberhelman SM: The interpretation of prescriptive dreams in ancient Greek medicine. **J Hist Med Allied Sci** 1981 Oct;36(4):416–24
Wooten CW: Unnoticed medical language in Demosthenes. **Hermes** 1979;107:157–60

**India**

Filliozat J: Sur l'identification des maladies dans l'Ayurveda. In Mazars G, ed: Les médecines traditionnelles de l'Asie. Strasbourg, Université Louis Pasteur, 1981. p. 140–9.
Lienhard S: Remarks on the early history of Indian medical terminology. **Sci Orient** 1979;16:9–20
Raison A, ed: La Haritasamhita: texte médical sanskrit; avec un index de nomenclature ayurvédique. Pondichéry, Institut français d'indologie, 1974. xlvi, 396 p. (Publications de l'Institut français d'indologie; no. 52).
Singh R, Singh AN: Socio-economic and trade relations of ancient India with the western world as reflected in plant names with particular reference to saffron (Kunkum/Kesara). **Stud Hist Med** 1981 Sep;5(3):228–32

**Rome**

Dirckx JH: Dermatologic terms in the De Medicina of Celsus. **Am J Dermatopathol** 1983 Aug;5(4):363–9
Pearcy LT: Melancholy rhetoricians and melancholy rhetoric: 'black bile' as a rhetorical and medical term in the second century A.D. **J Hist Med Allied Sci** 1984 Oct;39(4):446–56

**500 A.D.–1450**

Barcia Goyanes JJ: Dos nombres enigmaticos del trocanter mayor: tharuca y carchametra; two enigmatic names of the greater trochanter: tharuca and carchametra. **Med Esp** 1980 Nov–Dec;79:1–11
Daems WF: Synonymenvielfalt und Deutungstechnik bei den nomina plantarum medievalia. In Dilg P, et al., ed: Perspektiven der Pharmaziegeschichte. Graz, Austria, Akademische Druck- u. Verlagsanstalt, 1983. p. 29–37.
Gerhardt C: Kröte und Igel in schwankhafter Literatur des späten Mittelalters. **Medizinhist J** 1981;16(4):340–57
Hirth W: Popularisierungstendenzen in der mittelalterlichen Fachliteratur. **Medizinhist J** 1980;15(1/2):70–89
Jackson SW: Acedia the sin and its relationship to sorrow and melancholia in medieval times. **Bull Hist Med** 1981 Summer;55(2):172–85
Kottek SS: 'Mater puerorum'. A medieval naming for an enigmatic children's disease. **Eur J Pediatr** 1981 Sep;137(1):75–9
Leibowitz JO: Jewish translators of medical works in the Middle Ages. In International Congress of the History of Medicine, 27th, Barcelona, 1980. Actas. Barcelona, Académia de Ciències Mèdiques de Catalunya i Balears, 1981. p. 276–80.
Maragi M: Le glossaire latin–allemand d'anatomie de Walfridus Strabo (IXème siècle). In International Congress of the History of Medicine, 27th, Barcelona, 1980. Actas. Barcelona, Académia de Ciències Mèdiques de Catalunya i Balears, 1981. p. 304–15.
Trynková O: Některé metody středověkého léčení podle mistra rhazesa a mistra Salicettiho. III. Výběr z anatomických pojmu užívaných ve středověké medicíně. **Sb Lek** 1982 Feb;84(2):59–63

**Arabic**

Carreras Panchón A: Sobre el concepto de pestilencia (WABA') en el Canon de Avicena. **Asclepio** 1981;33:265–73
Ghalioungui P: Hunayn Ibn Ishaq, translator and medical writer. In International Congress of the History of Medicine, 27th, Barcelona, 1980. Actas. Barcelona, Académia de Ciències Mèdiques de Catalunya i Balears, 1981. p. 245–8.

**France**

Norwood FE, ed: The fourteenth-century medico-botanical glossary of Raimon de Castelnou. Leeds, W. S. Maney for the Leeds Philosophical and Literary Society, 1974. (Proceedings of the Leeds Philosophical and Literary Society, Literary and Historical Section, Vol. XV, Part VI, pp. 135–225).

**Germany**

Hirth W: Corpusbildung in der deutschsprachigen medizinischen Fachliteratur des Mittelalters. **Suhoffs Arch** 1982;66(3):239–75

**Great Britain**

Bierbaumer P: Der botanische Wortschatz des Altenglischen. 1. Teil: Das Laeceböc. Bern, Herbert Lang; Frankfurt, Peter Lang, 1975. xv, 168 p. (Grazer Beiträge zur Englischen Philologie, Bd. 1).

**India**

Rama Rao B: Abhidhanaratnamala; a work with a new classification of Dravyas. **Bull Inst Hist Med (Hyderabad)** 1973 Oct;3(4):165–8

**Yugoslavia**

Katić RV: Naknadno prikupljeni termini Srpske srednjovekovne medicine. **Srp Arh Celok Lek** 1984 Mar;112(3):373–93

**1450–1700**

Barcia Goyanes JJ: Los arabismos en las ediciones latinas del libro I del Colliget de Averroes. **Med Esp** 1984 Jan–Feb;83:9–29
Barcia Goyanes JJ: Los terminos osteologicos de la Fabrica y la evolucion del lenguaje anatomico hebreo en la Edad Media. **Sefarad** 1982;42:299–326
Goldwyn RM: Port wine stain. **Plast Reconstr Surg** 1980 Oct;66(4):647
Gysel C: Les implications cartésiennes de la nosologie bucco-dentaire de Pierre Fauchard (1678–1761–1978). **Rev Belge Med Dent** 1979;34(3):313–20
Slaughter MM: Universal languages and scientific taxonomy in the seventeenth century. Cambridge, Cambridge University Press, 1982. x, 277 p.
Telle J: Die Schreibart des Paracelsus im Urteil deutscher Fachschriftsteller des 16. und 17. Jarhunderts. **Medizinhist J** 1981;16(1–2):78–100
Walter JD: More on 'hare-lip'. **Cleft Palate J** 1984 Jan;21(1):44

**Great Britain**

Cule J: Medical translations in sixteenth century Wales. In International Congress of the History of Medicine, 27th, Barcelona, 1980. Actas. Barcelona, Académia de Ciències Mèdiques de Catalunya i Balears, 1981. p. 233–7.
Jucovy PM: Circle and circulation: the language and imagery of William Harvey's discovery. **Perspect Biol Med** 1976 Autumn;20(1):92–107
McConchie RW: Additions to OED from John Cotta's Ignorant Practisers of Physicke, 1612. **Notes Queries** 1981 Dec;28(6):490–3
Niebyl PH: Science and metaphor in the medicine of Restoration England. **Bull Hist Med** 1973 Jul–Aug;47(4):356–74
Teigen KH: A note on the origin of the term 'nature and nurture': not Shakespeare and Galton, but Mulcaster. **J Hist Behav Sci** 1984 Oct;20(4):363–4

**Hungary**

Lázár Szini K: Adalékok a XVI. századi Ars Medica vizsgálatához. **Orvostort Kozl** 1982;92(4):133–46

**Italy**

Graziani R: Fracastoro's 'syphilis' and Priapus. **Clio Med** 1981 Dec;16(2/3):93–9

**Mexico**

López Austin A: Textos acerca de las partes del cuerpo humano y de las enfermedades y medicinas en los primeros memoriales de Sahagún. **Estud Cult Nahuatl** 1972;10:129–53
Torre JM: Los balbuceos de la cardiologia mexicana. **Bol Soc Mex Hist Filos Med** 1980 Sep–Dec;5(32–33):109–22

**Netherlands**

Beukers H: Mechanistische principes bij Franciscus dele Boë, Sylvius. **Tijdschr Geschied Geneeskd** 1982;5(1):6–15
Jarcho S: Blankaart's Dictionary, an index to 17th century medicine. **Bull NY Acad Med** 1982 Sep;58(6):568–77

**Poland**

Roeske W: Lexicon Synonymorum Mineralo-Chymico-Pharmaceuticorum Trilingue Latino-Germano-Polonicum Collectum et Conscriptum a Johanne Stanko anno MCDLXXII (1472). In Hickel E, Schröder G, ed: Neue Beiträge zur Arzneimittelgeschichte. Festschrift für Wolfgang Schneider zum 70. Geburtstag. Stuttgart, Wissenschaftliche Verlagsgesellschaft, 1982. p. 29–39.

**Spain**

Sanchez-Moscoso Hermida A: Distinción entre alimento y medicamento en un texto médico del siglo XVI. **Bol Soc Esp Hist Farm** 1980 Oct;31(123):151–90

**Switzerland**

Braun L: Vom Wesen des Grundes bei Paracelsus. **Salzburger Beitr Paracelsusforsch** 1984;23:27–35

Lenzen W: Mentis Laesiones, Psychopathologie bei Felix Platter (1536–1614). Diss. Bonn, 1982. 151 p.

**1700 to Present**

Adams MB: From 'Gene Fund' to 'Gene Pool': on the evolution of evolutionarylanguage. **Stud Hist Biol** 1979;3:241–85

Anderson WC: Translating the language of chemistry: Priestley and Lavoisier. **Eighteenth Cent Theory Interpret** 1981;22(1):21–31

Arnold HL: How 'indeterminate' leprosy got its name. **Int J Dermatol** 1981 Jun;20(5):393–5

Benedek TG, Rodnan GP: The early history and nomenclature of scleroderma and of its differentiation from sclerema neonatorum and scleroedema. **Semin Arthritis Rheum** 1982 Aug;12(1):52–67

Berciano J, Rebollo M, Coria F, et al: Heredoataxia de Marie. Nuevas consideraciones sobre su uso e independencia nosológica. **Med Clin (Barc)** 1983 Apr 2;80(11):506–8

Bernhard JD, Elliot AD: A letter from Darier to Bowen on the naming of Bowen's disease. **Arch Dermatol** 1983 Mar;119(3):261–2

Biraben JN: Histoire des classifications de causes de décès et de maladies aux XVIIIe et XIXe siècles. In Imhof AE, ed: Mensch und Gesundheit in der Geschichte. Husum, Matthiesen, 1980. p. 23–34.

Bleker J: Die historische Pathologie, Nosologie und Epidemiologie im 19. Jahrhundert. **Medizinhist J** 1984;19(1–2):33–52

Comiti VP: Histoire des maladies et diagnostic médical historique. **Gaz Med Fr** 1981 Jun 5;88(21):3087–90

Côté RA, Robboy S: Progrès dans la gestion de l'information médicale. La nomenclature systématisée de la médecine (Snomed). **Union Med Can** 1980 Sep;109(9):1243–52

Côté RA, Robboy S: Progress in medical information management. Systematized nomenclature of medicine. **JAMA** 1980 Feb 22–29;243(8):756–62

Cowen DL: A note on pharmaceutical literature and the introduction of the new chemical nomenclature. **Beitr Gesch Pharm** 1981;11:84–5

Diara A: Sens et definition du mot 'espece' dans l'oeuvre biologique de Felix Le Dantec. **Rev Synth (Paris)** 1981;102(101–102):73–86

Federspil G, Scandellari C: La malattia da Morgagni a oggi. **Veltro** 1982;26(5–6):417–34

Fiks A: Cystosarcoma phyllodes of the mammary gland--Müller's tumor. For the 180th birthday of Johannes Müller. **Virchows Arch [Pathol Anat]** 1981;392(1):1–6

Forrester J: Language and the origins of psychoanalysis. London, Macmillan, 1980. xvi, 285 p.

Ganzinger K: Zur Geschichte der chemischen Nomenklatur in den amtlichen Arzneibüchern. **Beitr Gesch Pharm** 1980;31(5):33–7

Gras VW: Myth and the reconciliation of opposites: Jung and Lévi-Strauss. **J Hist Ideas** 1981 Jul–Sep;42(3):471–88

Gravitz MA, Gerton MI: Origins of the term hypnotism prior to Braid. **Am J Clin Hypn** 1984 Oct;27(2):107–10

Haffter C: Die Entstehung des Begriffs der Zivilisationskrankheiten. **Gesnerus** 1979;36(3–4):228–37

Hahn von Dorsche H: Die Nomenklaturen der Anatomen. Ein historischer Uberblick. **Anat Anz** 1981;150(1–2):11–43

Haller JS: With a spoonful of sugar. The art of prescription writing in the late 19th and early 20th century. **Pharm Hist** 1984;26(4):171–8

Holubar K: Terminology and iconography of lupus erythematosus. A historical vignette. **Am J Dermatopathol** 1980 Fall;2(3):239–42

Johnson DE: A concordance of abbreviations used in references to reviews in botanical bibliographies by Cobres (1782), Bohmer (1787), and Militz (1829). **Huntia** 1979;3(2):103–14

Karlson P: Was sind Hormone? Der Hormonbegriff in Geschichte und Gegenwart. **Naturwissenschaften** 1982 Jan;69(1):3–14

Lepore FE: Toward a definition of papilledema: a historical review, 1851–1911. **Surg Neurol** 1982 Mar;17(3):178–80

Lerman SJ: Why is chickenpox called chickenpox? **Clin Pediatr (Phila)** 1981 Feb;20(2):111–2

Levin S: Mongolian spot; Afro-Asian stain; sacral stain. **S Afr Med J** 1981 Jul 25;60(4):123–4

Lindenmann J: Origin of the terms 'antibody' and 'antigen'. **Scand J Immunol** 1984 Apr;19(4):281–5

Livianos Aldana L, Rojo Moreno L, Rojo Moreno J, et al: La nosología psiquiátrica y las taxonomías numéricas. **Actas Luso Esp Neurol Psiquiatr** 1984 Jan–Feb;12(1):63–72

Lundström R: Rubella under graviditet--historik och nomenklatur. **Lakartidningen** 1979 Oct 10;76(41):3512–3

Mahony P: Freud as a writer. New York, International Universities Press, 1982. xv, 227 p.

Meadow R, Lennert T: Munchausen by proxy or Polle syndrome: which term is correct? **Pediatrics** 1984 Oct;74(4):554–6

Menzel I: Vive la berloque. Etymologische Betrachtungen zur Berlocke-Dermatitis. **Hautarzt** 1980 Oct;31(10):558–9

Merton RK, Sills DL, Stigler SM: The Kelvin dictum and social science: an excursion into the history of an idea. **J Hist Behav Sci** 1984 Oct;20(4):319–31

Monteil RA, Knoche JF: Etude de l'évolution du terme odontome depuis sa création jusqu'au concept anatomo-patholgique actuel. **Actual Odontostomatol (Paris)** 1980;(132):583–95

Morer G: Naissance d'un vocable. **Hist Sci Med** 1984;18(2):165–71

Neville RG, Smeaton WA: Macquer's Dictionnaire de Chymie: a bibliographical study. **Ann Sci** 1981;38(6):613–62

Parkes D: History of narcolepsy. In Rose FC, Bynum WF, ed: Historical aspects of the neurosciences. New York, Raven, 1982. p. 151–63.

Postel J: Les névroses. Evolution historique du concept de 1769 à nos jours. **Soins Psychiatr** 1982 Feb;(16):13–9

Ryalls J: Where does the term 'aphasia' come from? **Brain Lang** 1984 Mar;21(2):358–63

Sartorius N: La classification: une optique internationale. **Acta Psychiatr Belg** 1983 Mar–Apr;83(2):88–103

Scadding JG: The eponymy of sarcoidosis. **J R Soc Med** 1981 Feb;74(2):147–57

Schiller F: When is posterior not dorsal but medial? **Neurology** 1984 Apr;34(4):511–4

Schurig V: Die Eingliederung des Begriffs 'Ethologie' in das System der Biowissenschaften im 19. Jahrhundert. **Sudhoffs Arch** 1984;68(1):94–104

Severova EIa: O proiskhozhdenii i ispol'zovanii termina 'lekarstvennaia bolenzn". **Sov Med** 1982;(5):113–5

Teich M: Ferment or enzyme: what's in a name? **Hist Philos Life Sci** 1981;3(2):193–215

Trüb CL: Die Terminologie und Definition Sozialmedizin und Sozialhygiene in den literarischen Sekundärquellen der Jahre 1900 bis 1960. Opladen, Westdeutscher Verlag, 1978. 87 p.

Whitrow M: A classification scheme for the history of science, medicine and technology. In Forbes EG, ed: Human implications of scientific advance. Edinburgh, Edinburgh University Press, 1978. p. 518–30.

Zacharias KL: The construction of a primate order: taxonomy and comparative anatomy in establishing the human place in nature, 1735–1916. Ph.D. diss. The Johns Hopkins University. Baltimore, 1980. 464 leaves.

Zülch KJ: Historical development of the classification of brain tumours and the new proposal of the World Health Organization (WHO). **Neurosurg Rev** 1981;4(3):123–7

**China**

Ho PY: Chinese scientific terminology. **Pap Far East Hist** 1974;(9):1–14

**Czechoslovakia**

Bunčáková V, Bednárová E, Ivanová A, et al: Vývoj slovenskej lekárskej terminológie od vzniku Bratislavských lekárskych listov a Lekárskej fakulty Univerzity Komenského. **Bratisl Lek Listy** 1983 Aug;80(2):221–35

Simon F: Latinčinár ako historik medicíny. **Cas Lek Cesk** 1984 Oct 12;123(40–41):1250

**France**

Albury WR: French nosologies around 1800 and their relationship with chemistry. In Forbes EG, ed: Human implications of scientific advance. Edinburgh, Edinburgh University Press, 1978. p. 502–17.

Eisele FR: Origins of 'gerontocracy'. **Gerontologist** 1979 Aug;19(4):403–7

Fanti PA, Varotti C: 'Les eczématides'. Historical review of the term. **Am J Dermatopathol** 1984 Oct;6(5):437–40

Hooton A, Hooton C: A critical analysis of French psychiatric nosology. **Can J Psychiatry** 1981 Mar;26(2):120–5

Huard P, Imbault-Huart MJ: Vicq d'Azyr et la nomenclature moderne des nerfs crâniens. In: Congrès National des Sociétés Savantes, 105e, Caen, 1980. Comptes Rendus, Paris, 1980. Section des Sciences, Fasc. V. p. 61–83.

Picheau P: Diagnostika i klassifikatsiia psikhicheskikh rasstroĭstv vo Frantsii (istoriia, sovremennye vzgliady i terminologicheskie sopostavleniia). **Zh Nevropatol Psikhiatr** 1982;82(8):103–10

Pichot PJ: The French approach to psychiatric classification. **Br J Psychiatry** 1984 Feb;144:113–8

A propos du syndrome de Turner: **LARC Med** 1981 Oct;1(1):63

Schiller J: Henri Dutrochet et la terminologie scientifique. In: Congrès National des Sociétés Savantes, 97e, Nantes, 1972. Comptes Rendus. Paris, 1976. Section des Sciences, Tome 1. p. 83–9.

**Germany**

Heimann H: Nosologie und Pathophysiologie in der Psychiatrie--Aspekte der Krankheitslehre Kraepelins heute. **Confin Psychiatr** 1980;23(4):262-74
Kempler K: Az elemek rendszerezésének kezdetei (Megemlékezés Johann Wolfgang Döbereiner születésének 200. évfordulóján). **Orv Hetil** 1981 Jan 11;122(2):101-3
Klingmüller G: Treponema pallidum oder Spirochaeta pallida? **Hautarzt** 1983 Dec;34(12):628-31
Kobes LW: Quellenstudie zu Petrus Camper und der nach ihm benannten Schädelebene. **Dtsch Zahnarztl Z** 1983;38(3):268-70
Larson JL: An alternative science, Linnaean natural history in Germany, 1770-1790. **Janus** 1979;66(4):267-83
Morowitz HJ: How E. coli got its name. **Hosp Pract** 1982 Dec;17(12):58-9
Poggi I: Wundt e il linguaggio dei gesti. **Stor Crit Psicol** 1981;2(2):297-314
Rödel V: Johann Christoph Gatterers 'Linnaeismus graphicus'. Klassifikation und Universalismus im 18. Jahrhundert. **Medizinhist J** 1982;17(3):215-38
Schierhorn H: Die Multinationalität der Anatomischen Gesellschaft und die Mehrsprachigkeit ihrer Versammlungen. **Anat Anz** 1980;148(2):168-206
Suárez CV: Ampulla of Vater---a misnomer. **Mt Sinai J Med (NY)** 1980 Jul-Aug;47(4):373-85
Wahl RW: Eponym: the loop of Henle. **South Med J** 1984 Apr;77(4):494-5

**Great Britain**

Beatty J: What's in a word? Coming to terms in the Darwinian revolution. With a comment by D. Hull. In M. Ruse, ed: Nature animated. Historical and philosophical case studies in Greek medicine, nineteenth-century and recent biology, psychiatry, and psychoanalysis. Volume II. Dordrecht, D. Reidel, 1983. p. 79-111.
Bell C: A hundred years of Lancet language. **Lancet** 1984 Dec 22;2(8417-18):1453
Shuttleworth SA: The language of science and psychology in George Eliot's Daniel Deronda. In Paradis J, Postlewait T, ed: Victorian science and Victorian values: literary perspectives. New York, New York Academy of Sciences, 1981. p. 269-98.

**Hungary**

Az orvosi ismeretek elavulásáról és revíziójának szkségességéröl: **Orv Hetil** 1984 Jun 10;125(24):1475-6
Szîlási A: A magyar nyelvü belgyógyászati oktatás kezdete. **Orv Hetil** 1979 Oct 7;120(40):2435-7

**Italy**

Altieri Biagi ML: L'episteme stillistica di Lazzaro Spallanzani. **Intersezioni** 1981;1:575-99

**Japan**

Marui E: Public health and 'Koshu-Eisei'. Speciality and universality of the modern Japanese public health. In Ogawa T, ed: Public health. Tokyo, Saikon, 1981. p. 99-107.

**Luxembourg**

Nahas GG: Bilinguisme médical: vingt cinq ans d'expérience. **Bull Soc Sci Med Grand Duche Luxemb** 1979;116(1):83-7

**Romania**

Manoliu E, Manoliu V: The history of medical terminology in Romania. In: Congrès international d'histoire de la médecine, XXVe, Québec, 1978. Actes. Québec, 1977. p. 951-6.

**Spain**

Del E, María Suñé J. La 'Farmacopea Matritense en Castellano' y la 'Farmacopea en Castellano o colección de las fórmulas más usuales y acreditadas de la matritense y española'. **Bol Soc Esp Hist Farm** 1984 Jun;35(138):69-87

**Sweden**

Broberg G: Homo sapiens; Linnaeus's classification of man. In Frängsmyr T, ed: Linnaeus, the man and his work. Berkeley, University of California Press, 1983. p. 156-94.
Leikola A: Zeus Faber--antiikin tarustoa eläinkunnassa. **Hist Arkisto (Finl)** 1978;(73):110-19
Schramm E: Linné, Gedner und die biologische Kontrolle. **Medizinhist J** 1984;19(3):244-9

**United States**

Bayer R, Spitzer RL: Edited correspondence on the status of homosexuality in DSM-III. **J Hist Behav Sci** 1982 Jan;18(1):32-52
Rák K: Korunk orvosi szakirodalma és a klinikai medicina. **Orv Hetil** 1980 Sep 14;121(37):2243-8
Reddy CP, Surawicz B: Terminology of tachycardias: historical background and evolution. **PACE** 1983 Sep;6(5 Pt 2):1123-42
Rudolph ED: The introduction of the Natural System of classification of plants to nineteenth century American students. **Arch Nat Hist** 1982 Apr;10(3):461-8
Smith DC: The rise and fall of typhomalarial fever: I. origins. **J Hist Med Allied Sci** 1982 Apr;37(2):182-220
Tamony P: Tripping out from San Francisco. **Am Speech** 1981;56(2):98-103

**USSR**

Belitskaia EI: Systema morborum (klassifikatsiia bolezneĭ) I. I. Diad'kovskogo (k 150-letiiu opublikovaniia). **Sov Zdravookhr** 1983;5:63-6
Carlisle R: Arterial sounds by phases: an object lesson in terminological confusion? **J R Soc Med** 1981 Mar;74(3):212-8
Stepanov PF, Romanov NA: Istoriko-leksikologicheskiĭ aspekt russkoĭ anatomicheskoĭ terminologii. **Arkh Anat Gistol Embriol** 1980 Jun;78(6):111-5

**Yugoslavia**

Djordjević S: Iz istorije rada na medicinskom jeziku i terminologiji u nas. **Srp Arh Celok Lek** 1981;109(12):1675-8
Posinovec J: O hrvatskom stomatološkom nazivlju u drugoj polovici XIX. stoljeca. **Lijec Vjesn** 1980 May;102(5):282-3

# THERAPEUTIC CULTS

Bankhofer H: Die grossen Naturheiler. Ihr Leben - ihre Lehren. Frankfurt, Ullstein, 1982. 359 p.
Das S: Zur Stellung der Naturheilverfahren in der Allgemeinmedizin. **ZFA (Stuttgart)** 1983 Apr 10;59(10):575-84

**India**

Kakar S: Shamans, mystics, and doctors: a psychological inquiry into India and its healing traditions. New York, Knopf, 1982. x, 306 p.
Venkat Rao B: Development of naturopathy in Andhra Pradesh. **Bull Indian Inst Hist Med (Hyderabad)** 1979;9:41-5

**Before 500 A.D.**

Kádár Z: Gyógyító istenségek tisztelete Pannóniában topográfiai adatok tükrében. **Orvostort Kozl** 1981;93-96(27 No 1-4):63-78

**1450-1700**

**Ireland**

Breathnach CS: Biographical sketches no. 32--Greatrakes. **Ir Med J** 1983 Sep;76(9):402

**1700 to Present**

Albanese CL: The poetics of healing: root metaphors and rituals in nineteenth-century America. **Soundings** 1980;63(4):381-406
Rothschuh KE: Aus der Geschichte der Naturheilbewegung (I). Ueber den 'Naturismus' als die weltanschauliche Grundlage der Naturheilbewegung. **ZFA (Stuttgart)** 1981 May 10;57(13):1011-8
Rothschuh KE: Aus der Geschichte der Naturheilbewegung (VII). Die Heilkräfte von Licht, Luft und Erde. Arnold Rikli, Adolf Just und Pastor Felke. **ZFA (Stuttgart)** 1983 Jun 10;59(16):933-40
Rothschuh KE: Die Konzeptualisierung der Naturheilkunde im 19. Jahrhundert. **Gesnerus** 1981;38:175-90
Seidler E: Die Naturheilkundebewegung, ihre Systeme und Motive. In Dilg P, et al., ed: Perspektiven der Pharmaziegeschichte. Graz, Austria, Akademische Druck- u. Verlagsanstalt, 1983. p. 331-41.
Sizer SS: New spirit, new flesh: the poetics of nineteenth-century mind-cures. **Soundings** 1980;63(4):407-22

**Costa Rica**

Low SM: Dr. Moreno Cañas: a symbolic bridge to the demedicalization of healing. **Soc Sci Med** 1982;16(5):527-31

**France**

Léonard J: Les guérisseurs en France au XIXe siècle. **Rev Hist Mod Contemp** 1980 Jul-Sep;27:501-16

# THERAPEUTIC CULTS

**Germany**

Müller R: Wandlung zur Ganzheit: die Initiatische Therapie nach Karlfried Graf Dürckheim und Maria Hippius. Freiburg, Herder, 1981. 328 p.
Rothschuh KE: Aus der Geschichte der Naturheilbewegung (II). Die Entwicklung allgemeiner theoretischer Grundsätze in der Naturheilkunde des 19. Jahrhunderts. **ZFA (Stuttgart)** 1981 May 20;57(14):1091-100
Rothschuh KE: Aus der Geschichte der Naturheilbewegung (IX). Körperkultur (Kleiderreform, Nacktkultur) aus dem Geiste der Lebensreform. **ZFA (Stuttgart)** 1983 Oct 10;59(28):1570-8
Rothschuh KE: Aus der Geschichte der Naturheilbewegung (VI). Zur Fortentwicklung und Pflege der Naturheilverfahren in der zweiten Hälfte des 19. Jahrhunderts. **ZFA (Stuttgart)** 1983 Apr 10;59(10):585-91
Rothschuh KE: Aus der Geschichte der Naturheilbewegung (VIII). Von der Naturheilbewegung zur Lebensreform. **ZFA (Stuttgart)** 1983 Sep 20;59(26):1446-53
Rothschuh KE: Naturheilbewegung, Reformbewegung, Alternativbewegung. Stuttgart, Hippokrates, 1983. 148 p.
Unschuld PU: The issue of structured coexistence of scientific and alternative medical systems: a comparison of East and West German legislation. **Soc Sci Med [Med Anthropol]** 1980 Feb;14B(1):15-24
Warner E: The role of belief in healing. **Can Med Assoc J** 1983 May 1;128(9):1107-9

**Great Britain**

Barrow L: Democratic epistemology: mid-19th-century plebeian medicine. **Soc Soc Hist Med Bull (Lond)** 1981 Dec;29:25-9
Brown PS: Herbalists and medical botanists in mid-nineteenth-century Britain with special reference to Bristol. **Med Hist** 1982 Oct;26(4):405-20
Brown PS: The vicissitudes of herbalism in late nineteenth- and early twentieth-century Britain. **Med Hist** 1985 Jan;29(1):71-92
Cooter R: Interpreting the fringe. **Soc Soc Hist Med Bull (Lond)** 1981 Dec;29:33-6
Price R: Hydropathy in England 1840-70. **Med Hist** 1981 Jul;25(3):269-80
Sigsworth EM, Swan P: Para-medical provision in the West Riding. **Soc Soc Hist Med Bull (Lond)** 1981 Dec;29:37-9

**United States**

Berman A: The eclectic 'concentrations' and American pharmacy (1847-1861). **Pharm Hist** 1980;22(3):91-103
Bonnabeau RC: Samuel Thomson and Thomsonian medicine. The near-destruction of American medicine. **Minn Med** 1984 May;67(5):285-7
Cottam C, Smith EM: The roots of cranial manipulation: Nephi Cottam and 'craniopathy'. **Chiropr Hist** 1981;1(1):31-5
Kaufman M: Orthodoxy in medicine. In Reich WT, et al, ed: Encyclopedia of bioethics, v.3. New York, Free Press, 1978. p. 1173-6.
Keeney EB, Lederer SE, Minihan EP: Sectarians and scientists: alternatives to orthodox medicine. In Numbers RL, Leavitt JW, ed: Wisconsin medicine. Historical perspectives. Madison, University of Wisconsin Press, 1981. p. 47-74.
King LS: Medicine in the USA: historical vignettes. III. Medical sects and their influence. **JAMA** 1982 Sep 10;248(10):1221-4
Miller NJ, Howard-Ruben J: Unproven methods of cancer management part I: background and historical perspectives. **Oncol Nurs Forum** 1983 Fall;10(4):46-52
Peitzman SJ: 'Thoroughly practical': America's polyclinic medical schools. **Bull Hist Med** 1980 Summer;54(2):166-87
Petrisko TW: Schism and suppression: the elimination of medical protest schools, 1846-1939. **Chiropr Hist** 1982;2(1):35-9
Silberger J: On the psychology of the aging woman. Mourning and transformation: how Mary Baker Eddy found in middle age a way of making a new life for herself. **J Geriatr Psychiatry** 1979;12(1):9-25
Swan R: Faith healing, Christian Science, and the medical care of children. **N Engl J Med** 1983 Dec 29;309(26):1639-41
Wallace DJ: Thomsonians: the people's doctors. **Clio Med** 1980 Jul;14(3-4):169-86
Whorton JC: 'Physiologic optimism': Horace Fletcher and hygienic ideology in progressive America. **Bull Hist Med** 1981 Spring;55(1):59-87

# THERAPEUTICS

See also **Drugs and Chemicals; Pharmacology; The Various Medical Specialities**

Akahori A: Chapters of 'Huang-ti-nei-ching-su-wen' derived from 'Yin-yang-shih-i-mo-chiu-ching'. (Jpn) **Nihon I-Shigaku Zasshi** 1979;25:277-89
Albarracín Teulón A: La terapeutica clinica como experimento. **Asclepio** 1981;33:243-9
Bennion E: Phlebotomy: the art, practice & instruments. **MD** 1981;25(8):43-6
Berg AO: The placebo effect reconsidered. **J Fam Pract** 1983 Oct;17(4):647-50
Bossy J: Acupuncture et organisation nerveuse periphérique, segmentaire et intersegmentaire. In Mazars G, ed: Les médecines traditionnelles de l'Asie. Strasbourg, Université Louis Pasteur, 1981. p. 41-8.
Brain P: In defence of ancient bloodletting. **S Afr Med J** 1979 Jul 28;56(4):149-54
Brody H: Placebos and the philosophy of medicine: clinical, conceptual and ethical issues. Chicago and London, University of Chicago Press, 1980. vii, 164 p.
Brody H: The lie that heals: the ethics of giving placebos. **Ann Intern Med** 1982 Jul;97(1):112-8
Chuang Y: The historical development of acupuncture. Los Angeles, Oriental Healing Arts Institute, 1982. 83 p.
Davis A, Appel T: Bloodletting instruments in the National Museum of History and Technology. Washington, Smithsonian Institution Press, 1979. 103 p.
de Moulin D: The value of tobacco smoke in the treatment of intussusception. **Neth J Surg** 1984 Apr;36(2):57-9
Estes JW: Making therapeutic decisions with protopharmacologic evidence. **Trans Stud Coll Physicians Phila** 1979 Jun;5(1 no 2):116-37
Galzigna L, Galzigna M: La produzione del corpo curabile. **Acta Med Hist Patav** 1982-83;29:29-65
Garnuszewski Z: Historia akupunktury. **Arch Hist Med (Warsz)** 1980;43(2):147-61
Gast W, Barth J, Rytter M: Der lange Weg zur PUVa-Therapie. **Dermatol Monatsschr** 1983;169(9):594-600
Gibson HB: Pain and its conquest. London, Boston, Peter Owen, 1982. 224 p.
Glaser FB: The origins of the drug-free therapeutic community. **Br J Addict** 1981 Mar;76(1):13-25
Grmek MD: La moxibustion en Méditerranée et en Extrême-Orient. **Clio Med** 1981 Dec;16(2/3):113-22
Grmek MD: La moxibustion en méditerranée et en extrème-orient. In Mazars G, ed: Les médecines traditionnelles de l'Asie. Strasbourg, Université Louis Pasteur, 1981. p. 60-74.
Haas H: History of antipyretic analgesic therapy. **Am J Med** 1983 Nov 14;75(5A):1-3
Heissig W: Die Heilung der 'Weissen' Arznei in der mongolischen Heldendichtung. **Asiat Forsch** 1980;71:30-5
Heppner F: Die heilende Hitze. **Fortschr Med** 1983 Apr 14;101(14):621-3
Homblé AG: De echel of bloedzuiger in de volksgeneeskunde. **Oostvlaam Zanten** 1980;55(1):1-32
Ivanov VI: O sochetannom primenenii akupunktury i medikamentoznoĭ terapii. **Voen Med Zh** 1982 Feb;(2):49-51
Jalil A: Mermas and acupuncture points, a comparative study. **Stud Hist Med** 1981 Mar;5(1):18-34
James T: A history of bloodletting. **Adler Mus Bull** 1983 Nov;Spec issue:21-8
Jordi Gonzalez R: Oportunas consideraciones sobre la auto--medicacion. **An Med Cir** 1979 Apr-Jun;(256):99-114
Jüttner G: Alchemie und Sympathielehre in der Therapie der frühen Neuzeit. In: Der Uebergang zur Neuzeit und die Wirkung von Traditionen. VortrAB/age, gehalten auf der Tagung der Joachim-Jungius-Gesellschaft der Wissenschaften, Hamburg, am 13. und 14. Oktober 1977. Göttingen, Vandenhoeck & Ruprecht, 1978. p. 130-140.
Koelbing HM: Lehren aus der Therapiegeschichte--der therapeutische Optimismus und seine Tücken. **Schweiz Med Wochenschr** 1983 Oct 1;113(39):1378-84
Kouskoukis CE, Leider M: Cupping. The art and the value. **Am J Dermatopathol** 1983 Jun;5(3):235-9
Laín Entralgo P: History of the [therapeutic] relationship. In Reich WT, et al, ed: Encyclopedia of bioethics, v.4. New York, Free Press, 1978. p. 1655-63.
Lecomte J: L'acupuncture: approche historique et applications. **Cah Clio** 1981;67:17-21
Lee RV: The generalist: a jaundiced view. **Am J Med** 1983 Apr;74(4):532-4
Leupold-Kirschneck D: Das Handauflegen. Eine ärztliche Urgebärde in Geschichte und Gegenwart. Basel/Stuttgart, Schwabe, 1981. 81 p. (Basler Veröffentlichungen zur Geschichte der Medizin und der Biologie, 33).
Lomax E: Historical development of concepts of thermoregulation. In P. Lomax, E. Schönbaum, ed: Body temperature: regulations, drug effects, and therapeutic implications. New York, Basel, Marcel Dekker, 1979. p. 1-23.
Lu Gwei-djen, Needham J: Celestial lancets: a history and rationale of acupuncture and moxa. Cambridge, Cambridge University Press, 1980. xxi, 427 p.
Maibaum EA: Der therapeutische Aderlass von der Entdeckung des Kreislaufs bis zum Beginn des 20. Jahrhunderts - Versuch einer kritischen Neubewertung. Herzogenrath, Murken-Altrogge, 1983. 104 p. (Studien zur Medizin-, Kunst und Literaturgeschichte, Bd. 2).
Martiny M: Geschichte der Akupunktur. In Sournia JC, Martiny M, Poulet J, ed: Illustrierte Geschichte der Medizin. Salzburg, Andreas, 1980. Vol. 8. p. 3081-91.
Meyer JL: Hyperthermia as an anticancer modality--a historical perspective. **Front Radiat Ther Oncol** 1984;18:1-22
Orosz JJ: A short history of bloodletting. **Artif Organs** 1981 Aug,5(3):226-8
Pasqualini RQ: La vigencia de los remedios. **Medicina (B Aires)**

1983;43(4):463-5
Payton BW: An historical survey of illustrations of the medicinal leech. **J Audiov Media Med** 1984 Jul;7(3):105-12
Phillips WR: Patients, pills, and professionals: the ethics of placebo therapy. **Pharos** 1981 Winter;44(1):21-5
Romm S: Rejuvenation revisited. **Aesthetic Plast Surg** 1983;7(4):241-8
Seigworth GR: Bloodletting over the centuries. **NY State J Med** 1980 Dec;80(13):2022-8
Smirnova LI: Girudoterapiia. **Feldsher Akush** 1983;48(1):58-60
Stoeckle DB, Carter RD: Cupping in New York State--1978; historic review. **NY State J Med** 1980 Jan;80(1):117-20
Storm FK, Morton DL: Localized hyperthermia in the treatment of cancer. **CA** 1983 Jan-Feb;33(1):44-56
Stout G: Any old iron. **MIMS Mag** 1981 Sept 1;:48-9
Szentgyörgyvölgyi G: Erdélyi történetírók egészségügyi közlései a török idökböl. **Orv Hetil** 1984 Apr 1;125(14):837-41
Tellenbach H, ed: Psychiatrische Therapie heute. Antike Diaita und moderne Therapeutik. Ein Symposium in Salzburg 1979. Stuttgart, Ferdinand Enke, 1982. 135 p. Contributions by P. L. Entralgo, D. Gracia-Guillen, H. Schipperges, W. Schmitt, K. P. Kisker, D. Wyss, W. Blankenburg.
Turk JL, Allen E: Bleeding and cupping. **Ann R Coll Surg Engl** 1983 Mar;65(2):128-31
Vidal F: Les saignées dan la médecine des XVIIe et XVIIIe siècles. **Chir Dent Fr** 1982 Dec 2;52(181):25-35
Vidal F: Odontoiatria del passato. Salasso e mal di denti nel XVII e nel XVIII sécolo. **Dent Cadmos** 1981 Mar;49(3):59-63
Vogt H: Das Bild des Kranken. Die Darstellung äusserer Veränderungen durch innere Leiden und ihrer Heilmassnahmen von der Renaissance bis in unsere Zeit. 2d. ed. München, Bergmann, 1980. 384 p.
Wei Jia: [A brief discussion of Gehong's achievement in the science of acupuncture and moxibustion] (Chi). **Chung I Tsa Chih** 1979;20(9):48-50
Weiers M: Fragment einer Anweisung zur Moxibustion oder Akupunktur in Mandschurischer Sprache. **Asiat Forsch** 1980;71:139-44
Zhuo O: Chinese traditional medicine: its contribution to physical rehabilitation. **Arch Phys Med Rehabil** 1982 Oct;63(10):499-500

**Africa**

Ademuwagun ZA, et al, ed: African therapeutic systems. Waltham, Massachusetts, Crossroads Press of the African Studies Association, 1979. vii, 273 p.

**China**

Chen chiu shih hua: Hong Kong, I yao wei sheng ch'u pan she, 1977. 54 p.
Huard P: La thérapeutique chinoise d'hier et d'aujourd'hui. **Sci Orient** 1978;9:1-18
Jonecko A, Stasienko J, Jonecko U: Historia akupunktury chińskiej w średniowieczu i w czasach nowożytnych. **Wiad Lek** 1982 Dec 15;35(23-24):1593-601
Jonecko A, Stasienko J, Jonecko U: Zarys historii akupunktury chińskiej w średniowieczu i w czasach nowozytnych. **Arch Hist Med (Warsz)** 1984;47(3):417-27
Li Q: [Discussion on the time of formation of the theoretical system of Ziwuliuzhu (Selection of acupoint for treatment varied with the circadian changes of vital energy and blood flow in the channels and collaterals relevant to heavenly stem and earthly branches)] (Chi). **Chung Hua I Shih Tsa Chih** 1984;14(2):85-9
Needham J: Science in traditional China. A comparative perspective. Cambridge, Harvard University Press; Hong Kong, The Chinese University Press, 1981. x, 134 p.
Ren M: [The therapeutic custom handed down from the Meng He School] (Chi). **Chung Hua I Shih Tsa Chih** 1984;14(2):72-4
Soulie de Morant G: Acuponcture. (Communications 1929-1951). Avant-propos par N. Soulié de Morant. Paris, Guy Trédaniel, 1979. 234 p.
Wang Xuetai: [Research on the origin and development of acupuncture and moxibustion in China] (Chi). **Chung I Tsa Chih** 1979;20(8):59-64
Wei J. [History of the prevention and treatment of rabies by acupuncture and moxibustion, a review and prospect] (Chi). **Chung Hua I Shih Tsa Chih** 1984 Jan;14(1):14-5
Werner R: Offentliches Gesundheitswesen, traditionelle chinesische Medizin, westliche Medizin, Barfussärzte und Heilmittelkunde in der Volksrepublik China. 1. Teil. **Off Gesundheitswes** 1981 Oct;43(10):480-99
Wong M: Histoire du massage en Chine. In M. Wong: Les massages en médecine traditionnelle chinoise. Paris, Masson, 1984. p. 7-29.

**Europe**

Feucht G: Die Geschichte der Akupunktur in Europa. Heidelberg, Haug, 1977. 31 p.

**Finland**

Strandberg H: Cupping, an old popular method of healing - a Finnish 20th century survival of ancient humoral pathology. In International Congress of the History of Medicine. 26th, Plovdov, 1978. Actes du Congress. Sofia, 1981. Volume II. p. 206-7.
Vaskilampi T, Hänninen O: Cupping as an indigenous treatment of pain syndromes in the Finnish culture and social context. **Soc Sci Med** 1982;16(21):1893-901

**France**

Vidal F: [Bloodletting and dentistry in the 17th and 18th centuries.] (Fre). **Inf Dent** 1980;62:4059-64

**Germany**

Arnold HJ: Die Geschichte der Akupunktur in Deutschland. Heidelberg Haus, 1976. 128 p.

**Great Britain**

Clough M: Early healing. In Passmore R, ed: Proceedings of the Royal College of Physicians of Edinburgh Tercentenary Congress, 1981. Edinburgh, Royal College of Physicians of Edinburgh, 1982. p. 181-9.

**Hungary**

Szentgyörgyvölgyi G: Szemelvények Debrecen gyógyítástörténeti múltiából. **Orv Hetil** 1982 May 2;123(18):1114-6

**Japan**

Ohya Z: Moxas et acupuncture au Japon. In: Congrès international d'histoire de la médecine, XXVe, Québec, 1976. Actes. Québec, 1977. p. 1026-30.

**United States**

Kuhns WJ: Blood letting and early blood transfusion in the Carolinas. **NC Med J** 1983 Jun;44(6):385-8
Schmidt PJ, Changus JE: The bloodletters of Florida. **J Fla Med Assoc** 1980 Aug;67(8):743-7

**Before 500 A.D.**

**China**

Akahori A: Medical manuscripts found in Han Tomb No. 3 at Ma-wang-tui. **Sudhoffs Arch** 1979;63(3):297-300
Epler DC: Bloodletting in early Chinese medicine and its relation to the origin of acupuncture. **Bull Hist Med** 1980 Fall; 54(3):337-67
Jonecko A, Stasienko J, Jonecko U: Najdawniejszs historia akupunktury chińskiej. **Wiad Lek** 1981 Apr 15;34(8):703-9

**Greece**

Kudlien F: A new testimony for Erasistratus? **Clio Med** 1981 Apr;15(3-4):137-42
Oberhelman SM: The interpretation of prescriptive dreams in ancient Greek medicine. **J Hist Med Allied Sci** 1981 Oct;36(4):416-24

**Rome**

Dolzani C: Un 'prelievo' di sangue adombrato in una poesia di Giovanni Pascoli? **Acta Med Hist Patav** 1982-83;29:25-8

**500 A.D.-1450**

**Arabic**

Faruqi AH: Use of leeches in Greco-Arab medicine. **Stud Hist Med** 1982 Jun;6(2):137-40
Kataye S: L'hémostase dans la médecine arabe. In International Congress of the History of Medicine. 26th, Plovdiv, 1978. Actes du Congress. Sofia, 1981. Volume II. p. 122-4.
Rama Rao GS: Contribution of Avicenna in therapeutics reflecting on modern medicine. **Bull Indian Inst Hist Med (Hyderabad)** 1981;1-4:118-22

**China**

Wan Fang: Two questions about the Tian Sheng bronze statue for acupuncture of the Sung dynasty. (Chi). **Chin J Med Hist** 1981;11(1):62-4

**Great Britain**

Cohen VL: Bleeding monks. **Lancet** 1981 Jul 18;2(8238):158

**Mexico**

Prygova NM: Metody i vidy lecheniia u atstekov. **Klin Med (Mosk)** 1982 Feb;60(2):110–2

**Spain**

Labarta A: Textos para el estudio de la terapéutica entre los moriscos valencianos. **Dynamis** 1981;1:275–319

**1450–1700**

Boss J: The methodus medendi as an index of change in the philosophy of medical science in the sixteenth and seventeenth centuries. **Hist Philos Life Sci** 1979;1(1):13–42

Halleux R: L'usage des pierres précieuses dans la thérapeutique aux XVIe et XVIIe siècles. In International Congress of the History of Medicine. 26th, Plovdiv, 1978. Actes du Congress. Sofia, 1981. Volume II. p. 106–8.

**France**

Guyotjeannin C: Un aperçu de la thérapeutique au XVIIe siècle. **Monit Pharm Lab** 1981 Apr–May;1465–6:1677–8, 1680–1, 1845, 1847–8

Swinton WE: Rabelais' coarse humour was therapy for his patients. **Can Med Assoc J** 1981 Feb 15;124(4):500–4

**Great Britain**

Kaplan BB: Greatrakes the stroker: the interpretations of his contemporaries. **ISIS** 1982 Jun;73(267):178–85

Steneck NH: Greatrakes the stroker: the interpretations of historians. **ISIS** 1982 Jun;73(267):161–77

**Hungary**

Sipos G: Egy 1495–re szóló érvágó kalendárium a fövárosi Szabó Ervin könyvtárban. **Magy Konyvsz** 1977;93(1):43–6

**1700 to Present**

Alberti PW: Tracheotomy versus intubation. A 19th century controversy. **Ann Otol Rhinol Laryngol** 1984 Jul–Aug;93(4 Pt 1):333–7

Bartecchi CE: Intravenous therapy: from humble beginnings through 150 years. **South Med J** 1982 Jan;75(1):61–4

Bloom SW: Sociohistorical perspectives [on the therapeutic relationship]. In Reich WT, et al, ed: Encyclopedia of bioethics, v.4. New York, Free Press, 1978. p. 1663–68.

Cartwright FF: Pneumatic medicine. **Pharm Hist (London)** 1970 Jun;1(5):4–6

Crellin JK: Internal antisepsis or the dawn of chemotherapy? **J Hist Med Allied Sci** 1981 Jan;36(1):9–18

Curry R, Johnston L: Percutaneous transluminal angioplasty. **Ulster Med J** 1982;51(1):59–66

Dauber LG: Compound X given intravenously. On the history of the nitrogen mustards. **NY State J Med** 1984 Mar;84(3 pt 1):122–4

Dixon B: Tissue therapy. **Br J Hosp Med** 1979 Nov;22(5):512

Dotter CT: Two decades of transluminal angioplasty. An overview. **J Mal Vasc** 1982;7 Suppl 4:357–61

Dreznik A, Falk RE, Howard V, et al: Hyperthermia as a treatment for neoplasia. **Can J Surg** 1982 Nov;25(6):603–8

Dunea G: Maintenance dialysis after 20 years. **JAMA** 1980 Jul 4;244(1):67

Dwyer JM: Thirty years of supplying the missing link. History of gamma globulin therapy for immunodeficient states. **Am J Med** 1984 Mar 30;76(3A):46–52

Estes JW: The protopharmacological basis of therapeutics. **Pharmacologist** 1984;26(1):25–30

Evans GS: A great therapeutic age. **Br Med J** 1979 Oct 20;2(6196):981

Farrell K: Hyperthermia for malignant disease--a history of medicine note--the work of Georges Lakhovsky. **Adv Exp Med Biol** 1982;157:9–10

Forman R: Medical resistance to innovation. **Med Hypotheses** 1981 Aug;7(8):1009–17

Girdwood RH: Developments in therapeutics in the past fifty years. **Scott Med J** 1981 Jan;26(1):53–8

Goodwin JS, Goodwin JM: The tomato effect. Rejection of highly efficacious therapies. **JAMA** 1984 May 11;251(18):2387–90

Grefberg N, Nilsson P: Peritonealdialys--60-års jubileum och expansion genom CAPD. **Nord Med** 1983;98(11):260–2

Gross R, Claus O: Chemotherapie von Tumorleiden: Vergangenheit und Gegenwart. **Med Welt** 1982 Nov 5;33(44):1531–8

Guillerme J: Oxygène et thérapeutique. **Dix-huit Siecle** 1982;14:27–43

Hahn FE: Virus chemotherapy: the problem, its development and nature. In Hahn FE, ed: Virus chemotherapy. Basel, New York, Karger, 1980. p. 1–21. (Antibiotics and chemotherapy, v. 27).

Haller JS: Use of surface irritants in nineteenth century medicine. **NY State J Med** 1980 Jul;80(8):1314–23

Iveson-Iveson J: The art of observation. 2. Shock treatment. **Nurs Mirror** 1982 Sep 1;155(9):26

Kempler K: A kemoterápia haladása napjainkig. **Orv Hetil** 1982 Apr 4;123(14):861–4

Lee JA: Sydney Ringer (1834–1910) and Alexis Hartmann (1898–1964). **Anaesthesia** 1981 Dec;36(12):1115–21

Mann WE, Hoffman E: The man who dreamed of tomorrow. A conceptual biography of Wilhelm Reich. Los Angeles, Tarcher, 1980. 295 p.

Pratt EL: Development of parenteral fluid therapy. **J Pediatr** 1984 Apr;104(4):581–4

Scarano GB: Considerazioni storiche sull'uso dei sali d'oro nell'artrite reumatoide. **Med Secoli** 1982 May–Aug;19(2):175–91

Schiller F: Reverend Wesley, Doctor Marat and their electric fire. **Clio Med** 1981 Apr;15(3–4):159–76

Schwan HP: Ultrasound and electromagnetic radiation in hyperthermia--a historical perspective. **Br J Cancer** 1982 Mar;45(5)Suppl:84–92

Stevenson LG: Exemplary disease: the typhoid pattern. **J Hist Med Allied Sci** 1982 Apr;37(2):159–81

Stevenson LG: Joseph Dietl, William Osler and the definition of therapeutic nihilism. In Ganzinger K, Skopec M, Wyklicky H, ed: Festschrift für Erna Lesky zum 70. Geburtstag. Wien, Brüder Hollinek, 1981. p. 149–52.

Taylor E: The electrified hand--psychotherapeutic implications. **Med Instrum** 1983 Jul–Aug;17(4):281–2

Wallerström A: Levande tärd av maskar--terapeutisk användning av fluglarver. **Nord Medicinhist Arsb** 1980;:136–46

Wilson C: The quest for Wilhelm Reich. Garden City, N.Y., Anchor, 1981. xv, 272 p.

Zubrod CG: The cure of cancer by chemotherapy - reflections on how it happened. (The fifth Myron Karon Memorial Lecture). **Med Pediatr Oncol** 1980;8:107–14

**Africa**

Feierman S: History of pluralistic medical systems. Change in African therapeutic systems. **Soc Sci Med [Med Anthropol]** 1979 Dec;13B(4):277–84

Janzen JM: Ideologies and institutions in the precolonial history of equatorial African therapeutic systems. **Soc Sci Med [Med Anthropol]** 1979 Dec;13B(4):317–26

Kiernan J: Saltwater and ashes: instruments of curing among some Zulu zionists. **J Relig Afr** 1978;9:27–32

**Austria**

Gross-Bachmann M: Daniel Sailer, Leben und Wirken eines Idealisten. **Tirol Heimat** 1976;40:163–90

Sakula A: Joseph Skoda 1805–81: a centenary tribute to a pioneer of thoracic medicine. **Thorax** 1981 Jun;36(6):404–11

**Belgium**

Colard A: Evocation du passé: les débuts de l'oxygénothérapie. **Rev Med Brux** 1983 Feb;4(2):98–100

Colard A: Evocation du passé. Propos d'un vieux médecin sur la thérapeutique. **Rev Med Brux** 1981 Jan;2(1):39–41

Havelange C: Pléthore et art de guérir. Le malaise des médecins liégeois au XIXe siècle. **Rev Med Liege** 1984 Oct 1;39(19):676–95

**Bulgaria**

Furnadzhiev G: Razvitie i segashno sŭstoianie na Katedrata p farmakologiia i fitoterapiia. **Vutr Boles** 1981;20(6):22–6

**China**

Grover Y: La correspondance scientifique du P. Dominique Parrenin (1665–1741). In: France: Centre de Recherches interdisciplinaires de Chantilly (CERIC). Les rapports entre la Chine Sinologie (16–18 septembre 1977). Chantilly, Paris, Les Belles Lettres, 1980, 83–99.

**Cuba**

Deschamps Chapeaux P: El negro en la economía Habanera del siglo XIX. Flebotomianos y dentistas. **Rev Bibl Nac Jose Marti** 1971;13(1):75–86

**Finland**

Hänninen O, Vaskilampi T: Cupping as a part of living Finnish traditional healing. A remedy against pain. **Acupunct Electrother Res** 1982;7(1):39–50

**France**

Benguigui I: La théorie de l'électricité de Nollet et son application en médecine à travers sa correspondance: inédite avec Jallabert. **Gesnerus** 1981;38:225–35

Charroppin P: L'escargot contre la hernie? **Rev Hist Pharm (Paris)** 1983 Sep;30(258):215–9

Colard A: Evocation du passé: propos d'un vieux médecin sur la

thérapeutique. **Rev Med Brux** 1983 May;4(5):391–3
Dodin A: Ephéméride 1884–1934–1984. **Bull Soc Pathol Exot Filiales** 1984 Jan–Feb;77(1):6–8

**Germany**

Parascandola J: The theoretical basis of Paul Ehrlich's chemotherapy. **J Hist Med Allied Sci** 1981 Jan;36(1)19–43
Rothschuh KE: Therapia rationalis systematica bei Friedrich Hoffmann (1660–1742). In Dilg P, et al., ed: Perspektiven der Pharmaziegeschichte. Graz, Austria, Akademische Druck- u. Verlagsanstalt, 1983. p. 269–80.
Schröder G: Die Wiederbelebung der Phytotherapie im Zusammenhang mit den Reformbestrebungen der NS-Pharmazie. In Hickel E, Schröder G, ed: Neue Beiträge zur Arzneimittelgeschichte. Festschrift für Wolfgang Schneider zum 70. Geburtstag. Stuttgart, Wissenschaftliche Verlagsgesellschaft, 1982. p. 111–28.
Simmer HH: Organotherapie mit Ovarialpräparaten in der Mitte der neunziger Jahre des 19. Jahrhunderts; Medizinische und pharmazeutische Probleme. In Hickel E, Schröder G, ed: Neue Beiträge zur Arzneimittelgeschichte. Festschrift für Wolfgang Schneider zum 70. Geburtstag. Stuttgart, Wissenschaftliche Verlagsgesellschaft, 1982. p. 229–64.
Wentges RT: Wilhelm Fliess en de nasale reflexneurose. **Ned Tijdschr Geneeskd** 1981 Feb 14;125(7):278–84

**Great Britain**

Cooter R: Open-air therapy and the rise of open-air hospitals. **Soc Soc Hist Med Bull (Lond)** 1984 Dec;35:44–6
Henkelmann T: Zur Geschichte des pathophysiologischen Denkens. John Brown (1735–1788) und sein System der Medizin. Berlin, New York, Springer, 1981. 104 p.
Levere TH: Dr. Thomas Beddoes: the interaction of pneumatic and preventive medicine with chemistry. **Interdiscip Sci Rev** 1982;7:137–47
Scott EL: The origins of 'pneumatic medicine' and its practice in Manchester. **Mem Proc Manch Lit Philos Soc** 1974–75;117:75–92
Warner JH: Physiological theory and therapeutic explanation in the 1860s: the British debate on the medical use of alcohol. **Bull Hist Med** 1980 Summer;54(2):235–57
Warner JH: Therapeutic explanation and the Edinburgh bloodletting controversy: two perspectives on the medical meaning of science in the mid-nineteenth century. **Med Hist** 1980 Jul;24(3):241–58

**Hungary**

Az orvosi ismeretek elavulásáról és revíziójának szkségességéről: **Orv Hetil** 1984 Jun 10;125(24):1475–6
Balogh J: A befecskendezéses kezelés kezdetei Magyarországon. **Orvostort Kozl** 1980;89–91(26 no 1–3):111–23
Pisztora F, Ungvári G: A gyógyítással és az orvostudomány haladásával kapcsolatos inventorius téveseszmék a XX. század elsö fel'eben. **Orv Hetil** 1980 Mar 23;121(12):716–7

**Italy**

Cremona GF: L'elettroterapia nel XVIII secolo. Ricerche di elettrofisiolgia e di elettroterapia di studiosi piemontesi. **Ann Osp Maria Vittoria Torino** 1981 Jan–Jun;24(1–6):167–77
Fink M: Meduna and the origins of convulsive therapy. **Am J Psychiatry** 1984 Sep;141(9):1034–41

**Netherlands**

de Knecht-van Eekelen A: Abraham Pieter Fokker (1840–1906) en de serumtherapie bij difterie. **Tijdschr Geschied Geneeskd Natuurwet Wiskd Tech** 1984;7(4):161–71

**Sweden**

Ahlström CG: Om spansk fluga och dess medicinska användning i Lund. **Sydsven Medicinhist Sallsk Arsskr** 1984;21:49–61

**United States**

Andrew ER: A historical review of NMR and its clinical applications. **Br Med Bull** 1984 Apr;40(2):115–9
Austin D, Hunnicutt BK: National Therapeutic Recreation Society: the first twelve years. **Ther Recreation J** 1978 3d Quarter;12(3):4–14
Brewer LA: A historical account of the 'wet lung of trauma' and the introduction of intermittent positive-pressure oxygen therapy in World War II. **Ann Thorac Surg** 1981 Apr;31(4):386–93
Chow EP: Acupuncture: its history and educational significance to health practices in the United States. Ph.D. Diss., The Fielding Institute. Santa Barbara, 1975. 156 leaves.
Davies NE, Davies GH, Sanders ED: William Cobbett, Benjamin Rush, and the death of General Washington. **JAMA** 1983 Feb 18;249(7):912–5
Detre KC, Frank T, Kniazzeh CR, et al: Roots of art therapy. Margaret Naumburg (1890–1983) and Florence Cane (1882–1952). A family portrait. **Am J Art Ther** 1983 Jul;22(4):111–23
Hercher GP: The work cure at Devereux Mansion. **Essex Inst Hist Collect** 1980;116(2):101–10
Loewen SL: The art of bloodletting: as practiced by my father. **J Am Hist Soc Ger Russ** 1980;3(2):13–7
McDonell KM: 'One bold incision': Dr. William A. Lindsay's radical cure. **Indiana Med Hist Q** 1980;6(3):3–23
Pellegrino ED: The sociocultural impact of twentieth-century therapeutics. In Vogel MJ, Rosenberg CE, ed: The therapeutic revolution. Philadelphia, 1979. p. 245–266.
Poirier S: The Weir Mitchell rest cure: doctor and patients. **Womens Stud** 1983;10(1):15–40
Pollack CV: Electronic therapeutics of Albert Abrams, M.D. **Pharm Hist** 1984;26(2):109–13
Ransom JF: The origins of chiropractic physiological therapeutics: Howard, Forester and Schulze. **Chiropr Hist** 1984;4(1):47–52
Rosenberg CE: The therapeutic revolution: medicine, meaning, and social change in nineteenth-century America. **Perspect Biol Med** 1977 Summer;20(4):485–509
Rosenberg CE: The therapeutic revolution: medicine, meaning, and social change in nineteenth-century America. In Vogel MJ, Rosenberg CE, ed: The therapeutic revolution. Philadelphia, 1979. p. 3–25.
Ruderman FA: A placebo for the doctor. **Commentary** 1980;69(5):54–60
Santos GW: History of bone marrow transplantation. **Clin Haematol** 1983 Oct;12(3):611–39
Savitt TL: Understanding the medical past through literature: bloodletting and the Louisiana swamp doctor. **J Okla State Med Assoc** 1982 Jul;75(7):174–7
Schneck JM: Elisha Dick, Benjamin Rush, and George Washington. **JAMA** 1983 Jul 8;250(2):164
Siddall AC: Bloodletting in American obstetric practice, 1800–1945. **Bull Hist Med** 1980 Spring;54(1):101–10
Whorton JC: 'Antibiotic abandon': the resurgence of therapeutic rationalism. In Parascandola J, ed: The history of antibiotics. Madison, American Institute of the History of Pharmacy, 1980. p. 125–136.
Wortis J: How shock treatment came to America: what history teaches. **Biol Psychiatry** 1982 Nov;17(11):1203–5
100 years ago: household medicine and treatment: the gospel according to Dr. Chase: **One One** 1981 May–Jun;3(3):4–5

**USSR**

Egaĭ VS, Kuimov AD: K istorii stanovleniia nauchnoĭ terapevticheskoĭ kliniki Sibiri (k 400-letiiu prisoedineniia Sibiri k Rossii). **Ter Arkh** 1982;54(12):122–3
Egaĭ VS: Razvitie terapii v Sibiri: M. G. Kurlov i ego shkola. M. G. Kurlov i ego shkola. Novosibirsk, Nauka, Sibirskoe otd-nie, 1981. 112 p.
IAstreb NI: Razvitie terapii v Ukrainskoĭ SSR. Kiev, Zdorov'ia, 1978. 165 p.
Obrosov AN: Etapy razvitiia metoda impul'snoĭ terapii v SSSR. **Vopr Kurortol Fizioter Lech Fiz Kult** 1980 Mar–Apr;(2):4–10
Piaĭ LT, Kalnin VV: Razvitie terapii v Tartuskom universitete. **Ter Arkh** 1984;56(3):44–6
Revutskiĭ EL: 50 let Respublikanskogo nauchnogo obshchestva terapevtov USSR. **Vrach Delo** 1981 Oct;(10):120–1
Sapińska I: Rozwój refleksoterapii (akupunktury) w Zwiazku Radzieckim. **Wiad Lek** 1984 Aug 1;37(15):1233–7
Shostak NA, Gorelova LE: Kafedra fakul'tetskoĭ terapii II Moskovskogo meditsinskogo instituta im. I. N. Pirogova (k 70-letiiu so dnia osnovaniia). **Vopr Revm** 1980 Jan–Mar;(1):66–9
Shul'tsev GP: Vklad uchenykh Tsentral'nogo ordena Lenina instituta usovershenstvovaniia vracheĭ v razvitie sovetskoĭ terapii (k 50-letiiu instituta). **Klin Med (Mosk)** 1980 Jun;58(6):8–11
Smirnov AN: Razvitie terapii v SSSR. **Feldsher Akush** 1982;47(12):14–9

**Zambia**

Prins G: Disease at the crossroads: towards a history of therapeutics in Bulozi since 1876 [1]. **Soc Sci Med [Med Anthropol]** 1979 Dec;13B(4):285–315

## TOXICOLOGY

Casarett LJ, Bruce MC: Origin and scope of toxicology. In Doull J, Klaassen CD, Amdur MO, ed: Casarett and Doull's Toxicology: the basic science of poisons. 2d. ed. New York, Macmillan, 1980. p. 3–10.
Eckert WG: Historical aspects of poisoning and toxicology. **Am J Forensic Med Pathol** 1981 Sep;2(3):261–4
Girard P: Toxiques et poisons dans le passé pharmaceutique de la Savoie. **Rev Hist Pharm (Paris)** 1983 Dec;71(30):287–95
Willett LB, Schanbacher FL, Teske RH: Toxicology and the dairy industry: will problems outrun solutions? **J Dairy Sci** 1981 Jun;64(6):1483–93

# TOXICOLOGY

**Luxembourg**

Wennig R: Histoire de la toxicologie au Luxembourg. **Bull Soc Sci Med Grand Duche Luxemb** 1984;121(2):39–52

**Before 500 A.D.**

Ericson JE, Coughlin EA: Archaeological toxicology. **Ann NY Acad Sci** 1981;376:393–403

**Greco–Roman**

Schmidt V: Zu dem medizinischen Traktat Pap. Laur. 68. **Z Papyrologie Epigraphik** 1977;24:151–4

**1450–1700**

**Switzerland**

Maehle AH: Johann Jakob Wepfer (1620–1695) als Toxikologe. Diss., Rheinische Friedrich-Wilhelms-Universität. Bonn, 1983. 202 p.

**1700 to Present**

Fabre M, Boudet F, Boe M, et al: Intoxications par le phosgène. **Toxicol Eur Res** 1983 Jul;5(4):185–8

Kotwas J, Meyer-Wilmes J, Ohlendorf D, ed: Pharmazie und Medizin--Grenzen und Möglichkeiten. Verhandlungsbericht über eine Internationale Tagung der Arbeitsgemeinschaft Deutscher Krankenhausapotheker in Zusammenarbeit mit der Bayerischen Internistenvereinigung München, 18.–19.April 1980. Berlin, Acron, 1981. 152 p. Contributions by R. Winau, D. Ohlendorf, A.G. Hildebrandt, W. Weissauer, R. Quintiliani, D.D. Breimer, R. Preisig, T. Zysset, D. Adam, H. Remmer, G. Dirheimer, K.H. Beyer, H.P.T. Ammon.

Krister CJ: Safety evaluation ... it ain't all science. **Vet Hum Toxicol** 1980 Jun;22(3):156–9

Müller RK: Zur Entwicklung der toxikologischen Denkweise anfangs des 19. Jahrhunderts. **Z Gesamte Hyg** 1983 Jun;29(6):348–50

**France**

Delaveau P: Sur le 'registre pour l'inscription des poisons' d'un pharmacien tourangeau (1833–1841). **Rev Hist Pharm (Paris)** 1984 Jun;31(261):144–50

**Great Britain**

Neuberger A, Smith RL: Richard Tecwyn Williams: the man, his work, his impact. **Drug Metab Rev** 1983;14(3):559–607

Proudfoot AT: The development of clinical toxicology in Edinburgh. In Passmore R, ed: Proceedings of the Royal College of Physicians of Edinburgh Tercentenary Congress, 1981. Edinburgh, Royal College of Physicians of Edinburgh, 1982. p. 204–10.

**Italy**

Knoefel PK: Felice Fontana on Poisons. **Clio Med** 1980;15(1/2):35–65

**Japan**

Suzuki T, Hongo T, Yamamoto R: Hair mercury levels of Japanese women during the period 1881 to 1968. **J Appl Toxicol** 1984 Apr;4(2):101–4

**Netherlands**

Wit JG: Institute of Veterinary Pharmacology, Pharmacy, and Toxicology: its research (1961–1980). **Tijdschr Diergeneeskd** 1981 Oct;106(20):suppl 3:169–75

**Poland**

Kieć E, et al: Prof. Dr. Leon Cholewa. **Przegl Lek** 1984;41(7):465–76

**Spain**

Bertrán Capella A, Huguet Ramia E: La aportacion de Pedro Mata a la toxicologia. **Asclepio** 1980;32:53–63

**United States**

Autian J, Wood G: The role of toxicology in the pharmacy curriculum. **Am J Pharm Educ** 1976 Nov,;40(4):378–82

Niyogi SK: Historic development of forensic toxicology in America up to 1978. **Am J Forensic Med Pathol** 1980 Sept;1(3):249–64

**USSR**

Kakhn KhA: Razvitie ėksperimental'noĭ i klinicheskoĭ toksikologii v Estonskoĭ SSR. **Gig Tr Prof Zabol** 1983 Oct;:(10):3–5

Korbakova AI, Ulanova IP: Nauchnaia deiatel'nost' vydaiushchegosia sovetskogo toksikologa N. S. Pravdina i razvitie ego ideĭ v mashi dni. **Gig Tr Prof Zabol** 1983 Feb;(2):44–5

Nikolaĭ Sergeevich Pravdin (k 100–letiiu so dnia rozhdeniia): **Farmakol Toksikol** 1983 May–Jun;46(3):127–8

Stepanskiĭ GA, Fomenko VN: Sovetskaia toksikologicheskaia nauka i deiatel'nost' moskovskikh toksikologov (k 15–letiiu toksikologicheskoĭ sektsii Moskovskogo nauchnogo obshchestva farmakologov). **Farmakol Toksikol** 1980 Nov–Dec;43(6):747–50

# TRANSPORTATION OF PATIENTS

See also **Emergency Medical Services; Red Cross**

Karbowski J: Tecza nad Solferino. Warszawa, Państwony Zakład Wydawn. Lekarskich, 1973. 211 p.

Simon P, Seifert E: Rollende Hilfsmittel fur Körperbehinderte als Gegenstand in der bildenden Kunst. In KF Schlegel, ed: Der Körperbehinderte in Mythologie und Kunst. Stuttgart, New York, Thieme, 1983. p. 89–125.

**1700 to Present**

Jones DR: Aeromedical transportation of psychiatric patients: historical review and present management. **Aviat Space Environ Med** 1980 Jul;51(7):709–16

**Cuba**

Torres Medina J: Los barcos hospitales en la campaña de Cuba. **Rev Hist Mil** 1970;14(29):161–86

**France**

Brown GC, ed: With the ambulance service in France: the wartime letters of William Gorham Rice, jr. **Wis Mag Hist** 1981;64(4):278–93

Delaby PA: Un groupe de brancardiers pendant la bataille de Verdun. **Hist Sci Med** 1980;14:293–303

**Germany**

Schmidt R, Kludas A: Die deutschen Lazarettschiffe im Zweiten Weltkrieg. Stuttgart, Motorbuch, 1978. 174 p.

**Great Britain**

Collacott RA: The air-ambulance: Orkney's experience. **J R Coll Gen Pract** 1984 Mar;34(260):163–5

Fletcher I: Aid, first and foremost: a brief outline history of the St John Ambulance Association and Brigade. **Injury** 1979 Nov;11(2):104–9

Macdonald RC, Banks JG, Ledingham IM: Transportation of the injured. **Injury** 1980 Nov;12(3):225–33

Mathews M, Harris M: The Royal Naval Medical Air Evacuation Unit. **J R Nav Med Serv** 1980 Summer;66(2):147–51

**Hungary**

Bencze B: Emlékezés Orovecz Bélára az Országos Mentöszolgálat megszervezöjére (1909–1967). **Orv Hetil** 1979 Nov 18;120(46):2819–20

**Italy**

Orsini M, Piroli AT, Gaudiosi O: Gli eliporti ospedalieri nell'organizzazione sanitaria militare: l'eliporto dell'ospedale militare di Caserta. **Riv Mil** 1973;29(5):614–26

**Poland**

Moskwa Z: Początki Warszawskiego Pogotowia Ratunkowego. **Wiad Lek** 1982 Jan 1;35(1):81–3

Wankiewicz R: Służba zdrowia Wojska Polskiego w bitwie nad Bzura. **Przegl Lek** 1984;41(1):68–79

**Spain**

Soteras Elía B: Centenario de la batalla de Oroquieta: primera actuacion de los camilleros de la Cruz Roja. **Pregon** 1972;(111):n p

**United States**

Brady ER: The thread of a concept. **Marine Corps Gaz** 1971;55(5):35–42

Dolphin J: Private ambulance. **Emerg Med Serv** 1977 Nov–Dec;6(6):155–6

Hirschman JC, Nagel EL: Prehospital mobile emergency care in Miami, Florida. An historical commentary. **J Fla Med Assoc** 1981 Aug;68(8):624–34

Murphy EF: Reflections on automotive adaptive equipment--an essay.

**Bull Prosthet Res** 1979 Fall;16(2):191–207
Quilali air strip: **Marine Corps Gaz** 1970;54(11):41–3
A report on the quality of ambulance service as observed in 1862 by S. L. Abbot, Francis Minot. Transactions of the New York State Medical Society, 1863: **NY State J Med** 1982 Mar;82(3):393–4
Stewart MJ: Moving the wounded. Litters, cacolets and ambulance wagons, U. S. Army, 1776–1876. Ft. Collins, Colorado, Old Army Press, 1979. 134 p.

#### USSR

Bak M: Kórházvonatos tapasztalatok a II. világháború fertözö betegségeiröl. **Orv Hetil** 1983 Oct 16;124(42):2568–70
Baranovskiĭ GIa, Kapitonov GI: Nakotorye osobennosti meditsinskoĭ évakuatsii v Stalingradskoĭ bitve. (K 40–letiiu Stalingradskoĭ bitvy). **Voen Med Zh** 1983;(1):71–4
Baranovskiĭ GIa, Kapitonov GI: Nekotorye voprosy podgotovki i organizatsii raboty sanitarno–transportnykh sudov v period Velikoĭ Otechestvennoĭ voiny. **Voen Med Zh** 1984 May;(5):25–8
Baranovskiĭ GIa, Kapitonov GI: Ob évakuatsii ranenykh i bol'nykh zheleznodorozhnym transportom vo vremia Velikoĭ Otechestvennoĭ voĭny. **Voen Med Zh** 1981 Mar;(3):9–10
Borodin VG: Nekotorye voprosy organizatsii lecheniia i voenno–vrachebnoĭ ékspertizy ranenykh i bol'nykh v évakuatsionnykh gospitaliakh Urala vo vremia Velikŏ Otechestvennoi voiny. **Voen Med Zh** 1983 Mar;(3):71–4
Bragin AI, Ivanov NM: Evakuatsiia ranenykh i grazhdanskogo naseleniia iz Leningrada v tyl strany v period blokady (1941–1943 gg.). **Zdravookhr Ross Fed** 1980;(5):9–11
Ermakov MA: Iz istorii organizatsii évakuatsii ranenykh i bol'nykh partizan na Bol'shuiu zemliu. **Med Sestra** 1982 Mar;41(3):43–5
Germanov GP: Opyt évakuatsii ranenykh i bol'nykh rechnym transportom v gody Velikoĭ Otechestvennoĭ voĭny. **Voen Med Zh** 1983 Sep;9:9–11
Gladkikh PF: Ob évakuatsii ranenykh i bol'nykh iz gospital'noĭ bazy Leningradskogo fronta v period polnoĭ blokady Leningrada. **Voen Med Zh** 1983 Feb;(2):70–3
Granat NE: K 35–letiiu pobedy (vospominaniia o sluzhbe v voenno–sanitarnom poezde). **Med Sestra** 1980 May;39(5):7–11
Ivan'kovich FA: Opyt évakuatsii ranenykh i bol'nykh voenno–sanitarnymi letuchkami vo vremia Stalingradskoĭ bitvy. **Voen Med Zh** 1983 Feb;(2):68–70
Selivanov VI, Tkhostov DR, Selivanov EF: Lechbno– evakuatsionnaia kharakteristika ranenykh i bol'nykh, lechivshikhsia v gospital'noi baze tyla strany. **Voen Med Zh** 1980 Jun;(6):20–3
Voĭtenko MF, Zil'berberg LB: Organizatsiia raboty DMP pri massovom postuplenii ranenykh v period Velikoĭ Otechestvennoĭ voiny. **Voen Med Zh** 1983 Nov;(11):15–8

## TRAVEL

Cohn RL, Jensen RA: The determinants of slave mortality rates on the middle passage. **Explor Econ Hist** 1982;19(3):269–82
Habrich C: Die Ausstattung von Haus– und Reise–apotheken in ihrer pharmazie– und medizinhistorischen Bedeutung. **Pharm Ztg** 1979 Jun 14;124(24):1151–5
Laissus Y: Les voyageurs naturalistes du Jardin du roi et du Muséum d'histoire naturelle: essai de portrait–robot. **Rev Hist Sci (Paris)** 1981 Jul–Oct;34(3–4):259–317
Mazzei Uzcátegui M: Los medicos en la aventura y en la exploracion. **Rev Soc Venez Hist Med** 1972–73;20–21(34–35):161–96

#### Americas

Beddall BG: Essay review: Spanish science and the New World. **J Hist Biol** 1983 Fall;16(3):433–40

#### Argentina

Kohn Loncarica AG: Historia de la inmigracion medica en la republica Argentina. Tesis, Universidad de Buenos Aires, 1971–1981. 442 leaves.

#### Great Britain

Matthews LG: Medical men as mapmakers. **Pharm Hist (London)** 1975 Aug;5(2):2–4

#### Italy

Premuda L: Schweizer Medizinstudenten und Arzte im Gebiet zwischen Padua und Triest. **Gesnerus** 1984;41(3–4):299–321

#### Spain

Jetter D: Neue Funde zur Geschichte der alten Pilgerherberge in Santiago de Compostela. In Seidler E, Schott H, ed: Bausteine zur Medizingeschichte. Stuttgart, Steiner, 1984. p. 52–64.

#### Yugoslavia

Glesinger L: Strani liječnici u našoj zemlji. **Saopcenja** 1978;24(3–4):275–84

### 500 A.D.–1450

#### Asia

Lindgren U: The problems of being a foreigner: Ruy Gonzáles de Clavijo's journey to Samarkand. **Clio Med** 1980 Jul;14(3–4):225–34

#### France

Mason E: 'Rocamadour in Quercy above all other churches': the healing of Henry II. In Sheils WJ, ed: The Church and healing. Papers read at the twentieth summer meeting and the twenty–first winter meeting of the Ecclesiastical History Society. Oxford, Basil Blackwell for the Society, 1982. p. 39–54.

### 1450–1700

Bourilkova L, Israel S: Données sur la médecine et l'hygiène dans les terres bulgares d'après la description du voyageur Ogier Ghiselin de Busbecq (1522–1592). In International Congress of the History of Medicine. 26th, Plovdiv, 1978. Actes du Congress. Sofia, 1981. Volume II. p. 62–3.
Cooke MA: Richard Surflet, translator and practitioner in physic. **Med Hist** 1981 Jan;25(1):41–56
Levental Z: Medizinisches in den Schriften Edward Brownes (1642–1708). **Gesnerus** 1982;39(2):215–35
Mistler J: Voyageurs d'autrefois. **Nouv Rev Deux Mondes** 1977;(2):265–75;(3):519–27
Rosner E: Hohenheims Weg von St. Gallen nach Augsburg (1531–1536). Wien, 1977. 91 p. (Salzburger Beiträge zur Paracelsusforschung, 16).

#### Americas

Alegría C: Medicos que estimularon a Cristobal Colón en su actividad precursora al descubrimiento de America. **Rev Soc Venez Hist Med** 1969–71;17–19(31–33):199–203
Brotóns Picó J: Un medico en el descubrimiento de America. **Rev Gen Mar** 1980 Jul;199:3–11
Cardenas J de: Primera parte de los problemas y secretos maravillosos de las Indias. Edicion, estudio preliminar y notas para X. Lozoya. Mexico, Academia Nacional de Medicina, 1980. 320 p.

#### Asia

Bowers JZ, Carrubba RW: Exotic antidotes in seventeenth century Asia: two assays from the Amoenitatum Exoticarum of Engelbert Kaempfer. **Clio Med** 1980 May;14(2):129–40
Kaempfer E: Amoenitatum Exoticarum Politico–physico–medicarum. Fasciculi V, Quibus Continentur Variae Relationes, Observationes and Descriptiones Rerum Persicarum and Ulterioris Asiae (Lemgo: Meyeri, 1712). **J Hist Med Allied Sci** 1978 Jul;33(3):320–43
Kraft ES: Andreas Cleyer. In Balde JH, Schmiking W, ed: Festschrift zum 86. Deutschen Arztetag in Kassel. Kassel, Arztevereins, 1983. p.40.

#### Belgium

De Poorter DA: David Lipsius Iscanius, 17e–eeuws doctor medicus afkomstig uit Overijse. **Periodiek** 1980;35:16–22

#### Europe

Hakulinen E: Hälsoråd till tidigare resenärer. **Nord Med** 1984;99(10):266–7

#### Great Britain

Alsop JD: Some notes on seventeenth–century continental hospitals. **Br Libr J** 1981;7(1):70–4

#### Greece

Tomasi LT: L'isola dei semplici. **Kos** 1984 Jun;1(5):61–84

#### Iran

Carrubba RW: The first detailed report on Persian mummy. **Physis** 1981;23(4):461–71

#### Italy

Berti–Bock G., et al: Le séjour de William Harvey à Padoue. **Hist Sci Med** 1980;14:317–24

# TRAVEL

**Mexico**

Fastlicht S: Spain's first scientific expedition to Mexico in the XVI century: the tragic story of Francisco Hernandez. **Bull Hist Dent** 1980 Apr;28(1):3-10

**Netherlands**

Poorter DA de: David Lipsius Iscanius, 17e-eeuws doctor medicus afkomstig uit Overijse. **Periodiek** 1980;35:16-22

**Saudi Arabia**

Faust E: Arabien 1680. Olfert Dappers Arabienbuch und seine Quellen, geprüft an Nachrichten über Kaffee, Sesam und Träumen. Köln, Universität zu Köln, 1977, 256 p. (Kölner medizinhistorische Beiträge, 5; also Diss).

**USSR**

Appleby JH: Dr. Arthur Dee: merchant and litigant. **Slav East Eur Rev** 1979;57(1):32-55

**1700 to Present**

Ash MG: Disziplinentwicklung und Wissenschaftstransfer--Deutschsprachige Psychologen in der Emigration. **Ber Wissenschaftsgesch** 1984;7(4):207-26
Bender GA: Henry Hurd Rusby: scientific explorer, societal crusader, scholastic innovator. **Pharm Hist** 1981;23(2):71-85
Bowman IA: Books by physician travelers. **Bookman** 1984 May-Jun;11(3):3-9
Chaigneau M: Christophe-Augustin Lamare-Picquot, pharmacien, naturaliste, explorateur. **Rev Hist Pharm (Paris)** 1982 Mar;29(252):5-26
Craig D: History of medicine: observation and theory: some reflections occasioned by reading Nansen's 'Farthest North'. **Practitioner** 1980 Feb;224(1340):219-22
Dodin A: Pourquoi les pandémies cholériques? **Bull Soc Pathol Exot Filiales** 1984 Mar-Apr;77(2):127-34
Edwards PI: Robert Brown (1773-1858) and the natural history of Matthew Flinders' voyage in H.M.S. Investigator, 1801-1805. **J Soc Bibliogr Nat Hist** 1976;7(4):385-407
Herbert S, ed: The red notebook of Charles Darwin. Ithaca and London, Cornell University Press and British Museum (Natural History), 1980. 164 p.
Kaiser W, Völker A: Johann Reinhold Forster (1729-1798) als Ordinarius in Halle. **Wiss Z Martin Luther Univ (Math)** 1981;30(2):61-79
Keys A: From Naples to seven countries--a sentimental journey. **Prog Biochem Pharmacol** 1983;19:1-30
Morton G: Henderson Wightman, R. N., 1810-16. **Ir Sword** 1980;14(54):69-72
Pankhurst R: The medical activities in eighteenth century Ethiopia of James Bruce the explorer. **Medizinhist J** 1982;17(3):256-76
Riley JC: Mortality on long-distance voyages in the eighteenth century. **J Econ Hist** 1981;41(3):651-6
Rosales VJ: The medicotrophic syndrome: an acute modern phenomenon. **Unitas** 1970;43(4):30-59
Sokal MM, ed: An education in psychology: James McKeen Cattell's journal and letters from Germany and England. 1880-1888. Cambridge, Mass., MIT Press, 1981, xxvii, 372 p.
Thiel C: Folgen der Emigration deutscher und österreichischer Wissenschaftstheoretiker und Logiker zwischen 1933 und 1945. **Ber Wissenschaftsgesch** 1984;7(4):227-56
Vetter T: Témoignages du Strasbourgeois Victor Stoeber sur la médecine parisienne (1824-1825). **Gesnerus** 1983;40(1-2):215-22
Vondráček V: Lékař dále vzpromíná (1920-1938). Praha, Avicenum, 1977. 481 p.

**Africa**

Leblond S: Le Dr James Douglas, de Québec, remonté le Nil en 1860-61. **Cah Dix** 1979;42:101-23
Lefevre P: Les voyages de la Marine Royale Belge au Sénégal, en Gambie et en Basse Guinée. Récits des médecins qui accompagnèrent les navires de guerre belges 'Louise-Marie' et 'Duc de Brabant' (1847-1856) dans le cadre de la tentative de colonisation au Rio Nunez. **Rev Belge Hist Milit** 1978-79;22-23:647-68, 39-64, 137-48
Logeay R: Le voyage de René Caillé à Tombouctou; ce qu'il lui en a coûté. **Hist Sci Med** 1982;16(4):273-83

**Americas**

Bernstein RE: Historical vignette: Harvey Pirie (1879-1965) and the Falklands. **S Afr Med J** 1983 Jan 29;63(5):169-70
Parrilla Hermida M: Biografia del doctor Jose Salvany Lleopart. **Asclepio** 1980;32:303-10
Szallasi A: Reports by Hungarian physicians on North America in the nineteenth century. In: Congrès international d'histoire de la médecine, XXVe, Québec, 1976. Actes. Québec, 1977. p. 1341-6.

**Asia**

Moseley JE: Travels of Alexandre Yersin: letters of a pastorian in Indochina, 1890-1894. **Perspect Biol Med** 1981 Summer;24(4):607-18

**Austria**

Brătescu C, Gheorghiu E: Vizita unei misiuni austriece la carantinele româneşti în 1849. **Rev Ig [Bacteriol]** 1982 Jul-Sep;27(3):217-21
Hubenstorf M: Osterreichische Arzteemigration 1934-1945--Zwischen neuem Tätigkeitsgebiet und organisierten Rückkehrplänen. **Ber Wissenschaftsgesch** 1984;7(2):85-107

**Canada**

Rousseau J: Dièreville. In Dictionary of Canadian biography, 1701 to 1740. Volume 2, 1969. p. 188-9.

**Chile**

Costa-Casaretto C: Marañon y los chilenos. **Rev Med Chil** 1980 Mar;108(3):277-81

**China**

Hummel D: Som läkare vid hedinexpeditionen till Kina 1927-31. **Nord Medicinhist Arsbok** 1983;:155-44

**Czechoslovakia**

Káš S: Cestopisy v díle ceských lékařu spisovatelu. **Cas Lek Cesk** 1983 Mar 4;122(9):278-9

**Ecuador**

Humble RM: The Gill-Merrill expedition: penultimate chapter in the curare story. **Anesthesiology** 1982 Dec;57(6):519-26

**Europe**

Mann G: Franz Joseph Galls kranioskopische Reise durch Europa (1805-1807). Fundierung und Rechtfertigung neuer Wissenschaft. **Nachrichtenbl Dtsch Ges Gesch Med Naturwiss Tech** 1984;34(3):86-114
Sydow C von: Notiser från Frans von Sydows utrikes studieresor 1861-1886. **Nord Medicinhist Arsb** 1984;:117-28

**France**

Boschung U: Ein Brief Albrecht Hallers über seinen Aufenthalt in Paris und Strassburg (1728). **Physis** 1977;19(1-4):185-96
Carson G: The dentist and the empress. The adventures of Dr. Tom Evans in gas-lit Paris. Boston, Houghton Mifflin, 1983. xiii, 222 p.
Estes JW, Kuhnke L: French observations of disease and drug use in late eighteenth-century Cairo. **J Hist Med Allied Sci** 1984 Apr;39(2):121-52
Sicard A: L'aide des médecins de la Salpêtrière à la première expédition polaire de Jean-Baptiste Charcot. **Hist Sci Med** 1983;17(2):129-33
Thunberg CP: Ma visite à l'Ecole Vétérinaire d'Alfort en 1771. **Hist Med Vet** 1977;2(4):123-6

**Germany**

Baader G: Politisch motivierte Emigration deutscher Arzte. **Ber Wissenschaftsgesch** 1984;7(2):67-84
Loetzke HH: Die wissenschaftlichen Arbeiten des polnischen Histologen Władysław Szymonowicz während seiner Studienaufenthalthe 1895 und 1896 in Berlin. **Arch Hist Med (Warsz)** 1979;42(3):359-64
Rocchietta S: Vita avventurosa di Johann Andreas Eisenbarth (1663-1727), chirurgo e medico girovago. **Minerva Med** 1981 Jan 28;72(3):173-4

**Great Britain**

Bernstein RE: Dr Harvey Pirie and the Scottish National Antartic Expedition (1902-4). Scottish science and medicine in the Falklands and Antarctica. **Scott Med J** 1983 Jan;28(1):75-9
Forbes EG: Liebig in Grossbritannien. **Nachrichtenbl Dtsch Ges Gesch Med Naturwiss Tech** 1983 Winter;33(3):115-33
Smith DG: The voyage of the challenger. **Bookman** 1983 Apr;10(2):3-9

**Greece**

Wegner PC: Le docteur Gall à Cynthère. **Medizinhist J** 1984;19(3):233-43

**Hungary**

Csorba H: Rola polskich lekarzy na Wegrzech 1939–1945. **Arch Hist Med (Warsz)** 1984;47(2):207–19

Csorba T: Głosy polskich lekarzy o pobycie na Wegrzech 1939–1945. **Arch Hist Med (Warsz)** 1984;47(2):221–37

Naiken VS: Richard Bright, physician and budding socio-cultural anthropologist. In: Congrès international d'histoire de la médecine, XXVe, Québec, 1976. Actes. Québec, 1977. p. 999–1001.

Nikodemusz I: Közlekedésünk egészségügye a múltban. **Orv Hetil** 1984 Apr 29;125(18):1084–5

**Indonesia**

Lysaght A: A letter from Sydney Parkinson in Batavia to Dr. John Fothergill. **Notes Rec R Soc Lond** 1981;36(1):79–81

**Japan**

Hesekiel T, ed: Ein deutscher Chirurg und seine Frau in Japan vor 100 Jahren. Briefe von Dr. Wilhelm Schultze und seiner Frau Emma geb. Wegscheider an die Eltern Dr. Wegscheider in Berlin aus Japan 1878–1881. Lübeck, (the author), 1980. 316 p.

**Korea**

Hall S: With stethoscope in Asia: Korea. McLean, Virginia, MCL Associates, 1978, xiv, 637 p.

**New Guinea**

Gajdusek DC: Journal of further explorations in the Kuru region and in the Kukukuku country, eastern highlands of eastern New Guinea and of a return to West New Guinea, December 25, 1963 to May 4, 1964. Bethesda, National Institutes of Health, 1980. [36 leaves], 235 p.

**Philippines**

Harvey AM: Johns Hopkins's pioneer venture into international medicine: the commission to the Philippine Islands. **Johns Hopkins Med J** 1980 Jul;147(1):13–27

**Polar Regions**

Bernstein RE: Dr. Harvey Pirie: versatile man of science and pioneer explorer of sub-antarctic regions eighty years ago. **Adler Mus Bull** 1984 Mar;10(1):4–10

Johnson RE: Isaac Israel Hayes. In Dictionary of Canadian biography, 1881–1890. 1982;11:393–4.

Johnson RE: Robert McCormick. In Dictionary of Canadian biography, 1881–1890. 1982;11:543–4.

Szállási A: A fagyvilágmagyar orvosvándora. **Orv Hetil** 1984 Apr 1;125(14):835–7

**South Africa**

Gandevia B: A surgeon's view of Cape Town in 1787. **Adler Mus Bull** 1983 Nov;Spec issue:9–12

**Sweden**

Sparre A: Dagboksanteckningar från 1858. **Sydsven Medicinhist Sallsk Arsskr** 1981;:132–50

**United States**

Bang F: From a visit in America. **Hist Med Vet** 1979;4(2):25–30

Barnett RD: Dr. Samuel Nunes Ribeiro and the settlement of Georgia. In: Migration and settlement. London, Jewish Historical Society of England, 1971. p. 63–100.

Beatty WK: Nicholas Senn -- surgeon and traveler. **Proc Inst Med Chic** 1980 Jan–Mar;33(1):8–9

Beaver H: Parkman's crack-up: a Bostonian on the Oregon Trail. **N Engl Q** 1975;48(1):84–103

Berkeley E, Berkeley DS: The life and travels of John Bartram: from Lake Ontario to the River St. John. Tallahassee, University Presses of Florida, 1982. xvi, 376 p.

Chuinard EG: Only one man died: the medical aspects of the Lewis and Clark Expedition. Glendale, Clark, 1980, 444 p.

Cohen SS: Two refugee chemists in the United States, 1794: how we see them. **Proc Am Philos Soc** 1982 Aug;126(4):301–15

Cowen DL: The nineteenth century German immigrant and American pharmacy. In Dilg P, et al., ed: Perspektiven der Pharmaziegeschichte. Graz, Austria, Akademische Druck- u. Verlagsanstalt, 1983. p. 13–28.

Fortuine R: Ships' surgeons and naturalists in the early history of Alaska. **Alaska Med** 1984 Apr–Jun;26(2):57–61

Fox SD: Healing, imagination, and New Mexico. **NM Hist Rev** 1983;58(3):213–37

Hammarsten JF, Caylor JA: Physicians and the Lewis and Clark expedition. **Trans Am Clin Climatol Assoc** 1979;91:115–27

Hendrick W, Hendrick G, ed: On the Illinois frontier. Dr. Hiram Rutherford 1840–1848. Carbondale and Edwardsville, Southern Illinois University Press, 1981. xxv, 155 p.

Hood B: 'This worry I have': Mary Herren journal. **Oreg Hist Q** 1979;80(3):228–57

Jensen JE: A Med–Chi physician's travelog 1860–62 (Dr. H. Willis Baxley). **Md State Med J** 1984 Feb;33(2):90–2

Kidd CV: The movement of younger scientists into and out of the United States from 1967 to 1980: some aspects of the international movement of scientific knowledge. **Minerva** 1983 Winter;21(4):387–409

King LS: Medicine in the USA: historical vignettes. XXIII. The automobile makes an impact. **JAMA** 1984 May 11;251(18):2352–5

Lesky E: American medicine as viewed by Viennese physicians, 1893–1912. **Bull Hist Med** 1982 Fall;56(3):368–76

O'Neill YV: Jose Maria Benites' informe--alta California's first medical account. In International Congress of the History of Medicine, 27th, Barcelona, 1980. Actas. Barcelona, Académia de Ciències Médiques de Catalunya i Balears, 1981. p. 203–6.

Pearle KM: Arzteemigration nach 1933 in die USA: der Fall New York. **Medizinhist J** 1984;19(1–2):112–37

Smith JM: Thomas Huxley in Nashville. **Tenn Hist Q** 1974;33(2):191–203;(3):322–41

Szállási A: Nendtvich Károly orvosvegyész amerikai utazása 1855-ben. **Orv Hetil** 1984 Sep 2;125(36):2205–6, 2209–10

Wilber JA: The founding of Georgia and the discovery of blood pressure. **J Med Assoc Ga** 1981 May;70(5):333

**USSR**

Krombach JD: A foreign physician in Russia in the 1930s. **NY State J Med** 1984 Jun;84(6):317–8

Krüger M: Uber progressive Traditionen in der haltung bürgerlicher deutscher ärzte der 20er Jahre gegenüber der Sowjetunion und ihrer Medizin am Beispiel des Hämatologen Viktor Schilling. **Wiss Z Univ Rostock** 1971;20(5):329–32

Matusov AL: Iz istorii meditsinskogo obespecheniia russkikh morskikh i poliarnykh ekspeditsiĭ. Leningrad, Gidrometeoizdat, 1972. 118 p.

Müller-Dietz H: Friedrich Joseph Haass als Arzt in Moskau: biographische Skizzen. Berlin, Osteuropa-Institut, 1980. 133 p.

Palkin BN: S. S. Andreevskiĭ v Astrakhani. **Sov Zdravookhr** 1981;(6):66–8

Tansey EM: The life and works of Sir Alexander Crichton, F.R.S. (1763–1856): a Scottish physician to the Imperial Russian Court. **Notes Rec R Soc Lond** 1984;38(2):241–59

Veselov EI, Belevitin AB: A. V. Eliseev--vrach, puteshestvennik, uchenyĭ (k 125-letiiu so dnia rozhdeniia). **Voen Med Zh** 1984 Sep;(9):68–9

Wagner D: Zu August Hirschs epidemiologischer Reise an die Wolga im Jahre 1879 (ein Beispiel russisch-deutscher Zusammenarbeit auf medizinischem Gebiet. **Z Gesamte Hyg** 1980;26(5):377–8

## TROPICAL MEDICINE

See also **Parasitology**

Blanc F, Blanc FP, Blanc B: Geschichte der Tropenkrankheiten. In Sournia JC, Martiny M, Poulet J, ed: Illustrierte Geschichte der Medizin. Salzburg, Andreas, 1980. Vol. 7. p. 2609–47.

Harrison G: Mosquitoes, malaria, and man: A history of the hostilities since 1880. New York, Dutton, 1978. 314 p.

Kean BH, Mott K, Russell AJ: Tropical medicine and parasitology: classic investigations. 2 v. Ithaca, N. Y., Cornell Univ. Press, 1978. xxiii, 677 p.

Kupferschmidt HG: 'Exotische' Krankheiten--einst und heute. **Z Arztl Fortbild (Jena)** 1983;77(1):33–6

**France**

Chippaux C: Le Service de Santé des troupes de Marine. **Med Trop (Mars)** 1980 Nov–Dec;40(6):605–30

**Great Britain**

Glanville VJ: British books on tropical medicine. **Br Book News** 1980 Nov;:645–9

**India**

Jaggi OP: Western medicine in India: epidemics and other tropical diseases. Delhi, Atma Ram, 1979. xii, 331 p.

**500 A.D.–1450**

**Portugal**

Reis CS, Jans GJ: Sessão comemorativa do 7.o centenário de Pedro

Hispano -- 20 de Maio de 1977. **An Inst Hig Med Trop (Lisb)** 1977-1978;5(1-4):3-19

### 1450-1700

#### Jamaica

Ashcroft MT: Tercentenary of the first English book on tropical medicine, by Thomas Trapham of Jamaica. **Br Med J** 1979 Aug 25;2(6188):475-7

### 1700 to Present

Beauperthuy de Benedetti R: Laveran y Beauperthuy. **Acta Med Venez** 1981 Jan-Mar;28(1):47-52
Boyd J: Sir Neil Hamilton Fairley. In Dictionary of national biography, 1961-1970. Suppl. 8, 1981. p. 344-6.
Browne SG: The contribution of medical missionaries to tropical medicine. **Trans R Soc Trop Med Hyg** 1979;73(4):357-60
Bruce-Chwatt LJ: Franco-British cooperation in tropical medicine. **Bull Soc Pathol Exot Filiales** 1983 Nov;76(5):713-5
Chernin E: Sir Patrick Manson: an annotated bibliography and a note on a collected set of his writings. **Rev Infect Dis** 1983 Mar-Apr;5(2):353-86
Chesterman C: The medical missionary. **Trans R Soc Trop Med Hyg** 1979;73(4):360-1
Collier LH: Recherches sur les Chlamydia - une vue rétrospective. **Rev Int Trach Pathol Ocul Trop Subtrop Sante Publique** 1982;(2-3):17-23
Duffy J, ed: Ventures in world health; the memoirs of Fred Lowe Soper. Washington, Pan American Health Organization, 1977. 365 p. (Scientific Publ. No. 355).
Frank SB: International Society of Tropical Dermatology in perspective. **Int J Dermatol** 1981 Jan-Feb;20(1):69-71
Goodwin LG: New drugs for old diseases. **Trans R Soc Trop Med Hyg** 1980;74(1):1-7
Hackett CJ: McLetchie on mass campaigns. **Trop Doct** 1982 Jan;12(1):35-8
Kluxen G: Augenheilkunde deutscher Tropenärzte vor 1918. Düsseldorf, Triltsch Druck, 1980. 50 p. (Düsseldorfer Arbeiten zur Geschichte der Medizin, Beiheft V).
McRobert G: Sir Leonard Rogers. In Dictionary of national biography, 1961-1970. Suppl. 8, 1981. p. 891-3.
Majoor CL, Hafkenscheid JC, Van Dijk C: Enkele kernpunten uit de geschiedenis van cardiale beriberi, die voor de praktisch werkzame arts van betekenis lijken. **Ned Tijdschr Geneeskd** 1982 Apr 24;126(17):771-5
Paddison RM, Skinner RE, ed: Antonie Wouter Voors, M.D., M.P.H., D.P.H. A biographical sketch and a bibliography of his work. New Orleans: History of Medicine Club of Louisiana State University Medical Center, 1983. 23 p.
Parish LC: The history of tropical dermatology and the 1907 International Congress of Dermatology. **Int J Dermatol** 1980 Oct;19(8):474-7
Sandbach FR: The history of schistosomiasis research and policy for its control. **Med Hist** 1976 Jul;20(3):259-75
Stroppiana L: Correspondencia cientifica de 1858 entre el doctor Beauperthuy de Caracas y el doctor Socrate Cadet de Roma. **Rev Soc Venez Hist Med** 1979;28(42):37-44
Warren KS: The bench and the bush in tropical medicine. **Am J Trop Med Hyg** 1981 Nov;30(6):1149-58

#### Africa

Eddy TP: The evolution of British colonial hospitals in West Africa. **Trans R Soc Trop Med Hyg** 1983;77(4):563-4
Wirz A: Malaria-Prophylaxe und kolonialer Städtebau: Fortschritt als Rückschritt? **Gesnerus** 1980;37(3/4):215-34

#### Caribbean

Reusch C: Die medizinische Versorgung auf den französischen Westindischen Inseln im 18. Jhd. im Spiegel des Werkes von J.B. Dazille 'Les Maladies des Nègres, leurs causes, leur traitement, et les moyens de les prévenir.' Diss., Universität Düsseldorf. Düsseldorf, 1982. 117 p.

#### Cuba

Delgado García G: Libros de texto cubanos sobre parasitología y enfermedades tropicales. Comentarios bibliográficos. Primera et segunda parte. **Rev Cubana Med Trop** 1982 Sep-Dec;34(3):327-41
Guerra FS, Flores GK: Carlos J. Finlay y Barrés (1833-1915). **Trans R Soc Trop Med Hyg** 1983;77(6):850
Perspectivas de desarrollo del Instituto de Medicina Tropical 'Pedro Kourí': **Rev Cubana Med Trop** 1979 Sep-Dec;31(3):161-3

#### Czechoslovakia

Felsenfeld O: Selected bibliography O. Felsenfeld. **Acta Trop (Basel)** 1979 Jun;36(2):193-8

#### France

Bruce-Chwatt LJ: 'Ecole du Pharo' in Marseille. **Trans R Soc Trop Med Hyg** 1981;75(1):131-2
Courtois D: Naissance de l'Institut de Médecine Tropicale du Service de Santé des Armées. **Med Trop (Mars)** 1980 Nov-Dec;40(6):631-4
Dodin A: Ephéméride 1884-1934-1984. **Bull Soc Pathol Exot Filiales** 1984 Jan-Feb;77(1):6-8
Nicolle P: Un événement capital dans la vie passionnée de Charles Nicolle: le Prix Nobel de physiologie ou médecine. Souvenirs évoqués par Pierre Nicolle. **Bull Soc Pathol Exot Filiales** 1981 Jan-Feb;74(1):101-18
Tachon J: La revue 'Médecine Tropical'--retrospective. **Med Trop (Mars)** 1980 Nov-Dec;40(6):639-41
Voelckel J: L'école du Pharo. Tradition-permanence-avenir. **Med Trop (Mars)** 1980 Nov-Dec;40(6):635-8
75ème anniversaire de l'Institut de Médecine Tropicale du Service de Santé des Armées (le Pharo Marseille).: **Med Trop (Mars)** 1980 Nov-Dec;40(6):591-604

#### Great Britain

Duggan AJ: Henry Wellcome: architect of tropical opportunities. **Trans R Soc Trop Med Hyg** 1981;75(4):477-83
Duggan AJ: Medicine and health in the tropics: a brief history of Britain's role with a comment on its future. **Trans R Soc Trop Med Hyg** 1981;75 Suppl:5-8
Durrant GR: Griffith Evans--a pioneer in tropical medicine. **Br Army Rev** 1980;65:66-8
Garnham PC: Some contributions of Scotland to tropical medicine. In Passmore R, ed: Proceedings of the Royal College of Physicians of Edinburgh Tercentenary Congress, 1981. Edinburgh, Royal College of Physicians of Edinburgh, 1982. p. 128-42.
Manson-Bahr PE, Willmott S: Dermatology and the Royal Society of Tropical Medicine and Hygiene. **Int J Dermatol** 1981 Jul-Aug;20(6):429-30
Mulligan HW: Tropical medicine and research in British territories overseas. **Trans R Soc Trop Med Hyg** 1981;75 Suppl:9-11
Rook A: William Tilbury Fox (1836-1879): his contribution to tropical dermatology. **Int J Dermatol** 1981 Mar;20(2):140-2
Schram R: Britain's contribution to health and medicine in tropical countries through medical missions. **Trans R Soc Trop Med Hyg** 1981;75 Suppl:56-8
Sinclair KB: Britain's role in tropical veterinary medicine: past, present and future. **Trans R Soc Trop Med Hyg** 1981;75 Suppl:32-4

#### Liberia

Kálmán G: Libéria egykori magyar minisztere Fuszek Rudolf dr. **Orv Hetil** 1984 Apr 1;125(14):841-2

#### Mali

Saint André P: The Marchoux Institute. **Lepr Rev** 1980 Mar;51(1):35-42

#### Panama

Filós-Díaz JA: Histoplasmosis en Panamá. Revisión histórica y nota de actualización. **Rev Med Panama** 1984 Jan;9(1):8-21
Ocaña G: La misión del 'Smithsonian Tropical Research Institute' (STRI) en Panamá y en el trópico en general. **Rev Med Panama** 1981 Jan;6(1):3-12

#### Poland

Brodniewicz A: Józef Jakóbkiewicz M.D., pioneer of maritime and tropical medicine in Poland. **Bull Inst Marit Trop Med Gdynia** 1980;31(1-2):5-13

#### Portugal

Sassão solene comemorativa do 75.o aniversário do Instituto de Higiene e Medicina Tropical--14 de Novembro de 1977: **An Inst Hig Med Trop (Lisb)** 1977-1978;5(1-4):21-35
Sessão solene de homenagem ao Prof. Dr. Francisco Cambournac, por ocasião da atribuição do prémio e medalha da Fundação Léon Bernard pela Organização Mundial de Saúde--22 de Junho de 1978: **An Inst Hig Med Trop (Lisb)** 1977-1978;5(1-4):37-53

#### Puerto Rico

Bibliography of the scientific works of Dr. Ramón M. Suárez. **Bol Asoc Med PR** 1983 Nov;75(11):521-5
García Palmieri MR: Observaciones sobre la contribución del Dr. Ramón M. Suárez al reconocimiento de la cardiopatía reumática en el trópico. **Bol Asoc Med PR** 1983 Nov;75(11):503-5

South Africa

Barker A: A Zulu contribution. **Trans R Soc Trop Med Hyg** 1979;73(4):364–5

United States

Chernin E: Josiah Clark Nott, insects, and yellow fever. **Bull NY Acad Med** 1983 Nov;59(9):790–802

Kiple KF, King VH: Another dimension to the black diaspora: diet, disease, and racism. Cambridge, Cambridge University Press, 1981. 295 p.

USSR

Askarov UA: Znachenie trudov Akademika AMN SSSR I. A. Kassirskogo v nauchnoĭ razrabotke uzlovykh problem kraevoĭ patologii Uzbekistana (k 10-letiiu so dnia smerti). **Ter Arkh** 1982;54(2):150–2

# UROLOGY

Benjamin JA, Tobin CE: The fasciae of the genito-urinary organs: historical, anatomical, and clinical aspects. **Trans Stud Coll Physicians Phila** 1981 Dec;5(3 no 4):264–79

Brummer P: Uroskopi-föregångare till vår tids laboratorieundersökningar. **Nord Med** 1981 Dec;96(12):325

Dufour A: Geschichte der Urologie. In Sournia JC, Martiny M, Poulet J, ed: Illustrierte Geschichte der Medizin. Salzburg, Andreas, 1980. Vol. 4. p. 1429–81.

Ek A, Bradley WE: History of cystometry. **Urology** 1983 Sep;22(3):335–50

Grossman E, Posner NA: Surgical circumcision of neonates: a history of its development. **Obstet Gynecol** 1981 Aug;58(2):241–6

Grossman EA, Posner NA: The circumcision controversy: an update. **Obstet Gynecol Annu** 1984;13:181–95

Hackett E: The foreskin saga. **Med J Aust** 1984 Aug 4;141(3):187–9

James T: Eunuchs and eunuchism--an historical discourse. **Adler Mus Bull** 1981 Oct;7(3):2–7

James T: Eunuchs and eunuchism - an historical discourse. Part II - Civil law. **Adler Mus Bull** 1982 Nov;8(2):3–7

Knell AJ: Liver function and failure: the evolution of liver physiology. **J R Coll Physicians Lond** 1980 Jul;14(3):205–8

Meier RY, ed: The Joseph H. Kiefer catalog of history of urology and medicine. Chicago, Library of the Health Sciences, University of Illinois at the Medical Center, 1981. ix, 207 p. (Special collections catalog).

Opitz JM, Pallister PD: Brief historical note: the concept of 'gonadal dysgenesis'. **Am J Med Genet** 1979;4(4):333–43

Otten HH: Die operative Behandlung der Prostata. Ein historischer Rückblick. In Göpfert W, Otten HH, ed: Metavoeite: wandelt euch durch neues Denken. Düsseldorf, Triltsch, 1983. p. 213–24.

Schultze-Seemann F: The historical evolution of the internal urethrotomy. **Eur Urol** 1982 Jan–Feb;8(1):54–60

Tkachuk VN: Znamenatel'nye i iubileĭnye daty v istorii urologii i pogranichnykh oblasteĭ v 1984 godu. **Urol Nefrol (Mosk)** 1984 Jan–Feb;(1):72–4

Tucker RA: History of sizing of genitourinary instruments. **Urology** 1982 Sep;20(3):346–9

Zglinicki F von: Die Uroskopie in der bildenden Kunst: eine kunst- und medizinhistorische Untersuchung über die Harnschau. Darmstadt, G-I-T Verlag Giebeler, 1982. 173 p.

Germany

Schneider HJ, Doberentz D: Zur Geschichte der Jenaer Harnsteinforschung. Mit einem vollständigen Abdruck der Dissertationsschrift Arno Krüches 'Ueber Struktur und Entstehung der Uratsteine' aus dem Jahre 1879. Jena, Friedrich-Schiller-Universität, 1979. 84, 42 p. (Jenaer Reden und Schriften).

Italy

Mellicow MM: Castrati singers and the lost 'cords'. **Bull NY Acad Med** 1983 Oct;59(8):744–64

Before 500 A.D.

Gentile DP: 'Urethrolithotomy': an ingenious approach of the ancients. **J Urol** 1984 Aug;132(2):359–60

Kook H: Introduction to the history of urology in the Bible and Talmud. **Koroth** 1979 Nov;7(9–10):CCXIX–CCXX(710–15)

Greece

Dimopoulos C, Gialas A, Likourinas M, et al: Hippocrates: founder and pioneer of urology. **Br J Urol** 1980 Apr;52(2):73–4

India

Das S: Shusruta of India: pioneer in vesicolithotomy. **Urology** 1984 Mar;23(3):317–9

Rome

Rubin JP: Celsus' decircumcision operation: medical and historical implications. **Urology** 1980 Jul;16(1):121–4

500 A.D.–1450

Winter G: Zur Wirkungsgeschichte des frühmittelalterlichen 'Harnregelnkatalogs.' Diss., Universität Würzburg. Würzburg, 1981. 95 p.

Arabic

Mukhtarov AM, Bolgarskiĭ IS: Voprosy urologii v trudakh Abu Ali Ibn-Siny. **Urol Nefrol (Mosk)** 1980 Nov–Dec;(6):52–5

1700 to Present

Aterman K: Connective tissue: an eclectic historical review with particular reference to the liver. **Histochem J** 1981 May;13(3):341–96

Bukhman AA, Novak GIa: Khirurgicheskoe lechnenie bolezni Peĭroni (obzor literatury). **Khirurgiia (Mosk)** 1981 Jul;(7):108–10

Caldamone AA: Theodor Billroth: the urologist. **Urology** 1981 Sep;18(3):316–24

Devlesaver P: Néphrostomies transcutanées. **Acta Urol Belg** 1983;51(4):473–83

Donovan MG, Barrett DM: Ureteral prostheses. **Semin Urol** 1984 Aug;2(3):158–66

Friedman EA, Lundin AP: Dialysate delivery: historical, theoretical, and practical aspect. **Kidney Int [Suppl]** 1980 Sep;Suppl 10:S33–43

Gow JG: The evolution of modern endoscopic photography. **Eur Urol** 1984;10(2):133–8

Herman JR: Autourotherapy; the water of life. **NY State J Med** 1980 Jun;80(7 Pt 1):1149–54

Herman JR: Urethral forceps. **Urology** 1983 Jan;21(1):60C

Hingston WH: La lithotritie et la lithotomie. **Union Med Can** 1981 Dec;110(12):1050

Jantsch M: Zur Geschichte der Röntgendiagnostik in der Urologie. **Wien Klin Wochenschr** 1984 Sep 14;96(17):637–42

Kaleli A, Ansell JS: The artificial bladder: a historical review. **Urology** 1984 Nov;24(5):423–8

Kolle P: Entwicklung, Stand und Zukunft der Urologie. **MMW** 1980 Nov 7;122(45):1575–6

Küss R: Urologie. Introduction. **Rev Prat** 1981 Jun 21;31(35):2477–8, 2481–2

Lindstedt E, Lundquist SB: Utveckling av den transurethrala kirurgien. **Sydsven Medicinhist Sallsk Arsskr** 1980;:94–111

Lippert GP: Xenogener Uretherersatz in Tierversuch unter besonderer Berücksichtigung der historischen Entwicklung von Ureterbioprothesen. Diss. Mainz, 1979. 43 p.

Marshall VF: A urological perspective. **Urol Surv** 1981 Jun;31(3):55–60

Merrill JP: A historical perspective of renal trasplantation. **Proc Clin Dial Transplant Forum** 1979;9:221–5

Mielke HP: Brustgläser, Uringläser und Urinale. Zur Typologie dreier im medizinischen Gebrauch beheimateter Gläser. In Göpfert W, Otten HH, ed: Metavoeite: wandelt euch durch neues Denken. Düsseldorf, Triltsch, 1983. p. 209–12.

Moulin AM, Löwi I: La double nature de l'immunologie: histoire de la transplantation rénale. **Fundam Sci** 1983;4(3/4):201–18

Pérez Castro E: Antologia urologica: Profesor Alexander von Lichtenberg (1880–1980). **Arch Esp Urol** 1980 Nov–Dec;33(6):529–38

Redman JF: Partial nephretomy. **Urol Clin North Am** 1983 Nov;10(4):677–84

Rickham PP, Stauffer UG: Exstrophy of the bladder progress of management during the last 25 years. **Prog Pediatr Surg** 1984;17:169–88

Rubin LP: A young woman taken to the doctor by her family. Mezzotint by Johann Andreas Pfeffel after an original painting by Jan Josef Horemans. **J Hist Med Allied Sci** 1981 Oct;36(4):489

Ryall RL, Marshall VR: Measurement of urinary flow rate. **Urology** 1983 Nov;22(5):556–64

Schuur KH: Radiological visualization of the portal venous system. A historical review. **Diagn Imag Clin Med** 1984;53(4):173–6

Stephen RL: Artificial kidneys: past, present and future. **Ann Biomed Eng** 1980;8(4–6):487–502

Timio M: Il rene artificiale: la storia di uno strumento per una vita semiartificiale. **Med Secoli** 1982;19(3):273–301

Válek A, Wing AJ: Development of dialysis and transplant activity in the world during the seventies of the 20th century. **Z Exp Chir Transplant Kunstliche Organe** 1984;17(2):69–78

Zorgniotti AW: Suprapubic prostatectomy: an Anglo-American success story. In Hinman F., Boyarsky S, ed: Benign prostatic hypertrophy. New York, Springer-Verlag, 1983. p. 45–58.

# UROLOGY

**Australia**

Murphy LJ: Harry Harris and his contribution to suprapubic prostatectomy. **Aust NZ J Surg** 1984 Dec;54(6):579–88

**Austria**

Haschek H: 108 years of urology at the Poliklinik of Vienna. **Urology** 1981 Jan;17(1):113–7
Watschinger B: Klinische Nephrologie (Entwicklung und Aufgaben). **Wien Med Wochenschr** 1984 Jun 30;134(12):275–9

**Canada**

Collins WE: Urology in the Ottawa valley. **Can J Surg** 1983 Sep;26(5):423–6
Hill C: On becoming the first woman urologist in Canada. **Can Med Assoc J** 1980 Feb 9;122(3):356

**Cuba**

Pytel' AIa: Ioakhim Al'barran i ego rol' v razvitii urologii. **Urol Nefrol (Mosk)** 1981 Nov–Dec;(6):56–61

**Czechoslovakia**

Válek A: Ceskoslovenské nefrologické společnosti je dvacet let. **Cas Lek Cesk** 1982 May 7;121(18):568–71

**France**

Brøndum N: Et kirurgisk indgreb skildret i musik. **Dan Medicinhist Arbog** 1983;12:170–4
Mirouze J: Les transformations en un quart de siècle de l'insuffisance rénale aiguë. **Nephrologie** 1981;2(1):20–2
Rothman CM: The varicocele--1800. **Urology** 1980 Jan;15(1):99–100
Shaw R, Stubenbord WT: Alexis Carrel, M.D.; contribution to kidney transplantation and preservation. **NY State J Med** 1980 Aug;80(9):1438–42
Zorgniotti AW: Bladder cancer in the pre-cystoscopic era. **Prog Clin Biol Res** 1984;162A:1–9

**Germany**

Anger G, Adler G: Die Entwicklung der Urologie in Halle. **Wiss Z Martin Luther Univ (Math)** 1977;26(3):133–44
Bach H: Die Entwicklung der künstlichen Niere aus Hydrodiffusion und Hämodialyse, von J. A. Nollet bis G. Haas. Der Ursprung des ersten Künstlichen inneren Organs. Giessen, Schmitz, 1983. 334 p. (Arbeiten zur Geschichte der Medizin in Giessen, Bd. 7)
Lopatkin NA, Shchabad AL: Die Zystoskopie und ihre Bedeutung in der Urologie. **Z Urol Nephrol** 1979 Jul;72(12):517–22
Oehler D, Weiner R: Entwicklung und Differenzierung der operativen Therapie urologischer Patienten im Krankenhaus St. Georg, Leipzig, in den letzten 65 Jahren. **Z Urol Nephrol** 1980 Mar;73(3):171–80
Prentner H: Geschichte der Urologie in Würzburg. Diss. Würzburg, 1981. 68 p.
Schober KL, Simon G: Vor etwa hundert Jahren (26). Exstirpation einer Niere bei Steinkranheit. **Zentralbl Chir** 1981;106(3):183–6
Weise M: Experimental and clinical aspects of proteinuria. Introduction. **Contrib Nephrol** 1981;24:VI–IX
Winau R: James Israel, 1848–1926. Wiesbaden, F. Steiner, 1983. 256 p.

**Hungary**

Balogh F: A magyar urológia fejlödése a két világháború között. **Orv Hetil** 1984 Jan 8;125(2):101–8
Pintér J: Az urológia fejlódéséról 25 éves tapasztalat alapján. **Orv Hetil** 1980 Nov 2;121(44):2685–9
Vértes L: Dr. Ivanchich Viktor. **Orv Hetil** 1984 Sep 16;125(38):2321–4

**Italy**

Valvo JR, Cos LR, Cockett AT: Giovanni Battista Morgagni: his contributions to urology. **Urology** 1983 Oct;22(4):452–7

**Netherlands**

Karthaus PP, Brongersma LD: H. R. G. J. Brongersma en de Nederlandse Vereniging voor Urologie. **Ned Tijdschr Geneeskd** 1983 Sep 3;127(36):1642–3

**Poland**

Cendrzak E: Alfred Obaliński--prekursor urologii w Polsce. **Arch Hist Med (Warsz)** 1984;47(2):239–48
Milik JR: W XXX rocznicę śmierci Wacława Lilpopa i założenia polskiego towarzystwa urologicznego. **Wiad Lek** 1979 Nov 1;32(21):1569–71

**Portugal**

Lach E: The circumcision of the child on the eighth day...An anonymous engraving after a design by Bernard Picart. **J Hist Med Allied Sci** 1982 Apr;37(2):221

**Romania**

Spielmann J: Ein siebenbürgischer Pionier der Nephrektomie: Josef Brandt (1838–1912). **Sudhoffs Arch** 1980;64(2):151–62

**United States**

Barrett DM, Donovan MG: Prosthetic bladder augmentation and replacement. **Semin Urol** 1984 Aug;2(3):167–75
Bush RB: Philadelphia surgeon - lithotomists 1750–1810. Their training, their practice and their teaching. In: Congrès international d'histoire de la médecine, XXVe, Québec, 1976. Actes. Québec, 1977. p. 522–36.
Carson RB: Fifty years of history: Southeastern Section, American Urological Association, 1931–1981. The Section, 1981. 119 p.
Evans JA: Landmark perspective: Roentgenography of the urinary tract. **JAMA** 1983 Nov 25;250(20):2854–5
Herman JR: Hot water bag for diseased prostate. **Urology** 1979 Dec;14(6):545–V
Kiefer JH: History of the Division of Urology of the University of Illinois College of Medicine. **IMJ** 1983 Dec;164(6):498–508
Kunitomo T: Development of new artificial kidney systems (Carl W. Walter). **Am J Surg** 1984 Nov;148(5):594–8
Murphy WP: Carl Walter: a pioneer in shaping the medical device industry. **Am J Surg** 1984 Nov;148(5):590–3
Starzl TE: The landmark identical twin case. **JAMA** 1984 May 18;251(19):2572–3
Zorgniotti AW: The Civiale Remedial Agency. Urologic quackery in the gay nineties. **Urology** 1981 Jan;17(1):109–12

**USSR**

Abramian AIa, Trapeznikova MF: K 50-letiiu urologicheskoĭ MONIKI im. M. F. Vladimirskogo. **Urol Nefrol (Mosk)** 1981 Jul–Aug;(4):64–8
Gusakov NI: K 200-letiiu ucheniia A.M. Schumlianskogo o pochke (1782–1982). **Sov Med** 1983;(4):117–8
Karpenko VS, Kamyshan IS, Kobiakova LF: Razvitie ftiziourologii na Ukraine (1922–1982). **Probl Tuberk** 1984 Jul;(7):75–8
Mirski MB: [The history of the problem of kidney transplantation in Soviet medicine (Rus). **Orvostort Kozl** 1980;89–91(26 no 1–3):125–36
Suslov VV, Gusakov NI: K 200-letiiu ucheniia A. M. Shumlianskogo o pochke (1782–1982). **Urol Nefrol (Mosk)** 1983 Jan–Feb;(1):61–3

**Yugoslavia**

Sariić P: Je li Zabrebački kirurg Dragutin Schwarz uradio prvu nefrektomiju u Hrvatskoj? **Lijec Vjesn** 1980 Apr;102(4):205–7

# VETERINARY MEDICINE

See also **Animals**

Adamson PB: The relationship between medical and veterinary surgeons from Sumer to the present. **Vet Hist** 1983 Summer;3(1):16–24
Daems WF: Die Apoteca ein 'Stall' und die 'Stall-Apotheke'. **Sudhoffs Arch** 1978;62(1):95–6
Driesch A von den: Falkenheilkunde--ein historischer Uberblick. **Tierarztl Prax** 1983;11(1):53–66
Fischer KD: 'Three lexicographical notes.' **Glotta** 1979;57:224–6
Fischer KD: Wege zum Verständnis antiker Tierkrankheitsnamen. **Hist Med Vet** 1977;2(4):106–11
Gerweck U: Die Huf- und Hufeisensammlung des Instituts für Tiermedizin und Tier-hygiene mit Tierklinik der Universität Hohenheim, zugleich ein Rückblick auf die historische Entwicklung des Hufeisens. Diss. Hannover, 1979. 139p.
Leclainche E: Die Veterinärmedizin vom Mittelalter bis zum Ende des 18. Jahrhunderts. In Sournia JC, Martiny M, Poulet J, ed: Illustrierte Geschichte der Medizin. Salzburg, Andreas, 1980. Vol. 5. p. 1779–1827.
Lochmann EH: Das 16. Internationale Symposion der Welt-Gesellschaft für Geschichte der Veterinärmedizin, 21.-24. Mai 1980 in Bärau, Schweiz. **Ber Wissenschaftsgesch** 1980;3(3–4):207–13
Schwabe CW: Cattle, priests, and progress in medicine. Minneapolis, University of Minnesota Press, 1978. xiii, 277 p.
Senczek D: Zur frühgeschichtlichen Entwicklung der tierärztlichen Nahrungsmittelhygiene aus freiberuflicher Sicht. **Z Ernaehrungwiss** 1980 Mar;19(1):40–6
Shoshan A: Rift Valley Fever and its relation to the 4th plague. **Koroth** 1980 Jun;7(11–12):810–3
Simić V: About correct and incorrect terminology in veterinary medicine. **Hist Med Vet** 1979;4(1):1–7

Steele JH: International and world developments in veterinary public health with a comment on historical developments. **Int J Zoonoses** 1979 Jun;6(1):1-32
Verwer MA: Diergeneeskunde--diergeneeskunst. **Tijdschr Diergeneeskd** 1983 Dec 15;108(24):964-9
Wilkinson L: Veterinary cross-currents in ideas on infectious diseases since Aristotle. **Vet Hist** 1980/81;1(n.s.):149-52
Wilkinson L: Veterinary cross-currents in the history of ideas on infectious disease. **J R Soc Med** 1980 Nov;73(11):818-27
Willett LB, Schanbacher FL, Teske RH: Toxicology and the dairy industry: will problems outrun solutions? **J Dairy Sci** 1981 Jun;64(6):1483-93

**Bulgaria**

Kalupov I: Khiliadoletie Bulgarska veterinarna meditsina. **Vet Med Nauki** 1981;18(7):3-9

**Czechoslovakia**

Böhm R: Weniger bekannte historische Schriften aus der CSSR. **Hist Med Vet** 1977;2(2):56-7

**Denmark**

Rose CH, Nansen P, Jørgensen RJ, et al: Sheep farming in Greenland. Its history, managemental practices and disease problems. **Nord Vet Med** 1984 Mar-Apr;36(3-4):65-76

**Europe**

Brøndegaard VJ: Das Wurzelstechen. **Sudhoffs Arch** 1983;67(2):199-209

**Germany**

Holste T, Keil G: Tierheilkundliches im altdeutschen Theriak-Traktat. **Hist Med Vet** 1979;4(1):18-21

**Great Britain**

Cooper JE: Surgery of the foot in falcons: a historic operation. **Ann R Coll Surg Engl** 1980 Nov;62(6):445-8
Ingram A: The country animal doctor. Aylesbury, Bucks, Shire, 1979. 32 p. (Shire album; no. 40).
Penn RG: Veterinary drugs: the beginnings of legislative control in the U.K. **Vet Res Commun** 1983 Dec;7(1-4):377-81

**Hungary**

Oláh A: Althergebrachte Tierheilpraktiken im Komitat Békés, Ungarn. **Ethnomedizin** 1978-79;5(3-4):301-18

**India**

Driesch A von den: Hastividyarnava, eine assamesische Handschrift über Elefantologie. **Ethnomedizin** 1978-79;5(3-4):341-8

**Japan**

Kagoshima J: Kachiku hoken eiseijo no ayumi. Kagoshima, Japan, Kagoshima-ken Noseibu, Showa 51 nen, 1976. 226 p.

**Before 500 A.D.**

Fischer KD, ed: Pelagonii Ars Veterinaria. Leipzig, Teubner, 1980. xlv, 203 p. (Bibliotheca Teubneriana).
Leclainche E: Die Tierheilkunde in der Antike. In Sournia JC, Martiny M, Poulet J, ed: Illustrierte Geschichte der Medizin. Salzburg, Andreas, 1980. Vol. 2. p. 539-87.

**Bulgaria**

Popov M: Novi materiali za istoriiata na veterinarnata meditsina u nas. **Vet Med Nauki** 1979;16(2):93-7

**Great Britain**

Noddle B: Livestock at Garton Slack 2000 years ago. **Vet Hist** 1983 Summer;3(1):9-15
Wright RP: A Roman veterinary physician from the Thames Valley. **Britannia** 1977;8:279-82

**Greco-Roman**

Fischer KD: The first Latin treatise on horse medicine and its author Pelagonius Saloninus. **Medizinhist J** 1981;16(3):215-26
Fischer KD: Two notes on the Hippiatrica. **Greek Roman Byz Stud (Cambridge, Mass.)** 1979;20:371-9

**Rome**

Amberger G: Die Mulomedicina Chironis, ein Buch über Pferdeheilkunde aus dem 4. Jahrhundert n. Chr. **Ethnomedizin** 1978-79;5(3-4):233-61
Fischer KD: Palladius, De vet. med. 14. 15, 5. **Liverp Classical Mon** 1979;4:73-4
Hausmann W: Bericht über einen Fund in Sezze Romano. **Tierarztl Prax** 1980;8(4):417-8
Janiszewski J: Veterinärmedizin Catos des Aelteren. **Hist Med Vet** 1979;4(2):42-5
Richter W: Palladius und sein Columella - Text im Buch über die Tiermedizin. **Wien Stud Z Klass Philol** 1978;12:249-71

**500 A.D.-1450**

**Byzantium**

Fischer KD, Sonderkamp JA: Ein byzantinischer Text zur Altersbestimmung von Pferden; aus Ambrosianus H 2 inf. **Sudhoffs Arch** 1980;64(1):55-68

**Germany**

Bauer B: Studien zum ersten altdeutschen Pferdearzneibuch des anonymen Kopenhagener Ms. Thott Nr. 202. DMV Diss. Hannover, 1980. 99 p.

**Great Britain**

Svinhufvud AC: A Late Middle English treatise on horses edited from British Library Ms. Sloane 2584 ff 102-117b. **Acta Univ Stockh** 1978;47:1-281
Voigts LE: British Library, Cotton Vitellius C. III, f. 82. **Old Engl Newsl** 1978 Fall;12(1):12-3

**1450-1700**

**Denmark**

Andersen S: Simon Paulli. Betaenkning over en Kongelig Ridehest. **Dan Medicinhist Arbog** 1979;9-97
Nansen P: En sygdomsbeskrivelse fra 1600-tallets Danmark. **Nord Vet Med** 1980 Jan;32(1):38-45
Vial G: Studien zum ersten altdeutschen Pferdearzneibuch des dänischen Lehnsmannes Mogens Sehestedt (1598-1657). Diss. Hannover, 1978. 272 p.

**Great Britain**

Cooke MA: Richard Surflet, translator and practitioner in physic. **Med Hist** 1981 Jan;25(1):41-56

**Italy**

Fehringer WT: Studien zum altitalienischen Pferdearzneibuch des Carlo Bartolomeo Rinaldi (1655). Diss. Hannover, 1978, 247 p.

**1700 to Present**

Barone R: L'Association Mondiale des Anatomistes Vétérinaires: 1955-1980. **Anat Histol Embryol** 1980;9(3):280-8
Brown F: A quarter of a century in foot-and-mouth disease research. **Zentralbl Veterinarmed [B]** 1984 Oct;31(9):646-8
Buchsteiner W: Studien zu Texten zur Bujatrik von 1687-1825. Diss. Hannover, 1981. 189 p.
Comben N: Book values and the book market; some hints for collectors. **Vet Hist** 1982/83;NS2(4):151-60
De Wailly P, Crawford LM: The life of Alexandre Liautard. **Hist Med Vet** 1978;3(2):47-9
Engelbrecht H: Taenia saginata, eine entdeckungsgeschichtliche und ökologisch-epidemiologische Betrachtung. **Angew Parasitol** 1984 Mar;25(1):17-26
Ewald BH, Gregg DA: Animal research for animals. **Ann NY Acad Sci** 1983;406:48-58
Fankhauser R: Hundestaupe--Geschichte einer Krankheit. **Schweiz Arch Tierheilkd** 1982 May;124(5):245-56
Fenner F: Mousepox (infectious ectromelia): past, present, and future. **Lab Anim Sci** 1981 Oct;31(5 Pt 2):553-9
Francis J: International (World) Veterinary Congress. **Aust Vet J** 1983 Aug;60(8):249-50
Hall LW: Equine anaesthesia: discovery and rediscovery. **Equine Vet J** 1983 Jul;15(3):190-5
Jukes TH: Early studies on nicotinic acid in animal nutrition. **Fed Proc** 1981 Apr;40(5):1536-7
Katić I: Dansk-russiske veterinaere forbindelser 1796-1976. **Nord Vet Med** 1982;34 Suppl 1:1-319

# VETERINARY MEDICINE

Leach DH, Dagg AI: Evolution of equine locomotion research. **Equine Vet J** 1983 Apr;15(2):87-92

Nicol L: Geschichte der Tiermedizin von der Mitte des 19. Jahrhunderts bis zur Gegenwart. In Sournia JC, Martiny M, Poulet J, ed: Illustrierte Geschichte der Medizin. Salzburg, Andreas, 1980. Vol. 7. p. 2681-709.

Niemi SM: Early veterinary biologics. **Mod Vet Pract** 1980 Nov;61(11):926-9

Ruckebusch Y: An historical profile of veterinary pharmacology and therapeutics. **J Vet Pharmacol Ther** 1982 Mar;5(1):1-20

Sackmann W: Der Arzt und Biochemiker Emil Abderhalden (1877-1950) und seine Beziehungen zur Tiermedizin. **Schweiz Arch Tierheilkd** 1982 Jan;124(1):1-10

Scholz G: Vom Hufbeschlag zur Huforthopädie. **DTW** 1981 Nov 5;88(11):475-9

Schürch A: Zur Geschichte der Anwendung antimikrobieller Stoffe in der Tierernährung. **Schweiz Arch Tierheilkd** 1983 Apr;125(4):169-74

**Australia**

Beveridge WI: The origin and early history of the Mules operation. **Aust Vet J** 1984 May;61(5):161-3

Fisher JR: Foot-and-mouth disease in Australia. **Aust Vet J** 1984 May;61(5):158-61

Hill JR: Cruelty reviewed. **Aust Vet J** 1984 Aug;61(8):245-7

Smith WS: History of the control of some diseases of sheep and cattle in South Australia. **Aust Vet J** 1983 Apr;60(4):122-3

Underwood EJ: The contribution of H. W. Bennetts to the solution and control of animal disease problems in Western Australia. **Hist Rec Aust Sci** 1980;5(1):59-67

**Austria**

Wyklicky H: Maria Theresia und Joseph II. als Reformatoren des Gesundheitswesens in Oesterreich. **Wien Tierarztl Monatsschr** 1981;68(1):3-7

**Belgium**

Marchal P, Roland JL, Thill G: Le symptôme vétérinaire. **Esprit** 1981;12:80-98

**Botswana**

Falconer J: History of the Botswana veterinary services--1905-66. **Botsw Notes Rec** 1971;3:74-8

**Brazil**

Souza LC: João Moniz Barreto de Aragão-médico militar e pioneiro da veterinária brasileira. **Rev Inst Hist Georgr Bras** 1974;305:51-68

**Bulgaria**

Dimitrov D: Iz istoriiata na veterinarnomeditsinskoto obrazo vanie. **Vet Med Nauki** 1981;18(7):112-5

Dimitrov D: 50 godini Raĭonen veterinarnomeditsinski institut vŭv Veliko Tŭrnovo. **Vet Med Nauki** 1982;19(9):113-4

Dzhankov I, Vitkov M: Petdeset godini raĭonen nauchnoizsledovatelski veterinaren institut v Stara Zagora. **Vet Med Nauki** 1982;19(5):3-6

Gŭdev Kh, Iliev N: Pŭrvi rŭkopisen uchebnik po veterinarana medistina za kusistite ot Voennoto veterinarnofeldshersko uchilishte v Sofiia. **Vet Med Nauki** 1980;17(9-10):84-8

Kalapow I: Die historische Rolle des Kampfes gegen die Rinderpest in den Jahren 1913 - 1914 in Bulgarien. **Hist Med Vet** 1977;2(3):76-81

Kalŭdov I, et al: Prof. Dr. George Pavlov (a centennial of his birth). **Vet Med Nauki** 1981;18(2):3-89

Kalŭpov I: Edin vek veterinarnomeditsinska nauka v Bŭlgariia. **Vet Med Nauki** 1982;19(7):6-13

Prakhov R, Doĭchev S: Vŭrkhu istoriiata na izkustvenoto osemeniavane na selskostopanskite zhivotni v Bŭlgaiia. **Vet Med Nauki** 1980;17(5):90-5

Rachev RI: Nachalo i razvitie na izkustvenoto osemeniavane na zhivoti v Shumenski okrŭg. **Vet Med Nauki** 1980;17(5):96-8

Shestdeset godini Vissh veterinarnomeditsinski institut: **Vet Med Nauki** 1982;19(7):3-5

Shestdeset godini Vissh veterinarnomeditsinski institut: **Vet Med Nauki** 1984;21(1):3-5

Shterev I: 35 let samootverzhennogo truda. **Veterinariia** 1979 Nov;(11):12-4

**Canada**

Teigen PM: William Osler and comparative medicine. **Can Vet J** 1984;25:400-5

**Cyprus**

Crowther RW, Gambles RM: Anthrax eradication in Cyprus: an historical survey. **Trop Anim Health Prod** 1983 May;15(2):103-5

**Czechoslovakia**

Holub A: Dvacet pět let Výzkumného ústavu veterinárního lékařstvví v Brně. **Vet Med (Praha)** 1982 May;27(5):257-66

Kubícek A: Z historie veterinární mediciny. Pardubice, Státní veterinární správa MZVz CSR, Oddelení veterinární osvety, 1980 69 p.

**Denmark**

Harrison JD: Professor E. Viborg and therapeutic parotid ductal ligation. **Hist Med Vet** 1977;2(2):42-9

Nansen P: A Danish pathography from the 16th century. **Hist Med Vet** 1979;4(4):73-81

Rasmussen PG: The history of veterinary roentgenology in Denmark 1895 - 1975. **Hist Med Vet** 1977;2(3):65-8

With TK: Thirty years with biochemistry and clinic of porphyrias in man and animals. **Int J Biochem** 1980;12(5-6):985-8

**Europe**

Kiessling W: Der Tierarzt in der bildenden Kunst seit Gründung der tierärztlichen Bildungsstätten. Diss. Hannover, 1981. 385 p.

**Finland**

Klatt CH: Die ersten Doktoranden der Veterinärmedizin in Finnland. **DTW** 1981 Apr 5;88(4):142-3

Klatt CH: Im 19. Jahrhundert nach Finnland zugezogene und dort zugelassene Tierärzte (Kurzmitteilung). **DTW** 1980 Nov 5;87(11):414

**France**

Blin PC: Bourgelat, founder of veterinary teaching, 1712-1779. **Comp Immunol Microbiol Infect Dis** 1980;3(1-2):xiii-xvi

Delaunay A, ed: Présence de Pasteur. Paris, Fayard, 1973. 225 p. Includes contributions by P. Bidan, A. Gamet, J. Guillaume, L. Léger, J. Piton, J. De Rosnay, R. Scriban, C. Vago.

Kostychev SP: Pasteur: his life and achievements. Annotated translation from the Russian by S. A. Wilde. New Delhi, Oxford & IBH Publishing Co., 1978. 96 p.

Léonard J: Pasteur, un vétérinaire qui ira loin. **Histoire** 1979;12:78-80

Mammerickx M: André-Marie Ampère et Claude-Julien Bredin, I. Ampère, Bredin et la philosophie, ou la belle histoire d'une amitié. **Hist Med Vet** 1977;2(1):11-19

Thunberg CP: Ma visite à l'Ecole Vétérinaire d'Alfort en 1771. **Hist Med Vet** 1977;2(4):123-6

Vallat F: Histoire de l'illustration dans l'anatomie vétérinaire française. Bayeux, Bayeusaine, 1973. 157 p.

Varenne E: Traitée de médecine vétérinaire et de chirurgie par Bardon Jean, Maréchal-ferran à Cours. Explications de ce qui m'arrive dans mes exercices de vétérinaire. - Année 1870. Première partie: un maréchal-ferrand vétérinaire de la fin du XIX siècle. **Quercy Rech** 1982;(45-6):36-47

Villemin M: Les vétérinaires français au XIXe siècle. Maisons-Alfort, Editions du point vétérinaire, [1982]. 319 p.

**Germany**

Behrens H: Die Entstehung der Schweinegesundheitsdienste in Deutschland bis 1945 und in der Bundesrepublik Deutschland. **DTW** 1980 Dec 5;87(12):455-60

Behrens H: Geschichte und Aufgaben der deutschen Tiergesundheitsämter. **DTW** 1981 Aug 5;88(8):325-32

Efkes F: Entstehung und Entwicklung der studentischen Korporationen an der Tierärztlichen Hochschule Hannover im 19. Jahrhundert. Diss. Hannover, 1978. 227 p.

Enigh K: Als Parasitologe im Veterinärdienst des Heeres. **DTW** 1981 Nov 5;88(11):479-83

Enigk K: Abriss der Geschichte der deutschen vet. med. Parasitologie. **Berl Munch Tierarztl Wochenschr** 1982 Oct 1;95(19):374-82

Feige W: Leben und Schaffen des Schlachthofdirektors Oberveterinärrat Dr. med. vet. Hugo Andreas Heiss, Straubing (1863-1936). Diss., Tierärztliche Hochschule. Hannover, 1982. 163 p.

Frielinghaus E: Initiativen des Veterinär-Inspekteurs der deutschen Wehrmacht auf dem Gebiet der Pferdezucht im Kriege 1939-45. **DTW** 1981 Nov 5;88(11):457-61

Fritzsche K: Erfahrungen bei der Tätigkeit in zwei 'Beweglichen Veterinär-Untersuchungsstellen' an der Ost- und Westfront während des letzten Weltkrieges. **DTW** 1982 Feb 5;89(2):65-70

Grapentin F: Veterinärärztliches Gerät im Zweiten Weltkrieg. **DTW** 1981 Nov 5;88(11):473-5

Härtl J: Prof. Dr. phil. et Dr. med. h.c. Johann Martin Kreutzer, märtyrer oder rebell? **Hist Med Vet** 1977;2(4):112-22

Heckmann G: Anzeigepflichtige Tierseuchen in der Bundesrepublik Deutschland von 1950 bis 1983, unter besonderer Darstellung des Zeitabschnittes von 1970 bis 1983 in Zahlen und Grafiken. Berlin, Parey, 1984. 123 p.

Hepding L: Das Rossarzneibuch des Scharfrichters Johannes Deigendesch von 1716. **DTW** 1983 Apr 6;90(4):147-50
Hofschulte B: Die Geschichte des Schlacht- und Viehhofes der Stadt Karlsruhe bis zum Jahre 1927. Diss., Tierärzliche Hochschule Hannover. Hannover, 1983. 226 p.
Jaeger F: Die Tierärztekammer niedersachsen, 1945-1982. Diss. Hannover, 1984. 192 p.
Johannes A: Zur Geschichte der Tierärztlichen Hochschule Hannover während der ersten 200 Jahre ihres Bestehens. II. Die Klinik für Geburtshilfe und Gynäkologie des Rindes und ihre Vorläufer. Diss. Hannover, 1983. 148 p.
Kaemmerer K: Die Arzneimittel des Veterinärdienstes im Zweiten Weltkrieg. **DTW** 1981 Nov 5;88(11):461-73
Krumholz W: Eugen Woldemar Bostroem (1850-1928), Lehrer der Bathologie und Förderer der Medizin in Giessen. Giessen, Schmitz, 1983. 311 p. (Arbeiten zur Geschichte der Medizin in Giessen, Bd. 8)
Lechtenböhmer S: Die Dissertationen aus dem Institut für Pathologie der Tierärztlichen Hochschule Hannover seit Erteilung des Promotionsrechtes im Jahre 1910 bis Ende 1980. Diss., Tierärzliche Hochschule Hannover. Hannover, 1983. 162 p.
Marx S: Zwei Kollegmitschriften nach den Vorlesungen von August Conrad Havemann, geschrieben 1799 und 1818 an der Tierärztlichen Hochschule Hannover. Diss. Hannover, 1981. 360 p.
Mayr T: Martin Lerche--in memoriam. **Zentralbl Veterinarmed [A]** 1981;28(1):1-17
Meyer A: Zur Geschichte der Tierärztlichen Hochschule Hannover während der ersten 200 Jahre ihres Bestehens. I. Die Entwicklung der pathologischen Thematik und des Institutes für Pathologie. Diss. Hannover 1980. 207 p.
Mocek R: Wilhelm Roux--Hans Driesch. Zur Geschichte der Entwicklungsphysiologie der Tiere ['Entwicklungsmechanik']. Jena, Fischer, 1974. 229 p. (Biographien bedeutender Biologen, Band 1).
Neumann D: Reformbestrebungen zum Viehgewährschaftsrecht (Viehmängelhaftungsrecht). Historische Entwicklung und die Kritik aus tierärztlicher Sicht. Diss., Tierärztliche Hochschule Hannover. Hannover, 1983. 294 p.
Ostermann E: 25 Jahre Auslandsbeziehungen der Tierärztlichen Hochschule Hannover. Bericht über den Zeitraum von 1958-1983. Diss. Hannover, 1984. 123 p.
Reimer H: Robert Koch und die Rindertuberkulose. **Z Gesamte Hyg** 1982 Mar;28(3):156-60
Schliesser T: Die Rindertuberkulose im Wandel der letzten 100 Jahre (1882-1982). **Prax Klin Pneumol** 1982 Mar;36(3):151-6
Schliesser T: Zur Geschichte und Entwicklung der Rindertuberkulose-Bekämpfung. **Zentralbl Bakteriol Mikrobiol Hyg [A]** 1982 Mar;251(3):326-40
Schulze W: Conrad Felixmüller 1897 - 1977--ein Maler der Tierärzte. **Hist Med Vet** 1977;2(2):51-5
Stähle R: Verlauf und Verbreitung der Rinderpest im Herzogtum Bremen und Verden von 1715 bis 1781. Diss. Hannover, 1981. 147 p.
Voss HJ: Beitrag zur Seuchenlage in den Pferdebeständen einer Armee 1940/41 und zur Erfahrung als Leiter eines Seuchenlazarettes für Pferde. **DTW** 1981 Nov 5;88(11):483-6
Wens HM: Johann Adam Kerstings Neujahrs-Kolleg an der Thierarzney-Schule (TAS), Hannover vom 3. Januar 1784. **DTW** 1981 Jan 5;88(1):35-8
Wimmel B, Geus A, ed: Die tiermedizinischen Zeitschriften des 18. Jahrhunderts. Stuttgart, Hiersemann, 1981. 200 p. (Indices naturwissenschaftlich-medizinischer Periodica bis 1850, 3).
Zieger W: Zur 100. Wiederkehr des Geburtstages von Generaloberstabsveterinär Professor Dr. Curt Schulze. **DTW** 1981 Nov 5;88(11):449-52

### Ghana

Patterson KD: The veterinary department and the animal industry in the Gold Coast, 1909-1955. **Int J Afr Hist Stud** 1980;13(3):457-91

### Great Britain

Alder GJ: Moorcroft's life in England; some new evidence. **Vet Hist** 1979-80;1(3):78-93
Andrews AH: A century of cattle practice. **Vet Rec** 1982 Jun 26;110(26):598-601
Bell JC, Palmer SR: Control of zoonoses in Britain: past, present, and future. **Br Med J [Clin Res]** 1983 Aug 27;287(6392)591-3
Brander GC: The pharmaceutical industry and the veterinary profession: 100 years of symbiosis. **Vet Rec** 1982 Sep 18;111(12):255-8
BVA centenary: One hundred years of farm animal practice. **Vet Rec** 1982 Jun 26;110(26):596-612
Carter HE: Historical cases. Illustrations of the distemper of dogs. By William Youatt. **J Small Anim Pract** 1981 Apr;22(4):207-11
Carter HE: Who needs veterinary history? **J Small Anim Pract** 1981 Apr;22(4):175-6
Catton R: The early history of the library of the Royal Veterinary College. **Vet Hist** 1982 Summer;2(3):91-9
Cule J: Griffith Evans (1835-1935) and his trypanosome. **Vet Hist** 1979-80;1(3):94-101
Duncan A: The Royal Counties Veterinary Association 1883-1983. **Vet Rec** 1983 Dec 10;113(24):552-3
Fisher J: Professor Gamgee and the farmers. **Vet Hist** 1979-80;1(2):47-63
Fisher JR: The economic effects of cattle disease in Britain and its containment, 1850-1900. **Agric Hist** 1980;54(2):278-94
Formston C: A veterinary student's experience of the general strike. **Vet Hist** 1983 Summer;3(1):25-9
Hall SA: The skeleton of Eclipse. **Vet Hist** 1984;3(3):94-100
Hartley JC: The centenary of the Lincolnshire Veterinary Medical Society **Vet Hist** 1983 Summer;3(1):33-6
Heinecke H: Die Kontrolle im Tierversuch--eine historische Studie über Tierversuche von G. F. Fordyce. **Z Versuchstierkd** 1983;25(4):223-6
Henderson WM: A history of the ARC's support of veterinary research. **Vet Rec** 1981 Jul 11;109(2):29-34
Henderson WM: Wellcome research: virology and the promotion of animal health. **Vet Rec** 1980 Oct 11;107(15):347-50
Hickman J: Sir Frederick Smith--his life and work. **Equine Vet J** 1984 Sep;16(5):403-10
Jones DM: The veterinary surgeon in the zoo world. **Vet Rec** 1982 Dec 4;111(23):526-8
Kirkness JM: A history of the Animal Health Register. London, The Association of the British Pharmaceutical Industry, 1981?. 39 p.
MacKay IM: Zoonoses in South Wales, 1875-1915. **Vet Hist** 1980/81;N.Ser.,1:137-45
Oxford Street memorial to pioneer veterinarian (William Moorcroft): **Vet Rec** 1982 Oct 2;111(14):313
Pattison I: The Veterinary Surgeons Act, 1881. **Vet Rec** 1981 Feb 21;108(8):157-60
Rees WH: The State Veterinary Service. **Vet Rec** 1982 Jun 26;110(26):606-10
Salsbury D: Step into the twenties with Jen-Sal's veterinary display. [An early 20th cent. veterinarian's office.] **Found News** 1979 Nov;:12-13
Salter AL: Veterinary life in the Boer War 1899-1902. Correspondence of James William Hall Masheter M.R.C.V.S. **Vet Hist** 1984;3(3):87-92
Sinclair KB: Britain's role in tropical veterinary medicine: past, present and future. **Trans R Soc Trop Med Hyg** 1981;75 Suppl:32-4
Singleton WB: The decade preceding the B.S.A.V.A. **Vet Hist** 1982/83;NS2(4):161-4
Smith RN: D. J. A. McBride, MRCVS, 1843?-1889, itinerant professor extraordinary. **Vet Hist** 1981 N.Ser;2(1):3-25
Snodgrass N: BVA centenary. One Hundred years of Congress. **Vet Rec** 1982 Sep 18;111(12):251-4
Snodgrass N: BVA Centenary. The British Veterinary Association: an historical note. **Vet Rec** 1982 Mar 20;110(12):279-88
Turner T, Lane D: One hundred years of small animal practice. **Vet Rec** 1982 Dec 4;111(23):519-23
Vogel C: From firing to phenylbutazone in equine practice. **Vet Rec** 1982 Dec 4;111(23):523-5
Ware J, Hunt H: The several lives of a Victorian vet. London, Bachman and Turner, 1979. 213 p.
Warin RP: Medicine and Bristol Zoo. **Bristol Med Chir J** 1982 Jul-Oct;97(363-364):4-11
Watt JA: Sheep medicine: a century of progress. **Vet Rec** 1982 Jun 26;110(26):602-3
West GP, Ware F: A history of the overseas veterinary services. London, British Veterinary Assn., 1961-1973. 2 v.

### Hungary

Hajnóczkyné ME: Adalékok az állatorvostudományi egyetem történetéből (1919-1969). **Agratort Sz** 1977;19(1-2):251-7
Kapronczay K: Az állatgyógyászat múltjából Magyarországon (a Semmelweis Orvostörténeti Múzeum új időszakos kiállítása. **Orv Hetil** 1980 Aug 10;121(32):1859-60
Karasszon D: As összehasonlító orvostudomány története hazánkban. **Orv Hetil** 1982 Mar 21;123(12):737-40

### India

Alder GJ: The origins of 'the Pusa experiment': the East India Company and horse-breeding in Bengal, 1793-1808. **Bengal Past Present** 1979;98(1):10-32

### Italy

Théodoridès J: Sebastiano Rivolta (1832-1893) parasitologiste et microbiologiste. **Hist Sci Med** 1980;14(2):227-32

### Netherlands

Bool PH: 75 Jaar Centraal Diergeneeskundig Instituut. **Tijdschr Diergeneeskd** 1980 Aug 1;105(15):583-6
Smits WH: Prof. W.J. Roepke: Forty year link between science and practice. **Vet Q** 1984 Jul;6(3):105-6
Van Bekkum JG: 75 jaar C. D. I. Ter introduktie. **Tijdschr Diergeneeskd** 1980 Aug 15;105(16):631-5

# VETERINARY MEDICINE

Wit JG: Institute of Veterinary Pharmacology, Pharmacy, and Toxicology: its research (1961–1980). **Tijdschr Diergeneeskd** 1981 Oct;106(20):suppl 3:169–75

**Nigeria**

Field HI: The development of veterinary education in Nigeria. **Vet Hist** 1982 Summer;2(3):112–23

**Norway**

Excerpt of a letter from veterinary surgeon Haldoe Dahl: from the Diocese of Trondheim to Professor E. Viborg. **Hist Med Vet** 1977;2(1):4–9

**Poland**

Turek K: Działalność weterynaryjna fizyków szczecińskich w XVIII i XIX wieku. **Arch Hist Med (Warsz)** 1980;43(4):407–13

Wyrost P: A hundred years of Lvov-Wrocxaw veterinary anatomy (1881–1981). **Folia Morphol (Warsz)** 1982;41(1):5–16

**Romania**

Iscru GD: Prima carte de cunoştinţe veterinare tiparita şi difuzata in tara Romaneasca. **An Univ Bucur Istor** 1978;27:69–71

**South Africa**

The eradication of East Coast fever in South Africa: **J S Afr Vet Assoc** 1981 Mar;52(1):71–3

Gutsche T: There was a man. The life and times of Sir Arnold Theiler K.C.M.G. of Onderstepoort. Cape Town, Timmins, 1979. 487 p.

Le Roux JM: Beskouings oor die Fakulteit Veeartsenykunde, Universiteit van Pretoria. **J S Afr Vet Assoc** 1982 Sep;53(4):136–40

**Spain**

Crawford LM: Maestro Domingo Royo and the Llave de Albeyteria. **Hist Med Vet** 1977;2(2):33–6

García Alfonso C, Pérez García JM: Académicos veterinarios en la Real Academia Nacional de Medicina. **An R Acad Nac Med (Madr)** 1982;99(4):671–704

Pérez García JM: Los origenes de la Escuela de Veterinaria de Zaragoza. **Asclepio** 1982;34:101–80

Saturno Hernández PJ: Los veterinarios de la comarca de la huerta de Murcia. Numero, distribucion espacial, movilidad, tipo de ejercicio, edad y años de colegiacion. Evolucion de 1960 a 1975. **Asclepio** 1980;32:433–52

**Sudan**

Wilson RT: The incidence and control of livestock diseases in Darfur, Anglo-Egyptian Sudan, during the period of the condominium, 1916–1956. **Int J Afr Hist Stud** 1979;12(1):62–82

**Sweden**

Brogården in Skaba – the cradle of Swedish veterinary medicine: **Vet Hist** 1982 Summer;2(3):124–7

**Switzerland**

Fankhauser F: Prof. Dr. Alfred Leuthold, Bern, 1901–1982. **Schweiz Arch Tierheilkd** 1982 Sep;124(9):473–8

Fankhauser R: Dem 125. Bande zum Geleit. **Schweiz Arch Tierheilkd** 1983 Jan;125(1):1–15

Fankhauser R: Joseph Guillerey, Porrentruy: premier Dr méd. vét. suisse. Un jubilé passé inaperçu. **Schweiz Arch Tierheilkd** 1983 Dec;125(12):871–5

Fankhauser R, Hörning B: Zum hundertsten Todestag David von Niederhäusern's. **Schweiz Arch Tierheilkd** 1982 Feb;124(2):53–68

Fankhauser R, Hörning B: 175 Jahre tierärztliche Lehranstalt zu Bern. **Schweiz Arch Tierheilkd** 1980 Feb;122(2):57–94

Veterinär-Medizinische Fakultät der Universität Zürich, 1902–1977: Jubiläumsschrift zum 75-jährigen Bestehen: [Zürich, Veterinär-Medizinische Fakultät, Universität Zürich, 1977?].

Zerobin K, Senn C: Rudolf Zangger, Direktor der Tierarzneischule in Zürich (26. November 1826–6, März 1882). **Schweiz Arch Tierheilkd** 1982 Mar;124(3):111–9

**Turkey**

Erk N: Adil Mustafa (Adil-Bey), a pioneer veterinary bacteriologist in Turkey. **Hist Med Vet** 1977;2(4):99–101

**United States**

American Animal Hospital Association: [Fifty years of the American Animal Hospital Association. Mishawaka, Indiana, AAHA, 1983]. 64 p.

Bang F: From a visit in America. **Hist Med Vet** 1979;4(2):25–30

Bierer BW: American veterinary history. [Madison, Wis., Carl Olson, 1980]. 222 leaves.

Brown M: History of the formation of the UW School of Veterinary Medicine. **J Vet Med Educ** 1982;8:105–8

Faler K: The conquest of tuberculosis. A contribution of American veterinary medicine to human welfare. **Mod Vet Pract** 1984 Jan;65(1):51–3

Gaunt RN: Three perspectives on the political history of Virginia's veterinary school. Ph.D. Diss., University of Virginia. Charlottesville, 1980. xi, 378 p.

Goodger WJ, Ruppanner R: Historical perspective on the development of dairy practice. **J Am Vet Med Assoc** 1982 Jun 1;180(11):1294–7

Hansel W, Leonard EP, Dukes HH: A backward look from far above Cayuga's waters. **Physiologist** 1982 Dec;25(6):469–74

Hinshaw WR: The history of avian medicine in the United States. VII. Developments in avian pathology with emphasis on avian practice. **Avian Dis** 1982 Jul–Sep;26(3):462–72

Knowles RC: An overview of equine infectious anemia control and regulation in the United States. **J Am Vet Med Assoc** 1984 Feb 1;184(3):289–92

Lemonds LL: A century of veterinary medicine in Nebraska. Henderson, Nebraska, Service Press, 1982. 395 p.

Leonard EP: A Cornell heritage: veterinary medicine 1868–1908. Ithaca, New York State College of Veterinary Medicine, 1979. xix, 288 p.

Leonard EP: In the James Law tradition, 1908–1948. Ithaca, New York State College of Veterinary Medicine, 1982. xviii, 342 p.

Lutz R: A century of progress. A look at the past 100 years of veterinary medicine in Iowa. [Des Moines, Iowa Veterinary Medical Association, 1981?] 112 p.

Miller EB: Comparative medicine: American experience with equine tetanus – from Benjamin Rush to Toxoid. **Bull Hist Med** 1983;57(1):81–92

Miller EB: Nonacademic influences on education of the veterinarian in the United States, 1887–1921. **J Am Vet Med Assoc** 1979 Nov 15;175(10):1106–10

Miller EB: Petition for a Federal Veterinary Sanitary Bureau. **J Am Vet Med Assoc** 1984 May 15;184(10):1224–5

Miller EB: Private veterinary colleges in the United States, 1852–1927. **J Am Vet Med Assoc** 1981 Mar 15;178(6):583–93

Morgan GR: 'Sugar bowls' (Clematis hirsutissima): a horse restorative of the Nez Perces. **J Ethnopharmacol** 1981 Jul;4(1):117–20

Niemi SM: D. E. Salmon and the first bacterin. **Mod Vet Pract** 1981 Dec;62(12):913–7

Pilling R: A horse on the street is a rare sight. **Am Hist Illus** 1982;17(6):42–4

Pocius GL: Veterinary folk medicine in Susquehanna County, Pennsylvania. **Pa Folklife** 1976;25(4):2–15

Smithcors JF: Discovery of the arthropod vector of disease. **Mod Vet Pract** 1981 May;62(5):371–4

Stalheim OH: Contributions of the Bureau of Animal Industry to the veterinary profession. **J Am Vet Med Assoc** 1984 May 15;184(10):1222–4

Stalheim OH: Daniel Elmer Salmon, the National Veterinary College, and veterinary education. **J Am Vet Med Assoc** 1983 Jan 1;182(1):33–6

Stockton JJ, ed: A century of service. Veterinary medicine in Indiana, 1884–1984. Indianapolis, Indiana Veterinary Medical Association, 1984. 199 p.

Trout GM: The American Dairy Science Association: the third twenty-five years, 1957–1981. **J Dairy Sci** 1981 Jun;64(6):876–99

Whitaker AH: Pesticide use in early twentieth century animal disease control. **Agric Hist** 1980;54(1):71–81

Wolff E: The history and development of surgical tables for large animals. **VM SAC** 1981 Jul;76(7):1033–5

Wood C: Science and politics in the war on cattle diseases: the Kansas experience, 1900–1940. **Agric Hist** 1980;54(1):82–92

75 years of dedication and progress: American Dairy Science Association: **J Dairy Sci** 1981 Jun;64(6):875–1526

**USSR**

Balashov IuS: Razvitie meditsinskoĭ i veterinarnoĭ arakhnoéntomologii v SSSR. **Parazitologiia** 1982 Nov–Dec;16(6):441–4

Danilevskiĭ VM, Luk'ianovskiĭ VA, Migalatiuk DIa, et al: Shest'desiat trudovykh vakht. **Veterinariia** 1979 Dec;(12):9–14

Dobin MA: Veterinarnoe obrazovanie v Rossii. **Veterinariia** 1980 Jan;(1):76–7

Goregliad KhS, Tuzova RV: K istorii bor'by s tuberkulezom sel'skokhoziaĭstvennykh zhivotnykh. **Probl Tuberk** 1983 Nov;(11):71–3

Kalugin VI: Gody stanovleniia. **Veterinariia** 1980 Apr;(4):72–4

Panosian GA, Shakarian GA: Vuz vstrechaet iubileĭ. **Veterinariia** 1979 Nov;(11):18–20

Saunders LZ: Veterinary pathology in Russia, 1860–1930. Ithaca, Cornell University Press, 1980. xxi, 327 p.

Shishkov VP, Poliakov AA: Vsesoiuznyĭ tsentr sel'skokhoziaĭstvennoĭ nauki (k 50-letiiu VASKhNIL). **Veterinariia** 1979 Dec;(12):5–8

Tovmasian DA: 50 let--45 vypuskov. **Veterinariia** 1979 Nov;(11):14–8

**Yugoslavia**

Dolenc M: Bolezni vimena v ljudskem živinozdravništvu. **Kronika (Yugosl)** 1980;28(1):26–31

Rapić S: O zivotu i radu Ferde Kerna. In: I simpozij o historiji mikrobiologije i imunologije u Hrvatskoj do 1923. godine. Zagreb, Jugoslavenskoj akademiji, 1973. p. 85–93.

Topolnik E: Razvoj veterinarske bakteriologije i imunologije u Hrvatskoj do god. In: I simpozij o historiji mikrobiologije i imunologije u Hrvatskoj do 1923. godine. Zagreb, Jugoslavenskoj akademiji, 1973. p. 119–26.

**Zambia**

Perry BD, Hedger RS: History and epidemiology of foot-and-mouth disease in Zambia: a review. **Trop Anim Health Prod** 1984 May;16(2):107–14

## WAR

See also **Aerospace Medicine; Military Medicine; Naval Medicine**

Beswick FW: Chemical agents used in riot control and warfare. **Hum Toxicol** 1983 Apr;2(2):247–56

Green LC: War law and the medical profession. **Leg Med Q** 1979;3(3):175–96

Hauben DJ, Sonneveld GJ: The influence of war on the development of plastic surgery. **Ann Plast Surg** 1983 Jan;10(1):65–9

Histoire de la médecine aux armées: Tome 1. De l'Antiquité à la Révolution. Paris, Charles Lavauzelle, 1982. 513 p.

Jonsen AR, Sagan L: Torture and the ethics of medicine. **Man Med** 1978;3(1):33–49

Kessler RH: Gunpowder altered the physician's wartime role. Should nuclear weapons change it again? **Arch Intern Med** 1983 Apr;143(4):784–6

Kirby NG: How fertile the blood of warriors. **J R Coll Surg Edinb** 1981 Jan;26(1):1–11

Sidel VW, Sidel M: Biomedical science and war. In Reich WT, et al, ed: Encyclopedia of bioethics, v.4. New York, Free Press, 1978. p. 1699–1704.

Vastyan EA: Medicine and war. In Reich WT, et al, ed: Encyclopedia of bioethics, v.4. New York, Free Press, 1978. p. 1695–9.

**Algeria**

Friedman EG: Trinitarian hospitals in Algiers: an early example of health care for prisoners of war. **Cathol Hist Rev** 1980;66(4):551–64

**Spain**

Guerra F: Las heridas de guerra. Contribución de los cirujanos Españoles en la evolución de su tratamiento. Santander, Catedra de Historia de la Medicina, Universidad de Santander, 1981. XVI, 237 p.

**USSR**

Voronkov OV: Iz istorii sozdaniia sapasov meditsinskogo imushchestva dlia obespecheniiavoĭsk na sluchaĭ voĭny (soobshchenie pervoe). **Voen Med Zh** 1984 Feb;(2):72–3

**Before 500 A.D.**

Grmek M: Les ruses de guerre biologiques dans l'antiquité. **Rev Etud Grec** 1979;92:142–63

**Greece**

Coulomb J: La mort d'Alexandre Le Grand. **Hist Sci Med** 1984;18(2):137–45

**500 A.D.–1450**

Griffiths RA: The interaction of war and plague in the later middle ages. In J. Cule, ed: Wales and medicine. London, British Society for the History of Medicine, 1975. p. 127–40.

**1700 to Present**

Adams P: Health of the state. New York, N.Y., Praeger, 1982. x, 198 p.

Agafonov VI: Nekotorye uroki iz opyta Velikoĭ Otechestvennoĭ voĭny 1941–1945 gg. i zadachi po dal'neĭshemu sovershenstvovaniiu protivoépidemicheskoĭ raboty. **Zh Mikrobiol Epidemiol Immunobiol** 1980 May;(5):3–6

Curtis DE: Nurses and war. The way it was. **Am J Nurs** 1984 Oct;84(10):1253–4

Francis TJ: Non freezing cold injury: a historical review. **J R Nav Med Serv** 1984 Winter;70(3):134–9

Gibelli A: La guerra laboratorio: eserciti e igiene sociale verso la guerra totale. **Mov Operaio Soc** 1982;5(3):335–49

Glaser S: L'arma batteriologica secondo la convenzione 1971. **Riv Mil** 1975;98(4):56–62

Henry WD: The case of Captain Colthurst. **Practitioner** 1981;225:418–20

Hoffman LE: War, revolution, and psychoanalysis: Freudian thought begins to grapple with social reality. **J Hist Behav Sci** 1981;17:251–69

Huard P, Rousseau A, Wong M: Les prisonniers de guerre aux XVIIIe et XIXe siècles. In: Congrès National des Sociétés Savantes, 91e, Rennes, 1966. Comptes Rendus. Paris, 1967. Section des Sciences, Tome 1. p. 87–91.

Ingraham LH, Manning FJ: Psychiatric battle casualties: the missing column in a war without replacements. **Milit Rev** 1980;60(8):18–29

Johnson JP: Herbert Hoover: the orphan as children's friend. **Prologue J Nat Arch** 1980;12(4):193–206

Jones DP: American chemists and the Geneva protocol. **Isis** 1980 Sep;71(258):426–40

Keystone J: The physical health of the Indochinese refugees. In Adelman, Howard, ed: The Indochinese Refugee Movement: The Canadian Experience (Toronto: Operation Lifeline, 1980): 163–5.

Kleber BE, Birdsell D: The unused weapon. **Milit Rev** 1965;45(1):54–62

Kornfeld H: Nuclear weapons and civil defense. The influence of the medical profession in 1955 and 1983. **West J Med** 1983 Feb;138(2):207–12

Lifton RJ: The concept of the survivor. In Dimsdale, Joel E., ed: Survivors, victims, and perpetrators. Essays on the Nazi Holocaust. Washington, Hemisphere Publ., 1980. p. 113–26.

Liston SL: Traumatic amputation of the external ear: the War of Jenkins' Ear and George Washington. **Am J Surg** 1984 Nov;148(5):599–601

Meselson M: Gas warfare and the Geneva protocol of 1945. **Bull At Sci** 1972;28(2):33–7

Nutton V: Galeno salvato dalle acque. **Kos** 1984 Mar;1(2):33–50

Popp L: Die Fleckfieber-Epidemie in Kulmbach im Jahre 1793. **Medizinhist J** 1981;16(3):257–69

Romm S, Zacher J: Anna Coleman Ladd: maker of masks for the facially mutilated. **Plast Reconstr Surg** 1982 Jul;70(1):104–11

Russell A: Late effects--influence on the children of the concentration camp survivor. In Dimsdale, Joel E., ed: Survivors, victims, and perpetrators: Essays on the Nazi holocaust. Washington, Hemisphere Publ., 1980. p. 175–204.

Sandoz Y: Le droit d'initiative du Comité International de la Croix-Rouge. **Ger Yearb Int Law** 1979;22:352–73

Schwaber P: Freud and the twenties. **Mass Rev** 1981;22(1):133–51

Siniak KM: Epidemicheskie posledstviia vremennoĭ fashistskoĭ okkupatsii Ukrainskoĭ SSR i mery po ikh preodoleniiu. **Zh Mikrobiol Epidemiol Immunobiol** 1982 May;(5):11–4

Stembrowicz W: Pruski kordon sanitarny w okresie wojny Polsko-Rosyjskiej (1830–1831). **Arch Hist Med (Warsz)** 1982;45(1–4):39–44

Swann JP: The search for synthetic penicillin during World War II. **Br J Hist Sci** 1983 Jul;16(53 Pt 2):154–90

Vanes JM: The Indiana University School of Dentistry in times of war. **Bull Hist Dent** 1980 Oct;28(2):91–5

Westing AH: Research communication: war as a human endeavor: the high-fatality wars of the twentieth century. **J Peace Res** 1982;19(3):261–70

Whymant R: The Butchers of Harbin. Experimentation on POWs--Japan, World War II. **Conn Med** 1983 Mar;47(3):163–5

Zabłotniak R: Polskie Towarzystwo Pomocy Ofiarom Wojny w Rosji (1914–1919). **Arch Hist Med (Warsz)** 1981;44(3/4):345–54

**Asia**

Bowie DC: Captive surgeon in Hong Kong: the story of the British Military Hospital, Hong Kong 1942–1945. **J Hong Kong Branch R Asiat Soc** 1975;15:150–290

**Austria**

Spiro HM: Eppinger of Vienna: scientist and villain? **J Clin Gastroenterol** 1984 Dec;6(6):493–7

**Belgium**

Gotovitch J: Quelques données relatives à l'extermination des Tsiganes de Belgique. **Cah Hist Seconde Guerre Mond** 1976;4:161–80

**Canada**

Fahrni GS: Contributions made to Canadian medicine during World War II. **Can Med Assoc J** 1981 Apr 15;124(8):1095, 1098–9, 1101–2

Roland CG: War amputations in Upper Canada. **Archivaria** 1980 Summer;10:73–84

**China**

Socknat TP: The Canadian contribution to the China convoy. **Quaker Hist** 1980;69(2):69–90

# WAR

**Cyprus**

Volkan VD: Cyprus--war and adaptation: a psychoanalytic history of two ethnic groups in conflict. Charlottesville, University Press of Virginia, 1979. xxviii, 192 p.

**Czechoslovakia**

Bolecek O: Protifašistický odboj na zdravotnické frontě. Vzpomínky na ilegální činnost za okupace na Bulovce. **Cas Lek Cesk** 1980 May 9;119(19):538–42

Remišová M, Janec M, Bruchác D, et al: Medici v Slovenskom národnom povstaní. **Bratisl Lek Listy** 1984 Sep;82(3):1142–52

**Ethiopia**

Hulin I: Háborús koponyasérülések. Tapasztalatok az ogadeni és eritreai háborúkból. I. rész. Neurotraumatológiai sérültek statisztikája. **Magy Traumatol Orthop Helyreallito Sebesz** 1982;25(4):273–9

**Europe**

Rosenzweig KA: Dental health service in the Cyprus detention camps, 1946–1948. **Bull Hist Dent** 1982 Oct;30(2):92–5

**France**

Baumont M: Maurice Barrès et les morts de la guerre de 1914–18. **Inf Hist** 1969;31(1):30–5

Beauquier JP: Quelques aspects de la démographie et de la santé à Marseille pendant la seconde guerre mondiale. **Provence Hist** 1983;33(134):439–47

Bevan-John P: Down memory lane: escape from Alsace. **Nurs Mirror** 1980 Sept 25;151(13):34

Dillemann G: Les écoles de médecine des départements annexés de l'an XI (1803) à 1814. Le cas de l'école de Mayence. **Hist Sci Med** 1984;18(1):45–51

Lanari A: La batalla de Valmy y la medicina. **Medicina (B Aires)** 1981;41(2):257–8

Lefebvre P, Barbas S: L'hystérie de guerre. Etude comparative de ses manifestations au cours des deux derniers conflits mondiaux. **Ann Med Psychol (Paris)** 1984 Feb;142(2):262–6

Livet JM: Les années terribles: l'Ecole libre de Médecine de Strasbourg de 1870 à 1872. In Livet G, Schaff G, ed: Médecine et assistance en Alsace, XVIe-XXe siècle. Strasbourg, Istra, 1976. p. 265–86.

Miączyński A: Szpital polski na emigracji w Aix-les-Bains. **Przegl Lek** 1980;37(1):158–62

Ryan S: Reflections on the psychohistory of France, 1919–1940. **J Psychohist** 1983 Fall;11(2):225–41

Scherrer P: La débâcle de 1940: recueil des malades mentaux à l'Hôpital Psychiatrique d'Auxerre. **Ann Med Psychol (Paris)** 1984 Feb;142(2):266–70

**Germany**

Bräutigam W: Rückblick auf das Jahr 1942. Betrachtungen eines psychoanalytischen Ausbildungskandidaten des Berliner Instituts der Kriegsjahre. **Psyche (Stuttg)** 1984 Oct;38(10):905–14

Broszat M: Hitler und die Genesis der 'Endlösung.' Aus Anlass der Thesen von David Irving. **Vierteljahrsh Zeitgesch** 1977;25(4):739–75

Cieply J: Warunki sanitarne w zastepcym wiezieniu policyjnym w Mysłowicach. **Przegl Lek** 1981;38(1):95–107

Cieślawski M: Z przezyć dzieci i matek-robotnic przymusowych na Pomorzu Zachodnim. **Przegl Lek** 1981;38(1):121–4

Groehler O: Die Entwicklung der technischen Mittel des chemischen Krieges im imperialistischen Deutschland 1915–1945. **Militaergesch** 1976;15(6):718–28

Hahn L: 'Was tut denn der noch da?' Ein Beitrag zum Thema 'Euthanasie'. **Krankenpfl J** 1982 Jan 15;20(1):11

Jagoda Z, Kłodzinski S, Masłowski J: Stosunek ofiar Oświecimia-Brzezinki do prześladowców. **Przegl Lek** 1981;38(1):37–62

Jeśman C: Organizacja niemieckiej Izby Aptekarskiej i gospodarka lekami w tzw. Generalnym Gubernatorstwie w latach 1939–1945. **Arch Hist Med (Warsz)** 1984;47(3):403–15

Marasanov RA, Mel'nichuk AN: Meditsinskoe obespechenie nemetskogo naseleniia na zavershaiushchem ėtape Velikoĭ Otechestvennoĭ voĭny i posle ee okonchaniia. **Voen Med Zh** 1981 Jun;(6):16–9

Perl G: I was a doctor in Auschwitz. New York, Arno Press, 1979. 189 p.

Sons HU: Lebensbedingungen in Nordrhein-Westfalen nach dem Zweiten Weltkrieg. Teil 1: Die Situation. **Fortschr Med** 1984 Apr 5;102(13):93–5 (cont)

Späte HF, Thom A: Psychiatrie im Faschismus--Bilanz der historischen Analyse. **Z Gesamte Hyg** 1980;26(8):553–60

Szemraj-Lochynska A, Kempisty C: Stan adaptacji do zycia na emeryturze nauczycieli akademickich represjonowanych przez hitleryzm. **Przegl Lek** 1981;38(1):33–6

Wolfensberger W: The extermination of handicapped people in World War II Germany. **Ment Retard** 1981 Feb;19(1):1–7

Wondrák E: Medicína na scestí. **Cas Lek Cesk** 1982 Jul;121(28):882–5

**Great Britain**

Allison RS: The second world war 1939–45: an RNVR medical officer's view. **J R Nav Med Serv** 1982;68(2):102–9

Lerner JC: The public and private management of death in Britain, 1890–1930. Ph.D. Diss., Columbia University. New York, 1981. iv, 309 leaves.

Murley R: Peace and strife in Hunter's time. (Part I). **Ann R Coll Surg Engl** 1982 Jan;64(1):20–8

Newcombe N, Lerner JC: Britain between the wars: the historical context of Bowlby's theory of attachment. **Psychiatry** 1982 Feb;45(1):1–12

Nicholson AN: Long-range air capability and the South Atlantic Campaign. **Aviat Space Environ Med** 1984 Apr;55(4):269–70

Owen-Smith MS: A computerized data retrieval system for the wounds for war: the Northern Ireland casualties. **J R Army Med Corps** 1981 Feb;127(1):31–54

Sinclair HM: Sherrington and industrial fatigue. **Notes Rec R Soc Lond** 1984 Sep;39(1):91–104

Weller B: The spy who nursed me (Edith Cavell). **Nurs Times** 1984 Oct 17–23;80(42):18–9

Winter JM: Aspects of the impact of the first world war on infant mortality in Britain. **J Eur Econ Hist** 1982;11(3):713–38

**Hungary**

Kapronczay K, Szemkeö E: A betegápolás szervezése a szabadságharc idején. **Orvostort Kozl** 1981;93–96(27 No 1–4):113–22

Kapronczay K: Az 1848/49-es magyar szabadságharc egészségügyének szervezete. **Orv Hetil** 1984 Jun 10;125(24):1454–6

**India**

Broehl WG, McGee VE: Content analysis in psychohistory: a study of three lieutenants in the Indian mutiny, 1857–58. **J Psychohist** 1981 Winter;8(3):281–306

**Italy**

Morgan K: No boots in Sicily. **Nurs Mirror** 1983 Nov 2;157(18):42

**Japan**

Errera M, Einstein A: Effets à court terme d'explosions nucléaires. **Bull Mem Acad R Med Belg** 1982;137(8–9):560–8

Tubiana M: Effets à long terme observés chez les survivants des explosions d'Hiroshima et Nagasaki. Implications pour l'évaluation des risques d'un guerre atomique. **Bull Mem Acad R Med Belg** 1982;137(8–9):533–41

Uchibori C: [Problems faced by public health nurses during World War II] (Jpn). **Hokenfu Zasshi** 1982 Aug;38(8):694–6

Warren S: Shields Warren, M.D.: Excerpts from 'Medical aspects of the atomic bombings'. 1946. **Am J Forensic Med Pathol** 1980 Dec;1(4):303–7

Yavenditti MJ: The Hiroshima maidens and American benevolence in the 1950's. **Mid-Am** 1982;64(2):21–39

**Korea**

Cowdrey AE: 'Germ warfare' and public health in the Korean conflict. **J Hist Med Allied Sci** 1984 Apr;39(2):153–72

**Malta**

Waterman BB: Memories of Malta 1940–42. **J R Nav Med Serv** 1984 Winter;70(3):182–5

**Norway**

Bang HO, Dyerberg J: Personal reflections on the incidence of ischaemic heart disease in Oslo during the Second World War. **Acta Med Scand** 1981;210(4):245–8

Eitinger L: The concentration camp syndrome and its late sequelae. In Dimsdale, Joel E., ed: Survivors, victims and perpetrators: Essays on the Nazi holocaust. Washington, Hemisphere Publ., 1980. p. 127–62.

**Pacific Islands**

Rallu JL: La dépopulation des archipels du Pacifique: l'exemple de quatre villages de l'île Malekula. **Population** 1981;36(3):519–40

**Poland**

Basinski J: Zachorowalność i obrazenia wojenne w Powstaniu Wielkopolskim. Czas od 27.12.1918 do 13.11.1919 roku. **Arch Hist Med (Warsz)** 1979;42(2):177–87

Bayer S: Z dziejów konspiracyjnej służby zdrowia w Warszawie

(1939-1944). **Przegl Lek** 1980;37(1):131-7
Bogdanow: Wrzesień w Lublinie. **Pieleg Polozna** 1979;(9):26-7
Bojanowski T: Zdrowotne warunki pracy polaków zatrudnionych w przemyśle łódzkim podczas okupacji hitlerowskiej. **Przegl Lek** 1981;38(12):869-72
Borkowski W: Wspomnienia z 'Krankenbau' w Oświecimiu. **Przegl Lek** 1984;41(1):100-8
Chylińska M: Refleksje z obozu w Brzezince. **Przegl Lek** 1984;41(1):115-20
Csorba H: Rola polskich lekarzy na Wegrzech 1939-1945. **Arch Hist Med (Warsz)** 1984;47(2):207-19
Csorba I: Głosy polskich lekarzy o pobycie na Wegrzech 1939-1945. **Arch Hist Med (Warsz)** 1984;47(2):221-37
Dwudziesty trzeci zeszyt poświęcony zagadnieniom lekarskim okresu Hitlerowskiej okupacji: **Przegl Lek** 1983;40(1):1-247
Foster GM: Typhus disaster in the wake of war: the American-Polish relief expedition, 1919-1920. **Bull Hist Med** 1981 Summer;55(2):221-32
Frenk S: Non omnis moriar. A cuarenta años de distancia de las investigaciones clínicas sobre el hambre realizadas en 1942 en el gueto de Varsovia. **Gac Med Mex** 1982 Dec;118(12):509-13
Górski M: Wspomnienia wojenne. **Arch Hist Med (Warsz)** 1983;46(1):91-112
Jaroszewski Z, Tarmanowska B: Dzieci w Instytucie Higieny Psychicznej (w Warszawie, 1943-1944). **Przegl Lek** 1981;38(1):152-5
Kasperek J: Zarys organizacji służby zdrowia w Lublinie w okresie okupacji hitlerowskiej. **Przegl Lek** 1980;37(1):149-57
Klodziński S: Dr Józef Gałka. **Przegl Lek** 1981;38(1):184-7
Kłodziński S: Dr. Stefania Perzanowska. **Przegl Lek** 1981;38(1):189-97
Kłodziński S: Kilka uwag o KZ-syndromie. **Przegl Lek** 1984;41(1):17-21
Kłodziński S: Lek. Zbigniew Sobieszczański. **Przegl Lek** 1984;41(1):131-6
Kłodziński S, Masłowski J: Patologia pracy w Oświecimiu-Brzezince. **Przegl Lek** 1984;41(1):37-54
Kłodziński S: Ppłk lek. med. Jan Zielina. **Przegl Lek** 1981;38(1):202-6
Kłodziński S: Prof. dr Włodzimierz Lawkowicz. **Przegl Lek** 1981;38(1):197-202
Kretowski J, Killar M, Znosko K, et al: Pomoc społeczna i lekarska kombatantom w Białymstoku. **Przegl Lek** 1981;38(1):30-3
Kroszczor H: Służba zdrowia w getcie warszawskim. **Biul Zydowskiego Inst Hist Pol** 1978;35(3-4):107-13
Leśniak E, Leśniak R, Ryn Z: Nurt oświecimski w twórczości Antoniego Kępińskiego. **Przegl Lek** 1983;40(12):849-54
Lisowski W: Sanitariuszki walczącej Warszawy. **Pieleg Polozna** 1979;(9):23-5
Maisel W: Plany Hitlerowskie w odniesieniu do chorych na gruźlicę Polaków w Wartegau. **Przegl Zachod** 1981;37(3-4):99-106
Marczyński A: Dr Artur Karol Werner. **Przegl Lek** 1981;38(1):206-9
Marczyński A: Dr Tadeusz Boczoń. **Przegl Lek** 1984;41(1):127-31
Maslowski J: Antoni Kepiński w latach 1939-1947. **Przegl Lek** 1981;38(1):126-37
Masłowski J: Okupacyjna tematyka lekarska w polskich publikacjach z roku 1979. **Przegl Lek** 1980;37(1):213-28
Masłowski J: Okupacyjna tematyka lekarska w polskich publikacjach z roku 1983. **Przegl Lek** 1984;41(1):159-77
Meclewski E: Der faschistische völkermord in polen. **Dtsch Aussenpolit** 1967;12(2):169-76
Micheva Z: Shesta sesiia na Bulgaro-Polskata Komisiia na istoritsite. **Istor Pregl** 1978;34(5):162-4
Monkiewicz W, Kretowski J: Los chorych psychicznie, kalek i starców w okupowanym Białostockiem. **Przegl Lek** 1984;41(1):80-4
Ostromęcka H: Z badań nad dziejami polskiego wydziału lekarskiego przy Uniwersytecie w Edynburgu. **Kwart Hist Nauki Tech** 1982;27(2):291-311
Petelski M: Dr Józef Bednarz. **Przegl Lek** 1981;38(1):173-5
Przychodzki M: Dr Stanislaw Janiszewski. **Przegl Lek** 1981;38(1):180-2, 187-9
Przychodzki M: Lekarze Poznanscy w latach hitlerowskiej okupacji 1939-1945. **Przegl Zachod** 1977;33(1):106-39
Przychodzki M: Płk dr Eugeniusz Parczewski. **Przegl Lek** 1981;38(1):177-9
Ryn Z, Kłodziński S: Głód w obozie koncentracyjnym. **Przegl Lek** 1984;41(1):21-37
Ryn Z: Zakopiańskie placówki słyzby zdrowia podczas okupacji hitlerowskiej. **Przegl Lek** 1981;38(1):114-21
Sembol J: Dr Wacław Olszak. **Przegl Lek** 1981;38(1):169-73
Sikorski J, Kłodiński S: Mjr dr Marian Gustek. **Przegl Lek** 1981;38(1):182-4
Sikorski J: Płk dr Jan Bularski. **Przegl Lek** 1981;38(1):175-7
Sobolewicz T: Wieźniowie w oświecimskiej kuchni obozowej. **Przegl Lek** 1984;41(1):111-5
Sobolewicz T: Z przeżyć w rewirze oświecimskim. **Przegl Lek** 1984;41(1):108-10
Strzelecka I: Pierwszy szpital obozowy w Brzezince. **Przegl Lek** 1984;41(1):88-93
Strzelecka I: Rozwój szpitali obozowych w Oświecimiu-Brzezince. **Przegl Lek** 1984;41(1):84-8
Strzelecki A: O postawach wieźniów konspiratorów w Oświecimiu. **Przegl Lek** 1984;41(1):93-6
Tomaszewski W: The Polish School of Medicine at the University of Edinburgh: an album. Edinburgh, W. Tomaszewski, 1983. 164 p.
Treść poprzednich zeszytów 'Przegladu lekarskiego' poświeconych zagadnieniom lekarskim okupacji hitlerowskiej: **Przegl Lek** 1984;41(1):178-202
Truck B: Mengele, l'ange de la mort. La vie diabolique du docteur Josef Mengele, médecin-chef du camp d'extermination d'Auschwitz. Paris, Presses de la cité, 1976. 248 p.
Urbanek B: Godzina W na Ochocie. **Pieleg Polozna** 1979;(8):25-6
Urbanek B: Z konspiracyjnej działalności sanitariuszek i pielęgniarek w okupowanej Warszawie. **Przegl Lek** 1980;37(1):137-41
Walter-Janke Z: Z dziejów służby zdrowia okupowanego Sląska. **Przegl Lek** 1980;37(1):104-12

**Senegal**

Bouche D: Dakar pendant la deuxième guerre mondiale: problèmes de surpeuplement. **Rev Fr Hist Outre Mer** 1978;65(3):423-48

**Singapore**

Masaki T: [Department of dentistry at Singapore University during the war] (Jpn). **Dent Outlook** 1978;52(2):277

**Spain**

Grande Covian F: Vitamin deficiencies during the Spanish Civil War in Madrid: a reminiscence. **Acta Vitaminol Enzymol** 1982;4(1-2):99-103
Jordi González FR: Recetas en circulación en Barcelona durante la Guerra Civil de 1936-1939. **Circ Farm** 1979 Nov;11(120):40-5
Jordi González FR: Un desconocido anteproyecto de confederación de farmacias nacido en Barcelona durante la guerra civil de 1936-1939. **Circ Farm** 1979 Dec;11(121):54-8
Jordi González R: Notas sobre la economía de una farmacia barcelonesa colectivizada durante la guerra civil española. **Circ Farm** 1980;12(122):51-67
Riera J: José Masdevall y la medicina española ilustrada (Enseñanza, epidemias y guerra a finales del siglo XVIII). Valladolid, Universidad de Valladolid, 1980. 257 p. (Acta Historico-Medica Vallisoletana, Monografias, X)
Shapiro MF: Medical aid provided by American, Canadian and British Nationals to the Spanish Republic during the Civil War, 1936-1939. **Int J Health Serv** 1983;13(3):443-58
Soteras Elía B: Centenario de la batalla de Oroquieta: primera actuacion de los camilleros de la Cruz Roja. **Pregon** 1972;(111):n p

**Switzerland**

Ettlinger L: Wartime research on penicillin in Switzerland and antibiotic screening. In Parascandola J, ed: The history of antibiotics. Madison, American Institute of the History of Pharmacy, 1980. p. 57-67.
Schettler G: Atherosclerosis during periods of food deprivation following World Wars I and II. **Prev Med** 1983 Jan;12(1):75-83

**United States**

Adams RR: Dr. James Craik, George Washington's physician and friend. **Record** 1980 May, Sep;1-4,1-3
Carnegie ME: Nurses and war. Black nurses at the front. **Am J Nurs** 1984 Oct;84(10):1250-2
Conn HJ: The history of the Stain Commission. V. War and its consequences. **Stain Technol** 1981 May;56(3):135-42
Courtwright DT: Opiate addiction as a consequence of the Civil War. **Civ War Hist** 1978;24(2):101-11
Downs F, Meshad S, Krieger D: The anguish of the veterans. **Cent Mag** 1979;12(4):27-36
Foster GM: The limitations of federal health care for freed men, 1862-1868. **J South Hist** 1982;48(3):349-72
Ginneken J van: Bacteriological warfare. **J Contemp Asia** 1977;7(2):130-52
Helfand WH, Woodruff HB, Coleman KM, et al: Wartime industrial development of penicillin in the United States. In Parascandola J, ed: The history of antibiotics. Madison, American Institute of the History of Pharmacy, 1980. p. 31-56.
Holcombe HW: Patent medicine tax stamps. A history of the firms using United States private die proprietary medicine tax stamps. Ed. G. B. Griffenhagen. Lawrence, Quarterman, 1979. xxv, 604 p. Reprinted articles from various journals.
Imber M: The First World War, sex education, and the American Social Hygiene Association's campaign against venereal disease. **J Educ Adm Hist** 1984;16(1):47-56
Jacobson LO: From atom to eve. **Perspect Biol Med** 1981 Winter;24(2):195-216
Jensen JE: 166 years ago this month ... William Beanes: the doctor behind 'The Star-Spangled Banner'. **Md State Med J** 1980 Sep;29(9):60-5
McGrath MH: Scalping: the savage and the surgeon. In Romm S, ed: Symposium on historical perspectives of plastic surgery. Philadelphia, Saunders, 1983. p. 679-88.
McSherry JA: Reiter's syndrome and the American revolutionary war. **Practitioner** 1982 Apr;226(1366):794-5
Marshall JR: Political integration and the effect of war on suicide: United States, 1933-76. **Soc Forces** 1981;59(3):771-85

## WAR

Quart L, Auster A: The wounded vet in postwar film. **Soc Policy** 1982;13(2):24–31
Steinfeld JL, Summers N, Schoenberg BS: Southern medicine in the Civil War. **South Med J** 1980 Apr;73(4):497–8
Straight WM: Florida medicine and the war between the states. **J Fla Med Assoc** 1980 Aug;67(8):748–60
Taylor B: Free state physicians who served the confederacy: Medical doctors of Maryland in the CSA, by Daniel D. Hartzler. **Md State Med J** 1980 Apr;29(4):35–8
Thomasson WA: Deadly legacy: dioxin and the Vietnam veteran. **Bull At Sci** 1979;35(5):15–19
Trice ER: Theodorick Bland, Jr: Virginia physician, cuirassier. **Va Med** 1980 Feb;107(2):88–9
Van Ginneken J: Bacteriological warfare. **J Contemp Asia** 1977;7(2):130–52
Wasserman H, Solomon N, Alvarez R, et al: Killing our own: the disaster of America's experience with atomic radiation. New York, Dell, 1982. xiii, 368 p.

**USSR**

Abramov VV: O geroizme meditsinskikh rabotnikov v period oborony Kerchenskikh kamenolomen v 1942 g. **Voen Med Zh** 1982 May;(5):71–3
Agafonov VI, Perepelkin VS: Opyt protivoépidemicheskoĭ raboty v gody voĭny i ego znachenie v sovremennykh usloviiakh. **Voen Med Zh** 1980 May;(5):57–60
Altynbekov MA: Zdravookhranenie Chimkentskoĭ oblasti v gody Velikoĭ Otechestvennoĭ voĭny. **Sov Zdravookhr** 1980;(8):51–3
Bragin AI, Ivanov NM: Evakuatsiia ranenykh i grazhdanskogo naseleniia iz Leningrada v tyl strany v period blokady (1941–1943 gg.). **Zdravookhr Ross Fed** 1980;(5):9–11
Chaĭka NA: Deiatel'nost' Leningradskogo nauchno-issledovatel'skogo instituta épidemiologii i mikrobiologii im. Pastera v gody Velikoĭ Otechestvennoĭ voĭny. **Sov Zdravookhr** 1980;(8):47–51
Garshin VG: Tam, gde smert' pomogaet zhizni. **Arkh Patol** 1984;46(5):83–8
Germanov GP: Opyt évakuatsii ranenykh i bol'nykh rechnym transportom v gody Velikoĭ Otechestvennoĭ voĭny. **Voen Med Zh** 1983 Sep;9:9–11
Gilbrin E: Le docteur Paul Caujole: l'hôpital français d'Oumiah (septembre 1917 - avril 1918). **Hist Sci Med** 1980;14(2):155–64
Gladkikh PF: Rabota psikhiatricheskikh uchrezhdeniĭ v Leningrade vo vremia blokady. **Zh Nevropatol Psikhiatr** 1980;80(5):760–1
Iarovinskiĭ MI: Zdravookhranenie Moskvy v gody Velikoĭ Otechestvennoĭ voĭny. **Sov Zdravookhr** 1983;(7):63–7
Kantorovich MM: Oni zashchishchali Leningrad (k 40-letiiu sniatiia blokady Leningrada). **Med Sestra** 1984 Jan;43(1):46–9
Kirsanov NA, Razumov VI: Iz istorii organizatsii massovogo donorskogo dvizheniia v gody velikoi otechestvennoi voiny. **Vestn Mosk Univ Ser 8 Istor** 1980;(5):32–41
Koval' MV: Tovarsystvo chervonoho khresta i chervonoho pivmisiatsia ursr-frontu i tylu (1941–1945). **Ukr Istor Zh** 1975;(4):78–87
Kovanov VV: Po Dorogam voĭny. **Voen Med Zh** 1980 May;(5):69–73
Kulagina AA: O geroizme medikov Bashkirii v gody Velikoĭ otechestvennoĭ voĭny. **Sov Zdravookhr** 1981;(1):59–60
Kuz'menko VI: Uchastie meditsinskikh rabotnikov Belorussii v partizanskom dvizhenii. **Sov Zdravookhr** 1980;(9):49–53
Lebedev NI: Epidemicheskie posledstviia nemetsko-fashistkoĭ okkupatsii Belorussii v 1941–1944 gg. i mery po ikh likvidatsii. **Zh Mikrobiol Epidemiol Immunobiol** 1982 Jul;(7):106–10
Letavet AA: K 35-letiiu Velikoĭ Pobedy. **Gig Tr Prof Zabol** 1980 May;(5):1–3
Lopatenok AA, Fisher AM: Deiatel'nosti M. D. Tushinskogo v blokirovannom Leningrade. **Klin Med (Mosk)** 1982 Jan;60(1):112–4
Makhrova A: Patrioticheskoe dvizhenie za podgotovku medsester v krasnoi armii i na flote(1938–1940 gg). **Voen Istor Zh** 1974;(3):93–6
Menshutin AA: 'Krasnogvardeets' v gody Velikoĭ Otechestvennoĭ. **Med Tekh** 1980 May–Jun;(3):3–7
Meshkov VV: Podvig sovetskikh medikov ne pomerknet v vekakh. **Feldsher Akush** 1980;45(5):3–7
Radlitzki T: Reshimot mimei hakibush hagermani Be-lvov (Lemberg), 1941–1943. **Yalkut Moreshet Period** 1976;21:7–34
Shereshkov GM, Leont'ev PA: Velikiĭ podvig sovetskogo naroda. **Vopr Okhr Materin Det** 1980 May;25(5):3–6
Shmidt AA: Stranitsy vospominanii o blokade goroda Lenina. **Latv PSR Zinat Akad Vestis** 1975;(5):10–7
Smirnov EI, Garin NS: Voĭna i protivoépidemicheskaia zashchita. **Zh Mikrobiol Epidemiol Immunobiol** 1980 May;(5):6–10
Stegunin SI, Razumov VI: Pomoshch' narodov SSSR ranenym i bol'nym voinam Krasnoĭ Armii (1941–1945). **Sov Zdravookhr** 1982;(8):59–62
Sukhanov NV: Meditsinakaia i trudovaia reabilitatsiia ranenykh v gospitaliakh Zapadnoĭ Sibiri v period Velikoĭ Otechestvennoĭ voiny. **Voen Med Zh** 1981;(7):72–4
Tepun PD: Deiatel'nost' partiĭnykh organizatsiĭ i naseleniia Severnogo Kavkaza po okazaniiu pomoshchi ranenym v gody Velikoĭ Otechestvennoĭ voĭny. **Sov Zdravookhr** 1980;(5):61–3
Voronkov OV: Remont meditsinskogo imushchestva vo vremia Velikoĭ Otechestvennoĭ voĭny. **Voen Med Zh** 1982 May;(5):73–5
Weinrib A: Zikhronot shel rofe migetto Vilna. **Yalkut Moreshet Period** 1979;(27):7–60
Zabłotniak R: Polacy studiujący medycynę i farmację w Kownie (1940–1944). **Przegl Lek** 1980;37(1):101–4

**Yugoslavia**

Cernozubov N: Osvrt na dosadašnji rad civilnog saniteta u NO-pokretu. **Lijec Vjesn** 1979 Nov;101(11):694–7
Dragić M: Zdravstvene prilike u Beogradu za vreme okupacije u prvom svetskom ratu i spanski grip 1918–1919. godine. **Srp Arh Celok Lek** 1980 Sep;108(9):969–74
Harmsen H: Demografische Verluste Kroatien 1941 bis 1946. **Donauraum** 1978;23(4):154–7
Južnič M: Razvoj partizanskog saniteta u Sloveniji u toku nardnooslobodilačkog rata (II). **Vojnosanit Pregl** 1982 Mar–Apr;39(2):127–42
Katan E: Napori za ublažavanje oskudice i očuvanje sanitetskih sredstava u toku bitaka na Neretvi i Sutjesci. **Vojnosanit Pregl** 1984 Jan–Feb;41(1):49–53
Kosić I: Rad civilne zdravstvene službe području kotara Korenica i Udbina u odredenom razdoblju NOB-e. **Lijec Vjesn** 1979 Nov;10(11):682–4
Kralj I: Zdravstvo u NOB uoči prvog kongresa liječnika NOF Hrvatske. **Lijec Vjesn** 1979 Nov;101(11):656–62
Rakić L: Prilog proučuvanju zdravstvenih prilika u Backoj posle revolucije 1848–1849. **Naucni Sastanak Zb Rad Naucno Drus Istor Zdrav Kult Jugosl** 1980;21:149–52

## WITCHCRAFT

See also **Magic and Occult**

Crowe MJ, ed: Witchcraft: catalogue of the witchcraft collection in Cornell University Library. Millwood, N. Y., KTO Press, 1977. xxcviii, 644 p.
Daněk K: Pul tisíciletí 'čarodějnické' buly. Pokus o přehled lékařsko-historických aspektu 'čarodějnické' pověry. **Cas Lek Cesk** 1984 Nov 23;123(47):1444–9
Lebrun F: Se soigner autrefois. Médecins saints et sorciers aux 17e et 18e siècles. Paris, Temps Actuels, 1983. 206 p. (La passion de l'histoire).
Shephard L, ed: Encyclopedia of occultism and parapsychology. A compendium of information on the occult sciences, magic, demonology, superstitions, spiritism, mysticism, metaphysics, psychical science, and parapsychology, with biographical and bibliographical notes and comprehensive indexes. Detroit, Gale, 1978. Two volumes.
Sormani E: Il fondo sulla stregoneria della Biblioteca Angelica di Roma. **Mem Riv Stor Donne** 1981;(1):114–5
Spanos NP, Gottlieb J: Demonic possession, mesmerism, and hysteria: a social psychological perspective on their historical interrelations. **J Abnorm Psychol** 88(5):527–46, Oct 79
Stöber O: Drudenfuss-Monographie. Linz, Stadt-Verlag Neydharting, 1981. 460 p.

**Americas**

Silverblatt I: The evolution of witchcraft and the meaning of healing in colonial Andean society. **Cult Med Psychiatry** 1983 Dec;7(4):413–27
Simmons M: Witchcraft and black magic: an interpretive view. **Palacio** 1974;80(2):5–11

**Europe**

Ben-Yehuda N: The European witch craze of the 14th to 17th centuries: a sociologist's perspective. **Am J Sociol** 1980 Jul;86(1):1–31
Hook D, Ben-Yehuda N: [European witch-hunts: two perspectives]. **Am J Sociol** 1983;88(6):1270–9
Tamáska P: A boszorkányüldözések gazdasági és társadalmi háttere. **Orv Hetil** 1983 Sep 18;124(38):2322, 2325

**Germany**

Lehmann H: Hexenverfolgungen und Hexenprozesse im alten Reich zwischen Reformation und Aufklärung. **Jahrb Inst Dtsch Gesch** 1978;7:9–70

**Great Britain**

Garrett C: Women and witches: patterns of analysis. **Signs** 1977;3(2):461–70
Larner C: Enemies of God: the witch-hunt in Scotland. Baltimore, Johns Hopkins Univ. Press, 1981. x, 244 p.
McLachlan HV, Swales JK: Stereotypes and Scottish witchcraft. **Contemp Rev** 1979:234(1357):88–94
Matalene C: Women as witches. **Int J Womens Stud** 1978;1(6):573–87

**Italy**

Accati L: Lo spirito della fornicazione: virtù dell'anima e virtù del corpo in Friuli, fra '600 e '700. **Quad Stor** 1979;14(2):644–72

**United States**

Kerr H, Crow CL, ed: The occult in America: new historical perspectives. Urbana, Chicago, University of Illinois Press, 1983. 246 p.
Snyderman GS: Witches, witchcraft, and Allegany Seneca medicine. **Proc Am Philos Soc** 1983;127(4):263–77
Tierney GD: Botany and witchcraft. **Palacio** 1974;80(2):44–50

**500 A.D.–1450**

**Czechoslovakia**

Sindelář B: Carodějnictví a jeho pronásledování u nás do r. 1526. **Sb Pr Filos Fak Brnenske Univ Rada Hist** 1981;30(28):177–206

**1450–1700**

Andreski S: The syphilitic shock: a new explanation of the 'great witch craze' of the 16th and 17th centuries in the light of medicine and psychiatry. **Encounter (Lond)** 1982;58(5):7–26
Bergamaschi MT, et al: Streghe e raccoglitrici di bambori: al confine tra la medicina colta, empiria e pratiche magiche (XV–XVI secolo). **Mem Riv Stor Donne** 1981;(1):106–13
Easlea B: Witch hunting, magic, and the new philosophy: an introduction to debates of the scientific revolution, 1450–1750. Brighton, Sussex, Harvester Press, 1980. xii, 283 p.
Estes LL: The medical origins of the European witch craze: a hypothesis. **J Soc Hist** 1983;17:271–84
Fischer-Homberger E: The medicalization of demonology––the contribution of forensic medicine to early modern psychiatry. In International Congress of the History of Medicine, 27th, Barcelona, 1980. Actas. Barcelona, Académia de Ciències Médiques de Catalunya i Balears, 1981. p. 69–73.
Horsley RA: Who were the witches? The social roles of the accused in the European witch trials. **J Interdiscip Hist** 1979;9(4):689–715
Kirsch I: Demonology and science during the scientific revolution. **J Hist Behav Sci** 1980 Oct;16(4):359–68
Monter EW: Witchcraft in France and Switzerland: the borderlands during the Reformation. Ithaca, Cornell University Press, 1976. 232 p.

**Austria**

Nagl H: Der Zauberer-Jackl-Prozess: Hexenprozesse im erzstift Salzburg 1675–1690. **Mitt Ges Salzburger Landeskd** 1972–73;112–113(2):385–539

**Canada**

Pearl JL: Witchcraft in New France in the seventeenth century: the social aspect. **Hist Reflect** 1977;4(2):191–205

**Europe**

Horsley RA: Further reflections to witchcraft and European folk religion. **Hist Relig** 1979;19(1):71–95

**France**

Billich A: Un procès de sorcellerie à Turckheim en 1628. In: Congrès National des Sociétés Savantes, 104e, Bordeaux, 1979. Actes. Paris, 1981. Histoire Moderne et Contemporaine, Tome 2. p. 407–10.
Soman A: La sorcellerie vue du Parlement de Paris au début du XVIIe siècle. In: Congrès National des Sociétés Savantes, 104e, Bordeaux, 1979. Actes. Paris, 1981. Histoire Moderne et Contemporaine, Tome 2. p. 393–405.

**Great Britain**

Geis G, Bunn I: Sir Thomas Browne and witchcraft: a cautionary tale for contemporary law and psychiatry. **Int J Law Psychiatry** 1981;4(1–2):1–11
Jobe TH: The devil in Restoration science: the Glanvill-Webster witchcraft debate. **Isis** 1981 Sep;72(263):343–56
Matossian MK: Bewitched or intoxicated? The etiology of witch persecution in early modern England. **Medizinhist J** 1983;18(1–2):33–42

**Portugal**

Pereira I da R: Processos de feitiçaria e de bruxaria na Inquisiçao de Portugal. **An Acad Port Hist** 1977;24(2):83–178

**United States**

Bolkhovitinoe NN: Sielemskaia ved'ma. **Vopr Istor** 1982;(10):187–9
Demos J: Entertaining Satan. **Am Heritage** 1978;29(5):14–23
Demos JP: Entertaining Satan. Witchcraft and the culture of early New England. New York, Oxford, Oxford University Press, 1982. xiv, 543 p.
Green SA: Salem witchcraft: a biopsychosocial analysis. **Pharos** 1982 Summer;45(3):9–13
Painter F: An early 18th century witch bottle: a legacy of the wicked witch of Pungo. **Chesopiean** 1980;18(3–6):62–71
Spanos NP: Ergotism and the Salem witch panic: a critical analysis and an alternative conceptualization. **J Hist Behav Sci** 1983 Oct;19(4):358–69

**USSR**

Zguta R: Was there a witch craze in Muscovite Russia? **South Folkl Q** 1977;41:119–28

**1700 to Present**

**Austria**

Auer G: Reste des hexenglaubens in Donnerskirchen. **Burgenl Heimatbl** 1973;35(3):109–24

**France**

Maire CL: Les possédées de Morzine (1857–1873). Lyon, Presses Universitaires, 1981. 134 p.
Wilkins KS: Attitudes to witchcraft and demonic possession in France during the 18th century. **J Eur Stud** 1973;3(4):348–62

**Ivory Coast**

Walker SS: Witchcraft and healing in an African church. **J Relig Afr** 1979;10(2):127–138

**Kenya**

Brantley C: An historical perspective of the Giriama and witchcraft control. **Africa (Gt Brit)** 1979;49(2):112–33

**Nigeria**

Latham AJ: Witchcraft accusations and economic tension in precolonial old Calabar. **J Afr Hist** 1972;13(2):249–60

**United States**

Blanchard D: Who or what's a witch: Iroquois persons of power. **Am Indian Q** 1982;6(3–4):218–37
Carey GG: Folklore from the printed sources of Essex County, Massachusetts. **South Folkl Q** 1968;32(1):17–43
Davis J: Witchcraft and superstitions of Torrance County. **NM Hist Rev** 1979;54(1):53–9
Hurt WR: Witchcraft in New Mexico. **Palacio** 1974;80(2):12–20
Milspaw YJ: Witchcraft belief in a Pennsylvania German family. **Pa Folklife** 1978;27(4):14–24
Welsh ME: A selected bibliography [on witchcraft]. **Palacio** 1974;80(2):51–4
Witter DA: Witchcraft along the Rio Grande. **Palacio** 1974;80(2):21–37

## WOMEN

See also **Nursing**

Barcs-Masson ML: Les femmes et la pharmacie. Nice, Belisane, 1977. 149 p.
Burlingame LJ: The history of women in medicine. **Md Hist** 1978;9(2):51–62
Cunin OE: Femmes dentistes, femmes de dentistes. **Hist Sci Med** 1980;14(2):207–12
Kanei H: [The role of women and nursing - a lesson in folk medicine. 3]. **Sogo Kango** 1982;17(1):79–89
Knibiehler Y, Fouquet C: La femme et les médecins. Analyse historique. [Paris], Hachette, 1983. 333 p.
Melzer R: The housewife doctor. **Adler Mus Bull** 1984 Jun;10(2):1–2
Merchant C: Isis' consciousness raised. **Isis** 1982 Sep;73(268):398–409
Nadelson CC, Notman MT: [History of] women as health professionals. In Reich WT, et al, ed: Encyclopedia of bioethics, v.4. New York, Free Press, 1978. p. 1713–20
Penneau D, Loriot J, Proteau J, et al: La femme médecin à travers les âges et les pays. **Hist Sci Med** 1981;15(4):335–43
Rothman BK: In labor. Women and power in the birthplace. New York, London, W.W. Norton, 1982. 320 p.

**Canada**

Bernier H: Charlotte Gallard. In Dictionary of Canadian biography, 1701 to 1740. Volume 2, 1969. p. 235–6.
Bernier H: Marie Morin. In Dictionary of Canadian biography, 1701 to 1740. Volume 2, 1969. p. 489–92.
Campeau L: Jeanne-Françoise Juchereau de la Ferté. In Dictionary of

Canadian biography, 1701 to 1740. Volume 2, 1969. p. 302-3.

**Great Britain**

Crawford P: Printed advertisements for women medical practitioners in London, 1670–1710. **Soc Soc Hist Med Bull (Lond)** 1984 Dec;35:66–70
Wyman AL: The surgeoness: the female practitioner of surgery 1400–1800. **Med Hist** 1984 Jan;28(1):22–41

**Iceland**

Helgadóttir GP: Kvinner og legekunst i fornsagaene. **Nord Medicinhist Arsb** 1984;:35–47

**Mexico**

Juan López M, Berumen Amor E, Trejo Rayón S, et al: La mujer en las acciones de atención a la salud en México. **Salud Publica Mex** 1984 Nov–Dec;26(6):537–45

**United States**

Leavitt JW, ed: Women and health in America: historical readings. Madison, University of Wisconsin Press, 1984. ix, 526 p. (Previously published articles by various authors)
Mathes VS: Native American women in medicine and the military. **J West** 1982;21(2):41–8

**Before 500 A.D.**

Nickel D: Berufsvorstellungen über weibliche Medizinalpersonen in der Antike. **Klio** 1979;61:515–8

**China**

Zeng Shixin: Bao Gu, the distinguished woman physician of the Jin Dynasty. **Chung Hua I Shih Tsa Chih** 1981;11:75–7

**Greece**

Pomeroy SB: Plato and the female physician ('Republic', 454d 2). **Am J Philol** 1978;99:496–500

**500 A.D.–1450**

**Italy**

Caffaratto TM: Rilettura e commento dell'opera 'De Mulierum passionibus' di Trotula de Ruggiero, o Trocta Salernitana. **Minerva Med** 1981 Nov 17;72(46):3123–31

**1450–1700**

Bergamaschi MT, et al: Streghe e raccoglitrici di bambori: al confine tra la medicina colta, empiria e pratiche magiche (XV–XVI secolo). **Mem Riv Stor Donne** 1981;(1):106–13

**Canada**

Bernier H: Françoise Maumousseau. In Dictionary of Canadian biography, 1701 to 1740. Volume 2, 1969. p. 466–7.
Bernier H: Marie-Madeleine Maufils. In Dictionary of Canadian biography, 1701 to 1740. Volume 2, 1969. p. 466.
Paquin M: Louise Soumande. In Dictionary of Canadian biography, 1701 to 1740. Volume 2, 1969. p. 613.
Voisine N: Marguerite Bourdon. In Dictionary of Canadian biography, 1701 to 1740. Volume 2, 1969. p. 92–3.

**Great Britain**

Rawlings FH: Two 17th century women apothecaries. **Pharm Hist (London)** 1984 Sep;14(3):7

**1700 to Present**

Barker JT: Women as leaders in the field of rehabilitation. **J Rehabil** 1982 Jan–Mar;48(1):9–18, 68–70
Bauer C, Ritt L: 'The little health of ladies.' An anatomy of female invalidism in the nineteenth century. **J Am Med Wom Assoc** 1981 Oct;36(10):300–6
Beauperthuy de Benedetti R: La mujer y la medicina. **Rev Soc Venez Hist Med** 1969–71;17–19(31–33):135–51
Brogan DR: Women in medicine: Australia, New Zealand, Canada, and United States. **Women Health** 1982 Spring;7(1):5–14
Buckley NL: Women psychoanalysts and the theory of feminine development: a study of Karen Horney, Helene Deutsch, and Marie Bonaparte. Ph.D. Diss., University of California. Los Angeles, 1982. 178 p.
Dumont-Johnson M: Les infirmières: cols roses? **Nurs Que** 1981 Sep–Oct;1(6):10–9
Hoff SG: Frieda Fromm-Reichmann. In Dictionary of American Biography, Suppl. 6, 1956–1960. p. 219–20, 1980.
Mandelbaum DR: Women in medicine. **Signs** 1978;4(1):136–45
O'Connell AN, Russo NF, ed: Models of achievement. Reflections of eminent women in psychology. New York, Columbia University Press, 1983. xiii, 338 p.
Rosenthal MM: Perspectivenes on women physicians in the USA through cross-cultural comparison: England, Sweden, USSR. **Int J Womens Stud** 1979;2(6):528–40
Smith KM: Dr. James Barry: military man--or woman? **Can Med Assoc J** 1982 Apr 1;126(7):854–7
Vaksman IA, Popugaĭlo VM: Zhenshchiny mediki na pochtovykh markakh mira. **Feldsher Akush** 1984 Jul;49(7):38–43
Yoshikawa R: [Biography of Nightingale published in the early Meiji era - on 'Self-Help for Women'] (Jpn). **Sogo Kango** 1982;17(1):91–102

**Austria**

Aigner R: Die Grazer Aerztinnen aus der Zeit der Monarchie. **Z Hist Ver Steiermark** 1979;70:45–70

**Brazil**

Lobo FB: Duas pioneiras–Madame Dubocher, Rita Lobato. **Rev Inst Hist Geogr Bras** 1980;(328):53–6

**Canada**

Ames EW: The status of women in Canadian psychology: a case study of women in science. **Int J Womens Stud** 1981;4(4):431–40
Ducharme J: Marie-Catherine-Françoise Céloron. In Dictionary of Canadian biography, 1801 to 1820. Volume 5, 1983. p. 174.
Hill C: On becoming the first woman urologist in Canada. **Can Med Assoc J** 1980 Feb 9;122(3):356
Plamondon L: Marie-Catherine Payen de Noyan. In Dictionary of Canadian biography, 1801 to 1820. Volume 5, 1983. p. 661–2.
Rousseau F: Marie-Geneviève Parent. In Dictionary of Canadian biography, 1801 to 1820. Volume 5, 1983. p. 658–9.
Rousseau F: Marie-Vénérande Melançon. In Dictionary of Canadian biography, 1801 to 1820. Volume 5, 1983. p. 587–8.
Séguin G: Marie-Angélique Dussaus. In Dictionary of Canadian biography, 1801 to 1820. Volume 5, 1983. p. 293.
Smith K: Dr. Augusta Stowe-Gullen: a pioneer of social conscience. **Can Med Assoc J** 1982 Jun 15;126(12):1465–7
Vachon A: Marguerite Dizy. In Dictionary of Canadian biography, 1701 to 1740. Volume 2, 1969. p. 189–90.

**Chile**

Costa-Casaretto C: Dra. Eloísa Díaz. Centenario del ingreso de la mujer chilena al estudio de las profesiones universitarias. **Rev Med Chil** 1981 Apr;109(4):355–66

**Denmark**

Britze N: Da en kvindelig tandlaege kun behandlede kvinder og børn. **Tandlaegebladet** 1982 Nov;86(20):714–5

**Finland**

Tallberg M: Sophie Mannerheim: en historisk beskrivning och analys av hennes verksamhet 1904–1928. **Vard Nord Utveckl Forsk** 1983 Spring;3(4):123–30

**France**

Dentistry in folk art XI: L'arracheuse de dents (The tooth puller): **Bull Hist Dent** 1980 Oct;28(2):87
Fouré J: A French woman dentist who gave her life as a freedom fighter against the Nazis. **Bull Hist Dent** 1984 Oct;32(2):133–4
Largillière A: Madeleine Pelletier, femme, médecin, féministe. **Penelope** 1981;(5):68–72
Manevy JV: Nicole Grasset, médecin du bout du monde. [Paris?], Balland, 1982. 245 p.
Poirier J, Nahon R: L'accession des femmes à la carrière médicale (à la fin du XIXe siècle). In Poirier J, Poirier JL, ed: Médecine et philosophie à la fin du XIXe siècle. Paris, Université de Paris XII - Val de Marne, [1980?]. p. 23–46.
Schmid-Kitsikis E: Un certain regard sur l'oeuvre de N. Galifret-Granjon. **Psychiatr Enfant** 1984;27(1):35–48
Sicard A: Un doyen misogyne et un recteur féministe. **Hist Sci Med** 1982;16(1):15–20

**Germany**

Albisetti JC: The fight for female physicians in Imperial Germany. **Cent Eur Hist** 1982;15:99–123
Erxleben DC: Gründliche Untersuchung der Ursachen, die das weibliche Geschlecht vom Studieren abhalten. Reprint of the Berlin, 1742, ed., mit einem Nachwort von G. Rechenberg. Hildesheim, New York, Olms, 1977. [68], 250 p.
Froböse HH: Die Tagung des preussischen Apothekerrates im Jahre 1897--ein Beitrag zur Frage der Zulassung der Frauen zur Pharmazie. **Pharmazie** 1982 Aug;37(8):596–9
Garrison D: Karen Horney and feminism. **Signs** 1981;6(4):672–91
Hamburger V: Hilde Mangold, co-discoverer of the organizer. **J Hist Biol** 1984 Spring;17(1):1–11
Kaiser W: Die ersten promovierten Aerztinnen. Zum 225. Jahrestag der halleschen Graduierung von Dorothea Christian Erxleben (1715–1762). **Z Gesamte Inn Med** 1980 Feb 15;35(4):176–83
McKale D: Purging Nazis: the postwar trials of female German doctors and nurses. **Proc SC Hist Assoc** 1981;:156–70
Martha Schmidtmann (4. 8. 1892 bis 28. 4. 1981): **Verh Dtsch Ges Pathol** 1981;65:571–5
Pfister G: The influence of women doctors on the origins of women's sports in Germany. In Borms J, Hebbelinck M, Venerando A, ed: Women and sport. Basel, Karger, 1981. p. 58–65.

**Great Britain**

Barnes M, Pratt PK: Women sanitary inspectors. **Hist Workshop J** 1978;6:225
Cohen IB: Florence Nightingale. **Sci Am** 1984 Mar;250(3):128–37
Craddock S: Retired except on demand: the life of Dr. Cicely Williams. Oxford, Green College, 1983. 198 p.
Evans B: Freedom to choose: the life and work of Dr. Helena Wright, pioneer of contraception. London, Bodley Head, 1984. 285 p.
Fee E: Science and the 'woman question', 1860–1920: a study of English scientific periodicals. Ph. D. Diss., Princeton University. Princeton, 1978. v, 351 leaves.
Gaffney R: Women as doctors and nurses. In Checkland O, Lamb M, ed: Health care as social history; the Glasgow case. Aberdeen, Aberdeen University Press, 1982. p. 134–48.
Gardner of Parkes: 'Fair to the fair'. **Br Dent J** 1982 Aug 3;153(3):117–9
Hebert RG: Florence Nightingale: saint, reformer or rebel? Malabar, Florida, Robert E. Krieger, 1981. 236 p.
Jones EW: Addysg feddygol i ferched: cyfraniadau o gymru at agor y cyndyn ddorau. **Cylchgrawn Llyfrgell Genedlaethol Cymru** 1976;19(3):249–92
Kalisch BJ, Kalisch PA: Heroine out of focus: media images of Florence Nightingale. Part I. Popular biographies and stage productions. **Nurs Health Care** 1983 Apr;4(4):181–7
Karll A: Florence Nightingale. **Nurs J India** 1983 May;74(5):110
Lebovici S: L'oeuvre D'Anna Freud (1895–1982). **Psychiatr Enfant** 1984;27(1):5–34
MacLeod R, Moseley R: Fathers and daughters: reflections on women, science, and Victorian Cambridge. **Hist Educ** 1979;8:321–33
Matthews DA: Dr. Marjory Warren and the origin of British geriatrics. **J Am Geriatr Soc** 1984 Apr;32(4):253–8
Palmer IS: Florence Nightingale: the myth and the reality. **Nurs Times** 1983 Aug 3–9;79(31):40–2
Schnorrenberg BB: Is childbirth any place for a woman? The decline of midwifery in eighteenth-century England. **Stud Eighteenth Cent Cult** 1981;10:393–408
Shannon R: [Re-evaluation of Florence Nightingale: a review of 'Florence Nightingale: Reputation and Power' by F. B. Smith] (Jpn). **Kango Kyoiku** 1982 Nov;23(11):677–85
Shellard EJ: Some early women research workers in British pharmacy 1886–1912. **Pharm Hist (London)** 1982 Aug;12(2):2–3
Smith FB: Florence Nightingale. Reputation and power. London, Canberra, Croom Helm, 1982. xii, 216 p.
Smith FT: [Florence Nightingale: early feminist] (Jpn). **Kango Kyoiku** 1982 Nov;23(11):671–6
Southgate MT: A summer's reading: Virginia Woolf and her granddaughters. **Conn Med** 1981 Aug;45(8):483–6
Stewart J: Women pioneers of medicine. **Midwife Health Visit Community Nurse** 1983 Jun;20(6):240, 242
Walton RG: Women in social work. London, Boston, Routledge and Kegan Paul, 1975. xvi, 308 p.

**Hungary**

Szállási A: 100 éve szerzett oklevelet az elsö magyar orvosnö. **Orv Hetil** 1979 Aug 19;120(32):1950–2
Szekér E: Hugonnaie Vilma balatonfüredi emlékezete. **Orv Hetil** 1982 Mar 7;123(10):611–2

**Italy**

Borsarelli F: Storia della Associazione Italiana Donne Medico--A.I.D.M. Affiliata alla Medical Women's International Association--M.W.I.A. Torino, Edizioni Minerva Medica, 1977. 55 p.

**New Zealand**

Pack AR: Women in New Zealand dentistry, 1880–1980. **NZ Dent J** 1981 Jan;77(347):19–25

**Norway**

Alvsvåg H: Sykepleiens historie og kvinnesynet. **Sykepleien** 1982 Oct 5;69(17):6–10, 29

**South Africa**

Barlow MR: Women doctors of South Africa. **S Afr Med J** 1983 Jun 29;Spec No:29–32

**Sweden**

Malmstedt J: Hon förlöste vävarnas barn--barnmorskan Anna Norin. **Jordemodern** 1982 Oct;95(10):341–4

**United States**

Abram RJ: Documenting our past. Daughters of Aesculapius. **J Am Med Wom Assoc** 1983 May–Jun;38(3):71–2, 82
Agris J: Stamps commemorating medicine. 'Dr. Mary Edwards Walker' (1832–1919). **J Dermatol Surg Oncol** 1982 Nov;8(11)::926
Alexander LL: Early medical heroes: Susan Smith McKinney-Steward, M.D., 1847–1918. **Crisis** 1980;87(1):21–3
Allen M: Charlotte Bertha Bühler. In: Notable American women. The modern period. Cambridge, Mass., Belknap-Harvard Univ. Press, 1980. 4:119–21.
Antler J: Medical women and social reform--a history of the New York Infirmary for Women and Children. **Women Health** 1976 Jul–Aug;1(4):11–15,18
Apple RD: Lillie Rosa Minoka-Hill. In: Notable American women. The modern period. Cambridge, Mass., Belknap-Harvard Univ. Press, 1980. 4:481–3.
Axinn J: Jessie Taft. In: Notable American women. The modern period. Cambridge, Mass., Belknap-Harvard Univ. Press, 1980. 4:673–5.
Bardell EB: America's only school of pharmacy for women. **Pharm Hist** 1984;26(3):127–33
Barlow W, Powell DO: A case for medical coeducation in the 1870s. **J Am Med Wom Assoc** 1980 Dec;35(12):285–8
Barlow W, Powell DO: Homeopathy and sexual equality: the controversy over coeducation at Cincinnati's Pulte Medical College, 1873–1879. **Ohio Hist** 1981 Spring;90(2):101–13
Baserga SJ: The early years of coeducation at the Yale University School of Medicine. **Yale J Biol Med** 1980 May–Jun;53(3):181–90
Batchelor AJ: AMWA's founder--the 'red headed dynamo'. **J Am Med Wom Assoc** 1984 Jul–Aug;39(4):123, 139
Beatty WK: Mary Harris Thompson--pioneer surgeon and hospital founder. **Proc Inst Med Chic** 1981 Jul–Sep;34(3):83–6
Beatty WK: Sarah Hackett Stevenson--concerned practitioner and social activist. **Proc Inst Med Chic** 1982 Jul–Sep;35(3):99–101
Bendiner E: Past and present: Elizabeth Blackwell: 'heresy with intelligence'. **Hosp Pract** Jun;15(6):1821–1910
Bendiner E: The 'derailment' that spurred a feminist revolution in medicine. **Hosp Pract** 1983 Mar;18(3):225, 228, 233–40 passim
Blount M: Surpassing obstacles: black women in medicine. **J Am Med Wom Assoc** 1984 Nov–Dec;39(6):192–5
Bogardus CR: Kentucky's first woman dentist (Lucy Dupuy Montz). **Ky Dent J** 1984 Mar–Apr;36(2):23–5
Bonsett CA: Mary Frame Thomas, M.D. (1816–1888). **J Indiana State Med Assoc** 1980;73:270
Brandt AM: Virginia Kneeland Frantz. In: Notable American women. The modern period. Cambridge, Mass., Belknap-Harvard Univ. Press, 1980. 4:247–8.
Brieger GH: Florence Rena Sabin. In: Notable American women. The modern period. Cambridge, Mass., Belknap-Harvard Univ. Press, 1980. 4:614–7.
Brinkhous KM: Judith Graham Pool. In: Notable American women. The modern period. Cambridge, Mass., Belknap-Harvard Univ. Press, 1980. 4:553–4.
Briscoe AM: Diary of a mad feminist chemist. **Int J Womens Stud** 1981;4(4):420–30
Brody SI: Lady physicians. **RI Med J** 1980 Apr;63(4):95
Brooks P: Rachel Louise Carson. In: Notable American women. The modern period. Cambridge, Mass., Belknap-Harvard Univ. Press, 1980. 4:138–41.
Bruch H: Personal reminiscences of Frieda Fromm-Reichmann. **Psychiatry** 1982;45(2):98–104
Bullough B, Bullough V: Education problems in a woman's profession. **JNE** 1981 Sep;20(7):6–17
Bullough VL: Female physiology, technology and women's liberation. In

Trescott, Martha Moore, ed. Dynamos and Virgins revisited: Women and technological change in history. Metuchen, N. J., Scarecrow Pr., 1979. p. 236–51.
Burnham JC: Augusta Fox Bronner. In: Notable American women. The modern period. Cambridge, Mass., Belknap–Harvard Univ. Press, 1980. 4:108–10.
Burns C, Nelson M: Mary Elizabeth Bass. In: Notable American women. The modern period. Cambridge, Mass., Belknap–Harvard Univ. Press, 1980. 4:63–5.
Callan CM: A leader in psychiatry--Carol Nadelson, M.D. **Conn Med** 1981 Aug;45(8):491–2
Calmes SH: Virginia Apgar: a woman physician's career in a developing specialty. **J Am Med Wom Assoc** 1984 Nov–Dec;39(6):184–8
Cangi EC: Patrons and proteges: Cincinnati's first generation of women doctors 1875–1910. **Cinci Hist Soc Bull** 1979;37(2):89–114
Chaff SL: Archives and special collections on women in medicine. **J Am Med Wom Assoc** 1983 May–Jun;38(3):73–4
Christie J: Mary Elizabeth Switzer. In: Notable American women. The modern period. Cambridge, Mass., Belknap–Harvard Univ. Press, 1980. 4:669–70.
Clar R: First Jewish women physician of Los Angeles. **West States Jew Hist Q** 1981;14(1):66–75
Cohen RA: Notes on the life and work of Frieda Fromm–Reichmann. **Psychiatry** 1982;45(2):90–8
Conable CW: Louise Stanley. In: Notable American women. The modern period. Cambridge, Mass., Belknap–Harvard Univ. Press, 1980. 4:657–9.
Corner GW: Louise Pearce. In: Notable American women. The modern period. Cambridge, Mass., Belknap–Harvard Univ. Press, 1980. 4:531–2.
Cowan RS: Lillian Evelyn Moller Gilbreth. In: Notable American women. The modern period. Cambridge, Mass., Belknap–Harvard Univ. Press, 1980. 4:271–3.
Crooks JB: The role of women in volunteerism: a short history. **Volunt Action Leadersh** 1981 Summer;22–8
Crowley RM: Frieda Fromm–Reichmann: recollections of a student. **Psychiatry** 1982;45(2):105–7
Crumpacker L: The art of the healer: women in the fiction of Sarah Orne Jewett. **Colby Libr Q** 1983;19(3):155–66
Curtis J, Curtis B: Illness and the Victorian lady: the case of Jeannie Sumner. **Int J Womens Stud** 1981;4(5):527–43
Drachman VG: Female solidarity and professional success: the dilemma of women doctors in late nineteenth-century America. **J Soc Hist** 1982;15(4):607–19
Dubos R: Hattie Elizabeth Alexander. In: Notable American women. The modern period. Cambridge, Mass., Belknap–Harvard Univ. Press, 1980. 4:10–1.
Dwork D: Elsie Strang L'Esperance. In: Notable American women. The modern period. Cambridge, Mass., Belknap–Harvard Univ. Press, 1980. 4:417–9.
Dwork D: Sophia Josephine Kleegman. In: Notable American women. The modern period. Cambridge, Mass., Belknap–Harvard Univ. Press, 1980. 4:398–400.
Easley EB: The female medical student in the 30's. **NC Med J** 1983 May;44(5):307–8
Etheridge EW: Grace Arabell Goldsmith. In: Notable American women. The modern period. Cambridge, Mass., Belknap–Harvard Univ. Press, 1980. 4:283–4.
Farley F: Two generations of women physicians: the New York Infirmary, 1870–1899. **J Am Med Wom Assoc** 1984 Nov–Dec;39(6):189–91
Ferguson A: The sweetheart of the PSC--Mabel Heath Palmer: the early years. **Chiropr Hist** 1984;4(1):25–8
Fischoff E: Elizabeth Blackwell: first woman M.D. **Pearson Mus Monogr Ser** 1981;4:1–22
Freudenberg N: Alice Hamilton 1869-1970. **Women Health** 1976 Sep–Oct;1(5):1–2
Friedell JN: Blanche Ames Ames. In: Notable American women. The modern period. Cambridge, Mass., Belknap–Harvard Univ. Press, 1980. 4:15–6.
Fullard J: Ann Preston: pioneer of medical education and women's rights. **Pa Herit** 1982;8(1):9–14
Garber E: Marie Gertrude Rand. In: Notable American women. The modern period. Cambridge, Mass., Belknap–Harvard Univ. Press, 1980. 4:565.
Gilbo PF: Candid 'cranky' Clara Barton gave us the Red Cross. **Smithsonian** 1981;12(2):126–42
Gordon L: Lena Levine. In: Notable American women. The modern period. Cambridge, Mass., Belknap–Harvard Univ. Press, 1980. 4:419–20.
Grayson VS: Mary Cromwell Jarrett. In: Notable American women. The modern period. Cambridge, Mass., Belknap–Harvard Univ. Press, 1980. 4:377–9.
Green D, Murdock ME, ed: The Margaret Sanger Centennial Conference, November 13 & 14, 1979. Northampton, Smith College, 1982. 68 p. Contributions by J. K. Conway, A. Harper, L. Gordon, J. Reed, E. Fee.
Gunst VK: Memoirs–Professional and personal: a decade with Frieda Fromm–Reichmann. **Psychiatry** 1982;45(2):107–15
Hamilton WA, Hamilton PR: Sex and the dental practice: a reinterpretation of the history of dental hygienists. **Bull Hist Dent** 1980 Oct;28(2):64–8
Hancock V: Women in Arizona medicine: Mary Lawson Neff, M.D. **Ariz Med** 1984 Nov;41(11):750–4; Dec;41(12):819–21
Haraway DJ: Ethel Browne Harvey. In: Notable American women. The modern period. Cambridge, Mass., Belknap–Harvard Univ. Press, 1980. 4:319–21.
Haycock CE: Women physicians of New Jersey: the early era. **J Med Soc NJ** 1984 Sep;81(9):773–7
Hazzard FW: Eliza Maria Mosher, MD (1846–1928). **Women Health** 1982 Summer;7(2):1–4
Hofer K: Dr. Lucy Hobbs Taylor, first woman dentist. **CAL** 1981 Oct;45(4):13–5, 18
Hoobler IG: Boundless horizons. Portrait of a pioneer woman scientist. Smithtown, N. Y., Exposition Press, 1982. 197 p.
Horn M: 'Sisters worthy of respect': family dynamics and women's roles in the Blackwell family. **J Fam Hist** 1983 Winter;8(4):367–82
Hunt M: Woman's place in medicine: the career of Dr. Mary Hancock McLean. **Bull Mo Hist Soc** 1980;36(4):255–63
Ihde AJ: Lydia Jane Roberts. In: Notable American women. The modern period. Cambridge, Mass., Belknap–Harvard Univ. Press, 1980. 4:580–1.
Jacob KA: The Mosher report. **Am Heritage** 1981;32(4):56–64
Jerrido MJ: In recognition of...early black women physicians. **Women Health** 1980 Fall;5(3):1–3
Johnson EE: Ida Henrietta Hyde: early experiments. **Physiologist** 1981 Dec;24(6):10–1
Kaiser RM, Chaff SL, Peitzman SJ: A Philadelphia medical student of the 1890's: the diary of Mary Theodora McGavran. **Pa Mag Hist Biogr** 1984 Apr;108(2):217–36
Kampmeier RH: Women in medical school. **South Med J** 1984 Sep;77(9):1217
Kathren RL: Elda Emma Anderson. In: Notable American women. The modern period. Cambridge, Mass., Belknap–Harvard Univ. Press, 1980. 4:20–1.
Keyfitz N: Irene Barnes Taeuber. In: Notable American women. The modern period. Cambridge, Mass., Belknap–Harvard Univ. Press, 1980. 4:672–3.
Kohlstedt SG: In from the periphery: American women in science, 1830–1880. **Signs** 1978;4(1):81–96
Lahiri K: Clara Swain, MD (1834–1910) and her work in India. **Women Health** 1983 Spring;8(1):3–6
Leavitt JW: Birthing and anesthesia: the debate over twilight sleep. **Signs** 1980;6(1):147–64
Lengeler J: Barbara McClintock und die Entdeckung der beweglichen Gene. **MMW** 1983 Nov 25;125(47):1095–7
Levin BS: Women and medicine. Metuchen, N. J., London, Scarecrow, 1980. vii, 257 p.
Lewis BE: A tradition of exceptional women. **J Am Med Wom Assoc** 1983 May–Jun;38(3):75–6, 82
Lockwood A: Pantsuited pioneer of women's lib, Dr. Mary Walker. **Smithsonian** 1977;7(12):113–9
Loevy HT: M. Evangeline Jordon, pioneer in pedodontics. **Bull Hist Dent** 1984;32(1):19–26
Lynaugh J: Katherine Berry Richardson, MD (1858–1933). **Women Health** 1982 Spring;7(1):1–3
McGovern CM: Doctors or ladies? Women physicians in psychiatric institutions, 1872–1900. **Bull Hist Med** 1981 Spring;55(1):88–107
Machol L: Dorothy Hansine Andersen. In: Notable American women. The modern period. Cambridge, Mass., Belknap–Harvard Univ. Press, 1980. 4:18–20.
McPherson MP: 'On the same terms precisely': the women's medical fund and the John Hopkins School of Medicine. **J Am Med Wom Assoc** 1981 Feb;36(2):37–40
Malinsky BJ: The (Woman's) Medical College of Pennsylvania. **Women Health** 1979 Fall;4(3):217–21
Marrett CB: Influences on the rise of new organizations: the formation of women's medical societies. **Adm Sci Q** 1980 Jun;25(2):185–99
Marrett CB: On the evolution of women's medical societies. **Bull Hist Med** 1979 Fall;53(3):434–48
Mathes VS: Susan La Flesche Picotte: Indian physician. **Masterkey Ind Lore Hist** 1983;57(1):10–4
Mathes VS: Susan La Flesche Picotte: Nebraska's Indian physician, 1865–1915. **Nebr Hist** 1982;63(4):502–30
Mehler B: Madge Thurlow Macklin. In: Notable American women. The modern period. Cambridge, Mass., Belknap–Harvard Univ. Press, 1980. 4:451–2.
Mennel RM: Ethel Sturges Dummer. In: Notable American women. The modern period. Cambridge, Mass., Belknap–Harvard Univ. Press, 1980. 4:208–10.
Minot WS: Millay's 'Ungrafted tree'; the problem of the artist as woman. **New Engl Q** 1975;48(2):260–69
Moldow G: 'For women, by women': women's dispensaries and clinics in Washington, 1882–1900. **Rec Columb Hist Soc** 1980;50:290–308
Morantz RM: Bertha van Hoosen. In: Notable American women. The modern period. Cambridge, Mass., Belknap–Harvard Univ. Press, 1980. 4:706–7.
Morantz RM: Feminism, professionalism, and germs: the thought of Mary Putnam Jacobi and Elizabeth Blackwell. **Amer Q** 1982;34:459–78
Morantz RM, Pomerleau CS, Fenichel CH, ed: In her own words: oral

histories of women physicians. Westport, Conn., Greenwood, 1982. xiv, 284 p. (Contributions in Medical History, 8).
Morantz RM, Zschoche S: Professionalism, feminism, and gender roles: a comparative study of nineteenth-century medical therapeutics. **J Am Hist** 1980 Dec;67(3):568-88
Morantz RM: Women in the medical profession: why were there so few? **Rev Am Hist** 1978;6(2):163-70
Noble I: Contemporary women scientists in America. New York, Messner, 1979. 158 p.
Nursing revisited: Mary M. Riddle (1856-1936). **Mass Nurse** 1983 Oct;52(10):4
O'Hern EM: Alice Catherine Evans. In: Notable American women. The modern period. Cambridge, Mass., Belknap-Harvard Univ. Press, 1980. 4:219-21.
Parascandola J: Gerty Theresa Radnitz Cori. In: Notable American women. The modern period. Cambridge, Mass., Belknap-Harvard Univ. Press, 1980. 4:165-7.
Parascandola J: Maud Caroline Slye. In: Notable American women. The modern period. Cambridge, Mass., Belknap-Harvard Univ. Press, 1980. 4:651-2.
Peitzman SJ: The quiet life of a Philadelphia medical woman: Mary Willits (1855--1902). **J Am Med Wom Assoc** 1979 Dec;34(12):443-6, 448, 450, passim
Perry HS: Clara Mabel Thompson. In: Notable American women. The modern period. Cambridge, Mass., Belknap-Harvard Univ. Press, 1980. 4:680-3.
Phillips CJ: Rosetta Sherwood Hall. In: Notable American women. The modern period. Cambridge, Mass., Belknap-Harvard Univ. Press, 1980. 4:299-301.
Powell RC, Hoff SG: Frieda Fromm-Reichmann. In: Notable American women. The modern period. Cambridge, Mass., Belknap-Harvard Univ. Press, 1980. 4:252-5.
Powell RC: (Helen) Flanders Dunbar. In Dictionary of American Biography, Suppl. 6, 1956-1960. p. 180-1, 1980.
Powsner R: Women physicians--expanding the domain. **Mich Med** 1983 Aug;82(37):483-4, 502
Punnett L: Marie Elizabeth Zakrzewska 1829-1902. **Women Health** 1976 Jul-Aug;1(4):1-2
Punnett L: Women-controlled medicine--theory and practice in 19th century Boston. **Women Health** 1976 Jul-Aug;1(4)3-11
Raacke ID: Agnes Fay Morgan. In: Notable American women. The modern period. Cambridge, Mass., Belknap-Harvard Univ. Press, 1980. 4:495-7.
Raacke ID: Jane Anne Russell. In: Notable American women. The modern period. Cambridge, Mass., Belknap-Harvard Univ. Press, 1980. 4:610-1.
Raacke ID: Marjorie Maxine Nelson. In Dictionary of American biography, 1961-1965. Suppl. 7, 1981. p. 568-9.
Rabe V: Ida Sophia Scudder. In: Notable American women. The modern period. Cambridge, Mass., Belknap-Harvard Univ. Press, 1980. 4:634-6.
Radbill SX: Remarks on the Kate Hurd Mead lectures. **Trans Stud Coll Physicians Phila** 1977 Apr;44(4):179-81
Reed J: Katharine Dexter McCormick. In: Notable American women. The modern period. Cambridge, Mass., Belknap-Harvard Univ. Press, 1980. 4:440-2.
Reed J: Louise Frances Stevens Bryant. In Dictionary of American Biography, Suppl. 6, 1956-1960. p. 80-2, 1980.
Reed J: Margaret Sanger. In: Notable American women. The modern period. Cambridge, Mass., Belknap-Harvard Univ. Press, 1980. 4:623-7.
Remley ML: Jessie Hubbell Bancroft. In: Notable American women. The modern period. Cambridge, Mass., Belknap-Harvard Univ. Press, 1980. 4:46-7.
Robinton ED: Anna Wessels Williams. In: Notable American women. The modern period. Cambridge, Mass., Belknap-Harvard Univ. Press, 1980. 4:737-9.
Robinton ED: Dorothy Reed Mendenhall. In: Notable American women. The modern period. Cambridge, Mass., Belknap-Harvard Univ. Press, 1980. 4:468-70.
Romanofsky P: Ellen Culver Potter. In Dictionary of American Biography, Suppl. 6, 1956-1960. p. 515-16, 1980.
Rosenkrantz BG: Sara Claudia Murray Jordan. In: Notable American women. The modern period. Cambridge, Mass., Belknap-Harvard Univ. Press, 1980. 4:387-8.
Rosenthal PA, Eaton J: Women MDs in America: 100 years of progress and backlash. **J Am Med Wom Assoc** 1982 May;37(5):129-33
Rossiter MW: Women scientists in America. Struggles and strategies to 1940. Baltimore, London, Johns Hopkins University Press, 1982. xviii, 439 p.
Rossiter MW: 'Women's work' in science, 1880-1910. **Isis** 1980 Sep;71(258):381-98
Rubin LP: Elizabeth Lee Hazen. In: Notable American women. The modern period. Cambridge, Mass., Belknap-Harvard Univ. Press, 1980. 4:326-8.
Rubins JL: Karen Danielson Horney. In: Notable American women. The modern period. Cambridge, Mass., Belknap-Harvard Univ. Press, 1980. 4:351-4.
Saltzman BB: Saga of America's first woman dental graduate. **Dent Stud** 1983 Oct;62(1):24-5
Schmidt WM: Ethel Collins Dunham. In: Notable American women. The modern period. Cambridge, Mass., Belknap-Harvard Univ. Press, 1980. 4:212-3.
Schroeder MJ: Manuscript collections: The Jeannette Dean-Throckmorton papers. **Ann Iowa** 1979;44(7):551-4
Scully AL: How the West was won ... by women doctors. **J Am Med Wom Assoc** 1982 Feb;37(2):36-7
Selavan IC: Angel in hell-with-the-lid-off. **Am J Nurs** 1980;80:2064-5
Sicherman B: Alice Hamilton. In: Notable American women. The modern period. Cambridge, Mass., Belknap-Harvard Univ. Press, 1980. 4:303-6.
Sloan JB: The founding of the Naples Table Association for promoting scientific research by women, 1897. **Signs** 1978;4(1):208-16
Smith D: A persistent rebel. **Am Hist Illus** 1981;15(9):28-35
Smith MB: Else Frenkel-Brunswik. In: Notable American women. The modern period. Cambridge, Mass., Belknap-Harvard Univ. Press, 1980. 4:250-2.
Smith NB: The women who went to the war: the Union Army nurse in the Civil War. Ph.D. Diss., Northwestern Univ. Evanston, 1981. 183 p.
Spalding P: Women in the Medical College of Georgia. **South Med J** 1981 Feb;74(2):221-4
Stanton AH: Frieda Fromm-Reichmann, MD: her impact on American psychiatry. **Psychiatry** 1982;45(2):121-7
Stevens R: The changing idea of a medical specialty. **Trans Stud Coll Physicians Phila** 1980 Sep;5(2 no 3):159-77
Stewart S: Sharing more than marble palaces. **DAR Mag** 1981;115(3):188-91
Stokes GA: Helen Flanders Dunbar. In: Notable American women. The modern period. Cambridge, Mass., Belknap-Harvard Univ. Press, 1980. 4:210-2.
Takaki R: Aesculapius was a white man: antebellum racism and male chauvinism at Harvard Medical School. **Phylon** 1978;39(2):128-34
Thomas CB: Fulfilling the promise: Hopkins women before World War II. **J Am Med Wom Assoc** 1981 Feb;36(2):40-3
Thomson EH: Esther Pohl Lovejoy. In: Notable American women. The modern period. Cambridge, Mass., Belknap-Harvard Univ. Press, 1980. 4:424-6.
Trecker JL: Katharine Blunt. In: Notable American women. The modern period. Cambridge, Mass., Belknap-Harvard Univ. Press, 1980. 4:87-8.
Tucker GS: Ida Henrietta Hyde: the first woman member of the society. **Physiologist** 1981 Dec;24(6):1-9
Turner TB: Women in medicine--a historical perspective. **J Am Med Wom Assoc** 1981 Feb;36(2):33-7
Twin SL: Ethel Perrin. In: Notable American women. The modern period. Cambridge, Mass., Belknap-Harvard Univ. Press, 1980. 4:539-41.
Vickers ED: F. Elisabeth Cromwell: Pensacola's pioneer nurse. **J Fla Med Assoc** 1983 Aug;70(8):642-6
Waldinger RJ: Virginia Apgar. In: Notable American women. The modern period. Cambridge, Mass., Belknap-Harvard Univ. Press, 1980. 4:27-8.
Wall HM: Feminism and the New England Hospital, 1949-1961. **Am Q** 1980;32(4):435-52
Walsh MR: The rediscovery of the need for a feminist medical education. **Harv Educ Rev** 1979;49(4):447-66
Wardell D: Margaret Sanger: birth control's successful revolutionary. **Am J Public Health** 1980 Jul;70(7):736-42
Waugh ES, McGoldrick KE: On the history of JAMWA. **J Am Med Wom Assoc** 1980 Jun;35(6):137-9
Weaver B: Should women be admitted to medical school? The issue in the late 19th century. **South Med J** 1984 May;77(5):623-5
Weaver BL, Thompson JA: Women in medicine and the issue in late nineteenth-century Alabama. **Ala Hist Q** 1981;43(4):292-314
Weissman MB: Elizabeth Burchenal. In: Notable American women. The modern period. Cambridge, Mass., Belknap-Harvard Univ. Press, 1980. 4:121-2.
Wolf TH: Florence Laura Goodenough. In: Notable American women. The modern period. Cambridge, Mass., Belknap-Harvard Univ. Press, 1980. 4:284-6.
Women in medicine: **South Med J** 1981 Jun;74(6):775
Women in psychiatry--a quiet revolution: **Psychiatr News** 1980 Jul 18;15(14):7, 20-1
Woolverton DK: Taking stock: Med-Chi and its women members. **Md State Med J** 1983 Oct;32(10):787-91
Young JH: Adelle Davis. In: Notable American women. The modern period. Cambridge, Mass., Belknap-Harvard Univ. Press, 1980. 4:179-80.

**USSR**

Brzheskiĭ VCh: A. A. Sakhnovskaia (k stoletiiu so dnia rozhdeniia). **Vestn Dermatol Venerol** 1983 May;(5):73-4
Dionesov SM: K istorii zhenskogo meditsinskogo obrazovaniia v Rossii. **Feldsher Akush** 1983 Dec;48(12):44-5
Dionesov SM: Zhenskie vrachebnye kursy pri Peterburgskom nikolaevskom voennom gospitale. **Sov Med** 1982;(6):117-9
Engel BA: Women medical students in Russia, 1872-1882: reformers or rebels? **J Soc Hist** 1979;12(3):394-415
Gan'zha SV: U istokov zhenskogo meditsinskogo obrazovaniia. **Med Sestra** 1984 Feb;43(2):45-7

Ionov IuV: Narodovolets Sof'ia Perovskaia i ee meditsinskaia deiatel'nost'. **Feldsher Akush** 1982;47(10):41-2

Kocere V: Latvijas PSR Zinātnu akademijas akademike Rita Kukaine: biobibliogrāfiskais rāditājs. Riga, Zinātne, 1982. 129 p.

Kravchenko AT: Pamiati professora Glotovoĭ Eleny Vladimirovny (k 100-letiiu so dnia rozhdeniia). **Zh Mikrobiol Epidemiol Immunobiol** 1983 Mar;(3):112-3

Malozemova AI: Zhenshchiny-mediki v politicheskikh protsessakh 1881 g. (k 100-letiiu protsessov). **Sov Zdravookhr** 1981;(7):54-9

Tikotin MA: Peterburgskiĭ zhenskiĭ meditsinskiĭ institut v revoliutsionnom dvizhenii. **Sov Zdravookhr** 1981;(7):51-4

Zabludovskiĭ PE: N. I. Pirogov i meditsinskiĭ trud zhenshchin. **Feldsher Akush** 1981;46(11):53-4

**Yugoslavia**

Berić BM: Dr Eva Haljecka (18??-1947) prva žena akušer-ginekolog u jugoslovenskim zemljama. **Jugosl Ginekol Opstet** 1983 May-Aug;23(3-4):95-9

# PART III. AUTHORS

## A

**[A century of euthanasia] (Dut): Geneeskd Gids** 1978;141:150–60

**A. L. Copley: curriculum vitae and publications: Biorheology** 1981;18(3–6):703––23

**[A meeting to commemorate the 100th anniversary of Ms. Haya Ishibashi, a pioneer in psychiatric nursing] (Jpn): Kango** 1980 Jun;32(6):88

**Aalto SK** see **Brooks GP**

**Aaraas O:** Demografishe kriser i Norge: hunger eller sykdom? **Socialmed Tidsskr** 1979;56

**Aarli JA:** History of myasthenia gravis. In Rose FC, Bynum WF, ed: Historical aspects of the neurosciences. New York, Raven, 1982. p. 223–34.

**Aaron C** see **Huard P**

**Aaron PG, Clouse RG:** Freud's psychohistory of Leonardo de Vinci: A matter of being right or left. **J Interdiscip Hist** 1982;13(1):1–16

**Aasveien J:** A vaere sykepleier for 50 år siden. **Sykepleien** 1984 Aug 20;71(14):14–5, 23

**Abarracín Teulón A:** Santiago Ramón y Cajal, o la pasión de España. Barcelona, Editorial Labor, [1978?] 319 p.

**Abate Y:** Population growth and urbanization in Africa. **Curr Hist** 1980;78(455):102–6, 132–3

**Abbott A:** Religion, psychiatry, and problems of everyday life. **Sociol Anal** 1980;41(2):164–71

**Abbott D:** The biographical dictionary of scientists: biologists. London and New York, Blond Educational and Bedrick, 1984. 182 p.

**Abbott EC:** Composers and tuberculosis: the effects on creativity. **Can Med Assoc J** 1982 Mar 1;126(5):534, 536–8, 543–4

**Abbott JA** see **Vandam LD**

**Abbott P, Wertheimer R:** Philosophers and the abortion question. **Polit Theory** 1978;6(3):313–44

**Abbott SA** see **Wood BA**

**Abbott WF:** The density-pathology hypothesis in comparative perspective: density, status and pathology in prerevolutionary Moscow. **Int J Comp Sociol** 1982;23(1–2):17–33

**Abdalla IH:** Islamic medicine and its influence on traditional Hausa practitioners in northern Nigeria. Ph.D. Diss., University of Wisconsin. Madison, 1981. vii, 240 p.

**Abdellah FG:** [Nursing in the world: 35 years of development after World War II. Changes affecting nursing in the United States 1949–1984] (Jpn). **Kango** 1984 Jul;36(8):2–10

**Abdrakhimov BE** see **Suleĭmenov AA**

**Abdul Ali:** Contribution of Islam to the development of medical science. **Stud Hist Med** 1980 Mar;4(1):44–52

**Abdul Hai Farooqi:** Dafi al-Amrad; an important medical manuscript. **Stud Hist Med** 3(3):199–203, Sep 79

**Abdul-Rauf M:** Contemporary Muslim perspective [on medical ethics]. In Reich WT, et al, ed: Encyclopedia of bioethics, v. 2. New York, Free Press, 1978. p. 892–5.

**Abdullaev MS:** Anatomiia v trudakh Aristotelia. **Arkh Anat Gistol Embriol** 1984 Mar;86(3):95–9

**Abdullaev MS:** Aristotel'i razvitie predstavleniĭ o nervnoĭ sisteme. **Arkh Anat Gistol Embriol** 1984 Sep;87(9):97–103

**Abdullaev MS:** Vklad V. I. Razumovskogo v istoriiu otechestvennoĭ anatomii (k 125-letiiu so dnia rozhdeniia). **Arkh Anat Gistol Embriol** 1982 Aug;83(8):96–100

**Abdullaev RA:** Uspekhi i perspektivy vnutrenneĭ meditsiny v Uzbekskoĭ SSR. **Ter Arkh** 1982;54(12):7–11

**Abdullaev AKh, Sharafiddinov TA:** Abu Ali Ibn-Sina (Avitsenna) o lepre. **Vestn Dermatol Venerol** 1981 May;(5):76–9

**Abdullokhodzhaev ZI:** G. P. Rudnev: 1899–1970. Moskva, Meditsina, 1981. 70 p.

**Abdurasulov DM:** Osnoynye étapy razvitiia i nauchnye dostizheniia meditsinskoĭ radiologii i rentgenologii v Uzbekskoĭ SSR za 60 let. **Med Radiol (Mosk)** 1982 Dec;27(12):21–6

**Abe HR, Tiedt N:** August Friedrich Hecker (1763–1811) und die Anfänge der modernen Pathophysiologie. **Beitr Gesch Univ Erfurt** 1979–83;19:165–85

**Abe HR:** Aus der Frühgeschichte der deutschen Impfgesetzgebung. **Z Gesamte Hyg** 1980;26(5):373–4

**Abe HR:** Der soziale Aspekt im ärztlichen Wirken des grossen deutschen Gallenchirurgen Dr. Hans Kehr. **Beitr Gesch Univ Erfurt** 1979–83;19:241–58

**Abe HR:** Die internationale Ausstrahlung der Kehr-Rohdenschen Privatklinik in Halberstadt (1890–1910). Ein Beitrag zur Geschichte der modernen Gallenwegschirurgie. In International Congress of the History of Medicine. 26th, Plovdiv, 1978. Actes du Congress. Sofia, 1981. Volume II. p. 78–80.

**Abe HR:** Die Medizinische Akademie Erfurt und ihre progressiven Traditionen. **Beitr Gesch Univ Erfurt** 1979–83;19:9–51

**Abe HR, Schmidt H:** Dr. med. Marie-Elise Kayser (1885–1950) - ein Leben für die Kinder. **Beitr Gesch Univ Erfurt** 1979–83;19:293–8

**Abe HR, Kaiser L:** Ferdinand Sauerbruch und Erfurt. **Beitr Gesch Univ Erfurt** 1979–83;19:271–81

**Abe HR:** Zum Leben und Werk bedeutender Thüringischer Apotheker. **Pharmazie** 1981 Jun;36(6):435–7

**Abe HR:** Zur Biographie von Hans Kehr (1862–1916). **Beitr Gesch Univ Erfurt** 1979–83;19:233–40

**Abe HR:** Zur medizinhistorischen Topographie und ihrer Bedeutung für die Pflege fortschrittlicher Traditionen auf dem Gebiet des Gesundheitswesens. **Z Gesamte Hyg** 1984 May;30(5):298–301

**Abe HR:** Zur Sicherstellung des Nachlasses von Prof. Dr. Hans Kehr. **Beitr Gesch Univ Erfurt** 1979–83;19:259–64

**Abe HR** see **Güthert H**

**Abebe W:** Traditional pharmaceutical practice in Gondar region, northwestern Ethiopia. **J Ethnopharmacol** 1984 Jun;11(1):33–47

**Abeele R van den:** Jan Albert Roselt, plattelandschirurgijn te Machelen (1714–1785). **Jaarb Kunst Oudheidk Kring Deinze** 1978;:83–117

**Abel EL:** Marihuana. The first twelve thousand years. New York, London, Plenum Press, 1980. xi, 289 p.

**Abel EL:** Marijuana on trial: the Panama Canal Zone Report. **Int J Addict** 1982 May;17(4):667–78

**Abel GB:** The subapical segment: a historical note. **NZ Med J** 1980 Jul 9;92(663):24–6

**Abelanet R** see **Castaigne P**

**Abelanet R** see **Signoret JL**

**Abelshausen M:** De Antwerpse Werkhuizen van Liefdadigheid (1802–1870): weldadigheidsinstelling of fabriek? **Ann Soc Belg Hist Hop** 1982;20:61–108

**Abelson PH, Kulstad R, et al:** Science centennial––3 July 1880 to 4 July 1980. **Science** 1980 Jul 4;209(4452):19–198

**Abend SM:** Charles Brenner. An appreciation. **Psychoanal Q** 1984 Jan;53(1):1–12

**Aberbach D:** Freud's Jewish problem. **Commentary** 1980;69(6):35–9

**Aberg S:** Tämäkin on yhteinen asiamme. **Katilolehti** 1982 May;87(5):172–3

**Aberg S:** Uusi tarkastaja Lääkintöhallituksessa. **Katilolehti** 1980 Feb;85(2):56–7

**Abir-Am P:** Beyond deterministic sociology and apologetic history: reassessing the impact of research policy upon new scientific disciplines (Reply to Fuerst, Bartels, Olby and Yoxen). **Soc Stud Sci** 1984 May;14(2):252–63

**Abir-Am P:** From biochemistry to molecular biology: DNA and the acculturated journey of the critic of science Erwin Chargaff. **Hist Philos Life Sci** 1980;2(1):3–60

**Abir-Am P:** The discourse of physical power and biological knowledge in the 1930s: a reappraisal of the Rockefeller Foundation's 'policy' in molecular biology. **Soc Stud Sci** 1982 Aug 3;12(3):341–82

**Abir-Am P** see **Bartels D**

**Abir-Am P** see **Fuerst JA**

**Abir-Am P** see **Olby R**

**Abir-Am P** see **Yoxen EJ**

**Abir-Am PG:** Essay review: how scientists view their heroes: some remarks on the mechanism of myth construction. **J Hist Biol** 1982 Summer;15(2):281–315

Abish M: A guest's column. Urology 1979 Dec;14(6):545-P, 545-V
Abraham EP: Ernst Chain and Paul Garrod. J Antimicrob Chemother 1980 Jul;6(4):423-4
Abraham EP: Fleming's discovery. Rev Infect Dis 1980 Jan-Feb;2(1):129-140
Abraham EP: Leonard Colebrook. In Dictionary of national biography, 1961-1970. Suppl. 8, 1981. p. 230-2.
Abraham HJ: Religion, medicine, and the state: reflections on some contemporary issues. J Church State 1980;22(3):423-36
Abrahams HJ: A medicine for 'Sickness of the spirit.' Trans Stud Coll Physicians Phila 1977 Apr;44(4):202-3
Abrahams HJ: Lavoisier and his contemporaries debate the supply of water for Paris. Bull NY Acad Med 1981 Jun;57(5):355-69
Abram RJ: Documenting our past. Daughters of Aesculapius. J Am Med Wom Assoc 1983 May-Jun;38(3):71-2, 82
Abramenko VV, Gendel' MG: Rol' A. Ia. Krassovskogo v razvitii operativnogo akusherstva. Akush Ginekol (Mosk) 1984 Jan;(1):67-9
Abramian AIa, Trapeznikova MF: K 50-letiiu urologicheskoĭ MONIKI im. M. F. Vladimirskogo. Urol Nefrol (Mosk) 1981 Jul-Aug;(4):64-8
Abramov VV: O geroizme meditsinskikh rabotnikov v period oborony Kerchenskikh kamenolomen v 1942 g. Voen Med Zh 1982 May;(5):71-3
Abramov ShI: Iubileĭ pervoĭ kafedry. Vestn Rentgenol Radiol 1980 Jan-Feb;(1):89-91
Abrams HL see Snellen HA
Abrams RA, Drake CW, Segal H: Dr. Sanford C. Barnum and the invention of the rubber dam. Gen Dent 1982 Jul-Aug;30(4):320-2
Abramson DJ: The surgical residency, the surgical clinic at the Walter Reed Army Medical Center. Milit Med 1982 Dec;147(12):1025-8
Abramson HA: The historical and cultural spectra of homosexuality and their relationship to the fear of being a lesbian. J Asthma Res 1980 Jul;17(4):177-88
Abreu Fialho S de: O Instituto Imperial dos Meninos Cegos. Rev Inst Hist Geogr Bras 1977;315:201-31
Abse D, ed: My medical school. London, Robson, 1978. 211 p.
Absher RR: The history of the Indiana State Board of Health from 1922 to 1954. Diss. Indiana University. [Bloomington], 1978. 323 leaves.
Absolon KB: Ein einmaliger Brief - Der zwanzigjährige Billroth beschreibt seine Reise durch Thüringen im Jahre 1849. Pommern 1982;4:18-27
Absolon KB: The surgeon's surgeon. Theodor Billroth 1829-1894. Vol. I. Lawrence, Kansas, Coronado Press, 1979. xxi, 282 p.
Absolon KB: The surgeon's surgeon. Theodor Billroth 1829-1894. Volume II. Lawrence, Kansas, Coronado Press, 1981. 232 p.
Absolon KB: Theodor Billroth and cardiac surgery. J Thorac Cardiovasc Surg 1983 Sep;86(3):451-2
Abu-Shwairb 'Abd al-Karim: Mushahadati haul al-tib al-sha'bi fi Fazan (tarjamah wa-taqdim limushahadat tabib Turki). Majallat al-Puhuth al-Tarikhiya (Lybia) 1979;1(2):37-50
Academia Nacional de Medicina: Libro conmemorativo del primer centenario. México, Comité Editorial de la Comisión Organizadora del Congreso del Centenario, 1964. 2 v. (xxxii, 454 p.; xxxix, 719 p.).
Accardo PJ: An early case report of muscular dystrophy. A footnote to the history of neuromuscular disorders. Arch Neurol 1981 Mar;38(3):144-6
Accardo PJ: Deformity and character. Dr. Little's diagnosis of Richard III. JAMA 1980 Dec 19;244(24):2746-7
Accardo PJ: Freud on diplegia. Commentary and translation. Am J Dis Child 1982 May;136(5):452-6
Accati L: Lo spirito della fornicazione: virtù dell'anima e virtù del corpo in Friuli, fra '600 e '700. Quad Stor 1979;14(2):644-72
Acceptance of the Gold Headed Cane Award: Am J Pathol 1979 Aug;96(2):368-71
Acevedo Z: Abortion in early America. Woman Health 1979 Summer;4(2):121-33
Aceves S: Contribuciones de México a la cardiología. Breve síntesis de la historia de la cardiología mexicana. In Academia Nacional de Medicina. Libro conmemorativo del primer centenario. México, Comité Editorial de la Comisión Organizadora del Congreso del Centenario, 1964. Tome 2. p. 535-46.
Achard A: 'La nourrice sur place'. Ann Demogr Hist (Paris) 1984;:259-68
Achard E: 1956--numéro 1 des 'Annales de Chirurgie Plastique'. Ann Chir Plast 1980;25(2):191-2
Acharya AM: The first Indian War of Independence and military surgery. Bull Indian Inst Hist Med (Hyderabad) 1975 Oct;5(4):225-39
Achenbaum WA: Old age in a new land: the American experience since 1970. Baltimore, Johns Hopkins Univ. Press, 1978. xiii, 237 p.
Achievements in the normal and pathological morphology in Romania: Morphol Embryol (Bucur) 1981 Apr-Jun;27(2):105-8
Achté K, Turunen S: Den första psykiatriska artikeln i Finland. Dan Medicinhist Arbog 1983;12:74-81
Achté K: Döden i den fornfinska kulturen. Tron påsjälens odödlighet. Dan Medicinhist Arbog 1983;12:82-90
Achterberg E: Albert Schweitzer: ein Leben in der Zeitenwende. Hameln, Soltsien, 1968. 88 p.
Ackerknecht E see Wallace ER
Ackerknecht EH: A short history of medicine. Rev. ed. Baltimore and London, Johns Hopkins University Press, 1982. xx, 277 p.
Ackerknecht EH: Causes and pseudocauses in the history of diseases. In Stevenson LG, ed: A celebration of medical history. Baltimore, Johns Hopkins University Press, 1982. (The Henry E. Sigerist supplements to the Bulletin of the History of Medicine; new ser., no. 6). p. 19-31. With commentary by C. E. Rosenberg, 'The history of disease: now and in the future,' p. 32-6.
Ackerknecht EH: Charles Meryon and physicians. J Hist Med Allied Sci 1984 Oct;39(4):462-4
Ackerknecht EH: Diathesis: the word and the concept in medical history. Bull Hist Med 1982 Fall;56(3):317-25
Ackerknecht EH: From barber-surgeon to modern doctor. Bull Hist Med 1984 Winter;58(4):545-53
Ackerknecht EH: Great doctors and scientists as freemasons. Clio Med 1982 Dec;17(2-3):145-56
Ackerknecht EH: Jüdische Arzte als Gestalter der Weltmedizin. Gesnerus 1981;38:127-33
Ackerknecht EH: La médecine française de 1790 à 1850. Bull Acad Natl Med (Paris) 1981 Feb 17;Spec No:27-30
Ackerknecht EH: La médecine française de 1790 à 1850. Bull Acad Natl Med (Paris) 1981 Feb;165(2):225-8
Ackerknecht EH: The history of psychosomatic medicine. Psychol Med 1982 Feb;12(1):17-24
Ackerknecht EH: The history of the drug treatment of mental diseases. Trans Stud Coll Physicians Phila 1979 Sep;5(1 No 3):161-70, Sep 79
Ackerknecht EH: Wilhelm Reich (1897-1957). In Ganzinger K, Skopec M, Wyklicky H, ed: Festschrift für Erna Lesky zum 70. Geburtstag. Wien, Brüder Hollinek, 1981. p. 5-12.
Ackerknecht EH: Zur Geschichte der Krebsbehandlung. Gesnerus 1980;37(3/4):189-97
Ackerknecht EH see George Rosen: In Memoriam
Ackerman C: The rural demography of medieval England. Ethnohistory 1976 Spring;23:105-15
Ackerman EB: The activities of a country doctor in New York State: Dr. Elias Cornelius of Somers, 1794-1803. Hist Reflect 1982 Spring-Summer;9:181-93
Ackerman EB: Use by patients of a French provincial hospital, 1895-1923. Bull Hist Med 1980 Summer;54(2):188-203
Ackerman FK: The Geisinger Medical Center. Natl Forum Hosp Health Aff 1978;:9-18
Ackerman LV: Dr. Evarts Graham and surgical pathology. J Thorac Cardiovasc Surg 1984 Nov;88(5 Pt 2):851-3
Ackerman LV: H. P. Smith Award lecture. Tumor pathologists I have known. Am J Clin Pathol 1982 Apr;77(4):385-90
Ackerman RH: Joubert's 'Erreurs populaires'. An insight into some aspects of sixteenth century health care. In: Congrès international d'histoire de la médecine, XXVe, Québec, 1976. Actes. Québec, 1977. p. 455-60.
Ackerman SH: Herbert Weiner 'at home'. Psychosom Med 1982 Mar;44(1):5-17
Ackermann EB: L'Hôpital de Mantes dans la première moitié du XIXe siècle. Ann Hist Mantois 1979;6:65-73
Ackner D: The crime of incest. Med Leg J 1980;48(pt 3):79-91
Acosta Rodríguez, Antonio see Holmes JD
Across the channel: catalogue of an exhibition. London, Royal College of Physicians of London, 1982. iii, 24 p.
The ACT Foundation: ten years of service to EMS: J Emerg Med Serv JEMS 1981 Oct;6(10):35-7
Acuña HR: Aedes aegypti, dengue y fiebre amarilla. Bol Of Sanit Panam 1982 Dec:93(6):503-5
Acuña HR: El Boletín de la Oficina sanitaria panamericana: a los sessenta años. Bol Of Sanit Panam 1982 May;92(5):377-8
Acuña HR: Etica médica y educación médica. Bol Of Sanit Panam 1981 Jun;90(6):471-7
Acuña HR: La medicina y el estado. Recuento histórico y problemas acutales de la cirugía. Bol Of Sanit Panam 1981 Oct;91(4):283-8
Acworth GW: Acworth Leprosy Hospital, Bombay. Lepr Rev 1984 Mar;55(1):77-8
ADA historical report--dental insurance: how it started and where it is today: Employ Benefit Plan Rev 1978 Nov;33(5):94, 96
Adacher S, Bernabò M, Sesti E: I manoscritti medici della Biblioteca Laurenziana di Firenze. Kos 1984 Feb;1(1):113-21
Adacher S, Orofino G: I manoscritti medici dell'Archivio dell'Abbazia di Montecassino. Kos 1984 Jun;1(5):5-16
Adam D see Kotwas J
Adam J, Fikentscher E, Liebner K: Untersuchungen zur sexuellen Entwicklung. Wiss Z Martin Luther Univ (Math) 1976;25(3):81-91
Adamczyk A: Ostatnie dni w szpitalu obozu w Litomierzycach. Przegl Lek 1980;37(1):184-6
Adamec J: Jan Janský. Cas Lek Cesk 1983 Sep 23;122(38):1180-2
Adamec J: Lékařská na stránkách Casopisu lékařu českých v prvním pulstoletí jeho existence. Cas Lek Cesk 1981;120(52):1589-93
Adamec J, Petrásek J: Reforma lékařského studia v roce 1953 a okolnosti jejího vzniku. Cesk Zdrav 1981 Dec;29(12):508-14
Adamec J: Z historie výuky I. interní kliniky v Praze. Cas Lek Cesk 1981;120(49):1475-7
Adamec J see Hlaváčková L
Adamec J see Petrásek J
Adamec J see Rozsívalová E
Adams DB: Abdominal gunshot wounds in warfare: a historical review. Milit Med 1983 Jan;148(1):15-20
Adams DP: The penicillin mystique and the popular press (1935-1950). Pharm Hist 1984;26(3):134-42
Adams MB: Biology after Stalin: a case study. Survey 1977-78;23(1):53-80
Adams MB: From 'Gene Fund' to 'Gene Pool': on the evolution of evolutionarylanguage. Stud Hist Biol 1979;3:241-85
Adams MB see Mayr E
Adams P: Health of the state. New York, N.Y., Praeger, 1982. x, 198

p.
**Adams P:** Mortality crises in nineteenth century France. In: Les Grandes mortalités: étude méthodologique des crises démographiques du passé. H. Charbonneau et A. LaRose, ed. Liège, U.I.E.S.P., 1979, p. 29-31.
**Adams RE:** Social structural consequences of population growth. **J Biosoc Sci** 1981 Jan;13(1):107-22
**Adams RR:** Dr. James Craik, George Washington's physician and friend. **Record** 1980 May, Sep;1-4,1-3
**Adams S:** Medical bibliography in an age of discontinuity. Chicago, Medical Library Association, 1981. xviii, 224 p.
**Adamson J:** 75th Anniversary of the Royal Australian Nursing Federation. **Australas Nurses J** 1980 Nov;9(12):3-4
**Adamson PB:** Anatomical and pathological terms in Akkadian. **J R Asiat Soc GB Irel** 1974;102-6: 1979;2-8: 1981;125-32.
**Adamson PB:** Medical practice in the ancient Near East, with particular reference to Mesopotamia. **Med Secoli** 1982 May-Aug;19(2):163-73
**Adamson PB:** The military surgeon: his place in history. **J R Army Med Corps** 1982 Feb;128(1):43-50
**Adamson PB:** The relationship between medical and veterinary surgeons from Sumer to the present. **Vet Hist** 1983 Summer;3(1):16-24
**Addington WW** see **Leff A**
**Addison NV:** Abdominal tuberculosis--a disease revived. **Ann R Coll Surg Engl** 1983 Mar;65(2):105-11
**Adelman H:** Hitler and Gandhi: the will as spirit and as flesh. **Psychoanal Rev** 1980 Winter;67(4):543-61
**Adeloye A:** Nigerian pioneers of modern medicine. Selected writings. Ibadan, Nigeria, Ibadan University Press, 1977. xiv. 299 p.
**Adelsen CE:** The last days of Adam Mickiewicz, poet of freedom. **Mankind** 1976;5(5):16-20, 60-1
**Adelson R** see **Walsh JP**
**Ademuwagun ZA, et al, ed:** African therapeutic systems. Waltham, Massachusetts, Crossroads Press of the African Studies Association, 1979. vii, 273 p.
**Ader R, Schmale AH:** George Libman Engel: on the occasion of his retirement. **Psychosom Med** 1980;42(1 Suppl):79-101
**Adham MN** see **Teimourian B**
**Adjusting the dental chair: J Am Dent Assoc** 1984 Apr;108(4):490-1
**Adlakha AL** see **Jain AK**
**Adler C:** Dr. Charles Porter. **Adler Mus Bull** 1984 Jun;10(2):9-14
**Adler C:** Historical perspectives. A corner of history in South Africa: the Adler Museum. **Prev Med** 1984 Mar;13(2):226-30
**Adler C:** René Théophile Hyacinthe Laënnec (1781-1826), inventor of the stethoscope. **Adler Mus Bull** 1981;7(2):3-7
**Adler C:** Why a medical historical museum? **Tydskr Tandheelkd Ver S Afr** 1982 Apr;37(4):261-3
**Adler G** see **Anger G**
**Adler HE:** Vicissitudes of Fechnerian psychophysics in America. In R. W. Rieber, K. Salzinger, ed: Psychology: theoretical-historical perspectives. New York, Academic Press, 1980. p. 11-23.
**Adler KA:** A personal autobiography. **J Individ Psychol** 1981 Nov;37(2):196-204
**Adler MW:** Academic Department of Genitourinary Medicine, Middlesex Hospital Medical School, London. **Br Med J** 1980 Jul 19;281(6234):206-11
**Adler MW:** History of the development of a service for the venereal diseases. **J R Soc Med** 1982 Feb;75(2):124-8
**Adler S:** The operation on President McKinley. In Plesur M, ed.: An American Historian: essays to honor Selig Adler (Buffalo: State U. of N.Y., 1980): 37-49.
**Adler C, ed** see **Cowley J**
**Adly A, ed:** The history of medicinal and aromatic plants. Proceedings of the Second International Congress organised by The Arab Society for the History of Pharmacy in co-operation with The World Union of Societies of the History of Pharmacy, Alexandria - Egypt, December 15th to 19th, 1980. Karachi, Hamdard Foundation Press, 1982. 216 p.
**Ado AD:** A. A. Bogomolets i sovremennaia allergologiia. **Patol Fiziol Eksp Ter** 1981 Mar-Apr;(2): 70-3
**Ado AD:** Razvitie ideĭ A. A. Bogomol'tsa v sovremennoĭ allergologii. **Fiziol Zh** 1981 May-Jun;27(3):354-7
**Adolph EF:** Growing up in the American Physiological Society. **Physiologist** 1979 Oct;22(5):11-5
**Adonajło A:** Włośnica. **Przegl Epidemiol** 1980;34(2):213-5
**Adour KK, Diamond C:** Decompression of the facial nerve in Bell's palsy: a historical review. **Otolaryngol Head Neck Surg** 1982 Jul-Aug;90(4):453-60
**Adranvala TK:** Vital aspects of nursing: the historical perspective. **Nurs J India** 1982 May;73(5):125-8
**Advances in immunology: a meeting in honor of Sir Peter Medawar: Cell Immunol** 1981 Aug;62(2):233-310
**Aellen HP:** Dr. Med. Armin Emil Elsaesser (1875-1952), Schueler von Theodor Kocher: sein Werden und Wirken in der Schweiz und in den Vereinigten Staaten von Amerika. Bern, [s.n.], 1982. x, 187 p.
**Aernouts R:** L'eau de Lourdes est-elle un médicament? **Rev Hist Pharm (Paris)** 1980 Mar;27(244):5-7
**Aeschlimann J:** Rudolf Brun (1885-1969). Leben und Werk des Zürcher Neurologen, Psychoanalytikers and Entomologen. Zürich, Juris, 1980. 70p. (Zürcher medizingeschichtliche Abhandlungen. Neue Reihe, Nr. 144).
**Afanas'ev IuI, Belova TI, Fel'dman NG:** Boris Innokent'evich Lavrent'ev (k 90-letiiu so dnia rozhdeniia). **Arkh Anat Gistol Embriol** 1983 Nov;85(11):98-101
**Afanas'eva AV** see **Uglov FG**
**Afanas'eva GM:** Demograficheskaia kharakteristika Avamskikh Nganasan po istochnikam XVIII-XIX. **Sov Etnogr** 1980;2:25-34
**Afaq SH** see **Khan AB**
**Afek-Kamińska M** see **Rozwadowska-Dowzenko M**
**Affeldt JE:** Voluntary accreditation. **Proc Acad Polit Sci** 1980;33(4):182-91
**Africa TW:** Worms and the death of kings: a cautionary note on disease and history. **Classical Antiq** 1982;1(1):1-17
**Afseth J:** 20 Jahre skandinavische Plaquepharmakologie. **Schweiz Monatsschr Zahnmed** 1984 Jan;94(1):86-90
**After seventy-five years, 1890-1965:** Baltimore, Waverly Press, William & Wilkins, 1965. 46 p.
**Afzelius BA:** Half a century of electron microscopy: the early years. **Ultrastruct Pathol** 1981 Jul-Sep;2(3):309-11
**Agababov SV, Savinov VA:** Vklad russkikh uchenykh XIX veka v sozdanie i razvitie ucheniia o revmatizme. **Ter Arkh** 1983;55(11):139-44
**Agafonov VI:** Nekotorye uroki iz opyta Velikoĭ Otechestvennoĭ voĭny 1941-1945 gg. i zadachi po dal'neĭshemu sovershenstvovaniiu protivoépidemicheskoĭ raboty. **Zh Mikrobiol Epidemiol Immunobiol** 1980 May;(5):3-6
**Agafonov VI, Perepelkin VS:** Opyt protivoépidemicheskoĭ raboty v gody voĭny i ego znachenie v sovremennykh usloviiakh. **Voen Med Zh** 1980 May;(5):57-60
**Agamova KA:** Razvitie tsitologicheskoĭ diagnostiki opukholĭ cheloveka. **Sov Med** 1982;(6):65-9
**Agård S:** Mandlernes historie 1953-1983. **Sygeplejersken** 1984 Mar 21;84(12):23-4
**Agarkov VA** see **Dunaev PV**
**Agass M** see **Shipley M**
**Agins TC:** Collector's item. Americana. **NY J Dent** 1983 Nov;53(7):317
**Agins TC:** Year of the twenty-dollar gold piece. **NY J Dent** 1980 Apr;50(4):123-6
**Agnew LR:** An 18th century amputation (Lady Anne Dawson). **Lancet** 1983 Nov 5;2(8358):1074-5
**Agogino GA, Ferguson B:** Curanderismo: the folk healer in the Spanish-speaking community. **Masterkey Ind Lore Hist** 1983;57(3):101-6
**Agostoni G, Berti Bock G, Favero GA:** Il concetto di miocardite nell'Ottocento. **Acta Med Hist Patav** 1979-80;26:9-27
**Agranenko VA** see **Fedotenkov AG**
**Agrimi J:** Malato, medico, e medicina nel Medioevo. Torino, Loescher Editore, 1980. 301 p.
**Agris J:** 'Henry Dearborn'. Physician, soldier, civil servant, diplomat. **J Dermatol Surg Oncol** 1979 Sep;9(5):677
**Agris J:** 'Jane Addams'. Medical student, social worker and activist, humanitarian. **J Dermatol Surg Oncol** 1979 Dec;5(12):936
**Agris J:** 'John McLoughlin' physician, pioneer, fur trader, settler. **J Dermatol Surg Oncol** 1979 Oct;5(10):760
**Agris J:** Stamps commemorating medicine. 'American Red Cross'. **J Dermatol Surg Oncol** 1981 Sep;7(9):697
**Agris J:** Stamps commemorating medicine. 'Dr. Charles R. Drew'. **J Dermatol Surg Oncol** 1982 Feb;8(2):96
**Agris J:** Stamps commemorating medicine. 'Dr. Crawford Williamson Long' the father of anesthesia. **J Dermatol Surg Oncol** 1980 May;6(5):415
**Agris J:** Stamps commemorating medicine. 'Dr. Mary Edwards Walker' (1832-1919). **J Dermatol Surg Oncol** 1982 Nov;8(11)::926
**Agris J:** Stamps commemorating medicine: Emily Bissell. **J Dermatol Surg Oncol** 1980;6(9):705
**Agris J:** Stamps commemorating medicine: 'Ephraim McDowell' (1771-1830). **J Dermatol Surg Oncol** 1980 Aug;6(8):621
**Agris J:** Stamps commemorating medicine. 'Honoria Acosta Sison' pioneer gynecologist and obstetrician. **J Dermatol Surg Oncol** 1980 Mar;6(3):178
**Agris J:** Stamps commemorating medicine: 'Indian folk art: the medicine man'. **J Dermatol Surg Oncol** 1981;7(1):82
**Agris J:** Stamps commemorating medicine. 'The Doctors William James and Charles Horace Mayo'. **J Dermatol Surg Oncol** 1980 Jul;6(7):523
**Agüero AL:** La Sanidad Militar Argentina en la guerra con el territorio del Brasil. In Congreso de Historia de la Medicina Argentina [Transactions], 5th, Mendoza, 1983. p. 79-101.
**Agüero I, Rey AO:** La evolución reciente de la fecundidad en España. **Rev Esp Invest Sociol** 1980;(10):121-50
**Aguilar Ruíz J** see **Torres Ramírez C**
**Aguilar Ruiz J** see **Zuluaga Gómez A**
**Aguilera Guirao A** see **Vidal Casero MC**
**Aguirre Zozaya F, Iglesias M, Reyes RM, et al:** Aspectos históricos, culturales, legales, psicosociales y educativos del aborto inducido. **Ginecol Obstet Mex** 1980 Aug;48(286):111-35
**Aharonowitz Y, Cohen G:** Les micro-organismes et l'industrie pharmaceutique. **Pour Sci** 1981;49:92-105
**Ahearn FL:** Disaster mental health: a pre- and post-earthquake comparison of psychiatric admission rates. **Urban Soc Change Rev** 1981;14(2):22-8
**Ahearn FL:** Puerto Ricans and mental health: some socio-cultural considerations. **Urban Soc Change Rev** 1979;12(2):4-9
**Ahlin JH:** The historical development of Maxillofacial orthopedic technique. **Bull Hist Dent** 1982 Oct;30(2):96-107
**Ahlquist RP:** Historical perspective. Classification of adrenoreceptors. **J Auton Pharmacol** 1980 Nov;1(1):101-6
**Ahlrichs EL:** Dr. D. A. Wittop Koning 70 jaar. **Pharm Weekbl** 1981 Nov 6;116(45):1365-9
**Ahlrichs EL:** Van leerjongen tot meester-apotheker (VII). **Pharm Weekbl** 1981 Nov 6;116(45):1369-73
**Ahlström CG, Ekström P, Persson O:** Cartesius' kranium.

**Sydsven Medicinhist Sallsk Arsskr** 1983;:23–50
**Ahlström CG:** Ett gammalt museum berättar; glimtar från patologiska institutionens museum i Lund. **Sydsven Medicinhist Sallsk Arsskr** 1982;:15–31
**Ahlström CG:** Om spansk fluga och dess medicinska användning i Lund. **Sydsven Medicinhist Sallsk Arsskr** 1984;21:49–61
**Ahlström CG:** Patologisk anatomi i Lund, 1668–1962. Lund, 1983. 155 p. (Sydsvenska Medicinhistoriska Sällskapets Arsskrift, Suppl. 2, 1983).
**Ahlström CG:** Uppfattningen om cancer i äldre tider; en översikt med särskild hänsyn till Sverige. **Sydsven Medicinhist Sallsk Arsskr** 1980;:10–39
**Ahmad Y** see **Said HM, ed**
**Ahmed M:** Bengal famine of 1943: British responsibility and social consequences. **Dacca Univ Stud [A]** 1978;(28):68–80
**Ahrens EH** see **Trends in biomedical research, 1901–1976**
**Aiache JM, Dussaud MD:** Ordonnancier et préparations magistrales de 1906 à 1960. **Rev Hist Pharm (Paris)** 1984 Jun;31(261):151–7
**Aĭdaraliev AA:** Kirgizskomu gosudartsvennomu meditsinskomu institutu––40 let. **Zdravookhr Kirg** 1980;(1):3–6
**Aidoo TA:** Rural health under colonialism and neocolonialism: a survey of the Ghanaian experience. **Int J Health Serv** 1982;12(4):637–57
**Aigner R:** Die Grazer Aerztinnen aus der Zeit der Monarchie. **Z Hist Ver Steiermark** 1979;70:45–70
**Aiken J:** Leon Battista Alberti's system of human proportions. **J Warburg Courtauld Inst** 1980;43:68–96
**Aiken KG:** From mission to hospital: the Detroit Florence Crittenton Organization, 1897–1930. **Detroit Perspect** 1982 Spring;6:50–60
**Aiken L** see **Durbin PT, ed**
**Aïrapetova RA, Kiazimov RA, ed:** M. A. Topchibashev. Baku, Izd-vo Akademii nauk Azerbaĭdzhanskoĭ SSR, 1965. 66 p.
**Aissar A** see **Berrance de Castro J**
**Ait Khaled N, Oussedik N, Chaulet P:** Evolution du coût des médicaments antituberculeux de 1964 à 1980; son influence dans le choix d'une politique de traitement de la tuberculose en Algérie. **Bull Int Union Tuberc** 1981 Sep–Dec;56(3–4):170–4
**Aitken R:** A historical dispute. **Clin Sci** 1981 Sep;61(3):360–2
**Ajuriaguerra J de:** L'enfant dans l'histoire–––problèmes psychologiques. **Psychiatr Enfant** 1979;22(1):101–26
**Akademii meditsinskikh nauk SSSR––40 let: Med Radiol (Mosk)** 1984 Jun;29(6):3–6
**Akahori A:** Chapters of 'Huang-ti-nei-ching-su-wen' derived from 'Yin-yang-shih-i-mo-chiu-ching'. (Jpn) **Nihon I-Shigaku Zasshi** 1979;25:277–89
**Akahori A:** Medical manuscripts found in Han Tomb No. 3 at Ma-wang-tui. **Sudhoffs Arch** 1979;63(3):297–300
**Akçiçek E:** Islâm tibbinda hemşirelik. **Turk Hemsire Derg** 1983;33(3):23–4
**Akdogan C:** Optics in Albert the Great's De sensu et sensato; an edition, English translation, and analysis. Ph.D. Diss., University of Wisconsin. Madison, 1978. iv, 267 leaves.
**Aker F, Schroeder DC, Baycar RS:** Cause and prevention of maxillofacial war wounds: a historical review. **Milit Med** 1983 Dec;148(12):921–7
**Aker F, Cecil JC:** The influence of disease upon European history. **Milit Med** 1983 May;148(5):441–6
**Akerman S:** En befolkning före den demografiska revolutionen. **Karolinska Forb Arsb** 1977;66–113
**Akert K** see **Milos G**
**Akhapkin IA, ed:** Leninskie dekrety po zdravookhraneniiu. Moskva, Meditsina, 1980. 510 p.
**Akhmedov AA:** K istorii organizatsii Azerbaĭdzhanskogo nauchnogo obshchestva stomatologov. **Stomatologiia (Mosk)** 1980 Jun;59(3):89–91
**Akhtar MS** see **Said HM, ed**
**Aki M:** The history of neurology in Japan, with special reference to its postwar period. In Rose FC, Bynum WF, ed: Historical aspects of the neurosciences. New York, Raven, 1982. p. 451–62.
**Aki-gun Ishikaishi Hensan Iinkai:** Aki-gun Ishikai shi. Kaida-machi, Japan, Aki-gun Ishikai, Showa 52 nen, 1977. 769 p.
**Akighir A:** Traditional and modern psychiatry: a survey of opinions and beliefs amongst people in plateau state, Nigeria. **Int J Soc Psychiatry** 1982 Autumn;28(3):203–9
**Akimov GA, Arkhangel'skiĭ AE:** K istorii deiatel'nosti Leningradskogo nauchnogo obshchestva nevropatologov i psikhiatrov (pervye gody). **Zh Nevropatol Psikhiatr** 1983;83(7):1067–9
**Akiyoshi T, Takai S, Esaki H:** [Old medical books of the Oda family in Kashima, Saga] (Jpn). **Igaku Kenkyu** 1983 Jun;53(3):167–73
**Akiyoshi T** see **Noriyasu S**
**Akopov AI** see **Akopov VI**
**Akopov VI, Akopov AI:** Iz istorii otechestvennykh sudebno-meditsinskikh zhurnalov. **Sud Med Ekspert** 1982 Jan–Mar;25(1):53–5
**Akpabio SP:** World Health Organisation. **Br Dent J** 1983 Feb 5;154(3):83–4
**Akpata ES:** Endodontic treatment in Nigeria. **Int Endod J** 1984 Jul;17(3):139–51
**Akulov KI, Shlepnina TG:** Nauchnoe obosnovanie standartizatsii kachestva pit'evoĭ vody v trudakh prof. S. N. Cherkinskogo. **Gig Sanit** 1982 Aug;(8):50–3
**Akulov KI, Korol'kov AA:** Pervaia piateletka strany Sovetov i stanovlenie gosudarstvennogo sanitarnogo nadzora. **Gig Sanit** 1982 Sep;(9):45–8
**Akupunktur––en framtidsmetod med gamla anor: Odontol Foren Tidskr** 1980 Nov;44(4):47–50
**Alagna SW** see **Moriarty KM**
**Alajouanine T, Signoret JL:** Paul Broca et l'aphasie. **Bull Acad Natl Med (Paris)** 1980;164(6):545–51
**Alameida BC:** Underdevelopment in a 'developing' nation: a quantitative study of health and medicine in Brazil, 1950–1975. Ph. D. Diss., University of California. Los Angeles, 1980. 338 leaves.
**Alarco F:** La psicoterápia dinámica y José Carlos Mariátegui. **Rev Neuropsiquiatr** 1979 Sep–Dec;42(3–4):145–64
**Alarcon-Segovia D:** Descriptions of therapeutic arthrocenthesis and of synovial fluid in a Nahuatl text from prehispanic Mexico. **Ann Rheum Dis** 1980 Jun;39(3):291–3
**Alarcón-Segovia D:** Descriptions of therapeutic arthrocenthesis and of synovial fluid in a Nahuatl text from prehispanic Mexico. **Bol Soc Mex Hist Filos Med** 1979 Sep;4(28):105–12
**Alarcón-Segovia D, Laffón A, Alcocer-Varela J:** Probable depiction of juvenile arthritis by Sandro Botticelli. **Arthritis Rheum** 1983 Oct;26(10):1266–8
**Alarcón-Segovia D** see **Fuente JR de la**
**Alarcon-Segovia D** see **Schumacher HR**
**Alarcón-Segovia D** see **Treviño-García Manzo N**
**Alawneh I:** Historische Bemerkungen über Gallenwegtrauma. **Aktuel Traumatol** 1981 Dec;11(6):231–3
**Alba F:** La fecundidad entre los mexicano-norteamericanos en relacion a los cambiantes patrones reproductivos en Mexico y los Estados Unidos. **Demogr Econ** 1982;16(2):236–49
**Albanese CL:** The poetics of healing: root metaphors and rituals in nineteenth-century America. **Soundings** 1980;63(4):381–406
**Albarello B, Collorio C:** Analisi dei collegamenti tra l'opera freudiana e il positivismo ottocentesco. **Acta Med Hist Patav** 1982–83;29:9–18
**Albarello B:** Il concetto di regressione in Freud. **Minerva Psichiatr** 1984 Jan–Mar;25(1):23–36
**Albarracín A:** Gaspar Casal y el concepto moderno de especie morbosa. **Asclepio** 1983;35:189–95
**Albarracín A:** Ramón y Cajal entre los poderes y los saberes. **Med Hist (Barc)** 1984;4:1–16
**Albarracín Teulón A:** Cajal y el problema del conocimiento cientifico. **Asclepio** 1980;32:7–17
**Albarracín Teulón A:** La terapeutica clinica como experimento. **Asclepio** 1981;33:243–9
**Albarracín Teulón A, López Piñero JM, Granjel LS, ed:** Medicina e historia. Madrid, Editorial de la Universidad Complutense 1980. 387 p. Contributions by P. Laín Entralgo, J. A. Paniagua, E. Balguer Perigüell, R. Ballester Añon, A. Lafuente, J. Riera, A. Carreras Panchón, D. García Guerra, J. L. Peset, M. Luz Terrada, P. Marset.
**Albasanz Gallan JL:** La digital, en su segundo centenario. **An R Acad Nac Med (Madr)** 1983;100(2):181–208
**Albee GW** see **Kasschau RA**
**Albemarle-Charlottesville Health Department:** The history of the Albemarle-Charlottesville Health Department. Charlottesville, Va., Jefferson Printing, 1973. 42 p.
**Alberdi RM:** La enfermería profesión femenina? **Rev Enferm** 1983 Apr;6(57):21–6
**Alberman ED** see **Pharoah PO**
**Albert DM:** 400th anniversary of Batisch's Der Augendienst. **Arch Ophthalmol** 1983 Dec;101(12):1857
**Albert DM** see **Fournier GA**
**Albert DM** see **Lamping KA**
**Albert-Puleo M:** The obstetrical use in ancient and early modern times of Convolvulus scammonia or Scammony: another non-fugal source of ergot alkaloids? **J Ethnopharmacol** 1979 Apr;1(2):193–5
**Albert-Puleo M:** Van Gogh's vision: thujuone intoxication. **JAMA** 1981 Jul 3;246(1):42
**Alberti H:** Die heiligen Kosmas und Damian auf einer Prozessionsfahne im Deutschen Apotheken-Museum. **Dtsch Apoth Ztg** 1979 Jun 14;119(24):948–50 (also in Pharm Ztg 1979 Jun 14;24:1155–7
**Alberti PW:** Tracheotomy versus intubation. A 19th century controversy. **Ann Otol Rhinol Laryngol** 1984 Jul–Aug;93(4 Pt 1):333–7
**Alberti Fidanza A** see **Fidanza F**
**Albertini H** see **Puech PF**
**Alberts WJ:** Armen- en ziekenzorg in Gelre en Limburg, 15de - 19de eeuw. **Spiegel Hist** 1982;17(5):278–84
**Albin M, Devlin RJ, Heeger G, ed:** New directions in psychohistory. The Adelphi papers in honor of Erik H. Erikson. Lexington, Toronto, D. C. Heath, 1980. xx, 217 p. Includes contributions by E. S. Wolf, M. F. Shore, G. M. Platt, H. Feinstein, S. H. Rudolph, L. I. Rudolph.
**Albini G:** A proposito di studi recenti die storia della salute nel medioevo e nell'età moderna. **Nuova Riv Stor** 1980;64(1–2):143–63
**Albisetti JC:** The fight for female physicians in Imperial Germany. **Cent Eur Hist** 1982;15:99–123
**Al'bitskiĭ VIu:** K 150-letiiu so dnia rozhdeniia Nikolaia Andreevicha Vinogradova - uchenika S. P. Botkina. **Klin Med (Mosk)** 1982 Sep;60(9):121–3
**Al'bitskiĭ VIu** see **Kalnin VV**
**Albrecht U** see **Klessen D**
**Albrecht von Haller, 1708–1777:** Zehn Vorträge gehalten am Berner Haller-Symposion vom 6. bis 8. Oktober 1977. Basel, Birkhäuser, 1978. x, 182 p. With contributions by M. Stettler, K. S. Guthke, U. Im Hof, N. Mani, L. Premuda, H. Zoller, R. Toellner, A. Lindt, W. Zimmerli, W. Killy.
**Albritton RB, Bahry D:** Effects of public and private sector decisions on health care costs. **Policy Stud J** 1979;7(4):762–9
**Albury WR:** French nosologies around 1800 and their relationship with chemistry. In Forbes EG, ed: Human implications of scientific advance. Edinburgh, Edinburgh University Press, 1978. p. 502–17.

**Albury WR:** Going beyond the introduction: Claude Bernard scholarship in the 1970s, an essay review. **Bull Hist Med** 1982 Summer;56(2):271-5
**Albury WR:** Heart of darkness: J. N. Corvisart and the medicalization of life. **Hist Reflect** 1982;9(1-2):17-31.
**Alcauskas ES, ed** see **Tyson RA**
**Alcocer J:** El archivo historico de la secretaria de salubridad y asistencia. **Bol Soc Mex Hist Filos Med** 1980 Sep-Dec;5(32-33):103-7
**Alcocer Andalón A:** La cirugia potosina de 1592 a 1911. **Bol Soc Mex Hist Filos Med** 1981 Jun;5(35):171-88
**Alcócer Bernés JM:** El Hospital del Divino Salvador. **Salud Publica Mex** 1983 Sep-Oct;25(5):525-30
**Alcocer-Varela J** see **Alarcón-Segovia D**
**Aldea PA** see **Teichman SL**
**Alder GJ:** Moorcroft's life in England; some new evidence. **Vet Hist** 1979-80;1(3):78-93
**Alder GJ:** The origins of 'the Pusa experiment': the East India Company and horse-breeding in Bengal, 1793-1808. **Bengal Past Present** 1979;98(1):10-32
**Alderson JD** see **Padfield A**
**Aldis AS:** Cardiff Royal Infirmary, 1883-1983. Cardiff, University of Wales Press, 1984. v, 52 p.
**Aldrete JA, Marron GM, Wright AJ:** The first administration of anesthesia in military surgery: on occasion of the Mexican-American War. **Anesthesiology** 1984 Nov;61(5):585-8
**Aldrich JE:** Nova Scotia's pioneers in radiology. **Can Med Assoc J** 1984 Aug 15;131(4):376-80
**Aldrich M:** Determinants of mortality among New England cotton mill workers during the Progressive era. **J Econ Hist** 1982;42(4):847-63
**Aldrich M:** Mortality from byssinosis among New England cotton mill workers. 1905-1912. **J Occup Med** 1982 Dec;24(12):977-80
**Aldrich M:** Progressive economics, and scientific racism: Walter Willcox and black Americans, 1895-1910. **Phylon** 1979;40(1):1-14
**Aldrich R:** Homosexuality in France. **Contemp Fr Civiliz** 1982;7(1):1-10
**Aldridge WN:** Insecticides, past, present and future: practice and the understanding of mechanisms. **Ann Occup Hyg** 1979;22(4):407-9
**Alegre Pérez E, González García M:** Estudio de la vida y obra científica de D. Manuel Jiménez Murillo. **Bol Soc Esp Hist Farm** 1983;34(136):185-201
**Alegre Perez E, Andres Turrion L de:** La altea en las prescripciones hechas a la Real familia durante el reinado de Carlos IV (1788-1808). In Hickel E, Schröder G, ed: Neue Beiträge zur Arzneimittelgeschichte. Festschrift für Wolfgang Schneider zum 70. Geburtstag. Stuttgart, Wissenschaftliche Verlagsgesellschaft, 1982. p. 159-63.
**Alegre Pérez E:** La asistencia social en la Real Botica durante el último cuarto del siglo XVIII. **Bol Soc Esp Hist Farm** 1984 Sep;35(139):199-210
**Alegre Perez E, Caraballo Ortega T:** Utilización de las aguas de 'El Molar' por las reales personas durante los años 1841, 42, 43 y 1851. **Bol Soc Esp Hist Farm** 1981 Sep;32(127):115-36
**Alegre Perez ME, Santonja R:** Delito o previsión de futuro? **Bol Soc Esp Hist Farm** 1980 Mar-Jun;31(121-2):31-7
**Alegre Perez ME, Fuente Souviron E:** Noticias sobre los farmaceuticos habilitados para atender por cuenta de la Real Hacienda a los individuos del Real Servicio y personas agraciadas por los Reyes (Reinado de Fernando VII). **Bol Soc Esp Hist Farm** 1982 Mar;33(130):113-22
**Alegre Perez ME, Andres Turrion ML de:** Polémica surgida con motivo de la convocatoria a oposiciones para la Real Botica, en el año 1816. **Bol Soc Esp Hist Farm** 1980/81 Dec-Mar;31-32(124-5):35-45
**Alegría C:** Doctor Gaspar Marcano; médico y antropólogo de gran prestigio. **Rev Soc Venez Hist Med** 1972-73;20-21(34-35):151-60
**Alegría C:** Dos medicos en la aurora de la gesta emancipadora de Venezuela. **Rev Soc Venez Hist Med** 1969-71;17-19(31-33):29-48
**Alegría C:** Medicos que estimularon a Cristobal Colón en su actividad precursora al descubrimiento de America. **Rev Soc Venez Hist Med** 1969-71;17-19(31-33):199-203
**Alegría E** see **Barba J**
**Aleksandrovskiĭ BN, Shchetova GA:** K istorii russko-nemetskikh nauchnykh sviazeĭ v oblasti épidemiologii i gigieny. **Sov Zdravookhr** 1982;(1):61-5
**Aleksandrovskiĭ BN, Shchepetova GA:** P. H. Sokolov--vidnyĭ organizator zdravookhraneniia Saratova. **Sov Zdravookhr** 1979;(11):55-9
**Aleksandrow D, Aleksandrow W:** Osiagni ecia i niepowodzenia intensywnej terapii kardiologicznej za okres 13 lat (doświadczenia własne). **Kardiol Pol** 1980;23(2):103-10
**Aleksandrow W** see **Aleksandrow D**
**Aleksandrowicz JW, Bomba J, Broszkiewicz E, et al:** Kępiński jako klinicysta. **Przegl Lek** 1983;40(12):843-8
**Aleksandrowicz R:** From the history of the Polish Anatomical Society and the International Federation of Anatomical Societies. **Folia Morphol (Warsz)** 1980;39(4):393-5
**Aleksanian IV, Knopov MSh:** Akhutinskoe dvizhenie. **Voen Med Zh** 1981;(7):74-5
**Aleksanian IV, Knopov MSh:** K 125-letiiu so dnia rozhdeniia G. I. Turnera. **Khirurgiia (Mosk)** 1984 Jan;(1):154-5
**Aleksanian IV, Kulish IM:** Sanitarno-gigienicheskoe i protivoé pidemicheskoe obespechenie voĭsk v gody Velikoĭ Otechestvennoĭ voĭny.
**Aleksanian IV:** Sovetskaia voennaia meditsina v Velikoĭ Otechestvennoĭ voĭne (k 35-letiiu pobedy nad fashistskoĭ Germanieĭ). **Sov Zdravookhr** 1980;(5):3-6
**Aleksanian IV, Knopov MSh:** Vidnyĭ sovetskiĭ khirurg V. S. Levit (k 100-letiiu so dnia rozhdeniia). **Klin Khir** 1983 Jun;6:58-60
**Aleksanian IV, Knopov MSh:** Vladimir Semenovich Levit (k 100-letiiu so dnia rozhdeniia). **Voen Med Zh** 1983 Jun;6:72-3
**Alekseev GA, Sergeev TS, Galkina ND:** N. K. Adrianov--pervyĭ vrach-chuvash. **Sov Zdravookhr** 1981;(11):65-7
**Alekseev GA:** Pervye lekari srednego povolzhia. **Sov Zdravookhr** 1983;(4):68-70
**Alekseev GA, Alekseev VA, Gunin GP:** Razvitie sovetskogo zdravookhraneniia v Chuvashii za 60 let avtonomii. **Sov Zdravookhr** 1980;(7):52-4
**Alekseev GA, Butsevitskiĭ VS, Galkina ND:** Revoliutsionnaia deiatel'nost' vracha A.A. Buĭnovskogo. **Sov Zdravookhr** 1979;(8):54-5
**Alekseev GA:** Zarozhdenie organizatsii okhrany zdorov'ia v Srednem Povolzh'e (XVII vek). **Sov Zdravookhr** 1984;(9):49-52
**Alekseev GA** see **Zasukhin DN**
**Alekseev MA, Person RS:** I. M. Sechenov i nekotorye voprosy fiziologii dvizheniĭ. **Usp Fiziol Nauk** 1979 Jul-Sep;10(3):15-25
**Alekseev VA** see **Alekseev GA**
**Alekseeva IN** see **Il'chevich NV**
**Alekseeva LP:** Z. G. Frenkel'. Moskva, Meditsina, 1971. 126 p.
**Aleksentsev AI:** Otchet o deiatel'nosti prodovol'stvennoi armii za pervyi god ee sushchestvovaniia. **Sov Arkh** 1981;5:33-8
**Aleskerov DSh** see **Bakhshiev BA**
**Aleskerov DSh** see **Ragumov RN**
**Alewitz S:** Ezra Mundy Hunt--physician, writer, humanitarian. **J Med Soc NJ** 1981 May;78(5):381-5
**Alewitz S:** Sanitation and public health: Philadelphia, 1870-1900. Ph.D. Diss., Case Western Reserve University. Cleveland, 1981. vii, 421 p.
**Alewitz S:** The life and times of Camden. **J Med Soc NJ** 1984 Sep;81(9):740-6
**Alex W:** The significance of Erich Neuman in Jungian psychology. **Isr Ann Psychiatry** 1979 Dec;17(4):263-8
**Alexa I:** La 100 ani de la naşterea doctorului Mihai Ciucă (1883-1983). **Rev Med Chir Soc Med Nat Iasi** 1983 Oct-Dec;87(4):731-6
**Alexander E:** Archaeology: the big neurosurgical dig. **Clin Neurosurg** 1981;28:323-73
**Alexander E, Alexander E (3d):** German influences on the work of Harvey Cushing, the pioneer of neurosurgery in America. **Neurosurgery** 1981 Nov;9(5):501-5
**Alexander E (3d)** see **Alexander E**
**Alexander ER:** Inactivated poliomyelitis vaccination. Issues reconsidered. **JAMA** 1984 May 25;251(20):2710-2
**Alexander J** see **Mertens C. de**
**Alexander JT:** Bubonic plague in early modern Russia; public health & urban disaster. Baltimore and London, Johns Hopkins University Press, 1980. xviii, 385 p.
**Alexander JT:** Catherine the great and public health. **J Hist Med Allied Sci** 1981 Apr;36(2):185-204
**Alexander JT:** Communicable disease, anti-epidemic policies, and the role of medical professionals in Russia, 1725-62. **Can Am Slav Stud** 1978;12(1):154-69
**Alexander JT:** Ivan Vien and the first comprehensive plague tractate in Russian. **Med Hist** 1980;24(4):419-31
**Alexander JT:** Medical professionals and public health in 'Doldrums' Russia (1725-62). **Can Am Slav Stud** 1978;12(1):116-35
**Alexander L** see **Krupinski J**
**Alexander LB:** Social work's Freudian deluge: myth or reality? **Soc Serv Rev** 1972;46(4):517-38
**Alexander LL:** Early medical heroes: Susan Smith McKinney-Steward, M.D., 1847-1918. **Crisis** 1980;87(1):21-3
**Alexander M:** 'The rigid embrace of the narrow house': premature burial & the signs of death. **Hastings Cent Rep** 1980 Jun;10(3):25-31
**Alexander RS:** History of the Cardiovascular Section. **Physiologist** 1984 Apr;27(2):67-8
**Alexander RS:** Pitts and urine acidification. **Physiologist** 1983 Dec;26(6):364-6
**Alexander SF, Nevins MA:** Home care delivery in Bergen County in the 19th century. **J Med Soc NJ** 1983 Apr;80(4):283-7
**Alexander SF:** Samuel Alexander, M.D., and the Uniform Medical Practice Act. **J Med Soc NJ** 1984 Sep;81(9):759-62
**Alexander TG:** The word of wisdom: from principle to requirement. **Dialogue J Mormon Thought** 1981;14(3):78-88
**Alexander Mitscherlich:** Aus der Analyse eines Gummi-Fetischisten. **Psyche (Stuttg)** 1983 Oct;37(10):867-904
**Alexander Mitscherlich:** Zur Dynamik des Wechsels von Depression und organischem Symptom. **Psyche (Stuttg)** 1983 Oct;37(10):905-20
**Alexandru O:** Nicolae Ionescu Sisesti, neurolog, 1888--1954 (91 ani de la naşterea sa). **Rev Med Interna [Neurol Psihiatr]** 1979 Apr-Jun;24(2):143-6
**Alfonso Galán MT** see **Sánchez-Moscoso Hermida A**
**Alford JA:** Medicine in the Middle Ages: the theory of a profession. **Centen Rev** 1979;23(4):377-96
**Alfred A. Angrist: NY State J Med** 1983 May;83(6):809-11, 872-6
**Alfredsson JH, Gudmundsson SP, Snaedal G:** Artificial insemination by donor with frozen semen. **Obstet Gynecol Surv** 1983 Jun;38(6):305-13
**Algeorge G, Jemna I:** Dezvoltarea micobacteriologici pe plan internaţional şi in ţara noastră. **Rev Ig [Pneumoftiziol]** 1982 Oct-Dec;31(4):291-5
**Algeorge G:** La 100 de ani de la descoperirea de către Robert Koch a agentului etiologic al tuberculozei. **Rev Ig [Pneumoftiziol]** 1982 Jan-Mar;31(1):13-7
**Algería C:** 'El vejamen' y 'El hucusque' en la universidad colonial. **Rev Soc Venez Hist Med** 1972-73;20-21(34-35):29-34
**Alho Filho JL** see **Seibel SD**
**Ali MI** see **Bano M**

Ali SS see **Said HM, ed**
**Ali WM:** The establishment and practice of forensic medicine in Iraq. **Am J Forensic Med Pathol** 1980 Mar;1(1):81–4
**Aliev MA, Ioffe LTs, Chekurov PR, et al:** Razvitie nekotorykh vidov spetsializirovannoĭ khirurgicheskoĭ pomoschi v Kazakhstane. **Vestn Khir** 1983 Mar;130(3):17–23
**Alikhanian SI:** Kafedra genetiki Moskovskogo gosudartsvennogo universiteta imeni M. V. Lomonosova--1930–1948 gg. **Genetika (Moskva)** 1981;17(7):1320–7
**All India Institute of Hygiene & Public Health golden jubilee, 1932–1982:** [New Delhi], Ministry of Health & Family Welfare, Government of India; Calcutta, The Institute, 1982. 25, 4 p.
**Allaire C** see **Quinn S, ed**
**Allan N:** Illustrations from the Wellcome Institute Library: a Jewish physician in the seventeenth century. **Med Hist** 1984 Jul;28(3):324–8
**Allan N:** Some early medical contacts with the Kalmuck tribes of Siberia. **Med Hist** 1983 Jul;27(3):305–9
**Allan N:** The oriental collections in the Wellcome Institute for the History of Medicine, London. **J R Asiat Soc GB Irel** 1981;1:10–25
**Allan N:** The Wellcome Institute and its Library with special reference to South East Asia. **Southeast Asia Libr Group Newsl** 1980;22:1–4
**Allan N** see **Symons H**
**Allan NM:** Gustave Alexandre Liétard, orientalist and physician. **Med Hist** 1981 Jan;25(1):85–8
**Allan P, Jolley M, ed:** Nursing, midwifery and health visiting since 1900. London, Faber and Faber, 1982. 316 p. With contributions by R. H. Pyne, B. Watkin, V. H. Darling, M. E. Lee, C. R. Kratz, G. M. Owen, R. Everest, P. D. Birchenall, D. M. Saunders, B. M. Slaney, D. Blenkinsop, M. D. Green, C. M. Chapman, E. A. Bent, J. C. Hayward, S. R. Lelean, A. V. Cowie, S. Quinn, I. S. Palmer, D. H. Rye.
**Allard GH** see **Sutto C, ed**
**Allderidge P** see **Webster C, ed**
**Allen B:** David Stewart: first professor of pharmacy in America. **Md Pharm** 1982 Feb;:4–8
**Allen BF:** Formation of the Maryland State Pharmaceutical Association. **Med Pharm (Tokyo)** 1982 Apr;:4–7
**Allen BF:** Maryland College of Pharmacy and the doctor of pharmacy degree. **Md Pharm** 1982 Mar;:12–4
**Allen BW, Hinkes WF:** Koch's cultivation of tubercle bacilli. **Med Lab Sci** 1983 Jan;40(1):85–7
**Allen BW, Hinkes WF:** La coloration de Koch pour les bacilles de la tuberculose. **Bull Int Union Tuberc** 1982 Sep–Dec;57(3–4):194–6
**Allen C:** The schizophrenia of Joan of Arc. **Hist Med (Lond)** 1975 Autumn–Winter;6(3–4):4–9
**Allen CR:** A survey of medical numismatics. Medicina in Nummis. **JAMA** 1981 Nov 20;246(20):2347–9
**Allen DE:** Hospital planning: the development of the 1962 hospital plan. London, Pitman Medical, 1979. 191 p.
**Allen DE:** James Edward Smith and the Natural History Society of Edinburgh. **J Soc Bibliogr Nat Hist** 1978;8(4):483–93
**Allen DE:** The plagiarisms of Thomas Henry Cooper. **J Soc Bibliogr Nat Hist** 1979 Nov;9(3):275–9
**Allen DL:** The history and current status of curriculum length in the United States dental schools. **J Dent Educ** 1981 Oct;45(10):702–5
**Allen E, Cooper JE:** A Hunterian account of human rabies. **Vet Hist** 1980/81,n.s.;1:146–8
**Allen E, Turk JL:** Microscopes in the Hunterian Museum. **Ann R Coll Surg Engl** 1982 Nov;64(6):414–8
**Allen E** see **Turk JL**
**Allen FH** see **Grob GN, ed**
**Allen G:** The transformation of a science: T. H. Morgan and the emergence of a new American biology. In Oleson A, Voss J, ed: The organization of knowledge in modern America, 1860–1920. Baltimore and London, Johns Hopkins University Press, 1979. p. 173–210.
**Allen G** see **Beatty J**
**Allen G** see **Bird RD**
**Allen GE:** Essay review: the roots of biological determinism. **J Hist Biol** 1984 Spring;17(1):141–5
**Allen GE:** Morphology and twentieth-century biology: a response. **J Hist Biol** 1981 Spring;14(1):159–76
**Allen GE:** Naturalists and experimentalists: the genotype and the phenotype. **Stud Hist Biol** 1979;3:179–209
**Allen GE** see **Mayr E**
**Allen JC:** The history of Cornell University - New York Hospital School of Nursing, 1942–1979. Ed.D. Diss., Columbia University Teachers College. New York, 1982.
**Allen JG:** First blood bank, first blood banker Oswald Hope Robertson, M.D. **Lab World** 1981 Feb;:20–3
**Allen L, Carmichael E:** The first sixty-two years: Methodist Hospital, Lubbock, Texas, 1918–1980. Lubbock, Methodist Hospital, 1980. 265 p.
**Allen M:** Charlotte Bertha Bühler. In: Notable American women. The modern period. Cambridge, Mass., Belknap–Harvard Univ. Press, 1980. 4:119–21.
**Allen R:** The evolution of pediatric surgery. **J Pediatr Surg** 1980 Dec;15(6):711–8
**Allen TD:** Lest we forget. **South Med J** 1983 Jun;76(6):699–700
**Allen VR:** Medical practices and health in the Choctaw Nation. 1831–1885. **Chron Okla** 1970;48(1):60–73
**Allen WR:** All the names of death: Walker Percy and Hemingway. **Miss Q** 1982–83;36(1):3–19
**Allen GE, et al** see **Caspari EW**
**Allgöwer M, Border JR:** Advances in the care of the multiple trauma patient--introduction. **World J Surg** 1983 Jan;7(1):1–3
**Allgöwer M, Tröhler U:** Biographical note on Theodor Billroth. **Br J Surg** 1981 Oct;68(10):678–9
**Allgöwer M:** Die Behandlung der Tibiaschaftfraktur im Wandel der Zeit. **Hefte Unfallheilkd** 1982;158:417–21
**Alliez J:** Jean-Baptiste Lautard et la 'maison des fous' de Marseille. **Marseille** 1981;127:44–9
**Alliez J, Cain JR, Thermoz P:** L'assistance aux malades mentaux dans le Sud-Est méditerranéen aux XVIIe et XVIIIe siècles: les 'asiles' de Saint-Paul-de-Mausole et de Saint-Pierre-de-Canon, à Saint-Rémy et à Aurons, en Provence. **Ann Med Psychol (Paris)** 1982 Dec;140(10):1122–8
**Alliez J, Huber JP:** L'assistance aux malades mentaux en Provence au XVIIIe siècle. **Ann Med Psychol (Paris)** 1984 Mar;142(3):321–42
**Allison DJ:** Christopher Columbus: first case of Reiter's disease in the Old World? **Lancet** 1980 Dec 13;2(8207):1309
**Allison HM:** Doctor Amos Twitchell: pioneer surgeon. **Hist NH** 1978;33(2):167–79
**Allison MJ, Gerszten E, Munizaga J, et al:** Metastatic tumor of bone in a Tiahuanaco female. **Bull NY Acad Med** 1980 Jul–Aug;56(6):581–7
**Allison MJ:** Paleopathology in Peru. **Nat Hist** 1979;88(2):74–82
**Allison MJ** see **Sawyer DR**
**Allison RS:** The second world war 1939–45: an RNVR medical officer's view. **J R Nav Med Serv** 1982;68(2):102–9
**Allman J:** The demographic transition in the Middle East and North Africa. **Int J Middle East Stud** 1980;12(3):277–301
**Alloway DN** see **Cordasco F**
**Alloway WJ, Ronkin ME:** The social anthropology of chiropractic in Washington, D.C.: project DC/DC. **Chiropr Hist** 1982;2(1):7–11
**Allwork SP:** Maladie du Roger 1879: a new translation for the centenary. **Am Heart J** 1979 Sep;98(3):307–11
**Almada Bay I** see **Canales Muñoz JL**
**Almagro BR:** From clay tablets to electronic publications: the history of medical books. **Ariz Med** 1984 Jan;41(1):31–4
**Almoyna CM** see **Almoyna JM**
**Almoyna JM, Almoyna CM:** Continencia anal. Antecedentes históricos. **Rev Esp Enferm Apar Dig** 1983 Dec;64(6):549–55
**Almquist HJ:** Vitamin K; discovery, identification, synthesis, functions. **Fed Proc** 1979 Dec;38(13):2687–9
**Alonso HO:** La enfermedad cardíaca de Gustav Mahler. **Medicina (B Aires)** 1981;41(3):373–7
**Aloush N** see **Ober WB**
**Aloysius DJ, Ranasinghe L:** Historical perspective of the Sri Lanka Medical Association. **Ceylon Med J** 1981 Mar;26(1):8–34
**Aloysius DJ** see **Uragoda CG**
**Alper TG:** Psychology in New England: a retrospective look -- a woman's point of view. **J Hist Behav Sci** 1980 Jul;16(3):220–4
**Alpern M:** Presentation of the Procter Medal for Research in vision and Ophthalmology to Gerald Westheimer. **Invest Ophthalmol Vis Sci** 1979 Sep;18(9):883–92
**Alpert RT:** From Jewish science to rabbinical counseling. Philadelphia. [s.n.], 1977. 200 leaves.
**Als Aerzte den Modeschöpfern ins Handwerk pfuschten: MMW** 1980 Feb 1;122(5):56–7
**Als die Zahnheilkunde ihre Lehrzeit absolvierte: Zahnarztl Mitt** 1983 Dec 16;73(24):2766–7
**Alsina i Bofill J:** De la medicina d'ahir a la medicina de demà. In Congrés International d'Història de la Medicina Catalana, 2nd, Barcelona, 1975. Llibre d'Actes. Barcelona, Socitra, 1977. p. 139–46.
**Alsobrook DE:** Mobile v. Birmingham: the Alabama Medical College controversy, 1912–1920. **Ala Rev** 1983;36(1):37–56
**Alsop J:** A private consultation by Dr. William Harvey in 1642. **Med Hist** 1980 Jan;24(1):93–8
**Alsop JD:** A footnote on the circulation of the blood: Joseph Colston and Harvey's discovery in 1642. **J Hist Med Allied Sci** 1981 Jul;36(3):331–4
**Alsop JD:** Some notes on seventeenth-century continental hospitals. **Br Libr J** 1981;7(1):70–4
**Alsop JD:** The fatal illness of the antiquary William Burton (1609–57). **Notes Queries** 1979 Oct;26(5):424–5
**Alsop JD:** Two letters on the cuticular glove: keratolysis of 1769. **J Hist Med Allied Sci** 1984 Apr;39(2):224–5
**Alstermark H:** Das Arzneibuch des Johan van Segen. Stockholm, Almquist & Wiksell, 1977. 174 p. (Acta Universitatis Stockholmiensis. Stockholmer germanistische Forschungen, 22)
**Alt K:** In der Weimarer Zeit war der Rundfunk ein beliebtes Fortbildungs-Instrument. **Zahnarztl Mitt** 1984 Oct 16;74(20):2325–6
**Altaffer LF:** Penis captivus and the mischievous Sir William Osler. **South Med J** 1983 May;76(5):637–41
**Altchek ED:** Plus ça change. **Plast Reconstr Surg** 1980 Jun;65(6):849–50
**Altemeier WA:** Perspectives in surgical infections. **Surg Clin North Am** 1980 Feb;60(1):5–13
**Altemeier WA:** Sepsis in surgery. **Arch Surg** 1982 Feb;117(2):107–12
**Altenstetter C, Bjorkman JW:** Federal-state health policies and impacts: the politics of implementation. Washington, University Press of America, 1978. xi, 116 p.
**Alter G:** Plague and the Amsterdam annuitant: a new look at life annuities as a source for historical demography. **Popul Stud** 1983 Mar;37(1):23–41
**Alteras I:** Jewish physicians in Southern France during the thirteenth and fourteenth centuries. **Jew Q Rev** 1978 Apr;68–209–23

**Althoff A:** Wissenschaftlicher Briefwechsel von und mit Theodor Bilharz. Düsseldorf, Triltsch, 1980. 133 p. (Düsseldorfer Arbeiten zur Geschichte der Medizin, 56; also Diss.) **Dusseld Arb Gesch Med Hefte** 1980;56:1–133

**Altholz JL:** The Huxley–Wilberforce debate revisited. **J Hist Med Allied Sci** 1980 Jul;35(3):313–16

**Altieri Biagi ML:** L'episteme stillistica di Lazzaro Spallanzani. **Intersezioni** 1981;1:575–99

**Alting MP, Waterbolk TW:** New light on the anatomical errors in Rembrandt's Anatomy Lesson of Dr. Nicolass Tulp. **J Hand Surg** 1982 Nov;7(6):632–4

**Altman D:** Health care for the poor. **Ann Am Acad Polit Soc Sci** 1983;(468):103–21

**Altman SB:** A brief history of South Dakota Academy of Ophthalmology and Otorhinolaryngology. **SD J Med** 1981 May;34(5):39

**Altschule MD:** Invalidity of using so-called Starling curves in clinical medicine. **Perspect Biol Med** 1983 Winter;26(2):171–87

**Altschule MD:** Occasional notes. A near miss--Osler's early description of Cushing's syndrome with, regrettably, no post-mortem examination. **N Engl J Med** 1980 May 15;302(20):1153–5

**Altschuller GI, Keenan WA:** History of the development of painless surgery in Russia. **Bull NY Acad Med** 1982 Jun;58(5):493–502

**Al'tshular NS, Mikhaĭlov FA:** Pervaia otechestvennaia dissertatsiia po tuberkulezu. **Probl Tuberk** 1983 May;(5):70–2

**Al'tshuler NS:** Iz istorii razvitiia bor'by s tuberkulezom v SSSR (1918–1924). **Probl Tuberk** 1980 May;(5):72–4

**Al'tshuler NS:** Voprosy bor'by s tuberkulezom v deiatel'nosti peredovoĭ meditsinskoĭ obshchestvennosti v dorevoliutsionnoĭ Rossii. **Probl Tuberk** 1979 Dec;(12):62–5

**Altŭnkov P:** D-r Vladimir Petrov Glavchev (1878–1915 g.). **Khirurgiia (Sofiia)** 1982;35(6):632

**Altŭnkov P** see **Lukanov A**

**Altwerden in der Bundesrepublik Deutschland: Geschichte – Situationen – Perspektiven:** Berlin, Deutsches Zentrum für Altersfragen, 1982. 3 volumes (Beiträge zur Gerontologie und Altenarbeit).

**Altynbekov MA:** Zdravookhranenie Chimkentskoĭ oblasti v dorevoliutsionnyĭ period. **Sov Zdravookhr** 1981;(8):63–5

**Altynbekov MA:** Zdravookhranenie Chimkentskoĭ oblasti v gody Velikoĭ Otechestvennoĭ voĭny. **Sov Zdravookhr** 1980;(8):51–3

**Altynbekov MA:** Zdravookhranenie Chimkentskoĭ oblasti v poslevoennyĭ period. **Sov Zdravookhr** 1981;(3):57–9

**Alumäe N:** Eesti NSV teaduste akadeemia aastail 1965–1972. [toimetuskolleegium N. Alumäe ... et al.]. Tallinn, The Academy, 1973. 274 p.

**Alvaer I:** Sykepleier i 'de gode, gamle dager'. **Sykepleien** 1981 Dec 5;68(21):8–11

**Alvarado JM:** El primer episodio psiquiátrico de la conquista hispana. **Acta Psiquiatr Psicol Am Lat** 1979 Sep;25(3):225–8

**Alvares AP:** Cytochrome P-450s: research highlights of the last two decades. **Drug Metab Rev** 1981;12(2):431–6

**Alvarez C** see **Valverde JL**

**Alvarez PJ:** Doctor J. M. de los Ríos: precursor de la pediatria en Venezuela. **Rev Sos Venez Hist Med** 1972–73;20–21(34–35):15–20

**Alvarez R** see **Wasserman H**

**Alvarez Amézquita J:** Influencia de la salud pública en el desarrollo social. In Academia Nacional de Medicina. Libro conmemorativo del primer centenario. México, Comité Editorial de la Comisión Organizadora del Congreso del Centenario, 1964. Tome 2. p. 630–40.

**Alvarez de Abajo M, Frances Causape MC:** La inspeccion de boticas en el Obispado de Malaga entre 1824 y 1830. **Bol Soc Esp Hist Farm** 1981 Dec;32(128):251–63

**Alvarez de Morales C, Irueste FG:** Medicina creencial y medicina racional en la España arabe del siglo IX: el Mujtasar Fi L-tibb (compendio de medicina) de 'Abd al-Malik Ibn Habib al-Ilbiri (c. 790–854). **Asclepio** 1982;34:283–94

**Alvarez-Klein L** see **Frenk J**

**Alves M:** Dr. Arthur Neiva. **Rev Inst Hist Geogr Bras** 1979;325:123–31

**Alvi MA** see **Rahman A**

**Alvsvåg H:** Sykepleiens historie--er den objektiv? **Sykepleien** 1983 Feb 7;70(3):20–1

**Alvsvåg H:** Sykepleiens historie og kvinnesynet. **Sykepleien** 1982 Oct 5;69(17):6–10, 29

**Alwin M. Pappenheimer, Jr: Cell Immunol** 1982 Jan 1;66(1):3–8

**Al'zhanov AG:** Iz istorii podgotovki fel'dsherov v dorevoliutsionnom Kazakhstane. **Feldsher Akush** 1982;47(12):38–40

**Amadeo EM:** Recordando a un maestro de la odontología internacional y pionero de la endodoncia: Henry Lentulo 1889–1981. **Rev Asoc Odontol Argent** 1983 Sep;71(5):150–2

**Amadi GI:** Healing in 'The Brotherhood of the Cross and Star'. In Sheils WJ, ed: The Church and healing. Papers read at the twentieth summer meeting and the twenty-first winter meeting of the Ecclesiastical History Society. Oxford, Basil Blackwell for the Society, 1982. p. 367–83.

**Amakoue A:** Médecine et pharmacopée traditionnelle en Afrique. **Dialogue J Mormon Thought** 1978 Nov–Dec;46–70

**Amalric P:** Claude Bernard et l'ophtalmologie. **Bull Soc Ophtalmol Fr** 1979 Nov–Dec;79(11–12):995–7

**Amalric P:** De l'Hôpital de la Grave à la Grande Armée. L'ophtalmologie de Dominique Larrey. **Bull Soc Ophtalmol Fr** 1979 Feb;79(2):151–4

**Amalric P:** Dominique Anel et les Quinze Vingts de Paris. **Bull Soc Ophtalmol Fr** 1982 Jan;82(1):87–90

**Amalric P:** La Clinique Ophtalmologique de l'Hôtel Dieu à 100 ans. **Bull Soc Ophtalmol Fr** 1980 Dec;80(12):1177–80

**Amalric P:** La naissance de la neuro-ophtalmologie à Montpellier au XVIIme siècle à travers l'oeuvre de Raymond Vieussens et de Guilhem Briggs. **Bull Soc Ophtalmol Fr** 1983 Jan;83(1):83–8

**Amalric P:** La naissance et les premiers pas de l'ophtalmoscopie binoculaire. **Bull Soc Ophthalmol Fr** 1982 Nov;82(11):1469–71

**Amalric P:** L'influence de Guy de Chauliac à Toulouse au XVIIe siècle. A propos d'un petit livre inédit. **Bull Soc Ophtalmol Fr** 1980 Jun–Jul;80(6–7):617–8

**Amalric P:** Ophtalmoscopie et périphérie rétinienne. Quelques aperçus historiques. **Bull Soc Ophtalmol Fr** 1980 Jun–Jul;80(6–7):595–7

**Amalric P** see **Royer J**

**Aman A:** Det sociala tvånget. **Sven Tidskr** 1979;66(1):30–3

**Aman MG:** Hyperactivity: nature of the syndrome and its natural history. **J Autism Dev Disord** 1984 Mar;14(1):39–56

**Amann A, Majce G:** A short history of the development of social-scientific research on aging in Austria. **ZFA** 1984 Jan–Feb;39(1):9–15

**Amat N:** El médico y el acceso a la información bibliográfica en biomedicina. Guía metodológica para la utilización de fuentes de información. La National Library of Medicine: Index Medicus y Medlars. **Med Clin (Barc)** 1982 Apr 16;78(8):344–50

**Amberger G:** Die Mulomedicina Chironis, ein Buch über Pferdeheilkunde aus dem 4. Jahrhundert n. Chr. **Ethnomedizin** 1978–79;5(3–4):233–61

**Ambrosoli C** see **Armocida G**

**Ambrus O:** Historie a přehled lázeňské péče v psychiatrii v Ceskoslovensku. **Fysiatr Reumatol Vestn** 1982 Apr;60(2):105–7

**Ambrusová L** see **Krahulec I**

**Amdisen A** see **Johnson FN**

**Amelung P:** Dinckmuts Drucke des Regimen sanitatis. **Gutenberg Jahrb** 1979;:58–71

**American Academy of Arts and Sciences, American Philosophical Society:** Survey of sources for the history of biochemistry and molecular biology. **Surv Sources Newsl** 1975–1981;1(1–10):various pagings

**American Animal Hospital Association:** [Fifty years of the American Animal Hospital Association. Mishawaka, Indiana, AAHA, 1983]. 64 p.

**The American Dental Association in 1982: Tic** 1982 Nov;41(11):1–3

**American Dental Association 1859–1880: J Am Dent Assoc** 1984 Apr;108(4):479–89, 492

**American Dental Association 1881–1917: J Am Dent Assoc** 1984 Apr;108(4):497–510

**American Dental Association 1918–1928: J Am Dent Assoc** 1984 Apr;108(4):515–9, 522

**American Dental Association 1929–1945: J Am Dent Assoc** 1984 Apr;108(4):527–33, 535–6

**American Dental Association 1946–1962: J Am Dent Assoc** 1984 Apr;108(4):541–51, 554–6

**American Dental Association 1963–1984: J Am Dent Assoc** 1984 Apr;108(4):561–71, 574–9

**The American Institute of Pharmacy: 50th anniversary: Am Pharm** 1984 Aug;NS24(8):suppl 1–16

**American Nurses' Association:** A force through history. **Nurs Careers** 1982 May–Jun;3(3):3

**The American Radium Society: Am J Clin Oncol** 1982 Apr;5(2):99–100

**American Red Cross celebrates 100th anniversary: Am Nurse** 1981;13(5):15, 17

**Ames EW:** The status of women in Canadian psychology: a case study of women in science. **Int J Womens Stud** 1981;4(4):431–40

**Ames KL:** Ideologies in stone: meanings in Victorian gravestones. **J Pop Cult** 1981;14(4):641–56

**Ames SR:** Karl Ernest Mason (1900–1978): a biographical sketch. **J Nutr** 1984 Mar;114(3):463–6

**Amin M** see **Said HM, ed**

**Aminev AM:** 125 let so dnia rozhdeniia Vasiliia Ivanovicha Razumovskogo. **Vestn Khir** 1983 May;130(5):137–9

**Amiot M, Béguinot P:** L'alimentation en eau potable de la ville de Dijon et son assainissement. **Mem Acad Sci Arts B-Lett Dijon** 1977;122:551–602

**Amitai M, Cremerius J:** Dr. med. Arthur Muthmann. Ein Beitrag zur Frühgeschichte der Psychoanalyse. **Psyche (Stuttg)** 1984 Aug;38(8):738–53

**Ammar S:** Introduction à l'étude de la médecine arabo-islamique. **Tunis Med** 1980 Jul–Aug;58(4):544–55, 562–77

**Ammar S:** Le message hippocratique à travers la médecine arabe. **Tunis Med** 1981 Nov–Dec;59(6):498–504

**Ammon HP, Kemper FH:** Ayurveda: 3000 Jahre indische traditionelle Medizin. **Med Welt** 1982 Jan 29;33(4):148–53

**Ammon HP** see **Kotwas J**

**Amoh T** see **Fujimori K**

**Amoroso EC:** George Bernays Wislocki. In Dictionary of American Biography, Suppl. 6, 1956–1960. p. 703–5, 1980.

**Amos DB:** Peter Alfred Isaac Gorer. In Dictionary of national biography, 1961–1970. Suppl. 8, 1981. p. 443–5.

**Amsel E, ed** see **Broughton JM**

**Amstutz P:** Für Gesundheitsschutz am Arbeitsplatz: Die Fachkommission der Schweizerischen Gesellschaft für Arbeitsmedizin, Arbeitshygiene und Arbeitssicherheit. **Soz Praventivmed** 1981 Jul;26(3):120–5

**Amulree L:** Pergamum. **Hist Med (Lond)** 1975 Autumn–Winter;6(3–4):15–22

**Amundsen DW:** Casuistry and professional obligations: the regulation of physicians by the court of conscience in the late Middle Ages. Part II. **Trans Stud Coll Physicians Phila** 1981 Jun;3(2):93–112

**Amundsen DW:** [History of medical ethics]: ancient Greece and Rome [and]

medieval Europe. In Reich WT, et al, ed: Encyclopedia of bioethics, v.3. New York, Free Press, 1978. p. 930–51.
**Amundsen DW:** [Medical ethics in the] ancient Near East. In Reich ET, et al, ed: Encyclopedia of bioethics, v. 2. New York, Free Press, 1978. p. 880–3.
**Amundsen DW:** Medicine and faith in early Christianity. **Bull Hist Med** 1982 Fall;56(3):326–50
**Amundsen DW, Ferngren GB:** The forensic role of physicians in Roman Law. **Bull Hist Med** 1979 Spring;53(1):39–56
**Amundson LH:** The roots of family practice in South Dakota. **SD J Med** 1981 May;34(5):43–8
**Amundson R:** E. C. Tolman and the intervening variable: a study in the epistemological history of psychology. **Philos Sci** 1983;50:268–82
**Anagnostopoulos CE** see **Sanderson CJ**
**Anand RM** see **Gurjar GK**
**Anan'ev BV** see **Moikin IuV**
**Anan'ev BV** see **Tarasenko NIu**
**Ananthanarayan R:** Robert Koch's contribution to microbiology. **Indian J Pathol Microbiol** 1982 Apr;25(2):169–71
**ANA's economic and general welfare program: a historical perspective: ANA Publ** 1981;(EC–143):1–10
**Anastasatu C:** Aportul lui Iacob Felix la combaterea tuberculozei în țara noastră (cu acasia aniversarii a 150 de ani de la naștere). **Rev Ig [Pneumoftiziol]** 1983 Oct–Dec;32(4):379–80
**Anastasatu C:** Centenarul descoperirii bacilului Koch. **Rev Ig [Pneumoftiziol]** 1982 Jan–Mar;31(1):1–3
**Anastasatu C:** 200 de ani de la nașterea lui Laennec. **Rev Ig [Pneumoftiziol]** 1981 Oct–Dec;30(4):250–1
**Anastassiou A:** Zur hippokratischen Schrift De locis in homine und zum Hippokratesglossar des Galen. **Rheinisches Mus Philol** 1982;125:193–201
**Anastassiou A** see **Grmek MD, ed**
**An ancient art revived: Gastrointest Endosc** 1979 Feb;25(1):28–9
**Andelic P, Balevic M, Nikolin P, et al:** Razvoj stomatološke službe u regionu istočnog Srema. **Med Pregl** 1982;35(11–12):495–6
**Ander Z:** Quo vadis medicina legalis? In: International Congress of the History of Medicine, 26th, Plovdiv (Bulgaria), 1978. Actes du Congres, Vol. 1. Sofia, 1980. p. 82–3.
**Andersen O:** A malaria epidemic in Denmark. In Charbonneau H, Larose A, ed: The great mortalities: methodological studies of demographic crises in the past. Liège, Belgium, Ordina Editions, 1980. p. 33–49.
**Andersen O:** The development in Danish mortality 1735–1850. **Scand Popul Stud** 1979;5:9–21
**Andersen S:** Simon Paulli. Betaenkning over en Kongelig Ridehest. **Dan Medicinhist Arbog** 1979;9–97
**Andersen S** see **Carmelli D**
**Andersen SR, Geertinger P:** Moselig i retsmedicinsk belysning. **Dan Medicinhist Arbog** 1982;:23–42
**Andersen S, ed:** Simonis Paulli velmenende råd gennem hvilke formedelst Guds hjaelp en højadelig person lykkeligt blev kureret da han i året 1668 i Paris blev ramt af slag. **Dan Medicinhist Arbog** 1982;:73–91
**Anderson AB:** Vanishing spas. Dorchester, [Eng.], Friary Press, 1974. 103 p.
**Anderson BA** see **Coale AJ**
**Anderson CM:** Measles mortality and ethnic groups. **S Afr Med J** 1982 Jul 17;62(3):86–8
**Anderson DA:** Dental health services and the Northern Territory of Australia. A short review of people, places, and programmes to 1981. **Aust Dent J** 1982 Dec;27(6):345–51
**Anderson DE** see **Howell JB**
**Anderson DL, Anderson GT:** Nostalgia and malingering in the military during the Civil War. **Perspect Biol Med** 1984 Autumn;28(1):156–66
**Anderson GT** see **Anderson DL**
**Anderson J** see **Gay EC**
**Anderson J** see **Llewelyn DE**
**Anderson JA** see **Wangensteen OW, ed**
**Anderson JQ** see **Hand WD, ed**
**Anderson JR:** Acayatl, ancient Aztec sorcerer. **Ala Med** 1984 Feb;53(8):14, 17–8, 20
**Anderson JR:** An old medical specialty puts on a new face...and head...and neck. **South Med J** 1980 Aug;73(8):1058–62
**Anderson JW:** In search of Mary James. **Psychohist Rev** 8(1–2):63–70, Summer–Fall 79
**Anderson JW:** The methodology of psychological biography. **J Interdiscip Hist** 1981;11:455–75
**Anderson JW:** 'The worst kind of melancholy': William James in 1869. **Harv Libr Bull** 1982 Oct;30(4):369–86
**Anderson NE:** The historical development of American nursing education. **JNE** 1981 Jan;20(1):18–36
**Anderson NF:** The 'marriage with a deceased wife's sister bill' controversy: incest anxiety and the defense of family purity in Victorian England. **J Br Stud** 1982;21(2):67–86
**Anderson O:** Did suicide increase with industrialization in Victorian England? **Past Present** 1980;86:149–73
**Anderson O:** Suicide in Victorian London; an urban view. **Soc Soc Hist Med Bull (Lond)** 1980 Jun;26:18–21
**Anderson PG:** The spa, the fairgrounds, and the psychiatric hospital: the 21st General Hospital in World War II. **Outlook Mag** 1982 Spring;19(1):2–8
**Anderson PG** see **Hoolihan C**
**Anderson RA:** Chiropractic in American history: the ins and outs of museums. **Chiropr Hist** 1982;2(1):15–9
**Anderson RH, Becker AE:** Stanley Ken and accessory atrioventricular connections. **J Thorac Cardiovasc Surg** 1981 May;81(5):649–58
**Anderson RJ, Reed WG, Hillis LD, et al:** History, epidemiology, and medical complications of nasal inhaler abuse. **J Toxicol Clin Toxicol** 1982 Mar;19(1):95–107
**Anderson TH:** Becoming sane with psychohistory. **Historian** 1978;41(1):1–20
**Anderson WC:** Translating the language of chemistry: Priestley and Lavoisier. **Eighteenth Cent Theory Interpret** 1981;22(1):21–31
**Andersson L, Kinn AC:** Njursten och blåssten––en medicinhistorisk översikt. **Nord Medicinhist Arsb** 1982;:76–85
**Andersson N** see **Marks S**
**Anderton DL** see **Mineau GP**
**Andorka R:** A család és háztartás nagysága és összetétele 1800 körül két déldunántúli faluban (Alsónyéken és Kölkeden). Kisérlet P. Laslett elemzési módszerének felhasználására. **Tort Stat Tanulm** 1977;3:215–36
**Andorka R:** Birth control in the eighteenth and nineteenth centuries in some Hungarian villages. **Local Popul Stud (Matlock)** 1979;22:38–43
**Andrä A:** Zur Entwicklung der Kieferchirurgie in Rostock. **Zahn Mund Kieferheilkd** 1982;70(1):4–9
**Andral G:** Pathological hematology: an essay on the blood in disease. Reprint of the 1844 ed. With a historical introduction by L. A. May. Oceanside, N. Y. Dabor Science Publications, 1977. 129 p.
**André J** see **Bernier JJ**
**Andre JM:** La notion de Pestilentia à Rome: du tabou religieux à l'interprétation pré-scientifique. **Latomus** 1980;39:2–16
**Andre P:** Schumann. Les chants de l'ombre. Paris, Jean-Claude Lattes, 1982. 225 p.
**Andre P** see **Ashton RE**
**André R:** Etude régionale de la natalité et de la fécondité des populations belge et étrangère. **Rev Inst Sociol** 1969;3:569–86
**André R:** La mortalité de la population de nationalité belge. **Rev Inst Sociol** 1969;2:305–24
**André R, Pereira-Roque J:** La mortalité infantile au Portugal. **Rev Inst Sociol** 1972;3:573–91
**André R, Gyselings R:** Variation saisonnière de la mortalité infantile en Belgique. **Rev Inst Sociol** 1970;3:587–97
**André-Leicknam B:** Les premiers écrits médicaux. Le sang en Mésopotamie. **Nouv Rev Fr Hematol** 1983;25(2):141–4
**Andreano R:** Some personal observations on health policy in Iran, 1973–1978. **Soc Sci Med** 1984;19(1):1–7
**Andreasen NC** see **Trautmann J, ed**
**Andree C:** Theodor Billroth (1829–1894) zum 150. Geburtstag. **Med Welt** 1979 Dec 7;30(49):1857–62
**Andree C** see **Kudlien F**
**Andree C** see **Mann G, ed**
**Andreeva VN, Kosmachevskaia EA:** Ocherk razvitiia fiziologii krovoobrashcheniia v laboratoriiakh Mediko-khirurgicheskoĭ (Voenno-meditsinskoĭ) akademii v XIX veke (K istorii vzaimosviazi teorii i praktiki v issledovatel'skoĭ rabote). **Fiziol Zh SSSR** 1981 Jun;67(6):934–50
**Andrejew A:** Wacław Koler, sławny medyk Krakowski w świetle swego inwentarza. **Arch Hist Med (Warsz)** 1984;47(1):39–47
**Andres Turrion L de** see **Alegre Perez E**
**Andrés Turrión ML de:** Normativa sobre la confección de recetas en la Real Botica durante el siglo XIX. **Bol Soc Esp Hist Farm** 1984 Jun;35(138):89–102
**Andres Turrion ML de** see **Alegre Perez ME**
**Andreski S:** The syphilitic shock: a new explanation of the 'great witch craze' of the 16th and 17th centuries in the light of medicine and psychiatry. **Encounter (Lond)** 1982;58(5):7–26
**Andreski S:** The syphilitic shock: puritanism, capitalism, and a medical factor. **Encounter (Lond)** 1980;55(4):76–81
**Andrew ER:** A historical review of NMR and its clinical applications. **Br Med Bull** 1984 Apr;40(2):115–9
**Andrewes CH:** Alick Isaacs. In Dictionary of national biography, 1961–1970. Suppl. 8, 1981. p. 569–70.
**Andrews AH:** A century of cattle practice. **Vet Rec** 1982 Jun 26;110(26):598–601
**Andrews BF:** William Harvey in perinatal perspective. In Smith GF, Smith PN, Vidyasagar D, ed: Historical review and recent advances in neonatal and perinatal medicine. [Chicago?], Mead Johnson Nutritional Division, 1983. Vol. II. p. 165–78.
**Andrews BF** see **Smith GF**
**Andrews J** see **El-Najjar MY**
**Andrews LB, Levin LS:** Self-care and the law. **Soc Policy** 1979;9(4):44–9
**Andrews MW:** Medical attendance in Vancouver, 1886–1920. **BC Stud** 1978–79(40):32–56
**Andrews MW:** Medical services in Vancouver, 1886–1920. A study in the interplay of attitudes, medical knowledge, and administrative structures. Ph.D. Diss. The University of British Columbia. Victoria, 1979.
**Andrews MW:** St. Luke's Home, Vancouver, 1888–1936: a transitional hospital. **J Can Church Hist Soc** 1982,24(2):90–8
**Andrews P** see **McHenry HM**
**Andrews WH:** A perspective review of the development of AOAC microbiological methods. **J Assoc Off Anal Chem** 1984 Jul–Aug;67(4):661–73
**Andrian-Werburg K von:** Das Gesundheits- und Medizinalwesen in Sachsen-Coburg und das Coburger Landkrankenhaus. **Jahrb Coburg Landesstift** 1977;:13–94
**Andrianov VL, Veselov NG, Kapitanaki IA:** Leningradskiĭ

nauchno-issledovatel'skiĭ detskiĭ ortopedicheskiĭ institut im. G.I. Turnera i ego rol' v okhrane zdorov'ia deteĭ (k 50-letiiu so dnia organizatsii). **Pediatriia** 1983 Nov;(11):74-5

**Andrianov VL:** Leningradskomu nauchno-issledovatel'skomu detskomu ortopedicheskomu institutu im. G. I. Turnera 50 let. **Ortop Travmatol Protez** 1983 Mar;(3):56-60

**Andrianov VL** see **Tkachenko SS**

**Andrianova IG** see **Bogomolova LG**

**Andrienko AP** see **Dumbrov DA**

**Andrieu L:** Les fous de Saint-Aubin-la-Campagne. In Congrès National des Sociétés Savantes, 102e, Limoges, 1977. Actes. Paris, 1978. Tome I, p. 9-21.

**Andrievskiĭ VA** see **Popushoĭ EP**

**Andrik P, Stukovský R:** K otázkám terminálnej redukcie chrupu. **Cesk Stomatol** 1980 Jul;80(4):242-5

**Androutsos G** see **Dimopoulos C**

**Anees MA:** History of Islamic medicine and pharmacy: contribution of Sami Hamarneh. **Hamdard** 1983 Apr-Jun;26(2):67-75

**Angel JL:** History and development of paleopathology. **Am J Phys Anthropol** 1981 Dec;56(4):509-15

**Angel JL:** Physical anthropology: determining sex, age, and individual features. In A. Cockburn, E. Cockburn, ed: Mummies, disease, and ancient cultures. Cambridge, Cambridge University Press, 1980. p. 241-57.

**Angelescu B** see **Ioanid N**

**Angeli I:** 50 éve halt meg Oskar Minkowski a pancreas-diabetes felfedezöje. **Orv Hetil** 1981 Jul 12;122(28):1726-9

**Angelini A:** Wilhelm Reich nel dibattito psicoanalitico degli anni Trenta. **Stor Crit Psicol** 1984;5(2):373-88

**Angelis E de:** Rapporti tra mente e corpo dall'eta' classica al XIX secolo. **Med Secoli** 1982 May-Aug;19(2):193-213

**Anger G, Adler G:** Die Entwicklung der Urologie in Halle. **Wiss Z Martin Luther Univ (Math)** 1977;26(3):133-44

**Anger P, Wenz W:** Aus der Pionierzeit der Arteriographie. **Radiologe** 1981 Feb;21(2):65-71

**Angers D:** La vicomté de Bayeux au bas Moyen-Age: esquisse d'histoire démographique. **Francia** 1979;7:141-72

**Angevine E:** History of the National Consumers League, 1899-1979. Washington, The League, 1979. 69 leaves.

**Angevine JB** see **Livingston KE**

**Anglin B:** Twenty-five years of growing together. A history of the Ontario Association for the Mentally Retarded, 1978. 92, x p.

**Angolotti E:** La fiebre amarilla. Historia y situación actual. La fiebre amarilla en la Barcelona de 1821. **Rev Sanid Hig Publica (Madr)** 1980 Jan-Feb;54(1-2):89-102

**Angorn RA** see **Shapiro LJ**

**Angot J:** Un crâne à face décorée de la civilisation mixtèque. **Hist Sci Med** 1984;18(3):255-9

**Angot JL:** Pierre Fauchard (1677?-1761). Expert pour les dents, et maître chirurgien de Saint-Côme de Paris. **Clio Med** 1983 Mar;17(4):207-21

**Angulo Arvelo LA:** Acerca de la probable causa de la muerte de Alejandro el Grande. **Rev Soc Venez Hist Med** 1981;30(45-46):105-10

**Angus MS:** Harriet (Cartwright) Dobbs. In Dictionary of Canadian biography, 1881-1890. 1982;11:265-6.

**Angus MS:** Horatio Yates. In Dictionary of Canadian biography, 1881-1890. 1982;11:940-1.

**Angus MS:** John Robinson Dickson. In Dictionary of Canadian biography, 1881-1890. 1982;11:263-4.

**Anholm JD** see **Maud PJ**

**Anic N** see **Dragic D**

**Animalcular and cryptogamic theories on the origins of fevers. Reprinted works by John Kearsley Mitchell (1849), John L. Riddell (1836), Josiah Clark Nott (1848). New York, Arno, 1977. Various paginations.:**

**Anis AY:** Principles and evolution of intraocular lens implantation. **Int Ophthalmol Clin** 1982 Summer;22(2):1-13

**Anisimov VE:** Nikolaĭ Andreevich Vinogradov (k 150-letiiu so dnia rozhdeniia). **Klin Med (Mosk)** 1982 Mar;60(3):118-9

**Anisimov VE:** Professor L. E. Pikulin (1784-1824) (k 200-letiiu so dnia rozhdeniia). **Sov Zdravookhr** 1984;(10):75-6

**Anisimov VE:** Ucheniki i psoledovateli S. P. Botkina v. Kazani. **Klin Med (Mosk)** 1982 Sep;60(9):113-6

**Anjard R:** Mayan dental wonders. **J Oral Implantol** 1981;9(3):423-6

**Annas GJ:** The case of Karen Silkwood. **Am J Public Health** 1984 May;74(5):516-8

**Annear MW:** Some healing and holy wells of Wales. In J. Cule, ed: Wales and medicine. London, British Society for the History of Medicine, 1975. p. 185-89.

**Annegers JH:** Department of Physiology Northwestern University Medical School. **Physiologist** 1983 Jun;26(3):120-1

**Anner E:** Gelöbnisse der Medizinalpersonen im Kanton Zürich seit 1798. Zürich, Juris, 1979. 76 p. (Zürcher Medizingeschichtliche Abhandlungen, Neue Reihe Nr. 135).

**Anning S:** Yorkshire apothecaries. **Pharm Hist (London)** 1980 Dec;10(3):3-4

**Anning ST, Walls WK:** A history of the Leeds School of Medicine: one and a half centuries, 1831-1981. [Leeds], Leeds University Press, 1982. xiv, 170 p.

**Anning ST:** A medical case book: Leeds, 1781-84. **Med Hist** 1984 Oct;28(4):420-31

**Anning ST:** The history of medicine in Leeds. Leeds, Maney, 1980. 218 p.

**Anning ST:** William Hey, F.R.S.: the father of Leeds surgery. **Proc Leeds Philos Lit Soc (Lit Hist Sect)** 1980;17(5):101-11

**Anokhin AM** see **Tsaregorodtsev GI**

**Anokhin VN:** K 20-letiiu zhurnala 'Voprosy revmatizma'. **Vopr Revm** 1981 Apr-Jun;(2):3-4

**Anoshina AA** see **Tkachenko BI**

**Anoshkin IG** see **Lomakina NM**

**Ansbacher HL:** Discussion of Alfred Alder's preface to The Diary of Vaslav Nijinsky. **Arch Gen Psychiatry** 1981 Jul;38(7):834-41

**Ansbacher HL:** Psychology: a way of living. **J Individ Psychol** 1981 Nov;37(2):153-95

**Ansbacher HL:** 'To love and to work'. Adlerian thoughts on an anecdote about Freud. **Bull Menninger Clin** 1981 Sep;45(5):439-41

**Ansell JS** see **Kaleli A**

**Anselmi S, Sorcinelli P:** Epidemie e rivalità commerciali nelle piazze maritime marchigiane (secoli XVI-XIX). **Econ Stor** 1977;24(3):293-310

**Antal G:** Freud in Hungary. An interview with Imre Hermann, the psychoanalyst. **New Hung Q** 1982;23(85):88-95

**Antall J:** Az orvostörténelem helyzete Magyarországon. **Orv Hetil** 1981 Mar 8;122(10):555-60

**Antall J:** Der Einfluss der Apotheker auf das öffentliche Leben Ungarns im 19. Jahrhundert. **Pharm Acta Helv** 1979;54(9-10):295-8

**Antall J:** Entwicklungstendenzen des Apothekerberufs in Ungarn. **Pharm Ztg** 1981;126:417-23

**Antall J:** Gesundheitliche Aufklrung und Gesundheitserziehung in Ungarn im 18-19. Jahrhundert. **Orvostort Kozl** 1979;86(24 no 4):25-37

**Antall J:** Herausbildung der wissenschaftlichen Pharmazie in Ungarn und die Pester Medizinische Schule. In Hein WH, ed: Pharmaziehistorischer Kongress, Budapest, 1981. Stuttgart, Wissenschaftliche Verlagsgesellschaft, 1983. p. 101-4.

**Antall J, Kapronczay K:** Jan Nepomuk Czermak in Hungary. In E. Schultheisz, ed: History of physiology. Oxford, Elmsford, New York, Pergamon, 1981. xvi, 208 p. (Advances in Physiological Sciences. Proceedings of the 28th International Congress of Physiological Sciences, Budapest, 1980, Volume 21), p. 77-84.

**Antall J:** Organisatorische Reformbestrebungen im militärärztlichen Dienst des ungarischen Freiheitskampfes 1848/49. In: International Congress of the History of Medicine, 26th, Plovdiv (Bulgaria), 1978. Actes du Congres, Vol. 1. Sofia, 1980. p. 83-5.

**Antall J:** Pictorial history of European medicine and pharmaceutics. Budapest, Corvina Kiadó, 1981. 21, [121] p.

**Antall J, Kapronczay K:** Toldy Ferenc az orvos. **Orvostort Kozl** 1979;87-88(25 no 1-2):105-22

**Antall J:** Wien und Budapest im Lebenswerk Semmelweis'. **Wien Med Wochenschr** 1982 Apr 15;132(7):161-7

**Antall J:** Wien und Budapest im Lebenswerk Semmelweis'. In Ganzinger K, Skopec M, Wyklicky H, ed: Festschrift für Erna Lesky zum 70. Geburtstag. Wien, Brüder Hollinek, 1981. p. 13-23.

**Antall J** see **Habrich C**

**Antepowicz J:** Historia leczenia przetoki okołloodbytniczej. **Wiad Lek** 1981 May 15;34(10):863-6

**Antepowicz J:** Historia leczenia przetoki okołoodbytniczej w piśmiennictwie polskim. **Wiad Lek** 1981 Jun 1;34(11):957-61

**Anthony D** see **Robbins T**

**Antic D** see **Sarac S**

**Antipenko E** see **Kuzin M**

**Antiseri D:** Metaphysical ideas and the development of science. **Riv Biol** 1981 Winter;74(4):529-42

**Antiseri D** see **Epistemologia, metodologia clinica e storia della scienza medica, 1**

**Antiseri D** see **Epistemologia, metodologia clinica e storia della scienza medica, 2**

**Antler J:** Medical women and social reform--a history of the New York Infirmary for Women and Children. **Women Health** 1976 Jul-Aug;1(4):11-15,18

**Antman EM** see **Lamas GA**

**Antoine JP:** 'Les horreurs' anatomiques de Florence. **Histoire** 1980;26:96-8

**Antoine ME, Waquet J:** La médecine civile en France a l'époque napoléonienne et le legs du XVIIIe siècle: étude d'un recrutement professionnel. **Rev Inst Napoleon (Paris)** 1976;(132):67-90

**Antón Fructuoso P:** Las ideas biológicas en la psiquiatría de ayer. **Rev Med Univ Navarra** 1981 Sep;25(3):59-62

**Anton'ev AA, Milich VM, Suvorova KN:** K 50-letiiu tsentral'nogo ordena Lenina instituta usovershenstvovaniia vracheĭ. **Vestn Dermatol Venerol** 1980 Aug;(8):33-8

**Antonina M** see **Spor E, ed**

**Antonov AM:** Kafedre patologicheskoĭ anatomii Saratovskogo ordena Trudovogo Krasnogo Znameni meditsinskogo instituta 70 let (1911-1981). **Arkh Patol** 1981;43(7):80-3

**Antonov VB** see **Petrov NS**

**Antonovich T:** Ima podviga--gumanizm. **Med Sestra** 1981 Dec;40(12):41-4

**Antoszewski Z:** Krótki rys historyczny rozwoju pozaustrojowego krażenia krwi i niektórych aparatórych aparatów sztuczne 'płuco-serce'. **Przegl Lek** 1979;36(12):869-72

**Antunovic-Mikačič S:** O počecima mikrobiološke dijagnostike u Dalmaciji do 1923. g. In: I simpozij o historiji mikrobiologije i imunologije u Hrvatskoj do 1923. godine. Zagreb, Jugoslavenskoj akademiji, 1973. p. 5-15.

**Anufrieva VN** see **Kupriianova ES**

**Anvaripour P** see **Blum L**

**Anzieu D, Carapanos F, Gillibert J, et al:** Psychanalyse et culture grecque. Paris, Société d'Edition 'Les Belles Lettres,' 1980. 243 p.

**Anzures y Bola/ac/nos MC** see **Esteyneffer J de**

**Aoki N:** [Aging report: an observation on geriatric care in England. 4. History of geriatric care] (Jpn). **Kangogaku Zasshi** 1982 Apr;46(4):466-8

**Apeldoorn J:** Cook Islanders' attitude toward excessive drinking of alcohol. **Int J Addict** 1983 May;18(4):583-7

**Apffelstaedt G:** Militärlazarette während des Bürgerkrieges in den USA anhand von Beispielen aus den Bezirken Washington, District of Columbia, Baltimore, Maryland, Philadelphia, Pennsylvanien und New York. Münster, Murken-Altrogge, 1981. 203 p. (Studien zur Geschichte des Krankenhauswesens, 6)

**Aponte GE** see **Brooks JJ**

**Apostolopoulos DG:** Alexandros Maurokordatos. **Ellenika** 1976;29:311-5

**Apostolov M:** D-r Robert Iur'evich Berzin (1887-1950 g.) i bolnitsata na ruskiia Cherven krust v Sofiia. **Khirurgiia (Sofiia)** 1982;35(2):223-7

**Apostolov M, Kodov H:** The Hilendar medical collection. In International Congress of the History of Medicine. 26th, Plovdiv, 1978. Actes du Congress. Sofia, 1981. Volume II. p. 55-7.

**Apostolov MA:** Pervaia Bolgarskaia khirurgicheskaia shkola. **Klin Med (Mosk)** 1984 Oct;62(10):149-51

**Apothekerspotten:** Apothecary jars. The Hague, Gemeentemuseum, 1979. [59] p.

**Appel T** see **Davis A**

**Appel TA:** The archives of the American Physiological Society. **Physiologist** 1984 Jun;27(3):131-2

**Appel TA:** The 1941-42 search for an APS emblem. **Physiologist** 1984 Apr;27(2):69-70

**Appelboom T, Boelpaepe C de, Ehrlich GE, et al:** Rubens and the question of antiquity of rheumatoid arthritis. **JAMA** 1981 Feb 6;245(5):483-6

**Appelgryn MS:** Die siektetoestand en laaste dae van president T. F. Burgers. **Kleio (S Afr)** 1980;12(1-2):18-31

**Appell RA:** Medical aspects of the Confederacy (1861--1865). **South Med J** 1980 Jun;73(6):784-6

**Appels A:** Cultural aspects of coronary prone behavior. An approach from the history of art. **Adv Cardiol** 1982;29:32-6

**Apple RD:** 'How shall I feed my baby?' Infant feeding in the United States, 1870-1940. Ph. D. Diss., University of Wisconsin. Madison, 1981. xxxiii, 428 p.

**Apple RD:** Lillie Rosa Minoka-Hill. In: Notable American women. The modern period. Cambridge, Mass., Belknap-Harvard Univ. Press, 1980. 4:481-3.

**Apple RD:** 'To be used only under the direction of a physician': commercial infant feeding and medical practice, 1870-1940. **Bull Hist Med** 1980 Fall;54(3):402-17

**Apple RD, comp:** Illustrated catalogue of the slide archive of historical medical photographs at Stony Brook; Center for Photographic Images of Medicine and Health Care. Westport, Conn., Greenwood, 1984. xi, 442 p.

**Appleby A** see **Charbonneau H**

**Appleby AB:** Epidemics and famine in the little ice age 1550-1700. **J Interdiscip Hist** 1980;10:643-63

**Appleby AB:** Famine in Tudor and Stuart England. Stanford, Stanford Univ. Press, 1978. 250 p.

**Appleby AB:** The disappearance of plague: a continuing puzzle. **Econ Hist Rev** 1980;33(2):161-73

**Appleby AB** see **Webster C, ed**

**Appleby JH:** Doctor Christopher Reitinger and a seal of Tsar Boris Godunov. **Oxf Slav Pap** 1979;12:32-9

**Appleby JH:** Dr. Arthur Dee: merchant and litigant. **Slav East Eur Rev** 1979;57(1):32-55

**Appleby JH:** Ginseng and the Royal Society. **Notes Rec R Soc Lond** 1983 Mar;37(2):121-45

**Appleby JH:** Ivan the Terrible to Peter the Great: British formative influence on Russia's medico-Apothecary system. **Med Hist** 1983 Jul;27(3):289-304

**Appleby JH:** New light on John Woodall, surgeon and adventurer. **Med Hist** 1981 Jul;25(3):251-68

**Appleby JH:** 'Rhubarb' Mounsey and the Surinam toad--a Scottish physician--naturalist in Russia. **Arch Nat Hist** 1982 Oct;11(1):137-52

**Appleby JH, Cunningham A:** Robert Erskine and Archibald Pitcairne: two Scottish physicians' outstanding libraries. **Bibliotheck** 1982;11:3-16

**Appleby JH:** Robert Erskine--Scottish pioneer of Russian natural history. **Arch Nat Hist** 1982 Apr;10(3):377-98

**Applegryn MS:** Die ontstaan van die eerste gesondheitskomitee van Johannesburg. **Kleio (S Afr)** 1971;3(2):1-7

**Appleyard RT:** Economic demography of the twentieth century. In Stanley NF, Joske RA, ed: Changing disease patterns and human behaviour. London, New York, Academic Press, 1980. p. 389-401.

**Arabian medicine in the Middle Ages: J R Soc Med** 1984 May;77(5):438

**Aracil P** see **Remy C**

**Aragon F:** La politica cientifica en la España del s. XVIII a traves de la revista 'Anales de Ciencias Naturales', Madrid, 1799-1804. **Llull (Spain)** 1978;2:19-25

**Aragon R** see **Canalis RF**

**Aragon RM** see **Canalis RF**

**Araki S** see **Kato M**

**Arana Soto S:** El Hospital de Puerto Rico. San Juan de Puerto Rico, [s.n.], 1976. 296 p.

**Arana Soto S:** La oftalmología en Puerto Rico hasta el 1898. [s.l., s. n.], 1977. 61 p.

**Arata LA:** Nostalgia: the medicine show. **J Indiana State Med Assoc** 1980 Jun;73(6):353

**Aráujo A, Ferreira LF, Confalonieri UE, et al:** Eggs of Diphyllobothrium pacificum in precolumbian human coprolites. **Paleopathol Newsl** 1983 Mar;41:11-3

**Araújo AJ, Confalonieri UE, Ferreira LF:** Oxyurid infestations in small animals from 9,000 B.P. in Brazil. **Paleopathol Newsl** 1980 Sep;(31):13-14

**Aráujo AJ de** see **Ferreira LF**

**Arbini R:** Did Descartes have a philosophical theory of sense perception? **J Hist Philos** 1983;21:317-37

**Arbouet C** see **Buffat JJ**

**Arcamone F** see **Di Marco A**

**Arce J:** De Feijoo a Quintana. Testimonios lingüistico-literarios sobre inoculación y vacuna. **Bol Cent Estud Siglo XVIII** 1978;6:3-18

**Arceneaux MG:** Acadian to Cajun: population, family, and wealth in southwest Louisiana, 1765-1854. Ph.D. Diss., Brigham Young University, Provo, 1982. xii, 436 p.

**Archer S:** Historical perspective on the chemistry and development of naltrexone. **Natl Inst Drug Abuse Res Monogr Ser** 1981;28:3-10

**Archi A:** La peste presso gli Ittiti. **Parola Passato** 1978;179:81-9

**Archibald RM:** A short historical note on the Conjoint DIH. **J Soc Occup Med** 1984 Aug;34(3):80

**Archila R:** Discurso de orden pronunciado el 23 de junio de 1982 con motivo del traslado de los restos del Doctor Luis Razetti al Panteón Nacional. Caracas, Miguel Angel Garcia, 1982. 18 p.

**Archila R** see **Bowers JZ**

**Archinard M:** Nouvelle salle de microscopes au Musée d'histoire des Sciences. **Mus Geneve** 1982;224:7-13

**Archives and manuscripts [in] The Alan Mason Chesney Medical Archives, The Johns Hopkins Medical Institutions:** Baltimore, The Johns Hopkins University and The Johns Hopkins Hospital, 1980. 64 p.

**Arcuri EA:** Conheça um pouco de sua opção: enfermagem. **Rev Esc Enferm USP** 1982 Aug;16(2):127-36

**Ardelt R:** Geschichte des Konventes und Krankenhauses der Elisabethinen zu Linz. **Hist Jahrb Stadt Linz** 1978;:95-146

**Arderne J:** A fourteenth-century description of rectal cancer. **World J Surg** 1983 Mar;7(2):304-7

**Ardila R:** La Psicologia contemporanea. Buenos Aires, Paidos, 1972. 212 p.

**Ardila R** see **Brozek J**

**Ardolino F:** The saving hand of God: the significance of the emblematic frontispiece of the Religio medici. **Engl Lang Notes** 1977;15:19-23

**Ardry R:** Alchimie, une odeur de soufre. **Rev Hist Pharm (Paris)** 1984 Mar;31(260):13-7

**Ardry R:** Alchimie, une odeur de soufre. **Rev Hist Pharm (Paris)** 1984 Jun;31(261):121-30

**Arechabaleta G de:** Historia de la antropología física en Venezuela. Caracas, Universidad Central de Venezuela, Facultad de Ciencias Económicas y Sociales, División de Publicaciones, 1973. 30 p.

**Arena JM:** Medical student life at Duke fifty years ago. **NC Med J** 1983 Apr;44(4):235-7

**Arena JM:** The pediatrician's role in the poison control movement and poison prevention. **Am J Dis Child** 1983 Sep;137(9):870-3

**Arenander E:** Kirurgi under föranestetisk tid--ur anteckningar efter Anders Johan Hagströms Operations Collegium. **Nord Medicinhist Arsb** 1981;:88-105

**Arendarevskiĭ LF** see **Pozmogov AI**

**Arendt A:** Die Rolle der Neuropathologie in der Allgemeinen Pathologie und Speziellen Pathologischen Anatomie. **Zentralbl Neurochir** 1983;44(2):113-20

**Arendt H** see **Spicker SF, ed**

**Arendt HJ:** Eine demokratische Massenbewegung unter Führung der KPD im Frühjahr 1931. **Z Geschichtswiss** 1971;19(2):212-23

**Argemi-Lloveras J** see **Marinesco M**

**Arianoff AA:** Historique de la chirurgie biliaire. A propos du centenaire de la première cholécystectomie. **Acta Chir Belg** 1983 Jul-Aug;(4):241-52

**Arias O:** Evolución natural de la sífilis y del mal del pinto. In Academia Nacional de Medicina. Libro conmemorativo del primer centenario. México, Comité Editorial de la Comisión Organizadora del Congreso del Centenario, 1964. Tome 2. p. 83-6.

**Arias S:** In connection with the Waardenburg commemoration, Dr. Sergio Arias has submitted the following correspondence. **Am J Med Genet** 1980;7(1):41-5

**Aries NR:** Abortion clinics and the organization of work: a case study of Charles Circle. **Rev Radic Polit Econ** 1980;12(2):53-62

**Ariès P:** Døden i historien. **Samtiden (Norway)** 1980;89(3):7-14

**Ariès P:** Invisible Death. **Wilson Q** 1981;5(1):105-15

**Ariès P:** La contraception autrefois. **Histoire** 1978;1:36-44

**Ariès P:** L'homme devant la mort. Paris, Seuil, 1977. 641 p.

**Ariès P:** The hour of our death. New York, Knopf, 1981. xvii, 651 p.

**Aring CD:** A medical perspective. **Neurology** 1984 Oct;34(10):1357-61

**Aring CD:** The Boston City Hospital days with Drs. Merritt and Putnam. **Epilepsia** 1983;24 Suppl 1:S1-3

**Arion R:** Prof. C. Ionescu-Mihăieşti, o personalitate de însemnătate fundamentală în istoria medicinii preventive din România. **Rev Ig [Bacteriol]** 1984 Jan-Mar;29(1):89-95

**Arisi F** see **De Leo D**

**Arjona Castro A:** La poblacion de Córdoba en el siglo XIX. Sanidad y crisis demográfica en la Córdoba decimonónica. Córdoba, Instituto de Historia de Andalucia, Universidad de Córdoba, 1979. 184 p.

**Arkhangel'skaia LN** see **Roshchin AV**

**Arkhangel'skiĭ AE** see **Akimov GA**

**Arkhangel'skiĭ GA:** N. A. Belogolovyĭ--obshchestvennyĭ vrach, zhurnalist

(k 150–letiiu so dnia rozhdeniia). **Sov Zdravookhr** 1984;(10):67–70
**Arkhangel'skiĭ GV:** A. I. Gertsen i S. P. Botkin. **Klin Med (Mosk)** 1982 Nov;60(11):118–20
**Arkhangel'skiĭ GV:** K istorii izucheniia neĭromaliarii i soliarnogo sindroma. **Zh Nevropatol Psikhiatr** 1982;82(7):128–30
**Arkhangel'skiĭ GV:** K prioritetu opisaniia akademikom V. M. Bekhterevym khoreicheskoĭ paducheĭ. **Zh Nevropatol Psikhiatr** 1981;81(6):929–30
**Arkhangel'skiĭ GV:** L.F. Zmeev–vydaiushchiĭsia otechestvennyĭ istorik meditsiny i bibliograf. **Sov Zdravookhr** 1979;(8):64–7
**Arkhangel'skiĭ GV:** Moskovskiĭ vrach–gumanist Fedor Petrovich Gaaz (1780–1853) i ego znachenie v razvitii otechestvennoĭ meditsiny. **Klin Med (Mosk)** 1981 Feb;59(2):118–20
**Arkhangel'skiĭ GV:** N. S. Leskov o problemakh zdravookhraneniia (k 150–letiiu so dnia rozhdeniia pisatelia). **Sov Zdravookhr** 1981;(10):63–5
**Arkhangel'skiĭ GV:** Primenenie naukovedcheskikh metodov vi istorii meditsiny. **Sov Zdravookhr** 1981;(3):70–3
**Arkhangel'skiĭ GV:** S. P. Botkin i M. E. Saltykov–Shchedrin. **Klin Med (Mosk)** 1982 Oct;60(10):114–8
**Arkhangel'skii GV:** S. P. Botkin i otechestvennye deiateli muzykal'noĭ i khudozhestvennoĭ kul'tury. **Klin Med (Mosk)** 1982 May;60(5):112–7
**Arkhangel'skiĭ GV:** S. P. Botkin i pisateli–revoliutsionery demokraty. **Sov Zdravookhr** 1983;(2):60
**Arkhangel'skiĭ GV:** Teoreticheskie vzgliady S. P. Botkina po klinicheskim i obshchepatologicheskim voprosam meditsiny (k 150–letiiu so dnia rozhdeniia). **Klin Med (Mosk)** 1981 Nov;59(11):109–13
**Arkhangel'skiĭ GV:** V. E. Larionov––odin iz osnovopolozhnikov otechestvennoĭ otonevrologii. **Vestn Otorinolaringol** 1984 Mar–Apr;(2):88–93
**Arkhangel'skiĭ GV:** V. M. Bekhterev––vydaiushchiĭsia deiatel' otechestvennoĭ nauki (k 125–letiiu so dnia rozhdeniia). **Klin Med (Mosk)** 1983 Feb;61(2):106–10
**Arkhangel'skiĭ GV:** Vklad Akademika G.I. Markelova v teoriiu otechestvennoĭ nevrologii (k 100–letiiu so dnia rozhdeniia). **Klin Med (Mosk)** 1980 Oct;58(10):114–8
**Arkhangel'skiĭ GV:** Vrachebnoe okruzhenie vydaiusnchegosia Russkogo poéta V. A. Zhukovskogo (k 200–letiiu so dnia rozhdeniia). **Klin Med (Mosk)** 1984 May;62(5):139–44
**Arkhangel'skiĭ GV:** Vrachi meditsina v tvorchestve N. S. Leskova (k 150–letiiu so dnia rozhdeniia pisatelia). **Klin Med (Mosk)** 1981;59(10):114–7
**Arkhangel'skiĭ GV:** Znachenie S. P. Botkina v razvitii otechestvennoĭ nevrologii. **Klin Med (Mosk)** 1983 Apr;61(4):105–9
**Arkhangel'skiĭ GV** see **Lisitsyn IuP**
**Arlow JA** see **Ostow M**
**Armagnac C, Retel–Laurentin A:** Relations between fertility, birth intervals, foetal mortality and maternal health in Upper Volta. **Popul Stud** 1981 Jul;35(2):217–34
**Armas Cruz R:** Alguna meditaciones sobre la medicina actual. **Rev Med Chil** 1980 Apr;108(4):338–50
**Armelagos GJ, Carlson DS, Van Gerven DP:** The theoretical foundations and development of skeletal biology. In F. Spencer, ed: A history of American physical anthropology, 1930–1980. New York, Academic Press, 1982. p. 305–28.
**Armelagos GJ** see **Bassett EJ**
**Armelagos GJ** see **Goodman AH**
**Armelagos GJ** see **Lovejoy CO**
**Armelagos GJ** see **Martin DL**
**Armendares S** see **Campillo–Sainz C**
**Armocida G:** Annotazioni sull'ospedalità privata per malati di mente nella prima metà dell'800: l'esempio di Milano. In International Congress of the History of Medicine, 27th, Barcelona, 1980. Actas. Barcelona, Académia de Ciències Médiques de Catalunya i Balears, 1981. p. 23–6.
**Armocida G, Ambrosoli C, Finavera L, et al:** Gli 'ospizi privati per i pazzi' in Milano nel 1846. **Minerva Psichiatr** 1980 Jan–Mar;21(1):57–62
**Armocida G, Ambrosoli C, Majeron MA:** Note biografich intorno a Vincenzo Racchetti (1777–1819). Contributo alla storia della neurologia. **Minerva Med** 1980 Apr 21;71(16):1221–6
**Armoroli M, ed:** Le cere anatomiche Bolognesi del settecento. Catalogo della mostra organizzata Settembre–Novembre 1981. Bologna, Università degli Studi di Bologna, Accademia delle Scienze, 1981. 97 p. Contributions by R. A. Bernabeo, L. Bonuzzi, F. Ruggeri.
**Armstrong C:** Federalism and government regulation: the case of the Canadian insurance industry, 1927–34. **Can Public Adm** 1976;19(1):88–101
**Armstrong D:** Child development and medical ontology. **Soc Sci Med [Med Psychol Med Sociol]** 1979 Jan;13(1):9–12
**Armstrong D:** Political anatomy of the body. Medical knowlege in Britain in the twentieth century. Cambridge, Cambridge University Press, 1983. xii, 146 p.
**Armstrong D:** The doctor–patient relationship: 1930–80. In P. Wright, A. Treacher, ed: The problem of medical knowledge. Examining the social construction of medicine. Edinburgh, Edinburgh University Press, 1982. p. 109–22.
**Armstrong D:** The invention of the normal child. **Soc Soc Hist Med Bull (Lond)** 1980;27:32
**Armstrong D:** The Peckham key: ideal project and terrifying dream. **Soc Soc Hist Med Bull (Lond)** 1983 Dec;33:9–10
**Armstrong L:** The cradle of sexual politics. **Frontiers** 1981;6(1–2):19–25
**Armstrong PB** see **Smith JH, ed**
**Armstrong PC, Beary JF:** Office of the Assistant Secretary of Defense for Health Affairs: a history. **Milit Med** 1983 Aug;148(8):637–43
**Armstrong WA:** The trend of mortality in Carlisle between the 1780s and the 1840s: a demographic contribution to the standard of living debate. **Econ Hist Rev** 1981;34(1):91–114
**Armytage WH:** Issue at stake: the biosocial background. **Hist Educ** 1981;10(3):183–94
**Arnaiz Bonilla A:** Las afamadas boticas burgalesas de los hospitales de San Juan y San Julian y San Quirce (Barrantes). Burgos, Exma. Diputacíon Provincial de Burgos, [1981]. 152 p.
**Arnaldez R:** The theory and practice of science according to Ibn Sina and al–Biruni. **Stud Philos Med** 1977 Mar;1(1):58–69
**Arnau de Vilanova** see **Paniagua Arellano JA**
**Arnaud G** see **Lagier R**
**Arnaud P:** Le Corps en mouvement: précurseurs et pionniers de l'éducation physique. Toulouse, Privat, 1981. 314 p.
**Arnaud S** see **Lagier R**
**Arndal S:** Krop, sjael og ånd Georg Ernst Stahls og Christian Friedrich Richters medicinske antropologi. **Dan Medicinhist Arbog** 1980;:126–66
**Arndt C** see **Arndt KH**
**Arndt KA:** Archives of Dermatology. Second century. **Arch Dermatol** 1984 Jan;120(1):42–3
**Arndt KH, Arndt C:** Die Medizin bei Olympia. **Z Arztl Fortbild (Jena)** 1980 Apr 15;74(8):389–92
**Arney WR:** Power and the profession of obstetrics. Chicago, London, University of Chicago Press, 1982. xi, 290 p.
**Arnold E:** La lutte contre la tuberculose. **Rev Med Swisse Romande** 1982 Mar;102(3):231–9
**Arnold E** see **Bernische Liga gegen die Tuberkulose 1930–1980**
**Arnold G:** Breve storia delle estrazioni dentarie dall'antichità ai nostri giorni. **Dent Cadmos** 1980 Dec;48(12):61–3
**Arnold HJ:** Die Geschichte der Akupunktur in Deutschland. Heidelberg Haus, 1976. 128 p.
**Arnold HL:** How 'indeterminate' leprosy got its name. **Int J Dermatol** 1981 Jun;20(5):393–5
**Arnold HL:** Landmark perspective: penicillin and early syphilis. **JAMA** 1984 Apr 20;251(15):2011–2
**Arnold HL:** Udo Julius Wile, A.B., M.D., LL.D. (1882–1965). **J Am Acad Dermatol** 1984 Jan;10(1):157–62
**Arnold LJ:** Valentine Greatrakes, a seventeenth–century 'touch–doctor'. **Eire Irel** 1976;11:3–12
**Arnold O:** Charité et maladie dans la 1re moitié du XIXe siècle. **Penelope** 1981;(5):41–4
**Arnold P:** The education of the deaf child: for integration or autonomy? **Am Ann Deaf** 1984 Feb;129(1):29–37
**Arnoulet F:** L'oeuvre hospitalière des Trinitaires et des Capucine dans le Régence de Tunis. **Cah Tunis** 1978;26(3–4):35–48
**Arntzenius AC, ed** see **Snellen HA**
**Arnulf G:** A propos de la naissance de la radiologie en France. L'oeuvre d'Etienne Destot à Lyon. **Bull Acad Natl Med (Paris)** 1981 Oct;165(7):955–9
**Aron E:** Bretonneau et sa légende. **Hist Sci Med** 1980;14(2):187–91
**Aron E:** Louis XI et ses guérisseurs. Chambray, C. L. D., [1983]. 197 p.
**Aron E** see **Histoire culturelle de la maladie**
**Aron JP:** Le régime des nourrices au début du XIXe siècle à Paris. In: Congrès National des Sociétés Savantes, 93e, Tours, 1968. Actes. Paris, 1971. Section d'Histoire Moderne et Contemporaine, Tome 1. p. 207–15.
**Aron JP:** Odontoiatria del passato. Mutamenti del 'potere medico' in Francia dalla rivoluzione ad oggi. **Dent Cadmos** 1982 Mar;50(3):65–9
**Aron JP** see **Forster R**
**Aronsfeld CC:** 'Perish Judah': Nazi Extermination Propaganda 1920–1945. **Patterns Prejudice** 1978:12(5):17–26
**Aronson ME:** Sherlock Holmes, father of forensic pathology. **Trans Stud Coll Physicians Phila** 1978 Jul;45(5):258–61
**Aronson N:** Nutrition as a social problem: a case study of entrepreneurial strategy in science. **Soc Probl** 1982;29(5):474–87
**Aronson N:** Social factors in the development of nutrition studies: 1880–1920. **J NAL Assoc** 1980;5(1–2):32–7
**Aronson SM:** Lead and the demon rum in colonial America. **RI Med J** 1983 Jan;66(1):37–40
**Aroua A:** Hygiene et prevention médicale chez Ibnou Sina (Avicenne). Alger, S.N.E.D., [1974?]. 106 p.
**Aroua A:** L'hygiène et la prevention chez Ibn Sina. **Tunis Med** 1980 Jul–Aug;58(4):556–61
**Arouca AS:** El trabajo médico, la producción capitalista y la viabilidad del proyecto de prevención. **Rev Mex Cienc Polit Soc** 1976;22(84):33–56
**Arques J, Suñe JM:** Razones que motivaron la individualizacion de la Catedra de Historia de la Farmacia de la Universidad Central, en 1896. **Bol Soc Esp Hist Farm** 1983 Mar–Jun;34(133–134):3–10
**Arquiola E:** Anatomia y antropologia en el positivismo frances. **Asclepio** 1978–79;30–31:19–32
**Arquiola E:** Anatomía y antropología en la obra de Olóriz. **Dynamis** 1981;1:165–77
**Arquiola E:** Anatomia y antropologia fisica en el positivismo español. **Asclepio** 1981;33:3–22
**Arquiola E:** Darwinism in the Société d'Anthropologie de Paris. **Clio Med** 1980 May;14(2):119–28
**Arquiola E:** La antropologia criminal y la 'Societe d'Anthropologie' de Paris. **Asclepio** 1978–79;30–31:63–82
**Arquiola E:** La enfermedad en la antropología física francesa durante el positivismo. **Asclepio** 1983;35:217–26
**Arquiola E:** La lesión neurologica en 'De sedibus et causis morborum' de Morgagni. In: Congrès international d'histoire de la médecine, XXVe, Québec, 1976. Actes. Québec, 1977. p. 461–8.

**Arquiola E:** Topinard: medico y antropologo fisico. **Asclepio** 1978–79;30–31:41–61
**Arquiola E** see **Peset JL**
**Arquiola E** see **Peset M**
**Arrebola Nacle P** see **Valverde JL**
**Arreguín E:** Datos historicos sobre la fundacion de la escuela medica de Michoacan. **Bol Soc Mex Hist Filos Med** 1980 Sep–Dec;5(32–33):57–65
**Arrieta JA** see **Barba J**
**Arrigoni T:** Fra la curiosità e la scienza. **Kos** 1984 May;1(4):47–64
**Arseneau JC, Thigpen JT:** The new quack--pseudoscience, public relations and politics. **J Miss State Med Assoc** 1981 Aug;22(8):202–7
**Arseni C, Ciurea AV:** The history of Romanian neurosurgery. Bucharest, Medical Publishing House, 1981. 21 p.
**Arsuaga JL** see **Pérez PJ**
**Arsuaga JL de** see **Pérez PJ**
**Arthur AR** see **Johannes Adelphus**
**Arthurs R:** The man who played doctor. **Civ War Times Illus** 1980;19(5):36–8
**Artía A:** Centenario de la fundación de la Sociedad Alemana de Pediatría. Influencia de ésta en la pediatría chilena. **Rev Chil Pediatr** 1983 Nov–Dec;54(6):387–9
**Articus R:** Geschichte der alten Husumer Apotheken: ein Beitrag zur Geschichte des Gesundheitswesens in Schleswig-Holstein. Husum, Schwan-Apotheke, 1981. 76 p.
**Artiges A:** L'institution de la Pharmacopée Européenne: un bilan à l'issue de la première édition. **Inf Pharm** 1980 Apr;(232):506–44
**Artiukhov SA:** Sochinskaia gospital'naia baza v gody Velikoĭ Otechestvennoĭ voĭny. **Voen Med Zh** 1981 Mar;(3):70–2
**Artiukhov SA:** Sochinskaia gospital'naia baza v gody Velikoĭ Otechestvennoĭ voĭny. **Sov Zdravookhr** 1981;(9):66–7
**Arton M:** Children first and always. **Nurs Times** 1982 Oct 6–12;78(40):1687–8
**Arton M:** The development of psychiatric nursing education in England and Wales. **Nurs Times** 1981 Jan 15;77(3):124–7
**Arts en sameleving. Medical history contributions by H. W. Pleket, J. Van Herwaarden, W. Frijhoff, C. Offringa, M. J. Van Lieburg, C. Bakker-Van der Kooij: Tijdschr Geschied Geneeskd** 1983;96:323–475
**Arturson G:** The history of burns treatment in Sweden. **Scand J Plast Reconstr Surg** 1984;18(1):11–20
**Aruffo C** see **Escobar A**
**Arvanitakis K** see **Goldman DL**
**Arvy L:** Clara Louise Maass (1876–1901) et la fièvre jaune. **Clio Med** 1979 May;13(3–4):277–82
**Arvy L, Rivet R:** Dupuytren (1777–1835) face à l'énigme qu'était la fièvre jaune en 1826. In: Congrès National des Sociétés Savantes, 102e, Limoges, 1977. Comptes Rendus. Paris, 1977. Section des Sciences, Fasc. III. p. 27–32.
**Arvy L:** Jean-Baptiste Marcellin Bory de Saint-Vincent (1778–1846) et les 'Animaux Spermatiques'. In: Congrès National des Sociétés Savantes, 104e, Bordeaux, 1979. Comptes Rendus. Paris, 1979. Section des Sciences, Fasc. IV. p. 21–5.
**Arzhantsev PZ:** Etapy razvitiia spetsializirovannoĭ stomatologicheskoĭ pomoshchi v GVKG imeni N. N. Burdenko. **Voen Med Zh** 1980 Feb;(2):78–80
**Arzua Zulaica E de:** Historia del fibroscopio. **Rev Esp Enferm Apar Dig** 1980 Jan;57(1):77–80
**Arzumetov IuS:** Ibn Sina--vrach-éntsiklopedist i nekotorye osnovy ego ucheniia o zdorov'e i bolezni (k 1000-letiiu so dnia rozhdeniia). **Fiziol Zh SSSR** 1980 Sep;66(9):1273–7
**Arzumetov IuS:** Voprosy gepatologii v 'Kanone vrachebnoĭ nauki' Ibn-Sina. **Sov Zdravookhr** 1980;(5):67–9
**As I remember: Clarence R. Straatsma: Ann Plast Surg** 1981 Oct;7(4):327–32
**As I remember Earl C. Padgett: Ann Plast Surg** 1981 Feb;6(2):142–57
**As I remember. T. P. Kilner.: Ann Plast Surg** 1980 Apr;4(4):328–36
**Asahino SN** see **Suyehiro H**
**Asatiani DK** see **Kurchishvili IB**
**Asbell MB:** The dental art and its practitioners in colonial Philadelphia. **Bull Phila Cty Dent Soc** 1981 Mar;46(6):6–11
**Ascenzi A, Cockburn A, Kleiss E:** Miscellaneous mummies. In A. Cockburn, E. Cockburn, ed: Mummies, disease, and ancient cultures. Cambridge, Cambridge University Press, 1980. p. 224–38.
**Ascuasiati de Alfau C:** Efémerides en la historia de la parasitología. [Santo Domingo], Dept. de Microbiología y Parasitología, Universidad Autónoma de Santa Domingo, 1982. 24 p.
**Asdonk J:** Die Physikalische Lymphdrainage- und Odemtherapie der Feldbergklinik. Eine historische Ubersicht über den derzeitigen Stand der physikalisch-lymphologischen Medizin. **Z Lymphol** 1983 Jul;7(1):40–6
**Asendorf MI:** Die gelehrten Arzte Joseph und Karl Wenzel, ihr Leben und Werk in Mainz und Frankfurt am Main. Diss. Mainz, 1981. 269 p.
**Ash L, Murray MA, ed:** Serial publications containing medical classics. An index to citations in Garrison/Morton (3rd edition, 1970). 2nd ed., revised and enlarged. Bethany, Connecticut, The Antiquarium, 1979, x, 169 p.
**Ash MG:** Academic politics in the history of science: experimental psychology in Germany, 1879–1941. **Cent Eur Hist** 1980;13(3):255–86
**Ash MG:** Disziplinentwicklung und Wissenschaftstransfer--Deutschsprachige Psychologen in der Emigration. **Ber Wissenschaftsgesch** 1984;7(4):207–26
**Ash MG:** The emergence of Gestalt theory: experimental psychology in Germany 1890–1920. Ph.D. Diss., Harvard University. Cambridge, 1982. xlii, 613 p.
**Ash MG** see **Brozek J**
**Ashby E:** The politics of clean air. Oxford, Clarendon Press, 1981. viii, 178 p.
**Ashby JK:** De aurium doloris et vitium curis or concerning the care of pain and troubles of the ears. **J Speech Hear Disord** 1980 Aug;45(3):424–5
**Ashcraft ML, Berki SE:** Health maintenance organizations as Medicaid providers. **Ann Am Acad Polit Soc Sci** 1983;(468):122–31
**Ashcroft MT:** Tercentenary of the first English book on tropical medicine, by Thomas Trapham of Jamaica. **Br Med J** 1979 Aug 25;2(6188):475–7
**Asherson N:** The age of John Hunter's golden guineas (1763–93). **Ann R Coll Surg Engl** 1982 Jul;64(4):262–5
**Ashmianskas IuI:** Prepodavanie gigieny pitaniia v Vil'niusskom universitete. **Gig Sanit** 1980 Jan;(6):42–3
**ASHP Research and Education Foundation dedicates the Donald E. Francke Memorial Library: Am J Hosp Pharm** 1982 Jul;39(7):1206–10
**Ashraf M** see **Said HM, ed**
**Ashton N:** Ophthalmological Societies of the United Kingdom. Centenary Meeting, April 1980. **Trans Ophthalmol Soc UK** 1980 Apr;100(pt 1):1–8
**Ashton RE, Andre P, Lowe NJ, et al:** Anthralin: historical and current perspectives. **J Am Acad Dermatol** 1983 Aug;9(2):173–92
**Ashton RM:** The Royal College of Midwives: past, present and future. **Int J Gynaecol Obstet** 1979–80 Sep–Oct;17(2):124–7
**Ashworth B:** The Bramwells and neurology in Edinburgh. **Scott Med J** 1981 Oct;26(4):364–70
**Asif M** see **Khan AB**
**Asimov I:** A short history of biology. Westport, Conn., Greenwood Press, 1980. ix, 189 p.
**Asimov I:** Asimov's biographical encyclopedia of science and technology. The lives and achievements of 1510 great scientists from ancient times to the present chronologically arranged. Second revised edition. Garden City, New York, Doubleday, 1982. xxxv, 941 p.
**Asimov MS, et al:** Avicenna. **Unesco Cour** 1980 Oct;33:1–46
**Asimov MS, et al:** [On the 1000th anniversary of Avicenna] (Rus). **Vopr Istor Estestvozn Tekh** 1980,4:69–76
**Asimova MZ, Kuznetsov VK, Piotrovskiĭ SM:** Abu Ali Ibn-Sina i znachenie ego nauchnogo naslediia v istorii akusherstva. **Feldsher Akush** 1980;45(5):59–61
**Askari H, Cummings J:** Food shortages in the Middle East. **Middle East Stud** 1978;14(3):326–51
**Askarov UA:** Znachenie trudov Akademika AMN SSSR I. A. Kassirskogo v nauchnoĭ razrabotke uzlovykh problem kraevoĭ patologii Uzbekistana (k 10-letiiu so dnia smerti). **Ter Arkh** 1982;54(2):150–2
**Askenasi R:** Plaidoyer pour une nouvelle spécialité. **Acta Clin Belg** 1983;38(4):265–70
**Askew M:** 'I have hay fever: I love you. George.' **Practitioner** 1979 Jun;222(1332):866–8
**Askew M:** The health of General Douglas MacArthur. **Practitioner** 1982 Oct;226(1372):1814–5
**Askienazy S** see **Huard P**
**Aslam M, Bano H, Vohora SB:** Sartan (cancer) and its treatment in Unami Medicine. **Am J Chin Med** 1981 Summer;9(2):95–107
**Asliddinov IF** see **Kadyrov AA**
**Asper SP, Haddad FS:** [History of medical ethics in the] contemporary Arab world. In Reich WT, et al, ed: Encyclopedia of bioethics, v. 2. New York, Free Press, 1978. p. 888–91.
**Aspinwall B:** Social Catholicism and health: Dr. and Mrs. Thomas Low Nichols in Britain. In Sheils WJ, ed: The Church and healing. Papers read at the twentieth summer meeting and the twenty-first winter meeting of the Ecclesiastical History Society. Oxford, Basil Blackwell for the Society, 1982. p. 249–70.
**Aspirin-bewährt: Krankenpfl J** 1982 Oct 15;20(10):14–5
**Asplund J:** The Scandinavian Association of Obstetricians and Gynecologists 1933–1983. **Acta Obstet Gynecol Scand [Suppl]** 1984;120:9–26
**Asquith GH:** Anton T. Boisen and the study of 'living human documents.' **J Presbyt Hist** 1982;60(3):244–65
**Asratian EA, Shingarov GKh:** Leninskaia teoriia otrazheniia i uchenie I. P. Pavlova o vyssheĭ nervnoĭ deiatel'nosti (k 110-i godovshchine so dnia rozhdeniia V. I. Lenina). **Zh Vyssh Nerv Deiat** 1980 Mar–Apr;30(2):227–34
**Assefi V:** Le lèpre en Iran. **Acta Leprol (Geneve)** 1982 Nov–Dec;(89):53–60
**Assennato G, Navarro V:** Workers' participation and control in Italy: the case of occupational medicine. **Int J Health Serv** 1980;10(2):217–32
**Assistance et charité:** Toulouse, Privat, 1978. 435 p. (Cahiers de Fanjeaux, Collection d'Histoire religieuse du Languedoc au XIIIe et début du XIVe siècles, 13).
**Astapenko VG:** Belorusskoe Nauchnoe Meditsinskoe Obshchestvo Khirurgov (k 50-letiiu obrazovaniia obshchestva). **Khirurgiia (Mosk)** 1980;1:113–4
**Astaurov BL:** Problemy obshcheĭ biologii i genetiki. Moskva, Nauka, 1979. 292 p.
**Astor G:** The disease detectives. Deadly medical mysteries and the people who solved them. New York, Scarborough, Ont., NAL Books, 1983. 216 p.
**Astrow A:** Anxiety - frustration - repressed hostility. An original drawing, painted in gouache, by Boris Artzybasheff. **J Hist Med Allied Sci** 1980 Oct;35(4):453
**Astrup P:** Blutgase und medizinische Säure-Basen-Chemie einst und jetzt. I. Blutgase. **Z Med Lab Diagn** 1984;25(6):299–306

**At the turn-of-the-decade: J Iowa Med Soc** 1980 Apr;70(4):144–58
**Ata-ur-Rahim M:** Medical literature on Pakistan from 1840–1947. **JPMA** 1980 Dec;30(12):281–2 concl
**Ata-ur-Rahim M:** The contribution of Muslim medical scientists during British period in India -- a bibliography. **JPMA** 1980 Apr;30(4):102–5 contd.
**Atabaev ShT, Babakhodzhaev NK, Il'inskiĭ II:** Gigiencheskie vzgliady Abu Ali ibn-Siny (k 1000-letiiu so dnia rozhdeniia). **Gig Sanit** 1979 Dec;(12):36–40
**Atallah W:** L'intérêt des traductions arabes dans l'édition des textes hippocratiques. In La collection hippocratique et son rôle dans l'histoire de la médecine. Colloque de Strasbourg (23–27 octobre 1972) organisé par le Centre de Recherches sur la Grèce Antique, avec le concours des Facultés de Philosophie et des Langues Classiques. Leiden, E. J. Brill, 1975. p. 19–33.
**Aterman K:** Connective tissue: an eclectic historical review with particular reference to the liver. **Histochem J** 1981 May;13(3):341–96
**Aterman K, MacSween HM, Perry PE, et al:** Recurrent infections, diarrhea, ascites and phonophobia in a 57-year-old man. **Can Med Assoc J** 1982 Mar 15;126(6):623–8
**Aterman K, Grimaud JA:** The brothers Lumière. Pioneers in medical photography. **Am J Dermatopathol** 1983 Oct;5(5):479–81
**Aterman K:** The development of the concept of lysosomes. A historical survey, with particular reference to the liver. **Histochem J** 1979 Sep;11(5):503–41
**Atherton DJ:** Joseph Towne: wax modeler extraordinary. **J Am Acad Dermatol** 1980 Sep;3(3):311–6
**Atiyeh M:** Arab hospitals in history. **King Faisal Spec Hosp Med J** 1982 Apr;2(2):121–6
**Atkins E:** Fever: its history, cause, and function. **Yale J Biol Med** 1982 May–Aug;55(3–4):283–9
**Atkins E:** Fever: the old and the new. **J Infect Dis** 1984 Mar;149(3):339–48
**Atkins H:** Memoirs of a surgeon. London, Springwood, 1977. xiv, 265 p.
**Atkinson P:** Fitness, feminism and schooling. In Sara Delamont, Lorna Duffin ed: The 19th-century woman: her cultural and physical world. London, Croom Helm, New York, Barnes & Noble, 1978. p. 92–133
**Atomic Bomb Casualty Commission:** The Atomic Bomb Casualty Commission, 1947–1975. [Hiroshima?] The Commission, [1978?] vi, 240 p.
**Atropine poisoning in Hawthorne's the Scarlet Letter: N Engl J Med** 1984 Nov 29;311(22):1438–41
**Attreed LC:** Preparation for death in sixteenth-century northern England. **Sixteenth Century J** 1982;13(3):37–66
**Attwood HD:** Matthew Baillie--a possible early description of amniotic fluid embolism. **Aust NZ J Obstet Gynaecol** 1979 Aug;19(3):176–7
**Attwood HD:** Patients, pathologists and practice. **Aust NZ J Obstet Gynaecol** 1982 Feb;22(1):11–4
**Attwood HD** see **Gault EW**
**Atwater EC:** 'Making fewer mistakes': a history of students and patients. **Bull Hist Med** 1983 Summer;57(2):165–87
**Atwater EC** see **Mazumdar PM**
**Atwater EC** see **Numbers RL, ed**
**Atwood GE:** The pursuit of being in the life and thought of Jean-Paul Sartre. **Psychoanal Rev** 1983 Summer;70(2):143–62
**Atwood GE** see **Goldberg A, ed**
**Atwood GE** see **Stolorow RD**
**Aucoin P:** Public policy analysis and the Canadian health care system. **Can Public Adm** 1980;23(1):166–74
**Audet LP:** Louis Giard. In Dictionary of Canadian biography, 1881–1890. 1982;11:345–6.
**Audet-Lapointe P, Perrault JL, Deslauriers L, et al:** L'Hôpital Notre-Dame de Montréal. **Union Med Can** 1980 Jan;109(1):16–8
**Aue-Hauser G** see **Bergman P**
**Auer EM:** 80 Geburtsbriefe aus den Büchern des Vizedomamtes in Oesterreich unter der Enns. **Jahrb Landeskd Niederoesterr** 1961–63;35:50–105
**Auer G:** Reste des hexenglaubens in Donnerskirchen. **Burgenl Heimatbl** 1973;35(3):109–24
**Auerbach C:** A pilgrim's progress through mutation research. **Perspect Biol Med** 1978 Spring;21(3):319–34
**Aufderheide AC, Neiman FD, Wittmers LE, et al:** Lead in bone II: skeletal-lead content as an indicator of lifetime lead ingestion and the social correlates in an archaeological population. **Am J Phys Anthropol** 1981 Jul;55(3):285–91
**Aufderheide AC** see **Streitz JM**
**Aufranc OE:** Trends in contemporary practice. Prefatory chapter. **Clin Orthop** 1983 May;(175):2–7
**Aufricht G:** Story of the foundation of the Plastic and Reconstructive Surgery journal and reminiscences of the early formative years of plastic surgery as a specialty. **Plast Reconstr Surg** 1981 Sep;68(3):370–5
**Augensen K, Koller O, Bergsjø P:** Mødredødelighet i Norge 1951–1980. **Tidsskr Nor Laegeforen** 1983 Feb 20;103(5):525–30
**Augusto León C** see **McCullough LB**
**Aul DJ:** Margaret Sanger labeled 'racist'. **Am J Public Health** 1981 Jan;71(1):91
**Aulas JJ:** La folie dans le cinéma allemand (1913–1933). **Ann Med Psychol (Paris)** 1980;138(8):925–38
**Aulas JJ** see **Simeoni CE**
**Aulie RP:** Evolution and special creation: historical aspects of the controversy. **Proc Am Philos Soc** 1983 Dec 30;127(6):418–62
**Aulizio F:** Come si estraevano i denti un tempo. Lo strumentario dentistico della Fondazione Putti ... Bologna. **Strenna Stor Bolognese** 1979;29:29–41
**Aulizio F:** Ideas for a renewed methodology in the research and in teaching the history of medicine. In: International Congress of the History of Medicine, 26th, Plovdiv (Bulgaria), 1978. Actes du Congres, Vol. 1. Sofia, 1980. p. 113–4.
**Aulizio F:** Il bambino nel passato e nel presente. **Minerva Pediatr** 1980 Jul 31;32(14):881–5
**Aulizio F:** Is the Hippocratic oath still uptodate today? In International Congress of the History of Medicine, 27th, Barcelona, 1980. Actas. Barcelona, Académia de Ciències Mèdiques de Catalunya i Balears, 1981. p. 441–5.
**Aulizio F:** Principi per una rinnovato metodologia nella ricerca e nell' insegnamento della storia della medicina. **Med Secoli** 1980 Jan–Apr;17(1):129–34
**Auman C, et al:** A state mental hospital and public welfare team up. **Public Welf** 1969;27(1):59–65
**Aumont B:** La situation démographique en USSR. **Contrat Soc** 1968;12(4):219–22
**Aumüller G:** Benedict Stillings (1810–1879) Untersuchungen über das Rückenmark--ein Wendepunkt in der neuroanatomischen Forschung. **Medizinhist J** 1984;19(1–2):53–69
**Aurach G:** Le jardin de richesses. Texte calligraphié et préface par B. Biebel. Neuilly-sur-Seine, Arma Artis, 1978. xix, 83 p.
**Aurel D:** De l'histoire des relations médicales franco-roumaines -- au 120e anniversaire de la mort de François Achard -- l'activité de François Achard en Roumanie. **Soc Fr Hist Art Dent** 1979 Sep–Dec;(5–6):30–3
**Aus dem Archiv der Psychoanalyse:** Carl Müller-Braunschweig: Psychoanalyse und Weltanschauung. **Psyche (Stuttg)** 1983 Dec;37(12):1136–45
**Aus dem Archiv der Psychoanalyse. John F. Rittmeister: Voraussetzungen und Konsequenzen der Jungschen Archetypenlehre: Psyche (Stuttg)** 1982 Nov;36(11):1032–44
**Ausman RK, Bellamy D Jr:** Problems and resolutions in the development of the flexible plastic blood container (Carl W. Walter). **Am J Surg** 1984 Nov;148(5):559–61
**Aussedat M** see **Picard JM**
**Austen R:** Stoddard's little tricks in South Sea Idyls. **J Homosex** 1983 Spring–Summer;8(3–4):73–81
**Austen WG:** Cardiovascular surgery: past, present, and future. **Cardiovasc Res Cent Bull** 1979 Jan–Mar;17(3):56–65
**Auster A** see **Quart L**
**Austin AL:** Isabel Maitland Stewart. In: Notable American women. The modern period. Cambridge, Mass., Belknap-Harvard Univ. Press, 1980. 4:660–2.
**Austin D, Hunnicutt BK:** National Therapeutic Recreation Society: the first twelve years. **Ther Recreation J** 1978 3d Quarter;12(3):4–14
**Austin F, Jones B:** The Clifts and the arts. **Ann R Coll Surg Engl** 1984 Jan;66(1):63–70
**Austin F:** The Letters of William Home Clift, 1803–1832. Dorset, Meldon House, 1983. ix, 115 p.
**Austin F, Jones B:** William Home Clift: the first assistant Conservator of the Hunterian Museum. **Ann R Coll Surg Engl** 1980 Jul;62(4):299–303
**Austin JH:** Chase, chance, and creativity: the lucky art of novelty. New York, Columbia Univ. Press, 1978. xvii, 237 p.
**Austin RT:** Treatment of broken legs before and after the introduction of gypsum. **Injury** 1983 Mar;14(5):389–94
**Austin Bradford Hill: Stat Med** 1982 Oct–Dec;1(4):305–9
**Austoni M** see **Epistemologia, metodologia clinica e storia della scienza medica, 2**
**Austrian R:** Perrin Hamilton Long. In Dictionary of American biography, 1961–1965. Suppl. 7, 1981. p. 477–8.
**Austrian R:** Pneumococcus: the first one hundred years. **Rev Infect Dis** 1981 Mar–Apr;3(2):183–9
**Austrian R:** Pneumonia in the later years. **J Am Geriatr Soc** 1981 Nov;29(11):481–9
**Austrian R:** Tracking the identity of Lister's pneumococcal groups T and V (Danish types 45 and 46). **Yale J Biol Med** 1982 May–Aug;55(3–4):173–8
**Autian J, Wood G:** The role of toxicology in the pharmacy curriculum. **Am J Pharm Educ** 1976 Nov,;40(4):378–82
**Autopsy: necessity or anachronism?: MD** 1980 Dec;24(12):75–8
**Avdeeva TA, Khazenson LB:** Osnovnye itogi 60-letnykh issledovaniĭ Leningradskogo Instituta épidemiologii i mikrobiologii imeni Pastera po ostrym kishechnym infektsiiam (1923–1983). **Zh Mikrobiol Epidemiol Immunobiol** 1984 Jan;(1):115–9
**Avellano E, Bedault M, Bedrani R, et al:** Un mémoire sur la contraception. **Soins Gynecol Obstet Pueric Pediatr** 1982 Jul–Aug;(14–15):55–61
**Avenarius R** see **Janzarik W ed**
**Averill LA:** Recollections of Clark's G. Stanley Hall. **J Hist Behav Sci** 1982 Oct;18(4):341–6
**Averill LC:** St. George's Hospital, the first fifty years. Christchurch, St. George's Hospital Executive, 1978. 169 p.
**Avery RC** see **Haines MR**
**El avicenismo: Med Tradic** 1980;3(10):33–6
**Avilov EN** see **Norovpil TS**
**Avilov EN** see **Zhamba G**
**Awad EA** see **Hamarneh SK**
**Axdorph S:** Den första 'röntgenblicken' - en studie av Leonardo da Vincis anatomiska bilder. **Lakartidningen** 1983 Dec 21;80(51):5005–8
**Axinn J:** Jessie Taft. In: Notable American women. The modern period.

Cambridge, Mass., Belknap-Harvard Univ. Press, 1980. 4:673-5.
**Axthelm H:** Fortbildung aus der Sicht einer 50 jährigen Praxistätigkeit. **Zahnarztl Mitt** 1984 Feb 1;74(3):227-30, 235
**Ayala FJ:** Darwin y la idea de progreso. **Arbor** 1982;113(441-2):59-75
**Ayd FJ** see **Settle EC**
**Ayer E, Montandon D:** Pierre Franco (1506-1580) and the treatment of a cheek ulcer. **Chir Plast** 1980;5(4):289-93
**Aymard M** see **Forster R**
**Aymonin GG:** Lamarck et son herbier. **Hist Nat** 1980-81;17-18:13-7
**Aymonin GG:** L'herbier de Lamarck. **Rev Hist Sci (Paris)** 1981;34:25-58
**Ayvasian LF:** American Thoracic Society: the fifty-five Trudeau medalists (1926-1980): a seventy-fifty anniversary review. **Am Rev Respir Dis** 1980 Apr;121(4):753-75
**Az Orvosi Hetilap múltjából: Orv Hetil** 1982 Jan 10;123(2):111
**Az Orvosi Hetilap múltjából: Orv Hetil** 1982 Apr 18;123(16):992-3 (continued periodically)
**Az Orvosi Hetilap múltjából: Orv Hetil** 1982 May 16;123(20):1250-1
**Az Orvosi Hetilap 125. évfordulója: Orv Hetil** 1982 Jan 3;123(1):3-4
**Az orvosi ismeretek elavulásáról és revíziójának szkségességéröl: Orv Hetil** 1984 Jun 10;125(24):1475-6
**Azar HA:** Arthur Purdy Stout (1885-1967). The man and the surgical pathologist. **Am J Surg Pathol** 1984 Apr;8(4):301-7
**Azeez Pasha M:** Biography of the Unani physician Arestu. **Bull Indian Inst Hist Med (Hyderabad)** 1978;8(1-4):26-31
**Azeez Pasha M:** Bukhrat (Hippocrates); the most famous physician of Yunan (Greece). **Bull Indian Inst Hist Med (Hyderabad)** 1975 Jul;5(3):129-42
**Azeez Pasha M:** Jalinoos [Galen] the famous physician of Yunan (Greece). **Bull Indian Inst Hist Med (Hyderabad)** 1975 Oct;5(4):211-24
**Azeez Pasha M:** Yusrul Ilaj; a Persian medical manuscript compiled in India by Hakeem Hidaetullah, in 1731 A.D. **Bull Inst Hist Med (Hyderabad)** 1973 Oct;3(4):201-6
**Azemar R:** Les causes de décès à La Roque-Sainte-Marguerite, en sud-Rouergue, de 1721 à 1742. **Ann Demogr Hist (Paris)** 1984;:239-58
**Azhenov MS:** Razvitie sotsial'noi struktury Kazakhstana v usloviiakh sotsializma. **Vopr Filos** 1980;8:44-51
**Aznar B:** Personalidad biologica de Azorín. Salamanca, Universidad de Salamanca, 1973. 73p. (Cuadernos de Historia de la Medicina Española, Monografias, 23).
**Aznarez EP:** Historia de la Facultad de Ciencias Médicas de Córdoba. **Medicina (B Aires)** 1982;42(2):204-12
**Aznárez EP:** Juan Bialet Massé, ilustre médico catalán emigrado a la Argentina. In International Congress of the History of Medicine, 27th, Barcelona, 1980. Actas. Barcelona, Académia de Ciències Médiques de Catalunya i Balears, 1981. p. 165-7.
**Azouvi F:** Irritabilité et magnétisme animal: une lettre inédite de J.-M.-A. Servan. **Dix-huit Siecle** 1982;14:191-7
**Azouvi F:** La peste, la mélancolie et le diable, ou l'imaginaire réglé. **Diogenes** 1979 Oct-Dec
**Azouvi F** see **Tissot SA**
**Azzaroli ML, Lanza B:** La Venere scomponibile. **Kos** 1984 May;1(4):65-81
**Azzi Visentini M:** Il giardino dei semplici die Padova: un prodotto della cultura del Rinascimento. **Comunita** 1980;34(182):259-338
**Azzone GF:** L'opinione di studiosi sulla vivisezione. **Minerva Med** 1980 May 7;71(18):1334-5

# B

**Baader G:** Der ärztliche Stand in der Antike. **Jahrb Univ Dusseld** 1977-78;:301-15
**Baader G:** Handschrift und Frühdruck als Ueberlieferungsinstrumente der Wissenschaften. **Ber Wissenschaftsgesch** 1980;3(1-2):7-22
**Baader G:** Medizinisches Reformdenken und Arabismus im Deutschland des 16. Jahrhunderts. **Sudhoffs Arch** 1979;63(3):261-96
**Baader G:** Naturwissenschaft und Medizin im 12. Jahrhundert und Hildegard von Bingen. **Arch Mittelrheinischen Kirchengesch** 1979;31:33-54
**Baader G:** Politisch motivierte Emigration deutscher Arzte. **Ber Wissenschaftsgesch** 1984;7(2):67-84
**Baader G:** Zu den Aufgaben der medizinhistorischen Forschung auf dem Gebiet der Geschichte der mittelalterlichen Medizin in der Gegenwart. In: International Congress of the History of Medicine, 26th, Plovdiv (Bulgaria), 1978. Actes du Congres, Vol. 1. Sofia, 1980. p. 85-8.
**Baader G** see **Habrich C**
**Baasher T:** Promotion and development of research in traditional medicine: the WHO role in countries of the Eastern Mediterranean Region. **J Ethnopharmacol** 1980 Mar;2(1):75-9
**Baatz D:** Das Badegebäude des Limeskastells Walldürn (Odenwaldkreis). **Saalburg Jahrb** 1978;35:61-107
**Babakhodzhaev NK** see **Atabaev ShT**
**Babayan R:** Reduktionsplastik der Mamma. **Med Welt** 1980 Nov 28 and Dec 19;31(48, 51-52):1873-6, 1767-9
**Babé J:** Amigdalectomía extracapsular con reconstrucción de la celda amigdalina. **An Otorrinolaringol Ibero Am** 1983;10(1):19-50
**Babecki JW:** Ze wspomnień czerwonokrzyskich na emigracji podczas II wojny światowej. **Arch Hist Med (Warsz)** 1980;43(3):317-22
**Babes V:** Opere alese. Vol. I. Bucuresti, Editura Academiei Republicii Socialiste Romania, 1979. 330 p. Biographical contributions by B. Dutescu, N. Marcu, and I. Moraru.
**Babeş VT:** Recent research on viral hepatitis performed in the 'Stefan S. Nicolau' Institute of Virology. **Virologie** 1984 Oct-Dec;35(4):251-7
**Babeş VT:** Some less well-known priorities of Victor Babeş. **Virologie** 1979 Jul-Sep;30(3):235-6
**Babic N** see **Beric B**
**Babic-Ilic N** see **Beric B**
**Babin E** see **Wackenheim A**
**Babin VP:** Iz opyta organizatsii lecheniia legkoranenykh v mediko-sanitarnom batal'one mekhanizirovannogo korpusa v gody Velikoĭ Otechestvennoĭ voĭny. **Voen Med Zh** 1981 Jun;(6):73-4
**Babin VP:** Mediki 554-go mediko-sanitarnogo batal'ona v bitve za Dnepr. **Voen Med Zh** 1983 Oct;10:63-4
**Babin VP:** Nekotorye osobennosti raboty mediko-sanitarnogo batal'ona mekhanizirovannogo korpusa v period Velikoĭ Otechestvennoĭ voĭny. **Voen Med Zh** 1982 Feb;(2):74-6
**Babin VP:** O travmaticheskikh povrezhdeniiakh u lits letnogo sostava v period Velikoĭ Otechestvennoĭ voĭny. **Voen Med Zh** 1980 Jul;(7):19-21
**Babini J:** Historia de la ciencia versus historia de la medicina. **Medicina (B Aires)** 1980 Jul-Aug;40(4):486-8
**Babini J:** Para una bibliografía de Aldo Mieli. **Physis** 1979;21(1-4):357-424
**Babini VP:** La 'Riforma' di Maine de Biran e i dibattiti sulla folia e il sogno all'Académie Impériale de Médecine. **Atti Accad Sci Ist Bologna** 1979, reçu 1980;67(1):199-222
**Babini VP, Cotti M, Minuz F, et al:** La storia della psichiatria nell'Ottocento: i contributi italiani nell'ultimo decennio (1968-1978). **Stor Crit Psicol** 1980;1(2):177-96
**Babini VP, Cotti M, Minuz F, et al:** Tra sapere e potere. La psichiatria italiana nella seconda metà dell'Ottocento. Bologna, Società Editrice il Mulino, 1982. 272 p. (Studi e Ricerche, CLV).
**Babini VP:** Tra sapere e potere: la psichitria italiana nella seconda metà dell'Ottocento. Bologna, Società editrice il mulino, 1982. 272 p.
**Babushkin A:** Razvedka khimicheskikh sredstv protivnika (po opytu v 1944-1945 gg.). **Voen Istor Zh** 1973;(1):85-9
**Bacchi W:** Su alcune note sperimentali inedite di Francesco Redi. **Ann Ist Mus Stor Sci Fir** 1982;7(1):35-56
**Bach A, Simon K:** Sterblichkeit des Menschen im historischen Verlauf unter besonderer Berücksichtigung ihrer Geschlechtsspezifik. **Alt-Thueringen** 1978;15:7-17
**Bach H:** Die Entwicklung der künstlichen Niere aus Hydrodiffusion und Hämodialyse, von J. A. Nollet bis G. Haas. Der Ursprung des ersten Künstlichen inneren Organs. Giessen, Schmitz, 1983. 334 p. (Arbeiten zur Geschichte der Medizin in Giessen, Bd. 7)
**Bach I:** Karl Gottlob Springsfeld--Arzt, Gelehrter und Akademiemitglied in der Zeit der Aufklärung. **Z Arztl Fortbild (Jena)** 1984;78(19):829-32
**Bachev VI:** K metodike izucheniia memuarno-épistoliarnykh proizvedeniĭ. **Sov Zdravookhr** 1980;(3):60-1
**Bachev VI:** Klassifikatsiia istoriko-meditsinskikh istochnikov sovetskogo perioda. **Sov Zdravookhr** 1983;9:58-9
**Bachev VI:** Kompleksnyĭ podkhod k izucheniiu istoriko-meditsinskikh istochnikov sovetskogo perioda. **Sov Zdravookhr** 1984;(7):56-8
**Bachev VI:** Mestnaia periodicheskaia pechat' kak istoriko-meditsinkiĭ istochnik. **Sov Zdravookhr** 1981;(6):56-8
**Bächi H:** Das Universitätsspital Zürich im Wandel der Zeit 1204-1980. Zürich, Schulthess, 1981. 61 p.
**Bachinskiĭ IuS** see **Kunovskiĭ BV**
**Bachmann R:** Samuel Thomas von Sömmerring - 18. Januar 1755 bis 2. März 1830. Gedenken zum 150. Todestag. **Verh Anat Ges** 1981;75(Pt 1):33-46
**Bachoffner P:** Le premier règlement des apothicaires de Strasbourg (vers 1500). **Rev Hist Pharm (Paris)** 1981;28(248):35-8
**Bachoffner P:** Vulgarisation thérapeutique à travers la 'Materia Medica' de Georges-Henri Behr, médecin strasbourgeois. In Livet G, Schaff G, ed: Médecine et assistance en Alsace, XVIe-XXe siècle. Strasbourg, Istra, 1976. p. 145-53.
**Bachrach A** see **Fournier GA**
**Bachrach B** see **Kroll J**
**Bacin F, Gibert C:** Activité chirurgicale d'un ophthalmologiste clermontois de 1934 à 1938. **Bull Soc Ophtalmol Fr** 1981 Oct;81(10):771-4
**Back F, Ritter L:** Adatok a magyar proctológia történetéhez (1700-1847). **Orv Hetil** 1983 Jun 26;124(26):1581-82
**Back KW** see **Talmor E, ed**
**Bacq ZM:** Le centenaire de la mort de Claude Bernard. **Rev Med Liege** 1979 Jun 1;34(11):525-8
**Bacq ZM:** Les expériences de W. Feldberg en l'année 1932. **Bull Mem Acad R Med Belg** 1982;137 Suppl:9-30
**Bacq ZM:** Marcel Florkin. Harvard et Californie 1929-1930. **Rev Med Liege** 1983 Apr 1;38(7):257-60
**Bacq ZM:** Marcel Florkin, 1900-1979. In Florilège des Sciences en Belgique - II. Bruxelles, Académie Royale de Belgique, 1980. p. 675-78.
**Bacq ZM** see **Lecomte J**
**Bacsa S:** Morfinszármazékok adásának veszélye pancreatitisben. **Orv Hetil** 1982 May 30;123(22):1387-8
**Bădărău GH, Ciurea D, Pirozynski T, et al:** Societatea de Medici si Naturalisti din Iasi la a 150-a aniversare (1830-1980). **Rev Med Chir Soc Med Nat Iasi** 1980 Oct-Dec;84(4):601-11
**Bădărău Gh:** Sesiunea stiintifică jubiliară Medicina progresului si umanismul medical. La 150 de ani de activitate a Societatii de Medici si Naturalisti (1830-1980) Iasi, 4 Octombrie 1980. **Rev Med Chir Soc Med Nat Iasi** 1980 Oct-Dec;84(4):613-24
**Bader A** see **Janzarik W ed**
**Badr SM:** Women and sports in Egypt: history and problems. In Borms J, Hebbelinck M, Venerando A, ed: Women and sport. Basel, Karger, 1981. p. 45-51.

**Baechler J:** Mourir à Jonestown. **Eur J Sociol** 1979;20(2):173-210
**Baer ED:** The conflictive social ideology of American nursing: 1893, a microcosm. Ph.D. Diss , New York University. New York, 1982. vii, 237 p.
**Baer HA:** A historical overview of British and European chiropractic. **Chiropr Hist** 1984;4(1):11-5
**Baer HA:** Prophets and advisors in black spiritual churches: therapy, palliative, or opiate? **Cult Med Psychiatry** 1981 Jun;5(2):145-70
**Baer HA:** The organizational rejuvenation of osteopathy: a reflection of the decline of professional dominance in medicine. **Soc Sci Med [A]** 1981 Sep;15(5):701-11
**Baer HA:** Toward a systematic typology of black folk healers. **Phylon** 1982;43(4):327-43
**Baer KE von:** Reden gehalten in wissenschaftlichen Versammlungen und kleinere Aufsätze vermischten Inhalts. With an introduction by K. B. Sterling. New York, Arno Press, 1978. Three volumes in two. (Reprint. St. Petersburg, 1864/1876/1873).
**Baer RL, Kopf AW:** Marion B. Sulzberger (1895-1983). **J Am Acad Dermatol** 1984 Jun;10(6):91A-96A
**Baerentsen K:** Gamle Apoteker Krukker. Kobenhavn, Danmarks Apotekerforening, 1980. 65 p.
**Baerentsen K** see **Bruun NW**
**Baerentsen K** see **Retzius AJ**
**Baetjer AM:** The early days of industrial hygiene--their contribution to current problems. **Am Ind Hyg Assoc J** 1980 Nov;41(11):773-7
**Baetjer AM:** The early days of industrial hygiene - their contribution to current problems. **Am Ind Hyg Assoc J** 1980;41:773-7
**Baev AA:** Sovremennaia biologiia kak sotsial'noe iavlenie. **Vopr Filos** 1981;3:17-26
**Baeyer W** see **Janzarik W ed**
**Baeyer WR von, Pongratz LJ, ed:** Psychiatrie in Selbstdarstellungen. Bern, Huber, 1977. 516 p.
**Baffa Filho O** see **Mascarenhas S**
**Bagchi AK:** Indian influences on Arabic and Moorish medicine. **Phronesis** 1978;37:3-12
**Bagchi AK:** Sanskrit and modern medical vocabulary. A comparative study. Calcutta, RDDHI-India, 1978. 119 p.
**Bagchi AK:** The evolution and chronology of ancient Indian medical sciences. **Bull Indian Inst Hist Med (Hyderabad)** 1979;9:21-6
**Bagdasar'ian SM:** Velikiĭ russkiĭ khirurg N. I. Pirogov (k 100-letiiu so dnia smerti). **Klin Med (Mosk)** 1982 Jul;60(7):111-5
**Bagdasarian SM:** Velikiĭ Russkiĭ klinitsist S. P. Botkin (k 150-letiiu so dnia rozhdeniia). **Klin Med (Mosk)** 1982 Dec;60(12):94-9
**Bagdasar'ian SM:** Voennye vrachi--veterany pervoĭ piatiletki. **Voen Med Zh** 1982 Jun;(6):75-6
**Bagdasar'ian SM:** Vydaiushchiĭsia sovetskiĭ uchenyĭ (k 40-letiiu prisvoeniia zvaniia Geroia Sotsialisticheskogo Truda N. N. Burdenko). **Voen Med Zh** 1983 May;5:64-8
**Baggiolini M:** Phagozyten und Phagozytose hundert Jahre nach Metschnikoff. Ein aktuelles Bild des neutrophilen Leukozyten. **Schweiz Med Wochenschr** 1982 Oct;112(41):1403-11
**Baglaĭ EB:** Formirovanie predstavleniĭ o prichinakh individual'nogo razvitiia: istoricheskiĭ ocherk. Moskva, Nauka, 1979. 152 p.
**Baglaĭ EB:** [The first attempt to prove the dominant role of the nucleus in heredity.] (Rus). **Istor Biol Issled** 1978;7:156-62
**Bagley C:** Social policy and development: the case of child welfare, health and nutritional services in India. **Plural Soc** 1979;10(1):3-26
**Bagnara S, Biocca M, Mazzonis DG:** Consiglio Nazionale delle Ricerche, Rome, Italy. **Int J Health Serv** 1981;11(3):431-50
**Bagne C** see **Greenberg ER**
**Bagot D'Arc M** see **Portmann M**
**Báguena Cervellera J, Gener Galbis C:** La triquinosis en la España del siglo XIX a través de la obra de Antonio Suárez: de las trichinas y de la trichinosis en España. **Med Hist (Barc)** 1984;3:1-26
**Baguenier-Desormeaux L:** Henry Drysdale Dakin à Compiègne, en 1915. **Rev Hist Pharm (Paris)** 1981 Jun;28(249):79-88
**Bagur D:** Sociedad odontologica del Rio de la Plata, periodo 1897-98. **Rev Asoc Odontol Argent** 1980 Nov;68(7):464-7
**Bagur DB:** Sociedad odontologica del Rio de la Plata: periodo 1899-1902. **Rev Asoc Odontol Argent** 1981 May;69(3):147-50
**Bagur DB** see **Muñoz Al**
**Bagwell CE:** Ambröise Paré and the renaissance of surgery. **Surg Gynecol Obstet** 1981 Mar;152(3):350-4
**Bahn C** see **Davey H**
**Bahnson HT:** Classics in thoracic surgery. **Ann Thorac Surg** 1982 Jan;33(1):96-8 (continued regularly)
**Bahr G von:** Den fysiologiska optikens utveckling i Sverige. **Nord Medicinhist Arsb** 1982;:66-75
**Bahr G von:** Mannen bakom Graefes symtom: dog ung, men ändå ett världsnamn inom oftalmologin. **Lakartidningen** 1984 Mar 21;81(12):1168
**Bahr G von:** Upsala Läkare Klubb (ULK)--ur en gammal protokollsbok. **Nord Medicinhist Arsb** 1981;:172-5
**Bahr G von:** Upsala Läkareförening 150 år. **Ups J Med Sci [Suppl]** 1982;35:1-33
**Bahrani AS** see **Orr JF**
**Bahry D** see **Albritton RB**
**Baicu G** see **Samborschi E**
**Baillargeat R, et al:** Les invalides: trois siècles d'histoire. Paris, Musée de l'armée, 1974. 600 p.
**Bailliart JP, Royer J, Faure MH, ed:** L'ophtalmologie des origines à nos jours. Tome 2. Annoynay, France, Laboratoires H. Faure, 1979. 191 p. Selections by various authors.
**Bailliart JP:** Quelques uns des liens privilégiés unissant les ophtalmologies grecque et française. **Bull Soc Ophtalmol Fr** 1980 Oct;80(10):807-9
**Bainton DF:** The discovery of lysosomes. **J Cell Biol** 1981 Dec;91(3 pt 2):66s-76s
**Bair B:** 'The full light of the dawn': Congressman John Fogarty and the historical cycle of community mental health policy in Rhode Island. **RI Hist** 1982;41(4):127-38
**Bair B:** The parents council for retarded children and social change in Rhode Island, 1951-1970. **RI Hist** 1981;40(4):144-59
**Bairati A:** Ultrastructure of the protoplasm. The 'pioneer' work by A. Bairati and F. E. Lehmann revisited. **J Submicrosc Cytol** 1981 Apr;13(2):117-25
**Baird ND:** A Kentucky physician examines Memphis. **Tenn Hist Q** 1978;37(2):190-202
**Baird ND:** David Wendel Yandell, physician of old Louisville. Lexington: University Press of Kentucky, 1978. x, 116 p.
**Baird ND:** Luke Pryor Blackburn: physician, governor, reformer. Lexington, University Press of Kentucky, 1979. viii, 127 p.
**Baird ND:** There is no Sunday in the army: Civil War letters of Lunsford P. Yandell, 1861-62. **Filson Club Hist Q** 1979;53(4):317-27
**Baird WD:** Medical education in Arkansas, 1879-1978. Memphis, Memphis State University Press, 1979. 505 p.
**Baird WD, ed:** Years of discontent. Doctor Frank L. James in Arkansas, 1877-1878. Memphis, Memphis State University Press, 1977. xxviii, 84 p.
**Baĭsogolov GD:** Rol' zhurnala 'Meditsinskaia Radiologiia' v razvitii luchevoĭ terapii v SSSR. **Med Radiol (Mosk)** 1982 Apr;27(4):3-6
**Baissette G:** Die Medizin bei den Griechen. In Sournia JC, Martiny M, Poulet J, ed: Illustrierte Geschichte der Medizin. Salzburg, Andreas, 1980. Vol. 1. p. 179-99.
**Baĭtinger VF** see **Zadorozhnyĭ AA**
**Bak M:** Kórházvonatos tapasztalatok a II. világháború fertözö betegségeiröl. **Orv Hetil** 1983 Oct 16;124(42):2568-70
**Bak M:** Lux Jakab dr. (1822-1876) munkássága mai orvosi szemléletünkben. **Orv Hetil** 1984 Apr 29;125(18):1082-4
**Bakalar JB** see **Grinspoon L**
**Bakalkin GIa, Taborko MM:** Neĭropeptidy: istoriia izucheniia i perspektivy primeneniia v meditsine. **Bol Serv Odontol Saint (Porto Alegre)** 1981;4(2):100-5
**Bakalova L, Draganova T:** Stomatologichni retsepti vuv vuzrozhdenski lekarstven spravochnik ot 1870 g. **Stomatologiia (Sofiia)** 1979;(3):203-6
**Bakan D:** Freud e la tradizione mistica ebraica: psicoanalisi e cabala. **Comunita** 1976;39(176):206-44
**Bakan D:** Politics and American psychology. In R. W. Rieber, K. Salzinger, ed: Psychology: theoretical-historical perspectives. New York, Academic Press, 1980. p. 125-44.
**Bakanova DI** see **Kochemasova ZN**
**Bakay L:** The ancient fear of trephining through the cranial sutures. **Orvostort Kozl** 1982;28(1-3):15-22
**Bakay L:** The danger of trephining through the cranial sutures. **Surg Neurol** 1982 Oct;18(4):284-5
**Bakdash H:** Perspectives in international neurosurgery: neurosurgery in Syria. **Neurosurgery** 1979 Dec;5(6):759-60
**Baker AL:** The San Francisco evolution debates: June 13-14, 1925. **Advent Herit** 1975;2(2):23-32
**Baker C:** The Government Medical Service in Malawi: an administrative history, 1891-1974. **Med Hist** 1976 Jul;20(3):296-311
**Baker DC, Murphy JL:** Myles Blomefylde, Elizabethan physician, alchemist and book collector: a sketch of a life. **Bodleian Libr Rec** 1982 Nov;11(1):35-46
**Baker GL:** The medical curriculum--from the 70's into the 80's. **J Iowa Med Soc** 1980 Apr;70(4):159-60
**Baker HC:** Patent medicine in Pennsylvania before 1906: a history through advertising. **Pa Folklife** 1977-78;27(2):20-33
**Baker HW:** The general surgeon and cancer. **Am J Surg** 1980 May;139(5):606-7
**Baker J:** Animal diseases in archaeology. London, New York, Academic Press, 1980. ix, 235 p.
**Baker JW:** A historical overview of surgical decompression in advanced intestinal obstruction. **Surg Gynecol Obstet** 1984 Jun;158(6):593-8
**Baker M:** Midwifery by gaslight. **Nurs Times** 1984 Aug 29-Sep 4;80(35):40-3
**Baker M:** The development of the office of a permanent medical health officer for St. John's, Newfoundland, 1826-1905. **HSTC** 1983 May;24(7 No 2):98-105
**Baker M:** Thomas Howley. In Dictionary of Canadian biography, 1881-1890. 1982;11:429-30.
**Baker PQ:** Memories of medicine. **Nebr Med J** 1983 Oct;68(10):338-9
**Baker PT:** Human population biology: a viable transdisciplinary science. **Hum Biol** 1982 May;54(2):203-20
**Baker SG** see **Torrington M**
**Baker SL:** Physician licensure laws in the United States, 1865-1915. **J Hist Med Allied Sci** 1984 Apr;39(2):173-97
**Baker TC:** Half a century of medical practice in East London. **S Afr Med J** 1983 Jun 29;Spec No:23
**Baker TS, Eveleth PB:** The effects of funding patterns on the development of physical anthropology. In F. Spencer, ed: A history of American physical anthropology, 1930-1980. New York, Academic Press, 1982. p. 31-48.
**Baker-Jones DL:** 'To supply the sick poor'. **Carmarthensh Hist** 1978;:15

**Bakhshiev BA, Beĭbutov ShM, Aleskerov DSh, et al:** Istoriia razvitiia radiologii v Azerbaĭdzhane. **Med Radiol (Mosk)** 1982 Dec;27(12):18–21
**Bakhtadze G:** Akademik Aleksandr Stepanovich Aladashvili: zhizn' i deiatel'nost. Tbilisi, Metsniereba, 1980. 147 p.
**Bakker EJ** see **Horstmanhoff HF, ed**
**Bakker EJ** see **Horstmanhoff HF, et al**
**Bakker-van der Kooij C:** De zoekende zusters. Enige beschouwingen naar aanleiding van de herdruk van de roman 'Zuster Bertha', geschreven door Arnold Aletrino en voor het eerst uitgegeven in 1891. **Tijdschr Ziekenverpl** 1983 Apr 26;36(9):275–8
**Bakker-van der Kooij C:** Honderd jaar krankzinnigheid. **Tijdschr Ziekenverpl** 1984 Aug 21;37(17):545–8
**Bakker-Van der Kooij C** see **Arts en sameleving. Medical history contributions by H. W. Pleket, J. Van Herwaarden, W. Frijhoff, C. Offringa, M. J. Van Lieburg, C. Bakker-Van der Kooij**
**Baklykov LI** see **Odonchiméd L**
**Bala P:** The Ayurvedic system of medicine: its fate in medieval India. **Bull Indian Inst Hist Med Hyderabad** 1982;12(1–4):22–7
**Balaguer i Perigüell E, Ballester i Añón R, Bujosa i Homar F, et al:** Els impresos científics a Catalunya en els segles XV i XVI. In Congrés International d'Història de la Medicina Catalana, 2nd, Barcelona, 1975. Llibre d'Actes. Barcelona, Socitra, 1977. p. 185–96.
**Balaguer Perigüell E, Ballester Añon R:** El colegio di cirugía de Zaragoza, intento de renovación de las instituciones médicas aragonesas. 2. Jornadas sobre el estado actual de los Estudios sobre Aragón, diciembre de 1979, Esp. 1980: 713–8.
**Balaguer Perigüell E:** La historia en la medicina. **Real Acad Med Zaragoza** 1980;34, Curso 1979;:100–16
**Balaguer Perigüell E, Ballester Añón R:** Repercusiones de la epidemia de peste de Zaragoza de 1652. In: Sociedad Española de Historia de la Medicina. V Congreso Nacional. Madrid, 1977. **Asclepio** 1977;29:67–72
**Balaguer Perigüell E** see **Albarracín Teulón A**
**Balák K:** Třicet let výzkumného ústavu MZ CSR. **Cesk Gynekol** 1982 Mar;47(2):81–112
**Balan B:** L'ordre et le temps. L'anatomie comparée et l'histoire des vivants au XIXe siècle. Paris, Vrin, 1979. 610 p.
**Balanski R** see **Rusanov GA**
**Balas V:** I. chirurgická klinika a její vliv na rozvoj chirurgie v Ceskoslovensku. **Rozhl Chir** 1983 Apr;62(4):289–307
**Balas V:** 100 years of Czech surgery. **Sb Lek** 1983 Apr;85(4):97–104
**Balasalle NM:** A history of public policy for the education of handicapped children in Massachusetts. Ed.D. Dissertation, Harvard University. Cambridge, 1980. viii, 273 p.
**Balasheva II, Zhukova IV:** K 90-letiiu kafedry pediatrii Tomskogo meditsinskogo instituta. **Pediatriia** 1982;(9):71–3
**Balashov IuS:** Issledovaniia parazitícheskikh chlenistonogikh i perenoschikov v Zoologicheskom institute AN SSSR. **Parazitologiia** 1982 Sep–Oct;16(5):428–31
**Balashov IuS:** Razvitie meditsinskoĭ i veterinarnoĭ arakhnoéntomologii v SSSR. **Parazitologiia** 1982 Nov–Dec;16(6):441–4
**Balbo T:** In memoria di Edoardo Perroncito nel centenario di fondazione della prima Cattedra di Parassitologia. **Parassitologia** 1980 Dec;22(3):233–7
**Balch P** see **Spaulding J**
**Baldacci G, Frontali L, Lattanzi A:** The debate on spontaneous generation and the birth of microbiology. **Fundam Sci** 1981;2(2):123–36
**Balde JH:** Dreizehn biographische Skizzen. In Balde JH, Schmiking W, ed: Festschrift zum 86. Deutschen Arztetag in Kassel. Kassel, Arztevereins, 1983. p. 51–86.
**Balde JH, Schmiking W, ed:** Festschrift zum 86. Deutschen Aerztetag in Kassel. Kassel, Der Arzteverein, 1983. 112 p.
**Baldini M** see **Epistemologia, metodologia clinica e storia della scienza medica, 1**
**Baldock D:** Early midwifery: one of the oldest professions. **Nurs Mirror** 1981 Jul 15;153(3):40–2
**Baldwin J:** The Nichols: 100 years of Ohio dentistry. **Ohio Dent J** 1980 May;54(5):22–3
**Baldwin K:** 'The lumberjack and the deaf tree': images of the deaf in folk narrative. **Ky Folkl Rec** 1982;28(1–2):6–11
**Baldwin RS:** The fungus fighters: two women scientists and their discovery. Ithaca, Cornell University Press, 1981. 212 p.
**Bal'dysh G:** Bekhterev v Peterburge-Leningrade. Leningrad, Lenizdat, 1979. 318 p.
**Balevic M** see **Andelic P**
**Balickij KP** see **Kaveckij RE**
**Balikhin LN:** 50 let proizvodstva meditsinskikh instrumentov na Mozhaĭskom mediko-instrumental'nom zavode im. P. V. Gusenkova. **Med Tekh** 1981 Sep–Oct;(5):15–7
**Balius R:** Hitos de la historia de la educacion fisica española. **Apuntes Med Deportiva** 1975;12:215–20
**Baljet B:** Willem Vrolik als teratoloog. **Ned Tijdschr Geneeskd** 1984 Aug 11;128(32):1530–4
**Balk MM** see **Bringmann WG**
**Ball T:** Platonism and penology: James Mill's attempted synthesis. **J Hist Behav Sci** 1982 Jul;18(3):222–9
**Balla J:** 50 éves a mátraházai gyógyintézet. **Orv Hetil** 1983 Mar 20;124(12):712–3
**Ballantine HT:** 'Sciatica' and the neurosurgeon: historical perspectives and personal reminiscenses. **Clin Neurosurg** 1980;27:541–52
**Ballantyne GH:** Review of sigmoid volvulus: history and results of treatment. **Dis Colon Rectum** 1982 Jul–Aug;25(5):494–501
**Ballantyne GH:** The meaning of ileus. Its changing definition over three millennia. **Am J Surg** 1984 Aug;148(2):252–6
**Ballas C:** Greek co-operatives of the 18th century and social welfare in Ampelakia of Thessaly. In: International Congress of the History of Medicine, 26th, Plovdiv (Bulgaria), 1978. Actes du Congres, Vol. 1. Sofia, 1980. p. 88–90.
**Ballas CN** see **Marketos SG**
**Ballbé R:** El psiquiatra y el hombre contemporáneo. **Actas Luso Esp Neurol Psiquiatr** 1981 Mar–Apr;9(2):89–102
**Ballentine C:** Taste of raspberries, taste of death: the 1937 elixir sulfanilamide incident. **FDA Consum** 1981 Jun;15(5):18–21
**Ballester R, Bujosa F, Olagüe G:** Colección historicomédica de la Facultad de Medicine de Valencia. Valencia, Càtedra e Instituto de Historia de la Medicina, 1976. 54 p. (Cuadernos Valencianos de Historia de la Medicina y de la Ciencia, 18, Serie A (Monografías)).
**Ballester R:** Factores biológicos y actitudes vigentes frente a la infancia en la sociedad española del antiguo régimen. **Asclepio** 1983;35:343–57
**Ballester R:** La utilizacion de los clasicos en la obra pediatrica de Luis Mercado (1525–1611). **Asclepio** 1978–79;30–31:307–18
**Ballester Añon R** see **Albarracín Teulón A**
**Ballester Añón R** see **Balaguer Perigüell E**
**Ballester i Añón R** see **Balaguer i Perigüell E**
**Ballesteros S** see **Villarroel H**
**Ballesteros Rodríguez J:** La peste en Córdoba. Córdoba, Excma. Diputación Provincial de Córdoba, Servicio de Publicaciones, 1982. 238 p.
**Ballowitz L** see **Smith GF**
**Ballstadt C, Peterman M, Hopkins E:** 'A glorious madness': Susanna Moodie and the spiritualist movement. **J Can Stud** 1982–83;17(4):88–100
**Balmary M:** Psychoanalyzing psychoanalysis--Freud and the hidden fault of the father. Baltimore, Johns Hopkins University Press, 1982. xxiii, 184 p.
**Balmer H:** Walliser Naturforscher. **Gesnerus** 1979;36(1/2):35–49
**Balmukhanov SB** see **Suleĭmenov AA**
**Balner H, Marquet RL:** Transplantation biology--past and present: reappraisal of 'breakthroughs' since 1955. **Transplant Proc** 1981 Mar;13(1 pt 1):13–8
**Balog CE:** History, medicine, and culture: history for science students. **Indiana Soc Stud Q** 1980–81;33(3):53–62
**Balogh F:** A magyar urológia fejlödése a két világháború között. **Orv Hetil** 1984 Jan 8;125(2):101–8
**Balogh J:** A befecskendezéses kezelés kezdetei Magyarországon. **Orvostort Kozl** 1980;89–91(26 no 1–3):111–23
**Balogh J, Sükösd L:** Manninger Vilmos akadémiai pályadíjának 80 éves évfordulójára. **Orv Hetil** 1983 Oct 30;124(44):2693–5
**Balon LR:** N. I. Pirogov--osnovopolozhnik otechestvennoĭ vosstanovitel'noĭ khirurgii. **Vestn Khir** 1983 Jun;130(6):93–7
**Balóné Fleischmann M:** A rehabilitáció hazai úttöröje Gárdi Jenö dr. (1886–1944). **Orv Hetil** 1984 Feb 19;125(8):470–2
**Baltes PB** see **Lerner RM, ed**
**Baly M:** A leading light. **Nurs Mirror** 1982 Nov 10;155(19):49–51
**Baly M:** A new history of nursing. Three. The nurse élite (Florence Nightingale). **Nurs Times** 1984 Oct 17–23;80(42):55–7
**Baly M:** Care or cure? **Nurs Mirror** 1982 Sep 22;155(12):43–4
**Balzac et la médecine de son temps:** [Paris], Maison de Balzac, [1976?]. [98] p.
**Balzani A:** Primi interventi di bonifica dello stato unitario nella campagna romana. **Studi Romani** 1980;28(1):47–67
**Bammi V:** Nutrition, the historian, and public policy: a case study of U. S. national nutrition policy in the 20th century. **J Soc Hist** 1980;14(4):627–48
**Bancaud J** see **Postel J**
**Bancroft PM:** Rickets and solar radiation – medicine's debt to Professor Frank Mussehl. **Nebr Med J** 1982 Jul;67(7):184–5
**Bandera B:** La Academia Nacional de Medicina y la evolución de la anestesia en México. In Academia Nacional de Medicina. Libro conmemorativo del primer centenario. México, Comité Editorial de la Comisión Organizadora del Congreso del Centenario, 1964. Tome 2. p. 546–52.
**Bandi W** see **Willenegger H**
**Bandyopadhyay J** see **Shiva V**
**Bandyopadhyaya K:** The Chinese food-grain crisis: 1959–61--some explanations. **China Rep (India)** 1971;7(3):16–25
**Banerjee B, Hazra J:** Geo-ecology of leprosy with special reference to West Bengal. **Geogr Med** 1982;12:26–58
**Bang F:** From a visit in America. **Hist Med Vet** 1979;4(2):25–30
**Bang HO, Dyerberg J:** Personal reflections on the incidence of ischaemic heart disease in Oslo during the Second World War. **Acta Med Scand** 1981;210(4):245–8
**Banga I:** A Magyar Elettani Társaság 50 éves jubileuma. **Orv Hetil** 1981 Dec 13;122(50):3093–6
**Banga I:** Az izomkutatás eredményei. **Orv Hetil** 1983 Oct 2;124(40):2440–3
**Bangs JD:** Andries Salomonsz, a converted 'Rabbi and Doctor' in Leiden (1553–1561). **Jew Soc Stud** 1978;40(3–4):271–86
**Bankhofer H:** Die grossen Naturheiler. Ihr Leben – ihre Lehren. Frankfurt, Ullstein, 1982. 359 p.
**Banks CS:** Two pioneer physicians of San Antonio. **Friends P. I. Nixon Med Hist Libr** 1973 Oct;2:2–17
**Banks DE, Barkman HW:** Silicosis epidemic reported in 1900. **JAMA** 1984 Jan 13;251(2):217
**Banks JA:** Victorian values: secularism and the size of families. London,

Boston, Routledge & Kegan Paul, 1981. ix, 203 p.
**Banks JG** see **Macdonald RC**
**Banks A, ed:** Monumental stone. Barre, Vermont, 1939 and 1940. In her: First-person America. New York, Knopf, 1980. p. 93–119.
**Bannister T, Ireland T:** 'Hospitality' in the Middle Ages. **Mich Hosp** 1983 Dec;19(12):31–5
**Bano H** see **Aslam M**
**Bano M, Ali MI:** Cosmetics according to Avicenna. **Bull Indian Inst Hist Med (Hyderabad)** 1981;1–4:110–7
**Bano-Fleischmann M, Zalai K:** Gegenstände der Erinnerung an Kosma und Damian in Ungarn. **Ther Hung** 1981;29(3):152–6
**Bánóczy J, Borós S:** A Semmelweis Orvostudományi Egyetem Konzerváló Fogászati Klinika negyedszázados története és munkássága. **Fogorv Sz** 1984 Nov;77(11):321–3
**Bánóczy J:** Visszapillantás. **Fogorv Sz** 1980 Dec;73(12):354–5
**Baños G** see **Franco Grande A**
**Banta HD, Burns AK, Behney CJ:** Policy implications of the diffusion and control of medical technology. **Ann Am Acad Polit Soc Sci** 1983;(468):165–81
**Banta HD** see **Thacker SB**
**Banta JE:** International health: challenges to the basic sciences. **Trans Stud Coll Physicians Phila** 1982 Dec;5(4 no 4):291–303
**Banziger G:** Intergenerational communication in prominent western drama. **Gerontologist** 1979 Oct;19(5 pt 1):471–80
**Baradel Y:** Quelques aspects de la médecine à Belfort au XVIIIe siècle. In Livet G, Schaff G, ed: Médecine et assistance en Alsace, XVIe–XXe siècle. Strasbourg, Istra, 1976. p. 135–44.
**Barahona Fernándes H:** O sentido actual de obra de K. Kleist e as repercusões nos países Ibero-Americanos. **Actas Luso Esp Neurol Psiquiatr** 1979 Nov–Dec;7(6):341–52
**Baraka A:** Anesthesiology is the 'Critical Care of the Surgical Patient'. **Middle East J Anaesthesiol** 1982 Jun;6(5):237–9
**Baraka A:** Evolution of anaesthesia circuits **Middle East J Anaesthesiol** 1979 Jun;5(4):225–7
**Baraka A:** Historical aspects of opium. **Middle East J Anaesthesiol** 1982 Jun;6(5):289–302
**Baran D:** Istoriografie. **Rev Med Chir Soc Med Nat Iasi** 1981 Jul–Sep;85(3):468, 472, 510
**Baranova EV** see **Kuznetsov VK**
**Baranovskiĭ GIa, Kapitonov GI:** Nakotorye osobennosti meditsinskoĭ évakuatsii v Stalingradskoĭ bitve. (K 40-letiiu Stalingradskoĭ bitvy). **Voen Med Zh** 1983;(1):71–4
**Baranovskiĭ GIa, Kapitonov GI:** Nekotorye voprosy podgotovki i organizatsii raboty sanitarno-transportnykh sudov v period Velikoĭ Otechestvennoĭ voiny. **Voen Med Zh** 1984 May;(5):25–8
**Baranovskiĭ GIa, Kapitonov GI:** Ob évakuatsii ranenykh i bol'nykh zheleznodorozhnym transportom vo vremia Velikoĭ Otechestvennoĭ voĭny. **Voen Med Zh** 1981 Mar;(3):9–10
**Baraut C:** Un manuscrit llatí de medicina de l'Arxiu Capitular de la Seu d'Urgell. In Congrés International d'Història de la Medicina Catalana, 2nd, Barcelona, 1975. Llibre d'Actes. Barcelona, Socitra, 1977. p. 273–94.
**Barba J, Arrieta JA, Perugachi C, et al:** Espasma arterial coronario. Antecedentes históricos. **Rev Med Univ Navarra** 1982 Jun;26(2):12–3
**Barbachano AE:** Datos prehispanicos del tabaquismo en America. **Bol Soc Mex Hist Filos Med** 1982 Jun;6(39):29–42
**Barbaix M, Clotuche J, Jonckere P de, et al:** Naissance et développement de l'Oto-rhino-laryngologie dans l'histoire de la médecine. **Acta Otorhinolaryngol Belg** 1981;35 Suppl 2:1–392
**Barbaix M, Clotuche J, De Jonckere P, et al:** Naissance et développement de l'oto-rhino-laryngologie dans l'histoire de la médecine. (Suite). **Acta Otorhinolaryngol Belg** 1981;35 Suppl 4:1045–622 contd
**Barbakow F** see **Schmid R**
**Barbas S** see **Lefebvre P**
**Barbeau A, Sadibelouiz M, Roy M, et al:** Origin of Friedreich's disease in Quebec. **Can J Neurol Sci** 1984 Nov;11(4 Suppl):506–9
**Barber CL:** Some implications of declining birth rates in developed countries. **Trans R Soc Can** 1979;17:174–85
**Barber D:** Secret operation on US president. **Probe (Lond)** 1982 May;23(11):415–6
**Barber DN:** Doc Holliday, the wildest dentist of the West. **Probe (Lond)** 1984 Mar;25(9):301–2
**Barber GO:** The diverse uses of glycerine in pre-antibiotic days. **MIMS Mag** 1981 Apr 15;:46–7
**Barber LH** see **Skudder S**
**Barber M:** Lepers, Jews and Moslems: the plot to overthrow Christendom in 1321. **History** 1981;66:1–17
**Barbier F:** Les caractères généraux de la démographie de Valenciennes au XIXe siècle. **Rev Nord** 1983;65(258):567–79
**Barblan MA:** Journalisme médical et échanges intellectuels au tournant du XVIIIe siècle: le cas de la Bibliothèque Britannique. **Arch Sci** 1977;30(3):283–398
**Barblan MA** see **Cramer M**
**Barbor PR** see **Child abuse: historical perspective**
**Barbu G:** Din istoria combaterii epidemiilor în țara noastră. (I). Frățiile milosteniei. **Rev Ig [Bacteriol]** 1984 Apr–Jun;29(2):189–92
**Barbu G:** Din istoria luptei antiepidemice în România (II). Completări la istoricul spitalului Dudești. **Rev Ig [Bacteriol]** 1984 Jul–Sep;29(3):283–7
**Barbu G:** Medici sub steagul revoluției în tara românească. **Rev Arhiv** 1973;35 suppl:153–69
**Barbu O** see **Samborschi E**
**Barcaro U:** Galileo e il mondo biologico. **Physis** 1982;24(3):357–79
**Bárcena A, Barrera A, Ruiz E, et al:** Interpretación etnobotánica de la iconografía del Códice de la Cruz-Badiano. **An Soc Mex Hist Cienc Tec** 1979;5:35–48
**Barchenko LI** see **Il'chevich NV**
**Barcia D:** La significacion de la antropologia medica de Lain Entralgo para la psiquiatria actual. **Asclepio** 1980;32:19–45
**Barcia Goyanes JJ:** Dos nombres enigmaticos del trocanter mayor: tharuca y carchametra; two enigmatic names of the greater trochanter: tharuca and carchametra. **Med Esp** 1980 Nov–Dec;79:1–11
**Barcia Goyanes JJ:** Las correcciones de Vesalio a la anatomia de Galeno. **Med Esp** 1980;79:1–16
**Barcia Goyanes JJ:** Los albores del lenguaje anatómico en las lenguas neolatinos. La traduccion del inventarium de Guy de Chauliac por Bernat de Casaldovol. **Med Esp** 1980;79:235–49
**Barcia Goyanes JJ:** Los arabismos en las ediciones latinas del libro I del Colliget de Averroes. **Med Esp** 1984 Jan–Feb;83:9–29
**Barcia Goyanes JJ:** Los nombres medievales del 'infundibulum'. **Med Esp** 1981;80:139–44
**Barcia Goyanes JJ:** Los terminos osteologicos de la Fabrica y la evolucion del lenguaje anatomico hebreo en la Edad Media. **Sefarad** 1982;42:299–326
**Barcia Goyanes JJ:** Onomatologia anatomica nova: historia del lenguaje anatomico. Tomo VI. Nares–Profundus. Valencia, Universidad de Valencia, 1983. 467 p.
**Barcia Goyanes JJ:** Onomatologia anatomica nova; historia del lenguaje anatómico. Tomos I–III. Valencia, Universidad de Valencia, 1978.
**Barcia Goyanes JJ:** Un extraño nombre del apendice xifoides: 'malum punicum'; a strange name of the xiphoid process: 'malum punicum'. **Med Esp** 1981;80:105–11
**Barciszewski J:** Transferowe kwasy rybonukleinowe--dwadzieścia pieć lat badań. **Postepy Biochem** 1983;29(3–4):255–60
**Barckley V:** The best of times and the worst of times. Historical reflections from an American Cancer Society national nursing consultant. **Oncol Nurs Forum** 1982 Summer;9(3):54–6
**Barclay WR:** Landmark perspective: Asbestos. An industrial asset with a health cost. **JAMA** 1984 Jul 6;252(1):96
**Barcs-Masson ML:** Les femmes et la pharmacie. Nice, Belisane, 1977. 149 p.
**Bardeau F:** Les clefs secrètes de la chimie des anciens. Paris, Laffont, 1975. 204 p.
**Bardell D:** An 1898 report by Gamaleya for a lytic agent specific for Bacillus anthracis. **J Hist Med Allied Sci** 1982 Apr;37(2):222–5
**Bardell D:** Antoni van Leeuwenhoek's explanation in 1704 of the function of eyelids. **J Hist Med Allied Sci** 1984 Oct;39(4):464–7
**Bardell D:** The roles of the sense of taste and clean teeth in the discovery of bacteria by Antoni van Leeuwenhoek. **Microbiol Rev** 1983 Mar;47(1):121–6
**Bardell EB:** America's only school of pharmacy for women. **Pharm Hist** 1984;26(3):127–33
**Bardell EB:** Dame Agatha's dispensary. **Pharm Hist** 1984;26(1):13–9
**Bardet JP, Lynch KA, Mineau GP, et al:** La mortalité maternelle autrefois: une étude comparée (de la France de l'ouest à l'Utah). **Ann Demogr Hist (Paris)** 1981;:31–48
**Bárdos V, Schulz F:** Výskyt škvrnitého týfu na východnom Slovensku v rokoch 1939–1945. **Bratisl Lek Listy** 1982 Aug;78(2):235–42
**Barer GM** see **Norovpil TS**
**Barer R:** Cosslett's contribution to microscopy (Ellis Cosslett). **J Microsc** 1979 Sep;117(1):5–10
**Barg L:** Andrzej Krupiński (1744–1783). W dwusetną rocznicę śmierci. **Arch Hist Med (Warsz)** 1983;46(3):347–53
**Barg L, Szpilczynski S:** Elements of methodology and searching directions in Polish medical historiography till 1939. In International Congress of the History of Medicine. 26th, Plovdiv, 1978. Actes du Congress. Sofia, 1981. Volume II. p. 72–3.
**Barg L:** O poprawną bio-bibliografię Teodora Tomasza Weichardta kandydata na profesora patologii i terapii akademii krakowskiej w 1783 roku. **Arch Hist Med (Warsz)** 1980;43(3):289–304
**Barger AC:** New technology for a new century: Walter B. Cannon and the invisible rays. **AJR** 1981 Jan;136(1):187–95
**Barger AC:** Some of Carl Walter's contributions to Harvard Medical School and Hospitals. **Am J Surg** 1984 Nov;148(5):578–80
**Barger AC:** The meteoric rise and fall of William Townsend Porter, one of Carl J. Wigger's 'Old Guard'. **Physiologist** 1982 Oct;25(5):407–13
**Barger AC** see **Benison S**
**Barger J:** Origin of flight nursing in the United States Army Air Forces. **Aviat Space Environ Med** 1979 Nov;50(11):1176–8
**Barile MF:** A brief history of the IOM. **Yale J Biol Med** 1983 Sep–Dec;56(5–6):353–4
**Barker A:** A Zulu contribution. **Trans R Soc Trop Med Hyg** 1979;73(4):364–5
**Barker AE:** The Kelsale wonder. **Local Popul Stud (Matlock)** 1981 Spring;26:43
**Barker DJ:** Geographical variations in disease in Britain. **Br Med J** 1981;283:398–400
**Barker JT:** Women as leaders in the field of rehabilitation. **J Rehabil** 1982 Jan–Mar;48(1):9–18, 68–70
**Barker LF:** History of internal medicine. **Md State Med J** 1981 May;30(5):43–4, 47–8, 50, passim
**Barker P** see **Olsen O**
**Barker R:** The local study of plague. **Local Hist** 1981;14(6):332–40
**Barker WH, Jonas S:** The teaching of preventive medicine in American

medical schools, 1940–1980. **Prev Med** 1981 Nov;10(6):674–88
**Barker-Benfield GJ:** A historical perspective on women's health care--female circumcision. **Women Health** 1976 Jan–Feb;1(1):13–15,18–20
**Barker-Benfield GJ** see **Fellman AC**
**Barkley S:** A nurse who made a difference. **Pulse** 1984 May;20(5):1–2
**Barkman HW** see **Banks DE**
**Barkóczi I:** On outstanding achievements of Soviet general psychology. **Ann Univ Sci Budap Rolando Eotvos Nominatae** 1979;6:61–9
**Barlay OS:** Boldizsár Batthyány und sein Humanisten-Kreis. Die ersten Jahrzehnten der Güssinger Bibliothek. **Magy Konyvsz** 1979;95(3):231–51
**Barlow J, Richardson C:** China doctor of John Day. Portland, Bonford & Mort, 1979. ix, 118 p.
**Barlow K:** The pioneer health centre at Peckham. **Soc Soc Hist Med Bull (Lond)** 1984 Dec;35:47
**Barlow MR:** Women doctors of South Africa. **S Afr Med J** 1983 Jun 29;Spec No:29–32
**Barlow T** see **Solomon R**
**Barlow W, Powell DO:** A case for medical coeducation in the 1870s. **J Am Med Wom Assoc** 1980 Dec;35(12):285–8
**Barlow W, Powell DO:** Homeopathy and sexual equality: the controversy over coeducation at Cincinnati's Pulte Medical College, 1873–1879. **Ohio Hist** 1981 Spring;90(2):101–13
**Barlow W, Powell DO:** Ixodes as a source of conflict: Otis E. Hunt vs. J. Mason Warren. **J Hist Med Allied Sci** 1981 Apr;36(2):221–4
**Barlow W, Powell DO:** The cure of Rachel Baker's 'Devotional Somnium' (Sleep-preaching). **Acad Bookman** 1978;31(1–2):3–10
**Barlow W, Powell DO:** To find a stand: New England physicians on the western and southern frontier, 1790–1840. **Bull Hist Med** 1980 Fall; 54(3):386–401
**Barmatoski SP** see **Barnhart MI**
**Barmina NM** see **Blokhin NN**
**Barnard EE:** Physiological aspects of naval problems. **J R Nav Med Serv** 1980 Spring;66(1):23–5
**Barnard K:** Research designs: the historical method. **MCN** 1981 Nov–Dec;6(6):391
**Barnard PD:** Review of activities and progress, 1962–1972, Dental Health Education and Research Foundation. Sydney, Dental Health Education and Research Foundation, Univ. of Sydney, [1972?] 30 p.
**Barnard TC:** Sir William Petty: his Irish estates and Irish population. **Ir Econ Soc Hist** 1979;6
**Barnartt SN, Harris RJ:** Recent changes in predictors of abortion attitudes. **Sociol Soc Res** 1982;66(3):320–34
**Barner S:** Die Entwicklung der Kinderpsychiatrie in Frankreich von den Anfängen bis 1948. Freiburg, Schulz 1980. 300 p. (Freiburger Forschungen zur Medizingeschichte, Neue Folge, 11).
**Barnes AM** see **Tomich PQ**
**Barnes J:** Aristotle's de Motu Animalium. **Classical Rev** 1980;30(2):222–6
**Barnes M, Pratt PK:** Women sanitary inspectors. **Hist Workshop J** 1978;6:225
**Barnes P** see **The preservation of medical and public health records**
**Barnet MC:** Life in 19th century York. **Pharm Hist (London)** 1984 Jun;14(2):3–5
**Barnett GH, Hardy RW:** Gardner tongs and cervical traction. **Med Instrum** 1982 Nov–Dec;16(6):291–2
**Barnett R:** Dr. Jacob de Castro Sarmento and Sephardim in medical practice in 18th-century London. **Trans Jew Hist Soc Engl** 1978–80, paru 1982;27:84–114
**Barnett RD:** Dr. Samuel Nunes Ribeiro and the settlement of Georgia. In: Migration and settlement. London, Jewish Historical Society of England, 1971. p. 63–100.
**Barnhart MI, Barmatoski SP, Goodman M, et al:** Tissue vestiges of an ancient Magadan mammoth calf. **Scan Electron Microsc** 1980;(pt 2):163–70
**Barnhart RJ:** Cesarean section: changing indications, 1968–1977. **J Kans Med Soc** 1980 Feb;81(2):57–62, 78
**Barnhill JF:** An epoch of medical education. **Indiana Med Hist Q** 1975;3(1):53–63
**Baroian OV:** Aspects épidémiologiques de l'immunologie contemporaine. Moscou: [s.n.], 1972 (Cahors: Tardy-Quercy-Auvergne, 1976) 378 p.
**Barometer on baromedicine: MD** 1978 Jun;22(6):53–5, 57
**Baron A, Baron P:** Du charlatan au chirurgien-dentiste. **Inf Dent** 1983 Jan 13;65(2):123–4
**Baron F** see **Paracelsus in der Tradition**
**Baron JB:** Etienne-Jules Marey. **Acta Belg Med Phys** 1983 Oct–Dec;6(4):187–97
**Baron JH:** James Lind would not have approved. **Lancet** 1982 Jun 5;1(8284):1313
**Baron P** see **Baron A**
**Barón Fernández J:** La faceta medica del gran patriota Filipino Jose Rizal. **Asclepio** 1980;32:47–52
**Barondess JA:** The doctor, the patient, and the system: reflections on education for clinical careers. **Perspect Biol Med** 1983 Winter;26(2):205–18
**Barone R:** L'Association Mondiale des Anatomistes Vétérinaires: 1955–1980. **Anat Histol Embryol** 1980;9(3):280–8
**Barootes EW:** Dr. Norman Bethune: inspiration for a modern China. **Can Med Assoc J** 1980 May 24;122(10):1176–84
**Barr HH, Barrie FH:** Edward G. McGavran: guardian of the body politic. Chapel Hill, School of Public Health, Univ. of North Carolina at Chapel Hill, 1979. xii, 177 p.
**Barr JW:** Canadian Forces medicine: 25 years of unified service. **Can Med Assoc J** 1984 Apr 15;130(8):1061–5
**Barr MB:** Looking back: Guy's Hospital. **Lamp** 1980 Aug;37(8):49–51
**Barr MB:** Looking back. Some London hospitals: St Bartholomew's Hospital. **Lamp** 1980 Jun;37(6):59–61
**Barr MB:** Looking back: St Thomas's Hospital. **Lamp** 1980 Aug;37(8):51–2
**Barr ML:** A century of medicine at Western. A centennial history of the Faculty of Medicine, University of Western Ontario. London, Canada, University of Western Ontario, 1977. xiv, 672 p.
**Barr ML:** James Bertram Collip (1892–1965): a Canadian pioneer in endocrinology. In: Congrès international d'histoire de la médecine, XXVe, Québec, 1976. Actes. Québec, 1977. p. 469–76.
**Barraco RA:** Paleobiochemistry. In A. Cockburn, E. Cockburn, ed: Mummies, disease, and ancient cultures. Cambridge, Cambridge University Press, 1980. p. 312–26.
**Barraco RA** see **Cockburn A**
**Barraquer JI:** The history of the microscope in ocular surgery. **J Microsurg** 1980 Jan–Feb;1(4):288–99
**Barraquer i Bordás L, Gutiérrez Gómez D:** En el centenario de la neurología clínica española. **Arch Neurobiol (Madr)** 1982 Mar–Apr;45(2):157–62
**Barré R:** Dieppe, l'assistance et la charité au cours des âges. [France? s. n., 1972?]. 20 p.
**Barrera A** see **Bárcena A**
**Barrett DM, Donovan MG:** Prosthetic bladder augmentation and replacement. **Semin Urol** 1984 Aug;2(3):167–75
**Barrett DM** see **Donovan MG**
**Barrett G:** Delegate John M. Bernhisel, Salt Lake physician following the Civil War. **Utah Hist Q** 1982;50(4):354–60
**Barrett HH, Hawkins WG, Joy ML:** Historical note on computed tomography. **Radiology** 1983 Apr;147(1):172
**Barrett LE** see **Hand WD, ed**
**Barrett RE:** Short-term trends in bastardy in Taiwan. **J Fam Hist** 1980 Fall;5(3):293–312
**Barrick ME:** Cumberland county death lore. **Pa Folklife** 1979;28(4):37–46
**Barrie FH** see **Barr HH**
**Barrie HJ:** Sir William Boyd: a legacy in print. **Can Med Assoc J** 1982 Feb 15;126(4):421,423–4
**Barron FL:** The American origins on the temperance movement in Ontario, 1828–1850. **Can Rev Am Stud** 1980;11(2):131–50
**Barrow L:** Anti-establishment healing: spiritualism in Britain. In Sheils WJ, ed: The Church and healing. Papers read at the twentieth summer meeting and the twenty-first winter meeting of the Ecclesiastical History Society. Oxford, Basil Blackwell for the Society, 1982. p. 225–47.
**Barrow L:** Democratic epistemology: mid-19th-century plebeian medicine. **Soc Soc Hist Med Bull (Lond)** 1981 Dec;29:25–9
**Barrow L:** Deviants in death? Plebeian secularists and spiritualists c. 1860–1910. **Soc Soc Hist Med Bull (Lond)** 1980 Jun;26:22–4
**Barrow MV:** Early history of medicine in Alachua County. **J Fla Med Assoc** 1982 Aug;69(8):670–80
**Barrow MV, Stetson CA:** Origin and development of University of Florida College of Medicine. **J Fla Med Assoc** 1980 Mar;67(3):279–82
**Barrow MV:** Self-treatment practices in North Florida. **J Fla Med Assoc** 1979 Aug;66(8):840–4
**Barrows S:** After the commune: alcoholism, temperance, and literature in the early Third Republic. In Merriman, John M., ed: Consciousness and class experience in nineteenth-century Europe. New York, Holmes and Meier, 1979. p. 205–18.
**Barrucand D:** Bernheim. Importance historique et actualité de l'Ecole de Nancy. In: Congrès National des Sociétés Savantes, 103e, Nancy, 1978. Comptes Rendus. Paris, 1978. Section des Sciences, Fasc. V. p. 75–86.
**Barry J:** Guide to sources and writings on the history of medicine in Bristol, 1600–1900. **Soc Soc Hist Med Bull (Lond)** 1984 Dec;35:48–52
**Barry M, Stansfield SK, Bia FJ:** Haiti and the Hôpital Albert Schweitzer. **Ann Intern Med** 1983 Jun;98(6):1018–20
**Barry PS, Connolly R:** Lead concentrations in mediaeval bones. **Int Arch Occup Environ Health** 1981;48(2):173–7
**Barsukov MI:** Zdravookhranenie v gody Velikoĭ Otechestvennoĭ voĭny 1941–1945. Sbornik dokumentov i materialov. Moskva, Meditsina, 1977. 575 p.
**Bart C:** L'astronome Nicolas Copernic a-t-il été médecin? In: Congrès international d'histoire de la médecine, XXVe, Québec, 1976. Actes. Québec, 1977. p. 477–86.
**Bart P** see **Scully D**
**Barta T:** História otolaryngologickej starostlivosti v Bratislave. **Cesk Otolaryngol** 1984 Jul;33(4):268–71
**Barta T, Klačanský I:** Tridsat rokov Slovenskej otolaryngologickej spoločnosti. **Cesk Otolaryngol** 1984 Feb;33(1):47–51
**Bartecchi CE:** Cardiopulmonary resuscitation--an element of sophistication in the 18th century. **Am Heart J** 1980 Oct;100(4):580–1
**Bartecchi CE:** Historical beginnings of the mitral valve prolapse syndrome. **Am J Cardiol** 1984 Nov 1;54(8):1165–6
**Bartecchi CE:** Intravenous therapy: from humble beginnings through 150 years. **South Med J** 1982 Jan;75(1):61–4
**Bartecchi CE:** Primary cardiac tumors· historically elusive lesions. **South Med J** 1982 Oct;75(10):1249–50
**Bartels D:** The Rockefeller Foundation's funding policy for molecular biology: success or failure? **Soc Stud Sci** 1984 May;14(2):238–43
**Bartels K:** Apotheker-Dienstbriefe. In Dilg P, et al., ed: Perspektiven der Pharmaziegeschichte. Graz, Austria, Akademische Druck- u. Verlagsanstalt, 1983. p. 1–12.
**Bartels K:** Die ersten Apotheken und Apotheker Coburgs. Ergänzungen

zur Geschichte des Coburger Apothekenwesens I. **Pharm Ztg** 1980;125:457–60

**Bartels K:** Ein vielseitiger Apotheker der ersten Hälfte des 19. Jahrhunderts: Anselm Franz Strauss. **Beitr Gesch Pharm** 1979;31(4):26–30

**Bartels K:** Miscellanea civitatis et ducatus Coburgiae pharmaceutica. Ergänzungen zur Coburger Apothekengeschichte II. **Pharm Ztg** 1980;125:1780–4

**Bartels M, ed:** Mensch und Tod: Totentanzsammlung der Universität Düsseldorf. Eine Ausstellung. Düsseldorf, Goethe-Museum, [1978?] 111 p. Einführung von H. Schadewaldt.

**Barth J** see **Gast W**

**Barthel I:** Arzneimittelversuche des 19.Jahrhunderts am gesunden Menschen im deutschsprachigen Raum. Diss., Universität Düsseldorf. Düsseldorf, 1982. 105 p.

**Barthelmé E:** Histoire de la notion du cancer. **Hist Sci Med** 1981;15(2):167–72

**Barthelme E:** Sur la fièvre miliaire ardente, a propos de la mort de Mozart. **Hist Sci Med** 1983;17(1):23–8

**Barthes R** see **Forster R**

**Bartholomew S** see **Watne Al**

**Bartlett EE** see **Reid RA**

**Bartlett RM:** Meditation on the subject of holes in the head. **Pharos** 1980 Spring;43(2):19

**Bartley M:** Coronary heart disease: a disease of affluence or a disease of industry? **Soc Soc Hist Med Bull (Lond)** 1983 Dec;33:50–1

**Bartley RL, Kucewicz WP:** 'Yellow rain' and the future of arms agreements. **Foreign Aff** 1983;61(4):805–26

**Bartók I:** A magyar szemészet legrégibb emlékei. **Orvostort Kozl** 1981;93–96(27 No 1–4):211–7

**Barton D** see **Wolkinson BW**

**Barton M:** Painful duties: art, character, and culture in Confederate letters of condolence. **South Q** 1979;17(2):123–34

**Barton M** see **Blain D**

**Barton NJ:** Hand markings of the Shroud of Turin. **Hand** 1980;12:323

**Bartos I:** Társadalombiztosításunk 30 éve. **Orv Hetil** 1981 Mar 22;122(12):679–80

**Bartrip P:** Workmen's compensation in British law, society and politics, 1897–1946. **Soc Soc Hist Med Bull (Lond)** 1983 Dec;33:30–2

**Bartrip PW, Fenn PT:** The administration of safety: the enforcement policy of the early factory inspectorate, 1844–64. **Public Adm** 1980;58(1)

**Bartsocas CS:** An introduction to ancient Greek genetics and Skeletal Dysplasias. **Prog Clin Biol Res** 1982;104:3–13

**Bartsocas CS:** Paleodermatoglyphics. **Prog Clin Biol Res** 1982;84:139–43

**Bartunek A, Petrociová O:** Vzájomné vztahy medzi levočským a prešovským lekárenstvom v 17. až 19. storočí. **Cesk Farm** 1984 Sep;33(7):308–11

**Baruch JZ:** Maimonides as a physician. **Gesnerus** 1982;39(3–4):347–57

**Baruchin A** see **Hauben DJ**

**Baruk H:** Actualité du traitement moral et de la nosographie de Pinel. **Ann Med Psychol (Paris)** 1982 Apr;140(4):442–7

**Baruk H:** Die französische und europäische Psychiatrie von Pinel bis heute. In Sournia JC, Martiny M, Poulet J, ed: Illustrierte Geschichte der Medizin. Salzburg, Andreas, 1980. Vol. 6. p. 2034–43.

**Baruk H:** La médecine et la Torah. **Rev Hist Med Heb** 1981 Jul;34(2):19–22

**Baruk H:** La médecine et la Torah. **Rev Hist Med Heb** 1981 Oct;34(3):35–9

**Baruk H:** La médecine hebraïque face à la médecine hippocratique. In La collection hippocratique et son rôle dans l'histoire de la médecine. Colloque de Strasbourg (23–27 octobre 1972) organisé par le Centre de Recherches sur la Grèce Antique, avec le concours des Facultés de Philosophie et des Langues Classiques. Leiden, E. J. Brill, 1975. p. 291–303.

**Baruk H:** L'Ecole de Nancy et la découverte de la psychothérapie. La régression psychanalytique à l'ancienne hystérie. In: Congrès National des Sociétés Savantes, 103e, Nancy, 1978. Comptes Rendus. Paris, 1978. Section des Sciences, Fasc. V. P. 71–4.

**Baruk H:** L'hôpital psychiatrique d'hier et de demain. **Ann Med Psychol (Paris)** 1980 Jun;138(6):700–7

**Baruk H:** Moïse, Freud et le veau d'or. **Rev Hist Med Heb** 1984 Jul;37(2):19–23

**Baruk H:** Quelques réflexions sur l'histoire de la psychiatrie. **Hist Sci Med** 1984;18(3):205–7

**Baruk H:** Vers la résurrection de la civilisation hébraïque. La psychiatrie hébraique. **Rev Hist Med Heb** 1983 Jul;36(145):25–7

**Baruk H:** Viktor Frankl et la psychanalyse. **Ann Med Psychol (Paris)** 1982 Apr;140(4):438–42

**Baruk H** see **Vié J**

**Barz H:** Psychologische Probleme des Unbewussten: C.G. Jung und sein Lebenswerk für die moderne Psychologie. **Universitas (Stuttg)** 1980;35(3):275–82

**Barzó M:** Zur Entwicklung der Dokumentation und Auswertung der stationären Morbidität in Ungarn. **Z Gesamte Hyg** 1980 Apr;26(4):275–80

**Basante Pol RM, Garcia Ada R:** La botica del Colegio Imperial de Madrid. **Bol Soc Esp Hist Farm** 1982 Mar;33(132):219–36

**Basante Pol RM, Castillo Tello MM:** La correspondencia dirigida a D. Casimiro Gomez Ortega, desde Valencia en el periodo comprendido entre 1783–1788. **Bol Soc Esp Hist Farm** 1982 Mar;33(130):131–44

**Basante Pol RM, Castillo Tello MM:** La correspondencia dirigida a D. Casimiro Gómez Ortega por D. Cándido M.a Trigueros. **Bol Soc Esp Hist Farm** 1981 Sep;32(127):137–47

**Basante Pol RM:** La farmacia en los monasterios, hospitales y hospederías del Bierzo. **Bol Soc Esp Hist Farm** 1984 Sep;35(139):165–86

**Basante Pol RM:** La real oficina de farmacia en las postrimerias del reinado de Isabel II (1843–1868). **Bol Soc Esp Hist Farm** 1983 Mar–Jun;34(133–134):11–23

**Basante Pol RM:** Notas sobre algunos de los boticarios madrileños de los primeros años de siglo XVIII. **Bol Soc Esp Hist Farm** 1980 Oct;31(123):235–58

**Basante Pol RM** see **Folch Jou G**

**Basas M:** La epidemia del cólera morbo de 1854–1855 en Bilbao y otras noticias de este tiempo. **Estud Duesto** 1969;17:135–73

**Basch MF:** Selfobject disorders and psychoanalytic theory: a historical perspective. **J Am Psychoanal Assoc** 1981;29(2):337–51

**Basch MF** see **Goldberg A, ed**

**Baserga A, Zavagli G:** Ferrata's stem cells: an historical review on hemocytoblasts and hemohistioblasts. **Blood Cells** 1981;7(3):537–45

**Baserga A:** Le anemie: passato, presente e futuro. **Recenti Prog Med** 1983 Jan;74(1):1–10

**Baserga A:** Una descrizione della forma dei globuli rossi dell'emolisi nella Pavia del settecento. **Haematologica (Pavia)** 1980 Feb;65(1):131–34

**Baserga SJ:** The early years of coeducation at the Yale University School of Medicine. **Yale J Biol Med** 1980 May–Jun;53(3):181–90

**Basham AL:** Hinduism [and Hindu medicine]. In Reich WT, et al, ed: Encyclopedia of bioethics, v. 2. New York, Free Press, 1978. p. 661–66.

**Bashtanova LV** see **Verenkina TN**

**Basich Z, et al:** Testimonios sobre medicina de los antiguos mexicanos. México, Instituto Mexicano del Seguro Social, 1980. n. p.

**Bäsig W:** Die Philatelie im Dienste der Rehabilitation. **Rehabilitation (Stuttg)** 1981 May;20(2):86–9

**Basileios Stephanopoulos–Vrettos: mia alesmonete mneme: Stomatologia (Athenai)** 1980 Nov–Dec;37(6):5–48

**Basilevsky A** see **Hum D**

**Basinski J:** Leczenie rannych i chorych w przebiegu Powstania Wielkopolskiego. Czas od 27.12.1918 do 13.11.1919. **Arch Hist Med (Warsz)** 1979;42(2):189–204

**Basiński J:** Organizacja i działalność słuzby zdrowia w pierwszym okresie powstania Wielkopolskiego. **Arch Hist Med (Warsz)** 1979;42(1):1–18

**Basinski J:** Zachorowalność i obrazenia wojenne w Powstaniu Wielkopolskim. Czas od 27.12.1918 do 13.11.1919 roku. **Arch Hist Med (Warsz)** 1979;42(2):177–87

**Basinski J:** Zaplecze i środki sanitarno–medyczne wojsk sanitarnych Powstańczej Armii Wielkopolskiej. Czas od 16.01.1919 do 13.11.1919. **Arch Hist Med (Warsz)** 1979;42(2):161–76

**Bass J:** Strike at Charleston. **New South** 1969;24(3):35–44

**Bass P** see **Palm LC**

**Bass WM** see **Gregg JB**

**Basset A:** Aperçu sur l'épidémiologie de la lèpre en France au cours de ces cinquante dernières années. **Bull Mem Acad R Med Belg** 1984;139(2):156–64

**Basset A, Burgun R:** Geschichte der Dermatologie. In Sournia JC, Martiny M, Poulet J, ed: Illustrierte Geschichte der Medizin. Salzburg, Andreas, 1980. Vol. 4. p. 1547–73.

**Bassett EJ, Keith MS, Armelagos GJ, et al:** Tetracycline-labeled human bone from ancient Sudanese Nubia (A.D. 350). **Science** 1980 Sep 26;209(4464):1532–4)

**Bassis M, Delpech G:** Discovery of the red blood cell with notes on priorities and credits of discoveries, past, present and future. **Blood Cells** 1981;7(3):447–80

**Bast G:** Viktor Schilling 1883–1983. Selbstzeugnisse und Erinnerungen an den Altmeister der morphologischen Hämatologie. **Folia Haematol (Leipz)** 1983;110(5):617–29

**Bastenchuk AZ, Vladova MI, Siur HA, et al:** Dosiahnennia aptechnoiï sluzhby Zaporiz'koï oblasti z chasu pryïniattia dekretu pro natsionalizatsiiu aptek na Ukraïni. **Farm Zh** 1979;(6):9–11

**Bastenie PA:** Le vieillissement. Vers une nouvelle source de jeunesse. Paris, Flammarion, 1983. 270 p. (De La Science à l'Homme).

**Bastholm E:** Laennec og stetoskopet. **Dan Medicinhist Arbog** 1982;:112–35

**Bastholm E, ed** see **Skov H**

**Bastien JW:** Exchange between Andean and Western medicine. **Soc Sci Med** 1982;16(7):795–803

**Bastien JW:** Herbal curing by Qollahuaya Andeans. **J Ethnopharmacol** 1982 Jul;6(1):13–28

**Bastien JW:** Pharmacopeia of Qollahuaya Andeans. **J Ethnopharmacol** 1983 Jul;8(1):97–111

**Bastin R:** Méningites purulentes. Rappel historique. **Rev Prat** 1981 Jun 11;31(33):2343–4, 2347

**Bataille G** see **Bernard J**

**Batári G:** Az elsö gyógyászati szakfolyóiratok magyarországon. **Magy Konyvsz** 1982;98(1):72–5

**Batári G:** Az Erdélyi Orvosok Egyesülete (1833–1836). **Orv Hetil** 1981 Jul 12;122(28):1732

**Batari G:** Az orvosi sajtóreferálás kezdetei Magyarországon. **Orv Hetil** 1982 Oct 17;123(42):2611–3

**Batári G:** Erik Ingman finn orvos látogatása Pesten Bugát Pálnál 1847–ben. **Orvostort Kozl** 1981;93–96(27 No 1–4):189–92

**Batári G:** Schmidt Béla és az erdélyi Magyar Népegészségügyi Szemle. **Orv Hetil** 1982 Oct 31;123(44):2737–8

**Batári G:** Schwartzer Ottó mint az orvosi sajtóreferálás kezdeményezöje. **Orv Hetil** 1979 Jul 1;120(26):1586–7

**Batchelor AJ:** AMWA's founder--the 'red headed dynamo'. **J Am Med Wom Assoc** 1984 Jul–Aug;39(4):123, 139

**Batchen LS:** La curandera. **Palacio** 1975;81(1):20–5

**Bates DB** see **Webster C**

**Bates DG:** Sydenham and social history.
**Soc Soc Hist Med Bull (Lond)** 1980;27:27-9
**Bates DG:** Teaching and research in the history of medicine in China. **Bull Hist Med** 1979 Spring;53(1):128-39
**Bates DG:** Teaching medical history to medical students: the McGill experience, 1966-1981. With a commentary by L.G. Stevenson. In J. J. Bylebyl, ed: Teaching the history of medicine at a medical center. Baltimore, London, Johns Hopkins University Press, 1982. (The Henry E. Sigerist supplements to the Bulletin of the History of Medicine; new ser., no. 7). p. 121-38.
**Bates EM:** A consumer's view of the Australian experience in health insurance. **Lancet** 1980 Jul 5;2(8184):26-8
**Bates JD:** The extraction debate of 1911. **New Dent** 1980 Jan;10(5):36-7
**Bates SS** see **Buchanan AV**
**Bateson W:** Problems of genetics. Reprint of 1913 ed. Historical introduction by G. E. Hutchinson and S. Rachootin. New Haven and London, Yale University Press, 1979. xxii, 258 p.
**Bath CR:** Health and environmental problems: the role of the border in El Paso-Ciudad Juarez coordination. **J Interam Stud World Aff** 1982;24(3):375-92
**Batiashvili OG:** I. K. Abakeliia--osnovopolozhnik ftiziatrii i organizator bor'by s tuberkulezom v Gruzii (k 100-letiiu dnia rozhdeniia). **Probl Tuberk** 1983 Jul;(7):73-4
**Bator PA:** Saving lives on the wholesale plan: public health reform in the city of Toronto, 1900-1930. Ph. D. Diss. University of Toronto. Toronto, 1979.
**Bator PA:** 'The struggle to raise the lower classes': public health reform and the problem of poverty in Toronto, 1910 to 1921. **J Can Stud** 1979;14(1):43-9
**Battin J:** Le sentiment de l'enfance. In: Congrès National des Sociétés Savantes, 104e, Bordeaux, 1979. Comptes Rendus. Paris, 1979. Section des Sciences, Fasc. IV. p. 319-27.
**Battistella R, Eastaugh SR:** Health cost containment.
**Proc Acad Polit Sci** 1980;33(4):192-205
**Battle JD Jr:** The 'periodical head-achs' of Thomas Jefferson.
**Cleve Clin Q** 1984 Fall;51(3):531-9
**Battocletti JH, Halbach RE, Salles-Cunha SX, et al:** The NMR blood flowmeter--theory and history. **Med Phys** 1981 Jul-Aug;8(4):435-43
**Batty Shaw A:** Knappers' rot; silicosis in East Anglian flint-knappers. **Med Hist** 1981 Apr;25(2):151-68
**Batuev AS:** Fiziologicheskaia nauchnaia shkola Leningradskogo universiteta. **Fiziol Zh SSSR** 1984 Oct;70(10):1353-60
**Baud CA** see **Kramar C**
**Baud CA** see **Lagier R**
**Baudin C:** Pasteur: un homme, une oeuvre. **Chir Dent Fr** 1983 Jul 7;53(211):23-5
**Baudis P:** Franz Köstl a jeho práce s epidemiologickým zaměřením. **Cesk Psychiatr** 1979 Apr;75(2):144-7
**Baudot G** see **Histoire culturelle de la maladie**
**Baudot M** see **La médecine hospitalière française au XVIIIème siècle**
**Baudry FD:** Adolescent love and self-analysis as contributors to Flaubert's creativity. **Psychoanal Study Child** 1980;35:377-416
**Baudry FD:** Problems in the application of psychoanalysis to Mary Shelley's Frankenstein. **Int J Psychoanal Psychother** 1982-83;9:647-56
**Baue AE:** Landmark perspective: Evarts A. Graham and the first pneumonectomy. **JAMA** 1984 Jan 13;251(2):260-4
**Baue AE:** 60 years of the Archives of Surgery. July 1920-July 1980. **Arch Surg** 1980 Jul;115(7):809-11
**Bauer A:** Das öffentliche Krankenhaus als wissenschaftliche Bildungs-Anstalt. In Seidler E, Schott, ed: Bausteine zur Medizingeschichte. Stuttgart, Steiner, 1984. p. 9-27.
**Bauer A:** Rudolf Virchow: der politische Arzt. Berlin, Stapp, 1982. 131 p. (Preussische Köpfe, 6).
**Bauer B:** Studien zum ersten altdeutschen Pferdearzneibuch des anonymen Kopenhagener Ms. Thott Nr. 202. DMV Diss. Hannover, 1980. 99 p.
**Bauer C, Ritt L:** 'The little health of ladies.' An anatomy of female invalidism in the nineteenth century. **J Am Med Wom Assoc** 1981 Oct;36(10):300-6
**Bauer G:** Das 'Haager Aderlassbüchlein'. (Studien zum ärztlichen Vademecum des Spätmittelalters, 1). Pattensen/Hannover, 1978. 198 p. (Würzburger medizinhistorische Forschungen, 14). Also Diss. Würzburg, 1978.
**Bauer G:** Sven Johanssons betydelse för höftfrakturernas behandling. **Sydsven Medicinhist Sallsk Arsskr** 1981;:12-29
**Bauer GH** see **Stambolian G**
**Bauer KH:** Die Deutschen Chirurgenkongresse seit der 50. Tagung aus der Sicht ihrer Vorsitzenden. Berlin, New York, Springer-Verlag, 1983. ix, 262 p.
**Bauer Y:** Genocide: was it the Nazis' original plan.
**Ann Am Acad Polit Soc Sci** 1980;450:35-45
**Bauerndoktor und Volksmedizin. 1. Ausstellung anlässlich des 800-jährigen Bestehens von Stainz. Sonderausstellung: Juni bis Okt. 1977. Katalog: Nr. 3. Maria Kundegraber, unter Mitarb. v. Bernd Mader. Steiermark, Landesmuseum Joanneum, 1977. 63 p.:**
**Baugut G** see **Bredy E**
**Baum L:** Gold foil. **Oper Dent** 1984 Spring;9(2):42-9
**Bauman M:** Intrepid nurses faced the challenges. **Alaska J** 1980;10:36-42
**Baumann HU:** Ueber Mehrfachentdeckungen. Eine Darstellung des allgemeinen Problems mit Beispielen aus drei Teilgebieten der theoretischen Medizin. Diss. Münster, 1972. 133 p.
**Baumann J:** Das Stadtkrankenhaus Kassel während der Jahre 1942 bis 1965. In Balde JH, Schmiking W, ed: Festschrift zum 86. Deutschen Arztetag in Kassel. Kassel, Arztevereins, 1983. p. 89-98.
**Baumann J:** Destinée de la méthode anatomo-clinique.
**Bull Acad Natl Med (Paris)** 1981 Feb 17;Spec No:45-50
**Baumberger HR:** Carl Liebermeister 1833-1901. Zürich, Juris, 1980. 181 p (Zürcher Medizingeschichtliche Abhandlungen, Neue Reihe, 137).
**Baume LG, Treccani A:** La biologia della polpa dentaria e della dentina: storia delle scoperte istologiche (parte I). **Riv Ital Stomatol** 1983 Oct;52(10):799-803
**Baume LJ:** Centenaire de l'Ecole dentaire de Genève. La biologie pulpo-dentinaire au temps de la création d l'Ecole dentaire de Genève (21 octobre 1881). **Swiss Dent** 1981 Dec;2(12):16-8, 20-2
**Baume LJ:** Evolution de la médecine dentaire opératoire.
**Rev Belge Med Dent** 1983 Mar;38(2):33-7
**Baume LJ:** Vers le centenaire de notre Société.
**Schweiz Monatsschr Zahnmed** 1984 Oct;94(10):1061-2
**Baumel HB:** Biology: its historical development. New York, Philosophical Library, 1978. 101 p.
**Baumer G, Greulich G:** Otto Rank. In J. Rattner, ed: Wandlungen der Psychoanalyse. Wien, Europaverlag, 1980. p. 31-52.
**Baumgartner L:** Two hundred years of children.
**Trans Stud Coll Physicians Phila** 1977 Apr;44(4):165-78
**Baumgartner R:** Fussprothese aus einem frühmittelalterlichen Grab aus Bonaduz. **Helv Archaeol** 1982;13(51-2):155-62
**Bäumler E:** Paul Ehrlich, Forscher für das Leben. Frankfurt, Societäts-Verlag, 1979. 370 p.
**Baumont M:** Maurice Barrès et les morts de la guerre de 1914-18. **Inf Hist** 1969;31(1):30-5
**Baur FJ, Parker WA:** The aflatoxin problem: industry-FDA-USDA cooperation. **J Assoc Off Anal Chem** 1984 Jan-Feb;67(1):3-7
**Baur O, Bott B, Braunfels-Esche S, et al:** Leonardo da Vinci Anatomie, Physiognomik, Proportion und Bewegung. Köln, 1984. 343 p. (Kölner medizinhistorische Beiträge: Arbeiten der Forschungsstelle des Instituts für Geschichte der Medizin der Universität zu Köln, Band 23/1)
**Bauriedel K:** Early continuing medical education in dermatology. **Int J Dermatol** 1981 Nov;20(9):614-5
**Bautista T** see **Valverde JL**
**Bautista Méndez JL** see **Valverde JL**
**Bautista Mendez MT** see **Valverde JL**
**Bautista Mendez T** see **Valverde JL**
**Bauwens P:** La peste à Huy au XVIIe siècle. Fédération des Cercles d'Archéologie et d'Histoire de Belgique. 44e session. Congrès de Huy, 1976. Annales. Tielt, 1978. p. 235-9.
**Bawden CR:** W. A. Unkrig's correspondence with the British and Foreign Bible Society. A contribution to ... printing in Mongolian.
**Zentralasiat Stud** 1980;14(1):65-108
**Baxby D:** A death from inoculated smallpox in the English Royal Family. **Med Hist** 1984 Jul;28(3):303-7
**Baxby D:** An unauthorized contemporary reprinting of Jenner's paper on the cuckoo. **J Hist Med Allied Sci** 1981 Apr;36(2):218-9
**Baxby D:** Jenner's smallpox vaccine. The riddle of vaccinia virus and its origin. London, Heinemann Educational Books, 1981. xiv, 214 p.
**Baxter AL:** E. B. Wilson's 'Destruction' of the germ-layer theory. **Isis** 1977 Sep;68(243):363-74
**Baxter EG:** Dr. Jephson of Leamington Spa. Edited by J. Lane and R. Bearman. Leamington Spa, Warwickshire Local History Society, 1980. xii, 104 p.
**Bay A:** Chemical warfare: perspectives and potentials. **Strategy Tactics** 1980;81:23-33
**Bay E:** Neurologie im Wandel. **Jahrb Univ Dusseld** 1977-78;:135-52
**Bay E:** Sigmund Freud's contribution to the early history of aphasiology. In Rose FC, Bynum WF, ed: Historical aspects of the neurosciences. New York, Raven, 1982. p. 103-7.
**Baycar RS** see **Aker F**
**Bayer FW:** Der Merck'sche Jahresbericht als Quelle zur Geschichte der Therapie. **Pharm Ind** 1980;42(7):701-6
**Bayer H:** Walter Stoeckel--Leben und Werk. **Zentralbl Gynakol** 1983;105(1):52-5
**Bayer R, Spitzer RL:** Edited correspondence on the status of homosexuality in DSM-III. **J Hist Behav Sci** 1982 Jan;18(1):32-52
**Bayer RA:** Q fever as an occupational illness at the National Institutes of Health. **Public Health Rep** 1982 Jan-Feb;97(1):58-60
**Bayer S:** Z dziejów konspiracyjnej służby zdrowia w Warszawie (1939-1944). **Przegl Lek** 1980;37(1):131-7
**Bayertz K:** Naturwissenschaft und Sozialismus: Tendenzen der Naturwissenschafts-Rezeption in der deutschen Arbeiterbewegung des 19. Jahrhunderts. **Soc Stud Sci** 1983 Aug;13(3):355-94
**Bayliss JH:** The earliest British medical practitioner? **Lancet** 1984 Dec 22;2(8417-18):1458
**Bayliss JH:** The extinction of bubonic plague in Britain. **Endeavour** 1980;4(2):58-66
**Bayliss RA:** Andrew Moir: an Aberdeen anatomist. **Scott Med J** 1980;25:315-9
**Bayliss RA, Ellis CW:** Neil Arnott, F.R.S., reformer, innovator and popularizer of science, 1788-1874. **Notes Rec R Soc Lond** 1981;36(1):103-24
**Bayliss RA:** The Round Table Club, Edinburgh. **Practitioner** 1980 Apr;224(1342):438-40
**Baylon H:** L'oeuvre du Service de Santé des Armées en Afrique noire d'expression française. **Bull Acad Natl Med (Paris)** 1981 Apr;165(4):449-60

Rev Soc Venez Hist Med 1981;30(45-46):111-4
**Beaujón O:** La salud y el pensamiento militar y politico del General San Martín. **Bol Acad Nac Hist (Caracas)** 1979;62(245):35-56
**Beaulieu A** see **Levere TH, ed**
**Beaune C** see **Guillemain B**
**Beauperthuy de Benedetti R:** Au sujet des quatre faits importants de la medecine au Venezuela. In: International Congress of the History of Medicine, 26th, Plovdiv (Bulgaria), 1978. Actes du Congres, Vol. 1. Sofia, 1980. p. 90-2.
**Beauperthuy de Benedetti R:** Beauperthuy. La herpetología y Venuzuela. In International Congress of the History of Medicine, 27th, Barcelona, 1980. Actas. Barcelona, Académia de Ciències Médiques de Catalunya i Balears, 1981. p. 454-7.
**Beauperthuy de Benedetti R:** Beauperthuy y su microscopio. **Rev Soc Venez Hist Med** 1978;27(41):59-64
**Beauperthuy de Benedetti R:** Bref commentaire à un travail de Sir William Osler et sa reconnaissance de la théorie scientifique de Beauperthuy sur la fièvre jaune. In: Congrès international d'histoire de la médecine, XXVe, Québec, 1976. Actes. Québec, 1977. p. 487-92.
**Beauperthuy de Benedetti R:** Informe sobre la publicacion del señor Cesar Rodriguez Exposito. **Rev Soc Venez Hist Med** 1972-73;20-21(34-35):141-50
**Beauperthuy de Benedetti R:** La mujer y la medicina. **Rev Soc Venez Hist Med** 1969-71;17-19(31-33):135-51
**Beauperthuy de Benedetti R:** Laveran y Beauperthuy. **Acta Med Venez** 1981 Jan-Mar;28(1):47-52
**Beauperthuy de Benedetti R:** Repercusion en la Argentina en 1871 del descubrimiento del vector de la fiebre amarilla realizado por Beauperthuy en Venezuela. **Rev Soc Venez Hist Med** 1980;29(43-44):87-93
**Beauperthuy de Benedetti R:** Resonancia del descurbrimiento del agente transmisor de la fiebre amarilla que hizo Beauperthuy en Venezuela. **Rev Soc Venez Hist Med** 1972-73;20-21(34-35):67-77
**Beauperthuy de Benedetti R:** Un cirujano y un medico de Montpellier en el siglo pasado en Caracas. **Rev Soc Venez Hist Med** 1979;28(42):29-30
**Beauperthuy de Benedetti R** see **Sociedad Venezolana de Historia de la medicina**
**Beauquier JP:** Quelques aspects de la démographie et de la santé à Marseille pendant la seconde guerre mondiale. **Provence Hist** 1983;33(134):439-47
**Beaver H:** Parkman's crack-up: a Bostonian on the Oregon Trail. **N Engl Q** 1975;48(1):84-103
**Beaver WT:** Analgesic development: a brief history and perspective. **J Clin Pharmacol** 1980 Apr;20(4 Pt 2):213-5
**Beavert CS** see **Hessler RK**
**Beawer D de B:** The American scientific community, 1800-1860; a statistical-historical study (Doctoral Dissertation, Yale University, 1966). New York, Arno Press, 1980. 379 p.
**Bebear JP** see **Portmann M**
**Bec A** see **Bec M**
**Bec M, Bec A:** Ignacy Schuch -- lekarz sandomierski. **Arch Hist Med (Warsz)** 1984;47(3):383-7
**Bec P:** Le prochain centenaire de la société française d'ophtalmologie (1883-1983). **J Fr Ophtalmol** 1980;3(5):313-4
**Bečer A, Tichý M:** Začiatky otolaryngológie na lekárskej fakulte UK v Bratislave. **Bratisl Lek Listy** 1983;79(3):369-74
**Bechtel W:** The evolution of our understanding of the cell: a study in the dynamics of scientific progress. **Stud Hist Philos Sci** 1984 Dec;15(4):309-56
**Bechtereva NP, Bundzen PV, Malyshev VN:** [Sechenov's tradition in the development of physiology of mental activity, its origins and perspectives] (Rus). **Istor Biol Issled** 1980;8:163-72
**Beck A:** Medicine, tradition, and development in Kenya and Tanzania, 1920-1970. Waltham, Crossroads Press, 1981. viii, 114 p.
**Beck A:** Priorities in biological research at Amani, 1902-1914. **Tanzan Notes Rec** 1981;(86-87):13-6
**Beck A:** Recent changes in attitude toward medicine in East Africa. In: Congrès international d'histoire de la médecine, XXVe, Québec, 1976. Actes. Québec, 1977. p. 493-501.
**Beck AM** see **Worth D**
**Beck IT:** Canadian gastroenterology: yesterday, today and tomorrow. **Clin Invest Med** 1982;5(2-3):93-107
**Beck JM:** George Murray. In Dictionary of Canadian biography, 1881-1890. 1982;11:633-4.
**Beck LA** see **Blakely RL**
**Beck WC** see **Meyer KK**
**Beck-Mannagetta P:** Zum 300. Todestag des Johann Wilhelm Ritter von Mannagetta und seinem Wirken in Niederösterreich. **Unsere Heimat** 1966;37(4-6):125-9
**Bečka J:** Otec lékařu Avicenna v naší vědě a kultuře. Abú Alí ibn Síná (980-1037). **Cas Lek Cesk** 1980 Jan 5;119(1):17-23
**Becke U:** Eine hinterlassene psychiatrische Studie Paul Johann Reiters über Luther. **Z Kirchengesch** 1979;90(1):85-95
**Becker A:** Radiological pioneers in Saskatoon. **Sask Hist** 1983;36(1):31-7
**Becker AE** see **Anderson RH**
**Becker C, Martin V:** Les premiers recensements au Sénégal; le Sénégal centre-ouest et son évolution démographique. **Ann Demogr Hist (Paris)** 1981;:367-86
**Becker H:** Helmuth von Moltke als Beobachter der hygienischen und medizinischen Situation im osmanischen Kaiserreich (1835-39). In Göpfert W, Otten HH, ed: Metavoeite: wandelt euch durch neues Denken. Düsseldorf, Triltsch, 1983. p. 147-59.
**Becker H:** Roter Graben 10: ausgewählte Kapital aus der Pharmaziegeschichte, 1790-1870. Herzogenrath [Germany], Murken-Altrogge, [1982]. 288 p.
**Becker J:** Die Geschichte des Rheinischen Landeskrankenhauses Düsseldorf-Grafenberg von 1876 bis 1918. Diss. Düsseldorf, 1978. 212 p.
**Becker K:** 100 Jahre gesetzliche Krankenversicherung. Entwicklung, Krise, Lösungsansätze in der Krankenversicherung der Rentner. (Mit einem Beitrag von Jens Jessen, Programmierter Kollaps der GKV?) Mainz, MPS, 1980. 74 p.
**Becker KF:** Kirche und Alter in Geschichte Gegenwart. **Z Gerontol** 1984 Jan-Feb;17(1):32-8
**Becker KH, Schmidt HD:** Uber eine bisher unerschlossene Quelle der Preyer-Forschung. **Z Psychol** 1984;192(2):182-91
**Becker KP, Sovák M:** Lehrbuch der Logopädie. 2. Auflage. Königstein/Ts., Verlagsgruppe Athenäum, Hain, Scriptor, Hanstein, 1979. Historical section, p. 31-48.
**Becker KP:** 30 Jahre Lehre, Forschung und Wissenschaftsentwicklung im Dienste der Bildung, Erziehung und Rehabilitation Geschädigter. **Wiss Z Humboldt Univ Berl [Gesellschaftswiss Sprachwiss Reihe]** 1979;28(2):157-64
**Becker RA:** The John Jacob Abel papers--primary sources for the history of American pharmacology. **Pharm Hist** 1982;24(3):115-6
**Becker S** see **Brede K**
**Becker T:** Das chirurgische Erbe. Erwin Payr zum Gedenken. **Zentralbl Chir** 1981;106(23):1563-8
**Becker V:** Carl Ruge: 100 Jahre Stückchen-Diagnose. **Arch Gynecol** 1979 Sep;227(3):193-204
**Beckett JV:** An eighteenth-century case history: Carlisle Spedding 1738. **Med Hist** 1982 Jul;26(3):303-6
**Beckett JV:** Illness and amputation in the eighteenth century: the case of Sir James Lowther (1673-1755). **Med Hist** 1980 Jan;24(1):88-92
**Beckh-Widmannstetter HA:** Zur Geschichte der Individualpsychologie: Julius Wagner-Jauregg über Alfred Adler. **Unsere Heimat** 1965;36(10-12):182-8
**Beckham SD** see **Wilson LG, ed**
**Beckmann P, Kirchhoff HW:** Heilkunst und Heilkunde am Beispiel des Pfarrers Sebastian Kneipp. **Ther Ggw** 1980 Aug;119(8):945-53
**Beckwith CI:** The introduction of Greek medicine into Tibet in the seventh and eighth centuries. **J Am Orient Soc** 1979;99:297-313
**Bedault M** see **Avellano E**
**Beddall BG:** Essay review: Spanish science and the New World. **J Hist Biol** 1983 Fall;16(3):433-40
**Beddings A** see **Cremone JC**
**Bedford J:** Prostitution in Calgary 1905-1914. **Alberta Hist** 1981;29(2):1-11
**Bedini SA:** Derek J. de Solla Price (1922-1983). **Technol Cult** 1984 Jul;25(3):701-5
**Bedini SA:** Derek J. DeSolla Price. **Ann Ist Mus Stor Sci Fir** 1984;9(1):95-115
**Bednář B** see **Mířejovský P**
**Bednarczyk A:** Antymechanicyzm w osiemnastowiecznej filozofii medycyny: Georg Ernst Stahl (1659-1734) i animizm. **Arch Hist Med (Warsz)** 1981;44(2):163-87
**Bednarczyk A:** Pierre Louis Moreau de Maupertuis (1698-1759) atomizm biologiczny i panpsychizm. **Kwart Hist Nauki Tech** 1981;26(2):335-62
**Bednárová E** see **Bunčáková V**
**Bednarski Z:** Robert Koch (1843-1910). **Wiad Lek** 1983 Mar 1;36(5):425-7
**Bednarski Z:** Sto lat od odkrycia prątka gruźlicy (1882-1982) przez Roberta Kocha: szybka reakcja w polskich czasopismach lekarskich. **Pol Tyg Lek** 1983 Mar 28;38(13):419-21
**Bedrani R** see **Avellano E**
**Bedrin AV, Medvinskaia KG:** Sverdlovskomu nauchno-issledovatel'skomu institutu tuberkuleza 50 let. **Probl Tuberk** 1982 May;(5):75-8
**Bedwell SF:** D'Anville's doom--a neurological vignette from historic Halifax. **Can J Neurol Sci** 1980 Feb;7(1):1-8
**Beebe RT:** Albany Medical College and Albany Hospital: a history, 1839-1982. Albany, N. Y., New Art Printing, 1983. xxv, 458 p.
**Beecher DM:** The history of dental health on Guam. **Bull Hist Dent** 1983 Oct;31(2):108-12
**Beeching BW:** Historical background to radiation safety of dental x-ray sets in the English speaking countries. **Dentomaxillofac Radiol** 1981;10(2):85-92
**Beeck M:** Merkmale epileptischer Bildnerei: mit Pathographie Van Gogh. Bern, Huber, 1982. 134 p.
**Beer AE** see **Billingham RE**
**Beer CG:** Darwin, instinct, and ethology. **J Hist Behav Sci** 1983 Jan;19(1):68-80
**Beer FJ:** Le souvenir d'Henri-Ernest Sigerist (1891-1957). **Hist Sci Med** 1982;16(1):49-53
**Beer G:** Anxiety and interchange: Daniel Deronda and the implications of Darwin's writing. **J Hist Behav Sci** 1983 Jan;19(1):31-44
**Beer H, Dorolle P, Howard-Jones N:** Geschichte der internationalen Gesundheitsbehörden. In Sournia JC, Martiny M, Poulet J, ed: Illustrierte Geschichte der Medizin. Salzburg, Andreas, 1980. Vol. 8. p. 3109-39.
**Beer H, Dorolle P, Howard-Jones N:** Histoire des institutions médicales internationales. In: Histoire de la médecine, de la pharmacie, de l'art dentaire, et de l'art véterinaire. Tome VIII. Paris, Albin Michel, Laffont, Tchou, 1980. p. 327-41.
**Beer M:** Suicidio e inettitudine: nota sui romanzi femminili Italiani del ventennio 1880-1890. **Mem Riv Stor Donne** 1981;(2):76-88
**Beere P** see **Sanderson CJ**
**Beerens J:** Ombre et lumière sur la médecine. **Cah Biloque** 1980;30:41-53,

81–96
**Beering SC:** 'The spark within.' **J Indiana State Med Assoc** 1982 Jan;75(1):22–4
**Beerli UP:** Medizinisches in Scheuchzers Physica sacra oder Kupferbibel. Zürich, Juris, 1980. 89p. (Zürcher medizingeschichtliche Abhandlungen, Neue Reihe, Nr. 143).
**Beerman H:** Frederick Deforest Weidman, M.D. **J Am Acad Dermatol** 1983 Sep;9(3):479–86
**Beerman H:** John Hinchman Stokes, M.D. An appreciation. **J Am Acad Dermatol** 1983 Aug;9(2):321–34
**Beerman H:** My half century in dermatopathology (1928–1978). **Am J Dermatopathol** 1979 Fall;1(3):237–43
**Beerman H:** Sherlock Holmes and medical history. **Trans Stud Coll Physicians Phila** 1978 Jul;45(5):243–8
**Beerman H** see **Shelley WB**
**Beeson PB:** Some diseases that have disappeared. **Am J Med** 1980 Jun;68(6):806–11
**Beg MH:** Muslim contribution to surgery. **JPMA** 1984 Jul;34(7):218–21
**Beg MH:** Zaheeruddin Mohammad Babar. **JPMA** 1981;31(5):114–7
**Béguinot P** see **Amiot M**
**Behan PO, Behan WM:** Sir Robert Carswell: Scotland's pioneer pathologist. In Rose FC, Bynum WF, ed: Historical aspects of the neurosciences. New York, Raven, 1982. p. 273–92.
**Behan WM** see **Behan PO**
**Behbehani AM:** The smallpox story: life and death of an old disease. **Microbiol Rev** 1983 Dec;47(4):455–509
**Behbehani AM:** The smallpox story: man finally defeats an old adversary. **J Kans Med Soc** 1980 Oct;81(10):447–56, 474
**Behlmer GK:** Child abuse and moral reform in England, 1870–1908. Stanford, Stanford University Press, 1982. viii, 320 p.
**Behn RD, Sperduto K:** Medical Schools and the 'entitlement ethic'. **Public Interest** 1979;57:48–68
**Behney CJ** see **Banta HD**
**Behnke O, Wieth JO:** Laegeuddannelsen i København 1479–1979. **Nord Med** 1979 Dec;94(12):321–4
**Behnke O:** Review of the history of the University of Copenhagen and the Faculty of Medicine. **Dan Med Bull** 1980 May;27(Suppl 1):1–4
**Behrens H:** Die Entstehung der Schweinegesundheitsdienste in Deutschland bis 1945 und in der Bundesrepublik Deutschland. **DTW** 1980 Dec 5;87(12):455–60
**Behrens H:** Geschichte und Aufgaben der deutschen Tiergesundheitsämter. **DTW** 1981 Aug 5;88(8):325–32
**Behrens V** see **Taylor W**
**Behrman S:** Congestion of the brain. In Rose FC, Bynum WF, ed: Historical aspects of the neurosciences. New York, Raven, 1982. p. 179–84.
**Beĭbutov ShM** see **Bakhshiev BA**
**Beierlein C:** Zum Leben und Schaffen von Sigmund Freud (1856–1939) im Umfeld seiner Zeit. **Wiss Z Martin Luther Univ (Math)** 1984;33(2):101–12
**Beighton PH** see **Hayden MR**
**Beĭlikhis GA:** Ob issledovaniiakh po gigienie truda v XVII–XVIII vekakh v Rossii. **Gig Tr Prof Zabol** 1980 Aug;(8):40–2
**Béjin A** see **Dupâquier J**
**Bek V:** Postgraduální výchovně vzdělávací proces v klinické onkologii. Přehled činnosti katedry klinické onkologie u příležitosti 30. výročí Institutu pro další vzdělávání lékařu a farmaceutu v Praze. **Cas Lek Cesk** 1983 Nov 25;122(47):1457–60
**Beklemishev VN:** Problemy épidemiologii i épizootologii kleshchevogo éntsefalita (po neopublikovannym materialam iz arkhiva V. N. Beklemisheva). **Med Parazitol (Mosk)** 1983 Jan–Feb;52(1):66–74
**Bel E, María Suñé J:** La 'Farmacopea Matritense en Castellano' y la 'Farmacopea en Castellano o colección de las fórmulas más usuales y acreditadas de la matritense y española'. **Bol Soc Esp Hist Farm** 1984 Jun;35(138):69–87
**Bel-Haj Mahmoud N:** La psychologie des animaux chez les arabes, notamment à travers le kitab al-hayawan de Djahiz. Paris, Klincksieck, 1977. xxiii, 231 p. (Etudes arabes et islamiques, Série 3; Etudes et documents, 8).
**Bélanger LF:** On a nickel and a prayer. Ottawa, University of Ottawa Press, 1978. 146 p.
**Belanger M:** Une nouvelle branche du droit international: le droit international de la sante. **Etud Int** 1982;13(4):611–32
**Belda W:** Aspectos da hanseníase na área urbana do município de São Paulo - Hanseníase indiferenciada, 1963–1977. **Hansenol Int** 1981 Jun;6(1):23–50
**Belda W** see **Siqueira LF**
**Belevitin AB** see **Veselov EI**
**Belguedj S:** La Collection hippocratique et l'embryologie coranique. In La collection hippocratique et son rôle dans l'histoire de la médecine. Colloque de Strasbourg (23–27 octobre 1972) organisé par le Centre de Recherches sur la Grèce Antique, avec le concours des Facultés de Philosophie et des Langues Classiques. Leiden, E. J. Brill, 1975. p. 321–33.
**Beliaev DK:** Vydaiushchiesia sovetskie genetiki: sbornik biograficheskikh ocherkov. Moskva, Nauka, 1980. 147 p.
**Beliakov VD:** Uchenie L. V. Gromashevskogo ob épidemicheskom protsesse i razvitie étogo ucheniia na sovremennom étape. **Zh Mikrobiol Epidemiol Immunobiol** 1984 Jul;(7):115–8
**Beliaskiĭ EA** see **Zakharov BI**
**Beliatskiĭ DP:** K istorii razvitiia zdravookhraneniia BSSR na osnove printsipov leninskoĭ natsional'noĭ politiki KPSS. **Sov Zdravookhr** 1982;(11):57–60
**Belic N, Gardin JM:** Implantable cardiac pacemakers--an overview. **Int J Dermatol** 1982 Nov;21(9):543–50
**Belicza B:** Liječnička udruženja i razvoj medicinske periodike s posebnim osvrtom na 'Liječnički vjesnik' Glasilo Zbora liječnika Hrvatske (1877–1977). **Saopcenja** 1978;21(1–2):133–56
**Belicza B:** Ranarnici u zdravstvenoj povijesti hrvatske. **Saopcenja** 1973;16(4):213–23
**Belicza B:** U povodu stote obljetnice Zbora Liječnika Hrvatske (1874–1974). **Saopcenja** 1974;17(1):55–74
**Belicza B:** Zagreb u borbi protiv kolere. In: I simpozij o historiji mikrobiologije i imunologije u Hrvatskoj do 1923. godine. Zagreb, Jugoslavenskoj akademiji, 1973. p. 17–29.
**Belino ED** see **Umoh JU**
**Belitskaia EI:** Systema morborum (klassifikatsiia bolezneĭ) I. I. Diad'kovskogo (k 150–letiiu opublikovaniia). **Sov Zdravookhr** 1983;5:63–6
**Belitskaia EIa:** Gigienicheskie i sotsial'no–gigienicheskie vzgliady S. P. Botkina (k 150–letiiu so dnia rozhdeniia). **Gig Sanit** 1982 Jul;(7):34–8
**Belitskaia EIa, Zhuravleva KI:** K 60–letiiu Kafedry sotsial'noĭ gigieny i organizatsii zdravookhraneniia Leningradskogo sanitarno–gigienicheskogo meditsinskogo instituta. **Sov Zdravookhr** 1982;(7):61–3
**Belitskaia EIa:** O sotsial–gigieniste A. V. Korchake–Chepurkovskom (K 125–letiiu so dnia rozhdeniia). **Sov Zdravookhr** 1982;(6):66–8
**Belitskaia EIa:** V. I. Lenin on voprosakh narodnonaseleniia. **Sov Zdravookhr** 1980;(4):8–10
**Belitskaia EIa:** V. V. Paevskiĭ i ego kniga 'Elementy statistiki' (k 50–letiiu opublikovaniia). **Sov Zdravookhr** 1981;(6):64–6
**Beljan JR:** Medical education: historical perspectives and future directions. **Aviat Space Environ Med** 1979 Nov;50(11):1161–5
**Belke I:** Die Begründung der Völkerpsychologie in Deutschland: Eine Alternative zur etablierten Geschichtswissenschaft? **Riv Filos** 1982;73:192–233
**Belkin J:** Eucharius Rösslin des Jüngeren Lebensgeschichte. **Gutenberg Jahrb** 1978;96–105
**Belkin NL:** Textiles as aseptic barriers: the past, present, and future. **Med Instrum** 1980 Jul–Aug;14(4):233–6
**Bell A** see **Shipley M**
**Bell BA:** A history of the study of cerebral edema. **Neurosurgery** 1983 Dec;13(6):724–8
**Bell BA:** A history of the study of the cerebral circulation and the measurement of cerebral blood flow. **Neurosurgery** 1984 Feb;14(2):238–46
**Bell C:** A hundred years of Lancet language. **Lancet** 1984 Dec 22;2(8417–18):1453
**Bell C:** Implementing safety and health regulations for women in the workplace. **Feminist Stud** 1979;5(2):286–301
**Bell FG:** Surgeon's saga. Wellington, Reed, [1968] 216 p.
**Bell G** see **Johnson EA**
**Bell J:** Crisis at Gettysburg. **Nurs Times** 1981 Feb 12;77(7):294–5
**Bell JC, Palmer SR:** Control of zoonoses in Britain: past, present, and future. **Br Med J [Clin Res]** 1983 Aug 27;287(6392)591–3
**Bell JD:** Giving birth to the new Soviet man: politics and obstetrics in the USSR. **Slavic Rev** 1981;40(1):1–16
**Bell LV:** Treating the mentally ill: from colonial times to the present. New York, Praeger, 1980. xi, 245 p.
**Bell LV** see **Tyor PL**
**Bell M:** On the move. **Ulster Med J** 1979;48(1):1–18
**Bell MJ:** The relation of mentality to race: William Wells Newell and the Celtic hypothesis. **J Am Folkl** 1979;92(363):25–43
**Bell S:** George Henry Lewes: a man of his time. **J Hist Biol** 1981 Fall;14(2):278–98
**Bell SK:** Plus ça change, plus c'est la même chose: CPhA 1907–1982. **Can Pharm J** 1982 Oct;115(10):367–8
**Bell WJ:** George W. Corner (1889–1981): historian. **Bull Hist Med** 1982 Spring;56(1):93–8
**Bell WJ, Butterfield LH, ed:** My dearest Julia: the love letters of Dr. Benjamin Rush to Julia Stockton. New York, Neale Watson Academic Publications, 1979. xvii, 62 p.
**Bell WJ:** Private physicians and public collections: medical libraries in the United States before 1900. In Stevenson LG, ed: A celebration of medical history. Baltimore, Johns Hopkins University Press, 1982. (The Henry E. Sigerist supplements to the Bulletin of the History of Medicine; new ser., no. 6). p. 85–102.
**Bell WJ** see **Cash P**
**Bellaby P** see **Davies C, ed**
**Bellagarda G** see **Bellagarda M**
**Bellagarda M, Trisoglio M:** Il contributo della scienza e dell'odontostomatologia in particolare alla scoperta ed al progresso dell'anestesia. **Minerva Med** 1981 Apr 7;72(14):897–902
**Bellagarda M, Bellagarda G:** L'attività storico–scientifica di Luigi Casotti (1891–1959). **Minerva Med** 1984 Nov 17;75(44):2695–704
**Bellamy D Jr** see **Ausman RK**
**Bellet P:** Les membres résidents de la Société, puis Académie de Pharmacie. **Rev Hist Pharm (Paris)** 1981 Jun;28(249):118–20
**Bellettini A, Samoggia A:** Evolution différentielle et mouvement saisonnier de la mortalité infantile et enfantine dans la banlieue de Bologne (XVIIe–XIXe siècles). **Ann Demogr Hist (Paris)** 1983;:195–207
**Bellinazzi P:** Panpsichismo e psicologia nel pensiero di Ernst H. Haeckel. **Stor Crit Psicol** 1982 Dec;3(2):281–99
**Bellizzi R** see **Cruse WP**
**Belloni L:** Ancora sul manoscritto 'De dissensionibus, et controversis

anatomicis' di Bartolomeo Eustachi. **Physis** 1981;23(4):581-7

**Belloni L:** Bartolomeo Eustachi, anatomico del cinquecento, al lume di recenti ricerche. **Arch Int Hist Sci (Paris)** 1979 Jun-Dec;29(104):5-10

**Belloni L:** Claudius Aubrius a Francesco M. Fiorentini sull'assunzione di latte da parte del feto nell'utero. **Physis** 1977;19(1-4):378-82

**Belloni L:** Der Beitrag von Francesco Buzzi zur Entdeckung der 'Macula lutea' under 'Fovea centralis' des menschlichen Auges. **Gesnerus** 1983;40(1-2):23-30

**Belloni L:** Hermann Helmholtz und Franz Boll. **Medizinhist J** 1982;17(1/2):129-37

**Belloni L:** Il Morgagni tra il Malpighi e il Cotugno. **Gesnerus** 1982;39(2):195-213

**Belloni L:** Konsilien von Professoren aus Neapel und Padua gegen die Sehstörungen von G. V. Pinelli. **Gesnerus** 1981;38:135-42

**Belloni L:** Leeuwenhoek's Sehversuch am zusammengesetzten Auge und die entsprechende Beobachtung Boll's an der Stäbchenschicht der Netzhaut. **Janus** 1980;67(1-2-3):59-61

**Belloni L:** The discovery of duodenal ancylostoma and of its pathogenic power. In M. D. Grmek, R. S. Cohen, G. Cimino, ed: On scientific discovery. The Erice Lectures 1977. Dordrecht, D. Reidel, 1981. p. 261-79. (Boston Studies in the Philosophy of Science, v. 34).

**Belloni L:** Un circolo bernardiano in Italia: la Società delle Scienze Biologiche in Torino. Luigi Vella de la curaroterapia del tetano. **Physis** 1981;23(3):301-10

**Belloni L:** Zur Deutung zweier pathologischer Stellen (eine mit Zeichnung) aus der Anatomie von Leonardo: Lungenechinococcus, Halslymphdrüsenverkalkung. **Gesnerus** 1980;37(1/2):139-44

**Belloni L:** Zur Entdeckung des Eisens im Organismus. In Ganzinger K, Skopec M, Wyklicky H, ed: Festschrift für Erna Lesky zum 70. Geburtstag. Wien, Brüder Hollinek, 1981. p. 25-30.

**Belloni L see Habrich C**

**Belloni L see Libri e manoscritti di Haller, 1777-1977**

**Bellows B:** 'Insanity is the disease of civilization': the founding of the South Carolina Lunatic Asylum. **SC Hist Mag** 1981;82(3):263-72

**Bellucci G:** Storia della Società Italiana di Anestesia ed Analgesia, Società Italiana di Anestesiologia, Società Italiana di Anestesia e Rianimazione, Società Italiana di Anestesiologia, Analgesia, Rianimazione e Terapia Intensiva. **Minerva Anestesiol** 1980 Jul;46(7):733-56

**Bellush J:** A municipal hospital system: myths and realities. **Natl Civ Rev** 1980;69(6):313-20

**Bellush J:** Indispensable facilities: in defense of municipal hospitals. **NY Aff** 1979;5(4):111-19

**Beloborodova NL:** Moskovskiĭ vospitatel'nyĭ dom i ego rol' v istorii zdravookhraneniia Rossii. **Sov Zdravookhr** 1984;(7):58-61

**Beloborodova NL:** Moskovskoe otdelenie mediko-khirurgicheskoĭ akademii v Otechestvennuiu voinu 1812 goda. **Voen Med Zh** 1982 Nov;(11):66-7

**Beloff M:** Dr. Darlington's provocative work: the genetic approach to world history. **Encounter (Lond)** 1970;35(4):85-8

**Belolapotkova AV:** Voprosy stomatologii v 'Kanone vrachebnoĭ nauki' Ibn-Siny. **Stomatologiia (Mosk)** 1980 Nov-Dec;59(6):69-70

**Belous VI, Mesiats NK:** S. M. Ter-Arutiuniants--osnovatel' glaznoĭ sluzhby na Zhitomirshchine. **Oftalmol Zh** 1984;(1):63-4

**Belov SI:** Vrachebnaia étika v kurse istorii meditsiny. **Sov Med** 1981;(6):116-7

**Belova LV, Mirakhmedov UM:** Vklad Abu Ali ibn-Sina v dermato-venerologiiu. **Vestn Dermatol Venerol** 1983 Dec;(12):60-4

**Belova LV:** Vklad Abu Ali ibn-Siny v kosmetologiiu. **Sov Zdravookhr** 1984;(9):53-6

**Belova LV:** Znachenie tvochestva Ibn Sina dlia sovremennoĭ meditsiny. **Med Sestra** 1983 Nov;42(11):46-51

**Belova TI see Afanas'ev IuI**

**Belozerov VN:** 150-letie so dnia rozhdeniia Karlosa Kh. Finleia. **Parazitologiia** 1983 Nov-Dec;17(6):498-9

**Belozerov VV, Galin LL:** Zhurnal dlia ranenykh i bol'nykh krasnoarmeĭtsev. **Voen Med Zh** 1984 Apr;(4):65-9

**Beltrán E:** Conmemoración del descubrimiento de uno de los gérmenes patogénicos del paludismo. **Gac Med Mex** 1981 May;117(5):195-201

**Beltran E:** La protozoología médica en México. In Academia Nacional de Medicina. Libro conmemorativo del primer centenario. México, Comité Editorial de la Comisión Organizadora del Congreso del Centenario, 1964. Tome 1. p. 109-12.

**Beltrán E:** Notas de historia protozoológica V. el renacimiento de la protozoología. Siete fecundos lustros: 1941-1976. **An Soc Mex Hist Cienc Tec** 1979;5:91-114

**Beltrán E:** Notas de historia protozoológica VI. la regeneración en los protozoarios. **An Soc Mex Hist Cienc Tec** 1979;5:115-26

**Beltrán E:** Reflexiones sobre historiografía de la biología en México. **An Soc Mex Hist Cienc Tec** 1979;5:1-19

**Beltrán E:** Una polémica sobre Francisco Hernández y su obra en 1785. **An Soc Mex Hist Cienc Tec** 1979;5:49-73

**Beltrán GA see Flores y Troncoso FA**

**Belykh AI see Danilevskiĭ VM**

**Ben-Hur N, Converse JM:** The impact of plastic surgery on transplantation from skin graft to microsurgery. **Transplant Proc** 1980 Dec;12(4):616-20

**Ben Milad A:** Biographie des médécins arabes: Ishaq Ibn Omrane. **Tunis Med** 1979 Nov-Dec;57(6):378-9

**Ben Yedder W:** Enseignement para-médical en Tunisie. L'école professionnelle de la santé publique de Tunis 'Avicenne'. **Tunis Med** 1981 Jan-Feb;59(1):874-5

**Ben-Yehuda N:** The European witch craze of the 14th to 17th centuries: a sociologist's perspective. **Am J Sociol** 1980 Jul;86(1):1-31

**Ben-Yehuda N see Hook D**

**Ben-Zeev A:** J. J. Gibson and the ecological approach to perception. **Stud Hist Philos Sci** 1981 Jun;12(2):107-39

**Benaim F:** Thirty years at the service of the burned in Argentina and South America. **J Trauma** 1981 May;21(5):356-63

**Bénard JC:** Fille ou garçon à volonté: un aspect du discours médical au XIXe siècle. **Ethnol Fr** 1981;11:63-76

**Benavente Barreda JM:** Evolución biológica y herencia natural. **Arbor** 1982;113(441-2):111-25

**Benayahu M:** Rabbi Abraham Hacohen of Zante and the Padua group of doctor-poets. **Hasifrut** 1978;26:108-40

**Benayahu M:** Rabbi Samson Morpurgo. **Sinai** 1979;84:134-65

**Bencivenni M:** Il Principe dello Studiolo. **Kos** 1984 Jul-Aug;1(6):52-78

**Bencze B:** Emlékezés Orovecz Bélára az Országos Mentöszolgálat megszervezöjére (1909-1967). **Orv Hetil** 1979 Nov 18;120(46):2819-20

**Bendall DS, ed:** Evolution from molecules to men. Cambridge, Cambridge University Press, 1983. xiii, 594 p.

**Bender AE:** Importance of proteins and protein quality. **Bibl Nutr Dieta** 1983;(32):55-66

**Bender AE:** The future of our food supplies. **R Soc Health J** 1981 Aug;101(4):158-62

**Bender GA:** Henry Hurd Rusby: scientific explorer, societal crusader, scholastic innovator. **Pharm Hist** 1981;23(2):71-85

**Bender GA:** Nineteenth century pharmaceutical research into plants of the southwestern deserts. **Pharm Hist** 1980;22(2):49-59

**Bender GA see Parascandola JL**

**Bender MB, Shanzer S:** History of binocular movements. In Rose FC, Bynum WF, ed: Historical aspects of the neurosciences. New York, Raven, 1982. p. 45-54.

**Bender TR see Michael JM**

**Bendiner E:** A rebellious Breton who revolutionized medicine. **Hosp Pract** 1983 Nov;18(11):205-7, 210-1, 214 passim

**Bendiner E:** Avery: making sense of a 'stupid tetranucleotide'. **Hosp Pract** 1982 Oct;17(10):195, 199, 202-3 passim

**Bendiner E:** Baron von Pirquet: the aristocrat who discovered and defined allergy. **Hosp Pract** 1981 Oct;16(10):137, 141, 144 passim

**Bendiner E:** Ehrlich: immunologist, chemotherapist, prophet. **Hum Dev** 1980 Nov;15(11):129, 133, 138-9 passim

**Bendiner E:** Enders, Weller, and Robbins: the trio that 'fished in troubled waters'. **Hosp Pract** 1982 Jan;17(1):163, 169, 174-5 passim

**Bendiner E:** From barbershop to battlefield--Paré and the renaissance of surgery. **Hosp Pract** 1983 Aug;18(8):193-5, 199, 202 passim

**Bendiner E:** Jenner: from folklore to scientific triumph. **Hosp Pract [Off]** 1984 Apr;19(4):183-7, 190-1, 196, passim

**Bendiner E:** Korczak: pediatrician on the road to hell. **Hosp Pract** 1981 Jul;16(7):125-8, 132-4, 138-9 passim

**Bendiner E:** Marcello Malpighi: a life of passionate exploration. **Hosp Pract** 1980 Jul;15(7):109-36

**Bendiner E:** Noguchi: many triumphs and a brilliant failure. **Hosp Pract [Off]** 1984 Feb;19(2):222-3, 227, 231 passim

**Bendiner E:** Past and present: Elizabeth Blackwell: 'heresy with intelligence'. **Hosp Pract** Jun;15(6):1821-1910

**Bendiner E:** Philippe Pinel: reason for the unreasoning. **Hosp Pract** 1981 Jun;16(6):76E-76P

**Bendiner E:** Salk: adulation, animosity, and achievement. **Hosp Pract** 1983 Jun;18(6):194-6, 200-1, 204-5 passim

**Bendiner E:** The Curies: pioneers and victims of the atomic era. **Hosp Pract** 1981 Dec;16(12):80, 82-4 passim

**Bendiner E:** The 'derailment' that spurred a feminist revolution in medicine. **Hosp Pract** 1983 Mar;18(3):225, 228, 233-40 passim

**Bendiner E:** The descent of man and the ascent of the Darwins. **Hosp Pract** 1982 Dec;17(12):160, 165, 173-4 passim

**Bendiner E:** The Dublin school: from poverty, a rich legacy. **Hosp Pract [Off]** 1984 Jun;19(6):221-47

**Bendiner E:** The man who did not invent the microscope. **Hosp Pract [Off]** 1984 Aug;19(8):139, 144-5, 149 passim

**Bendixen HH:** Respirators and respiratory care. **Acta Anaesthesiol Scand** 1982 Jun;26(3):279-86

**Benedek I:** Semmelweis. Budapest, Gondolat, 1980. 269 p.

**Benedek I:** Semmelweis' Krankheit. Budapest, Akadémiai Kiadó, 1983. 110 p. (Hungarian version published 1978 in Communicationes de historia artis medicinae, Nos. 83-84)

**Benedek TG, Rodnan GP:** A brief history of the rheumatic diseases. **Bull Rheum Dis** 1982;32(6):59-68

**Benedek TG:** A comparison of the medical writings of two humanists: F. Petrarca and W. Pirckheimer. In: Congrès international d'histoire de la médecine, XXVe, Québec, 1976. Actes. Québec, 1977. p. 502-6.

**Benedek TG:** Subcutaneous nodules and the differentiation of rheumatoid arthritis from rheumatic fever. **Semin Arthritis Rheum** 1984 May;13(4):305-21

**Benedek TG, Rodnan GP:** The early history and nomenclature of scleroderma and of its differentiation from sclerema neonatorum and scleroedema. **Semin Arthritis Rheum** 1982 Aug;12(1):52-67

**Benedek TG:** The gout of Desiderius Erasmus and Willibald Pirckheimer: medical autobiography and its literary reflections. **Bull Hist Med** 1983 Winter;57(4):526-44

**Benedek TG see Radcliff-Umstead D, ed**

**Benedek TG see Rodnan GP**

**Benedek-Jaszmann LJ:** Hendrik van Deventer (1651-1724); the silversmith who became the co-founder of modern obstetrics. **Orvostort Kozl** 1980;89-91(26 no 1-3):241-9

**Benedetti G:** Die neurotische Lebensproblematik Nietzsches als eine Wirkkraft und eine Grenze seiner Philosophie. **Gesnerus** 1984;41(1/2):111-32
**Benedetti G** see **Fischle-Carl H, ed**
**Benedetti Y:** Les fondations hospitalières pisanes en Corse (XIIIe-XVe siècles). Maîtrise. Univ. d'Aix-en-Provence, 1976, 166 p.
**Benedum J, Michler M:** Das Siegel der Medizinischen Fakultät Giessen. Giessen, Universitätsbibliothek, 1982. 47 p., [18 leaves]. (Berichte und Arbeiten aus der Universitätsbibliothek Giessen, no. 35).
**Benedum J:** Die Augenanomalie an einem römischen Bildnis. **Medizinhist J** 1981;16(4):446-52
**Benedum J, Giese C:** Die Professoren der Medizin in der giessener Gemäldegalerie. Giessen, Schmitz, 1983. 230 p. (Arbeiten zur Geschichte der Medizin in Giessen, Bd. 5)
**Benedum J:** Vom Giessener pharmakologischen Institut unter Rudolf Buchheim und Karl Gaehtgens (1867-1898). **Medizinhist J** 1980;15(1/2):103-19
**Benedum J:** Zur lydischen Arztinschrift IGRR IV 1359. **Z Papyrologie Epigraphik** 1978;29:115-21
**Benedum J:** 375 Jahre Medizin in Giessen: eine Bild- und Textdokumentation: Katalog zur Ausstellung anlässlich der 375 - Jahrfeier im Institut für Anatomie und Zytobiologie, vom 11.5.-30.6. 1982. Giessen, Schmitz, 1982. 186 p.
**Benedum J** see **Grmek MD, ed**
**Benejeam M** see **Thiveaud D**
**Benencia JA:** Los restos del general D. Juan Galo de Lavalle. **Historia (Argentina)** 1965;10(39):84-5
**Benenson AS:** Immunization and military medicine. **Rev Infect Dis** 1984 Jan-Feb;6(1):1-12
**Benes V, Benesová Z:** Horsleyv vosk. **Rozhl Chir** 1982 Feb;61(2):141-3
**Benesová Z** see **Benes V**
**Benfey OT:** Spinach is an alchemical antidote to heavy metal poisoning. **Kagakushi Kenkyu** 1981;15:8-12
**Benge MO:** Midwifery history: How to bring away the after-burden. **Nurs Times** 1984 Oct 10-16;80(41):37
**Benguigui I:** La théorie de l'électricité de Nollet et son application en médecine à travers sa correspondance: inédite avec Jallabert. **Gesnerus** 1981;38:225-35
**Benham L:** The labor market for registered nurses: a three equation model. **Rev Econ Stat** 1971;53(3):246-52
**Beniak M:** Sociálna podmienenost tuberkulózy na Slovensku pred prvou svetovou vojnou. **Bratisl Lek Listy** 1984 Mar;81(3):376-81
**Beniak M** see **Moravec R**
**Beniak M** see **Tichý M**
**Benison S:** Celebration and history: the centenary of Robert Koch's discovery of the tubercle bacillus. **Bull Hist Med** 1982 Summer;56(2):157-9
**Benison S, Barger AC, Wolfe EL:** Changing of the guard. **Harv Med Alumni Bull** 1982 Spring;56(2):34-41
**Benison S:** Ideology über alles: an essay review. **J Hist Med Allied Sci** 1982 Jan;37(1)83-90
**Benison S:** International medical cooperation: Dr. Albert Sabin, live poliovirus vaccine and the Soviets. **Bull Hist Med** 1982;56(4):460-83
**Benison S:** Technology the dehumanizer. **Rev Am Hist** 1979;7(4):477-9
**Benison S** see **George Rosen: In Memoriam**
**Benison S** see **Trends in biomedical research, 1901-1976**
**Benitez J** see **El-Najjar MY**
**Benitez JT, Lynn GE:** Temporal bone studies. In A. Cockburn, E. Cockburn, ed: Mummies, disease, and ancient cultures. Cambridge, Cambridge University Press, 1980. p. 301-11.
**Benítez RF:** Historia de la deficiencia mental endemica en la region Andina. **Asclepio** 1982;34:339-76
**Benjamin B:** Changes in public health in London in the past fifty years. **R Soc Health J** 1981 Dec;101(6):245-60
**Benjamin B** see **Sorsby A**
**Benjamin H:** Georg Benjamin: eine Biographie. 2d ed. Leipzig, S. Hirzel, 1982. 363 p.
**Benjamin JA, Tobin CE:** The fasciae of the genito-urinary organs: historical, anatomical, and clinical aspects. **Trans Stud Coll Physicians Phila** 1981 Dec;5(3 no 4):264-79
**Benjamin LT, Jones MR:** From motivational theory to social cognitive development: twenty-five years of the Nebraska Symposium. **Nebr Symp Motiv** 1978;26:ix-xix
**Benjamin LT** see **Brozek J**
**Benkö F:** A vatta hazai elötörténete. **Orv Hetil** 1984 Nov 25;125(48):2965
**Benko F:** Die Gemälde der Apotheke zum Goldenen Einhorn im Debrecziner Déri Museum. In Hein WH, ed: Pharmaziehistorischer Kongress, Budapest, 1981. Stuttgart, Wissenschaftliche Verlagsgesellschaft, 1983. p. 85-96.
**Benna P** see **Bergamini L**
**Bennahum DA:** Intimations of mortality reconsidered: terminal care. **Am J Med** 1980 Oct;69(4):488-90
**Bennett AE:** Historical development of somatic therapies in affective disorders. **Int Pharmacopsychiatry** 1979;14(2):85-93
**Bennett AG** see **Sorsby A**
**Bennett DH:** Francis Everett Townsend. In Dictionary of American Biography, Suppl. 6, 1956-1960. p. 645-7, 1980.
**Bennett F:** A Canterbury tale. The autobiography of Dr. Francis Bennett. Wellington, Oxford University Press, 1980. 249 p.
**Bennett HS:** A perception of histochemistry. **J Histochem Cytochem** 1983 Jan;31(1A Suppl):127-30
**Bennett HS** see **Porter KR**
**Bennett JL:** Room M-112: Medical Sciences Building. **J Fla Med Assoc** 1980 Mar;67(3):251-7
**Bennett JP:** Aspects of the history of plastic surgery since the 16th century. **J R Soc Med** 1983 Feb;76(2):152-6
**Bennett JP:** Sir William Fergusson and the Indian Rhinoplasty. **Ann R Coll Surg Engl** 1984 Nov;66(6):444-8
**Bennett RB** see **Whittaker DK**
**Bennett SM** see **Owsley DW**
**Bennich HH** see **Johansson SG**
**Bennion E:** Phlebotomy: the art, practice & instruments. **MD** 1981;25(8):43-6
**Benoliel JQ:** The historical development of cancer nursing research in the United States. **Cancer Nurs** 1983 Aug;6(4):261-8
**Bensley EH:** James Grant: ship's surgeon on the ill-fated Empress of Ireland. **Can Med Assoc J** 1982 Feb 1;126(3):318-9
**Bensley EH:** John Poad Drake (1794-1883), the first artist to portray the Hospital. **Montreal Gen Hosp News** 1981;19(1):8-9
**Bensley EH:** Pages of history. Montreal, [Montreal General Hospital], 1981. 40 p.
**Bensley EH:** Robert Palmer Howard. In Dictionary of Canadian biography, 1881-1890. 1982;11:428-9.
**Bensley EH:** The great remove [1955]. **Montreal Gen Hosp News** 1980;18(2):12-3
**Benson B, Wall R:** Historical demography in the nineteenth and twentieth centuries in the absence of the civil registers. **Local Popul Stud (Matlock)** 1981 Spring;26:14-28
**Benson CD:** The astrological medicine of Chaucer's physician and Nicholas of Lynn's Kalendarium. **Am Notes Queries** 1984 Jan-Feb;22(5-6):62-6
**Benson ES:** Laboratory medicine in the United States--the dream and the reality. **Am J Clin Pathol** 1981 Jul;76(1):1-7
**Benson ES** see **Wangensteen OW, ed**
**Benson F:** Blood tests showing nonpaternity-conclusive or rebuttable evidence? The Chaplin case revisited. **Am J Forensic Med Pathol** 1981 Sep;2(3):221-3
**Benson KR:** Problems of individual development: descriptive embryological morphology in America at the turn of the century. **J Hist Biol** 1981 Spring;14(1):115-28
**Benson KR:** William Keith Brooks (1848-1908): a case study in morphology and the development of American biology. Ph.D. Diss. Oregon State University. Corvallis, 1979. 356 leaves.
**Benson KR:** 'William Keith Brooks (1848-1908): primary resource material'. **Mendel Newsl** 1983 Nov;23:7-11
**Benson PR:** Labeling theory and community care of the mentally ill in California: the relationship of social theory and ideology to public policy. **Hum Organ** 1980;39(2):134-41
**Benson RP:** Organized medicine in the Eastern Cape. **S Afr Med J** 1981 Oct 17;60(16):631-8
**Bent EA:** From three hours to three days in 101 years. **Midwife Health Visit Community Nurse** 1983 Jul;20(7):267-73
**Bent EA** see **Allan P**
**Bentham A:** Down Memory Lane: as it happened. **Nurs Mirror** 1982 Aug 11;155(6):28-30
**Benzinger TH, ed:** Temperature, part 1: arts and concepts. Stroudsburg, Pa., Dowden, Hutchinson & Ross, 1977. viii, 353 p. (Benchmark Papers in Human Physiology, 9).
**Ber A:** Les avatars d'une recherche sur l'hystérie. **Penelope** 1983;(8):15-19
**Beran M** see **Tomiček F**
**Berar L:** History of ophthalmology in stamps. **Metab Pediatr Syst Ophthalmol** 1982;6(3-4):367-9
**Berber S:** Istorija zdravstvene kulture u Somboru. Sombor, Dispanzer za kardiovaskularne bolesti, 1980. 95 p.
**Bercherie P:** Le concept de folie hystérique avant Charcot. **Rev Int Hist Psychiatr** 1983;1(1):47-58
**Berciano J, Rebollo M, Coria F, et al:** Heredoataxia de Marie. Nuevas consideraciones sobre su uso e independencia nosológica. **Med Clin (Barc)** 1983 Apr 2;80(11):506-8
**Bercovy D:** Quelques Juifs à Malte. **Rev Hist Med Heb** 1984 Jul;37(2):24-5
**Bercuş CI** see **Miloşescu P**
**Bercus CI, ed:** Spitalul Coltea: Două sute saptezeci si cinci ani de existentă, 1704-1979. Bucuresti, Spitalul Clinic Coltea, 1979. 582 p.
**Bercuson DJ:** Tragedy at Bellevue: anatomy of a mine disaster. **Labour** 1978;3:221-31
**Berdyshev GD** see **Golda DM**
**Berelowitch W:** L'évolution de la fécondité légitime à Saint-Petersbourg-Petrograd-Leningrad (1869-1926). **Ann Demogr Hist (Paris)** 1982;:243-65
**Berenbrinker A:** Die zahnmedizinische Karikatur I: 1780-1840. Köln, 1982. 227 p. (Arbeiten der Forschungsstelle des Instituts für Geschichte der Medizin der Universität zu Köln, Band 25).
**Berenholc C, Martin C:** Du rotatif au manuel. Considerations sur l'utilisation du mouvement en endodontie. **Chir Dent Fr** 1982 Oct 7;52(173):29-33
**Berenholc C:** L'amalgame d'argent, obturation provisoire de longue durée. **Chir Dent Fr** 1981 Feb;51(98):37-42 contd.
**Berenshteĭn GF** see **Karavaev AG**
**Berentson L:** Florence Nightingale: change agent. **RN Id** 1982 Apr-May;6(2):3, 7
**Berezhnaia NM:** Uchenie o reaktivnosti A. A. Bogomolets i razvitie sovremennoĭ allergologii. **Fiziol Zh** 1981 May-Jun;27(3):358-68
**Berezhniak AP:** Polirabotniki meditsinskikh chasteĭ i uchrezhdeniĭ v gody Velikoĭ Otechestvennoĭ voĭny. **Voen Med Zh** 1981 Sep;(9):70-1

**Berezin IV, Osipova TA, Figurovsky NA:** The development of investigation of immobilized enzymes in the USSR. **Istor Biol Issled** 1983;9:113–26
**Berezovskiĭ VA:** Ivan Mikhaĭlovich Sechenov. Kiev, Nauk. dumka, 1981. 173 p.
**Berezovskiĭ VA, Nazarenko AI:** Krupnyĭ vklad v gepatologiiu. **Fiziol Zh** 1980 Mar–Apr;26(2):244–9
**Berezovskiĭ VA:** Ritmy biologicheskikh protsessov kak proiavlenie individual'noĭ reaktivnosti i konstitutsii individa. **Patol Fiziol Eksp Ter** 1981 May–Jun;(3):3–7
**Berezowski S:** Ceský vědecký přínos v programech sjezdu polských lékařu a přírodovědcu 100. Výročí prvního sjezdu polských lékařu a přírodovědcu. **Cas Lek Cesk** 1979 Nov 23;118(47):1463–5
**Berezowski S:** Jan Dolliner--chirurg bocheński (przyczynek do historii zdobywania doktoratów chirurgii w Uniwersytecie Jagiellońskim). **Pol Tyg Lek** 1979 Aug 27;34(35):1403–5
**Berezowski S:** Joseph Dietl, a great Polish physician of the 19th century. In International Congress of the History of Medicine. 26th, Plovdiv, 1978. Actes du Congress. Sofia, 1981. Volume II. p. 64–5.
**Berg AO:** The placebo effect reconsidered. **J Fam Pract** 1983 Oct;17(4):647–50
**Berg G** see **Spicker SF**
**Berg RL:** The life and research of Boris L. Astaurov. **Q Rev Biol** 1979 Dec;54(4):397–419
**Berg S:** Die Bedeutung der Rechtsmedizin für die Archäologie. **Beitr Gerichtl Med** 1982;40:287–96
**Berg A, ed:** Lanfranks 'Chirurgia parva' in der Abschrift Konrad Schrecks von Aschaffenburg. Diss. Würzburg 1975, 145 S. (Altdeutsche Lanfrank-Uebersetzungen III).
**Berg-Schorn E** see **Landsberger M**
**Bergalli L** see **Praderi RC**
**Bergamaschi MT, et al:** Streghe e raccoglitrici di bambori: al confine tra la medicina colta, empiria e pratiche magiche (XV–XVI sécolo). **Mem Riv Stor Donne** 1981;(1):106–13
**Bergamini L, Benna P:** Social aspects of epilepsy. **Prog Clin Biol Res** 1983;124:325–30
**Bergasse JD:** Jean Anglade (1698–1764) et la fondation de l'hôpital rural de Cazouls-les-Béziers au XVIIIe siècle. Bergasse (ed.) Hommage à Jacques Fabre de Morlhon. Albi, O.J.S., 1978. p. 133–47.
**Bergemann H:** Drachenzähne und Opfergaben. **Zahnarztl Mitt** 1980 May 16;70(10):655–7
**Bergemann H:** Zahnheilkunde zwischen Magie und Grobschmied. **Zahnarztl Mitt** 1981 Jul;71(14):856–7
**Bergen SS:** Medical education of New Jersey: the development of UMDNJ. **J Med Soc NJ** 1984 Sep;81(9):791–7
**Bergener M:** Gestalt-wandel in der Psychiatrie. **MMW** 1980 Jan 11;122(2):41–2
**Bergenheim AL:** Jubileumsår i NSF. **Sykepleien** 1982 Apr 5;69(7):5
**Berger C:** Science, God, and nature in Victorian Canada. Toronto; Buffalo, University of Toronto Press, 1983. xiv, 92 p.
**Berger H:** Kurzer historischer Rückblick auf den Beginn der 'Ernährungsprobleme bei frühgeborenen Kindern'. **Padiatr Padol** 1983;18(2):99–103
**Berger J:** New views on the Biblical Joseph. **Am J Psychoanal** 1981 Fall;41(3):277–82
**Berger LR, Johansson SR:** Child health in the workplace: the Supreme Court in Hammer v. Dagenhart (1918). **J Health Polit Policy Law** 1980 Spring;5(1):81–97
**Berger M:** The 'scientific approach' to intelligence: an overview of its history with special reference to mental speed. In H. J. Eysenck, ed: A model for intelligence. Berlin, Springer-Verlag, 1982. p. 13–43.
**Berger RL, Clem TR, Harden VA, et al:** Historical development and newer means of temperature measurement in biochemistry. **Methods Biochem Anal** 1984;30:269–331
**Berger W** see **Jung R**
**Berges P:** Grenzen sollte man vergessen. [S.l., s.n., 1981?] 32 p.
**Berges PH:** Goldene Zwanziger? Not der Krankenkassen und Arzneimittelsubstitution. **Beitr Gesch Pharm** 1983;31(18/19):155–9
**Berges PH:** Mäusedreck für Pfeifer... Der Apotheker und die Substitution. Ein kleines Mosaik. **Dtsch Apoth Ztg** 1981 Jan 8;121(2):53–9
**Berges PH, ed:** Internationaler Kongress für Geschichte der Pharmazie in Basel/Lausanne, vom 13. bis 19. Juni 1979. [Summary of events plus abstracts of papers] Sonderdruck aus: Deutsche Apotheker Zeitung 119 (1979): 973–976, 1081–1084, 1133–1138, 1170–1173.
**Berghaus A:** Die Entwicklung der Methoden zur physiologischen Wertbestimmung von Digitalispräparaten. Husum, Matthiesen, 1982. 135 p. (Abhandlungen zur Geschichte der Medizin und der Naturwissenschaften, 42).
**Berghaus A, Winau R:** Probleme der Standardisierung von Digitalispräparaten. In Hickel E, Schröder G, ed: Neue Beiträge zur Arzneimittelgeschichte. Festschrift für Wolfgang Schneider zum 70. Geburtstag. Stuttgart, Wissenschaftliche Verlagsgesellschaft, 1982. p. 265–79.
**Bergman A:** Pobeg V. S. Mitskevicha-Kapsukasa iz suvalkskoi bol'nitsy v 1906 G. **Vopr Istor** 1965;(3):74–6
**Bergman LE, Hansson T:** Hard tissue changes of the temporomandibular joint in an archaeo-osteological material from the 11th century. **Swed Dent J** 1979;3(5):149–55
**Bergman P, Aue-Hauser G:** Methodische Beiträge zu kraniometrischen Studien einiger frühmittelalterlicher Populationen des oberen Donauraumes. I. Die gebräuchlichsten Schädelindices als Grundlage für Populationsvergleiche (graphische und Approximationsverfahren). **Anthropol Anz** 1980 Nov;38(4):251–64
**Bergman P, Hauser G:** Methodische Beiträge zu kraniometrischen Studien einiger frühmittelalterlicher Populationen des oberen Donauraumes. II. Vergleich der frümittelalterlichen Populationen anhand absoluter Schädelmasse. **Anthropol Anz** 1982 Sep;40(3):173–84
**Bergman R:** [Israel nursing--35 years of evolutionary change] (Jpn). **Kango** 1984 Jul;36(8):44–9
**Bergmann H:** Neufunde zum Pesttraktat Jakob Engelins von Ulm. **Sudhoffs Arch** 1978;62(3):282–93
**Bergmann MS** see **Ostow M**
**Bergmar M:** Stor förändring i nya, självständiga Zimbabwe: en sjukvård som gäller alla – inte går efter hudfärg. **Vardfacket** 1981 Apr 9;5(7):64–6
**Bergmark M:** Medevi 300 år. Ett nytt blad i vår svenska hydroterapis historia. **Nord Medicinhist Arsb** 1980;Suppl 6:122–8
**Bergoglio RM:** En el centenario del nacimiento de Carlos Chagas. **Rev Fac Cien Med Univ Nac Cordoba** 1981 Jan–Dec;39(1–4):87–9
**Bergoglio RM:** Tétanos neonatorum. Intentos históricos de su prevención en América Latina. **Medicina (B Aires)** 1982;42 Suppl 1:77–81
**Bergsjø P, Ulstein M:** Jørgen Løvset 1896–1981. **Acta Obstet Gynecol Scand** 1982;61(3):193–4
**Bergsjø P** see **Augensen K**
**Bergstrand A, Ostman J:** Männen bakom syndromet: Paul Kimmelstiel och Clifford Wilson. Tysk och engelsman som möttes vid Harvard – först att beskriva speciell glomerulusskada. **Lakartidningen** 1984 Jan 25;81(4):227–8
**Bergstrand CR:** Big profit in private hospitals. **Soc Policy** 1982;13(2):50–4
**Bergström CO:** Den sjuka människan i Hjalmar Bergmans diktning. **Nord Medicinhist Arsb** 1984;:165–73
**Bériac F:** L'Hôpital Saint-Julien de Bordeaux, XIIIe–XVIe siècle. **Rev Hist Bordeaux Dep Gironde** 1975, 1977;24:47–74
**Bériac JP:** Le Parlement, la Jurade et l'hôpital Saint-André de Bordeaux face à 'l'effrénée multitude des pauvres' au XVIe siècle et au début du XVIIe. **Rev Hist Bordeaux Dep Gironde** 1977, reçu 1980;26:41–58
**Beric B, Babic N:** Dr. Antun Lobmayer (1844–1906) pionir savremenog akušerstva i školovanja primalja u Hrvatskoj. **Jugosl Ginekol Opstet** 1979;19(1–2):113–8
**Beric B, Rajkovic D, Babic-Ilic N:** Dr Nikola Hadži-Nikolić (1855–1915) prvi akušer-ginekolog u Srbiji i Njegov značaj za razvoj akušerstva i ginekologije u Srbiji. **Jugosl Ginekol Opstet** 1981 Dec;21(5–6):143–8
**Beric B, Miskov D:** Pregled istorije bolnice u Novom Sadu (1730–1980). **Med Pregl** 1981;34(5–6):259–65
**Beric BM:** Dr Eva Haljecka (18??–1947) prva žena akušer-ginekolog u jugoslovenskim zemljama. **Jugosl Ginekol Opstet** 1983 May–Aug;23(3–4):95–9
**Beric BM, Beric ML:** Društvo lekara iz Vojvodine (1919–1929). **Med Pregl** 1983;36(5–6):253–7
**Beric BM:** Prvi ginekolog-akušer u Vojvodini--dr Aleksander Sosberger (1873–1944). **Jugosl Ginekol Opstet** 1984 May–Aug;24(3–4):71–2
**Beric ML** see **Beric BM**
**Beritic T:** Carl Prausnitz Giles i saga or reaginima. **Lijec Vjesn** 1981 Jul;103(7):312–4
**Berjón Rufes JJ:** Cómo vio el siglo XX nacer y evolucionar a una nueva enfermedad: la hernia hiatal. **Rev Esp Enferm Apar Dig** 1982 Feb;61(2):169–81
**Berk DW:** Adventism on the picture post card. **Advent Herit** 1978;5(2):48–53
**Berk JB:** Antiquarian antisepsis. **Contemp Surg** 1980 Jun;16(6):62–3
**Berk RN:** Gallstones: diagnostic imaging in historical perspective. **Pharos** 1983 Winter;46(1):30–4
**Berk SL:** Bacterial pneumonia in the elderly: the observations of Sir William Osler in retrospect. **J Am Geriatr Soc** 1984 Sep;32(9):683–5
**Berkay F:** Perspectives in international neurosurgery: neurosurgery in Turkey. **Neurosurgery** 1980 Oct;7(4):419–22
**Berkel K van** see **Palm LC**
**Berkeley DS** see **Berkeley E**
**Berkeley E, Berkeley DS:** The life and travels of John Bartram: from Lake Ontario to the River St. John. Tallahassee, University Presses of Florida, 1982. xvi, 376 p.
**Berkelhamer JE, Noyes EJ, Chen RT:** Child health policy–an overview of federal involvement. **Adv Pediatr** 1982;29:211–8
**Berkey LG:** History of the Ninth District Dental Society, 1909–1984. **Bull Ninth Dist Dent Soc** 1984 Jun;68(6):11pp
**Berki SE** see **Ashcraft ML**
**Berkowitz E, McQuaid K:** Welfare reform in the 1950s. **Soc Serv Rev** 1980 Mar;54(1):45–58
**Berkowitz ED:** Rehabilitation: the federal government's response to disability, 1935–1954. New York, Arno, 1980. xv, 339 p. (The Physically Handicapped in Society.) Also Ph.D. Diss., Northwestern University. Evanston, 1976.
**Berkowitz ED:** The federal government and the emergence of rehabilitation medicine. **Historian** 1981;43(4):530–45
**Berkowitz ED:** The historian as policy analyst: the challenge of HEW. **Public Hist** 1979;1(3):17–25
**Berkowitz ED:** The politics of mental retardation during the Kennedy Administration. **Soc Sci Q** 1980;61(1):128–43
**Berkowitz M:** Occupational safety and health. **Ann Am Acad Polit Soc Sci** 1979;443:41–53
**Berkutov AN:** Das chirurgische Erbe. N.I. Pirogov und die gegenwärtige Chirurgie. **Zentralbl Chir** 1984;109(17):1149–52
**Berkutov AN:** Zavety N. I. Pirogova i sovremennaia khirurgiia. **Vestn Khir** 1982 May;128(5):125–7

**Berkutov AN** see **Deriabin II**

**Berlan JP:** The world food problem: Malthus, Marx and their epigones. **Mon Rev** 1980;31(10):20–32

**Berle EJ:** Legenden om en senantikk bentransplantasjon. **Sydsven Medicinhist Sallsk Arsskr** 1984;21:135–40

**Berlin JB:** Richard Beer-Hofmann and Theodor Reik: a letter in exile. **Psychoanal Rev** 1981–82 Winter;68(4):479–86

**Berliner AK:** Psychoanalysis and society. The social thought of Sigmund Freud. Washington, D.C., University Press of America, 1983. x, 205 p.

**Berliner H:** Medical modes of production. In P. Wright, A. Treacher, ed: The problem of medical knowledge. Examining the social construction of medicine. Edinburgh, Edinburgh University Press, 1982. p. 162–73.

**Berliner N** see **Dotz W**

**Berlot J:** Razvitak mikrobiologije i imunologije u Hrvatskoj do 1923. god. In: I simpozij o historiji mikrobiologije i imunologije u Hrvatskoj do 1923. godine. Zagreb, Jugoslavenskoj akademiji, 1973. p. 31–45.

**Berman A:** An unpublished letter from Eugene Soubeiran to Antoine Portal, June 3, 1828. **Pharm Hist** 1982;24(1):32–7

**Berman A:** The eclectic 'concentrations' and American pharmacy (1847–1861). **Pharm Hist** 1980;22(3):91–103

**Berman DM:** Death on the job. Occupational health and safety struggles in the United States. New York, Monthly Review Press, 1978. xii, 260 p.

**Berman DM:** Worker's compensation: preventive care for industry. **Health PAC Bull** 1976 Jul–Aug;(71):9–14

**Berman IW:** Musicogenic epilepsy. **S Afr Med J** 1981 Jan 10;59(2):49–52

**Berman MC:** The clinical investigator: a tribute to the late Professor Bernard Pimstone. **S Afr Med J** 1983 Mar 5;63(10):366–71

**Bermúdez RH** see **Ramírez Ronda Ch**

**Bermudez de Castro JM** see **Pérez PJ**

**Bernabeo R:** La gotta. Presupposti storici alle concezioni moderne. **Minerva Med** 1980 Oct 6;71(38):2739–43

**Bernabeo RA, ed:** Il ferro chirurgico nella raccolta Vittorio Putti di Bologna. Bologna, Università degli Studi di Bologna, 1981. 14 p. (Catalog of an exhibit Sept.–Nov. 1981).

**Bernabò M:** La 'Rinascenza Macedone' e l'arte dei bendaggi. **Kos** 1984 Jun;1(5):45–51

**Bernabò M** see **Adacher S**

**Bernand C:** El caso Manuel: enfermedad y fatalidad en los Andes. **Asclepio** 1983;35:265–73

**Bernard CA:** Dickens and Victorian dream theory. In Paradis J, Postlewait T, ed: Victorian science and Victorian values: literary perspectives. New York, New York Academy of Sciences, 1981. p. 197–216.

**Bernard H:** L'histoire de la psychiatrie selon Ey (sa forme et son sens, le mythe). **Rev Int Hist Psychiatr** 1983;1(1):59–77

**Bernard J:** Authority, autonomy, and radical commitment: Stephen and Abby Kelley Foster. **Proc Am Antiq Soc** 1980:90(2):347–86

**Bernard J:** Création poétique et création cientifique. **Bull Assoc Guillaume Bude** 1981;3:275–83

**Bernard J:** Evolution de l'hématologie. **Nouv Rev Fr Hematol** 1980 Dec;22(4):453–8

**Bernard J:** Hématologie et transfusion sanguine. **Nouv Rev Fr Hematol** 1982;24(5):277–9

**Bernard J, Druon M:** La langue française et la médecine dans le monde. **Rev Deux Mondes** 1979;:45–51

**Bernard J:** Laennec et la médecine moderne. **Nouv Rev Deux Mondes** 1981;4:13–9

**Bernard J:** Lasthénie de Ferjol, Marie de Saint-Vallier, Emilie de Tourville ou le romancier et l'anémie. **Nouv Rev Fr Hematol** 1982;24(1):43–4

**Bernard J, Wintrobe M, Faure E, et al:** Le sang d'Altamira ou la naissance de l'hématologie. **Nouv Rev Fr Hematol** 1981;23(4):249–51

**Bernard J:** Le sang et l'histoire. Paris, Buchet/Chastel, 1983. 157 p.

**Bernard J:** Les progrès de la biologie et la définition de l'homme. **Rev Med Suisse Romande** 1984 Mar;104(3):239–48

**Bernard J:** L'espérance, ou le nouvel état de la médecine. Paris, Editions Buchet/Chastel, 1978. 255 p.

**Bernard J:** Robert Debré: l'humanisme et les académies. **Bull Acad Natl Med (Paris)** 1982 Dec;166(9):1281–4

**Bernard J:** The American drinking tradition. **Rev Am Hist** 1980;8(2):206–14

**Bernard J** see **Bessis M**

**Bernard J** see **Robin ED, ed**

**Bernard M, Pociello C, Vigarello G:** Itinéraire d'un concept. **Esprit** 1975;(5):704–23

**Bernardi L:** La diaspora dotanique polonaise. **Mus Geneve** 1981;216:11–6

**Bernasconi M, Carminati A, Tamburini C:** Panorama storico sulla patalogia del cancro. Lotta tra due vite. **Krankenpflege (Bern)** 1983 Nov;76(11):70–1

**Bernays EL:** Uncle Sigi. **J Hist Med Allied Sci** 1980 Apr;35(2):216–23

**Berndt H:** Emile Roux zum 50. Todestag. **Z Arztl Fortbild (Jena)** 1983;77(3):126–7

**Berndt T:** Bite mark science. Forensic dentistry's hottest frontier. **Fla Dent J** 1982 Spring;53(1):22–4, 42–3

**Berneaud-Kötz G:** Wilhelm Conrad Röntgen: aus den Erinnerungen des Schweizer Ophthalmologen Ernst Wölfflin. **Klin Monatsbl Augenheilkd** 1982 Aug;181(2):138–41

**Berner P:** Zur Geschichte der Psychiatrie in Wien: eine Bilddokumentation. Wien, C. Brandstätter, 1983. 143 p.

**Berner P** see **Peters UH, ed**

**Berner P** see **Postel J**

**Berner P** see **Zur Geschichte der Psychiatrie in Wien**

**Berney B:** The rise and fall of the UMW Fund. **South Exposure** 6(2):95–102, 1978

**Bernfeld S:** Freuds früheste Theorien und die Helmholtz-Schule (1944). **Psyche (Stuttg)** 1981 May;35(5):435–55

**Bernhard CM:** Dr. Ephraim McDowell: father of abdominal surgery. **Am Surg** 1980 Jan;46(1):1–5

**Bernhard JD, Elliot AD:** A letter from Darier to Bowen on the naming of Bowen's disease. **Arch Dermatol** 1983 Mar;119(3):261–2

**Bernier H:** Charlotte Gallard. In Dictionary of Canadian biography, 1701 to 1740. Volume 2, 1969. p. 235–6.

**Bernier H:** Françoise Maumousseau. In Dictionary of Canadian biography, 1701 to 1740. Volume 2, 1969. p. 466–7.

**Bernier H:** Marie-Madeleine Maufils. In Dictionary of Canadian biography, 1701 to 1740. Volume 2, 1969. p. 466.

**Bernier H:** Marie Morin. In Dictionary of Canadian biography, 1701 to 1740. Volume 2, 1969. p. 489–92.

**Bernier J:** François Blanchet et le mouvement réformiste en médecine au début du XIXe siècle. **Rev Hist Am Fr** 1980;34(2):223–44

**Bernier J:** La standardisation des études médicales et la consolidation de la profession dans la deuxième moitié du XIXe siècle. **Rev Hist Am Fr** 1983;37(1):51–65

**Bernier J:** Le corps médical québecois à la fin du XVIIIe siècle. In Roland CG, ed: Health, disease and medicine. Toronto, Hannah Institute for the History of Medicine, 1984. p. 36–64.

**Bernier J:** Les practiciens de la santé à Québec, 1871–1921: quelques données statistiques. **Rech Sociogr** 1979;20(1):41–58

**Bernier J:** L'integration du corps médical Quebeçois à la fin du XIXe siècle. **Hist Reflect** 1983;10(1):91–113

**Bernier J:** Philippe-Louis-François Badelard. In Dictionary of Canadian biography, 1801 to 1820. Volume 5, 1983. p. 46–7.

**Bernier J:** Pierre Beaubien. In Dictionary of Canadian biography, 1881–1890. 1982;11:57–8.

**Bernier J:** Vers un nouvel ordre médical: les origines de la Corporation des Médecins et Chirurgiens du Quebec. **Rech Sociogr** 1981;22(3):307–30

**Bernier JJ, Chevallier P, Teysseire D, et al:** La maladie de Louis XIII. Tuberculose intestinale ou maladie de Crohn? **Nouv Presse Med** 1981 Jun 20;10(27):2243, 2247–50

**Bernier R:** Aux sources de la biologie. 1. Les vingt premiers siècles. La classification. Montrèal, Presses de l'Université du Québec – Paris, Masson, 1975. xii, 264 p.

**Bernier R:** Histoire institutionnelle et sociale de l'hôpital de Tulle sous l'Ancien Régime. Mémoire de fin d'assistanat à l'Ecole Nationale de la Santé Publique de Rennes, 1976, 8 n.p., 114 p.

**Bernier R:** Les mesures publique d'assistance à la fin de l'Ancien régime dans la généralité de Caen. D.E.S. d'histoire du droit et des faits sociaux, Univ. de Caen, 1972 vii, 89, 56 p.

**Bernische Liga gegen die Tuberkulose 1930–1980:** Festschrift zum 50jährigen Jubiläum 20. Juni 1980 in Bern. Bern, 1980? 72 p. Contributions by S. Weiss, E. R. Mordasini, E. Arnold, R. Keller.

**Bernos M:** Une 'suscitation' au Buis-les-Baronnies en 1699. Nouvelle contribution à l'étude des sanctuaires 'a répit'. **Ann Midi** 1980;92(146):87–93

**Bernoulli R:** A propos d'une vieille querelle: Montaigne était-il hypocondriaque? **Hist Sci Med** 1982;16(3):145–9

**Bernoulli R:** Montaigne: ein Medizinprogramm im sechzehnten Jahrhundert. **Gesnerus** 1981;38:119–26

**Bernoulli R:** Un grand méconnu: Gustave Roussy. **Gesnerus** 1980;37(1/2):34–46

**Bernsmeier H** see **Kluxen G**

**Bernstein BJ:** On mass inoculation, who should be heard? **Cent Mag** 1981;14(5):56–61

**Bernstein BJ:** The swine flu vaccination campaign of 1976: politics, science, and the public. **Congr Pres J Cap Stud** 1983;10(1):95–103

**Bernstein NR:** The first one hundred years. Essays on the history of the American Public Health Association. Washington, American Public Health Assn., 1972. 97 p.

**Bernstein RE:** Darwin's alter ego: co-originator Alfred Wallace. **Perspect Biol Med** 1984;27(2):234–8

**Bernstein RE:** Darwin's illness: Chagas' disease resurgens. **J R Soc Med** 1984 Jul;77(7):608–9

**Bernstein RE:** Dr Harvey Pirie and the Scottish National Antartic Expedition (1902–4). Scottish science and medicine in the Falklands and Antarctica. **Scott Med J** 1983 Jan;28(1):75–9

**Bernstein RE:** Dr. Harvey Pirie: versatile man of science and pioneer explorer of sub-antarctic regions eighty years ago. **Adler Mus Bull** 1984 Mar;10(1):4–10

**Bernstein RE:** Historical vignette: Harvey Pirie (1879–1965) and the Falklands. **S Afr Med J** 1983 Jan 29;63(5):169–70

**Bernstein RE:** Homeopathic 'firsts' in South Africa. **S Afr Med J** 1981 Jun 27;59(27):968

**Bernstein RE:** What was Charles Darwin's illness? **S Afr Med J** 1982 Jun 19;61(25):939

**Bernstein S** see **Simmons GB**

**Bernstein BJ, et al:** The artificial heart program. **Cent Mag** 1981;14(3):22–41

**Berntsen B:** Fra Malthus til befolkningsåret 1974. **Samtiden (Norway)** 1973;82(4):232–9

**Bernus A von:** Alchymie und Heilkunst. Nürnberg, Carl, 1981. 243 p.

**Bernus A von, ed:** Alt-Kräuterbüchlein. Nach dem 'New-Kreüterbüchlein' des Leonhart Fuchs. Mit einem Nachwort von E. Mittler. Frankfurt am Main, Insel, 1980. 153 p.

**Bernus-Taylor M, Kalus L:** Musée du Louvre, département des Antiquités orientales. Un vase d'apothicaire islamique. **Rev Louvre Mus Fr** 1980;30(2):95–101

**Berrance de Castro J, Scarano JM, Aissar A:** A mortalidade entre os filhos de trabalhadores pretos e brancos estrangeiros numa regiõ cafeeira paulista: 1875–1930. **Rev Hist (Brazil)** 1973;46(94):603–17
**Berridge V:** Drugs and social policy: the establishment of drug control in Britain 1900–30. **Br J Addict** 1984 Mar;79(1):17–29
**Berridge V:** Opiate use in England, 1800–1926. **Ann NY Acad Sci** 1982;398:1–11
**Berridge V:** Opium and oral history. **Oral Hist** 1979;7(2):48–58
**Berridge V, Edwards G:** Opium and the people. Opiate use in nineteenth-century England. London and New York; Allen Lane and St. Martin's Press; 1981. 369 p.
**Berridge V:** Victorian opium eating: response to opiate use in nineteenth century England. **Victorian Stud** 1978;21(4):437–61
**Berrios GE:** Delirium and confusion in the 19th century: a conceptual history. **Br J Psychiatry** 1981 Nov;139:439–49
**Berrios GE:** Descriptive psychopathology: conceptual and historical aspects. **Psychol Med** 1984 May;14(2):303–13
**Berrios GE:** Epilepsy and insanity during the early 19th century. A conceptual history. **Arch Neurol** 1984 Sep;41(9):978–81
**Berrios GE:** Stupor: a conceptual history. **Psychol Med** 1981 Nov;11(4):677–88
**Berrios GE:** Tactile hallucinations: conceptual and historical aspects. **J Neurol Neurosurg Psychiatry** 1982 Apr;45(4):285–93
**Berriot-Salvadore E:** La femme soignante à la Renaissance: de la profession médicale à la vocation charitable. **Penelope** 1981;(5):24–8
**Berry EM:** The evolution of scientific and medical journals. **N Engl J Med** 1981;305:400–2
**Berry H** see **Fernandes L**
**Berry J Jr, Malt RA:** Appendicitis near its centenary. **Ann Surg** 1984 Nov;200(5):567–75
**Berryman JW, Brislin J:** The ladies' department of the American Farmer, 1825–1830. A locus for the advocacy of family health and exercise. **J NAL Assoc** 1977;2(2):8–15
**Bersch MC:** Notre revue a 75 ans. **Krankenpflege (Bern)** 1983 Jan;(1):18–22
**Bert P:** La pression barométrique. Recherches de physiologie expérimentale. Facsimile of 1878 edition. Biographical introduction by P. Dejour. Paris, Editions du Centre National de la Recherche Scientifique, 1979. viii, 1183 p.
**Bertaux P:** Der Wandel der Auffassungen über Hölderlins Krankheit. War Hölderlin geisteskrank? **Med Welt** 1980 Mar 28;31(13):486–90
**Bertelli G, Foà V:** Ramazzini, cinquanta anni dopo, su 'la medicina del lavoro'. **Med Lav** 1983 Nov–Dec;74(6):423–5
**Berthe JP:** Les epidémies au Mexique au XVIe siècle. **Asclepio** 1983;35:257–63
**Berthe M** see **Guillemain B**
**Berti Bock G, Vial F, Heymans G, et al:** Considerazioni critiche sull'opera di Carlo Forlanini (1847–1918). **Minerva Med** 1980 Jun 30;71(26):1879–83
**Berti Bock G** see **Agostoni G**
**Berti Bock G** see **Heymans G**
**Berti-Bock G., et al:** Le séjour de William Harvey à Padoue. **Hist Sci Med** 1980;14:317–24
**Bertier J** see **Grmek MD, ed**
**Bertier de Sauvigny RP:** Témoignages américains sur la médecine parisienne (1815–1848). **Hist Sci Med** 1980;14:439–47
**Bertini RC:** The American Red Cross-- a centennial year. **RI Med J** 1981 Apr;64(4):183–4
**Bertoye A** see **Woehrle R**
**Bertram E, Wengenmayer M:** Ein Dezennium Lungenchirurgie. Operative Therapie am Krankengut der Jahre 1958 bis 1967. **Prax Klin Pneumol** 1980 May;34(5):282–94
**Bertrán Capella A, Huguet Ramia E:** La aportacion de Pedro Mata a la toxicologia. **Asclepio** 1980;32:53–63
**Bertrand G** see **Olivier A**
**Bertrand G** see **Picard C**
**Bertrand M** see **Robin ED, ed**
**Berumen Amor E** see **Juan López M**
**Berzi A, Cipriani C, Poggesi M:** Florentine scientific museums. **J Soc Bibliogr Nat Hist** 1980 Apr;9(4):413–25
**Bescherer J:** Krankheitsbilder und Verhaltensweisen bei langfristigen Schülern in Klinik und Körperbehindertenschule--Eindrücke und Erfahrungen eines Sonderschullehrers aus 40 Berufsjahren. Zugleich ein Beitrag zur Geschichte der Pädiatrie und der Sonderpädagogik. **Arztl Jugendkd** 1984 Apr;75(2):88–102
**Beshkov L:** Stranitsi ot istoriiata na tolbukhinskata bolnitsa. Tolbukhin, [s.n.], 1967 (Tolbukhin: SPP Kiro Stefanov). 255 p.
**Beslin M:** 30 godina neuropsyhijatrijske bolnice 'Dr Slavoljub Bakalović' Vršac. **Med Pregl** 1984;37(1–2):71–4
**Besombes A:** Die Zahnheilkunde vom Mittelalter bis zum achtzehnten Jahrhundert. In Sournia JC, Martiny M, Poulet J, ed: Illustrierte Geschichte der Medizin. Salzburg, Andreas, 1980. Vol. 6. p. 2045–73.
**Besombes A:** Die Zahnmedizin vom 18. Jahrhundert bis zur Gegenwart. In Sournia JC, Martiny M, Poulet J, ed: Illustrierte Geschichte der Medizin. Salzburg, Andreas, 1980. Vol. 8. p. 3053–79.
**Besombes A:** La triste fin de Pierre-Nicolas Gaulard (1713–1740) 'élève-associé de Fauchard'. **Hist Sci Med** 1980;14(2):213–20
**Besombes A:** Odonto-stomatologie et diplomatie de l'Impératrice Eugénie à Clemenceau. **Hist Sci Med** 1983;17(1):13–22
**Besscho C:** [Life of Mrs. Seki Hora, the founder of Japanese public health nursing] (Jpn). **Kango** 1980 Jun;32(6):112–20
**Besser FS:** Notes on Dr. Charles West and his grave in Chislehurst (Kent). **Hist Med (Lond)** 1975 Autumn–Winter;6(3–4):47–50
**Bessho C:** [Nursing as image. From nurses' point of view: nurses of past and present] (Jpn). **Kango** 1984 Aug;36(9):20–6
**Bessis M, Bernard J:** Remissions after exchange transfusions in acute leukemia. On the possible antileukemic properties of normal blood. Historical notes and recent reflections. **Blood Cells** 1983;9(1):75–82
**Bessis M, Delpech G:** Sickle cell shape and structure: images and concepts (1840–1980). **Blood Cells** 1982;8(2):359–435
**Bessler O, Kaiser W:** Hallesche und wittenbergische Absolventen in der Frühgeschichte des Pharmakopöewesens. **Wiss Z Martin Luther Univ (Math)** 1973;22(5):139–46
**Besson A:** The Medico-Legal Tracts Collection of Dr. A. S. Taylor, FRCP. **J R Coll Physicians Lond** 1983 Apr;17(2):147–9
**Best MR:** Medical use of a sixteenth-century herbal: Gervase Markham and the Banckes herbal. **Bull Hist Med** 1979 Fall;53(3):449–58
**Besterman E:** Waller before Einthoven in the clinical development of noninvasive ECG. **Am Heart J** 1982 Apr;103(4 pt 1):572
**Besterman EM** see **Vecht RJ**
**Beswick FW:** Chemical agents used in riot control and warfare. **Hum Toxicol** 1983 Apr;2(2):247–56
**Bethge R:** Erstes orthopädisches Lehrbuch der Welt für den Gebrauch der Arzte. Zum 200. Geburtstage von Johann Christian Gottfried Jörg. **Beitr Orthop Traumatol** 1979 Sep;26(9):520–4
**Bethge R, Knöfler EW:** 30 Jahre Gesellschaft für Orthopädie der DDR--Zur Erinnerung an ihren Mitbegründer und ersten Vorsitzenden Friedrich Loeffler. **Beitr Orthop Traumatol** 1983 May;30(5):233–6
**Bethge R, Knöpfler EW:** 50 Jahre Orthopädische Klinik der Karl-Marx-Universität Leipzig. **Beitr Orthop Traumatol** 1980 Oct;27(10):545–52
**The Bethlem Royal Hospital and the Maudsley Hospital--a glance at the future...and a look at the past.: Nurs Times** 1980 Sep 4;76(36):1558–62
**Bethmann W, Hampel H, Knöfler W:** Zur Problematik der stomatologischen Implantation. Die historische Betrachtung der Implantologie-Forschung mit dem Versuch einer Periodizierung nach wissenschaftlichen Gesichtspunkten. **Stomatol DDR** 1981;31(2):100–7
**Bethune manuscripts in the Osler Library: HSTC Bull** 1980;15/16:3
**Betke K:** 125 Jahre Pädiatrie. **MMW** 1983 Jul 1;125(26):619–20
**Bettelheim B:** Reflections: Freud and the Soul [as perceived in America]. **New Yorker** 1982;68(2):52–93
**Betteridge KJ:** An historical look at embryo transfer. **J Reprod Fertil** 1981 May;62(1):1–13
**Bettermann A:** Das Attribut des Asklepios. Versuch über das Zeichen des ärztlichen Standes. **ZFA (Stuttgart)** 1982 Dec 20;58(35–36):1903–7
**Bettex M, Oesch I:** The hiatus hernia saga. Ups and downs in gastroesophageal reflux: past, present, and future perspectives. **J Pediatr Surg** 1983 Dec;18(6):670–80
**Bèttica-Giovannini R:** Giuseppe Berruti e l'Ospizio Marino Piemontese per ragazzi scrofolosi poveri con una nota su la fondazione dell'Ospedale Maria Vittoria di Torino (1887). **Ann Osp Maria Vittoria Torino** 1977 Jul–Dec;20(7–12):227–340
**Bèttica-Giovannini R:** Il contributo 1958–1977 degli Annali Dell'Ospedale Maria Vittoria Di Torino alla storia della medicina. **Ann Osp Maria Vittoria Torino** 1980 Jan–Jun;23(1–6):175–223
**Bèttica-Giovannini R:** Il malgoverno dell'Ospedale di Chivasso dal Cinquecento al Settecento. **Ann Osp Maria Vittoria Torino** 1983 Jan–Jun;26(1–6):183–96
**Bèttica-Giovannini R:** La preghiera di Blaise Pascal per il buon uso delle malattie. **Ann Osp Maria Vittoria Torino** 1979 Jul–Dec;22(7–12):420–5
**Bèttica-Giovannini R:** La sfida di Peano: matematica e paranoia. **Ann Osp Maria Vittoria Torino** 1982 Jul–Dec;25(7–12):241–4
**Bèttica-Giovannini R:** Terra di Castagneto Po e acqua di San Genesio presso Chivasso. **Ann Osp Maria Vittoria Torino** 1981 Jan–Jun;24(1–6):217–27
**Bèttica-Giovannini R** see **Bazzi F**
**Bettini S** see **Pampiglione S**
**Beukers H:** De beginjaren van de microscopie aan de geneeskundige faculteiten te Utrecht en Leiden. **Tijdschr Geschied Geneeskd** 1983;6(2):65–81
**Beukers H:** De tijdschriften van Willem van Ranouw. **Ned Tijdschr Geneeskd** 1981 Oct 3;125(40):1613–7
**Beukers H:** Het laboratorium van Sylvius. **Tijdschr Geschied Geneeskd** 1980;3(1):28–36
**Beukers H:** Mechanistische principes bij Franciscus dele Boë, Sylvius. **Tijdschr Geschied Geneeskd** 1982;5(1):6–15
**Bevan PG:** Generalism and specialisation in surgery. **Ann R Coll Surg Engl** 1981 Nov;63(6):383–5
**Bevan-John P:** Down memory lane: escape from Alsace. **Nurs Mirror** 1980 Sept 25;151(13):34
**Beveridge WI:** The origin and early history of the Mules operation. **Aust Vet J** 1984 May;61(5):161–3
**Bevilacqua P:** Emigrazione transoceanica e mutamenti dell'alimentazione contadina calabrese fra otto e novecento. **Quad Stor** 1981;16(2):520–55
**Beya Alonso E:** Boticarios de Gerona en el siglo XV. **Bol Soc Esp Hist Farm** 1979 Dec;30(120):337–42
**Beya Alonso E:** La dietetica en los cartujos. **Bol Soc Esp Hist Farm** 1982 Sep;33(131):185–92
**Beya Alonso E:** La farmacia en la trapa. **Bol Soc Esp Hist Farm** 1983 Sep;135:85–94
**Beya Alonso E:** 'Los ingenieros industriales como Analistas Clínicos'. **Bol Soc Esp Hist Farm** 1981 Jun;32(126):91–3
**Beya Alonso E:** Un comentario sobre los 'Elementos de Farmacia', de Carbonell. **Bol Soc Esp Hist Farm** 1980/81

Dec–Mar;31–32(124–5):315–22
**Beya y Alonso E:** Prescripciones medicas y sanitarias en la Regla de San Benito. **Bol Soc Esp Hist Farm** 1984;35(137):61–7
**Beyer C:** Temperaturmessung. **Pharm Unserer Zeit** 1983 Jul;12(4):97–110
**Beyer KH** see **Kotwas J**
**Beynon JH:** The history of mass spectrometry and the search for zero. **Biomed Mass Spectrom** 1981 Sep;8(9):380–3
**Beyria B** see **Fabre M**
**Beyt JP:** La médecine de bienfaisance et d'assistance dans le Pas-de-Calais, 1856–1914. **Rev Nord** 1983;65(259):683–9
**Bezel E:** Johann Jakob Steger, 1798–1857. Beispiel eines Medizinstudiums im frühen 19. Jahrhundert nach den Briefen an seine Eltern. Zürich Juris, 1981. 156 p. (Zürcher medizingeschichtliche Abhandlungen, Neue Reihe, Nr. 147).
**Bezkorovainy A:** Ophthalmologic research in pre-World War I Russia. **Bull Hist Med** 1979 Winter;53(4):593–605
**Bezkorovainy A:** Science and medicine in Imperial Russia. Chicago, (The Author), 1980. 271 p.
**Bharadwaj LK** see **Peck DL**
**Bhat PS** see **Mishra SK**
**Bhatta BR** see **Mishra SK**
**Bhattacharyya NN:** Indian puberty rites. Second edition, revised and enlarged. New Delhi, Munshiram Manoharlal, 1980. 124 p.
**Bhatty MK** see **Said HM, ed**
**Bia FJ** see **Barry M**
**Biadała E:** Opis zatrucia jadem kiełbasianym z 1822 roku. **Wiad Lek** 1981 Jul 15;34(14):1223–5
**Biadała E:** Sztuczne oddychanie metodą usta-usta i pobudzanie prądem elektrycznym akcji serca opisane przed 200 laty. **Wiad Lek** 1981 Sep 1;34(17):1471–7
**Biadała E:** Wiadomości o strzykawkach stosowanych do leczenia chorych z 1820 r. **Wiad Lek** 1980 Nov 15;33(22):1849–50
**Bialasiewicz AA** see **Silverstein AM**
**Białowąs M:** Z rozmyślańo śmierci. **Wiad Lek** 1981 Sep 15;34(18):1581–3
**Bianco L:** Birth control in China: local data and their reliability. **China Q** 1981;(85):119–37
**Bianco L:** Voyage en Chine. **Esprit** 1973; (4):595–604
**Biaudet JC:** Mathias Mayor (1775–1847). **Rev Med Suisse Romande** 1984 May;104(5):343–7
**Bibbings J:** Honey, lizard dung and pigeons' blood. **Nurs Times** 1984 Nov 28–Dec 4;80(48):36–8
**Bibel DJ:** Sternberg, Metchnikoff, and the phagocytes. **Milit Med** 1982 Jul;147(7):550–3
**Bibel DJ:** The discovery of the oral flora--a 300-year retrospective. **J Am Dent Assoc** 1983 Oct;107(4):569–70
**Bibergeil H:** Vom Diabetikerheim zum Diabetes-Forschungsinstitut--50 jähriges Jubiläum im Zentralinstitut für Diabetes 'Gerhardt Katsch' Karlsburg. **Z Gesamte Inn Med** 1981 Jan 1;36(1):1–3
**Bibliografia biezaca: Historii Nauki i Techniki: Kwart Hist Nauki Tech** 1984;29(Suppl 3–4):1–29
**Bibliographie des travaux de P. Broca consacrés à l'aphasie.: Rev Neurol (Paris)** 1980;136(10):663–4
**Bibliography:** Publications (in English) of Sir Austin Bradford Hill. **Stat Med** 1982 Oct–Dec;1(4):369–75
**Bibliography of Dr. E. H. Lambert: Muscle Nerve** 1982;5(9S):S166–72
**Bibliography of original works on orthopaedic surgery, traumatology and related sciences, 1872–1972.:** Belgrade, Yugoslav Association for Orthopaedic Surgery and Traumatology, 1980. 251 p.
**Bibliography of the history of medicine:** no. 14--1978. Bethesda, National Library of Medicine, 1979. 224 p. (NIH Publication No. 80–315).
**Bibliography of the history of medicine, No. 15, 1975–1979:** Bethesda, National Library of Medicine, 1981. lxxii, 924 p. (NIH Publication No. 81–1224).
**Bibliography of the history of medicine, No. 16, 1980:** Bethesda, National Library of Medicine, 1982. xi, 305 p. (NIH Publication No. 82–315).
**Bibliography of the history of medicine, No. 17, 1981:** Bethesda, National Library of Medicine, 1983. xi, 240 p. (NIH Publication No. 83–315).
**Bibliography of the history of medicine, No. 18, 1982:** Bethesda, National Library of Medicine, 1983. ix, 305 p. (NIH Publication No. 84–315).
**Bidan P** see **Delaunay A, ed**
**Bidault R, Ledoux A:** La vie médicale bisontine et comtoise à l'aube de l'ère pasteurienne (2ème moitié du XIXe siècle). In: Congrès National des Sociétés Savantes, 99e, Besançon, 1974. Comptes Rendus. Paris, 1976. Section des Sciences, Fasc. V. p. 161–70.
**Bideau A:** A demographic and social analysis of widowhood and remarriage: the example of the castellany of Thoissey-en-Dombes, 1670–1840. **J Fam Hist** 1980 Spring;5(1):28–43
**Bideau A:** Accouchement 'Naturel' et accouchement à 'haut risque'. **Ann Demogr Hist (Paris)** 1981;:49–66
**Bideau A, Poulain M:** De la généalogie à la démographie historique: généalogie ascendante et analyse démographique. **Ann Demogr Hist (Paris)** 1984;:55–68
**Bideau A:** Présentation. **Ann Demogr Hist (Paris)** 1981;:23–30
**Bideau A:** Variables familiales de la mortalité infantile. In Imhof AE, ed: Mensch und Gesundheit in der Geschichte. Husum, Matthiesen, 1980. p. 223–50.
**Bideau A, et al:** Démographie historique et génétique des populations: la concentration géographique d'une maladie héréditaire rare. **Ann Econ Soc Civilis** 1979;34:85–105
**Biebel B** see **Aurach G**
**Biéder J:** L'odyssée d'Ulysse Trélat (1795–1879). **Ann Med Psychol (Paris)** 1984 Jan;142(1):128–41
**Biéder J:** Un aliéniste du XIXe siècle: Louis-Antoine Evrat (1797–1876). **Ann Med Psychol (Paris)** 1983 Jan;141(1):122–33
**Biéder J:** Un président de la Société Médico-Psychologique: Prosper Lucas (1808–1885). **Ann Med Psychol (Paris)** 1983 Sep–Oct;141(8):908–15
**Bieder RE:** Scientific attitudes toward Indian mixed-bloods in early nineteenth century America. **J Ethn Stud** 1980;8(2):17–30
**Biedermann H:** Medicina magica. Metaphysische Heilmethoden in spätantiken und mittelalterlichen Handschriften. 2. Auflage. Graz, Akademische Druck- u. Verlagsanstalt, 1978. 107 p.
**Biedowa J:** Morfologia zębów trzonowych na tle ich tendencji ewolucyjnych. **Czas Stomatol** 1980 Mar;33(3):191–6
**Bielewicz A:** Przemiany struktury spożycia napojów alkoholowych w Polsce. **Psychiatr Pol** 1983 Mar Apr;17(2):171–8
**Bienengräber A:** Wilhelm Busch und die Medizin. **Zentralbl Chir** 1980;105(24):1644–52
**Biener K** see **Häusermann R**
**Bienia BH** see **Bienia RA**
**Bienia RA, Stein E, Bienia BH:** United States Public Health Service hospitals (1798–1981)--the end of an era. **N Engl J Med** 1983 Jan 20;308(3):166–8
**Bierbaum M, Faller A:** Niels Stensen. Anatom, Geologe und Bischof, 1638–1686. 2d ed. Münster, Aschendorff, 1979. xi, 203 p. Includes Thomasen AL, Der Wandel des Stensenbildes.
**Bierbaumer P:** Der botanische Wortschatz des Altenglischen. 1. Teil: Das Laeceböc. Bern, Herbert Lang; Frankfurt, Peter Lang, 1975. xv, 168 p. (Grazer Beiträge zur Englischen Philologie, Bd. 1).
**Bierer BW:** American veterinary history. [Madison, Wis., Carl Olson, 1980]. 222 leaves.
**Biermann KR:** Alexander von Humboldt in seinem Verhältnis zur Leopoldina und zu anderen Akademien. **Acta Hist Leopoldina** 1980;13:39–49
**Biesterfeldt HH:** Some opinions on the physician's remuneration in medieval Islam. **Bull Hist Med** 1984 Spring;58(1):16–27
**Biget JL, Tricard J:** Livres de raison et démographie familiale en Limousin au XVe siècle. **Ann Demogr Hist (Paris)** 1981;:321–63
**Biglow LA:** Medical record education: an historical perspective. **J Am Med Rec Assoc** 1982 Aug;53(4):50–8
**Bignall JR:** A century of treating tuberculosis. **Tubercle** 1982 Mar;63(1):19–22
**Bigot A:** La médecine française à Pondichéry aux XVIIIe et XIXe siècles. In: Congrès National des Sociétés Savantes, 91e, Rennes, 1966. Comptes Rendus. Paris, 1967. Section des Sciences, Tome 1. p. 31–46.
**Bigwood J** see **Chilton WS**
**Bijok H:** Adolph Carl Gustav Wernher (1809–1883); Sein Leben und Wirken am Giessener Akademischen Hospital. Giessen, Schmitz, 1979. 235 p. (Arbeiten zur Geschichte der Medizin in Giessen, Band 1).
**Biklen D** see **Bogdan R**
**Bilaĭ VI** see **Smirnov VV**
**Bilas I:** Pierre-Etienne Fortin. In Dictionary of Canadian biography, 1881–1890. 1982;11:320–1.
**Bílek V, Niklíček L:** Dílo Alfreda Grotjahna a jeho vliv na vývoj sociálního lékařství v Cechách. Cást I. **Cesk Zdrav** 1982 Apr;30(4):145–56
**Bílek V, Niklíček L:** K hlavním otázkám historie Ceskoslovensko-sovětských lékářských styku vletech 1918–1952. **Cesk Zdrav** 1981 Apr;29(4):133–46
**Bilikiewicz A:** Problematyka psychiatryczna w polskiej epileptologii ostatniego 35-lecia. **Psychiatr Pol** 1981 Mar–Apr;15(2):189–93
**Biliński Z:** Przyczynek do poznania zjawiska szerzenia się chorób wenerycznych-w oparciu o problem występowania prostytucji w Jarosławiu w okresie zaboru austriackiego (1895–1916). **Przegl Dermatol** 1982 Jan–Apr;69(1–2):113–5
**Billanovich MC:** I libri di Benedetto Greco da Salerno, studente a Padova in medicina (1401). **Quad Stor Univ Padova** 1974;7:1–15
**Biller P:** Curate infirmos: the medieval waldensian practice of medicine. In Sheils WJ, ed: The Church and healing. Papers read at the twentieth summer meeting and the twenty-first winter meeting of the Ecclesiastical History Society. Oxford, Basil Blackwell for the Society, 1982. p. 55–57.
**Billich A:** Un procès de sorcellerie à Turckheim en 1628. In: Congrès National des Sociétés Savantes, 104e, Bordeaux, 1979. Actes. Paris, 1981. Histoire Moderne et Contemporaine, Tome 2. p. 407–10.
**Billick G ed.:** References for the history of human nutrition in America, 1600 to the present: a selected bibliography. **J NAL Assoc** 1980;5(1–2):45–61
**Billig M:** The origins of race psychology - I. **Patterns Prejudice** 1982;16(3):3–16
**Billingham RE, Beer AE:** Reproductive immunology: past, present, and future. **Perspect Biol Med** 1984;27(2):259–75
**Billioud J:** Les Saints de la Peste. Une grande page de solidarité. **Marseille** 1983;(132–133):56–63
**Bilson G:** A darkened house: cholera in nineteenth century Canada. Toronto, Buffalo, University of Toronto Press, 1980. 222 p.
**Bilson G:** Canadian doctors and the cholera. **Hist Pap Can Hist Assoc** 1977:104–19
**Bilson G:** Cholera and public health in Canada. **Can J Public Health** 1984 Sep–Oct;75(5):352–5
**Bilson G:** 'Muscles and health': health and the Canadian immigrant, 1867–1906. In Roland CG, ed: Health, disease and medicine. Toronto, Hannah Institute for the History of Medicine, 1984. p. 398–411.
**Bilyk VD, Klantsa PA, Kul'chitskiĭ KI, et al:** Zaslugi N. I. Pirogova v sozdanii i razvitii material'no-tekhnicheskoĭ bazy vysshego

meditsinskogo obrazovaniia. **Klin Khir** 1983 Mar;(3):55-7
**Binder G:** Penal reform and progressive ideology. **Rev Am Hist** 1981;9(2):224-32
**Bindra JS, Lednicer D, ed:** Chronicles of drug discovery. Volume 1. New York, John Wiley & Sons, 1982. xiii, 283 p.
**Binet JL:** Aspect des cellules sanguines au XIXe siècle. **Clio Med** 1982 Dec;17(2-3):133-44
**Binet JL:** Dessins et traités d'anatomie. Paris, Chêne, 1980. 247 p.
**Binet JL:** Histoire de la sphèrocytose congénitale. **Nouv Rev Fr Hematol** 1981 Sep;23(3):177-84
**Binet JL:** Historical notes on quantitative blood cell measurements. **Blood Cells** 1980 Jun;6(3):507-11
**Binet JL:** Les premiers clichès du sang. **Nouv Rev Fr Hematol** 1981;23(2):135-7
**Binet JL** see **Bernard J**
**Binet JL** see **Golliet P**
**Binford CH, Reich CV:** Ricardo S. Guinto, M.D., M.P.H., epidemiologist-leprologist, 1907-1983. In appreciation of 50 years dedicated to research in leprosy. **Int J Lepr** 1983 Dec;51(4):587-91
**Binford CH** see **Skinsnes AV**
**Binford Ch:** Esmond Ray Long, M.D., Ph. D., 1890-1979, Editor, International Journal of Leprosy, 1964-1968. **Int J Lepr** 1980 Sep;48(3):322-6
**Bing F** see **Postel J**
**Bing FC, Prebluda HJ:** E. V. McCollum: pathfinder in nutrition investigations and world agriculture. **Agric Hist** 1980;54(1):157-66
**Bing FC:** Emma Kohman and the early history of nutritional edema. **J Am Diet Assoc** 1983 Jun;82(6):605-9
**Bing FC:** James Lawder Gamble (1883-1959). A biographical sketch. **J Nutr** 1981;111:203-7
**Bing FC:** Vincent du Vigneaud (1901-1978): a biographical sketch. **J Nutr** 1982 Aug;112(8):1463-73
**Bing RJ:** Carrel: a personal reminiscence. **JAMA** 1983 Dec 23-30;250(24):3297-8
**Bing RK:** Nationally speaking--living forward, understanding backwards, Part I. **Am J Occup Ther** 1984 Jun;38(6):363-6
**Bingham M:** Medical education at Hartford Hospital: an historical review. **Conn Med** 1979 Nov;43(11):683-6
**Bingham S:** Ministering angels. Oradell, New Jersey, Medical Economics Company, 1979. 224p.
**Biniek EM:** Psychotherapie mit gestalterischen Mitteln. Eine Einführung in die Gestaltungstherapie. (Die Medizin) Darmstadt, Wissenschaftliche Buchgesellschaft, 1982. 169 p.
**Binneveld JM:** Van bewaarplaats tot geneeskundig gesticht. **Spiegel Hist** 1981;16(5):267-73
**Binnie GA:** George Johnston: 1797-1855. **Br Med J [Clin Res]** 1982 Oct 9;285(6347):1014-6
**Biocca E:** Problemi parassitologici in rapporto ad una politica dell'ambiente. **Parassitologia** 1979;21(1-3):1-9
**Biocca M** see **Bagnara S**
**Biographical sketch:** Dr. Israel Michael Rabbinowicz (1818--1893). **Koroth** 1979 Nov;7(9-10):CCXXIII-CXXIV(717-9)
**Biographical sketches no. 31--Lasèque: Ir Med J** 1983 Aug;76(8):367
**Biondani P, Frazzingaro S:** Evoluzione storica del concetto di aggressività in psicoanalisi ed etologia. **Acta Med Hist Patav** 1981/82;28:9-20
**Biraben JN:** André Armengaud, 1920-1980. **Ann Demogr Hist (Paris)** 1980;:7-10
**Biraben JN:** Essai sur l'évolution du nombre des hommes. **Population** 1979;34(1):13-24
**Biraben JN:** Histoire des classifications de causes de décès et de maladies aux XVIIIe et XIXe siècles. In Imhof AE, ed: Mensch und Gesundheit in der Geschichte. Husum, Matthiesen, 1980. p. 23-34.
**Biraben JN:** La diffusion de la vaccination en France au 19e siècle. **Ann Bretagne** 1979;86(3):265-76
**Biraben JN:** Les hommes et la peste en France et dans les pays européens et méditeranéens. Tome II. Les hommes face à la peste. Paris, Mouton, 1976. 416 p.
**Biraben JN** see **Charbonneau H**
**Biraben JN** see **Flinn MW**
**Birch CA:** Names we remember: 56 eponymous medical biographies. Beckenham, Kent: Ravenswood, 1979. xi, 165 p.
**Birchall S:** A disowned apothecary. **Pharm Hist (London)** 1984 Sep;14(3):8
**Birchenall PD** see **Allan P**
**Bircher M:** Deutsche Drucke des Barock 1600-1720 in der Herzog August Bibliothek Wolfenbüttel. Abteilung A: Bibliotheca Augusta. Band 2: Arithmetica, Astronomica, Bellica, Geographica, Geometrica, Medica, Oeconomica, Physica. Nendeln, KTO Press, 1979. 408 p.
**Bird DT:** A catalogue of sixteenth-century medical books in Edinburgh libraries. Edinburgh, Royal College of Physicians of Edinburgh, 1982. xxxii, 298 p.
**Bird J** see **Turner CG**
**Bird JR:** Group approaches and Army health. **J R Army Med Corps** 1980 Oct;126(3):112-9
**Bird PD:** The development of dental radiology. The realisation of a scientific dream. **Br Dent J** 1981 Jul 7;151(1):28-30
**Bird RD, Allen G:** The J.H.B. Archive report: the papers of Harry Hamilton Laughlin, eugenicist. **J Hist Biol** 1981 Fall;14(2):339-53
**Birdsell D** see **Kleber BE**
**Birken W:** Dr. John King (1614-1681) and Dr. Assuerus Regemorter (1615-1650). Brethren in the Dutch Church and in the Royal College of Physicians of London, with added references to other 'Dutch' congregants in the Royal College, Dr. Baldwin Hamey and Dr. George Ent. **Med Hist** 1976 Jul;20(3):276-95
**Birken WJ:** The Royal College of Physicians of London and its support of the parliamentary cause in the English civil war. **J Br Stud** 1983;23(1):47-62
**Birkett DA** see **Hart GD, ed**
**Biró I:** A szemészet haladása Helmholtztól napjainkig. **Orv Hetil** 1982 Feb 21;123(8):475-8
**Bíró I:** Babits Mihály szenvedései. **Orv Hetil** 1983 Nov 27;124(48):2937-9
**Biró I:** Rekviem a Grósz-iskoláért. **Orv Hetil** 1979 Dec 30;120(52):3183-4
**Bíró I:** Szily Adolf, Szily Aurél. **Orv Hetil** 1983 Aug 21;124(34):2065-6
**Biron H:** Antoine Chaudillon. In Dictionary of Canadian biography, 1701 to 1740. Volume 2, 1969. p. 140-1.
**Biron H:** Pierre Baudeau. In Dictionary of Canadian biography, 1701 to 1740. Volume 2, 1969. p. 47-48.
**Birtalan G:** Adatok a két világháború között Magyarországon végzett szervezett egészségvédelmi munkáról, különös tekintettel az Oki tevékenységére. **Orvostort Kozl** 1979;87-88(25 no 1-2):181-218
**Birtalan G:** Avicenna Kánonja és az európai orvostudomány. **Orvostort Kozl** 1980;89-91(26 no 1-3):25-43
**Birtalan G:** Dobrudscha in den 60-er Jahren des 19. Jahrhunderts in den Augen eines ungarischen Arztes. In International Congress of the History of Medicine. 26th, Plovdiv, 1978. Actes du Congress. Sofia, 1981. Volume II. p. 103-5.
**Birtalan G:** Klinisch-ätiologische Konzeptionen der achtziger Jahre des 19. Jahrhunderts im Spiegel der ungarischen Fachliteratur. **Wiss Beitr Martin Luther Univ Halle Wittenberg** 1983;5-R80:123-7
**Birtalan G:** Laennec and Skoda, classics of internal diagnostics. **Orvostort Kozl** 1982;28(1-3):33-41
**Birtalan G:** Személyi egeszségvédelem és mentálhygiéne a 18. században. **Orv Hetil** 1982 Mar 7;123(10):607-10
**Birtasevic B:** Razvoj naše vojne preventivne medicine. **Vojnosanit Pregl** 1981 Sep-Oct;38(5):308-13
**Bischof K** see **Ross HE**
**Bischoff P, Speiser P:** Mittelalterliche Augenheilkunde im Kloster St. Gallen. **Gesnerus** 1982;39(1):47-52
**Biserte G:** Les grands fondamentalistes médicaux lillois du début du siècle. **Hist Sci Med** 1980;14(1):115-21
**Biserte G:** L'Histoire de la Faculté Mixte de Médecine et de Pharmacie de Lille. (2 vols). Vol I. Lille, l'Association Corporative des Etudiants en Médecine de Lille, 1975. 169 p.
**Bishop B** see **Gordon G**
**Bishop C:** Hsien Wu (1893-1959): a biographical sketch. **Clin Chem** 1982 Feb;28(2):378-80
**Bishop DW:** H. Burr Steinbach: Prosit! **Soc Gen Physiol Ser** 1981;36:xi-xiv
**Bishop MG:** The celestial family: early Mormon thought on life and death, 1830-1846. Ph.D. Diss., Southern Illinois University. Carbondale, 1981. viii, 165 leaves.
**Bishop PJ:** Evolution of the stethoscope. **J R Soc Med** 1980 Jun;73(6):448-56
**Bishop PJ:** Laennec: a great student of tuberculosis. **Tubercle** 1981 Jun;62(2):129-34
**Bishop PJ:** Reception of the stethoscope and Laënnec's book. **Thorax** 1981 Jul;36(7):487-92
**Bishop PJ:** The history of the Brompton Hospital. **Trans Stud Coll Physicians Phila** 1979 Sep;5(1 No 3):171-82
**Bishop PJ** see **Grange JM**
**Bisset NG:** Arrow poisons in China. Part I. **J Ethnopharmacol** 1979 Dec;1(4):325-84
**Bitensky L** see **Chayen Y**
**Bithell TC:** Hereditary dysfibrinogenemia--the first 25 years. **Acta Haematol (Basel)** 1984;71(3):145-9
**Bitterling K:** Zwei bisher unbeachtete Fragmente der mittelenglischen Uebersetzung von Bartholomaeus Anglicus, 'De rerum proprietatibus'. **Neuphilol Mitt** 1977;78:47-56
**Bitty L** see **Bornstein S**
**Bixler RH:** The Psychology Department at the University of Louisville, 1907-1953. **Filson Club Hist Q** 1983;57(3):253-69
**Bizière JM:** 'Before and after': essai de psycho-histoire. **Rev Hist Mod Contemp** 1980 Apr-Jun;27:177-207
**Bizière JM:** Psychohistory and histoire des mentalités. **J Psychohist** 1983 Summer;11(1):89-109
**Bizière JM:** Une psycho-histoire, pourquoi faire? **Bull Soc Hist Mod** 1980;79(6):11-5
**Biziuliavichius SK, Galvonaïte AL:** Razvitie meditsiny v Vil'niusskom Universitete (k 200-letiiu vysshego meditsinskogo obrazovaniia v Litve). **Sov Zdravookhr** 1982;(4):54-8
**Bjarke B:** Mannen bakom syndromet: Arthur Fallot. En medicinens 'doldis'--fransmannen vars namn alla känner men få vet någonting om. **Lakartidningen** 1984 Oct 24;81(43):3934-5
**Bjarnason O:** Epidemics in Iceland in the 18th century. **Nord Medicinhist Arsb** 1980;Suppl 6:76-81
**Bjork DW:** The compromised scientist: William James in the development of American psychology. New York, Columbia University Press, 1983. xiv, 221 p.
**Björk VO:** The development of the Björk-Shiley artificial heart valve. **Clin Cardiol** 1984 Jan;7(1):3-5
**Björk VO:** The development of the Björk-Shiley artificial heart valve. **Clin Physiol** 1984 Feb;4(1):1-4
**Björkholm M:** Mannen bakom syndromet: Thomas Hodgkin. Temperamentsfull föregångare inom patologin och kämpe för rättvisa

åt förtryckta folk. **Lakartidningen** 1983 Feb 2;80(5):334–5
**Bjorkman JW** see **Altenstetter C**
**Björnberg A:** Ansiktsmutilationer inom Mochicakonsten. **Sydsven Medicinhist Sallsk Arsskr** 1982;19:32–44
**Black D:** The spirit of occupational medicine. **Br Med J** 1979 Dec 22–29;2(6205):1622–6
**Black D:** The story of nephrology. **J R Soc Med** 1980 Jul;73(7):514–8
**Black DW:** Psychosurgery. **South Med J** 1982 Apr;75(4):453–7
**Black E:** Dealing with the doctors: the Canadian experience. **Mon Rev** 1981;33(4):27–35
**Black E:** The great contact-lens con. **Wash Mon** 1980;12(7):23–9
**Black EF, Libby LM:** Commercial food irradiation. **Bull At Sci** 1983;39(6):48–50
**Black FL:** Modern isolated pre-agricultural populations as a source of information on prehistoric epidemic patterns. In Stanley NF, Joske RA, ed: Changing disease patterns and human behaviour. London, New York, Academic Press, 1980. p. 37–54.
**Black GW:** American science and technology; a bicentennial bibliography. Carbondale, Ill., Southern Illinois University Press, 1979. xi, 170 p.
**Black H:** Doctor and teacher, hospital chief. Dr. Samuel Proger and the New England Medical Center. Chester, Connecticut, Globe Pequot Press, 1982. xii, 210 p.
**Black J, Sholtes V:** Biomaterial aspects of surface replacement arthroplasty of the hip. **Orthop Clin North Am** 1982 Oct;13(4):709–28
**Black JJ:** A stitch in time--1. The history of sutures. **Nurs Times** 1982 Apr 14–20;78(15):619–23
**Black LT:** Volcanism as a factor in human ecology: the Aleutian case. **Ethnohistory** 1981;28(4):313–40
**Black MM, Drury PJ, Tindale WB:** Twenty-five years of heart valve substitutes: a review. **J R Soc Med** 1983 Aug;76(8):667–80
**Black NA:** Is glue ear a modern phenomenon? A historical review of the medical literature. **Clin Otolaryngol** 1984 Jun;9(3):155–63
**Black SE:** Pseudopods and synapses: the amoeboid theories of neuronal mobility and the early formulation of the synapse concept, 1894–1900. **Bull Hist Med** 1981 Spring;55(1):34–58
**Black SP:** Wilfred Trotter. **Surg Neurol** 1983 Mar;19(3):199–204
**Blackden S:** The Poor Law and wealth: a survey of parochial medical aid in Glasgow, 1845–1900. In: The search for wealth and stability. Ed. by T. C. Smout. London, Macmillan, 1979.
**Blackden SM:** The development of public health administration in Glasgow, 1842–1872. Ph.D. thesis, Univ. of Edinburgh, 1976.
**Blackwood L:** Alaska native fertility trends, 1950–1978. **Demography** 1981 May;18(2):173–9
**Blahd WH:** History of external counting procedures. **Semin Nucl Med** 1979 Jul;9(3):159–63
**Blain D, Barton M:** The history of American psychiatry: a teaching and research guide. Washington, American Psychiatric Association, 1979. iv, 44 p. Contributions by D. F. Musto, G. Mora, E. T. Carlson.
**Blain D:** Twentieth century psychiatry--living history in the life of Kenneth E. Appel, M.D., 1896–1979. **Trans Stud Coll Physicians Phila** 1980 Jun;5(2 no 2):144–54
**Blair GW:** The history of rheology. **Biorheology** 1982;19(1/2):231–5
**Blair RD, Vogel RJ:** A survivor analysis of commercial health insurers. **J Bus** 51(3):521–9, 1978
**Blair WG:** The chiropractic story. [s.l., s.n.], 1973. 17 p.
**Blake JB:** Homeopathy in American history; a commentary. **Trans Stud Coll Physicians Phila** 1981 Jun;3(2):83–92
**Blake JB:** Medicine and the Revolution. **Milit Med** 1984 Apr;149(4):189–95
**Blake JB** see **Numbers RL, ed**
**Blake TM:** Myocardial infarction and electrocardiography in historical perspective. **South Med J** 1983 Dec;76(12):1470–2
**Blake JB, ed:** Centenary of Index Medicus, 1879–1979. Bethesda, National Library of Medicine, 1980. viii, 115 p. (NIH Publication No. 80–2068; Order from U.S. Government Printing Office). Contributions by C. E. Rosenberg, G. Miller, F. B. Rogers, W. B. Bean, E. Wolf, K. G. Huston, S. Jarcho.
**Blakeley PR:** Francis Green: 'a suffering loyalist and friend to the British government. **NS Hist Q** 1979;9(1):1–14
**Blakely RL, Beck LA:** Trace elements, nutritional status, and social stratification at Etowah, Georgia. **Ann NY Acad Sci** 1981;376:417–31
**Blalock JB:** History and evolution of peptic ulcer surgery. **Am J Surg** 1981 Mar;141(3):317–22
**Blamire RV:** Meat hygiene: the changing years. **J R Soc Health** 1984 Oct;104(5):180–5
**Blanc B** see **Blanc F**
**Blanc F, Blanc FP, Blanc B:** Geschichte der Tropenkrankheiten. In Sournia JC, Martiny M, Poulet J, ed: Illustrierte Geschichte der Medizin. Salzburg, Andreas, 1980. Vol. 7. p. 2609–47.
**Blanc FP** see **Blanc F**
**Blanc O:** La natalité vaudoise: deux cents ans d'histoire. **Schweiz Z Gesch** 1981;31(2):144–73
**Blanchard D:** Who or what's a witch: Iroquois persons of power. **Am Indian Q** 1982;6(3–4):218–37
**Blancher DA:** Workshops of the bacteriological revolution: a history of the laboratories of the New York City Department of Health, 1892–1912. Ph.D. Diss., City University of New York. New York, 1979. xiv, 311 leaves.
**Blanchet D:** Evolution de la fécondite des régions françaises depuis 1960. **Population** 1981;36(4–5):817–44
**Blanckaert C:** Médecine et histoire naturelle de l'homme: l'anthropologie française dans la seconde moitié du XIXe siècle. In Poirier J, Poirier JL, ed: Médecine et philosophie à la fin du XIXe siècle. Paris, Université de Paris XII - Val de Marne, [1980?]. p. 101–16
**Blanckaert C:** Réflexions sur la détermination de l'espèce en anthropologie (XVIII–XIX siècles). **Doc Hist Vocab Sci** 1983;(4):43–80
**Blanco MA, Melnikov VP:** On the history of application of isotopes in biochemical research. **Istor Biol Issled** 1983;9:85–98
**Blanco RL:** American army hospitals in Pennsylvania during the Revolutionary War. **Pa Hist** 1981;48(4):347–68
**Blanco RL:** Medicine in the Continental Army, 1775–1781. **Bull NY Acad Med** 1981 Oct;57(8):677–704
**Blanco RL:** Military medicine in northern New York, 1776–1777. **NY Hist** 1982;63(1):39–58
**Blanco RL:** Physician of the American revolution, Jonathan Potts. New York, Garland STPM Press, 1979. xv, 276 p.
**Blanco RL:** The diary of Jonathan Potts: a Quacker medical student in Edinburgh (1766–67). **Trans Stud Coll Physicians Phila** 1977 Jan;44(3):119–30
**Bland CS:** The Halsted mastectomy: present illness and past history. **West J Med** 1981 Jun;134(6):549–55
**Bland EF:** The first ductus revisited. **N Engl J Med** 1984 Jun 28;310(26):1749
**Blaney R:** Henry Maunsell (1806–1879): an early community physician. **Ir J Med Sci** 1984 Jan;153(1):42–3
**Blank H:** 'The treatment of dermatomycoses with orally administered griseofulvin' by Blank and Roth, March 1959. Commentary: Treatment of dermatomycoses with griseofulvin. **Arch Dermatol** 1982 Oct;118(10):827–36
**Blank RH, Ostheimer JM:** Biomedical policy. **Policy Stud Rev** 1982;1(4):789–99
**[Blank MI]:** Research on the mental health of the aging 1960–1976. Rockville, Md., National Institute of Mental Health, 1977 (and 1981), xii, 69 p.
**Blankaart S:** Den Nederlandschen Herbarius. Facsimile of 1698 ed. Edited by D. A. Wittop Koning. Alphen, Stafleu Brussel. 621 p.
**Blankenburg W:** Unausgeschöpftes in der Psychopathologie von Karl Jaspers. **Nervenarzt** 1984 Sep;55(9):447–60
**Blankenburg W** see **Kraus A, ed**
**Blankenburg W** see **Tellenbach H, ed**
**Blanpain J, Delesie L, Nys H:** National health insurance and health resources. Cambridge, Harvard Univ. Press, 1978. xiv, 294 p.
**Blantz TE:** Thomas Anthony Dooley. In Dictionary of American biography, 1961–1965. Suppl. 7, 1981. p. 190–1.
**Blardone G:** Rapports entre alimentation et types de développements. **Acquis Med Recent** 1981;198:35–55
**Blaschko H:** Frederick Hughes Scott and his contribution to the early history of the transmitter concept. **Notes Rec R Soc Lond** 1983 Mar;37(2):235–47
**Blaschko H:** Hans Krebs: nineteen nineteen and after. **FEBS Lett** 1980 Aug 25;117 Suppl:K11–15
**Blasco A:** Berre et la peste de 1720. Berre-L'Etang, Association sciences et culture, 1983. 114 p.
**Blaser R** see **Domandl S, ed**
**Blaser RH:** Paracelsus in Basel. Festschrift für Professor Dr. Robert-Henri Blaser zum 60. Geburtstag. Herausgegeben von der Schweizerischen Paracelsus-Gesellschaft. Biographical introduction by K. Goldammer. Muttenz/Basel, St. Arbogast Verlag, 1979. 210 p. (Reprint of 7 works by Blaser).
**Blaser RH:** Paracelsus und die Basler Apotheker. **Pharm Acta Helv** 1979;54(9–10):281–5
**Blaser RH:** Paracelsus und die Dichter. **Salzburger Beitr Paracelsusforsch** 1984;23:9–26
**Blaser RH:** Ulrich Gyger, sin diener. Versuch einer biographischen Rekonstruktion. **Medizinhist J** 1981;16(1–2):53–66
**Blasi A:** Der Kochsche Grundversuch und seine gegenwärtigen experimentellen Varianten. **Z Erkr Atmungsorgane** 1983;161(1):51–5
**Bläsig W:** Die Sondermarken zum Internationalen Jahr der Behinderten - geordnet nach Gesichtspunkten der Rehabilitation. **Rehabilitation (Stuttg)** 1983 Nov;22(4):162–5
**Blasius D:** Der verwaltete Wahnsinn: eine Sozialgeschichte des Irrenhauses. Frankfurt am Main, Fischer, 1980. 201 p.
**Blasius D:** Psychiatrische Versorgung in Preussen, 1880–1910. **Sudhoffs Arch** 1982;66(2):105–28
**Blaskovič D:** Twenty-five years of Acta Virologica. **Acta Virol (Praha)** 1982 Sep;26(5):408–16
**Blaták F, Valenčik J:** Historické podmínky budování moravakých ústavu pro duševně choré v druhé polovině 19. století. **Cesk Psychiatr** 1981 Oct;77(5):348–51
**Blatt A:** Panchayati raj and the mobilisation of the periphery: the case of the location of a primary health centre. **J Commonw Polit Stud** 1972;10(2):130–48
**Blaufox MD, Constable AR:** Antique hazards: a latter day encounter with radium. **J Nucl Med** 1983 Jan;24(1):79–82
**Blaurock-Busch E** see **Sollmann AH**
**Blauth W, Donner K:** Zur Geschichte der Arthroplastik. **Z Orthop** 1979 Dec;117(6):997–1006
**Blaxter K:** Cervinus annos vivere: an account of opinion about the length of life of the deer. **Br Vet J** 1979 Nov–Dec;135(6):591–9
**Blaydes JE** see **Hughes WL**
**Blayo C** see **Calot G**
**Blayo Y** see **Laslett P**
**Blažekovic T:** Entwicklung und Stand der wissenschaftlichen Bibliotheken

in Kroatien. **Biblos (Vienna)** 1978;27(1):5-29
**Blázy A:** Az 1855. évi kolerajárvány hatása Zala megye lakosságára. [Effect of the 1855 cholera epidemic on the population of Zala county.] (Hun) MTA Pécsi és Veszprémi Akadémiai Bizottságának Ertesitője. (Proceeding of the Conference on the History of Settlements, Székeféhérvár 24-25 May, 1978). 1978; 3:105-113.
**Blázy A:** Die Namensgebung der Apotheken in Ungarn in Vergangenheit und Gegenwart. In Hein WH, ed: Pharmaziehistorischer Kongress, Budapest, 1981. Stuttgart, Wissenschaftliche Verlagsgesellschaft, 1983. p. 105-10.
**Bleich JD, Harakas SS, Hehir JB, et al:** Population ethics: religious traditions. In Reich WT, et al, ed: Encyclopedia of bioethics, v.3. New York, Free Press, 1978. p. 1250-73.
**Bleich JD, ed** see **Rosner F**
**Bleiker MA** see **Sutherland I**
**Bleker J:** Die historische Pathologie, Nosologie und Epidemiologie im 19. Jahrhundert. **Medizinhist J** 1984;19(1-2):33-52
**Bleker J:** Die Naturhistorische Schule 1825-1845. Ein Beitrag zur Geschichte der klinischen Medizin in Deutschland. Stuttgart, New York, Fischer, 1981. ix, 174 p.
**Bleker J:** Die Stadt als Krankheitsfaktor; eine Analyse ärztlicher Auffassungen im 19. Jahrhundert. **Medizinhist J** 1983;18(1-2):118-36
**Bleker J** see **Konrad M**
**Blenkinsop D** see **Allan P**
**Bleser C, ed:** The Hammonds of Redcliffe. New York, Oxford, Oxford University Press, 1981. xxii, 421 p.
**Bleuler M:** Eugen Bleuler and schizophrenia. **Br J Psychiatry** 1984 Mar;144:327-8
**Bleuler M, ed:** Beiträge zur Schizophrenielehre der Zürcher Psychiatrischen Universitätsklinik Burghölzli (1902-1971). Einleitende Uebersicht und gekürzter Nachdruck von Veröffentlichungen. Darmstadt, Wissenschaftliche Buchgesellschaft, 1979. vii, 358 p.
**Bliakher LI:** Ia. A. Borzenkov-istorik biologii. **Vopr Istor Estestvozn Tekh** 1982;1:36-44
**Blicksilver J:** Kinship and friendship in the emergence of a family-controlled southern enterprise: Life Insurance Company of Georgia, 1891-1950. In: Greenfield, Sidney M.; Strickon, Arnold; Aubey, Robert T., ed. Entrepreneurs in Cultural Context. Albuquerque, U. of New Mexico Pr., 1979. p. 9-121.
**Blight JG:** Jonathan Edwards's theory of the mind: its applications and implications. In J. Brozěk, ed: Explorations in the history of psychology in the United States. Lewisburg, Bucknell University Press, 1984. p. 61-120.
**Blin PC:** Bourgelat, founder of veterinary teaching, 1712-1779. **Comp Immunol Microbiol Infect Dis** 1980;3(1-2):xiii-xvi
**Blinderman A:** Isaac Bashevis Singer; medicinal fiction. **NY State J Med** 1981 Aug;81(9):1382-91
**Blinderman CS:** Unnatural selection: creationism and evolutionism. **J Church State** 1982;24(1):73-86
**Bliquez LJ:** An unidentified Roman surgical instrument in Bingen. **J Hist Med Allied Sci** 1981 Apr;36(2):219-20
**Bliquez LJ:** Classical prosthetics. **Archaeology** 1983 Sep-Oct;36(5):25-9
**Bliquez LJ, Kazhdan A:** Four testimonia to human dissection in Byzantine times. **Bull Hist Med** 1984 Winter;58(4):554-7
**Bliquez LJ:** Roman surgical instruments in the Johns Hopkins University Institute of the History of Medicine. **Bull Hist Med** 1982 Summer;56(2):195-217
**Bliss EL:** History of anorexia nervosa. In Gross M, ed: Anorexia nervosa. A comprehensive approach. Lexington, D. C. Heath, 1982. p. 5-7.
**Bliss M:** The aetiology of the discovery of insulin. In Roland CG, ed: Health, disease and medicine. Toronto, Hannah Institute for the History of Medicine, 1984. p. 333-46.
**Bliss M:** The discovery of insulin. Chicago, University of Chicago Press, 1982. 304 p.
**Bliss M, ed:** Banting's, Best's, and Collip's accounts of the discovery of insulin. **Bull Hist Med** 1982;56(4):554-68
**Bliumel' NF** see **Suvorov VIu**
**Bloch H:** Discovery of blood circulation; Some dependence factors in evolution of a discovery. **NY State J Med** 1979 Nov;79(12):1940-3
**Bloch H:** Francis Bacon (1561-1626), his interest and influence in education, science, and medicine. **NY State J Med** 1981 Jun;81(7):1120-2
**Bloch H:** Guillaume Dupuytren, M.D. (1777-1835). Surgeon of Hôtel Dieu and his American students. **NY State J Med** 1981 Feb;81(2):259-60
**Bloch H:** Jan Baptiste Van Helmont, M.D. (1579-1644); religion, mysticism, and science in a century of change. **NY State J Med** 1980 Sep;80(10):1631-3
**Bloch H:** Man's reasoning about diseases. Time and place. **NY State J Med** 1980 Nov;80(12):1888-91
**Bloch H:** Medical botany; note on Constantine Samuel Refinesque (1784-1841). **NY State J Med** 1979 Sep;79(10):1610-1
**Bloch H:** Nicholas Culpeper, M.D. (1616 to 1654). Medical maverick in seventeenth-century England. **NY State J Med** 1982 Dec;82(13):1865-7
**Bloch H:** Smallpox: a disease that disappeared. **Clin Pediatr (Phila)** 1984 May;23(5):290-1
**Bloch H:** William Charles Wells, M.D., F.R.S., 1757-1817. An American physician-scientist America almost forgot. **NY State J Med** 1983 Feb;83(2):248-50
**Bloch RH:** Untangling the roots of modern sex roles: a survey of four centuries of change. **Signs** 1978;4(2)
**Block K:** Feodor Lynen: Architekt der klassischen Biochemie. **Max Planck Ges Ber Mitt** 1980;2:21-30
**Block P:** Podiatric medicine in Britain and the United States: contrasts in development. **Milit Med** 1981 Mar;146(3):205-10
**Blodi FC:** Ophthalmology and philately. **Arch Ophthalmol** 1982 Mar;100(3):425,44 (continuing periodically)
**Blodi FC:** Ophthalmology and philately: I. Ophthalmologist on stamps--M.R. de Gama Pinto (1853-1945). **Arch Ophthalmol** 1980 Jan;98(1):143
**Blodi FC:** Ophthalmology and philately: I. Ophthalmologists on stamps--Ricardo Vertiz. **Arch Ophthalmol** 1979 Sep;97(9):1706 (continued periodically)
**Blodi FC:** Ophthalmology and philately: II. Ophthalmologists who became famous in other areas of endeavor--Carlos Finlay (1833-1915). **Arch Ophthalmol** 1980 Oct;98(10):1763
**Blodi FC:** Ophthalmology and philately: V. The diagnosis and treatment of occular diseases.--Eye banks. **Arch Ophthalmol** 1982 Nov;100(11):1794
**Blodi FC:** Was Mozart cross-eyed? **Arch Ophthalmol** 1981 May;99(5):823
**Blodi FC** see **Hirschberg J**
**Blodi FC** see **Newell FW**
**Blohmke M:** Stadt-Land-Unterschiede im Gesundheitszustand historischer und heutiger Bevölkerungen. In Imhof AE, ed: Leib und Leben in der Geschichte der Neuzeit. Berlin, Duncker & Humblot, 1983. p. 63-75.
**Blokhin NN, Napalkov NP:** Razvitie onkologii v SSSR. **Vopr Onkol** 1982;28(12):3-9
**Blokhin NN, Trapeznikov NN, Chaklin AV, et al:** Vsesoiuznomu onkologicheskomu naushnomu tsentru AMN SSSR 30 let. **Vopr Onkol** 1981;27(12):81-7
**Blokhin NN:** 60-letie Soiuza Sovetskikh Sotsialisticheskikh Respublik i razvitie Sovetskoĭ meditsinskoĭ nauki. **Vestn Akad Med Nauk SSSR** 1983;6:3-5
**Blom JJ, ed:** Descartes, his moral philosophy and psychology. Hassocks, Sussex, Harvester Press, 1978. xxi, 288 p.
**Blombäck B, Copley AL:** Hymie Nossel (11 July 1930-8 October 1983). **Thromb Res** 1984 Apr 1;34(1):1-7
**Blömer H:** 20 Jahre Herzschrittmacher-therapie. **ZFA (Stuttgart)** 1982 Jan 10;58(1):19-25
**Blomquist C** see **McCullough LB**
**Blönningen J:** Die Osteomalazie als Indikation für eine bilaterale Oophorektomie im späten 19. und frühen 20. Jahrhundert. Ergebnisse und Erklärungsversuche. Diss. Erlangen-Nürnberg, 1980. 113 p.
**Bloodgood FF** see **Jenner CL, ed**
**Bloom DE:** What's happening to the age at first birth in the United States? A study of recent cohorts. **Demography** 1982 Aug;19(3):351-70
**Bloom L:** Notes for a history of speech pathology: an addendum. **Folia Phoniatr (Basel)** 1982 Nov-Dec;34(6):296-9
**Bloom SW:** Sociohistorical perspectives [on the therapeutic relationship]. In Reich WT, et al, ed: Encyclopedia of bioethics, v.4. New York, Free Press, 1978. p. 1663-68.
**Bloomfield DK:** Early work on external electrical defibrillation. **N Engl J Med** 1980 Dec 4;303(23):1366-7
**Bloomfield RL** see **Chandler ET**
**Bloor DU:** Club practice. **J R Coll Gen Pract** 1982 May;32(238):310-5
**Bloor DU:** The certifying surgeons. **J R Coll Gen Pract** 1981 Jan;31(222):33-7
**Blos D:** 100 Jahre Rotes Kreuz. **Fortschr Med** 1983 Mar 31;101(12):524-6
**Blotzer JW:** Systemic lupus erythematosus I: historical aspects. **Md State Med J** 1983 Jun;32(6):439-41
**Blouin CB** see **Bourget P**
**Blount M:** Surpassing obstacles: black women in medicine. **J Am Med Wom Assoc** 1984 Nov-Dec;39(6):192-5
**Blue plaques: London houses of medicohistorical interest: Br Med J [Clin Res]** 1983 Feb 19;286(6365):641
**Bluefarb SM:** Dermatologists on postage stamps (Hulusi Behçet, Ruzar Briffa). **Int J Dermatol** 1982 Jan-Feb;21(1):54
**Bluemle LW:** Jefferson College and Thomas Jefferson University. In Medical-Science colloquium. Special edition of Topic: a journal of the liberal arts. Washington, Pennsylvania, Washington and Jefferson College, 1983. p. 39.
**Bluemle LW:** John Morgan--the father of American medicine. In Passmore R, ed: Proceedings of the Royal College of Physicians of Edinburgh Tercentenary Congress, 1981. Edinburgh, Royal College of Physicians of Edinburgh, 1982. p. 159-61.
**Blum A:** Alton Ochsner, MD, 1896-1981. He cleared the air. **NY State J Med** 1983 Dec;83(13):1251
**Blum A:** Fleeting hopes and promises of advertising. **Med J Aust** 1982 May 29;1(11):485
**Blum A:** Les établissements d'assistance en Basse-Alsace au début du XVIIe siècle. In Livet G, Schaff G, ed: Médecine et assistance en Alsace, XVIe-XXe siècle. Strasbourg, Istra, 1976. p. 71-86.
**Blum L, Slater S, Reuben D, et al:** A consideration of current clinical thermometry. **Bull NY Acad Med** 1982 Oct;58(7)621-7
**Blum L:** An eighteenth century health care provider and medical entrepreneur. **Bull NY Acad Med** 1984 Nov;60(9):944-7
**Blum L:** The youth of geriatrics. **Mt Sinai J Med (NY)** 1983 Nov-Dec;50(6):476-82
**Blum MH:** Toscanini's relation to his orchestra. **Hillside J Clin Psychiatry** 1983;5(1):91-127
**Blum RH:** Psychological processes in preparing contemporary biography. **Biography** 1981;4(4):293-311
**Blum W:** Der Apotheker und Chemiker Otto A. Ziurek (1821-1886) und die Apothekenreformbewegung von 1848. Braunschweig, 1980. 110 p. (Veröffentlichungen aus dem Pharmaziegeschichtlichen Seminar der

Technischen Universität Braunschweig, 22).
**Blumberg LU:** The significance of the alcohol prohibitionists for the Washington temperance societies; with special reference to Paterson and Newark, New Jersey. **J Stud Alcohol** 1980 Jan;41(1):37–77
**Blumenthal AL:** Wilhelm Wundt and early American psychology: a clash of cultures. In R. W. Rieber, K. Salzinger, ed: Psychology: theoretical-historical perspectives. New York, Academic Press, 1980. p. 25–42.
**Blumenthal AL:** Wundt – revisions and reappraisals. In K. Salzinger, ed: Psychology in progress: an interim report. (Annals of the New York Academy of Sciences, vol. 270). New York, New York Academy of Sciences, 1976. p. 21–9.
**Blumenthal AL** see **Rieber RW, ed**
**Blumenthal-Barby K:** Gedanken zu Sterben und Tod in der Belletristik. **ZFA** 1983 Sep–Oct;38(5):395–8
**Blustein BE:** A New York medical man: William Alexander Hammond, M.D. (1828–1900), Neurologist. Ph.D. Diss. University of Pennsylvania. Philadelphia, 1979. 418 leaves.
**Blustein BE:** The Philadelphia Biological Society, 1857–61: a failed experiment? **J Hist Med Allied Sci** 1980 Apr;35(2):188–202
**Blustein BE** see **Scull A, ed**
**Bluszcz G, Ciszek Z:** Leptospirozt w materiale chorych oddziału zakaźnego w Raciborzu w latach 1966–1977. **Przegl Epidemiol** 1979;33(4):515–8
**Blyth** see **McKinney HL, ed**
**Blythe WB, et al:** Walter Reece Berryhill. **NC Med J** 1984 Oct;45(10):615–29
**Boa YH** see **Zheng GZ**
**Boag JW:** Silvanus Phillips Thompson--some studies in the 'prehistory' of X rays. **Br J Radiol** 1984 Jan;57(673):1–15
**Boas Hall M:** Renaissance science and professionalisation. **Ann Ist Mus Stor Sci Fir** 1982;7(2):53–64
**Boas Hall M** see **Hall AR**
**Boase J:** Regulation and the paramedical professions: an interest group study. **Can Public Adm** 1982;25(3):332–53
**Boatman BE:** On American nostrum making and quackery. **J Okla State Med Assoc** 1982 Jan;75(1):3–7
**Boatner EB:** Captioned films of the deaf. **Am Ann Deaf** 1981 Aug;126(5):520–5
**Boaz NT:** A hominoid clavicle from the Mio-Pliocene of Sahabi, Libya. **Am J Phys Anthropol** 1980 Jul;53(1):49–54
**Boaz NT:** American research on Australopithecines and early Homo, 1925–1980. In F. Spencer, ed: A history of American physical anthropology, 1930–1980. New York, Academic Press, 1982. p. 239–60.
**Boaz NT** see **Cronin JE**
**Bobbio S:** Sorano de Efeso. **Femina** 1979;7:791–6
**Bobbioni MT:** Strutture demografiche e strutture sociali in una comunità rurale tra '500 e '600: il caso di s. secondo (prime indagini). **Genus** 1979;35(1–2):237–43
**Bober H, McKinney LC:** La prima autopsia. **Kos** 1984 Mar;1(2):51–60
**Bobkov AG, Mikhaĭlov VP:** Nauchnaia deiatel'nost' V. G. Garshina (1887–1956) i razvitie nauchnykh kontseptsiĭ v rabotakh sovetskikh morfologov. **Arkh Patol** 1983;45(4):77–80
**Bobková M** see **Mucha V**
**Bobon D** see **Mormont C**
**Bobrik II, Chernyshenko LV:** Istoriia anatomicheskikh muzeev na Ukraine i ikh znachenie dlia ateisticheskoĭ propagandy i populiarizatsii dostizheniĭ nauki. **Vrach Delo** 1984 Feb;(2):119–22
**Bobrik II, Chernyshenko LV:** Istoriia anatomii na Ukraine v gody Sovetskoĭ vlasti. **Arkh Anat Gistol Embriol** 1983 Jan;84(1):95–8
**Bobrik II, Chernyshenko LV:** 140 let kafedry anatomii Kievskogo meditsinskogo instituta. **Vrach Delo** 1982 Feb;(2):1–2
**Bocharov VJ** see **Speransky LS**
**Bochin A:** Et si nous visitions l'Hôpital Saint-Roch de Buzançais? **Bull Soc Fr Hist Hop** 1979;(39):32–49
**Bochkov NP:** V. D. Timakov (1905--1977). Moskva, Meditsina, 1982. 62 p.
**Bochkov NP:** Vklad s. n. Davidenkova v razrabotku probelmy nasledstvennykh nervynkh i psikhicheskikh zabolevaniĭ. **Zh Nevropatol Psikhiatr** 1982;82(3):1–4
**Bock HE:** Franz Volhard: Erinnerungen. Stuttgart, New York, Schattauer, 1982. xi, 345 p.
**Bock HE:** Pflanzen und Pflanzliches in Geschichte und Gegenwart der Medizin. **Universitas (Stuttg)** 1981;4
**Bock HE, ed, Hildebrand KH, ed, Sarre HJ, ed:** Franz Volhard, Erinnerungen. Stuttgart and New York, Schattauer, 1982. 345 p.
**Bockemühl J:** Die Typhus-Schutzimpfung gestern und heute. **Immun Infekt** 1983 Jan;11(1):16–22
**Bocock R:** Freud and modern society. An outline and analysis of Freud's sociology. New York, Holmes & Meier, 1978. xv, 200 p.
**Bocock R:** Sigmund Freud. Chichester, Horwood; London; New York, Tavistock, 1983. 145 p.
**Bocquet JP** see **Chabert JM**
**Bodarev VKh:** Tuberkulez vchera i segodnia (material dlia besed). **Feldsher Akush** 1979 Oct;44(10):13–6
**Bodde D:** Forensic medicine in pre-imperial China. **J Am Orient Soc** 1982;102:1–15
**Boddy FA** see **Butler JR**
**Bode UK:** Frühe histologische Krebsforschung in Deutschland, Frankreich und Oesterreich. Köln, 1979. 208 p. (Kölner medizinhistorische Beiträge. Arbeiten der Forschungsstelle des Instituts für Geschichte der Medizin der Universität zu Köln, Band 12).
**Bodemer CW:** Baron Dominique Jean Larrey, Napoleon's surgeon. **Bull Am Coll Surg** 1982 Jul;67(7):18–21
**Bodemer CW:** France, the fundament, and the rise of surgery. **Dis Colon Rectum** 1983 Nov;26(11):743–50
**Boden IM:** Fifty years of pharmaceutical development. **Practitioner** 1980 May;224(1343):513–5
**Boden MA:** Jean Piaget. New York, Viking, 1979. xii, 176 p.
**Boden RT:** Public health and physical planning--a time to reconsider? **S Afr Med J** 1981 Oct 10;60(15):582–8
**Bodenham DC:** In quest of perfection: training in plastic surgery. (McIndoe Memorial Lecture, 1980). **Ann R Coll Surg Engl** 1981;63:233–8
**Bodian D:** Normand Louis Hoerr. In Dictionary of American Biography, Suppl. 6, 1956–1960. p. 295–6, 1980.
**Bodó L** see **Orsós S**
**Bodosi M** see **Frankl J**
**Bodson L:** Aristotle's statement on the reproduction of sharks. **J Hist Biol** 1983 Fall;16(3):391–407
**Bodson L:** Des animaux parmi les hommes. L'ethnozoologie appliquée à l'Antiquité gréco-romaine. **Cah Clio** 1979;:9–16
**Bödvarsdóttir I:** Apoteks oprettelse og de første apotekere i Island. **Nord Medicinhist Arsb** 1982;:157–61
**Boe M** see **Fabre M**
**Boehm EH, Pope BH, Ensign MS, ed:** Historical periodicals directory. Volume 3: Europe: East and Southeast; USSR. Santa Barbara, Oxford, ABC-Clio, 1984. xv, 252 p. (Clio Periodicals Directories).
**Boelpaepe C de** see **Appelboom T**
**Boer C** see **Ficino M**
**Boesiger E** see **Mayr E**
**Boewe C:** Editing Rafinesque's holographs: the case of the short letters. **Filson Club Hist Q** 1980;54(1):37–49
**Bofill Pellicer C** see **Carmona Cornet AM**
**Bogard MO, Higby GJ:** A look at covered mortars and pestles. **Pharm Hist** 1984;26(2):106–8
**Bogard MO:** Colored glass in pharmacy. **Pharm Hist** 1984;26(1):20–7
**Bogard MO:** Eighteenth-century poison phials. **Pharm Hist** 1984;26(4):183–4
**Bogard MO:** Facts about artifacts; drugstore perfumes in the 1890s. **Pharm Hist** 1983;25(2):80–2
**Bogard MO:** Peoria's pioneer druggists, the Farrells, and Farrell's Arabian liniment. **Pharm Hist** 1982;24(3):99–105
**Bogard MO:** Vials and bottles for peppermint and other essences. **Pharm Hist** 1983;25(3):142–6
**Bogardus CR:** Kentucky's first woman dentist (Lucy Dupuy Montz). **Ky Dent J** 1984 Mar–Apr;36(2):23–5
**Bogatyrev MF:** Meditsinskoe obespechenie 25-i Krasnoznamennoĭ gvardeĭskoĭ Sinel'nikovskoĭ strelkovoĭ divizii v Budapeshtskoĭ nastupatel'noĭ operatsii. **Voen Med Zh** 1983 Oct;10:64–6
**Bogdan J:** Care or cure? Childbirth practices in 19th-century America. **Feminist Stud** 1978;4(2):92–9
**Bogdan R, Biklen D, Shapiro A, et al:** The disabled: media's monster. **Soc Policy** 1982;13(2):32–5
**Bogdan R** see **Taylor SJ**
**Bogdan TT:** Poluvekovoĭ opyt khirurgii raka legkogo. **Vestn Khir** 1984 Apr;132(4):69–71
**Bogdanov EA:** 50 Let travmatologicheskomu punktu Moskovskogo raĭona Leningrada. **Ortop Travmatol Protez** 1982 Dec;(12):61–3
**Bogdanov OV:** Vklad D. A. Biriukova v émbriofiziologiiu i dal'neĭshee razvitie ego ideĭ. **Fiziol Zh SSSR** 1984 Sep;70(9):1248–55
**Bogdanow:** Wrzesień w Lublinie. **Pieleg Polozna** 1979;(9):26–7
**Boggs DR:** Experimental hematology and bone marrow transplantation. **Exp Hematol** 1984 Mar;12(3):147–51
**Boglioni P** see **Sutto C, ed**
**Bognitskaia TN** see **Komarov BD**
**Bogolepova LS** see **Izmerov NF**
**Bogoliubov VM, Sokolova NF:** [Department of Physiotherapy of the Order of Lenin Central Institute of Physician Advanced Training in preparing medical personnel] (Rus). **Vopr Kurortoi Fizioter Lech Fiz Kult** 1980;6:62–3
**Bogoliubov VM:** V. I. Lenin i razvitie sanatorno-kurortnogo dela v SSSR. **Vopr Kurortol Fizioter Lech Fiz Kult** 1980 Mar–Apr;(2):1–3
**Bogoliubov VM:** Vklad russkikh uchenykh v razvitie kurortologii v Gruzii. **Vopr Kurortol Fizioter Lech Fiz Kult** 1984 Mar–Apr;(2):5–9
**Bogomolova LG, Andrianova IG, Selivanov EA:** Zaslugi A. N. Filatova v razvitie problemy sozdaniia lechebnykh preparatov krovi i krovezamenitelei. **Vestn Khir** 1982 Oct;129(10):9–13
**Bogovski P:** Historical perspectives of occupational cancer. **J Toxicol Environ Health** 1980 Sep–Nov;6(5–6):921–39
**Bogush LK:** Razvitie i dostizheniia khirurgii tuberkuleza legkikh v SSSR. **Probl Tuberk** 1983 Oct;10:3–7
**Bogusz J:** Uwagi lekarza o martyrologii Zydów polskich. **Przegl Lek** 1984;41(1):54–62
**Bogusz J:** Wpływ norymberskiego procesu lekarzy hitlerowskich na kształtowanie sie pojeć o dokonywaniu badań na ludziach. **Przegl Lek** 1981;38(1):72–9
**Boguszaková J:** Třicet let oftalmologické katedry institutu pro další vzdělávání lékařu a farmaceutu v Praze. **Cesk Oftalmol** 1983 May;39(3):145–8
**Bohland J** see **Knox PL**
**Böhm R:** Weniger bekannte historische Schriften aus der CSSR. **Hist Med Vet** 1977;2(2):56–7
**Böhme G:** Medizinische Porträts berühmter Komponisten: Wolfgang

Amadeus Mozart, Ludwig van Beethoven, Carl Maria von Weber, Frédéric Chopin, Peter Iljitsch Tschaikowski, Béla Bartók. 2. verbesserte und erweiterte Auflage. Stuttgart, New York, Gustav Fischer Verlag, 1981. xi, 199 p.
**Böhme K** see **Kulessa C**
**Bohme FG, ed:** Twenty censuses: population and housing questions 1790–1980. Washington, Bureau of the Census, 1979. 91 p.
**Böhmer W:** Der Wittenberger Kaiserschnitt von 1610. **Zentralbl Gynakol** 1983;105(19):1265–70
**Böhmer W, Helmbold P:** Die reproduktionsbedingte Mortalität während früherer Jahrhunderte. **Zentralbl Gynakol** 1984;106(13):939–46
**Böhmer W, Kirsten F:** Reformatorische Ausstrahlungen Martin Luthers auf das Gesundheitswesen seiner Zeit. **Z Gesamte Inn Med** 1983 Oct 15;38(20):546–51
**Boianov B:** Iubileina godishnina na purvata doktorska disertatsiia v oblastta na stomatologiiata. **Stomatologiia (Sofiia)** 1979 Jul–Aug;61(4):256–9
**Boic V:** Hematologija u prvoj polovici našega stoljeća. **Lijec Vjesn** 1980 Feb;102(2):107–8
**Bois P:** Le centenaire de l'Hôpital Notre-Dame. **Union Med Can** 1980 Jan;109(1):157–8
**Boisanger B de, Cudennec Y, Buffe P:** Aperçu sur la médecine de soins et la médecine du travail, dans une plantation de Guyane au XVIIIe siècle. **Hist Sci Med** 1984;18(3):215–21
**Boisseau-Lebreuil MT** see **Doby JM**
**Boissonnault CM:** Antoine Forestier. In Dictionary of Canadian biography, 1701 to 1740. Volume 2, 1969. p. 226.
**Boissonnault CM:** Michel Bertier. In Dictionary of Canadian biography, 1701 to 1740. Volume 2, 1969. p. 60.
**Boisvert DJ:** Florence Nightingale's cap. **N Engl Galaxy** 1978;20(2):42–51
**Boisvert H:** Etudes sur la rage (1925–1935). **Hist Sci Med** 1984;18(2):129–35
**Boisvert H** see **Saenz A**
**Bojanowski T:** Zdrowotne warunki pracy polaków zatrudnionych w przemyśle łódzkim podczas okupacji hitlerowskiej. **Przegl Lek** 1981;38(12):869–72
**Bojczuk H:** Stanisław Konopka (1896–1982), historyk medycyny, bibliotekarz i bibliograf, twórca polskiej bibliografii lekarskiej. **Arch Hist Med (Warsz)** 1983;46(4):439–51
**Bokeriia LA:** Leninskie dekrety v oblasti zdravookhraneniia. **Anesteziol Reanimatol** 1980 Mar–Apr;(2):3–5
**Bolander V:** A preliminary examination of John Wesley's 'Primitive physick'. **Bookman** 1983 Jul–Aug;10(4):3–10
**Boldyrev AA:** 55 let otechestvennoĭ biokhimii. **Biol Nauki** 1982;(5):107–8
**Bolecek O:** Protifašistický odboj na zdravotnické frontě. Vzpomínky na ilegální činnost za okupace na Bulovce. **Cas Lek Cesk** 1980 May 9;119(19):538–42
**Boletín panamericano de sanidad de la Oficina sanitaria internacional: Bol Of Sanit Panam** 1982 May;92(5):429–48
**Bolgarskiĭ IS** see **Mukhtarov AM**
**Boliukh BA** see **Nechiporuk VM**
**Bolkhovitinoe NN:** Sielemskaia ved'ma. **Vopr Istor** 1982;(10):187–9
**Bollen KA, Phillips DP:** Imitative suicides: a national study of the effects of television news stories. **Am Sociol Rev** 1982;47(6):802–9
**Bollen KA:** Temporal variations in mortality: a comparison of U. S. suicides and motor vehicle fatalities, 1972–1976. **Demography** 1983 Feb;20(1):45–59
**Bollet AJ:** A report of reactive arthritis following dysentery in 1743. **Arthritis Rheum** 1981 Jun;24(6):860
**Bollet AJ:** The rise and fall of disease. **Am J Med** 1981 Jan;70(1):12–6
**Bollet AJ:** Toxic shock syndrome: a new disease but an old phenomenon. **Conn Med** 1981 Apr;45(4):223–4
**Bollet AJ:** Wounded presidents: 1981 almost repeats the events of 1881. **Med Times** 1981 Jul;109(7):19–23
**Bollinelli R, Carles P:** Geschichte der Lungenheilkunde. In Sournia JC, Martiny M, Poulet J, ed: Illustrierte Geschichte der Medizin. Salzburg, Andreas, 1980. Vol. 8. p. 2795–825.
**Bologa VL:** Nils Rosen Rosenstein über die Erbsyphilis. **Acta Hist Rerum Nat Tech** 1972;6:77–82
**Bolton C, Leasure JW:** Evolution politique et baisse de la fécondité en occident. **Population** 1979;34(4–5):825–43
**Bolton G, Dean M:** Nursing history: women of good character. **Nurs Mirror** 1980 Nov 20;151(21):24–7
**Bolton G** see **Davies C, ed**
**Bolton S, Null G, Troetel WM:** The medical uses of garlic--fact and fiction. **Am Pharm** 1982 Aug;22(8):40–3
**Bolyki J:** Komáromi Csipkés György: Pestis pestise (1664). **Orvostort Kozl** 1979;86(24 no 4):81–9
**Bolz KD** see **Ostensen H**
**Bolzinger A:** Jalons pour une histoire de la psychiatrie à travers la Revue de Neuropsychiatrie infantile. **Neuropsychiatr Enfance Adolesc** 1981 Mar;29(3):127–40
**Bolzinger R, Beau A:** L'hôpital militaire d'instruction de Metz. In: Congrès national des Sociétés Savantes, 103e, Nancy, 1978. Comptes rendus. Paris, Section des Sciences, Fasc. V. p. 11–8.
**Bolzinger R, Gilbrin E, Lorrang F:** L'hôpital Saint-Nicolas de Metz avant la révolution. Sa fondation laïque, ses singulières prérogatives financières. **Hist Sci Med** 1979;13(4):369–77
**Bomba J** see **Aleksandrowicz JW**
**Bonadies A:** Manuel Diaz Rodriguez: maestro del estilismo y medico. **Rev Soc Venez Hist Med** 1969–71;17–19(31–33):109–15
**Bonalumi F:** Il medico di Balzac e il curato di Ravizza. **Aevum** 1979;53(3):519–32
**Bonard EC:** L'anémie du Saint-Gothard. **Rev Med Suisse Romande** 1980 Dec;100(12):1055–60
**Bonard EC:** Variole. **Rev Med Suisse Romande** 1980 Dec;100(12):1051–4
**Bonard JF:** 1980---Année du centenaire de la 'Revue médicale de la Suisse Romande'. **Rev Med Suisse Romande** 1980 Jan;100(1):1–3
**Boncompagni R:** Problemi relativi all'interpretazione e alla composizione del Regime delle malattie acute (Acut.). In La collection hippocratique et son rôle dans l'histoire de la médecine. Colloque de Strasbourg (23–27 octobre 1972) organisé par le Centre de Recherches sur la Grèce Antique, avec le concours des Facultés de Philosophie et des Langues Classiques. Leiden, E. J. Brill, 1975. p. 195–207.
**Bond JR, Johnson CA:** Implementing a permissive policy: hospital abortion services after Roe V. Wade. **Am J Pol Sci** 1982;26(1):1–24
**Bond JR** see **Johnson CA**
**Bond GR, et al:** Mended hearts: a self-help case study. **Soc Policy** 1979;9(4):50–7
**Bondar PN:** O role uchenykh Kievskogo meditsinskogo instituta v razvitii éndokrinologii. **Vrach Delo** 1981 Aug;(8):124–5
**Bondarenko NS** see **Korzh AA**
**Bonduelle M:** Sclérose latérale amyotrophique. **Rev Neurol (Paris)** 1982;138(12):1027–39
**Bondurant S:** Some means by which medical schools adapt to changing needs. **Bull NY Acad Med** 1984 Apr;60(3):271–80
**Bondy PK:** What's so special about Osler? **Yale J Biol Med** 1980 May–Jun;53(3):213–7
**Bonelli ML, Helden A van:** Divini and Campani: a forgotten chapter in the history of the Academia del Cimento. **Ann Ist Mus Stor Sci Fir** 1981;6(1):3–176
**Bonenfant JL:** La pathologie à l'âge des incertitudes. **Union Med Can** 1984 May;113(5):352–4
**Bonenfant-Feytmans AM:** Les organisations hospitalières vues par Jacques de Vitry (1225). **Ann Soc Belg Hist Hop** 1980;18:17–45
**Bonequi CC:** La huella del Hospital Infantil de México en la pediatría. Cuarenta años de vida institucional. **Bol Med Hosp Infant Mex** 1983 Aug;40 Suppl 2:1–10
**Bongiovi V** see **Harper RG**
**Bonica JJ:** History, current status and future of regional anesthesia. **Ann Chir Gynaecol** 1984;73(3):108–17
**Bonica JJ:** Pain. **Res Publ Assoc Res Nerv Ment Dis** 1980;58:1–17
**Bonifas V:** Alexandre Yersin (1863–1943). **Rev Med Suisse Romande** 1984 May;104(5):349–51
**Bonilauri F:** Museo e città. Le collezioni Spallanzani e chierici a Reggio Emilia. Firenze, Olschki, 1978. 199 p. (Biblioteca della 'Rivista di Storia delle Scienze Mediche e Naturali').
**Bonin M:** Depuis l'Institut Marguerite-d'Youville, 50 ans d'études supérieures au Québec. **Infirm Can** 1984 Oct;26(9):31–4
**Bonink K** see **Mann G, ed**
**Bonn G:** Der wissenschaftliche Nachlass des lippischen Forschungsreisenden Engelbert Kaempfer im Britischen Museum. **Lipp Mitt Gesch Landeskd** 1979;48:69–116
**Bonnabeau MM** see **Bonnabeau RC**
**Bonnabeau RC:** Edward Jenner and the advent of vaccination. **Minn Med** 1983 May;66(5):331–3
**Bonnabeau RC:** Hippocratic medicine. **Minn Med** 1984 Jul;67(7):389–91
**Bonnabeau RC:** Samuel Thomson and Thomsonian medicine. The near-destruction of American medicine. **Minn Med** 1984 May;67(5):285–7
**Bonnabeau RC:** The development of inhalation anesthesia. **Minn Med** 1984 Sep;67(9):507–8
**Bonnabeau RC:** The Royal College of Physicians and the apothecaries in the 17th century. A dispute for all seasons. **Minn Med** 1983 Sep;66(9):565–7
**Bonnabeau RC:** The school at Alexandria and the vascular system. The circulation near miss. **Minn Med** 1983 Feb;66(2):100–1
**Bonnabeau RC, Bonnabeau MM:** William Harvey revisited 1578–1978. **Minn Med** 1981 Jan;64(1):28–33
**Bonnaud L:** Pierre ophtalmiques en Haut-Limousin. **Bull Soc Archeol Hist Limousin** 1978;105:164–70
**Bonneau E, Moreau R, Vaillant JM:** Notions de craniométrie anthropologique. **Actual Odontostomatol (Paris)** 1983 Jun;142:319–40
**Bonnefoy JP** see **Petitjean F**
**Bonnemain H:** François Magendie et ses perspectives pharmacologiques. **Hist Sci Med** 1983;17(4):333–43
**Bonnemain H:** La Faculté de Pharmacie de Paris depuis cent ans Avenue de de l'Observatoire. **Rev Hist Pharm (Paris)** 1982 Mar;29(252):39–48
**Bonnemain H:** La Société d'Histoire de la Pharmacie; sa création – son développement – ses activités. In: Vorträge des Internationalen Pharmaziehistorischen Kongresses Innsbruck 1977. Stuttgart, Wissenschaftliche Verlagsgesellschaft, 1979. p. 81–90.
**Bonnemain H:** Un recueil de recettes 'éprouvées'. **Rev Hist Pharm (Paris)** 1982;29(252):160–4
**Bonnemain H:** Une famille médico-pharmaceutique: les Augiéras-Bernou. **Rev Hist Pharm (Paris)** 1981;28(248):14–20
**Bonnemain H** see **Boussel P**
**Bonner JT** see **Darwin CR**
**Bonnet JC** see **Forster R**
**Bonneval G:** Prévention réele de l'amblyopie strabique. Historique et perspectives. **Bull Soc Ophtalmol Fr** 1982 Mar;82(3):345–8
**Bonnevie O** see **Ostensen H**
**Bonnevie P:** Dermatologi og dermatologer – før og nu. **Dan Medicinhist Arbog** 1982;:137–52
**Bonnevie P:** Dermatology in Denmark. **Int J Dermatol** 1983

Apr;22(3):193–200

**Bonnin P, Lavat P:** A propos d'un cas d'épithéliopathie en plaques de Gass en 1860. **Bull Soc Ophtalmol Fr** 1983 Jan;83(1):49–52

**Bonnot I:** Du clystère au quinquina. Pour une étude des comptes d'apothicaires aux XVIIe et XVIIIe siècles. **Bull Liaison Assoc Amis Mus Pharm Montp** 1983;:(8):61–75

**Bono JJ, Schmitt CB:** An unknown letter of Jacques Daléchamps to Jean Fernel: local autonomy versus centralized government. **Bull Hist Med** 1979 Spring;53(1):100–27

**Bonora F:** Compiti e ruoli attuali della storia della medicina. **Med Secoli** 1982;19(3):249–63

**Bonsdorff B von:** Smittämnenas historia; en översikt. **Nord Medicinhist Arsbok** 1983;:89–101

**Bonsett CA:** Dr. G. W. H. Kemper and his work in indexing the Transactions of the Indiana State Medical Society. **J Indiana State Med Assoc** 1980 Sept;73(9):561

**Bonsett CA:** G. W. H. Kemper, M.D. (1839–1927), Indiana medical historian. **J Indiana State Med Assoc** 1980 Jul;73(7):424

**Bonsett CA:** Mary Frame Thomas, M.D. (1816–1888). **J Indiana State Med Assoc** 1980;73:270

**Bonsett CA:** Medical museum notes. **J Indiana State Med Assoc** 1981 Dec;74(12):770

**Bonsett CA:** Medical museum notes: Indianapolis City Hospital. **J Indiana State Med Assoc** 1983 Oct;76(10):657

**Bonsett CA:** Medical museum notes: The Indiana Medical History Society. **J Indiana State Med Assoc** 1982 Dec;75(12):839

**Bonsett CA:** Medical museum notes: Thomas B. Harvey. **J Indiana State Med Assoc** 1983 Jun;76(6):371

**Bonsett CA:** Museum notes [John Shaw Billings' birthplace] **J Indiana State Med Assoc** 1981;74:348

**Bonsett CA:** Mystery photo: why was it shown to med students? **J Indiana State Med Assoc** 1980 Mar;73(3):123

**Bonsett CA:** Physician ads of yesteryear lacked scruples. **J Indiana State Med Assoc** 1983 Apr;76(4):229, 246

**Bonsett CA:** The world's first gall bladder surgeon was a Hoosier. **J Indiana State Med Assoc** 1980 Apr;73(4):201

**Bonsiepen W** see **Hasler L, ed**

**Bonte FJ:** The notorius decontamination caper. **Semin Nucl Med** 1979 Jul;9(3):218–9

**Bonuzzi L:** Alberto Brighenti nella storia della fisiologia. **Acta Med Hist Patav** 1981/82;28:21–8

**Bonuzzi L:** Per l'iconologia della melancolia. **Acta Med Hist Patav** 1980–81;27:55–80

**Bonuzzi L** see **Premuda L**

**Böök JA** see **Modrzewska K**

**Bool PH:** 75 Jaar Centraal Diergeneeskundig Instituut. **Tijdschr Diergeneeskd** 1980 Aug 1;105(15):583–6

**Boon LJ:** 'Utrechtenaren': de sodomieprocessen in Utrecht, 1730–1732. **Spiegel Hist** 1982;17(11):553–8

**Boone JO** see **Collins WE**

**Boone MS:** A socio-medical study of infant mortality among disadvantaged Blacks. **Hum Organ** 1982;41(3):227–36

**Boor M:** Effects of United States presidential elections on suicide and other causes of death. **Am Sociol Rev** 1981;46(5):616–8

**Boorman WH:** Local history and the pharmacist. **Pharm Hist (London)** 1968 Mar;1(2):3–6

**Booth CC:** Clinical science in the age of reason. **Perspect Biol Med** 1981 Autumn;25(1):93–114

**Booth CC:** Medical communication: the old and new. The development of medical journals in Britain. **Br Med J [Clin Res]** 1982 Jul 10;285(6335):105–8

**Booth CC:** Robert Willan and his kinsmen. **Med Hist** 1981 Apr;25(2):181–96

**Booth D** see **Higgs R**

**Booyens J** see **Gathiram P**

**Boozer JS:** Children of Hippocrates: doctors in Nazi Germany. **Ann Am Acad Polit Soc Sci** 1980;450:83–97

**Boray JC:** Obituary: Georg Lämmler. **Int J Parasitol** 1981 Oct;11(5):335–40

**Borch-Johnsen K:** Byliv og lungecancer. En kvantitativ og kvalitativ vurdering af den urbane faktor. **Ugeskr Laeger** 1982 Jun 7;144(23):1713–8

**Border JR** see **Allgöwer M**

**Bordes F:** Le livre des remèdes de Labadie. Contribution à l'histoire de la médecine populaire landaise au XVIIIe siècle. **Bull Soc Borda** 1982;107(387):399–412

**Bordley JE:** History of research training. **Arch Otolaryngol** 1982 Oct;108(10):612–5

**Bordley JE:** The American Rhinologic Society: its foundation and its future responsibilities. **Laryngoscope** 1980 May;90(5 Pt 1):876–9

**Borek F:** Eighty years of Ehrlich's side-chain theory. **J Immunol Methods** 1980;33(4):393

**Borell M:** D'Arsonval's calorimeter: measurement of animal heat, 1877. **Med Instrum** 1982 Nov–Dec;16(6):307–8

**Borell U:** Opening speech at the 50th anniversary congress of the Scandinavian Association of Obstetricians and Gynecologists in Stockholm, January 28–29, 1983. **Acta Obstet Gynecol Scand [Suppl]** 1984;120:5–7

**Bores LD:** Historical review and clinical results of radial keratotomy. **Int Ophthalmol Clin** 1983 Fall;23(3):93–118

**Borggrefe M** see **Seipel L**

**Borgoño JM:** Control de las enfermedades transmisibles. Chile, 1952–1977. **Rev Med Chil** 1977 Oct;105(10):696–700

**Bori PC:** Materiale storico-religioso nella biblioteca di Sigmund Freud: alcuni rilievi sul catalogo. **Ann Ist Stor Italo-Ger** 1975;1:281–9

**Borich I:** O zhurnale 'Meditsinskaia sestra'. **Med Sestra** 1982 Aug;41(8):42–4

**Borie J:** Les dents de la mer: Notes sur le rôle du médecin dans l'idéologie scientifique au 19e siècle. **Stanford Fr Rev** 1978 Fall;2:159–92

**Borie J:** Mythologies de l'hérédité au XIXe siècle. Paris, Editions Galilée, 1981. 215 p.

**Bořík O, Khel R, Zdichynec B:** Několik poznámek k ušnímu onemocnění Bedřicha Smetany. **Cesk Otolaryngol** 1983 Nov;32(6):367–71

**Bořík O:** Vstřebávací schopnost anatomick ych část i ucha pro léčiva jako jev známý již v historické medicíně. **Cesk Fysiol** 1979;28(5):463–70

**Borisenko NF, Gabovich RD, Goncharuk EI, et al:** Osnovnye itogi deiatel'nosti sanitarno-gigienicheskogo fakul'teta Kievskogo meditsinskogo instituta (k 140-letiiu osnovaniia instituta i 50-letiiu osnovaniia fakul'teta. **Gig Sanit** 1982 Oct;(10):48–51

**Borisenko NF, Slepushkina II, Rakitskaia TV:** Stanovlenie i razvitie sanitarnoĭ sluzhby po gigiene deteĭ i podrostkov na Ukraine (1919–1938 gg.). **Gig Sanit** 1983 Aug;(8):38–41

**Borisenko NF, Slepushkina II, Proklina TL, et al:** Stanovlenie i razvitie sanitarnoĭ sluzhby po gigiene deteĭ i podrostkov na Ukraine (1938–1945 gg.). **Gig Sanit** 1984 Aug;(8):44–8

**Borisenkova RV, Egorov IuL, Pal'tsev IuP:** Vklad Moskovskogo instituta gigieny im. F. F. Erismana v gigienu truda (k 60-letiiu so dnia osnovaniia instituta). **Gig Tr Prof Zabol** 1981 Jul;(7):39–43

**Borisenkova RV** see **Shitskova AP**

**Borisev V, Savic K, Jovanovic D:** Spina bifida sa istorijskog aspekta. **Med Pregl** 1984;37(1–2):75–6

**Borisov EN, Stepanov AA, Voronkov OV, et al:** Organizatsiia meditsinskogo snabzheniia Krasnoĭ Armii. **Voen Med Zh** 1980 May;(5):61–4

**Borisov P:** Od ranocelnistva do zacetkov znanstvene kirurgije na Slovenskem. Ljubljana, Slovenska akademija znanosti in umetnosti, 1977. 339 p.

**Borisov P:** Slovensko-Hrvatske medicinske veze u prošlosti. **Lijec Vjesn** 1981 Oct;103(10):472–4

**Borisov PU:** Die Wiener medizinische Fakultät und die Arzte im ehemaligen Krain. **Wien Med Wochenschr** 1981;131(13–14):357–61

**Borisov VA:** Okruzhnomu voennomu gospitaliu Krasnoznamennogo Zakavkazskogo Boennogo Okruga--175 let. **Voen Med Zh** 1983 Jul;(7):74–5

**Borisova MA, Bychkovskiĭ AV:** Vklad Sergeia Petrovicha Bokina v izuchenie infektsionnykh bolezneĭ (k 150-letiiu so dnia rozhdeniia). **Vrach Delo** 1982 Sep;(9):116–9

**Borit A:** History of tumors of the pineal region. **Am J Surg Pathol** 1981 Sep;5(6):613–20

**Bork K:** Dermatologisches im Werk der Hildegard von Bingen. **Hautarzt** 1980 Jul;31(7):381–3

**Borkenhagen R, Hipskind M, Lewy R:** Reminiscences of otorhinolaryngology from Loyola University and Hines Veterans Hospital. **Proc Inst Med Chic** 1982 Apr–Jun;35(2):51–2

**Borkowski W:** Wspomnienia z 'Krankenbau' w Oświecimiu. **Przegl Lek** 1984;41(1):100–8

**Borman SA:** Origins of risk assessment. **Anal Chem** 1983 Dec;55(14):1438A–1440A

**Borms J, Hebbelinck M, Venerando A, ed:** Women and sport: an historical, biological, physiological and sportsmedical approach. Basel, Karger, 1981. 229 p. (Medicine and sport, Vol. 14)

**Born GV:** The effect of the scientific environment in Britain on refugee scientists from Germany and their effects on science in Britain. **Ber Wissenschaftsgesch** 1984;7(3):129–43

**Bornemissza G:** [Péan and his accomplishments.] (Hun). **Orv Hetil** 1980;121:2951–2

**Bornside GH:** Jaime Ferran and preventive inoculation against cholera. **Bull Hist Med** 1981 Winter;55(4):516–32

**Bornside GH:** Waldemar Haffkine's cholera vaccines and the Ferran-Haffkine priority dispute. **J Hist Med Allied Sci** 1982 Oct;37(4):399–422

**Bornstein S, Bitty L:** Essai sur folie et roman: un auteur en quête de psychiatres. **Ann Med Psychol (Paris)** 1983 Nov;141(9):957–67

**Borob'ev RI:** I. A. Kassirskiĭ i razvitie Sovetskoĭ meditsiny. **Ter Arkh** 1982;54(2):148–50

**Borodiĭ MK:** Do istoriï aptechnoï spravy na Ukraïni u druhiĭ polovyni XVIII storichchia. **Farm Zh** 1980;(2):76–9

**Borodiĭ MK:** Do istoriï aptechnoï spravy na Ukraïni v pershiĭ polovyni XVIII storichchia. **Farm Zh** 1980;(1):77–9

**Borodiĭ NK:** A.F. Maslovskiĭ--vydaiushchiĭsia Ukrainskiĭ vrach XVIII v. **Sov Zdravookhr** 1984;(5):70–2

**Borodiĭ NK:** I. A. Poletika--vydaiushchiĭsia ukrainskiĭ vrach i uchenyĭ XVIII st. **Mikrobiol Zh** 1982 May–Jun;44(3):90–4

**Borodiĭ NK:** K biografii N. M. Maksimovicha-Ambodika. **Akush Ginekol (Mosk)** 1982;(8):60–1

**Borodiĭ NK:** Karantinnaia sluzhba i protivoépidemicheskie meropriiatiia na Ukraine v XVIII veke. **Zh Mikrobiol Epidemiol Immunobiol** 1980 May;(5):117–20

**Borodiĭ NK:** Mediki na Ukraine v XVIII veke. **Sov Zdravookhr** 1980;(9):64–7

**Borodiĭ NK:** O razvitii meditsiny Ukrainy v XVIII veke. **Sov Zdravookhr** 1981;(11):53–6

**Borodin VG:** Govorit veteran Velikoĭ Otechestvennoĭ. **Voen Med Zh** 1984 May;(5):66–9

**Borodin VG:** Nekotorye voprosy organizatsii lecheniia i voenno-vrachebnoĭ ékspertizy ranenykh i bol'nykh v évakuatsionnykh gospitaliakh Urala vo vremia Velikŏ Otechestvennoi voiny.

Voen Med Zh 1983 Mar;(3):71-4
**Borodulin VI:** A. L. Miasnikov i ego rol' v formirovanii kardiologii v SSSR. **Kardiologiia** 1979;19(12):99-101
**Borodulin VI, Gogin EE, Martynov IV, et al:** Iz istorii klinicheskogo prepodavaniia (k 275-letiiu Glavnogo voennogo klinicheskogo gospitalia im. N. N. Burdenko). **Klin Med (Mosk)** 1984 Feb;62(2):141-4
**Borodulin VI:** Klinicheskaia shkola Korvizara i ee rol' v razvitii ucheniia o bolezniakh serdtsa (k 100-letiiu so dnia smerti Zhana Batista Buĭo). **Kardiologiia** 1982 Jan;22(1):113-5
**Borodulin VI:** Stanovlenie kardiologii v SSSR. **Kardiologiia** 1982 Dec;22(12):96-9
**Borodulin VI:** T. Sidengam i razvitie klinicheskoĭ meditsiny (k 300-letiiu opisaniia podagry). **Ter Arkh** 1984;56(1):135-8
**Borodulin VI, Martynov IV:** Uchenie M. V. Ianovskogo o 'perifericheskom serdtse' i razvitie predstavleniĭ o klinicheskom znachenii sosudistoi periferii. **Klin Med (Mosk)** 1982 May;60(5):9-12
**Borodulin VI:** Vydaiushchiĭsia terapevt V. F. Zelenin i ego rol' v razvitii sovetskoĭ meditsiny. **Feldsher Akush** 1982;47(3):52-4
**Borodulin VI** see **Martynov IV**
**Borodyi MK:** Arkhivni dzerela z istorii medytsyny na livoberezhnyi ukraini u XVIII st. **Ukr Istor Zh** 1981;(9):137-41
**Boron WF** see **Roos A**
**Borós S** see **Bánóczy J**
**Borowitz HO:** A medical tour through The Cleveland Museum of Art. **Cleve Clin Q** 1983 Winter;50(4):417-38
**Borsarelli F:** Storia della Associazione Italiana Donne Medico--A.I.D.M. Affiliata alla Medical Women's International Association--M.W.I.A. Torino, Edizioni Minerva Medica, 1977. 55 p.
**Borst HG, Hetzer R:** Die Rolle des Experiments in der Kardiovaskularchirurgie. **Fortschr Med** 1982 Nov 4;100(41):1889-92
**Borst HG** see **Zenker R**
**Bosch K:** Zur Vorgeschichte chemiatrischer Pharmakopöepräparate im 16./17. Jahrhundert. Braunschweig, 1980. 223 p. (Veröffentlichungen aus dem Pharmaziegeschichtlichen Seminar der Technischen Universität Braunschweig, 21).
**Boschung U:** Chirurgiemechanik im 18. Jahrhundert. **Medita** 1980;10:14
**Boschung U:** Ein Brief Albrecht Hallers über seinen Aufenthalt in Paris und Strassburg (1728). **Physis** 1977;19(1-4):185-96
**Boschung U:** Geburtshilfliche Lehrmodelle. Notizen zur Geschichte des Phantoms und der Hysteroplasmata. **Gesnerus** 1981;38:59-68
**Boschung U:** Gustav Adolf Wehrli (1888-1949), Gründer der Medizinhistorischen Sammlung der Universität Zürich. **Gesnerus** 1980;37(1/2):91-103
**Boschung U, Rüttimann B:** Herrn Professor Dr. med. H. M. Koelbing zum 60. Geburtstag. **Gesnerus** 1983;40(1-2):3-13
**Boschung U:** Iatromechanik and Chirurgie bei Lorenz Heister. **Gesnerus** 1983;40(1-2):31-41
**Boschung U:** Johannes von Muralt, 1645-1733: Arzt, Chirurg, Anatom, Naturforscher, Philosoph. Zürich, Rohr, 1983. 105 p.
**Boschung U:** Medizinische Lehrmodelle. **Medita** 1980;10(Geschichte der Medizin, 4):xv
**Boschung U:** Medizinstudium im Zeitalter der Aufklärung. **Schweiz Rundsch Med Prax** 1983 Dec 20;72(51-52):1607-15
**Bose AK:** Aphrodisiacs - a psychosocial perspective. **Indian J Hist Sci** 1981;16(1):100-3
**Bosk CL:** The doctors. **Wilson Q** 1980;4(2):75-86
**Bosman-Jelgersma HA:** De functie van de hofapotheker. **Pharm Weekbl** 1981 Nov 6;116(45):1373-9
**Bosman-Jelgersma HA:** 'Gräfinnenpulver'. In Hickel E, Schröder G, ed: Neue Beiträge zur Arzneimittelgeschichte. Festschrift für Wolfgang Schneider zum 70. Geburtstag. Stuttgart, Wissenschaftliche Verlagsgesellschaft, 1982. p. 165-71.
**Bosman-Jelgersma HA:** Vijf eeuwen delftse apothekers, een bronnenstudie over de geschiedenis van de farmacie in een hollandse stad. Amsterdam, Ronald Meesters, 1979. xx, 446 p. (Thesis, Amsterdam).
**Bosnak R** see **Wallace ER**
**Bosredon J** see **Moretti G**
**Boss J:** An early eighteenth-century criticism of clinical medicine as experimental philosophy. **Koroth** 1980 Jun;7(11-12):CCLXV-CCLXXV
**Boss J:** Helmont, Glisson, and the doctrine of the common reservoir in the seventeenth-century revolution in physiology. **Br J Hist Sci** 1983 Nov;16(54 Pt 3):261-72
**Boss J:** Richard Bright's Reports of Medical Cases (1827): a sesquicentennial note. **Bristol Med Chir J** 1978 Jan-Apr;93(345-346):5-6, 18
**Boss J:** The methodus medendi as an index of change in the philosophy of medical science in the sixteenth and seventeenth centuries. **Hist Philos Life Sci** 1979;1(1):13-42
**Boss J:** The relation of clinical to non-clinical medicine according to Thomas Sydenham (1624-1689). In E. Schultheisz, ed: History of physiology. Oxford, Elmsford, New York, Pergamon, 1981. xvi, 208 p. (Advances in Physiological Sciences. Proceedings of the 28th International Congress of Physiological Sciences, Budapest, 1980. Volume 21). p. 9-21.
**Boss JM:** 'Doctrina de circulatione sanguinis haud immutat antiquam Medendi Methodum': an unpublished manuscript (1662) by Francis Glisson (1597-1677) on the implications of Harvey's physiology. **Physis** 1978;20(1-4):309-35
**Boss M:** Entwicklung der Psychotherapie im 20. Jahrhundert. **Universitas (Stuttg)** 1981;6:
**Boss M:** Exposé sur le développement de la psychothérapie au XXe siècle. **Schweiz Arch Neurol Neurochir Psychiatr** 1981;128(2):183-96
**Bossard E** see **Nauroy J**
**Bosshardt HG:** Hans Hörmann (1924-1983). **Arch Psychol (Frankf)** 1983;135(3):163-73
**Bossy J:** Acupuncture et organisation nerveuse periphérique, segmentaire et intersegmentaire. In Mazars G, ed: Les médecines traditionnelles de l'Asie. Strasbourg, Université Louis Pasteur, 1981. p. 41-8.
**Bossy J** see **Histoire culturelle de la maladie**
**Bossy J** see **Huard P**
**Boström H:** Internmedicinen - en produkt av vårt eget århundrade. **Lakartidningen** 1983 Nov 16;80(46):4405-7
**Boswell J:** Christianity, social tolerance, and homosexuality: gay people in Western Europe from the beginning of the Christian era to the fourteenth century. Chicago and London, University of Chicago Press, 1980. xviii, 424 p.
**Boswell JE:** Expositio and oblatio: the abandonment of children and the ancient and medieval family. **Am Hist Rev** 1984;89(1):10-33
**Böszörményi E:** Hódmezövásárhelyi öngyilkosságok. **Tort Stat Tanulm** 1977;3:237-304
**Botella Llusiá J:** La ginecología de Cataluña vista por un madrileño. In Congrés International d'Història de la Medicina Catalana, 2nd, Barcelona, 1975. Llibre d'Actes. Barcelona, Socitra, 1977. p. 163-84.
**Botevgard District Hospital:** 90 years (1892-1982). Botevgard, [s.n.], 1982. 25 p.
**Botey i Puig A:** L'obra del Dr. Ricard Botey i Ducoing. In Congrés Internacional d'Historie de la Medicina Catalana, 1st, Barcelona-Montpellier, 1970. Barcelona, Editorial Scientia, 1971. v 4, p. 20-6.
**Botha JL** see **Torrington M**
**Bott B** see **Baur O**
**Botterell EH:** Kenneth George McKenzie, M.D., F.R.C.S., 1923-1963. **Surg Neurol** 1982 Feb;17(2):81-9
**Böttiger LE:** På spaning i 'På spaning': om homosexualiteten i Prousts verk. **Sydsven Medicinhist Sallsk Arsskr** 1984;21:99-108
**Bottius R** see **Avellano E**
**Bouček K:** Problematika zdraví v pracích českých utopistu. **Cas Lek Cesk** 1983 Oct 7;122(40):1217-20
**Bouchard CB:** Consanguinity and noble marriages in the tenth and eleventh centuries. **Speculum** 1981 Apr;56(2):268-87
**Bouchard G:** Démographie et société rurale au Saguenay, 1851-1935. **Rech Sociogr** 1978;19(1):7-31
**Bouchard G, Brard P:** Le programme de reconstitution automatique des familles saguenayennes: données de base et resultats provisoires. **Soc Hist (Canada)** 1979;12(23):170-85
**Bouchard G:** Nouvelles perspectives pour les recherches génétiques. Le fichier-réseau de la population du Saguenay. **Ann Demogr Hist (Paris)** 1984;:81-8
**Bouchard JP** see **Barbeau A**
**Bouche D:** Dakar pendant la deuxième guerre mondiale: problèmes de surpeuplement. **Rev Fr Hist Outre Mer** 1978;65(3):423-48
**Boucher M:** The Cape passage: some observations on health hazards aboard Dutch East Indiamen outward-bound. **Historia (S Afr)** 1981;26(1):24-36
**Bouchet A:** Geschichte der Chirurgie vom Ende des 18. Jahrhunderts bis zur Gegenwart. In Sournia JC, Martiny M, Poulet J, ed: Illustrierte Geschichte der Medizin. Salzburg, Andreas, 1980. Vol. 7. p. 2541-607.
**Bouchet A, Masson JL:** Les localisations anatomiques de l'âme au cours des siècles. **Hist Sci Med** 1980;14(1):95-106
**Bouchet A** see **Forgue E**
**Bouchier IA:** Some experiences of ships' surgeons during the early days of the sperm whale fishery. **Br Med J [Clin Res]** 1982 Dec 18-25;285(6357):1811-3
**Bouckaert A:** Le paludisme, maladie professionnelle du soldat belge avant 1900. **Rev Belge Hist Milit** 1980;23:525-8
**Boudet F** see **Fabre M**
**Boudreau F:** The Quebec psychiatric system in transition: a case study in psychopolitics. **Can Rev Sociol Anthropol** 1980;17(2):122-37
**Boudreaux AM:** Les remèdes du vieux temps: remedies and cures of the Kaplan area in southwestern Louisiana. **South Folkl Q** 1971;35(2):121-40
**Bouffard P:** Historique du strabisme et de la vision binoculaire. Paris, Editions du C.E.R.E.S., 1983. 64 p.
**Bougard JP:** La fécondité au Borinage au XVIIe et au début du XIXe siècle. **Popul Famille** 1979;:109-46
**Bougard JP:** La formation de la classe ouvrière dans le borinage au XVIIIème et au début du XIXème siècle. La cas de Wasmes et de Warquignies. **Rev Nord** 1981;63:248:157-68
**Bouissy A:** Pirandello, 'psychologue de décadence'. **Rev Etud Ital** 1981;26(2-4):173-94
**Boulanger JB:** Dissidences, sécessions et défections dans l'histoire du mouvement psychanalytique. **Union Med Can** 1983 Aug;112(8):744-6
**Boulanger M** see **Paiement B**
**Boulle L:** La médicalisation des hôpitaux Parisiens dans la première moitié du xixème siècle. **Hist Reflect** 1982;9(1-2):33-44
**Boulle L, Grmek MD, Lupovici C, et al:** Laennec, Catalogue des manuscrits scientifiques. Paris, Masson, 1982. 316 p.
**Boulton TB:** The rise and fall of general anaesthesia in the dental chair. **SAAD Dig** 1980 Jul;4(7):156-65
**Bound JP, Harvey PW, Brookes DM, et al:** The incidence of anencephalus in the Fylde peninsula 1956-76 and changes in water hardness. **J Epidemiol Community Health** 1981 Jun;35(2):102-5
**Bouquet A:** Note sur la pharmacopée traditionnelle d'une province française. **Rev Hist Pharm (Paris)** 1981 Jun;28(249):100-2

**Bour P:** L'apport de Jacob Lévy Moréno. **Ann Med Psychol (Paris)** 1983 Dec;141(10):1079-87
**Boura AL, Green AF:** Noradrenergic neurone blocking agents. **J Auton Pharmacol** 1981 Jun;1(3):255-67
**Bourassa MG, Goulet C:** L'évolution de la recherche à l'Institut de Cardiologie de Montréal. **Union Med Can** 1979 Oct;108(10):1128-38
**Bourbeau R, Légaré J:** Evolution de la mortalité au Canada et au Québec, 1831-1931. Essai de mesure par génération. Montreal, Les Presses de l'Universite de Montreal, 1982. 140 p.
**Bourdais A** see **Buffat JJ**
**Bourgeois M:** Jules Cotard et son syndrome cent ans après. **Ann Med Psychol (Paris)** 1980 Dec;138(10);1165-80
**Bourgeois M** see **Furukawa F**
**Bourgeois P:** Laennec et son temps. **Sem Hop Paris** 1981 Dec 18-25;57(47-48):2047-56
**Bourgeois-Pichat J:** Recent demographic change in Western Europe: an assessment. **Popul Dev Rev** 1981;7(1):19-42
**Bourget P:** Histoire de la médecine depuis 1940: plus de progrès en 40 ans qu'en siècles. [Paris], Presses de la cité, 1983. 254 p.
**Bourget P, Blouin CB:** Histoire de la médecine depuis 1940. Plus de progrès en 40 ans qu'en 40 siècles. Paris, Presses de la Cité, 1983. 254 p.
**Bourgey L, Martiny M:** Hippokrates und die griechische Medizin des klassischen Zeitalters. In Sournia JC, Martiny M, Poulet J, ed: Illustrierte Geschichte der Medizin. Salzburg, Andreas, 1980. Vol. 1. p. 301-49.
**Bourgey L:** La relation du médecin au malade dans les écrits de l'Ecole de Cos. In La collection hippocratique et son rôle dans l'histoire de la médecine. Colloque de Strasbourg (23-27 octobre 1972) organisé par le Centre de Recherches sur la Grèce Antique, avec le concours des Facultés de Philosophie et des Langues Classiques. Leiden, E. J. Brill, 1975. p. 209-27.
**Bourgey L** see **Grmek MD, ed**
**Bourguignon A:** Certains problèmes épistemologiques évoqués par Claude Bernard. In Poirier J, Poirier JL, ed: Médecine et philosophie à la fin du XIXe siècle. Paris, Université de Paris XII - Val de Marne, [1980?]. p. 85-100.
**Bourguignon A:** Geschichte der Psychoanalyse. In Sournia JC, Martiny M, Poulet J, ed: Illustrierte Geschichte der Medizin. Salzburg, Andreas, 1980. Vol. 7. p. 2403-29.
**Bourguignon A** see **Manus A**
**Bouriez J:** Lens, trois savants oubliés: Auguste Behal, Amand Valeur, Raymond Delaby. [France], Société de recherches historiques de la région d'Henin-Carvin, [1981] 69 leaves.
**Bourilkova L, Israel S:** Données sur la médecine et l'hygiène dans les terres bulgares d'après la description du voyageur Ogier Ghiselin de Busbecq (1522-1592). In International Congress of the History of Medicine. 26th, Plovdiv, 1978. Actes du Congress. Sofia, 1981. Volume II. p. 62-3.
**Bourlière F:** Geschichte der Pflege und Behandlung des alten Menschen. In Sournia JC, Martiny M, Poulet J, ed: Illustrierte Geschichte der Medizin. Salzburg, Andreas, 1980. Vol. 6. p. 2075-101.
**Bournique CP:** La S.H.P. a Douai, Seclin et Lille. **Rev Hist Pharm (Paris)** 1981;28(248):5-13
**Bourquelot L:** Le congrès médical de France: défense d'und profession libérale sous la Monarchie de Juillet. **Ann Bretagne** 1979,86(3):301-12
**Bourrus R:** Le Docteur Bourrus, professeur et médecin à Mont-de-Marsan (1820-1897). **Bull Soc Borda** 1982;107(386):197-200
**Bousigue JY:** Les lésions axiales du traumatisme crânien. Evolution des idées depuis un siècle. **Neurochirurgie** 1983;29(5):365-9
**Boussel P:** Dorvault, sa vie et son oeuvre. Honfleur [France], Editions de la porte verte, 1979. 301 p.
**Boussel P:** Histoire de la médecine et de la chirurgie de la grande peste à nos jours. Paris, Editions de la Porte Verte, 1979. 283 p.
**Boussel P, Bonnemain H, Bove FJ:** Histoire de la pharmacie et de l'Industrie pharmaceutique. Paris, Editions de la Porte Verte, 1982. 287 p.
**Boussel P, Bonnemain H, Bové FJ:** History of pharmacy and pharmaceutical industry. Paris, Lausanne, Asklepios, 1983. 285 p.
**Boute P:** De ontwikkeling van de tandheelkunde aan de VUB - van 1950-'68 in het kader van de unitaire ULB - van 1969-heden: als zelfstandige universiteit. **Rev Belge Med Dent** 1981;36(3):120-3
**Bouvenot G, Delboy C:** Geschichte der grossen physiologischen Konzepte. In Sournia JC, Martiny M, Poulet J, ed: Illustrierte Geschichte der Medizin. Salzburg, Andreas, 1980. Vol. 8. p. 2881-909.
**Bouvrain Y:** La thérapeutique cardiologique au XIXe siècle. **Ann Cardiol Angeiol (Paris)** 1983 Mar-Apr;32(2):79-82
**Bouwsma WJ:** John Calvin's anxiety. **Proc Am Philos Soc** 1984 Sep;128(3):252-6
**Bouza Brey F:** Las enfermedades infantiles de Rosalia de Castro y los ritos de medicina magica en Galicia. **Cuad Estud Gallegos** 1967;22(67):183-97
**Bove FJ** see **Boussel P**
**Bovee EC:** Theodore Louis Jahn. 1905-1979. In memoriam. **J Protozool** 1979 Nov;26(4):527-9
**Bovy A** see **Moermans JP**
**Bowditch HP:** The life and writings of Henry Pickering Bowditch. 2 vols. New York, Arno Press, 1980. Various paginations.
**Bowen P:** The early days of postgraduate medical television in London. **J Audiov Media Med** 1980 Oct;3(4):134-5
**Bowen TE:** William Crawford Gorgas, physician to the world. **Milit Med** 1983 Dec;148(12):917-20
**Bower B:** St. Elizabeths Museum. **Psychiatr News** 1982 Mar 19;17(6):6-7
**Bower EM, ed:** The handicapped in literature. A psychosocial perspective. Denver, Love, 1980. xi, 407 p.
**Bowers DF:** Return of the worm. **Ohio Dent J** 1984 Sep;58(9):9-10
**Bowers DF:** W. D. Miller: a second pilgrimage to his home. **Ohio Dent J** 1982 Mar;56(3):15-23
**Bowers F** see **James W**
**Bowers JZ:** A note on the history of medical education in the United States. **Dan Med Bull** 1980 May;27(Suppl 1):4-5
**Bowers JZ:** Alpha Omega Alpha program of audiovisual memoirs of leaders in American medicine. **Bull Hist Med** 1973 Jul-Aug;47(4):409-16
**Bowers JZ, Purcell EF, ed:** Aspects of the history of medicine in Latin America. [Report of a conference held 10-13 October 1971 in Antigua, Guatemala.] New York, Josiah Macy, Jr. Foundation, 1979. viii, 196 p. Contributions by F. Guerra, F. Cabieses, C. Tejada, E. C. Long, J. M. Gomez, L. C. Santos Filho, D. B. Cooper, A. Seriano Lleras, G. V. Palau, C. R. Boxer, R. Archila.
**Bowers JZ, Carrubba RW:** Exotic antidotes in seventeenth century Asia: two assays from the Amoenitatum Exoticarum of Engelbert Kaempfer. **Clio Med** 1980 May;14(2):129-40
**Bowers JZ:** Shields Warren's exemplary sanitary survey. **Am J Forensic Med Pathol** 1980 Dec;1(4):365-6
**Bowers JZ:** The adoption of German medicine in Japan: the decision and the beginning. **Bull Hist Med** 1979 Spring;53(1):57-80
**Bowers JZ, King EE:** The conquest of yellow fever: the Rockefeller Foundation. **J Med Soc NJ** 1981 Jul;78(7):539-41
**Bowers JZ:** The odyssey of smallpox vaccination. **Bull Hist Med** 1981 Spring;55(1):17-33
**Bowers JZ:** Truants from medicine. **Perspect Biol Med** 1979 Autumn;23(1):83-91
**Bowers JZ:** When the twain met. The rise of western medicine in Japan. Baltimore, London, The Johns Hopkins Univ. Press, 1980. xi, 173 p. (Henry E. Sigerist Supplements to the Bulletin of the History of Medicine, n.s., no. 5).
**Bowers JZ:** Yale and the Atomic Bomb Casualty Commission. **Yale J Biol Med** 1983 Jan-Feb;56(1):39-45
**Bowers JZ** see **George Rosen: In Memoriam**
**Bowers RA:** Frederick B. Kilmer: a notable New Jersey pharmacist. **J Med Soc NJ** 1984 Sep;81(9):765-8
**Bowie DC:** Captive surgeon in Hong Kong: the story of the British Military Hospital, Hong Kong 1942-1945. **J Hong Kong Branch R Asiat Soc** 1975;15:150-290
**Bowler PJ:** Biology and social thought. **Can Rev Am Stud** 1980;11(1):87-94
**Bowler PJ:** E. W. MacBride's Lamarckian eugenics and its implications for the social construction of scientific knowledge. **Ann Sci** 1984 May;41(3):245-60
**Bowler S:** Nursing Mirror midwifery forum. 3. Survival test for babies. **Nurs Mirror** 1983 Mar 16;156(11):viii
**Bowles G:** National Health Dental Services 1948-1955. **Soc Soc Hist Med Bull (Lond)** 1981 Dec;29:1-6
**Bowman AO** see **Lester JP**
**Bowman FP** see **Stambolian G**
**Bowman IA:** Anatomical illustrations with superimposed flaps. **Bookman** 1981 Jul-Aug;9(6):3-7
**Bowman IA:** Books by physician travelers. **Bookman** 1984 May-Jun;11(3):3-9
**Bowman IA:** Herbal medicines and the midwife. **Bookman** 1982 Jul-Aug;9(6):3-9
**Bowman IA:** History of medical instrumentation. **Bookman** 1982 Dec;9(10):3-8
**Bowman IA:** 'My life'; an important Ellis manuscript. **Bookman** 1981 Apr;8(4):3-7
**Bowman IA:** Ottoman and European diet in the fifteenth century **Bookman** 1981 Mar;8(3):3-9
**Bowman IA:** Prostitution and the medical profession in the nineteenth century. **Bookman** 1982 Jan;9(1):3-9
**Bowman IA:** The image of the nurse on international postage stamps, 1920-1970. In Jones AH, ed: Images of healers. Albany, State University of New York, Press, 1983. p. 91-100.
**Bowman IA:** Thomas Cogan on studying. **Bookman** 1980 Feb;7(2):5-10
**Bowman IA:** Was it yellow fever? **Bookman** 1981 Feb;8(2):3-4
**Bowman WC:** Drugs ancient and modern. **Scott Med J** 1979 Apr;24(2):131-40
**Bowman IA, ed:** Child health on postage stamps. **Bookman** 1982 Feb;9(2):3-7
**Bowman IA, ed:** John Sealy Hospital Training School for Nurses. **Bookman** 1982 Oct;9(8):3-11
**Bowman IA, ed:** The care of the insane in Texas. **Bookman** 1984 Mar-Apr;11(2):3-9
**Bowman IA, ed:** UTMB: eighty years ago. **Bookman** 1983 May-Jun;10(3):3-10
**Bown TM** see **Fleagle JG**
**Box JF:** R. A. Fisher: the life of a scientist. New York, Wiley, 1978. xii, 512 p.
**Boxer CR** see **Bowers JZ**
**Boyd DP:** A half century of publishing. **Chest** 1984 Nov;86(5):654-5
**Boyd DP:** Doctor Lahey and his clinic. **Postgrad Med** 1984 Feb 15;75(3):14-6, 18
**Boyd DR:** The conceptual development of EMS systems in the United States, Part I. **Emerg Med Serv** 1982 Jan-Feb;11(1):19-23
**Boyd E, Scammon RE:** Origins of the study of human growth. Ed. Savara BS, Schilke JF. [Eugene], University of Oregon Health Sciences Center Foundation, 1980. 676 p.
**Boyd J:** Sir Neil Hamilton Fairley. In Dictionary of national biography, 1961-1970. Suppl. 8, 1981. p. 344-6.

**Boyd J:** Sir William Porter MacArthur. In Dictionary of national biography, 1961–1970. Suppl. 8, 1981. p. 688–9.
**Boyd M:** Coping with Samoan restistance after the 1918 influenza epidemic: Colonel Tate's problems and perplexities. **J Pac Hist** 1980;15(3):155–74
**Boyd MA** see **Teteruck WR**
**Boyd TJ:** 70 years of NHI. **Hosp Financ Manage** 1976 Oct;30(10):20–2, 24, 26 passim
**Boyer LB:** Die Psychoanalyse in der Ethnologie. Ein Literaturbericht. **Psyche (Stuttg)** 1980 Aug;34(8):694–715
**Boyer M:** Hier et aujourd'hui: l'école d'infirmières de La Source. **Krankenpflege Soins Infirm** 1984 May;77(5):38–43
**Boyer S:** This is the final issue of The Johns Hopkins Medical Journal [editorial]. **Johns Hopkins Med J** 1982 Dec;151(6):263–82
**Boyett GW:** Aging in seventeenth-century New England. **N Engl Hist Geneal Regist** 1980 Jul;134:181–93
**Boylan M:** Mechanism and teleology in Aristotle's biology. **Apeiron** 1981, reçu 1982;15(2):96–102
**Boylan M:** The digestive and 'circulatory' systems in Aristotle's biology. **J Hist Biol** 1982 Spring;15(1):89–118
**Boylan M:** The Galenic and Hippocratic challenges to Aristotle's conception theory. **J Hist Biol** 1984 Spring;17(1):83–112
**Boyland E:** The history and future of chemical carcinogenesis. **Br Med Bull** 1980 Jan;36(1):5–10
**Boyle JD:** Morton I. Grossman, M.D., Ph.D.: an oral history. **Gastroenterology** 1982 Jul;83(1 Pt 2):285–324
**Boziian KA:** Razvitie zdravookhraneniia v Nagorno-Karabakhskoĭ Avtonomnoĭ oblasti. **Sov Zdravookhr** 1983;7:69–71
**Božovic B:** Osvrt na nedostatke u dosadašnjem radu našeg vojnog saniteta. **Lijec Vjesn** 1979 Nov;101(11):690–3
**Brace CL, Nagai M:** Japanese tooth size: past and present. **Am J Phys Anthropol** 1982 Dec;59(4):399–411
**Brace CL:** The roots of the race concept in American physical anthropology. In F. Spencer, ed: A history of American physical anthropology, 1930–1980. New York, Academic Press, 1982. p. 11–29.
**Bracegirdle B:** Displaying the history of medicine: the Wellcome Museum in the Science Museum. **J Audiov Media Med** 1982 Oct;5(4):124–9
**Bracegirdle B:** The Wellcome Museum of the History of Medicine. **J Audiov Media Med** 1980 Apr;3(2):59–63
**Braceland FJ:** Psychiatry, medicine's erring sibling, returns: a history and a prophecy. **Trans Stud Coll Physicians Phila** 1981 Sep;5(3 no 3):181–94
**Brach CC** see **Orofino G**
**Bracher MD, Santow G:** Breast-feeding in Central Java. **Popul Stud** 1982 Nov;36(3):413–29
**Brachet J:** Esquisse d'une histoire de la biochimie de la biologie cellulaire et de la biologie moléculaire en Belgique. In Florilège des Sciences en Belgique - II. Bruxelles, Académie Royale de Belgique, 1980. p. 289–314.
**Brachet J:** Marcel Florkin. **Bull Cl Sci Acad R Belg** 1980;5(66):188–94
**Brachet J:** Un demi siècle de recherches en embryologie et en cytologie. **Comp Biochem Physiol** 1980;67B:367–72
**Brachman PS:** Inhalation anthrax. **Ann NY Acad Sci** 1980;353:83–93
**Bradburne P, Williams PO:** The Wellcome Trust story. **Grants Mag** 1978 Sep;1(3):196–205
**Brade AE:** The Danish folk medicine. A research project. In International Congress of the History of Medicine, 27th, Barcelona, 1980. Actas. Barcelona, Académia de Ciències Médiques de Catalunya i Balears, 1981. p. 458–61.
**Bradford DE:** Viral haemorrhagic fevers. **J R Army Med Corps** 1983 Jun;129(2):120–1
**Brading DA, Wu C:** Population growth and crisis: León, 1720–1860. **J Lat Am Stud** 1973;5(1):1–36
**Bradley BE:** The historic use of diazepam in dentistry. **Anesth Prog** 1981 Mar–Apr;28(2):38–40
**Bradley DJ** see **Sabben-Clare EE**
**Bradley JP:** Shaping administrative policy with the aid of congressional oversight: the Senate Finance Committee and Medicare. **West Polit Q** 1980;33(4):492–501
**Bradley L:** Review essay: The population history of England 1541–1871: a reconstruction. **Local Popul Stud (Matlock)** 1981;27:53–64
**Bradley LE** see **Frayer DW**
**Bradley WE** see **Ek A**
**Brady AP:** Medical achievements this century--high technology or community health approach. **Ir J Med Sci** 1983 Nov;152(11):413–9
**Brady ER:** The thread of a concept. **Marine Corps Gaz** 1971;55(5):35–42
**Brady GM:** Lou Gehrig: the iron man. **Manuscripts** 1980;32(2):84–9
**Braekman WL:** Recepten en pokkentraktaat uit een Middelnederlands handschrift. **Volkskunde** 1977;78:177–98
**Braff SM:** Contact lens horizons. **Am J Optom Physiol Opt** 1983 Oct;60(10):851–8
**Bragg DG** see **El-Najjar MY**
**Bragg TA:** The McLean Hospital archives. **Mass Nurse** 1984 Sep;54(8):3
**Bragin AI, Ivanov NM:** Evakuatsiia ranenykh i grazhdanskogo naseleniia iz Leningrada v tyl strany v period blokady (1941–1943 gg.). **Zdravookhr Ross Fed** 1980;(5):9–11
**Bragin AM:** I. M. Sechenov i otechestvennaia meditsina (k 150-letiiu so dnia rozhdeniia. **Klin Med (Mosk)** 1980 Jun;58(6):113–7
**Brahma B, Singh M:** The man behind the name: Ernest William Hey Groves 1872–1944. **NATNEWS** 1982 Jun;19(6):26
**Brahma B, Singh M:** The man behind the name: Eugene Louis Doyen 1859–1916. **NATNEWS** 1981 Dec;18(12):14
**Brahma B, Singh M:** What lies behind a name? (Sir Thomas Spencer Wells 1818–1897). **NATNEWS** 1981 Jul;18(7):15
**Brahmaji Rao U:** Avicenna's contribution to the understanding of anatomy and pathology of heart. **Bull Indian Inst Hist Med (Hyderabad)** 1981;1-4:91–4
**Brain JB, Brain P:** Nostalgia and alligator bite--morbidity and mortality among Indian migrants to Natal, 1884–1911. **S Afr Med J** 1984 Jan 21;65(3):98–102
**Brain JB, Brain P:** The health of indentured Indian migrants to Natal, 1860–1911. **S Afr Med J** 1982 Nov 6;62(20):739–42
**Brain P:** In defence of ancient bloodletting. **S Afr Med J** 1979 Jul 28;56(4):149–54
**Brain P** see **Brain JB**
**Brainard MD, Plyer CO:** Historical perspectives in family practice. **J Fla Med Assoc** 1980 Sep;67(9):812–6
**Brainin E, Kaminer IJ:** Psychoanalyse und Nationalsozialismus. **Psyche (Stuttg)** 1982 Nov;36(11):989–1012
**Braithwaite PA, Shugg D:** Rembrandt's Bathsheba: the dark shadow of the left breast. **Ann R Coll Surg Engl** 1983 Sep;65(5):337–8
**Brajkovich HL:** Dr. Snellen's 20/20: the development and use of the eye chart. **J Sch Health** 1980 Oct;50(8):472–4
**Brambe R:** Rigas pilsetas iedzìvotàju skaita dinamika no 1787. lidz 1860. gadam. **Latv PSR Zinat Akad Vestis** 1972;8:55–66
**Bramberga VM:** Stanovlenie, sovremennoe sostoianie i perspektivy razvitiia onkologii v Latviiskoĭ SSR. **Vopr Onkol** 1982;28(10):8–13
**Branca P, ed:** The medicine show. Patients, physicians and the perplexities of the health revolution in modern society. New York, Science History Publications, 1977. viii, 280 p. (Mostly articles reprinted from Journal of Social History, vol. 10, Summer 1977).
**Brand JL:** Evolutionary years of American neurology, 1865–1875. In: Congrès international d'histoire de la médecine, XXVe, Québec, 1976. Actes. Québec, 1977. p. 507–21.
**Brand JL** see **Numbers RL, ed**
**Brand JW** see **Rudney JD**
**Brand U:** Aerztliche Ethik im 19. Jahrhundert. Der Wandel ethischer Inhalte im medizinischen Schrifttum. Ein Beitrag zum Verständnis der Arzt-Patient-Beziehung. Freiburg, Schulz, 1977. 224 p. (Freiburger Forschungen zur Medizingeschichte, Neue Folge, 5).
**Brandchaft B** see **Goldberg A, ed**
**Brandenburg D:** Das Portrait des Ibn Sînâ (Avicenna). **Med Welt** 1983 Jun 10;34(23):682–4
**Brandenburg D:** Medizin und Magie. Heilkunde und Geheimlehre des islamischen Zeitalters. Berlin, Hessling, 1975. 159 p. (Medizingeschichtliche Miniaturen, Band 1).
**Brandenburg D:** Medizinisches bei Herodot. Eine literaturhistorische Studie zur antiken Heilkunde. Berlin, Hessling, 1976. 176 p. (Medizingeschichtliche Miniaturen, Band 2).
**Brandenburg D:** Theriak. Ein Beitrag zur Arzneimittellehre des europäischen und orientalischen Mittelalters. **Med Welt** 1982 Aug 20;33(33):1137–40
**Brander GC:** The pharmaceutical industry and the veterinary profession: 100 years of symbiosis. **Vet Rec** 1982 Sep 18;111(12):255–8
**Brandl E, Spitzy KH:** Chemotherapie in Osterreich. Geschichte und Ausblick. **Wien Med Wochenschr** 1983;133 Suppl 1:3–10
**Brandon E** see **Hand WD, ed**
**Brändström A, Broström G, Persson LA:** The impact of feeding patterns on infant mortality in a nineteenth century Swedish parish. **J Trop Pediatr** 1984 Jun;30(3):154–9
**Brändstrom, Anders** see **Imhof AE**
**Brandt AM:** Herbert Spencer Gasser. In Dictionary of American biography, 1961–1965. Suppl. 7, 1981. p. 279–81.
**Brandt AM:** James Angus Doull. In Dictionary of American biography, 1961–1965. Suppl. 7, 1981. p. 194–5.
**Brandt AM:** Polio, politics, publicity, and duplicity: ethical aspects in the development of the Salk vaccine. **Conn Med** 1979 Sep;43(9):581–7, 589–90
**Brandt AM:** Virginia Kneeland Frantz. In: Notable American women. The modern period. Cambridge, Mass., Belknap-Harvard Univ. Press, 1980. 4:247–8.
**Brandt EN:** Medical education: the past 80 years. **Tex Med** 1980 May;76(5):4–5
**Brandt L, Pokar H, Schütte H:** 100 Jahre Intubationsnarkose. William Macewen, ein Pionier der endotrachealen Intubation. **Anaesthesist** 1983 May;32(5):200–4
**Brandt L** see **Ljunggren B**
**Brandt P:** The Howard Bishop Lewis papers. **Surv Sources Newsl** 1976 Dec;4:5–7
**Brann NL:** Melancholy and the divine frenzies in the French Pléiade: their conflicting roles in the art of 'beaux exercices spirituels.' **J Mediev Renaiss Stud** 1979;9:81–100
**Brann NL:** Was Paracelsus a disciple of Trithemius? **Sixteenth Century J** 1979;10(1):71–82
**Brannan J** see **Notle A**
**Brannan JH:** A history of health education at the Ohio State University, 1872–1981. Ph.D. Diss., Ohio State University. Columbus, 1981. xi, 579 p.
**Brannon WL** see **Massey EW**
**Branovački D, Maric D:** Razvoj stomatološke delatnosti na teritoriji SAP Vojvodine posle II svetskog rata. **Med Pregl** 1980;33(11–12):447–8
**Brantigan CO, Grow JB:** Cricothyroidotomy revisited again. **Ear Nose Throat J** 1980 Jul;59(7):289–95
**Brantley C:** An historical perspective of the Giriama and witchcraft control. **Africa (Gt Brit)** 1979;49(2):112–33
**Brănzei P:** Secvențe din viața spitalului 'Socola' sau despre viitorul

psihiatriei. Adaptare - integrare - recuperare.
**Rev Med Chir Soc Med Nat Iasi** 1981;85(1):153–7
**Brard P** see **Bouchard G**
**Brasseaux CA:** Acadians, Creoles, and the 1787 Lafourche smallpox outbreak. **Rev Louisiane–LA Rev** 1979;8(1):55–58
**Brătescu C, Gheorghiu E:** Vizita unei misiuni austriece la carantinele româneşti în 1849. **Rev Ig [Bacteriol]** 1982 Jul–Sep;27(3):217–21
**Brătescu G:** Aerul, soarele şi apa în igiena populară. **Viata Med [Medii Sanit]** 1983 May;31(5):119–20
**Brătescu G:** Charles Davila et l'organisation sanitaire moderne de la Roumanie. **Sante Publique (Bucur)** 1982;25(1):33–43
**Bratescu G:** Des préliminaires de la création des Facultés de Médecine de Bucarest et de Jassy. **Noesis** 1981;7:63–7
**Brătescu G:** Eléments archaïques dans la médecine hippocratique. In La collection hippocratique et son rôle dans l'histoire de la médecine. Colloque de Strasbourg (23–27 octobre 1972) organisé par le Centre de Recherches sur la Grèce Antique, avec le concours des Facultés de Philosophie et des Langues Classiques. Leiden, E. J. Brill, 1975. 41–9.
**Brătescu G:** Preocupări epidemiologice ale doctorului V. Voiculescu. **Rev Ig [Bacteriol]** 1980 Jan–Mar;25(1):59–61
**Brătescu G, Gheorghiu E:** Vizita unei misiuni austriece la carantinele româneşti in 1849. **Rev Ig [Bacteriol]** 1982 Jan–Mar;27(1):53–7
**Brătescu G** see **Grmek MD, ed**
**Bratescu G** see **Habrich C**
**Bratton TL:** The identity of the plague of Justinian [part II]. **Trans Stud Coll Physicians Phila** 1981 Sep;5(3 no 3):174–80
**Bratus' VD:** Khirurgiia v Kieve (K 1500–letiiu goroda). **Klin Khir** 1982 May;(5):1–7
**Braucher CL** see **Francis WR**
**Braude RM:** Medical librarians and the White House Conference: from complacency, to concern, to commitment. **Bull Med Libr Assoc** 1981 Apr;62(2):231–5
**Bräuer G:** Die morphologischen Affinitäten des jungpleistozänen Stirnbeines aus dem Elbmündungsgebiet bei Hahnöfersand. **Z Morphol Anthropol** 1980;71(1):1–42
**Braun AD, Vereninov AA, Kaulin AB:** Afanasiĭ Semenovich Troshin (k 70–letiiu so dnia rozhdeniia). **Tsitologiia** 1983 Jun;25(6):726–32
**Braun L:** Nature et philosophie. **Medizinhist J** 1981;16(1–2):140–50
**Braun L:** Paracelse, commentateur des Aphroismes d'Hippocrate. In La collection hippocratique et son rôle dans l'histoire de la médecine. Colloque de Strasbourg (23–27 octobre 1972) organisé par le Centre de Recherches sur la Grèce Antique, avec le concours des Facultés de Philosophie et des Langues Classiques. Leiden, E. J. Brill, 1975. p. 335–46.
**Braun L:** Paracelse: nature et philosophie. Strasbourg, Association des Publications près les Universités de Strasbourg, 1981. 176 p.
**Braun L:** Paracelsus und die Philosophiegeschichte. Eine systematische Betrachtung. Wien, 1965. 26 p. (Salzburger Beiträge zur Paracelsusforschung, 5).
**Braun L:** Vom Wesen des Grundes bei Paracelsus. **Salzburger Beitr Paracelsusforsch** 1984;23:27–35
**Braun L** see **Domandl S, ed**
**Braun L** see **Paracelsus in der Tradition**
**Braun M:** Classics in Oncology. Idipathic multiple pigmented sarcoma of the skin by Kaposi. **CA** 1982 Nov–Dec;32(6):340–7
**Braun RN:** Allgemeinmedizin zwischen gestern und morgen. **Fortschr Med** 1983 Mar 10;101(9):343–4
**Braun–Falco O:** 50 Jahre Dermatologie im Städtischen Krankenhaus Thalkirchnerstrasse - Rückblick und Ausblick. **Hautarzt** 1980 Jan;31(1):37–41
**Braun L, et al:** Paracelse. Paris, Albin Michel, 1980. 280 p. (Cahiers de l'Hermétisme).
**Braunfels–Esche S** see **Baur O**
**Braunstein AY:** The main stages of enzymatic transfer of amino groups studies. **Istor Biol Issled** 1983;9:16–50
**Braunwald E:** Thirty–five years of progress in cardiovascular research. **Circulation** 1984 Nov;70(5 Pt 2):III8–25
**Bräutigam W:** Die Erkrankung Goyas von 1792. **Nervenarzt** 1980 Apr;51(4):233–8
**Bräutigam W:** Rückblick auf das Jahr 1942. Betrachtungen eines psychoanalytischen Ausbildungskandidaten des Berliner Instituts der Kriegsjahre. **Psyche (Stuttg)** 1984 Oct;38(10):905–14
**Bräutigam W** see **Fischle–Carl H, ed**
**Braverman IM:** 'Cutaneous manifestations of internal malignant tumors' by Becker, Kahn and Rothman, June 1942. Commentary: Migratory necrolytic erythema. **Arch Dermatol** 1982 Oct;118(10):784–98
**Bravo C:** Hospitales de La Paz, datos historicos. **Illimani** 1974;(6):47–63
**Bravo JL:** Bosquejo histórico de la cirugía de la ulcera péptica. **Rev Gastroenterol Mex** 1981 Apr–Jun;46(2):63–70
**Bravo Lozano J:** La visita del hospital real de San Lázaro de Córdoba (1599–1603). **Hispania** 1979;39(143):639–70
**Bravo Peña F:** Nociones de historia de la enfermeria. 7a. ed: México, Porrúa, 1980. 191 p.
**Brayshay M, Pointon VF:** Local politics and public health in mid–nineteenth–century Plymouth. **Med Hist** 1983 Apr;27(2):162–78
**Brazier MA:** A history of neurophysiology in the 17th and 18th centuries: from concept to experiment. New York, Raven Press, 1984. xiii, 230 p.
**Brazier MA:** Challenges from the philosophers to the neuroscientists. In Brain and mind. Ciba Foundation Symposium 69 (new series). Amsterdam, Oxford, New York, Excerpta Medica, 1979. p. 5–43.
**Brazier MA:** Pioneers in the discovery of evoked potentials. **Electroencephalogr Clin Neurophysiol** 1984 Feb;59(1):2–8
**Brazier MA:** The birth of the International Brain Research Organization: a tribute to Henri Gastaut. **Electroencephalogr Clin Neurophysiol** 1982;35:13–4
**Brazier MA:** The problem of neuromuscular action: two 17th century Dutchmen. In Rose FC, Bynum WF, ed: Historical aspects of the neurosciences. New York, Raven, 1982. p. 13–22.
**Brea Tavárez CA:** 80 años de instruccion odontologica en la Universidad Autonoma de Santo Domingo. Primera parte. **Rev Dent (St Domingo)** 1979 Jun–Dec;22(1–2):35–45
**Breakwell J:** Birmingham General Hospital and the Birmingham Music Festivals. **Practitioner** 1979 Sep;223(1335):406–10
**Breathnach CS:** Biographical sketches No. 18--Flemming. **Ir Med J** 1982 Jun;75(6):177
**Breathnach CS:** Biographical sketches No. 26--W. Hunter. **Ir Med J** 1983 Feb;76(2):59
**Breathnach CS:** Biographical sketches No. 27--Ringer. **Ir Med J** 1983 Mar;76(3):119
**Breathnach CS:** Biographical sketches no. 28 -- Graham. **Ir Med J** 1983 Apr;76(4):167
**Breathnach CS:** Biographical sketches No. 29--Papanicolaou. **Ir Med J** 1983 May;76(5):220
**Breathnach CS:** Biographical sketches no. 32--Greatrakes. **Ir Med J** 1983 Sep;76(9):402
**Breathnach CS:** Biographical sketches no. 33--Papez. **Ir Med J** 1983 Oct;76(10):441
**Breathnach CS:** Biographical sketches No. 34--Magendie. **Ir Med J** 1983 Nov;76(11):471
**Breathnach CS:** Biographical sketches no. 36 -- Sims. **Ir Med J** 1984 Jan;77(1):27
**Breathnach CS:** Golgi. **Ir Med J** 1983 Jun;76(6):298
**Breathnach CS:** John William Moore. **Ir J Med Sci** 1983 Jan;152(1):69–71
**Breccia P** see **Quinn S, ed**
**Brecher G:** A further note on red cell discoveries. William B. Castle's contribution to the discovery of hemoglobin S. **Blood Cells** 1982;8(2):471–2
**Brecher G:** A red cell discovery of the 20th century: hemoglobin S. **Blood Cells** 1981;7(3):481–3
**Brecilj B:** Medicinska doktrina u NOR u Sloveniji. **Vojnosanit Pregl** 1982 Mar–Apr;39(2):121–6
**Brede J** see **Lohmann HM, ed**
**Brede K, Irion U, Lohmann HM, et al:** Mitscherlich, Alexander, 1908–19821700 to PresentGermany **Psyche (Stuttg)** 1984 Nov;38(11):1023–52
**Bredin TF:** Henry Septimus Beddome. In Dictionary of Canadian biography, 1881–1890. 1982;11:63–4.
**Bredy E, Baugut G:** Der offene Biss - eine historische Betrachtung. **Fortschr Kieferorthop** 1982 Apr;43(2):110–26
**Breed W:** The Negro and fatalistic suicide. **Pac Sociol Rev** 1970;13(3):156–62
**Breeden JO:** Andersonville--a southern surgeon's story. **Bull Hist Med** 1973 Jul–Aug;47(4):317–43
**Breeden JO:** 'Medicine in the West'--an introduction. **J West** 1982 Jul;21(3):3–4
**Breeden JO:** 'The case of the miraculous bullet' revisited. **Milit Aff** 1981;45(1):23–6
**Breen RE, Garnjobst W:** Surgical procedures for carcinoma of the rectum. A historical review. **Dis Colon Rectum** 1983 Oct;26(10):680–5
**Breeze E** see **Holland WW**
**Bregadze IL:** Novoe v pokazaniiakh k khirurgicheskim vmeshatel'stvam pri vnutrennikh zabolevaniiakh (k 40–letiiu so dnia smerti M. P. Konchalovskogo). **Klin Med (Mosk)** 1981;59(10):78–9
**Bregante–Marsili D** see **Marsili A**
**Brégeat P:** Antoine Portal, fondateur de l'Académie de médecine. **Bull Acad Natl Med (Paris)** 1982 Dec;166(9):1304–16
**Bréhant J:** La médecine, dans la vie et l'oeuvre de Voltaire (deuxième partie). **Bull Acad Natl Med (Paris)** 1980 Oct;164(7):675–81
**Bréhant J:** La médecine dans la vie et l'oeuvre de Voltaire (Première partie). **Bull Acad Natl Med (Paris)** 1980 Oct;164(7):659–64
**Bréhant J:** Un visage peu connu de Voltaire: le Voltaire biologiste (ses expériences de décapitation des gastéropodes). **Bull Mem Acad R Med Belg** 1981;136(12):580–8
**Bréhant J:** Voltaire et la médecine. **Sem Hop Paris** 1982 Dec 23;58(47):2792–801
**Breidenbach PS:** 'Sunsum edwuma': the limits of classification and the significance of an event. **Soc Res (NY)** 1979;46(1):63–87
**Breimer DD** see **Kotwas J**
**Breimer L, Sourander P:** The discovery of the parathyroid glands in 1880: triumph and tragedy of Ivar Sandström. **Bull Hist Med** 1981 Winter;55(4):558–63
**Breit DH, Wunder JF:** The history of radiology in South Dakota. **SD J Med** 1981 May;34(5):56–8
**Breitenbach W:** Sons of the fathers: temperance reformers and the legacy of the American Revolution. **J Early Repub** 1983;3(1):69–82
**Breitenecker MT:** [Biographical] Lexikon. In Sournia JC, Martiny M, Poulet J, ed: Illustrierte Geschichte der Medizin. Salzburg, Andreas, 1984. Vol. 9. p. 3201–503.
**Breithardt G** see **Seipel L**
**Breitwieser MR:** Cotton Mather's pharmacy. **Early Am Lit** 1981;16(1):42–9
**Bremner RH** see **Breul FR**

**Brendel W** see **Habrich C**
**Breneman JC:** Overview of food allergy: historical perspective. **Ann Allergy** 1983 Aug;51(2 Pt 2):220–1
**Brennan JF:** History and systems of psychology. Englewood Cliffs, Prentice-Hall, 1982. x, 374 p.
**Brennan JF, Zieliński K:** Science in Poland. The Nencki Institute of Experimental Biology. **Pavlov J Biol Sci** 1981 Apr–Jun;16(2):118–23
**Brent RL:** Biography of Josef Warkany. **Teratology** 1982 Apr;25(2):137–51
**Brent RL:** Comments on the history of teratology. **Teratology** 1979 Oct;20(2):199–200
**Brentini P:** Die Institutiones medicinae des Daniel Sennert (1572–1637). Zürich, Juris, 1971. 69 p. (Diss., Zürich).
**Bresgen C:** Homo omnis creatura. Arcimboldo und Paracelsus - eine Gegenüberstellung aus der Sicht des Künstlers. **Salzburger Beitr Paracelsusforsch** 1984;23:36–49
**Breslow L:** From cancer research to cancer control. **Prog Clin Biol Res** 1983;120:1–19
**Bresnihan B** see **Cassidy M**
**Brest AN, Goldberg S:** Coronary thrombosis: historic aspects. **Cardiovasc Clin** 1983;14(1):5–8
**Brestkin AP:** Iz vospominanii ob akademike L. A. Orbeli: vstrechi i besedy v sviazi s issledovaniiami po fiziologii vodolaznogo truda. **Vopr Istor Estestvozn Tekh** 1982;2:27–37
**Bretey J:** Robert Koch et son bacille. Un reportage. **Bull Acad Natl Med (Paris)** 1982 Mar;166(3):399–406
**Breton Y** see **Dupâquier J**
**Breuer R:** Berufskrankheiten von Instrumentalmusikern aus medizinhistorischer Sicht (vom 15. Jahrhundert bis 1930). Diss., Johannes Gutenberg-Universität. Mainz, 1982. 110 p.
**Breul FR, Diner SJ, ed:** Compassion and responsibility. Readings in the history of social welfare policy in the United States. Chicago, London, University of Chicago Press, 1980. 372 p. Contributions by R. E. Pumphrey, C. A. Chambers, M. W. Jernegan, E. Wisner, D. M. Schneider, E. Parkhurst, B. J. Klebaner, M. B. Treudley, N. K. Teeters, W. I. Trattner, S. W. Manning, J. H. Franklin, R. H. Bremner, A. F. Davis, G. C. White, M. H. Leff, J. L. Castrovinci, J. L. Kreader, L. Gordon, B. McArthur.
**Breustedt A:** 30 Jahre DDR--30 Jahre Mitarbeit der stomatologisch-wissenschaftlichen Gesellschaften bei der Gestaltung des sozialistischen Gesundheitswesens in der DDR. **Stomatol DDR** 1979;29(10):729–34
**Brevnov VP:** M. Ia. Mudrov v bor'be s kholernoĭ épidemieĭ v Rossii (1830–1831 gg.). **Feldsher Akush** 1981;46(11):54–6
**Brewer AF:** U.S. philately in medicine. **J Fla Med Assoc** 1979 Aug;66(8):866–70
**Brewer C, Lait J:** Can social work survive? London, Temple Smith, 1980. Historical chapters, p. 11–85.
**Brewer LA:** A historical account of the 'wet lung of trauma' and the introduction of intermittent positive-pressure oxygen therapy in World War II. **Ann Thorac Surg** 1981 Apr;31(4):386–93
**Brewer LA:** Historical notes on lung cancer before and after Graham's successful pneumonectomy in 1933. **Am J Surg** 1982 Jun;143(6):650–9
**Brewer LA:** History of surgery of the esophagus. **Am J Surg** 1980 Jun;139(6):730–43
**Brewer LA:** Open heart surgery and myocardial revascularization. Historical notes. **Am J Surg** 1981 Jun;141(6):618–31
**Brewer LA:** Sphygmology through the centuries. Historical notes. **Am J Surg** 1983 Jun;145(6):696–702
**Brewer LA:** The contributions of the Second Auxiliary Surgical Group to military surgery during World War II with special reference to thoracic surgery. **Ann Surg** 1983 Mar;197(3):318–26
**Brewer LA:** The failing myocardium. Historical notes. **Am J Surg** 1984 Jun;147(6):712–8
**Brewer LA:** The first pneumonectomy. Historical notes. **J Thorac Cardiovasc Surg** 1984 Nov;88(5 Pt 2):810–26
**Brewer NR:** Personalities in the early history of laboratory animal science and medicine. **Lab Anim Sci** 1980 Aug;30(4 pt 2):741–58
**Brewer NR, et al:** The origins of laboratory animal science and medicine: proceedings of a symposium ... American Association for Laboratory Animal Science ... 1979. **Lab Anim Sci** 1980;30:737–800
**Breyer H:** Johann Peter Frank. 'Fürst unter den Arzten Europas.' Leipzig, S. Hirzel, 1983. 184 p.
**Breyer H:** Max von Pettenkofer: Arzt im Vorfeld der Krankheit. Leipzig, Hirzel, 1980. 234 p.
**Březina Z:** Péče o děti v CSSR před dvaceti lety. **Cesk Zdrav** 1984 Feb;32(2):92–3
**Březina Z:** Sociální pediatrie v Ostravě. **Cesk Zdrav** 1982 Nov;30(11):480–3
**Brian VA:** Infant welfare in the Bible. **Nurs Times** 1980 Dec 18–25;76(51):2230–1
**Briceño-Maaz T:** Dos nombres en la dermatologia venezolana. **Rev Soc Venez Hist Med** 1972–73;20–21(34–35):87–98
**Briceño Maaz T:** Im-Hotep: dios egipcio de la medicina. **Rev Soc Venez Hist Med** 1969–71;17–19(31–33):75–82
**Briceño Maaz T:** La isla de Cos y el santuario de esculapio. **Rev Soc Venez Hist Med** 1977;25(39):9–47
**Briceño Maaz T:** Santuario de Esculapio en Epidauro. **Rev Soc Venez Hist Med** 1972–73;20–21(34–35):51–65
**Briceño-Maaz T:** Sobre Axel Munthe y su libro 'La Historia de San Michele'. **Rev Soc Venez Hist Med** 1969–71;17–19(31–33):121–30
**Briceño Romero G:** Discurso del doctor Gabriel Briceño Romero al tomar posesion de la presidencia de la Sociedad Venezolana de Historia de la Medicina. **Rev Soc Venez Hist Med** 1972–73;20–21(34–35)79–86
**Briceño Romero G** see **Sociedad Venezolana de Historia de la medicina**
**Bricker EM:** Evarts A. Graham and the American College of Surgeons. **J Thorac Cardiovasc Surg** 1984 Nov;88(5 Pt 2):834–41
**Brickman JP:** Mother love - mother death. Maternal and infant care: social class and the role of government. Ph.D. Diss., City University of New York. New York, 1978. vii, 750 leaves. (2 v.).
**Bridgforth LR:** Heroics and heretics: medical practice in antebellum Mississippi. **J Miss State Med Assoc** 1984 Jan;25(1):8–12
**Bridgforth LR:** Medical education in Mississippi. Ph.D. Diss., Memphis State University. Memphis, 1982. vii, 400 p.
**Bridgman RF:** La formation de la théorie médicale en Chine à l'occasion de la récente découverte de manuscrits à Ma Wang Dui. In Mazars G, ed: Les médecines traditionnelles de l'Asie. Strasbourg, Université Louis Pasteur, 1981. p. 5–12.
**Bridgman RF:** Les fonctions physiologiques chez l'homme dans la Chine antique. **Hist Philos Life Sci** 1981;3(1):3–17
**Bridson GD, Phillips VC, Harvey AP, ed:** Natural history manuscript resources in the British Isles. London, Mansell; New York, Bowker, 1980. xxxiv, 473 p.
**A brief history of the European meetings on electroencephalography and epileptology better known as the 'Colloques de Marseille': Electroencephalogr Clin Neurophysiol** 1982;(35):VIII–XI
**[Brief history of the Japan Society of Medical Electronics and Biological Engineering] (Jpn): Iyodenshi To Seitai Kogaku** 1982 Dec;20(7):486–98
**Brieger GH:** Early ambulation. A study in the history of surgery. **Ann Surg** 1983 Apr;197(4):443–9
**Brieger GH:** Fielding H. Garrison: the man and his book. **Trans Stud Coll Physicians Phila** 1981 Mar;3(1):1–21
**Brieger GH:** 'Fit to study medicine': notes for a history of pre-medical education in America. **Bull Hist Med** 1983;57(1):1–21
**Brieger GH:** Florence Rena Sabin. In: Notable American women. The modern period. Cambridge, Mass., Belknap-Harvard Univ. Press, 1980. 4:614–7.
**Brieger GH:** History [of human experimentation]. In Reich WT, et al, ed: Encyclopedia of bioethics, v. 2. New York, Free Press, 1978. p. 684–90.
**Brieger GH:** Medical education in the Far West. **J West** 1982 Jul;21(3):42–8
**Brieger GH:** The diseases of runners: a view from the eighteenth century--a commentary. **Pharos** 1980 Fall;43(4):29–32
**Brieger GH:** The history of health and disease for health professionals: the case study approach. With a commentary by G.B. Risse. In J. J. Bylebyl, ed: Teaching the history of medicine at a medical center. Baltimore, London, Johns Hopkins University Press, 1982. (The Henry E. Sigerist supplements to the Bulletin of the History of Medicine; new ser., no. 7). p. 13–30.
**Brieger GH:** The history of medicine and the history of science. **Isis** 1981 Dec;72(264):537–40
**Brieger GH** see **Durbin PT, ed**
**Brieger GH** see **Numbers RL, ed**
**Bright P:** Dr. Richard Bright (1789–1858). London, Bodley Head, 1983. 312 p.
**The bright side of dentistry: J Am Dent Assoc** 1984 Apr;108(4):520–1
**Brihaye J:** Celebration of the 10th anniversary of the European Association of Neurosurgical Societies. **Acta Neurochir (Wien)** 1982;60(1–2):1–6
**Brihaye J:** History of the European Association of Neurosurgical Societies. **Neurosurgery** 1984 Aug;15(2):262–4
**Brill H:** Notes on the history of social psychiatry. **Compr Psychiatry** 1980 Nov–Dec;21(6):492–9
**Brill RE:** The Sabbath-day summer: Madison, Indiana, and the 1849 cholera epidemic. **Indiana Hist Soc** 1982 Sep;8(3):3–16
**Brillante C, Laffi GC:** Profilo storico-sintetico della malattia diabetica (dal papiro di Ebers a Banting e Best. **Minerva Med** 1982 Apr 21;73(17):1087–106
**Brimley R:** Health visiting as it was. Interview by Shirley Goodwin. **Nurs Mirror** 1981 Jul 22;153(4):22–4
**Bringmann W** see **Brozek J**
**Bringmann WG, Ungerer GA:** The establishment of Wilhelm Wundt's Leipzig laboratory. **Stor Crit Psicol** 1980;1(1):11–28
**Bringmann WG, Balk MM:** Wilhelm Wundt's publication record: a re-examination. **Stor Crit Psicol** 1983;4(1):61–86
**Brink A:** Depression and loss: a theme in Robert Burton's 'Anatomy of melancholy' (1621). **Can J Psychiatry** 1979 Dec;24(8):767–72
**Brink A:** Love and conflict in Bertrand Russell's letters. **Queens Q** 1979;86(1):1–15
**Brink TL:** History and depth psychology: some reconsiderations. **Historian** 1979;41(4):738–53
**Brinkhous KM:** Judith Graham Pool. In: Notable American women. The modern period. Cambridge, Mass., Belknap-Harvard Univ. Press, 1980. 4:553–4.
**Brinkhous KM:** W. W. Duke and his bleeding time test. A commentary on platelet function. **JAMA** 1983 Sep 2;250(9):1210–14
**Brinkman AA:** Chemie in de Kunst. Amsterdam, Rodopi, 1975. 69 p.
**Brinkman AA:** De alchemist in de prentkunst. Amsterdam, Rodopi, 1982. 69 p. Reprint of several articles. (Nieuwe Nederlandse Bijdragen tot de Geschiedenis der Geneeskunde en der Natururwetenschappen, no. 5).
**Brinkmann A:** Streiftog i cellehistorie. **Tidsskr Nor Laegeforen** 1981 Jan 20;101(2):147–50
**Brinnin JM:** The sway of the grand saloon: queasy come, queasy go. **Am Heritage** 1971;22(6):16–9, 98–9
**Briot A:** Die japanische Medicine. In Sournia JC, Martiny M, Poulet J,

ed: Illustrierte Geschichte der Medizin. Salzburg, Andreas, 1980. Vol. 2. p. 655–85.

**Briscoe AM:** Diary of a mad feminist chemist. **Int J Womens Stud** 1981;4(4):420–30

**Briskman AM:** O 'khoreicheskoĭ paducheĭ' Bekhtereva i mioklonus-épilepsii. **Zh Nevropatol Psikhiatr** 1984;84(1):122–5

**Brislin J** see **Berryman JW**

**Brison M:** L'école et l'enfant à Lyon: le problème de l'alimentation dans les cantines scolaires. **Rev Hist Deuxieme Guerre Mond** 1982;32(125):37–71

**Brister L:** J. G. Zimmermanns Essay 'Von der Erfahrung in der Arzneikunst': Ein Beitrag zur rationalen Medizin. **Schweiz Med Wochenschr** 1980 Apr 19;110(16):615–9

**Britt MC** see **Weaver D**

**Britz KK** see **Stieber MT**

**Britze N:** Da en kvindelig tandlaege kun behandlede kvinder og børn. **Tandlaegebladet** 1982 Nov;86(20):714–5

**Brix J:** Laegevirke i Sønderjylland før 1864. **Dan Medicinhist Arbog** 1980;:9–10

**Brix M** see **Remisová M**

**Brncic D:** El desarrollo de la biología general en la Facultad de Medicina y su impacto en la actividad científica nacional. **Rev Med Chil** 1982 Aug;110(8):801–5

**Broad WJ:** Sir Isaac Newton: mad as a hatter. **Science** 1981 Sep 18;213(4514):1341–2, 1344

**Broadbent DE:** Sir Frederic Charles Bartlett. In Dictionary of national biography, 1961–1970. Suppl. 8, 1981. p. 77–9.

**Broadi TA** see **Glover JL**

**Broadley ME:** Patients come first: nursing at 'The London' between the two World Wars. London, London Hospital Special Trustees, 1980. 282 p.

**Broager B:** Perspectives in international neurosurgery: neurosurgery in Denmark. **Neurosurgery** 1980 Nov;7(5):529–30

**Broberg G.** Homo sapiens, Linnaeus's classification of man. In Frängsmyr T, ed: Linnaeus, the man and his work. Berkeley, University of California Press, 1983. p. 156–94.

**Broberg G** see **Frängsmyr T, ed**

**Brocas R** see **La Salpêtrière**

**Brock CH:** Dr. Thomas Bond of Philadelphia and his 'Worm'. **Trans Stud Coll Physicians Phila** 1981 Sep;5(3 no 3):209–13

**Brock CH:** Dr. William Hunter's Museum, Glasgow University. **J Soc Bibliogr Nat Hist** 1980 Apr;9(4):403–12

**Brock CH:** James Douglas (1675–1742), botanist. **J Soc Bibliogr Nat Hist** 1979 Apr;9(2):137–45

**Brock CH:** William Hunter, 1718–1783: a memoir. East Kilbride, University of Glasgow Press, 1983. xviii, 81 p.

**Brock CH** see **Cash P**

**Brock WH:** Liebigiana: old and new perspectives. **Hist Sci** 1981 Sep;19(45 pt 3):201–18

**Brocklies LW:** Medical teaching at the University of Paris, 1600–1720. **Ann Sci** 1978;35–221–51

**Brockway LH:** Science and colonial expansion. The role of the British Royal Botanic Gardens. New York, Academic Press, 1979. 215 p. (Studies in Social Discontinuity).

**Brod J:** Nephrology in the past, in the present and perspectives in the future. **Minerva Nefrol** 1983 Jan–Mar;30(1):1–6

**Brod J:** The history of medicine at Charles University. **J R Coll Physicians Lond** 1982 Jul;16(3):195–8

**Brod RL, May PA, Stewart TJ:** Recruitment and retention of federal physicians on the Navajo Reservation. **Soc Sci J** 1982;19(4):47–66

**Broda E:** Ludwig Boltzmann als evolutionistischer Philosoph. **Ber Wissenschaftsgesch** 1983;6(1–4):103–14

**Broder LIa:** K istorii primeneniia zakisi azota v Rossii. **Anesteziol Reanimatol** 1983 Mar–Apr;(2):f73

**Brodhead MJ** see **Cutright PR**

**Brodie B:** Children: a glance at the past. **MCN** 1982 Jul–Aug;7(4):219–25

**Brodie B:** One long step: Virginia nursing moves into the university setting. **Va Nurse** 1983 Winter;51(4):201–4

**Brodin MB:** William Osler and dermatology, pathology, and dermatopathology. **Am J Dermatopathol** 1981 Fall;3(3):261–4

**Brodkey C, Gaydos JC:** United States Army guidelines for troop living space: a historical review. **Milit Med** 1980 Jun;145(6):418–21

**Brodman E:** A medical dynasty in New Jersey. **J Med Soc NJ** 1984 Sep;81(9):779–84

**Brodman E:** Education and attitudes of early medical librarians to their work: a discussion based on the oral history project of the Medical Library Association. **J Libr Hist** 1980;15(2):167–82

**Brodman E:** Possible uses of MLA's oral history taped interviews. **Bull Med Libr Assoc** 1981 Jan;69(1):34–6

**Brodman E** see **Teigen PM, ed**

**Brödner E:** Zur Entwicklungsgeschichte des Bades, 2. Teil. **Antike Welt** 1978;9(1):47–57

**Brodniewicz A:** Józef Jakóbkiewicz M.D., pioneer of maritime and tropical medicine in Poland. **Bull Inst Marit Trop Med Gdynia** 1980;31(1–2):5–13

**Brody BA:** Law and morality [in bioethics]. In Reich WT, et al, ed: Encyclopedia of bioethics, v. 2. New York, Free Press, 1978. p. 817–21.

**Brody GS** see **Meals RA**

**Brody H:** Placebos and the philosophy of medicine: clinical, conceptual and ethical issues. Chicago and London, University of Chicago Press, 1980. vii, 164 p.

**Brody H:** The lie that heals: the ethics of giving placebos. **Ann Intern Med** 1982 Jul;97(1):112–8

**Brody J, Field J, ed:** A catalogue of books printed before 1641 in the Science Museum Library. [London], Science Museum, 1979. ii, 43 p. (4 p. supplement to 1981 attached)

**Brody M:** Trial of Daniel M'Naghten. Insanity defense, and its well-kept secret. **NY State J Med** 1982 Mar;82(3):381–6

**Brody SI:** Lady physicians. **RI Med J** 1980 Apr;63(4):95

**Broedner E:** Zur Entwicklungsgeschichte des Bades. **Antike Welt** 1977;8(4):45–56

**Broehl WG, McGee VE:** Content analysis in psychohistory: a study of three lieutenants in the Indian mutiny, 1857–58. **J Psychohist** 1981 Winter;8(3):281–306

**Brogan DR:** Women in medicine: Australia, New Zealand, Canada, and United States. **Women Health** 1982 Spring;7(1):5–14

**Brogården in Skaba – the cradle of Swedish veterinary medicine: Vet Hist** 1982 Summer;2(3):124–7

**Broggi M:** Progressos assolits en sanitat militar durant la guerra civil espanyola (1936–39). In International Congress of the History of Medicine, 27th, Barcelona, 1980. Actas. Barcelona, Académia de Ciències Mèdiques de Catalunya i Balears, 1981. p. 168–71.

**Bromage TG, Horne PD:** Stafne defect: a histological approach. **Paleopathol Newsl** 1981 Jan;33:7–9

**Bromberg W:** Psychiatry between the wars, 1918–1945. A recollection. Westport, London, Greenwood Press, 1982. xxxii, 184 p. (Contributions in Medical History, No. 10).

**Brome V:** Ernest Jones, Freud's alter ego. London, Caliban Books, 1982. 250 p.

**Brome V:** Havelock Ellis, philospher of sex: a biography. London, Boston, Routledge & Kegan Paul, 1979. xiv, 271 p.

**Bromley LL** see **Vecht RJ**

**Bron B:** Depression und Glaube bei Hiob. **Schweiz Arch Neurol Neurochir Psychiatr** 1983;133(1):159–74

**Bron B:** Zur Psychopathologie und Verkündigung des Propheten Ezechiel. Zum Phänomen der prophetischen Ekstase. **Schweiz Arch Neurol Neurochir Psychiatr** 1981;128(1):21–31

**Brøndegaard VJ:** Das Wurzelstechen. **Sudhoffs Arch** 1983;67(2):199–209

**Brøndegaard VJ:** Ethnomedizinische Cusucuta – Applikationen. **Ethnomedizin** 1978–79;5(1–2):47–56

**Brøndum N:** Et kirurgisk indgreb skildret i musik. **Dan Medicinhist Arbog** 1983;12:170–4

**Brøndum N:** Tandforhold i det klassiske Rom. **Dan Medicinhist Arbog** 1983;12:164–8

**Bronfenbrenner U** see **Lerner RM, ed**

**Brongersma LD** see **Karthaus PP**

**Brońka E** see **Sawicki B**

**Bronsen D** see **Spicker SF**

**Bronswijk JE van** see **Palm LC**

**Brooke JH** see **Forgan S, ed**

**Brookes B:** Housewives' depression: the debate over abortion and birth control in the 1930's. **NZ J Hist** 1981;15(2):115–34

**Brookes B** see **Lewis J**

**Brookes DM** see **Bound JP**

**Brooks CM:** An event in the history of physiology. Transfer of Aristotelian corpus of science and the Hippocratic-Galenic corpus of medicine to the Islamic world by the Nestorians. In E. Schultheisz, ed: History of physiology. Oxford, Elmsford, New York, Pergamon, 1981. xvi, 208 p. (Advances in Physiological Sciences. Proceedings of the 28th International Congress of Physiological Sciences, Budapest, 1980. Volume 21). p. ix–xvi.

**Brooks CM, Seller H:** Early and late contributions to our knowledge of the autonomic nervous system and its control made by German scientists. **J Auton Nerv Syst** 1981 Apr;3(2–4):105–19

**Brooks CM:** Origin, essence and survival of physiology: queen of sciences. **Isr J Med Sci** 1982 Jan;18(1):3–7

**Brooks CM:** Walter Joseph Meek: August 15, 1878–February 15, 1963. **Biogr Mem Natl Acad Sci** 1983;54:251–68

**Brooks GE** see **Knapp DA**

**Brooks GP, Aalto SK:** The rise and fall of moral algebra: Frances Hutcheson and the mathematization of psychology. **J Hist Behav Sci** 1981;17:343–56

**Brooks HG:** A visit to Dr. Unna's clinic in Hamburg. an excerpt: British Journal of Dermatology 1890. **Am J Dermatopathol** 1982 Jun;4(3):225–8

**Brooks JA, Kleine-Kracht AE:** Evolution of a definition of nursing. **ANS** 1983 Jul;5(4):51–85

**Brooks JJ, Enterline HT, Aponte GE:** The final diagnosis of President Cleveland's lesion. **Trans Stud Coll Physicians Phila** 1980 Mar;(2 no 1):1–25

**Brooks JR:** Carl W. Walter, MD: surgeon, inventor, and industrialist. **Am J Surg** 1984 Nov;148(5):555–8

**Brooks P:** Rachel Louise Carson. In: Notable American women. The modern period. Cambridge, Mass., Belknap-Harvard Univ. Press, 1980. 4:138–41.

**Brooks PM:** Anti-rheumatic therapy through the ages. **Australas Nurses J** 1980 Mar;9(4):19–20

**Broome JD:** L-Asparaginase: discovery and development as a tumor-inhibitory agent. **Cancer Treat Rep** 1981;65 Suppl 4:111–4

**Brophy L:** Towards a golden jubilee. The Career of 'Caritas' through a half-century. **Caritas** 1983–84;49(49):4–6

**Broquist HP, Olson RE:** Progress in nutrition research: 1942–1982. **Nutr Rev** 1982 Nov;40(11):343–8

**Broshevan VM:** Pikluvannia partiinykh, radians'kykh i viis'kovykh orhaniv

Krymu pro okhoronu zdorov'ia osobovoho skladu chervonoi armii. **Ukr Istor Zh** 1981;(12):64–8
**Brossollet J:** Quelques aspects religieux de la grande peste du XIVe siècle. **Rev Hist Philos Relig** 1984 Jan–Mar;64(1):53–66
**Broström G** see **Brändström A**
**Broszat M:** Hitler und die Genesis der 'Endlösung.' Aus Anlass der Thesen von David Irving. **Vierteljahrsh Zeitgesch** 1977;25(4):739–75
**Broszinski H:** Medizinische Handschriften in Kassel. In Balde JH, Schmiking W, ed: Festschrift zum 86. Deutschen Arztetag in Kassel. Kassel, Arztevereins, 1983. p. 5–24.
**Broszkiewicz E** see **Aleksandrowicz JW**
**Brotherston JH:** James Macalister Mackintosh. In Dictionary of national biography, 1961–1970. Suppl. 8, 1981. p. 698–9.
**Brotóns Picó J:** Un medico en el descubrimiento de America. **Rev Gen Mar** 1980 Jul;199:3–11
**Broughton JM:** Psychology and the history of the self: from substance to function. In R. W. Rieber, K. Salzinger, ed: Psychology: theoretical-historical perspectives. New York, Academic Press, 1980. p. 81–99.
**Broughton JM, Leadbeater B, Amsel E, ed:** Reflections on Piaget: proceedings of the Jean Piaget Memorial Conference. **Teach Coll Rec** 1981;83(2):151–217
**Broughton R:** A brief outline of the career and accomplishments of Henri Gastaut. **Electroencephalogr Clin Neurophysiol** 1982;35:XII–XV
**Broughton R** see **Gastaut H**
**Brown A:** COHSE: pioneers from the past. **Nurs Mirror** 1980 Jul 10;151(2):8
**Brown AB:** Assessment of paleonutrition from skeletal remains. **Ann NY Acad Sci** 1981;376:405–16
**Brown AS:** Caroline Bartlett Crane and urban reform. **Mich Hist** 1972;56(4):287–301
**Brown BI:** Gerty Theresa Radnitz Cori. In Dictionary of American Biography, Suppl. 6, 1956–1960. p. 126–7, 1980.
**Brown BS** see **Lindemann E**
**Brown CL:** Fifty years of psychiatry. **J Med Assoc State Ala** 1981 Aug;51(2):40–3
**Brown CL:** The Four Horsemen of amateur psychiatry, class of '46 [interview by William H McDonald] **J Med Assoc State Ala** 1980 Nov;50(5):8–10, 15
**Brown CL:** Thomas Wolfe: a psychiatric view. **J Med Assoc State Ala** 1981 Oct;51(4):11–5
**Brown D** see **Vahey T**
**Brown DC:** Health of farm children in the South, 1900–1950. **Agric Hist** 1979;53(1):170–87
**Brown DH** see **Buchanan WW**
**Brown EA:** Death and the human body in the later Middle Ages: the legislation of Boniface VIII on the division of the corpse. **Viator** 1981;12:221–70
**Brown EG:** Notes on the University Hospital: the early decades. **Mich Q Rev** 1964;3(1):8–17
**Brown EM:** Neurology and spiritualism in the 1870s. **Bull Hist Med** 1983 Winter;57(4):563–77
**Brown ER:** Exporting medical education: professionalism, modernization and imperialism. **Soc Sci Med [Med Psychol Med Sociol]** 1979 Nov;13A(6):585–95
**Brown ER:** He who pays the piper: foundations, the medical profession, and medical education. In Reverby S, Rosner D, ed: Health care in America. Philadelphia, Temple University Press, 1979. p. 132–54.
**Brown ER:** Rockefeller medicine men. Medicine and capitalism in America. Berkeley, University of California Press, 1979. xii, 283 p.
**Brown ER** see **Benison S**
**Brown F:** A quarter of a century in foot-and-mouth disease research. **Zentralbl Veterinarmed [B]** 1984 Oct;31(9):646–8
**Brown HM:** Reminiscences of Dr. Senn. **Milw Hist** 1981;4(3–4):87–94
**Brown HP:** Sir Alexander Carr-Saunders. In Dictionary of national biography, 1961–1970. Suppl. 8, 1981. p. 175–6.
**Brown JE, Finder JG, Lidge RT:** The Clinical Orthopaedic Society, Inc.: an informal history, 1912–1981. Brunswick, Ga., Glover Printing Co., [1982?]. vii, 288 p.
**Brown JM:** History of masters education in nursing in the United States, 1945–1969. Ed.D. Diss., Columbia University. New York, 1979. 225 leaves.
**Brown JS:** Of battle and disease: the East African Campaign of 1914–18. **Parameters** 1982;12(2):16–24
**Brown JS** see **Hearst E, ed**
**Brown JV:** The professionalization of Russian psychiatry: 1857–1911. Ph.D. Diss., Univ. of Pennsylvania. Philadelphia, 1981. 431 p.
**Brown KA:** The identification of Linda Agostini: the significance of dental evidence in the Albury Pyjama Girl case. **Am J Forensic Med Pathol** 1982 Jun;3(2):131–41
**Brown KS:** Evolution and development of the dentition. **Birth Defects** 1983;19(1):29–66
**Brown LD:** Competition and health care policy: experience and expectations. **Ann Am Acad Polit Soc Sci** 1983;(468):48–59
**Brown M:** History of the formation of the UW School of Veterinary Medicine. **J Vet Med Educ** 1982;8:105–8
**Brown MC:** The health care crisis in historical perspective. **Can J Public Health** 1979 Sep–Oct;70(5):300–6
**Brown P:** Couching a cataract. **Med Instrum** 1982 Mar–Apr;16(2):123
**Brown P:** National celebrities brought cheer to young patients at Riley Hospital (I. U. Medical Center) in the 1930's. **Indiana Med Hist Q** 1976;2(4):65–9
**Brown PS:** Defining the medical profession in mid-nineteenth century Bristol. **Bristol Med Chir J** 1981 Jan–Apr;96(357–358):4–7
**Brown PS:** Herbalists and medical botanists in mid-nineteenth-century Britain with special reference to Bristol. **Med Hist** 1982 Oct;26(4):405–20
**Brown PS:** Mesmerism, galvanism and quackery. **Bristol Med Chir J** 1983 Apr;98(366):61–4
**Brown PS:** Some treatments of skin disease in eighteenth century Bath. **Int J Dermatol** 1982 Nov;21(9):555–9
**Brown PS:** The providers of medical treatment in mid-nineteenth-century Bristol. **Med Hist** 1980 Jul;24(3):297–314
**Brown PS:** The venders of medicines advertised in eighteenth-century Bath newspapers. **Med Hist** 1975 Oct;19(4):352–69
**Brown PS:** The vicissitudes of herbalism in late nineteenth- and early twentieth-century Britain. **Med Hist** 1985 Jan;29(1):71–92
**Brown R** see **Kasschau RA**
**Brown RD** see **Cash P**
**Brown RH:** The development of methods for the determination of hazardous substances in factory atmospheres: an historical perspective. **Ann Occup Hyg** 1984;28(2):183–8
**Brown RW, Henderson JH:** The mass production and distribution of HeLa cells at Tuskegee Institute, 1953–55. **J Hist Med Allied Sci** 1983 Oct;38(4):415–31
**Brown SE:** Sexuality and the slave community. **Phylon** 1981;42(1):1–10
**Brown SL** see **Stool SE**
**Brown T:** Shell shock in the Canadian Expeditionary Force, 1914–1918: Canadian psychiatry in the Great War. In Roland CG, ed: Health, disease and medicine. Toronto, Hannah Institute for the History of Medicine, 1984. p. 308–32.
**Brown T:** The mechanical philosophy and the 'animal oeconomy'. New York, Arno Press, 1981. viii, 419 p.
**Brown TE:** The mental hospital and its historians. **Bull Hist Med** 1982 Spring;56(1):109–14
**Brown TM:** The changing self-concept of the 18th-century London physician. **Eighteenth Cent Life** 1982;7(2):31–40
**Brown VK:** A cathedral of healing: the story of Wesley Memorial Hospital. Chicago, Northwestern Memorial Hospital, 1981.
**Brown GC, ed:** With the ambulance service in France: the wartime letters of William Gorham Rice, jr. **Wis Mag Hist** 1981;64(4):278–93
**Browne AD:** The section of obstetrics and obstetric and gynaecological development over the century. **Ir J Med Sci** 1983 Jan;152(1):26–38
**Browne EG:** Arabian medicine. The FitzPatrick lectures delivered at the College of Physicians in November 1919 and November 1920. Westport, Hyperion, 1983. x, 138 p. Reprint of four lectures.
**Browne EJ** see **Bynum WF**
**Browne HJ:** A century of changing fashions in peptic ulcer surgery. **Ir Med J** 1979 Nov 30;72(11):458–69
**Browne HS:** Newport's revolutionary physicians. **Newport Hist** 1981;54(1):4–34
**Browne J:** Darwin's botanical arithmetic and the 'principle of divergence,' 1854–1858. **J Hist Biol** 1980 Spring;13(1):53–89
**Browne J:** Essay review: new developments in Darwins studies? **J Hist Biol** 1982 Summer;15(2):275–80
**Browne SG:** How old is leprosy? **Int J Dermatol** 1980 Nov;19(9):530–2
**Browne SG:** The contribution of medical missionaries to tropical medicine. **Trans R Soc Trop Med Hyg** 1979;73(4):357–60
**Browning DS:** Homosexuality, theology, the social sciences and the church. **Encounter (Lond)** 1979;40(3):223–43
**Brozěk J:** David Jayne Hill: between the old and the new psychology. In J. Brozěk, ed: Explorations in the history of psychology in the United States. Lewisburg, Bucknell University Press, 1984. p. 121–47.
**Brozek J, Pongratz LJ, ed:** Historiography of modern psychology: aims, resources, approaches. Toronto, Hogrefe, 1980. 336 p. Contributions by R. Ardila, M. G. Ash, L. T. Benjamin, W. Bringmann, R. León, B. Ross, M. Sokal, H. Thomae, G. A. Ungerer, R. I. Watson, M. Wertheimer, W. Woodward, L. J. Pongratz.
**Brozek J, Evans RB, ed:** R. I. Watson's selected papers on the history of psychology. Hanover, University of New Hampshire, 1977. xiii, 393 p.
**Brożek J** see **Robert I. Watson and the development of the history of psychology: a symposium**
**Brożek K:** Dr med. Karol Zahorski (1879--1970) lekarz-społecznik w Zagłębiu Dąbrowskim (w 100-lecie urodzin). **Pol Tyg Lek** 1979 Jun 25;34(26):1057–9
**Brożek K:** Ruch naukowy towarzystw medycznych w regionie śląsko-dąbrowskim. **Wiad Lek** 1980 Aug 1;33(15):1265–9
**Brożek K:** Społeczne tradycje medycyny w regionie śląsko-dąbrowskim (1901–1950). **Kult Spoleczenstwo** 1979;23(3):67–78
**Brozěk J, ed:** Explorations in the history of psychology in the United States. Lewisburg, [Pa.], Bucknell University Press, 1984. 333 p. Contributions by R. B. Evans, J. G. Blight, W. R. Woodward, J. A. Popplestone, M. W. McPherson, M. M. Sokal.
**Bru Villaseca L:** Física del frío y medicina. **An R Acad Nac Med (Madr)** 1983;100(2):243–78
**Bruce FE:** Water supply and waste disposal [in the twentieth century]. In Williams TI, ed: A history of technology. Vol. VII. The twentieth century, ca. 1900 to ca. 1950, Part II. Oxford, Clarendon, 1978. p. 1363–98.
**Bruce J:** Of sugar and salt and things in the cellar and sun: food preservation in Jackson County in the 1850's. **Mo Hist Rev** 1981;75(4):417–47
**Bruce MC** see **Casarett LJ**
**Bruce NG:** Searching the history of the health sciences.

**Med Ref Serv Q** 1982 Fall;1(3):13–35

**Bruce-Chwatt LJ:** Alphonse Laveran's discovery 100 years ago and today's global fight against malaria. **J R Soc Med** 1981 Jul;74(7):531–6

**Bruce-Chwatt LJ:** 'Ecole du Pharo' in Marseille. **Trans R Soc Trop Med Hyg** 1981;75(1):131–2

**Bruce-Chwatt LJ:** Franco-British cooperation in tropical medicine. **Bull Soc Pathol Exot Filiales** 1983 Nov;76(5):713–5

**Bruce-Chwatt LJ:** George Bate--Cromwell's devious physician. **J R Coll Physicians Lond** 1983 Apr;17(2):144–6

**Bruce-Chwatt LJ:** Jacopone da Todi's mystical pathology. **Br Med J [Clin Res]** 1982 Dec 18–25;285(6357):1803–4

**Bruce-Chwatt LJ:** Ludovicus Nonnius, M.D., 1553–1645. **Bull NY Acad Med** 1984 Nov;60(9):938–43

**Bruce-Chwatt LJ:** Man against malaria: conquest or defeat. **Trans R Soc Trop Med Hyg** 1979;73(6):605–17

**Bruce-Chwatt LJ:** Medical sense and nonsense in biography. **Br Med J [Clin Res]** 1983 Apr 16;286(6373):1281

**Bruce-Chwatt LJ:** Myth of quartan malaria. **Trans R Soc Trop Med Hyg** 1982;76(1):133–4

**Bruce-Chwatt LJ, Zulueta J de:** The rise and fall of malaria in Europe; a historico-epidemiological study. Oxford, Oxford University Press, 1980, xvi, 240 p.

**Brucer M:** Historical note. Elizabeth Rona 1890–1981. **Health Phys** 1982 Apr;42(4):405–6

**Brucer M, Harris CC, MacIntyre WJ, et al:** The heritage of nuclear medicine. Commemorating the 25th anniversary of the Society of Nuclear Medicine, 1954–1979. New York, Society of Nuclear Medicine, 1979. xxvi, 167 p. Reprints of various articles.

**Bruch H:** Personal reminiscences of Frieda Fromm-Reichmann. **Psychiatry** 1982;45(2):98–104

**Bruchâč D** see **Remisová M**

**Brück C:** Tidsbilder kring en läkargeneration för 100 år sedan. Efter ett föredrag av Johan Hellström 1935. **Nord Medicinhist Arsb** 1984;:141–52

**Brück C:** Vaccination och smittskoppor--ett livs erfarenhet. **Nord Medicinhist Arsb** 1982;:122–36

**Brücke EW von:** Briefe an Emil Du Bois-Reymond. Ed. H. Brücke, W. Hilger, W. Höflechner, W. W. Swoboda. Erster Teil. Graz, Akademische Druck- und Verlagsanstalt, 1978. 308 p. (Publikationen aus dem Archiv der Universität Graz, Band 8/1).

**Brudnjak Z:** Razvoj virologije u Hrvatskoj do god. 1940. **Lijec Vjesn** 1982 Oct;104(10):448–51

**Brudnoy D:** An untarnished youth in the gilded age: Theodore Schroeder of Wisconsin and Dakota territory. **ND Hist** 1972;39(4):17–25, 34

**Bruesch SR:** Yellow fever in Tennessee in 1878. Part I. **J Tenn Med Assoc** 1978 Dec;71(12):887–96

**Brügelmann J:** Medikalisierung von Säuglings- und Erwachsenenalter in Deutschland zu Beginn des 19. Jahrhunderts aufgrund von medizinischen Topographien. In Imhof AE, ed.: Leib und Leben in der Geschichte der Neuzeit. Berlin, Duncker & Humblot, 1983. p. 177–92.

**Brügelmann J:** Observations on the process of medicalization in Germany, 1770–1830, based on medical topographies. **Hist Reflect** 1982;9(1–2):131–49

**Brugsch T:** Arzt seit fünf Jahrzehnten. Berlin, Rütten & Loening, 1978. 390 p.

**Brühlmann-Jecklin E:** Zehn Jahre Gesellschaft für Muskelkrankheiten. Fachleute und Betroffene am gleichen Strick. **Krankenpflege Soins Infirm** 1984 Jun;77(6):34–6

**Bruhn JG** see **Holmstedt B**

**Bruhn JG, et al:** The tobacco from Niño Korin: identification of nicotine in a Bolivian archaeological collection. **Goteb Ethnogr Mus** 1976;:45–8

**Bruijn J:** Abortus in de 19de eeuw. **Spiegel Hist** 1980;15(9):463–5

**Brulin F, Doual A, Gysel C:** Evolution des rapports de la psychologie et de l'odontologie. **Orthod Fr** 1980;51:197–202

**Brullard P:** Pierre Christophe (1758–1826), médecin, soldat et humaniste. In: Congrès National des Sociétés Savantes, 103e, Nancy, 1978. Comptes Rendus. Paris, 1978. Section des Sciences, Fasc. V. p. 43–53.

**Brumberg JJ:** Chlorotic girls, 1870–1920: a historical perspective on female adolescence.

**Brumgardt JR, ed:** Civil war nurse. The diary and letters of Hannah Ropes. Knoxville, University of Tennessee Press, 1980. 149 p.

**Brumley WC, Sphon JA:** Regulatory mass spectrometry. **Biomed Mass Spectrom** 1981 Sep;8(9):390–6

**Brummer P:** Uroskopi-föregångare till vår tids laboratorieundersökningar. **Nord Med** 1981 Dec;96(12):325

**Brumpt L:** Eloge de Pierre Huard (1901–1983). **Bull Acad Natl Med (Paris)** 1984 Jan–Feb;168(1–2):181–7

**Brumpt L:** Epidémiologie de la maladie de Chagas. **Bull Acad Natl Med (Paris)** 1980 Nov;164(8):782–5

**Brumpt L:** L'oeuvre de Laveran en protozoologie et ses conséquences. **Bull Acad Natl Med (Paris)** 1980 Jan;164(1):88–93

**Brun D:** Les sources infantiles de la théorie chez Freud. Une scène d'enfance dans l'après-coup. **Rev Fr Psychanal** 1982;46(3):583–99

**Brunclík J:** Freud o dostojevském - či naopak. **Cas Lek Cesk** 1982 Aug 13;121(32):1015–6

**Bruneel C:** La mortalité dans les campagnes: Le Duché de Brabant aux XVIIe et XVIIIe siècles. Louvain, Bureau du Recueil, Bibliothèque de l'Université, et Editions Nauwelaerts, 1977. lxiv, 777 p. and atlas, 97 p. (Université de Louvain, Recueil de Travaux d'Histoire et de Philologie, 6e série, Fasc. 10).

**Bruneel C:** L'epidemie de dysenterie de 1779 dans les Pays-Bas autrichiens. **Bull Comm R Hist** 1979;145(3–4):191–395

**Bruneel C:** Malades et défunts au Grand Hôpital de Louvain (1767–1796). **Ann Soc Belg Hist Hop** 1978;16:3–33

**Bruneel C:** Répertoire des thèses imprimées de l'Université de Louvain (1425–1797). Louvain, Université Catholique de Louvain, 1977. xxv, 113 p. (Catalogues, inventaires et répertoires de la Bibliothèque Centrale. III.).

**Bruneel C:** Un problème de gouvernement: le pouvoir face à l'epidémie de fièvre putride à Bruxelles en 1772–1773. In Imhof AE, ed: Mensch und Gesundheit in der Geschichte. Husum, Matthiesen, 1980. p. 199–221.

**Brunel G, Morissette L:** Guérison et ethno-étiologie populaire. **Anthropologica** 1979;21(1):43–72

**Brunet F:** Die spätantike und die byzantinische Medizin. In Sournia JC, Martiny M, Poulet J, ed: Illustrierte Geschichte der Medizin. Salzburg, Andreas, 1980. Vol. 2. p. 441–71.

**Brunet G:** Un bourg rural de la Dombes au XVIIIe et XIXe siècles: Saint-Trivier-sur-Moignans. Démographie, société et mentalités, 2 volumes. Lyon II. Thèse de doct de 3e cycle 1979. 128 p.

**Brunet J** see **La Salpêtrière**

**Bruneteau C:** John Arbuthnot (1667–1735) et les idées au début XVIIIe siècle. Univ. de Paris III, 1973. 949 p.

**Brunner TF:** Marijuana in ancient Greece and Rome? the literary evidence. **Bull Hist Med** 1973 Jul–Aug;47(4):344–55

**Brunner-Wildisen B:** Medizinisches aus den Schriften des Renward Cysat, 1545–1614. Zürich, Juris, 1980. 75 p. (Zürcher Medizingeschichtliche Abhandlungen, Neue Reihe, Nr. 138).

**Brunswick AF:** Social meanings and developmental needs: perspectives on black youth's drug abuse. **Youth Soc** 1980;11(4):449–73

**Brunyate M:** Montaigne and medicine. In K. Cameron, ed: Montaigne and his age. Univ. of Exeter, 1981. p. 26–38, 170–71.

**Bruton EM, ed:** M A S H: binding up the wounds. An exhibition at the National Museum of American History, Smithsonian Institution, Washington, D.C. New York, George Fenmore Associates, 1983. 32 p.

**Bruun NW, Baerentsen K, Jensen VG:** Anders Jahan Retzius: 'Fragmentum historiae pharmaceutices veterum'. Med dansk oversaettelse, biografiske noter og kommentarer. **Theriaca** 1981;20:5–151

**Bruun NW** see **Retzius AJ**

**Bruyn GW:** The seat of the soul. In Rose FC, Bynum WF, ed: Historical aspects of the neurosciences. New York, Raven, 1982. p. 55–81.

**Bryan CS** see **Wickwar H**

**Bryan SA:** Pioneering specialists: a history of the American Academy of Ophthalmology and Otolaryngology. San Francisco, American Academy of Ophthalmology, Rochester, Minn.: American Academy of Otolaryngology–Head and Neck Surgery, 1982. viii, 305 p.

**Bryant AW:** A history of medicine in Atlanta and Fulton County, Georgia. Part I: Terminus to the turn of the century. **J Med Assoc Ga** 1980 Apr;69(4):273–9

**Bryant AW:** A history of medicine in Atlanta and Fulton County. Part II. **J Med Assoc Ga** 1980 Jul;69(7):589–95 (continued)

**Bryant BJ:** The Harvard residency program in otolaryngology: an overview. **Am J Otol** 1979 Jul;1(1):60–3

**Bryant BJ:** The residency program in otolaryngology at Baylor College of Medicine. **Am J Otol** 1979 Oct;1(2):132–4

**Bryc S:** Thirty five years of activities of the Lublin Medical Centre. **Ann Univ Mariae Curie Sklodowska [Med]** 1979;34:1–5

**Bryce DP, Nuis DB, ed:** The American Laryngological Association, 1878–1978. Washington, American Laryngological Assn., 1978. xiv, 152 p.

**Bryce TR:** Burial practices in Lycia. **Mankind Q** 1980 Winter;21(2):165–78

**Bryder L:** 'Lessons' of the 1918 influenza epidemic in Auckland. **NZ J Hist** 1982;16(2):97–121

**Bryder L:** Papworth Village Settlement--a unique experiment in the treatment and care of the tuberculous? **Med Hist** 1984 Oct;28(4):372–90

**Bryder L:** Tuberculosis, silicosis, and the slate industry in North Wales: Medical examinations of the high tuberculosis death rates in the North Wales slate mining and quarrying districts, 1927–1939. **Soc Soc Hist Med Bull (Lond)** 1983;33:43–6

**Brygoo E:** Les médecins de Montpellier et le Jardin du Roi à Paris. **Hist Nat** 1979;(14):3–29

**Brzeziński T:** Die Entwicklung des medizinhistorischen Unterrichts in Polen. **NTM** 1981;18(2):98–108

**Brzeziński T:** Problemy nauczania historii medycyny w Polsce. **Arch Hist Med (Warsz)** 1979;42(3):379–82

**Brzeziński T:** Problemy robotnicze w pismach lekarzy Polskich przełomu XIX i XX wieku. **Arch Hist Med (Warsz)** 1984;47(1):75–83

**Brzeziński T:** Słuzba Zdrowia i Dywizji Piechoty im. T. Kościuszki i jej udział w bitwie pod Lenino. **Arch Hist Med (Warsz)** 1978;41(4):413–22

**Brzheskiĭ VC:** Neskol'ko slov o zabytom prioritete. **Grudn Khir** 1983 May–Jun;3:82–3

**Brzheskiĭ VCh:** A. A. Sakhnovskaia (k stoletiiu so dnia rozhdeniia). **Vestn Dermatol Venerol** 1983 May;(5):73–4

**Brzheskiĭ VCh:** Imena khirurgov v pamiati sovetskogo naroda. **Klin Khir** 1979 Nov;(11):64–70

**Brzheskiĭ VCh, Evdokimov PP:** K istorii bolezni V.G. Belinskogo. **Klin Med (Mosk)** 1984 Aug;62(8):150–2

**Brzheskiĭ VCh:** K istorii pervoĭ v mire kafedry oftal'mologii. **Vestn Oftalmol** 1981 Sep–Oct;(5):69–70

**Brzheskiĭ VCh:** Mestnaia pechat' - o meditsinskikh rabotnikakh. **Sov Zdravookhr** 1983;6:70–1

**Brzheskiĭ VCh:** O znakakh, uvekovechivaiushchikh imia N. I. Pirogova v strane. **Khirurgiia (Mosk)** 1980 Feb;(2):105–6

**Brzheskiĭ VCh:** Uvekovechennye imena otechestvennykh

uchenykh--morfologov. **Arkh Anat Gistol Embriol** 1981 Jan;80(1):108-9
**Brzozowski R, Piątkiewicz W:** Sztuczna wątroba--historia idzień dzisiejszy. **Pol Arch Med Wewn** 1980 Nov;64(5):457-65
**Bubis M:** Petroleum in Talmudic sources. **Koroth** 1981;8(1-2):41-4
**Buchanan AV, Weiss KM, Schwartz RJ, et al:** Reconstruction of genealogies from vital records: the Laredo Epidemiology Project. **Comput Biomed Res** 1984 Aug;17(4):326-51
**Buchanan AV** see **Schwartz RJ**
**Buchanan DJ:** Huron District Medical Society (No. 5). **SD J Med** 1981 May;34(5):15-7
**Buchanan I:** Infant mortality and social policy: the eugenists and the social ameliorators, 1900-1914. **Soc Soc Hist Med Bull (Lond)** 1980;27:5-7
**Buchanan M:** The sick child. **Nurs Times** 1983 Feb 23-Mar 1;79(8):66-9
**Buchanan PD** see **Hunt LB**
**Buchanan R:** Fighting the ubiquitous monarch, disease: the 1866 report on the Sanitary Relations of Kansas. **J Hist Med Allied Sci** 1983 Jan;38(1):78-83
**Buchanan WW, Brown DH:** Joseph Black (1728-1799): Scottish physician and chemist. **Practitioner** 1980 Jun;224(1344):663-6
**Buchanan WW, Kean WF:** Robert Burn's illness revisited. **Scott Med J** 1982 Jan;27(1):75-88
**Buchanan WW, Kraag GR, Palmer DG, et al:** The first recorded case of osteitis fibrosa cystica. **Can Med Assoc J** 1981 Mar 15;124(6):812-5
**Buchanan WW** see **Kean WF**
**Buchanan WW** see **Spencer DG**
**Bucher S:** Die Pest in der Ostschweiz. In: Historischer Verein des Kantons St. Gallen, 119. Neujahrsblatt. St. Gallen, Stehle, 1979. p. 7-58.
**Bucher S:** Die Pest in der Ostschweiz. St. Gallen [Switzerland], Historischer Verein des Kantons St. Gallen, 1979. 90 p.
**Buchet C** see **Guillemain B**
**Buchet L:** Médecine et chirurgie pendant les premiers siècles du Moyen Age. Présentation de quelues vestiges anthropologiques. **Rev Archeol Centre France** 1983;22(Dec):273-81
**Buchholz R:** Famous physicians and scientists in the history of the Medical School of Marburg. **Birth Defects** 1979;15(4):1-4
**Büchi J:** Das Dispensatorium Medicum seu Pharmacopoea Noşocomii Thuricensis 1757. **Pharm Acta Helv** 1981;56(4-5):101-5
**Büchi J:** Die Arzneiversorgung und der Sanitätsdienst der schweizerischen Truppen vom 15.-18. Jahrhundert. Stuttgart, Wissenschaftliche Verlagsanstalt, 1981. 94 p. (Veröffentlichungen der Internationalen Gesellschaft für Geschichte der Pharmazie, Neue Folge, 49).
**Büchi J:** Die wiederaufgefundene 'Pharmacia contracta' des Johann Jakob Scheuchzer (1672-1733). **Gesnerus** 1982;39(2):145-69
**Buchin ID, Peck S:** Harvey Peck, 1937-1981. **Angle Orthod** 1982 Jan;52(1):3-5
**Büchner F:** Der junge Rudolf Virchow. **Verh Dtsch Ges Pathol** 1981;65:458-61
**Buchsteiner W:** Studien zu Texten zur Bujatrik von 1687-1825. Diss. Hannover, 1981. 189 p.
**Buchvald J** see **Ozorovský V**
**Buchvarova N:** Mezhdunaroden Kongres po istoriia na meditsinata. **Istor Pregl** 1978;34(6):148-52
**Buchwald H, Rucker RD:** The history of metabolic surgery for morbid obesity and a commentary. **World J Surg** 1981 Nov;5(6):781-7
**Buchwald H:** The scientist-surgeon. **Am J Surg** 1981 Aug;142(2):245-6
**Buck BA:** Ancient technology in contemporary surgery. **West J Med** 1982 Mar;136(3):265-9
**Buck DD:** Imperially inspired philanthropy in the Ch'ing: the case of granaries in the eighteenth century. **Bull Inst Mod Hist Acad Sin** 1982;11:225-50
**Buck MR:** Medicinischer Volksglauben u. Volksaberglauben aus Schwaben. Eine kulturgeschichtliche Skizze. 4. Auflage. (Reprint, originally published 1865.) Riedlingen, Ulrich, 1981. vi, 72 p.
**Buck P:** American science and modern China, 1876-1936. Cambridge, Cambridge University Press, 1980. viii, 283 p.
**Buck P:** People who counted: political arithmetic in the eighteenth century. **Isis** 1982 Mar;73(266):28-45
**Buckley AD:** Unofficial healing in Ulster. **Ulster Folklife** 1980;26:15-34
**Buckley KW:** Behaviorism and the professionalization of American psychology: a study of John Broadus Watson, 1878-1958. Ph.D. Diss., University of Massachusetts. Amherst, 1982. vii, 313 p.
**Buckley KW:** The selling of a psychologist: John Broadus Watson and the application of behavioral techniques to advertising. **J Hist Behav Sci** 1982 Jul;18(3):207-21
**Buckley NL:** Women psychoanalysts and the theory of feminine development: a study of Karen Horney, Helene Deutsch, and Marie Bonaparte. Ph.D. Diss., University of California. Los Angeles, 1982. 178 p.
**Buckley P, Galanter M:** Altered states of consciousness during psychotherapy: a historical and cultural perspective. **Int J Soc Psychiatry** 1979 Summer;25(2):118-24
**Buckley RH:** Presidential address. Reflections on the 1970s and a look to the future. **J Allergy Clin Immunol** 1980 Dec;66(6):432-7
**Buckley S:** Efforts to reduce infant maternity mortality in Canada between the two world wars. **Atlantis** 199;2 (2 pt 2):76-84
**Buckley S, McGinnis JD:** Venereal disease and public health reform in Canada. **Can Hist Rev** 1982;63(3):337-54
**Bucklin R:** The Shroud of Turin: a pathologist's viewpoint. **Leg Med** 1982;:33-9
**Bucklin R:** The Shroud of Turin: a pathologist's viewpoint. **J Miss State Med Assoc** 1983 Apr;24(4):95-8
**Buckwalter KC, Church OM:** Euphemia Jane Taylor: an uncommon psychiatric nurse. **Perspect Psychiatr Care** 1979 May-Jun;17(3):125-31
**Buckwalter KC** see **Church OM**
**Bucy PC:** 'Ancora imparo'--'I continue to learn'. **Neurol Med Chir (Tokyo)** 1981 Jul;21(7):629-34
**Bucy PC:** The pioneers of neurology and neurosurgery in the world and their contributions. A lecture for young Japanese neurosurgeons. **No Shinkei Geka** 1982 May;10(5):490-8
**Buda B** see **Füredi J**
**Budernik A:** Die zweite Türkenbelagerung Wiens, mit besonderer Berücksichtigung der sanitären Verhältnisse vor und während dieser Zeit. **Wien Klin Wochenschr** 1983 Oct 14;95(19):688-92
**Bud'ko VI** see **Bastenchuk AZ**
**Budnick LD:** The spirit of Chadwick. **NY State J Med** 1983 Dec;83(13):1345-6
**Budnikowski A, Rusiński M:** O skutkach ekonomicznych przeciwdziałani zanieczyszczeniu środowiska w krajach kapitalistycznych. **Ekonomista** 1974;(2):401-14
**Buell FD:** Nineteenth century surgeon: Dr. Alden March, founder, Albany Medical College, 1795-1869. Albany, Albany Medical College, 1981. 12 p.
**Buelvas Acosta E** see **Ordosgoitia Yarzagaray E**
**Bueno AG:** La flora de Aragon: notas a un proyecto de Francisco Loscos y Jose Pardo. **Bol Soc Esp Hist Farm** 1984;35(137):23-33
**Buerki RA, ed:** Survey of instructional resources in history of pharmacy undergraduate courses. [Columbus, Ohio], Ohio State University, [1981?]. x, 160 p.
**Buess H, Portmann ML:** Berühmte Schweizer Arzte. **Gesnerus** 1980;37(3/4):289-306
**Buess H:** Der Wiener Sozialmediziner Ludwig Teleky (1872-1957) und seine 'History of factory and mine hygiene'. **Wien Med Wochenschr** 1981 Oct 15;131(19):479-83
**Buess H:** Der Wiener Sozialmediziner Ludwig Teleky (1872-1957) und seine 'History of Factory and Mine Hygiene'. In Ganzinger K, Skopec M, Wyklicky H, ed: Festschrift für Erna Lesky zum 70. Geburtstag. Wien, Brüder Hollinek, 1981. p. 31-7.
**Buess H:** Henry E. Sigerist (1891-1957) und die erste medizinhistorische Konferenz in Pura (Tessin); zur Erinnerung an den 25./26. März 1950. **Gesnerus** 1980;37(1/2):104-12
**Buess H:** Nikolaus Senn (1844-1908), ein schweizerischer Pionier der Chirurgie in den USA. **Gesnerus** 1979;36(3-4):238-45
**Buess H:** Prof. Dr. med. Dr.h.c. Walter Pagel (1898-1983). **Gesnerus** 1984;41(3-4):359-63
**Buettner J:** Why the history of our discipline should be discussed in this journal. **J Clin Chem Clin Biochem** 1981;19:309-10
**Buffat JJ, Thonnier C, Bourdais A, et al:** Anesthésie et odonto-stomatologie. **Actual Odontostomatol (Paris)** 1982;36(139)303-13
**Buffat M:** Diderot, le corps le la machine. **Rev Sci Hum** 1982-3;186-7:185-97
**Buffe P** see **Boisanger B de**
**Bugaj R:** Koncepcje elementów ognia i powietrza u Arystotelesa i ich rola w procesach spalania i oddychania. **Kwart Hist Nauki Tech** 1980;25(1):89-103
**Bugbee G:** George Bugbee: a first-person profile (Part 2). **Health Serv Res** 1981 Winter;16(4):459-66
**Bugyi B:** A hazai anthropológia néhány korai írása. **Orvostort Kozl** 1979;87-88(25 no 1-2):261-8
**Bugyi B:** Akit indokolatlanul elfelejtettek: Schnirch Emil (1822-1884). **Orv Hetil** 1982 Oct 17;123(42):2613-4
**Bugyi B:** Az elsö 'népszerü orvostan' föiskolai tanszék (1834-1852) történetéböl. **Orvostort Kozl** 1981;93-96(27 No 1-4):225-35
**Bugyi B:** Az iskolázottak betegségeiröl. **Magy Konyvsz** 1976;92(4):397-401
**Bugyi B:** Az orvosi sajtó etikájáról--hetven évvel ezelött. **Orv Hetil** 1979 Dec 30;120(52):3184-6
**Bugyi B:** Bausner Bertalan (1629-1682). **Orv Hetil** 1984 Jul 22;125(30):1831-2
**Bugyi B:** Csehov, az orvos. **Orv Hetil** 1980 Nov 16;121(46):2834-7
**Bugyi B:** G. Flaubert (1821-1880) és az orvosok. **Orv Hetil** 1980 Jun 1;121(22):1339-40
**Bugyi B:** Genersich Antal vasutépítés orvosakénti tevékenységéröl. **Orv Hetil** 1983 Jul 24;124(30):1825-6
**Bugyi B:** Lichtenthal Péter, egy elfelejtett nagy magyar orvos-zenetudós.
**Bugyi B:** Medical geography of Moldavia: historical contribution. **Geogr Med** 1979;9:109-15
**Bugyi B:** Medical topography of Bulgaria and Serbia in the third quarter of the 19th century. **Geogr Med** 1981;11:158-61
**Bugyi B:** N. J. Jacquin, the first medical doctor-chemist in Hungary. **Ther Hung** 1979;27(4):192-3
**Bugyi B:** Orvosi helyleírásunk történetéhez. **Orvostort Kozl** 1981;93-96(27 No 1-4):219-24
**Bugyi B:** Tagung der Deutschen Gesellschaft für Geschichte der Medizin und der Naturwissenschaften im Jahre 1929 zu Budapest. **Orvostort Kozl** 1979;86(24 no 4):65-71
**Bugyi I:** Az antisepsistöl a hyperasepsisig. **Orv Hetil** 1981 Feb 8;122(6):345-7
**Buianov MI:** Vrach-puteshestvennik A. V. Eliseev. **Klin Med (Mosk)** 1982;60(8):113-4
**Buican D:** Histoire de la génétique et de l'évolutionnisme en France. Paris, Presse universitaires de France, 1984. 421 p.
**Buican D:** La génétique classique en France devant le neo-lamarckisme tardif. **Arch Int Hist Sci (Paris)** 1983 Dec;33(111):300-24

**Buican D:** Lucien Cuénot et la redécouverte de la génétique. **Pour Sci** 1981;45:21-9
**Buican D:** Milestones in the philosophic and historical framework of the development of biology in France. **Scientia** 1982;117(9-12):609-21
**Buick R** see **Groves D**
**Buikstra JE:** Prehistoric tuberculosis in the Americas. Evanston, Northwestern University, Archeological Program, 1981. xii, 182 p.
**Buikstra JE, Gordon CC:** The study and restudy of human skeletal series: the importance of long term curation. **Ann NY Acad Sci** 1981;376:449-65
**Buikstra JE** see **Cook DC**
**Buikstra JE** see **Lambert JB**
**Bujałowska B:** Recepcja poglądów hipokratesa w polsce na tle dziejów medycyny powszechnej. **Pol Tyg Lek** 1983 Aug 15;38(33-34):1063-6
**Bujosa F** see **Ballester R**
**Bujosa F** see **López Piñero JM**
**Bujosa Homar F** see **López Piñero JM**
**Bujosa i Homar F:** La afasia y su historiografía. **Dynamis** 1981;1:131-63
**Bujosa i Homar F:** Reconsiderations on the history of aphasia. In International Congress of the History of Medicine, 27th, Barcelona, 1980. Actas. Barcelona, Académia de Ciències Médiques de Catalunya i Balears, 1981. p. 27-38.
**Bujosa i Homar F** see **Balaguer i Perigüell E**
**Bukharov PL** see **Kuz'min MK**
**Bukhman AA, Novak GIa:** Khirurgicheskoe lechnenie bolezni Peĭroni (obzor literatury). **Khirurgiia (Mosk)** 1981 Jul;(7):108-10
**Bukov VA:** Opyt meditsinskogo obespecheniia 13-ĭ armii. Soobshchenie vtoroe. Meditsinskoe obespechnie armii v khode operatsioi. **Voen Med Zh** 1982 Aug;(8):12-7
**Bukov VA:** Opyt meditsinskogo obespecheniia 13-ĭ armii v bitve pod Kurskom. **Voen Med Zh** 1982;(7):14-9
**Bukowiecki H, Kuznicka B:** The pharmacy in the Warsaw royal castle. A monument of pharmaceutical culture. **Q J Hist Sci Technol (Polish Acad Sci)** 1980;25(4):755-67
**Bukowiecki H, Kuźnicka B:** The pharmacy in the Warsaw Royal Castle - a monument of pharmaceutical culture. **Kwart Hist Nauki Tech** 1980;25(4):755-67
**Büky B:** Rejtett orvosi vonatkozások régi szavainkban. **Orvostort Kozl** 1979;87-88(25 no 1-2):223-8
**Bulber M:** The slow and uneven growth of sociology in Great Britain. **Minerva** 1983 Summer-Autumn;21(2-3):338-47
**Bülbring E, Walker JM:** Joshua Harold Burn: 6 March 1892-13 July 1981. **Biogr Mem Fellows R Soc** 1984;30:45-89
**Bulferetti L:** Quantification in the historiography of sciences and techniques. **Organon** 1980/81;16-17:19-41
**Bulgaro PJ, Webb AY:** Federal-state conflicts in cost control. **Proc Acad Polit Sci** 1980;33(4):93-110
**Bulger MA:** American sportswomen in the 19th century. **J Pop Cult** 1982;16(2):1-16
**Bulhan HA:** Frantz Fanon: the revolutionary psychiatrist. **Race Cl** 1980 Winter;21:251-72
**Bulhof IN:** From psychotherapy to psychoanalysis: Frederik van Eeden and Albert Willem van Renterghem. **J Hist Behav Sci** 1981;17:209-21
**Bulhof IN:** Psychoanalysis in the Netherlands. **Comp Stud Soc Hist** 1982;24(4):572-88
**Bulkina ZP** see **Diadiusha GF**
**Bull JW:** The history of neuroradiology. In Rose FC, Bynum WF, ed: Historical aspects of the neurosciences. New York, Raven, 1982. p. 255-64.
**Bulla A:** Reîntîlnire cu opera ştiinţfică a lui Robert Koch. **Rev Ig [Pneumoftiziol]** 1982 Jan-Mar;31(1):5-11
**Bulla A:** Revue de la morbidité et de la mortalité par tuberculose d'après les données officiellement rapportées dans le monde (1967-1971-1977). **Bull Int Union Tuberc** 1981 Sep-Dec;56(3-4):122-8
**Bullitt WC** see **Freud S**
**Bullock A:** Francis Schlatter: a fool for God. **Palacio** 1975;83(1):38-45
**Bullock MB:** An American transplant: the Rockefeller Foundation and Peking Union Medical College. Berkeley, University of California Press, 1980. xxvii, 280 p.
**Bullough B, Bullough V:** Education problems in a woman's profession. **JNE** 1981 Sep;20(7):6-17
**Bullough B, Bullough VL, Elcano B:** Nursing. A historical bibliography. New York, London, Garland, 1981. xxiv, 408 p. (Garland reference library of social science, v. 66).
**Bullough B** see **Bullough VL**
**Bullough V, Campbell C:** Female longevity and diet in the Middle Ages. **Speculum** 1980 Apr;55(2):317-25
**Bullough V** see **Bullough B**
**Bullough VL:** A brief note on rubber technology and contraception: the diaphragm and the condom. **Technol Cult** 1981;22(1):104-11
**Bullough VL:** Age at menarche: a misunderstanding. **Science** 1981 Jul 17:209(4505):365-6
**Bullough VL, Elcano BW, Legg WD, et al:** An annotated bibliography of homosexuality. 2 vols. Vol. I. New York, Garland, 1976. xxxvii, 405 p.
**Bullough VL:** Bottle feeding: an amplification. **Bull Hist Med** 1981 Summer;55(2):257-9
**Bullough VL:** Female physiology, technology and women's liberation. In Trescott, Martha Moore, ed. Dynamos and Virgins revisited: Women and technological change in history. Metuchen, N. J., Scarecrow Pr., 1979. p. 236-51.
**Bullough VL:** Homosexuality: a history. New York, New American Library, 1979. ix, 196 p.
**Bullough VL, Groeger S:** Irving W. Potter and internal podalic version: the problems of disciplining a skilled but heretical doctor. **Soc Probl** 1982;30(1):109-16
**Bullough VL, Bullough B:** Prostitution--an illustrated social history. New York, Crown Publishers, 1978. xii, 336 p.
**Bullough VL, Bullough B:** Sin, sickness and sanity. New York, Garland, 1977. ix, 276 p.
**Bullough VL:** Transvestites in the middle ages. **Am J Sociol** 1974 May;79(6):1381-94
**Bullough VL** see **Bullough B**
**Bulmer M:** Quantification and Chicago social science in the 1920s: a neglected tradition. **J Hist Behav Sci** 1981;17:312-31
**Bulmer M:** The early institutional establishment of social science research: the local community research committee at the University of Chicago, 1923-30. **Minerva** 1980 Spring;18(1):51-110
**Bulst N:** Der Schwarze Tod. Demographische, wirtschafts- und kulturgeschichtliche Aspekte der Pestkatastrophe von 1347-1352. Bilanz der neueren Forschung. **Saeculum (Freiburg)** 1979;30(1):45-67
**A bulwark against mighty woes:** The hundredth anniversary of the American Red Cross. **Am Heritage** 1981;32(2):81-91
**Buma S:** De ontwikkeling van het verpleegkundig beroep op Curaçao, I--Van de vroegste periode tot 1940. **Tijdschr Ziekenverpl** 1980 Feb 12;33(4):150-6
**Buma S:** De ontwikkeling van het verpleegkundig beroep op Curaçao. II. Het einde van het Missietijdperk en de introductie van de opleidingen; van 1940 tot heden. **Tijdschr Ziekenverpl** 1980 Feb 26;33(5):210-8
**Bumbaširevic Z:** Sedamdeset pet godina ortopedske hirurgije u Srbiji. **Srp Arh Celok Lek** 1981 Mar;109(3):425-38
**Bumosa F** see **López Piñero JM**
**Bumpass LL** see **Rindfuss RR**
**Bunčáková V, Bednárová E, Ivanová A, et al:** Vývoj slovenskej lekárskej terminológie od vzniku Bratislavských lekárskych listov a Lekárskej fakulty Univerzity Komenského. **Bratisl Lek Listy** 1983 Aug;80(2):221-35
**Bunchuk NV, Vasil'ev VI, Trusova TM:** Razvitie otechestvennoĭ revmatologii za gody sovetskoĭ vlasti. **Vestn Akad Med Nauk SSSR** 1981;(6):4-7
**Bundzen PV** see **Bechtereva NP**
**Bunge M:** The limits on science. **Physiologist** 1980 Feb;23(1):7-13
**Buniiatov ZM, Kagramanov KM:** O 30-m traktate Abu-l-kasima Khalafa Ibn Abbasa Az-Zakhravi. **Vestn Akad Med Nauk SSSR** 1980;9:75-8
**Bunn I** see **Geis G**
**Bunnell JB:** Respiratory assistance: a review of techniques, rationale, and problems with a glimpse at the future. **Ann Biomed Eng** 1982;9(5-6):645-67
**Bunnell WW** see **Paul JR**
**Buño W** see **Gil L**
**Burak GG** see **Ibragimova ZI**
**Buranchiev AB, Sizov IE:** K 40-letiiu kafedry kozhnykh i venericheskikh bolezneĭ Kirgizskogo meditsinskogo instituta. **Vestn Dermatol Venerol** 1980 Nov;(11):27-9
**Burbick J:** Emily Dickinson and the revenge of the nerves. **Womens Stud** 1980;7(1-2):95-109
**Burch CB:** Huygens' pulse models as a bridge between phenomena and Huygens' mechanical foundations. **Janus** 1981;68:53-64
**Burch M:** 'I don't know only what we hear': the soldiers' view of the 1918 influenza epidemic. **Indiana Med Hist Q** 1983 Dec;9(4):23-7
**Burchall JJ:** The development of the diaminopyrimidiness. **J Antimicrob Chemother** 1979 Nov;5(B):3-14
**Burchardt J:** List Witelona do Ludwika we Lwowku Slaskim. Problematyka teorioporznawcza, kosmologiczna i medyczna. Wroclaw, Polish Academy of Sciences, 1979. 225 p. (Studia Copernicana, 19).
**Burchell H:** Sir Thomas Lewis: his impact on American cardiology. **Br Heart J** 1981 Jul;46(1):1-4
**Burchell HB:** Contributions of the basic sciences to successful clinical application of cardiopulmonary bypass. **Mayo Clin Proc** 1980 Dec;55(12):754-7
**Burchell HB:** Digitalis poisoning: historical and forensic aspects. **J Am Coll Cardiol** 1983 Feb;1(2 Pt 1):506-16
**Burchell HB:** Important events in cardiology, 1940-1982 a retrospective view. **JAMA** 1983 Mar 4;249(9):1197-200
**Burchell HB:** Mechanical and hydraulic analogies in Harvey's discovery of the circulation. **J Hist Med Allied Sci** 1981 Jul;36(3):260-77
**Burchell HB:** The investigator as volunteer subject. **Mayo Clin Proc** 1982 Jul;57 Suppl:28-33
**Burchell HB:** The QT interval historically treated. **Pediatr Cardiol** 1983 Apr-Jun;4(2):139-48
**Burchinskiĭ GI:** Razvitie kliniki vnutrennikh bolezneĭ v USSR za 60 let. **Klin Med (Mosk)** 1982 Dec;60(12):22-9
**Burd JG:** Forty years on the same job (or orthopedic surgery can be fun). **J Tenn Med Assoc** 1979 Jul;72(7):534-6
**Burdeĭ GD** see **Speranskiĭ VS**
**Burdon JG, Kramer H:** Early history of penicillin. **Med J Aust** 1982 Dec 11-25;2(12):555-6
**Burdov VS, Nemchaninov SK, Miziak AN:** K istorii okruzhnogo voennogo gospitala Belorusskogo voennogo okruga. **Voen Med Zh** 1984 Aug;(8):71-3
**Burenkov SP:** Torzhestvo leninskikh ideĭ v zdrakhookhranenii. **Sov Zdravookhr** 1980;(11):3-8
**Burenkov SP:** 60-letie obrazovaniia SSSR i zadachi Sovetskogo zdravookhraneniia. **Vestn Akad Med Nauk SSSR** 1983;6:5-13

Burg AM: Les archives hospitalières de Haguenau. In Livet G, Schaff G, ed: Médecine et assistance en Alsace, XVIe–XXe siècle. Strasbourg, Istra, 1976. p. 113–5.
Burg BR: Ho hum, another work of the devil. Buggery and sodomy in early Stuart England. **J Homosex** 1980–81 Fall–Winter;6(1–2):69–78
Burg BR: Sodomy and the perception of evil: English sea rovers in the seventeenth-century Caribbean. New York, New York University Press, 1983. xxxiii, 215 p.
Burg BR: The sick and the dead: the development of psychological theory on necrophilia from Krafft-Ebing to the present. **J Hist Behav Sci** 1982 Jul;18(3):242–54
Burg P: Demographie und Geschichte. **Rheinische Vierteljahrsbl** 1978;(42):298–383
Burgasov PN: Itogi i perspektivy profilaktiki infektsionnykh bolezneĭ. **Zh Mikrobiol Epidemiol Immunobiol** 1982 Dec;(12):3–7
Burgasov PN: Shest'desiat let SSSR: itogi i perspektivy raboty parazitologov nasheĭ strany. **Med Parazitol (Mosk)** 1982 Nov–Dec;60(6):3–9
Bürgel JC: Islam [and Arabic medicine]. In Reich WT, et al, ed: Encyclopedia of bioethics, v. 2. New York, Free Press, 1978. p. 785–9.
Burgel JC: Musicotherapy in the Islamic Middle Ages as reflected in medical and other sources. **Stud Hist Med** 1980 Mar;4(1):23–8
Burgener L: Pestalozzi et l'education physique. **Paedagog Hist** 1977;17(2):516–18
Burger A: Drug development: challenges and hurdles. **Va Q Rev** 1981;57(3):420–39
Burger G: Nerven- und Geisteskrankheiten als Indikationen für eine bilaterale Oophorektomie im späten 19. Jahrhundert. Diss. Erlangen–Nürnberg, 1984. 185 p.
Burgess R: The dance of Death. An iconographic interpretation of the popular theme of death through five centuries. **Soc Soc Hist Med Bull (Lond)** 1980 Jun;26:25–37
Burguéz NA: Los pioneros de la medicina en San Juan de la frontera la institucionalizacion de la medicina en la accíon de los pioneros Sanjuaninos del siglo XIX. In Congreso de Historia de la Medicina Argentina [Transactions], 5th, Mendoza, 1983. p. 183–96.
Burgun R, Laugier P: Die Geschichte der Syphilis in Strassburg. In Sournia JC, Martiny M, Poulet J, ed: Illustrierte Geschichte der Medizin. Salzburg, Andreas, 1980. Vol. 4. p. 1517–45.
Burgun R: Mesures de protection contre la lèpre et la syphilis à Strasbourg au cours des siècles. In Livet G, Schaff G, ed: Médecine et assistance en Alsace, XVIe–XXe siècle. Strasbourg, Istra, 1976. p. 53–67.
Burgun R see **Basset A**
Burgun R see **Laugier P**
Burhol PG see **Ostensen H**
Burilkova L see **Habrich C**
Burius A: Lings gymnastik och homeopatien. **Nord Medicinhist Arsb** 1980;:99–123
Burka AA see **Kovalev MM**
Burke CB: American collegiate population: a test of the traditional view. New York, London, New York Univ. Press, 1982. ix, 373 p.
Burke G: Disease, labour migration and technological change: the case of the Cornish miners. **Soc Soc Hist Med Bull (Lond)** 1983 Dec;33:37–9
Burke G, Richardson P: The profits of death: a comparative study of miners' phthisis in Cornwall and the Transvaal, 1876–1918. **J South Afr Stud** 1978;4(2):147–71
Burke GW, Shepard FE: Edgar Allan Poe: Richmond's bright star. **Va Dent J** 1980;57(2):12–8
Burke J, Mortelmans J: Rol van België in de strijd tegen de slaapziekte en de dierlijke trypanosomiases en hun studie. **Bull Seances Acad R Sci Outre Mer** 1980 Suppl.;1:111–35
Burke JA: The Dominican nun's school for the deaf and dumb in New South Wales. **J R Aust Hist Soc** 1973;59(4):270–85
Burke JF: Ashley A. Miles and the prevention of infection following surgery. **Arch Surg** 1984 Jan;119(1):17–9
Burke JT: Bref historique de la pharmacovigilance du maléate de perhexiline. **Therapie** 1981 May–Jun;36(3):279–80
Burkhardt C: Euthanasie – 'Vernichtung lebensunwerten Lebens' im Spiegel der Diskussionen zwischen Juristen und Medizinern von 1900 bis 1940. Diss., Johannes-Gutenberg-Universität. Mainz, 1981. 221 p.
Burkhardt FH see **James W**
Burkhardt R, Kienle G: Controlled clinical trials and drug regulations: a report of recent developments in the Federal Republic of Germany. **Controlled Clin Trials** 1980 Sep;1(2):153–66
Burkhardt RW: Closing the door on Lord Morton's mare: the rise and fall of telegony. **Stud Hist Biol** 1979;3:1–21
Burkhardt RW see **Mayr E**
Burkhart LL: The good fight: medicine in colonial Pennsylvania, 1681–1765. Ph.D. Diss., Lehigh University. Bethlehem, 1982. 348 p.
Burkinshaw SM: A look at Kingston General Hospital's archives. **Dimens Health Serv** 1982 Nov;59(11):20–1
Burkitt DP: The discovery of Burkitt's lymphoma. **Cancer** 1983 May 15;51(10):1777–86
Burleigh R, Zivanovic S: Radiocarbon dating of a Cro-Magnon population from Padina, Yugoslavia, with some general recommendations for dating human skeletons. **Z Morphol Anthropol** 1980;70(3):269–74
Burlingame LJ: The history of women in medicine. **Md Hist** 1978;9(2):51–62
Burlingame VS: The family therapy tapestry: a multi-disciplinary history of the family therapy movement in the United States from 1900 to 1957. Ph.D. Diss., Northwestern University. Evanston, 1982. vii, 608 p.
Burmeister KH: Achilles Gasser als Stadtarzt von Feldkirch. **Montfort** 1968;20(3):326–42
Burmeister KJ, Lange-Pfautsch R: Maxim Zetkin--Kommunist und Arzt (1883-1965). **Z Arztl Fortbild (Jena)** 1983;77(16):695–7
Burnby J: House and home for apothecaries and druggists. **Pharm Hist (London)** 1978 Dec;8(3):2–3
Burnby J: Medals for British rhubarb. **Pharm Hist (London)** 1971 Dec;2(3):6–7
Burnby J: Robert Uredale (1642–1722) botanist. **Pharm Hist (London)** 1974 Jul;4(2):4–5
Burnby J: Some provincial apothecaries. **Pharm Hist (London)** 1978 Mar;8(1):5–6,4
Burnby J: The mortar of Charles Angibaud. **Pharm Hist (London)** 1979 Apr;9(1):6–8
Burnby J: The Raggs of Edmonton Green. **Pharm Hist (London)** 1975 Dec;5(3):2–3
Burnby J: The Thomas Fautrart pill tile. **Pharm Hist (London)** 1977 Dec;7(3):6
Burnby J: Three 17th century London apothecaries; Richard Meynell, Charles Needham, William Booker. **Pharm Hist (London)** 1975 May;5(1):2–3
Burnby JG: A study of the English apothecary from 1660 to 1760. London, Wellcome Institute for the History of Medicine, 1983. 128 p. (Medical History, Suppl. no. 3).
Burnby JG: Pharmacy and the cocoa bean. **Pharm Hist (London)** 1984 Jun;14(2):9–12
Burnby JG: Robert Drane: no ordinary pharmacist. **Pharm Hist (London)** 1984 Dec;14(4):3–6
Burnby JG: Some Derbyshire apothecaries. **Pharm Hist (London)** 1970 Dec;1(6):5–8
Burnet M: Biomedical research: changes and opportunities. **Perspect Biol Med** 1981;24:511–24
Burnett CS: The impact of Arabic science on western civilisation in the Middle Ages. **Bull Br Assoc Orient** 1979–80 N.Ser;11:40–51
Burnett J: The Giustiniani medicine chest. **Med Hist** 1982 Jul;26(3):325–33
Burnett JW: Reflections of a dermatology professor. **Cutis** 1984 May;33(5):471–4
Burney LE: Policy over politics. The first statement on smoking and health by the Surgeon General of the United States Public Health Service. **NY State J Med** 1983 Dec;83(13):1252–3
Burnham JC: American medicine's golden age: what happened to it? **Science** 1982 Mar 19;215(4539):1474–9
Burnham JC: Augusta Fox Bronner. In: Notable American women. The modern period. Cambridge, Mass., Belknap-Harvard Univ. Press, 1980. 4:108–10.
Burnham JC: Change in the popularization of health in the United States. **Bull Hist Med** 1984 Summer;58(2):183–97
Burnham JC, McGuire W: Jelliffe: American psychoanalyst and physician & his correspondence with Sigmund Freud and C. G. Jung. Chicago, University of Chicago Press, 1983. xx, 324 p. With contributions by A. R. D'Amore and J. E. Sauer.
Burnham JC: John Broadus Watson. In Dictionary of American Biography, Suppl. 6, 1956–1960. p. 670–3, 1980.
Burnham JC: The acceptance of psychoanalysis in Western cultures: an afterword on its comparative history. **Comp Stud Soc Hist** 1982;24(4):603–10
Burnham JC: The founding of the Archives of Neurology and Psychiatry; or, what was wrong with the Journal of Nervous and Mental disease? **J Hist Med Allied Sci** 1981 Jul;36(3):310–24
Burnham JC: Will medical history join the American mainstream? **Rev Am Hist** 1978;6(1):43–9
Burningham RL: The evolution of the dental office. **Bull Hist Dent** 1980 Apr;28(1):21–8
Burns AK see **Banta HD**
Burns C, Nelson M: Mary Elizabeth Bass. In: Notable American women. The modern period. Cambridge, Mass., Belknap-Harvard Univ. Press, 1980. 4:63–5.
Burns CR: Locating sources in the history of medicine and health care: a guide for students and faculty at UTMB. **Bookman** 1984;11(5):3–9
Burns CR: Medical history and medical humanities: some new styles of learning and teaching. With a commentary by T.L. Savitt. In J. J. Bylebyl, ed: Teaching the history of medicine at a medical center. Baltimore, London, Johns Hopkins University Press, 1982. (The Henry E. Sigerist supplements to the Bulletin of the History of Medicine; new ser., no. 7). p. 31–45.
Burns CR: Richard Cabot and 'The American type' of psychotherapy. In International Congress of the History of Medicine, 27th, Barcelona, 1980. Actas. Barcelona, Académia de Ciències Médiques de Catalunya i Balears, 1981. p. 39–41.
Burns CR see **McCullough LB**
Burns CR see **Numbers RL, ed**
Burns LS: Noise. **Horizon** 1977;20(1):66–9
Burns PE: Log-linear analysis of dental caries occurrence in four skeletal series. **Am J Phys Anthropol** 1979 Nov;51(4):637–47
Burns SB: Early medical photography in America (1839–1883). **NY State J Med** 1980 Aug;80(9):1444–69 (continued regularly)
Burns SB: Early medical photography in America (1839--1883); IV. Early wet-plate era. **NY State J Med** 1979 Nov;79(12):1931–8
Burns SB: Early medical photography in America (1839–1883) V. Beginnings of psychiatric photography. **NY State J Med** 1980 Feb;80(2):270–82

**Burns SB:** Early medical photography in America (1839–1883). VII. American medical publications with photographs. **NY State J Med** 1981 Jul;81(8):1126–64
**Burr GO:** The essential fatty acids fifty years ago. **Prog Lipid Res** 1981;20:xxvii–xxix
**Burri R:** Die Delfter Pest von 1557 nach den Beobachtungen von Petrus Forestus. Zürich, Juris Druck, 1982. III, 219 p. (Zürcher Medizingeschichtliche Abhandlungen, Neue Reihe Nr. 151).
**Burridge J** see **Taylor PJ**
**Burrow GN, Hazlett BE, Phillips MJ:** A case of diabetes mellitus. **N Engl J Med** 1982 Feb 11;306(6):340–3
**Burrow JG:** [History of] organized medicine. In Reich WT, et al, ed: Encyclopedia of bioethics, v.3. New York, Free Press, 1978. p. 1034–42.
**Burrows A, Schumacher I:** Doktor Diamonds Bildnisse von Geisteskranken. Transl. of Doctor Diamond's portraits of the insane. Frankfurt am Main, Syndikat, 1979. 159 p.
**Burrows GE:** Lead toxicosis in domestic animals: a review of the role of lead mining and primary lead smelters in the United States. **Vet Hum Toxicol** 1981 Oct;23(5):337–43
**Burrus O:** Les aventures d'un curiste..de Napoléon III à la Belle Epoque. **Rev Infirm** 1982 Mar;32(6):26–8
**Burst HV:** The influence of consumers on the birthing movement. **Top Clin Nurs** 1983 Oct;5(3):42–54
**Burstein SS:** Prepaid health care in the United States. **IMJ** 1981 Aug;160(2):83–5
**Burstyn HL** see **Rice AL**
**Burt BA:** The epidemiological basis for water fluoridation in the prevention of dental caries. **J Public Health Policy** 1982 Dec;3(4):391–407
**Burton N** see **Day M**
**Bury C:** Workers' health protection as an issue of industrial hygiene and occupational medical science in the early Kaiserreich (1871–84). **Soc Soc Hist Med Bull (Lond)** 1983 Dec;33:34–6
**Busacchi V:** Marcello Malpighi (1628–1694), lettore a Bologna, Pisa e Messina, archiatra pontificio. **Strenna Stor Bolognese** 1978;28:81–98
**Buscaglia M** see **Vidal F**
**Buscaino GA, Guadagnino M:** Ulteriore contributo a 'orientamenti teorici e pratici della psichiatria italiana'. Dal 1950 al 1976. **Acta Neurol [Quad]** 1978;37:131–59
**Buscaino GA** see **Guadagnino M**
**Busch C** see **Edwards G**
**Buschauer W:** Homöopathie als Vollendung der Hippokratischen Medizin. Heidelberg, Haug, 1982. Historical sections, p. 9–79.
**Buser BN:** The evolution of school health services: New York and nationwide. **J Sch Health** 1980 Oct;50(8):475–7
**Bush LE:** Mormon 'physiology' 1850–1875. **Bull Hist Med** 1982 Summer;56(2):218–37
**Bush LE:** The word of wisdom in early nineteenth-century perspective. **Dialogue J Mormon Thought** 1981;14(3):46–65
**Bush RB:** Max Thorek. In Dictionary of American Biography, Suppl. 6, 1956–1960. p. 631–2, 1980.
**Bush RB:** Philadelphia surgeon - lithotomists 1750–1810. Their training, their practice and their teaching. In: Congrès international d'histoire de la médecine, XXVe, Québec, 1976. Actes. Québec, 1977. p. 522–36.
**Bushnell OA:** 'Our good friend Mr. Stevenson'. **Biography** 1982;5(2):118–28
**El-Bushra ES:** Some demographic indicators for Khartoum Conurbation, Sudan. **Middle East Stud** 1979;15(3):295–309
**Büsing W:** Bedeutende Apotheker aus fünf Jahrhunderten im Weser-Ems-Raum. **Dtsch Apoth Ztg** 1979 Nov 22;119(47):1913–9
**Buslaeva MM, Volodina MN:** Pervaia Mezhdunarodnia konferentsiia po izucheniiu raka (k 75-letiiu so dnia provedeniia). **Vopr Onkol** 1981;27(11):90–2
**Buslaeva MM** see **Puchkov IuG**
**Busnardo AC, DiDio LJ, Tidrick RT, et al:** History of the pancreas. **Am J Surg** 1983 Nov;146(5):539–50
**Busó R:** Fundación de Investigaciones Clínicas. (Pro Deus, patriae eus scientia). **Bol Asoc Med PR** 1983 Nov;75(11):500
**Buss FL:** La partera, story of a midwife. Ann Arbor, University of Michigan Press, 1980. viii, 137 p.
**Bussarsky VA** see **Petrov P**
**Busse H:** Christoph Wilhelm Hufeland: der berühmte Arzt der Goethezeit, Leibarzt der Königin Luise. St. Michael, Bläschke, 1982. 334 p.
**Busse H, Hollwich F, Jünemann G:** Plastische und rekonstruktive Chirurgie der Tränenwege. **Ber Zusammenkunft Dtsch Ophthalmol Ges** 1979;(77):111–21
**Bustamante M:** Nicolás Achúcarro: el hombre y su obra. **Arch Neurobiol (Madr)** 1982 Jan–Feb;45(1):55–72
**Bustamante ME:** Hechos sobresalientes en la historia de la Secretaría de Salubridad y Asistencia. **Salud Publica Mex** 1983 Sep–Oct;25(5):465–82
**Bustamante ME:** Historia de la Secretaría de Salubridad y Asistencia. **Salud Publica Mex** 1983 Sep–Oct;25(5):461–4
**Bustamante ME:** La coordinación de los servicios sanitarios federales y locales como factor de progreso higiénico en México. Su evolución y desarrollo de 1934 a 1964. In Academia Nacional de Medicina. Libro conmemorativo del primer centenario. México, Comité Editorial de la Comisión Organizadora del Congreso del Centenario, 1964. Tome 2. p. 652–64.
**Bustamante ME:** La medicina preventiva. In Academia Nacional de Medicina. Libro conmemorativo del primer centenario. México, Comité Editorial de la Comisión Organizadora del Congreso del Centenario, 1964. Tome 2. p. 640–2.
**Bustamante ME:** La necesidad para los historiadores de saber leer y de poder leer. **Bol Soc Mex Hist Filos Med** 1979 Dec;4(29):141–52
**Bustamante ME:** Supervivencia y muerte de los Jesuitas de la Provincia de Mexico entre 1767 y 1820. **Bol Soc Mex Hist Filos Med** 1983;6(45):235–63
**Bustamante O'Leary J:** La Academia de Ciencias Médicas, Físicas y Naturales de la Habana. **Conf Estud Hist Organ Cienc** 1979;11:1–19
**Bustamente ME:** La primera enfermera en la historia de la salud pública, Isabel Cendala y Gómez. **Rev Col Nac Enferm** 1980 Jul, 1981 Feb;27–28(107):7–12
**Busvine JR:** The evolution and mutual adaptation of insects, microorganisms and man. In Stanley NF, Joske RA, ed: Changing disease patterns and human behaviour. London, New York, Academic Press, 1980. p. 55–68.
**Butcher HR:** Evarts Graham and surgical residency education. **J Thorac Cardiovasc Surg** 1984 Nov;88(5 Pt 2):848–50
**Butcher HR:** What's past is prologue. **Arch Surg** 1980 Apr;115(4):371–6
**Butenandt O:** Pädiatrie vor 100 Jahren. Aus Berichten des 'Jahrbuches für Kinderheilkunde', Band 18, 1882. **Fortschr Med** 1983 Feb 17;101(7):251–4
**Butenandt O:** 100 Jahre Endokrinologie. **Fortschr Med** 1982 Dec 16;100(47–48):2194–8
**Butkus DE:** Post-traumatic acute renal failure in combat casualties: a historical review. **Milit Med** 1984 Mar;149(3):117–24
**Butler J:** Mediaeval midwifery. **Nurs Times** 1981 Oct 7–13;77(41):1762–3
**Butler JR, Boddy FA:** The evolution of health services research in Britain. **Community Med** 1983 Aug;5(3):192–9
**Butler M** see **Hirschman C**
**Butler RA:** Basic science researcher in otolaryngology at the University of Chicago. **Ann Otol Rhinol Laryngol [Suppl]** 1983 Jan–Feb;102:27–9
**Butler RA** see **Mhoon EE**
**Butler SV:** From physician to scientist: changing styles of thought in late Victorian physiology. **Soc Soc Hist Med Bull (Lond)** 1980 Jun;26:7–10
**Butler SV** see **Pickstone JV**
**Butler T:** Plague and other Yersinia infections. New York, London, Plenum Medical Book Co., 1983. xii, 220 p. (Current Topics in Infectious Disease).
**Butsevitskiĭ VS** see **Alekseev GA**
**Butterfield LJ** see **Smith GF**
**Butterfield LH, ed** see **Bell WJ**
**Buttermann G:** Lungenszintigraphie. Entwicklung, gegenwärtiger Stand und Zukunftsperspektiven. **Fortschr Med** 1983 Mar 17;101(10):403–8
**Butterworth VE:** The girls in white. Independence, Mo., Herald Publishing House, 1979. 176 p.
**Buttet H de:** Les Invalides en 1709. In: Congrès National des Sociétés Savantes, 97e, Nantes, 1972. Actes. Paris, 1977. Histoire Moderne et Contemporaine, Tome 1. p. 55–65.
**Büttner J:** Evolution of clinical enzymology. **J Clin Chem Clin Biochem** 1981 Aug;19(8):529–38
**Büttner J:** From chemistry of life to chemistry of disease: the rise of clinical biochemistry. **Clin Biochem** 1980 Oct;13(5):232–5
**Büttner J:** Interrelationships between clinical medicine and clinical chemistry, illustrated by the example of the German-speaking countries in the late 19th century. **J Clin Chem Clin Biochem** 1982 Jun;20(6):465–71
**Büttner L, Meyer B:** Karl Marx und die Begründung der Gesundheitspolitik der revolutionären Arbeiterbewegung I. Vormarxistische Kritik der bürgerlichen Gesundheitspolitik. **Z Arztl Fortbild (Jena)** 1983;77(17):743–8
**Büttner L, Meyer B:** Karl Marx und die Begründung der Gesundheitspolitik der revolutionären Arbeiterbewegung. II. Marx' Aufdeckung des Klasseninhalts der bürgerlichen Gesundheitspolitik. **Z Arztl Fortbild (Jena)** 1983;77(19):819–23
**Büttner L, Meyer B:** Zur Herausbildung und Entwicklung der Gesundheitspolitik der SED nach 1945. **Wiss Z Martin Luther Univ (Math)** 1975;24(3):5–14
**Büttner J, ed:** History of clinical chemistry. Berlin, New York, Walter de Gruyter, 1983. 91 p. Various reprints from the Journal of Clinical Chemistry and Clinical Biochemistry. Contributions by N. Mani, J.S. Fruton, E. Hickel, H.H. Simmer, W.T. Caraway.
**Butts HF:** Frantz Fanon's contribution to psychiatry: the psychology of racism and colonialism. **J Natl Med Assoc** 1979 Oct;71(10):1015–8
**Buus S, Florentine M, Redden RB:** The SISI test: a review. Part I. **Audiology** 1982;21(4):273–93
**Buyssens E** see **Riese W**
**Buzinkay G:** Az egyetemi nyomda és orvosi-természettudományos szakirodalmunk kialakulása. **Magy Konyvsz** 1977;93(1):25–37
**Buzsàki G:** Situational conditional reflexes. Physiologic studies of the higher nervous activity of freely moving animals: P. S. Kupalov. **Pavlov J Biol Sci** 1983 Jan–Mar;18(1):13–21
**BVA centenary:** One hundred years of farm animal practice. **Vet Rec** 1982 Jun 26;110(26):596–612
**Byard PJ:** Population history, demography, and genetics of the St. Lawrence Island Eskimos. Ph.D. Diss., University of Kansas. Lawrence, 1981. v, 143 leaves.
**Bychkovskiĭ AV** see **Borisova MA**
**Bye Ba Rin Bsrel:** Instructions of the great Zur-mkhar Mñam-ñid-rdo-rje on medical treatment comprising the Ma yig, Bu yig, and Kha 'thor collections. (Tib) Reproduced from a print from the Tsharon Sman-dgon blocks. Leh, Ladakh, Tashigangpa, 1974. np (Smanrtsis Shesrig Spendzod, Vol. 58).
**Byers E:** Fertility transition in a New England commercial center: Nantucket, Massachusetts, 1680–1840. **J Interdiscip Hist** 1982;13(1):17–40

**Bykhovskaia-Pavlovskaia IE:** Istoriia otkrytiia Sharlem Nikollem puti zarazheniia sypnym tifom. **Parassitologia** 1981 Jan-Feb;15(1):87-91

**Bykov GV, Trifonov DN:** Issledovaniia po istorii khimii. **Vopr Istor Estestvozn Tekh** 1981;2:33-8

**Byl S:** Note sur huit recentiores du livre IV Du régime. **Rev Philol (Paris)** 1978;52:37-49

**Byl S** see **Grmek MD, ed**

**Bylebyl J** see **Ebbert A, et al**

**Bylebyl JJ:** Boyle and Harvey on the valves in the veins. **Bull Hist Med** 1982 Fall;56(3):351-67

**Bylebyl JJ:** The growth of Harvey's De Motu Cordis. **Bull Hist Med** 1973 Sep-Oct;47(5):427-70

**Bylebyl JJ** see **Premuda L**

**Bylebyl JJ** see **Webster C, ed**

**Bylebyl JJ, ed:** Teaching the history of medicine at a medical center. Baltimore, London, Johns Hopkins University Press, 1982. 162 p. (The Henry E. Sigerist supplements to the Bulletin of the History of Medicine; new ser., no. 7).

**Bylebyl JJ, ed:** William Harvey and his age: the professional and social context of the discovery of the circulation. Baltimore, Johns Hopkins University Press, 1979. xii, 154 p. (Henry E. Sigerist Supplements to the Bulletin of the History of Medicine, n.s., 2). Includes contributions by S. Jarcho, C. Webster, R. G. Frank.

**Bynum WF:** Alcoholism and degeneration in 19th century European medicine and psychiatry. **Br J Addict** 1984 Mar;79(1):59-70

**Bynum WF:** Darwin and the doctors: evolution, diathesis, and germs in 19th-century Britain. **Gesnerus** 1983;40(1-2):43-53

**Bynum WF, Browne EJ, Porter R, ed:** Dictionary of the history of science. Princeton, Princeton University Press, 1981. [xxxiv], 494 p.

**Bynum WF:** Health, disease and medical care. In G. S. Rousseau, R. Porter, ed. The ferment of knowledge. Studies in the historiography of eighteenth-century science. Cambridge, Cambridge University Press, 1980. p. 211-53.

**Bynum WF:** Themes in British psychiatry, J. C. Prichard (1786-1848) to Henry Maudsley (1835-1918). With comments by S. Poggi. In M. Ruse, ed: Nature animated. Historical and philosophical case studies in Greek medicine, nineteenth-century and recent biology, psychiatry, and psychoanalysis. Volume II. Dordrecht, D. Reidel, 1983. p. 225-66.

**Bynum WF:** Theory and practice in British psychiatry from J. C. Prichard (1785-1848) to Henry Maudsley (1835-1918). **Nihon I-Shigaku Zasshi** 1981;27(1):94-73

**Bynum WF** see **Scull A, ed**

**Bynum WF, ed** see **Rose FC**

**Byre CS** see **Mullner R**

**Byrne E:** Historical and current concepts in mitochondrial myopathies. **Aust NZ J Med** 1983 Jun;13(3):299-305

**Byrne JJ:** Lengthening shadows. **N Engl J Med** 1981 Oct 29;305(18):1051-9

**Byrne R:** Keynote address--50th anniversary BPA meeting, Boston, Massachusetts. **J Biol Photogr** 1981 Apr;49(2):39-44

**Byrnes DP:** Perspectives in international neurosurgery: neurosurgery in Ireland. **Neurosurgery** 1983 May;12(5):585-8

**Bystryn MH** see **Greenberg DF**

**Bywaters EG:** Historical aspects of ankylosing spondylitis. **Rheumatol Rehabil** 1979 Nov;18(4):197-203

**Bywaters EG:** Historical perspectives in the aetiology of ankylosing spondylitis. **Br J Rheumatol** 1983 Nov;22(4 Suppl 2):1-4

# C

**C[one] TE:** A plea to give weakly children a fair chance, by William Farr (1865). **Pediatrics** 1981;68:49

**C[one] TE:** Early viability of the fetus - an extraordinary case (1845). **Pediatrics** 1981;67:903

**C[one] TE:** Jeremy Bentham's list of data needed to understand the growth and development of children (1797). **Pediatrics** 1981;68:447

**C[one] TE:** Mrs. Nathaniel Hawthorne's invalidism, until her marriage at age 31, was attributed to difficult teething in infancy. **Pediatrics** 1981;67:606

**C[one] TE:** On the proper treatment of infants according to David Ramsay of South Carolina (1790). **Pediatrics** 1981;68:353

**C[one] TE:** The appalling industrial hazards to which American working children were exposed in 1900. **Pediatrics** 1981;68:378

**C[one] TE:** William Douglass on the first reported cases of scarlet fever in New England, 1736. **Pediatrics** 1981;68:230

**Cabal Gonzalez M:** Historia de los boticarios de Oviedo en el siglo XIX. Oviedo, Instituto de Estudios Asturianos, 1979. 107 p.

**Caballero O:** De milagros, medicina onírica y curanderos. **Rev Enferm** 1982 Sep;5(50):64-6

**Caban J:** Znaczenie badań nad tężcem J. K. Kostrzewskiego po dwudziestu latach. **Przegl Epidemiol** 1980;34(2):191-2

**Cabanne F, Gérard-Marchant R, Destaing F:** Geschichte des Krebses. In Sournia JC, Martiny M, Poulet J, ed: Illustrierte Geschichte der Medizin. Salzburg, Andreas, 1980. Vol. 8. p. 2849-79.

**Cabanne F:** Pierre Masson. Précurseur et rénovateur (1880-1959). **Ann Pathol** 1983;3(1):95-7

**Cabarrocas Gafarot E** see **Miguel Martínez J**

**Cabello de la Torre P:** El herbario medico medieval Macer Floridus en la medicina de la baja edad media. **Asclepio** 1978-79;30-31:157-65

**Cabieses F** see **Bowers JZ**

**Cabieses F** see **Canalis RF**

**Cabourdin G:** Introduction aux problèmes de la démographie de la période 1500-1670. **Ann Demogr Hist (Paris)** 1980;:13-8

**Cabrillana N:** Repoblación y despoblación en Almería (1572-1599). **Rev Arch Bibl Mus** 1977;80(4):703-29

**Caccialanza E:** Il problema delle cranioplastiche dal punto di vista storico ed etio-patogenetico. **Minerva Chir** 1983 Jun 30;38(12):815-8

**Caceres B:** La coca, el mundo andino y los extirpadores de idolatrías de siglo XX. **Am Indig** 1978;38(4):769-85

**Cachinero Sánchez B:** El modelo europeo de matrimonio, evolucion, determinantes y consecuencias. **Rev Esp Invest Sociol** 1981;15:33-58

**Cadden J:** A matter of life and death: water in the natural philosophy of Albertus Magnus. **Hist Philos Life Sci** 1980;2(2):241-52

**Cadden J:** Albertus Magnus' universal physiology: the example of nutrition. In Weisheipl JA, ed: Albertus Magnus and the sciences. Toronto, Pontifical Institute of Mediaeval Studies, 1980. 321-39.

**Cadden J:** The medieval philosophy and biology of growth: Albertus Magnus, Thomas Aquinas, Albert of Saxony and Masilius of Inghen on Book I, Chapter V, of Aristotle's 'De generatione et corruptione.' With translated texts of Albertus Magnus and Thomas Aquinas. Ph. D. Diss. Indiana University. Bloomington, 1971. vii, 267 leaves.

**Cade JF:** Mending the mind. A short history of twentieth-century psychiatry. Melbourne, Sun Books, 1979. 108 p.

**Cadmus RR:** Intensive care reaches silver anniversary. **Hospitals** 1980 Jan 16;54(2):98-102

**Cadotte M:** A propos de la description par Jacques Cartier d'une 'grosse maladie' survenue au cours de son deuxième voyage au Canada. **Union Med Can** 1984 Aug;113(8):651-5

**Cadotte M:** Historique du laboratoire de pathologie de l'Hôtel-Dieu de Montréal: de sa création en 1896, à l'arrivée du professeur Pierre Masson en 1928. **Union Med Can** 1979 May;108(5):479-94

**Cadotte M, Lessard R:** Jean-Baptiste Rieutord. In Dictionary of Canadian biography, 1801 to 1820. Volume 5, 1983. p. 712-3.

**Cadotte M:** L'héritage scientifique du professeur Pierre Masson. **Union Med Can** 1984 May;113(5):344-5

**Cady B, Sedgwick CE:** History of thyroid and parathyroid surgery. **Major Probl Clin Surg** 1980;15:1-5

**Caen JP:** A propos du hasard et de la nécessité: la découverte du facteur Fletcher (prékallikréine). **Nouv Rev Fr Hematol** 1981 Dec;23(5):309-10

**Caen JP:** Heparin: a 70 year history from 1914 to 1984. **Nouv Rev Fr Hematol** 1984;26(4):209-10

**Caffaratto A:** Storia della legislazione sanitaria ed igienica in Piemonte da Amedeo VIII all'Unità d'Italia. Parte I. **Minerva Med** 1979 Nov 3;70(48):3315-21 (contd)

**Caffaratto A:** Storia della legislazione sanitaria ed igienica in Piemonte da Amedeo VIII all'Unità d'Italia. Parte II, III. **Minerva Med** 1979;70(51,54):3511-23, 3729-34 (continued)

**Caffaratto A:** Storia della legislazione sanitaria ed igienica in Piemonte da Amedeo VIII all'Unità d'Italia. Parte III. **Minerva Med** 1979 Dec 1;70(54):3729-43

**Caffaratto AT:** La raccolta di fotografie segnaletiche del Museo di Antropologia Criminale di Torino: la fotografia come documento e testimonianza dell'opera di Cesare Lombroso. **Ann Osp Maria Vittoria Torino** 1980 Jul-Dec;23(7-12):295-332

**Caffaratto TM:** Aspetti medico-sociali delle malattie dei lavoratori piemontesi della terra, nella seconda metà del secolo XIX. **Minerva Med** 1984 Apr;75(14-15):842-51; (17):999-1012; (18):1079-88

**Caffaratto TM:** Breve storia delle ostetriche. **Minerva Ginecol** 1981 Sep;33(9):867-80

**Caffaratto TM:** Dalle origini. **Minerva Ginecol** 1984 Sep;36(9):541-66

**Caffaratto TM:** Elogio dell'olio medicinale. **Minerva Med** 1983 Mar 31;74(13):747-55

**Caffaratto TM:** Fantasia e realtà nella storia della medicina. Il diavolo, la strega, il medico. **Minerva Med** 1981 Oct 32;72(42):2837-5

**Caffaratto TM:** Il Libro Lunghetto, ricettario del '600 dell'Ospedale Mauriziano di Torino. **Minerva Med** 1980 Apr 2;71(13):981-7

**Caffaratto TM:** La più grande nemica del genere umano: la peste. **Minerva Ginecol** 1980 Oct;32(10):945-7

**Caffaratto TM:** Le antiche radici della riforma sanitaria. **Minerva Med** 1982 Jun 30;73(27):1905-16

**Caffaratto TM:** Moda e medicina. **Minerva Ginecol** 1980 Sep;32(9):843-6

**Caffaratto TM:** Rilettura e commento dell'opera 'De Mulierum passionibus' di Trotula de Ruggiero, o Trocta Salernitana. **Minerva Med** 1981 Nov 17;72(46):3123-31

**Caffaratto TM:** Storia dell'Ospedale Maggiore di Torino della Religione ed Ordine dei SS. Maurizio e Lazzaro--dal secolo XVI al secolo XX. **Ann Osp Maria Vittoria Torino** 1979 Jul-Dec;22(7-12):365-419

**Caffaratto TM:** Storia dell'Ospedale Mauriziano di Lanzo. **Ann Osp Maria Vittoria Torino** 1982 Jan-Jun;25(1-6):97-148

**Caffaratto TM:** Una pagina di storia per l'herpes progenitalis. **Minerva Med** 1984 May 7;75(19):1159-61

**Cafiso, LM:** Storia della teoria sulla generazione spontanea: Redi, Spallanzani, Pasteur. **Cult Sc** 1981;20(80):236-43

**Cahall JB:** The history of occupational health nursing. **Occup Health Nurs** 1981 Oct;29(10):11-3

**Cahill LS:** Within shouting distance: Paul Ramsey and Richard McCormick on method. **J Med Philos** 1979 Dec;4(4):398-417

**Cahn JD:** A doctor's legacy: Dr. John E. T. Camper and the MeDeSo. **J Natl Med Assoc** 1980 Mar;72(3):283-7

**Cahn LR:** Some notes on Sir Jonathan Hutchinson (1828-1913). **Am J Surg Pathol** 1979 Dec;3(6):563-6

**Cahow CR:** People, patients and politics: the history of the North Carolina mental hospitals, 1848-1960. New York, Arno Press, 1980. vii, 254 p

(Ph.D. Diss., Duke University, 1967).
**Cain AJ:** Zoological ideas 1831-1981. **Nature** 1981 Sep 3;293(5827):15-6
**Cain JR** see **Alliez J**
**Cain LP:** An economic history of urban location and sanitation. **Res Econ Hist** 1977;2:337-89
**Cain LP:** Child abuse: historical precedent and legal ramifications. **Health Soc Work** 1980 Aug;5(3):61-7
**Cain LP:** Sanitation strategy for a lakefront metropolis. The case of Chicago. DeKalb, Northern Illinois University Press, 1978. xv, 173 p.
**Cain LP:** The creation of Chicago's sanitary district and construction of the Sanitary and Ship Canal. **Chic Hist** 1979;8(2):98-110
**Cain AM, ed:** A catalog of the Percival Bailey collection of neurology & psychiatry. Chicago, Library of the Health Sciences, University of Illinois at the Medical Center, Chicago, 1973. viii, 230 p.
**Caire JB:** A holographic model of a psychosomatic pattern: Freud's specimen dream re-interpreted. **Psychother Psychosom** 1981;36(2):132-42
**Cairns RB** see **Hearst E, ed**
**Caissie F:** Joseph-Godric Blanchet. In Dictionary of Canadian biography, 1881-1890. 1982;11:85-6.
**Cajal N:** 1949-1984: 35 years devoted to the study of viruses in the 'Stefan S. Nicolau' Institute of Virology. **Virologie** 1984 Oct-Dec;35(4):247-50
**Calabrese MC:** La politica di planificazione familiare in Egitto fino al 1977. **Oriente Mod** 1978;58(1-3):97-107
**Calabuig J** see **Barba J**
**Calagan JL:** The conjoined twins born near Worms, 1495. **J Hist Med Allied Sci** 1983 Oct;38(4):450-1
**Calame A:** Etre prématuré: hier, aujourd'hui, demain. **Rev Med Suisse Romande** 1983 Apr;103(4):319-31
**Calatrava Páramo DL:** La boca en lo social, la salud, la enfermedad y lo legal. **An R Acad Nac Med (Madr)** 1982;99(1):91-108
**Calatrava Páramo L:** La llamada enfermedad de los Habsburgo: datos históricos, su tratamiento actual y resultados. **An R Acad Nac Med (Madr)** 1979;96(4):557-74
**Calciu M:** La 125 de ani de la naşterea lui V. Babes (1854-1979). contribuţiile lui Victor Babes la edificarea ftiziologiei ştiinţifice. **Rev Ig [Pneumoftiziol]** 1979 Jul-Sep;28(3):187-91
**Calcoen R:** George Sarton. **Handel Maatsch Geschied Oudheidk Gent** 1980;N.R.,34:181-91
**Calcraft LG:** Aldous Huxley and the Sheldonian hypothesis. **Ann Sci** 1980 Nov;37(6):657-71
**Caldamone AA:** Theodor Billroth: the urologist. **Urology** 1981 Sep;18(3):316-24
**Calder A** see **Pretty GL**
**Caldera R** see **Sociedad Venezolana de Historia de la medicina**
**Caldwell GG, Kelley D, Zack M, et al:** Mortality and cancer frequency among military nuclear test (Smoky) participants, 1957 through 1979. **JAMA** 1983 Aug 5;250(5):620-4
**Caldwell JC:** The mechanisms of demographic change in historical perspective. **Popul Stud** 1981 Mar;35(1):5-27
**Caldwell JC, Reddy PH, Caldwell P:** The social component of mortality decline: an investigation in South India employing alternative methodologies. **Popul Stud** 1983 Jul;37(2):185-205
**Caldwell JR** see **Morse D**
**Caldwell P** see **Caldwell JC**
**Calhoun D:** On the psychohistory of childhood. **Hist Educ Q** 1974;14(3):371-7
**Callaghan JC:** Early experiences in the study and development of an artificial electrical pacemaker for standstill of the heart: view from 1949. **PACE** 1980 Sep;3(5):618-9
**Callahan JA, Key JD, Keys TE:** Sir Thomas Lewis: the centennial of a medical human dynamo. **Mayo Clin Proc** 1981 Dec;56(12):749-52
**Callahan JA** see **Key JD**
**Callan CM:** A leader in psychiatry--Carol Nadelson, M.D. **Conn Med** 1981 Aug;45(8):491-2
**Callaway JL:** Saga of a North Carolina dermatologist. An autobiographical experience. **J Am Acad Dermatol** 1980 Nov;3(5):544-50
**Callery BG:** Ancients, moderns and reliable friends: stated sources of some English herbals. **J Soc Bibliogr Nat Hist** 1978;8(4):435-44
**Callmer C:** Tre bilder av grekiska läkare. **Sydsven Medicinhist Sallsk Arsskr** 1981;:30-8
**Callmer C:** Ur arkiater-titelns historia. **Sydsven Medicinhist Sallsk Arsskr** 1980;:40-80
**Calmes SH:** Virginia Apgar: a woman physician's career in a developing specialty. **J Am Med Wom Assoc** 1984 Nov-Dec;39(6):184-8
**Calmy C:** La sexualité au XIXe siècle: entretien avec Alain Corbin. **Histoire** 1979;12:80-2
**Calne RY:** The development of immunosuppressive therapy. **Transplant Proc** 1981 Mar;13(1):44-9
**Calo AA:** Notes on a bygone practice in a North African country. **J Med Soc NJ** 1981 Aug;78(9):606-10
**Calogirou DK:** L'Asclêpieion de Cos, Hippocrate et la maladie des coronaires. **Hist Sci Med** 1979;13(4):427-39
**Calot G:** Données comparées sur l'évolution de la fécondité selon le rang de naissance en Allemagne Fédérale et en France (1950-1977). **Population** 1979;34(Special):1291-347
**Calot G:** Le mouvement journalier des naissances à l'intèrieur de la semaine. **Population** 1981;36(3):477-504
**Calot G:** L'observation de la fécondité à court et moyen terme. **Population** 1981;36(1):9-40
**Calot G, Blayo C:** Recent course of fertility in Western Europe. **Popul Stud** 1982 Nov;36(3):349-72
**Calton S:** Nursing past, present and future: keeping pace with the times. **Nurs Mirror** 1980 Jan 31;150(5):36-7
**Calvi G:** L'oro, il fuoco, le forche: la peste napoletana del 1656. **Arch Stor Ital** 1981;139(3):405-58
**Calwell HG:** Care of sick children in Belfast in the nineteenth century. **J R Soc Med** 1979 Sep;72(9):706-8
**Calwell HG:** W. J. Wilson and the Weil-Felix reaction. **Ulster Med J** 1980;49:169-70
**Cambiano G** see **Grmek MD, ed**
**Cambier J:** De la mort de Louis XV à la vaccination du roi de Rome. **Nouv Presse Med** 1980 Jun 7;9(25):1746
**Cambier J:** Le syndrome de Déjerine-Roussy. **Rev Neurol (Paris)** 1982;138(12):979-88
**Cambrosio A:** Quand la psychologie fait son entrée à l'usine: sélection et contrôle des ouvriers aux Etats-Unis pendant les années 1910. **Mouvement Soc** 1980;113:37-65
**Cambrosio A, Keating P:** The disciplinary stake: the case of chronobiology. **Soc Stud Sci** 1983 Aug;13(3):323-53
**Camelin A:** Considérations biographiques sur Alphonse Laveran (1845-1922). **Hist Sci Med** 1980;14:377-82
**Camerino G, Darbon P, Graber E, et al:** I manoscritti medici della Osterreichische Nationalbibliothek di Vienna. **Kos** 1984 Mar;1(2):12-9
**Cameron D, Jones IG:** John Snow, the broad street pump and modern epidemiology. **Int J Epidemiol** 1983 Dec;12(4):393-6
**Cameron JE:** The Tallapoosa County Medical Society. **J Med Assoc State Ala** 1982 Jul;52(1):20-3
**Cameron JM:** The medico-legal expert--past, present and future. **Med Sci Law** 1980 Jan;20(1):3-13
**Cameron N:** Ceremony of presentation of diplomates. **Ann R Coll Surg Engl** 1981 Nov;63(6):447-9
**Cameron N:** The growth of London schoolchildren 1904-1966: an analysis of secular trend and intra-county variation. **Ann Hum Biol** 1979 Nov-Dec;6(6):505-25
**Cameron S, Falk LA:** Some black medical history: Dr. Martin R. Delany's Canadian years as medical practitioner and abolitionist (1856-1864). In: Congrès international d'histoire de la médecine, XXVe, Québec, 1976. Actes. Québec, 1977. p. 537-45.
**Camisa C** see **Weissmann A**
**Camp FR:** Forensic serology in the United States. I. Blood grouping and blood transfusion--historical aspects. **Am J Forensic Med Pathol** 1980 Mar;1(1):47-55
**Camp J:** One hundred years of medical murder. London, Bodley Head, 1982. 221 p.
**Campan L:** A propos du centenaire de la mort de Charles Thomas Jackson (1805-1880). **Ann Anesthesiol Fr** 1981;22(1):3-7
**Campan L:** Le tricentenaire de Morgagni (1682-1721). **Agressologie** 1982;23(7):291-2
**Campan L:** Naissance, vie, mort et survie de la cocaïne. **Agressologie** 1979;20(3):135-47
**Campan L** see **Lazorthes G**
**Campbell A:** Some general questions about movable elements and their implications. **Cold Spring Harbor Symp Quant Biol** 1980;45(1):1-9
**Campbell BJ:** Springhill's first doctor. **NS Hist Q** 1979;9(4):297-312
**Campbell C** see **Bullough V**
**Campbell DB** see **Mishler W**
**Campbell DT:** On the conflicts between biological and social evolution and between psychology and moral tradition. **Zygon** 1976;11:167-208
**Campbell EK:** Beyond anthropocentrism. **J Hist Behav Sci** 1983 Jan;19(1):54-67
**Campbell H:** Mary Lambie: a biography. Wellington, New Zealand Nursing Education and Research Foundation, 1976. x, 100 p.
**Campbell J:** Smallpox in aboriginal Australia, 1829-31. **Hist Stud** 1983;20:536-56
**Campbell JM:** Dentistry then and now. Revised and enlarged Third edition of From a trade to a profession. [S.l. : s.n.], 1981 (Glasgow: Bell & Bain). xvi, 395 p.
**Campbell M:** Mendel's theory: its context and plausibility. **Centaurus** 1982;26(1):38-69
**Campbell M:** The concepts of dormancy, latency, and dominance in nineteenth-century biology. **J Hist Biol** 1983 Fall;16(3):409-31
**Campbell N, Smellie RM:** The Royal Society of Edinburgh (1783-1983). The first two hundred years. Edinburgh, The Society, 1983. xvi, 186 p.
**Campbell P:** Medical education for an African colonist. **Md Hist Mag** 1970;65(2):130-7
**Campbell R:** Sir David Brewster (1781-1868). Edinburgh, History of Medicine and Science Unit, University of Edinburgh, [1982?] [12] p.
**Campbell RJ:** Flashbacks: scenes from psychiatry's revolutions. **Bull NY Acad Med** 1984 Jun;60(5):479-93
**Campbell WA:** Joseph Priestley's soda water. **Endeavour** 1983;7(3):141-3
**Campbell WA:** Library resources for the history of science in Newcastle upon Tyne. **Br J Hist Sci** 1982 Nov;15(51 pt 3):281-4
**Campbell WA:** Oxalic acid, epsom salt and the poison bottle. **Hum Toxicol** 1982 Mar;1(2):187-93
**Campbell WC:** History of trichinosis: Paget, Owen and the discovery of Trichinella Spiralis. **Bull Hist Med** 1979 Winter;53(4):520-52
**Campeau L:** Jeanne-Françoise Juchereau de la Ferté. In Dictionary of Canadian biography, 1701 to 1740. Volume 2, 1969. p. 302-3.
**Campenhausen C von** see **Mann G, ed**
**Campiglio L:** La dinamica degli infortuni sul lavoro nel periodo 1951-1970. **Riv Int Sci Sociali** 1973;81(1-2):134-65

Campillo D, Viñas R: Contribución a la paleopatología a través del arte rupestre. In International Congress of the History of Medicine, 27th, Barcelona, 1980. Actas. Barcelona, Académia de Ciències Médiques de Catalunya i Balears, 1981. p. 462–71.
Campillo D, Turbón D: Cráneo trepanado de la Bauma dels Ossos. In International Congress of the History of Medicine, 27th, Barcelona, 1980. Actas. Barcelona, Académia de Ciències Médiques de Catalunya i Balears, 1981. p. 472–9.
Campillo D: Estudio etiopatogenico de la lesion encontrada en un craneo procedente del Yacimiento Talayotico de cales coves en Menorca (146, L. P.). Asclepio 1980;32:77–85
Campillo D: Los traumatismos en la prehistoria y en los tiempos antiguos. Med Hist (Barc) 1984;2:1–16
Campillo D: Malformacion vertebral en un individuo perteneciente a la cultura Talayotica Menorquina (L. P. 147). Asclepio 1980;32:65–76
Campillo D: Neurosurgical pathology in prehistory. Acta Neurochir (Wien) 1984;70(3–4):275–90
Campillo D: Paleopatologia del craneo en Cataluña, Valencia y Baleares. Barcelona, Editorial Montblanc-Martin, 1977. 630 p.
Campillo D see Vives E
Campillo-Sainz C, Xirau R, Armendares S, et al: La indentidad del hombre. Gac Med Mex 1982 Sep;118(9):366–78
Campillo Sainz C see Somolinas Palencia J
Campillo-Sainz C, et al: Homenaje al Doctor Erich Fromm. Gac Med Mex 1980;116:431–45
Campillo-Serrano C see Campillo-Sainz C
Campo Posada A: Una vida, un médico. Bogota, Colombia, Ediciones Fondo Cultural Cafetero, [1982]. 248 p.
Campos J, Miguel JM de: Sociologos-de-bata-blanca y medicos-con-barba: relaciones entre las ciencias sociales y la medicina en España. Rev Esp Invest Sociol 1981;15:133–41
Camps F: Sir Sydney Alfred Smith. In Dictionary of national biography, 1961–1970. Suppl. 8, 1981. p. 963–4.
Campusano C see Villarroel H
Camus CH: La psychoanalyse, avènement d'une connaissance originale (Sigmund Freud). Soins Psychiatr 1980 Dec;(6):3–8
Canada's amazing health history: let's murder the medical officer: Can J Public Health 1984 Sep–Oct;75(5):344–7
Canales López LG see Carrada Bravo T
Canales Muñoz JL, Almada Bay I, Narro Robles J: La mortalidad en una población rural de México y su relación con el uso de los servicios médicos antes de la muerte. Salud Publica Mex 1984 Jul–Aug;26(4):404–14
Canalis RF, Aragon RM, Cabieses F, et al: Fibrous dysplasia: findings in a pre-Columbian skull. Am J Otolaryngol 1980 Feb;1(2):131–5
Canalis RF: Laryngeal ventricle. Historical features. Ann Otol Rhinol Laryngol 1980 Mar–Apr;89(2 Pt 1):184–7
Canalis RF, Cabieses F, Hemenway WG, et al: Prehistoric trephination of the frontal sinus. Ann Otol Phinol Laryngol 1981 Mar–Apr;90(2 pt 1):186–9
Canard J: Les pestes en Beaujolais, Forez, Jarez, Lyonnais; du XIVème au XVIIIème siècle. [France: s.n.], 1979. (Règny, Imprimerie de l'Abbaye de Pradines). 121, A–I p.
Cancro R see Tobach E
Canelón JS: Dos artículos odontológicos en la 'Gaceta Cientifica de Venezuela' de 1877. Acta Odontol Venez 1980 Jan–Apr;18(1):87–95
Canelon JS: Hacia una historia social de la odontológia latinoamericana. Acta Odontol Venez 1982 Jan–Apr;20(1):55–63
Canetta R: Mortalità ed epidemie nello stato di Milano durante l'ultimo terzo del Settecento nelle valutazioni dei pubblici amministratori. Econ Stor 1978 Jan–Mar;25:52–64
Cangi EC: Abraham Flexner's philanthrophy: the full-time system in the department of surgery at the University of Cincinnati College of Medicine, 1910–1930. Bull Hist Med 1982 Summer;56(2):160–74
Cangi EC: Patrons and proteges: Cincinnati's first generation of women doctors 1875–1910. Cinci Hist Soc Bull 1979;37(2):89–114
Canham JE see Levenson SM
Cannell H: Struck by lightning -- the effects upon the men and the ships of HM Navy. J R Nav Med Serv 1979;65(3):165–70
Cannell H: Struck by lightning -- the effects upon the men and the ships of HM Navy. J R Nav Med Serv 1980 Spring;66(1):71–6
Cannell H: Struck by lightning--the effects upon the men and the ships of HM Navy. J R Nav Med Serv 1980 Summer;66(2):152–6
Cannon B: External esophageal construction remembered. Plast Reconstr Surg 1983 Apr;71(4):540–2
Cannon B: Walter Bradford Cannon, M. D.: Reflections on the physician, the man, and his contributions. Gastrointest Radiol 1982;7(1):1–6
Cannon JE: Rhode Island's health: yesterday, today, tomorrow. RI Med J 1979 Aug;62(8):297–307
Cannon SF: Science in culture: the early Victorian period. Kent, Eng., Dawson; New York, Science History Publications, 1978. xii, 296 p.
Cannon SF see Schweber SS
Cano-Valle F see Kuthy-Porter J
Canon BC, Jaros D: The impact of changes in judicial doctrine: the abrogation of charitable immunity. Law Soc Rev 1979;13(4):969–86
Cáňová E: Mor v čechách v roce 1680. Sb Arch Pr 1981;31(2):265–339
Cáňová E: Vývoj úmrtnosti od poloviny 17. do poloviny 19. století. Arch Cas 1977;27(4):222–5
Cantarel-Besson Y: Les morts exemplaires dans la peinture militaire sous le consulat et l'empire. Rev Inst Napoleon (Paris) 1977;(133):97–105
Cantwell JD: Angina: from Heberden to Prinzmetal. South Med J 1984 Jul;77(7):896–9
Cantwell JD: Osler: a role model for today's physician. J Med Assoc Ga 1983 Jul;72(7)::493–4
Capdebielle A: L'activité médicale à l'Hôtel des Invalides. Med Armees 1981;9:631–8
Cape RD see Kirshen AJ
Capildeo R: Charcot in the 80s. In Rose FC, Bynum WF, ed: Historical aspects of the neurosciences. New York, Raven, 1982. p. 383–96.
Capildeo R see Steiner TJ
Caplan AL see Markle GE
Caplan RL: Pasteurized patients and profits: the changing nature of self-care in American medicine. Ph.D. Diss., University of Massachusetts. Amherst, 1981. xi, 463 p.
Caplan RM: On the creation of a new medical museum. J Iowa Med Soc 1983 Jun;73(6):229
Caplan RM: The circumstances of the missing biographer or why Watson didn't narrate these four Sherlock Holmes stories. J Am Acad Dermatol 1982 Jun;6(6):1112–4
Caplan RM: 'The Lion's Mane'. Concerning the diagnostic acumen of Sherlock Holmes. Am J Dermatopathol 1983 Dec;5(6):577–9
Cappelletti AJ: El sentido del gusto, segun Aristoteles. Rev Soc Venez Hist Med 1978;27(41):41–57
Cappelletti AJ: El sentido del olfato, segun Aristoteles. Rev Soc Venez Hist Med 1978;27(41):9–40
Cappelletti AJ: Lamettrie medico y filosofo del hombre. Rev Soc Venez Hist Med 1972–73;20–21(34–35):211–27
Cappelletti AJ: Servet, teologo, filosofo y medico. Rev Soc Venez Hist Med 1975–76;23(37):147–61
Cappelletti V: Aspects of German biology. From Virchow to Driesch. Riv Biol 1981 Winter;74(4):479–502
Cappelletti V: Bernard, oltre meccanicismo e vitalismo. Med Secoli 1979 Jan–Apr;16(1):5–11
Cappelletti V: Claude Bernard between history and the 'principles' of science. Riv Biol 1980 Spring;73(1):21–33
Capper J, Power G, Shivers FR: Chesapeake waters. Pollution, public health, and public opinion, 1607–1972. Centreville, Maryland, Tidewater Publishers, 1983. xii, 201 p.
Capper WM, Johnson D, ed: The faith of a surgeon. Belief and experience in the life of Arthur Rendle Short. Exeter, England, Paternoster Press, 1976. 156 p.
Capps D: Psychohistory in religious studies. Group Psychol Hist Newsl 1974;3(2):4–8
Caprioli MP: Il patrimonio del povero. L'inchiesta sulle Opere Pie del 1861. Quad Stor 1980;15(3):918–41
Capron AM: Death and the law: a decade of change. Soundings 1980;63(3):290–320
Cara M: Le Service d'Aide Médicale Urgente (SAMU) de Paris. Bull Acad Natl Med (Paris) 1981 Mar;165(3):365–72
Caraballo Ortega T see Alegre Perez E
Caracci P: Vicende de una farmacopea di stato della serenissima repubblica di Venezia. Acta Med Hist Patav 1981/82;28:29–38
Caramelli N: Introduzione a Piaget. Stor Crit Psicol 1981;2(1):5–85
Carapanos F see Anzieu D
Caravati CM: President Andrew Jackson: despite infirmities, a strong leader. Va Med 1983 Mar;110(3):194–5
Caraway WT: Major developments in clinical chemical instrumentation. J Clin Chem Clin Biochem 1981 Jul;19(7):491–6
Caraway WT see Büttner J, ed
Carbonell JA: Rafael Rangel. Rev Soc Venez Hist Med 1975–76;23(37):129–33
Cardenas J de: Primera parte de los problemas y secretos maravillosos de las Indias. Edicion, estudio preliminar y notas para X. Lozoya. Mexico, Academia Nacional de Medicina, 1980. 320 p.
Cardenas M see Dobkin de Rios M
Cárdenas-de la Peña E: La sección de historia de la medicina, de la Academia Nacional de Medicina. Síntesis histórica. Gac Med Mex 1980 Feb;116(2):77–91
Cárdenas de la Peña E: Médicos y medicina en la vida de un libro. Gac Med Mex 1983 Sep;119(9):370–82
Cardiel JR: Sociobiología. La última forma de darwinismo. Arbor 1982;113(441–2):87–98
Cardwell D, Mottram J: Fresh light on John Dalton. Notes Rec R Soc Lond 1984 Sep;39(1):29–40
Carey AB see Kass EH
Carey GG: Folklore from the printed sources of Essex County, Massachusetts. South Folkl Q 1968;32(1):17–43
Caricote N: Formacion odontopediatrica del odontologo general en la UCV. Acta Odontol Venez 1980 Jan–Apr;18(1):69–85
Carles J: Monogenisme ou polygenisme: les leçons de la génétique. Etudes (Fr) 1983;358(3):355–66
Carles P see Bollinelli R
Carley CD: Historical and archaeological evidence of 19th century fever epidemics and medicine at Hudson's Bay Company's Fort Vancouver. Hist Archaeol 1981;15(1):19–35
Carlini EA: Homeopatia: ontem, hoje e amanhã. AMB 1983 Nov–Dec;29(11–12):210–4
Carlisle CH see Dodson G
Carlisle R: Arterial sounds by phases: an object lesson in terminological confusion? J R Soc Med 1981 Mar;74(3):212–8
Carlson DG: African fever, a study of British science, technology, and politics in West Africa, 1787–1864. New York, Science History Pub.,

1981.

**Carlson DG:** Drug supply systems in West Africa; a historical overview with particular reference to Nigeria. **Pharm Hist** 1982;24(2):73–82

**Carlson DS** see **Armelagos GJ**

**Carlson EA:** Genes, radiation, and society. The life and work of H. J. Muller. Ithaca, Cornell University Press, 1981. xiv, 457 p.

**Carlson ET, Quen JM:** American psychoanalysis: origins and development. New York, Brunner/Mazel, 1978.

**Carlson ET:** Benjamin Rush and his friends on human nature. **Psychiatr Q** 1979 Winter;51(4):300–6

**Carlson ET, Wollock JL, Noel PS, ed:** Benjamin Rush's Lectures on the mind. Philadelphia, American Philosophical Society, 1981. xix, 735 p. (Memoirs of the American Philosophical Society, 144).

**Carlson ET:** The history of multiple personality in the United States: I: The beginnings. **Am J Psychiatry** 1981 May;138(5):666–8

**Carlson ET:** The history of multiple personality in the United States: Mary Reynolds and her subsequent reputation. **Bull Hist Med** 1984 Spring;58(1):72–82

**Carlson ET** see **Blain D**

**Carlson ET** see **Kane A**

**Carlson ET** see **Wallace ER**

**Carlson PA:** Three contributors to cardiac catheterization. **J Thorac Cardiovasc Surg** 1980 May;79(5):782–8

**Carlson RJ:** Holism and reductionism as perspectives in medicine and patient care. **West J Med** 1979 Dec;131(6):466–70

**Carlson WB:** Innovation in medical technology: Elihu Thomson, General Electric, and X rays in 1896. **Med Instrum** 1982 Jul–Aug;16(4):218

**Carlström S:** Första insulinbehandlingen av diabetes i Lund––ett beriktigande. **Sydsven Medicinhist Sallsk Arsskr** 1980;:49–51

**Carlton C:** Three British revolutions and the personality of kingship. In Pocock, JG. ed: Three British revolutions: 1641, 1688, 1776. Princeton, N.J., Princeton U. Press, 1980. p. 165–207.

**Carlton C:** Towards a psychobiography of Charles I. **J Psychohist** 1984 Spring;11(4):513–31

**Carmelli D, Andersen S:** A longevity study of twins in the Mormon genealogy. **Prog Clin Biol Res** 1981;69 pt C:187–200

**Carmelli D, Hasstedt S, Andersen S:** Demography and genetics of human twinning in the Utah Mormon Genealogy. **Prog Clin Biol Res** 1981;69A:81–93

**Carmen IH:** The constitution in the laboratory: recombinant DNA research as 'free expression.' **J Polit** 1981;43(3):737–62

**Carmen Frances M del:** El aloes en las farmacopeas nacionales Espanolas. In Hickel E, Schröder G, ed: Neue Beiträge zur Arzneimittelgeschichte. Festschrift für Wolfgang Schneider zum 70. Geburtstag. Stuttgart, Wissenschaftliche Verlagsgesellschaft, 1982. p. 149–57.

**Carmichael AG:** Plague legislation in the Italian Renaissance. **Bull Hist Med** 1983 Winter;57(4):508–25

**Carmichael AG:** The Lindsay–Stipp debate. **Indiana Med Hist Q** 1981;7(4):6–19

**Carmichael E:** Dr. Papanicolaou and the Pap smear. **Ala J Med Sci** 1984 Jan;21(1):101–4

**Carmichael E** see **Allen L**

**Carmichael EB:** The pellagra story in the U.S. **J Med Assoc State Ala** 1980 Jan;49(7):11–7

**Carmichael EB:** The pellagra story in the United States of America. **J Med Assoc State Ala** 1980 Mar;49(9):23, 31, 33

**Carmichael JL:** Dr. James Monroe Mason, Jr. and his era in medicine. **J Med Assoc State Ala** 1982 May;51(11):30–7

**Carmichael JL:** Medical reminiscences. **Ala Med** 1984 Jun;53(12):16–27; July;54(1):13–5, 17

**Carmichael SW:** The adrenal chromaffin vesicle: an historical perspective. **J Auton Nerv Syst** 1983 Jan;7(1):7–12

**Carmichael AG, ed:** [John S. Bobbs]. **Indiana Med Hist Q** 1982;8(2):3–24

**Carminati A** see **Bernasconi M**

**Carmona–Cornet AM:** Actuación de la comisión regia de reforma de los reglamentos de la ciencia de curar (1790–1840). In International Congress of the History of Medicine, 27th, Barcelona, 1980. Actas. Barcelona, Acadèmia de Ciències Mèdiques de Catalunya i Balears, 1981. p. 480–5.

**Carmona Cornet AM:** Ensayo sobre la medicina naval del año 1847. In International Congress of the History of Medicine, 27th, Barcelona, 1980. Actas. Barcelona, Acadèmia de Ciències Mèdiques de Catalunya i Balears, 1981. p. 369–72.

**Carmona Cornet AM, Gómez Caamaño JL:** Historia de la Cátedra de técnica física aplicada a la Farmacia y análisis químico y en particular de los alimentos, medicamentos y venenos de la Facultad de Farmacia de la Universidad de Barcelona (1886–1936). **Bol Soc Esp Hist Farm** 1984 Jun;35(138):125–37

**Carmona Cornet AM, Bofill Pellicer C:** Instruments i operacions farmacéutiques del segle XIX a Catalunya: creació d'un aparell destl.latori de vapor per a ús farmacéutic. **Bol Soc Esp Hist Farm** 1980/81 Dec–Mar;31–32(124–5):275–82

**Carnegie ME:** Nurses and war. Black nurses at the front. **Am J Nurs** 1984 Oct;84(10):1250–2

**Carney AL:** Vertebral artery surgery: historical development, basic concepts of brain hemodynamics, and clinical experience of 102 cases. **Adv Neurol** 1981;30:249–82

**Caroli F** see **Petitjean F**

**Carotenuto A:** A secret symmetry: Sabina Spielrein between Jung and Freud. New York, Pantheon Books, 1982. xix, 250 p.

**Caroti S:** La biblioteca di un medico fiorentino [Simone de Cinozzo di Giovanni Cini]. **Bibliofilia** 1978;80:123–38

**Caroti S:** Problèmes textuels et lexicographiques dans l'oeuvre scientifique d'Albert le Grand. **Ann Ist Mus Stor Sci Fir** 1981;6(1):187–202

**Carpenter CB:** Clinical histocompatibility testing: a brief historical perspective. **Transplant Proc** 1981 Mar;13(1):55–60

**Carpenter CC:** Myths, mandarins and molecules: the cautionary tale of cholera. **Trans Am Clin Climatol Assoc** 1980;92:167–93

**Carpenter EM** see **Parker JK**

**Carpenter M:** Unity in action. **Nurs Times** 1980 Jul 10;76(28):1204–5

**Carpenter M:** William Farr: a pioneer of public health. **Nurs Times** 1983 Jun 15–21;79(24):9–11

**Carpenter M** see **Davies C, ed**

**Carpi D:** R. Yehuda Messer Lion vepe'ulato kerofe. **Michael Hist Jews Diaspora** 1972;1:277–301

**Carpinteri F:** Sociologia sanitaria a Siracusa ed in altre città della Sicilia: Mali, medici, medicine e terapie: casistiche documentate dal 1728 al 1833. **Cah Int Hist Econ Soc** 1980;12:288–322

**Carr JD:** History of dental education in Indiana. **Indiana Med Hist Q** 1978;4(3):4–20

**Carr JD:** The great radiology debate: the letters of C. Edmund Kells and Howard R. Raper. **Bull Hist Dent** 1981 Oct;29(2):69–73

**Carr JG:** Microbes I have known: a study of those associated with fermented products. **J Appl Bacteriol** 1983 Dec;55(3):383–401

**Carr MW:** Thomas W. Evans: his life and influence on the development of dentistry as a learned profession. **J Am Coll Dent** 1979 Apr;46(2):87–100

**Carr N:** The fascinating story of X–rays. **Br Dent Surg Assist** 1980 Sept–Oct;39(5):92–3

**Carr V:** The concept of clinical state in psychiatry: a review. **Compr Psychiatry** 1983 Jul–Aug;24(4):370–91

**Carrada Bravo T:** Datos para la epidemiología del sarampión en la República Mexicana. Investigación preliminar. **SPM** 1979 Sep–Oct;21(5):497–519

**Carrada Bravo T, Velázquez Díaz G:** El impacto del sarampión en México. **Salud Publica Mex** 1981 Jul–Aug;22(4):359–408

**Carrada Bravo T, Gómez Orozco J, Luna Martínez J, et al:** La tosferina y la vacunación antitosferinosa. Trabajo para conmemorar el 40 aniversario de la vacunación antitosferinosa en México, Junio 13 de 1940. **Salud Publica Mex** 1982 Jul–Aug;24(4):399–465

**Carrato Ibáñez A:** Cajal y su Instituto. **Trab Inst Cajal Invest Biol** 1979;70(3):181–94

**Carré A:** Aspects médicaux de la Campagne de l'Inde. **Rev Hist Armees** 1983;(153):50–61

**Carré A:** Essai de synthèse des maladies des gens de mer au XVIIIe siècle et leur évolution au début du XIXe siècle. In: Congrès National des Sociétés Savantes, 91e, Rennes, 1966. Comptes Rendus. Paris, 1967. Section des Sciences, Tome 1. p. 11–29.

**Carré A:** La révolution colbertienne et l'assistance aux familles maritimes des origines à 1673. In: Congrès National des Sociétés Savantes, 97e, Nantes, 1972. Comptes Rendus. Paris, 1976. Section des Sciences, Tome 1. p. 227–48.

**Carré A:** L'évolution du système classes–invalides de 1673 (Edit de Nancy) à 1784 (Réformes de Castries). In: Congrès National des Sociétés Savantes, 97e, Nantes, 1972. Comptes Rendus. Paris, 1976. Section des Sciences, Tome 1. p. 249–67.

**Carré A:** Scorbut marin historique et biologie moderne. In: Congrès National des Sociétés Savantes, 104e, Bordeaux, 1979. Comptes Rendus. Paris, 1979. Section des Sciences, Fasc. IV. p. 219–30.

**Carre A** see **Curet M**

**Carré A** see **La médecine hospitalière française au XVIIIème siècle**

**Carreras i Roca M:** La introducció del positivisme mèdic a Catalunya. In Congrés International d'Història de la Medicina Catalana, 2nd, Barcelona, 1975. Llibre d'Actes. Barcelona, Socitra, 1977. p. 7–18.

**Carreras Panchón A:** El ejercicio profesional segun el testimonio de Gaspar Tristan. **Asclepio** 1980;32:87–92

**Carreras Panchon A:** El problema del niño exposito en la España ilustrada. Salamanca, 1977. 94 p. (Cuadernos de Historia de la Medicina Española, Monografias, 32).

**Carreras Panchon A:** La obra de Juan de Villarreal y otros estudios historico–medicos. Salamanca, Ediciones Universidad de Salamanca, 1978. 69 p. (Cuadernos de Historia de la Medicina Española, Mongrafias, XXXIII).

**Carreras Panchón A:** Las epidemias de peste en la España del Renacimiento. In: Sociedad Española de Historia de la Medicina. V Congreso Nacional. Madrid, 1977. **Asclepio** 1977;29:5–15

**Carreras Panchón A:** Perez Cascales y la clinica del garrotillo. **Asclepio** 1978–79;30–31:319–22

**Carreras Panchón A:** Sobre el concepto de pestilencia (WABA') en el Canon de Avicena. **Asclepio** 1981;33:265–73

**Carreras Panchón A** see **Albarracín Teulón A**

**Carreras Verdaguer A:** La dermatología en la medicina catalana. Su contribución a la medicina mundial. **Actas Dermosifiliogr** 1980 Nov–Dec;71(11–12):487–94

**Carrick PJ:** Ancient Greek ethical perspectives on abortion and euthanasia. Ph.D. Diss., Temple University. Philadelphia, 1982. vii, 346 p.

**The carrier state. New York, Arno, 1977. Various paginations. Four reprinted papers on microbiology by William H. Park and George Soper, 1895–1919.:**

**Carrillo JL, Castellanos J, Ramos MD:** Enfermedad y sociedad en la Malaga de Comienzos del siglo XIX: el Diálogo de los muertos en la epidemia de Málaga (c. 1803). Introducción y Transcripción. Málaga, Universidad de Málaga, 1980. 41 p.

**Carrillo JL, Garcia–Ballester L:** Enfermedad y sociedad en la Málaga de

los siglos XVIII y XIX. I. La fiebre amarilla (1741-1821). Málaga, Universidad de Málaga, 1980. 199 p.
**Carrillo JL, Paz Torres M:** Ibn Al-Baytar y el arabismo español del XVIII. Edicion trilingüe del prologo de su 'Kitab al-chami.' Benalmádena, Ayuntamiento de Benalmádena, 1982. 57 p.
**Carrillo JL:** La dialectica ciencia--creencia y su manifestacion en la Malaga de 1803: el conflicto del cierre de los templos. **Jabega (Malaga)** 1979;26(2):3-8
**Carrillo JL, Olagüe G:** La enseñanza de la anatomia comparada en la Inglaterra de comienzos del siglo XIX: a proposito de las Lectures de Everard Home (1756-1832). **Asclepio** 1978-79;30-31:83-8
**Carrillo JL, Gago R:** Memoria sobre una nueva y metodica clasificacion de los fluidos elasticos permanentes y gaseosos de Juan Manuel de Arejula (1755-1830). Introduccion, transcripcion y notas. Malaga, Universidad de Malaga, 1980. 47 p.
**Carrillo JL, García Ballester L:** Repercusiones sociales de la epidemia de fiebre amarilla de Malaga (1803-1804): posturas tradicionales e ilustradas en el estamento eclesiastico. In: Sociedad Española de Historia de la Medicina. V Congreso Nacional. Madrid, 1977. **Asclepio** 1977;29:73-99
**Carrillo JL** see **Gago R**
**Carrillo Broatch A:** Aspectos del linde de la psiquiatría y la terapéutica biológica. **Rev Neuropsiquiatr** 1980 Jun;43(2):87-96
**Carrillo-Rascón J:** Escherichia coli: historia de una hipótesis. **Bol Med Hosp Infant Mex** 1983 Aug;40 Suppl 2:28-33
**Carroll D:** The contribution of the Johns Hopkins University School of Medicine. **Md State Med J** 1981 Oct;30(10):76-8
**Carroll D:** The state of medical knowledge in Maryland, 1870s. **Md State Med J** 1980 Sep;29(9):12-5
**Carroll D:** The University of Maryland School of Medicine, 1807-1920. **Md State Med J** 1981 Jun;30(6):35-50
**Carroll DG:** Medical education in Maryland: cottage industry to university. **Md State Med J** 1980 Feb;29(2):21-5
**Carroll MA, Humphrey RH:** Moral problems in nursing: case studies. Washington, University Press of America, 1979. Historical chapters, p. 6-28.
**Carroll PT:** Academic chemistry in America, 1876-1976: diversification, growth, and change. Ph.D. Diss., University of Pennsylvania. Philadelphia, 1982. xviii, 551 p.
**Carroll PT** see **Kevles DJ**
**Carrubba RW:** The first detailed report on Persian mummy. **Physis** 1981;23(4):461-71
**Carrubba RW:** The first report of the harvesting of Asafetida in Iran. **Agric Hist** 1979;53(2):451-61
**Carrubba RW:** The Latin document confirming the date and institution of Wilhem ten Rhyne's M.D. **Gesnerus** 1982;39(3-4):473-6
**Carrubba RW** see **Bowers JZ**
**Carson CC:** Charles Horace Mayo (1865-1939). **Invest Urol** 1981;18:313-4
**Carson G:** The dentist and the empress. The adventures of Dr. Tom Evans in gas-lit Paris. Boston, Houghton Mifflin, 1983. xiii, 222 p.
**Carson HL** see **Mayr E**
**Carson J** see **Clark G**
**Carson RA:** Selzer's surgeon as seer. **Perspect Biol Med** 1981 Winter;24(2):284-9
**Carson RB:** Fifty years of history: Southeastern Section, American Urological Association, 1931-1981. The Section, 1981. 119 p.
**Carson SL:** Presidential children: abandonment, hysteria and suicide. **J Psychohist** 1984 Spring;11(4):533-44
**Carstensen G:** Die Chirurgie in der Kunst. Düsseldorf, Econ, 1983. 206 p.
**Carswell H:** 'Elephant Man' had more than neurofibromatosis. **JAMA** 1982 Sep 3;248(9):1032-3
**Carter EC** see **Stapleton DH**
**Carter HE:** Historical cases. Illustrations of the distemper of dogs. By William Youatt. **J Small Anim Pract** 1981 Apr;22(4):207-11
**Carter HE:** Identification and synthesis of threonine. **Fed Proc** 1979 Dec;38(13):2684-6
**Carter HE:** Who needs veterinary history? **J Small Anim Pract** 1981 Apr;22(4):175-6
**Carter JH** see **Lyles MR**
**Carter JT:** Vitiated air: a Victorian villain? **J R Soc Med** 1981 Dec;74(12):914-9
**Carter KC:** Germ theory, hysteria, and Freud's early work in psychopathology. **Med Hist** 1980 Jul;24(3):259-74
**Carter KC:** Ignaz Semmelweis, Carl Mayrhofer, and the rise of germ theory. **Med Hist** 1985 Jan;29(1):33-53
**Carter KC:** Infantile hysteria and infantile sexuality in late nineteenth-century German-language medical literature. **Med Hist** 1983 Apr;27(2):186-96
**Carter KC:** Nineteenth-century treatments for rabies as reported in the Lancet. **Med Hist** 1982 Jan;26(1):67-78
**Carter KC:** Semmelweis and his predecessors. **Med Hist** 1981 Jan;25(1):57-72
**Carter KC:** Semmelweis's possible influence on Karl Mayrhofer and on those who subsequently developed nineteenth century etiological theories. **Orvostort Kozl** 1982;28(1-3):23-31
**Carter L:** Down Memory Lane: debut of a drug. **Nurs Mirror** 1982 Nov 3;155(18):21-2
**Carter L:** Down memory lane: the bottomless pit. **Nurs Mirror** 1982 Jan 27;154(4):26-7
**Carter L:** Snatching the thyroid. **Nurs Times** 1984 Mar 7-13;80(10):38
**Carter RB:** Descartes' medical philosophy. The organic solution to the mind-body problem. Baltimore, London, Johns Hopkins University Press, 1983. xi, 301 p.
**Carter RB:** Gilbert and Descartes: the science of conserving the compound body. **Z Allg Wissenschaftstheorie** 1982;13(2):224-33
**Carter RD** see **Stoeckle DB**
**Cartier M:** Quand la Chine avait cent millions d'habitants. **Histoire** 1980;24:87-9
**Cartmill M:** Basic primatology and prosimian evolution. In F. Spencer, ed: A history of American physical anthropology, 1930-1980. New York, Academic Press, 1982. p. 147-86.
**Cartwright FF:** Pneumatic medicine. **Pharm Hist (London)** 1970 Jun;1(5):4-6
**Cartwright FF** see **Hart GD, ed**
**Cartwright MF:** The filthy state of Cape Town in 1858. **Q Bull S Afr Libr** 1978;33(2):53-6
**Cartwright ML:** Sir Edward Foyle Collingwood. In Dictionary of national biography, 1961-1970. Suppl. 8, 1981. p. 232-4.
**Cartwright RA:** Historical and modern epidemiological studies on populations exposed to N-substituted aryl compounds. **Environ Health Perspect** 1983 Mar;49:13-9
**Carty MA:** The examination of a young surgeon. Hand-colored etching by George Cruikshank, from The Scourge, 1811. **J Hist Med Allied Sci** 1981 Apr;36(2):214
**Carvalho AC de:** Escola de Enfermagem da Universidade de São Paulo. Resumo histórico 1942-1980. **Rev Esc Enferm USP** 1980 Aug;14 Suppl:1-271
**Casado Llopmart JR:** La microfusion como principio de los colados en protesis estomatologica. **Rev Esp Estomatol** 1982 Mar-Apr;30(2):113-22
**Casal A:** Hace cien años, 1881-1981--Billroth y la primera gastrectomía. **Acta Gastroenterol Latinoam** 1981;11(2):326-8
**Casal MA:** Hace cien años: 1882-1982. 'Carl Langenbuch, la primera colecistectomía y breve historia de una polémia famosa. **Acta Gastroenterol Latinoam** 1982;12(2):181-4
**Casales Ortiz G** see **Peña Páez I de la**
**Casanovas J:** La enfermedad ocular de Francisco de Asís. **Klin Oczna** 1980 May;82(5):243-4
**Casarett LJ, Bruce MC:** Origin and scope of toxicology. In Doull J, Klaassen CD, Amdur MO, ed: Casarett and Doull's Toxicology: the basic science of poisons. 2d. ed. New York, Macmillan, 1980. p. 3-10.
**Casaretto CC:** Juan Ignacio Molina (Huaraculén 1740 - Bolonia 1829), fundador de la patografia y de la autopatografia en Chile. **Rev Med Chil** 1979 Nov;107(11):1053-61
**Casaux-Bussière M:** Georges Denigès (1859-1951). Essai biographique. Thèse, Bordeaux II, 1981. 374 leaves.
**A case of diabetes mellitus: N Engl J Med** 1982 Jul 8;307(2):127-8
**Casetta A** see **Hand WD**
**Casey A:** A history of dentistry in Northern Ireland 1920-1973. Part I. **J Ir Dent Assoc** 1982 May-Jun;28(3):53-7
**Casey AE, Copeland H, Downey-Prince EL, et al:** Differential craniometry: (A) Maori 3000 BC--Thera? (B). Ptolemaic Egyptians--New Guinea, America. **Ala J Med Sci** 1979 Oct;16(4):382-9
**Casey AJ:** A history of dentistry in Northern Ireland 1920-1973. Part II. **J Ir Dent Assoc** 1982 Sep-Oct;28(5):113-5
**Casey AJ:** A history of dentistry in Northern Ireland 1920-1973. Part IV. **J Ir Dent Assoc** 1983 Jan-Feb;29(1):9-11
**Casey KF** see **Jain KM**
**Casey M:** 50 years of general practice. **Ir Med J** 1981 Jun;74(6):155-8
**Cash P:** An analysis of the social, political and professional impact of the Revolution upon the Boston medical community. (1759-1789). In: Congrès international d'histoire de la médecine, XXVe, Québec, 1976. Actes. Québec, 1977. p. 546-59.
**Cash P, Pine C:** John Jeffries and the struggle against smallpox in Boston (1775-1776) and Nova Scotia (1776-1779). **Bull Hist Med** 1983;57(1):93-7
**Cash P, Christianson EH, Estes JW, ed:** Medicine in colonial Massachusetts 1620-1820. A conference held 25 & 26 May 1978 by the Colonial Society of Massachusetts. Boston, Colonial Society of Massachusetts, 1980. xxiii, 425 p. (Publications, Vol. 57) Contributions by R. D. Brown, C. H. Brock, G. B. Warden, W. J. Bell, J. C. Greene, D. L. Jones, W. C. Wigglesworth, J. H. Cassedy, G. E. Gifford.
**Cash P:** Pride, prejudice and politics. **Harv Med Alumni Bull** 1980 Dec;54(6):20-5
**Cash P:** The phoenix and the eagle: The founding of the Boston and Massachusetts Medical Societies in 1780 and 1781. **N Engl J Med** 1981 Oct 29;305(18):1033-9
**Caspari EW, Allen GE, et al:** Controversial geneticist and creative biologist. [Richard B. Goldschmidt] A critical review on his contributions. **Experientia [Suppl]** 1980;Suppl 35:1-154
**Cassar P:** Impact of British pharmacy in Malta. **Pharm Hist (London)** 1978 Mar;8(1):2-4
**Cassebaum H:** Neues über die Entdeckung von Säuren in organischem Material durch C.W. Scheele. **Pharmazie** 1981;36(2):135-8
**Cassedy JH:** American medicine and statistical thinking, 1800-1860. Cambridge, Mass., Harvard University Press, 1984. x, 306 p.
**Cassedy JH:** An American clerical crisis: ministers' sore throat 1830-1860 (the Fielding H. Garrison Lecture). **Bull Hist Med** 1979 Spring;53(1):23-38
**Cassedy JH:** Charles V. Chapin re-visited: an appreciation. **RI Med J** 1983 Jan;66(1):41-4
**Cassedy JH:** Church record-keeping and public health in early New England. In: Medicine in Colonial Massachusetts 1620-1820. (Publications of the Colonial Society of Massachusetts, vol. 57), 1980. p. 249-62.

**Cassedy JH:** Highlights in the development of medical history in the United States. (Materials from an exhibit). Bethesda, National Library of Medicine, 1984. 30 p.
**Cassedy JH:** The flourishing and character of early American medical journalism, 1797–1860. **J Hist Med Allied Sci** 1983 Apr;38(2):135–50
**Cassedy JH** see **Cash P**
**Cassell EJ:** Changing ideas of causality in medicine. **Soc Res (NY)** 1979;46(4):728–43
**Cassell EJ** see **Spicker SF, ed**
**Cassidy M, Jacobs A, Bresnihan B:** The use of unproven remedies for rheumatoid arthritis in Ireland. **Ir Med J** 1983 Nov;76(11):464–5
**Cassinelli G** see **Di Marco A**
**Cassone E:** Historia de la Cirugia en Mendoza. In Congreso de Historia de la Medicina Argentina [Transactions], 5th, Mendoza, 1983, p. 69–78.
**Cassorla RM:** Suicídio e adolescência. I--Incidência, histórico e fatores suicidógenos. **Acta Psiquiatr Psicol Am Lat** 1979 Dec;25(4):288–95
**Castagnino HE, Thompson AC:** Sufrió Darwin la enfermedad de Chagas? **Medicina (B Aires)** 1981;41(2):263–4
**Castagnola L, Garberoglio U:** Breve cronistoria dei materiali e delle metodiche di impronta. **Riv Odontoiatr Amici Brugg** 1983 Apr–Jun;2(2):101–2
**Castaigne P:** Centenaire de la Clinique des maladies du système nerveux de la Salpêtrière. Introduction. **Rev Neurol (Paris)** 1982;138(12):879–86
**Castaigne P, Lhermitte F, Signoret JL, et al:** Description et étude scannographique du cerveau de Leborgne. La découverte de Broca. **Rev Neurol (Paris)** 1980;136(10):563–83
**Castaigne P:** Photographies et tomodensitométrie des deux cerveaux sur lesquels Broca fonda sa conception anatomoclinique de l''aphémie'. **Bull Acad Natl Med (Paris)** 1979 Oct;163(7):663–7
**Castaigne P** see **La Salpêtrière**
**Castaigne P** see **Signoret JL**
**Castaing L, Chapman C, Rooker C, et al:** This I remember...An informal history of Louisiana State University School of Medicine. New Orleans, Louisiana State University School of Medicine, 1983. xi, 83 p.
**Castañeda H** see **Fernández del Castillo F**
**Castel F, Castel R, Lovell A:** La société psychiatrique avancée. Paris, Grasset, 1979. 365 p.
**Castel F** see **Castel R**
**Castel R:** L'ordre psychiatrique: l'âge d'or de l'aliénisme. Paris, Editions de Minuit, 1976. 334 p.
**Castel R, Castel F, Lovell A:** The psychiatric society. La société psychiatrique avancée. New York, Columbia University Press, 1982. xxiii, 358 p.
**Castel R** see **Castel F**
**Castel R** see **Mitchell H**
**Castellani C:** Appunti per uno studio della biologia post–Spallanazaniana: 1780–1820. **Physis** 1978;20(1–4):5–29
**Castellani C:** Fra preformismo e epigenesi: le teorie di Prevost e Dumas. **Hist Philos Life Sci** 1980;2(2):253–68
**Castellani C:** Ontogenesi di una dissertazione: le 'osservazioni e sperienze sui vermicelli spermatici ...' di L. Spallanzani. **Hist Philos Life Sci** 1982;4(1):125–57
**Castellani C:** Ricognizione di alcuni inediti spallanzaniani, con particolare riguardo agli studi sui pipistrelli (1793–1794). La Memoria sul volo cieco dei pipistrelli dedicata al Senebier nelle due versioni: testo e considerazioni. **Physis** 1984;26(3):433–83
**Castellani C:** Una rilettura ottocentesca di Spallanzani: la nouvelle théorie de la génération di Prévost e Dumas (1824). **Hist Philos Life Sci** 1979;1(2):215–59
**Castellanos J, Reguero MA:** La peste en la Malaga del siglo XVII (1637): approximacion a su historia social. In: Sociedad Española de Historia de la Medicina. V Congreso Nacional. Madrid, 1977. **Asclepio** 1977;29:101–18
**Castellanos J** see **Carrillo JL**
**Castelli MC** see **Pinto–Cisternas J**
**Castillo A:** Algunas anotaciones demográficas sobre Cádiz en los primeros siglos del Imperio romano. **Hispania** 1978 Jul–Aug;38:235–57
**Castillo Tello MM** see **Basante Pol RM**
**Castle M, Klimek JJ:** From newsletter to journal: a 10–year review. **Am J Infect Control** 1982 Aug;10(3):79–83
**Castle WB** see **Finland M**
**Castleman B, Sutton SB, Crockett DC:** The Massachusetts General Hospital, 1955–1980. Boston, Little, Brown, 1983. xxii, 410 p.
**Castleman B** see **Sweeney RE**
**Castner CJ:** Epicurean Hetairai as dedicants to healing deities? **Greek Roman Byz Stud (Cambridge, Mass.)** 1982;23:51–7
**Castorina JA, Lerner BD:** Comentarios sobre la investigación clínica en Freud y Piaget. **Acta Psiquiatr Psicol Am Lat** 1983 Jun;29(2):85–95
**Castro F de:** Historia da vida e obras de S. Joao de Deus. Translation and notes by Foâo Gameiro, OH. Montemor–O–Novo, Editorial Franciscana, 1982. 166 p.
**Castro JM de:** Etude anthropologique de la denture de la population préhispanique de l'Ile de Grande Canarie. **Bull Group Int Rech Sci Stomatol Odontol** 1984 Jan;27(1):11–29
**Castro M de:** Johannes Aegidii Zamorensis, OFM, contra venena et animalia venenosa. Introducción edición y notas. **Arch Iberoam** 1976;36:3–116
**Castro–Vázquez A:** The dawn of neuroendocrinology: conquest and heroes. **Acta Physiol Lat Am** 1981;31(3):151–9
**Castrodeza C:** La importancia práctica del darwinismo. **Arbor** 1982;113(441–2):127–36
**Castroviejo R** see **Hughes WL**
**Castrovinci JL** see **Breul FR**
**Casula D:** I cinquanti'anni della Società Italiana di Medicina del Lavoro e Igiene Industriale. **Med Lav** 1980 Mar–Apr;71(2):115–8
**Catahier S:** A l'occasion du millénaire de la mort d'Ibnoul–Jazzar (Algizar). **Hist Sci Med** 1984;18(3):247–53
**Català F:** Autour d'une consultation par correspondance sous l'Empire. In Congrés International d'Història de la Medicina Catalana, 2nd, Barcelona, 1975. Llibre d'Actes. Barcelona, Socitra, 1977. p. 133–7.
**Catalogus van de Bibliotheek der Nederlandsche Maatschappij tot Bevordering der Geneeskunst, in bruikleen verenigd met de Bibliotheek der Universiteit van Amsterdam:** Vol. III. Amsterdam, Rodopi, 1980. 966 columns.
**Catchpole HR:** Growth hormone. **JAMA** 1980 Feb 15;243(7):652
**Catchpole P** see **Shipley M**
**Cates GL:** 'The seasoning': disease and death among the first colonists of Georgia. **Ga Hist Q** 1980;64(2):146–58
**Cates W:** Abortion attitudes of black women. **Women Health** 1979 Nov–Dec;2(3):3–9
**Cathelin M:** Les insensés au XVIIIe siècle: naissance de la solution asilaire. **Bull Soc Fr Hist Hop** 1983;46:21–35
**Catlin FI:** Pioneers in stapedectomy. **Am J Otolaryngol** 1983 May–Jun;4(3):217
**Catlin FI:** Pulmonary complications of tonsillectomy as originally described by Samuel J. Crowe, M.D. **Laryngoscope** 1981 Jan;91(1):52–61
**Catterall RD:** The emergence of a specialty. **Sex Transm Dis** 1983 Apr–Jun;10(2):85–92
**Catton R:** The early history of the library of the Royal Veterinary College. **Vet Hist** 1982 Summer;2(3):91–9
**Caudill RP:** Soviet naval medicine: Military Medical Order of Lenin Medical Academy Imeni S. M. Kirov (VNEA). **US Navy Med** 1980;71(10):16–7
**Caulfield E** see **Matossian MK**
**Cavaliere F** see **Zigiotti GL**
**Cavallo C, Cei A:** Pinel e il magnetismo animale. **Stor Crit Psicol** 1984 Jun;5(1):91–109
**Cavallo D:** Sexual politics and social reform: Jane Addams, from childhood to Hull House. In: Albin, Mel, ed. New Directions in Psychohistory: The Adelphi Papers in Honor of Erik H. Erikson. Lexingon, Mass., Health, 1980: 161–82.
**Cavallo GP** see **Martinetto P**
**Cavanagh GS:** A new view of the Vesalian landscape. **Med Hist** 1983 Jan;27(1):77–9
**Cavanaugh G:** The corruptions of science. **Dissent** 1981;28(2):195–202
**Cavanaugh JC:** Early developmental theories: a brief review of attempts to organize developmental data prior to 1925. **J Hist Behav Sci** 1981 Jan;17(1):38–47
**Cavanha AO:** La revolucion biologica. **CERON** 1980 Dec;5(3):29–32
**Cavazza M:** Bologna and the Royal Society in the seventeenth century. **Notes Rec R Soc Lond** 1980 Dec;35(2):105–23
**Cave AJ:** A constellation of conservators. **Ann R Coll Surg Engl** 1980 Jan;62(1):66–70
**Cawson RA, Stocker IP:** The early history of fluorides as anti–caries agents. **Br Dent J** 1984 Dec 8;157(11):403–4
**Caylor JA** see **Hammarsten JF**
**Cazort AG, Gordon VH:** History of allergy. University of Arkansas School of Medicine. **J Arkansas Med Soc** 1980 Oct;77(5):197–8
**Céard J** see **Margolin JC**
**Cebe B, Rozear MP, ed:** E. A. Stead, Jr.: what this patient needs is a doctor. Durham, N. C., Carolina Academic Press, 1978. xii, 244 p.
**Cecconi:** Le Marais et le mal de dents. **Soc Fr Hist Art Dent** 1979 Sep–Dec;(5–6):18–21
**Cech S:** Milan Dvorzhak (k 50–letiiu so dnia rozhdeniia). **Arkh Anat Gistol Embriol** 1980 Jul;79(7):121–5
**Cecil JC** see **Aker F**
**Cecil R:** Holy dying: evangelical attitudes to death. **Hist Today** 1982 Aug;32:30–4
**Cegielka L:** A sound investment. The Department of Dental Science at the Royal College of Surgeons of England. **Br Dent J** 1983 Jul 9;155(1):30–1
**Cei A** see **Cavallo C**
**Cela CJ:** Marañon, el hombre. In Congrés International d'Història de la Medicina Catalana, 2nd, Barcelona, 1975. Llibre d'Actes. Barcelona, Socitra, 1977. p. 59–71.
**Celani AM** see **Salemme MA**
**Celant E:** L'empirico dei mali e dei rimedi. Palermo, 'Il Vespro', 1979. 173 p.
**Cendrzak E:** Alfred Obaliński--prekursor urologii w Polsce. **Arch Hist Med (Warsz)** 1984;47(2):239–48
**Cendrzak E** see **Jamróg–Cendrzak A**
**Centenaire de la Société Française d'Ophtalmologie:** **Bull Mem Soc Fr Ophtalmol** 1983;95:clxxxiii–cxcix
**Centenario del descubrimiento del agente trasmisor de la fiebre amarilla:** **Rev Cubana Med Trop** 1981 Jan–Apr;33(1):3–7
**Centenarul Institutului de Medicină şi Farmacie din Iasi (1879–1979):** **Rev Med Chir Soc Med Nat Iasi** 1979 Oct–Dec;83(4):727–32
**Centenary issue: 1880–1980.:** **Br Dent J** 1980 Jul 1;149(1):1–36
**Centenary of a medical journal.:** **S Afr Med J** 1979 Sep 8;56(11):419–20
**Centennial edition: The South Dakota State Medical Association:** **SD J Med** 1981 May;34(5):1–80
**Centennial: Koch's discovery of the tubercle bacillus:** **MMWR** 1982 Mar

19;31(10):121-3
**Centennial of Koch's bacillus: NZ Med J** 1982 Jun 9;95(709):384
**A century of dental education in Indiana. 1879-1979: Alumni Bull Sch Dent Indiana Univ** 1979 Spring;:5-146
**A century of health care: Med J Aust** 1982 Jul 24;2(2):98-9
**Cepeda Adán J:** Enfermos and enfermedades en el siglo XVII: el marqués y la Marquesa de San Leonardo. **Rev Univ Complut Madr** 1978;27(112):165-84
**Cernáček J:** Počiatky neurológie na Slovensku. **Bratisl Lek Listy** 1982 Sep;78(3):363-9
**Cernoch A:** Třicet pět let československěho porodnictví. **Cesk Gynekol** 1980 Jun;45(5):281-4
**Cernovodeanu D:** Din corespondenta inedită a medicului militar Nicolae Stonescu in timpul Războiului de Independenta. **Rev Istor** 1977;30(6):1051-70
**Cernozubov N:** Osvrt na dosadašnji rad civilnog saniteta u NO-pokretu. **Lijec Vjesn** 1979 Nov;101(11):694-7
**Cervantes V:** 'Ensayo a la materia medica vegetal de Mexico' (Introduccion). **Med Tradic** 1982;3(11):34-6
**Cerveňanská N:** Ian Cherveniankskiĭ--osnovopolozhnik chekhoslovatsko-sovetskikh sviazeĭ v ortopedii. **Ortop Travmatol Protez** 1983 Apr;(4):68-71
**Cerveňanská N:** Príspevok k histórii Slovensko-sovietskych stykov v medicíne. **Bratisl Lek Listy** 1982 Jan;77(1):85-105
**Cerveňanská N:** 60 rokov Ortopedickej kliniky University Komenského. **Acta Chir Orthop Traumatol Cech** 1983 Dec;50(6):485-90
**Cervenka J:** African mask with cleft lip and palate. **Cleft Palate J** 1984 Jan;21(1):38-40
**Cervený J** see **Subrtová A**
**Cervera S:** La influencia de los acontecimientos de la vida en los trastornos psiquiátricos: planteamiento del problema. **Rev Med Univ Navarra** 1982 Sep;26(3):147-9
**César R** see **La Salpêtrière**
**Cesnokova S** see **Lindemann M**
**Cesnys G:** Lietuvos didžiosios kunigaikštystes demografiniai rodikliai 1790m. gyventoju surašymo duomenimis. **Liet Istor Metrast** 1980:5-16
**Cetrdeset godina Vojnosanitetskog pregleda: Vojnosanit Pregl** 1984 Sep-Oct;41(5):315-9
**Ceypek T:** Uzupełnienie do artykułu pt. 'Klinika Laryngologii w 30-leciu Slaskiej Akademii Medycznej'. **Otolaryngol Pol** 1979;33(6):671-2
**Chabbert P, Mangin P:** Les premières publications de Philippe Pinel consacrées à la médecine mentale. In International Congress of the History of Medicine, 27th, Barcelona, 1980. Actas. Barcelona, Académia de Ciències Médiques de Catalunya i Balears, 1981. p. 42-7.
**Chabbert P:** Maxence Audouard (1776-1856). In: Congrès National des Sociétés Savantes, 96e, Toulouse, 1971. Comptes Rendus. Paris, 1974. Histoire des Sciences, Tome 1. p. 83-97.
**Chabbert P:** Problèmes scientifiques évoqués à l'Académie de Castres (1648-1670). In: Congrès National des Sociétés Savantes, 100e, Paris, 1975. Actes. Paris, 1976. Histoire Moderne et Contemporaine et Histoire des Sciences. p. 21-9.
**Chabert JM, Bocquet JP:** A propos d'un denier de la république romaine. **Hist Sci Med** 1982;16(2):89-92
**Chaboche R:** Le clergé de France et l'assistance aux invalides de guerre au XVIIe siècle. In: Congrès National des Sociétés Savantes, 97e, Nantes, 1972. Actes. Paris, 1977. Histoire Moderne et Contemporaine, Tome 1. p. 31-47.
**Chabot CB:** Freud on Schreber. Psychoanalytic theory and the critical act. Amherst, University of Massachusetts Press, 1982. 171 p.
**Chacón Jiménez F** see **Marset Campos P**
**Chadney JG:** Sikh family patterns and ethnic adaptation in Vancouver. **Amerasia J** 1980;7(1):31-50
**Chaff SL:** Archives and special collections on women in medicine. **J Am Med Wom Assoc** 1983 May-Jun;38(3):73-4
**Chaff SL** see **Kaiser RM**
**Chaff SL** see **Mandelbaum DR**
**Chagin KP:** Rol' akademika E. N. Pavlovskogo v izuchenii épidemiologii parazitarnykh i transmissivnykh bolezneĭ (k 100-letiiu so dnia rozhdeniia). **Zh Mikrobiol Epidemiol Immunobiol** 1984 Jun;(6):117-20
**Chagin KP** see **Pervomaĭskiĭ GS**
**Chaïa J:** A propos des malheurs de l'escadre du Duc D'Anville (1746). In: Congrès National des Sociétés Savantes, 107e. Brest, 1982. Comptes Rendus, Paris, 1983. Section des Sciences, Fasc. IV. p. 333-9.
**Chaïa J:** Contrat d'un chirurgien d'une plantation de Cayenne au XVIIe siècle. In: Congrès National des Sociétés Savantes, 93e, Tours, 1968. Comptes Rendus. Paris, 1971. Section des Sciences, Tome II. p. 51-4.
**Chaïa J:** Sur une correspondance, entre 1739 et 1749, de Duhamel du Monceau avec J.-F. Artur, médecin du roy a Cayenne. In: Congrès National des Sociétés Savantes, 102e, Limoges, 1977. Comptes Rendus. Paris, 1977. Section des Sciences, Fasc. III. p. 21-6.
**Chaia J:** Vicq d'Azyr, la Société Royale de Médecine et la Guyane. In: Congrès National des Sociétés Savantes, 105e, Caen, 1980. Comptes Rendus, Paris, 1980. Section des Sciences, Fasc. V. p. 9-15.
**Chaïa J** see **Huard P**
**Chaigneau M:** Christophe-Augustin Lamare-Picquot, pharmacien, naturaliste, explorateur. **Rev Hist Pharm (Paris)** 1982 Mar;29(252):5-26
**Chaĭka NA:** Deiatel'nost' Leningradskogo nauchno-issledovatel'skogo instituta épidemiologii i mikrobiologii im. Pastera v gody Velikoĭ Otechestvennoĭ voĭny. **Sov Zdravookhr** 1980;(8):47-51
**Chain E:** A short history of the penicillin discovery from Fleming's early observations in 1929 to the present time. In J. Parascandola, ed: The history of antibiotics. Madison, American Institute of the History of Pharmacy, 1980. p. 15-29.
**Chaklin AV** see **Blokhin NN**
**Chakraborty R** see **Weiss KM**
**Chakravorty RC:** Charles Richard Drew (1904-1950). **Scalpel Tongs** 1981;25:69-70
**Chakravorty RC:** Girolamo Fracastoro, a man of the Renaissance. **Hist Med (Lond)** 1975 Autumn-Winter;6(3-4):65-7
**Chakravorty RC:** Management of clean wounds and abscesses as described in the Sushrutasamhita. In: Congrès internationale d'histoire de la médecine, XXVe, Québec, 1976. Actes. Québec, 1977. p. 560-3.
**Chakravorty RC:** Medical ethics in ancient India. In International Congress of the History of Medicine, 27th, Barcelona, 1980. Actas. Barcelona, Académia de Ciències Médiques de Catalunya i Balears, 1981. p. 486-9.
**Chakravorty RC:** Philip Mazzei - physician, statesman, horticulturist, citizen of the world. **Scalpel Tongs** 1981;25:50-1
**Chalat NI:** Jean Marc Gaspard Itard - 1774-1838. **Laryngoscope** 1982 Jun;92(6 Pt 1):627-9
**Chalat NI:** Sir Morell Mackenzie revisited. **Laryngoscope** 1984 Oct;94(10):1307-10
**Chalat NI:** Some psychologic aspects of deafness: Beethoven, Goya, and Oscar Wilde. **Am J Otol** 1980 Apr;1(4):240-6
**Chalat NI:** Who was Prosper Menière and why am I still so dizzy? **Am J Otol** 1979 Jul;1(1):52-6
**Chalbert P:** Une lignée d'apothicaires et de pharmaciens languedociens: les Audouard, d'Agde, Béziers et Castres. **Rev Hist Pharm (Paris)** 1980 Sep;27(246):175-88
**Chaldecott JA:** Wedgwood's ceramic wares for chemical use, production and supply from 1779-1794. **Ambix** 1981 Nov;28(3):184-205
**Challinor JR:** The aged in families: a retrospective view. **Long Term Care Health Serv Adm Q** 1978 Sep;2(3)189-96
**Chalmers TC:** The clinical trial. **Milbank Mem Fund Q** 1981 Summer;59(3):324-39
**Chamberlain RW:** Arbovirology--then and now. **Am J Trop Med Hyg** 1982 May;31(3 Pt 1):430-7
**Chambers CA, Romanofsky P, ed:** Social service organizations. 2 v. Westport, Conn., Greenwood Press, 1978. xxxiii, 843 p.
**Chambers CA** see **Breul FR**
**Chambers EB** see **Miller B**
**Chambers R** see **McKinney HL, ed**
**Chambers RW, Durkin JT, ed:** Papers of the Alexis Carrel centennial conference, Georgetown University June 28, 1973. Washington, Georgetown University, 1973. 107 p. Contributions by C. A. Lindbergh, A. Gros, S. Maggio, L. G. Walker, C. A. Hufnagel, T. I. Malinin.
**Chambers WL:** Contributions to American history by physicians. **Am J Surg** 1981 Dec;142(6):640-5
**Chambonnet F:** Les faiences pharmaceutiques conservées dans les établissements hospitaliers de la région lyonnaise. Le Puy-en-Velay, [s.n.], 1978. 213 p. (Thèse, Lyon).
**Chamings PA** see **Ham LM**
**Chamorro G:** El Dr. Hernán Alessandri y el desarrollo de la medicina interna en el Hospital de Salvador. **Rev Med Chil** 1979 May;107(5):438-40
**Chamorro G:** Uso y abuso de la digital. **Rev Med Chil** 1982 Apr;110(4):361-7
**Champ JF:** Bishop Milner, Holywell, and the cure tradition. In Sheils WJ, ed: The Church and healing. Papers read at the twentieth summer meeting and the twenty-first winter meeting of the Ecclesiastical History Society. Oxford, Basil Blackwell for the Society, 1982. p. 153-64.
**Champagne MT:** Innovation in nurse education: a history of the Associate degree program, 1940-1964. Ph.D. Diss., University of Texas. Austin, 1981. xvi, 474 p.
**Champion GD:** Gold compounds in rheumatic diseases--1. **Med J Aust** 1984 Jan 21;140(2):73-7
**Chan H:** [A description of demographic cognition during the Ch'ing Dynasty] (Chi). **Ssu yu Yen** 1973;10(6):425-31
**Chandler DL:** Health and slavery in colonial Colombia. New York, Arno Press, 1981. iv, 307 p. (Ph.D. Diss., Tulane 1972).
**Chandler DP:** Folk memories of the decline of Angkor in nineteenth-century Cambodia: the legend of the leper king. **J Siam Soc** 1979;67(1):54-62
**Chandler ET, Bloomfield RL:** Salernitan wisdom. **South Med J** 1983 Jul;76(7):913-5
**Chandpuri K:** Hakim Aziz al-Din; foreign minister of the Sikh kingdom. **Stud Hist Med** 1979 Sep;3(3):178-80
**Chandrasekhar S:** 'A dirty, filthy book.' The writings of Charles Knowlton and Annie Besant on reproductive physiology and birth control and an account of the Bradlaugh-Besant trial. With the definitive texts of Fruits of philosophy by Charles Knowlton; The law of population by Annie Besant; Theosophy and the law of population by Annie Besant. Berkeley, University of California Press, 1981. xi, 217 p.
**Chandrasena RD:** Phenomenology and nosology of schizophrenia: historical review. **Psychiatr J Univ Ottawa** 1983 Jun;8(2):17-24
**Chaney JA:** Birthing in early America. **J Nurse Midwife** 1980 Mar-Apr;25(2):5-13
**Chang CT** see **Cho LJ**
**Chang JK** see **Chang S**
**Chang MC:** [History and background of research on fertilization in mammals] (Chi). **Sheng Li Ko Hsueh Chin Chan** 1983 Oct;14(4):289-93
**Chang MC:** The meaning of sperm capacitation. A historical perspective. **J Androl** 1984 Mar-Apr;5(2):45-50
**Chang MC** see **Freedman R**
**Chang NJ** see **Yan YB**

**Chang S, Chang JK:** A historical review of echocardiographic detection of pericardial effusion. **Jpn Heart J** 1981 Sep;22(5):789–800
**Chang S:** In memory of our visiting professor: Walter B. Cannon at Peking. **Physiologist** 1980 Jun;23(3):39–40
**Changeux JP** see **Robin ED, ed**
**The changing look of dental assisting: Dent Assist** 1984 Sep–Oct;53(5):23–6
**Changus JE** see **Schmidt PJ**
**Channick BJ** see **Kessler RK**
**Chanoit PF** see **Richou H**
**Chantraine P:** Remarques sur la langue et le vocabulaire du Corpus Hippocratique. In La collection hippocratique et son rôle dans l'histoire de la médecine. Colloque de Strasbourg (23–27 octobre 1972) organisé par le Centre de Recherches sur la Grèce Antique, avec le concours des Facultés de Philosophie et des Langues Classiques. Leiden, E. J. Brill, 1975. p. 35–40.
**Chao TC:** Coroner's practice in Singapore. **Ann Acad Med Singapore** 1982 Jul;11(3):469–72
**Chao You Chen:** [A study of the ancient medical manuscript 'Tsu-pei-shih-i-mo-chiu-ching' recently found in Ma-wang-t'ui, China.] (Jpn). **Nihon I-Shigaku Zasshi** 1981;27(1):1–5
**Chapel A, Mehregan AH, Reyman TA:** Histologic findings in mummified skin. **J Am Acad Dermatol** 1981 Jan;4(1):27–30
**Chapin G, Wasserstrom R:** Pesticide use and malaria resurgence in Central America and India. **Soc Sci Med** 1983;17(5):273–90
**Chaplin, JP, Krawiec TS:** Systems and theories of psychology. New York, Holt, Rinehart and Winston, 1979. viii, 651 p.
**Chaplinskiĭ VV, Iatsekevich IaE:** L'vovskomu nauchnomu obshchestvu travmatologov-ortopedov 25 let. **Ortop Travmatol Protez** 1982 Dec;(12):60–1
**Chapman A** see **Webster C, ed**
**Chapman AH, Vieira e Silva D:** Base para uma psiquiatria científica: os conceitos de Harry Stack Sullivan. **Arq Neuropsiquiatr** 1980 Mar;38(1):76–80
**Chapman C** see **Castaing L**
**Chapman CB:** An aspect of medical publication: 1846 and 1982. **N Engl J Med** 1982 Dec 9;307(24):1531
**Chapman CB:** Stratton vs. Swanlond: the fourteenth-century ancestor of the law of malpractice. **Pharos** 1982 Fall;45(4):20–4
**Chapman CB:** The importance of being ethical. **Perspect Biol Med** 1981 Spring;24(3):422–39
**Chapman CM** see **Allan P**
**Chapman EM:** History of the discovery and early use of radioactive iodine. **JAMA** 1983 Oct 21;250(15):2042–4
**Chapman ID, Farina C:** Accountability and the science research board. **J Can Stud** 1982–83;17(4):3–9
**Chapman JE** see **Lostetter JO**
**Chapman JS:** Forts and fevers: medicine on the Texas frontier. **Friends P. I. Nixon Med Hist Libr** 1979 Oct;8:1–8
**Chapman PD:** Schools as sorters: testing and tracking in California, 1910–1925. **J Soc Hist** 1981;14(4):701–17
**Chapman RF:** Leonard Wood and leprosy in the Philippines: the Culion Leper Colony, 1921–1927. [Washington, D. C.], University Press of America, 1982. xviii, 219 p.
**Chappert A:** L' autobiographical sketch de Thomas Young. **Rev Hist Sci (Paris)** 1981 Apr;34(2):137–8
**Charap MH:** The periodic health examination: genesis of a myth. **Ann Intern Med** 1981 Dec;95(6):733–5
**Charbit Y** see **Dupâquier J**
**Charbit Y** see **Leridon H**
**Charbonneau H, Larose A, ed:** The great mortalities: methodological studies of demographic crises in the past. Liège, Belgium, Ordina Editions, [1980]. 373 p. Includes contributions by A. Appleby, S. Sogner, J. N. Biraben. Text in English or French.
**Charbonneau H** see **Jette R**
**Charbonnel A:** Histoire de l'oto-neuro-ophtalmologie. **Rev Otoneuroophtalmol** 1979 Oct–Dec;51(5):399–416
**Charbusky K:** Zur Geschichte des Vöslauer Thermalbades. **Jahrb Landeskd Niederoesterr** 1964;36:425–44
**Chardack WM:** Recollections--1958–1961. **PACE** 1981 Sep;4(5):592–6
**Charkes MD** see **Kessler RK**
**Charkviani LI:** Zakavlazskie konferentsii onkologov. **Vopr Onkol** 1981;27(9):48–52
**Charle C:** Histoire professionnelle, histoire sociale? Les médecins de l'ouest au XIXe siècle. **Ann Econ Soc Civilis** 1979;34(4):787–93
**Charles AD:** History of dentistry in South Carolina. Greenville, S.C., [s.n.], 1982. viii, 124 p.
**Charles AD:** History of dentistry in South Carolina. Ph.D. Diss., University of South Carolina. Columbia, 1981. v, 222 leaves.
**Charles AD:** The story of dental amalgam. **Bull Hist Dent** 1982 Apr;30(1):2–7
**Charles DC, Charles LA:** Charles Dickens' old people. **Int J Aging Hum Dev** 1979–80;10(3):231–7
**Charles LA** see **Charles DC**
**Charles Darwin, 1809–1882; Anton Dohrn, 1840–1909:** Correspondence. Napoli, Macchiaroli, 1982. 118 p.
**Charlton C:** The fight against vaccination: the Leicester demonstration of 1885. **Local Popul Stud (Matlock)** 1983 Spring;30:60–66
**Charlton C:** The National Health Society Almanack, 1883. **Local Popul Stud (Matlock)** 1984;32:54–7
**Charlton C, Drake M, Gwynne T, et al:** The Registrar General's indexes and registers: microfilm copies may be available. **Local Popul Stud (Matlock)** 1984;32:4–11
**Charmasson T:** L'établissement d'un almanach médical pour l'année 1437. In: Congrès National des Sociétés Savantes, 99e, Besançon, 1974. Comptes Rendus. Paris, 1976. Section des Sciences, Fasc. V. p. 217–34.
**Charmasson T:** Roland l'Ecrivain, médecin des Ducs de Bourgogne. In: Congrès National des Sociétes Savantes, 101e, Lille, 1976. Comptes Rendus. Paris, 1976. Section des Sciences, Fasc. III. p. 21–32.
**Charnley J:** Evolution of total hip replacement. **Ann Chir Gynaecol** 1982;71(2):103–7
**Charpin J:** Goyrand, d'Aix, un académicien de province au XIX siècle (1803–1866). **Bull Acad Natl Med (Paris)** 1982 Jun;166(6):787–90
**Charpin J:** Laënnec et l'asthme. **Rev Fr Mal Respir** 1981;9(2):151–3
**Charroppin P:** L'escargot contre la hernie? **Rev Hist Pharm (Paris)** 1983 Sep;30(258):215–9
**Charuty G:** La folie féminine dans la société languedocienne traditionnelle. Les effets de la psychiatrisation. **Penelope** 1983;(8):36–9
**Charuty G:** La psychiatrisation des croyances: savoir médical et savoirs surnaturels en Languedoc, 1850–1940. **Asclepio** 1983;35:197–215
**Chase A:** Jerome Frank and American psychoanalytic jurisprudence. **Int J Law Psychiatry** 1979;2(1):29–54
**Chase A:** Magic shots: a human and scientific account of the long and continuing struggle to eradicate infectious diseases by vaccination. New York, Morrow, 1982. 576 p.
**Chase A:** The legacy of Malthus: the social costs of the new scientific racism. Urbana, University of Illinois Press, 1980. xxix, 686, xviii p.
**Chase A** see **Tobach E**
**Chase MW:** Irreverent recollections from Cooke and Coca, 1928–1978. **J Allergy Clin Immunol** 1979 Nov;64(5):306–20
**Chase RA:** The development of tissue transfer in hand surgery. **J Hand Surg [Am]** 1984 Jul;9(4):463–77
**Chasis H:** History of collaboration by Department of Physiology at New York University School of Medicine. **Physiologist** 1983 Apr;26(2):64–70
**Chasseguet-Smirgel J:** De Sade: Der Körper und der Mord an der Realität. **Psyche (Stuttg)** 1981 Mar;35(3):237–52
**Chatelaine KL:** Harry Stack Sullivan, the formative years. Washington, D.C., University Press of America, 1981. xxiv, 553 p.
**Chato JC:** Reflections on the history of heat and mass transfer in bioengineering. **J Biomech Eng** 1981 May;103(2):97–101
**Chatterjee PK:** Medical education in India since independence. **J Indian Med Assoc** 1981 Sep;77(5–6):91–5
**Chatters LM** see **Jackson JS**
**Chaturvedi GN, Tiwari SK, Rai NP:** Medicinal use of opium and cannabis in Medieval India. **Indian J Hist Sci** 1981, reçu 1982;16(1):31–5
**Chaturvedi GN** see **Rai NP**
**Chauhan DK, Singh RN:** Contribution of Medieval India to Ayurvedic Materia Medica. **Indian J Hist Sci** 1982;16(1):17–21
**Chaulet P** see **Ait Khaled N**
**Chauleur P:** Développement et problèmes démographiques Africains. **Etudes (Fr)** 1981;354(4):437–49
**Chaunu P, Dupâquier J, Chesnais JC:** La dénatalité. Analyse historique du présent: la dénatalité. 'La vie c'est bon.' Les retournements de l'avenir. **Histoire** 1978;(3,6):62–6, 62–5
**Chaunu P, et al.** see **Guillemain B**
**Chausovskaia MM** see **Poletaev SD**
**Chave SP:** Duncan of Liverpool--and some lessons for today. **Community Med** 1984 Feb;6(1):61–71
**Chave SP:** The rise and fall of the medical officer of health. **Community Med** 1980 Feb;2(1):36–45
**Chaves-Carballo E:** Samuel T. Darling: studies on malaria and the Panama Canal. **Bull Hist Med** 1980 Spring;54(1):95–100
**Chávez I:** Historia de la cardiologia, raíces, desarrollo y perspectivas. **Bol Soc Mex Hist Filos Med** 1980 Jun;5(31):25–35
**Chavez I:** La evolución de la medicina en México. **Cuad Am** 1980;229(2):155–67
**Chávez I:** La moral médica frente a la medicina de nuestro tiempo. In Academia Nacional de Medicine. Libro conmemorativo del primer centenario. México, Comité Editorial de la Comisión Organizadora del Congreso del Centenario, 1964. Tome 2. p. 668–73.
**Chávez I:** Reflexiones de un clinico en torno de los momentos culminantes de la cardiologia. **Bol Soc Mex Hist Filos Med** 1980 Jun;5(31):37–55
**Chavkin W:** Occupational hazards to reproduction: a review essay and annotated bibliography. **Feminist Stud** 1979;5(2):310–25
**Chawla PL:** Child psychiatry--historical perspective. **Indian J Pediatr** 1984 Mar–Apr;51(409):191–2
**Chayen Y, Bitensky L:** Modern cytological techniques in biological and medical research. **Acta Med Pol** 1982;23(3–4):127–39
**Chazaud J:** Les contestations actuelles de la psychanalyse. Toulouse, Privat, 1974. 227 p.
**Chebotarev DF:** Idei A. A. Bogomol'tsa razvitie sovremenno i gerontologii. **Fiziol Zh** 1981 May–Jun;27(3):400–6
**Chebotarev DF, Duplenko IuK:** Vklad A. A. Bogomol'tsa v razrabotku aktual'nyk problem medikobiologicheskoĭ nauki (k 100-letiiu so dnia rozhdeniia). **Vrach Delo** 1981 May;(5):6–10
**Chebotarev DF:** 25 let deiatel'nosti Instituta gerontologii AMN SSSR v razvitii nauki o starenii. **Vestn Akad Med Nauk SSSR** 1984;(3):3–9
**Chebotarev RS:** Ocherki po istorii meditsinskoĭ i veterinarnoĭ parazitologii. Minsk, Nauka i tekhnika, 1977. 308 p.
**Chechenkina OI:** Progress zdravookhraneniia c respublikakh Sredneĭ Azii i Kazakhstane - rezul'tat Leninskoĭ natsional'noĭ politiki. **Sov Zdravookhr** 1982;(11):49–51
**Checkland O, Lamb M, ed:** Health care as social history; the Glasgow

case. Aberdeen, Aberdeen University Press, 1982. xix, 285 p.
**Checkland O:** Maternal and child welfare. In Checkland O, Lamb M, ed: Health care as social history; the Glasgow case. Aberdeen, Aberdeen University Press, 1982. p. 117-33.
**Checkland S:** British urban health in general and in a single city. In Checkland O, Lamb M, ed: Health care as social history; the Glasgow case. Aberdeen, Aberdeen University Press, 1982. p. 170-90.
**Chekareva GA:** I. V. Davydovskiĭ, 1887-1968. Moskva, Meditsina, 1980. 79 p.
**Chekurov PR** see **Aliev MA**
**Cheli E:** Le decisioni d'interesse pediatrico del Consiglio Superiore di Sanita'. **Minerva Med** 1979 Nov 3;70(48):XVI-XIX
**Chelius JR:** Economic and demographic aspects of the occupational injury problem. **Q Rev Econ Bus** 1979;19(2):65-70
**Chemerisski IA:** Kommunisticheskaia partiia: organizator bor'by s golodom (1921-1922 gg). **Vopr Istor KPSS** 1971;11:42-53
**Chemin A, Ganry C:** Approche systémique et thérapie familiale. Place et histoire du mouvement systémique. **Soins Psychiatr** 1983 Dec;(38):3-7
**Chen BH:** Neurosurgery in China. (A report presented in the Italian Cities of Turin, Padua and Florence in October, 1981). **J Neurosurg Sci** 1982 Oct-Dec;26(4):273-7
**Chen CY** see **Hsu HY**
**Chen JY** see **Lin CC**
**Chen KJ:** Certain progress in the treatment of coronary heart disease with traditional medicinal plants in China. **Am J Chin Med** 1981 Autumn;9(3):193-6
**Chen KJ:** [Historical data of medicine in Qing Dynasty: case records of westerners treated by traditional Chinese medicine] (Chi). **Chung Hsi I Chieh Ho Tsa Chih** 1981;1(2):122
**Chen KK:** Two pharmacological traditions: notes from experience. **Annu Rev Pharmacol Toxicol** 1981;21:1-6
**Chen LB, Hung T:** [Scanning electron microscopic view of parasitic worm ova in an ancient corpse (author's transl)] (Chi). **Chung Kuo I Hsueh Ko Hsueh Yuan Hsueh Pao** 1981 Mar;3(1):64-5
**Chen MC** see **Yang KL**
**Chen RT** see **Berkelhamer JE**
**Chen W:** [A history of the discovery of cholera pathogen] (Chi). **Chung Hua I Shih Tsa Chih** 1984;14(2):104-6
**Chen WY** see **Yang KL**
**Chen YZ:** A brief introduction to the ancient history of eye injuries in China. **Chin Med J [Engl]** 1980 Mar;93(3):164-8
**Chen YZ:** Ramble in Chinese ophthalmology, past and present. **Chin Med J [Engl]** 1981 Jan;94(1):1-4
**Chen YZ:** The courageous and brilliant blind monk Jianshen. **Chin Med J [Engl]** 1980 Feb;93(2):130-3
**Chen ZS** see **Yang KL**
**Chen chiu shih hua:** Hong Kong, I yao wei sheng ch'u pan she, 1977. 54 p.
**Chen Menglai:** [Ly Yanshi, life and medical achievements.] (Chi). **Chin J Med Hist** 1981;11:93-4
**Chené-Williams A** see **Sutto C, ed**
**Cheney RA** see **Condran GA**
**Cheng M:** The Medical Library in the University of Singapore. **Singapore Libr** 1975;5:50-3
**Cheng TO:** Glimpses of the past from the recently unearthed ancient corpses in China. **Ann Intern Med** 1984 Nov;101(5):714-5
**Cheng Zhifan:** [Galen's thought, physiology and anatomy as taught by him] (Chi). **Chin J Med Hist** 1980;10:92-5
**Chepik IK:** Moral'nyi zakon nashei zhizni (obzor dokumentov Moskovskoi oblastnoi Partiinoi organizatsii vtorogo perioda velikoi otechestvennoi voiny o pomoshchi sem'iam zashchitnikov rodiny i invalidam voiny). **Sov Arkh** 1975;(6):75-80
**Chepulis SP, Tertsionas PV:** Nekotorye aspekty razvitiia stomatologii v Litve. **Stomatologiia (Mosk)** 1982;(6):10-1
**Cherkasov SV:** Leninskoe uchenie ob istine i problema kriteriia praktiki v diagnostike. **Klin Khir** 1980 Jun;(6):1-6
**Cherkasov SV:** Leninskoe uchenie ob istine i probleme kriterii praktiki v diagnostike. **Ter Arkh** 1980;52(7):146-40
**Cherlin AJ:** Explaining the postwar baby boom. **Soc Sci Res Counc Items** 1981;35(4):57-63
**Chernenko VD, Shtel'makh NI:** K 100-letiiu osnovaniia kafedry propevtiki vnutrennikh bolezneĭ lechebnogo fakul'teta Khar'kovskogo meditsinskogo instituta. **Vrach Delo** 1984 Aug;(8):119-21
**Chernetskiĭ OE:** Meditsinskie sestry na pochtovykh markakh. **Med Sestra** 1980 Apr;39(4):53-6
**Chernick V** see **Smith GF**
**Chernin E:** Josiah Clark Nott, insects, and yellow fever. **Bull NY Acad Med** 1983 Nov;59(9):790-802
**Chernin E:** Sir Patrick Manson: an annotated bibliography and a note on a collected set of his writings. **Rev Infect Dis** 1983 Mar-Apr;5(2):353-86
**Chernin E:** Sir Patrick Manson's studies on the transmission and biology of filariasis. **Rev Infect Dis** 1983 Jan-Feb;5(1):148-66
**Chernin E:** The curious case of the lateral-spined egg: schistosoma mansoni. **Trans R Soc Trop Med Hyg** 1983;77(6):847-50
**Chernin E:** Two physicians, a landscape architect, and malaria. **Bull NY Acad Med** 1984 Nov;60(9):932-7
**Chernobrov IV:** Vrach-revoliutsioner N. A. Alekseev. **Sov Zdravookhr** 1983;(11):57-9
**Chernok NB:** Nursing homes--response to a need. **J Long Term Care Adm** 1978 Winter;6(4):41-50
**Chernomas R:** A comparative view of the relationship between the business cycle and mortality, 1871-1900. **Int J Health Serv** 1984;14(1):127-46
**Chernov AZ:** Aleksandr Filippovich Samoĭlov. **Klin Med (Mosk)** 1983 Jan;61(1):116-20
**Chernov PA:** Sanitarno-épidemiologicheskaia sluzhba Kirgizskoĭ SSR. **Gig Sanit** 1982 Dec;(12):43-5
**Chernukh AM, Morozov BV, Pogodaev GV:** O povyshenii éffektivnosti prioritetnykh issledovaniĭ v nauchnykh uchrezhdeniiakh AMN SSSR. **Vestn Akad Med Nauk SSSR** 1980;(4):22-8
**Chernukh AM:** Ocherki obshcheĭ (teoreticheskoĭ) patologii. **Patol Fiziol Eksp Ter** 1983 May-Jun;3:51-78
**Chernyĭ VP:** Znamenitye patsienty N. I. Pirogova. **Feldsher Akush** 1983 Sep;48(9):34-7
**Chernyshenko LV** see **Bobrik II**
**Cherokov VS:** Mediki Krasnoznamennoĭ Ladozhskoĭ voennŏi flotilii. **Voen Med Zh** 1980 Jan;(1):66-7
**Cherry R:** Biology and sociology and economics: an historical analysis. **Rev Soc Econ** 1980;38(2):141-54
**Cherry S:** The hospitals and population growth: part 1. The voluntary general hospitals, mortality and local populations in the English provinces in the eighteenth and nineteenth centuries. **Popul Stud** 1980 Mar;34(1):59-75
**Chertok L:** Hypnosis and suggestion in a century of psychotherapy: an epistemological assessment. **J Am Acad Psychoanal** 1984 Apr;12(2):211-32
**Chertok L:** La riabilitazione dell'inconscio in Unione Sovietica: il Convegno internazionale di Tbilisi. **Stor Crit Psicol** 1982 Jun;3(1):41-62
**Chertok L:** On the centenary of Charcot: hysteria, suggestibility and hypnosis. **Br J Med Psychol** 1984 Jun;57(Pt 2):111-20
**Chertok L, De Saussure R:** The therapeutic revolution from Mesmer to Freud. New York, Brunner/Mazel, 1979. xiii, 226 p. Translation of French ed., 1973.
**Chertok L:** 30 ans après. La petite histoire de la découverte des neuroleptiques. **Ann Med Psychol (Paris)** 1982 Nov;140(9):971-6
**Cherubini A:** Medicina e lotte sociali (1900-1920). Roma, Il Pensiero Scientifico, 1980. 358 p.
**Chervakova TV** see **Manuilova IM**
**Cheshko VT:** The development of ideas on nature of heterosis in biochemical genetics (1940-1970). **Istor Biol Issled** 1983;9:186-90
**Chesley LC:** Evolution of the Department of Obstetrics and Gynecology at Downstate, 1860-1980. [New York?, s.n., 1982?] 96 p.
**Chesnais JC:** La baisse de la natalite et ses consequences pour la planification sectorielle dans les pays capitalistes developpes. **Population** 1982;37(6):1133-58
**Chesnais JC:** La hausse de la mortalité infantile en Union Sovietique. **Population** 1981;36(6):1176-80
**Chesnais JC:** La notion de cycle en démographié: la fécondité post-transitionnelle est-elle cyclique? **Population** 1983;38(2):361-90
**Chesnais JC** see **Chaunu P**
**Chess S** see **Schopler E**
**Chessick RD:** Freud teaches psychotherapy. Indianapolis, Cambridge, Hackett, 1980. viii, 342 p.
**Chessick RD:** Socrates: first psychotherapist. **Am J Psychoanal** 1982 Spring;42(1):71-83
**Chesterman C:** The medical missionary. **Trans R Soc Trop Med Hyg** 1979;73(4):360-1
**Cheung WY:** Discovery and recognition of calmodulin: a personal account. **J Cyclic Nucleotide Res** 1981;7(2):71-84
**Cheung YW** see **New PK**
**Chevalier P** see **Rullière R**
**Chevalier PA, ed:** The heart and circulation. Stroudsburg, Pennsylvania, Dowden, Hutchinson & Ross, 1976. xix, 385 p. (Benchmark Papers in Human Physiology, 8).
**Chevallier P** see **Bernier JJ**
**Chew CH** see **Teo SK**
**Cheymol J:** Hôpitaux des pèlerins de Saint-Jacques-de-Compostelle. **Hist Sci Med** 1980;14:387-97
**Cheymol J:** Hôpitaux des pèlerins de Saint-Jacques-de-Compostelle. IV. Sur la route du Puy: l'hospice de Pradelles. V. L'hôpital de Saint-Géraud et la confrérie des pèlerins d'Aurillac. **Hist Sci Med** 1981;15(1):99-107
**Cheymol J:** Hôpitaux et confrérie des pèlerins de Saint-Jacques-de-Compostelle à Paris. **Hist Sci Med** 1980;14(1):29-42
**Cheymol J:** L'hôpital de la Trinité en la rue Saint-Denis à Paris (1201-1790). **Hist Sci Med** 1983;17(2):159-70
**Cheymol J:** L'hôpital Sainte-Catherine à Paris (1181-1794). **Hist Sci Med** 1982;16(4):239-51
**Chi nien Pai Ch'iu-en:** in memory of Norman Bethune. Pei-ching, Jen min ch'u pan she, 1979. 285 p.
**Chia T:** Chung-kuo i hsüeh shih lüeh. Taiyüan, Shan-hsi jen min ch'u pan she, 1979. 4, 316 p.
**Chiacone FM:** Appunti per uno studio sulla vitaminologia in Italia. **Acta Vitaminol Enzymol** 1979;1(1-6):33-109
**Chiba M** see **Franz MM**
**Chiba Daigaku Igakubu Hyakushunen Kinenshi Henshu Iinkai:** Chiba Daigaku Igakubu hyakushunen kinenshi. Chiba, Japan, Chiba Daigaku Hyakushunen Kinenkai, Showa 53 nen, 1978. xv, 686 p.
**Chico C** see **Thompson RL**
**Chien S** see **Skalak R**
**Chikamori K** see **Fujimori K**
**Chikin SIa:** Leninskie printsipy okhrany narodnogo zdorov'ia. **Vestn Akad Med Nauk SSSR** 1980;(4):3-9
**Chikin SIa:** Razvitie zdravookhraneniia SSSR v period mezhdu XXI i

XXVI s'ezdami KPSS. **Med Sestra** 1981 Feb;40(2):3-7
**Chikin SIa:** Sotsial'no-gigienicheskie idei K. Marksa (k 100-letiiu so dnia smerti). **Sov Med** 1983;(3):75-8
**Chikin SIa:** 60-letie obrazovaniia SSSR i uspekhi razvitiia sovetskogo zdravookhraneniia. **Sov Med** 1982;(12):3-10
**Child abuse: historical perspective:** In D. N. Jones, J. Pickett, M. R. Oates, P. R. Barbor, ed: Understanding child abuse. Kent, Hodder and Stoughton, 1982. p. 38-50.
**Children's Bureau studies:** Introduction by W. M. Schmidt. New York, Arno, 1974. Reprinted works by various authors.
**Chilton WS, Bigwood J, Jensen RE:** Psilocin, bufotenine and serotonin: historical and biosynthetic observations. **J Psychedelic Drugs** 1979 Jan-Jun;11(1-2):61-9
**Chinard FP:** Edward Miller--American physician (1760-1812) **J Med Soc NJ** 1981 Apr;78(4):296-9
**Chippaux C:** Le Service de Santé des troupes de Marine. **Med Trop (Mars)** 1980 Nov-Dec;40(6):605-30
**Chirico F:** Spunti per un'interpretazione medica del mito egiziano di Horus er Seth. **Acta Med Hist Patav** 1981/82;28:41-57
**Chirkov AI:** Meditsinskoe snabzhenie russkoĭ armii v voĭnakh XVIII veka. **Voen Med Zh** 1981 Aug;(8):74-6
**Chirkov AI:** Organizatsiia meditsinskogo snabzheniia russkoĭ armii v Otechestvennuiu voĭnu 1812 goda. **Voen Med Zh** 1982 Apr;(4):70-2
**Chiropractors -- healers or quacks? Part 1: The 80-year war with science: Consum Rep** 1975 Sep;40(9):542-7
**Chissov VI, Demidov VP, Kapatsinskiĭ EV, et al:** Rol' Moskovskogo nauchno-issledovatel'skogo instituta im. P. A. Gertsena Minzdrava RSFSR v razvitii otechestvennoĭ onkologii. **Vopr Onkol** 1983;29(11):3-7
**Chitnis AC:** Universities, medicine and science. In his: The Scottish Enlightenment: a social history. 279 pp. London: Croom Helm; Totawa, N.J.: Rowman & Littlefield, 1976. p. 124-94.
**Chitwood WR:** Ludlow's esophageal diverticulum: a preternatural bag. **Surgery** 1979 May;85(5):549-53
**Chiyo:** [Illustrated history of nursing] (Jpn). **Kango Kyoiku** 1984 Feb;25(2):95-102 contd
**Chlumský J:** Třicet let Institutu pro další vzdělávání lékařu a farmaceutu. **Cesk Gastroenterol Vyz** 1983 Nov;37(6-7):361-3
**Chmielewska-Szlajfer M** see **Suchodolski B**
**Cho LJ, Kobayashi K, ed:** Fertility transition of the East Asian populations. Honolulu, University Press of Hawaii, 1979. vi, 300 p. (Monographs of the Center for Southeast Asian Studies, Kyoto University). Contributions by A. J. Coale, S. B. Hanley, Y. Tsubouchi, H. Y. Lee, P. E. Perry, T. H. Sun, Y. L. Soong, P. K. Liu, B. Mok, V. T. Palan, Y. J. Takeshita, C. T. Chang, C. Tuan, R. Freeman.
**Chodkowski EG** see **Goss CM**
**Choi SY** see **Lee S**
**Chojna JW:** Pierwsza próba opracowania metodologii historii medycyny w piśmiennictwie polskim. **Arch Hist Med (Warsz)** 1981;44(1):77-84
**Chojna JW:** Piśmiennictwo lekarskie związane z epidemia cholery na ziemiach polskich w czasie powstania listopadowego. **Arch Hist Med (Warsz)** 1981;44(2):143-55
**Chojna JW:** Warszawskie lazarety wojskowe w czasie powstania listopadowego. **Arch Hist Med (Warsz)** 1981;44(3/4):277-308
**Chojna JW:** Warszawskie lazarety wojskowe w czasie powstania listopadowego. **Arch Hist Med (Warsz)** 1983;46(1):1-19
**Chojna JW:** Warszawskie lazarety wojskowe w czasie Powstania Listopadowego. **Arch Hist Med (Warsz)** 1980;43(4):353-75
**Chokin AR, Ibragimov NG:** Obshchestvenno-politicheskaia deiatel'nost' progressivnykh medikov dorevoliutsionnogo Kazakhstana i Bashkirii. **Sov Zdravookhr** 1981;(7):59-62
**Chokin AR, Ibragimov NG:** Okhrana materinstva i detstva v Kazakhstane i Bashkirii v pervoe desiatiletie Sovetskoĭ vlasti. **Sov Zdravookhr** 1984;(3):55-9
**Chokin AR, Kabykenov PS:** Voprosy zdorav'ia i meditsiny v trudakh izvestnykh Kazakhskikh prosvetiteleĭ. **Sov Zdravookhr** 1983;6:71-4
**Chokin AR** see **Klebanov IaA**
**Chomakhashvili AI** see **Kurchishvili IB**
**Chopchik DI** see **Orzheshkovskiĭ VV**
**Chorover SL:** From genesis to genocide. The meaning of human nature and the power of behavior control. Cambridge, Mass., MIT Press, 1979. xiii, 238 p.
**Chothia C** see **Dodson G**
**Chow EP:** Acupuncture: its history and educational significance to health practices in the United States. Ph.D. Diss., The Fielding Institute. Santa Barbara, 1975. 156 leaves.
**Chow KW** see **Khoo FY**
**Chow Tse-Tsung:** The childbirth myth and ancient Chinese medicine: a study of aspects of the 'wu' tradition. In D. T. Roy, T. Tsien, ed: Ancient China. Hong Kong, 1978. p. 43-89.
**Chrástek J** see **Horák J**
**Chrétien J, Marsac J:** La sarcoïdose. Rappel historique et évolution des concepts. **Rev Prat** 1983 Sep 11;33(39):2011-4, 2017-9
**Chrétien J:** La sarcoïdose un siècle après Besnier: de l'approche descriptive à l'approche pathogénique. **Ann Med Interne (Paris)** 1984;135(2):89-90
**Christen AG:** Charles C. Bass, M.D.--1875-1975: that cantankerous genius of preventive dentistry. **Bull Hist Dent** 1982 Apr;30(1):8-18
**Christen AG:** Orally used smokeless tobacco as advertised in the metamorphic trade cards of 1870-1900. **Bull Hist Dent** 1983 Oct;31(2):82-6
**Christen AG, Swanson BZ, Glover ED, et al:** Smokeless tobacco: the folklore and social history of snuffing, sneezing, dipping, and chewing. **J Am Dent Assoc** 1982 Nov;105(5):821-9
**Christen AG:** The oral history interview: a treasurehouse for present and future dental historiographers. **Bull Hist Dent** 1981;29(1):8-14
**Christen AG** see **Forrest WR**
**Christensen AL:** 'Og så gjekk me og så på lik'. **Samtiden (Norway)** 1980;89(3):23-9
**Christensen HA, Fairchild GB, Herrer A, et al:** The ecology of cutaneous leishmaniasis in the Republic of Panama. **J Med Entomol** 1983 Oct 5;20(5):463-84
**Christensen HT:** Mormon sexuality in cross-cultural perspective. **Dialogue** 1976;10(2):62-75
**Christensen OS:** Modellen af Domus Anatomica. **Dan Medicinhist Arbog** 1980;:169-79
**Christenson CV:** Alfred Charles Kinsey. In Dictionary of American Biography, Suppl. 6, 1956-1960. p. 342-4, 1980.
**Christiansen PA:** Bibliotek for Laeger 175 år. **Ugeskr Laeger** 1983 Jun 27;145 Spec No:3-4
**Christianson EH:** The colonial surgeon's rise to prominence: Dr. Silvester Gardiner (1707-1786) and the practice of lithotomy in New England. **N Engl Hist Geneal Regist** 1982 Apr;136:104-14
**Christianson EH:** The conditions for science in the academic department of Transylvania University, 1799-1857. **Regist Ky Hist Soc** 1981;79(4):305-25
**Christianson EH:** The emergence of medical communities in Massachusetts, 1700-1794: the demographic factors. **Bull Hist Med** 1980 Spring;54(1):64-77
**Christianson EH:** Wound management advice in antebellum America. In Romm S, ed: Symposium on historical perspectives of plastic surgery. Philadelphia, Saunders, 1983. p. 671-7.
**Christianson EH** see **Cash P**
**Christianson EH** see **Romm S, ed**
**Christie AB:** Infection in Britain yesterday. **J R Coll Physicians Lond** 1981 Apr;15(2):95-7
**Christie J:** Mary Elizabeth Switzer. In: Notable American women. The modern period. Cambridge, Mass., Belknap-Harvard Univ. Press, 1980. 4:669-70.
**Christie JR, Golinski JV:** The spreading of the word: new directions in the historiography of chemistry 1600-1800. **Hist Sci** 1982 Dec;50(4):235-66
**Christoffersen JC:** L. L. Jacobson (1783-1843). **Invest Urol** 1980;18:227
**Christol D:** Historique et définitions de l'antisepsie et de la désinfection. Leurs frontières. Position actuelle du problème. **Rev Prat** 1980 Jun 11;30(33):2159-65
**Christophers BE:** Gout and its sufferers. **Med J Aust** 1979 Sep 22;2(6):311
**Christozov C:** Histoire de la psychiatrie infantile en Bulgarie. **Acta Paedopsychiatr (Basel)** 1981 Jan;46(4):207-11
**Christozov C:** Histoire de la psychiatrie infantile en Bulgarie. In International Congress of the History of Medicine. 26th, Plovdiv, 1978. Actes du Congress. Sofia, 1981. Volume II. p. 65-6.
**Christy NP:** Harvey Cushing as clinical investigator and laboratory worker. **Am J Med Sci** 1981 Mar-Apr;281(2):79-96
**Christy TE:** Clinical practice as a function of nursing education: an historical analysis. **Nurs Outlook** 1980 Aug;28(8):493-7
**Christy TE:** The need for historical research in nursing. **Res Nurs Health** 1981 Jun;4(2):227-8
**Chromý K:** Masturbace a historie psychiatrie. **Cesk Psychiatr** 1984 Jun;80(3):180-3
**A chronology of health legislation in the U.S., 1798-1983: Conn Med** 1984 Apr;48(4):251-7
**Chróścicki A:** Osłuchiwanie serca--od stetoskopu do ultradźwi eków. **Pediatr Pol** 1979 Oct;54(10):1095-100
**Chrzanowski A:** Dar Narodowy dla pani Marii Skłodowska-Curie. **Nowotwory** 1980 Jan-Mar;30(1):93-7
**Chrzanowski A:** Instytut Curie w Krakowie, pierwszy zakład leczenia radem w Polsce. **Nowotwory** 1979 Jul-Sep;29(3):239-41
**Chrzanowski A:** Rozwój Instytutu Radowego w Warszawie w okresie 1932-1939. **Nowotwory** 1980 Jul-Sep;30(3):305-9
**Chrześciewski L:** Filozofia medycyny Władysława Szumowskiego (1875-1954). **Wiad Lek** 1984 Apr 15;37(8):653-4
**Chrześciewski L:** Filozofia medycyny Wøadysøawa Szumowskiego (1875-1954). **Wiad Lek** 1984 Feb 15;37(4):321-2
**Chrzęściewski L:** Jędrzej śniadecki (1768-1838) - prekursor współczesnej myśli pedagogicznej w medycynie. **Arch Hist Med (Warsz)** 1983;46(1):29-38
**Chrzęściewski L:** Pierwsze domy opieki dla dzieci psychicznie chorych w Krakowie. **Psychiatr Pol** 1982 Sep-Dec;16(5-6):437-8
**Chu Tinxiang:** [A sketch of the life of Lu Liuliang.] (Chi). **Chin J Med Hist** 1981;11:89-90
**Chuan-Kui H, Da-Ding F, Gan-Yun Y:** Some sketches on the history of Chinese dermatology. **Arch Dermatol Res** 1982;272(1-2):185-90
**Chuang Y:** The historical development of acupuncture. Los Angeles, Oriental Healing Arts Institute, 1982. 83 p.
**Chubin DE** see **Studer KE**
**Chudacoff HP:** The life course of women: age and age consciousness, 1865-1915. **J Fam Hist** 1980 Fall;5(3):274-92
**Chudańska T** see **Stefański K**
**Chuinard EG:** Only one man died: the medical aspects of the Lewis and Clark Expedition. Glendale, Clark, 1980, 444 p.
**Chun SC:** [Historical review of the nurses' status in Korea] (Kor). **Taehan Kanho** 1983 Sep 20;22(3):30-41
**Church LE:** The ancestors we never knew. **J Md State Dent Assoc** 1983

Dec;26(3):122-3
**Church OM, Buckwalter KC:** Harriet Bailey---a psychiatric nurse pioneer. **Perspect Psychiatr Care** 1980 Mar-Apr;18(2):62-6
**Church OM:** Preparation in historiography in nursing research. **NLN Publ** 1983;(41-1935):54-6
**Church OM** see **Buckwalter KC**
**Churchill FB:** In search of the new biology: an epilogue. **J Hist Biol** 1981 Spring;14(1):177-91
**Churchill FB:** Sex and the single organism: biological theories of sexuality in mid-nineteenth century. **Stud Hist Biol** 1979;3:139-77
**Churchill FB:** The Weismann-Spencer controversy over the inheritance of acquired characters. In Forbes EG, ed: Human implications of scientific advance. Edinburgh, Edinburgh University Press, 1978. p. 451-68.
**Churchill FB** see **Mayr E**
**Churg J:** Diffuse collagen disease. **JAMA** 1984 Nov 16;252(19):2702
**Churg J** see **Selikoff IJ**
**Chylińska M:** Refleksje z obozu w Brzezince. **Przegl Lek** 1984;41(1):115-20
**Chylińska M:** W kregu reakcji obronnych. **Przegl Lek** 1984;41(1):121-6
**Chyrek-Borowska S:** XXX lat Akademii Medycznej im. J. Marchlewskiego w Białymstoku. Białystok, Krajowa Agencja Wydawnicza, 1980. 87 p.
**Ciardi RP:** Fra pelle e ossa. **Kos** 1984 Mar;1(2):93-117
**Cibic B** see **Musič D**
**Cibois P:** La natalisme national. **Esprit** 1982;10:76-96
**Cicu N** see **Marinescu I**
**Cid F:** Broussais, su concepto de irritación en el cuadro de la locura durante el siglo XIX. **Med Hist (Barc)** 1984;(5):3-7
**Cieply J:** Warunki sanitarne w zastepcym wiezieniu policyjnym w Mysłowicach. **Przegl Lek** 1981;38(1):95-107
**Cierny G:** O vývoji a dalších perspektívach teoretických medicínskych odborov lekárskej fakulty Univerzity Komenského v Bratislave. **Cas Lek Cesk** 1979 Dec 21;118(51):1571-3
**Cieślawski M:** Z przezyć dzieci i matek-robotnic przymusowych na Pomorzu Zachodnim. **Przegl Lek** 1981;38(1):121-4
**Cifuentes Delatte L:** Historia del estudio microscópico de los cálculos del aparato urinario en el siglo XIX. **Arch Esp Urol** 1981 Sep-Oct;34(5):375-84
**Cilenti V, Milasi G, Jori A:** Evoluzione storica del concetto di dolore. **Med Secoli** 1982 May-Aug;19(2):225-30
**Cimini TA, Wong A:** The historical development of federal involvement in health care. **Am Arch Rehabil Ther** 1979 Spring;27(1):4-6
**Cimino G:** Claude Bernard sulle 'funzioni del cervello'. **Physis** 1980;22(1):85-119
**Cimino G, ed** see **Grmek MD**
**Cina C:** Social science for whom? A structural history of social psychology. Ph.D. Diss., State University of New York. Stony Brook, 1981. xiii, 417 leaves.
**Cinquantenaire de la Société d'Oto-Rhino-Laryngologie de Lyon et de la Région. Le ler mars 1931: J Fr Otorhinolaryngol** 1982 Jun;31(6):389-96
**Cinti DC** see **Hawkins HB**
**Ciochon RL** see **Corruccini RS**
**Cipolla C:** Peste del 1630--31 nell' Empolese. **Arch Stor Ital** 1978;136:469-81
**Cipolla CM:** A plague doctor. In Miskimin HA, et al, ed.: the medieval city. New Haven. Yale Univ. Press, 1977. p. 65-72
**Cipolla CM:** Cristofano e la peste. Bologna, Il Mulino, 1976. 157 p.
**Cipolla CM:** Faith, reason and the plague in seventeenth-century Tuscany. Ithaca, Cornell University Press, 1979. 113 p.
**Cipolla CM:** Fighting the plague in seventeenth-century Italy. Madison, University of Wisconsin Press, 1981, xi, 123 p. (Merle Curti Lectures, 1978).
**Cipolla CM:** Peste del 1630-31 nel'Empolese. **Arch Stor Ital** 1978;136(3-4):469-82
**Cipriani C** see **Berzi A**
**Cirillo VJ:** Edward Bliss Foote: pioneer American advocate of birth control. **Bull Hist Med** 1973 Sep-Oct;47(5):471-9
**Cirillo VJ:** Nineteenth-century views on blood fluidity. **J Med Soc NJ** 1983 Jul;80(7):535-9
**Cirn JT:** The birth throes of the Wisconsin Medical Practice Act: the physicians versus the newspaper editors. **Wis Med J** 1980 May;79(5):12-4
**Cislaghi:** Storia dei denti artificiali. Analisi dei materiali e delle tecniche di costruzione dai Fenici agli attuali orientamenti biomeccanici. Pisa, Mariotti, 1968. 84 p. (Clinica Odonto-Protesica Stomatologica, Monografie, 1; Supplemento alla Rivista Clinica Odonto-Protesica Stomatologica, 14, 1968).
**Ciszek Z** see **Bluszcz G**
**Ciucura TB:** Dissent, law and psychiatry in the Soviet Union. **Can Slavonic Pap** 1979;21(1):98-108
**Ciuffreda KJ:** Astigmatic amblyopia: George Martin. 1890. Translation. **Am J Optom Physiol Opt** 1978 Feb;55(2):133-6
**Ciulei SG:** Robert Koch (1843-1910), membru de onoare al Societății de Medici şi Naturalişti din Iaşi. **Rev Med Chir Soc Med Nat Iasi** 1983 Jul-Sep;87(3):503-4
**Ciurea AV** see **Arseni C**
**Ciurea D:** Societatea de Medici şi Naturalişti din Iaşi (1830-1980). **Rev Med Chir Soc Med Nat Iasi** 1980 Jul-Sep;84(3):587-92
**Ciurea D** see **Bădărău GH**
**Civatte J:** Jean Darier: a memoir. **Am J Dermatopathol** 1979 Spring;1(1):57-60
**Ciźmář J:** Botanist Carl Theimer (1823--1870) in the cultural context of Brno during the period of Mendel's research. **Folia Mendeliana** 1979;14:265-70
**Ciźmář J:** Závodní časopisy Mediky. **Cesk Farm** 1982 Dec;31(10):393-5
**Clagett GP** see **Rich NM**
**Clagett M:** Lynn Thorndike. In Dictionary of American biography, 1961-1965. Suppl. 7, 1981. p. 741-2.
**Clagett M:** The life and works of Giovanni Fontana. **Ann Ist Mus Stor Sci Fir** 1976;1(1):5-28
**Clair G** see **Delaveau P**
**Claman G:** A typhoid fever epidemic and the power of the press in Denver in 1879. **Colo Mag** 1979 Summer-Fall;56:143-60
**Clanet M** see **Rascol A**
**Clar R:** First Jewish women physician of Los Angeles. **West States Jew Hist Q** 1981;14(1):66-75
**Clark AJ:** Book catalogue of the Library of the Royal Society. University Publication of America, 1982. 5 v.
**Clark CW:** The Zodiac man in medieval medical astrology. Ph.D. Diss., University of Colorado. Boulder, 1979. 440 p.
**Clark D, Hyde GL:** A brief history of the University of Kentucky Department of Surgery. **J Ky Med Assoc** 1984 Jul;82(7):343-7
**Clark D:** Jules Tinel and Tinel's sign. In Romm S, ed: Symposium on historical perspectives of plastic surgery. Philadelphia, Saunders, 1983. p. 627-8.
**Clark D** see **Romm S, ed**
**Clark E** see **Neuburger M**
**Clark EW:** A brief history of lanolin. **Pharm Hist (London)** 1980 Dec;10(3):5-6
**Clark G, White E, White D, et al:** Bibliography of biomedical ultrasound from 1 January 1971, No. 20. **Ultrasound Med Biol** 1980;6(1):63-85
**Clark H:** Foiling the pirates: the preparation and publication of Andreas Vesalius's De humani corporis fabrica. **Libr Q** 1981;51(3):301-11
**Clark LC:** Measurement of oxygen tension: a historical perspective. **Crit Care Med** 1981 Oct;9(10):690-2
**Clark MJ:** 'A plastic power ministering to organisation': interpretations of the mind-body relation in late nineteenth-century British psychiatry. **Psychol Med** 1983 Aug;13(3):487-97
**Clark MJ** see **Scull A, ed**
**Clark RB:** John J. McAlmont, M.D. 1821-1896. **J Arkansas Med Soc** 1984 Apr;80(11):552
**Clark RW:** Freud: the man the cause. New York, Random House, 1980. 652 p.
**Clark RW:** Sigmund Freud's sortie to America. **Am Heritage** 1980;3(3):34-43
**Clark SG:** Farewell to the SBA. **J R Nav Med Serv** 1984 Spring;70(1):3-8
**Clark WD, Quinn FB:** Erroneous reporting of errors. **JAMA** 1984 Jul 13;252(2):207-8
**Clarke AM:** Psychology and education. **Br J Educ Stud** 1982;30(1):43-56
**Clarke B:** Mental illness and rehabilitation in early nineteenth-century Ireland; the case of Charles Stock. **Psychol Med** 1983 Nov;13(4):727-34
**Clarke J:** Dr. Max Herz. Sydney, Alternative Publishing Co-operative, 1976. xv, 184 p.
**Clarke JH:** Increased student participation in a dental history course after changing the grading method. **Bull Hist Dent** 1980 Apr;28(1):44-6
**Clarke JM:** Surgery in Jehovah's witnesses. **Br J Hosp Med** 1982 May;27(5):497-500
**Clarke JN:** Medicalization and secularization in selected English Canadian fiction. **Soc Sci Med** 1984;18(3):205-10
**Clarke JW:** American assassins: an alternative typology. **Br J Polit Sci** 1981;11(1):81-104
**Clarke K:** Infanticide, illegitimacy and the medical profession in nineteenth century England. **Soc Soc Hist Med Bull (Lond)** 1980 Jun;26:11-14
**Clarke MC:** Some medical customs of the Cocos-Keeling Islanders. **Aust Nurses J** 1979 Oct;9(4):42-4, 50
**Clarke SK:** Early childhood morbidity trends in prehistoric populations. **Hum Biol** 1980 Feb;52(1):79-85
**Clarke SS:** Hyman J Weiner's use of systems and population approaches: their relevance to social work practice in health care today. **Soc Work Health Care** 1983 Winter;9(2):5-14
**Clarkson BD:** The elusive goal. **Cancer Res** 1981 Dec;41(12 pt 1):4865-84
**Clarkson TB:** Evolution and history of training and academic programs in laboratory animal medicine. **Lab Anim Sci** 1980 Aug;30(4 pt 2):790-2
**Clary DA, ed:** 'I am already quite a Texan': Albert J. Myer's letters from Texas. **Southwest Hist Q** 1978;82(1):25-76
**Clasen U:** Deutsche und deutschstämmige Arzte in New South Wales und South Australia zwischen 1846 und 1911. Diss., Universität Düsseldorf. Düsseldorf, 1982. 66 p.
**Clasen U** see **Gandevia B**
**Classic articles in colonic and rectal surgery: Dis Colon Rectum** 1981 Jul-Aug;24(5):408-10 (continued periodically)
**Classic articles in colonic and rectal surgery:** James Young Simpson 1811-1870. **Dis Colon Rectum** 1982 Sep;25(6):611-22
**Classic articles in colonic and rectal surgery:** John Arderne 1307-1380 (?). **Dis Colon Rectum** 1982 Nov-Dec;25(8):832-40
**Classic articles in colonic and rectal surgery. Owen Harding Wangensteen 1899-1981: Dis Colon Rectum** 1982 Jan-Feb;25(1):65-78
**Classic articles in colonic and rectal surgery. Robert Fulton Weir 1838-1927:** An improved method of treating high-seated cancers of the rectum. **Dis Colon Rectum** 1982 Jul-Aug;25(5):503-7
**The classics: Clin Orthop** 1982 May;(165):6-32 (continued regularly)
**Classics in infectious diseases:** A contribution to human helminthology: Theodore Bilharz (1825-1862). **Rev Infect Dis** 1982 May-Jun;4(3):727-32
**Classics in infectious diseases:** Excerpts from the Natural History of Pliny.

Rev Infect Dis 1982 Nov–Dec;4(6):1266–9

**Classics in infectious diseases. Letter from Theobald Smith to Edward Krumbhaar: Rev Infect Dis** 1984 Mar–Apr;6(2):280–1

**Classics of infectious diseases: Rev Infect Dis** 1981 Mar–Apr;3(2):372–95 (continued regularly)

**Claude Bernard fut-il un médecin praticien?:** Entretiens de Bichat, Faculté de médecine, Pitié-Salpêtrière, Paris, 29 septembre–8 Octobre 1978. [France], Expansion scientifique, 1978 printing. [32] p.

**Claus LM:** The development of medical sociology in Europe. **Soc Sci Med** 1983;17(21):1591–7

**Claus O** see **Gross R**

**Clausen C, ed** see **Waserman M**

**Clawson DK:** The founding of the Association of Orthopaedic Chairmen. **Clin Orthop** 1983 Dec;181:298–303

**Claxton AC:** An early dental identification of a corpse. **Br Dent J** 1984 Aug 25;157(4):122

**Clayman CB** see **Zucker GM**

**Clean water and the health of the cities:** New York, Arno, 1977. Various paginations. Facsimile reprints of works by William T. Sedgwick (1893), George C. Whipple (1907), and J. Scott MacNutt (1910).

**Cleeland C** see **Zimmermann G**

**Cleghorn RA:** Cardiovascular failure in experimental adrenal insufficiency: a historical rivival. **Perspect Biol Med** 1983 Autumn;27(1):135–55

**Cleghorn RA:** The emergence of psychiatry at McGill. **Can J Psychiatry** 1984 Nov;29(7):551–6

**Cleland WP:** The evolution of cardiac surgery in the United Kingdom. **Thorax** 1983 Dec;38(12):887–96

**Clem TR** see **Berger RL**

**Clemedson CJ:** Berömda svenska böcker inom medicin och farmaci. **Nord Medicinhist Arsb** 1980;Suppl 6:35–51

**Clemedson CJ** see **Habrich C**

**Clement A:** André Boucher. **Bull Acad Chir Dent (Paris)** 1981–82;27(27):99–102

**Clément PP:** Quelques aspects de la vie et de l'oeuvre de Jean-Jacques Rousseau: s'oublier--se surveiller--fixer par l'écriture. **Univ Ottawa Q** 1979;49(3–4):292–9

**Clemmensen O:** Hutchinson's freckle. **Am J Dermatopathol** 1982 Oct;4(5):425–8

**Clemmesen J:** Johannes Fibiger. Copenhagen, Munksgaard, 1978. 13 p.

**Clendennen GW:** Livingstone's second book. **Bibliotheck** 1980;10(1):10–9

**Clerc B, Hanne M:** La Croix-Rouge et l'Afrique: essai bibliographique. **Geneva Afr** 1970;9(1):94–101

**Cleveland AB** see **Gorevic PD**

**Cleveland FP:** History of environmental pathology. **Am J Forensic Med Pathol** 1983 Dec;4(4):331–6

**Cliche MA:** Les attitudes devant la mort d'après les clauses testamentaires dans le gouvernement de Québec sous le régime français. **Rev Hist Am Fr** 1978;32(1):57–94

**Cliff A, Haggett P:** Island epidemics. **Sci Am** 1984 May;250(5):138–47

**Clifford S** see **Gregg JB**

**Clifford T:** Tibetan Buddhist medicine and psychiatry: the diamond healing. Introduction by Lokesh Chandra. York Beach, Me., S. Weiser, 1983. xx, 268 p.

**The clinic at Beech Fork--its 57-year history is a mini-history of FNS: Front Nurs Serv Q Bull** 1984 Summer;60(1):1–10

**Clocotici L:** Asociaţia naţională a surorilor de ocrotire din românia, cadru de acţiune pentru dezvoltarea şi afirmarea profesiei (partea a ii-a). **Viata Med [Medii Sanit]** 1982 Nov;30(11):257–61

**Clocotici L:** Aspecte din tecutul profesiei de moaşă. **Viata Med [Medii Sanit]** 1983 Nov;31(11):261–4

**Clocotici L:** Organiza tii profesionale ale personalului sanitar mediu III. **Viata Med [Medii Sanit]** 1980 Jan;28(1):19–21

**Clocotici L:** Organizaţii profesionale ale personalului sanitar mediu (I). **Viata Med [Medii Sanit]** 1979 Jul;27(7):163–6

**Clocotici L:** Organizaţii profesionale ale personalului sanitar mediu (II). **Viata Med [Medii Sanit]** 1979 Nov;27(11):261–4

**Clocotici L:** Sănătatea este un mod de a exista. **Viata Med [Medii Sanit]** 1981 Nov;29(11):259–60

**Clocotici L:** Sora de ocrotire. **Viata Med [Medii Sanit]** 1982 Sep;30(9):213–6

**Clodius L** see **Martin O**

**Close HG:** A genetic Odyssey. **S Afr Med J** 1982 Jun 26;61(26):1010–2

**Clotuche J** see **Barbaix M**

**Clough M:** Early healing. In Passmore R, ed: Proceedings of the Royal College of Physicians of Edinburgh Tercentenary Congress, 1981. Edinburgh, Royal College of Physicians of Edinburgh, 1982. p. 181–9.

**Clouse RG** see **Aaron PG**

**Cloutier RJ:** Florence Kelley and the radium dial painters. **Health Phys** 1980 Nov;39(5):711–6

**Clowes GH:** George Henry Alexander Clowes, PhD, DSc, LLD (1877–1958): a man of science for all seasons. **J Surg Oncol** 1981;18(2):197–217

**Cluchard J:** Quelques aspects de la vie sociale des apothicaires bordelais au XVIIIe siècle. Thèse. Bordeaux, 1982. in various pagings.

**Clyde WA, Fernald GW:** Mycoplasmas: the pathogens' pathogens. **Cell Immunol** 1983 Nov;82(1):88–97

**Coale AJ, Anderson BA, Härm E:** Human fertility in Russia since the nineteenth century. Princeton, N. J., Princeton Univ. Press, 1979. xxiii, 285 p.

**Coale AJ** see **Cho LJ**

**Coatsworth JH:** Anotaciones sobre la producción de alimentos durante el Porfiriato. **Hist Mex** 1976;26(2):167–87

**Cobanovic K** see **Hadjivukovic S**

**Cobb AB, Riecken WE:** Public health in Mississippi. **J Miss State Med Assoc** 1981 Dec;22(12):319–24

**Cobb HV, Gray MZ, et al:** Mental retardation: past and present. Washington, President's Committee on Mental Retardation, 1977. viii, 276 p.

**Cobb WM:** Edwin Bentley, MD, 1824–1917: Connecticut Yankee in Washington and Little Rock. **J Natl Med Assoc** 1980;72:1012–4

**Cobb WM:** Forward--the only way. **J Natl Med Assoc** 1984 May;76(5):487–97

**Cobb WM:** Man, the slow learner. **J Natl Med Assoc** 1981 Oct;73(10):973–86

**Cobb WM:** The Black American in medicine. **J Natl Med Assoc** 1981 Dec;73 Suppl:1185–244

**Cobo Cobo J** see **Puerto Sarmiento FJ**

**Coburn D, Torrance GM, Kaufert JM:** Medical dominance in Canada in historical perspective: the rise and fall of medicine? **Int J Health Serv** 1983;13(3):407–32

**Coccanari MA:** Les plantes et leur action sur le cerveau et sur la psiche: science et magie. **Med Secoli** 1982 May–Aug;19(2):215–9

**Cochran WG** see **Hilts VL**

**Cochrane RC:** The National Academy of Sciences: the first hundred years, 1863–1963. Washington, D.C., National Academy of Sciences, 1978. xv, 694 p.

**Cochrane RG:** Notes concerning the formation of the International Leprosy Association. **Int J Lepr** 1981 Mar;49(1):67–71

**Cock AG:** Chauvinism and internationalism in science: The International Research Council, 1919–1926. **Notes Rec R Soc Lond** 1983 Mar;37(2):249–88

**Cock AG:** Faking and the intent to deceive. **Br Med J** 1980 Nov 1;281(6249):1214–5

**Cock AG:** William Bateson's pilgrimages to Brno. Cesty Williama Batesona do Brna. **Folia Mendeliana** 1980;65(15):243–50

**Cock AG:** William Bateson's rejection and eventual acceptance of chromosome theory. **Ann Sci** 1983 Jan;40:19–59

**Cockburn A, Peck WH, Barraco RA, et al:** A classic mummy: PUM II. In A. Cockburn, E. Cockburn, ed: Mummies, disease, and ancient cultures. Cambridge, Cambridge University Press, 1980. p. 52–70.

**Cockburn A:** Ancient parasites on the West Bank of the Nile. **Lancet** 1981 Oct 24;2(8252)938

**Cockburn A, Cockburn E:** Autopsies in mummies. **N Engl J Med** 1981 Dec 17;305(25):1534

**Cockburn A, Cockburn E, ed:** Mummies, disease, and ancient cultures. Cambridge, Cambridge University Press, 1980. x, 340 p.

**Cockburn A** see **Ascenzi A**

**Cockburn A** see **Vreeland JM**

**Cockburn E, Reyman TA:** Paleopathology. **JAMA** 1982 Jul 23;248(4):472–3

**Cockburn E** see **Cockburn A**

**Cockburn E, ed** see **Cockburn A**

**Cockcroft IG:** They did not leave the valley. **Nada** 1969;10(1):50–3

**Cocker W:** A history of the university chemical laboratory, Trinity College, Dublin. **Hermathena** 1978;124:58–76

**Cockerham WC:** The state of medical sociology in the United States, Great Britain, West Germany and Austria: applied vs pure theory. **Soc Sci Med** 1983;17(20):1513–27

**Cockett AT** see **Saraf PG**

**Cockett AT** see **Valvo JR**

**Cockett FB:** The statue of Sir Robert Clayton. **St Thomas Hosp Gaz** 1981;79:52–5

**Cocks GC:** Psychoanalyse, Psychotherapie und Nationalsozialismus. **Psyche (Stuttg)** 1983 Dec;37(12):1057–106

**Cockshott WP:** Old medical societies. **N Engl J Med** 1980 Dec 4;303(23):1371

**Cockshott WP** see **Buchanan WW**

**Cockx-Indestege E:** Cornelis Schuute en de onlangs ontdekte almanak voor 1551. Biekorf, Westvlaams Archief, 1981. 12 p.

**Cody CA:** Slave demography and family formation: a community study of the Ball Family plantations, 1720–1896. Ph.D. Diss., University of Minnesota. Minneapolis, 1982. xiv, 429 p.

**Cofer CN:** The history of the concept of motivation. **J Hist Behav Sci** 1981 Jan;17(1):48–53

**Cofer CN** see **Hearst E, ed**

**Cofer CN, ed** see **Kasschau RA**

**Coghi Ruggiero T.** L'antica spezieria del monastero di San Giovanni Evangelista in Parma: un libro mastro de 1588 e una controversia del 1722. **Arch Stor Prov Parmensi** 1980;32:231–44

**Cohen A:** Prophecy and madness: women visionaries during the Puritan Revolution. **J Psychohist** 1984 Winter;11(3):411–30

**Cohen B:** A tale of two paintings. **Ann R Coll Surg Engl** 1982 Jan;64(1):4–12

**Cohen B:** An inquiry into the decay of teeth. **Ann R Coll Surg Engl** 1982 Nov;64(6):375–82

**Cohen B:** Erasmus Darwin's observations on rotation and vertigo. **Hum Neurobiol** 1984;3(3):121–8

**Cohen B:** John Hunter's application of science to surgery. **Ann R Coll Surg Engl** 1984 Jan;66(1):59–62

**Cohen CB:** 'Quality of life' and the analogy with the Nazis. **J Med Philos** 1983 May;8(2):113–35

**Cohen D:** J. B. Watson, the founder of behaviourism: a biography. London, Routledge and Kegan Paul, 1979. vi, 297 p.

**Cohen D:** Social medicine: amputating the wrong leg. **Work Pap Mag** 1981;8(6):17–20

Cohen D: The last 100 years, medicine. New York, M. Evans, 1981. 192 p.
Cohen G see Aharonowitz Y
Cohen IB: Florence Nightingale. Sci Am 1984 Mar;250(3):128–37
Cohen IB: From Leonardo to Lavoisier 1450–1800. New York, Scribner's, 1980. xiii. 298 p. (Album of Science).
Cohen IB see Levere TH, ed
Cohen IB see Recollections & reflections
Cohen J: Death and the Danse Macabre. Hist Today 1982 Aug;32:35–40
Cohen J see Kohn D
Cohen JS see Portugal FH
Cohen LA: Een curieus geval van schijndood in 1857. Ned Tijdschr Geneeskd 1983 Dec 10;127(50):2304
Cohen LJ: Bayesianism versus Baconianism in the evaluation of medical diagnoses. Br J Philos Sci 1980;31(1):45–62
Cohen LK: Dentistry and the behavioral/social sciences: an historical overview. J Behav Med 1981 Sep;4(3):247–56
Cohen MR: A tribute to Martin J. Clyman, M.D., 1914–1979. J Reprod Med 1983 Apr;28(4):233–4
Cohen MS: American civilization in three dimensions: the evolution of the Museum of History and Technology of the Smithsonian Institution. Ph.D. Diss., George Washington University. Washington, D.C., 1980. iv, 349 leaves.
Cohen PC: A calculating people. The spread of numeracy in early America. Chicago, London, Univ. of Chicago Press, 1982. ix, 271 p.
Cohen RA: Cyrus Fay, a pioneer in forceps design. Bull Hist Dent 1983 Apr;31(1):32–3
Cohen RA: Notes on the life and work of Frieda Fromm-Reichmann. Psychiatry 1982;45(2):90–8
Cohen RS, Laudan L, ed: Physics, philosophy and psychoanalysis. Essays in honor of Adolf Grünbaum. Dordrecht, D. Reidel, 1983. xviii, 339 p. (Boston Studies in the Philosophy of Science, v. 76).
Cohen RS see Grmek MD
Cohen S: The mental hygiene movement, the development of personality and the school: the medicalization of American education. Hist Educ Q 1983;23(2):123–49
Cohen SG: In memoriam. Marion B. Sulzberger (1895–1983). A dermatologist's contributions to allergy. J Allergy Clin Immunol 1984 Dec;74(6):855–60
Cohen SS: Two refugee chemists in the United States, 1794: how we see them. Proc Am Philos Soc 1982 Aug;126(4):301–15
Cohen SS see Robin ED, ed
Cohen VL: Bleeding monks. Lancet 1981 Jul 18;2(8238):158
Cohen W: The blackest hour. Synthesis 1980;5(1):2–12
Cohen WJ see Numbers RL, ed
Cohen YA: Shrinking households. Society 1981;18(2):48–52
Cohen EP, ed: Medicine in transition: the centennial of the University of Illinois College of Medicine: a symposium in Chicago, October 1–2, 1981. [Chicago], University of Illinois College of Medicine, and University of Illinois Press, 1981. 340 p.
Cohen IB, ed: Studies on William Harvey. New York, Arno Press, 1981. 572 p. in various pagings. (A collection of previously published articles and short works by various authors).
Cohen IB, ed: The career of William Beaumont and the reception of his discovery. New York, Arno Press, 1980. Various pagings. Reprint of G. Miller: William Beaumont's formative years: two early notebooks 1811–1821 (1946); G. Rosen: The reception of William Beaumont's discovery in Europe (1942); G. Rosen: Notes on the reception and influence of William Beaumont's discovery (1943). (Three centuries of Science in America).
Cohen IB, ed: The life and scientific and medical career of Benjamin Waterhouse: with some account of the introduction of vaccination in America. 2 vols. New York, Arno Press, 1980. Reprints of various works. Various paginations.
Cohen IB, ed: Thomas Jefferson and the sciences. New York, Arno Press, 1980. Reprints of various works. Various paginations. (Three Centuries of Science in America).
Cohen RA, et al: The British Dental Association. The advance of the dental profession; a centenary history 1880–1980. London, British Dental Association, 1979. ix, 289 p.
Cohn DF: Joseph Babinski and his reflex (1857–1932). Koroth 1982 Aug;8(3/4):191–4
Cohn J: Misbruk og mishandling av barn – før og nå. Dan Medicinhist Arbog 1981;:158–68
Cohn M: An introduction to 'Le Pap'. Cell Immunol 1982 Jan 1;66(1):11–6
Cohn RL, Jensen RA: The determinants of slave mortality rates on the middle passage. Explor Econ Hist 1982;19(3):269–82
Cohn V: Sister Kenny's fierce fight for better polio care. Smithsonian 1981;12(8):180–200
Coignerai-Devillers L: Médecine, diététique et santé à la cour de Louis XIV d'après les lettres de la princesse Palatine (1652–1722). Rev Hist Pharm (Paris) 1983 Dec;71(30):265–74
Coin rubbing and related folk medicine: JAMA 1981 May 8;245(18):1819
Coing H: Remarks on the history of foundations and their role in the promotion of learning. Minerva 1981 Summer;19(2):271–81
Colaert J see Schyns C
Colangelo G, Luzi V, Mattioni R: Analisi craniometrica comparativa tra crani etruschi e moderni. Dent Cadmos 1982 Jan;50(1):47–51
Colapinto L: Il Nobile Collegio Chimico Farmaceutico Romano. Cenni storici. Roma, Stomygen, 1979, 30 p.
Colard A: En chirurgie, Ambroise Paré n'a pas innové la ligature vasculaire. Rev Med Brux 1980; NS 1;687–9
Colard A: Evocation du passé: des bons soins que donna Ambroise Paré à un Prince en Hainaut et du succès qu'il en advint. Rev Med Brux 1980 Jun;1(6):405–8
Colard A: Evocation du passé en chirugie. Ambroise Paré n'a pas innové la ligature vasculaire. Rev Med Brux 1980 Dec;1(10):687–9
Colard A: Evocation du passé. Jehan Yperman et l'éthique médicale. Rev Med Brux 1982 Mar;3(3):171–2
Colard A: Evocation du passé: les débuts de l'oxygénothérapie. Rev Med Brux 1983 Feb;4(2):98–100
Colard A: Evocation du passé. Propos d'un vieux médecin sur la thérapeutique. Rev Med Brux 1981 Jan;2(1):39–41
Colard A: Evocation du passé: propos d'un vieux médecin sur la thérapeutique. Rev Med Brux 1983 May;4(5):391–3
Colard A: Evocation du passé: sur le professeur Baron Seutin et sa méthode amovo-inamovible. Rev Med Brux 1983 Jan;4(1):39–44
Colas des Francs G: L'oeuvre de Jules Amar entre 1914 et 1918. Thèse, Université René-Descartes, Faculté Cochin-Port-Royal. Paris, 1984. 21, 29, 7, 70 p.
Colbert L: Amish attitudes and treatment of illness. Pa Folklife 1980;30(1):9–15
Cole BL, Vingrys AJ: A survey and evaluation of lantern tests of color vision. Am J Optom Physiol Opt 1982 Apr;59(4):346–74
Cole DR: Helping: origins and development of the major psychotherapies. Toronto, Butterworths, 1982. xv, 390 p.
Cole M see Luria AR
Cole RA, Rudnicky AI: What's new in speech perception? The research and ideas of William Chandler Bagley, 1874–1946. Psychol Rev 1983 Jan;90(1):94–101
Cole RB: Noonan's syndrome: a historical perspective. Pediatrics 1980 Sep;66(3):468–9
Cole S see Luria AR
Cole T: The ideology of old age and death in American history. Am Q 1979;31(2):223–31
Cole TR: The prophecy of Senescence: G. Stanley Hall and the reconstruction of old age in America. Gerontologist 1984 Aug;24(4):360–6
Cole WH: Some ether anecdotes. Anaesth Intensive Care 1981 May;9(2):174–6
Cole WH: The development of cholecystography. J Thorac Cardiovasc Surg 1984 Nov;88(5 Pt 2):827–33
Coleman CM see Miller B
Coleman FC: A brief look at the sociopolitical and economic history of pathology in the United States. J Fla Med Assoc 1980 Feb;67(2):89–96
Coleman FC: The legislative history of Medicare. Pathologist 1981 Feb;35(2):97–9
Coleman FC: The legislative history of Medicare: Part II. Pathologist 1981 Mar;35(3):156–8
Coleman KM see Helfand WH
Coleman SR: Historical context and systematic functions of the concept of the operant. Behaviorism 1981;9:207–26
Coleman W: Bergmann's rule: animal heat as a biological phenomenon. Stud Hist Biol 1979;3:67–88
Coleman W: Death is a social disease. Public health and political economy in early industrial France. Madison, University of Wisconsin Press, 1982. xxi, 322 p. (Wisconsin Publications in the History of Science and Medicine, 1).
Coleman W: L'hygiène et l'état selon Montyon. Dix-Huit Siecle 1977;9:101–8
Coleman W: Medicine against Malthus: François Mélier on the relation between subsistence and mortality (1843). Bull Hist Med 1980 Spring;54(1):23–42
Coleman W: The Queen's women. Bull Hist Med 1981 Winter;55(4):580–9
Coleman W see Mayr E
Coles R: Flannery O'Connor's lupus. A commentary on her collected letters, The habit of being. JAMA 1980 Sep 26;244(13):1441–2
Coles R: William Carlos Williams. A writing physician. JAMA 1981 Jan 2;245(1):41–2
Coley NG: Physicians and the chemical analysis of mineral waters in eighteenth-century England. Med Hist 1982 Apr;26(2):123–44
Coley NG: The preparation and uses of artificial mineral waters (ca. 1680–1825). Ambix 1984;31(1):32–48
Colin J: Geschichte der Luftfahrtmedizin. In Sournia JC, Martiny M, Poulet J, ed: Illustrierte Geschichte der Medizin. Salzburg, Andreas, 1980. Vol. 8. p. 3025–51.
Collacott RA: Hereditary physicians of the Scottish islands. Scott Med J 1983 Oct;28(4):377–81
Collacott RA: Neonatal tetanus in St. Kilda. Scott Med J 1981 Jul;26(3):224–7
Collacott RA: The air-ambulance: Orkney's experience. J R Coll Gen Pract 1984 Mar;34(260):163–5
Collado Lopez O see Rivero de la Calle M
Coller BS: Bizzozero and the discovery of the blood platelet. Lancet 1984 Apr 7;1(8380):804
Collet AJ: Luis Vaz de Camões. Scalpel Tongs 1981;25:52
Collet AJ: Luiz Vaz de Camões (1524?–1580). Scalpel Tongs 1981;25:44–5
Collier LH: Recherches sur les Chlamydia – une vue rétrospective. Rev Int Trach Pathol Ocul Trop Subtrop Sante Publique 1982;(2–3):17–23
Collier LH see Wylie JA
Collier RJ: From Pap to ApUp. Cell Immunol 1982 Jan 1;66(1):17–23
Collière MF: La profession infirmière en quête de son histoire 1870–1980. Rev Infirm 1980 Dec;30(10):13–24

**Collière MF:** Promouvoir la vie. Paris, Inter-Editions, 1982. Historical chapters, p. 23–35, 125–87.
**Collingridge D, Douglas J:** Three models of policymaking: expert advice in the control of environmental lead. **Soc Stud Sci** 1984 Aug;14(3):343–70
**Collins BC:** A round of calomel. **J Tenn Med Assoc** 1983 Sep;76(9):609–10
**Collins DT:** Gustav Mahler's summer of 1910. **Bull Menninger Clin** 1982 May;46(3):255–79
**Collins HM:** The place of the 'core-set' in modern science: social contingency with methodological propriety in science. **Hist Sci** 1981;19:6–19
**Collins J** see **Horowitz M**
**Collins J** see **Smith JH, ed**
**Collins JJ:** The contribution of medical measures to the decline of mortality from respiratory tuberculosis: an age-period-cohort model. **Demography** 1982 Aug;19(3):409–27
**Collins JL:** Psychiatry in China. **J Natl Med Assoc** 1982 Oct;74(10):993–8
**Collins K** see **Harrison G**
**Collins LD, Higgins D, ed:** The politics of abortion: trends in Canadian fertility policy. **Atlantis** 1982;7(2):2–20
**Collins P** see **MacLeod RM**
**Collins R, Restivo S:** Development, diversity, and conflict in the sociology of science. **Sociol Q** 1983;24(2):185–200
**Collins SM:** Nursing--the next 100 years. **J Adv Nurs** 1981 May;6(3):165–71
**Collins TF:** John Max Mehliss, M.D. A Transvaal medical pioneer. **S Afr Med J** 1983 Jun 29;Spec No:14–6
**Collins TF:** The history of southern Africa's first tuberculosis epidemic. **S Afr Med J** 1982 Nov 13;62(21):780–8
**Collins WE, Boone JO, VanDeventer AD:** The selection of air traffic control specialists: history and review of contributions by the Civil Aeromedical Institute, 1960–80. **Aviat Space Environ Med** 1981 Apr;52(4):217–40
**Collins WE:** Urology in the Ottawa valley. **Can J Surg** 1983 Sep;26(5):423–6
**Collis JL:** The history of British oesophageal surgery. **Thorax** 1982 Nov;37(11):795–802
**Collomb P:** La diffusion des méthodes contraceptives modernes en France de 1971 à 1978. **Population** 1979;34(6):1045–65
**Collorio C** see **Albarello B**
**Colmin J:** L'aventure du quartier ney. Paris, Editions du Scarabée, 1980. 167 p.
**Colombo B:** La tradizione italiana negli studi biodemografici. **Genus** 1979;35(3–4):7–22
**Colombo MO** see **Marcondes CH**
**Colón Roure C, Rivera Nieves M:** La intervención del terapista ocupacional en el equipo interdisciplinario en el area de la salud mental. **Bol Asoc Med PR** 1984 Jul;76(7):319–22
**Colonel Leverett Hubbard's address to the Society at their meeting Feby 2d 1784: Conn Med** 1984 Sep;48(9):557
**Colotla VA, Jurado S:** Contributions to the history of psychology: XXXIV. Enrique O. Aragon, a pioneer in Mexican psychology. **Percept Mot Skills** 1983 Dec;57(3 Pt 1):1013–4
**Colp R:** Charles Darwin, Dr. Edward Lane, and the 'Singular Trial' of Robinson v. Robinson and Lane. **J Hist Med Allied Sci** 1981 Apr;36(2):205–13
**Colp R:** [Charles Darwin: Essay-Review] **Trans Stud Coll Physicians Phila** 1983 Dec;5(5 no 4):353–75
**Colp R:** Charles Darwin's coffin, and its maker. **J Hist Med Allied Sci** 1980 Jan;35(1):59–74
**Colp R:** Charles Darwin's reprobation of nature. 'Clumsy, wasteful, blundering low and horribly cruel.' **NY State J Med** 1981 Jun;81(7):1116–9
**Colp R:** Dr. Erasmus Darwin consults with another physician. **Radic Hist Rev** 1979 Spring/Summer;Spec:66–71
**Colp R:** 'I was born a naturalist': Charles Darwin's 1838 notes about himself. **J Hist Med Allied Sci** 1980 Jan;35(1):8–39
**Colp R:** The Darwin exhibition at the Cambridge University Library. **Bull NY Acad Med** 1983 Jun;59(5):526–8
**Colp R Jr:** Notes on Dr. William S. Halsted. **Bull NY Acad Med** 1984 Nov;60(9):876–87
**Coltart WD** see **Watson-Jones R**
**Colton T** see **Greenberg ER**
**Columbus: was it Reiter's disease?: Lancet** 1981 Jan 10;1(8211):94–5
**Comadrán Ruiz J:** Evolución demográfica argentina durante el périodo hispano, 1535–1810. Buenos Aires, Editorial Universitaria de Buenos Aires, 1969. xi, 120 p.
**Comaroff J:** Medicine: symbol and ideology. In P. Wright, A. Treacher, ed: The problem of medical knowledge. Examining the social construction of medicine. Edinburgh, Edinburgh University Press, 1982. p. 49–68.
**Comas J:** Influencia de la farmacopea y terapéutica indígenas de Nueva España en la obra de Juan de Barrios (1607). **An Antropol** 1971;8:125–50
**Comben N:** Book values and the book market; some hints for collectors. **Vet Hist** 1982/83;NS2(4):151–60
**Combes RE:** J. C. Sharland's pharmacy at Apothecaries' Hall. **J Auckl Waikato Hist Soc** 1979;34:31–4
**Combs MW, Welch S:** Blacks, Whites, and attitudes toward abortion. **Public Opin Q** 1982;46(4):510–20
**Comelles JM:** El tratamiento moral en Catalunya (I): el 'Proyecto médico razonado' de Emili Pi i Molist (1860). In International Congress of the History of Medicine, 27th, Barcelona, 1980. Actas. Barcelona, Académia de Ciències Mèdiques de Catalunya i Balears, 1981. p. 48–55.
**Comelles JM, Prat Caros J, Pujadas Muñoz JJ:** La medicina tradicional en el Estado español y la antropología cultural. In International Congress of the History of Medicine, 27th, Barcelona, 1980. Actas. Barcelona, Académia de Ciències Mèdiques de Catalunya i Balears, 1981. p. 490–4.
**Comer GM** see **Morse D**
**Comiti V** see **La médecine hospitalière française au XVIIIème siècle**
**Comiti VP:** Evolution de la pathologie française au XXe siècle. **Bull Sect Geogr Com Trav Hist Sci** 1978;83(2):11–28
**Comiti VP:** Histoire des maladies et diagnostic médical historique. **Gaz Med Fr** 1981 Jun 5;88(21):3087–90
**Comiti VP:** Importance des connaissances médico-biologiques actuelles pour une étude critique de pathocénose historique. In Imhof AE, ed: Mensch und Gesundheit in der Geschichte. Husum, Matthiesen, 1980. p. 35–43.
**Comiti VP:** Intérêts et apports d'une étude historique des maladies aux XVIIIe et XIXe siecles. **Hist Sci Med** 1980;14(2):201–6
**Comiti VP:** Intoxications non microbiennes et epidemies infectieuses historiques. In International Congress of the History of Medicine, 27th, Barcelona, 1980. Actas. Barcelona, Académia de Ciències Mèdiques de Catalunya i Balears, 1981. p. 495–8.
**Comiti VP:** La fièvre à la fin du XVIIe siècle. **Gaz Med Fr** 1980;87:2159–60
**Comiti VP:** La fièvre et les fièvres. **Doc Hist Vocab Sci** 1983;(5):91–5
**Comiti VP:** La géographie médicale de la Corse à la fin du XVIIIe siècle. Genève, Droz, 1980. 142 p. (Centre de Recherches d'Histoire et de Philologie de la IVe Section de l'Ecole pratique des Hautes Etudes; Hautes Etudes Médiévales et Modernes, 41).
**Comiti VP:** Les maladies d'autrefois. **Recherche** 1980 Oct;115:1044–51
**Comiti VP:** Les maladies et le travail lors de la révolution industrielle française. **Hist Philos Life Sci** 1980;2(2):215–39
**Comiti VP** see **Huard P**
**Commémoration du bicentenaire de la naissance de M.T.H. Laennec 1781–1826: Bull Acad Natl Med (Paris)** 1981 Feb 17;Spec no.:1–61
**Commémoration du centenaire de la mort de Paul Broca: Chirurgie** 1980;106(10):773–93
**Commemorative coin for Dr. Zamenhof: Newsl Optom Hist Soc** 1981;12(1):6
**Compton A:** Developments of skills in physiotherapy over the last 60 years. **Midwife Health Visit Community Nurse** 1980 Oct;16(10):412–4
**Comroe JH:** Exploring the heart: discoveries in heart disease and high blood pressure. New York, Norton, 1983. 348 p.
**Comroe JH:** Pay dirt: the story of streptomycin. Part II. Feldman and Hinshaw; Lehmann. **Am Rev Respir Dis** 1978 May;117(5):957–68
**Comroe JH:** Roast pig and scientific discovery. Part II. **Am Rev Respir Dis** 1977 Jun;115(6):1035–44
**Comtor JH:** Harvey's 1651 perfusion of the pulmonary circulation of man. **Circulation** 1982 Jan;65(1):1–3
**Conable CW:** Louise Stanley. In: Notable American women. The modern period. Cambridge, Mass., Belknap-Harvard Univ. Press, 1980. 4:657–9.
**Concepcion R:** Medical ethics in connection with torture of prisoners and other persons under some form of detention. **Unitas** 1976;49(4):542–92
**Condon AG:** John Caleff. In Dictionary of Canadian biography, 1801 to 1820. Volume 5, 1983. p. 134–5.
**Condon RE** see **Fraser ID**
**Condran GA, Crimmins E:** A description and evaluation of mortality data in the federal census: 1850–1900. **Hist Methods Newsl** 1979;12(1):1–23
**Condran GA:** An evaluation of estimates of underenumeration in the census and the age pattern of mortality, Philadelphia, 1880. **Demography** 1984 Feb 1;21(1):53–69
**Condran GA, Seaman J:** Linkage of the 1880–81 Philadelphia death register to the 1880 manuscript census: a comparison of hand and machine-record linkage techniques. **Hist Methods** 1981;14(2):73–84
**Condran GA, Crimmins E:** Mortality differentials between rural and urban areas of states in the Northeastern United States 1890–1900. **J Hist Geogr** 1980;6(2):179–202
**Condran GA, Cheney RA:** Mortality trends in Philadelphia: age- and cause--specific death rates 1870–1930. **Demography** 1982 Feb;19(1):97–123
**Condran GA** see **Crimmins EM**
**Cone RO, Danzig L, Resnick D, et al:** The bicipital groove: radiographic, anatomic, and pathologic study. **AJR** 1983 Oct;141(4):781–8
**Cone TE:** A rachitic infant painted by Burgkmair 136 years before Dr. Whistler described rickets. **Clin Pediatr (Phila)** 1980 Mar;19(3):194
**Cone TE:** Abraham Jacobi on medical specialization, as viewed in 1880. **Pediatrics** 1981;67:481
**Cone TE:** Abraham Jacobi on the establishment of systematic instruction in the diseases of childhood in the United States. **Pediatrics** 1981;67:357
**Cone TE:** Daniel Defoe on the deplorable effect of the great London plague of 1665 on women with child. **Pediatrics** 1981;67:221
**Cone TE:** Eighth century Irish rules regarding the care of a sick person. **Pediatrics** 1981;67:795
**Cone TE:** History of American pediatrics. Historical introduction by S. X. Radbill. Boston, Little, Brown, 1979. xiv, 278 p.
**Cone TE:** History of infant and child feeding: from the earliest years through the development of scientific concepts. In Bond JT, et. al., ed: Infant and child feeding. New York, Academic Press, 1981. p. 3–34.
**Cone TE:** Is this the first published report on the diagnostic value of the telephone in pediatric practice (1879)? **Pediatrics** 1981;68:321
**Cone TE:** On dressing the American newborn infant a century ago. **Pediatrics** 1981;67:268
**Cone TE:** Overdosing with opium, a serious pediatric problem in England a century and a half ago. **Pediatrics** 1981;68:86
**Cone TE:** 'The boke of children' (1544) by Thomas Phaire [Phaer], the first pediatric text published in English. **Pediatrics** 1981;68:182
**Cone TE:** The first journal devoted exclusively to pediatrics (1834).

Pediatrics 1981;68:321
**Cone TE:** The first journal devoted to the diseases of children. **Pediatrics** 1981;67:810
**Cone TE:** The first published report of an incubator for use in the care of the premature infant (1857). **Am J Dis Child** 1981 Jul;135(7):658–60
**Cone TE:** The nursing bottle caries syndrome. **JAMA** 1981 Jun 12;245(22):2334
**Cone TE** see **Smith GF**
**Confalonieri UE** see **Aráujo A**
**Confalonieri UE** see **Araújo AJ**
**Confalonieri UE** see **Ferreira LF**
**Conger DJ, Luan DC:** Dynamic properties of Taiwanese fertility, 1950–1972. **Stud Comp Int Dev** 1979 Summer;14:54–74
**Congrès international d'histoire de la médecine, XXVe, Québec, 1976:** Actes. Québec, 1977. 3 vols. 1403 p.
**Conk Z:** Cumhuriyet dönemi ve hemşirelik. **Turk Hemsire Derg** 1983;33(4):3–5
**Conlins J:** Beans, bacon, and galantine truffles: the food of the Western miners. **Ariz West** 1981;23(1):29–52
**Conn HJ:** The history of the Stain Commission. **Stain Technol** 1980 Sep;55(5):269–79
**Conn HJ:** The history of the Stain Commission. II. Organization 1921–2. **Stain Technol** 1980 Nov;55(6):327–52
**Conn HJ:** The history of the Stain Commission. III. Birth of the Stain Commission. 1922–3. **Stain Technol** 1981 Jan;56(1):1–17
**Conn HJ:** The history of the Stain Commission IV. Expansion of the work, 1924–39. **Stain Technol** 1981 Mar;56(2):59–66
**Conn HJ:** The history of the Stain Commission. V. War and its consequences. **Stain Technol** 1981 May;56(3):135–42
**Conn JH:** Nature of magnetic treatment. **J Am Soc Psychosom Dent Med** 1982;29(2):44–53
**Conn JH:** Unusual features of Anna O. 's illness. **Am J Psychiatry** 1980 Jan;138(1):123
**Connaugton D:** Alton Ochsner: not as a legend. **Bull Am Coll Surg** 1981;66(5):27, 31–2
**Connell MT:** Feminine consciousness and the nature of nursing practice: a historical perspective. **Top Clin Nurs** 1983 Oct;5(3):1–10
**Connell–Tatum EB** see **Tatum HJ**
**Connelly DM** see **Stieber MT**
**Connolly DC, Mann RJ:** Dominic J. Corrigan (1802–1880) and his description of the pericardial knock. **Mayo Clin Proc** 1980 Dec;55(12):771–3
**Connolly GP:** Little brother be at peace: the priest as holy man in the nineteenth–century ghetto. In Sheils WJ, ed: The Church and healing. Papers read at the twentieth summer meeting and the twenty–first winter meeting of the Ecclesiastical History Society. Oxford, Basil Blackwell for the Society, 1982. p. 191–206.
**Connolly JF:** Wound management and the legacy of H. Winnett Orr. **Nebr Med J** 1982 Mar;67(3):60–1
**Connolly MP:** Health visiting 1850–1900: a review. **Midwife Health Visit Community Nurse** 1980 Jul;16(7):282–5
**Connolly MP:** Health visiting 1900–1910: a review. **Midwife Health Visit Community Nurse** 1980 Sep;16(9):375–8
**Connolly R** see **Barry PS**
**Connolly SJ:** Illegitimacy and pre–nuptial pregnancy in Ireland before 1864: the evidence of some Catholic parish registers. **Ir Econ Soc Hist** 1979;6:5–23
**Connor LH:** Ships of fools and vessels of the divine: mental hospitals and madness, a case study. **Soc Sci Med** 1982;16(7):783–94
**Connors DM:** Doctors afield in early Wisconsin. **Wis Med J** 1980 Mar;79(3):14–6
**Conquest R:** Forced labour statistics: some comments. **Sov Stud** 1982;34(3):434–9
**Conrad B:** Genius and intemperance. **Horizon** 1980;23(12):33–40
**Conrad GB von:** The first eighty years: the history of Lutheran Medical Center School of Nursing, 1898–1978. Ph.D. Diss., Saint Louis University. Saint Louis, 1980. 157 p.
**Conroy BF:** The history of faciel prostheses. In Romm S, ed: Symposium on historical perspectives of plastic surgery. Philadelphia, Saunders, 1983. p. 689–707.
**Conroy BF** see **Romm S, ed**
**Conroy GC:** Evolutionary significance of cerebral venous patterns in paleoprimatology. **Z Morphol Anthropol** 1980;71(2):125–34
**Conroy MS:** Malaria in late Tsarist Russia. **Bull Hist Med** 1982 Spring;56(1):41–55
**Conry Y:** L'idée d'une 'marche de la nature' dans la biologie prédarwinienne au XIXe siècle. **Rev Hist Sci (Paris)** 1980 Apr;33(2):97–149
**Conry Y:** Organisme et organisation: de Darwin à la génétique des populations. In Actes du Colloques R.A. Fisher.... Paris, 5–6 déc. 1979. p. 291–330. **Rev Synth (Paris)** 1981;102(103–104)
**Constable AR** see **Blaufox MD**
**Constantikes A** see **Yeazell RB**
**Constantin–Lhuillery A:** Les enfants du bureau des pauvres de Chartres (1693–1715). Mém. de maîtrise. Univ. de Tours, 1976, 213 p
**Constantine J** see **Kessler RK**
**Contento I:** Thinking about nutrition education: what to teach, how to teach it, and what to measure. **Teach Coll Rec** 1980;81(4):421–47
**Conti Bizzarro F, et al:** Per l'edizione dei libri medicinali di Aezio Amideno. **Koinonia** 1978;2:169–97
**Continenza B:** Darwin e la psicologia. **Stor Crit Psicol** 1981;2(1):99–105
**Continenza B:** L'effetto Baldwin. **Stor Crit Psicol** 1982 Dec;3(2):335–42
**Continenza B, Gagliasso E:** Ricerche pre–etologiche sul comportamento sociale animale e umano. **Physis** 1980;22(3–34):355–78
**Contreni JJ:** The study and practice of medicine in Northern France during the reign of Charles the Bald. **Stud Mediev Cult** 1976;6–7:43–54
**Contreras Dueñas F:** La lepra se cura cada vez con mayor frecuencia. De acuerdo con los recientes progresos científicos tienen que terminar todas las enfermedades incurables.
**Contreras Mas A:** Legislacion frente a la peste en Mallorca bajomedieval 'Ordinations; capitols del morbo de la ciutat e regna de Mallorques'. **Asclepio** 1978–79;30–31:167–76
**Contreras Mas A:** Notas para la historia de la psiquiatría Bajomedieval en Mallorca. In International Congress of the History of Medicine, 27th, Barcelona, 1980. Actas. Barcelona, Acadèmia de Ciències Mèdiques de Catalunya i Balears, 1981. p. 56–63.
**Contreras Poza L:** La Torre de Babel del léxico sanitario. **Rev Sanid Hig Publica (Madr)** 1982 Mar–Apr;56(3–4):311–40
**Converse JM:** Alexis Carrel: the man, the unknown. **Plast Reconstr Surg** 1981 Oct;68(4):629–39
**Converse JM:** Experimental human skin allografts, the hla complex, and a Nobel prize. **Plast Reconstr Surg** 1982 Aug;70(2):255–62
**Converse JM:** The extraordinary career of Doctor Varaztad Hovhannes Kazanjian. **Plast Reconstr Surg** 1983 Jan;71(1):138–43
**Converse JM** see **Ben–Hur N**
**Conway JK** see **Green D**
**Cook AL:** Liverpool's Northern Hospital, 1834–1978. Liverpool, Liverpool Area Health Authority (Teaching), 1981. v, 141 p.
**Cook BW:** The historical denial of lesbianism. **Radic Hist Rev** 1979 Spring/Summer;Spec:60–5
**Cook CS:** Clark Bentom. In Dictionary of Canadian biography, 1801 to 1820. Volume 5, 1983. p. 68–9.
**Cook D:** The story of inhalation anaesthesia. **Br Dent Surg Assist** 1981 Sep–Oct;40(5):103–5; Nov–Dec;40(6):111–3
**Cook DC, Buikstra JE:** Health and differential survival in prehistoric populations: prenatal dental defects. **Am J Phys Anthropol** 1979 Nov;51(4):649–64
**Cook DC:** Hereditary enamel hypoplasia in a prehistoric Indian child. **J Dent Res** 1980 Sep;59(9):1522
**Cook DC:** Koniag Eskimo tooth ablation: was Hrdlička right after all? **Curr Anthropol** 1981;22(2):159–63
**Cook G** see **Lakie MH**
**Cook HJ, Steneck NH, Vander AJ, et al:** Early research on the biological effects of microwave radiation: 1940–1960. **Ann Sci** 1980 May;37(3):323–51
**Cook HJ:** The regulation of medical practice in London under the Stuarts, 1607–1704. Ph.D. Diss., University of Michigan. Ann Arbor, 1981. 438 p.
**Cook HJ** see **Steneck NH**
**Cook LG:** A 17th century drug account. **Pharm Hist (London)** 1974 Jul;4(2):2–4
**Cook MS, Repetto R:** The relevance of the developing countries to demographic transition theory: further lessons from the Hungarian experience. **Popul Stud** 1982 Mar;36(1):105–28
**Cook ND:** Population data for Indian Peru: sixteenth and seventeenth centuries. **Hisp Am Hist Rev** 1982;62(1):73–120
**Cook TM:** Samuel Hahnemann. The founder of homoeopathic medicine. Wellingborough, Northamptonshire, Thorsons, 1981. 192 p.
**Cooke AM:** Queen Victoria's medical household. **Med Hist** 1982 Jul;26(3):307–20
**Cooke AM:** Sir Hans Sloane and the Philosophical Transactions. **J R Coll Physicians Lond** 1984 Jul;18(3):170–1
**Cooke BE:** History of oral medicine. **Br Dent J** 1981 Jul 7;151(1):11–3
**Cooke MA:** Richard Surflet, translator and practitioner in physic. **Med Hist** 1981 Jan;25(1):41–56
**Cooke RG:** Los hábitos alimentarios de los indígenas precolombinos de Panamá. **Rev Med Panama** 1981 Jan;6(1):65–89
**Coombs WH:** Recollections of a veteran [interview by Peter Center]. **Radiography** 1983 Oct;49(586):235–8
**Coon DJ:** Eponymy, obscurity, Twitmyer, and Pavlov. **J Hist Behav Sci** 1982 Jul;18(3):255–62
**Coon LJ:** Orthokeratology: part I historical perspective. **J Am Optom Assoc** 1982 Mar;53(3):187–95
**Cooney RS, Min K:** Demographic characteristics affecting living arrangements among young currently unmarried Puerto Rican, non–Spanish black, and non–Spanish white mothers. **Ethnicity** 1981;8(2):107–20
**Cooney RS, Rogler LH, Schroder E:** Puerto Rican fertility: an examination of social characteristics, assimilation and minority status variables. **Soc Forces** 1981;59(4):1094–1113
**Cooper AJ** see **Perry HO**
**Cooper AM:** Psychoanalysis at one hundred: beginnings of maturity. **J Am Psychoanal Assoc** 1984;32(2):245–67
**Cooper AM** see **Frances A**
**Cooper AM** see **Goldberg A, ed**
**Cooper DB:** The Royal College of Physicians of London during the reign of the House of Stuart (1603–1714). **Trans Stud Coll Physicians Phila** 1983 Sep;5(5 No 3):191–211
**Cooper DB** see **Bowers JZ**
**Cooper EL:** L'évolution de l'immunité. **Recherche** 1979;103:824–33
**Cooper EL:** Prix D'Immunologie Behring–Metschnikoff. **Dev Comp Immunol** 1982 Summer;6(3):389–90
**Cooper IS:** Sir Victor Horsley: father of modern neurological surgery. In

Rose FC, Bynum WF, ed: Historical aspects of the neurosciences. New York, Raven, 1982. p. 235-8.
**Cooper JE:** Some aspects of John Hunter's work on the diseases of birds of prey. **Ann R Coll Surg Engl** 1982 Sep;64(5):345-7
**Cooper JE:** Surgery of the foot in falcons: a historic operation. **Ann R Coll Surg Engl** 1980 Nov;62(6):445-8
**Cooper JE** see **Allen E**
**Cooper JK** see **Johnson TP**
**Cooper R:** A note on the biologic concept of race and its application in epidemiologic research. **Am Heart J** 1984 Sep;108(3 Pt 2):715-22
**Cooper R:** Rising death rates in the Soviet Union. The impact of coronary heart disease [1960-77]. **N Engl J Med** 1981;304:1259-65
**Cooper T, Stucki JC:** Commentary on 'animal research - for and against: a philosophical, social, and historical perspective'. **Perspect Biol Med** 1983 Autumn;27(1):18-21
**Cooper T, Olimpio NA:** Medical education. **Proc Acad Polit Sci** 1980;33(4):32-44
**Cooper WM, Platt H:** John Sebastian Bach Stopford. In Dictionary of national biography, 1961-1970. Suppl. 8, 1981. p. 985-7.
**Cooper WC, ed** see **Manson Thomas ML**
**Cooter R:** Anticontagionism and history's medical record. In P. Wright, A. Treacher, ed: The problem of medical knowledge. Examining the social construction of medicine. Edinburgh, Edinburgh University Press, 1982. p. 87-108.
**Cooter R:** Interpreting the fringe. **Soc Soc Hist Med Bull (Lond)** 1981 Dec;29:33-6
**Cooter R:** Open-air therapy and the rise of open-air hospitals. **Soc Soc Hist Med Bull (Lond)** 1984 Dec;35:44-6
**Cooter R:** The politics of brain: phrenology in Birmingham. **Soc Soc Hist Med Bull (Lond)** 1983 Jun;32:34-6
**Cooter R** see **Scull A, ed**
**Cope FW:** In memoriam . . . B. David Polis--mitochondrial biochemist, discoverer of polymeric prostaglandin PGBx for prevention and therapy of damaged mitochondrial oxidative phosphorylation. **Physiol Chem Phys** 1980;12(6):541-4
**Cope I** see **McDonald IA**
**Cope JC:** Roman medical instruments. **Mo Med** 1980 Sep;77(9):574
**Copeland H** see **Casey AE**
**Copenhaver BP:** Symphorien Champier and the reception of the occultist tradition in Renaissance France. The Hague, New York, Mouton, 1978. 368 p.
**Copley AL:** The endo-endothelial fibrin lining. A historical account. **Thromb Res [Suppl]** 1983;5:1-26
**Copley AL** see **Blombäck B**
**Coppleson VM:** Australian Postgraduate Federation in Medicine. The development of graduate education with particular reference to Australia. [s.l.: s.n.], 1964. 46 leaves.
**Coppock JB:** Food technology [in the twentieth century]. In Williams TI, ed: A history of technology. Vol. VII. The twentieth century, ca. 1900 to ca. 1950. Part II. Oxford, Clarendon, 1978. p. 1399-445.
**Coppola G:** Condizioni materiali e problemi sociali in Lombardi tra '700 e '800. **Ann Ist Stor Italo-Ger** 1976;2:553-61
**Corbella Corbella J:** El crecimiento del saber medico legal en España en el siglo XVI. **Asclepio** 1978-79;30-31:323-37
**Corbella Corbella J:** Notas sobre la historia de la medicina en la comarca del Bagés. **Ascleopio** 1980;32:93-101
**Corbella Corbella J, Doménech Llabería E:** Notas sobre medicos de la comarca del Priorato en el siglo XIX. **Asclepio** 1980;32:103-9
**Corbella Corbella J, Martí Amengual G:** Recuerdo de la obra de Pedro Mata y Fontanet (1811-1877) en su centenario. **Asclepio** 1980;32:111-9
**Corbett M:** The emblematic title-page to Stirpium Adversaria nova by Petro Pena and Mathias de L'Obel (1570). **Arch Nat Hist** 1981 Apr;10(1):111-7
**Corbett ME, Hardwick JL:** The investigation of dental disease in exhumed remains. **J Dent** 1981 Dec;9(4):302-10
**Corbin A:** L'hérédosyphilis ou l'impossible rédemption: contribution à l'histoire de l'hérédité morbide. **Romantisme** 1981;31:131-49
**Corbin A** see **Calmy C**
**Corcos A** see **Monaghan F**
**Corcos AF:** Reproduction and heredity beliefs of the Hindus based on their sacred books. **J Hered** 1984 Mar-Apr;75(2):152-4
**Cordasco F:** Laughlin Macleane's Expediency of Inoculation (1756): a checklist of deposit locations. **Am Notes Queries** 1981 Jan-Feb;19(5/6):75
**Cordasco F, Alloway DN:** Medical education in the United States. A guide to information sources. Detroit, Gale Research, 1980. xx, 393 p. (Education Information Guide Series, v. 8).
**Cordell LS** see **Devor EJ**
**Cordera-Pastor A, Corvera-Bernardelli J:** A propósito de la deshumanización de la medicina. **Gac Med Mex** 1982 Nov;118(11):431-8
**Cordeschi R:** Craik e la psicologia meccanicistica. **Stor Crit Psicol** 1984 Jun;5(1):161-75
**Cordeschi R:** Dal comportamentismo alla simulazione del comportamento. **Stor Crit Psicol** 1983;4(1):87-113
**Cordoliani A:** L'hôpital militaire du Val de Grâce dans la vie sociale parisienne. In Congrès National des Sociétés Savantes, 103e, Nancy-Metz, 1978. Actes. Paris, 1979. Tome I, p. 607-24.
**Cordoliani A** see **Dostatni P**
**Córdova Alvelais LT:** El surgimiento de la medicina mexicana comtemporánea. **Arch Inst Cardiol Mex** 1981 Jan-Feb;51(1):103-8
**Corgan JX:** A preliminary catalog of the scientific and technical societies of Antebellum East Tennessee. **East Tenn Hist Soc Publ** 1976(issued Feb 80);48:21-8
**Corgan JX:** Richard Owen Currey, a little known intellectual figure of antebellum Tennessee. **East Tenn Hist Soc Publ** 1978;50:58-70
**Coria F** see **Berciano J**
**Corlieu P** see **Huard P**
**Cormack AM:** Early two-dimensional reconstruction and recent topics stemming from it. **Med Phys** 1980 Jul-Aug;7(4):277-82
**Cormack AM:** Early two-dimensional reconstruction and recent topics stemming from it. **Science** 1980 Sep 26;209(4464):1482-6
**Cormack AM:** Early two-dimensional reconstruction (CT scanning) and recent topics stemming from it. **J Comput Assist Tomogr** 1980 Oct;4(5):658-64
**Cormack AM:** Recollections of my work with computer assisted tomography. **Mol Cell Biochem** 1980 Sep 15;32(2):59-61
**Cormier C:** Jacques Bourgeois. In Dictionary of Canadian biography, 1701 to 1740. Volume 2, 1969. p. 94.
**Corn JK:** Byssinosis--an historical perspective. **Am J Ind Med** 1981;2(4):331-52
**Corn JK:** 'Dark as a dungeon': environment and coal miners' health and safety in nineteenth century America. **Environ Rev** 1983;7(3):257-68
**Corn M** see **Rose JC**
**Cornacchia P, et al:** I funghi magici: farmacologia, tossicologia e tecnologia dell'estasi chimica. Milano, Editiemme, 1980. 174 p.
**Cornand G:** Trachome et armées. **Rev Int Trach Pathol Ocul Trop Subtrop** 1979;56(3-4):99-110
**Cornell JF:** Analogy and technology in Darwin's vision of nature. **J Hist Biol** 1984 Fall;17(3):303-44
**Cornell JF:** From creation to evolution: Sir William Dawson and The idea of design in the nineteenth century. **J Hist Biol** 1983 Spring;16(1):137-70
**Corner GW:** Leo Loeb. In Dictionary of American Biography, Suppl. 6, 1956-1960. p. 385-7, 1980.
**Corner GW:** Louise Pearce. In: Notable American women. The modern period. Cambridge, Mass., Belknap-Harvard Univ. Press, 1980. 4.531-2.
**Corner GW:** The seven ages of a medical scientist, an autobiography. Philadelphia, University of Pennsylvania Press, 1981. xi, 411 p.
**Corner GW:** Thomas Milton Rivers. In Dictionary of American biography, 1961-1965. Suppl. 7, 1981. p. 648-9.
**Cornesco M:** American-Romanian cooperation in the study of and fight against scarlet fever. In International Congress of the History of Medicine, 27th, Barcelona, 1980. Actas. Barcelona, Académia de Ciències Médiques de Catalunya i Balears, 1981. p. 499-502.
**Cornet A:** François Moutier médecin et poète (1881-1961). **Hist Sci Med** 1983;17(2):171-9
**Cornet AM, Sagrera JE de:** En memoria de nuestro maestro: José Luis Gómez-Caamaño (1909-1984). **Bol Soc Esp Hist Farm** 1984;35(137):1-22
**Corney G:** Sir Francis Galton, 1822-1911. **Acta Genet Med Gemellol (Roma)** 1984;33(1):13-8
**Cornforth J:** Portrait of Dorothy Hodgkin, O.M., F.R.S. **Notes Rec R Soc Lond** 1982 Aug;37(1):1-4
**Corning M:** Redes de información biomédica: experiencia de la Biblioteca Nacional de Medicina de los Estados Unidos de América. **Educ Med Salud** 1981;15(4):424-41
**Corning ME:** A review of the United States role in international biomedical research and communications: international health and foreign policy. Bethesda, National Library of Medicine, 1980. xxvii, 436 p. (NIH Publication No. 80-1638).
**Cornudella J:** L'obra mèdica del Dr. Joan Freixas i Freixas. In Congrés Internacional d'Historie de la Medicina Catalana, 1st, Barcelona-Montpellier, 1970. Llibr d'Actes. Barcelona, Editorial Scientia, 1971. v 4, p. 362-5.
**Cornwell JB, Davis HN:** Historical perspective, current applications: the chest cuirass. **Respir Ther** 1979 Jan-Feb;9(1):87-9, 90
**Corps de mère, corps d'enfant:** Paris, Stock, 1980. 223 p.
**Corrêa JV:** Podagra--uma tese de 1788. **Rev Hosp Clin Fac Med Sao Paulo** 1981 Feb;36(1):1-6
**Correa Vázquez ME:** Capital monopolista, estado e instituciones estatales de salud en Mexico, 1940-1978. **Invest Econ** 1981;40(158):57-83
**Corrigan D:** Irish Ethno-botany by Michael Moloney--an early contribution to the concept of ethnopharmacology. **J Ethnopharmacol** 1981 Nov;4(3):343-5
**Corrigan TJ:** Biographia Literaria and the language of science. **J Hist Ideas** 1980 Jul-Sep;41(3):399-419
**Corruccini RS, Handler JS, Mutaw RJ, et al:** Osteology of a slave burial population from Barbados, West Indies. **Am J Phys Anthropol** 1982 Dec;59(4):443-59
**Corruccini RS, Ciochon RL:** Primate facial allometry and interpretations of australopithecine variation. **Nature** 1979 Sep 6;281(5726):62-4
**Corruccini RS, Handler JS:** Temporomandibular joint size decrease in American Blacks: evidence from Barbados. **J Dent Res** 1980 Sep;59(9):1528
**Corruccini RS** see **McHenry HM**
**Corsano A:** Medicina e teologia nel pensiero rinascimentale. La fisiologia di Michele Serveto. **G Crit Filos Ital** 1975;6(1):84-8
**Corsi P, Weindling P, ed:** Information sources in the history of science and medicine. London, Boston, Butterworth Scientific, 1983. xvi, 531 p. (Butterworth Guides to Information Sources).
**Corsini CA, Delille G:** La peste de 1656 dans le diocese de Salerne quelques resultats et problemes. In Charbonneau H, Larose A, ed: The great mortalities: methodological studies of demographic crises in the past. Liège, Belgium, Ordina Editions, 1980. p. 51-60.

**Cortes KF:** Democracy in the American Public Health Association: a historical analysis. [New York?, s.n.], 1976. 362 leaves.
**Cortez P, Sărmăşeanu-Cortez ML:** Un psihiatru în căutarea propriului său destin. Dr. Anastse Andrei Periclis Dosis (1900–1974). **Rev Med Interna [Neurol Psihiatr]** 1980 Jul–Sep;25(3):231–7
**Cortez P** see **Sărmăşanu-Cortez ML**
**Cortez PP** see **Sărmăşanu-Cortez ML**
**Corvera-Bernardelli J** see **Cordera-Pastor A**
**Corvera-Bernardelli J** see **Kuthy-Porter J**
**Corvera-Bernardelli J** see **Somolinos-Palencia J**
**Cos LR** see **Valvo JR**
**Cosma-Muller P:** Entre science et commerce: les eaux minerales en France a la fin de l'ancien regime. **Hist Reflect** 1982;9(1–2):249–62
**Cosmacini G:** Scienza medica e giacobinismo in Italia: l'impresa politico-culturale di Giovanni Rasori (1796–1799). Milano, F. Angeli, 1982. 130 p.
**Cosman MP:** A feast for Aesculapius: historical diets for asthma and sexual pleasure. **Annu Rev Nutr** 1983;3:1–33
**Cosman MP:** Machaut's medical musical world. In Cosman MP, Chandler B, ed: Machaut's world: science and art in the fourteenth century. New York, New York Academy of Sciences, 1978. (Annals of the New York Academy of Sciences, v. 314). p. 1–36.
**Cosman MP:** The medieval medical third party: compulsory consultation and malpractice insurance. **Ann Plast Surg** 1982 Feb;8(2):152–62
**Costa C:** Prehistoria de la cátedra de histología de la Universidad de Chile (1872–1881). Parte I. El affaire Magalhaes. **Rev Med Chil** 1980 Apr;108(4):367–73
**Costa C:** Prehistoria de la cátedra de histología de la Universidad de Chile (1872–1881) Parte II. Microscopio e histología en Chile antes de 1873. **Rev Med Chil** 1980 May;108(5):463–9
**Costa O:** Storie sommerse di biologia e medicina. **Scientia** 1980;115:215–25
**Costa RL:** Periodontal disease in the prehistoric Ipiutak and Tigara skeletal remains from Point Hope, Alaska. **Am J Phys Anthropol** 1982 Sep;59(1):97–110
**Costa V:** HEMOPE, luta pelo sangue. Recife, Fundação de Ensino Superior de Pernambuco, 1979. 129 p.
**Costa-Casaretto C:** Centenario del título de profesor extraordinario de la Universidad de Chile. **Rev Med Chil** 1980 Feb;108(2):161–71
**Costa-Casaretto C:** Chile en dueda con el Doctor Francisco Fonck. **Rev Med Chil** 1981 Nov;109(11):1119–25
**Costa-Casaretto C:** Cincuentenario de la penicilina. **Rev Med Chil** 1979 Jun;107(6):549–56
**Costa-Casaretto C:** Condiciones de la asistencia psiquiátrica en Chile durante el último cuarto del siglo XIX. **Rev Med Chil** 1980 Jul;108(7):657–65
**Costa-Casaretto C:** Don Diego Portales y el Dr. Guillermo C. Blest. **Rev Med Chil** 1984 Jun;112(6):625–31
**Costa-Casaretto C:** Dra. Eloísa Díaz. Centenario del ingreso de la mujer chilena al estudio de las profesiones universitarias. **Rev Med Chil** 1981 Apr;109(4):355–66
**Costa-Casaretto C:** El Dr. D. Jose de Passamán. **Rev Med Chil** 1984 May;112(5):503–8
**Costa-Casaretto C:** El 'origen real' de la enseñanza para graduados en la Facultad de Medicina de la Universidad de Chile. **Rev Med Chil** 1981 Oct;109(10):1013–23
**Costa-Casaretto C:** Enseñanza libre contra estado docente: un episodio de la historia educacional chilena (1972–73). **Rev Med Chil** 1981 Jun;109(6):573–81
**Costa-Casaretto C:** Esomenología (en vez del híbrido futurología) médica. Una visita de médico en 1978, soñada en ... 1878. **Rev Med Chil** 1981 Sep;109(9):901–9
**Costa-Casaretto C:** Ideario psiquiátrico del médico de la Casa de Locos de Santiago en 1862. **Rev Med Chil** 1980 Jun;108(6):559–67
**Costa-Casaretto C:** La cátedra de neuropsiquiatría de la Universidad de Chile desde 1891 hasta 1906. **Rev Med Chil** 1980 Sep;108(9):855–62
**Costa-Casaretto C:** La descripción de la viruela--su viruela--por el estudiante jesuita Juan Ignacio Molina (1761). **Rev Med Chil** 1979 Dec;107(12):1141–51
**Costa-Casaretto C:** La enseñanza para graduados en la Facultad de Medicina de la Universidad de Chile. I. Antecedentes próximos y no tan próximos. **Rev Med Chil** 1981 Jan;109(1):73–80
**Costa-Casaretto C:** Las enfermedades venéreas en Chile desde el descubrimiento hasta la colonia. **Rev Med Chil** 1980 Oct;108(10):969–76
**Costa-Casaretto C:** Los primeros becarios chilenos en Europa (1874). **Rev Med Chil** 1979 Sep;107(9):886
**Costa-Casaretto C:** Los primeros becarios chilenos en Europa (1874). Alborada de la docencia y la práctica médicas actuales. **Rev Med Chil** 1979 May;107(5):432–7
**Costa-Casaretto C:** Marañon y los chilenos. **Rev Med Chil** 1980 Mar;108(3):277–81
**Costa-Casaretto C:** Nonagésimo aniversario de la Escuela de Medicina de la Avenida Independencia. Testimonios de una odisea. **Rev Med Chil** 1979 Aug;107(8):761–70
**Costa-Casaretto C:** Nonagésimo aniversario del primer Congreso Médico Chileno. **Rev Med Chil** 1979 Sep;107(9):865–75
**Costa-Casaretto C:** Ochenta y cinco años de radiología chilena. Su partida de nacimiento y su fe de beautismo. **Rev Med Chil** 1981 Jul;109(7):669–78
**Costa-Casaretto C:** Por que se les otorgo el Premio Nobel de medicina y fisiologia a Ehrlich y a Metchnikoff en 1908? **Rev Med Chil** 1980;108:775–6
**Costa-Casaretto C:** Presentacion del Dr. Guillermo C. Blest. **Rev Med Chil** 1983 Apr;111(4):364–7
**Costa-Casaretto C:** Presentación del Dr. Lorenzo Sazié. **Rev Med Chil** 1983 Dec;111(12):1289–98
**Costa-Casaretto C:** Presentación del Dr. Pedro Morán (1771–1840). **Rev Med Chil** 1984 Jul;112(7):729–38
**Costa-Casaretto C:** Primeros proyectos de organización sanitaria y de campaña antivenerea después de la emancipación politica de Chile. **Rev Med Chil** 1980 Dec;108(12):1161–9
**Costa-Casaretto C:** Recuerdos olvidados de los orígenes de la Sociedad Médica de Santiago y del la 'Revista Médica de Chile'. **Rev Med Chil** 1979 Jul;107(7):663–72
**Costa-Casaretto C:** Septuagésimo aniversario de la asistencia pública de Santiago. **Rev Med Chil** 1981 Aug;109(8):795–803
**Costa-Casaretto C:** Sobre el. Dr. Carlos Sazie, primer profesor de neurología y segundo de psiquiatria en la universidad de Chile (1881–1891). **Rev Med Chil** 1980 Aug;108(8):749–56
**Costa Filho M:** O Erário mineral de Luiz Gomes Ferreira. **Rev Inst Hist Geogr Bras** 1957;235:331–40
**Costea V:** Cîteva date din activitatea primilor trei profesori titulari ai clinicii dermato-venerologice: Gh. Demetriade, E. I. Mironescu şi Gh. Nastase (1901–1962). **Rev Med Chir Soc Med Nat Iasi** 1983 Jan–Mar;87(1):149–55
**Coston TO:** A personal sketch of Frank Burton Walsh. **Surv Ophthalmol** 1983 Jul–Aug;28(1):50–4
**Côté RA, Robboy S:** Progrès dans la gestion de l'information médicale. La nomenclature systématisée de la médecine (Snomed). **Union Med Can** 1980 Sep;109(9):1243–52
**Côté RA, Robboy S:** Progress in medical information management. Systematized nomenclature of medicine. **JAMA** 1980 Feb 22–29;243(8):756–62
**Cote RJ** see **Sanderson CJ**
**Cotereau Y:** L''Officine' de Dorvault. **Rev Hist Pharm (Paris)** 1980 Jun;27(245):95–107
**Cotinat L:** Les vases de pharmacie à l'exposition de faïences françaises du Grand-Palais (juin-août 1980). **Rev Hist Pharm (Paris)** 1981;28(248):49–53
**Cotinat L:** Vases de l'hôpital Saint-Joseph de Moulins. **Rev Hist Pharm (Paris)** 1980 Mar;27(244):11–14
**Cotrău M, Gheorghiţă I:** Prescriptii medicale in manuscrisul inedit de la Spitalul Se. Spiridon Iasi, din secolul al XVIII-LEA (IV). **Rev Med Chir Soc Med Nat Iasi** 1983 Apr–Jun;87(2):307–12
**Cotrău M, Gheorghiţă I:** Prescripţii medicale în manuscrisul inedit de la spitalul SF. Spiridon Iaşi, din secolul al XVIII-lea. **Rev Med Chir Soc Med Nat Iasi** 1983 Jan–Mar;87(1):113–6
**Cotrău M, Gheorghiţă I:** Prescripţii medicale în manuscrisul inedit de la Spitalul Sf. Spiridon Iaşi, din secolul al XVIII-lea (I). **Rev Med Chir Soc Med Nat Iasi** 1982 Jul–Sep;86(3):501–3
**Cotrău M, Gheorghiţă I:** Prescripţii medicale în manuscrisul inedit de la Spitalul Sf. Spiridon Iaşi, din secolul al XVIII-lea. (II). **Rev Med Chir Soc Med Nat Iasi** 1982 Oct–Dec;86(4):673–6
**Cotrău M:** Procesful cottorului Carol Davila (Iaşi, 1872). **Rev Med Chir Soc Med Nat Iasi** 1980 Apr–Jun;84(2):325–6
**Cott NF:** Passionlessness: an interpretation of Victorian sexual ideology, 1790–1850. **Signs** 1978;4(2):219–36
**Cottam C, Smith EM:** The roots of cranial manipulation: Nephi Cottam and 'craniopathy'. **Chiropr Hist** 1981;1(1):31–5
**Cotter JV, Patrick LL:** Disease and ethnicity in an urban environment. **Ann Assoc Am Geogr** 1981;71(1):40–9
**Cotterman CW:** Relationship and probability in Mendelian populations. **Am J Med Genet** 1983 Nov;16(3):393–440
**Cottet J:** Evolution de la consommation du sel en France. **Bull Mem Acad R Med Belg** 1981;136(11):556–65
**Cotti C:** Il femminismo come caso letterario: un'inchiesta di inizio '900 su amore e sessualita. **Mem Riv Stor Donne** 1981;(2):112–8
**Cotti M** see **Babini VP**
**Cotuţiu C** see **Munteanu A**
**Coudurier P:** Les prix de journée: détermination et contentieux. Nancy, Berger-Levrault, 1978. 225 p.
**Coughlin EA** see **Ericson JE**
**Coulanges P:** Cinquantenaire du vaccin antipesteux EV (Girard et Robic). **Bull Soc Pathol Exot Filiales** 1983 Mar–Apr;76(2):114–20
**Coulanges P:** Cinquantenaire du vaccin antipesteux EV (Girard et Robic). **Arch Inst Pasteur Madagascar** 1982;50(1):169–84
**Coulanges P, Rakotonirina-Randriambeloma PJ:** Epidémiologie de la rage à Madagascar. **Arch Inst Pasteur Tunis** 1982 Mar;59(1):47–74
**Coulanges P** see **Zeller H**
**Coulomb J:** La mort d'Alexandre Le Grand. **Hist Sci Med** 1984;18(2):137–45
**Coulomb J:** Les Minoens et l'anatomie humaine. **Hist Sci Med** 1981;15(1):81–9
**Coulter HL:** Divided legacy: the conflict between homoeopathy and the American Medical Association. Science and ethics in American medicine 1800–1914. 2d ed. Richmond, California, North Atlantic Books, 1982. 552 p.
**Coulter HL:** Homoeopathy and modern medical science. **J Am Inst Homeopath** 1980 Jun;73(2):7–28
**Coulter HL:** Homoeopathy and modern medical science. **J Am Inst Homeopath** 1980 Sept–Dec;73(3–4):17–38, 23–50
**Coulthard SW** see **Titche LL**
**The Council at midcentury--:** the reach for growth and status 1934–1950. **Except Child** 1981 Jan;47(4):286–96
**Counihan HE:** Corrigan on pulmonary disease.

**J Ir Coll Physicians Surg** 1980 Jul;10(1):38–40
**Countryman BA** see **Riordan J**
**Coura SH** see **Seibel SD**
**Cournand A** see **Robin ED, ed**
**Cournut J:** L'innocence de la Marquise ou spécificités et vicissitudes de l'après-coup dans la théorie freudienne et la pratique analytique. **Rev Fr Psychanal** 1982;46(3):535–57
**Court WE:** The pharmaceutical society's collection of materia medica and herbaria. **Pharm Hist (London)** 1980 Dec;10(3):2–3
**Courtine JC:** L'Armée d'Afrique et l'anesthésie-réanimation: de Baudens (1853) au Corps expéditionnaire française à la Première Armée (1942–1945) et à la guerre d'Algérie. **Hist Sci Med** 1983;17(4):411–17
**Courtivron I de** see **Stambolian G**
**Courtois D:** Naissance de l'Institut de Médecine Tropicale du Service de Santé des Armées. **Med Trop (Mars)** 1980 Nov–Dec;40(6):631–4
**Courtois JE:** Le pharmacien Jacques Personne (1816–1880) pionnier de la chimie analytique. **Rev Hist Pharm (Paris)** 1980 Dec;247(68 no 27):263–71
**Courtwright D:** Opiate addiction in the American West, 1850–1920. **J West** 1982 Jul;21(3):23–31
**Courtwright DT:** Dark paradise: opiate addiction in America before 1940. Cambridge, London, Harvard Univ. Press, 1982. 270 p.
**Courtwright DT, Joseph H, Des Jarlais DC:** Memories from the street: oral histories of elderly methadone patients. **Oral Hist Rev** 1981;9:47–64
**Courtwright DT:** Opiate addiction as a consequence of the Civil War. **Civ War Hist** 1978;24(2):101–11
**Courtwright DT:** The female opiate addict in 19th-century America. **Essays Arts Sci** 1982;10:161–72
**Courtwright DT:** The hidden epidemic: opiate addiction and cocaine use in the South, 1860–1920. **J South Hist** 1983;49(1):57–72
**Cousins N, ed:** The physician in literature. Philadelphia, Saunders, 1982. xxiii, 477 p. Selections from many authors.
**Coussement A** see **Lalanne C**
**Couto R:** Property, pinmakers, and physicians: liberal myths and American health care anomalies. **Soundings** 1979;62(3):275–92
**Couturier P** see **Le Fichoux Y**
**Covell RM:** The impact of regulation on health care quality. **Proc Acad Polit Sci** 1980;33(4):111–25
**Coventry JB:** The dental estimates board. Thirty-three years at Eastbourne. **Br Dent J** 1981 Jul 7;151(1):33–4
**Covert C:** A view of the press in the twenties. **Journalism Hist** 1975;2(3):66–7, 92–6
**Covert HH, Kay RF:** Dental microwear and diet: implications for determining the feeding behaviors of extinct primates, with a comment on the dietary patterns of Sivapithecus. **Am J Phys Anthropol** 1981 Jul;55(3):331–6
**Cowan CL Jr** see **Young RC Jr**
**Cowan JC** see **Trautmann J, ed**
**Cowan RS:** Lillian Evelyn Moller Gilbreth. In: Notable American women. The modern period. Cambridge, Mass., Belknap-Harvard Univ. Press, 1980. 4:271–3.
**Cowan RS** see **Stafleu FA**
**Cowan WM:** Jerzy E. Rose. **J Comp Neurol** 1980 Aug 1;192(3):401–6
**Cowan RS, ed** see **Stafleu FA**
**Coward DA:** Attitudes to homosexuality in eighteenth century France. **J Eur Stud** 1980;10(4):231–55
**Coward J:** Birth under-registration in the Republic of Ireland during the twentieth century. **Econ Soc Rev (Irel)** 1982;14(1):1–27
**Coward J:** Recent characteristics of Roman Catholic fertility in Northern and Southern Ireland. **Popul Stud** 1980 Mar;34(1):31–44
**Cowdrey AE:** 'Germ warfare' and public health in the Korean conflict. **J Hist Med Allied Sci** 1984 Apr;39(2):153–72
**Cowell B, Wainwright D:** Behind the blue door: the history of the Royal College of Midwives, 1881–1981. London, Baillière Tindall, 1981. 111 p.
**Cowell B:** Royal College of Midwives: one hundred years young! **Nurs Mirror** 1981 Jul 15;153(3):18–20
**Cowell B, Wainwright D:** The battle for status. **Nurs Times** 1981 Jul 15–21;77(29):1237–8
**Cowell HR:** Osteomyelitis revisited: a 19th century case report. **Del Med J** 1982 May;54(5):263–5
**Cowen DL:** A century of American pharmacy. **Carol J Pharm** 1980 May;60(5):5,7,9–10. Also in: Md Pharm 1981;57(1–3):8–9 and 58(4):8–9. Ala Pharm 1981 Aug–Oct;13(2–4). LA Pharm 1982 Jan–Feb;11(1–2)
**Cowen DL:** A century of American pharmacy. In Alabama Pharmaceutical Association: Centennial celebration, 1881–1981. (Birmingham?), Alabama Pharmaceutical Association, 1981. 11 p.
**Cowen DL:** A note on pharmaceutical literature and the introduction of the new chemical nomenclature. **Beitr Gesch Pharm** 1981;11:84–5
**Cowen DL, Segelman AB, ed:** Antibiotics in historical perspective. [Rahway, New Jersey], Merck, Sharp & Dohme, 1981. 225 p.
**Cowen DL, King LD, Lordi NG:** Drug use in the 19th century: a computer analysis. In Hickel E, Schröder G, ed: Neue Beiträge zur Arzneimittelgeschichte. Festschrift für Wolfgang Schneider zum 70. Geburtstag. Stuttgart, Wissenschaftliche Verlagsgesellschaft, 1982. p. 59–67.
**Cowen DL:** Fifty years of the New Jersey Journal of Pharmacy. **NJ J Pharm** 1977 Oct;50(10):14–17
**Cowen DL:** Louisiana--pioneer in the regulation of pharmacy. **La Pharm** 1982 Apr;41(4):4–9
**Cowen DL:** New Jersey medical historiography, 1964–1984. **J Med Soc NJ** 1984 Sep;81(9):807–10
**Cowen DL, King LD, Lordi NG:** Nineteenth century drug therapy: computer analysis of the 1854 prescription file of a Burlington pharmacy. **J Med Soc NJ** 1981 Oct;78(11):758–61
**Cowen DL:** Pharmacy and freedom. **Pharm Hist** 1984;26(2):70–82
**Cowen DL:** Pharmacy and freedom. **Am J Hosp Pharm** 1984 Mar;41(3):459–67
**Cowen DL:** Robert P. Fischelis 1891–1981. **NJ J Pharm** 1982 Feb;55(2):12–4
**Cowen DL:** The historical collections of the Pharmacist Institute of New Jersey. **NJ J Pharm** 1980 Oct;53(10):15 and 1982 Jan;55(1):8–9
**Cowen DL:** The history of pharmacy and the history of the Jews. In H.R. Fehlmann, F. Ledermann, ed: Festschrift für A. Lutz und J. Büchi. Zürich, Juris Druck, 1983. p. 67–83. (Veröffentlichungen der Schweizerischen Gesellschaft fur Geschichte der Pharmazie, Bd. 2).
**Cowen DL:** The influence of the Edinburgh Pharmacopoeia and the Edinburgh Dispensatories. **Pharm Hist (London)** 1982;12(3):2–4
**Cowen DL:** The nineteenth century German immigrant and American pharmacy. In Dilg P, et al., ed: Perspektiven der Pharmaziegeschichte. Graz, Austria, Akademische Druck- u. Verlagsanstalt, 1983. p. 13–28.
**Cowen DL, Helfand WH:** The progressive movement and its impact on pharmacy. **Pharm Acta Helv** 1979;54(11):317–23
**Cowen DL, Helfand WH:** The Progressive Movement and its impact on pharmacy. **Pharm Acta Helv** 1979;(11):1–6
**Cowen DL:** The trustees' garden at Savannah. **Ga Pharm Q** 1983 Spring;60(2):5–3
**Cowen DL:** Tying the knot - secundum artem. **NJ J Pharm** 1983;56(3):6
**Cowen DL** see **Helfand WH**
**Cowen DL** see **Numbers RL, ed**
**Cowen D, ed** see **Wankmüller A**
**Cowgill UM:** Marriage and its progeny in the city of York, 1538–1751. **Kroeber Antropol Soc Pap** 1970;(42):47–87
**Cowie AV** see **Allan P**
**Cowley J, Adler C, ed:** A descriptive catalogue of early medical books in the Adler Museum of the History of Medicine and the University of the Witwatersrand Medical Library. Johannesburg, University of the Witwatersrand Library, 1982. x, 145 p.
**Cowlishaw G:** Infanticide in aboriginal Australia. **Oceania** 1978;48:262–83
**Cox EG:** Sir William Kershaw Slater. In Dictionary of national biography, 1961–1970. Suppl. 8, 1981. p. 955–6.
**Cox JS:** Die Entwicklung der amerikanischen Tierkörperverwertungs-industrie. **Zentralbl Bakteriol [B]** 1980 Mar;170(3–4):217–21
**Cox MK:** Victory through defeat: a character analysis of Robert E. Lee. **Psychoanal Rev** 1980 Winter;67(4):443–63
**Cox WW, Evans RJ:** Health practices in Collier County: a study in diversity and contrast. **J Fla Med Assoc** 1982 Aug;69(8):695–701
**Coyle G** see **Liberti L**
**Cozens DD** see **Palmer AK**
**Craddock D** see **Maddern GJ**
**Craddock S:** Retired except on demand: the life of Dr. Cicely Williams. Oxford, Green College, 1983. 198 p.
**Crafts NF:** Illegitimacy in England and Wales in 1911. **Popul Stud** 1982 Jul;36(2):327–31
**Craggs J:** Simple method for auto-ophthalmoscopy. **Br J Ophthalmol** 1983 May;67(5):330–1
**Craig B:** Smallpox in Ontario: public and professional perceptions of disease, 1884–1885. In Roland CG, ed: Health, disease and medicine. Toronto, Hannah Institute for the History of Medicine, 1984. p. 215–49.
**Craig D:** History of medicine: observation and theory: some reflections occasioned by reading Nansen's 'Farthest North'. **Practitioner** 1980 Feb;224(1340):219–22
**Craig GM:** Michael Barrett. In Dictionary of Canadian biography, 1881–1890. 1982;11:53–4.
**Craig P:** Medical topography. **Soc Soc Hist Med Bull (Lond)** 1984 Dec;35:33–4
**Craig P:** The 'biographical memoirs' of the Bristol Infirmary. **Soc Soc Hist Med Bull (Lond)** 1984 Dec;35:53–4
**Craig P:** The first B.M.A. meeting in Bristol. **Bristol Med Chir J** 1983 Jul;98(367):104–8
**Craig RB:** Human rights and Mexico's antidrug campaign. **Soc Sci Q** 1980;60(4):691–701
**Craig RB, Turner MA:** International control of narcotics and dangerous drugs: a synopsis. **Indian Pol Sci Rev** 1977;11(1):33–47
**Craig RP:** Military cold injury during the war in the Falkland Islands 1982: an evaluation of possible risk factors. **J R Army Med Corps** 1984 Jun;130(2):89–96
**Crainz F:** The editions and translations of Dr. Matthew Baillie's Morbid Anatomy. **Med Hist** 1982 Oct;26(4):443–52
**Cramer CH:** The story of dentistry and the school in University Circle. Cleveland, School of Dentistry, Case Western Reserve University, 1982. x, 235 p.
**Cramer JA** see **Smith DB**
**Cramer M, Starobinski J, ed, Barblan MA:** Centenaire de la Faculté de Médecine de l'Université de Genève. Genève, Editions Médecine et hygiène, 1978. xvi, 165 p.
**Cramp R** see **Hart GD, ed**
**Cranach M von:** Die Münchner Klinik und die psychiatrische Diagnostik. **MMW** 1981 May 8;123(19):777–80
**Crandell CE, ed** see **Knudtzon K**
**Crane D:** Invisible colleges: diffusion of knowledge in scientific

communities. Chicago, University of Chicago Press, 1972. x, 213 p.
**Crane D** see **Durbin PT, ed**
**Cranefield PF:** Alfred Einstein Cohn. In Dictionary of American Biography, Suppl. 6, 1956–1960. p. 117–18, 1980.
**Cranefield PF, ed:** Two great scientists of the nineteenth century. Correspondence of Emil Du Bois-Reymond and Carl Ludwig. Collected by Estelle Du Bois-Reymond. Foreword, notes, and indexes by Paul Diepgen. Translation of 1927 German ed. Baltimore, London, Johns Hopkins Univ. Press, 1982. xix, 183 p.
**Cravens H:** Robert Mearns Yerkes. In Dictionary of American Biography, Suppl. 6, 1956–1960. p. 717–19, 1980.
**Cravens H:** Samuel Cate Prescott. In Dictionary of American biography, 1961–1965. Suppl. 7, 1981. p. 629–30.
**Cravens H:** The triumph of evolution: American scientists and the heredity-environment controversy 1900–1941. [Philadelphia], University of Pennsylvania Press, 1978. xvi, 351 p.
**Crawford LM:** Maestro Domingo Royo and the Llave de Albeyteria. **Hist Med Vet** 1977;2(2):33–6
**Crawford LM** see **De Wailly P**
**Crawford P:** Attitudes to menstruation in seventeenth-century England. **Past Present** 1981;91:47–73
**Crawford P:** Attitudes to pregnancy from a woman's spiritual diary, 1687–8. **Local Popul Stud (Matlock)** 1978;21:43–5
**Crawford P:** Printed advertisements for women medical practitioners in London, 1670–1710. **Soc Soc Hist Med Bull (Lond)** 1984 Dec;35:66–70
**Crawford R:** Individual responsibility and health politics in the 1970s. In Reverby S, Rosner D, ed: Health care in America. Philadelphia, Temple University PRess, 1979. p. 247–68.
**Crawford RJ:** Missionary accounts of fofo mo'omo'o. **J Polynesian Soc** 1977;86(4):531–4
**Crawford S:** Health science libraries in the United States: I. Overview of the post-World War II years. **Bull Med Libr Assoc** 1983 Jan;71(1):16–20
**Crawford S:** Health science libraries in the United States: III. Hospital health science libraries, 1969–1979. **Bull Med Libr Assoc** 1983 Jan;71(1):30–6
**Crawford S:** Health sciences libraries in the United States: II. Medical school libraries, 1960–1980. **Bull Med Libr Assoc** 1983 Jan;71(1):21–9
**Crawford WL:** On the movements of the iris, and, incidentally, on the essential portion of the organ of vision. **Am J Optom Physiol Opt** 1979 Oct;56(10):658–60
**Crawford WM:** More on the ether operation. **N Engl J Med** 1984 Feb 23;310(8):534
**Craytor JK:** Highlights in education for cancer nursing. **Oncol Nurs Forum** 1982 Fall;9(4):51–9
**Crellin J:** Selected items from the history of pathology. **Am J Pathol** 1980 Jan;98(1):60
**Crellin J:** 'The past recaptured'...five North Carolina pharmacies. **Pharm Hist** 1980;22(2):77–8
**Crellin J:** Théophile Bonet (1620–1689). **Am J Pathol** 1980 Jan;98(1):212
**Crellin JK:** Alcoholism and drug addiction in the 'nineties: an American in London. **Br J Addict** 1980 Jun;75(2):153–62
**Crellin JK:** Antibiosis in the nineteenth century. In J. Parascandola, ed: The history of antibiotics. Madison, American Institute of the History of Pharmacy, 1980. p. 5–13.
**Crellin JK:** Internal antisepsis or the dawn of chemotherapy? **J Hist Med Allied Sci** 1981 Jan;36(1):9–18
**Crellin JK:** Medical care in pioneer Illinois. Springfield, Pearson Museum, Southern Illinois University, School of Medicine, 1982. xi, 128 p.
**Crellin JK, Helfand WH:** Medical care in the 20th century. Facets of change illustrated by American and British postcards. Durham, Duke University Medical Center, 1982. 106 p. (Readings and Perspectives in Medicine, Booklet Number 3).
**Crellin JK:** Pharmacies as general stores in the 19th century. **Pharm Hist (London)** 1979 Apr;9(1):5–6
**Crellin JK, Helfand W:** Picture postcards; a resource for social history of pharmacy. **Pharm Hist** 1983;25(3):116–30
**Crellin JK:** The surgical teaching of Philip Syng Physick. Durham, Medical History Program and the Trent Collection, Duke University Medical Center, 1981 vi, 101 p.
**Crellin JK** see **Helfand WH**
**Crellin JK** see **Parascandola J**
**Crellin JK, ed:** Plants in medicine: from yesterday to today. Durham, Duke University Medical Center, 1982. 114 p. Readings and Perspectives in Medicine, Booklet Number 2.
**Cremer T** see **Kirkwood TB**
**Cremerius J:** Die ödipal verkleidete präödipale Liebe oder Feydeaus professionelles Missverständnis. **Psyche (Stuttg)** 1981;35:253–67
**Cremerius J:** Die Reszeption der Psychoanalyse in der Soziologie, Psychologie und Theologie im deutschsprachigen Raum bis 1940. Frankfurt am Main, Suhrkamp, 1981. 339 p.
**Cremerius J:** 'Die Sprache der Zärtlichkeit und der Leidenschaft'. Reflexionen zu Sándor Ferenczis Wiesbadener Vortrag von 1932. **Psyche (Stuttg)** 1983 Nov;37(11):988–1015
**Cremerius J:** Freuds Sterben--Die Identität von Denken, Leben und Sterben. **Psychother Psychosom Med Psychol** 1983 Sep;33(5):163–6
**Cremerius J:** Robert Musil. Das Dilemma eines Schriftstellers vom Typus 'poeta doctus' nach Freud. **Psyche (Stuttg)** 1979 Aug;33(8):733–72
**Cremerius J** see **Amitai M**
**Cremerius J** see **Fischle-Carl H, ed**
**Cremerius J** see **Lohmann HM, ed**
**Cremona GF:** Cenni sullo sviluppo della ginnastica educativa e medica in Italia. **Ann Osp Maria Vittoria Torino** 1981 Jan–Jun;24(1–6):210–6
**Cremona GF:** La bioclimatologia medica: aspetti dell'evoluzione storica, con particolare riguardo al contributo degli scienziati piemontesi. **Ann Osp Maria Vittoria Torino** 1982 Jul–Dec;25(7–12):245–58
**Cremona GF:** L'elettroterapia nel XVIII secolo. Ricerche di elettrofisiolgia e di elettroterapia di studiosi piemontesi. **Ann Osp Maria Vittoria Torino** 1981 Jan–Jun;24(1–6):167–77
**Cremona GF:** Studi di biologia e medicina nell'opera del fisico piemontese G. B. Beccaria. **Ann Osp Maria Vittoria Torino** 1982 Jul–Dec;25(7–12):259–68
**Cremone JC, Beddings A:** Aesthetic reconstruction [letter]. **Plast Reconstr Surg** 1983 Mar;71(3):440–2
**Cremone JC:** The anatomy lesson of Dr. Nicolaas Tulp. **J Hand Surg** 1982 Sep;7(5):530
**Cremone JC:** Thinking before incising. **Plast Reconstr Surg** 1984 Mar;73(3):500
**Crespo Cossio P:** Aportes acerca de la incidencia de la epidemia de cólera de 1867 en el Departamento Totoral y población del mismo nombre. **Rev Fac Cien Med Univ Nac Cordoba** 1980;38(1–4):41–2, 45
**Creteanu G, Teodorovici G:** Revista Medico-chirurgicală si contributia sa la progresul asistentei medicale. **Rev Med Chir Soc Med Nat Iasi** 1980 Oct–Dec;84(4):625–9
**Criado FJ, Wilson TH:** Posterior transsphincteric approach for surgery of the rectum: the Bevan operation. **Dis Colon Rectum** 1981;24:145–50
**Crick F:** Crick looks back on DNA. **Science** 1979 Nov 9;206(4419):667
**Crider S:** Anesthesia. A history of Simpson's discovery of chloroform. **J Kans Med Soc** 1983 Mar;84(3):143–6
**Crile G:** Breast cancer. A personal perspective. **Surg Clin North Am** 1984 Dec;64(6):1145–9
**Criley JM, Niemann JT, Rosborough JP:** Cardiopulmonary resuscitation research 1960–1984: discoveries and advances. **Ann Emerg Med** 1984 Sep;13(9 Pt 2):756–8
**Crimmins E** see **Condran GA**
**Crimmins EM, Condran GA:** Mortality variation in U.S. cities in 1900: a two-level explanation by cause of death and underlying factors. **Soc Sci Hist** 1983;7(1):31–60
**Crimmins EM:** The changing pattern of American mortality decline, 1940–1977, and its implications for the future. **Popul Dev Rev** 1981;7(2):229–54
**Crimmins EM:** The completeness of 1900 mortality data collected by registration and enumeration for rural and urban parts of states: estimates using the Chandra Sekar-Deming technique. **Hist Methods** 1980;13(3):163–9
**Crisan E:** Aspekte der ärztlichen Betreuung der Eisenbahnarbeiter im XIX. Jahrhundert (Rom) **Acta Mus Napocensis (Cluj)** 1978;15:461–5
**Crişan V:** Herbert Olivecrona (1891–1980). **Rev Med Interna [Neurol Psihiatr]** 1981 Oct–Dec;26(4):307–10
**Crisan V:** Neurochirurgische Beiträge über die Benutzung der keltischen Sägen, sowie die in Galatii Bistritei in Rumanien gefundene Säge. In: International Congress of the History of Medicine, 26th, Plovdiv (Bulgaria), 1978. Actes du Congres, Vol. 1. Sofia, 1980. p. 93–6.
**Crisciani C:** Valeurs éthiques et savoir médical entre le XIIe et le XIVe siècle. Problèmes et thèmes d'une recherche. **Hist Philos Life Sci** 1983;5(1):33–52
**Crisp KA:** Chiropractic lyceums: the colorful origins of chiropractic continuing education. **Chiropr Hist** 1984;4(1):17–22
**Crispell KR:** Beaumont and Dunglison: who was Dunglison? **Trans Am Clin Climatol Assoc** 1980;92:194–8
**Crissey JT, Parish LC:** Ferdinand Hebra: a reexamination of his contributions to dermatology. **Int J Dermatol** 1980 Dec;19(10):585–8
**Crissey JT, Parish LC:** The dermatology and syphilology of the nineteenth century. New York, Praeger, 1981. viii, 439 p.
**Crissey JT:** William Allen Pusey. **J Am Acad Dermatol** 1984 Oct;11(4 Pt 1):702–8
**Crissey JT** see **Parish LC**
**Cristoffanini AP:** El internado en los estudios médicos. **Educ Med Salud** 1982;16(2):134–50
**Critchley M:** Dax's law. **Int J Neurol** 1978;11(4):404–11
**Crockett DC** see **Castleman B**
**Croft C:** The confinement and death of Princess Charlotte. **St Thomas Hosp Gaz** 1981;79:46–9
**Croix A:** L'homme et son corps dans l'Au-delà. In Imhof AE, ed: Leib und Leben in der Geschichte der Neuzeit. Berlin, Duncker & Humblot, 1983. p. 155–62.
**Crombie AC:** James Sterling Wilkie: 1906–1982. **Br J Hist Sci** 1984 Nov;17(57 pt 3):310–1
**Crombie AC:** Science and the arts in the Renaissance: the search for truth and certainty, old and new. **Hist Sci** 1980 Dec;18(42 pt 4):233–46
**Crombie AC** see **Recollections & reflections**
**Crombie DH:** The founding staff of Hartford Hospital and its legacy. **Conn Med** 1979 Nov;43(11):682–3
**Cromley RG** see **Shannon GW**
**Crompton L:** Don Leon, Byron, and homosexual law reform. **J Homosex** 1983 Spring-Summer;8(3–4):53–71
**Crompton L:** The myth of lesbian impunity: capital laws from 1270 to 1791. **J Homosex** 1980–81 Fall-Winter;6(1–2):11–25
**Crompton R, Gall D:** Georgi Markov--death in a pellet. **Med Leg J** 1980;48(2):51–62
**Cronholm B:** Från långbad och isolering till farmakoterapi och rehabilitering. **Nord Medicinhist Arsb** 1981;:133–50
**Cronin JE, Boaz NT, Stringer CB, et al:** Tempo and mode in hominid

evolution. **Nature** 1981 Jul 9;292(5819):113–22
**Cronin JE** see **Goodman M**
**Crook DP:** Darwinism – the political implications. **Hist Eur Ideas** 1981;5:99–139
**Crookes GP:** Communication in ophthalmology. **Trans Ophthalmol Soc UK** 1981;101 (Pt 4):409–21
**Crooks JB:** The role of women in volunteerism: a short history. **Volunt Action Leadersh** 1981 Summer;22–8
**Crosby AW:** God... would destroy them, and give their country to another people. **Am Heritage** 1978;29(6):38–43
**Crosby AW:** The early history of syphilis: a reappraisal. **Am Anthropol** 1969;71(2):218–27
**Crosby WH:** An historical sketch of splenic function and splenectomy. **Lymphology** 1983 Jun;16(2):52–5
**Crosby WH:** Landmark perspective. Pernicious anemia. **JAMA** 1983 Dec 23–30;250(24):3336–8
**Crosby WH, Haubrich WS:** The death of Walter Reed. **JAMA** 1982 Sep 17;248(11):1342–5
**Crosby WH:** The golden age of the Army Medical Corps: a perspective from 1901. **Milit Med** 1983 Sep;148(9):707–11
**Crosland M:** Chemistry and the chemical revolution. In G. S. Rousseau, R. Porter, ed: The ferment of knowledge. Studies in the historiography of eighteenth-century science. Cambridge, Cambridge University Press, 1980. p. 389–416.
**Crosland M:** Explicit qualifications as a criterion for membership of the Royal Society: a historical review. **Notes Rec R Soc Lond** 1983 Mar;37(2):167–87
**Crosland M:** From prizes to grants in the support of scientific research in France in the nineteenth century: the Montyon legacy. **Minerva** 1979 Autumn;17(3):355–80
**Crosland M:** The library of Gay-Lussac. **Ambix** 1981 Nov;28(3):158–70
**Crosland M** see **Forgan S, ed**
**Cross HE:** Dieta y nutricion en el medio rural de Zacatecas y San Luis Potosi (siglos XVIII y XIX). **Hist Mex** 1981;31(1):101–16
**Cross SJ:** John Hunter, the animal oeconomy, and late eighteenth-century physiological discourse. **Stud Hist Biol** 1981;5:1–110
**Cross W, Moses J:** 'My God, sir, I think the president is doomed!' [Grover Cleveland's cancer surgery] **Am Hist Illus** 1982 Nov;17:40–5
**Crossgrove W:** Ein frühes Zeugnis für Ortolfs Arzneibuch. **Z Dtsch Altert Dtsch Lit** 1979;108:234–9
**Crosskey RW, Post RJ:** Which cytospecies of the Simulium damnosum complex did Blacklock incriminate in the transmission of Onchocerca volvulus? **Ann Trop Med Parasitol** 1981 Oct;75(5):569–71
**Crouch HE:** History of basal cell carcinoma and its treatment. **J R Soc Med** 1983 Apr;76(4):302–6
**Crow JF:** Sewall Wright, the scientist and the man. **Perspect Biol Med** 1982 Winter;25(2):279–94
**Crow CL, ed** see **Kerr H**
**Crowder EM:** Nursing in Texas: a pictorial history. Waco, Texas, Texian Press, 1980, ix, 184 p.
**Crowdy JP:** The science of the soldier's food. **Army Q Def J** 1980;110(3):266–79
**Crowe MJ, ed:** Witchcraft: catalogue of the witchcraft collection in Cornell University Library. Millwood, N. Y., KTO Press, 1977. xxcviii, 644 p.
**Crowley JE, Shapiro D:** Aspirations and expectations of youth in the United States: part I. Education and fertility. **Youth Soc** 1982;13(4):391–422
**Crowley JW:** Dating Howells' adolescent breakdown. **Old Northwest** 1982;8(1):13–22
**Crowley RM:** Frieda Fromm-Reichmann: recollections of a student. **Psychiatry** 1982;45(2):105–7
**Crowley RM:** Harry Stack Sullivan as social critic. **J Am Acad Psychoanal** 1981 Apr;9(2):211–26
**Crowley RM:** William V. Silverberg as teacher and colleague. **J Am Acad Psychoanal** 1981 Oct;9(4):493–500
**Crowther MA:** Family responsibility and state responsibility in Britain before the welfare state. **Hist J (Gt Brit)** 1982;25(1):131–45
**Crowther MA:** Paupers or patients? Obstacles to professionalization in the Poor Law medical service before 1914. **J Hist Med Allied Sci** 1984 Jan;39(1):33–54
**Crowther RW, Gambles RM:** Anthrax eradication in Cyprus: an historical survey. **Trop Anim Health Prod** 1983 May;15(2):103–5
**Croxatto H:** Homenaje al Dr. Teodoro Muhm (1869–1939). **Rev Med Chil** 1984 Jan;112(1):81–8
**Croxson LJ:** The dentist and society: a symbiosis? **Ann R Australas Coll Dent Surg** 1977 Jun;5:109–17
**Crozier WL:** A people apart: a census analysis of the Polish community of Winona, Minnesota, 1880–1905. **Pol Am Stud** 1981;38(1):5–22
**Cruft GE, Humphreys JW, Hermann RE, et al:** Recertification in surgery, 1980. **Arch Surg** 1981 Aug;116(8):1093–6
**Crugnola A, ed:** Scholia in Nicandri Theriaka, cum glossis. Varese-Milano, Istituto Editoriale Cisalpino, 1971. 329 p.
**Crul JF:** [History of anesthesiology]. (Ita) **Minerva Anestesiol** 1979 Sep;45(9):721–9
**Crul JF:** Relaxant drugs: from native drugs to the selective agents of today. **Acta Anaesthesiol Scand** 1982 Aug;26(4):409–15
**Crump T:** Translation of case reports in Ueber die multiplen Fibrome der Haut und ihre Beziehung zu den multiplen Neuromen by F. v. Recklinghausen. **Adv Neurol** 1981;29:259–75
**Crumpacker L:** The art of the healer: women in the fiction of Sarah Orne Jewett. **Colby Libr Q** 1983;19(3):155–66
**Cruse P:** Florence Nightingale. **Surgery** 1980 Sep;88(3):394–9
**Cruse WP, Bellizzi R:** A historic review of endodontics, 1689–1963, part 1–3. **J Endod** 1980;6(3–5):495–9,532–5,576–80
**Crutcher JC:** A memorial lecture for Dr. Ben Wells. **Ala J Med Sci** 1979 Oct;16(4):346–9
**Cruz FO** see **Aráujo A**
**Cruz WL** see **Tiglao T**
**Cruz-Coke R:** Centenario de la muerte de Mendel. **Rev Med Chil** 1984 Jan;112(1):61–4
**Cruz-Coke R:** El plan Garretón-Alessandri. **Rev Med Chil** 1980 Nov;108(11):1073–5
**Cruz-Coke R:** Los profesores de la Escuela de Medicina y la historia política nacional (1833–1983). **Rev Med Chil** 1983 Apr;111(4):380–7
**Cruz Dones A:** Escuela de Enfermería de la Clínica Díaz García. **Bol Col Prof Enferm PR** 1982 Sep;8(31):23
**Csanak DF:** Teleki József Szerepe egy XVIII. századi francia tudományos vitaban. **Szazadok** 1974;108(2):406–22
**Csiky CE** see **Csiky K**
**Csiky K, Csiky CE, Grecu G:** Electroşocul în psihiatrie. **Rev Med Interna [Neurol Psihiatr]** 1981 Oct–Dec;26(4):259–66
**Csillag I:** Az elsö magyar orthopédiai intézet. **Orv Hetil** 1982 May 2;123(18):1111–4
**Csillag I:** David Gruby. **Orvostort Kozl** 1982;28(1–3):177–86
**Csillag I:** Eckstein Ferenc és a hadisebészet a Napóleon elleni háborúban. **Orv Hetil** 1984 Feb 19;125(8):467–70
**Csillag I:** Elfelejtett kórházak nyomában. Balassa és Semmelweis a régi zsidó kórházban. **Orv Hetil** 1981 Feb 22;122(8):463–5
**Csillag I:** L'ancien hôpital juif de Pest. **Rev Hist Med Heb** 1980;33(4):73–4
**Csillag I:** Quelques médecins juifs hongrois et les événements viennois de 1848. **Rev Hist Med Heb** 1984;37(1):7–9
**Csillik B:** Prof. Dr. Ambrus Abrahám. **Acta Biol Acad Sci Hung** 1983;34(2–3):131–5
**Csorba H:** Rola polskich lekarzy na Wegrzech 1939–1945. **Arch Hist Med (Warsz)** 1984;47(2):207–19
**Csorba S:** Kölcsey Ferenc hibás szemének kérdéséhez. **Orvostort Kozl** 1982;28(1–3):191–9
**Csorba T:** Głosy polskich lekarzy o pobycie na Wegrzech 1939–1945. **Arch Hist Med (Warsz)** 1984;47(2):221–37
**Cuciureanu R** see **Năstasă V**
**Cudennec Y** see **Boisanger B de**
**Cueva J, Ramírez Oviedo A:** Historia de la alergia en México. In Academia Nacional de Medicina. Libro conmemorativo del primer centenario. México, Comité Editorial de la Comisión Organizadora del Congreso del Centenario, 1964. Tome 2. p. 552–8.
**Cule J:** A doctor for the people: 2000 years of general practice in Britain. London and Boston, Update, 1980. 145 p.
**Cule J:** Catheters: forerunners of Foley. **Nurs Mirror** 1980 Feb 21;150(8):Suppl i–vi
**Cule J:** Griffith Evans (1835–1935) and his trypanosome. **Vet Hist** 1979–80;1(3):94–101
**Cule J:** Medical translations in sixteenth century Wales. In International Congress of the History of Medicine, 27th, Barcelona, 1980. Actas. Barcelona, Académia de Ciències Mèdiques de Catalunya i Balears, 1981. p. 233–7.
**Cule J:** Pestis flava: y fad felen. In J. Cule, ed: Wales and medicine. London, British Society for the History of Medicine, 1975. p. 141–55.
**Cule J:** Wales and medicine. A source-list for printed books and papers showing the history of medicine in relation to Wales and Welshmen. [Aberystwyth], National Library of Wales, 1980. xvii, 229 p.
**Cule J:** William Price of Llantrisant--1800-1893. **Br Med J [Clin Res]** 1982 Feb 13;284(6314):483–4
**Cule J, ed:** Wales and medicine. An historical survey from papers given at the Ninth British Congress on the History of Medicine at Swansea & Cardiff, 4–8th September, 1973. London, British Society for the History of Medicine, 1975. xi, 249 p.
**Culik H:** Mindful of the body: medical allusions in Beckett's Murphy. **Eire-Irel** 1977 Spring;14:84–101
**Cullen JP:** Chimborazo Hospital: 'That charnal house of living sufferers.' **Civ War Times Illus** 1981;19(9):36–42
**Cullinan J:** The roses of no man's land. **Nurs Times** 1980 Oct 16;76(42):1823–5
**Cultures industrielles au pays des collines: plantes médicinales, chicorée, tabac (1890–1914):** Ath [Belgium], 1982. 146 p.
**Cumberland WH:** Epidemic! Iowa battles the Spanish influenza. **Palimpsest** 1981;62(1):26–32
**Cumming E, Lazer C:** Kinship structure and suicide: a theoretical link. **Can Rev Sociol Anthropol** 1981;18(3):271–82
**Cummings J** see **Askari H**
**Cummings MM:** Comments on John Shaw Billings. **J Indiana State Med Assoc** 1981 Oct;74(10):638
**Cummings MM:** Index Medicus, 1879–1979. **Milit Med** 1979 Dec;144(12):829–30
**Cummins CJ:** A history of medical administration in New South Wales 1788–1973. Sydney, Health Commission of New South Wales, 1979. 223 p.
**Cundey B:** Artificial teeth: a bit of a mouthful. **Nurs Mirror** 1981 Apr 9;152(15):30–2
**Cunha AS:** Algumas considerações sobre medicina dentária forense e o seu início em Portugal. **Rev Port Estomatol Cir Maxilofac** 1980 Apr–Jun;22(2):187–200
**Cunha BA:** Typhoid fever, the typhus-like disease: historical perspective. **NY State J Med** 1982 Mar;82(3):321–4

**Cunha-Melo JR** see **Earlam R**
**Cunha Rodrigues MR da:** A morte da Imperatriz Leopoldina (11-XII-1826). **Rev Hist (Brazil)** 1971;43(88):345-52
**Cunin OE:** Femmes dentistes, femmes de dentistes. **Hist Sci Med** 1980;14(2):207-12
**Cunningham A** see **Appleby JH**
**Cunningham DJ:** Claude Gordon Douglas. In Dictionary of national biography, 1961-1970. Suppl. 8, 1981. p. 303-4.
**Cunningham RJ:** James Moore Hickson and spiritual healing in the American Episcopal church. **Hist Mag Protest Episc Church** 1970;39(1):2-16
**Cunningham SG, Mitchell PH:** The use of animals in nursing research. **ANS** 1982 Jul;4(4):72-84
**Cunningham W:** The control of woolsorter's disease. **Pharm Hist (London)** 1975 May;5(1):4-5
**Cuny J** see **Kernéis JP**
**Cuppy D** see **Dockery JL**
**Curelaru I, Sandu L:** Eugen Bogdan Aburel (1899-1975). The pioneer of regional analgesia for pain relief in childbirth. **Anaesthesia** 1982 Jun;37(6):663-9
**Curet M, Carre A, Henaff R:** Les écoles de chirurgie et de médecine navales. **Med Armees** 1980;8(10)spec:797-800
**Curet M, Carre A, Henaff R:** Les hôpitaux des ports. **Med Armees** 1980;8(10)spec:795-6
**Curet M, Huard P, Carre A, et al:** Les traditions de la marine: une médecine de la mer. **Med Armees** 1980;8(10)spec:787-94
**Curran AS:** Lead poisoning: a historical overview. **NY State J Med** 1984 Sep;84(9):437-8
**Curran CE:** Roman Catholicism [and the history of bioethics]. In Reich WT, et al, ed: Encyclopedia of bioethics, v.4. New York, Free Press, 1978. p. 1522-34.
**Curran DJ:** Symbolic solutions for deadly dilemmas: an analysis of federal coal mine health and safety legislation. **Int J Health Serv** 1984;14(1):5-29
**Curran JA:** Founders of the Harvard School of Public Health, with biographical notes, 1909-1946. New York, Josiah Macy, Jr. Foundation, 1970. xviii, 294 p.
**Curran WJ:** An historical perspective on the law of personality and status with special regard to the human fetus and the rights of women. **Milbank Mem Fund Q** 1983 Winter;61(1):58-75
**Curriculum vitae:** Thomas Bernard Fitzpatrick. **J Invest Dermatol** 1983 Jun;80 Suppl:6s-11s
**Curriculum vitae and writings: Niels Hjorth.: Acta Derm Venereol [Suppl] (Stockh)** 1979;59(85):5-9
**Currie BS** see **Spicker SF, ed**
**Currie R, Driedger L, Linden R:** Abstinence and moderation: mixing Mennonite drinking norms. **Mennon Q Rev** 1979;53(4):263-81
**Curry D** see **Heirs of Hippocrates**
**Curry R, Johnston L:** Percutaneous transluminal angioplasty. **Ulster Med J** 1982;51(1):59-66
**Curtis AC, Owens BB:** Centennial paper: Beta dimethylaminoethyl benzhydryl ether hydrochloride (benadryl) in treatment of urticaria by Arthur C. Curtis and Betty Brechner Owens. **Arch Dermatol** 1983 May;119(5):438-41
**Curtis B** see **Curtis J**
**Curtis CH:** Autotransfusion in gynecologic hemoperitoneum. **Am J Obstet Gynecol** 1983 Jul 1;146(5):501-4
**Curtis DE:** Nurses and war. The way it was. **Am J Nurs** 1984 Oct;84(10):1253-4
**Curtis FB:** William Blake and eighteenth-century medicine. **Blake Stud** 1979;8:187-99
**Curtis J, Curtis B:** Illness and the Victorian lady: the case of Jeannie Sumner. **Int J Womens Stud** 1981;4(5):527-43
**Curtis JB, Miller D, Simpson D:** The Neurosurgical society of Australasia: the first forty years. **Aust NZ J Surg** 1980 Aug;50(4):434-7
**Curtis P:** Three hundred years of family health care: some perspectives. **J Fam Pract** 1981 Feb;12(2):323-7
**Curtis RI:** Salted fish products in ancient medicine. **J Hist Med Allied Sci** 1984 Oct;39(4):430-45
**Curtius F:** Richard Siebeck (1883-1965). **Med Welt** 1983 Mar 18;34(11):347-53
**Cushman P:** Amos Evans, M.D.; surgeon on U.S.S. Constitution in War of 1812. **NY State J Med** 1980 Oct;80(11):1753-6
**Cushman P:** Medicine at turn of century. Perspectives from press. **NY State J Med** 1982 Jan;82(1):81-4
**The cutaneous punch by Edward L. Keyes (J Cutan Genitourin Dis, March 1887): Arch Dermatol** 1982 Nov;118(11):940-2
**Cuthbertson DP:** Symposium on 'surgery and nutrition'. Historical approach. **Proc Nutr Soc** 1980 May;39(2):101-5
**Cutright P, Shorter E:** The effects of health on the completed fertility of nonwhite and white U.S. women born from 1867 through 1935. **J Soc Hist** 1979;13(2):191-218
**Cutright PR, Brodhead MJ:** Elliott Coues: naturalist and frontier historian. Urbana, University of Illinois Press, 1981. xv, 509 p.
**Cyprian T:** Problem Karalności zagrożenia w sprawach o wypadki drogowe. **Panstwo Prawo** 1965;20(2):273-9
**Cyr C** see **Mathieu J**
**Czapska I:** Whołdzie najlepszym (Anita Zofia Brodniewicz). **Pieleg Polozna** 1983;(6):28-9
**Czapska I, Kamińska A:** Whołdzie najlepszym (Halina Bandurska). **Pieleg Polozna** 1983;(5):27, 31
**Czarnetzki A:** Menschen des Frühen Mittelalters im Spiegel der Anthropologie und Medizin: Begleitheft zur Ausstellung. Stuttgart, Würtemmbergisches Landesmuseum Stuttgart, 1982. 103 p.
**Czarnetzki A** see **Riethe P**
**Czehák J:** November 7: Gondolatok az egészségügy és a társadalom kapcsolatáról. **Orv Hetil** 1983 Nov 6;124(45):2723-4
**Czeisler CA, Guilleminault C:** 250 years ago: tribute to a new discipline (1729--1979). **Sleep** 1979;2(2):155-60
**Czeizel A:** A historical evaluation of the doctrine of heredodegeneration. **Orvostort Kozl** 1979;87-88(25 no 1-2):157-79
**Czeizel A:** Life and death [of] Tutankhamun from human genetic aspects. **Ther Hung** 1980;28(1):40-3
**Czeizel A:** Ludwig van Beethoven. **Ther Hung** 1982;30(1):43-7
**Czeizel E:** A genetika fejlödésének belsö ellentmondása. **Orv Hetil** 1982 Feb 7;123(6):349-57
**Czeizel E:** Tage Kemp, a nagy dán orvos-genetikus, az elsö gentikai tanácsadó megalapítója. **Orv Hetil** 1980 Jun 15;121(24):1460-2
**Czeley-Wybieralska M:** Early medical books in the Jesuits' Library, Małopolska Province, Cracow. **Arch Hist Med (Warsz)** 1980;43:461-3
**Czeley-Wybieralska M:** Nieznana relacja obdukcyjna (visum repertum) z 1853 r. zachowana w aktach państwowego Archiwum w Lublinie. **Arch Hist Med (Warsz)** 1981;44(1):111-3
**Czeley-Wybieralska M:** Nobilitacje lekarzy i aptekarzy w Królestwie Polskim w latach 1817-1861. **Arch Hist Med (Warsz)** 1983;46(2):205-4
**Czeley-Wybieralska M:** O ogłoszeniach lekarskich w Polsce. **Arch Hist Med (Warsz)** 1983;46(3):315-23
**Czeley-Wybieralska M:** Starodruki medyczne w ksiegozbiorze OO. Bonifratrów w Krakowie. **Arch Hist Med (Warsz)** 1982;45(1-4):85-92
**Czeley-Wybieralska M** see **Kaminska-Axer M**
**Czigány LG:** The use of hallucinogens and the shamanistic tradition of the Finno-Ugrian people. **Slav East Eur Rev** 1980;58(2):212-7
**Czygan FC:** Atherische Ole und Duft kulturhistorisch betrachtet. **Pharm Unserer Zeit** 1981 Jul:10(4):109-21
**Czyrek G** see **Maciałek E**

# D

**D. D.'s first book: Chiropr Hist** 1874;4(1):6-10
**Da-Ding F** see **Chuan-Kui H**
**Al-Dabbagh F:** Aksel Mentah, nafsani Suwidi, wa-mu'allif qissat San Mishel. **Al-Arabi** 1973;179:60-3
**Dabrowski S:** Wspomnienia z okresu studiów na wydziale lekarskim uniwersytetu poznańskiego (1935-1945). **Arch Hist Med (Warsz)** 1983;46(1):67-90
**Dąbska M** see **Sieiński W**
**Dačev B** see **Georgieva K**
**Dacie J:** Evolution of ideas on the life-span of the red blood cell. **J R Soc Med** 1979 Jun;72(6):447-52
**Dacquino G:** Psicoanalisi e ipnosi nella dottrina e nella pratica clinica. **Minerva Med** 1982 Nov 24;73(45):3207-12
**Dae Woo Han** see **Rindfuss RR**
**Daem M:** Van baardemaker tot barbier (Gentse chirurgijn-barbiers). Brussel, Aurelia Books, 1976. 170 p. (Aureliae Folklorica, no. 9).
**Daems WF:** Die Apoteca ein 'Stall' und die 'Stall-Apotheke'. **Sudhoffs Arch** 1978;62(1):95-6
**Daems WF:** Ermengald Blasius' Tabellen zum 'Antidotarium Nicolai'. **Pharm Acta Helv** 1979;54(4):101-5
**Daems WF:** Heilpflanzenkunde in Vergangenheit, Gegenwart und Zukunft. **Drei Z Wiss Kunst Soz Leben** 1978;11:642-57
**Daems WF:** Himmel und Erde schaffen den Menschen. Zur Faksimile-Ausgabe eines astromedizinischen Hausbuches (Kodex Schurstab, Zürich, Zentralbibl. Ms. C. 54). **Drei Z Wiss Kunst Soz Leben** 1981;51:177-94
**Daems WF:** Radix Ratanhiae, die Droge mit einer gesicherten Geschichte. **Dtsch Apoth Ztg** 1981 Jan 8;121(2):46-52
**Daems WF:** Renward Cysat und Paracelsus. **Gesnerus** 1982;39(3-4):469-72
**Daems WF:** Stimmi, Stibium, Antimon: eine substanzhistorische Betrachtung. Arlesheim (Schweiz), Weleda, 1976. 35 p.
**Daems WF:** Synonymenvielfalt und Deutungstechnik bei den nomina plantarum medievalia. In Dilg P, et al., ed: Perspektiven der Pharmaziegeschichte. Graz, Austria, Akademische Druck- u. Verlagsanstalt, 1983. p. 29-37.
**Daems WF, Keil G:** Zum Ansehen des Apothekers im spätmittelalterlichen Deutschland. **Sudhoffs Arch** 1980;64(1):86-9
**Daeschner CW:** Education for primary care of children. A report to Abraham and Mary Jacobi. **Am J Dis Child** 1983 Jun;137(6):566-71
**Dagen G** see **David T**
**Dagg AI** see **Leach DH**
**Daglio P:** L'epistemologia medica: nuova filosofia della medicina. **Minerva Med** 1982 Dec 8;73(47):3359-67
**Daglio P:** San Benedetto da Norcia patrono d'Europa, nella medicina e nella storia. **Minerva Med** 1982 Sep 8;73(34):2193-8
**Daglio P:** Vincenzo Tiberio e la scoperta della penicillina. Una grande conquista a cavallo di due secoli. **Minerva Med** 1982 Jul 14;73(28-29):2005-9
**Dagosto M** see **Szalay FS**
**Dagsland H, Lysnes M:** Sykepleiens historie--forskning og objektivitet. **Sykepleien** 1983 Mar 7;70(5):17-9
**Dagurov VG:** Razvitie farmakologii v Moskovskom universitete vo vtoroĭ polovine XIX veka. **Farmakol Toksikol** 1983 Jan-Feb;46(1):92-8
**Dagurov VG, Miazdrikova AA:** Stanovlenie farmakologii v Moskovskom universitete. **Farmakol Toksikol** 1981 Nov-Dec;;44(6):733-7

**Dahl T** see **Forsdahl A**

**Dahlberg AA** see **Morse D**

**Dahlerup T:** Den sociale forsorg og reformationen i Danmark. **Historie** 1979;13(1-2):194-207

**Dahlin DC:** James Watson Kernohan: 1896-1981. **Surg Neurol** 1984 Feb;21(2):107-9

**Dahlin M:** Perspectives on the family life of the elderly in 1900. **Gerontologist** 1980 Feb;20(1):99-107

**Dahlström G:** Johannes Raicus' tankar om lungsoten. **Nord Medicinhist Arsb** 1984;:63-70

**Dahlström G:** Medicinsk utveckling och grundforskning i historiskt perspektiv. **Nord Medicinhist Arsbok** 1983;:117-25

**Dahm I, Schorr R, Niehoff JU:** Zum 50. Todestag von Alfred Grotjahn. **Z Arztl Fortbild (Jena)** 1981 Sep 15;75(16):878-81

**Dahm S:** Fruhe Krankenbildnisse: Alibert Esquirol Baumgartner. Köln, 1981. (Kölner medizinhistorische Beiträge; Arbeiten der Forschungsstelle des Instituts für Geschichte der Medizin der Universität zu Köln, Band 21).

**Dahmer H, Rosenkötter L:** Jasager und Weisswäscher. **Psyche (Stuttg)** 1983 Dec;37(12):1146-53

**Dahmer H:** Kapitulation vor der 'Weltanschauung'. Zu einem Aufsatz von Carl Müller-Braunschweig aus dem Herbst 1933. **Psyche (Stuttg)** 1983 Dec;37(12):1116-35

**Dahmer H:** 'Psychoanalyse unter Hitler'--Rückblick auf eine Kontroverse. **Psyche (Stuttg)** 1984 Oct;38(10):927-42

**Dailey RD** see **Morse D**

**Dain N:** Clifford W. Beers: advocate for the insane. Pittsburgh, Univ. of Pittsburgh Press, 1980. xxix, 392 p.

**Dainton C:** Bart's Hospital, from its refoundation by Henry VIII. **Hist Today** 1978;28(12):810-6

**Dainton C:** Mustard, vinegar, and hog's grease: a short history of St. Thomas's Hospital. **Br Hist Illus** 1979;6(3):16-26

**Dainton C:** The age of specialisation. **Br Herit** 1981;2(2):56-65

**Dainton C:** The years of reform. **Br Herit** 1981-82;3(1):22-31

**Dake WJ:** Het medische werk van de zending in Nederlands-Indië. Kampen, Kok, 1972. 235 p.

**Dakpa N:** La folie d'après un commentaire du Rgyud-bži, les quatre tantra. **Sci Orient** 1979;16:31-9

**Dakpa N:** La Sphygnologie tibétaine. In Mazars G, ed: Les médecines traditionnelles de l'Asie. Strasbourg, Université Louis Pasteur, 1981. p. 23-9.

**Dal' MK:** Zdorov'e N. I. Pirogova v razlichnom vozraste i ego posledniaia. bolezn'. **Klin Khir** 1981 Mar;(3):59-60

**Dalat J:** Un chirurgien de mer à la fin du XVIIIe siècle. **Rev Hist Pharm (Paris)** 1983 Dec;71(30):275-81

**Dalcq A:** Pol Gérard, 1886-1961. In Florilège des Sciences en Belgique - II. Bruxelles, Académie Royale de Belgique, 1980. p. 609-16.

**Dale DC** see **Gray L**

**Dale JG:** Orthodontics: past, present and future? **Can Dent Assoc J** 1982 Mar;48(3):180-2

**Dalessio DJ:** Trigeminal neuralgia, Cushing. **JAMA** 1983 Jul 22-29;250(4):529-31

**Daley EA:** The Royal Flying Doctor Service of Australia. **Victorian Hist Mag** 1970;41(3-4):375-95

**Dalhoff A:** Fünfzig Jahre Penicilline. Eine Ubersicht über Struktur-Wirkungsbeziehungen der Beta-Laktamantibiotika und ihre mikrobiologische sowie klinische Relevanz. **Infection** 1979;7(6):294-302

**Dalitz RH, Stone GC:** Doctor Bernard Connor: physician to King Jan III Sobieski and author of the History of Poland (1698). **Oxf Slav Pap** 1981;14:14-35

**d'Allaines C:** Alexis Carrel (1873-1944), visionnaire de la chirurgie cardio-vasculaire. **Arch Mal Coeur** 1984 Sep;77(9):1074-7

**Dallett JB:** Paracelsus in Moronia. Bischof Joseph Halls satirische Darstellung von 'Bustius Hohenheimius' und dessen Collegium. Wien, 1976. 20 p. (Salzburger Beiträge zur Paracelsusforschung, 14).

**Dallett JB:** Woldemar Nürnbergers Paracelsus-Roman. **Salzburger Beitr Paracelsusforsch** 1984;23:50-60

**Dalsimer K:** Female adolescent development. A study of the Diary of Anne Frank. **Psychoanal Study Child** 1982;37:487-522

**Daly LW:** Miltiades. Aratus and compound fractures. **Am J Philol** 1980;101:59-60

**Daly RJ:** Samuel Pepys and post-traumatic stress disorder. **Br J Psychiatry** 1983 Jul;143:64-8

**Daly WJ:** A personal testament--reflections on the Tower of Babel. **J Lab Clin Med** 1982 Jan;99(1):10-4

**Damadian R:** In memoriam--Freeman Widener Cope--1930-1982. **Physiol Chem Phys** 1982;14(5):411-4

**D'Amato NA:** Nathaniel Chapman: first president of the American Medical Association. **Va Med** 1984 Nov;111(11):708-10

**D'Amato NA:** William Edmonds Horner: anatomist, educator, author. **Va Med** 1982 Mar;109(3):209-10

**Dammann G:** Pictorial encyclopedia of Civil War medical instruments and equipment. Missoula, Mont., Pictorial Histories Pub. Co., 1983. iv, 100 p.

**Dammann GE:** Dental care during the Civil War. **Ill Dent J** 1984 Jan-Feb;53(1):12-7

**Dammin GJ:** Transplantation, 1950s. **Transplant Proc** 1981 Mar;13(1):16-23

**Damodar Joshi:** Mercury in Indian medicine. **Stud Hist Med** 1979 Dec;3(4):234-97

**D'Amore AR:** Ernest Jones: founder of the American Psychoanalytic Association. **Int J Psychoanal** 1979;60(Pt 3)287-90

**D'Amore AR:** Psychoanalysis in America: 1930-1939. **Psychoanal Q** 1981;50(4):570-86

**D'Amore AR** see **Burnham JC**

**D'Amore C, Radice A, Schiano Di Zenise M:** Studio radiologico del cranio 1 della necropoli di Madonna delle Grazie a Mirabella Eclano (Avellino). **Radiol Med (Torino)** 1981 Jul-Aug;67(7-8):503-8

**Damsteegt BC** see **Palm LC**

**Damsteegt PG:** Health reform and the Bible in early Sabbatarian Adventism. **Advent Herit** 1978;5(2):13-21

**Danchin A:** Une révolution lamarckienne en immunologie. **Recherche** 1981;12(118):84-5

**Danckaert L, De Smet A, ed:** Notes bibliographiques [on the history of science in Belgium], 89. [Brussels], Comité belge d'histoire des sciences, 1979. 24 p.

**Danda J:** K devadesátým narozeninám prof. MUDr. K. Hübschmanna, DrSc. **Cesk Dermatol** 1980 Oct;55(5):289-94

**Daněk K:** Bernard Bolzano v historii medicíny. **Cas Lek Cesk** 1981 Sep 24;120(38)1160-3

**Daněk K:** Incitabilita, stenie a astenie. K 200. výročí Brownových Základu medicíny. **Cas Lek Cesk** 1980 Jul 11;119(27-28):774-6

**Daněk K:** Lyžování v dějinách lékařství. K 90. vtoči začátku lyžování na Vysŏ cinĕ. **Cas Lek Cesk** 1982 Apr 9;121(14):437-40

**Daněk K:** Pul tisíciletí 'čarodějnické' buly. Pokus o přehled lékařsko-historických aspektu 'čarodějnické' pověry. **Cas Lek Cesk** 1984 Nov 23;123(47):1444-9

**Daněk K:** Skiing in and through the history of medicine. **Nord Medicinhist Arsb** 1982;:86-100

**Daněk K:** Sto let zdravotnických obvodu na Moravě. Z historie československých priorit ve zdravotnictví. **Cas Lek Cesk** 1984 Feb 3;123(5):133-6

**Daněk K:** The many facets of nostalgia in the history of medicine. **Nord Medicinhist Arsb** 1984;:71-81

**Danforth DM** see **Miller MK**

**Daniel TM:** Robert Koch, tuberculosis, and the subsequent history of medicine. **Am Rev Respir Dis** 1982 Mar;125(3 Pt 2):1-3

**Danielson L, Mann E:** The first American account of cerebrospinal meningitis. **Rev Infect Dis** 1983 Sep-Oct;5(5):969-72

**Danilevskiĭ NF, Sakharchuk IM:** Druzhba narodov SSSR--reshaiushchiĭ faktor vosstanovleniia stomatologicheskikh kadrov na Ukraine. **Stomatologiia (Mosk)** 1982;(6):7-10

**Danilevskiĭ VM, Luk'ianovskiĭ VA, Migalatiuk DIa, et al:** Shest'desiat trudovykh vakht. **Veterinariia** 1979 Dec;(12):9-14

**Danilichev VF** see **Volkov VV**

**Danilischina EI, Schneck P:** D. O. Ott (1855-1929) und die russisch-deutschen medizinischen Beziehungen. **Z Arztl Fortbild (Jena)** 1981 Oct 1;75(19):924-7

**Danilishina EI:** Ernst Bumm (k 125-letiiu so dnia rozhdeniia). **Akush Ginekol (Mosk)** 1984 Jan;(1):69-70

**Danilishina EI, Dzhalalova KM:** Materinskaia smertnost' i boriba s neĭ v SSSR v 20-30-e gody. **Sov Zdravookhr** 1983;(8):51-4

**Danilishina EI:** Razvitie okhrany materinstva i detstva v SSSR. **Sov Zdravookhr** 1983;(1):61-4

**Danilishina EI:** Rol' Narkomzdrava RSFSR v stanovlenii okhrany zdorov'ia materi i rebenka. **Sov Zdravookhr** 1983;(7):59-63

**Danilishina EI** see **Vengrova IV**

**Daniuk GI** see **Palkin BN**

**Daniushevskiĭ SM:** Leninskaia zabota o detiakh. **Sov Zdravookhr** 1980;(4):10-4

**Dann G, Higby G:** Bibliography of the publications of George Urdang on his birth centenary. **Pharm Hist** 1982;24(3):106-14

**Dannenbaum J:** The crusade against drink. **Rev Am Hist** 1981;9(4):497-502

**Dannenfeldt KH:** Ambergris: the search for its origin. **Isis** 1982 Sep;73(268):382-97

**Dannheim E:** Orthoptische Uebungsbehandlung des Binokularsehens. Ein geschichtlicher Ueberblick. **Klin Monatsbl Augenheilkd** 1981 Mar;178(3):212-5

**Danon J:** Enseñanza de la historia de la medicina en España durante el siglo XIX. In: International Congress of the History of Medicine, 26th, Plovdiv (Bulgaria), 1978. Actes du Congres, Vol. 1. Sofia, 1980. p. 97-100.

**Danón J:** Un brote de fiebre amarilla en el puerto de Barcelona, en 1803. In: Sociedad Española de Historia de la Medicina. V Congreso Nacional. Madrid, 1977. **Asclepio** 1977;29:119-25

**Danon y Bretos J:** Visió històrica de l'Hospital General de Santa Creu de Barcelona. Barcelona, Fundació Salvador Vives Casajuana, 1978. 207 p.

**D'Antonio WV, Stack S:** Religion, ideal family size, and abortion: extending Renzi's hypothesis. **J Sci Stud Relig** 1980;19(4):397-408

**Dányi D:** AZ 1964-1976. Evi termékenység elemzése kísírlet II. **Demografia** 1978;21(4):452-66

**Danzig L** see **Cone RO**

**Danziger K** see **Rieber RW, ed**

**Danzin A:** Data, evolution and entropy. **Methods Inf Med** 1980 Jan;19(1):2-6

**Danzinger K:** The history of introspection reconsidered. **J Hist Behav Sci** 1980 Jul;16(3):241-62

**Danzinger R, Lyon G:** Das Beratungszentrum für psychische und sociale Fragen in Graz. Wien, Osterreichische Akademie der Wissenschaften, 1982. 140 p.

**Dar-mo Sman-ram Blo-bzan-chos-grags:** Dar Mo Bka' Brgya Ma. Man nag zab mo kun gyi snin khu bsdus pa dar-mo sman-rams-pa'i gdams

nag bka rgya ma. A collection of profound instructions on the methods and rituals of Tibetan healing transmitted by the physician of the 5th Dalia Lama. Reproduced from a print from the Sde-Dge blocks, 2 vols; and from the Ska-' Bum blocks, 2 vols. Leh, Ladakh, T. S Tashigangpa, 1978. n.p. (Smanrtsis Shesrig Spendzog, Vols. 88-91).
**D'Arbon P:** Rehabilitation yesterday and today. **Lamp** 1980 Dec;37(12):16-8
**Darbon P** see **Camerino G**
**Darby WJ:** A perspective on food legislation. **Nutr Rev** 1981 Nov;39(11):413-6
**Darby WJ:** Folic acid and macrocytic anemias. **South Med J** 1983 Nov;76(11):1341-3
**Darby WJ:** The Nutrition Foundation: 1942-1982. **Nutr Rev** 1982 Nov;40(11):348-52
**Darby WJ** see **Totter JR**
**D'Arcy E:** [History of the theory of] natural law [in bioethics]. In Reich WT, et al, ed: Encyclopedia of bioethics, v.3. New York, Free Press, 1978. p. 1131-7.
**Darga LL, Klauenberg S, Davis KF:** The cultural model of the menstrual cycle. **Mich Acad** 1981;13(4):475-84
**Dargan A** see **Jenner CL, ed**
**Darius J:** Radiography of the living brain. **Nature** 1984 Mar 15-21;308(5956):225
**Darling AI** see **Levers BG**
**Darling VH** see **Allan P**
**Darlington C** see **Beloff M**
**Darlington CD** see **Mayr E**
**Darmon P:** Le mythe de la procréation a l'âge baroque. [Paris], Pauvert, 1977. 283 p.
**Darmon P:** Les vols de cadavres et la science (XVIIe-XIXe siècles). **Histoire** 1982;48:30-7
**Darnés C, Solé A:** Influencia de las comunidades religiosas en la enfermería de Cataluña. **Rev Enferm** 1981 Dec-1982 Jan;5(42-43):61-2
**Darquenne R:** Controverses sur la nocivité du charbon de terre (18e-19e siècles). **Ann Soc Belg Hist Hop** 1981;:33-45
**Darquenne R:** Médecine et chirurgie hainuyères au siècle des lumières. **Ann Cerc Archeol Mons** 1976-77;70:139-76
**Darquenne R:** Remous autour de la Pharmacopée Montoise (1755). **Mem Publ Soc Sci Arts Lett Hainaut** 1981-82;92:169-201
**Darracq PJ:** Les chirurgiens à Bordeaux au XVIIIe siècle. **Hist Sci Med** 1981;15(4):299-303
**Darsel J:** L'assistance sociale dans la marine sous l'Ancien Régime en la Province de Bretagne. In: Congrès National des Sociétés Savantes, 97e, Nantes, 1972. Comptes Rendus. Paris, 1976. Section des Sciences, Tome 1. p. 293-309.
**Darwin C** see **McKinney HL, ed**
**Darwin CR:** The descent of man, and selection in relation to sex. 2 vols in 1. Reprint of 1871 ed, with historical introduction by J. T. Bonner and R. M. May. Princeton, Princeton University Press, 1981. xli, 475, x, p.
**Das S:** Shusruta of India: pioneer in vesicolithotomy. **Urology** 1984 Mar;23(3):317-9
**Das S:** Shusruta of India, the pioneer in the treatment of urethral stricture. **Surg Gynecol Obstet** 1983 Dec;157(6):581-2
**Das S:** Zur Stellung der Naturheilverfahren in der Allgemeinmedizin. **ZFA (Stuttgart)** 1983 Apr 10;59(10):575-84
**Dash B, ed** see **Sharma RK**
**da Silva LJ:** Sobre a antigüidade de alguns focos de esquistossomose do Estado de São Paulo. **Rev Bras Malariol Doencas Trop** 1983;35:73-8
**Daston LJ** see **Park K**
**Dastugue J:** Die Paläopathologie. In Sournia JC, Martiny M, Poulet J, ed: Illustrierte Geschichte der Medizin. Salzburg, Andreas, 1980. Vol. 1. p. 19-47.
**Dastugue J:** Les maladies de nos ancêtres. **Recherche** 1982;(136):980-8
**Date K:** ['Eisei-Shinpen'--Ogai Mori as a physician (II)] (Jpn). **Igakushi Kenkyu** 1978;51:26-41
**Datta B, Gupta D:** The age of menarche in classical India. **Ann Hum Biol** 1981 Jul;8(4):351-9
**Datta C** see **Sharma RK**
**Dätwyler B, Schmidhofer M, L'adrach U:** Unterricht in 'Geschichte der Krankenpflege' oder Hilfe zur Selbsthilfe. **Krankenpflege (Bern)** 1983 May;(5):62
**Daubenton F:** Professor Cuthbert Crichton--the man and his times. **S Afr Med J** 1979 Dec 15;56(25):1064-75
**Dauber LG:** Compound X given intravenously. On the history of the nitrogen mustards. **NY State J Med** 1984 Mar;84(3 pt 1):122-4
**Dauber LG:** Dickens and doctors; physicians in fiction of Charles Dickens. **NY State J Med** 1981 Sep;81(10):1522-6
**Dauber LG:** Peter Blood and the Brethren of the Coast. Fictional physicians afield. **NY State J Med** 1982 Jun;82(7):1107-9
**D'Aubigné RM:** Notre orthopédie, hier...et demain. **Rev Chir Orthop** 1980;66 Suppl 2:13-20
**D'Aubigné RM:** Paul Broca et la chirurgie de l'appareil moteur. **Chirurgie** 1980;106(10):791-3
**Daudistel HC** see **Hedderson J**
**Daumard A:** Les généalogies sociales: un des fondements de l'histoire sociale comparative et quantitative. **Ann Demogr Hist (Paris)** 1984;:9-24
**Daumas F:** Réflexion sur la médecine égyptienne. **Bull Liaison Assoc Amis Mus Pharm Montp** 1978 Dec 10;:23-40
**Dausset J:** The birth of MAC. **Vox Sang** 1984;46(4):235-7
**Dausset J:** The challenge of the early days of human histocompatibility. **Immunogenetics** 1980;10(1):1-5
**Dauven J:** La genèse de la psychanalyse (Freud, Wagner, et la Walkyrie Materna). Paris, Nouvelles Editions latines, 1979. 163 p.
**Davanzo J, Haaga J:** Anatomy of a fertility decline: Peninsular Malaysia, 1950-1976. **Popul Stud** 1982 Nov;36(3):373-93
**Davenport HW:** Carbonic anhydrase, or, the strange case of the disappearing scientist. **Physiologist** 1980 Apr;23(2):11-5
**Davenport HW:** Physiology, 1850-1923. The view from Michigan. **Physiologist** 1982 Feb;24(1 Suppl):1-96
**Davenport HW:** Signs of anxiety, rage, or distress. **Physiologist** 1981 Oct-Nov;24(5):1-5
**Davenport HW:** The early days of research on carbonic anhydrase. **Ann NY Acad Sci** 1984;429:4-9
**Davey H:** The law relating to the mentally defective. The Mental Deficiency Act, 1913. 2nd ed. Reprint of 1914 ed., with a new introduction by C. Bahn. New York, Da Capo, 1981. x, xxvii, 568 p.
**Davic P, Popov K, Popov-Dragin O:** Prve babice i razvoj akušerske službe u Somboru u XVIII veku. **Med Pregl** 1982;35(1-2):59-67
**Davico R:** La morte barocca: popolazione, quartieri e campagne Messina nella rivolta del 1674-1678. La rivolta di Messina e il mondo Mediterraneo nella seconda metà del seicento, Cosenza, Pelligrini, 1979, p. 359-394.
**David A:** A medical sermon of R. Gedalya ibn Yahya. **Koroth** 1982;8(3-4):187-9
**David M:** A case of scleroderma mentioned by Hippocrates in his aphorisms. **Koroth** 1981;8(1-2):61-3
**David M:** Critical edition of Hippocrates' Aphorisms translated into Hebrew by J.S. Delmedigo (1591-1655), sections IV, V. **Koroth** 1979 Nov;7(9-10):680-709
**David M:** Critical edition of Hippocrates' Aphorisms, translated into Hebrew by J. S. Delmedigo (1591-1655), sections VI-VIII (cont. and end). **Koroth** 1980 Jun;7(11-12):764-94
**David M** see **Wertheimer P**
**David SI:** To lift a heavy burden: the story of the Medicare and Medicaid law. Ph.D. Diss., City University of New York. New York, 1982. viii, 312 p.
**David T, Dagen G, Gauval VB:** Les dents de Louis XIV. **Soc Fr Hist Art Dent** 1979 Sep-Dec;(5-6):6-10
**David-Danel ML:** Un ex-libris non professionnel à l'effigie de saint Côme. **Rev Hist Pharm (Paris)** 1982;29(252):171-2
**David, Goliath, et al.:** **N Engl J Med** 1984 Mar 22;310(12):790
**David GR, ed:** The manuscript papers of British scientists, 1600-1940. London, H.M.S.O., 1982. 109 p.
**David-Peyre Y:** Manuel Alvares, ou la synthèse de la littérature médicale sur la préservation contre la peste. **Bull Etud Port Bres** 1965;26:67-87
**David Shakow, Ph.D., 1901-1981:** In Memoriam. **Schizophr Bull** 1981;7(3):383-7
**Davidenko OS** see **Siniak KM**
**Davidenkova EF:** Zanchenie nauchnogo naslediia S. N. Davidenkova v razvitii klinicheskoĭ genetiki (k 100-letiiu so dnai rozhdeniia). **Klin Med (Mosk)** 1981;59(4):112-6
**Davidiuk VG** see **Verenkina TN**
**Davidson AT:** The role of the historic black colleges in the training of black professionals. **J Natl Med Assoc** 1983 Oct;75(10):1019-22
**Davidson JR, Ortiz de Montellano BR:** The antibacterial properties of an Aztec wound remedy. **J Ethnopharmacol** 1983 Aug;8(2):149-61
**Davidson M:** Ancient references to dentistry and 'Biblical bites'. **Bull Hist Dent** 1983 Apr;31(1):30-1
**Davidson N:** Cottage hospital. Just like home. (Meynell Ingram Cottage Hospital, Yoxall, Staffs). **Health Soc Serv J** 1981 Aug 21;:1018-9
**Davidson WD, Montville JV:** Foreign policy according to Freud. **Foreign Policy** 1981-82;45:145-57
**Davidson WS:** Havens of refuge. Nedlands, Univ. of Western Australia Press, 1978. xii, 188 p.
**Davies B:** The first patient to receive lithium. **Aust NZ J Psychiatry** 1983 Dec;17(4):366-8
**Davies C:** Making sense of the census in Britain and the U.S.A.: the changing occupational classification and the position of nurses. **Sociol Rev** 1980;28(3):581-610
**Davies C:** Past and present in nursing education. **Nurs Times** 1980 Sep 25;76(39):1703-7
**Davies C:** Where next for nursing history? **Nurs Times** 1980 May 22;76(21):920-2
**Davies GC:** The Welsh doctor as a poet: Henry Vaughan-Silurist. In J. Cule, ed: Wales and medicine. London, British Society for the History of Medicine, 1975. p. 112-18.
**Davies GH** see **Davies NE**
**Davies GR:** The invasion of Normandy--D-day. **NATNEWS** 1984 Sep;21(9):24-6
**Davies HE, Owen ME:** Meddygon Myddfai. In J. Cule, ed: Wales and medicine. London, British Society for the History of Medicine, 1975. p. 156-68.
**Davies J:** Cambridge Museum of Technology. **Ind Archaeol** 1980;15(4):335-55
**Davies J:** David Lloyd George and the National Insurance Act of 1911. In J. Cule, ed: Wales and medicine. London, British Society for the History of Medicine, 1975. p. 1-9.
**Davies JB:** Onchocerciasis vector control--50 years ago. **Trans R Soc Trop Med Hyg** 1983;77(1):139-40
**Davies JN:** Pestilence and disease in the history of Africa. Johannesburg, Witwatersrand University Press, for The Institute for the Study of Man in Africa, 1979. 20 p.

historisch overzicht. **Rev Belge Med Dent** 1981;36(3):101–2

**De Bondt J:** Historische overzicht van de dienst stomatologie en tandheelkunde aan de Katholieke Universiteit te Leuven. **Rev Belge Med Dent** 1981;36(3):111–4

**Debras C** see **Kunegel JM**

**Debré M:** Robert Debré, réformateur. **Bull Acad Natl Med (Paris)** 1982 Dec;166(9):1295–303

**De Bruijn J:** Geschiedenis van de abortus in Nederland. Een analyse van opvattingen en discussies, 1600–1979. Amsterdam, Van Gennep, 1979. 330 p.

**Debus AG:** History with a purpose: the fate of Paracelsus. **Pharm Hist** 1984;26(2):83–96

**Debus AG:** Scientific truth and occult tradition: the medical world of Ebenezer Sibly (1751–1799). **Med Hist** 1982 Jul;26(3):259–77

**Debus AG:** The Arabic tradition in the medical chemistry of the scientific revolution. In: International Symposium for the History of Arabic Science, 1st, University of Aleppo, 1976. Proceedings. Aleppo, Syria, 1976. Papers in European Languages, Vol. II. p. 275–90.

**Debus AG:** The chemical philosophy. Paracelsian science and medicine in the sixteenth and seventeenth centuries. 2 vols. New York, Science History Publications, 1977. xv, 606 p.

**Debus AG:** The Paracelsians in eighteenth century France: a Renaissance tradition in the age of the Enlightenment. **Ambix** 1981 Mar;28(1):36–54

**Debus AG:** Thomas Sherley's philosophical essay (1672): Helmontian mechanism as the basis of a new philosophy. **Ambix** 1980 Jul;27(2):124–35

**Debus AG:** Walter Pagel (1898–1983). **Bull Hist Med** 1983 Winter;57(4):611–5

**A decade of health development in South-East Asia, 1968–1977:** New Delhi, NHO Regional Office for South-East Asia, 1978. xx, 418 p.

**A decade of open heart surgery at the University Hospital of the West Indies, Kingston, Jamaica, 1968–1978: West Indian Med J** 1980 Dec;29 Suppl:299–345

**De Carneri I:** Un secolo di ricerche di parassitologia umana in Italia: riflessioni e prospettive. **Parassitologia** 1981 Dec;23(1–3):1–30

**Decaux A:** Napoléon III et la chirurgie. **Chirurgie** 1984;110(1):23–8

**Dechaume M, Huard P:** Paul Broca (1824–1880). Stomatologiste ou la stomatologie du siècle dernier. **Actual Odontostomatol (Paris)** 1980;(132):537–43

**Dechêne L, Robert JC:** Le choléra de 1832 dans le Bas-Canada: mesure des inegalités devant la mort. In Charbonneau H, Larose A, ed: The great mortalities: methodological studies of demographic crises in the pase. Liège, Belgium, Ordina Editions, 1980. p. 229–56.

**Decker DL:** Sociological theory and the social position of the aged. **Int J Contemp Sociol** 1978;15(3–4):303–17

**Decker H** see **Wallace ER**

**Decker HS:** Freud and Dora: constraints on medical progress. **J Soc Hist** 1981;14(3):445–64

**Decker HS:** Psychoanalysis and the Europeans. In J. M. Quen, E. T. Carlson, ed: American psychoanalysis: origins and development. The Adolf Meyer seminars. New York, Brunner/Mazel, 1978. p. 1–19.

**Decker HS:** The choice of a name: 'Dora' and Freud's relationship with Breuer. **J Am Psychoanal Assoc** 1982;30(1):113–36

**Decker HS:** The historical evolution of dementia praecox. In Fann, et al, ed: Phenomenology and treatment of schizophrenia. New York, Spectrum, 1978. p. 301–309.

**Decker HS:** The reception of psychoanalysis in Germany. **Comp Stud Soc Hist** 1982 Oct;24(4):589–602

**Decker-Hauff HM** see **Paracelsus in der Tradition**

**Declaración sobre el aborto provocado:** Sagrada Congregación para la Doctrina de la Fe **Rev Med Univ Navarra** 1982 Dec;26(4):255–60

**Decourt J:** Aragon, tendre et fidèle. **Sem Hop Paris** 1983 May 12;59(19):1489–92

**Decourt P:** Les zymases ou ferments solubles de Béchamp à la lumière des connaissances du XXe siècle. **Hist Sci Med** 1984;18(2):147–51

**Decourt P:** L'oeuvre de James Reilly. **Hist Sci Med** 1983;17(1):29–35

**Decourt P** see **Nonclercq M**

**Dedek J** see **Ozorovský V**

**Dedek J** see **Tichý M**

**Dedet JP** see **Desjeux P**

**Dedieu H:** Notes sur les pertes humaines subies par les communautés religieuses de Séville durant l'epidémie de 1649. **Arch Franciscanum Hist** 1978;71(3–4):462–68

**Dedov II** see **Shlykov IP**

**De Duve C, Beaufay H:** A short history of tissue fractionation. **J Cell Biol** 1981 Dec;91(3 pt 2):293s–99s

**De Duve C:** Le développement de centrifugeuses à haute vitesse et leurs applications au fractionnement cellulaire. Un demi-siècle de collaboration entre la Belgique et l'Institut Rockefeller. **Bull Cl Sci Acad R Belg** 1980;5(66):470–2

**Deeley TJ:** A brief history of cancer. **Clin Radiol** 1983 Nov;34(6):597–608

**Deeley WS:** Greeks, Romans applied science to knowledge of the oral cavity. **Dent Stud** 1976 Jun;54(9):38–40

**Defalque RJ:** The first experiment in obstetrical anesthesia. **Anesth Analg (Cleve)** 1983 Dec;62(12):1136

**De Fréminville B:** La raison du plus fort. Paris, Editions du Seuil, 1977. 189 p.

**DeFriese GH, Woomert A:** The policy implications of self-care. **Soc Policy** 1982;13(2):55–8

**DeFronzo J:** Female labor force participation and fertility in 48 states: cross-sectional and change analyses for the 1960–1970 decade. **Sociol Soc Res** 1980;64(2):263–78

**Dega W:** Profesor dr Ireneusz Wierzejewski jako prekursor rehabilitacji. (Z okazji setnej rocznicy jego urodzin). **Chir Narzadow Ruchu Ortop Pol** 1981;46(6):599–602

**Dega W:** Zapiski do autobiografii moja droga zyciowa do wiedzy i zawodu. **Kwart Hist Nauki Tech** 1984;29(2):259–322

**Degen R:** The Kitab al-Aghdhiya of Hunayn ibn Ishaq. In: International Symposium for the History of Arabic Science, 1st, University of Aleppo, 1976. Proceedings. Aleppo, Syria, 1976. Papers in European Languages, Vol. II. p. 291–9.

**Degeorges M:** De l'auscultation médiate à l'auscultation intra-cardiaque. Les avatars de la découverte de Laennec. **Rev Palais Decouv** 1981;10(92):17–8

**Deghaye P** see **Braun L, et al**

**DeGiorgio M:** Primi sintomi di un carattere appassionato: dal collegio. **Mem Riv Stor Donne** 1981;(1):94–102

**Degler C:** Can a historian or social scientist learn anything from sociobiology? An attempt at an answer. **Hist Methods** 1981;14(4):173–9

**Degleris N:** Contribution à l'étude des relations Franco-Helleniques au point de vue de la presse neuro-psychiatrique française (1880–1914); les membres associés grecs de la Société Médico-Psychologique. Mémoire pour le titre d'assistant étranger, Université Paris V, René Descartes, Faculté de Médecine Cochin-Port Royal, Paris, 1984. 96 leaves.

**Degleris N, Rozos B:** L'Academie Ionienne, la première faculté de médecine dans les Balkans. Athènes, Université d'Athènes, Chaire de l'Histoire de la Médecine, 1979. 24 p.

**Degleris N:** [The 19th-century Greek medical journals index: sources of information--results] (Gre). Athens, Athens University Medical Faculty, 1980. 171 p.

**Degleris NE, Rozos BP:** [Public health, medical education and social care of Ionian Isles in the middle of the 19th century (press documents)] (Gre). **Arch Hyg** 1980;:90–101

**De Haen P:** New drug parade: a historical minireview, 1954–1982. Englewood, Colo., Paul de Haen International, 1983. 36 p.

**Dehillerin B, Goubert JP:** A la conquete du monopole pharmaceutique: le College de Pharmacie de Paris (1777–96). **Hist Reflect** 1982;9(1–2):233–48

**Dehillerin B:** Le Collège de Pharmacie de Paris: du régime des corporations au régime de germinal ou de l'étonnante vitalité du modèle parisien. Th. doct. 3e cycle. Paris, Univ. Paris I, 1981. 346 leaves.

**Dehillerin B:** Les maîtres apothicaires de Paris au XVIIIe siècle: le Collège de Pharmacie. Mém. de maîtrise. Paris, Univ. Paris I, 1976. 333 leaves.

**Deich I:** The redistribution of authority in national laboratories in Western Germany. **Minerva** 1979 Autumn;17(3):413–44

**Deichgräber K:** Der hippokratische Eid. Text griechisch und deutsch - Interpretation - Nachleben. 4., erweiterte Auflage. Stuttgart, Hippokrates Verlag, 1983. 92 p.

**Deichgraber K:** Die Patienten des Hippokrates. Historisch-prosopographische Beiträge zu den Epidemien des Corpus Hippocraticum. Mainz, Akademie der Wissenschaften und der Literatur, 1982. 41 p. (Abhandlungen der Geistes- und Sozialwissenschaftlichen Klasse, Jahrgang 1982. Nr. 9).

**Deikman AJ:** The observing self. Mysticism and psychotherapy. Boston, Beacon Press, 1982. xiii, 194 p.

**Deines H von, Grapow H, Westendorf W:** Grundriss der Medizin der alten Agypter, IX. Ergänzungen: Drogenquanten, Sachgruppen, Nachträge, Bibliographie, Generalregister. Berlin, Akademie Verlag, 1973. 241 p.

**De Jonckere P** see **Barbaix M**

**DeJong CJ:** Een verklaring door Anthony van Riebeeck als scheepschirurgijn in 1636. **Historia (S Afr)** 1973;18(4):231–3

**DeJong RN:** A history of American neurology. New York, Raven Press, 1982. 157 p.

**Dejour P** see **Bert P**

**Dejussieu J:** Note sur le jardin botanique de la Marine à Rochefort-sur-Mer. In: Congrès National des Sociétés Savantes, 91e, Rennes, 1966. Comptes Rendus. Paris, 1967. Section des Sciences, Tome 1. p. 129–33.

**De Keyzer W:** L'évolution de la léproserie Saint-Ladre de Mons aux XIIIe et XIVe siècles. Fédération des Cercles d'Archéologie et d'Histoire de Belgique. 44e session. Congrès de Huy, 1976. Annales. Tielt, 1978. p. 174–6.

**Dekhtsunian KM:** Nauchnaia deiatel'nost' Armianskogo ordena Trudovogo Krasnogo Znameni NII épidemiologii, virusologii i meditsinskoĭ parazitologii im. A. B. Aleksaniana (k 60-letiiu so dnia osnovaniia instituta). **Zh Mikrobiol Epidemiol Immunobiol** 1984 Feb;(2):114–7

**de Knecht-van Eekelen A:** Abraham Pieter Fokker (1840–1906) en de serumtherapie bij difterie. **Tijdschr Geschied Geneeskd Natuurwet Wiskd Tech** 1984;7(4):161–71

**Dekosky RK:** The history of science in a history department. **Hist Teacher** 1980;13(3):371–8

**De la Broquerie F:** Les débuts de la pédiatrie à Québec 1892 à 1929. **Union Med Can** 1983 Jul;112(7):656–63

**de la Fuente R** see **Somolinos-Palencia J**

**Delaby PA:** Appareillages de réanimation. **Hist Sci Med** 1980;14(2):153–4

**Delaby PA:** Le doyen Guillaume Valette (1902–1982). **Hist Sci Med** 1982;16(2):65–79

**Delaby PA:** Un groupe de brancardiers pendant la bataille de Verdun. **Hist Sci Med** 1980;14:293–303

**Delaby PA:** Une 'marmotte' de pâtes et pastilles selon le Codex de 1908. **Rev Hist Pharm (Paris)** 1983 Sep;30(258):191–8

**De Lacy PH:** Galen's concept of continuity. **Greek Roman Byz Stud (Cambridge, Mass.)** 1979;20:355–69

**Delage J:** Cinquante ans de pédopsychiatrie à Quebec. De l'Ecole La Jemmerais à la Chaire de Psychiatrie infantile et juvénile (Hôtel-Dieu du Sacré-Coeur). **Neuropsychiatr Enfance Adolesc** 1980 Jun;28(6):239–41
**Delahaye MC:** L'absinthe. Histoire de la fée verte. Paris, Berger-Levrault, 1983. 128 p.
**Delahousse J:** Gregory Bateson et les Alcooliques Anonymes. **Soins** 1984 Jan;(421–422):52–3
**Delaide J** see **Quinn S, ed**
**Delaney JJ:** Edward Jackson. **Colo Med** 1983 Apr;80(4):116–7
**Delaney JJ:** Hubert Work. **Colo Med** 1983 Oct;80(10):285–6
**Delaney JJ:** Leonard Freeman. **Colo Med** 1983 Aug;80(8):219–20
**Delaney JJ:** The doctors Amesse. **Colo Med** 1984 Mar;81(3):77–9
**Delannoy Y:** Une épidémie de choléra à Enghien (1849). **Ann Cerc Archeol Enghien** 1977;18:279–307
**Delaporte F:** Nature's second kingdom. Explorations of vegetality in the eighteenth century. Cambridge, London, MIT Press, 1982. xii, 266 p. (Originally published in France under the title Le second règne de la nature, 1979).
**Delaporte F:** Theories of osteogenesis in the eighteenth century. **J Hist Biol** 1983 Fall;16(3):343–60
**Delarue NC:** Lung cancer in historical perspective: lessons from the past, implications of present experience, challenges for the future. **Can J Surg** 1980 Nov;23(6):549–57
**Delatte L, Opsomer-Halleux C:** Ancient medical recipes and the computer: the Theorema project. **Pharm Hist** 1981;23(2):87–9
**Delatte L, Halleux R:** Recettes médicales anciennes et ordinateur: le projet Theorema. **Rev Hist Pharm (Paris)** 1980 Sep;27(246):155–160
**Delaunay A** see **Fasquelle R**
**Delaunay P:** Médecins de jadis et d'aujourd'hui; souvenirs des hôpitaux et de la Faculté de Paris de 1895 à 1905. **Hist Sci Med** 1981;15(4):307–20
**Delaunay A, ed:** Présence de Pasteur. Paris, Fayard, 1973. 225 p. Includes contributions by P. Bidan, A. Gamet, J. Guillaume, L. Léger, J. Piton, J. De Rosnay, R. Scriban, C. Vago.
**Delaveau P:** Histoire et renouveau des plantes médicinales. Paris, Albin Michel, 1982. 354 p.
**Delaveau P:** Le ginseng, drogue ancestrale d'Extrême Orient, devant la critique expérimentale. In Mazars G, ed: Les médecines traditionnelles de l'Asie. Strasbourg, Université Louis Pasteur, 1981. p. 75–84.
**Delaveau P:** Les fonds des pharmacopées traditionnelles et l'expérimentation. **Sci Orient** 1977;12:1–16
**Delaveau P:** Sur le 'registre pour l'inscription des poisons' d'un pharmacien tourangeau (1833–1841). **Rev Hist Pharm (Paris)** 1984 Jun;31(261):144–50
**Delaveau P, Paris RR, Clair G:** The Museum of Materia Medica of Paris. **Pharm Hist** 1984;26(3):143–5
**Delboy C** see **Bouvenot G**
**Delbrel R:** Asclépios et les secrets d'epidaure. **Atlantis** 1981 Jan–Feb;:173–247
**DelCastillo AR:** Sterilization: an overview. In Mora, Magdalena and DelCastillo, Adelaida R., ed. Mexican Women in the United States: Struggles past and present. Los Angeles, U. of California Chicano Studies Res. Center, 1980. p. 65–70.
**DelChicca S, Tedeschi J:** L'insonnia di Galileo in una lettera inedita di Francesco Redi. **Arch Stor Ital** 1979;173(4):615–8
**De Leo D, Arisi F, Magni G:** Difficoltà interpretative e problemi terapeuti nella neurastenia. Rassegna storica. **Minerva Psichiatr** 1982 Apr–Jun;23(2):75–81
**Delesie L** see **Blanpain J**
**Delgado B:** La revista de psicologia i pedagogia de Barcelona (1933–1937). **Perspect Pedagog (Barc)** 1982;12(49):47–70
**Delgado Escueta AV** see **Smith DB**
**Delgado García G:** Libros de texto cubanos sobre parasitología y enfermedades tropicales. Comentarios bibliográficos. Primera et segunda parte. **Rev Cubana Med Trop** 1982 Sep–Dec;34(3):327–41
**Delille G** see **Corsini CA**
**Delion P:** Aperçu historico-clinique sur la schizophrénie. Etat des différentes recherches à son sujet. **Soins Psychiatr** 1981 Dec;(14):3–5
**Delion P:** Freud, l'hystérique et la psychanalyse. **Soins Psychiatr** 1983 Jan;(27):7–10
**Dell RB** see **Winters RW**
**Della Peruta F:** Fonti a stampa relative alla storia della sanità in Lombardia, 1816–1859. **Soc Stor** 1978;:369–92
**Della Peruta F:** Infanzia e famiglia nella prima metà dell'ottocento. **Studi Stor** 1979;20(3):473–91
**Della Peruta F:** Sanità pubblica e legislazione sanitaria dall'unità a Crispi. **Studi Stor** 1980;21(4):713–59
**Dellamonica P** see **Le Fichoux Y**
**Dellamora R:** An essay in sexual liberation, Victorian style: Walter Pater's 'Two early French stories'. **J Homosex** 1983 Spring–Summer;8(3–4):139–50
**DellaPergola S:** Patterns of American Jewish fertility. **Demography** 1980 Aug;17(3):261–73
**Delmas A:** Geschichte der Anatomie. In Sournia JC, Martiny M, Poulet J, ed: Illustrierte Geschichte der Medizin. Salzburg, Andreas, 1980. Vol. 3. p. 871–929.
**Delmas A:** L'anatomiste devant les problèmes du langage. **Bull Assoc Anat (Nancy)** 1980;64:313–47
**Delmas A:** Paul Broca et l'anatomie. **Bull Acad Natl Med (Paris)** 1980;164(6):552–6
**Delmas A:** Paul Broca (1824–1880). Esquisse biographique. Le chirurgien et l'anatomiste. **Cah Anthropol** 1980;1–2:15–45
**Delmas J:** Le travail des enfants dans les manufactures de 1841 à 1914. **Bull Soc Fr Hist Hop** 1980;(41):17–25
**Del Nero CR:** De polícia médica à medicina social: uma análise genética. **AMB** 1980 Jul;26(7):255–6
**Delon M:** Le prétexte anatomique. **Dix-Huit Siecle** 1980;12:35–48
**Deloncle J:** Sobre la terapèutica a través dels sants a Catalunya Nord. In Congrés International de la Història de la Medicina Catalana, 2nd, Barcelona, 1975. Llibre d'Actes. Barcelona, Socitra, 1977. p. 129–32.
**Delooz F:** Petites touches sur le portrait de Saint-Etienne-aux-Clos: Antoine Trappe, médecin (1767–1847). **Lemouzi** 1981;80:411–30
**Delori FC** see **Nussbaum JJ**
**Del Panta L, Livi-Bacci M:** Chronology, intensity and diffusion of mortality in Italy, 1600–1850. In Charbonneau H, Larose A, ed: The great mortalities: methodological studies of demographic crises in the past. Liège, Belgium, Ordina Editions, 1980. p. 69–81.
**Delpech G** see **Bassis M**
**Delpech G** see **Bessis M**
**Del Prado S:** Einblick in eine Krankenpflegehilfe--Schule (Ausbildung). Der historische Weg zum Selbstverständnis in der Krankenpflegehilfe. **Krankenpflege (Frankfurt)** 1982 Jul–Aug;36(7–8):260–2
**Delprato DJ:** The reactional biography concept: early contribution to a perspective for the psychology of aging. **Hum Dev** 1980;23(5):314–22
**del Regato JA:** Isadore Lampe. **Int J Radiat Oncol Biol Phys** 1984 Feb;10(2):173–83
**Del Regato JA:** Jean Frederic Joliot. **Int J Radiat Oncol Biol Phys** 1980 May;6(5):621–40
**Del Regato JA:** The tracks of the Compton effect. **Med Phys** 1981 Nov–Dec;8(6):761–5
**Del Regato JA:** William Henry Bragg. **Int J Radiat Oncol Biol Phys** 1981 Jan;7(1):83–97
**del Regato JA** see **Franklin J**
**Delumeau J:** L'age d'or de la melancolie. **Histoire** 1982;42:28–37
**del Villar R:** La otología en el Hospital Infantil de México; evolución y enseñanza. **Bol Med Hosp Infant Mex** 1983 Aug;40 Suppl 2:22–7
**De Maar FE:** The toothpick carvers of Lorvao. **Bull Hist Dent** 1980 Apr;28(1):11–15
**Demain Al, Solomon NA:** Industrial microbiology. **Sci Am** 1981 Sep;245(3):67–75
**Demaitre L, Travill AA:** Human embryology and development in the works of Albertus Magnus. In Weisheipl JA, ed: Albertus Magnus and the sciences. Toronto, Pontifical Institute of Mediaeval Studies, 1980. p. 405–40.
**Demaitre LE:** Doctor Bernard de Gordon: professor and practitioner. Toronto, Pontifical Institute of Mediaeval Studies, 1980. xii, 236 p.
**Demal J:** Paul Debaisieux, 1886–1978. In Florilège des Sciences en Belgique - II. Bruxelles, Académie Royale de Belgique, 1980. p. 617–23.
**Demandt A:** Natur- und Geschichtswissenschaft im 19. Jahrhundert. **Ber Wissenschaftsgesch** 1983;6(1–4):59–78
**Démant F:** Vplyv Vel'kej októbrovej socialistickej revolúcie na starostlivost' o diet'a ZSSR. **Cesk Pediatr** 1979 Dec;34(12):697–8
**De Marco O, Nebbia G, Pizzoli Mazzacane EM:** Ibn Jazla et les connaissances de l'Islam médiéval en sciences naturelles. **Rev Hist Pharm (Paris)** 1979 Dec;26(243):249–58
**DeMark JL:** Chasing the cure--a history of healthseekers to Albuquerque, 1902–1940. **J West** 1982 Jul;21(3):49–58
**de Marneffe R:** Albin Lambotte, pionnier de l'ostéosynthèse moderne. **Rev Med Brux** 1982 Sep;3(7):493–5
**DeMause L:** Foundations of psychohistory. New York, Creative Roots, 1982. v, 336 p.
**deMause L:** The making of a fearful leader: 'Where's the rest of me?' **J Psychohist** 1984 Summer;12(1):5–21
**Dembińska M:** Dieetvoedsel en medicijnen voor kinderen in Polen van de 16de tot de 19de eeuw. **Spiegel Hist** 1981;16(11):623–6
**Dembińska M:** Pożywienie dziecka w polskich żródlach historycznych. **Kwart Hist Kultury Mater** 1980;28(4):481–99
**Dembińska M:** Z badań nad dziennymi racjami żywnościowymi rabotników przemysłowych w królestwie polskim w drugiej poł. XIX w. (próba interpretacji zródeł). **Kwart Hist Kultury Mater** 1979;27(2):145–56
**Demel M:** Wysoko jak król Zygmunt. Zycie i dzieło dra Stanisława Markiewicza. Warszawa, Państwowy Zakład Wydawn. Lekarskich, 1977. 102 p.
**Dement'ev IuG:** V. M. Velichkina (Bonch-Bruevich)--organizator sluzhby okhrany materinstva i detstva. **Pediatriia** 1979 Nov;(11):53–4
**Demerson P:** Le chirurgien Larrey et 'l'invasion française' à l'academie de médecine de Madrid. **Melanges Casa Velasquez** 1973;9:483–501
**De Messemaeker-De Wilde G:** De parochiale armenzorg te Gent in de late middeleeuwen. **Ann Soc Belg Hist Hop** 1980;18:47–58
**De Mey A** see **Moermans JP**
**De Meyts P, Rousseau GG:** Receptor concepts. A century of evolution. **Circ Res** 1980 Jun;46(6 Pt 2):13–9
**Demidov VP** see **Chissov Vi**
**Demidova NI:** Telefonicheskie issledovaniia v élektrofiziologii. **Zh Vyssh Nerv Deiat** 1982 Jul–Aug;32(4):783–5
**Demidova NI:** [The role of I. M. Sechenov's school in the development of electrophysiology] (Rus). **Istor Biol Issled** 1980;8:156–62
**Demin VN:** 50 let prepodavaniia onkologii v ordena Lenina Gosudarstvennom institute dlia usovershenstvovaniia vracheĭ im. S. M. Kirova. **Vopr Onkol** 1981;27(4):98–100
**Demin VT** see **Pozmogov AI**
**Demirhan A:** Ibn Sina's canon and some patterns. **Med Bull Istanbul Med Fac** 1979;12:158–62
**Demirhan A:** Pediatrics and history of medicine. In: Congrès international

d'histoire de la médecine, XXVe, Québec, 1976. Actes. Québec, 1977. p. 564–69.
**Demirhan A:** The development of education of pathology and anatomy in Ottoman Turks. **Stud Hist Med** 1981 Jun;5(2):160–6
**Demirhan A:** The theriacs in the history of medicine. **Med Bull Istanbul Med Fac** 1976;9:151–8
**De Mitcheli A:** Libros médicos italianos en la antigua Universidad de México. **Prensa Med Mex** 1979 Jul–Aug;44(7–8):152–6
**Demling L** see **Lux G**
**De mortuis nil nisi bonum: J Am Acad Dermatol** 1982 May;6(5):968–76
**Demos J:** Entertaining Satan. **Am Heritage** 1978;29(5):14–23
**Demos J:** Old age in early New England. In Demos, J, Boocock, SS, ed.: Turning points: historical and sociological essays on the family. Chicago, U. of Chicago Press, 1978. p. 248–87.
**Demos JP:** Entertaining Satan. Witchcraft and the culture of early New England. New York, Oxford, Oxford University Press, 1982. xiv, 543 p.
**Demoulin B:** Bossuet et la Mort. In Congrès National des Sociétés Savantes, 102e, Limoges, 1977. Actes. Paris, 1978. Tome I, p. 263–79.
**De Moulin D:** Gerrit Arie Lindeboom and the history of medicine in the Netherlands. **Janus** 1980;67(1–2–3):1–6
**De Moulin D:** Historical notes on breast cancer, with emphasis on the Netherlands. I. Pathological and therapeutic concepts in the seventeenth century. **Neth J Surg** 1980;32(4):129–34
**De Moulin D:** Medizinische und naturwissenschaftliche Aspekte der Regierungszeit des Grafen Johann Moritz von Nassau als Gouverneur in Brasilien (1637–1644). In: Soweit der Erdkreis reicht. J. M. von Nassau-Siegen 1604–1679. Kleve: Städtisches Museum Haus Koekkoek. 1979. pp. 33–46.
**De Moulin D:** On the early history of antisepsis. **Arch Chir Neerl** 1979;31(4):197–201
**de Moulin D:** The value of tobacco smoke in the treatment of intussusception. **Neth J Surg** 1984 Apr;36(2):57–9
**Dence CS:** Herbs and spices through the ages. 5. **Herbal Rev** 1979;4(2):4–9
**Deneke JF:** Das Gesundheitswesen der ersten Hälfte des 19.Jahrhunderts im Spiegel der Amts- und Intelligenzpresse. Düsseldorf, Triltsch, 1983. 161 p. (Düsseldorfer Arbeiten zur Geschichte der Medizin, Beiheft IX).
**Deneke JF:** Vorbeugende Massnahmen gegen Kindesmord im 19. Jahrhundert. **Krankenpfl J** 1984 May 1;22(5):36–8
**Dénes J:** A Semmelweis Orvostudományi Egyetem Gyermekfogászati és Fogszabályozási Klinikájának negyedszázados története és munkássága. **Fogorv Sz** 1984 Sep;77(9):258–9
**De Neve M:** E. J. Marey, inventieve registrator van de fysiologische fenomenen. **Acta Belg Med Phys** 1983 Oct–Dec;6(4):153–5
**Deniker P:** Psychopharmacologie et psychiatrie biologique rappel historique. **Soins Psychiatr** 1983 Nov;(37):5–6
**DeNiro MJ** see **Schoeninger MJ**
**Denis G** see **Le Fichoux Y**
**Denis MN:** Un problème de moeurs dans l'Alsace rurale traditionnelle: naissances illégitimes et conceptions prénuptiales à Bosselshausen (Bas-Rhin) de 1738 à 1838. In Congrès National des Sociétés Savantes, 103e, Nancy–Metz, 1978. Actes. Paris, 1979. Tome II, p. 57–69.
**Denisenko PP, Nuraliev IuN:** Abu Ali Ibn-Sina i farmakologiia; k 1000–letiiu so dnia rozhdeniia Avitsenny. **Farmakol Toksikol** 1980 Nov–Dec;43(6):753–4
**Denisenko VZ:** 60 Let na strazhe zdorov'ia voennosluzhashchikh. **Voen Med Zh** 1982;(9):78–9
**Denisiako EI** see **Maïatruk PN**
**Denisova TP** see **Korol' GG**
**Denko CW:** Chernogubov's syndrome: a translation of the first modern case report of the Ehlers–Danlos syndrome. **J Rheumatol** 1978 Fall;5(3):347–52
**Dennell RW:** Prehistoric diet and nutrition: some food for thought. **World Archaeol** 1979;11:121–35
**Dennis C:** The role of dingaka tsa setswana from the 19th century to the present. **Botsw Notes Rec** 1978;10:53–66
**Dennis PM:** The Edison questionnaire. **J Hist Behav Sci** 1984 Jan;20(1):23–37
**Denny FW:** Atypical pneumonia and the Armed Forces Epidemiological Board. **J Infect Dis** 1981 Mar;143(3):305–16
**Denny-Brown D:** The development of procedures in clinical neurology. **Trans Stud Coll Physicians Phila** 1980 Mar;5(2 no 1):26–30
**Denoix P:** Paul Broca. L'anatomie pathologique, le cancer, la statistique. **Chirurgie** 1980;106(10):787–90
**The Dental Corps of the United States Navy:** Washington, Bureau of Medicine and Surgery, Navy Dept. 73 p.
**A dental laboratory's catalog:** from before the turn of the century. **Bull Hist Dent** 1980 Apr;28(1):47–8
**Dentistry--for music's sake. I. How dental 'miracles' helped jazz greats with their careers (Buck Clayton): Tic** 1979 Dec;38(12):1–3
**Dentistry in folk art XI: L'arracheuse de dents (The tooth puller): Bull Hist Dent** 1980 Oct;28(2):87
**Dentistry in Japan: Br Dent J** 1983 Aug 20;155(4):136
**Deodhar NS:** Primary health care in India. **J Public Health Policy** 1982 Mar;3(1):76–99
**de Pasquale A:** Pharmacognosy: the oldest modern science. **J Ethnopharmacol** 1984 Jun;11(1):1–16
**De Poorter DA:** David Lipsius Iscanius, 17e-eeuws doctor medicus afkomstig uit Overijse. **Periodiek** 1980;35:16–22
**Depp ME** see **Golovin GV**
**Dequeker J:** Arthritis in the paintings of Sandro Botticelli. **Arthritis Rheum** 1984 Oct;27(10):1196–7
**Dequeker JV:** Polymyalgia rheumatica with temporal arteritis, as painted by Jan van Eyck in 1436. **Can Med Assoc J** 1981 Jun 15;124(12):1597–8
**De Quervain's stenosing tenovaginitis: Fritz de Quervain, 1868–1940: Orthop Nurs** 1982 Sep–Oct;1(5):24–5
**Der dreifache Fluch: Jüdin, Intellektuelle, Sozialistin: Lebenserinnerungen einer Arztin in Deutschland und im Exil:** Frankfurt/Main, New York, Campus Verlag, 1981. 320 p.
**Der Marderosian A** see **Liberti L**
**Deranian HM:** An historical overview of American dentistry. **Compend Contin Educ Dent** 1984 Jul–Aug;5(7):592–9
**Deranian HM:** The miracle man of the western front: the story of Dr. Varaztad Kazanjian. **Bull Hist Dent** 1984 Oct;32(2):85–103
**Derbenev NE:** Zdravnitsa dlia ranenykh voinov. **Voen Med Zh** 1980 Jul;(7):21–2
**DeRemee RA** see **Gracey DR**
**Dergacheva TI** see **Kupriianova ES**
**Deriabin II, Berkutov AN:** Razvitie voenno-polevoï khirurgii za 60 let Soiuza SSR. **Vestn Khir** 1983 Feb;2:3–7
**Dermott R:** 'A great black book': East of Eden and Gunn's New family physician. **Am Stud** 1981;22(2):41–57
**Derogatis LR, et al:** The Hopkins symptom checklist (HSCL): a self-report symptom inventory. **Behav Sci** 1974;19(1):1–15
**De Rosa A** see **Vizioli R**
**Dérot M:** Perspectives en diabétologie (d'hier à demain). **Bull Mem Acad R Med Belg** 1981;136(8–9):435–42
**Derouet B:** Une démographie sociale différentielle: clés pour un système auto-régulateur des populations rurales d'Ancien Régime. **Ann Econ Soc Civilis** 1980;35(1):3–41
**Derrick AA:** Old volumes provide links with medicine of today. **J Miss State Med Assoc** 1981 Dec;22(12):331–2
**Derums VJ:** Extensive trepanation of the skull in ancient Latvia. **Bull Hist Med** 1979 Fall;53(3):459–64
**Derums VIa, Pfafrod GO, Vilks IuK:** Dinamika strukturnykh i biomekhanicheskikh izmeneniï bedrennoï. **Arkh Anat Gistol Embriol** 1980 Aug;79(8):78–84
**Dérums VIa:** Rentgenomorfologicheskaia kharakteristika travmaticheskikh povrezhdeniï i raneniï kosteï zhiteleï drevneï Pribaltiki. **Arkh Patol** 1980;42(2):64–8
**Dervin D:** Michael Balint's contributions to the psychoanalysis of literature. **Psychoanal Rev** 1979–80 Winter;66(4):553–70
**Dervin D:** Rainbow, phoenix, and plumed serpent: D. H. Lawrence's great composite symbols and their vicissitudes. **Psychoanal Rev** 1980 Winter;67(4):515–41
**Des Cilleuls J:** L'inspecteur général Jacques de Villemanzy, Sénateur et Pair de France (1751–1830). **Hist Sci Med** 1979;13(4):379–81
**Des Jarlais DC** see **Courtwright DT**
**De Saint-Maur PP:** Que pensait Laennec de l'anatomie pathologique? **Ann Pathol** 1981;1(4):249–50
**Desaive JP:** L'alimentation populaire d'après les archives de l'Académie de Médecine (1774–1794). In: Congrès National des Sociétés Savantes, 93e, Tours, 1968. Actes. Paris, 1971. Section d'Histoire Moderne et Contemporaine, Tome 1. p. 39–53.
**Desaive JP:** Médecins, climat et épidémies à la fin du XVIIIe siècle. Paris, Mouton, [1972]. 254 p.
**de San Eustaquio Tudanca F** see **Parra Hidalgo P**
**De Saussure R** see **Chertok L**
**Deschamps A:** Aspects de la coca. **Decouv Civilis** 1974 Dec;7–8:31–46
**Deschamps Chapeaux P:** El negro en la economía Habanera del siglo XIX. Flebotomianos y dentistas. **Rev Bibl Nac Jose Marti** 1971;13(1):75–86
**Desgraves L, ed:** Répertoire bibliographique des livres imprimés en France au XVIIe siècle. Tome VI. Baden-Baden, Koerner, 1982. 248 p. (Bibliotheca Bibliographica Aureliana, XCI).
**d'Eshougues JR:** Gicht und Rheumatismus. In Sournia JC, Martiny M, Poulet J, ed: Illustrierte Geschichte der Medizin. Salzburg, Andreas, 1980. Vol. 6. p. 2319–49.
**De Silva A, Uragoda CG:** Traditional methods of snake-bite treatment in Sri Lanka. **Ceylon Med J** 1983 Sep;28(3):170–4
**Desjardins E:** Jacques Dénéchaud. In Dictionary of Canadian biography, 1801 to 1820. Volume 5, 1983. p. 248–9.
**Desjardins E:** Joseph Emery-Coderre. In Dictionary of Canadian biography, 1881–1890. 1982;11:302–3.
**Desjardins E:** Le docteur Jean-Baptiste Jobert (1733--1792). **Union Med Can** 1979 Feb;108(2):200
**Desjeux P, Waroquy L, Dedet JP:** La leishmaniose cutanée humaine en Afrique de l'ouest. **Bull Soc Pathol Exot Filiales** 1981 Jul–Aug;74(4):414–25
**Deslauriers L** see **Audet-Lapointe P**
**De Smet A, ed** see **Danckaert L**
**Desnick RJ:** Gaucher disease: a century of delineation and understanding. **Prog Clin Biol Res** 1982;95:1–30
**Desnick RJ:** Gaucher disease (1882–1982): centennial perspectives on the most prevalent Jewish genetic disease. **Mt Sinai J Med (NY)** 1982 Nov–Dec;49(6):443–55
**Desowitz RS:** New Guinea tapeworms and Jewish grandmothers. Tales of parasites and people. New York, London, W. W. Norton, 1981. 224 p.
**De Spiegeler P:** La léproserie de Cornillon et la cité de Liège (XIIe–XVe siècle). **Ann Soc Belg Hist Hop** 1980;18:3–16
**Desrosiers G:** Evolution de la médecine et répercussion sur la formation médicale en Amérique du Nord. **Union Med Can** 1981 Sep;110(9):817–20

**Desrosiers G:** Histoire de la santé publique au Québec. **Can J Public Health** 1984 Sep–Oct;75(5):359–63
**Destaing F** see **Cabanne F**
**Detinova TS** see **Kupriianova ES**
**Detlefsen EG:** Abraham Stone. In Dictionary of American Biography, Suppl. 6, 1956–1960. p. 602–3, 1980.
**Detlefsen EG:** George Edward Pfahler. In Dictionary of American Biography, Suppl. 6, 1956–1960. p. 505–6, 1980.
**Detlow-Berg AL:** Omvårdnad i Vadstena kloster. **Dan Medicinhist Arbog** 1983;12:65–73
**Detragiache D:** Un aspect de la politique demographique de l'Italie fasciste: la repression de l'avortement. **Melanges Archeol Hist Ec Fr Rome** 1980;92(2):691–735
**Detre KC, Frank T, Kniazzeh CR, et al:** Roots of art therapy. Margaret Naumburg (1890–1983) and Florence Cane (1882–1952). A family portrait. **Am J Art Ther** 1983 Jul;22(4):111–23
**Detti T:** Medicina, democrazia e socialismo in Italia tra '800 e '900. **Mov Operaio Soc** 1979;2(1):3–49
**Deutsch Delanoy G:** Quelques ephemera des cent ans écoulés. **Rev Hist Pharm (Paris)** 1980 Sep;27(246):189–98
**Deutsch-Delanoy G:** Un catalogue de la 'Pharmacie Universelle', à Paris, vers 1900. **Rev Hist Pharm (Paris)** 1982 Mar;29(252):31–6
**Deutsch-Kasimir M:** Die Heilige Apollonia. **Quintessenz J** 1982 Nov;12(11):1025–6
**De Vahl Davis V:** A history of the Walter and Eliza Hall Institute of Medical Research, 1915–1978. Ph.D. Diss. University of New South Wales. Sydney, 1979.
**DeValk A:** Understandable but mistaken: law, morality and the Canadian Catholic Church 1966–1969. **Can Cathol Hist Assoc Study Sess** 1982;49:87–109
**Devance L** see **Dupâquier J**
**Devaraj TL:** A bird's eye view of history of ayurveda in Karnataka State. **Sachitra Ayurved** 1981 Mar;:185–9
**De Vásquez Am** see **Christensen HA**
**Devauchelle D, Pezin M:** Un papyrus médical démotique. **Chron Egypte** 1978 Jan;53:57–66
**Devaux G:** Pharmaciens éponymes des rues de l'agglomération bordelaise. **Rev Hist Pharm (Paris)** 1983 Dec;71(30):299–304
**Devaux G:** Saint Michel, patron des apothicaires de Bordeaux et d'autres lieux. **Rev Hist Pharm (Paris)** 1982;29(252):151–9
**De Vaux de Foletier F:** Anoblissements de médecins et chirurgiens de Louis XIV à Louis XVI. **Hist Sci Med** 1982;16(3):163–6
**De Vecchi P** see **Schmid R**
**The development of social insurance in Hungary over three decades. [Budapest?], The Administration, [1975?]. 114 p.:**
**Devereux G:** The family: historical function, dysfunction, lack of function, and schizophrenia. **J Psychohist** 1980;8:183–93
**Devevey J** see **Rochefort R**
**Deviatova LN:** Itogi profilaktiki infektsionnykh zabolevaniĭ i bor'by s infektsiiami v SSSR. **Feldsher Akush** 1982;47(12):9–13
**Deviatova LN** see **Kovaleva EP**
**Devick WS** see **Tomich PQ**
**Deville JC:** Analyse harmonique dul calendrier de constitution des familles en France. Disparités sociales et évolution de 1920 à 1960. **Population** 1977;32(1):17–63
**De Villiers JC, Munnik LA, Luyt R, et al:** Jan Hendrik Louw. **S Afr Med J** 1980 Mar;57(16):605–12
**De Villiers JC:** Perspectives in international neurosurgery: neurosurgery in South Africa. **Neurosurgery** 1983 Nov;13(5):609–10
**Devine P:** Mental retardation: an early subspecialty in psychiatric nursing. **J Psychosoc Nurs Ment Health Serv** 1983 Mar;21(3):21–30
**De Vinuesa FS** see **Valverde JL**
**Deviri E** see **Yechezkel M**
**Devitt N:** The statistical case for elimination of the midwife: fact versus prejudice, 1890–1935. **Women Health** 1979;4:81–96, 169–86
**Devitt N:** The statistical case for elimination of the midwife: fact versus prejudice, 1890–1935 (part 2). **Women Health** 1979 Summer;4(2):121–33
**Devitt N:** The transition from home to hospital birth in the United States, 1930–1960. **Birth Fam J** 1977;4(2):47–58
**Devlesaver P:** Néphrostomies transcutanées. **Acta Urol Belg** 1983;51(4):473–83
**Devlin J:** Nurses join the stamp set. **Nurs Times** 1984 May 2–8;80(18):40–1
**Devlin R:** A new look at old wives. **Nurs Mirror** 1981 Sep 16;153(12):8–9
**Devlin R:** The VADs nursing in no man's land. **Nurs Mirror** 1980 Oct 23;151(17):8–9
**Devlin RJ** see **Albin M**
**Devor EJ, Cordell LS:** Neural-tube defects in a prehistoric south-western Indian population. **Ann Hum Biol** 1981 Jan–Feb;8(1):65–75
**Devos D, Devos JC:** L'hôpital militaire de Barèges (Hautes-Pyrénées) du debut du XVIIIe siècle à la fin du Premier Empire. In: Congrès National des Sociétés Savantes, 97e, Nantes, 1972. Actes. Paris, 1977. Histoire Moderne et Contemporaine, Tome 1. p. 105–13.
**Devos JC** see **Devos D**
**De Vos R** see **Van der Haegen H**
**De Vos S** see **Knodel J**
**DeVries PA:** The surgery of anorectal anomalies: its evolution, with evaluations of procedures. **Curr Probl Surg** 1984 May;21(5):1–75
**Devyatova LN** see **Ermakov VV**
**Dew WC:** John Ross Callahan: a man, a memorial, an award. **Ohio Dent J** 1982 Jul–Aug;56(7–8):46–52
**deWachter MA:** Is death and dying merely an ethical issue? **Ann Am Acad Polit Soc Sci** 1980;447:78–88
**De Wailly P, Crawford LM:** The life of Alexandre Liautard. **Hist Med Vet** 1978;3(2):47–9
**Dewan L:** St. Albert, the sensibles, and spiritual being. In Weisheipl JA, ed: Albertus Magnus and the sciences. Toronto, Pontifical Institute of Mediaeval Studies. p. 291–320.
**Dewel BF:** Orthodontics: midcentury recollections. **Eur J Orthod** 1981;3(2):77–87
**Dewel BF:** The ribbon arch. Its influence in the development of orthodontic appliances. **Angle Orthod** 1981 Oct;51(4):263–8
**Dewey FL:** Thomas Jefferson's law practice: the Norfolk anti-inoculation riots. **Va Mag Hist Biogr** 1983;91(1):39–53
**Dewey PE:** Food production and policy in the United Kingdom, 1914–1918. **Trans R Hist Soc** 1980;(30):71–89
**Dewhurst J:** Royal confinements. **Ala J Med Sci** 1982 Oct;19(4):443–52
**Dewhurst J:** Royal midwives of former times. **Midwife Health Visit Community Nurse** 1983 Oct;19(10):386–92
**Dewhurst J:** Royal twins. **Br Med J [Clin Res]** 1983 Dec 24–31;287(6409):1937–9
**Dewhurst J:** The alleged miscarriages of Catherine of Aragon and Anne Boleyn. **Med Hist** 1984 Jan;28(1):49–56
**Dewhurst K:** Thomas Willis and the foundations of British neurology. In Rose FC, Bynum WF, ed: Historical aspects of the neurosciences. New York, Raven, 1982. p. 327–46.
**Dewhurst K:** Thomas Willis's Oxford Lectures. Oxford, Sandford, 1980. x, 182 p.
**Dewhurst K, ed:** Willis's Oxford casebook (1650–52). Oxford, Sanford, 1981 xi, 199 p.
**Dews PB:** Pavlov and psychiatry. **J Hist Behav Sci** 1981;17:246–50
**Dexter L** see **Snellen HA**
**Dexter RW:** The impact of evolutionary theories on the Salem group of Agassiz zoologists (Morse, Hyatt, Packard, Putnam). **Essex Inst Hist Collect** 1979;115(3):144–71
**Dey DL:** Penicillin in Australia. **Med J Aust** 1982 Aug 21;2(4):172
**Deyts S** see **Patrimoine hospitalier de la Bourgogne**
**Dezsö D:** Az 1964–1976, évi termékenység elemzése, kísérlet i. **Demografia** 1978;21(2–3):221–43
**Dezsö D:** Népességi nézetek és népesedéspolitika Magyarországon a kapitalizmus korában. **Demografia** 1962;5(2):143–64
**De Zulueta J:** La introducción del 'Plasmodium falciparum' en la Europa del Mediterráneo: passado y presente. **Rev Sanid Hig Publica (Madr)** 1982 Jul–Aug;56(7–8):693–8
**Dhoore L, Halter S:** Secretaris-generaal van het Ministerie van Volksgezondheid en van het Gezin, Prof. Dr. S. Halter. **Arch Belg Med Soc** 1981 Jul;39(7)Suppl:1–64
**Di Benedetto V** see **Grmek MD, ed**
**Di Giandomenico M** see **Epistemologia, metodologia clinica e storia della scienza medica, 2**
**D'iachenko DP:** Pervaia bol'nitsa Kamchatskoĭ gubernii (K 75-letiiu Petropavlovsk-Kamchatskoĭ gorodskoĭ bol'nitsy No. 1). **Sov Zdravookhr** 1984;(3):60–2
**Diachenko SS:** Iz istorii izucheniia semeĭstva kishechnykh bakteriĭ v Ukrainskoĭ SSR. **Mikrobiol Zh** 1982 Jan–Feb;44(1):95–9
**Diachenko SS:** Stanovlenie i razvitie meditsinskoĭ virusologii v Ukraine. **Mikrobiol Zh** 1980 Nov–Dec;42(6):798–802
**Diachenko SS:** U istochnikov meditsinskoĭ mikrobiologii v Kieve. **Mikrobiol Zh** 1982 Mar–Apr;44(2):5–10
**D'iachkov VI:** Revoliutsionnoe proshloe pervogo meditsinskogo uchebnogo zavedeniia v Sibiri (o Tobol'skoĭ povival'noĭ shkole). **Feldsher Akush** 1984 Mar;49(3):55–6
**Diadiusha GF, Turkevich NM, Bulkina ZP:** Vklad R. E. Kavetskogo v razvitie onkologii (k 80-letiiu so dnia rozhdeniia). **Vopr Onkol** 1979;25(11):102–10
**Diamant H:** Robert Bárány och Nobel-priset. **Sydsven Medicinhist Sallsk Arsskr** 1984;21:123–8
**Diamond BE** see **Wegner PN**
**Diamond BL:** The psychiatrist as expert witness. **Psychiatr Clin North Am** 1983 Dec;6(4):597–609
**Diamond C** see **Adour KK**
**Diamond LK:** Milestones in blood transfusion and blood banking. **Pharos** 1982 Spring;45(2):7–10
**Diamond LK:** The Rh problem: (an example of the tsunami phenomenon in medicine). **Turk J Pediatr** 1982 Jan–Mar;24(1):35–47
**Diamond P:** The natural theologians and Darwin: a case of divergent evolution in the history of ideas. **Aust J Polit Hist** 1980;26(2):204–11
**Diamond S:** Buckle, Wundt, and psychology's use of history. **Isis** 1984 Mar;75(276):143–52
**Diamond S:** Francis Galton and American psychology. In R. W. Rieber, K. Salzinger, ed: Psychology: theoretical-historical perspectives. New York, Academic Press, 1980. p. 43–55.
**Diamond S:** Sigmund Freud, his Jewishness, and scientific method: the seen and the unseen as evidence. **J Hist Ideas** 1982 Oct–Dec;43(4):613–34
**Diamond S** see **Rieber RW, ed**
**Diara A:** Sens et definition du mot 'espece' dans l'oeuvre biologique de Felix Le Dantec. **Rev Synth (Paris)** 1981;102(101–102):73–86
**Dias JR:** Famine and disease in the history of Angola, C. 1830–1930. **J Afr Hist** 1981;22(3):349–78
**Diaz CM:** Perspectives in international neurosurgery: neurosurgery in Honduras. **Neurosurgery** 1982 Feb;10(2):277–8
**Díaz F:** Influencia de San Juan de Dios en la enfermería. **Rev Enferm** 1982 Mar;5(45):12–4

**Díaz JL:** Ethnopharmacology and taxonomy of Mexican psychodysleptic plants. **J Psychedelic Drugs** 1979 Jan–Jun;11(1–2):71–101
**Díaz-Briquets S, Pérez L:** Fertility decline in Cuba: a socioeconomic interpretation. **Popul Dev Rev** 1982;8(3):513–37
**Díaz-Briquets S:** The health revolution in Cuba. Austin, University of Texas Press, 1983. xvii, 227 p.
**Diaz Garcia A:** Three medical recipes in Codex Biblioteca Medicea-Laurenziana Or. 215. **J Hist Arabic Sci** 1980;4:265–86
**Díaz-Jano-Sov C:** Feminism and the evolution of the profession of nursing. **Bol Col Prof Enferm PR** 1981 Jun;7(26):6–12
**Díaz y de Ovando C:** Odontología y publicidad en la prensa mexicana del siglo XIX. **Bol Soc Mex Hist Filos Med** 1984 Jun;7(47):325–46
**Di Benedetto V:** De la maladie au malade particulier: changement de perspective de la médecine du Ve siècle avant Jésus-Christ. In La collection hippocratique et son rôle dans l'histoire de la médecine. Colloque de Strasbourg (23–27 octobre 1972) organisé par le Centre de Recherches sur la Grèce Antique, avec le concours des Facultés de Philosophie et des Langues Classiques. Leiden, E. J. Brill, 1975. p. 51–5.
**Dibold H** see **Schönbauer D**
**Dickerson LA** see **McBryde AM**
**Dickey B:** Care for the aged poor in Australia, 1788–1914. **Community Health Stud** 1983 Oct;7(3):247–55
**Dickey B:** No charity there: a short history of social welfare in Australia. Melbourne, Nelson, 1980. xix, 252 p.
**Dickey B:** St. Vincent's Hospital, Sydney: a note. **J R Aust Hist Soc** 1978;64(2):131–33
**Dickey B:** The sick poor in New South Wales, 1840–1880: colonial practice in an amateur age. **J R Aust Hist Soc** 1973;59(1):16–28
**Dickman SR:** The search for the specific factor in scurvy. **Perspect Biol Med** 1981;24:382–95
**Dickson DF** see **Morse D**
**Dickson I:** Early history of CPA. The Canadian Psychiatric Association. **Can J Psychiatry** 1980 Feb;25(1):86–97
**Dickson P:** Passage of the lines. **Army Q Def J** 1982;112(2):199–204
**Dickstein-Bernard C:** Genèse del'hôpital universitaire, 1834–1935. **Rev Med Brux** 1984 May;5(5):315–8
**Dickstein-Bernard C:** La pratique de la chirurgie dans les hôpitaux bruxellois au XIXe siècle. **Ann Soc Belg Hist Hop** 1981;:69–94
**DiCori P:** Come controllare i sentimenti: tra scienza delle emozioni e identita di genere all'inizio del '900. **Mem Riv Stor Donne** 1981;(1):26–32
**Diculescu I, Onicescu D:** At the hundredth anniversary of the Department of Histology of the Bucharest Faculty of Medicine. **Morphol Embryol (Bucur)** 1980 Jul–Sep;26(3):199–204
**Diczfalusy E:** Gregory Pincus and steroidal contraception revisited. **Acta Obstet Gynecol Scand [Suppl]** 1982;105:7–15
**Diczfalusy E:** The early history of estriol. **J Steroid Biochem** 1984 Apr;20(4B):945–53
**Didi-Huberman G:** Invention de l'hystérie: Charcot et l'iconographie photographique de la Salpêtrière. Paris, Macula, 1982. 303 p.
**Didier C:** Aperçu sur les médecins et chirurgiens à Colmar au XVIIIe siècle. In Livet G, Schaff G, ed: Médecine et assistance en Alsace, XVIe–XXe siècle. Strasbourg, Istra, 1976. p. 87–111.
**DiDio LJ** see **Busnardo AC**
**Die Alte Kunst des Apothekers:** Wiederentdeckt bei einem Besuch im Deutschen Apotheken-Museum in Heidelberg. Mannheim, Boehringer Mannheim, 1980. 39 p.
**Die Deutsche Gesellschaft für Zahn-, Mund- und Kieferheilkunde:** Vom Zentralverein 1859 bis heute; ein weiter und erfolgreicher Weg. **ZWR** 1981 Apr;90(4):10–6
**Die französische Medizin im Mittelalter:** In Sournia JC, Martiny M, Poulet J, ed: Illustrierte Geschichte der Medizin. Salzburg, Andreas, 1980. Vol. 2. p. 755–65.
**Dieck M:** Residential and community provisions for the frail elderly in Germany: current issues and their history. **Gerontologist** 1980 Jun;20(3 Pt 1):260–72
**Dieckhöfer K:** Aspekte einer rudimentären Psychologie, Psychopathologie und Psychotherapie bei Seneca. In: Congrès international d'histoire de la médecine, XXVe, Québec, 1976. Actes. Québec, 1977. p. 579–95.
**Dieckhöfer K:** Der flämische Schriftsteller Hendrik Conscience (1812–1883) und die psychisch Kranken von Geel. **Z Psychosom Med Psychoanal** 1984;30(2):179–90
**Dieckhöfer K:** El desarrollo de la psiquiatría en España. Aspectos históricos y culturales. **Actas Luso Esp Neurol Psiquiatr** 1983 Jul–Aug;11(4):333–42
**Dieckhöfer K:** El desarrollo de la psiquiatría en España. Aspectos historicos y culturales. **Actas Luso Esp Neurol Psiquiatr** 1983 Nov–Dec;11(6):487–96
**Dieckhöfer K:** Frühe Formen der Antipsychiatrie und die Reaktion der Psychiatrie. **Medizinhist J** 1984;19(1–2):101–11
**Dieckhöfer K:** Geistesgeschichtliche Strömungen in der Biographik—ein kulturhistorischer Abriss. **Z Psychosom Med Psychoanal** 1980 Jul–Sep;26(3):275–81
**Dieckhöfer K:** II. El desarrollo de la psiquiatría en España. Aspectos históricos y culturales. **Actas Luso Esp Neurol Psiquiatr** 1983 Sep–Oct;11(5):407–22
**Dieckhöfer K:** Juan Huarte de San Juan, precursor de la psicología diferencial. In International Congress of the History of Medicine, 27th, Barcelona, 1980. Actas. Barcelona, Académia de Ciències Médiques de Catalunya i Balears, 1981. p. 64–8.
**Dieckhöfer K:** Menschliches, Allzumenschliches—zur verstehenden Psychologie bei Nietzsche. **Z Klin Psychol Psychother** 1980;28(2):101–5
**Dieckhöfer K:** Psychohygienische Konzepte in der römischen Kaiserzeit. **Ther Ggw** 1981;120(1):80–95
**Dieckhöfer K:** Zur Rolle einer Psychohygiene im Griechenland des 5. vorchristlichen Jahrhunderts bis zur Zeitenwende. **Clio Med** 1982 Dec;17(2–3):81–94
**Dieckmann I:** Untersuchungen des menschlichen Endometriums durch Hanns Kundrat (1845–1893) und George Julius Engelmann (1847–1903). Diss. Erlangen-Nürnberg, 1980. 73 p.
**Dieffenbach VC:** Powwowing among the Pennsylvania Germans. **Pa Folklife** 1975–76;25(2):29–46
**Diehl B:** Der Wandel der Historiographie von Medizin und Naturwissenschaften in ihrer gesellschaftlichen Bedingtheit. **Sudhoffs Arch** 1982;66(3):276–300
**Diels H** see **Durling R**
**Diemath HE:** Perspectives in international neurosurgery: neurosurgery in Austria. **Neurosurgery** 1981 Nov;9(5):604–5
**Diener L:** Från antikonception till amning – om tillökning i familjen i det faraoniska Egypten. **Nord Medicinhist Arsbok** 1983;:41–58
**Diener L:** Hygieniska förhållanden i det faraoniska Egypten. **Nord Medicinhist Arsb** 1982;:41–55
**Diener L:** Osteologi och historia—röntgenologiska aspekter. **Nord Medicinhist Arsb** 1980;Suppl 6:112–7
**Diener L:** Skönhet, skönhetsvård och skönhetsmedel i det faraoniska Egypten. **Nord Medicinhist Arsb** 1980;:38–52
**Diener L, ed:** Röster ur Riksgropen. **Nord Medicinhist Arsb** 1984;:49–61
**Diener L, et al:** Nutida folkmedicin. **Nord Medicinhist Arsb** 1981;:193–202
**Dienstbier E:** Prof. MUDr. Roman Kadlický. Jeho život a dílo. **Cas Lek Cesk** 1980 Aug 22;119(33–34):915–20
**Dienstbier Z:** Třicet let Ustavu biofyziky a nukleární medicíny FVL KU. **Sb Lek** 1983 Mar;85(3):65–7
**Dienstbier Z:** 25 let Ceskoslovenské společnosti nukleární medicíny a radiační hygieny. **Cas Lek Cesk** 1981 Aug 13;120(31–32):963–7
**Dienstbier Z:** 25 years of the Czechoslovak Society for Nuclear Medicine and Radiation Hygiene. **Czech Med** 1981;4(3):97–106
**Dieppe P** see **Rogers J**
**Dierauer U:** Tier und Mensch im Denken der Antike: Studien zur Tierpsychologie, Anthropologie, und Ethik. Amsterdam, Grüner, 1977. xvii, 320 p. (Studien zur antiken Philosophie, 6.).
**Diercksen G, et al:** Aus der Chronik der Aerzteschaft Karlsruhe, 1715–1977: nach alten Aufzeichnungen, aktuellen Berichten, Biographien und Presseveröffentlichungen. Karlsruhe, Aerzteschaft Karlsruhe, 1978. 519, 8 p.
**Dierżykray-Rogalski T:** Historia Badán szczątków kostnych Jana z Czarnolasu Kochanowskiego. **Kwart Hist Nauki Tech** 1983;28(2):425–35
**Diesbachs A von** see **Jaeschke G**
**Dietemann J** see **Wackenheim A**
**Diethelm O** see **Peck W**
**Dietrich DJ:** Psychohistory: Clio on the couch – or off? **Hist Methods** 1982;15(2):83–90
**Dietrich U** see **Casey AE**
**Dietsch H:** Die Altershygiene Kants. **Med Welt** 1982 Apr 16;33(15):570–2
**Dietsch H:** Von der Metamorphose zur Homologie. Zum 150. Todestag Goethes. **Med Welt** 1982 Dec 3;33(48):1767–8
**Dietz G:** Abriss der Entwicklung der Endodontie. **Zahnarzt** 1983 Dec;27(12):780–4
**Dietzch S** see **Hasler L, ed**
**Dietzsch HJ:** 50 Jahre Kinderklinik der Medizinischen Akademie 'Carl Gustav Carus' Dresden und ihre Vorgeschichte. **Kinderarztl Prax** 1981 Jun;49(6):318–26
**Different letters from the past:** Tobias Smollett to William Hunter. **Ann R Coll Surg Engl** 1980 Mar;62(2):146–9
**Different letters from the past. 4) Horatio, Viscount Nelson to Earl Spencer.: Ann R Coll Surg Engl** 1980 Sep;62(5):388–9
**Digby A:** Changes in the asylum: the case of York, 1777–1815. **Econ Hist Rev** 1983;36:218–39
**Digby A:** The York Retreat: the growing ascendancy of medicine, 1796–1914. **Pharm Hist (London)** 1984 Jun;14(2):2–3
**Digby A** see **Dupâquier J**
**DiGeronimo EM, Marraccini P:** Body-mind sculpture: battle of the titans. **Plast Reconstr Surg** 1984 Feb;73(2):324–5
**Di Giacomo V:** A case of Takayasu's disease occurred over two hundred years ago. **Angiology** 1984 Nov;35(11):750–4
**DiGioia JM, Rocko JM, Swan KG:** Baron Larrey. Modern military surgeon. **Am Surg** 1983 May;49(5):226–30
**Di Gioia JM** see **Rocko JM**
**Di Gregorio MA:** In search of the natural system: problems of zoological classification in Victorian Britain. **Hist Philos Life Sci** 1982;4(2):225–54
**Di Gregorio MA:** Order or process of nature: Huxley's and Darwin's different approaches to natural sciences. **Hist Philos Life Sci** 1981;3(2):217–41
**Di Gregorio MA:** The dinosaur connection: a reinterpretation of T. H. Huxley's evolutionary view. **J Hist Biol** 1982 Fall;15(3):397–418
**Dikova S:** The Bulgarian Red Cross and the development of blood donation in Bulgaria. In International Congress of the History of Medicine. 26th, Plovdiv, 1978. Actes du Congress. Sofia, 1981. Volume II. p. 220.
**Dikshteĭn EA, Orlova NL:** Kafedre patologicheskoĭ anatomii Donetskogo meditsinskogo instituta 50 let. **Arkh Patol** 1984;46(1):73–4
**Dilg P:** Die 'Reformation der Apotecken' (1536) des Berner Stadtarztes Otto Brunfels. **Gesnerus** 1979;36(3–4):181–205
**Dilg P:** Examen pharmacopoeorum vulgare. Aus einer Handschrift des Laurentius Blumentrost d. A. (1619–1705). In Dilg P, et al., ed: Perspektiven der Pharmaziegeschichte. Graz, Austria, Akademische

Druck- u. Verlagsanstalt, 1983. p. 39–64.
**Dilg P:** Vom Ansehen der Arzneikunst; historische Reflexionen in Kräuterbüchern des 16. Jahrhunderts. **Sudhoffs Arch** 1978;62(1):64–79
**Dilg P:** Zur Geschichte des 'alteren deutschen Apothekenwesens', XVI. Die Strassburger Apothekerordnung (um 1500). **Pharm Ztg** 1979;124:2664–70
**Dilg-Frank R:** Alexandre Yersin als Medizinstudent in Marburg. **Alma Mater Philipp** 1978–1979;19–23
**Dilg-Frank R** see **Braun L, et al**
**Dilg-Frank R** see **Paracelsus in der Tradition**
**Dilg, P, et al., ed:** Perspektiven der Pharmaziegeschichte: Festschrift für Rudolf Schmitz zum 65. Geburtstag. Bibliography by F. J. Kühlen. Graz, Austria, Akademische Druck- u. Verlagsanstalt, 1983. xviii, 497 p.
**Dill DB, Gordon AS:** Background on manual artificial respiration and mouth-to-mouth resuscitation. Addendum: Background on cardiopulmonary resuscitation. **Physiologist** 1980 Jun;23(3):33–7
**Dill DB:** International high altitude expedition to Chile, 1935. **Prog Clin Biol Res** 1983;136:201–4
**Dillemann G:** Die französische Pharmazie vom 3. Jahrhundert bis zur Gegenwart. In Sournia JC, Martiny M, Poulet J, ed: Illustrierte Geschichte der Medizin. Salzburg, Andreas, 1980. Vol. 5. p. 1723–77.
**Dillemann G:** Histoire de l'enseignement pharmaceutique en France. **Pharm Acta Helv** 1979;54(9–10):269–72
**Dillemann G:** La difficile conquête des prérogatives universitaires par les pharmaciens. **Rev Hist Pharm (Paris)** 1982 Sep;29(254):155–63
**Dillemann G, Michel ME:** La réception des pharmaciens en France de la Révolution à l'application de la loi du 21 germinal an XI (1791–1813). **Rev Hist Pharm (Paris)** 1984;31(260):42–61
**Dillemann G:** Le Doyen Guillaume Valette (1902–1982). **Rev Hist Pharm (Paris)** 1982 Jun;29(253):83–6
**Dillemann G:** Le monopole pharmaceutique et le décret du 2 mars 1791. **Rev Hist Pharm (Paris)** 1980 Dec;247(68 no 27):235–8
**Dillemann G:** L'éloge de Magendie par Claude Bernard. **Hist Sci Med** 1983;17(4):345–9
**Dillemann G:** Les cumuls d'emplois en 1821. **Rev Hist Pharm (Paris)** 1981 Jun;28(249):109–11
**Dillemann G:** Les dénominations successives des établissements autonomes d'enseignement pharmaceutique. **Bull Liaison Assoc Amis Mus Pharm Montp** 1983;:(8):77–82
**Dillemann G:** Les écoles de médecine des départements annexés de l'an XI (1803) à 1814. Le cas de l'école de Mayence. **Hist Sci Med** 1984;18(1):45–51
**Dillemann G:** Les illustres pharmaciens dont les noms ont été donnés aux amphithéatres de la Faculté de Pharmacie de Paris. **Bull Ordre Natl Pharm** 1979 Apr;221:517–41
**Diller H:** Das Selbstverständnis der griechischen Medizin in der Zeit des Hippokrates. In La collection hippocratique et son rôle dans l'histoire de la médecine. Colloque de Strasbourg (23–27 octobre 1972) organisé par le Centre de Recherches sur la Grèce Antique, avec le concours des Facultés de Philosophie et des Langues Classiques. Leiden, E. J. Brill, 1975. p. 77–93.
**Dilman I:** Freud and human nature. Oxford, Basil Blackwell, 1983. 207 p.
**Di Marco A, Cassinelli G, Arcamone F:** The discovery of daunorubicin. **Cancer Treat Rep** 1981;65 Suppl 4:3–8
**Di Matteo J:** Les Archives des maladies du coeur et des vaisseaux. **Arch Mal Coeur** 1980 Jun;73(6):563–84
**Dimic CA:** Gide et la maladie. **Studi Francesi** 1979;23(67):62–75
**Dimitrov D:** Iz istoriiata na veterinarnomeditsinskoto obrazo vanie. **Vet Med Nauki** 1981;18(7):112–5
**Dimitrov D:** 50 godini Raĭonen veterinarnomeditsinski institut vŭv Veliko Tŭrnovo. **Vet Med Nauki** 1982;19(9):113–4
**Dimitrov D** see **Nikolaeva I**
**Dimitrov TS:** Istoricheski danni za balkanskata endemichna nefropatiia. **Vutr Boles** 1982;21(2):74–7
**Dimopoulos C, Gialas A, Likourinas M, et al:** Hippocrates: founder and pioneer of urology. **Br J Urol** 1980 Apr;52(2):73–4
**Dinel G** see **Mathieu J**
**Diner SJ, ed** see **Breul FR**
**Dinet D:** Mourir en religion aux dix-septième et dix-huitième siècles; la mort dans quelques couvents des dioceses d'Auxerre, Langres et Dijon. **Rev Hist (Paris)** 1978;259(3):29–54
**Dinet D** see **LeBras H**
**Dinet-Lecomte MC:** Les bâtiments hospitaliers de Blois aux XVIIe et XVIIIe siècle (1). **Bull Soc Fr Hist Hop** 1983;46:14–20
**Dingle AE:** 'The monster nuisance of all': landowners, alkali manufacturers, and air pollution, 1828–64. **Econ Hist Rev** 1982;35(4):529–48
**Dinning JS:** Reflections on Nutrition Reviews from an international nutritionist. **Nutr Rev** 1982 Nov;40(11):328–30
**Dionesov SM:** K istorii zhenskogo meditsinskogo obrazovaniia v Rossii. **Feldsher Akush** 1983 Dec;48(12):44–5
**Dionesov SM:** Stranitsa iz istorii Pervogo s'ezda Russkogo soiuza psikhiatrov i nevropatologov. **Zh Nevropatol Psikhiatr** 1981;(5):744–5
**Dionesov SM:** Vrachebnoe obshchestvo v Derpte. **Sov Zdravookhr** 1983;5:62–3
**Dionesov SM:** Zhenskie vrachebnye kursy pri Peterburgskom nikolaevskom voennom gospitale. **Sov Med** 1982;(6):117–9
**Di Pietro P:** La 'storia naturale del mare' di Lazzaro Spallanzani. **Thalassia Salentina** 1978;8:53–62
**Diraison Y** see **Buffat JJ**
**Dirckx JH:** Armand J. Quick: pioneer and prophet of coagulation research. **Ann Intern Med** 1980 Apr;92(4):553–8
**Dirckx JH:** Dermatologic terms in the De Medicina of Celsus. **Am J Dermatopathol** 1983 Aug;5(4):363–9
**Dirckx JH:** Doctor Watson's brothers. **Pharos** 1981 Summer;44(3):24–7
**Dirckx JH:** Graham Greene's doctors. **Pharos** 1983 Spring;46(2):27–9
**Dirckx JH:** Hannibal's ophthalmia. **Pharos** 1983 Fall;46(4):28–30
**Dirckx JH:** New meanings for old words. A gentle introduction to semantics. **Am J Dermatopathol** 1983 Jun;5(3):249–54
**Dirckx JH:** Ovid's dermatologic formulary. **Am J Dermatopathol** 1980 Winter;2(4):327–32
**Dirckx JH:** Peter Juliani, physician and pope. **Pharos** 1980 Fall;43(4):8–13
**Dirckx JH:** Scientific and medical terms and references in the writings of St. Luke. **Am J Dermatopathol** 1983 Oct;5(5):491–9
**Dirckx JH:** Sir Thomas Browne (1605–1682). A model for medical humanists. **JAMA** 1982 Oct 15;248(15):1845–7
**Dirckx JH:** The pied piper of Hamelin. A medical-historical interpretation. **Am J Dermatopathol** 1980 Spring;2(1):39–45
**Dirckx JH:** Virgil and medicine. **JAMA** 1981 Sep 18;246(12):1326–9
**Dirckx JH:** Virgil on anthrax. **Am J Dermatopathol** 1981 Summer;3(2):191–5
**Dirckx JH:** Voltaire on the pox. **Am J Dermatopathol** 1983 Dec;5(6):581–4
**Dirheimer G** see **Kotwas J**
**Disertori B, Piazza M:** Felice Fontana precursore delle moderne neuroscienze. **Ann Osp Maria Vittoria Torino** 1981 Jan–Jun;24(1–6)178–209
**Disertori B, Piazza M:** L'epilettologia di Apuleio. **Ann Osp Maria Vittoria Torino** 1977 Jul–Dec;20(7–12):341–53
**Dishman M:** Coleman Hall. A monument to Indiana medicine. **Indiana Med** 1984 Aug;77(8):622–3
**Dishong A:** Highlights of twenty years' research at the University of Florida College of Medicine. **J Fla Med Assoc** 1980 Mar;67(3):288–93
**Distinguished contribution for applications in psychology award for 1978 (Alphonse Chapanis).: Am Psychol** 1979 Jan;34(1):48–55
**Distinguished contribution to psychology in the public interest.: Am Psychol** 1979 Jan;34(1):65–8
**Distinguished Professional Contribution Award for 1978:** (Arthur L. Benton). **Am Psychol** 1979 Jan;34(1):56–64
**Distinguished scientific contribution awards for 1978 (Julian Hochberg, Philip Teitelbaum, Robert B. Zajonc).: Am Psychol** 1979 Jan;34(1):35–47
**Ditchburn RW:** Newton's illness of 1692–3. **Notes Rec R Soc Lond** 1980 Jul;35(1):1–16
**Di Trocchio F:** Paul-Joseph Barthez e l' 'Encyclopédie'. **Physis** 1980;22(3–4):379–92
**Dittmann S:** Die Welt ist pockenfrei--Durchführung und Erfolg eines grandiosen Programms. **Z Gesamte Inn Med** 1980 Dec 15;35(24):858–63
**Dittmann S, Paulenz H, Scheel G, et al:** 30 Jahre Staatliche Hygieneinspektion der DDR. **Z Gesamte Hyg** 1983 Oct;29(10):584–8
**Dittmer I:** James Marion Sims. 1813–1883. **MMW** 1984 Feb 10;126(6):159–60
**Dittrich HM:** Die Pavlov-Lehre im Forschungsprogramm von Gerhardt Katsch. **Z Gesamte Inn Med** 1983 Apr 1;38(7):230–2
**Dittrich HM** see **Dorsche HH von**
**Dittrich M:** Der Darwinist Fritz Müller (1822–1897) und sein Medizinstudium in Greifswald. Analyse der Motive seiner progressiven Haltung. In: International Congress of the History of Medicine, 26th, Plovdiv (Bulgaria), 1978. Actes du Congres, Vol. 1. Sofia, 1980. p. 100–1.
**Divett RT:** His chastening rod: cholera epidemics and the Mormons. **Dialogue J Mormon Thought** 1979;12(3):6–15
**Divett RT:** Medicine and the Mormons. An introduction to the history of Latter-Day Saint health care. Bountiful, Utah, Horizon, 1981. 222 p.
**Dixon B:** Spontaneous generation. **New Sci** 1981;91:553
**Dixon B:** Tissue therapy. **Br J Hosp Med** 1979 Nov;22(5):512
**Dixon LS:** Alchemical imagery in Bosch's Garden of Delights. Ann Arbor, UMI Research Press, 1981. xxii, 225 p. (Studies in the Fine Arts: Iconography, no. 2).
**Dixon RA** see **Lerner RM, ed**
**Dixon RB:** Hallelujah the pill? **Trans Action** 1970;8(1/2):44–9, 92
**Dizdar A:** Der türkische Arzt Serafeddin Sabuncuoğlu (1385–1472) und seine Verdienste um die Zahnheilkunde. Diss. Würzburg, 1981. 68 p.
**Djhnga S:** Perspectives in international neurosurgery: neurosurgery in Zaire. **Neurosurgery** 1983 Jul;13(1):95–7
**Djordjevic M:** [Surgeon and gerontologist Dr. Adolf L. Vischer: a contribution to Serbo-Swiss relations] (Serbo-Croat). **Srp Arh Celok Lek** 1979;107:1079–92
**Djordjevic S:** Dr. George N. Papanicolaou (13. V 1883--19. II 1962). **Srp Arh Celok Lek** 1983 May;111(5):699–703
**Djordjevic S:** Iz istorije rada na medicinskom jeziku i terminologiji u nas. **Srp Arh Celok Lek** 1981;109(12):1675–8
**Djordjevic SP:** Akademik prof. dr Dušan Borić (1. IX 1889-3. IX 1978). **Srp Arh Celok Lek** 1980 May;108(5):541–53
**Djordjevic SP:** General Prof. Dr. Vladimir S. Stanojević (3. III 1886 - 5. VI 1978. **Srp Arh Celok Lek** 1980 Mar;108(3):281–92
**Djordjevic SP:** Hilandarski medicinski kodeks. **Srp Arh Celok Lek** 1980 Sep;108(9):961–7
**Djordjevic SP:** Prof. dr Julije Budisavljević (2. III 1882--5. V 1981). **Srp Arh Celok Lek** 1983 Jun;111(6):861–4
**Djordjevic SP:** Prvo Otorinolaringološko odeljenje u Srbiji u Opštoj državnoj bolnici u Beogradu, i prvi otorinolaringolog dr Dragoljub Sraga. **Srp Arh Celok Lek** 1982 Oct;110(10):1245–60
**Djordjevic SP:** Sećanja na rad u vojnom sanitetu Srbije u toku II balkanskog

rata 1913. godine. Iz sećanja dr Julija Budisavljevinja i njegovih kolega iz Hirurške klinike u Insbruku. **Srp Arh Celok Lek** 1983 Jun;111(6):853–9
**Djordjevic SP:** Stampani radovi i prikazi bolesnika prvog otorhinolaringologa u Beogradu i Srbiji dr Dragoljuba Srage. **Srp Arh Celok Lek** 1982 Oct;110(10):1261–6
**Djuretic V:** Socijalno–zdravstvena i kulturno–prosvjetna aktivnost organa vlasti u bosni i hercegovini izmedju drugog i trećeg zasjedanja zavnobih–a. **God Drus Istor Bosne Herceg** 1976;21–27:239–67
**Djuric L:** Vojno–teritorijalna sanitetska služba na baniji u toku nor–a. **Vojnois Glas** 1971;22(3):191–206
**Dmitriev VG:** 'Nauka o babich'em dele' i ee avtor. (N. Maksimovich–Ambodik). **Feldsher Akush** 1984 Feb;49(2):50–1
**Do JP, Lacombe M:** Approche philosophique et historique à un enseignement des droits de l'homme. **Acta Med Leg Soc (Liege)** 1980;30(1):233–40
**Dobbs R, Robinson R, MacCarthy D, et al:** Douglas Gairdner, editor of the Archives 1964–79. **Arch Dis Child** 1979 Nov;54(11):813, 815–21
**Dobek R, Kolmsee P:** Maxim Zetkin--Arzt, Kriegschirurg und Kommunist. **Militaergesch** 1978;17(5):595–603
**Dobell AR:** John H. Gibbon, Jr. Part II. Personal reminiscenses. **Ann Thorac Surg** 1982 Sep;34(3):342–4
**Doberentz D** see **Schneider HJ**
**Doberneck RC, Kleinman R:** The surgical garb. **Surgery** 1984 Jun;95(6):694–8
**Dobiás J, Marek J:** Dr. Václav Treitz (1819–1872). K 110. výročí úmrtí a 125. výročí vybudování patologickoanatomického ústavu v Praze. **Cas Lek Cesk** 1983 Apr 1;122(13):405–7
**Dobiás J, Marek J:** Patologická anatomie na pražské univerzitě před rokem 1882. **Cesk Patol** 1984 Feb;20(1):1–10
**Dobin MA:** Veterinarnoe obrazovanie v Rossii. **Veterinariia** 1980 Jan;(1):76–7
**Dobísek K:** První čtyři primáři Pražského ústavu choromyslných. 2. Josef Pelikan. **Cesk Psychiatr** 1981 Dec;77(6):414–9
**Dobísek K:** První čtyři primáři pražského ústavu choromyslných. 3. Karl Damian Schroff, medicinae Doctor et Chirurgae magister. **Cesk Psychiatr** 1982 Feb;78(1):61–6
**Dobísek K:** První čtyři primáři pražského ústavu choromyslných. 4. Wenzel Friedrich Rilke, Medicinae et Chirurgiae doctor. **Cesk Psychiatr** 1983 Aug;79(4):275–82
**Dobísek K:** První čyři primáři pražského ústavu choromyslných. **Cesk Psychiatr** 1980 Aug;76(4):270–5
**Dobkin de Rios M:** Plant hallucinogens, sexuality and shamanism in the ceramic art of ancient Peru. **J Psychoactive Drugs** 1982 Jan–Jun;14(1–2):81–90
**Dobkin de Rios M, Cardenas M:** Plant hallucinogens, shamanism and Nazca ceramics. **J Ethnopharmacol** 1980 Sept;2(3):233–46
**Dobras W:** Cosmas und Damian in oberbayerischen Kirchen. **Pharm Ztg** 1981 Dec 24;126(52–53):2715–6
**Dobrescu AL:** Dermato–venerologia ieşeană in ultimii 20 de ani (1962–1982). **Rev Med Chir Soc Med Nat Iasi** 1983 Jan–Mar;87(1):156–66
**Dobrescu G** see **Munteanu A**
**Dobrin L:** Origin and evolution of the walkerette. **Mt Sinai J Med (NY)** 1980 Mar–Apr;47(2):172–4
**Dobrowolska J:** Wspomnienia z pracy w Warszawskim Towarzystwie Lekarskim. **Wiad Lek** 1980 Jun 1;33(11):927–30
**Dobrowolska–Nowak J:** XXV–lecie Studium Nauczycielskiego Szkół Medicznych w Waszawie. **Pieleg Polozna** 1982;(6):19–20
**Dobrý E:** 35 let transfúzní služby v CSSR. **Vnitr Lek** 1984 Sep;30(9):833–5
**Dobrzyniecki Z:** 'Dzieje Polskie' Jana Długosza jako źródło do dziejów medycyny w Polsce w XIV i XV w. **Arch Hist Med (Warsz)** 1981;44(3/4):265–76
**Dobson J, Walker RM:** Barbers and barber–surgeons of London: a history of the barbers' and barber–surgeons' companies. Oxford, Blackwell Scientific Publications for the Worshipful Company of Barbers, 1979. xix, 171 p.
**Dobson J:** Some associations of St. Thomas's Hospital with the Company of Barber–Surgeons of London. **St Thomas Hosp Gaz** 1981;79:73–8
**Dobson J** see **Hart GD, ed**
**Dobson M:** Marsh fever: the geography of malaria in England. **J Hist Geogr** 1980;6(4):357–89
**Dobson MJ:** Environments of disease and mortality in the New World and the Old World. **Soc Soc Hist Med Bull (Lond)** 1984 Dec;35:7–10
**Dobson C., et al:** Winchester in the 18th century. **Pharm Hist (London)** 1981 Apr;11(1):4–6
**Doby JM, Le Duigou D, Guiguen C, et al:** Le favus en Bretagne. Etude historique à propos d'un cas autochtone. **Ann Dermatol Venereol** 1983;110(11):925–31
**Doby T:** A tribute to Sven–Ivar Seldinger. **AJR** 1984 Jan;142(1):1–4
**Doby T:** History of cardiovascular catheterization. In: Congrès international d'histoire de la médecine, XXVe, Québec, 1976. Actes. Québec, 1977. p. 596–602.
**Dobyns HF:** Their number become thinned: native American population dynamics in eastern North America. Knoxville, University of Tennessee Press, 1983. 378 p.
**Dobzhansky T** see **Mayr E**
**Dochev D:** Razvitie i segashno sŭstoianie na Katedrata po klinichna laboratoriia. **Vutr Boles** 1981;20(6):15–22
**Dockery JL, Deal WB, Cuppy D, et al:** The University of Florida College of Medicine's alumni during the school's first twenty years. **J Fla Med Assoc** 1980 Mar;67(3):283–7
**Documents in Hopi Indian sexuality:** Imperialism, culture and resistance. **Radic Hist Rev** 1979 Spring/Summer;Spec:99–130
**Dodd BE:** Early work on the Rh factor including the finding of anti–E. **Vox Sang** 1984;47(6):449–51
**Dodd BE:** First tests with anti–human globulin on the red cells of patients suffering from haemolytic anaemia. **Vox Sang** 1984;46(3):183–4
**Dodds WR:** From medicine to president [Sun Yat Sen]. **Practitioner** 1981 Sep;225(1359):1342–3
**Dodge NN:** Population estimates for the Malay Peninsula in the nineteenth century, with special reference to the East Coast States. **Popul Stud** 1980;34(3):437–75
**Dodi Osnaghi L:** Aspetti della condizione operaia e della nocività attarverso le riviste di medicina del lavoro. **Ann Ist Giangiacomo Feltrinelli** 1979–80;20:231–83
**Dodin A:** Albert Calmette. Président de la Société de Pathologie Exotique. **Bull Soc Pathol Exot Filiales** 1983 May–Jun;76(3):211–4
**Dodin A:** Ephéméride 1884–1934–1984. **Bull Soc Pathol Exot Filiales** 1984 Jan–Feb;77(1):6–8
**Dodin A:** Historique des vaccinations. **Ther Umsch** 1983 Mar;40(3):184–6
**Dodin A:** Pourquoi les pandémies cholériques? **Bull Soc Pathol Exot Filiales** 1984 Mar–Apr;77(2):127–34
**Dodoens R:** Histoire des plantes. Traduction française, suivie du Petit recueil, auquel est contenue la description d'aucunes gommes et liqueurs etc., par Charles de l'Escluse (1557). Fac–similé avec introduction, commentaires et la concordance avec la terminologie scientifique moderne, par J.–E. Opsomer. Bruxelles, Centre National d'Histoire des Sciences, 1978. 78, 584 p. (Publications du Centre National d'Histoire des Sciences, V).
**Dodson G, Chothia C:** Fifty years of pepsin crystals [news] **Nature** 1984 May 24–30;309(5966):309
**Dodson G, Glusker JP, Sayre D, ed:** Structural studies on molecules of biological interest. A volume in honour of Professor Dorothy Hodgkin. Oxford, Clarendon, 1981. xviii, 610 p. Historical and biographical chapters by M. F. Perutz, D. Phillips, D. P. Riley, F. Welch, C. H. Carlisle, L. Pauling, T. You–chi, J. H. Robertson, D. F. Steiner, J. G. White, J. D. Dunitz.
**Dodt E:** Die erste Beschreibung des Knicks in der Dunkeladaptationskurve durch H. Aubert (1865). **Klin Monatsbl Augenheilkd** 1983 Jan;182(1):107–8
**Doederlein G:** Arzneiapplikationen in der antiken Chirurgie. **Dtsch Apoth Ztg** 1979 Jun 14;119(24):936–8
**Doenicke A:** Zum 200. Geburtstag von Friedrich Wilhelm Adam Sertürner. **Anaesthesist** 1983 Jun;32(6):239–41
**Doering D:** Die Logotherapie Viktor Emil Frankls. Köln, 1981, 272 p. (Kölner medizinhistorische Beiträge; Arbeiten der Forschungsstelle des Instituts für Geschichte der Medizin der Universität zu Köln, Band 19).
**Doern GB:** Science and technology in the nuclear regulatory process: the case of Canadian uranium miners. **Can Public Adm** 1978;21(1):51–82
**Doerner K:** Madmen and the bourgeoisie. A social history of insanity and psychiatry. (First published in German as Bürger und Irre, 1969.) Oxford, Basil Blackwell, 1981 vi, 361 p.
**Doerner WG:** Why does Johnny Reb die when shot? The impact of medical resources upon lethality. **Sociol Inq** 1983;53(1):1–15
**Doerr W:** Bedürfen wir einer Bio–Ethik? In Seidler E, Schott H, ed: Bausteine zur Medizingeschichte. Stuttgart, Steiner, 1984. p. 18–26.
**Doerr W:** Evolutionstheorie und pathologische Anatomie. **Verh Dtsch Ges Pathol** 1983;67:663–84
**Doerr W:** Gestalt theory and morbid anatomy. **Virchows Arch** [A] 1984;403(2):103–15
**Dogel' LV, Shalagina TL:** S. N. Davidenkov v Leningradskom gosudarstvennom institute usovershenstvovaniia vracheĭ. **Zh Nevropatol Psikhiatr** 1982;82(3):107–9
**Dogle NV:** Issledovaniia F. F. Erismana v Moskovskoĭ gubernii i sovremennost'. **Gig Tr Prof Zabol** 1983 Jul;(7):38–41
**Dohnal K:** Deset let léčeben pro dlouhodobě nemocné v CSR. **Cas Lek Cesk** 1984 Aug 17;123(33):1027–30
**Dohnany L:** Der Sanitätsdienst bei den Militär– und Partisaneneinheiten im Slowakischen Nationalaufstand des Jahres 1944. In International Congress of the History of Medicine. 26th, Plovdiv, 1978. Actes du Congress. Sofia, 1981. Volume II. p. 69–71.
**Dohnány L:** L. N. Tolsztoj az egészségügyröl. **Orv Hetil** 1982 Aug 8;123(32):1985–8
**Döhner L:** Die Kochschen Postulate und die Virologie. **Z Erkr Atmungsorgane** 1983;161(1):21–4
**Doĭchev S** see **Prakhov R**
**Doig FK:** Sexualverhalten im alten Peru. Lima, Kompaktos, 1979. 189 p.
**Doise W:** Dalla filosofia alla psicologia sociale. Una 'lettura' di Carlo Cattaneo. **Stor Crit Psicol** 1983;4(1):117–29
**Dôke T:** Yôan Udagawa: a pioneer scientist of early 19th century feudalistic Japan. **Jpn Stud Hist Sci** 1973;12:99–120
**Dolabjian ZL:** The International Congress on Electrocardiography: a brief history. **J Electrocardiol** 1984 Jul;17(3):307–8
**Dolan JA:** Nursing in society, a historical perspective. 14th ed. Philadelphia, Saunders, 1978. viii, 402 p.
**Dolan JP, Holmes GR:** Some important epochs in medicine. **South Med J** 1984 Aug;77(8):1022–6
**Dolan KD** see **Bean WB**
**Dolan–Leclerc C** see **Sutto C, ed**
**Dolenc A:** Medizinische Fragen und Aspekte des mittelalterlichen Totentanzes (Ein Beitrag aus Jugoslawien). **Beitr Gerichtl Med** 1980;38:347–52
**Dolenc M:** Bolezni vimena v ljudskem živinozdravništvu.

**Kronika (Yugosl)** 1980;28(1):26-31
**Dolenc M:** Medicinsko bukovništvo na Koroškem, Stajerskem in Prekmurju. **Cas Zgodovino Narodop** 1978;14(1):82-91
**Dolenc M:** 'Nova Gronat-Jabuka'-rokopisne ljudskomedicinske bukve iz 1751. leta. **Cas Zgodovino Narodop** 1980;16(2):311-21
**Dolev E:** [A twelfth century hospital in Jerusalem] (Heb). **Harefuah** 1980 Sep;99(5-6):136-7
**Doležal A:** Císařský řez na živé v Cechách v roce 1789. **Cesk Gynekol** 1982 Jul;47(6):436-41
**Dolgikh VP** see **Zadorozhnyĭ AA**
**Dolgoleev NF:** Brianskoe meditsinskoe uchilishche No. 1. **Feldsher Akush** 1983 Sep;48(9):41-2
**Dolgova SP:** Zapiski ochevidtsa o chumnom bunte v Moskve v 1771 godu. **Sov Arkh** 1976;(6):66-70
**Dolique R:** Sur les projets de masse pour l'Ecole de Pharmacie de Montpellier (en 1809) et la Faculté de Pharmacie (en 1966). **Bull Liaison Assoc Amis Mus Pharm Montp** 1979;4:1-6
**Doll EE:** Deborah Kallikak: 1889-1978, a memorial. **Ment Retard** 1983 Feb;21(1):30-2
**Doll R:** Back to Methuselah? Opportunities for preventive medicine. **Ir J Med Sci** 1983 Jan;152(1):64-8
**Doll R:** Clinical trials: retrospect and prospect. **Stat Med** 1982 Oct-Dec;1(4):337-44
**Doll R:** Green College, Oxford: its contribution to clinical medicine. **Br Med J [Clin Res]** 1982 Dec 18-25;285(6357):1805-6
**Doll R:** Smoking and death rates. **JAMA** 1984 Jun 1;251(21):2854-7
**Doll R:** The controlled trial. **Postgrad Med J** 1984 Nov;60(709):719-24
**Doll R:** The route back to Methusaleh. **Trans Hunter Soc** 1978-80;37-38:161-74
**Doll R:** William Michael Court Brown. In Dictionary of national biography, 1961-1970. Suppl. 8, 1981. p. 152-3.
**Dollfus MA:** Geschichte der Augenheilkunde. In Sournia JC, Martiny M, Poulet J, ed: Illustrierte Geschichte der Medizin. Salzburg, Andreas, 1980. Vol. 4, p. 1211-49
**Dolman CE:** Hideyo Noguchi (1876-1928): his final effort in West Africa. In: Congrès international d'histoire de la médecine, XXVe, Québec, 1976. Actes. Québec, 1977. p. 603-24.
**Dolman CE:** 'That impudent fellow Hill'. **Ann Sci** 1983 May;40(3):281-8
**Dolphin J:** Private ambulance. **Emerg Med Serv** 1977 Nov-Dec;6(6):155-6
**Dols MW:** The leper in medieval Islamic society. **Speculum** 1983 Oct;58(4):891-916
**Dols MW:** The second plague pandemic and its recurrences in the Middle East: 1347-1894. **J Econ Soc Hist Orient (Netherl)** 1979;22(2):162-89
**Dolzani C:** Un 'prelievo' di sangue adombrato in una poesia di Giovanni Pascoli? **Acta Med Hist Patav** 1982-83;29:25-8
**Domandi S:** Hohenheims De natura rerum. Eine Einführung in die geistige Welt des Paracelsus. **Salzburger Beitr Paracelsusforsch** 1984;23:61-88
**Domandl S:** Erziehung und Menschenbild bei Paracelsus. Anfänge einer verantwortungsbewussten Pädagogik. Wien, Notring, 1970. 144 p. (Salzburger Beiträge zur Paracelsusforschung, 9).
**Domandl S:** Paracelsus und Paracelsustradition in Salzburg (1524-1976). Ein Beitrag zur Kultur- und Zeitgeschichte. Wien, 1977. (Salzburger Beiträge zur Paracelsusforschung, 17), p. 9-44, 48-59. Includes O. Kostenzer: Das Paracelsusgrabmal in Stams, p. 45-48.
**Domandl S** see **Paracelsus-Forschung heute**
**Domandl S** see **Paracelsus in der Tradition**
**Domandl S, ed:** Paracelsus im Blickfeld heutiger wissenschaftsgeschichtlicher Betrachtung (ein Rundgespräch). Wien, 1974. 59 p. (Salzburger Beiträge zur Paracelsusforschung, 12). Contributions by L. Braun, A. W. Gutsch, V. Bazala, K. Goldammer, H. Goerke, W. Schneider, R. Blaser, KH Weimann, G. Harrer, A. Dyk.
**Domanowski GF** see **Spiegel AD**
**Dombrowski DA:** Vegetarianism and the argument from marginal cases in Porphyry. **J Hist Ideas** 1984 Jan-Mar;45(1):141-3
**Domen RE:** Paleopathological evidence of rheumatoid arthritis. **JAMA** 1981 Oct 23-30;246(17):1899
**Doménech Llabería E:** Las ideas de Pedro Mata en el campo de la psicologia de su tiempo. **Asclepio** 1980;32:137-50
**Doménech Llabería E** see **Corbella Corbella J**
**Domergue D:** [French sanitary services on the Ivory Coast.] (Fre). **Rev Fr Hist Outre Mer** 1979;65
**Domergue D:** La lutte contre la trypanosomiase en Côte d'Ivoire, 1900-1945. **J Afr Hist** 1981;22(1):63-72
**Domergue D:** Les vingt premières années de l'action sanitaire en Côte d'Ivoire. **Rev Fr Hist Outre Mer** 1978;65(1):40-63
**Dominguez XA:** Conocimientos médicos de los mayas, aztecas, tarascos y la herbolaria médica mexicana. **Guatem Indig** 1978;13(1/2):220-38
**Dominguez Alcon C:** Les soins et la profession d'infirmière en Espagne. Une étude de sociologie de la connaissance appliquée. Thèse de doct 3e cycle. Paris, Ecole des hautes études en sciences sociales, 1983. 437 p.
**Dominik K:** Dwusetna rocznica rozpoczecia na ziemiach polskich uniwersyteckich wykładów ze stomatologii. **Arch Hist Med (Warsz)** 1984;47(3):395-401
**Domino EF, ed:** PCP (phencyclidine): historical and current perspectives. Ann Arbor, Mich., NPP Books, 1981. xx, 537 p. Historical chapters by V. H. Maddox and D. A. McCarthy.
**Domínquez Alcón C:** Historia de la enfermería Catalana. **Rev Enferm** 1981 Dec-1982 Jan;5(42-43):57-8
**Dommisse J:** Gestational age--fact or fallacy? **S Afr Med J** 1980 Sep 13;58(11):449-50
**Don RS** see **Menczer LF**
**Donaghy RM:** The history of microsurgery in neurosurgery. **Clin Neurosurg** 1979;26:619-25
**Donahue EM:** Preserving history through oral history reflections. **J Gerontol Nurs** 1982 May;8(5):272-8
**Donahue MP:** Isabel Maitland Stewart's philosophy of education. **Nurs Res** 1983 May-Jun;32(3):140-6
**Donahue MP:** [Isabel Maitland Stewart's philosophy of education] (Jpn). **Kango Kyoiku** 1984 Oct;25(10):611-21
**Donahue P:** Nursing history in the undergraduate curriculum. **NLN Publ** 1983;(41-1935):38-44
**Donald AG:** James Higgins Mcintosh, M.D.: an archetype for the family practitioner? **J SC Med Assoc** 1980 May;76(5):245-8
**Donald KW:** Submarine escape breathing air. A review and analysis of animal and human experiments by the Royal Navy. **Bull Physiopathol Respir (Nancy)** 1979 Sep-Oct;15(5):739-54
**Donaldson JA:** Ars scientia mores. **Br Dent J** 1980 Dec 2;149(11):335-6
**Donaldson JA:** The life and times of Sidney Spokes. **J R Soc Med** 1981 Jul;74(7):537-9
**Donaldson JA:** The use of gold in dentistry: an historical overview. **Gold Bull** 1980;13(3):117-24; (4),160-5
**Donaldson PJ, Nichols DJ:** The changing tempo of fertility in Korea. **Popul Stud** 1978;32(2):231-50
**Donaldson PJ** see **Goldstein MS**
**Donat K:** Goethe aus ärztlicher Sicht. **Fortschr Med** 1982 May 13;100(18):852-8
**Donáth T:** Dr. Péterfi Tibor (1883-1953). **Orv Hetil** 1983 Dec 11;124(50):3061-2
**Donáth T:** Egy évforduló ürügyén. **Orv Hetil** 1984 Sep 30;125(40):2441-4
**Donáth T:** Nagy anatómusok jubileuma. **Orv Hetil** 1984 Feb 5;125(6):344-6
**Donato A:** Waring Historical Library, Charleston, South Carolina. **J SC Med Assoc** 1981 Dec;77(12):638
**Donato AK:** Waring historical library. **South Med J** 1980 Mar;73(3):369-70
**Donato L:** Twenty-five years of nuclear medicine. **J Nucl Med Allied Sci** 1981 Oct-Dec;25(4):195-200
**Donatucci CF:** In anticipation of Flexner. **Trans Stud Coll Physicians Phila** 1978 Jul;45(5):280-9
**Donchenko GP** see **Potemkin NT**
**Dondelinger R:** La tomodensitométrie des années 80. **Bull Soc Sci Med Grand Duche Luxemb** 1980;117(2):23-7
**Dondi RF:** Uno strumento chirurgico dimenticato: le forbici del Valtolini. **Ann Osp Maria Vittoria Torino** 1980 Jul-Dec;23(7-12):289-94
**Dondi RF:** Vicende dell'Universita' degli Studi di Ferrara nella seconda meta' dell'ottocento. **Ann Osp Maria Vittoria Torino** 1980 Jul-Dec;23(7-12):333-42
**Donegan H** see **Dockery JL**
**Dong Renda:** [Textual research - on records of ancient Chinese medical history.] (Chi). **Chin J Med Hist** 1981;11:82-3
**Dongier M:** Briquet and Briquet's syndrome viewed from France. **Can J Psychiatry** 1983 Oct;28(6):422-7
**Donizetti P:** I cacciatori d'ombre: storia della radiologia. Milano, Mondadori. 1978. 275 p.
**Donnellan WL:** Medicine and society in the sixteenth and seventeenth centuries: their influence on the life and work of Herman Boerhaave, 1668-1738. Ph.D. Diss., Northwestern University. Evanston, 1981. vii, 483 p.
**Donnelley S** see **Spicker SF, ed**
**Donnelly B:** The great famine and the literary imagination. **Studies** 1980;69(275-6):260-72
**Donnelly FK:** The destruction of the Sheffield School of Anatomy in 1835: a popular response to class legislation. **Trans Hunter Archaeol Soc** 1975;10:167-72
**Donnelly PG:** The origins of the Occupational Safety and Health Act of 1970. **Soc Probl** 1982 Oct;30:13-25
**Donner K** see **Blauth W**
**Donner L:** Ctyřicet let od vydání prvé české klinické hematologie. **Vnitr Lek** 1983 Feb;29(2):184-9
**Donner MW:** Der Weg der amerikanischen Radiologie zu ihrer jetzigen Stellung. **Radiologe** 1982 Jan;22(1):1-6
**Donoso V:** La industria farmacéutica en España. Oligopolio y colonización. **Rev Fom Soc** 1978;129:79-90;130:187-201;131:287-302
**Donovan AJ:** Surgical treatment of portal hypertension: a historical perspective. **World J Surg** 1984 Oct;8(5):626-45
**Donovan MG, Barrett DM:** Ureteral prostheses. **Semin Urol** 1984 Aug;2(3):158-66
**Donovan MG** see **Barrett DM**
**Dons R:** Projet d'établissement d'un jardin botanique à Saint-Gilles-Bruxelles en 1789. **Folkl Brabancon** 1980;227-228:310-22
**Dooley B** see **Hughes ES**
**Doolittle IG:** The effects of the Plague on a provincial town in the sixteenth and seventeenth centuries. **Med Hist** 1975 Oct;19(4):333-41
**Doona ME:** At least as well cared for ... Linda Richards and the mentally ill. **Image J Nurs Sch** 1984 Spring;16(2):51-6
**Doona ME:** District nurses celebrate nursing's past. **Mass Nurse** 1983 Nov;52(11):9
**Doona ME:** Nursing at Boston College: glimpses of the past. **Mass Nurse** 1983 Dec;52(12):6-7, 20
**Doona ME:** Nursing revisited: Mary Gerrin and the idea of nursing. **Mass Nurse** 1984 Feb;53(2):5
**Doona ME:** Nursing revisited: memories - Armistice and suffrage. **Mass Nurse** 1983 Nov;52(11):15

**Doona ME:** Nursing revisited: nursing at the winter's solstice. **Mass Nurse** 1983 Dec;52(12):1, 3
**Doona ME:** Nursing revisited: the Massachusetts General Hospital, Base Hospital No. 6. **Mass Nurse** 1984 Apr;53(4):9
**Doona ME:** Nursing revisited: the Worcester State Hospital and nursing. **Mass Nurse** 1984 Jan;53(1):19
**Doona ME:** Nursing revisited: the 1903 convention. **Mass Nurse** 1984 Jun;54(6):6
**Doona ME:** The cause is just: Mary E. P. Davis. **Mass Nurse** 1982 Jul;51(7):4–6
**Doona ME:** The Lucy Lincoln Drown Nursing History Society. **Mass Nurse** 1984 Feb;53(2):6
**Doona ME:** The Massachusetts Nurses Association eighty years young. **Mass Nurse** 1983 Feb;52(2):8–9
**Dooner H:** Los ultimos cincuenta años del Hospital San Borja. **Rev Med Chil** 1982 Jul;110(7):698–701
**Doornaert JP:** Vesalius. **Plast Reconstr Surg** 1984 Nov;74(5):726
**Dopis prof. J. Trapla prof. L. Havláskovi: Cesk Gynekol** 1983 Feb;48(1):51–5
**Dopp C** see **Schadewaldt H**
**Dopson L:** Celebrating 75 years. **Nurs Times** 1980 May 22;76(21):923–36
**Dopson L:** From workhouse to workshop. **Nurs Times** 1984 Aug 15–21;80(33):16–7
**Dopson L:** Hospital history in miniature. **Nurs Times** 1982 Jun 23–29;78(25):1078–9
**Dopson L:** One hundred years on. **Nurs Times** 1982 May 12–18;78(19):781–2
**Dopson L:** 'Sick Kids'—100 years on. **Nurs Times** 1983 Mar 30–Apr 5;79(13):8–9
**Dopson L:** The cut-throat world of nursing politics - 18th century-style. **Nurs Times** 1984 Apr 25–May 1;80(17):19–20
**Dopson L:** The new breed of nurse historian. **Nurs Times** 1984 Sep 19–25;80(38):16–7
**Dopson L:** The QA museum. **Nurs Times** 1981 Nov 11–17;77(46):1974
**Dopson L:** Volunteer nurses. One. VADs at war. **Nurs Times** 1984 Aug 1–7;80(31):36–8
**Dopson L:** 100 years of ophthalmic nursing. **Nurs Times** 1981 Jun 11;77(24):1043–4
**Dor J:** Jean Bobon et la psychopathologie du langage. **Acta Psychiatr Belg** 1983 May–Jun;83(3):197–206
**Dorazilová V** see **Mířejovský P**
**Dorche J:** Une institution lyonnaise: les religieuses au service des malades dans les hospices civils de Lyon 1500–1950. **Lyon Pharm** 1981 Apr;32(3):155–60
**Dorczak W:** Ostre zatrucia w latach 1972—1977 we Wrocławiu. **Pol Tyg Lek** 1979 Aug 13;34(33):1309–10
**Dore MM** see **McConnell NF**
**Dörffel EW, Held F, Oelssner W:** Zum 30. Jahrestag der Gründung der Deutschen Demokratischen Republik. Die Bedeutung Fritz Gietzelts für die Radiologie und Geschwulst-bekämpfung. **Radiobiol Radiother (Berl)** 1979 Oct;20(5):621–6
**Döring GK:** Ist das Kondom heute besser als sein Ruf? **Fortschr Med** 1980 Jan 31;98(4):113–7
**Dorjee P, Richards E:** Cures & concepts of Tibetan medicine. **Tibetan Med** 1981;2:1–83
**Dorkins HR:** Suxamethonium—the development of a modern drug from 1906 to the present day. **Med Hist** 1982 Apr;26(2):145–68
**Dorokhov II:** Iz istorii kafedry patologicheskoĭ anatomii Rostovskogo meditsinskogo instituta. **Arkh Patol** 1984;46(1):69–73
**Dorokhov II:** Sravnitel'nyĭ amaliz sektsionnykh materialov Rostova-na-Donu za dovoennyĭ i poslevoennyĭ periody. **Arkh Patol** 1980;42(8):29–33
**Dorolle P** see **Beer H**
**Dorosevich AE:** Professor Petr L'vovich Poznanin—predstavitel' moskovskoĭ shkoly patologoanatomov. **Arkh Patol** 1983;45(1):79–80
**Dorozhkova IR** see **Kochemasova ZN**
**Dörr-Zegers O** see **Janzarik W ed**
**d'Ors A:** Cuatro precursores de la ciencia española de nuestro tiempo. **Rev Med Univ Navarra** 1980 Dec;24(4):55–60
**Dorsche HH von, Dittrich HM:** Die Diabetesforschung in Greifswald im 19. Jahrhundert und am Beginn des 20. Jahrhunderts in ihrer Bedeutung für die Diabetologie. **Anat Anz** 1982;152(5):435–48
**Dorsey JM:** University Professor John M. Dorsey. Detroit, Wayne State University Press, 1980. 282 p.
**Dorsz-Szteke E:** Nauczanie medycyny na Pomorzu Zachodnim w i poł. XVIII wieku. **Arch Hist Med (Warsz)** 1980;43(3):305–16
**Dorsz-Szteke E, Maciejewska-Dorsz K:** O cholerze w Szczecinie w i poł. xix wieku. **Wiad Lek** 1981 Oct 1;34(19):1657–9
**Dorsz-Szteke E, Maciejewska-Dorsz K:** O opiece nad psychicznie chorymi w Szczecinie w XIX wieku. **Wiad Lek** 1980 Sep 15;33(18):1509–10
**Dorsz-Szteke E, Maciejewska-Dorsz K:** Pomoc wojskowej służby zdrowia dla ludności cywilnej Pomorza Zachodniego w latach 1945–1946. **Wiad Lek** 1981;34(7):615–8
**Dortmund EK:** Daniel Paul Schreber: a case study of private fate as public possibility. **Res Stud** 1978;46(3):141–55
**Dose K:** Ernst Haeckel's concept of an evolutionary origin of life. **Biosystems** 1981;13(4):253–8
**Dosne Pasqualini C** see **Pavlovsky S**
**Dossetti M:** La demografia delle valli Valdesi dal 1686 al 1800. **Boll Stori Bibliogr Subalpino** 1981;79(2):535–602
**Dostatni P, Cordoliani A:** L'histoire de la médecine et la recherche documentaire automatisée. **Hist Sci Med** 1984;18(1):25–32
**Doszkoos TE, Rapp BA, Schoolman HM:** Automated information retrieval in science and technology. **Science** 1980 Apr 4;208(4439):25–30
**Dotter CT:** Two decades of transluminal angioplasty. An overview. **J Mal Vasc** 1982;7 Suppl 4:357–61
**Dotz W:** Albrecht Dürer. Depictions of facies as expressions of personality. **Am J Dermatopathol** 1981 Spring;3(1):59–65
**Dotz W:** Jan Vermeer and his alopecic models. **Am J Dermatopathol** 1983 Jun;5(3):245–8
**Dotz W:** Jean Paul Marat. His life, cutaneous disease, death, and depiction by Jacques Louis David. **Am J Dermatopathol** 1979 Fall;1(3):247–50
**Dotz W, Berliner N:** Rhinophyma. A master's depiction, a patron's affliction. **Am J Dermatopathol** 1984 Jun;6(3):231–5
**Dotz W:** St. Anthony's fire. **Am J Dermatopathol** 1980 Fall;2(3):249–53
**D'où nous viennent la d'emence précoce et la schizophrénie?: Acta Psychiatr Belg** 1982 May–Jun;82(3):243–76
**Doual A** see **Brulin F**
**Doubrovsky S** see **Stambolian G**
**Doughty J:** The dentist in comic postcards. **Br Dent J** 1984 Mar 10;156(5):186–7
**Douglas A:** Promises to keep. **Thorax** 1984 Jul;39(7):481–6
**Douglas DM:** Sir James Rögnvald Learmonth. In Dictionary of national biography, 1961–1970. Suppl. 8, 1981. p. 638–40.
**Douglas H:** Burke and Hare. **Br Hist Illus** 1978–79;5(5):32–43
**Douglas J** see **Collingridge D**
**Dourson ML, Stara JF:** Regulatory history and experimental support of uncertainty (safety) factors. **Regul Toxicol Pharmacol** 1983 Sep;3(3):224–38
**Douville R:** Jacques Dugay. In Dictionary of Canadian biography, 1701 to 1740. Volume 2, 1969. p. 202–3.
**Dow D:** The archives of the Greater Glasgow Health Board. In Checkland O, Lamb M, ed: Health care as social history; the Glasgow case. Aberdeen, Aberdeen University Press, 1982. p. 158–69.
**Dowd AM** see **Reyman TA**
**Dowdall GW** see **Marshall JR**
**Dowling HF:** City hospitals. The undercare of the underprivileged. Cambridge, Mass., London, Harvard University Press, 1982. vii, 245 p.
**Dowling J:** Smallpox and literature in eighteenth-century Spain. **Stud Eighteenth Cent Cult** 1979;9:59–77
**Downey-Anderson C:** The 'Coggins Affair': desegregation and Southern mores in Madison County, Florida. **Fla Hist Q** 1981 Apr;59:464–72
**Downey-Prince EL** see **Casey AE**
**Downie AW:** Sir Samuel Phillips Bedson. In Dictionary of national biography, 1961–1970. Suppl. 8, 1981. p. 86–7.
**Downing J:** An outline of the history of dental mechanics (1). **Dent Tech** 1984 Mar;37(3):17–8 (cont)
**Downing PB:** Bargaining in pollution control. **Policy Stud J** 1983;11(4):577–86
**Downing R:** Historical review of pancreatic islet transplantation. **World J Surg** 1984 Apr;8(2):137–42
**Downs F, Meshad S, Krieger D:** The anguish of the veterans. **Cent Mag** 1979;12(4):27–36
**Downs RB:** Landmarks in science, Hippocrates to Carson. Littleton, Colo., Libraries Unlimited, 1982. 305 p.
**Downs WG:** A new look at yellow fever and malaria. **Am J Trop Med Hyg** 1981 May;30(3):516–22
**Downs WG:** History of epidemiological aspects of yellow fever. **Yale J Biol Med** 1982 May–Aug;55(3–4):179–85
**Downs WG:** The Rockefeller Foundation virus program: 1951–1971 with update to 1981. **Annu Rev Med** 1982;33:1–29
**Doyle CC:** The power of not thinking: a jocular toothache cure. **Ky Folkl Rec** 1983;29(1–2):24–9
**Doyle JS:** Corrigan on fever. **J Ir Coll Physicians Surg** 1980 Jul;10(1):44–5
**Doyle WP:** James Crawford (1682–1731), M. D. Edinburgh, University of Edinburgh, [1981]. 10 p. (Scottish men of science).
**Doyle WP:** Thomas Charles Hope M.D., F.R.S.E., F.R.S. (1766–1844). Edinburgh, University of Edinburgh, 1982. [12 p.] (Scottish Men of Science).
**Dr. Alexis Carrel and tissue culture: JAMA** 1984 Jul 6;252(1):44–5
**Dr. Frederick Banting getting out of town: Can Med Assoc J** 1984 May 1;130(9):1215–23
**Dr. Guggenbühl's Hospice for cretins on the Abendberg in Switzerland (1840): Pediatrics** 1983 Mar;71(3):452
**Dr. Harold P. Rusch and the Wisconsin Clinical Cancer Center: Wis Med J** 1979 Jun;78(6):96–7
**Dr. Marcolino Gomes Candau (30.05.1911—23.01.1983): Rev Bras Malariol Doencas Trop** 1982;34:119–22
**Dr. med. Willy Bircher-Schwarzenbach (1898–1970):** s. l., s. n., 1970?. 28 p.
**Dr. Zdeněk Fencl 1922–1981: Folia Microbiol (Praha)** 1982;27(5):285–94
**Drábek P:** Casopis českého lékárnictva a jeho předchudci. **Cesk Farm** 1982 May;31(3–4)85–96
**Drábek P:** Dějiny Státního ústavu pro kontrolu léčiv (1918–1983). II. Vývoj Státního ústavu pro kontrolu léčiv (1952–1983). **Cesk Farm** 1984 Jun;33(5):201–9
**Drabik R:** Die Entwicklung des Leistungspotentials der Krankenhausmedizin im 20.Jahrhundert in Deutschland. Diss., Universität Düsseldorf. Düsseldorf, 1982. 98 p.
**Drachman VG:** Female solidarity and professional success: the dilemma of women doctors in late nineteenth-century America. **J Soc Hist** 1982;15(4):607–19
**Drachman VG:** The Loomis trial: social mores and obstetrics in the mid-nineteenth century. In Reverby S, Rosner D, ed: Health care in

America. Philadelphia, Temple University Press, 1979. p. 67–83.
**Draganova T** see **Bakalova L**
**Dragic D:** Drug tito i njegov doprinos razvoju vojnomedicinske misli. **Vojnosanit Pregl** 1980 May;37:54–7
**Dragic D:** Hronologija značajnijih dogadaja za sanitetsku službu u toku NOR-a 1941–1945. **Vojnosanit Pregl** 1981 Nov–Dec;38(6):423–8
**Dragic D, Anic N:** Nastanak i razvoj sanitetskih jedinca sa hronologijom dogadjaja iz sanitetske službe u narodnooslobodilačkom ratu. **Vojnois Glas** 1981;32(1):181–94
**Dragic D:** Sanitetska služba u Bosni i Hercegovini u vreme održavanja Prvog kongresa partizanskih lekara. **Vojnosanit Pregl** 1983 Sep–Oct;40(5):386–94
**Dragic M:** Dr. Janko i hjegove zasluge za nauku, književnost i prosvety u Srbiji. **Srp Arh Celok Lek** 1981 Aug;109(8):1101–8
**Dragic M:** Dr. Vladan Djordjević i zakon o zaštiti narodnog zdravlja u Srbiji iz 1881. godine. **Srp Arh Celok Lek** 1982 Jun;110(6):791–8
**Dragic M:** Higijenske prilike u Beogradskoj tvrdjavi i Beogradu 1829. godine (prema putopisu Ota Dubislava Pirha). **Srp Arh Celok Lek** 1982 Jul–Aug;110(7–8):951–7
**Dragic M:** Povodom stogodišnjice osnivanja časopisa 'Zdravlje' dr Milana Jovanović-Batuta. **Srp Arh Celok Lek** 1980 Apr;108(4):391–5
**Dragic M:** Razvoj i pioniri socijalno-medicinskih ideja u Srbiji. **Srp Arh Celok Lek** 1982 Nov;109(11):1543–53
**Dragic M:** Zdravstvene prilike u Beogradu za vreme okupacije u prvom svetskom ratu i spanski grip 1918–1919. godine. **Srp Arh Celok Lek** 1980 Sep;108(9):969–74
**Dragin O** see **Protic M**
**Dragsted PJ:** Avendelse af edb i sundhedsvaesenet--det historiske forløb i Danmark. **Nord Med** 1981 Oct;96(10):235–6
**Drahota Z:** Třicet let Fyziologického ústavu CSAV. **Cesk Fysiol** 1984;33(4):289–92
**Drake CG:** Aneurysm surgery: past, present, and future. **Int Anesthesiol Clin** 1982 Summer;20(2):1–9
**Drake CW** see **Abrams RA**
**Drake DF:** The cost of hospital regulation. **Proc Acad Polit Sci** 1980;33(4):45–59
**Drake M** see **Charlton C**
**Drake S** see **Levere TH, ed**
**Drane JF** see **Rosenbaum M, ed**
**Drazan JG:** The nightmare: a checklist of the world literature to 1976. Palo Alto, R & E Research Associates, 1979.
**Dreifuss JJ:** W. L. Gaines, précurseur du concept de réflexe neuroendocrine. **Gesnerus** 1981;38(3/4):331–8
**Dreiling DA:** The first fifty years--a history of evolution of the American College of Gastroenterology as a Society for Clinical Gastroenterology. **Am J Gastroenterol** 1983 Mar;78(3):138–9
**Drell MJ:** Hermine Hug-Hellmuth, a pioneer in child analysis. **Bull Menninger Clin** 1982 Mar;46(2):139–50
**Dressendörfer W:** Drogeneinkaufsmengen einer Münchener Apotheke um die Mitte des 15. Jahrhunderts. Beiträge zur Geschichte des Arzneimittelhandels im Mittelalter. 1. Mitteilung. **Beitr Gesch Pharm** 1982;31(14):105–7
**Dressendörfer W:** Französische Apothekendarstellungen aus dem 13. Jahrhundert. **Beitr Gesch Pharm** 1980;31(8):57–61
**Dressendörfer W:** Spätmittelalterliche Arzneitaxen des Münchner Stadtarztes Sigmund Gotzkircher aus dem Grazer Codex 311. Ein Beitrag zur Frühgeschichte des süddeutschen Apothekenwesens. Pattensen/Hannover, Wellm, 1978. 327 p. (Würzburger medizinhistorische Forschungen, 15). Also Diss. (Pharm) München.
**Dresslerová I** see **Krahulec I**
**Drew GR:** The Dr. Charles R. Drew stamp. **J Afro-Am Hist Geneol Soc** 1981;2(4):139–42
**Drew-Bear A:** Face-painting scenes in Ben Jonson's plays. **Stud Philol** 1980 Fall;47(4):338–401
**Drews FH, Guenter M:** Die herrschaftliche Apotheke. 400 Jahre Pharmazie in Celle. Celle, Löwen-Apotheke, 1980. 65 p.
**Drews J:** Ein Kratersturz ins Unbewusste. Zur Konstruktion von Traum und Tagtraum [in] Arno Schmidts Roman 'Kaff auch Mare Crisium' (1960). **Psyche (Stuttg)** 1981 Dec;35(12):1103–21
**Drews RC:** The Barraquer experience with intraocular lenses. 20 years later. **Ophthalmology (Rochester)** 1982 Apr;89(4):386–93
**Drey RE:** A dated slipware drug jar. **Pharm Hist (London)** 1975 May;5(1):1
**Drey RE:** Drug jars from hospitals and from royal pharmacies. **Pharm Hist (London)** 1971 Dec;2(3):11–12
**Drey RE:** Drug jars from the Convent of St. Saviour of Jerusalem. **Pharm Hist (London)** 1984;14(1):11–2
**Drey RE:** Les vases de pharmacie de l'Hôpital majeur de Novare. **Rev Hist Pharm (Paris)** 1979 Dec;26(243):259–62
**Drey RE:** Trois familles nobles de Florence et leur vases de pharmacie. **Rev Hist Pharm (Paris)** 1982 Sep;29(254):177–9
**Dreyer WP:** The history of periodontology in South Africa. **Tydskr Tandheelkd Ver S Afr** 1981 Apr;36(4):271–2, 274–5
**Dreyfus G:** Médecine scientifique et art médical. Une controverse à propos de Claude Bernard. **Sem Hop Paris** 1983 May 19;59(20):1569–71
**Dreznik A, Falk RE, Howard V, et al:** Hyperthermia as a treatment for neoplasia. **Can J Surg** 1982 Nov;25(6):603–8
**Driedger L** see **Currie R**
**Driesch A von den:** Falkenheilkunde--ein historischer Uberblick. **Tierarztl Prax** 1983;11(1):53–66
**Driesch A von den:** Hastividyarnava, eine assamesische Handschrift über Elefantologie. **Ethnomedizin** 1978–79;5(3–4):341–8
**Drinnan AJ:** Odontophilately. **NY State Dent J** 1980 Apr;46(4):173
**Drinnan AJ:** Odontophilately. **NY State Dent J** 1980 Feb;46(2):73
**Drinnan AJ:** Odontophilately (Abul Kasim). **NY State Dent J** 1979 Aug–Sep;45(7):332
**Drinnan AJ** see **Froriep R**
**Driver WJ:** Forty-fifth anniversary of social security. **Soc Secur Bull** 1980;43(8):3–5
**Drobizhev VZ:** Organizatsiia ucheta estestvennogo dvizheniia naseleniia SSSR v 1917–1926 gg. **Vestn Mosk Univ Ser 8 Istor** 1978;3:27–33
**Drobizhev VZ:** Stanovlenie politiki sovetskogo gosudarstva v oblasti estestvennogo dvizheniia naseleniia. **Vestn Mosk Univ Ser 8 Istor** 1981;1:17–26
**Drobizhev VZ** see **Vdovin AI**
**Drössler K:** Robert Koch--auch ein Pionier der Immunitätsforschung? **Allerg Immunol (Leipz)** 1982;28(1):13–20
**Droz R:** Aperçu sur les dentistes strasbourgeois aux XVIIIe et XIXe siècles. In Livet G, Schaff G, ed: Médecine et assistance en Alsace, XVIe–XXe siècle. Strasbourg, Istra, 1976. p. 209–23.
**Droz R:** Dentistes et dentisteries à Strasbourg au XVIIIe siècle. **Annu Soc Amis Vieux Strasb** 1977;7:29–51
**Drozdowski P, Fortuna D, Nieniewska M, et al:** Dr med. Małgorzata Dominik (1941–1979). **Psychiatr Pol** 1980 Sep–Oct;14(5):549–54
**Drozdowski P, Kokoszka A:** Psychoterapia według Antoniego Kępińskiego. **Przegl Lek** 1983;40(12):877–80
**Drucker E** see **Tobach E**
**Druett H:** David Willis Wilson Henderson. In Dictionary of national biography, 1961–1970. Suppl. 8, 1981. p. 504–6.
**Drummond CG:** Adam Drummond of Megginch, surgeon-apothecary. **Pharm Hist (London)** 1971 Dec;2(3):3–5
**Drummond CG:** Charles Wilson (1804–1884). In Passmore R, ed: Proceedings of the Royal College of Physicians of Edinburgh Tercentenary Congress, 1981. Edinburgh, Royal College of Physicians of Edinburgh, 1982. p. 199–203.
**Druon M** see **Bernard J**
**Drury MI:** Diabetes in pregnancy--Matthews Duncan revisited. **Ir J Med Sci** 1984 Apr;153(4):144–51
**Drury MI:** The history of medicine in Dublin. **Q J Med** 1981 Autumn;50(200):485–92
**Drury PJ** see **Black MM**
**Drury RA:** The golden ages of histological technique. **Malays J Pathol** 1979 Aug;2:33–7
**Drury VW:** Foxglove and chips. **J R Coll Gen Pract** 1984 Mar;34(260):129–39
**Druzhinina LV:** Razvitie detskikh doshkol'nykh uchrezhdeniĭ v SSSR. **Pediatriia** 1982;(9):3–7
**Drygas A:** Uprawnienia rektorów Uniwersytetu Krakowskiego w zakresie kontroli aptek krakowskich w XV i XVI wieku w świetle źródeł i prezekazów pośrednich. **Arch Hist Med (Warsz)** 1983;46(2):183–203
**Drygas A:** Walka z partactwem aptekarskim i medycznym. **Arch Hist Med (Warsz)** 1981;44(3/4):329–43
**Drysdale A:** The regional equalization of health care and education in Syria since the Ba'thi revolution. **Int J Middle East Stud** 1981;13(1):93–111
**Du Toit DA:** Die hospitaal as 'n burokrasie. **Curationis** 1983 Jun;6(2):11–8
**du Toit ML:** A mission doctor's experiences in West Africa. **S Afr Med J** 1984 Nov 17;66(20):775–8
**Duan Yishan:** [Examples of special literary problems of ancient medical classics.] (Chi). **Chin J Med Hist** 1981;11:120–3
**Dub O:** 100 let od narození George N. Papanicolaua. **Cas Lek Cesk** 1983 Oct 28;122(43):1337
**Dubarry JJ:** J. Vincent Laborde et son procédé de réanimation par tractions rythmées de la langue; la survie neuro-musculaire après décapitation. **Hist Sci Med** 1980;14(1):77–82
**Dubarry JJ:** Le curriculum universitaire d'un étudiant en médecine en U.R.S.S. **Hist Sci Med** 1980;14:383–6
**Dubb A:** Medical philately. Doctors in politics. **S Afr Med J** 1980 Aug 23;58(8):326–9
**Dubb A:** Medical philately: Robert Koch (1843–1910) the man, his germ and history. **Adler Mus Bull** 1984 Mar;10(1):16–22
**Dubb A:** Medical philately: sport and medicine. **S Afr Med J** 1981 Jul 25;60(4):144–6
**Dubb A:** Medical philately: The pen and the scalpel -- the story of medicine and literature. **S Afr Med J** 1979 Nov 17;56(21):847–50
**Dube CB, Kansal CM:** Diseases due to deficiencies of vital principles in the body. **Indian J Hist Sci** 1981;16(1):104–7
**Dube WF:** Medieval medicine in middle high German epics. Ph.D. Diss. Indiana University. [Bloomington], 1981. 295 leaves.
**Dübec I:** Jordemødre i retshistorisk belysning. **Historie** 1973;10(3):337–90
**Dübeck I:** Jordemødre og jura: en retshistorisk studie. **Tidsskr Rettsvitenskap** 1973;(5):729–57
**Duberman MB:** 'Writhing bedfellows': 1826. Two young men from antebellum South Carolina's ruling elite share 'extravagant delight'. **J Homosex** 1980–81 Fall–Winter;6(1–2):85–101
**Dubin JL, Roney JL:** The public welfare project on aging. **Public Welf** 1971;29(4):439–46
**Dubinin NP, ed:** Nauchno-teoreticheskaia konferentsiia 'Perspektivy razvitiia genetiki v SSSR v svete soedineniia uspekhov nauchno-tekhnicheskoĭ revoliutsii s preimushchestvami sotsializma', Moscow?, 1976?
**Dubois A:** La lèpre au Congo avant les sulfones. **Bull Seances Acad R Sci Outre Mer** 1965;11(2):640–51
**Dubois CG:** Isomorphisme de deux constructions imaginaires: le grand

oeuvre alchmique et la grand oeuvre de Dieu. **Aust J Fr Stud** 1980;17(1):73–85
**Dubois E:** How to face the plague: some seventeenth-century practices. **Newsl Soc 17th Century Fr Stud** 1980;2:29–36
**Dubos R:** Hattie Elizabeth Alexander. In: Notable American women. The modern period. Cambridge, Mass., Belknap-Harvard Univ. Press, 1980. 4:10–1.
**Dubos R:** Peyton Rous. **J Exp Med** 1979 Oct 1;150(4):735–7
**Dubost C:** First successful resection of an aneurysm of the abdominal aorta with restoration of the continuity by a human arterial graft. **World J Surg** 1982 Mar;6(2):256–7
**Dubovsky H:** John Keats (1795–1821)--poet, physician and tuberculosis patient. **S Afr Med J** 1981 Jun 6;59(24):875–8
**Dubovsky H:** Robert Koch (1843–1910)--the man and his work. **S Afr Med J** 1982 Nov 17;Spec No:3–5
**Dubovsky H:** Tuberculosis and art. **S Afr Med J** 1983 Nov 12;64(21):823–6
**Dubowitz V:** History of muscle disease. In Rose FC, Bynum WF, ed: Historical aspects of the neurosciences. New York, Raven, 1982. p. 213–22.
**Dubrov AP** see **Durinian RA**
**Dubrulle C:** Soins infirmiers, rétrospective, perspectives. **Soins** 1980 Jul 5–20;25(13–14):67–72
**Duburcq P:** Ambroise Paré et l'odontologie. **Chir Dent Fr** 1982 Mar–Apr;52(151–3):21–38
**Duburcq P:** Odontoiatria del passato. Ambroise Paré e l'odontoiatria. I. 'Io l'ho curato d Dio l'ha guarito'. **Dent Cadmos** 1982 Jun–Jul;50(6–7):75–9, 87–9
**Duburcq P:** Odontoiatria del passato. Ambroise Paré l'odontoiatria. III. **Dent Cadmos** 1982 Aug;50(8):83–5
**Duburq P:** Ambroise Paré et l'odontologie. **Chir Dent Fr** 1982 Mar 18;52(150):41–9 contd.
**Ducable G:** L'art de guérir en Mésopotamie ancienne. **Hist Sci Med** 1982;16(1):23–7
**Ducable G** see **Maitre AM**
**Ducatillon J:** Polémiques dans la collection hippocratique. Lille, Atelier de Reproduction des Thèses; Paris, Librairie Honore Champion, 1977. 382 p. (Thèse, Paris, 1976).
**Ducatillon J** see **Grmek MD, ed**
**Ducharme J:** Marie-Catherine-Françoise Céloron. In Dictionary of Canadian biography, 1801 to 1820. Volume 5, 1983. p. 174.
**Duchatel F:** Insertion vélamenteuse du cordon ombilical et hémorragie de Benckiser. **Hist Sci Med** 1982;16(3):185–92
**Duchatel F:** L'auscultation obstétricale de Philippe Le Goust au monitorage foetal. **Hist Sci Med** 1982;16(1):37–47
**Duchatel F:** Paul Portal (1630? - ler juillet 1703): un accoucheur méconnu du XVIIe siècle. **Hist Sci Med** 1980;14:407–18
**Duchemin A:** F. V. Raspail, l'apôtre du camphre. **Bull Liaison Assoc Amis Mus Pharm Montp** 1979;4:7–14
**Duchesne R:** La bibliothèque scientifique de l'Abbé Léon Provancher. **Rev Hist Am Fr** 1981;34(4):535–56
**Duchesne R:** Magasin de curiosités ou musée scientifique? Le musée d'histoire naturelle de Pierre Chasseur à Québec (1824–1854). **HSTC** 1983 May;24(7 No 2):59–79
**Duchesne R:** Science et société coloniale: les naturalistes du Canada français et leurs correspondants scientifiques (1860–1900). **HSTC Bull** 1981;5:99–139
**Duchesneau F:** De Boerhaaave et Baglivi à Haller: vers un concept 'analytique' de la structure organique. **Arch Int Hist Idees** 1982;95:103–40
**Duchesneau F:** De l'épigenèse au vitalisme (C. F. Wolff et Blumenbach). **Arch Int Hist Idees** 1982:95:312–60
**Duchesneau F:** G. E. Stahl: antimécanisme et concept d'organisme. **Arch Int Hist Idees** 1982;95:1–31
**Duchesneau F:** G. E. Stahl: Antimécanisme et physiologie. **Arch Int Hist Sci (Paris)** 1976;26:3–26
**Duchesneau F:** La physiologie des lumières. Empirisme, modèles et théories. The Hague, Martinus Nijhoff, 1982. xxi, 611 p. (International Archives of the History of Ideas, no. 95).
**Duchesneau F:** La théorie physiologique de Haller: irritabilité et sensibilité. **Arch Int Hist Idees** 1982;95:141–70
**Duchesneau F:** Le système mécaniste de Friedrich Hoffmann. **Arch Int Hist Idees** 1982;95:32–64
**Duchesneau F:** Monades, molécules organiques et ordre physiologique: de Maupertuis et Buffon à Haller. **Arch Int Hist Idees** 1982;95:235–311
**Duchesneau F:** Sensibilité et structure organique: l'alternative Whytt-Haller. **Arch Int Hist Idees** 1982;95:171–234
**Duchesneau F:** Vers une théorie analytique de l'organisme (Bichat). **Arch Int Hist Idees** 1982;95:431–76
**Dückert M** see **Gehrke H**
**Duckett SJ:** Structual interests and Australian health policy. **Soc Sci Med** 1984;18(11):959–66
**Ducommun C:** Paul Dubois (1848–1918). Sa place dans l'histoire de la psychothérapie. **Gesnerus** 1984;41(1/2):61–99
**Ducourtioux JC** see **Marain Y**
**Ducrocq F:** Des thérapeutes du corps médical. **Penelope** 1981;(5):45–9
**Duda M, Serý Z:** Geschichte und Stand der Chirurgie der Hiatushernien und der Refluxkrankheit des Osophagus. **Dtsch Z Verdau Stoffwechselkr** 1980;40(5):177–83
**Duda M, Serý Z:** Historie a současnost chirurgie hiátových hernií a refluxní nemoci jícnu. **Cesk Gastroenterol Vyz** 1979 Sep;33(6):332–41
**Duda R:** Spitalul comunal Tutova, Jud. Vaslui 75 ani de activitate. **Rev Med Chir Soc Med Nat Iasi** 1983 Oct–Dec;87(4):667–8
**Dudchenko MA:** Aleksandr Mikhaĭlovich Shumlianskiĭ. **Klin Med (Mosk)** 1983 Jan;61(1):114–6
**Dudgeon JA:** Immunization in times ancient and modern. **J R Soc Med** 1980 Aug;73(8):581–6
**Dudley HA:** From Edinburgh, an academic surgeon. **Aust NZ J Surg** 1981 Jun;51(3):247–50
**Dudrick SJ** see **Rhoads JE**
**Dudziński W:** Choroba i zgon króla Augusta III Sasa. **Wiad Lek** 1981 Sep 1;34(17):1479–84
**Dudziński W:** Choroba i zgon króla Michała Korybuta Wiśniowieckiego. **Wiad Lek** 1979 Jan 1;32(1):55–8
**Dudziński W:** Choroby i zgon króla Aleksandra Jagiellończyka. **Wiad Lek** 1981 Jul 15;34(14):1227–32
**Dudziński W:** Choroby i zgon króla Jana Kazimierza. **Wiad Lek** 1980 Jan 1;33(1):61–5
**Dudziński W:** Choroby i zgon króla Władysława Jagiełły. **Wiad Lek** 1981 May 15;34(10):859–61
**Dudziński W:** Choroby i zgon króla Zygmunta Augusta. **Wiad Lek** 1981 Aug 15;34(16):1411–6
**Dudziński W:** Choroby i zgon króla Zygmunta Starego. **Wiad Lek** 1981 Aug 1;34(15):1317–22
**Dudziński W:** Choroby zgon króla Jana Olbrachta. **Wiad Lek** 1981 Jul 1;34(13):1131–5
**Dudziński W:** Epigramaty i sentencje łacińskie na tematy medyczne. **Pol Tyg Lek** 1980 Dec 1;35(48):1883–6
**Dudziński W:** Medicinalia w pierwszej ojczystej gazecie 'Merkuriuszu Polskim'. **Wiad Lek** 1981 Oct 1;34(19):1653–5
**Dudziński W:** Smierć króla Kazimierza Jagiellończyka. **Wiad Lek** 1981 Jun 15;34(12):1041–4
**Dudziński W:** Smierć króla Władysława Warneńczvka. **Wiad Lek** 1981 Jun 1;34(11):953–5
**Duerr HP, ed:** Der Wissenschaftler und das Irrationale. Band 1. Beiträge aus Ethnologie und Anthropologie. Frankfurt am Main, Syndikat, 1981. 692 p.
**Duerr HP, ed:** Der Wissenschaftler und das Irrationale. Band 2. Beiträge aus Philosophie und Psychologie. Frankfurt am Main, Syndikat, 1981. 679 p.
**Dufek WM:** Der Internist Otto Naegeli, 1871–1938. Zürich, Juris Druck, 1983. 76 p. (Zürcher Medizingeschichtliche Abhandlungen, Neue Reihe, Nr. 160).
**Duff W:** An essay on original genius and its various modes of exertion in philosophy and the fine arts, particularly in poetry (1767). Facsimile. Ed. by J. L. Mahoney. Delmar, New York, Scholars' Facsimiles and Reprints, 1978. ix, 296 p.
**Duffy J:** American perceptions of the medical, legal, and theological professions. **Bull Hist Med** 1984 Spring;58(1):1–15
**Duffy J:** An unnoticed copy of Hippocrates' prognosticon. **Scriptorium** 1982;36(1):89–90
**Duffy J:** Haven Emerson. In Dictionary of American Biography, Suppl. 6, 1956–1960. p. 192–3, 1980.
**Duffy J:** Medicine in the West: an historical overview. **J West** 1982 Jul;21(3):5–14
**Duffy J:** Rudolph Matas. In Dictionary of American Biography, Suppl. 6, 1956–1960. p. 434–5, 1980.
**Duffy J:** School vaccination: the precursor to school medical inspection. **J Hist Med Allied Sci** 1978 Jul;33(3):344–55
**Duffy J:** The American medical profession and public health: from support to ambivalence. **Bull Hist Med** 1979 Spring;53(1):1–22
**Duffy JM:** Stephanus the philosopher: lectures on the Prognosticon of Hippocrates. Critical text and translation. Ph. D. Diss., State University of New York, Buffalo, 1975. xxi, 449 p.
**Duffy RJ, Liles BZ:** A translation of Finkelnburg's (1870) lecture on aphasis as 'asymbolia' with commentary. **J Speech Hear Disord** 1979 May;144(2):156–68
**Duffy S:** The origin of speeches: Inherit the Wind, Irving Stone and the Scopes trial. **Am Notes Queries** 1983 Sep–Oct;22(1–2):14–7
**Duffy TP:** Sir William Osler revisited. **Yale J Biol Med** 1980 May–Jun;53(3):219–24
**Duffy J, ed:** Ventures in world health; the memoirs of Fred Lowe Soper. Washington, Pan American Health Organization, 1977. 365 p. (Scientific Publ. No. 355).
**Duffy JT, et al:** 'Days of darkness – days of hope' [special issue on the mentally retarded]. **RI Hist** 1981 Nov;40:107–59
**Dufour A:** Geschichte der Urologie. In Sournia JC, Martiny M, Poulet J, ed: Illustrierte Geschichte der Medizin. Salzburg, Andreas, 1980. Vol. 4. p. 1429–81.
**Dufour D, Péron Y:** Vingt ans de mortalité au Québec: les causes de décés, 1951–1971. Montréal, Presses de l'Université de Montréal, 1979. 204 p. (Collection 'Démographie canadienne, 4). 204 p.
**Dufour P, Hamelin J:** Pierre de Sales Laterrière. In Dictionary of Canadian biography, 1801 to 1820. Volume 5, 1983. p. 735–8.
**Dufourmentel C:** Reconstruction du sein après mastectomie. Historique, état actuel, perspectives d'avenir. **Bull Acad Natl Med (Paris)** 1981 Jan;165(1):103–8
**Dugački V:** 'Hrvatsko društvo za čuvanje narodnog zdravlja' i njegov časopis 'Zivot i zdravlje'. **Lijec Vjesn** 1982 May;104(5):208–10
**Dugacki V:** Le traitement des maladies oculaires dans la medecine populaire yougoslave. In International Congress of the History of Medicine. 26th, Plovdiv, 1978. Actes du Congress. Sofia, 1981. Volume II. p. 85–8.
**Dugački V:** Počeci organizirane skrbi za slijepe u Hrvatskoj. Prosvećeno Medunarondoj godini invalida. **Lijec Vjesn** 1981 Nov;103(11):531–3

**Dupâquier J, Hollingsworth TH, Köllmann W:** Bibliographie internationale sur les crises de mortalité. In Charbonneau H, Larose A, ed: The great mortalities: methodological studies of demographic crises in the past. Liège, Belgium, Ordina Editions, 1980. 257–70.
**Dupâquier J:** De l'animal à l'homme: le mécanisme autorégulateur des populations traditionnelles. **Rev Inst Sociol** 1972;2:177–211
**Dupâquier J, Lachiver M:** Du contresens à l'illusion technique, suivi d'une réponse de John Knodel à Jacques Dupâquier. **Ann Econ Soc Civilis** 1981;36(3):489–92
**Dupâquier J:** Etude comparative des données sur la fécondité dans 25 monographies concernant le bassin parisien à la fin du XVIIe siècle et au début du XVIIIe siècle. In Leridon H, Menken J, ed: Fécondité naturelle, U. T. E. S. P., 1979, p. 409–39.
**Dupaquier J:** L'analyse statistique des crises de mortalite. In Charbonneau H, Larose A, ed: The great mortalities: methodological studies of demographic crises in the past. Liège, Belgium, Ordina Editions, 1980. p. 83–112.
**Dupâquier J, Fauve-Chamoux A, Grebenik E, ed:** Malthus past and present. London; New York, Academic Press, 1983. xix, 416 p. Contributions by A. Béjin, Y. Breton, Y. Charbit, L. Devance, A. Digby, M. W. Flinn, R. E. Frisch, M. Godelier, L. Gordon, P. Guillaume, G. Heinsohn, T. H. Hollingsworth, P. A. Jewell, N. Keyfitz, R. Keynes, H. Le Bras, M. Perrot, F. Rausky, M. Rebérioux, R. Remond, F. Ronsin, G. R. Searle, B. Stapleton, O. Steiger, P. Vallin, E. Van de Walle, A. Waterman, J. Wolff, E. A. Wrigley, V. Wynne-Edwards.
**Dupâquier J** see **Chaunu P**
**Dupaquier M:** La famille Bertillon et la naissance d'une nouvelle science sociale: la démographie. **Ann Demogr Hist (Paris)** 1983;:293–310
**Dupèbe J** see **Margolin JC**
**Duplenko KF, Leonenko NA, Kogan VIa, et al:** Organizatsiia istoriko-meditsinskikh isslevaniĭ v Ukrainskoĭ SSR. **Sov Zdravookhr** 1981;(5):57–9
**Duplenko IûK:** Die russisch-deutschen naturwissenschaftlichen Kontakte in der Diskussion über die Zellmechanismen des Alterns und der Lebensdauer. **Z Alternsforsch** 1980;35:239–43
**Duplenko IuK:** Istoki sovremennogo razvitiia fiziologii stareniia na Ukraine. **Fiziol Zh** 1984 Jan-Feb;30(1):102–6
**Duplenko IuK** see **Chebotarev DF**
**DuPlessis RB, Friedman SS:** 'Woman is perfect': H. D.'s debate with Freud. **Feminist Stud** 1981;7(3):407–30
**Dupont J:** At long last 'The TMC Story: premieres'. **EITV** 1984 Mar;16(3):52–4
**DuPont RL** see **Martin WR**
**Dupré J:** Les enfants abandonnés à l'hospice civil et militaire de Châteauroux de 1805 à 1820 inclusivement. **Bull Soc Fr Hist Hop** 1980;(41):9–16
**Dupré P:** Les stations bainéaires de la côte du Calvados: Genèse et développement. **Ann Normandie** 1983;33(3):239–58
**Dupree AH:** The rise and fall of the American establishment. **Minerva** 1984 Spring;22(1):116–24
**Dupuis M:** Etienne-Jules Marey, le photographe du mouvement. **Sci Avenir** 1980;400:95–100
**Dupuis M** see **Audet-Lapointe P**
**Dupuy WL** see **Holstein J**
**Duquénois P:** Devenir des plantes médicinales et des médications végétales aux XVIIIe et XIXe siècles sous l'influence de la chimie moderne. In Livet G, Schaff G, ed: Médecine et assistance en Alsace, XVIe-XXe siècle. Strasbourg, Istra, 1976. p. 227–39.
**Durand J, Hampartzoumian A:** Les manuscrits de la faculté de médecine de Montpellier. **Connaiss Pays Occident** 1981;49:26–31
**Durand M** see **Huard P**
**Durant JR:** Innate character in animals and man: a perspective on the origins of ethology. In C. Webster, ed: Biology, medicine and society 1840–1940. Cambridge, Cambridge University Press, 1981. p. 157–92.
**Durbin PT, ed:** A guide to the culture of science, technology, and medicine. New York, Free Press, 1980. xl, 723 p. Contributions by A. Thackray, C. W. Pursell, G. H. Brieger, A. C. Michalos, C. Mitcham, H. T. Engelhardt, J. Gaston, L. Aiken, D. Crane.
**Durcan J:** The Penrose Cancer Hospital. The first thirty-five years, 1941–1976. Colorado Springs, Century One Press, 1976. 120 p.
**Durey M:** The return of the plague. British society and the cholera 1831–2. Dublin, Gill and Macmillan, 1979. 269 p.
**Durfee HA** see **Smith JH, ed**
**Durinian RA, Dubrov AP:** Leninskaia teoriia otrazheniia i metodologicheskie problemy fiziologii i refleksoterapii. **Vestn Akad Med Nauk SSSR** 1981;(4):41–5
**Durkin JT, ed** see **Chambers RW**
**Durley MS:** Dr. Edmund Bailey O'Callaghan, his early years in medicine, Montreal, 1823–1828. **Study Sess Can Cathol Hist Assoc** 1980;47:23–40
**Durling R:** Corrigenda and addenda to Diels' Galenica: II. codices miscellanei. **Traditio** 1981;37:373–81
**Durling RJ:** Konrad Gessner's Briefwechsel. In: Schmitz R, Krafft F, ed: Humanismus und Naturwissenschaften. Boppard, Boldt, 1979? p. 101–111. (Beiträge zur Humanismusforschung, Band VI).
**Durling RJ:** Lexicographical notes on Galen's pharmacological writings. **Glotta** 1979;57(3–4):218–24
**Durling RJ:** Lexicographical notes on Galen's writings. **Glotta** 1981;59:108–16
**Durling RJ:** Lexicographical notes on Galen's writings (part II). **Glotta** 1980;58(3–4):260–5
**Durling RJ** see **Teigen PM, ed**
**Durnin E:** Cancels unite world against malaria. **Scalpel Tongs** 1981;25:49
**Durr M:** Contribution à l'étude démographique d'une paroisse de l'ancien Tournugeois: Préty-Lacrost-La Truchère, 1678–1752 (3e partie). **Soc Amis Arts Sci Tournus** 1978;77:92–112
**Durrant GR:** Griffith Evans--a pioneer in tropical medicine. **Br Army Rev** 1980;65:66–8
**Durrany KS, Uddin Siddiqui T:** Al-Adwiyat al-Qalbiya. **Stud Hist Med** 1980 Mar;4(1):29–38
**Durrany KS:** Ibn Sinā's concept of man. **Stud Hist Med** 1982 Sep;6(3):161–94
**Dürrigl T:** Počeci auroterapije u Jugoslaviji. **Reumatizam** 1982;29(2):37–9
**Dushmanov SKh, Dushmanova TB:** Zdravookhranenie Ural'skoĭ oblasti. **Sov Zdravookhr** 1983;6:66–9
**Dushmanova TB** see **Dushmanov SKh**
**Dusmuratov MD, Semeniuta AIa:** Travmatologiia i ortopediia v Uzbekskoĭ SSR (istoriia, sostoianie i perspektivy razvitiia). **Ortop Travmatol Protez** 1982 Dec;(12):4–7
**Dussaud MD** see **Aiache JM**
**Dussault G, Sheiham A:** Medical theories and professional development. The theory of focal sepsis and dentistry in early twentieth century Britain. **Soc Sci Med** 1982;16(15):1405–12
**Dusseau JL:** Tertium Quid: a third something in a muddied puzzle. **Perspect Biol Med** 1982 Winter;25(2):238–53
**Dustan A, ed:** In memoriam Wallace O. Fenn 1893–1971. [S.l., s.n.] 1979? [127] p.
**Dustin P:** Cinquante années de progrès des sciences biologiques. **Rev Med Brux** 1984 Mar;5(3):115–9
**Dustin P:** Die pathologische Anatomie. In Sournia JC, Martiny M, Poulet J, ed: Illustrierte Geschichte der Medizin. Salzburg, Andreas, 1980. Vol. 6. p. 2103–47.
**Dustmann HO, Ebel V:** Darstellungen von Fussdeformierungen und deren Behandlung in der Kunst. In KF Schlegel, ed: Der Körperbehinderte in Mythologie und Kunst. Stuttgart, New York, Thieme, 1983. p. 41–56.
**Dustmann HO:** Das Bildnis des Amputierten in der Kunst. In KF Schlegel, ed: Der Körperbehinderte in Mythologie und Kunst. Stuttgart, New York, Thieme, 1983. p. 57–87.
**Dutescu B** see **Babes V**
**Duthoit JP:** La Marquise de Sévigné et quelques aspects de la thérapeutique médicale au XVIIe siècle. Lille, 1980. 110, 8 p.
**Dutkevich IG** see **Golovin GV**
**Dutkevich IG** see **Uglov FG**
**Dutkiewicz M:** Ubiór służby zdrowia Wojska Polskiego w okresie Królestwa Polskiego i wojny 1830–1831 roku. **Arch Hist Med (Warsz)** 1981;44(2):157–62
**Dutkiewicz M, Felchner A, Kuna M:** Wystawa czasowa 'Starodruki medyczne w zbiorach łodzkich bibliotek naukowych' zorganizowana w dziesieciolecie Muzeum Polskiej Wojskowej Słuzby Zdrowia WAM. **Arch Hist Med (Warsz)** 1982;45(1–4):93–100
**Dutkiewicz M:** Z dziejów munduru i symboli słuzby zdrowia Wojska Polskiego. **Arch Hist Med (Warsz)** 1984;47(1):85–90
**Dutra FR:** Electrical burns of the skin. Medicolegal investigation. **Am J Forensic Med Pathol** 1981 Dec;2(4):309–12
**Dutton JC:** Causes of Soviet adult mortality increases. **Sov Stud** 1981;33(4):548–59
**Duve C de:** Le lysosome: essai d'une esquisse historique et évolutive. **Arch Biol (Liege)** 1980;91(2):175–91
**Duvoisin RC** see **Plaitakis A**
**Duxbury ML:** Nursing in neonatology. In Smith GF, Smith PN, Vidyasagar D, ed: Historical review and recent advances in neonatal and perinatal medicine. [Chicago?], Mead Johnson Nutritional Division, 1983. Vol. I. p. 107–22.
**Duxbury ML** see **Smith GF**
**Dwivedi RB** see **Mishra SK**
**Dwork D:** Elsie Strang L'Esperance. In: Notable American women. The modern period. Cambridge, Mass., Belknap-Harvard Univ. Press, 1980. 4:417–9.
**Dwork D:** Health conditions of immigrant Jews on the Lower East Side of New York: 1880–1914. **Med Hist** 1981 Jan;25(1):1–40
**Dwork D:** Koch and the Colonial Office: 1902–1904; the second South Africa Expedition. **NTM** 1983;20(1):67–74
**Dwork D:** Sophia Josephine Kleegman. In: Notable American women. The modern period. Cambridge, Mass., Belknap-Harvard Univ. Press, 1980. 4:398–400.
**Dworkin AG, Stephen RC:** Mexican-American adolescent inhalant abuse: a proposed Model. **Youth Soc** 1980;11(4):493–506
**Dwudziestolatka: Pieleg Polozna** 1982;(3):21
**Dwudziesty drugi zeszył poświęcony zagadnieniom lekarskim okresu hitlerowskiej okupacji: Przegl Lek** 1982;39(1–3):1–267
**Dwudziesty trzeci zeszyt poświęcony zagadnieniom lekarskim okresu Hitlerowskiej okupacji: Przegl Lek** 1983;40(1):1–247
**Dwyer E:** Mental health care in early twentieth century Indiana and the limits of reform. **Indiana Med Hist Q** 1983 Mar;9(1):23–7
**Dwyer JM:** Thirty years of supplying the missing link. History of gamma globulin therapy for immunodeficient states. **Am J Med** 1984 Mar 30;76(3A):46–52
**Dwyer JT, Oiso T:** Changing food patterns. **Prog Clin Biol Res** 1981;77:509–25
**Dyck P:** Lumbar nerve root: the enigmatic eponyms. **Spine** 1984 Jan-Feb;9(1):3–6
**Dyck RG:** Health care planning in Slovenia. **Pap Slov Stud** 1977;105–23
**Dye D, Tarpey K:** Maternity and infant care services in

Chicago--retrospectus: our legacy, our challenge. In Smith GF, Smith PN, Vidyasagar D, ed: Historical review and recent advances in neonatal and perinatal medicine. [Chicago?], Mead Johnson Nutritional Division, 1983. Vol. II. p. 139–58.
**Dye D** see **Smith GF**
**Dye NS:** History of childbirth in America. **Signs** 1980;6(1):97–108
**Dye NS:** Mary Breckinridge, the Frontier Nursing Service and the introduction of nurse-midwifery in the United States. **Bull Hist Med** 1983 Winter;57(4):485–507
**Dyer JA:** Corneal contact lenses in perspective 1948–1981. **Contact Intraocular Lens Med J** 1982 Jan–Mar;8(1):3–8
**Dyer L:** Rock or sand? **Physiotherapy** 1982 Jun;68(6):177–81
**Dyer NA:** The artificial eye. **Aust J Ophthalmol** 1980 Nov;8(4):325–7
**Dyerberg J** see **Bang HO**
**Dyhouse C:** Working-class mothers and infant mortality in England, 1895–1914. **J Soc Hist** 1978;12(2):248–67
**Dyhouse C:** Working-class mothers and infant mortality in England, 1895–1914. In C. Webster, ed: Biology, medicine and society 1840–1940. Cambridge, Cambridge University Press, 1981. p. 73–98.
**Dyk A** see **Domandl S, ed**
**Dyk A** see **Paracelsus-Forschung heute**
**Dyk A** see **Paracelsus in der Tradition**
**Dykhno MM** see **Kochemasova ZN**
**Dymarskiĭ LIu:** K istorii razvitiia khirurgicheskogo lecheniia raka molochnoĭ zhelezy, nachinaia s drevnego Egipta i do nashikh dneĭ. **Khirurgiia (Mosk)** 1981 Apr;(4):111–6
**Dymarskiĭ LIu:** Taĭna 'Virsavii', kartiny Rembrandta. **Vopr Onkol** 1984;30(10):90–101
**Dymond D:** The famine of 1527 in Essex. **Local Popul Stud (Matlock)** 1981 Spring;26: 29–40
**Dynamite doctors: Practitioner** 1980 Feb;224(1340):119–20
**Dyrskjøt I:** Familien Friis har haft tandklinik i Hjørring i 100 år. **Tandlaegebladet** 1983 Jan;87(1):29–32
**Dyrvik S:** Marriage and social norms: a study of Etne, 1715–1801. **Tidsskr Samfunnsforskning** 1970;11(4):285–300
**Dyshlebyi PS** see **Sytnik KM**
**Dyskin EA, Klishov AA:** O roli Voenno-meditsinskoĭ akademii im. S. M. Kirova v podgotovke vysokokvalifitsirovannykh kadrov anatomov i gistologov SSSR. **Arkh Anat Gistol Embriol** 1983 Mar;84(3):90–6
**Dyskin EA:** Stanovlenie i razvitie prepodavaniia anatomii v Peterburge v XVIII v. **Arkh Anat Gistol Embriol** 1984 Feb;86(2):96–101
**Dželajlija S, Debijadi R:** Razvoj sanitetske službe u RV i PVO. **Vojnosanit Pregl** 1982 Nov–Dec;39(6):408–11
**Dzhalalova KM** see **Danilishina EI**
**Dzhamadze ShV:** Tuberkuleznomu sanatoriiu im. V. I. Lenina v Gul'ripshi - 80 let. **Probl Tuberk** 1983 Feb;(2):73–4
**Dzhanelidze MB:** O 'Lechebnoĭ knige-karabadine' i ee avtore Zaze Panaskerteli-Tsitsishvili (k 550-letiiu so dnia rozhdeniia). **Sov Zdravookhr** 1981;(5):67–8
**Dzhankov I, Vitkov M:** Petdeset godini raĭonen nauchnoizsledovatelski veterinaren institut v Stara Zagora. **Vet Med Nauki** 1982;19(5):3–6
**Dzhoshibaev SD:** Razvitie serdechnoĭ khirurgii v Kirgizii. **Zdravookhr Kirg** 1980 Mar–Apr;2:7–11
**Dzhuraev IN** see **Tashmukhamedov IR**
**Dziak A:** Zainteresowania ortopedyczne niektórych chirurgów polskich wieku XIX. **Chir Narzadow Ruchu Ortop Pol** 1980;45(1):95–102
**Dzierzykray-Rogalski T:** Un cas de la lèpre à un stade avancé découvert dans la nécropole musulmane de Kôm El-Dikka, à Alexandrie. **Afr Bull** 1978;28:140–6
**Dziob JS:** Ten years before 'M A S H'. **RI Med J** 1982 Dec;65(12):499–506

# E

**Eades CG** see **Martin WR**
**Eadie MJ:** A. W. Campbell: Australia's first neurologist. **Clin Exp Neurol** 1980;17:27–35
**Eagle M** see **Ross JM**
**Eagle MN:** The epistemological status of recent developments in psychoanalytic theory. In R.S. Cohen, L. Laudan, ed: Physics, philosophy and psychoanalysis. Dordrecht, D. Reidel, 1983. p. 31–55.
**Eakins WA:** Thomas Crawford, regimental medical officer in the Crimea, 1855. **Ulster Med J** 1982;51(1):46–51
**Eamon W:** Arcana disclosed: the advent of printing, the books of secrets tradition and the development of experimental science in the sixteenth century. **Hist Sci** 1984;22(pt 2):111–50
**Eamon W:** The tale of Monsieur Gout. **Bull Hist Med** 1981 Winter;55(4):564–7
**Earl JW:** The role of the men's hall in the development of the Anglo-Saxon superego. **Psychiatry** 1983 May;46(2):139–60
**Earlam R, Cunha-Melo JR:** Benign oesophageal strictures; historical and technical aspects of dilatation. **Br J Surg** 1981 Dec;68(12):829–36
**Earle C:** Environment, disease and mortality in early Virginia. **J Hist Geogr** 1979;5(4):365–90
**Earle CV:** Environment, disease, and mortality in early Virginia. In Tate, TW, Ammerman, DL, ed. The Chesapeake in the seventeenth century: essays on Anglo-American society (Chapel Hill, U. of North Carolina Press for the Institute of Early American History and Culture, 1979):96–125.
**Earle DP:** A history of malaria and its ironies. **Trans Am Clin Climatol Assoc** 1979;90:1–26
**Earle DP:** An eighteenth century suggestion for peritoneal dialysis? **Int J Artif Organs** 1980 Mar;3(2):67–8
**Earle RM:** Prevention of alcoholism in the United States and the National Council on Alcoholism: 1944–1950. **Int J Addict** 1982 May;17(4):679–702
**Earles MP:** Cutting the tapestry. **Pharm Hist (London)** 1972 Sep;2(4):1–4
**Earles MP:** Four eighteenth century experimental studies of crude curare. In Hickel E, Schröder G, ed: Neue Beiträge zur Arzneimittelgeschichte. Festschrift für Wolfgang Schneider zum 70. Geburtstag. Stuttgart, Wissenschaftliche Verlagsgesellschaft, 1982. p. 175–84.
**Earles MP:** The Pharmacopoeia Londinenis 1618. A new look at an old problem. **Pharm Hist (London)** 1982 Aug;12(2):4–5
**Early S** see **Witt M**
**Early history of the South Dakota Dental Society: Northwest Dent** 1983 Jul–Aug;62(4):17–22
**Earwicker R:** A study of the BMA-TUC Joint Committee on Medical Questions, 1935–1939. **J Soc Policy** 1979;8:335–56
**Earwicker R:** Miners' medical services before the First World War: the South Wales coalfield. **Llafur J Soc Stud Welsh Labour Hist** 1981;3(2):39–52
**Earwicker R:** The emergence of a medical strategy in the Labour Movement 1906–1919. **Soc Soc Hist Med Bull (Lond)** 1981 Dec;29:6–9
**Easlea B:** Witch hunting, magic, and the new philosophy: an introduction to debates of the scientific revolution, 1450–1750. Brighton, Sussex, Harvester Press, 1980. xii, 283 p.
**Easley EB:** The female medical student in the 30's. **NC Med J** 1983 May;44(5):307–8
**East-west discord over the prince of scholars [Avicenna]: New Sci** 1981;91:395
**Eastaugh SR** see **Battistella R**
**Eastcott HH** see **Vecht RJ**
**Easterlin RA:** Population issues in American economic history: a survey and critique. **Res Econ Hist** 1977;(supplement 1):131–58
**Eastman JW:** 'Doctors' orders': the American medical profession and the origins of automobile design for crash protection, 1930–1955. **Bull Hist Med** 1981;55(3):407–24
**Easton L:** Hermann Johannes Pfannenstiel (1862–1909). **Br J Obstet Gynaecol** 1984 Jun;91(6):538–41
**Eastwood B:** Directory of audio-visual sources. History of science, medicine, and technology. New York, Science History Publications, 1979. 41, [108] p.
**Eastwood BS:** Cosmology and physiology in Galenic visual theory: Hunayn Ibn Ishaq. **Trans Stud Coll Physicians Phila** 1980 Dec;5(2 no 4):276–83
**Eastwood BS:** Galen on the elements of olfactory sensation. **Rheinisches Mus Philol** 1981;124:268–90
**Eastwood BS:** The elements of vision: the micro-cosmology of Galenic visual theory according to Hunayn Ibn Ishaq. Philadelphia, American Philosophical Society, 1982. 59 p. (Transactions of the American Philosophical Society, Vol. 72, pt. 5).
**Eastwood BS:** The place of medicine in a hierarchy of knowledge: the illustration in Lyon Palais des Arts, ms. 22, f. lr, from the eleventh century. **Sudhoffs Arch** 1982;66(1):20–37
**Eaton J** see **Rosenthal PA**
**Eaves TC** see **Kimpel BD**
**Eaves Walton PM, et al.:** The 250th and 100th anniversaries of the Royal Infirmary of Edinburgh and the 100th anniversary of the Simpson Memorial Maternity Pavilion. Edinburgh, Royal Infirmary of Edinburgh, 1979. 53 p.
**Eavey RD:** First operation under ether anesthesia: a correction. **N Engl J Med** 1983 Oct 20;309(16):990–1
**Ebbert A, et al:** [Reminiscences and appreciations of Madeline E. Stanton] Contributions by L. G. Wilson, L. G. Stevenson, T. R. Forbes, S. B. Nuland, F. Gyorgyey, J. Bylebyl, G. L. Geison, W. Le Fanu, G. Robinson. **J Hist Med Allied Sci** 1981 Apr;36(2):129–50
**Ebbs JH:** The Canadian Paediatric Society: its early years. **Can Med Assoc J** 1980 Dec 20;123(12):1235–7
**Ebel H:** Notes toward a psychohistory of the movies. **Psychoanal Rev** 1983 Spring;70(1):121–4
**Ebel V** see **Dustmann HO**
**Ebel H, et al:** The psychohistory of history: a symposium. **J Psychohist** 1981 Winter;8(3):259–79
**Eberhard W** see **Trüb CL**
**Eberhard Altenähr (4. 12. 1940 bis 5. 4. 1981): Verh Dtsch Ges Pathol** 1981;65:561–70
**Eberhardt-Müller R:** Pankreasforschung im XVII. Jahrhundert. Diss., Bonn. Hatten, 1982. 151 p.
**Eberle MW:** Lucas Cranach's cupid as honey thief paintings: allegories of syphilis? **Com J Mediev Renaiss Stud** 1979–80;10:21–30
**Ebers GC, Stewart J:** In defence of Osler. **J R Soc Med** 1982 Dec;75(12):989
**Eberson F:** Apostles and prophets. Medicine for society's ills. Hicksville, Exposition Press, 1977. xi, 106 p.
**Eberson F:** Early physicians of the West. Forerunners of modern medicine. St. Petersburg, Valkyrie Press, 1979. ix, 140 p.
**Eberson F:** Eradication of hookworm disease in Florida. **J Fla Med Assoc** 1980 Aug;67(8):736–42
**Eberson F:** Profiles, giants in social medicine. St. Petersburg, Valkyrie Press, 1980. 103 p.
**Eberson FW:** Kentucky biographical notebook: Dr. Frederick Ridgely, 1757–1824. **Filson Club Hist Q** 1983;57(2):223–5
**Eberstadt N:** America and world hunger. **Wilson Q** 1981;5(3):138–46
**Eberstein IW, Pol LG:** Mexican-American ethnicity, socioeconomic status, and infant mortality: a county-level analysis. **Soc Sci J** 1982;19(2):61–71
**Ebert RV:** The First Aspen Conference in retrospect. **Chest** 1984 Jun;85(6

Suppl):2S-3S
**Ebling E** see **Ebling FJ**
**Ebling FJ:** Homage to Paul Langerhans. **J Invest Dermatol** 1980 Jul;75(1):3-5
**Ebling FJ, Ebling E:** The contribution of Paul Langerhans (1847-1888) to tuberculosis research. **Wiss Beitr Martin Luther Univ Halle Wittenberg** 1983;5-R80:261-72
**Ebner H:** Die Lungenabteilung des Pflegeheimes der Stadt Wien-Lainz im Wandel der Zeit. **Wien Med Wochenschr** 1980 Feb 29;130(4):147-8
**Ebnöther D** see **Farley J**
**Ebon M:** Why did Hitler hate the Jews? **Midstream** 1979;25(8):19-24
**Eccles A:** Obstetrics and gynaecology in Tudor and Stuart England. Kent, Kent State University Press, 1982. 145 p.
**Eccles JC, Gibson WC:** Sherrington: his life and thought. Berlin, New York, Springer International, 1979. xv, 269 p.
**Echemendia V:** Zum 100. Jahrestag der Entdeckung des Vektors des Gelbfiebers durch den kubanischen Gelehrten Carlos J. Finlay. **Z Gesamte Hyg** 1983 Jan;29(1):35-6
**Echkardt G:** Die Gründung der psychologischen Anstalt in Jena (1923). **Wiss Z Friedrich Schiller Univ (Gesellsch)** 1973;22(4):517-59
**Eckardt G:** Einleitung: Bemerkungen zum Anliegen psychologiegeschichtlicher Forschung. In Eckardt G, ed: Zur Geschichte der Psychologie, Berlin, VEB Deutscher Verlag der Wissenschaften, 1970. p. 7-20.
**Eckardt G, ed:** Zur Geschichte der Psychologie. Berlin, VEB, 1979. 128 p.
**Eckart W:** 'Machiavellus Medicus': eine satirischkritische Schrift zur medizinischen 'Politik' des ausgehenden 17. Jahrhunderts. **Nouv Repub Lett** 1982;(1):97-125
**Eckart W:** 'Medicus Politicus' oder 'Machiavellus Medicus'? Wechselwirkungen von Ideal und Realität des Arzttypus im 17. Jahrhundert. **Medizinhist J** 1984;19(3):210-24
**Eckart WU:** Zur Funktion der Abbildung als Medium der Wissenschaftsvermittlung in der medizinischen Literatur des 17. Jahrhunderts. **Ber Wissenschaftsgesch** 1980;3(1-2):35-53
**Eckenhoff EA, Harasymiw SJ:** Contributors to research literature: 1948-1973. **Hosp Health Serv Adm** 1979 Summer;24(3):11-20
**Ecker A:** The discovery of human cerebral arterial spasm in angiograms: an autobiographical note.. **Neurosurgery** 1982 Jan;10(1):90
**Ecker HA, Epsteen CM:** The American Society of Maxillofacial Surgeons. Williamsport, Pa., Grit Pub. Co., 1978. 69 p.
**Eckert C:** Evarts A. Graham and the American Board of Surgery. **J Thorac Cardiovasc Surg** 1984 Nov;88(5 Pt 2):842-7
**Eckert EA:** Seasonality of plague in early modern Europe: Swiss epidemic of 1628-1630. **Rev Infect Dis** 1980 Nov-Dec;2(6):952-9
**Eckert EA:** Spatial and temporal distribution of plague in a region of Switzerland in the years 1628 and 1629. **Bull Hist Med** 1982 Summer;56(2):175-94
**Eckert WG:** Advances in American forensic sciences. California's role. **Am J Forensic Med Pathol** 1981 Jun;2(2):155-61
**Eckert WG, Kaye S:** Alexander O. Gettler (1883-1983). A centennial of his birth. **Am J Forensic Med Pathol** 1983 Dec;4(4):297-301
**Eckert WG:** American forensic sciences 1776-1976. **Am J Forensic Med Pathol** 1982 Mar;3(1):57-62
**Eckert WG:** Catastrophes et morts collectives. Recent American experiences in mass deaths. **Am J Forensic Med Pathol** 1980 Mar;1(1):77-9
**Eckert WG:** Dr. Benjamin M. Vance (1886-1962). **Am J Forensic Med Pathol** 1980 Mar;1(1):73-6
**Eckert WG:** Dr. Harrison Stanford Martland (1883-1954). **Am J Forensic Med Pathol** 1981 Mar;2(1):83-4
**Eckert WG:** Fatal commercial air transport crashes, 1924-1981. Review of history and information on fatal crashes. **Am J Forensic Med Pathol** 1982 Mar;3(1):49-56
**Eckert WG:** Historical aspects of poisoning and toxicology. **Am J Forensic Med Pathol** 1981 Sep;2(3):261-4
**Eckert WG:** History of the U.S. Army Graves Registration Service (1917-1950s). **Am J Forensic Med Pathol** 1983 Sep;4(3):231-43
**Eckert WG:** Identification of the remains of John Paul Jones: a look at early methods. **Am J Forensic Med Pathol** 1982 Jun;3(2):143-52
**Eckert WG:** Medicolegal investigation in New York City. History and activities 1918-1978. **Am J Forensic Med Pathol** 1983 Mar;4(1):33-54
**Eckert WG:** Physician crimes and criminals. The historical and forensic aspects. **Am J Forensic Med Pathol** 1982 Sep;3(3):221-30
**Eckert WG, Garland N:** The history of the forensic applications in radiology. **Am J Forensic Med Pathol** 1984 Mar;5(1):53-6
**Eckert WG:** The Lindbergh case. A triumph in forensic investigation. **Am J Forensic Med Pathol** 1980 Jun;1(2):151-3
**Eckert WG:** The murder masquerade. The Domer case. **Am J Forensic Med Pathol** 1980 Mar;1(1):71-2
**Eckert WG:** The Rockne crash. American commercial air crash investigation in the early years. **Am J Forensic Med Pathol** 1982 Mar;3(1):17-27
**Eckert WG:** The St. Valentine's Day massacre. **Am J Forensic Med Pathol** 1980 Mar;1(1):67-70
**Eckert WG:** The Whitechapel murders: the case of Jack the Ripper. **Am J Forensic Med Pathol** 1981 Mar;2(1):53-60
**Eckert WG:** The writings of Sir Bernard Spilsbury: Part I. **Am J Forensic Med Pathol** 1984 Sep;5(3):231-8
**Eckhardt G, ed:** Zur Geschichte der Psychologie. Berlin, VEB Deutscher Verlag der Wissenschaften, 1979. 128p. Mit Beiträgen von H. Hiebsch, F. Klix, W. Schreier, und L. Sprung.
**Eckstaedt A:** 'Mimi überreicht Madam Grenouillet einen Blumenstrauss'. Eine psychoanalytische Studie über den Weg der Phantasie des vierjährigen Paul Klee anhand einer Kinderzeichnung. **Psyche (Stuttg)** 1980 Dec:34(12):1123-44
**Eddleman WL** see **Rich NM**
**Eddy JH:** Buffon, organic alterations, and man. **Stud Hist Biol** 1984;7:1-45
**Eddy TP:** The evolution of British colonial hospitals in West Africa. **Trans R Soc Trop Med Hyg** 1983;77(4):563-4
**Edel A:** Science: ethical implications. In Reich WT, et al, ed: Encyclopedia of bioethics, v.4. New York, Free Press, 1978. p. 1535-41.
**Edel A** see **Tobach E**
**Edelman DA** see **Goldsmith A**
**Edelman F:** Nicotiana, les botanistes et le tabac, des premiers herbiers à nos jours. **Flammes Fumees** 1977;(79):65-128
**Edelston H:** A psychiatrist in Youth Aliah (1956-57). **Midstream** 1981;27(9):42-5
**Eden AR, Opland J:** Bartolommeo Eustachio's De Auditus Organis and the unique murder plot in Shakespeare's Hamlet. **N Engl J Med** 1982 Jul 22;307(4):259-61
**Eder NR:** Medical opinion and the first year of national health insurance in Britain. **Albion** 1979;11(2):157-71
**Eder NR:** National health insurance, social politics and medical practice in Britain, 1913-1939. Ph.D. diss. University of Illinois. Chicago, 1980. 375 leaves.
**Ederer F:** Jerome Cornfield's contributions to the conduct of clinical trials. **Biometrics** 1982 Mar;38 Suppl:25-32
**Edgar II:** A history of early Jewish physicians in the State of Michigan. New York, Philosophical Library, 1982. 249 p.
**Edgar II:** Dr. Louis Jacob Hirshman. **Mich Jew Hist** 1980;20(2):5-10
**Edgar RK:** An annotated bibliography of the American microscopist and diatomist Jacob Whitman Bailey (1811-1857). **Occas Pap Farlow Herb Cryptogam Bot Harv Univ** 1977;11:1-26
**Edgar RS:** Max Delbrück. **Annu Rev Genet** 1982;16:501-5
**Edgcumbe R:** Anna Freud--child analyst. **Int J Psychoanal** 1983;64 (Pt 4):427-33
**Ediger EM:** Influences on the origin and development of Mennonite mental health centers. **Mennon Q Rev** 1982;56(1):32-46
**Edlich RF:** Reflections on Wangensteen's academic village. **Am J Surg** 1981 May;141(5):601-4
**Edmonds-Seal J, Mitchell JV:** The Oxford training scheme in anaesthesia and other matters. **Anaesthesia** 1979 Sep;34(8):776-83
**Edmondson CM:** An enquiry into the termination of Soviet famine relief programmes and the renewal of grain export, 1922-23. **Sov Stud** 1981;33(3):370-85
**Edmondson CM:** The politics of hunger: the Soviet response to famine. **Sov Stud** 1977;29(4):506-18
**Edmonson JM:** Surgical garb, 1870-1920. Cleveland, Cleveland Health Sciences Library, 1982. 20 p. (Occasional contributions to the history of the health sciences from the Historical Division of the Cleveland Health Sciences Library, no. 1).
**Edmunds LH:** A historical review of shunts for cyanotic heart disease. In B. L. Tucker, G. G. Lindesmith, ed: First clinical conference on congenital heart disease. New York, Grune & Stratton, 1979. p. 207-17.
**Edredge N:** I manoscritti medici della Osterreichische Nationalbibliothek di Vienna. (contd). **Kos** 1984 Apr;1(3):7-13
**Edsall JT:** Essay review; Horace Judson and the molecular biologists. **J Hist Biol** 1980 Spring;13(1):141-58
**Edsall JT:** Marcel Florkin, August 15, 1900--May 3, 1979. **Isis** 1980 Jun;71(257):286-8
**Edsall JT:** Some perspectives on carbonic anhydrase since 1960. **Ann NY Acad Sci** 1984;429:18-25
**Edsall JT:** Stabilization of serum albumin to heat, and inactivation of the hepatitis virus. **Vox Sang** 1984;46(5):338-40
**Edsall JT:** The forgotten paper on buffer values: Koppel and Spiro, 1914. **Surv Sources Newsl** 1981;10:11
**Edsall JT:** The Journal of Biological Chemistry after seventy-five years. **J Biol Chem** 1980 Oct 10;255(19):8939-51
**Edsall JT:** The papers of W.T. Astbury and J.D. Bernal. **Surv Sources Newsl** 1981 Apr;10:2-6
**Edsall JT:** The William Mansfield Clark papers: a second installment. **Surv Sources Newsl** 1981;10:1
**Edsall JT:** William Mansfield Clark papers. **Surv Sources Newsl** 1978 Mar;7:2-5
**Edsall JT** see **Recollections & reflections**
**Edsall JT, ed** see **Bearman D**
**Education of a provincial apothecary: Pharm Hist (London)** 1978 Jul;8(2):5-6
**Edwards A, Yerkovic L, Santamaría J:** La tuberculosis y el Hospital San José de Santiago. **Rev Med Chil** 1983 Mar;111(3):315-9
**Edwards CL:** Tumor-localizing radionuclides in retrospect and prospect. **Semin Nucl Med** 1979 Jul;9(3):186-9
**Edwards G, Busch C:** Drug problems in Britain: a review of ten years. London, Academic Press, 1981. 333 p.
**Edwards G:** William Ernest Henley: early impressions. **Nurs Mirror** 1981 Jun 17;152(25):33-4
**Edwards G** see **Berridge V**
**Edwards GA:** Causation of insanity in nineteenth century Australia. **Aust NZ J Psychiatry** 1982 Mar;16(1):53-62
**Edwards GA, Hall W:** The case of William Chidley: a study in psychiatry, morality and lunacy law. **Aust NZ J Psychiatry** 1980 Jun;14(2):133-9
**Edwards GA:** The mental illness of Captain Hyndman.

**Aust NZ J Psychiatr** 1979 Jun;13(2):147-52
**Edwards GT:** Bella Coola: Indian and European medicines. **Beaver** 1980;311(3):4-11
**Edwards H** see **Gathiram P**
**Edwards I** see **Whittaker DK**
**Edwards IG:** Down memory lane: burial at sea. **Nurs Mirror** 1980 Jul 3;150(21):36-7
**Edwards PI:** Robert Brown (1773-1858) and the natural history of Matthew Flinders' voyage in H.M.S. Investigator, 1801-1805. **J Soc Bibliogr Nat Hist** 1976;7(4):385-407
**Edwards R:** Graham-Kellogg, early American contributors to health education. **J Sch Health** 1981 Nov;51(9):589-91
**Edwards RH** see **Mond HG**
**Edwards S:** Science and secular idealism. **Midwest Q** 1980;22(1):21-31
**Edwards SS:** Femina sexualis: medico-legal control in Victoriana. **Soc Soc Hist Med Bull (Lond)** 1981 Jun;28:17-20
**Edwards WS:** Alexis Carrel's contributions to thoracic surgery. **Ann Thorac Surg** 1983 Jan;35(1):111-4
**Eerenbeemt HF van den:** De 'Rode dood' in stad en meierij van 's-Hertogenbosch: een dysenterie-epidemie in de jaren 1779-1783. **Econ Soc Hist Jaarb** 1973;36:75-101
**Eerie murder in Shakespeare's Hamlet: N Engl J Med** 1982 Dec 9;307(24):1531
**Efimov AE:** Neizvestnoe pis'mo N. I. Pirogova. **Sov Zdravookhr** 1983;(8):61-2
**Efkes F:** Entstehung und Entwicklung der studentischen Korporationen an der Tierärztlichen Hochschule Hannover im 19. Jahrhundert. Diss. Hannover, 1978. 227 p.
**Efremov VV:** K istorii otkrytiia vitaminov N. I. Luninym. **Vopr Pitan** 1982 May-Jun;(3):68-72
**Efremov VV, Shtenberg AI:** 50-letnii put' Instituta pitaniia AMN SSSR: ego sozdanie, stanovlenie i razvitie. **Vopr Pitan** 1980 Sept-Oct;(5):4-9
**Eftychiadis A** see **Marketos SG**
**Eftychiadis AC, Marketos SG:** [Geriatrics in Byzantium.] (Gre). **Mater Med Greca** 1981;9:217-20
**Eftychiadis AC, Marketos SG:** [The treatment of mental disorders ... in Byzantium.] (Gre). **Mater Med Greca** 1981;9:221-5
**Egaĭ VS, Kuimov AD:** K istorii stanovleniia nauchnoĭ terapevticheskoĭ kliniki Sibiri (k 400-letiiu prisoedineniia Sibiri k Rossii). **Ter Arkh** 1982;54(12):122-3
**Egaĭ VS:** Razvitie terapii v Sibiri: M. G. Kurlov i ego shkola. M. G. Kurlov i ego shkola. Novosibirsk, Nauka, Sibirskoe otd-nie, 1981. 112 p.
**Egan MC:** Public health nutrition services: issues today and tomorrow. **J Am Diet Assoc** 1980 Oct;77(4):423-7
**Egeblad K:** Militaerkirurgen Dominique Jean Larrey: Om pesten i felttoget til Aegypten og Syrien 1798-1801. **Dan Medicinhist Arbog** 1979;132-59
**Egerton FN:** The history of ecology: achievements and opportunities, part one. **J Hist Biol** 1983 Summer;16(2):259-310
**Egerton FN** see **Greene EL**
**Egger E:** Die Standardisierungskonzeption diagnostischer Laboratoriumsmethoden in der DDR. **Z Med Lab Diagn** 1983;24(7):401-7
**Eggert GH:** Wernicke's works on aphasia. The Hague, New York, Mouton, 1977. xiii, 307 p.
**Egglmaier HH:** Das medizinisch-chirurgische Studium in Graz. Ein Beispiel für den Wandel staatlicher Zielvorstellungen im Bildungs- und Medizinalwesen. Diss. Graz. 1980. xi, 599 p. (Dissertationen der Universität Graz, 50).
**Egli H:** The situation of the haemophiliac: yesterday and today. **Haemostasis** 1981;10 Suppl 1:1-10
**Egon S:** Az európai országok termékenységét közvetlenül, vagy közvetve befolyásoló törvények. **Demografia** 1973;16(1):114-8
**Egorov IuL** see **Borisenkova RV**
**Egorysheva IV:** Novye dannye iz istorii Krasnogo Kresta v dorevoliutsionnoĭ Rossii. **Sov Zdravookhr** 1981;(2):57-60
**Egorysheva IV, Rabinovich RS, Serdiuk GV, et al:** Zhamenatel'nye iubileĭnye daty istorii khirurgii 1983 g. **Khirurgiia (Mosk)** 1982 Nov;(11):103-5
**Egorysheva IV** see **Lotova EI**
**Egorysheva IV** see **Rabinovich RS**
**Egorysheva IV** see **Vengrova IV**
**Egozcue J:** Darwin y el origen del hombre. **Arbor** 1982;113(441-2):77-86
**Egremy JL** see **Juan López M**
**Egri B:** Arab triangulum **Orv Hetil** 1981 Jun 28;122(26):1595-600
**Egri B:** Keleti géniusz. Emlékezés Avicennára, születésének 1000. évfordulóján. **Orv Hetil** 1980 Dec 28;121(52):3207-12
**Egri B:** Mecsnyikov a cambridge-i Darwin-emlékünnepségekröl. **Orv Hetil** 1982 Nov 14;123(46):2858-60
**Egri B:** Talmud-tradiciók magyarul. **Orv Hetil** 1984 May 27;125(22):1333-5
**Ehlers AP:** Medizinisches und Pharmazeutisches in Bernal Diaz del Castillos, 'Historia verdadera de la conquista de la Nueva-España,' Madrid, 1632. Diss. Düsseldorf, 1980. 118 p.
**Ehlers H:** Bjerrum's Clinic. **Surv Ophthalmol** 1981 Sep-Oct;26(1):101-2
**Ehni G:** Seeking the hidden flaw. **Spine** 1981 Jul-Aug;6(4):369-74
**Ehrhardt H:** 130 Jahre Deutsche Gesellschaft für Psychiatrie und Nervenheilkunde. Wiesbaden, Steiner, 1972. 125 p.
**Ehrhardt JP:** L'Ecole du Service de Santé de la Marine de Bordeaux des origines à nos jours. In Congrès National des Sociétés Savantes, 103e, Nancy-Metz, 1978. Actes. Paris, 1979. Tome I, p. 9-21.
**Ehrhardt JP:** Les médecins naturalistes de 'La Coquille' et de 'L'Astrolabe', ex-gabare 'La Coquille'. In: Congrès National des Sociétés Savantes, 104e, Bordeaux, 1979. Comptes Rendus. Paris, 1979. Section des Sciences, Fasc. IV. p. 205-17.
**Ehrlich GE:** Landmark perspective. Diffuse collagen disease. **JAMA** 1984 Mar 23-30;251(12):1595-6
**Ehrlich GE** see **Appelboom T**
**Eich W, Seidler E:** Historische Modelle der Prognostik in der Heilkunde. **Internist (Berlin)** 1981 Mar;22(3):118-23
**Eich W:** 18th and 19th century medical semiotics; a contribution to medical theory. In International Congress of the History of Medicine, 27th, Barcelona, 1980. Actas. Barcelona, Académia de Ciències Médiques de Catalunya i Balears, 1981. p. 503-5.
**Eichberg H:** Leistung zwischen Wänden--Die sportive Parzellierung der Körper. In Imhof AE, ed: Leib und Leben in der Geschichte der Neuzeit. Berlin, Duncker & Humblot, 1983. p. 119-39.
**Eicher CK:** Facing up to Africa's food crisis. **Foreign Aff** 1982;61(1):151-74
**Eichhorn H:** Ernst Gottlob Pienitz und die Heil- und Verpflegungsanstalt Sonnenstein. **Psychiatr Neurol Med Psychol (Leipz)** 1982 Jan;34(1):60-3
**Eichler W, Jahn I:** Fritz Peus 1904--1978. **Angew Parasitol** 1979 Oct;20(3):164-72
**Eichler W:** Nachruf auf Günter Timmermann (zugleich eine wissenschaftsgeschichtliche Studie zum Disput um die Fahrenholzsche Regel). **Angew Parasitol** 1981 Feb;22(1):53-6
**Eichwald EJ, Silmser CR:** H-Y and serendipity. **Hum Genet** 1981;58(1):6-8
**Eigen JP:** Historical developments in psychiatric forensic evidence: the British experience. **Int J Law Psychiatry** 1983;6(3-4):423-9
**Eigler J, Müller B:** Die Patienten des ersten Jahres (1813-1814) im Allgemeinen Krankenhaus München. **MMW** 1982 Apr 30;124(17):429-33
**Eimas R** see **Heirs of Hippocrates**
**Einarsdóttir ES:** Midwifery education in Iceland: yesterday and today. **J Nurse Midwife** 1983 Nov-Dec;28(6):31-2
**Einstein A** see **Errera M**
**Eisele FR:** Origins of 'gerontocracy'. **Gerontologist** 1979 Aug;19(4):403-7
**Eiseley L:** Darwin and the mysterious Mr. X: new light on the evolutionists. New York and London, Harcourt Brace Jovanovich, 1981. xii, 278 p.
**Eisenberg D** see **King DF**
**Eisenberg I:** A history of rhinoplasty. **S Afr Med J** 1982 Aug 21;62(9):286-92
**Eisenberg L:** Rudolf Ludwig Karl Virchow, where are you now that we need you? **Am J Med** 1984 Sep;77(3):524-32
**Eisenberg L** see **Schopler E**
**Eisenbud M:** Environment, technology, and health: human ecology in historical perspective. New York, New York University Press, 1978. x, 384 p.
**Eisenbud M:** Origins of the standards for control of beryllium disease (1947-1949). **Environ Res** 1982 Feb;27(1):79-88
**Eisenbud M** see **Morandi M**
**Eisenring R:** La médecine dentaire à l'Université de Liège. **Rev Belge Med Dent** 1981;36(3):137-40
**Eisenstein EL:** The printing press as an agent of change. Communications and cultural transformations in early-modern Europe. 2 vols. Cambridge, Cambridge University Press, 1979. xxi, 794 p.
**Eisinger J:** Lead and wine. Eberhard Gockel and the colica Pictonum. **Med Hist** 1982 Jul;26(3):279-302
**Eisnerova V:** The anatomy of plants and its contribution to the origin of cellular theory in the early 19th century. **Acta Hist Rerum Nat Tech** 1971;5:269-333
**Eissler KR:** Freud und Wagner-Jauregg vor der Kommission zur Erhebung militärischer Pflichtverletzungen. Wien, Löcker, 1979. 333 p.
**Eissler KR:** K. R. Eissler on errors regarding Freud. **Int J Psychoanal** 1981;62(3):371-2
**Eissler KR:** Victor Tausk's suicide. New York, International Universities Press, 1983. 322 p.
**Eitinger L:** The concentration camp syndrome and its late sequelae. In Dimsdale, Joel E., ed: Survivors, victims and perpetrators: Essays on the Nazi holocaust. Washington, Hemisphere Publ., 1980. p. 127-62.
**Eitner S:** Das gerontologische Engagement von Maxim Zetkin in seinen späten Lebensjahren. **ZFA** 1984 Jan-Feb;39(1):5-8
**Ek A, Bradley WE:** History of cystometry. **Urology** 1983 Sep;22(3):335-50
**Ekbom K:** Mannen bakom syndromen: Jean-Martin Charcot. Under hans inspirerande ledning skapades den klassiska franska neurologin. **Lakartidningen** 1984 Jun 6;81(23):2363-4
**Ekbom K, Waldenlind E:** Mannen bakom syndromet: Bayard T. Horton. En pionjär inom huvudvärksforskningen. **Lakartidningen** 1982 Sep 15;79(37):3187
**Eklund J** see **Hansson O**
**Ekstein R:** As I remember her: Anna Freud, 1895-1982. **Adolesc Psychiatry** 1983;11:5-8
**Ekström P** see **Ahlström CG**
**Ekström S:** Jöns Jacob Berzelius--ett 200-årsminne. **Sven Farm Tidskr** 1979;83:635-51
**Elaut LJ:** Een epos: het Gentse Akademisch Ziekenhuis. Antwerpen, Nederlandsche Boekhandel, 1977. 83 p. (VVA monografie; 3).
**El'baum RN** see **Krasil'shchikov MI**
**Elcano B** see **Bullough B**
**Elcano BW** see **Bullough VL**
**Elcock H:** Regional government in action: the members of two regional health authorities. **Public Adm** 1978 Winter;56:379-97
**Elder GH:** Scarcity and prosperity in postwar childbearing: explorations from a life course perspective. **J Fam Hist** 1981 Winter;6(4):410-31
**Eldredge N, Tattersall I:** The myths of human evolution. New York, Columbia University Press, 1982. 197 p.
**Eleínikova VS:** Uchebnye plany, programmy i prepodavanie istorii

meditsiny. **Sov Zdravookhr** 1984;(1):43-6
**Elferink JG:** The narcotic and hallucinogenic use of tobacco in Pre-Columbian Central America. **J Ethnopharmacol** 1983 Jan;7(1):111-22
**Elferink JG:** The significance of the pre-Columbian pharmaceutical knowledge for European medicine in the XVIth century. **Pharm Acta Helv** 1979;54(9-10):299-302
**Elgjo RF:** Hospice-bevegelsen. **Tidsskr Nor Laegeforen** 1982 Sep 20;102(26):1352-4
**Eliasson Orn:** Farmer's lung disease: a new historical perspective from Iceland. **J Hist Med Allied Sci** 1982 Oct;37(4):440-4
**Elinov NP:** 60 let Leningradskomu khimiko-farmatsevticheskomu institutu. **Farmatsiia** 1979 Nov-Dec;28(6):49-56
**Eliot's farewell address, May 1, 1909: Harv Med Alumni Bull** 1982 Spring;56(2):14-6
**Elizaveta Nikolaevna Oleneva (k 60-letiiu so dnia rozhdeniia): Arkh Anat Gistol Embriol** 1984 Mar;86(3):107-9
**Elizondo RS, Jacobs N, Moore WW:** Physiology at Indiana University-Bloomington. A history. **Physiologist** 1984 Oct;27(5):319-24
**Elkana Y:** The discovery of the conservation of energy. Cambridge, Mass., Harvard University Press, 1974. xiv, 213 p.
**Elkhadem H:** Une nouvelle conception de l'hygiène et de la diététique au XIe siècle. **Technologia** 1982;5(3-4):61-73
**Elkin II:** Leninskiĭ étap v razvitii épidemiologii. **Zh Mikrobiol Epidemiol Immunobiol** 1981 Jan;(1):3-8
**Elkin II:** Nauchnyĭ podvig L. A. Gromashevskogo. **Zh Mikrobiol Epidemiol Immunobiol** 1982 Jan;(1):113-7
**Elkin II, Frolova VV:** Rol' N. I. Pirogova v podgotovke I. I. Mechnikova k nauchnoĭ deiatel'nosti (k 135-letiiu so dnia rozhdeniia I. I. Mechnikova. **Zh Mikrobiol Epidemiol Immunobiol** 1980 Sep;(9):114-8
**Elkin II:** Voenno-épidemicheskaia doktrina (po opytu protivoėpidemicheskoĭ zashchity voĭsk v Velikuiu Otechestvennuiu voinu 1941-1945). **Zh Mikrobiol Epidemiol Immunobiol** 1980 May;(5):11-7
**Elkind MM:** Radiobiology in radiotherapy: a personal history. **Int J Radiat Oncol Biol Phys** 1984 Jul;10(7):1143-8
**Ell SR:** Five hundred years of specialty certification and compulsory continuing medical education. Venice 1300-1801. **JAMA** 1984 Feb 10;251(6):752-3
**Ell SR:** Interhuman transmission of medieval plague. **Bull Hist Med** 1980 Winter;54(4):497-510
**Ell SR:** Some evidence for interhuman transmission of medieval plague. **Rev Infect Dis** 1979 May-Jun;1(3):563-6
**Ell SR:** The two medicines: some ecclesiastical concepts of disease and the physician in the high Middle Ages. **Janus** 1981;68:15-25
**Ellacuría I:** Seguridad social y solidaridad humana: aproximacion filosofica al fenomeno de la seguridad social. **Estud Cent Am** 1969;24(253):357-66
**Elleder M** see **Mířejovský P**
**Ellenberger H:** Le secret pathogène et son traitement. **Rev Int Hist Psychiatr** 1983;1(1):5-22
**Ellenberger M:** Fragonard, l'anatomiste. **Pour Sci** 1982;53:98-108
**Ellencweig AY, Yoshpe RB:** Definition of public health. **Public Health Rev** 1984;12(1):65-78
**Elliot AD** see **Bernhard JD**
**Elliott A, Freeling P, Owen J:** District nurse training. **J R Coll Gen Pract** 1980 Feb;30(211):69-74
**Elliott CA:** Models of the American scientist: a look at collective biography. **Isis** 1982 Mar;73(266):77-93
**Elliott CK:** Bonesetters. **Practitioner** 1981 Feb;225(1352):253-5
**Elliott FA:** Biological roots of violence. **Proc Am Philos Soc** 1983 Apr 20;127(2):84-94
**Elliott J:** Orthopedist is pioneer in prosthetic design. **JAMA** 1976 Oct 26;242(17):1831-3, 1837
**Elliott J:** The rod and the staff. **Ulster Med J** 1979;48(1):32-42
**Elliott LS:** A pictorial history of mechanical respiration devices. **Respir Ther** 1979 Jan-Feb;9(1):52-4
**Ellis CG:** The king's evil. A case of scrofula. **Practitioner** 1981 Oct;225(1360):1519
**Ellis CW** see **Bayliss RA**
**Ellis FR:** Waterton's wourali. **Can Anaesth Soc J** 1983 Jan;30(1):110
**Ellis H:** A history of bladder stone. **J R Soc Med** 1979 Apr;72(4):248-51
**Ellis H:** Cutting for the stone. **Aust NZ J Surg** 1980 Feb;50(1):4-7
**Ellis H:** The bladder stone of the Emperor Napoleon III. **Chirurgie** 1984;110(4):370-1
**Ellis J:** The responsibility of medical schools for teaching hospitals and the provision of clinical services. **Med Educ** 1981 May;15(3):171-83
**Ellis JH:** Business leadership in Memphis public health reform, 1880-1900. **West Tenn Hist Soc Pap** 1965;19:94-104
**Ellis PS:** The origins of the war neuroses. **J R Nav Med Serv** 1984 Winter;70(3):168-77 contd
**Ellis R:** Pharmacy in Stamford a century ago. **Pharm Hist (London)** 1967 Oct;1(1):4-8
**Ellis RH** see **Sykes WS**
**Ellison RG:** Paul C. Samson, M.D., 1905-1982. Part I. His contributions to the Society of Thoracic Surgeons. **Ann Thorac Surg** 1983 Nov;36(5):500-1
**Ellison RG:** The Society of Thoracic Surgeons: the first twenty years. **Ann Thorac Surg** 1984 Jan;37(1):1-8
**Ellison RC, ed:** A pioneer Alabama doctor's ledger. **Ala Hist Q** 1981;43(4):315-32
**Ellman MH:** William Crawford Gorgas and the American Medical Association. **JAMA** 1980 Feb 15;243(7):659-60
**Elmore JA:** Frances Elliott Davis. In: Notable American women. The modern period. Cambridge, Mass., Belknap-Harvard Univ. Press, 1980. 4:180-2.
**Elmore R:** View from the Rive Gauche: a comment on Annales Historiography. **Psychohist Rev** 1978;7(2):30-5
**Elmqvist R:** Review of early pacemaker development. **PACE** 1978 Oct;1(4):535-6
**Elmslie R:** The colonial career of James Patrick Murray. **Aust NZ J Surg** 1979 Feb;49(1):154-62
**Elmslie RG:** Our honoured anatomists. **Aust NZ J Surg** 1981 Oct;51(5):415-9
**Elom-Ntouzo'o E:** Médecine, pharmacopées traditionelles et développement en Afrique. **Presence Afr** 1978;108:38-49
**Elósegui J:** Un guipuzcoano benemérito del siglo XVIII, Manuel Bernardino de Aranguren, médico (1743-1794). **Bol Real Soc Vascongada Amigos Pais** 1973;29(1-3):171-91
**Elsas M:** Archives: the 'memory of man.' **Pharm Hist (London)** 1968 Dec;1(3):1-3
**Elstad JI:** Helsetilstand og dødelighet i Sogn og Fjordane og Finnmark i sosiologisk perspektiv. **Tidsskr Samfunnsforskning** 1982;23(1):49-70
**Elster R:** Porträt unserer Zeitschrift. **Krankenpflege (Frankfurt)** 1981 Jan;35(1):7-10
**Elster R** see **Quinn S, ed**
**Elting JJ, Starna WA:** A possible case of pre-Columbian treponematosis from New York State. **Am J Phys Anthropol** 1984 Nov;65(3):267-73
**Elton GR:** The real Thomas More? **Psychol Med** 1980 Nov;10(4):611-7
**Elvin M, et al:** The work of Joseph Needham. **Past Present** 1980;87:17-53
**Elwood JH:** Thomas Carnwath. **Ulster Med J** 1982;51(2):98-109
**Elzay RP** see **Sawyer DR**
**Elzinga A:** Christiaan Huygens' theory of research. **Janus** 1980;67:281-300
**Emanuel DA, Kryda MJ:** Farmer's lung disease. **Clin Rev Allergy** 1983 Dec;1(4):509-32
**Emblin RI** see **Quinn S, ed**
**Emboden WA:** The mushroom and the water lily: literary and pictorial evidence for Nymphaea as a ritual psychotogen in Mesoamerica. **J Ethnopharmacol** 1982 Mar;5(2):139-48
**Emboden WA:** Transcultural use of narcotic water lilies in ancient Egyptian and Maya drug ritual. **J Ethnopharmacol** 1981 Jan;3(1):39-83
**Emboden WA** see **Hand WD, ed**
**Emch-Dériaz AS:** L'inoculation justifiee-or was it? **Eighteenth Cent Life** 1982;7(2):65-72
**Emeksuzian VS:** A. P. Golubkov v sibirskoĭ ssylke. **Sov Zdravookhr** 1981;(11):59-62
**Emerit M:** Un curé de l'aude atteint du mal du siècle: Jean Terson. In Congrès National des Sociétés Savantes, 102e, Limoges, 1977. Actes. Paris, 1978. Tome I, p. 351-60.
**Emerson RL:** The Philosophical Society of Edinburgh 1748-1768. **Br J Hist Sci** 1981 Jul;14(pt 2 no 47):133-76
**Emerson RM, Rochford EB, Shaw LL:** Economics and enterprise in Board and Care Homes for the mentally ill. **Am Behav Sci** 1981;24(6):771-85
**Emerson RS:** Olympics and sports medicine. **NY State J Med** 1980 May;80(6):992-4
**Emerson RS, Schwartz RM:** Professional liability. **NY State J Med** 1983 Jan;83(1):69-74
**Emerson GM, ed:** Aging. Stroudsburg, Pa., Dowden, Hutchinson & Ross, 1977. xii, 372 p. (Benchmark Papers in Human Physiology, 11).
**Emery PJ** see **Phelps PD**
**Emling RC:** Historical overview of causes and treatment of dental hypersensitivity. **Compend Contin Educ Dent** 1982;(Suppl 3):S92-4
**Emmerick RE:** Arsenic and sida. In Mazars G, ed: Les médecines traditionnelles de l'Asie. Strasbourg, Université Louis Pasteur, 1981. p. 93-102.
**Emmerick RE:** Contributions to the study of the 'Jivaka-pustaka'. **Bull Sch Orient Afr Stud** 1979;42:235-43
**Emmerick RE:** On the indexation of Sanskrit medical verses and prescriptions. **Sci Orient** 1979;16:3-8
**Emmerick RE:** Some lexical items from the rGyud-bźi. In: Proceedings of the Csoma de Körös Memorial Symposium ... Matrafüred ... 1976. Budapest: Akad. Kiadó. 1978. pp.101-108.
**Emmerson JS, ed:** Catalogue of the Pybus collection of medical books, letters and engravings, 15th-20th centuries, held in the University Library, Newcastle upon Tyne. Newcastle Upon Tyne, Manchester University Press, for the University Library, 1981. xiv, 270 p.
**Emmons J:** The medical career of Samuel H. Stout. **J Med Assoc Ga** 1980 Nov;69(11):904-10, 1981 Mar;80(3):169-77
**Emmons RW** see **Reeves WC**
**Emslie RD:** A century of British periodontology. **Br Dent J** 1980 Jul 1;149(1):3-4
**Emslie RD:** A history of oral hygiene measures. **Community Dent Oral Epidemiol** 1980;8(5):225-9
**Emson HE:** The case of Emmett-Dunne. A personal reminiscence. **Am J Forensic Med Pathol** 1983 Sep;4(3):255-8
**En el milenario de Avicena: Med Tradic** 1980;2(8):5-9
**Enarson HL:** Perspectives on college health in the 80's: a president's view. **J Am Coll Health Assoc** 1981 Aug;30(1):11-3
**Ende A:** Children in history: a personal review of the past decade's published research. **J Psychohist** 1983 Summer;11(1):65-88
**Endicott SL:** Germ warfare and 'plausible denial': the Korean war, 1952-1953. **Mod China** 1979;5(1):79-104
**Endo E:** [Nurse's images in the Taisho period; nurses described in women's magazines] (Jpn). **Igakushi Kenkyu** 1980;54:28-35
**Endo E:** [Visiting nurse after the World War II] (Jpn).

**Igakushi Kenkyu** 1978;49:22-6

**Endo E:** [Visiting nursing in 1926-1945] (Jpn). **Igakushi Kenkyu** 1977;48:30-8

**Endrei W:** Egy korai magyar nyelvü orvoslevél. **Orvostort Kozl** 1980;89-91(26 no 1-3):267-8

**Endres L:** Entwicklung der Artikulatoren. **Zahntechnik (Geneve)** 1980;38(4):334-5

**Endtz LJ:** La neurologie et l'illustration photographique du livre médical. **Rev Neurol (Paris)** 1983;139(6-7):439-44

**Endtz LJ** see **Schulte BP**

**Enfermería y sociedad (notas para una historia social de la enfermería): Rev Enferm** 1981 Feb;4(31):35-44

**Eng E:** Locke's Tabula Rasa and Freud's 'Mystic writing pad.' **J Hist Ideas** 1980 Jan-Mar;41(1):133-40

**Engel A:** Hälsan före födelsen. Prenatal forskning i Sverige. Stockholm, 1981. 128 p. (Nordisk Medicinhistorisk Arsbok, Supplementum, VIII).

**Engel BA:** Women medical students in Russia, 1872-1882: reformers or rebels? **J Soc Hist** 1979;12(3):394-415

**Engel BF:** Why so doleful? The funereal poetry of the early Midwest. **Old Northwest** 1981;7(2):147-59

**Engel C:** Leben und Werk des Bonner Frauenarztes Gustav von Veit. Diss., Rheinische Friedrich-Wilhelms-Universität. Bonn, 1983. 141 p.

**Engel K:** Der Gräfenberg-Ring. Zu seiner Vorgeschichte, Entwicklung, Anwendung und frühen Rezeption. Diss. Erlangen-Nürnberg, 1979. 137 p.

**Engel M:** Das Dahlem-Projekt und sein Scheitern. Ein wissenschaftspolitischer Modellfall medizinischer Forschung an der Schwelle zum 20. Jahrhundert - Zur Geschichte des Robert-Koch-Instituts und der Charité. **Fortschr Med** 1982 Jun3;100(21):1009-12

**Engelbrecht H:** Taenia saginata, eine entdeckungsgeschichtliche und ökologisch-epidemiologische Betrachtung. **Angew Parasitol** 1984 Mar;25(1):17-26

**Engelbrecht H, Gräfner G, Müller P, et al:** 20 Jahre Parasitologische Gesellschaft der DDR. **Angew Parasitol** 1981 Nov;22(4):185-92

**Engelhardt A** see **Engelhardt R, ed**

**Engelhardt D von:** Das literarische Kunstwerk als Therapeutikum. **Dtsch Apoth Ztg** 1981;33:292-302

**Engelhardt D von, Schipperges H:** Die inneren Verbindungen zwischen Philosophie und Medizin im 20. Jahrhundert. Darmstadt, Wissenschaftliche Buchgesellschaft, 1980. vii, 190 p.

**Engelhardt D von, Henkelmann T:** Eine medizinhistorische Exkursion in die Renaissance der Toskana. **Wolfenbutteler Renaiss Mitt** 1980;4:87-92

**Engelhardt D von:** Historisches Bewusstein in der Medizin der Romantik. In Seidler E, Schott H, ed: Bausteine zur Medizingeschichte. Stuttgart, Steiner, 1984. p. 26-34.

**Engelhardt D von:** Medizin und Philosophie - Positionen und Gegenstand in der Entwicklung der Neuzeit. **MMG** 1980;5:94-100

**Engelhardt D von:** Polemik und Kontroversen um Haeckel. **Medizinhist J** 1980;15(3):284-304

**Engelhardt D von** see **Hasler L, ed**

**Engelhardt D von** see **Mann G, ed**

**Engelhardt DV, Henkelmann T:** Una excursión de história de la medicina con el renacimiento de la toscana. **Folia Hum (Barc)** 1981;19(216):49-56

**Engelhardt DV:** Virchow et Haeckel et la liberté de la science. In Poirier J, Poirier JL, ed: Médecine et philosophie à la fin du XIXe siècle. Paris, Université de Paris XII - Val de Marne, [1980?]. p. 117-25.

**Engelhardt HT:** Clinical judgement. **Metamedicine** 1981;2:301-17

**Engelhardt HT:** Philosophical perspectives [of health and disease]. In Reich WT, et al, ed: Encyclopedia of bioethics, v. 2. New York, Free Press, 1978. p. 599-605.

**Engelhardt HT, Erde EL:** [Philosophy of medicine]. In Reich WT, et al, ed: Encyclopedia of bioethics, v.3. New York, Free Press, 1978. p. 1049-54.

**Engelhardt HT** see **Durbin PT, ed**

**Engelhardt R, ed:** Das römische Aerzte-Instrumentarium. Bingen, Engelhardt, 1974. 47 p. (Binger Annalen, IV) Contributions by C. Palm, K. M. Heidecker, P. Nahm, E. Naujack, A. Engelhardt.

**Engelman E:** Berggasse 19, Sigmund Freud's home and offices, Vienna, 1938: the photographs of Edmund Engelman. Chicago, University of Chicago Press, 1981. 153 p.

**Engels D:** The problem of female infanticide in the Greco-Roman world. **Classical Philol** 1980;75:112-20

**Engels W:** Zur Geschichte des Verstaatlichungsgedankens im deutschen Apothekenwesen. Stuttgart, Deutscher Apotheker Verlag, 1984. 261 p. (Quellen und Studien zur Geschichte der Pharmazie, Bd. 28).

**Engerman SL:** Changes in black fertility, 1880-1940. In T. K. Hareven and M. A. Vinovskis, ed: Family and population in nineteenth-century America. Princeton, Princeton University Press, 1978. p. 126-53.

**Engerman SL** see **Fogel RW**

**Engle EK, Lott AS:** Man in flight: biomedical achievements in aerospace. Annapolis, Md., Leeward, 1979. xxvii, 396 p.

**Engle EK:** Medic. New York, Day, [c 1967]. 255 p.

**Engle MA:** Biographies of great American pediatricians--Helen Brooke Taussig: the mother of pediatric cardiology. **Pediatr Ann** 1982 Jul;11(7):629-31

**Englisch F:** Die Döblinger Privatirrenanstalt. **Wien Geschichtsbl** 1969;24(1):398-406

**English EB:** Women and sport during the Renaissance. In Borms J, Hebbelinck M, Venerando A, ed: Women and sport. Basel, Karger, 1981. p. 24-30.

**English PC:** Pediatrics and the unwanted child in history: foundling homes, disease, and the origins of foster care in New York City, 1860 to 1920. **Pediatrics** 1984 May;73(5):699-711

**English PC, Grossman H:** Radiology and the history of child abuse. **Pediatr Ann** 1983 Dec;12(12):870-4

**English PC:** Shock, physiological surgery, and George Washington Crile. Medical innovation in the Progressive era. Westport, Connecticut, and London, Greenwood, 1980. xi, 271 p. (Contributions in medical history, 5)

**English TA:** Heart transplantation---1979. **Trans Hunter Soc** 1978-80;37-38:143-51

**Engquist-Seidenberg G:** The States' role in health care cost containment. **Policy Stud Rev** 1981;1(2):275-87

**Engrand C:** Les abandons d'enfants à Amiens vers la fin de l'Ancien Régime. **Rev Nord** 1982;64(252):73-92

**Engström A:** Reflexioner kring våra matvanor förr och nu. **Nord Medicinhist Arsb** 1984;:83-90

**Enigh K:** Als Parasitologe im Veterinärdienst des Heeres. **DTW** 1981 Nov 5;88(11):479-83

**Enigk K:** Abriss der Geschichte der deutschen vet. med. Parasitologie. **Berl Munch Tierarztl Wochenschr** 1982 Oct 1;95(19):374-82

**Enjoubault:** Petite histoire de l'anesthésie. **Infirm Fr** 1982 Jul;(237):27-30

**Enoch JM:** Joseph Le Conte. **Am J Optom Physiol Opt** 1983 Dec;60(12):1003

**Enoch JM:** To woo a Helmholtz. **Am J Optom Physiol Opt** 1982 Oct;59(10):843

**Enríquez Morales MJ, Gelabert González JE:** Un aspecto del consumo alimentico en la España de la secunda mitad del siglo XIX. **Hispania** 1978;38(140):617-35

**Ensign MS, ed:** Historical periodicals directory. Volume 1: USA and Canada. Santa Barbara, Oxford, ABC-Clio, 1981. xii, 180 p. (Clio Periodicals Directories).

**Ensign MS, ed** see **Boehm EH**

**Ensley PC:** Indiana and the influenza pandemic of 1918. **Indiana Med Hist Q** 1983 Dec;9(4):3-15

**Enterline HT** see **Brooks JJ**

**Entin MA:** Med-Chi is 140 years old: a historical sketch of the Montreal Medical Chirurgical Society. **Can J Surg** 1983 Nov;26(6):563-5

**Entralgo PL** see **Tellenbach H, ed**

**Epifanov NS:** I. F. Zemmel'veis. **Med Sestra** 1983 Aug;42(8):50-1

**Epifanov NS:** I. K. Spizharnyĭ v Viatskoĭ ssylke (materialy biografii). **Sov Zdravookhr** 1983;(2):70-1

**Epifanov NS:** Khirurg, uchenyĭ, patriot (k110-letiiu so dnia rozhdeniia V.A. Oppelia). **Khirurgiia (Mosk)** 1982 Nov;(11):101-3

**Epifanov NS:** Nastavnik pervykh russkikh meditsinskikh sester. **Med Sestra** 1983 Mar;42(3):48-50

**Epifanov NS:** Neustannyĭ borets s tiazhelym nedugom (k 100-letiiu so dnia rozhdeniia P. G. Korneval). **Feldsher Akush** 1983 Sep;48(9):37-8

**Epifanov NS:** Vasiliĭ Ivanovich Razumovskiĭ (k 125-letiiu so dnia rozhdeniia). **Feldsher Akush** 1982;47(7):42-3

**Epistemologia, metodologia clinica e storia della scienza medica, 1:** Roma, Cossidente, 1977. xliii, 225 p. (Collana di Studi Epistemologici). Introduction by D. Antiseri. Contributions by D. Antiseri, G. Giunchi, M. Baldini, O. Todisco, M. D. Grmek, P. Potestà, V. Scalera.

**Epistemologia, metodologia clinica e storia della scienza medica, 2:** Roma, Cossidente, 1978. 172 p. (Collana di Studi Epistemologici). Introduction by D. Antiseri. Contributions by V. Mathieu, V. Tomini, E. Urbani, V. Somenzi, G. Federspil, C. Scandellari, M. Austoni, M. Di Giandomenico, E. Riverso, E. Garulli.

**Epler DC:** Bloodletting in early Chinese medicine and its relation to the origin of acupuncture. **Bull Hist Med** 1980 Fall; 54(3):337-67

**Epsteen CM** see **Ecker HA**

**Epstein D:** Hayehudi hayehidi (ha'ayarah Libishei bashoah). **Yalkut Moreshet Period** 1975;20:7-34

**Epstein R** see **Skinner BF**

**Epstein WL:** 'Multiple benign sarkoid of the skin' by Boeck, December 1899. Commentary: What begot Boeck? **Arch Dermatol** 1982 Oct;118(10):711-22

**The eradication of East Coast fever in South Africa: J S Afr Vet Assoc** 1981 Mar;52(1):71-3

**Eramo S:** L'odontoiatria nell'arte. Su un affresco raffigurante S. Apollonia nella Basilica di Santa Maria di Collemaggio a l'Aquila. **Dent Cadmos** 1984 Apr;52(4):135-7

**Ercoli N:** L'antimonio da Basilio Valentino all'anno duemila. **Acta Med Hist Patav** 1979-80;26:47-61

**Erde EL** see **Engelhardt HT**

**Erdemir-Demirhan A:** The evolution and characteristics of important Turkish medical manuscripts by Anatolian Turks. In International Congress of the History of Medicine, 27th, Barcelona, 1980. Actas. Barcelona, Académia de Ciències Médiques de Catalunya i Balears, 1981. p. 238-44.

**Erdheim M:** Freuds Grössenphantasien, sein Konzept des Unbewussten und die Wiener Décadence. **Psyche (Stuttg)** 1981 Oct;35(10):857-74;Nov;35(11):1006-33

**Erdt T:** Jonathan Edwards: art and the sense of heart. Amherst, University of Massachusetts Press, 1980. xiv, 123 p.

**Eremenko SA** see **Sosnovskiĭ AT**

**Eremin VM** see **Onopchenko NA**

**Erez S:** Ottoman medicine viewed through Western eyes. **Hexagon Roche** 1981;9(3):Suppl I-IV

**Ergetowski R:** Akta personalne prof. Antoniego Stanisława Jurasza w

Heidelbergu i Karlsruhe. **Arch Hist Med (Warsz)** 1983;46(2):215–35
**Ergetowski R:** Uzupełniajace studia H. Kadyi'ego w Uniwersytecie Lipskim w 1879 r. **Arch Hist Med (Warsz)** 1979;42(3):309–15
**Erichsen SW:** Dronning Caroline Mathildes reiseapotek og litt om Stadsfysikus Johan Gotfried Erichsen. **Aust Agder Arv** 1977–78;:55–69
**Erichsen-Brown C:** Use of plants for the past 500 years. Aurora, Ont., Breezy Creeks Press, 1980, xxii, 512 p.
**Erickson GE** see **Spencer F**
**Erickson P:** The anthropology of Charles Caldwell, M.D. **ISIS** 1981 Jun;72(262):252–6
**Erickson RC, Hyerstay BJ:** Historical perspectives on the treatment of the mentally ill. In Gibbs M, et al., ed: Community psychology: theoretical and empirical approaches. New York, Gardner, 1980. p 29–63.
**Erickson RP:** Ohrwall, Henning and von Skramlik; the foundations of the four primary positions in taste. **Neurosci Biobehav Rev** 1984 Spring;8(1):105–27
**Ericson JE, Coughlin EA:** Archaeological toxicology. **Ann NY Acad Sci** 1981;376:393–403
**Ericsson R:** Mineralvatten på svenska apotek--en svunnen epok. **Nord Medicinhist Arsb** 1980;Suppl 6:129–38
**Erikson B:** Sjuksköterskeutbildningen i Sverige genom tiderna. **Nord Medicinhist Arsb** 1980;Suppl 6:69–75
**Erikson GE** see **Geist DC**
**Eriksson B:** A lesbian execution in Germany, 1721: the trial records. **J Homosex** 1980–81 Fall–Winter;6(1–2):27–40
**Eriksson E:** Ivar Palmer, a great name in the history of cruciate ligament surgery. **Clin Orthop** 1983 Jan–Feb;(172):3–10
**Eriksson G:** Linnaeus the botanist. In Frängsmyr T, ed: Linnaeus, the man and his work. Berkeley, University of California Press, 1983. p. 63–109.
**Eriksson G:** Om ingenting. Olof Rudbeck föreläsningsprogram 1679. **Lychnos** 1979–80;:79–108
**Eriksson G** see **Frängsmyr T, ed**
**Erk N:** Adil Mustafa (Adil-Bey), a pioneer veterinary bacteriologist in Turkey. **Hist Med Vet** 1977;2(4):99–101
**Erlen J:** Medicine in literature: theses; a survey of secondary sources. **Watermark** 1983 Summer;7(1):1–3
**Ermakov MA:** Iz istorii organizatsii évakuatsii ranenykh i bol'nykh partizan na Bol'shuiu zemliu. **Med Sestra** 1982 Mar;41(3):43–5
**Ermakov ME:** Meditsinskiĭ punkt partizanskogo otriada. **Feldsher Akush** 1983;48(5):47–9
**Ermakov VV, Devyatova LN:** The experience and the stages of development in USSR of the WHO English International Courses for epidemiology (1969–1978). **Sante Publique (Bucur)** 1980;23(1):3–14
**Ermakov VV** see **Serenko AF**
**Ermolaev GT** see **Makovskiĭ ChN**
**Ermolaev MM:** Vklad A. N. Marzeeva v stanovlenie i razvitie sanitarnogo prosveshcheniia na Ukraine. **Vrach Delo** 1983 Jan;(1):118–21
**Ernst CB** see **Rutkow IM**
**Ernst EA:** John A. Kennicott of the Grove: physician, horticulturist, and journalist in nineteenth-century Illinois. **J Ill State Hist Soc** 1981;74(2):109–18
**Ernst K:** Geisteskrankheit ohne Institution. Eine Feldstudie im Kanton Fribourg aus dem Jahr 1875. **Schweiz Arch Neurol Neurochir Psychiatr** 1983;133(2):239–62
**Eron C:** The virus that ate cannibals. New York, Macmillan, 1981. xii, 1983 p.
**Erös F:** Cooperation, legitimation and some aspects of the history of social psychology. **Stor Crit Psicol** 1981;2(1):87–96
**Erosa Barbachano A:** Historia de la medicina en Yucatan. **Bol Soc Mex Hist Filos Med** 1984 Dec;7(49):399–404
**Eross B** see **Grenvik A**
**Errera M, Einstein A:** Effets à court terme d'explosions nucléaires. **Bull Mem Acad R Med Belg** 1982;137(8–9):560–8
**Erspamer V:** Half a century of comparative research on biogenic amines and active peptides in amphibian skin and molluscan tissues. **Comp Biochem Physiol [C]** 1984;79(1):1–7
**Ertl JW von:** Die Versorgung von Amputationsstümpfen durch Osteo-Myoplastik nach v. Ertl. **Z Plast Chir** 1981 Sep;5(3):184–9
**Erxleben DC:** Gründliche Untersuchung der Ursachen, die das weibliche Geschlecht vom Studieren abhalten. Reprint of the Berlin, 1742, ed., mit einem Nachwort von G. Rechenberg. Hildesheim, New York, Olms, 1977. [68], 250 p.
**Erzinçlioğlu YZ:** The application of entomology to forensic medicine. **Med Sci Law** 1983 Jan;23(1):57–63
**Esaki H** see **Akiyoshi T**
**Esakov VD:** Soobshchenie N. M. Tulaikova ob otkrytii N. I. Vavilovym Zakona gomologicheskikh riadov. **Vopr Istor Estestvozn Tekh** 1981;4:111–3
**Eşanu V:** Research in the field of antiviral chemotherapy performed in the 'Stefan S. Nicolau' Institute of Virology. **Virologie** 1984 Oct–Dec;35(4):281–93
**Eschebach H:** Schola labri. Die Entwicklung der Schola labri in den Vesuvstädten, dargestellt am Labrum des Männercaladariums der Stabianer Thermen in Pompeji. **Cron Pompeiane** 1977;3:156–76
**Escobar A, Aruffo C:** La paleoneurología y el desarrollo del cerebro en los homínidos. **Gac Med Mex** 1980 Mar;116(3):115–32
**Escoe R:** A new look at John Greenwood's denture for George Washington. **Bull Hist Dent** 1981;29(1):37–43
**Escourolle R, Gray F, Hauw JJ:** Les atrophies cérébelleuses. **Rev Neurol (Paris)** 1982;138(12):953–65
**Escudero JC:** Desnutrición en América Latina, su magnitud (una primera aproximación). **Rev Mex Cienc Polit Soc** 1976;22(84):83–130
**Escudero Mendo A, Sagrera JE de:** El Rosario de los filósofos: una copia en castellano del siglo XIII (I). **Bol Soc Esp Hist Farm** 1983;34(136):151–66
**Eshraghi R:** [History of medical ethics in] Persia. In Reich WT, et al, ed: Encyclopedia of bioethics, v. 2. New York, Free Press, 1978. p. 884–7.
**Eskes TK:** Classic illustration. Figure showing the relationship between malformations of the thalidomide type and the sales of thalidomide. **Eur J Obstet Gynecol Reprod Biol** 1984 Jan;16(5):365
**Eskes TK:** Classic illustrations: Researches on prenatal life. **Eur J Obstet Gynecol Reprod Biol** 1981 May;11(6):435–6
**Esman AH:** Henri Dagonet. Pioneer of psychiatric photography. **NY State J Med** 1984 Feb;84(2):79–81
**Esman AH:** The study of lives: discussion of Tashjian and Shaw. **Adolesc Psychiatry** 1982;10:99–105
**Esoavelomandroso F:** Résistance à la médecine en situation coloniale: la peste à Madagascar. **Ann Econ Soc Civilis** 1981;36(2):168–90
**Espejo Maldonado E** see **Zuluaga Gómez A**
**Esping-Anderson G** see **Starr P**
**Espinosa JC** see **Tjarks G**
**Espinosa JM** see **Salazar JG**
**Espinosa RE, Vlietstra RE, Mann RJ:** J. B. A. Chauveau, E. J. Marey, and their resolution of the apex beat controversy through intracardiac pressure recordings. **Mayo Clin Proc** 1983 Mar;58(3):197–202
**Espinosa de los Reyes V:** El doctor Isidro Espinosa de los Reyes y los inicios de la atención materno-infantil en México. **Gac Med Mex** 1981 Feb;117(2):81–7
**Espinosa Iborra J:** El enfermo mental al final del Antiguo Régimen. **Asclepio** 1983;35:277–85
**Espinosa Ramos E** see **Esteva de Sagrera J**
**Espinosa y León VM:** Reseña histórica de los roedores domésticos. **Salud Publica Mex** 1984 Jan–Feb;26(1):77–81
**Espinoza Guadamuz JC** see **Tjarks GO**
**Esplugues J:** Tradición farmacológica valenciana: sus momentos estelares. Valencia, Real Academia de Medicina de Valencia, 1975. 71 p.
**Essen-Möller E:** The psychology and psychiatry of Henrik Sjöbring (1879–1956). **Psychol Med** 1980 May;10(2):201–10
**Establishment of the American Board of Oral and Maxillofacial Radiology.: Oral Surg** 1980 Jun;49(6):549–51
**Estes CL** see **Lee PR**
**Estes JW:** An account of the foxglove in America. **Bull Hist Med** 1973 Jul–Aug;47(4):394–408
**Estes JW, Kuhnke L:** French observations of disease and drug use in late eighteenth-century Cairo. **J Hist Med Allied Sci** 1984 Apr;39(2):121–52
**Estes JW:** Hall Jackson and the purple foxglove: medical practice and research in revolutionary America 1760–1820. Hanover, NH, University Press of New England, 1979. xvi, 291 p.
**Estes JW:** Making therapeutic decisions with protopharmacologic evidence. **Trans Stud Coll Physicians Phila** 1979 Jun;5(1 no 2):116–37
**Estes JW:** Medical skills in colonial New England. **N Engl Hist General Regist** 1980 Oct;134:259–75
**Estes JW:** Naval medicine in the age of sail: the voyage of the New York, 1802–1803. **Bull Hist Med** 1982 Summer;56(2):238–53
**Estes JW:** The practice of medicine in 18th-century Massachusetts: a bicentennial perspective. **N Engl J Med** 1981 Oct 29;305(18):1040–7
**Estes JW:** The protopharmacological basis of therapeutics. **Pharmacologist** 1984;26(1):25–30
**Estes LL:** The medical origins of the European witch craze: a hypothesis. **J Soc Hist** 1983;17:271–84
**Estes WK** see **Hearst E, ed**
**Estes JW, ed** see **Cash P**
**Estestvennye i preformirovannye fizicheskie faktory vo vrachebnoĭ deiatel'nosti Abu-Ali Ibn-Siny (k 1000-letiiu so dnia rozhdneiia): Vopr Kurortol Fizioter Lech Fiz Kult** 1981 Jan–Feb;(1):64–6
**Esteva J:** La historia y el actual debate epistemológico. **Bol Soc Esp Hist Farm** 1980/81 Dec–Mar;31–32(124–5):287–97
**Esteva de Sagrera J:** Alquimia seudoluliana y medicina. In Congrés International d'Història de la Medicina Catalana, 2nd, Barcelona, 1975. Llibre d'Actes. Barcelona, Socitra, 1977. p. 301–3.
**Esteva de Sagrera J:** Aplicación del 'Ars' luliana a la medicina. In Congrés International d'Història de la Medicina Catalana, 2nd, Barcelona, 1975. Llibre d'Actes. Barcelona, Socitra, 1977. p. 295–300.
**Esteva de Sagrera J, Espinosa Ramos E:** El proceso inquisitorial de Proust y el protagonismo cultural de Feijoo en el panorama científico de la ilustracion española. **Bol Soc Esp Hist Farm** 1982 Mar;33(129):77–92
**Esteva de Sagrera J:** Influencia decisiva de la biografía y la filosofía de Ramón Llull en su obra médica. In Congrés International d'Historia de la Medicina Catalana, 2nd, Barcelona, 1975. Llibre d'Actes. Barcelona, Socitra, 1977. p. 305–7.
**Esteva de Sagrera J:** La farmacia española frente al cambio político. Barcelona, Ketres, 1978. 102 p.
**Esteva de Sagrera J, Espinosa Ramos E:** Los trociscos de vibrora en la obra de Luís de Oviedo, Gerónimo de la Fuente Piérola y Félix Palacios. **Unifarma** 1980 Jun 13;:244–51
**Esteva de Sagrera J:** Una obra inédita y desconocida de Agustín Yáñez y Girona. **Bol Soc Esp Hist Farm** 1979 Dec;30(120):295–304
**Estévez R:** Sir James Paget. **Rev Med Chil** 1984 Jul;112(7):740–3
**Estévez Cordovez R:** El Hospital San Francisco de Borja. **Rev Med Chil** 1982 Jul;110(7):694–8
**Estévez González A:** Anotaciones a la historia de la neuropsicoloía.

**Arch Neurobiol (Madr)** 1980 Nov–Dec;43(6):401–20
**Estévez González A:** El cerebro frontal y motor, según Luria. Su patologia, síndromes y afasias. **Arch Neurobiol (Madr)** 1981 Mar–Apr;44(2):75–94
**Esteyneffer J de:** Florilegio medicinal. Edicion, estudio preliminar, notas, glosario e indice analitico by M. del Carmen Anzures y Bolaños. México, Academía Nacional de Medicina, 1978. 2 v. xxiii, 973 p.
**Estienne P** see **Naranjo B**
**Estrin GB:** Voprosy khirurgii i travmatologii v zhurnale 'Vrach' V. A. Manasseina (1880–1901 gg.). **Vestn Khir** 1981 Oct;127(10):142–4
**Etchegoyen RH:** Fifty years after the mutative interpretation. **Int J Psychoanal** 1983;64 ( Pt 4):445–59
**Etessami S:** La contraction musculaire: de l'antiquité jusqu'à nos jours. In: Congrès international d'histoire de la médecine, XXVe, Québec, 1976. Actes. Québec, 1977. p. 644–9.
**Etheridge EW:** Grace Arabell Goldsmith. In: Notable American women. The modern period. Cambridge, Mass., Belknap–Harvard Univ. Press, 1980. 4:283–4.
**Ethridge RF:** Tobacco among the Cherokees. **J Cherokee Stud** 1978;3(2):77–86
**Etiología de la tuberculosis: Dr. Roberto Koch: Salud Publica Mex** 1982 May–Jun;24(3):241–57
**Ettling J:** The germ of laziness. Rockefeller philanthropy and public health in the new South. Cambridge, Harvard, 1981. x, 263 p.
**Ettlinger L:** Wartime research on penicillin in Switzerland and antibiotic screening. In Parascandola J, ed: The history of antibiotics. Madison, American Institute of the History of Pharmacy, 1980. p. 57–67.
**Etzioni A:** How much is a life worth? **Soc Policy** 1979;9(5):4–8
**Etziony M:** History of psychosomatic medicine: semantic and philosophic bird's eye view. **Koroth** 1979 Nov;7(9–10):CCIX–CCX(658–66)
**Etzkowitz H:** Entrepreneurial scientists and entrepreneurial universities in American academic science. **Minerva** 1983 Summer–Autumn;21(2–3):198–233
**Eule H:** Die Auswirkung der Entdeckung und der Arbeiten Robert Kochs auf die Entwicklung der Therapie der Tuberkulose. **Z Erkr Atmungsorgane** 1982;158(1–2):155–62
**Euler US von:** Chemical neurotransmission––yesterday and today. **Ciba Found Symp** 1982;(91):3–12
**Euler US von:** History and development of prostaglandins. **Gen Pharmacol** 1983;14(1):3–6
**Euler US von:** Prostaglandin, historical remarks. **Prog Lipid Res** 1981;20:xxxi–xxxv
**Eulner HH, Hoepke H, ed:** Der Briefwechsel zwischen Rudolph Wagner und Jacob Henle 1838–1862. Göttingen, Vandenhoeck & Ruprecht, 1979. 115 p. (Arbeiten aus der Niedersächsischen Staats- und Universitätsbibliothek Göttingen, Band 16).
**Eulner HH:** Zur Geschichte der Meeresheilkunde: Georg Christoph Lichtenberg und das Seebad Cuxhaven. **Medizinhist J** 1982;17(1/2):115–28
**Eva D** see **Gillespie B**
**Evans AE:** Leukemia: historical development of cancer therapy. The first battle is won. **Front Radiat Ther Oncol** 1981;16:18–29
**Evans AS** see **Richmond PA**
**Evans B:** Freedom to choose: the life and work of Dr. Helena Wright, pioneer of contraception. London, Bodley Head, 1984. 285 p.
**Evans B, Waites B:** IQ and mental testing. An unnatural science and its social history. London, Macmillan, 1981. x, 228 p. (Critical social studies).
**Evans C:** Thomas Graham Brown. In Dictionary of national biography, 1961–1970. Suppl. 8, 1981. p. 151–2.
**Evans D:** Alexander Thomas Glenny. In Dictionary of national biography, 1961–1970. Suppl 8, 1981. p. 434–5.
**Evans EC:** Physiognomics in the ancient world. Philadelphia, American Philosophical Society, 1969. 101 p. (Transactions of the American Philosophical Society, n. s., Vol. 59, Part 5).
**Evans GS:** A great therapeutic age. **Br Med J** 1979 Oct 20;2(6196):981
**Evans GT:** On-line library networking: a bibliographic essay. **Bull Am Soc Inf Sci** 1979 Jun;5(5):11–4
**Evans H** see **Knightley P**
**Evans JA:** Landmark perspective: Roentgenography of the urinary tract. **JAMA** 1983 Nov 25;250(20):2854–5
**Evans LT:** Darwin's use of the analogy between artificial and natural selection. **J Hist Biol** 1984 Spring;17(1):113–40
**Evans M:** Medicine and stamps. **Hist Med (Lond)** 1981;9(1):21–2
**Evans N:** Charitable bequests and their recipients. **Local Hist** 1982;15(4):225–6
**Evans N:** 'The first charity in Wales'. Cardiff Infirmary and South Wales Society, 1837–1914. **Welsh Hist Rev** 1979;9(3):n.p.
**Evans P** see **Williams JE**
**Evans PE:** Cerclage fixation of a fractured humerus in 1775. Fact or fiction? **Clin Orthop** 1983 Apr;(174):138–42
**Evans PR:** Infantile scurvy: the centenary of Barlow's disease. **Br Med J [Clin Res]** 1983 Dec 17;287(6408):1862–3
**Evans RB, Talmadge P:** Dial access: a history of the Southern Medical Association's newest contribution to continuing medical education. **South Med J** 1980 Apr;73(4):489–96
**Evans RB, MacLeod RB:** Foreword to Systematic psychology: Prolegomena by Edward Bradford Titchener. Ithaca, London, Cornell University Press, 1972. v–xvi.
**Evans RB:** The origins of American academic psychology. In J. Brozěk, ed: Explorations in the history of psychology in the United States. Lewisburg, Bucknell University Press, 1984. p. 17–60.
**Evans RB** see **James W**
**Evans RB** see **Robert I. Watson and the development of the history of psychology: a symposium**
**Evans RD:** Inception of standards for internal emitters, radon and radium. **Health Phys** 1981 Sep;41(3):437–48
**Evans RI:** B. F. Skinner, the man and his ideas: dialogue with B. F. Skinner. New York, Praeger, 1981. xiv, 140 p.
**Evans RI:** Dialogue with C. G. Jung. New York, Praeger, 1981. xi, 241 p.
**Evans RI:** Dialogue with Carl Rogers. New York, Praeger, 1981. lxxxviii, 195 p.
**Evans RI:** Dialogue with Erik Erikson. New York, London, Harper & Row, 1967. xvi, 142 p.
**Evans RI:** Dialogue with Gordon Allport. New York, Praeger, 1981. xxv, 157 p.
**Evans RI:** Dialogue with Jean Piaget. New York, Praeger, 1981. lxi, 189 p. (Dialogues in Contemporary Psychology Series).
**Evans RI:** Dialogue with R. D. Laing. New York, Praeger, 1981. lxxv, 170 p. (Reprint of 1976 ed; with new introduction).
**Evans RJ** see **Cox WW**
**Evans WG** see **Pereira CB**
**Evans RB, ed** see **Brozek J**
**Evdokimov PP, Kulak VM:** [D. I. Ul'ianov in Simbirsk] (Rus). **Med Sestra** 1981;40(1):42–3
**Evdokimov PP:** K istorii bolezni F. I. Shaliapina. **Klin Med (Mosk)** 1983 May;61(5):115–6
**Evdokimov PP:** Lechashchie vrachi sem'i I.N. Ul'ianova. **Sov Zdravookhr** 1980;(11):64–5
**Evdokimov PP:** Mediki, privlekaemye i sudimye po 'Delu 193-kh'. **Sov Zdravookhr** 1980;(6):61–3
**Evdokimov PP, Kulak VM:** Pervye s'ezdy vracheĭ v Povolzh'e. **Sov Zdravookhr** 1983;9:70–2
**Evdokimov PP:** Uchastie studentov–medikov Kazani v revoliutsionnom dvizhenii 1870–1880 gg. **Sov Zdravookhr** 1981;(1):60–2
**Evdokimov PP** see **Brzheskiĭ VCh**
**Evdokimov PP** see **Kulak VM**
**Eveleth PB** see **Baker TS**
**Evens L:** History of strabismus treatment. **Bull Soc Belge Ophtalmol** 1981;195:19–52
**Everest R** see **Allan P**
**Everett DE:** Dr. Pat Ireland Nixon: letters to and from his book-loving friends. **Friends P. I. Nixon Med Hist Libr** 1974 Oct;3:1–13
**Everett M** see **Levy JE**
**Everett MA:** Anne-Charles Lorry. The first French dermatologist. **Int J Dermatol** 1979 Nov;18(9):762–4
**Everett MA:** Jean Louis Alibert. The father of French dermatology. **Int J Dermatol** 1984 Jun;23(5):351–6
**The evolution of Mohs' surgery: J Dermatol Surg Oncol** 1982 Aug;8(8):650–4
**The evolution of the O. R.: Hosp Adm Can** 1978 Apr;20(4):38–9
**Evoluzione dell'anestesiologia in Italia: Minerva Anestesiol** 1984 Jun;50(6):285–92
**Evrard E:** Chirurgiens militaires britanniques à la bataille de Waterloo et dans les hôpitaux de Bruxelles en juin 1815. **Rev Belge Hist Milit** 1982;24(5):425–64
**Evrard E:** Le service de santé militaire hollando-belge à la bataille de Waterloo et dans les hôpitaux de Bruxelles en juin 1815. **Rev Belge Hist Milit** 1983;25(1):61–96
**Ewald BH, Gregg DA:** Animal research for animals. **Ann NY Acad Sci** 1983;406:48–58
**Ewalt DJ:** Patients, politics and physicians: the struggle for control of State Lunatic Asylum No. 1, Fulton, Missouri. **Mo Hist Rev** 1983 Jan;77:170–88
**Ewan J:** Five pupils of Benjamin Smith Barton: the men and their minds. **Trans Stud Coll Physicians Phila** 1983 Dec;5(5 no 4):309–20
**Ewart WB:** Causes of mortality in a subarctic settlement (York Factory, Man.), 1714–1946. **Can Med Assoc J** 1983 Sep 15;129(6):571–4
**Ewerbeck H:** Die Gesundheit des Kindes im Laufe des 20. Jahrhunderts. **Off Gesundheitswes** 1979 Sep;41 Suppl 1:1–6
**Ewert G:** Auffassungen der Sozialhygiene zum Organisationsaspekt im Gesundheitswesen. **Z Gesamte Hyg** 1980 Apr;26(4):280–3
**Ewert G, Rothe J:** K vývoji sociální hygieny v Německé Demokratické Republice. **Cesk Zdrav** 1979 Oct;27(10):391–8
**Ewert G:** Kratkiĭ obzor o razvitii sotsial'noĭ gigieny v GDR. **Sov Zdravookhr** 1980;(3):45–9
**Ewert G** see **Rothe J**
**Excerpt of a letter from veterinary surgeon Haldoe Dahl:** from the Diocese of Trondheim to Professor E. Viborg. **Hist Med Vet** 1977;2(1):4–9
**Exposition 'enfants des montagnes' au musée dauphinois à Grenoble: Bull Soc Fr Hist Hop** 1980;(41):32–5
**Expósito CR:** Dr. Félix Figueredo y Diaz (Un hombre del 68 y de la Protesta de Baraguá). Habana, Organismos, 1973. 417 p. (Cuadernos de Historia de la Salud Pública, 55).
**Extracts from the last century:** Dental preventive medicine. **Br Dent J** 1981 Jul 7;151(1):23
**Ey H:** Naissance de la médecine. Paris, New York, Masson, 1981. viii, 230 p.
**Eyckmans L:** Le problème du choléra en Afrique de l'Est. **Bull Seances Acad R Sci Outre Mer** 1979;(3):445–50
**Eyler JM:** The conceptual origins of William Farr's epidemiology: numerical methods and social thought in the 1830s. In Lilienfeld AM, ed: Times, plaes, and persons. Baltimore, London, Johns Hopkins Univ. Press, 1980. (Sigerist suppl. to the Bull Hist Med, n.s., no 4) p. 1–21.

Eyler JM: The conversion of Angus Smith: the changing role of chemistry and biology in sanitary science, 1850-1880. **Bull Hist Med** 1980 Summer;54(2):216-34
**Eyman E:** Alfred Barring Garrod--pionier badán nad dną (1819--1907). **Reumatologia** 1980;18(2):189-90
**Eyquem A:** L'immuno-pathologie de l'auto-immunisation 1900-1980. **Arch Inst Pasteur Tunis** 1981 Sep-Dec;58(3):281-95
**Ezell MD:** Early attitudes toward alcoholic beverages in the South. **Red River Val Hist Rev** 1982;7(1):64-70
**Ezrahi Y:** Utopian and pragmatic rationalism: the political context of scientific advice. **Minerva** 1980 Spring;18(1):111-31

# F

**Fabbi A:** La scuola chirurgica di Preci. Preci [s.n.], 1974. 213 p.
**Faber JF:** Life tables for the United States: 1900-2050. Actuarial Study No. 87. Washington, D.C., Social Security Administration, 1982. ii, 86 p. (SSA Pub. No. 11-11534).
**Faber-Castell, K von:** Arzt, Krankheit und Tod im erzählerischen Werk Theodor Fontanes. Zürich, Juris Druck, 1983. 97 p. (Zürcher Medizingeschichtliche Abhandlungen, Neue Reihe, Nr. 157).
**Fabian B, Spieckermann ML:** Deutsche Uebersetzungen englischer humanmedizinischer Werke 1680-1810. Eine vorläufige Bibliographie. **Medizinhist J** 1980;15(1/2):154-71
**Fábián T:** A Semmelweis OTE fogpótlástani klinikájának negyedszázados története és munkássága. **Fogorv Sz** 1984 Oct;77(10):289-91
**Fábián T:** 75 éves a Fogorvosi Szemle. **Fogorv Sz** 1982 Jan;75(1):1-3
**Fabre A:** Les traditions de la médecine de l'avant. **Med Armees** 1980;8(10)spec:781-6
**Fabre M, Boudet F, Boe M, et al:** Intoxications par le phosgène. **Toxicol Eur Res** 1983 Jul;5(4):185-8
**Fabre A, ed:** Histoire de la médecine aux armées. Tome 2. De la Révolution française au conflit mondial de 1914. Paris, Charles-Lavazelle, 1984. 491 p.
**Faculdade de Odontologia da Universidade de São Paulo, 1934-1974:** São Paulo, Faculdade, [1974?]. 60 p.
**The faculty of medicine at Harvard College:** **N Engl J Med** 1983 Feb 3;308(5):288-9
**Fadiga E:** Giulio Cesare Pupilli. Milano, 5-10-1893-Pescia (PT), 17-8-1973. **Arch Fisiol** 1979 Jun 30;71(1-4):3-22
**Fagan RW, Mauss AL:** Padding the revolving door: an initial assessment of the uniform alcoholism and intoxication treatment act in practice. **Soc Probl** 1978;26(2):232-47
**Fagerheim E:** Lars Levi Laestadius' teologiske studier. **Nor Teol Tidsskr** 1972;73(1):35-50
**Fagermoen MS:** From apprenticeship to study--the development of nursing education in Norway. **Int J Nurs Stud** 1984;21(3):165-75
**Fagot A:** La philosophie de l'hygiène en 1878. In Poirier J, Poirier JL, ed: Médecine et philosophie à la fin du XIXe siècle. Paris, Université de Paris XII - Val de Marne, [1980?]. p. 61-84.
**Fagot AM:** Medicina e probabilità. **Kos** 1984 Feb;1(1):24-31
**Fagrell B:** Först med stort patientmaterial på rökbetingad allergi. **Lakartidningen** 1982 Oct 13;79(41):3669-7
**Fähndrich E, Helmchen H, Hippius H:** The history of the AMDP-System. **Mod Probl Pharmacopsychiatry** 1983;20:1-9
**Fahnestock J:** The heroine of irregular features: physiognomy and conventions of heroine description. **Victorian Stud** 1981;24(3):325-50
**Fahrni GS:** Contributions made to Canadian medicine during World War II. **Can Med Assoc J** 1981 Apr 15;124(8):1095, 1098-9, 1101-2
**Fahrni GS:** Prairie surgeon. Winnipeg, Queenston House, 1976. vi, 138 p.
**Fair MF** see **Ryan MT**
**Fairbanks B, Scharfman B:** The cervical cap: cap and current experience. **Women Health** 1980 Fall;5(3):61-80
**Fairbanks RJ:** The Journal of Pastoral Care: an historical perspective. **J Pastoral Care** 1975 Sep;29(3):204-6
**Fairchild GB** see **Christensen HA**
**Falcao RF:** A proposito do quarto centenario de publicão do 'Tratado de las drogas' de Cristóvão da Costa. **Rev Port Farm** 1980;30:234-44
**Falconer J:** History of the Botswana veterinary services--1905-66. **Botsw Notes Rec** 1971;3:74-8
**Faler K:** The conquest of tuberculosis. A contribution of American veterinary medicine to human welfare. **Mod Vet Pract** 1984 Jan;65(1):51-3
**Faletti HE** see **Radcliff-Umstead D, ed**
**Falise C:** Le choléra à Bruxelles en 1866. **Ann Soc Belg Hist Hop** 1979;17:81-104
**Falk A:** Moshe Dyan: the infantile roots of political action. **J Psychohist** 1983 Fall;11(2):271-88
**Falk D:** Primate neuroanatomy: an evolutionary perspective. In F. Spencer, ed: A history of American physical anthropology, 1930-1980. New York, Academic Press, 1982. 75-103.
**Falk H** see **Caldwell GG**
**Falk IS:** Some lessons from the fifty years since the CCMC final report, 1932. **J Public Health Policy** 1983 Jun;4(2):135-61
**Falk LA:** Black Abolitionist doctors and healers, 1810-1885. **Bull Hist Med** 1980 Summer;54(2):258-72
**Falk LA** see **Cameron S**
**Falk LA** see **George Rosen: In Memoriam**
**Falk RE** see **Dreznik A**
**Falke TH, Ziedses des Plantes BG, Voorthuisen AE van:** The Netherlands' initial experience with NMR imaging. **Diagn Imaging** 1984;53(1):43-52
**Falkiewiczowa S:** Kronika Wrocławskiej Kliniki Neurologicznej. **Neurol Neurochir Pol** 1984 May-Jun;18(3):303-9
**Falkiewiczowa S, Świątkowski S, Teppa S:** Neurologia lwowska. **Neurol Neurochir Pol** 1982 Jan-Jun;16(1-3):85-107
**Falkmer S:** Patologi i Umeå. **Nord Medicinhist Arsb** 1980;:147-76
**Falkowski W:** W Bielsku Podlaskim. **Pieleg Polozna** 1984;(2):26-7
**Faller A:** Die Präparation der weissen Substanz des Gehirns bei Stensen, Willis und Vieussens. **Gesnerus** 1982;39(2):171-93
**Faller A:** Die 'Tetralogie von Fallot'; zur geschichtlichen Entwicklung von Diagnose und Therapie eines kongenitalen Herzsyndroms von Niels Stensen bis zur modernen Herzchirurgie. **Gesnerus** 1982;39(3-4):321-46
**Faller A:** Elemente einer Wissenschaftslehre und einer Wissenschaftskritik in den Schriften von Niels Stensen (1638-1686). **Gesnerus** 1980;37(3/4):169-88
**Faller A:** Welchen Platz nimmt Stensens anatomische Forschung in Lorenz Heisters Chirurgie und Anatomie ein? **Gesnerus** 1983;40(1-2):55-66
**Faller A:** Wertschätzung von Stensens 'Discours sur l'anatomie du cerveau' im Verlaufe von drei Jahrhunderten. Aarau, Verlag Sauerländer, 1981. 96 p. (Veröffentlichungen der Schweizerischen Gesellschaft für Geschichte der Medizin und der Naturwissenschaften, 35).
**Faller A** see **Bierbaum M**
**Fäller J** see **Takáts L**
**Fallis AM:** John L. Todd: Canada's first professor of parasitology. **Can Med Assoc J** 1983 Sep 1;129(5):486, 488-90
**Famaey JP** see **Appelboom T**
**Fan CC:** T'i yü ti li shih. **Shih-ta Hsüeh-pao** 1977;22:417-40
**Fan Chêng-chih:** Chung-kuo t'i-yu ti shih-hsueh Yan-chiu. **Shih-ta Hsueh-pao** 1981;26:117-58
**Fancher RE:** Alphonse de Candolle, Francis Galton, and the early history of the nature-nurture controversy. **J Hist Behav Sci** 1983 Oct;19(4):341-52
**Fancher RE:** Francis Galton's African ethnography and its role in the development of his psychology. **Br J Hist Sci** 1983 Mar;16(12 No. 1):67-79
**Fankhauser F:** Prof. Dr. Alfred Leuthold, Bern, 1901-1982. **Schweiz Arch Tierheilkd** 1982 Sep;124(9):473-8
**Fankhauser R:** Dem 125. Bande zum Geleit. **Schweiz Arch Tierheilkd** 1983 Jan;125(1):1-15
**Fankhauser R:** Hundestaupe--Geschichte einer Krankheit. **Schweiz Arch Tierheilkd** 1982 May;124(5):245-56
**Fankhauser R:** Joseph Guillerey, Porrentruy: premier Dr méd. vét. suisse. Un jubilé passé inaperçu. **Schweiz Arch Tierheilkd** 1983 Dec;125(12):871-5
**Fankhauser R, Hörning B:** Zum hundertsten Todestag David von Niederhäusern's. **Schweiz Arch Tierheilkd** 1982 Feb;124(2):53-68
**Fankhauser R, Hörning B:** 175 Jahre tierärztliche Lehranstalt zu Bern. **Schweiz Arch Tierheilkd** 1980 Feb;122(2):57-94
**Fanti PA, Varotti C:** 'Les eczématides'. Historical review of the term. **Am J Dermatopathol** 1984 Oct;6(5):437-40
**Fantini B:** Chemical and biological classification of proteins. **Hist Philos Life Sci** 1983;5(1):3-32
**Fantini B:** La genetica classica. Torino, Loescher, 1979. 293 p. (Storia della Scienza, 5).
**Fantini B** see **Grmek MD**
**Farahani EM:** Abridged life tables of Iran, 1956-1966. **Genus** 1978;34(1-2):215-26
**Farber SJ:** A tribute to Lewis Thomas. **Cell Immunol** 1983 Nov;82(1):21-2
**Farber W:** Drogerien in Babylonien und Assyrien. **Iraq** 1977;2:223-8
**Farcnik F, Vrbic V:** Stomatološka klinika včeraj, danes, jutri. **Zobozdrav Vestn** 1981 Summer;36(3-4):81-7
**Fardeau M** see **Sorrel-Dejerine Y**
**Farge A** see **Forster R**
**Farina C** see **Chapman ID**
**Farina G:** Interpretazioni cartesiane. **Med Secoli** 1982 May-Aug;19(2):221-4
**Farina P:** Il corpuscolarismo di Henricus Regius: materialismo e medicina in un cartesiano olandese del Seicento. In: Ricerche sull'atomismo del Seicento. Florence: La Nuova Italia, 1977. p. 119-78.
**Farkas G:** Eclampsia in the course of times. In: Congrès international d'histoire de la médecine, XXVe, Québec, 1976. Actes. Québec, 1977. p. 650-3.
**Farkas G, Farkas G Jr:** People's customs related to pregnancy and delivery in former Transylvania. In: Congrès international d'histoire de la médecine, XXVe, Québec, 1976. Actes. Québec, 1977. p. 654-8.
**Farkas G Jr** see **Farkas G**
**Farkas J, Pisztora F, Martos G:** Történeti szocio-kulturpsychiátriai vizsgálatok egy zárt faluközösségre, a mezökövesdi matyó populációra vonatkozóan 1895 és 1945 között. **Orvostort Kozl** 1982;92(4):127-31
**Farkas J** see **Martos G**
**Farley F:** Two generations of women physicians: the New York Infirmary, 1870-1899. **J Am Med Wom Assoc** 1984 Nov-Dec;39(6):189-91
**Farley J:** Gametes & spores. Ideas about sexual reproduction, 1750-1914. Baltimore, London, Johns Hopkins University Press, 1982. x, 299 p.
**Farley J, Geison GL, Ebnöther D:** Le débat entre Pasteur et Pouchet: science, politique et génération spontanée, au 19e siècle en France. **Pandore** 1982;special number
**Farley M, Keel O, Limoges C:** Les commencements de l'administration montréalaise de la santé publique (1865-1885). **HSTC** 1982 May;21(6 no 2):85-109
**Farley M, Keel O, Limoges C:** Les commencements de l'administration montrèalaise de la santé publique (1865-1885)--I. **HSTC** 1982 Jan;20(6

no 1):24–46

**Farley MA:** [History of] sexual ethics. In Reich WT, et al, ed: Encyclopedia of bioethics, v.4. New York, Free Press, 1978. p. 1575–89.

**Farley MF:** Stranger's fever. **SC Hist Illus** 1970;1(1):54–61

**Farmer ED:** Dental education in Europe. **J R Soc Med** 1984 Jun;77(6):452–8

**Farmer HF:** The germ of laziness: a Florida historical perspective. **J Fla Med Assoc** 1983 Aug;70(8):659–62

**Farmer RD** see **Low AA**

**Farnham TJ:** New Haven, 1784. **Conn Med** 1984 Sep;48(9):563–5

**Farnsworth N:** Sobre la preparacion de extractos de plantas para su evaluacion farmacologica en animales. **Med Tradic** 1982;3(11):27–33

**Farolfi B:** Dall'antropometria militare alla storia del corpo. **Quad Stor** 1979;14(3):1056–91

**Farquhar J, Gajdusek DC, ed:** Kuru: Early letters and field notes from the collection of D. Carleton Gajdusek. New York, Raven Press, 1981. xxviii, 338 p.

**Farr AD:** Early opposition to obstetric anaesthesia. **Anaesthesia** 1980 Sept;35(9):896–907

**Farr AD:** Learn, that you may improve: the history of the Institute of Medical Laboratory Sciences. Sussex, Denley Instruments, 1982. xi, 214 p.

**Farr AD:** Religious opposition to obstetric anaesthesia: a myth? **Ann Sci** 1983 Mar;40(2):159–77

**Farr AD:** The first human blood transfusion. **Med Hist** 1980 Apr;24(2):143–62

**Farr AD:** The Marquis de Sade and induced abortion. **J Med Ethics** 1980 Mar;6(1):7–10

**Farr AD:** Treatment of haemophilia by transfusion: the first recorded case. **J R Soc Med** 1981 Apr;74(4):301–5

**Farrah MA:** Andrew Carnegie: a psychohistorical sketch. D. A. Diss. Carnegie-Mellon University. Pittsburgh, 1982. ix. 183 p.

**Farrar GE:** Advances in pharmacology––the golden age of therapeutics. **Penn Med** 1983 Dec;86(12):48–9

**Farrar WE:** Parzival's pericardial puncture. **Ann Intern Med** 1980 May;92(5):640

**Farrell JJ:** Inventing the American way of death, 1830–1920. Philadelphia, Temple University Press, 1980 viii, 287 p.

**Farrell JJ:** The dying of death: the meaning and management of death in America, 1830–1920. Ph.D. diss. University of Illinois, Urbana, Ill., 1980. 329 p.

**Farrell K:** Hyperthermia for malignant disease––a history of medicine note––the work of Georges Lakhovsky. **Adv Exp Med Biol** 1982;157:9–10

**Farsund O:** Fra hjerte til hjerte: om blod og blodoverføring. **Sykepleien** 1980 Jun 5;67(10):11–5

**Faruqi AH:** Use of leeches in Greco-Arab medicine. **Stud Hist Med** 1982 Jun;6(2):137–40

**Fasella P** see **Passi S**

**Fasol E:** Der Internist Hermann Eichhorst, 1849–1921. Zürich, Juris Druck, 1983. 98 P. (Zürcher Medizingeschichtliche Abhandlungen, Neue Reihe, Nr. 159).

**Fasquelle J** see **150e année**

**Fasquelle R, Delaunay A:** Geschichte der Mikrobiologie. In Sournia JC, Martiny M, Poulet J, ed: Illustrierte Geschichte der Medizin. Salzburg, Andreas, 1980. Vol. 7. p. 2459–97.

**Fasquelle R:** Pasteur et l'épopée pasteurienne. **Sem Hop Paris** 1983 Dec 22;59(48):3395–404

**Fasquelle R** see **150e année**

**Fassler B:** Theories of homosexuality as sources of Bloomsbury's androgyny. **Signs** 1979;5(2):237–51

**Fastlicht S:** Spain's first scientific expedition to Mexico in the XVI century: the tragic story of Francisco Hernandez. **Bull Hist Dent** 1980 Apr;28(1):3–10

**Fastlicht S:** Tooth mutilations and dentistry in pre-Columbian Mexico. Berlin, Buch- und Zeitschriften-Verlag 'Die Quintessenz', 1976. 164 p.

**Fath H:** A dream come true: the story of St. Jude Children's Research Hospital and ALSAC. Memphis, TN, ALSAC, 1983. 214 p.

**Faulkner TC:** Computer applications for an edition of Robert Burton's The anatomy of melancholy: a system for scholarly publishing. **Comput Hum** 1981 Nov;15(3):163–82

**Faure E** see **Bernard J**

**Faure O:** A l'hôpital, avant les infirmières: les soeurs hospitalières de Lyon au début du XIXe siècle. **Penelope** 1981;(5):52–5

**Faure O:** L'hôpital et la médicalisation au début du 19e siècle: l'exemple lyonnais (1800–1830). **Ann Bretagne** 1979;86(3):277–90

**Faure O:** Médecins, médecine et hôpital à Lyon au début du XIXe siècle. **Bull Soc Fr Hist Hop** 1981;(42):15–24

**Faure MH, ed** see **Bailliart JP**

**Faust DG:** Mary Breckinridge. In: Notable American women. The modern period. Cambridge, Mass., Belknap-Harvard Univ. Press, 1980. 4:103–5.

**Faust E:** Arabien 1680. Olfert Dappers Arabienbuch und seine Quellen, geprüft an Nachrichten über Kaffee, Sesam und Träumen. Köln, Universität zu Köln, 1977, 256 p. (Kölner medizinhistorische Beiträge, 5; also Diss).

**Fautrez J:** Les Archives de Biologie, les fondateurs et les éditeurs de la revue. **Arch Biol (Liege)** 1980;91(2):133–40

**Fauve-Chamoux A** see **Dupâquier J**

**Favaloro RG:** The present era of myocardial revascularization––some historical landmarks. **Int J Cardiol** 1983 Oct;4(3):331–44

**Favazza AR:** Behind the sickness of Hitler. **MD** 1981;25(5):37–8;25(7):15

**Favazza AR:** Hitler's encephalitis? **Am J Psychiatry** 1981 Jul;138(7):999–1000

**Favero GA:** Odontoiatria del passato. La stomatologia nelle opere di Cessare Cavina (1888–1935). **Dent Cadmos** 1982 Oct;50(10):83–91

**Favero GA** see **Agostoni G**

**Favez G:** Charlotte Olivier (1864–1945). **Rev Med Suisse Romande** 1984 May;104(5):353–68

**Favorova LA:** Uchenie L. V. Gromashevskogo i problema likvidatsii infekstionnykh bolezneĭ. **Zh Mikrobiol Epidemiol Immunobiol** 1984 Jul;(7):119–23

**Favre R:** De 'médico-topographique' à Lyon en 1783. **Dix-Huit Siecle** 1977;9:151–9

**Favre R:** La mort dans la littérature et la pensée française au siècle des lumières. Lyon, Presses universitaires de Lyon, 1978. 640 p.

**Fawaz G:** Whither AUB? An excursion through the campus lasting five-score years and ten. **Middle East J Anaesthesiol** 1983 Feb–Jun;7(1–2):9–19

**Fay FR:** History of medical congresses in Tasmania. **Med J Aust** 1980 May 3;1(9):414–6, 437

**Fay-Sallois F:** Les nourrices à Paris au XIXe siècle. Paris, Payot, 1980. 284 p.

**Fayle R:** Introducing the history of Russian pharmacy. **Pharm Hist (London)** 1975 Dec;5(3):1

**Fazekas A:** A magyar nyelvu herbárium irodalomról. **Orvostort Kozl** 1982;28(1–3):43–64

**Fazekas A:** Jósa András 150 éve született (1834. nov. 30.–1918. szept. 6.). **Orv Hetil** 1984 Sep 30;125(40):2444–6

**Fazekas A:** Lencsés György és az elsö magyar nyelvü kéziratos orvosi könyv 1577–böl. **Egeszsegneveles** 1982;23:79–81

**Fazekas A:** Szabolcsi adatok a pestisjárványok történetéhez. **Orvostort Kozl** 1979;86(24 no 4):91–106

**Fazekas A:** 100 éve volt az eszlári per –nem ölték meg, a tiszának ment Solymosi Eszter–. **Orv Hetil** 1982 Jul 25;123(30):1870–2

**Fearon Z:** Patients and doctors. History of their roles and relationships. **Consum Health Perspect** 1982 Oct;9(2):1–3

**Febres-Cordero F:** Acerca de la 'Desmonopolizacion' en odontologia. **Acta Odontol Venez** 1979 May–Dec;17(2–3):3–11

**Febres-Cordero F:** Acerca de la fundacion de la Escuela Dental en Venezuela. **Acta Odontol Venez** 1980 Jan–Apr;18(1):7–35

**Fébres-Cordero F:** Algunos aspectos de la medicina venezolana del siglo XIX y su relación con el período histórico a que corresponde. **Tec Hosp** 1981 Mar–Jun;28(1–2)41–7

**Febres-Cordero F:** Bibliografía Odontólogica Venezolana. **Acta Odontol Venez** 1982 Sep–Dec;20(3):183–91

**Febres-Cordero F:** Cirujanos y odontologos proceden de los barberos medievales? **Acta Odontol Venez** 1981 Sep–Dec;19(3):283–304

**Febres-Cordero F:** Datos sobre el estado de la salud dentaria del Libertador. Caracas, 1983. [2 p.]

**Febres-Cordero F:** Datos sobre el estado de salud dentaria del Libertador. **Thorax** 1979;6(1):29–31

**Febres-Cordero F:** Fue Hugues Planque autorizado para ejerceer en Venezuela 'su industria de dentista'? **Acta Odontol Venez** 1982 Jan–Apr;20(1):39–52

**Fébres-Cordero F:** Hoja de servicios (1929–1979). Datos biográficos, actividades, labor intelectual y algunos juicios y comentarios sobre la obra realizada. Caracas, Publicaciones del Consejo de Profesores Universitarios Jubilados, 1979. 256 p.

**Febres-Cordero F:** Incorrecciones en el lenguaje de medicos y odontologos. Trabajo presentado en el X Congreso Venezolano de Ciencias Medicas. Caracas, 8 de marzo de 1983. 19 p.

**Febres-Cordero F:** La creacion de la Facultad de Odontologia. **Acta Odontol Venez** 1980 May–Aug;18(2):293–305

**Febres-Cordero F:** La enseñanza en Venezuela de la historia de la odontologia. **Acta Odontol Venez** 1979 May–Dec;17(2–3):210–11

**Febres-Cordero F:** La odontologia andina prehispanica. **Acta Odontol Venez** 1984;22(1):39–73

**Febres-Cordero F:** La odontologia, es una 'profesion' o un oficio? **Acta Odontol Venez** 1980 May–Aug;18(2):337–52

**Febres Cordero F:** La odontologia venezolana ante la historia. **Acta Odontol Venez** 1980 Jan–Apr;18(1):175–90

**Febres-Cordero F:** Publicaciones periodicas odontologicas de Venezuela. **Acta Odontol Venez** 1983;21(2):129–47; 21(3):237–59

**Fechner MU** see **Fechner PU**

**Fechner PU, Fechner MU, Reis H:** Der Okulist Tadini. Zur Geschichte der künstlichen Augenlinse. **Klin Monatsbl Augenheilkd** 1980 Jun;176(6):1003–11

**Fechner PU, Fechner MU:** Tadini, the man who invented the artificial lens. **J Am Intraocul Implant Soc** 1979 Jan;5(1):22–3

**Feckenstein KJ:** The rheoscopic frog and the study of animal electricity. **Med Instrum** 1983 May–Jun;17(3):235–6

**Federn E:** On the difficulty of writing history of ideas: a reply. **J Hist Behav Sci** 1980 Jan;16(1):45–9

**Federn E:** Psychoanalyse und Sozialarbeit in Osterreich. **Zeitgesch** 1980;7(5):141–9

**Federn E** see **Lohmann HM, ed**

**Federspil G, Scandellari C:** La malattia da Morgagni a oggi. **Veltro** 1982;26(5–6):417–34

**Federspil G:** Lo sviluppo delle teorie sulla glicogenesi e il diabete in Claude Bernard e oggi. **Med Secoli** 1979 Jan–Apr;16(1):31–50

**Federspil G** see **Epistemologia, metodologia clinica e storia della scienza medica, 2**

**Fedo DA:** Liberal arts and pharmacy education: where do we now stand? **Pharm Hist** 1980;22(2):60–8

Fedorov NA, Movshed BE: Teoriia A. A. Bogomol'tsa o kolloidoklazii v mekhanizme deĭstviia perelivaniia krovi i ee sovremennoe razvitie. Probl Gematol Pereliv Krovi 1981 May;26(5):5-13
Fedorova ZD: Osnovnye napravleniia rabot A. N. Filatova po probleme svertyvaniia krovi. Vestn Khir 1982 Oct;129(10):13-6
Fedotenkov AG, Agranenko VA: Sluzhba krovi i transfuziologiia k 60-letiiu obrazovaniia SSSR. Probl Gematol Pereliv Krovi 1982 Dec;27(12):3-11
Fedotov V: Zabota partii i naroda o ranenykh v gody voiny. Voen Istor Zh 1977;6:90-4
Fee E: Competition for the first school of hygiene and public health. Bull Hist Med 1983 Fall;57(3):339-63
Fee E: Nineteenth-century craniology: the study of the female skull. Bull Hist Med 1979 Fall;53(3):415-33
Fee E: Psychology, sexuality, social control in Victorian England. Soc Sci Q 1978;58(4):632-46
Fee E: Science and the 'woman question', 1860-1920: a study of English scientific periodicals. Ph. D. Diss., Princeton University. Princeton, 1978. v, 351 leaves.
Fee E, Wallace M: The history and politics of birth control: a review essay. Feminist Stud 1979;5(1):201-15
Fee E: William Henry Howell: physiologist and philosopher of health. Am J Epidemiol 1984 Mar;119(3):293-300
Fee E see Green D
Feery B: Impact of immunization on disease patterns in Australia. Med J Aust 1981 Aug 22;2(4):172-6
Fegersten S: Crude death rate and infant mortality (1840-1900) in Norway, Sweden, Denmark, England and Wales with particular attention to the relationship between mortality and population density-urbanisation. Scand Popul Stud 1979;5:83-97
Feggetter G: Suicide in opera. Br J Psychiatry 1980 Jun;136:552-7
Fehlmann HR: Bearbeitung des pharmazeutischen Reiseführers Schweiz. In: Vorträge des Internationalen Pharmaziehistorischen Kongresses Innsbruck 1977. Stuttgart, Wissenschaftliche Verlagsgesellschaft, 1979. p. 165-70.
Fehlmann HR: Beziehungen zwischen Arzt und Apotheker im 16. bis 18. Jahrhundert in der Schweiz. Gesnerus 1983;40(1-2):67-74
Fehlmann HR: Ceratum Galeni. Zur Geschichte von Unguentum leniens. In Dilg P, et al., ed: Perspektiven der Pharmaziegeschichte. Graz, Austria, Akademische Druck- u. Verlagsanstalt, 1983. p. 65-77.
Fehlmann HR: 'Herrn Adams äusseres Augenmittel.' Eine Frankfurter Merkwürdigkeit aus dem Jahre 1794. Pharm Ztg 1980;125:407-8
Fehr AM: Geschichte des Winterthurer Spitals. Gesnerus 1982;39(1):89-95
Fehrenbacher DE: In quest of the psychohistorical Lincoln. Rev Am Hist 1983;11(1):12-9
Fehringer WT: Studien zum altitalienischen Pferdearzneibuch des Carlo Bartolomeo Rinaldi (1655). Diss. Hannover, 1978, 247 p.
Fehrman C: Esaias Tegnér and psychiatry: history of literature from medical view-point. Sydsven Medicinhist Sallsk Arsskr 1984;21:47-8
Feibel RM: Edward J. Curran and the concept of relative pupillary block. Surv Ophthalmol 1981 Jan-Feb;25(4):270-8
Feibel RM: Historical error. Ophthalmology (Rochester) 1983 Jul;90(7):857
Feibel RM: John Vetch and the Egyptian ophthalmia. Surv Ophthalmol 1983 Sep-Oct;28(2):128-34
Feierman S: History of pluralistic medical systems. Change in African therapeutic systems. Soc Sci Med [Med Anthropol] 1979 Dec;13B(4):277-84
Feierman S see Janzen JM
Feierman S, ed: Health and society in Africa: a working bibliography. Waltham, Mass., Crossroads Press, 1979. xii, 210 p.
Feige W: Leben und Schaffen des Schlachthofdirektors Oberveterinärrat Dr. med. vet. Hugo Andreas Heiss, Straubing (1863-1936). Diss., Tierärztliche Hochschule. Hannover, 1982. 163 p.
Feigenbaum B see Lindsay CM
Feinberg M, Pegeron JP, Steiner M: The effect of morphine on symptoms of endogenous depression. Natl Inst Drug Abuse Res Monogr Ser 1983 Apr;43:245-50
Feindel W: The contributions of Wilder Penfield and the Montreal Neurological Institute to Canadian neurosciences. In Roland CG, ed: Health, disease and medicine. Toronto, Hannah Institute for the History of Medicine, 1984. p. 347-58.
Feindel W: The contributions of Wilder Penfield to the functional anatomy of the human brain. Hum Neurobiol 1982;1(4):231-4
Feinleib M: History of the genetic epidemiology of coronary heart disease. Prog Clin Biol Res 1984;147:1-7
Feinmann J: How a lunatic fared in 1781. Med News 1981;13(22):22-3
Feinstein H see Albin M
Feinstein HM: Family therapy for the historian?--The case of William James. Fam Process 1981 Mar;20(1):97-107
Feinstein HM: The 'crisis' of William James: a revisionist view. Psychohist Rev 1981;10(2):71-80
Feinstein HM: The sins of the fathers. Psychoanal Rev 1983 Spring;70(1):95-100
Feinstein HM: The therapeutic fantasy of psychohistorian. Psychoanal Rev 1982 Summer;69(2):221-8
Feinstein HM: The use and abuse of illness in the James family circle: a view of neurasthenia as a social phenomenon. Psychohist Rev 1979;8(1-2):6-14
Feinstein SC: Why they were afraid of Virginia Woolf: perspectives on juvenile manic-depressive illness. J Adolesc 1980 Sep;3(3):187-96
Feinstein SC: Why they were afraid of Virginia Woolf: perspectives on juvenile manic-depressive illness. Adolesc Psychiatry 1980;8:332-43
Feitknecht-Gallati S: Wandel in der medizinischen Versorgung des Oberwallis in den Jahren 1930-1980. Diss. Bern, 1984. 91 p.
Fekete J: Dr. Selig Arpád (1880-1929). Orv Hetil 1980 Jan 13;121(2):98-101
Fel' II, Truman GL: A. M. Aliev--vydaiushchiĭsia pertiĭnyĭ, gosudarstvennyĭ deiatel', organizator zdravookhraneniia i meditsinskoĭ nauki v Sovetskom Azerbaĭdzhane. Sov Zdravookhr 1982;(8):57-9
Fel' II, Truman GL: Meditsinskiĭ fakul'tet Bakinskogo (Azerbaĭdzhanskogo) universiteta i rol' russkikh uchenykh v stanovlenii i razvitii vyshego meditsinskogo obrazovaniia i meditsinskoĭ nauki v Sovetskom Azerbaĭdzhane (k 60-letiiu obrazovaniia Azerbaĭdzhanskoĭ SSR). Sov Zdravookhr 1980;(5):64-7
Fel'berg MB see Safarov RN
Fel'berg MV: S. S. Iudin v 'Zakhar'ine'. Sov Zdravookhr 1983;(3):71-3
Felchner A, Pepłowska E: Polski Komitet Pomocy Sanitarnej jednym z prekursorów świeckiego pielegniarstwa w Polsce. Arch Hist Med (Warsz) 1984;47(1):91-7
Felchner A see Dutkiewicz M
Feldberg W: Sir Henry Hallett Dale. In Dictionary of national biography, 1961-1970. Suppl. 8, 1981. p. 262-5.
Feldberg W: Sir John Henry Gaddum. In Dictionary of national biography, 1961-1970. Suppl. 8, 1981. p. 412-3.
Feldberg WS: Fifty years on--looking back on some developments in neurohumoral physiology. Liverpool, Liverpool University Press, 1982. xiii, 106 p.
Feldenkirchen W: Aspekte der Bevölkerungs- und Sozialstruktur der Stadt Köln in der französischen Zeit (1794-1814). Rheinische Vierteljahrsbl 1979;43:182-227
Feldman A, Ford P: Scientists & inventors. New York, Facts On File, 1979. 336 p.
Feldman M: Rafael Rangel y la crisis del medico. Rev Soc Venez Hist Med 1979;28(42):13-24
Fel'dman NG see Afanas'ev IuI
Feldman R, Scheffler R: The union impact on hospital wages and fringe benefits. Ind Labor Relat Rev 1982;35(2):196-206
Feldman S see Rieber RW, ed
Feldman SA: Anesthesia's debt to science and its contribution to medicine. Acta Anaesthesiol Belg 1979;30 Suppl:13-21
Feldmann H: Development of diagnostic hearing tests. Audiology 1983;22(4):393-403
Felici L: L'opera medica die Teofane Nonno in manoscritti inediti. Acta Med Hist Patav 1981/82;28:59-74
Felig P: Landmark perspective: Protamine insulin. Hagedorn's pioneering contribution to drug delivery in the management of diabetes. JAMA 1984 Jan 20;251(3):393-6
Feliksiakowa J: Stand der biologischen Bibliographie in Polen in den Jahren 1945-1970. Hist Philos Life Sci 1981;3(1):115-31
Felix RH see Martin WR
Felker M: The political economy of sexism in industrial health. Soc Sci Med 1982;16(1):3-13
Feller I: Die zahnmedizinische Karikatur II: 1840-1880. Köln, 1983. 284 p. (Arbeiten der Forschungsstelle des Instituts für Geschichte der Medizin der Universität zu Köln, Band 26).
Fellman AC, Fellman M: Making sense of self. Medical advice literature in late nineteenth-century America. Philadelphia, University of Pennsylvania Press, 1981. 198 p.
Fellman AC, Fellman M: Man amuck. Rev Am Hist 1976;4(4):558-64
Fellman G: Leaf in a storm: Jayaprakash Narayan as politician and as saint. Psychohist Rev 1981;9(3):183-213
Fellman M see Fellman AC
Fellner R, Höflechner W: Die Augenheilkunde an der Universität Graz. Graz, Akademische Druck- u. Verlagsanstalt, 1973. ix, 180 p. (Publikationen aus dem Archiv der Universität Graz, Bd. 2).
Felsenfeld O: Selected bibliography O. Felsenfeld. Acta Trop (Basel) 1979 Jun;36(2):193-8
Felson B see Bean WB
Felstein I, Naqvi N: Samuel Taylor Chadwick: 1809-73. Br Med J [Clin Res] 1983 Jun 25;286(6383):2031-2
Felton BJ, Shinn M: Ideology and practice of deinstitutionalization. J Soc Issues 1981;37(3):158-72
Felton JS: Classical syndromes in occupational medicine: Phosphorus necrosis--a classical occupational disease. Am J Ind Med 1982;3(1):77-120
Felton JS: Industrial medicine to occupational health and safety: a 50-year retrospective. Occup Health Saf 1982 Sep;51(9):14-22
Felts JH: Browne spots. NC Med J 1982 Aug;43(8):591
Felts JH: On epidemics, metaphors and madness. NC Med J 1980 Apr;41(4):221-3
Fenaroli G, Garibaldi U, Penco MA: Giochi, scommesse sulla vita, tabelle di mortalità, nascita del calcolo probabilistico, statistica e teoria delle popolazioni. Arch Hist Exact Sci 1981;25(4):329-41
Fenaroli G, Penco MA: Le prime analisi di problemi di mortalità in termini probabilistici. Physis 1981;23(1):115-34
Feng WH see Zheng GZ
Fenichel O: Psychoanalyse und Gesellschaftswissenschaften (1938). Psyche (Stuttg) 1981 Nov;35(11):1055-71
Fenichel CH, ed see Morantz RM
Fenn D: White slaves. Wash Mon 1981;13(9):21-8
Fenn JE: Some observations on the evolution of current aortic aneurysm management. Conn Med 1979 Dec;43(12):783-9
Fenn PT see Bartrip PW
Fennel ML, Rodin MB, Kantor GK: Problems in the work setting, drinking,

and reasons for drinking. **Soc Forces** 1981;60(1):114–32
**Fenner ET:** Rasayana Siddhi: medicine and alchemy in the Buddhist tantras. Ph.D. diss. University of Wisconsin. Madison, 1979. 272 leaves.
**Fenner F:** Mousepox (infectious ectromelia): past, present, and future. **Lab Anim Sci** 1981 Oct;31(5 Pt 2):553–9
**Fenner F:** Smallpox and its eradication. In Stanley NF, Joske RA, ed: Changing disease patterns and human behaviour. London, New York, Academic Press, 1980. p. 215–29.
**Fenner F:** Sociocultural change and environmental diseases. In Stanley NF, Joske RA, ed: Changing disease patterns and human behaviour. London, New York, Academic Press, 1980. p. 7–26.
**Fenton P:** L'importance de la guenizah du Caire pour l'histoire de la médecine. **Rev Hist Med Heb** 1980 Mar–Apr;33(1):21–2
**Fenton P:** The importance of the Cairo Genizah for the history of medicine. **Med Hist** 1980 Jul;24(3):347–8
**Fenton PB:** The importance of the Cairo Genizah for the history of medicine. **J Hist Arabic Sci** 1980;4:330–1
**Fenton WN:** The 'Great Good Medicine.' **NY State J Med** 1979 Sep;79(10):1603–9
**Ferenczy M:** Csokonai Vitéz Mihály egészségügyi tanácsai. **Orv Hetil** 1982 Nov 28;123(48):2973–4
**Ferenczy M:** Izzasztó fürdök és testedzés otthon. **Orv Hetil** 1983 Mar 20;124(12):713–4
**Ferguson A:** The sweetheart of the PSC--Mabel Heath Palmer: the early years. **Chiropr Hist** 1984;4(1):25–8
**Ferguson AE:** Commercial pharmaceutical medicine and medicalization: a case study from El Salvador. **Cult Med Psychiatry** 1981 Jun;5(2):105–34
**Ferguson B** see **Agogino GA**
**Ferguson D:** Civilisation for Africa: a study of the impact of modern scientific medicine on Africa. Port Elizabeth, South Africa, E. H. Walton Co., 1981. 160 p.
**Ferguson JP:** The College library. In Passmore R, ed: Proceedings of the Royal College of Physicians of Edinburgh Tercentenary Congress, 1981. Edinburgh, Royal College of Physicians of Edinburgh, 1982 p. 103–15.
**Ferguson M:** Reflections on teaching a history of nursing. **Nurs Times** 1979 Nov;75(46–47):suppl 29–30:117–20, 121–2
**Ferguson RA:** Yellow fever and Charles Brockden Brown: the contest of the emerging novelist. **Early Am Lit** 1979–80;14(3):293–305
**Ferguson TB:** Evarts A. Graham--the man. **J Thorac Cardiovasc Surg** 1984 Nov;88(5 Pt 2):803–9
**Fergusson IL, Taylor RW, Watson JM, ed:** Records and curiosities in obstetrics and gynaecology. London, Baillière Tindall, 1982. x, 115 p.
**Ferke A** see **Földes V**
**Ferkó S:** Pálfyn Johann (1650–1730) a szülészeti fogó egyik feltalálója halálának 250. évfordulójára. **Orv Hetil** 1980 Mar 17;121(10):585–6
**Fernald GW** see **Clyde WA**
**Fernandes JJ:** Thomas Hopkins Gallaudet on language and communication: a reassessment. **Am Ann Deaf** 1983 Aug;128(4):467–73
**Fernandes L, Berry H, Hamilton E:** Historical perspectives on penicillamine. **Cah Haut Marnais** 1980;14(2):130–6
**Fernandes R:** Jose Martins da Cruz Jobim, um fundador da Academia Nacional de Medicina. **Rev Inst Hist Geogr Bras** 1980;327:247–68
**Fernandez C:** Pioneers in research in otolaryngology at the University of Chicago. **Ann Otol Rhinol Laryngol [Suppl]** 1983 Jan–Feb;102:23–6
**Fernandez C** see **Mhoon EE**
**Fernandez D:** Francois Carlier, La Prostitution antiphysique (1857). Précédé de La Pederastie (1887) par Ambroise Tardieu. Paris, Le Sycomore, 1981. ix, 250 p.
**Fernández DW:** Manuel Pantoja. **Bol Acad Nac Hist (Caracas)** 1982;65(259):685–8
**Fernández DW:** Marcos Jordan. **Rev Soc Venez Hist Med** 1979;28(42):25–7
**Fernández FM** see **Tjarks G**
**Fernandez G:** The social structure of the medical model of madness and the physician's role. **Psychiatry** 1981 Aug;44(3):241–52
**Fernández PL, Quindós LS, Soto J, et al:** Radiation exposure levels in Altamira Cave. **Health Phys** 1984 Feb;46(2):445–7
**Fernandez-Conde A:** One Cuban physician's odyssey. **J Fla Med Assoc** 1979 Aug;66(8):845–52
**Fernández de Castro J:** Historia de la oncocercósis. **SPM** 1979 Nov–Dec;21(6):683–96
**Fernández del Castillo F:** El expediente médico de Valentín Gómez Farias. **Bol Inst Invest Bibliogr** 1970;(4):125–9
**Fernández del Castillo F, Castañeda H:** El Museo de la Medicina. **Salud Publica Mex** 1982 Sep–Oct;24(5):509–21
**Fernández del Castillo F** see **Somolinos D'Ardois G**
**Fernández Felgueroso E, Torcida Valiente I, Rodero Vicente B:** Alcoholismo y sociedad. **Rev Sanid Hig Publica (Madr)** 1981 Nov–Dec;55(11–12):1277–94
**Fernández García A:** Enfermedad y sociedad: la epidemia de cólera de 1865 en Madrid. **Cuad Invest Hist** 1979;3:155–86
**Fernández García A:** Repercusiones sociales de las epidemias de colera del siglo XIX. In: Sociedad Española de Historia de la Medicina. V Congreso Nacional. Madrid, 1977. **Asclepio** 1977;29:127–45
**Fernández González M, Gago Bohórquez R:** La medicina en la obra cientifica de Francisco de Paula Montells y Nadal (1813–1893). **Asclepio** 1980;32:151–9
**Fernández Pérez DW** see **Sociedad Venezolana de Historia de la medicina**
**Fernández Picón L:** Concepcion Arenal en la historia de la medicina. Ideas medicas de Concepcion Arenal. **Asclepio** 1980;32:161–70
**Ferngren GB:** A Roman declamation on vivisection. **Trans Stud Coll Physicians Phila** 1982 Dec;5(4 no 4):272–90
**Ferngren GB** see **Amundsen DW**
**Ferrand F:** L'hôpital de Goncelin (Isère) 1658–1793. In Congrès National des Sociétés Savantes, 98e, Saint-Etienne, 1973. Actes. Paris, 1975. Tome II, p. 319–27.
**Ferrándiz Araujo C:** El Hospital de la Caridad de Cartagena. Murcia, Imprenta Provincial, 1981. 286 p.
**Ferrandiz Araujo C** see **Marset Campos P**
**Ferrari Sacco A, Oliaro T:** A cent'anni dalla scoperta del micobatterio della tbc. (1822–1982). Robert Koch autore della grande scoperta. **Minerva Med** 1982 Sep 8;73(34):2199–202
**Ferrari Sacco A:** Benedetto da Norcia e la medicina conventuale in Europa (nel 1500th anniversario della nascita). **Minerva Med** 1981 Mar 10;72(9):585 7
**Ferreira LF, Ribeiro Filho BM, Araújo AJ de, et al:** Enterobius vermicularis eggs in preColumbian human coprolites from Chile. **Paleopathol Newsl** 1984;46:4–5
**Ferreira LF, Aráujo AJ de, Confalonieri UE:** The finding of eggs and larvae of parasitic helminths in archaeological material from Unai, Minas Gerais, Brazil. **Trans R Soc Trop Med Hyg** 1980;74(6):798–800
**Ferreira LF, Araújo AJ de, Confalonieri UE:** The finding of helminth eggs in a Brazilian mummy. **Trans R Soc Trop Med Hyg** 1983;77(1):65–7
**Ferreira LF** see **Aráujo A**
**Ferreira LF** see **Araújo AJ**
**Ferreira França M:** Panorama medico dos seculos XVI e XVII. **Rev Inst Hist Geogr Bras** 1970;288:255–74
**Ferrer D:** Dictamen solicitando la erección de los actuales edificios de la Facultad de Medicina y Hospital Clínico de Barcelona. In Congrés International d'Història de la Medicina Catalana, 2nd, Barcelona, 1975. Llibre d'Actes. Barcelona, Socitra, 1977. p. 249–58.
**Ferrer D:** La sanidad en las 'Leyes de los reinos de las indias'. In International Congress of the History of Medicine, 27th, Barcelona, 1980. Actas. Barcelona, Académia de Ciències Médiques de Catalunya i Balears, 1981. p. 172–6.
**Ferrer D:** Las ordenanzas de la Universidad del Estudio General de la ciudad de Barcelona, 1596. **Asclepio** 1978–79;30–31:339–58
**Ferrer D:** Representación para el establecimiento de un Colegio de Ciruxia en Barcelona a la manera del de Cádiz (1759). In Congrés International d'Història de la Medicina Catalana, 2nd, Barcelona, 1975. Llibre d'Actes. Barcelona, Socitra, 1977. p. 259–61.
**Ferrer M:** The Royal College of Midwives 1881 - 1981. **Midwife Health Visit Community Nurse** 1981 Jul;17(7):288–94
**Ferrières M:** Les Donatifs Comtadins: une iconographie hospitalière méconnue. **Bull Soc Fr Hist Hop** 1980;(40):23–8
**Ferrone V:** Il dibattito su probabilità e scienze sociali nel secolo XVIII. **Physis** 1980;22(1):27–71
**Ferroni G:** Nota sull' Erbolato. **Rass Lett Ital** 1979;7(1–2):202–14
**Ferru M:** La faillite du BCG. Poitiers, Ferru, 1977. 274 p.
**Ferruzzi F** see **Dazzi N**
**Ferry AP, Ferry MK:** Dr. Isaac Thompson and his celebrated eye water. **Ophthalmology** 1984 May;91(5):528–37
**Ferry MK** see **Ferry AP**
**Fershee NF:** Dental hygiene in Michigan--our 'roots'. **Bull Mich Dent Hyg Assoc** 1984 Sep;14(3):4–7
**Ferwerda H** see **Gregg JB**
**Feshbach M** see **Davis C**
**Festschrift in honor of David W. Smith: J Pediatr** 1982 Nov;101(5):797–804
**Festschrift in honor of Robert A. Good on the occasion of his 60th birthday: Clin Immunol Immunopathol** 1982 May;23(2):155–61
**Festschrift Otto Thalhammer zum 60. Geburtstag: Padiatr Padol** 1982;17(2):127–548
**Festschrift to Dr. Samuel R. Powers, Jr. September 25, 1919 - March 27, 1980: Arch Surg** 1981 Oct;116(10):1241–1356
**Festy M:** Les internements psychiatriques en Norvège. **Population** 1981;36(2):317–36
**Festy P, Rallu JL:** Constitution et reconstitution des familles françaises: état civil et recensements de 1968 et 1975. **Population** 1981;36(1):63–92
**Festy P:** La fécondité des pays occidentaux de 1870 à 1970. Paris, I.N.E.D., Presses Universitaires de France, 1979. 390 p. (Travaux et documents, cahier no 85).
**Festy P:** La fécondité en Amérique du nord: vingt années de baisse. **Population** 1979;34(4–5):767–99
**Fetgatter GL** see **Liston SE**
**Fetscher I:** Alexander Mitscherlich--zur Pathologie der bundesdeutschen Gesellschaft. **Psyche (Stuttg)** 1983 Apr;37(4):298–310
**Fetterman GH:** Maud L. Menten (1879–1960). **Perspect Pediatr Pathol** 1984 Spring;1(1):5–7
**Fetzer W:** Pharmazie: Historisches aus Museen und Sammlungen der DDR. Leipzig, VEB Deutscher Verlag für Grundstoffindustrie, 1983. 279 p.
**Feucht G:** Die Geschichte der Akupunktur in Europa. Heidelberg, Haug, 1977. 31 p.
**Feuereisl R:** 30 years of the Research Institute of Tuberculosis and Respiratory Diseases in Prague. **Czech Med** 1983;6(4):193–5
**Feurstein G:** Vorarleberg: das familienfreundlichste Bundesland Oesterreichs. **Montfort** 1979;31(2–3):135–41
**Feyereisen P** see **Seron X**
**Fich S, Li JK:** Aorto-ventricular dynamics: theories, experiments, and instrumentation. **Crit Rev Biomed Eng** 1983;9(3):245–85
**Fichtner G:** Christus als Arzt: Ursprünge und Wirkungen eines Motivs. **Fruhmittelalt Stud** 1982;16:1–18
**Fichtner G, Siefert H, ed:** Padua. Stuttgart, New York, Schattauer, 1978.

224 p. (Medizinhistorische Reisen, Band 2).
**Fichtner G:** Psychiatrie zur Zeit Hölderlins: Ausstellung anlässlich der 63. Jahrestagung der Deutschen Gesellschaft für Geschichte der Medizin, der Naturwissenschaften und Technik in Tübingen, Universitätsbibliothek Tübingen, Bonatzbau 27. September bis 30. Oktober 1980. Tübingen, Universitätsbibliothek, 1980. 99 p.
**Fichtner G, ed:** Index wissenschaftshistorischer Dissertationen (IWD). Verzeichnis abgeschlossener Dissertationen auf dem Gebiet der Geschichte der Medizin, der Pharmazie, der Naturwissenschaften und der Technik. Nr. 1:1970–1980. Tübingen, Institut für Geschichte der Medizin, 1981. 285 p.
**Fichtner G, ed:** Laufende wissenschaftshistorische Dissertationen (LWD). Verzeichnis in Bearbeitung befindlicher Dissertationen auf dem Gebiet der Geschichte der Medizin, der Pharmazie, der Naturwissenschaften und der Technik. Nr. 1, Tübingen, Institut für Geschichte der Medizin, 1981. 125 p.
**Ficino M:** The book of life. A translation by Charles Boer of Liber de Vita (or De Vita Triplici). Irving, Texas, Spring Publications, 1980. xix, 217 p.
**Fickeissen JL:** A history lesson for today: the creation of the State Board. **NJ Nurse** 1983 Nov–Dec;13(6):20–1
**Fickeissen JL:** New Jersey State Nurses' Association. **J Med Soc NJ** 1984 Sep;81(9):805–6
**Fidanza F, Alberti Fidanza A:** Attempts to improve food habits in rapidly changing societies; e.g. Italy. **Bibl Nutr Dieta** 1983;(32):32–9
**Fiedler LA:** Images of the nurse in fiction and popular culture. In Jones AH, ed: Images of healers. Albany, State University of New York Press, 1983. p. 79–90.
**Field HI:** The development of veterinary education in Nigeria. **Vet Hist** 1982 Summer;2(3):112–23
**Field J** see **Talmor E, ed**
**Field MH:** Social casework practice during the 'psychiatric deluge'. **Soc Serv Rev** 1980;54(4):482–507
**Field J, ed** see **Brody J**
**Fielding A** see **Portwood D**
**Fielding J:** Corrigan on abdominal disease. **J Ir Coll Physicians Surg** 1980 Jul;10(1):41–3
**Fielding J:** History of penicillin. **Lancet** 1980 Jan 5;1(8158):43–4
**Fielding JH:** Crohn's disease in London in the latter half of the nineteenth century. **Ir J Med Sci** 1984 Jun;153(6):214–20
**Fields K, Kontrovitz M:** An invisible art blazes into life under microscope. **Smithsonian** 1980;11(7):109–13
**Fierz M:** Girolamo Cardano (1501–1576): Arzt, Naturphilosoph, Mathematiker, Astronom, und Traumdeuter. Basel, Birkhäuser, 1977. 138 p.
**Fierz M:** Girolamo Cardano, 1501–1576. Physician, natural philosopher, mathematician, astrologer, and interpreter of dreams. Boston, Birkhäuser, 1983. xxii, 202 p.
**Fiessinger JN** see **Roncière J de la**
**Fieve RR, Jamison KR:** Rubidium: overview and clinical perspectives. **Mod Probl Pharmacopsychiatry** 1982;18:145–63
**Fife AE** see **Hand WD, ed**
**Fifteen years of the Otological Research Laboratory, Baylor College of Medicine: Acta Otolaryngol [Suppl] (Stockh)** 1983;393:1–112
**Fiftieth anniversary:** American College of Gastroenterology. Reprints. The American Journal of Gastroenterology celebrates the Golden Anniversary of the College. **Am J Gastroenterol** 1982 Oct;77(10):701–832
**Fifty years of cephalometric radiography: Angle Orthod** 1981 Apr;51(2):88–171
**Fifty years of chemotherapy: Endeavour** 1982;6(4):145
**Fifty years of psychoanalysis in Israel: past, present and future: Isr J Psychiatry Relat Sci** 1983;20(1–2):1–203
**Figallo Espinal L:** Vejez y envejecimiento (resumen historico). **Rev Soc Venez Hist Med** 1980;29(43–44):39–53
**Figarella J:** Jacques Daviel à Marseille. **Hist Sci Med** 1979;13(4):347–62
**Figarella J:** Jacques Daviel, chirurgien marseillais. **Marseille** 1978;113:42–56
**Figarella J:** La Provence et la peste de 1720. **Marseille** 1978;112:13–23
**Figarella J:** L'art médical au temps du Roi René. **Marseille** 1981;126:10–7
**Figa'Talamanca I, Galmacci G:** Infant mortality and economic stability. An analysis of the last century. **Nuovi Ann Ig Microbiol** 1979 Mar–Apr;30(2):107–26
**Figlio K:** How does illness mediate social relations? Workmen's compensation and medico-legal practices, 1890–1940. In P. Wright, A. Treacher, ed: The problem of medical knowledge. Examining the social construction of medicine. Edinburgh, Edinburgh University Press, 1982. p. 174–224.
**Figlio K, Weindling P:** Was social medicine revolutionary? Rudolf Virchow and the revolutions of 1848. **Soc Soc Hist Med Bull (Lond)** 1984 Jun;34:10–8
**Figlio K:** What is an accident? **Soc Soc Hist Med Bull (Lond)** 1983 Dec;33:27–9
**Figueiredo JM de:** Ayurvedic medicine in Goa according to European sources in the sixteenth and seventeenth centuries. **Bull Hist Med** 1984 Summer;58(2):225–35
**Figueredo Díaz F:** La guerra de Cuba en 1878 (La protesta de Baragua). Habana, Organismos, 1973. 338 p. (Cuadernos de Historia de la Salud Pública, 56).
**Figueroa L:** Betances, el irreductible. **Atenea (Puerto Rico)** 1972;9(3–4):29–39
**Figueroa Marroquin H:** De qué murió Simon Bolivar? **Bol Soc Mex Hist Filos Med** 1981 Dec;5(37):217–47
**Figueroa Marroquín H:** De que murio Simon Bolivar? **Bol Hist Antig (Bogota)** 1981;68(733):385–419
**Figuerola I** see **Figuerola JE**
**Figuerola JE, Figuerola I:** La cuenta de medicinas administradas a la hija del Marques de la Quadra. **Bol Soc Esp Hist Farm** 1980 Mar–Jun;3(121–2)
**Figurovsky NA** see **Berezin IV**
**Fijałek J:** Dr. N. Med. Jerzy Kasznicki (3.1.1934--20.VII.1979). **Arch Hist Med (Warsz)** 1980;43(2):121–5
**Fijałek J:** Kasa Chorych--pierwowzór społecznego, samorzadowego lecznictwa pracowniczego w Polsce. **Arch Hist Med (Warsz)** 1984;47(1):99–106
**Fijałek J:** Problemy badań naukowych i kształcenia kadry naukowej w dziedzinie historii medycyny w Polsce. **Arch Hist Med (Warsz)** 1979;42(3):383–8
**Fijałek J, Machalski J:** Publiczna opieka zdrowotna u poczatków Polski Niepodległej. **Arch Hist Med (Warsz)** 1978;41(4):393–404
**Fijałkowski W:** 50 lat naturalnego planowania rodziny. **Ginekol Pol** 1979 Nov;50(11):909–16
**Fikentscher E** see **Adam J**
**Fiks A:** Cystosarcoma phyllodes of the mammary gland--Müller's tumor. For the 180th birthday of Johannes Müller. **Virchows Arch [Pathol Anat]** 1981;392(1):1–6
**Filatov VG:** Gistoricheskie i évoliutsionnye predposylki stanovleniia landshaftnoĭ épidemiologii gel'mintozov. **Parassitologia** 1981 Jan–Feb;15(1):3–9
**Filatov VI:** K stoletiiu otechestvennogo protezirovaniia (1883–1983). **Ortop Travmatol Protez** 1983 March;(3):61–3
**Fildes V:** Neonatal feeding practices and infant mortality during the 18th century. **J Biosoc Sci** 1980 Jul;12(3):313–24
**Fildes V:** The age of weaning in Britain 1500–1800. **J Biosoc Sci** 1982 Apr;14(2):223–40
**Fildes V:** The early history of the infant feeding bottle. **Nurs Times** 1981 Jan 15 and 22;77(3–4):128, 168–9
**Fildes V:** Weaning: on the bottle again. **Nurs Mirror** 1980;151(24):18–21
**Fildes V:** Weaning the Elizabethan child. **Nurs Times** 1980 July–Aug 7;76:31–32:1357–9,1402–3
**Filimonov AR:** Pervyi tom zhurnala 'Vestnik oftal'mologii: (1884 g.). **Vestn Oftalmol** 1984 Jul–Aug;(4):5–7
**Filimonov AR:** 'Vestnik oftal'mologii' 50 let nazad. **Vestn Oftalmol** 1984 Nov–Dec;(6):6–8
**Filimonov AR:** 'Vestnik oftal'mologii' 75 let nazad. **Vestn Oftalmol** 1984 Sep–Oct;(5):7–8
**Filip M:** 25 rokov katedry sociálneho lekárstva Lekárskej fakulty UPJS v Košiciach. **Cesk Zdrav** 1980 Oct;28(10):397–402
**Filipe NF:** S. João de deus um homem que soube amar. 2. edição. Lisboa, Edições Paulistas, [198–?]. 150 p.
**Filipowicz W** see **Szafrański P**
**Filippova LF:** K stanovleniiu kombustiologii na Ukraine. **Klin Khir** 1980 May;(5):72–3
**Filliozat J:** La doctrine classique de la médecine indienne: ses origines et ses parallèles grecs, Paris, Ecole française d'Extrême-Orient, 1975. vii, 230 p. (also Thèse 1946).
**Filliozat J, Raison A:** Problèmes d'identification de la matière médicale indienne. **Sci Orient** 1979;16:41–50
**Filliozat J:** Sur l'identification des maladies dans l'Ayurveda. In Mazars G, ed: Les médecines traditionnelles de l'Asie. Strasbourg, Université Louis Pasteur, 1981. p. 140–9.
**Filliozat J:** The expansion of Indian medicine abroad. **Sachitra Ayurved** 1981 Mar;:171–3
**Filliozat J:** Yogaśataka, texte médical attribué à Nagārjuna. Textes sanskrit et tibétain, traduction française, notes, indices. **Publ Inst Fr Indologie** 1979;62:1–206
**Filliozat J** see **La médecine hospitalière française au XVIIIème siècle**
**Filliozat J, ed:** Yogaśataka. Texte médical attribué à Nagarjuna. Textes sanskrit et tibétain; traduction française. Pondichéry, Institut Français d'Indologie, 1979. xxxviii, 206 p.
**Filós-Díaz JA:** Histoplasmosis en Panamá. Revisión histórica y nota de actualización. **Rev Med Panama** 1984 Jan;9(1):8–21
**Finavera L** see **Armocida G**
**Finby N** see **Kraft E**
**Finck J:** Thomas Mann et la psychanalyse. Précédé de Thomas Mann et l' irrationnel par J-M Palmier. Paris, Société d'Edition 'Les Belles Lettres', 1982. 216 p. (Confluents Psychanalytiques).
**Finckh E:** Tibetan medicine, theory and practice. In: Tibetan studies in honor of H. E. Richardson. Warminster, Aris and Phillips, 1980. p. 103–10.
**Findeisen DG:** Tuberkulose und Allergie. Erkenntnisschritte von der Entdeckung des Mycobacterium tuberculosis durch Robert Koch (24 März 1882). Zu einer umfassenden Immundiagnostik, Immuntherapie und Immunprophylaxe. **Allerg Immunol (Leipz)** 1982;28(1):3–12
**Finder JG** see **Brown JE**
**Finderle V:** Mobilne kirurške ekipe. **Lijec Vjesn** 1979 Nov;101(11):706
**Findlay GH:** Alphonse Loewenthal (1903–1983)--the uncrowned king of dermatology in Africa. **S Afr Med J** 1983 Dec 24;64(27):1064–7
**Findlay GH:** South African tick-bite fever (1931–1981). **S Afr Med J** 1981 Dec 26;60(26):998–1000
**Fine DJ, Meyer ER:** Quality assurance in historical perspective. **Hosp Health Serv Adm** 1983 Nov–Dec;28(6):94–121
**Fine PE:** John Brownlee and the measurement of infectiousness: an historical study in epidemic theory. **J R Stat Soc** 1979;142:347–62
**Fine-Souriac A:** La limitation des naissances dans le sud-ouest de la France:

fécondité, allaitement et contraception au pays de Sault du milieu du XVIIIe siècle à 1914. **Ann Midi** 1978;90(2):155–88

**Fingerland A:** Iaroslav Glava--osnovatel' chekhoslovatskoĭ shkoly patologoanatomov. **Arkh Patol** 1981;43(10):62–6

**Fingerland A:** 100. Výroči rozdělení Karlovy univerzity na českou a německou. Následný vliv na československou patologii. **Cesk Patol** 1983 Aug;19(3):129–32

**Fink A:** Historie českého porodnictví, a to nedávná aneb jak je to s českými mezikrajovými semináři. **Cesk Gynekol** 1983 Apr;48(3):230–3

**Fink L, Greenberg B:** Organizing Montefiore: labor militancy meets a progressive health care empire. In Reverby S, Rosner D, ed: Health care in America. Philadelphia, Temple University Press, 1979. p. 226–44.

**Fink M:** Meduna and the origins of convulsive therapy. **Am J Psychiatry** 1984 Sep;141(9):1034–41

**Finland M:** Doting: my early experiences at Boston City Hospital. **Pharos** 1982 Summer;45(3):17–22

**Finland M:** Empiric therapy for bacterial infections: the historical perspective. **Rev Infect Dis** 1983 Mar–Apr;5 Suppl 1:S2–8

**Finland M:** Gaps in therapy for infectious diseases: a historical perspective. **J Infect Dis** 1982 Mar;145(3):401–7

**Finland M, Castle WB:** The Harvard Medical Unit at Boston City Hospital. Boston, Harvard Medical School: Distributed by the University Press of Virginia for The Francis A. Countway Library of Medicine, 1982–83. 2 volumes in 3.

**Finlay IM:** Craniometry and cephalometry: a history prior to the advent of radiography. **Angle Orthod** 1980 Oct;50(4):312–21

**Finlay R:** Differential child mortality in pre-industrial England: the example of Cartmel, Cumbria, 1600–1750. **Ann Demogr Hist (Paris)** 1981;:67–80

**Finlay R:** Distance to church and registration experience. **Local Popul Stud (Matlock)** 1980 Spring;24:26–40

**Finlay R:** Health and mortality in London 1580–1650. **Soc Soc Hist Med Bull (Lond)** 1981 Jun;28:1–5

**Finlay R:** Population and metropolis. The demography of London, 1580–1650. Cambridge, New York, Cambridge University Press, 1981. xii, 188 p.

**Finlay Seiglie A:** Datos interesantes y anecdóticos sobre el sabio cubano Carlos J. Finlay, descubridor del agente trasmisor de la fiebre amarilla. **Rev Cubana Med Trop** 1981 Jan–Apr;33(1):8–12

**Finlayson G:** Osteopathic hospitals and AOHA. United in progress for 50 years. **OH** 1984 Sep;28(8):12–4

**Finlayson G:** The birth of a profession: osteopathic medicine. **OH** 1984 Sep;28(8):16–7

**Finn R:** Salt and hypertension: discussion paper. **J R Soc Med** 1983 Oct;76(10):853–8

**Finn WF:** Maternal Welfare--Nassau County, New York, 1957–1981. **Obstet Gynecol Surv** 1984 Mar;39(3):127–33

**Finnane M:** Insanity and the insane in post-famine Ireland. London, Croom Helm; and Totowa, New Jersey, Barnes & Noble, 1981. 241 p.

**Finnane M:** The popular defence of Chidley. **Labour Hist** 1981;41:57–73

**Finnäs F** see **Hoem JM**

**Finot A:** Les premiers élèves et collaborateurs (surtout Bretons) de Laennec. In: Congrès National des Sociétés Savantes, 91e, Rennes, 1966. Comptes Rendus. Paris, 1967. Section des Sciences, Tome 1. p. 181–9.

**Fiori L:** Les origines du CICIAMS et son évolution pendant 50 ans. **Nouv Com Int Cathol Infirm Assist Med Soc** 1983;(3):41–8

**Firebaugh G:** Population density and fertility in 22 Indian villages. **Demography** 1982 Nov;19(4):481–94

**Firman JP** see **Vladeck BC**

**Firmin F:** Cancer de la joue et autoplastie en l'an 1838. Opération de génioplastie pratiquée par M. Roux de Brignolles. **Ann Chir Plast** 1982;27(1):91–3

**Firmin F:** De la réunion immédiate de quelques doigts amputés. **Ann Chir Plast** 1980;25(2):187–90

**Firmin F:** Quelques reconstructions palpébrales au XIXe siècle. **Ann Chir Plast** 1981;26(1):77–81

**Firoiu I:** Istoria ochelarilor. **Rev Chir [Oftalmol]** 1983 Jul–Sep;27(3):231–4

**The first American Medical Association reports on public hygiene in American cities. Twelve reports reprinted from the Transactions of the American Medical Association, Vol. II, 1849. New York, Arno, 197. P. 431–634.:**

**The first fifty years 1931–1981: Dent Assist** 1981 Jan–Feb;50(1):24–6

**The first report on Semmelweis' discovery of the cause and prevention of childbed fever:** Most important experiences about the etiology of puerperal fevers epidemic in birthing institutions. **Infect Control** 1982 Nov–Dec;3(6):478–9

**Fisch L:** Development of school screening audiometry. **Br J Audiol** 1981 May;15(2):87–95

**Fischbach H:** Coping with the aflatoxin problem in the early years. **J Assoc Off Anal Chem** 1984 Jan–Feb;67(1):1–3

**Fischenich J** see **Ingram J**

**Fischer AK** see **Srole L**

**Fischer C:** Bog bodies of Denmark. In A. Cockburn, E. Cockburn, ed: Mummies, disease, and ancient cultures. Cambridge, Cambridge University Press, 1980. p. 177–93.

**Fischer CH:** Die Entwicklung der japanisch-deutschen Beziehungen aus zahnärztlicher Sicht. **Zahnarztl Mitt** 1981;71(5):292–4

**FiscHer H:** Der deutsche Sanitätsdienst, 1921–1945: Organisation, Dokumente und persönliche Erfahrungen. Band 1. Osnabrück, Biblio, 1982. viii, 289 p.

**Fischer H:** Der Streit um das Arzneimittel im Spiegel frühzeitlicher Antimonliteratur. **Beitr Gesch Pharm** 1983;31(18/19):150–4

**Fischer H:** Die Apothekenanfänge in Bayreuth bis zum Beginn des 18. Jahrhunderts und die Entwicklung des Apothekenrechts in der Markgrafschaft bis um 1800. **Arch Gesch Oberfranken** 1978;57–58:187–271

**Fischer H:** Zur Entwicklung Bayreuths. Das Hospital und seine Kirche bis zum Ende des 16. Jahrhunderts. **Arch Gesch Oberfranken** 1979;59:41–88

**Fischer JL:** Etienne Geoffroy Saint-Hilaire (1772–1844) face au problème du déterminisme du sexe. **Hist Philos Life Sci** 1979;1(2):261–83

**Fischer JL, Smith J:** French embryology and the 'Mechanics of development' from 1887 to 1910: L. Chabry, Y. Delage & E. Bataillon. **Hist Philos Life Sci** 1984;6(1):25–39

**Fischer JL:** L'aspect social et politique des relations épistolaires entre quelques savants français et la Station zoologique de Naples de 1878 à 1912. **Rev Hist Sci (Paris)** 1980 Jul;33(3):225–51

**Fischer JL:** L'hybridologie et la zootaxi du Siècle des Lumières à l'Origine des espèces. **Rev Synth (Paris)** 1981;102(101–102):47–72

**Fischer JL:** Yves Delage (1854–1920): l'epigenèse néo-lamarckienne contre la prédétermination weismannienne. **Rev Synth (Paris)** 1979;100(95–6):443–61

**Fischer KD:** Antike Verse in medizinischen Schriften des Mittelalters. **Gesnerus** 1982;39(3–4):443–50

**Fischer KD, Sonderkamp JA:** Ein byzantinischer Text zur Altersbestimmung von Pferden; aus Ambrosianus H 2 inf. **Sudhoffs Arch** 1980;64(1):55–68

**Fischer KD:** Palladius, De vet. med. 14. 15, 5. **Liverp Classical Mon** 1979;4:73–4

**Fischer KD:** Seneca d. A., Controversiae 10,5,17: ein übersehenes Zeugnis zur Geschichte der antiken Anatomie. **Sudhoffs Arch** 1984;68(1):110–2

**Fischer KD:** The first Latin treatise on horse medicine and its author Pelagonius Saloninus. **Medizinhist J** 1981;16(3):215–26

**Fischer KD:** 'Three lexicographical notes.' **Glotta** 1979;57:224–6

**Fischer KD:** Two notes on the Hippiatrica. **Greek Roman Byz Stud (Cambridge, Mass.)** 1979;20:371–9

**Fischer KD:** Wege zum Verständnis antiker Tierkrankheitsnamen. **Hist Med Vet** 1977;2(4):106–11

**Fischer RP** see **Gervin AS**

**Fischer W:** Der Psychiater Heinroth--eine kritische Betrachtung. **Psychiatr Neurol Med Psychol (Leipz)** 1983 Oct;35(10):623–8

**Fischer W:** Die Psychiatrie des Mediziners J.C. Reil--eine kritische Betrachtung. **Psychiatr Neurol Med Psychol (Leipz)** 1984 Apr;36(4):229–35

**Fischer W:** Franz Joseph Gall und Johann Kaspar Spurzheim--Vorläufer einer biologischen Psychiatrie. **Psychiatr Neurol Med Psychol (Leipz)** 1984 Jul;36(7):433–7

**Fischer-Homberger E:** Aerztliche Ethik und ärztliche Standespolitik--ein Aspekt der Geschichte der ärztlichen Ethik. **Bull Schweiz Akad Med Wiss** 1980 Nov;36(4–6):395–410

**Fischer-Homberger E:** Die gerichtsmedizinische Wundbegutachtung vom 16. zum 18. Jahrhundert. **Gesnerus** 1983;40(1–2):75–80

**Fischer-Homberger E:** Herr und Weib: Zur Geschichte der Beziehung zwischen ordnendem Geist und anderen Impulsen. In Fischer-Homberger E: Krankheit Frau. Zur Geschichte der Einbildungen. Darmstadt, Sammlung Luchterhand, 1984. p. 92–121.

**Fischer-Homberger E:** 'Krankheit Frau'. In Imhof AE, ed: Leib und Leben in der Geschichte der Neuzeit. Berlin, Duncker & Humblot, 1983. p. 215–29.

**Fischer-Homberger E:** Medizin vor Gericht: Gerichtsmedizin von der Renaissance bis zur Aufklärung. Bern, H. Huber, 1983. 487 p.

**Fischer-Homberger E:** On the medical history of the doctrine of imagination. **Psychol Med** 1979 Nov;9(4):619–28

**Fischer-Homberger E:** Psychiatrie im Wandel der Zeit. **Schweiz Spital** 1980;44(2):24–7

**Fischer-Homberger E:** The medicalization of demonology--the contribution of forensic medicine to early modern psychiatry. In International Congress of the History of Medicine, 27th, Barcelona, 1980. Actas. Barcelona, Acadèmia de Ciències Mèdiques de Catalunya i Balears, 1981. p. 69–73.

**Fischer-Homberger E:** Vergiftungen in der Gerichtsmedizin vom 16. bis zum 18. Jahrhundert. **Schweiz Aerzteztg** 1980;61(51):3399–406

**Fischer KD, ed:** Pelagonii Ars Veterinaria. Leipzig, Teubner, 1980. xlv, 203 p. (Bibliotheca Teubneriana).

**Fischle-Carl H, ed:** Theorie und Praxis der Psychoanalyse. Fellbach, Bonz, 1979. Historical contributions p. 7–132, by H. Thomä, J. Cremerius, A. Dührssen, P. Kutter, W. Bräutigam, G. Benedetti.

**Fischmann E:** Retracing Röntgen's discovery. **Diagn Imaging** 1979;48(5):294–303

**Fischoff E:** Elizabeth Blackwell: first woman M.D. **Pearson Mus Monogr Ser** 1981;4:1–22

**Fisenne IM, Keller HW:** A short history of ZnS on Mylar as an alpha-scintillation detector. **Health Phys** 1981 May;40(5):739–41

**Fish WR:** Changing food use patterns in Brazil. **Luso-Braz Rev** 1978;15(1):69–89

**Fishbein L:** Freud and the radicals: the sexual revolution comes to Greenwich Village. **Can Rev Am Stud** 1981;12(2):173–89

**Fishbein L:** The snake pit (1948): the sexist nature of sanity. **Am Q** 1979;31(5):641–65

**Fishchenko AIa** see **Klantsa PA**

**Fisher AM** see **Lopatenok AA**

**Fisher D:** The role of philanthropic foundations in the reproduction and

production of hegemony: Rockefeller foundations and the social sciences. **Sociology** 1983;17(2):206–33
**Fisher DA:** The Endocrine Society: past and present. **J Clin Endocrinol Metab** 1984 Dec;59(6):1229–33
**Fisher DJ:** Lacans's ambiguous impact on French psychoanalysis. **Contemp Fr Civiliz** 1981–82;6(1–2):89–114
**Fisher GT, Fisher JB, Stark RB:** Origin of the use of subcuticular sutures. **Ann Plast Surg** 1980 Feb;4(2):144–8
**Fisher J:** Professor Gamgee and the farmers. **Vet Hist** 1979–80;1(2):47–63
**Fisher JB** see **Fisher GT**
**Fisher JR:** Foot-and-mouth disease in Australia. **Aust Vet J** 1984 May;61(5):158–61
**Fisher JR:** The economic effects of cattle disease in Britain and its containment, 1850–1900. **Agric Hist** 1980;54(2):278–94
**Fisher JW:** The influence of Dorpat on modern pharmacology. **Pharmacologist** 1984;26(1):31–6
**Fisher S:** The pastoral interest and Sydney's public health. **Hist Stud** 1982;20(78):73–89
**Fisher S, Greenberg RP, ed:** The scientific evaluation of Freud's theories and therapy; a book of readings. New York, Basic Books, 1978. xv, 446 p. (Reprinted articles of various authors).
**Fisher SH:** An accumulation of misery? **Labour Hist** 1981;40:16–28
**Fishman AP, Richards DW:** Circulation of the blood: men and ideas. Bethesda, American Physiological Society, 1982. xx, 859 p.
**Fishman AP:** Hail and farewell. **Am J Physiol** 1981 May;240(5):C161–3
**Fishman N:** John Bell, MD--teacher to William Osler. **Can Med Assoc J** 1981 Nov 1;125(9):1042, 1044
**Fishman S:** The history of childhood sexuality. **J Contemp Hist** 1982;17(2):269–83
**Fishman SH** see **Rooks JB**
**Fitch NE:** Statistical and mathematical methods for historians: an annotated bibliography of selected books and articles. **Hist Methods** 1980;13(4):222–31
**Fitchen JF:** The problem of ventilation through the ages. **Technol Cult** 1981 Jul;22(3):485–511
**Fitness for Canadians 1909–1983: Can J Public Health** 1983 May–Jun;74 Suppl 1:1–45
**Fitz-Hugh GS:** Anesthesia in otolaryngology: historical overview. **Otolaryngol Clin North Am** 1981 Aug;14(3):467–81
**Fitzgerald GF:** Le Canada et le développement du droit international: la contribution de l'affaire de la fonderie de Trail à le formation du nouveau droit de la pollution atmosphérique transfrontière. **Etud Int** 1980;11(3):393–420
**Fitzgerald M:** A 50 years' overview of paediatric nursing practice. **Aust Nurses J** 1982 Aug;12(2):63–4
**Fitzgerald PJ:** Medical anecdotes concerning some diseases of the pancreas. **Monogr Pathol** 1980;21:1–29
**Fitzgerald RH:** Disaster relief after the Charleston earthquake of 1886. **J SC Med Assoc** 1981 Dec;77(12):607–8
**Fitzgerald RH:** What is the Dukes' system for carcinoma of the rectum? **Dis Colon Rectum** 1982 Jul–Aug;25(5):474–7
**Fitzpatrick JJ:** Suicidology and suicide prevention: historical perspectives from the nursing literature. **J Psychosoc Nurs Ment Health Serv** 1983 May;21(5):20–8
**Fitzpatrick ML:** A history of the National Organization for Public Health Nursing, 1912–1952. [New York, N. Y., s. n.], 1973. 3, vi, 451 leaves.
**Fitzpatrick ML:** Nursing. **Signs** 1977;2(4):818–34
**Fitzpatrick ML:** Nursing history: route to professional identity. **NLN Publ** 1983;(41–1935):27–38
**Fitzpatrick SA:** Only the poor in a gilded age: public health care for the poor in St. Louis, 1890–1900. Ph.D. diss. Saint Louis University. St. Louis, 1979. 157 leaves.
**Fitzpatrick TP:** The Lenape contribution to New Jersey medicine. **J Med Soc NJ** 1984 Sep;81(9):701–6
**Fiumara NJ:** A restrospective approach to syphilis in the 1970s. **Int J Dermatol** 1982 Sep;21(7):400–3
**Fiziologiia v SSSR: Fiziol Zh SSSR** 1982 Dec;68(12):1593–630
**Fjeld C** see **Sommer R**
**Flahaut S:** Le pharmacien Charles-Louis Cadet de Gassicourt, bâtard de Louis XV, et sa famille. **Rev Hist Pharm (Paris)** 1980 Mar;27(244):53–61
**Flameng F:** La journée d'un médecin de Bruxelles en 1830. **Folkl Brabancon** 1979 Jun;222:171–214
**Flamm ES:** The decline of osteology and the rise of surgical neurology in the management of head injuries. In Rose FC, Bynum WF, ed: Historical aspects of the neurosciences. New York, Raven, 1982. p. 243–53.
**Flanagan OJ:** Psychology, progress and the problem of reflexivity: a study in the epistemological foundations of psychology. **J Hist Behav Sci** 1981;17:375–86
**Flanagan TE:** Problems of psychobiography. **Queens Q** 1982;89(3):596–610
**Flanagan L, ed:** One strong voice: the story of the American Nurses' Association. Kansas City, Mo., American Nurses' Assn., 1976. xiii, 692 p.
**Flandrin JL:** Repression and change in sexual life of young people in medieval and early modern times. In R. Wheaton, T. K. Hareven, ed: Family and sexuality in French history. Philadelphia. University of Pennsylvania Press, 1980. p. 27–48.
**Flandrin JL** see **Margolin JC**
**Flatau E** see **Kohn D**
**Flaumenhaft E:** Asian medicinal plants in 17th century French literature. **Econ Bot** 1982;36:147–62
**Flavin TH:** The Clinical Center: twenty-five years of research for people. **Conn Med** 1979 Sep;43(9):563–7
**Fleagle JG, Jungers WL:** Fifty years of higher primate phylogeny. In F. Spencer, ed: A history of American physical anthropology, 1930–1980. New York, Academic Press, 1982. p. 187–230.
**Fleagle JG, Bown TM:** New primate fossils from late Oligocene (Colhuehuapian) localities of Chubut Province, Argentina. **Folia Primatol (Basel)** 1983;41(3–4):240–66
**Fleck L:** Genesis and development of a scientific fact. Edited by T. J. Trenn and R. K. Merton. Chicago, Univ. of Chicago Press, 1979. xxviii, 203 p.
**Fleck L** see **McCullough LB**
**Fleck L** see **Sadegh-Zadeh K**
**Fleck L** see **Trenn TJ**
**Fleckenstein K:** Etienne Marey and the electric torpedo fish. **Med Instrum** 1984 Sep–Oct;18(5):288–9
**Fleckenstein K:** The early ECG in medical practice. **Med Instrum** 1984 May–Jun;18(3):191–2
**Flegenheimer WV:** Techniques of brief pschotherapy. New York, London, Jason Aronson, 1982. xiii, 206 p.
**Flegg AT:** Inequality of income, illiteracy and medical care as determinants of infant mortality in underdeveloped countries. **Popul Stud** 1982 Nov;36(3):441–58
**Flehr H:** Geschichte des Arztlichen Vereins in Frankfurt am Main und sein standespolitisches Wirken. Diss. Mainz, 1982. 144 p.
**Fleischhauer K:** In memoriam Philipp Stöhr jr. **Anat Anz** 1981;150(3):239–47
**Fleischhauer K:** In memoriam Wolfgang Bargmann. **Anat Anz** 1979;146(8):209–34
**Fleishmann-Bánó M, Zalai K:** St. Cosmas and St. Damian relics in Hungary. **Ther Hung** 1981;29(3):142–6
**Fleiss JL:** Multicentre clinical trials: Bradford Hill's contributions and some subsequent developments. **Stat Med** 1982 Oct–Dec;1(4):353–9
**Fleissner RF:** Putting Falstaff to rest: 'tabulating' the facts. **Shakespeare Stud** 1983;16:57–74
**Fleming AF:** HTLV from Africa to Japan. **Lancet** 1984 Feb 4;1(8371):279
**Fleming DW:** The founders of the college: Western Australia. **Aust NZ J Surg** 1981 Dec;51(6):623–4
**Fleming M** see **Sirkin M**
**Fleming y la penicilina: Rev Col Nac Enferm** 1979 Aug–Dec;26(105):16–8
**Fletcher C:** Mastectomy in the 1880s. **Br Med J [Clin Res]** 1983 Mar 19;286(6369):966–7
**Fletcher G, Harris JI:** Pharmacy in Bath during the Regency period. **Pharm Hist (London)** 1970 Jun;1(5):2–4
**Fletcher GF:** The history of exercise in the practice of medicine. **J Med Assoc Ga** 1983 Jan;72(1):35–40
**Fletcher I:** Aid, first and foremost: a brief outline history of the St John Ambulance Association and Brigade. **Injury** 1979 Nov;11(2):104–9
**Fletcher JC:** The evolution of the ethics of informed consent. **Prog Clin Biol Res** 1983;128:187–228
**Fletcher RH** see **Fletcher SW**
**Fletcher SW, Fletcher RH, Greganti MA:** Clinical research trends in general medical journals, 1946–1976. In E. B. Roberts, et al, ed: Biomedical innovation. Cambridge, London, MIT Press, 1981. p. 284–300.
**Fleurentin J, Mazars G, Pelt JM:** Additional information on the cultural background of drugs and medicinal plants of Yemen. **J Ethnopharmacol** 1983 Sep;8(3):335–44
**Fleurentin J, Mazars G, Pelt JM:** Cultural background of the medicinal plants of Yemen. **J Ethnopharmacol** 1983 Mar;7(2)183–203
**Flick C:** The movement for smoke abatement in 19th-century Britain. **Technol Cult** 1980 Jan;21(1):29–50
**Flinn D:** John Macculloch, M.D., F.R.S., and his geological map of Scotland: his years in the Ordnance. 1795–1826. **Notes Rec R Soc Lond** 1981;36(1):83–101
**Flinn MW:** Plague in Europe and the Mediterranean countries. **J Eur Econ Hist** 1979;8(1):131–48
**Flinn MW:** The European demographic system, 1500–1820. Baltimore, Johns Hopkins Univ. Press, 1981. 175 p.
**Flinn MW** see **Dupâquier J**
**Flint EP** see **Williams D**
**Florence Nightingale:** the original geriatric nurse. **Okla Nurse** 1980 May;25(4):6
**Florentine M** see **Buus S**
**Flores D:** Historia de la sanidad publica de Bolivia, durante los primeros años de la republica. **Illimani** 1974;(5):22–38
**Flores GK** see **Guerra FS**
**Flores y Troncoso FA:** Historia de la medicina en México desde la época de los indios hasta la presente. Facsimile of 1886 ed. plus new indices. 4 vols. México, Instituto Mexicano del Seguro Social, 1982. Various pagings. Historical and biographical chapters by V. M. Ruiz Naufal, A. G. Medrano, C. Viesca, G. A. Beltrán, J. S. Palencia, J. S. Riquer, B. F. Hernández.
**Floriano AC:** En torno a la enfermedad y muerte del príncipe Don Carlos (hijo de Felipe II). In: Homenaje al Profesor Carriazo. Seville, Univ. of Seville, 1973. vol. 2. p. 203–31.
**Florkin M:** A history of biochemistry. Part IV. Early studies of biosynthesis. Amsterdam, Elsevier, 1977. xx, 362 p. (Comprehensive biochemistry, Vol. 32).
**Florkin M, Théodoridès J:** Henri de Lacaze-Duthiers et Léon Fredericq: correspondance (1876–1900). **Arch Int Physiol Biochim** 1982 Jul;90(2):Suppl 1–94
**Florkin M:** L'Ecole Liégeoise de Physiologie et son Maître Léon Fredericq

(1851-1935), pionnier de la zoologie chimique. Liège, Vaillant-Carmanne, 1979. 211 p. (Publication des Archives Internationales de Physiologie et de Biochimie, Médecine et Médicins au Pays de Liège, IV).

**Flowers RB:** Freedom of religion versus civil authority in matters of health. **Ann Am Acad Polit Soc Sci** 1979;446:149-61

**Flynn JP:** Maryland physicians in World War II. **Md State Med J** 1984 Jun;33(6):455

**Flynn RJ:** The founding and early history of the American Association for Laboratory Animal Science. **Lab Anim Sci** 1980 Aug;30(4 pt 2):765-79

**Foà V** see **Bertelli G**

**Foão Gameiro OH** see **Castro F de**

**Fock G:** Om sköterskor, havandeskap, förlossning samt barnsäng i Finland på Elias Lönnrots tid. **Kätilölehti** 1982 Jan;87(1):11-4

**Fockert JA de:** De klinisch geriatrische afdeling in een ziekenhuis: officële erkenning als experiment. **Tijdschr Ziekenverpl** 1982 Sept 21;35(19):621-5

**Focus on the Bahamas: Jamaican Nurse** 1982;22(1):19-22

**Fodor B:** 100 Jahre 'Fortschritte der Medizin'--Höhepunkte der Medizin 1882-1982. **Fortschr Med** 1982 Dec 16;100(47-48):2207-13

**Fodor F:** 100 de ani de la introducerea procedeului profilactic Crédé. **Rev Chir [Oftalmol]** 1981 Jul-Sep;25(3):161-3

**Fodor J, Malott JC, King AY:** The radiographic investigation of two Egyptian mummies. **Radiol Technol** 1983 Jul-Aug;54(6):443-8

**Fodstad H:** Carl Peter Thunberg: Swedish pioneer of Occidental medicine in Japan. **Neurol Med Chir (Tokyo)** 1982 Jul;22(7):577-81

**Foege WH:** Centers for disease control. **J Public Health Policy** 1981 Mar;2(1):8-18

**Foege WH** see **Ravenholt RT**

**Foerster I, Kirschke S:** Soziobiologie oder Biosoziologie? **Wiss Z Martin Luther Univ (Math)** 1984;33(4):51-67

**Fogarty RS, Grant HR:** Free love in Ohio: Jacob Beilhardt and the Spirit Fruit Colony. **Ohio Hist** 1980;89(2):206-21

**Fogel RW, Engerman SL, Trussell J:** Exploring the uses of data on height: the analysis of long-term trends in nutrition, labor welfare, and labor productivity. **Soc Sci Hist** 1982;6(4):401-21

**Fogel RW, Engerman SL:** Recent findings in the study of slave demography and family structure. **Sociol Soc Res** 1979;63(3):566-89

**Fogel RW, et al:** The economics of mortality in North America, 1650-1910: a description of a research project. **Hist Methods Newsl** 1978;11(2):75-108

**Foglia VG:** The history of Bernardo A. Houssay's research laboratory, Instituto de Biologia y Medicina Experimental: the first twenty years, 1944-1963. **J Hist Med Allied Sci** 1980 Oct;35(4):380-96

**Foisil M:** Louis XIII à travers le stethoscope. **Histoire** 1982;42:76-8

**Fokina EN:** Fedor Petrovich Gaaz i ego issledovaniia po izucheniiu lechebnykh mineral'nykh istochnikov Kavkaza. **Vopr Kurortol Fizioter Lech Fiz Kult** 1980 Sep-Oct;(5):65-6

**Fokina NS** see **Sukharev AG**

**Folb PI:** The thalidomide disaster and its impact on modern medicine. Cape Town, Univ. of Cape Town, 1977. 11 p.

**Folch i Pi A** see **Puche J**

**Folch Jou G, Muñoz Calvo S:** Aportación de Olmedilla y Puig al desarrollo de la historiografía farmacéutica en España. **Bol Soc Esp Hist Farm** 1980 Oct;31(123):205-34

**Folch Jou G, Muñoz Calvo S:** Catalogo de los documentos conservados en el Archivo de la Real Academia de Farmacia. **An R Acad Farm (Madr)** 1978;44(2):199-351

**Folch Jou G, Muñoz Calvo S:** Datos para la historia del Colegio de Boticarios de Madrid. Actos con motivo de la preparacion de la Triaca en el siglo XVIII. **An R Acad Farm (Madr)** 1979;45(4):599-606

**Folch Jou G, Muñoz Calvo S:** El concepto de 'Legislacion Farmaceutica' a traves de la Historiografia Universitaria de la Facultad de Farmacia de Madrid (1884-1965). **Bol Soc Esp Hist Farm** 1982 Mar;33(131):145-61

**Folch Jou G, Basante Pol RM, Sanchez-Villacañas CM:** La farmacia madrileña de la plaza de Santo Domingo num. 6. **Bol Soc Esp Hist Farm** 1983;34(136):111-37

**Folch Jou G, Puerto Sarmiento FJ:** Las Cantaridas en Espana. In Hickel E, Schröder G, ed: Neue Beiträge zur Arzneimittelgeschichte. Festschrift für Wolfgang Schneider zum 70. Geburtstag. Stuttgart, Wissenschaftliche Verlagsgesellschaft, 1982. p. 131-47.

**Folch Jou G:** L'influence de Dorvault en Espagne. **Rev Hist Pharm (Paris)** 1980 Jun;27(245):109-18

**Folch Jou G, Javier Puerto F:** Los medicamentos incluidos en los formularios del Hospital General de Madrid (Siglos XVIII y XIX). **Bol Soc Esp Hist Farm** 1982 Mar;33(129):49-76

**Folch Jou G, Sanz Diaz L, Puerto Sarmiento FJ:** Los proyectos de socialización de la farmacia durante la Segunda República española. **Pharm Acta Helv** 1979;54(9-10):286-94

**Folch Jou G:** Medicamentos empleados por los`árabes y su influencia en la farmacia de occidente en especial española. **Bol Soc Esp Hist Farm** 1979 Dec;30(120):319-35

**Folch Jou G:** Medicamentos empleados por los arabes y su posible influencia en la introduccion de la quimica en la Farmacia. **Asclepio** 1978-79;30-31:177-86

**Folch Jou G, Nuñez Varela V:** Un examen de farmaceutico por comisionados del protomedicato en la Andalucia del siglo XIX. **Bol Soc Esp Hist Farm** 1982 Sep;33(131):193-8

**Folch Jou G, Muñoz Calvo S:** Un intento de reforma legislativa en la Farmacia Española del siglo XIX: J. Guerrero Fernández y su 'Proyecto de Servicio Farmacéutico'. **Bol Soc Esp Hist Farm** 1980/81 Dec-Mar;31-32(124-5):299-314

**Földes F:** Az aneaesthesiológia szerepe a betegellátásban, orvosképzésben és az orvostudomány fejlödéséven **Orv Hetil** 1981 Feb 15;122(7):375-9

**Földes V, Kósa F, Virágos-Kis E, et al:** Atomabsorptions-spektrophotometrische Untersuchung des Gehaltes an anorganischen Substanzen von Skelettbefunden zur Ermittlung der Dauer des Begrabenseins in der Erde. **Arch Kriminol** 1980 Sep-Oct;166(3-4):105-11

**Foley GP:** A treasury of dentistry. **J Am Coll Dent** 1983 Spring;50(1):42-3

**Foley GP:** A treasury of dentistry. Early offices were a dangerous place to practice. **J Am Coll Dent** 1983 Summer;50(2):24-5

**Foley GP:** A treasury of dentistry. Henry Cogswell. **J Am Coll Dent** 1984 Summer;51(2):20-1

**Foley GP:** A treasury of dentistry: John B. Rich, pioneer dental leader. **J Am Coll Dent** 1982 Summer;49(2):28-9

**Foley GP:** A treasury of dentistry. Royal extractions. **J Am Coll Dent** 1984 Fall;51(3):22-3

**Foley GP:** A treasury of dentistry. The dental attraction of the Wells Cathedral. **J Am Coll Dent** 1983 Fall;50(3):16-7

**Foltyn W:** Biblioteka Towarzystwa Lekarskiego Warszawskiego w latach 1821-1944. **Arch Hist Med (Warsz)** 1983;46(2):151-82

**Fomenko VN** see **Stepanskiĭ GA**

**Fomina IP** see **Navashin SM**

**Fonareva KS:** K istorii izucheniia kozhnogo leĭshmanioza v Rossii. **Med Parazitol (Mosk)** 1983 Mar-Apr;52(2):84-6

**Fondiller S:** Nursing history in undergraduate curriculum: renewal and relevance. **Deans List** 1983 Mar;4(4):1-2

**Fondiller SH:** The entry dilemma: the National League for Nursing and the higher education movement, 1952-1972, with an epilogue to 1983. New York, N.Y., National League for Nursing, 1983. vii, 136 p.

**Fontaine M:** From the physiology of marine organisms to oceanographic physiology or physiological oceanography. In Sears M, Merriman D, ed: Oceanography, the past. New York, Springer, 1980. p. 353-59.

**Fontaine M:** The history of comparative physiology. In E. Schultheisz, ed: History of physiology. Oxford, Elmsford, New York, Pergamon, 1981. xvi, 208 p. (Advances in Physiological Sciences. Proceedings of the 28th International Congress of Physiological Sciences, Budapest, 1980. Volume 21). p. 23-28.

**Fontaine MM** see **Margolin JC**

**Fontaine O:** Introduction aux thérapies comportementales (behavior therapies). Historique, bases théoriques, pratique. Bruxelles, Mardaga, 1978. 299 p. (Psychologie et sciences humaines).

**Fontaine-Levent P:** Prunelle et la bibliothèque de la Faculté de médecine de Montpellier. **Hist Sci Med** 1980;14(2):241-3

**Fontanille MT:** Avortement et contraception dans la médecine gréco-romaine. Paris, Laboratoires Searle, 1977. 233 p.

**Foraker AG:** A reluctant surgeon at sea. **JAMA** 1981 Jun 12;245(22):2302-3

**Forbes EG:** Liebig in Grossbritannien. **Nachrichtenbl Dtsch Ges Gesch Med Naturwiss Tech** 1983 Winter;33(3):115-33

**Forbes EG:** Scientific archives in the Federal Republic of Germany. **Ber Wissenschaftsgesch** 1979;2(3-4):197-201

**Forbes TR:** Births and deaths in a London parish: the record from the registers, 1654-1693 and 1729-1743. **Bull Hist Med** 1981;55(3):371-91

**Forbes TR:** Books and broadsides: what Colonial physicians read. **Conn Med** 1984 Sep;48(9):566-8

**Forbes TR:** Coroners' inquisitions on the deaths of prisoners in the hulks at Portsmouth, England, in 1817-27. **J Hist Med Allied Sci** 1978 Jul;33(3):356-66

**Forbes TR:** Early forensic medicine in England: the Angus murder trial. **J Hist Med Allied Sci** 1981 Jul;36(3):296-309

**Forbes TR:** John Hunter as expert witness. **Trans Stud Coll Physicians Phila** 1980 Jun;5(2 no 2):75-80

**Forbes TR:** Mortality at St. Bartholomew's Hospital, London, 1839-72. **J Hist Med Allied Sci** 1983 Oct;38(4):432-49

**Forbes TR:** 'To be dissected and anatomized.' **J Hist Med Allied Sci** 1981 Oct;36(4):490-2

**Forbes TR:** When did Lionel Wafer die? **J Hist Med Allied Sci** 1981 Jan;36(1)69-70

**Forbes TR** see **Ebbert A, et al**

**Forbes TR** see **Hand WD, ed**

**Forbes TR** see **Webster C, ed**

**Forbes EG, ed:** Human implications of scientific advance. Proceedings of the XVth International Congress of the History of Science, Edinburgh 10-15 August 1977. Edinburgh, Edinburgh University Press, 1978. 596 p. (This volume includes papers delivered at ten special symposia)

**Force JE:** Hume and the relation of science to religion among certain members of the Royal Society. **J Hist Ideas** 1984 Oct-Dec;45(4):517-36

**Ford BJ:** Bacteria and cells of human origin on van Leeuwenhoek's sections of 16741,2. **Trans Am Microsc Soc** 1982 Jan;101(1):1-9

**Ford BJ:** Correlated optical and electron microscopy of Leeuwenhoek's elder-pith sections. **J Microsc** 1982 Nov;128 Pt 2:211-3

**Ford BJ:** Cytological examination of Leeuwenhoek's first microbial specimens. **Tissue Cell** 1982;14(2):207-17

**Ford BJ:** Found - van Leeuwenhoek's original specimens. **New Sci** 1981;91:301

**Ford BJ:** Leeuwenhoek's specimens discovered after 307 years [news]. **Nature** 1981 Jul 30;292(5822):407

**Ford BJ:** Revelation and the single lens. **Br Med J [Clin Res]** 1982 Dec 18-25;285(6357):1822-4

**Ford BJ:** The van Leeuwenhoek specimens. **Notes Rec R Soc Lond** 1981;36(1):37-59

**Ford EB** see **Mayr E**

Ford J: Ideas which have influenced attempts to solve the problems of African trypanosomiasis. **Soc Sci Med [Med Anthropol]** 1979 Dec;13B(4):269–75
**Ford JM:** Apothecaries' roles reassessed. **J R Soc Med** 1983 Aug;76(8):634
**Ford JM:** Medical indications for taking the waters of Tunbridge Wells. **J R Soc Med** 1984 Nov;77(11):955–9
**Ford P** see **Feldman A**
**Ford P** see **Howell M**
**Ford RI** see **Hand WD, ed**
**Fordham EW** see **Ram PC**
**Fordham M:** Analytical psychology in England. **J Anal Psychol** 1979 Oct;24(4):279–97
**Foreman T, Gordon B, Weese WC:** In honor of Robert Koch, M.D. **Ariz Med** 1983 Mar;40(3):149
**Forgan S, ed:** Science and the sons of genius: studies on Humphry Davy. London, Science Reviews, 1980. xii, 247 p. Contributions by M. Neve, T. H. Levere, J. Z. Fullmer, M. Crosland, J. H. Brooke, R. Siegfried, D. Knight, E. B. Smith.
**Forget M:** La fondation Roguet à Clichy. **Bull Soc Fr Hist Hop** 1978;(36–37):31–9
**Forgue E, Bouchet A:** Die Chirurgie bis zum Ende des 18. Jahrhunderts. In Sournia JC, Martiny M, Poulet J, ed: Illustrierte Geschichte der Medizin. Salzburg, Andreas, 1980. Vol. 3. p. 931–1021.
**Forman R:** Medical resistance to innovation. **Med Hypotheses** 1981 Aug;7(8):1009–17
**Formston C:** A veterinary student's experience of the general strike. **Vet Hist** 1983 Summer;3(1):25–9
**Fornaciari G:** Natural mummies in central Italy: a preliminary survey. **Paleopathol Newsl** 1982 Dec;40:11–2
**Fornaciari G:** The mummies of the Abbey of Saint Domenico Maggiore in Naples. **Paleopathol Newsl** 1984 Sep;(47):10–4
**Foronda MA:** An army doctor in Leyte. **Leyte-Samar Stud** 1980;14(1):1–37
**Forrai G:** Noah or the legend of albinism. **Ther Hung** 1980;28(2):87–9
**Forrest RD:** Development of wound therapy from the Dark Ages to the present. **J R Soc Med** 1982 Apr;75(4):268–73
**Forrest RD:** Early history of wound treatment. **J R Soc Med** 1982 Mar;75(3):198–205
**Forrest WR, Christen AG:** Recollections of a dental researcher. Fifty years at the U. S. Bureau of Standards: Interviews with George C. Paffenbarger. Part I. **J Ala Dent Assoc** 1982 Summer;66(3):24–8
**Forrest WR, Christen AG:** Recollections of a dental researcher. Fifty years at the U.S. National Bureau of Standards: interviews with George C. Paffenbarger, D.D.S., D.Sc. Part II. **J Ala Dent Assoc** 1982 Fall;66(4):36–8
**Forrest WR, Christen AG:** Recollections of a dental researcher. Fifty years at the U.S. National Bureau of Standards: interviews with George C. Paffenbarger, D.D.S., D.Sc. Part VI. **J Ala Dent Assoc** 1984 Spring;68(2):29–31, 34–7
**Forrester J:** Language and the origins of psychoanalysis. London, Macmillan, 1980. xvi, 285 p.
**Forrester J:** Michel Foucault and the history of psychoanalysis. **Hist Sci** 1980 Dec;18(42 pt 4):286–303
**Forschbach G:** Tuberculosis and creative man. **Bull Int Union Tuberc** 1984 Mar–Jun;59(1–2):104–7
**Forsdahl A, Dahl T:** Spedalske i brønnøy legedistrikt i forrige århundre. **Tidsskr Nor Laegeforen** 1983 Oct 30;103(30):2024–7
**Forsey RR:** One hundred years ago. A century of hospital administrators. **Montreal Gen Hosp News** 1981;19(1):9
**Forster FM:** B. Fawcett, a nineteenth–century Australian quack doctor. **J R Aust Hist Soc** 1981;67(3):272–82
**Forster FM:** Benjamin Fawcett, a 19th century Australian quack–doctor. In: International Congress of the History of Medicine, 26th, Plovdiv (Bulgaria), 1978. Actes du Congres, Vol. 1. Sofia, 1980. p. 111–2.
**Forster FM:** David D. Davis' Obstetric Atlas in Tasmania in 1846. Edmund Bowden's gift to Robert Officer. **Aust NZ J Obstet Gynaecol** 1983 May;23(2):88–92
**Forster FM** see **McDonald IA**
**Forster R, Ranum O, ed:** Food and drink in history. Selections from the Annales economies, sociétés, civilisations. Volume 5. Baltimore, London, Johns Hopkins University Press, 1979. xiii, 173 p. Reprinted articles by M. Aymard, M. Morineau, J. Revel, JJ. Hémardinquer, W. Frijhoff, JC. Bonnet, R. Barthes, D. Julia, J. Leclant, J.P. Aron, G. Thuillier, J. Soler.
**Forster R, Ranum O, ed:** Medicine and society in France. Selections from the Annales -- Economies, Sociétés, Civilisations. Baltimore and London, Johns Hopkins University Press, 1980. ix, 176 p. Reprinted articles by J. P. Goubert, J. Léonard, M. F. Morel, D. Roche, A. Farge, M. Joerger, M. Laget.
**Forsythe-Jauch WE:** L Cpl Joseph John Farmer, VC, AHC. Centenary of the battle of Majuba 1881. **J R Army Med Corps** 1981 Jun;127(2):100–2
**Fortič B:** Sesdeset godina stručnog rada i razvoja Golnika. **Plucne Bolesti Tuberk** 1981 Oct–Dec;33(4):197–215
**Fortique JR:** Hernán Pérez de la Muela, primer médico europeo establecido en Venezuela. **Bol Acad Nac Hist (Caracas)** 1979;62(245):147–58
**Fortuine R:** Ships' surgeons and naturalists in the early history of Alaska. **Alaska Med** 1984 Apr–Jun;26(2):57–61
**Fortuine R:** Ships' surgeons and naturalists in the early history of Alaska. Parts 2 and 3. **Alaska Med** 1984 Jul–Sep;26(3):82–6; Oct–Dec;26(4):117–21
**Fortuine R:** Traditional surgery of the Alaska natives. **Alaska Med** 1984 Jan–Mar;26(1):22–5
**Fortuna D, Nieniewska M, Szymusik A:** Kępiński jako nauczyciel i wychowawca. **Przegl Lek** 1983;40(12):837–41
**Fortuna D** see **Drozdowski P**
**Forty A:** The modern hospital in England and France: the social and medical uses of architecture. In King, Anthony D., ed. Buildings and society: essays on the social development of the built environment. London, Routledge and Kegan Paul, 1980. p. 61–93.
**Forum: the place of prevention in medical education: past, present, and future: Prev Med** 1981 Nov;10(6):661–740
**Fossa A** see **Schyns C**
**Fossard J:** Aperçus médico-politiques en Provence orientale à la Belle Epoque. **Hist Sci Med** 1982;16(4):267–72
**Fossard J:** Faut-il rendre à Gamelin l'Ecorché de Bayonne attribué à Géricault? **Hist Sci Med** 1984;18(2):153–8
**Fossard J:** Un inédit d'un fondateur de la Société française d'histoire de la médecine, le docteur Paul Delaunay. **Hist Sci Med** 1981;15(4):305–6
**Fossgreen J:** Manuel medicin. Historie og nutid. **Ugeskr Laeger** 1982 May 24;144(21):1545–7
**Foster C** see **Maud PJ**
**Foster CC** see **Sugar HS**
**Foster GM:** Applied anthropology and international health: retrospect and prospect. **Hum Organ** 1982;41(3):189–97
**Foster GM:** The limitations of federal health care for freed men, 1862–1868. **J South Hist** 1982;48(3):349–72
**Foster GM:** Typhus disaster in the wake of war: the American–Polish relief expedition, 1919–1920. **Bull Hist Med** 1981 Summer;55(2):221–32
**Foster HL:** The history of commercial production of laboratory rodents. **Lab Anim Sci** 1980 Aug;30(4 pt 2):793–8
**Foster J, Sheppard J:** British archives. A guide to archive resources in the United Kingdom. Surrey, Macmillan, 1982. xxv, 533 p.
**Foster J** see **Davies C, ed**
**Foster JB:** History of syringomyelia. In Rose FC, Bynum WF, ed: Historical aspects of the neurosciences. New York, Raven, 1982. p. 205–7.
**Foster NI** see **Heindel ND**
**Foster R:** United States place names and Sherlock Holmes. **Trans Stud Coll Physicians Phila** 1978 Jul;45(5):249–51
**Foster WD:** Edward Gibbon's health. **Br Med J** 1979 Dec 22–29;2(6205):1633–5
**Foster WD:** The Church Missionary Society and modern medicine in Uganda. The life of Sir Albert Cook, K.C.M.G., 1870–1951. Newhaven, Sussex, [The author], 1978. 234 p.
**Foster Z, Wald FS, Wald HJ:** The hospice movement: a backward glance at its first two decades. **New Physician** 1978 May;27(5):21–4
**Foster GM, et al:** El legado hipocratico latinoamericano: 'caliente' y 'frio' en la medicina popular contemporanea. **Med Tradic** 1979;2(6):5–24
**Fothergill J:** Observations on the recovery of a man dead in appearance by distending the lungs with air. Facsimile of London 1745 edition, with biographical note by K. G. Huston. Van Nuys, California, Hoffman, 1980. 13 p.
**Foucault M:** El nacimiento de la medicina social. **Med Tradic** 1982;3(11):3–16
**Foucault MJ:** The history of sexuality. Histoire de la sexualité. La volonté de savoir. v. 1. London, Lane, 1978. 168 p.
**Foulds WS:** The changing pattern of eye surgery. **Br J Anaesth** 1980 Jul;52(7):643–7
**Fouquet C:** Le cas de l'épilepsie. **Penelope** 1983;(8):10–2
**Fouquet C** see **Knibiehler Y**
**Four from '44: the Winslow editorials: J Public Health Policy** 1980 Mar;1(1):15–24
**Fourastié J:** Réflexions sur la science d'aujourd'hui. **Chirurgie** 1981;107(1):23–5
**Fourcroy JL:** L'éternel couteau: review of female circumcision. **Urology** 1983 Oct;22(4):458–61
**Fouré J:** A French woman dentist who gave her life as a freedom fighter against the Nazis. **Bull Hist Dent** 1984 Oct;32(2):133–4
**Fouré J:** Talma - the dentist who became the greatest French actor of all times. **Bull Hist Dent** 1983 Apr;31(1):3–10
**Fourest HP, Sainte-Fare-Garnot PN:** Les pots de pharmacie: Paris et l'Ile-de-France. Paris, Dacosta, 1981. 229 p.
**Fournier GA, Albert DM, Bachrach A, et al:** Symbol of Boston's Museum of Science has eye tumor. **N Engl J Med** 1983 Mar 31;308(13):782–3
**Fournier GA** see **Lamping KA**
**Fournier M:** Hoofdlijnen van de microscopie in de negentiende eeuw. **Tijdschr Geschied Geneeskd** 1983;6(2):59–64
**Fournier M:** Huygens' microscopical researches. **Janus** 1981;68:199–209
**Fournier M:** Jan Swammerdam en de 17e eeuwse microscopie. **Tijdschr Geschied Geneeskd** 1981;4(2)74–86
**Fournier M:** 'Ontdeckte onsightbaarheden'. **Spiegel Hist** 1982;17(2):612–8
**Fournier R:** La médicine ancienne dans le centre-ouest. Coutumes populaires disparues et survivances. Poitiers, Brissaud, 1979. 170 p.
**Fournier Villada R:** Miguel Jiménez y su contribución al estudio del absceso hepático. In Academia Nacional de Medicina. Libro conmemorativo del primer centenario. México, Comité Editorial de la Comisión Organizadora del Congreso del Centenario, 1964. Tome 2. p. 558–60.
**Fourquet F:** Histoire de la psychiatrie de secteur. Paris, Recherches, 1980. viii, 338 p.
**Foussereau J:** History of epicutaneous testing: the blotting-paper and other methods. **Contact Dermatitis** 1984 Oct;11(4):219–23
**Fowlie W** see **Stambolian G**
**Fox A:** Obstetrics and Gynecology in Macbeth. **Shakespeare Stud** 1979;12:127–41
**Fox B, Maddick I:** A century of dental myths and messages.

**Soc Soc Hist Med Bull** 1980;27:47–53
**Fox B, Maddick I:** A hundred years of dental health education. **Br Dent J** 1980 Jul 1;149(1):28–32
**Fox BW:** Dental school circa 1920. **CAL** 1983 Dec;47(6):9–11, 21
**Fox BW:** Turn of the century dentistry. **CAL** 1983 Aug;47(2):18–9, 21–4
**Fox C** see **Wallace ER**
**Fox D:** Henryson's 'Sum Practysis of Medecyne'. **Stud Philol** 1972;69:453–60
**Fox DM:** Abraham Flexner's unpublished report: foundations and medical education, 1909–1928. **Bull Hist Med** 1980 Winter;54(4):475–96
**Fox DM, Stone JF:** Black lung: miners' militancy and medical uncertainty, 1968–1972. **Bull Hist Med** 1980 Spring;54(1):43–63
**Fox DM:** Economists and health care. From reform to relativism. With commentaries. New York, Prodist, 1979.
**Fox DM:** The decline of historicism: the case of compulsory health insurance in the United States. **Bull Hist Med** 1983 Winter;57(4):596–610
**Fox DM** see **Terry JS**
**Fox ER:** Mrs. Laennec and the stethoscope. **West J Med** 1981 Jan;134(1):73–4
**Fox ER:** The face of medicine. **West J Med** 1981 Nov;135(5):424–5
**Fox R, Weisz G:** The institutional basis of French science in the nineteenth century. In R. Fox, G. Weisz, ed: The organization of science and technology in France 1808–1914. Cambridge, Cambridge University Press, 1980. p. 1–28.
**Fox R:** The organization of science and technology in France, 1808–1914. Cambridge, New York, Cambridge University Press, 1980. x, 355 p.
**Fox RC, Swazey JP:** Critical care at Tianjin's First Central Hospital and the fourth modernization. **Science** 1982 Aug 20;217(4561):700–5
**Fox RC, Swazey JP:** Medical morality is not bioethics--medical ethics in China and the United States. **Perspect Biol Med** 1984 Spring;27(3):336–60
**Fox RC:** The sting of death in American society. **Soc Serv Rev** 1981;55(1):42–59
**Fox RW** see **Rosenkrantz BG**
**Fox SD:** Healing, imagination, and New Mexico. **NM Hist Rev** 1983;58(3):213–37
**Fox VC, Quitt MH, ed:** Loving, parenting and dying: the family cycle in England and America, past and present. New York, Psychohistory Press, 1980. v, 488 p. Includes original essays by the editors, by M. A. Glendon, and A. Macfarlane. Also includes numerous previously published articles by various other authors.
**Fox W:** Přerušovaná chemoterapie plicní tuberkulózy. Se zvláštním zřetelem k přínosu Střediska SZO spolupracujícím na chemoterapii tuberkulózy v Praze. **Cas Lek Cesk** 1984 Feb 10;123(6):153–7
**Fozzard JA:** Professors of anatomy in the University of Cambridge: the first two hundred and sixty-one years of the Cambridge University Department of Anatomy, 1707–1968. Cambridge, FOSSLIA, 1983. 87 p.
**Frable WJ:** Fine-needle aspiration biopsy: a review. **Hum Pathol** 1983 Jan;14(1):9–28
**Fracard ML:** L'organisation hospitalière des Frères de Saint-Jean-de-Dieu à Niort (Poitou) dans la seconde moitié du XVIIIe siècle. In: Congrès National des Sociétés Savantes, 97e, Nantes, 1972. Actes. Paris, 1977. Histoire Moderne et Contemporaine, Tome 1. p. 299–327.
**Frädrich G** see **Scheld HH**
**Fraenkel-Conrat H:** Portraits of viruses: tobacco mosaic virus. **Intervirology** 1981;15(4):177–89
**Fraga C:** Vida e obra de Osvaldo Cruz. Rio de Janeiro, Livraria José Olympio Editôra em convênio com o Instituto Nacional do Livro, [1972]. 186 p.
**Fraga M, Tenenbaum L:** Florence Nightingale--model for today's nurse. **Fla Nurse** 1981 May;29(5):11
**Fragnul de Nieto MS** see **Muñoz AI**
**Fragoso Uribe R:** Algunas observaciones que apoyan el origen precolombino de la 'enfermedad de Robles' en América. **SPM** 1979 Nov-Dec;21(6):697–706
**Fraider CT:** Arthroscopic surgery of the knee: history and state of the art. **JAOA** 1981 Aug;80(12):817–22
**Fraikor AL:** Fiddling on a drifting roof: genetic implications of Jewish settlement patterns and life style. **Prog Clin Biol Res** 1982;95:535–47
**Francavilla A** see **Starzl TE**
**Frances A, Cooper AM:** Descriptive and dynamic psychiatry: a perspective on DSM-III. **Am J Psychiatry** 1981 Sep;138(9):1198–202
**Francés C:** Manuel Hernández de Gregorio: a Spanish pharmacist dedicated to science and the history of pharmacy. In: Vorträge des Internationalen Pharmaziehistorischen Kongresses Innsbruck 1977. Struttgart, Wissenschaftliche Verlagsgesellschaft, 1979. p. 181–6.
**Frances M del C:** Problemática sobre la botica de Villaluenga de la Sagra a fines del siglo XVIII. **Bol Soc Esp Hist Farm** 1980/81 Dec-Mar;31–32(124–5):283–5
**Frances MC:** Contrata suscrita entre José Terraza y el partido de Beteta en el siglo XIX. **Bol Soc Esp Hist Farm** 1981 Sep;32(127):207–16
**Frances MC:** Noticias de farmacéuticos que ejercieron en Buendía (Cuenca) en el siglo XVIII. **Bol Soc Esp Hist Farm** 1980 Mar-Jun;3(121–2):139–46
**Frances MC** see **Herrero P**
**Francès Causapè MC, Zubiri García MD:** Estudio de la 'revista popular de conocimientos utiles', años 1880–1885, desde el punto de vista sanitario. **Bol Soc Esp Hist Farm** 1983 Sep;135:69–83
**Frances Causape MC** see **Alvarez de Abajo M**
**Franche M:** Omagiu Profesorului Mihai Ciucă, la 100 ani de la naştere. Profesorul Mihai Ciucă şi spitalul clinic de boli contagioase 'izolarea' Iaşi. **Rev Med Chir Soc Med Nat Iasi** 1983 Oct-Dec;87(4):726–8
**Franchi J** see **La Salpêtrière**
**Franciosi RA:** Evolution of SIDS diagnosis. **Minn Med** 1983 Jul;66(7):411–3
**Francis H:** The reorganisation of the National Health Service in 1974. **Soc Soc Hist Med Bull (Lond)** 1981 Dec;29:9–20
**Francis H** see **The preservation of medical and public health records**
**Francis J:** International (World) Veterinary Congress. **Aust Vet J** 1983 Aug;60(8):249–50
**Francis TJ:** Non freezing cold injury: a historical review. **J R Nav Med Serv** 1984 Winter;70(3):134–9
**Francis WR, Gammill CG, Braucher CL:** The MAC concept: a historical perspective. **Med Mark Media** 1980 Sep;15(9):56–68
**Francke OC:** Svenska Tandläkare-Sällskapets samlingar. **Nord Medicinhist Arsb** 1980;Suppl 6:143–6
**Francke OC:** Tandbehandling för 100 år sedan och Mark Twain som patient. **Nord Medicinhist Arsb** 1984;:137–40
**Francke OC:** The dental turbine handpiece, a Swedish invention. **Bull Hist Dent** 1981 Oct;29(2):91–3
**Franco Grande A, Martinón JM, Pombo MV, et al:** Evolución histórica de la intubación tráqueal. A porpósito de Franz Kuhn en el aniversario de su muerte. **Rev Esp Anestesiol Reanim** 1979 May;26(3):243–54
**Franco Grande A, Ginesta Galán F, Martinón Sanchez JM:** Primeras tesis doctorales sobre anestesia en lengua castellana. **Rev Esp Anestesiol Reanim** 1980 Jul;27(4):357–61
**Francome C:** Abortion politics in the United States. **Polit Stud** 1980;28(4):613–21
**Frängsmyr T, ed:** Linnaeus. The man and his work. Berkeley, University of California Press, 1983. xii, 203 p. With contributions by S. Lindroth, G. Eriksson, G. Broberg.
**Frank A** see **Zimmermann G**
**Frank DH** see **Lee S**
**Frank JB:** Moses Maimonides: rabbi of medicine. **Yale J Biol Med** 1981 Jan-Feb;54(1):79–88
**Frank N:** From criminal to civil penalties in the history of health and safety laws. **Soc Probl** 1983;30(5):532–44
**Frank RG:** Harvey and the Oxford physiologists: scientific ideas and social interaction. Berkeley, University of California Press, 1980. xviii, 368 p.
**Frank RG:** The physician as virtuoso in seventeenth-century England. In Shapiro, Barbara and Frank, Robert G., Jr. ed: English scientific virtuosi in the 16th and 17th centuries. Los Angeles, William Andrews Clark Memorial Lib., U. of California, 1980. p. 57–114.
**Frank RG** see **Bylebyl JJ, ed**
**Frank RG** see **Mani N**
**Frank RG** see **Shapiro B**
**Frank SB:** International Society of Tropical Dermatology in perspective. **Int J Dermatol** 1981 Jan-Feb;20(1):69–71
**Frank T** see **Detre KC**
**Frank Netter:** The man, the artist, the surgeon. **Med Times** 1981;109(1):31–3
**Franke H:** Materialien zur Arzneimittelgesetzgebung der Yüan-Zeit. **Asiat Forsch** 1980;71:22–9
**Franke JL** see **Lester JP**
**Franke NH:** James Bell Heyl, Bermuda's pharmacist-photographer. **Pharm Hist** 1982;24(3):117–9
**Franke OC:** Wilhelm Conrad Roentgen and other X-ray pioneers. **Bull Hist Dent** 1983 Apr;31(1):11–7
**Frankel DA:** Human experimentation: codes of ethics. **Leg Med Q** 1977 Mar;1(1):7–14
**Franken FH:** Krankheit und Tod grosser Komponisten. Baden-Baden, New York, Witzstrock, 1979. 280 p.
**Franken FH:** Mozarts Todeskrankheit. **Fortschr Med** 1980 Mar 6;98(9):301–2
**Frankena WK** see **Temkin O**
**Frankenberg R:** Man, society and health: towards the definition of the role of sociology in the development of Zambian medicine. **Afr Soc Res** 1969;(8):573–87
**Frankenburg F:** The 1978 Ontario Mental Health Act in historical context. **RSTC** 1982;22(6 No 3):172–7
**Frankenburg FR:** The history of the confinement of the mentally ill in Ontario. **Psychiatr J Univ Ottawa** 1982 Dec;7(4):240–3
**Frankl J:** Adatok Kaposi Móricz professzor magyarságához. **Orv Hetil** 1982 Jan 10;123(2):110–1
**Frankl J, Bodosi M:** Csorba József emlékezete. **Orv Hetil** 1984 Aug 19;125(34):2087–9
**Frankl J:** Entz Béla professzor tudomanyos müködése. **Orvostort Kozl** 1979;86(24 no 4):107–11
**Frankl J:** Faber Tamás dr., Somogy els ó megyei orvosa. **Orv Hetil** 1983 Feb 20;124(8):466–7
**Frankl J:** Somogy megyei adatok az abszolutizmus orvostörténelméhez. **Orv Hetil** 1982 Aug 22;123(34):2117–20
**Frankl J:** 150 éves orvosi vélemény a dohányzásról. **Orv Hetil** 1980 Dec 14;121(50):3078–9
**Frankl J** see **Holubar K**
**Franklin EC** see **Gorevic PD**
**Franklin J, Sutherland J, del Regato JA:** Yellow fever research. **Science** 1984 Jun 8;224(4653):1043–4, 1128
**Franklin JH** see **Breul FR**
**Franklin WE:** Thomas Blackwood, frontier physician. **Mich Hist** 1970;54(4):216–30
**Franz ML von:** Alchemy: an introduction to the symbolism and the psychology. Toronto, Inner City Books, 1980. 280 p. (Studies in Jungian Psychology, 5).

**Franz MM, Chiba M:** Abortion, contraception, and motherhood in post-war Japan and the United States. **Int J Womens Stud** 1980;3(1):66-75

**Franzini C:** La evoluzione del concetto di stress in fisiologia. **Arch Sci Biol (Bologna)** 1978 Jan-Dec;62(1-4):131-7

**Frascani P:** Il medico nell'ottocento. **Studi Stor** 1982;23(3):617-37

**Frascani P:** Medicina e statistica nella formazione del sistema santiario italiano: l'inchiesta del 1885. **Quad Stor** 1980;15(3):942-65

**Fraser A:** King Charles II, 'The Father of His People'. In Passmore R, ed: Proceedings of the Royal College of Physicians of Edinburgh Tercentenary Congress, 1981. Edinburgh, Royal College of Physicians of Edinburgh, 1982. p. 23-43.

**Fraser A:** RCM supplement. The modest midwife. **Nurs Times** 1984 Jul 18-24;80(29):suppl 20-1

**Fraser I:** An historical perspective on mechanical aids in intestinal anastomosis. **Surg Gynecol Obstet** 1982 Oct;155(4):566-74

**Fraser I:** Sir William MacCormac and his times. **Ann R Coll Surg Engl** 1983 Sep;65(5):339-46

**Fraser I:** Steinach operation. **Br Med J [Clin Res]** 1984 Jan 21;288(6412):242

**Fraser ID, Condon RE:** Sutureless bowel anastomosis -- an historical perspective. **Wis Med J** 1980 May;79(5):16-8

**Fraser KJ:** Anglo-French contributions to the recognition of rheumatoid arthritis. **Ann Rheum Dis** 1982 Aug;41(4):335-43

**Fraser SM:** Dr William Johnston (1846-1900) of Leicester--an unknown Victorian general practitioner. **J R Coll Gen Pract** 1983 Jun;33(251):369-71

**Fraser SM:** Leicester and smallpox: the Leicester method **Med Hist** 1980 Jul;24(3):315-32

**Frassetto F:** Le cose son numeri. **Riv Biol** 1981 Autumn;74(3):402-8

**Fraudet JR:** La pression antéro-postérieure des lèvres sur l'arcade dentaire inférieure à l'époque néolithique. **Rev Stomatol Chir Maxillofac** 1984;85(5):438-40

**Fraundorf KC:** Organized dentistry and the pursuit of entry control. **J Health Polit Policy Law** 1984 Winter;8(4):759-81

**Frayer DW, Bradley LE:** A late woodland burial from Platte County, Missouri. **Plains Anthropol** 1979;24(83):21-27

**Frazzingaro S** see **Biondani P**

**Frederick W** see **Graner JL**

**Fredga A:** Varför lärdomshistoria? **Nord Medicinhist Arsb** 1980;Suppl 6:22-4

**Fredga A** see **Holmstedt B**

**Fredgant D:** Antique pharmacy bottles: sources and pricing. **Pharm Hist** 1984;26(1):46-9

**Fredrickson DS:** Biomedical research in the 1980s. **N Engl J Med** 1981 Feb 26;304(9):509-17

**Fredrickson JM:** Otoneurology. **Ann Otol Rhinol Laryngol [Suppl]** 1983 Jan-Feb;102:17-9

**Fredrickson JM** see **Mhoon EE**

**Fredy D** see **Huard P**

**Freeden M:** Eugenics and progressive thought: a study in ideological affinity. **Hist J (Gt Brit)** 1979;22(3):645-72

**Freedman BJ:** For debate ... Caucasian. **Br Med J [Clin Res]** 1984 Mar 3;288(6418):696-8

**Freedman DS** see **Freedman R**

**Freedman GS:** Radionuclide tomography. **Semin Nucl Med** 1979 Jul;9(3):201-2

**Freedman R, Freedman DS, Thornton AD:** Changes in fertility expectations and preferences between 1962 and 1977: their relation to final parity. **Demography** 1980 Nov;17(4):365-78

**Freedman R, Chang MC, Sun TH:** Household composition, extended kinship and reproduction in Taiwan: 1973-1980. **Popul Stud** 1982 Nov;36(3):395-411

**Freedman R** see **Spicker SF**

**Freeling P** see **Elliott A**

**Freeman D:** The evolutionary theories of Charles Darwin and Herbert Spencer. **Curr Anthropol** 1974;15(3):211-21

**Freeman E** see **The preservation of medical and public health records**

**Freeman EJ** see **Teigen PM, ed**

**Freeman FW, Law A:** Allan Ramsay's first published poem: the poem to the memory of Dr. Archibald Pitcairne. **Bibliotheck** 1979;9:153-60

**Freeman JT:** Aging: its history and literature. New York, Human Sciences Press, 1979. 161 p.

**Freeman JT:** Collecting books on old age. **Spec Collect** 1982;1(3-4):131-48

**Freeman JT:** Some notes on the history of the National Institute on Aging. **Gerontologist** 1980 Oct;20(5 pt 1):610-4

**Freeman L, Strean HS:** Freud and women. New York, Frederick Ungar, 1981. xiii, 238 p.

**Freeman R** see **Cho LJ**

**Freeman RB:** The works of Charles Darwin: an annotated bibliographical handlist. 2d. ed. Folkestone, England, Dawson, 1977. 235 p.

**Freeman RG:** History of the American Society of Dermatopathology. **Am J Dermatopathol** 1984 Feb;6(1):25-33

**Freeman RH** see **Davis JO**

**Freeman T:** Anna Freud--psychiatrist. **Int J Psychoanal** 1983;64 (Pt 4):441-4

**Freerksen E:** Die Atiologie der Tuberkulose--Der Weg dahin und die Folgen. **Prax Klin Pneumol** 1982 Mar;36(3):122-34

**Frei E:** Intramural therapeutic research at the National Cancer Institute, Department of Medicine: 1955-1965. **Cancer Treat Rep** 1984 Jan;68(1):21-30

**Freier EF** see **Rausch VL**

**Freilich AR:** Tzaraat--'biblical leprosy'. **J Am Acad Dermatol** 1982 Jan;6(1):131-4

**Freimanis I, Starr A:** The unnatural history of valvular heart disease: late results with silastic ball valve prostheses. **J Cardiovasc Surg (Torino)** 1984 May-Jun;25(3):191-8

**Freimuth HC:** Alexander O. Gettler (1883-1968). A reflection. **Am J Forensic Med Pathol** 1983 Dec;4(4):303-5

**Freire-Maia A:** Historical note: the extraordinary handless and footless families of Brazil--50 years of acheiropodia. **Am J Med Genet** 1981;9(1):31-41

**Freire-Maia DV:** Bócio endêmico: classificação e histórico. **AMB** 1981 Mar;27(3):111-2

**Freireich E:** Landmark perspective: Nitrogen mustard therapy. **JAMA** 1984 May 4;251(17):2262-3

**Freitas CA de:** A memória de Oswaldo Cruz. **Rev Bras Malariol Doencas Trop** 1978;30:129-33

**Freitas DG de:** La médecine sociale dans la plus grande et plus populeuse ville du Brésil: Sao Paulo. In: Congrès international d'histoire de la médecine, XXVe, Québec, 1976. Actes. Québec, 1977. p. 77-97.

**Frenay C:** Histoire d'un hôpital: Hôtel-Dieu de Villefranche-sur-Saône. Villefranche-en-Beaujolais, Du Cuvier, 1980. 238 p.

**French J:** Nurses in society: far from home. **Nurs Mirror** 1984 May 23;158(21):32

**French RK:** An origin for the bone text of the 'five-figure series'. **Sudhoffs Arch** 1984;68(2):143-56

**French RK, Lloyd GE:** Greek fragments of the lost books of Galen's Anatomical procedures. **Sudhoffs Arch** 1978;62(3):235-49

**Frenckell R von** see **Mormont C**

**Frenckner B:** Pionjär för pediatrisk forskning - omtyckt kliniker, mindre värderad föreläsare. **Lakartidningen** 1983 Nov 30;80(48):4664-5

**Frenk J, Hernández-Llamas H, Alvarez-Klein L:** Análisis histórico del internado rotatorio de pregrado en México. **Gac Med Mex** 1983 Feb;119(2):87-96

**Frenk J, Hernández-Llamas H, Alvarez-Klein L:** El mercado de trabajo médico. II. Evolución histórica en México. **Gac Med Mex** 1980 Jun;116(6):265-84

**Frenk S:** Historia reciente de la asistencia materno-infantil en México. **Salud Publica Mex** 1983 Sep-Oct;25(5):513-7

**Frenk S:** Non omnis moriar. A cuarenta años de distancia de las investigaciones clínicas sobre el hambre realizadas en 1942 en el gueto de Varsovia. **Gac Med Mex** 1982 Dec;118(12):509-13

**Frenk S:** Raquitismo, una enfermedad social. **Bol Med Hosp Infant Mex** 1984 Mar;41(3):129-39

**Frenk SF:** El raquitismo: un hito en la historia de la pediatria. **Bol Soc Mex Hist Filos Med** 1982 Dec;6(41):89-104

**Frenzen PD, Hogan DP:** The impact of class, education, and health care on infant mortality in a developing society: the case of rural Thailand. **Demography** 1982 Aug;19(3):391-408

**Fréor P:** Médecins, chirurgiens, épidémies. In: Congrès National des Sociétés Savantes, 97e, Nantes, 1972. Comptes Rendus. Paris, 1976. Section des Sciences, Tome 1. p. 433-44.

**Fréour P:** Du pneumo-thorax vu par Th. Laënnec. **Rev Fr Mal Respir** 1981;9(3):265-9

**Freour P** see **Histoire culturelle de la maladie**

**Freshwater MF:** Priorities in plastic surgery. **Plast Reconstr Surg** 1984 Jun;73(6):987-90

**Freud S, Bullitt WC:** Thomas Woodrow Wilson, twenty-eighth President of the United States: a psychological study. Boston, Houghton Mifflin; and Cambridge, Riverside, 1967. 307 p.

**Freudenberg N:** Alice Hamilton 1869-1970. **Women Health** 1976 Sep-Oct;1(5):1-2

**Freundt EA:** Derrick Graham ffarington Edward: a pioneer in mycoplasmology. **Rev Infect Dis** 1982 May-Jun;(4 Suppl):S3-7

**Freundt EA:** Mycoplasma hominis: historical outline and taxonomy. **Sex Transm Dis** 1983 Oct-Dec;10(4 Suppl):226-9

**Frey EF:** Early eighteenth-century French medicine: setting the stage for revolution. **Clio Med** 1982 May;17(1):1-13

**Frey EF:** Saints in medical history. **Clio Med** 1979 Jul;14(1):35-70

**Frey EF:** The earliest Egyptian medical texts. **Bookman** 1984 Nov-Dec;11(6):3-7

**Frey EF:** The herbal in the healing arts. In: Congrès international d'histoire de la médecine, XXVe, Québec, 1976. Actes. Québec, 1977. p. 659-79.

**Frey EF:** The influence of Rabelais on medicine and its reform. **Clio Med** 1980;15(1/2):25-33

**Frey EF:** The physician in nineteenth-century English and American literature. **Bookman** 1981 May-Jun;8(5):3-8

**Frey EF:** The regulations of patent medicines in the United States and France. **Bookman** 1983 Jan-Feb;10(1):3-6

**Frey EF:** Voltaire's relation to the discipline of medicine. **Bookman** 1982 May-Jun;9(5):3-7

**Frey-Rohn L:** Von Freud zu Jung. Eine vergleichende Studie zur Psychologie des Unbewussten. (2. überarbeitete Ausgabe) Zürich, Daimon Verlag, 1980?. 456 p.

**Freydank WF:** Zwei medizinische Texte aus Assur. **Schr Gesch Kult Alten Orients** 1977;5:255-8

**Freymann JG:** American health care system: its genesis and trajectory. new ed. Huntington, N. Y., Krieger, 1980. xxiii, 407 p.

**Freymann JG:** The origins of disease orientation in American medical education. **Prev Med** 1981 Nov;10(6):663-73

**Frick K:** Dr. Med. Johann Gottfried Kumpf (1781-1862) und die ägyptische Augenkrankheit in Kärnten. **Carinthia** 1966;156:670-712

**Frick K:** Michael Ferdinand Wittmann (1755-1826) Magister und Doktor

der Chirurgie, der erste graduierte Chirurg in Kärnten. **Carinthia** 1968;158:643–62
**Fricke A:** Die thematische Entwicklung unserer Zeitschrift; Rückblick--Gegenwart--Ausblick. **Krankenpflege (Frankfurt)** 1981 Jan;35(1):11–5
**Fried Y** see **Peters UH, ed**
**Frieda Fromm-Reichmann:** A seminar in the history of psychiatry. **Psychiatry** 1982 May;45(2):89–136
**Frieda Fromm-Reichmann discusses the 'Rose garden' case: Psychiatry** 1982 May;45(2):128–36
**Friedberg SA:** The memorable life of Hosmer A. Johnson, early midwestern laryngologist. **Ann Otol Rhinol Laryngol** 1983 Sep–Oct;92(5 Pt 1):470–2
**Friedberger M:** The decision to institutionalize: families with exceptional children in 1900. **J Fam Hist** 1981 Winter;6(4):396–409
**Friedell JN:** Blanche Ames Ames. In: Notable American women. The modern period. Cambridge, Mass., Belknap-Harvard Univ. Press, 1980. 4:15–6.
**Friedemann H:** Zur Entwicklung der disziplinären Verantwortlichkeit für die Organisation des Gesundheitswesens in einigen internationalen Gesundheitssystemen. **Z Gesamte Hyg** 1980 Apr;26(4):283–90
**Frieden NM:** Child care: medical reform in a traditionalist culture. In Ransel DL, ed: The family in Imperial Russia: new lines of historical research. Urbana, University of Illinois Press, 1978. p. 236–59.
**Frieden NM:** Russian physicians in an era of reform and revolution, 1856-1905. Princeton, Princeton University Press, 1981. xvii, 378 p.
**Frieden NM:** The roots of Russian zemstvo medicine. In: Congrès international d'histoire de la médecine, XXVe, Québec, 1976. Actes. Québec, 1977. p. 99–120.
**Friedländer S:** History and psychoanalysis. An inquiry into the possibilities and limits of psychohistory. New York and London, Holmes & Meier, 1978. 175 p. (Translation of French edition, 1975)
**Friedländer S:** L'extermination des Juifs d'Europe: pour une etude historique globale. **Rev Etud Juives** 1976;135(1–3):113–44
**Friedman A:** Nursing revisited: oral history in nursing, Mary A. Maher. **Mass Nurse** 1984 May;53(5):7, 28
**Friedman AP:** Houston Merritt. In Rose FC, Bynum WF, ed: Historical aspects of the neurosciences. New York, Raven, 1982. p. 379–82.
**Friedman BL:** Productivity gains in the drugstore industry, 1958–79. **Mon Labor Rev** 1980;103(11):18–22
**Friedman EA, Lundin AP:** Dialysate delivery: historical, theoretical, and practical aspect. **Kidney Int [Suppl]** 1980 Sep;Suppl 10:S33–43
**Friedman EG:** Trinitarian hospitals in Algiers: an early example of health care for prisoners of war. **Cathol Hist Rev** 1980;66(4):551–64
**Friedman GC:** The heights of slaves in Trinidad. **Soc Sci Hist** 1982;6(4):482–515
**Friedman JB:** The monstrous races in medieval art and thought. Cambridge, London, Harvard University Press, 1981. xiii, 268 p.
**Friedman L** see **Goldberg A, ed**
**Friedman L** see **Ross JM**
**Friedman LI** see **Rechsteiner J**
**Friedman LJ, Shaffer AH:** History, politics, and health in early American thought: the case of David Ramsay. **J Am Stud** 1979;13(1):37–56
**Friedman M** see **Sharkey PW, ed**
**Friedman SS** see **DuPlessis RB**
**Friedrich C, Seidlein HJ:** Beiträge zur Geschichte der Pharmazeutischen Wissenschaft. **Pharmazie** 1984 May;39(5):340–5
**Friedrich C, Seidlein HJ:** Beiträge zur Geschichte der Pharmazeutischen Wissenschaft. 11. Mitteilung: Die Bedeutung Johannes (Hans) Valentin für die Entwicklung der Pharmazeutischen Wissenschaft. **Pharmazie** 1984 Apr;39(4):262–9
**Friedrich C, Langer H, Seidlein HJ:** Beiträge zur Geschichte der Pharmazeutischen Wissenschaft 3. Mitteilung: Christian Ehrenfried von Weigel -- Seine Bedeutung für die Entwicklung der Pharmazeutischen Wissenschaft. Teil 1: Herkunft und Entwicklung. **Pharmazie** 1982 Apr;37(4):290–3
**Friedrich C, Langer H, Seidlein HJ:** Beiträge zur Geschichte der Pharmazeutischen Wissenschaft. 4. Mitteilung: Christian Ehrenfried von Weigel--Seine Bedeutung für die Entwicklung der Pharmazeutischen Wissenschaft. Teil 2: Christian Ehrenfried von Weigel als Hochschullehrer. **Pharmazie** 1982 Jun;37(6):446–50
**Friedrich C, Langer H, Seidlein HJ:** Beiträge zur Geschichte der Pharmazeutischen Wissenschaft. 5. Mitteilung: Christian Ehrenfried von Weigel--Seine Bedeutung für die Entwicklung der pharmazeutischen Wissenschaft. **Pharmazie** 1982 Jul;37(7):514–7
**Friedrich C, Seidlein HJ:** Otto Anselmino--Seine Bedeutung für die Entwicklung der Pharmazeutischen Wissenschaft, insbesondere an der Universität Greifswald. **Pharmazie** 1981 Dec;36(12):846–52
**Friedrich I:** 18. századi magyar nyelvu orvosi könyvek az 'ügyefogyott szegények' szolgálatában. **Magy Konyvsz** 1978;94(2):158–67
**Friedsam HJ:** The coming on of years: social science perspectives on aging and death. **Soc Sci Q** 1970;51(1):120–8
**Friel PB:** Death and dying. **Ann Intern Med** 1982 Nov;97(5):767–71
**Frielinghaus E:** Initiativen des Veterinär-Inspekteurs der deutschen Wehrmacht auf dem Gebiet der Pferdezucht im Kriege 1939–45. **DTW** 1981 Nov 5;88(11):457–61
**Fries SD:** The ideology of science during the Nixon years: 1970–76. **Soc Stud Sci** 1984 Aug;14(3):323–41
**Friesen JD:** The emergence of the new genetics. In J. G. Little, ed: Prospects for man: genetic engineering. Toronto, Centre for Research on Environmental Quality, Faculty of Science, York University, 1979. p. 1–23.
**Frijhoff W** see **Arts en sameleving. Medical history contributions by H. W. Pleket, J. Van Herwaarden, W. Frijhoff, C. Offringa, M. J. Van Lieburg, C. Bakker-Van der Kooij**
**Frijhoff W** see **Forster R**
**Frileck SP:** More on Robert Abbe's contributions to the field of plastic surgery. **Ann Plast Surg** 1979 Oct;3(4):357–60
**Frisbie CJ:** Burial as a disposition mechanism for Navajo jish or medicine bundles. **Am Indian Q** 1978;4(4):347–66
**Frisch H:** Die Entwicklung der Neonatologie in Tirol von 1968 bis 1978 und deren Einfluss auf die Morbidität und Mortalität von Früh- und Neugeborenen. **Wien Klin Wochenschr** 1980;92(116):1–58
**Frisch RE** see **Dupâquier J**
**Frischauer W:** The clinic. London, Frewin, 1976. 200 p.
**Fritsche C:** Wandlungen in Struktur und Funktion der Psychotherapie ab 1933. **Z Gesamte Hyg** 1984 Feb;30(2):115–7
**Fritsche H:** Samuel Hahnemann: Idee und Wirklichkeit der Homöopathie. Göttingen, Verlag für homöopathische Literatur, 1982. 366 p.
**Fritts HW:** Are we Socratic teachers? **Trans Am Clin Climatol Assoc** 1979;90:109–15
**Fritz G:** Analysis of human skeletal remains from the Montgomery farm, Barry County, Missouri. **Arkansas Archeol** 1979;20:69–78
**Fritzsche K:** Erfahrungen bei der Tätigkeit in zwei 'Beweglichen Veterinär-Untersuchungsstellen' an der Ost- und Westfront während des letzten Weltkrieges. **DTW** 1982 Feb 5;89(2):65–70
**Froböse HH:** Beiträge des Apothekers zur Therapieoptimierung--ein Rückblick. **Pharmazie** 1983 Sep;38(9):618–20
**Froböse HH:** Die Tagung des preussischen Apothekerrates im Jahre 1897--ein Beitrag zur Frage der Zulassung der Frauen zur Pharmazie. **Pharmazie** 1982 Aug;37(8):596–9
**Froch W** see **Kobylińska-Szymańska M**
**Froggatt P:** The resignation of Robert Little from the chair of midwifery at Inst [Academical Institution, Belfast] **Ulster Med J** 1979;48(1):19–31
**Frohn Villeneuve W** see **Grmek MD, ed**
**Frolov IT, Pastushnyi SA:** Dialektika istoricheskoi formny i soderzhaniia otkrytiia G. Mendelia. **Vopr Istor Estestvozn Tekh** 1981;(4):20–8
**Frolov VA:** K razvitiiu nauki v SSSR. **Med Sestra** 1982 Dec;41(12):7–9
**Frolov VA:** K 40-letiiu sozdaniia Akademii meditsinskikh nauk USSR. **Patol Fiziol Eksp Ter** 1984 Jul–Aug;(4):3–9
**Frolova OG** see **Muchiev GS**
**Frolova VV** see **Elkin II**
**From Gazette to Review: 1904–1979: Hosp Health Serv Rev** 1980 Jan;76(1):19–22
**Fröml F:** Pod dohledem městského fyzika. **Cas Lek Cesk** 1982 Jan 15;121(2):58–60
**Fröml F:** Poslední léta městských chirurgu v Prostějově. **Cas Lek Cesk** 1981;120(51):1573–4
**Fröml F:** První skolní lékař na Moravě. **Cas Lek Cesk** 1982 Jun 11;121(23):724–5
**Fröml F:** Venkovský lékař a ranhojič na konci 19. století. **Cas Lek Cesk** 1979 May 25;118(21):662–4
**Fromm H:** Virginia Woolf: art and sexuality. **Va Q Rev** 1979;55(3):441–59
**Frommknecht M:** Frieda Fromm-Reichmann. In J. Rattner, ed: Wandlungen der Psychoanalyse. Wien, Europaverlag, 1980. p. 115–39.
**Fronsini R** see **Ronchi L**
**Frontali L** see **Baldacci G**
**Froriep R:** Aspects of tongue (1828). Original Latin text edited and translated by C. Garton, J. D. Gerencser, A. J. Drinnan. Buffalo, Dept. of Classics, State University of N. Y., 1982. xix, 109, 108a p. (Arethusa Monographs IX).
**Frost SB:** Alexander Skakel, LL.D.: a founder, M.G.H. governor, and a many sided man. **Montreal Gen Hosp News** 1980;18(2):3–5
**Frost SB:** Science education in the 19th century: The Natural History Society of Montreal, 1827-1925. **McGill J Educ** 1982;17(1):31–48
**Fruchtbaum H:** [History of] public health. In Reich WT, et al, ed: Encyclopedia of bioethics, v.3. New York, Free Press, 1978. p. 1392–99.
**Fruton JS:** A bio-bibliography for the history of the biochemical sciences since 1800. Philadelphia, American Philosophical Society, 1982. xiii, 885 p.
**Fruton JS:** Biochemistry and clinical chemistry--a retrospect. **J Clin Chem Clin Biochem** 1982 Apr;20(4):243–52
**Fruton JS:** Marcel Florkin, 1900–1979, historian of biochemistry. **Hist Philos Life Sci** 1980;2(1):167–71
**Fruton JS** see **Büttner J, ed**
**Fruton JS** see **Robin ED, ed**
**Fry G** see **El-Najjar MY**
**Fry J, Hunt JH, Pisent RJ, ed:** A history of the Royal College of General Practitioners. The first 25 years. Lancaster, Boston, MTP Press, 1983. xiii, 270 p.
**Fry J:** First David Bruce lecture in the David Bruce tradition. The evolution of general practice in the British Army. **J R Army Med Corps** 1982 Oct;128(3):152–9
**Fry J, Hunt JH, Pinsent RJ:** The Royal College of General Practitioners: the first 25 years.
**Fryer JG, et al:** Comparing the early mortality rates of the local authorities of England and Wales. **J R Stat Soc** 1979;142(2)
**Fuchs C** see **Struck HG**
**Fuchs M:** Dr. Matthew O'Connor: the unhealthy healer of Djuna Barnes's Nightwood. In Jones AH, ed: Images of healers. Albany, State University of New York Press, 1983. p. 125–34.
**Fuchsová V** see **Rozsívalová E**
**Fuente JR de la, Alarcón-Segovia D:** Depression as expressed in

pre-Columbian Mexican art. **Am J Psychiatry** 1980 Sep;137(9):1095-8
**Fuente Souviron E** see **Alegre Perez ME**
**Fuerst JA:** The definition of molecular biology and the definition of policy: the role of the Rockefeller Foundation's policy for molecular biology. **Soc Stud Sci** 1984 May;14(2):225-37
**Fuhrmeister H:** Hallesche Duplikate der Majolikareliefs vom Berliner Albrecht-von-Graefe-Denkmal. **Klin Monatsbl Augenheilkd** 1980 May;176(5):867-9
**Fujimori K, Chikamori K, Matsubara H, et al:** Human bones from three burial mounds in Tokushima. **Tokushima J Exp Med** 1979 Dec;26(3-4):73-9
**Fujimori K** see **Yamada M**
**Fujita S:** Die Bedeutung Robert Kochs für die japanische Medizin--Tuberkuloseforschung in Japan. **Prax Klin Pneumol** 1982 Mar;36(3):111-5
**Fujita S:** Robert Kochs Bedeutung für die japanische Medizin--Tuberkuloseforschung in Japan. **Prax Klin Pneumol** 1983 Oct;37 Suppl 1:423-9
**Fukase Y:** [Tezuka Ryosen, army doctor-in-chief of the infantry regiment.] (Jpn). **Nihon I-Shigaku Zasshi** 1981;27(1):21-34
**Fukuyama K, Yasuda T:** Outstanding contributions by Japanese dermatologists. **J Am Acad Dermatol** 1982 Feb;6(2):173-8
**Fukuyama Y:** A quarter-century of the Japanese Society of Child Neurology. **Brain Dev** 1984;6(2):109-18
**Fukuyama Y:** [Progress of the Japanese Society of Pediatric Neurology in the past quarter of a century] (Jpn). **No To Hattatsu** 1984;16(3):179-88
**Fullard J:** Ann Preston: pioneer of medical education and women's rights. **Pa Herit** 1982;8(1):9-14
**Fuller MB:** Alexander Hollaender Papers (1898- ). **Mendel Newsl** 1984;(24):5-7
**Fuller MB:** Theodosius Dobzhansky Papers. **Mendel Newsl** 1980 Jun;(18):1-8
**Fuller MB:** Thomas Hunt Morgan papers at the American Philosophical Society. **Mendel Newsl** 1981 Nov;21:6-8
**Fuller RC:** Mesmerism and the American cure of souls. Philadelphia, University of Pennsylvania Press, 1982. xvi, 227 p.
**Fuller WC** see **Bean DW**
**Fullinwider SP:** Sigmund Freud, John Hughlings Jackson, and speech. **J Hist Ideas** 1983 Jan-Mar;44(1):151-8
**Fullinwider SP:** Technicians of the finite. The rise and decline of the schizophrenic in American thought 1840-1960. Westport, Conn., Greenwood, 1982. ix, 253 p. (Contributions in Medical History, 9).
**Fullmer JZ** see **Forgan S, ed**
**Fulton JF:** History of medicine-Arnold Klebs and Harvey Cushing at the 1st International Neurological Congress at Berne in 1931. **Int J Neurol** 1980;14(1):103-15
**Fulton MW:** Hartley D. Price: his contributions to physical education and gymnastics. Ph.D. Diss., Florida State University. Tallahassee, 1981. xvii, 171 leaves.
**Fulton T:** Through the artist's eyes. **Ulster Med J** 1982;51(1):1-22
**Funder W:** Uber eine bisher unbekannte ophthalmologische Monographie von Jakob Rüff (um 1500-1558). **Klin Monatsbl Augenheilkd** 1981 Oct;179(4):297-8
**Funk TG:** Uterine Fibromyome und Blutungen als Indikation für eine bilaterale Oophorektomie im späten 19. Jahrhundert. Diss. Erlangen-Nürnberg,1984. 158 p.
**Fürderer C:** Medizin- und geistesgeschichtliche Vorläufer klinisch-psychiatrischer Biographik in der Epoche der Aufklärung und Romantik. Diss. Bonn, 1981. 151 p.
**Füredi J, Buda B:** A pszichiátria önállósodásának problémája Magyarországon. **Orv Hetil** 1980 May 11;121(19):1115-20
**Furkalo NK:** Osnovnye étapy razvitiia kardiologii. **Vrach Delo** 1980 Aug;(8):5-9
**Furmaga S:** 30 lat Polskiego Towarzystwa parazytologicznego. **Wiad Parazytol** 1980;26(4-5):293-8
**Furmanchuk VM:** Podvigi meditsinskikh sester v pervyĭ period Velikoĭ Otechestvennoĭ voĭny. **Med Sestra** 1980 Oct;37(10):60-2
**Furmanchuk VM:** Uchastie rabochikh sester i sanitarok v Oktiabr'skoĭ revoliutsii. **Med Sestra** 1982 Apr;41(4):49-51
**Furnadzhiev G:** Razvitie i segashno sŭstoianie na Katedrata p farmakologiia i fitoterapiia. **Vutr Boles** 1981;20(6):22-6
**Furness DA:** Asthma -- a note on its history. **Hist Med (Lond)** 1980 Jan-Feb;8(1):26
**Fürst L:** O Březnické lékárně a lékárnících. **Cesk Farm** 1979 Mar;28(2):82-7
**Furukawa A:** [The rod of Asklepios and Hygieia's cup--medico-dental and pharmacological symbols] (Jpn). **Shikai Tenbo** 1981 Nov;58(5):977-86
**Furukawa F, Bourgeois M:** Délires de possession par le renard au Japon (ou délire de Kitsune-Tsuki). **Ann Med Psychol (Paris)** 1984 May;142(5):677-87
**Furukawa T:** [Development of neurophysiology in Japan brought by introduction of microelectrodes] (Jpn). **Nippon Seirigaku Zasshi** 1984;46(1):5-7
**Fusayama T:** [Progress in operative dentistry in the past 30 years] (Jpn). **Shikai Tenbo** 1982 Jun;59(7):1375-85
**Fuse S:** Ishi no rekishi: sono Nihonteki tokucho. Tokyo, Chuo Koronsha, 1979. ii, 213 p.
**Fusé T:** Modernization and suicide in Japan: a comparative approach. **Cult Dev** 1980;12(1):45-80
**Fusswerk-Fursay J:** A propos d'un inédit de Pierre Janet sur les croyances. **Ann Med Psychol (Paris)** 1984 May;142(5):703-10
**Fuster P:** Análisis bibliográfico de las psicosis infantiles. **Asclepio** 1980;32:171-94
**Füves O:** Orvosi vonatkozású feljegyzések egy kecskeméti görög naplójában. **Orvostort Kozl** 1979;87-88(25 no 1-2):301-2
**Fuwa K:** Metallothionein: historical aspects of trace spectrochemical. **Dev Toxicol Environ Sci** 1982;9:1-10
**Fye WB:** Acute coronary occlusion always results in death--or does it? The observations of William T. Porter. **Circulation** 1985 Jan;71(1):4-10
**Fye WB:** Coronary arteriography--it took a long time! **Circulation** 1984 Nov;70(5):781-7
**Fye WB:** Ernest Henry Starling, his law and its growing significance in the practice of medicine. **Circulation** 1983 Nov;68(5):1145-8
**Fye WB:** Heparin: the contributions of William Henry Howell. **Circulation** 1984 Jun;69(6):1198-203
**Fye WB:** Librarians in the history of the health sciences: challenges and opportunities in the 80's. **Watermark** 1983 Apr;6(4):14-8
**Fye WB:** S. Weir Mitchell, Philadelphia's 'lost' physiologist. **Bull Hist Med** 1983 Summer;57(2):188-202
**Fye WB:** Sydney Ringer, calcium, and cardiac function. **Circulation** 1984 Apr;69(4):849-53
**Fye WB:** Why a physiologist?--the case of Henry P. Bowditch. **Bull Hist Med** 1982 Spring;56(1):19-29
**Fyler DC:** The history of treatment of patent ductus arteriosus. In B. L. Tucker, G. G. Lindesmith, ed: First clinical conference on congenital heart disease. New York, Grune & Stratton, 1979. p. 3-11.
**Fyrand O:** The history of Norwegian dermato-venereology during the last two centuries. **Int J Dermatol** 1983 Dec;22(10):593-7
**Fysikatsdistrikter i det sønderjyske område indtil 1864: Dan Medicinhist Arbog** 1980;:66-78

## G

**Gabaeva NS** see **Tokin BP**
**Gabaldon A:** Malaria eradication in Venezuela: doctrine, practice, and achievements after twenty years. **Am J Trop Med Hyg** 1983 Mar;32(2):203-11
**Gabbay J:** Asthma attacked? Tactics for the reconstruction of a disease concept. In P. Wright, A. Treacher, ed: The problem of medical knowledge. Examining the social construction of medicine. Edinburgh, Edinburgh University Press, 1982. p. 23-48.
**Gabellon S** see **Rich NM**
**Gaberthüel M:** Krankengeschichten und Operationsberichte 1784-1811 nach den Aufzeichnungen von Johann Heinrich Steger (1767-1842) und Johann Jakob Steger (1798-1857). Zürich, Juris, 1980. 121 p. (Zürcher Medizingeschichtliche Abhandlungen, Neue Reihe, 140).
**Gabler K:** Das Krankenhauswesen der Stadt Krefeld im 19. Jahrhundert. Herzogenrath, Murken-Altrogge, 1983. 405 p. (Studien zur Geschichte des Krankenhauswesens, Band 19)
**Gabovich RD** see **Borisenko NF**
**Gabovich RD** see **Maĭstruk PN**
**Gabriel A:** Sir Arthur Conan Doyle: to see and to be seen. **Bull Menninger Clin** 1982 Nov;46(6):530-8
**Gach J** see **Wallace ER**
**Gachnochi G:** La violence de l'antisémitisme. **Ann Med Psychol (Paris)** 1979 Oct;137(8):807-16
**Gadacz-Grünefeld G:** Die Medizinalentwicklung im Kreise Aurich im 19. und 20. Jahrhundert. Münster, Murken-Altrogge, 1979. 282 p. (Studien zur Geschichte des Krankenhauswesens, 9).
**Gadamer HG** see **Kraus A, ed**
**Gade DW:** Inca and colonial settlement, coca cultivation and endemic disease in the tropical forest. **J Hist Geogr** 1979 Jul;5:263-80
**Gädeke R:** Ein medizingeschichtliches Panorama der akuten Eisenvergiftung. **Klin Paediatr** 1979 Sep;191(5):442-6
**Gadeyne G:** De plaatselijke commissies van geneeskundkig toevoorzicht in Oost-Vlaanderen (1818-1830). **Handel Maatsch Geschied Oudheidk Gent** 1979;33:175-220
**Gadeyne G:** Oostvlaamse medici en parochiepriesters, slachtoffers van de tyfusepidemie, 1847-48: een episode uit de sociale geschiedenis. **Handel Maatsch Geschied Oudheidk Gent** 1980;34:167-79
**Gadomska H:** Ocena częstości wyst ępowania osteosarcoma na tle innych postaci nowotdworów złośliwych kości, Warszawa 1963-1974. **Nowotwory** 1979;Suppl:13-21
**Gadomska H** see **Olakowski T**
**Gadow S** see **Spicker SF**
**Gaebel RE:** Saturnine gout among Roman aristocrats. **N Engl J Med** 1983 Aug 18;309(7):431
**Gaertner H:** Adam Marian Langie. **Klin Oczna** 1982 Apr;84(4):131-4
**Gaertner H:** Kazimierz Karelus, Stefan Pasierbiński, Ignacy Chrzanowski i Czesław Klinowski--ordynatorzy i konsulenci okulistyki krakowskiego szpitala Braci Miłosiernych (obecnie im. E. Biernackiego). **Klin Oczna** 1983 Mar;85(3):129-32
**Gaertner H:** Ordynatorzy oddziału chirurgicznego Krakowskiego Szpitala Braci Miłosiernych (obecnie im. Edmunda Biernackiego). **Nasza Przeslosc** 1979;(51):179-204
**Gaffney R:** Poor law hospitals 1845-1914. In Checkland O, Lamb M, ed: Health care as social history; the Glasgow case. Aberdeen, Aberdeen University Press, 1982. p. 44-58.
**Gaffney R:** Women as doctors and nurses. In Checkland O, Lamb M, ed: Health care as social history; the Glasgow case. Aberdeen, Aberdeen University Press, 1982. p. 134-48.
**Gagliano JA:** La medicina popular y la coca en el Perú: un análisis histórico de actitudes. **Am Indig** 1978;38(4):789-805

**Gagliasso E** see **Continenza B**
**Gagnière S, Julien P:** Panneaux peints de la pharmacie de l'hôpital de Valréas. **Rev Hist Pharm (Paris)** 1981;28(248):21–4
**Gago R, Olagüe G, Carrillo JL:** Aportación al estudio del movimiento novator en España: el Laboratorio Químico del Palacio Real (1694) y la obra del boticario aragonés Juan del Bayle (fl. 1698). **Bol Soc Esp Hist Farm** 1981 Jun;32(126):95–107
**Gago R, Olagüe G, Carrillo JL, et al:** El plan de estudios del rector Blasco (1786) y la renovacion de las disciplinas cientificas en la Universidad de Valencia: la quimica y la enseñanza clinica. **Estudis** 1977;6:157–65
**Gago R, Carrillo JL:** La obra fisiológica de Ignacio María Ruiz de Luzuriaga (1763–1822) y su plagio del cientifico británico Adair Crawford (1748–1795). **Dynamis** 1981;1:87–100
**Gago R** see **Carrillo JL**
**Gago Bohórquez R** see **Fernández González M**
**Gai L:** Interventi rinascimentali nello spedale del Ceppo di Pistoia. Ridefinizione nell'attività pistoiese di Michelozzo architetto. **Boll Stor Pistoiese** 1977;12(1–2):72–155
**Gaïev A:** Suicides d'écrivains sovietiques. **Contrat Soc** 1968;12(4):237–41
**Gaignault JC:** Alfred Houdé. Un bel exemple de fondateur d'une industrie pharmaceutique française au XIXe siècle. **Bull Ordre Natl Pharm** 1980 Dec;239:1816–26
**Gaillard J:** Le médecin et l'avortement au XIXe siècle. **Histoire** 1979;16:35–7
**Gaillard J** see **Patrimoine hospitalier de la Bourgogne**
**Gaĭsinovich AE:** K. F. Vol'f i ego rol' v istorii embriologii i anatomii (k 250-letiiu so dnia rozhdeniia). **Arkh Anat Gistol Embriol** 1984 Aug;87(8):90–6
**Gaissinovitch AE:** The origins of Soviet genetics and the struggle with Lamarckism, 1922–1929. **J Hist Biol** 1980 Spring, 13(1):1–51
**Gaitonde PD:** Portuguese pioneers in India: spotlight on medicine. Bombay, Popular Prakashan, 1983. xv, 188 p.
**Gajda Z:** Niektórzy historycy wobec historii medycyny kilka refleksji sceptycznych. **Arch Hist Med (Warsz)** 1984;47(1):1–10
**Gajdusek DC:** Journal of further explorations in the Kuru region and in the Kukukuku country, eastern highlands of eastern New Guinea and of a return to West New Guinea, December 25, 1963 to May 4, 1964. Bethesda, National Institutes of Health, 1980. [36 leaves], 235 p.
**Gajdusek DC, ed** see **Farquhar J**
**Gajeerski SF:** Szpitale Zydowskie na Rusi czerwonej w XVI–XVIII w. **Biul Zydowskiego Inst Hist Pol** 1979;(4):25–33
**Galaburda AM:** La région de Broca: observations anatomiques faites un siècle après la mort de son découvreur. **Rev Neurol (Paris)** 1980;136(10):609–16
**Galaĭ IuG:** Novye dokumenty o vrache-pisatele S. Ia. Elpat'evskom. **Sov Zdravookhr** 1983;(9):59–62
**Galakhov EV** see **Orlov DA**
**Galan V:** 'Seneca oil'. **Rev Ig [Pneumoftiziol]** 1980 Apr–Jun;29(2):127–8
**Galand A:** Historique de la chirurgie transsclérale. **J Fr Ophtalmol** 1980 Dec;3(12):763–4
**Galand R** see **Stambolian G**
**Galanos AN** see **Pappas DG**
**Galanter M** see **Buckley P**
**Galati D:** Lacan: un ritorno a Freud? **Stor Crit Psicol** 1980;1(1):79–91
**Galaziĭ GI:** Istoriia botanicheskikh issledovaniĭ na Baĭkale: itogi i perspektivy ekologo-botanicheskikh rabot. Novosibirsk, Nauka, Sibirskoe otd-nie, 1982. 152 p.
**Galdston I:** Social and historical foundations of modern medicine. New York, Brunner/Mazel, 1981. xiv, 147 p. (Reprinted articles from various sources)
**Gale EF:** Donald Devereux Woods. In Dictionary of national biography, 1961–1970. Suppl. 8, 1981. p. 1102–3.
**Gale GL:** The changing years. The story of Toronto Hospital and the fight against tuberculosis. Toronto, West Park Hospital, 1979. xvii, 134 p.
**Gale GL:** Tuberculosis in Canada: a century of progress. **Can Med Assoc J** 1982 Mar 1;126(5):526–9
**Gale TS:** Segregation in British West Africa. **Cah Etud Afr** 1980;20(4):495–507
**Galen:** On the doctrines of Hippocrates and Plato. Edition, translation and commentary by P De Lacy. Second Part: Books VI–IX. Berlin, Akademie Verlag, 1980. p. 361–609. (Corpus Medicorum Graecorum, V, 4, 1, 2).
**Galérant G:** Deux toulousains et un rouennais contre Pasteur au sujet de la génération spontanée. In: Congrès National des Sociétés Savantes, 96e, Toulouse, 1971. Comptes Rendus. Paris, 1974. Histoire des Sciences, Tome 1. p. 193–200.
**Galginaitis C:** An analysis of dental practice from 1952 to 1976. Council on Dental Practice and Bureau of Economic and Behavioral Research. **J Am Dent Assoc** 1980 Jan;100(1):89–96
**Galiev VZ:** Meditsinskaia deiatel'nost' ssyl'nykh revoliutsionerov v Kazakhstane (vtoraia polovina XIX veka). Alma-Ata, Kazakhstan, 1982. 158 p.
**Galin LL:** Deiatel'nost' voenno-sanitarnoĭ sluzhby v gody Velikoĭ Otechestvennoĭ voĭny (po materialam 'Voenno-meditsinskogo zhurnala'). **Sov Zdravookhr** 1984;(5):58–61
**Galin LL:** Gotov k trudu i oborone SSSR (k 50-letiiu vvedeniia Vsesouiznogo fizkul'turnogo kompleksa). **Voen Med Zh** 1981 Jun;(6):75–6
**Galin LL:** Publikatsii N. I. Pirogova na stranitsakh 'Voenno--meditsinskogo zhurnala. **Voen Med Zh** 1980 Nov;(11):69–71
**Galin LL:** Shina Diterikhsa. **Feldsher Akush** 1983 Nov;48(11):46–8
**Galin LL:** Vklad P. P. Potiralovskogo v razvitie organizatsionnykh voprosov voennoĭ meditsiny. **Voen Med Zh** 1982 Apr;(4):68–70
**Galin LL, Pal'chikov PA:** Vklad 'Voenno-Meditsinskogo Zhurnala' v razvitie voennoĭ meditsiny. **Sov Zdravookhr** 1983;(2):63–7
**Galin LL** see **Belozerov VV**
**Galin LL** see **Gladkikh PF**
**Galiński J, Hebanowski M, Lipińska-Namysł E:** Serotypy uropatogenne Escherichia coli w materiałach z klinik i przychodni gdańskich w latach 1973–1976. **Przegl Epidemiol** 1980;34(2):155–61
**Galishoff S:** Germs know no color line: black health and public policy in Atlanta, 1900–1918. **J Hist Med Allied Sci** 1985 Jan;40(1):22–41
**Galishoff S:** The Passaic Valley trunk sewer. **NJ Hist** 1970;88(4):197–214
**Galishoff S** see **Melosi MV, ed**
**Galkina ND** see **Alekseev GA**
**Gall D** see **Crompton R**
**Gall YM:** [I. I. Schmalhausen and the problem of the causes of evolution] (Rus). **Istor Biol Issled** 1980;8:106–23
**Gallagher HG:** FDR: handicapped American. **Public Welf** 1984 Spring;42(2):6–18
**Gallagher JR:** The origins, development, and goals of adolescent medicine. **J Adolesc Health Care** 1982 Aug;3(1):57–63
**Gallagher N:** Late contributions to Arabic medicine: a treatise on cholera. In: International Symposium for the History of Arabic Science, 1st, University of Aleppo, 1976. Proceedings. Aleppo, Syria, 1976. Papers in European Languages, Vol. II. p. 300–3.
**Gallagher NE:** Arabic medical manuscripts at the University of California, Los Angeles. Malibu, Undena Publications, 1983. xix, 24 p. (Aids and Research Tools in Middle East Studies, v. 1).
**Gallagher NE:** Medicine and power in Tunisia, 1780–1900. Cambridge; New York, Cambridge University Press, 1983. xii, 145 p.
**Galle P:** Fortschritte in der operativen Behandlung hüftgelenksnaher Frakturen seit W. Denk. **Wien Klin Wochenschr** 1982 Apr 2;94(7):185–9
**Galle P** see **Spängler H**
**Gallegos AJ:** The zoapatle I—a traditional remedy from Mexico emerges to modern times. **Contraception** 1983 Mar;27(3):211–25
**Gallent M:** Control social de la ciencia medica en Valencia durante el S. XV. **Llull (Spain)** 1978;2:95–105
**Gallistel CR:** Bell, Magendie, and the proposals to restrict the use of animals in neurobehavioral research. **Am Psychol** 1981 Apr;36(4):357–60
**Gallman JM:** Determinants of age at marriage in colonial Perquimans County, North Carolina. **William Mary Q** 1982;39(1):176–91
**Gallman JM:** Mortality among white males: colonial North Carolina. **Soc Sci Hist** 1980;4(3):295–316
**Galloway J** see **Low MD**
**Galmacci G** see **Figa'Talamanca I**
**Galvao CA** see **Pereira CB**
**Gálvez Rodríguez E:** Problematica de la medicina en la Baja Edad Media. **Asclepio** 1978–79;30–31:187–97
**Galvonaĭte AL** see **Biziuliavichius SK**
**Galzigna L, Galzigna M:** La produzione del corpo curabile. **Acta Med Hist Patav** 1982–83;29:29–65
**Galzigna M** see **Galzigna L**
**Gamba A:** Un ritratto inedito di Giambattista Morgagni. **Acta Med Hist Patav** 1982–83;29:67–74
**Gamberale M:** La genealogia de Ippocrate di Cos e gli Asclepiadi di Rodi. **Accad Naz Lincei Rome** 1980, Ser 8;35(1–2):109–16, 119
**Gambill J:** Potential problems of detecting and treating psychosis in the White House. Potential psychosis in the White House. **Int J Soc Psychiatry** 1980;26(4):255–62
**Gambles RM** see **Crowther RW**
**Gamet A** see **Delaunay A, ed**
**Gamez GL:** Drug abuse: an overview. **Unitas** 1972;45(3):11–23
**Gamlen C** see **Gould ME**
**Gammill CG** see **Francis WR**
**Gan-Yun Y** see **Chuan-Kui H**
**Ganapathi K:** Medicine in social development. **Hindustan Antibiot Bull** 1979 Feb;21(3):102–8
**Ganapini L:** Provvedimenti della pietà e della scienza: il frenocomio di Trieste (1908–1914). **Mov Operaio Soc** 1980;3(4):423–39
**Gandevia B:** A surgeon's view of Cape Town in 1787. **Adler Mus Bull** 1983 Nov;Spec issue:9–12
**Gandevia B:** Childhood mortality in Australia from 1788. In International Congress of the History of Medicine. 26th, Plovdiv, 1978. Actes du Congress. Sofia, 1981. Volume II. p. 100–3.
**Gandevia B:** Dr. John Hutchinson: the inventor of the spirometer. **Aust Fam Physician** 1981 Jul;10(7):574–8
**Gandevia B, Clasen U:** James George Beaney: his authorship. **Med J Aust** 1981 Aug 8;2(3):160
**Gandevia B:** The historical role of Australian medical libraries. **Aust Libr J** 1974 Dec;23(11):391–7
**Gandilhon R:** La bouse de vache. Etude d'ethnologie. **Mem Soc Agric Commer Sci Arts Marne** 1978;271–306
**Gandillac M de** see **Margolin JC**
**Gandziuk VM** see **Gordeev VI**
**Gangadaharan N:** The state of Ayurvada in the eighteenth and nineteenth centuries. **Indian J Hist Sci** 1982;17(1):154–63
**Gangadharam V, Sudhakara Reddy P, Subba Reddy BV:** Concept of disease and folk therapy in a village of Andhra Pradesh. **Bull Indian Inst Hist Med (Hyderabad)** 1978;8(1–4):44–50
**Gangler P:** Endodontic treatment in the GDR. **Int Endod J** 1984 Jul;17(3):152–62

**Ganguin HG:** Beitrag der medizinisch-wissenschaftlichen Gesselschaft für Bronchopneumonologie der DDR und ihrer Sektionen zur Entwicklung des Fachgebietes Bronchopneumonologie. **Z Erkr Atmungsorgane** 1979 Apr;153(11):5–13
**Gani L:** Jules Guesde, Paul Lafargue et les problèmes de population. **Population** 1979;34(4):1023–1044
**Ganiage J:** La population du Beauvaisis: transformations économiques et mutations démographiques (1790–1975). **Ann Geogr** 1980;89(491):1–36
**Gann LH, Gelfand M:** Huggins of Rhodesia. London, Allen & Unwin [1964]. 285 p.
**Gannon JR:** Deaf heritage. A narrative history of deaf America. Silver Spring, National Associaton of the Deaf, 1981. xxxi, 483 p.
**Ganong A** see **Viney W**
**Ganry C** see **Chemin A**
**Ganschow TW** see **Spicker SF**
**Gantt DG:** A method of interpreting enamel prism patterns. **Scan Electron Microsc** 1979;(3):491–6
**Gantt WH:** E. Cowles Andrus (1896––1978), eighth president of the Pavlovian Society. **Pavlov J Biol Sci** 1979 Jan–Mar;14(1):74–5
**Gantt WH:** Review of the shaping of a behaviorism (B.F. Skinner). **Pavlov J Biol Sci** 1980 Jan–Mar;15(1):42–4
**Gan'zha SV:** U istokov zhenskogo meditsinskogo obrazovaniia. **Med Sestra** 1984 Feb;43(2):45–7
**Ganzinger K:** Der Lippe-Detmoldische Leibarzt Johann Christian Friedrich Scherf (1750–1818) als Medizinalpolitiker und Reformator der Pharmazie. **Beitr Gesch Pharm** 1981;31(10):73–8
**Ganzinger K:** Die 'Oesterreichische pharmazeutische Gesellschaft' 1873 bis 1938. **Osterr Apoth Ztg** 1980;34:3–6
**Ganzinger K, Skopec M, Wyklicky H, ed:** Festschrift für Erna Lesky zum 70. Geburtstag. Wien, Brüder Hollinek, 1981. 212 p.
**Ganzinger K:** Johann Peter Frank und die Apothekerordnung für die österreichische Lombardei. **Osterr Apoth Ztg** 1981;35:410–4
**Ganzinger K:** Johann Peter Frank und die Apothekerordnung für die österreichische Lombardei. In Ganzinger K, Skopec M, Wyklicky H, ed: Festschrift für Erna Lesky zum 70. Geburtstag. Wien, Brüder Hollinek, 1981. p. 39–47.
**Ganzinger K:** Naturwissenschaften und Pharmazie unter Maria Theresia und Joseph II. **Osterr Apoth Ztg** 1980;34:361–5
**Ganzinger K:** Zur Geschichte der chemischen Nomenklatur in den amtlichen Arzneibüchern. **Beitr Gesch Pharm** 1980;31(5):33–7
**Ganzinger K:** Zur Geschichte der Universitätsapotheke. In Dilg P, et al., ed: Perspektiven der Pharmaziegeschichte. Graz, Austria, Akademische Druck- u. Verlagsanstalt, 1983. p. 79–88.
**Ganzinger K, ed:** Die Vorträge des Internationalen Pharmaziehistorischen Kongresses Innsbruck 1977. Stuttgart, Wissenschaftliche Verlagsgesellschaft, 1979. 213 p. (Veröffentlichungen der Internationalen Gesellschaft für Geschichte der Pharmazie, Neue Folge, 47).
**Gara PF de:** In celebration of the 75th birthday of 'allergy'. **J Asthma** 1982;19(1):3–4
**Garbelotto N:** Teoria e politica nella psicosociologia di E. Mayo. **Stor Crit Psicol** 1980;1(1):61–78
**Garber E:** Marie Gertrude Rand. In: Notable American women. The modern period. Cambridge, Mass., Belknap-Harvard Univ. Press, 1980. 4:565.
**Garberoglio U** see **Castagnola L**
**García JC:** Historia de las instituciones de investigación en salud en América Latina, 1880–1930. **Educ Med Salud** 1981;15(1):71–90
**García JC:** Medicina y sociedad. Las corrientes de pensamiento en el campo de la salud. **Educ Med Salud** 1983;17(4):363–97
**Garcia JC:** The laziness disease. **Hist Philos Life Sci** 1981;3(1):31–59
**García MM:** History and design of artifical heart valves. **Bol Asoc Med PR** 1981 Nov;73(11):567–73
**Garcia Ada R** see **Basante Pol RM**
**García-Alejo RH:** Enfermedad osea de Paget: comentarios a sus primeras descripciones y evolucion historica de su etiopatogenia. **Asclepio** 1982;34:181–97
**García Alfonso C, Pérez García JM:** Académicos veterinarios en la Real Academia Nacional de Medicina. **An R Acad Nac Med (Madr)** 1982;99(4):671–704
**García-Argüelles R:** De la digital de ayer a los lanatosidos de hoy. Una breve historia de los cardiotonicos. **Asclepio** 1980;32:195–9
**García Ballester L:** Evolucion y problematica de las investigaciones sobre historia de la medicina bajomedieval en España. **Asclepio** 1978–79;30–31:121–56
**García Ballester L:** Experiencia y especulación en el diagnóstico galénico. **Dynamis** 1981;1:203–23
**García Ballester L:** Factores sociomédicos en el proceso de constitución de las especialidades médicas: el caso de la otología. In Albarracin Teulon A, et al, ed: Medicina e Historia. Madrid, Edic. Univ. Comp., 1973. p. 321–38.
**García Ballester L:** In memoriam Dr. Vicente Peset Llorca (1914–1981). **Dynamis** 1981;1:221–2
**García Ballester L, García-González G:** Nota sobre la asistencia a los locos y 'desfallecidos de seso' en la Cordoba medieval: el Hospital de Jesucristo (1419). **Asclepio** 1978–79;30–31:199–207
**García-Ballester L:** Studies on Hippocrates and Galen in modern Spain. **Trans Stud Coll Physicians Phila** 1979 Sep;5(1 No 3):215–29
**Garcia-Ballester L:** The circulation and use of medical manuscipts in ARabic in 16th century Spain. **J Hist Arabic Sci** 1979;3(2):183–99
**García Ballester L** see **Carrillo JL**
**Garcia Ballester L** see **Gago R**
**Garcia-Ballester L** see **Grmek MD, ed**
**García del Carrizo San Millán MG:** Breve apunte sobre los estudios histologicos en el departamento de anatomia de San Carlos hasta la creacion de la catedra de histologia. **Asclepio** 1978–79;30–31:89–97
**Garcia del Carrizo San Millan MG:** Obras de interes medico y cientifico en las bibliotecas universitaria y de Santa Cruz de Valladolid (hasta 1877). Valladolid, Universidad de Valladolid, 1981. 172 p. (Acta Historico-Medica Vallisoletana, Monografias, XI)
**Garcia Gamboa MA:** Estudio retrospectivo de los forceps de Tarnier 1862–1877. La evolucion de la traccion axial y los forceps curvos tractores sobre su eje sin tractores. 2 vols. 2a. ed. [Rio Piedras, Puerto Rico, Universidad de Puerto Rico, Escuela de Medicina, 1981. 359 leaves.
**Garcia Gamboa MA:** La cesarea abdominal: historia y evolucion. [Río Piedras] Universidad de Puerto Rico, Recinto de Ciencias Medicas, Escuela Medicina, 1982. 139 p.
**Garcia-Godoy F:** Caries dental en cráneos primitivos de la Isla Santo Domingo. **Rev Asoc Odontol Argent** 1978 Jul–Sep;66(3):147–50
**García-González G** see **García Ballester L**
**Garcia Gonzalez R, Prieto Cantero A:** Licenciados en medicina y cirugia graduados en la Universidad de Valladolid (1871–1936). Vallodolid, Universidad de Valladolid, 1979. 383 p. (Acta Historico-Medica Vallisoletana, Monografias, IX)
**García Guerra D:** El hospital real de Santiago en el siglo XVIII; aspects del ejercicio médico. **Asclepio** 1980;32:211–28, 492–503
**García Guerra D:** Epidemiologia gallega del siglo XVIII. Su repercusión sobre el Hospital Real de Santiago. In: Sociedad Española de Historia de la Medicina. V Congreso Nacional. Madrid, 1977. **Asclepio** 1977;29:147–65
**García Guerra D:** La asistencia médica en el Hospital Real de Santiago al final del Antiguo Régimen. **Asclepio** 1983;35:287–300
**García Guerra D:** La 'Disertacion medica' de Fernando Oxea. Un testimonio de auscultacion inmediata del torax en el siglo XVIII. **Asclepio** 1980;32:201–9
**García Guerra D** see **Albarracín Teulón A**
**García Iglesias L:** La edad difícil y la sexualidad adolescente en la España visigoda. **Hisp Antiq** 1976;6:79–96
**García Palmieri MR:** Observaciones sobre la contribución del Dr. Ramón M. Suárez al reconocimiento de la cardiopatía reumática en el trópico. **Bol Asoc Med PR** 1983 Nov;75(11):503–5
**García-Palmieri MR** see **Torres-Gómez JM**
**García Peña de Alexander M del P:** Nota biográfica sobre el Doctor Francisco de Asís Pons i Freixa. In Congrés Internacional d'Historie de la Medicina Catalana, 1st, Barcelona-Montpellier, 1970. Barcelona, Editorial Scienta, 1971. v 4, p. 81–6.
**García Prieto A** see **Ortega Millán A**
**García Ramos JA:** Datos originales del folklore medico almeriense. **Asclepio** 1981;33:275–314
**García-Sainz M:** El Sistema Internacional de Unidades en la prática médica. I. **Gac Med Mex** 1981 Dec;117(12):479–83
**Garcia Sanchez J:** Contribución a la historia de la botica del Hospital de la Pasión, de Ciudad Rodrigo. **Bol Soc Esp Hist Farm** 1980/81 Dec–Mar;31–32(124–5):1–7
**García Sanz A, Pérez Moreda V:** Análisis histórico de una crisis demográfica: Villacastín de 1466 a 1800. **Estud Segov** 1972;(70):119–46
**Gardin JM** see **Belic N**
**Gardiner JF:** C. Edmund Kells: New Orleans' gift to dentistry. **Bull Hist Dent** 1981;29(1):2–7
**Gardiner JF:** Solyman Brown and his epic poem 'Dentologia'. **Bull Hist Dent** 1984;32(1):44–51
**Gardner AL:** Padua, Italy: the renaissance of medicine. **J Indiana State Med Assoc** 1983 Dec;76(12):842–5
**Gardner B:** Economic aspects of the fertility of rural-farm and urban women. **South Econ J** 1972;38(4):518–24
**Gardner KD:** Looking upon the water: in which we return to the Civil War. **Am J Kidney Dis** 1984 Sep;4(2):101–2
**Gardner R:** Miracles of healing in Anglo-Celtic Northumbria as recorded by the venerable Bede and his contemporaries: a reappraisal in the light of twentieth century experience. **Br Med J [Clin Res]** 1983 Dec 24–31;287(6409):1927–33
**Gardner of Parkes:** 'Fair to the fair'. **Br Dent J** 1982 Aug 3;153(3):117–9
**Gareau S:** L'organisation hospitalière dans le nord-ouest Quebeçois. **Can Cathol Hist Assoc Study Sess** 1982;49:35–58
**Garfield E:** W hołdzie Hilaremu Koprowskiemu: uczonemu, muzykowi i przyjacielowi. **Pol Tyg Lek** 1983 Sep 5;38(36):1119–23
**Garfield R, Salmon JW:** Struggles over health care in the People's Republic of China. **J Contemp Asia** 1981;11(1):91–103
**Garfield SL:** Psychotherapy. A 40-year-appraisal. **Am Psychol** 1981 Feb;36(2):174–83
**Garfinkel L:** A tribute to Harold S. Diehl (1891–1973) – changing patterns of smoking and disease. **CA** 1981;31:114–9
**Garfinkel L:** Asbestos: historical perspective. **CA** 1984 Jan–Feb;34(1):44–7
**Garfinkel PE** see **Kaplan AS**
**Garg MG:** IMA: its origin, role and prospects. **J Indian Med Assoc** 1983 Oct;81(7–8):142–7
**Garg NK, Nigam SK:** Interaction in chemistry and medicine between India and Europe in 18th–19th century. **Indian J Hist Sci** 1981;16(2):145–55
**Gargan L:** [The libraries of Guglielmino de Treviso, Pasquale da Villorba & Niccolo Cesi da Mignagola.] (Ita) In: Cultura et arte nel Veneto al tempo del Petrarca. (Studi sul Petrarca, 5.) Padua, 1978;:101–12, 198–211.
**Garibaldi U** see **Fenaroli G**
**Garibdzhanian LL** see **Kirienko AI**

**Gariepy TP:** Hyacum, et lues venerea. **J Hist Med Allied Sci** 1981 Jul;36(3):325
**Garin AM** see **Perevodchikova NI**
**Garin JP** see **Woehrle R**
**Garin NS** see **Smirnov EI**
**Garland J:** Jerome Van Crowningshield Smith. **N Engl J Med** 1970 Aug 6;283:303-4
**Garland JE:** The centennial history of the Boston Medical Library 1875-1975. Boston, Boston Medical Library, 1975. xiv, 223 p.
**Garland N** see **Eckert WG**
**Garmash VIa, Ushmarov AK:** Znachenie ucheniia I. P. Pavlova dlia kliniki vnutrennikh bolezneĭ. **Med Sestra** 1981 Feb;40(2):8-10
**Garmasheva NL, Konstantinova NN:** Osnovnye étapy razvitiia perinatologii v SSSR. **Akush Ginekol (Mosk)** 1982;(7):7-10
**Garmier JF:** Soufflot et Mâcon: La charité, l'Hotel-Dieu. **Cah Rech Archit** 1980;6-7, Suppl:142-51
**Garn SM:** The growth of growth. **Am J Phys Anthropol** 1981 Dec;56(4):521-30
**Garner J:** Burroughs and Wellcome: American architects of a British empire. **Can Pharm J** 1980 Dec;:417-9
**Garner J:** Louis Hébert: his pharmaceutical skills helped Canada's first permanent settlement to survive. **Can Pharm J** 1982 Oct;115(10):380-1
**Garnerus K:** Die Versammlungen Deutscher Narturforscher und Arzte--Medaillen berichten. **Naturwissenschaften** 1982 Apr;69(4):158-61
**Garnham PC:** Some contributions of Scotland to tropical medicine. In Passmore R, ed: Proceedings of the Royal College of Physicians of Edinburgh Tercentenary Congress, 1981. Edinburgh, Royal College of Physicians of Edinburgh, 1982. p. 128-42.
**Garnham PC:** The present state of malaria research: an historical survey. **Experientia** 1984 Dec 15;40(12):1305-10
**Garnjobst W** see **Breen RE**
**Garnot NS, Simon N:** Parigi degli ospedali. **Kos** 1984 May;1(4):95-114
**Garnuszewski Z:** Historia akupunktury. **Arch Hist Med (Warsz)** 1980;43(2):147-61
**Garrafa V:** Epidemiología: desarrollo histórico de su concepto. **CERON** 1979 Apr;4(1):23-7
**Garrafa V:** Epidemiologia: desenvolvimento histórico do seu conceito. **Rev Assoc Paul Cir Dent** 1980 May-Jun;34(3):196-202
**Garralda Hualde ME:** El modelo inglés de formación en psiquiatría infantil. **Actas Luso Esp Neurol Psiquiatr** 1981 Mar-Apr;9(2):103-12
**Garrett C:** Women and witches: patterns of analysis. **Signs** 1977;3(2):461-70
**Garrett CG:** Anton Julius Carlson. In Dictionary of American Biography, Suppl. 6, 1956-1960. p. 99-100, 1980.
**Garrett CG:** Frederick George Novy. In Dictionary of American Biography, Suppl. 6, 1956-1960. p. 481-2, 1980.
**Garrett CG:** Robert Russell Bensley. In Dictionary of American Biography, Suppl. 6, 1956-1960. p. 53-4, 1980.
**Garretta M** see **Muller A**
**Garriott JC** see **Anderson RJ**
**Garrison D:** Karen Horney and feminism. **Signs** 1981;6(4):672-91
**Garrison FH** see **Ash L**
**Garshin VG:** Tam, gde smert' pomogaet zhizni. **Arkh Patol** 1984;46(5):83-8
**Gartner LM:** Neonatal jaundice: a selected retrospective. In Smith GF, Smith PN, Vidyasagar D, ed: Historical review and recent advances in neonatal and perinatal medicine. [Chicago?], Mead Johnson Nutritional Division, 1983. Vol. I. p. 87-97.
**Gartner LM** see **Smith GF**
**Garton C** see **Froriep R**
**Garulli E** see **Epistemologia, metodologia clinica e storia della scienza medica, 2**
**Gasparini F** see **Premuda L**
**Gass RS:** Codes and statements related to medical ethics. In Reich WT, et al, ed: Encyclopedia of bioethics, v.4. New York, Free Press, 1978. p. 1721-1815.
**Gassiev VI:** Iz istorii zdravookhraneniia Iuzhnoĭ Osetii. **Sov Zdravookhr** 1983;(2):61-3
**Gassiev VI:** Zdravookhranenie Iuzhnoĭ Osetii v gody Velikoĭ Otechestvennoĭ voĭny. **Sov Zdravookhr** 1983;5:55-8
**Gast W, Barth J, Rytter M:** Der lange Weg zur PUVa-Therapie. **Dermatol Monatsschr** 1983;169(9):594-600
**Gastão M:** S. João de Deus: sua vida-sua obra. Lisboa, Centro do Livro Brasileiro, 1982. 733 p.
**Gastaut H, Gastaut Y, Broughton R:** Gustave Flaubert's illness: a case report in evidence against the erroneous notion of psychogenic epilepsy. **Epilepsia** 1984 Oct;25(5):622-37
**Gastaut H, Gastaut Y:** La maladie de Gustave Flaubert. **Rev Neurol (Paris)** 1982;138(6-7):467-92
**Gastaut H:** New comments on the epilepsy of Fyodor Dostoevsky. **Epilepsia** 1984 Aug;25(4):408-11
**Gastaut Y** see **Gastaut H**
**Gaston J** see **Durbin PT, ed**
**Gataullin MM:** Razvitie psikhiatrii v Bashkirii (k 425-letiiu dobrovol'nogo prisoedineniia Bashkirii k ruskomu gosudarstvu (1557-1982 gg.). **Zh Nevropatol Psikhiatr** 1982;82(12):99-102
**Gates BT:** Suicide and the Victorian physicians. **J Hist Behav Sci** 1980 Apr;16(2):164-74
**Gathiram P, Katzeff IE, Edwards H, et al:** Dynamic electrocardiography IV. The 'imaginary cardiac vector' hypothesis: the evolution of the vectorcardiographic inverse solution. **Med Hypotheses** 1981 Jul;7(7):825-62
**Gatterman MI:** W. A. Budden: the transition through proprietary education, 1924-1954. **Chiropr Hist** 1982;2(1):21-5
**Gatz M, Gease EI, Tyler FB, et al:** Psychosocial competence characteristics of black and white women: the constraining effects of 'triple jeopardy'. **Black Scholar** 1982;13(1):5-12
**Gaucher D:** La formation des hygiénistes à l'Université de Montréal, 1910-1975: de la santé publique à la médecine préventive. **Rech Sociogr** 1979;20(1):59-85
**Gaucher disease:** A century of delineation and research. **Prog Clin Biol Res** 1982;95:1-740
**Gaude W:** Die alte Apotheke. Eine tausendjährige Kulturgeschichte. Stuttgart, Deutscher Apotheker Verlag, 1979. 219 p.
**Gaude W:** Zur Krankengeschichte Martin Luthers. **Beitr Gesch Univ Erfurt** 1979-83;19:113-63
**Gaudiosi O** see **Orsini M**
**Gaudiot C:** Le Service de Santé dans la bataille de Verdun. **Hist Sci Med** 1980;14(2):193-200
**Gaukroger S:** Aristotle on the function of sense perception. **Stud Hist Philos Sci** 1981 Mar;12(1):75-89
**Gault EW, Attwood HD:** Medical men in the early history of the Austin Hospital. Five doctors of widely varying ages and backgrounds were associated with the formative years of the Austin Hospital. **Med J Aust** 1981 Dec 12-26;2(12-13):680-3
**Gaumer B:** Contribution de Ernest Conseil à la naissance de l'épidémiologie en Tunisie. **Arch Inst Pasteur Tunis** 1983 Mar-Sep;60(1-2):49-64
**Gaunt D:** Historisk demografi eller demografisk historia? En översikt och ett debattinlägg om ett tvärvetenskapligt dilemma. **Hist Tidskr** 1973;93(3):382-405
**Gaunt D** see **Laslett P**
**Gaunt KL:** Colorado hospitals of the 1800's. **Denver West Roundup** 1979 Sep-Oct;35:3-19
**Gaunt RN:** Three perspectives on the political history of Virginia's veterinary school. Ph.D. Diss., University of Virginia. Charlottesville, 1980. xi, 378 p.
**Gause GF:** Gramicidin S and early antibiotic research in the Soviet Union. In J. Parascandola, ed: The history of antibiotics. Madison, American Institute of the History of Pharmacy, 1980. p. 91-5.
**Gaustad ES:** George Berkeley in America. New Haven, Yale University Press, 1979. xi, 225 p.
**Gautier A:** Heurs et malheurs politiques d'une loi fédérale sur les épidémies. **Rev Med Suisse Romande** 1980 Dec;100(12):1061-2
**Gautier J:** Freud a menti. Périgny-sur-Yerres, Mandres-les-Roses, Edition de 'La vie claire, 1977. vii, 566 p.
**Gautier JC:** Accidents vasculaires. **Rev Neurol (Paris)** 1982;138(12):939-51
**Gauval VB:** Détails piquants sur la vie d'un des praticiens du Roi et de ses honoraires. **Soc Fr Hist Art Dent** 1979 Sep-Dec;(5-6):11-14
**Gauval VB, Vidal F:** Etiologie et pathogénie du mal scorbutique chez les médecins des XVIIe et XVIIIe siècles. **Chir Dent Fr** 1984 Jul 12-19;54(258-259):23-8
**Gauval VB** see **David T**
**Gavazzi C:** Odontoiatria del passato. I denti umani fossili di Salto (Valle Orco). **Dent Cadmos** 1981 Oct, Nov;49(10,11):59-63 contd, 71-9
**Gavin WJ:** Vagueness and empathy: a Jamesian view. **J Med Philos** 1981 Feb;6(1):45-65
**Gavrilov OK:** Meditsinskaia nauka k 60-ĭ godoshchine obrazovaniia Soiuza Sovetskikh Sotsialisticheskikh Respublik. **Sov Zdravookhr** 1982;(8):3-8
**Gavrilovic VS:** Doprinos Mihajla Pupina svetskoj medicinskoj nauci. **Srp Arh Celok Lek** 1981 Feb;109(2):293-302
**Gavriushova LP** see **Matveev MP**
**Gawel M:** The development of concepts concerning cerebral circulation. In Rose FC, Bynum WF, ed: Historical aspects of the neurosciences. New York, Raven, 1982. p. 171-8.
**Gay EC, Anderson J, Graham SS:** An old medical specialty puts on a new face ... and head ... neck. **J Arkansas Med Soc** 1982 Feb;78(9):359-62
**Gay EW:** Atlanta's city hospital had a rough beginning. **J Med Assoc Ga** 1983 Nov;72(11):781-4
**Gay EW:** Francis O. Ticknor, 19th century physician-poet--Part I and II. **J Med Assoc Ga** 1981;70(7):499-503, (8):561-4
**Gay EW:** The medical profession in Georgia, 1733-1983. Atlanta, Auxiliary to the Medical Association of Georgia, 1983. xvi, 447 p.
**Gay GR:** You've come a long way, baby! Coke time for the new American lady of the Eighties. **J Psychoactive Drugs** 1981 Oct-Dec;13(4):297-318
**Gay P:** On the bourgeoisie: a psychological interpretation. In Merriman, John M., ed: Consciousness and class experience in nineteenth-century Europe. New York, Holmes and Meier, 1979. p. 187-203.
**Gay P:** Victorian sexuality: old texts and new insights. **Am Scholar** 1980;49(3):372-8
**Gayda M** see **Vacola G**
**Gaydos JC** see **Brodkey C**
**Gaye P:** La médecine sociale en Afrique de l'ouest (historique, situation actuelle et perspective d'avenir). In: Congrès international d'histoire de la médecine, XXVe, Québec, 1976. Actes. Québec, 1977. p. 121-40.
**Gazenko OG, Genin AM, Gurovskiĭ NN, et al:** Pervyĭ kosmicheskiĭ polet cheloveka. **Kosm Biol Aviakosm Med** 1981 Mar-Apr;15(2):5-7
**Gear JH:** Studies of the rickettsial diseases at the South African Institute for Medical Research: epidemic louse-borne typhus fever. **Adler Mus Bull** 1984 Nov;10(3):8-15
**Gear JH:** The Anglo-Boer War of 1899-1902:enteric fever and Captain Maxwell Louis Hughes. **Adler Mus Bull** 1981;7(1):10-3
**Gear JH:** The 1918 influenza epidemic. **Adler Mus Bull** 1983 Nov;Spec issue:13-20
**Gease EI** see **Gatz M**

**Gebauer C:** Die Lindenburg zu Köln (1848-1965). Beispiel eines grossen Klinikum-Neubaus zu Beginn des 20. Jahrhunderts. Köln, 1979. 340 p. (Kölner medizinhistorische Beiträge, Band 11)
**Gebbie DA:** Reproductive anthropology--descent through woman. New York, Wiley, 1981. 371 p.
**Gebhard B** see **Hand WD, ed**
**Gebhardt O, Kubik G:** Zur Bündnispolitik der Arbeiterklasse und ihrer marxistisch-leninistischen Partei mit der medizinischen Intelligenz. **Med Ges** 1978;(3):28-47
**Gedalia I** see **Meir E**
**Geddes LA:** A short history of the electrical stimulation of excitable tissue. Including electrotherapeutic applications. **Physiologist** 1984 Feb;27(1 Suppl):S1-47
**Geertinger P** see **Andersen SR**
**Geerts A, Kornblith BA, Urmson WJ:** Compensation for bodily harm. L'indemnisation des lésions corporelles à travers les siècles. Brussels, Fernand Nathan, Labor, 1977. 213 p.
**Gegenheimer E:** Selected letters of Humphrey Hood, Litchfield physician. **J Ill State Hist Soc** 1979;72:193-212, 243-56
**Gegesi Kiss P:** Bókay János junior a tanítvány szemével. **Orv Hetil** 1983 May 29;124(22):1329-34
**Geha AS** see **Hammond GL**
**Gehrie MJ** see **Ross JM**
**Gehrke H, Dückert M:** Gesundheitspolitik der deutschen Arbeiterklasse und ihre Unterstützung durch die fortschrittlichsten Vertreter der medizinischen Intelligenz. **Z Arztl Fortbild (Jena)** 1983;77(12):530-4
**Geiger A:** Lorenz Heister als Geburtshelfer und gynäkologischer Chirurg. Vergleichende Untersuchung anhand der verschiedenen Auflagen seiner 'Chirurgie'. Zürich, Juris Druck, 1983. 140 p. (Zürcher Medizingeschichtliche Abhandlungen, Neue Reihe, Nr. 162).
**Geiger I:** Das Leben und Werk von Wilhelm Tönnis unter besonderer Berücksichtigung seiner Würzburger Zeit. Diss. Würzburg, 1981. 109 p.
**Geiler G:** Bedeutungsvolle Leistungen des Pathologischen Instituts Leipzig zur experimentell-theoretischen Pathologie und ätiopathogenetischen Forschung. **Zentralbl Allg Pathol** 1982;126(3-4):237-44
**Geis G, Bunn I:** Sir Thomas Browne and witchcraft: a cautionary tale for contemporary law and psychiatry. **Int J Law Psychiatry** 1981;4(1-2):1-11
**Geiser E:** Emile Magitot (1834-1897)--ein Lebensbild. **Schweiz Monatsschr Zahnmed** 1984 Sep;94(9):813-20
**Geison GL:** Divided we stand: physiologists and clinicians in the American context. In Vogel MJ, Rosenberg CE, ed: The therapeutic revolution. Philadelphia, 1979. p. 67-90.
**Geison GL:** Pasteur on vital versus chemical ferments: a previously unpublished paper on the inversion of sugar. **Isis** 1981 Sep;72(263):425-45
**Geison GL:** Scientific change, emerging specialties, and research schools. **Hist Sci** 1981;19(1):20-40
**Geison GL** see **Ebbert A, et al**
**Geison GL** see **Farley J**
**Geist DC:** William Williams Keen, M.D. (1837-1932), surgeon and author. **Trans Stud Coll Physicians Phila** 1977 Apr;44(4):182-93
**Gejrot T:** Frans Vilhelm Törne. **Sydsven Medicinhist Sallsk Arsskr** 1984;21:129-34
**Gejrot T:** Medikofilosofisk examen; om medikofilare och medikofilen. **Sydsven Medicinhist Sallsk Arsskr** 1982;19:45-53
**Gejvall NG:** Skelettmaterial från utgrävningar som bidrag till medicinhistorisk forkning. **Nord Medicinhist Arsb** 1980;Suppl 6:106-11
**Gejvall NG:** Swedenborg--a man with head enough for two. **Ossa** 1978;5:123-31
**Gejvall NG** see **Hart GD, ed**
**Gelabert González JE** see **Enríquez Morales MJ**
**Gelabert i Mas A, Gironella i Coll J:** El papa Inocencio XI: approximación etiológica a su patología renal. In International Congress of the History of Medicine, 27th, Barcelona, 1980. Actas. Barcelona, Acadèmia de Ciències Mèdiques de Catalunya i Balears, 1981. p. 506-10.
**Gelberman RH:** Microsurgery and the development of the operating microscope. **Contemp Surg** 1978 Dec;13(6):43-6
**Gelbier S, Randall SB:** Charles Edward Wallis and London's Toothbrush Clubs: 1909 style. **Dent Health (London)** 1982;21(1):12-5
**Gelbier S, Randall S:** Charles Edward Wallis and the rise of London's school dental service. **Med Hist** 1982 Oct;26(4):395-404
**Gelbier S:** Frederick Breese and London's first school dental clinic. **Br Dent J** 1981 Nov 3;151(9):309-11
**Gelbier S:** Some early dental history. **Dent Health (London)** 1982;21(6):6-7
**Geldard FA:** The Southern Society for Philosophy and Psychology at midstream. **J Hist Behav Sci** 1984 Jan;20(1):60-2
**Gelfand M:** African customs in relation to preventive medicine. **Cent Afr J Med** 1981 Jan;27(1):1-8
**Gelfand M:** Joseph Lister. **Cent Afr J Med** 1981 Feb;27(2):31-4
**Gelfand M:** The N'anga, the guardian of the Shona way of life, its ethics and behaviour. **Cent Afr J Med** 1981 Jul;27(7):146-8
**Gelfand M** see **Gann LH**
**Gelfand T:** Chirurghi dei Lumi. **Kos** 1984 Feb;1(1):51-73
**Gelfand T:** Demystification and surgical power in the French Enlightenment. **Bull Hist Med** 1983 Summer;57(2):203-17
**Gelfand T:** Deux cultures, une profession: les chirurgiens français au XVIIIe siècle. **Rev Hist Mod Contemp** 1980 July-Sep;27:468-84
**Gelfand T:** Gestation of the clinic. **Med Hist** 1981 Apr;25(2):169-80
**Gelfand T:** Les caractères originaux d'un hospice parisien à la fin de l'Ancien Régime. In Imhof AE, ed: Mensch und Gesundheit in der Geschichte. Husum, Matthiesen, 1980. p. 339-55.
**Gelfand T:** Medicine in New France: les francais look at les canadiens during the seven years' war. In International Congress of the History of Medicine, 27th, Barcelona, 1980. Actas. Barcelona, Académia de Ciències Mèdiques de Catalunya i Balears, 1981. p. 511-6.
**Gelfand T:** Professionalizing modern medicine: Paris surgeons and medical science and institutions in the 18th century. Westport, Connecticut, Greenwood Press, 1980. xviii, 271 p. (Contributions in medical history, 6)
**Gelfand T:** Public medicine and medical careers in France during the reign of Louis XV. **Soc Soc Hist Med Bull (Lond)** 1979 Dec;25:48-51
**Gelfand T:** Public medicine and medical careers in France during the reign of Louis XV. In Russell AW, ed: The town and state physician in Europe from the Middle Ages to the Enlightenment. Wolfenbüttel, Herzog August Bibliothek, 1981. p. 99-122 (Wolfenbütteler Forschungen, 17).
**Gelfand T:** The Annales and the history of medicine. **Bull Hist Med** 1981 Winter;55(4):589-93
**Gelfand T:** The gestation of the clinic. In: Congrès international d'histoire de la médecine, XXVe, Québec, 1976. Actes. Québec, 1977. p. 680-98.
**Gelfand T:** The hospice of the Paris College of Surgery (1774-1793), 'a unique and invaluable institution.' **Bull Hist Med** 1973 Jul-Aug;47(4):375-93
**Gelfand T:** Two cultures, one profession: the surgeons of France in the eighteenth century. In the consortium on Revolutionary Europe: Proceedings, 1978, 1980. p. 171-87. French language version, Rev Hist Mod Contemp 1980 Jul-Sep; 27:468-84.
**Gelfand T:** Who practised medicine in New France?: a collective portrait. In Roland CG, ed: Health, disease and medicine. Toronto, Hannah Institute for the History of Medicine, 1984. p. 16-35.
**Gelfand T** see **Greenbaum LS**
**Gelfand T** see **Jones C**
**Gel'fman AA:** Fel'dshera-iskrovtsy v revoliutsionnom dvizhenii. **Feldsher Akush** 1984 Apr;49(4):49-50
**Gelis J:** De la matrone à la sage-femme: les transformations de l'accoucheuse de campagne au XVIIIe siècle. **Penelope** 1981;(5):33-6
**Gélis J:** La Pierre et le saint: recours populaires pour la guérison des petits enfants (XVIIe-XIXe siècles). **Asclepio** 1983;35:129-58
**Gélis J:** La pratique obstétricale dans la France moderne: les carnets du chirurgien accoucheur Pierre Robin (1770-1797). **Ann Bretagne** 1979;86:191-210
**Gélis J:** L'enquête de 1786 sur les sages-femmes du royaume. **Ann Demogr Hist (Paris)** 1980;:301-43
**Gélis J:** Miracle et medecine aux siècles classiques: le corps medical et le retour temporaire a la vie des mort-nes. **Hist Reflect** 1982;9(1-2):85-101
**Gélis J:** Obstétrique et classes sociales en milieu urbain aux XVIIe et XVIIIe siècles: évolution d'une pratique. **Hist Sci Med** 1980;14:425-33
**Gélis J:** Quand les femmes accouchaient sans médecin. **Histoire** 1981;34:105-12
**Gélis J:** Regard sur l'Europe médicale des Lumières: la collaboration internationale des acchoucheurs et la formation des sages-femmes au XVIIIe siècle. In Imhof AE, ed: Mensch und Gesundheit in der Geschichte. Husum, Matthiesen, 1980. p. 279-99.
**Gella Iturriaga J:** El médico mayor de la escuadra del pacífico: Oliva Muñoz. **Rev Gen Mar** 1980 Aug;199:3-14
**Geller B** see **Greydanus DE**
**Geller SA:** Autopsy. **Sci Am** 1983 Mar;248(3):124-9, 132, 135-6
**Geller SA:** Autopsy. **Mt Sinai J Med (NY)** 1984 Jan-Feb;51(1):77-81
**Geller SA:** Brown's (Cushing's) syndrome. **N Engl J Med** 1983 Jun 9;308(23):1425
**Geller SA:** Comments on the anniversary of the description of Hodgkin's disease. **Mt Sinai J Med (NY)** 1982 Jul-Aug;49(4):308-10
**Geller SA:** Comments on the anniversary of the description of Hodgkin's disease. **J Natl Med Assoc** 1984 Aug;76(8):815-7
**Gellhorn A:** The evolving post-Flexnerian model of medical education. In: Congrès international d'histoire de la médecine, XXVe, Québec, 1976. Actes. Québec, 1977. p. 141-59.
**Gembitskiĭ EV:** Opyt raboty terapevtov v boevykh usloviiakh i ego znachenie dlia razvitiia voenno-polevoĭ terapii. **Voen Med Zh** 1980 May;(5):46-9
**Gembitskiĭ EV:** S. P. Botkin kak voennyĭ terapevt. **Klin Med (Mosk)** 1982 Sep;60(9):22-7
**Gençer AI:** Istanbul tersansesinde acilan ilk tib mektebi **Tarih Dergesi (Turkey)** 1977;31:301-16
**Gendel' MG** see **Abramenko VV**
**Gener Galbis C** see **Báguena Cervellera J**
**Genesse J** see **Hudson T**
**Genest J:** A satellite view of hypertension. **Clin Invest Med** 1983;6(3):229-41 .
**Genest J:** L'assureur-vie dans la cité. **Action Natl** 1981;70(7):601-12
**Genesté B:** La biotechnologie: un domaine de recherche particulièrement fécond et porteur d'espoir. **Rev Palais Decouv** 1983;11(107):18-45
**Genet-Varcin E** see **Tillier AM**
**Genin AM** see **Gazenko OG**
**Genné WH:** Sex, marriage and family: an update from Amsterdam. **J Ecumenical Stud** 1979;16(1):154-60
**Genschorek W:** Christoph Wilhelm Hufeland. Der Arzt, der das Leben verlängern half. Leipzig, Hirzel, 1976. 202 p.
**Genschorek W:** Christoph Wilhelm Hufeland: der Arzt, der das Leben verlängern half. Leipzig, Hirzel, 1982. 215 p.
**Genschorek W:** Ernst Ludwig Heim. Das Leben eines Volksarztes. Leipzig,

S. Hirzel, 1982. 226 p.
**Genschorek W:** Robert Koch. Selbstloser Kampf gegen Seuchen und Infektionskrankheiten. Leipzig, Hirzel, 1981. 224 p. (Hervorragende Arzte im Dienste des Menschen).
**Genschorek W:** Wegbereiter der Chirurgis: Johann Friedrich Dieffenbach, Theodor Billroth. Leipzig, Hirzel, Teubner, 1983. 252 p.
**Gentile DP:** 'Urethrolithotomy': an ingenious approach of the ancients. **J Urol** 1984 Aug;132(2):359–60
**Geoffroy G** see **Barbeau A**
**George O:** Eskimo medicine man. [Portland], Oregon Historical Society, 1978. xi, 278 p.
**George W:** Darwin. Glasgow, Fontana Paperbacks, 1982. 160 p.
**George W:** The Mendel enigma, the farmer's son: the key to Mendel's motivation. **Arch Int Hist Sci (Paris)** 1982 Dec;32(109):177–83
**George Rosen: In Memoriam:** With contributions by S. Benison, E. H. Ackerknecht, J. Z. Bowers, L. A. Falk, G. A. Silver, O. H. Wangensteen, A. J. Viseltear, E. H. Thomson. **J Hist Med Allied Sci** 1978 Jul;33(3):244–317
**George Sarton's correspondence: Isis** 1984 Mar;75(276):33–62
**Georgiev I:** Development and scientific research activity achievements in the higher medical institute 'I. P. Pavlov' - Plovdiv. **Folia Med (Plovdiv)** 1981;23(3-4):5–23
**Georgieva K, Dačev B:** 100 godini obstesyveno zdraveopazvane. **Stomatologiia (Sofiia)** 1979 Nov–Dec;61(6):337–41
**Georgievski M:** Zdravstveni radnici--narodni heroji. **Lijec Vjesn** 1983 Feb–Mar;105(2-3):99–104
**Georgievskiĭ AS, Lobanov GP:** Meditsinskoe obespechnenie Rzhevsko-Sychevskoĭ nastupatel'noĭ operatsii. **Voen Med Zh** 1982 Oct;(10):62–6
**Georgievskiĭ AS, Tel'iatev IV:** Sistemnyĭ podkhod v istoriko-meditsinskikh issledovaniiakh. **Sov Zdravookhr** 1981;(6):52–5
**Georgievskiĭ AS:** Vklad russkikh voennykh vracheĭ v stanovlenie i razvitie profilakticheskogo napravleniia meditsiny. **Sov Zdravookhr** 1982;(10):66–70
**Georgievskiĭ AS:** Vklad S. P. Botkina v razvitie otechestvennoĭ voennoĭ meditsiny. **Sov Zdravookhr** 1983;6:62–6
**Georgievskiĭ AS** see **Gurvich MM**
**Georgievskiĭ AS** see **Ivanov NG**
**Georgievskiĭ AS** see **Petrov NS**
**Georgotas A, Gershon S:** Historical perspectives and current highlights on lithium treatment in manic-depressive illness. **J Clin Psychopharmacol** 1981 Jan;1(1):27–31
**Geppert W, Hartmann E, Hennis I, et al:** Die Entwicklung dentaler Technologien, dargestellt am Bestand einer historischen Sammlung. (II). **Quintessenz Zahntech** 1982 Nov;8(11):1261–70
**Geppert W, Hartmann E, Hennis I, et al:** Die Entwicklung dentaler Technologien, dargestellt am Bestand einer historischen Sammlung (III). **Quintessenz** 1983 Mar;34(3):543–9
**Gepts-Friedenreich E:** Ziekenhuishygiëne vroeger en nu. **FNIB** 1981 Apr;59(2):7–15
**Gerard A:** Chronique médico-chirurgicale Lilloise sous la Révolution et l'Empire. **Lille Med** 1979 Dec;24(10):774–83
**Gérard A:** De la gastro-entérologie à la politique: la fistule du Grand Roi. **LARC Med** 1983 May;3(5):341–8
**Gerard A, Milot J:** Histoire médicale du Camp de Boulogne d'après les papiers du général Vandamme. **Hist Sci Med** 1982;16(1):29–36
**Gérard A:** Quelques aspects du fonctionnement des hospices civils de Lille de 1793 à 1815. **Rev Nord** 1982;64(254-255):803–21
**Gerard J:** Histoire des médecins belges. [S. l.], Wesmael-Charlier, 1981. 107 p.
**Gérard-Marchant R** see **Cabanne F**
**Gerasimovich GT:** Belorusskomu Nauchnomu Meditsinskomu obshchestvu Akusherov-Ginekologov 50 let. **Akush Ginekol (Mosk)** 1981 Sep;(9):59–61
**Gercke H, Jarchov I, ed:** Die Prinzhorn-Sammlung. Bilder, Skulpturen, Texte aus psychiatrischen Anstalten (ca. 1890–1920). Königstein/Taunus, Athenäum Verlag, 1980. 312 p.
**Gerdts WH:** The art of healing: medicine and science in American art. [Birmingham, Alabama], Birmingham Museum of Art, 1981. 119 p. (Exhibit, Birmingham, 1981).
**Gerebtzoff MA:** Recherches sur la structure du système nerveux et ses modifications expérimentales publiées dans les Archives de Biologie de 1880 à 1900. Analyse critique. **Arch Biol (Liege)** 1980;91(2):223–42
**Gerecke K, Richter J, Koch H:** Třicet let Německé demokratické republiky a jejich přínos mezinárodímu vývoji farmacie. **Cesk Farm** 1981 Jun;30(5):142–6
**Gereffi G:** Drug firms and dependency in Mexico: the case of the steroid hormones industry. **Int Organ** 1978;32:237–86
**Gerencser JD** see **Froriep R**
**Gerevich J:** Az elemebeteggé minösítés szépirodalmi modelljei. **Orv Hetil** 1982 Nov 28;123(48):2971–2
**Gerevich J:** Gulácsy Lajos festömüvész akut pszichózisa (adalék heveny téboly genezisének kérdéséhez). **Orv Hetil** 1981 May 3;122(18):1083–6
**Gergely J:** Az onallosodott immunbiologia: eredmenyek-perspektivak. **Magy Tud** 1981;26(2):93–101
**Gergely J:** Ehrlich 'varázslövedéke' a megvalósulás útján (gyógyszerek irányított célbajuttatása specifikus ellenanyagokkal). **Orv Hetil** 1982 Sep 19;123(38):2331–6
**Gerhardt C:** Kröte und Igel in schwankhafter Literatur des späten Mittelalters. **Medizinhist J** 1981;16(4):340–57
**Gerhardt RE:** The first teaching hospital. **N Engl J Med** 1983 May 19;308(20):1230
**Gerhartl G:** Dr. med. Franz Lorenz (1805–1883). **Mitt Krems Stadtarch** 1971;11:107–14
**Gerichter CB** see **Goldblum N**
**Gericke D:** '100 Jahre Dienst am Menschen'. Meilensteine der Pharma-Hoechst. **Fortschr Med** 1984 May 24;102(20):75–7
**Gerish AG:** P. P. Kashchenko: 1859–1920. Moskva, Meditsina, 1980. 77 p.
**Gerlach J:** Hartwig Kuhlenbeck--60 Jahre vergleichend neuroanatomische Forschung. **J Hirnforsch** 1979;20(2):107–13
**Gerlach J:** Perspectives in international neurosurgery: neurosurgery in West Germany. **Neurosurgery** 1982 Jun;10(6 Pt 1):785–7
**Gerlach LP:** The flea and the elephant: infant formula controversy. **Society** 1980;17(6):51–7
**Germain CP:** Nursing the dying: implications of Kübler-Ross' staging theory. **Ann Am Acad Polit Soc Sci** 1980;447:46–58
**Germain J, Solís J:** José Miguel Sacristán (1887–1956). **Arch Neurobiol (Madr)** 1982 Jul–Aug;45(4):299–319
**Germanov GP:** Opyt évakuatsii ranenykh i bol'nykh rechnym transportom v gody Velikoĭ Otechestvennoĭ voĭny. **Voen Med Zh** 1983 Sep;9:9–11
**Gerngross R:** Ein bayerischer Arzt in China. **MMW** 1980 Jan 25;122(4):141–2
**Gersdorff M:** Evolution des techniques d'audiométrie objective de 1970 à 1980. **Acta Otorhinolaryngol Belg** 1981;35(3-4):274–80
**Gershenowitz H:** Chauncey Wright's views on Lamarck. **Indian J Hist Sci** 1979, reçu 1982:14(1):16–24
**Gershenowitz H:** Gavin De Beer and the Neo-Lamarckians. **Indian J Hist Sci** 1978, reçu 1982;13(1):23–7
**Gershenowitz H:** George Gaylord Simpson and Lamarck. **Indian J Hist Sci** 1978, reçu 1982;13(1):56–61
**Gershenowitz H:** George Henslow: true Darwinist. **Indian J Hist Sci** 1979, reçu 1982;14(1):25–30
**Gershenowitz H:** Napoleon and Lamarck. **Indian J Hist Sci** 1980;15:204–9
**Gershenowitz H:** The influence of Lamarckism on the development of Freud's psychoanalytic theory. **Indian J Hist Sci** 1979 Nov;14(2):105–13
**Gershenowitz H:** The treatment of Lamarckism as found in forty-one college textbooks. **Indian J Hist Sci** 1978, reçu 1982;13(2):144–50
**Gershon ES:** The historical context of Franz Kallmann and psychiatric genetics. **Arch Psychiatr Nervenkr** 1981;229(4):273–6
**Gershon S** see **Georgotas A**
**Gershon S** see **Kelwala S**
**Gerstein DR:** Cultural action and heroin addiction. **Sociol Inq** 1981;51(3-4):355–70
**Gersuny C:** New England mill casualties: 1890–1910. **N Engl Q** 1979;52(4):467–82
**Gerszten E** see **Allison MJ**
**Gerton MI** see **Gravitz MA**
**Gervin AS, Fischer RP:** Resuscitation of trauma patients with type-specific uncrossmatched blood. **J Trauma** 1984 Apr;24(4):327–31
**Gerweck U:** Die Huf- und Hufeisensammlung des Instituts für Tiermedizin und Tier-hygiene mit Tierklinik der Universität Hohenheim, zugleich ein Rückblick auf die historische Entwicklung des Hufeisens. Diss. Hannover, 1979. 139p.
**Gerwel T:** Słuzba zdrowia Marynarki Wojennej w konspiracji 1941–1945. **Przegl Lek** 1981;38(1):92–5
**Gerwel T:** Słuzba zdrwia w obronie Wybrzeza w r. 1939. **Przegl Lek** 1981;38(1):80–92
**Geschichte der Tuberkulose - philatelistisch illustriert: MMW** 1982 Apr 23;124(16):92–3
**Geselvich AM:** Letopis' zhizni N.I. Pirogova, 1810–1881. Moskva, Meditsina, 1976. 97 p.
**Gęsicka T** see **Sobień-Kopczyńska S**
**Gestewitz HR, Steiner ER, et al:** Historische Entwicklung und Charakteristik der Militärmedizin. In their: Militärmedizin: Hochschullehrbuch für Studenten der Medizin und Stomatologie. 2. Auflage. Berlin, Militärverlag der Deutschen Demokratischen Republik, 1981. p. 13–49.
**Gettings F:** Dictionary of occult, hermetic and alchemical sigils. London, Routledge & Kegan Paul, 1981. 410 p.
**Getty IA** see **Rasporich AW**
**Getz FM:** Anatomia del medioevo. **Kos** 1984 May;1(4):33–46
**Getz FM:** Gilbertus Anglicus anglicized. **Med Hist** 1982 Oct;26(4):436–42
**Geus A** see **Sajner J**
**Geus A, ed** see **Wimmel B**
**Geuter U:** Die Professionalisierung der deutschen Psychologie im Nationalsozialismus. Frankfurt am Main, Suhrkamp, 1984. 592 p.
**Geuter U, Mattes P:** Historiography of psychology in West Germany: approaches from social history. A review of the past ten years. **Stor Crit Psicol** 1984 Jun;5(1):111–26
**Gevitz N:** The D.O.'s Osteopathic medicine in America. Baltimore, London, Johns Hopkins University Press, 1982. x, 183 p.
**Gewargis AA:** Gynäkologisches aus dem Kamil as-Sina a At Tibbiya des Ali ibn Al-Abbas Al-Magusi. Die Abschnitte über Anatomie, Pathologie und konservative Therapie des nichtschwangeren Uterus. Diss. Erlangen-Nürnberg, 1980. 153 p.
**Geyman JP:** The Oslerian tradition and changing medical education: a reappraisal. **West J Med** 1983 Jun;138(6):884–8
**Geymonat M, ed:** Scholia in Nicandri Alexipharmaca, cum glossis. Milan, Cisalpino-Goliardica, 1974. 218 p.
**Ghalioungui P:** A naval physician in ancient Egypt. In International Congress of the History of Medicine, 27th, Barcelona, 1980. Actas.

Barcelona, Académia de Ciències Médiques de Catalunya i Balears, 1981. p. 373–5.
**Ghalioungui P:** Four landmarks of Egyptian cardiology. **J R Coll Physicians Lond** 1984 Jul;18(3):182–6
**Ghalioungui P:** Hunayn Ibn Ishaq, translator and medical writer. In International Congress of the History of Medicine, 27th, Barcelona, 1980. Actas. Barcelona, Académia de Ciències Médiques de Catalunya i Balears, 1981. p. 245–8.
**Ghalioungui P:** Medical services throughout Egyptian history. In: Congrès international d'histoire de la médecine, XXVe, Québec, 1976. Actes. Québec, 1977. p. 161–69.
**Ghalioungui P:** The last day of Psametik, physician to Pharoah. A tale. **Trans Stud Coll Physicians Phila** 1980 Jun;5(2 no 2):90–111
**Ghalioungui P:** The persistence and spread of some obstetric concepts held in ancient Egypt. **Ann Serv Antiq Egypte** 1977;62:141–54
**Ghalioungui P** see **Hunayn Ibn Ishak, al-Ibadi**
**Ghalioungui [:** On the necessity of medical-archaeological cooperation. In: Congrès international d'histoire de la médecine, XXVe, Québec, 1976. Actes. Québec, 1977. p. 699–705.
**Gheorghiţă I** see **Cotrău M**
**Gheorghiu E:** Opinions on old pharmacopeias integration into modern therapy. **Sante Publique (Bucur)** 1984;27(1):83–8
**Gheorghiu E** see **Brătescu C**
**Gheorghiu E** see **Brătescu G**
**Gheorghiu T** see **Munteanu A**
**Ghiselin MT** see **Mayr E**
**Ghoneim M:** Antoine-Barthelemy Clot créateur de l'école de médecine. **Cah Hist** 1969;11:125–36
**Giacinto M:** A modern anaesthesia kialakuklása, jelene és perspektívái. **Orv Hetil** 1979 Oct 28;120(43):2593–7
**Gialas A** see **Dimopoulos C**
**Giampalmo A:** Patologia renale. Riferimenti e riflessioni. **Pathologica** 1983 Sep–Oct;75(1039):607–18
**Giannattasio ME, Nencini R:** Il mito jacksoniano. **Stor Crit Psicol** 1982 Dec;3(2):315–27
**Gibbons LK:** La investigación en enfermería: un campo interdisciplinario. **Educ Med Salud** 1980;14(1):76–94
**Gibbons RW:** Chiropractic in America: the historical conflicts of cultism and science. **J Pop Cult** 1977;10:720–31
**Gibbons RW:** Forgotten parameters of general practice: the chiropractic obstetrician. **Chiropr Hist** 1982;2(1):27–33
**Gibbons RW:** Physician-chiropractors: medical presence in the evolution of chiropractic. **Bull Hist Med** 1981 Summer;55(2):233–45
**Gibbons RW:** Solon Massey Langworthy: keeper of the flame during the 'lost years' of chiropractic. **Chiropr Hist** 1981;1(1):15–21
**Gibbs RC:** Portrait of a dermatologist as an artist. **Am J Dermatopathol** 1984 Feb;6(1):73–9
**Gibelli A:** Emarginati e classi lavoratrici: le ragioni di un nodo storiografico. **Mov Operaio Soc** 1980;3(4):361–7
**Gibelli A:** La guerra laboratorio: eserciti e igiene sociale verso la guerra totale. **Mov Operaio Soc** 1982;5(3):335–49
**Gibert C** see **Bacin F**
**Gibson HB:** Pain and its conquest. London, Boston, Peter Owen, 1982. 224 p.
**Gibson HL:** The Biological Photographic Association, its half century. The era of maturation, 1965–1980. **J Biol Photogr** 1980 Apr;48(2):41–86
**Gibson II:** Illness of Dorothy Wordsworth. **Br Med J [Clin Res]** 1982 Dec 18–25;285(6357):1813–5
**Gibson JR:** Smallpox on the Northwest Coast. **BC Stud** 1982–83;(56):61–81
**Gibson ME:** The identification of kala azar and the discovery of Leishmania donovani. **Med Hist** 1983 Apr;27(2):203–13
**Gibson R:** Little grains of sand. **Br Med J [Clin Res]** 1981 Dec 19;283(6307):1647–50
**Gibson R:** The family doctor: his life and history. London, Boston, Allen & Unwin, 1981. xv, 214 p.
**Gibson SS:** Scientific societies and exchange: a facet of the history of scientific communication. **J Libr Hist** 1982 Spring;17(2):144–63
**Gibson T:** The Royal College of Physicians and Surgeons of Glasgow: a short history based on the portraits and other memorabilia. Edinburgh, Macdonald Publishers, 1983. 301 p.
**Gibson WC:** Oxford revisited. **JAMA** 1980 Aug 8;244(6):577–9
**Gibson WC:** Some British contributors to cortical localization. In Rose FC, Bynum WF, ed: Historical aspects of neurosciences. New York, Raven, 1982. p. 109–13.
**Gibson WC:** The cost of not doing medical research. **JAMA** 1980 Oct 17;244(16):1817–9
**Gibson WC** see **Eccles JC**
**Gibson WP:** The operating microscope and the development of ear surgery. **J R Soc Med** 1980 Jan;73(1):53–5
**Gichlhorn R:** Eine Episode aus S. Freuds Mittelschulzeit. **Unsere Heimat** 1965;36(1–3):18–24
**Gichon M:** Roman baths, Erets, Israel. (Heb) **Qadmoniot** 1978;11(2–3):37–53
**Gicklhorn R, Göpfert W, Müller I, et al:** Bemerkungen zur Geschichte und Ikonographie des Drachenbaumes. **Dtsch Apoth Ztg** 1980 Jul 3;120(27):1260–6
**Gidney RD, Millar WP:** The origins of organized medicine in Ontario, 1850–1869. In Roland CG, ed: Health, disease and medicine. Toronto, Hannah Institute for the History of Medicine, 1894. p. 65–95.
**Giebel A:** Drei Generationen Constantini als Hofapotheker in Rotenburg a. d. Fulda. **Hess Familienkd** 1977;13:445–8
**Giebel G, Rimpler M:** Klebungen am Skellettsystem: Klebstoffe, 50 Jahre Hilfsstoffe für den Chirurgen (Teil 1). **Biomed Tech (Berlin)** 1981 Mar;26(3):35–40
**Giedke A:** Die Liebeskrankheit in der Geschichte der Medizin. Diss., Universität Düsseldorf, Düsseldorf, 1983. 205 p.
**Gieger G:** Schwachsinnigenfürsorge und Hilfe für das geistig behinderte Kind. Eine Analyse der 'Zeitschrift für das Idiotenwesen' (1880–1934). Freiburg, Schulz, 1977. 245 p. (Freiburger Forschungen zur Medizingeschichte, Neue Folge, 6).
**Gielen JE, Laduron P, Lapière CM:** Receptors in classical pharmacology and cell biology. A report of a symposium held on the occasion of the 25th anniversary of the first publication of Biochemical Pharmacology. **Biochem Pharmacol** 1983 Dec 15;32(24):3891–2
**Gielow V:** Daniel David Palmer: rediscovering the frontier years, 1845–1887. **Chiropr Hist** 1981;1(1):11–3
**Gierek T, Namysłowski G, Kondracka E:** Nowotwory złośliwe ucha leczone w i klinice ORL Śląskiej Akademii Medycznej w okresie od 1967 do 1977 r. **Otolaryngol Pol** 1980;34(1):11–6
**Giese C** see **Benedum J**
**Giese KP** see **Semm K**
**Giesinger A:** Conditions in the Volga region 1919–1922. **J Am Hist Soc Ger Russ** 1982;5(1):7–10
**Gifford G** see **Wallace ER**
**Gifford GE:** A medical tour of Boston. **JAMA** 1981 May 15;245(19):1931–5
**Gifford GE:** James de Berty Trudeau: physician-naturalist. **Bull Hist Med** 1980 Spring;54(1):78–94
**Gifford GE:** Magdeleine of Martinique. **Int J Dermatol** 1980 Mar;19(2):107–10
**Gifford GE:** Medicine and science in early America. Being the collected essays of George Edmund Gifford, Jr., 1930–1981. Edited by Dorothy I. Lansing. Devon, Pa., Published by the friends of George E. Gifford, Jr., 1982. ix, 388 p.
**Gifford GE:** The medical botany of the New England area, 1782–1842. **Proc Camb Mass Hist Soc 1973–5** [1980];43:127–40
**Gifford GE** see **Cash P**
**Gifu Seishin Byoin:** Soritsu gojisshunenshi. Gifu, Japan, Gifu Seishin Byoin, Showa 53 nen, 1978. 283 p.
**Giglio JN:** Voluntarism and public policy between World War I and the New Deal: Herbert Hoover and the American Child Health Association. **Pres Stud Q** 1983;13(3):430–52
**Gil L, Buño W:** La medicina, los médicos y las enfermedades en el epistolario de Manuel Marti. **Med Esp** 1980;79:261–72
**Gilbert AN:** Conceptions of homosexuality and sodomy in Western history. **J Homosex** 1980–81 Fall-Winter;6(1–2):57–68
**Gilbert AN:** Masturbation and insanity: Henry Maudsley and the ideology of sexual repression. **Albion** 1980;12(3):268–82
**Gilbert AN:** Sodomy and the law in eighteenth- and early nineteenth-century Britain. **Societas** 1978;8(3):225–41
**Gilbert B:** The cry was: go west, young man, and stay healthy. **Smithsonian** 1983;13(12):138–49
**Gilbert DL:** The first documented description of mountain sickness: the Andean or Pariacaca story. **Respir Physiol** 1983 Jun;52(3):327–47
**Gilbert DL:** The first documented report of mountain sickness: the China or Headache Mountain story. **Respir Physiol** 1983 Jun;52(3):315–26
**Gilbert GN, Mulkay M:** Warranting scientific belief. **Soc Stud Sci** 1982 Aug 3;12(3):383–408
**Gilbert R:** La nouvelle morale sociale et l'état surveillant. In: Congrès international d'histoire de la médecine, XXVe, Québec, 1976. Actes. Québec, 1977. p. 171–92.
**Gilbert SF, Greenberg JP:** Intellectual traditions in the life sciences. II. Stereocomplementarity. **Perspect Biol Med** 1984 Autumn;28(1):18–34
**Gilbert SF:** Owen's vertebral archetype and evolutionary genetics -- a Platonic appreciation. **Perspect Biol Med** 1980 Spring;23(3):475–88
**Gilbo PF:** Candid 'cranky' Clara Barton gave us the Red Cross. **Smithsonian** 1981;12(2):126–42
**Gilbo PF:** The American Red Cross. The first century. New York, Harper & Row, 1981 ix, 246 p.
**Gilbrin E:** Gaston Ramon (1886–1963). Le soixantième anniversaire des anatoxines. **Hist Sci Med** 1984;18(1):53–60
**Gilbrin E:** Le docteur Paul Caujole: l'hôpital français d'Oumiah (septembre 1917 - avril 1918). **Hist Sci Med** 1980;14(2):155–64
**Gilbrin E:** Les médecins français au Sseu Tch'ouan au début du XXe siècle; l'hopital de Tch'eng Tou. **Hist Sci Med** 1982;16(3):199–204
**Gilbrin E:** Les médecins français au Sseu Tch'ouan au début du XXe siècle; l'hôpital de Tch'eng Tou. **Hist Sci Med** 1983;17(1):105–10
**Gilbrin E:** Les médecins français au Sseu Tch'ouan au début du XXe siècle; l'hôpital de Tch'ong King. **Hist Sci Med** 1982;16(2):125–30
**Gilbrin E** see **Bolzinger R**
**Gilbrin E** see **Hillemand P**
**Gilbrin E** see **Histoire culturelle de la maladie**
**Gilchrist LD, Schinke SP:** Teenage pregnancy and public policy. **Soc Serv Rev** 1983;57(2):307–22
**Gildea M** see **Wallace ER**
**Gilder SB:** A Norwegian centenary. **Tidsskr Nor Laegeforen** 1981 Jan;101(1):70–1
**Gilder SS:** Leipoldt the editor. **S Afr Med J** 1980 Dec 6;58(23):926–32
**Gilder SS:** Mavericks in medicine. **S Afr Med J** 1984 Aug 18;66(7):252–5
**Gilder SS:** South African medicine in the 1880s. **S Afr Med J** 1984 Aug 18;66(7):247–9
**Gilder SS:** South African medicine in the 1890s. **S Afr Med J** 1983 Jun 29;Spec No:4–7
**Gilder SS:** South African patients and their diseases in the 1880s.

S Afr Med J 1984 Aug 18;66(7):250–2

**Gilderdale S** see **Levine HM**

**Gilgen AR:** American psychology since World War II. A profile of the discipline. Westport, Connecticut, London, Greenwood Press, 1982. xiii, 272 p.

**Gill D:** Quest, the life of Elisabeth Kübler-Ross. New York, Harper & Row, 1980. xiv, 329 p.

**Gill D:** The dueling doctors of Stockton. **Pac Hist** 1981;25(1):52–8

**Gill M:** Smallpox. **Midwife Health Visit Community Nurse** 1982 Nov;18(11):491–2

**Gill MM:** David Rapaport. In Dictionary of American Biography, Suppl. 6, 1956–1960. p. 526–8, 1980.

**Gillespie B, Eva D, Johnston R:** Carcinogenic risk assessment in the United States and Great Britain: the case of Aldrin/Dieldrin. **Soc Stud Sci** 1979;9(3):265–301

**Gillespie JS:** Antagonists of alpha adrenoceptors and adrenergic transmission. **Bull Mem Acad R Med Belg** 1982;137 Suppl:45–55

**Gillespie RR:** The early development of the scientific movement in Australian education - child study. **Anzhes J** 1982;11(2):1–14

**Gillespie SA:** Childbirth in the 1980s: what are the options? **Issues Health Care Women** 1981 Mar–Apr;3(2):101–28

**Gillett MC:** Medicine in the United States in the late eighteenth century. In Medical-Science colloquium. Special edition of Topic: a journal of the liberal arts. Washington, Pennsylvania, Washington and Jefferson College, 1983. p. 13–25.

**Gillett MC:** The Army Medical Department 1775–1818. Washington, Center of Military History, U. S. Army, 1981. xiii, 299 p.

**Gillett MC:** Thomas Lawson, second Surgeon General of the U. S. Army: a character sketch. **Prologue J Nat Arch** 1982 Spring;14(1):15–24

**Gilliand E:** The legalization of chiropractic in the state of Louisiana. **North La Hist Assoc J** 1981;12(2–3):104–10

**Gillibert J** see **Anzieu D**

**Gillies K:** Out of the past. Diamond jubilee 1909–1984. **Fla Nurse** 1984 Sep;32(9):4, 12

**Gilliland M:** The FMA Auxilliary––a half century of progress and accomplishment. **J Fla Med Assoc** 1981 Mar;68(3):166–8

**Gillingham FJ:** The influence of Harvey Cushing on British and European neurosurgery. **Surg Neurol** 1982 May;17(5):344–9

**Gilly C:** Zwischen Erfahrung und Spekulation. Theodor Zwinger und die religiöse und kulturelle Krise seiner Zeit. **Basler Z Gesch Altertumskd** 1977;77:57–137

**Gilman SC:** Degeneracy and race in the nineteenth century: the impact of clinical medicine. **J Ethn Stud** 1983;10(4):27–50

**Gilman SL:** Den Geisteskranken sehen: Mackenzie, Kleist, William James. **Confin Psychiatr** 1979;22(3):127–44

**Gilman SL:** Freud and the prostitute: male stereotypes of female sexuality in fin-de-siècle Vienna. **J Am Acad Psychoanal** 1981 Jul;9(3):337–60

**Gilman SL:** Madness and racial theory in I. J. Singer's The family Carnovsky. **Mod Jud** 1981;1(1):90–100

**Gilman SL:** Seeing the insane: a cultural history of madness and art in the western world, showing how the portrayal of stereotypes has both reflected and shaped the perception and treatment of the mentally disturbed. New York, Wiley; Brunner/Mazel, 1982. xiii, 241 p.

**Gilman SL:** The Nietzsche murder case. **New Lit Hist** 1983;14(2):359–72

**Gilman SL:** Zur Physiognomie des Geisteskranken in Geschichte und Praxis, 1800–1900. **Sudhoffs Arch** 1978;62(3):209–34

**Gilmore WJ:** Media resources available for teaching psychohistory. **Group Psychol Hist Newsl** 1975;3(4):15–20

**Gilson AG:** A group of Roman surgical and medical instruments from Cramond, Scotland. **Medizinhist J** 1983;18(4):384–93

**Ginalska A:** 35 lat minełо. Szkole Pielegniarstwa w Chełmie. **Pieleg Polozna** 1984;(4):26–8

**Ginesta V** see **Franco Grande A**

**Ginesta Galán F** see **Franco Grande A**

**Gineste T, Postel J:** J. M. G. Itard et l'enfant connu sous le nom de 'sauvage de l'Aveyron'. **Psychiatr Enfant** 1980;23(1):251–307

**Gineste T:** Naissance de la psychiatrie de l'enfant. De l'idiotie aux psychoses infantiles. **Soins Psychiatr** 1982 Feb;(16):21–6

**Gineste T:** Une histoire de la psychiatrie de l'enfant. Janvier 1800 - novembre 1800: Découverte d'une 'créature très intéressante', l'enfant connu sous le nom de Sauvage de l'Aveyron. Mém. pour le diplôme de psychiatrie. Univ. de Paris XI, 1977. 233 p, 8 n.p.

**Gineste T:** Victor de L'Aveyron: dernier enfant sauvage, premier enfant fou. Paris, Le Sycomore, 1981. 327 p.

**Gingerich PD:** Dental and cranial adaptations in Eocene Adapidae. **Z Morphol Anthropol** 1980;71(2):135–42

**Gingold N:** Data concerning the foundation of the Romanian Society of Hematology. **Med Interne** 1981 Jan–Mar;19(1):99–100

**Ginneken J van:** Bacteriological warfare. **J Contemp Asia** 1977;7(2):130–52

**Ginott N** see **Winter ST**

**Ginsberg CA** see **Hammel EA**

**Ginzberg E:** How many physicians are enough? **Ann Am Acad Polit Soc Sci** 1983;(468)::205–15

**Ginzberg E:** The public stake in health policy. **J Med Soc NJ** 1979 Aug;76(9):599–601

**Ginzburg C:** Morelli, Freud and Sherlock Holmes: clues and scientific method. **Hist Workshop J** 1980;9:5–36

**Giordano A:** Morgagni and the first steps of a European pathology. A brief historical report. **Pathol Res Pract** 1984 Jul;178(6):642–3

**Giorgino R:** Nicola Pende: medico, ricercatore, maestro. **G Clin Med** 1981 Nov;62(11):747–57

**Giovanni Alessandro Brambilla nella cultura medica del Settecento Europeo:** Milano, Istituto Editoriale Cisalpino–La Goliardica, 1980. 371 p.

**Giran Irueste F:** La medicina practica en la España arabe del siglo XII: El 'Kitab al-Yami fi-l-asriba wa-l-Ma ayin de Abu Marwan abd al-Malik ibn Zuhr (Avenzoar). Edicion, traduccion y comentarios. Resumen of Diss. 209. Granada, 1978. 33 p.

**Girard A, Roussel L:** Ideal family size, fertility, and population policy in Western Europe. **Popul Dev Rev** 1982;8(2):323–45

**Girard A:** Le nouveau régime démographique et la crise des valeurs. **Etudes (Fr)** 1979;350(1):7–23

**Girard DE:** The history of Osler's Principles and practice of medicine. **Med Times** 1981 Jul;109(7):1s–4s, 13s

**Girard LJ:** Contributions to ophthalmology by contact lens research and development. **Contact Intraocular Lens Med J** 1982 Apr–Jun;8(2):77–80

**Girard P:** Geschichte der Neurologie. In Sournia JC, Martiny M, Poulet J, ed: Illustrierte Geschichte der Medizin. Salzburg, Andreas, 1980. Vol. 3. p. 1125–88.

**Girard P:** Toxiques et poisons dans le passé pharmaceutique de la Savoie. **Rev Hist Pharm (Paris)** 1983 Sep;30(258):177–90

**Girard P:** Toxiques et poisons dans le passé pharmaceutique de la Savoie. **Rev Hist Pharm (Paris)** 1983 Dec;71(30):287–95

**Girard R:** Force et tension psychologique selon Pierre Janet. **Schweiz Arch Neurol Neurochir Psychiatr** 1981;128(1):33–51

**Girardot NJ:** Taoism [and the history of Chinese medicine]. In Reich WT, et al, ed: Encyclopedia of bioethics, v.4. New York, Free Press, 1978. p. 1631–8.

**Girden E:** Conditioning decorticate canines in Culler's laboratory: some reflexions and second thoughts. **Am J Psychol** 1983 Summer;96(2):243–52

**Girdwood RH:** Developments in therapeutics in the past fifty years. **Scott Med J** 1981 Jan;26(1):53–8

**Girdwood RH:** Doctors, pharmacists and the public. In Passmore R, ed: Proceedings of the Royal College of Physicians of Edinburgh Tercentenary Congress, 1981. Edinburgh, Royal College of Physicians of Edinburgh, 1982. p. 190–8.

**Girdwood RH:** The Royal Infirmary of Edinburgh 1729–1979. Its influence on medicine overseas. **Scott Med J** 1979 Apr;24(2):154–8

**Girdwood RH:** Three hundred years of the Royal College of Physicians of Edinburgh. **Br Med J [Clin Res]** 1981 Sep 5;283(6292):651–4

**Girin VN:** Sokrovishchnitsa meditsinskikh znaniĭ (k 50-letiiu Respublikanskoĭ nauchnoĭ meditsinskoĭ biblioteki imeni D. I. Ul'ianova). **Vrach Delo** 1980 Jul;(7):1–4

**Girod C:** Die Geschichte der Histologie. In Sournia JC, Martiny M, Poulet J, ed: Illustrierte Geschichte der Medizin. Salzburg, Andreas, 1980. Vol. 5. p. 1877–937.

**Girod C:** Geschichte der Embryologie. In Sournia JC, Martiny M, Poulet J, ed: Illustrierte Geschichte der Medizin. Salzburg, Andreas, 1980. Vol. 5. p. 1939–87.

**Giron F:** Nota sobre un supuesto hospital arabe en Algeciras. **Llull (Spain)** 1978;2:113–5

**Girón Irueste F:** En torno al Maristan (hospital arabe) de Granada. **Asclepio** 1978–79;30–31:223–31

**Girón Irueste F:** Los medicos mozarabes y el proceso de constitucion de la medicina arabe en al-Andalus. Siglos VIII–X. **Asclepio** 1978–79;30–31:209–22

**Girón Irueste F** see **Pena Munoz C**

**Gironella i Coll J** see **Gelabert i Mas A**

**Girre L:** La médecine par les plantes, à travers les âges. Rennes, Ouest-France. 1981, 187 p.

**Girstenbrey W:** Robert Koch und sein Erbe. Bedingungen, Konsequenzen und aktuelle Bedeutung einer historischen Leistung für Medizin und Gesundheitspolitik. **Fortschr Med** 1982 Mar 25;100(12):541, 544–6

**Girstenbrey W:** Soll und Haben eines pharmazeutischen Evergreens. **Fortschr Med** 1983 Jul 28;101(27–28):1294–7

**Gish O:** The political economy of primary care and 'health by the people': an historical explanation. **Issue** 1979 Fall;9:6–13

**Gish O:** The political economy of primary care and 'health by the people': an historical exploration. **Soc Sci Med** 1979 Dec;13C(4):203–11

**Gitelman Z:** Poriyut hayehudim bivrit hamo'atsot. **Shvut (Israel)** 1977;5:7–20

**Gittings CL:** Arizona's reputation as a health spa. **Ariz Med** 1983 Mar;40(3):150–3

**Gittings R:** Edward Osler and John Keats. In J. Cule, ed: Wales and medicine. London, British Society for the History of Medicine, 1975. p. 107–11.

**Gittings R:** Keats and medicine. **Contemp Rev** 1971;219(1268):138–42

**Giuffré R:** Successful radical removal of an intracranial meningioma in 1835 by Professor Pecchioli of Siena. **J Neurosurg** 1984 Jan;60(1):47–51

**Giuffrè R** see **Guidetti B**

**Giulio L:** Un tema ricorrente nello Zibaldone: la memoria. **Stor Crit Psicol** 1982 Jun;3(1):27–40

**Giunchi G** see **Epistemologia, metodologia clinica e storia della scienza medica, 1**

**Giura V:** Note sulle caratteristiche demografiche della comunità Ebraica di Napoli nel '700. **Genus** 1979;35(1–2):259–63

**Giusberti F:** Tra povertà e malattia: il Sant'Orsola a Bologna dal XVII al XVIII secolo. **Ann Fond Luigi Einaudi** 1979;13:117–50

**Giuseppe Capailla D:** El psiquiatra frente a los derechos del hombre. **An R Acad Nac Med (Madr)** 1981;98(3):463–72

**Giusti GV:** Leone Lattes: Italy's pioneer in forensic serology. **Am J Forensic Med Pathol** 1982 Mar;3(1):79–81

**Giustini PA:** Museografia e storia del pensiero scientifico. **Med Secoli**

1982;19(3):265-71

**Given FT:** Dr. John Pott: maligned early patriot. **Am J Obstet Gynecol** 1983 Sep 15;147(2):115-20

**Gizella M:** Termékenységi vizsgálat három generáción keresztül a Mezökövesdi népességben. **Demografia** 1980;23(4):370-96

**Gladfelter BG** see **Singer R**

**Gladkikh PF, Galin LL:** K istorii teoreticheskoi razrabotki sistemy étapnogo lecheniia ranenykh i bol'nykh. **Voen Med Zh** 1984 May;(5):74-5

**Gladkikh PF:** Meditsinskoe obespechenie 2-ĭ udarnoĭ armii v period proryva blokady Leningrada. **Voen Med Zh** 1981 Feb;(2):71-3

**Gladkikh PF:** Ob évakuatsii ranenykh i bol'nykh iz gospital'noĭ bazy Leningradskogo fronta v period polnoĭ blokady Leningrada. **Voen Med Zh** 1983 Feb;(2):70-3

**Gladkikh PF:** Perestroĭka sistemy podgotovki voenno-meditsinskikh kadrov v tridtsatye gody. **Voen Med Zh** 1983 Sep;9:70-2

**Gladkikh PF:** Rabota psikhiatricheskikh uchrezhdeniĭ v Leningrade vo vremia blokady. **Zh Nevropatol Psikhiatr** 1980;80(5):760-1

**Gladkikh PF:** Zabota M. I. Kutuzova o zdorov'e Russkogo soldata (k 170-letiiu so dnia Borodinskogo srazheniia). **Sov Zdravookhr** 1983;(3):68-70

**Gladstein GA:** The historical roots of contemporary empathy research. **J Hist Behav Sci** 1984 Jan;20(1):38-59

**Gladstone W:** Early medical photography in America (1839-1883); VI. Civil war medical photography. **NY State J Med** 1981 Jan;81(1):5, 8

**Gladwin LA:** Tobacco and sex: some factors affecting nonmarital sexual behavior in colonial Virginia. **J Soc Hist** 1978;12(1):57-75

**Gładykowska-Rzeczycka J:** Dislocation of the hip joint (probably congenital) in the woman from the mediaeval burial ground in Poland. **Folia Morphol (Warsz)** 1980;39(2):211-4

**Glandien O:** Franz Xaver Messerschmidt (1736-1783) - Ausdrucksstudien und Charakterköpfe, Köln: 1981. 205 p. (Kölner medizinhistorische Beiträge: Arbeiten der Forschungsstelle des Instituts für Geschichte der Medizin der Universität zu Köln, Band 20).

**Glantz LH:** The role of personhood in treatment decisions made by courts. **Milbank Mem Fund Q** 1983 Winter;61(1):76-100

**Glanville VJ:** British books on tropical medicine. **Br Book News** 1980 Nov;:645-9

**Glas E:** Chemistry and physiology in their historical and philosophical relations. Delft, Delft University Press, 1979. 199 p.

**Glaser FB:** Samuel Johnson: sometimes abstemious, always intemperate. **J Addict Res Found** 1981;10(9):11

**Glaser FB:** The origins of the drug-free therapeutic community. **Br J Addict** 1981 Mar;76(1):13-25

**Glaser S:** L'arma batteriologica secondo la convenzione 1971. **Riv Mil** 1975;98(4):56-62

**Glass B:** A hidden chapter of German eugenics between the two world wars. **Proc Am Philos Soc** 1981;125(5):357-67

**Glass B:** The preservation of historical materials in genetics. **Bull Hist Med** 1983;57(1):98-105

**Glass E:** Chemistry and physiology in their historical and philosophical relations. Delft, Delft University Press, 1979. xiii, 199 p.

**Glass H:** [The Canadian nursing scene] (Jpn). **Kango** 1984 Jul;36(8):11-9

**Glassberg D:** The design of reform: the public bath movement in America. **Am Stud** 1979;20(2):5-21

**Glatzel J:** Die Psychopathologie Karl Jaspers' in der Kritik. **Nervenarzt** 1984 Jan;55(1):10-7

**Glatzel J** see **Janzarik W ed**

**Glaus B:** Autographen und Manuskripte zur ETH- und zur Wissenschaftsgeschichte. **Gesnerus** 1982;39(3-4):437-42

**Glavchev P:** Pogled vŭrkhu istoriiata na Druzhestvoto na internistite v Bŭlgariia (po sluchaĭ 50 godini ot osnovavaneto mu). **Vutr Boles** 1984;23(2):140-3

**Glazer I:** A brief history of the Israel Society of Aerospace Medicine--a 1981 affiliate of the Aerospace Medical Association. **Aviat Space Environ Med** 1983 Apr;54(4):371-2

**Glazer J:** Ancestors. **J Am Dent Assoc** 1984 Jul;109(1):17

**Gleason ML:** The Royal Society of London: years of reform, 1827-1847. Ph.D. Diss. Harvard University. Cambridge, Mass. 1979.

**Glendinning V:** A gentle probe into dentistry 1770-1970. **Dent Tech** 1980 Feb;33(2):9-12

**Glendon MA** see **Fox VC**

**Glenn J:** 'The open-air closet'. **Am J Psychoanal** 1980 Summer;40(2):165-8

**Glenn ND, Weaver CN:** Education's effects on psychological well-being. **Public Opin Q** 1981;45(1):22-39

**Glenn WW:** Some account of the early years of cardiac surgery. **Conn Med** 1980 Jun;44(6):338-44

**Glenn WW:** The lymphatic system. Some surgical considerations. **Arch Surg** 1981 Aug;116(8):989-95

**Glenn J, ed** see **Kanzer M**

**Glenn J, ed., et al** see **Kanzer M**

**Glesinger L:** Der Humanist Andreas Dudith im Kreise der Antiparacelsisten. Wien, 1967. (Salzburger Beiträge zur Paracelsusforschung, 7). p. 3-12.

**Glesinger L:** Der Ursprung der Pestepidemien und deren Vorbeugungsmethoden im Alten Dubrovnik. In Radovi sa Medunarodnog simpozija u povodu sestote obljetnice Dubrovacke karantene. Dubrovnik, 29 i 30. rujna 1977. Zagreb, 1980. p. 93-102.

**Glesinger L:** Medicine in old Dubrovnik. In Veteris ragusae medicina et pharmacia. Zagreb, PLIVA, n.d. p. 35-48.

**Glesinger L:** Povijest kirurgije u Hrvatskoj do sredine XIX stoljeća. **Acta Chir Iugosl** 1967;14:121-35

**Glesinger L:** Strani liječnici u našoj zemlji. **Saopcenja** 1978;24(3-4):275-84

**Glesinger L:** Uloga stranih liječnika i prirodoslovaca u istraživanju i suzbijanju zaraznih bolesti u Hrvatskoj. In: I simpozij o historiji mikrobiologije i imunologije u Hrvatskoj do 1923. godine. Zagreb, Jugoslavenskoj akademiji, 1973. p. 47-61.

**Glick PC** see **Spanier GB**

**Glick TF:** The naked science: psychoanalysis in Spain. **Comp Stud Soc Hist** 1982;24(4):533-71

**Glinka J** see **Rassengeschichte der Menschheit**

**Glinski J:** 70 lat walki z gruźliçą w Rudce. **Pneumonol Pol** 1980 Jul;48(7):491-2

**Gliński S, Majewska E:** Powstanie i działalność szpitala powiatowego w lasinie do roku 1945. **Arch Hist Med (Warsz)** 1984;47(2):249-68

**The global eradication of smallpox:** Final report of the Global Commission for the certification of smallpox eradication, Geneva, December 1979. Geneva, World Health Organization, 1980. 122 p.

**Głośnicka R** see **Gruszkiewicz E**

**Glover DW:** Model No. 110 Kreiselman Resuscitator. **Respir Care** 1977 Feb;22(2):203

**Glover ED** see **Christen AG**

**Glover J:** Health and disease in Birmingham, 1770-1830. **Warwickshire Hist** 1978-9;4:40-55

**Glover JL, Broadi TA:** Intraoperative autotransfusion. **Prog Clin Biol Res** 1982;108:151-70

**Głowacki WW:** Ein verlorenes pharmazeutisches Wörterbuch des siebzehnten Jahrhunderts aus Schlesien. **Pharmazie** 1983 Nov;38(11):759-61

**Głowacki WW:** Ustawy medyczne Królestwa Sycylii z lat 1140-1241. **Arch Hist Med (Warsz)** 1983;46(2):137-47

**Glowatzki G:** Das Magische im menschlichen Denken. Seine Auswirkungen auf die Medizin. **Ther Ggw** 1980 Oct;119(10):1107-28

**Glowatzki G:** Der Mesmerismus--und seine Spuren in der heutigen Medizin. **ZFA (Stuttgart)** 1983 Sep 10;59(25):1360-6

**Glowatzki G** see **Kloiber A**

**Glowatzki G** see **Ulrich-Bochsler S**

**Gluckman LK:** Abortion in the nineteenth century Maori: a historical and ethnopsychiatric review. **NZ Med J** 1981 Jun 10;93(685):384-6

**Gluckman LK:** Aspects of early medical organisation in Auckland, New Zealand. **NZ Med J** 1980 Mar 26;91(656):224-6

**Gluckman LK:** Dr. Carl Fischer MD and the history of homeopathy in Auckland in the 19th century. **NZ Med J** 1979 Jul 25;90(640):66-9

**Gluckman LK:** Dr. Carl Frank Fischer M.D.: an early Auckland physician, botanist and viticulturalist. **J Auckl Waikato Hist Soc** 1980;(37):18-20

**Glueck HI:** Twenty years of funding of research by the National Institute of Health grant 02904 entitled 'Determination of Natural Clotting Factors'. **J Am Med Wom Assoc** 1980 Jun;35(6):141-4

**Gluecksohn-Waelsch S:** Fifty years of developmental genetics. **Trans NY Acad Sci** 1983;41:243-51

**Glukhen'kiĭ TT:** Petr Vasil'evich Nikol'skiĭ (k 125-letiiu so dnia rozhdeniia). **Vestn Dermatol Venerol** 1984 Jan;(1):69-70

**Glupker DF:** The yesteryear of orthopaedic nursing (Agnes Hunt). **Orthop Nurs** 1984 Nov-Dec;3(6):48

**Glushakova TI:** Razvitie predstavleniĭ ob individual'nosti khromosom. Moskva, Nauka, 1983. 119 p.

**Glusker JP** see **Dodson G**

**Glymour C:** The theory of your dreams. In R.S. Cohen, L. Laudan, ed: Physics, philosophy and psychoanalysis. Dordrecht, D. Reidel, 1983. p. 57-71.

**Gmelin OF:** Anti-Freud: von der Psychoanalyse zur Medienwissenschaft. Mit einem Beitrag von Helene Saussure. Frankfurt am Main, Haag and Herchen, 1979. 175 p.

**Gnesda L:** Gli 'ospizi' nelle Dolomiti. Firenze, Olschki, 1979. 81 p. (Comitato dei Geografi Italiani, 4).

**Godber G:** Looking back on the NHS. **Hosp Health Serv Rev** 1979 Jan;75(1):23-4

**Godber G:** The British health system: achievements and limitations. **Isr J Med Sci** 1982 Mar;18(3):365-73

**Godber G:** The Domesday Book of British hospitals. **Soc Soc Hist Med Bull (Lond)** 1983 Jun;32:4-13

**Godber G:** The NHS in an international setting. **Health Bull (Edinb)** 1982 Mar;40(2):67-76

**Godber GE:** Sir Arthur Salusbury MacNalty. In Dictionary of national biography, 1961-1970. Suppl. 8, 1981. p. 706-7.

**Goddard CH:** A history of firearms identification to 1930. **Am J Forensic Med Pathol** 1980 Jun;1(2);155-68

**Gödde G:** Theodor Reik. In J. Rattner, ed: Wandlungen der Psychoanalyse. Wien, Europaverlag, 1980. p. 87-113.

**Godelier M** see **Dupâquier J**

**Godfrey CM:** Medicine for Ontario: a history. Belleville, Ont., Mika Pub. Co., 1979. 302 p.

**Godfrey CM:** Theophilus Mack. In Dictionary of Canadian Biography, 1881-1890. 1982;11:558-9.

**Godisen zbornik na medicinskiot fakultet vo Skopje:** **God Zb Med Fak Skopje** 1979 Jan;25:1-536

**Godlewski G:** Chopin génie asexué. **Sem Hop Paris** 1979 Dec 18-25;55(43-44):2051-63

**Godlewski G:** De l'Académie de médecine à l'Académie française. **Bull Acad Natl Med (Paris)** 1982 Mar;166(3):407-13

**Godlewski G:** Flaubert l'inassouvi. **Sem Hop Paris** 1980 Dec 18-25;56(47-68):2051-62

**Godlewski G:** Le Docteur Clemenceau. **Sem Hop Paris** 1981 Dec

18-25;57(47-48):2057-71
**Godlewski G:** Le docteur Combes, pourfendeur de l'Eglise. **Sem Hop Paris** 1982 Dec 23;58(47):2802-13
**Godlove C, Mann A:** Thirty years of the welfare state: current issues in British social policy for the aged. **Aged Care Serv Rev** 1980;2(1):1, 3-13
**Godon A** see **Lefebvre P**
**Godonnèche J:** A propos d'une thèse de médecine à Paris en 1809. In: Congrès National des Sociétés Savantes, 97e, Nantes, 1972. Comptes Rendus. Paris, 1976. Section des Sciences, Tome 1. p. 331-6.
**Godonnèche J:** La dégradation de la santé des gens de lettres d'après Tissot. In: Congrès National des Sociétés Savantes, 99e, Besançon, 1974. Comptes Rendus. Paris, 1976. Section des Sciences, Fasc. V. p. 235-41.
**Godonnèche J:** La Doulou: auto-observation d'Alphonse Daudet. **Hist Sci Med** 1981;15(4):321-5
**Godonnèche J:** Médecins hydrologues à Châtelguyon au XIXe siècle. In: Congrès National des Sociétés Savantes, 93e, Tours, 1968. Comptes Rendus. Paris, 1971. Section des Sciences, Tome II. p. 193-200.
**Godtfredsen E:** Forbraendigens forudsaetninger i medicinsk-historisk lys. **Dan Medicinhist Arbog** 1981;:142-56
**Godwin J:** Robert Fludd: hermetic philosopher and surveyor of two worlds. London, Thames and Hudson, 1979. 96 p. An annotated collection of plates from Fludds's works.
**Goedde AG:** Internal diversification and US regulatory controls in the pharmaceutical industry. **Q Rev Econ Bus** 1982;22(1):101-10
**Goergen A:** L'art de guérir et la santé publique dans le grand-duché de Luxembourg. Luxembourg, Cour Victor Buck, 1916. [5], 383 p.
**Goering JD:** Sigmund Freud, Carl Jung and religion. **Mennon Q Rev** 1982;56(1):47-56
**Goerke H:** Carl von Linné als Marinearzt (1739-1741). In Göpfert W, Otten HH, ed: Metavoeite: wandelt euch durch neues Denken. Düsseldorf, Triltsch, 1983. p. 89-94.
**Goerke H:** Grandi ospedali in Germania: ieri e oggi. **Acta Med Hist Patav** 1979-80;26:81-93
**Goerke H:** Linné und die Pharmacopoea Svecica (1775). In Dilg, P, et al., ed: Perspektiven der Pharmaziegeschichte. Graz, Austria, Akademische Druck- u. Verlagsanstalt, 1983. p. 89-96.
**Goerke H:** 150 Jahre Arztlicher Verein München. Rückschau auf Gründung, Aufgaben und Leistungen. **MMW** 1983 Oct 14;125(41):906-10
**Goerke H** see **Domandl S, ed**
**Goerke H, ed:** Berliner Aerzte. 2d ed. Berlin, Berlin Verlag, 1984. 328 p.
**Goertzel MG** see **Goertzel TG**
**Goertzel TG, Goertzel MG, Goertzel V:** Linus Pauling: the scientist as crusader. **Antioch Rev** 1980;38(3):371-82
**Goertzel V** see **Goertzel TG**
**Goethe H, Vuksanovic P:** Bei Seeleuten häufig vorkommende Erkrankungen. In Göpfert W, Otten HH, ed: Metavoeite: wandelt euch durch neues Denken. Düsseldorf, Triltsch, 1983. p. 69-78.
**Goethe H, Rodegra H:** The history of nautical medicine in Hamburg at the time of Bernhard Nocht around 1900. In International Congress of the History of Medicine, 27th, Barcelona, 1980. Actas. Barcelona, Académia de Ciències Mèdiques de Catalunya i Balears, 1981. p. 376-83.
**[Goethe Link. Includes text of two of his talks.]: Indiana Med Hist Q** 1977;3(4):63-71
**Goetz CG, Klawans HL:** Gilles de la Tourette on Tourette syndrome. **Adv Neurol** 1982;35:1-16
**Gofman VR** see **Gorokhov AA**
**Gogin EE** see **Borodulin VI**
**Gögler E:** Notarztsysteme in der Bundesrepublik Deutschland. Geschichtlicher Rückblick. **MMW** 1982 Dec 3;124(48):1083-6
**Gogun KV** see **Gordeev VI**
**Goh HH** see **Ratnam SS**
**Goic A:** 150 años de educación médica formal en Chile (1833-1983). **Rev Med Chil** 1983 Apr;111(4):343-9
**Gojunen no kaiko:** Tokyo, Do Dosokai, Showa 53 nen. [1978]. 2 v.
**Golbeck AL:** Quantification in ethnology and its appearance in regional culture trait distribution studies (1888 to 1939). **J Hist Behav Sci** 1980 Jul;16(3):225-7
**Gol'braĭkh VR:** U istokov stomatologicheskogo obrazovaniia (k 100-letiiu pervoĭ zubovrachebnoĭ shkoly v Rossii). **Stomatologiia (Mosk)** 1982 Jul-Aug;61(4):64-5
**Gol'braĭkh VR:** Velikiĭ khirurg N. I. Pirogov--osnovopolozhnik khirurgii cheliustno-litsevoĭ oblasti (k 100-letiiu so dnia smerti). **Stomatologiia (Mosk)** 1982 Jul-Aug;61(4):66-7
**Gol'braĭkh VR** see **Gruzdev NA**
**Gol'd E IU:** M. N. Solov'ev: 1886-1980. Moskva, Meditsina, 1982. 60 p.
**Gold RD:** Cardiac pacing--from then to now. **Med Instrum** 1984 Jan-Feb;18(1):15-21
**Gold SI:** Early origins of hydrogen peroxide use in oral hygiene. A historical note. **J Periodontol** 1983 Apr;54(4):247
**Gold SI:** Robert Neumann: a pioneer in periodontal flap surgery. **J Periodontol** 1982 Jul;53(7):456-9
**Gol'd EIu, Ladnyĭ ID:** S. V. Suvorov i ego rol' v istorii sovetskoĭ protivochumnoĭ organizatsii. **Zh Mikrobiol Epidemiol Immunobiol** 1979 Nov;(11):106-9
**Golda DM:** Iu. A. Filipchenko--osnovopolozhnik otechestvennoĭ genetiki (1882-1930 gg.). **Tsitol Genet** 1982;16(1):73 passim
**Golda DM, Berdyshev GD:** Prepodavanie genetiki v Kievskom universitete (k 150-letiiu KGU). **Tsitol Genet** 1984 Sep-Oct;18(5):393-4
**Goldammer K:** Neues zur Frage der Paracelsischen Spuria. **Sudhoffs Arch** 1984;68(2):235-9
**Goldammer K:** Paracelsus, Humanisten und Humanismus. Ein Beitrag zur kultur- und geistesgeschichtlichen Stellung Hohenheims. Wien, 1964. 32 p. (Salzburger Beiträge zur Paracelsusforschung, 4).
**Goldammer K:** Paracelsus in der deutschen Romantik. Eine Untersuchung zur Geschichte der Paracelsus-Rezeption und zu geistesgeschichtlichen Hintergründen der Romantik. Mit einem Anhang über die Entstehung und Entwicklung der Elementargeister-Vorstellungen seit dem Mittelalter. Wien, 1980. 212 p. (Salzburger Beiträge zur Paracelsusforschung, 20).
**Goldammer K:** Zur philosophischen und religiösen Sinngebung von Heilung und Heilmittel bei Paracelsus. In Dilg P, et al., ed: Perspektiven der Pharmaziegeschichte. Graz, Austria, Akademische Druck- u. Verlagsanstalt, 1983. p. 113-29.
**Goldammer K** see **Blaser RH**
**Goldammer K** see **Braun L, et al**
**Goldammer K** see **Domandl S, ed**
**Goldammer K** see **Habrich C**
**Goldammer K** see **Paracelsus-Forschung heute**
**Goldberg A:** A Committee on Safety of Medicines. **Health Bull (Edinb)** 1981 Nov;39(6):393-7
**Goldberg A:** Ten years of The Medicines Act. **Br J Clin Pharmacol** 1981 Oct;12(4):447-8
**Goldberg BA:** Horseshoers, doctors and judges and the law on medical competence. **Spec Law Dig Health Care (Mon)** 1980 May;2(3):3-41
**Goldberg H:** An early psychologist of the unconscious. **J Hist Ideas** 1982 Apr-Jun;43(2):269-84
**Goldberg HI, Rodrigues W, Thome AM, et al:** Infant mortality and breast-feeding in North-Eastern Brazil. **Popul Stud** 1984 Mar;38(1):105-15
**Goldberg J** see **Latimer D**
**Goldberg MF:** Cocaine: the first local anesthetic and the 'third scourge of humanity'. A centennial melodrama. **Arch Ophthalmol** 1984 Oct;102(10):1443-7
**Goldberg S** see **Brest AN**
**Goldberg A, ed:** The future of psychoanalysis. Essays in honor of Heinz Kohut. New York, International Universities Press, 1983. xx, 514 p. Contributions by A. M. Cooper, R. S. Wallerstein, W. W. Meissner, R. D. Stolorow, G. E. Atwood, A. H. Modell, R. Michels, L. Friedman, J. S. Grotstein, J. D. Lichtenberg, M. Kanzer, P. Tolpin, E. Schwaber, E. S. Wolf, B. Brandchaft, M. Tolpin, A. Ornstein, B. E. Litowitz, N. S. Litowitz, M. F. Basch, P. H. Knapp, N. J. London, C. B. Strozier.
**Goldblith SA:** Samuel Cate Prescott: - pioneer food technologist -gifted teacher. **Adv Food Res** 1981;27:1-21
**Goldblum N, Swartz T, Gerichter CB, et al:** The natural history of poliomyelitis in Israel, 1949-1982. **Prog Med Virol** 1984;29:115-23
**Golden HH** see **Wilcox J**
**Golden J, Schneider EC:** Custody and control: the Rhode Island Hospital for Mental Diseases, 1870-1970. **RI Hist** 1982;41(4):113-25
**Golden RL:** A 'forgotten' clinic of Sir William Osler. **JAMA** 1981 Feb 6;245(5):500-1
**Golden RL:** Medallic tributes to Sir William Osler and their historical associations. **JAMA** 1979 Dec 28;242(26):2862-7
**Golden RL:** Osler and Oriental medicine: a discursive review. Princeton, Science Press Associates, 1982. iii, 93 p.
**Golden RL:** Osler, 'E. Y. D.,' and hysteria. **JAMA** 1982 May 21;247(19):2698-9
**Golden J, ed** see **Merrington M**
**Goldfischer S, Janis M:** A 42-year-old king with a cavitary pulmonary lesion and intestinal perforation. **Bull NY Acad Med** 1981 Mar;57(2):139-43
**Goldhaft TM:** Historical note on the origin of the LaSota strain of Newcastle disease virus. **Avian Dis** 1980 Apr-Jun;24(2):297-301
**Goldhagen E:** Nazi sexual demonology. **Midstream** 1981;27(5):7-15
**Goldhahn WE:** Die interdisziplinären Verbindungen der Neurochirurgie in Vergangenheit, Gegenwart und Zukunft. **Zentralbl Neurochir** 1983;44(4):295-301
**Goldie I:** Progress in Sweden. **Clin Orthop** 1984 Dec;(191):2-3
**Goldin G:** A protohospice at the turn of the century: St. Luke's House, London, from 1893 to 1921. **J Hist Med Allied Sci** 1981 Oct;36(4):383-415
**Golding PS:** The development of the toothbrush. A short history of tooth cleansing. Part 1. **Dent Health (London)** 1982;21(4):25-7
**Goldman AB** see **Cone RO**
**Goldman DL, Arvanitakis K:** D. Ewen Cameron's Day Hospital and the day hospital movement. **Can J Psychiatry** 1981 Aug;26(5):365-8
**Goldman HH:** Integrating health and mental health services: historical obstacles and opportunities. **Am J Psychiatry** 1982 May;139(5):616-20
**Goldman HH** see **Morrissey JP**
**Goldman L:** Diagnostic advances v the value of the autopsy, 1912-1980. **Arch Pathol Lab Med** 1984 Jun;108(6):501-5
**Goldman L:** Portrait of an elderly woman with a nodular eruption. What was it? **Am J Dermatopathol** 1982 Aug;4(4):353
**Goldman L:** Pre-Columbian leishmaniasis. **Arch Dermatol** 1983 Jul;119(7):540
**Goldman L** see **Wright RC**
**Goldman RH** see **Reich MR**
**Goldman WD** see **Pomerantz MB**
**Goldsmith A, Edelman DA:** Métodos anticonceptivos de barrera. **Reproduccion** 1982 Jul-Dec;6(3-4):185-92
**Goldsmith WN:** Sir Archibald Montague Gray. In Dictionary of national biography, 1961-1970. Suppl. 8, 1981. p. 452-3.
**Goldstein A** see **Goldstein S**

**Goldstein HB:** Sir James Paget. **Am J Dermatopathol** 1980 Spring;2(1):27–31
**Goldstein J:** Anna Freud in law. **Psychoanal Study Child** 1984;39:3–13
**Goldstein J:** The hysteria diagnosis and the politics of anticlericalism in late nineteenth-century France. **J Mod Hist** 1982;54(2):209–39
**Goldstein LM:** The life and death of John Lambe. **Guildhall Stud Lond Hist** 1979;4(1):19–32
**Goldstein MS, Donaldson PJ:** Exporting professionalism: a case study of medical education. **J Health Soc Behav** 1979 Dec;20(4):322–37
**Goldstein PJ:** Birth asphyxia. In Smith GF, Smith PN, Vidyasagar D, ed: Historical review and recent advances in neonatal and perinatal medicine. [Chicago?], Mead Johnson Nutritional Division, 1983. Vol. I. p. 177–84.
**Goldstein PJ** see **Smith GF**
**Goldstein RL:** Sigmund Freud: forensic psychiatrist. **Bull Am Acad Psychiatry Law** 1983;11(3):273–7
**Goldstein S, Goldstein A:** The impact of migration on fertility: an 'own children' analysis for Thailand. **Popul Stud** 1981;35(2):265–84
**Goldstein-Préaud T:** Albert le Grand et les questions du XIIIe siècle sur le De animalibus d'Aristote. **Hist Philos Life Sci** 1981;3(1):61–71
**Goldsworthy BM:** The end of an era--the story of mass miniature chest radiography in the Royal Navy. **J R Nav Med Serv** 1981;67(1):32–6
**Goldwert M:** Toynbee and Jung: the historian and analytical psychology--a brief comment. **J Anal Psychol** 1983 Oct;28(4):363–6
**Goldwyn RM:** Carl August Burow. **Plast Reconstr Surg** 1984 Apr;73(4):687–90
**Goldwyn RM:** Is there plastic surgery in the Edwin Smith Papyrus? **Plast Reconstr Surg** 1982 Aug;70(2):263–4
**Goldwyn RM:** Keloid. **Plast Reconstr Surg** 1981 Oct;68(4):640–1
**Goldwyn RM:** Port wine stain. **Plast Reconstr Surg** 1980 Oct;66(4):647
**Goldwyn RM:** 'Surgeon'. **Plast Reconstr Surg** 1983 Aug;72(2):229–30
**Goldwyn RM:** The paraffin story. **Plast Reconstr Surg** 1980 Apr;65(4):517–24
**Goldwyn RM:** Transition. **Plast Reconstr Surg** 1980 Jan;65(1):70–1
**Goldzieher JW:** Estrogens in oral contraceptives: historical perspectives. **Johns Hopkins Med J** 1982 May;150(5):165–9
**Gołębiowski SZ:** Bogusław palicki, lekarz i działacz społeczny w wielkopolsce (1813–1868). **Arch Hist Med (Warsz)** 1983;46(2):249–53
**Gołebiowski SZ:** Niemiecki lekarz Jan Metzig (1804--1868) przyjacielem Polaków. **Arch Hist Med (Warsz)** 1979;42(3):295–301
**Golenkov AK, Zaslavskaia LA:** Oftal'mologiia na tselinnoĭ zemle. **Vestn Oftalmol** 1980 Mar–Apr;(2):3–4
**Golikov VIa** see **Krotkov FG**
**Golinski JV** see **Christie JR**
**Golinski JV** see **Wood PB**
**Golliet P, Binet JL:** Deux historiens du sang, ou Réponse de Lucien Lévy-Bruhl et de Wifredo Lam à Jean Bernard. **Nouv Rev Fr Hematol** 1983;25(5):337–41
**Golosov BA:** Ob organizatsii meditsinskogo obespecheniia voĭsk v bitve pod Kurskom (K 40-letiiu bitvy pod Kurskom). **Voen Med Zh** 1983 Jul;(7):17–21
**Golovin GV, Depp ME, Dutkevich IG:** Vydaiushchiĭsia sovetskiĭ khirurg i transfuziolog (k 80-letiiu so dnia rozhdeniia A. N. Filatova). **Vestn Khir** 1982 Oct;129(10):3–8
**Golovin GV** see **Uglov FG**
**Golovteev VV, Korchagin VP:** [Rates and proportions of the development of prophylactic medical care in the USSR] (Rus). **Sov Zdravookhr** 1980;12:9–13
**Goltz D** see **Schouten J**
**Goltz RW:** WWII, the 147th General hospital & Harry Arnold. **Hawaii Med J** 1982 Nov;41(11):410
**Golub S:** Coping with cancer: Freud's experiences. **Psychoanal Rev** 1981 Summer;68(2):191–200
**Golubev LV** see **Kamalov MKh**
**Gomberg ES:** Historical and political perspective: women and drug use. **J Soc Issues** 1982;38(2):9–23
**Gomberg SJ:** Colonial cultivation and concoctions. **MCVQ** 1981;16(3):113–7
**Gómez EA:** El problema del enfermo mental crónico indigente: un análisis histórico. **Acta Psiquiatr Psicol Am Lat** 1983 Sep;29(3):213–22
**Gómez EA:** El problema del liderazgo en psicoanalisis. **Rev Neuropsiquiatr** 1978 Sep–Dec;41(3–4):92–100
**Gomez JM** see **Bowers JZ**
**Gómez P, Rosado A:** Unidad de Investigación Clínica, Hospital de Oncología, Centro Médico Nacional, IMSS. **Arch Invest Med (Mex)** 1981;12(3):361–75
**Gómez Caamaño JL:** Historiographie pharmaceutique Catalane-Balear par un groupe universitaire. In: Vorträge des Internationalen Pharmaziehistorischen Kongresses Innsbruck 1977. Stuttgart, Wissenschaftliche Verlagsgesellschaft, 1979. p. 173–8.
**Gomez Caamaño JL, Rof Carballo MC:** Los boticarios catalanes de la ilustración. **Bol Soc Esp Hist Farm** 1980 Mar–Jun;3(121–2):39–50
**Gómez Caamaño JL** see **Carmona Cornet AM**
**Gómez Orozco J** see **Carrada Bravo T**
**Gómez-Santos M:** Vida de Gregorio Marañón. Esplugas de Llobregat, Plaza & Janés, 1977. 478 p.
**Gomez-Villalba Ballesteros R** see **Valverde Lopez JL**
**Gomołka B:** On the authorship of an astrologico-medical calendar for 1474. (Pol) **Biul Bibl Jagiellon** 1978;28(1–2)
**Gömöri G:** Bejegyzések Bánfihunyadi János oxfordi bibliájában és adalekok Angliai múködéséhez. **Magyar Könyvsz** 1978;94(1):93–9
**Gonçalves J:** Endocardite infecciosa. Sete décadas de evolução. **Acta Med Port** 1979 Mar–Apr;1(2):267–77
**Goncharov NI** see **Speransky LS**
**Goncharov NP** see **Klebanov IaA**
**Goncharova SG** see **Iarovinskiĭ MIa**
**Goncharuk EI** see **Borisenko NF**
**Gong Chun:** [Army medical organization of Qing Dynasty after the Opium War] (Chi). **Chin J Med Hist** 1980;10:86–9
**Gonthier N:** Les hôpitaux et les pauvres à la fin du moyen âge: l'exemple de Lyon. **Moyen Age** 1978;84:279–308
**Gonvers JJ:** L'ulcère: un passé célèbre, un avenir incertain? **Rev Med Suisse Romande** 1984 May;104(5):387–94
**González AD:** La mision de Carlos M. Ramirez al Brasil y el convenio sanitario de 1887. **Bol Acad Nac Hist (Argentina)** 1964;35:327–53
**González E** see **Tjarks G**
**González JL:** La medicina militar en la guerra del Paraguay. In Congreso de Historia de la Medicina Argentina [Transactions], 5th, Mendoza, 1983. p. 103–10.
**González-Angulo A** see **Campillo-Sainz C**
**Gónzalez Blasco P, Jiménez Blanco J, López Piñero JM:** Historia y sociología de la ciencia en España. Madrid, Alianza, 1979. 195 p.
**González Galván A:** Aspectos sociales de la lepra. **Prensa Med Mex** 1978 Sep–Oct;43(9–10):261–3
**González García M** see **Alegre Pérez E**
**Gonzalez Iglesias J:** Los Borbones y el desarrollo de la odontologia en Espãna. **Bol Inf Dent (Madr)** 1978;Spec no:63–92
**Gonzalez Iglesias J:** Los dentistas Catalanes de finales del siglo XIX. Su influencia en el desarrollo de la odonto-estomatologia en España. **Rev Esp Estomatol** 1979 May–Jun;27(3):164–82
**Gonzalez Iglesias J** see **Moreno Gonzalez JP**
**González-Pedrero E:** La medicina del siglo XX y su proyección futura. III. Salud, sociedad y política. **Gac Med Mex** 1981 Nov;117(11):428–33
**González-Polo I:** La ciudad de México a fines del siglo XVIII-disquisiciones sobre un manuscrito anónimo. **Hist Mex** 1976;26(1):29–47
**Gooch PS** see **Hart GD, ed**
**Good AE:** Reiter's disease: modern concepts. **Cutis** 1979 Nov;24(5):514–23
**Good RA** see **Wangensteen OW, ed**
**Gooddy W:** Charles Edward Brown-Séquard. In Rose FC, Bynum WF, ed: Historical aspects of the neurosciences. New York, Raven, 1982. p. 371–8.
**Gooddy W:** Dr. Brown-Sequard in space and time. **Trans Hunter Soc** 1978–80;37–38:153–9
**Gooddy W** see **Riese W**
**Goodger WJ, Ruppanner R:** Historical perspective on the development of dairy practice. **J Am Vet Med Assoc** 1982 Jun 1;180(11):1294–7
**Goodheart WB:** C. G. Jung's first 'patient': on the seminal emergence of Jung's thought. **J Anal Psychol** 1984 Jan;29(1):1–34
**Goodlin RC:** Why fetal monitoring. **Semin Perinatol** 1981 Apr;5(2):105–7
**Goodman AH, Armelagos GJ, Rose JC:** Enamel hypoplasias as indicators of stress in three prehistoric populations from Illinois. **Hum Biol** 1980 Sept;52(3):515–28
**Goodman AH, Armelagos GJ, Rose JC:** The chronological distribution of enamel hypoplasias from prehistoric Dickson Mounds populations. **Am J Phys Anthropol** 1984 Nov;65(3):259–66
**Goodman ES** see **Robert I. Watson and the development of the history of psychology: a symposium**
**Goodman LR:** Nursing administration in psychiatric hospitals. **J Psychosoc Nurs Ment Health Serv** 1983 Aug;21(8):26–34
**Goodman M, Cronin JE:** Molecular anthropology: its development and current directions. In F. Spencer, ed: A history of American physical anthropology, 1930–1980. New York, Academic Press, 1982. p. 105–46.
**Goodman M** see **Barnhart MI**
**Goodman M** see **Reyman TA**
**Goodman N:** Congenital syphilis in the Burgas area in Bulgaria about 1930. A suppressed report of the health organisation of the League of Nations. In International Congress of the History of Medicine. 26th, Plovdiv, 1978. Actes du Congress. Sofia, 1981. Volume II. p. 168–70.
**Goodman WS, Wallace IR:** Tympanoplasty--25 years later. **J Otolaryngol** 1980 Apr;9(2):155–64
**Goodwin B** see **Webster G**
**Goodwin JC** see **Stephens SD**
**Goodwin JM** see **Goodwin JS**
**Goodwin JS, Goodwin JM:** Failure to recognize efficacious treatments: a history of salicylate therapy in rheumatoid arthritis. **Perspect Biol Med** 1981 Autumn, 25(1):78–92
**Goodwin JS, Goodwin JM:** The tomato effect. Rejection of highly efficacious therapies. **JAMA** 1984 May 11;251(18):2387–90
**Goodwin LG:** New drugs for old diseases. **Trans R Soc Trop Med Hyg** 1980;74(1):1–7
**Goodwin WE:** Recollections: early experiences in kidney transplantation. **Transplant Proc** 1981 Mar;13(1):29–31
**Goose DH:** Changes in human face breadth since the Mediaeval period in Britain. **Arch Oral Biol** 1981;26(9):757–8
**Goossens FA** see **van Ijzendoorn MH**
**Göpfert W, Otten HH, ed:** Metavoeite: wandelt euch durch neues Denken: Festschrift für Professor Hans Schadewaldt zur Vollendung des 60. Lebensjahres. Düsseldorf, Triltsch, 1983. 226 p.
**Göpfert W** see **Gicklhorn R**
**Góral R:** Akademia Medyczna w Poznaniu--osiągniecia : perspektywy rozwoju. **Nauka Pol** 1977;25(4):55–72
**Gorbunov VP:** 50 let na strazhe zdorov'ia voĭnov. **Voen Med Zh** 1984

Aug;(8):76-8
**Gorceix B** see **Braun L, et al**
**Gorchakova GA:** Osnovnye vekhi razvitiia nauchnykh issledovaniĭ po kurortologii v USSR. **Vopr Kurortol Fizioter Lech Fiz Kult** 1982 Nov-Dec;(6):16-8
**Gordan GS:** Fuller Albright and postmenopausal osteoporosis: a personal appreciation. **Perspect Biol Med** 1981 Summer;24(4):547-60
**Gordeev VI, Gogun KV, Gandziuk VM:** Vydaiushchiesia vrachi-khirurgi Khersonshchiny. **Klin Khir** 1983 Jun;(6):56-8
**Gordienko SM:** Stoletniĭ put' razvitiia teorii fagotsitoza. Sovremennye predstavleniia o roli fagotsitov v nespetsificheskom kletochnom immunitete. **Ter Arkh** 1983;55(8):144-50
**Gordis L:** Symposium in honor of Abraham M. Lilienfeld. Chronic disease epidemiology at the threshold of a new decade. **Am J Epidemiol** 1980 Aug;112(2):169-77
**Gordon AS** see **Dill DB**
**Gordon B:** Maryland section's ACD day. **J Am Coll Dent** 1984 Summer;51(2):27-32
**Gordon B** see **Foreman T**
**Gordon CC** see **Buikstra JE**
**Gordon D** see **Litchfield RB**
**Gordon DA:** The growth of rheumatology. **J Rheumatol** 1981 Jan-Feb;8(1):4-5
**Gordon E, Kraiuhin C, Kelly P, et al:** The development of hysteria as a psychiatric concept. **Compr Psychiatry** 1984 Sep-Oct;25(5):532-7
**Gordon EW, Rubain TJ:** Bias and alternatives in psychological testing. **J Negro Educ** 1980;49(3):350-60
**Gordon G, Bishop B:** Community control, Cuban style. **Freedomways** 1981;21(3):194-200
**Gordon L:** Lena Levine. In: Notable American women. The modern period. Cambridge, Mass., Belknap-Harvard Univ. Press, 1980. 4:419-20.
**Gordon L:** The long struggle for reproductive rights. **Radic Am** 1981;15(1-2):75-88
**Gordon L** see **Breul FR**
**Gordon L** see **Dupâquier J**
**Gordon L** see **Fee E**
**Gordon L** see **Green D**
**Gordon MD:** How socially distinctive is cognitive deviance in an emergent science? The case of parapsychology. **Soc Stud Sci** 1982 Feb;12(1):151-65
**Gordon RA:** Forty years onward. **Can Anaesth Soc J** 1983 Sep;30(5):460-5
**Gordon RL:** The development of Louisiana's public mental institutions, 1735-1940. 2 vols. in 1. Ph.D. Diss., Louisiana State University. Baton Rouge, 1978, 498 leaves.
**Gordon S:** Motherhood is powerful. **Work Pap Mag** 1982;9(2):15-9
**Gordon VH** see **Cazort AG**
**Gordon DB, ed:** Hypertension: the renal basis. Stroudsburg, Pa, Dowden, Hutchinson & Ross, 1980. xvi, 432 p. (Benchmark Papers in Human Physiology, 13).
**Gordon S, ed:** All our lives. A centennial history of Michael Reese Hospital and Medical Center, 1881-1981. Chicago, Michael Reese Hospital and Medical Center, 1981. vii, 210 p.
**Goregliad KhS, Tuzova RV:** K istorii bor'by s tuberkulezom sel'skokhoziaĭstvennykh zhivotnykh. **Probl Tuberk** 1983 Nov;(11):71-3
**Gorelick L** see **Gwinnett AJ**
**Gorelova LE** see **Korotkikh RV**
**Gorelova LE** see **Shostak NA**
**Gorevic PD, Cleveland AB, Franklin EC:** The biologic significance of amyloid. **Ann NY Acad Sci** 1982;389:380-94
**Gorham E:** Robert Angus Smith, F.R.S., and 'Chemical climatology'. **Notes Rec R Soc Lond** 1982 Feb;36(2):267-72
**Gorham J:** A medical triumph: the iron lung. **Respir Ther** 1979 Jan-Feb;9(1):71-3
**Gorham J:** Commercial development of the oxygen tent. **Respir Ther** 1979 Jan-Feb;9(1):48-9
**Gorham JD** see **Silvers DN**
**Gorin OZ** see **Zhamba G**
**Gorizontov PD:** K 130-letiiu so dnia rozhdeniia I. P. Pavlova (vstupitel'noe slovo k Pervym Pavlovskim chteniiam). **Zh Vyssh Nerv Deiat** 1980 May-Jun;30(3):627-30
**Gorizontov PD:** Patologicheskaia fiziologiia v SSSR (k 60-letiiu obrazovaniia SSSR). **Patol Fiziol Eksp Ter** 1983 May-Jun;3:14-22
**Gormakh SIa:** Razvitie zdravookhraneniia Rovenskoĭ oblasti za gody Sovetskoĭ vlasti. **Vrach Delo** 1979 Nov;(11):1-5
**Gorman BM, McKinzie RD, Wilson TA:** From shamans to specialists: a history of medicine and health care in Jackson County, Missouri. Kansas City, Mo., Jackson County Medical Society, 1981. 240 p.
**Gorman M:** Pre-war conformity research in social psychology: the approaches of Floyd H. Allport and Muzafer Sherif. **J Hist Behav Sci** 1981 Jan;17(1):3-14
**Gorman M:** Sir William B. O'Shaughnessy, pioneer chemical educator in India. **Ambix** 1983 Jul;30(2):107-16
**Gorman M:** Sir William Brooke O'Shaughnessy, F.R.S. (1809-1889), Anglo-Indian forensic chemist. **Notes Rec R Soc Lond** 1984 Sep;39(1):51-64
**Gorney JE:** The clinical application of Lacan in the psychoanalytic situation. **Psychoanal Rev** 1982 Summer;69(2):241-8
**Gornostaeva RM** see **Kupriianova ES**
**Gorodniaia VN** see **Shumada IV**
**Gorog F, Leguil F:** Histoire de l'hystérie. **Soins Psychiatr** 1983 Jan;(27):3-6
**Gorokhov AA, Gofman VR:** K istorii razvitiia spetsializirovannoĭ otorinolaringologicheskoĭ pomoshchi. **Voen Med Zh** 1981 Aug;(8):76-7
**Gorokhova EM** see **Poletaev SD**
**Górski M:** Wspomnienia wojenne. **Arch Hist Med (Warsz)** 1983;46(1):91-112
**Gorskiĭ AN** see **Makovoz AA**
**Gortner SR:** The history and philosophy of nursing science and research. **ANS** 1983 Jan;5(2):1-8
**Görtz R:** Esculape ou Prométhée: les mutations de la médecine du thaumaturge au démiurge. **Arch Belg Med Soc** 1980 Oct;38(8):479-516
**Goscilo H:** Lermontov's debt to Lavater and Gall. **Slav East Eur Rev** 1981;59(4):500-15
**Goss CM, Chodkowski EG:** 'On Bones for Beginners' by Galen of Pergamon: a translation with commentary. **Am J Anat** 1984 Jan;169(1):59-74
**Goszczyńska W:** Szkoła im. piel ęgniarek Warszawy. **Pieleg Polozna** 1979;(9):20-2
**Gotch FA:** The evolution of the society. **Trans Am Soc Artif Intern Organs** 1979;25:534-8
**Gotenba-shi I:** Gotenba-shi Ishikai shi. [Gotenba, Japan], Do Ishikai, Showa 53 nen, [1978]. 680, [35] p.
**Gotovitch J:** Quelques données relatives à l'extermination des Tsiganes de Belgique. **Cah Hist Seconde Guerre Mond** 1976;4:161-80
**Gots IuD** see **Borisenko NF**
**Gott VL:** Extracorporeal circulation: 1970-1982. **Trans Am Soc Artif Intern Organs** 1982;28:17-9
**Gottdenker P:** Francesco Redi and the fly experiments. **Bull Hist Med** 1979 Winter;53(4):575-92
**Gottdenker P:** Three clerics in pursuit of 'little animals.' **Clio Med** 1980 Jul;14(3-4):213-24
**Gottesman II:** James Shields, 1918-1978. **Acta Genet Med Gemellol (Roma)** 1979;28(1):83-90
**Gottfried RS:** Bury St. Edmunds and the populations of late medieval English towns, 1270-1530. **J Br Stud** 1980;20(1):1-31
**Gottfried RS:** English medical practitioners, 1340-1530. **Bull Hist Med** 1984 Summer;58(2):164-82
**Gottfried RS:** The black death. Natural and human disaster in Medieval Europe. New York, London, Free Press, 1983. xvii, 203 p.
**Gottheil E:** An introduction to the evaluation of alcoholism outcome studies. **Curr Alcohol** 1979;7:275-85
**Gottlieb G** see **Hearst E, ed**
**Gottlieb J** see **Spanos NP**
**Gottschalk E:** Quo vadit chirurgia paediatrica? **Beitr Gesch Univ Erfurt** 1979-83;19:361-7
**Gottsegen R:** Periodontics 1950-1980 **NY J Dent** 1980 Apr;50(4):132-3
**Gotz I:** Untersuchungen an drei Schädeln des 14./15. Jahrhunderts aus einem mittelfränkischen Rittergeschlecht. **ZWR** 1982 Sep;91(9):62-4
**Götz W:** Die Bedeutung Johann Bartholomäus Trommsdorffs für die Entwicklung der Chemie in Deutschland zu Beginn des 19. Jahrhunderts. Ein Versuch anhand seiner Korrespondenz mit Justus von Liebig und Heinrich Emanuel Merck. In Dilg P, et al., ed: Perspektiven der Pharmaziegeschichte. Graz, Austria, Akademische Druck- u. Verlagsanstalt, 1983. p. 97-112.
**Götz W:** Die Briefe Jacques Peschiers aus Genf an Joh. Barth. Trommsdorff, Erfurt, als Beispiel für internationale pharmazeutische Kontakte zu Beginn des 19. Jahrhunderts. **Pharm Acta Helv** 1979;54(9-10):303-7
**Götz W:** J. B. Trommsdorffs 'Chemische Receptirkunst'. Bisher unbekannte Übersetzungen und Ausgaben. **Beitr Gesch Pharm** 1982;31(14):107-10
**Gotzkowsky B** see **Johannes Adelphus**
**Gøtzsche I:** Andelig omsorg/7. Kristendommens indflydelse på sundhedsvaesenet. **Sygeplejersken** 1983 Mar 9;83(10):12-6
**Goubert JP:** A 'quiet revolution': the coming of pure water to contemporary France. **Soc Soc Hist Med Bull (Lond)** 1984 Dec;35:28-9
**Goubert JP:** Die Medikalisierung der französischen Gesellschaft am Ende des Ancien Régime: die Bretagne als Beispiel. **Medizinhist J** 1982;17(1/2):89-114
**Goubert JP:** La médicalisation de la société française à la fin de l'Ancien Régime. **Francia** 1980, paru 1981;8:245-56
**Goubert JP:** La médicalisation de la société française, 1770-1830. **Hist Reflect** 1982;9:1-304
**Goubert JP:** La médicalisation de la société française, 1770-1830. Waterloo, Ont., Historical Reflections Press, 1982. 304 p.
**Goubert JP:** La pénétration du médecin dans le corps social en France (1770-1850). **Hist Sci Med** 1980;14:435-8
**Goubert JP, Lepetit B:** Les niveaux de medicalisation des villes Françaises à la fin de l'ancien régime. **Hist Reflect** 1982;9(1-2):45-67
**Goubert JP:** L'hygiène de l'eau dans la France contemporaine d'après le thèses de doctorat de la Faculté de Médecine de Paris (1830-1940). In Imhof AE, ed: Mensch und Gesundheit in der Geschichte. Husum, Matthiesen, 1980. p. 59-78.
**Goubert JP:** Ordre et désordre: l'origine aquatique de la fièvre typhoïde. **Asclepio** 1983;35:161-70
**Goubert JP:** Réseau médical et médicalisation en France à la fin du 18e siècle. **Ann Bretagne** 1979;86(3):221-9
**Goubert JP:** The medicalization of French society at the end of the Ancien Régime. With commentary by C. Hannaway, p. 173-9. In Stevenson LG, ed: A celebration of medical history. Baltimore, Johns Hopkins University Press, 1982. (The Henry E. Sigerist supplements to the Bulletin of the History of Medicine; new ser., no. 6). p. 173-9.
**Goubert JP:** 1770-1830: la premiere croisade medicale. **Hist Reflect** 1982;9(1-2):3-13
**Goubert JP:** 1789: le corps médical et le changement. **Hist Sci Med**

1982;16(2):99–105
**Goubert JP** see **Dehillerin B**
**Goubert JP** see **Forster R**
**Gouch JB:** Lavoisier's memoirs on the nature of water and their place in the chemical revolution. **Ambix** 1983 Jul;30(2):89–106
**Goudreault L:** Naissance de la statistique alieniste au Canada jusqu'en 1867. In: Congrès international d'histoire de la médecine, XXVe, Québec, 1976. Actes. Québec, 1977. p. 706–26.
**Gould F, Roweth B:** Public spending and social policy: the United Kingdom 1950–1977. **J Soc Policy** 1980 Jul;9(3):337–57
**Gould KH:** Family planning and abortion policy in the United States. **Soc Serv Rev** 1979;53(3):452–63
**Gould ME, Gamlen C:** [A woman of parts. Florence Nightingale]. (Jpn) **Sogo Kango** 1980;15(1):95–9
**Gould MH:** The administrative units used for water supply purposes in Northern Ireland from 1828. **R Soc Health J** 1981 Jun;101(3):119–22
**Gould SJ:** Darwinism and the expansion of evolutionary theory. **Science** 1982 Apr 23;216(4544):380–7
**Gould SJ:** Ever since Darwin. Reflections in natural history. New York, W. W. Norton, 1977. 285 p.
**Gould SJ:** The mismeasure of man. New York, London, W.W., Norton & Co., 1981. 352 p.
**Gould SJ** see **Hamrum CL, ed**
**Gould SJ** see **Mayr E**
**Goulet C** see **Bourassa MG**
**Gourevitch D, Gourevitch M:** Chronique anachronique III. Simulation. **Evol Psychiatr (Paris)** 1981;46(1):205–9
**Gourevitch D** see **Grmek MD, ed**
**Gourevitch M:** Coup d'oeil sur la naissance de la psychiatrie à Paris. **Soins Psychiatr** 1982 Feb;(16):9–11
**Gourevitch M:** Esquirol et la medicalisation de la psychiatrie: théorie médicale et pratique clinique. In International Congress of the History of Medicine, 27th, Barcelona, 1980. Actas. Barcelona, Académia de Ciències Médiques de Catalunya i Balears, 1981. p. 74–7.
**Gourevitch M:** Le musée Adler d'histoire de la médecine à Johannesburg. **Hist Sci Med** 1982;16(1):21–2
**Gourevitch M** see **Gourevitch D**
**Gove WR, Hughes M:** Beliefs vs. data: more on the illness behavior of men and women. **Am Sociol Rev** 1981;46(1):123–8
**Gove WR, Hughes M:** Possible causes of the apparent sex differences in physical health: an empirical investigation. **Am Sociol Rev** 1979;44(1):126–46
**Govier WM:** A helminthic tale. **Perspect Biol Med** 1984 Autumn;28(1):104–6
**Govinda Reddy C:** Recent Indian medical historiography; bibliography for 1973. **Bull Indian Inst Hist Med (Hyderabad)** 1975 Oct;5(4):253–68
**Govinda Reddy C:** Recent Indian medical historiography: bibliography for 1975. **Bull Indian Inst Hist Med (Hyderabad)** 1978;8(1–4):63–87
**Govyrin VA, Grigor'ian RA:** Akademik L. A. Orbeli: étapy zhizni i nauchnoĭ deiatel'nosti (k 100–letiiu so dnia rozhdeniia). **Usp Fiziol Nauk** 1982 Jun–Sep;13(3):3–8
**Gow CE:** The dentitions of the Tritheledontidae (therapsida: cynodontia). **Proc R Soc Lond [Biol]** 1980 Jul 17;208(1173):461–81
**Gow JG:** The evolution of modern endoscopic photography. **Eur Urol** 1984;10(2):133–8
**Goyan JE:** Dr. Harvey Wiley's brainchild, 75 years later. **J Assoc Off Anal Chem** 1981 Mar;64(2):256–9
**Goyan JE:** FDA at 75--failure, symbiosis, convergence. In Young JH, ed: The early years of federal food and drug control. Madison, American Institute of the History of Pharmacy, 1982. p. 53–60.
**Goznyĭ AD:** K istorii perelivaniia posmertnoĭ krovi. **Feldsher Akush** 1980;45(12):58–9
**Graaff MG:** Milieuvervuiling: een oud probleem. **Spiegel Hist** 1982;17(2):86–96
**Grabarits I:** A kalocsai érseki könyvtár orvosi könyvritkaságai. **Orv Hetil** 1982 May 30;123(22):1369–70
**Grabarits I:** Der Arzneischatz des Herbariums von Melius. In Hein WH, ed: Pharmaziehistorischer Kongress, Budapest, 1981. Stuttgart, Wissenschaftliche Verlagsgesellschaft, 1983. p. 49–56.
**Grabarits I:** Die Klassifizierung des ungarischen Arzneischatzes im 18. Jahrhundert. In Hickel E, Schröder G, ed: Neue Beiträge zur Arzneimittelgeschichte. Festschrift für Wolfgang Schneider zum 70. Geburtstag. Stuttgart, Wissenschaftliche Verlagsgesellschaft, 1982. p. 87–105.
**Graber E** see **Camerino G**
**Grabham AH:** Precepts and practice: Charles Hastings's vision and reality. **Br Med J [Clin Res]** 1982 Dec 18–25;285(6357):1789–92
**Grabner E:** Zwischen Wunderbuch und Rezeptbuchweisheit. Zum Aussagewert eines handschriftlichen burgenländischen Arzneibuches aus der ersten Hälfte des 19. Jahrhunderts. **Ethnomedizin** 1978–79;5(1–2):25–43
**Grabowski HG, Vernon JM, Thomas LG:** Estimating the effects of regulation on innovation: an international comparative analysis of the pharmaceutical industry. **J Law Econ** 1978;21(1):133–63
**Grace E:** House-staff officers: collective bargaining in the health care system. **J Leg Med (Chicago)** 1981 Sep;2(3):415–31
**Gracey DR, DeRemee RA:** The University of Vienna Medical School. **Mayo Clin Proc** 1981 Oct;56(10):634–8
**Grachev AI, Zhalkovskiĭ BV:** Istoriia sozdaniia i deiatel'nosti Odesskoĭ stantsii skoroĭ meditsinskoĭ pomoshchi. **Klin Khir** 1983 Dec;(12):56–8
**Grachev AI:** Zainteresovannost' N. I. Pirogova istorieĭ i arkheologieĭ. **Vrach Delo** 1980 Jan;(1):114–6
**Gracheva AG:** Sistema okhrany zdorov'ia deteĭ v Rossiiskoĭ Federatsii. **Pediatriia** 1982 Dec;(12):9–11
**Gracia D, Vidal JL:** Avicena, sobre el corazón. In International Congress of the History of Medicine, 27th, Barcelona, 1980. Actas. Barcelona, Académia de Ciències Médiques de Catalunya i Balears, 1981. p. 711–22.
**Gracia D, Vidal JL:** Avicena, sobre la definición de la medicina. In International Congress of the History of Medicine, 27th, Barcelona, 1980. Actas. Barcelona, Académia de Ciències Médiques de Catalunya i Balears, 1981. p. 723–30.
**Gracia D:** Chirino en el Retablo de las Maravillas. **Asclepio** 1978–79;30–31:265–76
**Gracia D:** El orden médico. La ética médica de Thomas Percival. **Asclepio** 1983;35:227–55
**Gracia D:** En torno al averroismo medico latino. **Asclepio** 1978–79;30–31:233–64
**Gracia D:** The structure of medical knowledge in Aristotle's philosophy. **Sudhoffs Arch** 1978;62(1):1–36
**Gracia-Guillen D** see **Tellenbach H, ed**
**Gráda CO:** The population of Ireland 1700–1900: a survey. **Ann Demogr Hist (Paris)** 1979;:281–99
**Graebner W:** Doing the world's unhealthy work: the fiction of free choice. **Hastings Cent Rep** 1984 Aug;14(4):28–37
**Graebner W:** The unstable world of Benjamin Spock: social engineering in a democratic culture, 1917–1950. **J Am Hist** 1980 Dec;67(3):612–29
**Graepel PH:** Die Calwer Apothekerfamilie Gärtner im Bild. **Beitr Gesch Pharm** 1981;31(12):92–5
**Graeser F, Keil G:** Die Pestrezepte des Fuldaer Kodex Aa 129. **Z Dtsch Altert Dtsch Lit** 1980;109(1):72–85
**Gräfner G** see **Engelbrecht H**
**Grafton TS:** The founding and early history of the National Society for Medical Research. **Lab Anim Sci** 1980 Aug;30(4 pt 2):759–64
**Grage TB** see **Reed K**
**Graham AN:** Contribution of the International Journal of Social Psychiatry. **Int J Soc Psychiatry** 1979;25(4):238–9
**Graham EE:** A probable submandibular gland defect in a prehistoric mandible. **Oral Surg** 1980 Aug;50(2):187–9
**Graham FE, Wright RJ:** The American College of Medical Group Administrators: twenty-five years in brief perspective. **Med Group Manage** 1981 Sep–Oct;28(5):60–2, 64, 66
**Graham JB:** James Bell Bullitt, M.D., 1874–1964: a University of North Carolina medical giant. **NC Med J** 1984 Feb;45(2):88–92
**Graham JC:** The French connection in the early history of canning. **J R Soc Med** 1981 May;74(5):374–81
**Graham JS** see **Hand WD, ed**
**Graham L:** Biomedicine and the politics of science in the USSR. **Sov Union** 1981;8(2):147–58
**Graham LR:** Between science and values. New York, Columbia University Press, 1981. x, 449 p.
**Graham PW:** A mirror for medicine: Richard Selzer, Michael Crichton, and Walker Percy. **Perspect Biol Med** 1981 Winter;24(2):229–39
**Graham RM:** Music therapy: the state of the field. **J Natl Assoc Priv Psychiatr Hosp** 1979;11(2):32–9
**Graham S:** Notes on nursing, 1860–1980. Angels of plain speech. **Nurs Times** 1980 Oct 23;76(43):1874
**Graham SD:** Ephraim McDowell (1771–1830). The President's lithotomist. **Invest Urol** 1981 Nov;19(3):216–7
**Graham SH** see **Wood BA**
**Graham SN** see **Tolnay SE**
**Graham SS** see **Gay EC**
**Graham TR:** The courage of his diversity: medicine, writing and William Carlos Williams. In Jones AH, ed: Images of healers. Albany, State University of New York Press, 1983. p. 9–20.
**Graham TR:** William Carlos Williams: biographical note. In Jones AH, ed: Images of healers. Albany, State University of New York Press, 1983. p. 1–2.
**Graham TR:** William Carlos Williams. In Dictionary of American biography, 1961–1965. Suppl. 7, 1981. p. 788–91.
**Grainger CR:** Leprosy and Curieuse Island. **Lepr Rev** 1981 Jun;52(2):151–4
**Grainger CR:** Leprosy in the Seychelles. **Lepr Rev** 1980;51(1):43–9
**Grainger RG:** Intravascular contrast media--the past, the present and the future. **Br J Radiol** 1982 Jan;55(649):1–18
**Grainger RG** see **Veiga-Pires JA**
**Gramling LG:** A history of pharmacy in Florida. Gainesville, Ewing Printing, 1973. iv, 225 p.
**Gran P:** Medical pluralism in Arab and Egyptian history: an overview of class structures and philosophies of the main phases. **Soc Sci Med [Med Anthropol]** 1979 Dec;13B(4):339–48
**Granat NE:** K 35-letiiu pobedy (vospominaniia o sluzhbe v voenno-sanitarnom poezde). **Med Sestra** 1980 May;39(5):7–11
**Granat NE:** K 40-letiiu Ukaza Prezidiuma Verkhovnogo Soveta SSSR ob okhrane materinstva i detstva. **Med Sestra** 1984 Jun;43(6):6–10
**Granat NE:** O 1-ĭ obshchegorodskoĭ nauchno-prakticheskoĭ konferentsii akusherok i meditsinskikh sester akushersko-ginekologicheskikh uchrezhdeniĭ Leningrada (1939 g.). **Med Sestra** 1980 Jun;39(6):40–2
**Granat NE:** 'Skorbnyĭ list' ginekologicheskoĭ bol'noĭ kontsa XIX stoletiia. **Med Sestra** 1979 Dec;38(12):51–5
**Granat NE:** Zhurnal 'Akusherka' (po stranitsam starinnogo zhurnala). **Feldsher Akush** 1983;48(4):58–60
**Grande Covian F:** Vitamin deficiencies during the Spanish Civil War in Madrid: a reminiscence. **Acta Vitaminol Enzymol** 1982;4(1–2):99–103

**Grando AA, Makarenko IM, Polianskiĭ AA:** Kafedre sotsial'noĭ gigieny i organizatsii zdravookhraneniia Kievskogo meditsinskogo instituta--60 let. **Sov Zdravookhr** 1984;(3):52-3

**Grando AA, Mezhirov LS:** Muzeĭ meditsiny Ukrainskoĭ SSR. **Sov Zdravookhr** 1984;(8):59-62

**Grando AA, Kogan Via:** Rol' Narkomzdrava RSFSR v stanovlenii zdravookhraneniia Sovetskoĭ Ukrainy. **Sov Zdravookhr** 1983;9:55-7

**Graner JL:** An introduction to the writings of Egerton Yorrick Davis. **IMJ** 1983 Jul;164(1):47-8

**Graner JL, Frederick W:** William Halsted's cocaine habit. **Arch Ophthalmol** 1984 Dec;102(12):1746

**Graney CM** see **Graney MJ**

**Graney MJ, Graney CM:** Colorectal surgery from antiquity to the modern era. **Dis Colon Rectum** 1980 Sep;23(6):432-41

**Grange JM:** Koch's Tubercle Bacillus a centenary reappraisal. **Zentralbl Bakteriol Mikrobiol Hyg [A]** 1982 Mar;251(3):297-307

**Grange JM, Bishop PJ:** 'Uber Tuberkulose'. A tribute to Robert Koch's discovery of the tubercle bacillus, 1882. **Tubercle** 1982 Mar;63(1):3-17

**Granger BH** see **Hand WD, ed**

**Granger R:** Histoire de la chimie organique à la Faculté de Pharmacie de Montpellier. **Trav Soc Pharm Montp** 1978;38:301-8

**Granier-Doyaux M** see **Sociedad Venezolana de Historia de la medicina**

**Graninger W** see **Zazgornik J**

**Granjel LS:** El libro medico en España (1808-1936). Salamanca, 1975. 111 p (Cuadernos de Historia de la Medicina Española, Monografias, 28).

**Granjel LS:** La medicina española antigua y medieval. Salamanca, Ediciones Universidad de Salamanca, 1981. 184 p. (Historia general de la medicina española. I.).

**Granjel LS:** La medicina española del siglo XVII. Salamanca, Ediciones Universidad de Salamanca, 1978. 250 p.

**Granjel LS:** La medicina española del siglo XVIII. Salamanca, Ediciones Universidad de Salamanca, 1979. 285 p. (Historia general de la medicina española, IV).

**Granjel LS:** La medicina española renacentista. Salamanca, Ediciones Universidad de Salamanca, 1980. 289 p. (Historia general de la medicina española, II).

**Granjel LS:** Las epidemias de peste en la España del siglo XVII. In: Sociedad Española de Historia de la Medicina. V Congreso Nacional. Madrid, 1977. **Asclepio** 1977;29:17-36

**Granjel LS:** Literatura historico-medica Española de postguerra (1940-1975). Salamanca, 1977. 71 p. (Cuadernos de Historia de la Medicina Española, Monografias, 30).

**Granjel LS, ed** see **Albarracín Teulón A**

**Granshaw LP:** St. Thomas's Hospital, London, 1850-1900. Ph.D. Diss., Bryn Mawr College. Bryn Mawr, 1981 v, 564 leaves.

**Grant AA:** A century of change in prosthetic dentistry. **Br Dent J** 1980 Jul 1;149(1):9-12

**Grant AS:** The RCM--the first 100 years: some things never change. **Midwives Chron** 1981 Oct;95(1125):348-50

**Grant HR** see **Fogarty RS**

**Grant PG:** A prehistoric case of congenital radioulnar synostosis. **Ossa** 1978;5:13-15

**Grant RE:** Tuuhikya: the Hopi healer. **Am Indian Q** 1982;6(3-4):291-304

**Grantham JJ** see **Terreros DA**

**Grapentin F:** Veterinärärztliches Gerät im Zweiten Weltkrieg. **DTW** 1981 Nov 5;88(11):473-5

**Grapow H** see **Deines H von**

**Gras VW:** Myth and the reconciliation of opposites: Jung and Lévi-Strauss. **J Hist Ideas** 1981 Jul-Sep;42(3):471-88

**Grass U:** Zu Leben und Werk von Jakob Reinbold Spielmann (1722-1783). Stuttgart, Deutscher Apotheker, 1983. 254 p. (Quellen und Studien zur Geschichte der Pharmazie, Bd. 20).

**Grasshoff K:** Leibesübungen und Gesellschaft im Gemälde 'Melancolia 1558' des Mathias Gerung. **Stadion** 1977;3(1):44-59

**Grassi C:** Influence de l'oeuvre de Laénnec sur la médecine italienne. **Rev Fr Mal Respir** 1981;9(5):421-6

**Grau C** see **Komkov GD**

**Graveley A:** Midwives celebrate century of professional advancement. **Australas Nurses J** 1981 Mar;10(3):8-9

**Gravenstein JS:** A perspective on science. The language and history of anesthesia. **Ala J Med Sci** 1984 Jul;21(3):304-10

**Gravenstein JS:** The history of drug inhalation: a brief overview. **Anesth Analg (Cleve)** 1980 Feb;59(2):140-5

**Graves V:** Graves Medical Audiovisual Library: 1957-82. **Br Med J [Clin Res]** 1982 Dec 4;285(6355):1627-8

**Graves V:** Twenty-five audiovisual years (the story of GMAL). **J Audiov Media Med** 1983 Jan;6(1):25-7

**Gravitz MA:** An early case of investigative hypnosis: a brief communication. **Int J Clin Exp Hypn** 1983 Oct;31(4):224-6

**Gravitz MA:** Bibliographic sources of nineteenth century hypnosis literature. **Am J Clin Hypn** 1981 Jan;23(3):217-9

**Gravitz MA, Gerton MI:** Freud and hypnosis: report of post-rejection use. **J Hist Behav Sci** 1981 Jan;17(1):68-74

**Gravitz MA, Gerton MI:** Origins of the term hypnotism prior to Braid. **Am J Clin Hypn** 1984 Oct;27(2):107-10

**Gravitz MA, Gerton MI:** Polgar as Freud's hypnotist? contrary evidence. **Am J Clin Hypn** 1982 Apr;24(4):272-6

**Gray AS** see **McCombie F**

**Gray C:** Osteopathy: is there a place in Canadian medicine? **Can Med Assoc J** 1981 Jul 1;125(1):108-11

**Gray C:** The remarkable surgical collection of John Hunter. **Can Med Assoc J** 1983 May 15;128(10):1225-8

**Gray C:** The Wellcome library: reflection of an insatiable collector. **Can Med Assoc J** 1982 Mar 15;126(6):712, 716-20

**Gray C:** Travelling archives depict early days in Canadian medicine. **Can Med Assoc J** 1980 Sep 6;123(5):426, 430, 432

**Gray F** see **Escourolle R**

**Gray JA:** Ivan Pavlov. New York, Viking Press, 1979. vii, 153 p.

**Gray JA:** The elderly in Scandinavia: demographic, economic, social and health conditions in 1834. **Scand J Soc Med** 1984;12(2):65-8

**Gray L, Rodriguez K, Dale DC:** University of Washington School of Medicine. **West J Med** 1984 May;140(5):803-11

**Gray TC:** 'Another side of Mars'. **J R Army Med Corps** 1984 Feb;130(1):3-11

**Gray MZ, et al** see **Cobb HV**

**Grayson RS:** Collection of psychoanalytic classics. **J Am Psychoanal Assoc** 1979;27(4):913-20

**Grayson VS:** Mary Cromwell Jarrett. In: Notable American women. The modern period. Cambridge, Mass., Belknap-Harvard Univ. Press, 1980. 4:377-9.

**Graziani R:** Fracastoro's 'syphilis' and Priapus. **Clio Med** 1981 Dec;16(2/3):93-9

**The great famine in Ukraine: a journalist's eyewitness account: Ukr Rev (Lond)** 1979;27(2):87-97

**Greb FL** see **Spor E, ed**

**Greben SE:** CPA--yesterday and today. **Can J Psychiatry** 1980 Feb;25(1):27-9

**Grebenev AL:** S. P. Botkin o N. I. Pirogove. **Klin Med (Mosk)** 1982 Sep;60(9):108-10

**Grebeneva LS:** K 150-letiiu opisaniia Kruivel'e prostoĭ khronicheskoĭ iazvy zheludka. **Klin Med (Mosk)** 1981 May;59(5):112-4

**Grebenik E, ed** see **Dupâquier J**

**Grecu G** see **Csiky K**

**Greeff K, Schadewaldt H:** Introduction and remarks on the history of cardiac glycosides. In Greeff K, ed: Handbook of experimental pharmacology. Berlin, Springer, 1981. p. 1-12 (Vol. 56/I)

**Greeff K:** Therapie der Myokardinsuffizienz, gestern und heute. **Z Kardiol** 1982 Mar;71(3):139-41

**Greeff K:** Zur 48. Jahrestagung der Deutschen Gesellschaft für Herz- und Kreislaufforschung. Eröffnungsansprache. **Verh Dtsch Ges Herz Kreislaufforsch** 1982;48:XI-XX

**Green A** see **Anzieu D**

**Green AF:** The discovery of bretylium and bethanidine. **Br J Clin Pharmacol** 1982 Jan;13(1):25-34

**Green AF** see **Boura AL**

**Green BF:** Three decades of quantitative methods in psychology. **Am Behav Sci** 1980;23(6):811-34

**Green D, Murdock ME, ed:** The Margaret Sanger Centennial Conference, November 13 & 14, 1979. Northampton, Smith College, 1982. 68 p. Contributions by J. K. Conway, A. Harper, L. Gordon, J. Reed, E. Fee.

**Green D:** The Medvedev experience: 1984 and medicine. **Perspect Biol Med** 1976 Autumn;20(1):145-55

**Green DM:** William John Tulloch. In Dictionary of national biography, 1961-1970. Suppl. 8, 1981. p. 1019-20.

**Green E:** U. S. population policies, development, and the rural poor of Africa. **J Mod Afr Stud** 1982;20(1):45-67

**Green E** see **Myles J**

**Green H:** Some things that happened on Lew Thomas' floor. **Cell Immunol** 1983 Nov;82(1):98-101

**Green HP:** The recombinant DNA controversy: a model of public influence. **Bull At Sci** 1978;34(9):12-16

**Green LC:** War law and the medical profession. **Leg Med Q** 1979;3(3):175-96

**Green M, Rieber RW:** The assimilation of psychoanalysis in America. In R. W. Rieber, K. Salzinger, ed: Psychology: theoretical-historical perspectives. New York, Academic Press, 1980. p. 263-304.

**Green MD** see **Allan P**

**Green MH:** John Edgar Hubble, M.D., a rare physician and surgeon. Van Nuys, California, Hoffman, 1979. 61 p.

**Green MW:** Epilogue, prologue: from the past comes the future: the first 75 years of the National Association of Boards of Pharmacy. Chicago, National Association of Boards of Pharmacy, 1979. ix, 109 p.

**Green P:** Ars gratia cultus: Ovid as beautician. **Am J Philol** 1979;100:381-92

**Green SA:** Salem witchcraft: a biopsychosocial analysis. **Pharos** 1982 Summer;45(3):9-13

**Green M, ed** see **Rieber RW**

**Greenacre P:** A historical sketch of the use and disuse of reconstruction. **Psychoanal Study Child** 1980;35:35-40

**Greenacre P:** Hans Christian Andersen and children. **Psychoanal Study Child** 1983;38:617-35

**Greenbaum LS:** Medicine in revolution: an essay review. **J Hist Med Allied Sci** 1982 Jan;37(1):90-5

**Greenbaum LS:** Nurses and doctors in conflict: piety and medicine in the Paris Hôtel-Dieu on the eve of the French Revolution. **Clio Med** 1979 May;13(3-4):247-67

**Greenbaum LS:** Science, medicine, religion: three views of health care in France on the eve of the French Revolution. **Stud Eighteenth Cent Cult** 1981;10:373-91

**Greenbaum LS:** Scientists and politicians: hospital reform in Paris on the eve of the French Revolution. **Proc Consort Revolutionary Eur** 1973:168-91

**Greenberg B** see **Fink L**
**Greenberg DF, Bystryn MH:** Christian intolerance of homosexuality. **AJS** 1982 Nov;88(3):515–48
**Greenberg ER, Colton T, Bagne C:** Measurement of cancer incidence in the United States: sources and uses of data. **JNCI** 1982 May;68(5):743–50
**Greenberg HR, Greenberg RR:** 'A bintel brief;' the editor as compleat therapist. **Psychiatr Q** 1980 Fall;52(3):222–30
**Greenberg JH:** Bureau of Laboratories created for protection of public health. **Tex Med** 1980 May;76(5):50
**Greenberg JP** see **Gilbert SF**
**Greenberg L:** Serratia marcescens in human affairs. **Drug Intell Clin Pharm** 1978 Nov;12(11):674–9
**Greenberg M:** Classical syndromes in occupational medicine: the Montague Murray case. **Am J Ind Med** 1982;3(3):351–6
**Greenberg M, O'Neill TF:** Solid waste: the end of the bottomless pit. **NY Aff** 1978;5(2):114–29
**Greenberg MH:** Neonatal feeding. In Smith GF, Smith PN, Vidyasagar d, ed: Historical review and recent advances in neonatal and perinatal medicine. [Chicago?], Mead Johnson Nutritional Division, 1983. Vol. I. p. 55–85.
**Greenberg MH** see **Smith GF**
**Greenberg MR:** A note on the changing geography of cancer mortality within metropolitan regions of the United States. **Demography** 1981 Aug;18(3):411–20
**Greenberg RR** see **Greenberg HR**
**Greenberg SC:** The entry of microbiology into clinical medicine. **Conn Med** 1980 Oct;44(10):641–3
**Greenberg RP, ed** see **Fisher S**
**Greenblatt RB:** The humiliating demise of Lord Randolph Churchill, 1849–1895. **Postgrad Med** 1984 Jan;75(1):129–31, 134
**Greene EL:** Landmarks of botanical history. Ed., F. N. Egerton, with contributions by R. P. McIntosh and R. McVaugh. 2 vols. Stanford, Stanford University Press, 1983. 1139 p. (Vol. I first published 1909)
**Greene J:** Hospital heritage: on the tile trail. **Health Soc Serv J** 1982 Feb 11;92(4783):182–3
**Greene J:** Where now for psychiatric nursing? Steps along the way. **Nurs Mirror** 1980 Jun 26;150(20):suppl iv–vii
**Greene JC:** American science in the age of Jefferson. Ames, Iowa State University Press, 1984. xiv, 484 p.
**Greene JC:** Science, ideology, and world view: essays in the history of evolutionary ideas. Berkeley/Los Angeles, Univ. of California Press, 1981. x, 202 p.
**Greene JC** see **Cash P**
**Greene JC** see **Wilson LG, ed**
**Greene M** see **Spicker SF, ed**
**Greene NM:** Anesthesia and the development of surgery (1846–1896). **Middle East J Anaesthesiol** 1979 Oct;5(5):309–23
**Greene VW:** Cleanliness and the health revolution. New York, Soap and Detergent Association, 1984. vii, 68 p.
**Greener EH:** Amalgam -- yesterday, today, and tomorrow. **Oper Dent** 1979 Winter;4(1):24–35
**Greenfield GM:** The development of the underdeveloped city: public sanitation in São Paulo, Brazil, 1885–1913. **Luso-Braz Rev** 1980;17(1):107–18
**Greenhouse SW:** Jerome Cornfield's contributions to epidemiology. **Biometrics** 1982 Mar;38 Suppl:33–45
**Greenland C, Griffin JD:** The Honorable Mary Macdonald: a lesson in attitude. **Can Med Assoc J** 1981 Aug 1;125(3):305–8
**Greenland C:** William George Metcalf. In Dictionary of Canadian biography, 1881–1890. 1982;11:590–1.
**Greenland C** see **Griffin JD**
**Greenman PE:** Osteopathic medicine--origins and outlook. **Postgrad Med** 1980 Nov;68(5):31, 33
**Greenough PR:** Indian famines and peasant victims: the case of Bengal in 1943–44. **Mod Asian Stud** 1980;14(2):205–35
**Greenough PR:** Variolation and vaccination in South Asia, c. 1700–1865: a preliminary note. **Soc Sci Med [Med Geogr]** 1980 Sep;14D(3):345–7
**Greenstone JD:** Dorothea Dix and Jane Addams: from transcendentalism to pragmatism in American social reform. **Soc Serv Rev** 1979;53(4):527–59
**Greenwald GI, Greenwald MW:** Medicolegal progress in inquest of felonious deaths: Westminster, 1761–1866. **J Leg Med (Chicago)** 1981 Jun;2(2):193–264
**Greenwald GI** see **Greenwald MW**
**Greenwald MW, Greenwald GI:** Coroner's inquests. A source of vital statistics: Westminster, 1761–1866. **J Leg Med (Chicago)** 1983 Mar;4(1):51–86
**Greenwald MW** see **Greenwald GI**
**Greenwalt TJ:** Rh immunization. The importance of a critical case study. **JAMA** 1984 Mar 9;251(10):1318–20
**Greenway G** see **Resnick D**
**Greenwood RD:** Operation for Aneurism of the Axillae'--1834, a historical notation. **J Med Assoc State Ala** 1982 May;51(11):57
**Greenwood RD:** Surgical treatment for facial hemangioma, 1834. **Ala Med** 1984 Sep;54(3):27
**Greenwood RD:** 19th century medicine in Indiana. An 1869 clinical report by J. S. Bobbs. **Indiana Med** 1984 Jun;77(6):476
**Grefberg N, Nilsson P:** Peritonealdialys--60-års jubileum och expansion genom CAPD. **Nord Med** 1983;98(11):260–2
**Greffe F** see **La Salpêtrière**
**Greganti MA** see **Fletcher SW**
**Gregg DA** see **Ewald BH**
**Gregg JB, Zimmerman LJ, Steele JP, et al:** Ante-mortem osteopathology at Crow Creek. **Plains Anthropol** 1981;26(94 pt 1):287–300
**Gregg JB, Zimmerman L, Clifford S, et al:** Craniofacial anomalies in the Upper Missouri River over a millennium: archeological and clinical evidence. **Cleft Palate J** 1981 Jul;18(3):210–22
**Gregg JB, Steele JP:** Mastoid development in ancient and modern populations. A longitudinal radiological study. **JAMA** 1982 Jul 23;248(4):459–64
**Gregg JB, Reed A:** Monostotic fibrous dysplasia in the temporal bone: a late prehistoric occurrence. **Am J Phys Anthropol** 1980 May;52(4):587–93
**Gregg JB, Steele JP, Zimmerman L, et al:** Otolaryngic osteopathology in 14th century mid-America. The crow creek massacre. **Ann Otol Rhinol Laryngol** 1981 May–Jun;90(3 pt 1):288–93
**Gregg JB, Steele JP, Bass WM:** Unusual osteolytic defects in ancient South Dakota skulls. **Am J Phys Anthropol** 1982 Jul;58(3):243–54
**Gregg JB** see **Zimmerman LJ**
**Gregg PS** see **Gregg JB**
**Gregg PS** see **Zimmerman LJ**
**Gregg JB, et al:** Possible treponematosis in fourteenth century Dakota territory: a progress report. **Paleopathol Newsl** 1981 Jun;34:5–6
**Gregl A, Heyden D von, Muschter R:** Diagnostik peripherer Odeme in der Praxis und in der Klinik. **Z Lymphol** 1982 Jun;6(1):25–32
**Grégoire-Reiters M** see **Hélin E**
**Gregor Johann Mendel 1822–1884. In centenary commemoration: Hereditas** 1984;100(1):2–13
**Gregory CJ:** Elfrida K. Berzins: world record holder, olympic athlete, concert soloist, author, and pioneer physical educator. **Can J Hist Sport Phys Educ** 1979;10(2):1–14
**Gregory JW, Piché V:** African population: reproduction for whom? **Daedalus** 1982 Spring;:179–209
**Gregory RL:** Bacon's last egg?--the Exploratory. **Perception** 1982;11(4):371–5
**Gregory RL:** Forty years on: Kenneth Craik's The Nature of Explanation (1943). **Perception** 1983;12(3):233–7
**Gregory RL:** French without fears: Denis Diderot. **Perception** 1983;12(5):509–12
**Gregory RL:** Gnomenclature of magic mechanisms (2). **Perception** 1982;11(1):1–3
**Gregory RL:** Mind in science. A history of explanations in psychology and physics. Cambridge, New York, Cambridge University Press, 1981. xi, 641 p.
**Gregory RL:** The oldest optical society in the world. **Perception** 1979;8(3):245–6
**Gregory RL:** The 4th dimension of 3-D. **Perception** 1980;9(6):613–6
**Gregory RL:** Two pins and a length of string: Kepler's vision. **Perception** 1983;12(4):371–4
**Greiner JR** see **Rosenthal MM**
**Greisman HC:** Social structure, psychoanalysis, and collective aggression. **Hist Eur Ideas** 1981;2(1):35–48
**Greisman HC:** Tycho Brahe: astronomer of renaissance Denmark. In Romm S, ed: Symposium on historical perspectives of plastic surgery. Philadelphia, Saunders, 1983. p. 629–33.
**Greisman HC:** Wound management and medical organization in the Civil War. **Surg Clin North Am** 1984 Aug;64(4):625–38
**Greisman HC** see **Romm S, ed**
**Greither A:** Otto Pankok und Düsseldorf; der Akademieprofessor Otto Pankok und seine Kunst. **Jahrb Univ Dusseld** 1977–78;:249–57
**Grellet I, Kruse C:** Histoires de la tuberculose. Les fièvres de l'âme 1800–1940. Paris, Ramsay, 1983. 333 p.
**Grenander ME:** Of graver importance than history: psychiatry in fiction. **J Libert Stud** 1978;2(1):29–44
**Grenander ME:** Psychiatry's sacred cow. **Reason** 1979;10(11):30–1, 34
**Grendel E:** Het had een excursie van de Kring kunnen zijn. **Pharm Weekbl** 1981 Nov 6;116(45):1383–6
**Grene M** see **Spicker SF, ed**
**Grenier JY:** Quelques éléments pour une étude des liens entre conjoncture économique et conjoncture démographique aux XVIIe et XVIIIe siècles. **Ann Demogr Hist (Paris)** 1984;:175–99
**Grenon-Plante D:** La contraception: oui, mais à quel prix? **Infirm Can** 1982 Nov;24(10):27–31
**Grensemann H:** Das 24. Kapitel von 'De aeribus, aquis, locis' und die Einheit der Schrift. **Hermes** 1979;107:423–41
**Grensemann H:** Eine jüngere Schicht in den gynäkologischen Schriften. In La collection hippocratique et son rôle dans l'histoire de la médecine. Colloque de Strasbourg (23–27 octobre 1972) organisé par le Centre de Recherches sur la Grèce Antique, avec le concours des Facultés de Philosophie et des Langues Classiques. Leiden, E. J. Brill, 1975. p. 151–69.
**Grensemann H** see **Grmek MD, ed**
**Grensemann H, ed:** Hippokratische Gynäkologie. Die gynäkologischen Texte des Autors C nach den pseudohippokratischen Schriften De muliebribus I, II, und De sterilibus. Wiesbaden, Steiner, 1982. 191 p.
**Grenvik A, Eross B, Powner D:** Historical survey of mechanical ventilation. **Int Anesthesiol Clin** 1980 Summer;18(2):1–10
**Greulich G** see **Baumer G**
**Grey-Turner E:** The British Medical Association and its South African branches. **S Afr Med J** 1983 Jun 29;Spec No:2–3
**Greydanus DE, Geller B:** Masturbation; historic perspective. **NY State J Med** 1980 Nov;80(12):1892–6
**Gribanov ED:** Emblemy meditsiny. Tbilisi, Sabchota Sakartvelo, 1979. 111

p.
Gribanov ED, Sgibova LI: Leonardo da Vinchi kak anatom. **Feldsher Akush** 1982;47(7):43-6
**Gribanov ED:** Memorial'nye medali N. I. Pirogova (k 100-letiiu so dnia smerti). **Feldsher Akush** 1981;46(12):42-5
**Gribanov ED:** Muzeĭ Tsentral'nogo ordena Lenina instituta usovershenstvovaniia vracheĭ. **Sov Zdravookhr** 1982;(8):77-8
**Gribanov ED:** Rol' Tsentral'nogo instituta usovershenstvovaniia vracheĭ v podgotovke kadrov istorikov meditsiny. **Sov Zdravookhr** 1979;(10):60-1
**Gribanov ED** see **Soloveĭ MG**
**Gribanov ED** see **Vladimirova LB**
**Gridgeman NT:** A semicentennial. The NRCC research journals 1929-1979. **Can J Physiol Pharmacol** 1979 Jul;57(7):i-xiv; Also in Can J Biochem 1979 Jul;57(7):iv-xvi; Also in Can J Zool 1979 Jul; 57(7):i-xiv
**Grieman R** see **Teplitsky PE**
**Grieshaber EP:** Survival of Indian communities in nineteenth-century Bolivia: a regional comparison. **J Lat Am Stud** 1980;12(2):223-69
**Griffenhagen G:** Drug and underprints from France. [Laboratoire Veyron-Froment, Marseilles.] **Scalpel Tongs** 1981;25:61-3
**Griffenhagen G:** Pharmacy centennials in Australia and New Zealand. **Scalpel Tongs** 1981;25:75
**Griffenhagen GB** see **Holcombe HW**
**Griffin JD, Greenland C:** Asylum at lower Fort Garry, 1874-1886. **Beaver** 1980;310(4):18-23
**Griffin JD, Greenland C:** Institutional care of the mentally disordered in Canada--a 17th century record. **Can J Psychiatry** 1981 Jun;26(4):274-8
**Griffin JD, Greenland C:** Manifestations of madness in New France. In: Congrès international d'histoire de la médecine, XXVe, Québec, 1976. Actes. Québec, 1977. p. 727-45.
**Griffin JD:** The amazing careers of Hincks and Beers. **Can J Psychiatry** 1982 Dec;27(8):668-71
**Griffin JD** see **Greenland C**
**Griffin JR:** Historical summary of visual fields methods. **J Am Optom Assoc** 1980 Sep;51(9):833-5
**Griffin R** see **Silvay G**
**Griffin RJ:** Herbal medicine revisited: science looks anew at ancient Chinese pharmacology. **Am Pharm** 1979 Sep;19(10):16-22
**Griffin RJ:** New approaches to an ancient disease: leprosy. **Am Pharm** 1981 Sep;21(9):18-23
**Griffith DP:** Urolithiasis. **J Urol** 1981 Oct;126(4):431
**Griffith WP:** Priestley in London. **Notes Rec R Soc Lond** 1983 Aug;38(1):1-16
**Griffiths CT** see **Winfree LT**
**Griffiths J:** Doctor Thomas Dimsdale, and smallpox in Russia. The variolation of the Empress Catherine the Great. **Bristol Med Chir J** 1984 Jan;99(369):14-6
**Griffiths RA:** The interaction of war and plague in the later middle ages. In J. Cule, ed: Wales and medicine. London, British Society for the History of Medicine, 1975. p. 127-40.
**Grigg D:** Modern population growth in historical perspective. **Geography** 1982;67(2):97-108
**Grigg ER** see **Murphy BE**
**Grigorash FF, Tsudechkis LM, Grigor'ev IuP:** K istorii bor'by alkogolizmom v Latvii. **Sov Zdravookhr** 1981;(6):58-60
**Grigorenko GF:** K 110-letiiu Vladivostokskogo voenno-morskogo gospitalia. **Vestn Khir** 1983 May;130(5):142-3
**Grigor'ev IuP** see **Grigorash FF**
**Grigor'eva VA:** Tvorcheskiĭ vklad v biokhimiiu myshts. **Ukr Biokhim Zh** 1980 Nov-Dec;52(6):783-8
**Grigorewitsch A:** Prinzipien in der Behandlung Geisteskranker im Russland des 19. Jahrhunderts. **Psychiatr Neurol Med Psychol (Leipz)** 1980 Jul;32(7):424-9
**Grigorian NA:** I. M. Sechenov i razvitie nauki v Rossii (k 150-letiiu so dnia rozhdeniia). **Sov Zdravookhr** 1979;(10):50-4
**Grigorian NA:** [I. M. Sechenov on science and its history] (Rus). **Istor Biol Issled** 1980;8:173-87
**Grigor'ian NA:** I. P. Pavlov o nauke i sotsial'noĭ otvetvennosti uchenogo. **Sov Zdravookhr** 1984;(2):58-61
**Grigorian NA:** Rol' uchenykh Kazanskogo universiteta v razvitii obshchestvennoĭ meditsiny. **Sov Zdravookhr** 1981;(7):48-51
**Grigor'ian RA** see **Govyrin VA**
**Grigori'ian NA:** Razvitie ucheniia o vyssheĭ nervnoĭ deiatel'nosti v trudakh L. A. Orbeli. **Zh Vyssh Nerv Deiat** 1982 Nov-Dec;32(6):1011-9
**Grimaud JA** see **Aterman K**
**Grimm H:** Carl Heinrich Stratz (1858 bis 1924) als Mitbegründer einer ärztlichen Jugendkunde. Zeittafeln zu seinem Leben und seiner Wirksamkeit. **Aerztl Jugendkd** 1979 Jun;70(3):177-92
**Grimm H:** Neue Hinweise auf ur- und frühgeschichtliches sowie mittelalterliches Vorkommen der Rachitis und ähnlicher Mineralisationsstörungen. **Arztl Jugendkd** 1984 Jun;75(3):168-77
**Grimm H:** Paläopathologische Befunde an Menschenresten der römischen Kaiserzeit und Völkerwanderungszeit in der DDR. **Ausgrab Funde** 1979;24:267-74
**Grimm H:** Was wissen wir über ur- und frühgeschichtliche Kindernahrung? **Aerztl Jugendkd** 1981;72(3):170-3
**Grimm H:** Weibliche Figurinen als Zeugnisse vorgeschichtlicher Jugendweihe-Riten? **Aerztl Jugendkd** 1982 Mar;73(1):40-3
**Grimm H:** Zur historischen Vertiefung der Akzelerationsforschung. **Aerztl Jugendkd** 1982;73(3):182-93
**Grimm M:** Frakturen und Frakturheilung in der Ur- und Frühgeschichte. **Beitr Orthop Traumatol** 1982 Feb;29(2):61-70
**Grims F** see **Heilmittel aus Pflanzen und Tieren**
**Grin' NV** see **Vankhanen VD**
**Grin' V:** Organizatsiia meditsinskogo obespecheniia v oboronitel'nykh operatsiiakh pervogo perioda voiny. **Voen Istor Zh** 1978;3:101-6
**Grin' VA:** O meditsinskom obespechenii bitvy pod Kurskom. **Voen Med Zh** 1980 Apr;(4):21-6
**Grin' VA** see **Iurov IA**
**Grinberg L, Rodríguez JF:** The influence of Cervantes on the future creator of psychoanalysis. **Int J Psychoanal** 1984;65(Pt 2):155-68
**Grinder RD** see **Melosi MV, ed**
**Grindstaff CF** see **Trovato F**
**Grinker RR:** Fifty years in psychiatry. Springfield, Ill., Thomas, 1979. xiii, 263 p.
**Grinspoon L, Bakalar JB:** Coca and cocaine as medicines: an historical review. **J Ethnopharmacol** 1981 Mar-May;3(2-3):149-59
**Grinstein A:** Sigmund Freud's dreams. New York, International Universities Press, 1980. 486 p.
**Grisanti A:** La medicina, libertada por el libertador. **Rev Soc Venez Hist Med** 1972-73;20-21(34-35):203-5
**Grist NR:** Pandemic influenza 1918. **Br Med J** 1979 Dec 22-29;2(6205):1632-3
**Gritsiute LA** see **Telichenas AI**
**Gritskevich VP:** Istoriko-meditsinskoe istochnikovedenie. **Sov Zdravookhr** 1980;(9):56-8
**Grivaux M:** Soixante-quinzième anniversaire de l'Associaton d'Enseignement médical des Hôpitaux de Paris (1907-1982). **Sem Hop Paris** 1983 Mar 31;59(13):865-7
**Grivetti LE:** Cultural nutrition: anthropological and geographical themes. **Annu Rev Nutr** 1981;1:47-68
**Grmek M:** La vita, la morte, la malattia nel mondo di Omero. **Intersezioni** 1983;3:243-64
**Grmek M:** Les ruses de guerre biologiques dans l'antiquité. **Rev Etud Grec** 1979;92:142-63
**Grmek MD:** A plea for freeing the history of scientific discoveries from myth. In M. D. Grmek, R. S. Cohen, G. Cimino, eds: On scientific discovery. The Erice Lectures 1977. Dordrecht, D. Reidel, 1981. p. 9-42. (Boston Studies in the Philosophy of Science, v. 34).
**Grmek MD:** La légende et la réalité de la nocivité des fèves. **Hist Philos Life Sci** 1980;2(1):61-121
**Grmek MD:** La moxibustion en Méditerranée et en Extrême-Orient. **Clio Med** 1981 Dec;16(2/3):113-22
**Grmek MD:** La moxibustion en méditerranée et en extrème-orient. In Mazars G, ed: Les médecines traditionnelles de l'Asie. Strasbourg, Université Louis Pasteur, 1981. p. 60-74.
**Grmek MD:** La réalité nosologique au temps d'Hippocrate. In La collection hippocratique et son rôle dans l'histoire de la médecine. Colloque de Strasbourg (23-27 octobre 1972) organisé par le Centre de Recherches sur la Grèce Antique, avec le concours des Facultés de Philosophie et des Langues Classiques. Leiden, E. J. Brill, 1975. p. 239-55.
**Grmek MD:** Le concept d'infection dans l'Antiquité et au Moyen Age, les anciennes mesures sociales contre les maladies contagieuses et la fondation de la première quarantaine à Dubrovnik (1377). In Radovi sa Medunarodnog simpozija u povodu sestote obljetnice Dubrovacke karantene. Dubrovnik, 29 i 30. rujna 1977. Zagreb, 1980. p. 9-54.
**Grmek MD:** Le médecin au service de l'hôpital médiéval en Europe occidentale. **Hist Philos Life Sci** 1982;4(1):25-64
**Grmek MD, Fantini B:** Le rôle du hasard dans la naissance du modèle de l'opéron. **Rev Hist Sci (Paris)** 1982 Jul;35(3):193-215
**Grmek MD, Cohen RS, Cimino G, ed:** On scientific discovery. The Erice Lectures 1977. Dordrecht, D. Reidel, 1981. 333 p. (Boston Studies in the Philosophy of Science, v. 34).
**Grmek MD:** Planung und Zufall in der Forschung-eine historische Betrachtung. In R. Wittern, ed: Jahrbuch des Instituts für Geschichte der Medizin der Robert Bosch Stiftung. Stuttgart, Hippokrates Verlag, 1984. Bd. 1. p. 9-27.
**Grmek MD:** Vestigia della chirurgia greca: il Codice di Niceta e i suoi discendenti. **Kos** 1984 Jun;1(5):52-60
**Grmek MD** see **Boulle L**
**Grmek MD** see **Epistemologia, metodologia clinica e storia della scienza medica, 1**
**Grmek MD** see **Huard P**
**Grmek MD, ed:** Hippocratica. Actes du Colloque hippocratique de Paris (4-9 septembre 1978). Paris, Editions du Centre National de la Recherche Scientifique, 1980. 486 p. (Colloques Internationaux du C.N.R.S., No. 583). Contributions by A. Anastassiou, J. Benedum, J. Bertier, L. Bourgey, G. Brătescu, S. Byl, G. Cambiano, V. Di Benedetto, J. Ducatillon, M. P. Duminil, L. Garcia-Ballester, D. Gourevitch, H. Grensemann, G. Harig, J. Irigoin, C. Irmer, D. Irmer, R. Joly, J. Jouanna, H. M. Koelbing, V. Langholf, C. Lichtenthaeler, G. Maloney, W. Frohn Villeneuve, J. Mansfeld, P. Manuli, P. Mudry, J. M. Pigeaud, C. Sandulesco, W. D. Smith, A. Thivel, M. Vegetti.
**Grob GN:** Abuse in American mental hospitals in historical perspective: myth and reality. **Int J Law Psychiatry** 1980;3(3):295-310
**Grob GN:** Historical origins of deinstitutionalization. **New Dir Ment Health Serv** 1983 Mar;(17):15-29
**Grob GN:** Mental illness and American society, 1875-1940. Princeton, Princeton University Press, 1983. xiii, 428 p.
**Grob GN:** Rediscovering asylums: the unhistorical history of the mental hospital. In Vogel MJ, Rosenberg CE, ed: The therapeutic revolution. Philadelphia, 1979 p. 135-157.
**Grob GN, ed:** American perceptions of drug addiction: five studies,

1872–1912. New York, Arno Press, 1981. 1 v. (various pagings).
**Grob GN, ed:** Epidemiology of drug addiction: three studies, 1924–1926. New York, Arno, 1981 various pagings. Reprinted works.
**Grob GN, ed:** Mental hygiene in twentieth century America: four studies, 1921–1924. New York, Arno Press, 1979. Separate paginations.
**Grob GN, ed:** Narcotic addiction and American foreign policy: seven studies, 1924–1938. New York, Arno Press, 1981. 276 p. in various pagings. (Reprinted works).
**Grob GN, ed:** Nineteenth-century medical attitudes toward alcoholic addiction: six studies, 1814–1867. New York, Arno. 1981. various pagings (Reprinted works).
**Grob GN, ed:** Origins of medical attitudes toward drug addiction in America: eight studies, 1791–1858. New York, Arno Press, 1981. 1 v. (various pagings).
**Grob GN, ed:** Public policy and mental illness. Four investigations, 1915–1939. New York, Arno, 1980. Separate paginations.
**Grob GN, ed:** Public policy and the problem of addiction: four studies, 1914–1924. New York, Arno Press, 1981. 1 v. (various pagings).
**Grob GN, ed:** The beginnings of American psychiatric thought and practice. Five accounts, 1811–1830. New York, Arno, 1973. Various paginations. Includes Account of the rise and progress of the Asylum . . . near Philadelphia (1814), and works by Theodric Romeyn Beck (1811); Thomas Eddy (1815); George Parkman (1814); and Rufus Wyman (1830).
**Grob GN, ed:** The beginnings of mental hygiene in America. Three selected essays 1833–1850. New York, Arno, 1973. Various paginations. Includes works by Amariah Brigham (1833); William Sweetser (1850); Samuel B. Woodward (1840).
**Grob GN, ed:** The medical professions and drug addiction: six studies, 1882–1832. New York, Arno, 1981. various pagings. Reprinted works.
**Grobbelaar WC:** Die gemeenskapsverpleegkundige in perspektief. **Curationis** 1982 Sep;5(3):44–9
**Grobler SA:** Hemofilie--'n koninklike siekte. **S Afr Med J** 1981 Jul 25;60(4):143–4
**Grodum T:** Sindssygehuset i Slesvig. **Dan Medicinhist Arbog** 1983;12:122–43
**Grodzicka-Królak H** see **Horbowska-Marzec H**
**Groeben C, ed:** Guida alla Mostra allestita nella Sala degli Affreschi della Stazione Zoologica nella Villa Comunale (6 luglio – 30 settembre 1982) su Charles Darwin e la Stazione Zoologica di Napoli.
**Groeger S** see **Bullough VL**
**Groehler O:** Die Entwicklung der technischen Mittel des chemischen Krieges im imperialistischen Deutschland 1915–1945. **Militaergesch** 1976;15(6):718–28
**Groh F:** Zu einigen Aspekten der Mortalitäts- und Todesursachenstatistik. **Wiss Z Martin Luther Univ (Math)** 1978;27(6):121–32
**Gromala T:** Broadsides, epigrams, and testimonials: the evolution of chiropractic advertising. **Chiropr Hist** 1984;4(1):41–5
**Gromov AP, Panov IE, Panfilenko OA:** Razvitie sudebno-meditsinskoĭ sluzhby v SSSR. **Sud Med Ekspert** 1982 Oct–Dec;25(4):6–9
**Gronski P, Seiler FR:** Spezifische Serumtherapie gestern und heute von Antikörper-Präparaten Teil 1: Der Weg zur therapeutischen Anwendung. **Fortschr Med** 1983 Jan 27;101(4):103–6
**Groos KS:** Enkele opmerkingen met betrekking tot het graf van Herman Boerhaave in de Pieterskerk te Leiden. **Tijdschr Geschied Geneeskd** 1979;2(4):176–81
**Gros A** see **Chambers RW**
**Gröschel DH, Hornick RB:** Who introduced typhoid vaccination: Almroth Wright or Richard Pfeiffer? **Rev Infect Dis** 1981 Nov–Dec;3(6):1251–4
**Gross EG, Long JP:** Pharmacology at Iowa 1920–1980. **Life Sci** 1980 Dec 22–29;27(25–26):2423–6
**Gross G:** Medizin zwischen Wissenschaft und Spekulation. Die Phrenologie des Dr. Johann Kaspar Spurzheim aus Longwich. **Kurtrier Jahrb** 1977;17:35–52
**Gross HP:** Medical mission to Nepal. **SD J Med** 1983 Jan;36(1):5–7
**Gross J** see **Pfäfflin F**
**Gross R, Claus O:** Chemotherapie von Tumorleiden: Vergangenheit und Gegenwart. **Med Welt** 1982 Nov 5;33(44):1531–8
**Gross-Bachmann M:** Daniel Sailer, Leben und Wirken eines Idealisten. **Tirol Heimat** 1976;40:163–90
**Grosse SD:** The politics of family planning in the Maghrib. **Stud Comp Int Dev** 1982;17(1):22–48
**Grosse-Brockhoff F:** Herzbehandlung mit dem 'Fingerhut' einst und jetzt. Opladen, Westdeutscher Verlag, 1980. 58 p. (Rheinisch-Westfälische Akademie der Wissenschaften; Natur-, Ingenieur- und Wirtschaftswissenschaften, Vorträge N 293).
**Grossgebauer K** see **Pohle HD**
**Grosshans OR:** Biographical research in health education. **Health Educ (Wash)** 1981 Sep–Oct;12(5):40–1
**Grossi Turchetti ML:** La dotazione libraria di un collegio universitario del Quattrocento. **Physis** 1980;22(3–4):463–75
**Grossinger R:** Planet medicine. From stone age shamanism to post-industrial healing. Revised edition. Boulder, London, Shambhala, 1982. xviii, 436 p.
**Grossinger R, ed:** Alchemy; pre-Egyptian legacy, millennial promise. Richmond, California, North Atlantic Books, 1979. 253 p.
**Grosskurth P:** Havelock Ellis: biography. New York, Knopf, 1980. xvi, 492 p.
**Grossman E, Posner NA:** Surgical circumcision of neonates: a history of its development. **Obstet Gynecol** 1981 Aug;58(2):241–6
**Grossman EA, Posner NA:** The circumcision controversy: an update. **Obstet Gynecol Annu** 1984;13:181–95
**Grossman H** see **English PC**
**Grossman LI:** A personal history of dental practice: 1920–1980. **J Am Dent Assoc** 1981;102:360–5
**Grossman LI:** In the interest of historical fact. **J Endod** 1984 Apr;10(4):168
**Grossman LT:** A personal history of dental practice: 1920–1980. **J Am Dent Assoc** 1981 Mar;102(3):360–5
**Grossmann T:** Die hl. Ottilie, Patronin der Augenkranken. Eine ungewöhnliche Abbildung am Gnadenstuhlaltar von Bad Aussee mit Krebsscherenattribut. **Klin Monatsbl Augenheilkd** 1981 Jun;178(6):480–1
**Grote J** see **Mitcham C**
**Groth CG:** Kidney transplantations in the Nordic countries 1956–1980. **Scand J Urol Nephrol** 1981;64:12–5
**Grotjahn M:** Remembering Theodor Reik and the third ear. **Psychoanal Rev** 1981–82 Winter;68(4):473–6
**Grotstein JS** see **Goldberg A, ed**
**Grover Y:** La correspondance scientifique du P. Dominique Parrenin (1665–1741). In: France: Centre de Recherches interdisciplinaires de Chantilly (CERIC). Les rapports entre la Chine Sinologie (16–18 septembre 1977). Chantilly, Paris, Les Belles Lettres, 1980, 83–99.
**Groves D, Dunlop J, Buick R:** Les premières traces de vie. **Pour Sci** 1981;50:22–35
**Grow JB** see **Brantigan CO**
**Grozdanova E:** Za demografskoto sustoianie na karnobatsko i aitosko prez 17 i 18 vek. **Istor Pregl** 1976;32(6):81–8
**Grubb JM:** The first successful cesarean section and the first oophorectomy in the Americas. **W Va Med J** 1984 Oct;80(10):221–3
**Grubb R:** The discovery of the genetic markers of human immunoglobulins. **Vox Sang** 1983;45(1):89–90
**Gruber B:** Anatomist, scholar and gentleman: Arthur V. Nilsson–a legend in his own time. **Chiropr Hist** 1984;4(1):31–8
**Gruber B** see **Heilmittel aus Pflanzen und Tieren**
**Gruber B** see **Napolitano EG**
**Gruber HE, Keegan RT, ed:** Charles Darwin and the human sciences. Special issue. **J Hist Behav Sci** 1983 Jan;19(1):3–113
**Gruber HE:** Cognitive psychology, scientific creativity, and the case study method. In M. D. Grmek, R. S. Cohen, G. Cimino, ed: On scientific discovery. The Erice Lectures 1977. Dordrecht, D. Reidel, 1981. p. 295–322. (Boston Studies in the Philosophy of Science, v. 34).
**Gruber HE:** Darwin on man: a psychological study of scientific creativity. 2d. ed. Chicago, University of Chicago Press, 1981. xxvii, 310 p.
**Gruber HE:** Darwin on psychology and its relation to evolutionary thought. In R. W. Rieber, K. Salzinger, ed: Psychology: theoretical-historical perspectives. New York, Academic Press, 1980. p. 145–74.
**Gruber HE:** History and creative work: from the most ordinary to the most exalted. **J Hist Behav Sci** 1983 Jan;19(1):4–14
**Gruber HE:** Piaget's mission. **Soc Res (NY)** 1982;49(1):239–64
**Gruber HE:** The evolving systems approach to creative scientific work: Charles Darwin's early thought. In T. Nickles, ed: Scientific discovery: case studies. Dordrecht, D. Reidel, 1980. (Boston Studies in the Philosophy of Science, v. 60). p. 113–30.
**Gruber HE** see **Keegan RT**
**Gruber W** see **Gürtler LG**
**Grubmüller K:** Ein Arzt als Literat: Hans Hartlieb. In Honemann V, Ruh K, et al: Poesie und Gebrauchsliteratur im deutschen Mittelalter. Würzburger Colloquium 1978. Tûbingen, Niemeyer, 1979. p. 14–36.
**Grubrich-Simitis I:** Siegfried Bernfeld: Historiker der Psychoanalyse und Freud-Biograph. **Psyche (Stuttg)** 1981 May;35(5):397–434
**Grucci J de:** Consideraciones sobre Historia de la Gastroenterologia. (Tercer Congreso Nacional de Historia de la Medicina Argentina, 1973). **Sem Med** 1973;79(Aniversario):251–6
**Gruenbaum ER:** Medical anthropology, health policy and the state: a case study of Sudan. **Policy Stud Rev** 1981;1(1):47–65
**Grujic M:** Stogodišnjica otkrića bacila tuberkuloze. Zivot i delo Roberta Kocha. **Plucne Bolesti Tuberk** 1982 Jan–Jun;34(1–2):5–7
**Grujic V:** Nekolike korespondentne veze ismedju Vladana Djordjevića i Valtazara Bogišića. **Srp Ark Celok Lek** 1981 Jan;109(1):161–8
**Gruman GF** see **Spicker SF**
**Gruman GJ, ed:** Roots of modern gerontology and geriatrics. Frederic D. Zeman's 'Medical history of old age' and selected studies by other writers. New York, Arno, 1979. Various paginations.
**Gruman GJ, ed:** The 'Fixed period' controversy: prelude to modern ageism. New York, Arno Press, 1979. Various paginations. Reprint of passages by George M. Beard, William Osler, and James Crichton-Browne.
**Grumbach MM:** Herbert McLean Evans, revolutionary in modern endocrinology: a tale of great expectations. **J Clin Endocrinol Metab** 1982 Dec;55(6):1240–7
**Grünberg A:** Entwicklungen im Krankenhausbau in Deutschland unter Berücksichtigung funktioneller und hygienischer Aspekte. Diss. Mainz, 1981. 98 p.
**Grundy JH:** The evolution and impact of medical entomology. **J R Army Med Corps** 1980 Oct;126(3):140–50
**Grundy JH:** The evolution and impact of medical entomology. In Burgess NR, ed: John Hull Grundy's Arthropods of medical importance. Watch Cottage, Chilbolton, Hampshire, Noble Books, 1981. p. 13–25.
**Grunebaum A** see **Siegler AM**
**Grunert J:** Zur Geschichte der Psychoanalyse in München. **Psyche (Stuttg)** 1984 Oct;38(10):865–904
**Grünfeld B, Maltau JM:** Et helsepolitisk perspektiv på fruktbarhetsutviklingen i Norge 1880–2000. **Tidsskr Nor Laegeforen** 1983 Mar 20;103(8–9):795–9

**Grünfeld B** see **Maltau JM**
**Grunze H, Spriggs AI:** History of clinical cytology: a selection of documents. Darmstadt, Giebeler, 1980. 185 p.
**Grupe G:** Die Identifikation des Skelettes von Georg Christoph Lichtenberg. **Anthropol Anz** 1984 Mar;42(1):1–9
**Grüsser OJ:** J.E. Purkyně's contributions to the physiology of the visual, the vestibular and the oculomotor systems. **Hum Neurobiol** 1984;3(3):129–44
**Gruszkiewicz E, Głośnicka R, Kunikowska D:** Seroreactions in detecting Yersinia enterocolitica and Yersinia pseudotuberculosis in the Gdánsk region, years 1973–1976. **Bull Inst Marit Trop Med Gdynia** 1980;31(1–2):97–102
**Grützmacher KH** see **Klessen D**
**Gruzdev NA, Gol'braĭkh VR:** Voprosy istorii klinicheskoĭ stomatologicheskoĭ anatomii. **Stomatologiia (Mosk)** 1981 May–Apr;60(2):59–60
**Gruzinski S:** La mère dévorante: alcoolisme, sexualité et déculturation chez les mexicas (1500–1550). **Cah Am Lat** 1979;20:5–36
**Gryfe CI:** James E. Kadwo Kwegyir Aggrey, D.D., D.O., 1875–1927. **Scalpel Tongs** 1981;25:53–5
**Gryfe CI:** John Jeffries: the first flying physician. **Scalpel Tongs** 1981;25:80–2
**Grynaeus T, Papp J:** Régi magyar (gyógy) növénynevek mutatója, 15–17. század. **Orvostort Kozl** 1979;86(24 no 4):131–7
**Grzegorczyk L:** Uwagi na temat sytuacji epidemiologicznej w zakresie chorób zawodowych skóry w Polsce w latach 1971–1977. **Przegl Dermatol** 1980 Jul–Aug;67(4):455–7
**Gsell O:** Die Geschichte der Pneumonien--Wandel vom 19. zum 21. Jahrhundert. **Prax Klin Pneumol** 1984 Sep;38(9):379–88
**Gsell O:** Geschichte der Pneumonie. **Sudhoffs Arch** 1984;68(2):182–216
**Gsell O:** Geschichte und Bedeutung der Pneumonie im hohen Alter. **Z Gerontol** 1982 Nov–Dec;15(6):325–31
**Gsell O:** Hundert Jahre innere Medizin. Eröffnungsreden der Vorsitzenden der Deutschen Gesellschaft für innere Medizin. I. Teil 1882–1932. **Med Welt** 1983 Apr 8;34(14):428–33
**Gsell O:** Hundert Jahre innere Medizin. Eröffnungsreden der Vorsitzenden der Deutschen Gesellschaft für innere Medizin. II. Teil 1933–1982. **Med Welt** 1983 Apr 15;34(15):462–5
**Gsell O:** The history of leptospirosis: 100 years. **Zentralbl Bakteriol Mikrobiol Hyg [A]** 1984 Sep;257(4):473–8
**Guadagnino M, Buscaino GA:** Un secondo contributo a 'orientamenti teorici e pratici della psichiatria italiana dal 1950 al 1970'. **Acta Neurol [Quad]** 1978;37:116–30
**Guadagnino M** see **Buscaino GA**
**Gual Castro C:** Informe de labores con motivo del XXXV aniversario de la fundación del instituto Nacional de la Nutrición Salvador Zubirán. **Rev Invest Clin** 1982 Jan–Mar;34(1):85–9
**Guan JH** see **Neumeyer JL**
**Guardia CA:** Salud pública y saneamiento en la Zona del Canal de Panamá: un recuento histórico, 1880–1915. **Bol Of Sanit Panam** 1983 Jul;95(1):62–73
**Guardia y Pascual del Pobil R de la:** Los servicios de sanidad de la Armada en la Aeronautica Naval. **Rev Gen Mar** 1978 Aug–Sep;195:109–23
**Guarner V:** El conocimiento de la historia de la medicina en la educacion del cirujano. **Bol Soc Mex Hist Filos Med** 1979 Mar;4(26):73–87
**Guarner V, Ortiz-Monasterio F, Somolinos-Palencia J:** El enfermo en la historia de la medicina. **Gac Med Mex** 1983 Aug;119(8):301–14
**Guarner V:** El pequeño farabeuf, aquel gigante de mi vida estudiantil. **Bol Soc Mex Hist Filos Med** 1982 Mar;6(38):15–22
**Guarner V:** Louis-Hubert Farabeuf (1841–1910). **Gac Med Mex** 1982 Dec;118(12):505–8
**Guarner V** see **Jinich H**
**Guarner V** see **Somolinos-Palencia J**
**Guarnieri E:** La medicina a Firenze durante il governo dei Medici: 1440–1748. **Agressologie** 1981 Dec;22(F):7–9
**Gubéran E:** Tendances de la mortalité en Suisse. 2. Maladies infectieuses 1876–1977. **Schweiz Med Wochenschr** 1980 Apr 12;110(15):574–83
**Gubko AT:** Le rôle de l'Académie de Kiev dans la naissance de la science psychologique en Ukraine. (Rus) **Vopr Psikhol** 1980;(1):82–93
**Gŭdev Kh, Iliev N:** Pŭrvi rŭkopisen uchebnik po veterinarana medistina za kusistite ot Voennoto veterinarnofeldshersko uchilishte v Sofiia. **Vet Med Nauki** 1980;17(9–10):84–8
**Gudmundsson SP** see **Alfredsson JH**
**el-Guebaly A** see **el-Guebaly N**
**el-Guebaly N, el-Guebaly A.** Alcohol abuse in ancient Egypt: the recorded evidence. **Int J Addict** 1981 Oct;16(7):1207–21
**Guédès M:** Qu'est-ce qu'un mendélien? **Hist Nat** 1980–81;17–18:69–75
**Guédès M:** Une variante de la page de titre du De historia stirpium de L. Fuchs (1542). **J Soc Bibliogr Nat Hist** 1974;7(1):81–5
**Guéguen E:** Les jardins botaniques de Bretagne aux XVIIIe et XIXe siècles. In: Congrès National des Sociétés Savantes, 97e, Nantes, 1972. Comptes Rendus. Paris, 1976. Section des Sciences, Tome 1. p. 377–83.
**Gueniot-Le Minor G:** La peste des chiffonniers à Paris en 1920. Diss. Paris, 1980. 83 lv.
**Guenter M** see **Drews FH**
**Guenzi A:** Processo popolare in Piazza Maggiore: la carestia del 1648 a Bologna. **Archiginnasio (Italy)** 1979;74:161–80
**Guerini V:** Historia tes odontiatrikes. **Odontostomatol Proodos** 1981 Nov–Dec;35(6):198–204 contd
**Guerlac H:** Essays and papers in the history of modern science. Baltimore, London, Johns Hopkins University Press, 1977. xix, 540 p.
**Guerlac H:** Theological voluntarism and biological analogies in Newton's physical thought. **J Hist Ideas** 1983 Apr–Jun;44(2):219–29
**Guerra F:** El medico politico. Estudios biográficos sobre la influencia del médico en la Historia Politica de Hispanoamérica y Filipinas. Madrid, Afrodisio Aguado, 1975. 350 p.
**Guerra F:** Historia de la medicina. Tomo I. Madrid, Ediciones Norma, 1982. ix, 387 p.
**Guerra F:** La cirurgía catalana y contemporánea y la cirugía castellana del Renacimiento. In Congrés International d'Història de la Medicina Catalana, 2nd, Barcelona, 1975. Llibre d'Actes. Barcelona, Socitra, 1977. p. 49–58.
**Guerra F:** La evaluacion farmacológica de las fuentes históricas sobre la medicina precolombina. **Guatem Indig** 1978;13(1/2):175–85
**Guerra F:** La neurosis del exilio en Mariano Batllés, 1827. In International Congress of the History of Medicine, 27th, Barcelona, 1980. Actas. Barcelona, Académia de Ciències Médiques de Catalunya i Balears, 1981. p. 177–80.
**Guerra F:** La tradicion medieval en la cirugia española del siglo XVI. **Asclepio** 1978–79;30–31:359–63
**Guerra F:** Las heridas de guerra. Contribución de los cirujanos Españoles en la evolución de su tratamiento. Santander, Catedra de Historia de la Medicina, Universidad de Santander, 1981. XVI, 237 p.
**Guerra F:** Les médecins patriotes. In: Congres international d'histoire de la médecine, XXVe, Québec, 1976. Actes. Québec, 1977. p. 746–54.
**Guerra F:** Medicine in Dutch Brazil 1624–1654. In: Johan Maurits van Nassau-Siegen 1604–1679 ... Essays on the ... tercentenary of his death. Ed. by E. van den Boogaart et al. The Hague, J. M. van Nassau-Siegen Stichting, 1979. p. 472 ff.
**Guerra F:** The description of syphilis in Avicenna. In International Congress of the History of Medicine, 27th, Barcelona, 1980. Actas. Barcelona, Académia de Ciències Médiques de Catalunya i Balears, 1981. p. 731–3.
**Guerra F:** The historical cycles in traditional medicine. **Stud Hist Med** 1980 Mar;4(1):57–63
**Guerra F:** Three battles that changed military surgery: Avigliana 1536. Moscow 1812. Ebro 1938. In International Congress of the History of Medicine. 26th, Plovdiv, 1978. Actes du Congress. Sofia, 1981. Volume II. p. 82–3.
**Guerra F** see **Bowers JZ**
**Guerra F** see **Hand WD, ed**
**Guerra F** see **Sanchez Tellez MC**
**Guerra FS, Flores GK:** Carlos J. Finlay y Barrés (1833–1915). **Trans R Soc Trop Med Hyg** 1983;77(6):850
**Guerra M:** Corino Andrade na história da medicina Portuguesa. **Acta Med Port** 1983 Apr–May;4(4–5):239–43
**Guerra M:** Origens do ensino da história da medicina em Portugal. **Acta Med Port** 1980 Sep–Dec;2(5–6):335–6
**Guerra M:** Os primeiros passos na clínica de há 70 anos descritos por Romão Loff. **Acta Med Port** 1983 Jul–Aug;4(7–8):379–80
**Guerrand RH:** L'âge d'or du bidet. **Histoire** 1983;(57):84–7
**Guerrand RH:** Petite histoire du quotidien: l'avènement de la chasse d'eau. **Histoire** 1982;43:96–9
**Guerrero AC:** The superego concept. Part I: historical review; object relations approach. **Psychoanal Rev** 1981 Fall;68(3):321–42
**Guerrier Y, Mounier-Kuhn P:** Histoire des maladies de l'oreille, du nez et de la gorge. Les grandes étapes de l'otorhino-laryngologie. Paris, Dacosta. 1980. 492 p.
**Guerrier Y** see **Mounier-Kuhn P**
**Guerrino AA:** Las traducciones médicas hasta el renacimiento. In International Congress of the History of Medicine, 27th, Barcelona, 1980. Actas. Barcelona, Académia de Ciències Médiques de Catalunya i Balears, 1981. p. 249–52.
**Guesdon C:** Contribution à l'étude de l'évolution de la pharmacie rouennaise: les différents titulaires d'une officine rue du Gros-Horloge. Thèse Dipl. d'Etat Dr. en Pharm., Université Rouen. Rouen, 1982. 65 (13) leaves.
**Guess HA:** Bernoulli's cost-benefit analysis of smallpox immunization. **N Engl J Med** 1981 Aug 6;305(6):347
**Guest AM:** Fertility variation among the U.S. foreign stock population in 1900. **Int Migr Rev** 1982;16(3):577–94
**Guest AM:** Social structure and U. S. inter-state fertility differentials in 1900. **Demography** 1981 Nov;18(4):465–86
**Guest AM** see **Tolnay SE**
**Guest C:** The Pied Piper of Hamelin. **Lancet** 1984 Dec 22;2(8417–18):1454–5
**Guest-Gornall RG:** Good servants are scarce. **Br Med J [Clin Res]** 1981 Dec 19;283(6307):1674–5
**Guggenbühl-Craig A:** Geschichtliche Entwicklung des Begriffes der Psychopathie. In his: Seelenwüsten. Betrachtungen über Eros und Psychopathie. Zürich, Schweizer Spiegel Verlag, 1980. p. 50–68.
**Guggenheim KY:** Nutrition and nutritional diseases. The evolution of concepts. Lexington, Massachusetts, Toronto, D.C. Heath and Company, 1981. xii, 378 p.
**Guggenheim YK:** Forerunners of the vitamin doctrine. **Koroth** 1979 Nov;7(9–10):CLXXXI–CXCIV(634–43)
**Guggenheim YK:** Jonathan Pereira's contribution to the science of nutrition. **Koroth** 1982 Aug;8(3/4):123–34
**Guggenheim YK:** [Joseph Goldberger's contributions to pellagra research] (Heb). **Harefuah** 1980;99(5–6):134–6
**Guggenheim YK:** Leonardo da Vinci's views on nutrition. **Koroth** 1981;8(1–2):31–9
**Guha M, Wood M:** Does health visiting have a history? **Health Visit** 1981

Dec;54(12):540

**Guidetti B:** Francesco Durante. June 29, 1844 to October 2, 1934. **Surg Neurol** 1983 Jul;20(1):1-3

**Guidetti B, Giuffrè R, Valente V:** Italian contribution to the origin of neurosurgery. **Surg Neurol** 1983 Oct;20(4):335-46

**Guidotti A:** Frequencies of cribra orbitalia in central Italy (19th century) under special consideration of their degrees of expression. **Anthropol Anz** 1984 Mar;42(1):11-6

**Guiguen C** see **Doby JM**

**Guillat JC:** La contraception: introduction. **Soins Gynecol Obstet Pueric Pediatr** 1982 Jul-Aug;(14-15):3-4

**Guillat JC:** L'histoire de la contraception à travers les textes officiels. **Soins Gynecol Obstet Pueric Pediatr** 1982 Jul-Aug;(14-15):53-4

**Guillaume J** see **Delaunay A, ed**

**Guillaume M** see **Patrimoine hospitalier de la Bourgogne**

**Guillaume P:** Malades, médecine et médecins à Bordeaux au 19e siècle. **Ann Bretagne** 1979;86(3):291-300

**Guillaume P** see **Dupâquier J**

**Guillemain B, Chaunu P, et al.:** La mort au moyen âge. Colloque de l'Association des Historiens médiévistes fraçais rèunis à Strasbourg en Juin 1975 au Palais Universitaire. Strasbourg, Istra, 1975. 152 p. Contributions by J. Le Goff, J. P. Sodini, P. C. Timbal, L. Buchet, C. Lorren, J. C. Schmitt, F. Rapp, M. Berthe, P. Vaillant, P. Paravy, H. Martin, C. Beaune, F. Thiriet.

**Guillemin J:** La maladie de Richard Wagner. Pour le centenaire de sa mort à Venise. **Sem Hop Paris** 1983 May 12;59(19):1493-6

**Guillemin R** see **Robin ED, ed**

**Guilleminault C** see **Czeisler CA**

**Guillermand J:** La tradition hospitalière militaire. **Med Armees** 1980;8(10)spec:817

**Guillermand J:** Un anniversaire et une tradition: l'Académie Royale de Chirurgie. **Med Armees** 1981;9:807-11

**Guillerme A:** Medical topography and the rebuilding of Le Mans. **Soc Soc Hist Med Bull (Lond)** 1984 Dec;35:26-7

**Guillerme J:** Oxygène et thérapeutique. **Dix-huit Siecle** 1982;14:27-43

**Guillerot E:** Réflexion historique sur le traitement préventif des phlébites des membranes inférieurs selon Nard et Chalier. **Phlebologie** 1984 Jan-Mar;37(1):13-6

**Guillon J:** Un aspect de la population pendant la Révolution. Les entrées à l'Hôtel-Dieu de Paris, ler novembre 1791 - 10 novembre 1799. Maîtrise. Univ. de Paris I, 1976. 104 p.

**Guillory F:** Family planning in Louisiana. **New South** 1971;26(4):29-34

**Guinsberg E** see **Langer M**

**Guinsburg AM:** Paracelsian magic and theology; a case study of the Matthew commentaries. **Medizinhist J** 1981;16(1-2):125-39

**Guirao Pérez M** see **Zuluaga Gómez A**

**Guliaeva SE:** K istorii izucheniia épilepsii Kozhevnikova. **Zh Nevropatol Psikhiatr** 1984;84(6):919-29

**Gulida MV:** Ialtinskomu protivotuberkuleznomu dispanseru 60 let. **Probl Tuberk** 1984 Mar;(3):71-2

**Gulida MV:** Razvitie sanatorno-kurortnogo lecheniia bol'nykh tuberkulezom na iuzhnom beregu Kryma. **Probl Tuberk** 1981;(7):65-8

**Gumpert M:** Hölle im Paradies. Selbstdarstellung eines Arztes. Hildesheim, Gerstenberg, 1983. xxiii, 280 p. (Exilliteratur, Band 17) Reprint of 1939 ed., with new biographical forward by F. Trapp.

**Gumpert TE:** Recollected in tranquillity. Sheffield, [Eng.], Walker and Carson, 1978. 168 p.

**Gunawardena DC:** Medicinal and economic plants of the Musaeum Zeylanicum of Paul Hermann. **J Sri Lanka Branch R Asiat Soc** 1975;19:33-48

**Gunby P:** 'Air therapy' history offers lessons for clinicians today. **JAMA** 1981 Sep 4;246(10):1064, 1066

**Guncheon KF:** Diagnostic imaging: an inside look. **Hospitals** 1981 Jan 1;55(1):86-8, 95

**Gundel HG, ed:** Die ältesten Statuten der Giessener Medizinischen Fakultät: Leges et Statuta Collegii Medici. Giessen, Universitätsbibliothek, 1979. 32 p.

**Gundersen A:** Appendicitis. **Wis Med J** 1981 Dec;80(12):23-8

**Gundlach JL:** Prof. Dr Stefan Furmaga (1924-1983). Wspomnienie pośmiertne. **Wiad Parazytol** 1984;30(3):385-91

**Gunev V:** Chetvŭrt vek spisanie 'Akusherstvo i ginekologiia'. **Akush Ginekol (Sofiia)** 1983;22(3):242-3

**Gunin GP** see **Alekseev GA**

**Gun'ko MA** see **Onopchenko NA**

**Gunn RA:** Botulism: from van Ermengem to the present. A comment. **Rev Infect Dis** 1979 Jul-Aug;1(4):720-1

**Gunnell JG:** The technocratic image and the theory of technocracy. **Technol Cult** 1982 Jul;23(3):392-16

**Gunst VK:** Memoirs-Professional and personal: a decade with Frieda Fromm-Reichmann. **Psychiatry** 1982;45(2):107-15

**Gunter PA:** Bergson and Jung. **J Hist Ideas** 1982 Oct-Dec;43(4):635-52

**Günther B:** Génesis del de homeostasis: de Claude Bernard a Walter Cannon. **Rev Med Chil** 1981 May;109(5):484-5

**Günther M:** Die Institutionalisierung der Rassenhygiene an den deutschen Hochschulen vor 1933. Diss., Johannes Gutenberg-Universität, Mainz, 1982. 148 p.

**Guntrip G:** The unknown Edith Cavell. **Nurs Times** 1984 Apr 25-May 1;80(17):63-4

**Guo Chengyu:** [Yang Tianhui and his 'Records on Radix aconitinum'] (Chi). **Chin J Med Hist** 1981;11(1):48-50

**Gupta AD:** Catastrophes and their population symptoms. In Charbonneau H, Larose A, ed: The great mortalities: methodological studies of demographic crises in the past. Liège, Belgium, Ordina Editions, 1980. p. 61-8.

**Gupta BL:** Surgery in angina. **Indian Heart J** 1980;(9):415-24

**Gupta D** see **Datta B**

**Gurauskas VB, Miashka VA:** Razvitie kurortologii v Litve za gody Sovetskoĭ vlasti. **Vopr Kurortol Fizioter Lech Fiz Kult** 1982 Nov-Dec;(6):18-20

**Gurd DP:** As it was in the beginning. . . **J R Nav Med Serv** 1980 Summer;66(2):140-6

**Gurd DP:** Australia and around the world. **J R Nav Med Serv** 1982 Winter;68(3):159-66 contd

**Gurd DP:** Headquarters Queen Anne's Mansions. **J R Nav Med Serv** 1983 Winter;69(3):161-6

**Gurd DP:** Mediterranean memories. **J R Nav Med Serv** 1981;67(3):169-76 contd.

**Gurevich NM:** Dinamika rosta naseleniia zarubezhnoi Azii v nashei ere. **Nar Azii Afriki** 1975;(4):69-80

**Gurevich SA:** Aktual'nye problemy psikhiatrii v 'Vestnike klinicheskoĭ i sudebnoĭ psikhiatrii i nevropatologii' (k 100-letiiu osnovaniia otechestvennoĭ psikhiatricheskoĭ periodiki). **Zh Nevropatol Psikhiatr** 1983;83(8):1236-40

**Gurevich SA:** Lev Tolstoĭ i psikhiatriia. **Zh Nevropatol Psikhiatr** 1981;81(9):1386-9

**Gurevich SA:** Problemy épileptologii v otechestvennoĭ psikhiatrii XIX veka (po materialam pervykh psikhiatricheskikh zhurnalov). **Zh Nevropatol Psikhiatr** 1983;83(6):914-7

**Gurevitsh SA:** [The pathographic method in the history of medicine.] (Rus). **Orvostort Kozl** 1981;93-96(27 No 1-4):155-69

**Gurgenidze GS** see **Iaroshevski MG**

**Gurjar GK, Anand RM:** Apurva Vaidya of Vagbhata. **Bull Indian Inst Hist Med (Hyderabad)** 1975 Oct;5(4):207-10

**Gurovskiĭ NN** see **Gazenko OG**

**Gurría Lacroix J:** La población de la provincia de Tabasco durante el virreinato. **Estud Hist Novohisp** 1978;6:65-88

**Gürtler LG, Jäger V, Gruber W, et al:** Presence of proteins in human bones 200, 1200 and 1500 years of age. **Hum Biol** 1981 Feb;53(1):137-50

**Guru LV** see **Singhal GD**

**Gurvich KI:** Uchastiie meditsinskikh rabotnikov v revoliutsionnom dvizhenii v Rossii XIX- nachala XX veka. **Vopr Istor** 1972;4:203-6

**Gurvich MM, Georgievskiĭ AS:** Nekotorye uroki organizatsii meditsinskogo obespecheniia voĭsk Zapadnogo i Kalininskogo frontov v kontrnastuplenii (k 40-letiiu razgroma nemetsko-fashistskikh voĭsk pod Moskvoĭ). **Voen Med Zh** 1982 Jan;(1):14-9

**Gusakov NI:** K 200-letiiu ucheniia A.M. Schumlianskogo o pochke (1782-1982). **Sov Med** 1983;(4):117-8

**Gusakov NI** see **Suslov VV**

**Gusakov IuA** see **Savich VI**

**Gusdorf G:** Médecine romantique. **Etud Philos** 1983;:11-23

**Gusdorf G:** Médecine romantique. A la mémoire du Pr Marc Klein. **Etud Philos** 1981;(1):11-23

**Güse HG, Schmacke N:** Psychiatrie zwischen bürgerlicher Revolution und Faschismus. Kronberg, Ger., Athenäum Verlag, 1976.

**Güse HG, Schmacke N:** Psychiatry and the origins of Nazism. **Int J Health Serv** 1980;10(2):177-96

**Guseĭnov DIa, Guseĭnova ZN:** Razvitie farmakologii v Azerbaĭdzhane (k 60-letiiu Azerbaidzhanskoi SSR). **Farmakol Toksikol** 1980 Jul-AUg;43(4):443-5

**Guseĭnova ZN** see **Guseĭnov DIa**

**Gusev AV:** Commemorating the 100th birthday of Valentin Aleksandrovich Dogiel (1882-1955). **J Parasitol** 1982 Dec;68(6):1188-9

**Gusev AV:** 150 Jahre Zoologisches Institut der Akademie der Wissenschaften der UdSSR. **Angew Parasitol** 1982 May;23(2):109-11

**Gusev MI** see **Shitskova AP**

**Gus'kov EN, Mustaev RK:** Dostizheniia dermato-venerologicheskoĭ sluzhby v Mordovskiĭ ASSR za 50 let. **Vestn Dermatol Venerol** 1980;(5):35-6

**Gusmão HH:** Indústria e Comércio de Minérios S.A.--ICOMI, Rio de Janeiro, Brazil. **Am J Trop Med Hyg** 1982 Jul;31(4):705-10

**Gussow JD:** Food and nutrition education: a redefinition. **Teach Coll Rec** 1980;81(4):411-6

**Gussow JD:** Who pays the piper? **Teach Coll Rec** 1980;81(4):448-66

**Gustafsson RA:** Omvårdnadsforskning. Forskningen startade på läkarnas villkor. **Vardfacket** 1981 Aug 27;5(15):6-10

**Gustavson KH:** Mannen bakom syndromet: John Down. Banade väg för den kliniska kromosomforskningen. **Lakartidningen** 1984 May 30;81(22):2261-3

**Guten G** see **Maud PJ**

**Guter P:** Die Krankenversicherung. Vertrags- und Honorarsituation seit 1935. **Zahnarzt** 1980 Jan;24(1):12-20 contd.

**Gütgemann A:** In Memoriam Freiherr von Redwitz. Bonn, Hanstein, 1966. 40 p.

**Guth JL:** Herbert Hoover, the U. S. Food Administration, and the dairy industry, 1917-1918. **Bus Hist Rev** 1981;55(2):170-87

**Güthert H, Abe HR:** Zur Entstehungsgeschichte der Medizinisch-wissenschaftlichen Gesellschaft an der Medizinischen Akademie Erfurt - Gedanken, Reflexionen, Erinnerungen. **Beitr Gesch Univ Erfurt** 1979-83;19:339-59

**Guthke KS:** Haller im Halblicht. Vier Studien. Bern, München, Francke, 1981. 72 p. (Sonderdruck aus Das Abenteuer der Literatur).

**Guthke KS** see **Albrecht von Haller, 1708-1777**

**Guthorn PJ:** William Augustus Newell, M.D., and the Life Saving Service. **J Med Soc NJ** 1984 Sep;81(9):769–72
**Guthrie MW:** Misi Utu, Dr. D. W. Hoodless and the development of medical education in the South Pacific. Suva, Fiji Institute of Pacific Studies, 1979. vi, 60 p.
**Gutiérrez A** see **Lara–Terrazas A**
**Gutiérrez C:** The birth and growth of neuroradiology in the USA. **Neuroradiology** 1981;21(4):227–37
**Gutierrez D:** D. H. Lawrence and modern destructiveness. **Suicide Life Threat Behav** 1980 Winter;10(4):219–29
**Gutierrez H:** Evolution de la population totale et qualité des previsions démographiques à court terme, par dpartements de la région Midipyrenées, 1821–1976. **Population** 1981;36(1):182–7
**Gutierrez H** see **Houdaille J**
**Gutiérrez Avila JH** see **Marcial LD**
**Gutiérrez Gómez D** see **Barraquer i Bordás L**
**Gutina VN:** Pasteur's views on the science. **Istor Biol Issled** 1983;9:134–44
**Gutman RA:** Renal dialysis for kidney failure in North Carolina: history, practice, and lessons. **NC Med J** 1984 Jun;45(6):359–63
**Gutmann A:** Freud versus feminism. **Dissent** 1979;26(2):204–12
**Gutmann MP, Walle E van de:** New sources for social and demographic history: the Belgian population registers. **Soc Sci Hist** 1978;2(2):121–43
**Gutmann MR, Wyrick R:** Adapting methods to needs: studying fertility and nuptiality in seventeenth- and eighteenth-century Belgium. **Hist Methods** 1981;14(4):163–71
**Gutmann R:** Une lettre signée de Larrey, Desgenettes, Coste et Parmentier, à propos d'une épidémie de fièvre jaune en Espagne. **Hist Sci Med** 1980;14:337–41
**Gutmann RA:** Une lettre de Marjolin sur ses rapports avec Dupuytren. **Hist Sci Med** 1981;15(2):123–7
**Gutmann WF** see **Mann G, ed**
**Gutner R, Miller D:** Inside the fundus camera. **Ann Ophthalmol** 1983 Jan;15(1):13–6
**Gutsch AW** see **Domandl S, ed**
**Gutsche T:** There was a man. The life and times of Sir Arnold Theiler K.C.M.G. of Onderstepoort. Cape Town, Timmins, 1979. 487 p.
**Gutt RW:** Historia Recentiorum. (Próba oceny osiągnięć medycyny od zakończenia i Wojny do r. 1950.) **Arch Hist Med (Warsz)** 1981;44(3/4):355–62
**Gutt RW:** Jöns Jacob Berzelius (1779–1848) i poczatki chemii fizjologicznej). **Arch Hist Med (Warsz)** 1979;42(1):83–92
**Gutt RW:** O medycynie w Polsce XVIII–wiecznej. Próba wprowadzenia. **Arch Hist Med (Warsz)** 1979;42(2):211–15
**Gutt RW:** Refleksje na temat XXV–lecia Polskiego Towarzystwa Historii Medycyny. **Arch Hist Med (Warsz)** 1982;45(1–4):5–10
**Gutt RW:** Rozważania o historii, filozofii i socjologii medycyny, (artykuł dyskusyjny). **Arch Hist Med (Warsz)** 1981;44(1):85–91
**Gutt RW:** The development of hematology. **Hexagon Roche** 1981;9(3):9–16
**Gutt RW:** W setna rocznice określenia czynności wydzielniczej komórek błony śluzowej zoładka. **Arch Hist Med (Warsz)** 1978;41(4):479–81
**Guttentag OE** see **Spicker SF, ed**
**Güttler F:** Fölling's sygdom: 50 år og stadig katalysator for nye medicinske opdagelser. **Nord Med** 1984;99(3):78–81
**Guttman FM, Guttman HA:** Historical note on embryo transfer: 599 B. C (with apologies to drs. Steptoe and Edwards). **Fertil Steril** 1980 Nov;34(5):513–5
**Guttman HA** see **Guttman FM**
**Gutzke DW:** 'The cry of the children': the Edwardian medical campaign against maternal drinking. **Br J Addict** 1984 Mar;79(1):71–84
**Guy A:** Donner corps à la voix. **Esprit** 1982;2:200–5
**Guy JR:** Archbishop Secker as a physician. In Sheils WJ, ed: The Church and healing. Papers read at the twentieth summer meeting and the twenty–first winter meeting of the Ecclesiastical History Society. Oxford, Basil Blackwell for the Society, 1982. p. 127–35.
**Guy JR:** Doctor's recipe book? **Pharm Hist (London)** 1984;14(1):6–8
**Guy JR:** Surgeons and surgery in Victorian Yeovil. **Bristol Med Chir J** 1984 Apr;99(370):48–50
**Guy JR:** The episcopal licensing of physicians, surgeons and midwives. **Bull Hist Med** 1982;56(4):528–42
**Guy Y:** Sur les origines possibles de la ségrégation des Cagots. **Hist Sci Med** 1983;17(1):85–93
**Guyotjeannin C:** A propos des préservatifs. **Monit Pharm Lab** 1983;37(1566):2364–5
**Guyotjeannin C, Lehuenen J:** Contribution à l'étude de la pathologie aux îles Saint–Pierre–et–Miquelon (XIXe siècle – début du XXe siècle). **Hist Sci Med** 1984;18(1):61–5
**Guyotjeannin C:** Les médicaments de Marcel Proust. **Monit Pharm** 1983 Sep 10;37(1577):3423, 3425, 3427; 1983 Oct 15;37(1582):3987–8
**Guyotjeannin C:** Les médicaments de Tchékhov. **Monit Pharm** 1983;37(1557):1248–50
**Guyotjeannin C, Lehuenen J:** Quelques documents inédits concernant les thérapeutiques utilisées aux îles Saint–Pierre–et–Miquelon (XIXe siècle – début XXe siècle). **Hist Sci Med** 1984;18(2):159–64
**Guyotjeannin C:** Remèdes d'autrefois aux îles Saint–Pierre–et–Miquelon. **Rev Hist Pharm (Paris)** 1984 Jun;31(261):115–20
**Guyotjeannin C:** Un aperçu de la thérapeutique au XVIIe siècle. **Monit Pharm Lab** 1981 Apr–May;1465–6:1677–8, 1680–1, 1845, 1847–8
**Guyton AC** see **Snellen HA**
**Guzek JW:** Profesor Franciszek Venulet (1878–1967) w 15 rocznice śmierci. **Arch Hist Med (Warsz)** 1982;45(1–4):27–38
**Guzek JW:** Professor Karol Klecki 1866–1931. **Przegl Lek** 1981;38(12):873–4
**Guzek JW:** Two hundred years of the pathologic physiology in Poland--a survey of its past and its present status. **Acta Physiol Pol** 1983 Jan–Feb;34(1):1–4
**Guzmán–Flores C:** El Doctor Efrén C. Del Pozo, Fisiólogo y Maestro. **Bol Estud Med Biol** 1980 Jul–Oct;31(3–4):116–26
**Guzmán Tirado MG:** Dengue. I. Antecedentes históricos; agentes etiológicos; cuadro clínico. **Rev Cubana Med Trop** 1980 May–Aug;32(2):123–30
**Guzzon V** see **Montorsi W**
**Gvozdev MP, Petrov VA:** Iustin Iulianovich Dzhanelidze (K 100–letiiu so dnia rozhdeniia). **Voen Med Zh** 1983 Aug;(8):72–4
**Gvozdják J** see **Reinis Z**
**Gwinnett AJ, Gorelick L:** Inlayed teeth of ancient Mayans: a tribological study using the SEM. **Scan Electron Microsc** 1979:(3);575–80
**Gwynne T** see **Charlton C**
**Gyárfás A:** Gálfalvi Domby Sámuel, Borsod vármegye föorvosa (1729–1807)]. **Orv Hetil** 1982 Aug 22;123(34):2123–5
**Gyenes G:** Adatok a magyarországi Hodgkin–kór kutatáshoz. **Orv Hetil** 1979 Nov 18;120(46):2812–4
**Gyenes G:** Adatok a splenectomia történetéhez Magyarországon. **Orv Hetil** 1980 Apr 6;121(14):853–4
**Gyenes G:** Adatok Babits betegségéhez. **Orv Hetil** 1983 Nov 27;124(48):2942–6
**Gyenes G:** Adatok Babits Mihaly betegségéhez. **Orvostort Kozl** 1981;93–96(27 No 1–4):193–200
**Gyenes G:** Klinische, physikalische und biologische Grundlagen der modernen Strahlentherapie. **Radiobiol Radiother (Berl)** 1980;21(3):208–17
**Gyenes G:** 65 éves az elsö magyar röntgen tankönyv. **Orv Hetil** 1983 Jul 24;124(30):1829–30
**Gyokaishi Henshu Iinkai** see **Nihon Shika Kigyo Kyogikai**
**Gyöngyössy A:** Kovács Ferenc (1890–1974). **Orv Hetil** 1984 Aug 19;125(34):2085–6
**Gyorgyey F** see **Ebbert A, et al**
**Gysel C:** Anomalies, mélanodontie et orthodontie dans le traité de pathologie dentaire (1778) de Joseph Jakob Plenk (1732–1807). **Orthod Fr** 1979;50:769–88
**Gysel C:** Appréciation d'Urbain Hémard et de sa 'Recherche de la vraye anatomie des dents'. **Actual Odontostomatol (Paris)** 1982;36(139):395–410
**Gysel C:** Arnoldus Senguerdius (1610–1668) en zijn wijsgerige verhandeling 'De Dentibus'. **Ned Tijdschr Tandheelkd** 1978 Nov;85(11):468–70
**Gysel C:** Bernardin Martin et sa 'dissertation sur les dents' (1679–1979). **Actual Odontostomatol (Paris)** 1980;34(129):59–72
**Gysel C:** Cartesianisme en tandheelkunde bij Henricus Regius (1598--1679--1979). **Rev Belge Med Dent** 1979;34(2):213–22
**Gysel C:** Conférence autour de Camper (1722–1789) et de 'son' angle facial. **Orthod Fr** 1980;51:LIX-XCVII
**Gysel C:** Daubenton (1716–1800) et ses recherches sur le trou occipital. **Orthod Fr** 1979;50:377–92
**Gysel C:** De ontwikkeling van de tandheelkunde in België van 1830 tot 1930. **Rev Belge Med Dent** 1981;36(3):103–10
**Gysel C:** De tandheelkunde van Adrianus Spigelius Bruxellensis (1578–1625–1978). **Rev Belge Med Dent** 1979;34(1):99–120
**Gysel C:** Dentistry and Cartesianism (1637–1650). **Dent Cadmos** 1980;48(3):53–5
**Gysel C:** Een vulgarisator van de anatomie van het kauwstelsel: Gerard Blasius (1626–1682–1982). **Ned Tijdschr Tandheelkd** 1984 Jun;91(6):153–8
**Gysel C:** Helmontianisme en odontologie (I). **Rev Belge Med Dent** 1979;34(3):295–312
**Gysel C:** Helmontianisme en odontologie (II). 3. Van Helmont en het nagerslacht. **Rev Belge Med Dent** 1979;34(4):385–96
**Gysel C:** Il dentista Fauchard. **Dent Cadmos** 1980 Jan;48(1):61–3. Feb;48(2):49–52
**Gysel C:** Jan Swammerdam (1637–1680–1980), zijn Cartesianism en de fysiologie van het kauwstelsel (I). **Ned Tijdschr Tandheelkd** 1981 Jun;88(6):238–41
**Gysel C:** Jan Swammerdam (1637–1680–1980), zijn Cartesianisme en de fysiologie van het kauwstelsel (II). **Ned Tijdschr Tandheelkd** 1981 Jul–Aug;88(7–8):274–7
**Gysel C:** Jan Swammerdam (1637– 1680– 1980), zijn Cartesianisme en de fysiologie van het kauwstelsel (SLOT). **Ned Tijdschr Tandheelkd** 1981 Nov;88(11):414–6
**Gysel C:** Jean–Baptiste Van Helmont (1579–1644), le baroque et les dents. **Rev Belge Med Dent** 1979;34(4):397–404
**Gysel C:** Les implications cartésiennes de la nosologie bucco–dentaire de Pierre Fauchard (1678–1761–1978). **Rev Belge Med Dent** 1979;34(3):313–20
**Gysel C:** Les relations du jeune Blumenbach avec Camper vieillissant. **Hist Sci Med** 1983;17(2):135–9
**Gysel C:** L'odonto–stomatologie d'après les 'vrais et solides fondements de la médecine', établis par Louis du Gardin, professeur à l'université de Douai, sous le règne d'Albert et d'Isabelle. **Rev Belge Med Dent** 1982 Jul;37(4):164–71
**Gysel C:** L'odonto–stomatologie formellement scolastique de Paul de Sorbait (1624–1691). **Rev Belge Med Dent** 1983 Mar;38(2):55–62
**Gysel C:** L'odontologie à la fin de la Renaissance, sous le règne de Galien et des deux Riolan. **Actual Odontostomatol (Paris)** 1981;(135):373–90
**Gysel C:** Odontoiatria del passato. L'odontostomatologia nel contesto delle 'vere e solide fondamenta della medicine', definite da Louis Du Gardin, Professore all'Universitá di Douai, sotto il regno di Alberto ed Isabella. **Dent Cadmos** 1983 Apr;51(4):91–5 contd

**Gysel C:** Odontoiatria e cartesianesimo nascente (1637–1650). **Dent Cadmos** 1980 Mar;48(3):53–5
**Gysel C:** Odontologie et cartesianisme naissant (1637--1650). **Rev Belge Med Dent** 1979;34(2):223–30
**Gysel C:** Renaissance, filosofie en geneeskunde. **Rev Belge Med Dent** 1983 Jan;38(1):16–20
**Gysel C:** Thomas Bartholinus (1616–1680–1980), zijn nederlandse relaties en de tandheelkunde (II). **Ned Tijdschr Tandheelkd** 1982 Oct;89(10):414–9
**Gysel C:** Thomas Bartholinus (1616–1680–1980), zijn Zederlandse relaties en de tandheelkunde (I). **Ned Tijdschr Tandheelkd** 1982 Jan;89(1):39–43
**Gysel C:** Umanesimo e odontoiatria: Harvey e Spigelius, due vite parallele. **Dent Cadmos** 1981 Jan;49(1):61–6
**Gysel C:** Un siècle d'ephémérides médico-dentaires belges (1830–1930). **Rev Belge Med Dent** 1981;36(3):124–7
**Gysel C:** Un tricentenaire: la prophylaxie dentaire du Sieur de Fleurimont (1682–1982) (I). **Med Hyg (Geneve)** 1983 Jul 15;41(1525):2549–50; Jul 30;41(1526):2622–3
**Gysel C:** W. Harvey (1578–1657) et A. van den Spiegel (1578–1625), l'humanisme et l'odontologie. **Rev Belge Med Dent** 1979;34(1):121–6
**Gysel C** see **Brulin F**
**Gysel G:** Odontoiatria del passato. L'odontostomatologia nel contesto delle 'vere e solide fondamenta della medicina', definite da Louis Du Gardin, Professore all'Università di Douai, sotto il regno di Alberto ed Isabella. II. **Dent Cadmos** 1983 May;51(5):107–9, 112
**Gysel G:** Renaissance, 'Republique des lettres' et médecine. **Rev Belge Med Dent** 1984 Jun;39(3):99–105
**Gyselings R** see **André R**
**Gyug R:** The effects and extent of the Black Death of 1348: new evidence for clerical mortality in Barcelona. **Mediaev Stud** 1983;45:385–98

# H

**Haabala SH, Kopper JA, Mann RJ, et al:** 'Say please!' A study in library cooperation. **Hosp Libr** 1979 Winter;4(4):26–31
**Haag JE, Jackson LH:** The acceptance of chaplains in mental hospitals. **Am Benedictine Rev** 1981;32(4):328–35
**Haaga J** see **Davanzo J**
**Haage BD:** Das alchemistische Bildgedicht vom 'Nackten Weib' in seiner bisher ältesten Uberlieferung. **Centaurus** 1982–3;26(2–3):204–14
**Haage B, ed:** Das 'Kunstbüchlein' des Alchemisten Caspar Hartung vom Hoff. Göppingen, Kümmerle, 1975. 141 p.
**Haan H de:** Fertiliteit in pre-industriële samenlevingen. **Spiegel Hist** 1980;15(10):554–60
**Haas GE** see **Tomich PQ**
**Haas H:** History of antipyretic analgesic therapy. **Am J Med** 1983 Nov 14;75(5A):1–3
**Haas JD:** The development of research strategies for studies of biological variation in living human populations. In F. Spencer, ed: A history of American physical anthropology, 1930–1980. New York, Academic Press, 1982. 435–46.
**Haas WH de:** Vincent van Gogh, zijn lichamelijke ziekten, verwondingen en zelfmoord. **Ned Tijdschr Geneeskd** 1983 Dec 24;127(52):2390–2
**Haase HH:** Max von Pettenkofer--einige Gedanken zu Leben, Werk und Hinterlassenschaft. **Z Gesamte Hyg** 1980;26(10):697–9
**Haase HH:** Uber einige Auswirkungen Robert Kochs und seiner Lehre auf die Entwicklung der Allgemeinen und Kommunalen Hygiene. **Z Gesamte Hyg** 1982 Mar;28(3):154–6
**Haase J** see **Müller-Ruchholtz ER**
**Haavisto H** see **Niemineva K**
**Habacher M:** Auf der suche nach dem 'Od'; Karl Ludwig Freiherr von Reichenbach (1788–1869) und Karl Wilhelm Mayrhofer (1806–1853), zwei Verbündete contra Justus von Liebig. **Clio Med** 1980 May;14(2):105–18
**Habacher M:** Homöopathische Fernbehandlung durch Samuel Hahnemann. **Medizinhist J** 1980;15(4):385–91
**Habeck C** see **Habeck JO**
**Habeck JO, Habeck C:** Die Auskultation der Darmgeräusche -- Geschichte und Entwicklungsmöglichkeiten. **Z Arztl Fortbild (Jena)** 1980 Jun 15;74(12):596–9
**Habel G:** Zur Geschichte der Säuglingspylorusstenose. **Padiatr Grenzgeb** 1983;22(2–3):203–5
**Haber C:** Beyond sixty-five: the dilemma of old age in America's past. Cambridge, New York, Cambridge University Press, 1983. ix, 181 p.
**Haber C:** Geriatrics: a specialty in search of specialists. **Z Gerontol** 1984 Jan–Feb;17(1):26–31
**Habermann G:** Max Joseph Oertel 1835–1897. **Folia Phoniatr (Basel)** 1983;35(1–2):91
**Habermas J:** Bemerkungen zu Alexander Mitscherlichs analytischer Socialpsychologie. **Psyche (Stuttg)** 1983 Apr;37(4):352–63
**Habert R** see **Laforest NL**
**Habib KM:** Pharmacology and materiae medicae in the medical formulary of Al-Kindi. **Hamdard** 1981;24(1–2):92–101
**Habib KM** see **Said HM, ed**
**Habibullah CM:** Avicenna, a physician and his approach to medicine. **Bull Indian Inst Hist Med (Hyderabad)** 1981;1–4:75–7
**Habrich C:** Die Ausstattung von Haus- und Reise-apotheken in ihrer pharmazie- und medizinhistorischen Bedeutung. **Pharm Ztg** 1979 Jun 14;124(24):1151–5
**Habrich C:** Mediziner und Medizinisches am Hofe des Grafen Casimir zu Sayn-Wittgenstein (1687–1741). **Beitr Gesch Pharm** 1983;31(18/19):138–44
**Habrich C, Marguth F, Wolf JH, et al:** Medizinische Diagnostik in Geschichte und Gegenwart. Festschrift für Heinz Goerke zum sechzigsten Geburtstag. München, Fritsch, 1978. 656 p. Historical contributions by J. Antall, G. Baader, V. Bazala, L. Belloni, G. Bratescu, W. Brendel, L. Burilkova, C. J. Clemedson, K. Goldammer, H. Henne, S. Hofmann, G. Keil, K. P. Killian, W. Klinner, W. Kloppe, M. Knedel, W. Kock, F. Köcher, H. M. Koelbing, K. S. Kolta, E. Kreuzer, V. Krizek, O. Larsen, B. I. Lindskog, N. Mani, V. Møller-Christensen, Y. Otsuka, G. Preiser, L. Premuda, E. Püschel, H. Röhrich, E. Rosner, G. Rudolph, J. Sájner, H. Schadewaldt, H. Schipperges, H. H. Simmer, J. Spielmann, M. Stürzbecher, A. Terzioglu, R. Winau, N. Plovdiv. (Neue Münchner Beiträge zur Geschichte der Medizin und Naturwissenschaften, Medizinhistorische Reihe, Band 7/8).
**Habrich C:** Therapeutische Grundsätze pietistischer Arzte des 18. Jahrhunderts. **Beitr Gesch Pharm** 1982;31(16):121–3
**Habs H:** Die sogenannte Pest des Thukydides: Versuch einer epidemiologischen Analyse. Berlin, New York, Springer-Verlag, 1982. 46 p.
**Habs H:** Immunologische Begriffe bei Thukydides. **Zentralbl Bakteriol Mikrobiol Hyg [A]** 1982 Jun;252(2):143–6
**Hachinski V:** Cerebral arteriosclerosis and dementia: evolution of a misconception. In: Congrès international d'histoire de la médecine, XXVe, Québec, 1976. Actes. Québec, 1977. p. 755–60.
**Hachinski V:** Transient cerebral ischemia: a historical sketch. In Rose FC, Bynum WF, ed: Historical aspects of the neurosciences. New York, Raven, 1982. p. 185–93.
**Hackett CJ:** McLetchie on mass campaigns. **Trop Doct** 1982 Jan;12(1):35–8
**Hackett CJ:** Private medical practice and anti-yaws campaigns in South Eastern Nigeria 1925–1950. **Trop Doct** 1980 Jul;10(3):129–32
**Hackett CJ** see **Hart GD, ed**
**Hackett E:** The foreskin saga. **Med J Aust** 1984 Aug 4;141(3):187–9
**Hackett R:** Recent developments in the healing concepts and activities of the Aladura churches. **Afr Notes** 1981;8(2):55–8
**Hackmann WD:** Early societies popularize scientific research. **Med Instrum** 1983 Sep–Oct;17(5):338
**Haddad FS, Richter-Bernburg L:** A hitherto unknown eighth-century commentary on Avicenna's 'Kulliyyat'. **J Hist Arabic Sci** 1980;4:253–8
**Haddad FS:** Arab medical ethics. **Stud Hist Med** 1982 Jun;6(2):122–36
**Haddad FS:** Arab medical manuscripts in the Sami I. Haddad memorial library. In International Congress of the History of Medicine, 27th, Barcelona, 1980. Actas. Barcelona, Académia de Ciències Médiques de Catalunya i Balears, 1981. p. 253–8.
**Haddad FS:** Arabic medical manuscripts in the Sami I Haddad Memorial Library. **Clio Med** 1981 Dec;16(2/3):123–7
**Haddad FS:** Gleanings of anaesthesia in Lebanon. **Middle East J Anaesthesiol** 1980 Oct;5(8):553–6
**Haddad FS:** History of anesthesia in Lebanon 1800–1914. **Middle East J Anaesthesiol** 1982 Jun;6(5):241–80
**Haddad FS** see **Asper SP**
**Hadingham E** see **Wildgoose M**
**Hadjioloff A, Valtchev A:** Problèmes de la médecine et de la santé publique bulgare dans les rapports des semaines médicales balkaniques / 1962–1977. In International Congress of the History of Medicine. 26th, Plovdiv, 1978. Actes du Congress. Sofia, 1981. Volume II. p. 105–6.
**Hadjivukovic S, Cobanovic K:** Prirodno kretanje stanovništva jugoslavije, socialističkih republika i autonomnih pokrajina u posleratnom periodu. **Zb Drus Nauke** 1978;(65):107–22
**Hadju SI:** A note on the history of Carbowax in cytology. **Acta Cytol (Baltimore)** 1983 Mar–Apr;27(2):204–6
**Hadley GG:** Loma Linda University School of Medicine. **West J Med** 1983 May;138(5):742–5
**Hadwiger DF:** Nutrition, food safety, and farm policy. **Proc Acad Polit Sci** 1982;34(3):79–88
**Hadžiomeragic M:** Prikaz znanja o bolestima jezika prije 1000 godina. **Stomatol Vjesn** 1983;12(3–4):147–51
**Hadžiomeragic M:** Prvi zubni lijecnik kod nas (1493. god.). **Stomatol Vjesn** 1978;7(3–4):89–92
**Haeberle EJ:** Human rights and sexual rights. The legacy of René Guyon. **Med Law** 1983;2(2):159–72
**Haeberle EJ:** 'Stigmata of degeneration'. Prisoner markings in Nazi concentration camps. **J Homosex** 1980–81 Fall–Winter;6(1–2):135–9
**Haebertin HK** see **Rieber RW, ed**
**Haeger K** see **Haeger-Aronsen B**
**Haeger-Aronsen B, Haeger K:** Porfyri hos Mary Stuarts efterkommande: en historisk-medicinsk tvistefråga. **Sydsven Medicinhist Sallsk Arsskr** 1984;21:63–75
**Haenel T:** Die Bewertung des Suizides im Laufe der Geschichte. **Medizinhist J** 1983;18(3):213–26
**Haenel T:** Die Suizidproblematik bei Stefan Zweig. **Schweiz Arch Neurol Neurochir Psychiatr** 1981;129(2):297–314
**Haenel T:** Jakob Klaesi--Schlafkur und Antieidodiathese. **Gesnerus** 1979;36(3–4):246–65
**Haenel T:** Zur Geschichte der Psychiatrie: Gedanken zur allgemeinen und Basler Psychiatriegeschichte. Basel; Boston, Birkhäuser Verlag, 1982. 249 p.
**Haenel T:** Zur Geschichte der Psychiatrischen Poliklinik Basel. **Schweiz Arch Neurol Neurochir Psychiatr** 1979;124(2):335–50
**Haensch WG:** Die menschlichen statuetten des mittleren Jungpaläolithikums aus der sicht der Somatischen Anthropologie. Bonn, Habelt, 1982. 294 p. (Antiquitas, 2).
**Haesenne-Peremans N:** Les asiles pour malades, vieillards et orphelins dans

l'arrondissement de Liège au début du XIXe siècle. **Bull Inst Archeol Liegeois** 1979;91:85–157
**Haesenne-Peremans N:** Les Hospices et Orphelinats de la région Verviétoise au début du XIXe siècle. **Ann Soc Belg Hist Hop** 1978;16:35–56
**Haeublein HG:** Early studies of miners and smelters. **Am J Ind Med** 1982;3(3):357–8
**Haffen M:** Structures de l'homéopathie en France: (1919–1982). Paris, Editions médicales internationales, 1982. 158 p.
**Haffter C:** Die Entstehung des Begriffs der Zivilisationskrankheiten. **Gesnerus** 1979;36(3–4):228–37
**Hafkenscheid JC** see **Majoor CL**
**Häfner H** see **Janzarik W ed**
**Haga S** see **Tsuboi Y**
**Hagen JB:** Experimental taxonomy, 1930–1950: the impact of cytology, ecology, and genetics on ideas of biological classification. Ph.D. Diss., Oregon State University. Corvallis, 1982. 226 leaves.
**Hagen W:** Auftrag und Wirklichkeit: Sozialarzt im 20. Jahrhundert. München-Gräfelfing, Werk-Verlag, 1978. 253 p.
**Hagenfeldt K:** Dramatiskt minskad mödramortalitet. Framsynta åsikter i abortfrågan. **Lakartidningen** 1983 Nov 9;80(45):4299–302
**Hagerman PJ** see **Hagerman RJ**
**Hagerman RJ, McBogg P, Hagerman PJ:** The fragile X syndrome: history, diagnosis, and treatment. **JDBP** 1983 Jun;4(2):122–30
**Hägermark O:** Beläst, försynt invärtesmedicinare – piojär även inom lumbalpunktionsteknik och lungkirurgi. **Lakartidningen** 1983 Nov 16;80(46):4429–30
**Hagger J:** Australian colonial medicine. Adelaide, Rigby, 1979. xii, 219 p.
**Haggerty L:** Nursing revisited: Strong public health nurse leader and educator. **Mass Nurse** 1984 Jul–Aug;54(7):7
**Haggett P** see **Cliff A**
**Hagman HC:** Artic-u-logic. **Dent Lab Rev** 1981 Feb;56(2):18–21
**Hagman HC:** George S. Monson, DDS. **Dent Lab Rev** 1982 Mar;57(3):36
**Hagman HC:** Gnathology and its originators. **Dent Lab Rev** 1982 Jul;57(7):20–1
**Hagman HC:** History: Charles Goodyear. **Dent Lab Rev** 1981 Aug;56(8):33
**Hagman HC:** History of articulators. **Dent Lab Rev** 1980 Feb;55(2):28–31
**Hagman HC:** History of ceramics, part II. **Dent Lab Rev** 1980 Dec;55(3):34–6
**Hagman HC:** History of ceramics, part 1. **Dent Lab Rev** 1980 Nov;:34, 36
**Hagman HC:** History of crown and bridgework, part I. **Dent Lab Rev** 1980 May;55(5):20–4
**Hagman HC:** History of partial dentures, part 1. **Dent Lab Rev** 1980;55(8):28–9
**Hagman HC:** History roots. **Dent Lab Rev** 1981 Jul;56(7):30
**Hagman HC:** Prosthetic memoirs. **Dent Lab Rev** 1979 Sep–Oct;54(10–11):12–3, 54; 40–2
**Hagman HC:** Prosthetic memoirs, part III. **Dent Lab Rev** 1979 Dec;54(13):22–6
**Hagman HC:** The elusive condyles, part I. **Dent Lab Rev** 1982 Oct;57(10):33
**Hagman HC:** The evolution of dental castings. **Dent Lab Rev** 1979 Jul;54(8):28–33
**Hagman HC:** The history of dentures. **Dent Lab Rev** 1979 Mar;54(3):24–9 (continued periodically)
**Hagman HC:** 3,000 years of dental gold. **Dent Lab Rev** 1979 Jun;54(7):28–30
**Hagman HS:** History of partical dentures, part 1. **Dent Lab Rev** 1980 Jul;55(8):28–9
**Hahn FE:** Virus chemotherapy: the problem, its development and nature. In Hahn FE, ed: Virus chemotherapy. Basel, New York, Karger, 1980. p. 1–21. (Antibiotics and chemotherapy, v. 27).
**Hahn G:** Zwanzig Jahre des Ungarischen Gesundheitswesens. Budapest: Ministerium für Gesundheitswesen, 1965. 116 p.
**Hahn H:** Paternalism and public policy. **Society** 1983;20(3):36–46
**Hahn L:** 'Was tut denn der noch da?' Ein Beitrag zum Thema 'Euthanasie'. **Krankenpfl J** 1982 Jan 15;20(1):11
**Hahn R:** A bibliography of quantitative studies on science and its history. Berkeley, Office for History of Science, 1980. 84 p. (Berkeley Papers in History of Science, 3).
**Hahn S:** Der 'Lübecker Totentanz' (1930), ein Beispiel für ethische Debatten zum Problem der Tuberkulose. **Wiss Beitr Martin Luther Univ Halle Wittenberg** 1983;5–R80:91–8
**Hahn S:** Die Herausbildung progressiver bürgerlicher Auffassungen zur lebensbewahrenden Aufgabe der Medizin und zur Betreuung Sterbender zu Beginn des 19. Jahrhunderts in Deutschland. **Z Gesamte Inn Med** 1982 Dec 15;37(24):857–62
**Hahn S:** Martin Luther--was sagt er uns Arzten heute? **Z Gesamte Inn Med** 1983 Oct 15;38(20):551–4
**Hahn S:** Positionen der Kommunistischen Partei Deutschlands zur lebensbewahrenden Aufgabe der Medizin in der Zeit der Weimarer Republik. **Z Exp Chir** 1982 Jul;28(7):468–71
**Hahn S:** Schwerpunkte ethischer Diskussionsentwicklung um die Tuberkulose-Bekämpfung in fachwissenschaftlichen Veröffentlichungen von 1900 bis 1932. **Z Gesamte Hyg** 1982 Mar;28(3):193–201
**Hahn U:** Die Entwicklung des Tierschutzgedankens in Religion und Geistesgeschichte. DMV Diss. Hannover, 1980. 192 p.
**Hahn von Dorsche H:** Die Nomenklaturen der Anatomen. Ein historischer Uberblick. **Anat Anz** 1981;150(1–2):11–43
**Hahnloser P, Pugin P:** La formation des thromboses et des embolies paradoxales par un shunt interauriculaire. Commentaires sur les articles de F. Wilh. Zahn: de la formation des thrombus, état actuel de cette question. Thrombose de plusieurs branches de la veine cave inférieure avec embolies consécutives dans les artères pulmonaire, splénique, rénale et iliaque droite. **Rev Med Suisse Romande** 1980 Dec;100(12):1103–8
**Hahoda M:** Aus den Anfängen der sozialwissenschaftlichen Forschung in Osterreich. **Zeitgesch** 1981;8(4):133–41
**Haide M:** Leprosy control in China 1981. **East Horiz** 1981;20(9):18–21
**Haight V:** A brief history of hemoglobinometry. **Am J Med Technol** 1983 Feb;49(2):127–8
**Hailsham:** The British Academy of Forensic Sciences. The Inaugural Lund Lecture: legal aid. **Med Sci Law** 1982 Jul;22(3):169–77
**Haines MR:** Age specific and differential fertility in Durham and Easington registration districts, England, 1851 and 1861. **Soc Sci Hist** 1977;2(1):23–52
**Haines MR:** Fertility and marriage in a nineteenth century industrial city. Philadelphia, 1850–1880. **J Econ Hist** 1980;40(1):151–8
**Haines MR:** Recent developments in historical demography: a review of the European fertility project with some comparisons from Japan. **Hist Methods** 1978;11(4):162–73
**Haines MR, Avery RC:** The American life table of 1830–1860: an evaluation. **J Interdiscip Hist** 1980;11(1):73–95
**Hainsworth M** see **Bardet JP**
**Hair PE:** A note on Jean Barbot (1655–1713). **Proc Huguenot Soc Lond** 1981;23:295–308
**Hajal F:** Galen's ethical psychotherapy: its influence on a medieval Near Eastern physician. **J Hist Med Allied Sci** 1983 Jul;38(3):320–33
**Hajal F:** Psychological treatment of anorexia: a case from the ninth century. **J Hist Med Allied Sci** 1982 Jul;37(3):325–8
**Hájek P:** 10 let Kroměřížského psychoterapeutického oddělení. **Cesk Psychiatr** 1982 Jun;78(3):196–8
**Hajnóczkyné ME:** Adalékok az állatorvostudományi egyetem történetéből (1919–1969). **Agratort Sz** 1977;19(1–2):251–7
**Hajnsek F:** Osnivanje i razvitak antiepileptičke službe u SR Hrvatskoj (1956–1981). **Lijec Vjesn** 1982 May;104(5):212–4
**Hakfoort C:** Wetenschapshistorische etiketten en de gevaren van polaire analyses. **Tijdschr Geschied Geneeskd** 1982;5(1):1–5
**Hakme F:** Abdominoplasty: peri- and supra-umbilical lipectomy. **Aesthetic Plast Surg** 1983;7(4):213–20
**Hakulinen E:** Hälsoråd till tidigare resenärer. **Nord Med** 1984;99(10):266–7
**Hakulinen E:** Mannen bakom syndromet: Richard Bright. En av de stora inom njurforskningen--hans 'Reports of medical cases' epokgörande. **Lakartidningen** 1984 Apr 25;81(17):1722–3
**Hal G** see **Lukázs J**
**Halaburt H, Langfeldt B, Rasmussen P:** Computerized tomography (CT-scan) of a 2,500-year-old Danish 'Queen'. **Acta Neurochir (Wien)** 1981;56(3–4):153–5
**Halas MA:** Sexism in women's medical care. **Frontiers** 1979;4(2):11–5
**Halbach RE** see **Battocletti JH**
**Halberg E** see **Halberg F**
**Halberg F, Halberg E:** Circadian rhythms in the mammalian central nervous system, blood pressure and parasites – hobbies of Rudolf Engel. **Int J Chronobiol** 1979;7(1):1–16
**Halberg E, et al:** Forging chronobiology and pediatrics as well as geriatrics – a birthday greeting for Theodor Hellbrugge. **Int J Chronobiol** 1979;6:135–43
**Halberstadt-Freud HC:** Proust and perversion: some clinical and theoretical consideration. **Int J Psychoanal** 1980;61(3):403–10
**Halberstein RA, Saunders AB:** Traditional medical practices and medicinal plant usage on a Bahamian Island. **Tex Stud Lit Lang** 1978;2:177–203
**Halbert MR** see **Hartmann K**
**Haldipur CV:** Madness in ancient India: concept of insanity in Charaka Samhita (1st century A.D.). **Compr Psychiatry** 1984 May–Jun;25(3):335–44
**Hale DK:** Cyrus N. Ray: the Abilene man. **West Tex Hist Assoc Yearb** 1979;55:17–36
**Hale M:** Human science and social order: Hugo Münsterberg and the origins of applied psychology. Philadelphia, Temple University Press, 1980. xii, 239 p.
**Hale M:** Psychology and social order: an intellectual biography of Hugo Münsterberg. Ph.D. Diss. University of Maryland. College Park, 1977. ix, 444 leaves.
**Hale NG** see **Federn E**
**Hale NG** see **Roazen P**
**Haley B:** The healthy body and Victorian culture. Cambridge, Massachusetts, Harvard University Press, 1978. 296 p.
**Haliţa M:** Cinci decenii de la o afirmare a medicinii româneşti. **Rev Med Interna [Med Interna]** 1980 Mar–Apr;32(2):189–92
**Hall AP:** Exotic infectious diseases: malaria. **R Soc Health J** 1980 Apr;100(2):57–61
**Hall AP** see **Recollections & reflections**
**Hall AR:** Homo fabricator: a new species. **Hist Philos Life Sci** 1980;2(2):193–14
**Hall AR:** On Whiggism. **Hist Sci** 1983 Mar;21(51 Pt 1):45–59
**Hall AR, Boas Hall M:** The first human blood transfusion: priority disputes. **Med Hist** 1980;24(4):461–5
**Hall BM, Sheil AG:** Transplantation in Australia and New Zealand. **Transplant Proc** 1984 Aug;16(4):925–6
**Hall BS** see **Levere TH, ed**
**Hall CA:** Doctors afield: John Calef, M.D. **N Engl J Med** 1981 Oct 29;305(18):1048–51
**Hall CP:** Medical malpractice problem. **Ann Am Acad Polit Soc Sci**

1979;443:82-93
**Hall D:** Ointment of love: Oliver E. Comstock and Tuscon's [sic] tent city. **J Ariz Hist** 19(2):111-30, 1978
**Hall DL:** Why do animals breathe? New York, Arno Press, 1981. xviii, 296 p.
**Hall EJ:** Particles in radiation therapy--Part III. **Int J Radiat Oncol Biol Phys** 1982 Dec;8(12):2041-4
**Hall EJ:** The contribution of the physical sciences to the development of radiation therapy. **J Surg Oncol** 1983 Dec;24(4):248-57
**Hall EM:** In the ward next door to Sister Kenny. **Aust Nurses J** 1981 May;10(10):57-8
**Hall IS:** John Robert Hume: personal physician to the first Duke of Wellington. **J R Coll Surg Edinb** 1980 Jul;25(4):219-32
**Hall LA:** The Stopes collection in the Contemporary Medical Archives Centre at the Wellcome Institute for the History of Medicine. **Soc Soc Hist Med Bull (Lond)** 1983 Jun;32:50-1
**Hall LW:** Equine anaesthesia: discovery and rediscovery. **Equine Vet J** 1983 Jul;15(3):190-5
**Hall MB:** The Royal Society and Italy 1667-1795. **Notes Rec R Soc Lond** 1982 Aug;37(1):63-81
**Hall MB:** The Royal Society in Thomas Henry Huxley's time. **Notes Rec R Soc Lond** 1984;38(2):153-8
**Hall R:** Henry James: interpreting an obsessive memory. **J Homosex** 1983 Spring-Summer;8(3-4):83-97
**Hall S:** With stethoscope in Asia: Korea. McLean, Virginia, MCL Associates, 1978, xiv, 637 p.
**Hall S** see **Landes RR**
**Hall SA:** The skeleton of Eclipse. **Vet Hist** 1984;3(3):94-100
**Hall TD, Lindsay CM:** Medical schools: producers of what? sellers to whom? **J Law Econ** 1980;23(1):55-80
**Hall VM:** The role of force or power in Liebig's physiological chemistry. **Med Hist** 1980 Jan;24(1):20-59
**Hall W** see **Edwards GA**
**Haller JS:** Aconite: a case study in doctrinal conflict and the meaning of scientific medicine. **Bull NY Acad Med** 1984 Nov;60(9):888-904
**Haller JS:** American medicine in transition, 1840-1910. Urbana, University of Illinois Press, 1981. xii, 457 p.
**Haller JS:** Hypodermic medication; early history. **NY State J Med** 1981 Oct;81(11):1671-9
**Haller JS:** Opposition to compressed tablets in 19th and early 20th century medicine. **NY State J Med** 1984 Nov;84(11):554-8
**Haller JS:** Sampson of the terebinthinates: medical history of turpentine. **South Med J** 1984 Jun;77(6):750-4
**Haller JS:** Smut's dark poison: ergot in history and medicine. **Trans Stud Coll Physicians Phila** 1981 Mar;3(1):62-79
**Haller JS:** The foul tongue: a 19th century index of disease. **West J Med** 1982 Sep;137(3):258-64
**Haller JS:** The United States Pharmacopoeia: its origin and revision in the 19th century. **Bull NY Acad Med** 1982 Jun;58(5):480-92
**Haller JS:** Use of surface irritants in nineteenth century medicine. **NY State J Med** 1980 Jul;80(8):1314-23
**Haller JS:** With a spoonful of sugar. The art of prescription writing in the late 19th and early 20th century. **Pharm Hist** 1984;26(4):171-8
**Haller alla 'Charité' con Ledran: Dent Cadmos** 1979 Feb 2;47(2):54-6
**Hallett GE:** Progress of children's dentistry. **Br Dent J** 1980 Jul 1;149(1):13-6
**Hallett JP:** Something in excess? Priapea 50, 2. **Mnemosyne** 1978;31:203-6
**Halleux R:** Gnose et expérience dans la philosophie chimique de Jean-Baptiste Van Helmont. **Bull Cl Sci Acad R Belg** 1979;65:217-27
**Halleux R:** Les alchimistes grecs. Tome I. Papyrus de Leyde, Payrus de Stockholm, Fragments de Recettes. Paris. Les Belles Lettres, 1981. xv, 235 p.
**Halleux R:** Les textes alchimiques. Turnhout, Brepols, 1979. 153 p. (Typologie des sources du Moyen Age occidental, fasc. 32).
**Halleux R:** L'usage des pierres précieuses dans la thérapeutique aux XVIe et XVIIe siècles. In International Congress of the History of Medicine. 26th, Plovdiv, 1978. Actes du Congress. Sofia, 1981. Volume II. p. 106-8.
**Halleux R:** Marcellin Berthelot, historien de l'alchimie. In: Congrès National des Sociétés Savantes, 104e, Bordeaux, 1979. Comptes Rendus. Paris, 1979. Section des Sciences, Fasc. IV. p. 169-80.
**Halleux R** see **Barbaix M**
**Halleux R** see **Delatte L**
**Halleux-Opsomer C:** Les herbiers comme source pour l'histoire de la pathologie et de la thérapeutique au Moyen Age. In International Congress of the History of Medicine. 26th, Plovdiv, 1978. Actes du Congress. Sofia, 1981. Volume II. p. 91-3.
**Halleux-Opsomer C:** Un herbier médicinal du haut moyen âge: l'alfabetum Galieni. **Hist Philos Life Sci** 1982;4(1):65-97
**Halmai J:** Beiträge zur Geschichte der Pharmazie in Burgenland bis 1918. **Burgenl Heimatbl** 1969;31(4):181-7
**Halpern AL:** Elimination of the exculpatory insanity rule. A modern societal need. **Psychiatr Clin North Am** 1983 Dec;6(4):611-27
**Halpern I:** [Rush marriages among Eastern European Jews] (Heb). **Zion** 1962;27(1-2):36-58
**Halpert BP:** Development of the term 'senility' as a medical diagnosis. **Minn Med** 1983 Jul;66(7):421-4
**Halstead SB, Papaevangelou G:** Transmission of dengue 1 and 2 viruses in Greece in 1928. **Am J Trop Med Hyg** 1980 Jul;29(4):635-7
**Halter S** see **Dhoore L**
**Halub MA:** The catheter--a historical perspective. **AUAA J** 1983 Apr-Jun;3(4):7-9
**Ham LM, Chamings PA:** Nursing history: our wasted asset. **Nurs Health Care** 1982 Oct;3(8):434-7
**Ham LM:** Reflections of nursing: portrait or carricature? **Image (IN)** 1981 Feb;13(1):9-12
**Hamada T, Namba T:** [Pharmacognostical studies on the molluscan drugs (14). Historical and herbological investigations on 'Tianluo' and 'Luosi'] (Jpn). **Yakushigaku Zasshi** 1983;18(2):53-64
**Hamanaka Y:** [Basic neuropsychologic concepts and their origins (conclusion)] (Jpn). **No To Shinkei** 1983 Mar;35(3):310-1
**Hamanaka Y:** [Jackson's theory of stratification of neurological functions--a controversy involving Broca at a symposium (1868) at Norwich] (Jpn). **No To Shinkei** 1982 Oct;34(10):1018-9
**Hamann P:** Peter Willers Jessens ehemaliges Asyl Hornheim in Kiel. Ein Beitrag zur Psychiatriegeschichte Schleswig-Holsteins. **Hist Hosp** 1979-80;13:69-95
**Hamarneh NT** see **Hamarneh SK**
**Hamarneh S:** Arabic manuscripts of the National Library of Medicine, Washington, D.C. **J Hist Arabic Sci** 1977 May;1(1):72-108
**Hamarneh S:** Medical technology in Ibn al-Quff's surgery. In I. El-Sayyad, ed: Papers presented to the First International Conference on Islamic Medicine, celebrating the advent of the fifteenth century hijri. Kuwait, Ministry of Public Health. National Council for Culture, Arts and Letters, 1981. p. 140-7.
**Hamarneh S:** Sarton (1884-1956) and the Arabic-Islamic legacy. **J Hist Arabic Sci** 1977 Nov;1(2):299-318
**Hamarneh SK:** Al-Biruni, the father of Arabic pharmacy and marine biology as demonstrated in al-Saydanah. In: International Congress held in Pakistan on the occasion of Millenary of Abu Raihan Muhammad ibn Ahmad al-Biruni (973-ca 1051 A.D.) November 26, 1973 thru December 12, 1973. Proceedings. Karachi, Hamdard National Foundation, 1979. p. 479-500.
**Hamarneh SK:** Arabic-Islamic alchemy--three intertwined stages. **Ambix** 1982 Jul;29(2):74-87
**Hamarneh SK, Awad EA:** Early surgical instruments excavated in old Cairo, Egypt. In: Congrès international d'histoire de la médecine, XXVe, Québec, 1976. Actes. Québec, 1977. p. 761-4.
**Hamarneh SK:** Ibn Al-Quff's writings on hygienic regulations and the preservation of health. In A. Hadidi, ed: Studies in the history and archaeology of Jordan. Amman, Department of Antiquities, 1982. p. 373-83.
**Hamarneh SK:** Introduction to the history and philosophy of Arabic-Islamic medicine and allied sciences. **Stud Hist Med** 1982 Sep;6(3):195-213
**Hamarneh SK:** Jabir, Jildki and Ibn-Sallum, and Arabic-Islamic Alchemy. **Mesopotamia Q** 1980;8(29,30):110-22, 225-41
**Hamarneh SK:** Majusi's observations and instructions on medicine and public health. **Hamdard** 1980 Jan-Mar;23(1):3-35
**Hamarneh SK, Stieb EW:** Pharmacy museums and historical collections on public view in the United States and Canada. Madison, American Institute of the History of Pharmacy in cooperation with the National Museum of American History. Washington, D.C., Smithsonian, 1981. 144 p. (Publication/American Institute of the History of Pharmacy, new series, no. 6).
**Hamarneh SK, Hamarneh NT:** The physician-surgeon al-Zahrawi and the natural origins and manufacture of drugs. In A. R. El-Gindy, ed: Proceedings of the Second International Conference on Islamic Medicine. No. IV. Kuwait, Islamic Medicine Organization, 1982. (Bulletin of Islamic Medicine, v. 2). p. 375-82, 401-406.
**Hamarneh SK** see **Said HM, ed**
**Hambridge RA:** 'Empiricomany, or an infatuation in favour of Empiricism or Quackery': the socio-economics of eighteenth-century quackery. In S. Soupel, R. A. Hambridge: Literature and science and medicine. Los Angeles, William Andrews Clark Memorial Library, UCLA, 1982. p. 45-102.
**Hambsch K, Treutler H, Pietruschka WD:** Profil und Aufgabenstellung einer medizinischen Universitätspoliklinik in Vergangenheit und Gegenwart am Beispiel des Medizinisch-Poliklinischen Institutes der Karl-Marx-Universität Leipzig. **Z Gesamte Inn Med** 1981 Mar 15;36(6):186-9
**Hamburger J:** Le journal d'Harvey. Paris, Flammarion, 1983. 339 p.
**Hamburger J:** Note préliminaire sur les greffes rénales. **Nephrologie** 1982;3(1):2-5
**Hamburger J:** Past, present, and future of transplantation. **Transplant Proc** 1981 Mar;13(1):41-3
**Hamburger V:** Hilde Mangold, co-discoverer of the organizer. **J Hist Biol** 1984 Spring;17(1):1-11
**Hamburger V:** S. Ramón y Cajal, R. G. Harrison, and the beginnings of neuroembryology. **Perspect Biol Med** 1980;23(4):600-16
**Hamburger V:** Trophic interactions in neurogenesis: a personal historical account. **Annu Rev Neurosci** 1980;3:269-78
**Hamburger V** see **Mayr E**
**Hameed A:** A historian of medicine, Major General (Dr) S. L. Bhatia, passes away. **Stud Hist Med** 1981 Sept;5(3):239-41
**Hameed A:** Attemperament in medicine. **Stud Philos Med** 1977 Mar;1(1):31-9
**Hameed A:** Medical ethics in Islam. **Stud Hist Med** 1981 Jun;5(2):133-59
**Hameed A:** Medical ethics in Medieval Islam. **Stud Philos Med** 1977 Mar;1(1):108-24
**Hameed HA, Reyaz Ali Parvaz S:** Source material of Arab medicine. **Stud Hist Med** 1979 Dec;3(4):225-33
**Hamel P:** Le remède et l'apparence. Plan de la Tour, Editions

d'aujourd'hui, 1981. 128 p.
**Hamelin J** see **Dufour P**
**Hamelmann H:** Zur Geschichte der Vereinigung Nordwestdeutscher Chirurgen: zur 125. Tagung 12.–14. Juni 1980. Lübeck, Wullenwever, 1980?. 103 p.
**Hamersley H:** Radiation science and Australian medicine, 1896–1914. **Hist Rec Aust Sci** 1982;5(3):41–63
**Hamilton D, Lamb M:** Surgeons and surgery. In Checkland O, Lamb M, ed: Health care as social history; the Glasgow case. Aberdeen, Aberdeen University Press, 1982. p. 74–85.
**Hamilton D:** The early history of the Highlands and Islands Medical Scheme. **Scott Med J** 1979 Jan;24(1):64–8
**Hamilton D:** The healers: a history of medicine in Scotland. Edinburgh, Canongate, 1981. xiii, 318 p.
**Hamilton D:** The nineteenth-century surgical revolution--antisepsis or better nutrition? **Bull Hist Med** 1982 Spring;56(1):30–40
**Hamilton DG:** Hand in hand. Sydney, Ferguson, 1979. 338 p.
**Hamilton DG:** Whooping cough immunization. **Med J Aust** 1979 Dec 15;2(12):651
**Hamilton DG:** 100 years of paediatric surgery in Sydney. **Med J Aust** 1980 Dec 27;2(13):721–6
**Hamilton DN, Reid WA:** Yu. Yu. Voronoy and the first human kidney allograft. **Surg Gynecol Obstet** 1984 Sep;159(3):289–94
**Hamilton DN** see **McWhinnie DL**
**Hamilton E** see **Fernandes L**
**Hamilton HD, Lander BG:** Public policy analysis: water and sewers for McElrath Park. **Phylon** 1979;40(1)41–51
**Hamilton M:** Opposition to the Contagious Diseases Act, 1864–1886. **Albion** 1978;10:14–27
**Hamilton PR** see **Hamilton WA**
**Hamilton WA, Hamilton PR:** Sex and the dental practice: a reinterpretation of the history of dental hygienists. **Bull Hist Dent** 1980 Oct;28(2):64–8
**Hamilton WM** see **Shamansky SL**
**Hamlin C:** Edward Frankland's early career as London's official water analyst, 1865–1876: the context of 'previous sewage contamination'. **Bull Hist Med** 1982 Spring;56(1):56–76
**Hamlin CS:** What becomes of pollution? Adversary science and the controversy of self-purification of rivers in Britain, 1850–1900. Ph.D. Diss., University of Wisconsin. Madison, 1982. vi, 618 p.
**Hamlin H:** Oskar Hirsch. **Surg Neurol** 1981 Dec;16(6):391–3
**Hamm WG:** The development of plastic surgery during the past sixty years. **Ann Plast Surg** 1984 Feb;12(2):102–4
**Hammarsten JE** see **Hammarsten JF**
**Hammarsten JF, Caylor JA:** Physicians and the Lewis and Clark expedition. **Trans Am Clin Climatol Assoc** 1979;91:115–27
**Hammarsten JF:** The contributions of Idaho physicians to knowledge of Rocky Mountain Spotted Fever. **Trans Am Clin Climatol Assoc** 1982;94:27–43
**Hammarsten JF, Tattersall W, Hammarsten JE:** Who discovered smallpox vaccination? Edward Jenner or Benjamin Jesty? **Trans Am Clin Climatol Assoc** 1979;90:44–55
**Hammel EA, Johansson SR, Ginsberg CA:** The value of children during industrialization: sex ratios in childhood in nineteenth-century America. **J Fam Hist** 1983 Winter;8(4):346–66
**Hammer B:** Die Geschichte der Computertomographie (anlässlich von 10 Jahren klinischer Computertomographie). **Computertomographie** 1982 Jun;2(2):59–61
**Hammer SN, ed:** Symposium for the 75th Anniversary of the Food, Drug & Cosmetic Act, Meat Inspection Act, 1906–1981. Monday, June 8, 1981. Washington, D.C. **Food Drug Cosmet Law J** 1982 Jan;37(1):3–149
**Hammersmith SK** see **Weinberg MS**
**Hammett HB:** The historical context of the origins of CPE. **J Pastoral Care** 1975 Jun;29(2):76–85
**Hammett JY:** A second drink at the well: theological and philosophical context of CPE origins. **J Pastoral Care** 1975 Jun;29(2):86–9
**Hammond DC:** Myths about Erickson and Ericksonian hypnosis. **Am J Clin Hypn** 1984 Apr;26(4):236–45
**Hammond EA:** Dr. Newton D. Phillips, Florida Medical Association's eleventh president. **J Fla Med Assoc** 1982 Aug;69(8):683–7
**Hammond EC** see **Selikoff IJ**
**Hammond GL, Laks H, Geha AS:** Development of aortic valve prostheses. **Conn Med** 1980 Jun;44(6):348–52
**Hammond JH:** Camera, camera, camera. **J Audiov Media Med** 1984 Jan;7(1):19–20
**Hammond M:** The expulsion of the Neanderthals from human ancestry: Marcellin Boule and the social context of scientific research. **Soc Stud Sci** 1982 Feb;12(1):1–36
**Hamoir M** see **Barbaix M**
**Hamowy R:** Medicine and the crimination of sin: 'self-abuse' in the 19th century America. **J Libert Stud** 1977;1(3):229–70
**Hamowy R:** The early development of medical licensing laws in the United States, 1875–1900. **J Libert Stud** 1979;3(1):73–119
**Hampartzoumian A** see **Durand J**
**Hampel H, Knöfler W:** Stand und Entwicklung der stomatologischen enossalen Hemiimplantologie an der Karl-Marx-Universität Leipzig. **Stomatol DDR** 1980 Jul;30(7):457–61
**Hampel H** see **Bethmann W**
**Hampel J:** Medizin der Zoroastrier im vorislamischen Iran. Husum, Matthiesen, 1982. 142 p. (Abhandlungen zur Geschichte der Medizin und der Naturwissenschaften, Heft 45).
**Hampel RL:** Diversity in early temperance reform; another look at the Massachusetts Society for the Suppression of Intemperance, 1813–1825. **J Stud Alcohol** 1982 May;43(5):453–68
**Hamrum CL, ed:** Darwin's legacy. Nobel Conference XVIII, Gustavus Adolphus College. St. Peter, Minnesota, held October 5–6, 1982. San Francisco, Harper & Row, 1983. 125 p. Contributions by S. J. Gould, I. Stone, R. E. Leakey, P. B. Medawar, E. O. Wilson, J. Pelikan.
**Hanafee WN** see **Canalis RF**
**Hanafy HM:** Sex aids: 'energising ring' and 'surgical splints' for treatment of impotence. **Urology** 1980 May;15(5):478E, 478F
**Hanajima T** see **Uzawa Y**
**Hanan R:** A dentist at large. Christchurch, N. Z. Merivale, 1977. 181 p.
**Hanashima T** see **Kishi Y**
**Hanashima T** see **Tanaka K**
**Hanawalt L:** The doctors' war in the Michigan legislature, 1835–1861. **Mich Hist** 1979;63(1):29–43
**Hanawalt LL** see **Kaufman M**
**Hanbury J:** A reminiscence: pharmacy in the first half of the 20th century. **Pharm Hist (London)** 1978 Jul;8(2):2–4
**Hanckel RW:** A brief history of otolaryngology and head and neck surgery in South Carolina. **J SC Med Assoc** 1984 Aug;80(8):376–7
**Hancock RG** see **Lewin PK**
**Hancock V:** Women in Arizona medicine: Mary Lawson Neff, M.D. **Ariz Med** 1984 Nov;41(11):750–4; Dec;41(12):819–21
**Hancock WG:** John Waldron. In Dictionary of Canadian biography, 1801 to 1820. Volume 5, 1983. p. 837–9.
**Hand WD:** Magical medicine: the folkloric component of medicine in the folk belief, custom, and ritual of the peoples of Europe and America: selected essays. Berkeley, University of California Press, 1980. xxvii, 345 p.
**Hand WD:** Medical science's legacy of outmoded doctrines to folk and primitive medicine. In International Congress of the History of Medicine, 27th, Barcelona, 1980. Actas. Barcelona, Acadèmia de Ciències Mèdiques de Catalunya i Balears, 1981. p. 517–21.
**Hand WD, Casetta A, Thiederman SB, ed:** Popular beliefs and superstitions. A compendium of American folklore from the Ohio Collection of Newbell Niles Puckett. 3 volumes. Boston, G. K. Hall, 1981.
**Hand WD, ed:** American folk medicine; a symposium. Berkeley, University of California Press, 1976. viii, 347 p. Contributions by C. H. Talbot, T. R. Forbes, S. X. Radbill, J. Puhvel, D. B. Price, D. J. Hufford, B. Gebhard, B. G. Myerhoff, L. J. Bean, V. J. Vogel, R. I. Ford, W. A. Emboden, F. Guerra, J. S. Graham, B. H. Granger, L. Lacourcière, E. Brandon, D. Yoder, J. A. Hostetler, B. Jackson, A. E. Fife, L. E. Barrett, M. O. Jones, J. Q. Anderson.
**Handa H:** [Percival Bailey (author's transl)] (Jpn). **No Shinkei Geka** 1981 Mar;9(4):538–41
**Handbook of Physiology 1959–1978.: Physiologist** 1980 Oct;23(5):14–6
**Handelman H:** Cuban food policy and popular nutritional levels. **Cuban Stud** 1981–82;11–12(2–1):127–46
**Handelsman A:** Le médecin hydropathe---color lithograph by Honoré Daumier. **J Hist Med Allied Sci** 1981 Jan;36(1)63
**Handler CE** see **Perkin GD**
**Handler JS** see **Corruccini RS**
**Handloff R:** Prayers, amulets and charms: health and social control. **Afr Stud Rev** 1982;25(2–3):185–94
**Handrack C:** Georg Friedrich Wilhelm Balser (1780–1846). Giessen, Schmitz, 1979. 388 p. (Arbeiten zur Geschichte der Medizin in Giessen, 2).
**Handsher R** see **Goldblum N**
**Haneveld GT:** Bij het eeuwfeest van de gonokok: het belang van zijn ontdekking en de ontvangst daarvan in Nederland (Ludwig Sigesmund Albert Neisser). **Ned Tijdschr Geneeskd** 1979 Oct 27;123(43):1875–8
**Haneveld GT:** De antieke reisapotheek. **Arts Auto** 1981;47:896–9
**Haneveld GT:** De ledezetters van Jisp. **Spiegel Hist** 1977;12(100):514–17
**Haneveld GT:** 'De secrete' toiletfacilities in sea-going vessels. In International Congress of the History of Medicine, 27th, Barcelona, 1980. Actas. Barcelona, Acadèmia de Ciències Mèdiques de Catalunya i Balears, 1981. p. 384–6.
**Haneveld GT:** Early Dutch contributions on Peyronie's disease. **Arch Chir Neerl** 1979;31(3):123–9
**Haneveld GT:** Koning Willem I en de aankoop van anatomische kabinetten. **Spiegel Hist** 1978;13(7–8):488–95
**Haneveld GT:** Medische aspecten van de slag bij Doggersbank. **Tijdschr Geschied Geneeskd** 1982;5(2):78–88
**Haneveld GT:** Oude medische gebouwen van Nederland. Amsterdam, Meesters, 1976. 218 p.
**Haneveld GT:** Pathologische Anatomie in Utrecht, circa 1800–1850. Amsterdam, Meesters, 1978. x, 371 p.
**Haneveld GT:** Pott's disease before Pott. **Neth J Surg** 1980;32(1):2–7
**Hangorsky C:** Juvenile periodontitis/periodontosis: historical overview and update. **Dent Hyg (Chic)** 1982 Jun;56(6):29–32, 34
**Hankart R:** L'hôpital Saint-Michel dit des Communs Pauvres-en-Ile à Liège. Histoire de ses origines (XIIe–XVe siècles). **Bull Inst Archeol Liegeois** 1978;90:157–95 Also in Bull Soc R Vieux Liege 1977–79;9:281–7, 385–94
**Hankins TL:** Prosopography of the British Association: an essay review. **J Hist Med Allied Sci** 1982 Oct;37(4):451–4
**Hankiss J:** A tudományos teljesítmény értékelése. Fleming felfedezése tükrében. **Orv Hetil** 1980 Jan 13;121(2):95–8
**Hankoff LD, Munver UL:** Prenatal experience in Hindu mythology. **NY State J Med** 1980 Dec;80(13):2006–14
**Hanley PH:** Colon and rectal surgery. Our heritage.

**Dis Colon Rectum** 1983 Feb;26(2):81-4
**Hanley SB, Yamamura K:** Economic and demographic change in preindustrial Japan, 1600-1868. Princeton, N. J., Princeton University Press, 1977. xiii, 409 p.
**Hanley SB** see **Cho LJ**
**Hanlon CR:** The surgical presidency. **Ann Surg** 1982 Sep;196(3):233-8
**Hannaway C:** Abraham M. Lilienfeld (1920-1984). **Bull Hist Med** 1984 Winter;58(4):558-9
**Hannaway C:** From private hygiene to public health: a transformation in Western medicine in the eighteenth and nineteenth centuries. In Ogawa T, ed: Public health. Tokyo, Saikon, 1981. p. 108-28.
**Hannaway C** see **Goubert JP**
**Hannaway C** see **Lilienfeld DE**
**Hanne M** see **Clerc B**
**Hannemann EA:** Little Laura and others like her. Health care of American Colonial children. **Indiana Med** 1984 Jan;77(1):48-52
**Hanngren A:** R. T. H. Laënnec, lungmedicinens fader, 1781-1826. **Kvartalsskr Sven Hjart Lungsjukdomor** 1981;76:73-82
**Hanngren A:** René Théophile Hyacinthe Laennec (1781-1826). **Nord Medicinhist Arsb** 1981;:106-19
**Hänninen O, Vaskilampi T:** Cupping as a part of living Finnish traditional healing. A remedy against pain. **Acupunct Electrother Res** 1982;7(1):39-50
**Hänninen O** see **Vaskilampi T**
**Hannon TF** see **Sammons JH**
**Hanron J:** Nursing revisited: Clarissa Harlow Barton. **Mass Nurse** 1983 Sep;52(9):9, 27
**Hans-Jürgen Mohr (1. 11. 1922 bis 7. 6. 1982): Verh Dtsch Ges Pathol** 1983;67:762-71
**Hansch-Mock B:** Arbeitshygiene in schweizerischen Kalendern des 19. Jahrhunderts. **Gesnerus** 1981;38:165-74
**Hänsel D:** Die 'Physiologische Erziehung' der Schwachsinningen. Edouard Séguin (1812-1880) und sein Konzept einer medizinischen Pädegogik. Freiburg, Schulz, 1974. 329 p. (Freiburger Forschungen zur Medizinigeschichte, Neue Folge, 3).
**Hansel W, Leonard EP, Dukes HH:** A backward look from far above Cayuga's waters. **Physiologist** 1982 Dec;25(6):469-74
**Hansell P:** A backward glance -- 2. **J Audiov Media Med** 1979 Jul;2(3):107-11
**Hansen AC:** Black Americans in medicine. **J Natl Med Assoc** 1984 Jul;76(7):693-5
**Hansen B:** The historical construction of homosexuality. **Radic Hist Rev** 1979;20:66-73
**Hansen B:** The historical construction of homosexuality. **Radic Hist Rev** 1979 Spring/Summer;Spec:66-73
**Hansen C:** Willowbrook: try, try again. **Soc Policy** 1979;10(3):41-5
**Hansen E:** 'Overlaying' in 19th-century England: infant mortality in infanticide? **Hum Ecol** 1979;7:333-52
**Hansen GA, Watt FB, ed:** The memories and reflections of Dr. G. Armauer Hansen. Würzburg, German Leprosy Relief Association, 1976. 135 p.
**Hansen H, Susser M:** Historic trends in death from chronic kidney disease in the United States and Britain. **Am J Epidemiol** 1971 Jun;93:413-24
**Hansen H** see **Moss C**
**Hansen HO:** A comparison of empirical life tables for Iceland 1785-1860 with selected model life tables. **Scand Popul Stud** 1979;5:22-37
**Hansen HO:** Some age structural consequences of mortality variations in pre-transitional Iceland and Sweden. In: Charbonneau H., La Rose A., ed.: The great mortalities: methodological studies of demographic crises in the past. Liège, Ordina, 1979, p. 113-32.
**Hansen HO:** Some age structural consequences of mortality variations in pre-transitional Iceland and Sweden. In Charbonneau H, Larose A, ed: The great mortalities: methodological studies of demographic crises in the past. Liège, Belgium, Ordina Editions, 1980. p. 113-32.
**Hansen JR:** Scientific fellowship in a Swiss community enlightenment: a history of Zurich's Physical Society, 1746-1798. Ph.D. Diss., Ohio State University. Columbus, 1981. viii, 264 leaves.
**Hansen KJ:** Mormon sexuality and American culture. **Dialogue** 1976;10(2):45-56
**Hansen SB:** State implementation of supreme court decision: abortion rates since Roe v. Wade. **J Polit** 1980;42(2):372-95
**Hansen E, et al, ed:** Seit über einem Jahrhundert ...: Verschüttete Alternativen in der Sozialpolitik. Sozialer Fortschritt, organisierte Dienstleistermacht und nationalsozialistische Machtergreifung: der Fall der Ambulatorien in den Unterweserstädten und Berlin. 100 Jahre kaiserliche Botschaft zur Sozialversicherung: Eine Festschrift. Köln, Bund-Verlag, 1981. 618 p.
**Hansluwka H** see **Ruzicka LT**
**Hanson AE:** Hippocrates: Diseases of women. 1. **Signs** 1975;1:567-84
**Hanson AL** see **Wolff M**
**Hanson CL, Owsley DW:** Frontal sinus size in Eskimo populations. **Am J Phys Anthropol** 1980 Aug;53(2):251-5
**Hanson JR:** Structure and complexity of medicine bundle systems of selected Plains Indian tribes. **Plains Anthropol** 1980;25(89):199-216
**Hanson LA, Kallós P:** Host parasite relationships in gram-negative infections. **Prog Allergy** 1983;33:1-8
**Hanson RD:** Medical services at Chatham Dockyard 1625-1984. **J R Nav Med Serv** 1984 Spring;70(1):38-40
**Hansson O, Eklund J:** A historical review of hydrocolloids and an investigation of the dimensional accuracy of the new alginates for crown and bridge impressions when using stock trays. **Swed Dent J** 1984;8(2):81-95
**Hansson T** see **Bergman LE**
**Hantsche HJ:** Die Entwicklung der wissenschaftlichen Zahnheilkunde in Halle/Saale vor 100 Jahren. **Zahntechnik (Berl)** 1983 Oct;24(10):415-6
**Hanzlíček Z:** Dějiny Státního ústavu pro kontrolu léčiv (1918-1983). Dějiny ustavu pro zkoumáni léčiv (1918-1952). **Cesk Farm** 1984 Mar;33(2):83-91
**Hanzlíček Z:** Ostatní Ceské farmaceutické časopisy. (Příspěvek k dějinám českého farmaceutického periodického tisku). **Cesk Farm** 1982 Dec;31(10):384-92
**Hanzlíček Z:** První česká lékárna v Chicagu. **Cesk Farm** 1981 May;30(3-4):125-30
**Hanzlíček Z:** Redaktoři Casopisu českého lékárnictva. **Cesk Farm** 1982 May;31(3-4):97-109
**Hanzlíček Z:** Sto let českých farmaceutických časpisu. **Cesk Farm** 1982 May;31(3-4):83-4
**Hao B, et al:** [My new opinion on the date of writing of the 'Seven Grand Chapters' in Internal Classics of Yellow Emperor: exploration based on the origin and evolution of the historical materials of ancient records on astronomy, classical music and calendar] (Chi). **Chung Hua I Shih Tsa Chih** 1984 Jan;14(1):46-50
**Haq I** see **Said HM, ed**
**Harada M:** A brief history of hospital dentistry in the United States. **Bull Hist Dent** 1982 Apr;30(1):46-54
**Harakas SS** see **Bleich JD**
**Harasymiw SJ** see **Eckenhoff EA**
**Haraway D:** The biological enterprise: sex, mind, and profit from human engineering to sociobiology. **Radic Hist Rev** 1979 Spring/Summer;Spec:206-37
**Haraway DJ:** Ethel Browne Harvey. In: Notable American women. The modern period. Cambridge, Mass., Belknap-Harvard Univ. Press, 1980. 4:319-21.
**Haraway DJ:** In the beginning was the word: the genesis of biological theory. **Signs** 1981;6(3):469-81
**Harbison SF, Weishaar ME:** Samoan migrant fertility: adaptation and selection. **Hum Organ** 1981;40(3):268-73
**Harboe M:** The work and concepts of Armauer Hansen: how do they stand today? **Ethiop Med J** 1983 Apr;21(2):123-6
**Harden VA** see **Berger RL**
**Hardesty FP:** Louis William Stern: a new view of the Hamburg years. In K. Salzinger, ed: Psychology in progress: an interim report. (Annals of the New York Academy of Sciences, 1976. p. 31-44.
**Hárdi I:** Ferenczi Sándor jelentösége a mai orvostudomány számára. **Orv Hetil** 1983 Aug 21;124(34):2067-70
**Hárdi I:** Hollós István (születésének 110-ik évfordulójára). **Orv Hetil** 1982 Dec 12;123(50):3099-100
**Hardin RC:** An Iowa contribution to blood banking. **J Iowa Med Soc** 1983 Oct;73(10):399-404
**Harding PM:** A Red Cross nurse in Belgrade: Mary Gladwin saw World War I from the inside of a hospital. Her battles were no easier than those of the soldiers. **Am Hist Illus** 1982;17(1):41-7
**Harding RM, Mills FJ:** Special form of flight. I: Balloons, gliders, and hang gliders. **Br Med J [Clin Res]** 1983 Jul 23;287(6387):277-8
**Hardwick JL** see **Corbett ME**
**Hardy A:** Smallpox in London: factors in the decline of the disease in the nineteenth century. **Med Hist** 1983 Apr;27(2):111-38
**Hardy A:** Water and the search for public health in London in the eighteenth and nineteenth centuries. **Med Hist** 1984 Jul;28(3):250-82
**Hardy G:** William Rathbone and the early history of district nursing. Ormskirk, Hesketh, 1981. 54 p.
**Hardy HL** see **Stoeckle JD**
**Hardy JD:** Landmark perspective. Transplantation of blood vessels, organs, and limbs. **JAMA** 1983 Aug 19;250(7):954-7
**Hardy JH:** Royal Army Dental Corps diamond jubilee (1921-1981). **Br Dent J** 1981 Nov 17;151(10):351-2
**Hardy JL** see **Reeves WC**
**Hardy L, Rafferty AM:** Nursing and history. **Nurs Times** 1982 Sep 15-21;78(37):1564-5
**Hardy RW** see **Barnett GH**
**Hardy SB** see **Spira M**
**Hare E:** Great books in psychiatry. **Br J Psychiatry** 1981 Mar;138:261-3
**Hare E:** The two manias: a study of the evolution of the modern concept of mania. **Br J Psychiatry** 1981 Feb;138:89-99
**Hare E:** Was insanity on the increase? The fifty-six Maudsley Lecture. **Br J Psychiatry** 1983 May;142:439-55
**Hare E** see **Scull A**
**Hare EH, Moran PA, Macfarlane A:** The changing seasonality of infant deaths in England and Wales 1912-78 and its relation to seasonal temperature. **J Epidemiol Community Health** 1981 Jun;35(2):77-82
**Hare HJ:** First graduate--USD School of Medicine. Lyle Hare, M.D., family practitioner. **SD J Med** 1981 May;34(5):70-1
**Hare R:** The scientific activities of Alexander Fleming, other than the discovery of penicillin. **Med Hist** 1983 Oct;27(4):347-72
**Hareven TK:** Cycles, courses and cohorts: reflections on theoretical and methodological approaches to the historical study of family development. **J Soc Hist** 1978;12(1):97-109
**Hareven TK, Vinovskis MA:** Patterns of childbearing in late nineteenth-century America: the determinants of marital fertility in five Massachusetts towns in 1880. In their: Family and population in nineteenth-century America. Princeton, Princeton University Press, 1978. p. 85-125.
**Hargreaves AS:** Old bones are brittle. **Dent Tech** 1980 Sept;33(9):5-9
**Hargreaves AS:** The development of denture design. **Br Dent J** 1981 Aug

4;151(3):101-2
**Hargreaves H:** 'De spermate hominis': a Middle English poem on human embryology. [Nat. Libr. Scotland, Advocates' MS. 23.7.11]. **Mediaev Stud** 1977;39:506-10
**Harig G:** Bemerkungen zum medizinhistorischen Unterricht in der DDR. **Z Gesamte Hyg** 1980;26(5):383-5
**Harig G, Kollesch J:** Der hippokratische Eid. **Philologus** 1978;122:157-76
**Harig G:** Die philosophischen Grundlagen des medizinischen Systems des Asklepiades von Bithynien. **Philologus** 1983;127:43-60
**Harig G, Kollesch J:** Galen und Hippokrates. In La collection hippocratique et son rôle dans l'histoire de la médecine. Colloque de Strasbourg (23-27 octobre 1972) organisé par le Centre de Recherches sur la Grèce Antique, avec le concours des Facultés de Philosophie et des Langues Classiques. Leiden, E. J. Brill, 1975. p. 257-74
**Harig G:** Mittelalterliche und antike Traditionen in der ärztlichen Ausbildung der Renaissance. **Klio** 1979;61:525-32
**Harig G:** Soziale Aspekte der antiken medizinischen Deontologie. **Orvostort Kozl** 1981;93-96(27 No 1-4):37-45
**Harig G:** Zu den Aufgaben der medizinhistorischen Forschung auf dem Gebiet der antiken Medizin in der Gegenwart. In International Congress of the History of Medicine. 26th, Plovdiv, 1978. Actes du Congress. Sofia, 1981. Volume II. p. 109-11.
**Harig G** see **Grmek MD, ed**
**Harig G** see **Tutzke D, ed**
**Harigaya K** see **Kageyama K**
**Harington JS, McGlashan ND:** Migrant workers and cancer patterns in South Africa. **J South Afr Stud** 1976;3(1):92-101
**Harkness B:** Greene's old-fashioned remedy in the heart of the matter. **Am Notes Queries** 1982 Mar-Apr;20(7-8):115-6
**Harland KM:** A short history of Queen Alexandra's Royal Naval Nursing Service. **J R Nav Med Serv** 1984 Summer;70(2):59-65
**Harley D:** Religious and professional interests in northern spa literature, 1625-1775. **Soc Soc Hist Med Bull (Lond)** 1984 Dec;35:14-6
**Harley DN:** Ignorant midwives--a persistent stereotype. **Soc Soc Hist Med Bull (Lond)** 1981 Jun;28:6-9
**Harley JM:** The Royal Maternity Hospital, Belfast. Fifty glorious years 1933-1983. **Ulster Med J** 1984;53(1):1-17
**Härm E** see **Coale AJ**
**Harmand L:** Une ambulance militaire ouverte par le curé d'une paroisse messine durant les batailles sous Metz (août-décembre 1870). In: Congrès National des Sociétés Savantes, 97e, Nantes, 1972. Actes. Paris, 1977. Histoire Moderne et Contemporaine, Tome 1. p. 121-8.
**Harmarneh SK:** Ibn al-Ayn Zarbi and his definitions of diseases and their diagnoses. In: International Symposium for the History of Arabic Science, 1st, University of Aleppo, 1976. Proceedings. Aleppo, Syria, 1976. Papers in European Languages, Vol. II. p. 305-23.
**Harmat P, Hebenstreit G:** Freud, Ferenczi und die Psychoanalyse in Ungarn. **Wien Med Wochenschr** 1982 Feb 15;132(3):63-6
**Harmat P:** Psychoanalyse und Marxismus in Ungarn (1900-1980). **Psyche (Stuttg)** 1984 Mar;38(3):254-69
**Harmat P, Hebenstreit G:** Sándor Ferenczis theoretisches Werk. **Wien Med Wochenschr** 1984 Jan 31;134(2):49-53
**Harmer M:** The forgotten hospital: an essay. Chichester, Springwood Books, 1982. 170 p.
**Harmon MD:** The evolution of nursing education in the U.S. **Nev Rnformation** 1984 May;:6
**Harmon SD:** Florence Kelley in Illinois. **J Ill State Hist Soc** 1981;74(3):162-78
**Harms H:** Zum 100. Geburtstag von Walther Löhlein. **Klin Monatsbl Augenheilkd** 1983 Jun;182(6):585-90
**Harmsen H:** Demografische Verluste Kroatien 1941 bis 1946. **Donauraum** 1978;23(4):154-7
**Harper A** see **Green D**
**Harper AB, Laughlin WS:** Inquiries into the peopling of the new world: development of ideas and recent advances. In F. Spencer, ed: A history of American physical anthropology, 1930-1980. New York, Academic Press, 1982. p. 281-304.
**Harper AB:** Istoriia Aleutskoi populiatsii. **Sov Etnogr** 1980;(6):50-60
**Harper AB** see **Laughlin WS**
**Harper AE:** McCollum and directions in the evaluation of protein quality. **J Agric Food Chem** 1981 May-Jun;29(3):429-35
**Harper AE:** Reflections on Nutrition Reviews from a university professor. **Nutr Rev** 1982 Nov;40(11):330-1
**Harper DS:** Footnotes on allergy. Uppsala, Pharmacia AB, 1980. 103 p.
**Harper E:** The sailor's surgeon (James Yonge). **J R Nav Med Serv** 1979 Spring;65(1):35-7
**Harper JP:** Be fruitful and multiply: origins of legal restrictions on planned parenthood in nineteenth-century America. In Berkin, C. R., Norton, M. B. ed: Women of America: a history. Boston, Houghton Mifflin, 1979: 245-69.
**Harper JP:** 'Be fruitful and multiply': the reaction to family limitation in nineteenth-century America. Ph.D. Dis., Columbia University, New York, 1975. 273 leaves.
**Harper R:** A psychoanalytic geronimo. **Queen Q** 1981;88(2):256-63
**Harper RG, Kenigsberg K, Sia CG, et al:** Xiphopagus conjoined twins: a 300-year review of the obstetric, morphopathologic, neonatal, and surgical parameters. **Am J Obstet Gynecol** 1980 Jul 1;137(5):617-29
**Harper AB, ed** see **Laughlin WS**
**Harrauer H, Sijpesteijn PJ, ed:** Medizinische Rezepte und Verwandtes. Wien, Brüder Hollinek, 1981. xv, 56 p. (Mitteilungen aus der Papyrussammlung der Osterreichischen Nationalbibliothek (Papyrus Erzherzog Rainer), Neue Serie, 13. Folge).
**Harrell GT:** Grace Revere Osler: a turn of the century professor's wife. **Ann Intern Med** 1980 Sep;93(3):504-5
**Harrell GT:** Lady Osler. **Bull Hist Med** 1979 Spring;53(1):81-99
**Harrell GT:** Osler's practice. **Bull Hist Med** 1973 Nov-Dec;47(6):545-68
**Harrell GT:** Pediatrics in an academic health center. **J Fla Med Assoc** 1984 Mar;71(3):163-6
**Harrell GT:** The early years at Bowman Gray. **NC Med J** 1983 Dec;44(12):805-7
**Harrell GT:** The first years of the University of Florida College of Medicine. **J Fla Med Assoc** 1980 Mar;67(3):247-50
**Harrell GT:** The Osler-endowed Tudor and Stuart Club. **Pharos** 1984 Summer;47(3):23-6
**Harrell GT:** The Osler family. **JAMA** 1982 Jul 9;248(2):203-9
**Harrer G** see **Domandl S, ed**
**Harries LL** see **Titche LL**
**Harries WG:** Bened Feddyg: a Welsh medical practitioner in the late medieval period. In J. Cule, ed: Wales and medicine. London, British Society for the History of Medicine, 1975. p. 169-84.
**Harrington A:** After the impossible happened. **Synthesis** 1982;5(2):2-21
**Harris CC** see **Brucer M**
**Harris CD:** Dental electrosurgery. **Georgetown Dent J** 1979 Jul;53(2):45-53
**Harris CM:** The GP and the medical student. The background. **Br Med J [Clin Res]** 1983 Jan 8;286(6359):111-2
**Harris J:** William Beveridge. A biography. Oxford, Clarendon Press, 1977. 488 p.
**Harris J** see **Iskander Z**
**Harris JE, Wente EF:** An X-ray atlas of the royal mummies. Chicago, University of Chicago Press, 1980. xix, 403 p.
**Harris JE, Ponitz PV:** Dental health in ancient Egypt. In A. Cockburn, E. Cockburn, ed: Mummies, disease, and ancient cultures. Cambridge, Cambridge University Press, 1980. p. 45-51.
**Harris JI** see **Fletcher G**
**Harris M:** Facts about artifacts [in the history of pharmacy]. **Pharm Hist** 1980;22(3):126-7 (continued periodically)
**Harris M** see **Mathews M**
**Harris MH, Davis DG:** American library history. Austin, Univ. of Texas Press, 1978. xix, 260 p.
**Harris MR:** Abraham Flexner. In Dictionary of American Biography, Suppl. 6, 1956-1960. p. 207-9, 1980.
**Harris P, Ross JC, et al:** [Ludwig Guttmann - special issue]. **Paraplegia** 1979 May;17(1): passim
**Harris R:** An excursion in serendipity--the conquest of pain. **Ann R Australas Coll Dent Surg** 1979 Nov;6:103-11
**Harris R:** Centenary of the British Dental Association. **Aust Dent J** 1980 Jun;25(3):169-70
**Harris RJ** see **Barnartt SN**
**Harris SE:** History of health insurance. In his: The economics of health care; finance and delivery. Berkeley, McCutchan, 1975. p. 333-92.
**Harrison B:** Women's health and the women's movement in Britain: 1840-1940. In C. Webster, ed: Biology, medicine and society 1840-1940. Cambridge, Cambridge University Press, 1981. p. 15-71.
**Harrison DB** see **Parrott JR**
**Harrison DC:** Coronary bypass: the first 10 years. **Hosp Pract** 1981 Jun;16(6):49-56
**Harrison DF:** Neurochemistry and Sherrington's enchanted loom. **J R Soc Med** 1984 Aug;77(8):706-7
**Harrison F:** The dark angel: aspects of Victorian sexuality. New York, Universe, 1977. 288 p.
**Harrison G, Collins K:** In memoriam Joseph Sydney Weiner (1915-1982). **Ann Hum Biol** 1982 Nov-Dec;9(6):583-92
**Harrison G:** Mosquitoes, malaria, and man: A history of the hostilities since 1880. New York, Dutton, 1978. 314 p.
**Harrison GA:** The past fifty years of human population biology in North America: an outsider's view. In F. Spencer, ed: A history of American physical anthropology, 1930-1980. New York, Academic Press, 1982. p. 467-72.
**Harrison JA:** Military medicine in the United Kingdom: similarities and differences with respect to the United States and other NATO allies. **Milit Med** 1980 Jun;145(6):388-92
**Harrison JA:** Military medicine in the United Kingdom: similarities and differences with respect to the United States and other NATO allies. **J R Nav Med Serv** 1980 Winter;66(3):173-9
**Harrison JD:** Professor E. Viborg and therapeutic parotid ductal ligation. **Hist Med Vet** 1977;2(2):42-9
**Harrison JN** see **Levison CH**
**Harrison M:** Fire from heaven: a study of spontaneous combustion in human beings. Rev. ed. New York, Methuen, 1978. xvi, 295 p.
**Harrison MR:** Unborn: historical perspective of the fetus as a patient. **Pharos** 1982 Winter;45(1):19-24
**Harrison PH:** Salute to some nursing pioneers. **Curationis** 1979 Sep;2(2):53-5
**Harrison RC, Mills F:** Canadian contributions toward the comprehension of hyperinsulinism: the first successful excision of an insulinoma. **Can J Surg** 1980 Jul;23(4):401-3
**Harrison SH:** Accident surgery--the life and times of William Gissane. **Injury** 1984 Nov;16(3):145-54
**Harrod DC:** Chelsea physic garden tercentenary. **Pharm Hist (London)** 1974 Jan;4(1):4-5
**Harsch OM:** Philatelistisch-Odontologises Panopticum. **Zahnarztl Mitt** 1983 Jul 1;73(13):1470-1 contd

Harstad PT: Frontier medicine in the Territory of Wisconsin. In Numbers RL, Leavitt JW, ed: Wisconsin medicine. Historical perspectives. Madison, University of Wisconsin Press, 1981. p. 13-23.
Hart AW: Religion and education: the Scopes controversy in Utah. **Utah Hist Q** 1983;5(2):183-98
**Hart BL:** Neurosurgery for behavioral problems. A curiosity or the new wave? **Vet Clin North Am [Small Anim Pract]** 1982 Nov;12(4):707-14
**Hart ED:** Conan Doyle as rheumatologist. **Ann Rheum Dis** 1982 Aug;41(4):437-8
**Hart FD:** The British rheumatological journals. **Br J Rheumatol** 1984 Aug;23(3):164-5
**Hart FD:** William Harvey and his gout. **Ann Rheum Dis** 1984 Apr;43(2):125-7
**Hart G:** A medical caduceus from Roman London. **Trans Med Soc Lond** 1979;95:99-105
**Hart GD:** Anemia in ancient times. **Blood Cells** 1981;7(3):485-93
**Hart GD, Millett N, Scott J:** Paleopathology and the autopsy of an Egyptian mummy. In: Congrès international d'histoire de la médecine, XXVe, Québec, 1976. Actes. Québec, 1977. p. 765-70.
**Hart GD** see **Millet NB**
**Hart H:** Some notes on the sponsoring of patients for hospital treatment under the voluntary system. **Med Hist** 1980;24(4):447-60
**Hart JA:** The ethnobotany of the Northern Cheyenne Indians of Montana. **J Ethnopharmacol** 1981 Jul;4(1):1-55
**Hart PD:** Berustten de armen in Nederland omstreeks 1800 eerbiedig in hun lot? **Spiegel Hist** 1982;17(3):148-55
**Hart PD:** Waren de armen in Nederland omstreeks 1800 zorgeloze klaplopers? **Spiegel Hist** 1982;17(2):62-8
**Hart GD, ed:** Disease in ancient man. An international symposium held in London, 1979. Toronto, Clarke Irwin, 1983. 297 p. Contributions by D. A. Birkett, F. F. Cartwright, R. Cramp, J. Dobson, A. J. Duggan, N. G. Gejvall, P. S. Gooch, C. J. Hackett, P. D. Horne, P. Janssens, B. Knight, A. K. Knowles, N. B. Millet, V. Møller-Christensen, W. J. Moore, R. Perrot, F. D. Pooley, D. F. Rideout, A. Rook, W. M. Russell, P. Slack, W. E. Swinton, H. A. Waldron.
**Hartemann J:** Geschichte der Geburtshilfe vom 18. Jahrhundert bis zur Gegenwart. In Sournia JC, Martiny M, Poulet J, ed: Illustrierte Geschichte der Medizin. Salzburg, Andreas, 1980. Vol. 4. p. 1359-427.
**Harthorne JW:** Historic milestones of electrotherapy and cardiac pacing. **Prog Cardiovasc Dis** 1981 May-Jun;23(6):389-92
**Härtl J:** Prof. Dr. phil. et Dr. med. h.c. Johann Martin Kreutzer, märtyrer oder rebell? **Hist Med Vet** 1977;2(4):112-22
**Hartl P:** Vývoj pedagogické psychologie a její význam pro oblast výchovy a vzdělávání dospělých. **Acta Univ Carol [Hist] (Praha)** 1977;5:25-52
**Hartley F:** Pharmacy in the time of John Hunter (1728-1793). **Trans Hunter Soc** 1978-80;37-38:99-107
**Hartley H:** Douglas McKie. In Dictionary of national biography, 1961-1970. Suppl. 8, 1981. p. 695-7.
**Hartley H:** Humphry Davy. London, Nelson, 1966. viii, 160 p.
**Hartley JC:** The centenary of the Lincolnshire Veterinary Medical Society. **Vet Hist** 1983 Summer;3(1):33-6
**Hartley S** see **Laslett P**
**Hartman B** see **Schulz R**
**Hartmann E** see **Geppert W**
**Hartmann F:** Homo patiens. Zur ärztlichen Anthropologie von Leid und Mitleid. In Seidler E, Schott H, ed: Bausteine zur Medizingeschichte. Stuttgart, Steiner, 1984. p. 35-44.
**Hartmann K, Margolin L:** The Nebraska Asylum for the Insane, 1870-1886. **Nebr Hist** 1982;63(2):164-83
**Hartmann K, Halbert MR, Margolin L:** Treatment at the Nebraska asylum for the insane a century ago. **Nebr Med J** 1982 May;67(5):131-3
**Hartog AP den:** Werklozen en hun voeding in de jaren 1930-1939. **Spiegel Hist** 1982;17(9):445-51
**Hartree EF:** David Keilin. In Dictionary of national biography, 1961-1970. Suppl. 8, 1981. p. 604-5.
**Hartree EF:** Ethics for authors: a case history of acrosin. **Perspect Biol Med** 1976 Autumn;20(1):82-91
**Hartshorne C** see **Spicker SF, ed**
**Hartung K:** Einhundert Jahre schulärztlicher Dienst--ein beinahe vergessenes Jubiläum. **Off Gesundheitswes** 1983 Dec;45(12):615-7
**Hartwell SW:** From horse and buggy practice to world-renowned medical center. History of the Cleveland Clinic Foundation. **Postgrad Med** 1984 May;75(6):14-6, 21-6
**Hartwig GW:** Demographic considerations in East Africa during the nineteenth century. **Int J Afr Hist Stud** 1979;12(4):653-72
**Hartwig GW:** Economic consequenses of long-distance trade in East-Africa: the disease factor. **Afr Stud Rev** 1975;18(2):63-77
**Hartwig GW:** Smallpox in the Sudan. **Int J Afr Hist Stud** 1981;14(1):5-33
**Harty FJ:** Endodontic treatment in England. **Int Endod J** 1984 Jul;17(3):106-12
**Harty FJ** see **Watson RM**
**Hartzler DD** see **Taylor B**
**Harvey AD:** Prosecutions for sodomy in England at the beginning of the nineteenth century. **Hist J (Gt Brit)** 1978;21(4):939-48
**Harvey AM:** Alfred Blalock. In Dictionary of American biography, 1961-1965. Suppl. 7, 1981. p. 59.
**Harvey AM:** Amebic dysentery gets its name: the story of William Thomas Councilman. **Johns Hopkins Med J** 1980 May;146(5):185-92, 199-201
**Harvey AM:** Classics in clinical science. **Am J Med** 1980 Jan;68(1):6-8 (continued periodically)
**Harvey AM:** Clinical investigation of chronic diseases: its successful pursuit in an outpatient setting. **J Chronic Dis** 1980;33(9):529-66
**Harvey AM:** David Marine: America's pioneer thyroidologist. **Am J Med** 1981 Mar;70(3):483-5
**Harvey AM:** Francis Weld Peabody: the blending of general internal medicine and clinical science. **Pharos** 1981 Summer;44(3):6-8
**Harvey AM:** George Canby Robinson. In Dictionary of American Biography, Suppl. 6, 1956-1960. p. 546-7, 1980.
**Harvey AM:** Henry M. Thomas: Johns Hopkins's first neurologist. **Johns Hopkins Med J** 1982 Jan;150(1):11-21
**Harvey AM:** Henry Mills Hurd: the first superintendent of the Johns Hopkins Hospital and the first professor of psychiatry. **Johns Hopkins Med J** 1981 Mar;148(3):135-48
**Harvey AM:** James Howard Means and his romance with the thyroid gland. **Am J Med** 1981 Jun;70(6):1158-60
**Harvey AM:** Johns Hopkins and yellow fever: a story of tragedy and triumph. **Johns Hopkins Med J** 1981 Jul;149(1):25-39
**Harvey AM:** Johns Hopkins's pioneer venture into international medicine: the commission to the Philippine Islands. **Johns Hopkins Med J** 1980 Jul;147(1):13-27
**Harvey AM:** Joseph Charles Aub: applying the tools of the basic sciences to clinical investigation. **Am J Med** 1981 Jul;71(1):13-5
**Harvey AM:** Louis Harry Newburgh: compleat clinical investigator with a passion for measurement. **Am J Med** 1981 Apr;70(4):759-61
**Harvey AM:** Orthopaedic surgery at Johns Hopkins: a heritage of excellence in clinical practice, training and research. **Johns Hopkins Med J** 1982 Jun;150(6):221-45
**Harvey AM:** Research and discovery in medicine. Contributions from Johns Hopkins. Baltimore and London, Johns Hopkins University Press, 1981. xiii, 322 p. [Collected historical papers reprinted from various journals].
**Harvey AM:** Samuel J. Meltzer: pioneer catalyst in the evolution of clinical science in America. **Perspect Biol Med** 1978 Spring;21(3):431-40
**Harvey AM:** Science at the bedside. Clinical research in American medicine, 1905-1945. Baltimore, London, Johns Hopkins University Press, 1981. xix, 554 p.
**Harvey AM:** Science at the bedside: the footprints of Yale and Johns Hopkins. **Yale J Biol Med** 1979 Nov-Dec;52(6):569-79
**Harvey AM:** Science at the bedside: the story of Warfield Theobald Longcope. **Trans Stud Coll Physicians Phila** 1981 Sep;5(3 no 3):161-73
**Harvey AM:** Stanhope Bayne-Jones, 1886-1970: the story of a lifetime devoted to country and to medicine. **Johns Hopkins Med J** 1981 Oct;149(4):150-66
**Harvey AM:** The conquest of scarlet fever: some Johns Hopkins contributions. **Johns Hopkins Med J** 1980 Aug;147(2):53-63
**Harvey AM:** The influence of William Stewart Halsted's concepts of surgical training. **Johns Hopkins Med J** 1981 May;148(5):215-36
**Harvey AM:** The Interurban Clinical Club (1905-1976): a record of achievement in clinical science. [s.l.], Interurban Clinical Club, 1978. xiii, 573 p.
**Harvey AM** see **Trends in biomedical research, 1901-1976**
**Harvey HR:** Public health in Aztec society. **Bull NY Acad Med** 1981 Mar;57(2):157-65
**Harvey KA:** Practicing medicine at the Baltimore Almshouse, 1828-1850. **Md Hist Mag** 1979;74(3):223-37
**Harvey PW** see **Bound JP**
**Harvey WL, Hatch R:** Articulators--a perspective: wristolator to robots. **J Colo Dent Assoc** 1981 Nov-Dec;60(3):3-5
**Harvey AP, ed** see **Bridson GD**
**Harvey W. Wiley and the Pure Food and Drug Act: Nutr Hist Notes** 1981;11:2-4
**Harwood J:** The IQ in history. **Soc Stud Sci** 1983 Aug;13(3):465-77
**Harwood J:** The reception of Morgan's chromosome theory in Germany: inter-war debate over cytoplasmic inheritance. **Medizinhist J** 1984;19(1-2):3-32
**Harwood JH:** The history of genetics in Germany. **Mendel Newsl** 1984;(24):1-3
**Harwood-Nash DC:** Computed tomography of ancient Egyptian mummies. **J Comput Assist Tomogr** 1979 Dec;3(6):768-73
**Has the Republic no need of learning?: J Hist Med Allied Sci** 1981 Jul;36(3):257-9
**Hasáková E** see **Krahulec I**
**Haschek H:** 108 years of urology at the Poliklinik of Vienna. **Urology** 1981 Jan;17(1):113-7
**Haschen RJ:** Entwicklung der Forschung auf dem Gebiet der Pathologischen und Klinischen Biochemie. **Z Med Lab Diagn** 1983;24(7):381-6
**Hasegawa A:** [Social events in the history of nursing after World War II. I. Hospital and nurses on strike] (Jpn). **Kango** 1984 Aug;36(9):126-44
**Hasegawa M:** [Changes in oral (endodontic) treatment] (Jpn). **Shikwa Gakuho** 1983 May;83(5):587-97
**Hasegawa M:** [History of endodontics (1)] (Jpn). **Nippon Shika Hyoron** 1983 Feb;(484):135-45
**Haskins CP:** The changing environments of science. **Daedalus** 1965;94(3):682-712
**Hasler L, ed:** Schelling: seine Bedeutung für eine Philosophie der Natur und der Geschichte. Referate und Kolloquien der Internationalen Schelling-Tagung Zürich 1979. Stuttgart-Bad Cannstaff, Frommann-Holzboog, 1981. 319 p. Includes contributions by H. Krings, D. von Engelhardt, R. Löw, N. Tsouyopoulos, R. Toellner, H. Poser, H. Querner, K. E. Rothschuh, F. Moiso, S. Dietzch, D. v. Uslar, W. Bonsiepen.
**Hassani AM:** The appearance of scientific naturalism in Syria and Egypt.

**J Hist Arabic Sci** 1977 Nov;1(2):284–98
**Hassel FJ, Künzl E:** Ein römisches Arztgrab des 3. Jahrhunderts n. Chr. aus Kleinasien. **Medizinhist J** 1980;15(4):403–21
**Hässig A:** 40 Jahre Blutspendedienst des Schweizerischen Roten Kreuzes. **Ther Umsch** 1984 Aug;41(8):533–5
**Hassler WW:** Dr. Hunter Holmes McGuire: surgeon to Stonewall Jackson, the Confederacy, and the Nation. **Va Cavalcade** 1982;32(2):52–61
**Hasson GS:** Health and welfare of freedmen in reconstruction Alabama. **Ala Rev** 1982;35(2):94–110
**Hasson GS:** The medical activities of the Freedmen's Bureau in Reconstruction Alabama, 1865–1868. Ph.D. Diss, University of Alabama, University, 1982. 252 p.
**Hasstedt S** see **Carmelli D**
**Hast A:** Robert Anderson Cooke. In Dictionary of American Biography, Suppl. 6, 1956–1960. p. 123–4, 1980.
**Hastings DW** see **Levison CH**
**Hastreiter RJ:** Fluoridation conflict: a history and conceptual synthesis. **J Am Dent Assoc** 1983 Apr;106(4):486–90
**Hastrup JL** see **McMahon CE**
**Hatate M** see **Miura F**
**Hatch CE:** New Jersey's Reaction to the Tennesse evolution trial. **NJ Hist** 1972;90(4):226–41
**Hatch R** see **Harvey WL**
**Hatcher J:** Simon Flexner. **Gaz Inst Med Lab Sci** 1981;25:317–8
**Hatfield FM:** Analysis and remediation of aphasia in the U.S.S.R: the contribution of A. R. Luria. **J Speech Hear Disord** 1981 Nov;46(4):338–47
**Hatfield G:** Robert Brown A.M., F.R.S.E. (1773–1858). Edinburgh, History of Medicine and Science Unit, University of Edinburgh, [1981?]. [11] p.
**Hau FR:** Die Bildung des Arztes im Islamischen Mittelalter. **Clio Med** 1979 May;13(3–4):175–200
**Hau FR:** Die Bildung des Arztes im Islamischen Mittelalter. **Clio Med** 1979 Jul;14(1):7–33
**Hau T:** The surgical practice of Dominique Jean Larrey. **Surg Gynecol Obstet** 1982 Jan;154(1):89–94
**Hauben D:** Die Geschichte der gespaltenen Gaumen. **Z Plast Chir** 1981 Dec;5(4):228–33
**Hauben DJ:** Aulus (Aurelius) Cornelius Celsus (25 v.u.Z.–50 n.u.Z.) – Vater der plastischen Chirurgie. **Zentralbl Chir** 1984;109(6):441–3
**Hauben DJ:** Carl Ferdinand von Graefe (1787–1840). **Zentralbl Chir** 1984;109(14):950–1
**Hauben DJ:** Das chirurgische Erbe. Bernhard Rudolf Conrad Langenbeck (1810–1887). **Zentralbl Chir** 1984;109(20):1338–9
**Hauben DJ:** Das chirurgische Erbe. Guillaume Dupuytren (1777–1835). **Zentralbl Chir** 1984;109(11):765–6
**Hauben DJ:** Das chirurgische Erbe. Pioniere der plastischen Chirurgie der Renaissance (1). **Zentralbl Chir** 1984;109(9):631–7
**Hauben DJ:** Die Geschichte der Rhinoplastik. **Laryngol Rhinol Otol (Stuttg)** 1983 Feb;62(2):53–5
**Hauben DJ:** Ernst Blasius's contributions to plastic surgery. **Plast Reconstr Surg** 1984 Oct;74(4):561–70
**Hauben DJ:** Jacques Joseph (1865–1934). **Laryngol Rhinol Otol (Stuttg)** 1983 Feb;62(2):56–7
**Hauben DJ, Baruchin A, Mahler A:** On the history of the free skin graft. **Ann Plast Surg** 1982 Sep;9(3):242–5
**Hauben DJ:** Plastic surgery - historical aspects. **Koroth** 1981;8(1–2):71–7
**Hauben DJ:** Robert Liston's life and work in the renaissance of plastic surgery. **Ann Plast Surg** 1983 Jun;10(6):502–9
**Hauben DJ:** Sushruta Samhita (Sushruta's Collection) (800–600 B.C.?). Pioneers of plastic surgery. **Acta Chir Plast (Prague)** 1984;26(2):65–8
**Hauben DJ, Sonneveld GJ:** The influence of war on the development of plastic surgery. **Ann Plast Surg** 1983 Jan;10(1):65–9
**Hauberg P:** Laegebøger med tilknytning til Henrik Harpestraeng. **Theriaca** 1982 Jun;22:1–362
**Haubrich WS** see **Crosby WH**
**Haugejorden O** see **Helöe LA**
**Haugen A:** Sanderud: sykehus i 175 år: psykiatrisk sykehus i 70 år. [s.L.]. Elverum trykk, 1978. 132 p.
**Haugen LK:** Darwin, evolusjonen og medisinen. **Tidsskr Nor Laegeforen** 1982 Dec 10;102(34–36):1835–8
**Haugen LK:** The human upper and middle face. A morphological investigation in a Norwegian medieval population. **Acta Morphol Neerl Scand** 1980 Jun;18(23):93–112,113–23
**Haugh MC:** The Doulton story (Henry Doulton). **Nurs Times** 1979 Jul 19;75(29):1207–8
**Haugwitz T von:** Ophthalmologisch-optische Untersuchungsgeräte. Entwicklung und gegenwärtiger Stand. **Buch Augenarzt** 1981;(85):1–226
**Hauk J:** Carl Harko Hermann Johannes von Noorden (1858–1944), sein Leben und Werk unter besonderer Berücksichtigung seiner Theorien über die Ursachen des Diabetes mellitus. Diss. Mainz, 1980. 288 p.
**Hauptman LM:** Smallpox and American Indian; depopulation in colonial New York. **NY State J Med** 1979 Nov;79(12):1945–9
**Hauser G** see **Bergman P**
**Häusermann R, Koelbing H, Biener K:** Präventivmedizin in den alten Religionen. **Soz Praventivmed** 1984;29(2):72–7
**Hausman A:** Historique et activités du C.C.R. **Rev Inst Hyg Mines (Hasselt)** 1983;38(2):138–9
**Hausmann J:** Die Syndrome 'Manie' und 'Melancholie' an der Wende zum 18. Jahrhundert. Dargestellt an zwei zeitgenössischen Dissertationen. Diss., Rheinische Friedrich-Wilhelms-Universität. Bonn, 1982. 148 p.
**Hausmann W:** Bericht über einen Fund in Sezze Romano. **Tierarztl Prax** 1980;8(4):417–8
**Hausmann W:** Chironica ars-- antike Autoren über Cheiron. **DTW** 1982 Oct 5;89(10):407–11
**Hausmann W:** Christliche Votivtäfelchen aus Metall. **Tierarztl Prax** 1981;9(1):3–8
**Hausmann W:** Der Becher des Gudea. **Tierarztl Prax** 1979;7(2):141–3
**Hausmann W:** Der Stier als Fruchtbarkeitssymbol. Ein Bericht über Funde aus mehreren Ländern. **DTW** 1982 Feb 5:89(2):86–8
**Hausmann W:** Medizinhistorische Antiquitäten aus Indien. **Tierarztl Prax** 1981;9(4):421–5
**Hausmann W:** Weibliche Fruchtbarkeitssymbole der Quanchen und Tarasken. **Tierarztl Prax** 1983;11(3):417–20
**Hausmann WO:** Die medizinische Höhlenschule des Cheiron. **Berl Munch Tierarztl Wochenschr** 1982 Mar 1;95(5):94–5
**Häussermann E:** Für den Zahnarzt im Dichter-Schloss nur ein kleines Mansarden-Zimmer. **Zahnarztl Mitt** 1983 Sep 16;73(18):1990, 1993–4
**Häussler S:** Johannes Kepler und die Allgemeinmedizin. **ZFA (Stuttgart)** 1982 May 31;58(15):I–1037–8
**Haustein KO:** Digitalis. **Pharmacol Ther** 1982;18(1):1–89
**Haustein UF** see **Schreier J**
**Haut J** see **Royer J**
**Hauw JJ** see **Escourolle R**
**Havelange C:** Médecine traditionnelle ou exercice illégal de l'art de guérir? Les empiriques liégeois au dix-neuvième siècle. **Rev Med Liege** 1983 Nov 15;38(22):860–8
**Havelange C:** Pléthore et art de guérir. Le malaise des médecins liégeois au XIXe siècle. **Rev Med Liege** 1984 Oct 1;39(19):676–95
**Haven M:** La vie et les oeuvres de Maître Arnaud de Villenauve. Genève, Slatkine Reprints, 1972. [192] p.
**Havens LL:** Twentieth-century psychiatry: a view from the sea. **Am J Psychiatry** 1981 Oct;138(10):1279–87
**Havighurst W:** The mind of John Shaw Billings. In his: Men of old Miami, 1809–1873, a book of portraits. New York, Putnams, 1974. p. 189–207.
**Haviland CF** see **Grob GN, ed**
**Havránek J:** Ustavení Ceské university a její lékařské fakulty v letech 1882 a 1883. **Cas Lek Cesk** 1983 Feb 18;122(7):193–5
**Hawker R:** Rules to control visitors, 1746–1900. **Nurs Times** 1984 Mar 21–27;80(12):48–51
**Hawkins A:** Two pathographies: a study in illness and literature. **J Med Philos** 1984 Aug;9(3):231–52
**Hawkins H:** Transatlantic discipleship: two American biologists and their German mentor. **Isis** 1980 Jun;71(257):197–210
**Hawkins HB, Cinti DC:** Magnetic resonance imaging. Where did it come from? What is it? Where is it going? Part I. History and physical principles. **Conn Med** 1984 Sep;48(9):575–7
**Hawkins MJ:** Reason and sense perception in Comte's theory of mind. **Hist Eur Ideas** 1984;5:149–63
**Hawkins WG** see **Barrett HH**
**Hay GW** see **Szarek WA**
**Hayami A** see **Laslett P**
**Hayashi J:** [History of graphs and the basic rules in drawing] (Jpn). **Josanpu Zasshi** 1983 Dec;37(12):1035–9
**Hayashi T:** [Reflection on my research in bacteriology] (Jpn). **Nippon Saikingaku Zasshi** 1984 Mar;39(2):81–4
**Haycock CE:** The female athlete and sportsmedicine in the 70's. **J Fla Med Assoc** 1980 Apr;67(4):411–4
**Haycock CE:** Women physicians of New Jersey: the early era. **J Med Soc NJ** 1984 Sep;81(9):773–7
**Hayden GF, Saulsbury FT:** A review of The Journal of Pediatrics: the first 50 years. **J Pediatr** 1982 Jul;101(1):5–11
**Hayden GF:** Clinical research in Southern Medical Journal: current trends. **South Med J** 1983 Dec;76(12):1473–6
**Hayden J:** Niels Bjorn Jorgensen: painless dentist. **Advent Herit** 1979;6(2):44–8
**Hayden MR, Hopkins HC, Macrea M, et al:** The origin of Huntington's chorea in the Afrikaner population of South Africa. **S Afr Med J** 1980 Aug 2;58(5):197–200
**Hayes AH:** Food and drug regulation after 75 years. **JAMA** 1981 Sep 11;246(11):1223–6
**Hayes AH:** Science and public policy. **J Assoc Off Anal Chem** 1982 Mar;65(2):202–5
**Hayes B:** Ventilation and ventilators. **J Med Eng Technol** 1982 Sep–Oct;6(5):177–92
**Hayler B:** Abortion. **Signs** 1979;5(2):307–23
**Hayles AB, Key JD:** Adventures of two prairie pioneers. **Minn Med** 1981 Oct;64(10):629–32
**Hayles AB:** Gigantism. **Pediatr Ann** 1980 Apr;9(4):163–9
**Hayman J:** Mycobacterium ulcerans: an infection from Jurassic time? **Lancet** 1984 Nov 3;2(8410):1015–6
**Hayman R:** Nietzsche's madness. **Partisan Rev** 1980;47(1):29–44
**Haynes DM:** History of placental studies. **Obstet Gynecol Annu** 1983;12:1–14
**Haynes R:** The Society for Psychical Research, 1882–1982: a history. London, Macdonald, 1982. xv, 240 p.
**Hayward JC** see **Allan P**
**Haywood A:** The National Health Survey--in the beginning. **Public Health Rep** 1981 May–Jun;96(3):195–9
**A hazai porcragasztás prioritásáról: Orv Hetil** 1984 Dec 16;125(51):3150
**Hazard JB:** An introduction to the history of surgical pathology. **Am J Clin Pathol** 1981 Mar;75(3 Suppl):444–6
**Hazelrigg C:** Central State Hospital. Part 2. **Indiana Med Hist Q**

1981;7(3):3–23
**Hazlett BE** see **Burrow GN**
**Hazra J** see **Banerjee B**
**Hazzard FW:** Eliza Maria Mosher, MD (1846–1928). **Women Health** 1982 Summer;7(2):1–4
**He A:** [Exploration on the date of birth and death of Chunyu Yi] (Chi). **Chung Hua I Shih Tsa Chih** 1984;14(2):80–4
**He Zongyu:** [Translation, interpretation and textual research of medical works unearthed in Ma Wang Dui.] (Chi). **Chin J Med Hist** 1981;11:125–7
**Head ES** see **Smith EB**
**The healing art: Am Heritage** 1981;32(4):16–27
**Health care and its costs:** The development of the National Health Service in England. London, H. M. S. O., 1983. 51 p.
**Health care planning in urban areas: Zagreb: World Hosp** 1978 May;14(2):123–9
**Health in the southern United States:** New York, Arno, 1977. Various paginations. Facsimiles of works by David Ramsay (1790 and 1796), Josiah C. Nott (1847), Edward H. Barton (1851), Wickliffe Rose (1910), Joseph Goldberger (1916).
**The health of women and children. New York, Arno, 1977. Varius paginations. Five reprinted articles by various authors, 1909–1953.:**
**'Health Physics': 25th anniversary issue commemorating the founding of the Health Physics Society 1955–1980.: Health Phys** 1980 Jun;38(6):883–1209
**Healthy people:** The Minnesota experience. Minnesota Center for Health Statistics, 1982. [xix], 168 p.
**Hearnshaw LS:** Cyril Burt, psychologist. Ithaca, Cornell University Press, 1979. xi, 370 p.
**Hearst E, ed:** The first century of experimental psychology. Hillsdale, N.J., Erlbaum, 1979. xxiii, 693 p. Contributions by R. A. Littman, J. Hochberg, G. Gottlieb, H. M. Jenkins, J. S. Brown, G. Mandler, C. N. Cofer, M. I. Posner, G. L. Shulman, R. F. Thompson, D. N. Robinson, R. B. Cairns, P. A. Ornstein, I. D. Steiner, B. A. Maher, W. B. Maher, W. K. Estes.
**Heath A** see **Salsburg D**
**Heath CW** see **Caldwell GG**
**Heath G:** The illusory freedom. London, Heinemann, 1978. 131 p.
**Heaton KW:** T. L. Cleave and the fibre story. **J R Nav Med Serv** 1980;66(1):5–10
**Hebanowski M** see **Galiński J**
**Hebb DO:** Neuropsychology: retrospect and prospect. **Can J Psychol** 1983 Mar;37(1):4–7
**Hebbelinck M** see **Borms J**
**Hebbert FJ:** Belle-Ile and the secret expedition. **Trans Hunter Soc** 1978–80;37–38:193–210
**Hebenstreit G** see **Harmat P**
**Hebert M** see **Muller A**
**Hébert M** see **Sutto C, ed**
**Hebert RG:** Florence Nightingale: saint, reformer or rebel? Malabar, Florida, Robert E. Krieger, 1981. 236 p.
**Hécaen H:** L'evolution et les perspectives de la neuropsychologie. **Acta Neurol Latinoam** 1980;26(2):75–102
**Hécaen H:** Storia dell'afasia. **Kos** 1984 Mar;1(2):118–27
**Hecht A:** Wesen und geistige Wurzeln der Leipziger Pathologischen Anatomie. **Zentralbl Allg Pathol** 1982;126(3–4):229–36
**Hecht J:** Johann Peter Sussmilch, point alpha ou omega de la science démographique naïve? **Ann Demogr Hist (Paris)** 1979;:101–34
**Heck CV:** Fifty years of progress: in recognition of the 50th anniversary of the American Academy of Orthopaedic Surgeons. Chicago, American Academy of Orthopaedic Surgeons, 1983. vi, 361 p.
**Heck J:** Leishmaniasis und Fruchtbarkeitskult. **Dtsch Med Wochenschr** 1982 Jun 4;107(22):872–4
**Heckelsberg LF:** Historical note: thermoluminescent dosimetry (LiF) 1950–51. **Health Phys** 1980 Sep;39(3):391–3
**Heckmann G:** Anzeigepflichtige Tierseuchen in der Bundesrepublik Deutschland von 1950 bis 1983, unter besonderer Darstellung des Zeitabschnittes von 1970 bis 1983 in Zahlen und Grafiken. Berlin, Parey, 1984. 123 p.
**Heckmann K:** Die Entwicklung der Schlitzaufnahmen. **Rontgenblatter** 1984 Jan;37(1):29–39
**Hed H:** Opportunity for selection during the 17th–19th centuries in the diocese of Linköping as estimated with Crow's index in a population of clergymen's wives. **Hum Hered** 1984;34(6):378–87
**Hed HM, Rasmuson M:** Cohort study of opportunity for selection on two Swedish 19th century parishes with a survey of other estimates. **Hum Hered** 1981;31(2):78–83
**Hedderson J, Daudistel HC:** Infant mortality of the Spanish surname population. **Soc Sci J** 1982;19(4):67–78
**Hedenvind A:** Födelseår 1903. **Arbetarrörel Arsb** 1975;:32–42
**Hedfors E:** Mannen bakom syndromet: Augustus Roi Felty. Fann ovanlig symtomkonstellation: artrit, splenomegali, leukopeni. **Lakartidningen** 1983 Sep 14;80(37):3281
**Hedger RS** see **Perry BD**
**Hedman D:** Medicinhistoriska synpunkter på avhuggna näsor och andra näsdefekter. **Nord Medicinhist Arsb** 1981;:40–51
**Heeger G, ed** see **Albin M**
**Heeney B:** Opposition to state medicine and state education: an historical analogy. **Queens Q** 1968;75(1):72–89
**Heer K de:** Zur Pathogenität der Galle. Historisches und neue experimentelle Ergebnisse. **Med Welt** 1981 Aug 28;32(35):1292–6
**Heerden JA van:** First encounters with pheochromocytoma. The story of Mother Joachim. **Am J Surg** 1982 Aug;144(2):277–9
**Hefner LL:** The National Women's Relief Society and the U.S. Sheppard–Towner Act. **Utah Hist Q** 1982;50(3):255–67
**Hegedüs L:** Zwei berühmte ungarische Arcana aus dem 14. und 15. Jahrhundert. In Hein WH, ed: Pharmaziehistorischer Kongress, Budapest, 1981. Stuttgart, Wissenschaftliche Verlagsgesellschaft, 1983. p. 41–7.
**Heggelbacher O:** Geisteskrankheit und kirchenrechtliche Verantwortlichkeit. **Osterr Arch Kirchenr** 1967;18(1):3–16
**Hehir JB** see **Bleich JD**
**Hehrlein FW** see **Mulch J**
**Hehrlein FW** see **Scheld HH**
**Heidecker KM** see **Engelhardt R, ed**
**Heidel G:** Zur wahrscheinlich ältesten deutschen Ubersetzung des Syphilisgedichtes von Girolamo Fracastoro. **Dermatol Monatsschr** 1983;169(2):130–5
**Heidelberger M:** A 'pure' organic chemist's downward path: chapter 3--'retirement'. **Perspect Biol Med** 1981 Summer;24(4):619–36
**Heidelberger M:** Recognition of antibodies as labeled globulins. **Ann NY Acad Sci** 1983;420:1–4
**Heidelberger M** see **Trends in biomedical research, 1901–1976**
**Heidenheimer AJ:** Organized medicine and physician specialization in Scandinavia and West Germany. **West Eur Polit** 1980;3(3):373–87
**Heifets L:** Centennial of Metchnikoff's discovery. **J Reticuloendothel Soc** 1982 May;31(5):381–91
**Heifets L:** Metchnikoff's recollections of Robert Koch. **Tubercle** 1982 Jun;63(2):139–41
**Heikkinen R:** Lönnrot Kajaanin piirin ja linnan lääkärinä. **Duodecim** 1983;99(23–24):1726–9
**Heilmann K:** Gesundheitstechnologien. [Köln?], Deutscher Instituts-Verlag, 1984. 56 p.
**Heilmittel aus Pflanzen und Tieren:** Ausstellung des Oberösterreichischen Landesmuseums im Schlossmuseum zu Linz vom 9. 5. bis 3. 8. 1980. Linz, Landesmuseum, 1980. 359 p. (Katalog des Oberösterr. Landesmuseums, 105). Contributions by W. Kubelka, R. Schmidt, F. Speta, H. Heltmann, B. Kopp, B. Gruber, E. Speta, R. Steinwendtner. K. Rumpler, A. Kump, F. Grims, B. Heinzl.
**Heilwagen W:** Das Kasseler Gesundheitswesen der Gegenwart. In Balde JH, Schmiking W, ed: Festschrift zum 86. Deutschen Arztetag in Kassel. Kassel, Arztevereins, 1983. p. 105–12.
**Heim LR:** Birth and development of a scientific journal, and a society. **Exp Hematol** 1983 Nov;11(10):907–13
**Heimann H:** De Kraepelin au sytème AMDP. **Acta Psychiatr Belg** 1983 Mar–Apr;83(2):147–54
**Heimann H:** Nosologie und Pathophysiologie in der Psychiatrie--Aspekte der Krankheitslehre Kraepelins heute. **Confin Psychiatr** 1980;23(4):262–74
**Heimans J:** Hugo De Vries and the gene theory. In Forbes EG, ed: Human implications of scientific advance. Edinburgh, Edinburgh University Press, 1978. p. 469–80.
**Heimbuch RC** see **Laitman JT**
**Heimrath T:** Ewolucja doboru pozycji podczas rodzenia. **Wiad Lek** 1984 May 15;37(10):797–9
**Heimrath T, Smereka J:** Lekarze polscy wykształceni we wrocławskiej Klinice Kobiecej w latach 1811--1918. **Arch Hist Med (Warsz)** 1979;42(3):345–9
**Heimrath T:** Organizacja wrocławskiej kliniki Kobiecej jako wyraz poglądów medycznych epoki (1890 r.). **Arch Hist Med (Warsz)** 1981;44(3/4):381–4
**Heimrath T:** Położnictwo i genekologia w Akademii Medycznej we Wrocławiu w latach 1945–1980. **Ginekol Pol** 1982 Jul–Aug;53(7–8):563–8
**Hein G** see **Tautz P**
**Hein J:** Ludolph Brauer--Der Wegbereiter der modernen Pneumologie. **Prax Klin Pneumol** 1984 Oct;38(10):471–3
**Hein JW:** The industrial contribution to safe and effective dentifrices. **Community Dent Oral Epidemiol** 1980;8(5):230–6
**Hein WH, Wittop Koning AW:** Apothekengefässe der Durlacher Fayence-Fabrik. **Pharm Ztg** 1980;125:25–7
**Hein WH, Schwarz HD, ed:** Deutsche Apotheker-Biographie. Band II, M–Z. Stuttgart, Wissenschaftliche Verlagsgesellschaft, 1978. p. 393–788. (Veröffentlichungen der Internationalen Gesellschaft für Geschichte der Pharmazie, Neue Folge, Band 46).
**Hein WH:** Die ephesische Diana als Natursymbol bei Alexander von Humboldt. In Dilg P, et al., ed: Perspektiven der Pharmaziegeschichte. Graz, Austria, Akademische Druck- u. Verlagsanstalt, 1983. p. 131–46.
**Hein WH:** Ein arabisches Apothekeninterieur vom Jahre 1222. **Pharm Ztg** 1979 Jan 4;124(1):3–4
**Hein WH:** Fälschungen deutscher Apothekengläser. **Beitr Gesch Pharm** 1982;31(15):113–16
**Hein WH:** Historische und kritische Betrachtungen zu den Veröffentlichungen der Gesellschaft. In: Vorträge des Internationalen Pharmaziehistorischen Kongresses Innsbruck 1977. Stuttgart, Wissenschaftliche Verlagsgesellschaft, 1979. p. 15–22.
**Hein WH:** Sur le frontispice de la Pharmacopée de Milan de 1698. **Rev Hist Pharm (Paris)** 1982 Jun;29(253):87–90
**Hein WH:** Zum Curarebericht des Jesuitenpaters Franz Xaver Veigl. **Beitr Gesch Pharm** 1981;11:81–4
**Hein WH, ed:** Pharmaziehistorischer Kongress, Budapest, 1981. I. Vorträge zur ungarischen Pharmaziegeschichte. II. Vorträge in Zusammenfassungen. Stuttgart, Wissenschaftliche Verlagsgesellschaft, 1983. 191 p. (Veröffentlichungen der Internationalen Gesellschaft für Geschichte der Pharmazie e. V., 52).
**Heindel ND, Foster NI:** Medicine, music and 'Money' Munyon.

**Pa Folklife** 1982;32(1):44–8
**Heindel ND, Foster NI:** The Allentown Academy: America's first German medical school. **Pa Folklife** 1980;30(1):2–8
**Heinecke H:** Die Kontrolle im Tierversuch--eine historische Studie über Tierversuche von G. F. Fordyce. **Z Versuchstierkd** 1983;25(4):223–6
**Heinecke K** see **Opitz R**
**Heinecke P** see **Opitz R**
**Heinemeyer W, Pünder T:** 450 Jahre Psychiatrie in Hessen. Marburg, Elwert (Kommissionsverlag), 1983. x, 461 p.
**Heinl E:** Třicet let výchovně vzdělávací činnosti Institut pro další vzdělávání lékařu a farmaceutu. **Cas Lek Cesk** 1983 Oct 21;122(42):1286–90
**Heinrich J:** Historical perspectives on public health nursing. **Nurs Outlook** 1983 Nov–Dec;31(6):317–20
**Heinrich P** see **Neumann A**
**Heinrich WL:** Richard Walther Darré und der Hegehofgedanke. Diss. Mainz, 1980. 161 p.
**Heinrichs HJ:** Bibliographie der Schriften von Jacques Lacan. **Psyche (Stuttg)** 1980 Oct;34(10):958–73
**Heinrichs HJ:** Harold Linckes Versuch einer Vermittlung von Natur- und Geisteswissenschaften. **Psyche (Stuttg)** 1980 Feb;34(2):152–67
**Heins M:** Landmark perspective: The 'battered child' revisited. **JAMA** 1984 Jun 22–29;251(24):3295–300
**Heinsohn G** see **Dupâquier J**
**Heintel B, Heintel H:** Historische Stätten der Neurologie in Baden-Württemberg. Stuttgart and New York, Fischer, 1982. n.p.
**Heintel B:** Historische Stätten der Neurologie in Baden-Württemberg. Stuttgart; New York, G. Fischer, 1982. [66] p.
**Heintel H:** Die Fallhaube: eine Erfindung des 16. Jahrhunderts? **Medizinhist J** 1984;19(3):273–6
**Heintel H:** Ein unbekanntes Porträt des Hirnforschers Oskar Vogt (1870–1959). **Medizinhist J** 1984;19(3):277–9
**Heintel H:** Hermann Andreas Reimer und seine 1855 eröffnete 'Heilanstalt für Epileptische' in Görlitz. **Medizinhist J** 1982;17(1/2):156–60
**Heintel H:** Moritz Schiffs gescheiterter Habilitationsversuch an der Universität Göttingen im Jahre 1855. **Medizinhist J** 1980;15(4):378–84
**Heintel H** see **Heintel B**
**Heinzl B** see **Heilmittel aus Pflanzen und Tieren**
**Heird WC** see **Winters RW**
**Heirs of Hippocrates:** The development of medicine in a catalogue of historic books in the Health Sciences Library, The University of Iowa. Compiled by R. Eimas, E. Holtum, D. Curry. Iowa City, Friends of the University of Iowa Libraries, 1980. xiv, 474 p.
**Heischkel-Artelt E:** Kurort, Patient und Badearzt in ihrem Zusammenwirken, gezeigt an historischen Beispielen. **Z Angew Bader Klimaheilkd** 1978;25:318–25
**Heissig W:** Die Heilung der 'Weissen' Arznei in der mongolischen Heldendichtung. **Asiat Forsch** 1980;71:30–5
**Heithersay GS:** Endodontic treatment in Australia. **Int Endod J** 1984 Jul;17(3):125–38
**Heitz R:** Leonardo da Vinci did not invent contact lenses. **CLAO J** 1983 Oct–Dec;9(4):313–6
**Heitz RF:** The invention of contact lenses by August Müller (1887). **CLAO J** 1984 Jan–Mar;10(1):88–95
**Hejny J** see **Linkesch W**
**Hekma G:** Homoseksualiteit: van zonde tot geaardheid. **Spiegel Hist** 1980;15(9):484–91
**Helbling M:** Der altägyptische Augenkranke, sein Arzt und seine Götter. Zürich, Juris, 1980. 78 p. (Zürcher medizingeschichtliche Abhandlungen, Neue Reihe, Nr. 141) Also Diss., Zürich.
**Held AJ:** A propos de dentifrices et du Dr Albert Senn (1869–1934)--notice historique. **SSO Schweiz Monatsschr Zahnheilkd** 1981 Apr;91(4):218–20
**Held AJ:** Chronique des Ecoles universitaires suisses de médecine dentaire. **SSO Schweiz Monatsschr Zahnheilkd** 1982 Aug;92(8):711–9
**Held AJ:** L'enseignement de la médecine dentaire à Genève. A la recherche d'une voie. **Med Hyg (Geneve)** 1981 Oct 7;39(1440):3282–95
**Held AJ:** Un demi-siècle de parodontologie. **Rev Belge Med Dent** 1983 Mar;38(2):30–3
**Held AJ:** Une gestation longue et un enfantement laborieux: la médecine dentaire d'aujourd'hui en Swisse. **SSO Schweiz Monatsschr Zahnheilkd** 1981 Oct;91(10):769–857
**Held AJ:** 100e anniversaire de la fondation de l'Ecole de Médecine dentaire de l'Université de Genève (1881–1981). Sommaire bilan d'un premier siècle. **SSO Schweiz Monatsschr Zahnheilkd** 1981 Oct;91(10):764–8
**Held F** see **Dörffel EW**
**Helden A van** see **Bonelli ML**
**Helfand W** see **Crellin JK**
**Helfand W** see **Jenner CL, ed**
**Helfand WH, Cowen DL:** American pharmaceutical posters. In W.H. Hein, G. Schramm, ed: Die Vorträge des Internationalen Pharmaziehistorischen Kongresses Basel 1979. Stuttgart, Wissenschaftliche Verlagsgesellschaft, 1981. (Veröffentlichungen der Internationalen Gesellschaft für Geschichte der Pharmazie e.V., Neue Folge, Bd. 50).
**Helfand WH, Cowen DL:** Evolution of a revolutionary oral dosage form. **Pharm Int** 1982 Dec;3(12):393–5
**Helfand WH, Crellin JK:** The pharmacy in comic postcards. **Pharm Hist** 1981;23(3):107–13
**Helfand WH, Woodruff HB, Coleman KM, et al:** Wartime industrial development of penicillin in the United States. In Parascandola J, ed: The history of antibiotics. Madison, American Institute of the History of Pharmacy, 1980. p. 31–56.
**Helfand WH** see **Cowen DL**
**Helfand WH** see **Crellin JK**
**Helfant RH** see **Weintraub WS**
**Helgadóttir GP:** Kvinner og legekunst i fornsagaene. **Nord Medicinhist Arsb** 1984;:35–47
**Helies JC:** Aperçu historique sur les hôpitaux de Carcassonne, des origines à la fin du XIXe siècle. Thèse méd., Toulouse, 1977. 94 p.
**Helin E:** A la recherche d'une mesure de la léthalité des épidémies: les désignations de tuteurs pour les orphelins servent-elles d'indicateur? **Ann Demogr Hist (Paris)** 1980;:67–78
**Hélin E, Lebrun M, Grégoire-Reiters M:** Bibliographie internationale de démographie historique, 1981. **Ann Demogr Hist (Paris)** 1981;:v–cxii
**Hélin E, Lebrun M, Grégoire-Reiters M:** International bibliography of historical demography, 1980. **Ann Demogr Hist (Paris)** 1980;:I–CXI
**Hell W:** Research on monocular depth perception between 1884 and 1914: influence of the German Unfallversicherungsgesetz and of the jurisdiction of the Reichsversicherungsamt. **Perception** 1982;10(6):683–94
**Hellbrügge T:** Anwalt des praktizierenden Arztes: 100 Jahre 'Fortschritte der Medizin'. **Fortschr Med** 1982 Apr 15;100(14):613–4
**Hellbrügge T:** Zum 100jährigen Jubiläum der Deutschen Gesellschaft für Kinderheilkunde. **Fortschr Med** 1983 Sep 8;101(34):1513–6
**Heller G:** Idéologie et rituels de la propreté aux XIXe et XXe siècles. In Imhof AE, ed: Leib und Leben in der Geschichte der Neuzeit. Berlin, Duncker & Humblot, 1983. p. 193–202.
**Heller R:** Johann Christian Reil's training scheme for medical auxiliaries. **Med Hist** 1975 Oct;19(4):321–32
**Heller S:** Boerhaaves Schweizer Studenten: ein Beitrag zur Geschichte des Medizinstudiums. Zürich, Juris, 1984. 111 p. (Zürcher Medizingeschichtliche Abhandlungen, Neue Reihe, Nr. 169)
**Heller SA:** A Public Health Service wife. Rockville, Printex, 1978. [144] leaves.
**Heller WM:** Dispensing in 1982. **Drug Intell Clin Pharm** 1983 Jul–Aug;17(7–8):570–3
**Hellinger J, Hornuf H:** Zum Einfluss Dresdner Arzte und Wissenschaftler auf die Entwicklung der Orthopädie. **Beitr Orthop Traumatol** 1981 Dec;28(12):637–44
**Helliwell PJ:** Henry Walter Featherstone, first President of the Association of Anesthetists of Great Britain and Ireland (1932–34). **Anaesthesia** 1982 Apr;37(4):394–7
**Helliwell PJ:** The Association of Anaesthetists of Great Britain and Ireland. **Anaesthesia** 1982 Sep;37(9):913–23
**Hellman C** see **Maud PJ**
**Hellman I:** Work in the Hampstead war nurseries. **Int J Psychoanal** 1983;64 (Pt 4):435–9
**Hellman LM:** A history and reminiscence of the office of the Deputy Assistant Secretary for Population Affairs, Department of Health, Education and Welfare, 1969–1977. **Bull Hist Med** 1982 Spring;56(1):77–87
**Hellmich J** see **Hellmich S**
**Hellmich S, Hellmich J:** Der Zwischenkieferknochen und Goethes Mephistopheles. **Laryngol Rhinol Otol (Stuttg)** 1982 Oct;61(10):552–6
**Hellmuth H:** Heinrich Wilhelm Ferdinand Wackenroder 8. März 1798--14. September 1854. **Pharmazie** 1980;34(5–6):321–3
**Hellström S, Stenfors LE:** The original description of Shrapnell's membrane reviewed in the light of recent experimental studies. **J Laryngol Otol** 1983 Nov;97(11):985–9
**Helm D:** Die Cholera in Lübeck. Epidemieprophylaxe und -bekämpfung im 19. Jahrhundert. Neumünster, Wachholtz, 1979. 81 p. (Kieler Beiträge zur Geschichte der Medizin und Pharmazie, 16).
**Helm S, Prydsö U:** Assessment of age-at-death from mandibular molar attrition in medieval Danes. **Scand J Dent Res** 1979 Apr;87(2):79–90
**Helm S, Prydsö U:** Prevalence of malocclusion in medieval and modern Danes contrasted. **Scand J Dent Res** 1979 Apr;87(2):91–7
**Helmbold P** see **Böhmer W**
**Helmchen H** see **Fähndrich E**
**Helmer F:** Das chirurgische Erbe. Der Einfluss Theodor Billroths auf die heutige Abdominalchirurgie. **Zentralbl Chir** 1982;107(22):1469–80
**Helmrich HE:** Spagyrik. Alter Wein in neuen Schläuchen. Heidelberg, Haug, 1977. 253 p.
**Helöe LA, Haugejorden O:** 'The rise and fall' of dental caries: some global aspects of dental caries epidemiology. **Community Dent Oral Epidemiol** 1981 Dec;9(6):294–9
**Helpern M:** History of the methods of detecting murder. **Am J Forensic Med Pathol** 1981 Mar;2(1):61–5
**Heltmann H** see **Heilmittel aus Pflanzen und Tieren**
**Helvétius CA:** Anfänge der Erziehung. Claude Adrien Helvétius (1772). **Krankenpfl J** 1984 Mar 1;22(3):30–1
**Hémardinquer JJ** see **Forster R**
**Hemenway WG** see **Canalis RF**
**Hemmingsen R** see **Kramp P**
**Hemminki E:** Quality of clinical trials--a concern of three decades. **Methods Inf Med** 1982 Apr;21(2):81–5
**Henaff R** see **Curet M**
**Henderson AH** see **Christen AG**
**Henderson AR:** A centennial remembrance of Koch's discovery of the tubercle bacillus. **Md State Med J** 1982 May;31(5):47–51
**Henderson DA:** The deliberate extinction of a species. **Proc Am Philos Soc** 1982 Dec 17;126(6):461–71
**Henderson DA:** The history of smallpox eradication. In Lilienfeld AM, ed: Times, places, and persons. Baltimore, London, Johns Hopkins Univ.

Press, 1980. (Sigerist suppl. to the Bull Hist Med. n.s., no 4) p. 99–108.
**Henderson J:** Muldoon and Rowling: a preliminary analysis of contrasting personalities. **Pol Sci** 1980;32(1):26–46
**Henderson JH** see **Brown RW**
**Henderson JV:** The importance of operational definitions in design of a combat casualty information system. **J Med Syst** 1983 Oct;7(5):413–26
**Henderson M:** Royal Hospital for Sick Children. A 100-year-old gets a new lease on life. **Health Soc Serv J** 1983 Aug 11;93(4859):966–7
**Henderson P:** Psychohistorical perspectives on the presidency. **Mich J Polit Sci** 1981;1(1):1–11
**Henderson V:** Nursing--yesterday and tomorrow. **Nurs Times** 1980 May 22;76(21):905–7
**Henderson VW:** Jules Dejerine and the third alexia. **Arch Neurol** 1984 Apr;41(4):430–2
**Henderson WM:** A history of the ARC's support of veterinary research. **Vet Rec** 1981 Jul 11;109(2):29–34
**Henderson WM:** Wellcome research: virology and the promotion of animal health. **Vet Rec** 1980 Oct 11;107(15):347–50
**Henderson RW, ed:** Early American sport: a checklist of books by American and foreign authors published prior to 1860, including sporting songs. Third edition revised and enlarged. Rutherford, New Jersey, Fairleigh Dickinson University Press, 1977. 309 p.
**Hendrick W, Hendrick G, ed:** On the Illinois frontier. Dr. Hiram Rutherford 1840–1848. Carbondale and Edwardsville, Southern Illinois University Press, 1981. xxv, 155 p.
**Hendrick G, ed** see **Hendrick W**
**Hendrie HC:** Press coverage of Central State Hospital: alarms and excursions. **Indiana Med Hist Q** 1983 Mar;9(1):5–12
**Hendriks IH, Vries PA de:** Anticonceptie en abortus provocatus in de Grieks-Romeinse oudheid. **Groniek** 1978 Dec;60:1–11, 18
**Henisch BA:** Fast and feast: food in medieval society. University Park, Pennsylvania State University Press, 1976. 279 p.
**Henke W:** Das Calvarium von Binshof (Speyer) im Vergleich mit anderen Jungpaläolithikern. **Z Morphol Anthropol** 1980;70(3):275–94
**Henkel N:** Studien zum Physiologus im Mittelalter. Tübingen, Max Niemeyer, 1976. xi, 227 p. (Hermaea Germanistische Forschungen, N. F. xi, Bd. 38).
**Henkelmann T:** Die Struktur des Lebendigen. Die Fragmente zur Physiologie von Novalis. In Seidler E, Schott H, ed: Bausteine zur Medizingeschichte. Stuttgart, Steiner, 1984. p. 45–52.
**Henkelmann T:** Zur Geschichte des pathophysiologischen Denkens. John Brown (1735–1788) und sein System der Medizin. Berlin, New York, Springer, 1981. 104 p.
**Henkelmann T** see **Engelhardt D von**
**Henkelmann T** see **Engelhardt DV**
**Henker FO, Shorey JJ:** Dr. P. O. Hooper--father of Arkansas medicine. **J Arkansas Med Soc** 1981 Oct;78(5):189–92
**Henkind P:** An historical look at the retina, 1880–1980. **Trans Ophthalmol Soc UK** 1980 Apr;100(pt 1):20–4
**Henkind P** see **Newell FW**
**Henle M:** Robert M. Ogden and Gestalt psychology in America. **J Hist Behav Sci** 1984 Jan;20(1):9–19
**Henle M:** The influence of Gestalt psychology in America. In R. W. Rieber, K. Salzinger, ed: Psychology: theoretical-historical perspectives. New York, Academic Press, 1980. p. 177–90.
**Henle M:** Why study the history of psychology? In K. Salzinger, ed: Psychology in progress: an interim report. (Annals of the New York Academy of Sciences, vol. 270). New York, New York Academy of Sciences, 1976. p. 14–20.
**Henley KS:** History of fiberoptic endoscopy. **Gastroenterology** 1980 May;78(5 Pt 1):1123–4
**Henn V:** E. Mach on the analysis of motion sensation. **Hum Neurobiol** 1984;3(3):145–8
**Henne H** see **Habrich C**
**Henneberg G:** Das Robert Koch-Haus in Wollstein. **Med Welt** 1982 Mar 26;33(12):427
**Henneberg M** see **Piontek J**
**Hennebert GL:** Philibert Biourge, microbiologiste et mycologue (1864–1942). Colloque d'histoire des sciences III. Louvain, 1979. p. 61–98.
**Hennebert P** see **Barbaix M**
**Hennis I** see **Geppert W**
**Henrard G:** Histoire et medecine. **Cah Clio** 1981;67:22–31
**Henri Gastaut and the Marseilles school's contribution to the neurosciences:** Proceedings of the 25th and final Colloque de Marseille. **Electroencephalogr Clin Neurophysiol** 1982;35:1–447
**Henripin J** see **Kyriazis N**
**Henry L, Hurault J:** Mortalité de la population européenne de Guyane Française au début du XVIIIe siècle. **Population** 1979;34(6):1087–1100
**Henry LJ:** Florence Aby Blanchfield. In: Notable American women. The modern period. Cambridge, Mass., Belknap-Harvard Univ. Press, 1980. 4:83–5.
**Henry RL:** A recognition of the work of Walter H. Seegers in hemostasis and thrombosis. **Semin Thromb Hemostas** 1980;6(4):325–7
**Henry RL:** Paleoserology. In A. Cockburn, E. Cockburn, ed: Mummies, disease, and ancient cultures. Cambridge, Cambridge University Press, 1980. p. 327–34.
**Henry WD:** Stonewall Jackson--the soldier eccentric. **Practitioner** 1979 Oct;223(1336):580–7
**Henry WD:** The case of Captain Colthurst. **Practitioner** 1981;225:418–20
**Henschel WF, Kljucar S:** Intravenous anesthesia. Its development towards its position in today's anesthesia. **Acta Anaesthesiol Belg** 1980;31(3):195–205
**Hensel H** see **Mann G, ed**
**Henson PM:** Harold Fred Dorn. In Dictionary of American biography, 1961–1965. Suppl. 7, 1981. p. 191–3.
**Hepding L:** Das Rossarzneibuch des Scharfrichters Johannes Deigendesch von 1716. **DTW** 1983 Apr 6;90(4):147–50
**Hepp J:** Un grand chirurgien du début de ce siècle. **Sem Hop Paris** 1981 Jun 8–15;57(21–24):1049–54
**Hepplethwaite A:** Nursing in the thirties. **Nurs Times** 1984 Jul 11–17;80(28):40–2
**Heppner F:** Die heilende Hitze. **Fortschr Med** 1983 Apr 14;101(14):621–3
**Herbert V:** Landmark perspective: An 'extrinsic factor' and pernicious anemia. **JAMA** 1984 Jan 27;251(4):522–3
**Herbert S, ed:** The red notebook of Charles Darwin. Ithaca and London, Cornell University Press and British Museum (Natural History), 1980. 164 p.
**Herbison GJ:** Research: ends, setting, environment, activities, resources, creativity, health. **Arch Phys Med Rehabil** 1984 Mar;65(3):112–4
**Hercher GP:** The work cure at Devereux Mansion. **Essex Inst Hist Collect** 1980;116(2):101–10
**Heritage J:** The background to a royal commission. **Med Leg J** 1981;49(pt 2):58–71
**Héritier J:** La peste des chiffonniers. **Histoire** 1982;51:97–9
**Heritier J:** Le martyre des nez coupés: les débuts de la chirurgie esthétique. **Histoire** 1983;(57):68–71
**Herkov Z:** Srpska apotekarska funta. **Glas Srp Akad Nauka Umet** 1982;328(22):87–95
**Herlan RW:** Age at baptism in the London Parish of St. Olave, Old Jewry, 1645–1667. **Local Popul Stud (Matlock)** 1980 Spring;24:42–8
**Herlan RW:** Aspects of population history in the London parish of St. Olave, Old Jewry, 1645-1667. **Guildhall Stud Lond Hist** 1980;4(3):133–40
**Herlan RW:** Relief of the poor in Bristol from late Elizabethan times until the Restoration era. **Proc Am Philos Soc** 1982 Jun 8;126(3):212–28
**Herlant M:** Travaux consacrés aux glandes endocrines parus dans les Archives de Biologie entre 1880 et 1931. **Arch Biol (Liege)** 1980;91(2):243–65
**Herlant-Meewis H** see **Poll M**
**Hermalin AI** see **Knodel J**
**Herman BL:** Folk medical recipes in nineteenth-century American farm journals. **Pa Folklife** 1976;25(4):16–25
**Herman JK:** Home of BUMED, a hilltop in Foggy Bottom. **US Navy Med** 1982 Feb;73(2):9–15 contd.
**Herman JK:** Home of BUMED: a hilltop in Foggy Bottom. Controversy and transition, 1917–1942. **US Navy Med** 1983 Mar–Apr;74(2):8–17 concl
**Herman JK:** Home of BUMED: a hilltop in Foggy Bottom. The golden age (part 1). **US Navy Med** 1982 Jun;73(6):11–21
**Herman JK:** Home of BUMED: a hilltop in Foggy Bottom. Where medical college left off. The U.S. Naval Medical School and Naval Hospital 1902–1917. **US Navy Med** 1983 Jan–Feb;74(1):8–17 contd
**Herman JR:** Autourotherapy; the water of life. **NY State J Med** 1980 Jun;80(7 Pt 1):1149–54
**Herman JR:** Hot water bag for diseased prostate. **Urology** 1979 Dec;14(6):545–V
**Herman JR:** Old medical instruments. **Urology** 1984 Mar;23(3):301–B, 308–I
**Herman JR:** Operating furniture. 'Medical briefs'. **Urology** 1981 Sep;18(3):295 H
**Herman JR:** Rejuvenation: Brown-Sequard to Brinkley: monkey glands to goat glands. **NY State J Med** 1982 Nov;82(12):1731–9
**Herman JR:** The compleat English physician: or, the druggist's shop opened. **Urology** 1983 Mar;21(3):277H, 300D
**Herman JR:** Urethral forceps. **Urology** 1983 Jan;21(1):60C
**Hermanek P:** 90 Jahre Schnellschnitthistologie. **Pathologe** 1981 Dec;3(1):53–4
**Hermann A, Wankmüller A:** Physik, Physiologische Chemie und Pharmazie an der Universität Tübingen. Tübingen, J.C.B. Mohr, 1980. 181 p. (Contubernium, Bd. 21).
**Hermann EK:** Belizean nursing education in the 19th century. **Belizean Stud** 1979;7(4):16–24
**Hermann RE** see **Cruft GE**
**Hermanns LM:** John F. Rittmeister und C. G. Jung. **Psyche (Stuttg)** 1982 Nov;36(11):1022–31
**Hermelin R:** A law to last the century? **Spec Educ Forward Trends** 1981 Dec;8(4):6–7
**Hermelink H:** Zur Bestimmung von Birunis Todestag. **Sudhoffs Arch** 1977;61(3):298–300
**Hermosilla Molina A:** Epidemia de fiebre amarilla en Sevilla en el año 1800. Sevilla, Talleres Gráficos 'OIGA', 1978.
**Hernándex EI:** Sindrome de enclaustramiento. **Medicina (B Aires)** 1983;43(1):117–8
**Hernández BF** see **Flores y Troncoso FA**
**Hernández HH:** Historia de la Cirugia en Buenos Aires y Rosario. In Congreso de Historia de la Medicina Argentina [Transactions]. 5th. Mendoza, 1983. p. 33–68.
**Hernández PH:** Breve historia de la odontologia en Puerto Rico. **Rev Odontol PR** 1979 Nov–1980 May;17(1):2–15
**Hernández PH:** Cronología odontológica. **Rev Odontol PR** 1981 Feb–Apr;18(1):13–20 contd
**Hernandez S** see **Woodruff HB**
**Hernández de Alba G:** Una obra postuma cientifica monumental: la bibliografia medica Colombiana (1782–1976). **Bol Cult Bibliogr (Bogota)** 1976;16(7–8):176–9

**Hernández-Llamas H** see **Frenk J**
**Hernández-Morales F:** La contribución del Dr. Ramón M. Suárez a la investigación del esprú. **Bol Asoc Med PR** 1983 Nov;75(11):496-7
**Hernández Sánchez FA** see **Muñoz AL**
**Hernández Sánchez FA** see **Muñoz Al**
**Hernando y Ortega T:** Dos estudios históricos (vieja y nueva medicina). Madrid, Espasa-Calpe, 1982. 243 p.
**Heron JR:** Louis Pasteur: the nature of his illness. In Passmore R, ed: Proceedings of the Royal College of Physicians of Edinburgh Tercentenary Congress, 1981. Edinburgh, Royal College of Physicians of Edinburgh, 1982. p. 116-27.
**Herren R:** Freud und die Kriminologie: Einführung in die psychoanalytische Kriminologie. Stuttgart, Enke, 1973. x, 281 p.
**Herrer A** see **Christensen HA**
**Herrera M** see **Pacheco CR**
**Herrera MT** see **Vázquez de Benito C**
**Herrera Casado A:** Aportación francesa a la amigdalectomiá. **An Otorrinolaringol Ibero Am** 1981;8(6):487-94
**Herrera Casado A:** Vída y obra del doctor D. Juan Creus y Manso (1828-1897). **An Otorrinolaringol Ibero Am** 1980;7(2):109-32
**Herrerias Gutiérrez JM:** Promesas y realidades de la cimetidina. **Rev Esp Enferm Apar Dig** 1979 Oct;56(4):373-80
**Herrero P, Frances MC:** Influencia de la dosimetria en la farmacia española. **Bol Soc Esp Hist Farm** 1982 Mar;33(130):93-112
**Herrick JM:** Health care: the dilemma of delivery. **Aztlan** 1979;10:123-7
**Herring H:** The self and madness in Marlowe's 'Edward II' and Webster's 'The Duchess of Malfi'. **J Mediev Renaiss Stud** 1979;9:307-23
**Herring R:** Southern Baptist convention resolutions on the family. **Baptist Hist Heritage** 1982;17(1):36-45, 64
**Herrington JL, Sawyers JL:** Surgical management of alkaline reflux gastritis and esophagitis. **Surg Annu** 1981;13:341-59
**Herriott RM:** Life and contributions of Elmer V. McCollum. **Fed Proc** 1980 Aug;39(10):2713-5
**Herrmann B:** Zur Entstehung und Wirkung ästhetischer Prinzipien in der menschlichen Rassenkunde. In Imhof AE, ed: Leib und Leben in der Geschichte der Neuzeit. Berlin, Duncker & Humblot, 1983. p. 165-75.
**Herrmann EK:** Health care services in 19th century British Honduras. **Soc Sci Med [Med Psychol Med Sociol]** 1980 Jun;14(4):353-6
**Herrmann EK:** Strategies for teaching the history of nursing. **NLN Publ** 1983;(41-1935):57-65
**Herrnstein RJ:** Karl Spencer Lashley. In Dictionary of American Biography, Suppl. 6, 1956-1960. p. 367-8, 1980.
**Herschfeld JJ:** Bartholomeus Eustachius--the first great dental anatomist. **Bull Hist Dent** 1982 Oct;30(2):123-8
**Herschfeld JJ:** E. J. Greenfield and artificial implants. **Bull Hist Dent** 1984;32(1):33-41
**Herschfeld JJ:** G. V. Black and the search for a better amalgam. **Bull Hist Dent** 1980 Oct;28(2):76-82
**Herschfeld JJ:** John Hunter and his Practical treatise on diseases of the teeth. **Bull Hist Dent** 1981;29(1):32-6
**Herschfeld JJ:** Joseph Fox - pioneer dental investigator and author of The Natural History of the Human Teeth. **Bull Hist Dent** 1983 Oct;31(2):101-7
**Herschfeld JJ:** Nicholas Dubois de Chemant and the invention of mineral teeth. **Bull Hist Dent** 1982 Apr;30(1):40-3
**Herschfeld JJ:** Norman W. Kingsley and his pioneering techniques in the correction of cleft palate. **Bull Hist Dent** 1983 Apr;31(1):23-8
**Herschfeld JJ:** Sir John Tomes, dental pioneer. **Bull Hist Dent** 1981 Oct;29(2):94-8
**Herschfeld JJ:** W.G.A. Bonwill and the 'anatomical articulator.' **Bull Hist Dent** 1980 Apr;28(1):29-34
**Herschler R** see **Jacob SW**
**Hershey SG:** The Rovenstine inheritance--a chain of leadership. **Anesthesiology** 1983 Nov;59(5):453-8
**Hershkovitz P:** Comparative anatomy of platyrrhine mandibular cheek teeth dpm4, pm4, ml with particular reference to those of Homunculus (Cebidae), and comments on platyrrhine origins. **Folia Primatol (Basel)** 1981;35(2-3)179-217
**Hershkowitz L:** Powdered tin and rose petals: Myer Myers, Goldsmith, and Peter Middleton, physician. **Am Jew Hist** 1981;70(4):462-7
**Hershman D** see **Lieb J**
**Hershman MJ:** William Morrant Baker (1839-1896). **Int J Dermatol** 1980 Sep;19(7):409-12
**Herskovitz A** see **Terry JS**
**Hertig AT:** Early concepts of dysplasia and carcinoma in situ (a backward glance at a forward process). A brief historical review. **Obstet Gynecol Surv** 1979 Nov;34(11):795-803
**Hertz DG:** Pioneers and psychoanalysis: beginnings of the psychoanalytic movement in Eretz Israel. **Isr J Psychiatry Relat Sci** 1983;20(1-2):5-12
**Hertzberg R:** Bielschowsky's sign. Its genesis and other observations by Bielschowsky. **Aust J Ophthalmol** 1982 Nov;10(4):282-4
**Hertzberg R:** Ronald Francis Lowe. **Aust J Ophthalmol** 1980 May;8(2):109-15
**Hertzberg R:** Three great ophthalmologists (E. C. Temple-Smith, Norman Gregg, Arthur D'Ombrain). **Med J Aust** 1979 Dec 15;2(12):649-50
**Hertzka G:** Das Wunder der Hildegard-Medizin. Stein am Rhein, Christiana-Verlag, 1984. 236 p.
**Hervé Lelievre L:** La medicina hospitalaria have 50 años. Recuerdos del Hospital San Francisco de Borja. **Rev Med Chil** 1982 Jul;110(7):701-6
**Herzka HS, Otti L:** Geschichte der Kindheit--zum Belspiel: Industrialisierung. **Acta Paedopsychiatr (Basel)** 1984 May;50(1):5-6
**Herzlich C:** Malades d'hier, malades d'aujourd'hui: de la mort collective au devoir de guérison. Paris, Payot, 1984. 295 p.
**Herzlich C:** The evolution of relations between French physicians and the state from 1880 to 1980. **Sociol Health Illn** 1982 Nov;4(3):241-53
**Herzog H:** Wirklichkeit und Wahrheit--Weg und Ziel ärztlichen Wirkens. **Praxis** 1982 Aug 10;71(32):1254-61
**Hes HS:** Jewish physicians in the Netherlands 1600-1940. Assen, Van Gorcum, 1980. xxi, 206 p.
**Hes-Swartenberg HS:** Abraham Hartog Israels, M.D., 1822-1883: Netherlands' first professor in the history of medicine. **NY State J Med** 1979 Aug;79(9):1445-7
**Hesekiel T, ed:** Ein deutscher Chirurg und seine Frau in Japan vor 100 Jahren. Briefe von Dr. Wilhelm Schultze und seiner Frau Emma geb. Wegscheider an die Eltern Dr. Wegscheider in Berlin aus Japan 1878-1881. Lübeck, (the author), 1980. 316 p.
**Hess AJ:** History of medicine in Harrison County, West Virginia. Clarksburg, Harrison County Medical Society, 1978. xxiii, 662 p.
**Hess BB:** The politics of aging. **Society** 1978;15(5):22-3
**Hess WJ** see **MacPhail I**
**Hesse A:** Aerztliche Vereine und Standesorganisationen in Freiburg i. Br. Entwicklung und Struktur. Freiburg, Schulz, 1978. 321 p. (Freiburger Forschungen zur Medizingeschichte, Neue Folge, 8).
**Hesse PG:** Das erste staatliche zahnärztliche Institut Deutschlands und sein Gründer Friedrich Louis Hesse. **Stomatol DDR** 1983 Dec;33(12):861-3
**Hesse PG:** F. R. Shaudinn i jego dzieło. **Przegl Dermatol** 1983 May-Jun;70(3):303-6
**Hesse PG:** Współpraca naukowa Schaudinn--Siedlecki w roku 1897. **Przegl Dermatol** 1983 May-Jun;70(3):307-10
**Hesselnberg M:** Les thérapies familiales et leur histoire. **Soins Psychiatr** 1982 Jan;(15):41-4
**Hessler RK, Beavert CS:** Citizen participation in neighborhood health centers for the poor: the politics of reform organizational change, 1965-77. **Hum Organ** 1982;41(3):245-55
**Heston LL, Heston R:** The medical casebook of Adolf Hitler: his illnesses, doctors, and drugs. New York, Stein and Day, 1980. 184 p.
**Heston R** see **Heston LL**
**Hetzer H:** Kinder- und jugendpsychologische Forschung im Wiener Psychologischen Institut von 1922 bis 1938. **Z Entwicklungspsychol Padagog Psychol** 1982;14(3):175-224
**Hetzer H:** 100 Jahre kinderpsychologische Forschung. **Fortschr Med** 1983 Feb 17;101(7):255-8
**Hetzer R** see **Borst HG**
**Hevér O:** Max-Fernand Jayle, a haptoglobin felfedezöje. **Orv Hetil** 1979 Aug 26;120(34):2071-2
**Hevesy GC de:** Marie Curie and her contemporaries. **J Nucl Med** 1984 Jan;25(1):116-31
**Hewetson J:** Before and after the 'appointed day'. **Br Med J [Clin Res]** 1983 Oct 29;287(6401):1271-2
**Hexham I:** Some aspects of religion and spiritual healing in Cultsville, a contemporary North American city. In Sheils WJ, ed: The Church and healing. Papers read at the twentieth summer meeting and the twenty-first winter meeting of the Ecclesiastical History Society. Oxford, Basil Blackwell for the Society, 1982. p. 415-29.
**Heyd D:** The place of laughter in Hobbes's theory of emotions. **J Hist Ideas** 1982 Apr-Jun;43(2):285-95
**Heyd M:** Robert Burton's sources on enthusiasm and melancholy: from a medical tradition to religious controversy. **Hist Eur Ideas** 1984;5:17-44
**Heyden D von** see **Gregl A**
**Heydt H:** 30th year reunion of four scientists marks less tooth decay around the world--the monofluorophosphate story. **J Dent Assoc S Afr** 1980 Dec;35(12):837-9
**Heymans G, Vial F, Berti Bock G, et al:** Le peuple et la médecine au XVIIe siècle. **Acta Med Hist Patav** 1979-80;26:95-113
**Heymans G** see **Berti Bock G**
**Heymans G** see **Rullière R**
**Heymans H:** Eine Hülse mit Arztinstrumenten aus Maaseik (Belgien). **Archaeol Korrespbl** 1979;9:97-100
**Heyningen EB van:** The mysteries of the scarlet phial: spies and plague in Cape Town in 1907. **Q Bull S Afr Libr** 1979;34(2):53-8
**Heywood C:** D. H. Lawrence's 'blood consciousness' and the work of Xavier Bichat and Marshall Hall. **Etud Anglaises** 1979;32:397-413
**Heywood JS:** Childhood and society a hundred years ago. London, [1969]. 72 p.
**Hibberd D:** 'Problems A': the solution to Wilfred Owen's 'The Imbecile.' **Notes Queries** 1980 Jun;27(3):232-3
**Hibbott Y:** The collection of early printed books in the Medical School Library. **St Thomas Hosp Gaz** 1981;79:64-72
**Hickel E, Schröder G, ed:** Neue Beiträge zur Arzneimittelgeschichte. Festschrift für Wolfgang Schneider zum 70. Geburtstag. Stuttgart, Wissenschaftliche Verlagsgesellschaft, 1982. 285 p. (Veröffentlichungen der Internationalen Gesellschaft für Geschichte der Pharmazie e. V., Neue Folge, Band 51).
**Hickel E:** Pharmaziegeschichte als Wissenschafts- oder Sozialgeschichte? In: Vorträge des Internationalen Pharmaziehistorischen Kongresses Innsbruck 1977. Stuttgart, Wissenschaftliche Verlagsgesellschaft, 1979. p. 23-8.
**Hickel E:** The emergence of clinical chemistry in the 19th century: presuppositions and consequences. **J Clin Chem Clin Biochem** 1982 Jul;20(7):521-30
**Hickel E:** 1848 und 1871 als Epochen in der Entwicklung des modernen

Arzneimittelbegriffs. In Hickel E, Schröder G, ed: Neue Beiträge zur Arzneimittelgeschichte. Festschrift für Wolfgang Schneider zum 70. Geburtstag. Stuttgart, Wissenschaftliche Verlagsgesellschaft, 1982. p. 281-5.
**Hickel E** see **Büttner J, ed**
**Hickey T, Oriol WE:** New directions and societal responses to aging: a symposium in honor of Ollie A. Randall. Introduction. **Gerontologist** 1983 Aug;23(4):397-8
**Hickman J:** Sir Frederick Smith--his life and work. **Equine Vet J** 1984 Sep;16(5):403-10
**Hickman R:** The J. S. Marais Surgical Laboratory - 21 years old. **S Afr Med J** 1980 Mar;57(16):677-81
**Hicks R:** Rum regulation and riches. Sydney, Australian Hospital Association, 1981. vii, 231 p.
**Hicks TP:** The history and development of microiontophoresis in experimental neurobiology. **Prog Neurobiol** 1984;22(3):185-240
**Hickson FS, Newton VE:** Sound localization. Part I: a brief history. **J Laryngol Otol** 1981 Jan;95(1):29-40
**Hickson H ed** see **Myles J**
**Hidalgo J** see **Valverde JL**
**Hidgson C:** The social and political implications of tuberculosis among native Canadians. **Can Rev Sociol Anthropol** 1982;19(4):502-12
**Hidiroglou M:** The form and structure of the horse in Greek sculpture. **Hist Med Vet** 1977;2(2):37-41
**Hidiroglou M:** The horse in the low reliefs of the Parthenon. **Hist Med Vet** 1977;2(4):102-5
**Hídvégi J:** A száz éves JAMA-ról. **Orv Hetil** 1984 Jul 8;125(28):1705-7
**Hidvégi J:** Az ifjú Markusovszky világa. **Orv Hetil** 1982 Dec 26;123(52):3207-13
**Hidvegi J:** Die Resonanz der Kochschen Entdeckung in der medizinischen Fachpresse Ungarns. **Wiss Beitr Martin Luther Univ Halle Wittenberg** 1983;5-R80:87-90
**Hidvégi J:** Marx Károly betegsége és halála. **Orv Hetil** 1983 Mar 6;124(10):589-91
**Hidvégi J** see **Vas G**
**Hidvégi L:** Toldy Ferenc ceglédi iskolaéveiröl. **Orv Hetil** 1984 Sep 2;125(36):2203-5
**Hiebert EN:** Report on current activities in the history of science in the United States. **NTM** 1982;19(1):12-5
**Hiebert EN** see **Kieft L**
**Hiebsch H:** Ein Jahrhundert wissenschaftliche Psychologie. In Eckardt G, ed: Zur Geschichte der Psychologie. Berlin, VEB Deutscher Verlag der Wissenschaften, 1979. p. 21-31.
**Hiebsch/h** see **Eckhardt G, ed**
**Hieke M** see **Szymanski B**
**Hiepe T, Odening K, Vater G:** Georg Wildführ sen. zum 80. Geburtstag. **Angew Parasitol** 1984 Aug;25(3):117-20
**Hiepe T, Odening K:** Zur Entwicklung der Parasitologie in der DDR. **Angew Parasitol** 1979 Nov;20(4):177-85
**Hieronimi S:** Nationalsozialistische Vernichtungsaktionen an geistig Kranken im Spiegel psychiatrie-historischer Publikationen des Nachkriegsdeutschlands. Eine Auseinandersetzung mit psychiatrischen Positionen zur Geschichte der deutschen Psychiatrie 1933-1945. Diss. Mainz, 1981. 75 p.
**Hiestand WC:** History in graduate teaching. **NLN Publ** 1983;(41-1935):45-8
**Hiestand WC:** Midwife to nurse-midwife: a history. The development of nurse-midwifery education in the continental United States to 1965. Ed. D. Diss., Columbia University. New York, 1976. 294 p.
**Hiestand WC:** Nursing, the family, and the 'new' social history. **ANS** 1982 Apr;4(3):1-12
**Higa HH** see **Tomich PQ**
**Higashinakagawa T** see **Noriyasu S**
**Higby G** see **Dann G**
**Higby GJ:** Gold in medicine: a review of its use in the West before 1900. **Gold Bull** 1982;15(4):130-40
**Higby GJ:** Practical Pharmacy by Mohr, Redwood, and Procter: an international pharmacy textbook. **Pharm Hist** 1984;26(2):97-102
**Higby GJ** see **Bogard MO**
**Higgins A:** John Janvier Black (1837-1909): an ornament to his profession. **Del Med J** 1982 Apr;54(4):233-7
**Higgins GA:** Chirurgeon generalis--an endangered species. **Am Surg** 1984 Jan;50(1):1-5
**Higgins GA:** Problems in clinical trials: lessons from the 'tuck uppers'. **Cancer** 1981;47:2167-71
**Higgins PG, Wayland JR:** Labour and delivery in North America. **Nurs Times** 1981 Sept 16; Midwifery Suppl:4, 6, 8, 10
**Higgins D, ed** see **Collins LD**
**Higgs EJ:** Research into the history of alcohol use and control in England and Wales: the available sources in the Public Record Office. **Br J Addict** 1984 Mar;79(1):41-7
**Higgs R:** Cycles and trends of mortality in 18 large American cities, 1871-1900. **Explor Econ Hist** 1979;16(4):381-408
**Higgs R:** Edward Franklin Meeker (1943-1980). **Explor Econ Hist** 1981;18(2):209-10
**Higgs R, Booth D:** Mortality differentials within large American cities in 1890. **Hum Ecol** 1979;7:353-70
**High RP:** Shadworth Hodgson and William James's formulation of space perception: phenomenology and perceptual realism. **J Hist Behav Sci** 1981 Oct;17(4):466-85
**High RP, Woodward WR:** William James and Gordon Allport: parallels in their maturing conceptions of self and personality. In R. W. Rieber, K. Salzinger, ed: Psychology: theoretical-historical perspectives. New York, Academic Press, 1980. p. 57-79.
**High RP** see **Pastore N**
**Highlights of the Georgia Nurses Association in action 1907-1982: Ga Nurse** 1982 Dec;42(6):4-15
**Hightower CE:** Plants that kill and cure. **Vet Hum Toxicol** 1979 Oct;21(5):360-2
**Hightower F:** Surgeons of early North Carolina. **Ann Surg** 1981 May;193(5):525-38
**Higier J:** J. A. Kergaradec (1787-1877) - zapomniany odkrywca i pionier słuchawki położniczej. **Ginekol Pol** 1982;53(11):817-20
**Higier J:** Sto lat sporu o autorstwo (priorytet) operacji pośrodkowego zeszycia pochwy (colpocleisis mediana) 1881-1981. **Ginekol Pol** 1982;53(3)
**Higounet-Nadal A:** Périgueux aux XIVe et XVe siècles: étude de démographie historique. Bordeaux, Fédération historique du Sud-Ouest, 1978. 458 p.
**Hijazi AR:** L'anesthésie chez Avicenne et les techniques anesthésiques au XIe siècle. **Ann Fr Anesth Reanim** 1984;3(1):76-8
**Hijiya J:** American gravestones and attitudes toward death: a brief history. **Proc Am Philos Soc** 1983 Oct;127(5):339-63
**Hilario E:** Comfort and surroundings in hospitals. **Hosp Eng** 1979 Mar;33(2):20-2, 24-5
**Hilaski HJ, Wang CL:** How valid are estimates of occupational illness? **Mon Labor Rev** 1982;105(8):27-35
**Hildebrand R:** Beitrag der Würzburger Anatomie zur Entwicklung des mikroskopisch-anatomischen Unterrichts (1847 Kölliker--Petersen 1940). **Anat Anz** 1984;155(1-5):115-22
**Hildebrand R:** F. V. Raspail, Begründer der Histochemie und Wegbereiter der Zelltheorie, im Spiegel zeitgenössischer Medaillen. **Anat Anz** 1983;154(4):353-8
**Hildebrand KH, ed** see **Bock HE, ed**
**Hildebrandt AG** see **Kotwas J**
**Hildegard von Bingen:** Ursachen und Behandlung der Krankheiten (causae et curae). Ubersetzt von H. Schulz. 4. Auflage. Heidelberg, Haug, 1983. 373 p.
**Hilderbrand RM:** Dental remedies of the past. **Alumni Bull Sch Dent Indiana Univ** 1982 Spring;:25-31, 87
**Hildesheimer F, Robin G, Schenk J, ed:** Intendance sanitaire de Marseille. (Répertoire numérique de la sous série 200 E - Archives de la Région Provence-Alpes-Cote d'Azur et du Département des Bouches-du-Rhone). Marseille, Archives Departementales, 1979. 71 p.
**Hildesheimer F:** La protection sanitaire des côtes françaises au XVIIIe siècle. **Rev Hist Mod Contemp** 1980 Jul-Sep;27:443-67
**Hildesheimer F:** Le Bureau de la Santé de Marseille sous l'Ancien Régime. Le renfermement de la contagion. Marseille, Fédération historique de Provence, 1980. 256 p.
**Hildesheimer F:** Prévention de la peste et attitudes mentales en France au XVIIIe siècle. **Rev Hist (Paris)** 1981;265(1):65-79
**Hildreth ML:** The foundations of the modern medical system in France: physicians, public health advocates, and the medical legislation of 1892 and 1893. **Proc Annu Meet West Soc Fr Hist** 1980;8:311-27
**Hildreth PB:** Early Red Cross: the Howard Association of New Orleans, 1837-1878. **La Hist** 1979;20(1):77-92
**Hilgard ER:** Edward Chace Tolman. In Dictionary of American Biography, Suppl. 6, 1956-1960. p. 639-41, 1980.
**Hilgard ER:** The trilogy of mind: cognition, affection, and conation. **J Hist Behav Sci** 1980 Apr;16(2):107-17
**Hilgard ER** see **Robert I. Watson and the development of the history of psychology: a symposium**
**Hilgard E, ed:** American psychology in historical perspective: addresses of the presidents of the American Psychological Association, 1892-1977. Washington, D.C., The Association, 1978. viii, 558 p.
**Hilger W** see **Brücke EW von**
**Hilkemeyer R:** A historical perspective in cancer nursing. **Oncol Nurs Forum** 1982 Spring;9(2):47-56
**Hill AJ:** Nightingale, sainte ou diablesse? **Infirm Can** 1980 Nov;(10):34-6
**Hill BF:** The founding and early history of the Institute of Laboratory Animal Resources. **Lab Anim Sci** 1980 Aug;30(4 pt 2):780-5
**Hill C:** On becoming the first woman urologist in Canada. **Can Med Assoc J** 1980 Feb 9;122(3):356
**Hill D:** The changing role of psychiatry in medicine and society. **Br J Med Psychol** 1983 Mar;56(Pt 1):27-38
**Hill D:** The politics of schizophrenia: psychiatric oppression in the United States. Lanham, MD, University Press of America, 1983. xii, 577 p.
**Hill EC:** The Rubin test. **JAMA** 1983 Nov 4;250(17):2366-8
**Hill EK:** The fierce remedy: a note on The Passion. **Am Notes Queries** 1982 May-Jun;20(9-10):134-5
**Hill GB:** Counting cancers. **Can Med Assoc J** 1983 Dec 15;129(12):1262-3
**Hill IR:** The historical background to aerospace pathology. **Aviat Space Environ Med** 1982 Jan;53(1):1-5
**Hill JD:** John H. Gibbon, Jr. Part I. The development of the first successful heart-lung machine. **Ann Thorac Surg** 1982 Sep;34(3):337-41
**Hill JR:** Cruelty reviewed. **Aust Vet J** 1984 Aug;61(8):245-7
**Hill R:** Leslie William Mapson. In Dictionary of national biography, 1961-1970. Suppl. 8, 1981. p. 721-2.
**Hill TD:** VIII Genitus homo as a nomen sacrum in a twelfth-century Anglo-Latin fever charm. **Notes Queries** 1983 Dec;30(6):487-8
**Hillard D** see **Linet J**
**Hillel AD:** History of stapedectomy. **Am J Otolaryngol** 1983 Mar-Apr;4(2):131-40

**Hillemand P:** Geschichte der Magen-Darm-Heilkunde. In Sournia JC, Martiny M, Poulet J, ed: Illustrierte Geschichte der Medizin. Salzburg, Andreas, 1980. Vol. 5. p. 1829–75.

**Hillemand P, Gilbrin E, Segal A:** Le père Elisée et la réforme des études médicales. **Hist Sci Med** 1981;15(2):159–65

**Hillemand P, Gilbrin E:** Le Père Elisée, premier chirurgien de Louis XVIII et la création de l'Académie de Médecine. **Bull Acad Natl Med (Paris)** 1981 Jan;165(1):23–6

**Hillemand P, Gilbrin E:** Le père Elisée (1753–1817); premier chirurgien de Louis XVIII. **Hist Sci Med** 1980;14(2):233–40

**Hillemand P** see **Histoire culturelle de la maladie**

**Hiller I:** Betrachtungen zu medizinischen Aspekten des Umweltschutzes im 17. Jahrhundert. **Z Gesamte Hyg** 1983 Sep;29(9):560–3

**Hiller I:** Betrachtungen zu medizinischen Aspekten des Umweltschutzes im 17. Jahrhundert. **Z Gesamte Hyg** 1983 Sep;29(9):560–3

**Hiller I:** Ludwig Formeys 'Versuch einer medicinischen Topographie von Berlin' und kommunale Umweltproblematik im 18. Jahrhundert. **Z Exp Chir** 1982 Jul;28(7):474–6

**Hiller JK:** John Joseph Dearin. In Dictionary of Canadian biography, 1881–1890. 1982;11:239–40.

**Hillerdal O:** Robert Koch och hans 100-årsjubileer. **Nord Medicinhist Arsbok** 1983;:127–34

**Hilliard D:** Unenglish and unmanly: Anglo-Catholicism and homosexuality. **Victorian Stud** 1982;25(2):181–210

**Hillier SM, Jewell JA:** Health care and traditional medicine in China, 1800–1982. London, Routledge & Kegan Paul, 1983, xix, 453 p.

**Hillis LD** see **Anderson RJ**

**Hillman J** see **Osborn JW**

**Hillmar I** see **Gürtler LG**

**Hilloowala R:** Illustrations from the Wellcome Institute Library: the origin of the Wellcome anatomical waxes Albinus and the Florentine collection at La Specola. **Med Hist** 1984 Oct;28(4):432–7

**Hillson RM:** The Lancet 1823. **Lancet** 1983 Dec 24–31;2(8365–66):1507–8

**Hillyer GV:** Schistosomiasis in the Dominican Republic: a review. **Bol Asoc Med PR** 1983 Mar;75(3):114–7

**Hils HP:** Die Pestrezepte der Basler Handschrift D II 30. **Sudhoffs Arch** 1983;67(2):210–7

**Hils HP:** Konrad der Münzmeister oder Konrad der Apotheker? Zur Analyse eines spätmittelalterlichen Pesttraktates. **Sudhoffs Arch** 1984;68(1):105–9

**Hiltner S:** Fifty years of CPE. **J Pastoral Care** 1975 Jun;29(2):90–8

**Hilts V** see **Chappert A**

**Hilts VL:** Epidemiology and the statistical movement. In Lilienfeld AM, ed: Times, places, and persons. Baltimore, London, Johns Hopkins Univ. Press, 1980. (Sigerist suppl. to the Bull Hist Med, n.s., no 4) p. 43–55.

**Hilts VL:** History of science at the University of Wisconsin. **Isis** 1984 Mar;75(276):63–94

**Hilts VL:** Obeying the laws of hereditary descent: phrenological views on inheritance and eugenics. **J Hist Behav Sci** 1982 Jan;18(1):62–77

**Hilts VL:** Statist and statistician. New York, Arno, 1981. (Reprint of Ph.D. Diss., Harvard University, 1967). 647 p.

**Hilzinger F** see **Riall CT**

**Himelhoch MS, Shaffer AH:** Elizabeth Packard: nineteenth-century crusader for the rights of mental patients. **J Am Stud** 1979;13(3):343–75

**Himes JH:** An early hand-wrist atlas and its implications for secular change in bone age. **Ann Hum Biol** 1984 Jan–Feb;11(1):71–5

**Himmelsbach CK** see **Martin WR**

**Himmelstein JL:** The strange career of marihuana: politics and ideology of drug control in America. Westport, Greenwood, 1983. xii, 179 p.

**Himpens G:** Het Sint-Janshospitaal te Brugge en zijn landbouwbedrijf rond 1350. **Biekorf** 1980;80:93–6

**Himsel WL** see **Hughes WL**

**Himsworth H:** Bradford Hill and statistics in medicine. **Stat Med** 1982 Oct–Dec;1(4):301–3

**Himsworth H:** On the integration of expert knowledge into the machinery of government. **Br Med J** 1980 Nov 1;281(6249):1197–9

**Himsworth H:** Sir Geoffrey Jefferson. In Dictionary of national biography, 1961–1970. Suppl. 8, 1981. p. 580–1.

**Himsworth H:** Thomas Lewis and the development of support for clinical research. **Pharos** 1982 Spring;45(2):15–9

**Himsworth H:** Thomas Renton Elliott. In Dictionary of national biography, 1961–1970. Suppl. 8, 1981. p. 329–30.

**Hindermeyer J:** Geschichte der physikalischen Therapie und der Rehabilitation. In Sournia JC, Martiny M, Poulet J, ed: Illustrierte Geschichte der Medizin. Salzburg, Andreas, 1980. Vol. 7. p. 2649–79.

**Hindley-Smith D:** The General Dental Council. Twenty-five years on. **Probe (Lond)** 1981 Jul;23(1):29–30, 32

**Hindley-Smith D:** The general dental council. Twenty-five years on. **Br Dent J** 1981 Jul 7;151(1):31–2

**Hindmarch I:** A social history of the use of cannabis sativa. **Contemp Rev** 1972;220(1276):252–7

**Hine DC:** From hospital to college: black nurse leaders and the rise of collegiate nursing schools. **J Negro Educ** 1982 Summer;51:222–37

**Hine DC:** The Ethel Jones Report: black women in the nursing profession, 1925. **J Negro Hist** 1982 Fall;67:212–28

**Hine MK:** The status of the teaching of dental history: 1980. **Bull Hist Dent** 1981 Oct;29(2):102–4

**Hine WC:** Dr. Benjamin A. Boseman, Jr.: Charleston's black physician-politician. In Rabinowitz HN, ed: Southern Black leaders of the reconstruction era. Urbana, University of Illinois Press, 1982. p. 335–62.

**Hingston WH:** La lithotritie et la lithotomie. **Union Med Can** 1981 Dec;110(12):1050

**Hinkes WF** see **Allen BW**

**Hinman AR:** Mass vaccination against polio. **JAMA** 1984 Jun 8;251(22):2994–6

**Hinman AR:** Prospects for disease eradication or elimination. **NY State J Med** 1984 Oct;84(10):502–6

**Hino S, Konoshita K, Kitamura T:** HTLV and the propagation of Christianity in Nagasaki. **Lancet** 1984 Sep 8;2(8402):572–3

**Hinokida T:** T. Schwann's three preliminary articles on 'Cell theory'. **Kagakushi Kenkyu** 1983;22(145):35–43

**Hinsey JC** see **Wangensteen OW, ed**

**Hinshaw HC:** The dawn of chemotherapy of tuberculosis. **Indian J Chest Dis Allied Sci** 1982 Apr–Sep;24(2–3):179–83

**Hinshaw WR:** The history of avian medicine in the United States. VII. Developments in avian pathology with emphasis on avian practice. **Avian Dis** 1982 Jul–Sep;26(3):462–72

**Hinson G** see **Jenner CL, ed**

**Hinton BT:** Thomas Crapper (1837–1910). **Invest Urol** 1980 May;17(6):534–5

**Hinton RJ:** Differences in interproximal and occlusal tooth wear among prehistoric Tennessee Indians: implications for masticatory function. **Am J Phys Anthropol** 1982 Jan;57(1):103–15

**Hinton RJ:** Relationships between mandibular joint size and craniofacial size in human groups. **Arch Oral Biol** 1983 Jan;28(1):37–43

**Hinton RJ, Smith MO, Smith FH:** Tooth size changes in prehistoric Tennessee Indians. **Hum Biol** 1980 May;52(2):229–45

**Hinze E:** Feldscherer und Feldmedici in deutschen wie fremden Heeren und Flotten. (Biographisches Lexikon deutscher Militärärzte bis 1870) Band I. Hannover, Im Selbstverlag, 1979. 43 p.

**Hipp E:** 100 Jahre Orthopädie. **Fortschr Med** 1983 Feb 3;101(5):147–50, 179

**Hippius H:** Ziele und Wege der psychiatrischen Forschung. **MMW** 1981 May 8;123(19):770–1

**Hippius H** see **Fähndrich E**

**Hippocrates:** La nature de l'homme. Edité, traduit, et commenté par Jacques Jouanna. Berlin, Akademie Verlag, 1975. 331 p. (Corpus medicorum Graecorum, I, 1, 3). Includes Greek text.

**Hippocrates:** Ueber die Krankheiten, III, herausgegeben, übersetzt und erläutert von Paul Potter. Berlin, Akademie Verlag, 1980. 150 p. (Corpus medicorum Graecorum, I, 2, 3). Includes Greek text.

**Hippokrates:** Ueber Nachempfängnis, Geburtshilfe, und Schwangerschaftsleiden. Herausgegeben, übersetzt und erläutert von C. Lienau. Berlin, Akademie Verlag, 1973. 143 p. (Corpus Medicorum Graecorum, I, 2, 2).

**Hipskind M** see **Borkenhagen R**

**Hipskind MM:** A doctor's fifty year perspective. **Indiana Med Hist Q** 1983 Sep;9(3):4–15

**Hipwell J** see **Orner R**

**Hirsch B:** Geschichte der Nierentuberkulose. Köln, 1983. 183 p. (Kölner medizinhistorische Beiträge, Band 28)

**Hirsch EF:** Michael Servetus and the neoplatonic tradition: God, Christ and Man. **Bibl Hum Renaissance** 1980 Sep;42(3):561–75

**Hirsch HN:** Clio on the couch. **World Polit** 1980;32(3):406–24

**Hirsch JG:** The greatest success story in the history of medicine. **Med Times** 1980 Sep;108(9):36–43

**Hirsch PB:** Foreword: the Cosslett festschrift (Ellis Cosslett). **J Microsc** 1979 Sep;117(1):1–4

**Hirsch R, ed:** A catalogue of the manuscripts and archives of the Library of the College of Physicians of Philadelphia. Prepared by the Francis Clark Wood Institute for the History of Medicine. Philadelphia, University of Pennsylvania Press, 1983. xx, 259 p.

**Hirschberg J:** The history of ophthalmology. Translated from the German edition of 1899–1918 by F. C. Blodi. 11 vols. Bonn, Wayenborgh, 1982.

**Hirschberg JC:** History of child psychiatry. In H. I. Kaplan, et al, ed: Comprehensive textbook of psychiatry/III. Third edition. Baltimore, London, Williams and Wilkins, 1980. p. 2417–21.

**Hirschfeld J:** The discovery of the Gc system. **Vox Sang** 1984;46(2):122–4

**Hirschhorn B:** Richard Spencer Childs (1882–1978). His role in modernization of medicolegal investigation in America. **Am J Forensic Med Pathol** 1983 Sep;4(3):245–54

**Hirschhorn HH:** Botanical remedies of South and Central America, and the Caribbean: an archival analysis. Pt. 1. **J Ethnopharmacol** 1981;4:129–58

**Hirschhorn HH:** Ethnomedical acculturation of Florida Seminole Indians 1919–1952. **Ethnomedizin** 1981–82;7(1–4):127–47

**Hirschhorn K:** Overview and historical perspective of prenatal diagnosis. **Methods Cell Biol** 1982;26:1–9

**Hirschman A** see **Siegel RK**

**Hirschman AE** see **Siegel RK**

**Hirschman C, Butler M:** Trends and differentials in breast feeding: an update. **Demography** 1981 Feb;18(1):39–54

**Hirschman JC, Nagel EL:** Prehospital mobile emergency care in Miami, Florida. An historical commentary. **J Fla Med Assoc** 1981 Aug;68(8):624–34

**Hirst JD:** A failure 'without parallel': the School Medical Service and the London County Council 1907–12. **Med Hist** 1981 Jul;25(3):281–300

**Hirth W:** Corpusbildung in der deutschsprachigen medizinischen Fachliteratur des Mittelalters. **Suhoffs Arch** 1982;66(3):239–75

**Hirth W:** Popularisierungstendenzen in der mittelalterlichen Fachliteratur. **Medizinhist J** 1980;15(1/2):70–89

**Hirth W:** Uberlieferungen der pseudo-aristotelischen 'Secretum-secretorum'-Diätetik mit abweichenden Verfasserangaben. In International Congress of the History of Medicine, 27th, Barcelona, 1980. Actas. Barcelona, Acadèmia de Ciències Mèdiques de Catalunya i Balears, 1981. p. 259-63.
**Hirzel HO:** Der Weg zur modernen Kardiologie. **Praxis** 1983 Nov 29;72(48):1521-8
**Histoire culturelle de la maladie:** Toulouse, Privat, 1980. xvi. 454 p. Contributions by M. Sendrail, G. Baudot, G. Mazars, P. Huard, J. Bossy, P. Theil, P. Hillemand, E. Gilbrin, E. Aron, P. Freour.
**Histoire de la médecine aux armées:** Tome 1. De l'Antiquité à la Révolution. Paris, Charles Lavauzelle, 1982. 513 p.
**Historical review (Notre Dame Hospital).: Nurs Montreal** 1980 Jun;5(1):22-3
**Historical sketch: Loma Linda University School of Dentistry.: New Dent** 1979 Feb;9(3):28-9
**Histories of present dental schools in the United States: Dent Radiogr Photogr** 1981;54(4):Inside front cover, 79, 87-8 (continued regularly)
**Histories of present dental schools in the United States: Dent Radiogr Photogr** 1983;56(1):inside front cover, 19-20
**Histories of present dental schools in the United States:** Loma Linda University School of Dentistry. **Dent Radiogr Photogr** 1981;54(2),2,39-40
**Historik: Svenska Tandteknikerförbundet: Tandteknikern** 1981 Oct;50(10):500-23
**The history and future of psychiatric nursing: Can J Psychiatr Nurs** 1983 Oct-Nov;24(4):6-12
**History in the pharmaceutical press: Pharm Hist (London)** 1971 Mar;2(1):2-8
**History of accreditation of medical education programs: JAMA** 1983 Sep 23-30;250(12):1502-8
**History of FDA patient package insert requirements.: Am J Hosp Pharm** 1980 Dec;37(12):1660-1
**History of Pharmacy at the University of Granada: Pharm Hist** 1983;25(2):74-9
**[History of public health nursing activities among frontier farmers in Hokkaido] (Jpn): Hokenfu Zasshi** 1982 Jan;38(1):10-49
**The history of science:** A collection of manuscripts from the library of the Jewish Theological Seminary. An index to the microfilm collection, reels 1-17. Ann Arbor, University Microfilms, 1980. 79 p. (With Hebrew-English name index).
**A history of South Dakota Blue Shield: SD J Med** 1981 May;34(5):69
**History of South Dakota Society of Internal Medicine: SD J Med** 1981 May;34(5):63-4
**History of the American Geriatrics Society:** Malford W. Thewlis, J. Am. Geriatrics Soc. 1: 3, 1953. **J Am Geriatr Soc** 1981 Dec;29(12):544-9
**The history of the International Epidemiological Association brought up to date: Int J Epidemiol** 1984 Jun;13(2):139-41
**History of the Med-Chi Library: the first decade.: Md State Med J** 1980 Jun;29(6):38-45
**The history of the National Association of Operating Room Nurses: Va Nurse** 1982 Summer;50(2):43
**History of the provisions of the old-age, survivors, disability, and health insurance program: Soc Secur Bull** 1980;Suppl:19-40
**History of the provisions of the Supplemental Security Income program for the aged, blind, and disabled: Soc Secur Bull** 1980;Suppl:43-6
**History of the rising costs of the Medicare and Medicaid programs and attempts to control these costs:** Washington, U. S. General Accounting Office, 1976. iii, 126 p.
**History of the South Dakota State Department of Health (1891-1950): SD J Med** 1981 May;34(5):67-8
**History of writing and its relevance in dyslexia: J R Soc Med** 1982 Nov;75(11):917-8
**Hitchcock HP:** Contributions of orthodontists to organized dentistry. **J Am Dent Assoc** 1980 Jan;100(1):76-8
**Hitomi K:** [Historical progress and the present interpretation of schizophrenic theory held by Bleuler's school] (Jpn). **Seishin Shinkeigaku Zasshi** 1982;84(10):735-42
**Hitzig WH:** Conrad Gasser 1912-1982. **Schweiz Med Wochenschr** 1982 Oct 16;112(42):1486-7
**Hixson J:** The history of the human body. A 5000 year old mystery. New York, Cooper Square Publisher, 1966. 128 p.
**Hjort EF:** Rekruttering av Norges leger på 1800-tallet. **Tidsskr Nor Laegeforen** 1983 May 20;103(14):1149-54
**Hjort EF:** Vis medicatrix naturae og kirurgiens gjennombrudd i Norge. **Tidsskr Nor Laegeforen** 1981 Apr;101(11):641-5
**Hjorth N:** Geschichte der Kontaktdermatitis und ihr Einfluss auf die heutige Arbeitsdermatologie. **Hautarzt** 1980 Nov;31(11):621-6
**Hlaváčková L:** Budování klinických pracovišt české lékařské fakulty v době rozdělení pražské univerzity. II. Snahy o vybudování českých klinických pracovišt' před rozdělením univerzity. **Sb Lek** 1983 Apr;85(4):105-15
**Hlavácková L:** Budování klinických pracovišt Ceské Lékařské Fakulty v době rozdělení Pražské Univerzity. III. Budování českých klinických pracovišt' po rozdělení univerzity a lékařské fakulty. **Sb Lek** 1983 May;85(5):147 59
**Hlaváčková L:** Casopis lékařu českých a Spolek českých lékařu v boji za českou universitu a lékařskou fakultu. **Cas Lek Cesk** 1982 Dec 23;121(51):1569-73
**Hlaváčková L:** K stému výročí české výuky na I. interní klinice v. Praze. **Cas Lek Cesk** 1981 Nov 26;120(47):1478-82
**Hlaváčková L, Adamec J:** Sto let od zahájení výuky na české lékařské fakultě. **Cas Lek Cesk** 1983 Oct 14;122(41):1250-3
**Hlaváčková L:** Význam založení Casopisu lékařu českých v rámci rozvoje naší odborné publicistiky. **Cas Lek Cesk** 1981;120(52):1585-8
**Ho J:** Medical illustration in the Far East. **J Audiov Media Med** 1981 Apr;4(2):58-61
**Ho PY:** Chinese scientific terminology. **Pap Far East Hist** 1974;(9):1-14
**Hoagland M:** Discovery, the search for DNA's secrets. Boston, Houghton Mifflin, 1981. xiv, 198 p.
**Hoare CA:** Comparative aspects of human babesiosis. **Trans R Soc Trop Med Hyg** 1980;74(2):143-8
**Hobbs V:** But westward look: nursing in Western Australia, 1829-1979. [Perth], University of Western Australia Press, 1980. xvi, 256 p.
**Hobi F:** Zahnärztliche Röntgenologie von den Anfängen bis zum Jahre 1914: ihre Entwicklung in der Schweiz unter Berücksichtigung der im Ausland geschaffenen Voraussetzungen im Rahmen der Zahnheilkunde jener Zeit. Zürich, Juris, 1981. 126 p. (Zürcher medizingeschichtliche Abhandlungen, Neue Reihe, 145).
**Hoch SL:** Serf diet in nineteenth-century Russia. **Agric Hist** 1982;56(2):391-414
**Hochberg J** see **Hearst E, ed**
**Hochenegg H:** Tiroler Aerzte und Pharmazeuten als Künstler und Schriftsteller, Forscher und Volksvertreter. **Tirol Heimat** 1976;40:135-62
**Hochheiser S:** Synthetic food colors in the United States: a history under regulation. Diss. University of Wisconsin. [Madison, Wis.?: s.n.], 1982. v. 232 p.
**Hochheiser S:** The evolution of U. S. food color standards, 1913-1919. **Agric Hist** 1981;55(4):385-91
**Hochstadt S** see **Laslett P**
**Höcht B:** Operative Behandlung des Hodenhochstandes. Ein Rückblick auf die historische Entwicklung. **MMW** 1983 May 6;125(18):381-4
**Hockemeyer H:** Die Zeit seiner Schiffsarzttätigkeit in den Memoiren des napoleonischen Chirurgen Dominique-Jean Larrey. Diss., Universität Düsseldorf. Düsseldorf, 1982. 44 p.
**Hodge GP:** Medical illustration: our early years. Student days at Johns Hopkins, Evelyn Erickson Sullivan. **J Biocommun** 1982 Mar;9(1):18-22
**Hodge GP:** The drawings of Raynard N. LeNeil. **J Biocommun** 1983 Mar;10(1):24-9
**Hodge GP:** The preservation of scientific illustrations. **J Biocommun** 1980 Nov;7(3):28-31
**Hodge MJ:** Social forces, ideology, and the domain of mental health services. **Psychiatr Q** 1979 Winter;51(4):280-93
**Hodges HE, Lowe GD:** Race and change in rates of treatment and deaths due to alcoholism in a southern state: 1970-1974. **Phylon** 1977;38(2):152-9
**Hodges R:** Diet in the Dark Ages. **Nature** 1984 Aug 30-Sep 5;310(5980):726-7
**Hodgkin AL:** Some recollections of William Rushton and his contributions to neurophysiology. (1925-52). **Vision Res** 1982;22(6):623-5
**Hodgson CH** see **Wangensteen OW, ed**
**Hodgson ER:** Did early Spokane have a medical school? **Pac Northwest** 1983;27(2):93-6
**Hodgson GA:** The history of coal miners' skin diseases. In J. Cule, ed: Wales and medicine. London, British Society for the History of Medicine, 1975. p. 54-67.
**Hodgson MN:** The University of North Carolina Press may be a rare bargain. **NC Med J** 1983 May;44(5):315-6
**Hoeger K:** Medicinare som mördare. **Sydsven Medicinhist Sallsk Arsskr** 1981;:39-43
**Hoekelman RA:** Well-child visits revisited. **Am J Dis Child** 1983 Jan;137(1):17-20
**Hoem JM, Finnäs F:** Traek af fertilitetsfaldet i Danmark siden slutningen af tresserne. **Nationalocon Tidsskr** 1980;118(2):171-83
**Hoenig J:** Kurt Schneider and Anglophone psychiatry. **Compr Psychiatry** 1982 Sep-Oct;23(5):391-400
**Hoenig J:** The concept of Schizophrenia. Kraepelin-Bleuler-Schneider. **Br J Psychiatry** 1983 Jun;142:547-56
**Hoepke H:** Aus der Geschichte der Heidelberger Anatomie. **Ruperto Carola (Germany)** 1978;30(61):23-31
**Hoepke H, ed** see **Eulner HH**
**Hoerger H:** Mortalität, Krankheit und Lebenserwartung der Penzberger Bergarbeiterschaft im 19. und beginnenden 20. Jahrhundert. **Z Bayer Landesgesch** 1980;43(1):185-222
**Höfberg U:** 'Jungfru Mariae nycklar' och mödradödligheten genom två sekler. **Lakartidningen** 1982 Sep 1;79(35):2977-9
**Hofecker G, Seitelberger F:** The state and goals of basic research in gerontology in Austria. **ZFA (Dresden)** 1980;35(2):91-6
**Hofer K:** Dr. Lucy Hobbs Taylor, first woman dentist. **CAL** 1981 Oct;45(4):13-5, 18
**Höfer R** see **Thakur ML**
**Höfert R:** Krankenpflege im Spiegel der Zeiten. **Krankenpflege (Frankfurt)** 1983 Jan;37(1):6-8
**Hoff P:** Der Einfluss des Mesmerismus auf die Entwicklung der Suggestionstheorie in Deutschland. Diss. Mainz, 1980. 115 p.
**Hoff SG:** Frieda Fromm-Reichmann. In Dictionary of American Biography, Suppl. 6, 1956-1960. p. 219-20, 1980.
**Hoff SG** see **Powell RC**
**Hoffeld DR:** Mesmer's failure: sex, politics, personality, and the Zeitgeist. **J Hist Behav Sci** 1980 Oct;16(4):377-86
**Hoffenberg R:** Fiftieth anniversary. Medical Research Society. **Clin Sci** 1981 Sep;61(3):355-6
**Hoffer PC, Hull NE:** Murdering mothers: infanticide in England and New England 1558-1803. New York and London, New York University Press, 1981. xxii, 211 p. (New York University School of Law Series in Legal History, 2).

**Hoffer PC:** Psychohistory and empirical group affiliation: extraction of personality traits from historical manuscripts. **J Interdiscip Hist** 1978;9(1):131–45

**Hoffheimer MH:** Maupertuis and the eighteenth-century critique of preexistence. **J Hist Biol** 1982 Spring;15(1):119–44

**Hoffman E** see **Mann WE**

**Hoffman JH:** Dentistry is quack-less. **CAL** 1982 Apr;45(10):18–21

**Hoffman LE:** From instinct to identity: implications of changing psychoanalytic concepts of social life from Freud to Erikson. **J Hist Behav Sci** 1982 Apr;18(2):130–46

**Hoffman LE:** War, revolution, and psychoanalysis: Freudian thought begins to grapple with social reality. **J Hist Behav Sci** 1981;17:251–69

**Hoffman RJ:** Some cultural aspects of Greek male homosexuality. **J Homosex** 1980 Spring;5(3):217–26

**Hoffman W:** Der Zahnarzt in dieser Welt--gestern, heute und morgen. **Zahnarztliche Mitteilungen** 1980 Sep 1;70(17):1080–6

**Hoffman W, Shields J:** Doctors on the new frontier: breaking through the barriers of modern medicine. New York, Macmillan, 1981. xi, 207 p.

**Hoffmann H:** Urkundenregesten zur Geschichte des Juliusspitals in Würzburg 1576–1849 (Regesta Herbipolensia VI). Würzburg, Kommissionsverlag Ferdinand Schöningh, 1976. xxxi, 434 p. (Quellen und Forschungen zur Geschichte des Bistums und Hochstifts Würzburg, Band 29).

**Hoffmann H** see **Scheuch DW**

**Hoffmann P:** La théorie de l'âme dans la pensée médicale vers 1778. **Dix-Huit Siecle** 1979;11:201–12

**Hoffmann P:** Modèle mécaniste et modèle animiste. De quelques aspects de la représentation du vivant chez Descartes, Borelli et Stahl. **Rev Sci Hum** 1982–3;186–7:199–211

**Hoffmann WF:** Socrates revisited: his relevance today. **J Fam Pract** 1982 Jan;14(1):179–80

**Hoffmann-Axthelm:** 'Machtergreifung' vor 50 Jahren: Ein ausserst unerfreuliches Jubilaum. **Zahnarztl Mitt** 1983 Nov 16;73(22):2499–500, 2503

**Hoffmann-Axthelm W:** History of dentistry. Chicago, Quintessence, 1981. 435 p. (Translation of Die Geschichte der Zahnheilkunde.).

**Hoffmann-Axthelm W:** Karl August Lingner und die soziale Zahnmedizin. **Zahnarztl Mitt** 1983 Sep 16;73(18):1981–2, 1987–9

**Hoffmann-Axthelm W:** W. D. Miller - Ein Pionier der wissenschaftlichen Zahnheilkunde. **Quintessenz J** 1983 Oct;13(10):927–30

**Hoffmann-Axthelm W:** Wilhelm Dieck--Lehrer, Forscher und Standespolitiker. **Quintessenz** 1984 Feb;35(2):365–9

**Hoffmann-Axthelm W:** Zur Geschichte des Gaumenobturators. **Quintessenz Zahntech** 1980 Mar–Apr;6(3,4):85–93, 97–100

**Höflechner W** see **Brücke EW von**

**Höflechner W** see **Fellner R**

**Hofmann A:** How LSD originated. **J Psychedelic Drugs** 1979 Jan–Jun;11(1–2):53–60

**Hofmann B:** Kranker und Krankheit um 1500. Die Darstellung des Kranken im Zusammenhang mit den spätgotischen Bildnissen der Heiligen Elisabeth. Herzogenrath, Verlag Murken-Altrogge, 1983. 226 p. (Studien zur Medizin-, Kunst- und Literaturgeschichte, Bd. 3).

**Hofmann C:** Stimme und Konstitution im Werk Gregorio Marañóns. **Medizinhist J** 1984;19(3):259–66

**Hofmann S** see **Habrich C**

**Hofmann-Meier B:** Ein Geburtshelfer und Hebammenlehrer des 18. Jahrhunderts. Leben und Werk des Johann Philipp Hagen (1734–1792), Hebammenlehrer und Professor für Entbindungskunst in Berlin. Diss. Bern, 1982. 75 p.

**Hofmeister LH:** The Union Memorial Hospital. Its story...its people. 125 years of caring. Baltimore, Union Memorial Hospital, 1980. xi, 234 p.

**Höfner C:** Geschichte der Apotheke zu Rodach. **Jahrb Coburg Landesstift** 1978;23:1–34

**Hofschulte B:** Die Geschichte des Schlacht- und Viehhofes der Stadt Karlsruhe bis zum Jahre 1927. Diss., Tierärzliche Hochschule Hannover. Hannover, 1983. 226 p.

**Hofstadter L** see **Pfund N**

**Hofsten E, Lundström H:** Swedish population history. Main trends from 1750 to 1970. Stockholm, National Central Bureau of Statistics, 1976. 186 p. (Urval skriftserie utgiven av statistiska centralbyrån. Nummer 8).

**Hogan DP** see **Frenzen PD**

**Högberg U:** Allmogens förlossningsställningar. **Jordemodern** 1982 Jun;95(6):199–202

**Högberg U:** Förebyggande mödravård från kinesiska urkunder till moderna MVC. **Lakartidningen** 1983 Dec 21;80(51):5009–12, 5017

**Högberg U:** Mödradöd i förhistorisk tid. **Sydsven Medicinhist Sallsk Arsskr** 1983;:103–14

**Högberg U:** Mylingar, arsenik, fosfor och sonder--om aborter under gångna århundraden. **Lakartidningen** 1981 Aug 26;78(35):2951–2

**Hogenson GB:** Depth psychology, death and the hermeneutic of empathy. **J Med Philos** 1981 Feb;6(1):67–89

**Hogenson GB:** Jung's struggle with Freud. Notre Dame, London, University of Notre Dame Press, 1983. xi, 180 p.

**Hogue H:** Analyzing ossurary skeletal remains: techniques and problems. **South Indian Stud (NC)** 1977;29:2–22

**Hogye I:** 'Bábai mesterség' a Hegyalján (1711–1849). **Orvostort Kozl** 1982;28(1–3):201–8

**Hogye I:** Kazinczy Ferenc feljegyzései a betegségekrol. **Orvostort Kozl** 1982;28(1–3):241–3

**Hohmann E:** 100 Jahre Ausrüstungstechnik für die zahnärztliche Berufsarbeit. **Dent Echo (Heidelb)** 1980 Aug;50(5):36–58

**Hohmann E:** 100 years of equipment technology for the practice of dentistry. **Dent Echo (Heidelb)** 1981 May;50(3):89–109

**Hohorst G:** The decline of fertility once again: a critical note on John Knodel's book and standardized demographic indexes. **Hist Soc Res** 1982;22:50–62

**Hoiblain HG** see **Izmerov NF**

**Höjeberg P:** Mödrovård i Zambia. **Jordemodern** 1982 Jun;95(6):203–7

**Højgaard K:** Dentition on Bahrain, 2000 B.C. **Scand J Dent Res** 1980 Dec;88(6):467–75

**Højgaard K:** Dentition on Umm an-Nar (Trucial Oman), 2500 B.C. **Scand J Dent Res** 1980 Oct;88(5):355–64

**Hojgaard K:** Dilmun-tidens taender. Umm an-Nar (2500 f.v.t.). Al-Bahrain (2000 f.v.t.). **Tandlaegebladet** 1980 Sep;84(16):548

**Holaday B:** Changing views of infant care 1914–1980. **Pediatr Nurs** 1981 Jan–Feb;7(1):21–5

**Holbrook DM:** John Keats: student at the United Hospitals. **St Thomas Hosp Gaz** 1981;79(1):22–4

**Holck P:** Galls frenologi. **Tidsskr Nor Laegeforen** 1983 Sep 20;103(26):1805–7

**Holck P:** Harris' linjer. Røntgenfunn på et prehistorisk skjelett. **Tidsskr Nor Laegeforen** 1984 May 30;104(14):1028–31

**Holcombe HW:** Patent medicine tax stamps. A history of the firms using United States private die proprietary medicine tax stamps. Ed. G. B. Griffenhagen. Lawrence, Quarterman, 1979. xxv, 604 p. Reprinted articles from various journals.

**Holden C:** Bern Dibner: science bibliophile. **Science** 1980 May 30;208(4447):1012–4

**Holden C:** Paul MacLean and the triune brain. **Science** 1979 Jun 8;204(4397):1066–8

**Holden C:** The hospice movement and its implications. **Ann Am Acad Polit Soc Sci** 1980;447:59–63

**Holden JJ** see **White BN**

**Holder FL:** Søren Kierkegaard's final illness and death. **Anglican Theol Rev** 1979;61(4):508–14

**Holinka C:** Theodor Billroth: the life of a surgeon in the spirit of music. **Mt Sinai J Med (NY)** 1981 Jan–Feb;48(1):21–41

**Holladay AJ** see **Poole JC**

**Hollán SR:** An appreciation: J. J. van Loghem. **Haematologia (Budap)** 1980;13(1–4):5–22

**Hollán Z:** Rusznyák István utca. **Orv Hetil** 1983 Jun 26;124(26):1575–7

**Holland D:** Corrigan and The House of Industry Hospital. **J Ir Coll Physicians Surg** 1980 Jul;10(1):24–6

**Holland J:** A glorious anachronism: the American Philosophical Society. **Wilson Libr Bull** 1982;56(10):740–4

**Holland MM, Dean L:** Mother Joseph: founder, architect, beggar. **Hosp Prog** 1980 Apr;61(4):70–3

**Holland MR:** Chronology of dental history. **Northwest Dent** 1983 Mar–Apr;62(2):72–81

**Holland MR:** People, conditions, and activities in the 1880s and 1890s. **Northwest Dent** 1983 Mar–Apr;62(2):45–57

**Holland MR:** The Minnesota Dental Association: 1958–1983. **Northwest Dent** 1983 Mar–Apr;62(2):23–44

**Holland MR:** University of Minnesota School of Dentistry: a proud and productive history. **Northwest Dent** 1983 Mar–Apr;62(2):68–71

**Holland NN:** Freud, physics, and literature. **J Am Acad Psychoanal** 1984 Jul;12(3):301–20

**Holland PD:** The section of pathology and the development of pathology over the century. **Ir J Med Sci** 1983 Jan;152(1):50–6

**Holland WW, Breeze E, Swan AV:** Clinical trials: some reflections. **Stat Med** 1982 Oct–Dec;1(4):361–8

**Hollander A:** Betrachtungen über Paul Gerson Unna. **Z Hautkr** 1984 May 15;59(10):680–7

**Hollander A:** Geschichtliches aus vergangener Zeit: Politische Bekämpfung der Geschlechtskrankheiten? **Fortschr Med** 1981 Jun 25;99(24):927–8

**Hollander A:** Glimpses at the life and work of P. G. Unna. **Am J Dermatopathol** 1980 Summer;2(2):137–42

**Hollander A:** P. G. Unna revisited. **Am J Dermatopathol** 1981 Summer;3(2):187–9

**Hollander A:** Udo Julius Wile. **J Am Acad Dermatol** 1984 Jun;10(6):1071–2

**Hollander DH:** Etiogenesis of the European cystic fibrosis polymorphism: heterozygote advantage against veneral syphilis? **Med Hypotheses** 1982 Feb;8(2):191–7

**Hollander FP:** A giant step forward: dentistry in Connecticut a century ago. **Bull Hist Dent** 1980 Apr;28(1):35–7

**Hollander L** see **Stinaff R**

**Hollander R:** Life at the Washington asylum for the insane, 1871–1880. **Historian** 1982;44(2):229–41

**Hollander R:** Mental health policy in Washington territory, 1853–1875. **Pac Northwest Q** 1980;71(4):152–61

**Holle G:** Entwicklungslinien der morphologischen Forschung im Spiegel des Greifswalder Lehrstuhls für pathologische Anatomie. **Zentralbl Allg Pathol** 1982;126(5–6):417–23

**Holle S:** Die Widerlegung des Postulates von der Gleichzeitigkeit der Ovulation und Menstruation bei der Frau. Klinische und histologische Untersuchungen im frühen 20. Jahrhundert. Diss. Erlangen-Nürnberg, 1984. 100 p.

**Hollender MH:** The case of Anna O.: a reformulation. **Am J Psychiatry** 1980 Jul;137(7):797–800

**Hollerbach PE** see **Shedlin MG**

**Holley D** see **Brown DC**

**Holley HL:** Highlights in history of nineteenth century medicine in Alabama. **Ala J Med Sci** 1983 Jul;20(3):326–33

**Holley HL:** The history of medicine in Alabama. Birmingham, for University of Alabama School of Medicine, by University of Alabama Press, 1981. xiv, 418 p.

**Holling SA:** Medicine for heroes: a neglected part of pioneer life. [Mississauga, Ont.], Mississauga South Historical Society in association with the Boston Mills Press, 1981. 93 p.

**Hollingsworth DF:** Rationing and economic constraints on food consumption in Britain since the Second World War. **World Rev Nutr Diet** 1983;42:191–218

**Hollingsworth DF:** Sir Norman Charles Wright. In Dictionary of national biography, 1961–1970. Suppl. 8, 1981. p. 1115–6.

**Hollingsworth DR** see **Ney D**

**Hollingsworth R:** Causes and consequences of the American medical system. **Rev Am Hist** 1983;11(3):326–32

**Hollingsworth TH:** A preliminary suggestion for the measurement of mortality crises. In Charbonneau H, Larose A, ed: The great mortalities: methodological studies of demographic crises in the past. Liège, Belgium, Ordina Editions, 1980. p. 21–8.

**Hollingsworth TH** see **Dupâquier J**

**Hollister LE:** The pre-benzodiazepine era. **J Psychoactive Drugs** 1983 Jan–Jun;15(1–2):9–13

**Hollman A:** Sir Thomas Lewis (1881–1945). In J. Cule, ed: Wales and medicine. London, British Society for the History of Medicine, 1975. p. 203–7.

**Hollman A:** Thomas Lewis--the early years. **Br Heart J** 1981 Sep;46(3):233–44

**Hollmann W:** 100 Jahre Sportmedizin. **Fortschr Med** 1983 Oct 6;101(37):1660–3

**Hollmann W, Valentin H:** 50 Jahre Spiroergometrie 1929 bis 1979. **MMW** 1980 Feb 1;122(5):169–74

**Holloway L:** Medical obituaries: American physicians, biographical notices in selected medical journals before 1907. New York, Garland, 1982. xiv, 513 p.

**Holloway RL:** Exploring the dorsal surface of hominoid brain endocasts by stereoplotter and discriminant analysis. **Philos Trans R Soc Lond [Biol]** 1981 May 8;292(1057):155–66

**Holloway RL:** Indonesian 'Solo' (Ngandong) endocranial reconstructions: some preliminary observations and comparisons with Neandertal and Homo erectus groups. **Am J Phys Anthropol** 1980 Aug;53(2):285–95

**Holloway RL:** The O.H. 7 (Olduvai Gorge, Tanzania) hominid partial brain endocast revisited. **Am J Phys Anthropol** 1980 Aug;53(2):267–74

**Holloway RL:** Volumetric and asymmetry determinations on recent hominid endocasts: Spy I and II, Djebel Ihroud I, and the Sale Homo erectus specimens, with some notes on Neanderthal brain size. **Am J Phys Anthropol** 1981 Jul;55(3):385–93

**Holloway S:** Significance of the Apothecaries' Act, 1815. **Pharm Hist (London)** 1970 Jun;1(5):6–9

**Hollwich F** see **Busse H**

**Holmdahl MH** see **Nunn JB**

**Holmer PL** see **Smith JH, ed**

**Holmertz V:** Museet som berättar om m ormors sjukvård. **Vardfacket** 1982 May 13;6(9):8–9

**Holmes FL:** The fine structure of scientific creativity. **Hist Sci** 1981;19(1):60–70

**Holmes FL:** The history of biochemistry: a review of the literature of the field. **Spec Collect** 1982;1(2):7–15

**Holmes GL:** Roberts Bartholow. In search of anatomic localization. **NY State J Med** 1982 Feb;82(2):238–41

**Holmes GR** see **Dolan JP**

**Holmes JD:** A new look at Spanish Louisiana census accounts: the recent historiography of Antonio Acosta. **La Hist** 1980;21(1):77–86

**Holmes JH:** Diagnostic ultrasound during the early years of A.I.U.M. **JCU** 1980 Aug;8(4):299–308

**Holmes L:** Alabama granny midwife. **J Med Soc NJ** 1984 May;81(5):389–91

**Holmes WR:** The illness and death of Napoleon. **J Med Assoc Ga** 1983 Mar;72(3):201–4

**Holmstedt B, Bruhn JG:** Ethnopharmacology--a challenge. **J Ethnopharmacol** 1983 Sep;8(3):251–6

**Holmstedt B, Wassén SH, Schultes RE:** Jaborandi: an interdisciplinary appraisal. **J Ethnopharmacol** 1979 Jan;1(1):3–21

**Holmstedt B, Fredga A:** Sundry episodes in the history of coca and cocaine. **J Ethnopharmacol** 1981 Mar–May;3(2–3):113–47

**Holmstrup P, et al:** [J. J. Pindborg and Danish dentistry]. **Tandlaegebladet** 1981 Aug;85(13):380–408

**Holst JJ:** Tandlaegeskolen - Stormgade 17. **Tandlaegebladet** 1982 Dec;86(22):771–9

**Holste T, Keil G:** Tierheilkundliches im altdeutschen Theriak-Traktat. **Hist Med Vet** 1979;4(1):18–21

**Holstein J:** The first fifty years at the Jackson Laboratory. Edited by W. L. Dupuy. [Bar Harbor, Me.], Jackson Laboratory, 1979. xiii, 231 p.

**Holtkamp P:** Die Entwicklung der Bohrmaschine. **Quintessenz Zahntech** 1981 May;7(5):507–9

**Holtkamp P:** Fortschritte in der zahnärztlichen Prothetik durch die Einführung der Gusstechnik. **Quintessenz J** 1983 Jun;13(6):571–9

**Holtkamp P:** Narkosen mit 'Weingenuss bis zum Nasenbluten'. **Quintessenz J** 1981 Nov;11(11):995–6

**Holtkamp P:** 'Pastillen des Cosmus' zur Erhaltung wohlriechenden Atems. **Quintessenz J** 1981 Jun;11(6):559–61

**Holtkamp P:** Ringwerke--die erste Brückenprothetik. **Quintessenz Zahntech** 1981 Apr;7(4):401–3

**Holtmann HW** see **Poulet W**

**Holtom DB** see **Turner PJ**

**Holton S:** Social medicine in nineteenth century South Australia. **Community Health Stud** 1983;7(2):121–35

**Holtum E** see **Heirs of Hippocrates**

**Holtz W:** Bankrobbers, burkers and bodysnatchers. **Mich Q Rev** 1967;6(2):90–8

**Holtzman EM:** Marriage, sexuality, and contraception in the British middle class, 1918–1939: the correspondence of Marie Stopes. Ph.D. Diss., Rutgers University, The State Univ. of New Jersey. New Brunswick, 1982. v, 170 p.

**Holub A:** Dvacet pět let Výzkumného ústavu veterinárního lékařstvví v Brně. **Vet Med (Praha)** 1982 May;27(5):257–66

**Holubar K:** Die Dermatologie in Wien und die Deutsche Dermatologische Gesellschaft (DDG). Eine historische Perspektive. **Hautarzt** 1983;34(Suppl 6):xvii–xviii

**Holubar K:** Ferdinand von Hebra und das Allgemeine Krankenhaus in Wien. Uber die Domizilierung der beiden Hautkliniken um die Mitte des 19. Jahrhunderts und ihr Verhältnis zum II. Hof im Allgemeinen Krankenhaus. **Wien Med Wochenschr** 1982 Sep 30;132(18):423–6

**Holubar K, Frankl J:** Joseph Plenck (1735–1807). A forerunner of modern European dermatology. **J Am Acad Dermatol** 1984 Feb;10(2 pt 1):326–32

**Holubar K, Frankl J:** Moriz (Kohn) Kaposi. **Am J Dermatopathol** 1981 Winter;3(4):349–54

**Holubar K:** Terminology and iconography of lupus erythematosus. A historical vignette. **Am J Dermatopathol** 1980 Fall;2(3):239–42

**Holubar K:** The influence of the British School of Dermatology on the Vienna School in the first half of the 19th century. **Int J Dermatol** 1982 May;21(4):224–6

**Holubar K:** Vienna General Hospital--'Allgemeines Krankenhaus'--bicentennial. **Isr J Med Sci** 1984 Jun;20(6):553–4

**Holubar K** see **Kerl H**

**Holubar K** see **Tappeiner J**

**Hołyński J:** Wytwórczość przedprzemysłowa chemikaliów i środków leczniczych na przełomie XIX i XX wieku w Lodzi i regionie. **Arch Hist Med (Warsz)** 1983;46(3):273–84

**Holzberg CS:** Anthropology, life histories, and the aged: the Toronto Baycrest Centre. **Int J Aging Hum Dev** 1983–84;18(4):255–75

**Holzinger W:** A re-examination of charges of racism in the Converso controversy in the light of Medieval-Renaissance medical lore. **Rev Estud Hisp** 1978;12(3):337–52

**Hölzl N:** Zauberbücher, Vampire und einige vernünftige Köpfe. **Tirol Heimatbl** 1972;47(1–3):35–8

**Homans P:** A personal struggle with religion: significant fact in the lives and work of the first psychologists. **J Relig** 1982;62:128–44

**Hömberg W:** Bronzemörser für Apotheken Herstellung-Stilmerkmale-Fälschungen. **Beitr Gesch Pharm** 1983;31(21):33–40

**Homblé AG:** De echel of bloedzuiger in de volksgeneeskunde. **Oostvlaam Zanten** 1980;55(1):1–32

**Homble AG:** De medecijn Winckel van den verstandigen hovenier. **Brabantse Folkl** 1979 Sept;223:287–324

**Homblé AG:** Het keisnijden. Kwakzalverij of werkelijkheid? **Oostvlaam Zanten** 1980;55:105–14

**Homble AG:** Jan Albert Roselt, plattelandschirurgijn te Machelen. **Ons Heem** 1979;33:1–70

**Homburger F:** Carcinogenesis bioassay in historical perspective. **Prog Exp Tumor Res** 1983;26:182–6

**Home RW:** History of science in Australia. **Isis** 1982 Sep;73(268):337–42

**Homenaje al Doctor Erich Fromm: Gac Med Mex** 1980 Oct;116(10):431–45

**Homma K:** On the toothpick. In International Congress of the History of Medicine. 26th, Plovdiv, 1978. Actes du Congress. Sofia, 1981. Volume II. p. 111–4.

**Hommage au professeur Armand Delachaux à l'occasion de son 70e anniversaire: Soz Praventivmed** 1982 May;27(2–3):59–67

**Homolka J:** Třicet let Ceskoslovenské lékařské společnosti J.E. Purkyně. **Cas Lek Cesk** 1979 Dec 14;118(50):1541–7

**Homolka J:** Ze začátku historie Společnosti klinické biochemie. **Cas Lek Cesk** 1981 Jun 11;120(23):713–5

**Honda C** see **Kato M**

**Honegger C:** Uberlegungen zur Medikalisierung des weiblichen Körpers. In Imhof AE, ed: Leib und Leben in der Geschichte der Neuzeit. Berlin, Duncker & Humblot, 1983. p. 203–13.

**Honek K:** Die wissenschaftlichen Bibliotheken der Erzdiözese Wien. **Biblos (Vienna)** 1981;30(2):97–102

**Honeyman WP:** Myocardial infarction in Carlisle in 1783. **Br Med J [Clin Res]** 1982 Apr 10;284(6322):1113–4

**Hongo T** see **Suzuki T**

**Honigsbaum F:** Medical politics and the state: the part played by the medical profession in the development of the National Health Service. **Soc Soc Hist Med Bull (Lond)** 1981 Dec;29:20–1

**Honigsbaum F:** The BMA-TUC alliance and the Beveridge report. **Soc Soc Hist Med Bull (Lond)** 1983 Jun;32:19

**Honigsbaum F:** The division in British medicine. A history of the separation of general practice from hospital care 1911–1968. London, Kogan Page, 1979. xvi, 445 p.

**Honley SA:** A history of the 1873 yellow fever epidemic in Shreveport, Louisiana. **North La Hist Assoc** 1982;13(2–3):90–6

**Honti J, Szám I:** A budapesti Hann Fanny és a Hann syndroma (tranzitoricus diabetes insipidus). **Orv Hetil** 1984 Jun 24;125(26):1581–2

**Honti J:** A fiziológia az Orvosi Hetilap korai évfolyamaiban. **Orv Hetil** 1981 Aug 9;122(32):1979–80
**Honti J:** A magyar progresszió egészségpolitikai törekvései és a Nagy Októberi Szocialista Forradalom hatása. **Orvostort Kozl** 85(24 No 3):85–90, 1978
**Honti J:** Morgagni kórbonctana. **Orv Hetil** 1983 Jan;124(4):219–20
**Hoobler IG:** Boundless horizons. Portrait of a pioneer woman scientist. Smithtown, N. Y., Exposition Press, 1982. 197 p.
**Hood B:** 'This worry I have': Mary Herren journal. **Oreg Hist Q** 1979;80(3):228–57
**Hood TK** see **Myles J**
**Hood WH:** Physicians of Butte County, California, 1850–1900. Chico, Calif., W. H. Hood, 1980. 46 leaves.
**Hooff AJ van:** Oud-zijn in het oude Hellas. **Tijdschr Gerontol Geriatr** 1983 Aug;14(4):141–8
**Hoogland GA:** Some historical remarks on acoustic neuroma. **Adv Otorhinolaryngol** 1984;34:3–7
**Hoogstraal H:** Changing patterns of tickborne diseases in modern society. **Annu Rev Entomol** 1981;26:75–99
**Hook D, Ben-Yehuda N:** [European witch-hunts: two perspectives]. **Am J Sociol** 1983;88(6):1270–9
**Höök O:** Pehr Dubb -- en medicinsk storman inom västsvensk sjukvård på 1700-talet. **Lakartidningen** 1979 Dec 19;76(51):4710–3
**Hoolihan C, Anderson PG:** Special collections, Library, Washington University School of Medicine. St. Louis, [Washington University School of Medicine], 1981. iii, 66 p.
**Hooper A:** Further information on the prehistoric representations of human hands in the cave of Gargas. **Med Hist** 1980 Apr;24(2):214–16
**Hooper A** see **Wildgoose M**
**Hooper GS:** A regional blood program for Florida. **J Fla Med Assoc** 1980 Feb;67(2):146–8
**Hooper R:** Graeme Robertson and the golden age of neurology. **Proc Aust Assoc Neurol** 1978;15:1–10
**Hoopes J:** Jonathan Edwards's religious psychology. **J Am Hist** 1983;69(4):849–65
**Hoops R** see **Riese W**
**Hoorn CM van:** Willem Lemnius [William Lemnius]. **Spiegel Hist** 1980:15(2):111–4
**Hooton A, Hooton C:** A critical analysis of French psychiatric nosology. **Can J Psychiatry** 1981 Mar;26(2):120–5
**Hooton C** see **Hooton A**
**Hooykaas R:** Wissenschaftsgeschichte--eine Brücke zwischen Natur- und Geisteswissenschaften. **Ber Wissenschaftsgesch** 1982;5:153–72
**Hooykaas R** see **Van der Leun C, ed:**
**Hope RB:** Dateline--New Guinea 1942. **Forum Med** 1980 Aug;3(8):539–42
**Hope RB:** Pioneering in the delivery of health care. **Forum Med** 1979 Mar;2(3):218–22
**Hope-Simpson RE:** Recognition of historic influenza epidemics from parish burial records: a test of prediction from a new hypothesis of influenzal epidemiology. **J Hyg (Lond)** 1983 Oct;91(2):293–308
**Höpfinger E:** Höchster Anspruch an die Arbeit: Gesundheit bezahlbar machen. Rückblick auf eine langjährige Firmentradition der Boehringer Mannheim GmbH. **Fortschr Med** 1984 Apr 26;102(16):91–2
**Hopkins BS** see **Levenson SM**
**Hopkins E** see **Ballstadt C**
**Hopkins HC** see **Hayden MR**
**Hopkinson GD:** Alexander Dalmahoy: chemist to Her Majesty. **Pharm Hist (London)** 1984 Dec;14(4):8–11
**Hoppe B:** Adolf Windaus, Heinrich Wieland, Richard Kuhn, Leopold Ružička, Alexander Todd und Adolf Bunenandt. Die Erforschung der Vitamine und der Hormone. In: Die Grossen der Weltgeschichte. Zürich, Kindler, 1978. p. 336–81.
**Hoppe B:** Arbeit und Gesundheit; historische Aspekte ihrer gegenseitigen Beziehungen. Bericht über eine Tagung der 'International School of History of Biological Sciences' in Ischia/Neapel vom 29. Juni bis 12. Juli 1980. **Ber Wissenschaftsgesch** 1980;3(3–4):214–20
**Hoppe B:** Biologie, Wissenschaft von der belebten Materie von der Antike zur Neuzeit. Biologische Methodologie und Lehren von der stofflichen Zusammensetzung der Organismen. Wiesbaden, Steiner, 1976. vii, 368 p. (Sudhoffs Archiv, Beihefte, Heft 17)
**Hoppe B:** Biologische und technische Bewegungslehre. **Forschungsunternehm Fritz Thyssen Stift Stud Naturwiss Tech Wirtsch Neunzehn Jahrhundert** 1976;2:186–206
**Hoppe B:** Chemophysiologie zwischen vitalistischer und mechanistischer Biologie im 19. Jahrhundert. **Medizinhist J** 1983;18(3):163–83
**Hoppe B:** Darstellung der Alchemie in Gemälden von Jan Brueghel d. A. (1568–1625). **Beitr Gesch Pharm** 1983;31(18/19):144–9
**Hoppe B:** Die Biologie der Mikroorganismen von F. J. Cohn (1828–1898). **Sudhoffs Arch** 1983;67(2):158–89
**Hopps JA:** The development of the pacemaker. **PACE** 1981 Jan;4(1):106–8
**Hopstock C:** The Norwegian pharmacy museum; a presentation. In: Vorträge des Internationalen Pharmaziehistorischen Kongresses Innsbruck 1977. Stuttgart, Wissenschaftliche Verlagsgesellschaft, 1979. p. 141–5.
**Hör G, Munz DL:** Nuklearmedizin--einst und jetzt. Folge 1: Entwicklung, Aufgabenspektrum, Radiopharmazeutika, Messtechnik, Klinische Indikationen. **Fortschr Med** 1983 Mar 17;101(10):415–22
**Horák J, Chrástek J, Novotný V, et al:** 30 let práce Ustavu tělovýchovného lékařství fakulty všeobecného lékařství University Karlovy v Praze. **Sb Lek** 1980 Jan;82(1):30–2
**Horan MJ, Kennedy HL:** Ventricular ectopy. History, epidemiology, and clinical implications. **JAMA** 1984 Jan 20;251(3):380–6
**Horbowska-Marzec H, Grodzicka-Królak H, Wielopolska H:** Enterowirusy w przypadkach limfocytarnego zapalenia opon mózgowordzeniowych w Warszawie w latach 1963–1976. **Przegl Epidemiol** 1979;33(4):461–6
**Horbowska-Marzec H, Grodzicka-Królak H, Wielopolska H:** Wirusy ECHO-11 u chorych hospitalizowanych w Warszawie w latach 1968–1977. **Pediatr Pol** 1980 Feb;55(2):203–5
**Hörcsik E, Pisztora F:** Ritkuló és halványuló babonás hiedelmek valamint széles körben elterjedt technikai ismeretek napjaink pszichiátriai kórképeiben. **Orvostort Kozl** 1982;92(4):93–9
**Horden P:** Saints and doctors in the early Byzantine Empire: the case of Theodore of Sykeon. In Sheils WJ, ed: The Church and healing. Papers read at the twentieth summer meeting and the twenty first winter meeting of the Ecclesiastical History Society. Oxford, Basil Blackwell for the Society, 1982. p. 1–13.
**Horder J:** The origin of the Royal College of General Practitioners. **Soc Soc Hist Med Bull (Lond)** 1983 Dec;33:13–4
**Horder JP, Swift G:** The history of vocational training for general practice. **J R Coll Gen Pract** 1979 Jan;29(198):24–32
**Hordern A:** Changing pattern of health care in western countries. In Stanley NF, Joske RA, ed: Changing disease patterns and human behaviour. London, New York, Academic Press, 1980. p. 371–85.
**Hořejší J:** Jak u nás začínal a rozvíjel se výzkum jaterních chorob, zejména hepatitidy a její prevence. Retrospektivní pohled. **Cas Lek Cesk** 1981 Oct 1;120(39):1174–7
**Horelli HT** see **Jansen AA**
**Horgan J:** Corrigan on cardiac disease. **J Ir Coll Physicians Surg** 1980 Jul;10(1):27–31
**Hörger H:** Krankheit und religiöses Tabu--die Lepra in der mittelalterlich-frühneuzeitlichen Gesellschaft Europas. **Gesnerus** 1982;39(1):53–70
**Hörger H:** Mortalität, Krankheit und Lebenserwartung der Penzberger Bergarbeiterschaft im 19. und beginnenden 20. Jahrhundert. **Z Bayer Landesgesch** 1980:43(1);185–222
**Horibe H** see **Yamada M**
**Höring FO:** Kritischer Rückblick auf die Entwicklung der Immunitätslehre. **Z Gesamte Inn Med** 1981 Apr 1;36(7):229–35
**Horn D** see **Harper RG**
**Horn H, Winkler H:** 25 Jahre Institut für Allgemeine Hygiene der Medizinischen Akademie Erfurt. **Z Gesamte Hyg** 1984 Sep;30(9):529–30
**Horn H** see **Opitz R**
**Horn M:** 'Sisters worthy of respect': family dynamics and women's roles in the Blackwell family. **J Fam Hist** 1983 Winter;8(4):367–82
**Hornbein M:** Dr. Charles Spivak of Denver: physician, social worker, Yiddish author. **West States Jew Hist Q** 1979;11(3):195–211
**Hornbein M:** Dr. John Elsner, a Colorado pioneer. **West States Jew Hist Q** 1981;13(4):291–302
**Hornbein TF:** Everest without oxygen. **Prog Clin Biol Res** 1983;136:409–14
**Hornblower H:** Henry Furbush Howe. **Mass Hist Soc Proc** 1977,89:184–6
**Hornbrook MC:** Allocative medicine: efficiency, disease severity, and the payment mechanism. **Ann Am Acad Polit Soc Sci** 1983;(468):12–29
**Hornbrook MC:** Medicinal drugs: risks and regulations. **Curr Hist** 1980;78(457):201–5, 223–6
**Horne PD:** The prince of El Plomo. **Paleopathol Newsl** 1982 Dec;40:7–10
**Horne PD, Kawasaki SQ:** The Prince of El Plomo: a paleopathological study. **Bull NY Acad Med** 1984 Nov;60(9):925–31
**Horne PD** see **Bromage TG**
**Horne PD** see **Hart GD, ed**
**Horney theory and literature: a symposium: Am J Psychoanal** 1982 Spring;42(1):3–59
**Hornick RB** see **Gröschel DH**
**Hörning B** see **Fankhauser R**
**Hornowski J:** O obecnej siebzibie zarządu głownego Polskiego Towarzystwa Lekarskiego i Klubie Lekarza w Warszawie, Aleje Ujazdowskie nr. 24. **Wiad Lek** 1983 Jul 1;36(13):1127–35
**Hornowski J** see **Dawidowicz A**
**Hornuf H** see **Hellinger J**
**Hornykiewicz O, ed** see **Livingston KE**
**Horowitz M, Collins J:** A census of copies of the first edition of Andreas Vesalius' De humani corporis fabrica (1543), with a note on the recently discovered variant issue. **J Hist Med Allied Sci** 1984 Apr;39(2):198–221
**Horowitz M, ed** see **Palmer C**
**Horrax G:** Some of Harvey's Cushing's contributions to neurological surgery. **J Neurosurg** 1981 Apr;54(4):436–47
**Horsley RA:** Further reflections to witchcraft and European folk religion. **Hist Relig** 1979;19(1):71–95
**Horsley RA:** Who were the witches? The social roles of the accused in the European witch trials. **J Interdiscip Hist** 1979;9(4):689–715
**Horstmanhoff HF, ed:** [Ancient and medieval pestilences]. Includes contributions by R. A. Tybout, M. van Raalte, S. van der Lee, C. G. van Leijenhorst, E. J. Bakker, E. J. Schoten. **Hermeneus Tijdschr Antieke Cult** 1979;51(2):58–157
**Horstmanhoff HF, et al:** The plague and other pestilences in antiquity and the Middle Ages. Contributions by R. A. Tybout, M. van Raalte, S. van der Lee, C. G. van Leijenhorst, E. J. Bakker, E. J. Schoten. **Hermeneus Tijdschr Antieke Cult** 1979;51(2):58–117, 140–157
**Horton CE, Horton CE:** Dr. John Pott: America's first physician-governor and revolutionary. **Bull NY Acad Med** 1983 Sep;59(7):678–85
**Horton CE** see **Horton CE**
**Horton LE:** The boys in the club. **J Am Diet Assoc** 1982 Jul;81(1):17–25
**Horváth M:** Cigánycsecsmök halálozása Baranya megyében 1973–1977

között, városok és járások szerint. **Demografia** 1978;21(2-3):366-70
**Hosek E:** Dr. phil. PhMr. Ferdinand Daubrawa, světlý zjev mezi lékárníky Moravského venkova v 19. století. **Cesk Farm** 1979 Jun;28(5):223-4
**Hoshasen Igaku Sogo Kenkyusho 20-nenshi Hensan Iinkai:** Hoiken nijunenshi. Chiba, Japan, Do Kenkyusho, Showa 52 nen [1977]. 4, 349 p.
**Hosoi Y** see **Okamura H**
**Hosono K:** [The logical structure in the 'Notes on Nursing' (Florence Nightingale)] (Jpn). **Sogo Kango** 1982;16(4):51-60
**Hospital admission tickets: Profiles Hosp Mark** 1982 3rd Quarter;7:40-1
**Hoss J:** Albert Mooren: ein Augenarzt im 19. Jahrhundert. Düsseldorf, Triltsch, 1980. 183 p. (Düsseldorfer Arbeiten zur Geschichte der Medizin, 55).
**Hossard J:** Une rencontre inattendue: Flaubert et Dorvault. **Rev Hist Pharm (Paris)** 1980 Jun;27(245):119-22
**Hossard J, ed:** Flaubert et la médecine. [Catalog of an exhibition July 5-27, 1980.] Rouen, Musée Flaubert, Hôtel Dieu de Rouen, 1980. n. p.
**Hossli G:** Die historische Entwicklung der intravenösen Narkose. **Klin Anaesthesiol Intensivther** 1981;23:1-7
**Hostetler JA** see **Hand WD, ed**
**Hothersall D:** History of psychology. Philadelphia, Temple University Press, 1984. xx, 456 p.
**Hou HC:** Concerning the study of nutrition in China. **Proc Soc Exp Biol Med** 1982 Oct;171(1):1-6
**Houck PW:** A vanishing tribe: the Monacan Indians of Virginia. **Va Med** 1983 May;110(5):332-4
**Houdaille J, Gutierrez H:** Exploitation sommaire du recensement de Mexico en 1811. **Population** 1981;36(4-5):933-8
**Houdaille J:** La baisse de la fécondité en Belgique au XIXe siècle. **Population** 1980;35(2):450-56
**Houdaille J:** La fécondité en Allemagne avant 1850. **Population** 1979;34(3):695-705
**Houdaille J:** La Réunion, des origines à 1766: étude démographique. **Ann Demogr Hist (Paris)** 1980;:213-37
**Houdaille J:** Mortalité dans divers groupes de notables du XVIIe au XIXe siècles. **Population** 1980;35(4-5):966-8
**Houdaille J:** Mortalité des députés élus de 1789 à 1794. **Population** 1979;34(3):714-7
**Houdaille J:** Mouvement saisonnier des conceptions en France de 1740 à 1829. **Population** 1979;34(2):452-57
**Houdaille J:** Quelques aspects de la démographie ancienne de l'Acadie. **Population** 1980;35(3):581-602
**Houdart R:** Paul Broca, précurseur des disciplines neurologiques. **Chirurgie** 1980;106(10):783-6
**Hounsfield GN:** Computed medical imaging. **Med Phys** 1980 Jul-Aug;7(4):283-90
**Hounsfield GN:** Computed medical imaging. **J Comput Assist Tomogr** 1980 Oct;4(5):665-74
**Hourlier:** 7 juin 1983: Cérémonie d'hommage public à Calmette (Hôpital des Armées de Lorient). **Bull Soc Pathol Exot Filiales** 1983 May-Jun;76(3):312-6
**House RV:** A brief history of hookworm disease in North Carolina. **NC Med J** 1982 Nov;43(11):765-8
**Houser HR:** Wilderness doctor: the life and times of Dr. John Hole. [Centerville, Ohio], Centerville Historical Society, 1980. 32 p.
**Houstěk J:** Professor MUDr. Ján Birčák šedesátiletý. **Cesk Pediatr** 1983 Feb;38(2):117-9
**Houstěk J:** Professor MUDr. Otto Hrodek, DrSc., šedesátiletý. **Cesk Pediatr** 1983 Jan;38(1):58-60
**Houstěk J:** Sto let od narození profesora MUDr. Jiřího Brdlíka, DrSc., vedoucí osobnosti československé pediatrie (24. října 1883--6. července 1965). **Cesk Pediatr** 1983 Nov;38(11):680-1
**Houston CS:** New light on Dr. John Richardson. **Can Med Assoc J** 1984 Sep 15;131(6):653-4, 656-8, 660
**Houston CS:** The pressure chamber revisited. A look at the past. **Prog Clin Biol Res** 1983;136:213-20
**Houston CS:** The quest to understand high altitude. A trip back in time and a look ahead. **Postgrad Med** 1983 Jun;73(6):307-10, 313-4
**Houston RA:** Colliers with colic? **Local Popul Stud (Matlock)** 1979;22:57-9
**Houtzager HL:** A letter from Herman Boerhaave to Johan Philip Burggraaf jr. **Janus** 1980:67(1-2-3):201-5
**Houtzager HL:** Antonie van Leeuwenhoek. **Eur J Obstet Gynecol Reprod Biol** 1983 Jul;15(3):199-203
**Houtzager HL:** Cesarean section till the end of the 16th century. **Eur J Obstet Gynecol Reprod Biol** 1982 Feb;13(1):57-8
**Houtzager HL:** Dieren in Delft. **Tijdschr Geschied Geneeskd** 1979;2(2):52-61
**Houtzager HL:** Frederik Ruysch. **Eur J Obstet Gynecol Reprod Biol** 1982 May;13(3):199-201
**Houtzager HL:** Giles of Rome. **Eur J Obstet Gynecol Reprod Biol** 1981 Aug;12(2):127-9
**Houtzager HL:** Jacob Rueff. **Eur J Obstet Gynecol Reprod Biol** 1982 Mar;13(2):105-7
**Houtzager HL:** Jan Swammerdam [Jan Swammerdam]. **Spiegel Hist** 1980;15(5):295-300
**Houtzager HL:** Jean Louis Baudelocque. **Eur J Obstet Gynecol Reprod Biol** 1982 Aug;13(5):323-4
**Houtzager HL:** Medicyns, Vroedwyfs en Chirurgyns. Schets van de gezondheidszorg in Delft en beschrijving van het Theatrum Anatomicum aldaar in de 16e en 17e eeuw. Amsterdam, Rodopi, 1979. 133 p. (Serie-nitgave van het Genootschap Delfia Batavorum, 5).
**Hovell BC:** The Hull Royal Infirmary, 1782-1982. Hull, Hull Health Authority, [1982?]. 75 p.
**Hovesen E:** Ole Worm - aegtemand og husfader. **Dan Medicinhist Arbog** 1982;:93-111
**Hovesen E:** Ole Worm og familien i Arhus. **Dan Medicinhist Arbog** 1981;:9-23
**Hovesen E:** Slangen i laegekunsten. **Dan Medicinhist Arbog** 1983;12:105-21
**Hovland M:** Aberdeen District Medical Society (No. 1), 1957-1981. **SD J Med** 1981 May;34(5):8-9
**How the FAH began: Investor Owned Hosp Rev** 1976 Feb;9(1):43-4
**Howard A:** The power to heal in colonial Rotuma. **J Polynesian Soc** 1979;88(3):243-75
**Howard AN:** The historical development, efficacy and safety of very-low-calorie diets. **Int J Obes** 1981;5(3):195-208
**Howard J:** Darwin. New York, Hill and Wang, 1982. viii, 101 p.
**Howard JE:** Fuller Albright: the endocrinologists' clinical endocrinologist. **Perspect Biol Med** 1981 Spring;24(3):374-81
**Howard P:** From Concorde to the cosmos. **Trans Hunter Soc** 1978-80;37-38:37-48
**Howard R:** Medical politics and the founding of the Jardin des Plantes in Paris. **J Soc Bibliogr Nat Hist** 1980 Apr;9(4):395-402
**Howard RC:** The family of Guy de la Brosse, founder of the Jardin des Plantes in Paris. In: Conrès international d'histoire de la médecine, XXVe, Québec, 1976. Actes. Québec, 1977. p. 771-89.
**Howard RD** see **Leighton BD**
**Howard RN:** The founders of the College Victoria. **Aust NZ J Surg** 1981 Apr;51(2):227-38
**Howard RP:** 'The Chief'--Doctor William Osler. **Iowa Med** 1984 Apr;74(4):155-8
**Howard V** see **Castaing L**
**Howard V** see **Dreznik A**
**Howard-Jones N:** Cardiac catheterization, a historical note. **Bull Hist Med** 1973 Sep-Oct;47(5):524-6
**Howard-Jones N:** Expérimentation humaine et déontologie: une interprétation historique. In: Médicine et expérimentation. Québec, Les Presses de l'Université Laval, 1982. p. 39-65. (Cahiers de Bioethique, 4).
**Howard-Jones N:** Fake! **Br Med J [Clin Res]** 1982 Feb 13;284(6314):511
**Howard-Jones N:** Friedrich Wolter (1893?-1944): the last anticontagionist. **Br Med J** 1980 Feb 9;280(6211):372-3
**Howard-Jones N:** Human experimentation in historical and ethical perspectives. **Soc Sci Med** 1982;16(15):1429-48
**Howard-Jones N:** International public health: The organizational problems between the two World Wars (5). **WHO Chron** 1978 Mar;32(3):114-25
**Howard-Jones N:** Prelude to modern preventive medicine. In Stanley NF, Joske RA, ed: Changing disease patterns and human behaviour. London, New York, Academic Press, 1980. p. 69-80.
**Howard-Jones N:** Robert Koch and the cholera vibrio: a centenary. **Br Med J [Clin Res]** 1984 Feb 4;288(6414):379-81
**Howard-Jones N:** The Pan American Health Organization: origins and evolution (1). **WHO Chron** 1980 Oct;34(10):367-75 (contd)
**Howard-Jones N:** The Pan American Health Organization: origins and evolution (2). **WHO Chron** 1980 Nov;34(11):419-26 concl.
**Howard-Jones N:** The World Health Organization in historical perspective. **Perspect Biol Med** 1981 Spring;24(3):467-82
**Howard-Jones N** see **Beer H**
**Howard-Jones N** see **Subba Rao M**
**Howard-Ruben J** see **Miller NJ**
**Howe E** see **Millstein PL**
**Howell CD:** Elite doctors and the development of scientific medicine: the Halifax medical establishment and 19th century medical professionalism. In Roland CG, ed: Health, disease and medicine. Toronto, Hannah Institute for the History of Medicine, 1984. p. 105-22.
**Howell CD:** Reform and the monopolistic impulse: the professionalization of medicine in the Maritimes. **Acadiensis** 1981;11(1):3-22
**Howell JB, Anderson DE:** 'The basal-cell nevus' by Howell and Caro, January 1959. Commentary: The nevoid basal cell carcinoma syndrome. **Arch Dermatol** 1982 Oct;118(10):813-26
**Howell JD:** Early perceptions of the electrocardiogram: from arrhythmia to infarction. **Bull Hist Med** 1984 Spring;58(1):83-98
**Howell M, Ford P:** The true history of the elephant man. Harmondsworth, England, Penguin Books, 1980. 223 p.
**Howell R:** Women and sport: an historical overview. In Borms J, Hebbelinck M, Venerando A, ed: Women and sport. Basel, Karger, 1981. p. 11-5.
**Howells JG, Osborn ML:** A reference companion to the history of abnormal psychology. Westport, Conn., Greenwood Press, 1984. 2 v. xviii, 1141 p.
**Howells JG, Osborn ML:** The history of child psychiatry in the United Kingdom. **Acta Paedopsychiatr (Basel)** 1981 Jan;46(4):193-202
**Howells WW** see **Rassengeschichte der Menschheit**
**Howie J:** Gonorrhoea--a question of tactics. **Br Med J** 1979 Dec 22-29;2(6205):1631-2
**Howie WB:** Samuel Benion--Glasgow University's first Doctor of Medicine. **Scott Med J** 1979 Jan;24(1):76-9
**Höxtermann E:** Ein Halbjahrhundert Fortschritte der Zellphysiologie, Biochemie und Photobiologie - Otto Heinrich Warburg (1883 bis 1970). **NTM** 1983;20(2):1-24
**Hoy SM, Robinson MC, ed:** Public works history in the United States: a guide to the literature. Nashville, American Association for State and

Local History, 1982. Sections on water supply and waste disposal, p. 165–215.
**Hoy SM** see **Melosi MV, ed**
**Hoyt HF:** A frontier doctor. Ed. D. B. Nunis. Chicago, Donnelley -- Lakeside Press, 1979. liii, 518 p.
**Hrabovszky Z:** [Gyula Elischer: as seen by one of his students] (Hun). **Orv Hetil** 1980;121:2831–4
**Hradečná Z:** Pódíl Biofyzikálního ústavu CSAV na začátcích biofyzikálního výzkumu v CSSR. **Bratisl Lek Listy** 1984 Jan;81(1):106–8
**Hrazdira CL** see **Rektor I**
**Hrodek O, Kubát K:** Akademik Josef Houštěk sedmdesátiletý. **Cesk Pediatr** 1983 Aug;38(8):496–9
**Hromádková J:** Cesko-ruské lékařské vztahy na stránkách prvních dvaceti ročníku Casopisu lékařú českých. **Cas Lek Cesk** 1980 Nov 14;119(46):1259–61
**Hromádková J:** Medici v boji za českou universitu a lékařskou fakultu. **Cas Lek Cesk** 1983 Oct 14;122(41):1254–60
**Hromádková J:** Medici v boji za českou universitu a lékařskou fakultu. I. Medici a národnostní otázka v revolučních letech 1848–1849 a v období činnosti Klubu mediku českých (do roku 1868). **Sb Lek** 1983 Oct;85(9–10):277–84
**Hromádková J:** Medici v boji za Ceskou Univerzitu a Lékařskou Fakultu. II. Spolek českých mediku a jeho úloha v boji za českou lékařskou fakultu. **Sb Lek** 1984 Apr;86(4):119–28
**Hromis M** see **Protic M**
**Hrubisko M:** 30 rokov národnej transfúznej služby v CSSR. **Vnitr Lek** 1980 Feb;26(2):105–6
**Hruby K:** Das Auge war meine Welt: ein Leben als Augenarzt. Wien, W. Maudrich, 1983. x, 275 p.
**Hruby K:** Goethes Augenleiden. **Klin Monatsbl Augenheilkd** 1984 Jul;185(1):61–3
**Hrynyschyn K** see **Schlosser GA**
**Hsiung GD:** Progress in clinical virology--1960 to 1980: a recollection of twenty years. **Yale J Biol Med** 1980 Jan–Feb;53(1):1–4
**Hsu HY, Peacher WG:** Chen's history of Chinese medical science. Taipei, Modern Drug Publishers, 1977. 148 p.
**Hsu K:** [Tao Lieh---the pioneer in neurosciences of our country] (Chi). **Sheng Li Ko Hsueh Chin Chan** 1980 Apr;11(4):376–8
**Hsu-Yu H:** 100 Jahre Bekämpfung der Tuberkulose in China. Eine historische Kurzübersicht. **Prax Klin Pneumol** 1982 Mar;36(3):116–21
**HTLV missionaries and parasites: Lancet** 1984 Oct 20;2(8408):927–8
**Hu SY:** An enumeration of Chinese materia medica. Hong Kong, Chinese University Press, 1980. 287 p.
**Hu SY:** [Study on the parasite eggs in an ancient corpse from Zhangguo Chu Tomb No. 1 in Mashan brick-field of Jiangling County, Hubei] (Chi). **Chi Sheng Chung Hsueh Yu Chi Sheng Chung Ping Tsa Chih** 1984;2(1):8
**Hu WX** see **Wei DX**
**Hu ZY** see **Yang KL**
**Hu Naichang:** [Textual research on 'Xiao pin (short and miscellaneous) prescriptions'.] (Chi). **Chin J Med Hist** 1981;11:116–9
**Huang CS:** Medical education in China: historical background, present status, and further development. **Am J Surg** 1982 Jun;143(6):660–3
**Huang H:** [On the formation and development of the Meng He School of Jiangsu Province in traditional Chinese medicine] (Chi). **Chung Hua I Shih Tsa Chih** 1984;14(2):65–71
**Huang SQ** see **Wei DX**
**Huard P, Imbault-Huart MJ:** A propos du scorbut. In: Congrès National des Sociétés Savantes, 101e, Lille, 1976. Comptes Rendus. Paris, 1976. Section des Sciences, Fasc. III. p. 157–72.
**Huard P, Wong M:** Ablation d'un polype naso-pharyngien à la Trinité en 1812. In: Congrès National des Sociétés Savantes, 91e, Rennes, 1966. Comptes Rendus. Paris, 1967. Section des Sciences, Tome 1. p. 99–102.
**Huard P, Imbault-Huart MJ:** André Vesale, iconographie anatomique (Fabrica, Epitome, Tabulae sex). Paris, Dacosta, 1980. 255 p.
**Huard P:** Armel-Eugène Gripouilleau (1821–1909) officier de santé à Montlouis (Indre-et-Loire). In: Congrès National des Sociétés Savantes, 93e, Tours, 1968. Comptes Rendus. Paris, 1971. Section des Sciences, Tome II. p. 189–92.
**Huard P, Niaussat P:** Calendrier de l'évolution du stéthoscope. In: Congrès National des Sociétés Savantes, 106e, Perpignan, 1981. Comptes Rendus. Paris, Bibliothèque Nationale, 1982. Fasc. IV. p. 105–10.
**Huard P:** Claude Bernard et la chirurgie. In: Congrès National des Sociétés Savantes, 107e, Brest, 1982. Comptes Rendus. Paris, 1983. Section des Sciences, Fasc. IV. p. 267–71.
**Huard P:** Claude Bernard et la morphologie. In: Congrès National des Sociétés Savantes, 107e. Brest, 1982. Comptes Rendus, Paris, 1983. Section des Sciences, Fasc. IV. p. 273–9.
**Huard P:** Claude Bernard et le système vasculaire. In: Congrès National des Sociétés Savantes, 107e. Brest, 1982. Comptes Rendus, Paris, 1983. Section des Sciences, Fasc. IV. p. 281–6.
**Huard P, Grmek MD:** Coup d'oeil sur les élèves étrangers de Laennec. In: Congrès National des Sociétés Savantes, 97e, Nantes, 1972. Comptes Rendus. Paris, 1976. Section des Sciences, Tome 1. p. 21–35.
**Huard P, Niaussat PM:** Die Medizinisch-Chirurgische Schule der Marine in Brest. **Hist Hosp** 1979–80;13:147–52
**Huard P:** El problema de la representación del cuerpo humano. Su evolución en Eurasia. **Nueva Enferm** 1979 Dec;(7):3–6
**Huard P, Lefebvre P, Plessis JL:** François-Félix Jacquot (1819–1857). **Hist Sci Med** 1983;17(4):403–10
**Huard P, Imbault-Huart MJ:** Gabriel Andral (1797–1876). **Rev Hist Sci** 1982;35(2):131–53
**Huard P, Imbault-Huart MJ:** Geschichte der Militärmedizin. In Sournia JC, Martiny M, Poulet J, ed: Illustrierte Geschichte der Medizin. Salzburg, Andreas, 1980. Vol. 8. p. 2961–97.
**Huard P, Laplane R:** Histoire illustrée de la pédiatrie. Tome premier. Paris, Dacosta, 1981. 198 p.
**Huard P, Laplane R:** Histoire illustrée de la puériculture: aspects diététiques, socio-culturels et ethnologiques. Paris, Les Editions Roger Dacosta, 1979?, 196 p.
**Huard P:** II y a cent ans Constantin Paul présentait à l'Académie de Médecine son stéthoscope autostatique bi-auriculaire. **Bull Acad Natl Med (Paris)** 1981 Nov;165(8):1117–21
**Huard P:** Jacques Delpech (1777–1832). In: Congrès National des Sociétés Savantes, 96e, Toulouse, 1971. Comptes Rendus. Paris, 1974. Histoire des Sciences, Tome 1. p. 99–105.
**Huard P, Théodoridès J:** Jean-Baptiste Pipelet (1759–1823), Constance de Théis (1767–1845), Josef de Salm-Dyck (1773–1861) ou le chirurgien, la poétesse et le botaniste. In: Congrès National des Sociétés Savantes, 93e, Tours, 1968. Comptes Rendus. Paris, 1971. Section des Sciences, Tome II. p. 127–36.
**Huard P, Chaïa J:** La découverte du caoutchouc et ses premières applications médicales en France. In: Congrès National des Sociétés Savantes, 93e, Tours, 1968. Comptes Rendus. Paris, 1971. Section des Sciences, Tome II. p. 69–73.
**Huard P:** La gérontologie de J. M. Charcot. **Rev Neurol (Paris)** 1982;138(12):989–95
**Huard P, Nguyên Trân Huân:** La médecine vietnamienne au XVIIIe siècle. In: Congrès National des Sociétés Savantes, 101e, Lille, 1976. Comptes Rendus. Paris, 1976. Section des Sciences, Fasc. III. p. 61–8.
**Huard P, Aaron C, Askienazy S, et al:** La mort de Paul Broca (1824–1880). **Bull Acad Natl Med (Paris)** 1980 Oct;164(7):682–5
**Huard P, Imbault-Huart MJ:** La polémique Percy-Ollivier sur le typhus traumatique en 1822. In: Congrès National des Sociétés Savantes, 99e, Besançon, 1974. Comptes Rendus. Paris, 1976. Section des Sciences, Fasc. V. p. 243–9.
**Huard P, Lefebvre P, Nosny P, et al:** La scie ostéotome à chaîne de Bernhard-Franz Heine (1800–1846). **Hist Sci Med** 1983;17(2):147–57
**Huard P, Imbault-Huart MJ:** La stomatologie navale au XVIIIe siècle. In: Congrès National des Sociétés Savantes, 101e, Lille, 1976. Comptes Rendus. Paris, 1976. Section des Sciences, Fasc. III. p. 145–56. (also in 97e Congrès National des Sociétés Savantes, Nantes, 1972, Sciences, Tome I, p. 167–9).
**Huard P:** La thérapeutique chinoise d'hier et d'aujourd'hui. **Sci Orient** 1978;9:1–18
**Huard P, Imbault-Huart MJ:** L'Académie royale de chirurgie après le 8 aout 1793. In: Congrès National des Sociétés Savantes, 100e, Paris, 1975. Actes. Paris, 1976. Histoire Moderne et Contemporaine et Histoire des Sciences. p. 297–308.
**Huard P, Plessis JL:** L'amputation de jambe à la bordelaise. In: Congrès National des Sociétés Savantes, 104e, Bordeaux, 1979. Comptes Rendus. Paris, 1979. Section des Sciences, Fasc. IV. p 243–57.
**Huard P, Niaussat PM:** 'L'arsenal' du service de Santé de la Marine au XIXe siècle. In: Congrès National des Sociétés Savantes, 105e, Caen, 1980. Comptes Rendus, Paris, 1980. Section des Sciences, Fasc. V. p. 85–96.
**Huard P, Aaron C, Askienazy S, et al:** Le cerveau de Paul Broca (1824–1880). Confrontation anatomo-pathologique et tomo-densitométrique. **J Radiol** 1982 Mar;63(3):175–80
**Huard P, Imbault-Huart MJ:** Le concept d'Académie en France au XVIIIe siècle; son évolution face à la médecine et à la chirurgie. In: Congrès National des Sociétés Savantes, 100e, Paris, 1975. Actes. Paris, 1976. Histoire Moderne et Contemporaine et Histoire des Sciences. p. 289–96.
**Huard P, Imbault-Huart MJ:** Le professeur Georges Dieulafoy (1839–1911). In: Congrès National des Sociétés Savantes, 96e, Toulouse, 1971. Comptes Rendus. Paris, 1974. Histoire des Sciences, Tome 1. p. 201–5.
**Huard P, Rousseau A, Wong M:** Les bagnes et la médecine aux XVIIIe et XIXe siècles. In: Congrès National des Sociétés Savantes, 91e, Rennes, 1966. Comptes Rendus. Paris, 1967. Section des Sciences, Tome 1. p. 79–85.
**Huard P, Imbault-Huart MJ:** Les étapes du traitement des tumeurs par ischémie, priorité de Harvey. **Hist Sci Med** 1980;14(2):171–5
**Huard P:** Les facettes multiples de René Théophile Laennec (1781–1826). **Bull Acad Natl Med (Paris)** 1981 Feb 17;Spec No:51–6
**Huard P, Bossy J, Mazars G:** Les médecines de l'Asie. Paris, Editions du Seuil, 1978. 277 p.
**Huard P, Imbault-Huart MJ:** Les papiers d'Antoine Louis (1723–1792). In: Congrès National des Sociétés Savantes, 102e, Limoges, 1977. Comptes Rendus. Paris, 1977. Section des Sciences, Fasc. III. p. 7–14.
**Huard P, Rousseau A, Wong M:** Les prisonniers de guerre aux XVIIIe et XIXe siècles. In: Congrès National des Sociétés Savantes, 91e, Rennes, 1966. Comptes Rendus. Paris, 1967. Section des Sciences, Tome 1. p. 87–91.
**Huard P, Niaussat PM:** L'évolution du stéthoscope de Laennec à nos jours; son influence dans certains domaines des transmissions acoustiques. **Hist Sci Med** 1981;15(2):173–87
**Huard P, Niaussat P:** L'évolution du stéthoscope. In: Congrès National des Sociétés Savantes, 106e, Perpignan, 1981. Comptes Rendus. Paris, Bibliothèque Nationale, 1982. Fasc. IV. p. 91–104.
**Huard P:** L'oeuvre du Service de Santé de la Marine francaise au XIXe siècle. In: Congrès National des Sociétés Savantes, 91e, Rennes, 1966.

Comptes Rendus. Paris, 1967. Section des Sciences, Tome 1. p. 93–8.
**Huard P:** Marcel Florkin (1900–1979). **Clio Med** 1980 May;14(2):93–5
**Huard P, Lacombe C, Théodoridès J:** Marine et botanique aux XVIIIe et XIXe siècles; les jardins botaniques de la Marine. In: Congrès National des Sociétés Savantes, 91e, Rennes, 1966. Comptes Rendus. Paris, 1967. Section des Sciences, Tome 1. p. 109–27.
**Huard P:** Paul Broca anatomiste. **Chirurgie** 1980;106(10):774–6
**Huard P, Imbault-Huart MJ:** Percy, vénéréologue. In: Congrès National des Sociétés Savantes, 99e, Besançon, 1974. Comptes Rendus. Paris, 1976. Section des Sciences, Fasc. V. p. 259–64.
**Huard P, Comiti VP:** Quarantaine et lazarets en France. In Radovi sa Medunarodnog simpozija u povodu sestote obljetnice Dubrovacke karantene. Dubrovnik, 29 i 30. rujna 1977. Zagreb, 1980. p. 121–34.
**Huard P, Imbault-Huart MJ:** Travaux de Percy (1754–1825) sur l'hémostase des artères (1790–1810). In: Congrès National des Sociétés Savantes, 99e, Besançon, 1974. Comptes Rendus. Paris, 1976. Section des Sciences, Fasc. V. p. 251–7.
**Huard P:** Un traité chinois d'oculistique. **Rev Hist Sci (Paris)** 1984 Jan;37(1):71–4
**Huard P, Durand M:** Un traité de médecine sino-vietnamienne du XVIIIe siècle: La compréhension intuitive des recettes médicales de Hai-Thuong. **Sci Orient** 1976;:1–24
**Huard P:** Velpeau, cancérologue. In: Congrès National des Sociétés Savantes, 93e, Tours, 1968. Comptes Rendus. Paris, 1971 Section des Sciences, Tome II. p. 159–62.
**Huard P, Imbault-Huart MJ:** Vicq d'Azyr et la nomenclature moderne des nerfs crâniens. In: Congrès National des Sociétés Savantes, 105e, Caen, 1980. Comptes Rendus, Paris, 1980. Section des Sciences, Fasc. V. p. 61–83.
**Huard P** see **Curet M**
**Huard P** see **Dechaume M**
**Huard P** see **Histoire culturelle de la maladie**
**Huard P** see **La médecine hospitalière française au XVIIIème siècle**
**Huard P** see **Niaussat P**
**Huard P** see **Plessis JL**
**Huard PO, Imbault-Huart MJ:** Le cabinet de l'Académie Royale de Chirurgie. In: Congrès National des Sociétés Savantes, 102e, Limoges, 1977. Comptes Rendus. Paris, 1977. Section des Sciences, Fasc. III. p. 15–20.
**Hubault A:** Arthropathies nerveuses. **Rev Neurol (Paris)** 1982;138(12):1009–17
**Hubbard WN:** The role of controlled therapeutic investigations. **Prog Clin Biol Res** 1980;38:275–80
**Hubel DH:** Cortical neurobiology: a slanted historical perspective. **Annu Rev Neurosci** 1982;5:363–70
**Hubel DH:** Evolution of ideas on the primary visual cortex, 1955–1978: a biased historical account. **Biosci Rep** 1982 Jul;2(7):435–69
**Hubel DH:** Exploration of the primary visual cortex, 1955–78. **Nature** 1982 Oct 7;299(5883):515–24
**Hübener KH, Pahl WM:** Computertomographische Untersuchungen an altägyptischen Mumien. **ROFO** 1981 Aug;135(2):213–9
**Hubenstorf M:** Osterreichische Arzteemigration 1934–1945--Zwischen neuem Tätigkeitsgebiet und organisierten Rückkehrplänen. **Ber Wissenschaftsgesch** 1984;7(2):85–107
**Huber A:** W. R. Hess, the ophthalmologist. **Experientia** 1982 Dec 15;38(12):1397–400
**Huber A:** Walter Rudolf Hess als Ophthalmologe. **Gesnerus** 1982;39(2):287–93
**Huber G:** Die Bedeutung von Karl Jaspers für die Psychiatrie der Gegenwart. **Nervenarzt** 1984 Jan;55(1):1–9
**Huber G:** Erich Sternberg 1903–1980. **Arch Psychiatr Nervenkr** 1981;230(1):1–3
**Huber G** see **Janzarik W ed**
**Huber J:** Will U. S. fertility decline toward zero? **Sociol Q** 1980;21(4):481–92
**Huber JP** see **Alliez J**
**Huber R:** E. Werle's kallikrein inactivator, a model in biochemistry and biophysics. **Adv Exp Med Biol** 1983;156:29–36
**Huber W:** Psychoanalytische Pädagogik in der Zeit des Ständestaates. **Zeitgesch** 1979;6(11–12):386–400
**Hübner H, ed** see **Kaiser W**
**Hübschmann K:** History of Dermatology and Venerology from 1848 to the end of 1944 in Prague, Czechoslovakia. **Int J Dermatol** 1982 Jul–Aug;21(6):356–60
**Hübschmann K:** Sambergerovi současníci na klinice Janovského. **Cesk Dermatol** 1980 Oct;55(5):349–53
**Huch RK:** 'Typhoid' Truelsen, water and politics in Duluth, 1896–1900. **Minn Hist** 1981;47(5):189–99
**Huckbody E:** Dermatology throughout the dark ages. The interchange of experience. **Int J Dermatol** 1980 Jul–Aug;19(6):344–7
**Huckle P:** The womb factor: pregnancy policies and employment of women. **West Polit Q** 1981;34(1):114–26
**Hudson BL** see **Smith MT**
**Hudson RP:** Disease and its control. The shaping of modern thought. Westport, London, Greenwood Press, 1983. xvii, 259 p. (Contributions in Medical History, no. 12).
**Hudson RP:** Suicide: madness or the noble Roman way? **Pharos** 1982 Fall;45(4):14–7
**Hudson RP** see **Matossian MK**
**Hudson RP** see **Maulitz RC**
**Hudson T, Genesse J:** Hansen's Disease in the United States. **Soc Sci Med** 1982;16(9):997–1004
**Hudzenko PM:** Vtilennia ideï V. I. Lenina u spravu okhorony zdorov'ia baterynstva i dyttnstva. **Pediatr Akush Ginekol** 1980 Mar–Apr;(2):3–7
**Huertas Garcia G:** Bosquejo hist/BC/orico sobre endodoncia. **Rev Esp Endodoncia** 1983 Dec;1(3):123–33
**Hueston JT** see **Plant M**
**Huf EG:** Echoes of the past. Reflections on the early history of the concept of 'active transport'. **Physiologist** 1979 Dec;22(6):18–24
**Hufbauer K:** The formation of the German chemical community (1720–1795). Berkeley, University of California Press, 1982. viii, 312 p.
**Hufbauer K** see **Johnson MP**
**Huff DS, Scrinivasan B:** The oldest children's hospital building still in use in the United States? **J Pediatr** 1983 Jan;102(1):165–6
**Hufford DJ** see **Hand WD, ed**
**Hufnagel CA, Thorn GW:** Observations of a colleague (Carl W. Walter). **Am J Surg** 1984 Nov;148(5):581–3
**Hufnagel CA** see **Chambers RW**
**Hufschmidt HJ:** Das Rechts-Links-Profil im kulturhistorischen Längsschnitt. Ein Dominanzproblem. **Arch Psychiatr Nervenkr** 1980;229(1):17–43
**Hug H, ed:** Friedrich Liebling, 1893–1982, zum Gedenken: Gedenkfeier vom 28. März 1982. Zürich, Verlag Psychologische Menschenkenntnis, 1983. 140 p.
**Hügelow M:** Original-Lithographien speziell für Pharmazeuten: Historische Apothekergeräte und Heilpflanzen. **Pharm Unserer Zeit** 1984 Jul;13(4):97–101
**Huggins CB:** Peyton Rous and his voyages of discovery. **J Exp Med** 1979 Oct 1;150(4):733–4
**Huggins CG:** The first decade. **J Med Assoc State Ala** 1983 Feb;52(8):9–17
**Hughes AF:** The American biologist through four centuries. Springfield, Ill., Thomas, 1982. xvii, 386 p.
**Hughes B:** 75 years of Kai Tiaki. **NZ Nurs J** 1983 Jan;76(1):4–6
**Hughes E:** The fight against cholera: India 1812 - 1912. **Hist Med (Lond)** 1975 Autumn–Winter;6(3–4):68–74
**Hughes ES:** The development of a restorative operation for carcinoma of the rectum. **Aust NZ J Surg** 1981;51:117–9
**Hughes ES, Dooley B:** The Royal College of Surgeons in Ireland 1784–1984. **Aust NZ J Surg** 1984 Dec;54(6):502
**Hughes FN:** The Faculty of Pharmacy--a retrospective look. **Contin Pract** 1980;7(3):3–8
**Hughes JD:** The dreams of Alexander the Great. **J Psychohist** 1984 Fall;12(2):168–92
**Hughes JE:** A history of the Royal Adelaide Hospital. Second revised edition. Netley, South Australia, Board of Management of the Royal Adelaide Hospital, 1982. xvii, 240 p.
**Hughes JE** see **Skipper JK**
**Hughes JS:** In the law's darkness: insanity and the medical-legal career of Isaac Ray, 1707–1881. Ph.D. Diss., Rice University. Houston, 1982. xvii, 393 p.
**Hughes JT:** Miraculous deliverance of Anne Green: an Oxford case of resuscitation in the seventeenth century. **Br Med J [Clin Res]** 1982 Dec 18–25;285(6357):1792–3
**Hughes JT:** Spinal cord arteries described by Willis. In Rose FC, Bynum WF, ed: Historical aspects of the neurosciences. New York, Raven, 1982. p. 195–203.
**Hughes M** see **Gove WR**
**Hughes RE:** James Lind and the cure of scurvy: an experimental approach. **Med Hist** 1975 Oct;19(4):342–51
**Hughes RE, Scott LD:** The founding of San Diego's Red Cross. **J San Diego Hist** 1981;27(2):115–28
**Hughes SG:** The life and work of John Howard Mummery. **Bull Hist Dent** 1983 Oct;31(2):69–81
**Hughes TP:** Convergent themes in the history of science, medicine, and technology. **Technol Cult** 1981 Jul;22(3):550–8
**Hughes WL, Castroviejo R, Blaydes JE, et al:** The evolution of ophthalmic sutures. **Ann Plast Surg** 1981 Jan;6(1):48–65
**Hugly C:** L'argent dans la relation thérapeutique. **Rev Odontostomatol (Paris)** 1981 May–Jun;10(3):239–44
**Hugo WB:** Phenols: a review of their history and development as antimicrobial agents. **Microbios** 1978;23(92):83–5
**Huguet M:** Expérience mystique, pathologie mentale et condition féminine. **Penelope** 1983;(8):25–8
**Huguet Ramia E** see **Bertrán Capella A**
**Hühns E:** Der Berliner Totentanz. **Dtsch Jahrb Volkskd** 1968;14(2):235–46
**Huizink L:** Die Abhandlung über das Sehen von Hieronymus Fabricius ab Aquapendente (1537–1619): Ubersetzung von 'De actione oculorum' mit Kommentar. Zürich, Juris Druck, 1984. 58 p. (Zürcher Medizingeschichtliche Abhandlungen, Neue Reihe, Nr. 166).
**Hulin I:** Háborús koponyasérülések. Tapasztalatok az ogadeni és eritreai háborúkból. I. rész. Neurotraumatológiai sérültek statisztikája. **Magy Traumatol Orthop Helyreallito Sebesz** 1982;25(4):273–9
**Hulkonen DA** see **Levin HS**
**Hull D** see **Beatty J**
**Hull NE** see **Hoffer PC**
**Hullay J:** Perspectives in international neurosurgery: neurosurgery in Hungary. **Neurosurgery** 1981 May;8(5):627–8
**Hulse FS:** Habits, habitats, and heredity: a brief history of studies in human plasticity. **Am J Phys Anthropol** 1981 Dec;56(4):495–501
**Hülsmann WC** see **Zimmerman AN**
**Hum D, Basilevsky A:** Economic activity and cyclical variations in birthrates: some new evidence for Jamaica. **Soc Econ Stud**

1978;27(2):197–203
**Humberson C** see **Palmieri A**
**Humble RM:** The Gill-Merrill expedition: penultimate chapter in the curare story. **Anesthesiology** 1982 Dec;57(6):519–26
**Humm E:** Vinzenz von Paul und seine Aktualität. Sein Aufruf zur patientenorientierten Pflege. **Krankenpflege (Frankfurt)** 1982 Jan;36(1):3–4
**Hummel D:** Som läkare vid hedinexpeditionen till Kina 1927–31. **Nord Medicinhist Arsbok** 1983;:155–44
**Hummert JR, Van Gerven DP:** Tetracycline-labeled human bone from a medieval population in Nubia'Batn el Hajar (550–1450 A.D.). **Hum Biol** 1982 May;54(2):355–63
**Humphrey RH** see **Carroll MA**
**Humphreys JW** see **Cruft GE**
**Humphries SV:** Medical practice in the Australian outback 25 years ago. **Cent Afr J Med** 1982 Feb;28(2):45–7
**Humphries SV:** The place of the nurse in society. **Cent Afr J Med** 1981 Sep;27(9):187–9
**Hunayn Ibn Ishak, al-Ibadi:** Questions on medicine for scholars. Translated into English, with a preface and historical note, by P. Ghalioungui, M.D., from a critical edition by G. M. Moussa, Ph. D., of the ninth century. Arabic text 'Al Masa'il fi al-Tibb lil Muta'allimin.' Cairo, Al-Ahram Center for Scientific Translations, 1980. xlix, 162 p.
**Hundeiker M:** Wilhelm Knoth. **Verh Dtsch Ges Pathol** 1982;66:646–52
**Hünemörder C:** Aims and intentions of botanical and zoological classification in the Middle Ages and Renaissance. **Hist Philos Life Sci** 1983;5(1):53–67
**Hünemörder C:** Antike und mittelalterliche Enzyklopädien und die Popularisierung naturkundlichen Wissens. **Sudhoffs Arch** 1981;65(4):339–65
**Hung T** see **Chen LB**
**Hungate RE:** Evolution of a microbial ecologist. **Annu Rev Microbiol** 1979;33:1–20
**Hunger H:** 'Zoologie,' 'Botanik,' 'Mineralogie,' 'Alchemie,' and 'Medizin.' In: Die hochsprachliche profane Literatur der Byzantiner. Vol. II. Munich, Beck, 1978 (Part 5, Vol. 2 of the Byzantinisches Handbuch). p. 265–320.
**Hunger H:** Zum Badewesen in byzantinischen Klöstern. **Sitzungsber Oesterr Akad Wiss Philos Hist Kl** 1980;367:353–64
**Hungerland H:** Deutsche Universität einst und jetzt. **Med Welt** 1981 Apr 24;32(17):672–4
**Hunnicutt BK** see **Austin D**
**Hunnisett RF, ed:** Wiltshire coroners' bills, 1752–1796. Devizes, Wiltshire Record Society, 1981. liv, 239 p. (Wiltshire Record Society, v. 36).
**Hunstadbråten K:** Fluor i kariesprofylaksen omkring århundriskiftet. **Nor Tannlaegeforen Tid** 1981 May;91(7):227–31
**Hunstadbråten K:** Fluor in der Kariesprophylaxe der Jahrhundertwende. **Quintessenz J** 1984 Feb;14(2):147–51
**Hunstadbraten K:** Fluoride in caries prophylaxis at the turn of the century. **Bull Hist Dent** 1982 Oct;30(2):117–20
**Hunstadbraten K:** Kariesprophylaxe durch Fluoride um die Jahrhundertwende. **Zahnarztl Mitt** 1982 Nov 16;72(22):2537–9
**Hunt DM** see **Lewis D**
**Hunt H** see **Ware J**
**Hunt JC:** Pourquoi investir dans la recherche biomédicale? **Action Natl** 1980;69(5):372–83
**Hunt JH** see **Fry J**
**Hunt JM:** Toward equalizing the developmental opportunities of infants and preschool children. **J Soc Issues** 1982;38(4):163–91
**Hunt LB, Buchanan PD:** Richard Knight (1768–1844): a forgotten chemist and apparatus designer. **Ambix** 1984 Jul;31(2):57–67
**Hunt M:** A coming of age with pediatrics: Park Jerauld White, attending physician. **Outlook Mag** 1982 Spring;19(1):18–24
**Hunt M:** La charité maternelle aux Etats-Unis au 19e siècle: un cas d'étude institutionnelle, un hôpital pédiatrique. **Penelope** 1981;(5):50–1
**Hunt M:** Woman's place in medicine: the career of Dr. Mary Hancock McLean. **Bull Mo Hist Soc** 1980;36(4):255–63
**Hunt M:** Women and childsaving: St. Louis Children's Hospital 1879–1979. **Bull Mo Hist Soc** 1980;36(2, pt 1):65–79
**Hunt VR:** A brief history of women workers and hazards in the workplace. **Feminist Stud** 1979;5(2):274–85
**Hunter AR:** Anaesthesia for intracranial surgery: an autobiographical view. **Ann R Coll Surg Engl** 1981;63:316–21
**Hunter AR:** Zebulon Mennell. A pioneer of neurosurgical anaesthesia. **Anaesthesia** 1983 Dec;38(12):1214–6
**Hunter GM:** Pathologist turned general practitioner. Reflections of an ex-Army pathologist. **J R Army Med Corps** 1981 Jun;127(2):93–7
**Hunter JM, Thomas MO:** Hypothesis of leprosy, tuberculosis and urbanization in Africa. **Soc Sci Med** 1984;19(1):27–57
**Hunter KM:** The satiric image: healers in The House of God. In Jones AH, ed: Images of healers. Albany, State University of New York Press, 1983. p. 135–47.
**Hunter M:** Early problems in professionalizing scientific research: Nehemiah Grew (1641–1712) and the Royal Society with an unpublished letter to Henry Oldenburg. **Notes Rec R Soc Lond** 1982 Feb;36(2):189–209
**Hunter M:** Reconstructing restoration science: problems and pitfalls in institutional history. **Soc Stud Sci** 1982 Aug 3;12(3):451–66
**Hunter T:** Medical politics: decline in the hegemony of the Australian Medical Association? **Soc Sci Med** 1984;18(11):973–80
**Hunter T:** Pressure groups and the Australian political process: the case of the Australian Medical Association. **J Commonw Comp Polit** 1980;18(2):190–206
**Hunter WH:** South Carolina medicine 110 years ago. **J SC Med Assoc** 1984 Sep;80(9):459–60
**Hunter JA, ed:** Anna May: eighty-two years in New England. **Northeast Folkl** 1979;20:7–106
**Huntington R, Metcalf P:** Celebrations of death: the anthropology of mortuary ritual. Cambridge, New York, Cambridge University Press, 1979. xv, 230 p.
**Huntley FL:** 'Well Sir Thomas?': oration to commemorate the tercentenary of the death of Sir Thomas Browne. **Br Med J [Clin Res]** 1982 Jul 3;285(6334):43–7
**Hunyady G:** Történelem és pszichológia [History and psychology]. **Tortenelmi Sz** 1981;24(1):71–8
**Huppert J:** Somatic cell hybrids. **Folia Biol (Praha)** 1983;29(1):56–64
**Huppertz A:** Die Vertreter der Anatomie und des anatomischen Unterrichts in Giessen von 1702–1748. Giessen, Schmitz, 1982. 283 p. (Arbeiten zur Geschichte der Medizin in Giessen, 4).
**Hurault J** see **Henry L**
**Hureau JC** see **Monod T**
**Hurlburt J:** Midwifery in Canada: a capsule history. **Can Nurse** 1981 Feb;77(2):30–1
**Huron R:** La statistique medicale en France à l'époque romantique. **Mem Acad Sci Insc B-Lett Toulouse** 1976;138:121–39
**Hurst DL, Hurst MJ:** Bromide psychosis: a literary case. **Clin Neuropharmacol** 1984;7(3):259–64
**Hurst JW:** Landmark article (JAMA 1912). Clinical features of sudden obstruction of the coronary arteries. By James B. Herrick. **JAMA** 1983 Oct 7;250(13):1757–65
**Hurst LC:** Freud and the great neurosis: discussion paper. **J R Soc Med** 1983 Jan;76(1):57–61
**Hurst LC:** Porphyria revisited. **Med Hist** 1982 Apr;26(2):179–82
**Hurst LC:** What was wrong with Anna O? **J R Soc Med** 1982 Feb;75(2):129–31
**Hurst MJ** see **Hurst DL**
**Hurt WR:** Witchcraft in New Mexico. **Palacio** 1974;80(2):12–20
**Hurwic J:** Nieznany list Marii Skłodowskiej-Curie. **Kwart Hist Nauki Tech** 1984;29(3–4):557–8
**Husain SA:** Physicians of Hyderabad during Nizam II & III. **Bull Indian Inst Hist Med (Hyderabad)** 1980;10(1–4):40–7
**Husberg K, Räf L:** John Charnley efter 30 års arbete med höftledskirurgi: 'intuition och slump hjälpte fram genombrotten men protesens livslängd måste förbättras'. **Lakartidningen** 1982 Jun 9;79(23):2301–3
**Husfeldt E:** Traek af thoraxkirurgiens historie i Danmark. **Dan Medicinhist Arbog** 1982;:9–21
**Husing JM:** Brief historical background on the certification process in corrective therapy, and a policy statement regarding certification eligibility. **Am Correct Ther J** 1983 Nov–Dec;37(6):153–5
**Hussain SA:** Hakim Nizamuddin Ahmed Geelani; a physician of Qutub Shahi period. **Bull Indian Inst Hist Med (Hyderabad)** 1979;9:67–73
**Hussain SA:** Ilajul Atfal: a treatise on pediatrics by Fezl-e-Ali-Shifa-ee Khan. **Bull Indian Inst Hist Med Hyderabad** 1982;12(1–4):45–50
**Hussain SF** see **Said HM, ed**
**Hussenot C:** Sur un Erbier de Me Arnauld de Villeneuve (manuscrit médiéval). Thèse de doctorat, Université René-Descartes. Paris, 1983. 119 leaves. (U. E. R. des Sciences pharm. et biol. de Paris-Luxembourg, 1982–1983, no U 558).
**Hussey HH:** The hepatitis B saga. **JAMA** 1981 Apr 3;245(13):1317–8
**Husson B, ed:** Trois textes alchimiques inédits du XVIIe siècle. L'or potable des anciens; Lettres philosophiques; Le testament d'or. Paris, Librairie de Médicis, 1979. 101 p.
**Huston KG** see **Blake JB, ed**
**Huston KG** see **Fothergill J**
**Huston KG** see **MacLaglan D**
**Huszár G:** A budapesti Fogorvostudományi Kar negyedszázados története. **Fogorv Sz** 1980 Dec;73(12):356–8
**Huszár G:** A magyar fogászat feilódése Arkövytól napjainkig. **Orv Hetil** 1982 May 16;123(20):1243–6
**Huszár G:** A parodontológia magyar úttöröi. **Fogorv Sz** 1984 Apr;77(4):109–14
**Huszár G:** Abonyi József, a hazai protetika úttöröje. **Fogorv Sz** 1980 Jun;73(6):187–91
**Huszár G:** Ady Endre fogbántalmairól. **Orv Hetil** 1984 Oct 14;125(42):2575–6
**Huszár G:** Az önéletrajzok, mint fogorvostörténelmünk forrásai. **Orvostort Kozl** 1980;89–91(26 no 1–3):157–74
**Huszár G:** Emlékezés Simon Béla professzorra. **Fogorv Sz** 1983 May;76(5):151–5
**Huszár L, Varannai G:** Medicina in nummis: Hungarian medals relating to medicine. Budapest, Semmelweis Medical Historical Museum, Library, and Archives, 1977. 215 p.
**Hutch RA:** Explorations in character: Gamaliel Bradford and Henry Murray as psychobiographers. **Biography** 1981;4(4):312–25
**Hutchens KS:** The Indianapolis influenza epidemic of 1918. **Indiana Hist Soc** 1979 Dec;5(4):4–16
**Hutchinson F** see **McBryde AM**
**Hutchinson GE** see **Bateson W**
**Hutchinson JF:** Science, politics, and the alcohol problem in post-1905 Russia. **Slav East Eur Rev** 1980;58(2):232–54
**Hutchinson JF:** Society, corporation or Union? Russian physicians and the struggle for professional unity (1890–1913). **Jahrb Gesch Osteur** 1982;30(1):37–53

**Hutchison K:** What happened to occult qualities in the scientific revolution? **ISIS** 1982 Jun;73(267):233-53
**Huter F:** Apothekenwesen und Apothekerstudium in Tirol. **Anz Philol Hist Kl Osterr Akad Wiss** 1979;116:199-221
**Huter F:** Beiträge zur Geschichte des Apothekenwesens in Tirol [pt. 1]. **Tirol Heimat** 1977;41:5-43
**Huter F:** Beiträge zur Geschichte des Apothekerwesens in Tirol: I. Kapitel: Die voruniversitäre Periode. **Tirol Heimat** 1978;41:5-43
**Huter F:** Beiträge zur Geschichte des Apothekerwesens in Tirol (II). Von der Errichtung der Universität Innsbruck (1669) bis zu ihrer ersten Aufhebung (1782). **Tirol Heimat** 1978;42:5-51
**Huter F:** Die Wiedererrichtung des medizinisch-chirurgischen Studiums zu Innsbruck nach 1814. **Tirol Heimat** 1967-68;31-32:57-77
**Huter F:** Ein tiroler Student erlebt den Beginn der Wiener Märzrevolution. **Tirol Heimat** 1972;36:131-9
**Huter F:** Von der medizinischen Versorgung unserer alten Berggemeinden. **Tirol Heimat** 1975;39:5-31
**Huth EJ** see **Davis NE**
**Hutin S:** La vie quotidienne des alchimistes au moyen âge. Paris, Hachette, 1977. 254 p.
**Hutner G:** MSNJ: America's first and oldest medical society. **J Med Soc NJ** 1984 Sep;81(9):718-21
**Hutner R:** O rozwoju teorii pielęgnowania. **Pieleg Polozna** 1983;(6):8-9
**Hutt MS:** Historical introduction, Burkitt's lymphoma, nasopharyngeal carcinoma and Kaposi's sarcoma. **Trans R Soc Trop Med Hyg** 1981;75(6):761-5
**Hutt PB:** About fairness in applying the law. **FDA Consum** 1981 Jun;15(5):23-5
**Hutt PB:** Food and drug law: a strong and continuing tradition. In Hammer SN, ed: Symposium for the 75th Anniversary of the Food, Drug & Cosmetic Act, Meat Inspection Act, 1906-1981. Monday, June 8, 1981. Washington, D.C. **Food Drug Cosmet Law J** 1982 Jan;37(1):123-37
**Hutt PB:** Investigations and reports respecting FDA regulation of new drugs (Part I). **Clin Pharmacol Ther** 1983 Apr;33(4):537-48
**Hutter RV:** Classics in Oncology. Lobular carcinoma in situ by Foote and Stewart. **CA** 1982 Jul-Aug;32(4):232-7
**Huttmann A:** Eine imaginäre Krankheit: der Polyp des Herzens. **Medizinhist J** 1983;18(1-2):43-51
**Huttmann A:** Nichtärzte als erste Röntgenologen. **ROFO** 1982 Jan;136(1):85-8
**Hutton DA:** Cordial waters and cordial chests. **Pharm Hist (London)** 1973 Sep;3(2):6-8
**Hutton DA:** York bellfounders and their mortars. **Pharm Hist (London)** 1984 Sep;14(3):2-5
**Hutzinger O** see **Wijbenga A**
**Huusen AH:** Geboortenregeling in de moderne tijd. **Spiegel Hist** 1981;16(2):66-70
**Huyghe R** see **Bernard J**
**Huzel JP:** The demographic impact of the old poor law: more reflexions on Malthus. **Econ Hist Rev** 1980;33:367-81
**Hyatt R:** Chinese herbal medicine. **Herbal Rev** 1979;4(3):9-15
**Hyde A:** Hospital life: a breath of good sea air. **Health Soc Serv J** 1980 Jan 18;90(4676):78-9
**Hyde A:** Still set to serve the needy. **Health Soc Serv J** 1980 Mar 7;90(4683):314-5
**Hyde GL** see **Clark D**
**Hyerstay BJ** see **Erickson RC**
**Hylland RG:** Further evidence for plasmapheresis. **Arthritis Rheum** 1980 Jan;23(1):129
**Hyman HH:** Samuel Andrew Stouffer. In Dictionary of American Biography, Suppl. 6, 1956-1960. p. 604-6, 1980.
**Hyman V:** The autobiographical present in 'A Sketch of the Past'. **Psychoanal Rev** 1983 Spring;70(1):24-32
**Hyman VR:** Concealment and disclosure in Sir Leslie Stephen's mausoleum book. **Biography** 1980;3(2):121-31
**Hynes CJ:** The regulation of nursing homes: a case study. **Proc Acad Polit Sci** 1980;33(4):126-36
**Hynes J:** The remunerative advantages of ineffective medicines. **MIMS Mag** 1981 May 15;:70-3
**Hypnotherapy--past, present and future: Med J Aust** 1979 Sep 22;2(6):288
**Hyson JM:** William Saunders: the United States Army's first dentist--West Point's forgotten man. **Milit Med** 1984 Aug;149(8):435-41

# I

**I mutamenti del 'potere medico' in Francia dalla Rivoluzione ad oggi secondo Jean-Paul Aron: Minerva Med** 1982 Jul 14;73(28-29):2010-2
**I simpozij o historiji mikrobiologije i imunologije u Hrvatskoj do 1923. godine:** Zagreb, Jugoslavenskoj, akademiji, 1973. 126 p.
**Iafaev RKh** see **Rykushin IuP**
**Iancu-Agou D:** L'inventaire de la bibliothèque et du mobilier d'un médecin juif d'Aix-en-Provence au milieu du XVe siècle. **Rev Etud Juives** 1975;134(1-2):47-80
**Ianovskiĭ AG:** Fel'dshera i akusherki v revoliutsii 1905-1907 gg. **Feldsher Akush** 1980;45(11):41-4
**Ianushkevichus ZI, Krikshtopaĭtis MI:** O razvitii zdravookhraneniia Litovskoĭ SSR. **Klin Med (Mosk)** 1982 Dec;60(12):38-41
**Ianushkevichus ZI:** Razvitie ideĭ i rabot S. P. Botkina i ego shkoly v kardiologii i klinicheskoĭ farmakologii. **Vestn Akad Med Nauk SSSR** 1983;(3):14-7
**Iarchuk NI** see **Kozlov VA**
**Iaremchuk AIâ, et al:** [Importance of museums in optimizing the academic process and academic research work of students in a department of surgery.] (Rus). **Klin Khir** 1981;2:47-9
**Iarmonenko SP:** Klinicheskaia radiobiologiia--nauchnaia osnova luchevoĭ terapii opukholeĭ. **Med Radiol (Mosk)** 1982 Mar;27(3):6-9
**Iarochkin VS** see **Koziner VB**
**Iaroshevski MG, Gurgenidze GS:** L. S. Vygotski o prirode psikhiki. **Vopr Filos** 1981;(1):142-54
**Iaroshevskiĭ MG:** Genezis issledovatel'skoĭ programmy I. P. Pavlova (istoricheskoe znachenie madridskoĭ rechi I. P. Pavlova). **Zh Vyssh Nerv Deiat** 1984 Jan-Feb;34(1):3-13
**IAroshevskiĭ MG:** Uolter Kennon (1871-1945). Moskva, Nauka, 1976. 374 p.
**Iarovinskiĭ MI:** Zdravookhranenie Moskvy v gody Velikoĭ Otechestvennoĭ voĭny. **Sov Zdravookhr** 1983;(7):63-7
**Iarovinskiĭ MIa:** K otsenke pammiatnikov istorii meditsiny. **Sov Zdravookhr** 1981;(9):72-4
**Iarovinskiĭ MIa:** Rol' istorii meditsiny v deontologicheskoĭ podgotovke meditsinskikh rabotnikov. **Sov Zdravookhr** 1982;(4):51-3
**Iarovinskiĭ MIa, Goncharova SG:** Vklad medikov Moskvy v zdravookhranenie sredneaziatskikh respublik. **Sov Zdravookhr** 1983;(1):64-7
**Iarovinskiĭ MIa:** 100 let sanitarnoĭ organizatsii goroda Moskvy. **Sov Zdravookhr** 1984;(9):45-9
**Iartsev VV** see **Konovalov AN**
**Iarygin VN:** Nekotorye problemy darvinizma na sovremonnom étape. **Arkh Anat Gistol Embriol** 1982 Nov;83(11):7-17
**IAstreb NI:** Razvitie terapii v Ukrainskoĭ SSR. Kiev, Zdorov'ia, 1978. 165 p.
**Iastrebov VK:** Nauchnoe nasledie S. P. Karpova v oblasti prirodno-ochagovykh infektsiĭ. **Zh Mikrobiol Epidemiol Immunobiol** 1983 Oct;(10):113-5
**Iatsekevich IaE** see **Chaplinskiĭ VV**
**Ibarra LG:** Rehabilitationsdienste in territorialen Gesundheitseinrichtungen. **Z Gesamte Hyg** 1981;27(2):111-3
**Ibell BM:** The development of nursing as a profession. In her: Integrated basic theory and practice of nursing. Victoria, Pitmen, 1979. p. 65-75.
**Ibert M:** Contribution à l'étude historique de l'hôpital Ste-Marthe d'Avignon, période 1670-1740. Marseille, Pronto-Offset impr., 1979. 914 p. (Thèse, Marseille, 1979).
**Ibn Masawayh Y:** Le livre des axiomes médicaux (aphorismi). Edition du texte arabe et des versions latines avec traduction française et lexique par Danielle Jacquart et Gérard Troupeau. Geneva, Librairie Droz, 1980. iii, 368 p. (Centre de Recherches d'Histoire et de Philologie, II; Hautes Etudes Orientales, 14).
**Ibragimov NG:** Iz istorii podgotovki meditsinskikh sester v nasheĭ strane. **Med Sestra** 1982 Feb;41(02):55-7
**Ibragimov NG:** K istorii okhrany zdorov'ia neftianikov Bashkirii v 30-40-e gody. **Sov Zdravookhr** 1984;(4):65-8
**Ibragimov NG:** Meditsinskaia obshchestvennost' Bashkirii v gody grazhdanskoĭ i Velikoĭ Otechestvennoĭ voĭn. **Feldsher Akush** 1980;45(5):56-9
**Ibragimov NG:** Rol' obshchestvennosti v deiatel'nosti Ufimskogo gorodskogo Soveta po okhrane zdorov'ia naseleniia v pervye desiatiletiia Sovetskoĭ vlasti. **Sov Zdravookhr** 1981;(2):67-71
**Ibragimov NG:** Sanitarnyĭ aktiv Bashkirii v pervye desiatiletiia Sovetskoĭ vlasti. **Sov Zdravookhr** 1980;(7):56-60
**Ibragimov NG:** Stanovlenie i razvitie sotsial'nogo strakhovaniia v Bashkirii. **Sov Zdravookhr** 1983;5:58-61
**Ibragimov NG:** Uchastie obshchestvennosti v organizatsii okhrany zdorov'ia deteĭ v Bashkirii v pervoe desiatiletie Sovetskoĭ vlasti. **Sov Zdravookhr** 1979;(12):44-7
**Ibragimov NG** see **Chokin AR**
**Ibragimova ZI, Burak GG, Ol'shannikova VV, et al:** 50 let kafedre anatomii cheloveka Vitebskogo meditsinskogo instituta. **Arkh Anat Gistol Embriol** 1984 Jul;87(7):95-6
**Ibrahim MA, Kaplan BH, Patrick RC, et al:** The legacy of John C. Cassel. **Am J Epidemiol** 1980 Jul;112(1):1-7
**Ichinomiya-shi Ishikaishi Henshu Iinkai:** Ichinomiya-shi Ishikai shi. Ichinomiya, Japan, Ichinomiya-shi Ishikai, Showa 52 nen, 1977. 21, 1013 p.
**Idelberger K:** Erlebte Orthopädie (1937-1977). **Jahrb Univ Dusseld** 1977-78;:135-52
**Idel'chik KI:** A. P. Golubkov: 1880-1945. Moskva, Meditsina, 1980. 78 p.
**Idel'chik KhI:** Iz istorii meditsinskogo fakul'teta Moskovskogo universiteta. **Sov Zdravookhr** 1981;(2):60-4
**Idel'chik KhI:** K isotorii izdatel'stva 'Meditsina'. **Sov Zdravookhr** 1979;(10):54-9
**Idel'chik KhI:** K istorii izucheniia zdorov'ia rabochikh, zaniatykh v neftianoĭ promyshlennosti Azerbaĭdzhanskoĭ SSR v 20--30-e gody. **Sov Zdravookhr** 1982;(7):55-9
**Idel'chik KhI:** Nauchno-issledovatel'skie instituty gigieny truda i professional'nykh zabolevaniĭ v SSSR v 20--30-kh godakh (k 60-letiiu organizatsii pervogo instituta). **Gig Tr Prof Zabol** 1984 Sep;(9):30-2
**Idel'chik KhI:** Problema bor'by s alkogolizmom v nauchnoĭ obshchestvennoĭ deiatel'nosti professora L. S. Minora (k 125-letiiu so dnia rozhdeniia). **Sov Zdravookhr** 1981;(3):63-6
**Idel'chik KhI, Shtil'man NL:** Vazhnyĭ étap v razvitii russko-nemetskikh meditsinskikh sviazeĭ. **Sov Zdravookhr** 1982;(6):72-5
**Idel'chik KhI:** Vrachi-bol'sheviki S. I. Mitskevich i S. I. Chernomordik

u istokov Tsentral'nogo muzeia revoliutsii SSSR (k 60-letiiu muzeia). **Sov Zdravookhr** 1984;(9):56-9

**Idel'chik KhI** see **Lotova EI**

**Iftimovici R:** Constantin Levaditi, a forerunner of the modern research and interpretation of virus multiplication. **Virologie** 1979 Jul-Sep;30(3):237-42

**Igartua JE:** Le comportement démographique des marchands de Montréal vers 1760. **Rev Hist Am Fr** 1979;33(3):427-45

**Iglesias F:** Características de la población cubana en 1862. **Rev Bibl Nac Jose Marti** 1980;22(3):89-110

**Iglesias JG:** Origenes y evolucion de la odontoestomatologia en España. **Acta Odontol Venez** 1981 Sep-Dec;19(3):305-12

**Iglesias M** see **Aguirre Zozaya F**

**Ignatov D:** Istoricheski danni po vŭprosa za lechenieto na peritonita. **Probl Khig** 1980;8:154-63

**Ignatovich FI, Semeniuk SI:** Zh. E. Zhiliber i ego 'Flora Litvy'. **Sov Zdravookhr** 1981;(11):67-9

**Ihde AJ:** Conrad Arnold Elvehjem. In Dictionary of American biography, 1961-1965. Suppl. 7, 1981. p. 223-4.

**Ihde AJ:** Food controls under the 1906 act. In Young JH, ed: The early years of federal food and drug control. Madison, American Institute of the History of Pharmacy, 1982. p. 40-50.

**Ihde AJ:** Kurt Guenter Stern. In Dictionary of American Biography, Suppl. 6, 1956-1960. p. 595-6, 1980.

**Ihde AJ:** Lydia Jane Roberts. In: Notable American women. The modern period. Cambridge, Mass., Belknap-Harvard Univ. Press, 1980. 4:580-1.

**Ihde AJ** see **Kieft L**

**Iijima E:** [Records of hallucination: my attraction to Jung's world of hallucination]. (Jpn) **Kango Kyoiku** 1980 Feb;21(2):74-8

**Iio M:** Professor G. V. Hevesy, Doctor Y. Nishina and nuclear medicine in Japan. **Radiat Med** 1983 Jul-Sep;1(3):255-62

**Ikard RW:** The Nashville Academy of Medicine 'Yankee Gunboat' Gavel. **J Tenn Med Assoc** 1982 Aug;75(8):530-2

**Ikemi A** see **Ikemi Y**

**Ikemi Y, Ikemi A:** Psychosomatic medicine: a meeting ground of Eastern and Western medicine. **J Am Soc Psychosom Dent Med** 1983;30(1):3-16

**Ikeya M** see **Mascarenhas S**

**Ikezawa Y, Kono H:** [The starting point in nursing--an observation through the history of European ideology] (Jpn). **Kango Tenbo** 1981 Oct;6(10):905-13

**Ikic D** see **Kraljevic M**

**Ikonnikov MV** see **Miliavskiĭ VM**

**Il tripode si Sayre: Chir Organi Mov** 1981;66(2):279-81

**Ila B:** Contribution à l'histoire de la peste en Hongrie au XVIIIe siècle. In Charbonneau H, Larose A, ed: The great mortalities: methodological studies of demographic crises in the past. Liège, Belgium, Ordina Editions, 1980. p. 133-8.

**Il'chevich NV, Spasokukotskiĭ IuA, Alekseeva IN, et al:** Razvitie ideĭ A. A. Bogomol'tsa v oblasti ėksperimental'nogo izucheniia i primeneniia v praktike tsitotoksicheskikh syvorotok. **Fiziol Zh** 1981 May-Jun;27(3):339-46

**Iles JD:** Autopsy of an Egyptian mummy (Nakht--ROM I). **Can Med Assoc J** 1980 Mar 8;122(5):512-3

**Iles JD:** Velikovsky: psychiatrist, historian and catastrophist. **Can Med Assoc J** 1981 Sept 1;125(5):496-505

**Ilic D:** Conrad Meyer-Ahrens (1813-1872) und sein Werk über die Heilquellen und Kurorte der Schweiz. Zürich, Juris, 1975. 61 p.

**Iliescu R** see **Popa LM**

**Iliev N** see **Gŭdev Kh**

**Il'in AI:** Iz istorii sanitarno-statisticheskogo issledovaniia Vladimirskoĭ gubernii. **Gig Sanit** 1984 May;(5):35-7

**Il'in AI:** Iz istorii sanitarnogo prosveshcheniia vo Vladimirskoĭ gubernii v zemskiĭ period. **Gig Sanit** 1984 Jun;(6):32-5

**Il'in AI:** S. I. Sychugov--osnovopolozhnik sanitarnoĭ organizatsii Vladimirskoĭ gubernii. **Gig Sanit** 1983 Nov;:(11):53-5

**Il'in II, Preĭsman BS:** P. P. Zablotskiĭ-Desiatovskiĭ i ego rol' v razvitii venerologii v Rossii (k 100-letiiu so dnia smerti). **Vestn Dermatol Venerol** 1983 Dec;(12):59-60

**Il'inskiĭ II** see **Atabaev ShT**

**Illich I:** Medicalization and primary care. **J R Coll Gen Pract** 1982 Aug;32(241):463-70

**Illingworth C:** The sanguine mystery. 'This bloody and butcherly department of the healing art.' [London], Nuffield Provincial Hospitals Trust, 1970. 72 p.

**Illingworth R:** Historical concepts of spinal cord pathways subserving pain. In Rose FC, Bynum WF, ed: Historical aspects of the neurosciences. New York, Raven, 1982. p. 209-12.

**Illustrations from the Wellcome Institute Library:** A note on the botanical prints and drawings.

**Illustrations from the Wellcome Institute Library:** John Monro MD and Charles James Fox: etching by Thomas Rowlandson. **Med Hist** 1983 Jan;27(1):80-3

**Illustrations from the Wellcome Institute library:** The last moments of H. R. H. the Prince Consort. **Med Hist** 1982 Jul;26(3):321-4

**Ilnicki S:** Pomoc psychiatryczna na polu walki-ewolucja poglądów i metod postępowania. **Psychiatr Pol** 1980 Sep-Oct;14(5):539-46

**Im Hof U** see **Albrecht von Haller, 1708-1777**

**Imamuddin SM:** Maristan (Hospitals) in Medieval Spain. **Islam Stud** 1978;17(1):45-55

**Imanaga H:** [Honoring Theodor Billroth by attaining a hundred years since his first success in gastric cancer resection (author's transl)] (Jpn). **Nippon Gan Chiryo Gakkai Shi** 1981 Jun 20;16(3):405-8

**Imbault-Huart MJ:** La médecine au Moyen Age: à travers les manuscrits de la Bibliothèque Nationale. Paris, Editions de la porte verte: Bibliothèque nationale, 1983. 191 p.

**Imbault-Huart MJ:** La vieillesse: état pathologique ou ultime equilibre de vie? **Asclepio** 1983;35:301-15

**Imbault-Huart MJ:** Les chirurgiens et l'esprit chirurgical en France au XVIIIème siècle. **Clio Med** 1981 Apr;15(3-4):143-57

**Imbault-Huart MJ** see **Huard P**

**Imbault-Huart MJ** see **Huard PO**

**Imbault-Huart MJ** see **La médecine hospitalière française au XVIIIème siècle**

**Imbault-Huart MJ, ed:** Table ronde consacrée au recteur Pierre Huard (1901-1983). Contributions by J. L. Plessis, P. M. Niaussat, T. H. Nguyen, J. Théodoridès. **Hist Sci Med** 1983;17(4):381-402

**Imber M:** Analysis of a curriculum reform movement: the American Social Hygiene Association's campaign for sex education 1900-1930. Ph.D. Diss., Stanford University. Stanford, 1981. v, 173 leaves.

**Imber M:** The First World War, sex education, and the American Social Hygiene Association's campaign against venereal disease. **J Educ Adm Hist** 1984;16(1):47-56

**Imbert J, Mollat M:** Histoire des hôpitaux en France. Toulouse, Privat, 1982. 559 p.

**Imbert J:** L'assistance publique à Paris: le poids de l'histoire. **Rev Trav Acad Sci Morales Polit** 1978;131(2):675-89

**Imbroscio C:** Tissot e il suo tempo. **Atti Accad Sci Ist Bologna** 1978-1979, reçu 1980;67(1):323-43

**Imerti AD:** Vincenzo Catalani, Neapolitan Jacobin, jurist, reformer (1769-1843), with an appendix containing a translation of his work 'A digression on vaccination.' Lawrence, Kansas, Coronado Press, 1976. 155 p.

**Imhof A:** Les sermons funèbres comme source de la démographie historique pour la période de 1500 à 1650. **Ann Demogr Hist (Paris)** 1980;:79-86

**Imhof AE:** Die Uebersterblichkeit verheirateter Frauen im fruchtbaren Alter. Eine Illustration der 'condition féminine' im 19. Jahrhundert. **Z Bevoelkerungswiss** 1979;4:487-510

**Imhof AE:** Från ett osäkert till ett säkert liv. **Sydsven Medicinhist Sallsk Arsskr** 1983;:115-40

**Imhof AE:** La surmortalité des femmes mariées en age de procréation: un indice de la condition féminine au XIXe siècle. **Ann Demogr Hist (Paris)** 1981;:81-7

**Imhof AE:** Leib und Leben unserer Vorfahren: eine rhythmisierte Welt. In Imhof AE, ed: Leib und Leben in der Geschichte der Neuzeit. Berlin, Duncker & Humblot, 1983. p. 21-38.

**Imhof AE:** Man and body in the history of the modern age. Reflections on an International Symposium in Berlin, 1-3 December 1981. **Med Hist** 1983 Oct;27(4):394-406

**Imhof AE:** Mensch und Gesundheit in der Geschichte; Bericht über eine internationale Tagung in Berlin, 20.-23. September 1978. **Ber Wissenschaftsgesch** 1978;1(3-4):235-44

**Imhof AE:** Mensch und Gesundheit in Geschichte und Gegenwart. **Jahrb Gesch** 1979;1(3):29-33

**Imhof AE:** Recherches macroregionales sur la mortalité en Europe septentrionale sous l'ancien regime. In Charbonneau H, Larose A, ed: The great mortalities: methodological studies of demographic crises in the past. Liège, Belgium, Ordina Editions, 1980. p. 139-56.

**Imhof AE:** Säuglingssterblichkeit im europäischen Kontext, 17.-20 Jahrhundert. Ueberlegungen zu einem Buch von Anders Brändström. Umeå, Umeå University, 1984. 73 p. (Demographic Data Base, Newsletter No. 2)

**Imhof AE:** The analysis of eighteenth-century causes: some methodological considerations. **Hist Methods Newsl** 1978;2(1):3-36

**Imhof AE:** Ursachen und Folgen der zunehmenden durchschnittlichen Lebenserwartung seit dem 17. Jahrhundert; Bericht über eine interdisziplinäre Tagung an der Ecole des Hautes Etudes en Sciences Sociales, Paris, 24.-26. Oktober 1979. **Ber Wissenschaftsgesch** 1979;3(3-4):212-18

**Imhof AE:** Von der unsicheren zur sicheren Lebenszeit. Ein folgenschwerer Wandel im Verlaufe der Neuzeit. **Vierteljahrsschr Soz Wirtschgesch** 1984;71(2):175-98

**Imhof AE** see **Lindskog BI**

**Imhof P** see **Avellano E**

**Imhof AE, ed:** Leib und Leben in der Geschichte der Neuzeit: Vorträge eines internationalen Colloquiums. Berlin, Duncker & Humblot, 1983. 266 p. Text in German and French. (Berliner Historische Studien, Bd. 9. Einzelstudien 2).

**Imhof AE, ed:** Mensch und Gesundheit in der Geschichte. Vorträge eines Internationalen Colloquiums in Berlin vom 20. bis 23. September 1978. Husum, Matthiesen, 1980. viii, 415 p. (Abhandlungen zur Geschichte der Medizin und der Naturwissenschaften, 39).

**Immunology and virology--a 25 year retrospective:** Proceedings of the Silver Jubilee Symposium sponsored by The Wistar Institute in honor of Hilary Koprowski. **J Cell Physiol [Suppl]** 1982;2:1-147

**Impact of swine non-flu: Lancet** 1982 Nov 6;2(8306):1029

**Imperato PJ:** A historical overview of amebiasis. **Bull NY Acad Med** 1981 Apr;57(3):175-87

**Imperato PJ:** Early modern medical services at Moyale, Kenya. **East Afr Med J** 1983 Jun;60(6):367-73

**In honor of the memory of Ghislaine van Massenhove, international president of CICIAMS: Nouv Com Int Cathol Infirm Assist Med Soc** 1980;(1):1-24

**In memoriam. Dorothy Burlingham. 1891-1979.: Psychoanal Study Child**

1980;35:ix–xxii
**In memoriam Professor Dr. Marcel Florkin (1900–1979): Clio Med** 1980 May;14(2):89–90
**In the spirit of C.-E. A. Winslow: J Public Health Policy** 1980 Mar;1(1):3–5
**Inciardi JA:** The changing life of Mickey Finn: some notes on chloral hydrate down through the ages. **J Pop Cult** 1977;11(3):591–6
**The Indiana Medical History Museum: Indiana Med Hist Q** 1974;1(1):11–21
**Indretningen af Augustenborg Slot til lazaret i krigen 1848–1850 – en 'chronique scandaleuse'?: Dan Medicinhist Arbog** 1980;:91–123
**Ineson A** see **Thom D**
**Informazioni bibliografiche: Stor Crit Psicol** 1981;2(1):187–98
**Informe de labores con motivo del XXXIV aniversario del Instituto Nacional de la Nutricion: Rev Invest Clin** 1981 Jan–Mar;33(1):91–108
**Ingelfinger FJ:** Medicine. Status and future of applied sciences. **Science** 1980 Jul 4;209(4452):123–6
**Ingells DT:** Miss Cora Dow. **Cinci Hist Soc Bull** 1982;40(3):151–66
**Ingle ST:** Parliament and health policy: the role of MPs, 1970–75. Farnborough, Gower, 1981 vi, 171 p.
**Ingleby D:** The social construction of mental illness. In P. Wright, A. Treacher, ed: The problem of medical knowledge. Examining the social construction of medicine. Edinburgh, Edinburgh University Press, 1982. p. 123–43.
**Inglis B:** The diseases of civilisation. London, Hodder and Stoughton, 1981. xi, 371 p.
**Ingraham LH, Manning FJ:** Psychiatric battle casualties: the missing column in a war without replacements. **Milit Rev** 1980;60(8):18–29
**Ingraham RL:** Evolution in context. **San Jose Stud** 1982;8(3):4–19
**Ingram A:** The country animal doctor. Aylesbury, Bucks, Shire, 1979. 32 p. (Shire album; no. 40).
**Ingram J, Fischenich J:** Physician reimbursement. **Top Health Care Financ** 1982 Fall;9(1):32–52
**Inguaggiato B:** Evoluzione tecnologica del pace-maker. **Minerva Med** 1980 Oct 6;71(38):2793–6
**Inhelder B:** Genetic epistemology and developmental psychology. In R. W. Rieber, K. Salzinger, ed: Psychology: theoretical-historical perspectives. New York, Academic Press, 1980. p. 315–27.
**Inkster I:** Lunacy and the Industrial Revolution. Programme notes. **Soc Soc Hist Med Bull** 1980;27:43–6
**Inkster I, Morrell J:** Metropolis and province; science in British culture, 1780–1850. Philadelphia, University of Pennsylvania Press, 1983. 288 p.
**Inkster I:** Scientific culture and education in Nottingham, 1800–1843. **Trans Thoroton Soc** 1979;82
**Innes C** see **Langner SR**
**Innes J:** The Harveians of Edinburgh--their first two hundred years. **Scott Med J** 1983 Jul;28(3):285–9
**Inomata H:** Yoshiaki Taniguchi, M.D. **Jpn J Ophthalmol** 1983;27(1):1–8
**Inoue N, Kuo CH, Ito G, et al:** [Dental caries in Japanese remains (author's transl)] (Jpn). **Koku Eisei Gakkai Zasshi** 1981 Jul;31(2):90–7
**Inoue N:** [Dental diseases in Kamakura period (author's transl)] (Jpn). **Shikai Tenbo** 1980;(12):1009–18
**Inoue N:** [Historical view of maxilofacial development] (Jpn). **Nippon Shika Ishikai Zasshi** 1982;35(7):743–8
**Inque H:** Le problème de l'opium durant la période Jiaqing et Daoguang. **Toyoschi Kenkyu** 1982;41(1):58–83, 3–4
**Institut mikrobiologii i virusologii im. D. K. Zabolotnogo AN USSR--gorodu-iubiliaru: Mikrobiol Zh** 1982 Mar–Apr;44(2):3–4
**Institutu fiziologii imeni A. A. Bogomol'tsa Akademii nauk USSR--50 let: Neirofiziologiia** 1984;16(3):283–5
**The interaction of acoustical and electromagnetic fields with biological systems:** A collection of papers from the symposium honoring Professor Herman P. Schwan on the occasion of his 65th birthday. Philadelphia, November 24 and 25, 1980. **Prog Clin Biol Res** 1982;86:1–183
**Interferon: twenty-five years on: Philos Trans R Soc Lond [Biol]** 1982 Sep 24;299(1094):1–144
**International Congress of the History of Medicine, 26th, Plovdiv [Bulgaria], 20–25 August 1978:** Actes du Congres, 2 volumes. Sofia, 1980–81. Articles in Russian, French, English, German.
**International Congress of the History of Medicine, 27th, Barcelona, 1980: XXVII Congreso Internacional de Historia de la Medicina, 31 agosto – 6 septiembre 1980:** Actas. Barcelona, Acadèmia de Ciències Mèdique de Catalunya i Balears, 1981. 2 Vol., 799 p.
**The International Federation of Surgical Colleges:** 1958–1980. **Ann R Coll Surg Engl** 1981;63:290–2
**International Symposium on Cardiac Pacing, 5th, Tokyo, 1976:** Tawara memorial note. Tokyo, Organizing Committee of the Symposium, 1976. 28 p.
**Ioanid N, Angelescu B:** Fraţii Minovici. Bucureşti, Editura Ştiinţifică, 1970. 174 p.
**Ioffe LTs** see **Aliev MA**
**Ioksa VA** see **Popushoĭ EP**
**Ionasescu V** see **Zellweger H**
**Ionescu C:** Des 'remèdes' appliqués dans le district Prahova, par la médecine populaire, à fin du XIX siècle et le début du XX siècle. In: Congrès international d'histoire de la médecine, XXVe, Québec, 1976. Actes. Québec, 1977. p. 790–7.
**Ionescu C** see **Lazăr C**
**Ionov AIu** see **Ionov IuV**
**Ionov IuV, Ionov AIu:** A. P. Borodin – vrach, khimik, pedagog (k 150–letiiu so dnia rozhdeniia). **Sov Zdravookhr** 1984;(1):61–4
**Ionov IuV:** A. P. Chekhov i meditsina. **Feldsher Akush** 1980;45(6):51–4
**Ionov IuV, Ionov AIu:** Fel'dsher P. K. Beletskiĭ--pisatel', publitsist, étnograf, obshchestvennyĭ deiatel'. **Feldsher Akush** 1982;47(1):55–8
**Ionov IuV:** Fel'dshera i meditsinskie sestry--sportsmeny. **Feldsher Akush** 1980;45(7):5–7
**Ionov IuV:** Meditsinskie temy v proizvedeniiakh V. M. Garshina (k 125–letiiu so dnia rozhdeniia). **Klin Med (Mosk)** 1981 Jan;59(1):110–2
**Ionov IuV:** Narodovolets Sof'ia Perovskaia i ee meditsinskaia deiatel'nost'. **Feldsher Akush** 1982;47(10):41–2
**Ionov IuV:** Raboty Fridrikha Shellera kak vracha, ego meditsinskie dissertatsii i bolezn' (k 175–letiiu so dnia smerti). **Klin Med (Mosk)** 1981 Jun;59(6):112–5
**Ionov IuV:** Sal'vador Al'ende i ego meditsinskaia deiatel'nost'. **Feldsher Akush** 1981;46(2):39–41
**Ionov IuV, Ionov AIu:** Vklad russkikh vracheĭ v issledovanie Kamchatki i Dal'nego Vostoka v XIX veke. **Sov Zdravookhr** 1981;(10):59–62
**Ionov IuV, Ionov AIu:** Vrach I. L. Iavorskiĭ – issledovatel' Afganistana. **Sov Zdravookhr** 1983;(12):49–51
**Iorio M** see **Robetti I**
**Iqbal Ali M:** Contribution of Avicenna to medicine. **Bull Indian Inst Hist Med (Hyderabad)** 1981;1–4:139–45
**Irblich E** see **Camerino G**
**Ireland RL** see **Pike JS**
**Ireland T** see **Bannister T**
**Ireland and medicine: MD** 1979 Mar;23(3):81–93
**Irey TR:** Soldiering, suffering, and dying in the Mexican War. **J West** 1972;11(2):285–98
**Irgens LM:** The discovery of Mycobacterium leprae. A medical achievement in the light of evolving scientific methods. **Am J Dermatopathol** 1984 Aug;6(4):337–43
**Irgens LM:** Trafikkulykkenes epidemiologi: årsaksforhold og forebyggelse fra medisinsk synsvinkel. **Tidsskr Samfunnsforskning** 1981;22(1):17–38
**Iria A:** Evocação de Júlio Dantas no l. centenário do seu nascimento: duas raridades bibliográficas do médico militar. **An Acad Port Hist** 1979;25:359–84
**Iriarte DR:** [Public health in Venezuela]. **Rev Soc Venez Hist Med** 1975–76;23(37):107–21
**Irigoin J:** Tradition manuscrite et histoire du texte. Quelques problèmes relatifs à la collection hippocratique. In La collection hippocratique et son rôle dans l'histoire de la médecine. Colloque de Strasbourg (23–27 octobre 1972) organisé par le Centre de Recherches sur la Grèce Antique, avec le concours des Facultés de Philosophie et des Langues Classiques. Leiden, E. J. Brill, 1975. p. 3–18.
**Irigoin J** see **Grmek MD, ed**
**Irion U** see **Brede K**
**Irmer C** see **Grmek MD, ed**
**Irmer D** see **Grmek MD, ed**
**Irmer D** see **Strohmaier G**
**Irsigler FJ:** Evolution and hominization. **Mankind Q** 1981 Spring;21(3):211–26
**Irueste FG** see **Alvarez de Morales C**
**Irving D** see **Broszat M**
**Irwin LN:** Fulfillment and frustration: the confessions of a behavioral biochemist. **Perspect Biol Med** 1978 Spring;21(3):476–91
**Isaac O, Kristen G:** Alte und neue Wege der Kamillentherapie. Die Kamille als Beispiel für moderne Arzneipflanzenforschung. **Med Welt** 1980 Aug 8;31(31–32):1145–9
**Isaacs H:** European influences in Islamic medicine. In: Mashriq. Proc. of the Eastern Mediterranean Seminar ... 1977–1978. Manchester, University, 1980. p. 25–9.
**Isaacs H:** The impact of western medicine on Muslim physicians and their writings in the 17th century. **Bull Br Assoc Orient** 1979–80,N.Ser.;11:52–7
**Isacsson A:** A study of Louis J. Weichmann. **Lincoln Her** 1978;80(1):25–38
**Isambert FA:** Bio-éthique et techniques biomédicales. **Soc Sci Inf** 1983;22(1):125–37
**Isbell HS:** Development of concepts of ring conformation and neighboring group effects prior to 1940. In Harmon RE, ed: Asymmetry of carbohydrates. New York, Dekker, 1979. p 1–14.
**Isbell H, ed** see **Martin WR**
**Isbister JD, McGaw N:** Regulation of health care in the United States. **J Health Hum Resour Adm** 1978 Aug;1(1):11–29
**Isbister JP:** Direct blood transfusion. **Med J Aust** 1980 Feb 9;1(3):136
**Iscru GD:** Prima carte de cunoştinţe veterinare tiparita şi difuzata in tara Romaneasca. **An Univ Bucur Istor** 1978;27:69–71
**Iselin HK:** Zur Entstehung von C. G. Jungs 'Psychologischen Typen.' Der Briefwechsel zwischen C. G. Jung und Hans Schmid-Guisan im Lichte ihrer Freundschaft. Aarau, Sauerländer, 1982. 152 p. (Veröffentlichungen der Schweizerischen Gesellschaft für Geschichte der Medizin und der Naturwissenschaften, Bd. 38).
**Isenburg T:** Il dibattito su Malthus e sulla popolazione nell'Italia di fine '800. **Studi Stor** 1977;18(3):41–67
**Isetts CA:** Medical libraries in Cincinnati. **Cinci Hist Soc Bull** 1980 Spring;38(1):51–71
**Ishigaki Y, Uzawa Y:** [Historical review of continuing education in Hokkaido University Hospital] (Jpn). **Kango Tenbo** 1984 Nov;9(11):1021–32
**Ishigoro T:** [Historical background of the 'hara-obi' (a piece of cloth wrapped around the abdomen of a pregnant woman) and the origin of its name] (Jpn). **Josanpu Zasshi** 1984;38(4):336–9; (5):437–40; (6):519–23
**Ishiguro T:** [History of the abdominal binder. 4. Use of the abdominal binder by pregnant women: views by foreigners and opposition to its use] (Jpn). **Josanpu Zasshi** 1984 Jul;38(7):615–7
**Ishihara T** see **Kogiso M**

**Ishihara T** see **Miyasato K**
**Ishii A:** Seishin igaku shippeishi. Tokyo, Kongo Shuppan, [1981]. 161 p.
**Ishii T:** [Clinical pathology in the past 30 years] (Jpn) **Rinsho Byori** 1984 May;32(5):484–9
**Ishikawa E** see **Kageyama K**
**Ishikawa no kokuho yonjunen:** [Kanazawa, Japan], Ishikawa-ken, Showa 53 nen. [1978]. 221 p.
**Iskandar AZ:** An attempted reconstruction of the late Alexandrian medical curriculum. **Med Hist** 1976 Jul;20(3):235–58
**Iskandar AZ:** Another fragment from the autograph of Ibn Al-Tilmidh's 'Marginal commentary on Ibn Sina's Canon of medicine'. **Bull Sch Orient Afr Stud** 1981;44:253–61
**Iskander Z, Harris J, Shafik Farid:** Further evidence of dental prothesis in ancient Egypt. **Ann Serv Antiq Egypte** 1979;63(spécial);Mélanges Selim Hassan II:103–13
**Iskenderov AI** see **Bakhshiev BA**
**Iskhaki IuB, Kal'shteĭn LI:** Rol' Abu Ali Ibn-Siny v razvitii otorinolaringologii. **Vestn Otorinolaringol** 1980 Nov–Dec;(6):81–5
**Iskhakov SI:** Razvitie sanitarnogo prosveshcheniia v Tadzhikskoĭ SSR. **Feldsher Akush** 1982;47(11):26–9
**Isliker B:** Christian Ludwig Bachmanns Dissertation 'Uber die Wirkungen der Musik auf den Menschen' (Erlangen 1792). Zürich, Juris Druck, 1982. 76 p. (Zürcher Medizingeschichtliche Abhandlungen, Neue Reihe, Nr. 154).
**Ismail M, Raheem Rafeeq MA:** Anatomy of eye and the mechanism of vision according to Avicenna. **Bull Indian Inst Hist Med (Hyderabad)** 1981;1–4:146–51
**Ismét Luzsénszky Talmudja?:** **Orv Hetil** 1984 Aug 19;125(34):2086–7
**ISMS organization:** History of founding and expansion. **IMJ** 1981 Nov;160(5):297
**Isotani S** see **Noriyasu S**
**Ispirsky N:** Medical attendance for seafarers of the Bulgarian Marine from its establishments to present days. In International Congress of the History of Medicine. 26th, Plovdiv, 1978. Actes du Congress. Sofia, 1981. Volume II. p. 215–6.
**Israel L:** Le corps hystérique. **Soins Psychiatr** 1983 Jan;(27):15–9
**Israel S** see **Bourilkova L**
**Israelstam S, Lambert S:** Homosexuality as a cause of alcoholism: a historical review. **Int J Addict** 1983 Dec;18(8):1085–107
**Israili AH:** Humoral theory of Unani Tibb. **Indian J Hist Sci** 1981, reçu 1982;16(1):95–9
**Isser N** see **Schwartz LL**
**Issledovaniia po istorii estestvoznaniia i tekhniki v desiatoi piatiletke:** **Vopr Istor Estestvozn Tekh** 1981;1:3–12
**István L:** 1945. április 4. Korszakváltás kórházaink történetében. **Orv Hetil** 1983 Apr 3;124(14):803–5
**Ito G:** [Tooth to denture base discrepancy among Japanese during the Middle Ages] (Jpn). **Shikai Tenbo** 1980;(11):825–33
**Ito G** see **Inoue N**
**Ito H:** Health insurance policy development in Denmark and Sweden 1860--1950. **Soc Sci Med** 1979 Oct;13C(3):143–60
**Ito J:** [In search of educational humanity (5). Understanding of man in education (2): 'Emile' by Jean Jacques Rousseau] (Jpn). **Kango Kyoiku** 1983 May;24(5):310–4
**Iturralde G** see **Aguirre Zozaya F**
**Iudaev NA:** Sostoianie i puti razvitiia sovetskoĭ éndokrinologii. **Sov Med** 1982;(12):41–6
**Iudin KA** see **Speranskiĭ VS**
**Iuldashev KIu:** Vnutrenniaia meditsina Uzbekistana za 60 let. **Klin Med (Mosk)** 1982 Dec;60(12):29–32
**Iurikhin AP:** K 140-letiiu so dnia rozhdeniia Sergeia Petrovicha Kolomnina (1842–1886). **Klin Khir** 1982 Dec;(12):61–3
**Iurikhin AP:** N. I. Pirogov, ego ucheniki i posledovateli. **Klin Khir** 1984 May;(5):62–4
**Iurov IA, Grin' VA:** K 40-letiiu bitvy pod Moskvoĭ. **Voen Med Zh** 1981 Dec;(12):9–15
**Iurov IA, Grin' VA:** K 40-letiiu Stalingradskoĭ bitvy. **Voen Med Zh** 1982 Dec;(12):26–33
**Iurov IA, Grin' VA:** O meditsinskom obespechenii Belorusskoĭ operatsii. **Voen Med Zh** 1984 Jul;(7):8–16
**Iushkov MA** see **Lur'e GO**
**Ivan Luk'ianovich Bogdanov (k 80-letiiu so dnia rozhdeniia):** **Vrach Delo** 1983 Aug;(8):125–6
**Ivanenko AN** see **Dumbrov DA**
**Ivanhoe F:** Interglovular dentine in first and third molars: relation to hours of sunshine during growth in two archeological populations from England. **Calcif Tissue Int** 1982 Mar;34(2):136–44
**Ivaniushkin AIa:** Lenin--kul'tura--meditsina. **Farmakol Toksikol** 1980 May–Jun;43(3):261–5
**Ivan'kovich FA:** Opyt évakuatsii ranenykh i bol'nykh voenno-sanitarnymi letuchkami vo vremia Stalingradskoĭ bitvy. **Voen Med Zh** 1983 Feb;(2):68–70
**Ivanov C** see **Nikolaeva I**
**Ivanov EM:** Stanovlenie i razvitie otechestvennoĭ voenno-morskoĭ meditsiny. Leningrad, Meditsina, Leningradskoe otd-nie, 1976. 398 p.
**Ivanov IV** see **Nikulina TD**
**Ivanov NG, Georgievskiĭ AS:** Sergeĭ Petrovich Botkin i voenno-meditsinskaia akademiia. **Vestn Akad Med Nauk SSSR** 1983;(3):8–14
**Ivanov NG:** Sovetskoe voennoe zdravookhranenie nakanune i v gody Velikoĭ Otechestvennoĭ voĭny. **Sov Med** 1980;(5):3–10
**Ivanov NG:** Znachenie opyta Velikoĭ Otechestvennoĭ Voĭny dlia podgotovki voenno-meditsinskikh kadrov. **Voen Med Zh** 1980 May;(5):21–4
**Ivanov NM** see **Bragin AI**
**Ivanov S:** Razvitie i segashno sŭstoianie na Instituta po vŭtreshni bolesti. **Vutr Boles** 1981;20(6):1–6
**Ivanov VI:** O sochetannom primenenii akupunktury i medikamentoznoĭ terapii. **Voen Med Zh** 1982 Feb;(2):49–51
**Ivanová A** see **Bunčáková V**
**Ivanova K** see **Vutov M**
**Ivanovo-Kazas OM** see **Tokin BP**
**Ivanovskaia TE:** Patologicheskaia anatomiia bolezneĭ detskogo vozrasta na sovremennom étape. **Arkh Patol** 1983;45(10):3–8
**Ivashchenko IK:** Organizatsiia sanitarno-protivoépidemicheskikh meropriiatiĭ v voĭskakh Sibirskogo voennogo okruga v gody voĭny **Voen Med Zh** 1981 Mar;(3):11–2
**Ivern A:** El Muñiz de las Actas. (Tercer Congreso Nacional de Historia de la Medicina Argentina, 1973). **Sem Med** 1973;79(Aniversario):234–8
**Ivern A:** Muñiz presidente de la Facultad. (Tercer Congreso Nacional de Historia de la Medicina Argentina, 1973). **Sem Med** 1973;79(Aniversario):238–41
**Iveson-Iveson J:** A country midwife's tale. **Nurs Mirror** 1984 Apr 4;158(14):34–5
**Iveson-Iveson J:** A pin to see a peep show (Mary Seacole, Cicely Saunders). **Nurs Mirror** 1984 Mar 28;158(13):36
**Iveson-Iveson J:** Diploma of nursing. Part A: development of nursing as a profession. **Nurs Mirror** 1981 Feb 5;152(6):29–30
**Iveson-Iveson J:** History of nursing. **Nurs Mirror** 1982 Mar 24;154(12):34–6(continued periodically)
**Iveson-Iveson J:** History of nursing in the Air Force: string, sealing wax and individual daring. **Nurs Mirror** 1981 Jul 15;153(3):27–8
**Iveson-Iveson J:** History of the navy nurses: a life on the ocean waves. **Nurs Mirror** 1981 Jul 1;153(1):22–4
**Iveson-Iveson J:** Joined in parenthood. **Nurs Mirror** 1982 Sep 15;155(11):24
**Iveson-Iveson J:** Lesson from the past for trauma nursing. **Nurs Mirror** 1982 Jun 16;154(24):10
**Iveson-Iveson J:** Medical history. Napoleon: his final years. **Nurs Mirror** 1982 Aug 18;155(7):22–4
**Iveson-Iveson J:** Munchausen's syndrome: fantasy island (Rudolph Raspe). **Nurs Mirror** 1982 Jun 30;154(26):21
**Iveson-Iveson J:** Nurses in society: a legend in the breaking (Florence Nightingale). **Nurs Mirror** 1983 May 11;156(19):26–7
**Iveson-Iveson J:** Nursing Mirror midwifery forum. 10. Virgins and viragos. **Nurs Mirror** 1983 Nov 30;157(22):viii
**Iveson-Iveson J:** Profile: the forgotten heroine. (Mary Seacole). **Nurs Times** 1983 Sep 7;157(10):44–7
**Iveson-Iveson J:** St. David's day. **Nurs Mirror** 1984 Feb 29;158(9):16
**Iveson-Iveson J:** The art of observation. 2. Shock treatment. **Nurs Mirror** 1982 Sep 1;155(9):26
**Iveson-Iveson J:** The art of observation, 3. Attitudes to mental health. **Nurs Mirror** 1982 Sep 8;155(10):17
**Iveson-Iveson J:** Vampires: when fantasy meets reality. **Nurs Mirror** 1983 Jan 19;156(3):18–20
**Ivey-Davis EP:** Highland Hospital revisited. **NC Med J** 1980 Feb;41(2):85–9
**Ivic J:** Povodom 100-te obljetnice rodenja George N. Papanicolaoua 1883–1983. **Jugosl Ginekol Opstet** 1983 May–Aug;23(3–4):53–4
**Ivich Treviño MP** see **Rodriguez Arroyo JL**
**Iwai H, Morimoto I:** Reonarudo to kaibo. Leonardo anatomy. Tokyo, Iwasaki Bijutsusha, 1977. 171 p.
**Iwankiewicz S, Kossowski S:** Klinika Otolaryngologiczna AM we Wrocławiu (1948–1978). **Otolaryngol Pol** 1980;34(2–3):141–65
**Iwasaki T:** [Historical perspective on problems of the therapy, diagnosis and prevention of tuberculosis in Japan since 1886. (1)] (Jpn). **Kekkaku** 1982 Jun–Jul;57(6–7):357–62, 399–407
**Iwasaki T:** [History of tuberculosis in Japan--tuberculosis transmitted by Europeans?] (Jpn). **Kekkaku** 1981 Aug;56(8):407–22
**Izac R:** Du Rouergue en Moldavie; note sur Charles Maisonabe (1779–1851). **Hist Sci Med** 1979;13(4):451–8
**Izmerov NF, Hoiblain HG:** K 10-letiiu mezhdunarodnogo sotrudnichestva mezhdu SSSR i GDR po probleme 'Gigiena truda i profzabolevaniia'. **Gig Tr Prof Zabol** 1982 Jan;(1):3–6
**Izmerov NF, Bogolepova LS:** Sokhranit' i priumnozhit' nasledie gigieny truda. **Gig Tr Prof Zabol** 1980 Apr;(4):41–2
**Izmerov NF:** 60 let Nauchno-issledovatel'skomu institutu gigieny truda i professional'nykh zabolevaniĭ AMN SSSR. **Gig Tr Prof Zabol** 1983 Jun;(6):1–5
**Izmukhanov AK** see **Aliev MA**
**Izquierdo JJ:** Los laboratorios para la investigación, la formación y la especialización del profesorado, en la nueva Facultad de Medicina. In Academia Nacional de Medicina. Libro conmemorativo del primer centenario. México, Comité Editorial de la Comisión Organizadora del Congreso del Centenario, 1964. Tome 2. p. 561–5.
**Izquierdo JM:** Contribución a la historia de la neuropatología española. **Arch Neurobiol (Madr)** 1983 Sep–Oct;46(5):327–34
**Izquierdo Rojo JM:** Historia de la neurologia clinica Española (1882–1936). Madrid, Universidad Complutense-Madrid, 1978. 333 p.
**Izquierdo Rojo JM:** Wenceslao López Albo. **Arch Neurobiol (Madr)** 1983 Mar–Apr;46(2):131–46
**Izsák S:** Farmacia de-a lungul secolelor. Bucuresti, Editura Stiintifică si Enciclopediă, 1979. 418 p.
**Izsák S:** Gondolatok, szempontok és kutatások Pápai Páriz Ferenc 'Pax

Corporis'-ával kapcsolatban. **Orv Hetil** 1982 May 30;123(22):1365-8
**Iżycka J:** Międzynarodowa Rada Pielęgniarek. **Pieleg Polozna** 1982;(9):24-6

# J

**Jablońska D** see **Kucharz E**
**Jabłoński C:** Wymieralność w getcie w Brzezinach. **Przegl Lek** 1980;37(1):40-3
**Jaccard R:** Histoire de la psychanalyse. [France], Hachette, 1982. 2 v.
**Jachimowicz E:** Remember the nurses: Michael Reese Hospital School of Nursing, 1890-1981. **Chic Hist** 1981;10(2):96-8
**Jack D:** Rogues, rebels, and geniuses. The story of Canadian medicine. Toronto, Garden City, Doubleday, 1981. ix, 662 p.
**Jack DB:** Dastardly deeds at Dorpat. **Pharm Hist (London)** 1984 Sep;14(3):9-12
**Jack DB, Laugher SJ:** The earliest demonstration of the placental passage of morphine? **Pharm Hist (London)** 1982 Aug;12(2):7-8
**Jackes MK:** Osteological evidence for smallpox: a possible case from seventeenth century Ontario. **Am J Phys Anthropol** 1983 Jan;60(1):75-81
**Jackle P, Nittenwilm U, Steffens G, et al:** Alfred Gysi--ein Pionier der Zahnheilkunde und Zahntechnik. **Dent Labor (Muench)** 1982 Aug;30(8):1153-61
**Jackman SW:** The tribulations of an editor: Benjamin Silliman and the early days of the American Journal of Science and the Arts. **N Engl Q** 1979;52(1):99-106
**Jackson B:** The United Hospitals of the Borough. **St Thomas Hosp Gaz** 1981;79:56-61
**Jackson B** see **Hand WD, ed**
**Jackson BS:** Historical aspects of legal drafting in the light of modern theories of cognitive development. **Int J Law Psychiatry** 1980;3(4):349-69
**Jackson BS:** Nurses at work in America: a history of nursing's economic and general welfare posture. **Nurs Leadersh** 1983 Sep;6(3):93-9
**Jackson CO:** A difficult pill to swallow. **Rev Am Hist** 1981;9(4):516-20
**Jackson DJ:** Contributions to the history of psychology: XXXV. Dorothy Burlingham. **Psychol Rep** 1984 Jun;54(3):855-63
**Jackson DW:** The history of sports medicine. **Am J Sports Med** 1984 Jul-Aug;12(4):255-7
**Jackson E:** Treasures from the national collections. **Bull Hist Dent** 1982 Oct;30(2):121-2
**Jackson JJ:** Death rates of aged blacks and whites, United States, 1964-1978. **Black Scholar** 1982;13(1):36-48
**Jackson JS, Chatters LM, Neighbors HW:** The mental health status of older black Americans: a national study. **Black Scholar** 1982;13(1):21-35
**Jackson LH** see **Haag JE**
**Jackson R:** Historical outine of attempts to classify skin diseases. In: Congrès international d'histoire de la médecine, XXVe, Québec, 1976. Actes. Québec, 1977. p. 798-806.
**Jackson R:** How caustics were used to treat skin cancer. **J Dermatol Surg Oncol** 1979 Dec;5(12):949-50
**Jackson R:** Hutchinson on leprosy. **Int J Dermatol** 1982 Dec;21(10):614-9
**Jackson R:** Jonathan Hutchinson on syphilis. **Sex Transm Dis** 1980 Apr-Jun;7(2):90-6
**Jackson R:** Raynaud and Molière. **Arch Dermatol** 1983 Mar;119(3):263-6
**Jackson RH:** Epidemic disease and population decline in the Baja California Missions, 1697-1834. **South Calif Q** 1981;63(4):308-46
**Jackson RH:** The last Jesuit censuses of the Pimeria Alta Missions, 1761 and 1766. **Kiva** 1981;46(4):243-72
**Jackson S** see **Wallace ER**
**Jackson SW:** Acedia the sin and its relationship to sorrow and melancholia in medieval times. **Bull Hist Med** 1981 Summer;55(2):172-85
**Jackson SW:** Melancholia and mechanical explanation in eighteenth-century medicine. **J Hist Med Allied Sci** 1983 Jul;38(3):298-319
**Jackson SW:** Melancholia and the waning of the humoral theory. **J Hist Med Allied Sci** 1978 Jul;33(3):367-76
**Jackson WA:** Aether rounds. **Pharm Hist (London)** 1976 Aug;6(2):4
**Jackson WA:** Antiques of Mander, Weaver and Co., Wolverhampton. **Pharm Hist (London)** 1978 Dec;8(3):4-6
**Jackson WA:** Farr's Patent Ampulla. **Pharm Hist (London)** 1977 Dec;7(3):2-3
**Jackson WA:** Lupton of Levenshulme. **Pharm Hist (London)** 1977 Jul;7(2):2-4
**Jackson WA:** The Carbolic smoke ball. **Pharm Hist (London)** 1984;14(1):9-10
**Jacob KA:** The Mosher report. **Am Heritage** 1981;32(4):56-64
**Jacob M:** Science and social passion: the case of seventeenth-century England. **J Hist Ideas** 1982 Apr-Jun;43(2):331-9
**Jacob SW, Herschler R:** Dimethyl sulfoxide after twenty years. **Ann NY Acad Sci** 1983;411:xiii-xvii
**Jacob W** see **Kraus A, ed**
**Jacobs A** see **Cassidy M**
**Jacobs D:** Israel health stamps [on medicine bottles] **Scalpel Tongs** 1981;25:68-9
**Jacobs DE** see **Rose CH**
**Jacobs DW:** Mark Schwartz and the Biofeedback Certification Institute of America: an appreciation. **Biofeedback Self Regul** 1983 Jun;8(2):279-80
**Jacobs F:** Issac Ray and the profession of psychiatry. **RI Hist** 1979;38(4):99-111
**Jacobs M, Stevenson G:** Health and housing: a historical examination of alternative perspectives. **Int J Health Serv** 1981;11(1):105-22
**Jacobs N:** Les dents et la peinture classique et contemporaine. **Actual Odontostomatol (Paris)** 1981;136:631-51
**Jacobs N** see **Elizondo RS**
**Jacobs PA:** Human population cytogenetics: the first twenty-five years. **Am J Hum Genet** 1982 Sep;34(5):689-98
**Jacobs SE:** 'Our babies shall not die': a community's response to medical neglect. **Hum Organ** 1979;38(2):120-33
**Jacobson H:** The Egyptian plagues in the Palaea Historica. **Byzantion** 1977;47-363
**Jacobson HG:** A revisit with Leo M. Davidoff, M.D.--a titan of his time: some personal notes (1898-1975). **Neurosurgery** 1983 Nov;13(5):601-6
**Jacobson HG, Stern WZ:** Landmark perspective: The Graham-Cole 'test' revisited. The oral cholecystogram today. **JAMA** 1983 Dec 2;250(21):2977-82
**Jacobson LO:** From atom to eve. **Perspect Biol Med** 1981 Winter;24(2):195-216
**Jacobson W:** Gram's discovery of his staining technique. **J Infect** 1983 Sep;7(2):97-101
**Jacoby E:** Der Aufstieg ins Bürgertum und sein Preis. Charles Dickens als Beispiel. **Psyche (Stuttg)** 1982 Jul;36(7):609-29
**Jacoby MG:** The Fifth Plague of Egypt. **JAMA** 1983 May 27;249(20):2779-80
**Jacoby R:** Social amnesia: a critique of conformist psychology from Adler to Laing. Boston, Beacon, 1975. xxiii, 191 p.
**Jacquard A:** De la génétique des populations à la sociobiologie. In Actes du Colloque R.A. Fisher.... Paris, 5-6 déc. 1979. p. 405-31. **Rev Synth (Paris)** 1981;102(103-104)
**Jacquart D, Thomasset C:** Albert le Grand et les problèmes de la sexualité. **Hist Philos Life Sci** 1981;3(1):73-93
**Jacquart D:** La pratique médicale dans la région du nord au XVe siècle. In: Congrès National des Sociétés Savantes, 101e, Lille, 1976. Comptes Rendus. Paris, 1976. Section des Sciences, Fasc. III. p. 7-19.
**Jacquart D:** Le milieu médical en France du XIIe au XVe siècle: en annexe 2e supplément au 'Dictionnaire' d'Ernest Wickersheimer. Genève, Droz; Paris, Champion, 1981. 487 p. (Centre de recherches d'histoire et de philologie de la IVe section de l'Ecole pratique des hautes études. V, Hautes études médiévales et modernes ; 46)
**Jacquart D:** Le regard d'un médecin sur son temps: Jacques Despars (1380?-1458). **Bibl Ec Chartres** 1980;138:35-86
**Jacquart D:** Quelques réflexions sur la traduction du Kitab al-Mansuri de Rhazès par Gérard de Crémone. In International Congress of the History of Medicine, 27th, Barcelona, 1980. Actas. Barcelona, Académia de Ciències Mèdiques de Catalunya i Balears, 1981. p. 264-6.
**Jacquart D:** Un jalon dans l'histoire du syndrome hystérique. La 'suffocation de la matrice' dans la tradition médicale médiévale. **Penelope** 1983;(8):7-9
**Jacquart D** see **Ibn Masawayh Y**
**Jacquart D** see **Keil G**
**Jacquel R:** Trois Alsaciens et les débuts--modestes--de la médecine sociale en Pologne pendant l'époque des lumières (troisième tiers du XVIIIe siècle). Les médecins strasbourgeois Jacques Reinbold Spielmann (1722-1783) et Jean Boecler (1737-1808) et le savant mulhousien Jean-Henri Lambert (1728-1777). In Livet G, Schaff G, ed: Médecine et assistance en Alsace, XVIe-XXe siècle. Strasbourg, Istra, 1976. p. 155-200.
**Jacquemet G:** Urbanisme parisien: la bataille du tout-/AF/a-l'égout a la fin du XIXe siècle. **Rev Hist Mod Contemp** 1979;26(Oct-Dec):505-48
**Jacques E:** Médecine et spiritualité: un médecin belge oublié, ami de Port Royal, Philippe Ignace Save (1659-1702). **Rev Hist Eccles** 1980;75(2):322-42
**Jacques L** see **150e année**
**Jacquet-Ladrier F:** Les épidémies de peste à Namur aux XVIe et XVIIe siècles. Congrès de Comines, 1, 1980. Actes. p. 326-7.
**Jacquet-Ladrier F:** L'hôpital Saint-Roch et la lutte contre la peste à Namur, aux XVIIe et XVIIIe siècles. **Ann Soc Belg Hist Hop** 1980;18:59-70
**Jacyna LS:** Images of John Hunter in the nineteenth century. **Hist Sci** 1983 Mar;21(51 Pt 1):85-108
**Jacyna LS:** Immanence or transcendence; theories of life and organization in Britain, 1790-1835. **Isis** 1983 Sep;74(273):311-29
**Jacyna LS:** John Goodsir and the making of cellular reality. **J Hist Biol** 1983 Spring;16(1):75-99
**Jacyna LS:** Principles of general physiology: the comparative dimension to British neuroscience in the 1830s and 1840s. **Stud Hist Biol** 1984;7:47-92
**Jacyna LS:** Somatic theories of mind and the interests of medicine in Britain. **Med Hist** 1982 Jul;26(3):233-58
**Jacyna LS:** The physiology of mind, the unity of nature, and the moral order in Victorian thought. **Br J Hist Sci** 1981 Jul;14(pt 2 no 47):109-32
**Jacyna LS:** The romantic programme and the reception of cell theory in Britain. **J Hist Biol** 1984 Spring;17(1):13-48
**Jaeger F:** Die Tierärztekammer niedersachsen, 1945-1982. Diss. Hannover, 1984. 192 p.
**Jaeger M:** La profession d'infirmier psychiatrique: le poids de son passé. **Soins Psychiatr** 1984 Jun-Jul;(44-45):63-4
**Jaeger M:** Le d'esordre psychiatrique: des politiques de la santé mentale en France. Paris, Payot, 1981. 262 p.
**Jaeger W:** Die Ordnungsprinzipien der Farbsysteme des 17. Jahrhunderts. (Franciscus Aguilonius--Athanasius Kircher--Isaac Newton). **Klin Monatsbl Augenheilkd** 1984 Apr;184(4):321-5
**Jaeger W:** Sinnesphysiologische Forschungen der Jesuitengelehrten des 17. Jahrhunderts. **Klin Monatsbl Augenheilkd** 1981 Oct;179(4):288-96

**Jaeger W:** Symbolische Augendarstellungen in einer Ars Memorandi des 16. Jahrhunderts. **Klin Monatsbl Augenheilkd** 1983 Apr;182(4):337–40
**Jaeger W:** Wege der Forschung auf dem Gebiet der optischen Wahrnehmung. Ein wissenschaftshistorischer Rückblick. **MMW** 1982 Sep 10;124(36):785–8
**Jaeschke G, Diesbachs A von:** Berner 'Arzneibüchlein' in der Erlacher Fassung Daniel von Werdts (1658). Teil I: Text. Pattensen/Han., Wellm, 1978. 180 p. (Würzburger medizinhistorische Forschungen, Band 16).
**Jaffe A:** Addiction reform in the progressive age: scientific and social responses to drug dependence in the United States, 1870–1930. New York, Arno, 1981. vii, 358 p.
**Jaffé A:** Aufsätze zur Psychologie C. G. Jungs. Zürich, Daimon, 1982. 160 p.
**Jaffe JH** see **Martin WR**
**Jaffe M:** The evolution of ambulatory anesthesiology in dentistry **Anesth Prog** 1980 May–Jun;27(3):76–84
**Jaffe NC:** A second opinion on delusions and dreams. A reading of Freud's interpretation of Jensen. In Jones AH, ed: Images of healers. Albany, State University of New York Press, 1983. p. 101–7.
**Jagailloux S:** L'évolution de la chirurgie en Egypte au XIXe siècle. **Hist Sci Med** 1984;18(1):69–73
**Jäger V** see **Gürtler LG**
**Jäger-Sunstenau H:** Auswärtige in einem wiener Totenbuch 1687–1690. **Adler** 1967;7(13–14):205–8
**Jaggi OP:** Medicine in medieval India. Delhi, Atma Ram, 1977. 244 p.
**Jaggi OP:** Western medicine in India: epidemics and other tropical diseases. Delhi, Atma Ram, 1979. xii, 331 p.
**Jaggi OP** see **Unschuld PU**
**Jago JD:** Early dental charlatans and quacks. **Bull Hist Dent** 1984 Oct;32(2):118–25
**Jagoda Z, Kłodziński S, Masłowski J:** Agresja i agresywność w obozie oświęcimskim. **Przegl Lek** 1980;37(1):43–75
**Jagoda Z, Kłodzinski S, Masłowski J:** Stosunek ofiar Oświecimia–Brzezinki do prześladowców. **Przegl Lek** 1981;38(1):37–62
**Jagodic A** see **Musič D**
**Jahn AF:** Stapes surgery in the nineteenth century. **Am J Otol** 1981 Jul;3(1):74–8
**Jahn F:** Los cirujanos del ejercito libertador en la batalla de Carabobo. **Bol Acad Nac Hist (Caracas)** 1972;55(217):134–40
**Jahn I** see **Eichler W**
**Jahns CM:** Rudolf Virchow (1821–1902): Auswahlbibliographie. Berlin, Humboldt Universität, 1983. 87 p. (Schriftenreihe der Universitätsbibliothek Berlin, Nr. 42).
**Jahoda M:** La scuola psicoanalitica dalla Germania agli Stati Uniti. **Comunita** 1971;25(165):189–213
**Jährig K** see **Ratzmann GW**
**Jain AK, Adlakha AL:** Preliminary estimates of fertility decline in India during the 1970's. **Popul Dev Rev** 1982;8(3):589–606
**Jain KM, Swan KG, Casey KF:** Nobel Prize winner in surgery. Part 2. **Am Surg** 1982 May;48(5):191–6
**Jain KM, Swan KG, Casey KF:** Nobel prize winners in surgery. **Am Surg** 1982 Oct;48(10):495–500
**Jain KM, Swan KG, Casey KF:** Nobel prize winners in surgery. Part 3. (Frederick Grant Banting, Walter Rudolph Hess). **Am Surg** 1982 Jul;48(7):287–90
**Jaki SL:** The road of science and the ways to God. Chicago, London, Univ. of Chicago Press, 1978 vii, 478 p.
**Jakob Schoenmackers (26. 5. 1912 bis 22. 11. 1982): Verh Dtsch Ges Pathol** 1983;67:778–85
**Jakóbczyk W:** Karol Marcinkowski, 1800–1846. Warszawa; Poznań, Państwowe Wydawn. Nauk., Oddz. w Poznaniu, 1981. 189 p.
**Jakobi H:** Hermann Schwartze. 100 Jahre Ohrchirurgie in Halle/S. **Wiss Z Martin Luther Univ (Math)** 1976;25(2):109–12
**Jakobovits I:** Judaism [and medicine]. In Reich WT, et al, ed: Encyclopedia of bioethics, v. 2. New York, Free Press, 1978. p. 791–802.
**Jakobovits I:** Medical education––a Jewish perspective. **Isr J Med Sci** 1984 Jan;20(1):2–7
**Jakobsen J, Jorgensen JB, Kreiborg S, et al:** Kong Valdemar Atterdag: antropologiske fund under en odontologisk synsvinkel. **Tandlaegebladet** 1981 Jan;85(1):9–16
**Jakopič B:** Ob 80-letnici Centra za Rehabilitacijo Sluha in Govora v Ljubljani. **Kronika (Yugosl)** 1980;28(3):212–17
**Jakopič B:** Slušno in govorno prizadeti in gledališče. **Kronika (Yugosl)** 1978;26(2):100–3
**Jakopič B:** Zgodovina učnih načrtov in programov šol za gluhe na slovenskem. **Kronika (Yugosl)** 1979;27(3):185–92
**Jakubiak J** see **Stefański K**
**Jakubik A:** Antoni Kepiński: człowiek i dzieło. Warszawa, Państwowy Zakład Wydawn. Lekarskich, 1981. 426 p.
**Jakubik A:** Antoni Kępiński –– Twórca psychiatrii aksjologicznej. **Psychiatr Pol** 1980 Jul–Aug;14(4):403–7
**Jakubik A:** Psychiatria fenomenologiczna w ujęciu Antoniego Kępińskiego. **Psychiatr Pol** 1980 Jul–Aug;14(4):395–401
**Jalil A:** Mermas and acupuncture points, a comparative study. **Stud Hist Med** 1981 Mar;5(1):18–34
**Jaltel M:** La santé par les eaux. 2000 ans de thermalisme. Orleans, L'Instant Durable, 1983. 176 p.
**Jame DG:** Dr. Isambard Owen (1850–1927). In J. Cule, ed: Wales and medicine. London, British Society for the History of Medicine, 1975. p. 96–106.
**James DC:** Disease, debility and death in a Welsh Town: Cardiff 1845–65. **Public Health** 1984 May;98(3):157–62
**James DC:** Dr. Henry James Paine: medical officer of health for Cardiff 1853–1889. **Public Health** 1981 Jul;95(4):215–21
**James DC:** HLA–B27 in clinical medicine––historical reflections on the discovery of the disease association. **Br J Rheumatol** 1983 Nov;22(4 Suppl 2):20–4
**James DC:** The genesis of sanitary reform in Cardiff, 1774–1850. **Welsh Hist Rev** 1982;11(1):50–66
**James DG:** John Coakley Lettsom's Welsh connexions. In J. Cule, ed: Wales and medicine. London, British Society for the History of Medicine, 1975. p. 190–95.
**James DG** see **Bearn AG**
**James DG** see **Sharma OP**
**James EO:** Cultural and religious taboos related to food. **Prog Food Nutr Sci** 1979;3(3):67–77
**James JW:** Isabel Hampton and the professionalization of nursing in the 1890s. In Vogel MJ, Rosenberg CE, ed: The therapeutic revolution. Philadelphia, 1979. p. 201–244.
**James JW:** Lavinia Lloyd Dock. In: Notable American women. The modern period. Cambridge, Mass., Belknap-Harvard Univ. Press, 1980. 4:195–8.
**James JW:** Writing and rewriting nursing history: a review essay. **Bull Hist Med** 1984 Winter;58(4):568–84
**James P:** Population Malthus, his life and times. London, Routledge and Kegan Paul, 1979. xv, 524 p.
**James PJ:** 'A theory by which to work': Mr. Darwin reminisces. **Hist Philos Life Sci** 1982;4(2):255–70
**James PM:** One hundred years of dental public health. **Br Dent J** 1981 Jul 7;151(1):20–3
**James RL, May PR:** Diagnosing schizophrenia: Professor Kraepelin and the research diagnostic criteria. **Am J Psychiatry** 1981 Apr;138(4):501–4
**James T:** A history of bloodletting. **Adler Mus Bull** 1983 Nov;Spec issue:21–8
**James T:** A history of the medical branch of the Royal Air Force: part II aviation medicine. **Adler Mus Bull** 1984 Nov;10(3):2–7
**James T:** A history of the Medical Branch of the Royal Air Force, part 1. **Adler Mus Bull** 1984 Jun;10(2):3–8
**James T:** Dr. Alfred Cox and the South African Medical Association. **S Afr Med J** 1980 Mar 15;57(11):416–21
**James T:** Eunuchs and eunuchism––an historical discourse. **Adler Mus Bull** 1981 Oct;7(3):2–7
**James T:** Eunuchs and eunuchism – an historical discourse. Part II – Civil law. **Adler Mus Bull** 1982 Nov;8(2):3–7
**James T:** Medicine in Arabia Deserta. **Adler Mus Bull** 1981;7(2):13–6
**James TN:** Sir Thomas Lewis redivivus: from pebbles in a quiet pond to autonomic storms. **Br Heart J** 1984 Jul;52(1):1–23
**James TN:** The development of ideas concerning the conduction system of the heart. **Ulster Med J** 1982;51(2):81–97
**James W:** The principles of psychology. Edited and annotated by FH Burkhardt, F. Bowers and I. K. Skrupskelis. 3 vols. Cambridge, Mass. and London, Harvard University Press, 1981. lxviii, 1740 p. (The Works of William James) Introductory historical and biographical essays by G. E. Myers and R. B. Evans.
**James W** see **Rieber RW, ed**
**James WV** see **Orr JF**
**James Garber Galbraith, M.D.: Clin Neurosurg** 1982;29:xiii–xix
**Jameson MG:** Physicians and American political leadership. **JAMA** 1983 Feb 18;249(7):929–30
**Jameton AL** see **McCullough LB**
**Jamison KR** see **Fieve RR**
**Jamróg-Cendrzak A, Cendrzak E:** 100–lecie prac doświadczalnych nad dootrzewnowym przetaczaniem krwi. **Arch Hist Med (Warsz)** 1982;45(1–4):55–9
**Jan Z:** Biografija Bogomira Magajne. **Goriski Letnik** 1979;6:491–502
**Janda LH, Klenke-Hamel KE:** Human sexuality. New York, Van Nostrand, 1980. xv, 475 p.
**Janec M** see **Remisová M**
**Janeček M:** [The father of modern academic medicine (Jan D. Panýrek)] (Cze). **Cas Lek Cesk** 1980;119:1446–8
**Janet RJ:** Providence, prayer and cholera: the English general fast of 1832. **Hist Mag Protest Episc Church** 1982;51(3):297–317
**Janicki K:** Charakterystyka zachorowalności na białaczki w regionie krakowskim w latach 1961–1968 w świetle oceny prawdopodobieństwa według rozkładu Poissona. Doniesienie I: Analiza rozkładu częstości białaczek w 18 powiatowych jednostkach administracyjnych, przy założeniu równomiernego rozrzutu w całym regionie krakowskim. **Folia Med Cracov** 1979;21(2):275–94
**Janis M** see **Goldfischer S**
**Janisch R:** 60 let Ceskoslovenské biologické společnosti při CSAV v Brně. **Cas Lek Cesk** 1982 Nov;121(47):1467–8
**Janiszewski J:** Veterinärmedizin Catos des Aelteren. **Hist Med Vet** 1979;4(2):42–5
**Janko J:** From physiological chemistry to biochemistry. **Acta Hist Rerum Nat Tech** 1977;9:223–79
**Janowiec M, Pichulowa K:** Rozwój mikrobiologicznej diagnostyki gruźlicy w Polsce. **Pneumonol Pol** 1982 Nov;50(11):559–62
**Janowitz B** see **Goldberg HI**
**Janowitz HD:** Crohn and his disease. **Lancet** 1983 Nov 12;2(8359):1140
**Jans GJ** see **Reis CS**
**Jansen AA, Horelli HT:** Pellagra in Kenya. Past and present. **East Afr Med J** 1984 Mar;61(3):220–6

**Jansén C** see **Koulu L**
**Jansen JC:** Waanzin en verstoring der maatschappelijke orde. **Spiegel Hist** 1980;15(7-8):415-20
**Jansen PC:** Demografie in Nederland. **Kleio (Netherl)** 1979;20(8):353-7
**Janson G:** Charles Blake. In Dictionary of Canadian biography, 1801 to 1820. Volume 5, 1983. p. 88-9.
**Janson G:** Dominique Mondelet. In Dictionary of Canadian biography, 1801 to 1820. Volume 5, 1983. p. 599-600.
**Janson G:** Pierre-Joseph Compain. In Dictionary of Canadian biography, 1801 to 1820. Volume 5, 1983. p. 201-202.
**Janson I:** Kieferorthopädie gestern und heute. **Zahnarztl Prax** 1979 May 11;30(5):203-14
**Janssen G:** L'ingénieur hygiéniste à l'hôpital. **Soins** 1982 Jun;(384):29-30
**Janssen WF:** Cancer quackery: past and present. **FDA Consum** 1977 Jul-Aug;11(6):27-32
**Janssen WF:** FDLI's unforgettable character: Charles Wesley Dunn. **Food Drug Cosmet Law J** 1982 Oct;37(4):446-56
**Janssen WF:** Food and Drug Administration celebrates 75 years of consumer protection -- an album from the archives. **Public Health Rep** 1981 Nov-Dec;96(6):487-94
**Janssen WF:** Pharmacy .. and the Food and Drug Law. **Am Pharm** 1981 Apr;21(4):28-36
**Janssen WF:** The gadget quacks. **FDA Consum** 1977 Feb;11(1):4-11
**Janssen WF:** The story of the laws behind the labels. **FDA Consum** 1981 Jun;15(5):32-45
**Janssens P** see **Hart GD, ed**
**Janssens PA:** Antropologisch en paleopathologisch onderzoek van de beenderresten uit het centrale graf in de Onze-Lieve-Vrouwe-kerk te Brugge. De identificatie van de hertogin Maria van Bourgondie. **Verh K Acad Geneeskd Belg** 1981;43(4-5):213-70
**Janssens PA:** Medico-historische gegevens uit de 'Historia Francorum' van Gregorius van Tours. **Hades** 1977;16(30):1-53
**Janssens PG:** Parasitism, parasites and disease. **Ann Soc Belg Med Trop** 1982;62(3):183-212
**Janssens PG:** The colonial legacy: health and medicine in the Belgian Congo. **Trop Doct** 1981 Jul;11(3):132-40
**Janssens U:** Matthieu Maty and the adoption of inoculation for smallpox in Holland. **Bull Hist Med** 1981 Summer;55(2):246-56
**Jantsch M:** Zur Geschichte der Röntgendiagnostik in der Urologie. **Wien Klin Wochenschr** 1984 Sep 14;96(17):637-42
**Jantz RL, Owsley DW:** Temporal changes in limb proportionality among skeletal samples of Arikara Indians. **Ann Hum Biol** 1984 Mar-Apr;11(2):157-63
**Jantz RL** see **Owsley DW**
**Jantz RL** see **Ubelaker DH**
**Janzarik W:** Der schizoaffektive Zwischenbereich und die Lehre von den primären und sekundären Seelenstörungen. **Nervenarzt** 1980 May;51(5):272-9
**Janzarik W:** Jaspers, Kurt Schneider und die Heidelberger Psychopathologie. **Nervenarzt** 1984 Jan;55(1):18-24
**Janzarik W ed:** Psychopathologie als Grundlagenwissenschaft. Stuttgart, Ferdinand Enke, 1979. xi, 202 p. (Klinische Psychologie und Psychopathologie, Bd. 8). Contributions by H. Schipperges, H. D. Middelhoff, R. Avenarius, W. Schmitt, H. Kindt, W. Kretschmer, G. Huber, J. Glatzel, K. P. Kisker, H. Tellenbach, H. Häfner, A. Bader, L. Navratil, W. Baeyer, K. Koehler, O. Dörr-Zegers, B. Kimura.
**Janzen JM:** Ideologies and institutions in the precolonial history of equatorial African therapeutic systems. **Soc Sci Med [Med Anthropol]** 1979 Dec;13B(4):317-26
**Janzen JM, Feierman S:** The social history of disease and medicine in Africa. I. **Soc Sci Med [Med Anthropol]** 1979 Dec;13B(4):239-43
**Janzon B:** Idrott och ling-gymnastik i populär-medicinsk belysning. **Nord Medicinhist Arsb** 1980;:124-35
**Japan and dentistry: CAL** 1983 Jul;47(1):1, 3-4
**Japp PM:** Pioneer medicines: doctors, nostrums, and folk cures. **J West** 1982 Jul;21(3):15-22
**Jaques DA:** The fraternity of strangers. **Am J Surg** 1984 Oct;148(4):426-7
**Jaques LB:** The hemostasis paradigm in 1934 and in 1980. **Ann NY Acad Sci** 1981;370:1-4
**Jaqueti G:** Profesor José Gay Prieto. Maestro de dermatólogos (1905-1979). **Actas Dermosifiliogr** 1981 Jul-Aug;72(7-8):389-96
**Jarcho S:** Blankaart's Dictionary, an index to 17th century medicine. **Bull NY Acad Med** 1982 Sep;58(6):568-77
**Jarcho S:** Laveran's discovery in the retrospect of a century. **Bull Hist Med** 1984 Summer;58(2):215-24
**Jarcho S:** Some early Italian epidemiological maps. **Imago Mundi** 1983;35:9-19
**Jarcho S:** Some experiences with seminars in the history of medicine. In J. J. Bylebyl, ed: Teaching the history of medicine at a medical center. Baltimore, London, Johns Hopkins University Press, 1982. (The Henry E. Sigerist supplements to the Bulletin of the History of Medicine; new ser., no. 7). p. 115-20.
**Jarcho S:** Some historical problems connected with the study of Egyptian mummies. **Bull Inst Egypte (Cairo)** 1981;:58-9, 106-22
**Jarcho S:** Some Italian broadsides and passports of epidemiologic interest (1618-1723). **Trans Stud Coll Physicians Phila** 1981;Ser.5 3(1):40-52
**Jarcho S:** Some lost, obsolete, or discontinued diseases: Serous apoplexy, incubus, and retrocedent ailments. **Trans Stud Coll Physicians Phila** 1980 Dec;5(2 no 4):241-66
**Jarcho S:** The concept of heart failure from Avicenna to Albertini. Cambridge, Mass., and London, Harvard Univ. Press, 1980. 407 p.
**Jarcho S:** The Siamese twins of Santo Domingo. **Trans Stud Coll Physicians Phila** 1979 Jun;5(1 no 2):145-7
**Jarcho S** see **Blake JB, ed**
**Jarcho S** see **Bylebyl JJ, ed**
**Jarcho S** see **Woodward TE**
**Jarchov I, ed** see **Gercke H**
**Jardetzky O, Wade-Jardetzky NG:** Nuclear magnetic resonance as a structural method in molecular biology. **Rice Univ Stud** 1980;66(3):57-79
**Jarmer K:** Die Kurierfreiheit der Zahnärzte seit der Gewerbeordnung von 1869 und die Kämpfe der Zahnärzte mit ihren Konkurrenten. Teil I: Vorbemerkung und die Freigabe der Zahnheilkunde an jedermann. **Stomatol DDR** 1981;31(1):1-5
**Jarmer K:** I. Die Freigabe der Zahnheilkunde an jedermann. Fortsetzung von 'Die Kurierfreiheit der Zahnärzte...', siehe Heft 2/81, S. 119. 3. Die Freigabe der Zahnheilkunde an die eingewanderten Amerikaner, DDS. **Stomatol DDR** 1981 Mar;31(3):194-7
**Järnefelt J:** P. E. Simola ja sitruunahappokierto. **Duodecim** 1981;97(13):928-30
**Jaros D** see **Canon BC**
**Jarosz M:** Le suicide en Pologne. **Rev Etud Comp Est Ouest** 1978;9(4):65-101
**Jarosz M:** Manfred Bleuler i inni o wyst epowaniu prawidłowych stanów psychicznych u chorych na schizofrenię. **Psychiatr Pol** 1981 Jul-Dec;15(4-6):403-9
**Jaroszewski Z:** Działalność profesora Stanisława Batawii na polu alkohologii i walki z alkoholizmem. **Psychiatr Pol** 1979 Sep-Oct;13(5):445-9
**Jaroszewski Z, Tarmanowska B:** Dzieci w Instytucie Higieny Psychicznej (w Warszawie, 1943-1944). **Przegl Lek** 1981;38(1):152-5
**Jarrell RA:** Colonialism and the truncation of science in Ireland and French Canada during the nineteenth century. **HSTC** 1981 May;18(5 no 2):140-57
**Jarrick A:** Freud och historien. **Scandia** 1982;48(1):107-48
**Jasińska Z, Komorowska W:** Władysław Biegański (1857-1917). Spis prac w układzie chronologicznym. **Ann Univ Mariae Curie Sklodowska [Med]** 1978;33:15-27
**Jaskoski H:** 'My heart will go out': healing songs of native American women. **Int J Womens Stud** 1981;4(2):118-34
**Jasper HH, Sourkes TL:** Nobel laureates in neuroscience: 1904-1981. **Annu Rev Neurosci** 1983;6:1-42
**Jasser MT:** Anaesthesia and resuscitation in the history of Arabic medicine. In: International Symposium for the History of Arabic Science, 1st, University of Aleppo, 1976. Proceedings. Aleppo, Syria, 1976. Papers in European Languages, Vol. II. p. 324-5.
**Jastrzebowski Z:** Epidemie a rozwój ludności Królestwa Polskiego w latach 1815-1870. **Arch Hist Med (Warsz)** 1984;47(3):355-74
**Jastrzebowski Z:** Epidemie duru w Królestwie Polskim w latach 1815--1870. **Arch Hist Med (Warsz)** 1980;43(2):179-90
**Jastrzębowski Z:** Występowanie epidemii odry w Królestwie Polskim W XIX wieku (1815-1870). **Wiad Lek** 1983 Jul 1;36(13):1121-5
**Javier Puerto F:** La Farmacia de la Plaza de San Ildefonso (Madrid). **Bol Soc Esp Hist Farm** 1981 Sep;32(127):169-205
**Javier Puerto F, Sanz Diaz L:** Las ideas cientificas de Felix Palacios. **Bol Soc Esp Hist Farm** 1982 Mar;33(132):237-47
**Javier Puerto F:** Pedro Calvo Asensio (1821-1863): farmaceutico liberal. **Bol Soc Esp Hist Farm** 1983;34(136):203-28
**Javier Puerto F** see **Folch Jou G**
**Jaworska J:** Henryka Becka 'Bunkier 1944 roku'. Wrocław, Zakład Narodowy im. Ossolińskich, 1982. 119 p.
**Jaworska M** see **Jaworski Z**
**Jaworski Z:** Abrazja z ebów a zmiany w budowie anatomicznej żuchwy ludzi sprzed 3.000 lat z okolic Tarnobrzega. **Protet Stomatol** 1983 Jan-Feb;33(1):59-66
**Jaworski Z, Jaworska M:** Morfologia i topografia dna zatoki szczękowej w ciałopalnych szczątkach kostnych prasłowian. **Czas Stomatol** 1982 Apr;35(4):199-210
**Jaworski Z:** Morfologia zębów stałych z dziecięcych grobów ciałopalnych kultury łuzyckiej. **Czas Stomatol** 1981 May;34(5):487-92
**Jaworski Z:** Przyżyciowe braki zębowe w szczatkach kostnych z grobów ciałopalnych kultury łużyckiej. **Czas Stomatol** 1981 Oct;34(10):969-74
**Jaworski Z:** Sito zębodołowe a budowa żuchwy i choroby przyębia u prasłowian. Część II. **Czas Stomatol** 1983 May;36(5):333-8
**Jaworski Z:** Sito zębodołowe w szczątkach żuchw prasłowian z popielnicowych grobów ciałopalnych kultury łużyckiej. Część I. **Czas Stomatol** 1983 Apr;36(4):257-64
**Jaworski Z:** Szczątki szczęk i żuchw Prasłowian z grobów ciałopalnych kultury łużychiej. **Czas Stomatol** 1981 Sep;34(9):897-907
**Jay M, Phil M:** Nettleship's two pedigrees of retinitis pigmentosa: a historical postscript. **Surv Ophthalmol** 1983 Jan-Feb;27(4):264-8
**Jay M:** The Eisdell pedigree. Congenital stationary night-blindness with myopia. **Trans Ophthalmol Soc UK** 1983;103(Pt 2):221-6
**Jayatilaka AD:** Historical review of the study of anatomy. **Cent Afr J Med** 1983 Jul;29(7):147-53
**Jayawardane KW:** A bibliography of the history of medicine in Sri Lanka. **Ceylon Med J** 1979 Sep-Dec;24(3-4):71-8
**Jean R:** Communication sur la correspondance du docteur Guillard à sa femme lors du voyage à Sainte-Hélène: retour des cendres de Napoléon. **Hist Sci Med** 1980;14:271-6
**Jeanmart L:** Le radiodiagnostic de Roentgen à Hounsfield. **Flash Inf** 1983 May-Jun;:3-7
**Jeannerod M** see **Barbaix M**
**Jedlicka D** see **Reid JD**

**Jee BS:** A short history of Aryan medical science. Delhi, New Asian Publishers, 1978. 206 p., x.
**Jefferson A:** Geoffrey Jefferson 1886–1961. **Surg Neurol** 1984 Jul;22(1):1–4
**Jefferson JW** see **Strobusch AD**
**Jeffery R:** Indian medicine and the state. **Bull Br Assoc Orient** 1979–80 N.Ser;11:58–70
**Jeffery R:** Recognizing India's doctors: the institutionalization of medical dependency, 1918–1939. **Mod Asian Stud** 1979;13(2):301–26
**Jeffery T:** Mass-observation. **Soc Soc Hist Med Bull** 1980;27:8–14
**Jefferys M, Sachs H:** Re-thinking general practice: some issues of policy and practice in the 1970s illustrated by case study. **Soc Soc Hist Med Bull (Lond)** 1983 Dec;33:17–9
**Jeggle U:** Lebensalter und Körpererleben. In Imhof AE, ed: Leib und Leben in der Geschichte der Neuzeit. Berlin, Duncker & Humblot, 1983. p. 89–102.
**Jekel JF:** The 'Rainbow Reviews': publications of the National Center for Health Statistics. **J Chronic Dis** 1984;37(9–10):681–8
**Jelenko C, Matthews JB, Matthews JC:** Emergency medicine in colonial America: Revolutionary War casualties. **Ann Emerg Med** 1982 Jan;11(1):73–6
**Jelic R:** Zdravstvo u zadru i njegovu podrucju. Zadar, Narodni List, 1978. 383 p.
**Jelinek JE:** Jean-Paul Marat. The differential diagnosis of his skin disease. **Am J Dermatopathol** 1979 Fall;1(3):251–2
**Jemna I** see **Algeorge G**
**Jendrysik I:** 25 lat Koła PTP w Istebnej. **Pieleg Polozna** 1984;(5):30–1
**Jenkins C** see **Whittaker DK**
**Jenkins EW:** The development of school biology, 1918–1945. **Hist Educ** 1979;8(1):59–73
**Jenkins GN:** A century of oral physiology. **Br Dent J** 1981 Jul 7;151(1):6–10
**Jenkins HM** see **Hearst E, ed**
**Jenkins M:** Medicine and spices, with special reference to medieval monastic accounts. **Gard Hist** 1976;4:47–9
**Jenkins MT:** History of sequestered edema associated with surgical operations and trauma. **Contemp Anesth Pract** 1983;6:1 31
**Jenkins PR** see **Whittaker DK**
**Jenner H:** Organisation des Gesundheitswesens in Schleswig-Holstein in der ersten Hälfte des 19. Jahrhunderts. **Z Ges Schleswig Holstein Gesch** 1982;107:67–112
**Jenner CL, ed:** The Vi-Ton-Ka medicine show. American Place Theatre, 1983. 36 p. Contributions by B. McNamara, G. Hinson, F. F. Bloodgood, A. Dargan, C. Wolfe, J. H. Young, W. Helfand.
**Jennings M** see **Rowland B**
**Jennings WA:** When did you last see your röntgen?--The SI units and their use. **Phys Med Biol** 1984 Feb;29(2):131–7
**Jenny J:** An historic parallel: 19th century education, 20th century dental care. **J Public Health Dent** 1979 Fall;39(4):295–7
**Jenschorek N:** Robert Koch: Leben, Werk, Zeit. 2. durchgesehene Auflage. Leipzig, Hirzel, 1976. 247 p.
**Jensen E:** Et 125-arigt medicinsk bibliotek. **Bogens Verden** 1977;59(5):181–5
**Jensen E** see **Simmons GB**
**Jensen EV:** Steroid receptors in breast cancer: historical perspective. **Cancer** 1980 Dec 15;46(12 Suppl):2759–61
**Jensen JE:** A Med-Chi physician's travelog 1860–62 (Dr. H. Willis Baxley). **Md State Med J** 1984 Feb;33(2):90–2
**Jensen JE, Weisheit-Smith I:** History of the Library of the Medical and Chirurgical Faculty of the State of Maryland. **Md State Med J** 1980 Jun;29(6):35–7
**Jensen JE:** Manuscript notes of William Shippen, Jr., MD found in the Faculty Library. **Md State Med J** 1984 Jun;33(6):438–40
**Jensen JE:** More treasures. **Md State Med J** 1982 Nov;31(11):26–9
**Jensen JE:** Napoleonic medicine. **Md State Med J** 1981 Jul;30(7):66–8
**Jensen JE:** 166 years ago this month ... William Beanes: the doctor behind 'The Star-Spangled Banner'. **Md State Med J** 1980 Sep;29(9):60–5
**Jensen KR, Tkocz I:** Skeletmaterialet fra udgravningen af St. Jørgensgården i Odense. En foreløbig rapport. **Dan Medicinhist Arbog** 1983;12:52–64
**Jensen NS** see **Jakobsen J**
**Jensen OM, Larsen A:** Blaerecancer i Danmark 1943–1977. Kraeftstatistik 4. **Ugeskr Laeger** 1982 Nov 15;144(46):3458–60
**Jensen RA** see **Cohn RL**
**Jensen RE** see **Chilton WS**
**Jensen VG:** Poul Richard Hauberg, 1887–1959. **Theriaca** 1982 Jun;22:xi–xvi
**Jensen VG** see **Bruun NW**
**Jensen VG** see **Retzius AJ**
**Jensenius H:** Eutanasi -- historisk og aktuelt. **Dan Medicinhist Arbog** 1979;100–13
**Jenss H:** Jugendarbeitsschutz: von den Anfängen der Industrialisierung bis zur Gegenwart. Frankfurt, New York, Campus, 1980. xiv, 260 p.
**Jephcott A:** The Macintosh laryngoscope. A historical note on its clinical and commercial development. **Anaesthesia** 1984 May;39(5):474–9
**Jepson E:** Medicine from plants. **Trans Med Soc Lond** 1981–82;98:1–10
**Jéquier MC:** Auguste Tissot (1728–1797). **Rev Med Suisse Romande** 1984 May;104(5):337–41
**Jeřábek J:** 22 let trvání Katedry posudkového lékařství. **Cesk Zdrav** 1983 Sep;31(8–9):396–9
**Jernegan MW** see **Breul FR**
**Jerome Cornfield's publications: contributions to the literature as they appeared from 1941 through 1980: Biometrics** 1982 Mar;38 Suppl:47–52
**Jerrido MJ:** In recognition of...early black women physicians. **Women Health** 1980 Fall;5(3):1–3
**Jeśman C:** Organizacja niemieckiej Izby Aptekarskiej i gospodarka lekami w tzw. Generalnym Gubernatorstwie w latach 1939–1945. **Arch Hist Med (Warsz)** 1984;47(3):403–15
**Jette R, Charbonneau H:** Généalogie descendantes et analyse démographique. **Ann Demogr Hist (Paris)** 1984;:45–54
**Jetter D:** Die alten Hospitalpläne der Albertina in Wien. **Hist Hosp** 1979–80;13:29–45
**Jetter D:** Grundzüge der Geschichte des Irrenhauses. Darmstadt, Wissenschaftliche Buchgesellschaft, 1981. ix, 244 p.
**Jetter D:** Hospitäler in London; zur Typologie wohltätiger Einrichtungen im Spannungsfeld politischer Kräfte. **Sudhoffs Arch** 1978;62(3):250–81
**Jetter D:** Hospitäler in Salzburg. **Sudhoffs Arch** 1980;64(2):163–86
**Jetter D:** Klosterhospitäler; St. Gallen, Cluny, Escorial. **Sudhoffs Arch** 1978;62(4):313–38
**Jetter D:** Neue Funde zur Geschichte der alten Pilgerherberge in Santiago de Compostela. In Seidler E, Schott H, ed: Bausteine zur Medizingeschichte. Stuttgart, Steiner, 1984. p. 52–64.
**Jetter D:** Spanien von den Anfängen bis um 1500. Wiesbaden, Steiner, 1980. 239 p. (Geschichte des Hospitals. Band 4).
**Jetter D:** Wien von den Anfängen bis um 1900. Wiesbaden, Steiner, 1982. viii, 159 p. (Geschichte des Hospitals, Bd. 5).
**Jetter D:** Wiener Irrenhausprojekte. **Fortschr Neurol Psychiatr** 1981 Feb;49(2):43–52
**Jetter D:** Zur Typologie des Irrenhauses in Frankreich und Deutschland (1780–1840). Wiesbaden, Steiner, 1971. x, 206 p. (Geschichte des Hospitals, Band 2)
**Jewell JA** see **Hillier SM**
**Jewell PA** see **Dupâquier J**
**Ježek V:** Historický vývoi a současný stav výzkumu vztahu mezi plicní a systémovou cirkulací a funkcí obou srdečních komor. **Cesk Fysiol** 1981;30(2):103–6
**Jezierska ME:** Szpital obozu Buchenwald (na podstawie archiwaliów z okresu 3 IV – 20 VII 1945 r.). **Przegl Lek** 1980;37(1):76–85
**Jeziorski K, Matsumoto H:** Leczenie opiatowych zespołów odstawiennych (rys historyczny). **Pol Tyg Lek** 1984 Oct 22;39(43):1433–6
**Jhala HL:** Contribution of Bombay to progress of science of pathology. **Indian J Med Sci** 1980 Apr;34(4):65–71
**Jijlstra WG** see **Van Kampen EJ**
**Jilek-Aall L:** Acculturation, alcoholism and Indian-style Alcoholics Anonymous. **J Stud Alcohol [Suppl]** 1981 Jan;9:143–58
**Jiménez MR:** La epidemia de colera de 1834 en Zaragoza y su provincia. **Asclepio** 1982;34:3–31
**Jiménez Blanco J** see **Gónzalez Blasco P**
**Jiménez Herrero F:** La medicina y los médicos en el teatro de Casona. **Bol Inst Estud Asturianos** 1968;22(64–65):319–51
**Jimenez Muñoz JM, Riera J:** Bibliografía histórica en el siglo médico (1854–1936). Valladolid, Universidad de Valladolid, 1975. 107 p. (Acta Historico-Medica Vallisoletana, Monografias, VI)
**Jiménez Muñoz JM:** Salarios de medicos y cirujanos (I) (II). (Nóminas de Corte 1538–1629). **Asclepio** 1981;33:315–47
**Jiménez Muñoz JM** see **Riera J**
**Jiménez-Olivares E:** La demonología en el siglo XV. **Prensa Med Mex** 1979 Mar–Apr;44(3–4):72–4
**Jiménez-Olivares E:** La interpretación de los sueños en el México prehispánico. In International Congress of the History of Medicine, 27th, Barcelona, 1980. Actas. Barcelona, Académia de Ciències Mèdiques de Catalunya i Balears, 1981. p. 78–80.
**Jin Shiying:** [The influence of 'Pen tsao kang mu' in Japan.] (Chi). **Chin J Med Hist** 1981;11:102–5
**Jinich H:** La medicina del siglo XX y su proyección futura. IV. Rasgos esenciales de la medicina del siglo XX. **Gac Med Mex** 1981 Nov;117(11):434–8
**Jinich H, Pérez-Tamayo R, Sepúlveda B, et al:** La verdad y el error en medicina. **Gac Med Mex** 1984 Apr;120(4):133–44
**Jirka FJ:** One hundred years of American medicine. **J Tenn Med Assoc** 1983 Jul;76(7):450–1
**Jirous J:** Třicetiletá bilance a perspektivy Katedry sociálního lékařství a organizace zdravotnictví Institutu pro další vzdělávání lékařu a farmaceutu Praha. **Cesk Zdrav** 1983 Sep;31(8–9):360–7
**Jitariu P:** Societatea de Medici si Naturalisti si dezvoltarea stiintelor biologicie. **Rev Med Chir Soc Med Nat Iasi** 1980 Oct–Dec;84(4):636–42
**Joannis C:** Santé et sagesse traditionnelle. Le Puy, France, Bonneton, 1981. 127 p.
**Job R, Tabossi P:** Umana o artificiale, purché sia intelligenza. **Stor Crit Psicol** 1984 Jun;5(1):69–89
**Jobe TH:** The devil in Restoration science: the Glanvill-Webster witchcraft debate. **Isis** 1981 Sep;72(263):343–56
**Joblin J:** Monseigneur André Jacques Fougerat; ecclesiastical advisor of CICIAMS (1952–1982). **Nouv Com Int Cathol Infirm Assist Med Soc** 1983;(3):1–8
**Jobling IF:** The 'sporty' Australians: women and sport in Australian history. In Borms J, Hebbelinck M, Venerando A, ed: Women and sport. Basel, Karger, 1981. p. 66–72.
**Jochnowitz C** see **Lutzker E**
**Joerger M** see **Forster R**
**Johannes A:** Zur Geschichte der Tierärztlichen Hochschule Hannover während der ersten 200 Jahre ihres Bestehens. II. Die Klinik für Geburtshilfe und Gynäkologie des Rindes und ihre Vorläufer. Diss. Hannover, 1983. 148 p.
**Johannes Adelphus:** Ausgewählte Schriften. 3. Band. Das Buch des Lebens. Ed. A. R. Arthur, B. Gotzkowsky. Berlin, New York, De Gruyter, 1980. 413 p.

Johannessen CL: Folk medicine uses of melanotic Asiatic chickens as evidence of early diffusion to the New World. Soc Sci Med [D] 1981 Nov;15D(4):427–34
Johannisson K: Naturvetenskap på reträtt. En diskussion om naturvetenskapens status under svenskt 1700-tal. Lychnos 1979–80;:109–54
Johansen AH: Zur demographischen Entwicklung Kastiliens im 16. Jahrhundert. Gesammelte Aufs Kulturgesch Spaniens 1978;29:538–80
Johansen HC: Slave demography of the Danish West Indian Islands. Scand Econ Hist Rev 1981;29(1):1–20
Johansen O: Klipp fra 'Tidsskriftet' gjennom tidene. Tidsskr Nor Laegeforen 1981 Jan;101(1):25–35
Johanson C: Autocratic politics, public opinion, and women's medical education during the reign of Alexander II, 1855–1881. Slavic Rev 1979;38(3):426–43
Johanson DC see Kimbel WH
Johansson B: 'God bless you, my dear Miss Nightingale.' Letters from Emmy Carolina Rappe to Florence Nightingale 1867–1870. Stockholm, Almqvist & Wiksell International, 1977. 57 p. (Stockholm studies in English, 38).
Johansson BW, Nicol P: A Swedish report on acute myocardial infarction in 1859. Br Med J [Clin Res] 1982 Mar 20;284(6319):888–9
Johansson BW: Hjärtinfarkt--gammal sjukdom med nytt namn. Sydsven Medicinhist Sallsk Arsskr 1980;:57–79
Johansson SG, Bennich HH: The clinical impact of the discovery of IgE. Ann Allergy 1982 Jun;48(6):325–30
Johansson SR, Preston SH: Tribal demography: the Hopi and Navaho population as seen through manuscripts from the 1900 U.S. census. Soc Sci Hist 1978;3(1):1–33
Johansson SR see Berger LR
Johansson SR see Hammel EA
Johansson-Saleby E: I brottmål: Elsa Johansson-Saleby mot Svenska psykiaterkåren. Stockholm, Johansson-Salebys förlag, 1973. 101 p.
John S: Mitral valvotomy. Past and present. Indian J Chest Dis Allied Sci 1979 Oct-Dec;21(4):163–5
John Hull Grundy, artist and entomologist: J Audiov Media Med 1983 Jan;6(1):17–20
John Mitchell Bruce (1846–1929): Practitioner 1982 Apr;226(1366):800
John Paul II Pope: Discurso de Juan Pablo II a los profesores y estudiantes universitarios en la catedral de Colonia (Aalemania), 15.XI.1980. Rev Med Univ Navarra 1981 Jun;25(2):61–4
Johns HE: The physicist in cancer treatment and detection. Int J Radiat Oncol Biol Phys 1981 Jun;7(6):801–8
Johns OR: Essence of peppermint, a history of the medicine and its bottle. Hist Archaeol 1981;15(2):1–57
Johns RB see Williams JE
Johnsen B: Islands folkemedicin og Magnus Ketilsson. Dan Medicinhist Arbog 1982;:56–70
Johnsen B: Miasmer eller kontagion. Ginklofi (tetanus neonatorum) på Vestmannöerne og dr Peter Anton Schleisners indsats i dens bekaempelse. Nord Medicinhist Arsb 1982;:162–70
Johnson A: August Hoff--a Sydney dermatologist of the 1880's. Australas J Dermatol 1983 Apr;24(1):37–9
Johnson A: William John Munro (1863–1908). Am J Dermatopathol 1983 Oct;5(5):477–8
Johnson AW, Rose FL, Suckling CW: Alfred Spinks: 25 February 1917–11 February 1982. Biogr Mem Fellows R Soc 1984;30:567–94
Johnson BH: Doctors, druggists and dentists in the Oklahoma Territory, 1889–1907. Ariz West 1977;19:121–34
Johnson CA, Bond JR: Policy implementation and community linkages: hospital abortion services after Roe V. Wade. West Polit Q 1982;35(3):385–405
Johnson CA see Bond JR
Johnson CM see Christensen HA
Johnson CS: Anesthesia and photography. Harv Mag 1980 Jul-Aug;82(6):57
Johnson DA: History and the understanding of acupuncture anesthesia. South Med J 1983 Apr;76(4):497–8
Johnson DE: A concordance of abbreviations used in references to reviews in botanical bibliographies by Cobres (1782), Bohmer (1787), and Militz (1829). Huntia 1979;3(2):103–14
Johnson DL, Stratton RJ: Introduction to removable partial dentures. Quintessence Int 1979;10(10):55–62
Johnson DP: Dilemmas of charismatic leadership: the case of the People's Temple. Sociol Anal 1979;40(4):315–23
Johnson DR: The history of the 1906 Pure Food and Drugs Act and the Meat Inspection Act. In Hammer SN, ed: Symposium for the 75th Anniversary of the Food, Drug & Cosmetic Act, Meat Inspection Act, 1906–1981. Monday, June 8, 1981. Washington, D.C. Food Drug Cosmet Law J 1982 Jan;37(1):5–9
Johnson EA, Bell G: Whetstone Valley District Medical Society (No. 12). SD J Med 1981 May;34(5):32–4
Johnson EE: Ida Henrietta Hyde: early experiments. Physiologist 1981 Dec;24(6):10–1
Johnson FL: Marrow transplantation in the treatment of acute childhood leukemia. Historical development and current approaches. Am J Pediatr Hematol Oncol 1981 Winter;3(4):389–95
Johnson FN, Amdisen A: The first era of lithium in medicine. An historical note. Pharmacopsychiatria 1983 Mar;16(2):61–3
Johnson G: Micronesia: America's strategic trust. Bull At Sci 1979;35(2):10–15
Johnson G: Vistas in the management of bleeding esophageal varices. NC Med J 1982 May;43(5):353–7
Johnson JC: Emergency medicine in Indiana: past, present and future. J Indiana State Med Assoc 1980 Jun;73(6):354–6
Johnson JM: The water cure at 'the San.' NY Folkl Q 1966;22(3):201–5
Johnson JP: Herbert Hoover and David Copperfield: a tale of two childhoods. J Psychohist 1980 Spring;7(4):467–75
Johnson JP: Herbert Hoover: the orphan as children's friend. Prologue J Nat Arch 1980;12(4):193–206
Johnson JT: History of Protestant medical ethics. In Reich WT, et al, ed: Encyclopedia of bioethics, v.3. New York, Free Press, 1978. p. 1364–73.
Johnson KM, Scribner Cl, McCormick JB: Ecology of ebola virus: a first clue? J Infect Dis 1981 May;143(5):749–51
Johnson L see Smith GF
Johnson LL, Seibert S: Estimaciones de la población de Buenos Aires en 1744, 1778 y 1810. Desarrollo Econ 1979;19(73):107–19
Johnson LR: A footnote to modern gastroenterology. Gastroenterology 1982 Jun;82(6):1293–4
Johnson M see Castaing L
Johnson MP: Smothered slave infants; were slave mothers at fault? J South Hist 1981;47(4):493–520
Johnson MP, Hufbauer K: Sudden infant death syndrome as a medical research problem since 1945. Soc Probl 1982;30(1):65–81
Johnson NE: Minority-group status and the fertility of black Americans, 1970: a new look. Am J Sociol 1979;84(6):1386–1400
Johnson NE: Religious differentials in reproduction: the effects of sectarian education. Demography 1982 Nov;19(4):495–509
Johnson OS: A study of Chinese alchemy. New York, Arno, 1974. xi, 156 p.
Johnson RA: On the psychology of the aging woman. Mary Baker Eddy as a religious leader. J Geriatr Psychiatry 1979;12(1):27–35
Johnson RB: Pellagra, an historical review. J Okla State Med Assoc 1981 Dec;74(12):396–8
Johnson RE: Carlo Frank Consolazio: March 9, 1913--December 23, 1976. Prog Food Nutr Sci 1983;7(1–2):1–10
Johnson RE: Isaac Israel Hayes. In Dictionary of Canadian biography, 1881–1890. 1982;11:393–4.
Johnson RE: Robert McCormick. In Dictionary of Canadian biography, 1881–1890. 1982;11:543–4.
Johnson TP, Cooper JK: Physician shortage in Kentucky, 1930–1980. Am J Public Health 1982 Mar;72(3):257–60
Johnson VB: Drug product selection through the decades. Am Pharm 1980 Oct;20(10):20–4
Johnson D, ed see Capper WM
Johnston AJ: The frères de la charité and the Louisbourg Hôpital du Roi. Can Cathol Hist Assoc Study Sess 1981;48:5–25
Johnston EG: Medical services for the island of Guam until World War Two. Guam Rec 1971;1(1):38–46
Johnston FE, Selby H: Anthropology: the biocultural view. Dubuque, Iowa, Brown, 1978. Historical sections, p. 73–80, 125–213, 270–275.
Johnston GA: Tribute to a Chicago surgeon: Ulysses Grant Dailey. IMJ 1983 Jan;163(1):35–6
Johnston L see Curry R
Johnston R see Gillespie B
Johnston WD: [Scientific revolution in 18th century Japanese medicine: intellectual preconditions for the development of the Dutch school of medicine (Rampo).] (Jpn). Nihon I-Shigaku Zasshi 1981;27:131–156
Johnstone P: Aconite and its antidote in Arabic writings. J Hist Arabic Sci 1977 May;1(1):65–71
Johnstone P: Arab herbals and herbalists. In: Mashriq. Proc. of the Eastern Mediterranean Seminar ... 1977–1978. Manchester, University, 1980. p. 19–24.
Joiris A: Le vieux Bavière au XIXe siècle (1830–1895). Ann Soc Belg Hist Hop 1982;20:109–44
Jokisch R: Probleme der spanischen Wissenschaftsentwicklung. Die Institutionalisierung der spanischen Histologie im 19. Jahrhundert als Beispiel. In International Congress of the History of Medicine, 27th, Barcelona, 1980. Actas. Barcelona, Académia de Ciències Médiques de Catalunya i Balears, 1981. p. 522–9.
Jokl E: Medicine, science and sport. Trans Stud Coll Physicians Phila 1980 Jun;5(2 no 2):81–9
Jokl E: Sherrington, his life and thought: essay-review. Trans Stud Coll Physicians Phila 1980 Sep;5(2 no 3):223–35
Jolidon C, Zephir D, Ybert G: Considérations historiques sur la maladie de La Peyronie. Peu de choses ont changé! J Urol (Paris) 1984;90(5):365–6
Jolley M, ed see Allan P
Joly R: Hippocrates and the school of Cos. Between myth and skepticism. In M. Ruse, ed: Nature animated. Historical and philosophical case studies in Greek medicine, nineteenth-century and recent biology, psychiatry, and psychoanalysis. Volume II. Dordrecht, D. Reidel, 1983. p. 29–47.
Joly R: Le système cnidien des humeurs. In La collection hippocratique et son rôle dans l'histoire de la médecine. Colloque de Strasbourg (23–27 octobre 1972) organisé par le Centre de Recherches sur la Grèce Antique, avec le concours des Facultés de Philosophie et des Langues Classiques. Leiden, E. J. Brill, 1975. p. 107–27.
Joly R: L'école médicale de Cnide et son évolution. Antiq Class 1978;47:528–37
Joly R see Grmek MD, ed

**Jonas AM:** The mouse in biomedical research. **Physiologist** 1984 Oct;27(5):330–46
**Jonas S** see **Barker WH**
**Jonckere P de** see **Barbaix M**
**Jonecko A:** Drzeworyt ukazujący amputowane i protezowane podudzie w śląskim poemacie Roździeńskiego 'Officina ferraria' a roku 1612. **Wiad Lek** 1983 Jun 15;36(12):1025–31
**Jonecko A:** Drzeworyt ukazujacy amputowane i protezowane produdzie w ślaskim poemacie Roździeńskiego 'Officina Ferraria' z roku 1616. **Arch Hist Med (Warsz)** 1984;47(1):107–16
**Jonecko A, Stasienko J, Jonecko U:** Historia akupunktury chińskiej w średniowieczu i w czasach nowożytnych. **Wiad Lek** 1982 Dec 15;35(23–24):1593–601
**Jonecko A, Stasienko J, Jonecko U:** Najdawniejszs historia akupunktury chińskiej. **Wiad Lek** 1981 Apr 15;34(8):703–9
**Jonecko A:** Uwagi o podręczniku histochemii Freya z roku 1870 na tle osiągnięć histochemicznych połowy XIX wieku. **Wiad Lek** 1979 Dec 15;32(24):1811–4
**Jonecko A:** Wkład uczonych polskich do badań nad branchiogennymi odchyleniami rozwojowymi szyi na przełomie XIX i XX wieku. **Pol Przegl Chir** 1979 Sep;51(9):921–26
**Jonecko A, Stasienko J, Jonecko U:** Zarys historii akupunktury chińskiej w średniowieczu i w czasach nowozytnych. **Arch Hist Med (Warsz)** 1984;47(3):417–27
**Jonecko U** see **Jonecko A**
**Jones A:** In the children's aid: J. J. Kelso and child welfare in Ontario. Toronto, Buffalo, University of Toronto Press, 1981. viii, 210 p.
**Jones AG** see **Rice AL**
**Jones AH:** A commentary on 'Two pathographies: a study in illness and literature'. **J Med Philos** 1984 Aug;9(3):257–9
**Jones AH:** The healer-patient/family relationship in Vonda N. McIntyre's 'Of mist, and grass, and sand'. **Perspect Biol Med** 1983 Winter;26(2):274–80
**Jones AT:** The new medical centre and the development of medical education in Wales. In J. Cule, ed: Wales and medicine. London, British Society for the History of Medicine, 1975. p. 23–29.
**Jones B** see **Austin F**
**Jones BR:** Changing concepts of trachoma and its control. **Trans Ophthalmol Soc UK** 1980 Apr;100(pt 1):25–9
**Jones C:** 'Professionalizing modern medicine' in French hospitals. **Med Hist** 1982 Jul;26(3):341–9
**Jones C:** The coughing disease. **Health Visit** 1982 Dec;55(12):648–50
**Jones C:** The French Revolution, hospitals, and the medical profession. **Soc Soc Hist Med Bull (Lond)** 1984 Jun;34:6–9
**Jones C:** The 'new treatment' of the insane in Paris: the formation of the lunatic asylum under the French Revolution. **Hist Today** 1980 Oct;30:5–10
**Jones C, Sonenscher M:** The social functions of the hospital in 18th-century France: the case of the Hôtel-Dieu of Nîmes. **Fr Hist Stud** 1983;13:172–214
**Jones C:** The treatment of the insane in eighteenth- and early nineteenth-century Montpellier. A contribution to the prehistory of the lunatic asylum in provincial France. **Med Hist** 1980;24(4):371–90
**Jones DA:** Nicholas Culpeper and his Pharmacopoeia. **Pharm Hist (London)** 1980 Aug;10(2):9–10
**Jones DE, Ledingham KW:** Arsenic in Napoleon's wallpaper. **Nature** 1982 Oct 14;299(5884):626–7
**Jones DL** see **Cash P**
**Jones DM:** The veterinary surgeon in the zoo world. **Vet Rec** 1982 Dec 4;111(23):526–8
**Jones DN** see **Child abuse: historical perspective**
**Jones DP:** American chemists and the Geneva protocol. **Isis** 1980 Sep;71(258):426–40
**Jones DR:** Aeromedical transportation of psychiatric patients: historical review and present management. **Aviat Space Environ Med** 1980 Jul;51(7):709–16
**Jones DR** see **Low AA**
**Jones DR** see **Mills JG**
**Jones E:** Social class and psychotherapy: a critical review of research. **Psychiatry** 1974;37(4):307–20
**Jones EF:** The impact of women's employment on marital fertility in the U. S. 1970–1975. **Popul Stud** 1981;35(2):161–74
**Jones EF:** Ways in which childbearing affects women's employment: evidence from the U. S. 1975 national fertility study. **Popul Stud** 1982,36(1):5–14
**Jones EW:** Addysg feddygol i ferched: cyfraniadau o gymru at agor y cyndyn ddorau. **Cylchgrawn Llyfrgell Genedlaethol Cymru** 1976;19(3):249–92
**Jones EW:** Richard III's disfigurement: a medical postscript. **Folklore** 1980;91:211–27
**Jones EW:** Sir John Williams (1840–1926): his background and achievement. In J. Cule, ed: Wales and medicine. London, British Society for the History of Medicine, 1975. p. 86–95.
**Jones F:** John Clinch. In Dictionary of Canadian biography, 1801 to 1820. Volume 5, 1983. p. 189–190.
**Jones FA:** Presidential address. Lettsom, food and fibre. **Trans Med Soc Lond** 1977–78;94:1–14
**Jones G:** Alexander Fleming. **New Sci** 1981;91:349–51
**Jones GP:** The Welsh poet as a medical historian. In J. Cule, ed: Wales and medicine. London, British Society for the History of Medicine, 1975. p. 119–26.
**Jones GR:** The King Edward VII Welsh National Memorial Association, 1912–1948. In J. Cule, ed: Wales and medicine. London, British Society for the History of Medicine, 1975. p. 30–41.
**Jones GW:** George Edmund Gifford, jr. **Proc Am Antiq Soc** 1981;91(1):22–4
**Jones GW** see **Muthiah A**
**Jones IG:** Merthyr Tydfil: the politics of survival. **Llafur J Soc Stud Welsh Labour Hist** 1976;2(1):18–31
**Jones IG** see **Cameron D**
**Jones IH:** Menstruation: the history of sanitary protection. **Nurs Times** 1980 Mar 6;76(10):407–8
**Jones IH:** Wages through the ages. **Nurs Times** 1980 Jul 17;76(29):1279–80
**Jones IW:** Chloroform anaesthesia in Liverpool. **Anaesthesia** 1983 Jun;38(6):578–80
**Jones JE:** Parasites in Kentucky: the past seven decades. **J Ky Med Assoc** 1983 Aug;81(8):621–7
**Jones JH:** Alan Gregg. In Dictionary of American Biography, Suppl. 6, 1956–1960. p. 252–3, 1980.
**Jones JH:** Bad blood: the Tuskegee syphilis experiment. New York, Free Press; London, Collier Macmillan; 1981. xii, 272 p.
**Jones K:** Robert Gardiner Hill and the non-restraint movement. **Can J Psychiatry** 1984 Mar;29(2):121–4
**Jones MJ:** The Francis E. Fronczak Collection. **Niagara Frontier** 1978;25(4):96–9
**Jones MO** see **Hand WD, ed**
**Jones MR** see **Benjamin LT**
**Jones MV** see **Shoemaker P**
**Jones OP:** A peripatetic surgery in Valhalla (Frank Hastings Hamilton). **Am J Surg** 1982 Mar;143(3):370–3
**Jones OR:** Essense of peppermint: history of the medicine and its bottle. **Hist Archaeol** 1981;15(2):1–57
**Jones P:** Secreta Salernitana. **Kos** 1984 Feb;1(1):33–50
**Jones PG:** 'A man and his hospital'. **Aust Paediatr J** 1981 Mar;17(1):5–14
**Jones RE:** Moral treatment: the basis of private mental hospital care. **Psychiatr Hosp** 1983 Winter;14(1):5–9
**Jones RJ:** The NCCLS and medical devices. **JAMA** 1980 May 2;243(17):1748
**Jones RL:** A note on public health in early Galveston. **Bookman** 1982;9(9):3–7
**Jones TB:** Calvin Jones, M.D.: a case study in the practice of early American medicine. **NC Hist Rev** 1972;49(1):56–71
**Jones WB:** Mineral springs and medicine in North Carolina. **NC Med J** 1983 Sep;44(9):593–5
**Jones WL:** Ministering to minds diseases: a history of psychiatric treatment. London, W. Heinemann Medical Books, 1983. x, 157 p.
**Jones WR:** The clinic in three medieval societies. **Diogenes** 1983;122:86–101
**Jones AH, ed:** Images of healers. Albany, State University of New York Press, 1983. 160 p. (Literature and medicine, v. 2)
**Jongkees LB:** 125 jaar Nederlands Tijdschrift voor Geneeskunde, uit het verleden via het heden naar de toekomst. **Ned Tijdschr Geneeskd** 1982 Jan 2;126(1):1–3
**Jonsen AR:** Ethics as immunotherapy. **Forum Med** 1978 Oct;1(7):50–2
**Jonsen AR, Sagan L:** Torture and the ethics of medicine. **Man Med** 1978;3(1):33–49
**Jonsen AR** see **McCullough LB**
**Jonston WD:** [The scientific revolution in 18th century Japanese medicine – the ideal premise for the development of Dutch learning.] (Jpn). **Nihon I-Shigaku Zasshi** 1981;27(1):6–20
**Jopat PD:** Abstracts of medico historical articles in Hindi journals. **Bull Indian Inst Hist Med (Hyderabad)** 1978;8(1–4):51–62
**Jopat PD:** Abstracts of medico historical articles in Hindi journals. **Bull Indian Inst Hist Med (Hyderabad)** 1979;9:128–40
**Jopat PD:** Abstracts of medico-historical articles in Hindi journals. **Bull Indian Inst Hist Med Hyderabad** 1982;12(1–4):51–65
**Jopat PD:** Abstracts of select medico-historical articles in Hindi [1974]. **Bull Indian Inst Hist Med (Hyderabad)** 1975 Oct;5(4):249–52
**Jope EM:** The emergence of man: information from protein systems. **Philos Trans R Soc Lond [Biol]** 1981 May 8;292(1057):121–31
**Jopp R:** Einzelheiten zur Geschichte der Augenheilkunde von der Antike bis um 1800 am Beispiel von Köln. Köln, Universität zu Köln, 1980. 225 p. (Kölner medizinhistorische Beiträge, 16), (also Diss.).
**Joppich G:** Begegnung mit grossen Pädiatern aus der Frühzeit der deutschen Kinderheilkunde. **Monatsschr Kinderheilkd** 1984 Jun;1132(6):318–24
**Jorda V** see **Kolařik J**
**Jordan CA:** Graduate medical education in Mobile 1859–1981. **J Med Assoc State Ala** 1981 Oct;51(4):16, 18, 24–9
**Jordan TE:** Lancashire lasses and Yorkshire lads: childhood in the early nineteenth century. **R Soc Health J** 1982 Feb;102(1):14–20
**Jordan TG:** 'The roses so red and the lilies so fair': southern folk cemeteries in Texas. **Southwest Hist Q** 1980;83(3):227–58
**Jordanova L:** La donna di cera. **Kos** 1984 May;1(4):82–9
**Jordanova L:** Urban health in the French Enlightenment. **Soc Soc Hist Med Bull (Lond)** 1983 Jun;32:31–3
**Jordanova LJ:** Medical police and public health: problems of practice and ideology. **Soc Soc Hist Med Bull (Lond)** 1980;27:15–19
**Jordanova LJ:** Policing public health in France 1780–1815. In Ogawa T, ed: Public health. Tokyo, Saikon, 1981. p. 12–32.
**Jordanova LJ:** Romantic science? Michelet, morals, and nature. **Br J Hist Sci** 1980 Mar;13(43 pt 1):44–50
**Jordanova LJ:** Towards the light? Science, politics and the enlightenment. **Eur Stud Rev** 1982;12(4):479–88

**Jordanova L, ed:** Medical records newsletter. (Research Publications of the Wellcome Unit for the History of Medicine, Oxford. No. IV). Oxford, Wellcome Unit for the History of Medicine, 1980. viii, 42 p.
**Jorde LB** see **Skolnick MH**
**Jorden PJ:** Surgeon on safari. New York, Hawthorn, 1976. xiv, 173 p.
**Jordi FR:** Un capitulo de la propaganda farmacéutica: troquelados. **Circ Farm** 1981;12(134-5):58-61,68-72
**Jordi R:** Antonio Sala, un boticario barcelon/B//es aficionado a la botánica. **Farm Univers** 1980;13(1,2):10-7,78-82
**Jordi R:** Bases para un estudio de la evolución del medicamento en el Hospital de la Santa Cruz (1793-1796). Hospital General de Barcelona (1812-1814). Introducción. **Circ Farm** 1981 Jul;12(140):91-7
**Jordi R:** De los sabios de ayer al 'bichito' de hoy. **Periodico** 1981 Sep 5;4:883
**Jordi R:** Humor colérico. **Circ Farm** 1981 Apr;12(137):61-71
**Jordi R:** Legislación sanitaria marítima española en vigor durante el siglo XIX. **Circ Farm** 1981 Jun;12(139):75-84
**Jordi R:** Manuel Blasco, pintor, escritor y bohemio. **Circ Farm** 1981 Mar;12(136):83-8
**Jordi R:** Notas sobre terapéutica hospitalaria usada en una epidemia en Montblanc. Año 1725. **Circ Farm** 1981 May;12(138):38-73
**Jordi R:** Segundas nupcias de Catalina Barbara con Juan Vilarrubia. Inventario y Pacto. (3-10/ 3-11/ 11-11 de 1608). **Circ Farm** 1981 Aug-Sep;12(141-2)57-60, 56-66
**Jordi Gonzáles R:** Curiosas formulas de medicina popular pertenecientes al ultimo cuarto del siglo XV. **Offarm** 1982;1(4):239-46
**Jordi Gonzàlez FR:** Contribució a la genealogia dels farmacèutics catalans; consideracions sobre Narcís Viader i Font. Barcelona, the author, 1981. p. 4-10.
**Jordi González FR:** Notas legislativas sobre los estatutos de autonomia catalanes 1932/1979. **Circ Farm** 1979 Oct;11(119):19-27
**Jordi González FR:** Recetas en circulación en Barcelona durante la Guerra Civil de 1936-1939. **Circ Farm** 1979 Nov;11(120):40-5
**Jordi González FR:** Recuerdos para un Montepío. **Circ Farm** 1980 Dec;12(133):75-84
**Jordi González FR:** Un desconocido anteproyecto de confederación de farmacias nacido en Barcelona durante la guerra civil de 1936-1939. **Circ Farm** 1979 Dec;11(121):54-8
**Jordi Gonzàlez R:** Activitat del col.legi de Farmacèutics de Barcelona durant la Renaixença. **Figueres** 1981 (Separata: Ciència Renaixença Catalana)
**Jordi González R:** Anotaciones a los discursos botánicos del boticario barcelonés Antonio Sala Domènech. **An Med Cir** 1982;60(261):24-45
**Jordi González R:** Bibliotecas de boticarios catalanes: aportacion para un estudio. **Circ Farm** 1984;283:127-42
**Jordi González R:** Chocolate. De la taza a la farmacia. **Circ Farm** 1980 Jun;12(127):57-62
**Jordi Gonzalez R:** Cien año de vida farmacéutica barcelonesa (1830-1939). Barcelona, Circular Farmaceutica. [1982]. 615 p.
**Jordi González R:** Contribución para el estudio sociológico de la farmacia barcelonesa durante la guerra civil, a través de la prensa política. **Circ Farm** 1984;282:55-62
**Jordi González R:** Contribución para el estudio sociológico de la Farmacia barcelonesa durante la guerra civil, a través de la prensa política. (pt. I-VI). **Circ Farm** 1981-82 Dec, Jan, Feb, Mar, Jun, Sep;12-13:145-52
**Jordi González R:** Control de substancias medicinales por el colegio de boticarios de Barcelona en el siglo XVI (1531-1574). Federacion Farmaceutica, Sociedad Cooperative, Seccion Cienfica, 28th, Barcelona, April 7, 1983. 12 p.
**Jordi Gonzalez R:** Criterios basicos para una modificacion de los colegios de farmaceuticos catalanes. **Monit Farm Ter** 1980-81;2116-8:var. pagings
**Jordi González R:** Criterios del boticario y academico barcelones Jose Ignacio Mollar sobre la tinta de escribir. **Offarm** 1982;1(9):453-67
**Jordi González R:** Dos curiosos impresos, supuestos del siglo XIX. **Circ Farm** 1980 May;12(126):85-9
**Jordi González R:** Duedas y cuentas de boticarios: una reivindicación histórica obligada. [Barcelona], Réal Academía de Farmacía de Barcelona, 1985. 63 p.
**Jordi González R:** Formulas de medicina popular y supersticiosa pertenecientes a la primera mitad del siglo XVI (1504-1568). **Circ Farm** 1983;281:283-309
**Jordi González R:** Fórmulas medicinales populares y supersticiosas pertenecientes a la primera mitad del siglo XV (1417-1459). **Circ Farm** 1981 Oct-Dec;39(273):469-82
**Jordi González R:** Inventario incompleto perteneciente a la botica del hospital de Santa Cruz, de Barcelona (21-1-1585). **Circ Farm** 1982 Apr-Jun;40(275):211-21
**Jordi González R:** La tarifa del Colegio de Boticarios de Barcelona año 1588. **Circ Farm** 1982 Jul-Sep;40(276):313-25
**Jordi González R:** Nota sobre higiene ciudadana en la Barcelona de finales del siglo XVIII. **Circ Farm** 1980;12(124):61-4
**Jordi González R:** Notas dispersas sobre la Facultad de Farmacia de Barcelona. **Circ Farm** 1980 Apr;12(125):91-8
**Jordi González R:** Notas sobre boticarios y drogueros a finales del siglo XVI. Testigos en un pleito 1587-1589. In: Estudis històrics i documents dels arxius de protocols, VIII (1980). Barcelona, Col. Legi Notarial de Barcelona. 1980. p. 171-222.
**Jordi González R:** Notas sobre la clausura de una farmacia cooperativa, después del 6 de octubre de 1934. **Circ Farm** 1980 Feb;12(123):70-3
**Jordi González R:** Notas sobre la economía de una farmacia barcelonesa colectivizada durante la guerra civil española. **Circ Farm** 1980;12(122):51-67
**Jordi Gonzalez R:** Oportunas consideraciones sobre la auto--medicacion. **An Med Cir** 1979 Apr-Jun;(256):99-114
**Jordi Gonzalez R:** Reflexiones sobre el inventario de una botica barcelonesa del siglo XVIII. **Circ Farm** 1981;12(143):83-95
**Jordi González R:** Visita de boticas en Cataluña a principios del siglo XVIII (16-3-1710/10-4-1710). **Circ Farm** 1982 Jan-Mar;40(274):111-39
**Jordon RE:** 'An unusual type of pemphigus combining feature of lupus erythematosus' by Senear and Usher, June 1926. Commentary: Pemphigus erythematosus, a unique member of the pemphigus group. **Arch Dermatol** 1982 Oct;118(10):723-42
**Jorge H** see **Zambrano L**
**Jörgensen G:** Spiel und Sport aus genetisch-phylogenetischer Sicht. **MMW** 1981 Jun 19;123(25):1039-42
**Jorgensen JB** see **Jakobsen J**
**Jørgensen RJ** see **Rose CH**
**Jori A** see **Cilenti V**
**Joris I** see **Majno G**
**Joseph A:** Intelligence, IQ, and race: When, how, and why they became associated. San Francisco, R & E Research Associates, 1977. vii, 142 p.
**Joseph H** see **Courtwright DT**
**Josephson ME:** The AJC in March 1959. **Am J Cardiol** 1984 Mar 1;53(6):803-4
**Joshi D:** Concept of Rasa sala (pharmacy) in ancient India. **Nagarjun** 1978;22:88-90
**Joshi VK:** Evolution of the concept of Astavarga. **Indian J Hist Sci** 1983 May;18(1):9-14
**Josipovici J:** Franz Anton Mesmer, magnétiseur, médecin et franc-maçon. Monaco, Editions du Rocher, 1982. 200 p.
**Joske RA:** The physician and changing patterns of human disease and death. In Stanley NF, Joske RA, ed: Changing disease patterns and human behaviour. London, New York, Academic Press, 1980. p. 551-66.
**Jost A:** Commentaires sur les articles de Gustave Julliard. Fistule pyo-stercorale--laparotomie et suture de l'intestin--guérison par première intention. Hernio-laparotomie--résection de dix-huit centimètres d'intestin--guérison. **Rev Med Suisse Romande** 1980 Dec;100(12):1089-96
**Jost M:** Die Apoplexielehre Johann Jakob Wepfers (1620-1695). Diss., Rheinische Friedrich-Wilhelms-Universität, Bonn, 1982. 76 p.
**Jottras PL:** Jean Astruc, médecin humaniste. **Hist Sci Med** 1984;18(3):271-7
**Jouanna J:** Le schéma d'exposition des maladies et ses déformations dans les traités dérivés des Sentences cnidiennes. In La collection hippocratique et son rôle dans l'histoire de la médecine. Colloque de Strasbourg (23-27 octobre 1972) organisé par le Centre de Recherches sur la Grèce Antique, avec le concours des Facultés de Philosophie et des Langues Classiques. Leiden, E. J. Brill, 1975. p. 129-50.
**Jouanna J:** Le traité hippocratique du Régime dans les maladies aiguës: remarques sur la tradition manuscrite et sur le texte. **Rev Hist Textes (Paris)** 1976;6:1-30
**Jouanna J:** Une forme étymologique retrouvée: omelesis dans le Glossaire hippocratique de Galien et dans le traité hippocratique des Maladies II c, 31. **Rev Philol (Paris)** 1979;53:260-63
**Jouanna J** see **Grmek MD, ed**
**Jouanna J** see **Hippocrates**
**Joubert L:** Treatise on laughter. Translated and annotated by G. D. de Rocher. University, Alabama, University of Alabama Press, 1980. xv, 155 p.
**The Journal of the American Medical Association:** Reproduction of first issue Saturday, July 14, 1883. **JAMA** 1983 Jul 8;250(2):Centennial Issue.
**The Journal's 30th anniversary: J Prosthet Dent** 1980 Jan;43(1):4-8
**Jovanovic D** see **Borisev V**
**Jovanovič J:** Izvještaj ruskih ljekara o crnogorskim ranjenicima i borbama crnogoraca s turcima 1876. godine. **Istor Zapisi** 1979;32(3):77-88
**Jovanovic L** see **Sarac S**
**Jovin S:** Kolera u prošlosti Novog Sada. **Med Pregl** 1981;34(7-8):349-54
**Jovin S:** Uticaj zdravstvenih prilika na iščeznuce srpskog živla u selu Gložanu. **Naucni Sastanak Zb Rad Naucno Drus Iator Zdrav Kult Jugosl** 1977;15:161-66
**Joy ML** see **Barrett HH**
**Joy RJ:** Jonathan Letterman of Jefferson: medical director of the Army of the Potomac. In Medical-Science colloquium. Special edition of Topic: a journal of the liberal arts. Washington, Pennsylvania, Washington and Jefferson College, 1983. p. 26-38.
**Joy RJ:** Occupying the visual cortex: using slides to teach the history of medicine. In J. J. Bylebyl, ed: Teaching the history of medicine at a medical center. Baltimore, London, Johns Hopkins University Press, 1982. (The Henry E. Sigerist supplements to the Bulletin of the History of Medicine; new ser., no. 7). p. 103-14.
**Joy RJ:** Starting from scratch: installing a history of medicine program in a new medical school. With a commentary by L.G. Stevenson. In J. J. Bylebyl, ed: Teaching the history of medicine at a medical center. Baltimore, London, Johns Hopkins University Press, 1982. (The Henry E. Sigerist supplements to the Bulletin of the History of Medicine; new ser., no. 7). p. 139-51.
**Joyce RM:** Frontiers in Chemistry. **Science** 1980 Jul 4;209(4452):89-95
**Joynt RJ:** Landmark perspective: A new look at death. **JAMA** 1984 Aug 3;252(5):680-2
**Joynt RJ:** The great confrontation: the meeting between Broca and Jackson in 1868. In Rose FC, Bynum WF, ed: Historical aspects of the

neurosciences. New York, Raven, 1982. p. 99–102.
**Jozefíniová E** see **Bunčáková V**
**Juan López M, Berumen Amor E, Trejo Rayón S, et al:** La mujer en las acciones de atención a la salud en México. **Salud Publica Mex** 1984 Nov–Dec;26(6):537–45
**The jubilee year: NZ Dent J** 1980 Apr;76(344):47–8
**Jucker-Wannier E:** Zum Jubiläumsjahr der Ingenbohler Schwestern. Ein Rückblick auf Festfeiern und Ausstellung an der Schule für allgemeine Krankenpflege des Instituts Ingenbohl am St.-Clara-Spital Basel. **Krankenpflege (Bern)** 1980 Aug;(8):406–7
**Jucovy PM:** Circle and circulation: the language and imagery of William Harvey's discovery. **Perspect Biol Med** 1976 Autumn;20(1):92–107
**Judd CS:** Plantation health. **Hawaii Med J** 1982 Apr;41(4):116, 118
**Judd CS:** Some early physicians of Hawaii--1800s. **Hawaii Med J** 1984 Jul;43(7):250
**Judd CS Jr:** Leprosy in Hawaii, 1889–1976. **Hawaii Med J** 1984 Sep;43(9):328–9, 333–4
**Jude A** see **Nicolle P**
**Judkins BM:** Occupational health and the developing class consciousness of southern textile workers: the case of the Brown Lung Association. **Md Hist** 1982 Spring–Summer;13:55–71
**Judson H** see **Edsall JT**
**Judson HF:** Reflections on the historiography of molecular biology. **Minerva** 1980 Autumn;18(3):369–421
**Judson HF:** The eighth day of creation. New York, Simon and Schuster, 1979. 686 p.
**Juffermans P:** Economic crisis and health policy in the Netherlands. **Int J Health Serv** 1984;14(1):147–58
**Jugnot G** see **La Coste-Messelière R de**
**Juhász F:** Die Anfänge und spezifischen Züge der Persönlichkeitspädagogik im Ungarn der Jahrhundertwende. **Ann Univ Sci Budap Rolando Eotvos Nominatae** 1972;3:41–54
**Juhasz L:** Den selvregulerende mekanisme hos befolninger i eldre tid. **Heimen** 1974;16(5):255–8
**Juillet P:** Aspects évolutifs de la psychiatrie aux armées. In: Congrès National des Sociétés Savantes, 103e, Nancy, 1978. Comptes Rendus. Paris, 1978. Section des Sciences, Fasc. V. p. 99–111.
**Jukes TH:** A biochemical adventure--the hunt for vitamin D. **J Appl Biochem** 1983 Jun;5(3):147–8
**Jukes TH:** Early studies on nicotinic acid in animal nutrition. **Fed Proc** 1981 Apr;40(5):1536–7
**Jukes TH:** Living history: nutritional discoveries of the 1930's: introductory remarks. **Fed Proc** 1979 Dec;38(13):2679–80
**Jukes TH:** Philip Handler (1917–1981). A biographical sketch. **J Nutr** 1983 Jun;113(6):1086–94
**Julia D** see **Forster R**
**Julien P:** Culte et iconographie des saints médecins Come et Damien dans une province française. In International Congress of the History of Medicine, 27th, Barcelona, 1980. Actas. Barcelona, Académia de Ciències Médiques de Catalunya i Balears, 1981. p. 530–4.
**Julien P:** Deux saints médecins et pharmaciens, Côme et Damien. **Bull Liaison Assoc Amis Mus Pharm Montp** 1982;:(7):13–35
**Julien P:** La France envahie par Hunyadi János. In Hein WH, ed: Pharmaziehistorischer Kongress, Budapest, 1981. Stuttgart, Wissenschaftliche Verlagsgesellschaft, 1983. p. 111–28.
**Julien P:** Le Dr. Véron et Daumier, ou le fabricant de pâté pectorale en proie à la caricature. In: Congrès international d'histoire de la médecine, XXVe, Québec, 1976. Actes. Québec, 1977. p. 807–21.
**Julien P:** Le lunch des 12 millions. **Rev Hist Pharm (Paris)** 1980 Jun;27(245):91–3
**Julien P:** Le 'médecin de la montagne' Michel Schüppach (1707–1781): médecin ou charlatan? In International Congress of the History of Medicine. 26th, Plovdiv, 1978. Actes du Congress. Sofia, 1981. Volume II. p. 116–9.
**Julien P:** Le point sur les ex-libris professionnels à l'effigie des saints Côme et Damien. **Rev Hist Pharm (Paris)** 1982;29(252):176–8
**Julien P:** Les apothicaires et autres vendeurs de médicaments de la rue Dauphine, à Paris, dans la seconde moitié du XVIIIe siècle, et l'importation de produits pharmaceutiques. In Dilg P, et al., ed: Perspektiven der Pharmaziegeschichte. Graz, Austria, Akademische Druck- u. Verlagsanstalt, 1983. p. 165–79.
**Julien P:** Les 'Eléments de pharmacie' de Baumé et la contrefaçon. **Rev Hist Pharm (Paris)** 1981 Jun;28(249):103–6
**Julien P:** Médailles modernes à sujet pharmaceutique et médical. **Rev Hist Pharm (Paris)** 1980 Mar;27(244):39–47
**Julien P:** Pharmacie et philatélie. **Rev Hist Pharm (Paris)** 1981;28:69–73
**Julien P:** Remarque sur l'édition 1936 de 'l'Officine' de Dorvault. **Rev Hist Pharm (Paris)** 1982 Mar;29(252):37–8
**Julien P:** Sur le célèbre 'dentiste' ou 'pharmacien' de Pietro Longhi. **Pharm Weekbl** 1981 Nov 6;116(45):1389–92
**Julien P:** Trois expositions. **Rev Hist Pharm (Paris)** 1980 Dec;247(68 no 27):272–6
**Julien P:** Un empire industriel issu d'une droguerie pharmaceutique. **Rev Hist Pharm (Paris)** 1982 Sep;29(254):180–2
**Julien P:** Un psychanalyste, Jacques Lacan. **Etudes (Fr)** 1982;357(4):333–46
**Julien P:** Une miniature des saints Côme et Damien (fin XVe - début XVIe siècle). **Rev Hist Pharm (Paris)** 1982 Sep;29(254):175–6
**Julien P** see **Gagnière S**
**Jullien Y:** Histoire des benzodiazépines. **Ann Fr Anesth Reanim** 1984;3(3):153–4
**Junas J:** K rozvíjaniu sociálnolekárskych hl'adísk na Slovensku v 19. storočí. **Cesk Zdrav** 1983 Feb;31(2):65–70
**Junas J:** K starším dejinám psychiatrie na Slovensku. **Bratisl Lek Listy** 1981;76(3):383–7
**Junas J:** Prostredie štúdií a spoločenská aktivita slovenských medikov v 19. storočí. **Cas Lek cesk** 1980 Jul 25;119(29–30):820–2
**Junas J:** Z histórie česko-slovenských vztahov v medicíne a zdravotníctve. **Cesk Zdrav** 1983 Mar;31(3):114–8
**Juncà i Ramon JM:** L'Hospital de Sant Llàtzer: notes històriques. [S.l.]: J. M. Juncà Ramon, 1982. 47 p.
**Jünemann G** see **Busse H**
**Jünemann J:** Nachlese zu Rillen und Näpfchen auf sakralen Denkmalen (2). **Beitr Gesch Pharm** 1980;31(7):49–54
**Jung CG:** Erinnerungen, Träume, Gedanken. Olten, Walter-Verlag, 1984. 419 p.
**Jung CG:** The essential Jung. Princeton, Princeton University Press, 1983. 447 p.
**Jung R, Berger W:** Fünfzig Jahre EEG. Hans Bergers Entdeckung des Elektrenkephalogramms und seine ersten Befunde 1924--1931. **Arch Psychiatr Nervenkr** 1979 Dec;227(4):279–300
**Jung R:** Sinnesphysiologische Bemerkungen zu Thomas von Aquinos Maxime der Sinneserkenntnis. **Sudhoffs Arch** 1980;64(4):371–84
**Jung R:** W. R. Hess und das Ordnungsprinzip in der Physiologie. **Schweiz Arch Neurol Neurochir Psychiatr** 1983;132(2):277–308
**Jung R:** Walter R. Hess (1881–1973). **Rev Physiol Biochem Pharmacol** 1981;88:1–21
**Jung T:** X-rays in dentistry. **J Am Dent Assoc** 1982 Apr;104(4):438
**Jung-Merker L, Ruf E, ed:** C. G. Jung: Bibliographie. Olten [Switzerland], Walter-Verlag, 1983. 295 p. (C. G. Jung gesammelte Werke, 19)
**Jungers WL** see **Fleagle JG**
**Junghans RP:** Falstaff was drunker than he was fat. **N Engl J Med** 1983 Jun 16;308(24):1483
**Jungnickel C:** The Royal Saxon Society of Sciences: a study of nineteenth century German science. Ph.D. Diss., Johns Hopkins University. Baltimore, 1978. v, 222 leaves.
**Jungnitz B:** Die konfessionellen Krankenhäuser der Stadt Münster im achtzehnten und neunzehnten Jahrhundert. Herzogenrath, Verlag Murken-Altrogge, 1981. 304 p. (Studien zur Geschichte des Krankenhauswesens. 18).
**Junkte F:** Ueber Leonhard Thurneisser zum Thurn und seine deutschen Kalendar 1572–1584. **Arch Gesch Buchwes** 1978;19:1349–400
**Junkte F:** Ueber Leonhard Thurneisser zum Thurn und seine Schriften nach seine Flucht aus Berlin (1584). **Arch Gesch Buchwes** 1980;21:679–718
**Jurado S** see **Colotla VA**
**Juricic B:** Chile y las organizaciones internacionales de salud. **Rev Med Chil** 1977 Oct;105(10):674–9
**Jurion F, Parisel F:** Le troisième et dernier cimetière de l'hôpital Saint-Jean de Bruxelles (1704–1784). Etude paléopathologique des ossements du cimetière Saint-Jean. **Ann Soc Belg Hist Hop** 1982;20:2–60
**Jurkovic P** see **Stahan J**
**Jurmain R:** Human evolution: a century of research. **San Jose Stud** 1982;8(3):40–50
**Jurmain RD:** The pattern of involvement of appendicular degenerative joint disease. **Am J Phys Anthropol** 1980 Jul;53(1):143–50
**Jusatz HJ:** 150 Jahre pandemische Ausbreitung der asiatischen Cholera von 1831 bis 1981. **Zentralbl Bakteriol Mikrobiol Hyg [A]** 1982 Jun;252(2):257–67
**Just Viera JO:** Mitral valve commissurotomy by John Alexander: repeat surgery 28 years later. **Bol Asoc Med PR** 1981 Feb;73(2):56–8
**Justin-Besançon L** see **150e année**
**Juszczyński M:** Ostatnie osi ągni ęcia transplantacji serca i płuc. **Kardiol Pol** 1983;26(10):733–9
**Juszczyński M:** Piętnaście lat transplantacji serca. **Pol Tyg Lek** 1983 May 9;38(19):615–8
**Juszczyński M:** 15 lat transplantacji serca. **Pieleg Polozna** 1984;(2):16–7
**Jutikkala E:** Finnish mortality in the eighteenth century: the sources and the reality **Scand Econ Hist Rev** 1978;26(2):168–9
**Jüttner G:** Alchemie und Sympathielehre in der Therapie der frühen Neuzeit. In: Der Uebergang zur Neuzeit und die Wirkung von Traditionen. VortrAB/age, gehalten auf der Tagung der Joachim-Jungius-Gesellschaft der Wissenschaften, Hamburg, am 13. und 14. Oktober 1977. Göttingen, Vandenhoeck & Ruprecht, 1978. p. 130–140.
**Jüttner G:** Der Dialog in Pharmazie, Chemie und Botanik. Zum Anteil einer literarischen Gattung in der Darstellung, Vermittlung und im Unterricht der Naturwissenschaften. **Ber Wissenschaftsgesch** 1980;3(1–2):23–34
**Jüttner G:** Ein 'Pharmacopoeus spagyricus': Johann Conrad Barkhausen (1666–1723) und die Pharmazie. In Dilg P, et al., ed: Perspektiven der Pharmaziegeschichte. Graz, Austria, Akademische Druck- u. Verlagsanstalt, 1983. p. 147–64.
**Juvan V:** Djelatnost za zdravstvenu zaštitu žena Medicinskog centra u Varaždinu. **Jugosl Ginekol Opstet** 1978;18(5–6):445–53
**Južnič M:** Razvoj partizanskog saniteta u Sloveniji u toku nardnooslobodilačkog rata (II). **Vojnosanit Pregl** 1982 Mar–Apr;39(2):127–42
**Južnič M:** Razvoj partizanskog saniteta u Sloveniji za vreme Narodnooslobodilačkog rata. **Vojnosanit Pregl** 1981 Nov–Dec;38(6):412–22

# K


**K 100-letiiu so dnia rozhdeniia A. A. Bogomol'tsa: Klin Med (Mosk)** 1981 Nov;59(11):3-8
**K 100-letiiu so dnia rozhdeniia akademika A. A. Bogomol'tsa: Fiziol Zh** 1981 May-Jun;27(3):291-443
**K 100-letiiu so dnia smerti Charlza Darvina: Arkh Anat Gistol Embriol** 1982 Nov;83(11):5-6
**K 40-letiiu Akademii meditsinskikh nauk SSSR: Arkh Anat Gistol Embriol** 1984 Jun;86(6):5-10
**K 40-letiiu organov urpavleniia Tylom Vooruzhennykh Sil SSSR: Voen Med Zh** 1981 Aug;(8):7-11
**K 60. narodeninám doc. MUDr. Jána Simku, CSc: Cesk Gynekol** 1983 Mar;48(2):151-8
**K 80-letiiu zhurnala nevropatologii i psikhiatrii im. S. S. Korsakova: Zh Nevropatol Psikhiatr** 1981;81(1):3-5
**Kaba L:** Archers, musketeers, and mosquitoes: the Moroccan invasion of the Sudan and the Songhay resistance (1591-1612). **J Afr Hist** 1981;22(4):457-75
**Kabanov MM:** Razvitie v deiatel'nosti Leningradskogo nauchno-issledovatel'skogo psikhonevrologicheskogo instituta im. V. M. Bekhtereva ideĭ ego osnovatelia. **Zh Nevropatol Psikhiatr** 1982;82(11):1234-7
**Käbin I:** Medicinska fakulteten vid universitetet i Dorpat (Tartu) 1802-1940. **Nord Medicinhist Arsb** 1984;:91-103
**Kabir M:** Regional variations in nuptiality in England and Wales during the demographic transition. **Genus** 1980;36(3-4):171-87
**Kabykenov PS** see **Chokin AR**
**Kaczorowski W:** Choroba i prawdopodobna przyczyna zgonu Zygmunta III Wazy. **Arch Hist Med (Warsz)** 1982;45(1-4):45-54
**Kadankov D:** Usuvurshenstvuvane na Bulgarskite zubolekari (1890-1930). **Stomatologiia (Sofiia)** 1979 Jul-Aug;61(4):273-5
**Kádár Z:** Gyógyító istenségek tisztelete Pannóniában topográfiai adatok tükrében. **Orvostort Kozl** 1981;93-96(27 No 1-4):63-78
**Kádár Z, Szlatky M:** Orvosi könyvillusztrációk a 15--18. sz'azadban. **Orv Hetil** 1981 Mar 22;122(12):711-4
**Kádár Z:** Survivals of Greek zoological illuminations in Byzantine manuscripts. Budapest, Akadémiai Kiadó. 1978. 138 p. (With 232 half-tone illustrations and 10 color plates).
**Kadár Z, Vizkelety A:** Zu den Pflanzen- und Tierdarstellungen in einem mittelalterlichen deutschen Kodex zu Debrecen (Ungarn). In Hein WH, ed: Pharmaziehistorischer Kongress, Budapest, 1981. Stuttgart, Wissenschaftliche Verlagsgesellschaft, 1983. p. 35-40.
**Kadish SH** see **Temkin O**
**Kadlecová V, Matousek O:** Deník Dr. Med. Josefa A. Ryby. Překlad z Německého Rukopisu Věra Kadleová. **Cesk Oftalmol** 1981 Sep;37(5):383-8
**Kadlecová V, Malousek O, ed:** Deník Dr. Med. Josefa Ryby. Překlad z německého rukopisu. **Cesk Oftalmol** 1981 Jul;37(4):293-6
**Kadlecová V:** Počátky oční kliniky v Praze, Jej í první profesor J.N. Fischer a jeho asistenti. III. První profesor pražské oční kliniky J.N. Fischer: jeho život; Fischer - učitel, operatér, člověk. **Cesk Oftalmol** 1983 Jul;39(4):268-80
**Kadlecová V:** Počátky oční kliniky v Praze, její první profesor J. N. Fischer a jeho asistenti. **Cesk Oftalmol** 1983 Mar;39(2):131-8
**Kadlecová V:** Počátky oční kliniky v Praze, její první profesor J. N. Fischer a jeho asistenti. **Cesk Oftalmol** 1983 May;39(3):202-14
**Kadlecová V:** Počátky oční kliniky v Praze, její první profesor J. N. Fischer a jeho asistenti. IV. Asistenti pražké oční kliniky do r. 1847. **Cesk Oftalmol** 1983 Sep;39(5):357-64
**Kadlecová V** see **Kadlecová V**
**Kadunkov D:** Diplomirovani zubolekari v Bulgariia ot 1905 do 1914 g. **Stomatologiia (Sofiia)** 1979;(3):201-3
**Kadunkov D:** Niakoi danni za meditsinata zubolechenito prez vtoroto bulgarsko tsarstvo i srednovekov neto. **Stomatologiia (Sofiia)** 1979 Jan-Feb;61(1):68-9
**Kadŭnkov D:** Njakoi danni za zubloekarstvoto v Bulgarija (1911-1930). **Stomatologiia (Sofiia)** 1979 Sep-Oct;61(5):328-31
**Kadunkov D:** Purvite obstestveni zubolekarski kabineti v Bulgarija (1907-1971). **Stomatologiia (Sofiia)** 1979 Nov-Dec;61(6):405-8
**Kadunkov D:** Zubolecenieto v bulgariia prez bulgarskoto vuzrazdane do osvobozdenieto na bulgariia. **Stomatologiia (Sofiia)** 1979 Mar-Apr;61(2):130-3
**Kadyrov AA:** N. A. Semashko v Uzbekistane. **Sov Zdravookhr** 1984;(1):49-50
**Kadyrov AA, Madakhanov AS:** Pervyĭ meditsinskiĭ institut Uzbekistana. **Sov Zdravookhr** 1980;(6):57-8
**Kadyrov AA, Asliddinov IF:** Razvitie vysshego meditsinskogo obrazovaniia v respublikakh Sovetskogo Vostoka. **Sov Zdravookhr** 1984;(3):50-1
**Kaemmerer K:** Die Arzneimittel des Veterinärdienstes im Zweiten Weltkrieg. **DTW** 1981 Nov 5;88(11):461-73
**Kaempfer E:** Amoenitatum Exoticarum Politico-physico-medicarum. Fasciculi V, Quibus Continentur Variae Relationes, Observationes and Descriptiones Rerum Persicarum and Ulterioris Asiae (Lemgo: Meyeri, 1712). **J Hist Med Allied Sci** 1978 Jul;33(3):320-43
**Kaempffer AM:** Evolución de la salud materno infantil en Chile, 1952-1977. **Rev Med Chil** 1977 Oct;105(10):680-6
**Kafedre genetiki Moskovskogo gosudarstvennogo universiteta imeni M. V. Lomonosova--50 let: Genetika (Moskva)** 1981;17(7):1318-20
**Kagan A** see **Mitterauer M**
**Kagan J** see **Lerner RM, ed**
**Kagan J** see **Lomax EM**
**Kagan RL:** From trade to profession: surgical education in eighteenth-century Spain. **Hist Educ Q** 1978;18(2):195-200
**Kageyama K, Shimanine T, Ishikawa E:** A seventy-year history of the Japanese pathological society. **Acta Pathol Jpn** 1982;32 Suppl 1:1-21
**Kageyama K, Mikata A, Harigaya K:** [Studies of Hodgkin's disease in Japan: a historical survey] (Jpn). **Nippon Rinsho** 1983 Nov;41(11):2432-8
**Kagoshima J:** Kachiku hoken eiseijo no ayumi. Kagoshima, Japan, Kagoshima-ken Noseibu, Showa 51 nen, 1976. 226 p.
**Kagoshima-shi Ishikai:** Kagoshima-shi Ishikai sanjunenshi. [Thirty years' history of the Kagoshima City Medical Association]. (Jpn) Kagoshima, Japan, Ishikai, Showa 53 nen [1978]. 537 p.
**Kagramanov KM** see **Buniiatov ZM**
**Kahan A:** Social aspects of the plague epidemics in eighteenth-century Russia. **Econ Dev Cult Change** 1979;27(2):255-66
**Kahan BD:** Cosmas and Damian revisited. **Transplant Proc** 1983 Dec;15(4 Suppl 1-2):2211-6
**Kahle E:** Al-Magusi (Haly Abbas) über Kinderkrankheiten im Kamil as-sina'a at-tibbiya. Erlangen, Verlagsbuchhandlung Hannelore Lüling, 1980. 61, [6] p.
**Kahle E:** Avicenna (Ibn Sina) über Kinderkrankheiten im Kinderregimen seines Qanun. Erlangen, Verlagsbuchhandlung Hannelore Lüling, 1979. 53, [14] p.
**Kahle E:** Das Ammenregimen des Avicenna (Ibn Sina) in seinem Qanun. Erlangen, Verlagsbuchhandlung Hannelore Lüling, 1980. 45, [13] p.
**Kahle E:** Der Traktat über das Zusammenwirken der Naturen des Qustā Ibn Lūqā. In Keil G, et al., ed: Fachprosa-Studien. Beiträge zur mittelalterlichen Wissenschafts-und Geistesgeschichte. Berlin, Schmidt, 1982. p. 133-42.
**Kahle E, Stupp JA:** Hochschulschriften zur Geschichte der Medizin, Pharmazie, und Naturwissenschaften der Friedrich-Alexander-Universität Erlangen-Nürnberg 1885-1975. Erlangen, Verlagsbuchhandlung Hannelore Lüling, 1980. 94 p. (Medizinhistorische Materialien, 2).
**Kahle E:** Hochschulschriften zur Geschichte der Medizin Pharmazie und Naturwissenschaften der Julius-Maximilians-Universität Würzburg, 1885-1970. Medizinhistorische Materialien - 1. Erlangen, Verlagsbuchhandlung, 1979. 48 p.
**Kahle E:** Kleinwächter, Ludwig. In Neue Deutsche Biographie 12. 1980. p. 9-10.
**Kahle E:** Klinkosch, Joseph Thaddäus. In Neue Deutsche Biographie 12. 1980. p. 101-2.
**Kahle E:** Koelliker, Albert Ritter v. In Neue Deutsche Biographie 12. 1980. p. 322-3.
**Kahle E:** Kupffer. In Neue Deutsche Biographie 13. 1982. p. 319-20.
**Kahle E:** Laehr, Heinrich. In Neue Deutsche Biographie 13. 1982. p. 396-7.
**Kahle E:** Probleme bei der Ubersetzung mittelalterlicher arabischer pädiatrischer Texte. In International Congress of the History of Medicine, 27th, Barcelona, 1980. Actas. Barcelona, Académia de Ciències Médiques de Catalunya i Balears, 1981. p. 267-70.
**Kahlson G:** Upprustning av naturvetenskaplig och medicinsk forskning. **Sydsven Medicinhist Sallsk Arsskr** 1981;:44-52
**Kahn A:** A-Z in South African medical history. V. The Versveld family. **Adler Mus Bull** 1981;7(2):19-22
**Kahn A:** Highlights of the Adler Museum collections. **Adler Mus Bull** 1982 Nov;8(2):16-18
**Kahn A:** Highlights of the Adler Museum collections. **Adler Mus Bull** 1984 Nov;10(3):25-9
**Kahn A:** Highlights of the Adler Museum collections: the Jenner letter. **Adler Mus Bull** 1984 Jun;10(2):15-7
**Kahn A** see **Melzer R**
**Kahn AJ, Raisz LG:** Dedication to Donald G. Walker. **Metab Bone Dis Relat Res** 1981;3(2):77-80
**Kahn MF:** L'agent étiologique de la polyarthrite rhumatoïde: une hypothèse. **Rev Rhum Mal Osteoartic** 1979 Jul-Sep;46(7-9):510-1
**Kâhya E:** Bízde díseksíyon ne zaman ve nasil başladi? **Belleten (Turk)** 1979;43(172):739-59
**Kahya E:** Quand et comment la dissection a commencé chez nous. **Bell Turk Tarie Kŭrŭmŭ** 1979;43(172):739-60
**Kâhya E:** Renal calculi and their treatment in Ibn Sina. In International Congress of the History of Medicine, 27th, Barcelona, 1980. Actas. Barcelona, Académia de Ciències Médiques de Catalunya i Balears, 1981. p. 734-8.
**Kail AC:** Medicine in Shakespeare. The bard and the body. 2. Mental illness. **Med J Aust** 1983 Oct 15;2(8):399-405
**Kail AC:** Medicine in Shakespeare. The bard and the body. 6. Therapeutics. **Med J Aust** 1983 Dec 10-24;2(12):657-62
**Kail AC:** The bard and the body. 1. Shakespeare' physicians. **Med J Aust** 1983 Oct 1;2(7):338-44
**Kail AC:** The bard and the body. 3. Venereal disease--'the pox'. **Med J Aust** 1983 Oct 29;2(9):445-9
**Kail AC:** The bard and the body. 4. Drugs, herbs and poisons. **Med J Aust** 1983 Nov 12;2(10):515-9
**Kail AC:** The bard and the body. 5. Disease: its causes, diagnosis and cure. **Med J Aust** 1983 Nov 26;2(11):568-77
**Kaĭmakchieva R:** Belezhiti i iubileĭni dati po istoriia na meditsinata za 1969 godina. Sofiia, Meditsina i fizkultura, 1969. 38 p.
**Kaiser L** see **Abe HR**
**Kaiser LM:** Feriis Festisque Diebus: the salutatory oration of Elisha Cooke, Jr., 7 July 1697. **Harv Libr Bull** 1980 Oct;28(4):380-90
**Kaiser RM, Chaff SL, Peitzman SJ:** A Philadelphia medical student of

the 1890's: the diary of Mary Theodora McGavran. **Pa Mag Hist Biogr** 1984 Apr;108(2):217-36
**Kaiser W:** Athanasius Kircher (1602-1680) und die medizinisch-naturwissenschaftlichen Konzeptionen seiner Zeit. **Z Gesamte Inn Med** 1981 Jul 15;36(14):494-9
**Kaiser W, Trenckmann U:** Aus der Frühgeschichte der kardiologischen Diagnostik. **Z Gesamte Inn Med** 1980 Jun 1;35(11):454-62
**Kaiser W:** Bericht über die 61. Jahrestagung der Deutschen Gesellschaft für Geschichte der Medizin, Naturwissenschaft und Technik e. V. **Ber Wissenschaftsgesch** 1978;1(3-4):232-4
**Kaiser W, Trenckmann U:** Christian Friedrich Nasse (1778-1851). **Wiss Z Martin Luther Univ (Math)** 1980;29(2):65-89
**Kaiser W, Piechocki W:** Das hallesche Collegium Orientale und seine Ausstrahlung auf die medizinische Arabistik des 18. Jahrhunderts. **Wiss Z Martin Luther Univ (Math)** 1978;27(5):111-32
**Kaiser W, Völker A:** Das Medizinalwesen von Anhalt-Köthen im Einflussbereich des halleschen Pietismus. **Wiss Z Martin Luther Univ (Math)** 1983;32(2):61-87
**Kaiser W, Werner K:** Das Trinkwasser in der halleschen populärmedizinischen Aufklärungsliteratur des frühen 18. Jahrhunderts. **Z Gesamte Hyg** 1981;27(5):365-71
**Kaiser W, Völker A:** Der Arbeitskreis um den halleschen Physiologen Julius Bernstein (1839-1917) und seine Bedeutung für die klinische Medizin. **Wiss Z Martin Luther Univ (Math)** 1982;31(6):75-100
**Kaiser W, Völker A:** Die Aufgaben einer Medizinalbehörde im 19. Jahrhundert am Beispiel von Anhalt-Köthen. **Wiss Z Martin Luther Univ (Math)** 1983;32(2):39-69
**Kaiser W:** Die ersten promovierten Aerztinnen. Zum 225. Jahrestag der halleschen Graduierung von Dorothea Christian Erxleben (1715-1762). **Z Gesamte Inn Med** 1980 Feb 15;35(4):176-83
**Kaiser W, Simon A:** Die Geschichte der Gerichtsmedizin an der Universität Halle-Wittenberg. Halle, Martin-Luther-Universität Halle-Wittenberg, 1978. 81 p. (Beiträge zur Universitätsgeschichte, Nr. 12, Tome 25).
**Kaiser W, Träger O:** Die Geschichte des Bernburger Gesundheitswesens. Teil I. Von den Anfängen bis zur Mitte des 19. Jahrhunderts. Bernburg, Museum Schloss Bernburg, 1979. 142 p. (Veröffentlichungen zur Heimatgeschichte).
**Kaiser W:** Die hallisch-englischen Wissenschaftbeziehungen in der Medizin des 18. Jahrhunderts. **Wiss Z Martin Luther Univ (Math)** 1976;25(5):71-90
**Kaiser W, Völker A:** Die naturwissenschaftlichen Disziplinen im halleschen medizinischen Kollegeprogramm des 18. und 19. Jahrhunderts. **Z Gesamte Inn Med** 1983 Jul 15;38(14):375-82
**Kaiser W:** Dokumente zur halleschen Promotion polnischer Mediziner in den Jahren 1791 und 1792. **Wiss Z Martin Luther Univ (Math)** 1976;25(6):75-81
**Kaiser W:** Ein kurzer Abriss der Medizingeschichte in den Anhaltischen Territorien. **Wiss Z Martin Luther Univ (Math)** 1976;25(4):97-109
**Kaiser W:** Eisleben und das Mansfelder Land im medizinhistorischen Aspekt. Ein Beitrag zum Lutherjahr 1983. **Z Gesamte Inn Med** 1983 Oct 15;38(20):539-46
**Kaiser W:** Ernst Jeremias Neifeld (1721-1773), Herausgeber der ersten medizinischen Fachzeitschrift in Polen. **Wiss Z Martin Luther Univ (Math)** 1977;26(3):123-31
**Kaiser W:** Ernst Mach und das Mechanismusproblem in der Biologie. **Medizinhist J** 1982;17(3):179-94
**Kaiser W, Völker A:** Gedenktage 1980 aus der Geschichte der Medizinischen Fakultät Wittenberg (I): Die Chemie im medizinischen Ausbildungsprogramm des 17. und 18. Jahrhunderts. **Z Gesamte Inn Med** 1981 Feb 15;36(4):114-22
**Kaiser W, Völker A:** Gedenktage 1980 aus der Geschichte der Medizinischen Fakultät Wittenberg (II): Lehre und Forschung in der Amtsphase von Christian Vater (1651-1732) und Abraham Vater (1684-1751). **Z Gesamte Inn Med** 1981 May 15;36(10):325-32
**Kaiser W:** Georg Ernst Stahl (1659-1734)--Zur 250. Wiederkehr seines Todestages am 14. Mai 1984. **Z Gesamte Inn Med** 1984 Aug 1;39(15):371-6
**Kaiser W, Völker A:** Hygiene, Präventiv, und Unfallmedizin in den Schriften des halleschen Ordinarius Johann Heinrich Schulze (1687-1744). **Z Gesamte Hyg** 1981 Oct;27(10):779-84
**Kaiser W:** In memoriam Kurt Sprengel (1766-1833)--Zur 150. Wiederkehr seines Todestages am 15. März 1983. **Z Gesamte Inn Med** 1983 Feb 1;38(3):90-7
**Kaiser W:** Johann Friedrich Gottlieb Goldhagen (1742-1788) aus Nordhausen, Stadtphysikus und Ordinarius in Halle. **Beitr Heimatkd Stadt Kreis Nordhausen** 1978;(2-3):58-70
**Kaiser W, Völker A:** Johann Reinhold Forster (1729-1798) als Ordinarius in Halle. **Wiss Z Martin Luther Univ (Math)** 1981;30(2):61-79
**Kaiser W:** Johann Reinhold Forster (1729-1798) und Johann Georg Forster (1754-1794) in Halle. Zur 250. Wiederkehr des Geburtstages von Johann Reinhold Forster. **Z Gesamte Inn Med** 1979 Jul 15;34(14):373-81
**Kaiser W, Skrobacki A:** Królewieckie listy Jana Mukulicza de Fryderyka Althoffa. **Komun Mazursko Warm** 1975;4(130):455-65
**Kaiser W:** Leben und Werk des Basler Psychiaters und Psychoanalytikers Hans Christoffel (1888-1959. Zürich, Juris Druck, 1982. 267 p. (Zürcher Medizingeschichtliche Abhandlungen, Neue Reihe, Nr. 152.)
**Kaiser W, Voelker A:** Medizingeschichte und Populärwissenschaft bei Johann Heinrich Schulze. **Altertum** 1980;26:243-9
**Kaiser W:** Medizinhistorische Impressionen zum Karl-Marx-Jahr 1983. **Z Gesamte Inn Med** 1983 Dec 15;38(24):669-72
**Kaiser W:** Medizinisches Grundlagenstudium im frühen 18. Jahrhundert. Zur 300. Wiederkehr des Geburtstages von Georg Daniel Coschwitz (1679-1729). **Z Gesamte Inn Med** 1979 Aug 1;34(15):419-28
**Kaiser W:** Moritz O. Fränkel (1814-1902) als Mitarbeiter der 'Allgemeinen Zeitschrift für Psychiatrie'. **Wiss Z Martin Luther Univ (Math)** 1983;32(2):89-94
**Kaiser W, Völker A:** Oskar Minkowski (1858-1931). **Z Gesamte Inn Med** 1981 Dec 15;36(24):973-9
**Kaiser W, Skrobacki A:** Resonanz des polnischen Novemberaufstandes (1831) an der Königsberger Universität. **Arch Hist Med (Warsz)** 1979;42(3):281-4
**Kaiser W:** Robert Koch und die Entdeckung des Tuberkulose-Erregers. **Wiss Beitr Martin Luther Univ Halle Wittenberg** 1983;5-R80:31-9
**Kaiser W, Hübner H, ed:** Robert Koch (1843-1910). **Wiss Beitr Martin Luther Univ Halle Wittenberg** 1983;5-R80:3-321
**Kaiser W, Werner K, Rothe J:** Sozialmedizinische Konsequenzen aus dem Wirken von Robert Koch unter halleschem Aspekt. **Z Gesamte Hyg** 1982 Mar;28(3):179-84
**Kaiser W, Völker A:** Universität und Physikat in der Frühgeschichte des Amtsarztwesens. Halle, Martin-Luther-Universität, 1980. 95 p. (Beiträge zur Universitätsgeschichte: Wissenschaftliche Beiträge der Martin-Luther-Universität Halle-Wittenberg, 1980/53, T 39).
**Kaiser W:** Vertreter der Ars pharmaceutica im petrinischen und nachpetrinischen Russland. **Wiss Z Martin Luther Univ (Math)** 1973;22(5):147-52
**Kaiser W:** Vor 100 Jahren beschrieb Robert Koch den Tuberkulose-Erreger. **Z Gesamte Inn Med** 1982 Mar 1;37(5):137-44
**Kaiser W:** Wissenschaftsgeschichtliche Kooperation am Beispiel der slowakisch-ungarisch-halleschen Gemeinschaftsforschung zu Leben und Werk von Johann Andreas Segner und Johann Adam Reimann. **Wiss Z Martin Luther Univ (Math)** 1975;24(3):89-98
**Kaiser W, Pankiewicz H:** Zum Leben und Werk Franz Leopold de Lafontaine 1756--1812. **Arch Hist Med (Warsz)** 1979;42(2):231-9
**Kaiser W, Völker A:** Zur Geschichte der ärztlichen Fortbildung auf der Ebene regionaler Vereine und Gesellschaften. **Z Gesamte Inn Med** 1983 Jul 1;38(13):348-58
**Kaiser W:** Zur Geschichte des präakademischen medizinischen Unterrichts: Das Gymnasium illustre in Zerbst und das Philanthropinum in Dessau. **Z Gesamte Inn Med** 1983 Jan 1;38(1):22-9
**Kaiser W, Völker A:** Zur Mitgliedschaft ungarländischer Wissenschaftler in der Academia Naturae Curiosorum (17. und 18. Jahrhundert). **Orvostort Kozl** 1981;93-96(27 No 1-4):93-111
**Kaiser W:** 100 Jahre Universitätsklinikum Halle. Die Entwicklung der halleschen Universitätskliniken in den ersten Jahrzehnten ihres Bestehens. **Z Gesamte Inn Med** 1982 Jun 15;37(12):354-68
**Kaiser W:** 275 Jahre hallesche Medikamenten-Expedition. Aus der Frühgeschichte der pharmazeutischen Industrie in Deutschland. **Beitr Gesch Pharm** 1984;31(22):1-12
**Kaiser W:** 275 Jahre hallesche Medikamentenexpedition. **Z Gesamte Inn Med** 1984 Apr 1;39(7):125-33
**Kaiser W** see **Bessler O**
**Kaiser W** see **Rothe J**
**Kaishi Hensan Iinkai** see **Sakai-shi Ishikai**
**Kaishi Henshu Iinkai** see **Kumanoto-shi Ishikai**
**Kakar S:** Shamans, mystics, and doctors: a psychological inquiry into India and its healing traditions. New York, Knopf, 1982. x, 306 p.
**Kakhn KhA:** Razvitie ėksperimental'noĭ i klinicheskoĭ toksikologii v Estonskoĭ SSR. **Gig Tr Prof Zabol** 1983 Oct;:(10):3-5
**Kakhorov GK:** Gigienicheskie vzgliady Avitsenny. **Feldsher Akush** 1984 Feb;49(2):52
**Kaladze NN:** Nikolaĭ Fedorovich Golubov (k 125-letiiu so dnia rozhdeniia). **Klin Med (Mosk)** 1982 Nov;60(11):120-3
**Al-Kalai D** see **Shanks NJ**
**Kalankhodzhaev AA:** Istoriia organizatsii i razvitiia protivotuberkuleznoĭ sluzhby v Uzbekistane. **Probl Tuberk** 1983 Jul;(7):71-3
**Kalapow I:** Die historische Rolle des Kampfes gegen die Rinderpest in den Jahren 1913 - 1914 in Bulgarien. **Hist Med Vet** 1977;2(3):76-81
**Kalat JW:** Evolutionary thinking in the history of the comparative psychology of learning. **Neurosci Biobehav Rev** 1983 Fall;7(3):309-14
**Kalcher J:** Ambrosius war kein Dinosaurier--dem Hansischen Jugendbund nachträglich zum Geburtstag. Versuch einer Deutung. **Prax Kinderpsychol Kinderpsychiatr** 1979 Aug-Sep;28(6):212-24
**Kalderon AE:** The evolution of microscope design from its invention to the present days. **Am J Surg Pathol** 1983 Jan;7(1):95-102
**Kaleli A, Ansell JS:** The artificial bladder: a historical review. **Urology** 1984 Nov;24(5):423-8
**Kalevi Koski 60 years: Proc Finn Dent Soc** 1981;77(1-3):9-16
**Kalich R:** Aktuelle Ergebnisse auf dem Gebiet der Resistenzbestimmung von Mykobakterien. **Z Erkr Atmungsorgane** 1983;161(1):80-5
**Kalikow TJ:** Konrad Lorenz's ethological theory: explanation and ideology, 1938-1943. **J Hist Biol** 1983 Spring;16(1):39-73
**Kalin J:** Flintknapping and silicosis. **Flintknappers Exch** 1981;4(2):2-9
**Kalina GP:** Nekotorye voprosy istorii sanitarnoĭ mikrobiologii. **Gig Sanit** 1982 Nov;(11):47-50
**Kalinowsky LB:** The discoveries of somatic treatments in psychiatry: facts and myths. **Compr Psychiatry** 1980 Nov-Dec;21(6):428-35
**Kalis F:** Albert Leulier (1883-1957): a l'occasion du centenaire de sa naissance. Thèse, Univ. Claude-Bernard-Lyon I, U.E.R. de Pharm., 1983. 98 leaves.
**Kalis JB, Malkinson FD:** Landmark perspective: Dermatitis herpetiformis. A commentary. **JAMA** 1983 Jul 8;250(2):217-21
**Kalisch BJ, Kalisch PA, McHugh M:** Content analysis of film stereotypes of nurses. **Int J Womens Stud** 1980;3(6):531-58

Kalisch BJ, Kalisch PA: Heroine out of focus: media images of Florence Nightingale. Part I. Popular biographies and stage productions. **Nurs Health Care** 1983 Apr;4(4):181–7

**Kalisch BJ, Kalisch PA:** The Dionne quintuplets legacy: establishing the 'good doctor and his loyal nurse' image in American culture. **Nurs Health Care** 1984 May;5(5):242–51

**Kalisch BJ** see **Kalisch PA**

**Kalisch PA, Kalisch BJ, Scobey M:** Images of nurses on television. New York, Springer Pub. Co., 1983. ix, 214 p.

**Kalisch PA, Scobey M, Kalisch BJ:** Louyse Bourgeois and the emergence of modern midwifery. **J Nurse Midwife** 1981 Jul–Aug;26(4):3–17

**Kalisch PA:** Ordeal of the Oklahoma coal miners: coal mine disasters in the Sooner state, 1886–1945. **Chron Okla** 1979;48(3):331–40

**Kalisch PA, Kalisch BJ:** The image of nurses in novels. **Am J Nurs** 1982 Aug;82(8):1220–4

**Kalisch PA:** Tracadie and Penikese leprosaria: a comparative analysis of societal response to leprosy in New Brunswick, 1844–1880, and Massachusetts, 1904–1921. **Bull Hist Med** 1973 Sep–Oct;47(5):480–512

**Kalisch PA** see **Kalisch BJ**

**Kallee E:** Anamnese des Radioimmunassays. Eine historische Reminiszenz. **MMW** 1984 Jan 27;126(4):97–101

**Källén B, Löfkvist E:** Time trends of spina bifida in Sweden 1947–81. **J Epidemiol Community Health** 1984 Jun;38(2):103–7

**Kallinger W** see **Zazgornik J**

**Kallinich G, Schmidt-Glassner H:** Schöne alte Apotheken. 2. Auflage. München, Callwey, 1977. 251 p.

**Kallós P:** Immunity and concomitant immunity in infectious diseases. Introduction. **Prog Allergy** 1982;31:IX–XV

**Kallós P** see **Hanson LA**

**Kálmán G:** Libéria egykori magyar minisztere Fuszek Rudolf dr. **Orv Hetil** 1984 Apr 1;125(14):841–2

**Kálmán G:** Mészáros Kálmán emlékezete. **Orv Hetil** 1983 Apr;124(16):962–7

**Kalnin VV, Al'bitskiĭ VIu:** Iz istorii Tartuskogo i Kazanskogo universitetov. **Klin Med (Mosk)** 1981 Jan;59(1):108–10

**Kalnin VV:** U istokov nauchnoĭ meditsiny v Tartuskom universitete. **Sov Zdravookhr** 1982;(11):57–61

**Kalnin VV** see **Piaĭ LT**

**Kalok L:** Wilhelm Conrad Röntgen in Giessen, 1879–1888: Ausstellung in der Universitätsbibliothek Giessen vom 28. Juni–27. Juli 1979 aus Anlass der Berufung Röntgens nach Giessen vor 100 Jahren: Katalog. Giessen, Universitätsbibliothek, 1979. 34 p.

**Kal'shteĭn LI** see **Iskhaki IuB**

**Kalsner J:** The unique stress library of Dr. Hans Selye. **Can Med Assoc J** 1983 Aug 1;129(3):288–9

**Kaltenbach RF, Smith AA:** History of the Organization of Teachers of Dental Practice Administration. **J Dent Pract Adm** 1984 Jan–Mar;1(1):6–7

**Kaltreider S:** Tapping the tube. **MCVQ** 1981;16(3):106–12

**Kalŭdov I, et al:** Prof. Dr. George Pavlov (a centennial of his birth). **Vet Med Nauki** 1981;18(2):3–89

**Kalugai I:** Michel-Eugène Chevreul, 1786–1889. **Koroth** 1980 Jun;7(11–12):796–802

**Kalugin VI:** Gody stanovleniia. **Veterinariia** 1980 Apr;(4):72–4

**Kalŭpov I:** Edin vek veterinarnomeditsinska nauka v Bŭlgariia. **Vet Med Nauki** 1982;19(7):6–13

**Kalupov I:** Khiliadoletie Bulgarska veterinarna meditsina. **Vet Med Nauki** 1981;18(7):3–9

**Kalus L** see **Bernus-Taylor M**

**Kałużny J:** W 25-lecie redagowania Kliniki Ocznej przez prof. dra Witolda Orowskiego. **Klin Oczna** 1981;83(2):55–8

**Kälvemark AS:** Att vänta barn när man gifter sig. Föräktenskapliga förbindelser och giftermålsmönster i 800-talets Sverige. **Hist Tidskr** 1977;(2):181–99

**Kälvemark AS:** The country that kept track of its population: methodological aspects of Swedish population records. **Scand J Hist** 1977;2(3):211–30

**Kälvemark AS** see **Laslett P**

**Kalzinger W:** Das Fürsorgewesen der Stadt Linz bis zu Kaiser Josef II. **Hist Jahrb Stadt Linz** 1978;:11–94

**Kamalov MKh, Golubev LV, Petrov ME, et al:** K 60-letiiu iubileiu Bashkirskoĭ ASSR: sel'skoe zdravookhranenie Bashkirii i puti dal'neĭshego ego razvitiia. **Sov Med** 1980;(4):101–3

**Kamalov Mkh:** Zdravookhranenie Bashkirskoĭ ASSR. **Med Sestra** 1982 Dec;41(12):14–8

**Kamata H:** [The past and present of customs related to childbirth. 7. Ceremonial bathing of the infant] (Jpn). **Josanpu Zasshi** 1982 Jul;36(7):590–3

**Kamata H** see **Kogiso M**

**Kamavisdar SS:** Analytical studies in the evidences regarding chemico-culture in the history of Indian medicine in ancient period-allium series. **Indian J Hist Sci** 1980;15(2):210–22

**Kamegai T** see **Inoue N**

**Kameyama M:** Evaluation of the social position of the nurse in the modern history of nursing in Japan. Chapter 1. The Japan Red Cross and nurses (Jpn). **Kango** 1980 Jun;32(6):78–87 (continued periodically)

**Kamiide H** see **Makita K**

**Kamin L** see **Lewontin R**

**Kaminer IJ** see **Brainin E**

**Kamińska A** see **Czapska I**

**Kaminska-Axer M, Sosińska-Trawinska M:** Early medical books in the Capitular Library, Wrocław. **Arch Hist Med (Warsz)** 1981;44:119–26

**Kamińska-Axer M, Sosińska-Trawińska M:** Starodruki medyczne w Bibliotece Kapitulnej we Wrocławiu. **Arch Hist Med (Warsz)** 1979;42(3):393–402

**Kamińska-Axer M:** Starodruki medyczne w Bibliotece Seminaryjnej w Warszawie, druki XVII-wieczne (c.d.). **Arch Hist Med (Warsz)** 1978;41(4):483–91

**Kaminska-Axer M, Czeley-Wybieralska M:** Starodruki medyczne w ksiegozbiorze Biblioteki Seminaryjnej w Tarnowie. **Arch Hist Med (Warsz)** 1979;42(1):125–30

**Kamińska-Axer M, Sosińska-Trawińska M:** Starodruki medyczne z biblioteki kapitulnez we Wrocławiu XVII w. **Arch Hist Med (Warsz)** 1980;43(2):215–25

**Kamińska-Axer M:** Starodruki medyczne z Biblioteki Klasztoru ss Klarysek w Starym Saczu. **Arch Hist Med (Warsz)** 1979;42(3):389–91

**Kaminsky AP:** Morality legislation and British troops in late nineteenth century India. **Milit Aff** 1979;43(2):78–83

**Kämmerer EW** see **Braun L, et al**

**Kampmeier RH:** A century of the Tennessee Medical Association. **J Tenn Med Assoc** 1980 Mar;73(3):169–81

**Kampmeier RH:** Clarification of the systemic manifestations of syphilis, especially in the tertiary stage. **Sex Transm Dis** 1981 Apr–Jun;8(2):82–4

**Kampmeier RH:** Establishment of Treponema pallidum as the etiologic agent in general paralysis. **Sex Transm Dis** 1980 Oct–Dec;7(4):197–8

**Kampmeier RH:** Herpes genitalis: a clinical puzzle for two centuries. **Sex Transm Dis** 1984 Jan–Mar;11(1):41–5

**Kampmeier RH:** History of the American Venereal Disease Association. **Sex Transm Dis** 1984 Jul–Sep;11(3 Suppl):185–265

**Kampmeier RH:** Infection with Chlamydia trachomatis (TRIC agent). **Sex Transm Dis** 1984 Jul–Sep;11(3):169–72

**Kampmeier RH:** Introduction of sulfonamide therapy for gonorrhea. **Sex Transm Dis** 1983 Apr–Jun;10(2):81–4

**Kampmeier RH:** Medicine as an art: the history and physical examination. **South Med J** 1982 Feb;75(2):203–10

**Kampmeier RH:** Pernicious anemia. **South Med J** 1983 Feb;76(2):151–4

**Kampmeier RH:** Practice in Nashville--1905 and succeeding years. **J Tenn Med Assoc** 1983 Jan;76(1):9–15

**Kampmeier RH:** Seventy-five years of the journal. **J Tenn Med Assoc** 1983 Jul;76(7):431–8

**Kampmeier RH:** Syphilis and marriage by Alfred Fournier. **Sex Transm Dis** 1981 Jan–Mar;8(1):29–32

**Kampmeier RH:** The Asklepion Club of Nashville. **J Tenn Med Assoc** 1982 Feb;75(2):93–9

**Kampmeier RH:** The continuous treatment of early syphilis by arsphenamin and heavy metals. **Sex Transm Dis** 1981 Jul–Sep;8(3):224–6

**Kampmeier RH:** The demonstration of the immobilizing antibody for treponema pallidum (TPI test). **Sex Transm Dis** 1983 Oct–Dec;10(4):205–7

**Kampmeier RH:** The early history of medicine in Nashville. **J Tenn Med Assoc** 1983 Feb;76(2):89–96

**Kampmeier RH:** The establishment of lymphogranuloma inguinale (lymphopathia venereum) as a sexually transmitted disease. **Sex Transm Dis** 1982 Jul–Sep;9(3):146–8

**Kampmeier RH:** The evolution of the flocculation screening test for syphilis. **Sex Transm Dis** 1983 Jul–Sep;10(3):156–9

**Kampmeier RH:** The genito-anal-rectal syndrome: late manifestations of lymphogranuloma inguinale. **Sex Transm Dis** 1983 Jan–Mar;10(1):47–50

**Kampmeier RH:** The introduction of iodine in the treatment of syphilis: the writings of William Wallace, M.D., of Dublin. **Sex Transm Dis** 1980 Jan–Mar;7(1):26–8

**Kampmeier RH:** The introduction of penicillin for the treatment of syphilis. **Sex Transm Dis** 1981 Oct–Dec;8(4):260–5

**Kampmeier RH:** Venereal disease in the United States Army: 1775–1900. **Sex Transm Dis** 1982 Apr–Jun;9(2):100–3

**Kampmeier RH:** Wagner von Jauregg and the treatment of general paresis by fever. **Sex Transm Dis** 1980 Jul–Sep;7(3):142–4

**Kampmeier RH:** Women in medical school. **South Med J** 1984 Sep;77(9):1217

**Kamyshan IS** see **Karpenko VS**

**Kan SH, Kim Y:** Cause-structure of post-transitional mortality decline: the case of Utah. **Soc Sci J** 1982;19(1):63–71

**Kanagawa-ken I:** Kanagawa-ken Ishikai shi. Yokohama: Do Ishikai, Showa 52. 1977-. v.

**Kanai H:** [What Nightingale would have written about summer heat and nursing - a thought in connection with folk remedy] (Jpn). **Kango** 1982 Aug;34(9):4–14

**Kanai O:** [Chemotherapy for tuberculosis--experimental studies over the past 100 years. (1) Development of chemotherapy] (Jpn) **Kekkaku** 1982 Dec;57(12):643–51

**Kanaoka Y:** [The chemist in a biomedical environment: personal reflections on a quarter century of research at NIH] (Jpn) **Tanpakushitsu Kakusan Koso** 1979;24(14):1521–30

**Kanarek H** see **McCall N**

**Kandel E:** The origins of modern neuroscience. **Annu Rev Neurosci** 1982;5:299–303

**Kane A, Carlson ET:** A different drummer: Robert B. Carter and Nineteenth Century hysteria. **Bull NY Acad Med** 1982 Sep;58(6):519–34

**Kane GL** see **Cook HJ**

**Kane GL** see **Steneck NH**

**Kaneda H:** [Development of the concept on open system hospital in Japan] (Jpn). **Igakushi Kenkyu** 1978;50:60–4

**Kanei H:** [The role of women and nursing - a lesson in folk medicine. 3]. **Sogo Kango** 1982;17(1):79–89

**Kaneko M:** [An encounter with Nightingale] (Jpn) **Sogo Kango** 1980;15(4):22-8
**Kaneko M:** [The nature of observation expressed in the 'Observation of the sick' (Florence Nightingale)] (Jpn). **Sogo Kango** 1982;16(4):40-50
**Kanep VV:** Aktual'nye voprosy muzeevedeniia: iz opyta raboty Muzeia istorii meditsiny im. P. Stradynia : tezisy dokladov. Riga, Ministerstvo zdravookhraneniia Latviiskoi SSR, 1982. 195 p.
**Kanep VV:** Osnovnye tendentsii razvitiia meditsinskoi nauki i zdravo-okhraneniia latviiskoi SSR. **Latv PSR Zinat Acad Vestis** 1981;3:9-22
**Kanep VV:** Uspekhi v razvitii zdravookhraneniia Latviiskoi SSR. **Klin Med (Mosk)** 1982 Dec;60(12):33-7
**Kaneps V:** Padomju latvijas veselibas aizsardzibai 25 gadi. Riga, Izdevnieciba Zvaigzne, 1965. 157 p.
**Kania I:** Médecine tibétaine dans les collections du Musée Ethnographique de Cracovie. In: Proceedings of the Csoma de Körös Memorial Symposium....Matrafüred ... 1976. Budapest: Akad. Kiadó. 1978. pp. 153-160.
**Kanoh T** see **Kawai S**
**Kansal CM** see **Dube CB**
**Kanter DM:** The invisible monster. Investigations into the 1833 cholera epidemic in Southern Indiana. **Indiana Med Hist Q** 1978;4(4):4-13
**Kanterman CB:** Touch the tooth of a hanged man. **Tic** 1984 Oct;43(10):12-4
**Kantor GK** see **Fennel ML**
**Kántorová V** see **Tichý M**
**Kantorovich MM:** Neutomimye truzheniki--geroi Velikoi Otechestvennoi voiny. **Med Sestra** 1980 May;39(5):3-7
**Kantorovich MM:** Oni zashchishchali Leningrad (k 40-letiiu sniatiia blokady Leningrada). **Med Sestra** 1984 Jan;43(1):46-9
**Kantorovich MM** see **Selivanov EF**
**Kantrov I, Wittenstein K:** Mary Sewall Gardner. In: Notable American women. The modern period. Cambridge, Mass., Belknap-Harvard Univ. Press, 1980. 4:262-4.
**Kantrow L:** Philadelphia gentry: fertility and family limitation among an American aristocracy. **Popul Stud** 1980 Mar;34(1):21-30
**Kanzer M, Glenn J, ed., et al:** Freud and his patients. New York and London, Aronson, 1980. 452 p.
**Kanzer M, Glenn J, ed:** Freud and his self-analysis. New York and London, Aronson, 1979. x, 308 p. (Downstate Psychoanalytic Institute, Twenty-Fifth Anniversary Series, Vol. I). Includes reprinted papers by various authors.
**Kanzer M:** Freud, Theodor Lipps, and 'scientific psychology'. **Psychoanal Q** 1981;50(3):393-410
**Kanzer M** see **Goldberg A, ed**
**Kao FF** see **Unschuld PU**
**Kao JJ** see **Unschuld PU**
**Kao i ya i hsüeh hsi ch'eng li 20 chou nien t'e k'an:** Kaohsiung: Kao-hsiung i hsüeh yüan Ya i hsüeh hsi K'ou ch'iang i hsüeh hui Ting she, Min Kuo 66 nien, [1977]. 315 p.
**Kapatsinskii EV, Kozlova EV:** Rol' Moskovskogo nauchno-issledovatel'skogo onkologicheskogo instituta im. P. A. Gertsena v razvitii organizatsionnykh osnov onkologii. **Sov Zdravookhr** 1981;(11):50-2
**Kapatsinskii EV** see **Chissov Vi**
**Kapitanaki IA** see **Andrianov VL**
**Kapitanaki IA** see **Tkachenko SS**
**Kapitanenko AM:** Talantlivyi organizator, iskusnyi khirurg (k 100-letiiu so dnia rozhdeniia P. V. Mandryki). **Sov Zdravookhr** 1984;(10):58-60
**Kapitola J:** Dvacet let provozu radioizotopového oddělení III. interní kliniky FVL KU v Praze. **Sb Lek** 1983 Sep;85(7-8):211-5
**Kapitonov GI** see **Baranovskii GIa**
**Kaplan AH:** From discovery to validation: a basic challenge to psychoanalysis. **J Am Psychoanal Assoc** 1981;29(1):3-26
**Kaplan AS, Garfinkel PE:** Bulimia in the Talmud. **Am J Psychiatry** 1984 May;141(5):721
**Kaplan B:** 'Peopleware' and medical informatics. **JAMA** 1983 Feb 4;249(5):574-6
**Kaplan B** see **Lerner RM, ed**
**Kaplan BB:** Greatrakes the stroker: the interpretations of his contemporaries. **ISIS** 1982 Jun;73(267):178-85
**Kaplan BH** see **Ibrahim MA**
**Kaplan E:** E.R.N. Grigg, radiologist-historian. **Semin Nucl Med** 1979 Jul;9(3):149-50
**Kaplan HS:** Sexual medicine. A progress report. **Arch Intern Med** 1980 Dec;140(12):1575-6
**Kaplan MB** see **Movshovich IA**
**Kaplan MM:** Three decades of collaboration with Hilary Koprowski. **J Cell Physiol [Suppl]** 1982;2:1-6
**Kaplan SL:** Les subsistances et l'Ancien Régime: l'oeuvre de Jean Meuvret. **Ann Econ Soc Civilis** 1981;36(2):294-300
**Kappas A** see **Trends in biomedical research, 1901-1976**
**Kappers JA:** Short history of pineal discovery and research. **Prog Brain Res** 1979;52:3-22
**Kapronczay K, Szemkeö E:** A betegápolás szervezése a szabadságharc idején. **Orvostort Kozl** 1981;93-96(27 No 1-4):113-22
**Kapronczay K:** A krakkói orvosi kar 200 éves reformja. **Orv Hetil** 1980 Oct 19;121(42):2596-8
**Kapronczay K:** A magyar ápolón óképzés kezdetei. **Orv Hetil** 1983 Feb 6;124(6):344-50
**Kapronczay K:** A magyar kórházügy elsö reformja a XVIII. században. **Orv Hetil** 1981 May 31;122(22):1337-9
**Kapronczay K, Szemkeö E:** A magyar orvostársaságok kialakulása és fejlödése a 19-20. században. **Orvostort Kozl** 1979;87-88(25 no 1-2):141-55
**Kapronczay K:** A Magyar Vöröskereszt centenáriumára. **Orv Hetil** 1981 May 17;122(20):1197-9
**Kapronczay K:** A Magyar Vöröskereszt száz éve--idöszaki kiállítás a Semmelweis Orvostörténeti Múzeumban. **Orv Hetil** 1981 Nov 1;122(44):2732-3
**Kapronczay K:** A sebészeti eszközök fejlodése a XV-XVI. században. **Orvostort Kozl** 1982;28(1-3):141-50
**Kapronczay K:** A Spilenberger orvoscsalád. **Orv Hetil** 1980 Jul 27;121(30):1840-3
**Kapronczay K:** A vidéki orvosok társasága. **Orv Hetil** 1979 Jul 15;120(28):1703-5
**Kapronczay K:** Adatok a prágai egyetem magyar orvosi vonatkozásaihoz (1348-1850). **Orvostort Kozl** 1980;89-91(26 no 1-3):223-31
**Kapronczay K:** Adatok koraszülöttek inkubátoros ápolásának kezdeteiröl. **Orv Hetil** 1982 Oct 3;123(40):2487-90
**Kapronczay K:** Az állatgyógyászat múltjából Magyarországon (a Semmelweis Orvostörténeti Múzeum új idöszakos kiállítása. **Orv Hetil** 1980 Aug 10;121(32):1859-60
**Kapronczay K:** Az orvostörténelem oktatása a krakkói egyetemen. **Orv Hetil** 1979 Sep 23;120(38):2315-7
**Kapronczay K:** Az 1848/49-es magyar szabadságharc egészségügyének szervezete. **Orv Hetil** 1984 Jun 10;125(24):1454-6
**Kapronczay K:** Cesare Magati (1579-1647). **Orv Hetil** 1980 Feb 10;121(6):343-5
**Kapronczay K:** Einige alchimistische Werke aus der Raritätensammlung der Semmelweis-Bibliothek für Geschichte der Medizin. In Hein WH, ed: Pharmaziehistorischer Kongress, Budapest, 1981. Stuttgart, Wissenschaftliche Verlagsgesellschaft, 1983. p. 57-72.
**Kapronczay K:** Haberle Károly (1764-1832) emlékezete. **Orv Hetil** 1982 Nov 14;123(46):2860-1
**Kapronczay K:** Két kevéssé ismert 15. századi orvostörténeti munka. **Orv Hetil** 1983 Jul 10;124(28):1701-5
**Kapronczay K:** Magyar -- lengyel orvosi kapcsolatok a XV-XVI. században. **Orv Hetil** 1981 Feb 22;122(8):465-7
**Kapronczay K:** Magyar-lengyel orvosi kapcsolatok a XVI. században. **Orv Hetil** 1982 Jul 25;123(30):1867-70
**Kapronczay K:** Magyar-lengyel orvosi kapcsolatok a XVII-XIX. században. **Orv Hetil** 1981 Jul 12;122(28):1729-31
**Kapronczay K:** Magyar medikusok a bécsi egyetemen (1770-1848). **Orv Hetil** 1980 Oct 5;121(40):2467-9
**Kapronczay K:** Magyar medikusok a wittenbergi egyetemen Luther és Melanchton korában. **Orv Hetil** 1984 Apr 15;125(16):958-60
**Kapronczay K:** Magyar orvosok a török birodalomban a XIX. század közepén. **Orv Hetil** 1980 Mar 17;121(10):581-3
**Kapronczay K:** Markusovszky Lajos utolsó levele Fodor Józsefhez. **Orvostort Kozl** 1980;89-91(26 no 1-3):269-71
**Kapronczay K:** Markusovszky Lajos utolsó levele Fodor Józsefhez. **Orv Hetil** 1982 Dec 26;123(52):3213-4
**Kapronczay K:** Orvosi érdekvédelem a múlt század végén. **Orv Hetil** 1982 Sep 19;123(38):2373-5
**Kapronczay K:** Personalstand und territoriale Verteilung der ungarischen Apotheken am Ende des 18. Jahrhunderts. In Hein WH, ed: Pharmaziehistorischer Kongress, Budapest, 1981. Stuttgart, Wissenschaftliche Verlagsgesellschaft, 1983. p. 81-4.
**Kapronczay K:** The history of medicine with special regard to Hungarian studies. **Ther Hung** 1980;28(3):138-42
**Kapronczay K** see **Antall J**
**Kapsenberg JG:** Een halve eeuw modern influenza-onderzoek. **Ned Tijdschr Geneeskd** 1983 Sep 24;127(39):1780-1
**Kapuścik J:** Dr Adolf Rząśnicke - lekarz, uczony, artysta (w 30 rocznicę śmierci). **Arch Hist Med (Warsz)** 1983;46(2):237-48
**Kapustin AV, Panfilenko OA:** Osnovnye itogia nauchnoi deiatel'nosti Nauchno-issledovatel'skogo instituta sudebnoi meditsiny za 50 let. **Sud Med Ekspert** 1981 Oct-Dec;24(4):7-10
**Karamian AI:** Ivan Mikhailovich Sechenov i evoliutsionnaia neirofiziologiia. Leningrad, Nauka, Leningradskoe otd-nie, 1980. 112 p.
**Karamyan AI:** The importance of I. M. Sechenov's ideas on formation of human nervous and mental activity for evolutionary neurophysiology. **Hum Physiol** 1979 Nov-Dec;5(5):717-23
**Karasszon D:** As összehasonlító orvostudomány története hazánkban. **Orv Hetil** 1982 Mar 21;123(12):737-40
**Karasszon D:** Robert Kochs Forschungen zur Rinder-Tuberkulose. **Wiss Beitr Martin Luther Univ Halle Wittenberg** 1983;5-R80:111-6
**Karasszon Denes BB:** Militärärztliches zur ungarischen Legion im Kampfe der Vereinigung Italiens / Risorgimento/. In International Congress of the History of Medicine. 26th, Plovdiv, 1978. Actes du Congress. Sofia, 1981. Volume II. p. 58-59.
**Karavaev AG, Berenshtein GF:** Vydaiushchiisia épidemiolog (Vladimir Aaronovich Khavkin). **Med Sestra** 1981 Jul;40(7):55-7
**Karbe KH:** Das Betriebsarztsystem und zum Schicksal der Arbeitsmedizin im faschistischen Deutschland. **Z Gesamte Hyg** 1983 Oct;29(10):640-4
**Karbe KH:** Die Arbeitsmedizin als Gegenstand historischer Quellenforschung. In International Congress of the History of Medicine. 26th, Plovdiv, 1978. Actes du Congress. Sofia, 1981. Volume II. p. 120-2.
**Karbe KH:** Die 'Woche der Sowjet-Medizin' zu Berlin (28. November bis 2. Dezember 1932). **Z Gesamte Hyg** 1981 Oct;27(10):784-8
**Karbe KH:** Ein Leben für die soziale Medizin--Salomon Neumann zu seinem 75. Todestag. **Z Gesamte Hyg** 1983 Nov;29(11):696-8

**Karbe KH:** Ueber eine von Rudolf Virchow empfohlene anonyme Schrift aus dem Jahre 1848 zum Hungertyphus in Oberschlesien. **Arch Hist Med (Warsz)** 1979;42(3):291-4

**Karbe KH** see **Schreier J**

**Karbowski J:** Tecza nad Solferino. Warszawa, Państwony Zakład Wydawn. Lekarskich, 1973. 211 p.

**Karbowski J** see **Kretowski J**

**Kardashev TD, Velkov DL:** On the historical development of biophysics in Bulgaria. In International Congress of the History of Medicine. 26th, Plovdiv, 1978. Actes du Congress. Sofia, 1981. Volume II. p. 216.

**Kardinal CG:** Laetrile in historical perspective. **Mo Med** 1980 Sep;77(9):564-9

**Kardiner A:** My analysis with Freud. New York, Norton, 1977. 123 p.

**Karg AL** see **Stieber MT**

**Karger T:** A short history of the Karger Publishing firm. **Bull Med Libr Assoc** 1981 Apr;69(2):254-7

**Karger-Decker B:** Kräuter, Pillen, Präparate: Abenteuer der Arzneimittelforschung. Leipzig, Koehler & Amelang, 1981. 313 p.

**Karier C:** In praise of great men. **Hist Educ Q** 1980;20(4):473-86

**Kariev TM:** Razvitie khirurgicheskikh metodov lecheniia tuberkuleza legkikh v Uzbekskoĭ SSR. **Probl Tuberk** 1984 Jun;(6):69-71

**Kariev Mkh:** Istoriia i sostoianie neĭrokhirurgicheskoĭ sluzhby v respublikakh Sredneĭ Azii. **Zh Vopr Neirokhir** 1983 Sep-Oct;5:56-8

**Karim SM** see **Ratnam SS**

**Karinskaia GS** see **Shtern MI**

**Kark RM, Moore DT:** The life, work, and geological collections of Richard Bright, M.D. (1789-1858); with a note on the collections of other members of the family. **Arch Nat Hist** 1981 Apr;10(1):119-51

**Karker A:** Kong Frederik 2.s dod. **Jyske Saml** 1964;6(3):252-81

**Karl BD, Katz SN:** The American private philanthropic foundation and the public sphere 1890-1930. **Minerva** 1981 Summer;19(2):236-70

**Karl F** see **Weerda H**

**Karl Ernest Mason, 1900-1978.: Anat Rec** 1980 Sep;198(1):1-12

**Karl Menninger: a literary self-portrait:** A celebration issue for his 90th birthday. **Bull Menninger Clin** 1983 Jul;47(4):293-400

**Karlan MS:** An anatomic plate from Bartolomeo Eustachi. **J Hist Med Allied Sci** 1980 Jul;35(3):316-18

**Karlferdinand Kloos (17. 8. 1911 bis 29. 12. 1980): Verh Dtsch Ges Pathol** 1981;65:548-59

**Karll A:** Florence Nightingale. **Nurs J India** 1983 May;74(5):110

**Karlson P:** Was sind Hormone? Der Hormonbegriff in Geschichte und Gegenwart. **Naturwissenschaften** 1982 Jan;69(1):3-14

**Kármán T:** A nemzetközi összehasonlító népesedésstatisztika fejlödese a XIX. század utolsó negyedében (Luigi Bodio). **Demografia** 1978;21(4):493-504

**Karmi G:** State control of the physician in the Middle Ages: an Islamic model. In Russell AW, ed: The town and state physician in Europe from the Middle Ages to the Enlightenment. Wolfenbüttel, Herzog August Bibliothek, 1981. p. 63-84 (Wolfenbütteler Forschungen, 17).

**Karmi Ghada:** Arabic medicine in the 10th century---a study based on the book Ghina wa Muna by Abu Mansur al-Hasan b. Nuh al-Qumri. In: International Symposium for the History of Arabic Science, 1st, University of Aleppo, 1976. Proceedings. Aleppo, Syria, 1976. Papers in European Languages, Vol. II. p. 326-35.

**Karnani C:** William James and I. A. Richards. **Indian J Am Stud** 1980;10(1):78-82

**Karnoff EM:** Fifty years of the same thing. **NY J Dent** 1980 May;50(5):189-90

**Karnofsky ES:** The vision of Tainard, miraculum de quodam canonico Guatenensi per Sanctum Donatianum curato. In Sheils WJ, ed: The Church and healing. Papers read at the twentieth summer meeting and the twenty-first winter meeting of the Ecclesiastical History Society. Oxford, Basil Blackwell for the Society, 1982. p. 15-24.

**Karnovsky ML:** Metchnikoff in Messina: a century of studies on phagocytosis. **N Engl J Med** 1981 May 7;304(19):1178-80

**Karp LE:** Adrien Bleyer: in the right place at the wrong time. **Am J Med Genet** 1981;10(3):209-11

**Karp LE:** Eutelegenesis: a historical perspective. **Am J Med Genet** 1980;5(4):327-9

**Karp LE:** Genetic drift. A question of discovery: Part I. **Am J Med Genet** 1983 Jul;15(3):379-81

**Karp LE:** Genetic drift. A question of discovery: Part II. **Am J Med Genet** 1983 Aug;15(4):533-5

**Karp LE:** More on the Elephant Man. **Am J Med Genet** 1982 Nov;13(3):355

**Karp LE:** Past perfect: John Humphrey Noyes, stirpiculture, and the Oneida community - part II. **Am J Med Genet** 1982 Jun;12(2):127-30

**Karp LE:** The elephant man. **Am J Med Genet** 1981;10(1):1-3

**Kárpáti E:** Emlékezés Hamburger Jenöre (1883-1936). **Orv Hetil** 1983 Dec 11;124(50):3063-6

**Karpenko VS, Kamyshan IS, Kobiakova LF:** Razvitie ftiziourologii na Ukraine (1922-1982). **Probl Tuberk** 1984 Jul;(7):75-8

**Karpiński A:** Warunkizycia pensjonariuszy szpitali Warszawskich w XVI i w pierwszej połowie XVII wieku. **Kwart Hist Kultury Mater** 1977;25(1):43-62

**Karpov RS:** Vklad tomskikh uchenykh v razvitie otechestvennoĭ kardiologii. **Vestn Akad Med Nauk SSSR** 1981;(9):63-6

**Karrh BW:** The critical balance: the influence of government regulation, past and present. **J Occup Med** 1983 Jan;25(1):21-5

**Karsh E:** Taking the waters at Stafford Springs. The role of the Willard family in America's first health spa. In: Congrès international d'histoire de la médecine, XXVe, Québec, 1976. Actes. Québec, 1977. p. 822-39.

**Karsh E:** Taking the waters at Stafford Springs: the role of the Willard Family of Boston in America's first health spa. **Harv Libr Bull** 1980 Jul;28(3):264-81

**Kartasheva LA** see **Miliutina IK**

**Kartasheve LA** see **Duplenko KF**

**Karthaus PP, Brongersma LD:** H. R. G. J. Brongersma en de Nederlandse Vereniging voor Urologie. **Ned Tijdschr Geneeskd** 1983 Sep 3;127(36):1642-3

**Kartvelishvili EI** see **Tsitlanadze VG**

**Karush G:** Tierra, población y pobreza: las raíces de la crisis demográfica en El Salvador. **Estud Cent Am** 1977;32(350):893-910

**Karwat J:** Dręczyciele upośledzonych. **Psychiatr Pol** 1980 Jul-Aug;14(4):430-4

**Kás S:** Básnická tvorba v díle Ceských lékařu. **Cas Lek Cesk** 1983 May 6;122(18):568-70

**Kás S:** Cestopisy v díle ceských lékařu spisovatelu. **Cas Lek Cesk** 1983 Mar 4;122(9):278-9

**Kás S:** Dramatická tvorba v díle českých lékařu - spisovatelu. **Cas Lek Cesk** 1982 Dec 23;121(51):1592-4

**Kás S:** Medicínský humor v tvorbě českých lékařu - spisovatelu. **Cas Lek Cesk** 1983 Mar 18;122(11):344-5

**Kás S:** Románová tvorba českých lékařu--spisovatelu. **Cas Lek Cesk** 1983 Feb 25;122(8):244-6

**Kase NG:** Gynecologic endocrinology and infertility. A tribute to Martin J. Clyman, M.D. **J Reprod Med** 1983 Apr;28(4):231-2

**Käser O:** Zur Geschichte der Kontrazeption und ein Blick in die Zukunft. **Geburtshilfe Frauenheilkd** 1983 Jun;43 Suppl 1:2-7

**Kashida G** see **Kure S**

**Kashiwagi T:** [Hospice: report on the terminal care in England. 8. St Joseph Hospital. (1): its history and practice] (Jpn) **Kangogaku Zasshi** 1980 Aug;44(8):850-6

**Kashkin KA** see **Aliev MA**

**Kas'ianenko AM:** Sanitarno-épidemiologicheskaia sluzhba Sovetskoĭ Ukrainy. **Vrach Delo** 1983 Jan;(1):1-6

**Kas'ianenko AM:** Sanitarno-épidemiologicheskaia sluzhba Ukrainskoĭ SSR. **Gig Sanit** 1982 Dec;(12):22-5

**Kaspar R** see **Lorenz K, ed**

**Kasparova TIu** see **Kovaleva EP**

**Kasperek J:** Zarys organizacji służby zdrowia w Lublinie w okresie okupacji hitlerowskiej. **Przegl Lek** 1980;37(1):149-57

**Kasperek S:** Przymusowe sterylizacje w rejencji opolskiej 1934-1938. **Przegl Lek** 1980;37(1):33-9

**Kasperski A:** Występowanie raka krtani u chorych na obszarze byłego województwa bydgoskiego w latach 1955-1975 z uwzględnieniem niektórych czynników epidemiologicznych. **Otolaryngol Pol** 1980;34(1):125-6

**Kasprzyk Z:** Irena Chmielewska. **Acta Biochim Pol** 1982;29(1-2):3-5

**Kass AM, Kass EH:** Doctors afield. Martin Delany, Thomas Hodgkin, and the Black Nationalist movement. **N Engl J Med** 1981 Sep 17;305(12):682-4

**Kass AM:** Dr Thomas Hodgkin, Dr Martin Delany, and the 'Return to Africa'. **Med Hist** 1983 Oct;27(4):373-93

**Kass AM:** Dr. Thomas Hodgkin's friendship with Sir Moses Montefiore. **N Engl J Med** 1984 Feb 9;310(6):401-4

**Kass AM** see **Kass EH**

**Kass EH, Carey AB, Kass AM:** Thomas Hodgkin and Benjamin Harrison: crisis and promotion in academia. **Med Hist** 1980 Apr;24(2):197-208

**Kass EH** see **Kass AM**

**Kass LR** see **Spicker SF, ed**

**Kass N:** Abortion in Jewish law. **Koroth** 1983 Aug;8(7-8):323-31

**Kass N:** Sex determination--medically and in the Talmud. **Koroth** 1980 Jun;7(11-12):CCLXLIII-CCCI

**Kasschau RA, Cofer CN, ed:** Psychology's second century: enduring issues. New York, Praeger, 1981. 303 p. Historical contributions by G. W. Albee, R. Brown, K. H. Pribram, J. F. Rychlak, S. Toulmin.

**Kassirskaia NG** see **Kochemasova ZN**

**Kassler JC:** Man - a musical instrument: models of the brain and mental functioning before the computer. **Hist Sci** 1984 Mar;22(55 pt 1):59-92

**Kasten FH:** Ralph D. Lillie, 1896-1979. **Stain Technol** 1980 Jul;55(4):201-15

**Kastenbauer ER:** Zur Geschichte der Plastischen und Wiederherstellungschirurgie im Kopf- und Halsbereich. **Laryngol Rhinol Otol (Stuttg)** 1981 May;60(5):245-50

**Kästle O:** Zwei wiederentdeckte Rezensionen Sigmund Freuds von 1895. Wissenschaftlicher Kontext und biographischer Hintergrund. **Psyche (Stuttg)** 1983 Sep;37(9):805-27

**Kasumov TA:** Dostizheniia zdravookhraneniia Azerbaĭdzhana za 60 let i perspektivy ego razvitiia. **Sov Zdravookhr** 1980;(4):14-8

**Katan E:** Napori za ublažavanje oskudice i očuvanje sanitetskih sredstava u toku bitaka na Neretvi i Sutjesci. **Vojnosanit Pregl** 1984 Jan-Feb;41(1):49-53

**Katan E:** Sanitetsko snabdevanje Centralne bolnice Vrhovnog štaba i jedinica Glavne operativne grupe za vreme četvrte i pete ofanzive. **Vojnosanit Pregl** 1980 Nov-Dec;37(6):476-80

**Katan E:** Stručne publikacije sanitetske službe NOVJ izdavane pre Vojnosanitetskog pregleda. **Vojnosanit Pregl** 1984 Sep-Oct;41(5):424-30

**Katan E:** Ustanove za zbrinjavanje ranjenika NOVJ na području Beograda od 15. oktobra do kraja decembra 1944. godine. **Vojnosanit Pregl** 1980 Mar-Apr;37(2):121-5

**Kataya S:** Les Manuscrits Médicaux et Pharmaceutiques dans Les Bibliothèques publiques d'Alep. Alep, Université d'Alep, Institut du Patrimoine scientifique Arabe, 1976.

**Kataya S, ed.:** Quelle est la différence (Diagnostics Différentiels) de Abou-Bakr Zakaria Al-Razi (Rhazes). Edition Critique et commentaire de S. Kataya. Alep, Université d'Alep, Institut du Patrimoine Scientifique Arabe, 1978.

**Kataye S:** L'amygdalectomie dans la médecine arabe. **Hist Sci Med** 1979;13(4):419–25

**Kataye S:** L'hémostase dans la médecine arabe. In International Congress of the History of Medicine. 26th, Plovdiv, 1978. Actes du Congress. Sofia, 1981. Volume II. p. 122–4.

**Katchadourian H:** The historical background of psychiatry in Lebanon. **Bull Hist Med** 1980 Winter;54(4):544–53

**Katchalsky-Katzir A:** Some thoughts on the physics and biology of time. **Adv Biol Med Phys** 1977;16:289–322

**Kater MH:** Die 'Gesundheitsführung' des Deutschen Volkes. **Medizinhist J** 1983;18(4):349–75

**Kates M:** Adventures in membrane land. **Univ Ottawa Q** 1982;52(2):167–80

**Kathren RL:** Elda Emma Anderson. In: Notable American women. The modern period. Cambridge, Mass., Belknap-Harvard Univ. Press, 1980. 4:20–1.

**Kathren RL, ed** see **Ziemer PL**

**Katic I:** Dansk-russiske veterinaere forbindelser 1796–1976. **Nord Vet Med** 1982;34 Suppl 1:1–319

**Katic RV:** Naknadno prikupljeni termini Srpske srednjovekovne medicine. **Srp Arh Celok Lek** 1984 Mar;112(3):373–93

**Katic RV:** Srpske medicinske škole u srednjem veku. **Srp Arh Celok Lek** 1980 Nov;108(11):1193–1201

**Kato M, Araki S, Sadahiro U, et al:** [History of public health nursing in Hokkaido--through the war, postwar transition, repatriation, and reconstruction periods. A discussion] (Jpn). **Hokenfu Zasshi** 1982 Jan;38(1):58–75

**Kato N:** [Psychiatric treatment at Iwakura-Mura and in Kyoto] (Jpn). **Seishin Shinkeigaku Zasshi** 1982;84(11):889–94

**Kato S** see **Lifton RJ**

**Katori H:** [A special edition on 'the subject and the object'. Commentary: the history of objective conceptualization in psychology] (Jpn). **Kango Kenkyu** 1983 Summer;16(3):182–5

**Katsenovich RA, Mirzaev NL:** Kardiologicheskoe nasledie Abu Ali Ibn-Siny (k 1000-letiu so dnia rozhdeniia). **Kardiologiia** 1980 Nov;20(11):120–2

**Katslan IaD:** Iz istorii sozdaniia Glavnogo voennogo klinicheskogo gospitalia im. N. N. Burdenko i razvitiia v nem spetsializirovannoĭ terapevticheskoĭ pomoshchi. **Klin Med (Mosk)** 1983 Jan;61(1):107–10

**Katsnel'bogen AG:** Dekabrist G. S. Baten'kov. **Sov Zdravookhr** 1982;(8):62–7

**Katsnel'bogen AG:** Dekabristy i obshcestvennaia meditsina. **Sov Zdravookhr** 1979;(12):47–51

**Katsnel'bogen AG:** Dekabristy i obshchestvenno-meditsinskaia mysl' v Rossii. **Klin Med (Mosk)** 1981 Mar;59(3):115–8

**Katsnel'bogen AG:** Dekabristy i peredovaia meditsinskaia obshchestvennost' Rossii. **Sov Zdravookhr** 1980;(10):51–5

**Katsnel'bogen AG:** Delo o rassmotrenii lektsiĭ I. E. Diad'kovskogo. **Klin Med (Mosk)** 1981;59(4):116–8

**Katsnel'bogen AG:** Doktor N. V. Maĭer i dekabristy. **Sov Zdravookhr** 1980;(8):59–62

**Katsnel'bogen AG:** Idei Russkogo Prosveshcheniia i formirovanie obshchestvenno-meditsinskoĭ mysli vo vtoroĭ polovine XVIII veka. **Klin Med (Mosk)** 1984 Jan;62(1):146–51

**Katsnel'bogen AG:** M. Ia. Mudrov i voprosy vrachebnoĭ étiki. **Sov Zdravookhr** 1983;(10):58–61

**Katsnel'bogen AG:** Meditsinskaia zapiska dekabrista A. O. Kornilovicha. **Sov Zdravookhr** 1981;(11):62–4

**Katsnel'bogen AG:** N. I. Pirogov i brat'ia Pushchiny. **Sov Zdravookhr** 1983;(9):62–5

**Katsnel'bogen AG:** Neizuchennyĭ dokument dekabristov. **Sov Zdravookhr** 1980;(7):60–1

**Katsnel'bogen AG:** Neopublikovannaia rabota N. I. Pirogova. **Sov Zdravookhr** 1982;(11):61–4

**Katsnel'bogen AG:** Obshchestvenno-meditsinskaia deiatel'nost' Kh. I. Lodera. **Klin Med (Mosk)** 1982 Jun;60(6):117–20

**Katsnel'bogen AG:** Obshchestvenno-politicheskaia deiatel'nost' vracha-dekabrista F. B. Vol'fa. **Sov Zdravookhr** 1981;(1):66–70

**Katsnel'bogen AG:** Programmy zdravookhraneniia dekabristov (ot 'Zelenoĭ knigi' do 'Russkoĭ pravdy'). **Klin Med (Mosk)** 1979 Dec;57(12):97–101

**Katsnel'bogen AG, Stiazhkov AV:** Slavnye bol'shevichki--krasnye sestry miloserdiia. **Med Sestra** 1980 Nov;39(11):58–61

**Katsnel'bogen AG:** Vrachi-dekabristy. **Klin Med (Mosk)** 1980 Apr;58(4):107–10

**Katsnel'bogen AG:** Vzgliady P.I. Pestelia na meditsinu. **Klin Med (Mosk)** 1980 Aug;58(8):117–21

**Katsnel'son ZS:** Anton Vital'evich Nemilov (1879–1942), ego nauchnoe i pedagogicheskoe tvorchestvo (k 100-letiiu so dnia rozhdeniia). **Arkh Anat Gistol Embriol** 1981 Feb;80(2):108–16

**Katsuki B:** Medical men who helped to shape Hawaii. **Hawaii Med J** 1981 Oct;40(10):279–82

**Kattentidt B:** Erinnerungen eines alten Tuberkulosearztes. **Prax Klin Pneumol** 1982 Sep;36(9):404–7

**Kattermann R:** Walter Siegfried Loewe (1884–1963)). Sein Beitrag zur Analytik, Biologie und Pharmakologie der Sexualhormone. **J Clin Chem Clin Biochem** 1984 Aug;22(8):505–14

**Katus L:** A demográfiai átmenet kérdései magyarországon a 19. században. **Tortenelmi Sz** 1980;23(2):270–288

**Katz C:** The growth of group practice. **Postgrad Med** 1983 Feb;73(2):127–9

**Katz JL:** Three studies in psychosomatic medicine revisited: a tribute to the psychobiological perspective of Herbert Weiner. **Psychosom Med** 1982 Mar;44(1):29–42

**Katz MB, Stern MJ:** Fertility, class, and industrial capitalism: Erie County, New York, 1855–1915. **Am Q** 1981;33(1):63–92

**Katz MB, Stern MJ:** History and the limits of population policy. **Polit Soc** 1981;10(2):225–45

**Katz MB:** Poorhouses and the origins of the public old age home. **Milbank Mem Fund Q** 1984 Winter;62(1):110–40

**Katz O:** Der 'Führer' behandelte sich selbst. Aus jetzt verfügbaren Aufzeichnungen des Leibarztes Theo Morell werden realistische Konturen der geheimnisvollen Krankheiten Adolf Hitlers erkennbar (I). **Fortschr Med** 1984 Oct 4;102(37):70–1

**Katz O:** Prof. Dr. Med. Theo Morell: Hitlers Leibarzt. Bayreuth, Hestia, 1983. 397 p.

**Katz RV** see **Rudney JD**

**Katz S:** A new, informal glimpse of Dr. Frederick Banting. **Can Med Assoc J** 1983 Dec 1;129(11):1229–32

**Katz SI:** 'Sulfoxone (Diasone) sodium for dermatitis herpetiformis' by Cornbleet, December 1951. Commentary: Sulfoxone (Diasone) in the treatment of dermatitis herpetiformis. **Arch Dermatol** 1982 Oct;118(10):805–12

**Katz SN** see **Karl BD**

**Katzeff IE** see **Gathiram P**

**Kätzel S:** Individuum contra Gesellschaft? Ein Beitrag zur Kritik der Gesellschaftsauffassung von Sigmund Freud. **Wiss Z Karl Marx Univ Math Natur Wiss Reihe** 1973;22(5):467–82

**Katzenstein A, Thom A:** Die historische Leistung und die Grenzen des Werkes von Sigmund Freud (1856–1939). **Psychiatr Neurol Med Psychol (Leipz)** 1982 Feb;34(2):68–78

**Katzinger W:** Das Bürgerspital. **Hist Jahrb Stadt Linz** 1977:11–102

**Kaufert JM** see **Coburn D**

**Kauffman GB:** The mystery of Stephen H. Emmens: successful alchemist or ingenious swindler?. **Ambix** 1983 Jul;30(2):65–88

**Kauffman GB** see **Priebe PM**

**Kauffmann Doig F:** Comportamiento sexual en el antiguo Perú. Lima, Kompaktos G. S., [1978]. 189 p.

**Kaufman HJ** see **Kaufman M**

**Kaufman JA:** Francis H. Williams and the shadows of disease. **Conn Med** 1980 Apr;44(4):229–32

**Kaufman M, Hanawalt LL:** Body snatching in the Midwest. **Mich Hist** 1971;55(1):23–40

**Kaufman M, Kaufman HJ:** Henry Bergh, Kit Burns, and the sportsmen of New York. **NY Folkl Q** 1972;28(1):15–29

**Kaufman M:** Medicine and slavery: an essay review. **Ga Hist Q** 1979;64(3):380–90

**Kaufman M:** Medicine in America. **Can Rev Am Stud** 1983;14(3):287–96

**Kaufman M:** Orthodoxy in medicine. In Reich WT, et al, ed: Encyclopedia of bioethics, v.3. New York, Free Press, 1978. p. 1173–6.

**Kaufman M:** 'Step right up, ladies and gentlemen...': Patent medicines in 19th-century America. **Am Hist Illus** 1981;16(5):38–45

**Kaufman M** see **Numbers RL, ed**

**Kaufman P:** Burke, Freud, and the Gothic **Stud Burke Time** 1972;13(3):2179–92

**Kaufmann C:** La question de l'inoculation déférée à l'Eglise. **Asclepio** 1983;35:403–11

**Kaufmann E:** Gustav Jaeger, 1832–1917, Arzt, Zoologe und Hygieniker. Zürich, Juris, 1984. 67 p. (Zürcher Medizingeschichtliche Abhandlungen, Neue Reihe, 171)

**Kaufmann R** see **Müller-Ruchholtz ER**

**Kaul A, Smith GF:** Immunobiology of the fetus and newborn--historical perspectives and recent advances. In Smith GF, Smith PN, Vidyasagar D, ed: Historical review and recent advances in neonatal and perinatal medicine. [Chicago?], Mead Johnson Nutritional Division, 1983. Vol. I. p. 197–212.

**Kaul A** see **Smith GF**

**Kaulen DR:** Itogi i perspektivy deiatel'nosti nauchno-issledovatel'skogo instituta épidemiologii i mikrobiologii im. N. F. Gamalei AMN SSSR (k 90-letiiu so dnia osnovaniia). **Zh Mikrobiol Epidemiol Immunobiol** 1982 May;(5):116–20

**Kaulin AB** see **Braun AD**

**Kausar Chandpuri A:** Danish Nama-I Jehan. **Stud Hist Med** 1980 Mar;4(1):53–6

**Kaveckij RE, Balickij KP:** Les sciences médicales. (Rus). In: L'histoire de l'Académie des sciences d'Ukraine. 1919–1979. (Rus). Kiev: Naukova Dumka, 1979, Académie Ukrainienne des Sciences, URSS, 483–490.

**Kavtaradze VG:** O razvitii i sostoianii kardiologicheskoĭ pomoshchi v Gruzinskoĭ SSR. **Kardiologiia** 1982 Dec;22(12):16–8

**Kawai S, Kanoh T, Okada R:** [History of the etiological studies of myocardial infarction and angina pectoris] (Jpn). **Nippon Rinsho** 1983;41(2):265–70

**Kawakita Y:** [Nightingale in the history of medical philosophy--on the meaning of 'health'] (Jpn). **Kango** 1982 Feb;34(2):39–53

**Kawamura Z:** [Compilation of the history of public health nursing and observation of its significance] (Jpn). **Hokenfu Zasshi** 1981 Jul;37(7):570–86

**Kawasaki S** see **Ueda M**

**Kawasaki SQ** see **Horne PD**

**Kawasaki T, ed** see **Shigematsu I, ed**

**Kay CR:** James Mackenzie Lecture 1979. The happiness pill?

**Kelly TE:** Clinical genetics on the road: be Oslerian, young man. **Am J Med Genet** 1983 Aug;15(4):561-5

**Kel'ner MS** see **Kozlov AM**

**Kelwala S, Stanley M, Gershon S:** History of antidepressants: successes and failures. **J Clin Psychiatry** 1983 May;44(5 Pt 2):40-8

**Kemény P:** 50 éves a Madarász utcai Gyermekkórház. **Orv Hetil** 1979 Dec 30;120(52):3181-3

**Kempa K:** Tytus Chałubiński w opiniach współczesnych mu przedstawicieli literatury i sztuki. **Wiad Lek** 1980 Dec;33(23):1931-4

**Kempe C:** Detaljstudier av kromosomer en diagnostisk revolution. **Lakartidningen** 1980 Feb 13;77(7):503-4

**Kemper B** see **Stool SE**

**Kemper FH** see **Ammon HP**

**Kemper M** see **Stool SE**

**Kemper R:** Zur Syphillis-Erkrankung des Conrad Celtis zum 'Vaticinium' Ulsens und zum sogenannten 'Pestbild' Dürers. **Arch Kulturgesch** 1977;59:99-118

**Kempisty C** see **Szemraj-Lochynska A**

**Kempler K:** A gyógyszerészeti technológia hazai úttöröje Rozsnyay Mátyás. **Orv Hetil** 1984 Jul 22;125(30):1832-4, 1837

**Kempler K:** A kemoterápia haladása napjainkig. **Orv Hetil** 1982 Apr 4;123(14):861-4

**Kempler K:** A magyar kereskedelmi tengerjáró hajók kötelezö egészségügyi felszerelése a századfordulón. **Orvostort Kozl** 1981;93-96(27 No 1-4):171-82

**Kempler K:** Az alkaloida-kutatás kezdetei. **Orv Hetil** 1983 Jul 24;124(30):1821-5

**Kempler K:** Az elemek rendszerezésének kezdetei (Megemlékezés Johann Wolfgang Döbereiner születésének 200. évfordulóján). **Orv Hetil** 1981 Jan 11;122(2):101-3

**Kempler K:** Bonyodalmak a hazai kereskedelmi tengerhajózás egészségügyi ellátásáról szóló rendelet körül a szádfordulón. **Orv Hetil** 1980 Nov 30;121(48):2954-6

**Kempler K:** Hugó Issekutz, der Begründer der ersten ungarischen Universitätsapotheke. In Hein WH, ed: Pharmaziehistorischer Kongress, Budapest, 1981. Stuttgart, Wissenschaftliche Verlagsgesellschaft, 1983. p. 135-9.

**Kempler K:** Lex Szapáryana. **Acta Pharm Hung** 1980 Jul;50(4):166-72

**Kempler K:** Száz éves az elsö magyar gyógyszerkönyv kommentárja. Tallózás évszázados gyógyszerkincsünkben. **Orv Hetil** 1979 Dec 16;120(50):3055-7

**Kempler K:** Tervszerü kutatás, vagy véletlen? Gondolatok Fleming születésének centenáriumán. **Orv Hetil** 1981 Nov 29;122(48):2967-9

**Kempner W:** The Durham connection to Germany. **NC Med J** 1984 Jan;45(1):25-6

**Kendall KA:** A sixty-year perspective of social work. **Soc Casework** 1982 Sep;63(7):424-8

**Kendrew G:** Some remarks on the history of molecular biology. **Istor Biol Issled** 1983;9:127-34

**Kenéz J:** A fizikális mellkasvizsgálat és hazai úttöröi. **Orv Hetil** 1982 Oct 3;123(40):2483-7

**Kenéz J:** F. Esmarch jelentösége a hadisebészet fejlödésében. **Orv Hetil** 1984 Jul 8;125(28):1708-10

**Kenéz J:** Forradalmi átalakulás a medicinában a XIX. század elején. **Orv Hetil** 1984 May 27;125(22):1330-3

**Kenéz J:** H. Heine betegsége. Egy vita, mely a költ' ó halálának 125. évfordulója után sem zárult le. **Orv Hetil** 1982 May 16;123(20):1246-50

**Kenéz J:** Harvey Williams Cushing (1869-1939) und die moderne Hirnchirurgie. **Med Welt** 1980 Sep 5;31(36):1295-7

**Kenéz J:** Hitler patográfiája. Gastrointestinalis panaszok (carcinophobia). **Orv Hetil** 1983 Apr 3;124(14):835-6

**Kenéz J:** Hugó Richter, an outstanding Hungarian neurohistologist (1887--1945). **Ther Hung** 1979;27(2):99-100

**Kenéz J:** Joseph Babinski (1857-1932) a francia klinikai neurológia egyik úttöröje. **Orv Hetil** 1984 Jan 22;125(4):222-7

**Kenéz J:** József Tomcsik. Life and activity of an outstanding Hungarian microbiologist. **Ther Hung** 1980;28(4):189-90

**Kenéz J:** Results in drug treatment of tuberculosis (historical survey). **Ther Hung** 1982;30(3):151-5

**Kenéz J:** War Semmelweis geisteskrank? **Med Welt** 1981 Dec 25;32(51-52):1964-6

**Kenéz J:** 125 éve született Friedrich Kraus (1858-1936). **Orv Hetil** 1984 Oct 28;125(44):2691-3

**Kenigsberg K** see **Harper RG**

**Kennard JA:** The history of physical education. **Signs** 1977;2(4):835-42

**Kennedy DM:** Decrease and stultify: contraception and abortion in American society. **Rev Am Hist** 1979;7(1):18-25

**Kennedy DM** see **Lindemann C**

**Kennedy E:** Immigrants, cholera and the Saint John Sisters of Charity, 1854-64. **Can Cathol Hist Assoc Study Sess** 1977;44:25-44

**Kennedy H:** Anna Freud, 1895-1982. **Psychoanal Q** 1983 Oct;52(4):501-6

**Kennedy HC:** The 'Third sex' theory of Karl Heinrich Ulrichs. **J Homosex** 1980-81 Fall-Winter;6(1-2):103-11

**Kennedy HL** see **Horan MJ**

**Kennedy JE:** Jane Soley Hamilton, midwife. **NS Hist Rev** 1982;2(1):6-29

**Kennedy JG:** Poe and magazine writing on premature burial. **Stud Am Renaiss** 1977;165-78

**Kennedy JW:** Introduction of penicillin in syphilotherapy. **Ariz Med** 1982 Nov;39(11):730, 735

**Kennedy JW:** Publications of the Arizona Territorial Medical Society. **Ariz Med** 1981 Apr;38(4):290-3 contd

**Kennedy JW:** The California-Arizona Maneuver Area World War II. Some medical and nonmedical notes about this desert training center--1942-1944. Part I. **Ariz Med** 1983 Jul;40(7):484-7

**Kennedy JW:** The California-Arizona maneuver area World War II. Some medical and nonmedical notes about this desert training center--1942-1944. Part 2. **Ariz Med** 1983 Aug;40(8):571-5

**Kennedy JW:** The California-Arizona maneuver area, World War II. Some medical and nonmedical notes about this desert training center--1942-1944. Part 3. **Ariz Med** 1983 Sep;40(9):642-7

**Kennedy L:** Health planning in an age of austerity. **Policy Stud J** 1980-81;9(2):232-41

**Kenney AP:** The rhythm of life among the Hudson Valley Dutch in the eighteenth century. **Trans Stud Coll Physicians Phila** 1978 Apr;45(4):217-23

**Kenney JA:** The Department of Dermatology of the Howard University College of Medicine. **Cutis** 1983 Oct;32(4):336, 341

**Kennington R** see **Spicker SF, ed**

**Kenny PJ:** The founders of the College. **Aust NZ J Surg** 1981 Feb;51(1):95-101

**Kenny PJ, Miller ID:** The founders of the College. New South Wales. **Aust NZ J Surg** 1981 Jun;51(3):319-25

**Kent JR:** Population mobility and alms: poor migrants in the Midlands during the early seventeenth century. **Local Popul Stud (Matlock)** 1981;27:35-51

**Kent MC:** A satirical interpretation of the history of selected persons, events and organizations in American physical education. Ed.D. Diss., University of North Carolina. Greensboro, 1981. vi, 266 p.

**Kenyon FE:** Mary Baker Eddy, founder of Christian Science; the sublime hysteric. **Hist Med (Lond)** 1975 Autumn-Winter;6(3-4):29-46

**Kenyon J:** Brain stimulation and affective behavior: a note on an early demonstration of a 'reward center'. **J Hist Behav Sci** 1981;17:174-5

**Kenyon JR** see **Vecht RJ**

**Keough G:** History and heritage of the Veterans Administration Nursing Service 1930-1980. **League Exch** 1981;(127):i-vi, 1-16

**Keown KK:** A brief history of anesthesia and surgery of the heart and great vessels. **Can Anaesth Soc J** 1982 Jul;29(4):325-9

**Kępiński R** see **Stefański K**

**Kepler MO:** Medical stewardship: fulfilling the Hippocratic legacy. Westport, London, Greenwood Press, 1981. xviii, 280 p.

**Kepner J** see **Bullough VL**

**Kepner GR, ed:** Cell membrane permeability and transport. Stroudsburg, Pa., Dowden, Hutchinson & Ross, 1979. xiii, 410 p. (Benchmark Papers in Human Physiology, 12).

**Keppel Hesselink JM:** Some historical aspects of Parkinson's disease. The progression of insights in the period 1817-1868. **Janus** 1983;70(3-4):263-79

**Kerbrat G:** Laennec et ses combats (1781-1826). In: Congrès National des Sociétés Savantes, 107e. Brest, 1982. Comptes Rendus, Paris, 1983. Section des Sciences, Fasc. IV. p. 287-98.

**Kerekes L:** In memoriam Halász Géza (1816-1888). **Orvostort Kozl** 1979;86(24 no 4):113-22

**Kerekes L:** Miért vallott kudarcot Balogh Kálmán, a bakteriológia magyar úttöroje? **Orvostort Kozl** 1982;28(1-3):65-85

**Kerényi K:** Der göttliche Arzt. Studien über Asklepios und seine Kultstätten. Darmstadt, Wissenschaftliche Buchgesellschaft, 1975, 3rd ed. xxi, 113 p.

**Keresztes L** see **Lukázs J**

**Kerharo J:** Die traditionelle Medizin in Schwarzafrika. In Sournia JC, Martiny M, Poulet J, ed: Illustrierte Geschichte der Medizin. Salzburg, Andreas, 1980. Vol. 6. p. 2351-82.

**Kerherve J:** La peste à Moncontour en 1500. **Ann Bretagne** 1983;90(4):603-6

**Kerherve J:** Un accouchement dramatique à la fin du Moyen Age. **Ann Bretagne** 1982;89(3):391-6

**Kerkhoff AH:** Het eerste Nederlandstalinge tijdschrift op het terrein van gezondheids- voorlichting in de negentiende eeuw. **Ned Tijdschr Geneeskd** 1981 Nov 21;125(47):1935-40

**Kerkhoff AH:** Homerus Herbarius. **Janus** 1980:67(1-2-3):187-90

**Kerl H, Konrad K, Holubar K:** The Austrian Society of Dermatopathology. **Am J Dermatopathol** 1984 Jun;6(3):221-2

**Kermorvan F:** Les sirènes existent, l'histoire les a rencontrées. **Histoire** 1980;24:76-8

**Kern E:** Das chirurgische Erbe. Theodor Billroth und die Musik. **Zentralbl Chir** 1982;107(21):1408-16

**Kern E:** 100 Jahre Chirurgie. **Fortschr Med** 1982 Dec 16;100(47-48):2199-206

**Kern LJ:** Ideology and reality: sexuality and women's status in the Oneida community. **Radic Hist Rev** 1979 Spring/Summer;Spec:180-204

**Kern S:** The prehistory of Freud's dream theory: Freud's masterpiece anticipated. **Hist Med (Lond)** 1975 Autumn-Winter;6(3-4):83-92

**Kern SR:** Freud and the emergence of child psychology. [New York, s. n.], 1973. 3, vii, 415 leaves.

**Kernaghan LK:** Duncan Clark. In Dictionary of Canadian biography, 1801 to 1820. Volume 5, 1983. p. 187-8.

**Kernaghan LK:** John Philipps. In Dictionary of Canadian biography, 1801 to 1820. Volume 5, 1983. p. 670.

**Kernaghan LK:** William James Almon. In Dictionary of Canadian biography, 1801 to 1820. Volume 5, 1983. p. 23-4.

**Kernberg OF:** The contributions of Edith Jacobson: an overview. **J Am Psychoanal Assoc** 1979;27(4):793-819

**Kernëis JP:** Geschichte der Schiffahrtsmedizin am Beispiel der Schiffschirurgen. In Sournia JC, Martiny M, Poulet J, ed: Illustrierte

Geschichte der Medizin. Salzburg, Andreas, 1980. Vol. 8. p. 2999–3023.
**Kernéis JP, Rouzeau L, Cuny J:** L'histoire de la médecine navale à l'Université de Nantes. In: Congrès National de Sociétés Savantes, 97e, Nantes, 1972. Comptes Rendus. Paris, 1976. Section des Sciences, Tome 1. p. 149–64.
**Kerneis JP** see **La médecine hospitalière française au XVIIIème siècle**
**Kerner D:** Béla Bartóks Tod in New York. Zu seinem 100. Geburtstag am 25. März 1981. **MMW** 1981 Mar 27;123(13):525–9
**Kerner D:** Bellinis Tod in Paris. **Orchester** 1976;24:712–6
**Kerner D:** El último Brahms. **Folia Hum (Barc)** 1981;19:27–34
**Kerner K** see **Parssinen TM**
**Kerner S:** Samuel de Lion Benavente; chirurgien et lithotomiste (1643–1723). **Rev Hist Med Heb** 1981 Jul;34(2):29–30
**Kerr B:** Henry Moule and cholera in Dorset: nineteenth-century sanitary reform. **Hist Today** 1978;28(10):672–80
**Kerr H, Crow CL, ed:** The occult in America: new historical perspectives. Urbana, Chicago, University of Illinois Press, 1983. 246 p.
**Kerr LE:** Black lung. **J Public Health Policy** 1980 Mar;1(1):50–63
**Kerr LE:** The health of workers. **J Public Health Policy** 1981 Mar;2(1):3–7
**Kerr ME:** A capsule history of your journal. **Can Nurse** 1980 Mar;76(3):20–1
**Kerrigan W** see **Smith JH, ed**
**Kersley GD:** The history and effects of spa treatment. **Rev Environ Health** 1982;4(1):57–62
**Kersley GD:** The scope of rheumatology. **Ann Rheum Dis** 1981 Dec;40(6):631–2
**Kerson TS:** Almshouse to municipal hospital: the Baltimore experience. **Bull Hist Med** 1981 Summer;55(2):203–20
**Kerson TS:** Medical social work. New York, Irvington Publishers, 1980. 320 p.
**Kertész T:** Attila József (1905–1937). **Orv Hetil** 1980;121:2207–9
**Kessel AH:** Notes on ps.-Hippocrates De medico. **Mnemosyne** 1978;31:113–33
**Kessler N:** Die freie Heiltätigkeit im Gesundheitsgesetz des Kantons Appenzell Ausserrhoden. Zürich, Juris, 1981. 51 p. (Züricher medizingeschichtliche Abhandlungen, Neue Reihe Nr. 146).
**Kessler RC, McRae JA:** Trends in the relationship between sex and psychological distress: 1957–1976. **Am Sociol Rev** 1981;46(4):443–52
**Kessler RH:** Gunpowder altered the physician's wartime role. Should nuclear weapons change it again? **Arch Intern Med** 1983 Apr;143(4):784–6
**Kessler RK, Kessler WB, Constantine J, et al:** Sclerosis of thyroid cysts. **Arch Intern Med** 1984 Aug;144(8):1693, 1697
**Kessler WB** see **Kessler RK**
**Kestigian MC:** Early medical care in Deerfield. **Hist J West Mass** 1979;7(2):5–14
**Ketchum LD:** An historical account of the development of the calibrated dermatome. **Ann Plast Surg** 1978 Nov;1(6):608–11
**Kett JF:** Rites of passage. Adolescence in America, 1790 to the present. New York, Basic Books, 1977. ix, 327 p.
**Kett JF:** Temperance and intemperance as historical problems. **J Am Hist** 1981;67(4):878–85
**Kett JF:** The search for a science of infancy. **Hastings Cent Rep** 1984 Apr;14(2):34–9
**Kettel LJ:** University of Arizona, College of Medicine. **West J Med** 1983 Sep;139(3):395–9
**Kettle E:** That they might live. Sydney, F.P. Leonard, 1979. viii, 368 p.
**Kety SS:** The metamorphosis of a psychobiologist. **Annu Rev Neurosci** 1979;2:1–15
**Kevles DJ:** Genetics in the United States and Great Britain, 1890–1930: a review with speculations. **Isis** 1980 Sep;71(258):441–55
**Kevles DJ:** Genetics in the United States and Great Britain 1890–1930: a review with speculations. In C. Webster, ed: Biology, medicine and society 1840–1940. Cambridge, Cambridge University Press, 1981. p. 193–215.
**Kevles DJ, Sturchio JL, Carroll PT:** The sciences in America, circa 1880. **Science** 1980 Jul 4;209(4452):26–32
**Key JD, Keys TE, ed:** Classics and other selected readings in medical liberarianship. Huntington, N.Y., Krieger, 1980. xvii. 744 p.
**Key JD:** Osler's baby on the tracks. **Minn Med** 1983 Aug:66(8):515
**Key JD, Callahan JA, Nelson CW:** William J. Mayo--centennial notes. **Minn Med** 1982 Oct;65(10):636–8
**Key JD, Rodin AE:** William Osler and Arthur Conan Doyle versus the antivivisectionists: some lessons from history for today. **Mayo Clin Proc** 1984 Mar;59(3):189–96
**Key JD:** Winchell McKendree Craig. In Dictionary of American Biography, Suppl. 6, 1956–1960. p. 130–31, 1980.
**Key JD** see **Callahan JA**
**Key JD** see **Haabala SH**
**Key JD** see **Hayles AB**
**Key JD** see **Keys TE**
**Key JD** see **Mann RJ**
**Key JD** see **Rodin AE**
**Keyfitz N:** Irene Barnes Taeuber. In: Notable American women. The modern period. Cambridge, Mass., Belknap-Harvard Univ. Press, 1980. 4:672–3.
**Keyfitz N** see **Dupâquier J**
**Keynes G:** Dr. Martin Lister. A bibliography. Godalming, Surrey, St. Paul's Bibliographies, 1981. xii, 52 p.
**Keynes G:** The gates of memory. Oxford, Clarendon, 1981. xi, 428 p.
**Keynes M:** Handel's illnesses. **Lancet** 1980 Dec 20–27;2(8208–8209):1354–5
**Keynes M:** Medical sense and nonsense in biography. **Br Med J [Clin Res]** 1983 Mar 26;286(6370):1023–6
**Keynes M:** Sir Isaac Newton and his madness of 1692–93. **Lancet** 1980 Mar 8;1(8167):529–30
**Keynes R** see **Dupâquier J**
**Keys A:** From Naples to seven countries--a sentimental journey. **Prog Biochem Pharmacol** 1983;19:1–30
**Keys TE, Key JD:** An overlooked tribute for Dr. William Worrall Mayo. **Minn Med** 1984 Jul;67(7):375–8
**Keys TE:** Chauncey Depew Leake, 1896–1978: an appreciation. **J Hist Med Allied Sci** 1978 Jul;33(3):428–31
**Keys TE, Key JD:** Osler and Billings: their friendship and contributions to librarianship. **Am Coll Physicians Obs** 1981 Aug;1(8):1, 4–5
**Keys TE:** The Mayos: a historical vignette. **Adler Mus Bull** 1984 Nov;10(3):16–24
**Keys TE** see **Callahan JA**
**Keys TE, ed** see **Key JD**
**Keyser AL** see **Villiers JC de**
**Keystone J:** The physical health of the Indochinese refugees. In Adelman, Howard, ed: The Indochinese Refugee Movement: The Canadian Experience (Toronto: Operation Lifeline, 1980): 163–5.
**Khademol-Reza L:** Theories of dysmenorrhea. An historical review from 1850 to 1979. **J Kans Med Soc** 1983 Jun;84(6):335–40, 355–6
**Khadri SK:** 'Shaik -al - Rais' Abu Ali Ibn Sina (Avicenna) and his contribution to the science and art of medicine. **Bull Indian Inst Hist Med (Hyderabad)** 1981;1–4:130–8
**Khaidarov A:** On the isolation of crystalline oxidase in 1906. **Istor Biol Issled** 1983;9:158–66
**Khalatbari P, Müllen K, Strohbach E:** Népesedéspolitikai problémák a német demokratikus köztársaságban. **Demografia** 1972;15(2):184–94
**Khaleefathullah S:** Avicenna as a physician and medical writer. **Bull Indian Inst Hist Med (Hyderabad)** 1981;1–4:123–9
**Khalmuradov AG, Rybina AA:** Tvorcheskiĭ vklad akademika AN USSR R. V. Chagovtsa v razvitie biokhimii. **Ukr Biokhim Zh** 1984 Sep-Oct;56(5):576–86
**Khan AB, Tariq M, Afaq SH, et al:** Poisons and antidotes in Unani system of medicine. **Indian J Hist Sci** 1981, reçu 1982;16(1):57–63
**Khan AJ:** A survey of the concepts and measures developed by the Greco-Arab physicians related with the prevention and treatment of the infections and epidemic diseases. **Indian J Hist Sci** 1981;16(2):139–44
**Khan JA:** Atropine poisoning in Hawthorne's The Scarlet Letter. **N Engl J Med** 1984 Aug 9;311(6):414–6
**Khan MS:** An Arabic source for the History of Ancient Indian medicine. **Indian J Hist Sci** 1981, reçu 1982;16(1):47–56
**Khan Ghori SA** see **Rahman A**
**Khardori R:** The insulin controversy. **Ann Intern Med** 1980 Feb;92(2 Pt 1):267–8
**Kharshak EM:** Nauchnaia deiatel'nost' oblastnykh obshchestv otolaringologov v USSR za period 1957–1978 gg. (po protokolam i godovym otchetam obshchestv, opublikovannym v ZhUNGB s 1959 po 1978 g.). **Zh Ushn Nos Gorl Bolezn** 1980 May-Jun;(3):56–64
**Khazanov AI** see **Borodulin VI**
**Khazanov AT:** Iz istorii prozektury Obukhovskoĭ bol'nitsy. **Arkh Patol** 1983;45(5):68–73
**Khazenson LB** see **Avdeeva TA**
**Khel R** see **Bořík O**
**Khil'chenko MA** see **Mirskiĭ MB**
**Khilova IuK** see **Klishov AA**
**Khin Thet Htar:** Annotated bibliography of medical literature on Burma, 1866–1976. With supplement up to 1980. New Delhi, World Health Organization, South-East Asia Regional Office, 1981. vii, 484, 35 p. (WHO Regional Publications. South-East Asia series, no. 13).
**Khlebnikov GF:** Mediko-biologicheskaia podgotovka kosmonavtov (istoriia, soderzhanie, étpy, évoliustsiia i tendentsii razvitiia). **Kosm Biol Aviakosm Med** 1981 Mar-Apr;15(2):8–14
**Khmel'nitskiĭ OK:** Klavdiia Petrovna Ulezko-Stroganova (1856–1943). **Arkh Patol** 1981;43(8):72–4
**Khodorkov LA:** Meditsinskaia sluzhba Krasnoĭ Armii v operatsii na reke Khalkin-Gol. **Voen Med Zh** 1979 Aug;(8):76–8
**Khodos KhG:** Epidemicheskiĭ éntsefalit Ékonomo--nereshennaia nevrologicheskaia problema (k 60-letiiu opisaniia éntsefalita Ekonomo sovetskimi nevropatologami). **Zh Nevropatol Psikhiatr** 1981;81(2):124–7
**Khokhlov LK, Shipov VL:** K 200-letiiu Iaroslavskoĭ oblastnoĭ psikhiatricheskoĭ klinicheskoĭ bol'nitsy. **Zh Nevropatol Psikhiatr** 1980;80(9):1393
**Khokholia VP:** Nikolaĭ Markiianovich Volkovich (k 125-letiiu so dnia rozhdeniia). **Klin Khir** 1983 Dec;(12):55–6
**Khokholia VP, Stebliak AG:** Stranitsy iz istorii razvitiia khirurgii v Kieve. **Klin Khir** 1982 May;(5):65–7
**Khokholia VP** see **Rakovskaia GG**
**Khokholia VP** see **Shalimov AA**
**Khomniuk VF** see **Zheleznikov IG**
**Khoo FY, Chow KW:** The development of diagnostic radiology in Singapore. **Ann Acad Med Singapore** 1982 Jul;11(3):444–6
**Khromchenko OM, Sapegina AV:** Dvadtsatipiatletniĭ opyt usovershenstvovaniia rukovodiashchikh kadrov sanitarno-épidemiologicheskoĭ sluzhby v Tsentral'nom institute usovershenstvovaniia vracheĭ. **Gig Sanit** 1981 Mar;(3):51–3
**Khromov AS, Kutuzova EP:** Istoriia i sostoianie organizatsii bor'by protiv éndemicheskikh bolezneĭ v Respublike Bereg Slonovoĭ Kosti. **Med Parazitol (Mosk)** 1979 Nov-Dec;48(6):64–8
**Khurana SL:** Origin and development of nursing in India.

Nurs J India 1984 Jan;75(1):9-11
**Khusainova DZh:** Muzeĭnaia komnata 'Molodaia gvardiia' v meditsinskom uchilishche. **Med Sestra** 1982 Mar;41(3):56-7
**Khuton A, Khuton K:** Kriticheskiĭ analiz frantsuzskoĭ psikhiatricheskoĭ nozologii. **Zh Nevropatol Psikhiatr** 1982;82(4):121-3
**Khuton K** see **Khuton A**
**Kiazimov RA, ed** see **Aĭrapetova RA**
**Kibel MA:** Silver nitrate and the eyes of the newborn--a centennial. **S Afr Med J** 1981 Dec 26;60(26):979-80
**Kibre P:** Albertus Magnus on alchemy. In Weisheipl JA, ed: Albertus Magnus and the sciences. Toronto, Pontifical Institute of Mediaeval Studies 1980. p. 187-202.
**Kibre P:** Arts and medicine in the universities of the later Middle Ages. In Ijsewijn J, Paquet J, ed: The universities in the late Middle Ages. Leuven University Press, 1978. p. 213-27.
**Kibre P:** Hippocrates latinus: repertorium of Hippocratic writings in the Latin Middle Ages. **Traditio** 1977;33:253-95; 1978;34:193-226
**Kibre P:** Hippocrates latinus: repertorium of Hippocratic writings in the Latin Middle Ages. (VI). **Traditio** 1980;36:347-72
**Kibre P:** Hippocrates latinus: repertorium of Hippocratic writings in the Latin Middle Ages (VII). **Zwingliana** 1981;37:267-89
**Kibre P:** Hippocrates latinus: repertorium of Hippocratic writings in the Latin Middle Ages (VIII). **Traditio** 1982;38:169-71
**Kibre P** see **Witten LC**
**Kick H:** Antipsychiatrie um 1900: Zur Tradition des Konfliktes zwischen Psychiatrie und Presseberichterstattung. **Nervenarzt** 1982 May;53(5):299-300
**Kick H:** Der Forschungsansatz Kraepelins aus der Sicht seiner klinischen Praxis. **Fortschr Neurol Psychiatr** 1981 Jul;49(7):259-64
**Kidd CV:** The movement of younger scientists into and out of the United States from 1967 to 1980: some aspects of the international movement of scientific knowledge. **Minerva** 1983 Winter;21(4):387-409
**Kidd F, ed:** Profile of the Negro in American dentistry. Washington, Howard University Press, 1979. viii, 211 p.
**Kidwell R:** Handicapping an innovator. **Reason** 1981;13(4):39-46
**Kiec E, et al:** Prof. Dr. Leon Cholewa. **Przegl Lek** 1984;41(7):465-76
**Kiec-Swierczyńska M:** Uczuleniowy zawodowy wyprysk skóry rozpoznany w Instytucie Medycyny Pracy w Lodzi w latach 1972-1978. **Przegl Dermatol** 1980 Jul-Aug;67(4):449-53
**Kiefer JH:** History of the Division of Urology of the University of Illinois College of Medicine. **IMJ** 1983 Dec;164(6):498-508
**Kiefer JH, Wittman E:** University of Illinois College of Medicine centennial. **IMJ** 1981 Aug;160(2):92-5
**Kiefer WE:** The Gratiot County landfill: one of Michigan's foremost toxic waste sites. **Mich Acad** 1983;15(3):311-31
**Kieft L, Willeford BR, ed:** Joseph Priestley. Scientist, theologian, and metaphysician. A symposium celebrating the two hundredth anniversary of the discovery of oxygen by Joseph Priestley in 1774. Lewisburg, Bucknell University Press, 1980. 117 p. With contributions by E. N. Hiebert, A. J. Ihde, R. E. Schofield.
**Kielan-Jaworowska Z:** Polska Akademia Nauk, Zaklad Paleobiologii, Warsaw, Poland. **Nature** 1979 Feb 1;277(5695):402-3
**Kielanowski T:** My meetings with Ludwik Fleck in Lublin during the years 1945-1950. **Kwart Hist Nauki Tech** 1983;28(3-4):583-7
**Kielanowski T:** Powstanie i organizacja Akademii Medycznej w Białymtoku. **Kwart Hist Nauki Tech** 1980;25(2):299-318
**Kienle G** see **Burkhardt R**
**Kiermayer O:** Werke von Dr. h. c. Hans-Henning Heunert. **Mikroskopie** 1981 Feb;38(1-2):3-12
**Kiernan J:** Saltwater and ashes: instruments of curing among some Zulu zionists. **J Relig Afr** 1978;9:27-32
**Kierulf H:** Farsottenes rolle i dikteren Johan Falkbergets trilogi 'Christianus Sextus' (1720 årene). **Nord Medicinhist Arsb** 1980;Suppl 6:82-9
**Kierulf H:** L'ergotisme chez Bosch et Grünewald. **Nouv Presse Med** 1982 Oct 2;11(38):2803-9
**Kierulf H:** L'ergotisme chez Bosch et Grünewald. In International Congress of the History of Medicine, 27th, Barcelona, 1980. Actas. Barcelona, Acadèmia de Ciències Mèdiques de Catalunya i Balears, 1981. p. 81-90.
**Kiessling W:** Der Tierarzt in der bildenden Kunst seit Gründung der tierärztlichen Bildungsstätten. Diss. Hannover, 1981. 385 p.
**Kieta M:** Instytut higieny SS i Policji w Oświęcimiu. **Przegl Lek** 1980;37(1):172-6
**Kiger JC, ed:** Research institutions and learned societies. Westport, Conn., London, Greenwood Press, 1982. xxv, 551 p. (Greenwood Encyclopedia of American Institutions, no. 5).
**Kiikuni K:** The development of hospitals and clinics in Japan. In Ogawa T, ed: Public health. Tokyo, Saikon, 1981. p. 1-11.
**Kikuchi K:** Edo jidai ni okeru korera-byô - ne ryûkô - jiin kakochô ni yoru jisshô. **Jimbun Chiri** 1978;30(5):63-77
**Kikuchi S:** [The progress of 'Shigaku' in the past 70 years] (Jpn). **Shigaku** 1982 Jun;70(1):iii-ix
**Kikuchi Keifuen, Koshi, Japan:** Kanja Jichikai. Jichikai 50-nenshi Hensan Iinkai. Jichikai 50-nenshi. Koshimachi, Japan, Kikuchi Keifuen Kanja Jichikai, [1976]. 49, 228 p.
**Kilburn KH:** Chronic disease in the workplace and the environment. Lung disease: lessons from the past--keys to the future. **Arch Environ Health** 1984 May-Jun;39(3):139-43
**Kilimov N:** Georgi Uzunov. Sofiia, Izd-vo na Bŭlgarskata akademiia na naukite, 1978. 178 p.
**Killar M** see **Kretowski J**
**Killian H:** Meister der Chirurgie und die Chirurgenschulen im gesamten deutschen Sprachraum. 2., neubearbeitete Auflage. Stuttgart, Thieme, 1980. xii, 492 p.
**Killian KP** see **Habrich C**
**Killion G** see **Waller T**
**Killy W** see **Albrecht von Haller, 1708-1777**
**Kim DJ:** The influence of Western medicine, especially American medicine, on the development of medicine in Korea. **Trans Stud Coll Physicians Phila** 1977 Jan;44(3):131-4
**Kim JS, Pyo YS:** [Panel discussion: nurses' status in the community] (Kor). **Taehan Kanho** 1983 Sep 20;22(3):66-73, 41
**Kim SB** see **Sabagh G**
**Kim T:** Han'guk ŭihaksa: chŏn. Seoul, T'amgudang, 1975. xxi, 584 p.
**Kim Y** see **Kan SH**
**Kim YS:** Natural knowledge in a traditional culture: problems in the study of the history of Chinese science. **Minerva** 1982 Spring-Summer;30(1-2):83-104
**Kimbel WH, White TD, Johanson DC:** Cranial morphology of Australopithecus afarensis: a comparative study based on a composite reconstruction of the adult skull. **Am J Phys Anthropol** 1984 Aug;64(4):337-88
**Kimble C, et al:** Health in America. **Wilson Q** 1980 Spring;:60-101
**Kimbrough SO:** On the reduction of genetics to molecular biology. **Philos Sci** 1979;46:389-406
**Kimmel K, Steinkrüger F:** Der deutsche dental-medizinische Fachhandel. Geschichte--Aufgaben--Strukturen. **Dent Echo (Heidelb)** 1981 Dec;51(8):10-32
**Kimmel K, Steinkrüger F:** Der deutsche dental-medizinische Fachhandel (II). Geschichte--Aufgaben--Strukturen. **Dent Echo (Heidelb)** 1982 Feb;52(1):18-37
**Kimmel K, Steinkruger F:** Der deutsche dental-medizinische Fachhandel (III). Geschichte--Aufgaben--Strukturen. **Dent Echo (Heidelb)** 1982 Mar;52(2):14-33
**Kimmel K, Steinkruger F:** Der deutsche dental-medizinische Fachhandel. (IV). Geschichte--Aufgaben--Strukturen. **Dent Echo (Heidelb)** 1982 May;52(3):11-6, 18-21
**Kimmel K, Steinkrüger F:** Der deutsche dental-medizinische Fachhandel (V). Geschichte - Aufgaben - Strukturen. **Dent Echo (Heidelb)** 1982 Jun;52(4):36-52
**Kimmel K, Steinkrüger F:** Der deutsche dental-medizinische Fachhandel (VI). Geschichte - Aufgaben - Strukturen. **Dent Echo (Heidelb)** 1982 Aug;52(5):72-7, 80-2
**Kimmel K, Steinkrüger F:** Der deutsche dental-medizinische Fachhandel (VII). Geschichte - Aufgaben - Strukturen. **Dent Echo (Heidelb)** 1982 Nov;52(7):15-6, 19-20, 22-4 passim
**Kimmel K, Steinkrüger F:** Die Geschichte des deutschen dental-medizinischen Fachhandels. Geschichte--Aufgaben--Strukturen (I). **Dent Dienst** 1982 Feb;(2):8-9
**Kimmel K, Steinkrüger F:** Die Geschichte des deutschen dental-medizinischen Fachhandels (II). 1882-1939: Eine stürmische Epoche. **Dent Dienst** 1982 Mar;(3):14-7
**Kimmel K:** Was ist daraus geworden? (I) Ein Milchsauger und ein Kieferformer 25 Jahre nach ihrer Einführung. **ZWR** 1980 Feb;89(2):62-7
**Kimmelman BA:** The American Breeders' Association: genetics and eugenics in an agricultural context, 1903-13. **Soc Stud Sci** 1983 May;13(2):163-204
**Kimpel BD, Eaves TC:** More on Pound's prison experience. **Am Lit** 1981;53(3):469-76
**Kimpianga KM:** The religious therapeutic functions of the cemetery for the Kongo of Zaire. **Cah Relig Afr** 1978;12:107-24
**Kimura B** see **Janzarik W ed**
**Kimura B** see **Kraus A, ed**
**Kimura Y:** [Reflections on my research] (Jpn). **Nippon Saikingaku Zasshi** 1984 Jan;39(1):19-23
**Kinastowski W:** Próba analizy założeń weismannowskiej teorii dziedziczenia. Wrocław, Zakład Narodowy im. Ossolińskich, 1977. 42 p.
**Kinch MP:** Geographical distribution and the origin of life: the development of early nineteenth-century British explanations. **J Hist Biol** 1980 Spring;13(1):91-119
**Kindler H** see **Peters UH, ed**
**Kindt H** see **Janzarik W ed**
**Kindt H** see **Kloë E**
**Kindt H** see **Seidler E**
**Kindzel'skiĭ LP, Sivachenko TP:** Razvitie meditsinskoĭ radiologii v Ukrainskoĭ SSR. **Med Radiol (Mosk)** 1982 Dec;27(12):13-8
**King AY** see **Fodor J**
**King CG:** The isolation of vitamin C from lemon juice. **Fed Proc** 1979 Dec;38(13):2681-3
**King CW** see **Riddle JM**
**King DF:** A foot note to 'The tale of the psorosperm'. **Am J Dermatopathol** 1982 Aug;4(4):313-4
**King DF:** Chronic atypical epithelial proliferation of Bowen. A historical and biographical note. **Am J Dermatopathol** 1984 Feb;6(1):35-8
**King DF:** Gustav Simon. The father of dermatopathology. **Am J Dermatopathol** 1979 Fall;1(3):225-8
**King DF, King LA:** Jews in dermatology. **Am J Dermatopathol** 1984 Aug;6(4):415-6
**King DF, King LA:** Josef Plenck--grandfather of modern dermatology. **J Am Acad Dermatol** 1984 Jul;11(1):143-6
**King DF:** Modern textbooks of dermatopathology and acantholysis of

Auspitz. **J Am Acad Dermatol** 1984 Aug;11(2 Pt 1):301-3
**King DF, Eisenberg D:** Russell's fuchsine body. 'The characteristic organism of cancer.' **Am J Dermatopathol** 1981 Spring;3(1):55-8
**King DR:** The brutalization effect: execution publicity and the incidence of homicide in South Carolina. **Soc Forces** 1978;57(2):683-7
**King EE** see **Bowers JZ**
**King JC** see **Tobach E**
**King JM:** Historical review of early dermatology by J. M. King, MD, Nashville, Tenn. Originally published May 1927. **South Med J** 1983 Apr;76(4):426-36
**King JO:** The iron of melancholy: structures of spiritual conversion in America from the Puritan conscience to Victorian neurosis. Middletown, Conn., Wesleyan University Press, 1983. ix, 456 p.
**King LA** see **King DF**
**King LD** see **Cowen DL**
**King LS:** IX. The AMA gets a new code of ethics. **JAMA** 1983 Mar 11;249(10):1338-42
**King LS:** Medical education: the decade of massive change. **JAMA** 1984 Jan 13;251(2):219-24
**King LS:** Medical journalism, 1847-1883. **JAMA** 1983 Aug 12;250(6):744-8
**King LS:** Medical logic. **J Hist Med Allied Sci** 1978 Jul;33(3):377-85
**King LS:** Medical thinking, a historical preface. Princeton, Princeton University Press, 1982. vii, 336 p.
**King LS:** Medicine in the USA: Historical vignettes. II. Medical education: the early phases. **JAMA** 1982 Aug 13;248(6):731-4
**King LS:** Medicine in the USA: historical vignettes. III. Medical sects and their influence. **JAMA** 1982 Sep 10;248(10):1221-4
**King LS:** Medicine in the USA: historical vignettes. IV. The founding of the American Medical Association. **JAMA** 1982 Oct 8;248(14):1749-52
**King LS:** Medicine in the USA: Historical vignettes. VII. The painfully slow progress in medical education. **JAMA** 1983 Jan 14;249(2):270-4
**King LS:** Medicine in the USA: historical vignettes. VIII. Germ theory and its influence. **JAMA** 1983 Feb 11;249(6):794-8
**King LS:** Medicine in the USA: Historical vignettes. X. The changing scene. **JAMA** 1983 Apr 8;249(14):1897-900
**King LS:** Medicine in the USA: historical vignettes. XV. Clinical science gets enthroned. Part I. **JAMA** 1983 Sep 2;250(9):1169-72
**King LS:** Medicine in the USA: Historical vignettes. XVI. Clinical science gets enthroned. Part II. **JAMA** 1983 Oct 14;250(14):1847-50
**King LS:** Medicine in the USA: historical vignettes. XVII. Medical education: elitisms and reform. **JAMA** 1983 Nov 11;250(18):2457-61
**King LS:** Medicine in the USA: historical vignettes. XVIII. Medical education: the problems intensify. **JAMA** 1983 Dec 9;250(22):3100-4
**King LS:** Medicine in the USA: historical vignettes. XX. The Flexner report of 1910. **JAMA** 1984 Feb 24;251(8):1079-86
**King LS:** Medicine in the USA: historical vignettes. XXI. Medical practice: specialization. **JAMA** 1984 Mar 9;251(10):1333-8
**King LS:** Medicine in the USA: historical vignettes. XXII. Medical practice: making a living. **JAMA** 1984 Apr 13;251(14):1887-92
**King LS:** Medicine in the USA: historical vignettes. XXIII. The automobile makes an impact. **JAMA** 1984 May 11;251(18):2352-5
**King LS:** Medicine in the USA: historical vignettes. XXIV. The continuity of history. **JAMA** 1984 Jun 22-29;251(24):3233-6
**King LS:** The British background for American medicine. **JAMA** 1982 Jul 9;248(2):217-20
**King LS:** The 'old code' of medical ethics and some problems it had to face. **JAMA** 1982 Nov 12;248(18):2329-33
**King LS:** VI. Medical education: the AMA surveys the problems. **JAMA** 1982 Dec 10;248(22):3017-21
**King LS:** XI. Medicine seeks to be 'scientific'. **JAMA** 1983 May 13;249(18):2475-9
**King LS:** XII. Clinical laboratories become important, 1870-1900. **JAMA** 1983 Jun 10;249(22):3025-9
**King LS:** XIII. The founding of JAMA, 1883. **JAMA** 1983 Jul 8;250(2):177-80
**King P:** The contributions of Ernest Jones to the British Psycho-Analytical Society. **Int J Psychoanal** 1979;60(Pt 3):280-4
**King PH:** The life and work of Melanie Klein in the British Psycho-Analytical Society. **Int J Psychoanal** 1983;64 (Pt 3):251-60
**King RH:** From creeds to therapies: Philip Rieff's work in perspective. **Rev Am Hist** 1976;4(2):291-6
**King VH** see **Kiple KF**
**King WH:** Caroline Hampton Halsted and her family, revisited. **NC Med J** 1982 Jul;43(7):501-4
**King-Hele D, ed:** The letters of Erasmus Darwin. Cambridge, Cambridge University Press, 1981. xxxii, 363 p.
**Kingsbury M:** Book collector, bibliographer, and benefactor of libraries: Sir William Osler. **J Libr Hist** 1981 Winter;16(1):187-98
**Kingsdale JM:** The growth of hospitals: an economic history in Baltimore. Ph.D. Diss., University of Michigan. Ann Arbor, 1981. iv, 527 p.
**Kingsland S:** Raymond Pearl: on the frontier in the 1920's. Raymond Pearl memorial lecture, 1983. **Hum Biol** 1984 Feb;56(1):1-18
**Kingsley Brown A:** 'Mony a mickle...' **Trans Hunter Soc** 1978-80;37-38:7-33
**Kinloch J:** The Society and College of Radiographers--60 years on. **Radiography** 1980 Dec;46(552):271-87
**Kinn AC** see **Andersson L**
**Kinnaird DW:** Kentucky's Doctors Elkin contributions to growth of Emory's medical school. **J Ky Med Assoc** 1984 Jun;82(6):291-3
**Kinnear N:** The surgical section and surgical developments over the century. **Ir J Med Sci** 1983 Jan;152(1):44-8
**Kinney EL:** Smallpox in Provincetown, Massachusetts, 1872-73. **J Hist Med Allied Sci** 1981 Jul;36(3):334-6
**Kinney JR:** The first medical journal in Illinois. **J Hist Med Allied Sci** 1983 Apr;38(2):151-60
**Kinowskiej M** see **Majewska-Tronowicz J**
**Kinowskiej M** see **Michalczyk B**
**Kinross NJ:** Nursing education in New Zealand: a developmental perspective. **Int J Nurs Stud** 1984;21(3):193-9
**Kiple K, Kiple V:** The African connection: slavery, disease and racism. **Phylon** 1980;41(3):211-22
**Kiple KF, King VH:** Another dimension to the black diaspora: diet, disease, and racism. Cambridge, Cambridge University Press, 1981. 295 p.
**Kiple KF, Kiple VH:** Black tongue and black men: pellagra and slavery in the Antebellum South. **J South Hist** 1977 Aug;43(3):411-28
**Kiple KF, Kiple VH:** Deficiency diseases in the Caribbean. **J Interdiscip Hist** 1980 Autumn;11(2):197-215
**Kiple KF, Kiple VH:** Slave child mortality: some nutritional answers to a perennial puzzle. **J Soc Hist** 1977 Mar;10(3):284-309
**Kiple KF, Kiple VH:** The African connection: slavery, disease and racism. **Phylon** 1980 Fall;41(3):211-22
**Kiple KL, Kiple VH:** Black yellow fever immunities, innate and acquired, as revealed in the American South. **Soc Sci Hist** 1977;1(4):419-36
**Kiple V** see **Kiple K**
**Kiple VH** see **Kiple KF**
**Kiple VH** see **Kiple KL**
**Kirby NG:** How fertile the blood of warriors. **J R Coll Surg Edinb** 1981 Jan;26(1):1-11
**Kirchhoff H:** 40 Jahre miterlebte wissenschaftliche Forschung auf dem Gebiet der Gynäkologie und Geburtshilfe. **Ther Ggw** 1981 Jul;120(7):654-68
**Kirchhoff HW** see **Beckmann P**
**Kirchhoff KT** see **Rall P**
**Kir'iakulov GS** see **Zeligman SB**
**Kirienko AI, Garibdzhanian LL:** Embolektomiia iz legochnoĭ arterii. **Grudn Khir** 1983 Mar-Apr;(2):64-71
**Kirilenko TG:** Rol' Akademii meditsinskikh nauk SSSR v podgotovke mauchnykh kadrov. **Sov Zdravookhr** 1980;(2):64-7
**Kiriushchenkov AP:** Zabota Sovetskogo gosudarstva ob okhrane zdorov'ia materi i rebenka. **Feldsher Akush** 1982;47(8):3-9
**Kirkby B** see **Krag C**
**Kirklin JW:** Open-heart surgery at the Mayo Clinic. The 25th anniversary. **Mayo Clin Proc** 1980 May;55(5):339-41
**Kirkness JM:** A history of the Animal Health Register. London, The Association of the British Pharmaceutical Industry, 1981?. 39 p.
**Kirkpatrick DB:** The first primary brain-tumor operation. **J Neurosurg** 1984 Nov;61(5):809-13
**Kirkup J:** The history and evolution of surgical instruments. III. Handles. **Ann R Coll Surg Engl** 1983 Jul;65(4):269-73
**Kirkup J** see **Woodall J**
**Kirkup JR:** The history and evolution of surgical instruments. I. Introduction. **Ann R Coll Surg Engl** 1981 Jul;63(4):279-85
**Kirkup JR:** The history and evolution of surgical instruments. II Origins: function: carriage: manufacture. **Ann R Coll Surg Engl** 1982 Mar;64(2):125-32
**Kirkwood L:** Hier, aujourd'hui et demain. **Infirm Can** 1983 Oct;25(9):34-6
**Kirkwood TB, Cremer T:** Cytogerontology since 1881: a reappraisal of August Weisman and a review of modern progress. **Hum Genet** 1982;60(2):101-21
**Kirkwood K, ed** see **Sabben-Clare EE**
**Kirmse BH** see **Smith JH, ed**
**Kirn A** see **Keller F**
**Kirsanov NA, Razumov VI:** Iz istorii organizatsii massovogo donorskogo dvizheniia v gody velikoi otechestvennoi voiny. **Vestn Mosk Univ Ser 8 Istor** 1980;(5):32-41
**Kirsch I:** Demonology and science during the scientific revolution. **J Hist Behav Sci** 1980 Oct;16(4):359-68
**Kirsch J:** Jung's transference on Freud: its Jewish element. **Am Imago** 1984;41:63-84
**Kirschke G:** Die Ausbildung der Aerzte in Hyderabad (Indien). Köln, 1983. 213 p. (Kölner medizinhistorische Beiträge, Band 29)
**Kirschke S** see **Foerster I**
**Kirschner H:** Geneza i zadania medycyny społecznej. **Pol Arch Med Wewn** 1984 Jul-Aug;72(1-2):1-7
**Kirshen AJ, Cape RD:** A history of urinary incontinence: or, 400 years of incontinence--are we any drier? **J Am Geriatr Soc** 1984 Sep;32(9):686-8
**Kirshenblat IaD:** K istorii otkrytiia i izucheniia vozbuditelia adiaspiromikoza. **Mikrobiol Zh** 1980 Nov-Dec;42(6):781-2
**Kirsner JB:** Landmark perspective. Crohn's disease. **JAMA** 1984 Jan 6;251(1):80-1
**Kirsop W:** W. R. Greg and Charles Darwin in Edinburgh and after: an antipodean gloss. **Trans Camb Bibliogr Soc** 1979;7(3):376-90
**Kirsten F** see **Böhmer W**
**Kis J:** Der Knochenpathologe Emil Looser (1877-1936). Zürich, Juris, 1982. 68 p. Zürcher Medizingeschichtliche Abhandlungen, Neue Reihe, 149; also Diss.).
**Kiselev IN** see **Poliakov IA**
**Kiser TS:** A story of true devotion (Mary Breckinridge). **Front Nurs Serv Q Bull** 1981 Autumn;57(2):16-8
**Kishi Y, Uzawa Y, Hanashima T:** [Postwar transitions in the theories of nursing education: with special reference to the period between 1945 to 1955] (Jpn) **Kango Kyoiku** 1984 Sep;25(9):541-60

Kishkovskiĭ AN, Tiutin LA: K 50-letiiu kafedry rentgenologii i radiologii VMA imeni S.M. Kirov. **Voen Med Zh** 1980 Sep;(9):76-8
**Kisker KP** see **Janzarik W ed**
**Kisker KP** see **Tellenbach H, ed**
**Kiss A:** Medizinal-kultische Darstellungen und Hinweise altertümlicher Mosaiken. **Orvostort Kozl** 1981;93-96(27 No 1-4):79-82
**Kiss IN:** 'A kortól megtört, beteg, nyomorult személyek' összeírása Bártfa városában 1708-ban. **Orvostort Kozl** 1979;87-88(25 no 1-2):299-300
**Kiss PG:** János Bókay junior as seen by a disciple. **Acta Paediatr Hung** 1984;25(1-2):7-10
**Kissane JM:** Founders of Pediatric Pathology. Margaret G. Smith. 1896-1970. **Perspect Pediatr Pathol** 1982;7:v-viii
**Kiszely G:** Theodor Schwann. **Orv Hetil** 1983 Apr;124(16):959-62
**Kiszely G:** Visszaemlékezés a magyar humángenetika elmúlt 50 évére. **Orv Hetil** 1984 Mar 18;125(12):709-12
**Kitagawa EM:** New life-styles: marriage patterns, living arrangements, and fertility outside of marriage. **Ann Am Acad Polit Soc Sci** 1981;453:1-27
**Kitagawa JM** see **Unschuld PU**
**Kitahara I:** 'Kyoho' kikin to machikata segyo. **Nihonshi Kenkyu** 1981;228:1-38
**Kitamura T** see **Hino S**
**Kitchener RF:** Genetic epistemology, normative epistemology and psychologism. **Synthese** 1980;45(2):257-80
**Kitchener RF:** The nature and scope of genetic epistemology. **Philos Sci** 1981;48(3):400-15
**Kito O** see **Okamura H**
**Kitsuse JI:** Coming out all over: deviants and the politics of social problems. **Soc Probl** 1980;28(1):1-13
**Kitteringham G:** Science in provincial society: the case of Liverpool in the early nineteenth century. **Ann Sci** 1982;39:329-48
**Kittle CF:** Benjamin Rush--heritage and hope. **Proc Inst Med Chic** 1981 Apr-Jun;34(2):49-53
**Kittle CF:** Sir Arthur Conan Doyle--physician and detective. **Proc Inst Med Chic** 1981 Jan-Mar;34(1):7-11
**Kjellgren O:** The development of gynecological oncology in Scandinavia during the last 50 years. **Acta Obstet Gynecol Scand [Suppl]** 1984;120:27-34
**Klačanský I:** Rozvoj detskej otolaryngológie na Slovensku. **Cesk Otolaryngol** 1984 Jun;33(3):193-4
**Klačanský I** see **Barta T**
**Klafstad J:** Odontopathology of a Norwegian medieval population--a pilot study. **Ossa** 1978;5:43-55
**Klaĭshevich GI** see **Matveev MP**
**Klánova JV** see **Vlček J**
**Klantsa OP:** Zdravookhranenie na Podolii v period ustanovleniia Sovetskoĭ vlasti. **Sov Zdravookhr** 1983;(3):57-8
**Klantsa PA, Sobchuk GS, Fishchenko AIa:** Vishenskiĭ period deiatel'nosti N. I. Pirogova. **Khirurgiia (Mosk)** 1980 Feb;(2):106-10
**Klantsa PA** see **Bilyk VD**
**Klantsa PA** see **Kul'chitskiĭ KI**
**Klantsa PA** see **Sobchuk GS**
**Klapchuk VV:** Razvitie lechebnoĭ fizkul'tury na kurortakh Kryma (k 60-letiiu dekreta 'Ob ispol'zovanii Kryma dlia lechniia trudiahchikhsia'). **Vopr Kurortol Fizioter Lech Fiz Kult** 1981 Mar-Apr;(2):65-7
**Klapisch-Zuber C:** Genitori naturali e genitori di latte nella Firenze del quattrocento. **Quad Stor** 1980;15(2):543-63
**Klapisch-Zuber C:** Parents de sang, parents de lait: la mise en nourrice à Florence (1300-1530). **Ann Demogr Hist (Paris)** 1983;:33-64
**Klaschka F, Rauhut K, ed:** 100 Jahre Dermatologie in Berlin. Beiträge und Aufzeichnungen anlässlich der Festsitzung der Berliner Dermatologischen Gesellschaft am 12. und 13 Februar 1982. Berlin, Grosse Verlag, 1984. 152 p.
**Klasen EM:** Die Diskussion über eine 'Krise' der Medizin in Deutschland zwischen 1925 und 1935. Diss. Mainz, 1984. 169 p.
**Klasen HJ:** History of free skin grafting--knowledge or empiricism? Berlin, New York, Springer, 1981. 190 p.
**Klatt CH:** Die ersten Doktoranden der Veterinärmedizin in Finnland. **DTW** 1981 Apr 5;88(4):142-3
**Klatt CH:** Im 19. Jahrhundert nach Finnland zugezogene und dort zugelassene Tierärzte (Kurzmitteilung). **DTW** 1980 Nov 5;87(11):414
**Klauenberg S** see **Darga LL**
**Klausch B, Schwarz R:** Die Geschichte der Frauenklinik der Universität Rostock von den Anfängen bis zur Gegenwart. Rostock, Wilhelm-Pieck-Universität, 1980. 31 p.
**Klauss K:** Ein neuentdecktes frühes Dokument zur Geschichte der Erfindung des Augenspiegels durch Hermann v. Helmholtz. **NTM** 1981;18(1):58-61
**Klawans HL:** The acromegaly of Maximinus I: the possible influence of a pituitary tumor on the life and death of a Roman emperor. In Rose FC, Bynum WF, ed: Historical aspects of the neurosciences. New York, Raven, 1982. 317-26.
**Klawans HL:** The medicine of history. From Paracelsus to Freud. New York, Raven Press, 1982. ix, 238 p.
**Klawans HL** see **Goetz CG**
**Klawans HL** see **Tolosa ES**
**Klebaner BJ** see **Breul FR**
**Klebanov IaA, Goncharov NP, Chokin AR:** Sanitarno-ěpidemiologicheskaia sluzhba Kazakhskoĭ SSR. **Gig Sanit** 1982 Dec;(12):34-7
**Kleber BE, Birdsell D:** The unused weapon. **Milit Rev** 1965;45(1):54-62
**Kleber HD, Riordan CE:** The treatment of narcotic withdrawal: a historical review. **J Clin Psychiatry** 1982 Jun;43(6 Pt 2):30-4
**Kleberger E:** Fin Brillenfan des 16. Jahrhunderts. **Klin Monatsbl Augenheilkd** 1982 Sep;181(3):223-6
**Klee E:** 'Euthanasie' im NS-Staat: die 'Vernichtung lebensunwerten Lebens'. Frankfurt am Main, S. Fischer, 1983. 502 p.
**Kleeberg J:** A medical study of the story of Samson and Delilah. **Koroth** 1979 Nov;7(9-10):CXCV-CCII(644-9)
**Kleeberg J:** Goethe und die 'mal de rosa'. **Z Gastroenterol** 1983 May;21(5):241-3
**Kleeberg J:** Uber Ehrlichs Benzaldehyd-Reaktion (auf Urobilinogen) nach 80 Jahren. **Z Gastroenterol** 1982 Aug;20(8):424-8
**Kleeberg J, ed:** Eide und Bekenntnisse in der Medizin, eine Anthologie. Basel, München, Karger, 1979. 81 p.
**Klees L:** Quelques souvenirs des debuts du G.I.R.S.O. **Bull Group Int Rech Sci Stomatol Odontol** 1981 Jun;24(2):75-80
**Klein D:** Historical background and evidence for dominant inheritance of the Klein-Waardenburg syndrome (type III). **Am J Med Genet** 1983 Feb;14(2):231-9
**Klein DB:** Jewish origins of the psychoanalytic movement. New York, Praeger, 1981. xvi, 198 p.
**Klein E** see **Klein G**
**Klein F:** Janusz Korczak--Arzt und Erzieher--Ein Symbol gelebter Menschlichkeit für die heutige medizinische und heilpädagogische Praxis. **Off Gesundheitswes** 1984 May;46(5):244-8
**Klein G, Klein E:** Torbjörn Caspersson: some personal perspectives. **Cytometry** 1984 Jul;5(4):318
**Klein I:** Cholera: theory and treatment in nineteenth century India. **J Indian Hist** 1980;58(1-3):35-51
**Klein J:** Sir Francis Bacon's 'Valerius Terminus' (1603). **Sudhoffs Arch** 1982;66(1):38-69
**Klein JO:** Infectious diseases of the newborn infant--historical perspectives. In Smith GF, Smith PN, Vidyasagar D, ed: Historical review and recent advances in neonatal and perinatal medicine. [Chicago?], Mead Johnson Nutritional Division, 1983. Vol. I. p. 185-96.
**Klein JO** see **Smith GF**
**Klein P:** Die Infektionskrankheit im erzählerischen Werk Thomas Manns. **Medizinhist J** 1980;15(1/2):3-15
**Klein P:** 'Kognitive' Leistungen des Immunsystems. **Medizinhist J** 1983;18(1-2):3-20
**Klein P, Labisch A, Milles D, et al:** Zur Entwicklung der Arbeitsmedizin in Deutschland bis zum Ende der Weimarer Republik. **Arbeitsmed praventive Gesundheitspolitik** 1982;5:28-40
**Klein R:** Little 'hospital' on the prairie. Roughly the first hundred years of Rochester's Mayo Clinic. **Postgrad Med** 1984 Sep 1;76(3):15-6, 19, 22-4
**Klein-Franke F:** Die klassische Antike in der Tradition des Islam. Darmstadt, Wissenschaftliche Buchgesellschaft, 1980. ix, 181 p. (Erträge der Forschung, Band 136)
**Klein-Franke F:** The Arabic version of Galen's Periethon. **Jerus Stud Arabic Islam** 1979;1:125-50
**Klein-Franke F:** Vorlesungen über die Medizin im Islam. **Sudhoffs Arch Beih** 1982;23:1-146
**Kleine-Kracht AE** see **Brooks JA**
**Kleine-Natrop HE:** Theodor Grüneberg in der Tradition der halleschen Dermatologie. **Dermatol Monatsschr** 1981 Jun;167(6):393-5
**Kleiner SA:** Problem solving and discovery in the growth of Darwin's theories of evolution. **Synthese** 1981;47(1):119-62
**Kleinman LC, McHenry LC:** Fragments of neurologic history: phrenology's founders look at the spinal cord. **Neurology** 1984 Apr;34(4):505
**Kleinman R** see **Doberneck RC**
**Kleinmann R:** Facing cancer in the seventeenth century: the last illness of Anne of Austria, 1664-1666. **Adv Thanatol** 1978;4:37-55
**Kleiss E:** Medicine men and conditions of life in pre-Columbian Venezuela. **Arq Anat Antropol** 1978;3(3):83-112
**Kleiss E** see **Ascenzi A**
**Klemparskaya NN:** 100 years of the phagocytosis doctrine (Ilya Ilyich Mechnikov). **J Hyg Epidemiol Microbiol Immunol** 1983;27(3):249-52
**Klenke-Hamel KE** see **Janda LH**
**Klepinger LL:** The evolution of human disease: new findings and problems. **J Biosoc Sci** 1980 Oct;12(4):481-6
**Kler JH:** Along the path of modern medicine. **J Med Soc NJ** 1983 Jul;80(7):552
**Kler JH:** Medical philately. Missionary medicine. **J Med Soc NJ** 1983 Apr;80(4):302
**Kler JH:** Medical pioneers. **J Med Soc NJ** 1982 Dec;79(13):1025
**Kler JH:** Medicine and religion. **J Med Soc NJ** 1983 May;80(5):382
**Kler JH:** Pasteur. **J Med Soc NJ** 1981 Feb;78(2):121-4
**Klessen D, Albrecht U, Grützmacher KH, et al:** Stand und weitere Aufgaben der physikalischen Therapie in Berlin--Hauptstadt der DDR. **Sante Publique (Bucur)** 1981;24(4):347-57
**Klessen D:** Zur Entwicklung der Beziehungen zwischen Sozialhygiene und Organisation des Gesundheitswesens in der Sowjetunion. **Z Gesamte Hyg** 1980 Apr;26(4):290-4
**Klevay LM:** Changing patterns of disease: some nutritional remarks. **J Am Coll Nutr** 1984;3(2):149-58
**Kliachkin LM:** Ucheniki S. P. Botkina v. Saratove. **Klin Med (Mosk)** 1982 Sep;60(9):119-21
**Klickstein HS:** Wilhelm Conrad Röntgen: on a new kind of rays; a bibliographical study. [Philadelphia?], 1966. xvi, 129 p. (Mallinckrodt Classics of Radiology, v. 1).
**Klieneberger-Nobel E:** Pionierleistungen für die medizinische Mikrobiologie: Lebenserinnerungen. Stuttgart, New York, Fischer, 1977.

x, 144 p.

**Kligfield P:** Laennec and the discovery of mediate auscultation. **Am J Med** 1981 Feb;70(2):275–8

**Kligfield P:** The early pathophysiolic understanding of angina pectoris (Edward Jenner, Caleb Hillier Parry, Allan Burns). **Am J Cardiol** 1982 Dec;50(6):1433–5

**Kligfield P:** The frustrated benevolence of 'Dr. Anonymous'. **Am J Cardiol** 1981 Jan;47(1):185–7

**Kligfield PD:** A survey of variant title page vignettes in Lancisi's De subitaneis mortibus. **J Hist Med Allied Sci** 1983 Jul;38(3):336–9

**Klik J:** Pl Dobřany oslavuje stoleté výročí. **Cesk Psychiatr** 1980 Jun;76(3):204–6

**Kliks MM:** Parasites in archaeological material from Brazil. **Trans R Soc Trop Med Hyg** 1982;76(5):701

**Klimek JJ** see **Castle M**

**Kliminskiĭ IV** see **Maiat VS**

**Klimpel M:** F. von Hebra, Atlas der Hauterkrankungen (1856–1876). Köln, Universität zu Köln, 1980. 322 p. (Kölner medizinhistorische Beiträge, 17) (also Diss.).

**Kline DL:** Department of Physiology, University of Cincinnati, College of Medicine. **Physiologist** 1983 Dec;26(6):366–8

**Klingler M:** A glimpse into Roche research: antiparkinson treatment. **Int J Clin Pharmacol Ther Toxicol** 1982 Apr;20(4):190–3

**Klingmüller G:** Treponema pallidum oder Spirochaeta pallida? **Hautarzt** 1983 Dec;34(12):628–31

**'Klinicheskoĭ meditsine' 60 let!: Klin Med (Mosk)** 1980 Aug;58(8):4–6

**Klinkenberg HM:** Die historische Dimension der Umwelt. **Clio Med** 1980 Jul;14(3–4):187–211

**Klinner W** see **Habrich C**

**Kliorin AI:** N. I. Krasnogorskiĭ (k 100-letiiu so dnia rozhdeniia). **Pediatriia** 1983 May;5:76–8

**Klippe HJ, Löhr J, Kroeger C:** Historische Aspekte zur Entwicklung der endotrachealen Intubation. **Prax Klin Pneumol** 1981 Sep;35(9):413–20

**Klishov AA:** Istoriko-gnoseologicheskiĭ analiz poniatiia 'tkan''. **Arkh Anat Gistol Embriol** 1982 Jul;83(7):74–93

**Klishov AA:** N. M. Iakubovich--pervyĭ russkiĭ professor-gistolog. **Arkh Anat Gistol Embriol** 1981 Oct;81(10):105–15

**Klishov AA, Khilova IuK, Pankov EIa, et al:** Zhizn' i deiatel'nost' professora V. Ia. Rubashkina. **Arkh Anat Gistol Embriol** 1983 Nov;85(11):94–8

**Klishov AA** see **Dyskin EA**

**Klishov AA** see **Petlenko VP**

**Kliuzko AS** see **Shandala MG**

**Klix F:** Hermann Ebbinghaus---Ursprünge und Anfang psychologischer Forschungen an der Berliner Universität. In Eckardt G, ed: Zur Geschichte der Psychologie. Berlin, VEB Deutscher Verlag der Wissenschaften, 1979. p. 85–109.

**Klix F:** Hermann von Helmholtz' Beitrag zur Theorie der Wahrnehmung--Bleibendes und Vergängliches in einem grossen Lebenswerk. In Eckardt G, ed: Zur Geschichte der Psychologie. Berlin, VEB Deutscher Verlag der Wissenschaften, 1979. p. 45–59.

**klix F** see **Eckhardt G, ed**

**Kljucar S** see **Henschel WF**

**Kłodiński S** see **Sikorski J**

**Kłodziński S:** Dr Józef Gałka. **Przegl Lek** 1981;38(1):184–7

**Kłodziński S:** Dr. Stefania Perzanowska. **Przegl Lek** 1981;38(1):189–97

**Kłodziński S:** Kilka uwag o KZ-syndromie. **Przegl Lek** 1984;41(1):17–21

**Kłodziński S:** Lek. Zbigniew Sobieszczański. **Przegl Lek** 1984;41(1):131–6

**Kłodziński S, Masłowski J:** Patologia pracy w Oświecimiu-Brzezince. **Przegl Lek** 1984;41(1):37–54

**Kłodziński S:** Ppłk lek. med. Jan Zielina. **Przegl Lek** 1981;38(1):202–6

**Kłodziński S:** Prof. dr Włodzimierz Lawkowicz. **Przegl Lek** 1981;38(1):197–202

**Kłodzinski S:** Uwagi o sytuacji zdrwotnej robotników przymusowych w Niemczech hitlerowskich. **Przegl Lek** 1981;38(1):62–72

**Kłodziński S** see **Jagoda Z**

**Kłodziński S** see **Ryn Z**

**Kloë E:** Hysterie im Kindesalter. Zur Entwicklung des kindlichen Hysteriebegriffes. Freibug, Schulz, 1979. 181 p. (Freiburger Forschungen zur Medizingeschichte, Neue Folge, 9).

**Kloë E, Kindt H:** Zur Entstehung und Entwicklung des kindlichen Hysteriebegriffes. **Gesnerus** 1981;38(3/4):281–300

**Kloiber A, Glowatzki G, Mullis ML, et al:** Zur Identifizierung der mutmasslichen Gebeine des 'letzten Minnesängers', Oswald von Wolkenstein. **Anthropol Anz** 1982;40(4):285–98

**Klokke AH:** Antibakterielle Behandlung der erregerreichen Lepra. **Hautarzt** 1983 May;34(5):203–8

**Klonowicz S:** Excessive mortality of men. **Sante Publique (Bucur)** 1981;24(2–3):259–73

**Kloppe W** see **Habrich C**

**Klos SF:** Reform initiatives in American maternal health services: 1900–1940. Ed. D. Diss., Harvard University. Cambridge, 1979, vi, 182 p.

**Klosky BA:** Daring venture: a biography of Anne Austin Young, pioneer woman doctor. Columbia, S.C., Bryan, 1978. xiii, 193 p.

**Klotz P** see **Barbaix M**

**Kludas A** see **Schmidt R**

**Klukowski Z:** Szpital w Szczebrzeszynie. **Arch Hist Med (Warsz)** 1981;44(3/4):309–27

**Klumbies G:** Die Entwicklung der Hypnosetherapie in Europa. **Psychiatr Neurol Med Psychol (Leipz)** 1981;28:11–33

**Klutz M:** Die Rezepte in Oswald Crolls Basilica Chymica (1609) und ihre Beziehungen zu Paracelsus. Braunschweig, 1974. 124 p. (Veröffentlichungen aus dem Pharmaziegeschichtlichen Seminar der Technischen Universität Braunschweig, 14).

**Kluxen G:** Augenheilkunde deutscher Tropenärzte vor 1918. Düsseldorf, Triltsch Druck, 1980. 50 p. (Düsseldorfer Arbeiten zur Geschichte der Medizin, Beiheft V).

**Kluxen G, Bernsmeier H:** Die endemischen Augenkrankheiten in Samoa 1910 bis 1913. **Klin Monatsbl Augenheilkd** 1979 Dec;175(6):841–5

**Kluxen G, Bernsmeier H:** Endemic ocular infections of the South Seas in the German colonial era. **Papua New Guinea Med J** 1980 Dec;23(4):197–9

**Knapp DA, Knapp DE, Brooks GE:** Drug use in Australia and the United States as reflections of legislation and social attitudes. **Drug Intell Clin Pharm** 1977 May;11(5):298–303

**Knapp DE** see **Knapp DA**

**Knapp MR:** Economics of scale in sewage purification and disposal. **J Ind Econ** 1978 Dec;27:163–83

**Knapp PH** see **Goldberg A, ed**

**Knapp VJ:** Postmortems and the growth of modern medical knowledge in 19th century Europe. **J Okla State Med Assoc** 1983 Mar;76(3):73–6

**Knaus WA:** Claude Bernard fut-il l'inventeur de l'indice de gravité? **Presse Med** 1983 Jul 2;12(28):1755–6

**Knecht, van Eekelen A de:** Bakerboekjes in de 19e eeuw: en aanvulling. **Tijdschr Geschied Geneeskd** 1981;4(1):45–7

**Knedel M** see **Habrich C**

**Kneist W:** Arzte als Gesundheitserzieher von Kindern. **Z Gesamte Hyg** 1982 Apr;28(4):256–9

**Kneist W:** August Friedrich Heckers 'Die Kunst unsere Kinder zu gesunden Staatsbürgern zu erziehen...' (Erfurt 1805). **Beitr Gesch Univ Erfurt** 1979–83;19:187–204

**Kneist W:** Rauchen oder Gesundheit. Ein kulturhistorischer Rückblick. **Z Gesamte Hyg** 1981;27(6):477–80

**Kneist W:** Théophraste Renaudot und die Dispensairebetreuung. **Z Arztl Fortbild (Jena)** 1982 Mar 1;76(5):220–3

**Knell AJ:** Liver function and failure: the evolution of liver physiology. **J R Coll Physicians Lond** 1980 Jul;14(3):205–8

**Knel'ts VF:** Deiatel'nost' vracheĭ pervoĭ poloviny XIX veka na territorii sovremennoĭ Udmurtii. **Sov Zdravookhr** 1980;(10):55–7

**Knel'ts VF:** Pervyĭ s'ezd zemskikh vracheĭ i ego rol' v razvitii zdravookhraneniia Udmurtii. **Sov Zdravookhr** 1981;(7):62–3

**Knel'ts VF:** Revoliutsionnaia deiatel'nost' medikov Udmurtii v 1905–1907 gg. **Feldsher Akush** 1982;47(11):32–3

**Knel'ts VF:** Uchastie zemskikh vracheĭ Udmurtii v revoliutsionnom dvizhenii 1905–1907 gg. **Sov Zdravookhr** 1982;(6):64–6

**Knepper JD:** Use of human subjects in experimentation: a review of legal and ethical issues. **J Am Med Rec Assoc** 1982 Aug;53(4):62–7 contd.

**Kneževic S:** Gastroenterologija i njena povijest kao povod za razmišljanje o stanju suvremene medicinske znanosti. **Lijec Vjesn** 1981 Oct;103(10):421–4

**Kneževic S:** Iličijada i 'nakon' Ivana Ilića. **Lijec Vjesn** 1983 Sep;105(9):337–42

**Kniazzeh CR** see **Detre KC**

**Knibiehler Y, Fouquet C:** La femme et les médecins. Analyse historique. [Paris], Hachette, 1983. 333 p.

**Knibiehler Y:** La 'lutte antituberculeuse,' instrument de la médicalisation des classes populaires (1870–1930). **Ann Bretagne** 1979;86(3):321–36

**Knibiehler Y:** Les infirmières-visiteuses (1922–1938). **Penelope** 1981;(5):80–4

**Knigge KM:** Burton Lowell Baker 1912–1978. **Am J Anat** 1980 Aug;158(4):391–4

**Knight B** see **Hart GD, ed**

**Knight D** see **Forgan S, ed**

**Knight DM:** Chemistry, physiology and materialism in the romantic period. **Durham Univ J** 1972;64(2):139–45

**Knight IF:** Freud's 'Project': a theory for Studies on Hysteria. **J Hist Behav Sci** 1984 Oct;20(4):340–58

**Knight N:** Early moral and medical opposition to inhalation anesthesia and childbirth. In The history and sociology of technology: Proceedings of the 24th annual meeting of the Society for the History of Technology. Milwaukee, Milwaukee Public Museum, 1982. p. 29–37.

**Knightley P, Evans H, Potter E, et al:** Suffer the children: the story of thalidomide. New York, Viking Press, 1979. vi, 309 p.

**Knobel P:** Relations entre la psychiatrie francaise et le Brésil. **Ann Med Psychol (Paris)** 1984 Apr;142(4):499–503

**Knobil E:** William Harvey and the physiology of reproduction. **Physiologist** 1981 Feb;24(1):3–7

**Knobloch J:** Hrst vzpomínek na I. chirurgickou kliniku v době Jiráskově. **Cas Lek Cesk** 1983 Jul 15;122(28):871–5

**Knoche JF** see **Monteil RA**

**Knodel J, Hermalin AI:** Effects of birth rank, maternal age, birth interval, and sibship size on infant and child mortality: evidence from 18th and 19th century reproductive histories. **Am J Public Health** 1984 Oct;74(10):1098–106

**Knodel J:** Espacement des naissances et planification familiale: une critique de la méthode Dupâquier-Lachiver. **Ann Econ Soc Civilis** 1981;36(3):473–88

**Knodel J:** From natural fertility to family limitation: the onset of fertility transition in a sample of German villages. **Demography** 1979 Nov;16(4):493–521

**Knodel J, Van de Walle E:** Lessons from the past: policy implications of historical fertility studies. **Popul Dev Rev** 1979;5:217–45

**Knodel J, De Vos S:** Preferences for the sex of offspring and demographic behavior in eighteenth and nineteenth-century Germany: an examination of evidence from village genealogies. **J Fam Hist** 1980 Summer;5(2):145-66

**Knodel J:** Seasonal variation in infant mortality: an approach with applications. **Ann Demogr Hist (Paris)** 1983;:208-30

**Knodel J, Wilson C:** The secular increase in fecundity in German village populations: an analysis of reproductive histories of couples married 1750-1899. **Popul Stud** 1981 Mar;35(1):53-84

**Knodel J** see **Laslett P**

**Knoebel SB:** On the occasion of the 25th year of the Journal of the American College of Cardiology. **J Am Coll Cardiol** 1983 Jan;1(1):1-2

**Knoedler F:** De egestionibus. Texte und Untersuchungen zur spätmittelalterlichen Koproskopie. Diss., Würzburg. Pattensen/Han, Horst Wellm Verlag, 1979. 107 p. (Würzburger medizinhistorische Forschungen, Band 18).

**Knoefel PK:** Famine and fever in Tuscany. Eighteenth century Italian concern with the environment. **Physis** 1979;21(1-4):7-35

**Knoefel PK:** Felice Fontana: light thrown on his character by the case of the 'spazzino' Guidetti. **Med Secoli** 1981 May-Aug;18(2):229-42

**Knoefel PK:** Felice Fontana on Poisons. **Clio Med** 1980;15(1/2):35-65

**Knoepfmacher H:** Sigmund Freud in high school. **Am Imago** 1979 Fall;36(3):287-300

**Knöfler EW** see **Bethge R**

**Knöfler W** see **Bethmann W**

**Knöfler W** see **Hampel H**

**Knoke M:** Endotoxine in der Gastroenterologie--Ein medizinhistorischer Abriss. **Dtsch Z Verdau Stoffwechselkr** 1984;44(3):109-17

**Knoke M:** Viktor van der Reis--Wegbereiter der gastrointestinalen Mikroökologie des Menschen. **Nahrung** 1984;28(6-7):593-8

**Knoll J:** Deprenyl (selegiline): the history of its development and pharmacological action. **Acta Neurol Scand [Suppl]** 1983;95:57-80

**Knolle H:** Zur Pathomorphologie der Tuberkulose Erwachsener in der Gegenwart. **Wiss Beitr Martin Luther Univ Halle Wittenberg** 1983;5 R80:129 41

**Knöpfler EW** see **Bethge R**

**Knoplich J:** Cinqüentenário das Revista Paulista de Medicina. **Rev Paul Med** 1982 Nov-Dec;100(3):3-5

**Knopov MSh** see **Aleksanian IV**

**Knorr M:** Das Jahr 1882 - Anfang und Folgen einer neuren medizinischen Methodik um und von Robert Koch. **Zentralbl Bakteriol Mikrobiol Hyg [B]** 1982;176(5-6):413-24

**Knorr M, Schadewaldt H:** Infektiöse Erkrankungen im Wandel. Jahreszeitliche und säkulare Rhythmik von Infektionskrankheiten. Seasonal und periodic rhythms of infectious diseases. **Zentralbl Bakteriol [Orig B]** 1979;168(1-2):1-17

**Knorr M:** 1883-1983. Gedanken zum Jubiläumsband 177. **Zentralbl Bakteriol Mikrobiol Hyg [B]** 1983 Jan;177(1-2):i-iv

**Knorre G von, Paasch S:** Die Pest in Mitteldeutschland im 17. Jahrhundert. **Z Gesamte Inn Med** 1981 Aug 1;36(15):528-33

**Knowles AK** see **Hart GD, ed**

**Knowles RC:** An overview of equine infectious anemia control and regulation in the United States. **J Am Vet Med Assoc** 1984 Feb 1;184(3):289-92

**Knowles V:** Leaving with a red rose. A history of the Ottawa Civic Hospital School of Nursing. Ottawa, Ottawa Civic Hospital School of Nursing Alumnae Association, 1981. vi, 218 p.

**Knox PL:** Convergence and divergence in regional patterns of infant mortality in the United Kingdom from 1949-51 to 1970-72. **Soc Sci Med** 1981;15(3):323-8

**Knox PL, Bohland J, Shumsky NL:** The urban transition and the evolution of the medical care delivery system in America. **Soc Sci Med** 1983;17(1):37-43

**Knudson KG:** Walt Disney, dentistry and the armed forces during World War II. **Bull Hist Dent** 1984 Oct;32(2):112-7

**Knudtzon K, Crandell CE, ed:** From quonset hut to number one and beyond. A history of the UNC School of Dentistry. Chapel Hill, Univ. of North Carolina Dental Alumni Association, 1982. xxv, 426 p.

**Knuth H** see **Day RH**

**Koba F:** [History of school health nursing] (Jpn). **Kango** 1984 Jun;36(7):38-46

**Koba S, Koba-Ryszewska T:** Sylwetki zasłużonych lekarzy kieleckich z końca XIX i początku XX wieku. **Arch Hist Med (Warsz)** 1980;43(4):429-38

**Koba-Ryszewska T** see **Koba S**

**Kobarg I:** Das Leben und Werk von Sandor Rado. Diss. Mainz, 1979. 73 p.

**Kobayashi K, ed** see **Cho LJ**

**Kobe Daigaku Igakubu Shika Koko Geka gojisshunen kinen gyoseki shu:** Kobe, Japan, Do Geka, [1977]. 93 p.

**Kober R:** Abteilung Gesundheits- und Sozialwesen des Rates des Bezirkes Gera. **Z Arztl Fortbild (Jena)** 1979 Oct 1;73(19-20):983-6

**Kobes LW:** Quellenstudie zu Petrus Camper und der nach ihm benannten Schädelebene. **Dtsch Zahnarztl Z** 1983;38(3):268-70

**Kobiakova LF** see **Karpenko VS**

**Koblenzer PJ:** Edinburgh's influence on medicine in the new world. In Passmore R, ed: Proceedings of the Royal College of Physicians of Edinburgh Tercentenary Congress, 1981. Edinburgh, Royal College of Physicians of Edinburgh, 1982. p. 143-58.

**Kobuszewska-Faryna M:** Rok 1978--rokiem ważnych roczinic dla patomorfologów polskich. **Patol Pol** 1979 Apr-Jun;30(2):153-6

**Kobylińska-Szymańska M, Froch W:** Poczatki sztuki chirurgicznej w Lublinie i kształcenie jej adeptów (wiek XVI - XVIII). **Arch Hist Med (Warsz)** 1980;43(2):163-78

**Kocere V:** Latvijas PSR Zinātnu akademijas akademike Rita Kukaine: biobibliogrāfiskais rāditājs. Riga, Zinātne, 1982. 129 p.

**Koch CH:** Petrus Severinus, Francis Bacon og Naturiagttagelsen. **Dan Medicinhist Arbog** 1979;161-72

**Koch E:** Arzte, die Geschichte machten: Sternkunden der Heilkunde in 30 Lebensbildern. Augsburg, Hofmann, 1981. 195 p.

**Koch E** see **Schein CJ**

**Koch F:** Geschichte der Krankenpflege von 1930-1950. Bericht über ein Seminar im Bildungszentrum Essen (BZE) des DBfK. **Krankenpflege (Frankfurt)** 1984 Mar;38(3):85-6

**Koch G:** Euthanasie, Sterbehilfe. Eine dokumentierte Bibliographie. Erlangen, Palm und Enke, 1984. xvi, 300 p. (Bibliographica genetica medica, Vol. 18).

**Koch G:** Inhaltsreiche Jahre eines Humangenetikers: Mein Lebensweg in Bildern und Dokumenten. Erlangen, Perimed Fachbuchgesellschaft, 1982. 472 p.

**Koch H** see **Gerecke K**

**Koch HA:** Zum Nachweis einiger mikrobiologischer Probleme im Buch Leviticus (3. Buch Mose) des Alten Testamentes. **Mykosen** 1983 Mar;26(3):159-62

**Koch HT:** Julius Rosenbaum (1807-1874) als Medizinhistoriker. **NTM** 1981;18(1):84-90

**Koch HT:** Wilhelm Reil-Bey (1820-1880) und die Klimabehandlung der Tuberkulose. **Wiss Beitr Martin Luther Univ Halle Wittenberg** 1983;5-R80:251-60

**Koch R:** Classics in infectious diseases. The etiology of tuberculosis: Robert Koch. Berlin, Germany, 1882. **Rev Infect Dis** 1982 Nov-Dec;4(6):1270-4

**Koch T:** Gedanken zur 100. Wiederkehr des Tages der Entdeckung des Tuberkuloseerregers durch Robert Koch. **Gegenbaurs Morphol Jahrb** 1982;128(1):1-11

**Koch centennial supplement:** 100th anniversary of the announcement of the discovery of the tubercle bacillus by Robert Koch, March 24, 1882. **Am Rev Respir Dis** 1982 Mar;125(3 pt 2):1-132

**Kochemasova ZN, Dykhno MM, Dorozhkova IR, et al:** L-transformatsiia kak odin iz faktorov izmenchivosti vozbuditelia tuberkuleza (k 100-letiiu otkrytiia vozbuditelia tuberkuleza). **Sov Med** 1983;(3):20-3

**Kochemasova ZN, Dykhno MM, Dorozhkova IR, et al:** 100-letie so dnia otkrytiia R. Kokhom vozbuditelia tuberkuleza. **Klin Med (Mosk)** 1982 Nov;60(11):115-7

**Kochemasova ZN, Dykhno MM:** 60 let kafedre mikrobiologii i Moskovskogo meditsinskogo instituta im. I. M. Sechenova. **Zh Mikrobiol Epidemiol Immunobiol** 1981 May;(5):113-6

**Köcher F** see **Habrich C**

**Kocher JE:** Socio-economic development and fertility change in rural Africa. **Food Res Inst Stud** 1977;16(2):63-76

**Kochnova IE** see **Maiat VS**

**Koch's bacillus: Tubercle** 1982 Mar;63(1):1-2

**Kock W:** Ett filosofiskt tackbrev från Israel Hwasser. **Nord Medicinhist Arsb** 1980;:90-8

**Kock W:** Från Siukwakterska till sjuksköterska. **Nord Medicinhist Arsb** 1984;:129-35

**Kock W:** Hälsningsanförande. **Nord Medicinhist Arsb** 1980;Suppl 6:12-3

**Kock W:** Märkesdagar och märkesmän i svenska läkaresällskapet. **Lakartidningen** 1983 Nov 30;80(48):4667-70

**Kock W:** Medicinhistorisk krönika. **Nord Medicinhist Arsb** 1981;:5-23

**Kock W:** Nordens första medicinska Nobelpris. **Nord Medicinhist Arsb** 1982;:110-21

**Kock W:** Santiago Ramón y Cajal and the Nobel prize. In International Congress of the History of Medicine, 27th, Barcelona, 1980. Actas. Barcelona, Académia de Ciències Médiques de Catalunya i Balears, 1981. p. 550-6.

**Kock W:** Santiago Ramón y Cajal och Nobelpriset. **Nord Medicinhist Arsb** 1981;:151-9

**Kock W:** Sjuk i Sverige 1578-1978. **Nord Medicinhist Arsb** 1980;Suppl 6:57-66

**Kock W:** Sven Sköldberg och ovariotomien en pionjärinsats i svensk gynekologi. **Nord Medicinhist Arsbok** 1983;:103-16

**Kock W:** 80-talet: da å upptäcktes bisköldkörtlarna och då gjorde bakterierna sin entré. **Lakartidningen** 1979 Dec 19;76(51):4697-9

**Kock W** see **Habrich C**

**Kock W, ed** see **Nicou G**

**Kocsis SG, Marcsik A:** Zománcképzödmények a VII-VIII. századból származó koponýak fogain. **Fogorv Sz** 1981 Mar;74(3):89-93

**Kodama K:** [Care and cure defined in the 'Notes on Nursing' (Florence Nightingale)] (Jpn). **Sogo Kango** 1982;16(4):29-39

**Kodama K:** [From the old notes on Florence Nightingale] (Jpn) **Sogo Kango** 1980;15(4):12-7

**Kodama K:** [Scenes associated with Florence Nightingale] (Jpn) **Kango** 1980 Nov;32(11):48-59

**Kodama K** see **Usui T**

**Kodama K** see **Yumaki M**

**Kodov H** see **Apostolov M**

**Koehler K, Sass H:** Der Maniebegriff seit Kraepelin. **Nervenarzt** 1981 Jan;52(1):19-25

**Koehler K** see **Janzarik W ed**

**Koehler KG:** The Schreber case and affective illness: a research diagnostic re-assessment. **Psychol Med** 1981 Nov;11(4):689-96

**Koehler W, Mochmann H:** The development of the staining of bacteria up to the introduction of Gram's method in 1884. **Medicamentum**

1980;54:27-31; 55:29-31
**Koelbing H** see **Häusermann R**
**Koelbing HM:** Akademische Medizin und Offentlichkeit. Rektoratsreden von Zürcher Medizinern seit 1933. In Ganzinger K, Skopec M, Wyklicky H, ed: Festschrift für Erna Lesky zum 70. Geburtstag. Wien, Brüder Hollinek, 1981. p. 49-55.
**Koelbing HM:** 'De conceptu et generatione hominis' - die lateinische Fassung von Jakob Rueffs 'Trostbüchle', Zürich 1554. **Gesnerus** 1981;38:51-8
**Koelbing HM:** 'De conceptu et generatione hominis'. Die lateinische Fassung von Jakob Rueffs 'Trostbüchle', Zürich 1554. In International Congress of the History of Medicine, 27th, Barcelona, 1980. Actas. Barcelona, Académia de Ciències Mèdiques de Catalunya i Balears, 1981. p. 271-5.
**Koelbing HM:** Lehren aus der Therapiegeschichte--der therapeutische Optimismus und seine Tücken. **Schweiz Med Wochenschr** 1983 Oct 1;113(39):1378-84
**Koelbing HM:** Paracelsus. **Praxis** 1982 Dec 21;71(51):1973-6
**Koelbing HM:** The Hippocratic physician at his patient's bedside. **Practitioner** 1980 May;224(1343):551-4
**Koelbing HM:** Town and state physicians in Switzerland (16th-18th centuries). In Russell AW, ed: The town and state physician in Europe from the Middle Ages to the Enlightenment. Wolfenbüttel, Herzog August Bibliothek, 1981. p. 141-55 (Wolfenbütteler Forschungen, 17).
**Koelbing HM** see **Grmek MD, ed**
**Koelbing HM** see **Habrich C**
**Koelbing HM** see **Rösslin E**
**Koelbing HM** see **Rueff J**
**Koelbing HM** see **Wunderlich CA**
**Koelsch KA:** Die Entwicklukng der gastroenterologischen Endoskopie in der DDR während der letzten 10 Jahre, alte und neue Probleme. **Z Arztl Fortbild (Jena)** 1979 Oct 1;73(19-20):981-3
**Koenig GG:** Schamane und Schmied, Medicus und Mönch: ein Ueberblick zur Archäologie der merowingerzeitlichen Medizin im südlichen Mitteleuropa. **Helv Archaeol** 1982;13(51-2):75-154
**Koenigsberger D:** Renaissance man and creative thinking. A history of concepts of harmony 1400-1700. Hassocks, Sussex, Harvester Press, 1979. xiii, 282 p.
**Koerting W:** Die Deutsche Universität in Prag. München, Bayerische Landesärztekammer, 1968. 300 p.
**Koestler FA:** The unseen minority: a social history of blindness in the United States. New York, McKay, 1976. 559 p.
**Kofod H:** Danish contributions to the unicorn story. **Beitr Gesch Pharm** 1979;31(2):12-15
**Kogan VI, Petrova LF, Tarasenko IV:** Slavnaia stranitsa iz istorii sanitarnoĭ organizatsii Ukrainskoĭ SSR (k 60-letiiu sozyva I sessii Sanitarnogo soveta). **Gig Sanit** 1982 Jul;(7):32-4
**Kogan VIa:** II sessiia Vseukrainskogo tsentral'nogo komiteta i ee znachenie dlia razvitiia zdravookhraneniia Ukrainskoĭ SSR. **Sov Zdravookhr** 1984;(10):51-3
**Kogan VIa, Petrova LF:** Sanitarnye s'ezdy USSR i ikh sotsial'no-gigienicheskaia napravlennost'. **Sov Zdravookhr** 1983;(3):58-61
**Kogan VIa** see **Duplenko KF**
**Kogan Via** see **Grando AA**
**Kogan VIa** see **Shandala MG**
**Kogge D:** Zur geschichtlichen Entwicklung der Behandlungsmassnahmen bei Lippen-Kiefer-Gaumenspalten. Diss. Bonn, 1981. 84 p.
**Kogiso M, Ishihara T, Kamata H:** [On the history of midwifery. A discussion] (Jpn). **Josanpu Zasshi** 1981 Aug;35(8):562-76
**Koh TC:** Chinese medicine and martial arts. **Am J Chin Med** 1981 Autumn;9(3):181-6
**Köhbach M:** Europäische Aerzte im Osmanischen Reich am Beginn des 18. Jahrhunderts--der Fall Sinasi. **Sudhoffs Arch** 1980;64(1):79-85
**Kohl EW:** Virchow in Würzburg. Pattensen/Han., Wellm, 1976. 129 p. (Diss., Würzburg).
**Kohler RE:** From medical chemistry to biochemistry: the making of a biomedical discipline. Cambridge, New York, Cambridge University Press, 1982. ix, 399 p.
**Kohler RE:** Medical reform and biomedical science: biochemistry -- a case study. In Vogel MJ, Rosenberg CE, ed: The therapeutic revolution. Philadelphia, 1979. p. 27-66.
**Kohler RE:** Rudolf Schoenheimer, isotopic tracers, and biochemistry in the 1930's. **Hist Stud Phys Sci** 1977;8:257-98
**Kohler W** see **Mochmann H**
**Kohlhaas-Christ C:** Zur Geschichte des Apothekenwesens im Hamburg von den Anfängen bis zum Erlass der Medizinalordnung 1818. Stuttgart, Deutscher Apotheker Verlag, 1985. 279 p. (Quellen und Studien zur Geschichte der Pharmazie, Bd. 29)
**Kohlhauer CE:** Mediziner und Naturwissenschaftler im Fürstentum Ansbach. [Ansbach, s. n., 1964]. 30 p.
**Kohlhausen K:** 30 Jahre Bundesverband der Vertrauensärzte (jetzt: Bundesverband der Vertrauens- und Rentenversicherungsärzte e.V.). **Off Gesundheitswes** 1982 Apr;44(4):205-8
**Kohlstedt SG:** In from the periphery: American women in science, 1830-1880. **Signs** 1978;4(1):81-96
**Kohlstedt SG:** Science: the struggle for survival, 1880 to 1894. **Science** 1980 Jul 4;209(4452):33-42
**Kohn A:** Errors, fallacies, or deception? **Perspect Biol Med** 1978 Spring;21(3):420-30
**Kohn D, Stauffer RC, Smith S:** New light on The foundations of the origin of species: A reconstruction of the archival record. **J Hist Biol** 1982 Fall;15(3):419-42
**Kohn D, Weiss Z, Flatau E:** The history of malaria in the Jezreel Valley in the years 1922-1928 in En Harod. **Koroth** 1982 Aug;8(3/4):177-86
**Kohn D:** Theories to work by: rejected theories, reproduction, and Darwin's path to natural selection. **Stud Hist Biol** 1980;4:67-70
**Kohn D, Cohen J, Flatau E:** 60 years of medical activities in the Jezreel Valley. From the Archives of Central Emek Hospital in Afula. **Koroth** 1982 Aug;8(3/4):169-75
**Kohn Loncarica AG:** Contribuciones originales de la medicina argentina a la medicina universal. **Asclepio** 1981;33:411-24
**Kohn Loncarica AG:** Historia de la inmigracion medica en la republica Argentina. Tesis, Universidad de Buenos Aires, 1971-1981. 442 leaves.
**Kohn Loncarica AG:** La medicina en las campañas militares del siglo XIX. Las guerras de frontera. In Congreso de Historia de la Medicina Argentina [Transactions], 5th, Mendoza, 1983. p. 111-32.
**Kohn Loncarica AG** see **Pennini de Vega E**
**Kohnen N:** Arzt und Philosoph. Das Verhältnis von Medizin und Philosophie in seinem geschichtlichen Wandel. **Med Welt** 1981 Oct 16;32(42):1586-92
**Kohnen N:** Die Symbolkraft menschlicher Schädel und ihr ritueller Gebrauch. **Med Welt** 1983 May 6;34(18):552-6
**Kohnen N:** 'Ein und dasselbe ist Lebendiges und Totes ...'. Die enthaupteten Mutterschaftsfiguren aus Sawankhalok. **Dtsch Arztebl** 1982 Nov 5;79(44):83-7
**Kohnen N:** Geburtsbräuche bei den Kankanai-Igorot. Ein Beitrag zur 'natürlichen' Geburt. **Dtsch Med Wochenschr** 1983 Jul 29;108(30):1163-7
**Kohnen N:** Nationalheld und Wissenschaftler; der philippinische Arzt José Rizal. **Dtsch Arztebl** 1983 Apr 22;80(16):102-6
**Kohnen N:** Nicolai de Cusa. Liber quasi medicinalis: De staticis experimentis. In Göpfert W, Otten HH, ed: Metavoeite: wandelt euch durch Denken. Düsseldorf, Triltsch, 1983. p. 135-45.
**Kohut RI:** The clinical research of John Lindsay. **Ann Otol Rhinol Laryngol [Suppl]** 1983 Jan-Feb;102:20-2
**Kohut RI** see **Mhoon EE**
**Koĭchev K:** Po-vazhni momenti ot istoriiata i razvitieto na Katedrata po propodevtika na vŭtreshni bolesti. **Vutr Boles** 1981;20(6):12-5
**Koike A:** [Hitherto unknown profile of Florence Nightingale]. (Jpn) **Sogo Kango** 1980;15(1):100-8
**Koinange K:** Some reflections on development of health services in Kenya. **East Afr Med J** 1983 Sep;60(9):599-602
**Kokaska CJ, Woodward S, Tyler L:** Disabled people in the Bible. **Rehabil Lit** 1984 Jan-Feb;45(1-2):20-1
**Kokavec M, Tichý M, Porubský V, et al:** Vznik Ustavu súdneho lekárstva v Bratislave. **Soud Lek** 1983;28(1):1-6
**Kokhan AI:** Mediki-uzniki Petropavlovskoĭ kreposti. **Sov Zdravookhr** 1979;(12):52-5
**Kokhan AI, Miliavskiĭ VM:** Sestry miloserdiia v bor'be s épidemieĭ difterii. **Med Sestra** 1983 Oct;42(10):48-9
**Kokina NN:** P. K. Anokhin's concept of systems genesis and its subsequent development. **Neurosci Behav Physiol** 1980 Mar-Apr;10(2):142-6
**Kokoska U:** Johann Georg Noël Dragendorff (20.4.1836 - 7.4.1898): Sein Beitrag zur Gerichtsmedizin, Pharmakologie und Pharmazie an der Universität Dorpat. Diss. Berlin, 1983. 234 p.
**Kokoszka A** see **Drozdowski P**
**Kolář J, Michalková D:** Sedesát roku používání inzulínu v léčbě diabetes mellitus. **Cesk Pediatr** 1983 Jan;38(1):55-7
**Kolařik J, Jorda V:** Thirty-five years of the Faculty of Medicine at the reestablished university in Olomouc. **Acta Univ Palacki Olomuc Fac Med** 1982;103:7-21
**Kolarov NI:** Iz istoriiata na zhelezopŭtnata meditsinska sluzhba v Bŭlgariia, 1888-1944. Sofiia, Meditsina i fizkultura, 1978. 119 p.
**Kolarov P:** Sanitarnata sluzhba na internatsionalnite brigadi v ispaniia (1936-1938). **Izv Inst Istor Bkp** 1967;16:289-312
**Kolb A:** Sebastian Kneipp und Vorarlberg. **Montfort** 1971;23(2):158-62
**Kolb W** see **Ungethüm M**
**Kolbas V:** Marginalije u povodu dvadeset pete godišnjice 'Arhiva za zaštitu majke i djeteta'. **Lijec Vjesn** 1983 Jul-Aug;105(7-8):315-8
**Kolchinskiĭ EI:** [Development of the idea of transformation in evolution] (Rus). **Istor Biol Issled** 1978;7:25-45
**Kolesov VI:** Khirurgicheskomu obshchestvu Pirogova--100 let. **Vestn Khir** 1982 May;128(5):127-36
**Kolff WJ:** Artificial organs--forty years and beyond. **Trans Am Soc Artif Intern Organs** 1983;29:6-24
**Kolff WJ:** Past, present, and future of artificial kidneys. **Transplant Proc** 1981 Mar;13(1):35-40
**Koliadenko VG** see **Peleshchuk AP**
**Koliadich MN** see **Shirokov IuG**
**Koliadiuk IV, Mamontov AS, Kovaleva NS, et al:** Stranitsy nasheĭ istorii. **Sov Med** 1983;(12):111-3
**Kolin PC:** The Elizabethan stage doctor as a dramatic convention. Salzburg, Institut für englische Sprache und Literatur, Universität Salzburg, 1975. 212 p. (Salzburg studies in English literature; Elizabethan & Renaissance studies, 41).
**Kolisch P deR:** Paul Revere and medicine. **JAMA** 1984 Jun 22-29;251(24):3224
**Kollautz A:** Eine Episode aus der Praxis des Paracelsus. **Carinthia** 1967;157:578-87
**Kollberg H:** 1000 års erfarenhet av cystisk fibros--ett samlat 'testamente'. **Lakartidningen** 1981 Sep 16;78(38):3258-60
**Kolle P:** Entwicklung, Stand und Zukunft der Urologie. **MMW** 1980 Nov 7;122(45):1575-6

**Koller LR** see **Lamas GA**

**Koller M:** Kinderzahnmedizin im 18. und 19. Jahrhundert. **Swiss Dent** 1980 Dec;1(12):32–3

**Koller O** see **Augensen K**

**Kollesch J:** Aerztliche Ausbildung in der Antike. **Klio** 1979;61:507–13

**Kollesch J:** Antike Heilkunst: ausgewählte Texte aus dem medizinischen Schrifttum der Griechen und Römer. Leipzig, Reclam, 1981. 212 p.

**Kollesch J:** Das Berliner Corpus der antiken Aerzte. **Clio Med** 1981 Sep;16(1):45–7

**Kollesch J:** Galen als Vertreter der zweiten Sophistik. **Orvostort Kozl** 1981;93–96(27 No 1–4):47–54

**Kollesch J:** Papyri mit medizinischen, naturwissenschaftlichen und Mathematischen Texten. **Arch Papyrusforsch** 1978;26:141–8

**Kollesch J:** Zum Problem der Medizingeschichtsschreibung in der griechisch-römischen Antike. In International Congress of the History of Medicine. 26th, Plovdiv, 1978. Actes du Congress. Sofia, 1981. Volume II. p. 124–6.

**Kollesch J** see **Harig G**

**Kölli E:** 1920-luvun kätilön työstä. **Katilolehti** 1981 Dec;86(12):392–8

**Köllmann W** see **Dupâquier J**

**Kollmeier K:** Leben und Sterben in Pestzeiten. **Med Welt** 1983 Feb 11;34(6):186–91

**Kollmeier K:** Von der Ueberwasser-Elende zum Militärhospital. Die Entwicklung des militärischen Sanitätswesens in der Provinzhauptstadt Münster/Westfalen. **Hist Hosp** 1979–80;13:96–118

**Kolmsee P:** Nikolai Iwanowitsch Pirogow – Kriegschirurg und militärmedizinischer Organisator in Russland des 19. Jahrhunderts. **Militaergesch** 1981;20(5):536–45

**Kolmsee P** see **Dobek R**

**Kolod'ko ED** see **Kolontaĭ IuIu**

**Kołodziej J** see **Marek Z**

**Kołodziejska H:** Zarys historii Instytutu Radowego im. Marii Skłodowskiej-Curie. **Nowotwory** 1983 Jan–Mar;33(1):1–5

**Kolomiichenko MI:** Materialy X plenuma Nauchnogo obshchestva khirurgov USSR. Kiev, Zdorov'ia, 1967. 157 p.

**Kolontaĭ IuIu, Kondrashov AN, Kolod'ko ED:** 50 let kafedre travmatologii, ortopedii i voenno-polevoĭ khirurgii Dnepropetrovskogo ordena Trudovogo Krasnogo Znameni meditsinskogo instituta. **Ortop Travmatol Protez** 1980 Mar;(3):76–7

**Kolta KS:** Arzt und Hersteller von Heilmitteln im alten Aegypten. **Beitr Gesch Pharm** 1979;31(2):9–12

**Kolta KS:** Der Arzt und Hersteller von Heilmitteln im alten Agypten. In International Congress of the History of Medicine. 26th, Plovdiv, 1978. Actes du Congress. Sofia, 1981. Volume II. p. 127–8.

**Kolta KS, Rothe R:** Ein Bericht über die Röntgen- und Tomographiebefunde bei den Mumien der ägyptischen Staatssammlung in München. In International Congress of the History of Medicine, 27th, Barcelona, 1980. Actas. Barcelona, Acadèmia de Ciències Mèdiques de Catalunya i Balears, 1981. p. 557–9.

**Kolta KS:** Neue Erkenntnisse zur Medizin der Kopten. **Sudhoffs Arch** 1984;68(2):157–72

**Kolta KS** see **Habrich C**

**Kol'tsova MM:** Mekhanizmy integratsii uslovnykh refleksov v trudakh E. A. Asratiana. **Zh Vyssh Nerv Deiat** 1983 Mar–Apr;33(2):216–20

**Kolt'tsova MM** see **Volokhov AA**

**Komakhidze ME:** Ocherki o khirurgicheskoĭ rabote ofitserskogo gospitalia v period Velikoĭ Otechstvennĭ voĭny (1941–1955 gg.). Tbilisi, Metsniereba, 1977. 102 p.

**Komarov BD, Bognitskaia TN, Umanskaia VV:** Razvitie nauchnykh osnov neotlozhnoĭ khirurgii v Sovetskom Soiuze za 60 let. **Vestn Khir** 1982 Dec;129(12):10–3

**Komarov BD, Kustova EA:** 60 let skoroĭ meditsinskoĭ pomoshchi. **Sov Med** 1982;(12):25–9

**Komarov FI:** S. P. Botkin--vydaiushchiisia deiatel' otechestvennoi meditsiny. **Vestn Akad Med Nauk SSSR** 1983;(3):3–7

**Komarov FI:** Vklad voennykh medikov v pobedu nad vragom. **Voen Med Zh** 1980 May;(5):7–13

**Komatsu N:** [A study on Shimpei Goto/Part II & III. His basic idea on central and rural health organization] (Jpn). **Igakushi Kenkyu** 1980;53:10–21

**Komissarenko PV:** Znachenie issledovaniĭ A. A. Bogomol'tsa v razvitii sovremennoĭ ĕndokrinologii. **Fiziol Zh** 1981 May–Jun;27(3):388–93

**Komissarenko VP:** Idei A. A. Bogomol'tsa v razvitii sovremennoĭ ĕndokrinologii. **Patol Fiziol Eksp Ter** 1981 Mar–Apr;(2):82–9

**Komkov GD, Levsĭn BV, Semenov LK:** Geschichte der Akademie der Wissenschaften der UdSSR. Ed. C. Grau. Berlin, Akademie Verlag, 1981. 745 p. (Translation from the Russian edition of 1977)

**Komorowska W** see **Jasińska Z**

**Kon IS:** O sotsiologicheskoi interpretatsii seksual'nogo povedeniia. **Sotsiol Issled** 1982;(2):113–22

**Konami Y:** [Studies on Nightingale: the role of the matron] (Jpn) **Sogo Kango** 1980;15(4):29–36

**Konaréva N** see **Naidenov G**

**Konderska Z:** Drogi pielegniarstwa polskiego. **Pieleg Polozna** 1984;(7):16–8

**Konderska Z:** Powstanie Polskiego Towarzystwa Pielęgniarskiego. **Pieleg Polozna** 1982;(10):28–9

**Konderska Z:** Sprawa rodowodu. **Pieleg Polozna** 1981;(10–11–12):16–7, 27

**Konderska Z:** 25 lat Polskiego Towarzystwa Pielęgniarskiego. **Pieleg Polozna** 1982;(4–5):26–8, 31

**Kondracka E** see **Gierek T**

**Kondrashov AN** see **Kolontaĭ IuIu**

**Kondratas RA:** Biologics Control Act of 1902. In Young JH, ed: The early years of federal food and drug control. Madison, American Institute of the History of Pharmacy, 1982. p. 8–27.

**Kondrat'ev IM** see **Kosareva AA**

**Konev A:** Krasnaia gvardiia v bor'be za khleb. **Voen Istor Zh** 1978;3:78–83

**Kong YC:** Introduction to basic concepts in Chinese medicine. **Stud Hist Med** 1981 Mar;5(1):1–17

**König R:** Alexander Mitscherlich: Psychoanalyse und Zeitkritik (1969). **Psyche (Stuttg)** 1983 Oct;37(10):921–60

**König S:** Arzt und Medizin in der TIME 1971–1975. Diss. Düsseldorf, 1980. 205 p.

**König W** see **Schröder C**

**Konin GK:** Fel'dsher-revoliutsioner S. A. Gribov. **Feldsher Akush** 1982;47(11):33–5

**Koning A:** Die Pharmazie in der holländischen politischen Karikatur. **Pharm Acta Helv** 1979;54(9–10):308–10

**Koning AT:** De 'Kweekschool der Vroedkunde', de eerste verloskundige periodiek? **Ned Tijdschr Geneeskd** 1981 Aug 8;125(32):1299–302

**Koning AT:** Vijftig jaar Tijdschrift voor Kindergeneeskunde. **Tijdschr Kindergeneeskd** 1983 Feb;51(1):1–7

**Koning DA:** Grosse Funde in kleinen Museen. Einige Neuentdeckungen auf dem Gebiet der Apotheken-Fayencen. In Dilg P, et al., ed: Perspektiven der Pharmaziegeschichte. Graz, Austria, Akademische Druck- u. Verlagsanstalt, 1983. p. 431–39.

**Konjhodžic F, Simunovic V:** Prve operacije na glavi i mozgu u akufskoj bolnici u Sarajeve. **Med Arh** 1978 Sep–Oct;32(5):325–8

**Konkoly Thege A:** A Bergeni Orvosi Múzeum. **Orv Hetil** 1981 Nov 15;122(46):2858

**Kono H** see **Ikezawa Y**

**Kononov VS:** Perspektivy i problemy khirurgii detskogo vozrasta v Kirgizii. **Vestn Khir** 1982 Dec;129(12):14–8

**Konopka AF:** Problems, history, and dilemma. A case for science law. **Ala J Med Sci** 1981 Oct;18(4):352–3

**Konopka M** see **Bearman D**

**Konopka S:** Działalność naukowa, redakcyjna i wydawnicza prof. Adama Wrzoska w świetle jego wypowiedzi i listów nie ogłoszonych w druku. **Arch Hist Med (Warsz)** 1982;45(1–4):11–26

**Konopka S:** O źródłach do dziejów medycyny polskiej i o głównych przeszkodach, utrudniajacych rozwijanie badań naukowych z tej dziedziny. **Arch Hist Med (Warsz)** 1983;46(4):413–37

**Konopka S:** Odrodzenie się niektórych ważnych działów polskiej służby zdrowia w roku 1945. **Pol Tyg Lek** 1981 Sep 7;36(36):1369–75

**Konopka S:** Relacje profesorów Wydziału lekarskiego Uniwersytetu Jagiellonskiego o dziejach medycyny polskiej. **Arch Hist Med (Warsz)** 1979;42(1):107–24

**Konoshita K** see **Hino S**

**Konovalov AN, Iartsev VV:** Istoriia i perspektivy razvitiia sovetskoĭ neĭrokhirurgii. **Zh Vopr Neirokhir** 1982 Sep–Oct;(5):3–8

**Konovalov AN, Iartsev VV:** 50-letie Nauchno-issledovatel'skogo ordena Trudovogo Krasnogo Znameni instituta neĭrokhirurgii im. akad. N. N. Burdenko AMN SSSR. **Zh Vopr Neirokhir** 1981 Nov–Dec;(6):3–9

**Konovalov II:** A. S. Pushkin i M. Iu. Lermontov na Kavkazskikh Mineral'nykh Vodakh (k 200-letiiu Piatigorska). **Vopr Kurortol Fizioter Lech Fiz Kult** 1980 Sep–Oct;(5):68–70

**Konrad K** see **Kerl H**

**Konrad M, Bleker J:** Der Dr. med. dent. und die Medizingeschichte--Uber 1000 Dissertationen zur Geschichte der Zahnheilkunde seit 1919. **Dtsch Zahnarztl Z** 1983 May;38(5):590–1

**Konrády A:** A 75 éves Balassa kórház. **Orv Hetil** 1984 Jun 24;125(26):1577–8

**Konstantinov AA** see **Rosliakov AG**

**Konstantinova NN** see **Garmasheva NL**

**Konstantinova NP** see **Preobrazhenskiĭ NA**

**Kontrovitz M** see **Fields K**

**Kontúrová Z:** 30 rokov logopédie v zdravotníctve na Slovensku. **Cesk Otolaryngol** 1983 Jun;32(3):188–91

**Konyk IeB** see **Kvashenko BK**

**Konyshev VA** see **Shaternikov VA**

**Koo LC:** Camminare su due gambe: la medicina nella Cina moderna. **Mondo Cinese** 1974;2(8):100–17

**Kooij CG van der:** Rudolf de Mepsche en de Faanse processen. **Spiegel Hist** 1979;14(6):358–64

**Kook H:** Introduction to the history of urology in the Bible and Talmud. **Koroth** 1979 Nov;7(9–10):CCXIX–CCXX(710–15)

**Koop CE:** Pediatric surgery. the newest specialty for the youngest patient. **Trans Stud Coll Physicians Phila** 1981 Sep;5(3 no 3):195–208

**Kopanev VI:** [Role of the scientists of the S. M. Kirov Military Medical Academy in the development of aviation medicine]. (Rus) **Voen Med Zh** 1979 Dec;(12):63–5

**Kopanev VI:** The importance of K. E. Tsiolkovskii's ideas in the formation and development of space medicine. **Biol Bull Acad Sci USSR** 1979 Nov–Dec;6(6):764–71

**Kopelev L:** Der heilige Doktor Fjodor Petrowitsch: die Geschichte des Friedrich Joseph Haass, Bad Münstereifel 1780–Moskau 1853. 2. Aufl. Hamburg, Hoffmann und Campe, 1984. 231 p.

**Kopf AW** see **Baer RL**

**Koplin AN:** Anti-smoking legislation: the New Jersey experience. **J Public Health Policy** 1981;2(3):247–55

**Kopp B** see **Heilmittel aus Pflanzen und Tieren**

**Kopp C:** The Alfred E. Mirsky papers at the Rockefeller University Archives. **Mendel Newsl** 1983 Nov;23:1–4

**Kopp C:** The Edward Lawrie Tatum papers. **Mendel Newsl** 1981 Jul;20:1–2

**Kopp C:** The J. H. B. Archive report; the Edward Lawrie Tatum papers at the Rockefeller University Archives. **J Hist Biol** 1982 Spring;15(1):153–4
**Kopp C:** The origins of the American Scientific debate over fallout hazards. **Soc Stud Sci** 1979;9(4):403–22
**Köpp P:** Das Handbuch eines frühmittelalterlichen Arztes in der Stiftsbibliothek St. Gallen. **Helv Archaeol** 1982;13(51-2):163–75
**Köpp P:** Vademecum eines frühmittelalterlichen Arztes. Die gefaltete lateinische Handschrift medizinischen Inhalts im Codex 217 und der Fragmentensammlung 1396 der Stiftsbibliothek in St. Gallen. Aarau, Sauerländer, 1980. 128 p. (Veröffentlichungen der Schweizerischen Gesellschaft für Geschichte der Medizin und der Naturwissenschaften, 34).
**Køppe S:** The psychology of the neuron: Freud, Cajal and Golgi. **Scand J Psychol** 1983;24(1):1–12
**Kopper JA** see **Haabala SH**
**Kopsa H** see **Zazgornik J**
**Kopshitser IZ:** Trepanirovannyĭ cherep iz Dargavskogo nekropolia 'Goroda Mertvykh' v selenii Dargavs Severnoĭ Osetii. **Zh Vopr Neirokhir** 1983 Jul–Aug;4:61–2
**Kopzyński J** see **Mularczyk-Bal MU**
**Korarev II:** Evoliutsiia meditsinskogo éticheskogo kodeksa v SSSR i za rubezhom (printsipy i ikh realizatsiia). **Vestn Akad Med Nauk SSSR** 1980;(4):47–52
**Korbakova AI, Ulanova IP:** Nauchnaia deiatel'nost' vydaiushchegosia sovetskogo toksikologa N. S. Pravdina i razvitie ego ideĭ v mashi dni. **Gig Tr Prof Zabol** 1983 Feb;(2):44–5
**Körbler J:** Strahlen, Heilmittel und Gefahr. Wien, Ranner, 1977. 162 p.
**Korchagin VP** see **Golovteev VV**
**Korczak CW:** Jubileusz 80–lecia Polskiego Towarzystwa Higienicznego. **Pol Tyg Lek** 1979 Nov 12;34(46):1813–5
**Korczak CW:** 80–letie Pol'skogo Gigienicheskogo Obshchestva (1898–1978). **Gig Sanit** 1980 Mar;(3):58–9
**Korepanov VI:** Istoriia razvitiia lazernoĭ khirurgii. **Sov Med** 1984;(3):61–5
**Koretskii VI:** Smert' Groznogo Tsaria. **Vopr Istor** 1979;9:93–103
**Koritzer RT, St. Hoyme LE:** Extensive caries in early man circa 110,000 years before present. **J Am Dent Assoc** 1979 Oct;99(4):642–3
**Korn E:** Die Apotheke in Hovestadt. Werl, Dietrich–Coelde–Verlag, 1977. 87 p.
**Kornberg A:** Biochemistry evolving. **Can J Biochem** 1980 Feb;58(2):93–6
**Kornberg H, Williamson DH:** Hans Adolf Krebs: 25 August 1900–22 November 1981. **Biogr Mem Fellows R Soc** 1984;30:351–85
**Kornblith BA** see **Geerts A**
**Körner U** see **Löther R, ed**
**Kornfeld AD:** Hypnosis and behavior therapy: historical relationships. **Int J Psychosom** 1984;31(2):22–6
**Kornfeld H:** Nuclear weapons and civil defense. The influence of the medical profession in 1955 and 1983. **West J Med** 1983 Feb;138(2):207–12
**Korngold S:** Memories of the National Jewish Hospital of Denver in 1908. **West States Jew Hist Q** 1980;12(2):161–4
**Korol' GG, Denisova TP, Naumenko AM:** Iz istorii instituta im. N. V. Sklifosovskogo. **Sov Zdravookhr** 1984;(10):53–5
**Koroleva LN:** Znachenie bratskogo sotrudnichestva Sovetskikh narodov v podgotovke meditsinskikh kradov dlia zdravookhraneniia Kazakhstana (1928–1940). **Sov Zdravookhr** 1983;6:58–62
**Koroliuk AM:** K stoletiiu so dnia rozhdeniia Viacheslava Mikhaĭlovicha Aristovskogo. **Zh Mikrobiol Epidemiol Immunobiol** 1983 Mar;(3):109–12
**Korol'kov AA:** Iz istorii pervykh gigienicheskikh kafedr v Rossii. **Zdravookhr Ross Fed** 1980;(5):19–22
**Korol'kov AA** see **Akulov KI**
**Korostelev NB:** Osnovanie pervykh gigienicheskikh kafedr v Rossii. **Gig Sanit** 1984 Feb;(2):40–4
**Korostelev NB** see **Rumiantsev GI**
**Korotkikh RV, Gorelova LE, Shtil'man NL:** M. Tsetkin (k 100–letiiu so dnia rozhdeniia). **Sov Zdravookhr** 1983;(11):63–6
**Korotkikh RV:** N. I. Pirogov i voprosy vrachebnoĭ étiki. (K 100–letiiu so dnia smerti). **Sov Zdravookhr** 1981;(12)54–7
**Korotkikh RV:** Vklad A. F. Bilibina v razvitie problwm meditsinskoĭ deontologii. **Ter Arkh** 1982;54(10):103–6
**Korotkoff NS:** Experiments for determining the efficiency of arterial collaterals. Preface, biographical notes and editing of translation from Russian by H. N. Segall. Montreal, H. N. Segall, 1980. 265 p. (M. D. Thesis, Imperial Military Medical Academy, 1910).
**Korotkov AG, Valishin ES:** K 175–letiiu kafedry normal'noĭ anatomii cheloveka Kazanskogo meditsinskogo instituta. **Arkh Anat Gistol Embriol** 1982 Jan;82(1):110–4
**Korsun VF** see **Sosnovskiĭ AT**
**Korsunskiĭ MA:** Voennyĭ fel'dsher P. E. Lazimir. **Feldsher Akush** 1980;45(12):41–4
**Körtgen A:** Die Gesundheit des Fürsten. Diätetische Vorschriften für eine herausgehobene Menschengruppe von der Antike bis zum Anfang des zwanzigsten Jahrhunderts. Diss., Johannes Gutenberg - Universität in Mainz. Frankfurt am Main, Bern, Peter Lang, 1982. 231 p.
**Korting GW:** Atherom auf einem Olgemälde der Pinakothek in Brescia. **Hautarzt** 1984 Jun;35(6):321
**Kory WB:** Liberia's population figures. **Liberian Stud J** 1970–71;3(1):53–61
**Korzh AA, Simenach BI:** Kharkovskiĭ nauchno–issledovatel'skiĭ institut ortopedii i travmatologii im. prof. M.I. Sitenko. **Vestn Khir** 1983 Mar;130(3):23–5
**Korzh AA, Bondarenko NS:** Pamiati N. I. Pirogova (k 100–latiiu so dnia smerti). **Ortop Travmatol Protez** 1982 Apr;(4):56–9

**Kos J:** In memoriam Professor Karel Zlábek. **Anat Anz** 1984;156(5):345–50
**Kósa F** see **Földes V**
**Kosareva AA, Kondrat'ev IM:** 'Babii bunt' 1830 goda. **Vopr Istor** 1980;8:180–3
**Kosáry D:** Akadémiai tervek a 18. századi magyarországon. **Tortenelmi Sz** 1979;22(2):341–54
**Kościk–Grenda M** see **Kretowski J**
**Kościukiewicz–Michiewicz I:** Działalność i osiągnięcia Sekcji Ortodontycznej Polskiego Towarzystwa Stomatologicznego W latach 1951–1977. **Czas Stomatol** 1980 Jun;33(6):567–70
**Kosiakov PN:** K 100–letniu fagotsitarnoĭ teorii immuniteta I.I. Mechnikova. **Vopr Virusol** 1982 Sep–Oct;27(5):4–9
**Kosic I:** Rad civilne zdravstvene službe području kotara Korenica i Udbina u odredenom razdoblju NOB–e. **Lijec Vjesn** 1979 Nov;10(11):682–4
**Kosmachevskaia EA** see **Andreeva VN**
**Koss LG:** Analytical and quantitative cytology. A historical perspective. **Anal Quant Cytol** 1982 Dec;4(4):251–6
**Koss LG:** On the history of cytology. **Acta Cytol (Baltimore)** 1980 Nov–Dec;24(6):475–7
**Kössling FK, Prölss E:** Die Pathologie in Bremen. **Verh Dtsch Ges Pathol** 1980;64:XXIX–XXXV
**Kossowski S** see **Iwankiewicz S**
**Kostakopoulos A** see **Dimopoulos C**
**Kostal R** see **Solomon R**
**Kostandov EA** see **Volokhov AA**
**Kostenzer O:** Das Katharinenöl, ein altes Heilmittel. **Tirol Heimatbl** 1974;49(2):77–80
**Kostenzer O:** Dr. Johannes Cuefner aus Rattenberg (biographische Notizen). **Tirol Heimatbl** 1971;46(1–3):18–20
**Kostenzer O** see **Domandl S**
**Köster W:** Medizin–historische Studie über die Weiterführung der Vorstellungen von P. G. Unna in der Therapie und Biochemie von Hautkrankheiten in der Gegenwart. Therapie und Biochemie von Hautkrankheiten nach P. G. Unna. Berlin, Grosse, 1977. 161 p.
**Köstering B** see **Mulch J**
**Kostic AD:** Osvrt na ličnost prof. dr. Riharda Burijana i na vreme osnivanja medicinskog fakulteta univerziteta u Beogradu. **Srp Arh Celok Lek** 1982 Mar;110(3):387–98
**Kostowski W** see **Płaźnik A**
**Kostrouch Z** see **Mirejovský P**
**Kostrov NI:** Opyt sovetskoĭ voennoĭ otorinolaringologii v Velikoĭ Otechestvennoĭ voĭne. **Voen Med Zh** 1980 Aug;(8):17–9
**Kostrzewski J:** Swiat wolny od ospy. **Przegl Epidemiol** 1980;34(4):365–72
**Kostrzewski J** see **Rudowski W**
**Kostrzewski JK:** Rozwój nauk medycznych w Polsce na tle nauki światowej. **Nauka Pol** 1980;28(5):33–41
**Kostrzewski JK:** Stan zdrowia ludności Polski––dotychczasowe wyniki i dalsze kierunki badań. **Nauka Pol** 1979;27(4):3–18
**Kostychev SP:** Pasteur: his life and achievements. Annotated translation from the Russian by S. A. Wilde. New Delhi, Oxford & IBH Publishing Co., 1978. 96 p.
**Koszarowski T:** Udział Instytutu Onkologii im. Marii Skłodowskiej–Curie w rozwoju społecznej walki z chorobami nowotworowymi w Polsce w latach 1945–1982. **Nowotwory** 1983 Jan–Mar;33(1):7–12
**Kotani R** see **Ueda M**
**Kotarba JA:** Chronic pain center: A study of voluntary client compliance and entrepreneurship. **Am Behav Sci** 1981;24(6):786–800
**Kótay P:** István Weszprémi 1723–1799. **Orvostort Kozl** 1980;89–91(26 no 1–3):215–22
**Kötay P:** Rácz Sámuel és a magyar orvosi oktatás hajnala. **Orv Hetil** 1982 Jan 10;123(2):103–9
**Kotek S:** Geschichte der Kinderheilkunde von ihren Anfängen bis zum Ende des 18. Jahrhunderts. In Sournia JC, Martiny M, Poulet J, ed: Illustrierte Geschichte der Medizin. Salzburg, Andreas, 1980. Vol. 7. p. 2499–523.
**Kotek V, Niklíček L, Stein K:** K historii snah o postgraduální vzdělávání lékařu v Ceskoslovensku před rokem 1945. **Cas Lek Cesk** 1983 Oct 21;122(42):1308–12
**Kotek V** see **Niklíček L**
**Kotel'nikov VP:** F. P. Gaaz (k 200–letiiu so dnia roxhdeniia). **Klin Med (Mosk)** 1982 Jul;60(7):115–7
**Kotel'nikov VP:** Nauchnoe nasledie A. V. Martynova v izuchenii zabolevaniĭ podzheludochnoĭ zhelezy i zhelchevyvodiashchikh puteĭ. **Klin Med (Mosk)** 1983 Apr;61(4):117–9
**Kotel'nikov VP:** V. A. Oppel' i razvitie fiziologicheskoĭ khirurgii. **Klin Med (Mosk)** 1984 May;62(5):145–8
**Kotel'nikov VP:** Znachenie nauchnogo nslediia S. P. Botkina v khirurgii. **Klin Med (Mosk)** 1983 Jul;61(7):140–2
**Kotov GA** see **Kozlov VA**
**Kotovskaia AR** see **Gazenko OG**
**Kottayarikil C:** Sigmund Freud on religion and morality: a challenge to Christianity. Innsbruck, Resch, 1977. xx, 399 p.
**Kottek S:** Abraham Portaleone (1542–1612): an Italian Jewish physician of the Renaissance period. His life and his will; reflections on early burial. **Koroth** 1983 Aug;8(7–8):269–77
**Kottek S:** An oath taken by Jewish community physicians at Frankfort on Main, 1656. **Koroth** 1979 Nov;7(9–10):CCIII–CCVIII(650–7).
**Kottek S:** Aperçu sur l' 'introduction à la pratique médicale', (introitus medici ad praxin) de Zacutus Lusitanus, 1575 – 1642. **Rev Hist Med Heb** 1980 Mar–Apr;33(1):13–16
**Kottek S:** Aperçu sur l''introduction à la pratique médicale', (introitus

medici ad praxin) de Zacutus Lusitanus, 1575 - 1642. **Rev Hist Med Heb** 1980 Jul;33(2):35-8
**Kottek S:** Eléments de physiologie dans le 'Kusari' de Juda Halevi (Espagne, 12e siècle). In: Congrès international d'histoire de la médecine, XXVe, Québec, 1976. Actes. Québec, 1977. p. 840-7.
**Kottek S:** Jacob Rodriguez-Péreire (1715-1780); pionnier de l'éducation des sourds-muets: à l'occasion du 200e anniversaire de sa disparition. **Rev Hist Med Heb** 1981 Mar-Apr;34(1):5-8
**Kottek S:** Les Juifs et la médecine aux XVIIIe et XIVe siècles (1750-1850). **Rev Hist Med Heb** 1981 Dec;139(34 no 4):57-60
**Kottek S:** Medicine in Hebrew poetry: Judah al-Harizi. **Koroth** 1983 Aug;8(7-8):299-304
**Kottek S, Wilk D:** Professor Joshua O. Leibowitz; jubilee of his medico-historical activity. **Koroth** 1983 Aug;8(7-8):233-55
**Kottek S:** The humble physician, explanation of and notes on a Renaissance medal. **Koroth** 1980 Jun;7(11-12):747-53
**Kottek SS:** 'Andre Vesale'. Some remarks on a painting by E. J. C. Hamman. **Koroth** 1982 Aug;8(3/4):135-43
**Kottek SS, Seligman H:** Ecology in Talmudic sources. In H. Shuval, ed: Developments in arid zone ecology and environment quality. Philadelphia, Balaban ISS, 1981. p. 119-26.
**Kottek SS:** Embryology in Talmudic and Midrashic literature. **J Hist Biol** 1981 Fall;14(2):299-315
**Kottek SS:** [Jacob Rodriguez Pereire (1715-1780): an anniversary] (Heb). **Koroth** 1981;8(1-2):83-7; 79-81 [Engl. abstr.]
**Kottek SS:** Joseph ben Meir ibn Zabara of Barcelona (1140?-?) (his place in the history of medicine). In International Congress of the History of Medicine, 27th, Barcelona, 1980. Actas. Barcelona, Académia de Ciències Mèdiques de Catalunya i Balears, 1981. p. 181-7.
**Kottek SS, Metzger M, Metzger T:** Manuscrits hebraiques décorés ou illustrés du Canon d'Avicenne. In International Congress of the History of Medicine, 27th, Barcelona, 1980. Actas. Barcelona, Académia de Ciències Mèdiques de Catalunya i Balears, 1981. p. 739-45.
**Kottek SS:** 'Mater puerorum'. A medieval naming for an enigmatic children's disease. **Eur J Pediatr** 1981 Sep;137(1):75-9
**Kottek SS:** 'Medicina in Nummis': an exhibition of medical medals in the Hebrew University Hadassah Medical School--Jerusalem (May-June 1979). **Koroth** 1979 Nov;7(9-10):CCXXXI-CCXXXIV(722-3)
**Kottek SS:** 'The book of delights' by Joseph ben Meir ibn Zabara of Barcelona (12th cent.). **Koroth** 1981;8(1-2):21-6
**Kottek SS:** The hospital in Jewish History. **Rev Infect Dis** 1981 Jul-Aug;3(4):636-9
**Kottek SS:** The seat of the soul: contribution to the history of Jewish medieval psycho-physiology. **Clio Med** 1979 May;13(3-4):219-46
**Kottenkamp W:** 75 Jahre Niederrheinische Zahnärztliche Gesellschaft. **Dtsch Zahnarztl Z** 1981 Oct;36(10):610-3
**Kottler MJ:** Darwin, Wallace, and the origin of sexual dimorphism. **Proc Am Philos Soc** 1980 Jun;124(3):203-26
**Kotwas J, Meyer-Wilmes J, Ohlendorf D, ed:** Pharmazie und Medizin--Grenzen und Möglichkeiten. Verhandlungsbericht über eine Internationale Tagung der Arbeitsgemeinschaft Deutscher Krankenhausapotheker in Zusammenarbeit mit der Bayerischen Internistenvereinigung München, 18.-19.April 1980. Berlin, Acron, 1981. 152 p. Contributions by R. Winau, D. Ohlendorf, A.G. Hildebrandt, W. Weissauer, R. Quintiliani, D.D. Breimer, R. Preisig, T. Zysset, D. Adam, H. Remmer, G. Dirheimer, K.H. Beyer, H.P.T. Ammon.
**Kotze WJ:** Verpleegnavorsing in Suid-Afrika in historiese perspektief. **Curationis** 1984 Sep;7(3):11-8
**Koucky RW:** The buffalo disaster of 1882. **ND Hist** 1983;50(1):23-30
**Koudelka JB:** The genesis of the William H. Welch Medical Library and the Johns Hopkins Institute of the History of Medicine. In Stevenson LG, ed: A celebration of medical history. Baltimore, Johns Hopkins University Press, 1982. (The Henry E. Sigerist supplements to the Bulletin of the History of Medicine; new ser., no. 6). p. 69-76
**Koulu L, Jansén C:** Epidermiksen Langerhansin solu--ajankohtainen satavuotias. **Duodecim** 1980;96(23-24):1587-91
**Koupernik C:** Serbsky and czarist dissidents. **Arch Gen Psychiatry** 1983 Jun;40(6):697-8
**Kouřilová M** see **Bunčáková V**
**Kouskoukis CE, Leider M:** Cupping. The art and the value. **Am J Dermatopathol** 1983 Jun;5(3):235-9
**Koutras DA** see **Marketos SG**
**Kovačevic M:** Izrada i proizvodnja lekova u apotekarskoj službi NOVJ (JA). **Vojnosanit Pregl** 1981 Nov-Dec;38(6):404-11
**Kovách AG, Schultheisz E:** A physiologianak rövid sommája - a short summation of physiology. The first book of physiology in Hungarian. In E. Schultheisz, ed: History of physiology. Oxford, Elmsford, New York, Pergamon, 1981. xvi, 208 p. (Advances in Physiological Sciences. Proceedings of the 28th International Congress of Physiological Sciences, Budapest, 1980. Volume 21). p. 85-87.
**Kovachev VI** see **Tiurin EI**
**Kovacs E** see **Racz S**
**Koval' MV:** Tovarsystvo chervonoho khresta i chervonoho pivmisiatsia ursr-frontu i tylu (1941-1945). **Ukr Istor Zh** 1975;(4):78-87
**Kovalcik PJ:** Early history of regional enteritis. **Curr Surg** 1982 Nov-Dec;39(6):395-400
**Kovalev MM, Suslov VS:** Antonin Nikolaevich Filatov, ego rol' v razvitii sovremennoĭ khirurgii. **Klin Khir** 1983 Mar;(3):58-60
**Kovalev MM, Roĭ VP, Burka AA, et al:** Deviat'sot zasedaniĭ nauchnogo obshchestva khirurgov Kieva i Kievskoĭ oblasti. **Klin Khir** 1984 Apr;(4):58-61
**Kovalev MM** see **Shalimov AA**
**Kovaleva EP, Deviatova LN, Kasparova TIu, et al:** K 50-letiiu kafedry épidemiologii Tsentral'nogo instituta usovershenstvovaniia vracheĭ. **Zh Mikrobiol Epidemiol Immunobiol** 1981 Jun;(6):113-7
**Kovaleva EV** see **Lebedev DD**
**Kovaleva NS** see **Koliadiuk IV**
**Kovanov VV:** Po Dorogam voĭny. **Voen Med Zh** 1980 May;(5):69-73
**Kovanov VV:** V tylovom gospitale. **Voen Med Zh** 1980 Apr;(4):27-30
**Kováts Z:** A XVIII századi népesség-fejlödés kérdéséhez. **Agrartort Sz** 1969;11(1-2):218-27
**Kovel J:** Marx and Freud. In M. Albin, R. J. Devlin, G. Heeger, ed: New directions in psychohistory. The Adelphi papers in honor of Erik H. Erikson. Lexington, Toronto, D. C. Heath, 1980. p. 21-6.
**Kovrigina MD:** Tsentral'nomu ordena Lenina institutu usovershenstvovaniia vracheĭ 50 let. **Sov Zdravookhr** 1980;(11):13-6
**Kovrigina MD:** 50-letie Tsentral'nogo Instituta Usovershenstvovaniia Vracheĭ. **Klin Med (Mosk)** 1981 Jan;59(1):4-7
**Kovshilo VE:** K 60-letiiu so dnia priniatiia dekreta o sanitarnykh organakh RSFSR. **Gig Sanit** 1982 Sep;(9):4-6
**Kowalczyk M** see **Sobień-Kopczyńska S**
**Kowalczyk S:** Lubelskie Towarzystwo Lekarskie w Polsce Ludowej (1945-1951). **Ann Univ Mariae Curie Sklodowska [Med]** 1981;36:283-92
**Kowalewski D:** Politics and emotion in the thought of John Stuart Mill. **J Psychohist** 1980 Spring;7(4):455-66
**Kowieski L:** Działalność Wydziału Higieny Zawodowej i Przemysłu Oddziału Lubelskiego Warszawskiego Towarzystwa Higienicznego w latach 1903-1905. **Arch Hist Med (Warsz)** 1984;47(3):429-31
**Kowitz A:** Dentists of Chicago before the great fire. **Bull Hist Dent** 1984 Oct;32(2):126-30
**Kowitz A:** The earliest use of dental evidence in a courtroom: His Majesty's Advocate vs. Pattison et al, High Court of Justiciary, Edinburgh, Scotland, June 6-7, 1814. **Bull Hist Dent** 1981 Oct;29(2):82-7
**Kowitz A:** You don't have anything, do you? The historical resources of the American Dental Association. **Bull Hist Dent** 1980 Oct;28(2):69-75
**Kowitz A** see **Loevy HT**
**Koyama T:** [A history of pharmaceutical education in Okayama (I). Private Okayama pharmaceutical school (primary)] (Jpn). **Yakushigaku Zasshi** 1983;18(2):95-100
**Kozhokaru I, Maslev S:** Novootkriti dokumenti ot i za D-R Petur Beron. **Izv Inst Istor** 1968;20:229-341
**Kozik IV** see **Roshchin AV**
**Koziner VB, Iarochkin VS:** Razvitie problemy krovezameniteleĭ v trudakh akademika N. A. Fedorova i ego shkoly. **Gematol Transfuziol** 1984 Jan;29(1):12-6
**Kozliuk VM, Leonenko NA, Stefanovskaia NV:** O razvitii lechebno-profilakticheskoĭ pomoshchi naseleniiu USSR v 1917-1940 gg. **Vrach Delo** 1982 Apr;(4):3-7
**Kozlov AI** see **Nikitiuk BA**
**Kozlov AM, Kozlov IA:** Filosofskie vzgliady Gippokrata. **Klin Med (Mosk)** 1983 May;61(5):111-5
**Kozlov AM:** Genial'nyĭ myslitel', plamennyĭ revoliutsioner i velikiĭ chelovek (k 165-letiiu so dnia rozhdeniia i 100-letiiu so dnia smerti Karla Marksa). **Feldsher Akush** 1983;48(5):3-4
**Kozlov AM, Kel'ner MS, Losev NI:** K. Marks is problemy meditsiny (k 165-letiiu so dnia rozhdeniia K. Marksa). **Patol Fiziol Eksp Ter** 1983 May-Jun;3:3-9
**Kozlov AM:** Kliatva Gippokrata i ee vliianie na razvitie vrachebnoĭ étiki. **Sov Med** 1983;(3):79-82
**Kozlov IA** see **Kozlov AM**
**Kozlov II:** Dostizheniia kurortnogo dela v SSSR. **Vopr Kurortol Fizioter Lech Fiz Kult** 1982 Nov-Dec;(6):1-6
**Kozlov VA, Iarchuk NI, Kotov GA:** Razvitie cheliustno-litsevoĭ khirurgii c SSSR. **Vestn Khir** 1982 Nov;129(11):9-12
**Kozlova EV** see **Chissov Vi**
**Kozlova EV** see **Kapatsinskiĭ EV**
**Kozoll R** see **Reid RA**
**Kozovenko MN:** Rol' N. I. Pirogova v organizatsii truda meditsinskikh sester na voĭne. **Voen Med Zh** 1980 Nov;(11);72-3
**Kozubenko ID:** Partiĭnye organizatsii Dona vo glave razvitiia zdravookhraneniia v 1923-1924 gg. **Sov Zdravookhr** 1982;(6):56-9
**Kozubenko ID:** Uchastie meditsinskikh rabotnikov Dona v revoliutsionnoĭ bor'be. **Sov Zdravookhr** 1984;(1):47-8
**Kožuh-Novak M:** Kliničko istraživački rad Instituta za planiranje porodice na području intrauterine kontracepcije od 1964. do 1980. **Jugosl Ginekol Opstet** 1981 Jan-Apr;21(1-2):54-7
**Kozulin A:** Peter Blonsky and Russian progressivism: the early years. **Stud Sov Thought** 1982;24(1):11-21
**Kozulin A:** The influence of the personality of the scientist on his theorizing: I. P. Pavlov and the concept of human signal systems. **Stud Sov Thought** 1981;22(4):249-56
**Kraag GR** see **Buchanan WW**
**Kraatz H:** Gedanken zur Geschichte der Frauenheilkunde. **Zentralbl Gynakol** 1981;103(11):593-616
**Kraatz H:** Zwischen Klinik und Hörsaal. Ein Frauenarzt sieht sich in seiner Zeit. Berlin, Verlag der Nation, 1977. 351 p.
**Krachmer JH** see **Mannis MJ**
**Kraemer S:** A note on Spinoza's contribution to systemic therapy. **Fam Process** 1982 Sep;21(3):353-7
**Kraetschmer K:** Broca's localization theory reconsidered. **Br J Disord Commun** 1980 May;15(1):5-8
**Krafft F:** Der 'Historische Erfahrungsraum' der Entdeckung der

Kernspaltung. In Dilg P, et al., ed: Perspektiven der Pharmaziegeschichte. Graz, Austria, Akademische Druck- u. Verlagsanstalt, 1983. p. 209-24.

**Krafft F:** Forschungsberichte und Spezial-Bibliographien. **Ber Wissenschaftsgesch** 1980;3(3-4):127-88

**Krafft F** see **Rothschuh KE**

**Krafft M:** Die anthroposophische Heilmittellehre und ihre geistesgeschichtliche Beziehung zu Heilmittelkonzepten. des 19. Jahrhunderts. Stuttgart, Deutscher Apotheker Verlag, 1984. 210 p. (Quellen und Studien zur Geschichte der Pharmazie, Bd. 27).

**Kraft E, Finby N:** Beginning of radiology in 1896; first newspaper report of discovery of x-ray. **NY State J Med** 1981 Apr;81(5):805-6

**Kraft E, Finby N:** Röntgen's discovery of X-ray and Lenard's priority claim; award of first Nobel Prize in physics in 1901. **NY State J Med** 1980 Sep;80(10):1623-5

**Kraft ES:** Andreas Cleyer. In Balde JH, Schmiking W, ed: Festschrift zum 86. Deutschen Arztetag in Kassel. Kassel, Arztevereins, 1983. p.40.

**Kraft H:** Die Zeichnungen des Augustin Wilhelm. Psychopathologische Aspekte und kulturhistorische Vergleiche. **Confin Psychiatr** 1980;23(4):230-49

**Krag C, Kirkby B:** The deltopectoral flap: a historical review with comments on its role in neurovascular reconstruction. **Scand J Plast Reconstr Surg** 1980:14(2):145-50

**Kragt VE:** De ontwikkeling van het verpleegkundig beroep in Nederland (I). **Tijdschr Ziekenverpl** 1980 Aug 26;33(17):791-8

**Kragt VE:** De ontwikkeling van het verpleegkundig beroep in Nederland (II). **Tijdschr Ziekenverpl** 1980 Sep 9;33(18):853-60

**Krahulec I, Ambrusová L, Dresslerová I, et al:** Desat rokov činnosti Foniatrického pracoviska na otolaryngologickej klinike FN v Bratislave. **Cesk Otolaryngol** 1984 Jun;33(3):195-9

**Kraiuhin C** see **Gordon E**

**Krajinovic S:** Povodom stogodišnjice jednog izveštaja dr Vladana Djordjevića objavljenog y 'Srpskom Arhivu' 1883. godine. **Srp Arh Celok Lek** 1983 Jul;111(7):1005-8

**Krakovetskaia GA:** Gigienicheskie i lechebnye printsipy antichnoĭ meditsiny. **Gig Sanit** 1984 May;(5):37-40

**Krakówka P:** W 100-lecie odkrycia prątka gruźlicy. **Pneumonol Pol** 1982 Nov;50(11):557-8

**Kralj I:** O dostignućima sanitetske službe u NOB na teritoriji Hrvatske do jeseni 1942. godine. **Vojnosanit Pregl** 1983 Sep-Oct;40(5):379-85

**Kralj I:** Zdravstvo u NOB uoči prvog kongresa liječnika NOF Hrvatske. **Lijec Vjesn** 1979 Nov;101(11):656-62

**Kraljevic M, Rasuhin-Vekic N, Weisz-Maleček R, et al:** O razvoju vakcine i vakcinacije protiv variole (1890-1923). In: I simpozij o historiji mikrobiologije i imunologije u Hrvatskoj do 1923. godine. Zagreb, Jugoslavenskoj akademiji, 1973. p. 63-70.

**Kramar C, Baud CA, Lagier R:** Presumed calcified leiomyoma of the uterus. Morphologic and chemical studies of a calcified mass dating from the Neolithic period. **Arch Pathol Lab Med** 1983 Feb;107(2):91-3

**Kramar C** see **Lagier R**

**Kramer ES:** The history of art therapy in a large mental hospital. **Am J Art Ther** 1982 Apr;21(3):75-84

**Kramer H** see **Burdon JG**

**Kramer JC:** Opium rampant: medical use, misuse and abuse in Britain and the West in the 17th and 18th centuries. **Br J Addict** 1979 Dec;74(4):377-89

**Kramer JC:** The metapsychology of opium. **J Psychoactive Drugs** 1981 Jan-Mar;13(1):71-9

**Kramer JC:** The opiates: two centuries of scientific study. **J Psychedelic Drugs** 1980 Apr-Jun;12(2):89-103

**Kramer KW** see **Lester JP**

**Kramer MG:** Professionalism and principles of ethics--changing concepts for dentistry. **Pediatr Dent** 1980 Sep;2(3):245-51

**Kramer WG:** Das vindt man in der Appentegg. . . **Beitr Gesch Pharm** 1980;31(5):38

**Kramp P, Hemmingsen R:** Age distribution of patients with delirium tremens in Denmark 1836-1978. **Acta Psychiatr Scand** 1981 Mar;63(3):253-61

**Krampitz SD:** Historical development of baccalaureate nursing education in the American university: 1899-1935. **West J Nurs Res** 1983 Fall;5(4):371-80

**Krannich CR** see **Krannich RL**

**Krannich RL, Krannich CR:** Initiating a population revolution in Thailand: politics, bureaucracy, and social change. **Asian Profile** 1982;10(2):173-92

**Krantz JC:** An architect designs a needle. **W Va Med J** 1980 Apr;76(4):84-5

**Krantz JC, White JM:** Aspirin: four score and more. **South Med J** 1980 Dec;73(12):1630-4

**Krantz JC:** Recollections: a medical scientist remembers. Baltimore, Schneidereith, 1978. xvi, 185 p.

**Krasik ED, Minevich VB, Potapov AI:** Istoriia psikhiatricheskoi pomoshchi v Tomskoĭ oblasti. **Zh Nevropatol Psikhiatr** 1981;81(9):1393-9

**Krasil'shchik SI:** Zarubezhnye otzyvy o dostizheniiakh Sovetskoĭ meditsiny v gody Velikoĭ Otechestvennoĭ voĭny. **Voen Med Zh** 1984 May;(5):71-3

**Krasil'shchikov MI, Kulish EA, Rumer LZ, et al:** Tsentral'naia pechat' v propagande meditsinskikh i gigienicheskikh znaniĭ (1921-1932). **Sov Zdravookhr** 1983;(10):53-5

**Krasnick CL:** 'In charge of the loons': a portrait of the London, Ontario, Asylum for the Insane in the nineteenth century. **Ont Hist** 1982;74(3):138-84

**Krasnikov PG:** L. G. Belliarminov--vydaiushchiĭsia uchenyĭ, obshchestvennyĭ deiatel' i organizator oftal'mologicheskoĭ pomoshchi naseleniiu (k 125-letiiu so dnia rozhdeniia). **Vestn Oftalmol** 1984 Sep-Oct;(5):69-70

**Krasnikov PG:** Vydaiushcheesia izobretenie otechestvennogo oftal'mologa (100 let so vremeni sozdaniia applanatsionnogo tonometra Prof. A.N. Maklakova). **Vestn Oftalmol** 1984 Nov-Dec;(6):70-2

**Krasnogorskaia ES:** V armeĭskom gospitale. **Voen Med Zh** 1980 Mar;(3):69-70

**Krasnopeev II:** Blokadnyĭ vypusk vracheĭ Voenno-meditsinskoĭ akademii (K 40-letiiu sniatiia blokady Leningrada). **Voen Med Zh** 1984 Jan;(1):69-71

**Krasnov ML** see **Shul'pina NB**

**Krasnov MM:** Proshloe v nastoiashchem: Adrian Aleksandrovich Kriukov, redaktor 'Vestnika oftal'mologii' i osnovatel' Moskovskogo oftal'mologicheskogo veshchestva (k 75-letiiu zhurnala). **Vestn Oftalmol** 1984 Nov-Dec;(6):4-6

**Kratochvíl L, Lustig M:** K historii tzv. Batemanovy funkce. **Cesk Farm** 1984 Jun;33(5):210-2

**Kratochvil O:** 'X' disease in Australia (a historical story of medical detection). **Geogr Med** 1982;12:1-6

**Kratz C** see **Davies C, ed**

**Kratz CR** see **Allan P**

**Krauland W:** Die Deutsche Gesellschaft für Rechtsmedizin im Spiegel ihrer Tagungen. **Beitr Gerichtl Med** 1982;40:9-20

**Kraus B:** MUDR. Ferdinand Karafiát (1870-1928). Aliis serviendo consumor. **Cas Lek Cesk** 1983 Jul 1;122(26):830-1

**Kraus B:** MUDr. Jaroslav Mathon - chirurg, umělecký a památkový prαukopník. **Cas Lek Cesk** 1983 Sep 30;122(39):1214-5

**Kraus I:** Hermann Schelenz. In Balde JH, Schmiking W, ed: Festschrift zum 86. Deutschen Arztetag in Kassel. Kassel, Arztevereins, 1983. p. 41-9.

**Kraus S:** Stanford University School of Medicine. **West J Med** 1983 Aug;139(2):244-7

**Kraus A, ed:** Leib. Geist. Geschichte. Brennpunkte anthropologischer Psychiatrie. Festschrift zum 60. Geburtstag von Hubertus Tellenbach. With contributions by W. Baeyer, W. Blankenburg, H. G. Gadamer, W. Jacob, B. Kimura, H. Lang, A. Leder, G. Marcel, A Métraux, B. Pauleikhoff, H. Schipperges. Heidelberg, Hüthig, 1978. (Medizin im Wandel).

**Krause AK:** Introduction à l'étiologie de la tuberculose. **Bull Int Union Tuberc** 1981 Sept-Dec;56(3-4):110-4

**Krause RM:** A matter of opportunity. **J Allergy Clin Immunol** 1982 Jul;70(1):2-3

**Krause RM:** Koch's postulates and the search for the AIDS agent. **Rev Infect Dis** 1984 Mar-Apr;6(2):270-9

**Krause RM:** Koch's postulates and the search for the AIDS agent. **Public Health Rep** 1984 May-Jun;99(3):291-9

**Krause RM:** Philadelphia, the Founding Fathers, and systemic lupus erythematosus. **Arthritis Rheum** 1982 Jul;25(7):895-7

**Krause RM:** The restless tide. The persistent challenge of the microbial world. Washington, D. C., National Foundation for Infectious Diseases, 1981. 152 p.

**Krauss JB** see **Slavinsky AT**

**Krauss P:** Leiden und Hoffnung in der Sicht der Medizin. **Universitas (Stuttg)** 1980;35(3):511-8

**Krauss P:** 'Mediale' Psychotherapie einer depressiven Krise. Ein Kuriosum aus den Jahren 1833/34. **Psyche (Stuttg)** 1981 Oct;35(10):963-71

**Kravchenko AT:** Pamiati professora Glotovoĭ Eleny Vladimirovny (k 100-letiiu so dnia rozhdeniia). **Zh Mikrobiol Epidemiol Immunobiol** 1983 Mar;(3):112-3

**Kravchenko AT:** Razvitie ideĭ prof. I. L. Krichevskogo o priobretennom immuniteta (k 100-letiiu so dnia rozhdeniia I. L. Krichevskogo). **Zh Mikrobiol Epidemiol Immunobiol** 1984 Feb;(2):110-4

**Kravkov IuS:** Slavnyĭ jubileĭ. **Med Sestra** 1983 Apr;42(4):50-2

**Kravtsov DE:** Prosvetitel'skaia deiatel'nost' N. I. Pirogova v Kieve. **Voen Med Zh** 1982 Nov;(11):65-6

**Krawczyk K:** Rak płuc wśród chorych leczonych w oddziałach chorób płuc krakowskiego szpitala specjalistycznego im. dr Anki w latach 1956-1977. **Pneumonol Pol** 1979 Aug-Sep;47(7-8):573-80

**Krawiec TS** see **Chaplin, JP**

**Kraye J:** Francesco Filelfo on emotions, virtues and vices: a re-examination of his sources. **Bibl Hum Renaissance** 1981;43(1):129-40

**Kreader JL** see **Breul FR**

**Krebs H, Schmid R:** Otto Warburg: cell physiologist, biochemist, and eccentric. Oxford, Clarendon. 1981. x, 141 p.

**Krebs H:** Otto Warburg: Zellphysiologe--Biochemiker--Mediziner---1883-1970. Stuttgart, Wissenschaftliche Verlagsgesellschaft, 1979. 167 p. (Grosse Naturforscher, Band 41).

**Krebs H:** Reminiscenses and reflections. In collaboration with Anne Martin. Oxford, Clarendon Press, 1981. x, 298 p.

**Krebs H:** Wie ich aus Deutschland vertrieben wurde: Dokumente mit Kommentaren. **Medizinhist J** 1980;15(4):357-77

**Krebs LM** see **Terzioglu A**

**Krechmer MI** see **Sokolov EI**

**Krechmer MI** see **Troianskiĭ GN**

**Krehl WA:** Discovery of the effect of tryptophan on niacin deficiency. **Fed Proc** 1981;40:1527-30

**Kreibich H:** Betrachtungen zum 100. Jahrestag der Entdeckung des Mycobacterium tuberculosis durch Robert Koch. **Zentralbl Gynakol** 1982;104(5):258-67

**Kreiborg S** see **Jakobsen J**
**Kreis R:** The history of childhood through German literature: a psychogenic model. **J Psychohist** 1982 Winter;9(3):311-9
**Kreiser BR:** Miracles, convulsions, and ecclesiastical politics in early eighteenth-century Paris. Princeton, Princeton University Press, 1978. xvii, 485 p.
**Krekáň J** see **Tichý M**
**Krekeler G** see **Petsch K**
**Krell R:** At a children's hospital; a folklore survey. **West Folkl** 1980;39(3):223-31
**Kremenak N:** A centennial scrapbook. **Iowa Dent J** 1983 Jan;69(1):28-46
**Kremenak N:** John L. Naughton, inventor of the Den-Tal-Ez chair. An Iowa original. **Iowa Dent J** 1984 Oct;70(4):23-5
**Kremer J:** The significance of Antoni van Leeuwenhoek for the early development of andrology. **Andrologia** 1979;11:243-9
**Krenkel WA:** Masturbation in der Antike. **Wiss Z Univ Rostock** 1979;28(3):159-78
**Křepelka J** see **Tomiček F**
**Kretchmer N:** Science and scholarship in pediatrics. **Pediatr Res** 1980 Oct;14(10):1093-9
**Kretowski J, Killar M, Znosko K, et al:** Pomoc społeczna i lekarska kombatantom w Białymstoku. **Przegl Lek** 1981;38(1):30-3
**Kretowski J** see **Monkiewicz W**
**Kretschmer R** see **Campillo-Sainz C**
**Kretschmer W:** Psychiatrie in der Sowjetunion. **Osteuropa** 1978;28(4):317-20
**Kretschmer W** see **Janzarik W ed**
**Kretzmar N:** A half century of medical life in Kimberley. Personal reminiscences. **S Afr Med J** 1981 Aug 22;60(8):331-4
**Kretzoi M:** The significance of the Rudabánya prehominid finds in hominization research. **Acta Biol Acad Sci Hung** 1980;31(4):503-6
**Kreuzer DW** see **Miller GM**
**Kreuzer E** see **Habrich C**
**Krevans JR:** Transformation of medicine since 1945. **J Med Educ** 1984 Feb;59(2):75-8
**Kreyes E:** Die Geschichte der Wasserversorgung der Stadt Würzburg. Diss. Würzburg, 1969. 67 p.
**Kriegel L:** The wolf in the pit in the zoo. **Soc Policy** 1982;13(2):16-23
**Krieger D** see **Downs F**
**Kriel J, ed** see **Melzer R**
**Krikler DM:** Wolff-Parkinson-White syndrome: long follow-up and an Anglo-American historical note. **J Am Coll Cardiol** 1983 Dec;2(6):1216-8
**Krikshtopaĭtis MI** see **Ianushkevichus ZI**
**Krimsky S:** Genetic alchemy. The social history of the Recombinant DNA controversy. Cambridge, London, MIT Press, 1982. xiii, 445 p.
**Kringlen E:** Legemidler for behov eller profitt. **Samtiden (Norway)** 1970;79(9):546-63
**Kringlen E:** Personlighet og psykiatrisk teori. **Tidsskr Samfunnsforskning** 1980;21(2):179-85
**Krings H** see **Hasler L, ed**
**Krippner S, Winkelman M:** Maria Sabina: wise lady of the mushrooms. **J Psychoactive Drugs** 1983 Jul-Sep;15(3):225-8
**Krippner S:** Parapsychological research: a century of inquiry. **J Am Soc Psychosom Dent Med** 1982;29(4):121-7
**Kris AO:** The analyst's conceptual freedom in the method of free association. **Int J Psychoanal** 1983;64 (Pt 4):407-11
**Kris K:** A 70-year follow-up of a childhood learning disability. The case of Fanny Burney. **Psychoanal Study Child** 1983;38:637-52
**Krishan Y:** The doctrine of Karma and Ayurveda. **Bull Indian Inst Hist Med (Hyderabad)** 1980;10(1-4):34-9
**Krishan Y:** The meaning of prajnā-aparādha and karma in Ayurveda. **Bull Indian Inst Hist Med Hyderabad** 1982;12(1-4):28-33
**Krishnan P:** The historical demography of the Jews in India, 1881-1971. **Ann Demogr Hist (Paris)** 1983;:313-27
**Kristeller PO** see **Spicker SF, ed**
**Kristen G** see **Isaac O**
**Kristen KT, Reyman TA:** Radiographic examination of mummies with autopsy correlation. In A. Cockburn, E. Cockburn, ed: Mummies, disease, and ancient cultures. Cambridge, Cambridge University Press, 1980. p. 287-300.
**Krister CJ:** Safety evaluation ... it ain't all science. **Vet Hum Toxicol** 1980 Jun;22(3):156-9
**Kristiansen K:** Hospital services in Oslo. Oslo, Oslo City Hospital Board, 1979. p. 55-70.
**Kristiansen K:** Perspectives in neurosurgery: neurosurgery in Norway. **Neurosurgery** 1981 Jun;8(6):750-2
**Kritchevsky D:** Hilary Koprowski and The Wistar Institute. **J Cell Physiol [Suppl]** 1982;2:vi-viii
**Krivatsy P:** Medical incunabula and the diffusion of scientific knowledge. Incunabula in the National Library of Medicine. Published in conjunction with an exhibit at the National Library of Medicine, May-Oct. 1984. [Bethesda, National Library of Medicine, 1984.] 14 p.
**Krivobokov NG:** Shestidesiatiletie Piatigorskogo instituta kurotologii i fizioterapii. **Vopr Kurortol Fizioter Lech Fiz Kult** 1980 May-Jun;(3):67-8
**Krizay J:** Medicine and the market place. **Society** 1982;19(2):46-51
**Křížek V:** J.W. Goethe a ceské lázně. K 150. výročí básníkovy smrti 22. března 1832. **Cas Lek Cesk** 1982 Jun 4;121(22):695-8
**Křížek V, Nevoral V:** Jöns Jacob Berzelius a české minerální vody. **Fysiatr Reumatol Vestn** 1980 Aug;58(4):238-42
**Křížek V:** Samuel von Basch. Sto let od vynálezu nekrvavého měření krevního tlaku. **Cas Lek Cesk** 1980 Nov 28;119(48):1322-5
**Krizek V** see **Habrich C**
**Křížek V** see **Nevoral V**
**Kröber HL:** K. Schneiders Psychopathiebegriff als Hemmnis psychosomatischen Denkens. **Nervenarzt** 1984 Jan;55(1):25-9
**Kroc RL:** Relaxin--a perspective, or personal anecdotal recollections. **Ann NY Acad Sci** 1982;380:1-5
**Kroeger C** see **Klippe HJ**
**Krolenko SA** see **Vorob'ev VI**
**Królikowska M:** XXXV-lecie ginekologii i położnictwa w Akademii Medycznej w Lodzi. **Ginekol Pol** 1980 Nov;51(11):973-9
**Kroll J, Bachrach B:** Medieval visions and contemporary hallucinations. **Psychol Med** 1982 Nov;12(4):709-21
**Kroll J, Bachrach B:** Sin and mental illness in the Middle Ages. **Psychol Med** 1984 Aug;14(3):507-14
**Kroll J, Bachrach B:** Visions and psychopathology in the Middle Ages. **J Nerv Ment Dis** 1982 Jan;170(1):41-9
**Kroll RE:** Confines, wards, and dungeons. **NS Hist Soc Collect** 1980;40:93-107
**Krombach JD:** A foreign physician in Russia in the 1930s. **NY State J Med** 1984 Jun;84(6):317-8
**Krömer S:** Lärm als medizinisches Problem im 19. Jahrhundert. Diss. Mainz, 1981. 83 p.
**Kronenfeld MR** see **Thompson JA**
**Kronenthal RL** see **Hughes WL**
**Kronick DA:** Access to the medical journal literature of the 17th and 18th centuries through the Index catalogue. In International Congress of the History of Medicine. 26th, Plovdiv, 1978. Actes du Congress. Sofia, 1981. Volume II. p. 59-62.
**Kronick DA:** Artists and anatomists, some notes for an exhibit of anatomical atlases. **Friends P. I. Nixon Med Hist Libr** 1978 Oct;7:1-7
**Kronick DA:** Literature of the life sciences: the historical background. **Bull NY Acad Med** 1984 Nov;60(9):857-75
**Kronick DA:** The librarian's life, scholarship and librarianship. **Bull Med Libr Assoc** 1980 Oct;68(4):327-35
**Krook H:** Jacob Berzelius privat. **Nord Medicinhist Arsb** 1980;:81-9
**Krosnick A:** Moshe ben Maimon Ha-Sepharti (Maimonides). **J Med Soc NJ** 1979 Aug;76(9):569
**Krosnick A:** The art of Banting. **J Med Soc NJ** 1984 Feb;81(2):138-9
**Krosnick A:** The history of medical journalism in New Jersey. **J Med Soc NJ** 1984 Sep;81(9):723-6
**Krosnick A:** We are seventy-five. **J Med Soc NJ** 1979 Nov;76(12):809
**Kroszczor H:** Służba zdrowia w getcie warszawskim. **Biul Zydowskiego Inst Hist Pol** 1978;35(3-4):107-13
**Krótki KJ:** Some demographic, particularly fertility, correlates of female status in Eastern Europe and the Republics of the Soviet Union. In Yedlin, Tova, ed: Women in Eastern Europe and the Soviet Union, New York, Praeger, 1980. 239-69.
**Krotkov FG, Golikov VIa:** Gigienicheskaia nauka i klinicheskie distsipliny. **Klin Med (Mosk)** 1982 Dec;60(12):8-15
**Krotkov FG:** Lenin i sovetskoe zdravookhranenie. **Gig Sanit** 1980 Apr;(4):3-5
**Krotkov FG, Golikov VIa:** Profilakticheskaia meditsina i gigiena. **Gig Sanit** 1983 Feb;(2):24-8
**Krotoszynski BK** see **Moore JG**
**Kroupa J:** Dvacet pět let výzkumného ústavu traumatologického v brně. **Rozhl Chir** 1979;58(10):675-80
**Kroupa J:** Lékařský rod Rincolini v osvíceneckém Brně. **Cas Lek Cesk** 1982 Nov 19;121(46):1429-30
**Kroupa J:** 30 let trvání Výzkumného ústavu traumatologického v Brně. **Cas Lek Cesk** 1984 Jul 20;123(29):904-6
**Kroupa J:** 50 let od otevření úrazové nemocnice v Brně a 30 let činnosti Výzkumného ústavu traumatologického v Brně. **Rozhl Chir** 1984 Oct;63(10):633-42
**Krówczyński L:** Dorobek naukowy katedry i Zakładu Farmacji Stosowanej AM w Krakowie. **Folia Med Cracov** 1979;21(1):133-9
**Krueger HW** see **Sullivan CH**
**Krüger M:** Über progressive Traditionen in der haltung bürgerlicher deutscher ärzte der 20er Jahre gegenüber der Sowjetunion und ihrer Medizin am Beispiel des Hämatologen Viktor Schilling. **Wiss Z Univ Rostock** 1971;20(5):329-32
**Kruk R:** Aristoteles semitico-latinus. The Arabic version of Aristotle's Parts of animals. Book XI-XIV of the Kitab al-Hayawan. A critical edition with introduction and selected glossary. Amsterdam, Oxford, North-Holland Publishing Co., 1979. 96 [107] p.
**Krukoff S:** Utilisation, en craniologie, des vecteurs pour la mise en évidence du degré d'inclinaison du front et de la face chez le chimpanzé, l'homme actuel et fossile. **C R Seances Acad Sci [III]** 1981 May 11;292(17):969-74
**Krüll M:** Freud und sein Vater. München, Beck, 1979. 344 p.
**Krumholz W:** Eugen Woldemar Bostroem (1850-1928), Lehrer der Bathologie und Förderer der Medizin in Giessen. Giessen, Schmitz, 1983. 311 p. (Arbeiten zur Geschichte der Medizin in Giessen, Bd. 8)
**Krumova E** see **Vutov M**
**Krupinski J, Alexander L:** Patterns of psychiatric morbidity in Victoria, Australia, in relation to changes in diagnostic criteria 1848-1978. **Soc Psychiatry** 1983;18(2):61-7
**Krus S:** Sylwetki niektórych profesorów Warszawskiej Akademii Medycznej. Wystapienie na posiedzeniu Towarzystwa Lekarskiego Warszawskiego w dniu 24 IV 1980 r. **Pol Tyg Lek** 1980 Dec 15;35(50):1981-4
**Kruś S:** Tradycje historyczne Warszawskiej Akademii Medycznej. **Pol Tyg Lek** 1981 Jul 20;36(29):1123-7

**Kullberg G** see **Rabo M**
**Kullmann W:** Aristoteles' Grundgedanken zu Aufbau und Funktion der Körpergewebe. **Sudhoffs Arch** 1982;66(3):209–38
**Kullmann W:** Wesen und Bedeutung der 'Zweckursache' bei Aristoteles. **Ber Wissenschaftsgesch** 1982;5:25–39
**Kully RM** see **Sutto C, ed**
**Kulstad R, et al** see **Abelson PH**
**Külz J:** Interessantes und Amüsantes aus dem Nachlass von Karl Stolte. **Kinderarztl Prax** 1981 Nov;49(11):583–90
**Külz J:** 70 Jahre Pädiatrie als Lehrfach an der Universität Rostock. **Kinderarztl Prax** 1981 Feb;49(2):92–100
**Kumanoto-shi Ishikai, Kaishi Henshu Iinkai:** Kumamoto-shi Ishikai shi. Kumamoto, Japan, Do Ishikai, Showa 52 nen, 1977. 10, 465, 7 p.
**Kumar D:** Patterns of colonial science in India. **Indian J Hist Sci** 1980 May;15(1):105–13
**Kumate J:** Aparición declinación y reaparición de las enfermedades infecciosas del hombre. **Mem Col Nac (Mex)** 1979;9(2):19–41
**Kumate J:** La immunologia contemporánea. **Mem Col Nac (Mex)** 1978;8(4):11–24
**Kumate J:** Las herramientas de la inmunología contemporánea: nova et vetera. **Gac Med Mex** 1981 Sep;117(9):382–5
**Kumate J** see **Somolinas Palencia J**
**Kumate J** see **Treviño-García Manzo N**
**Kümmel WF** see **Nover A**
**Kump A** see **Heilmittel aus Pflanzen und Tieren**
**Kump WL:** The xenodochium of Pammachius. **Minn Med** 1982 Oct;65(10):633
**Kuna M** see **Dutkiewicz M**
**Kuna RR:** Hoodoo: the indigenous medicine and psychiatry of the black American. **Ethnomedizin** 1974–75;3(3–4):273–94
**Kunc Z:** Pěhled cinnosti neurochirurgické kliniky v Praze 1959--1978. **Cas Lek Cesk** 1979 Jul 20;118(29):897–901
**Kunčar K:** Olomoucкă psychiatrická klinika očima bývalých studentu. **Cesk Psychiatr** 1981 Oct;77(5):346–7
**Kundegraber M** see **Bauerndoktor und Volksmedizin. 1. Ausstellung anlässlich des 800-jährigen Bestehens von Stainz. Sonderausstellung: Juni bis Okt. 1977. Katalog: Nr. 3. Maria Kundegraber, unter Mitarb. v. Bernd Mader. Steiermark, Landesmuseum Joanneum, 1977. 63 p.**
**Kundsin RB:** Creative crusader against sepsis (Carl W. Walter). **Am J Surg** 1984 Nov;148(5):573–4
**Kunegel JM, Limoge A, Debras C:** Historique de l'électroanesthésie. **Inf Dent** 1982 Nov 18:64(40):3919–24
**Kung J:** Aristotle's De motu animalium and the separability of the sciences. **J Hist Philos** 1982;20:65–76
**Kuniak B, Strelka J:** Vývoj chirurgie strmienka pri otoskleróze na Slovensku. **Bratisl Lek Listy** 1983;79(2):222–6
**Kunichev LA:** Iz istorii lechebnogo massazha. **Feldsher Akush** 1981;46(2):43–5
**Kunikowska D** see **Gruszkiewicz E**
**Kunitomo T:** Development of new artificial kidney systems (Carl W. Walter). **Am J Surg** 1984 Nov;148(5):594–8
**Kunitsa LK, Mel'nik AN, Loboda VI:** K istorii razvitiia metoda tsitologicheskoĭ diagnostiki. **Vrach Delo** 1981 Jul;(7):123–5
**Kunitz SJ:** Efficiency and reform in the financing and organization of American medicine in the progressive era. **Bull Hist Med** 1981 Winter;55(4):497–515
**Kunitz SJ:** Mortality change in America, 1620–1920. **Hum Biol** 1984 Sep;56(3):559–82
**Kunitz SJ:** The historical roots and ideological functions of disease concepts in three primary care specialties. **Bull Hist Med** 1983 Fall;57(3):412–32
**Kunitz SJ:** Underdevelopment, demographic change, and health care on the Navajo Indian Reservation. **Soc Sci Med [Med Psychol Med Sociol]** 1981 Mar;15A(2):175–92
**Kunitz SJ** see **Levy JE**
**Kunitz SJ** see **Sorensen AA**
**Kunitzsch P:** Medizin, Naturwissenschaft und Technik im Mittelalter, Kontinuität und Wandel in Darstellung und Deutung: Die arabisch-islamische Welt. **Medizinhist J** 1982;17(1/2):54–62
**Kunovskiĭ BV, Bachinskiĭ IuS, Soroka AN:** K 100-letiiu otkrytiia vozbuditelia tuberkuleza. **Med Sestra** 1983 Feb;42(2):54–6
**Kuntz FJ:** Medizinisches bei Nikolaus Cusanus. **Mitt Forschungsbeitr Cusanus Ges** 1977;12:127–36
**Kunz K:** Chinese medicine: a history of revolution. **New Physician** 1979 Jan;28(1):28–30
**Kunze G:** Die Anfänge einer biomathematisch - biophysikalischen Denkweise in der Physiologie im Spiegel einiger Arbeiten Leonhard Eulers (1707–1783). Diss., Johannes-Gutenberg-Universität. Mainz, 1981. 182 p.
**Kunze J:** Ein geschichtlicher Beitrag zum Arbeitsschutz an der Porzellanmanufaktur zu Meissen um 1820. **Z Arztl Fortbild (Jena)** 1982 May 1;76(9):421–3
**Kunze M:** Strasse ins Feuer. Vom Leben und Sterben in der Zeit des Hexenwahns. München, Kindler, 1982. 397 p.
**Künzel W:** Die Gesellschaft für Stomatologie der DDR, 1964–1984. Leipzig, J. A. Barth, 1984. 187 p.
**Künzel W:** Stomatologie - eine neue Grundstudieneinrichtung an der Medizinischen Akademie Erfurt (1975–1980). **Beitr Gesch Univ Erfurt** 1979–83;19:305–37
**Künzel W:** Willoughby Dayton Miller zur 75. Wiederkehr des Todestages am 29. 7. 1982. **Zahn Mund Kieferheilkd** 1982;70(6):579–83
**Künzel W:** 20 Jahre Trinkwasserfluoridierung in der Deutschen Demokratischen Republik. **Stomatol DDR** 1979;29(10):743–52
**Künzl E** see **Hassel FJ**
**Kuo CH** see **Inoue N**
**Kuo P:** Lu-mu-ssu ti ch'e-ti ching-yen lun. **Bull Coll Lib Arts (Taiwan)** 1981;30:207–28
**Kuparinen E:** 'Enligt uppgift död i Sydafrika' - suomalaisten siirtolaisten terveydellinen ympäristö vuosisadan vaihteen etelä-Afrikassa. **Turun Hist Ark (Finl)** 1980;34:174–95
**Kuper A, Stone AA:** The dream of Irma's injection: a structural analysis. **Am J Psychiatry** 1982 Oct;139(10):1225–34
**Kupferschmidt HG:** 'Exotische' Krankheiten--einst und heute. **Z Arztl Fortbild (Jena)** 1983;77(1):33–6
**Kupperman KO:** Apathy and death in early Jamestown. **J Am Hist** 1979;66(1):24–40
**Kupriianov VV:** Otechestvennaia anatomiia na etapakh istorii. Moskva, Meditsina, 1981. 319 p.
**Kupriianov VV:** Vydaiushcheesia znachenie trudov Avitsenny dlia iatorii anatomii (k tysiacheletiiu so dnia rozhdeniia Ibn Siny). **Arkh Anat Gistol Embriol** 1980 Sep;79(9):109–11
**Kupriianova ES, Detinova TS, Anufrieva VN, et al:** Osnovnye napravleniia rabot V. N. Baklemisheva v oblasti meditsinskoĭ éntomologii i ikh znachenie v épidemiologii i profilaktike transmissivnykh bolezneĭ. **Med Parazitol (Mosk)** 1982 Jan–Feb;51(1):33–9
**Kupul Zh** see **Zhamba G**
**Kurashima K:** [Angle's orthodontics: a critical review. I. Angle's quest for science, and his classification of malocclusion] (Jpn). **Nippon Kyosei Shika Gakkai Zasshi** 1983 Sep;42(3):379–84
**Kurchishvili IB, Asatiani DK, Chomakhashvili AI:** Istoki meditsinskoĭ geografii v Gruzii. **Sov Zdravookhr** 1983;(12):51–3
**Kurdiumov NA, Novikova TP:** Kafedra normal'noĭ anatomii Dagestanskogo meditsinskogo instituta (k 50-letnemu iubileiu). **Arkh Anat Gistol Embriol** 1983 Dec;85(12):90–2
**Kure S, Kashida G:** Waga kuni ni okeru seishinbyo ni kansuru saikin no shisetsu. Tokyo, Seishin Igaku Shinkeigaku Koten Kankokai, [1977]. 270 p.
**Kurfess JF:** The legacy of Laplace. **J Ky Med Assoc** 1980 Apr;78(4):197–202
**Kuriloff P** see **Pittenger JC**
**Kuritz H:** The popularization of science in nineteenth-century America. **Hist Educ Q** 1981;21(3):259–74
**Kuriyama CB:** Hammer or anvil. Psychological patterns in Christopher Marlowe's plays. New Brunswick, Rutgers University Press, 1980. xiv, 240 p.
**Kurkotkin S:** Tyl sovetskikh vooruzhennykh sil v velikoi otechestvennoi voine. **Voen Istor Zn** 1975(5):44–52
**Kurpita PN:** Osobennosti sanitarno-gigienicheskogo obespecheniia na fronte i v tylu. **Voen Med Zh** 1980 May;(5):54–7
**Kursanova TA:** A. F. Fourcroy and zoochemistry in France at the beginning of the XIXth century. **Istor Biol Issled** 1983;9:176–86
**Kurtev V** see **Stamova N**
**Kurth DJ** see **Kurth RT**
**Kurth RT, Kurth DJ:** Oliver Wendell Holmes, M.D. (1809–1894); medical and literary knowledge intertwined. **NY State J Med** 1980 Jan;80(1):121–4
**Kurtz E:** Why A.A. works; the intellectual significance of Alcoholics Anonymous. **J Stud Alcohol** 1982 Jan;43(1):38–80
**Kurumada M:** ['Introductory notes on lying-in institutions' and problems of management--hospital management and Florence Nightingale] (Jpn). **Sogo Kango** 1983;18(1):107–19
**Kurz C:** De l'enfermement au secteur. **Soins Psychiatr** 1982 Feb;(16):2
**Kurzbauer E** see **Kurzbauer R**
**Kurzbauer R, Kurzbauer E, Sędzielowski Z:** Z historii electrostymulacji. **Pieleg Polozna** 1979;(10):3–4
**Kuś J, Miodoński A:** Kazimierz Kostranecki i jego uczniowie na tle epoki. **Przegl Lek** 1981;38(12):875–82
**Kuś J:** Profesor dr. Tadeusz Rogalski i jego działalność w czasie II wojny światowej (w stulecie jego urodzin). **Przegl Lek** 1982;39(10):683–9
**Kusakawa S, ed** see **Shigematsu I, ed**
**Kusevich GV:** Razvitie zadrvookhraneniia v g. Smele. **Med Sestra** 1981 Dec;40(12):3–5
**Kushner HI:** Americanization of the ego. **Can Rev Am Stud** 1979;10(1):95–101
**Kushner HI:** The suicide of Meriwether Lewis: a psychoanalytic inquiry. **William Mary Q** 1981;38(3):464–81
**Kuslan LI** see **Wilson LC, ed**
**Küss R:** Chirurgie générale ou chirurgie spécialisée. Une dualité dépassée? **Nouv Presse Med** 1980 Oct 11;9(37):2757–8
**Küss R:** Urologie. Introduction. **Rev Prat** 1981 Jun 21;31(35):2477–8, 2481–2
**Kustova EA** see **Komarov BD**
**Kutarňa A, Sajter V:** Subtrakcia a harmonizácia kontrastu röntgenového obrazu v diele prof. MUDr. Vojtecha Alexandra (1857–1916). **Bratisl Lek Listy** 1983 Dec;80(6):717–24
**Kutcher SP:** Toronto's metaphysicians: the social gospel and medical professionalization in Victorian Toronto. **HSTC Bull** 1981;5(1):41–51
**Kuthy-Porter J, Corvera-Bernardelli J, Martínez-Palomo A, et al:** Etica en la investigación clínica. **Gac Med Mex** 1983 Mar;119(3):97–112
**Kuthy-Porter J** see **Pacheco CR**
**Kutner NG:** Cost-benefit issues in U. S. national health legislation: the case of the end-stage renal disease program. **Soc Probl** 1982;30(1):51–64
**Kutorga VV** see **Siudikas VP**

**Kutter P** see **Fischle-Carl H, ed**
**Kuttler SL:** Dental hygiene: 70 years of growth and change taking a look at yesterday, today, and tomorrow. **Iowa Dent J** 1983 Oct;69(4):31-5
**Kuttner RE:** Protohistoric hepatomancy: an oracular form of pathology. **Proc Inst Med Chic** 1982 Jan-Mar;35(1):14
**Kutuzova EP** see **Khromov AS**
**Kuzin M, Antipenko E:** Zhizn' otdannaia nauke. **Voen Istor Zh** 1969;11(12):47-50
**Kuz'menko VI:** Uchastie meditsinskikh rabotnikov Belorussii v partizanskom dvizhenii. **Sov Zdravookhr** 1980;(9):49-53
**Kuzmin MK:** [Evolution of medicine in the principality of Moscow] (Rus). **Orvostort Kozl** 1979;87-88(25 no 1-2):91-104
**Kuz'min MK, Bukharov PL:** Ibn-Sina (Avitsenna) i narodnaia meditsina. **Feldsher Akush** 1981;46(3):50-2
**Kuzmin MK:** [Medicine in the Soviet Union and the impact of the scientific-technical revolution on its development.] (Rus). **Orvostort Kozl** 1981;93-96(27 No 1-4):201-10
**Kuz'min MK:** Muzhestvo i geroizm meditsinskikh rabotnikov. **Voen Med Zh** 1980 May;(5):65-8
**Kuz'min MK:** O proiskhozhdenii 'Prisiagi vracha Sovetskogo Soiuza'. **Sov Med** 1984;(8):117-9
**Kuz'min MK, Rumiantsev GI:** Razvitie osnovnykh napravleniĭ profilakticheskoĭ meditsiny na sanitarno-gigienicheskom fakul'tete (1930-1980). **Sov Med** 1981;(5):115-9
**Kuz'min MK:** Rol' sovetskikh uchenykh-medikov v Velikoĭ Otechestvennoĭ voĭne (k 35-letiiu Pobedy nad fashistskoĭ Germanieĭ). **Sov Med** 1980;(8):118-20
**Kuz'min MK:** Sovetskaia meditsina na razlichnykh étapakh sotsialisticheskogo stroitel'stva. **Sov Med** 1982;(12):10-6
**Kuz'min MK:** Sovetskaia meditsina v gody Velikoĭ Otechestvennoĭ voĭny ocherki. Moskva, Meditsina, 1979. 237 p.
**Kuz'min MK:** V. F. Zelenin i ego rol' v razvitii klinicheskoĭ élektrokardiografii i funktsional'noĭ diagnostike. **Klin Med (Mosk)** 1981 Aug;59(8):115-8
**Kuz'min MK:** Velikiĭ Russkiĭ khirurg N. I. Pirogov i sovremennost'. **Sov Med** 1983;(2):117-9
**Kuz'min MS:** Mezhnarodnye sviazi Narkomzdrava RSFSR v pervye gody Sovetskoĭ vlasti. **Sov Zdravookhr** 1984;(5):53-7
**Kuznetsov DN, Tikhonov AF:** V. I. Lenin i sovetskaia meditsina. **Vestn Khir** 1980 Apr;124(4):3-8
**Kuznetsov VK, Baranova EV:** Istoriia i sovremennoe sostoianie zakonodatel'stv ob absorte v stranakh mira. **Feldsher Akush** 1980;45(8):3-6
**Kuznetsov VK** see **Asimova MZ**
**Kuznetsova AI** see **Ponomareva PA**
**Kuznetsova MN** see **Koliadiuk IV**
**Kuźnicka B:** Kierunki rozwoju farmacji w Polsce epoki Oświecenia. Wrocław; Gdańsk, Zakład Narodowy im. Ossolińskich, Oddz. w Gdańsku, 1982. 172 p.
**Kuźnicka B:** The earliest printed herbals and evolution of pharmacy. **Organon** 1980/81;16-17:255-66
**Kuznicka B** see **Bukowiecki H**
**Kuźnicke L:** The Section of Biological Science of the Polish Academy of Sciences over the last 25 years. **Rev Pol Acad Sci (Warsz)** 1978;23:21-35
**Kuźnicki L, Radziwiłł M:** The section of biological science of the Polish Academy of Sciences over the last 25 years. **Rev Pol Acad Sci (Warsz)** 1978;23(1):21-35
**Kvarnes RG** see **Williman JP**
**Kvashenko BK, Konyk IeB:** [Obstetrical care in Rovno Province]. (Ukr) **Pediatr Akush Ginekol** 1979;(6):56-8
**Kvasnička J:** Sest' desat'roči Univerzity Komenského v Bratislave. **Cas Lek Cesk** 1979 Dec 21;118(51):1569-70
**Kvitnitskiĭ-Ryzhov IN:** Vydaiushchiĭsia issledovatel' otechestvennoĭ narodnoĭ meditsiny V. F. Demich (1858-1930). **Sov Zdravookhr** 1982;7:70-4
**Kvitnitskiĭ-Ryzhov IuN:** Iz istorii pervoĭ Kievskoĭ gistologicheskoĭ shkoly. **Arkh Anat Gistol Embriol** 1980 May;78(5):107-11
**Kvitnitskiĭ-Ryzhov IuN:** Iz istorii populiarizatsii meditsinskikh znaniĭ v Rosii. L.M. Chichagov i ego 'Meditsinskie besedy'. **Sov Zdravookhr** 1984;(8):66-70
**Kvitnitskiĭ-Ryzhov IuN:** Kievskie nekropoli v istoriko-meditsinskom aspekte (k 1500-letiiu Kieva). **Sov Zdravookhr** 1982;(9):65-8
**Kvitnitskiĭ-Ryzhov IuN:** O nekotorykh aktual'nykh voporosakh istorii morfologii (po povodu stateĭ V. Ch. Brzheskogo i V. P. Mikhaĭlova). **Arkh Anat Gistol Embriol** 1981 Aug;81(8):97-101
**Kvitnitskiĭ-Ryzhov IuN:** Zhizn' i deiatel'nost' ukrainskogo gistologa F. I. Lominskogo (k 125-letiiu so dnia rozhdeniia). **Arkh Anat Gistol Embriol** 1982 Apr;82(4):96-101
**Kvíz D:** Příspěvek k historiografii moravské gynekologie. **Cesk Gynekol** 1980 Mar;45(2):142-52
**Kyank H, Schwarz R:** Ergebnisse der Behandlung des Zervixkarzinoms an der Universitäts-Frauenklinik Rostock von 1959 bis 1972. **Zentralbl Gynakol** 1980;102(9):481-5
**Kyank H, Möbius W:** Zum 100. Geburtstag von Robert Schröder. **Zentralbl Gynakol** 1984;106(15):1092-8
**Kyle RA, Shampo MA:** [Historical aspects of medicine and philately]. **JAMA** 1982 Feb 12;247(6):796 (continued regularly)
**Kyle RA, Shampo MA, ed:** Medicine and stamps. Vol. 2. Huntington, New York, Krieger, 1980. xv, 209 p. (Reprinted articles from Journal of the American Medical Association).
**Kyle RA** see **Rehder K**
**Kyle RA** see **Shampo MA**
**Kylstra PH** see **Van der Leun C, ed:**
**Kyntera F:** Přínos vojenské epidemiologie za období 25leté existence Vojenského lékařského výzkumného a doškolovacího ústavu Jana Evangelisty Purkyně v Hradci Králové. **Cesk Epidemiol Mikrobiol Imunol** 1984 Jan;33(1):53-5
**Kyrge KKh:** K istorii transtorakal'nogo massazha serdtsa. **Klin Med (Mosk)** 1981 Jun;59(6):109-10
**Kyriazis N:** A parity-specific analysis of completed fertility in Canada. **Can Rev Sociol Anthropol** 1982;19(1):29-43
**Kyriazis N, Henripin J:** Women's employment and fertility in Québec. **Popul Stud** 1982 Nov;36(3):431-40

# L

**La Barre W:** Peyotl and mescaline. **J Psychedelic Drugs** 1979 Jan-Jun;11(1-2):33-9
**La Barre W:** Shamanic origins of religion and medicine. **J Psychedelic Drugs** 1979 Jan-Jun;11(1-2):7-11
**La Berge AF:** The early nineteenth-century French public health movement: the disciplinary development and institutionalization of hygiène publique. **Bull Hist Med** 1984 Fall;58(3):363-79
**La Coste-Messelière R de, Jugnot G, Treuille H:** Fonda des XVIIe-XVIIIe siècles et sources de l'histoire hospitalière médiévale XIIe-XIVe siècle. Toulouse, E. Privat, 1978. 283-318 p.
**La Coste Messelière R de:** Sources et illustrations de l'histoire des établissements hospitaliers et du pèlerinage de Saint-Jacques-de-Compostelle. **Bull Soc Hist Sci Deux Sevres** 1977;10:195-269
**La Croce E:** El concepto de locura en Grecia clásica. **Acta Psiquiatr Psicol Am Lat** 1981 Sep-Nov;27(4-5):285-91
**La información documental y su divulgación en medicina:** I. Breve reseña de los antecedentes y funciones del periodismo medico Mexicano. **Gac Med Mex** 1981 Apr;117(4):127-41
**La investigación biomédica en el Hospital Infantil de México: Bol Med Hosp Infant Mex** 1983 Nov;40 Suppl 3:3-23
**La médecine hospitalière française au XVIIIème siècle:** Colloque de l'Institut d'Histoire de la Médecine et de la Pharmacie de l'Université René Descartes, Paris, 6 octobre 1977. Strasbourg, Université Louis Pasteur, 1980. 213 p. Travaux d'histoire de la médecine et de la pharmacie, I. Contributions by P. Huard, M. J. Imbault-Huart, M. Baudot, J. Filliozat, P. Niaussat, A. Carré, J. P. Kerneis, V. Comiti
**La médicine populaire:** Exposition, 27 mars - 17 mai 1981. Bruxelles, Galerie CGER, 1981. 109 p.
**La Parra S** see **Peset JL**
**La Parra S** see **Peset M**
**La Peña Begué R de:** El uso de la coca en América. Según la legislación colonial y republicana. **Rev Esp Antropol Am** 1971;6:179-204
**La sagesse de la médecine traditionnelle Sino-Vietnamienne et les maladies de la femme. 2 vols. Paris, Centre de Thuyen d'Europe, 1978. 1260 p.:**
**La Salpêtrière:** Hier et aujourd'hui. (Numéro spécial hors série, L'Hôpital à Paris, Aout 1982.) 79 p. Contributions by G. Pallez, J. Brunet, R. Poujol, D. Puzin, R. César, F. Greffe, P. Castaigne, R. Brocas, J. Franchi.
**La tradition manuscrite des Quaestiones Nicolai peripatetici. In:** J.J.G. Alexander, M.T. Gibson (eds.) Medieval learning and literature: Essays presented to Richard William Hunt. Oxford: Clarendon Pr., 1976. p. 200-219.
**La Vergata A:** Claude Bernard, 'punti di vista fisiologici', ed economia della natura. **Riv Filos** 1982;73:361-95
**Labarbera M:** An ounce of prevention, and grandma tried them all. **NY Folkl Q** 1964;20(2):126-9
**Labarta A:** Textos para el estudio de la terapéutica entre los moriscos valencianos. **Dynamis** 1981;1:275-319
**Labazanov MM** see **Napalkov PN**
**Labaziewicz L:** Pisarstwo naukowe Ireneusza Wierzejewskiego. **Chir Narzadow Ruchu Ortop Pol** 1981;46(6):595-7
**LaBerge R:** Medicare is not the health charter for Canadians. **Can Labour** 1969;14(9):14-9
**Labhart A:** Diskursives Denken und Intuition in der medizinischen Forschung. **Helv Chir Acta** 1981 Feb;47(6):859-72
**Labisch A:** Alfred Grotjahn (1869-1931) und das gesundheitspolitische Programm der Mehrheitssozialdemokraten von 1922. **MMG** 1983;8:192-7
**Labisch A, Spree R, Weindling P:** Conference Report. Social history of nineteenth- and twentieth-century German medicine. **Soc Soc Hist Med Bull (Lond)** 1983;32:40-5
**Labisch A:** Das Krankenhaus in der Gesundheitspolitik der deutschen Sozialdemokratie vor dem Ersten Weltkrieg. **Med Soziol** 1981;1:127-51
**Labisch A:** Das Krankenhaus in der sozialdemokratischen Kommunalpolitik in Berlin um die Jahrhundertwende. **Hist Hosp** 1981-82;14:337-45
**Labisch A:** Entwicklungslinien des öffentlichen Gesundheitsdienstes in Deutschland. Vorüberlegungen zur historischen Soziologie öffentlicher Gesundheitsvorsorge. **Off Gesundheitswes** 1982 Nov;44(11):745-61
**Labisch A:** Gleiche Chance der medizinischen Versorgung; historischer Abriss über ein Leitmotiv in der Entwicklung der gesetzlichen Krankenversicherung. In Hauss, F., Naschold, F., Rosenbrock, R., ed: Schichtenspezifische Versorgungsprobleme im Gesundheitswesen. Bonn, Der Bundesminister für Arbeit und Sozialordnung, 1981. p. 32-50.
**Labisch A:** Krankenhauspolitik in der Krankenhausgeschichte. **Hist Hosp** 1979-80;13:217-33
**Labisch A:** Neue Quellen zum gesundheitspolitischen Programm der MSPD

von 1920/22. **Int Wiss Korresp Gesch Dtsch Arb-bew** 1980 June;16(2):231-47

**Labisch A, Spree R:** Neuere Ergebnisse und Entwicklungen einer Sozialgeschichte der Medizin und des Gesundheitswesens in Deutschland im 19. und 20. Jahrhundert. **Ber Wissenschaftsgesch** 1982;5(3):209-23

**Labisch A:** Recent trends in the social history of occupational medicine in the Federal Republic of Germany. **Soc Soc Hist Med Bull (Lond)** 1983 Dec;33:52-7

**Labisch A:** Selbsthilfe zwischen Auflehnung und Anpassung. Arbeiter-Sanitätskommission und Arbeiter-Samariterbund. **Jahrb Krit Med** 1983;77:11-26

**Labisch A:** The Workingmen's Samaritan Federation (Arbeiter-Samariter-Bund) 1888-1933. **J Contemp Hist** 1978;13:297-322

**Labisch A:** Zur Sozialgeschichte der Medizin. Methodologische Ueberlegungen und Forschungsbericht. **Arch Sozialgesch** 1980;20:431-70

**Labisch A, Tennstedt F:** 50 Jahre Gesetz über Vereinheitlichung des Gesundheitswesens. Dr. med. Arthur Gütt und die Gründung des öffentlichen Gesundheitsdienstes. **Off Gesundheitswes** 1984 Jul;46(7):291-8

**Labisch A** see **Klein P**

**Labor under ether:** Hilo, 1850. **Hawaii Med J** 1981 Oct;40(10):291-2

**Labreche J:** NRC: where science fiction often comes true. **Can Geogr** 1980;100(4):24-33

**Labrude P:** Albin Haller 1849-1925 pharmacien et chimiste. **Rev Hist Pharm (Paris)** 1982 Sep;29(254):207-9

**Labuda G, Rodzik I:** Scientists and scholars of Polish origin and Polish men of learning active abroad: their share in the development of science. **Rev Pol Acad Sci (Warsz)** 1980;25(1-2):105-23

**Lacan J:** The neurotic's individual myth. **Psychoanal Q** 1979 Jul;48(3):405-25

**Lacey JH:** Anorexia nervosa and a bearded female saint. **Br Med J [Clin Res]** 1982 Dec 18-25;285(6357):1816-7

**Lach E:** The circumcision of the child on the eighth day...An anonymous engraving after a design by Bernard Picart. **J Hist Med Allied Sci** 1982 Apr;37(2):221

**Lachiver M** see **Dupâquier J**

**L'acide barbiturique: Pour Sci** 1982;61:6

**Laclé A:** La falsa ciclotimia de Bolivar. **Rev Soc Bolivar Venez** 1979;36(121):71-3

**Lacombe C** see **Huard P**

**Lacombe M** see **Do JP**

**Lacorre B:** Role des savoirs constitués dans la justification de la notion d'inconscient psychique. In Poirier J, Poirier JL, ed: Médicine et philosophie à la fin du XIXe siècle. Paris, Université de Paris XII - Val de Marne, [1980?]. p. 127-40.

**Lacourcière L** see **Hand WD, ed**

**Lacroix MT:** L'hôpital Saint-Nicolas du Bruille (Saint-André) à Tournai de sa fondation à sa mutation en cloître (ca. 1230-1611). 2 tomes. Louvain, Université Catholique de Louvain, 1977. xxxvi, 892 p. (Publications de l'Institut d'Etudes Médiévales, 2e série, No. 1).

**Lactance:** L'ouvrage du Dieu créateur. 2 vols. Ed. par M. Perrin. Paris, Editions du Cerf, 1974. 456 p. (Sources Chrétiennes, No. 213, 214).

**Laczay A:** Történelmi tévedések a röntgendiagnosztikában és a tévedés etikája. **Orv Hetil** 1983 Dec 4;124(49):2999-3002

**Ladegaard Jakobsen AL:** A cripple from the late Middle Ages. **Ossa** 1978;5:17-24

**Ladendorf H:** Der alte Mensch in der Kunst. In Göpfert W, Otten HH, ed: Metavoeite: wandelt euch durch neues Denken. Düsseldorf, Triltsch, 1983. p. 55-68.

**Ladendorf H:** Leonardo da Vinci und die Wissenschaften: eine Literaturübersicht. Köln, 1984. 190 p. (Kölner medizinhistorische Beiträge: Arbeiten der Forschungsstelle des Instituts für Geschichte der Medizin der Universität zu Köln, Band 23/2)

**Ladendorf H** see **Baur O**

**Ladman AJ:** R. C. Truex memorial. **Anat Rec** 1981 Sep;201(1):3-11

**Ladnyĭ ID** see **Gol'd EIu**

**L'adrach U** see **Dätwyler B**

**Ladurie E LeRoy:** The territory of the historian. Translated from the French by B. and S. Reynolds. Hassocks, Sussex (England), Harvester Press, 1979. viii, 345 p.

**Ladurie EL:** Un concept: l'unification microbienne du monde (XIVe-XVIIe siècles). **Schweiz Z Gesch** 1973;23(4):627-94

**Laduron P** see **Gielen JE**

**Lady L:** Home visits by FNS nurses. **Front Nurs Serv Q Bull** 1980 Winter;56(3):35-41

**Laeger i Sønderjylland indtil 1864: Dan Medicinhist Arbog** 1980;:11-65

**Laffe F:** Médecins et société à Saint-Rémy de Provence au XVIIIe siècle. **Provence Hist** 1983;33(134):461-73

**Laffi GC** see **Brillante C**

**Laffón A** see **Alarcón-Segovia D**

**Lafon JC:** Le sourd et muet au XIXe siècle. **Bull Audiophonol** 1980;11(2):1-142

**Laforest NL:** L'art de soigner les pieds. Fac-simile de l'édition de 1782. Ed. R. Habert. Bruxelles, Caducea, 1979. 257 p.

**Lafosse A:** Les hôpitaux temporaires à Verviers durant les épidémies de choléra. **Ann Soc Belg Hist Hop** 1979;17:71-9

**Lafuente A** see **Albarracín Teulón A**

**Lage O da** see **Kelly C**

**Lagergren H:** Den implanterbara pacemakern 25 år. Utveckling och erfarenheter. **Lakartidningen** 1983 Oct 5;80(40):3688-91

**Laget M:** La césarienne ou la tentation de l'impossible, 17 et 18e siècle. **Ann Bretagne** 1979;86(3):177-89

**Laget M:** Naissances: l'accouchement avant l'âge de la clinique. Paris, Seuil, 1982. 346 p.

**Laget M:** Note sur la réanimation des nouveau-nés (XVIIIe-XIXe siècles). **Ann Demogr Hist (Paris)** 1983;:65-72

**Laget M** see **Forster R**

**Lagier R, Baud CA, Kramar C:** Brodie's abscess in a tibia dating from the Neolithic period. **Virchows Arch [A]** 1983;401(2):153-7

**Lagier R, Baud CA, Arnaud G, et al:** Lesions characteristic of infection or malignant tumor in Paleo-Eskimo skulls. An anatomical and radiological study of two specimens. **Virchows Arch [Pathol Anat]** 1982;395(3):237-43

**Lagier R** see **Kramar C**

**Lagnelius C:** Svenska röda korset som piojärorganisation. **Omvardaren** 1982;29(2):10-1

**Lagoutte J:** Claude Bernard, un physiologiste, un philosophe. Lyon, Centre régional de documentation pédagogique, 1978. 40 p.

**Laguna J** see **Somolinos-Palencia J**

**Lahaise R:** Marien Tailhandier. In Dictionary of Canadian biography, 1701 to 1740. Volume 2, 1969. p. 617-8.

**Laham J:** Le concept de bloc de branche. Evolution des idées (1910-1982). **Ann Cardiol Angeiol (Paris)** 1983 Jul-Sep;32(5):343-50

**Laher M, O'Brien E:** In search of Korotkoff. **Br Med J [Clin Res]** 1982 Dec 18-25;285(6357):1796-8

**Lahiri K:** Clara Swain, MD (1834-1910) and her work in India. **Women Health** 1983 Spring;8(1):3-6

**Lahmann F** see **Stam I**

**Laidig GL, et al:** Agricultural variation and human fertility in antebellum Pennsylvania. **J Fam Hist** 1981;6:195-204

**Laín Entralgo P:** Being healthy down through history. In Seidler E, Schott H, ed: Bausteine zur Medizingeschichte. Stuttgart, Steiner, 1984. p. 65-72.

**Laín Entralgo P:** History of the [therapeutic] relationship. In Reich WT, et al, ed: Encyclopedia of bioethics, v.4. New York, Free Press, 1978, p. 1655-63.

**Laín Entralgo P:** Los orígenes del diagnóstico medico. **Dynamis** 1981;1:3-15

**Lain-Entralgo P:** Quaestiones hippocraticae disputatae tres. In La collection hippocratique et son rôle dans l'histoire de la médecine. Colloque de Strasbourg (23-27 octobre 1972) organisé par le Centre de Recherches sur la Grèce Antique, avec le concours des Facultés de Philosophie et des Langues Classiques. Leiden, E. J. Brill, 1975. p. 305-19.

**Laín Entralgo P:** Relieves hipocráticos. **Med Hist (Barc)** 1984;1:1-16

**Laín Entralgo P** see **Albarracín Teulón A**

**Laine E:** Histoire de la chirurgie des anévrysmes cérébraux. **Bull Mem Acad R Med Belg** 1983;138(12):576-86

**Laird C:** Chemehuevi shamanism, sorcery, and charms. **J Calif Great Basin Anthropol** 1980;2(1):80-7

**Laird JD:** Thomas Young, M.D. (1773-1829). **Am Heart J** 1980 Jul;100(1):1-8

**Laird M:** Integrirovannye metody bor'by s perenoschikami i ugroza gemorragicheskoĭ likhoradlki Denge v tropicheskoĭ zone Tikhogo Okeana. **Parazitologiia** 1984 Mar-Apr;18(2):99-105

**Laissus J:** La succession de Le Monnier au Jardin du Roi: Antoine-Laurent de Jussieu et René Louiche-Desfontaines. In: Congrès National des Sociétés Savantes, 91e, Rennes, 1966. Comptes Rendus. Paris, 1967. Section des Sciences, Tome 1. p. 137-52.

**Laissus J:** Les conserves alimentaires: Nicolas Appert (1749-1841) bienfaiteur de l'humanité. In: Congrès National des Sociétés Savantes, 93e, Tours, 1968. Comptes Rendus. Paris, 1971. Section des Sciences, Tome II. p. 137-57.

**Laissus Y:** Les papiers du docteur J.-B. Mougeot (1776-1858): un fonds important pour l'histoire des sciences naturelles en Lorraine. In: Congrès National des Sociétés Savantes, 103e, Nancy, 1978. Comptes Rendus. Paris, 1978. Section des Sciences, Fasc. V. p. 233-40.

**Laissus Y:** Les voyageurs naturalistes du Jardin du roi et du Muséum d'histoire naturelle: essai de portrait-robot. **Rev Hist Sci (Paris)** 1981 Jul-Oct;34(3-4):259-317

**Laissus Y:** Lettres inédites de René Desfontaines à Louis-Guillaume le Monnier, conservées à la Bibliothèque centrale du Muséum national d'histoire naturelle. In: Congrès National des Sociétés Savantes, 91e, Rennes, 1966. Comptes Rendus. Paris, 1967. Section des Sciences, Tome 1. p. 153-69.

**Lait J** see **Brewer C**

**Laitman JT, Heimbuch RC:** The basicranium of Plio-Pleistocene hominids as an indicator of their upper respiratory system. **Am J Phys Anthropol** 1982 Nov;59(3):323-43

**Lake CR** see **Moriarty KM**

**Laker MR:** Newton's malady. **Science** 1982 Mar 5;215(4537):1185-6

**Lakie MH, Cook G, MacMurray D:** A 17th century poisoning case. **Pharm Hist (London)** 1976 Aug;6(2):2-3

**Lakosina ND:** Idei nevroticheskogo razvitiia v trudakh P. B. Gannushkina. **Zh Nevropatol Psikhiatr** 1982;82(11):127-9

**Laks H** see **Hammond GL**

**Lakshmipathi G:** Avicenna on ear, nose and throat diseases. **Bull Indian Inst Hist Med (Hyderabad)** 1981;1-4:79-82

**Lalanne C, Coussement A:** Geschichte der Radiodiagnostik. In Sournia JC, Martiny M, Poulet J, ed: Illustrierte Geschichte der Medizin. Salzburg, Andreas, 1980. Vol. 6. p. 2195-221.

**Lalic R** see **Sarac S**

**Lam CR:** Heart valve surgery at Henry Ford Hospital from a perspective

of thirty-two years. **Henry Ford Hosp Med J** 1982;30(3):170-1
**Lam CR:** The Central Surgical Association turns forty. Some highlights of the first twenty years. **Henry Ford Hosp Med J** 1982;30(2):77-80
**Lam D** see **Lee R**
**Lama S, Santra SC:** Development of Tibetan plant medicine. **Sci Cult** 1979;45(7):262-5
**Laman CA:** A prolegomenon to the history of perspectives in personality theory. Ph.D. Diss., Rice University. Houston, 1978. iv, 210 leaves.
**Lamarck JB** see **McKinney HL, ed**
**Lamare J, ed:** Médecine régionale: mystérieuse et pittoresque. Niort [France], Vernaculaires, 1981. 244 p.
**Lamarre C:** Vivre de charité à l'hôpital de Dijon au XVIIIe siècle: les secours aux enfants et aux viellards. **Bull Soc Fr Hist Hop** 1981;(42):25-35
**Lamarre-Tainturier C:** Les secours aux malades pauvres des campagnes dans la généralité de Bourgogne au XVIIIe siècle. In: Congrès National des Sociétés Savantes, 97e, Nantes, 1972. Actes. Paris, 1977. Histoire Moderne et Contemporaine, Tome 1. p. 499-511.
**Lamarre-Tainturier C** see **Patrimoine hospitalier de la Bourgogne**
**Lamas GA, Koller LR, Antman EM, et al:** Electrocardiogram by Einthoven 63 years earlier. **Am J Cardiol** 1984 Nov 1;54(8):1163-5
**Lamb M** see **Hamilton D**
**Lamb WK:** William Fraser Tolmie. In Dictionary of Canadian biography, 1881-1890. 1982;11:885-8.
**Lamb M, ed** see **Checkland O**
**Lambert D** see **Masters J**
**Lambert EI:** The United States labeling regulations for vegetable proteins: an historical perspective. **J Am Oil Chem Soc** 1979 Mar;56(3):234-7
**Lambert G:** Peter Wilson: colonial surgeon. Palmerston North, N.Z., Dunmore Press, 1981. 213 p.
**Lambert JB, Vlasak SM, Thometz AC, et al:** A comparative study of the chemical analysis of ribs and femurs in Woodland populations. **Am J Phys Anthropol** 1982 Nov;59(3):289-94
**Lambert M:** Jan Fryderyk Knolle's forgotten dissertation on osseous syphilis, 1763. **Sex Transm Dis** 1984 Jan-Mar;11(1):36-40
**Lambert M:** Udział niemieckich ośrodków naukowych w kształtowaniu polskiej myśli medycznej w czasach saskich (1697-1763). **Arch Hist Med (Warsz)** 1979;42(2):223-30
**Lambert S** see **Israelstam S**
**Lambertini G:** Die Schule von Salerno und die Universitäten von Bologna und Padua. In Sournia JC, Martiny M, Poulet J, ed: Illustrierte Geschichte der Medizin. Salzburg, Andreas, 1980. Vol. 2. p. 731-53.
**Lambertini G:** Il pensiero e i trovati di Angelo Ruffini nella sua opera 'Physiogeny'. [Italian and English] Padova, Piccin, 1980. 111 p.
**Lambiase M** see **Salomone G**
**Lamblin-Robert J, Lecomte D, Lathrop M, et al:** Epidemies virales et rapport de masculinité des naissances: des données divergentes. **Population** 1983;38(1):162-5
**Lambo TA:** Changing patterns of mental health needs in Africa. **Contemp Rev** 1973;222(1286):146-54
**Lambo TA:** Professor Gastaut and his contributions to the World Health Organization programme. **Electroencephalogr Clin Neurophysiol** 1982;35:3-6
**Lambrecht FL:** Notes on the history of sleeping sickness. **Botsw Notes Rec** 1968;1:41-9
**Lambrecht FL:** Palaeoecology of Tsetse flies and sleeping sickness in Africa. **Proc Am Philos Soc** 1980 Oct 10;124(5):367-85
**Lambrecht G:** Die Perikarditis-tuberkulosa-Diagnostik im ausgehenden 19. Jahrhundert. **Wiss Beitr Martin Luther Univ Halle Wittenberg** 1983;5-R80:117-22
**Lambrecht M:** A magyar klinikai oktatás hallei mint ája. Johann Juncker, az orvospedagógus. **Orv Hetil** 1982 Jul 11;123(28):1745-8
**Lambrecht M:** Die Krankheitsauffassung in der ätiologischen Ara. **Wiss Beitr Martin Luther Univ Halle Wittenberg** 1983;5-R80:63-70
**Lambrecht M:** Entz Béla, a klinikai pathológia egyik hazai úttörője. **Orv Hetil** 1984 Oct 28;125(44):2694-5
**Lambrecht M:** Gorka Sándor az elsö magyar biológusprofesszor. **Orv Hetil** 1979 Aug 19;120(32):1947-50
**Lambrecht M:** Virchow és Pertik. **Orvostort Kozl** 1980;89-91(26 no 1-3):233-9
**Lammel HU:** Virchow contra Koch? Neue Untersuchungen zu einer alten Streitfrage. **Z Gesamte Hyg** 1982 Mar;28(3):206-10
**Lämmer M:** Women and sport in ancient Greece; a plea for a critical and objective approach. In Borms J, Hebbelinck M, Venerando A, ed: Women and sport. Basel, Karger, 1981. p. 16-23.
**Lamothe MJ** see **Velter A**
**Lamoureux D:** La lutte pour le droit à l'avortement (1969-1981). **Rev Hist Am Fr** 1983;37(1):81-90
**Lampé L:** Egységes nemzetközi szülészeti adatgyüjtés (Tauffer nyomdokain). **Orv Hetil** 1982 Apr 11;123(15):895-903
**Lampé L:** Margaret Sanger munkássága és annak hatása a családtervezési mozgalomra. **Orv Hetil** 1984 Jan 22;125(4):221-2
**Lamperes BC** see **Tarr JA**
**Lampert RH:** Osler and his publishers. **Trans Stud Coll Physicians Phila** 1983 Sep;5(5 No 3):177-90
**Lamping KA, Albert DM, Snyder C, et al:** The Harrower collection and its place in the history of ophthalmic pathology. **Surv Ophthalmol** 1983 May-Jun;27(6):374-80
**Lamping KA** see **Fournier GA**
**Lamprecht-Naef E:** Albert Schweitzer und die Schweiz. Zürich, Juris Druck, 1982. 116 p. (Zürcher Medizingeschichtliche Abhandlungen, Neue Reihe, Nr. 153).
**Lampton DM:** Performance and the Chinese political system: a preliminary assessment of education and health policies. **China Q** 1978;(75):509-39
**Lampton DM:** The roots of interprovincial inequality in education and health services in China since 1949. **Am Pol Sci Rev** 1979,73(2):459-77
**Lamsfuss J** see **Swantes HJ**
**Lamur HE:** Demographic performance of two slave populations of the Dutch speaking Caribbean. **Bol Estud Latinoam Caribe** 1981;(30):87-102
**Lamy LH:** Sur un point particulier de la contribution de Robert Deschiens à la connaissance des amibes. **Bull Soc Pathol Exot Filiales** 1978;71 Spec No:502-8
**Lamy ML, Leridon H:** Les grossesses tardives donnant lieu à amniocentèse: enquête menée dans les trois centres de la région parisienne. **Population** 1981;36(1):174-82
**Lanari A:** La batalla de Valmy y la medicina. **Medicina (B Aires)** 1981;41(2):257-8
**Lancaster RK:** Green Mount: the introduction of the rural cemetry into Baltimore. **Md Hist Mag** 1979;74(1):62-79
**Lance D:** Meals on the mess deck: from canteen messing to professional catering. **Hist Today** 1978;28(7):476-9
**Lanchou G, Veron C:** Un évadé de la médecine: Jean-Baptiste Charcot (1867-1936). **Hist Sci Med** 1980;14(1):43-50
**Lanchy F:** La comtesse de Ségur et la santé des enfants. **Rev Hist Pharm (Paris)** 1982;29(252):179-85
**Lańcucki J:** Współczesne ziołolecznictwo. **Pol Tyg Lek** 1979 Jul 2;34(27):1095-8
**Land G** see **Numbers RL, ed**
**Land LC:** Hiran Hitchcock' legacy: the history of the Mary Hitchcock Memorial Hospital School of Nursing. Canaan, N. H., Phoenix Publishing for the Mary Hitchcock Memorial Hospital, 1980. x, 148 p.
**Landa LM:** Pomoshch' trudiashchikhsia turkestana golodaiushchemu naseleniiu RSFSR v 1921-1922 gg. **Istor SSSR** 1971;2:136-40
**Landáburu AJ** see **Pennini de Vega E**
**Landau RL:** Landmark perspective: treatment of hyperthyroidism. **JAMA** 1984 Apr 6;251(13):1747-8
**Landauer AA:** A note on the role of Karl Christian Wolfart (1778-1832) in the study of animal magnetism. **J Hist Behav Sci** 1981;17:206-8
**Landauer B:** Inhalationsanästhesie heute. Teil 1: Historische Entwicklung, allgemeine Tatsachen. **Fortschr Med** 1983 May 5;101(17):796-802
**Lander BG** see **Hamilton HD**
**Landes RR, Hall S:** A letter from Joseph Lister to Dr. David Walsh. **JAMA** 1984 Jun 15;251(23):3101-3
**Landi S:** Production and standardization of tuberculin (a brief history). **Indian J Chest Dis Allied Sci** 1982 Apr-Sep;24(2-3):78-87
**Landmann H:** Die Entwicklung der Tuberkulose in den letzten 100 Jahren unter besonderer Berücksichtigung der epidemiologischen Situation in der Deutschen Demokratischen Republik.
**Landmann H** see **Ocklitz HW**
**Landmann M** see **Spicker SF, ed**
**Landolt AM, Zachmann M:** The Irish giant: new observations concerning the nature of his ailment. **Lancet** 1980 Jun 14;1(8181):1311-2
**Landon SJ:** Giants of Paumanok. **York State Tradit** 1972;26(3):24-6, 48-54, 56, 64
**Landor JH:** Lester Reynold Dragstedt--physiologist-surgeon. **Gastroenterology** 1981 Apr;80(4):846-53
**Landsberger M:** Percussion discovered. **Trans Stud Coll Physicians Phila** 1981 Dec;5(3 no 4):255
**Landsberger M:** The story of the history of medicine: essay-review. **Trans Stud Coll Physicians Phila** 1980 Dec;5(2 no 4):315-8
**Lane AJ:** The politics of birth control. **Marx Perspect** 1979;2(3):160-9
**Lane D** see **Turner T**
**Lane J:** The medical practitioners of provincial England in 1783. **Med Hist** 1984 Oct;28(4):353-71
**Lane J:** The provincial practitioner and his services to the poor, 1750-1800. **Soc Soc Hist Med Bull (Lond)** 1981 Jun;28:10-4
**Lane J** see **Baxter EG**
**Lane R:** Suicide and the city. **Society** 1980;17(2):74-82
**Lane R:** Violent death in the city: suicide, accident, and murder in nineteenth-century Philadelphia. Cambridge, Mass., Harvard University Press, 1979. xiii, 193 p.
**Lang EF:** From earlier pages: the position and relationships of fragments in acute fractures. (E.H. Skinner). **AJR** 1980 Jan;134(1):206
**Lang H** see **Kraus A, ed**
**Lang HH** see **Nixon PI**
**Lang K:** Kritiker, Ketzer, Kämpfer: das Leben des Arbeiterarztes Fritz Brupbacher. Zürich, Limmat, 1983. 360 p.
**Langaney A** see **Lamblin-Robert J**
**Lange AB** see **Tamarina NA**
**Lange E:** Die Rodewischer Thesen 1963--Vermächtnis und Verpflichtung, Bekenntnis und Verwirklichung. **Psychiatr Neurol Med Psychol (Leipz)** 1979 Jul;31(7):385-92
**Lange FW:** Una reevalución de la población del norte de Yucatán en el tiempo del contacto Español: 1528. **Am Indig** 1971;31(1):117-39
**Lange FW** see **Corruccini RS**
**Lange G:** Die Vereinigung Westdeutscher Hals-, Nasen- und Ohrenärzte besteht im 85-sten Jahr. **HNO** 1982 Mar;30(3):114-5
**Lange J:** Humant spyt og auxiner--et historisk tilbagekig. **Tandlaegebladet** 1982 Oct;86(17):595
**Lange KA** see **Suvorov NF**
**Lange R:** Plagues and pestilence in Polynesia: the nineteenth-century Cook Islands experience. **Bull Hist Med** 1984 Fall;58(3):325-46
**Lange-Pfautsch R** see **Burmeister KJ**

**Langenwalter RE:** A possible shamans's cache from CA-RIV-102, Hemet, California. **J Calif Great Basin Anthropol** 1980;2(2):233–44
**Langer D:** Paul Ferdinand Schilder, Leben und Werk. Diss. Mainz, 1979. 259 p.
**Langer H** see **Friedrich C**
**Langer LN:** Plague and the Russian countryside: monastic estates in the late fourteenth and fifteenth centuries. **Can Am Slav Stud** 1976;10:351–68
**Langer M:** Memoria, historia y diálogo psicoanalítico. With Jaime del Palacio and Enrique Guinsberg. Mexico City. Folios Ediciones S. A., 1981. 240 p.
**Langer P** see **Macho L**
**Langfeldt B** see **Halaburt H**
**Langford C:** Fertility in Sri Lanka since the war: an analysis of the experience of different districts. **Popul Stud** 1981;35(2):285–306
**Langford CM:** A consideration of some retrospective data on breast-feeding in Great Britain. **J Biosoc Sci** 1978;10:389–400
**Langford CM:** Fertility change in Sri Lanka since the war: an analysis of the experience of different districts. **Popul Stud** 1981 Jul;35(2):285–306
**Langham-Carter RR:** The Caledon baths. **Adler Mus Bull** 1984 Jun;10(2):18–9
**Langham-Carter RR:** The death of the Duchesse de Nemours. **Adler Mus Bull** 1982 Nov;8(2):8–9
**Langholf V** see **Grmek MD, ed**
**Langley GE:** Sir John Charles Bucknill 1817–1897: our founder. **Br J Psychiatry** 1980;137:105–10
**Langley HD:** Edward Field: a pioneer practitioner of the old Navy. **Conn Med** 1982 Nov;46(11):667–72
**Langley HD:** Respect for civilian authority: the tragic career of Captain Angus. **Am Neptune** 1980;40(1):23–37
**Langmuir A** see **Eyler JM**
**Langner SR, Innes C:** Breathing, holism, and health. **Top Clin Nurs** 1980 Oct;2(3):1–10
**Langs R:** The psychotherapeutic conspiracy. New York, Aronson, 1982. xiii, 338 p.
**Langs R, ed:** Classics in psychoanalytic technique. New York, London, Jason Aronson, 1981. xii, 523 p. Contains 44 papers from various authors.
**Langsley DG:** Community psychiatry. In H. I. Kaplan, et al, ed: Comprehensive textbook of psychiatry/III. Third edition. Baltimore, London, Williams and Wilkins, 1980. p. 2836–54.
**Langston HT:** The first successful total repair of congenital atresia of the esophagus with tracheoesophageal fistula. **Ann Thorac Surg** 1984 Jul;38(1):72–4
**Langton J, Laxton P:** Parish registers and urban structure: the example of late-eighteenth century Liverpool. **Urban Hist Yearb** 1978:74–84
**Lankford ND:** The Victorian medical profession and military practice: army doctors and national origins. **Bull Hist Med** 1980 Winter;54(4):511–28
**Lansing DI, Penman WR, Davis DJ:** Puerperal fever and the Group B beta hemolytic streptococcus. **Bull Hist Med** 1983;57(1):70–80
**Lansing DI:** The coroner system and some ot its coroners in early Pennsylvania. **Trans Stud Coll Physicians Phila** 1977 Jan;44(3):135–40
**Lansing DI** see **Gifford GE**
**Lanteri-Laura G:** La constitution civile du cerveau. **Rev Int Hist Psychiatr** 1983;1(1):23–45
**Lanteri-Laura G:** Lecture des perversions: histoire de leur appropriation médicale. Paris, New York, Masson, 1979. 160 p.
**Lanteri Laura G:** L'hystérie. Matrice de la sémiologie neurologique. In Poirier J, Poirier JL, ed: Médecine et philosophie à la fin du XIXe siècle. Paris, Université de Paris XII - Val de Marne, [1980?]. p. 141–8.
**Lanthony P:** Daltonisme et peinture. **Bull Soc Ophtalmol Fr** 1982 Apr;82(4):509–13
**Lanthony P:** Daltonisme et peinture. **J Fr Ophtalmol** 1982;5(6–7):373–85
**Lantos PL:** Changing images of the brain. **Psychol Med** 1983 May;13(2):255–6
**Lanza B** see **Azzaroli ML**
**Lanzavecchia P, Lingua P, Sinigaglia G:** La popolazione manicomiale di Alessandria nella seconda metà dell'ottocento. **Mov Operaio Soc** 1980;3(4):405–22
**Lanzl EF, ed** see **Mhoon EE**
**Laor N:** Old whig psychiatry: the Szaszian variant. **Isr J Psychiatr Relat Sci** 1982;19(3):215–27
**Laor N:** Szasz, Feuchtersleben, and the history of psychiatry. **Psychiatry** 1982;45(4):316–24
**Laor N:** The myth of mental illness: the Feuchtersleben version. **Gesnerus** 1984;41(1/2):3–32
**LaPonna L:** La psychohistory: proposte e studi nella storiografia americana. **Quad Stor** 1981;16(2):574–605
**Lapière CM** see **Gielen JE**
**Lapiere CM** see **Pierard GE**
**Laplane R** see **Huard P**
**Laporte LF:** Simpson's Tempo and Mode in Evolution revisited. **Proc Am Philos Soc** 1983 Dec 30;127(6):365–417
**Laporte Y:** La sensibilité récurrente des racines rachidiennes antérieures. **Hist Sci Med** 1983;17(4):351–5
**Lapresle J:** La dystasie aréflexique héréditaire de Roussy-Lévy. Ses rapports historiques avec la maladie de Friedreich, l'atrophie Charcot-Marie=Tooth et la névrite hypertrophique de Dejerine-Sottas; l'état actuel de la famille originale; la place nosologique de cette entité. **Rev Neurol (Paris)** 1982;138(12):967–78
**Lara-Terrazas A, Ortega A, Gutiérrez A, et al:** El fenómeno de acoplamiento-excitación-contracción y relajacion cardíaca. Análisis retrospectivo. **Arch Inst Cardiol Mex** 1983 Jul-Aug;53(4):373–8
**Laragh JH:** Concept of anti-renin system therapy. Historic perspective. **Am J Med** 1984 Aug 20;77(2A):1–6
**Larcan A:** Le médecin inspecteur F. C. Maillot. In: Congrès National des Sociétés Savantes, 103e, Nancy, 1978. Comptes Rendus. Paris, 1978. Section des Sciences, Fasc. V. p. 19–30.
**Lardies González J:** Panorama historico de la psiquiatria argentina. **Asclepio** 1981;33:251–64
**Lardies González J** see **Pennini de Vega E**
**Lardinois R:** Une conjoncture de crise démographique en Indé du Sud au XIXe siècle: la famine de 1876–1878. **Population** 1982;37(2):371–404
**Lareng L** see **Fabre M**
**Largillière A:** Madeleine Pelletier, femme, médecin, féministe. **Penelope** 1981;(5):68–72
**Larner C:** Enemies of God: the witch-hunt in Scotland. Baltimore, Johns Hopkins Univ. Press, 1981. x, 244 p.
**Larocque R:** Les maladies chez les Iroquoiens pré-historique. **Rech Amerindiennes Que Bull Inf** 1980;10(3):165–80
**Larocque R:** L'introduction de maladies européennes chez les autochtones des XVIIe et XVIIIe siècles. **Rech Amerindiennes Que Bull Inf** 1982;12(1):13–24
**LaRose A:** Bibliographie courante sur l'histoire de la population canadienne et la démographie historique au Canada, 1977. **Soc Hist (Canada)** 1979;12(23):192–7
**Larose R:** The growth and development of the pharmaceutical industry in Montreal. **Can Pharm J** 1984;117:74–7
**Larose A, ed** see **Charbonneau H**
**Larsen A** see **Jensen OM**
**Larsen L** see **Willis FN**
**Larsen O:** Die Krankheitsauffassung und ihre historische Interpretation. Ein Auswertungsmodell aufgrund von norwegischen Medizinalberichten aus dem 19. Jahrhundert. In Imhof AE, ed: Mensch und Gesundheit in der Geschichte. Husum, Matthiesen, 1980. p. 45–58.
**Larsen O:** Eighteenth century diseases. Diagnostical trends and mortality. **Scand Popul Stud** 1979;5
**Larsen O:** Fårlig a vaere barneår og livesjanser. [Dangers of childhood--life prospects] (Nor). **Forskningsnytt (Norway)** 1979;24(4):14–9
**Larsen O:** Hundre år med sykdomsoppfatningen og dens konsekvenser. **Tidsskr Nor Laegeforen** 1981 Jan;101(1):11–4
**Larsen O:** Leben auf dem Lande: dem Körper nicht nur förderlich. In Imhof AE, ed: Leib und Leben in der Geschichte der Neuzeit. Berlin, Duncker & Humblot, 1983. p. 53–62.
**Larsen O** see **Habrich C**
**Larson JL:** An alternative science, Linnaean natural history in Germany, 1770–1790. **Janus** 1979;66(4):267–83
**Larsson E:** Malocclusions in a juvenile medieval skull material. **Swed Dent J** 1983;7(5):185–90
**Larsson J:** Hermann Boerhaave och 1700-talets Lund. **Sydsven Medicinhist Sallsk Arsskr** 1981;:53–64
**Larsson J:** Kirurgi och medicinsk teori vid Lunds Universitet under 1700-talet. En medicinhistorisk studie. (Supplementum nr 1). **Sydsven Medicinhist Sallsk Arsskr** 1982;Suppl V:1–262
**Lasagna L:** Analgesic methodology: a brief history and commentary. **J Clin Pharmacol** 1980 May-Jun;20(5–6 Pt 2):373–6
**Lasagna LC, Lindzey G:** Marijuana policy and drug mythology. **Society** 1983;20(2):67–78
**Lascaratos JG** see **Pentogalos GE**
**Lasch EE** see **Goldblum N**
**Lash JP:** Helen Keller. In: Notable American women. The modern period. Cambridge, Mass., Belknap-Harvard Univ. Press, 1980. 4:389–93.
**Lasiński W:** Achievements of the Polish morphology in 35 years of the Polish People's Republic. **Folia Morphol (Warsz)** 1981;40(3):205–16
**Lasky II:** A most benevolent Victorian (Sir Arthur Conan Doyle). **Md State Med J** 1982 Dec;31(12):22–4
**Lasky II:** Autopsy of Admiral John Paul Jones 113 years postmortem; historic and forensic aspects. **NY State J Med** 1982 Jun;82(7):1110–5
**Lasky II:** John Hunter, the Shakespeare of medicine. **Surg Gynecol Obstet** 1983 Apr;156(4):511–8
**Lasky II:** Medicine and music. **NY State J Med** 1982 Dec;82(13):1862–4
**Laslett P, Oosterveen K, Smith RM, ed:** Bastardy and its comparative history. Cambridge, Mass., Harvard University Press, 1980. xv, 431 p. Contributions by Y. Blayo, D. Gaunt, S. Hartley, A. Hayami, S. Hochstadt, A. S. Kälvemark, J. Knodel, D. Levine, A. Newman, A. Macfarlane, M. R. Matovic, J. Meyer, D. S. Smith, C. Smout, S. Stewart, E. van de Walle, R. V. Wells, K. Wrightson
**Laslett P:** The centrality of demographic experience. **Proc Annu Symp Eugen Soc** 1981;16:23–40
**Laslett P** see **Marshall TH**
**Lassen A:** Befolkningsudviklingen i Danmark 1660–1769. **Jyske Saml** 1960;5(2):173–97
**Lassig HE:** Etruskische Zahnärzte entwickelten eine sehr beachtliche Prothetik. **Zahnarztl Mitt** 1984 Sep 16;74(18):2015–9
**L'assistance médicale pendant 50 ans de Protectorat: Dr Mahmoud El Matri:** 'La Voie due Tunisien' le 11 mars 1931. **Tunis Med** 1982 Nov-Dec;60(6):378–9
**The last word:** Rabies control in olden times. **Mod Vet Pract** 1981 Dec;62(12):962
**Lastkov OA** see **Vankhanen VD**
**László G** see **Lénárt G**
**Laszlo J:** Two long-range clinical data bases are terminated: bang, whimper, or ripple? **J Clin Oncol** 1984 May;2(5):532–3

Latapí F, Ortiz Y: Historia de la dermatología en México. In Academia Nacional de Medicina. Libro conmemorativo del primer centenario. México, Comité Editorial de la Comisión Organizadora del Congreso del Centenario, 1964. Tome 2. p. 565–92.
Latapí F see Saúl A
Later-Chodyłowa E: Psychospołeczne podstawy więzi polonii z krajem pochodzenia. Przegl Zachod 1980;36(3):38–70
Latham AJ: Witchcraft accusations and economic tension in precolonial old Calabar. J Afr Hist 1972;13(2):249–60
Lathrop M see Lamblin-Robert J
Laties VG: I. V. Zavadskii and the beginnings of behavioral pharmacology: an historical note and translation. J Exp Anal Behav 1979 Nov;32(3):463–72
Latimer D, Goldberg J: Flowers in the blood; the story of opium. New York, Franklin Watts, 1981. 306 p.
Lattanzi A see Baldacci G
Lattimer GL: Legionnaires' disease legacies. JAMA 1980 Nov 28;244(21):2416
Lattimer JK: Lincoln did not have the Marfan Syndrome; documented evidence. NY State J Med 1981 Nov;81(12):1805–13
Lattimore MI: Early naval medical libraries, personal and corporate. J R Nav Med Serv 1983 Summer;69(2):107–11
Lattimore MI: Early naval medical libraries, personal and corporate. J R Nav Med Serv 1983 Winter;69(3):156–60
Lattimore MI: Sir David James Hamilton Dickson, MD (1780–1850). J R Nav Med Serv 1981;67(2):92–100
Lau I, ed see Spitzy KH, ed
Laubach GD: Federal regulation and pharmaceutical innovation. Proc Acad Polit Sci 1980;33(4):60–80
Laudan L: Progress and its problems. Toward a theory of scientific growth. Berkeley, Univ. of California Press, 1977. x, 257 p.
Laudan L, ed see Cohen RS
Lauer DJ: T. Lyle Hazlett: his role in industrial medicine, 1920–50. JOM 1979 Jun;21(6):403–6
Lauer HH: Ethik und ärztliches Denken im arabischen Mittelalter. In Seidler E, Schott H, ed: Bausteine zur Medizingeschichte. Stuttgart, Steiner, 1984. p. 72–86.
Laufman H: Carl Walter's half century of achievement in asepsis. Am J Surg 1984 Nov;148(5):565–70
Laufman H: Loyal Davis and the young surgeon. Surg Gynecol Obstet 1983 Aug;157(2):123–8
Laugher SJ see Jack DB
Laughlin JS: AAPM and RAMPS--antecedents and perspectives. Med Phys 1983 Jul–Aug;10(4):387–94
Laughlin WS, Harper AB, Thompson DD: New approaches to the pre- and post-contact history of Arctic peoples. Am J Phys Anthropol 1979 Nov;51(4):579–87
Laughlin WS, Harper AB, ed: The first Americans: origins, affinities, and adaptations. New York and Stuttgart, Fischer, 1979. xi, 340 p.
Laughlin WS see Harper AB
Laugier P, Burgun R: Die Geschichte der Geschlechtskrankheiten. In Sournia JC, Martiny M, Poulet J, ed: Illustrierte Geschichte der Medizin. Salzburg, Andreas, 1980. Vol. 4. p. 1483–516.
Laugier P see Burgun R
Laundon JR: The date of birth of Sir John Hill (1714–1775). Arch Nat Hist 1981 Apr;10(1):65–6
Laur WE: Christian science visited. South Med J 1980 Jan;73(1):71–4
Laur WE: Shave and a haircut--two sesterces: a brief account of men and their hair in Imperial Rome. Int J Dermatol 1981 Sep;20(7U):504–5
Laurell AC, et al: Enfermedad y desarrollo: análisis sociológico de la morbilidad en dos pueblos mexicanos. Rev Mex Cienc Polit Soc 1976;22(84):131–58
Lauren K see Seeman K
Laurence DR: Medicines then and now. Nature 1981 Sep 3;293(5827):13–5
Laurence JR, Perry C: Forensic hypnosis in the late nineteenth century. Int J Clin Exp Hypn 1983 Oct;31(4):266–83
Laurenti H: Une thèse de médecine sur Paul Valéry. Bull Etud Valeryennes 1980;(25):5–7
Laurig W: Feiert der Begriff 'Ergonomie' 1982 seinen 125. Geburtstag? Zentralbl Arbeitsmed Arbeitsschutz Prophyl Ergonomie 1982 Sep;32(9):341–4
Lauschke HP: Der Epileptologe Herrmann Andreas Reimer in Görlitz. Psychiatr Neurol Med Psychol (Leipz) 1982 Dec;34(12):745–8
Lauschner EA: The beginnings of aviation medicine in Germany. Aviat Space Environ Med 1984 May;55(5):355–7
Lauter H, Meyer JE: Mercy killing without consent. Historical comments on a controversial issue. Acta Psychiatr Scand 1982 Feb;65(2):134–41
Lautmann R: The pink triangle. The persecution of homosexual males in concentration camps in Nazi Germany. J Homosex 1980–81 Fall–Winter;6(1–2):141–60
Lavagne X, ed see Linet J
Laval E: Los alumnos del curso de medicina de 1833. Rev Med Chil 1984 Jan;112(1):65–71
Lavaque RJ: Botica publica de la capital de Don Felipe Vicente Reynoso. Bol Soc Esp Hist Farm 1983 Mar–Jun;34(133–134):35–7
Lavat P see Bonnin P
Lave JR, Silverman HA: Financing the health care of the aged. Ann Am Acad Polit Soc Sci 1983;(468):149–64
Lavely WR: The rural Chinese fertility transition: a report from Shifang Xian, Sichuan. Popul Stud 1984 Nov;38(3):365–84
Lavenne F: L'electrocardiographie et vectocardiographie. Rev Inst Hyg Mines (Hasselt) 1980;35(3):133–4
Laveran CL: Classics in infectious diseases: A newly discovered parasite in the blood of patients suffering from malaria. Parasitic etiology of attacks of malaria: Charles Louis Alphonse Laveran (1845–1922). Rev Infect Dis 1982 Jul–Aug;4(4):908–11
Laverychev VI: Gosudarstvenno-monopolisticheskie tendentsii pri organizatsii prodovol'stvennogo dela v Rossii (1914–fevral' 1917 g). Istor Zap Acad Nauk SSSR 1978;101:100–59
Laverychev VI: Krupnaia burzhuaziia i prodovol'stvennyi vopros v 1917 g. Istor Filol Zh 1977;99:312–21
Lavie P: Nasal obstructions, sleep, and mental function. Sleep 1983;6(3):244–6
Lavie P: Nothing new under the moon. Historical accounts of sleep apnea syndrome. Arch Intern Med 1984 Oct;144(10):2025–8
Lavoie R see Sutto C, ed
Lavoie Y see Mayer FM
Lavorel P see Signoret JL
Lavrik SS: Podgotovka vrachebnykh kadrov v Kievskom meditsinskom institute. Vrach Delo 1982 Jun;(6):5–9
Lavrik SS, Pogrebinskiĭ MB: Traditsii vuza i formirovanie kachestv sovetskogo vracha. Sov Zdravookhr 1981;(2):46–51
Lavrov BA: Ocherki po istorii sovetskoĭ vitaminologii, 1917–1967. Moskva, Meditsina, 1980. 199 p.
Law A see Freeman FW
Lawless DS: On Shakespeare's death, funeral, and burial. Notes Queries 1980 Apr;27(2):176–7
Lawrence C: Alfred Henry Garrod and the indirect measurement of the isometric period of the heart's contraction. Med Hist 1980 Jul;24(3):342–6
Lawrence C: Sanitary reformers and the medical profession in Victorian England. In Ogawa T, ed: Public health. Tokyo, Saikon, 1981. p. 145–68.
Lawrence C: Wellcome revisited. Nurs Times 1982 Dec 8–14;78(49):2089–90
Lawrence HS: An appreciation: notes of a Lewis Thomas-Watcher. Cell Immunol 1983 Nov;82(1):139–43
Lawrence HW: Southern spas: source of the American resort tradition. Landscape 1983;27(2):1–12
Lawrence M: Otologic research and the Zeitgeist. Ear Hear 1983 Mar–Apr;4(2):73–8
Lawrence SV: Modern ideas mix with history. Forum Med 1978 Nov;1(8):14–9
Lawrence W Jr: The scope of surgical oncology. Aust NZ J Surg 1982 Aug;52(4):325–30
Lawry JD: Guide to the history of psychology. Totowa, N. J., Littlefield, Adams, 1981. xi, 114 p.
Laws ER: Functional pituitary tumors. The neurosurgeon and neuroendocrinology. Clin Neurosurg 1980;27:3–18
Lawson I see Trautmann J, ed
Lawton H: The myth of altruism: a psychohistory of public agency social work. J Psychohist 1982 Winter;9(3):265–308
Laxenaire M, Marchand P: L'anorexie mentale a-t-elle changé? Ann Med Psychol (Paris) 1982 Apr;140(4):448–53
Laxton P see Langton J
Lay midwifery--still an 'illegal' profession: Women Health 1977 Nov–Dec;2(3):19–26
Layne GS: The Kirkbride-Langenheim collaboration: early use of photography in psychiatric treatment in Philadelphia. Pa Mag Hist Biogr 1981;105(2):182–202
Layzer D see Tobach E
Lazăr C, Ionescu C: Istoricul chirurgiei toraco-pulmonare din Moldova. Rev Med Chir Soc Med Nat Iasi 1980 Jul–Sept;84(3):575–7
Lázár Szini K: Adalékok a XVI. századi Ars Medica vizsgálatához. Orvostort Kozl 1982;92(4):133–46
Lazard M see Margolin JC
Lazer C see Cumming E
Lazo B see Villarroel H
Lazorthes G, Campan L: François Magendie (1783–1855). Bull Acad Natl Med (Paris) 1984 Jan–Feb;168(1–2):105–11
Lazorthes G, Campan L: Jean-Baptiste Morgagni (1682–1771), initiateur de la méthode anatomo-clinique. Bull Acad Natl Med (Paris) 1982 Dec;166(9):1317–21
Le Blevec D: Aux origines des hospitaliers de Saint-Jean de Jérusalem: Gérard dit 'Tenque' et l'établissement de l'Ordre dans le Midi. Ann Midi 1977;89:137–51
Le Bras H see Dupâquier J
Le Breton D: Apothicaires et moines à Bordeaux à la fin de l'Ancien Régime. Diss., Université de Bordeaux, II, 1983. 131 leaves.
'Le chirurgien-dentiste' di Pierre Fauchard, I and II: Dent Cadmos 1980 May;48(5):57–60, (6):53–7
Le Duigou D see Doby JM
Le Fanu W: Natural history drawings collected by John Hunter F.R.S. (1728–1793), at the Royal College of Surgeons of England. J Soc Bibliogr Nat Hist 1978;8(4):329–33
Le Fanu W see Ebbert A, et al
Le Fichoux Y, Marty P, Denis G, et al: Un ca d'ophtalmomyiase externe à oestrus ovis, linné, 1758 contractée sur la plage de Nice. Acta Trop (Basel) 1981 Dec;38(4):461–8
Le Goff A: La paroisse de Saint-Hélier de Rennes et sa démographie de 1711 à 1790. In Congrès National des Sociétés Savantes, 97e, Nantes, 1972. Actes. Paris, 1977. Tome II, p. 153–63.
Le Goff J see Guillemain B
Le Grand HE: Chemistry in a provincial context: the Montpellier Société Royale des Sciences in the eighteenth century. Ambix 1982

Jul;29(2):88–105
**Le Guen Y:** Etre infirmier en psychiatrie. **Rev Infirm** 1980 Nov;30(9):19–22
**Le Minor JM:** Origine et développement des pharmacies de l'arrondissement de Molsheim.
**Soc d'Hist d'Archeol Molsheim environs Annu** 1982;:129–44
**Le mouvement historique:** Bibliographie internationale d'histoire de la pharmacie et des sciences connexes. **Rev Hist Pharm (Paris)** 1982 Mar;29(252):60–76 (continued regularly)
**Le patrimoine hospitalier en Bourgogne: Bull Soc Fr Hist Hop** 1979;(39):8–9
**Le Roux JM:** Beskouings oor die Fakulteit Veeartsenykunde, Universiteit van Pretoria. **J S Afr Vet Assoc** 1982 Sep;53(4):136–40
**Le Scouëzec G:** La médecine en Gaule. Guipavas, Kelenn, 1976, 204 p.
**Le Tacon J:** La pleuroscopie. Rappel historique. **Poumon Coeur** 1981 Jan–Feb;37(1):5–6
**Le Traité de matière médicale de Dioscoride à la Renaissance:** Exposition d'exemplaires des XVe et XVIe siecles. Du 11 au 24 février 1984 à Louvain-en-Woluwe à la Bibliothèque de la Faculté de Médecine de l'U.C.L. Louvain, Université Catholique de Louvain, Centre d'Histoire de la Pharmacie et du Médicament, 1984. 40 p.
**Le Winn EB:** The steroidal actions of digitalis. **Perspect Biol Med** 1984;27(2):183–99
**Le 75e anniversaire de l'association des infirmières et infirmiers du Canada: Infirm Can** 1983 Oct;25(9):17–38
**Leach DH, Dagg AI:** Evolution of equine locomotion research. **Equine Vet J** 1983 Apr;15(2):87–92
**Leach RD:** Sir Gilbert Blane, Bart, MD FRS (1749–1832). **Ann R Coll Surg Engl** 1980 May;62(3):232–9
**Leadbeater B** see **Broughton JM**
**Leader JP:** The Pottawatomies and alcohol: an illustration of the illegal trade. **Kans Hist** 1979;2(3):157–65
**Leahey TH:** A history of psychology: main currents in psychological thought. Englewood Cliffs, Prentice-Hall, 1980. xii, 431 p.
**Leahey TH:** The mistaken mirror: on Wundt's and Titchener's psychologies. **J Hist Behav Sci** 1981;17:273–82
**Leahy PJ, Mazur A:** The rise and fall of public opposition in specific social movements. **Soc Stud Sci** 1980 Aug 3;10(3):259–84
**Leake ES:** The Henry Phipps Institute: recollections of a foreign research fellow. **Trans Stud Coll Physicians Phila** 1981 Dec;5(3 no 4):256–63
**Leakey RE** see **Hamrum CL, ed**
**Leakey RE** see **Walker A**
**Leaman A:** John Snow MD--his early days. **Anaesthesia** 1984 Aug;39(8):803–5
**Lear J:** Recombinant DNA: the untold story. New York, Crown, 1978. 280 p.
**Learmonth AT:** Reflections of the regional geography of disease in late colonial South Asia. **Soc Sci Med [Med Geogr]** 1980 Sep;14D(3):271–6
**Learning to deal with life and death: the story of becoming a doctor in Texas.: Tex Med** 1980 May;76(5):53–68
**Leary DE:** German idealism and the development of psychology in the nineteenth century. **J Hist Philos** 1980;18(3):299–317
**Leary DE:** Nature, art, and imitation: the Wild Boy of Aveyeron as a pivotal case in the history of psychology. **Stud Eighteenth Cult** 1984;13:155–72
**Leary DE:** The historical foundation of Herbart's mathematization of psychology. **J Hist Behav Sci** 1980 Apr;16(2):150–63
**Leary DE:** The psychology of Jakob Friedrich Fries (1773–1843): its context, nature, and historical significance. **Stor Crit Psicol** 1982 Dec;3(2):217–48
**Leasure JW:** La baisse de la fécondité aux Etats-Unis de 1800 à 1860. **Population** 1982;37(3):607–22
**Leasure JW** see **Bolton C**
**Leatham A:** Auscultation of the heart since Laënnec. **Thorax** 1981 Feb;36(2):95–8
**Leatherman GH:** Dentistry as I have seen it--1920 to 1984. **Br Dent J** 1984 Aug 25;157(4):141–6
**Leatherman GH:** Martin Rushton--the man, 1903 to 1970. **Br Dent J** 1983 Nov 5;155(9):315–7
**Leatherman GH:** The FDI: 1900–1980. **Probe (Lond)** 1981 Jul;23(1):5–10 (continued)
**Leatherman GH:** 80 Jahre FDI--eine Chronik moderner Gesundheitspolitik. **Zahnarztliche Mitteilungen** 1980 Sep 1;70(17):1070–9
**Leatherman GH:** 80 Jahre FDI-- 'Erntejahre' 1962–1980. **Zahnarztliche Mitteilungen** 1980 Nov 1;70(21):1392–7 concl
**Leatherman GH:** 80 Jahre FDI--1900–1980. Aktivitäten der Kommissionen 1962–1979. **Zahnarztliche Mitteilungen** 1980 Oct 16;70(20):1313–7 contd
**Leatherman GH:** 80 Jahre FDI--1900–1980. Die Zeit des Wiederaufbaus und der Reformen. **Zahnarztliche Mitteilungen** 1980 Sep 16;70(18):1172–8 contd
**Leatherman GH:** 80 years of the FDI. **Probe (Lond)** 1981 Aug;23(2):53–4 contd.
**Leatherman GH:** 80 years of the FDI. **Probe (Lond)** 1981 Oct;23(4):155–6, 161, Nov;23(5):203, 205–6, 208
**Leavesley J:** A history of general practice. **Med J Aust** 1984 Jul 21;141(2):107–9
**Leavesley J:** Cholera. **Med J Aust** 1984 Nov 10;141(10):659–61
**Leavesley J:** Malaria. **Med J Aust** 1984 Oct 13;141(8):523–5
**Leavitt DM:** Darwinism in the Arab world: the Lewis affair at the Syrian Protestant College. **Muslim World** 1981;71(2):85–98
**Leavitt JW:** Birthing and anesthesia: the debate over twilight sleep. **Signs** 1980;6(1):147–64
**Leavitt JW:** Health in urban Wisconsin: from bad to better. In Numbers RL, Leavitt JW, ed: Wisconsin medicine. Historical perspectives. Madison, University of Wisconsin Press, 1981. p. 155–75.
**Leavitt JW:** Politics and public health: small pox in Milwaukee, 1894–1895. In Reverby S, Rosner D, ed: Health care in America. Philadephia, Temple University Press, 1979. p. 84–101.
**Leavitt JW:** Public Health in Milwaukee 1867-1910. Ph.D. Diss., University of Chicago. Chicago, 1975. 363 leaves.
**Leavitt JW:** 'Science' enters the birthing room: obstetrics in America since the eighteenth century. **J Am Hist** 1983;70(2):281–304
**Leavitt JW, Numbers RL, ed:** Sickness and health in America. Readings in the history of medicine and public health. Madison, University of Wisconsin Press, 1978. ix, 454 p. Reprinted articles by various authors.
**Leavitt JW:** The healthiest city: Milwaukee and the politics of health reform. Princeton, Princeton University Press, 1982. xvii, 294 p.
**Leavitt JW:** The wasteland: garbage and sanitary reform in the nineteenth-century American city. **J Hist Med Allied Sci** 1980 Oct;35(4):431–52
**Leavitt JW:** Writing public health history: the need for a social scaffolding. **Rev Am Hist** 1976;4(2):150–7
**Leavitt JW** see **Numbers RL, ed**
**Leavitt JW, ed:** Women and health in America: historical readings. Madison, University of Wisconsin Press, 1984. ix, 526 p. (Previously published articles by various authors)
**Leavitt JW, ed** see **Numbers RL**
**Leavy BF:** Fathering and the British Mother's Magazine, 1845-1864. **Victorian Period Rev** 1980;13(1–2):10–7
**Lebedev BI:** O nekotorykh parasitologicheskikh uchrezhdeniaikh Iaaponii. **Parazitologiia** 1981 Jul–Aug;15(4):388–91
**Lebedev DD, Kovaleva EV, Semenova VN:** Nekotorye voprosy revmatizma, éndokrinnykh i nervnykh zabolevaniĭ u deteĭ v trudakh V.I. Molchanova i ego uchenikov (k 110-letiiu so dnia rozhdeniia). **Pediatriia** 1980 Aug;(8):64–7
**Lebedev KV:** Iz istorii Kazanskoĭ fiziologicheskoĭ shkoly. Kazan', Izd-vo Kazanskogo universiteta, 1978. 246 p.
**Lebedev NI:** Epidemicheskie posledstviia nemetsko-fashistkoĭ okkupatsii Belorussii v 1941–1944 gg. i mery po ikh likvidatsii.
**Zh Mikrobiol Epidemiol Immunobiol** 1982 Jul;(7):106–10
**Lebedev NI:** Istoricheskie preimushchestva sovetskoĭ épidemiologii v teorii i praktike profilaktiki infektsionnykh bolezneĭ.
**Zh Mikrobiol Epidemiol Immunobiol** 1981 Feb;(2):3–6
**Lebedev VV** see **Zefirova GS**
**Lebedeva NV** see **Shirokov IuG**
**Lebedkina ED:** International contacts of Soviet scientists during 1917–1924. **Sov Stud Hist** 1971–72;10(3):267–86
**Lebel M:** Editions, traductions et lexiques hippocratiques. Le docteur Louis Morin, (1635–1715) et son index des mots d'Hippocrate. In: Congrès international d'histoire de la médecine, XXVe, Québec, 1976. Actes. Québec, 1977. p. 848–65.
**Leblancné Kelemen M:** Adalékok a reformkori Nógrád megye egészségügyi helyzetéröl Baintner Ferenc megyei föorvos jelentései alapján. **Orvostort Kozl** 1979;87–88(25 no 1–2):269–75
**Leblond S:** James Douglas. In Dictionary of Canadian biography, 1881–1890. 1982;11:271–2.
**Leblond S:** Le Dr James Douglas, de Québec, remonté le Nil en 1860–61. **Cah Dix** 1979;42:101–23
**Leblond S:** Le mal de la baie était-il syphilis? In: Congrès international d'histoire de la médecine, XXVe, Québec, 1976. Actes. Québec, 1977. p. 866–72.
**Leboutte R:** Conditions d'hygiène et salubrité publique au siècle dernier. Neuf cents ans de vie autour de Saint Remacle au Pont, Liège, Soledi, 1979, p. 177–223.
**Leboutte R:** D'Austerlitz à Liège, mourir dans les armées de Bonaparte. **Tijdschr Geschied Geneeskd** 1978;91(3):429–46
**Leboutte R:** Les métaux et l'hygiène alimentaire: la vaisselle en zinc de l'abbé Dony. **Bull Soc R Vieux Liege** 1977–79;9:311–3
**Leboutte R:** L'infanticide dans l'est de la Belgique aux XVIIIe-XIXe siècles: une réalité. **Ann Demogr Hist (Paris)** 1983;:163–92
**Lebovici S:** Jacques Lacan and French psychiatry. **Psychol Med** 1983 Feb;13(1):9–13
**Lebovici S:** L'oeuvre D'Anna Freud (1895–1982). **Psychiatr Enfant** 1984;27(1):5–34
**LeBras H, Dinet D:** Mortalité des laïcs et mortalité des religieux: les Bénédictins de Saint-Maur aux XVIIe et XVIIIe siècles. **Population** 1980;35(2):347–83
**Lebrun F:** La grande dysenterie de 1779. **Histoire** 1981;39:17–24
**Lebrun F:** Les crises démographiques en France aux XVIIe et XVIIIe siècles. **Ann Econ Soc Civilis** 1980;35(2):205–34
**Lebrun F:** L'intervention des autorités face aux crises de mortalité dans la France d'ancien régime. In Imhof AE, ed: Leib und Leben in der Geschichte der Neuzeit. Berlin, Duncker & Humblot, 1983. p. 39–52.
**Lebrun F:** Quand un enfant sur deux mourait. **Histoire** 1982;42:78–81
**Lebrun F:** Se soigner autrefois. Médecins saints et sorciers aux 17e et 18e siècles. Paris, Temps Actuels, 1983. 206 p. (La passion de l'histoire).
**Lebrun M** see **Hélin E**
**Lebrun Y** see **Riese W**
**Lebzeltern G:** Ein vielsagender Irrtum S. Freuds.
**Z Klin Psychol Psychother** 1982;30(1):25–30
**Lebzeltern G:** Eine interessante Fehlleistung S. Freuds.
**Z Klin Psychol Psychother** 1980;28(1):14–20
**Lebzeltern G:** S. Freud und das Kokain. **Wien Klin Wochenschr** 1983 Nov 11;95(21):765–9

**Leca AP:** Die Medizin im Alten Agypten. In Sournia JC, Martiny M, Poulet J, ed: Illustrierte Geschichte der Medizin. Salzburg, Andreas, 1980. Vol. 1. p. 109–43.
**Lechat MF:** The International Leprosy Association at 50 years. **Int J Lepr** 1981 Mar;49(1):60–4
**Lechevalier HA:** The search for antibiotics at Rutgers University. In J. Parascandola, ed: The history of antibiotics. Madison, American Institute of the History of Pharmacy, 1980. p. 113–23.
**Lechner-Knecht S:** Ayurveda-Wissen vom langen Leben. Eine altindische 'Offenbarungsmedizin'. **Med Klin** 1979 Dec 14;74(50):1938–42
**Lechtenböhmer S:** Die Dissertationen aus dem Institut für Pathologie der Tierärztlichen Hochschule Hannover seit Erteilung des Promotionsrechtes im Jahre 1910 bis Ende 1980. Diss., Tierärzliche Hochschule Hannover. Hannover, 1983. 162 p.
**Leclainche E:** Die Tierheilkunde in der Antike. In Sournia JC, Martiny M, Poulet J, ed: Illustrierte Geschichte der Medizin. Salzburg, Andreas, 1980. Vol. 2. p. 539–87.
**Leclainche E:** Die Veterinärmedizin vom Mittelalter bis zum Ende des 18. Jahrhunderts. In Sournia JC, Martiny M, Poulet J, ed: Illustrierte Geschichte der Medizin. Salzburg, Andreas, 1980. Vol. 5. p. 1779–1827.
**Leclant J** see **Forster R**
**Leclercq-Kadaner J:** Physiologus de naturis animalium et bestiarum. Fédération des Cercles d'Archéologie et d'Histoire de Belgique. 44e session. Congrès de Huy, 1976. Annales. Tielt, 1978. p. 790–5
**L'ecole de soins infirmiers du CHUV:** Un cinquantenaire abondamment fêté. **Krankenpflege (Bern)** 1982 Aug;(8):73–4
**Lecomte D** see **Lamblin-Robert J**
**Lecomte J:** Apologie de Zénon Bacq 1903–1983. **Rev Med Liege** 1983 Sep 1;38(17):627–30
**Lecomte J:** L'acupuncture: approche historique et applications. **Cah Clio** 1981;67:17–21
**Lecomte J, Schoffeniels E:** L'oeuvre de Léon Frédéricq et son école (1853–1934) à travers les Archives de Biologie (1880–1904). **Arch Biol (Liege)** 1980;91(2):267–70
**Lecomte J, Bacq ZM:** Physiologie animale et humaine. In Florilège des Sciences en Belgique - II. Bruxelles Académie Royale de Belgique, 1980. p. 273–86.
**Lecomte J:** Sur l'homéopathie. **Rev Med Liege** 1980 May 1;35(9):354–62
**Lecomte MC:** Les enfants trouvés d'après les archives du bureau des pauvres de Chartres, de 1780 à 1792. Mém. de Maîtrise, Univ. de Tours, 1976. vii, 195 p.
**Lecuir J:** La médicalisation de la société français dans la deuxième moitié du 18e siècle en France: aux origin premiers traités de médecine légale. **Ann Bretagne** 1979;86(3):231–50
**Leden H von:** Laryngology: from Galen to Garcia. **Otolaryngol Head Neck Surg** 1982 Mar–Apr;90(2):226–32
**Leden I:** Antimalarial drugs--350 years. **Scand J Rheumatol** 1981;10(4):307–12
**Leden I:** Doubts about Sandro Botticelli's depiction of juvenile rheumatoid arthritis. **Arthritis Rheum** 1984 Oct;27(10):1197–8
**Leden I:** Kinabark--en historisk återblick. **Sydsven Medicinhist Sallsk Arsskr** 1980;:80–93
**Leden I:** Ledgångsreumatism och gikt - en historisk återblick. **Sydsven Medicinhist Sallsk Arsskr** 1981;:65–97
**Leden I:** Reumatologisk farmakoterapi ur historiskt/filatelistiskt perspektiv. **Lakartidningen** 1980 Dec 24;77(52):4943–6
**Leder A** see **Kraus A, ed**
**Lederberg J:** Edward Lawrie Tatum. **Annu Rev Genet** 1979;13:1–5
**Lederer SE:** 'The right and wrong of making experiments on human beings': Udo J. Wile and syphilis. **Bull Hist Med** 1984 Fall;58(3):380–97
**Lederer SE** see **Keeney EB**
**Lederman M:** The early history of radiotherapy: 1895–1939. **Int J Radiat Oncol Biol Phys** 1981 May;7(5):639–48
**Ledermann F:** El precio de los medicamentos en el canton de Neuchatel y en Suiza: 1930–1960. **Bol Soc Esp Hist Farm** 1982 Sep;33(131):163–72
**Ledermann F:** Faire de l'histoire de la pharmacie: pourquoi, comment? Quelques éléments historiographiques et théoriques en guise d'apologie. **Pharm Acta Helv** 1984;59(4):118–28
**Ledermann F:** Formation du pharmacien. Règlements, tendances, opinions. **Schweiz Apoth Ztg** 1979 Dec 13;117(24):664–8; 1980 Jan 10;118(1):11–15
**Ledermann F:** La dispensation des médicaments dans le canton de Neuchâtel (Suisse) 1930–1960. - S.l.n.n., 1978, in-4., 336 p., multigraphié. (Thèse doct. Univ., Pharm., Univ. René-Descartes, U.E.R. Sciences pharm. et biol. Paris-Luxembourg, 1978).
**Ledermann F:** La psychiatrie française et les médicaments: Pomme, Pinel, Esquirol, Morel. **Rev Hist Pharm (Paris)** 1982 Sep;29(254):189–206
**Ledermann F:** La thérapeutique médicamenteuse et la psychiatrie allemande du XIXe siècle: concordances, oppositions, indifférence? **Gesnerus** 1982;39(3–4):451–67
**Ledermann F:** L'histoire de la pharmacie dans les 'Pharmaceutica Acta Helvetiae', une bibliographie entre 1926 et 1979. **Pharm Acta Helv** 1981;56(3):93–6
**Ledingham IM** see **Macdonald RC**
**Ledingham KW** see **Jones DE**
**Lednicer D, ed** see **Bindra JS**
**Ledoux A** see **Bidault R**
**Lee AS, Lee ES:** The health of slaves and the health of freedmen: a Savannah study. **Phylon** 1977;38(2):170–80
**Lee D:** Jean Léger de la Grange. In Dictionary of Canadian biography, 1701 to 1740. Volume 2, 1969. p. 387–8.
**Lee DA:** Paul Broca and the history of aphasia. **Neurology** 1981 May;31(5):600–2
**Lee DH, Selikoff IJ:** Historical background to the asbestos problem. **Environ Res** 1979 Apr;18(2):300–14
**Lee ES, Roberts RE:** Ethnic fertility differentials in the Southwest: the case of Mexican Americans reexamined. **Sociol Soc Res** 1981;65(2):194–210
**Lee ES** see **Lee AS**
**Lee ES** see **Reid JD**
**Lee FR:** The 'silent art' of ancient China; Chung-kuo ku tai ssu hsiang: historical analysis of the intellectual and philosophical influences in the earliest medical corpus, Ling shu ching. Taipei, Linking Pub. Co., 1980. ii, 176 p.
**Lee HK:** Honoring the founder in his country: conception and struggle for Canada's Memorial College. **Chiropr Hist** 1981;(1):43–5
**Lee HY** see **Cho LJ**
**Lee J:** Food supply and population growth in southwest China, 1250–1850. **J Asian Stud** 1982;41(4):711–46
**Lee JA:** Anaesthesia. **Br Med J** 1979 Nov 10;2(6199):1192–4
**Lee JA:** Sydney Ringer (1834–1910) and Alexis Hartmann (1898–1964). **Anaesthesia** 1981 Dec;36(12):1115–21
**Lee M:** The 99 day Emperor, a misdiagnosis of historical importance. **Rostrum** 1981;(100):1–3
**Lee ME** see **Allan P**
**Lee PR:** Health policy and the health of the public. A two hundred year perspective. **Mobius** 1984 Jul;4(3):95–113
**Lee PR, Estes CL:** New federalism and health policy. **Ann Am Acad Polit Soc Sci** 1983;(468):88–102
**Lee PR** see **Silverman M**
**Lee R, Lam D:** Age distribution adjustments for English censuses, 1821–1931. **Popul Stud** 1983 Nov;37(3):445–64
**Lee RD:** Econometric studies of topics in demographic history. New York, Arno Press, 1978. 272 (12) p. (Ph.D. Diss, Harvard University, 1970).
**Lee RV:** Scurvy: a contemporary historical perspective. **Conn Med** 1983 Oct;47(10):629–32
**Lee RV:** Scurvy: a contemporary historical perspective (3). **Conn Med** 1984 Jan;48(1):33–5
**Lee RV:** The generalist: a jaundiced view. **Am J Med** 1983 Apr;74(4):532–4
**Lee RV:** The generalist: a jaundiced view. **Am J Med** 1983 Dec;75(6):902–5
**Lee RW:** Medicalisation and mortality trends in South Germany in the early 19th century. In Imhof AE, ed: Mensch und Gesundheit in der Geschichte. Husum, Matthiesen, 1980. p. 79–113.
**Lee S, Li SJ:** Clinical and experimental microsurgery in China: an historical note. **J Microsurg** 1982 Spring;3(3):180–3
**Lee S, Frank DH, Choi SY:** Historical review of small and microvascular vessel surgery. **Ann Plast Surg** 1983 Jul;11(1):53–62
**Lee S:** Vitiligo auf einem historischen Porträt. **Hautarzt** 1982 Jun;33(6):335–6
**Lee S van der** see **Horstmanhoff HF, ed**
**Lee S van der** see **Horstmanhoff HF, et al**
**Lee SH:** [Historical review of the nurses' status abroad] (Kor). **Taehan Kanho** 1983 Sep 20;22(3):42–8
**Lee SS:** Health policy, A social contract: a comparison of the United States and Canada. **J Public Health Policy** 1982 Sep;3(3):293–301
**Lee TC:** Van Gogh's vision. Digitalis intoxication? **JAMA** 1981 Feb 20;245(7):727–9
**Lee WR:** The mechanism of mortality change in Germany, 1750–1850. **Medizinhist J** 1980;15(3):244–68
**Lee YK:** Prostitution and venereal disease in early Singapore (1819–1889). **Singapore Med J** 1980;21:720–31
**Lee YK:** Prostitution and venereal disease in early Singapore (1819–1889)--Part II. **Singapore Med J** 1980 Dec;21(6):781–90
**Lee YK:** Singapore's pauper and Tan Tock Seng Hospitals. **J Malays Branch R Asiatic Soc** 1976;49(2):164–83 1977:50(2):111–35
**Lee YK:** The founding of the medical school in Singapore (Part I). **Singapore Med J** 1980 Jun;21(3):544–55
**Lee YK:** The founding of the medical school in Singapore (Part II). **Singapore Med J** 1980 Aug;21(4):666–76
**Lee YK:** The origins of medical registration in Singapore (Part I). **Singapore Med J** 1983 Oct;24(5):314–22
**Lee FR, ed** see **Saunders JB**
**Leebron WM:** Reflections on Hippocrates. **Am J Proctol Gastroenterol Colon Rectal Surg** 1982 Jun;33(6):7–8, 24
**Leeds JP:** Review of the Transactions of the American Academy of Optometry, 1922 to 1939. **Am J Optom Physiol Opt** 1982 Sep;59(9):735–7
**Leek FF:** Observations on a collection of crania from the mastabas of the reign of Cheops at Gîza. **J Egypt Archaeol** 1980;66:36–45
**Leek FF:** Palaeodontology of the Nile Valley. **Paleopathol Newsl** 1981 Jan;33:9–12
**Leelavathy S** see **Shankara MR**
**Leenhardt RH:** Un tournant de l'histoire de la nouvelle caledonie: Maurice Leenhardt (1878–1954). **Rev Fr Hist Outre Mer** 1978;65(2):236–52
**Lees FC** see **Relethford JH**
**LeFanu WR, ed** see **Ross JP**
**Lefebvre P:** Il y a deux siècles mourait Germain Pichault de la Martinière (1697–1783). **Chirurgie** 1983;109(10):805–8
**Lefebvre P:** La recherche par le clinicien: une activité inéluctable. **Bull Mem Acad R Med Belg** 1979 Nov 24;134(10):587–96
**Lefebvre P, Godon A:** Les cendres du baron Larrey. **Nouv Presse Med** 1982 Jan 30;11(4):235–9
**Lefebvre P:** L'hôpital Militaire Laveran de Constantine. **Med Trop (Mars)** 1980 Nov–Dec;40(6):645–9

**Lefebvre P, Barbas S:** L'hystérie de guerre. Etude comparative de ses manifestations au cours des deux derniers conflits mondiaux. **Ann Med Psychol (Paris)** 1984 Feb;142(2):262–6
**Lefebvre P:** Tradition de l'enseignement dans le Service de santé de l'armée de terre. **Med Armees** 1980;8(10)spec:827–44
**Lefebvre P** see **Huard P**
**Lefebvre P** see **Plessis JL**
**Lefemine AA:** A recollecton of men and events on the Thoracic Service of the Peter Bent Brigham Hospital: 1958–1966. **Artif Organs** 1980 Aug;4(3):210–8
**Lefèvre C:** Sur l'évolution d'Aristote en psychologie. Louvain, Editions de l'Institut supérieur de philosophie, 1972. ix, 345 p.
**Lefevre P:** Les voyages de la Marine Royale Belge au Sénégal, en Gambie et en Basse Guinée. Récits des médecins qui accompagnèrent les navires de guerre belges 'Louise–Marie' et 'Duc de Brabant' (1847–1856) dans le cadre de la tentative de colonisation au Rio Nunez. **Rev Belge Hist Milit** 1978–79;22–23:647–68, 39–64, 137–48
**Leff A, Lester TW, Addington WW:** Tuberculosis. A chemotherapeutic triumph but a persistent socioeconomic problem. **Arch Intern Med** 1979 Dec;139(12):1375–7
**Leff MH** see **Breul FR**
**Légaré J** see **Bourbeau R**
**Légaré J** see **Normandeau L**
**Légée G:** A. Vulpien (1826–1887), physiologiste élève de P. Flourens (1794–1867). In: Congrès international d'histoire de la médecine, XXVe, Québec, 1976. Actes. Québec, 1977. p. 873–80.
**Legée G:** Evolution de l'étude clinique, sociale et juridique de l'aliénation mentale, sous l'impulsion de Jean–Etienne–Dominique Esquirol (1772–1840), médecin aliéniste d'origine Toulousaine. In: Congrès National des Sociétés Savantes, 96e, Toulouse, 1971. Comptes Rendus. Paris, 1974. Histoire des Sciences, Tome 1. p. 63–81.
**Legée G:** Evolution de l'histologie du système nerveux au XIXe siècle; l'impulsion donnée par Camillo Golgi (1844–1926). **Clio Med** 1982 May;17(1):15–32
**Legée G:** Henri Ducrotay de Blainville (1777–1850) et la physiologie. In: Congrès National des Sociétés Savantes, 105e, Caen, 1980. Comptes Rendus, Paris, 1980. Section des Sciences, Fasc. V. p. 49–59.
**Legée G:** Influence du vitalisme montpelliérain sur la neurophysiologie de Pierre Flourens. **Hist Nat** 1982;21:13–45
**Legée G:** La découverte des fonctions des canaux semi–circulaires de l'oreille interne. In: Congrès National des Sociétés Savantes, 91e, Rennes, 1966. Comptes Rendus. Paris, 1967. Section des Sciences, Tome 1. p. 291–300.
**Legée G:** La notion de temps dans la physiologie neuro–musculaire au XIXe siècle. In: Congrès National des Sociétés Savantes, 99e, Besançon, 1974. Comptes Rendus. Paris, 1976. Section des Sciences, Fasc. V. p. 203–13.
**Legée G:** La place de Magendie dans la physiologie expérimentale du système nerveux. **Hist Sci Med** 1983;17(4):357–66
**Legée G:** L'activité parisienne d'un physiologiste languedocien Marie–Jean–Pierre Flourens (1794–1867). In: Congrès National des Sociétés Savantes, 96e, Toulouse, 1971. Comptes Rendus. Paris, 1974. Histoire des Sciences, Tome 1. p. 107–22.
**Legée G:** Les concepts de localisation et de coordination dans la neurophysiologie de Maire–Jean–Pierre Flourens (1794–1867). In: Congrès National des Sociétés Savantes, 96e, Toulouse, 1971. Comptes Rendus. Paris, 1974. Histoire des Sciences, Tome 1. p. 123–51.
**Legée G:** Les relations épistolaires de P. Flourens et de ses collègues de l'Institut de France. In: Congrès National des Sociétés Savantes, 106e, Perpignan, 1981. Comptes Rendus. Paris, Bibliothèque Nationale, 1982. Fasc. IV. p. 171–85.
**Legée G:** Lettres inédites des Félix Archimède Pouchet (1800–1872) au physiologiste Pierre Flourens (1794–1867). In International Congress of the History of Medicine. 26th, Plovdiv, 1978. Actes du Congress. Sofia, 1981. Volume II. p. 130–8.
**Legée G:** L'influence de la Société d'Auteuil sur les travaux des physiologistes. In: Congrès National des Sociétés Savantes, 100e, Paris, 1975. Actes. Paris, 1976. Histoire Moderne et Contemporaine et Histoire des Sciences. p. 229–42.
**Legee G:** P. Flourens, historien des sciences: valeur de son histoire de la découverte de la circulation du sang. In: Congrès National des Sociétés Savantes, 107e. Brest, 1982. Comptes Rendus, Paris, 1983. Section des Sciences, Fasc. IV. p. 313–31.
**Legée G:** P. Flourens (1794–1867) et la psychiatrie de son temps. In: Congrès National des Sociétés Savantes, 103e, Nancy, 1978. Comptes Rendus. Paris, 1978. Section des Sciences, Fasc. V. p. 113–23.
**Legée G:** Physiologie et phrenologie au temps du physiologiste Pierre Flourens (1794–1867). In International Congress of the History of Medicine, 27th, Barcelona, 1980. Actas. Barcelona, Académia de Ciències Médiques de Catalunya i Balears, 1981. p. 91–7.
**Legée G:** Schopenhauer (1788–1860) et les sciences de la nature. **Hist Nat** 1979;(14):39–62
**Léger JM:** Incidences de certaines croyances populaires (sorcellerie) sur la pratique médicale courante. **Rev Med Swisse Romande** 1982 Jun;102(6):629–39
**Leger L:** Allocution. **Chirurgie** 1980 Jan;106(1):3–10
**Léger L** see **Delaunay A, ed**
**Legg WD** see **Bullough VL**
**Legge D:** Peer review in the U.S.A.: an historical perspective. **Med J Aust** 1981 Jun 27;1(13):709–11
**Leggett CA:** The founders of the College. **Aust NZ J Surg** 1981 Oct;51(5):508–12
**Legrand J** see **Dumont GF**
**Legrenzi P, Sonino M:** Fisica ingenua a teoria cartesiana degli urti. **Stor Crit Psicol** 1984;5(2):213–28
**Legrenzi P:** L'uomo senza facoltà: modelli del comportamento in Musil. **Stor Crit Psicol** 1982 Dec;3(2):301–13
**Leguay JP:** Accidents du travail et maladies professionnelles au Moyen Age. **Inf Hist** 1981;43(5):223–33
**Leguil F** see **Gorog F**
**Lehmann H:** Hexenverfolgungen und Hexenprozesse im alten Reich zwischen Reformation und Aufklärung. **Jahrb Inst Dtsch Gesch** 1978;7:9–70
**Lehmann H:** Sickle cell anemia 35 years ago: reminiscence of early African studies. **Am J Pediatr Hematol Oncol** 1984 Spring;6(1):72–6
**Lehmann H:** The gradual understanding of thalassemia. **Prog Clin Biol Res** 1984;165:121–36
**Lehmann H:** The history of thalassemia. **Birth Defects** 1982;18(7):1–11
**Lehmann H:** Zur Geschichte der parenteralen Uebertragung der akuten ikterischen Virushepatitis. **Dtsch Med Wochenschr** 1981 Apr 17;106(16):517
**Lehmann HE:** De Binet et Wundt aux mesures neuropsychologiques et aux échelles de comportement. **Acta Psychiatr Belg** 1983 Mar–Apr;83(2):135–46
**Lehmann JF:** Rehabilitation medicine: past, present and future. **Arch Phys Med Rehabil** 1982 Jul;63(7):291–7
**Lehmann V:** Der Gebärstuhl--ein historisches Möbel oder eine sinnvolle Erneuerung. **Z Geburtshife Perinatol** 1983 Mar–Apr;187(2):55–64
**Lehmann V:** Der Gebärstuhl--ein historisches Möbel oder eine sinnvolle Erneuerung. **Arch Gynecol** 1983;235(1–4):XLVIII–LXIII
**Lehners JP:** Schwerpunkte historisch–demographischer Forschung in West– und Mitteleuropa. **Hist Soc Res** 1982;22:3–14
**Lehning JR:** The decline of marital fertility: evidence from a French department, la Loire (1851–1891). **Ann Demogr Hist (Paris)** 1984;:201–17
**Lehning JR:** The history of wet nursing and the history of the family. **Peasant Stud** 1982;9(4):250–7
**Lehoux F:** Le cadre de vie des médecins parisiens aux XVIe et XVIIe siècles. Paris, A. & J. Picard, 1976. x, 611 p.
**Lehrer PM:** How to relax and how not to relax: a re–evaluation of the work of Edmund Jacobson--I. **Behav Res Ther** 1982;20(5):417–28
**Lehuenen J** see **Guyotjeannin C**
**Leibecke–Englisch B:** Die lokale Wundbehandlung aus pharmakologischer and pharmazeutischer Sicht in der deutschsprachigen medizinischen Literatur von 1800 bis 1867. Diss. Mainz, 1979. 89p.
**Leibowitz JO:** Early accounts in geriatric pathology (Leonardo, Harvey, James Keill). **Koroth** 1980 Jun;7(11–12):CCLIII–CCLXIV
**Leibowitz JO:** Ibn Sina in Hebrew. **Koroth** 1981;8(1–2):3–8
**Leibowitz JO:** Jewish translators of medical works in the Middle Ages. In International Congress of the History of Medicine, 27th, Barcelona, 1980. Actas. Barcelona, Académia de Ciències Médiques de Catalunya i Balears, 1981. p. 276–80.
**Leibowitz JO:** Medical items in the book Torat ha–'Adam of Rabbi Moses ben Nahman (1194–1270). **Koroth** 1983 Aug;8(7–8):257–64
**Leibowitz JO:** R. Simon ben Zemah Duran (1361–1444) and his conception of metabolism in Magen Avot. **Koroth** 1979 Nov;7(9–10):CLXIX–XXIX(626–33)
**Leibowitz JO:** The final illness of Gotthold Ephraim Lessing. **Janus** 1980;67(1–2–3):21–30
**Leibowitz JO:** The idea of metabolism in the medical works of Maimonides. In: Congrès international d'histoire de la médecine, XXVe, Québec, 1976. Actes. Québec, 1977. p. 881–4.
**Leibowitz JO:** The ideal physician as revealed in the Zohar, book of Jewish mysticism. **Koroth** 1982 Aug;8(3/4):111–22
**Leibowitz JO:** The problem of medical license in Hebrew sources. In International Congress of the History of Medicine. 26th, Plovdiv, 1978. Actes du Congress. Sofia, 1981. Volume II. p. 139–40.
**Leibson L:** Endocrinology evolution and evolutionary endocrinology. **Perspect Biol Med** 1979 Autumn;23(1):25–43
**Leĭbson LG:** L. A. Orbeli i nekotorye aspekty ėvoliutsionnoĭ fiziologii. **Zh Evol Biokhim Fiziol** 1983 Jul–Aug;19(4):322–32
**Leiby J:** A history of social welfare and social work in the United States. New York, Columbia University Press, 1978. 426 p.
**Leider M** see **Kouskoukis CE**
**Leigh JP:** Education, working conditions, and worker's health. **Soc Sci J** 1983;20(2):99 107
**Leighton AH:** A recurrent millennium: the cure and prevention of mental illnesses. **Can Ment Health** 1982 Jun;30(2):2–5
**Leighton AH:** Caring for mentally ill people. Psychological and social barriers in historical context. Cambridge, Cambridge University Press, 1982. x, 277 p.
**Leighton BC:** The Dental Education Advisory Council: 50 years. **Br Dent J** 1980 Nov 4;149(9):267–8
**Leighton BD, Howard RD:** Orthodontics--the last hundred years. **Br Dent J** 1981 Jul 7;151(1):14–9
**Leijenhorst CG van** see **Horstmanhoff HF, ed**
**Leijenhorst CG van** see **Horstmanhoff HF, et al**
**Leikola A:** Alkmaion - den vetenskapliga medicinens pionjär. **Nord Medicinhist Arsbok** 1983;:59–63
**Leikola A:** The problem of generation in the 17th century Finnish university. A study in peripheralism. In International Congress of the History of Medicine, 27th, Barcelona, 1980. Actas. Barcelona, Académia de Ciències Médiques de Catalunya i Balears, 1981. p. 560–3.

**Leikola A:** Zeus Faber--antiikin tarustoa eläinkunnassa. **Hist Arkisto (Finl)** 1978;(73):110-19
**Leinfellner W** see **Lorenz K, ed**
**Leiser G:** Medical education in Islamic lands from the seventh to the fourteenth century. **J Hist Med Allied Sci** 1983 Jan;38(1):48-75
**Leisibach M:** Das Medizinisch-chirurgische Institut in Zürich, 1782-1833: Vorläufer der Medizinischen Fakultät der Universität Zürich. Zürich, Rohr, 1982. 136, [39] p.
**Leitner F** see **Takáts L**
**Leitner H:** Die jüdischen Arzte in Osterreich und ihr Beitrag zur medizinischen Wissenschaft. In K. Lohrmann, ed: 1000 Jahre Osterreichisches Judentum. Ausstellungskatalog. Eisenstadt, 1982. p. 161-92.
**Leitner J:** Leaders in medicine--George H. Garrison, MD. **J Okla State Med Assoc** 1981 Sep;74(9):298-304
**Lejman K:** Andrzej Badurski (1740-1789) jako założyciel szpitala akademickiego i inicjator klinicznego nauczania meydycyny. **Przegl Lek** 1981;38(7):567-70
**Lejmbach Z:** Myśl pediatryczna wśród pracowników szpitala im. Karola i Marii. **Pediatr Pol** 1984 Sep;59(9):701-3
**Lekisch K:** Drugs and politics. **Scalpel Tongs** 1981;25:93-4
**Leland TM:** Albertus Adair Moore, M.D. 1834-1910. **J SC Med Assoc** 1984 Jul;80(7):358
**Leland TM:** Anesthesiology in the Civil War (Dr. Julian John Chisolm). **J SC Med Assoc** 1981 Nov;77(11):524
**Leland TM:** DaVega's Floating Hospital. **J SC Med Assoc** 1984 Nov;80(11):581
**Leland TM:** 'First Physician in Spartanburg County' Andrew Barry Moore, M.D., 1771-1848. **J SC Med Assoc** 1983 May;79(5):299
**Leland TM:** Francis Lejan Parker, M.D. 1836-1913. **J SC Med Assoc** 1983 Feb;79(2):99
**Leland TM:** James Rufus Bratton 1821-1897. **J SC Med Assoc** 1984 Feb;80(2):84
**Lelean SR** see **Allan P**
**Lellouch A:** Histoire de l'angine de poitrine et du spasme artériel coronaire au travers de l'oeuvre de Prinzmetal. **Coeur Med Interne** 1980 Jan-Mar;19(1):85-90
**Lellouch A, Rullière R:** René Joseph Hyacinthe Bertin (1767-1827). **Hist Sci Med** 1980;14:325-36
**Lelu F:** La population des 'pauvres malades' de l'Hôtel-Dieu de Provins, de 1762 à 1791. Mém. de maîtrise. Univ. de Paris I, 1976. 13, 204 p.
**Lemaine G:** Perspectives on the emergence of scientific disciplines. Chicago, Aldine, 1976. xi, 281 p.
**Lemaire A:** Jacques Lacan. London and Boston, Rutledge and Kegan Paul, 1977. xxiv, 266 p.
**Lemaire A:** Les aléas de la découverte en thérapeutique ou l'aventure du médicament. **Bull Acad Natl Med (Paris)** 1981 Dec;165(9):1215-27
**Lemaire F** see **Rapin M**
**Lemaire JF:** A propos d'Antoine Portal. Le passé de la médecine et le regard de l'historien. **Hist Sci Med** 1980;14:399-406
**Lemaire JF:** Cent cinquante ans de médecine dans 'La Revue'. **Rev Deux Mondes** 1979 Oct;73-8
**Lemaire JF:** Gustave Flaubert, médecin passif. **Nouv Rev Deux Mondes** 1981;9:580-92
**Lemaire JF:** Le chirurgien-baron François Girardot (1773-1831) un oublié de l'histoire. **Hist Sci Med** 1980;14(1):107-14
**Lemaire JF:** 1696, l'irresponsabilité médicale momentanément consacrée. **Hist Sci Med** 1984;18(1):41-3
**Lemann N:** Let the nurses do it. **Wash Mon** 1979;11(2):29-36
**Lemay H:** The stars and human sexuality: some medieval scientific views. **Isis** 1980 Mar; 71(256):127-37
**Lemay JA, Rousseau GS:** The Renaissance man in the eighteenth century. Papers read at a Clark Library seminar, 9 October 1976. Los Angeles, William Andrews Clark Memorial Library, UCLA, 1978. xi, 139 p.
**Lembrych S:** 25-lecie działalności Opolskiego Oddziału Polskiego Towarzystwa Ginekologicznego. **Ginekol Pol** 1984 Jan;55(1):71-3
**Leme C de A:** Desenvolvimento histórico da eletrocardiografia. **Rev Hosp Clin Fac Med Sao Paulo** 1980 Aug;35(4):205-17
**Leme C de A:** História da eletrocardiografia no Brasil. **Rev Hosp Clin Fac Med Sao Paulo** 1981 Aug;36(4):179-83
**Lemeunier G** see **Marset Campos P**
**Lemieux B** see **Barbeau A**
**Lemoine P:** L'Organe permanent pour la sécurité et la salubrité dans les mines de houille et les autres industries extractives. **Rev Inst Hyg Mines (Hasselt)** 1983;38(2):140-2
**Lemoine P:** Une entreprise de répartition: l'Office Commercial Pharmaceutique de ses origines (1840) à 1965. **Rev Hist Pharm (Paris)** 1983 Mar;30(256):5-29
**Lemon HM:** Motivation in cancer education, with an appreciation of Dr. Henry Jackson, Jr., pioneer medical oncologist-hematologist (1892-1968). **Med Pediatr Oncol** 1980;8(4):407-22
**Lemon HM:** My specialty: oncology. **Nebr Med J** 1979 Aug;64(8):259
**Lemonds LL:** A century of veterinary medicine in Nebraska. Henderson, Nebraska, Service Press, 1982. 395 p.
**Lemos AA de:** Infra-estrutura da literatura biomédica: considerações acerca de um núcleo de revistas brasileiras do setor saúde. **Educ Med Salud** 1981;15(4):406-23
**Lemperier B:** Le système d'assistance dans la marine marchande. In: Congrès National des Sociétés Savantes, 97e, Nantes, 1972. Comptes Rendus. Paris, 1976. Section des Sciences, Tome 1. p. 311-7.
**Lempicki A:** Ireneusz Wierzejewski (1881-1930). **Chir Narzadow Ruchu Ortop Pol** 1981;46(6):589-93
**Lenarduzzi G, Pescarini L, Miotto D:** Un precursore dell'esame radiologico del tubo digerente: il prof. G. Vicentini. **Radiol Med (Torino)** 1980 Apr;66(4):263-4
**Lénárt G, László G:** Das Erleben der Verstümmelung in der alten Kunst. In KF Schlegel, ed: Der Körperbehinderte in Mythologie und Kunst. Stuttgart, New York, Thieme, 1983. p. 29-39.
**Lender ME:** Dictionary of American temperance biography: from temperance reform to alcohol research, the 1600s to the 1980s. Westport, Conn., Greenwood Press, 1984. xiv, 572 p.
**Lender ME, Martin JK:** Drinking in America: a history. New York, Free Press, London, Collier Macmillan, 1982. xv, 222 p.
**Lender ME:** Women alcoholics: prevalence estimates and their problems reflected in turn-of-the-century institutional data. **Int J Addict** 1981 Apr;16(3):443-8
**Leneman L:** The study of illegitimacy from kirk session records: two eighteenth-century Perthshire parishes. **Local Popul Stud** 1983 Autumn;31:29-33
**Lengeler J:** Barbara McClintock und die Entdeckung der beweglichen Gene. **MMW** 1983 Nov 25;125(47):1095-7
**Lengsfeld W:** La population allemande depuis un siècle. **Documents** 1979;34(3):61-70
**Lengsfeld W:** Un phénomène complexe: la fécondité. **Documents** 1979;34(3):79-85
**Lenhardt F:** Zur Ikonographie der Blutschau. **Medizinhist J** 1982;17(1/2):63-77
**Lenihan J:** Descartes versus Hippocrates--a conflict resolved? **Br J Radiol** 1984 Oct;57(682):861-5
**Lenihan J:** Paradox and partnership. The engineer's contribution to medicine. **Scott Med J** 1980 Apr;25(2):107-12
**Lenihan J:** The history of intensive care. **Nurs Focus** 1979 Oct;1(2):75-6
**Leninskaia zabota o blage naroda: Vopr Onkol** 1980;26(4):3-9
**Leninskie printsipy v rabote oftal'mologov: Vestn Oftalmol** 1980 May-Jun;(3):3-5
**Lennert T** see **Meadow R**
**Lennox J:** Teleology, chance, and Aristotle's theory of spontaneous generation. **J Hist Philos** 1981;19:219-38
**Lennox MA:** Professor Gastaut's contribution to the International League against Epilepsy. **Electroencephalogr Clin Neurophysiol** 1982;35:9-12
**Leno C** see **Berciano J**
**Lenoir T:** A history of biology: an essay review. **J Hist Med Allied Sci** 1983 Jul;38(3):348-51
**Lenoir T:** Kant, Blumenbach, and vital materialism in German biology. **Isis** 1980 Mar;71(256):77-108
**Lenoir T:** The Göttingen School and the development of transcendental Naturphilosophie in the Romantic Era. **Stud Hist Biol** 1981;5:111-205
**Lenoir T:** The strategy of life: teleology and mechanics in nineteenth century German biology. Dordrecht, Holland; Boston, Reidel, 1982. xii, 314 p.
**Lenský P:** Sclerosis multiplex. Nosologická identifikace před 150 lety. **Cas Lek Cesk** 1984 Jul 27;123(30):937-8
**Lenskyj H:** Femininity first, sport and physical education for Ontario girls, 1890-1930. **Can J Hist Sport Phy Educ** 1982;13(2):4-17
**Lentini J, Taure Gómez C, Leveroni J:** Conmemoración de un cincuentenario. In International Congress of the History of Medicine, 27th, Barcelona, 1980. Actas. Barcelona, Académia de Ciències Médiques de Catalunya i Balears, 1981. p. 564-9.
**Lenz F:** Theorie und Praxis in der Elektronenoptik. **Mikroskopie** 1982 Dec;39(11-12):359-73
**Lenz HG:** Der hessische Paracelsist Johann Thoelde. **Salzburger Beitr Paracelsusforsch** 1984;23:89-99
**Lenzen W:** Mentis Laesiones, Psychopathologie bei Felix Platter (1536-1614). Diss. Bonn, 1982. 151 p.
**Lenzi E:** Nota informativa sull'U.P.I.G.O. e sull'U.E.M.S. **Minerva Ginecol** 1981 Feb-Mar;33(2-3):153-5
**Léon A:** Psychopédagogie scientifique et humanisme dans l'oeuvre d'Henri Wallon (1879-1962). **Paedagog Hist** 1979;19(1):132-45
**León AP:** La brucelosis en México. In Academia Nacional de Medicina. Libro conmemorativo del primer centenario. México, Comité Editorial de la Comisión Organizadora del Congreso del Centenario, 1964. Tome 2. p. 527-32.
**Leon L:** Cos'è un ex libris. **Kos** 1984 Jun;1(5):112-6
**León R** see **Brozek J**
**Leonard AG:** Three score years and fifteen in the Philippines. **Br Dent J** 1983 Oct 22;155(8):284
**Leonard AS:** A tribute to Dr. Owen H. Wangensteen, 'the Chief'. **Surgery** 1981;89:402-6
**Leonard DC:** Harvard's first science professor: a sketch of Isaac Greenwood's life and work. **Harv Libr Bull** 1981 Apr;29(2):135-68
**Leonard EP:** A Cornell heritage: veterinary medicine 1868-1908. Ithaca, New York State College of Veterinary Medicine, 1979. xix, 288 p.
**Leonard EP:** In the James Law tradition, 1908-1948. Ithaca, New York State College of Veterinary Medicine, 1982. xviii, 342 p.
**Leonard EP** see **Hansel W**
**Léonard J:** A propos de l'hygiène navale sur les navires de guerre français dans la première moitié du XIXe siècle. In: Congrès National des Sociétés Savantes, 91e, Rennes, 1966. Comptes Rendus. Paris, 1967. Section des Sciences, Tome 1. p. 55-77.
**Léonard J:** La médecine entre les savoirs et les pouvoirs: histoire intellectuelle et politique de la médecine française au XIXe siècle. Paris, Aubier Montaigne, 1981. 384 p.

**Leonard J:** La médicalisation de l'Etat: l'exemple des premières décennies de la 3e République. **Ann Bretagne** 1979;86(3):313–20
**Léonard J:** La restauration et la profession médicale. **Hist Reflect** 1982;9(1–2):69–81
**Léonard J:** La vie quotidienne du médecin de province au XIXe siècle. Paris, Hachette, 1977. 285 p.
**Léonard J:** Le corps médical au début de la IIIe République ou l'heureux dénouement d'un malaise professionel. **Third Repub** 1978 Spring;5:94–113
**Leonard J:** Le corps médical au début de la IIIe République, ou l'heureux dénouement d'un malaise professionnel. In Poirier J, Poirier JL, ed: Médecine et philosophie à la fin du XIXe siècle. Paris, Université de Paris XII - Val de Marne, [1980?]. p. 9–21.
**Léonard J:** Le premier Congrès international d'eugénique (Londres, 1912) et ses conséquences françaises. **Hist Sci Med** 1983;17(2):141–6
**Léonard J:** Les débuts du 'Concours médical'. **Hist Sci Med** 1980;14:453–8
**Léonard J:** Les guérisseurs en France au XIXe siècle. **Rev Hist Mod Contemp** 1980 Jul–Sep;27:501–16
**Léonard J:** Les médecins au XIXe siècle. **Histoire** 1978;4:15–23
**Leonard J:** Les médecins de l'Ouest au XIXe siècle. **Ann Demogr Hist (Paris)** 1979;:337–45
**Leonard J:** Les medecins de l'ouest au XIXème siècle. Lille, Atelier reproduction des thèses, Univ. de Lille III; Paris, Champion, 1978. 3 vols. ccxl, 1570 p. (Thèse, Paris IV, 1976).
**Léonard J:** Pasteur, un vétérinaire qui ira loin. **Histoire** 1979;12:78–80
**Leonard J:** The ghost of Yellow Jack. **Harv Mag** 1981 Mar–Apr;83(4):20–7
**Léonard J** see **Charle C**
**Léonard J** see **Forster R**
**Leonard JC:** Thomas Bevill Peacock and the early history of dissecting aneurysm. **Br Med J** 1979 Jul 28;2(6184):260–2
**Leonard JC** see **Williams G**
**Leonard Tucker Skeggs--a multifaceted diamond: Clin Chem** 1981 Aug;27(8):1465–8
**Leonard Wood, M.D.:** Some Arizona Territory influences. **Ariz Med** 1982 Sep;39(9):593–6
**Leone LP** see **Wangensteen OW, ed**
**Leonenko NA** see **Duplenko KF**
**Leonenko NA** see **Kozliuk VM**
**Leonhard K:** Psychiatrische Behandlungsmethodik von Kraepelin nach seinen Lebenserinnerungen. **Psychiatr Neurol Med Psychol (Leipz)** 1984 Jul;36(7):395–405
**Leonnard P, Rommel J:** Lens implantation. Thirty years of progress. **Bull Soc Belge Ophtalmol** 1981;194:1–600
**Leonov IT:** Bol'sheviki–lenintsy--vospitanniki Voenno–meditsinskoĭ akademii. **Voen Med Zh** 1984 Oct;(10):62–5
**Leonov IT:** N. I. Pirogov i voennaia meditsina. **Feldsher Akush** 1981;46(11):51–3
**Leonov IT:** Vydaiushchiĭsia organizator meditsinskoĭ sluzhby i voenno–meditsinskogo obrazovaniia (k 90–letiiu so dnia rozhdeniia B. K. Leonardova). **Sov Zdravookhr** 1982;(9):60–2
**Leont'ev AA:** Lichnost' kak istoriko–etnicheskaia kategoriia. **Sov Etnogr** 1981;3:35–44
**Leont'ev PA** see **Shereshkov GM**
**Leontiuk AS, Lobko PI, Novikov II:** David Moiseevich Golub (k 80–letiiu so dnia rozhdeniia i 55–letiiu vrachebnoĭ, nauchnoĭ, pedagogicheskoĭ i obshchestvennoĭ deiatel'nosti). **Arkh Anat Gistol Embriol** 1981 Aug;81(8):122–6
**Leopold LA:** Radiology at the University of Pennsylvania 1890–1975. Philadelphia, University of Pennsylvania Press, 1981. xvi, 163 p.
**Leowski J:** Die Entwicklung des Gesundheitswesens in der VR Polen. **Med Ges** 1979;(6):99–109
**Lepetit B** see **Goubert JP**
**Lépine P:** Le secret de Madame Lafarge (lumières nouvelles sur une affaire célèbre). **Sem Hop Paris** 1983 Dec 22;59(48):3387–94
**Lépine P:** Un dossier contesté, l'affaire Lafarge. **Lyon Pharm** 1980 Jan 1;31(1):39–44
**Leplat G:** Hans de Winiwarter, 1875–1949. In Florilège des Sciences en Belgique - II. Bruxelles, Académie Royale de Belgique, 1980. p. 587–97.
**Lepore FE:** Neuro–ophthalmology according to Gordon Holmes. **Neurol Clin** 1983 Nov;1(4):789–805
**Lepore FE:** Toward a definition of papilledema: a historical review, 1851–1911. **Surg Neurol** 1982 Mar;17(3):178–80
**Lepore MJ:** Death of the clinician, requiem or reveille? Springfield, Thomas, 1982. xviii, 359 p.
**Lepow IH:** Louis Pillemer, Properdin, and scientific controversy. **J Immunol** 1980 Aug;125(2):471–5
**Leppard PI** see **Maddern GJ**
**Lequime J:** Marey et la cardiologie. **Acta Belg Med Phys** 1983 Oct–Dec;6(4):181–5
**Lerche C:** The National Institute of Public Health--fifty years of activity and development in retrospect. **NIPH Ann** 1979 Dec;2(2):3–10
**Leridon H, Charbit Y:** Patterns of marital unions and fertility in Guadeloupe and Martinique. **Popul Stud** 1981;35(2):235–46
**Leridon H** see **Lamy ML**
**Lerman SJ:** Why is chickenpox called chickenpox? **Clin Pediatr (Phila)** 1981 Feb;20(2):111–2
**Lerner BD** see **Castorina JA**
**Lerner EA:** Franz Gabriel Alexander. In Dictionary of American Biography, 1961–1965. Suppl. 7, 1981. p. 5–7.
**Lerner IJ:** The whys of cancer quackery. **Cancer** 1984 Feb 1;53(3 Suppl):815–9
**Lerner JC:** The public and private management of death in Britain, 1890–1930. Ph.D. Diss., Columbia University. New York, 1981. iv, 309 leaves.
**Lerner JC** see **Newcombe N**
**Lerner L:** Esther Menaker. **Psychoanal Rev** 1984 Spring;71(1):iii–viii
**Lerner RM, ed:** Developmental psychology: historical and philosophical perspectives. Hillsdale, N. J., London, Lawrence Erlbaum, 1983. xii, 274 p. Contributions by J. Kagan, S. H. White, P. B. Baltes, R. A. Dixon, J. R. Nesselroade. U. Bronfenbrenner, B. Kaplan.
**Leroi–Gouhran A** see **Bernard J**
**Leroux–Hugon V:** Infirmières des hôpitaux parisiens au début du siècle. **Penelope** 1981;(5):62–7
**Leroy D:** Laennec étudiant en médecine. **Bull Acad Natl Med (Paris)** 1979 Nov 6–27;163(8):849–56
**Leroy P:** L'ancien hôpital de la Charité de Senlis. Senlis, Société d'Histoire et d'Archéologie de Senlis, 1979? 20 p. (Collections Senlisiennes, no. 2).
**LeRoy Ladurie E:** Demographie et 'funestes secrets': le Languedoc (fin XVIIIe–debut XIXe siècle). **Ann Hist Revolut Fr** 1965;37(4):385–400
**LeRoy Ladurie E:** Pressure of numbers: medical evidence, changing attitudes and historical demography. In his: The territory of the historian. Hassocks, Sussex, England, Harvester Press, 1979. p. 221–84.
**Lert F:** Emergence et devenir du système de prise en charge de la tuberculose en France entre 1900 et 1940. **Soc Sci Med** 1982;16(23):2073–82
**Lerut T:** Groei en ontwekkeling van de slokdarmchirurgie. **Verh K Acad Geneeskd Belg** 1984;46(3):161–82
**Les enfants du Rouergue: Bull Soc Fr Hist Hop** 1980;(41):36
**Les pansements à la ouate de M. Alphonse Guérin: Union Med Can** 1981 May;110(5):464
**Les sociétés savantes: leur histoire: actes du 100e Congrès national des sociétés savantes, Paris, 1975, Section d'histoire moderne et contemporaine et Commission d'histoire des sciences et des techniques:** Paris, Bibliothèque nationale, 1976. 386 p.
**Lescarret JP:** Démographie et société dans le Haute–Lande depuis le XVIIIe siècle, Saugnac–le–Muret, 2 volumes. Univ. de Boredaux III. Thèse de doct. 1979. 642 p.
**Lesch JE:** Science and medicine in France: the emergence of experimental physiology, 1790–1855. Cambridge, Mass., Harvard University Press, 1984. viii, 276 p.
**Lesky E:** American medicine as viewed by Viennese physicians, 1893–1912. **Bull Hist Med** 1982 Fall;56(3):368–76
**Lesky E:** Das Portrait: Franz Joseph Gall 1758–1828. **Med Unserer Zeit** 1980;4(2):57–61
**Lesky E:** Der angeklagte Gall. **Gesnerus** 1981;38(3/4):301–11
**Lesky E:** Die Wiener Medizinische Schule im 19. Jahrhundert. Graz–Köln, Böhlaus, 1978. 660 p. (Studien zur Geschichte der Universität Wien, Band VI).
**Lesky E:** Die Wiener Medizinische Schule und die Donauländer. In Congress of History, Health, Culture of the Danubian Countries. 1. Novi Sad, 1975. p. 31–6.
**Lesky E:** Heilkunde und Gesundheitswesen unter Maria Theresia. **Osterr Apoth Ztg** 1980 May 17;34(20):357–60
**Lesky E:** Meilensteine der Wiener Medizin. Grosse Arzte Osterreichs in drei Jahrhunderten. Wien, Wilhelm Maudrich, 1981. 251 p.
**Lesky E:** Theorie und Praxis, aufgezeigt an den Wiener geburtshilflichen Lehrkanzeln 1752–1859. **Gesnerus** 1983;40(1–2):99–107
**Lesky E, ed:** Franz Joseph Gall, 1758–1828, Naturforscher und Anthropologe. Wien, Huber, 1979. (Hubers Klassiker der Medizin und der Naturwissenschaften, Band 15) 217 p.
**Leśniak E, Leśniak R, Ryn Z:** Nurt oświecimski w twórczości Antoniego Kępińskiego. **Przegl Lek** 1983;40(12):849–54
**Leśniak R** see **Leśniak E**
**Leśnikowska M:** Wspomnienia z tamtych lat. **Pieleg Polozna** 1980;(1):23–4, 26
**Lesný I:** Šílenství francouzského krále Karla VI. **Cas Lek Cesk** 1982 May 14;121(19):597–600
**Lessard R:** Alexandre Serres. In Dictionary of Canadian biography, 1801 to 1820. Volume 5, 1983. p. 752.
**Lessard R:** François–Michel Suzor. In Dictionary of Canadian biography, 1801 to 1820. Volume 5, 1983. p. 788–9.
**Lessard R** see **Cadotte M**
**Lessard S:** Busting our mental blocks on drugs and crime. **Wash Mon** 1971;3(4):6–18
**Lesson PA:** Notes sur les maladies des indigènes des iles Marquises en 1844. Manuscrit inédit. **Bull Soc Etud Oceaniennes** 1981;18(216):915–43
**Lester JF:** John Fiske's philosophy of science: the union of science and religion through the principle of evolution. Ph.D. Diss., Oregon State University, Corvallis, 1979. 275 leaves.
**Lester JP, Franke JL, Bowman AO, et al:** Hazardous wastes, politics, and public policy: a comparative state analysis. **West Polit Q** 1983;36(2):257–85
**Lester KS:** A short history of Westmead Centre Dental Clinical School. **Aust Dent J** 1981 Oct;26(5):321–7
**Lester TW** see **Leff A**
**Lesthaeghe R, Wilson C:** Les modes de production, la laïcisation et le rythme de la baisse de la fécondité en Europe de l'Ouest de 1870 à 1930. **Population** 1982;37(3):623–45
**Leszczak M:** 200 lat. **Pieleg Polozna** 1984;(3):30–1
**L'Etang H:** Fit to lead? London, Heinemann, 1980. 211 p.
**Letavet AA:** K 35–letiiu Velikoĭ Pobedy. **Gig Tr Prof Zabol** 1980 May;(5):1–3

**Letondal P:** Introduction à l'histoire de la pédiatrie au Canada français. In: Congrès international d'histoire de la médecine, XXVe, Québec, 1976. Actes. Québec, 1977. p. 885-94.

**Lett Z:** Anaesthesia in Hong Kong: evolution and present position. [Hong Kong], Centre of Asian Studies, University of Hong Kong, 1982. 36 p.

**Lett Z:** Anaesthesia in Hong Kong. Its history and present position. **Anaesthesia** 1980 Oct;35(10):993-8

**Letton AH:** Pyramids or Parthenons? **J Surg Oncol** 1983 Jun;23(2):63-9

**Leucah F:** Looking back: 'A psychological problem.' **Lamp** 1980 Dec;37(12):41-2

**Leuilliot P:** O współczesną historię medyczno-społeczną. **Kwart Hist Kultury Mater** 1975;23(2):255-67

**Leuilliot P:** Problèmes de méthode: histoire (et archives) de la santé. In Livet G, Schaff G, ed: Médecine et assistance en Alsace, XVIe-XXe siècle. Strasbourg, Istra, 1976. p. 11-17.

**Leupold-Kirschneck D:** Das Handauflegen. Eine ärztliche Urgebärde in Geschichte und Gegenwart. Basel/Stuttgart, Schwabe, 1981. 81 p. (Basler Veröffentlichungen zur Geschichte der Medizin und der Biologie, 33).

**Leupold-Löwenthal H:** Zur Geschichte der 'Frage der Laienanalyse'. **Psyche (Stuttg)** 1984 Feb;38(2):97-120

**Levenson SM, Hopkins BS, Waldron M, et al:** Early history of parenteral nutrition. **Fed Proc** 1984 Apr;43(5):1391-406

**Levenstein H:** The New England kitchen and the origins of modern American eating habits. **Am Q** 1980;32(4):369-86

**Levental Z:** Medizinisches in den Schriften Edward Brownes (1642-1708). **Gesnerus** 1982;39(2):215-35

**Lever WF:** Reminiscences about dermatopathology. **Am J Dermatopathol** 1979 Winter;1(4):313-7

**Lever WF:** Savary's 1814 article on the history of pemphigus related to contemporary views. **Int J Dermatol** 1979 Sep;18(7):584-5

**Levere TH:** Dr. Thomas Beddoes at Oxford: radical politics in 1788-1793 and the fate of the Regius Chair in Chemistry. **Ambix** 1981 Jul;28(2):61-9

**Levere TH:** Dr. Thomas Beddoes: the interaction of pneumatic and preventive medicine with chemistry. **Interdiscip Sci Rev** 1982;7:137-47

**Levere TH:** Dr. Thomas Beddoes (1750-1808): science and medicine in politics and society. **Br J Hist Sci** 1984 Jul;17(56 pt 2):187-204

**Levere TH:** Humphry Davy and the idea of glory. **Trans R Soc Can** 1980;18:247-61

**Levere TH:** Poetry realized in nature. Samuel Taylor Coleridge and early nineteenth-century science. Cambridge, Cambridge University Press, 1981. xiii, 271 p.

**Levere TH** see **Forgan S, ed**

**Levere TH, ed:** Editing texts in the history of science and medicine. Papers given at the seventeenth annual Conference on Editorial Problems, University of Toronto, 6-7 November 1981. New York, London, Garland, 1982. 190 p. Contributions by S. Drake, L. E. Voigts, B. S. Hall, A. Beaulieu, I. B. Cohen.

**Leveroni J** see **Lentini J**

**Levers BG, Darling AI:** Continuous eruption of some adult human teeth of ancient populations. **Arch Oral Biol** 1983;28(5):401-8

**Levers BG** see **Newman HN**

**Levertov D** see **Trautmann J, ed**

**Lévesque A, ed** see **Shephard DA**

**Levett JM** see **Sanderson CJ**

**Levey M:** Medical ethics on medieval Islam with special reference to Al-Ruhawi's 'Practical ethics of the physician.' Philadelphia, American Philosophical Society, 1967. 100 p. (Transactions of the American Philosophical Society, n.s., Vol. 57, Part 3, 1967).

**Levi F:** La cecita nella cultura. **Belfagor** 1982;37(5):569-80

**Levi M:** Functional redundancy and the process of professionalization: the case of registered nurses in the United States. **J Health Polit Policy Law** 1980 Summer;5(2):333-53

**Levien M, ed:** Naval surgeon. The voyages of Dr. Edward H. Cree, Royal Navy, as related in his private journals, 1837-1856. New York, E. P. Dutton, 1982. 275 p.

**Levin A:** Venel, Lavoisier, Fourcroy, Cabanis and the idea of scientific revolution: the French political context and the general patterns of conceptualization of scientific change. **Hist Sci** 1984 Sep;22(57 pt 3):303-20

**Levin AB** see **Sergeev VM**

**Levin BS:** Women and medicine. Metuchen, N. J., London, Scarecrow, 1980. vii, 257 p.

**Levin H:** Conservatism of social work. **Soc Serv Rev** 1982;56(4):605-15

**Levin HS, Peters BH, Hulkonen DA:** Early concepts of anterograde and retrograde amnesia. **Cortex** 1983 Dec;19(4):427-40

**Levin LS** see **Andrews LB**

**Levin MJ:** Psychology. A biographical approach. New York, McGraw-Hill, 1978. 662 p.

**Levin S:** Eshmun, healing of God of Sidon. **Adler Mus Bull** 1983 Nov;Spec issue:39-42

**Levin S:** Hebrew medical amulets. **Adler Mus Bull** 1981;7(2):8-12

**Levin S:** Landmark perspective: the atypical pneumonia syndrome. **JAMA** 1984 Feb 17;251(7):945-8

**Levin S:** Mongolian spot; Afro-Asian stain; sacral stain. **S Afr Med J** 1981 Jul 25;60(4):123-4

**Levine D:** Illiteracy and family life during the first industrial revolution. **J Soc Hist** 1980;14(1):25-44

**Levine D:** Siamese twins in the Parish Registers of Shepshed, Leicestershire. **Local Popul Stud (Matlock)** 1981 Spring;26:44-5

**Levine D** see **Laslett P**

**Levine ER:** Fifty years of respiratory therapy. **Respir Ther** 1979 Jan-Feb;9(1):57, 59-60

**Levine HG:** The alcohol problem in America: from temperance to alcoholism. **Br J Addict** 1984 Mar;79(1):109-19

**Levine HM, Gilderdale S:** Genetics and communism. **Colo Q** 1975;24(1):17-24

**Levine JR:** The true inventors of the keratoscope and photo-keratoscope. **Br J Hist Sci** 1965;2(8):324-42

**Levine M:** The history and politics of community mental health. New York, Oxford University Press, 1981. 232 p.

**Levine P:** Historical perspectives before 1945--updated. **Prog Clin Biol Res** 1980;43:3-11

**Levine P:** The discovery of Rh hemolytic disease. **Vox Sang** 1984;47(2):187-90

**Levine RE:** A historical perspective on professional values. **J Allied Health** 1983 Aug;12(3):183-91

**Levine RJ:** [History of biomedical research]. In Reich WT, et al, ed: Encyclopedia of bioethics, v.4. New York, Free Press, 1978. p. 1481-92.

**Levinger IM, ed:** 'Medizinisch-schwierige Talmudstellen' [by Karl Preis]. **Udim** 1977-78;7-8:95-107

**Levison CH, Hastings DW, Harrison JN:** The epidemiologic transition in a frontier town--Manti, Utah, 1849-1977. **Am J Phys Anthropol** 1981 Sep;56(1):83-93

**Levit AZ, Vankhanen NV:** V. I. Lenin o sotsial'nykh aspektakh narodnogo pitaniia. **Gig Sanit** 1981 Jan;(1):37-9

**Levit MM:** Metodologiia i metodika prepodavaniia istorii meditsiny. **Sov Zdravookhr** 1980;(3):54-7

**Levitin MN:** Stoĭkiĭ bol'shevik-leninets A. P. Golubkov. **Feldsher Akush** 1980;45(11):44-6

**Levitin NN:** Iz istorii bor'by s beshenstvom v Rossii. **Feldsher Akush** 1980;45(7):53-5

**Levitskaia SV** see **Matveev MP**

**Levsin BV** see **Komkov GD**

**Levtova KZ** see **Suvorov VIu**

**Lévy A:** Alphonse Laveran, initiateur de la pathologie coronaro-myocardique. **Nouv Presse Med** 1981 Mar 21;10(13):1015

**Lévy A:** Le rendez-vous manqué de la connaissance immédiate et du hasard. Contribution à l'historie de l'hypertension artérielle. **Coeur Med Interne** 1979 Oct-Dec;18(4):567-70

**Levy B:** Pharmacy graduates in use from 1880 to 1920. **Pharm Hist** 1984;26(3):150-4

**Levy C:** Essai d'estimation de la population handicapée en France. (Handicap sevère). **Population** 1983;38(1):178-84

**Lévy C:** La mortalité par accident des enfants et des adolescents dans huit pays développés. **Population** 1980;35(2):291-319

**Lévy J:** Magnétisme animal et médecine à Strasbourg à la fin du XVIIIe siècle. In Livet G, Schaff G, ed: Médecine et assistance en Alsace, XVIe-XXe siècle. Strasbourg, Istra, 1976. p. 201-7.

**Levy JE, Kunitz SJ, Everett M:** Navajo criminal homicide. **Southwest J Anthropol** 1969;25(2):124-52

**Levy M:** Intraperitoneal drainage. **Am J Surg** 1984 Mar;147(3):309-14

**Levy MJ** see **Yechezkel M**

**The Levy brothers: early San Francisco chiropodists, a picture story: West States Jew Hist Q** 1981;13(4):317-21

**Lewerenz-Steinsiepe M:** Fritz Ludwig Dumont: ein moderner Anaesthesist. **Anaesthesist** 1982 Jun;31(6):302-5

**Lewin PK, Hancock RG, Voynovich P:** Napoleon Bonaparte--no evidence of chronic arsenic poisoning. **Nature** 1982 Oct 14;299(5884):627-8

**Lewin PK** see **Millet NB**

**Lewin R:** Darwin died at a most propitious time. **Science** 1982 Aug 20;217(4561):717-8

**Lewinsohn R:** Carlos Chagas and the discovery of Chagas' disease (American trypanosomiasis). **J R Soc Med** 1981 Jun;74(6):451-5

**Lewis A** see **Maudsley H**

**Lewis BE:** A tradition of exceptional women. **J Am Med Wom Assoc** 1983 May-Jun;38(3):75-6, 82

**Lewis D, Hunt DM:** Hans Grüneberg: 26 May 1907-23 October 1982. **Biogr Mem Fellows R Soc** 1984;30:227-47

**Lewis ER:** Prairie state pharmacy. [Chicago?], Illinois Pharmacists Association, 1980. vi, 163 p.

**Lewis ER:** The anatomy of a pharmacist. **Pharm Hist** 1982;24(2):87-9

**Lewis IC:** The years of children. Part I. **Aust Nurses J** 1980 Jul;10(1):46-9

**Lewis J, Brookes B:** A reassessment of the work of the Peckham Health Centre, 1926-1951. **Milbank Mem Fund Q** 1983 Spring;61(2):307-50

**Lewis J:** The ideology and politics of birth control in inter-war Britain. **Womens Stud** 1979;2(l)

**Lewis J, Brookes B:** The Peckham Health Centre, 'Pep', and the concept of General practice during the 1930s and 1940s. **Med Hist** 1983 Apr;27(2):151-61

**Lewis J:** The politics of motherhood: child and maternal welfare in England, 1900-1939. London, Croom Helm, 1980. 235 p.

**Lewis JA:** Petit mal epilepsy. An early American report. **NY State J Med** 1983 Jul-Sep;83(8-10):1051-2

**Lewis JS:** Manners and medicine. Childbearing in the English aristocracy 1790-1840. Ph.D. Diss., Johns Hopkins University. Baltimore, 1979. vi, 301 leaves.

**Lewis JS:** Maternal health in the English aristocracy: myths and realities (1790-1840). **J Soc Hist** 1983;17:97-114

**Lewis JS:** Obstetric reminiscences in the course of general practice in Basutoland (over 50 years ago). **S Afr Med J** 1983 Jun 29;Spec No:20-2

**Lewis M:** Hospitalization for childbirth in Sydney, 1870–1939; the modern maternity hospital and the improvement in the health of women. **J R Aust Hist Soc** 1980;66(3):199–205
**Lewis M:** Milk, mothers, and infant welfare. In J. Roe, ed: Twentieth century Sydney: studies in urban and social history. Sydney, Hale & Iremonger for the Sydney Hist. Group, 1980. p. 193–207.
**Lewis M:** Some infant health problems in Sydney, 1880–1939. **J R Aust Hist Soc** 1982;68(1):67–73
**Lewis M:** The problem of infant feeding: the Australian experience from the mid-nineteenth century to the 1920s. **J Hist Med Allied Sci** 1980 Apr;35(2):174–87
**Lewis MJ:** Populate or perish: aspects of infant and maternal health in Sydney, 1870–1939. [S.l.:s.n.], 1976. xx, 365 p.
**Lewis N:** The interpretation of dreams and portents. Toronto, Sarasota, Stevens, 1976. xi, 167 p.
**Lewis OJ:** The joints of the evolving foot. Part III. The fossil evidence. **J Anat** 1980 Sep;131(Pt 2):275–98
**Lewis RK** see **Uphoff MJ**
**Lewis RW:** Evolution: a system of theories. **Perspect Biol Med** 1980;23(4):551–72
**Lewis TH:** Richard Carew on the treatment of a 'Franticke person' in Medieval Cornwall. **J Hist Med Allied Sci** 1981 Jan;36(1)64–6
**Lewis TH:** The changing practice of the Oglala medicine man. **Plains Anthropol** 1980;25(89):265–7
**Lewis Thomas: Cell Immunol** 1983 Nov;82(1):3–17
**Lewontin R, Rose S, Kamin L:** Bourgeois ideology and the origins of biological determinism. **Race Cl** 1982;24(1):1–16
**Lewontin RC, Moore JA, Provine WB, et al:** Dobzhansky's genetics of natural populations, I–XLIII. New York, Columbia University Press, 1981. xiv, 942 p. Includes Provine WB: Origins of the Genetics of natural populations series, p. 1–76.
**Lewontin RC** see **Mayr E**
**Lewy R** see **Borkenhagen R**
**Lex BW:** Neurological bases of revitalization movements. **Zygon** 1978;13(4):276–312
**L'Exposition Universelle de 1889:** Recherche des réponses au questionnaire et d'objets. **Bull Soc Fr Hist Hop** 1979;(39):19–21
**Ley H:** Ibn Sina (Avicenna, 980–1037): Gründe für 1000 Jahre Rückerinnerung. **Dtsch Z Philos** 1980;28(11):1309–23
**Leydon I** see **Quinn S, ed**
**Leyendecker CH:** Erfahrung und Theorie in der Sonderpädagogik Körperbehinderter--ein Diskurs zum Theorie-Praxis-Bezug. **Rehabilitation (Stuttg)** 1983 Aug;22(3):100–9
**Leyh F:** Hatte Rembrandt van Rijn eine Nickelallergie? **Hautarzt** 1984 Sep;35(9):472–3
**Leyh F, Wendt V:** Heinrich A. Gottron (1890–1974). **Am J Dermatopathol** 1983 Jun;5(3):241–3
**Leys R:** Background to the reflex controversy: William Alison and the doctrine of sympathy before Hall. **Stud Hist Biol** 1980;4:1–66
**Leys R:** Meyer's dealings with Jones: a chapter in the history of the American response to psychoanalysis. **J Hist Behav Sci** 1981 Oct;17(4):445–65
**Leyva Corzo A:** Toxoplasmosis: resumen histórico y revisión bibliográfica. **Rev Cubana Med Trop** 1979 May–Aug;31(2):141–58
**L'Héritier P:** Souvenirs d'un généticien. In Actes du Colloque R.A. Fisher.... Paris, 5–6 déc. 1979. p. 331–350. **Rev Synth (Paris)** 1981;102(103–104)
**Lhermitte F, Signoret JL:** L'aphasie de J. M. Charcot à Th. Alajouanine. **Rev Neurol (Paris)** 1982;138(12):893–919
**Lhermitte F** see **Castaigne P**
**Lhermitte F** see **Signoret JL**
**L'homme et son corps dans la société traditionelle:** Paris, Ministère de la culture et de la communication, Editions de la Réunion des musées nationaux, 1978. 144 p.
**L'Hôpital Des Enfants-Malades, the world's first children's hospital, founded in Paris in 1802: Pediatrics** 1981 May;67(5):670
**L'Hôtel-Dieu, le premier hôpital de Montréal: Auxiliaire** 1981 Mar–Apr;:13–5
**Li JK** see **Fich S**
**Li LM:** Food and famine in China. **Soc Sci Res Counc Items** 1981;35(1–2):11–4
**Li LM:** Workshop on food and famine in Chinese history. **Ch'ing-Shih Wen-t'i** 1980;4(4):90–100
**Li Q:** [Discussion on the time of formation of the theoretical system of Ziwuliuzhu (Selection of acupoint for treatment varied with the circadian changes of vital energy and blood flow in the channels and collaterals relevant to heavenly stem and earthly branches)] (Chi). **Chung Hua I Shih Tsa Chih** 1984;14(2):85–9
**Li SJ** see **Lee S**
**Li WB:** [History of epidemics in ancient China] (Chi). **Chung Hua Liu Hsing Ping Hsueh Tsa Chih** 1983 Oct;4(5):316–9
**Li Y:** [The discovery of paragonimiasis in Fujian Province] (Chi). **Chung Hua I Shih Tsa Chih** 1984 Jan;14(1):19–24
**Li Z:** [On Li Shizhen's contributions to the method of systematization of Chinese herbology] (Chi). **Chung Hua I Shih Tsa Chih** 1984 Jan;14(1):35–9
**Li ZY** see **Yang KL**
**Li Yousong:** [Exploration of the relationship between defeating Cao Cao in Chibi and schistosomiasis.] (Chi). **Chin J Med Hist** 1981;11:87–8
**Liamtseva GA** see **Shliakhtenko LI**
**Liashenko NI:** Aleksandr Porfir'evich Borodin (k 150 letiiu so dnia rozhdeniia). **Voen Med Zh** 1983 Nov;(11):66–9
**Liashenko NI** see **Shcherbina VP**
**Libánský J:** Vývoj hematologie od dob profesora Hynka a její další perspektivy. **Vnitr Lek** 1979 Sep;25(9):915–20
**Libby LM** see **Black EF**
**Liberti L, Coyle G, Der Marderosian A:** Historical pharmaceutical exhibits at PCP&S. **Pharm Hist** 1980;22(3):115–18
**Libicky H:** A personal sketch of Professor Anton Elschnig. **Surv Ophthalmol** 1982 Mar–Apr;26(5):266–8
**Libri e manoscritti di Haller, 1777–1977:** Nel II centenario della morte di Albrecht von Haller. Milano, Biblioteca Nazionale Braidense, 1977. 69 p.
**Licata SJ, Peterson RP ed:** Historical perspectives on homosexuality. **J Homosex** 1980–81 Fall–Winter;6(1–2):3–210
**Licata SJ:** Historical perspectives on homosexuality. New York, Haworth, 1981. 224 p.
**Lichello R:** Pioneer in blood plasma; Dr. Charles Richard Drew. New York, Messner, [1968]. 190 p.
**Lichtenberg JD** see **Goldberg A, ed**
**Lichtenthaeler C:** [A tribute to Hans Diller.] **Hermes** 1979;109:270–86
**Lichtenthaeler C:** Chronologische und gedankliche Bezugssysteme in und um 'Ueber die alte Medizin'. XI. Hippokratische Studie. Genève, Droz, 1980. 30 p. (Etudes d'histoire de la médecine, VI).
**Lichtenthaeler C:** Die sechs Leitgedanken von Magendies medizinischer Revolution. **Z Arztl Fortbild (Jena)** 1983;77(18):785–8
**Lichtenthaeler C:** Humanismus und Aufklärung aus der Sicht der allgemeinen Medizingeschichte. In: Aufklärung und Humanismus; hrsg. von R. Toellner. Heidelberg, Lambert Schneider, 1980. p. 235–49.
**Lichtenthaeler C:** Le serment d'Hippocrate: analyse d'ensemble. **Rev Med Suisse Romande** 1980 Dec;100(12):1001–11
**Lichtenthaeler C:** Outé gar iatori èrkoun to proton therapeuontes agnoia. **Hermes** 1979, 1978;107(3):270–86
**Lichtenthaeler C:** Préambule historique au 'baptême' des auditoires. **Rev Med Suisse Romande** 1984 May;104(5):335–6
**Lichtenthaeler C** see **Grmek MD, ed**
**Lick RF:** Geschichte der Magenchirurgie. **MMW** 1980 May 9;122(19):720–2
**Licorish KA:** Hypersensitivity pneumonitis--economic and legal aspects. **Clin Rev Allergy** 1983 Dec;1(4):487–96
**Lidge RT** see **Brown JE**
**Lidov IP:** Terapevty v Velikoĭ Otechestvennoĭ voĭne. **Ter Arkh** 1980;52(5):3–5
**Lie JT:** Carl Weigert (1845–1904), a pathfinder in medicine. **Mayo Clin Proc** 1980 Nov;55(11):716–20
**Lie JT, Mann RJ, Ludwig J:** The brothers von Winiwarter, Alexander (1848–1917) and Felix (1852–1931), and thromboangiitis obliterans. **Mayo Clin Proc** 1979 Dec;54(12):802–7
**Lieb J, Hershman D:** Isaac Newton: mercury poisoning or manic depression? **Lancet** 1983 Dec 24–31;2(8365–66):1479–80
**Liebel-Weckowicz H** see **Weckowicz TE**
**Liebenau J:** Charles Albert Browne (1870–1947). **Surv Sources Newsl** 1977 May;5:10–1
**Liebenau J:** The papers of Edmund Newton Harvey, (1887–1959). **Surv Sources Newsl** 1977 Nov;6:8–9
**Liebenau JM:** Medical science and medical industry, 1890–1929: a study of pharmaceutical manufacturing in Philadelphia. Ph. D. Diss., University of Pennsylvania. Philadelphia, 1981. vii, 489 p.
**Liebenau JM:** Medicine and technology. **Perspect Biol Med** 1983 Autumn;27(1):76–92
**Lieber Z:** Is there a relationship between illness and creativity? An analysis of the life and poetry of A. V. Koltsov. **Int J Soc Psychiatry** 1980;26(3):212–7
**Lieberman AN:** Adolph Hitler: his diaries and Parkinson's disease. **N Engl J Med** 1983 Aug 11;309(6):375–6
**Lieberman LM:** Itard: the great problem solver. **J Learn Disabil** 1982 Nov;15(9):566–8
**Liebert RS:** Michelangelo: a psychoanalytic study of his life and images. New Haven, Yale University Press, 1983. xxii, 447 p.
**Liebner K** see **Adam J**
**Liebow AA:** Encounter with disaster: a medical diary of Hiroshima, 1945. Condensed from the original publication, 1965. **Yale J Biol Med** 1983 Jan–Feb;56(1):23–38
**Lieburg MJ van:** De microscopie in het onderwijs van de klinische scholen in Nederland (1824–1865). **Tijdschr Geschied Geneeskd** 1983;6(2):82–98
**Lieburg MJ van:** De verpleegkundige literatuur in Nederland in de 19e eeuw. **Tijdschr Geschied Geneeskd** 1980;3(3):97–122
**Lieburg MJ van:** Het medisch Onderwijs te Rotterdam (1467–1967): een kort historisch Overzicht. Amsterdam, Rodopi, 1978. 111 p.
**Lienau C** see **Hippokrates**
**Lienhard S:** Remarks on the early history of Indian medical terminology. **Sci Orient** 1979;16:9–20
**Liepa A:** Ikh imena nosiat meditsinskie uchilischcha. **Med Sestra** 1980 Sep;37(9):54–6
**Lieth H** see **Schnitzler H**
**Lifton RJ:** Medicalized killing in Auschwitz. **Psychiatry** 1982;45(4):283–97
**Lifton RJ:** On the consciousness of holocaust. **Psychohist Rev** 1980;9(1):3–22
**Lifton RJ:** Psychohistory. In H. I. Kaplan, et al, ed: Comprehensive textbook of psychiatry/III. Third edition. Baltimore, London, Williams & Wilkins, 1980. p. 3104–12.
**Lifton RJ, Kato S, Reich MR:** Six lives, six deaths. Portraits from modern

Japan. New Haven and London, Yale University Press, 1979. xiii, 305 p.
**Lifton RJ:** The concept of the survivor. In Dimsdale, Joel E., ed: Survivors, victims, and perpetrators. Essays on the Nazi Holocaust. Washington, Hemisphere Publ., 1980. p. 113-26.
**Light TR:** Hands on stamps. **J Hand Surg** 1981 Sep;6(5):441
**Light TR:** Hands on stamps. **J Hand Surg** 1982 Jan;7(1):20
**Lightdale CJ:** Notes on the development of the American Society for Gastrointestinal Endoscopy. **Gastrointest Endosc** 1983 Feb;29(1):51-3
**Ligterink JH:** De apotheker en de zelfmedicatie. **Pharm Weekbl** 1981 Nov 6;116(45):1398-1400
**Likhachev AG:** Dostizheniia sovetskogo zdravookhraneniia. **Vestn Otorinolaringol** 1982 Nov-Dec;(6):3-8
**Likourinas M** see **Dimopoulos C**
**Liles BZ** see **Duffy RJ**
**Liles DM:** William Faulkner's Absalom, Absalom!: an exegesis of the homoerotic configurations in the novel. **J Homosex** 1983 Spring-Summer;8(3-4):99-111
**Lilienfeld AM:** Bradford Hill's influence on epidemiology. **Stat Med** 1982 Oct-Dec;1(4):325-8
**Lilienfeld AM:** Ceteris Paribus: the evolution of the clinical trial. (The Fielding H. Garrison Lecture). **Bull Hist Med** 1982 Spring;56(1):1-18
**Lilienfeld AM:** Epidemiology and health policy: some historical highlights. **Public Health Rep** 1984 May-Jun;99(3):237-41
**Lilienfeld AM, Lilienfeld DE:** Epidemiology and the public health movement: a historical perspective. **J Public Health Policy** 1982 Jun;3(2):140-9
**Lilienfeld AM, Lilienfeld DE:** John Snow, the Broad Street pump and modern epidemiology. **Int J Epidemiol** 1984 Sep;13(3):376-8
**Lilienfeld AM, Lilienfeld DE:** 'The epidemiologic fabric'. I--Weaving the threads. **Int J Epidemiol** 1980 Sep;9(3):199-206
**Lilienfeld AM, Lilienfeld DE:** 'The epidemiologic fabric'. II. The London Bridge--it never fell. **Int J Epidemiol** 1980 Dec;9(4):299-304
**Lilienfeld AM, Lilienfeld DE:** Threads of epidemiologic history. In their: Foundations of epidemiology. 2d ed. New York and Oxford, Oxford University Press, 1980. p. 23-45.
**Lilienfeld AM:** Wade Hampton Frost: contributions to epidemiology and public health. **Am J Epidemiol** 1983 Apr;117(4):379-83
**Lilienfeld AM** see **Lilienfeld DE**
**Lilienfeld DE:** Epidemiology 101: III. A 19th century example. **Int J Epidemiol** 1981 Mar;10(1):69-72
**Lilienfeld DE, Lilienfeld AM:** The French influence on the development of epidemiology. In Lilienfeld AM, ed: Times, places, and persons. Baltimore, London, Johns Hopkins Univ. Press, 1980. (Sigerist suppl. to the Bull Hist Med, n.s., no 4) p. 28-38.
**Lilienfeld DE** see **Lilienfeld AM**
**Lilienfeld AM, ed:** Times, places, and persons. Aspects of the history of epidemiology. Baltimore and London, Johns Hopkins University Press, 1980. 144 p. (Sigerist Supplements to the Bulletin of the History of Medicine, n.s., no. 4).
**Lilienthal G:** 'Rheinlandbastarde', Rassenhygiene und das Problem der rassenideologischen Kontinuität. Zur Untersuchung von Reiner Pommerin: 'Sterilisierung der Rheinlandbastarde'. **Medizinhist J** 1980;15(4):426-36
**Liljeblad S** see **Zimmermann G**
**Lillehei CW:** A personalized history of extracorporeal circulation. **Trans Am Soc Artif Intern Organs** 1982;28:5-16
**Lillehei RC:** History of vasodilation in treating shock and low flow states. **Adv Shock Res** 1978;1:1-17
**Lillehei RC:** The Wangensteen tradition: what it is and how can we perpetuate it? **Minn Med** 1981 Oct;64(10):626-8
**Lima JC** see **Veras RP**
**Limbrick E:** Franciscus Sanchez 'Scepticus': un médecin philosophe précurseur de Descartes (1550-1623). **Renaiss Reformation** 1982;18:264-72
**Limentani A:** Anna Freud's contribution to the work of the International Psychoanalytical Association. **Int J Psychoanal** 1983;64 (Pt 4):375-7
**Limoge A** see **Kunegel JM**
**Limoges C:** The development of the Muséum d'Histoire Naturelle of Paris, c. 1800-1914. In R. Fox, G. Weisz, ed: The organization of science and technology in France 1808-1914. Cambridge, Cambridge University Press, 1980. p. 211-40.
**Limoges C** see **Farley M**
**Limoges C** see **Mayr E**
**Limón E:** Homenaje al doctor Antonio Torres Estrada. **Gac Med Mex** 1984 May;120(5):205-12
**Lin CC, Chen JY:** [Development of natural crude drug resources from Taiwǎn (I). Pharmacognostical studies on the Chinese crude drug 'Hàn-lián-cǎo (1). The herbological studies] (Jpn). **Yakushigaku Zasshi** 1983;18(2):65-72
**Lin JI:** Virchow's pathological reports on Frederick III's cancer. **N Engl J Med** 1984 Nov 8;311(19):1261-4
**Lin P:** [Textual research on the date of birth and death of Chunyu Yi and his appointment] (Chi). **Chung Hua I Shih Tsa Chih** 1984;14(2):78-9
**Lin SP:** Family planning in Taiwan: its problems and solutions. **She Hui K'ohsueh Lun Ts'ung** 1978;27:109-51
**Lin Qianliang, Liu Zhengcai:** [Notions about gerontism, longevity and life span in ancient China.] (Chi). **Chin J Med Hist** 1981;11:84-6
**Linage Conde A:** Ibn Hazm de Cordoba y la neurosis. **Asclepio** 1981;33:349-77
**Linares Maza A:** La psiquiatría andaluza en la primera mitad de nuestro siglo. Personalidades destacadas. I. Miguel Prados Such (Málaga). **Arch Neurobiol (Madr)** 1983 Jan-Feb;46(1):59-66
**Lind J:** Researches in perinatal circulation. In Smith GF, Smith PN, Vidyasagar, D, ed: Historical review and recent advances in neonatal and perinatal medicine. [Chicago?], Mead Johnson Nutritional Division, 1983. Vol. II. p. 1-20.
**Lind J** see **Smith GF**
**Lindberg DC:** Theories of vision from Al-Kindi to Kepler. Chicago, London, University of Chicago Press, 1976. xii, 324 p.
**Lindberg DC, ed:** Opticae thesaurus. Alhazeni Arabis libri septem, nuncprimùm editi. Eiusdem liber De Crepusculis et nubium ascensionibus. Item Vitellonis Thuringopoloni libri X. Reprint of the 1572 ed. New York, Johnson Reprint Corp., 1972. xxxiv, 288, 474 p.
**Lindbergh CA** see **Chambers RW**
**Linde E:** Ernst von Bergmann. Rückblick auf das Leben anlässlich der Einweihung der Sanitätsakademie in München. **MMW** 1981 May 1;123(18):751-2
**Linde LM:** History of Northwest District Medical Association (No. 11). **SD J Med** 1981 May;34(5):31
**Lindeboom GA:** Anton de Heide als proefondervindelijk onderzoeker. **Tijdschr Geschied Geneeskd** 1983;6(3):121-34
**Lindeboom GA:** Cowper's brutale 'plagiaat' van Bidloo's Anatomische Atlas. **Ned Tijdschr Geneeskd** 1982 Oct 9;126(41):1878-82
**Lindeboom GA:** De ontdekking van het trilhaarepitheel door Antonius de Heide (1683). **Ned Tijdschr Geneeskd** 1980 May 24;124(21):839-41
**Lindeboom GA:** De verdiensten van Jan Swammerdam voor de medische wetenschap. **Ned Tijdschr Geneeskd** 1980 Dec 13;124(50):2135-41
**Lindeboom GA:** Descartes and medicine. Amsterdam, Rodopi, 1979. 134 p. (Nieuwe Nederlandse Bijdragen tot de Geschiedenis der Geneeskunde, No. 1).
**Lindeboom GA:** Euthanasie in Historisch Perspectief. Amsterdam, Rodopi, 1978. 47 p.
**Lindeboom GA:** Geschiedenis der geneeskunde: J. N. Ramaer (1817-1887) en zijn bibliotheek. **Ned Tijdschr Geneeskd** 1982 Aug 14;126(33):1504-10
**Lindeboom GA:** Jacob Voegen van Engelen, medisch journalist; 'De Surinaamsche Artz'. **Ned Tijdschr Geneeskd** 1981 Jun 27;125(26):1044-9
**Lindeboom GA:** Jan Swammerdam als microscopist. **Tijdschr Geschied Geneeskd** 1981;4(2):87-110
**Lindeboom GA:** Jan Swammerdam (1637-1680) and his Biblia Naturae. **Clio Med** 1982 Dec;17(2-3):113-31
**Lindeboom GA:** Nederlandse Bijdragen tot de ontwikkeling der moderne fysiologie. Voordracht gehouden op 20 mei 1976 bij de herdenking van het 25-jarig bestaan van het Fysiologisch Laboratorium aan de Vrije Universiteit te Amsterdam. Amsterdam, Laboratorium voor Fysiologie der Vrije Universiteit, 1978. 35 p.
**Lindeboom GA** see **Palm LC**
**Lindeboom GA, ed:** Boerhaave's correspondence. Part 3. Leiden, Brill, 1979. viii, 281 p. (Part 1 was published 1962, and Part 2 in 1964).
**Lindeboom GA, ed:** Haller in Holland: het dagboek van Albrecht von Haller van zijn verblijf in Holland (1725-1727). Amsterdam, Rodopi, 1979. 122 p.
**Lindeboom GA, ed:** Het cabinet van Jan Swammerdam (1637-1680). Facsimile reprinted from 1681 ed., Amsterdam, Rodopi, 1980. xxiv, 16 p.
**Lindell P:** Gastrostomi--enkel metod med många fördelar. **Lakartidningen** 1981 Jun 17;78(25):2473-5
**Lindemann C:** Margaret Sanger and the birth control movement. **Women Health** 1978 Mar-Apr;3(2):12-13,16-21
**Lindemann E:** Beyond grief: studies in crisis intervention. Ed. by E. B. Lindemann. Biographical introduction by B. S. Brown. New York and London, Aronson, 1979. 274 p.
**Lindemann EB** see **Lindemann E**
**Lindemann M:** Fürsorge für arme Wöchnerinnen in Hamburg um 1800: die Beschreibung eines 'Entbindungs-Winkels'. **Gesnerus** 1982;39(3-4):395-403
**Lindemann M:** Love for hire: the regulation of the wet-nursing business in eighteenth-century Hamburg. **J Fam Hist** 1981 Winter;6(4):379-95
**Lindemann M:** Maternal politics: the principles and practice of maternity care in eighteenth-century Hamburg. **J Fam Hist** 1984 Spring;9(1):44-63
**Lindemann M, Cesnokova S:** Wissenschaftliche Schulen in Deutschland im XIX. Jahrhundert und ihre Rolle für die Entwicklung der Physiologie in der Welt. In International Congress of the History of Medicine. 26th, Plovdiv, 1978. Actes du Congress. Sofia, 1981. Volume II. p. 140-3.
**Lindemann ME:** Producing policed man: poor relief, population policies and medical care in Hamburg, 1750-1806. Ph. D. Diss., University of Cincinnati. Cincinnati, 1980. vii, 386 p.
**Lindemayr W:** Die Bedeutung Albert Wiedmanns für die Entwicklung der Dermatologie in Wien nach 1945. **Wien Klin Wochenschr** 1981 Dec 25;93(24):735-9
**Linden R** see **Currie R**
**Linden SJ:** Alchemy and eschatology in seventeenth-century poetry. **Ambix** 1984 Nov;31(3):102-24
**Lindenbraten LD:** Voprosy prepodavaniia i podgotovki kadrov po rentgenologii i radiologii na stranitsakh zhurnala 'Meditsinskaia Radiologiia' (1956-1981). **Med Radiol (Mosk)** 1981;26(10):49-53
**Lindenmann J:** From interference to interferon: a brief historical introduction. **Philos Trans R Soc Lond [Biol]** 1982 Sep 24;299(1094):3-6
**Lindenmann J:** Origin of the terms 'antibody' and 'antigen'. **Scand J Immunol** 1984 Apr;19(4):281-5
**Lindenthal JJ:** Health and the eastern European Jewish immigrant.

**Am Jew Hist** 1981;70(4):420–41

**Linder SC:** Medicine in Marlboro County 1736 to 1980. Baltimore, Gateway, 1980. 206 p.

**Linder SC:** Pioneer physicians in Marlboro County, 1760–1824. **SC Hist Mag** 1980 Jul;81:232–44

**Linder SG:** Pioneer physicians in Marlboro County, 1760–1824. **SC Hist Mag** 1980;81(3):232–44

**Lindgren A:** Das Utrechter Arzneibuch (Ms. 1355,16 degrees, Bibliotheek der Rijksuniversiteit Utrecht). Stockholm, Almqvist & Wiksell, 1977. 199 p. (Acta Universitatis Stockholmiensis, Stockholmer Germanistische Forschungen, 21).

**Lindgren FT:** The plasma lipoproteins: historical developments and nomenclature. **Ann NY Acad Sci** 1980;348:1–15

**Lindgren G:** History and perspectives of social medicine. In: Congrès international d'histoire de la médecine, XXVe, Québec, 1976. Actes. Québec, 1977. p. 193–203.

**Lindgren S:** Ur svenska kirurgförbundets historia. **Nord Medicinhist Arsb** 1981;:160–71

**Lindgren S:** Utomäktenskaplig fertilitet i Helsingfors under 1800–talets senare del. **Hist Arkisto (Finl)** 1981;76:301–20

**Lindgren U:** The problems of being a foreigner: Ruy Gonzáles de Clavijo's journey to Samarkand. **Clio Med** 1980 Jul;14(3–4):225–34

**Lindholm RV:** Küntscher bone nailing – forecast and actuality. **Ann Chir Gynaecol** 1980;69(3):85–91

**Lindholm RV:** Küntscher bone nailing in Finland. Oulu, Finland, Univ. of Oulu, 1979. 35 p..

**Lindner H, et al, ed:** [Contemporary medical historiography in Germany]. **Nachrichtenbl Dtsch Ges Gesch Med Naturwiss Tech** 1980 Apr;30(1):1–64

**Lindop PJ, Rotblat J:** Radiation pollution of the environment. **Bull At Sci** 1971;27(7):17–24

**Lindroth S:** Medicinens historia som akademiskt undervisningsämne. **Nord Medicinhist Arsb** 1980;Suppl 6:25–9

**Lindroth S:** The two faces of Linnaeus. In Frängsmyr T, ed: Linnaeus, the man and his work. Berkeley, University of California Press, 1983. p. 1–62.

**Lindroth S** see **Frängsmyr T, ed**

**Lindsay CM, Seldon A, Feigenbaum B:** National health issues. [s.l.], Roche Laboratories, 1980. viii, 130 p.

**Lindsay CM** see **Hall TD**

**Lindskog BI:** Europeisk musei–konferens. **Sydsven Medicinhist Sallsk Arsskr** 1984;21:11–4

**Lindskog BI:** Mortalitätsanalyse einer südschwedischen Bevölkerung 1749–1818. In Imhof AE, ed: Mensch und Gesundheit in der Geschichte. Husum, Matthiesen, 1980. p. 163–73.

**Lindskog BI, Imhof AE:** Mortality in Scandinavia in the 18th century. In: Congrès international d'histoire de la médecine, XXVe, Québec, 1976. Actes. Québec, 1977. p. 205–15.

**Lindskog BI:** Otto Löfberg 1881–1954. **Sydsven Medicinhist Sallsk Arsskr** 1983;:65–76

**Lindskog BI** see **Habrich C**

**Lindskog GE:** Three generations of Doctors Bigelow at Harvard. **Conn Med** 1983 Dec;47(12):763–9

**Lindskog GE:** Two doctors Harvey: William (1578–1657); Samuel Clark (1886–1953). **Yale J Biol Med** 1979 Sep–Oct;52(5):467–82

**Lindstedt E, Lundquist SB:** Utveckling av den transurethrala kirurgien. **Sydsven Medicinhist Sallsk Arsskr** 1980;:94–111

**Lindsten J:** Sammanställde fall av kortvuxenhet och bristande ovariefunktion hos flickor. **Lakartidningen** 1983 Jul 13;80(28–29):2755

**Lindt A** see **Albrecht von Haller, 1708–1777**

**Lindy JD, Lindy JG:** Planning and delivery of mental health services in disaster: the Cincinnati experience. **Urban Soc Change Rev** 1981;14(2):16–21

**Lindy JG** see **Lindy JD**

**Lindzey G** see **Lasagna LC**

**Lineham PJ:** Restoring man's creative power: the theosophy of the Bible Christians of Salford. In Sheils WJ, ed: The Church and healing. Papers read at the twentieth summer meeting and the twenty–first winter meeting of the Ecclesiastical History Society. Oxford, Basil Blackwell for the Society, 1982. p. 207–23.

**Lines D:** 15th century ureteric reflux. **Lancet** 1982 Dec 25;2(8313):1473

**Linet J, Hillard D, Lavagne X, ed:** Catalogue des ouvrages imprimés au XVIe siècle, Bibliothèque Sainte–Geneviève, Paris: Sciences––Techniques––Médecine. Paris, New York, Saur, 1980. xvi, 493 p.

**Lingo AK:** The rise of medical practitioners in sixteenth–century France: the case of Lyon and Montpellier. Ph.D. diss. University of California. Berkeley, 1980. 318 leaves.

**Lingua P** see **Lanzavecchia P**

**Linhard J:** Aspectos sociales de los métodos naturales. **Reproduccion** 1981 Apr–Jun;5(2):95–104

**Link EP:** The Mayo family: a study in changing social ideas. In: Congrès international d'histoire de la médecine, XXVe, Québec, 1976. Actes. Québec, 1977. p. 895–916.

**Link K:** Potomac fever: the hazards of camp life. **Vt Hist** 1983;51(2):69–88

**Linkesch W, Urge L, Lukac J, et al:** Zur Geschichte der Tuberkulosebekämpfung in der CSSR: die ost–slowakischen Mykobakteriologie–Tbk–Seminare in Vysne Hagy und in Presov. **Wiss Beitr Martin Luther Univ Halle Wittenberg** 1983;5–R80:287–99

**Linn IJ** see **Wylie JA**

**Linss W:** Im memoriam Günther Geyer (25. 9. 1930––18. 6. 1980). **Anat Anz** 1981;149(3):193–209

**Linss W:** Karl von Bardeleben––der Begründer des 'Anatomischen Anzeigers'. **Anat Anz** 1981;150(1–2):5–10

**Linton SJ:** The man and the mind: Carl Emil Seashore, a pioneer on two frontiers. **Swed Pioneer Hist Q** 1980;31(2):122–8

**Lionel ND** see **Uragoda CG**

**Lipińska–Namysł E** see **Galiński J**

**Lipinski JK:** Some observations on early diagnostic radiology in Canada. **Can Med Assoc J** 1983 Oct 1;129(7):766–8

**Lipmann F:** A long life in times of great upheaval. **Annu Rev Biochem** 1984;53:1–33

**Lipmann F:** Hans Krebs and his metabolic cycles. **Naturwiss Rundsch** 1982;35:228–30

**Lipowski ZJ:** Holistic–medical foundations of American psychiatry: a bicentennial. **Am J Psychiatry** 1981 Jul;138(7):888–95

**Lipowski ZJ:** What does the word 'psychosomatic' really mean? A historical and semantic inquiry. **Psychosom Med** 1984 Mar–Apr;46(2):153–71

**Lippert GP:** Xenogener Ureterersatz in Tierversuch unter besonderer Berücksichtigung der historischen Entwicklung von Ureterbioprothesen. Diss. Mainz, 1979. 43 p.

**Lipps–Kant B:** Das ehemalige Oberamtskrankenhaus in Tettnang. Eine Anlage mit Zentralbau aus dem späten 19. Jahrhundert. **Hist Hosp** 1979–80;13:153–163

**Lipscomb JM:** New light on some Harvey portraits, in memoriam Sir Geoffrey Keynes. **Med Hist** 1983 Apr;27(2):197–202

**Lipton AA:** Was the 'nervous illness' of Schreber a case of affective disorder? **Am J Psychiatry** 1984 Oct;141(10):1236–9

**Lipton JD:** The rational evaluation of astrology in the period of Arabo–Latin translation ca. 1126–1187 AD. Ph.D. Diss., University of California. Los Angeles, 1978. 245 leaves.

**Lipton JS:** Oral surgery in Ancient Egypt as reflected in the Edwin Smith Papyrus. **Bull Hist Dent** 1982 Oct;30(2):108–14

**Lipton MA:** A letter from Anna Freud. **Am J Psychiatry** 1983 Dec;140(12):1583–4

**Lipton MA:** The evolution of the biological understanding of affective and schizophrenic disorders. In M. R. Zales, ed: Affective and schizophrenic disorders: new approaches to diagnosis and treatment. New York, Brunner/Mazel, 1983. p. 5–28.

**Lipton SD:** An addendum to 'The advantages of Freud's technique, as shown in his analysis of the Rat Man'. **Int J Psychoanal** 1979;60(pt2):215–6

**Lisanti L:** Urbanisation et folie São Paulo, 1852–1929. **Jahrb Gesch Staat Wirtsch Ges Lateinam** 1980;17:297–315

**Lise G:** Ceramica del '600 e farmacia / Giorgio Lise. Milano, Giuliani, 1974. 113 p.

**Lisfranc J:** Mémoire sur la rhynoplastie, ou l'art de refaire le nez. **Ann Chir Plast** 1982;27(2):189–93

**Lisiewicz J:** Jan Walenty Latos (1539––początek XVII w.) lekarz i astrolog Akademii Krakowskiej. **Wiad Lek** 1982 Dec 15;35(23–24):1589–91

**Lisiewicz J** see **Michalczak W**

**Lisitsyn KM:** Voenno–polevaia khirurgiia vo vremia Velikoĭ Otechestvennoĭ voĭny i perspektivy ee razvitiia. **Voen Med Zh** 1980 May;(5):42–5

**Lisitsyn IuP, Arkhangel'skiĭ GV:** S. P. Botkin––nevrolog. **Zh Nevropatol Psikhiatr** 1982;82(10):127–30

**Lisitsyn IuP:** V. I. Lenin i sovremennye voprosy sotsial'noĭ gigieny. **Zdravookhr Ross Fed** 1980;(4):3–9

**Lisowski FP:** Development of medicine in Japan. **East Horiz** 1980;19(3):29–34

**Lisowski FP:** The emergence and development of the barefoot doctor in China. **East Horiz** 1980;19(4):6–20

**Lisowski FP:** The evaluation of health care in China. **East Horiz** 1978;17(3):5–11

**Lisowski FP:** The evolution of health care in China (concluded). **East Horiz** 1978;17(4):16–21

**Lisowski FP** see **Oxnard CE**

**Lisowski W:** Sanitariuszki walczącej Warszawy. **Pieleg Polozna** 1979;(9):23–5

**Lissak K:** Tvorcheskoe sodruzhestvo vengerskikh i sovetskikh issledovateleĭ mozga. **Zh Vyssh Nerv Deiat** 1982 Nov–Dec;32(6):1183–4

**Lister J:** By the London post. The last post. **N Engl J Med** 1980 Dec 25;303(26):1528–31

**L'Istituto di Storia della Medicina dell'Università di Padova:** Un triennio di attività (Anni Acc. 1976–77/77–78/78–79). Padova, Tipografia 'La Garangola,' 1979. 23 p.

**Liston A:** To cure the sick and protect the healthy. In: Congrès international d'histoire de la médecine, XXVe, Québec, 1976. Actes. Québec, 1977. p. 217–28.

**Liston SE, Fetgatter GL:** The general essentials of accredited residencies in graduate medical education. **JAMA** 1982 Jun 4;247(21):3002–3

**Liston SL:** Traumatic amputation of the external ear: the War of Jenkins' Ear and George Washington. **Am J Surg** 1984 Nov;148(5):599–601

**Lisý Z** see **Horák J**

**Litchfield RB, Gordon D:** Closing the 'tour': a close look at the marriage market, unwed mothers, and abandoned children in mid–nineteenth century Amiens. **J Soc Hist** 1980;13(3):458–72

**Lithell UB:** Breast–feeding habits and their relation to infant mortality and marital fertility. **J Fam Hist** 1981;6:182–94

**Lithell UB:** Infant mortality rate and standards of living in the past. **Scand J Hist** 1981;6(4):297–315

**Lithium salts in the treatment of psychotic excitement: John F Cade:**

Aust NZ J Psychiatry 1982 Sep;16(3):129-33
**Lithner K:** Bilden i ögat. **Sydsven Medicinhist Sallsk Arsskr** 1983;:51-8
**Lithwick NH:** Science policy in Canada. **J Can Stud** 1968;3(3):29-38
**Litman DS** see **Litman RC**
**Litman RC, Litman DS:** Protection of the American consumer: the congressional battle for the enactment of the First Federal Food and Drug Law in the United States. **Food Drug Cosmet Law J** 1982 Jul;37(3):310-29
**Litoff JB:** Carolyn Conant van Blarcom. In: Notable American women. The modern period. Cambridge, Mass., Belknap-Harvard Univ. Press, 1980. 4:703-4.
**Litowitz BE** see **Goldberg A, ed**
**Litowitz NS** see **Goldberg A, ed**
**Little AC:** The eyes have it. **J Am Diet Assoc** 1980 Dec;77(6):688-91
**Little B:** Cheltenham: a gently sited town. **Contemp Rev** 1980;237(1377):191-3
**Little DA:** The relevance of prosthodontics and the science of dental materials to the practice of dentistry. **J Dent** 1982 Dec;10(4):300-10
**Little DM:** The founding of the specialty boards. **Anesthesiology** 1981 Sep;55(3):317-21
**Little MA:** The development of ideas on human ecology and adaptation. In F. Spencer, ed: A history of American physical anthropology, 1930-1980. New York, Academic Press, 1982. p. 405-33.
**Littlefield DC:** Plantations, paternalism, and profitability: factors affecting African demography in the old British Empire. **J South Hist** 1981;47(2):167-82
**Littman RA:** Psychology's histories: some new ones and a bit about their predecessors--an essay review. **J Hist Behav Sci** 1981 Oct;17(4):516-32
**Littman RA** see **Hearst E, ed**
**Littmann I:** A 125 éves Orvosi Hetilap és a modern sebészet kialakulása. Merre tart ma a sebészet? **Orv Hetil** 1982 Feb 7;123(6):323-6
**Littmann I:** Theodor Billroth (1829-1894). **Orvostort Kozl** 1979;87-88(25 no 1-2):123-39
**Littmann L** see **Robicsek F**
**Littmann SK:** King Saul: persecutor or persecuted? **Can J Psychiatry** 1981 Nov;26(7):464-7
**Litzinger WJ:** Ceramic evidence for prehistoric datura use in North America. **J Ethnopharmacol** 1981 Jul;4(1):57-74
**Liu B:** The costs of air quality deterioration and benefits of air pollution control: estimates of mortality costs for two pollutants in 40 U.S. metropolitan areas. **Am J Econ Sociol** 1979;38(2):187-95
**Liu PK** see **Cho LJ**
**Liu X:** Psychiatry in traditional Chinese medicine. **Br J Psychiatry** 1981 May;138:429-33
**Liu ZZ:** Shen Nong's Herbal, the earliest extant treatise on Chinese materia medica. **Chung Yao Tung Pao** 1982 Sep;7(5):43-5
**Liu Chi-Wan:** [The rite of a pestilence god in southern Taiwan] (Chi). **Bull Inst Ethnol Acad Sin** 1979;47:73-169
**Liu Zhengcai** see **Lin Qianliang**
**Livečka E:** Nástin konstituování gerontopedagogiky. **Acta Univ Carol Philos Hist** 1978;(4):41-76
**Lively CE:** Reminiscences of a state mental hospital attendant. **Indiana Med Hist Q** 1983 Mar;9(1):13-22
**Liveright T, Stanbury M:** An historical prospective study of mortality within a cohort of gas distribution workers. **Am J Ind Med** 1983;4(5):651-7
**Livesey SJ:** Metabasis: the interrelationship of the sciences in antiquity and the Middle Ages. Ph.D. Diss., University of California. Los Angeles, 1982. x, 742 p.
**Livesley CA:** 1839 advertisements. **Pharm Hist (London)** 1981 Apr;11(1):10-11
**Livet G, Schaff G, ed:** Médecine et assistance en Alsace, XVIe-XXe siècle. Recherches sur l'histoire de la santé. Strasbourg, Istra, 1976. 368 p. (Publications de la Sociéte Savante d'Alsace et des Régions de l'Est, Tome XI).
**Livet JM:** Les années terribles: l'Ecole libre de Médecine de Strasbourg de 1870 à 1872. In Livet G, Schaff G, ed: Médecine et assistance en Alsace, XVIe-XXe siècle. Strasbourg, Istra, 1976. p. 265-86.
**Livi-Bacci M** see **Del Panta L**
**Livianos Aldana L, Rojo Moreno L, Rojo Moreno J, et al:** La nosología psiquiátrica y las taxonomías numéricas. **Actas Luso Esp Neurol Psiquiatr** 1984 Jan-Feb;12(1):63-72
**Livingood CS:** History of the American Board of Dermatology, Inc. (1932-1982). **J Am Acad Dermatol** 1982 Dec;7(6):821-50
**Livingston KE, Hornykiewicz O, ed:** Limbic mechanisms. The continuing evolution of the limbic system concept. New York and London, Plenum, 1976. xv, 542 p. Tribute to James W. Papez; biographical contributions by P. D. MacLean, J. B. Angevine, P. I. Yakovlev.
**Livingston M:** LSD--a generation later. **Hawaii Med J** 1982 Dec;41(12):462, 464, 466 passim
**Livingston RH:** They comfort me. The history of nursing in Belfast. **Ulster Med J** 1981;50(1):33-45
**Livio JJ:** L'orthopédie, quelle place dans la société? **Rev Med Suisse Romande**
**Livock R:** Science, law and safety standards: a case study of industrial disease. **Br J Law Soc** 1979;6(2):172-99
**Ljungdell J:** Juglans regia L. - i den svenska farmakopéen och annorstädes. **Sydsven Medicinhist Sallsk Arsskr** 1982;19:54-62
**Ljunggren B, Säveland H, Brandt L:** Aneurysmal subarachnoid hemorrhage--historical background from a Scandinavian horizon. **Surg Neurol** 1984 Dec;22(6):605-16
**Ljunggren B:** Cushing och Sven Hedin. **Lakartidningen** 1982 Aug 11;79(32-33):2790-2
**Ljunggren B:** En stor man med en sjuk hjärna. **Sydsven Medicinhist Sallsk Arsskr** 1984;21:77-85
**Ljunggren B:** Harvey Cushing and Sven Hedin. **Surg Neurol** 1982 Mar;17(3):165-71
**Ljunggren B, Säveland H:** Hjärnpulsåderbråckens medicinska historia - ett långtifrån avslutat kapitel. **Sydsven Medicinhist Sallsk Arsskr** 1982;19:63-98
**Ljunggren B:** Pionjärer inom hjärnkirurgi. **Lakartidningen** 1982 Apr 7;79(14):1377-8
**Ljunggren B:** Reflexioner kring en hjärnsvulst hos 'En förnäm herre af 30 år'. **Sydsven Medicinhist Sallsk Arsskr** 1983;:87-102
**Ljunggren B:** The case of General Wood. **J Neurosurg** 1982 Apr;56(4):471-4
**Ljunggren B:** The case of George Gershwin. **Neurosurgery** 1982 Jun;10(6 Pt 1):733-6
**Ljunggren B:** The sleepy sea lord who was Churchill's friend. **Surg Neurol** 1982 Nov;18(5):307-19
**Ljunggren JG:** Vem var mannen bakom syndromet: ismail al-jurjani, testa, flagani, parry, graves eller basedow? **Lakartidningen** 1983 Aug 10;80(32-33):2902
**Llana JW:** Elements in eighteenth century French chemistry. Ph.D. diss. Indiana University. Bloomington, 1979. 226 leaves.
**Llaurado JG:** Role of the biomedical engineer in nuclear medicine. **J Clin Eng** 1981 Oct-Dec;6(4):269-76
**Llewelyn DE, Anderson J:** The historical development of the concepts of diagnosis and prognosis and their relationship to probabilistic inference. **Med Inf (Lond)** 1980 Oct-Dec;5(4):267-80
**Llewelyn JH** see **Whittaker DK**
**Llistosella Alberti R:** Evolucion historica de la ceramica. **Rev Esp Estomatol** 1983 Jan-Feb;31(1):27-30
**Llombart V:** Anotaciones a la introducción del 'ensayo sobre la población de Malthus en España. **Moneda Credito** 1973;126:79-86
**Lloyd C:** Cook and scurvy. **Mar Mirror** 1979 Feb;65:23-8
**Lloyd GA** see **Phelps PD**
**Lloyd GE:** Hippocratic problems. **Classical Rev** 1980;30(2):186-9
**Lloyd GE:** Magic, reason and experience. Studies in the origin and development of Greek science. Cambridge, New York, Cambridge University Press, 1979. xii, 335 p.
**Lloyd GE** see **French RK**
**Lloyd O:** Epidemiology: some early lessions. **Occup Health (Lond)** 1981 Jan;33(1):27-36
**Lloyd S:** The Ottawa typhoid epidemics of 1911 and 1912: a case study of disease as a catalyst for urban reform. **Urban Hist Rev** 1979;8(1):66-89
**Lloyd-Bostock SM:** Psychology and the law: a critical review of research and practice. **Br J Law Soc** 1981;8(1):1-28
**Lo WH, Wu M:** Medical genetics in China. **Am J Med Genet** 1981;10(3):257-60
**Loaring K, Wards M:** Brief history of Northfield. **Australas Nurses J** 1981 Apr;10(4):5-6, 8
**Lob M:** Aspects de la médecine du travail. **Soz Praventivmed** 1981 Jul;26(3):114-7
**Lobanov GP, Zhuravskiĭ VA:** Nekotorye voprosy organizatsii spetsial'noĭ podgotovki lichnogo sostava voenno-meditsinskoĭ sluzhby v period Voĭny. **Voen Med Zh** 1980 May;(5):28-33
**Lobanov GP:** Razvitie i sovershenstvovanie meditsinskoĭ sortirovki v period Velikoĭ Otechestvennoĭ Voĭny. **Voen Med Zh** 1983 May;5:15-20
**Lobanov GP** see **Georgievskiĭ AS**
**Lobastov OS:** Meditsinskoe obespechenie voĭsk vo frontovykh nastukpatel'nykh operatsiiakh na zavershaiuschchem étape Voĭny. **Voen Med Zh** 1980 May;(5):25-8
**Lobban RD:** Edinburgh and the medical revolution. Cambridge, Cambridge University Press, 1980. 48 p.
**Lobeck C:** UMC four-year medical school observes 25th anniversary. **Mo Med** 1981 Jun;78(6):293, 297
**Lobko PI** see **Leontiuk AS**
**Lobo F:** Perspectivas de la autorización de medicamentos en España. **Rev Sanid Hig Publica (Madr)** 1983 May-Jun;57(5-6):509-15
**Lobo FB:** Duas pioneiras-Madame Dubocher, Rita Lobato. **Rev Inst Hist Geogr Bras** 1980;(328):53-6
**Lobo FB:** Os professores de medicina e as conferencias da Gloria. **Rev Inst Hist Geogr Bras** 1980;(328):105-10
**Lobo FB:** Uma sede para a Faculdade de Medicina do Rio de Janeiro. **Rev Inst Hist Geogr Bras** 1977;315:158-88
**Loboda VI** see **Kunitsa LK**
**Lobzin VS, Pinchuk VK:** Pervaia v Rossii kafedra dlia usovershenstvovaniia nevropatologov. **Zh Nevropatol Psikhiatr** 1983;83(8):1240-5
**Loch W:** Alexander Mitscherlich und die Wiedergeburt der Psychoanalyse in Deutschland. **Psyche (Stuttg)** 1983 Apr;37(4):336-45
**Lochmann EH:** Das 16. Internationale Symposion der Welt-Gesellschaft für Geschichte der Veterinärmedizin, 21.-24. Mai 1980 in Bärau, Schweiz. **Ber Wissenschaftsgesch** 1980;3(3-4):207-13
**Lock MM:** East Asian medicine in urban Japan: varieties of medical experience. Berkeley, University of California Press, 1980. xiv, 311 p. (Comparative Studies of Health Systems and Medical Care, 4).
**Lock MM:** L'homme machine et l'homme-microcosme: l'approche occidentale et l'approche japonaise des soins médicaux. **Ann Econ Soc Civilis** 1980;35:1116-36
**Lock S:** A question of confidence. An editor's view. **Br Med J [Clin Res]** 1984 Jan 14;288(6411):123-5
**Lock S:** 'O that I were young again': Yeats and the Steinach operation.

**Br Med J [Clin Res]** 1983 Dec 24–31;287(6409):1964–8

**Lock W:** Die Schwerpunktbekämpfung der Tuberkulose im endemischen Stadium. **Z Erkr Atmungsorgane** 1983;161(1):100–2

**Lock W:** Robert Koch. Bemerkungen aus heutiger Sicht. **Prax Klin Pneumol** 1982 Mar;36(3):106–10

**Lock W:** Robert Koch, Leben und Werk. **Prax Klin Pneumol** 1983 Oct;37 Suppl 1:409–11

**Locke D:** Mind, matter, and the 'Meditations'. **Mind** 1981;90:343–66

**Lockhart J:** La historia del Hospital Maciel. Montevideo, Editora de Revistas, 1982. 244 p.

**Lockridge KA:** Historical demography. In Delzell, Charles F., ed.: the future of history: essays in the Vanderbilt University centennial symposium. Nashville, Vanderbilt U., 1977. p. 53–64.

**Lockwood A:** Pantsuited pioneer of women's lib, Dr. Mary Walker. **Smithsonian** 1977;7(12):113–9

**Lockyer WJ** see **Rechsteiner J**

**Lodge M:** How we ran the welfare. **Health Visit** 1983 Jul;56(7):244–6

**Löe HA:** Scientific revolutions in dentistry. **J Dent Res** 1979 Nov;58(Spec Issue D):2164–8

**Loebe FM:** Karl Eskuchen—ein fast vergessener Pionier der Liquorforschung. **Psychiatr Neurol Med Psychol (Leipz)** 1983 Sep;35(9):561–5

**Loehlin JC:** John Locke and behavior genetics. **Behav Genet** 1983 Jan;13(1):117–21

**Loehr WJ:** Civil war medicine in North Carolina. **NC Med J** 1982 Feb;43(2):120–1

**Loetzke HH:** Die wissenschaftlichen Arbeiten des polnischen Histologen Władysław Szymonowicz während seiner Studienaufenthalthe 1895 und 1896 in Berlin. **Arch Hist Med (Warsz)** 1979;42(3):359–64

**Loevy HT, Kowitz A:** Dentistry on stamps. **J Am Dent Assoc** 1980 Jun;100(6):917, 924

**Loevy HT, Kowitz A:** Dentistry on stamps. **J Am Dent Assoc** 1981 Jul;103(1):143

**Loevy HT, Kowitz A:** Dentistry on stamps. **J Am Dent Assoc** 1982 Jun;104(6):890

**Loevy HT, Kowitz A:** Dentistry on stamps. **J Am Dent Assoc** 1983 Oct;107(4):618 (continued periodically)

**Loevy HT, Kowitz A:** Dentistry on stamps (Dr. Kerstin Palm). **J Am Dent Assoc** 1984 Nov;109(5):755

**Loevy HT, Kowitz A:** Health science on stamps. **J Am Dent Assoc** 1980 Jan;100(1):86

**Loevy HT, Kowitz A:** Health science on stamps. **J Am Dent Assoc** 1980 Jul;101(1):156

**Loevy HT, Kowitz A:** Health science on stamps. **J Am Dent Assoc** 1984 May;108(5):797

**Loevy HT:** M. Evangeline Jordon, pioneer in pedodontics. **Bull Hist Dent** 1984;32(1):19–26

**Loevy HT, Kowitz A:** The Habsburgs and the 'Habsburg Jaw'. **Bull Hist Dent** 1982 Apr;30(1):19–23

**Loew ER:** Departmental history. Department of Physiology. Boston University School of Medicine (1873–1948). **Physiologist** 1984 Feb;27(1):4–12

**Loew FM:** Animal experimentation. **Bull Hist Med** 1982 Spring;56(1):123–6

**Loewen SL:** The art of bloodletting: as practiced by my father. **J Am Hist Soc Ger Russ** 1980;3(2):13–7

**Loewenberg P:** Decoding the past: the psychohistorical approach. New York, Knopf, 1983. xiv, 300 p.

**Loewenberg P:** Psychohistory. In M. Kammen, ed: The Past before us: contemporary historical writing in the United States. Ithaca, Cornell University Press, 1980. p. 408–32.

**Loewenberg P:** The graduate years: what kind of journey? **Group Psychol Hist Newsl** 1975;4(1):2–7

**Loewenstein G:** Kommunale Gesundheitsfürsorge und sozialistische Arztepolitik zwischen Kaiserreich und Nationalsozialismus. Bremen, Universität Bremen, 1980. v, 374 p.

**Löfkvist E** see **Källén B**

**Loftus MD:** St. Vincent Hospital and Health Care Center, Indianapolis, Indiana, 1881–1981. Indianapolis, Litho Press, 1981. xi, 191 p.

**Logan RD:** Charles Lindbergh and the 'right stuff'. **Aviat Space Environ Med** 1982 Jul;53(7):708–11

**Logan WP:** Cancer mortality by occupation and social class 1851–1971. **IARC Sci Publ** 1982;(36):1–253

**Logan WW** see **Sawyer DR**

**Logeay R:** Bonheurs et malheurs de la clinique Tarnier. **Hist Sci Med** 1984;18(3):261–70

**Logeay R:** Le voyage de René Caillé à Tombouctou; ce qu'il lui en a coûté. **Hist Sci Med** 1982;16(4):273–83

**Logue DC:** Treating the wounded abroad USS Monitor, 1862. **US Navy Med** 1982 Jan;73(1):4–5

**Lohff B:** Die Entwicklung des Experimentes im Bereich der Nervenphysiologie; Gedanken und Arbeiten zum Begriff der Irritabilität und der Lebenskraft. **Sudhoffs Arch** 1980;64(2):105–29

**Lohff B:** Johannes Müller, 'Jahresberichte zur Physiologie', in Müllers Archiv der Jahre 1834–1838. **Sudhoffs Arch** 1981;65(1):32–78

**Lohff B:** Zur Geschichte der Lehre von der Lebenskraft. **Clio Med** 1981 Dec;16(2/3):101–12

**Lohff B** see **Mann G, ed**

**Lohmann HM, Rosenkötter L:** Psychoanalyse in Hitlerdeutschland. Wie war es wirklich? **Psyche (Stuttg)** 1982 Nov;36(11):961–88

**Lohmann HM, Rosenkötter L:** Psychoanalyse in Hitlerdeutschland. Wie war es wirklich? Ein Nachtrag. **Psyche (Stuttg)** 1983 Dec;37(12):1107–15

**Lohmann HM:** Scheiden tut weh. **Psyche (Stuttg)** 1984 Oct;38(10):943–8

**Lohmann HM** see **Brede K**

**Lohmann HM, ed:** Die Psychoanalyse auf der Couch. Frankfurt am Main, Qumran, 1984. 330 p. Historical contributions by E. Federn, J. Cremerius, K. Brede, A. Lorenzer, M. Pohlen.

**Lohr CH:** Renaissance Latin Aristotle Commentaries: authors N–Ph. **Renaiss Q** 1979 Winter;32(4):529–80 (continued periodically)

**Lohr CH:** Renaissance Latin Aristotle commentaries: authors So–Z. **Renaiss Q** 1982 Summer;35(2):164–256

**Löhr HG:** Ein Vierteljahrhundert gemeinsamen Weges von Karl Marx und Friedrich Engels mit ihrem treuen Freund und Kampfgefährten Carl Schorlemmer. **Pharmazie** 1983 Nov;38(11):768–72

**Löhr J** see **Klippe HJ**

**Lohr W:** An historical view of the research on the behavioral and organizational factors related to the utilization of health services. [s.l.: s.n.], 1972. 67, 16 leaves.

**Loken MK, Williams LE:** A history of computers in nuclear medicine. **Semin Nucl Med** 1979 Jul;9(3):197–200

**Loker Z:** A Franco-Jewish physician—among the pioneers of medicine and science in Central America (Haiti). **Koroth** 1982 Aug;8(3/4):195–7

**Loker Z:** Docteur Michel Lopez de Paz, médecin et savant de Saint-Domingue. **Rev Hist Med Heb** 1980 Oct;134(33 no 3):55–7

**Lokhorst GJ:** An ancient Greek theory of hemispheric specialization. **Clio Med** 1982 May;17(1):33–8

**Lokhorst GJ:** The oldest printed text on hemispheric specialization. **Neurology** 1982 Jul;32(7):762

**Lolli G:** La tradizione scientifica italiana. **Scientia** 1980;115(9–12):713–23

**Lomakina NM, Merinov AP, Anoshkin IG:** Podvig medikov v Stalingradskoĭ bitve. **Voen Med Zh** 1980 Nov;(11):14–6

**Lomax E:** A mid-nineteenth century British pediatrician's interpretations of the mental peculiarities and disorders of childhood. **Clio Med** 1983 Mar;17(4):223–33

**Lomax E:** Changing attitudes during the past century as to the hazards of parental alcoholism to the progeny. In International Congress of the History of Medicine. 26th, Plovdiv, 1978. Actes du Congress. Sofia, 1981. Volume II. p. 144–7.

**Lomax E:** Charles West (1816–1898) on the mental peculiarieties and disorders of childhood. In International Congress of the History of Medicine, 27th, Barcelona, 1980. Actas. Barcelona, Académia de Ciències Médiques de Catalunya i Balears, 1981. p. 98–102.

**Lomax E:** Historical development of concepts of thermoregulation. In P. Lomax, E. Schönbaum, ed: Body temperature: regulations, drug effects, and therapeutic implications. New York, Basel, Marcel Dekker, 1979. p. 1–23.

**Lomax EM, Kagan J, Rosenkrantz BG:** Science and patterns of child care. San Francisco, W. H. Freeman, 1978. xiv, 247 p.

**Lombardi D:** 1629–1631: crisi e peste a Firenze. **Arch Stor Ital** 1979;137(1):3–50

**Lomnitz L:** Hierarchy and peripherality: the organisation of a Mexican research institute. **Minerva** 1979 Winter;17(4):527–48

**Lomonaco T:** Un medico fra gli aviatori. **Riv Med Aeronaut Spaz** 1980;Suppl:1–176

**London NJ** see **Goldberg A, ed**

**London P:** [History of] sexual behavior. In Reich WT, et al, ed: Encyclopedia of bioethics, v.4. New York, Free Press, 1978. p. 1560–9.

**London PS:** Inaugural William Gissane Lecture: man and memorial. **Injury** 1982 Nov;14(3):211–34

**Long EC** see **Bowers JZ**

**Long JP** see **Gross EG**

**Longfield-Jones GM:** A set of silver dental instruments from the New Milton Collection. **Med Hist** 1984 Jan;28(1):42–8

**Longley JD:** Ralph Dougall Lillie. 1896—1979. **J Histochem Cytochem** 1980 Apr;28(4):291–6

**Longmire WP:** Changing patterns of surgical training and practice. **Am J Surg** 1981 Jun;141(6):632–7

**Longmire WP:** Historic landmarks in biliary surgery. **South Med J** 1982 Dec;75(12):1548–50, 1552

**Longmire WP:** Loyal Davis' personal qualities and their influence on American surgery. **Surg Gynecol Obstet** 1983 Aug;157(2):114–7

**Longmire WP:** Surgical upbringing in America. **Bull Am Coll Surg** 1978 Sep;63(9):6–11

**Longmire WP:** Two great American surgeons, each with four aces. **Pharos** 1983 Summer;46(3):9–14

**Longo LD:** A short history of the Society for Gynecologic Investigation (1953–1983). Los Angeles, Calif., [s.n.], 1983. 70 p.

**Longo LD:** John Whitridge Williams and academic obstetrics in America. **Trans Stud Coll Physicians Phila** 1981 Dec;5(3 no 4):221–54

**Longo LD** see **Numbers RL, ed**

**Longrigg J:** Superlative achievement and comparative neglect: Alexandrian medical science and modern historical research. **Hist Sci** 1981 Sep;19(45 pt 3):155–200

**Longrigg J:** The great plague of Athens. **Hist Sci** 1980 Sep;18(41 pt 3):209–25

**Longrigg J:** Thucydides and the great plague of Athens. In International Congress of the History of Medicine, 27th, Barcelona, 1980. Actas. Barcelona, Académia de Ciències Médiques de Catalunya i Balears, 1981. p. 281–8.

**Longrigg J:** Two notes on Theophrastus 'De sensibus.' **Philologus** 1975;119:163–9

**Lonie IM:** Hippocrates the iatromechanist. **Med Hist** 1981 Apr;25(2):113–50

**Lonie IM:** The Hippocratic treatises: 'On Generation', 'On the Nature of the Child', 'Diseases IV'. A commentary. Berlin, New York, Walter de Gruyter, 1981. xxxix, 406 p. (Ars medica. II. Abteilung, Griechisch-lateinische Medizin; Bd. 7, 2).

**Lontainé SZ, Susa E, Varga T:** A Habsburgok József nádori ágához tartozók vércsoportvizsgálata. **Morphol Igazsagugyi Orv Sz** 1980 Oct;20(4):275-81

**Lôo P:** Plaidoyer pour la violence. **Ann Med Psychol (Paris)** 1979 Oct;137(8):836-9

**Look back to 1927:** The use of milk injections in pelvic inflammation. **East Afr Med J** 1980 Feb;57(2):71

**Looking back: the Australian army hospitals: Lamp** 1980 May;37(5):53-5

**Lopatenok AA, Fisher AM:** Deiatel'nosti M. D. Tushinskogo v blokirovannom Leningrade. **Klin Med (Mosk)** 1982 Jan;60(1):112-4

**Lopatenok AA:** M. D. Tushinskiĭ, 1882-1962. Moskva, Meditsina, 1983. 47 p.

**Lopatkin NA, Shchabad AL:** Die Zystoskopie und ihre Bedeutung in der Urologie. **Z Urol Nephrol** 1979 Jul;72(12):517-22

**Lopez D** see **Sabagh G**

**López G** see **Maibaum M**

**Lopez Andujar G** see **Valverde JL**

**Lopez Austin A:** Almas y experiencia entre los antiguos nahuas. **Bol Soc Mex Hist Filos Med** 1983;6(45):223-33

**López Austín A:** De las plantas medicinales y de otras cosas medicinales. **Estud Cult Nahuatl** 1971;9:125-230

**Lopez Austin A:** En defensa de la historia de la medicina. **Bol Soc Mex Hist Filos Med** 1984;7(50):467-75

**López Austin A:** Textos acerca de las partes del cuerpo humano y de las enfermedades y medicinas en los primeros memoriales de Sahagún. **Estud Cult Nahuatl** 1972;10:129-53

**López de Guereñu G:** Muerte, entierro y funerales in algunos lugares de Alava. **Bol Inst Sancho Sabio** 1978;22:189-242

**López de Hinojosos A:** Suma y recopilación de cirugía con un arte para sangrar muy útil y provechosa. Mexico, Academia Nacional de Medicina, 1977. xxiv, 227 p.

**López de la Osa Garcés L:** Estudio histórico de la evolución del tratamiento del carcinoma de cuello uterino. **Rev Esp Oncol** 1981;28(4):569-90

**López-Fanjul de Argüelles C:** El lamarckismo y algo sobre los neolamarckismos. **Arbor** 1982;113(441-2):41-57

**López Férez JA:** Algunos datos sobre la influencia de la teoria embriologica de Democrito en el corpus hippocraticum. Gemelos y abortos. **Asclepio** 1981;33:379-90

**López Férez JA:** El falso Demócrito y los escritos medicos pseudodemocritos. **An Hist Antigua Mediev** 1977-80;20:175-87

**López Férez JA:** Ideas embriologicas de Democrito. **Asclepio** 1982;34:317-26

**López Hermosa L, ed:** Bibliografía historica medica Mexicana 1970-1974. México, Sociedad Mexicana de Historia y Filosofía de la Medicina, (1978?). n.p.

**López Ibor JJ:** Egas Moniz, en su centenario. **Actas Luso Esp Neurol Psiquiatr** 1980 Jul-Aug;8(4):239-46

**López Ibor JJ:** Karl Jaspers en su centenario. **Actas Luso Esp Neurol Psiquiatr** 1982 Nov-Dec;10(6):321-30

**Lopez-Ibor Alino JJ:** Les développements récents de la politique psychiatrique en Espagne. **Ann Med Psychol (Paris)** 1980 Jun;138(6):716-21

**Lopez Lozano JF:** Articuladores. **Rev Esp Estomatol** 1980 May-Jun;28(3):145-54

**López McCabe A:** Francisco Javier Villanueva y Godoy: cirujano major de la armada. **Rev Mar** 1981;98(1):72-87

**López-Ochoterena E:** La décima octava carta de Leeuwenhoek. (Delft en Holanda, 9 octubre, 1676). **An Soc Mex Hist Cienc Tec** 1979;5:85-90

**López Piñero JM:** Ciencia y técnica en la sociedad española de los siglos XVI y XVII. Barcelona, Labor, 1979. 511 p.

**López Piñero JM, Bumosa F, Terrada ML:** Clásicos españoles de la anatomía patológica anteriores a Cajal. Spanish classics on pathology before Cajal. Valencia, Cátedra e Instituto de Historia de la Medicina, 1979. 254 p. (Cuadernos Valencianos de Historia de la Medicina y de la Ciencia, 21, Serie B).

**López Piñero JM, Bujosa F, Terrada ML, ed:** Clásicos españoles de la anatomía patológica anteriores a Cajal. Valencia, Cátedra e Instituto de Historia de la Medicina, 1979. xv, 254 p. (Cuadernos Valencianos de Historia de la Medicina y de la Ciencia, XXI, Serie B (Textos Clasicos)).

**López Piñero JM:** Diccionario histórico de la ciencia moderna en España. Barcelona, Peninsula, 1983. 2 v.

**López Piñero JM:** El estudio histórico de la medicina en la obra de Laín Entralgo. **Dynamis** 1981;1:231-9

**López Piñero JM:** Historical origins of the concept of neurosis. Cambridge, New York, Cambridge University Press, 1983. xi, 107 p.

**López Piñero JM:** La ciencia en la España de los siglos XVI y XVII. In Tuñón de Lara M, ed.: Historia de España. Tomo V. La frustración de un imperio (1476-1714). Barcelona, Labor, 1982. p. 355-423.

**Lopez Piñero JM, Terrada ML:** Las etapas históricas del periodismo médico en España. Estudio bibliométrico. **Med Esp** 1979:78:95-108

**Lopez Pinero JM:** Los estudios historicos sobre la actividad cientifica en la España de los siglos XVI y XVII. In: Coloquio sobre historia de la ciencia hispano-americana ... 1976. Madrid. 1977. pp. 133-166.

**López Piñero JM:** Medicina, historia, sociedad. Antología de clásicos médicos. 2a ed. Barcelona, Ariel, 1971. 352 p.

**López Piñero JM:** Medicina moderna y sociedad española (Siglos XVI-XIX). Valencia, Cátedra e Instituto de Historia de la Medicina, 1976. 326 p.

**López Piñero JM:** Social and economic factors in the translation of medical texts in Spain (16th-19th centuries). In International Congress of the History of Medicine, 27th, Barcelona, 1980. Actas. Barcelona, Académia de Ciències Médiques de Catalunya i Balears, 1981. p. 289-97.

**López Piñero JM:** The history of science and medicine in Spain. **Clio Med** 1980 Jul;14(3-4):295-9

**López-Piñero JM:** The medical profession in 16th century Spain. In Russell AW, ed: The town and state physician in Europe from the Middle Ages to the Enlightenment. Wolfenbüttel, Herzog August Bibliothek, 1981. p. 85-98 (Wolfenbütteler Forschungen, 17).

**Lopez Piñero JM, Bujosa Homar F:** Tradición y renovación de los saberes médicos en la España del siglo XVI. **Med Esp** 1978;77:355-66

**López Piñero JM, Bujosa Homar F:** Tradicion y renovacion en la medicina española del siglo XVI. **Asclepio** 1978-79;30-31:285-306

**López Piñero JM** see **Albarracín Teulón A**

**López Piñero JM** see **Gónzalez Blasco P**

**Lopez Sanchez J:** Carlos J. Finlay and the conception of contagion. **Indian J Hist Sci** 1981;16(2):156-68

**López Sánchez J:** Karlos KH. Finlai i teoriia peredachi infektsii. **Vopr Istor Estestvozn Tekh** 1981;(4):29-34

**López Segrera F:** Psicoanálisis de una generación. **Rev Bibl Nac Jose Marti** 1970;12(1,2):93-125, 101-52

**Loposzko T:** La famine à Rome en 57 avant J-Ch. **Quad Stor** 1979 Jul-Dec;5

**Loraine JA:** Alcoholism: a new pandemic. **Contemp Rev** 1981;238(1381):75-81

**Loraine JA:** Future patterns of disease: maladies of development. **Contemp Rev** 1983;242(1409):298-302

**Loraine JA:** Population and birth control in China. **Contemp Rev** 1981;239(1388):126-130

**Loraine JA:** Population perspectives in Asia. **Contemp Rev** 1979;235(1363):66-9

**Loraine JA:** The economics of fertility. **Midwife Health Visit Community Nurse** 1982 Jan;18(1):6-8

**Lordi NG** see **Cowen DL**

**Loré C, Piva I:** Pensiero e pratica psichiatrici in Toscana da chiarugi a livi. In International Congress of the History of Medicine, 27th, Barcelona, 1980. Actas. Barcelona, Académia de Ciències Médiques de Catalunya i Balears, 1981. p. 103-10.

**Lorensen M:** The contribution of the hospital to health care. **Nurs Times** 1983 Mar 9-15;79(10):42-4

**Lorenz B:** Il medico bibliofilo. **Kos** 1984 Jun;1(5):101-11

**Lorenz B:** Notizen zu Privatbibliotheken deutscher Arzte des 15.-17. Jahrhunderts. **Sudhoffs Arch** 1983;67(2):190-8

**Lorenz K, ed, Wuketits FM, ed:** Die Evolution des Denkens. München, Piper, 1983. 393 p. Contributions by G. Vollmer, R. Kaspar, R. Riedl, F. Seitelberger, G. P. Wagner, W. Leinfellner, E. Oeser, H. Mohr, R. Löw.

**Lorenzer A** see **Lohmann HM, ed**

**Lorenzo L** see **Bárcena A**

**Lorenzo Velázquez B:** Algunos recuerdos sobre Cajal en el XLVII aniversario de su muerte. **An R Acad Nacl Med (Madr)** 1981;98(4):663-88

**Lorenzo Velázquez B:** Presentación de dos formularios: 'Formulario de Terapéutica Clínica' (XV edición) y 'Formulario de Urgénica' (XVII edicion). **An R Acad Nac Med (Madr)** 1981;98(2):211-26

**Loretan S:** Das Antoniusspital in Brig. **Gesnerus** 1982;39(1):109-13

**Lorillot D:** 1789: les medecins ont la parole. **Hist Reflect** 1982;9(1-2):103-129

**Lorincz F:** A malária elleni küzdelem hazánkban az elso világháború után - visszaemlékzés. **Orvostort Kozl** 1982;28(1-3):251-4

**Loriot J** see **Penneau D**

**Lorrang F** see **Bolzinger R**

**Lorren C** see **Guillemain B**

**Lortie L:** François-Alexandre-Hubert La Rue. In Dictionary of Canadian biography, 1881-1890. 1982;11:495-7.

**Lortie L:** Joseph-Alexandre Crevier. In Dictionary of Canadian biography, 1881-1890. 1982;11:217-8.

**Los médicos en la batalla de Carabobo:** Caracas, Ministerio de Educación, Dirección General, Dept. de Publicaciones, 1972. 93 p.

**Losada J, Mayor J:** Esclavitud y psicología: una investigación interdisciplinaria. **Rev Bibl Nac Jose Marti** 1980;22(3):133-43

**Losee J:** Whewell and Mill on the relation between philosophy of science and history of science. **Stud Hist Philos Sci** 1983 Jun;14(2):113-26

**Losev NI** see **Kozlov AM**

**Losiowski Z:** Sanatorium w Zagórzu i jego rola w lecznictwie neurologicznym dzieci. **Pediatr Pol** 1980 Mar;55(3):379-84

**Lostetter JO, Chapman JE:** The participation of the United States government in providing financial support for medical education. **Health Policy Educ** 1979 Spring;1(1):27-65

**Lothane Z:** Listening with the Third Ear as an instrument in psychoanalysis: the contributions of Reik and Isakower. **Psychoanal Rev** 1981-82 Winter;68(4):487-503

**Löther I, Löther R:** Engels' 'Ludwig Feuerbach und der Ausgang der klassischen deutschen Philosophie', die Grundrichtungen des philosophischen Denkens und die Medizin. **Med Ges** 1979;(5):79-91

**Löther I:** Probleme der Wissenschaftlich-technischen Revolution und einige Aufgaben des sozialistischen Gesundheitsschutzes. **Med Ges** 1978;(3):69-78

**Löther I** see **Löther R, ed**

**Löther R:** Geschichte der Medizin und Theorie der Medizin. In International Congress of the History of Medicine. 26th, Plovdiv, 1978. Actes du Congress. Sofia, 1981. Volume II. p. 148-50.

**Löther R:** Lenins 'Zur Frage der Dialektik' und die Bedeutung dialektischen Denkens in der Medizin. **Med Ges** 1979;(5):106–12

**Löther R** see **Löther I**

**Löther R, ed:** Philosophische Schriften von Marx, Engels und Lenin und ihre Bedeutung für die Medizin heute. Jena, Fischer, 1979. 127 p. Contributions by U. Körner, I. Löther, P. W. Ruff, R. Stach, G. Straass.

**Lothian A, Short GR:** Angel design drug jars. **Pharm Hist (London)** 1977 Mar;7(1):1

**Lotova EI, Egorysheva IV:** Gigienist i obshchestvennyĭ deiatel' I. V. Bertenson (k 150–letiiu so dnia rozhdeniia). **Sov Zdravookhr** 1984;(1):57–60

**Lotova EI, Idel'chik KhI, Vengrova IV:** Mesto i rol' sotsial'no–gigienicheskikh issledovaniĭ v izuchenii zdorov'ia rabochikh v SSSR v 20–30–e gody. **Sov Zdravookhr** 1981;(12):51–4

**Lotsmanov IuA, Safin MS:** Bashkirskomu meditsinskomu institutu 50 let. **Sov Zdravookhr** 1982;(6):62–4

**Lott AS** see **Engle EK**

**Lotzová E:** Natural immunity. History, present, and future. **Nat Immun Cell Growth Regul** 1983–84;3(1):1–6

**Loudon B:** Pioneer pharmacist J. Walter Moyer's notes on Crawford and Fort Robinson in the 1890's. **Nebr Hist** 1977;58(1):89–117

**Loudon I:** How it strikes a historian. **Br Med J [Clin Res]** 1984 Jan 14;288(6411):125–6

**Loudon I:** Maternal mortality: an historical audit. **J R Coll Gen Pract** 1984 Nov;34(268):585–6

**Loudon I:** The concept of the family doctor. **Bull Hist Med** 1984 Fall;58(3):347–62

**Loudon I:** The consultation. **Br Med J [Clin Res]** 1983 Dec 24–31;287(6409):1970–1

**Loudon I:** The diseases called chlorosis. **Psychol Med** 1984 Feb;14(1):27–36

**Loudon I:** The nature of provincial medical practice in eighteenth–century England. **Med Hist** 1985 Jan;29(1):1–32

**Loudon I:** Two thousand medical men in 1847. **Soc Soc Hist Med Bull (Lond)** 1983 Dec;33:4–8

**Loudon IS:** A doctor's cash book: the economy of general practice in the 1830s. **Med Hist** 1983 Jul;27(3):249–68

**Loudon IS:** Chlorosis, anaemia, and anorexia nervosa. **Br Med J [Clin Res]** 1980 Dec 20–27;281(6256):1669–75

**Loudon IS:** Leg ulcers in the eighteenth and early nineteenth centuries. **J R Coll Gen Pract** 1981 May;31(226):263–73

**Loudon IS:** Leg ulcers in the eighteenth and early nineteenth centuries. II. Treatment. **J R Coll Gen Pract** 1982 May;32(238):301–9

**Loudon IS:** Sir Charles Bell and the anatomy of expression. **Br Med J [Clin Res]** 1982 Dec 18–25;285(6357):1794–6

**Loudon IS:** The origin of the general practitioner. **J R Coll Gen Pract** 1983 Jan;33(246):13–23

**Loudon IS:** The origins and growth of the dispensary movement in England. **Bull Hist Med** 1981;55(3):322–42

**Loughlin N:** The caesarean section: some historical qualifying perspectives. **Todays OR Nurse** 1981 Feb;2(12):7–10

**Loughman C:** Voices of the Wolf Man: the Wolf Man as autobiographer. **Psychoanal Rev** 1984 Sep;71(2):211–25

**Loughry CW:** Fifty years of surgical education at Akron City Hospital. **Ohio State Med J** 1982 Oct;78(10):723–6

**Louis A:** Mathieu de L'Obel 1538–1616. Episode de l'histoire de la botanique. Ghent/Louvain, Story–Scientia, 1980. 544 p.

**Louis R:** The anatomy of antiquity. **Anat Clin** 1983;5(3):139–40

**Louis R:** The anatomy of the Middle Ages. **Anat Clin** 1984;6(1):1–2

**Lounsbury JW, Roisum KG, Pokorny L, et al:** An analysis of topic areas and topic trends in the Community Mental Health Journal from 1965 through 1977. **Community Ment Health J** 1979 Winter;15(4):267–76

**Loustaud JP, Reboul G, Viroulet JJ:** Les thermes de la place de Jacobins à Limoges. **Archeologia** 1981;157:30–34

**Loutit JF:** Louis Harold Gray. In Dictionary of national biography, 1961–1970. Suppl. 8, 1981. p. 453–5.

**Louw JH:** A brief history of the Medical Faculty, University of Cape Town. **S Afr Med J** 1979 Nov 24;56(22):864–70

**Louw JH:** Leipoldt the paediatrician. **S Afr Med J** 1980 Dec 6;58(23):915–20

**Louw JH:** Professor Eric Cuthbert Crichton's contribution to the medical school. **S Afr Med J** 1979 Dec 15;56(25):1075–84

**Louw JH** see **Opie LH**

**Louw NS:** Hoe word die dokter betaal? **S Afr Med J** 1983 Jun 29;Spec No:40–2

**Loux F:** La femme soignante dans les traditions rurales du XIXe siècle. **Penelope** 1981;(5):37–40

**Loux F:** L'ogre et la dent. Pratiques et savoirs populaires relatifs aux dents. Paris, Berger–Levrault, 1981. 186 p.

**Loux F:** Recours convergents à la médecine officielle et à la médecine parallèle en matière de soins aux enfants en France (XIXe–XXe siècles). In Imhof AE, ed: Mensch und Gesundheit in der Geschichte. Husum, Matthiesen, 1980. p. 315–21.

**Lovaas OI:** Contrasting illness and behavioral models for the treatment of autistic children: a historical perspective. **J Autism Dev Disord** 1979 Dec;9(4):315–23

**Lovász A:** A konzerváló fogászati ellátás fejlödése az állami fogbetegellátásban 1951 és 1981 között a Központi Stomtologiai Intézet munkásságának tükrében. **Fogorv Sz** 1982;75(8):247–53

**Love R:** A note on courses taught by Australian psychology departments in the history and philosophy of psychology. **Newsl Australas Assoc Hist Philos Sci** 1975–6;7:28–33a

**Lovejoy CO, Mensforth RP, Armelagos GJ:** Five decades of skeletal biology as reflected in the American Journal of Physical Anthropology. In F. Spencer, ed: A history of American physical anthropology, 1930–1980. New York, Academic Press, 1982. p. 329–36.

**Lovel H, Mkandla M, Morley D:** Birth spacing in Zimbabwe a generation ago. **Lancet** 1983 Jul 16;2(8342):161–2

**Loveland LW:** A short history of continuing education in New York State dentistry. **NY State Dent J** 1984 Nov;50(9):614, 616

**Lovell A** see **Castel F**

**Lovell A** see **Castel R**

**Lovell RR:** The university medical presence in hospitals seventy years after Flexner and a look ahead. **Aust NZ J Med** 1983 Apr;13(2):187–94

**Low AA, Farmer RD, Jones DR, et al:** Suicide in England and Wales: an analysis of 100 years, 1876–1975. **Psychol Med** 1981 May;11(2):359 68

**Low MD, Purves SJ, Reeves B, et al:** Cerebral evoked potentials: a historical review of the marseilles contributions and a preliminary report on a study of the effects of various stimulus parameters on the P90 component of the pattern visual evoked potential. **Electroencephalogr Clin Neurophysiol** 1982;(35):369–79

**Löw R:** Pflanzenchemie zwischen Lavoisier und Liebig. Straubing und München, Donau Verlag, 1979. 404, 75 p. (Münchener Hochschulschriften, Reihe: Naturwissenschaften, 1).

**Löw R:** Philosophie des Lebendigen. Der Begriff des Organischen bei Kant, sein Grund und seine Aktualität. Frankfurt am Main, Suhrkamp, 1980. 358 p.

**Löw R:** Was hat die Pharmaziegeschichte der Wissenschaftstheorie zu sagen? In: Vorträge des Internationalen Pharmaziehistorischen Kongresses Innsbruck 1977. Stuttgart, Wissenschaftliche Verlagsgesellscaft, 1979. p. 29–38.

**Löw R** see **Hasler L, ed**

**Löw R** see **Lorenz K, ed**

**Low SM:** Dr. Moreno Cañas: a symbolic bridge to the demedicalization of healing. **Soc Sci Med** 1982;16(5):527–31

**Lowbury EJ:** Leonard Colebrook (1883–1967). **Br Med J [Clin Res]** 1983 Dec 24–31;287(6409):1981–3

**Lowe A** see **Spicker SF, ed**

**Lowe GD** see **Hodges HE**

**Lowe NJ** see **Ashton RE**

**Lowe RA:** Eugenicists, doctors and the quest for national efficiency: an educational crusade, 1900–1939. **Hist Educ** 1979;8(4):293–306

**Lowe RF:** An outline history of ophthalmology in Australia. **Aust J Ophthalmol** 1984 Feb;12(1):5–14

**Lowe RF:** Early Melbourne eye and ear hospital, and Dr. Turnbull's house at 101 (157) Spring Street. **Aust NZ J Surg** 1980 Oct;50(5):546–9

**Lowe RF:** John Box (1863–1934) and William Box (1905–1982). **Aust J Ophthalmol** 1983 Feb;11(1):51–3

**Lowe RF:** T. Aubrey Bowen and his house at 167 Collins Street East, Melbourne. **Aust NZ J Surg** 1981;51:102–5

**Lowe RF:** T. Aubrey Bowen, oculist, 1837–93. **Aust J Ophthalmol** 1981 May;9(2):155–62

**Lowe RF:** T. Aubrey Bowen, Oculist, 1837–93: his bequests to English charities. **Br J Ophthalmol** 1982 Oct;66(10):622–4

**Lowe RF:** T. Aubrey Bowen, oculist, 1837–93. His charitable bequest in Victoria. **Aust NZ J Surg** 1983 Apr;53(2):183–7

**Lowe RF:** The Conjoint Libraries of the Royal Victorian Eye and Ear Hospital and The Royal Australian College of Ophthalmologists. **Aust J Ophthalmol** 1983 May;11(2):127–32

**Lowe RF:** The Ophthalmological Society of Melbourne (1899–1913). **Aust J Ophthalmol** 1980 Aug;8(3):257–70

**Lowe RF:** William R. Wilde, Andrew S. Gray, and two eye and ear hospitals of very similar name. **Aust NZ J Surg** 1981 Dec;51(6):630–6

**Lowe TE:** The Thomas Baker, Alice Baker and Eleanor Shaw Medical Research Institute. [Melbourne], Trustees of the Institute, [1974?]. xii, 144 p.

**Lowell JD:** The ultraviolet environment in a nutshell (Carl W. Walter). **Am J Surg** 1984 Nov;148(5):575–7

**Lowenstam HA, Margulis L:** Evolutionary prerequisites for early Phanerozoic calcareous skeletons. **Biosystems** 1980;12(1–2):27–41

**Lowenstein JM:** Immunological reactions from fossil material. **Philos Trans R Soc Lond [Biol]** 1981 May 8;292(1057):143–9

**Lowenstein JM:** Species–specific proteins in fossils. **Naturwissenschaften** 1980 Jul;67(7):343–6

**Lowenstein JM** see **Prager EM**

**Lowenthal EG:** Zur Demographie der Juden im früheren Oberschlesien. **Z Ostforsch** 1979;28(1):81–4

**Lowenthal MN:** The yaws notebook of Dr. Acheson. **Trans R Soc Trop Med Hyg** 1982;76(5):627–9

**Löwi I** see **Moulin AM**

**Lowry LD:** Artificial larynges: a review and development of a prototype self–contained intra–oral artificial larynx. **Laryngoscope** 1981 Aug;91(8):1332–55

**Lowry RJ:** The evolution of psychological theory: a critical history of concepts and presuppositions. New York, Aldine Pub. Co., 1982. x, 246 p.

**Loza Colomer JC, Olascoaga ML:** La Sanidad del Ejército de los Andes. In Congreso de Historia de la Medicina Argentina [Transactions], 5th, Mendoza, 1983. p. 7–17.

**Lozina–Lozinsky LK, Zaar EI:** [To the history of the rise of exobiology] (Rus). **Istor Biol Issled** 1980;8:3–32

**Lozowski J:** Homeopatia (Samuela Hahnemanna). **Pieleg Polozna** 1982;4–5:16–7

**Lozoya M:** Antecedentes historicos de la diabetes Mellitus. **Med Tradic** 1980;3(10):5-9

**Lozoya X:** Fuentes bibliograficas de la herbolaria medicinal mexicana. **Med Tradic** 1980;3(10):69-71

**Lozoya X:** La herbolaria medicinal en Mexico y el Doctor Del Pozo. **Bol Soc Mex Hist Filos Med** 1980 Mar;5(30):11-6

**Lozoya X** see **Cardenas J de**

**Lu M:** History of plastic surgery in China. **Plast Reconstr Surg** 1982 Aug;70(2):273-4

**Lu YC:** The collective approach to psychiatric practice in the People's Republic of China. **Soc Probl** 1978;26(1):2-14

**Lu YF** see **Wei DX**

**Lu Gwei-djen, Needham J:** Celestial lancets: a history and rationale of acupuncture and moxa. Cambridge, Cambridge University Press, 1980. xxi, 427 p.

**Lu W, et al:** [A brief textual research on the life of Wang Shixiong, a renowned physician of Qing Dynasty] (Chi). **Chung Hua I Shih Tsa Chih** 1984 Jan;14(1):10-3

**Luan DC** see **Conger DJ**

**Lübbe H** see **Mann G, ed**

**Lübbers DW:** History of transcutaneous PO2 measurement. **Crit Care Med** 1981 Oct;9(10):693

**Lubchenco LO** see **Smith GF**

**Lubegina ZP:** K 50-letiiu Sverdlovskogo nauchno-issledovatel'skogo instituta travmatologii i ortopedii. **Ortop Travmatol Protez** 1981 Dec;(12):58-61

**Lubomudrov S:** Environmental politics in the Soviet Union: the Baikal controversy. **Can Slavonic Pap** 1978;20(4):529-43

**Lubove R** see **Numbers RL, ed**

**Lucas A:** Changing medical models in China: organizational options or obstacles? **China Q** 1980;(83):461-89

**Lucas A:** Chinese Medical Modernization. Comparative Policy Continuities, 1930s-1980s. New York, Praeger, 1982. xiii, 188 p.

**Lucas JR:** Wilberforce and Huxley: a legendary encounter. **Hist J (Gt Brit)** 1979;22(2):313-30

**Lucas MB:** Diamond jubilee medicine. The medical world of 1897 and 1898 seen in the pages of the South African Medical Journal. **S Afr Med J** 1979 Oct 20;56(17):688-94

**Lucaşciuc A:** Din istoricul ocrotirii mamei şi copilului în România (II). **Viata Med [Medii Sanit]** 1979 Oct;27(10):235-7

**Lucchetta F:** Girolamo Ramusio: profilo biografico. **Quad Stor Univ Padova** 1982;15:1-60

**Lucchetta F:** La data della morte di Andrea Alpago. **Quad Stor Univ Padova** 1982;15:147-8

**Lucchetta PM:** Nuovi documenti per la biografia di Antonio Vallisneri. **Quad Stor Univ Padova** 1982;15:131-45

**Lucchetti E:** Historical reconstitution of Varaita Valley population 1770-1970. **Acta Anthropogenet** 1981;5(4):255-70

**Luccio R:** De Sanctis e la psicologia italiana. **Stor Crit Psicol** 1981;2(2):317-68

**Luccio R:** La percezione della numerosità. **Stor Crit Psicol** 1983 Dec;4(2):215-83

**Luce EA:** The ordeal of Sigmund Freud. In Romm S, ed: Symposium on historical perspectives of plastic surgery. Philadelphia, Saunders, 1983. p. 715-6.

**Luce EA** see **Romm S**

**Luce EA** see **Romm S, ed**

**Luckin B:** Death and survival in the city: approaches to the history of disease. **Urban Hist Yearb** 1980;:53-62

**Luckin B:** States and epidemic threats. **Soc Soc Hist Med Bull (Lond)** 1984 Jun;34:25-7

**Luckin B:** The decline of small pox and the demographic revolution of the eighteenth century. **Soc Hist (Lond)** 1977;(6):793-97

**Ludlow MO:** A brief history of endodontics. **Chronicle** 1983 Mar;46(3):50-1

**Ludmerer KM:** Joseph Erlanger. In Dictionary of American biography, 1961-1965. Suppl. 7, 1981. p. 225-7.

**Ludmerer KM:** Reform at Harvard Medical School, 1869-1909. **Bull Hist Med** 1981;55(3):343-70

**Ludmerer KM:** Reform of medical education at Washington University. **J Hist Med Allied Sci** 1980 Apr;35(2):149-73

**Ludmerer KM:** The plight of clinical teaching in America. **Bull Hist Med** 1983 Summer;57(2):218-29

**Ludmerer KM:** The rise of the teaching hospital in America. **J Hist Med Allied Sci** 1983 Oct;38(4):389-414

**Ludmerer KM:** Writing the history of hospitals. An essay review. **Bull Hist Med** 1982 Spring;56(1):106-9

**Ludwig AM** see **Neill JR**

**Ludwig H:** Verhütung der Empfängnis--Verhängnis der Verhütung. Die Leistungen Ernst Gräfenbergs und die Reaktion der Gynäkologie seiner Zeit. **Zentralbl Gynakol** 1983;105(18):1197-205

**Ludwig J, Mann RJ:** Münchhausen versus Munchausen. **Mayo Clin Proc** 1983 Nov;58(11):767-9

**Ludwig J** see **Lie JT**

**Luft R:** Lysande upptäckter, men djup klyfta mellan forskningen och de sjukas situation. **Lakartidningen** 1984 Jun 27;81(26-27):2586-94

**Luft S:** Rys historyczny Instytutu Reumatologicznego. I. Lata 1948-1961. **Reumatologia** 1981;19(2):109-17

**Luft S** see **Małdyk E**

**Luger A:** 70 Jahre Krankenhaus Lainz. **Wien Klin Wochenschr** 1983 Jun 10;95(12):393-6

**Lugli T:** Hand diseases in early photographs. **Hand** 1980 Feb;12(1):97-104

**Lugnegård H:** Mannen bakom dupuytrens kontraktur: 'vilddjuret vid Seine' - sin tids mest namnkunnige kirurg. **Lakartidningen** 1983 Dec 28;80(52):5068-9

**Lugosi MM:** Die im Pray-Codex beschriebenen Heilpflanzen im späteren botanischen Lehrstoff der ersten ungarischen medizinischen Fakultät. In Hein WH, ed: Pharmaziehistorischer Kongress, Budapest, 1981. Stuttgart, Wissenschaftliche Verlagsgesellschaft, 1983. p. 97-9.

**Lukac J** see **Linkesch W**

**Lukács D:** Caspar Friedrick Wolff (1733-1794), a modern fejlödéstan megalapítója. **Orv Hetil** 1984 Aug 5;125(32):1962

**Lukács D:** Háromszázötven éve született Antony van Leeuwenhoek. **Orv Hetil** 1982 Oct 31;123(44):2732-7

**Lukács D:** Id. Jancsó Miklós malária kutatásai. **Orv Hetil** 1981 Jan 25;122(4):224-6

**Lukács D:** Pierre Paul Broca, az antropológia és a beszéd agykérgi központjának felfedezöje. **Orv Hetil** 1980 Aug 24;121(34):2081-2

**Lukács D:** Száz éve fedezte fel Charles Alphonse Louis Laveran a malária kórokozóit. **Orv Hetil** 1980 Dec 14;121(50):3076-8

**Lukacs JR:** Crown dimensions of deciduous teeth from prehistoric India. **Am J Phys Anthropol** 1981 Jun;55(2):261-6

**Lukanov A, Altŭnkov P:** Khirurgiiata v Bŭlgariia prez vekovete. **Khirurgiia (Sofiia)** 1982;35(1):100-7

**Lukas G:** Der Beitrag des Sports zur Persönlichkeitsentwicklung unter Berücksichtigung historischer Aspekte. **Wiss Z Martin Luther Univ (Sprachw)** 1975;24(3):29-35

**Lukas G:** Der Neuhumanismus in seiner Stellung zur Körpererziehung. **Wiss Z Martin Luther Univ (Sprachw)** 1978;27(1):47-54

**Lukas W:** Epidemiologie der Tuberkulose. Entwicklung seit Entdeckung des Erregers, gegenwärtige Situation in der Bundesrepublik und voraussichtliche Weiterentwicklung. **Med Welt** 1982 Mar 26;33(12):442-9

**Lukash AA:** 30 let deiatel'nosti Estonskogo otdeleniia Vsesouiznogo nauchnogo obshchestva sudebnykh medikov. **Sud Med Ekspert** 1982 Apr-Jun;25(2):57-9

**Lukavskiĭ MI, Ugulava SN:** Voenno-morskomu Krasnoznamennomu gospitaliu imeni akademika N. I. Pirogova--200 let. **Voen Med ZH** 1983 May;5:71-3

**Lukázs J, Keresztes L, Hal G, et al:** Die Entwicklung des Gesundheitswesens in der Ungarischen Volksrepublik. **Med Ges** 1979;(6):47-68

**Luke D** see **Spicker SF**

**Luk'ianovskiĭ VA** see **Danilevskiĭ VM**

**Lukic D:** Alkoholizam u vidjenju Dimitrija Tucovića. **Srp Arh Celok Lek** 1983 Mar;111(3):397-402

**Lukic D:** Gledišta Dimitrija Tucovića o tuberkulozi. **Srp Arh Celok Lek** 1981;109(12):1677-86

**Lukic D:** O narodnom zdravlju u delima Svetozara markovića. **Srp Arh Celok Lek** 1981 Apr;109(4):579-86

**Lumley JS:** Microsurgery. **Practitioner** 1982 Oct;226(1372):1723-6

**Lumpe A:** Zur Kulturgeschichte des Bades in der byzantinischen Ara. **Byzantinische Forsch** 1979;6:151-66

**Luna Martínez J** see **Carrada Bravo T**

**Lund HZ:** It was a long way to dermatopathology. **J Cutan Pathol** 1984 Apr;11(2):81-7

**Lund OE:** 125 Jahre Deutsche Ophthalmologische Gesellschaft. **MMW** 1982 Sep 10;124(36):761

**Lund P:** Sir Hans Krebs (1900-1981). **Clin Sci** 1982 Sep;63(3):225-30

**Lundberg GD:** One medical world. **JAMA** 1983 Jul 8;250(2):242-3

**Lunde AS:** Health in the United States. **Ann Am Acad Polit Soc Sci** 1981;453:28-69

**Lunde P** see **Stone C**

**Lundeen E:** [An interview with Miss Elizabeth Lundeen, a former GHQ nursing officer who contributed to the improvement of post-war Japanese nursing and recently visited Japan after 22 years] (Jpn) **Kango** 1982 Nov;34(12):76-7

**Lunden K:** Marknadsverdi i forhold til naeringsverdi av poteter og korn 1832-1865. **Hist Tidsskr** 1980;59(4):389-405

**Lundin AP** see **Friedman EA**

**Lundquist SB:** Blixtens inverkan på människan - magi och vetenskap. **Sydsven Medicinhist Sallsk Arsskr** 1981;:98-113

**Lundquist SB** see **Lindstedt E**

**Lundström B:** Medicinska aspekter på Lord Byron. **Sydsven Medicinhist Sallsk Arsskr** 1980;:112-23

**Lundström H** see **Hofsten E**

**Lundström R:** Rubella under graviditet--historik och nomenklatur. **Lakartidningen** 1979 Oct 10;76(41):3512-3

**Lungershausen M:** Unsere Rückblende aus dem Jahr 1952. Agnes Karll (25. 3. 1868 - 12. 2. 1927). **Krankenpflege (Frankfurt)** 1982 Feb;36(2):71-2

**Lunt R:** Bone and joint tuberculosis. **Br Med J** 1979 Oct 13;2(6195):907-9

**Lunzer EA** see **Varma VP**

**Luo GF** see **Yang KL**

**Luongo EP:** A biography of Wallace Mason Yater, M.D. [S.l., s.n.], 1982. iv, 180 p.

**Lupinc P:** Das zahnärztliche Lehrbuch des Wiener Militärarztes Joseph Georg Pasch 1767. Zürich, Juris Druck, 1984. 80 p. (Zürcher Medizingeschichtliche Abhandlungen, Neue Reihe, Nr. 165).

**Lupo G** see **Mazzola RF**

**Lupo O:** Sozialmedizin im alten Osterreich. Die Bekämpfung der Pellagra in der Bukowina zu Beginn dieses Jahrhunderts. **Osterr Osthefte** 1971;13(4):343-8

**Lupovici C** see **Boulle L**

**Lur'e GO, Savel'ev SA, Iushkov MA:** Iskusstvennoe krovoobrashchenie

v usloviiakh giperbaricheskoĭ oksigenatsii. **Anesteziol Reanimatol** 1982 Nov-Dec;(6):63-7
**Luria AR:** The making of mind. A personal account of Soviet psychology. Edited by M. Cole and S. Cole. Cambridge, London, Harvard University Press, 1979. 234 p.
**Lüst R:** Max Planck und die Max-Planck-Gesellschaft. **Gesch Wiss Unterr** 1979;30(9):527-37
**Lustig M** see **Kratochvíl L**
**Luten DB:** Ecological optimism in the social sciences: the question of limits of growth. **Am Behav Sci** 1980;24(1):125-51
**Lüth P:** Tagebuch eines Landarztes. Stuttgart, Deutsche Verlags-Anstalt, 1983. 303 p.
**Luthe R** see **Payne H**
**Luther E:** Gedanken zum 100. Geburtstag von Albert Schweitzer. **Wiss Z Martin Luther Univ (Math)** 1975;24(4):81-5
**Luther E:** Humanismus und gesellschaftliche Verantwortung. **Wiss Z Martin Luther Univ (Math)** 1984;33(2):122-7
**Luther E:** Theodor Brugsch und das ärztliche Ethos. **Wiss Z Martin Luther Univ (Math)** 1980;29(2):91-6
**Lutschg JH:** Why Uncle Sam is still smoking. **NY State J Med** 1983 Dec;83(13):1278-9
**Luttenberger F:** Hypnotisörernas tid. Hypnotismen i svensk medicin 1880-1900. **Lychnos** 1983;:90-119
**Lutz LA:** Shakespeare on plastic surgery. **Plast Reconstr Surg** 1984 Dec;74(6):841
**Lutz R:** A century of progress. A look at the past 100 years of veterinary medicine in Iowa. [Des Moines, Iowa Veterinary Medical Association, 1981?] 112 p.
**Lutzker E:** Cameron prizewinner: Waldemar M. Haffkine, C.I.E. **Clio Med** 1971 May;13(3-4):269-76
**Lutzker E:** From Malkowal to Calcutta: an historical appreciation of Haffkine's victorious struggle. **Adler Mus Bull** 1981;7(1):14-8
**Lutzker E:** From Malkowal to Calcutta: an historical appreciation of Haffkine's victorious struggle. In: Science and history: studies in honor of Edward Rosen. (Studia Copernicana, XVI.) Wrocław, Ossolineum, 1978. p. 543-53.
**Lutzker E:** Some unanswered questions in medical history. In: Congrès international d'histoire de la médecine, XXVe, Québec, 1976. Actes. Québec, 1977. p. 917-27.
**Lutzker E, Jochnowitz C:** The curious history of Waldemar Haffkine. **Commentary** 1980;69(6):61-4
**Lutzner MA:** The human papillomaviruses. A review. **Arch Dermatol** 1983 Aug;119(8):631-5
**Lux G, Demling L:** 100 Jahre Gastroskopie. **Fortschr Med** 1983 Jan 27;101(4):107-12
**Luxon SG:** A history of industrial hygiene. **Am Ind Hyg Assoc J** 1984 Nov;45(11):731-9
**Luyendijk W:** The arteries of the spinal cord. The history of a paradigmal shift. **Acta Neurochir (Wien)** 1982;61(1-3):25-41
**Luyendijk-Elshout AM:** Antoni van Leeuwenhoek (1632-1723) herdacht. **Ned Tijdschr Geneeskd** 1983 Jun 18;127(25):1111-2
**Luyendijk-Elshout AM:** Christiaan Huygens en de geneeskunde. **Spiegel Hist** 1979;14(4):230-33
**Luyendijk-Elshout AM:** Het medisch tijdschrift in Nederlands Oost-Indië (1844-1865). **Ned Tijdschr Geneeskd** 1981 Jun 6;125(23):923-6
**Luyendijk-Elshout AM:** Mechanicisme contra vitalisme de school van Herman Boerhaave en de beginselen van het leven. **Tijdschr Geschied Geneeskd** 1982;5(1):16-26
**Luyendijk-Elshout AM:** Samuel Musgrave's attack upon Stahl's and Boerhaave's doctrines in 1763. **Janus** 1980;67(1-2-3):141-56
**Luyendijk-Elshout AM:** The introduction of Juan Valverde's and Bartholomy Cabrol's anatomy into Low Countries between 1568-1633. In International Congress of the History of Medicine, 27th, Barcelona, 1980. Actas. Barcelona, Académia de Ciències Médiques de Catalunya i Balears, 1981. p. 298-303.
**Luyendijk-Elshout AM, ed** see **Kegel-Brinkgreve E**
**Luyt R:** The Medical School of the University of Cape Town. **S Afr Med J** 1979 Nov 24;56(22):861-2
**Luyt R** see **De Villiers JC**
**Luz Terrada M** see **Albarracín Teulón A**
**Luzi V** see **Colangelo G**
**Luzi von Scheid C:** Ueber die Entwicklung der Sanitätsgesetzgebung in Graubünden. Zürich, Bischofberger, 1970. 48 p. (Diss., Zürich).
**Lyba RM** see **Revenko TA**
**Lydecker M** see **Silverman M**
**Lyell A:** Daniel Turner (1667-1740) LRCP London (1711) M.D. honorary, Yale (1723) surgeon, physician and pioneer dermatologist: the man seen in the pages of his book on the skin. **Int J Dermatol** 1982 Apr;21(3):162-70
**Lyell A:** The staphylococcal scalded skin syndrome in historical perspective: emergence of dermopathic strains of Staphylococcus aureus and discovery of the epidermolytic toxin. A review of events up to 1970. **J Am Acad Dermatol** 1983 Aug;9(2):285-94
**Lyell C** see **McKinney HL, ed**
**Lyles MR, Carter JH:** Myth and strengths of the black family: a historical and sociological contribution to family therapy. **J Natl Med Assoc** 1982 Nov;74(11):1119-23
**Lynaugh J:** Katherine Berry Richardson, MD (1858-1933). **Women Health** 1982 Spring;7(1):1-3
**Lynch A** see **McCullough LB**
**Lynch EA:** An historical survey of the test services of the National League for Nursing. **NLN Publ** 1980;(17-1777):i-viii, 1-78
**Lynch KA:** Local and regional studies in historical demography. **Hist Methods** 1982;15(1):23-9
**Lynch KA** see **Bardet JP**
**Lynch M:** The 'Faithful Brethren' of Edinburgh: the acceptable face of Protestantism. **Bull Inst Hist Res** 1978;51(124):194-9
**Lyngdoh MG:** Life and works of Dr. Homiwell Lyngdoh. Shillong, Kyknsai M. Warjrie, 1980. 70 p.
**Lynn GE** see **Benitez JT**
**Lynn GE** see **El-Najjar MY**
**Lyon G** see **Danzinger R**
**Lyon TJ:** John Muir's enlightenment. **Pac Hist** 1981;25(2):50-7
**Lyons JB:** Letters to an editor. The William Doolin Memorial Lecture. **Ir Med J** 1980 Sep;73(9):323-30
**Lyons JB:** Sylvester O'Halloran's 'Treatise on the Air'. **Ir Med J** 1983 Jan;76(1):37-9
**Lyons JB:** The neurology of Robert Bentley Todd. In Rose FC, Bynum WF, ed: Historical aspects of the neurosciences. New York, Raven, 1982. p. 137-50.
**Lyons JB:** The section of medicine and medical developments over the century. **Ir J Med Sci** 1983 Jan;152(1):14-24
**Lyons M:** Death camps in the Congo: administrative responses to sleeping sickness 1903-1911. **Soc Soc Hist Med Bull (Lond)** 1984 Jun;34:28-31
**Lysaght A:** A letter from Sydney Parkinson in Batavia to Dr. John Fothergill. **Notes Rec R Soc Lond** 1981;36(1):79-81
**Lyskanowski M:** Medycyna i lekarze dawnej Warszawy. Warszawa, Państwowy Instytut Wydawniczy, 1976. 465 p.
**Lysnes M:** Marie Lysnes: sykepleie var vårt liv. **Sykepleien** 1984 Oct 5;71(17):22-7
**Lysnes M** see **Dagsland H**
**Lyte C:** Sir Joseph Banks, 18th century explorer, botanist and entrepreneur. London, David & Charles, 1980. 248 p.

## M

**Ma JH** see **Wei DX**
**Ma JX:** [An investigation on the dosage of herbal drug administration described in the medical works unearthed in Ma Wan Dui tomb of Han Dynasty (author's transl)] (Chi). **Chung Yao Tung Pao** 1982 May;6(3):41-3
**Ma Kanwen:** [An introduction to ancient Roman medicine] (Chi). **Chung Hua I Shih Tsa Chih** 1981;11:109-15
**Maas J:** Plant pathology: contributions in improving the American food supply. **J NAL Assoc** 1980;5(3-4):76-8
**Maat GJ:** Boerhaave en zijn tijdgenoten, en de betekenis van hun lichaamslengte (een fysisch-antropologisch onderzoek van begravenen in de Pieterskerk te Leiden). **Ned Tijdschr Geneeskd** 1982 Apr 17;126(16):705-12
**Macadam PS:** A small skeletal sample from northern Ghana. **Paleopathol Newsl** 1981 Jan;33:5-7
**McAllister TA:** Penicillins in perspective. **Scott Med J** 1982;27 Spec No.:S39-47
**MacAlpin RN:** Coronary arterial spasm: a historical perspective. **J Hist Med Allied Sci** 1980 Jul;35(3):288-311
**McArthur N:** And, behold, the plague was begun among the people. The Changing Pacific: Essays in honour of H. E. Maude. Melbourne, Oxford University Press, 1978. p. 273-84.
**McAuley CE** see **Ravitch MM**
**MacBeath G:** Philippe Enault de Barbaucannes. In Dictionary of Canadian biography, 1701 to 1740. Volume 2, 1969. p. 217.
**Macbeth R:** Sir Terence Edward Cawthorne. In Dictionary of national biography, 1961-1970. Suppl. 8, 1981. p. 179-80.
**Macbeth RA:** Medicine in French Canada from 1608 to 1763. In: Congrès international d'histoire de la médecine, XXVe, Québec, 1976. Actes. Québec, 1977. p. 931-43.
**McBogg P** see **Hagerman RJ**
**McBride DC, Page JB:** Adolescent Indian substance abuse: ecological and sociocultural factors. **Youth Soc** 1980;11(4):475-92
**McBride R:** The sceptical view of medicine and the comic vision in Molière. **Studi Francesi** 1979, 23(67):27-42
**McBryde AM, Pressly JA, Hutchinson F, et al:** North Carolina Orthopedic Hospital closes after 58 years of treatment of crippled children. **NC Med J** 1979 Dec;40(12):755-7
**McBryde B:** A nurse's war - 2. A trip to Rouen. **Nurs Times** 1979 Jul 5;75(26):1150-2
**McCall N, Kanarek H:** The Alan Mason Chesney Archives of the Johns Hopkins Medical Institutions. **Bull Hist Med** 1982 Spring;56(1):88-92
**McCall N:** The statue of the Christus Consolator at the Johns Hopkins Hospital: its acquisition and historic origins. **Johns Hopkins Med J** 1982 Jul;151(1):11-9
**McCallum DM:** A demographic study of the parishes of Bruton and Pitcombe in the County of Somerset. **Proc Somerset Archaeol Nat Hist Soc** 1977;121:77-87
**McCandless P:** 'Build! build!' the controversy over the care of the chronically insane in England, 1855-1870. **Bull Hist Med** 1979 Winter;53(4):553-74
**McCandless P:** 'Curses of civilization': insanity and drunkenness in Victorian Britain. **Br J Addict** 1984 Mar;79(1):49-58
**McCandless P:** Liberty and lunacy: the Victorians and wrongful confinement. **J Soc Hist** 1978;11(3):366-86
**McCann W:** (Austin) Merrill Moore. In Dictionary of American Biography, Suppl. 6, 1956-1960. p. 461-2, 1980.
**McCartan MA** see **Buchanan AV**

McCarthy CR: [History of biomedical research policy]. In Reich WT, et al, ed: Encyclopedia of bioethics, v.4. New York, Free Press, 1978. p. 1492–8.
McCarthy EF: Aseptic necrosis of bone. An historic perspective. Clin Orthop 1982 Aug;(168):216–21
McCarthy EF: Giant-cell tumor of bone: an historical perspective. Clin Orthop 1980 Nov–Dec;(153):14–25
McCarthy J see Watkins SC
McCarthy K: Early alcoholism treatment: the Emmanuel Movement and Richard Peabody. J Stud Alcohol 1984 Jan;45(1):59–74
McCarthy T: Freud and the problem of sexuality. J Hist Behav Sci 1981;17:332–9
McCarthy TG see Ratnam SS
MacCarthy D, et al see Dobbs R
McCarty DJ: The American Rheumatism Association and the Arthritis Foundation: commentary on 14 years of a happy union. Arthritis Rheum 1979 Dec;22(12):1394–5
McCarty M: Historical perspective on C-reactive protein. Ann NY Acad Sci 1982;389:1–10
McCarty M: Reminiscenses of the early days of transformation. Annu Rev Genet 1980;14:1–15
McCaughey D: Professional militancy: the Medical Defence Association vs. the College of Physicians & Surgeons of Ontario, 1891-1902. In Roland CG, ed: Health, disease and medicine. Toronto, Hannah Institute for the History of Medicine, 1984. p. 96–104.
McCauley HB: Professional dentistry and the University of Maryland at Baltimore. Bull Hist Dent 1982 Oct;30(2):73–91
McCauley HB: The century old Dental Department of the University of Maryland at Baltimore. J Md State Dent Assoc 1982 Dec;25(3):96–102
McCauley HB: The Maryland State Board of Dental Examiners. In the beginning. J Md State Dent Assoc 1984 Apr;27(1):22–9
McCauley HB: The Maryland State Dental Association: in the beginning. J Md State Dent Assoc 1983 Aug;26(2):74–8
Macchi G: Historia de la neuropatología italiana. Evolución de una problemática. Arch Neurobiol (Madr) 1984 Jan–Feb;47(1):45–8
McClary A: Don't go to Michigan, that land of ills. Mich Hist 1983;67(1):46–8
McClary A: 'Swat the Fly': popular magazines and the anti-fly campaign. Prev Med 1982 May;11(3):373–8
McClary A: The medicated woman: 1880. Pharos 1984 Summer;47(3):8–10
McClellan JE: The Académie Royale des Sciences, 1699–1793: a statistical portrait. Isis 1981 Dec;72(264):541–67
McClure RK: Coram's children, the London Foundling Hospital in the eighteenth century. New Haven, Yale University Press, 1981. xiii, 321 p.
McClure RK: Pediatric practice at the London Foundling Hospital. Stud Eighteenth Cent Cult 1981;10:361–71
McCollum RW: Some observations on viral hepatitis. Yale J Biol Med 1982 May–Aug;55(3–4):247–50
McCombie F, Gray AS: Dental public health in British Columbia. Can J Public Health 1984 Sep–Oct;75(5):368–9
McConchie RW: Additions to OED from John Cotta's Ignorant Practisers of Physicke, 1612. Notes Queries 1981 Dec;28(6):490–3
McConnell NF, Dore MM: Crittenton services, the first century, 1883–1983. Washington, D.C., National Florence Crittenton Mission, 1983. vi, 95 p.
McConville E: Oliver Harvey: 'Got to take some risks.' South Exposure 6(2):24–8, 1978
McCormick JB see Johnson KM
McCormick JP, Parascandola J: Dragon bones and drugstores: the interaction of pharmacy and paleontology in the search for early man in China. Pharm Hist 1981;23(2):55–70
McCormick JS: James Mackenzie and coronary heart disease. J R Coll Gen Pract 1981 Jan;31(222):26–30
McCormick RE see Maloney MT
McCormick WC see Shapiro LJ
McCoy DR: Jefferson and Madison on Malthus: population growth in Jeffersonian political economy. Va Mag Hist Biogr 1980;88(3):259–76
McCoy JJ: The cancer lady: Maud Slye and her heredity studies. Nashville, Nelson, 1977. 191 p.
McCracken D: A link with the past. Br Med J [Clin Res] 1981 Mar 21;282(6268):964–6
McCraw JB: The recent history of myocutaneous flaps. Clin Plast Surg 1980 Jan;7(1):3–7
McCray Beier L: The creation of the medical fringe 1500–1700. Soc Soc Hist Med Bull (Lond) 1981 Dec;29:29–31
McCuaig K: 'From social reform to social service': the changing role of volunteers: the anti-tuberculosis campaign, 1900–30. Can Hist Rev 1980;61(4):480–501
McCuaig K: Tuberculosis: the changing concepts of the disease in Canada 1900–1950. In Roland CG, ed: Health, disease and medicine. Toronto, Hannah Institute for the History of Medicine, 1984. p. 296–307.
McCue RJ: Did the word of wisdom become a commandment in 1851? Dialogue J Mormon Thought 1981;14(3):66–77
McCullagh KG, Silver IA: The actual cautery -- myth and reality in the art of firing. Equine Vet J 1981 Apr;13(2):81–4
McCulloch I: Nursing Mirror mental health forum. 3. From colony to community care. Nurs Mirror 1983 Apr 20:156(16):i–ii
McCullough LB, Page BB, Blomquist C, et al: [History of medical ethics in contemporary Europe and the Americas]. In Reich WT, et al, ed: Encyclopedia of bioethics, v.3. New York, Free Press, 1978. p. 975–1007.
McCullough LB, Jonsen AR, Burns CR, et al: [History of medical ethics in modern Europe and the Americas]. In Reich WT, et al, ed: Encyclopedia of bioethics, v.3. New York, Free Press, 1978. p. 951–75.
McCullough LB: Justice and health care: historical perspectives and precedents. In E. E. Shelp, ed: Justice and health care. Dordrecht, Reidel, 1981. (Philosophy and medicine, Vol. 8), p. 51–71.
McCullough LB: Thought-styles, diagnosis, and concepts of disease: commentary on Ludwig Fleck. J Med Philos 1981 Aug;6(3):257–61
McCurley J see Tarr JA
McDermott W: Colin Munro MacLeod: January 28, 1909–February 11, 1972. Biogr Mem Natl Acad Sci 1983;54:183–219
McDermott W, Rogers DE: Social ramifications of control of microbial disease. Johns Hopkins Med J 1982 Dec;151(6):302–12
McDermott WV: Endorphins, I presume. Lancet 1980 Dec 20–27;2(8208–8209):1353
Macdonald AA: Studies on the anatomy and physiology of the pig fetus and placenta: an historical review. In E. Schultheisz, ed: History of physiology. Oxford, Elmsford, New York, Pergamon, 1981. xvi, 208 p. (Advances in Physiological Sciences. Proceedings of the 28th International Congress of Physiological Sciences, Budapest, 1980. Volume 21). p. 53–60.
McDonald CJ: Seventh District Medical Society (Sioux Falls). SD J Med 1981 May;34(5):19–20
McDonald DI: The Newcastle Lunatic Asylum: so human a purpose. J R Aust Hist Soc 1980;66(1):20–38
MacDonald DM see White IR
Macdonald EM: World-wide conquests of disabilities. The history, development and present functions of the remedial services. London, Baillière Tindall, 1981. 299 p.
Macdonald EM: World-wide conquests of disabilities. The history, development and present functions of the remedial services. London, Baillière Tindall, 1981. 299 p.
Macdonald G: One hundred years Wellcome, 1880–1980: in pursuit of excellence. London, Wellcome Foundation, Ltd., 1980. 120 p.
MacDonald GM: Perspectives in international neurosurgery: the development of neurosurgical services in New Zealand. Neurosurgery 1980 Apr;6(4):466–7
McDonald IA, Cope I, Forster FM: Super Ardua. The Royal College of Obstetricians and Gynaecologists in Australia, 1929–1979. Melbourne, Australian Council RCOG, 1981. iv, 107 p.
McDonald JC: Louisiana's place in American surgery. J La State Med Soc 1984 Jan;136(1):3–8
MacDonald M: Insanity and the realities of history in early modern England. Psychol Med 1981 Feb;11(1):11–25
MacDonald M: Mystical bedlam: madness, anxiety, and healing in seventeenth-century England. Cambridge, Cambridge University Press, 1981. xvi, 323 p.
McDonald M: Religion, social change, and psychological healing in England, 1600–1800. In Sheils WJ, ed: The Church and healing. Papers read at the twentieth summer meeting and the twenty-first winter meeting of the Ecclesiastical History Society. Oxford, Basil Blackwell for the Society, 1982. p. 101–25.
McDonald MO, Utterback N, Wright RA: Medical malpractice and ordinary care in Kentucky. J Ky Med Assoc 1983 Jan;81(1):55–7
McDonald PR: Evolution of cataract surgery since the deSchweinitz era. Ophthalmic Surg 1979 May;10(5):44–52
Macdonald RC, Banks JG, Ledingham IM: Transportation of the injured. Injury 1980 Nov;12(3):225–33
MacDonald RR: Classic illustrations: From St. Anthony's fire to ergometrine (Ergonovine). Eur J Obstet Gynecol Reprod Biol 1982 Aug;13(5):325–7
McDonald WH: Country doctor: he can't go home again. J Med Assoc State Ala 1982 Oct;52(4):8–9, 12–4, 19–22
McDonald WH: Then and now. 75 years of Alabama medicine by father and son with comments on the birth of malpractice. J Med Assoc State Ala 1979 Jan;48(7):16–8
McDonald WI: Attitudes to the treatment of multiple sclerosis. Arch Neurol 1983 Oct 21;40(11):667–70
McDonell KM: Dr. William A. Lindsay, innovator, physician, enterpreneur. Indiana Med Hist Q 1980;6(1):5–23
McDonell KM: Medicine in antebellum Indiana: conflict, conservatism, and change. Indianapolis, Indiana Historical Society, 1984. 58 p. (Publications in Indiana Medical History, No. 1).
McDonell KM: 'One bold incision': Dr. William A. Lindsay's radical cure. Indiana Med Hist Q 1980;6(3):3–23
McDonell KM: Surgery in early nineteenth century Indiana. Indiana Med Hist Q 1980;6(4):3–23
McDonell KM: The Indianapolis City Hospital, 1833–1866. Indiana Med Hist Q 1983 June;9(2):3–23
McDonell KM: W. D. Allison: manufacturer of physicians' furniture. Snakeroot Extr 1984 Oct;(3):2–3
McDonell KM: William A. Lindsay in perspective. Indiana Hist Soc 1981 Jun;7(2):3–20
McDonell KM: Women and medicine in early nineteenth century Indiana. Indiana Med Hist Q 1980;6(2):3–23
MacDougall H: 'Enlightening the public': the views and values of the Association of Executive Health Officers of Ontario, 1886–1903. In Roland CG, ed: Health, disease and medicine. Toronto, Hannah Institute for the History of Medicine, 1984. p. 436–64.
MacDougall H: Public health in Toronto's municipal politics: the Canniff years, 1883–1890. Bull Hist Med 1981 Summer;55(2):186–202

**MacDougall HA:** The genesis of public health reform in Toronto, 1869–1890. **Urban Hist Rev** 1982;10(3):1–9

**McDougall IR:** Stanford University Medical School. **Scott Med J** 1979 Apr;24(2):159–62

**MacDougall JD:** Joseph Eastman, M.D., LL.D; citizen, soldier, surgeon and medical educator. **Indiana Med Hist Q** 1974;1(2):26–30

**McDowall DG:** The Yorkshire Connection--Priestley and Waterton. **Anaesth Intensive Care** 1982 Feb;10(1):4–8

**McDuff HC** see **Steinfeld AD**

**McEachern AC:** The founders of the College. **Aust NZ J Surg** 1981 Aug;51(4):400–5

**MacEntee MI:** The denturist movement in Canada. Part I: Growth and development in the western provinces. **Can Dent Assoc J** 1981 Aug;47(8):521–4

**McEntee MK:** The right to heritage: the teaching of deaf history. **Am Ann Deaf** 1981 Jun;126(4):402–3

**Macerak Z** see **Andelic P**

**McEvoy J:** The chronology of Robert Grosseteste's writings on nature and natural philosophy. **Speculum** 1983 July;58(3):614–55

**McEvoy JG:** Joseph Priestley, scientist, philosopher and divine. **Proc Am Philos Soc** 1984 Sep;128(3):193–9

**McEwin R:** Florey and Cairns--early work on penicillin. **Med J Aust** 1982 Jan 9;1(1):12–3

**McFadden ER:** Qualifying factors in the classification of asthma: how valuable they are to the clinician. **J Asthma** 1983;20 Suppl 1:5–8

**McFalls JA, Masnick GS:** Birth control and the fertility of the U. S. Black population, 1880 to 1980. **J Fam Hist** 1981 Spring;6(1):89–106

**Macfarlane A** see **Fox VC**

**Macfarlane A** see **Hare EH**

**Macfarlane A** see **Laslett P**

**Macfarlane RG:** Alexander Fleming: the man and the myth. London, Chatto & Windus, The Hogarth Press, 1984. xiv, 304 p.

**Macfarlane RG:** Howard Florey; the making of a great scientist. Oxford and New York, Oxford University Press, 1979. xvi, 396 p.

**Macfarlane RG:** Howard Walter Florey. In Dictionary of national biography, 1961–1970. Suppl. 8, 1981. p. 370–4.

**McFarlane W:** Beyond bedlam. **Work Pap Mag** 1982;9(2):10–4

**Macfie C:** Down Memory Lane: for king and country. **Nurs Mirror** 1982 Jul 21;155(3):41–4

**McGahan EW:** John Thomson. In Dictionary of Canadian biography, 1881–1890. 1982;11:878–9.

**McGahan EW:** Sylvester Zobieski Earle. In Dictionary of Canadian biography, 1881–1890. 1982;11:295–6.

**McGaw N** see **Isbister JD**

**McGee VE** see **Broehl WG**

**McGeown MG:** Twenty-first birthday of the Renal Unit at the Belfast City Hospital. **Ulster Med J** 1981;50(Suppl 1):2–3

**McGill University:** The Osler Library. Montreal, McGill University, 1979. 64 p.

**McGinnis JD:** 'Unclean, unclean': Canadian reaction to lepers and leprosy. In Roland CG, ed: Health, disease and medicine. Toronto, Hannah Institute for the History of Medicine, 1984. p. 250–75.

**McGinnis JD** see **Buckley S**

**McGinnis JP:** A city faces an epidemic. **Alberta Hist** 1976;24(4):1–11

**McGinnis JP:** Records of tuberculosis in Calgary. **Archivaria** 1980;10:173–89

**McGinnis JP:** The impact of epidemic influenza, Canada, 1918–1919. **Hist Pap Can Hist Assoc** 1977;:120–41

**McGinnis JP:** The impact of epidemic influenza: Canada, 1918–1919. **Can Hist Assoc Hist Pap** 1977;:121–40

**McGinnis JP:** The white plague in Calgary: sanatarium care in southern Alberta. **Alberta Hist** 1980;28(4):1–15

**McGinnis S:** History of nursing audit: a survey of the literature. **QRB** 1978;Spec No:2–4

**McGivering NJ:** View from childhood. **Br Med J** 1979 Oct 13;2(6195):909

**McGlashan ND** see **Harington JS**

**McGoldrick KE** see **Waugh ES**

**McGonagle RR:** Our golden age of orthodontics revisited. **Am J Orthod** 1980 Apr;77(4):461–4

**McGoon DC:** Cardiac surgery. Prologue: From Whence? **Cardiovasc Clin** 1981;12(3):1–8

**McGoon DC:** The dimensions of surgical progress in cardiac surgery. **Bol Asoc Med PR** 1983 Feb;75(2):80–2

**McGovern CM:** Doctors or ladies? Women physicians in psychiatric institutions, 1872–1900. **Bull Hist Med** 1981 Spring;55(1):88–107

**McGovern FH:** Sir Astley Cooper and his otological papers. **Ann Otol Rhinol Laryngol** 1984 Nov–Dec;93(6 Pt 1):531–3

**McGovern FH:** The elusive Henry Jones Shrapnell. **Laryngoscope** 1983 Jul;93(7):903–5

**McGovern JP, ed** see **Nation EF**

**McGrath MH:** Scalping: the savage and the surgeon. In Romm S, ed: Symposium on historical perspectives of plastic surgery. Philadelphia, Saunders, 1983. p. 679–88.

**McGregor IA:** Thomas Gibson's contribution to immunology. **Plast Reconstr Surg** 1983 Mar;71(3):440

**McGuckin A:** Nineteenth-century pharmacists of Newcastle. **Pharm Hist (London)** 1971 Jul;2(2):4–6

**McGuigan FJ, Szegal B:** Covert behavior and mental processes in Russian psychology. **Pavlov J Biol Sci** 1980 Jan–Mar;15(1):35–41

**McGuigan FJ:** The historical development of cognitive psychophysiology: theory and measurement. In E. Schultheisz, ed: History of physiology. Oxford, Elmsford, New York, Pergamon, 1981. xvi, 208 p. (Advances in Physiological Sciences. Proceedings of the 28th International Congress of Physiological Sciences, Budapest, 1980. Volume 21). p. 29–47.

**McGuiness-Scott J:** Benesh movement notation. An introduction to recording clinical data. Part 12: an historical perspective and clinical uses. **Physiotherapy** 1982 Jun;68(6):182–4

**McGuinness BF:** Freud e Wittgenstein. **Ann Sc Norm Super Pisa** 1979;9(1):409–24

**McGuire TM:** Ancient Maya mushroom connections: a transcendental interaction model. **J Psychoactive Drugs** 1982 Jul–Sep;14(3):221–38

**McGuire W** see **Burnham JC**

**Machado JT:** A doença que vitimou Herculano. **An Acad Port Hist** 1979;26(1):305–34

**Machalett G:** Ludwig Stromeyer--sein Beitrag zur Entwicklung der Militärmedizin in Deutschland. **Militaergesch** 1975;14(6):694–705

**Machalski J** see **Fijałek J**

**McHarg JF:** Dr. Johne Makluire and the 1630 attempt to establish the College. In Passmore R, ed: Proceedings of the Royal College of Physicians of Edinburgh Tercentenary Congress, 1981. Edinburgh, Royal College of Physicians of Edinburgh, 1982. p. 44–58.

**McHenry HM, Andrews P, Corruccini RS:** Miocene hominoid palatofacial morphology. **Folia Primatol (Basel)** 1980;33(4):241–52

**McHenry HM:** Relative cheek-tooth size in Australopithecus. **Am J Phys Anthropol** 1984 Jul;64(3):297–306

**McHenry LC:** L'idea e la mano. **Kos** 1984 Jul–Aug;1(6):79–90

**McHenry LC:** Neurology and Art. In Rose FC, Bynum WF, ed: Historical aspects of the neurosciences. New York, Raven, 1982. p. 481–519.

**McHenry LC** see **Kleinman LC**

**McHenry LC** see **Tyler KL**

**McHenry S:** The pox upon her. **Aramco World Mag** 1980, 31(4):13–21

**Macho L, Langer P:** 30 years of the Institute of Experimental Endocrinology. **Endocrinol Exp (Bratisl)** 1982 Nov;16(3–4):147–9

**Machol L:** Dorothy Hansine Andersen. In: Notable American women. The modern period. Cambridge, Mass., Belknap-Harvard Univ. Press, 1980. 4:18–20.

**Machovec FJ:** The cult of Asklipios. **Am J Clin Hypn** 1979 Oct;22(2):85–90

**Machtan L:** Workers' insurance versus protection of the workers. Remarks on state social policy in the early Kaiserreich. **Soc Soc Hist Med Bull (Lond)** 1983 Dec;33:33

**McHugh C:** Phrenology: getting your head together in ante-bellum America. **Midwest Q** 1981;23(1):65–77

**McHugh M** see **Kalisch BJ**

**McHugh P:** Prostitution and Victorian social reform. New York, St. Martin's Press, 1980. 306 p.

**McHugh PF:** The campaign against the Contagious Diseases Act: Some organizational aspects, 1869–1886. Ph.D thesis, Oxford Univ, 1976.

**Maciałek E, Sobocki S, Czyrek G:** Pięć wieków szpitalnictwa w Jarosławiu (1462–1977). **Ann Univ Mariae Curie Sklodowska [Med]** 1978;33:341–51

**Maciałek E** see **Sobocki S**

**Maciejewska-Dorsz K** see **Dorsz-Szteke E**

**McIlroy PD** see **Dundee JW**

**McIlwain H:** Neurochemistry and Sherrington's enchanted loom. **J R Soc Med** 1984 May;77(5):417–25

**McIntosh CA:** Demographic trends and policies in developed countries. **Int J Polit** 1982;12(3):3–26

**McIntosh K:** Folk obstetrics, gynecology, and pediatrics in Utica, New York. **NY Folkl** 1978;4(1–4):49–59

**McIntosh K:** Sense and nonsense in viral diagnosis--past, present, and future. **Curr Top Microbiol Immunol** 1983;104:1–6

**MacIntyre A:** Why is the search for the foundations of ethics so frustrating? **Hastings Cent Rep** 9(4):16–22, Aug 79

**McIntyre RJ:** The Bulgarian anomaly: demographic transition and current fertility. **Southeast Eur** 1980;7(2):147–70

**McIntyre RL:** Medical history museum. **J Med Soc NJ** 1982 Dec;79(13):1017

**MacIntyre WJ** see **Brucer M**

**Mack JE:** Psychoanalysis and biography: aspects of a developing affinity. **J Am Psychoanal Assoc** 1980;28(3):543–62

**McKale D:** Purging Nazis: the postwar trials of female German doctors and nurses. **Proc SC Hist Assoc** 1981;:156–70

**Mackay A:** Derek John de Solla Price: an appreciation. **Soc Stud Sci** 1984 May;14(2):315–20

**Mckay DR:** A history of the Nordrach Ranch: Colorado's first sanatorium of the open air. **Colo Mag** 1979 Summer–Fall;56:179–96

**McKay FW** see **Miller RW**

**MacKay IM:** Zoonoses in South Wales, 1875–1915. **Vet Hist** 1980/81;N.Ser.,1:137–45

**MacKay M:** The regulation of health insurance. **Proc Acad Polit Sci** 1980;33(4):81–91

**MacKay W:** Salesman surgeon. New York, McGraw-Hill, 1978. xii, 187 p.

**McKee GK:** Total hip replacement--past, present and future. **Biomaterials** 1982 Jul;3(3):130–5

**McKee HS** see **McKee ME**

**McKee ME, McKee HS:** E. Vieillard et E. Deplanche, deux grands botanistes collecteurs en Nouvelle-Calédonie. **Hist Nat** 1980–81;17–18:49–68

**Macken U:** Drug abuse in Ireland. Cork [Ire.]. Mercier Press, 1975. 132 p.

**McKenna EE:** Marriage and fertility in postfamine Ireland: a multivariate analysis. **Am J Sociol** 1974 Nov;80(3):688–705

MacKenna RM: Robert M. B. MacKenna. **J Am Acad Dermatol** 1982 Jan;6(1):135-44
McKenzie D: Die mediese fakulteit van die universiteit van Kaapstad. **S Afr Med J** 1979 Nov 24;56(22):862-3
MacKenzie D: Sociobiologies in competition: the biometrician-Mendelian debate. In C. Webster, ed: Biology, medicine and society 1840-1940. Cambridge, Cambridge University Press, 1981. p. 243-88.
McKenzie D see **De Villiers JC**
MacKenzie DA: Statistics in Britain, 1865-1930: the social construction of scientific knowledge. Edinburgh, Edinburgh University Press, 1981. viii, 306 p.
Mackenzie DB: The treatment of recurrent anterior shoulder dislocation by the modified Bristow-Helfet procedure. **S Afr Med J** 1984 Mar 3;65(9):325-30
McKenzie J see **Skreb N**
Mackenzie L: William James and the problem of interests. **J Hist Behav Sci** 1980 Apr;16(2):175-85
Mackenzie Hume WG: Aviation medicine? **Br Med J [Clin Res]** 1983 Dec 24-31;287(6409):1950-2
McKeown T: The direction of medical research. **Lancet** 1979 Dec 15;2(8155):1281-4
McKeown T: The role of medicine. Dream, mirage or nemesis? Princeton, Princeton University Press, Oxford, Basil Blackwell, 1979. xvi, 207 p.
Mackey LH see **Smith JH, ed**
McKinney LC see **Bober H**
McKinney HL, ed: Lamarck to Darwin: contributions to evolutionary biology 1809-1859. Contributions by J. B. Lamarck, W. C. Wells, P. Matthew, C. Lyell, E. Blyth, R. Chambers, A. R. Wallace, C. Darwin. Lawrence, Kansas, Coronado, 1971, 3rd printing R 75, 122 p.
McKinnon DA: Battalion surgeon on Iwo Jima. **Marine Corps Gaz** 1982;66(2):28-37
McKinzie RD see **Gorman BM**
Macklin R see **Sharkey PW, ed**
McKnight BE, ed: The washing away of wrongs: forensic medicine in thirteenth-century China. Ann Arbor, Center for Chinese Studies, University of Michigan, 1981. xv, 181 p.
Mackowiak K see **Wójciak L**
Mackowiak Z: Uwagi o życiu i działalności Witolda Chodźki (1875-1954). **Przegl Lek** 1980;37(4):437-40
McKusick VA: The human genome through the eyes of Mercator and Vesalius. **Trans Am Clin Climatol Assoc** 1980;92:66-90
McLachlan HV, Swales JK: Stereotypes and Scottish witchcraft. **Contemp Rev** 1979:234(1357):88-94
MacLaglan D: The ether song, 1850. With an introduction and notes by K. G. Huston. First printed in Edinburgh and now reprinted in Los Angeles, 1982. [12 p.].
McLaren A: A prehistory of the social sciences: phrenology in France. **Comp Stud Soc Hist** 1981;23(1):3-22
McLaren A: Abortion in nineteenth-century France. **Fr Hist Stud** 1978;10
McLaren A: Contraception and its discontents: Sigmund Freud and birth control. **J Soc Hist** 1979;12(4):513-29
McLaren A: Sexuality and social order: the debate over the fertility of women and workers in France, 1770-1920. New York, Holmes & Meier, 1982.
McLaren A: 'What has this to do with working class women?': Birth control and the Canadian left, 1900-1939. **Soc Hist (Canada)** 1981;14(28):435-54
McLaren D: Disease and dirty water in West Somerset in the late nineteenth century. **Soc Soc Hist Med Bull (Lond)** 1974 Dec;35:35-6
McLaughlin L: The pill, John Rock, and the church: the biography of a revolution. Boston, Little, Brown, 1982. 243 p.
McLaughlin P see **Rheinberger HJ**
McLaurin A: The influenza epidemic of 1918 in Shreveport. **North La Hist Assoc J** 1982;13(1):1-14
MacLaury J: The job safety law of 1970: its passage was perilous. **Mon Labor Rev** 1981;104(3):18-24
McLaury RL: A history of clinical thermometry. **J Okla State Med Assoc** 1983 Dec;76(12):420-6
Maclean I: The Renaissance notion of woman. A study in the fortunes of scholasticism and medical science in European intellectual life. New York, Cambridge University Press, 1980. VIII, 119p.
McLean JA: Direct blood transfusion. Its history, with special reference to the Alfred Hospital, Melbourne. **Med J Aust** 1979 Dec 15;2(12):625-8
MacLean LD, Rhode BM: The history of surgery for morbid obesity. **Can J Surg** 1984 Mar;27(2):126-7
MacLean PD see **Livingston KE**
McLean RB: Leonard D. Heaton--military surgeon. **Milit Med** 1982 Sep;147(9):717-27
Maclean V: A short-title catalogue of household and cookery books published in the English tongue 1701-1800. London, Prospect, 1981. 197 p.
McLeish J: The development of modern behavioural psychology. Calgary, Detselig Enterprises, 1981. 228 p.
McLellan I: Nineteenth century resuscitation apparatus. **Anaesthesia** 1981 Mar;36(3):307-11
McLendon WW: The Archives of Pathology and Laboratory Medicine. A new beginning. **Arch Pathol Lab Med** 1984 Jan;108(1):13-4
McLeod DC, Whitney HA: The legacy of Donald E. Francke: DICP--a fifteen-year commitment to clinical pharmacy. **Drug Intell Clin Pharm** 1981 Dec;15(12):990-1
McLeod K: Hallmarks of reform: social change and the new education in Canada. **Hist Educ Q** 1980;20(3):369-75
MacLeod R, Moseley R: Fathers and daughters: reflections on women, science, and Victorian Cambridge. **Hist Educ** 1979;8:321-33
MacLeod RB see **Evans RB**
MacLeod RM, Collins P: The parliament of science: the British Association for the Advancement of Science 1831-1981. London, Science Reviews, 1981. vi, 308 p.
McLetchie NG: Alloxan diabetes: the sorcerer and his apprentice. **Diabetologia** 1982 Jul;23(1):72-5
McLoughlin Q: History, science and psychohistory. **Psychohist Rev** 1980;8(4):22-31
McMahon CE, Oberg D: Functional illness and the status of psychosomatic concepts in nineteenth century medicine. **J Am Soc Psychosom Dent Med** 1983;30(4):156-61
McMahon CE, Hastrup JL: The role of imagination in the disease process: post-Cartesian history. **J Behav Med** 1980 Jun;3(2):205-17
McMahon M: Fairmount. **Am Heritage** 1979;30(3):100-7
McMahon SF: 'A comfortable subsistence': a history of diet in New England, 1630-1850. Ph.D. Diss., Brandeis University. Waltham, 1982. v, 351 p.
McManners J: Death and the Enlightenment. Changing attitudes to death among Christians and unbelievers in eighteenth-century France. Oxford, Clarendon Press; New York, Oxford University Press; 1981. vii, 619 p.
McMartin DA, MacOwan KJ, Swift LL: A century of classical contagious caprine pleuropneumonia: from original description to aetiology. **Br Vet J** 1980 Sep-Oct;136(5):507-15
McMichael J: Digitalis in the last half century. **Eur Heart J** 1982 Dec;3 Suppl D:3-4
McMichael J: History of atrial fibrillation 1628-1819 Harvey - de Senac - Laënnec. **Br Heart J** 1982 Sep;48(3):193-7
McMichael J: Sir Francis Richard Fraser. In Dictionary of national biography, 1961-1970. Suppl. 8, 1981. p. 393-4.
McMichael J: Sir James Mackenzie and atrial fibrillation--a new perspective. **J R Coll Gen Pract** 1981 Jul;31(228):402-6
McMillan CW: Evolution of modern concepts of hemostasis. A backward glance at the discoveries that made modern practice possible. **Am J Pediatr Hematol Oncol** 1981 Spring;3(1):97-103
McMillan M: Looking back: school nursing in England. **Lamp** 1980 Mar;37(3):69-71
Macmillan MB: Freud and Lindner on pleasure sucking. **Stor Crit Psicol** 1980;1(1):111-43
McMullin DR see **Stephan GE**
MacMurray D see **Lakie MH**
McMurry JF: Oskar Hirsch and surgery for exophthalmos. In Romm S, ed: Symposium on historical perspectives of plastic surgery. Philadelphia, Saunders, 1983. p. 649-52.
McNair EW see **Murphy LP**
McNamara DG: Landmark perspective: the Blalock-Taussig operation and subsequent progress in surgical treatment of cardiovascular diseases. **JAMA** 1984 Apr 27;251(16):2139-41
McNamara DG: Twenty-five years of progress in the medical treatment of pediatric and congenital heart disease. **J Am Coll Cardiol** 1983 Jan;1(1):264-73
MacNaughton NL see **Buchanan AV**
McNeil M: Medical theory and demographic concerns in early industrial England. **Soc Soc Hist Med Bull (Lond)** 1979 Dec;25:12-20
McNeill WH: Historical patterns of migration. **Curr Anthropol** 1979;20(1):94-8
McNeill WH: Migration patterns and infection in traditional societies. In Stanley NF, Joske RA, ed: Changing disease patterns and human behaviour. London, New York, Academic Press, 1980. p. 27-36.
MacOwan KJ see **McMartin DA**
MacPhail I, Hess WJ: The date of the Linnaean index in John Martyn's Historia plantarum rariorum. **Huntia** 1979;3(2):73-81
Macpherson AI: Blue babies before Fallot. **J R Coll Surg Edinb** 1984 Jul;29(4):199-204
Macpherson AI: Portal hypertension: a pilgrim's progress. **J R Coll Surg Edinb** 1979 Nov;24(6):317-35
McPherson CW: The origins of laboratory animal science at the National Institutes of Health. **Lab Anim Sci** 1980 Aug;30(4 pt 2):786-9
McPherson MP: 'On the same terms precisely': the women's medical fund and the John Hopkins School of Medicine. **J Am Med Wom Assoc** 1981 Feb;36(2):37-40
McPherson MW see **Poppleston JA**
McPherson MW see **Popplestone JA**
McPherson SD: A brief history of ophthalmology in North Carolina. **NC Med J** 1983 Oct;44(10):641-3
McPherson SD see **Hughes WL**
Macpike L: The social values of childbirth in the nineteenth-century novel. **Int J Womens Stud** 1980;3(2):117-30
McQuaid K see **Berkowitz E**
McQueen A: John Alexander Milne. **J Cutan Pathol** 1977 Dec;4(6):349-52
McQuillan K: Modes of production and demographic patterns in nineteenth-century France. **AJS** 1984;89(6):1324-46
McQuitty JL: The old Irish Bar and Bench. **Med Leg J** 1982;50(Pt 1):5-18
Macrae AD: Laboratory diagnosis of smallpox: role of the Virus Reference Laboratory, Colindale, 1947-70. **J Hyg (Lond)** 1982 Dec;89(3):399-407
McRae JA see **Kessler RC**
Macrea M see **Hayden MR**
McReynolds P: The clock metaphor in the history of psychology. In T. Nickles, ed: Scientific discovery: case studies. Dordrecht, D. Reidel,

1980. (Boston Studies in the Philosophy of Science, v. 60). p. 97–112.

**McRobert G:** Sir Leonard Rogers. In Dictionary of national biography, 1961–1970. Suppl. 8, 1981. p. 891–3.

**MacRoberts MH:** L. H. Bailey's citations to Gregor Mendel. **J Hered** 1984 Nov–Dec;75(6):500–1

**McSherry JA:** Reiter's syndrome and the American revolutionary war. **Practitioner** 1982 Apr;226(1366):794–5

**McSherry JA:** Some medical aspects of the Darien scheme: was it dengue? **Scott Med J** 1982 Apr;27(2):183–4

**MacSween HM** see **Aterman K**

**Macúch P:** K 30. výročí činnosti Institutu pro další vzdělávání lékařu a farmaceutu v Praze. **Cesk Zdrav** 1983 Sep;31(8–9):337–45

**Macúch P:** Třicet let činnosti Institutu pro další vzdělávání lékařu a farmaceutu v Praze integrální součást vývoje socialistického zdravotnictví v Ceskoslovensku. **Cas Lek Cesk** 1983 Oct 21;122(42):1281–4

**McVaugh M** see **Sider D**

**McVaugh MR:** The authorship of the Galenic compendium de interioribus, 'Quoniam diversitas...'. **Dynamis** 1981;1:225–9

**McVaugh MR** see **Mauskopf SH**

**McWhinnie DL, Hamilton DN:** The rise and fall of surgery for the 'floating' kidney. **Br Med J [Clin Res]** 1984 Mar 17;288(6420):845–7

**McWilliam CE:** The college buildings and their architects. In Passmore R, ed: Proceedings of the Royal College of Physicians of Edinburgh Tercentenary Congress, 1981. Edinburgh, Royal College of Physicians of Edinburgh, 1982. p. 92–102.

**Madai L:** Le premier enregistrement statistique des malades cancereux dans l'annee 1904, en hongrie. **Genus** 1981;37(3–4):227–40

**Madai L:** Les crises de mortalité en Europe dans la deuxième moitie cu XIXe siècle. In Charbonneau H, Larose A, ed: The great mortalities: methodological studies of demographic crises in the past. Liège, Belgium, Ordina Editions, 1980. p. 157–78.

**Madakhanov AS** see **Kadyrov AA**

**Maddern GJ, Craddock D, Leppard PI, et al:** Twelve years of coronary artery surgery in South Australia. **Med J Aust** 1984 Feb 4;140(3):136–40

**Maddick I** see **Fox B**

**Maddox K:** Schlink of Prince Alfred. A biography of Sir Herbert Schlink. Sydney, Royal Prince Alfred Hospital, 1978. vii, 283 p.

**Maddox RF:** The politics of World War II science: Senator Harley M. Kilgore and the legislative origins of the National Science Foundation. **W Va Hist** 1979;41(1):20–39

**Maddox VH:** The discovery of phencyclidine [proceedings]. **Psychopharmacol Bull** 1980 Oct;16(4):53–4

**Maddox VH** see **Domino EF, ed**

**Maddux JF** see **Martin WR**

**Madeira AA, Rosa JE:** [Historical background of dentistry teaching in the state of Santa Catarina] (Por). **Rev Catarinense Odontol** 1977;4(2):5–10

**Madeira AA, Rosa JE:** O curso de odontologia da Faculdade de Farmacia e Odontologia de Santa Catarina. **Rev Catarinense Odontol** 1979 Jul–Dec;6(2):9–20

**Madeira AA, Rosa JE:** O curso de odontologia do Instituto Polytechnico. **Rev Catarinense Odontol** 1978 Jan–Jun;5(2):7–17

**Madeira AA** see **Rosa JE**

**Mader B** see **Bauerndoktor und Volksmedizin. 1. Ausstellung anlässlich des 800-jährigen Bestehens von Stainz. Sonderausstellung: Juni bis Okt. 1977. Katalog: Nr. 3. Maria Kundegraber, unter Mitarb. v. Bernd Mader. Steiermark, Landesmuseum Joanneum, 1977. 63 p.**

**Mader FH:** Zur Geschichte der Famulatur bei Praktischen Aerzten. **ZFA (Stuttgart)** 1980 Aug 20;56(23):1415–8

**Mader G:** Studien zur Gesundheitsbildung und Ordnungslehre bei Sebastian Kneipp: ein Beitrag zur Frage 'machbarer' Gesundheit. Frankfurt am Main, Haag + Herchen, 1984. 198, 49 p.

**Mäder M:** Ludwig von Hoernigk: Arzt, Jurist und Bücherkommissar im 17. Jahrhundert. Diss. Bern, 1984. 77 p.

**Madrid Arias JL:** Evolución histórica de los agentes neurolíticos utilizados para tratamiento del dolor crónico. **Rev Esp Anestesiol Reanim** 1984 Sep–Oct;31(5):197–204

**Madsen CB** see **Sell A**

**Madsen CM** see **Roed–Petersen K**

**Madsen KE:** Dansk sundhedspolitik 1901–21. **Historie** 1982;14(2):239–71

**Madsen V:** Medicine in history. Dryden on the doctors and the death of Charles II. **J Dermatol Surg Oncol** 1981 May;7(5):366–9

**Madzhidova AT** see **Shamansurov SS**

**Maeder C:** Zur Geschichte der Psychiatrie. Umgang mit psychisch Kranken--gestern und heute. **Krankenpflege (Frankfurt)** 1984;38(5):155–8;(6):197–200

**Maeder C:** Zur Geschichte der Psychiatrie. Umgang mit psychisch Kranken--gestern und heute. **Krankenpflege (Frankfurt)** 1984 Apr;38(4):115–6, 121–2 contd

**Maeder C:** Zur Geschichte der Psychiatrie. Umgang mit psychisch Kranken--gestern und heute. 3. **Krankenpflege (Frankfurt)** 1984 Jul–Aug;38(7–8):247–50

**Maeder H:** Die Frau im 17. Jahrhundert im Spiegel der 'Quaestiones medico-legales' des Paolo Zacchia (1584–1659). Diss. Bern, 1981. 101 p.

**Maehle AH:** Johann Jakob Wepfer (1620–1695) als Toxikologe. Diss., Rheinische Friedrich–Wilhelms–Universität. Bonn, 1983. 202 p.

**Maeir DM:** The physician as a man . . . the man as a physician. A Jewish viewpoint. **NY State J Med** 1983 May;83(6):813–6

**Magalian P:** Florida Society of Hospital Pharmacists, Inc.: thirty–five years, 1947–1982. [Miami?], The Society, 1983. iii, 15 p.

**Magazov VS, Morogova VM:** 75 let Ufimskomu nauchno–issledovatel'skomu institutu vaktsin i syvorotok im. I. I. Mechnikova. **Zh Mikrobiol Epidemiol Immunobiol** 1981 Jan;(1):110–1

**Maggio S** see **Chambers RW**

**Maggs C:** A new history of nursing. Four. **Nurs Times** 1984 Nov 21–27;80(47):49–51

**Maggs C:** A new history of nursing. One. Changing perspectives. **Nurs Times** 1984 Sep 19–25;80(38):28–31

**Maggs C:** Control mechanisms and the 'new nurses' 1881–1914. **Nurs Times** 1981 Sep 2–8;77(36)suppl 25:97–100

**Maggs C:** The making of a history man [interview by Jane Salvage]. **Nurs Times** 1983 Aug 17–23;79(33):8–10

**Maggs C:** The register of nurses in the Scottish poor law service 1885–1919. **Nurs Times** 1981 Nov 25–Dec 1;77(48):suppl 33:129–32

**Maggs C** see **Davies C, ed**

**Maggs CJ:** Oral history and nursing history. **Nurs Times** 1983 Oct 19–25;79(42):55–7

**Magil'nitskiĭ SG:** Oftal'mologi–revoliutsionery. **Vestn Oftalmol** 1983 Nov–Dec;(6):72–5

**Magil'nitskiĭ SG:** Pervyĭ opyt otechestvennoĭ oftal'morentgenologii pri travmakh. **Oftalmol Zh** 1983;38(2):119–21

**Magil'nitskiĭ SG:** Raisa Vasil'evna Putiata--revoliutsionerka–oftal'molog. **Vestn Oftalmol** 1983;3:73–5

**Magil'nitskiĭ SG:** 'Vestniku oftal'mologii' – 100 let. **Vestn Oftalmol** 1984 May–Jun;(3):3–7

**Magil'nitskiĭ SG** see **Vipmanis VE**

**Magilton JR** see **Dawes JD**

**Magner LN:** A history of the life sciences. New York, Dekker, 1979. xi, 489 p.

**Magner LN:** Women and the scientific idiom: textual episodes from Wollstonecraft, Fuller, Gilman, and Firestone. **Signs** 1978;4(1):61–80

**Magni G** see **De Leo D**

**Magnus W** see **Spicker SF, ed**

**Magnussyni SS:** Den Isländska obstetrikens historia. **Katilolehti** 1983 Nov;88(11):310–4

**Magyar I:** Medical trends in interwar Hungary. **Orvostort Kozl** 1980;89–91(26 no 1–3):97–110

**Mahdihassan S:** A comparative study of the early system of Indian cosmology and the tridosa humoral doctrine. **Indian J Hist Sci** 1980;15:223–9

**Mahdihassan S:** A comparative study of the word sugar and of its equivalents in Hindustani as traceable to Chinese. **Am J Chin Med** 1981 Autumn;9(3):187–92

**Mahdihassan S:** Alchemy and its fundamental terms in Greek, Arabic, Sanskrit and Chinese. **Indian J Hist Sci** 1981;16(1):64–76

**Mahdihassan S:** Alembic and ambix as Sino–Arabic terms with an explanation of Mary's bath. **Stud Hist Med** 1980 Mar;4(1):39–43

**Mahdihassan S:** An analytical and comparative study of Indian and Chinese cosmologies. **Bull Indian Inst Hist Med Hyderabad** 1982;12(1–4):1–12

**Mahdihassan S:** Chinese alchemy in the light of its fundamental terms. **Am J Chin Med** 1980 Winter;8(4):307–12

**Mahdihassan S:** Chinese origin of the word alcohol. **Am J Chin Med** 1980 Autumn;8(3):239–44

**Mahdihassan S:** Indian alchemy or Rasayana in the light of asceticism [and] geriatrics. New Delhi, Vikas, 1979. x, 139 p.

**Mahdihassan S:** Indian and Chinese cosmic elements. **Am J Chin Med** 1979 Winter;7(4):316–23

**Mahdihassan S:** Interpreting Chinese cosmology and its association with the dualistic doctrine of Yin–Yang. **Stud Hist Med** 1982 Sep;6(3):214–24

**Mahdihassan S:** The tradition of alchemy in India. **Am J Chin Med** 1981 Spring;9(1):23–33

**Mahdihassan S** see **Said HM, ed**

**Maher B** see **Maher WB**

**Maher BA** see **Hearst E, ed**

**Maher MA** see **Friedman A**

**Maher WB, Maher B:** The ship of fools. Stultifera Navis or ignis fatuus? **Am Psychol** 1982 Jul;37(7):756–61

**Maher WB** see **Hearst E, ed**

**Mahler A** see **Hauben DJ**

**Mahler-Schachter E:** Svevo, Trieste and the Vienna Circle: Zeno's analyst analysed. **Eur Stud Rev** 1982;12(1):45–66

**Mahnke PF:** Die pathologisch–anatomische Schule Leipzig--ihre Stellung, Bedeutung und Wandlung in der klinischen Pathologie. Ein Beitrag zur Geschichte der Prosektur am Pathologisch–anatomischen Institut der Karl–Marx–Universität Leipzig. **Zentralbl Allg Pathol** 1982;126(3–4):245–52

**Mahoney ER** see **Tedrow LM**

**Mahoney JL** see **Duff W**

**Mahony P:** Freud as a writer. New York, International Universities Press, 1982. xv, 227 p.

**Mahta M:** The history of the Intractable Pain Society of Great Britain and Ireland. **Pain** 1980 Feb;8(1):121–2

**Mai A:** Diagnosestellung niedergelassener Arzte bei der Leichenschau im Vergleich zu den Ergebnissen der gerichtlichen Obduktion. Diss., Johannes Gutenberg – Universität in Mainz. Mainz, 1982. 143 p.

**Mai FM, Merskey H:** Briquet's concept of hysteria: an historical perspective. **Can J Psychiatry** 1981 Feb;26(1):57–63

**Mai FM:** Hysteria--100 years after Briquet. **Can J Psychiatry** 1983 Oct;28(6):417

**Mai FM:** Pierre Briquet: 19th century savant with 20th century ideas. **Can J Psychiatry** 1983 Oct;28(6):418–21

**Maiat KE** see **Maiat VS**

**Maiat VS, Kliminskiĭ IV, Maiat KE:** K istorii vagotomii. **Klin Med (Mosk)** 1980 Sep;58(9):105–11

**Maiat VS, Kochnova IE:** K 100–letiiu so dnia smerti N.I. Pirogova. **Klin Med (Mosk)** 1981 Nov;59(11):114–9

**Maiat VS:** Vladimir Semenovich Levit (K 100–letiiu so dnia rozhdeniia). **Khirurgiia (Mosk)** 1983 Jun;6:111–3

**Maĭatruk PN, Popik SIa, Petrun' AS, et al:** Stanovlenie, puti i perspektivy razvitiia gigieny pitaniia na Ukraine. **Vopr Pitan** 1982 Nov–Dec;(6):15–20

**Maibaum EA:** Der therapeutische Aderlass von der Entdeckung des Kreislaufs bis zum Beginn des 20. Jahrhunderts – Versuch einer kritischen Neubewertung. Herzogenrath, Murken–Altrogge, 1983. 104 p. (Studien zur Medizin–, Kunst und Literaturgeschichte, Bd. 2).

**Maibaum M, López G:** Drug abuse in the East Los Angeles Health District. **Aztlan** 1981;12(1):139–55

**Maĭboroda VS:** Sanitarno–épidemiologicheskaia sluzhba Tadzhikskoĭ SSR. **Gig Sanit** 1982 Sep;(9):15–6

**Maida AJ:** The new code of canon law: some historical perspectives. **Hosp Prog** 1982 Dec;63(12):10, 14

**Maienschein J:** Shifting assumptions in American biology: embryology, 1890–1910. **J Hist Biol** 1981 Spring;14(1):89–113

**Maienschein JA:** Ross Harrison's crucial experiment as a foundation for modern American experimental embryology. Ph.D. Diss., Indiana University. Bloomington, 1978. 252 leaves.

**Maier D:** Nineteenth–century Asante medical practices. **Comp Stud Soc Hist** 1979;21:63–81

**Maier–Bode S:** Die Stellung der lesbischen Frau in der heutigen Gesellschaft und in früheren Jahrhunderten. Diss., Rheinische Friedrich–Wilhelms–Universität. Bonn, 1983. 101 p.

**Maillé JG** see **Paiement B**

**Maillé–Virole C:** La naissance d'un personnage: le medecin Parisien à la fin de l'ancien régime. **Hist Reflect** 1982;9(1–2):153–79

**Maĭmonid kak estestvoispytaltel' i vrach: Ter Arkh** 1982;54(10):137–9

**Mainetti JA:** Leyendo con Freud La peau de chagrin de Balzac. **Asclepio** 1982;34:265–81

**Mainwaring M:** 'Phys/phren': why not to take each other at face value. **Smithsonian** 1980;11(8):193–212

**Maire CL:** Les convulsionnaires à Paris au XVIII siècle. **Penelope** 1983;(8):29–34

**Maire CL:** Les possédées de Morzine (1857–1873). Lyon, Presses Universitaires, 1981. 134 p.

**Maire M:** L'or du temps. Le musée de la chirurgie dentaire de la faculté d'odontologie de Lyon. **Chir Dent Fr** 1979 May 31;49(22):25–30

**Maire M:** Une mini histoire de la presse dentaire. **Chir Dent Fr** 1979 Dec 13;49(44):53–7

**Maisel AQ:** Miracles of military medicine. Freeport, N.Y., Books for Libraries Press, 1972. xiv, 373 p.

**Maisel W:** Plany Hitlerowskie w odniesieniu do chorych na gruźlicę Polaków w Wartegau. **Przegl Zachod** 1981;37(3–4):99–106

**Maison Nachet:** Catalogues de fonds de 1854 à 1910. Facsimile edition. Introduction par G. L'E. Turner. Paris, Brieux, 1979. Various paginations.

**Maĭstruk PN, Petrun' AS, Popik SIa, et al:** K istorii Kievskogo nauchno–issledovatel'skogo instituta gigieny pitaniia. **Vrach Delo** 1983 Apr;(4):1–5

**Maĭstruk PN, Popik SIa, Petrun' AS, et al:** Organizatsiia deiatel'nosti sanitarno–épidemiologicheskoĭ sluzhby v oblasti gigieny pitaniia na Ukraine v period stanovleniia Sovetskoĭ vlasti i v gody pervykh piatiletok. **Gig Sanit** 1982 Apr;(4):54–6

**Maitre AM, Ducable G:** Louis–René Villermé et le choléra en 1832. **Hist Sci Med** 1982;16(4):317–25

**Maizels M:** Medical literature in Yiddish. **Koroth** 1982 Aug;8(3/4):220–4

**Maizumi H:** [Early days of antibiotics] (Jpn). **Dent Outlook** 1979;53(2):307–12

**Maj M:** Evolution of the American concept of schizoaffective psychosis. **Neuropsychobiology** 1984;11(1):7–13

**Majce G** see **Amann A**

**Majdecki T:** Powstanie i rozwój w okresie miedzywojennym neurologicznego lecznictwa kolejowej służby zdrowia. **Neurol Neurochir Pol** 1984 Jan–Feb;18(1):87–91

**Majer EH:** Zur Geschichte der HNO–Heilkunde in Oesterreich. **Laryngol Rhinol Otol (Stuttg)** 1980 Jul;59(7):406–11

**Majeron MA** see **Armocida G**

**Majewska E** see **Gliński S**

**Majewska–Tronowicz J, Michalczyk B, Kinowskiej M:** Zeszyt 35/36 (VII–XII 1979). Dodatek do numeru 2/1980. Kwartalnika Historii Nauki i Techniki. **Kwart Hist Nauki Tech** 1980;25(2):Suppl.1–30

**Majewska–Tronowicz J, Michalczyk B, Kinowskiej M:** Zeszyt 37 (I–III 1980). Dodatek do numeru 3/1980. Kwartalnika Historii Nauki i Techniki. **Kwart Hist Nauki Tech** 1980;25(3):Suppl 1–28

**Majewski W:** Służba zdrowia l. armii Wojska Polskiego, 1943–1945. Warszawa, Wydawn. Ministerstwa Obrony Narodowej, 1976. 277 p.

**Majno G, Joris I:** Billroth and Penicillium. **Rev Infect Dis** 1979 Sep–Oct;1(5):880–4

**Majno G:** Inflammation and infection: historic highlights. **Monogr Pathol** 1982;(23):1–17

**Majnoni d'Intignano B, Stephan JC:** Hippocrate et les technocrates. Paris, Calmann–Lévy, 1983. 194 p.

**Majoor CL, Hafkenscheid JC, Van Dijk C:** Enkele kernpunten uit de geschiedenis van cardiale beriberi, die voor de praktisch werkzame arts van betekenis lijken. **Ned Tijdschr Geneeskd** 1982 Apr 24;126(17):771–5

**Major V:** Live in peace and joy. In: Congrès international d'histoire de la médecine, XXVe, Québec, 1976. Actes. Québec, 1977. p. 944–50.

**Majsec M, Manestar M:** Od kupališnog lječilišta do bolnice za reumatske bolesti i rehabilitaciju Krapinske Toplice. **Reumatizam** 1979;26(3):73–6

**Majtás J:** K dialektike zmien profesnej štruktúry vo vývine farmaceutického profesionalizmu. **Cesk Zdrav** 1984 Jan;32(1):18–22

**Makabe G:** [A visit at Kaiserwerth. (1) (Florence Nightingale)] (Jpn). **Sogo Kango** 1982;16(4):61–74

**Makabe G:** [Early nursing textbooks in Germany – 'Establishment of modern nursing' by Anna Sticker. (1)] (Jpn). **Sogo Kango** 1982 May;17(2):103–24

**Makabe G:** [Early nursing textbooks in Germany––'Establishment of Modern Nursing' by Anna Sticker. (2)] (Jpn). **Sogo Kango** 1982;17(3):59–77

**Makabe G:** [Foundation of nursing. Letter collection of Florence Nightingale] (Jpn). **Sogo Kango** 1982;17(4):8–34

**Makabe G:** [Nightingale's expectation on women––an impression of her writings] (Jpn) **Sogo Kango** 1980;15(4):70–2

**Makabe G:** [Visit to Kaiserwerth (2) (Florence Nightingale)]. (Jpn). **Sogo Kango** 1982;17(1):59–78

**Makarenko EM:** Molodoi Lafarg. **Vopr Istor** 1981;(6):115–22

**Makarenko IM** see **Grando AA**

**Makarenko IAO** see **Sheĭman IB**

**Makarov VA:** [I. M. Sechenov and the development of physiology in the Moscow University] (Rus). **Istor Biol Issled** 1980;8:138–55

**Makarov VA:** Razvitie I. M. Sechenovym ucheniia o edinstve organizma i sredy. **Usp Fiziol Nauk** 1979 Jul–Sep;10(3):5–14

**Makarov VA:** Uspekhi fiziologii v SSSR i perspektivy ee razvitiia (k 60–letiiu obrazovaniia Soiuza Sovetskikh Sotsialisticheskikh respublik). **Usp Fiziol Nauk** 1982 Oct–Dec;13(4):3–26

**Makarov VA:** 50 let kafecre normal'noĭ fiziologii 1–go Moskovskogo meditsinskogo instituta im. I. M. Sechenova (1930–1980). **Fiziol Zh SSSR** 1980 Dec;66(12):1860–4

**Makarova EP:** V. I. Razumovskiĭ––pervyĭ rektor Saratovskogo universiteta. **Vestn Khir** 1983 May;130(5):140–1

**Makechnie GK:** Optimal health: the quest. A history of Boston University's Sargent College of Allied Health Professionals, founded 1881, tendered to Boston University 1929. Boston, Boston University, 1979. x, 228 p.

**Makhmudov M:** Pervaia bol'nitsa v Khorezme. **Sov Zdravookhr** 1984;(1):67–9

**Makhmudov M:** Tashkentskiĭ meditsinskiĭ institut. **Sov Zdravookhr** 1980;(7):54–6

**Makhrova A:** Patrioticheskoe dvizhenie za podgotovku medsester v krasnoi armii i na flote(1938–1940 gg). **Voen Istor Zh** 1974;(3):93–6

**Makita K, Kamiide H:** Jido seishin igaku sosetsu. Tokyo, Yasuda Seimei Shakai Jigyodan, [1977]. 146 p.

**Makler PT:** New information on nutrition in ancient Greece. **Klio** 1980, reçu 1983;62(2):317–9

**Makliarski B:** Bor'ba s zagriaznenniem biosfery: ekonomicheskii i sotsial'nyi aspekt. **Mirovaia Ekon Mezhdunar Otnosheniia** 1974;(5):63–75

**Makovický E:** Desat rokov Katedry metodiky a plánovania dalšieho vzdelávania Inštitútu pre dalšie vzdelávanie lekárov a farmaceutov Praha. **Cesk Zdrav** 1983 Sep;31(8–9):346–9

**Makovický E:** Pätdesiat rokov Centrálneho inštitútu pre dalšie vzdelávanie lekárov, nositel'a Radu Lenina, v Moskve. **Vnitr Lek** 1981 May;27(5):417–20

**Makovoz AA:** D. V. Volchenetskiĭ––vydaiushchiĭsia vrach Rossii. **Feldsher Akush** 1983;48(4):57–8

**Makovoz AA, Gorskiĭ AN:** Muzei istorii meditsiny i zdravookhraneniia Kirovogradskoĭ oblasti. **Feldsher Akush** 1983;48(1):52–4

**Makovoz AA:** [Nikolai Ivanovich Pirogov in the Korovograd District] (Rus). **Sov Zdravookhr** 1981;3:59–60

**Makovoz AA:** O. A. Iunevich – vidnyĭ zemskiĭ vrach. **Sov Zdravookhr** 1984;(1):64–7

**Makovskiĭ ChN, Terent'eva LA, Ermolaev GT:** Kurorty Latviiskoĭ SSR. **Vopr Kurortol Fizioter Lech Fiz Kult** 1982 Nov–Dec;(6):21–2

**Makowiec J:** Kaliskie lecznictwo w latach 1874–1914. **Wiad Lek** 1984 Jul 15;37(14):1135–44

**Makowka V** see **Dreznik A**

**Makowski HM:** Georg Wilhelm Stein und die frühe Geburtshilfe in Bonn. Diss. Bonn, 1979. 110 p.

**Maksimov SS** see **Savich VI**

**Malamani A:** Medicina ottocentesca e medicina del lavoro: l'opera scientifico–sociale di Luigi Devoto a Pavia. **G Ital Med Lav** 1983 Jan;5(1):1–16

**Malamani A:** Notizie sul mal francese e gli ospedali degli incurabili in età moderna. **Crit Stor** 1978;15:193–216

**Malarewicz A:** 50 lat cytodiagnostyki ginekologicznej –– George Nicholas Papanicolaou. **Arch Hist Med (Warsz)** 1978;41(4):465–8

**Malát L:** 85 years of the hospital 'Na tabulovém Vrchu' and 35 years of its change into a faculty hospital. **Acta Univ Palacki Olomuk Fac Med** 1982;103:23–7

**Malcolm MT:** Foetal alcohol syndrome: historical aspects. **Alcohol Alcohol** 1984;19(3):261–2

**Małdyk E:** Osiągniecia zakładu anatomii patologicznej IR w zakresie patomorfologii chorób układu ruchu. **Reumatologia** 1981;19(2):123–9

**Małdyk E, Luft S:** Rys historyczny Instytutu Reumatologicznego II (lata 1962–1980). **Reumatologia** 1982;20(1–2):1–6

**Małdyk E:** 25 lat dzialalności Instytutu Rheumatologicznego. **Nauka Pol** 1976;24(9–10):77–83

**Małdykowa H:** Osiągnięcia Instytutu w zakresie diagnostyki i leczenia

układowych chorób tkani łącznej. **Reumatologia** 1981;19(2):119–22
**The male midwife.: Bygone Kent** 1980;1(9):532
**Malec J:** 100 let české oční kliniky. **Cas Lek Cesk** 1983 Nov 25;122(47):1466–7
**Malec J:** 100 let Ceské oční kliniky. **Sb Lek** 1984 Jan;86(1):27–30
**Málek P:** První sjezd ćeských lékařuv a přírodozpytcuv v Praze o letnicích roku 1880. **Cas Lek Cesk** 1980 Nov;119(45):1225
**Málek P:** Stoleté výroči obnovení činnosti české lékařské fakulty v Praze. **Cas Lek Cesk** 1984 Apr 6;123(14):425–8
**Malinas C, Malinas Y:** Emile Zola et la génétique. La nevrose des Rougon–Macquart. **J Genet Hum** 1981 Dec;29(5 Suppl):593–602
**Malinas Y** see **Malinas C**
**Malinin TI:** Surgery and life: the extraordinary career of Alexis Carrel. New York, Harcourt Brace Jovanovich, 1979. xiii, 242 p.
**Malinin TI** see **Chambers RW**
**Malinovich MM:** On Herbert Marcuse and the concept of psychological freedom. **Soc Res (NY)** 1982;49(1):158–80
**Malinsky BJ:** The (Woman's) Medical College of Pennsylvania. **Women Health** 1979 Fall;4(3):217–21
**Maliszewski B** see **Yeazell RB**
**Malkinson FD** see **Kalis JB**
**Malkinson FD** see **Newell LM**
**Mallach HJ:** Gibt es Ansätze zur Gerichtlichen Medizin in Friedrichs II. von Hohenstaufen Konstitutionen von Melfi? **Beitr Gerichtl Med** 1982;40:463–72
**Mallard J, Trott NG:** Some aspects of the history of nuclear medicine in the United Kingdom. **Semin Nucl Med** 1979 Jul;9(3):203–17
**Mallarino Paz A:** Sintesis historica de los programas de personal auxiliar de odontologia en Colombia. **Rev Fac Odontol Univ Nac Colomb** 1980 Jan–Mar;27(132):50–2
**Mallo N** see **Puigvert A**
**Malmoy CF, ed:** The French Protestant Hospital: extracts from the Archives of 'La Providence' relating to inmates and applicants for admission, 1718–1957, and to recipients of and applicants for the Coqueau Charity, 1745-1901. 2 vols. London, Huguenot Society of London, 1977.
**Malmstedt J:** Hon förlöste vävarnas barn--barnmorskan Anna Norin. **Jordemodern** 1982 Oct;95(10):341–4
**Maloney G:** Les particules dans trois traités d'Hippocrate. In: Mélanges d'études anciennes offerts à Maurice Lebel. St-Jean-Chrysostôme, Québec, 1980. p. 125–34.
**Maloney G** see **Grmek MD, ed**
**Maloney JM:** Recent developments in China's population planning: notes and comments. **Pac Aff** 1981;54(1):100–14
**Maloney MT, McCormick RE:** A positive theory of environmental quality regulation. **J Law Econ** 1982;25(1):99–123
**Malott JC** see **Fodor J**
**Malousek O, ed** see **Kadlecová V**
**Malozemova AI:** Revoliutsionery-mediki Pribylevy. **Sov Zdravookhr** 1984;(8):62–5
**Malozemova AI:** Uchastie meditsinskikh rabotnikov v 'Politicheskom Krasnom Kreste 'Nardonoĭ voli'. **Sov Zdravookhr** 1984;(4):59–63
**Malozemova AI:** Zhenshchiny-mediki v politicheskikh protsessakh 1881 g. (k 100-letiiu protsessov). **Sov Zdravookhr** 1981;(7):54–9
**Malt RA** see **Berry J Jr**
**Maltau JM, Grünfeld B:** Mødredødeligheten i Norge 1880–1979. Et medisinsk–historisk tilbakeblikk. **Tidsskr Nor Laegeforen** 1983 Feb 20;103(5):522–5
**Maltau JM** see **Grünfeld B**
**Maltby JR:** Charles Waterton (1782–1865): curare and a Canadian National Park. **Can Anaesth Soc J** 1982 May;29(3):195–202
**Malter R:** Schopenhauer und die Biologie: Metaphysik der Lebenskraft auf empirischer Grundlage. **Ber Wissenschaftsgesch** 1983;6(1–4):43–58
**Malter R** see **Mann G, ed**
**Malterre–Barthes A:** L'infirmière face aux problèmes de la prostitution. **Infirm Fr** 1981 May;(225):9–12 contd
**Malterre–Barthes A:** Un service bien particulier: les dispensaires antivénériens. **Soins Gynecol Obstet Pueric** 1981 Sep;(6):37–46
**Maluf NS:** Owen's gland. **Sudhoffs Arch** 1980;64(1):25–54
**Malvido E:** El abandono de los hijos--una forma de control del tamaño la familia y del trabajo indígena--Tula (1683–1730). **Hist Mex** 1980;29:521–61
**Malyshev VN** see **Bechtereva NP**
**Maman C:** Comment établir le moment de la mort. **Rev Hist Med Heb** 1980 Jul;33(2):27–34
**Mammerickx M:** André–Marie Ampère et Claude–Julien Bredin, I. Ampère, Bredin et la philosophie, ou la belle histoire d'une amitié. **Hist Med Vet** 1977;2(1):11–19
**Mammerickx M:** André–Marie Ampère et Claude–Julien Bredin, II. Ampère, Bredin et le magnétisme animal, ou la petite histoire d'une grande découverte. **Hist Med Vet** 1977;2(3):69–75
**Mamontov AS** see **Koliadiuk IV**
**Man–hung L:** Ch'ing mo pen kuo ya p'ien chih t'i tai chin k'ou ya p'ien (1858–1906). **Bull Inst Mod Hist Acad Sin** 1980;9:385–432
**Manafov IT:** N. Narimanov--vrach, revoliutsioner, partiĭnyi ĭ gosudarstvennyĭ deiatel'. **Sov Zdravookhr** 1982;(4):58–61
**Manafov IT:** Rol' Narkomzdrava Azerbaĭdzhanskoĭ SSR v stanovlenii Sovetskogo zdravookhraneniia v respublike. **Sov Zdravookhr** 1984;(5):67–70
**Manaka Y:** [The concept of Oriental medicine] (Jpn). **Kango** 1981 May;33(6):19–25
**Mancebo MF** see **Peset JL**
**Mancebo MF** see **Peset M**
**Manchester K:** Paleopathology of a royalist garrison. **Ossa** 1978;5:25–33
**Mancin S:** Days of darkness and hope at the State Hospital: a photographer's perspective. **RI Hist** 1982;41(4):139–41
**Mandák M:** K jubileu farmaceutického štúdia. **Cesk Farm** 1982 Jul;31(6):201–2
**Mande R:** Robert Debré et la pédiatrie sociale. **Bull Acad Natl Med (Paris)** 1982 Dec;166(9):1275–9
**Mandel ID:** Caries through the ages: a worm's eye view. **J Dent Res** 1983 Aug;62(8):926–9
**Mandel ID:** Dental caries. **Am Sci** 1979 Nov–Dec;67(6):680–8
**Mandel SL:** Chaucer's vivid medical word pictures (reflections of yore afflictions). **Int J Dermatol** 1983 Jun;22(5):329–31
**Mandelbaum DR:** Women in medicine. **Signs** 1978;4(1):136–45
**Mandelker IL:** Religion, sex, and utopia in nineteenth-century America. **Soc Res (NY)** 1982;49(3):730–51
**Mandell GL** see **Scheld WM**
**Manderson L:** Bottle feeding and ideology in colonial Malaya: the production of change. **Int J Health Serv** 1982;12(4):597–616
**Mandler G** see **Hearst E, ed**
**Mandrou R:** Un problème de diététique à l'Hôtel-Dieu de Paris à la veille de la Révolution. In: Congrès National des Sociétés Savantes, 93e, Tours, 1968. Actes. Paris, 1971. Section d'Histoire Moderne et Contemporaine, Tome 1. p. 125–37.
**Mandys V** see **Miřejovský P**
**Manestar M** see **Majsec M**
**Manevy JV:** Nicole Grasset, médecin du bout du monde. [Paris?], Balland, 1982. 245 p.
**Mangel C, Weisse AB:** Medicine: the state of the art. New York, Dial Press, 1984. 304 p.
**Mangin P** see **Chabbert P**
**Mangum BW** see **Berger RL**
**Manhart GB:** The Indiana Central Medical College, 1849–1852. **Indiana Hist Soc** 1982 Dec;8(4):3–13
**Mani N:** Biomedical thought in Glisson's hepatology and in Wepfer's work on apoplexy. With commentary by R. G. Frank, p. 84–8. In Stevenson LG, ed: A celebration of medical history. Baltimore, Johns Hopkins University Press, 1982. (The Henry E. Sigerist supplements to the Bulletin of the History of Medicine; new ser., no. 6). p. 37–63.
**Mani N:** Johann Jakob Wepfers Doktordisputation über das Herzklopfen (1647). **Gesnerus** 1981;38:143–7
**Mani N:** Neue Konzepte der Pathologie im 17. Jahrhundert. **Gesnerus** 1983;40(1–2):109–17
**Mani N:** Physiologische und medizinische Chemie zwischen 1800 und 1850. **Pharm Acta Helv** 1979;54(9–10):273–80
**Mani N:** The historical background of clinical chemistry. **J Clin Chem Clin Biochem** 1981 Jun;19(6):311–22
**Mani N:** Zur Geschichte der Hygiene. Kontinuität und Wandel hygienischer Vorstellungen von der Antike zum 19. Jahrhundert. **ZFA (Stuttgart)** 1981 Nov 20;57(32):2183–92
**Mani N** see **Albrecht von Haller, 1708–1777**
**Mani N** see **Büttner J, ed**
**Mani N** see **Habrich C**
**Manier E:** Darwin's language and logic. **Stud Hist Philos Sci** 1980;11:305–23
**Manier E:** History, philosophy and sociology of biology: a family romance. **Stud Hist Philos Sci** 1980 Mar;11(1):1–24
**Mann A** see **Godlove C**
**Mann E** see **Danielson L**
**Mann FD:** Ross Aiken Gortner and bound water, the water of life. **Perspect Biol Med** 1976 Autumn;20(1):142–4
**Mann FD** see **Mann RJ**
**Mann G:** Ernst Haeckel und der Darwinismus: Popularisierung, Propaganda und Ideologisierung. **Medizinhist J** 1980;15(3):269–83
**Mann G:** Franz Joseph Galls kranioskopische Reise durch Europa (1805–1807). Fundierung und Rechtfertigung neuer Wissenschaft. **Nachrichtenbl Dtsch Ges Gesch Med Naturwiss Tech** 1984;34(3):86–114
**Mann G:** Geschichte als Wissenschaft und Wissenschaftsgeschichte bei Du Bois–Reymond. **Hist Z** 1980;231:75–100
**Mann G:** Gunter Mann: Neovitalismus. **Medizinhist J** 1983;18(4):376–83
**Mann G:** Kreatur und Kosmos. Internationale Beiträge zur Paracelsus–Forschung. **Dtsch Arztebl** 1981;78:1020–2
**Mann G:** Teleologie und Evolutionslehre. **Ber Wissenschaftsgesch** 1982;5:83–96
**Mann G:** The Third International Eugenics Congress, 1932. **Medizinhist J** 1980;15(3):338–9
**Mann H** see **Schimming I**
**Mann L:** The wax block metaphor: Plato's views on learning disabilities. **J Learn Disabil** 1980 Oct;13(8):420–4
**Mann P:** Taking a look at 3,000–year–old teeth. **Br Dent J** 1980 Jul 15;149(2):57–8
**Mann R:** Philip Showalter Hench. In Dictionary of American biography, 1961-1965. Suppl. 7, 1981. p. 340–341.
**Mann RJ, Mann FD:** Emphysema. Era of Laennec; era of the cigarette. **Minn Med** 1984 Mar;67(3):142, 159–61
**Mann RJ, Key JD:** Joseph Bell, M.D., F.R.C.S.: 'notes on a case of paralysis following diphtheria'. **Pharos** 1982 Spring;45(2):27–9
**Mann RJ, Mann FD:** Laennec as a critical pathologist. **J Hist Med Allied Sci** 1981 Oct;36(4):446–54
**Mann RJ, Key JD:** The Osler Medical Historical Society. Mayo Foundation 'Chapter,' August 28, 1920–July 3, 1925. **Minn Med** 1980

May;63(5):348–54
**Mann RJ** see **Connolly DC**
**Mann RJ** see **Espinosa RE**
**Mann RJ** see **Haabala SH**
**Mann RJ** see **Lie JT**
**Mann RJ** see **Ludwig J**
**Mann WE, Hoffman E:** The man who dreamed of tomorrow. A conceptual biography of Wilhelm Reich. Los Angeles, Tarcher, 1980. 295 p.
**Mann WV:** G. V. Black revisited. **J Dent Educ** 1981 Jun;45(6):338–9
**Mann G, ed:** Naturwissen und Erkenntnis im 19. Jahrhundert: Emil Du Bois-Reymond. Hildesheim, Gerstenberg, 1981. 243 p. Contributions by K. E. Rothschuh, H. Hensel, R. Malter, C. von Campenhausen, B. Lohff, H. Lübbe, D. von Engelhardt, W. F. Gutmann, K. Bonink, C. Andree
**Manneville P:** Le poids des armées à l'hôpital du Havre à l'époque révolutionnaire. In Congrès National des Sociétés Savantes, 103e, Nancy–Metz, 1978. Actes. Paris, 1979. Tome I, p. 593–606.
**Manniche E:** Age at menarche: Nicolai Edvard Ravn's data on 3385 women in mid-19th century Denmark. **Ann Hum Biol** 1983 Jan–Feb;10(1):79–82
**Manniche E:** [History of induced abortion in Denmark from 1200 to 1979] (Jpn). **Josanpu Zasshi** 1982 Oct;36(10):842–7
**Manning FJ** see **Ingraham LH**
**Manning SW** see **Breul FR**
**Mannion RA:** Indiana medical history--the medical school at LaPorte. **Indiana Med Hist Q** 1975;2(1):70–1
**Mannis MJ, Krachmer JH:** Keratoplasty: a historical perspective. **Surv Ophthalmol** 1981 Mar–Apr;25(5):333–8
**Manoliu E, Manoliu V:** The history of medical terminology in Romania. In: Congrès international d'histoire de la médecine, XXVe, Québec, 1978. Actes. Québec, 1977. p. 951–6.
**Manoliu V:** History of medical societies in Romania. In: Congrès international d'histoire de la médecine, XXVe, Québec, 1976. Actes. Québec, 1977. p. 957–60.
**Manoliu V** see **Manoliu E**
**Manová L** see **Niklíček L**
**Mansfeld J:** Alcmaeon: 'Physikos' or physician? With some remarks on Calcidius' 'On vision' compared to Galen's Plac. Hipp. Plat. VII. In J. Mansfeld, L. M. de Rijk, eds. Kephalaion: Studies in Greek philosophy and its continuation. Assen, Van Gorcum, 1975. p. 26–38.
**Mansfeld J:** The historical Hippocrates and the origins of scientific medicine. In M. Ruse, ed: Nature animated. Historical and philosophical case studies in Greek medicine, nineteenth-century and recent biology, psychiatry, and psychoanalysis. Volume II. Dordrecht, D. Reidel, 1983. p. 49–76.
**Mansfeld J** see **Grmek MD, ed**
**Manski RJ:** A synopsis of recent literature concerning the dental implant. **J Oral Implantol** 1982;10(2):275–88
**Manson-Bahr PE, Willmott S:** Dermatology and the Royal Society of Tropical Medicine and Hygiene. **Int J Dermatol** 1981 Jul–Aug;20(6):429–30
**Manson Thomas ML, Cooper WC, ed:** Catalog of works in the neurological sciences collected by Cyril Brian Courville, M.D., representative of clinical neurology, neuroanatomy and neuropathology, with particular reference to head trauma, and books from historical medicine in the Medical Sciences Library, University of California, Irvine. Irvine, University of California, 1978. 239 p.
**Mansursov KhKh:** Vrachebnoe nasledie Ibn-Siny i sovremennaia klinicheskaia meditsina. **Ter Arkh** 1980;52(11):149–51
**Mantel N:** Jerome Cornfield and statistical applications to laboratory research: a personal reminiscence. **Biometrics** 1982 Mar;38 Suppl:17–23
**Manton KG:** Temporal trends in U. S. multiple cause of death mortality data: 1968 to 1977. **Demography** 1982 Nov,19(4):527–47
**Mäntylä I, Ylikahri R:** Mitä jokaisen välskärinkisällin tulee tietää? Lääketieteellinen kuulustelu vuonna 1751. **Duodecim** 1984;100(14):863–9
**Manuel DE:** Marshall Hall, F.R.S. (1790–1857); a conspectus of his life and work. **Notes Rec R Soc Lond** 1980 Dec;35(2):135–66
**Manuila A** see **Sournia JC**
**Manuilova IM, Chervakova TV:** Uspekhi otechestvennoï akushersko-ginekologicheskoï nauki k 60-letiiu obrazovaniia SSSR. **Sov Med** 1982;(12):35–41
**Manuli P, Vegetti M:** Cuore, sangue e cervello. Biologia e antropologia nel pensiero antico. Milano, Episteme, 1977. 241 p.
**Manuli P** see **Grmek MD, ed**
**Manus A, Bourguignon A:** Réflexions sur les limites de la psychiatrie. **Nouv Presse Med** 1979 Oct 8;8(38):3051–3
**Manuscripta alchemica der Sammlung Mellon: Bemerkungen zum Katalog: Sudhoffs Arch** 1981;65(1):79–96
**Manzi L:** Commento ad un consulto inedito di Francesco Roncati. **Minerva Med** 1982 Jan 28;73(3–4):133–6
**Manzi L:** I santi protettori degli artisti dello studio bolognese... Santi Cosma e Damiano. **Strenna Stor Bolognese** 1977;27:179–93
**Maracineanu G** see **Neagu I**
**Maragi M:** Le glossaire latin–allemand d'anatomie de Walfridus Strabo (IXème siècle). In International Congress of the History of Medicine, 27th, Barcelona, 1980. Actas. Barcelona, Académia de Ciències Mèdiques de Catalunya i Balears, 1981. p. 304–15.
**Marain Y, Ducourtioux JC:** Un 'règlement de police pour la maladie contagieuse' à Saint-Dizier en 1668. **Cah Haut Marnais** 1979;139:162–8
**Marangon P:** Il trattato 'De conservatione sanitatis' di Zanbonino da Gazzo (d. dopo il 1298). **Quad Stor Univ Padova** 1975;8:1–17
**Marasanov RA, Mel'nichuk AN:** Meditsinskoe obespechenie nemetskogo naseleniia na zavershaiushchem étape Velikoï Otechestvennoï voïny i posle ee okonchaniia. **Voen Med Zh** 1981 Jun;(6):16–9
**Marasanov RA, Mel'nichuk AN:** Meditsinskoe obespechenie ranenykh i bol'nykh nemetskikh voennoplennykh v gody Velikoï Otechestvennoï voïny. **Voen Med Zh** 1981 May;(5):19–22
**Marbach E:** Jean Piaget (1896–1980). **Z Allg Wissenschaftstheorie** 1981;12(1):1–27
**Marbach JU:** Domenico Cirillo; ein Lebenslauf, 1739–1799. **Gesnerus** 1980;37(3/4):257–69
**Marbach JU:** Wilhelm Bernhard, 1920–1978. **Gesnerus** 1979;36(3–4):303–11
**Marburger H:** 100 Jahre Kaiserliche Botschaft--zur Entwicklung des Leistungsrechts der Krankenversicherung von seinen Anfängen bis heute. **Off Gesundheitswes** 1982 Apr;44(4):247–51
**Marc JC:** Pharmaciens de la Marine et voyages de découvertes en océanie au XIXe siècle. In: Congrès National des Sociétés Savantes, 104e, Bordeaux, 1979. Comptes Rendus. Paris, 1979. Section des Sciences, Fasc. IV. p. 193–204.
**Marcadé J:** La 'peste' de Lisbonne en 1757 et ses conséquences dans le bas Poitou. **Bull Soc Antiq Quest Mus Poitiers** 1977;14:201–8
**Marcel G** see **Kraus A, ed**
**March JC:** Public issues and private problems: women and drug use. **J Soc Issues** 1982;38(2):153–65
**March SM** see **Taylor DC**
**Marchac D:** Julien Bourguet. The pioneer in aesthetic surgery of the neck. **Clin Plast Surg** 1983 Jul;10(3):363–5
**Marchais P:** Vers la fin de l'ère Kraepelinienne? **Ann Med Psychol (Paris)** 1980 Nov;138(9):1061–78
**Marchal P, Roland JL, Thill G:** Le symptôme vétérinaire. **Esprit** 1981;12:80–98
**Marchand H, Müller KP:** Der Berufsweg Robert Kochs bis zur Entdeckung des Tuberkelbakteriums. **Wiss Beitr Martin Luther Univ Halle Wittenberg** 1983;5–R80:99–109
**Marchand P** see **Laxenaire M**
**Marchenko MA:** Meditsinskaia sluzhba 4-ï Gvardeïskoï Apostolovskoï Krasnoznamennoï strelkovoï divizii v Iassko-Kishinevskoï operatsii. **Voen Med Zh** 1984 Aug;(8):15–8
**Marchette NJ, Stiller D:** Ecological relationships and evolution of the rickettsiae. Boca Raton, CRC Press, 1982. 2 v.
**Marchetti AG:** Wyatt v. Stickney: a historical perspective. **Appl Res Ment Retard** 1983;4(3):189–206
**Marchfield F** see **Moss C**
**Marcial LD, Gutiérrez Avila JH:** La vigilancia epidemiológica un siglo después. Nil novi sub sole? Comentarios al trabajo del Dr. Nicolás Ramírez de Arellano. **Salud Publica Mex** 1982 Sep–Oct;24(5):491–5
**Marcial LD:** Las publicaciones oficiales de la Secretaría de Salubridad y Asistencia. **Salud Publica Mex** 1983 Sep–Oct;25(5):489–97
**Marcilio ML:** Dos registros parroquiais a demografia historica no Brasil. **An Hist** 1970;2:81–100
**Marciniak W:** Zagadnienia wrodzonego zwichni ęcia biodra w pracach prof. dr Wiktora Degi – z okazji 85 rocznicy urodzin. **Chir Narzadow Ruchu Ortop Pol** 1982;47(3):219–23
**Marcondes CH, Colombo MO:** Irmandade da Santa Casa de Poços de Caldas. **Enfoque** 1984 Aug;12(1):15–8
**Marcos Martín A:** El sistemo hospitalario de Medina del Campo en el siglo XVI. **Cuad Invest Hist** 1978;2:341–62
**Marcotte JM** see **Skinner RE**
**Marcovich A:** Concerning the continuity between the image of society and the image of the human body – an examination of the work of the English physician, J. C. Lettsom (1746–1815). In P. Wright, A. Treacher, ed: The problem of medical knowledge. Examining the social construction of medicine. Edinburgh, Edinburgh University Press, 1982. p. 69–86.
**Marcsik A** see **Kocsis SG**
**Marcu N:** Viaţa si activitatea doctorului Constantin C. Pastia (1883–1926). **Rev Ig [Bacteriol]** 1983 Jan–Mar;28(1):89–95
**Marcu N** see **Babes V**
**Marcum JP:** Explaining fertility differences among U. S. protestants. **Soc Forces** 1981;60(2):532–43
**Marcum JP, Radosh M:** Religious affiliation, labor force participation and fertility. **Sociol Anal** 1981;42(4):353–62
**Marcus AC, Seeman TE:** Sex differences in health status: a reexamination of the nurturant role hypothesis. **Am Sociol Rev** 1981;46(1):119–23
**Marcus AI:** In sickness and in health: the marriage of the municipal corporation to the public interest and the problem of public health, 1820–1870. The case of Cincinnati. Ph.D. diss. University of Cincinnati. Cincinnati, 1979. 379 leaves.
**Marcus AI:** National history through local social evils and the origin of municipal services in Cincinnati. **Am Stud** 1981;22(2):23–39
**Marcus AI:** Professional revolution and reform in the Progressive era: Cincinnati physicians and the city elections of 1897 and 1900. **J Urban Hist** 1979;5(2):183–208
**Marcus AI:** The strange career of municipal health initiatives: Cincinnati and city government in the early nineteenth century. **J Urban Hist** 1980;7(1):3–29
**Marcus S** see **Mazzola RF**
**Marcusson H:** Zusammenhang zwischen Sozialpolitik und Gesundheitsschutz für Mutter und Kind--Ein Rückblick über 80 Jahre. **Z Gesamte Hyg** 1979 Oct;25(10):775–80
**Marczyński A:** Dr Artur Karol Werner. **Przegl Lek** 1981;38(1):206–9
**Marczyński A:** Dr Tadeusz Boczoń. **Przegl Lek** 1984;41(1):127–31
**Mardanov LM** see **Omirov RIu**
**Mardones F:** Historia y situación actual de la lactancia materna en Chile.

Rev Med Chil 1979 Aug;107(8):750–60
**Mardones J:** Orígen del Servicio Nacional de Salud. **Rev Med Chil** 1977 Oct;105(10):654–8
**Mardzhanian KS:** Stepanos Sharimanian. **Patma-Banasirakam Handes. Ist-Filol Zh** 1971;(3):236–46
**Marechal G:** De leprozen in de kwartieren Brugge en het Brugse Vrije. Nieuwe cijfers. **Ann Soc Emulation Bruges** 1979;116:147–62
**Marechal G:** De leprozen in de kwartieren Brugge en het Brugse vrije. Nieuwe cijfers. **Ann Soc Emulation Bruges** 1979;116:147–62
**Marechal G:** De zwarte dood te Brugge (1349–1351). **Biekorf** 1980;80:377–392
**Marechal G:** Het gebouw van de Brugse Leprozorie in de XVIe eeuw. **Biekorf** 1979;79:316–22
**Maréchal G:** Lepra in Vlaanderen. **Spiegel Hist** 1980;15(3):137–41
**Mareĭ AN:** 50 Let pervogo vypuska sanitarnykh vracheĭ. **Gig Sanit** 1982 Jul;(7):38–40
**Marek J** see **Dobiás J**
**Marek Z, Kołodziej J:** Samobójstwa w Krakowie w latach 1881–1980. **Przegl Lek** 1982;39(11):709–14
**Maren TH:** Carbonic anhydrase: the middle years, 1945–1960, and introduction to pharmacology of sulfonamides. **Ann NY Acad Sci** 1984;429:10–7
**Maret F:** Der Wein in der Medizingeschichte. **ZFA (Stuttgart)** 1980 May 10;56(13):887–97
**Marg E:** Is the animal model for stimulus deprivation amblyopia in children valid or useful? **Am J Optom Physiol Opt** 1982 Jun;59(6):451–64
**Margalith D:** Physicians, forerunners of modern Israel. Tel-Aviv, Jerusalem Academy of Medicine, 1973. 192, iv, 12 p.
**Margan V:** A case study of population change over two centuries: Blaris, Lisburn 1661–1848. **Ir Econ Soc Hist** 1976;3:5–16
**Marganne MH:** A propos du 'Médicinaire liégeois du XIIIe siècle' (manuscrit 815 de Darmstadt). 101. Congrès de Comines, 1, 1980. Actes. p. 348.
**Marganne MH:** Deux questionnaires d'ophtalmologie: P. Aberdeen 11 et P. Ross. Georg. 1.20. **Chron Egypte** 1978;53:313–20
**Marganne MH:** Glaucome ou cataracte? sur l'emploi des dérivés de GLAUKOS en ophtalmologie antique. **Hist Philos Life Sci** 1979;1(2):199–214
**Marganne MH:** Inventaire analytique des papyrus grecs de médecine. Genève, Droz, 1981. x, 406 p. (Centre des Recherches d'Histoire et de Philologie de la IVe Section de l'Ecole pratique des Hautes Etudes; Hautes Etudes du Monde Gréco-Roman, 12).
**Margo RA, Steckel RH:** Heights of native-born whites during the antebellum period. **J Econ Hist** 1983;43(1):167–74
**Margo RA, Steckel RH:** The heights of American slaves: new evidence on slave nutrition and health. **Soc Sci Hist** 1982;6(4):516–38
**Margolin JC:** L'histoire des lunettes à nez. **Histoire** 1980;21:14–21
**Margolin JC, Sauzet R, ed:** Pratiques et discours alimentaires à la Renaissance. Actes du colloque de Tours de mars 1979, Centre d'études supérieures de la Renaissance. Paris, Maisonneuve et Larose, 1982. 305 p. Contributions on medicine and diet by Y. Pélicier, J. Céard, M. de Gandillac, J. Dupèbe, M. M. Fontaine, M. Lazard, J. L. Flandrin, M. Reulos, M. C. Pouchelle-Peter.
**Margolin L** see **Hartmann K**
**Margolis M, Neary K:** Pressure politics revisited: the anti-abortion campaign. **Policy Stud J** 1980;8(5):698–716
**Margulis L** see **Lowenstam HA**
**Margulis ML:** An optometric detective: in search of antique eyewear. **J Am Optom Assoc** 1979 Dec;50(12):1337–42
**Marguth F** see **Habrich C**
**Marí VJ:** El martirio de Santa Agatha, un precedente de la mastectomia. Représentacion artistica con especial referencia a una coleccion de tallas. In International Congress of the History of Medicine. 26th, Plovdiv, 1978. Actes du Congress. Sofia, 1981. Volume II. p. 150–7.
**Marí Balcells VJ:** Tres historiadores de la medicina española: Villalba, Hernandez Morejon y Comenge, e influencia del primero en la obra de los otros dos. In: Sociedad Española de Historia de la Medicina. V Congreso Nacional. Madrid, 1977. **Asclepio** 1977;29:167–76
**Maria CI:** La disputa sulle scienze e la medicina come venne affrontata nel corso del XV secolo da Platonismo e Aristotelismo. **Med Secoli** 1982;19(3):323–8
**María Suñé J** see **Bel E**
**Mariátegui J:** Hermilio Valdizán, la psiquiatría comparativa y la medicina folklórica. **Acta Psiquiatr Psicol Am Lat** 1980 Jun;26(2):96–106
**Mariátegui J:** Hermilio Valdizán y la psiquiatriá peruana. **Rev Neuropsiquiatr** 1980 Mar;43(1):1–22
**Maric D:** Stomatologija--medicinska disciplina. **Med Pregl** 1981;34(1–2):91–4
**Maric D** see **Branovački D**
**Marie J:** Robert Debré (1882–1978): l'homme, le médecin, le professeur. **Bull Acad Natl Med (Paris)** 1982 Dec;166(9):1257–64
**Marin IM** see **Stamatin SI**
**Marín Fernández JL:** Aspectos bibliometricos de la obra de Roman Alberca Lorente (1903–1967). **Asclepio** 1980;32:229–53
**Marinesco G** see **Marinesco M**
**Marinesco M, Petresco A, Marinesco G:** Georges Marinesco et la France. **Hist Sci Med** 1984;18(1):13–8
**Marinesco M, Argemi-Lloveras J:** Georges Marinescu (Roumanie) et Santiago Ramon y Cajal; deux représentants du génie latin. In International Congress of the History of Medicine, 27th, Barcelona, 1980. Actas. Barcelona, Académia de Ciències Médiques de Catalunya i Balears, 1981. p. 570–4.
**Marinescu CG:** Concepțiile progresiste ale Doctorului N. Vasiliu. **Rev Med Chir Soc Med Nat Iasi** 1980 Jul-Sep;84(3)578–80
**Marinescu CG:** Concepțiile social-politice ale Profesorului Dr. E. I. Mironescu (II). **Rev Med Chir Soc Med Nat Iasi** 1979 Jan–Mar;83(1):159–62
**Marinescu CG, Stratone M, Teodorovici G:** Contributia unor medici la lupta pentru făurirea statului național unitar român. **Rev Med Chir Soc Med Nat Iasi** 1979 Jan–Mar;83(1):155–8
**Marinescu CG, Stratone N:** Contributii ale unor medici ieseni la promovarea gîndirii democratice si progresiste în perioada interbelică. **Rev Med Chir Soc Med Nat Iasi** 1979 Apr–Jun;83(2):341–5
**Marinescu CG, Vosniuc R:** Din istoricul Spitalului din Galați filiala epitropiei sf. spiridon. **Rev Med Chir Soc Med Nat Iasi** 1981 Apr–Jun;85(2):399–400
**Marinescu I, Cicu N, Mesaros E:** Románia népesedéspolitikájának néhány kérdése. **Demografia** 1972;15(2):195–201
**Marinescu M, Petrescu A:** Ecouri contemporane ale operei stiințifice a lui Gh. Marinescu. **Rev Med Interna [Neurol Psihiatr]** 1980 Oct–Dec;25(4):311–4
**Marinéskou-Chýmou M:** Ektor saraphídes: iatrós kaí lógis (1872–1950). **Epet Etaireias Stereoelladikon Meleton** 1974–75;5:547–52
**Maringer J:** Menschliche Unterkiefer und Zähne im Brauch und Glauben der vorgeschichtlichen Menschen. **Anthropol Anz** 1980 May;38(1):69–73
**Marini Bettolo GB:** Recent advances in the research on curare. **Verh K Acad Geneeskd Belg** 1981;43(3):185–212
**Marino H:** Reminiscences of the American Society of Plastic and Reconstructive Surgeons, Inc., and some of its members. **Plast Reconstr Surg** 1981 Sep;68(3):376–80
**Marino R:** Perspectives in international neurosurgery: neurosurgery in Brazil. **Neurosurgery** 1982 Sep;11(3):454–6
**Marinone N:** Galeno, De victu attenuante, 79 e 98. **Riv Filol Istruz Classica** 1976;104:328–36
**Marinovic I:** 'Balkanski okvir' (ram) ili 'Balkanska metoda' i njegov tvorac. **Srp Arh Celok Lek** 1984 Jan;112(1):127–36
**Marinow W:** Uber einige irrationale psychotherapeutische Heilmittel der Volksmedizin. In International Congress of the History of Medicine. 26th, Plovdiv, 1978. Actes du Congress. Sofia, 1981. Volume II. p. 80–1.
**Marion JF:** The fine old house. Philadelphia, Smith Kline Corp., 1980. 251 p.
**Marion P:** La polemica tra Henning e Bühler. **Stor Crit Psicol** 1980;1(2):297–310
**Marion P:** La psicologia del pensiero dalla polemica di Wundt alla Entwicklungspsychologie di Bühler. **Stor Crit Psicol** 1982 Dec;3(2):249–79
**Marion-Landais G:** The first European hospital in the Western Hemisphere. In: Congrès international d'histoire de la médecine, XXVe, Québec, 1976. Actes., Québec, 1977. p. 961–8.
**Marjanovic V:** Zdravstvena kultura Kragujevca u XIX veku. Kragujevac, Farmacija, 1979. 301 p.
**Mark B:** From 'lunatic' to 'client': 300 years of psychiatric patienthood. **J Psychiatr Nurs** 1980 Mar;18(3):32–6
**Mark LC** see **Papper EM**
**Markens IS:** De orthondontice ten tijde van de Renaissance. **Ned Tijdschr Tandheelkd** 1984 Sep;91(9):362–4
**Markens IS:** Een historisch overzicht van de ontwikkeling van de orthodontie tot aan de Middeleeuwen. **Ned Tijdschr Tandheelkd** 1983 Mar;90(3):154–60
**Marketos LJ:** [Recent data on the inoculation against smallpox in the Ionian Islands] (Gre). **Mater Med Greca** 1981;9:104–9
**Marketos S:** [The deep influence of ancient Greek civilization on the work of René Laënnec, inventor of the stethoscope.] (Gre). **Prakt Akad Athenon** 1981;56:132–8
**Marketos SG, Ballas CN:** Bronchial asthma in the medical literature of Greek antiquity. **J Asthma** 1982;19(4):263–9
**Marketos SG:** [René Théophile Laënnec (1781–1826)] (Gre). **Mater Med Greca** 1981;9:1–10
**Marketos SG:** [The concert for Laënnec's stethoscope] (Gre). **Mater Med Greca** 1981;9:125–34
**Marketos SG, Eftychiadis A, Koutras DA:** The first recognition of the association between goiter and exophthalmos. **J Endocrinol Invest** 1983 Oct;6(5):401–3
**Marketos SG** see **Eftychiadis AC**
**Marketos S, et al:** [René Théophile Laënnec. his relatively unknown research work] (Gre). **Mater Med Greca** 1981;9:249–57
**Markides A:** Some unusual cures of deafness. **J Laryngol Otol** 1982 Jun;96(6):479–90
**Markiewicz J:** Institute of Forensic Research in Cracow (Poland). Its history, organisation and activity. **Acta Med Leg Soc (Liege)** 1979;29(1):85–92
**Markina LZ** see **Verenkina TN**
**Markl H:** Tiere als Automaten oder als Verwandte? Descartes oder Darwin. **MMW** 1982 Nov 5;124(44):973–6
**Markle GE, Petersen JC, ed:** Politics, science, and cancer: the laetrile phenomenon. Boulder, Westview Press, for the American Association for the Advancement of Science, 1980. xiii, 190 p. (AAAS Selected Symposium, v. 46). Contributions by JH Young, RD Smith, RF Rich, GP Monaco, AI Caplan, D Nelkin.
**Markle GE** see **Petersen JC**
**Markolf AS:** Industrial nursing begins in Vermont. **Vt Regist Nurse** 1980 Jun;:15–7

al conocimiento y dominio del paludismo. **Gac Med Mex** 1981 May;117(5):209-14
**Martínez Báez M:** La obra hospitalaria del ilustrisismo Señor Don Vasco de Quiroga. **Mem Col Nac (Mex)** 1978;8(4):33-41
**Martínez Báez M:** Pasteur, maestro. **Mem Col Nac (Mex)** 1967-68;6(2-3):115-31
**Martinez Conesa JA:** Sobre 'De somniis' de Augerius Ferrerius. **Helmantica** 1975;26:341-55
**Martínez Cortés F:** Instituciones médicas de asistencia y de enseñanza. **Salud Publica Mex** 1983 Sep-Oct;25(5):499-503
**Martínez-Cortés F** see **Somolinos-Palencia J**
**Martínez-Fortún y Foyo O:** Dr. Claudio Delgado y su aportación al estudio de la fiebre amarilla. La Habana [Consejo Címentifico, Ministerio de la Salud Pública] 1967. 130 p.
**Martinez Marañón R:** Urna olmeca que podria representar la leishmaniasis tegumentaria diseminada. **Salud Publica Mex** 1982 Sep-Oct;24(5):497-507
**Martínez-Palomo A** see **Kuthy-Porter J**
**Martinez Ramos JM:** Articuladores: su influencia en la evolución de la propedeutica y terapeutica prostodoncica. **Estodont Press** 1983;1(1):32-5
**Martinez Torres JL** see **Torres Ramírez C**
**Martinon JF, Riou R:** Conditions de travail et de santé au XIX siècle: les verriers de Rive-de-Gier. **Cah Hist** 1981;26(1):27-39
**Martinón JM** see **Franco Grande A**
**Martinón Sanchez JM** see **Franco Grande A**
**Martiny M:** Geschichte der Akupunktur. In Sournia JC, Martiny M, Poulet J, ed: Illustrierte Geschichte der Medizin. Salzburg, Andreas, 1980. Vol. 8. p. 3081-91.
**Martiny M:** Geschichte der Homöopathie. In Sournia JC, Martiny M, Poulet J, ed: Illustrierte Geschichte der Medizin. Salzburg, Andreas, 1980. Vol. 6. p. 2295-317.
**Martiny M:** Laënnec et la pensée hippocratique. In La collection hippocratique et son rôle dans l'histoire de la médecine. Colloque de Strasbourg (23-27 octobre 1972) organisé par le Centre de Recherches sur la Grèce Antique, avec le concours des Facultés de Philosophie et des Langues Classiques. Leiden, E. J. Brill, 1975. p. 97-105.
**Martiny M:** Projet de loi présenté le 31 janvier 1923 par le député Edouard Grinda sur les assurances sociales. **Hist Sci Med** 1979;13(4):363-7
**Martiny M** see **Bourgey L**
**Martiny M** see **Sournia JC**
**Martorell R:** Notes on the history of nutritional anthropometry. **Fed Proc** 1981 Sep;40(11):2572-6
**Martos G, Farkas J, Pisztora F:** Szocio-kulturális tényezök hatása a mezökövesdi matyók pszichés sajátosságaira és megbetegedéseire a XVIII. és XIX. században. **Orvostort Kozl** 1982;92(4):119-26
**Martos G:** Termékenységi vizsgálat három generáción keresztül a mezökövesdi népességben. **Demografia** 1980;23(4):370-96
**Martos G** see **Farkas J**
**Martucci V:** Il discusso fascino di una ipotesi: la pangenesi di Darwin e gli studiosi italiani (1868-1888). **Hist Philos Life Sci** 1981;3(2):243-57
**Martucci V:** Sviluppo ontogenetico e citologia nell'ologenesi di Daniele Rosa. **Physis** 1980;22(1):73-84
**Marty ME:** Health/medicine and the faith traditions: an inquiry into religion and medicine. Philadelphia, Fortress Press, 1982. xii, 350 p.
**Marty P** see **Le Fichoux Y**
**Martynov IV, Borodulin VI:** Rol' V.F. Zelenina v otechestvennoĭ kardiologii. **Klin Med (Mosk)** 1981 Aug;59(8):118-20
**Martynov IV** see **Borodulin VI**
**Maruashvili GM:** Istoriia zavoza gambuzii v SSSR (k 100-letiiu so dnia rozhdeniia N. P. Rukhadze). **Med Parazitol (Mosk)** 1980 Jan-Feb;49(1):80-2
**Marui E:** Public health and 'Koshu-Eisei'. Speciality and universality of the modern Japanese public health. In Ogawa T, ed: Public health. Tokyo, Saikon, 1981. p. 99-107.
**Maruyama H, et al:** [My way of medical history study] (Jpn). **Igakushi Kenkyu** 1978;50:11-48
**Marvin HN:** Anatomy in Arkansas' Medical College 1879-1979. The history of a department. (continued) **J Arkansas Med Soc** 1980 Dec;77(7):253-64; 1981;77(8,9,10):305-12, 347-52, 386-419
**Marvitz L:** Manden bag navnet. **Tidsskr Tandlaeger** 1983 Apr;3:51
**Marvitz L:** Nanden bag navnet. Johann Jacob Joseph Serre. **Tidsskr Tandlaeger** 1982 Feb;2(1):35
**Marvitz L, Rasmussen EG:** Tandlaegeskaebner fra perioden 1790-1850. **Dan Medicinhist Arbog** 1983;12:23-36
**Marvitz L:** Theraphia antiqua. **Tidsskr Tandlaeger** 1981 Dec;1(3):36
**Marvitz L:** Therapia antiqua. **Tidsskr Tandlaeger** 1982 Dec;2(6):30
**Marvitz L:** Therapia antiqua. **Tidsskr Tandlaeger** 1983 Apr;3:48
**Marvitz L:** Therapia antiqua. **Tidsskr Tandlaeger** 1983 Jun;3(2-3):24
**Marvitz L:** Therapia antiqua. **Tidsskr Tandlaeger** 1983 Dec;3(4):23
**Marvitz L:** Therapia antiqua. **Tidsskr Tandlaeger** 1984 Jun;4(3):24
**Marwick CS:** Managing viral diseases--two centuries of progress. **Am Pharm** 1982 Apr;22(4):36-44
**Marx E:** The biography of a great man. **Z Gesamte Hyg** 1983 Oct;29(10):571-2
**Marx J:** Charles Bonnet contre les Lumières. 2 v. Oxford, Voltaire Foundation at the Taylor Institution, 1976. 782 p.
**Marx O** see **Wallace ER**
**Marx P:** Un procès médical en Normandie en 1730. **Hist Sci Med** 1981;15(4):293-8
**Marx R:** Angleterre: la legende noire des 'Asiles pour pauvres'. **Histoire** 1982;46:50-9
**Marx RS:** Rocky mountain spotted fever. **Compr Ther** 1983 May;9(5):43-8
**Marx S:** Zwei Kollegmitschriften nach den Vorlesungen von August Conrad Havemann, geschrieben 1799 und 1818 an der Tierärztlichen Hochschule Hannover. Diss. Hannover, 1981. 360 p.
**Marzec M:** Ksawery Lewkowicz (1869-1958) wybitny pediatra i bakteriolog. **Wiad Lek** 1982 Aug 15;35(13):845-7
**Marzocchi J:** Essais sur la médecine et la pharmacie à travers l'histoire de la Corse. [S.1], J. P. Marzocchi, [1978?].
**Mas i Perera P:** Tribut al Doctor Domènec Martí i Julià. **Xaloc** 1972;56:182-5
**Mas-Oliva J** see **Lara-Terrazas A**
**Masaki T:** [Department of dentistry at Singapore University during the war] (Jpn). **Dent Outlook** 1978;52(2):277
**Masaki T:** [Hideyo Noguchi and oral spirochaete]. (Jpn) **Dent Outlook** 1978;51(6):1265
**Mascarenhas S, Batta Filho O, Ikeya M:** Electron spin resonance dating of human bones from Brazilian shell-mounds (Sambaquís). **Am J Phys Anthropol** 1982 Dec;59(4):413-7
**Mascia AV:** In memoriam Israel Friedman (1906-1980). **J Asthma** 1982;19(1):59-60
**Masek J:** Zkoumání výživy dřive a dnes. **Cas Lek Cesk** 1983 May 27;122(21):645-8
**Mashkilleysson NA:** Four generations of dermatologists. **Int J Dermatol** 1983 Nov;22(9):546-7
**Masin SC:** Note on Eugenio Rignano as a forerunner of the 'New Look' theory of visual perception. **J Hist Behav Sci** 1980 Oct;16(4):313-6
**Maslev S** see **Kozhokaru I**
**Maslov AA:** Iz istorii narodnoĭ meditsiny Kabardiono-Balkarii. **Vopr Kurortol Fizioter Lech Fiz Kult** 1980 Sep-Oct;(5):66-8
**Maslov EV:** Iz istorii kliniki nervnykh i dushevnykh bolezniĭ Severo-Kavkazskogo meditsinskogo instituta (Rostov-na-Donu). **Zh Nevropatol Psikhiatr** 1983;83(4):601-3
**Maslowski J:** Antoni Kepiński w latach 1939-1947. **Przegl Lek** 1981;38(1):126-37
**Masłowski J:** Okupacyjna tematyka lekarska w polskich publikacjach z roku 1979. **Przegl Lek** 1980;37(1):213-28
**Masłowski J:** Okupacyjna tematyka lekarska w polskich publikacjach z roku 1983. **Przegl Lek** 1984;41(1):159-77
**Masłowski J:** Reakcje na twórczość Antoniego Kępińskiego. **Przegl Lek** 1983;40(12):861-4
**Masłowski J** see **Jagoda Z**
**Masłowski J** see **Kłodziński S**
**Masnick GS** see **McFalls JA**
**Mason AH:** Crime and anaesthesia -- robbery. **Hist Med (Lond)** 1980 Jan-Feb;8(1):18-19,32
**Mason E:** 'Rocamadour in Quercy above all other churches': the healing of Henry II. In Sheils WJ, ed: The Church and healing. Papers read at the twentieth summer meeting and the twenty-first winter meeting of the Ecclesiastical History Society. Oxford, Basil Blackwell for the Society, 1982. p. 39-54.
**Mason EM:** Some insights into the life of a country doctor. **Md State Med J** 1981 Nov;30(11):20-1
**Mason FM:** Charles Masterman and National Health Insurance. **Albion** 1978;10(1):54-75
**Mason LB:** Babies hospital, 1920-1978. **NC Med J** 1984 Jan;45(1):53-6
**Masoni A:** Continuita' e novita'. **G Ital Cardiol** 1979;9(1):1-3
**Masould N** see **Jackle P**
**Mass B:** Puerto Rico: a case study of population control. **Lat Am Perspect** 1977;4(4):66-82
**Massa F:** Alexandre Brethel, pharmacien et planteur au Carangolo: recherche sur sa correspondence brésilienne (1862-1901). Rennes, Université de Haute-Bretagne, Institut Armoricain de recherches économiques et humaines de Rennes, 1977. v, 462 p.
**Massachusetts Dental Society:** The story of dentistry in Massachusetts presented by the Massachusetts Dental Society on the occasion of its centennial, 1864-1964. Boston, The Society, 1964. 63 p.
**Massad PM, Sales BD:** Guardianship: an acceptable alternative to institutionalization? **Am Behav Sci** 1981;24(6):755-70
**Massé G, Petitjean F:** L'infirmier en psychiatrie. Loi du 30 juin 1838 -- 2e partie. **Infirm Fr** 1982 Jan;(231):3-4, 36 concl.
**Masse G** see **Petitjean F**
**Massey DS:** Residential segregation and spatial distribution of a non-labor force population: the needy elderly and disabled. **Econ Geogr** 1980;56(3):190-200
**Massey EW:** An interpretation of the hand and arm markings of the shroud of Turin. **Hand** 1980 Feb;12(1):75-80
**Massey EW:** Dr. Samuel Mudd: justice at last. **South Med J** 1980 Oct;73(10):1375-6
**Massey EW, Schoenberg B:** Foster Kennedy syndrome. **Arch Neurol** 1984 Jun;41(6):658-9
**Massey EW:** Joseph Bell, MD, FRCS - Mr. Sherlock Holmes? **South Med J** 1980;73:1635-6
**Massey EW:** North Carolina medical curiosities. **NC Med J** 1981 Apr;42(4):278-9
**Massey EW:** The heaviest man on record. **NC Med J** 1981 Mar;42(3):181-2
**Massey EW, Brannon WL, Riley TL:** The 'jerks': mass hysteria or epilepsy? **South Med J** 1981 May;74(5):607-9
**Massey EW** see **Massey JM**
**Massey JM, Massey EW:** Ergot, the 'jerks,' and revivals. **Clin Neuropharmacol** 1984;7(1):99-105
**Massey RU:** Reflections from the Dean's office. The cheerful physicians. **Conn Med** 1979 Nov;43(11):747

**Massie LB:** Celebrated celery city quacks. **Mich Hist** 1982;66(5):16–23
**Massironi M:** Considerazioni psicologiche su alcuni fenomeni della visione descritti nei trattati di prospettiva dei secoli XV–XVII. **Stor Crit Psicol** 1983 Dec;4(2):171–214
**Massmann J** see **Weidenbach H**
**Masson JL** see **Bouchet A**
**Massons JM:** El gobierno de las Hermandades de San Cosme y San Damián. In International Congress of the History of Medicine, 27th, Barcelona, 1980. Actas. Barcelona, Académia de Ciències Médiques de Catalunya i Balears, 1981. p. 580–5.
**Massons JM:** Los cirujanos madrileños del siglo XVIII ante el servicio militar. In International Congress of the History of Medicine, 27th, Barcelona, 1980. Actas. Barcelona, Académia de Ciències Médiques de Catalunya i Balears, 1981. p. 575–9.
**Masters A:** Bedlam, London, Michael Joseph, 1977. 206 p.
**Masters J, Lambert D, Paterson H:** Scientific prejudice, reproductive isolation, and apartheid. **Perspect Biol Med** 1984 Autumn;28(1):107–16
**Masters WH:** Half a century of unnecessary sexual myths. **JAMA** 1983 Jul 8;250(2):244
**Mastný A** see **Tiser H**
**Masuy-Stroobant G:** La surmortalité infantile des Flandres au cours de la deuxième moitié du XIXe siècle: mode d'alimentation ou mode de développement? **Ann Demogr Hist (Paris)** 1983;:231–56
**Matalene C:** Women as witches. **Int J Womens Stud** 1978;1(6):573–87
**Matalová A:** G. Mendel and the foundation of genetics. **Folia Mendeliana** 1983;18:277–85
**Matalová A:** Published primary sources to Gregor Mendel's biography. Mendelianum of the Moravian Museum, Brno. **Folia Mendeliana** 1981;16:239–51
**Matejček J:** K populačnímu vývoji severní Moravy a Slezska 1910–1921. **Slezsky Sb** 1978;76(1):43–63
**Matejski MP:** Nursing education, professionalism, and autonomy: social constraints and the Goldmark Report. **ANS** 1981;3(3):17–30
**Matheron A:** Spinoza et la sexualité. **G Crit Filos Ital** 1977;56:436–57
**Mathes VS:** Native American women in medicine and the military. **J West** 1982;21(2):41–8
**Mathes VS:** Susan La Flesche Picotte: Indian physician. **Masterkey Ind Lore Hist** 1983;57(1):10–4
**Mathes VS:** Susan La Flesche Picotte: Nebraska's Indian physician, 1865–1915. **Nebr Hist** 1982;63(4):502–30
**Mathews CL:** History of the Mississippi State Medical Association. **J Miss State Med Assoc** 1981 Dec;22(12):299–302
**Mathews CL:** The component society––a 'sine qua non' to membership. **J Miss State Med Assoc** 1981 Dec;22(12):303–5
**Mathews GS:** Contract medicine in Rhode Island. **RI Med J** 1983 Aug;66(8):323–6
**Mathews M, Harris M:** The Royal Naval Medical Air Evacuation Unit. **J R Nav Med Serv** 1980 Summer;66(2):147–51
**Mathews-Roth MM:** Carotenoid pigments and protection against photosensitization: how studies in bacteria suggested a treatment for a human disease. **Perspect Biol Med** 1984 Autumn;28(1):127–39
**Mathewson C:** Historical review of the San Francisco Surgical Society. **Am J Surg** 1982 Feb;143(2):246–51
**Mathieu J, Cyr C, Dinel G, et al:** Les alliances matrimoniales exogames dans le gouvernement de Québec 1700–1760. **Rev Hist Am Fr** 1981;35(1):3–32
**Mathieu V** see **Epistemologia, metodologia clinica e storia della scienza medica, 2**
**Mathisen DA:** Whatever happened to human body glue? **Reason** 1980;12(1):20–7
**Matiashina OM** see **Revenko TA**
**Matics KI:** Medical arts at Wat Phra Chetuphon: various Rishi statues. **J Siam Soc** 1977;65(2):145–52
**Mátiková M:** 30 rokov logopédie v zdravotníctve v Stredoslovenskom kraji. **Cesk Otolaryngol** 1984 Sep;33(5):313–5
**Matilla V:** Cuatro secretarios perpetuos ejemplares de la Real Academia Nacional de Medicina. **An R Acad Nac Med (Madr)** 1981;98(1):31–68
**Matilla Gómez V:** Presentación del libro 'Galería de Presidentes'. **An R Acad Nac Med (Madr)** 1982;99(1):31–40
**Matilla Gómez V:** Sesión necrológica del Excmo. Sr. D. Manuel Gómez Durán. Día 3 de abril de 1984. **An R Acad Nac Med (Madr)** 1984;101(2):273–88
**Matilla y Gómez V:** Avance de un trabajo sobre la historia de la Academia. **An R Acad Nac Med (Madr)** 1983;100(3):497–513
**Matinsen K:** Diakonissene––de første faglaerte sykepleiere. **Sykepleien** 1982 Apr 5;69(7):6–9
**Matiushkin DP:** Obzor: uchenie N. E. Vvedenskogo o vozbuzhdenii i tormozhenii v svete sovremennoĭ neĭrofiziologii. **Fiziol Zh SSSR** 1981 Mar;67(3):349–56
**Matkovskiĭ NI:** Vydaiushchiisia Sovetskiĭ terapevt–infektsionist Nikolaĭ Ivanovich Ragoza (k 100–letiiu so dnia rozhdeniia). **Klin Med (Mosk)** 1983 Oct;61(10):136–8
**Matossian MK:** Bewitched or intoxicated? The etiology of witch persecution in early modern England. **Medizinhist J** 1983;18(1–2):33–42
**Matossian MK:** Ergot and the Salem witchcraft affair. **Am Sci** 1982 Jul–Aug;70(4):355–7
**Matossian MK:** Mold poisoning: an unrecognized English health problem, 1550–1800. **Med Hist** 1981 Jan;25(1):73–84
**Matossian MK:** The throat distemper reappraised. **Bull Hist Med** 1980 Winter;54(4):529–43
**Matot JP:** Filiation problématique roman familial et secret (à propos de Louis Aragon. **Psychiatr Enfant** 1984;27(2):523–38
**Matousek O** see **Kadlecová V**
**Matovic MR** see **Laslett P**
**Matovinovic J:** David Marine (1880–1976): Nestor of thyroidology. **Perspect Biol Med** 1978 Spring;21(3):565–89
**Matsen HS:** Giovanni Garzoni (1419–1505) to Alessandro Achillini (1463–1512): An unpublished letter and defense. In Edward P Mahoney, ed. Philosophy and humanism: Renaissance essays in honor of Paul Oskar Kristeller. New York: Columbia Univ. Press, 1976. p. 518–530.
**Matsubara H** see **Fujimori K**
**Matsuda H:** [Madness described in essays during the Edo period] (Jpn). **Igakushi Kenkyu** 1980;53:1–9
**Matsuda H:** [Psychiatry in the early 19th century Japan] (Jpn). **Igakushi Kenkyu** 1978;49:18–21
**Matsuda K:** L'enseignement des sourds-muets et les philosophes au siècle de Lumières. **Zinbun** 1979;15:141–74
**Matsuda M** see **Tsuboi Y**
**Matsuda T:** [The Osaka Charity Hospital and private practitioner] (Jpn). **Igakushi Kenkyu** 1977;48:41–5
**Matsufuji G:** [Phosphor-poisoning in match factories and the Salvation Army General Booth] (Jpn). **Igakushi Kenkyu** 1980;54:1–6
**Matsufuji H:** [Chukichi Kubokawa and industrial Hygiene] (Jpn). **Igakushi Kenkyu** 1978;49:14–7
**Matsuhashi N:** [Introduction to immunology––history] (Jpn). **Shikai Tenbo** 1982 Jan;59(1):169–76
**Matsuki A:** [Current findings in the history of anesthesiology (17)––the first anesthesia-related fatalities in the world] (Jpn). **Masui** 1982 Apr;31(4):408–14
**Matsuki A:** [Current findings on the history of anesthesiology (11)––the Hannah Greener incident (1)] (Jpn). **Masui** 1980 Oct;29(10):1070–4
**Matsuki A:** [Current findings on the studies of the history of anesthesiology (8) –– Erwin Von Baelz and obstetrical anesthesia] (Jpn). **Masui** 1980 Mar;29(3):287–90
**Matsuki A:** [Current view of the studies on the history of anesthesiology (7)––Tekisai Okubo, a pioneer of the pain clinic in Japan] **Masui** 1980 Feb;29(2):182–4
**Matsuki A:** [Erwin von Baelz as a pioneer in obstetrical anaesthesia in Japan.] (Jpn). **Nihon I-Shigaku Zasshi** 1981;27(1):47–55
**Matsuki A:** Nothing new under the sun––a Japanese pioneer in the clinical use of intrathecal morphine. **Anesthesiology** 1983 Mar;58(3):289–90
**Matsuki A:** [Prevalence of scurvy among soldiers of the Hirosake feudal clan in Yezo area.] (Jpn). **Nihon I-Shigaku Zasshi** 1981;27(1):56–63
**Matsuki A:** [Recent findings in the history of anesthesiology] (Jpn). **Masui** 1981 Oct;30(10):1142–6 (continued regularly)
**Matsuki A:** [Recent findings in the history of anesthesiology (16) Tracing John Snow's work in London] (Jpn). **Masui** 1982 Mar;31(3):264–9
**Matsuki A:** [Recent findings in the history of anesthesiology (20) Discovery of muscle relaxant, magnocuraine in Japan. (Jpn). **Masui** 1982 Dec;31(12):1414–9
**Matsuki A:** [Recent findings in the study of anesthesiologic history (21). An etymological study of 'masui'.] (Jpn). **Masui** 1983 Aug;32(8):1012–7
**Matsumoto A:** [Current findings in the history of anesthesiology (12)] (Jpn) **Masui** 1980 Nov;29(12):1541–6
**Matsumoto A:** [Recent findings in the history of anesthesiology (10)––Khwada, a celebrated physician at the Han dynasty was a Persian] (Jpn). **Masui** 1980 Sep;29(9):946–8
**Matsumoto H** see **Jeziorski K**
**Matsumoto S:** [Maternal and child health in Japan during last 80 years (author's transl)] (Jpn). **Nippon Sanka Fujinka Gakkai Zasshi** 1980 Sep;32(9):1171–9
**Matsunaga F:** [80 years of the Japanese Society of Gastroenterology] (Jpn). **Nippon Shokakibyo Gakkai Zasshi** 1983 Jul;80(7):1395–409
**Matsuo Y:** [History and status of study on gastrointestinal hormones] (Jpn). **Nippon Naika Gakkai Zasshi** 1982 Mar 10;71(3):275–85
**Matsushita A:** [Recent findings in the history of anesthesiology (9); practice of the anesthetic method developed by Seishu Hanaoka] (Jpn). **Masui** 1980 Aug;29(8):828–30
**Matsushita T** see **Noriyasu S**
**Matsuyama K, Ogawa S:** [A historical study on expansive use of chloroquine] (Jpn). **Igakushi Kenkyu** 1980;53:22–29
**Mattar E:** Reminiscênias históricas da endocrinologia. Uma introdução à neuroendocrinologia e suas fronteiras. **Rev Hosp Clin Fac Med Sao Paulo** 1980 Aug;35(4):218–22
**Mattelaer B:** Le Benelux et son apport à l'histoire égyptienne et arabe de la pharmacie. **Bull Pharm** 1979;1–2:1–5
**Matteo J di:** Les 'Archives des Maladies du Coeur et des Vaisseaux'. Three-quarters of a century of cardiology. **Arch Mal Coeur** 1980;73:563–84
**Matteo J di:** L'oeuvre cardiologique de Laennec. **Bull Acad Natl Med (Paris)** 1981 Feb 17;Spec No:37–44
**Matter DE:** Biographical factors associated with longevity in male Kansas pioneers. **Psychol Rep** 1979 Dec;45(3):843–52
**Mattes P** see **Geuter U**
**Matthes T:** Die medizinisch-wissenschaftlichen Gesellschaften der DDR: Geschichte, Funktion, Aufgaben. Berlin, Volk und Gesundheit, 1981. 239 p., 371 p.
**Matthew P** see **McKinney HL, ed**
**Matthews DA:** Dr. Marjory Warren and the origin of British geriatrics. **J Am Geriatr Soc** 1984 Apr;32(4):253–8
**Matthews J:** Twenty five years of Asha. **ASHA** 1984 Sep;26(9):39–40
**Matthews JB** see **Jelenko C**

**Matthews JC** see **Jelenko C**
**Matthews JH:** Surrealism, insanity, and poetry. Syracuse, Syracuse University Press, 1982. xii, 154 p.
**Matthews LG:** Apothecaries' apprentices in Wiltshire and Surrey in the eighteenth century. **Pharm Hist (London)** 1971 Jul;2(2):7–8
**Matthews LG:** Apothecaries' memorials. **Pharm Hist (London)** 1968 Mar;1(2):2
**Matthews LG:** Apothecaries of the Spicers and Kings Lynn, Norfolk. **Pharm Hist (London)** 1971 Dec;2(3):9–10
**Matthews LG:** Italian charlatans in England. **Pharm Hist (London)** 1979 Apr;9(1):2–4
**Matthews LG:** Medical men as mapmakers. **Pharm Hist (London)** 1975 Aug;5(2):2–4
**Matthews LG:** The city of York's first spicers, grocers and apothecaries. **Pharm Hist (London)** 1967 Oct;1(1):2–3
**Matthews LG:** The History of Pharmacy Committee of the Pharmaceutical Society 1952–1967. **Pharm Hist (London)** 1976 Dec;6(3):3–4
**Matthews LG:** The pepperers, spicers, and apothecaries of London during the thirteenth and fourteenth centuries. London, The Faculty of the History and Philosophy of Medicine and Pharmacy of the Society of Apothecaries of London, 1980. 64 p.
**Matthews PB:** Evolving views on the internal operation and functional role of the muscle spindle. **J Physiol (Lond)** 1981 Nov;320:1–30
**Matthews WB:** Osler Oration. **J R Soc Med** 1982 May;75(5):307–14
**Matthies K:** Mary Breckinridge and the frontier nursing service. **DAR Mag** 1980;114(5):692–4
**Mattioli E:** Una prima analisi della struttura della mortalita' nelle province Italiane al 1960–62 ed al 1970–72. **Genus** 1980;36(1–2):23–57
**Mattioni R** see **Colangelo G**
**Mattis ER** see **Volkov MV**
**Mattmüller M:** Die Pest in Liestal. Notizen zu den demographischen Implikationen der frühneuzeitlichen Epidemien. **Gesnerus** 1983;40(1–2):119–28
**Mattmüller M:** Medizingeschichte und allgemeine Historie---Dialog und Zusammenarbeit auf dem Gebiet der modernen Sozialgeschichte. **Gesnerus** 1980;37(1/2):62–72
**Mattson RH** see **Smith DB**
**Mattsson V:** Ammor och barnafödande i Malmö 1750–1850. **Scandia** 1980;46(2):173–98
**Matulová V** see **Bunčáková V**
**Matumoto M:** [Ancient history of viral diseases in man] (Jpn). **Uirusu** 1983 Dec;33(2):79–86
**Matuschka ME:** Gynäkologische Sterilisationen zur Zeit des Hexenwahns. Eine Studie zur Geschichte der Human- und Veterinärmedizin sowie des zeitgenössischen Rechtsdenkens. Graz, Akademische Druck- u. Verlagsanstalt, 1981. 69 p.
**Matuschka MM:** Lambert van Velthuysens (1622–1685) Menstruationstheorie in ihrer wissenschaftshistorischen Bedeutung. Zur Vorgeschichte der Endokrinologie der Ovarien. Amsterdam, B. M. Israël, 1980. vii, 72 p.
**Matusov AL:** Iz istorii meditsinskogo obespecheniia russkikh morskikh i poliarnykh ekspeditsiĭ. Leningrad, Gidrometeoizdat, 1972. 118 p.
**Matveev MP, Klaĭshevich GI, Gavriushova LP, et al:** Rol' kafedry pediatrii v sisteme poslediplomnogo obucheniia pediatrov (k 50-letiiu Tsentral'nogo ordena V. I. Lenina instituta usovershenstvovaniia vracheĭ. **Pediatriia** 1981 Jul;(7):77–8
**Matveev MP:** Slovo o Georgii Nestoroviche Speranskom (K 110-letiiu so dnia rozhdeniia). **Pediatriia** 1983 Feb;(2):3–9
**Matysiak W:** Doktor Władysław Biegański -- żywa karta historii polskiej medycyny. **Ann Univ Mariae Curie Sklodowska [Med]** 1978;33:1–5
**Maud PJ, Pollock ML, Foster C, et al:** Fifty years of training and competition in the marathon: Wally Hayward, age 70--a physiological profile. **S Afr Med J** 1981 Jan 31;59(5):153–7
**Maudsley H:** The pathology of mind: a study of its distempers, deformities and disorders. Reprint of 1895 ed. Biographical introduction by A. Lewis. London, Friedmann, 1979. 571 p.
**Mauksch IG:** Nursing is coming of age--the journey from nursing service to nursing as a professional practice. **Fla Nurse** 1982 Nov;30(10):2–9
**Maulitz RC:** Channel crossing: the lure of French pathology for English medical students, 1816–36. **Bull Hist Med** 1981 Winter;55(4):475–96
**Maulitz RC:** Disciplinary perspectives in the history of medicine: a view from the 1980s. With a commentary by R.P. Hudson. In J. J. Bylebyl, ed: Teaching the history of medicine at a medical center. Baltimore, London, Johns Hopkins University Press, 1982. (The Henry E. Sigerist supplements to the Bulletin of the History of Medicine; new ser., no. 7). p. 46–61.
**Maulitz RC, Poses RM, Young MJ:** Medical history as an introduction to clinical reasoning. **J Med Educ** 1983 May;58(5):427–9
**Maulitz RC:** Metropolitan medicine and the man-midwife: the early life and letters of Charles Locock. **Med Hist** 1982 Jan;26(1):25–46
**Maulitz RC:** 'Physician versus bacteriologist': the ideology of science in clinical medicine. In Vogel MJ, Rosenberg CE, ed: The therapeutic revolution. Philadelphia, 1979. p. 91–107.
**Maulitz RC:** Robert Koch and American medicine. **Ann Intern Med** 1982 Nov;97(5):761–6
**Maulitz RC:** Robert Koch in the United States of America. **NTM** 1983;20(1):75–84
**Maulitz RC** see **Numbers RL, ed**
**Maull NL** see **Schaffner KF**
**Maultsby MC:** A historical view of Blacks' distrust of psychiatry. In Turner SM, Jones RT, ed: Behavior modification in Black populations; psychosocial issues and empirical findings. New York, Plenum, 1982. p. 39–55.
**Maumenee AE** see **Ryan SJ**
**Maurer HJ, Weber W:** Die Entdeckung der Röntgenstrahlen in der Trivialliteratur und der Fachpresse von 1896–1901. **Technikgeschichte** 1977;44:324–39
**Maurer HJ:** Die Entdeckung einer 'neuen Form von Strahlen' durch W. C. Röntgen im Spiegel der Presse. **Med Welt** 1982 Apr 8;33(14):520–4
**Maurissen AW:** De leprozerie van Molenbeek. **Eigen Schoon Brabander** 1979;62:29–40
**Maurizi AR, Moore RL, Shepard L:** Competing for professional control: professional mix in the eyeglass industry. **J Law Econ** 1981;24(2):351–64
**Mauskopf SH, Seymour H, McVaugh MR:** The elusive science: origins of experimental psychical research. Baltimore: Johns Hopkins University Press. 1980. xvi, 368 p.
**Mauss AL:** Shall the youth of Zion falter? Mormon youth and sex: a two-city comparison. **Dialogue** 1976;10(2):82–4
**Mauss AL** see **Fagan RW**
**Mauss EA** see **Tobach E**
**Mawas E** see **Mawas LJ**
**Mawas LJ, Mawas E, Weiss JB:** Dix siècles de diplopie physiologique d'al Hazen à nos jours (presentation d'instruments). **Bull Soc Ophtalmol Fr** 1981 Mar;81(3):281–6
**Mawas LJ, Mawas E, Weiss JB:** Intérêt en strabologie de la plaquette modifiée de Al Hazen. **Bull Soc Belge Ophtalmol** 1981;196:53–65
**Maxwell GP:** Iginio Tansini and the origin of the latissimus dorsi musculocutaneous flap. **Plast Reconstr Surg** 1980 May;65(5):686–92
**Maxwell MH** see **Marks LS**
**Maxwell RA:** Guanethidine after twenty years: a pharmacologist's perspective. **Br J Clin Pharmacol** 1982 Jan;13(1):35–44
**Maxwell VB:** The first 2 years--a brief history of the British Association of Aviation Medical Examiners. **Aviat Space Environ Med** 1983 May;54(5):xiii–xiv
**May BR:** Barbers, 'quacks,' and other early 'dentists'. **CAL** 1983 Feb;46(8):25–7
**May BR:** Curious dental practices of the Middle Ages. **CAL** 1979 Mar;42(9):23–4
**May CD:** Food allergy: lessons from the past. **J Allergy Clin Immunol** 1982 Mar;69(3):255–9
**May DL** see **Bean LL**
**May EL** see **Martin WR**
**May ET:** Sex in utopia: a review essay. **NY Hist** 1981;62(4):462–7
**May LA** see **Andral G**
**May PA** see **Brod RL**
**May PR** see **James RL**
**May R:** Freud and the phallic defense. **Psychiatry** 1979;42(2):147–56
**May R:** The discovery of being. Writings in existential psychology. New York, London, W.W. Norton, 1983. 192 p.
**May RM** see **Darwin CR**
**May LA, ed:** Classic descriptions of physical signs in medicine. Oceanside, N.Y., Dabor Science Publications, 1977. ix, 273 p.
**Mayall BH:** Torbjörn Oskar Caspersson: curriculum vitae and selected publications. **Cytometry** 1984 Jul;5(4):314–7
**Mayberry JF:** The dispensary and the infirmary, Cardiff. **Practitioner** 1980 Jul;224(1345):764–5
**Mayberry JF:** The Hamadryad Hospital Ship for Seamen, 1866–1905. **Br Med J [Clin Res]** 1980 Dec 20–27;281(6256):1690–2
**Mayberry JF:** The history of a hospital and its diagnostic index. **Public Health** 1979 Sep;93(5):311–6
**Mayberry WE:** The Mayo Clinic in 1984. Preserving the founding values amidst modern diversification. **Postgrad Med** 1984 Sep 1;76(3):13–5
**Mayer FM, Lavoie Y:** Généalogie, démographie et génétique; étude d'un cas: Saint-Barthélemy. **Ann Demogr Hist (Paris)** 1984;:89–102
**Mayer I** see **Meir E**
**Mayer J:** Quand Diderot corrige Diderot: l'élaboration des Eléments de physiologie. In J. Proust, ed: Recherches nouvelles sur quelques écrivains des lumières (II). Montpellier, Univ. Paul Valéry, 1979. p. 73–129.
**Mayer J:** The impact of Elmer Verner McCollum on national and global nutritional problems. **Trans Kans Acad Sci** 1982 Aug;85(3):142–51
**Mayer JR von:** Die Mechanik der Wärme: sämtliche Schriften. In Zusammenarbeit mit dem Stadtarchiv Heilbronn herausgegeben von Hans Peter Münzenmayer. Heilbronn, Stadtarchiv, 1978. 457 p. (Veröffentlichungen des Archivs der Stadt Heilbronn; 22).
**Mayer R:** Il y a cent ans, à Genève, au 4e Congrès international d'hygiène et de démographie, l''altercation' Pasteur - Koch. **Rev Med Suisse Romande** 1982 Aug;102(8):805–9
**Mayer R:** Il y a cent ans, Robert Koch découvrait le bacille de la tuberculose. **Rev Med Suisse Romande** 1982 Mar;102(3):199–226
**Mayer R:** Ils étaient trois! Jacques-Louis Reverdin, Jean-Louis Prévost et Constant Picot, fondateurs de la Revue médicale de la Suisse Romande. Evocation de la naissance d'une revue médicale et esquisse biographique de ses premiers rédacteurs. **Rev Med Suisse Romande** 1980 Dec;100(12):1013–41
**Mayer R:** L'enseignement de la médecine dentaire à l'Université Libre de Bruxelles. **Rev Belge Med Dent** 1981;36(3):130–6
**Mayer T:** Early history of heart surgery. **Pediatrics** 1980 May;65(5):1054
**Mayere JP** see **Buffat JJ**
**Maynard-Smith J:** The century since Darwin. **Nature** 1982 Apr 15;296(5858):599–601
**Mayne A:** City back-slums in the land of promise: some aspects of the

1876 report on overcrowding in Sydney. **Labour Hist** 1980;38:26-39
**Mayne AJ:** Fever, squalor and vice: sanitation and social policy in Victorian Sydney. St. Lucia, New York, University of Queensland Press, 1982. xviii, 263 p.
**Mayo Medical Library: selected milestones: Mayo Alumnus** 1982 Apr;:24-7
**Mayor J** see **Losada J**
**Mayoz de la Vega R:** La fotografía en medicina. Habana, Instituto del Libro Cubano, 1970. Historical sections, p. 271-304.
**Mayr E:** Reflections on human paleontology. In F. Spencer, ed: A history of American physical anthropology, 1930-1980. New York, Academic Press, 1982. p. 231-37.
**Mayr E, Provine WB, ed:** The evolutionary synthesis: perspectives on the unification of biology. Cambridge, Mass., and London, England, Harvard University Press, 1980. xi, 487 p. Contributions by M. B. Adams, G. E. Allen, E. Boesiger, R. W. Burkhardt, H. L. Carson, F. B. Churchill, W. Coleman, C. D. Darlington, T. Dobzhansky, E. B. Ford, M. T. Ghiselin, S. J. Gould, V. Hamburger, R. C. Lewontin, C. Limoges, B. Rensch, D. Shapere, G. L. Stebbins, A. Weinstein.
**Mayr E:** The growth of biological thought. Diversity, evolution, and inheritance. Cambridge, London, Harvard University Press, 1982. 974 p.
**Mayr E** see **Szyfman L**
**Mayr T:** Martin Lerche--in memoriam. **Zentralbl Veterinarmed [A]** 1981;28(1):1-17
**Mayrhofer VO:** Die Geschichte der Muskelvelaxanzien. **Klin Anaesthesiol Intensivther** 1980;22:1-9
**Maza Zorilla E:** [Population and plague of Vallalón 16-17 centuries.] (Spa) **Cuad Invest Hist** 1978;2
**Maza Zorrilla E:** Régimen demográfico de una villa castellana. La natalidad en Villalón de Campos durante los siglos XVI y XVII. **Invest Hist** 1979;1:69-97
**Maza Zorrilla E:** Villalón de Campos y la peste de 1599. Estudio demografico. **Cuad Invest Hist** 1978;2:363-86
**Mazal O:** Pflanzen, Wurzeln, Säfte, Samen: antike Heilkunst in Miniaturen des Wiener Dioskurides. Graz, Akademische Druck- u. Verlagsanstalt, 1981. 103 p.
**Mazars G:** Die altiranische Medizin. In Sournia JC, Martiny M, Poulet J, ed: Illustrierte Geschichte der Medizin. Salzburg, Andreas, 1980. Vol. 1. p. 165-77.
**Mazars G:** Die klassische indische Medizin. In Sournia JC, Martiny M, Poulet J, ed: Illustrierte Geschichte der Medizin. Salzburg, Andreas, 1980. Vol. 2. p. 631-53.
**Mazars G:** Die Medizin in den Weden. In Sournia JC, Martiny M, Poulet J, ed: Illustrierte Geschichte der Medizin. Salzburg, Andreas, 1980. Vol. 1. p. 145-63.
**Mazars G:** Jean Filliozat (1906-1982). **Watermark** 1983 Jan;12:3-7
**Mazars G** see **Fleurentin J**
**Mazars G** see **Histoire culturelle de la maladie**
**Mazars G** see **Huard P**
**Mazars G, ed:** Les médecines traditionnelles de l'Asie. Actes du colloque de Paris 11-12 Juin 1979. Strasbourg, Université Louis Pasteur, 1981. 162 p. (Publication du Séminaire sur les Sciences et les Techniques en Asie).
**Mazet P:** Points de vue théoriques en psychosomatique. Historique et actualité. **Sem Hop Paris** 1984 Mar 22;60(13):887-93
**Mazlish B:** The next 'next assignment': leader and led, individual and group. **Psychohist Rev** 1981;9(3):214-37
**Mazumdar PH** see **Trends in biomedical research, 1901-1976**
**Mazumdar PM:** Anatomical physiology and the reform of medical education: London, 1825-1835. **Bull Hist Med** 1983 Summer;57(2):230-46
**Mazumdar PM:** Karl Landsteiner and the problem of species 1838-1968. Ph.D. Diss., Johns Hopkins University. Baltimore, 1976. 725 leaves.
**Mazumdar PM:** The eugenists and the residuum: the problem of the urban poor. **Bull Hist Med** 1980 Summer;54(2):204-15
**Mazumdar PM:** The history of medicine in a medical context. With a commentary by E. C. Atwater. In J. J. Bylebyl, ed: Teaching the history of medicine at a medical center. Baltimore, London, Johns Hopkins University Press, 1982. (The Henry E. Sigerist supplements to the Bulletin of the History of Medicine; new ser., no. 7). p. 91-102.
**Mazur A:** The journalists and technology: reporting about Love Canal and Three Mile Island. **Minerva** 1984 Spring;22(1):45-66
**Mazur A** see **Leahy PJ**
**Mazur DP:** Procreation and new definitions in the role of women in a Soviet bloc country: the case of Poland. Yedlin Tova, ed. Women in Eastern Europe and the Soviet Union. New York, Praeger, 1980. p. 226-38.
**Mazurczak T, Wiśniewski L, Wald I, et al:** Rozwój i stan obecny diagnostyki prenatalnej w Polsce. **Ginekol Pol** 1983 Mar;54(3):141-5
**Mazurenko MD, Porksheian OKh, Servatinskiĭ GL, et al:** K 100-letiiu Leningradskogo Gosudarstvennogo ordena Lenina instituta usovershenstvovaniia vracheĭ im. S. M. Kirova i 60-letiiu kafedry sudebnoĭ meditsiny. **Sud Med Ekspert** 1984 Oct-Dec;27(4):57-9
**Mazurik EV:** O pedagogicheskoĭ deiatel'nosti N. I. Pirogova v Kamenets--Polol'ske i o ego sviaziakh s Obshchestvom polol'skikh vracheĭ (k 100-letiiu so dnia smerti N. I. Pirogova). **Sov Zdravookhr** 1981;(8):66-8
**Mazurik EV:** Pervye shagi nauchnoĭ deiatel'nosti D. K. Zabolotnogo. **Zh Mikrobiol Epidemiol Immunobiol** 1983 May;(5):99-101
**Mazurkiewicz B:** Polskie słownictwo pielęgniarskie. **Pieleg Polozna** 1980;(12):10-2
**Mazzei Uzcátegui M:** Cesar Lizardo, bondad y corazon. **Rev Soc Venez Hist Med** 1972-73;20-21(34-35):111-27
**Mazzei Uzcátegui M:** Dos figuras medicas venezolanas. **Rev Soc Venez Hist Med** 1969-71;17-19(31-33):163-94
**Mazzei Uzcátegui M:** Los medicos en la aventura y en la exploracion. **Rev Soc Venez Hist Med** 1972-73;20-21(34-35):161-96
**Mazzi MS** see **Panconesi E**
**Mazzola RF, Lupo G:** Evolving concepts in lip reconstruction. **Clin Plast Surg** 1984 Oct;11(4):583-617
**Mazzola RF, Marcus S:** History of total nasal reconstruction with particular emphasis on the folded forehead flap technique. **Plast Reconstr Surg** 1983 Sep;72(3):408-14
**Mazzolini RG:** Sugli studi embriologici di Albrecht von Haller negli anni 1755-1758. **Ann Ist Stor Italo-Ger** 1977;3:183-242
**Mazzolini RG:** The iris in eighteenth-century physiology. Bern, Hans Huber, 1980. 193 p. (Berner Beiträge zur Geschichte der Medizin und der Naturwissenschaften, n. F., Bd. 9).
**Mazzolini RG** see **Ongaro G**
**Mazzonis DG** see **Bagnara S**
**Mburu FM:** Socio-political imperatives in the history of health development in Kenya. **Soc Sci Med [A]** 1981 Sep;15(5):521-7
**McArthur B** see **Breul FR**
**McCandless P** see **Scull A, ed**
**McCarthy DA** see **Domino EF, ed**
**McCarthy VA** see **Smith JH, ed**
**McCarty M** see **Trends in biomedical research, 1901-1976**
**McCollister RJ** see **Wangensteen OW, ed**
**McCoy DS** see **Radcliff-Umstead D, ed**
**McCurley J** see **Melosi MV, ed**
**McDonald WH** see **Brown CL**
**McGrath MH** see **Romm S, ed**
**McGuire W** see **Wallace ER**
**McGuire W** see **Witten LC**
**McIntosh RP** see **Greene EL**
**McMurry JF** see **Romm S, ed**
**McNamara B** see **Jenner CL, ed**
**McPherson MW** see **Robert I. Watson and the development of the history of psychology: a symposium**
**McShane C** see **Melosi MV, ed**
**McVaugh R** see **Greene EL**
**Meadow R, Lennert T:** Munchausen by proxy or Polle syndrome: which term is correct? **Pediatrics** 1984 Oct;74(4):554-6
**Meadows AJ, ed:** Development of science publishing in Europe. Amsterdam, Elsevier Science, 1980. ix, 269 p.
**Meagher LR:** The influence of Darwinian theory upon biological research of the late nineteenth century. Ph.D. Diss., Duke University. Durham, 1979. xii, 329 leaves.
**Meals RA, Brody GS:** Gatewood and the first thenar pedicle. **Plast Reconstr Surg** 1984 Feb;73(2):315-9
**Means RK:** Historical perspectives on school health. Thorofare, New Jersey, Slack, 1975. 253 p.
**Meares R:** Body feeling in human relations: the possible examples of Brancusi and Giacometti. **Psychiatry** 1980 May;43(2):160-7
**Meares R** see **Gordon E**
**Measles and Indians: Br Med J [Clin Res]** 1982 Dec 18-25;285(6357):1762-3
**Mecacci L:** Brain and history. The relationship between neurophysiology and psychology in Soviet research. New York, Brunner/Mazel. 1977. xxiv, 198 p. (Translation of Cervello e storia).
**Mecacci L:** Il manifesto della scuola storico-culturale. **Stor Crit Psicol** 1980;1(2):263-95
**Mecacci L:** Koffka e la psicologia sovietica. **Stor Crit Psicol** 1980;1(1):95-109
**Mecacci L:** Le illusioni ottiche nell'Ottocento tra fenomenologia e neurofisiologia. **Stor Crit Psicol** 1983 Dec;4(2):287-9
**Mečíř J:** Dvě instrukce pro zaměstnance prvního ústavu pro choromyslné v Praze. **Cesk Psychiatr** 1984 Aug;80(4):215-9
**Mečíř J:** Vítězslav Hálek a jeho obec pomatených. **Cesk Psychiatr** 1983 Feb;79(1):60-3
**Mečíř J:** Z počátku sovětské dětské psychiatrie. **Cesk Psychiatr** 1979 Dec;75(6):402-7
**Mecke G:** Der Jäger Gracchus, Kafkas Geheimnis. **Psyche (Stuttg)** 1981 Mar;35(3):209-36
**Mecklinger L:** Robert Koch. **Bull Int Union Tuberc** 1982 Jun;57(2):109-10
**Mecklinger L:** Zum 100. Jahrestag der Entdeckung des Tuberkelbakteriums durch Robert Koch. **Z Gesamte Hyg** 1982 Dec 12;28(12):822-6
**Meclewski E:** Der faschistische völkermord in polen. **Dtsch Aussenpolit** 1967;12(2):169-76
**Medaer R:** Classics in neurology. Etching showing Claude Bernard doing an experiment surrounded by his colleagues. **Neurology** 1982 Oct;32(10):1145
**Medaer R:** Does the history of multiple sclerosis go back as far as the 14th century? **Acta Neurol Scand** 1979 Sep;60(3):189-92
**Medawar P:** Pluto's republic. Incorporating The art of the soluble and Induction and intuition in scientific thought. Oxford, New York, Oxford University Press, 1982. x, 351 p.
**Medawar PB** see **Hamrum CL, ed**
**Médecine et livre médical du XVIème au XIXème siècle:** Dunkerque, La Bibliothèque, 1983. 1 v. (various pagings).
**Médecine, villes d'eau, sanctuaires des eaux en Gaule dans l'Antiquité. Ve Partie: La médecine à la fin de l'Antiquité: Rev Archeol Centre France** 1983;22(Dec):259-82
**Medicaid: an historical perspective up to 1966: Mich Hosp** 1978

Oct;14(10):2-3

**Medical emergencies: MD** 1978 Nov;22(11):101-13

**Medical highlights in South Dakota--the first 100 years of the South Dakota State Medical Association: SD J Med** 1981 May;34(5):75-8

**Medical history without medicine: J Hist Med Allied Sci** 1980 Jan;35(1):5-7

**Medical instruments: MD** 1979 Nov;23(11):71-81

**Medical school reformer: MD** 1978 Jul;22(7):133-8

**Medici TC:** Das Gram-Präparat wird hundert Jahre alt. **Schweiz Rundsch Med Prax** 1983 Dec 13;72(50):1587-91

**Medicine and the law: Am Med News** 1981 Apr 17;24(15):3, 10

**Medieval woman's guide to health:** The first English gynecological handbook. Middle English text, with introduction and Modern English translation by B. Rowland. Kent, Kent State University Press, 1981. xvii, 192 p.

**Medik VA** see **Zakharov FG**

**Medina E:** Bibliografía comentada de la medicina tradicional chilena. **Med Tradic** 1982;3(11):17-26

**Medina E:** Contribución a la historia de la medicina chilena: 1930-1982. **Rev Med Chil** 1983 Apr;111(4):368-79

**Medina E:** Evolución de la salud pública en Chile en los últimos 25 años. **Rev Med Chil** 1977 Oct;105(10):739-45

**Médioni G:** Die griechische Medizin nach Hippokrates. In Sournia JC, Martiny M, Poulet J, ed: Illustrierte Geschichte der Medizin. Salzburg, Andreas, 1980. Vol. 1. p. 351-92.

**Medizingeschichte wird zum Kassenschlager:** Der Faksimile-Boom. **MMW** 1980 Apr 11;122(15):66-7

**Medizinischer Gedenkkalender 1984: Z Gesamte Hyg** 1984 Jan;30(1):54-9

**Medlen LM:** Health care in the Bible and the Talmud. **Curationis** 1980 Sep;3(2):28-31

**Medouze RM:** Histoire sociale et institutions hospitalières. De la fin de l'Ancient Régime à la veille de la Révolution de 1848. Quelques exemples pris à travers la Société lyonnaise et ses hôpitaus. D.E.S., Univ. des sciences sociales de Grenoble, 1976. 176 p.

**Medovy H:** Seven decades of service at the Children's Hospital of Winnipeg. **Can Med Assoc J** 1980 Dec 20;123(12):1259-61

**Medrano AG** see **Flores y Troncoso FA**

**Medvecká E** see **Medvecký J**

**Medvecký J, Medvecká E:** K histórii psychiatrického ústavníctva vo Východoslovenskom krji. **Cesk Psychiatr** 1981 Jun;77(3):209-12

**Medvedev VI:** I. M. Sechenov's ideas in modern physiology. **Hum Physiol** 1979 May-Jun;5(3):261-8

**Medvei VC:** A history of endocrinology. Lancaster, Boston, MTP Press, 1982. xviii, 913 p.

**Medvei VC:** Some notes on the history of neuroendocrinology. In Rose FC, Bynum WF, ed: Historical aspects of the neurosciences. New York, Raven, 1982. p. 307-15.

**Medvinskaia KG** see **Bedrin AV**

**Medzhidov BF:** Istoriia Nauchno-issledovatel'skogo instituta virusologii, mikrobiologii i gigieny imeni G. M. Musabekova. Baku, Azerbaidzhanskoe gos. izd-vo, 1968. 183 p.

**Meeker E:** The improving health of the United States, 1850-1915. **Explor Econ Hist** 1972;9(4):353-73

**Meeks HA:** Stagnant, smelly and successful: Vermont's mineral springs. **Vt Hist** 1979;47(1):5-20

**Meere J:** Het eerste receptarium uit Sumer. **Farm Tijdschr Belg** 1979;56:265-6

**Meerson FZ:** Razvitie nekotorykh ideĭ V. V. Parina v fiziologii i patofiziologii krovoobrashcheniia. **Usp Fiziol Nauk** 1983 Apr-Jun;14(2):7-27

**Meerwein P:** Der Krebspatient und sein Arzt im 19. Jahrhundert. Ursprünge der Psychoonkologie? Zürich, Juris, 1980. 97 p. (Zürcher Medizingeschichtliche Abhandlungen, Neue Reihe, 139).

**Mees LF:** Blessed by illness. Spring Valley, N.Y., Anthroposophic Press, 1983. Historical section, p. 29-91.

**Mees LF:** Kennis en wijsheid, herinneringen aan leermeesters. **Ned Tijdschr Geneeskd** 1980 Aug 9;124(32):1354-6

**Meeus M:** La peste à Tessenderlo au XVIIe siècle. Congrès de Comines, 1, 1980. Actes. p. 329-30.

**Megvinov LS:** Izgotovlenie anatomicheskikh muzeĭnykh preparatov s sokhraneniem ikh tsveta i konsistentsii. **Arkh Patol** 1981;43(8):71-2

**Mehler B:** Madge Thurlow Macklin. In: Notable American women. The modern period. Cambridge, Mass., Belknap-Harvard Univ. Press, 1980. 4:451-2.

**Mehlhose F:** Der gottesfürchtige Jung Stilling. Ein Pionier der Star-Extraktion. Düsseldorf, Triltsch, 1983. 63 p. (Düsseldorfer Arbeiten zur Geschichte der Medizin, Beiheft VII).

**Mehregan AH** see **Chapel A**

**Meier LA** see **Kenney AP**

**Meier P:** Jerome Cornfield and the methodology of clinical trials. **Controlled Clin Trials** 1981 May;1(4):339-45

**Meier P:** Paracelsus-Reminiszenzen--Arzt und Medizin im Werk von Reinhold Schneider. **Salzburger Beitr Paracelsusforsch** 1984;23:100-17

**Meier RY:** 'Sympathy' as a concept in early neurophysiology. Ph.D. Diss. The University of Chicago. Chicago, 1979.

**Meier RY:** 'Sympathy' in the neurophysiology of Thomas Willis. **Clio Med** 1982 Dec;17(2-3):95-111

**Meier RY, ed:** The Joseph H. Kiefer catalog of history of urology and medicine. Chicago, Library of the Health Sciences, University of Illinois at the Medical Center, 1981. ix, 207 p. (Special collections catalog).

**Meier-Seethaler C:** The child: Erich Neumann's contribution to the psychopathology of child development. **J Anal Psychol** 1982 Oct;27(4):357-79

**Meier-Sydow J** see **Schultze-Werninghaus G**

**Meiers J:** Joseph Meiers' autobiography 1894--an Adlerian physician's mostly non-medical life story. **J Individ Psychol** 1981 Nov;37(2):205-26

**Meigs JA:** Choosing your baby's sex - now and in the sixteenth century. **Tenn Folkl Soc Bull** 1982;48(4):111-6

**Meijer J:** De tuberkelbacterie een eeuw bekend; 1882 - 24 Maart - 1982 (Heinrich Hermann Robert Koch). **Ned Tijdschr Geneeskd** 1982 Mar 13;126(11):488-9

**Meijer J** see **Sutherland I**

**Meijler FL:** Vijftig jaar Nederlandse Vereniging voor Cardiologie of, Nederland, debakermat van de elektrocardiografie. **Ned Tijdschr Geneeskd** 1984 Mar 24;128(12):571-3

**Meilicke CA, ed, Storch J, ed:** Perspectives on Canadian health and social services policy. Edmonton, Faculty of Medicine, Univ. of Alberta, 1978. xii, 520 p.

**Meiling RL:** Reflections in a diamond year. **Ohio State Med J** 1980 Aug;76(8):481-3

**Meiling RL:** The United States Air Force medical service: tumultuous years of heritage and history. **Aviat Space Environ Med** 1984 Jul;55(7):642-56

**Meindl CO** see **Meindl JL**

**Meindl JL, Meindl CO:** Tuberculous meningitis in the 1830s. **Lancet** 1982 Mar 6;1(8271):554-5

**Meindl RS:** Components of longevity: developmental and genetic responses to differential childhood mortality. **Soc Sci Med** 1982;16(2):165-74

**Meinel C:** Die Chemie an der Universität Marburg seit Beginn des 19. Jahrhunderts. Ein Beitrag zu ihrer Entwicklung als Hochschulfach. Marburg, Elwert, 1978. xvi, 669 p. (Academia Marburgensis. Herausgegeben von der Philipps-Universität Marburg, Band 3).

**Meinel C:** Nationalismus und Internationalismus in der Chemie des 19. Jahrhunderts. In Dilg P, et al., ed: Perspektiven der Pharmaziegeschichte. Graz, Austria, Akademische Druck- u. Verlagsanstalt, 1983. p. 225-42.

**Meinel C:** Theory or practice? The eighteenth-century debate on the scientific status of chemistry. **Ambix** 1983 Nov;30(3):121-32

**Meininger JV, et al:** Geschiednis van Geneeskunde en Gezondheidszorg. Register van publicaties en Lopend Onderzoek. Onderzoek - onderwijs en overige activiteiten gedurende de jaren 1972-1977 in Nederland. Utrecht, Afdeling Maatschappelijke Gezondheidszorg van het Instituut voor Sociale Geneeskunde der Rijksuniversiteit te Utrecht, 1980. 70. p.

**Meinke H:** A short history of dental advertising. **Bull Hist Dent** 1983 Apr;31(1):36-42

**Meir E, Gedalia I, Smith P, et al:** Analysis for establishing chronological age of bone. **J Oral Rehabil** 1982 Jan;9(1):53-4

**Meisel P, ed:** Freud: a collection of critical essays. Englewood Cliffs, New Jersey, Prentice-Hall, 1981. 240 p. Reprinted works by literary figures.

**Meiser G** see **Meissner K**

**Meissen GJ** see **Lounsbury JW**

**Meissner K, Meiser G:** Primary open wound management after emergency laparotomies for conditions associated with bacterial contamination. Reappraisal of a historical tradition. **Am J Surg** 1984 Nov;148(5):613-7

**Meissner R:** Swiatowy priorytet Karola Mayera w dziedzinie radiodiagnostyki--przyczynek do dziejów tomografii. **Kwart Hist Nauki Tech** 1982;27(1):125-37

**Meissner RK:** In memoriam: Dr med. Edward Stocki (1909--1978), członek honorowy Polskiego Towarzystwa Historii Medycyny. **Arch Hist Med (Warsz)** 1979;42(2):141-55

**Meissner WW** see **Goldberg A, ed**

**Meissner WW** see **Smith JH, ed**

**Meites S:** Otto Folin's decade in Minnesota, 1882-1892: a brief review. **Clin Chem** 1982 Oct;28(10):2173-7

**Meites S:** The first call for clinical chemists in the United States. **Clin Chem** 1983 Oct;29(10):1852-3

**Mekhtyev MM:** K 50-letiiu kurorta 'Baĭram-Ali'. **Vopr Kurortol Fizioter Lech Fiz Kult** 1984 Jan-Feb;(1):66-8

**Mekie DE** see **Tansey V**

**Melchior JC, et al, ed:** Københavns Universitet 1479-1979. Bind VII. Det laegevidenskabelige Fakultet. København, Københavns Universitet, 1979. xi, 519 p.

**Melhado EM:** Jacob Berzelius. The emergence of his chemical system. Stockholm, Almqvist & Wiksell International; Madison, University of Wisconsin Press, 1981. 357 p. (Also published as 'Studies and sources published by the Swedish History of Science Society No. 34').

**Melichar B, Rusek V:** Příspěvek farmaceutické fakulty brněnské univerzity k vývoji farmaceutických věd. **Cesk Farm** 1983 Jul;32(6):201-4

**Melick DW:** Surgical therapy of pulmonary tuberculosis--a rare necessity of the 1980's. An historical review. **Ariz Med** 1983 Mar;40(3):158-9

**Melicow MM:** Castrati singers and the lost 'cords'. **Bull NY Acad Med** 1983 Oct;59(8):744-64

**Melikishvili MN** see **Tsitlanadze VG**

**Melkumian GA:** Hasarakakan kazmakerputyunneri dere kovkasyan banaki bezheshkakan spasarkmen gortsum arajin hamashkharhayin paterazmi tarinerin. **Patma Banasirakan Handes. Ist Filol Zh** 1977;3:221-34

**Mellett DJ:** Bureaucracy and mental illness: the Commissioner in Lunacy 1845-90. **Med Hist** 1981 Jul;25(3):221-50

**Mellett DJ:** The prerogative of asylumdom: social, cultural, and administrative aspects of the institutional treatment of the insane in nineteenth-century Britain. New York, Garland Pub. Co., 1982. 257 p.

**Mellgren A:** Grossesse nerveuse--en psykosomatisk sjukdom. **Nord Medicinhist Arsb** 1982;:101-9

**Mellin VM** see **Kovalev MM**
**Mellish FM:** The birth, growth and development and future dimensions of occupational health nursing. **Curationis** 1980 Sep;3(2):48–53
**Mel'man EP, Shutka BV:** Issledovanie V. Z. Golubevym mikroangioarkhitektoniki pochki. **Arkh Anat Gistol Embriol** 1983 Dec;85(12):87–9
**Mel'man EP:** N. V. Kondrat'ev i ego vklad v anatomiiu vegetativnoĭ nervnoĭ sistemy. **Arkh Anat Gistol Embriol** 1983 Nov;85(11):90–4
**Mel'man NIa** see **Pyrig LA**
**Mel'nichuk AN** see **Marasanov RA**
**Melnick JL:** Toward eradication of poliomyelitis by combined use of killed and liver vaccines. **Cardiovasc Res Cent Bull** 1982 Jan–Mar;20(3):49–60
**Melnick JL** see **Goldblum N**
**Melnick M:** Sakharov and genetic science in the Soviet Union [editorial] **J Craniofac Genet Dev Biol** 1984;4(3):171–2
**Mel'nik AN** see **Kunitsa LK**
**Melnikov VP** see **Blanco MA**
**Meloan SN** see **Puchtler H**
**Melosh B:** 'The physician's hand'. Work culture and conflict in American nursing. Philadelphia, Temple University Press, 1982. ix, 260 p.
**Melosi MV:** Battling pollution in the Progressive era. **Landscape** 1982;26(3):35–41
**Melosi MV:** Garbage in the cities. Refuse, reform, and the environment, 1880–1980. College Station, Texas A & M University Press, 1981. xvi, 268 p. (Environmental History Series, no. 4).
**Melosi MV:** Urban pollution: historical perspective needed. **Environ Rev** 1980;3(3):37–44
**Melosi MV, ed:** Pollution and reform in American cities, 1870–1930. Austin, Univ. of Texas Press, 1980. xii, 212 p. Contributions by S. Galishoff, J. A. Tarr, J. McCurley, T. F. Yosie, R. D. Grinder, R. W. Smilor, S. K. Schultz, C. McShane, S. M. Hoy.
**Melville ID:** The medical treatment of epilepsy: a historical review. In Rose FC, Bynum WF, ed: Historical aspects of the neurosciences. New York, Raven, 1982. p. 127–36.
**Melzer R:** A dark and terrible moment: the Spanish flu epidemic of 1918 in New Mexico. **NM Hist Rev** 1982;57(3):213–36
**Melzer R:** Centenary: Barberton Hospital. **Adler Mus Bull** 1984 Nov;10(3):30–2
**Melzer R:** Chekhov's doctors. **Adler Mus Bull** 1981 Oct;7(3):15–9
**Melzer R, Kahn A, Kriel J, ed:** Festschrift in honour of Dr. Cyril Adler on the occasion of his 80th birthday.
**Melzer R:** The housewife doctor. **Adler Mus Bull** 1984 Jun;10(2):1–2
**Melzer R:** William Osler's connection with South Africa. **S Afr Med J** 1983 Jun 29;Spec No.:8–13
**Mena CA:** Historia de la odontologia en Cuba. I. La colonia (1492–1898). Miami, Ediciones Universal, 1981. xxii, 395 p.
**Menaker E:** Otto Rank: a rediscovered legacy. New York, Columbia University Press, 1982. xvii, 166 p.
**Menárguez Carretero L:** Los avances de la cardiología en lo que va de siglo. **An R Acad Nac Med (Madr)** 1982;99(2):297–309
**Menczer LF, Mittelmann M, Don RS:** Pharmacy in Hartford's Historical Museum of Medicine and Dentistry. **Pharm Hist** 1984;26(3):156–7
**Mendelsohn R:** The condition of the people: social welfare in Australia, 1900–1975. Sydney, Allen and Unwin, 1979. 407 p.
**Mendelson BC:** The evolution of breast reconstruction. **Med J Aust** 1982 Jan 9;1(1):7–8
**Mendelson D** see **Mendelson G**
**Mendelson G, Mendelson D:** Psychological aspects of bronchial asthma in the writings of Isaac Babel. **Isr J Psychiatr Relat Sci** 1981;18(1):31–9
**Méndez I** see **Treviño–García Manzo N**
**Mendez Alvaro F:** Historia del periodismo medico y farmacéutico en España. Ed. J. Riera. Valladolid, Universidad de Valladolid, 1978. 179 p. (Acta Historico–Medica Vallisoletana, Monografias, VIII).
**Mendez–Bauer C** see **Roberts J**
**Mendo AE, Sagrera JE de:** El rosario de los filosofos: una copia en castellano del siglo XIII (II). **Bol Soc Esp Hist Farm** 1984;35(137):36–59
**Mendoza F:** Acerca del descubrimiento del bacilo de Koch. **Rev Med Chil** 1983 May;111(5):539–43
**Mendrina GI:** Von einer wenig bekannten Ubersetzung aus der 'Augenheilkunde' von Ali Abbas aus dem Latein ins Deutsche, die der russische Arzt gemacht hat. In International Congress of the History of Medicine, 27th, Barcelona, 1980. Actas. Barcelona, Acadèmia de Ciències Mèdiques de Catalunya i Balears, 1981. p. 316–20.
**Mendrina GI:** 100–letie Tomskogo universiteta. **Sov Zdravookhr** 1981;(2):64–7
**Menéndez EL:** Socioantropología del proceso de alcoholización en América Latina, 1970–1980 (Primera parte). **Acta Psiquiatr Psicol Am Lat** 1983 Dec;29(4):247–56
**Meneses MO de** see **Pina L de**
**Menini C:** Rapporto tra storia della medicina e medicina pratica: un contributo paradigmatico in tema di talassemia e favismo nella popolazione ferrarese. **Acta Med Hist Patav** 1978–79;25:40–54
**Menk R** see **Lagier R**
**Mennel RM:** Ethel Sturges Dummer. In: Notable American women. The modern period. Cambridge, Mass., Belknap–Harvard Univ. Press, 1980. 4:208–10.
**Menner O:** Kabay jános emléke képzömüvészeti alkotásokon. **Orvostort Kozl** 1981;93–96(27 No 1–4):237–49
**Menner O:** Menner Adolf dr. (1824–1901). **Orv Hetil** 1983 Jun 12;124(24):1451–3
**Menninger WC:** The Menninger Hospitals' Guide to the Order Sheet. **Bull Menninger Clin** 1982 Jan;46(1):1–112
**Menninger WW:** A psychiatric perspective of medical history. **J Okla State Med Assoc** 1980 Nov;73(11):386–90
**Mensforth RP** see **Lovejoy CO**
**Menshutin AA:** 'Krasnogvardeets' v gody Velikoĭ Otechestvennoĭ. **Med Tekh** 1980 May–Jun;(3):3–7
**Meny DJ** see **Dawson DA**
**Menza AJ:** Compulsoary commitment of the mentally ill: a study of the English law. **State Gov** 1977;50(4):255–61
**Menzel I:** Vive la berloque. Etymologische Betrachtungen zur Berlocke–Dermatitis. **Hautarzt** 1980 Oct;31(10):558–9
**Menzel W:** Klinische Rhythmusforschung unter A. Jores. **Dtsch Med Wochenschr** 1981;106:186–9
**Menzen KH:** Entwürfe subjektiver Totalität. Frankfurt am Main, Lang, 1980. 546 p.
**Menzen KH:** Zum Verhältnis von ästhetischer Theorie und ästhetischer Psychologie. **Ber Wissenschaftsgesch** 1981;4:143–8
**Merabishvili VM** see **Napalkov NP**
**Merani AL:** Freud y el Talmud: seguido de crítica de los fundamentos de la psicopatología. México, Grijalbo, 1974. 159 p.
**Merani AL:** Historia crítica de la psicología. Barcelona, Grijalbo, 1976. 671 p.
**Merbs CF** see **Tyson RA**
**Mercedes Gomez J:** La ciencia es la iniciacion del hombre en el conocimiento de la obra de dios. **Rev Soc Venez Hist Med** 1975–76;23(37):135–46
**Mercer AJ:** Risk of dying from tuberculosis or cancer: further aspects of a possible association. **Int J Epidemiol** 1981 Dec;10(4):377–80
**Mercer SR:** America's minority medical profession. In: Congrès international d'histoire de la médecine, XXVe, Québec, 1976. Actes. Québec, 1977. p. 969–79.
**Merchant C:** Isis' consciousness raised. **Isis** 1982 Sep;73(268):398–409
**Merchant C:** The death of nature. Women, ecology, and the scientific revolution. San Francisco, Harper & Row, 1980. xx, 348 p.
**Merchant C** see **Pagel W**
**Mercier C:** L'épidémiologie et la population. **Infirm Fr** 1983 Jun;(246):3–6
**Mercier P:** André Bocage et la naissance de la tomographie. **Bull Acad Natl Med (Paris)** 1979;3:188–91
**Mercier P:** Les instituts Pasteur d'outre–mer: leurs objectifs et moyens d'action. **Bull Acad Natl Med (Paris)** 1981 Apr;165(4):441–8
**Mercier P:** L'oeuvre scientifique de Robert Debré. **Bull Acad Natl Med (Paris)** 1982 Dec;166(9):1285–94
**Mercolli C:** Il Ticion del XIX. secolo ed il colera. **Krankenpflege (Bern)** 1982 Aug;(8):85–7
**Meredith EM** see **Meredith HV**
**Meredith HV, Spurgeon JH, Meredith EM:** Early seriatim research on human somatic growth. **Growth** 1981 Autumn;45(3):151–67
**Merényi O:** Berzsenyi Dániel (1776–1836) betegségéi és halála. **Orvostort Kozl** 1979;87–88(25 no 1–2):243–7
**Mereste U, Pullat R:** Tallinna elanikkonna kujune misest 18. sajandil ja aegridade rekonstrueerimis est ajaloolises demograafias (meetrikaraamatute andmeil). **Eesti NSV Tead Akad Toim** 1979;28(4):285–303
**Merger R:** Un grand médecin: Victor Hutinel, ancien élève du Collège de Chaumont, professeur de clinique des maladies des enfants (1849–1933).
**Merges RC:** Checking the cycle: the decline of community–based residential programs in New York State 1925 to 1950. **Ment Retard** 1982 Aug;20(4):180–2
**Mericle BP:** The male as psychiatric nurse. **J Psychosoc Nurs Ment Health Serv** 1983 Nov;21(11):28–34
**Mérida F:** Las enfermedades odontologicas y dermatologicas del Libertador. **Rev Soc Venez Hist Med** 1981;30(47):81–7
**Mérida F:** Semblanzas de Alejandro Prospero Révérend, primicias para calificar su actuacion frente a la ultima enfermedad del Libertador. **Rev Soc Venez Hist Med** 1981;30(47):71–80
**Mérida MT:** Las enfermedades odontológicas y dermatológicas del Liberatador. **Acta Odontol Venez** 1983 May–Aug;21(2):154–61
**Merigan TC:** Interferon–the first quarter century. **JAMA** 1982 Nov 19;248(19):2513–6
**Mérigot JG:** Le problème des naissances en France. **Def Natl** 1975;31(7):95–104
**Merikas G:** The philosophy of exercise. **Curr Probl Clin Biochem** 1982;11:13–23
**Merino Navarro JP** see **Sanz Sanjosé MG**
**Merinov AP** see **Lomakina NM**
**Merkulov VL:** I. P. Pavlov––organizator nauchnykh issledovaniĭ. Moskva, Nauka, Glav. red. vostochnoĭ lit–ry, 1971. 8 p.
**Merle d'Aubigné R:** Paul Broca (1824–1880). **Bull Soc Hist Protestantisme Fr** 1980;126(4):509–24
**Merle d'Aubigné R:** Surfing the wave: fifty years in the growth of French orthopedic surgery. **Clin Orthop** 1982 Nov–Dec;(171):3–23
**Merlen JF:** Pnénomène de Raynaud. Historique. **Rev Prat** 1981 Dec 1;31(55):3971–2, 3975–6
**Merlette B, Vial F, Rulliere R:** Le Marcellus de Laon: observations paléographiques et critiques. **Hist Sci Med** 1980;14(1):52–60
**Merlette B** see **Vial F**
**Merman MM:** Za kommunisticheskoe otnoshenie k zdorov'iu i trudu. **Feldsher Akush** 1983 Oct;48(10):3–8
**Merriam JC, et al** see **Tedeschi CG**
**Merriënboer FJ:** Eene buitenbaarmoederlijke zwangerschap, waar het

foetus na 18 Jaren bij de moeder vertoefd te hebben door de anus is ontlast, beschreven door C.H. van der Looy (1850). **Tijdschr Geschied Geneeskd** 1980;3(1):37-40
**Merrill JP:** A historical perspective of renal trasplantation. **Proc Clin Dial Transplant Forum** 1979;9:221-5
**Merrill JP:** Early days of the artificial kidney and transplantation. **Transplant Proc** 1981 Mar;13(1):4-8
**Merrington M, Golden J, ed:** A list of the papers and correspondence of Sir Francis Galton (1822-1911) held in the Manuscripts Room, The Library, University College London. London, Galton Laboratory University College London, 1978. 80 p.
**Merritt DH, ed:** Infant nutrition. Stroudsburg, Pennsylvania, Dowden, Hutchinson & Ross, 1976. xv, 431 p. (Benchmark Papers in Human Physiology, 7).
**Merskey H:** Hysteria: the history of an idea. **Can J Psychiatry** 1983 Oct;28(6):428-33
**Merskey H:** Some features of the history of the idea of pain. **Pain** 1980 Aug;9(1):3-8
**Merskey H** see **Mai FM**
**Mertens C. de:** An account of the plague which raged at Moscow, 1771. Facsimile of London, 1799, edition, with introduction and bibliography by J. Alexander. Newtonville, Mass., Oriental Research Partners, 1977. 39, 6, v, 122 p.
**Merton PA:** Neurophysiology on man. **J Neurol Neurosurg Psychiatry** 1981 Oct;44(10):861-70
**Merton PA** see **Whitteridge D**
**Merton RK:** George Alfred Léon Sarton. In Dictionary of American Biography, Suppl. 6, 1956-1960. p. 564-6, 1980.
**Merton RK, Sills DL, Stigler SM:** The Kelvin dictum and social science: an excursion into the history of an idea. **J Hist Behav Sci** 1984 Oct;20(4):319-31
**Merton RK** see **Fleck L**
**Mertz DP:** 'Bleigicht': Ursache oder Folge des Verfalls des Römischen Weltreiches? **Med Welt** 1983 Oct 14;34(41):1158-9
**Mertz DP:** 100 Jahre Gicht: Von Scharlatanerie und Hypotheses zur gezielten Therapie. **Fortschr Med** 1982 Apr 15;100(14):636-44
**Mervo Z:** A Hajdu-Bihar megyei tanács és Debrecen város egészségügyi szolgálatának ágazati felépítése, hataśköre 1950-1956 között. **Leveltari Sz** 1973;23(2):189-209
**Merwe DW van der:** Bochum-Blauberg: die ontstaan, stigting en ontwikkeling van die Helene Franz-Hospital, 1895-1935. **Kleio (S Afr)** 1978;10(1-2):2-20
**Mesa de discusion sobre la enseñanza de la historia y filosofia de la medicina en Mexico: Bol Soc Mex Hist Filos Med** 1984;7(50):439-65
**Mesaros E** see **Marinescu I**
**Meschig R, Schadewaldt H:** Schädeloperationen in Kenia. **Dtsch Med Wochenschr** 1981;106:157
**Meschig R, Schadewaldt H:** Skull trepanation in Eastern Africa. **Hexagon Roche** 1981;9(3):17-24
**Meschig R, Schadewaldt H:** Uvulektomie--ein Initiationsritus? **MMW** 1981;123(11):437-40
**Meschig R:** Zur Geschichte der Trepanation unter besonderer Berücksichtigung der Schädeloperationen bei den Kisii im Hochland Westkenias. Düsseldorf, Triltsch, 1983. xiii, 166 p. (Düsseldorfer Arbeiten zur Geschichte der Medizin, 57).
**Meselson M:** Gas warfare and the Geneva protocol of 1945. **Bull At Sci** 1972;28(2):33-7
**Mesgravis L:** O primeiro hospital do 'sertão' e a 'corrida do ouro'. **Rev Hist (Brazil)** 1973;46(94):549-62
**Meshad S** see **Downs F**
**Meshkov VV:** Podvig sovetskikh medikov ne pomerknet v vekakh. **Feldsher Akush** 1980;45(5):3-7
**Mesiats NK** see **Belous VI**
**Meskauskas JA** see **Cruft GE**
**Messel' AM** see **Dumbrov DA**
**Messerotti GF** see **Zigiotti GL**
**Messina AF:** Societa' ed epidemia. Il colera a Napoli nel 1836. Milano, Angeli, 1979. 174 p;
**Messina B:** Mariano Messini, il suo insegnamento: le basi scientifiche della terapia termale. **Clin Ter** 1982 Nov 30:103(4):351-6
**Mester AF, Stephens SD:** Development of the audiometer and audiometry. **Audiology** 1984;23(2):206-14
**Mester AF:** Six great men in Hungarian otorhinolaryngology. **Am J Otolaryngol** 1982 Jan-Feb;3(1):67-72
**Mészárosné Varga M:** A Magyar Tanácsköztársaság egészségügye Veszprém megyében - a korabeli sajtó alapján. **Orvostort Kozl** 1982;28(1-3):219-26
**Mészárosné Varga M:** Az 1831-es kolerajárvány Veszprém megyei története. **Orv Hetil** 1980 Jan 27;121(4):223-6
**Metcalf CD:** CAPS jottings on malaria. **Cent Afr J Med** 1979 Sep;25(9):207-11 (continued periodically)
**Metcalf P** see **Huntington R**
**Method HL:** Doctor Loyal Davis--the editor. **Surg Gynecol Obstet** 1983 Aug;157(2):144-6
**Metlin VN** see **Zykin LF**
**Métraux A** see **Kraus A, ed**
**Metz L** see **Neugebauer J**
**Metzger M** see **Kottek SS**
**Metzger T** see **Kottek SS**
**Meulemans A:** Dysenterie te Leuven in de XVIIe en de XVIIIe eeuw. **Farm Tijdschr Belg** 1979;56:267-77
**Meulenbeld GJ:** Observations on some medical authors called Madhava and their works. **Sci Orient** 1979;16:59-81
**Meulenbeld GJ:** Observations on the Arkaprakaśa, a medical Sanskrit Text ascribed to Ravana. In Mazars G, ed: Les médecines traditionnelles de l'Asie. Strasbourg, Université Louis Pasteur, 1981. p. 111-39.
**Meurer-Keldenich M:** Medizinische Literatur zur Bildnerei von Geisteskranken. Köln, 1979. 327 p. (Kölner medizinhistorische Beiträge, Band 14)
**Meuwissen E:** Les dépôts de mendicité au tribunal de l'histoire. **Ann Soc Belg Hist Hop** 1981;:47-67
**Meve EB:** Put' iskanii Roberta Kokha. **Klin Med (Mosk)** 1982 Nov;60(11):111-4
**Mevers FC, ed:** The papers of Josiah Bartlett, Hanover, University Press of New England, for the New Hampshire Historical Society, 1979. xxxvii, 477 p.
**Mews S:** The revival of spiritual healing in the Church of England 1920-26. In Sheils WJ, ed: The Church and healing. Papers read at the twentieth summer meeting and the twenty-first winter meeting of the Ecclesiastical History Society. Oxford, Basil Blackwell for the Society, 1982. p. 299-331.
**Meyburg P:** Ueber die Entwicklung des Operationstisches im 19. Jahrhundert. Diss. Mainz, 1980. 119 p.
**Meyer A:** Paul Flechsig's system of myelogenetic cortical localization in the light of recent research in neuroanatomy and neurophysiology. Part I. **Can J Neurol Sci** 1981 Feb;8(1):1-6
**Meyer A:** Paul Flechsig's system of myelogenetic cortical localization in the light of recent research in neuroanatomy and neurophysiology part II. **Can J Neurol Sci** 1981 May;8(2):95-104
**Meyer A:** The search for a morphological substrate in the brains of eminent persons including musicians: a historical review. In Critchley M, Henson RA, ed: Music and the brain: studies in the neurology of music. London, Heinemann, 1977. p. 255-81.
**Meyer A:** Zur Geschichte der Tierärztlichen Hochschule Hannover während der ersten 200 Jahre ihres Bestehens. I. Die Entwicklung der pathologischen Thematik und des Institutes für Pathologie. Diss. Hannover 1980. 207 p.
**Meyer B** see **Büttner L**
**Meyer BW:** An overview of thirty years of thoracic surgery. **J Thorac Cardiovasc Surg** 1982 Feb;83(2):163-7
**Meyer D:** Erforschung und Therapie der Oligophrenien in der ersten Hälfte des 19. Jahrhunderts. Berlin-Charlottenburg, Marhold, 1973. 174 p.
**Meyer ER** see **Fine DJ**
**Meyer F:** Gso-Ba Rig-Pa. Le système médical tibétain, Paris, Centre National de la Recherche Scientifique, 1981. 237 p.
**Meyer F:** Le système canalaire et la sphygmologie en médecine tibétaine d'après le rgyud-bži et son commentaire le Vaidurya snon-po (1). In Mazars G, ed: Les médecines traditionnelles de l'Asie. Strasbourg, Université Louis Pasteur, 1981. p. 30-40.
**Meyer F:** Médecine tibétaine--l'homme et son milieu. In: Ecologie et géologie de L'Himalaya. (Colloques int. du C.N.R.S., No. 268.) Paris, Centre National de la Recherche Scientifique, 1976. pp. 195-205.
**Meyer J:** Pierre Chaunu: la mort à Paris, XVIe, XVIIe, XVIIIe siècles. **Rev Hist (Paris)** 1980;263(2):403-16
**Meyer J** see **Laslett P**
**Meyer JE, Meyer R:** Selbstschilderungen eines Depressiven--Zur Pathobiographie William Cowper's. **Fortschr Neurol Psychiatr** 1984 Apr;52(4):107-12
**Meyer JE** see **Lauter H**
**Meyer JL:** Hyperthermia as an anticancer modality--a historical perspective. **Front Radiat Ther Oncol** 1984;18:1-22
**Meyer KK, Beck WC:** Mastectomy performed by Lawrence Heister in the eighteenth century. **Surg Gynecol Obstet** 1984 Oct;159(4):391-4
**Meyer L:** Cristofredo Jakob. A veinticinco años de su muerte. **Acta Psiquiatr Psicol Am Lat** 1981 Mar;27(1):13-4
**Meyer P:** L'homme et le sel. Réflexions sur l'histoire humaine et l'évolution de la médecine. Paris, Fayard, 1982. 171 p.
**Meyer R** see **Meyer JE**
**Meyer-Salzmann M:** Aus der medizinischen Vergangenheit in Langenthal. **Gesnerus** 1983;40(1-2):129-37
**Meyer-Salzmann M:** Die Spitalversorgung im Emmental. **Gesnerus** 1980;37(3/4):307-13
**Meyer-Salzmann M:** Michel Schüppach, 1707-1781. Ein Höhepunkt handwerklicher Heilkunst. Bern, Haupt, 1981. 135 p. (Berner Heimatbücher, 126).
**Meyer-Schwickerath G:** Das Annette von Droste-Hulshoff-Syndrom. **Klin Monatsbl Augenheilkd** 1984 Jun;184(6):574-7
**Meyer-Schwickerath G:** Die Geschichte der Photokoagulation und die Behandlung der intraocularen Tumoren mit dieser Methode. **Klin Oczna** 1981;83(2):59-61
**Meyer-Schwickerath GR:** Biometrical studies of the eye and retinal detachment. **Doc Ophthalmol** 1983 Dec 15;56(1-2):27-34
**Meyer v. Froreich H:** Zur Geschichte des Apothekenwesens der Grafschaft und des Fürstentums Lippe von den Anfängen bis zum Jahre 1918. Diss. rer. nat. Marburg, 1979. 437 p.
**Meyer-Wilmes J** see **Kotwas J**
**Meyers AR:** Famine relief and imperial policy in early modern Morocco: the political functions of public health. **Am J Public Health** 1981 Nov;71(11):1266-73
**Meyle E:** Sulfonamidtherapie gestern und heute. **Pharm Unserer Zeit** 1984 Nov;13(6):177-86
**Meynell G:** Banks papers in the Kent Archives Offices, including notebooks

by Joseph Banks and Francis Bauer. **Arch Nat Hist** 1981;10(1):77-88

**Meynell GG:** Freud translated: an historical and bibliographical note. **J R Soc Med** 1981 Apr;74(4):306-9

**Mez L** see **Olonetzky B**

**Mez-Mangold L:** Aus der Geschichte des Medikaments. Basel, Editiones 'Roche', 1980, 175 p.

**Mezhirov LS** see **Grando AA**

**Mezzetti MG:** Il massaggio cardiaco agli albori della tecnica. Uno strumento di dubbia utilità. **Minerva Anestesiol** 1981 Mar;47(3):123-5

**Mhoon EE, Lanzl EF, ed:** John Ralston Lindsay, MD, 1898-1981. Contributions by H. F. Schuknecht, J. M. Fredrickson, R. I. Kohut, C. Fernandez, R. A. Butler, R. F. Naunton. (Supplement 102). **Ann Otol Rhinol Laryngol [Suppl]** 1983 Jan-Feb;92(1 Pt.3):1-36

**Miączyński A:** Szpital polski na emigracji w Aix-les-Bains. **Przegl Lek** 1980;37(1):158-62

**Miagkaia IP:** Antiretikuliarnaia tsitotoksicheskaia syvorotka A. A. Bogomol'tsa kak sredstvo patogeneticheskoĭ terapii razlichnykh zabolevaniĭ. **Patol Fiziol Eksp Ter** 1981 Mar-Apr;(2):39-46

**Miagkaia IP:** Sovremennye predstavleniia o mekhanizme deĭstviia antiretikuliarnoĭ tsitotoksicheskoĭ syvorotki Bogomol'tsa. **Fiziol Zh** 1981 May-Jun;27(3):347-53

**Mianet JC:** Contribution à l'histoire des nerfs craniens. Diss. Paris V, René Descartes, 1981. 162, xiii leaves.

**Miashka VA** see **Gurauskas VB**

**Miazdrikova AA** see **Dagurov VG**

**Michael JM, Bender TR:** Fighting smallpox on the Texas border: an episode from PHS's proud past. **Public Health Rep** 1984 Nov-Dec;99(6):579-82

**Michael JM:** The Public Health Service leprosy investigation station on Molokai, Hawaii, 1909-13 -- an opportunity lost. **Public Health Rep** 1980 May-Jun;95(3):203-9

**Michaels T** see **Viney W**

**Michalany I:** Masson's contribution to pathology and to histological technique. With special reference to the discovery of argentaffin cells. **Ann Pathol** 1983;3(1):85-93

**Michalany J:** Masson que j'ai connu: mon maître et mon ami. **Union Med Can** 1984 May;113(5):386-9

**Michalczak W, Lisiewicz J:** Antoni Andrzejewski (1807-1883) -- lekarz powiatu kieleckiego. **Przegl Lek** 1980;37(10):717-8

**Michalczak W, Lisiewicz J:** Z dziejów budynków szpitalnych w Miechowie. **Przegl Lek** 1983;40(9):705

**Michalczyk B, Kinowskiej M:** Bibliografia biezaca historii nauki i techniki. **Kwart Hist Nauki Tech** 1984;29(2):Suppl 1-30

**Michalczyk B** see **Majewska-Tronowicz J**

**Michaličková J:** Vývoj a dalšie perspektívy rozvoja pediatrických odborov na lekárskej fakulte Univerzity Komenského v Bratislave. **Cas Lek Cesk** 1979 Dec 21;118(51):1581-3

**Michalková D** see **Kolář J**

**Michalos AC** see **Durbin PT, ed**

**Michalowski R:** Spital für Geschlechtskranke in Lublin 1832 bis 1982. **Dermatol Monatsschr** 1984;170(4):268-73

**Michałowski R:** Wspomnienie o 'Wiadomościach medycznych' (Warszawa 1934-1939) przez ich Redaktora Naczelnego w latach 1936-1938. **Arch Hist Med (Warsz)** 1981;44(3/4):369-79

**Michaud A:** Evolution du syndicalisme infirmier vis-à-vis les associations professionnelles. **Infirm Can** 1981 Jul-Aug;23(7):24-7

**Micheau F:** La formation des médecins arabes au Proche-Orient (Xe-XIIIe siècle). **Ann Est** 1982;34(1-2):105-25

**Michejda M:** Advances in fetal medicine. **J Med Primatol** 1983;12(3):117-23

**Michel B:** 'Familial benign chronic pemphigus' by Hailey and Hailey, April 1939. Commentary: Hailey-Hailey disease, familial benign chronic pemphigus. **Arch Dermatol** 1982 Oct;118(10):774-83

**Michel D:** Corps sauvages, corps étranges. **Dix-Huit Siecle** 1977;9:27-38

**Michel D:** 100 Jahre 'Fortschritte der Medizin'--100 Jahre Kardiologie. **Fortschr Med** 1982 Dec 16;100(47-48):2191-3

**Michel J:** Notice historique sur la création de l'orthophonie et de la phonologie par M. Colombat de l'Isère (1828). **J Fr Otorhinolaryngol** 1981 May;30(5):281-3

**Michel J:** Recherches historiques sur la découverte des maladies des sinus, le XIXe siècle. **J Fr Otorhinolaryngol** 1979 Nov;28(9):577-90

**Michel J:** Recherches historiques sur la découverte des maladies des sinus--le XIXe siècle. 2e partie: Les affections inflammatoires des sinus. **J Fr Otorhinolaryngol** 1979 Dec;28(10):669-85

**Michel J** see **Barbaix M**

**Michel ME:** Bibliographie internationale d'histoire de la pharmacie et des sciences connexes. **Rev Hist Pharm (Paris)** 1982 Sep;29(254):214-6

**Michel ME** see **Dillemann G**

**Micheli A de:** El sesquicentenario de la facultad de Medicina de la Universidad Nacional de México (la. parte: 1833-1859). **Arch Inst Cardiol Mex** 1983 May-Jun;53(3):271-6

**Micheli A de:** El sesquicentenario de la Facultad de Medicina de la Universidad Nacional de México (2a. parte: 1859-1945). **Arch Inst Cardiol Mex** 1983 Jul-Aug;53(4):379-84

**Micheli A de:** La inquisición y los médicos en la Nueva España. **Prensa Med Mex** 1979 Nov-Dec;44(11-12):273-7

**Micheli A de:** La inquisicion y los medicos en la Nueva España. **Bol Soc Mex Hist Filos Med** 1982 Sep;6(40):71-81

**Micheli A de:** La viruela en la Nueva España. **Prensa Med Mex** 1979 Sep-Oct;44(9-10):201-7

**Micheli A de:** Libros medicos italianos en la antigua universidad de Mexico. **Bol Soc Mex Hist Filos Med** 1979 Dec;4(29):129-39

**Micheli A de:** Libros médicos italianos en la antigua Universidad de México. **Prensa Med Mex** 1979;44:152-6

**Micheli A de:** Los balbuceos de la cardiologia en la medicina islamica. **Bol Soc Mex Hist Filos Med** 1982 Mar;6(38):5-13

**Micheli A de:** Los primeros libros médicos novohispanos. **Prensa Med Mex** 1979 Jan-Feb;43(1-2):25-30

**Micheli A de:** Los primeros libros médicos novohispanos. **Arch Inst Cardiol Mex** 1980 Jan-Feb;50(1):107-10

**Micheli A de:** Tópicos cardiológicos en la antigua medicina islámica. **Arch Inst Cardiol Mex** 1981 Sep-Oct;51(5):497-500

**Micheli Pellegrini V:** Histoire des glandes salivaires. **Acta Otorhinolaryngol Belg** 1981;35(2):351-92

**Michels R** see **Goldberg A, ed**

**Michetti D:** L'évolution des traitements de la tuberculose. **Rev Med Swisse Romande** 1982 Mar;102(3):227-9

**Micheva Z:** Shesta sesiia na Bulgaro-Polskata Komisiia na istoritsite. **Istor Pregl** 1978;34(5):162-4

**Michigan Department of Public Health:** The first 100 years. [Lansing, The Department, 1973?] 116 p.

**Michler M:** Aus der Geschichte der Gicht. **Orthop Prax** 1978;14(5):341-51

**Michler M:** Zur Entstehung des medizinischen Schmerzbegriffes. **Orthop Prax** 1979;15(5):347-50

**Michler M:** Zur Toposforschung in der medizinischen Literatur. In Ganzinger K, Skopec M, Wyklicky H, ed: Festschrift für Erna Lesky zum 70. Geburtstag. Wien, Brüder Hollinek, 1981. p. 57-65.

**Michler M** see **Benedum J**

**Michod RE:** Positive heuristics in evolutionary biology. **Br J Philos Sci** 1981;32(1):1-36

**Michod, RE:** Positive heuristics in evolutionary biology. **Br J Philos Sci** 1981;32:1-36

**Micic M:** Pharmaziegeschichtliche Museen und Sammlungen in Jugoslawien. In: Vorträge des Internationalen Pharmaziehistorischen Kongresses Innsbruck 1977. Stuttgart, Wissenschaftliche Verlagsgesellschaft, 1979. p. 107-25.

**Micic R:** General prof. dr Milan Arsenijević (24. III 1901 - 10. XI 1981). **Srp Arh Celok Lek** 1982 Sep;110(9):1109-13

**Miciotto RJ:** Anniversary 50: the birth and development of the LSU School of Medicine. The Murmur: LSU Medical Center Yearbook 1981 Fall; 13:34-41, 302-3.

**Miciotto RJ:** Carl Rokitansky: nineteenth-century pathologist and leader of the new Vienna school. Ph.D. diss. Johns Hopkins University, 1979. 301 leaves.

**Micoud M:** Die ansteckenden Krankheiten. In Sournia JC, Martiny M, Poulet J, ed: Illustrierte Geschichte der Medizin. Salzburg, Andreas, 1980. Vol. 6. p. 2243-93.

**Miczbán I:** A sejtkép szemléletének alakulása a XX. században. **Orvostort Kozl** 1982;92(4):9-16

**Middelhoff HD** see **Janzarik W ed**

**Middlebrook G:** Tuberculosis and medical science. **Am Rev Respir Dis** 1982 Mar;125(3 pt 2):4-7

**Middleton WE:** Some unpublished correspondence of Giovanni Alfonso Borelli. **Ann Ist Mus Stor Sci Fir** 1984;9(2):99-132

**Midelfort HC:** Madness and civilization in early modern Europe: a reappraisal of Michel Foucault. In Malament, Barbara C., ed. After the Reformation: Essays in honor of J. H. Hexter, Philadelphia; U. of Pennsylvania Press, 1980. p. 247-65.

**Midelfort HC:** Madness and the problems of psychological history in the sixteenth century. **Sixteenth Century J** 1981;12(1):5-12

**Midelfort HC:** The anthropological roots of Paracelsus' psychiatry. **Medizinhist J** 1981;16(1-2):67-77

**Midkiff VC:** The history of feed analysis, as chronicled in the development of AOAC official methods, 1884-1984. **J Assoc Off Anal Chem** 1984 Sep-Oct;67(5):851-60

**Mielke HP:** Brustgläser, Uringläser und Urinale. Zur Typologie dreier im medizinischen Gebrauch beheimateter Gläser. In Göpfert W, Otten HH, ed: Metavoeite: wandelt euch durch neues Denken. Düsseldorf, Triltsch, 1983. p. 209-12.

**Miert AS van:** Van Materia Medica tot rationele farmacotherapie. **Tijdschr Diergeneeskd** 1984 Jan 1;109(1):3-11

**Mierzecki H:** Czasy i klimaty. **Kwart Hist Nauki Tech** 1981;26(3-4):503-32

**Miętkiewskiego E:** XXX lat Pomorskiej Akademii Medycznej w Szczecinie. **Ann Acad Med Stetin** 1979;(Suppl 17):1-549

**Miéville C:** Fortbildungskurs der Schweizerischen Gesellschaft für Psychiatrie. Biologische Aspekte der Psychiatrie. Eröffnung. **Schweiz Arch Neurol Neurochir Psychiatr** 1979;125(2):187-91

**Migalatiuk DIa** see **Danilevskiĭ VM**

**Miguel A de:** La poblacion en Madrid en los primeros años del siglo. **Rev Esp Invest Sociol** 1982;(19):55-71

**Miguel J de:** Anotaciones al desenvolvimiento histórico de la cirugía de la úlcera péptica con especial referencia a la úlcera duodenal en los últimos 50 años. **Rev Esp Enferm Apar Dig** 1983 Jul;64(1):60-5

**Miguel JM de:** Siete tesis erróneas sobre la política sanitaria española y una alternativa sociológica crítica. **Rev Esp Invest Sociol** 1980;(9):53-80

**Miguel JM de** see **Campos J**

**Miguel Martínez J, Cabarrocas Gafarot E:** Bodas de plata de la associació catalana d'anestesiologia i reanimació (1953-1978). **Rev Esp Anestesiol Reanim** 1981 Mar;28(2):51-110

**Miguel Torre J:** Treinta años de vida de la Sociedad Potosina de Estudios Médicos. Una experiencia interesante. **Gac Med Mex** 1982 Apr;118(4):165-70

**Mihalcu F** see **Panaitescu D**

**Mihic DN:** Die erste orotracheale Intubation. **Anaesthesist** 1983

Sep;32(9):450–1

**Mijalkovic D:** Doprinos dr Laze K.Lazarevića infektologiji XIX veka. **Srp Arh Celok Lek** 1980 Jan;108(1):77–80

**Mijuskovic S:** Nastojanja kotorske opštine oko osnivanja centralne bolnice za boku sredinom XIX veka. **Istor Zapisi** 1972;25(3–4):443–52

**Mikata A** see **Kageyama K**

**Miké V:** Clinical studies in cancer: a historical perspective. In V. Miké, K. E. Stanley, ed: Statistics in medical research. Methods and issues, with applications in cancer research. New York, John Wiley & Sons, 1982. p. 111–55.

**Mikhail M, Rosen H:** History and etiology of myofascial paindysfunction syndrome. **J Prosthet Dent** 1980;44:438–44

**Mikhail Andreevich Sreseli (k 75–letiiu so dnia rozhdeniia): Arkh Anat Gistol Embriol** 1980 Apr;78(4):122–5

**Mikhail Grigor'evich Prives (k 75–letiiu so dnia rozhdeniia): Arkh Anat Gistol Embriol** 1980 Mar;78(3):120–1

**Mikhaĭlov AN:** Razvitie rentgenologii i radiologii v Belorusskoĭ SSR. **Vestn Rentgenol Radiol** 1982 Nov–Dec;(6):83–4

**Mikhailov C:** Etappes dans le développement de l'organisation de l'expertise médicale de la capacité de travail dans la republique populaire de Bulgarie. In International Congress of the History of Medicine. 26th, Plovdiv, 1978. Actes du Congress. Sofia, 1981. Volume II. p. 77–8.

**Mikhaĭlov FA:** Iz rasskazov o G. A. Zakhar'ine. **Klin Med (Mosk)** 1980 Jan;58(1):113–4

**Mikhaĭlov FA:** Rene Teofil' Giatsint Laénnek (1781–1826). **Klin Med (Mosk)** 1981 Dec;59(12):92–5

**Mikhaĭlov FA** see **Al'tshular NS**

**Mikhaĭlov GN:** Voprosy okhrany truda v rabotakh A. N. Sysina. **Gig Tr Prof Zabol** 1982 Oct;(10):41–3

**Mikhaĭlov VP:** Delo bol'shogo obshchestvennogo znacheniia (po povodu stat'i V. Ch. Brzheskogo). **Arkh Anat Gistol Embriol** 1981 Jan;80(1):109–13

**Mikhaĭlov VP:** Nikolaĭ Varnek i Karl Bér. **Arkh Anat Gistol Embriol** 1982 Apr;82(4):86–95

**Mikhaĭlov VP:** Pamiati Alekseia Georgievicha Knorre. **Arkh Anat Gistol Embriol** 1982 Feb;82(2):5–16

**Mikhaĭlov VP:** Zhurnal Rudneva (poluzabytaia glava v istorii otechestvennoĭ gistologii). **Arkh Anat Gistol Embriol** 1980 Feb;78(2):104–15

**Mikhaĭlov VP** see **Bobkov AG**

**Mikirtichan GL:** Iu. A. Mendeleva––vidnyĭ organizator sovetskogo zdravookhraneniia (1883–1959). **Sov Zdravookhr** 1983;(11):59–62

**Mikirtichan GL:** S. P. Botkin i okhrana zdorov'ia deteĭ (k 150–letiiu so dnia rozhdeniia). **Pediatriia** 1982 Oct;(10):62–4

**Mikirtichan GL** see **Suvorova RV**

**Mikoian AI:** Prodovol'stvie frontu. **Voen Istor Zh** 1978;1:63–71

**Mikolás M:** Gesztációs folyamatokra vonatkozó matematikai statisztikai vizsgálatok (Magyarország, 1931–1978). **Demografia** 1980;23(2–3):163–207

**Miksanek T:** Dostoevsky's The Idiot and psychic disorders in epilepsy. **Perspect Biol Med** 1982 Winter;25(2):231–7

**Mikulinskij SR, Markova LA, Starostin BA:** Alphonse de Candolle (1806–1893). Jena, Fischer, 1980. 224 p. (Biographien bedeutender Biologen, Band 3).

**Mikuz G:** Die Pathologie in Innsbruck. **Verh Dtsch Ges Pathol** 1981;65:XXI–XXVI

**Mikx F:** A. van Leeuwenhoek's microscopes: upside down? **Lancet** 1983 Jun 18;1(8338):1387–8

**Mikx F:** Antoni van Leeuwenhoek––300 sodina oralne mikrobiologije. **Acta Stomatol Croat** 1983;17(4):323–5

**Mikx FH:** Het tandplaque–onderzoek van Antoni van Leeuwenhoek in 1683. **Ned Tijdschr Tandheelkd** 1983 Sep;90(9):421–4

**Milad A ben:** Biographie des médécins arabes: Ishaq Ibn Omrane. **Tunis Med** 1979;57:378–9

**Milashkin AG:** Ispol'zovanie mazi Vishnevskogo v gody Velikoĭ Otechestvennoĭ voĭny. **Voen Med Zh** 1982 Feb;(2):76

**Milashkin AG:** Nauchno–issledovatel'skaia rabota po voprosam travmaticheskogo shoka v gody Velikoĭ Otechestvennoĭ voĭny. **Voen Med Zh** 1983 Aug;(8):74–5

**Milasi G** see **Cilenti V**

**Milbauer B, Obrentz BN:** The law giveth: legal aspects of the abortion controversy. New York, Atheneum, 1983. 363 p.

**Milcu SM:** Brief history of Romanian endocrinology. Bucharest, Medical Pub. House, 1981. 51 p.

**Milcu Sm:** The contributions made by Romanian physicians to the development of endocrinology. **Endokrinologie** 1981 Apr–Jun;19(2):81–6

**Milders JW:** Taking a look at the invisible. **Hindustan Antibiot Bull** 1982 Aug–Nov;24(3–4):93–6

**Mildner S** see **Winkelmann H**

**Miles A:** Reports by Louis Pasteur and Claude Bernard on the organization of scientific teaching and research. **Notes Rec R Soc Lond** 1982 Aug;37(1):101–18

**Miles DE:** The growth of suicide among black Americans. **Crisis** 1979;86(10):430–3

**Miles W** see **Pearson EF**

**Miles WD:** A history of the National Library of Medicine. The nation's treasury of medical knowledge. Bethesda, National Library of Medicine, 1982. viii, 531 p. (NIH Publication No. 82–1904).

**Milhomem AM, Suassuna I:** A imunidade na febre tifóide. I. A vacinação anti–tifoídica de Wright, 1896 a 1979. **Mem Inst Oswaldo Cruz** 1982 Jan–Mar;77(1):93–120

**Miliavskiĭ VM, Ikonnikov MV:** Fel'dsheritsa Liudmila Aleksandrovna Volkenshteĭn. **Feldsher Akush** 1983 Oct;48(10):42–3

**Miliavskiĭ VM:** K istorii prepodavaniia psikhiatrii v fel'dsherskikh shkolakh. **Feldsher Akush** 1982;47(4):53–4

**Miliavskiĭ VM, Ikonnikov MV:** K stoletiiu pervoĭ pnevmotomii v Rossii. **Klin Khir** 1983 Oct;:(10):73–4

**Miliavskiĭ VM:** Obshchestvo poltavskikh vracheĭ i 'Trudy post oiannoĭ meditsinskoĭ komissii pri Poltavskoĭ gubernnskoĭ zemskoĭ uprave'. **Sov Zdravookhr** 1981;(4):69–71

**Miliavskiĭ VM:** Znachenie 'Trudov postoiannoĭ meditsinskoĭ komissii pri Poltavskoĭ gubernskoĭ zemskoĭ uprave' dlia razvitiia zemskoĭ meditsiny v Rossii. **Sov Zdravookhr** 1984;(4):63–5

**Miliavskiĭ VM** see **Kokhan AI**

**Milic N:** Imunoproliferativne bolesti. Uvod. **Lijec Vjesn** 1983 Feb–Mar;105(2–3):105–6

**Milich VM** see **Anton'ev AA**

**Milik JR:** W XXX rocznicę śmierci Wacława Lilpopa i założenia polskiego towarzystwa urologicznego. **Wiad Lek** 1979 Nov 1;32(21):1569–71

**Milik JR:** W 20 rocznicę śmierci Bolesława Skarżyńskiego o jego zasługach w rozwoju historii medycyny w Polsce. **Wiad Lek** 1983 Sep 15;36(18):1561–2

**Milin M, Popescu A:** Sfîrsitul Lui Serban Cantacuzino. **Mag Istor** 1980;14(9):53–8

**Milio N:** Margaret Gene Arnstein. In: Notable American women. The modern period. Cambridge, Mass., Belknap–Harvard Univ. Press, 1980. 4:37–8.

**Miliutina IK, Kartasheva LA:** K voprosu informatsionnogo obespecheniia i informatisionnoĭ znachimosti istoriko–meditsinskikh issledovanii. **Sov Zdravookhr** 1981;(4):67–9

**Millar WP** see **Gidney RD**

**Miller B, Chambers EB, Coleman CM:** Indo–Chinese refugees: a national mental health need assessment. **Migr Today** 1981;9(2):26–31

**Miller B:** The incident. **Lincoln Her** 1980;82(1):342–3

**Miller BJ:** The development of heart lung machines. **Surg Gynecol Obstet** 1982 Mar;154(3):403–14

**Miller D** see **Curtis JB**

**Miller D** see **Gutner R**

**Miller DP:** The Royal Society of London 1800–1835: a study in the cultural politics of scientific organization. Ph. D. Diss., University of Pennsylvania, Philadelphia, 1981. vii, 422 leaves.

**Miller E:** The Browne doublet: 'Religio medici' in the history of English prose style. **Bull Res Humanit** 1979;82:213–21

**Miller EB:** Comparative medicine: American experience with equine tetanus – from Benjamin Rush to Toxoid. **Bull Hist Med** 1983;57(1):81–92

**Miller EB:** Nonacademic influences on education of the veterinarian in the United States, 1887–1921. **J Am Vet Med Assoc** 1979 Nov 15;175(10):1106–10

**Miller EB:** Petition for a Federal Veterinary Sanitary Bureau. **J Am Vet Med Assoc** 1984 May 15;184(10):1224–5

**Miller EB:** Private veterinary colleges in the United States, 1852–1927. **J Am Vet Med Assoc** 1981 Mar 15;178(6):583–93

**Miller EC** see **Miller JA**

**Miller ED** see **Bearn AG**

**Miller G:** Edward Jenner letters in Baltimore, Maryland. In International Congress of the History of Medicine. 26th, Plovdiv, 1978. Actes du Congress. Sofia, 1981. Volume II. p. 157–9.

**Miller G:** Henry Ernest Sigerist. In Dictionary of American Biography, Suppl. 6, 1956–1960. p. 580–1, 1980.

**Miller G:** In praise of amateurs: medical history in America before Garrison. **Bull Hist Med** 1973 Nov–Dec;47(6):586–615

**Miller G, Warriner CK:** Professional power and social change at the community level: the case of three prepaid health care programs. **Soc Sci J** 1980;17(3):1–19

**Miller G:** Putting Lady Mary in her place: a discussion of historical causation. **Bull Hist Med** 1981 Spring;55(1):2–16

**Miller G** see **Blake JB, ed**

**Miller G** see **Cohen IB, ed**

**Miller G** see **Henderson DA**

**Miller G** see **Numbers RL, ed**

**Miller G** see **Silverstein AM**

**Miller GH:** A drill in either hand. **CAL** 1981 Mar;44(9):14–5, 18–9

**Miller GH:** I remember Mama, too: a dentist's wife––circa 1900. **Tic** 1982 Mar;41(3):1–4

**Miller GM, Kreuzer DW:** The modified Hawley appliance: part I. **Int J Periodontics Restorative Dent** 1981;1(6):8–21

**Miller H:** 40 years of development in radioisotope non–imaging techniques. **Phys Med Biol** 1984 Feb;29(2):157–61

**Miller HD:** Patent license restrictions in the prescription drug industry. **Va Law Rev** 1967;53(6):1283–313

**Miller ID** see **Kenny PJ**

**Miller J:** A Gower Street scandal. The Samuel Gee lecture 1982. **J R Coll Physicians Lond** 1983 Oct;17(4):181–5, 188–91

**Miller J:** Interpretations of Freud's Jewishness, 1924–1974. **J Hist Behav Sci** 1981;17:357–74

**Miller JA, Miller EC:** Some historical aspects of N–aryl carcinogens and their metabolic activation. **Environ Health Perspect** 1983 Mar;49:3–12

**Miller JC:** The significance of drought, disease and famine in the agriculturally marginal zones of West–Central Africa. **J Afr Hist** 1982;23(1):17–61

**Miller JD** see **Sammons JH**

**Miller JM:** Copernicus, medicine, and the heliocentric concept.

**South Med J** 1983 Sep;76(9):1167–8
**Miller JM, Sakowski RA:** Doctors and the Declaration of Independence. **Surg Gynecol Obstet** 1980 Jun;150(6):903–5
**Miller JM:** Physicians and prose. **Md State Med J** 1982 Jan;31(1):43–7
**Miller JM:** Poisoning by antimony: a case report (Oliver Goldsmith). **South Med J** 1982 May;75(5):592
**Miller JM:** William Stewart Halsted and the use of the surgical rubber glove. **Surgery** 1982 Sep;92(3):541–3
**Miller L:** The role of a Braucher-chiropractor in an Amish community. **Mennon Q Rev** 1981;55(2):157–71
**Miller LE:** San Diego's early years as a health resort. **J San Diego Hist** 1982;28(4):232–47
**Miller LG:** Pain, parturition, and the profession: twilight sleep in America. In Reverby S, Rosner D, ed: Health care in America. Philadelphia, Temple University Press, 1979. p. 19–44.
**Miller M:** A. V. Hill papers. **Surv Sources Newsl** 1978 Oct;8:8–10
**Miller M:** Hans Thacher Clarke Papers. **Surv Sources Newsl** 1977 May;5:12–3
**Miller M:** The Max Bergmann papers. **Surv Sources Newsl** 1976Dec;4:7–8
**Miller M:** The Simon Flexner papers. **Surv Sources Newsl** 1979 Apr;9:2–4
**Miller M:** The Walter Bradford Cannon Papers. **Surv Sources Newsl** 1977 May;5:8–9
**Miller M** see **Bearman D**
**Miller MD:** Health care. **Proc Acad Polit Sci** 1979;33(3):82–90
**Miller MJ:** Tissue oxygenation in clinical medicine: an historical review. **Anesth Analg (Cleve)** 1982 Jun;61(6):527–35
**Miller MK, Voth DE, Danforth DM:** The medical care system and community malady: rural, urban, and suburban variations in impact. **Rural Sociol** 1982;47(4):634–54
**Miller NJ, Howard-Ruben J:** Unproven methods of cancer management part I: background and historical perspectives. **Oncol Nurs Forum** 1983 Fall;10(4):46–52
**Miller PJ:** Semmelweis. **Infect Control** 1982 Sep–Oct;3(5):405–9
**Miller RM:** Admission of foreign medical graduates to the U.S. **INS Rep** 1979;27(4):6–11
**Miller RR:** History of clinical pharmacy and clinical pharmacology. **J Clin Pharmacol** 1981 Apr;21(4):195–7
**Miller RW, McKay FW:** Decline in US childhood cancer mortality. 1950 through 1980. **JAMA** 1984 Mar 23–30;251(12):1567–70
**Miller S:** Glaucoma--then and now. **Trans Ophthalmol Soc UK** 1980 Apr;100(pt 1):17–9
**Miller VD, Pellicori SF:** Ultraviolet fluorescence photography of the Shroud of Turin. **J Biol Photogr** 1981 Jul;49(3):71–85
**Miller WH:** The habit of Sherlock Holmes. **Trans Stud Coll Physicians Phila** 1978 Jul;45(5):252–7
**Miller G, ed:** Letters of Edward Jenner and other documents concerning the early history of vaccination. From the Henry Barton Jacobs Collection in the William H. Welch Medical Library. Baltimore, London, Johns Hopkins University Press, 1983. xxix, 145 p. (Henry E. Sigerist Supplements to the Bulletin of the History of Medicine, n.s., no. 8).
**Miller-Guinsburg A** see **Paracelsus in der Tradition**
**Milles D:** From workers' diseases to occupational diseases: the causality of experts' evidence on liability in the development of social medicine. **Soc Soc Hist Med Bull (Lond)** 1983 Dec;33:58–62
**Milles D** see **Klein P**
**Millet NB, Hart GD, Reyman TA, et al:** ROM I: mummification for the common people. In A. Cockburn, E. Cockburn, ed: Mummies, disease, and ancient cultures. Cambridge, Cambridge University Press, 1980. p. 71–84.
**Millet NB** see **Hart GD, ed**
**Millett N** see **Hart GD**
**Milliez P:** La médecine socialisée. **Acquis Med Recent** 1978;:189–91
**Milling CJ:** Indian medicine. **SC Hist Illus** 1970;1(4):31–5
**Mills ES** see **Robert I. Watson and the development of the history of psychology: a symposium**
**Mills F** see **Harrison RC**
**Mills FJ** see **Harding RM**
**Mills GH:** Hawaiians and medicine. **Hawaii Med J** 1981 Oct;40(10):272–6
**Mills JG, Jones DR:** The adaptability rating for military aeronautics: an historical perspective of a continuing problem. **Aviat Space Environ Med** 1984 Jun;55(6):558–62
**Mills NL:** Valvular heart surgery--1984. **J La State Med Soc** 1984 Apr;136(4):43–6
**Mills R, O'Brien E:** Corrigan bibliography. **J Ir Coll Physicians Surg** 1980 Jul;10(1):50–4
**Mills R, O'Brien E:** Memorabilia and letters of Dominic Corrigan: catalogue of an exhibition. **J Ir Coll Physicians Surg** 1980 Jul;10(1):55–7
**Millstein CB:** W. D. Miller and the beginnings of occupational hygiene in dentistry. **Bull Hist Dent** 1984 Oct;32(2):135–6
**Millstein PL, Howe E:** A hundred years of dental history in a Boston building. **J Am Dent Assoc** 1984 Apr;108(4):641–2
**Milne GP:** The history of midwifery in Aberdeen. **Aberdeen Univ Rev** 1978;47:293–303
**Milner A:** The Franklin Institute: as diverse as its namesake. **Wilson Libr Bull** 1982;56(10):735–9
**Milner GR:** Epidemic disease in the postcontact southeast: a reappraisal. **Midcont J Archaeol** 1980;5(1):39–56
**Milner M:** Freud et l'interprétation de la littérature. Paris, Société d'édition d'enseignement supérieur, 1980. 328 p.
**Milos G, Akert K:** Die neurobiologischen Grundlagen der binoculären Raumwahrnehmung. Historische Übersicht über die Entwicklung der Vorstellungen und Erkenntnisse. **Schweiz Arch Neurol Neurochir Psychiatr** 1982;130(1):39–67
**Miloşescu P, Bercuş CI:** Constituirea otorinolaringologiei ca specialitate medicală în România. **Rev Chir [Otorinolaringol]** 1979 Apr–Jun;24(2):145–8
**Milosevic P:** Organizacija i razvoj partizanske zdravstvene službe u crnoj gori 1941–1942. godine. **Istor Zapisi** 1969;22(4):521–52
**Miłosz S, Stański M:** O niektórych tendencjach filozoficzno-metodologicznych medycyny w polsce na przełomie XIX i XX w. **Stud Filoz** 1977;11:127–38
**Milot J** see **Gerard A**
**Milspaw YJ:** Witchcraft belief in a Pennsylvania German family. **Pa Folklife** 1978;27(4):14–24
**Milstein S:** Domenico Cotugno. **Am J Otol** 1982 Jul;4(1):95–7
**Milstein S:** Otosclerosis. **Am J Otol** 1981 Jan;2(3):283–5
**Milstein S:** The history of mastoid surgery. **Am J Otol** 1980 Jan;1(3):174–8
**Miltényi K:** Uganda népesedésének néhány jellegzetessége. **Demografia** 1979;(2–3):228–36
**Miltényi M:** Emlékezés ifjú Bókay Jánosra. **Orv Hetil** 1983 May 29;124(22):1327–9
**Miltényi M:** Professor János Bókay, Jr. **Acta Paediatr Hung** 1984;25(1–2):3–5
**Miltner V:** [Ancient Indian concepts of the body and disease] (Cze). **Cas Lek Cesk** 1981 Jun 4;120(22):682–4
**Milza P:** La guerre froide à Paris: 'Ridgway la peste'. **Histoire** 1980;25:38–47
**Mims C:** The emergence of new infectious diseases. In Stanley NF, Joske RA, ed: Changing disease patterns and human behaviour. London, New York, Academic Press, 1980. p., 231–50.
**Min K** see **Cooney RS**
**Mina VA:** Estimaciones de los niveles, tendencias y diferenciales de la mortalidad infantil y en los primeros años de vida en México, 1940–77. **Demogr Econ** 1981;15(1):85–142
**Minami H:** [American nursing. Outline of the history of the development of studies in the United States. (I)] (Jpn). **Kango** 1982 Apr;34(5):46–54
**Minde K:** The scientific analyst -- a student's perspective. **Can J Psychiatry** 1979 Aug;24(5):498
**Minden K:** The development of early Chinese Communist health policy: health care in the border region, 1936–1949. **Am J Chin Med** 1979 Winter;7(4):299–315
**Mindham RH:** My father knew Adolf Meyer. The currency of Meyer's ideas in British psychiatry. **Br J Psychiatry** 1984 Mar;144:323–5
**Mineau GP:** A specification of marital fertility by parents' age, age at marriage and marital duration. **Demography** 1982 Aug;19(3):335–49
**Mineau GP, Anderton DL, Bean LL, et al:** Evolution différentielle de la fécondité et groupes sociaux religieux: l'exemple de l'Utah au XIXe siècle. **Ann Demogr Hist (Paris)** 1984;:219–36
**Mineau GP** see **Bardet JP**
**Mineau GP** see **Skolnick MH**
**Minęło 25 lat: Pieleg Polozna** 1983;(11):16–7
**Minevich VB** see **Krasik ED**
**Ming Wong** see **Théodoridès J**
**Miniati M:** Lo strumentario di G. A. Brambilla. **Kos** 1984 Feb;1(1):74–6
**Minihan EP** see **Keeney EB**
**Minot WS:** Millay's 'Ungrafted tree'; the problem of the artist as woman. **New Engl Q** 1975;48(2):260–69
**Mintz SW:** Time, sugar and sweetness. **Marx Perspect** 1979–80;2(4):56–73
**Minugh NS:** A brief survey of osteoarthritis outside of modern human populations. **J Am Podiatry Assoc** 1982 May;72(5):217–21
**Minuz F** see **Babini VP**
**Miodoński A** see **Kuś J**
**Miotto D** see **Lenarduzzi G**
**Mirakhmedov UM:** K 60-letiiu kafedry kozhnykh i venericheskikh bolezneĭ Tashkentskogo meditsinskogo instituta. **Vestn Dermatol Venerol** 1981 Nov;(11):74–6
**Mirakhmedov UM** see **Belova LV**
**Mirakian ME:** K istorii nauchnykh issledovaniĭ v oblasti otechestvennoĭ venerologii (XIX vek). **Vestn Dermatol Venerol** 1984 Jul;(7):72–5
**Miranda GE:** Gente de Razón marriage patterns in Spanish and Mexican California: a case study of Santa Barbara and Los Angeles. **South Calif Q** 1981;63(1):1–21
**Mirando EH:** Dr E. M. Wijerama. **Ceylon Med J** 1981 Mar;26(1):5–7
**Mieřejovský P, Bednář B, Elleder M, et al:** Současné zaměření a metodický základ poznávacího procesu v patologii. **Cas Lek Cesk** 1983 Oct 28;122(43):1317–9
**Miringoff ML:** The impact of population policy upon social welfare. **Soc Serv Rev** 1980;54(3):301–16
**Mironov BN:** Traditsionnoye Demograficheskoye povedeniye krest'yan v XIX - nachale XX V. Brachnost', Rozhdayemost', Smertnost', v Rossii i v sssr, (Vishnevskiy, A. G. ed.), Moskva, 1977, p. 83–104.
**Mironţov-Tuculescu V:** Homeopatia--specialitate sau metodă? **Rev Med Interna [Neurol Psihiatr]** 1981 Oct–Dec;26(4):247–9
**Mirouze J:** Les transformations en un quart de siècle de l'insuffisance rénale aiguë. **Nephrologie** 1981;2(1):20–2
**Mirouze J:** L'insuline: hier, aujourd'hui. **Rev Deux Mondes** 1982;10:81–98
**Mirski MB:** [The history of the problem of kidney transplantation in Soviet medicine (Rus). **Orvostort Kozl** 1980;89–91(26 no 1–3):125–36
**Mirskiĭ MB:** Dostizheniia sovetskoĭ transplantologii: nauchnyĭ obzor. Moskva, Vses. nauchno-issl. int med. i mediko-tekhn. informatsii, 1979. 96 p.
**Mirskiĭ MB:** Iu. K. Shimanovskiĭ i ego rol' v razvitii otechestvennoĭ

khirurgii i transplantologii (k 150-letiiu so dnia rozhdeniia). **Klin Khir** 1980 Mar;(3):68-71
**Mirskiĭ MB, Verbitskiĭ VM, Khil'chenko MA:** K 170-letiiu so dnia rozhdeniia A. A. Kitera. **Akush Ginekol (Mosk)** 1983 Sep;(9):72-3
**Mirskiĭ MB:** Khirurgi v épokhu srednevekov'ia. **Klin Med (Mosk)** 1984 Feb;62(2):144-7
**Mirskiĭ MB:** L. Oll'e i ego rol' v razvitii khirurgii i transplantologii (k 150-letiiu so dnia rozhdeniia). **Ortop Travmatol Protez** 1981 Oct;(10):75-6
**Mirskiĭ MB:** N. I. Pirogov--krupneĭshiĭ khirurg XIX veka. **Feldsher Akush** 1981;46(12):37-40
**Mirskiĭ MB:** Novye dokumenty o zhizni i nauchnoĭ deiatel'nosti I. I. Grekova (1867-1941). **Sov Zdravookhr** 1981;(5):64-7
**Mirskiĭ MB:** Pamiatnaia vekha v razvitii sovetskoĭ transplantologii (k 25-letiiu I Vsesoiuznoĭ konferentsii po probleme tkanevoĭ nesovmestimosti i transplantatsii organov i tkaneĭ. **Sov Zdravookhr** 1982;(10):70-2
**Mirskiĭ MB:** Pervaia peresadka pochki v klinike (k 50-letiiu operatsii sovetskogo khirurga Iu. Iu. Voronogo). **Klin Med (Mosk)** 1983 Nov;61(11):147-9
**Mirskiĭ MB, Khil'chenko MA:** Professor A. A. Kiter--pervyĭ uchenik Pirogova (k 170-letiiu so dnia rozhdeniia A. A. Kitera). **Sov Zhdravookhr** 1983;(11):68-71
**Mirskiĭ MB:** Teodor Bil'rot i ego vklad v khirurgiiu (k 150-letiiu so dnia rozhdeniia). **Klin Med (Mosk)** 1980 Sep;58(9):112-4
**Mirskiĭ MB:** V. I. Razumovskiĭ kak istorik khirurgii (k 125-letiiu so dnia rozhdeniia). **Sov Zdravookhr** 1983;5:66-70
**Mirskiĭ MB, Verbitskiĭ VM, Khil'chenko MA:** Vklad A. Ia. Krassovskiĭ v organizatsiiu rodovspomozheniia v Peterburge. **Sov Zdravookhr** 1984;(3):62-4
**Mirskiĭ MB:** Vklad Revedena v transplantologiiu i khirurgiiu. **Khirurgiia (Mosk)** 1980 Jun;(6):109-10
**Mirskiĭ MB:** Vydaiushchiĭsia russkiĭ khirurg E. I. Bogdanovskiĭ (k 150-letiiu so dnia rozhdeniia). **Vestn Khir** 1984 Mar;132(3):143-5
**Mirza GM** see **Retherford RD**
**Mirzaev NL** see **Katsenovich RA**
**Mirzoîan EN:** [Some trends in the development of biology in the XXth century] (Rus). **Istor Biol Issled** 1978:7:3-24
**Misaki K:** Diet in Provence in the late Middle Ages; an analysis according to the Annales School. **Shakai Keizai Shigaku** 1978;44(4):60-80
**Mish IR:** Nursing process--medieval style. **Nurs Forum** 1979;18(2):196-203
**Mishler W, Campbell DB:** The healthy state. Legislative responsiveness to public health care needs in Canada, 1920-1970. **Comp Pol** 1978 Jul;10:479-97
**Mishra SK, Bhatta BR, Bhat PS, et al:** Ideas of integration as a process of evolution of Indian system of medicine in the Medieval period. **Indian J Hist Sci** 1981, reçu 1982;16(1):36-40
**Mishura VI** see **Napalkov NP**
**Misiti R:** Ladygina-Kots and Soviet comparative psychology. **Stor Crit Psicol** 1982 Jun;3(1):109-12
**Misja V, Vejsiu Y:** Aspekte të zhvillimit të popullsisë në rps të shqipërisë. **Studime Hist** 1981;35(3):33-54
**Miskov D** see **Beric B**
**Missotten FE:** Historical review of pharyngo-oesophageal reconstruction after resection for carcinoma of pharynx and cervical oesophagus. **Clin Otolaryngol** 1983 Oct;8(5):345-62
**Mistler J:** Voyageurs d'autrefois. **Nouv Rev Deux Mondes** 1977;(2):265-75;(3):519-27
**Misurcová V:** K 150. výročí institucí předškolní výchovy. **Cesk Pediatr** 1983 Mar;38(3):177-9
**Mit Stücken von Silberteller füllte Zahnarzt kranke Zähne: Niedersachs Zahnarztebl** 1982 Sep;17(9):403
**Mitcham C, Grote J:** Philosophy of technology [and bioethics]. In Reich WT, et al, ed: Encyclopedia of bioethics, v.4. New York, Free Press, 1978. p. 1638-43.
**Mitcham C** see **Durbin PT, ed**
**Mitchell A:** Philippe Ariès and the French way of death. **Fr Hist Stud** 1978;10(4):684-95
**Mitchell FK:** The plague in Cape Town in 1901 and its subsequent establishment as an endemic disease in South Africa. **S Afr Med J** 1983 Jun 29;Spec No:17-9
**Mitchell H:** Politics in the service of knowledge: the debate over the administration of medicine and welfare in late eighteenth-century France. **Soc Hist (Lond)** 1981;6(2):185-207
**Mitchell H:** Politics, power and psychiatry: a review of L'Ordre psychiatrique: l'age d'or de l'aliénisme by Robert Castel. **Int J Law Psychiatry** 1979;2(2):249-61
**Mitchell H:** Rationality and control in French eighteenth-century medical views of the peasantry. **Comp Stud Soc Hist** 1979;21(1):82-112
**Mitchell H:** The passions according to Adam Smith and Pierre-Jean-Georges-Cabanis. Two sciences of man(1). **Soc Soc Hist Med Bull (Lond)** 1979 Dec;25:20-7
**Mitchell H** see **Hildreth ML**
**Mitchell JV:** Burma revisited. **Anaesthesia** 1979 Sep;34(8):811-21
**Mitchell JV** see **Edmonds-Seal J**
**Mitchell M:** History of the British Optical Association, 1895-1978: with additional material covering the founding of the British College of Ophthalmic Opticians (Optometrists) and the liquidation of the B.O.A. [London], The Association and the British Optical Association Foundation, [1982]. 304 p.
**Mitchell PH** see **Cunningham SG**
**Mitchell VL:** Louisiana health and the Civil Works Administration. **Red River Val Hist Rev** 1982;7(1):22-32
**Mitchinson W:** Causes of disease in women: the case of late 19th century English Canada. In Roland CG, ed: Health, disease and medicine. Toronto, Hannah Institute for the History of Medicine, 1984. p. 381-95.
**Mitchinson W:** Gynecological operations on insane women: London, Ontario, 1895-1901. **J Soc Hist** 1982;15(3):467-84
**Mitchinson W:** Gynecological operations on the insane. **Archivaria** 1980 Summer;10:125-44
**Mitchinson W:** Historical attitudes toward women and childbirth. **Atlantis** 1979;4(2 pt 2):13-34
**Mitchinson W:** R. M. Bucke: a Victorian asylum superintendent. **Ont Hist** 1981;73(4):239-54
**Mitchinson W:** The Woman's Christian Temperance Union: a study in organization. **Int J Womens Stud** 1981;4(2):143-56
**Mitic I:** Utjecaj kopnene trgovine na osnivanje dubrovačke karantene u XIV. In Radovi sa Medunarodnog simpozija u povodu sestote obljetnice Dubrovacke karantene. Dubrovnik, 29 i 30. rujna 1977. Zagreb, 1980. p. 85-90.
**Mito M:** [Lessons in Oriental medicine: its application in nursing] (Jpn). **Kango** 1981 May;33(6):26-30
**Mitra R:** Bakula, a reputed drug of Ayurveda, its history, uses in Indian medicine. **Indian J Hist Sci** 1981;16(2):169-80
**Mitrofanov VG:** K 90-letiiu so dnia rozhdeniia Mikhaila Semenovicha Lisitsyna. **Vestn Khir** 1983 May;130(5):141-2
**Mitrovic M:** Uticaj zdravsvenih prilika na privredni razvitak Pančeva 1792-1815. **Zb Istor** 1978;18:109-24
**Mitscherlich A:** Probleme und Standort der Psychoanalyse. **Universitas (Stuttg)** 1982;37(6):575-80
**Mitscherlich A:** Vor etwa 100 Jahren (7). Die Replantation und die Transplantation der Zähne. **Zentralbl Chir** 1979;104(9):612-4
**Mitsuhashi S:** [Recollection of my research activities in microbiology] (Jpn). **Nippon Saikingaku Zasshi** 1984 Jul;39(4):733-7
**Mitsura DI:** Vsegda riadom s voinom. **Med Sestra** 1981 Oct;40(10):58-62
**Mitteilung zur Tschirch Biographie: Schweiz Apoth Ztg** 1979;117:558 (continued irregularly here and in Pharm. Ztg, Dtsch Apoth Ztg, and Oesterr. Apoth Ztg)
**Mittelmann M** see **Menczer LF**
**Mitterauer M, Kagan A:** Russian and Central European family structures: a comparative view. **J Fam Hist** 1982 Spring;7(1):103-31
**Mitterstiller S:** 100 Jahre chirurgische Klinik in Innsbruck. **Tirol Heimat** 1970;:31-2
**Mitterstiller S:** 100 Jahre Chirurgische Klinik in Innsbruck. **Tirol Heimat** 1970;34:17-38
**Mittl RN** see **Ryan SJ**
**Mittler E** see **Bernus A von, ed**
**Mittwoch U:** Whistling maids and crowing hens--hermaphroditism in folklore and biology. **Perspect Biol Med** 1981 Summer;24(4):595-606
**Mitzman A:** Sartres Flaubert. **Psyche (Stuttg)** 1981 Mar;35(3):268-98
**Mitzman A:** The unstrung Orpheus: Flaubert's youth and the psycho-social origins of art for art's sake. **Psychohist Rev** 6(1):27-42, Summer 77
**Mitzscherling R:** Die Entwicklung der Allgemeinmedizin in der Deutschen Demokratischen Republik. **Z Arztl Fortbild (Jena)** 1983;77(6):268-71
**Miura F, Soma K, Hatate M:** [The orthodontic observation of ancient Peruvian calvaria--orthopedically induced deformity of the skull]. (Jpn) **Kokubyo Gakkai Zasshi** 1979 Sep;46(3):220-7
**Miura T, Richter J:** Changes in the seasonal distribution of births in Görlitz, Germany, during the period between 1657 and 1816. **Hum Biol** 1981 Feb;53(1):15-22
**Mixa J:** Neues über die Krankheit Wallensteins. **Medizinhist J** 1983;18(3):256-9
**Miyai M** see **Fujimori K**
**Miyamoto S:** Mori Ogai no Igakushiso (The medical thought of Ogai Mori). Tokyo, Keiso-shobo, 1979. iii, 264 p.
**Miyasato K, Ishihara T, Oshima K:** [Impression of the Symposium on the History of Obstetrics] (Jpn). **Josanpu Zasshi** 1983 Jul;37(7):566-77
**Miyasita S:** An historical analysis of Chinese drugs in the treatment of hormonal diseases, goitre and diabetes mellitus. **Am J Chin Med** 1980 Spring-Summer;8(1-2):17-25
**Miyasita S:** Honzo no'rui' gainen. (Categorization concepts in Chinese materia medica.) **Tohogaku** 1976;51:104-13
**Miyasita S:** Son Shibo no keikenbô. (Sun Ssu-mo's empirical remedies.) **Kampo No Rinsho** 1973;20:544-7
**Miyazaki M:** [On 'Chindoku' a toxicant in the oriental tradition] (Jpn). **Yakushigaku Zasshi** 1983;18(2):101-6
**Miziak AN** see **Burdov VS**
**Mkandla M** see **Lovel H**
**Mkrtchian LN:** Osnovnye étapy razvitiia onkologii i rentgenologii v Armianskoĭ SSR. **Vopr Onkol** 1982;28(12):20-4
**Mlosek K:** W 50 rocznicę polskiego czasopiśmiennictwa radiologicznego. **Pol Przegl Radiol** 1979 Nov-Dec;43(6):339-43
**Möbius W** see **Kyank H**
**Mocek R:** Robert Koch und die geistige Situation seiner Zeit. **Wiss Beitr Martin Luther Univ Halle Wittenberg** 1983;5-R80:15-29
**Mocek R:** Wilhelm Roux--Hans Driesch. Zur Geschichte der Entwicklungsphysiologie der Tiere ['Entwicklungsmechanik']. Jena, Fischer, 1974. 229 p. (Biographien bedeutender Biologen, Band 1).
**Moch LP:** Marriage, migration, and urban demographic structure: a case from France in the Belle Epoque. **J Fam Hist** 1981 Spring;6(1):70-88
**Mochmann H:** Biographische und literarische Notizen über Robert Koch aus Anlass des 100. Jahrestages -- 24. März 1982 -- seiner Bekanntgabe der Entdeckung des Tuberkelbazillus. **Padiatr Grenzgeb**

1982;21(2):83–112
**Mochmann H:** Die Entdeckung des Tuberkelbazillus vor 100 Jahren. **Kinderarztl Prax** 1982 Mar;50(3):113–6
**Mochmann H, Kohler W:** The clarification of the etiology of Asiatic cholera by the German cholera commission under the direction of Robert Koch in the year 1883--1884. **Indian J Public Health** 1983 Jan–Mar;27(1):6–20
**Mochmann H** see **Koehler W**
**Mociño JM:** Disertación de la fiebre epidémica que padeció Cádiz, Sevilla y la mayor parte de Andalucía desde el año 1800 y principalmente Ecixa el año 1804. México, Sociedad Mexicana de Historia y Filosofía de la Medicina, 1982. xxvi, 234 p.
**Mock HK** see **Rihm A**
**Modell AH** see **Goldberg A, ed**
**Modell J:** An ecology of family decisions: suburbanization, schooling, and fertility in Philadelphia, 1880–1920. **J Urban Hist** 1980;6(4):397–417
**Models for action: J Public Health Policy** 1980;1(2):103–9
**Modern midwives: MD** 1978 Oct;22(10):53–5
**Modestin J:** 30 Jahre Neuroleptika--Zeit zur kritischen Auseinandersetzung. **Dtsch Med Wochenschr** 1983 Sep 23;108(38):1446–51
**Modgil S, Modgil C, ed:** Jean Piaget. Consensus and controversy. New York, Praeger, 1982. 446 p.
**Modgil C, ed** see **Modgil S**
**Modig M:** Deutsches Apotheken-Museum i Heidelberg. **Sydsven Medicinhist Sallsk Arsskr** 1984;21:15–26
**Modig M:** Ex-libris de pharmaciens suédois. **Rev Hist Pharm (Paris)** 1980 Sep;27(246):162–4
**Modig M:** Karl XII:s siste fältskär. **Sydsven Medicinhist Sallsk Arsskr** 1983;:77–86
**Modig M:** Kungliga hus--och reseapotek. **Livrustkammaren** 1980;15(1):1–16
**Modig M:** Pharmacy ruins from 1600's excavated in Stockholm. **Pharm Hist** 1983;25(3):137–41
**Modig M:** Raritet från Rörstrand. Från luktvatten till syrgaskuddar–en inhalationshistorik. **Draco Med** 1983;24(7):14–5
**Modig M:** The allegory of Christ in a pharmacy. **Pharm Hist** 1984;26(1):44–5
**Modlin HC:** Contributions of the Menninger School of Psychiatry to psychiatric education. **Bull Menninger Clin** 1983 May;47(3):253–61
**Modlin HC:** Traumatic neurosis and other injuries. **Psychiatr Clin North Am** 1983 Dec;6(4):661–82
**Modlin M:** A history of urinary stone. **S Afr Med J** 1980 Oct 18;58(18):652–5
**Modrzewska K, Böök JA:** Sulla mortalita in un isolato della Svezia del nord, 1875–1975. **Genus** 1981;37(3–4):221–6
**Moe C:** Yellow fever in 19th century New Orleans: Necropolis of the South. Monticello, Illinois, Vance Bibliographies, 1979. (Public Administration Series: no. P–375).
**Moe GK:** Oscillating concepts in arrhythmia research; a personal account. **Int J Cardiol** 1984 Jan;5(1):109–13
**Moe K:** Should the Nazi research data be cited? **Hastings Cent Rep** 1984 Dec;14(6):5–7
**Moeller DD:** The odyssey of guaiac. **Am J Gastroenterol** 1984 Mar;79(3):236–7
**Moerchel J:** Sauerbruch und die Mayos. **Dtsch Med Wochenschr** 1980 May 9;105(19):697–9
**Moerchel J:** Simon Baruch (1840–1921) und die öffentliche Gesundheitspflege in New York. **Medizinhist J** 1982;17(1/2):138–47
**Moerchel J:** Soziale Bedingtheit von Gesundheit und Krankheit in Vergangenheit und Gegenwart. **Off Gesundheitswes** 1980 Nov;42(11):893–901
**Moerchel J:** The introduction of thoracic surgery into America. **Clio Med** 1980;15(1/2):67–73
**Moerman AK:** Daniël Joncktys--Dordts dokter en dichter. **Kwartaal Teken** 1979;5(3):5–10
**Moermans JP, Bovy A, De Mey A:** Aspects historiques des lambeaux libres. **Acta Chir Belg** 1982 May–Jun;82(3):213–8
**Moersch E:** Psychiatrie in Afrika zwischen Tradition und Moderne. **Psyche (Stuttg)** 1984 Aug;38(8):673–95
**Moes RJ:** The elusive Dr. Burrough: Alta California's first physician. **South Calif Q** 1982;64(4):265–80
**Mogilevskaia LN** see **Krasil'shchikov MI**
**Mohaghegh M:** The title of a work of Razi with reference to al–Tin al–Nishaburi. In: International Symposium for the History of Arabic Science, 1st, University of Aleppo, 1976. Proceedings. Aleppo, Syria, 1976. Papers in European Languages, Vol. II. p. 338–40.
**Mohanty JN** see **Spicker SF, ed**
**Mohler SR** see **Tipton DA**
**Mohlin B, et al:** The frequency of malocclusion and the craniofacial morphology in a medieval population in southern Sweden. **Ossa** 1978;5:57–84
**Mohr H** see **Lorenz K, ed**
**Mohr HJ:** Medizinische und legislatorische Probleme der inneren Leichenschau. **Pathologe** 1981 Jun;2(3):134–43
**Möhsen JK:** Beiträge zur Geschichte der Wissenschaften in der Marke Brandenburg; Leben Leonhard Thurneissers zum Thurn. München, Fritsch, 1976. 226 p.
**Moikin IuV, Tarasenko NIu, Anan'ev BV:** Znachenie naslediia I. M. Sechenova dlia razvitiia otechestvennoĭ fiziologii i gigieny truda. **Gig Tr Prof Zabol** 1980 Mar;(3):1–5
**Moĭkin IuV** see **Tarasenko NIu**
**Moĭkin IuV** see **Vorontsova EI**
**Moiseeva NI:** The role of I M. Sechenov's ideas in development of modern views on time perception. **Hum Physiol** 1979 Nov–Dec;5(5):723–7
**Moiso F** see **Hasler L, ed**
**Mok B** see **Cho LJ**
**Mokrovskaia AA** see **Vlasova NA**
**Molchanov VV, Kulikova TN:** K 70–letiiu kafedry nervnykh bolezneĭ Saratovskogo meditsinskogo instituta. **Zh Nevropatol Psikhiatr** 1983;83(9):1399–401
**Moldenhauer W:** Aufbau der Röntgendiagnostik an der Wilhelm–Pieck–Universität Rostock in den letzten 30 Jahren. **Wiss Z Univ Rostock** 1979;28(1–2):25–7
**Moldow G:** 'For women, by women': women's dispensaries and clinics in Washington, 1882–1900. **Rec Columb Hist Soc** 1980;50:290–308
**Moler CL:** The certification of radiological equipment specialists: a historical review. **Radiol Manage** 1980 Spring;2(4):9–13
**Molin C:** Karolinska sjukhusets avdelning för tand--och käksjukdomar--en tillbakablick efter fyrtio år. **Nord Medicinhist Arsb** 1981;:183–92
**Molina–Negro P:** Le rôle des neurostimulateurs dans le traitement de la douleur chronique rebelle. **Union Med Can** 1980 Jan;109(1):41–54
**Molinier A:** Une arme contre la famine: les greniers à blé du XVIIIe siècle. **Histoire** 1979;17:70–2
**Molino–Negro P:** Jules Hardy M.D. **Surg Neurol** 1984 Aug;22(2):109–12
**Moll J:** Das chirurgische Erbe. Ludwik Rydygier (1850–1920). **Zentralbl Chir** 1983;108(23):1532–5
**Mollaret HH:** Contribution à la connaissance des relations entre Koch et Pasteur. **NTM** 1983;20(1):57–65
**Mollaret P:** La découverte, par Alphonse Laveran de l'agent du paludisme. Constantine, 6 Novembre 1880. **Nouv Presse Med** 1980 Nov 1;9(41):3055–63
**Mollat M** see **Imbert J**
**Mollenhauer D:** Die Haeckel–Rezeption durch die Botanik. **Medizinhist J** 1980;15(3):305–36
**Möller HJ:** Die Begriffe 'Reizbarkeit' und 'Reiz': Konstanz und Wandel ihres Bedeutungsgehaltes sowie die Problematik ihrer exakten Definition. Stuttgart, Fischer, 1975. viii, 104 p. (Medizin in Geschichte und Kultur, 11).
**Møller–Christensen V** see **Hart GD, ed**
**Molleson T** see **Whittaker DK**
**Mollison PL:** The introduction of acidified citrate–glucose solutions as red cell preservatives. **Vox Sang** 1983;45(6):449–50
**Molmár ES:** Birth control, abortion and public opinion. **New Hung Q** 1982;23(85):125–30
**Molodtsova LI:** O chislennosti naseleniia knr. **Nar Azii Afriki** 1975;(4):81–91
**Moloney F, Worthington P:** The origin of the Le Fort I maxillary osteotomy: Cheever's operation. **J Oral Surg** 1981 Oct;39(10):731–4
**Molotkov VN:** Rol' Kievskogo ordena Trudovogo Krasnogo Znameni nauchno–issledovatel'skogo instituta tuberkuleza i grudnoĭ khirurgii im. F. G. Ianovskogo v razvitii ftiziatrii i pul'monologii. **Probl Tuberk** 1982 Dec;(12):18–22
**Mommaerts WF:** Gondolatok az izomkutatás történetéröl (A. Katschalsky–Katzir professzor emlékezetére). **Orv Hetil** 1983 Oct 2;124(40):2436–40
**Monaco GP** see **Markle GE**
**Monaghan F, Corcos A:** On the origins of the Mendelian laws. **J Hered** 1984 Jan–Feb;75(1):67–9
**Monckeberg F:** Lucha contra la desnutrición del niño en Chile, 1952–1977. **Rev Med Chil** 1977 Oct;105(10):687–95
**Mond HG, Sloman JG, Edwards RH:** The first pacemaker. **PACE** 1982 Mar;5(2):278–82
**Money J:** The genealogical descent of sexual psychoneuroendocrinology from sex and health theory: the eighteenth to the twentieth centuries. **Psychoneuroendocrinology** 1983;8(4):391–400
**Money R:** Early work on penicillin. **Med J Aust** 1982 May 1;1(9):367
**Monk BE:** Thomas Dover, physician and pirate. **J R Coll Physicians Lond** 1982 Jan;16(1):60–1
**Monkiewicz W, Kretowski J:** Los chorych psychicznie, kalek i starców w okupowanym Białostockiem. **Przegl Lek** 1984;41(1):80–4
**Monnier A:** Données récentes sur la population du Vietnam. **Population** 1981;36(3):610–19
**Monod H:** Evocation de d'Arsonval. **J Belge Med Phys Rehabil** 1981;4(3):103–15
**Monod H, Valentin M:** Les précurseurs de l'ergonomie. **Ergonomics** 1979 Jun;22(6):673–80
**Monod T, Hureau JC:** Un pharmacien niçois, Antoine Risso (1777–1845), sa vie et son oeuvre. In their: Antoine Risso, 1777–1845. Nice, Editions du Centre d'Etudes Méditerranéennes, 1977. pp. 9–28 (Annales du Muséum d'Histoire Naturelle de Nice, V, 1977).
**Monod–Broca P:** Anselme Schwartz 1872–1957. **Chirurgie** 1984;110(1):11–21
**Monod–Broca P:** Henri Redon, 1899–1974. **Chirurgie** 1983;109(1):15–22
**Monod–Broca P:** Henry Delagenière, 1858–1930. **Chirurgie** 1982;108(1):17–25
**Monod–Broca P:** Jacques Leveuf (1885–1948). **Chirurgie** 1980 Jan;106(1):18–25
**Monod–Broca P:** Louis Michon, 1892–1973. **Chirurgie** 1981;107(1):13–22
**Monod–Broca P:** Paul Broca (1824–1880). Le chirurgien, l'homme. **Bull Acad Natl Med (Paris)** 1980;164(6):536–44
**The monofluorophosphate story: Br Dent J** 1981 May 19;150(10):285–6
**Monory B:** Euthanasia – a pro és contra nézetek tükrében. **Orvostort Kozl** 1982;28(1–3):107–26

**Monroziès M:** Au service des femmes. Les services de gynécologie et d'obstétrique de l'hôpital de la Grave à Toulouse, 250 ans d'histoire 1729–1919. Toulouse, Privat, 1980. 88 p.
**Monsées Y:** 'Klinisches Ambulatorium' von Andor Dudits, 1890. **Medizinhist J** 1981;16(4):454–8
**Monserrat JT:** Medicina y médicos: Mallorca: siglo XIX. Palma de Mallorca, El autor, 1976. 98 p.
**Monson MC:** The dirty little secret behind our drug laws. **Reason** 1980;12(7):48–52
**Montag M** see **Rihm A**
**Montagne M** see **Vogt DD**
**Montague L:** Ambassadors of the king. **Nurs Times** 1983 Dec 14–20;79(50):57–60
**Montaña MT** see **Valverde JL**
**Montanari L, Ponci R:** I prezzi delle specialità medicinali in Italia--evoluzione storica della disciplina dei prezzi dei farmaci--attuale metodo per la determinazione dei prezzi delle specialità medicinali. **Farmaco [Prat]** 1982 Nov;37(11):343–64
**Montandon D:** History of plastic surgery of the orbital region. In S. J. Aston, et al., ed: Third international symposium of plastic and reconstructive surgery of the eye and adnexa. Baltimore, London, Williams & Wilkins, 1982. p. 2–10.
**Montandon D** see **Ayer E**
**Montarnal** see **Nardoux M**
**Monteil RA, Knoche JF:** Etude de l'évolution du terme odontome depuis sa création jusqu'au concept anatomo-patholgique actuel. **Actual Odontostomatol (Paris)** 1980;(132):583–95
**Monteiro LA:** Population policy and the press: the example of Brazil. **Contemp Rev** 1975;226(1309):76–81
**Montella M:** La malattia del Legionario: analisi descrittiva di un nuovo evento morboso. **Arch Monaldi** 1978 Sep–Dec;33(5–6):35–40
**Montenegro TH:** A tuberculose na vida e obra de Manuel Bandeira. **Interam Rev Bibliogr** 1969;19(3):278–300
**Monter EW:** Sodomy and heresy in early modern Switzerland. **J Homosex** 1980–81 Fall–Winter;6(1–2):41–55
**Monter EW:** Witchcraft in France and Switzerland: the borderlands during the Reformation. Ithaca, Cornell University Press, 1976. 232 p.
**Montès F:** La réinsertion professionnelle et sociale des handicapés. **Etudes (Fr)** 1981;354(4):467–83
**Montiel L:** El escritor y su enfermedad: patobiografía de Thomas Mann. In International Congress of the History of Medicine, 27th, Barcelona, 1980. Actas. Barcelona, Acadèmia de Ciències Mèdiques de Catalunya i Balears, 1981. p. 586–91.
**Montiel L:** El psicoanálisis en la Montaña mágica. In International Congress of the History of Medicine, 27th, Barcelona, 1980. Actas. Barcelona, Acadèmia de Ciències Mèdiques de Catalunya i Balears, 1981. p. 116–20.
**Montiel L:** Freud y el psicoanálisis en dos conferencias de Thomas Mann. In International Congress of the History of Medicine, 27th, Barcelona, 1980. Actas. Barcelona, Acadèmia de Ciències Mèdiques de Catalunya i Balears, 1981. p. 111–5.
**Montiel L:** La enfermedad como símbolo: la peste en la obra de Albert Camus. **Asclepio** 1983;35:171–6
**Montiel L:** La 'filosofía de la fisiologia' de Federico Schiller. **Asclepio** 1981;33:163–81
**Montiel L:** La influencia de la ideologia en la clinica medica del S. XIX español. La obra de Tomas Santero y Moreno (1817–1888). **Asclepio** 1981;33:127–42
**Montiel Llorente LE:** La ciencia medica en 'La montaña magica' de Thomas Mann. **Asclepio** 1980;32:271–85
**Montorsi W, Pezzuoli G, Guzzon V:** Influenza della farmacologia di Emilio Trabucchi nelle discipline chirurgiche e parachirurgiche. **Minerva Med** 1982 May 7;73(19):1255–68
**Montville JV** see **Davidson WD**
**Moogk PN:** Henri Lamarre. In Dictionary of Canadian biography, 1701 to 1740. Volume 2, 1969. p. 339–40.
**Moogk PN:** Simon Soupiran. In Dictionary of Canadian biography, 1701 to 1740. Volume 2, 1969. p. 613–4.
**Møoller-Christensen V** see **Habrich C**
**Mooney EC:** The white plague. **Am Heritage** 1979;30(2):54–9
**Mooney J:** Cherokee theory and practice of medicine. **J Cherokee Stud** 1982;7(1):25–9
**Mooney LR:** A middle English verse compendium of astrological medicine. **Med Hist** 1984 Oct;28(4):406–19
**Moore AF:** A review of the renin-angiotensin system: historical and methodological perspectives. **Methods Find Exp Clin Pharmacol** 1979;1(1):23–44
**Moore AM:** Sir Hugh Lett. In Dictionary of national biography, 1961–1970. Suppl. 8, 1981. p. 650–1.
**Moore C, Winer JL:** Dr. Peterson E. Harrison: pioneer traiblazer for mental health in West Texas. **West Tex Hist Assoc Yearb** 1979;55:49–58
**Moore DF:** The history and development of the BCG. **Practitioner** 1983 Feb;227(1376):i–iii
**Moore DT** see **Kark RM**
**Moore FD:** The changing mission and status of surgery 1780 to 1980. **Arch Surg** 1983 Sep;118(9):1013–8
**Moore FD:** Transplantation--a perspective. **Transplant Proc** 1980 Dec;12(4):539–50
**Moore FD:** Two hundred years ago: origins and early years of the Harvard Medical School. **Ann Surg** 1982 Nov;196(5):525–35
**Moore FD:** Zabdiel Boylston and colonial surgery. American surgery and public health in the early 18th century. **Bull Am Coll Surg** 1983 May;68(5):13–7
**Moore FD** see **Zook CJ**
**Moore JA** see **Lewontin RC**
**Moore JG, Krotoszynski BK, O'Neill HJ:** Fecal odorgrams. A method for partial reconstruction of ancient and modern diets. **Dig Dis Sci** 1984 Oct;29(10):907–11
**Moore JG** see **El-Najjar MY**
**Moore JT:** Battle for the Medical College: physicians, politicians, and the courts, 1882–1883. **Va Cavalcade** 1982;31(3):158–67
**Moore MJ:** Social work and social welfare: the organization of philanthropic resources in Britain 1900–1914. **J Br Stud** 1977;16:85–104
**Moore MJ** see **Patterson JN**
**Moore PV, Williamson GC:** Health promotion. Evolution of a concept. **Nurs Clin North Am** 1984 Jun;19(2):195–206
**Moore RD:** Zane Grey: dentist, novelist, baseball player, outdoors man. **Tic** 1982 Jul;41(7):5–7
**Moore RL** see **Maurizi AR**
**Moore TJ:** Credit for describing Cushing's syndrome. **N Engl J Med** 1983 Sep 22;309(12):735
**Moore WJ:** The role of sugar in the aetiology of dental caries. 1. Sugar and the antiquity of dental caries. **J Dent** 1983 Sep;11(3):189–90
**Moore WJ** see **Hart GD, ed**
**Moore WW** see **Elizondo RS**
**Moorefield WG** see **McBryde AM**
**Moorhead TF:** Chirurgia, medicina, dentrifricium. A brief trip into antiquity. **Br Dent J** 1983 May 21;154(10):340–2
**Mooring PK:** Residency training. **MD** 1978 Jul;22(7):23, 27
**Mora G:** Gregory Zilboorg. In Dictionary of American Biography, Suppl. 6, 1956–1960. p. 724–5, 1980.
**Mora G:** Mind-body concepts in the Middle Ages: part II. The Moslem influence, the great theological systems, and cultural attitudes toward the mentally ill in the late Middle Ages. **J Hist Behav Sci** 1980 Jan;16(1):58–72
**Mora G:** 1979 anniversaries. **Am J Psychiatry** 1980 Jan;137(1):56–60
**Mora C** see **Blain D**
**Mora G** see **Wallace ER**
**Mora X:** La medicina pre y post Colombina aplicada en la herborística. In Ureña Morales, Gabriel, ed. Memoria del Congreso Sobre el Mundo Centroamericano de su Tiempo: V. Centenario de Gonzalo Fernández de Oviedo. Nicoya, Costa Rica, Comisión Nac. Organizadora, 1980. p. 433–9.
**Mora Merida JA:** Freud: De la libido al eros. La coherencia del discurso freudiano. Malaga, Universidad de Malaga, 1979. 284 p.
**Morain WD:** History and plastic surgery: systems of recovering our past. In Romm S, ed: Symposium on historical perspectives of plastic surgery. Philadelphia, Saunders, 1983. p. 595–601.
**Morain WO** see **Romm S, ed**
**Morales Meneses J:** La congregación y Hospital de San Pedro. **Salud Publica Mex** 1984 Mar–Apr;26(2):190–4
**Morales y Morales A:** Francisco Antonio Solano, boticario revalidado. Asentista del Hospital Militar de Santa Cruz de Tenerife (1764–1771). **Bol Soc Esp Hist Farm** 1980 Mar–Jun;3(121–2):109–38
**Moran HM:** Looking back: Lister. **Lamp** 1981 Mar;38(3):57–60
**Moran JA** see **Gatz M**
**Moran PA** see **Hare EH**
**Morandi M, Eisenbud M:** Carbon monoxide exposure in New York City: a historical overview. **Bull NY Acad Med** 1980 Nov–Dec;56(9):817–28
**Morange M:** L'oeuvre scientifique de Jacques Monod. **Fundam Sci** 1982;3:396–404
**Morange M:** Schrödinger et la biologie moléculaire. **Fundam Sci** 1983;4(3/4):219–33
**Morani AD** see **Romm S, ed**
**Morantz RM:** Bertha van Hoosen. In: Notable American women. The modern period. Cambridge, Mass., Belknap-Harvard Univ. Press, 1980. 4:706–7.
**Morantz RM:** Feminism, professionalism, and germs: the thought of Mary Putnam Jacobi and Elizabeth Blackwell. **Amer Q** 1982;34:459–78
**Morantz RM, Pomerleau CS, Fenichel CH, ed:** In her own words: oral histories of women physicians. Westport, Conn., Greenwood, 1982. xiv, 284 p. (Contributions in Medical History, 8).
**Morantz RM, Zschoche S:** Professionalism, feminism, and gender roles: a comparative study of nineteenth-century medical therapeutics. **J Am Hist** 1980 Dec;67(3):568–88
**Morantz RM:** Women in the medical profession: why were there so few? **Rev Am Hist** 1978;6(2):163–70
**Moraru I** see **Babes V**
**Moravcová M** see **Moravec R**
**Moravec R, Tichý M, Moravcová M, et al:** Z dejín chirurgie v Bratislave. Profesor Kostlivý a začiatky chirurgickej kliniky na LFUK v Bratislava] **Rozhl Chir** 1984 Jul;63(7):526–31
**Moravia S:** The capture of the invisible. For a (pre)history of psychology in eighteenth-century France. **J Hist Behav Sci** 1983 Oct;19(4):370–8
**Moravia S:** The Enlightenment and the sciences of man. **Hist Sci** 1980 Dec;18(42 pt 4):247–68
**Morawski J** see **Zmudzki A**
**Moray G, Moray N:** A note on the basis of reversed perspective. **Perception** 1982;10(6):703–5
**Moray N** see **Moray G**
**Mordacq C:** Ecoles et soignants d'hier à demain, ou les sources du renouvellement d'une institution d'enseignement professionnel. **Krankenpflege (Bern)** 1981 Feb;(2):15–9

**Mordasini ER** see **Bernische Liga gegen die Tuberkulose 1930–1980**
**Mordier JP:** Les débuts de la psychanalyse en France 1895–1926. Paris, Francois Maspero, 1981. 275 p.
**Mordovtsev VN** see **Skripkin IuK**
**Moreau R** see **Bonneau E**
**Moreda VP:** The intensity of the mortality crises in Spain: an outline of their regional differences over time. In Charbonneau H, Larose A, ed: The great mortalities: methodological studies of demographic crises in the past. Liège, Belgium, Ordina Editions, 1980. p. 179–98.
**Morehead J:** Government involvement in programs for the handicapped. **Ser Libr** 1982;7(2):7–16
**Morehead RP:** The contribution of a great man to Wake Forest University and its Bowman Gray School of Medicine--Tinsley R. Harrison, M.D. **NC Med J** 1983 Dec;44(12):809–11
**Morel F** see **Robin ED, ed**
**Morel MF:** Health and illness in traditional rural France in the 18th and 19th centuries: the example of wet-nurses. **Soc Soc Hist Med Bull (Lond)** 1983 Dec;33:24–6
**Morel MF:** L'élevage des nourrissons dans la France d'autrefois XVIIIe–XIXe siècles. **Neuropsychiatr Enfance Adolesc** 1982 Apr–May;30(4–5):271–3
**Morel MF:** Les parents devant la maladie de leurs enfants dans la France moderne (XVIe–XVIIIe siècles). **Asclepio** 1983;35:359–74
**Morel MF:** Madame Roland, sa fille et les médecins: prime éducation et médicalisation à l'époque des lumières. **Ann Bretagne** 1979;86(3):211–9
**Morel MF:** Mère, enfant, médecin: la médicalisation de la petite enfance en France (XVIIIe–XIXe siècles). In Imhof AE, ed: Mensch und Gesundheit in der Geschichte. Husum, Matthiesen, 1980. p. 301–13.
**Morel MF:** Mères et nourrices au XVIIIe siècle: les soins aux jeunes enfants. **Penelope** 1981;(5):29–32
**Morel MF** see **Forster R**
**Moreno Gonzalez JP, Gonzalez Iglesias J:** Sorapan de Rieros y la odontologia. **Bol Inf Dent (Madr)** 1979 Sep–Oct;(302):37–44
**Morer G:** La découverte de Charles Krafft. **Hist Sci Med** 1984;18(1):33–40
**Morer G:** Naissance d'un vocable. **Hist Sci Med** 1984;18(2):165–71
**Moretti G, Bosredon J:** Le paludisme nautique tropical de la côte d'Afrique, hier et aujourd'hui. In: Congrès National des Sociétés Savantes, 104e, Bordeaux, 1979. Comptes Rendus. Paris, 1979. Section des Sciences, Fasc. IV. p. 309–17.
**Morfologiia v SSSR: Arkh Anat Gistol Embriol** 1982 Dec;83(12):9–35
**Morgan AH:** Is there a doctor in the house? or for the house? **Rev Am Hist** 1980;8(1):129–33
**Morgan CD** see **Anderson RJ**
**Morgan GR:** 'Sugar bowls' (Clematis hirsutissima): a horse restorative of the Nez Perces. **J Ethnopharmacol** 1981 Jul;4(1):117–20
**Morgan JG:** The place of nickel in the history of industrial disease. In J. Cule, ed: Wales and medicine. London, British Society for the History of Medicine, 1975. p. 68–74.
**Morgan JP:** The first reported case of electrical stimulation of the human brain. **J Hist Med Allied Sci** 1982 Jan;37(1):51–64
**Morgan K:** No boots in Sicily. **Nurs Mirror** 1983 Nov 2;157(18):42
**Morgan KO:** Dr. Christopher Addison and social reform. **Soc Soc Hist Med Bull (Lond)** 1981 Dec;29:21–5
**Morgan MW:** The Maddox classification of vergence eye movements. **Am J Optom Physiol Opt** 1980;57:537–9
**Morgan N:** The development of biochemistry in England through botany and the brewing industry (1870–1890). **Hist Philos Life Sci** 1980;2(1):141–66
**Morgan N:** William Dobinson Halliburton, F.R.S. (1860–1931) – pioneer of British biochemistry? **Notes Rec R Soc Lond** 1983 Aug;38(1):129–45
**Morgan RF:** The Fort McHenry General Hospital for plastic and maxillofacial surgery. **Plast Reconstr Surg** 1983 Aug;72(2):255–9
**Morgan RF** see **Nichter LS**
**Morgan RF** see **Romm S, ed**
**Morgan RF** see **Sargent LA**
**Morgan RJ:** William Smith. In Dictionary of Canadian biography, 1801 to 1820. Volume 5, 1983. p. 766–7.
**Morgan SP:** Parity-specific fertility intentions and uncertainty: the United States, 1970 to 1976. **Demography** 1982 Aug;19(3):315–34
**Morgan WG:** Mark Twain: behaviorist. **J Behav Ther Exp Psychiatry** 1984 Jun;15(2):99
**Morgan WT:** Arthur Wormall. In Dictionary of national biography, 1961–1970. Suppl. 8, 1981. p. 1110–1.
**Morgan HW, ed:** Yesterday's addicts. American society and drug abuse 1865–1920. Norman, University of Oklahoma Press, 1974. viii, 220 p. Collected documents.
**Morgan-Witts M** see **Thomas G**
**Morgenstern L:** The Virchow–Troisier node: a historical note. **Am J Surg** 1979 Nov;138(5):703
**Morgenstern S:** Henri Dunant and the Red Cross. **Bull NY Acad Med** 1979 Nov;55(10):949–56
**Morgenstern S:** Henri Dunant and the Red Cross. **Bull NY Acad Med** 1981 May;57(4):311–26
**Morgon A:** L'oto-rhino-laryngologie et la communication humaine. **J Fr Otorhinolaryngol** 1982 Jun;31(6):405–8
**Moriarty KM, Alagna SW, Lake CR:** Psychopharmacology. An historical perspective. **Psychiatr Clin North Am** 1984 Sep;7(3):411–33
**Moriceau JM:** Les crises démographiques dans le sud de la région parisienne de 1560 à 1670 **Ann Demogr Hist (Paris)** 1980;:105–23
**Morimoto I** see **Iwai H**
**Morimura K:** Advancement of the scientific character of Chinese materia medica from Ta-kuan pen-ts'ao to Pen-ts'ao kang-mu. In: International Congress for the History of Science, 14th, Tokyo, Kyoto, 1974. Proceedings. Tokyo, 1975. 3:323–326.
**Morin J:** Liveright Piuze. In Dictionary of Canadian biography, 1801 to 1820. Volume 5, 1983. p. 676.
**Morineau M** see **Forster R**
**Morison RS:** Is there a biological person? **Milbank Mem Fund Q** 1983 Winter;61(1):3–18
**Morison RS:** The Foundation interest. In Stevenson LG, ed: A celebration of medical history. Baltimore, Johns Hopkins University Press, 1982. (The Henry E. Sigerist supplements to the Bulletin of the History of Medicine; new ser., no. 6). p. 212–21.
**Morison RS** see **Trends in biomedical research, 1901–1976**
**Morissette L** see **Brunel G**
**Moritz AR:** Classical mistakes in forensic pathology. **Am J Forensic Med Pathol** 1981 Dec;2(4):299–308
**Moriyama N:** [Controversies on the Kul-Oba vase and its relation to the ancient Scythian dentistry (author's transl)] (Jpn). **Shikwa Gakuho** 1980 Apr;80(4):597–602
**Moriyama N, Takazoe I:** The historical relationship between Japanese dentistry and the Fédération Dentaire Internationale. **Bull Hist Dent** 1984 Oct;32(2):104–8
**Moriyama N:** The origin of the immediate root-canal filling. **Bull Hist Dent** 1982 Apr;30(1):34–9
**Morley D** see **Lovel H**
**Morley P, Wallis R, et al:** Culture and curing. Anthropological perspectives on traditional medical beliefs and practices. London, Owen, 1978. vii, 190 p.
**Morman ET:** Clinical pathology in America, 1865–1915: Philadelphia as a test case. **Bull Hist Med** 1984 Summer;58(2):198–214
**Mormont C, Bobon D, Frenckell R von, et al:** Introduction aux Journées AMDP d'hommage à Jean Bobon. **Acta Psychiatr Belg** 1982 Jul–Aug;82(4):367–70
**Morogova VM** see **Magazov VS**
**Morogues IM de:** N. S. Leskov: premieres polemiques. janvier 1860–mai 1862. **Cah Monde Russe Sovietique** 1982;23(2):243–55
**Morowitz HJ:** How E. coli got its name. **Hosp Pract** 1982 Dec;17(12):58–9
**Morowitz HJ:** Much ado about nothing. **Hosp Pract** 1982 Jul;17(7):215–6
**Morowitz HJ:** The mating poems of D. H. Lawrence. **Hosp Pract [Off]** 1984 May;19(5):233–5, 238
**Morowitz HJ:** Thoreau as a scientist. **Hosp Pract [Off]** 1984 Nov;19(11):143–6, 151
**Morowitz HJ** see **Smith TF**
**Morozov BV** see **Chernukh AM**
**Morozova VT:** Istoriia kafedry laboratornoĭ klinicheskoĭ diagnostiki Tsentral'nogo instituta usovershenstvovaniia vracheĭ. **Lab Delo** 1981;(6):375–8
**Morrant GA:** Eastman Dental Hospital/Institute of Dental Surgery. **Apex** 1979 Winter;11(3):80–4
**Morrant GA:** The Eastman reaches its half century. **Br Dent J** 1980 Oct 21;149(8):237–8
**Morrell J** see **Inkster I**
**Morrell JT:** Gentlemen of science: early years of the British Association for the Advancement of Science. Oxford, Clarendon Press; New York, Oxford University Press, 1981. xxiii, 592 p.
**Morricone A, Pedicino V:** Medici e guaritori in Sicilia: spunti di medicina popolare in un'opera diGiuseppe Pitré. In Congrès international d'histoire de la médecine, XXVe, Québec, 1976. Actes. Québec, 1977. p. 992–8.
**Morris AD:** Two Colliery doctors: the brothers Armstrong of Treorchy. In J. Cule, ed: Wales and medicine. London, British Society for the History of Medicine, 1975. p. 208–15.
**Morris AF:** Sports medicine today. **J Sports Med Phys Fitness** 1982 Jun;22(2):259–73
**Morris AG, Keen EN:** Lawrence Herbert Wells and the history of anatomical illustration. **S Afr Med J** 1982 Jan 9;61(2):40–3
**Morris E:** Lead poisoning: an historic view. **Occup Health (Lond)** 1980 Sep;32(9):449–59
**Morris GC:** A portrait of Thomas Hollier, Pepy's surgeon. **Ann R Coll Surg Engl** 1979 May;61(3):224–9
**Morris GC:** Which Molins treated Cromwell for stone--and did not prescribe for Pepys? **Med Hist** 1982 Oct;26(4):429–35
**Morris J:** The Gertrude Tuckwell collection (Trades Union Congress, Gt. Russell St., London, W.C.1.). **Hist Workshop J** 1978;5:155–62
**Morris JE** see **Sharkey PW, ed**
**Morris JP:** Emery Andrew Rovenstine. In Dictionary of American Biography, Suppl. 6, 1956–1960. p. 553–4, 1980.
**Morris JP:** Gordon Stifler Seagrave. In Dictionary of American biography, 1961–1965. Suppl. 7, 1981. 679–81.
**Morris JP:** Historical, medical, and social perspectives on the public's view of death. In Dempsey D., et al, ed: Death, the press, and the public. New York, Arno Press, 1982. p. 10–22.
**Morris JP:** Historical perspectives on educating the medical student in thanatology. In Schoenberg B., et al, ed: Educating medical students in thanatology. New York, Arno Press, 1981. p. 18–28.
**Morris JP:** Smallpox inoculation in the American colonies, 1763–1783. **Md Hist** 1977;8:47–58
**Morris JP:** Walter Timme. In Dictionary of American Biography, Suppl. 6, 1956–1960. p. 634–5, 1980.
**Morris JT:** Clinical notes on His Excellency James Elisha 'Big Jim' Folsom--Governor of Alabama (1947–1951 and 1955–1959). **J Med Assoc State Ala** 1982 Jan;51(7):36, 39–41, 46

**Morris L** see **Goldberg HI**
**Morris M:** Normandy 1944. One. D-Day diary. **Nurs Times** 1984;80(23):46-7; (24):44-5
**Morris N:** The cancer blackout: exposing the official blacklisting of beneficial cancer research, treatment and prevention. Los Angeles, Regent House, 1977. ix, 206 p.
**Morris RM:** The Umtali Hospitals. **Rhodesiana** 1979;40:29-33
**Morrison LR:** 'Nearer to the brute creation': the scientific defense of American slavery before 1830. **South Stud** 1980;19(3):228-42
**Morrissey JF:** Gastrointestinal endoscopy--20 years of progress. **Gastrointest Endosc** 1983 Feb;29(1):53-6
**Morrissey JP, Goldman HH:** Cycles of reform in the care of the chronically mentally ill. **Hosp Community Psychiatry** 1984 Aug;35(8):785-93
**Morrow CK:** Sick doctors: the social construction of professional deviance. **Soc Probl** 1982;30(1):92-108
**Morrow RB:** Family limitation in pre-industrial England: a reappraisal. **Econ Hist Rev** 1978;31(3):419-28
**Morrow RC:** On obeah, myalism and magical death in Jamaica. **West Indian Med J** 1983 Mar;32(1):4-6
**Morscher E:** Entwicklungen in der Chirurgie: das Department Chirurgie der Universität Basel 1967-1983. Basel, Schwabe, 1983. 192 p.
**Morse D:** Ancient disease in the Midwest. 2d ed. Springfield, Illinois, Illinois State Museum, 1978. xiii, 181 p. (Illinois State Museum Reports of Investigations, No. 15). Includes contributions by A. A. Dahlberg, D. Ubelaker, D. F. Dickson, J. R. Caldwell, R. C. Dailey, G. M. Comer.
**Morsy TA:** Cutaneous leishmaniasis in Egypt. Historical background and current knowledge. **J Egypt Soc Parasitol** 1983 Dec;13(2):597-611
**Morte PD:** Neurologic aspects of human anomalies. **West J Med** 1983 Aug;139(2):250-6
**Mortelmans J** see **Burke J**
**Mortimer R:** The Prior of Butley and the lepers of West Somerton. **Bull Inst Hist Res** 1980;53:99-103
**Morton AG:** History of botanical science. An account of the development of botany from ancient times to the present day. London, New York, N. Y., Academic Press, 1981. xii, 474 p.
**Morton AG:** Marginalia to Andrea Cesalpino's work on botany. **Arch Nat Hist** 1981 Apr;10(1):31-6
**Morton D:** 'Noblest and best': retaining Canada's war disabled 1915-23. **J Can Stud** 1981;16(3-4):75-85
**Morton DL** see **Storm FK**
**Morton G:** Henderson Wightman, R. N., 1810-16. **Ir Sword** 1980;14(54):69-72
**Morton LT** see **Ash L**
**Morton RS:** A reappraisal of non-specific genital infection with reference to the work of the late Dr. E. Weston Hurst. **Br J Vener Dis** 1983 Dec;59(6):394-6
**Moruzzi G:** In memoriam Lord Adrian (1889-1977). **Rev Physiol Biochem Pharmacol** 1980;87:1-24
**Mory B:** Dorvault et la 'Pharmacie centrale de France.' **Rev Hist Pharm (Paris)** 1980 Jun;27(245):79-90
**Morys P:** Medizin und Pharmazie in der Kosmologie Leonhard Thurneissers zum Thurn (1531-1596). Husum, Matthiesen, 1982. 179 p. (Abhandlungen zur Geschichte der Medizin und der Naturwissenschaften, 43).
**Mosadomi A** see **Sawyer DR**
**Mosch E:** Der Apotheker Pedro José da Silva, ein unbekannter Lebenslauf. **Beitr Gesch Pharm** 1980;31(9):65-71
**Moscheo R** see **Trevisani F**
**Moschke G:** Der Einfluss der Arbeiterklasse auf die Berufskrankheitengesetzgebung und Gewerbehygiene in der Weimarer Republik von 1925-1929. **Z Gesamte Hyg** 1981 Apr;27(4):307-9
**Moschke G:** Die Rolle des Sanitäts- und Hilfsdienstes bei der Gestaltung des Systems der medizinischen Versorgung in Leipzig von 1945-1948. **Z Gesamte Hyg** 1979;25(11):845-7
**Moschke G:** Die Stellung der KPD zur Berufskrankheitengesetzgebung in der Weimarer Republik. **Z Exp Chir** 1982 Jul;28(7):471-3
**Moschke G:** Samaritianskiĭ soiuz rabochikh Germanii--primer tvorcheskoĭ deiatel'nosti nemetskogo rabochego klassa v 1909-1930 gg. v bor'be protiv burzhuaznoĭ politiki zdravookhraneniia. **Sov Zdravookhr** 1981;(2):52-6
**Moschke G:** Zur Bedeutung des SMAD-Befehls Nr. 234 für die Entwicklung der Lehre über Sozialhygiene an der Leipziger Universität in den Jahren 1948 bis 1952. **Z Gesamte Hyg** 1983 Oct;29(10):620-3
**Moschner H:** Wissenschaftliche Arbeit und Lehre des Bonner Physiologen Eduard Friedrich Wilhelm Pflüger auf dem Gebiet des tierischen Stoffwechsels. Diss. Bonn, 1981. 233 p.
**Mosejczuk L** see **Walewski W**
**Mosek C:** Nutrition and fertility: a review essay. **Hist Methods** 1981;14(1):43-6
**Moseley J:** Alexis Carrel, the man unknown. Journey of an idea. **JAMA** 1980 Sep 5;244(10):1119-21
**Moseley JE:** Travels of Alexandre Yersin: letters of a pastorian in Indochina, 1890-1894. **Perspect Biol Med** 1981 Summer;24(4):607-18
**Moseley R:** From avocation to job: the changing nature of scientific practice. **Soc Stud Sci** 1979;9(4):511-22
**Moseley R** see **MacLeod R**
**Moses J** see **Cross W**
**Moses RJ:** Smallpox immunization in Alta California: a story based on José Estrada's 1821 postscript. **South Calif Q** 1979;61(2):125-45
**Mosher WD:** Demographic responses and demographic transitions: a case study of Sweden. **Demography** 1980 Nov;17(4):395-412
**Mosher WD:** The theory of change and response: an application to Puerto Rico, 1940 to 1970. **Popul Stud** 1980 Mar;34(1):45-58
**Moshkov VA:** Abu Ali Ibn-Sina (Avitsenna) o fizicheskikh uprazhneniiakh i massazhe. **Vopr Kurortol Fizioter Lech Fiz Kult** 1981 Jan-Feb;(1):66-7
**Mosk C:** Fertility and occupation: mining districts in prewar Japan. **Soc Sci Hist** 1981;5(3):293-316
**Mosk C:** Patriarchy and fertility: Japan and Sweden, 1880-1960. New York, Academic Press, 1983. xxii, 320 p.
**Mosk C:** Rural-urban fertility differences and the fertility transition. **Popul Stud** 1980;34(1):77-90
**Mosk C:** The evolution of the pre-modern demographic regime in Japan. **Popul Stud** 1981 Mar;35(1):28-52
**Moskoff W:** Pronatalist policies in Romania. **Econ Dev Cult Change** 1980;28(3):597-614
**Moskovskomu gorodskomu sovetu sanitarnykh fel'dsherov i laborantov 25 let: Feldsher Akush** 1980;45(2):57-9
**Moskow BS:** Dentistry in folk art, XIII: The dentist. **Bull Hist Dent** 1981 Oct;29(2):99
**Moskow BS:** Dentistry in folk art XV; Decamps--le dentiste. **Bull Hist Dent** 1982 Oct;30(2):128
**Moskow BS:** The dental cartoons of Honoré Daumier (1808-1879). **J Am Dent Assoc** 1981 Jan;102(1):82-6
**Moskow BS:** The iconography of the dental profession. **Quintessence Int** 1983 Oct;14(10):1072-3
**Moskow BS:** The iconography of the dental profession. **Quintessence Int** 1983 Nov;14(11):1184-5
**Moskow BS:** The iconography of the dental profession. **Quintessence Int** 1983 Dec;14(12):1278-9
**Moskow BS:** The iconography of the dental profession. **Quintessence Int** 1984 Apr;15(4):406-7
**Moskow BS:** The iconography of the dental profession. Der Zahnbrecher--the toothbreaker. Johannes Joachim Kändler (1706-1775). **Quintessence Int** 1984 Jan;15(1):40-1
**Moskow BS:** The iconography of the dental profession. Francisco Zurbarán (1598-1664). **Quintessence Int** 1984 Aug;15(8):814-5
**Moskow BS:** The iconography of the dental profession. Jean-Ignace-Isidore Gérard Grandville (1803-1847). **Quintessence Int** 1984 Oct;15(10):1028-9
**Moskow BS:** The iconography of the dental profession. Pietro Longhi (1702-1785). **Quintessence Int** 1984 Jul;15(7):728-9
**Moskwa Z:** Historia szczepień przeciwgruźliczych i powstanie szczepionki BCG. **Wiad Lek** 1983 Jan 1;36(1):81-5
**Moskwa Z:** Izby lekarskie--wczoraj i dziś. **Wiad Lek** 1984 Jul 1;37(13):1064-8
**Moskwa Z:** Opieka społeczna nad chorymi gruźliczymi na śląsku w latach 1928-1929. **Wiad Lek** 1983 Oct 1;36(19):1645-7
**Moskwa Z:** Pielęgniarstwo polskie w świetle ustawy z 1935 roku. **Wiad Lek** 1982 Sep 15;35(15-16):1017-9
**Moskwa Z:** Początki Warszawskiego Pogotowia Ratunkowego. **Wiad Lek** 1982 Jan 1;35(1):81-3
**Moskwa Z:** Powstańcza søużba zdrowia na Górnym Slasku w latach 1919-1921. **Wiad Lek** 1984 Feb 15;37(4):313-20
**Moskwa Z:** Publiczna służba zdrowia w świetle ustawy z 1939 roku. **Wiad Lek** 1983 Nov 1;36(21):1833-4
**Moskwa Z:** Tuberkulina. **Wiad Lek** 1983 Jun 15;36(12):1033-5
**Moskwa Z:** W setną rocznic e odkrycia prątka grużlicy. **Wiad Lek** 1983 May 1;36(9):799-802
**Moskwa Z:** Założenie kamienia wegielnego pod szpital Dzieciatka Jezus. **Wiad Lek** 1984 Mar 15;37(6):479-80
**Moskwa Z:** Zawód położnej w świetle rozporządzeń z lat 1928/29. **Wiad Lek** 1983 Jun 1;36(11):941-4
**Moss C, Marchfield F, Hansen H, et al:** A treasury of practice history. (Amy Elizabeth Pope). **Calif Nurse** 1983 Sep;79(3):6-7
**Moss HG** see **Trautmann J, ed**
**Moss JB:** Pathological images in the Quebec novel. **Am Rev Can Stud** 1980;10(1):39-47
**Moss JP:** Historical and current perspectives on surgical drainage. **Surg Gynecol Obstet** 1981 Apr;152(4):517-27
**Moss WG** see **Spicker SF**
**Mossakowski M** see **Rudowski W**
**Mössmer A:** Säuglingsflaschen aus Holz. In Göpfert W, Otten HH, ed: Metavoeite: wandelt euch durch neues Denken. Düsseldorf, Triltsch, 1983. p. 201-8.
**Mosteller JH:** 'Practices dentistry in Fayette, Alabama'. A tardy but sincere tribute to Claude Clenton Cannon. **J Ala Dent Assoc** 1977 Oct;61(4):19-24
**Moszyński J:** Galenus - De victu attenuante. **Arch Hist Med (Warsz)** 1982;45(1-4):61-75
**Mota Hernández F:** La implantación del expediente clínico organizado por problemas. **Bol Med Hosp Infant Mex** 1981 Jul-Aug;38(4):567-70
**Moteiunas LI:** Meditsinskiĭ fakul'tet Vil'niusskogo universiteta na poroge tret'ego stoletiia. **Zh Mikrobiol Epidemiol Immunobiol** 1983 Jan;(1):115-7
**Mothes K:** Pharmakognosie--gestern, heute, morgen. **Pharmazie** 1981 Mar;36(3):174-8
**Mothes K:** Zur Geschichte unserer Kenntnisse über die Alkaloide. **Pharmazie** 1981 Mar;36(3):199-209
**Motoyama S:** [Dental clinics in the Edo period] (Jpn). **Shikai Tenbo** 1984 Aug;64(2):353-61
**Mott K** see **Kean BH**
**Mottier G:** Histoire de l'Infirmerie de Lausanne et de La Source. **Krankenpflege (Bern)** 1983 Dec;76(12):27-30
**Mottram J** see **Cardwell D**

**Mottus JE:** New York Nightingales: the emergence of the nursing profession at Bellevue and New York Hospital, 1850–1920. Ann Arbor, Mich., UMI Research Press, 1981. xvii, 277 p. (Ph.D. Diss., New York University, 1980.

**Motulsky AG:** Impact of genetic manipulation on society and medicine. **Science** 1983 Jan 14;219(4581):135–40

**Moulin AM, Löwi I:** La double nature de l'immunologie: histoire de la transplantation rénale. **Fundam Sci** 1983;4(3/4):201–18

**Moulin D de:** A short history of breast cancer. Boston, Martinus Nijhoff, 1983. xiii, 124 p.

**Moulin D de:** Heelkundige onderwerpen in het Nederlandsch Weekblad voor Genesskundigen (1851–1856). **Ned Tijdschr Geneeskd** 1981 Aug 25;125(35):1427–30

**Moulin D de:** Historical notes on breast cancer, with emphasis on The Netherlands. II. Pathophysiological concepts, diagnosis and therapy in the 18th century. **Neth J Surg** 1981 Oct;33(4):206–16

**Moulin D de:** Historical notes on breast cancer, with emphasis on The Netherlands; III. The growth of scientific surgery in the 19th century. **Neth J Surg** 1982 Dec;34(5):193–200

**Moulin D de:** Microscopie en kankerdiagnostiek in de eerste helft van de negentiende eeuw. **Tijdschr Geschied Geneeskd** 1983;6(2):99–107

**Moulin D de:** Spontaneous human combustion. In: Congrès international d'histoire de la médecine, XXVe, Québec, 1976. Actes. Quebec, 1977. p. 570–8.

**Mounier-Kuhn P:** Un siècle d'oto-rhino-laryngologie. **J Fr Otorhinolaryngol** 1983 Jan;32(1):12–30

**Mounier-Kuhn P, Guerrier Y:** Vieussens et l'anatomie de l'oreille. **Acta Otorhinolaryngol Belg** 1982;36(6):1029–38

**Mounier-Kuhn P** see **Guerrier Y**

**Mourad K** see **Park WM**

**Mourant AE:** The discovery of the anti-globulin test. **Vox Sang** 1983;45(2):180–3

**Mouren MC** see **Simeoni CE**

**Mourgues G de:** Léopold Ollier, 1830–1900, père de la chirurgie orthopédique. **Rev Chir Orthop** 1979;65(11):2–3

**Mousnier R:** Réflexions d'un historien à la lecture d'un manuel de sociologie. **Rev Hist (Paris)** 1980;263(2):395–401

**Moussa GM** see **Hunayn Ibn Ishak, al-Ibadi**

**Moussaoui D, Touhami M, Msefer W:** Psychiatrie et psychosomatique dans la médecine arabe. **Ann Med Psychol (Paris)** 1980;138(8):967–74

**Mouton P:** La mort est venue de la mer. Paris, Pen Duick, 1982. 184 p.

**Movshed BE** see **Fedorov NA**

**Movshev BE:** Razvitie ucheniia A. A. Bogomol'tsa o mekhanizme deĭstviia perelivaniia krovi. **Gematol Transfuziol** 1984 Jan;29(1):6–12

**Movshovich IA, Kaplan MB:** 50 Let so dnia organizatsii travmatologicheskogo otdeleniia v bol'nitse im. S. P. Botkina. **Ortop Travmatol Protez** 1982 Jun;(6):74–5

**Mowat AG:** Strathpeffer Spa: Dr. William Bruce and polymyalgia rheumatica. **Ann Rheum Dis** 1981 Oct;40(5):503–6

**Mowrer OH:** Enuresis: the beginning work--what really happened. **J Hist Behav Sci** 1980 Jan;16(1):25–30

**Moya Pons F:** Datos para el estudio de la demografia aborigen en Santo Domingo. **Jahrb Gesch Staat Wirtsch Ges Lateinam** 1979;16:1–11

**Moylan TK:** Poverty, pigs and pestilence in medieval Dublin. **Dublin Hist Rec** 1978;31(4)

**Mozhaev VP:** Sanitarnye biulleteni o V. V. Maiakovskom. **Feldsher Akush** 1983 Dec;48(12):36–8

**Mozzhakov VI** see **Nguyen TK**

**Mozzhukhin AS:** [I. M. Sechenov - The founder of the first physiological school in Russia] (Rus). **Istor Biol Issled** 1980;8:124–37

**Mozzhukhin AS:** Rol' L. A. Orbeli v stanovlenii i razrabotke fiziologicheskikh problem radiobiologii. **Fiziol Zh SSSR** 1982 Jul;68(7):914–7

**Mřena V** see **Kubat R**

**Mrozowski K:** Wkład profesora doktora medycyny Witolda Eugeniusza Orłowskiego w zwalczaniu gruźlicy. **Pol Arch Med Wewn** 1981;65(5):385–9

**Mrtek RG:** Absent the incentive: an example of contemporary history. **Pharm Hist** 1981;23(4):145–51

**Msefer W** see **Moussaoui D**

**Muallem M:** Anesthesiology in the American University of Beirut 1922–1970. **Middle East J Anaesthesiol** 1982 Jun;6(5):281–8

**Mucha V, Bobková M:** K histórii poznatkov o Pseudomonas aeruginosa. **Bratisl Lek Listy** 1982 Feb;77(2):229–34

**Muchembled R:** Le corps, la culture populaire et la culture des élites en France (XVe-XVIIIe siècle). In Imhof AE, ed: Leib und Leben in der Geschichte der Neuzeit. Berlin, Duncker & Humblot, 1983. p. 141–53.

**Muchiev GS, Frolova OG:** Okhrana zdorov'ia ploda i novorozhdennogo v SSSR. Moskva, Meditsina, 1979. 207 p.

**Mück H:** Die rechtliche Entwicklung des Arzt-Patient-Verhältnisses in der DDR; vom Dienstvertrag zum medizinischen Betreuungsverhältnis. Köln, 1982. 322 p. (Kölner medizinhistorische Beiträge, Band 24)

**Mudry P:** Medicus amicus. Un trait romain dans la médecine antique. **Gesnerus** 1980;37(1/2):17–20

**Mudry P** see **Grmek MD, ed**

**Mueller I:** Krankheit und Heilmittel im Werk Hildegards von Bingen. In: Hildegard von Bingen. Festschrift 1179–1979. [1979] pp. 311–349.

**Mueller-Jahncke WD:** Der Höhepunkt der Iatromathematic. **Ber Wissenschaftsgesch** 1981;4(1/2):41–50

**Muerant J:** La Comité International de la Croix-Rouge et la protection des civils. **Rev Hist Deuxieme Guerre Mond** 1981;31(121):129–38

**Muestra en homenaje a los doctores Miguel Puiggari y Miguel Puiggari (h.): Publ Mus Farm** 1983 Jul-Sep;2(7–9):1–13

**Muggeridge JF:** Progress of optical discovery. **J R Soc Health** 1983 Aug;103(4):150–1

**Muggeridge JF:** The discovery of spectacles. **R Soc Health J** 1982 Aug;102(4):174

**Mugnai Carrara D:** Fra causalità astrologica e causalità naturale. Gli interventi di Nicolò Leoniceno e della sua scuola sul morbo gallico. **Physis** 1979;21(1–4):37–54

**Mugnai Carrara D:** Una polemica umanistico-scolastica circa l'interpretazione delle tre dottrine ordinate di Galeno. **Ann Ist Mus Stor Sci Fir** 1983;8(1):31–57

**Muhammad U:** Avicenna as a clinician. **Bull Indian Inst Hist Med (Hyderabad)** 1981;1–4:87–90

**Muhammad Abad al-Wahab Zahuri:** A medical treatise of the time of King Muhammad Tughlaq. **Stud Hist Med** 3(3):173–77, Sep 79

**Mühlemann H** see **Schmid R**

**Mühlemann HR:** 25 Jahre Schweizer Plaque-Pharmakologie. **Schweiz Monatsschr Zahnmed** 1984 Jan;94(1):91–101

**Muir CS:** Nasopharyngeal cancer--a historical vignette. **CA** 1983 May-Jun;33(3):180–5

**Muir IF:** The development of plastic surgery in the United Kingdom. **Ann Plast Surg** 1981 May;6(5):411–5

**Mukherjee JB:** History of forensic medicine. In his Forensic medicine and toxicology. Volume One. Calcutta, New Delhi, Academic Publishers, 1981. p. 1–6.

**Mukhitdinov BN:** Eticheskie printsipy Abu Ali Ibn-Siny (Avitsenny) i voprosy sovremennoĭ deontologii (k 1000-letiiu so dnia rozhdeniia). **Vestn Rentgenol Radiol** 1980 May-Jun;(3):80–2

**Mukhtarov AM, Bolgarskiĭ IS:** Voprosy urologii v trudakh Abu Ali Ibn-Siny. **Urol Nefrol (Mosk)** 1980 Nov-Dec;(6):52–5

**Mularczyk-Bal MU, Kopzyński J:** Smiertelność noworodków z niskim urodzeniowym ciężarem w latach 1970--1974 w szpitalach w Warszawie. **Pediatr Pol** 1980 Aug;55(8):957–63

**Mulch J, Scheld HH, Köstering B, et al:** 20 Jahre Herzklappenchirurgie. (1). Entwicklung der künstlichen Herzklappenventile. **ZFA (Stuttgart)** 1981 Mar 31;57(9):639–44

**Mulch J** see **Scheld HH**

**Mulder WJ:** De 'Anatomie clastique' van Dr. L. T. J. Anzoux. **Tijdschr Geschied Geneeskd** 1981:4(3):133–43

**Mulder WJ:** Microscopische preparaten van de praktizerend geneesheer G. J. Luchtmans. **Tijdschr Geschied Geneeskd** 1983;6(2):108–14

**Mul'diiarov PIa** see **Rebrikova NL**

**Müldner-Nieckowski P:** Dr. Jacek Machalski (2.VI.1926--3.X.1979). **Arch Hist Med (Warsz)** 1980;43(2):117–20

**Muldworf B:** Freud. Paris, Les Editeurs français réunis, 1976. 349 p.

**Mulhallen J, Wright DJ:** Samuel Johnson: amateur physician. **J R Soc Med** 1983 Mar;76(3):217–22

**Mulholland J:** Soma, an attempt to classify the plant and the drug. **J Asiat Soc** 1976;18(1–3):47–55

**Mulholland JA** see **Riddle JM**

**Mulinski TM** see **El-Najjar MY**

**Mulkay M** see **Gilbert GN**

**Mullaney MM:** Gender and revolution: Rosa Luxemburg and the female revolutionary personality. **J Psychohist** 1984 Spring;11(4):463–76

**Müllen K** see **Khalatbari P**

**Mullen PC:** Bitterroot enigma: Howard Taylor Ricketts and the early struggle against spotted fever. **Montana** 1983;32(1):2–13

**Mullen PC:** The commemoration of the Meckel bicentennial: Bozeman 1982. **Am J Med Genet** 1984 Aug;18(4):565–9

**Muller A, Garretta M, Hebert M:** Groupamatic system: overview, history of development and evaluation of use. **Vox Sang** 1981;40(3):201–13

**Müller B:** Franz Kiwisch, Ritter von Rotterau 1814–1851. Diss. Würzburg, 1980. 111 p.

**Müller B** see **Eigler J**

**Müller C, Nikliček L:** Der gegenwärtige Zustand und die Aufgaben des Unterrichts in der Geschichte der Medizin an der hygienischen medizinischen Fakultät der Karlsuniversität. In Congr. Hist. Sci., Prague 1981. p. 419–33. **Acta Hist Rerum Nat Tech** 1981;11, special number

**Müller C:** Historische Reminiszenz: die schizophrene Psychose der Kaiserin von Mexiko. **Fortschr Neurol Psychiatr** 1979 Oct;47(10):550–2

**Müller C:** Historische Vignette. August Forel und der Nationalsozialismus. **Nervenarzt** 1984 Sep;55(9):504–5

**Müller C, Nikliček L:** K postavení sociálního lékařství v historii systému výuky a výchovy lékařu na Univerzitě Karlově. **Cesk Zdrav** 1982 Jan;30(1):22–33

**Müller C:** Le Champ-de-l'Air, premier hôpital psychiatrique du Canton de Vaud. **Gesnerus** 1980;37(1/2):28–33

**Müller C, Niklícek L:** Třicet let lékařské fakulty hygienické Univerzity Karlovy. **Cesk Zdrav** 1982 Oct;30(10):402–7

**Müller C:** Un drame dans la famille d'Albrecht de Haller. **Gesnerus** 1984;41(1/2):133–6

**Müller C:** Zur Bevölkerungsentwicklung in Westberlin. **Wiss Z Humboldt Univ Berl [Gesellschaftswiss Sprachwiss Reihe]** 1979;28(1):105–13

**Müller C** see **Nikliček L**

**Muller CF:** 'N blad uit die joernaal van 'n sieketrooster, 1709–1710. **Historia (S Afr)** 1978;23(2):90–8

**Müller CW:** Die hippokratischen Schriften. In his: Gleiches zu Gleichem. Ein Prinzip frühgriechischen Denkens. Wiesbaden, Harrassowitz, 1965. p. 112–50. (Klassisch-philologische Studien, 31).

**Müller D** see **Rusek V**

**Muller E:** Bosquejo histórico de la Asociación Panamericana de Periodontología. **Acta Odontol Venez** 1983 May-Aug;21(2):173-9

**Müller E:** Die geschichtliche Entwicklung der Zahnheilkunde im Grossherzogtum Hessen-Darmstadt--einschliesslich seiner Vorgänger- und Nachfolgeterritorien--unter besonderer Berücksichtigung seiner Universitätsstadt Giessen. Giessen, Schmitz, 1981. 120 p. (Arbeiten zur Geschichte der Medizin in Giessen, 3).

**Müller H:** Die Anstalt in Kork (Baden). Von der 'Heil- und Pflegeanstalt für epileptische Kinder' zum 'Epilepsiezentrum Kork'. Freiburg, Schulz, 1979. 190 p. (Freiburger Forschungen zur Medizingeschichte, Neue Folge, 10).

**Müller HK:** Zur Entwicklung der medizinischen Wissenschaften in China. **Naturwissenschaften** 1980 Feb;67(2):55-60

**Müller I:** Die pflanzlichen Heilmittel bei Hildegard von Bingen. Salzburg, D. Müller, 1982. 215 p.

**Müller I:** Zur Theorie und Praxis der Antimontherapie. In Göpfert W, Otten HH, ed: Metavoeite: wandelt euch durch neues Denken. Düsseldorf, Triltsch, 1983. p. 173-88.

**Müller I** see **Gicklhorn R**

**Muller JE:** Coronary artery thrombosis: historical aspects. **J Am Coll Cardiol** 1983 Mar;1(3):893-6

**Muller JP:** Ego and subject in Lacan. **Psychoanal Rev** 1982 Summer;69(2):234-40

**Müller KP** see **Marchand H**

**Müller M:** Erinnerungen, erlebte Psychiatriegeschichte, 1920-1960. Berlin; New York, Springer-Verlag, 1982. 504 p.

**Muller M:** The health of nations. A North-South investigation. London, Faber and Faber, 1982. 255 p.

**Müller N:** Zur Entwicklung der Transfusionsmedizin. **MMW** 1979 Nov 9;121(45):1485-8

**Muller P:** Geschichte der Gynäkologie vom 18. Jahrhundert bis zur Gegenwart. In Sournia JC, Martiny M, Poulet J, ed: Illustrierte Geschichte der Medizin. Salzburg, Andreas, 1980. Vol. 4. p. 1311-37.

**Müller P** see **Engelbrecht H**

**Müller PK** see **Gürtler LG**

**Müller R:** Occupational health statistics in Germany and in the Federal Republic of Germany: a patient in need of care. Some contributions to the history of reporting of industrial pathology. **Soc Soc Hist Med Bull (Lond)** 1983 Dec;33:63-6

**Müller R:** Wandlung zur Ganzheit: die Initiatische Therapie nach Karlfried Graf Dürckheim und Maria Hippius. Freiburg, Herder, 1981. 328 p.

**Müller R** see **Klein P**

**Müller RA:** Mittelalterliches Konzil und Medizin. **MMW** 1983 Apr 1;125(13):263-4

**Müller RK:** Zur Entwicklung der toxikologischen Denkweise anfangs des 19. Jahrhunderts. **Z Gesamte Hyg** 1983 Jun;29(6):348-50

**Muller SA, Perry HO:** The Goeckerman treatment in psoriasis: six decades of experience at the Mayo Clinic. **Cutis** 1984 Sep;34(3):265-8, 270

**Müller W:** Geschichte der Universitätshautklinik Essen. **Hautarzt** 1982 Jan;33(1):26-9

**Müller W:** Vom Wöchnerinnenasyl zum Universitätsklinikum. Die Geschichte des Städtischen Krankenhauswesens in Essen. Münster, Murken-Altrogge, 1981. 364 p. (Studien zur Geschichte des Krankenhauswesens, 15)

**Müller-Dietz H:** Friedrich Joseph Haass als Arzt in Moskau: biographische Skizzen. Berlin, Osteuropa-Institut, 1980. 133 p.

**Müller-Dietz HE:** Aerzte im Russland des achtzehnten Jahrhunderts. Esslingen/Neckar, Robugen, 1973. 111 p.

**Müller-Dietz HE:** Friedrich Joseph Haass, ein deutscher Arzt in Moskau. **Clio Med** 1981 Apr;15(3-4):177-89

**Müller-Dietz HE:** Utländska läkare vid Lenins sjukbädd. **Sydsven Medicinhist Sallsk Arsskr** 1984;21:141-56

**Müller-Hermann E** see **Weerda H**

**Müller-Jahncke WD:** Agrippa von Nettesheim in Antwerpen. Ein Beitrag zur Geschichte des 'Englischen Schweiss'. In Dilg P, et al., ed: Perspektiven der Pharmaziegeschichte. Graz, Austria, Akademische Druck- u. Verlagsanstalt, 1983. p. 243-68.

**Müller-Jahncke WD:** Apothekerbildnisse auf Medaillen und Plaketten. 1. Deutschsprachiger Raum. Stuttgart, Wissenschaftliche Verlagsgesellschaft, 1980. 164 p. Veröffentlichungen der Internationalen Gesellschaft für Geschichte der Pharmazie, Neue Folge, 48).

**Müller-Jahncke WD:** Der Höhepunkt der Iatromathematik. **Ber Wissenschaftsgesch** 1981;4(1/2):41-50

**Müller-Jahncke WD:** Der 'latheinisch aussgestrichene Matthiolus' Landgraf Wilhelms IV von Hessen-Kassel und sein Schicksal. **Pharm Ztg** 1983 Feb 17;128(7):357-61

**Müller-Jahncke WD:** Die 'Magnarum Medicine partium herbariae et zoographiae imagines' von Georg Ollinger und Samuel Quicchelberg. **Beitr Gesch Pharm** 1982;31(17):129-33

**Müller-Jahncke WD:** In memoriam Walter Pagel (1898-1983). **Ber Wissenschaftsgesch** 1983;6(1-4):165-8

**Müller-Jahncke WD:** Kleiner Beitrag zum Prioritätenstreit um die Metoposkopie: Hájek contra Cardano. **Sudhoffs Arch** 1982;66(1):79-84

**Müller-Jahncke WD:** Weitere Apothekerbildnisse auf Medaillen und Plaketten des deutschsprachigen Raums. **Beitr Gesch Pharm** 1984;31(24):205-9

**Muller-Rensmann R:** Les trois grands pôles du miracle en France au 19e siècle, la médaille miraculeuse, Lourdes et Thérèse de Lisieux. **Penelope** 1981;(5):56-7

**Müller-Rohlfsen I:** Die lateinische Ravennatische Uebersetzung der hippokratischen Aphorismen aus dem 5./6. Jahrhundert n. Chr. Textkonstitution auf der Basis der Uebersetzungscodices. Hamburg, Lüdke, 1980. xlviii, 162 p. (Geistes- und Sozialwissenschaftliche Dissertationen, 55).

**Müller-Ruchholtz ER, Haase J, Kaufmann R:** Zwanzig Jahre Physiologisches Institut Düsseldorf. Bericht über die Arbeit des Institutes, Verzeichnis der Mitarbeiter und Verzeichnis der Veröffentlichungen 1970-1980. **Jahrb Univ Dusseld** 1977-78;209-47

**Mulligan G** see **Mulligan L**

**Mulligan HW:** Tropical medicine and research in British territories overseas. **Trans R Soc Trop Med Hyg** 1981;75 Suppl:9-11

**Mulligan L:** Puritans and English science: a critique of Webster. **Isis** 1980 Sep;71(258):456-69

**Mulligan L, Mulligan G:** Reconstructing restoration science: styles of leadership and social composition of the early Royal Society. **Soc Stud Sci** 1981;11(3):327-64

**Mullis ML** see **Kloiber A**

**Mullner R, Byre CS, Kubal JD:** Hospital closure in the United States, 1976-1980: a descriptive overview. **Health Serv Res** 1983 Fall;18(3):437-50

**Mulnard J:** Les vingt premières années des Archives de Biologie. **Arch Biol (Liege)** 1980;91(2):285-95

**Mumey N:** Ephraim McDowell, 1771-1830: a frontiersman who advanced the art of surgery. **Denver West Roundup** 1979 Jul-Aug;35:3-20

**Münchow W:** Albrecht von Graefe (1828-1870) in Memoriam. **Orvostort Kozl** 1979;86(24 no 4):55-64

**Munizaga J** see **Allison MJ**

**Munk F, ed:** Das medizinische Berlin um die Jahrhundertwende. 2d ed. München, Baltimore, Urban & Schwarzenberg, 1979. 182 p.

**Munnik LA** see **De Villiers JC**

**Muñoz AL, Hernández Sánchez FA:** 3 de Octubre: fecha rememorativa de la odontología y de la Confraternidad Odontológica Latinoamericana. **Salud Bucal** 1981 Oct-Nov;8(46):10-4, 73-7

**Muñoz P:** Origins of the caduceus. **Md State Med J** 1981 Oct;30(10):35-40

**Muñoz PE:** Psiquiatría social: un punto de vista sobre el enfermar. **Actas Loso Esp Neurol Psiquiatr** 1983 Mar-Apr;11(2):163-80

**Muñoz Al, Hernández Sánchez FA, Bagur DB, et al:** Jerarquización de la profesión odontológica. **Salud Bucal** 1981 Jun-Jul;8(44):23-38

**Muñoz Calvo S, Turegano Lopez A:** El control de alimentos del Laboratorio Químico Municipal de Madrid en el siglo XIX: contribución a su estudio. **Bol Soc Esp Hist Farm** 1981 Sep;32(127):149-67

**Muñoz Calvo S:** Notas para elaboracion de una sociologia farmaceutica en el sexenio revolucionario (1868-1874). **Bol Soc Esp Hist Farm** 1982 Sep;33(131):173-84

**Muñoz Calvo S:** Notas para un estudio historiográfico de la legislación farmacéutica en España. **Bol Soc Esp Hist Farm** 1979 Dec;30(120):305-17

**Muñoz Calvo S** see **Folch Jou G**

**Munoz CP, ed** see **Valverde JL**

**Muñoz-Perez F:** Douze ans d'avortement légal en Angleterre-Galles. **Population** 1981;36(6):1105-38

**Muñoz-Perez F:** L'évolution de la fécondité dans les pays industrialisés depuis 1971. **Population** 1982;37(3):483-512

**Munteanu A, Dobrescu G, Cotuțiu C, et al:** The 100th anniversary of the Jassy Faculty of Medicine and an historical approach to the evolution of its department of histology. **Morphol Embryol (Bucur)** 1980 Oct-Dec;26(4):371-3

**Munteanu M:** Inflințaree clinicii dermato-venerologice din Iaşi şi activitatea desfăşurată în perioada suplinirilor (1882-1901). **Rev Med Chir Soc Med Nat Iasi** 1983 Jan-Mar;87(1):141-8

**Muntner S** see **Rosner F**

**Muntschick W:** Ein Manuskript von Georg Meister, dem Kunst- und Lustgärtner, in der British Library. **Medizinhist J** 1984;19(3):225-32

**Müntzing A:** Analysen av människans kromosomer. **Sydsven Medicinhist Sallsk Arsskr** 1981;:116-31

**Munver UL** see **Hankoff LD**

**Munz DL** see **Hör G**

**Münzenmayer HP** see **Mayer JR von**

**Murakami S, ed:** Hokkaido baiyaku shi. [Sapporo, Japan], Hokkaido Haichi Kateiyaku Kyogikai, Showa 52 nen [1977]. 428 p.

**Muralt A von:** A life with several facets. **Annu Rev Physiol** 1984;46:1-13

**Murard L** see **Talmor E, ed**

**Muratori G:** I tumori delle ghiandole salivari. **Dent Cadmos** 1981 May;49(5):73-4

**Muratori G:** Odontoiatria del passato. I tumori della lingua. **Dent Cadmos** 1981 Apr;49(4):68-9

**Muratori G:** Odontoiatria del passato. I tumori delle labbra e della mucosa orale. **Dent Cadmos** 1981 May;49(5):71-2

**Muratori G:** Odontoiatria del passato. I tumori odontogeni. **Dent Cadmos** 1981 Apr;49(4):65-7

**Murav'ev EV:** Ugolok istorii. **Med Sestra** 1980 Oct;37(10):52-4

**Murav'ev MV:** K istorii stanovleniia sistemy usovershenstvovaniia vracheĭ v nasheĭ strane. **Sov Zdravookhr** 1980;(11):60-3

**Murav'ev MV:** K istorii vyezdnykh tsiklov--progressivnoĭ formy provysheniia kvalifikatsii vracheĭ. **Sov Zdravookhr** 1981;(4):59-63

**Murav'eva EF:** Meditsinskie temy v ékspozitsii Gosudarstvennogo Ermitazha. **Sov Zdravookhr** 1984;(9):62-5

**Murav'eva EF:** Unikal'nyĭ al'bom. **Sov Zdravookhr** 1980;(9):67-72

**Murdoch G:** Amputation revisited. **Prosthet Orthot Int** 1984 Apr;8(1):8-15

**Murdock ME, ed** see **Green D**

**Murken AH:** Das Krankenhaus im Wandel der Zeit ... 19. und 20. Jahrhunderts. **Neue Heimat** 1980;27(11/12):36-45

**Murken AH:** Die bauliche Entwicklung des deutschen Allgemeinen Krankenhauses im 19. Jahrhundert. Göttingen, Vandenhoeck & Ruprecht, 1979. 396 p. (Studien zur Medizingeschichte des neunzehnten Jahrhunderts, Bd. 9).
**Murken AH:** Die Entwicklung des Krankenhauses im 18. und 19. Jahrhundert. **Medita** 1980;10(3):i-xvi (Geschichte der Medizin)
**Murken AH:** Geschichte des Hospital- und Krankenhauswesens im deutschsprachigen Raum. In Sournia JC, Martiny M, Poulet J, ed: Illustrierte Geschichte der Medizin. Salzburg, Andreas, 1980. Vol. 5. p. 1595-1653.
**Murken AH:** Grundzüge des deutschen Krankenhauswesens von 1780 bis 1930 unter Berücksichtigung von Schweizer Vorbildern. **Gesnerus** 1982;39(1):7-45
**Murken AH:** Heilanstalten für Tuberkulöse. Zur Geschichte der Lungensanatorien und ihrer Therpiekonzeption im 19. Jahrhundert. In Göpfert W, Otten HH, ed: Metavoeite: wandelt euch durch neues Denken. Düsseldorf, Triltsch, 1983. p. 107-24.
**Murken AH:** Joseph Beuys und die Medizin. Münster, Coppenrath, 1979. 160 p. German and English.
**Murken AH, Rodegra H:** Krankenhausrundbauten in Vergangenheit und Gegenwart. Zur historischen Entwicklung von kreisförmigen Bettenhäusern und panoptisch angelegten Krankensälen. **Hist Hosp** 1979-80;13:197-216
**Murken AH:** Vom Armenhospital zum Grossklinikum. **Waage** 1980;19(1):25-37
**Murken AH, ed:** Kind, Krankheit und Krankenhaus im Bilderbuch von 1900 bis 1982. (Studien zur Medizin-, Kunst- und Literaturgeschichte. Band 5.). Herzogenrath, Verlag Murken-Altrogge, 1982. 238 p.
**Murley R:** John Hunter, velvet and vascular surgery. **Ann R Coll Surg Engl** 1984 May;66(3):214-8
**Murley R:** Peace and strife in Hunter's time. (Part I). **Ann R Coll Surg Engl** 1982 Jan;64(1):20-8
**Murley R:** Peace and strife in Hunter's time (part II). **Ann R Coll Surg Engl** 1982 Mar;64(2):81-90
**Murphey GT:** A Navy dentist's diary: from Okinawa to Viet Nam. (Griffin T. Murphey). **Dent Stud** 1979 Oct;58(2):52-4, 59, 67
**Murphey MG:** The psychodynamics of Puritan conversion. **Am Q** 1979;31(2):135-47
**Murphy BE, Grigg ER:** Radioassays. **Semin Nucl Med** 1979 Jul;9(3):169-72
**Murphy EA:** Skepsis, dogma, and belief. Uses and abuses in medicine. Baltimore, London, Johns Hopkins University Press, 1981. x, 176 p.
**Murphy EF:** Reflections on automotive adaptive equipment--an essay. **Bull Prosthet Res** 1979 Fall;16(2):191-207
**Murphy GK:** Death in the desert. The sabotage-derailment of 'The City of San Francisco'. **Am J Forensic Med Pathol** 1983 Jun;4(2):145-8
**Murphy GK:** The case of Stanley Setty. **Am J Forensic Med Pathol** 1980 Sep;1(3):245-7
**Murphy GP:** Landmark perspective: Bladder neoplasms. **JAMA** 1983 Sep 9;250(10):1326
**Murphy GP:** Roswell Park Memorial Institute, Genesis of a cancer center. **Oncology** 1980;37(6):426-8
**Murphy JA:** Tularemia and report of a case by Jerome A. Murphy. N. Y. State J. Med. 1928. **NY State J Med** 1983 Jul-Sep;83(8-10):1062
**Murphy JL** see **Baker DC**
**Murphy LJ:** Harry Harris and his contribution to suprapubic prostatectomy. **Aust NZ J Surg** 1984 Dec;54(6):579-88
**Murphy LP, McNair EW:** Summer program in medical school environment for undergraduate students: an evaluation. **J Negro Educ** 1981;50(4):407-14
**Murphy RL:** Auscultation of the lung: past lessons, future possibilities. **Thorax** 1981 Feb;36(2):99-107
**Murphy RL, Nodyne KR:** The healing science in the Mountain State: some notable medical personalities of West Virginia. **W Va Hist** 1981 Spring-Summer;42(3-4):285-306
**Murphy T:** The changing university. **Ir Med J** 1981 Jul;74(7):184-7
**Murphy TD:** Medical knowledge and statistical methods in early nineteenth-century France. **Med Hist** 1981 Jul;25(3):301-19
**Murphy WP:** Carl Walter: a pioneer in shaping the medical device industry. **Am J Surg** 1984 Nov;148(5):590-3
**Murray AE:** Bright delusion: Presbyterians and African colonization. **J Presbyt Hist** 1980;58(3):224-37
**Murray JE:** An interview with Joseph E. Murray, M.D. conducted by Joel M. Noe, M.D. **Ann Plast Surg** 1984 Jan;12(1):84-9
**Murray JE, Zollinger RM:** Carl Walter Appreciation Day: April 28, 1984. **Am J Surg** 1984 Nov;148(5):552-3
**Murray JE:** Reflections on the first successful kidney transplantation. **World J Surg** 1982 May;6(3):372-6
**Murray JE:** Remembrances of the early days of renal transplantation. **Transplant Proc** 1981 Mar;13(1):9-15
**Murray TJ:** Doctor Samuel Johnson's abnormal movements. **Adv Neurol** 1982;35:25-30
**Murray TJ:** The neurology of Alice in Wonderland. **Can J Neurol Sci** 1982 Nov;9(4):453-7
**Murray MA, ed** see **Ash L**
**Murrell TG:** A history of enteritis necroticans. **Papua New Guinea Med J** 1979 Mar;22(1):5-17
**Murthy CK:** Origin and slow progress of study of anatomy in ancient times. **Bull Indian Inst Hist Med (Hyderabad)** 1978;8(1-4):24-5
**Murthy CK:** Sculpture of fasting Buddha; artist's knowledge of anatomy in ancient India. **Bull Inst Hist Med (Hyderabad)** 1973 Oct;3(4):186-8
**Murthy SR:** An occurrence of cinnabar in Rasarnavakalpa. **Indian J Hist Sci** 1979 Nov;14(2):83-6
**Murthy SR:** Vagbhata on medicinal uses of gems. **Indian J Hist Sci** 1979 Nov;14(2):134-8
**Musaev TM:** Vzgliady Abu Ali Ibn Siny (Avitsenny) na opukholevye zabolevaniia. **Vopr Onkol** 1980;26(9):72-4
**Musallam BF:** Why Islam permitted birth control. **Arab Stud Q** 1981;3(2):181-97
**Musallam BF** see **Bleich JD**
**Musambachime MC:** The social and economic effects of sleeping sickness in Mweru-Luapula 1906-1922. **Afr Econ Hist** 1981;10:151-73
**Musatti C:** Freud e l'ebraismo. **Belfagor** 1980;35(6):687-96
**Muschter R** see **Gregl A**
**Musée de la Pharmacie:** Exposition: Montpellier: de l'apothicairerie à la pharmacie. Montpellier, Faculté de Pharmacie, n.d.
**Musiał G:** Historia operacji zaćmy. 1. Od czasów starożytnych do X wieku. **Klin Oczna** 1983 Aug-Sep;85(8-9):325-7
**Musiał G:** Historia operacji zaćmy. 2. Od średniowiecza do XVIII wieku. **Klin Oczna** 1983 Oct;85(10):371-3
**Musiał G:** Historia operacji zaćmy. 3. XIX iXX wiek. **Klin Oczna** 1983 Nov-Dec;85(11-12):439-41
**Musič D, Rakovec P, Jagodic A, et al:** The first description of syncopal attacks in heart block. **PACE** 1984 Mar;7(2):301-3
**Musick M, ed:** 'Glorious war': the diary of Westwood James, 16th Alabama. **Civ War Times Illus** 1978;17(6)34-42
**Musikterapi förr och nu för barn och vuxna: Lakartidningen** 1981;78(20):2045-55
**Muslin HL:** Romeo and Juliet: the tragic self in adolescence. **Adolesc Psychiatry** 1982;10:106-17
**Musset J:** L'intervention de l'administration en matière d'épidémie au XVIIIe siècle: l'élection de Saint-Lô en 1785. **Ann Normandie** 1978 Dec;28:344-6
**Musset J:** L'intervention de l'administration en matière d'épidémie, en milieu rural au XVIIIe siècle: l'élection de Saint-Lô (Généralité de Caen) en 1785. **Bull Soc Fr Hist Hop** 1979;(39):23-31
**Mustaev RK** see **Gus'kov EN**
**Musto DF:** Continuity across generations: the Adams Family myth. In M. Albin, R. J. Devlin, G. Heeger, ed: New directions in psychohistory. The Adelphi papers in honor of Erik H. Erikson. Lexington, Toronto, D. C. Heath, 1980. p. 117-29.
**Musto DF, Ramos MR:** Notes on American medical history: a follow-up study of the New Haven morphine maintenance clinic of 1920. **N Engl J Med** 1981 Apr 30;304(18):1071-7
**Musto DF:** Worthington Hooker (1806-1867): physician and educator. **Conn Med** 1984 Sep;48(9):569-74
**Musto DF** see **Blain D**
**Mutaw RJ** see **Corruccini RS**
**Muthiah A, Jones GW:** Fertility trends among overseas Indian populations. **Popul Stud** 1983 Jul;37(2):273-99
**Mutschlechner G:** Erde als Heilmittel für Mensch und Tier. **Tirol Heimatbl** 1974;49(1):23-7
**Mutschlechner G:** Vom Olbrennen und Olhandel im Zillertal. **Tirol Heimatbl** 1971;46(7-9):71-4
**Mutschmann H:** Milton's eyesight and the chronology of his works. New York, Haskell House, 1971. 50 p.
**Mutt V:** An appreciation of the work of Vittorio Erspamer. **Peptides (Fayetteville)** 1981;2(Suppl 2):3-6
**Muuss RE:** Peter Blos' modern psychoanalytic interpretation of adolescence. **J Adolesc** 1980 sep;3(3):229-52
**Muzrukova HB:** Chemistry and biology in the history of cellular's study. **Istor Biol Issled** 1983;9:51-65
**Myco F:** Eighteenth century medicine: of magic and mysticism. **Nurs Mirror** 1982 Sep 8;155(10):50-2
**Myer JS:** William Beaumont: a pioneer American physiologist. New ed. of his: Life and letters of Dr. William Beaumont. With historical introductions by E. Brodman and R. E. Shank. Includes reprint of 1833 ed. of Beaumont's Experiments and observations on the gastric juice and the physiology of digestion. St. Louis, Mosby, 1981. xi, 394 p.
**Myerhoff BG** see **Hand WD, ed**
**Myers GE** see **James W**
**Myers JA** see **Wangensteen OW, ed**
**Myers ML:** Centric relation records--historical review. **J Prosthet Dent** 1982 Feb;47(2):141-5
**Myers WA:** Mary Shelley's Frankenstein: creativity and the psychology of the exception. **Int J Psychoanal Psychother** 1982-83;9:625-45
**Myers WG:** Georg Charles de Hevesy: the father of nuclear medicine. **J Nucl Med** 1979 Jun;20(6):590-4
**Myers WG:** Historian's note: early experiences in nuclear medicine by John H. Lawrence, 1956. **J Nucl Med** 1979 Jun;20(6):560-4
**Myers WG:** PET = positrin+electron transmutation. **JNM** 1980;21:1200
**Myers WG:** The Anger scintillation camera becomes of age. **J Nucl Med** 1979 Jun;20(6):565-7
**Myers-Levin A:** Cerebral palsy: the early years of occupational therapy in Scotland. Edingburgh, Scottish Council for Spastics, 1978. xv, 131 p.
**Myhre BA:** Landmark perspective: the significance of Dr. Fantus' report. **JAMA** 1984 Feb 3;251(5):650-2
**Myhrman G:** Möte med en ny sjukdom--nephropathia epidemica. **Nord Medicinhist Arsb** 1984;:175-9
**Myíri JK:** Philosophy and suicide--statistics in Austria-Hungary. **East Cent Eur** 1978;5(1):69-89
**Mylenki M:** Historical collections in psychiatry and psychoanalysis.

**Libr Trends** 1982 Spring;:613–29
**Myles J, Green E, Hood TK, et al:** The doctor who never refused a call: [Arthur James] Hood, M.D. **Northeast Nev Hist Soc Q** 1980;(2):43–58
**Mysh VG:** L. R. Dragstedt (vklad v uchenie o patogeneze i lechenii iazvennoi bolezni). **Khirurgiia (Mosk)** 1983 Jul;7:140–1

# N

**Na strazhe Rodiny: Voen Med Zh** 1980 Feb;(2):3–6
**Naal W:** Arzt und ärztliche Versorgung auf dem Hunsrück seit dem 30jährigen Krieg beispielhaft dargestellt an der Familie Pies. Diss. Düsseldorf, 1979. 198 p.
**al-Naaman YD, Wada J:** The history of thoracic and cardiovascular surgery. **J Fac Med Baghdad** 1977;19(suppl):1–24
**Nabielek R:** Probleme bei der Edition der nur arabisch überlieferten pseudogalenischen Schrift De sommo et vigilia. **NTM** 1982;19(2):75–80
**Nabielek R:** Robert Koch und die Begründung des Lehrstuhls für Hygiene an der Berliner Universität. **Z Gesamte Hyg** 1982 Mar;28(3):185–93
**Nabielek R:** Zu den wichtigsten Veröffentlichungen des polnischen Histologen Henryk Fryderyk Hoyer (1834–1907) in deutschen Fachzeitschriften. **Z Mikrosk Anat Forsch** 1983;97(3):393–408
**Nabri IA:** El Zahrawi (936–1013 AD), the father of operative surgery. **Ann R Coll Surg Engl** 1983 Mar;65(2):132–4
**Nadal J:** L'última pandèmia de pesta a Catalunya, 1650–1654. In Congrés International d'Història de la Medicina Catalana, 2nd, Barcelona, 1975. Llibre d'Actes. Barcelona, Socitra, 1977. p. 19–38.
**Nadeau J:** La médecine populaire dans quatre paroisses du comté de Bellechasse. **Rev Ethnol Que** 1976;2(1):51–104
**Nadelson CC, Notman MT:** [History of] women as health professionals. In Reich WT, et al, ed: Encyclopedia of bioethics, v.4. New York, Free Press, 1978. p. 1713–20
**Nadig P, Wyatt BW:** A personal history of Bexar County medicine. **Friends P.I. Nixon Med Hist Libr** 1981;10:6–13
**Nagaev IM:** Krasnye medsestry na frontakh grazhdanskoĭ voĭny. **Med Sestra** 1980 Dec;39(12):41–2
**Nagai M** see **Brace CL**
**Nagaishi C:** A brief history of the Asia–Pacific Congress on Diseases of the Chest. **Chest** 1984 Nov;86(5):656–7
**Nagasaki-ken Yakuzaishikai, Yakushi Kenkyukai:** Nagasaki yakushi. Nagasaki, Nagasaki-ken Yakuzaishikai, Showa 53 nen, 1978. 502 p.
**Nagasawa Y:** [Encounter with Nightingale---a discovery of Nightingale in the field of hospital designs] (Jpn) **Sogo Kango** 1980;15(4):59–69
**Nagel A, Nagel R:** Von Arzten und Beamten. Ein Collegium Sanitatis für Kleve (1726). **Med Welt** 1983 Sep 16;34(37):1019–20
**Nagel EL** see **Hirschman JC**
**Nagel G:** Georges Vacher de Lapouge (1854–1936). Ein Beitrag zur Geschichte des Sozialdarwinismus in Frankreich. Freiburg, Schulz, 1975. 109 p. (Freiburger Forschungen zur Medizingeschichte, Neue Folge, 4).
**Nagel R** see **Nagel A**
**Nagl H:** Der Zauberer-Jackl-Prozess: Hexenprozesse im erzstift Salzburg 1675–1690. **Mitt Ges Salzburger Landeskd** 1972–73;112–113(2):385–539
**Nagy L:** Az 1713, évi pécsi pestisjárvány. **Orv Hetil** 1981 Oct 4;122(40):2488–90
**Nagy S:** Szépirodalom--orvostörténelem. **Orv Hetil** 1980 Sep 28;121(39):2421
**Nahas GG:** Bilinguisme médical: vingt cinq ans d'expérience. **Bull Soc Sci Med Grand Duche Luxemb** 1979;116(1):83–7
**Nahas GG:** Hashish in Islam 9th to 18th century. **Bull NY Acad Med** 1982 Dec;58(9):814–31
**Nahm PP** see **Engelhardt R, ed**
**Nahon R** see **Poirier J**
**Naidenov G, Konaréva N, Nikiforov N:** Hissar – station thermale de l'Antiquité jusqu'à nos jours. In International Congress of the History of Medicine. 26th, Plovdiv, 1978. Actes du Congress. Sofia, 1981. Volume II. p. 217–9.
**Naidis M:** 'Ants, muskeetoes, flies and stinking chints': the British battle against disease in India. **West Hum Rev** 1964;17(1):39–47
**Naiken VS:** Richard Bright, physician and budding socio-cultural anthropologist. In: Congrès international d'histoire de la médecine, XXVe, Québec, 1976. Actes. Québec, 1977. p. 999–1001.
**Naisawald LV:** Fanny Ricketts, nurse, diarist, devoted wife. **Va Cavalcade** 1972;21(3):14–21
**Najafi H:** Landmark perspective: Dr. Alexis Carrel and tissue culture. **JAMA** 1983 Aug 26;250(8):1086–9
**El Najjar M** see **Streitz JM**
**El-Najjar MY, Benitez J, Fry G, et al:** Autopsies on two native American Mummies. **Am J Phys Anthropol** 1980 Aug;53(2):197–202
**El-Najjar MY:** Human treponematosis and tuberculosis: evidence from the New World. **Am J Phys Anthropol** 1979 Nov;51(4):599–618
**El-Najjar MY, Andrews J, Moore JG, et al:** Iron deficiency anemia in two prehistoric American Indian skeletons: a dietary hypothesis. **Plains Anthropol** 1982;27(97):205–9
**El-Najjar MY, Mulinski TM:** Mummies and mummification practices in the southwestern and southern United States. In A. Cockburn, E. Cockburn, ed: Mummies, disease, and ancient cultures. Cambridge, Cambridge University Press, 1980. p. 103–17.
**Najman JM, Western JS:** A comparative analysis of Australian health policy in the 1970s. **Soc Sci Med** 1984;18(11):949–58
**Nakagawa Y:** [Medical history in the medical education] (Jpn). **Igakushi Kenkyu** 1978;50:2–10
**Nakajima M:** [Clinical study of pain]. Continued regularly. (Jpn). **Kangogaku Zasshi** 1984 May;48(5):569–72
**Nakamura T:** T. Willis' and Lower's physiology with special reference to the theory of heart movement. **Jpn Stud Hist Sci** 1977;16:23–41
**Nakazato T:** [The early days of modern nursing in Japan--the Kyoto School of Nursing] (Jpn). **Kango** 1981 Jan;33(1):70–83
**Nakazawa O:** The faith in Buddha of medicine in Japan. In: Congrès international d'histoire de la médecine, XXVe, Québec, 1976. Actes. Québec, 1977. p. 1002–8.
**Nakazawa S:** [Recent advances in neurological surgery (Jpn). **Nippon Ika Daigaku Zasshi** 1981 Dec;48(6):711
**Nalepka C:** Entry into professional nursing in the United States and in England viewed with a historical and comparative perspective. **Australas Nurses J** 1983 Jan–Feb;11(12):1–7
**Nally JN:** Développement scientifique de la prothèse dentaire et éthique médicale. **Schweiz Monatsschr Zahnmed** 1984 Jan;94(1):23–8
**Nalven J:** Health research on undocumented Mexicans. **Soc Sci J** 1982;19(2):73–88
**Nalven J:** Who benefits from knowledge about the health of undocumented Mexicans? **Policy Stud J** 1982;10(3):556–80
**Namba T** see **Hamada T**
**Namboodiri NK:** On factors affecting fertility at different stages in the reproduction history: an exercise in cohort analysis. **Soc Forces** 1981;59(4):114–29
**Namigohar F, Soltani A:** L'hygiène en Iran au temps d'Achemèdes. In International Congress of the History of Medicine. 26th, Plovdiv, 1978. Actes du Congress. Sofia, 1981. Volume II. p. 160–1.
**Namysłowski G** see **Gierek T**
**Nand Raj L:** Human experimentation of Drugs. **Bull Indian Inst Hist Med (Hyderabad)** 1980;10(1–4):53–61
**Nanetti L:** Su alcuni rapporti tra storia e medicina legale. **Acta Med Hist Patav** 1978–79;25:105–28
**Nansen P:** A Danish pathography from the 16th century. **Hist Med Vet** 1979;4(4):73–81
**Nansen P:** En sygdomsbeskrivelse fra 1600–tallets Danmark. **Nord Vet Med** 1980 Jan;32(1):38–45
**Nansen P** see **Rose CH**
**Napalkov NP, Mishura VI, Merabishvili VM, et al:** Razvitie ideĭ N. N. Petrova v oblasti organizatsii protivorakovoĭ bor'by. **Vopr Onkol** 1982;28(5):126–32
**Napalkov NP** see **Blokhin NN**
**Napalkov PN, Shafer II:** Professor Vasiliĭ Mikhaĭlovich Nazarov (k 100–letiiu so dnia rozhdeniia). **Vestn Khir** 1983 Mar;130(3):129–30
**Napalkov PN, Vigdorchuk IV, Labazanov MM:** Razvitie khirurgii v soiuznykh respublikakh za 60 let Soiuza SSR. **Vestn Khir** 1983;130(4):3–9
**Napodano RJ, Young LE:** The University of Rochester Associated Hospitals Programs in internal medicine. Seven years experience with an innovative city-wide residency for preparation of general internists. **Am J Med** 1982 Jun;72(6):945–50
**Napoli DS:** Architects of adjustment: the history of the psychological profession in the United States. Port Washington, N. Y., Kennikat Press, 1981. 176 p.
**Napolitano EG, Gruber B:** The struggle for accreditation in chiropractic: a unique history of educational bootstrapping. **Chiropr Hist** 1981;1(1):23–4
**Naquet R:** Gastaut and the EEG Federation. **Electroencephalogr Clin Neurophysiol** 1982;35:7–8
**Naqvi N** see **Felstein I**
**Naranjo B, Estienne P:** La mutation des comportements démographiques de la proche banlieue clermontoise: le rôle des étrangers. **Rev Auvergne** 1981;95(1):3–11
**Naranjo P:** Medicina indigena y popular de América Latina y medicina contemporánea. **Guatem Indig** 1978;13(1/2):186–219
**Naranjo P:** Social function of coca in pre-Columbian America. **J Ethnopharmacol** 1981 Mar–May;3(2–3):161–72
**Narbe S:** Egypten: på Ramses tid. **Odontol Foren Tidskr** 1981 Oct;45(4):30–2
**Nardoux M, Montarnal:** Carie--abrasion--dimension. Dents de la préhistoire. **Ligament (Montp)** 1980;137:88–91
**Narimanov ZM:** Dostizheniia gigieny truda i profpatologii v Sovetskoĭ Armenii. **Gig Tr Prof Zabol** 1982;(11):1–4
**Narro Robles J** see **Canales Muñoz JL**
**Nars PW:** Frühgeburten gestern und heute. **Praxis** 1981 Apr 21;70(17):757–62
**Nasemann T:** Der Morphologe Hermann Werner Siemens und seine Bemühungen um eine 'Allgemeine Dermatologie'. **Hautarzt** 1983 Nov;34(11):569–73
**Nash AE:** Mortality pattern of the Wiltshire lords of the manor, 1242–1377. **South Hist** 1979;2
**Naske CM:** Bob Bartlett and the Alaska Mental Health Act. **Pac Northwest Q** 1980;71(1):31–9
**Nasonova VA:** Razvitie ideĭ S. P. Botkina v sovremennoĭ revmatologii. **Vestn Akad Med Nauk SSSR** 1983;(3):41–6
**Nassimi MN:** The achievements of the Arab Prophet in the field of hygiene and preventive medicine. In: International Symposium for the History of Arabic Science, 1st, University of Aleppo, 1976. Proceedings. Aleppo, Syria, 1976. Papers in European Languages. Vol. II. p. 343–5.
**Năstasă V:** Activitatea ştiinţifică a farmaciştilor în cadrul 'societăţii de medici şi naturalişti' din iaşi. **Rev Med Chir Soc Med Nat Iasi** 1981;85(1):158–60
**Năstasă V, Sîrghie E, Cuciureanu R, et al:** Date istorice privind alimentarea cu apă potabilă a municipiului Iaşi, precum şi variaţiile cantitative şi

calitative ale acesteia. **Rev Med Chir Soc Med Nat Iasi** 1982 Jul–Sep;86(3):449–52

**Natadse R:** Die Rolle der Universität Tbilisi bei der entwicklung der Psychologie in Georgien. **Wiss Z Friedrich Schiller Univ (Gesellsch)** 1973;22(3):497–509

**Natadze TG:** O prioritete V. V. Voronina v nekotorykh oblastakh meditsiny i biologii (k 110–letiiu so dnia rozhdeniia V. V. Voronina). **Patol Fiziol Eksp Ter** 1981 May–Jun;(3):53–7

**Natadze TG:** Osnovnye dostizheniia gruzinskikh patofiziologov. **Patol Fiziol Eksp Ter** 1983 May–Jun;3:23–4

**Natali J:** Paul Broca, chirurgien vasculaire. **Chirurgie** 1980;106(10):777–82

**Nathans D:** The new genetics. **Trans Am Clin Climatol Assoc** 1979;91:75–97

**Nathanson N, Martin JR:** The epidemiology of poliomyelitis: enigmas surrounding its appearance, epidemicity, and disappearance. **Am J Epidemiol** 1979 Dec;110(6):672–92

**Nation EF, McGovern JP, ed:** Student and chief: the Osler–Camac correspondence. Pasadena, Castle Press, 1980. 131 p.

**National Institute of General Medical Sciences. Office of Research Reports:** Nobel prize laureates. [Bethesda, Md.], National Institutes of Health, Dept. of Health, Education, and Welfare. [1978]. 24 p.

**Natradze AG:** Russkie i sovetskie farmakopei. Moskva, Meditsina, 1978. 111 p.

**Natvig P:** Jacques Joseph, surgical sculptor. Philadelphia, Saunders, 1982. xiii, 264 p.

**Nauels I:** Arzt und Medizin in fünf Jahrgängen. Spiegel (1971–1975). Diss. Düsseldorf, 1981. 137 p.

**Nauert CG:** Caius Plinius Secundus. In Cranz FE, Kristeller PO, ed: Catalogus translationum et commentariorum: Mediaeval and Renaissance Latin translations and commentaries. Annotated lists and guides. Vol. IV. Washington, D.C., Catholic University of America Press, 1980. p. 297–422.

**Nauert CG:** The author of a Renaissance commentary on Pliny: Rivius, Trithemius or Aquaeus. **J Warburg Courtauld Inst** 1979;42:282–6

**Naujack E** see **Engelhardt R, ed**

**Naujoks R:** Zivilisation und Zahnheilkunde. **Dtsch Zahnarztl Z** 1980 Feb;35(2):156–61

**Naumann P** see **Schadewaldt H**

**Naumenko AM** see **Korol' GG**

**Naunton RF:** Clinical research in otolaryngology at the University of Chicago. **Ann Otol Rhinol Laryngol [Suppl]** 1983 Jan–Feb;102:30–1

**Naunton RF** see **Mhoon EE**

**Nauright L:** Politics and power: a new look at Florence Nightingale. **Nurs Forum** 1984;21(1):5–7

**Nauroy J:** L'équipement technique et le ravitaillement. **Med Armees** 1980;8(10)spec:845–50

**Nauroy J:** Les historiographes de la pharmacie militaire française. In: Vorträge des Internationalen Pharmaziehistorischen Kongresses Innsbruck 1977. Stuttgart, Wissenschaftliche Verlagsgesellschaft, 1979. p. 91–6.

**Nauroy J, Bossard E:** Louis–Marie Gessard, pharmacien et édile de Saint–Denis. **Rev Hist Pharm (Paris)** 1979 Dec;26(243):235–9

**Nauroy J:** Une pharmacienne confrontée malgré elle à la conspiration de Malet. **Rev Hist Pharm (Paris)** 1984 Mar;31(260):18–20

**Nauts HC:** Bacterial products in the treatment of cancer: past, present and future. In Jeljaszewicz J, Pulverer G, Roszkowski W, ed: Bacteria and cancer. London; New York, Academic Press, 1982. p. 1–25.

**Navarro P:** Lactancia mercenaria: hipocresía y exploitación. **Asclepio** 1983;35:375–87

**Navarro P:** The politics of air pollution. **Public Interest** 1980;59:36–44

**Navarro V:** Class struggle, the state and medicine. An historical and contemporary analysis of the medical sector in Great Britain. New York, Prodist, 1978. xviii, 156 p.

**Navarro V:** Medical history as justification rather than explanation: a critique of Starr's The Social Transformation of American Medicine. **Int J Health Serv** 1984;14(4):511–28

**Navarro V** see **Assennato G**

**Navarro Brotóns V:** Juan Bautista Corachán y la enseñanza universitaria. In: Estudios de historia de Valencia. Valencia, Universidad, Facultad de Derecho. 1978. p. 279–92.

**Navashin SM, Fomina IP:** Nauka ob antibiotikakh v SSSR – istoriia i perspektivy razvitiia. **Antibiotiki** 1982;27(12):5–9

**Naveau B** see **Ryckewaert A**

**Navratil L** see **Janzarik W ed**

**Navrátil M:** Padesát let Kojeneckého ústavu v Ostravě. **Cesk Pediatr** 1981 Aug;36(8):475–6

**Näyhä S:** Short and medium–term variations in mortality in Finland. A study on cyclic variations, annual and weekly periods and certain irregular changes in mortality in Finland during period 1868–1972. **Scand J Soc Med [Suppl]** 1981;(21):1–101

**Nayler WG:** Sydney Ringer––physician and scientist. **J Mol Cell Cardiol** 1984 Feb;16(2):113–6

**Naylor CD:** Canadian doctors and state health insurance, 1911–1918. **RSTC** 1982;22,6(3):127–50

**Naylor CD:** The CMA's first code of ethics: medical morality or borrowed ideology? **J Can Stud** 1982–83;17(4):20–32

**Naylor D:** Osler's first medical publications. **Can Med Assoc J** 1984 Oct 1;131(7):800–5

**Nazarenko AI** see **Berezovskiĭ VA**

**Nazarov VF:** K 60–letiiu organizatsii sanatorno–kurortnogo dela v Vooruzhennykh Silakh SSSR. **Voen Med Zh** 1982 Aug;(8):75–8

**Nazzaro–Porro M** see **Passi S**

**Ndetei DM:** Psychiatry in Kenya: yesterday, today and tomorrow. An overview. **Acta Psychiatr Scand** 1980 Sep;62(3):201–11

**Neagu I, Maracineanu G, Neagu M:** Contribution de la Société 'La Jeune Croix Rouge Américaine' au developpement de l'assistance médicale et sociale en Roumanie. In: Congrès international d'histoire de la médecine, XXVe, Québec, 1976. Actes. Québec, 1977. p. 1009–14.

**Neagu I, Neagu M:** Quelques données médico–historiques sur la 'Colonie Bulgare' de Ploiesti. In International Congress of the History of Medicine. 26th, Plovdiv, 1978. Actes du Congress. Sofia, 1981. Volume II. p. 161–3.

**Neagu I, Neagu M:** Vieux médicament utilisé dans la thérapeutique populaire de Roumanie. In: Congrès international d'histoire de la médecine, XXVe, Québec, 1976. Actes. Québec, 1977. p. 1015–25.

**Neagu M** see **Neagu I**

**Neale JM, Oltmanns TF:** Schizophrenia. New York, Wiley, 1980. Historical section, p. 2–16.

**Neary K** see **Margolis M**

**Nebbia G** see **De Marco O**

**Nechaev VV** see **Shliakhtenko LI**

**Nechaĭ AI, Sitenko VM:** Vladimir Nikolaevich Shamov (k 100–letiiu so dnia rozhdeniia). **Klin Khir** 1982 May;(5):62–4

**Nechaĭ AI** see **Samotokin BA**

**Nechiporenko PI:** Meditsinskaia émblema i ee istoriia. **Med Sestra** 1980 Feb;39(2):50–3

**Nechiporuk VM, Boliukh BA:** Iz istorii s'ézdov khirurgov USSR. **Klin Khir** 1979 Nov;(11):61–4

**Nedvei VC:** A history of endocrinology. Lancaster, Boston, MTP Press, 1982. xviii, 913 p.

**Needham J:** China and the origins of immunology. **East Horiz** 1980;19(1):6–12

**Needham J:** Science in traditional China. A comparative perspective. Cambridge, Harvard University Press; Hong Kong, The Chinese University Press, 1981. x, 134 p.

**Needham J:** The social position of scientific men and physicians in mediaeval China. In: International Congress for the History of Science, 14th, Tokyo, Kyoto, 1974. Proceedings. Tokyo, 1975. 4:19–34.

**Needham J** see **Lu Gwei–djen**

**Needleman J** see **Sharkey PW, ed**

**Neel JV:** Human evolution: many small steps, but not punctuated equilibria. **Perspect Biol Med** 1984 Autumn;28(1):75–103

**Neelavathi A:** A brief introduction of Siddha system of medicine. **Bull Indian Inst Hist Med (Hyderabad)** 1979;9:38–40

**Neelin JM:** Archibald Byron Macallum, pioneer of biochemistry in Canada. **Can J Biochem Cell Biol** 1984 Jun;62(6):viii–xi

**Neff DS:** "Extraordinary means': healers and healing in 'A Conversation with My Father'. In Jones AH, ed: Images of healers. Albany, State University of New York Press, 1983. p. 118–24.

**Neghme A:** La educación médica y el Servicio Nacional de Salud. **Rev Med Chil** 1977 Oct;105(10):668–73

**Neghme A:** La medicina chilena esta de duelo. **Rev Med Chil** 1980 May;108(5):399–406

**Neghme A:** La obra literaria de los médicos chilenos. **Rev Med Chil** 1981 Jun;109(6):557–64; Jul;109(7):683–91

**Neghme A:** La organización panamericana de la salud en su 75. aniversario. Tributo al Dr. Abraham B. Horwitz. **Rev Med Chil** 1977 Dec;105(12):950–2

**Neghme A:** Obra literaria de los médicos chilenos. (III, IV). **Rev Med Chil** 1981 Aug–Sep;109(8,9):789–93, 895–900 (continued periodically)

**Neghme A:** Semblanza del Dr. Carlos R. Chagas, figura señera de la medicina. **Rev Med Chil** 1979 Sep;107(9):876–8

**Neghme A:** Semblanza historica del Hospital San Francisco de Borja. **Rev Med Chil** 1982 Jul;110(7):693–4

**Neghme A:** Significado de la investigación biomédica en el desarrollo académico de una escuela de medicina. Remembranzas de un pasado no tan remoto. **Rev Med Chil** 1981 Sep;109(9):878–84

**Neghme A:** Vida y obra de Sir William Osler (1849–1919) y la fundación de la Escuela de Medicina en la Universidad de Johns Hopkins. **Rev Med Chil** 1983 Jan;111(1):83–92

**Negru I:** Aprovizionarea Bucureştilor cu apă prină in pragul secolului al XX–lea. **Viata Med [Medii Sanit]** 1983 Aug;31(8):185–90

**Negru I:** Carantinele Austriei şi rolul lor pe frontiera Dunării (Sec. XVIII–XIX). **Viata Med [Medii Sanit]** 1982 Jun;30(6):139–42

**Negru I:** Concepţia profesorului Victor Babeş asupra instruirii şi formării agentului sanitar. **Viata Med [Medii Sanit]** 1983 Sep;31(9):211–4

**Negru I:** Din primele realizări sanitare româneşti în Transilvania. **Viata Med [Medii Sanit]** 1980 Dec;28(12):281–4

**Negru I:** Informaţii asupra apariţiei şi răspîndirii luesului pe teritoriul Europei apusene. **Viata Med [Medii Sanit]** 1982 Jan;30(1):21–4

**Negru I:** Istoria medicinii: Sora de ocrotire––Teodora Gându. **Viata Med [Medii Sanit]** 1979 Apr;27(4):89–92

**Negru I:** Istoricul bolilor venerice in studiile clasice ale istoricilor medicinii ramâneşti. **Viata Med [Medii Sanit]** 1981 Dec;29(12):281–5

**Negru I:** Misiuni sanitare române în războiul balcanic din anul 1912. **Viata Med [Medii Sanit]** 1983 Apr;31(4):91–6

**Negru I:** Momente remarcabile din trecutul luptei împortriva cancerului în România. **Viata Med [Medii Sanit]** 1980 Sep;28(9):213–5

**Negru I:** Muzeul memorial 'Prof. dr. Gh. Marinescu'. **Viata Med [Medii Sanit]** 1981 Aug;29(8):187–90

**Negru I:** O şcoală de surori de ocrotire mai puţin cunoscută–şcoala din Timişoara (septembrie 1939–februarie 1942). **Viata Med [Medii Sanit]**

1984 Jul;32(7):163-6
**Negru I:** Originile medicinii române sti după dr. N. Vătămanu. **Viata Med [Medii Sanit]** 1980 Jun;28(6):141-4
**Negru I:** Primele anchete medico-sociale ale şcolii clujene de igienă. **Viata Med [Medii Sanit]** 1983 Jul;31(7):165-8
**Negru I:** Primele campanii antimalarice în România. **Viata Med [Medii Sanit]** 1982 Mar;30(3):71-2
**Negru I:** Prof. dr. Nicolae Gh. Lupu în lumina autobiografică şi a istoriei medicinii româneşti. **Viata Med [Medii Sanit]** 1983 Feb;31(2):45-7
**Negru I:** Profesorul Iuliu Moldovan creatorul primului Institut oncologic în România. **Viata Med [Medii Sanit]** 1982 Dec;30(12):281-6
**Negru I:** 'Secolul copilului' in discuţia congreselor medicale din România (1919 şi 1925). **Viata Med [Medii Sanit]** 1982 Feb;30(2):45-7
**Negru I:** Spitalul de tuberculoză de la 'Filaret' şi doctorul Stefan Irimescu. **Viata Med [Medii Sanit]** 1983 Mar;31(3):68-72
**Neguţ M** see **Panaitescu D**
**Néhány F:** Farkas Géza professzorról a tanítványai. **Orv Hetil** 1984 Nov 11;125(46):2817
**Neiburger EJ:** Lesions in a prehistoric bear: differential diagnosis. **Paleopathol Newsl** 1984 Dec;(48):8-11
**Neiburger EJ:** The evolution of human occlusion (II). **Quintessence Int** 1979 Jul;10(7):75-84
**Neibyl KH:** Science, medicine and the Puritan society. **J Eur Econ Hist** 1979;8(1):149-56
**Neighbors HW** see **Jackson JS**
**Neil G:** The Scott Memorial Hospital Scone: 90 years of nursing. **Lamp** 1982 Mar-Apr;39(2):19
**Neild FG:** James Neild (1744-1814) and prison reform. **J R Soc Med** 1981 Nov;74(11):834-40
**Neild FG:** Lieutenant Colonel C. T. Samman, OStJ, MRCS, LSA, DPH, Master of the Society of Apothecaries, 1928-31. **J R Army Med Corps** 1983 Oct;129(3):184-5
**Neill JR:** Adolf Meyer and American psychiatry today. **Am J Psychiatry** 1980 Apr;137(4):460-4
**Neill JR, Ludwig AM:** Psychiatry and psychotherapy: past and future. **Am J Psychother** 1980 Jan;34(1):39-50
**Neilson EA:** Reflections on health promotion through health education historical perspectives: options for the future. **Health Values** 1980 Jul-Aug;4(4):161-7
**Neilson JB** see **Paterson GR**
**Neiman FD** see **Aufderheide AC**
**Neĭman IM:** K 50-letiiu sozyva I Vsesoiuznogo s'ezda onkologov (iz vospominaniĭ uchastnika). **Vopr Onkol** 1981;27(11):88-9
**Neiman IM:** Predvidenie--osnovnaia osobennost' tvorchestva Aleksandra Aleksandrovicha Bogomol'tsa. **Fiziol Zh** 1981 May-Jun;27(3):307-10
**Neimann N, Pierson M:** Geschichte der Kinderheilkunde im 19. und 20. Jahrhundert. In Sournia JC, Martiny M, Poulet J, ed: Illustrierte Geschichte der Medizin. Salzburg, Andreas, 1980. Vol. 7. p. 2525-39.
**Neiss R:** Alfred Lorenzer. In J. Rattner, ed: Wandlungen der Psychoanalyse. Wien, Europaverlage, 1980. p. 233-56.
**Nel CJ:** Die departement chirurgie, universiteit van die oranje-vrystaat--die eerste tien jaar. **S Afr J Surg** 1980 Sep;19(3):81-6
**Nelken LE:** Reminiscences of my medical education (1916-1933) before emigrating to Palestine. **Koroth** 1981;8(1-2):51-6
**Nelkin D** see **Markle GE**
**Nelson CW** see **Key JD**
**Nelson EC:** 'In the Contemplation of Vegetables'--Caleb Threlkeld (1676-1728), his life, background and contribution to Irish botany. **J Soc Bibliogr Nat Hist** 1979 Nov;9(3):257-73
**Nelson EC:** The influence of Leiden on botany in Dublin in the early eighteenth century. **Huntia** 1982;4(2):133-46
**Nelson HE:** Disease, demography, and the evolution of social structure in Highland New Guinea. **J Polynesian Soc** 1971;80(2):204-16
**Nelson M** see **Burns C**
**Nelson NM** see **Smith GF**
**Nelson RB:** Occasional notes. Captains of an American credo: Walt and W. O. **N Engl J Med** 1981 Jul 9;305(2):110-2
**Nelson RB:** The final victory of General U. S. Grant. **Cancer** 1981 Feb 1;47(3):433-6
**Nelson RC** see **Tocus EC**
**Nelson TG:** Death, dung, the devil, and worldly delights: a metaphysical conceit in Harington, Donne, and Herbert. **Stud Philol** 1979 Summer;76(3):272-87
**Nelson VE** see **Schoen R**
**Nelson WE:** The first 50 years of The Journal of Pediatrics. **J Pediatr** 1982 Jul;101(1):1-4
**Nemchaninov SK** see **Burdov VS**
**Németh T, Nyárády I, Vadász I:** A gümökór epidemiológiai helyzete a világban és hazánkban (1882-1982). **Orv Hetil** 1983 May 29;124(22):1309-12
**Nemirovich LI** see **Pyrig LA**
**Nemitz K:** Die Bemühungen zur Schaffung eines Reichsgesundheitsministeriums in der ersten Phase der Weimarer Republik 1918-1922. **Medizinhist J** 1981;16(4):424-45
**Nemoianu V:** The semantics of Bramble's hypochondria: a connection between illness and style in the eighteenth century. **Clio (US)** 1979;9(1):39-51
**Nencini R** see **Giannattasio ME**
**Nepohoda-Seredenciuc I:** Our magazine is 25. **Sante Publique (Bucur)** 1983;26(1):3-8
**Ness DE:** C'est fini. . . .le pouls ne bat plus! Drawn by Paul Bernay, for Le Charivari, in 1872. **J Hist Med Allied Sci** 1980 Jul;35(3):312
**Nesselroade JR** see **Lerner RM, ed**
**Net echt!:** De anatomische wereld van Dr. Auzoux. [Exhibition, Museum Boerhaave, Leiden.] **Tijdschr Geschied Geneeskd** 1981;4(1):50-2
**Netolitzky A:** Marginalien über die Arecanuss im mittelalterlichen China. **Asiat Forsch** 1980;71:60-5
**Netzel Riera C:** Dirección de enfermería. Perspectiva histórica y encrucijada actual. **Rev Enferm** 1982 Dec;5(53):11-6
**Netzer C:** Annals of psychoanalysis: Ella Freeman Sharpe. **Psychoanal Rev** 1982 Summer;69(2):207-19
**Neu I:** Entwicklung und heutiger Stand der klinishen Neurologie. **Fortschr Med** 1980 Oct 2;98(37):1397-9
**Neu J:** One hundred fifth critical bibliography of the history of science and its cultural influences (to January 1980). **Isis** 1980;71(260):1 295
**Neubauer PB:** Anna Freud's legacy. **Psychoanal Q** 1983 Oct;52(4):507-13
**Neuberger A, Smith RL:** Richard Tecwyn Williams: the man, his work, his impact. **Drug Metab Rev** 1983;14(3):559-607
**Neuburger M:** The historical development of experimental brain and spinal cord physiology before Flourens. Edited by E. Clarke. Baltimore and London, Johns Hopkins University Press, 1981. xxiii, 391 p. (Trans. of 1897 ed).
**Neuerburg N:** An early California document. **Masterkey Ind Lore Hist** 1983;57(3):113-6
**Neufeld V:** The Mennonite mental health story. **Mennon Q Rev** 1982;56(1):18-31
**Neufeld VH, ed:** If we can love: the Mennonite mental health story. Newton, Kan., Faith and Life Press, 1983. xii, 340 p.
**Neugebauer J, Metz L:** 15 Jahre Gefässchirurgie am Städtischen Krankenhaus im Friedrichshain Berlin. **Z Arztl Fortbild (Jena)** 1979 Nov 1;73(21):1032-4
**Neugebauer R:** Application of a capture-recapture method (the Bernoulli census) to historical epidemiology. **Am J Epidemiol** 1984 Oct;120(4):626-34
**Neuhausen T:** Das Cholesterin. Vorstellungen über seine Rolle im Körper. Köln, Universität zu Köln, 1977. 187 p. (Kölner medizinhistorische Beiträge, 6).
**Neuhauser W:** Goethe sprach nie über die Leiden mit seinen Zähnen. **Zahnarztl Mitt** 1982 Aug 16;72(16):1735-43
**Neuhauser W:** Martin Luther bat Freund um Fürbitte bei heftigem Zahnschmerz. **Zahnarztl Mitt** 1983 Nov 1;73(21):2361-3
**Neuhauser W:** Zur Zeit der Bibel war der Zahn so viel wert wie das Leben selbst. **Zahnarztl Mitt** 1984 Apr 1;74(7):729-33
**Neuman RP:** Working class birth control in Wilhelmine Germany. **Comp Stud Soc Hist** 1978;20(3):408-28
**Neumann A, Heinrich P:** Die Bedeutung des Magdeburger Chirurgen Werner Hagedorn (1831 bis 1894) für die Einführung der Antiseptik auf dem europäischen Kontinent. **Zentralbl Chir** 1982;107(11):617-20
**Neumann D:** Reformbestrebungen zum Viehgewährschaftsrecht (Viehmängelhaftungsrecht). Historische Entwicklung und die Kritik aus tierärztlicher Sicht. Diss., Tierärztliche Hochschule Hannover. Hannover, 1983. 294 p.
**Neumann H:** Leben, wissenschaftliche Studien, Krankheiten und Tod Alfred Döblins. St. Michael [Austria], Bläschke, 1982. 110 p.
**Neumann J:** Eingeborenenheilkunde und Europäische Medizin in Kamerun. Arzt und Kranker in der Konfrontation zweier Kulturen. Freiburg, Schulz, 1978. 254 p. (Freiburger Forschungen zur Medizingeschichte, Neue Folge, 7).
**Neumann-Redlin von Meding E:** Ernst Neumann. Zum 150. Geburtstag des Königsberger Pathologen und Hämatologen am 30.1. 1984. **Pathologe** 1984 Jan;5(1):53-6
**Neumann-Redlin von Meding E:** Neumann' Zahnscheiden und Tomes' Zahnfasern. Zum 150. Geburtstag des Königsberger Pathologen Ernst Christian Neumann. **Dtsch Zahnarztl Z** 1984 Jan;39(1):65-9
**Neumärker KJ:** Zur Geschichte der Abteilung für Kinderneuropsychiatrie an der Berliner Charité. **Acta Paedopsychiatr (Basel)** 1982 Dec;48(6):297-305
**Neumeyer JL, Guan JH:** Pharmacy and the pharmaceutical industry, past, present and future, The People's Republic of China. **Am Pharm** 1982 Jan;22(1):14-21
**Neve M** see **Forgan S, ed**
**Neveux F:** Un établissement d'assistance en milieu rural au XIVe siècle: l'Hôtel-Dieu de Villers-Bocage. **Ann Normandie** 1977;1:3-17
**Neville RG, Smeaton WA:** Macquer's Dictionnaire de Chymie: a bibliographical study. **Ann Sci** 1981;38(6):613-62
**Neville W:** The birth rate in Singapore. **Popul Stud** 1978;32(1):113-4
**Nevins MA:** Bergen County's poet-physicians. **J Med Soc NJ** 1980 Nov;77(12):831-3
**Nevins MA** see **Alexander SF**
**Nevoral V, Křížek V:** J. J. Berzelius jako analytik minerálních vod. **Fysiatr Reumatol Vestn** 1980 Aug;58(4):244-7
**Nevoral V** see **Křížek V**
**Nevskiĭ NM:** O rabote frontovogo évakopunkta. **Voen Med Zh** 1980 Oct;(10):23-4
**New PK, Cheung YW:** Harvard Medical School of China, 1911--1916: an expanded footnote in the history of western medical education in China. **Soc Sci Med** 1982;16(12):1207-15
**The new Provident Medical Center: J Natl Med Assoc** 1983 Jul;75(7):727
**New Zealand Dental Journal. Seventy-fifth jubilee issue: NZ Dent J** 1980 Jul;76(345):107-48
**New Zealand Dept. of Health:** Health expenditures in New Zealand -- trends and growth patterns. Wellington, Management Services and

Research Unit, Department of Health, 1979. 62 p.
**Newbold M** see **Rook A**
**Newby MS:** Problems of teaching nursing history. 1. **Nurs Times** 1979 Nov 22;75(47):suppl 30:123–4 (continued periodically)
**Newcombe N, Lerner JC:** Britain between the wars: the historical context of Bowlby's theory of attachment. **Psychiatry** 1982 Feb;45(1):1–12
**Newell FW:** Centenary of Credé prophylaxis. **Am J Ophthalmol** 1980 Dec;90(6):874–5
**Newell FW, Blodi FC, Henkind P, et al:** In commemoration of 25 years of Survey of Ophthalmology. **Surv Ophthalmol** 1981 May–Jun;25(6):397–403
**Newell FW:** Pan-American Association of Ophthalmology––40 years. **Am J Ophthalmol** 1980 Mar;89(3):456–7
**Newell FW:** The first editor––Edward Jackson. **Am J Ophthalmol** 1982 Dec;94(6):809–10
**Newell FW:** The Ophthalmological Society of the United Kingdom: its first hundred years. **Am J Ophthalmol** 1980 Apr;89(4):605–7
**Newell LM, Malkinson FD:** 'Pyoderma (ecthyma) gangrenosum' by Brunsting, Goeckerman and O'Leary, October 1930. Commentary: Pyoderma gangrenosum. **Arch Dermatol** 1982 Oct;118(10):743–73
**Newman A** see **Laslett P**
**Newman C:** Nature of Samuel Pepys's 'wind colic'. **Br Med J [Clin Res]** 1980 Dec 20–27;281(6256):1716–7
**Newman CE:** The history of the College library, 1879–99. **J R Coll Physicians Lond** 1984 Jan;18(1):66–73
**Newman CE** see **Payne LM**
**Newman HN, Levers BG:** Tooth eruption and function in an early Anglo-Saxon population. **J R Soc Med** 1979 May;72(5):341–50
**Newman JL:** Acupuncture, anaesthesia, and all that. **NZ Med J** 1982 Jan 13;95(699):22
**Newman LF:** [Medical ethics in] primitive societies. In Reich WT, et al, ed: Encyclopedia of bioethics, v. 2. New York, Free Press, 1978. p. 877–9.
**Newman LM** see **Solnit AJ**
**Newman W:** Thomas Vaughan as an interpreter of Agrippa von Nettesheim. **Ambix** 1982 Nov;29(3):125–40
**Newmark P:** Thirty years of DNA. **Nature** 1983 Sep 29–Oct 5;305(5933):383–4
**Newton VE** see **Hickson FS**
**Ney D, Hollingsworth DR:** Nutritional management of pregnancy complicated by diabetes: historical perspective. **Diabetes Care** 1981 Nov–Dec;4(6):647–55
**Neyagawa-shi Ishikai no ayumi:** Neyagawa, Japan, Neyagawa-shi, [1977]. xxviii, 466 p.
**Nežic E:** Historijat endemske malarije u Dalmaciji do 1923. g. In: I simpozij o historiji mikrobiologije i imunologije u Hrvatskoj do 1923. godine. Zagreb, Jugoslavenskoj akademiji, 1973. p. 71–9.
**Ng CS** see **Ratnam SS**
**Ng SC** see **Ratnam SS**
**Ng VW:** Ch'ing laws governing the insane: an historical survey. **Ch'ing-Shih Wen-t'i** 1980;4(4):55–89
**Ngai SH** see **Papper EM**
**Nguyen TH** see **Imbault-Huart MJ, ed**
**Nguyen TK, Smirnov VS, Mozzhakov VI:** Tsentral'nomu voennomu gospitaliu v'et namskoĭ Narodnoĭ armii––30 let. **Voen Med Zh** 1981 Nov;(11):61–2
**Nguyen-Laissard M:** Note sur la pharmacie de l'hôpital de Nuits-Saint Georges. **Rev Hist Pharm (Paris)** 1980 Mar;27(244):15–16
**Nguyen-Laissard M:** Note sur l'hôpital de Moutiers-Saint-Jean et sa pharmacie. **Rev Hist Pharm (Paris)** 1983 Sep;30(258):233–4
**Nguyen-Tran-Huan:** La sphygmologie dans la médecine vietnamienne traditionnelle. Contribution à l'étude du traité 'Bin hú mài xué' de Lǐ Shí Zhen. In Mazars G, ed: Les médecines traditionnelles de l'Asie. Strasbourg, Université Louis Pasteur, 1981. p. 13–22.
**Nguyên Trân Huân** see **Huard P**
**Niaussat P:** Les 'coliques sèches' dans la Marine au XIXe siècle: Amédée Lefevre et son combat contre une tenace erreur médicale. In: Congrès National des Sociétés Savantes, 104e, Bordeaux, 1979. Comptes Rendus. Paris, 1979. Section des Sciences, Fasc. IV. p. 183–91.
**Niaussat P, Huard P:** Problèmes acoustiques communs à la médecine, à la marine et aux télécommunications, étudiés par le Docteur Paul Constantin. In: Congrès National des Sociétés Savantes, 106e, Perpignan, 1981. Comptes Rendus. Paris, Bibliothèque Nationale, 1982. Fasc. IV. p. 81–9.
**Niaussat P** see **Huard P**
**Niaussat P** see **La médecine hospitalière française au XVIIIème siècle**
**Niaussat PM:** Delioux de Savignac et le traitement des dysenteries. In: Congrès National des Sociétés Savantes, 107e. Brest, 1982. Comptes Rendus, Paris, 1983. Section des Sciences, Fasc. IV. p. 299–309.
**Niaussat PM:** L'activité scientifique des médecins et pharmaciens de la marine du XVIIe siècle à nos jours. **Med Armees** 1980;8(10)spec:800–6
**Niaussat PM:** Sociologie des médecins de marine au XIXe siècle. In Congrès National des Sociétés Savantes, 103e, Nancy-Metz, 1978. Actes. Paris, 1979. Tome I, p. 397–410.
**Niaussat PM** see **Huard P**
**Niaussat PM** see **Imbault-Huart MJ, ed**
**Niaussat PM** see **Valentin M**
**Nica-Udangiu S:** Henri Ey (1900–1977). **Rev Med Interna [Neurol Psihiatr]** 1984 Apr–Jun;29(2):151–6
**Nica-Udangiu S:** Hermann Rorschach (1884–1922). **Rev Med Interna [Neurol Psihiatr]** 1984 Jul–Sep;29(3):235–40
**Nica-Udangiu S:** J. Moreau de Tours (1804–1884). **Rev Med Interna [Neurol Psihiatr]** 1984 Jan–Mar;29(1):77–80
**Nica-Udangiu S:** Karl Jaspers (1883–1969). **Rev Med Interna [Neurol Psihiatr]** 1983 Oct–Dec;28(4):311–6
**Niccoli O:** 'Menstruum quasi monstruum': parti mostruosi e tabù mestruale nel '500. **Quad Stor** 1980;15(2):402–8
**Nice CM:** Medical images: past, present, and future. **CRC Crit Rev Diagn Imaging** 1980;14(1):73–109
**Nichik VM:** Filosofskie vzgliady A. A. Bogomol'tsa. **Patol Fiziol Eksp Ter** 1981 Mar–Apr;(2):20–30, also in Fiziol Zh 1981 May–Jun;27(3):302–6
**Nicholas RW:** The goddess Sitala and epidemic smallpox in Bengal. **J Asian Stud** 1981;41(1):21–45
**Nicholas S, Shergold PR:** The heights of British male convict children transported to Australia, 1825–1840. **Aust Paediatr J** 1982 Jun;18(2):76–83
**Nicholi AM:** Historical perspective––the long and colorful history of Erythoxylon coca. **J Am Coll Health** 1984 Jun;32(6):252–7
**Nicholl C:** The chemical theatre. London, Boston, Routledge and Kegan Paul, 1980. ix, 292 p.
**Nicholls A:** Atherosclerosis in chronic renal failure: a historical perspective. **Scott Med J** 1983 Jul;28(3):270–5
**Nichols BL:** Nurse practitioners: a national perspective. **J Fla Med Assoc** 1982 May;69(5):391–5
**Nichols DJ** see **Donaldson PJ**
**Nicholson AN:** Long-range air capability and the South Atlantic Campaign. **Aviat Space Environ Med** 1984 Apr;55(4):269–70
**Nicholson P:** Problems encountered by early endoscopists. **Urology** 1982 Jan;19(1):114–9
**Nichter LS, Morgan RF, Nichter MA:** The impact of Indian methods for total nasal reconstruction. In Romm S, ed: Symposium on historical perspectives of plastic surgery. Philadelphia, Saunders, 1983. p. 635–47.
**Nichter LS** see **Romm S, ed**
**Nichter MA** see **Nichter LS**
**Nichter MA** see **Romm S, ed**
**Nickel D:** Berufsvorstellungen über weibliche Medizinalpersonen in der Antike. **Klio** 1979;61:515–8
**Nickel D:** Galens Untersuchungen zur embryonalen Blutbewegung. **Orvostort Kozl** 1981;93–96(27 No 1–4):25–35
**Nickel D:** Medizingeschichtliches in den 'Fabulae' des Hyginus. In International Congress of the History of Medicine. 26th, Plovdiv, 1978. Actes du Congress. Sofia, 1981. Volume II. p. 170–3.
**Nicks R:** Australian surgeons and society. **Aust NZ J Surg** 1980 Dec;50(6):659–67
**Nicol L:** Geschichte der Tiermedizin von der Mitte des 19. Jahrhunderts bis zur Gegenwart. In Sournia JC, Martiny M, Poulet J, ed: Illustrierte Geschichte der Medizin. Salzburg, Andreas, 1980. Vol. 7. p. 2681–709.
**Nicol P** see **Johansson BW**
**Nicol W:** Exotic infectious diseases: smallpox. **R Soc Health J** 1980 Apr;100(2):41–7
**Nicola M, Stiebitz R:** Morphologische und pathologische Befunde von Zähnen und Kiefern aus der Mittleren Bronzezeit (Pitten, Niederösterreich). **Anthropol Anz** 1979 Oct;37(3):182–203
**Nicolai JP:** Earliest free muscle graft? **Br J Plast Surg** 1980 Jul;33(3):350–2
**Nicolai JP:** Facial paralysis –– 100 years of treatment. **Arch Chir Neerl** 1979;31(3):159–69
**Nicolaidis N** see **Anzieu D**
**Nicolás Marín ME** see **Marset Campos P**
**Nicolau A:** Practici empirice 'pentru aflarea şi tămăduirea boalelor minţii' în trecutul medicinii româneşti. **Rev Med Interna [Neurol Psihiatr]** 1983 Apr–Jun;28(2):153–60
**Nicolino F:** Trotskij e la psicoanalisi. **Nuova Riv Stor** 1978;62(5–6):605–25
**Nicolle P:** Alphonse Laveran et Charles Nicolle. **Arch Inst Pasteur Tunis** 1981 Sep–Dec;58(3):265–79
**Nicolle P, Jude A:** Réflexions sur les prix Nobel de physiologie ou médecine. **Hist Sci Med** 1980;14(1):83–93
**Nicolle P:** Un événement capital dans la vie passionnée de Charles Nicolle: le Prix Nobel de physiologie ou médecine. Souvenirs évoqués par Pierre Nicolle. **Bull Soc Pathol Exot Filiales** 1981 Jan–Feb;74(1):101–18
**Nicolov IC:** Doctors, participants in the national liberation movement of the Bulgarian people in Macedonia. In International Congress of the History of Medicine. 26th, Plovdiv, 1978. Actes du Congress. Sofia, 1981. Volume II. p. 167–8.
**Nicou G, Kock W, ed:** Från Gösta Forssells och den Svenska röntgenologiens ungdomstid. Södertälje, Sweden, Fingraf Tryckeri, 1984. 84 p. (Nordisk Medicinhistorisk Arsbok, Supplementum X, 1984)
**Niculescu SI:** Pe marginea corespondenţei dintre Harvey Cushing şi Dumitru Bagdasar. **Rev Med Interna [Neurol Psihiatr]** 1981 Jul–Sep;26(3):229–33
**Niebyl KH:** Science, medicine and the Puritan society. **J Eur Econ Hist** 1979;8(1):
**Niebyl PH:** Science and metaphor in the medicine of Restoration England. **Bull Hist Med** 1973 Jul–Aug;47(4):356–74
**Niebyl PH** see **Rather LJ**
**Niederland TR:** Desat rokov Slovenskej lekárskej spoločnosti a tridsat rokov Ceskoslovenskej lekárskej spoločnosti Jana E. Purkyne. **Cas Lek Cesk** 1979 Dec 14;118(50):1548–51
**Niederland TR:** Doterajší vývoj a perspektíva predklinických odborov na lekárskej fakulte Univerzity Komenského v Bratislave. **Cas Lek Cesk** 1979 Dec 21;118(51):1574–6
**Niederland WG:** Morbid conditions expressed in prehistoric art. **Am J Psychiatry** 1981 Jan;138(1):126–7
**Niehoff JU** see **Dahm I**

**Nielsen E:** Udgravningen af Odenses St. Jørgensgård. Foreløbige resultater. **Dan Medicinhist Arbog** 1983;12:39–51
**Nielsen J:** 125 års jubilaeum: fra Jydske asyl 1852 til Psykiatrisk hospital i Arhus 1977: [s. l.: s. n., 1977?]. 139 p.
**Nielsen JS:** Den patografiske tradition og metode. **Dan Medicinhist Arbog** 1983;12:91–104
**Nielzén S:** Ljudets väg från öra till perception; en sammanställning av biologiska bakgrunder till ljudupplevande bl.a. med utblick mot psykiatrin. **Sydsven Medicinhist Sallsk Arsskr** 1982;19:99–108
**Nielzén S:** Sjöbrings tankemodeller för personlighet och psykisk sjukdom. **Sydsven Medicinhist Sallsk Arsskr** 1980;:124–33
**Niemann H, Wiezorek WD:** Zur Geschichte der medizinischen Hochschulbildung in der Deutschen Demokratischen Republik. Teil I und II. **Z Arztl Fortbild (Jena)** 1980 Feb 1,74(3,4).115–22, 178–81
**Niemann JT** see **Criley JM**
**Niemi SM:** D. E. Salmon and the first bacterin. **Mod Vet Pract** 1981 Dec;62(12):913–7
**Niemi SM:** Early veterinary biologics. **Mod Vet Pract** 1980 Nov;61(11):926–9
**Niemineva K, Haavisto H, Perälä M:** Vanhoista Turkulaisia lääkemääräyksistä ja niiden kirjoittajista. **Turun Hist Ark (Finl)** 1979;33:146–63
**Nieniewska M** see **Drozdowski P**
**Nieniewska M** see **Fortuna D**
**Nierhaus G:** Ludwig von Bertalanffy 1901–1972. **Sudhoffs Arch** 1981;65(2):144–72
**Nieto D:** José Sanchís Banús. **Arch Neurobiol (Madr)** 1982 Sep–Oct;45(5):407–16
**Nigam SK** see **Garg NK**
**Nightingale F:** [Introductory notes on lying-in institutions (2)] (Jpn). **Sogo Kango** 1983 May 15;18(2):113–30
**Nightingale F:** [Introductory notes on lying-in institutions. 3] (Jpn). **Sogo Kango** 1983 Aug 15;18(3):89–104
**Nightingale F:** [Introductory notes on lying in institutions. 4] (Jpn). **Sogo Kango** 1983 Nov 15;18(4):93–113
**Nightingale TW:** A history of physical education, sport, recreation and amusement in Cincinnati, Ohio, in the nineteenth century. Ph.D. Diss., Ohio State University, Columbus, 1979. xi, 279 p.
**Nihlen B:** Fenomenala tandläkare - för 2500 år sedan! **Tandlakartidningen** 1982 Sep 15;74(18):999–1000
**Nihlén B:** Folkliga föreställningar om tandvärk och tandvård. **Tandlakartidningen** 1983 Mar 15;75(6):328, 330
**Nihlén B:** Medeltidsfynd avslojär: 55 av 100 människor led av tandsjukdomar. **Tandlakartidningen** 1982 Dec 15;74(24):1436–8
**Nihlén B:** 2 000-åriga skelett med perfekta tänder. **Tandlakartidningen** 1983 Dec 1;75(23):1356–7
**Nihon Chusha Kigu Kensa Kyokai 15-nenshi:** Chusha no rekishi to gyokai no ayumi. Tokyo, Do Kyokai, Showa 51 nen, [1976]. 187 p.
**Nihon Shika Kigyo Kyogikai, Gyokaishi Henshu Iinkai:** Nihon shika gyokai shi. Tokyo, Nihon Shika Kigyo Kyogikai, Showa 52, 1977– v.
**Niigata Daigaku Igakubu Shonikagaku Kyoshitsu shi:** [Niigata, Japan], Do Iinkai, Showa 52 nen [1977]. 180 p.
**Nikiforov N** see **Naidenov G**
**Nikitin DP:** Nauchno-issledovatel'skaia i proizvodstvennaia deiatel'nost' Moskovskogo nauchno-issledovatel'skogo instituta épidemiologii i mikrobiologii im. G. N. Gabrichevskogo. **Zh Mikrobiol Epidemiol Immunobiol** 1981 Mar;(3):102–5
**Nikitin EA:** Fel'dsher revoliutsionnogo korablia P. F. Glinkov. **Feldsher Akush** 1982;47(11):36–7
**Nikitin VN, Perskiĭ EE, Utevskiĭ LA:** Molekuliarnye mekhanizmy vozrastnogo razvitiia kollagenovykh struktur i teoriia stareniia A. A. Bogomol'tsa. **Fiziol Zh** 1981 May–Jun;27(3):407–12
**Nikitin VN, Perskiĭ EE, Utevskaia LA:** Uchenie A. A. Bogomol'tsa o roli soedinitel'noĭ tkani v starenii i sovremennye predstavleniia o mekhanizmakh vozrastnogo razvitiia kollagenovyk struktur. **Patol Fiziol Eksp Ter** 1981 Mar–Apr;(2):30–9
**Nikitin VN:** Vedushchie problemy sovremennykh vozrastnykh fiziologii, biokhimii i biofiziki i isledovaniia shkoly A. V. Nagornogo. **Usp Sovrem Biol** 1982 Nov–Dec;94(3):421–32
**Nikitiuk BA, Kozlov AI:** Nekotorye spornye polozheniia ucheniia ob antropogeneze v svete predstavlenii o destabiliziruiushchem otbore i dannykh sovremennoĭ paléoendokrinologii (k 100-letiiu so dnia rozhdeniia I. I. Shmal'gauzena). **Arkh Anat Gistol Embriol** 1984 Aug;87(8):5–14
**Niklíček L, Manová L:** Ceská hygiena a česká společnost na přelomu 19. a 20. století. **Cesk Zdrav** 1981 Apr;29(4):156–64
**Niklíček L, Stein K, Kotek V:** K historii postgraduální výchovy lékařu--zaměstnancu státní zdravotní správy v Ceskoslovensku před rokem 1938. **Cesk Zdrav** 1983 Dec;31(12):502–12
**Niklíček L, Müller C:** Uloha historie a historické methody v sociálním lékařství. **Cesk Zdrav** 1980 Oct;28(10):416–21
**Niklíček L** see **Bílek V**
**Niklíček L** see **Kotek V**
**Niklíček L** see **Müller C**
**Nikodemusz I:** Közlekedésünk egészségügye a múltban. **Orv Hetil** 1984 Apr 29;125(18):1084–5
**Nikolaeva I, Vassilev V, Ivanov C, et al:** Données statistiques sur l'activité l'hôpital 'Paraskeva Nikolaou' à Varna de 1879 à 1912. In International Congress of the History of Medicine. 26th, Plovdiv, 1978. Actes du Congress. Sofia, 1981. Volume II. p. 68–9.
**Nikolaeva I:** Istoriia na zdraveopazvaneto vüv Varna ot drevnostta do sotsialisticheskata revoliutsiia ot 9.IX.1944 g. Sofiia, Meditsina i fizkultura, 1980. 153 p.
**Nikolaĭ Ivanovich Ragoza (K 100-letiiu so dnia rozhdeniia):** **Voen Med Zh** 1983 Jul;(7):76
**Nikolaĭ Sergeevich Pravdin (k 100-letiiu so dnia rozhdeniia):** **Farmakol Toksikol** 1983 May–Jun;46(3):127–8
**Nikolai Wladimirovich Timof'eeff-Ressovsky, (1900–1981): Genetics** 1982 Jan;100(1):1–5
**Nikolic D:** Razvoj neonatalne službe bolnice u Vršcu (34-godišnji period: 1947–1981). **Med Pregl** 1982;35(9–10):383–5
**Nikolin P** see **Andelic P**
**Nikolov G:** Uiliam Kharveĭ, otkrivateliat na krüvoobrashtenieto. Sofiia, Meditsina i fizkultura, 1981. 74 p.
**Nikolov I** see **Zaprianov N**
**Nikonchik OK:** Razvitie sistemy okhrany materinstva i detstva v SSSR (1922–1982). **Akush Ginekol (Mosk)** 1982;(7):3–7
**Nikonova VA** see **Sergiev VP**
**Nikulin A:** U povodu 35-godišnjice rada Medicinskog fakulteta u Sarajevu. **Med Arh** 1981;35(5–6):245–7
**Nikulina TD, Ivanov IV:** Kuĭbyshevskoĭ oblastnoĭ tuberkuleznoĭ bol'nitse im. Z. P. Solov'eva 125 let. **Probl Tuberk** 1983 Apr;(4):69–71
**Niles AG:** The Dial Access Library for Health Professionals in Wisconsin: an historical account. [Madison,] University of Wisconsin-Extension, 1982. iv, 94 p.
**Nilius B:** Heuristische Aspekte im Verhältnis zwischen Philosophie und Einzelwissenschaft. **Wiss Z Martin Luther Univ (Math)** 1984;33(2):134–42
**Nilsen KH:** Det Norske Arbeiderparti og befolkningsspørsmålet i mellomkrigstida. **Hist Tidsskr** 1979;58(3):287–304
**Nilsson P** see **Grefberg N**
**Nimbkar KV:** A new life for the handicapped: a history of rehabilitation and occupational therapy in India. Bombay, Nimbkar Rehabilitation Trust, 1980. xviii, 374 p.
**Ninan R:** The lady with the lamp: a profile. **Nurs J India** 1982 Jun;73(6):151–5
**Ninomiya R** see **Unschuld PU**
**Nipe GM:** 'Jessee Bennett decided to operate on his wife at once'. **Va Med** 1979 Dec;106(12):884–5
**Nisbet NW, Woodruff M:** John Charnley: 29 August 1911–5 August 1982. **Biogr Mem Fellows R Soc** 1984;30:119–37
**Nishida A:** [In preparation of the key words for Nightingale's 'Notes on Nursing'--introduction to a humanistic theory] **Sogo Kango** 1980;15(4):46–58
**Nishida A:** [Understanding of man in the 'Notes on Nursing' (Florence Nightingale)] (Jpn). **Sogo Kango** 1982;16(4):9–22
**Nissen AJ:** Kvinneslektens hemmelige historie. **Samtiden (Norway)** 1979;88(1):99–103
**Nissen TP:** Musiktherapie. Ihre Ursprünge und modernen Formen. **Fortschr Med** 1983 Jun 2;101(21):972–8
**Nissenbaum S:** Sex, diet, and debility in Jacksonian America: Sylvester Graham and health reform. Westport, Connecticut, Greenwood, 1980. 198 p. (Contributions in Medical History, 4).
**Nitroglycerin--the first hundred years: Lancet** 1979 Dec 22–29;2(8156–8157):1340–1
**Nittenwilm U** see **Jackle P**
**Niven Mackay IM:** The relationship between human and animal health in nineteenth century Dublin. **Vet Hist** 1984;3(3):110–4
**Nixon PI:** Pat Nixon of Texas. Autobiography of a doctor. Ed. by H. H. Lang. College Station, Texas, and London, Texas A & M University Press, 1979. 288 p.
**Niyogi SK:** Historic development of forensic toxicology in America up to 1978. **Am J Forensic Med Pathol** 1980 Sept;1(3):249–64
**Nizard A, Vallin J:** Les causes de décès en France. II. couplage des 7e et 8e révisions de la classification internationale. Application à la période 1958–1974. **Population** 1980;35(6):1057–99
**Niziński J:** Z historii Towarzystwa Lekarskiego Zagłębia Dąbrowskiego. **Wiad Lek** 1980 Nov 15;33(22):1851–5
**NLN's 30th year - leading the way:** Renew the spirit! 1952–1982. **Nurs Health Care** 1982 Sep;3(5):398–9
**Nobel lectures in molecular biology, 1933–1975:** New York, Elsevier, 1977. ix, 534 p.
**Noble I:** Contemporary women scientists in America. New York, Messner, 1979. 158 p.
**Noble P:** Mental health services and legislation--an historical review. **Med Sci Law** 1981 Jan;21(1):16–24
**Nóbrega H:** As raízes das ciências da saúde na Paraíba: medicina, farmácia, odontologia e enfermagem. Joao Pessoa, Editora Universitária, 1979. 372 p.
**Nocon C:** Les médecins à Douai de 1900 à 1939. **Rev Nord** 1979;61(241):439–43
**Noddle B:** Livestock at Garton Slack 2000 years ago. **Vet Hist** 1983 Summer;3(1):9–15
**Nodyne KR:** Pioneer in oral surgery: Simon P. Hullihen. **J W Va Hist Assoc** 1982;6(1):41–8
**Nodyne KR** see **Murphy RL**
**Noel NL:** Nursing archives - preserving the profession's history. **Deans Notes** 1984 Mar;5(4):1–2
**Noel PS, ed** see **Carlson ET**
**Nogueira MJ:** A pesquisa em enfermagem no Brasil: retrospective histórica. **Rev Esc Enferm USP** 1982 Apr;16(1):17–26
**Noirfalise A:** Cent ans de bromatologie à l'Université de Liège. **Arch Belg** 1982;40(7–8):365–76

**Nojima Y:** [Nursing theory by Henderson. 4. Virginia Henderson and the history of nursing theory] (Jpn) **Kango Tenbo** 1979 Oct;4(10):949–57
**Nolan E:** Children's ward. Lithograph by Robert Riggs, ca. 1940–45. **J Hist Med Allied Sci** 1982 Jul;37(3):322
**Noland RW:** Psychobiography: case history of life history? **Midwest Q** 1978;20(1):7–17
**Nolding Gaffree A:** Ana Neri – la première infirmière militaire au Brésil. In: International Congress of the History of Medicine, 26th, Plovdiv (Bulgaria), 1978. Actes du Congres, Vol. 1. Sofia, 1980. p. 114–5.
**Nolen WA:** A short history of heart surgery. **Am Heritage** 1983;34(5):101–5
**Nomiyama K:** 'Kogai', environmental pollution and the related public nuisance. In Ogawa T, ed: Public health. Tokyo, Saikon, 1981. p. 82–98.
**Nonaka R** see **Seki M**
**Nonclercq M:** A. Béchamp, un' ingiustizia nella storia delle scienze. **Empedocle** 1983 Sep–Oct;1(1):39–49
**Nonclercq M:** Antoine Béchamp 1816–1908: l'homme et le savant originalité et fécondité de son oeuvre. Preface et note documentaire par le Docteur Philippe Decourt. Paris, Maloine, 1982. 249 p.
**Nonclercq M:** Un chapitre ignoré de l'histoire des sciences: l'oeuvre de Béchamp. In: Congrés National des Sociétés Savantes, 103e, Nancy, 1978. Comptes Rendus. Paris, 1978. Section des Sciences, Fasc. V. p. 157–69.
**Noorda S:** Illness and sin, forgiving and healing. The connection of medical treatment and religious beliefs in Ben Sira 38, 1–15. In: Studies in Hellenistic Religions; ed. by M. J. Vermaseren. Leiden, Brill, 1979. pp.215–224.
**Noore FD:** In medicina, veritas; the British and turbulent youth of the faculty of medicine and Harvard College. **N Engl J Med** 1982 Oct 7;307(15):917–25
**Norberg K:** Educating the poor: charity schools and charitable attitudes, Grenoble, 1600–1789. **Proc Annu Meet West Soc Fr Hist** 1980;8:181–90
**Nordau CG:** Grilles du temps jadis. **Monit Pharm Lab** 1980 Dec 6;34(1445):4363, 4365, 4367
**Nordbring F, Vahlquist B:** En sentida kommentar till en berättelse om en svår farsot i Uppsala 1742–1743. **Lakartidningen** 1979 Dec 19;76(51):4714–7
**Nordstrom WR:** How a dental museum – built and staffed by dental students – helps generate interest in dental history. **Bull Hist Dent** 1983 Apr;31(1):18–22
**Noreña CG:** Juan Luis Vives. The Hague, Nijhoff, 1970. xiii, 327 p.
**Norich I:** Kak lechili Toma Soïera. **Med Sestra** 1984 Feb;43(2):61–3
**Noriyasu S, Higashinakagawa T, Matsushita T, et al:** Human skeletal remains of the Yayoi Period excavated from the Tsumayama site, Saga Prefecture, Kyushu, Japan. **Fukuoka Igaku Zasshi** 1982 May;73(5):241–9
**Noriyasu S, Isotani S, Akiyoshi T:** Human skulls of the Yayoi Period excavated from Himekata site, Saga Prefecture, Kyushu, Japan. **Fukuoka Igaku Zasshi** 1982 May;73(5):232–40
**Norman C:** The unsung hero of yellow fever? **Science** 1984 Mar 30;223(4643):1370–2
**Norman EM:** Who and where are nursing's historians? **Nurs Forum** 1981;20(2):138–52
**Norman JE, Painter DM:** Hyperplasia of the mandibular condyle. A historical review of important early cases with a presentation and analysis of twelve patients. **J Maxillofac Surg** 1980 Aug;8(3):161–75
**Normand J:** Histoire d'une thérapeutique: la thérapeutique digitalique hier et aujourd'hui. **Ann Cardiol Angeiol (Paris)** 1982 Mar–Apr;31(2):89–95
**Normandeau L, Légaré J:** La mortalité infantile des Inuit du Nouveau-Quebec. **Can Rev Sociol Anthropol** 1979;16(3):260–74
**Norovpil TS, Avilov EN, Barer GM:** Razvitie stomatologicheskoĭ pomoshchi i podgotovka vracheĭ-stomatologov v Mongol'skoĭ Narodnoĭ Respublike. **Stomatologiia (Mosk)** 1981 Jan–Feb;60(1):91–2
**Norrby E:** Den medicinska betydelsen av rörliga strukturer i arvsmassan. **Lakartidningen** 1983 Oct 19;80(42):3911–3
**Norris J:** The country doctor in British Columbia: 1887–1975. **BC Stud** 1981;(49):15–39
**Norris J:** The 'scurvy disposition': heavy exertion as an exacerbating influence on scurvy in modern times. **Bull Hist Med** 1983 Fall;57(3):325–38
**Norris J:** Typhoid in the Rockies: epidemiology in a constrained habitat, 1883–1939. In Roland CG, ed: Health, disease and medicine. Toronto, Hannah Institute for the History of Medicine, 1984. p. 276–95.
**Norsk Farmasihistorisk Museum. Das Norwegische Pharmaziehistorische Museum (Apothekenmuseum). Le Musée norvégien de la pharmacie. Oslo, Norsk Folkemuseum, 1979, 16 p.:**
**Norsk Sykepleierforbund 70–års dag: historisk høytidsstund på Vettre:** 'Arhundrets sykepleier' har fått sitt monument. **Sykepleien** 1982 Oct 20;69(18):6–7, 31
**North E:** Classics in infectious diseases. Concerning the epidemic of spotted fever in New England: Elisha North, 1811. **Rev Infect Dis** 1980 Sep–Oct;2(5):811–6
**Northrup D:** African mortality in the suppression of the slave trade: the case of the bight of Biafra. **J Interdiscip Hist** 1978;9(1):47–64
**Northup GW:** Louisa Burns Memorial Lecture: Re––search. **J Am Osteopath Assoc** 1984 Sep;84(1):67–70
**Nortjé CJ:** Kefaloröntgenografie: 'n historiese literatuuroorsig. **Tydskr Tandheelkd Ver S Afr** 1979 Jun;34(6):327–33
**Norton B:** Fisher and the neo-Darwinian synthesis. In Forbes EG, ed: Human implications of scientific advance. Edinburgh, Edinburgh University Press, 1978. p. 481–94.
**Norton B:** La situation intellectuelle au moment des débuts de Fisher en génétique des populations. In Actes du Colloque R.A. Fisher.... Paris, 5–6 déc. 1979. p. 231–50. **Rev Synth (Paris)** 1981;102(103–104)
**Norton B:** Psychologists and class. In C. Webster, ed: Biology, medicine and society 1840–1940. Cambridge, Cambridge University Press, 1981. p. 289–314.
**Norwood WF:** The CME School of Medicine: its struggle for recognition and status, 1905–1915. **Advent Herit** 1979;6(2):15–24
**Norwood FE, ed:** The fourteenth-century medico-botanical glossary of Raimon de Castelnou. Leeds, W. S. Maney for the Leeds Philosophical and Literary Society, 1974. (Proceedings of the Leeds Philosophical and Literary Society, Literary and Historical Section, Vol. XV, Part VI, pp. 135–225).
**Nosal' VI:** Muzeĭ istorii zdravookhraneniia goroda. **Sov Zdravookhr** 1983;(4):44–5
**Nöske HD:** Lithotomia vesicae. München, Zuckschwerdt, 1982. v, 74 p.
**Nosny P:** Alphonse Laveran et la découverte de l'hématozoaire du paludisme. **Bull Acad Natl Med (Paris)** 1980 Jan;164(1):80–7
**Nosny P** see **Huard P**
**Nosov SD:** O nekotorykh tak nazyvaemykh novykh infektsionnykh bolezniakh. **Feldsher Akush** 1980;45(8):7–10
**Nossel HL, Spaet TH:** Clarence Merskey (1914–1982). **Thromb Res** 1983 Jun 1;30(5):401–5
**Nossik BM:** Albert Schweitzer. Ein Leben fur die Menschlichkeit. Leipzig, S. Hirzel, 1982. 372 p. (Humanisten der Tat. Hervorragende Arzte im Dienste des Menschen).
**[Notes on David Seixas and education of the deaf in Pennsylvania in the 1820's]** In: Myers, S. H. Handcraft to industry: Philadelphia ceramics. Washington, D. C., Smithsonian Institution Press, 1980. pp. 8–12 passim, 83–4.
**Notestein FW:** Demography in the United States: a partial account of the development of the field. **Popul Dev Rev** 1982;8(4):651–87
**Notle A, Brannan J:** Through the looking glass: health education curriculum. **Health Educ (Wash)** 1979 Nov–Dec;10(6):5–11
**Notman MT** see **Nadelson CC**
**Al-Nouri M** see **Maud PJ**
**Novák A:** Doc. MUDr. Eva Sedláčková, csc., a československá foniatrie. **Cesk Otolaryngol** 1982 Apr;31(2):68–71
**Novak DE:** Dental auxiliary evolution: a historical perspective. **Dent Assist** 1984 Sep–Oct;53(5):17–22
**Novák J:** Stočtyřicet let od narození prof. MUDr. Karla Chodounského. **Cas Lek Cesk** 1983 May 13;122(19):600–1
**Novak SJ:** Professionalism and bureaucracy: English doctors and Victorian public health administration. **J Soc Hist** 1973;6(4):440–62
**Novák VJ:** Zakladatel moderní biologie. Sto let od smrti Ch. R. Darwina. **Cas Lek Cesk** 1982 Apr 16;121(15):449–50
**Novak Z:** 30 godina 'Neuropsyhijatrije' i 'Neurologije'. **Neurologija** 1983;31(1–2):7–9
**Novak GIa** see **Bukhman AA**
**Novakova LIa:** Publikatsii o N. I. Pirogove v khirurgicheskom zhurnale Ukrainy. **Klin Khir** 1982 Feb;(2):49–50
**Novelli G:** Personal recollections to Fritz Lipmann during the early years of coenzyme A research. **Mol Biol Biochem Biophys** 1980;32:415–30
**Nover A, Kümmel WF:** Der Schnitt- und Augenarzt Caspar Stromayr und die ophthalmologischen Illustrationen in seiner 'Practica copiosa' (1559). **Klin Monatsbl Augenheilkd** 1984 Nov;185(5):321–3
**Nover A:** 100 Jahre Augenheilkunde. **Fortschr Med** 1982 Dec 16;100(47–48):2222–7
**Novich MM:** Early developments in sports medicine. **J Med Soc NJ** 1982 Apr;79(4):309–13
**Novichkova VG** see **Revenko TA**
**Novick DM** see **Pinsker H**
**Novikov FG, Tomashuk IP:** Iz istorii otechestvennoĭ voenno-polevoĭ khirurgii. **Klin Khir** 1980 May;(5):69–72
**Novikov II** see **Leontiuk AS**
**Novikov IV** see **Petrovskiĭ KS**
**Novikov IV** see **Shitskova AP**
**Novikov JV** see **Petrowskij KS**
**Novikova TP** see **Kurdiumov NA**
**Novikova ECh:** Okhrana zdorov'ia zhenshchin i deteĭ v strane v 60–iu godovshchinu obrazovaniia Soiuza Sovetskikh Sotsialisticheskikh Respublik. **Pediatriia** 1982 Dec;(12):3–8
**Novikova ECh:** V. I. Lenin i deti. **Vopr Okhr Materin Det** 1980 Apr;25(4):3–7
**Novoa Montero D:** El Profesor Luis Noguer Molins y la Universidad Venezolana. Nueva ed. Mérida, Venezuela, (The Author), 1980. 84 p.
**Novoa Montero D** see **Salfelder K**
**Novoselov VI:** Razvitie zakonodatel'stva o narodnom zdravookhranenii. **Sov Zdravookhr** 1980;(6):3–7
**Novotny A, Smith C, ed:** Images of healing. A portfolio of American medical & pharmaceutical practice in the 18th, 19th, & early 20th centuries. New York, Macmillan, 1980, 144 p.
**Novotný V** see **Horák J**
**Novy M** see **Radcliff-Umstead D, ed**
**Nowak JB:** Integration of nursing history into the nursing curriculum. **NLN Publ** 1983;(41–1935):49–53
**Nowak JB:** The forty-seven hundred. The story of the Mount Sinai Hospital School of Nursing. Canaan, N. H., Phoenix Pub., 1981. xii, 146 p.
**Nowotny E:** Die Gründung der Hofspitäler durch Ferdinand I. im 16. Jahrhundert mit besonderer Berücksichtigung des wiener Hofspitals. **Unsere Heimat** 1971;42(2):91–103
**Nowotny O:** De auro potabili. Wien, 1967. (Salzburger Beiträge zur Paracelsusforschung, 7). p. 13–23.

**Nowotny O:** Hans Heger und seine Bedeutung für die Geschichte der Pharmazie in Oesterreich. In: Vorträge des Internationalen Pharmaziehistorischen Kongresses Innsbruck 1977. Stuttgart, Wissenschaftliche Verlagsgesellschaft, 1979. p. 147–52.
**Noyes EJ** see **Berkelhamer JE**
**Nriagu JO:** Occupational exposure to lead in ancient times. **Sci Total Environ** 1983 Nov;31(2):105–16
**Nriagu JO:** Saturnine gout among Roman aristocrats. Did lead poisoning contribute to the fall of the Empire? **N Engl J Med** 1983 Mar 17;308(11):660–3
**Nriagu JO** see **Scarborough J**
**Nugent A:** Fit for work: the introduction of physical examinations in industry. **Bull Hist Med** 1983 Winter;57(4):578–95
**Nuis DD, ed** see **Dryce DP**
**Nuland SB:** 'A matter of great importance to mankind': the origins of the New Haven County Medical Association. **Conn Med** 1984 Sep;48(9):559–61
**Nuland SB:** Ingelfinger rule violated in 1846. **N Engl J Med** 1983 Apr 14;308(15):907
**Nuland SB:** The lymphatic contiguity of Hodgkin's disease: a historical study. **Bull NY Acad Med** 1981 Nov;57(9):776–86
**Nuland SB:** The origins of anesthesia. **Conn Med** 1984 Mar;48(3):171–4 contd
**Nuland SB:** The origins of anesthesia: part II. **Conn Med** 1984 Jun;48(6):379–83 contd
**Nuland SB:** The origins of anesthesia: Part III. **Conn Med** 1984 Sep;48(9):597–600
**Nuland SB** see **Ebbert A, et al**
**Null G** see **Bolton S**
**Numbers R** see **Shires GT**
**Numbers RL:** A note on medical education in Wisconsin. In Numbers RL, Leavitt JW, ed: Wisconsin medicine. Historical perspectives. Madison, University of Wisconsin Press, 1981. p. 177–84.
**Numbers RL:** Almost persuaded. American physicians and compulsory health insurance, 1912–1920. Baltimore and London, Johns Hopkins University Press, 1978. 158 p. (Henry E. Sigerist Supplements to the Bulletin of the History of Medicine, n.s., 1).
**Numbers RL:** Compulsory health insurance: the continuing American debate. Westport, Greenwood Press, 1982. xv, 172 p.
**Numbers RL:** Medicine in the New World: a comparison. In International Congress of the History of Medicine, 27th, Barcelona, 1980. Actas. Barcelona, Académia de Ciències Médiques de Catalunya i Balears, 1981. p. 592–5.
**Numbers RL:** Public protection and self-interest: medical societies in Wisconsin. In Numbers RL, Leavitt JW, ed: Wisconsin medicine. Historical perspectives. Madison, University of Wisconsin Press, 1981. p. 75–104.
**Numbers RL:** The third party: health insurance in America. In Vogel MJ, Rosenberg CE, ed: The therapeutic revolution. Philadelphia, 1979. p. 177–200.
**Numbers RL:** Together but not equal: amateurs and professionals in early American scientific societies. **Rev Am Hist** 1976;4(4):497–503
**Numbers RL, Orr WJ:** William Beaumont's reception at home and abroad. **Isis** 1981 Dec;72(264):590–612
**Numbers RL, Leavitt JW, ed:** Wisconsin medicine. Historical perspectives. Madison, University of Wisconsin Press, 1981. ix, 212 p.
**Numbers RL, ed:** Compulsory health insurance. The continuing American debate. Westport, Connecticut, London, Greenwood Press, 1982. xv, 172 p. With contributions by A. J. Viseltear, G. Land, T. R. Marmor, M. M. Poen, P. Starr, R. Lubove, W. J. Cohen. (Contributions in medical history, no. 11).
**Numbers RL, ed:** The education of American physicians: historical essays. [Preface includes biographical tribute to William F. Norwood]. Berkeley, University of California Press, 1980. xiii, 345 p. Contributions by L. G. Stevenson, M. Kaufman, J. B. Blake, J. H. Warner, J. Whorton, D. L. Cowen, R. C. Maulitz, E. C. Atwater, G. H. Brieger, L. D Longo, J. L. Brand, J. W. Leavitt, C R. Burns, G. Miller
**Numbers RL, ed** see **Leavitt JW**
**Nuñex D** see **Peset JL**
**Nunez D:** Anotaciones a un articulo de Ramon y Cajal. ['La sociedad del porvenir'. Vida Socialista, 1912, July 14.]. **Llull (Spain)** 1978;2:106–13
**Nuñez L** see **Aráujo A**
**Nuñez L** see **Ferreira LF**
**Nuñez Varela V** see **Folch Jou C**
**Nunis DB** see **Hoyt HF**
**Nunn JB, Holmdahl MH:** Henrik Enghoff and the volumen inefficax. **Ups J Med Sci** 1979;84(2):105–8
**Nuralev IuN:** Abu Ali Ibn-Sina i voprosy vrachebnoĭ étiki. **Klin Med (Mosk)** 1980 Oct;58(10):112–4
**Nuraliev IuN** see **Denisenko PP**
**Nurco DN:** Narcotic addiction over a quarter of a century in a major American city. Rockville, Md., U. S. Alcohol, Drug Abuse, and Mental Health Administration, 1979. vi, 92 p.
**Nursing hall of fame:** Kansas City, Mo., American Nurses' Association, 1982. 16 p.
**Nursing revisited:** Mary M. Riddle (1856–1936). **Mass Nurse** 1983 Oct;52(10):4
**Nursing revisited: Linda Richards (1841–1930): Mass Nurse** 1983 Jul;52(7):8
**Nursing revisited: Louisa May Alcott: Mass Nurse** 1983 Jun;52(6):13
**Nuseibeh S:** Avicenna: medicine and scepticism. **Koroth** 1981;8(1–2):9–20
**Nussbaum JJ, Pruett RC, Delori FC:** Historic perspectives. Macular yellow pigment. The first 200 years. **Retina** 1981;1(4):296–310
**Nussbaum MC** see **Barnes J**
**Nussbaum W:** Die Grippe-Epidemie 1918/1919 in der schweizerischen Armee. **Gesnerus** 1982;39(2):243–59
**Nussbaum MC, ed:** Aristotle's De motu animalium. Text with translation, commentary, and interpretive essays. Princeton, Princeton University Press, 1978. xxiii, 430 p.
**Nusynowitz ML:** The isolation of thyroxine (Edward C Kendall). **JAMA** 1983 Oct 21;250(15):2047–8
**Nuttali RH:** An early microscope by John Benjamin Dancer of Manchester. **Microscope** 1980;28(3/4):93–100
**Nuttall P:** Miss Florence Nightingale: 'the passionate statistician'. **Nurs J India** 1984 Jun;75(6):128–9
**Nuttall P:** The passionate statistician (Florence Nightingale). **Nurs Times** 1983 Sep 28–Oct 4;79(39):25–7
**Nuttall RH:** Microscopes from the Frank Collection 1800–1860. Illustrating the development of the achromatic instrument. Jersey, Channel Islands, A. Frank, 1979, 64 p.
**Nuttall RH:** The Department of Pure and Applied Chemistry: a history 1830–1980. Glasgow, University of Strathclyde, 1980. 16 p.
**Nutton V:** Conrad Gesner and the English naturalists. **Med Hist** 1985 Jan;29(1):93–7
**Nutton V:** Continuity or rediscovery? The city physician in classical antiquity and mediaeval Italy. In Russell AW, ed: The town and state physician in Europe from the Middle Ages to the Enlightenment. Wolfenbüttel, Herzog August Bibliothek, 1981. p. 9–46 (Wolfenbütteler Forschungen, 17).
**Nutton V:** Galen in the eyes of his contemporaries. **Bull Hist Med** 1984 Fall;58(3):315–24
**Nutton V:** Galeno salvato dalle acque. **Kos** 1984 Mar;1(2):33–50
**Nutton V:** Galen's autobiographies. In International Congress of the History of Medicine. 26th, Plovdiv, 1978. Actes du Congress. Sofia, 1981. Volume II. p. 173–5.
**Nutton V:** John Caius und Johannes Lange: medizinischer Humanismus zur Zeit Vesals. **NTM** 1984;21(2):81–7
**Nutton V:** Medicine in the age of Montaigne. In K. Cameron, ed: Montaigne and his age. Univ. of Exeter, 1981. p. 14–25, 163–70.
**Nutton V:** The seeds of disease: an explanation of contagion and infection from the Greeks to the Renaissance. **Med Hist** 1983 Jan;27(1):1–34
**Nutton V** see **Symons H**
**Nutton V, ed:** Galen On prognosis. Berlin, Akademie-Verlag, 1979. 262 p. (Corpus Medicorum Graecorum, vol. 5, pt. 8, fasc. 1).
**Nutton V, ed:** Karl Gottlob Kühn and his edition of the works of Galen. Oxford, Oxford Microform Publications, 1976. 35 p. (First published with the microfiche edition of Kühn's edition of The works of Galen, March 1976).
**Nwokedike A:** Folkmedicine in Iboland/Nigeria. Diss. Düsseldorf, 1980. 58 p.
**Nwoku AL** see **Sawyer DR**
**Nyárády I** see **Németh T**
**Nybäck H:** Mannen bakom syndromet: James Parkinson. Beskrev 'shaking palsy' 1817--i dag prövas transplantation som behandling. **Lakartidningen** 1982 Dec 29;79(52):4910
**Nyberg A:** Södertelge Lazarett--dess tillkomst och första verksamhetsår. **Nord Medicinhist Arsb** 1981;:120–32
**Nye MJ:** Scientific decline: is quantitative evaluation enough? **ISIS** 1984 Dec;75(279):697–708
**Nye RA:** Degeneration, hygiene and sports in fin-de-siècle France. **Proc Annu Meet West Soc Fr Hist** 1980;8:404–12
**Nyiri JK:** Philosophy and suicide--statistics in Austria-Hungary. **East Cent Eur** 1978;5(1):69–89
**Nyman GW, Solomon N:** Mental hygiene within the state health care delivery system: the Maryland perspective. **Md State Med J** 1980 Jun;29(6):62–6
**Nys H** see **Blanpain J**


# O


**Oakeley HF:** The end of my great ... grandfather's second wife, or chest medicine in Lambeth in 1671. **St Thomas Hosp Gaz** 1981;79:50–1
**Oakley A:** The relevance of the history of medicine to an understanding of current change: some comments from the domain of antenatal care. **Soc Sci Med** 1982;16(6):667–74
**Oakley CL:** Sir Gordon Roy Cameron. In Dictionary of national biography, 1961–1970. Suppl. 8, 1981. p. 167–9.
**Oaks BF:** 'Things fearful to name': sodomy and buggery in seventeenth-century New England. **J Soc Hist** 1978;12(2):268–81
**Oaks R:** Perceptions of homosexuality by justices of the peace in colonial Virginia. **J Homosex** 1979–80 Fall–Winter;5(1–2):35–41
**Oaks RF:** Defining sodomy in seventeenth-century Massachusetts. **J Homosex** 1980–81 Fall–Winter;6(1–2):79–83
**Oates MR** see **Child abuse: historical perspective**
**Obál F:** Emlékezés Charles Robert Darwin-ra (1809–1882) halála centenáriuma alkalmából. **Orv Hetil** 1982 Nov 14;123(46):2857–8
**Obayashi M:** [Historical background of the acceptance of induced abortion] (Jpn). **Josanpu Zasshi** 1982 Dec;36(12):1011–6
**Obe JM:** Oliver Goldsmith: doctor, poet, writer. **Cent Afr J Med** 1984 Mar;30(3):303–8
**Ober L:** Från förspelet till segern över de stora epidemierna. **Hist Foren Arsskr** 1972;:33–45
**Ober WB:** Boswell's clap and other essays. Medical analyses of literary

men's afflictions. Carbondale, Southern Illinois University Press; and London, Feffer & Simons, 1979. xiv, 291 p.

**Ober WB:** Bottoms up! The fine arts and flagellation. Part I. **Am J Dermatopathol** 1984 Oct;6(5):451-60

**Ober WB:** Can the leper change his spots? The iconography of leprosy. Part I. **Am J Dermatopathol** 1983 Feb;5(1):43-58

**Ober WB:** Can the leper change his spots? The iconography of leprosy. Part II. **Am J Dermatopathol** 1983 Apr;5(2):173-86

**Ober WB:** Emil Zuckerkandl and his delightful little organ. **Pathol Annu** 1983;18(Pt 1):103-19

**Ober WB:** Ghon but not forgotten: Anton Ghon and his complex. **Pathol Annu** 1983;18 (pt 2):79-85

**Ober WB:** History of the Brenner tumor of the ovary. **Pathol Annu** 1979;14 Pt 2:107-24

**Ober WB, Sciagura C:** Leydig, Sertoli, and Reinke: three anatomists who were on the ball. **Pathol Annu** 1981;16 Pt 1:1-13

**Ober WB:** Reuben's mandrakes: infertility in the Bible. **Int J Gynecol Pathol** 1984;3(3):299-317

**Ober WB, Aloush N:** The plague at Granada, 1348-1349: Ibn Al-Khatib and ideas of contagion. **Bull NY Acad Med** 1982 May;58(4):418-24

**Ober WB:** The sticky end of Frantisek Koczwara, composer of 'The Battle of Prague'. **Am J Forensic Med Pathol** 1984 Jun;5(2):145-9

**Oberg D** see **McMahon CE**

**Oberg L:** Malte Ljungdahl 1882-1957. **Sydsven Medicinhist Sallsk Arsskr** 1983;:59-64

**Oberg L:** Sjukdoms--och sjukvårdshistoriens källor. **Nord Medicinhist Arsb** 1980;Suppl 6:90-3

**Oberg L** see **Stolt CM**

**Oberhelman S:** Popular dream-interpretation in ancient Greece and Freudian psychoanalysis. **J Pop Cult** 1978;11:682-95

**Oberhelman SM:** Galen, On Diagnosis from Dreams. **J Hist Med Allied Sci** 1983 Jan;38(1):36-47

**Oberhelman SM:** The interpretation of prescriptive dreams in ancient Greek medicine. **J Hist Med Allied Sci** 1981 Oct;36(4):416-24

**Oberlander HP:** Aspects of public health in Toronto, in the 19th and early 20th centuries. **Can J Public Health** 1984 Sep-Oct;75(5):364-5

**Oberlé R:** Société et assistance à Mulhouse à la fin du XVIIIe siècle. In Livet G, Schaff G, ed: Médecine et assistance en Alsace, XVIe-XXe siècle. Strasbourg, Istra, 1976. p. 117-34.

**Obermajer J:** Endoskopie jako výtvarný motiv. **Cesk Gastroenterol Vyz** 1980 Jan;34(1):51-4

**Obermajer J:** Neznámé dopisy Purkyňova tchána K. A. Rudolphiho J. J. Berzeliovi. **Cas Lek Cesk** 1984 Feb 17;123(7):199-203

**Oberman HA:** The crossmatch. A brief historical perspective. **Transfusion** 1981 Nov-Dec;21(6):645-51

**Obermann CE:** A history of vocational rehabilitation in America. New York, Arno Press, 1980. 389 p.

**Obermeit W:** Die Wirklichkeit des Fiktiven. Literatur und Psychoanalyse. **Psyche (Stuttg)** 1981 Mar;35(3):193-208

**Obholzer K:** The Wolf-man. Conversations with Freud's patient--sixty years later. New York, Continuum, 1982. 250 p.

**Obituary William Albert Hugh Rushton F.R.S.: Vision Res** 1982;22(6):611-21

**Obradovic M** see **Puric J**

**Obrentz BN** see **Milbauer B**

**O'Brien E:** Corrigan's disease. **J Ir Coll Physicians Surg** 1980 Jul;10(1):32-7

**O'Brien E:** 'From the waters of Sion to Liffeyside'. The Jewish contribution: medical and cultural. **J Ir Coll Physicians Surg** 1981 Jan;10(3):10 p.

**O'Brien E:** Sir Dominic Corrigan (1802-1880). **J Ir Coll Physicians Surg** 1980 Jul;10(1):11-9

**O'Brien E:** The bicentenary of the Royal College of Surgeons in Ireland, 1784-1984. **Br Med J [Clin Res]** 1983 Dec 24-31;287(6409):1988-90

**O'Brien E:** The Lancet maketh the man? Sir Dominic John Corrigan (1802-80). **Lancet** 1980 Dec 20-27;2(8208-8209):1356-7

**O'Brien E** see **Laher M**

**O'Brien E** see **Mills R**

**O'Brien ET:** The man behind the eponym: Sir Dominic John Corrigan (1802-1880). **N Engl J Med** 1981 Feb 5;304(6):365-6

**O'Brien M:** Legal implications of the use of vaccines. **Med Leg J** 1979;47(4):152-9

**O'Brien ME:** Pragmatic survivalism: behavior patterns affecting low-level wellness among minority group members. **ANS** 1982 Apr;4(3):13-26

**O'Brien W:** The fevers of the Great Famine. **J Ir Coll Physicians Surg** 1980 Jul;10(1):46-9

**Obrosov AN:** Dostizheniia i perspektivy razvitiia nauchnoĭ kurortologii i fizioterapii. **Vopr Kurortol Fizioter Lech Fiz Kult** 1982 Nov-Dec;(6):6-12

**Obrosov AN:** Etapy razvitiia metoda impul'snoĭ terapii v SSSR. **Vopr Kurortol Fizioter Lech Fiz Kult** 1980 Mar-Apr;(2):4-10

**Ocaña G:** La misión del 'Smithsonian Tropical Research Institute' (STRI) en Panamá y en el trópico en general. **Rev Med Panama** 1981 Jan;6(1):3-12

**O'Carrigan C:** Two veteran nurses of World War I days (Sister Mary MacDonald, Sister Mary Vianney). **Med J Aust** 1984 Jun 23;140(13):782-4

**O'Carrigan C, ed** see **Pearn J**

**Ocherki istorii fiziologicheskikh nauk v SSSR:** Istoki i osobennosti razvitiia: materialy Pervoĭ Vsesoiuznoĭ konferentsii po istorii fiziologicheskikh nauk, Tartu, 1981. Leningrad, Nauka, Leningradskoe otd-nie, 1984. 287 p.

**Ochmann A:** Kritische Bemerkungen zur Gesundheitserziehung. **Off Gesundheitswes** 1982 Apr;44(4):230-1

**Ochoa FR:** Die Entwicklung des Gesundheitswesens in der Republik Kuba (1959-1973). **Med Ges** 1979;(6):84-98

**Ochoa S:** The thrill of discovery. **Boll Soc Ital Biol Sper** 1980 Sep 30;56(18 Pt 2):17-40

**Ochoa S:** The thrill of discovery. **Comp Biochem Physiol** 1980;67B:359-65

**Ochs S:** The early history of material transport in nerve. **Physiologist** 1979 Oct;22(5):16-9

**Ochsenhirt S:** The Archives of the History of American Psychology. **Stor Crit Psicol** 1982 Dec;3(2):329-32

**Ochsner A:** To our founder [Franklin H. Martin], with reflections. **Bull Am Coll Surg** 1981;66(5):26-30

**Ochsner SF:** Perspectives in radiology--1922 to 1982. **South Med J** 1983 Dec;76(12):1549-53

**Ocio León S** see **Ortega Millán A**

**Ocklitz HW, Landmann H:** Robert Koch und die Kindertuberkulose. **Kinderarztl Prax** 1982 Mar;50(3):117-29

**Ocklitz HW, Schmitz HH:** Unserem Lehrer Karl Stolte zum 100. Geburtstag. **Kinderarztl Prax** 1981 Nov;49(11):591-5

**O'Connell AN, Russo NF, ed:** Models of achievement. Reflections of eminent women in psychology. New York, Columbia University Press, 1983. xiii, 338 p.

**O'Connell M, Rogers CC:** Assessing cohort birth expectations data from the current population survey, 1971-1981. **Demography** 1983 Aug;20(3):369-84

**O'Connor TW:** A historical review of reversed gastric tube esophagoplasty. **Surg Gynecol Obstet** 1983 Mar;156(3):371-4

**Octavio O:** Algunos momentos familiares de Don Lisandro Alvarado. **Bol Acad Nac Hist (Caracas)** 1981;64(254):419-23

**Odajnyk VW:** Jung and politics. The political and social ideas of C. G. Jung. New York, New York University Press, 1976. xv, 190 p.

**Odegaard CE:** Minorities in medicine. From receptive passivity to positive action 1966-76. New York, Josiah Macy, Jr. Foundation, 1977. vii, 164 p.

**Odegård O:** Perspektiver efter 55 års psykiatrisk virksomhet. **Nord Med** 1982 Dec;97(12):310-3

**Odening K** see **Hiepe T**

**Odonchiméd L, Baklykov LI:** Razvite sanatorno-kurortnogo dela v Mongol'skoĭ Narodnoĭ Respublike. **Vopr Kurortol Fizioter Lech Fiz Kult** 1984 Jul-Aug;(4):40-3

**O'Donnell S:** Gilding the anemometer: Irish science of the past. **Eire Irel** 1982;17(4):148-51

**O'Donnell S:** Irish-American scientists. **Eire Irel** 1979;14(2):106-9

**Odontoiatria del passato:** Dei campanelli de Loreto. **Dent Cadmos** 1981 Jul;49(7):59-60

**Odontoiatria del passato:** La storia di De Trey. **Dent Cadmos** 1983 Mar;51(3):75-81

**Odrich J, Stanaland J:** Early development of dental hygiene. **NY J Dent** 1982 Apr;52(4):127 contd.

**Odrowaz-Szukiewicz H:** Wojskowa służba zdrowia na Sadybie podczas Powstania Warszawskiego. **Arch Hist Med (Warsz)** 1978;41(4):447-63

**O'Dwyer WF:** Corrigan and the Charitable Infirmary. **J Ir Coll Physicians Surg** 1980 Jul;10(1):21-3

**Oehler D, Weiner R:** Entwicklung und Differenzierung der operativen Therapie urologischer Patienten im Krankenhaus St. Georg, Leipzig, in den letzten 65 Jahren. **Z Urol Nephrol** 1980 Mar;73(3):171-80

**Oehme J:** Kinderkrankheiten und Kinderheikunde. **Klin Padiatr** 1984 Nov-Dec;196(6):325-6

**Oehme J:** Rückbesinnung zum 100 jährigen Bestehen der Deutschen Gesellschaft für Kinderheilkunde. **Klin Paediatr** 1983 Jan-Feb;195(1):1-3

**Oehme P:** Entwicklungstendenzen der Arzneimittelforschung. **Z Gesamte Inn Med** 1980 Jul 15;35(14):20-5

**Oei TI:** Over depressie (I). Enkele ontwikkelingen omtrent de depressie. **Tijdschr Ziekenverpl** 1983 Feb 15;36(4):105-8

**Oelssner W** see **Dörffel EW**

**Oesch I** see **Bettex M**

**Oeser E** see **Lorenz K, ed**

**Oesterreich K, Wagner O:** Psychopathologie des Alterns und der Voralterung--Historische Entwicklung der Begriffsbildung. **Z Gerontol** 1982 Nov-Dec;15(6):314-20

**O'Farrel P:** Whose reality?: The Irish famine in history and literature. **Hist Stud** 1982;20(78):1-13

**Ofcansky TP:** British colonial administration in the Fiji Islands during the 1875 measles epidemic. **Adler Mus Bull** 1984 Mar;10(1):23-7

**Ofcansky TP:** The life and times of Sir Albert Ruskin Cook. **J Hist Med Allied Sci** 1982 Apr;37(2):225-8

**Ofcansky TP:** The 1889-97 rinderpest epidemic and the rise of British and German colonialism in eastern and southern Africa. **J Afr Stud** 1981;8(1):31-8

**Offen K:** Depopulation, nationalism, and feminism in fin-de-siècle France. **Am Hist Rev** 1984;89(3):648-76

**The official publication of the American Association of Physical Anthropologists 1930-1980: Jubilee Issue: Am J Phys Anthropol** 1981 Dec;56(4):327-557

**Offret G:** Souvenirs sur une pathologie oculaire en voie d'extinction. **Bull Soc Ophtalmol Fr** 1980 Jan;80(1):43-5

**Offringa C** see **Arts en sameleving. Medical history contributions by H. W. Pleket, J. Van Herwaarden, W. Frijhoff, C. Offringa, M. J. Van Lieburg, C. Bakker-Van der Kooij**

**Ofosu-Amaah S:** The maternal and child health services in Ghana (their

origins and future). **J Trop Med Hyg** 1981 Dec;84(6):265-9
**Oganov RG:** Istoriia vsemirnykh kongressov kardiologov i uchastie v nikh sovetskikh uchenykh. **Kardiologiia** 1982 May;22(5):7-9
**Ogasawara K:** [Recollections on microbiological research] (Jpn). **Nippon Saikingaku Zasshi** 1982 Jul;37(4):757-9
**Ogata T** see **Sakurai K**
**Ogawa K:** Kohon Nippon gankagaku shi. Kyotol, Shibunkaku, [Showa 46 nen, 1971]. 218 p.
**Ogawa S** see **Matsuyama K**
**Ogawa S** see **Shibaike N**
**Ogawa T, ed:** Public health. Proceedings of the 5th International Symposium on the comparative history of medicine--East and West. Division of Medical History, The Taniguchi Foundation. Tokyo, Saikon, 1981. vi, 189 p.
**Ogle G:** The mysterious death of Mrs. Leland Stanford. **Pac Hist** 1981 Spring;25:1-7
**Ograjensek Z:** Raxvoj Instituta za planiranje porodice u Ljubljani. **Jugosl Ginekol Opstet** 1981 Jan-Apr;21(1-2):50-3
**Ogris A:** Zur Geschichte des Badens. Mit einem Exkurs über Warmbad Villach. **Wien Geschichtsbl** 1978;33(2):87-9
**Oguro M:** [Late Dr. Satoru Inagaki, a member of the Council of the Japan Society of Clinical Hematology: his life and contributions] (Jpn) **Rinsho Ketsueki** 1979 Nov;20(11):1532-3
**Oguse, D:** 'Socialisme et néo-malthusianisme', la Revue Socialiste, t. XLVI, juillet-décembre 1907, p. 27-124. **Ann Demogr Hist (Paris)** 1983;:371-89
**Ohadike DC:** The influenza pandemic of 1918-19 and the spread of cassava cultivation on the lower Niger: a study in historical linkages. **J Afr Hist** 1981;22(3):380-91
**O'Hern EM:** Alice Catherine Evans. In: Notable American women. The modern period. Cambridge, Mass., Belknap-Harvard Univ. Press, 1980. 4:219-21.
**Ohja J:** Chyavanaprasha: a scientific study. Varanasi [India], Tara Publications, 1978. x, 80 p.
**Ohlah A:** Changement des relations médecin-malade au cours des millenaires. Méthode socio-psychologique et histoire de la médecine. In International Congress of the History of Medicine. 26th, Plovdiv, 1978. Actes du Congress. Sofia, 1981. Volume II. p. 99-100.
**Ohlendorf D, ed** see **Kotwas J**
**Ohquist M:** Hälsosyster i Esbo på 1920-talet. **Hist Litteraturhist Studier (Finl)** 1979;54:201-38
**Ohry A:** A history of poliomyelitis research. **Koroth** 1979 Nov;7(9-10):CCXI-CCXVIII(668-679)
**Ohry A:** A short history of anaesthesia. **Koroth** 1983 Aug;8(7-8):281-3
**Ohry A:** Historical perspectives of medical rehabilitation. **Koroth** 1981;8(1-2):57-60
**Ohry A:** On pain. **Koroth** 1982;8(3-4):199-204
**Ohry A:** Respiratory items in Hippocratic medicine. **Koroth** 1980 Jun;7(11-12):CCLXXXV-CCLXLII
**Ohya Z:** Moxas et acupuncture au Japon. In: Congrès international d'histoire de la médecine, XXVe, Québec, 1976. Actes. Québec, 1977. p. 1026-30.
**Oide S:** Der Einfluss der galenischen Pneumatheorie auf die cusanische Spiritustheorie. Eine Anmerkung zu 'De quaerendo deum'. **Mitt Forschungsbeitr Cusanus Ges** 1978;13:198-207
**Oiso T** see **Dwyer JT**
**Ojeda Figueroa C:** Karl Jaspers: filosofía y psicoterapia. **Acta Luso Esp Neurol Psiquiatr** 1983 Mar-Apr;11(2):181-8
**Ojemann RG:** Biography of C. Miller Fisher, M.D. **Clin Neurosurg** 1983;31:xiii-xxviii
**Ojrzyński J** see **Kuchowicz Z**
**Okada M:** [Notes on 'Cassandra'. 1 (Florence Nightingale)] (Jpn) **Sogo Kango** 1984 Aug 15;19(3):63-78
**Okada R** see **Kawai S**
**Okada Y:** [Background of Rintaro Mori's debates on statistics] (Jpn). **Igakushi Kenkyu** 1978;49:1-13
**Okada Y:** [The incidence of Kakke-disease (beriberi) in pre-war mental hospitals] (Jpn). **Nihon I-Shigaku Zasshi** 1981;27:95-111
**Okamoto K:** [Historical significance of midwifery activities--with special reference to the Meiji period] (Jpn). **Josanpu Zasshi** 1981 Aug;35(8):577-99
**Okamoto Y:** [Nursing home: medical care a nursing practice in the United States. 8. Establishment of the system of nurses' registration and the history of the development of nursing assistants] (Jpn) **Kangogaku Zasshi** 1980 Aug;44(8):858-63
**Okamoto Y:** [Nursing homes. Status of medical care and nursing in the United States. 5. History of nursing homes]. **Kangogaku Zasshi** 1980 May;44(5):523-7
**Okamura A:** [A long road to the hospice movement--life of Mother Mary Aikenhead] (Jpn). **Kango Kyoiku** 1984 Jan;25(1):38-45;25(2):104-11 (continued periodically)
**Okamura A:** [Abnormal psychology and England from 1660 to 1760] (Jpn). **Kango Kyoiku** 1983 Jun;24(6):360-7
**Okamura A:** [Hospice and human rights movement. (2)] (Jpn). **Kango Kyoiku** 1983 May;24(5):294-302
**Okamura A:** [Let us take a walk in East Side: search of the background of the modern hospice, 3] (Jpn). **Kango Kyoiku** 1982 Oct;23(10):637-43
**Okamura A:** [Report on 19th century Dublin: the background of the modern hospice movement] (Jpn). **Kango Kyoiku** 1982 Nov;23(11):687-92
**Okamura H, Kito O, Sakamoto T, et al:** [History and prospect of hypothermia] (Jpn). **Rinsho Kyobu Geka** 1983 May;3(3):321-30
**Okasha A:** Mental disorders in Pharaonic Egypt. **J Egypt Med Assoc** 1978;61(Suppl 1-2):3-12
**Okazaki K:** Kusuri no rekishi. Tokyo, Kodansha, Showa 51 nen, [1976]. 324 p.
**Okazaki T** see **Stricevic MV**
**Okhrimenko NN:** Glavnyĭ voennyĭ gospital' i ego rol' v razvitii otechestvennoĭ voennoĭ nevrologii (k 275-letiiu so dnia osnovaniia Glavnogo. **Zh Nevropatol Psikhiatr** 1983;83(7):1069-71
**Okino S** see **Fujimori K**
**Okita S, ed:** Miyoshi-gun Ishikai shi. Ikeda-cho, Japan, Miyoshi-gun Ishikai, Showa 53 nen. [1978]. 568 p.
**Okuni M:** [A chronological table on district nurse (Hokenfu) in after the war. Part I] (Jpn). **Igakushi Kenkyu** 1977;48:39-40
**Olagüe G:** El discurso de Giovanni Maria Lancisi 'sobre la recta ordenacion de los estudios medicos segun la razon' (1715). **Asclepio** 1981;33:143-62
**Olagüe G:** El programa de reforma educativa de Giovanni Maria Lancisi: De recta medicorum studiorum ratione instituenda (1715). **Episteme** 1976 Jan-Dec;1-4:180-9
**Olagüe G:** La 'teoria fibrilar' en la obra de Giorgio Baglivi (1668-1707). Introduccion, traduccion de los capitulos I y II del libro I de su specimen Quatuor librorum de fibra motrice et morbosa (Perusa, 1700), y notas. **Morfol Norm Patol** 1979;3:335-56
**Olagüe G** see **Ballester R**
**Olagüe G** see **Carrillo JL**
**Olagüe G** see **Gago R**
**Olagüe de Ros G:** La epidemia europea de gripe de 1708-1709. Difusión témporo-espacial e interpretaciones contemporáneas: G. M. Lancisi, B. Ramazzini, K. F. Hoffmann. **Dynamis** 1981;1:51-86
**Olagüe i de Ros G** see **Balaguer i Perigüell E**
**Olague Ros G:** Biografia cientifica de Giovanni Maria Lancisi. **Med Esp** 1980;79:250-60
**Olagüe Ros G:** Elaboración y difusión de la medicina moderna en la Italia de los siglos XVI y XVII: la peculiaridad del ambiente científico romano (1548-1720). In Albarracin Teulon A, et al, ed: Medicina e Historia. Madrid, Edic. Univ. Comp., 1973. p. 265-90.
**Oláh A:** Althergebrachte Tierheilpraktiken im Komitat Békés, Ungarn. **Ethnomedizin** 1978-79;5(3-4):301-18
**Oláh A:** Zwiebel und Knoblauch in der Volksmedizin; das ungarische Theriak und Mithridaticum früher und heute. **Ethnomedizin** 1981-82;7(1-4):333-48
**Olakowski T, Rudzińska H, Gadomska H, et al:** Epidemiologia raka płuca w Polsce do roku 1977. **Pneumonol Pol** 1979 Aug-Sep;47(7-8):553-64
**Olarte J:** La bacteriología intestinal en México. In Academia Nacional de Medicina. Libro conmemorativo del primer centenario. México, Comité Editorial de la Comisión Organizadora del Congreso del Centenario, 1964. Tome 2. p. 521-3.
**Olascoaga ML** see **Loza Colomer JC**
**Olbort F:** Die Pestepidemie von 1653-1657 in Niederösterreich. **Unsere Heimat** 1974;45(1):11-23
**Olbort F:** Pestebild und Pestbekämpfung im Niederösterreich des 17. Jahrhunderts. **Unsere Heimat** 1977;48(1):13-29
**Olbort F:** 'Vergessene' Pestjahre. Die Seuche von 1653 bis 1656 in Wien. **Wien Geschichtsbl** 1973;28(1):10-14
**Olby R:** La theorie genetique de la selection naturelle vue par un historien. **Rev Synth (Paris)** 1981;102(103-104):251-89
**Olby R:** The sheriff and the cowboys: or Weaver's support of Astbury and Pauling. **Soc Stud Sci** 1984 May;14(2):244-7
**Olby RC:** The history of molecular biology. **Hist Philos Life Sci** 1980;2(2):299-310
**Olby RC:** The significance of the macromolecules in the historiography of molecular biology. **Hist Philos Life Sci** 1979;1(2):185-98
**Olch PD:** Evarts Ambrose Graham. In Dictionary of American Biography, Suppl. 6, 1956-1960. p. 245-7, 1980.
**Olch PD:** Medicine in the Indian-fighting army, 1866-1890. **J West** 1982 Jul;21(3):32-41
**Olch PD:** Owen H. Wangensteen (1898-1981). **Bull Hist Med** 1981;55:260-2
**Olch PD:** Robert Elman. In Dictionary of American Biography, Suppl. 6, 1956-1960. p. 189-90, 1980.
**Olch PD:** Some comments on the life of Emile Frederic Holman (1890-1977). **Bull Am Coll Surg** 1981;66(3):22-5
**The old pathology building (The Pathological Department of the Central Indiana Hospital for the Insane): Indiana Med Hist Q** 1974;1(1):7-10
**Oldenburg D:** Georg August Bertele (1767-1818) und die Arzneimittellehre der romantischen Naturphilosophie. **Medizinhist J** 1981;16(3):240-56
**Oldenburg D:** Romantische Naturphilosophie und Arzneimittellehre 1800-1840. Diss. (Doktor der Naturwissenschaften), Braunschweig, 1979. 267 p. (Veröffentlichungen aus dem Pharmaziegeschichtlichen Seminar der Technischen Universität Braunschweig, 20).
**Oldroyd D:** Gregor Mendel: founding-father of modern genetics? **Endeavour** 1984;8(1):29-31
**Oldroyd DR:** Darwinian impacts. An introduction to the Darwinian revolution. Atlantic Highlands, N. J., Humanities Press, 1980. xiv, 399 p.
**Oldroyd DR:** Some 'philosophical scribbles' attributed to Robert Hooke. **Notes Rec R Soc Lond** 1980 Jul;35(1):17-32
**Oleru UG** see **Sawyer DR**
**Olesińska-Serafin A:** Europejskie Stowarzyszenie Kształcenia Medycznego i jego wpływ na rozwój dydaktyki medycznej. **Pol Tyg Lek** 1984 Mar 26;39(13):453-5
**Oleson A, Voss J, ed:** The organization of knowledge in modern America, 1860-1920. Baltimore and London, Johns Hopkins University Press, 1979. xxi, 478 p.

**Oliaro A:** La chirurgia cento anni or sono. L'Anatomia Chirurgica del dott. **Minerva Chir** 1982 Dec 15-31;37(23-24):2159-79

**Oliaro T:** La funzione storica e didattica della Stampa Medica. **Minerva Med** 1983 Dec 15;74(47-48):2801-2

**Oliaro T:** La funzione storica e didattica della stampa medica. **Minerva Stomatol** 1984 May-Jun;33(3):536-7

**Oliaro T:** La medicina attraverso i tempi. Dalla bioritmologia alla cronobiologia. **Minerva Med** 1984 Jan 14;75(1-2):51-2

**Oliaro T:** Marco Aurelio Severino il perseguitato ricreatore della chirurgia italiana (1580-1656). **Minerva Chir** 1980 Sep 30;35(18 Suppl):32-4

**Oliaro T** see **Ferrari Sacco A**

**Olimpio NA** see **Cooper T**

**Oliveira JC de:** Em louvor de Koch. A propósito da descoberta do bacilo da tuberculose. **Acta Med Port** 1983 Mar;4(3):195-9

**Oliver G:** Le Service de santé militaire dans les Pyrénées-Orientales pendant la guerre de 1914-1918. In: Congrès National des Sociétés Savantes, 97e, Nantes, 1972. Comptes Rendus. Paris, 1976. Section des Sciences, Tome 1. p. 351-62.

**Oliver H:** The Shore Smith family library: Arthur Hugh Clough and Florence Nightingale. **Book Collect** 1979;28:521-9

**Oliver LC** see **Stoeckle JD**

**Oliver TP:** 67 years ago--the Journal of the Royal Naval Medical Service, Vol I. **J R Nav Med Serv** 1982 Winter;68(3):167-70

**Oliver TP:** 67 years ago--the Journal of the Royal Naval Medical Service Vol 1, No. 1. **J R Nav Med Serv** 1982;68(2):98-101

**Olivier A, Bertrand G, Picard C:** Discovery of the first human stereotactic instrument. **Appl Neurophysiol** 1983;46(1-4):84-91

**Olivier A** see **Picard C**

**Olivier AF:** In proper perspective: Daniel Hale Williams, M.D. **Ann Thorac Surg** 1984 Jan;37(1):96-7

**Olivier-Friguet G:** Les femmes du nord face à l'avortement (de 1975 à nos jours). **Rev Nord** 1981;63(250):775-800

**Ollero Granados D:** New light Celsus' 'De medicina'. **Sudhoffs Arch** 1978;62(4):359-77

**Olmedilla y Puig, J** see **Folch Jou G**

**Olmi G:** Farmacopea antica e medicina moderna: la disputa sulla teriaca nel cinquecento Bolognese. **Physis** 1977;19(1-4):197-246

**Olmi G:** Osservazione della natura e raffiguarazione in Ulisse Aldrovandi (1522-1605). **Ann Ist Stor Italo-Ger** 1977;3:105-81

**Olmos L** see **Barba J**

**Olness K:** Hypnosis in pediatric practice. **Curr Probl Pediatr** 1981 Dec;12(2):1-47

**Olonetzky B, Mez L:** Die Sammlung. Darstellung alter Arztinstrumente, Apotheker-Gefässe, Mikroskope, Einnehmelöffel, Terra sigillata, Amulette und anderer interessanter Gegenstände und Kuriositäten. Stuttgart, Thieme, 1980. 3 vol. in one. 123, 114, 127 p.

**Olsen AM:** ACCP International--'The world is our classroom'. **Chest** 1984 Nov;86(5):655-6

**Olsen O, Barker P:** Rabies archaeologorum. **Antiquity** 1980;54(210):15-20

**Olsen R** see **Trussell J**

**Ol'shannikova VV** see **Ibragimova ZI**

**Olson GD:** Dr. David Ramsay and Lt. Colonel Thomas Brown: patriot historian and loyalist critic. **SC Hist Mag** 1976;77:256-67

**Olson RE** see **Broquist HP**

**Olssen E:** Truby King and the Plunket Society: an analysis of a prescriptive ideology. **NZ J Hist** 1981;15(1):3-23

**Olsson JE, Reichard H:** Mannen bakom syndromet: Pierre Ménétrier. Tumörpatolog och mikrobiolog med tidig insikt om precancerösa förändringar. **Lakartidningen** 1984 Oct 10;81(41):3705-6

**Olsson L:** Altern im gesellschaftlichen Wandel--Ein interdisziplinäres Forschungsprojekt über Schweden im 19. und 20. Jahrhundert. **Z Gerontol** 1984 Jan-Feb;17(1):6-12

**Oltmanns TF** see **Neale JM**

**Om dårlige arbeidsrutiner. Med hilsen fra Florence Nightingale: Sykepleien** 1984 Sep 20;71(16):6-8, 30

**Omameuda M:** 1920 (sen-kyuhyaku niju) nen-dai ni okeru shokuryo seisaku no tenkai: kome-sodo-go no zosan seisaku to beikokuho. **Shigaku Zasshi** 1982;91(10):40-73

**Omar S:** Ibn Al-Haytham's theory of knowledge and its significance for later science. **Arab Stud Q** 1979;1(1):67-82

**Omirov RIu, Mardanov LM:** Nekotorye voprosy khirurgii v trudakh Abu Ali Ibn Siny (k 1000-letiiu so dnia rozhdeniia). **Klin Khir** 1980 Mar;(3):66-8

**Omiya Sekijui Byoin Yono, Japan:** Omiya Sekijuji Byoin yonjunenshi. Yono, Japan, Omiya Sekijuji Byoin, Showa 51 nen, 1976. 173 p.

**Omuro A:** X-sen igakukai no senkusha Miyahara Tatsutaro. Ichihara, Japan. Ichihara-shi Kyoiku Iinkai, Showa 50 nen [1975] 88 p.

**On the rôle of Laurence H. Synder in the development of human and medical genetics in the United States; an oral history tape interview: Am J Med Genet** 1981;8(4):449-68

**On the 125th anniversary of Victor Babeş birth: Virologie** 1979 Jul-Sep;30(3):169-70

**On the 35th anniversary of our journal: Virologie** 1984 Jan-Mar;35(1):3-4

**Oncel O:** Asepsis and antisepsis in the past and today. In International Congress of the History of Medicine. 26th, Plovdiv, 1978. Actes du Congress. Sofia, 1981. Volume II. p. 175-8.

**Ondrejička M:** 60 Rokov Bratislavských lekárskych listov. **Bratisl Lek Listy** 1982 Jan;77(1):3-5

**Ondrejička M:** 60 rokov internej medicíny na jubilujúcej lekárskej fakulte University Komenského v Bratizlave. **Vnitr Lek** 1979 Dec;25(12):1145-7

**Ondrejička M:** 60 rokov internistických disciplín na lekárskej fakulte University Komenského v Bratislave. **Cas Lek Cesk** 1979 Dec 21;118(51):1576-80

**O'Neil WM:** The beginnings of modern psychology. Brighton, Harvester Press; Atlantic Highlands, N.J., Humanities Press, 1982. x, 145 p.

**O'Neill HJ** see **Moore JG**

**O'Neill TF** see **Greenberg M**

**O'Neill YV:** An anatomical mystery with global dimensions. In: Congrès international d'histoire de la médecine, XXVe, Québec, 1976. Actes. Québec, 1977. p. 1031-44.

**O'Neill YV:** Jose Maria Benites' informe--alta California's first medical account. In International Congress of the History of Medicine, 27th, Barcelona, 1980. Actas. Barcelona, Acadèmia de Ciències Mèdiques de Catalunya i Balears, 1981. p. 203-6.

**O'Neill YV:** Ossa mandibulae inferioris duo. **Clio Med** 1980 May;14(2):97-104

**O'Neill YV:** Speech and speech disorders in Western thought before 1600. Westport, Connecticut, Greenwood, 1980. xii, 246 p. (Contributions in medical history, No. 3).

**Ongaro G, Mazzolini RG:** Quasi tradens se totum: i manoscritti morgagnani della Biblioteca Palatina di Parma. **Ann Ist Mus Stor Sci Fir** 1983;8(1):101-5

**Onicescu D** see **Diculescu I**

**Onishi W:** [A life among frontier farmers in Hokkaido: a public health nurse in a segment of history of the Showa era] (Jpn). **Kango** 1981 Aug;33(9):88-91

**Onishi W:** [Life among farmers of a reclamation project in Hokkaido: a life of a public health nurse in a segment of the history of the Showa period] (Jpn). **Kango** 1981 Dec;33(14):82-7

**Onishi W:** [Life among the frontier farmers of Hokkaido: public health nursing in the history of the Showa period. 10.] (Jpn). **Kango** 1982 Feb;34(2):65-71; 97-103

**Onishi W:** [Public health nurse working among the farmers in the Hokkaido Reclamation Project: a segment of the history of the Showa period] (Jpn). **Kango** 1981 Apr;33(4):73-9

**Onishi W:** [Public health nursing at land reclamation project in Hokkaido: a segment of the history of the Showa period] (Jpn). **Kango** 1981 Sep;33(10):98-103, Nov;33(12):81-91

**Ono H:** On Wells's (1792) law of visual direction. **Percept Psychophys** 1981 Oct;30(4):403-6

**Ono J:** Legacies of Jefferson men to Japanese medicine. **Ann Otol Rhinol Laryngol [Suppl]** 1981 Sep-Oct;90(5 pt 2 Suppl 87):1-10

**Ono K, Yamada S:** [Hygienic supplies for women used from the end of the Meiji era to the early Showa period: accounts by women who grew up in the Meiji period] (Jpn). **Josanpu Zasshi** 1983 Oct;37(10):819-27

**Ono Y:** [Human science. Religion (1). Religion as a psychological phenomenon--progress in religious psychology] (Jpn). **Kango Tenbo** 1981 Apr;6(4):350-6

**Onopchenko NA, Gun'ko MA, Eremin VM:** Nikolaĭ Fedotovich Mel'nikov-Razvedenkov--zamechatel'nyĭ organizator i vidnyĭ uchenyĭ-patologoanatom. **Arkh Patol** 1983;45(10):78-82

**Onsager LW:** That curious book 'The breath of life' by George Catlin. **Int J Oral Myol** 1980 Oct;6(4):7-10

**Onuigbo WI:** Historical notes on cancer in married couples. **Neth J Surg** 1984 Aug;36(4):112-5

**Onyemacke Ogum GE:** Fertility differentials in Nigeria. **Genus** 1980;36(3-4):203-13

**Oosterveen K** see **Laslett P**

**Opas T:** Dawne szpitale województwa Lubelskiego w świetle materiałów lustracyjnych z lat 1790-1791. **Kwart Hist Kultury Mater** 1972;20(2):267-82

**Opie LH, Louw JH:** John Hunter and angina pectoris. **Am J Cardiol** 1981 Nov;48(5):980

**Opitz JM, Pallister PD:** Brief historical note: the concept of 'gonadal dysgenesis'. **Am J Med Genet** 1979;4(4):333-43

**Opitz JM:** Cotterman and combinatorial genetics. **Am J Med Genet** 1983 Nov;16(3):389-92

**Opitz JM:** In memoriam: Petrus Johannes Waardenburg, 1886-1979. **Am J Med Genet** 1980;7(1):35-9

**Opitz JM:** Introduction of Sewall Wright on the occasion of receiving the first Meckel medal and prize in mammalian developmental genetics. **Am J Med Genet** 1984 Aug;18(4):587-90

**Opitz R, Horn H, Heinecke P, et al:** Robert Koch. Die Vorgeschichte der Berufung als ersten Ordinarius für Hygiene an die Universität Berlin. **MMW** 1981 Oct 16;123(42):1593-5

**Opland J** see **Eden AR**

**Oppenheim RW:** Laura Bridgeman's brain: an early consideration of functional adaptations in neural development. **Dev Psychobiol** 1979 Nov;12(6):533-7

**Oppenheimer JM:** Aristotle as a biologist. **Scientia** 1971;65(106):649-58

**Oppenheimer JM:** Asymmetry revisited. **Am Zool** 1974 Summer;14(3):867-79

**Oppenheimer JM:** Basic embryology and clinical medicine: a case history in serendipity. **Bull Hist Med** 1984 Summer;58(2):236-40

**Oppenheimer JM, Whitfield JB:** Biographical Memoirs: George Washington Corner (1889-1981). **Misc Am Philos Soc** 1982?;9 p.

**Oppenheimer JM:** Ernst Heinrich Haeckel as an intermediary in the transmutation of an idea. **Proc Am Philos Soc** 1982;126(5):347-55

**Oppenheimer JM:** Harvey, William. Disputations touching the generation of animals: essay review. **Trans Stud Coll Physicians Phila** 1982 Dec;4(4):306-9

**Oppenheimer JM:** Thomas Hunt Morgan as an embryologist: the view from Bryn Mawr. **Am Zool** 1983;23:845-54

**Oppenheimer JM:** Walter Landauer and developmental genetics. In Subtelny S, Abbott U, ed: Levels of genetic control in development. New York, Liss, 1981. p. 1-13.

**Oppenheimer JM, ed** see **Willier BH**

**Oppitz R:** Freiherr von Ehrenfels (1859-1932) und die Entwicklung des 'Neuen Menschen' zu Beginn des 20. Jahrhunderts. Diss. Mainz, 1980. 256 p.

**Opsomer C:** Les plantes exotiques du Livre des Simples Medecines de Lille. In: Congrès National des Sociétés Savantes, 101e, Lille, 1976. Comptes Rendus. Paris, 1976. Section des Sciences, Fasc. III. p. 33-44.

**Opsomer C:** Quelques somnifères de l'antiquité et du moyen âge. Fédération des Cercles d'Archéologie et d'Histoire de Belgique. 44e session. Congrès de Huy, 1976. Annales. Tielt, 1978. p. 589-92.

**Opsomer JE:** Problèmes d'identification de plantes dans les 'herbiers' anciens. Erreurs et confusions anciennes et récentes. Fédération des Cercles d'Archéologie et d'Histoire de Belgique. 44e session. Congrès de Huy, 1976. Annales. Tielt, 1978. p. 593-6.

**Opsomer JE** see **Dodoens R**

**Opsomer-Halleux C:** La diététique d'Ibn Butlan dans le manuscrit 887 (1041) de l'Université de Liège. Congrès de Comines, 1, 1980. Actes. p. 350.

**Opsomer-Halleux C** see **Delatte L**

**O'Rahilly R:** Plain words on planes and sections. **Radiol Technol** 1981 May-Jun;52(6):615-7

**O'Rahilly R:** The discovery of the parathyroid glands. **Bull Hist Med** 1982 Summer;56(2):263-4

**Oral history abstract catalog: Interviews 1969-1978. St. Louis, Archives Section, Washington Univ. School of Medicine Library, 1979. 15 p:**

**Oratovskaia NB** see **Revenko TA**

**Ordabekov S:** Zdravookhranenie Dzhambulskoĭ oblasti v dorevoliutsionnyĭ period. **Sov Zdravookhr** 1982;(4):64-5

**Ordina OM:** Professor V. P. Miroliubov (k 110-letiiu so dnia rozhdeniia). **Arkh Patol** 1982;44(7):80-3

**Ordosgoitia Yarzagaray E, Viaña Olaya R, Buelvas Acosta E:** Proceso historico de la Universidad de Carsagena. **Rev Fed Odontol Colomb** 1979 Jan-Mar;25(128):31-40

**Orenstein HH:** How excellent a showman: Joseph Eastman Sheehan, 1885-1951. **Bull NY Acad Med** 1983 Apr;59(3):327-30

**Oribabor P** see **Davies C, ed**

**Origin of the NSW Nurses' Association: Lamp** 1981 May;38(5 Suppl):9-10

**The origins of laboratory animal science and medicine: proceedings of a symposium presented at the 30th annual session of the American Association for Laboratory Animal Science, Atlanta, 16-21 September 1979.: Lab Anim Sci** 1980 Aug;30(4 pt 2):737-800

**Origins of the State Mental Hospital in America:** Reprints of six studies, 1837-1856. New York, Arno Press, 1973. Various pagings.

**Oring E:** The jokes of Sigmund Freud: a study in humor and Jewish identity. Philadelphia, University of Pennsylvania Press, 1984. xiii, 151 p.

**Oriol WE** see **Hickey T**

**Orlik-Grzybowska A:** Geneza powstania Sekcji Ortodontycznej Polskiego Tow. Stomat. i jej początkowa działalność w latach 1950-1955. **Czas Stomatol** 32(9):909-13, Sep 79

**Orlov DA, Galakhov EV, Zhiliaeva EP:** Uchastie mirovoĭ meditsinskoĭ obshchestvennosti v bor'be za mir i razoruzhenie. **Sov Zdravookhr** 1980;(10):38-44

**Orlova AN:** Vklad A. I. Nesterova v uchenie o mikrotsirkuliatsii (k 85-letiiu so dnia rozhdeniia A. I. Nesterova). **Vopr Revm** 1981 Jan-Mar;(1):58-61

**Orlova NL** see **Dikshteĭn EA**

**Orlova NV, Pariĭskaia TV, Vorob'ev AS:** 20 Let raboty po usovershenstvovaniiu znaniĭ pediatrov v oblasti kardiorevmatologii. **Pediatriia** 1982 Jun;(6):59-61

**Orlova RV** see **Shishkin NA**

**Orłowski WJ:** Patronka cierpiacych na oczy. **Klin Oczna** 1984 May;86(5):231-5

**Orłowski WJ:** Polska historiografia okulistyczna. **Klin Oczna** 1980;82(11):553-5

**Orłowski WJ:** Słowo wprowadzajqce do IX sympozjonu retinologicznego. **Klin Oczna** 1979 Dec;81(12):645-8

**Orłowski WJ:** Słowo wprowadzajqce do XI sympozjonu retinologicznego. **Klin Oczna** 1982 Sep;84(9):241-3

**Orłowski WJ:** Słowo wprowadzajqce do XII sympozjonu retinologicznego. **Klin Oczna** 1984 Jan;86(1):1-6

**Orłowski WJ:** W stulecie polskich zjazdów okulistycznych. **Klin Oczna** 1981 Oct-Dec;83(10-12):465-6

**Orłowski WJ:** Z teki szperacza-bibliografa. **Klin Oczna** 1984 Feb;86(2):90 contd

**Orłowski WJ:** Z teki szperacza-bibliografa (VIII). Przed 100 laty. **Klin Oczna** 1981;83(3):193-4

**Orłowski WJ:** Z teki szperacza-bibliografa (X). Przed 50 laty. **Klin Oczna** 1981;83(9):453-4

**Orłowski WJ:** Z teki szperacza-bibliografa (XIII). Przed 75 laty. **Klin Oczna** 1982 Apr;84(4):135-6

**Orłowski WJ:** Z teki szperacza--bibliografa (XVIII). Przed 50 laty. **Klin Oczna** 1983 Apr;85(4):189-91

**Orme JG, Stuart P:** The Habit Clinics: behavioral social work and prevention in the 1920s. **Soc Serv Rev** 1981;55(2):242-56

**Ormsbee RA:** A review: 'Studies in Pyroplasmosis hominis ('spotted fever' or 'tick fever' of the Rocky Mountains)' by Louis B. Wilson and William M. Chowning, published in The Journal of Infectious Diseases 1:31-57, 1904. **Rev Infect Dis** 1979 May-Jun;1(3):559-62

**Ormsby-Lennon H:** Radical physicians and conservative poets in Restoration England: Dryden among the doctors. **Stud Eighteenth Cent Cult** 1978;7:389-411

**Orner R, Hipwell J:** Njal's Saga: a 1000 year old record of premature ejaculation. **J Am Soc Psychosom Dent Med** 1980;27(1):10-2

**Ornowski J** see **Zajusz K**

**Ornstein A** see **Goldberg A, ed**

**Ornstein PA** see **Hearst E, ed**

**Orofino G, Brach CC:** Nel nome del bagno. **Kos** 1984 Apr;1(3):33-54

**Orofino G** see **Adacher S**

**Orosz JJ:** A short history of bloodletting. **Artif Organs** 1981 Aug;5(3):226-8

**Orosz L, Veress O:** Lassai levél... **Orv Hetil** 1980 Nov 2;121(44):2711-5

**O'Rourke DT:** John Houghton (1645-1705) Journalist, apothecary and F.R.S. **Pharm Hist (London)** 1979 Apr;9(1):2-3

**Orozco Acuaviva A:** Apuntes para la historia de la anatomia gaditana del siglo XIX. **Asclepio** 1978-79;30-31:99-116

**Orozco Acuaviva A:** El inventario de la botica del Convento-Hospital de San Juan de Dios de Cadiz, de 1822. **Bol Soc Esp Hist Farm** 1981 Dec;32(128):223-33

**Orozco Acuaviva A:** Historia de una enfermedad de los navegantes: el escorbuto. **An R Acad Med Cir Cadiz** 1979;15(1):7-30

**Orozco Acuaviva A:** La primera epidemia de 'Dengue' en España. In: Sociedad Española de Historia de la Medicina. V Congreso Nacional. Madrid, 1977. **Asclepio** 1977;29:209-15

**Orozco Acuaviva A:** Pedro María González y el tratado de las enfermedades de la gente del mar. In International Congress of the History of Medicine, 27th, Barcelona, 1980. Actas. Barcelona, Académia de Ciències Médiques de Catalunya i Balears, 1981. p. 394-8.

**Orozco Acuaviva A:** Sabater y el empirismo anatomopatológico en el Hospital de Bellavista del Callao. In International Congress of the History of Medicine, 27th, Barcelona, 1980. Actas. Barcelona, Académia de Ciències Médiques de Catalunya i Balears, 1981. p. 401-7.

**Orozco Acuaviva, A:** El 'Compendio de medicina práctica' de Josef Salvaresa del Real Colegio de Cirugía de Cádiz. In International Congress of the History of Medicine, 27th, Barcelona, 1980. Actas. Barcelona, Académia de Ciències Médiques de Catalunya i Balears, 1981. p. 387-93.

**Orr JF, James WV, Bahrani AS:** The history and development of artificial limbs. **Eng Med** 1982 Oct;11(4):155-61

**Orr MD:** Autotransfusion: intraoperative scavenging. **Int Anesthesiol Clin** 1982 Winter;20(4):97-119

**Orr N:** Why wear a mask in theatre? **NATNEWS** 1982 Jun;19(6):11-2

**Orr WJ** see **Numbers RL**

**Orsini M, Piroli AT, Gaudiosi O:** Gli eliporti ospedalieri nell'organizzazione sanitaria militare: l'eliporto dell'ospedale militare di Caserta. **Riv Mil** 1973;29(5):614-26

**Orsós S:** A megyei 'fogász-föorvostól' a stomatologus felügyelö szakföorvosig. **Fogorv Sz** 1984 Jun;77(6):165-9

**Orsós S, Bodó L:** Változások a fogorvosi szolgálat 25 éves dokumentációjában. **Forgorv SZ** 1982 May;75(5):135-9

**Ort-Wädensweiler L:** Johann Melchior Aepli: zur Verbesserung des Medizinalwesens in der Schweiz (1783/88). Zürich, Juris Druck, 1984. 70 p. (Zürcher Medizingeschichtliche Abhandlungen, Neue Reihe, Nr. 167).

**Ortega A** see **Lara-Terrazas A**

**Ortega Millán A, García Prieto A, Ocio León S:** Acercamiento a la vida y obra de Kafka. **Actas Luso Esp Neurol Psiquiatr** 1982 Jul-Aug;10(4):223-7

**Ortegón Páez R:** Vorágine alucinante en la historia de las drogas. Bogotá, Columbia, Ediciones Tercer Mundo, 1981. 417 p.

**Orticochea M:** History of the discovery of the musculocutaneous flap method as a substitute for the delay method. **Ann Plast Surg** 1983 Jul;11(1):63-8

**Ortiz Y** see **Latapí F**

**Ortiz de Montellano B:** Aztec medicine: empirical drug use. **Ethnomedizin** 1974-75;3(3-4):249-71

**Ortiz de Montellano BR** see **Davidson JR**

**Ortiz Gómez T:** El profesional medico en Andalucia: evolucion y distribucion de los medicos en la provincia de Granada (1901-1981). **Dynamis** 1982;2:325-51

**Ortiz--Monasterio F:** La medicina del siglo XX y su proyección futura. II. Los antecedentes. La medicina precientífica. **Gac Med Mex** 1981 Nov;117(11):426-8

**Ortiz-Monasterio F:** Labat and the three-lobed forehead flap. **Plast Reconstr Surg** 1984 Apr;73(4):705

**Ortiz-Monasterio F** see **Guarner V**

**Ortiz Monasterio J:** Analisis cuantitativo de la historiografia medica mexicana (1970-1974). **Bol Soc Mex Hist Filos Med** 1983 Mar;6(42):129-36

**Ortiz Monasterio J:** Reflexiones en torno a los origenes de la historiografia de la medicina. **Bol Soc Mex Hist Filos Med** 1980 Sep-Dec;5(32-33):83-92

**Ortiz Monasterio L:** La medicina mexicana en el Archivo General de la Nacion. **Bol Soc Mex Hist Filos Med** 1980 Sep-Dec;5(32-33):93-102

**Ortiz Monasterio L:** La medicina mexicana en el archivo general de la nación. **Prensa Med Mex** 1979 Jul-Aug;44(7-8):157-62

**Ortiz Picón JM:** Pío del Río Hortega. Un estudio biográfico. **Arch Neurobiol (Madr)** 1983 May-Jun;46(3):209-26

**Ortmann F:** Dietrich Georg Kieser (1779-1862)--nur ein romantischer **Z Gesamte Inn Med** 1979 Sep 1;34(17):486-9

**Outram D:** Politics and vocation: French science, 1793–1830. **Br J Hist Sci** 1980 Mar;13(43 pt 1):27–43

**Outram D:** The ordeal of vocation: the Paris Academy of Sciences and the Terror, 1793–95. **Hist Sci** 1983 Sep;21(53 pt 3):251–73

**Ouvrard J:** Perception de l'angoisse et de l'anxiété par quelques artistes à travers les siècles. **Actual Odontostomatol (Paris)** 1983 Dec;144:593–622

**Ouvry PA, Davy A:** De la vanité des incisions multiples dans la chirurgie des varices. **Phlebologie** 1982 Oct–Dec;35(4):851–5

**Ovchinnikov NM, Timchenko GF:** Dvadtsatiletniĭ opyt raboty Tsentral'nogo nauchno-issledovatel'skogo kozhnovenerologicheskogo instituta Minzdrava SSR po kontroliu i uluchsheniiu kachestva serologicheskikh laboratorii dermatovenerologicheskikh uchrezhdeniĭ SSSR. **Lab Delo** 1981;(2):120–2

**Ovchinnikov NM:** K 75-letiiu otkrytiia vozbuditelia sifilisa. **Vestn Dermatol Venerol** 1980 Mar;(3):74–8

**Over R:** The durability of scientific reputation. **J Hist Behav Sci** 1982 Jan;18(1):53–61

**Overbeek J, ed:** The evolution of population theory: a documentary sourcebook. Westport, Conn., Greenwood Press, 1977. x, 277 p.

**Overmier JA:** John Brown's Elementa medicinae: an introductory bibliographical essay. **Bull Med Libr Assoc** 1982 Jul;70(3):310–7

**Ovsiannikov SI:** Dokumenty orazvitii fizicheskoi kul'tury v krasnoi armii (1918–1919 gg). **Sov Arkh** 1977;4:73–8

**Owen CA:** H. P. Smith's place in the history of blood coagulation. **Am J Clin Pathol** 1984 Apr;81(4):424–6

**Owen CA:** The revolution of concepts of coagulation. **Ann NY Acad Sci** 1981;370:5–10

**Owen GM** see **Allan P**

**Owen J** see **Elliott A**

**Owen K:** John Hunter: a man of his age. **Trans Hunter Soc** 1978–80;37–38:85–97

**Owen M:** The archives of the Royal Australasian College of radiologists: guide to the history collection H706–H765 sundry accessions. **Australas Radiol** 1982 Mar;26(1):30–40

**Owen M:** The Journal of the Roentgen Society, Number 1, Volume 1: an outline. **Australas Radiol** 1983 Jul;27(2):170–3

**Owen MD:** The archives of the Royal Australasian College of Radiologists. **Australas Radiol** 1978 Sep;22(3):222–5

**Owen MD:** The archives of the Royal Australasian College of Radiologists. **Australas Radiol** 1979 Mar;23(1):15–9

**Owen ME** see **Davies HE**

**Owen-Smith MS:** A computerized data retrieval system for the wounds for war: the Northern Ireland casualties. **J R Army Med Corps** 1981 Feb;127(1):31–54

**Owens BB** see **Curtis AC**

**Owsley DW, Bennett SM, Jantz RL:** Intercemetery morphological variation in Arikara crania from the Mobridge Site (39WW1). **Am J Phys Anthropol** 1982 Jun;58(2):179–85

**Owsley DW** see **Hanson CL**

**Owsley DW** see **Jantz RL**

**Oxford Street memorial to pioneer veterinarian (William Moorcroft): Vet Rec** 1982 Oct 2;111(14):313

**Oxnard CE, Lisowski FP:** Functional articulation of some hominoid foot bones: implications for the Olduvai (hominid 8) foot. **Am J Phys Anthropol** 1980 Jan;52(1):107–17

**Ozaki NT:** Conceptual changes in Japanese medicine during the Tokugawa period. Ph.D. Diss., University of California. San Francisco, 1979. viii, 285 leaves.

**Ozawa S:** Hoigaku shiso Katayama Kunika/G. Tokyo, Shin Jinbutsu Oraisha, Showa 50 nen [1975]. 130 p.

**Ozbay F, Shorter FC:** Türkiye'de Aile plânlamasi uygulamalarinda 1963 ve 1968 yillari arasinda görülen degismeler. **Hacettepe Sosyal Bilimler Derg** 1970;2(2):194–211

**Ozbay K:** Türk asker hekimligi tarihi ve asker hastaneleri. 3 vols. in 4. Istanbul, Yörük Basimevi, 1976. 686, 349, 576, 493 p.

**Ozment S:** Luther and the family. **Harv Libr Bull** 1984 Winter;32(1):36–53

**Ozment S:** The family in Reformation Germany: the bearing and rearing of children. **J Fam Hist** 1983 Summer;8(2):159–76

**Ozorovský V, Tychý M, Buchvald J, et al:** Sociálne aspeckty začiatkov dermatovenerológie v Bratislave po roku 1918 a úloha professora Reinsberga. **Cesk Zdrav** 1982 Jul;30(7):319–25

**Ozorovský V** see **Tichý M**

# P

**Paál A:** Az aero-ionizáció orvos-biológiai felhasználásának lehetöségei a XVIII–XIX-ik században és mai idöszerüségük. **Orv Hetil** 1984 Mar 4;125(10):595–6, 599

**Páal A:** Orvostörténeti adatok a 'Magyar Faust', Hatvani istván professzor (1718–1786 ig) tanulmányairól és munkásságáról. **Orv Hetil** 1984 Aug 5;125(32):1957–8, 1961–2

**Paasch S** see **Knorre G von**

**Pabis-Braunstein M:** Aptekarstwo w Bieczu. Dzieje rodziny Fusków. **Arch Hist Med (Warsz)** 1984;47(2):191–206

**Pabis-Braunstein M:** Ponad stuletnie tradycje farmaceutycznej rodziny Nitribittów. **Arch Hist Med (Warsz)** 1983;46(3):295–313

**Pabis-Stachoń M:** Gremia aptekarskie w latach 1802–1939 na obszarach byłej Galicji Zachodniej. **Arch Hist Med (Warsz)** 1980;43(3):311–15

**Paborn K:** Något om barnavård år 1908. **Omvardaren** 1982;29(4):8–9

**Pace D:** Claude Lévi-Strauss, the bearer of ashes. Boston, Routledge & Kegan Paul, 1983. x, 263 p.

**Pace JL** see **Ramaswamy S**

**Pačes V:** Uvahy o nemoci Fryderyka Chopina. **Vnitr Lek** 1980 Oct;26(10):1027–31

**Pacheco CR, Quijano-Pitman F, Kuthy-Porter J, et al:** Centenario del descubrimiento del bacilo de la tuberculosis. **Gac Med Mex** 1982 Nov;118(11):439–48

**Pacheco CR:** Con motivo del centenario del descubrimiento del bacilo de la tuberculosis. **Salud Publica Mex** 1982 May–Jun;24(3):231–3

**Pacheco CR:** Influenza. **Gac Med Mex** 1982 Feb;118(2):78–82

**Pachella R** see **Manuscripta alchemica der Sammlung Mellon: Bemerkungen zum Katalog**

**Pachella R, ed** see **Witten LC**

**Paciorkiewicz M:** Izby lekarskie. Przyczynki do dziejów. **Pol Tyg Lek** 1982 Jul 5;37(21):621–4

**Paciorkiewicz M:** Z historii ... **Pieleg Polozna** 1984;(5):21–3

**Pack AR:** Women in New Zealand dentistry, 1880–1980. **NZ Dent J** 1981 Jan;77(347):19–25

**Pack RA:** Magister Iodocus: 'Regule phisonomie'. **Mediaev Stud** 1980;42:212–37

**Pack RA ed:** Pseudo-Aristotelis Epistola ad Alexandrum der regimine sanitatis a quodam Nicolao versificata. **Arch Hist Doctrinale Litt Moyen Age** 1978;53:307–25

**Packer H:** Memoirs of a venereologist. **J Tenn Med Assoc** 1979 Oct;72(10):731–8

**Pacovský V:** Universita a lékařská fakulta. **Cas Lek Cesk** 1983 Oct 14;122(41):1261–4

**Pacyńska M, Kedzia A, Smereka J:** Tematy neurologiczne w pracach doktorskich polaków studiujacych we Wrocławiu w XIX wieku. **Arch Hist Med (Warsz)** 1980;43(2):199–204

**Paddison RM, Skinner RE, ed:** Antonie Wouter Voors, M.D., M.P.H., D.P.H. A biographical sketch and a bibliography of his work. New Orleans: History of Medicine Club of Louisiana State University Medical Center, 1983. 23 p.

**Paddon A:** Public health in Sub-Arctic Labrador 1912–1978. **Can J Public Health** 1984 Sep–Oct;75(5):356–8

**Padfield A, Alderson JD:** Early days of anaesthesia in Sheffield. **Ann R Coll Surg Engl** 1984 Jul;66(4):293–6

**Padfield H** see **Tobach E**

**Padgug RA:** Sexual matters: on conceptualizing sexuality in history. **Radic Hist Rev** 1979;20:3–24

**Padis N:** The legacy of Byzantine medicine. In: Congrès international d'histoire de la médecine, XXVe, Québec, 1976. Actes. Québec, 1977. p. 1045–51.

**Pady DS:** A London medical satire of 1607. **J Hist Med Allied Sci** 1978 Jul;33(3):409–16

**Paediatrics and psychoanalysis--Miss Anna Freud: Arch Dis Child** 1983 Jun;58(6):472–3

**Paffenbarger GC:** Important accomplishments in dentistry, 1930–1980: a personal appraisal. **NY J Dent** 1980 May;50(5):190–1

**Pagán Ramos IH** see **Trías de Gómez L**

**Page BB** see **McCullough LB**

**Page IH:** A history of the Council for High Blood Pressure research. Past, imperfect, present indicative, and future perfect. **Hypertension** 1984 Mar–Apr;6(2 pt 2):208–10

**Page IH:** The discovery of serotonin. **Perspect Biol Med** 1976 Autumn;20(1):1–8

**Page JB** see **McBride DC**

**Page SL:** The law, the lawyer, and medical aspects of child abuse. In E. H. Newberger, ed: Child abuse. Boston, Little, Brown and Company, 1982. p. 105–35.

**Pagel G:** Narziss und Prometheus: die Theorie der Phantasie bei Freud und Gehlen. Würzburg, Königshausen & Neumann, 1984. 195 p. (Studien zur Anthropologie, Band 8).

**Pagel W:** Joan Baptista Van Helmont: reformer of science and medicine. Cambridge, Cambridge University Press, x, 1982. 219 p. (Cambridge monographs on the history of medicine).

**Pagel W:** Mother nature and the scientific revolution. **Hist Sci** 1981 Jun:19(44 pt 2):148–53

**Pagel W:** Paracelsus. An introduction to philosophical medicine in the era of the Renaissance, 2nd, revised edition. Basel, Karger, 1982. xii, 399 p.

**Pagel W:** The Paracelsian Elias Artista and the alchemical tradition. **Medizinhist J** 1981;16(1–2):6–19

**Pagel W:** The smiling spleen. In H. Lloyd-Jones, et al., ed. History and imagination: essays in honor of H. R. Trevor-Roper. New York, Holmes & Meier, 1982. p. 81–7.

**Pagel W** see **Paracelsus in der Tradition**

**Pagella P:** Il Susruta Samhita: un capitolo originale della chirurgia o una interdipendenza di valori nella storia della medicina? **Ann Osp Maria Vittoria Torino** 1977 Jul–Dec;20(7–12):354–63

**Pages from the past: NZ Nurs J** 1983 Jan;76(1):16–25

**Paglia L:** Odontoiatria del passato. Chi era Servet? **Dent Cadmos** 1984 Jan;52(1):79–81

**Pagni U:** Giovanbattista Cartegni da Bagnone lettore di medicina nello Studio di Pisa. **Arch Stor Prov Parmensi** 1979;31:91–102

**Pahl KP:** Life expectancy in ancient and modern man. **Acta Anthropogenet** 1981;5(2):119–28

**Pahl WM** see **Hübener KH**

**Paiement B, Boulanger M, Taillefer J, et al:** Anesthésie et cardiopathie: évolution des concepts et perspectives. **Union Med Can** 1979 Oct;108(10):1158–66

**Paillard E:** Louis Vassé, médecin à Chalôns. **Mem Soc Agric Commer Sci Arts Marne** 1975;90:109–29
**Painchaud R:** Théogène Fafard. In Dictionary of Canadian biography, 1881–1890. 1982;11:306–7.
**Painter DM** see **Norman JE**
**Painter F:** An early 18th century witch bottle: a legacy of the wicked witch of Pungo. **Chesopiean** 1980;18(3–6):62–71
**Pajorin K:** David Verbec könyvtárának töredéke a Semmelweis orvostörténeti könyvtárban. **Magy Konyvsz** 1978;94(3–4):314–21
**Pakhomov AF:** Peredovoi aviatsionnyi vrach. **Voen Med Zh** 1983 Aug;(8):7–10
**Pakkala K:** Kätilönä kolttien parissa. **Katilolehti** 1979 Dec;84(12):473–6
**Pakovich BI:** To commemorate the 80th year since discovery of conditional reflexes. **Pavlov J Biol Sci** 1983 Oct–Dec;18(4):175–80
**Pál E:** Habent sua fata libelli. Magyar orvosok és gyógyszerészek a nyelvújítás korában. **Orv Hetil** 1981 Feb 22;122(8):467–8
**Palabras pronunciadas por el doctor Mario Mazzei Uzcategui, con motivo de la colocacion del retrato del doctor Josa Maria Baptista, en la sede de la Sociedad Venezolana de Historia de la Medicina, en Caracas. Sesion del 8 de febrero de 1972.: Rev Soc Venez Hist Med** 1972–73;20–21(34–35):41–9
**Palacio J del** see **Langer M**
**Palafóx Marqués S:** Glosa al libro 'Galería de Presidentes. **An R Acad Nac Med (Madr)** 1982;99(2):147–65
**Palagin DA** see **Stegunin SI**
**Palan VT** see **Cho LJ**
**Palanichamy K:** Tamil medical manuscripts in Oriental Research Institute, S.V. University, Tirupati. **Bull Inst Hist Med (Hyderabad)** 1973 Oct;3(4):173–81
**Paläoimmunologie: Naturwissenschaften** 1980;67:560
**Pałasz M:** Eutanazja w świetle refleksji deontologicznej. **Pol Tyg Lek** 1981 Apr 27;36(17):611–13
**Palau GV** see **Bowers JZ**
**Pal'chikov PA:** Oni zhertvovali soboĭ radi pobedy. **Voen Med Zh** 1983 May;(5):68–70
**Pal'chikov PA** see **Galin LL**
**Palencia JS** see **Flores y Troncoso FA**
**Paleopathology Association: Ninth annual meeting and first Aidan Cockburn memorial symposium:** Mummies, disease, and ancient cultures: retrospect and prospect. Toledo, Paleopathology Association, 1982. 16 p.
**Palermo DS:** The history of the Boyd R. McCandless Young Scientist Awards: the first recipients. **Adv Child Dev Behav** 1982;16:1–6
**Paletta FX:** History of the American Society of Plastic and Reconstructive Surgeons, Inc., 1931–1981: its growth, change, unity. **Plast Reconstr Surg** 1981 Sep;68(3):292–369
**Palkin BN:** Gubernskaia reforma 1775 g. i organizatsiia grazhdanskoĭ meditsiny v Rossii. **Sov Zdravookhr** 1983;9:66–70
**Palkin BN, Daniuk GI:** Iz istorii akusherstva v Rossii kontsa XVIII–nachala XIX veka. **Feldsher Akush** 1983 Aug;48(8):44–6
**Palkin BN:** Iz istorii issledovaniia lepry v Astrakhanskoĭ gubernii v XVIII veke. **Vestn Dermatol Venerol** 1982 Aug;(8):72–4
**Palkin BN:** Nastavlenie doktora K. O. Iagel'skogo po profilaktike i lecheniiu chumy. **Zh Mikrobiol Epidemiol Immunobiol** 1982 Jan;(1):117–8
**Palkin BN:** Pervyĭ karantinnyĭ ustav v Rossii, sostavlennyĭ P. Z. Kondoidi. **Sov Zdravookhr** 1982;(9):63–5
**Palkin BN:** Reformy kontsa XVIII--nachala XIX stoletiia v oblasti meditsinskogo obrazovaniia v Rossii. **Sov Zdravookhr** 1981;(8):71–4
**Palkin BN:** Reformy v oblasti organizatsii meditsinskogo dela v Rossii kontsa XVII veka. **Sov Zdravookhr** 1981;(3):67–70
**Palkin BN:** S. S. Andreevskiĭ v Astrakhani. **Sov Zdravookhr** 1981;(6):66–8
**Palkin BN:** V. N. Tatishchev i zdravookhranenie Astrakhanskoĭ gubernii. **Sov Zdravookhr** 1982;(4):65–8
**Palkovich AM:** Demography and disease patterns in a protohistoric plains group: a study of the mobridge site (39WW1). **Plains Anthropol** 1981;26(94 pt 2):71–84
**Pallez G** see **La Salpêtrière**
**Pallis C:** From brain death to brain stem death. **Br Med J [Clin Res]** 1982 Nov 20;285(6353):1487–90
**Pallister JL** see **Pare A**
**Pallister PD** see **Opitz JM**
**Palloni A:** Mortality in Latin America: emerging patterns. **Popul Dev Rev** 1981;7(4):623–49
**Palm C** see **Engelhardt R, ed**
**Palm E:** Oftalmologin--perfekt och futurum. **Lakartidningen** 1980 Jun 11;77(24):2258–61
**Palm LC, Snelders HA, ed:** Antoni van Leeuwenhoek, 1632–1723. Studies on the life and work of the Delft scientist commemorating the 350th anniversary of his birthday. Amsterdam, Rodopi, 1982. 209 p. (Nieuwe Nederlandse Bijdragen tot de Geschiedenis der Geneeskunde en der Natuurwetenschappen, no. 8). Contributions by W. H. van Seters, B. C. Damsteegt, J. van Zuylen, P. Bass, J. E. van Bronswijk, G. A. Lindeboom, P. Smit, K. van Berkel.
**Palm LC:** Bij een beeld van Swammerdam. **Tijdschr Geschied Geneeskd** 1981;4:61–2
**Palm LC:** De paalwormepidemie van 1730. **Spiegel Hist** 1980;15(5):266–72
**Palm LC:** Van Leeuwenhoek en Swammerdam cartesiaanse microscopisten. **Spiegel Hist** 1979;14(4):223–9
**Palma Rodriguez F:** Vida y obra de Viana Mentesano. Salamanca, Universidad de Salamanca, 1977. 54 p. (Cuadernos de Historia de la Medicina Española, Monografias, XXXI).
**Palmer AK, Cozens DD:** Comments on the history of teratology testing. **Teratology** 1980 Apr;21(2):260
**Palmer BB:** The philosophy of dental health service: its relation to the changing social order. Advice from 1934. **J Am Coll Dent** 1981 Fall;48(3):179–92
**Palmer BD** see **Radcliff-Umstead D, ed**
**Palmer C, Horowitz M, ed:** Shaman woman, mainline lady: women's writings on the drug experience. New York, Morrow, 1982. 285 p.
**Palmer CA:** Public health in the South. **Rev Am Hist** 1982;10(2):229–33
**Palmer DG** see **Buchanan WW**
**Palmer IS:** Florence Nightingale and international origins of modern nursing. **Image (IN)** 1981 Jun;13(2):28–31
**Palmer IS:** Florence Nightingale: the myth and the reality. **Nurs Times** 1983 Aug 3–9;79(31):40–2
**Palmer IS:** Nightingale revisited. **Nurs Outlook** 1983 Jul–Aug;31(4):229–33
**Palmer IS:** [Nightingale revisited] (Jpn). **Kango** 1983 Nov;35(12):112–22
**Palmer IS** see **Allan P**
**Palmer R:** Physicians and the state in post-mediaeval Italy. In Russell AW, ed: The town and state physician in Europe from the Middle Ages to the Enlightenment. Wolfenbüttel, Herzog August Bibliothek, 1981. p. 47–61 (Wolfenbütteler Forschungen, 17).
**Palmer R:** The Church, leprosy and plague in medieval and early modern Europe. In Sheils WJ, ed: The Church and healing. Papers read at the twentieth summer meeting and the twenty-first winter meeting of the Ecclesiastical History Society. Oxford, Basil Blackwell for the Society, 1982. p. 79–99.
**Palmer R:** The influence of botanical research on pharmacists in sixteenth century Venice. **NTM** 1984;21(2):69–80
**Palmer R** see **Symons H**
**Palmer SR** see **Bell JC**
**Palmer VA:** Lenore H. Cawker, the animals' friend. **Milw Hist** 1979;2(2):43–8
**Palmer TY, ed:** The Palmer physicians. [s. l., s. n.], 1966. vii, 93 p.
**Palmier JM** see **Finck J**
**Palmieri A, Humberson C:** Medical incidents in the life of Dr. John H. Finfrock. **Ann Wyo** 1981;53(2):64–9
**Palmieri N:** Un antico commento a Galeno della scuola medica di Ravenna. **Physis** 1981;23:197–296
**Palmieri TJ:** Hands on coins. **Hand** 1982 Oct;14(3):341–2
**Palmieri TJ:** Scientists' hands on stamps. **J Hand Surg** 1983 Jan;8(1):3
**Palmore JA** see **Rindfuss RR**
**Palmquist PE:** Photography in medicine. **J West** 1982 Jul;21(3):59–64
**Pálos, S:** Chinesische Heilkunst: Einführung in die Theorie und Praxis der Naturheilkunde der Chinesen--Akupunktur, Moxibustion, Heilmassage, Heilgymnastik, Atemtherapie und Pharmakologie. Bern, Barth, 1984. 286 p.
**Paltrinieri M:** Cinquant'anni vissuti fra gli splendori dell'ortopedia. **Chir Organi Mov** 1982;67(1):1–6
**Pal'tsev IuP** see **Borisenkova RV**
**Paly D:** Portrait of William Norris. Broadside, 1815, with etched portrait (1814) entitled 'William Norris: confined in this manner in Bethlem Hospital'; George Arnald, A.R.A., artist, etcher, and publisher. **Radic Hist Rev** 1979 Spring/Summer;Spec:65
**Paly D:** The antiquaries' last will and testament; an etching with sepia wash by Thomas Rowlandson, 1814. **J Hist Med Allied Sci** 1980 Apr;35(2):215
**Pam DO:** The hungry years: the struggle for survival in Edmonton and Enfield before 1400. Enfield, Edmonton Hundred Historical Society, 1980. 31 p. (Occasional paper no. 42.)
**Pamiati Aleksandra Anatol'evicha Otelina: Arkh Anat Gistol Embriol** 1981 Sep;81(9):123–6
**Pampiglione S, Bettini S:** Bibliografia Italiana delle leishmaniosi dalle origini al 1980. **Ann Ist Super Sanita** 1981;17(1):1–150
**Pampiglione S:** Il contributo di Achille Breda alla conoscenza della leishmaniosi muco-cutanea americana. **Parassitologia** 1979 Dec;21(1–3):35–58
**Pan Chengxiang:** Origin and development of cytobilogy. (Chi) **Chin J Med Hist** 1981;11(1):11–7
**Panaitescu D, Mihalcu F, Neguț M:** Activitatea științifică a prof. Mihai Ciucă. **Rev Iq [Bacteriol]** 1984 Jan–Mar;29(1):80–8
**Panchenko DI, Vilenskiĭ IuG:** Leon Abgarovich Orbeli v Kieve (k 100-letiiu so dnia rozhdeniia). **Vrach Delo** 1982 Sep;(9):119–22
**Panchenko PM, Shereshevskiĭ AM:** V. M. Bekhterev i neĭrokhirurgiia (k 125-letiiu so dnia rozhdeniia). **Zh Vopr Neirokhir** 1982 Sep–Oct;(5):59–61
**Panconesi E, Mazzi MS:** The day syphilis came. **Int J Dermatol** 1984 May;23(4):284–6
**Pandey AN, Rama Rao B, Raghunathan K:** Gadadhara. **Bull Indian Inst Hist Med (Hyderabad)** 1975 Oct;5(4):193–7
**Pandey AN** see **Sastry VV**
**Pandya SK:** Medicine in Goa--a former Portuguese territory. **J Postgrad Med** 1982 Jul;28(3):123–48
**Pandya SK:** Medicine in Goa. Bombay, Dr. Ramesh Sanzgiri Foundation, 1980. n. p.
**Panebianco D** see **Bazzi F**
**Panel on dialysis: Transplant Proc** 1981 Mar;13(1):67–71
**Panfilenko OA** see **Gromov AP**
**Panfilenko OA** see **Kapustin AV**
**Paniagua JA:** Tradicion y renovacion en la obra del doctor Chanca. **Asclepio** 1978–79;30–31:365–9
**Paniagua JA** see **Albarracín Teulón A**
**Paniagua Arellano JA, Arnau de Vilanova:** El maravilloso regimiento y orden de vivir (una versión castellana del Regimen sanitatis ad regem

Aragonum). **Cuad Aragon Hist Med Cienc (B)** 1980;3:1-106
**Paniagua Vargas C** see **Tjarks GO**
**Panken S:** 'Working through and the novel. **Psychoanal Rev** 1983 Spring;70(1):4-23
**Pankey LD:** Evolution of a philosophy. **Continuum** 1980;:1-9
**Pankey LD:** The PMS technique: an historical perspective. **Continuum** 1981;:5-11
**Pankhurst R:** Le piaghe d'Etiopia. **Kos** 1984 Jul-Aug;1(6):33-50
**Pankhurst R:** The history of leprosy in Ethiopia to 1935. **Med Hist** 1984 Jan;28(1):57-72
**Pankhurst R:** The medical activities in eighteenth century Ethiopia of James Bruce the explorer. **Medizinhist J** 1982;17(3):256-76
**Pankiewicz H:** Prof. dr hab. Henryk Bukowiecki jako historyk farmacji. **Arch Hist Med (Warsz)** 1984;47(3):389-93
**Pankiewicz H** see **Kaiser W**
**Pankiewicz Z:** Cech chirurgów toruńskich w XVI, XVII i XVIII wieku. **Czas Stomatol** 1979;32(10):989-92
**Pankoke KT:** Im wilhelminischen Preussen nahm man sie ernst. Zur Geschichte der Jugendzahnpflege in Deutschland. **Zahnarzt** 1984 Aug;28(8):619-21
**Pankov EIa** see **Klishov AA**
**Panosian GA, Shakarian GA:** Vuz vstrechaet iubileĭ. **Veterinariia** 1979 Nov;(11):18-20
**Panouillé JP:** Et les Français prirent gout a l'absinthe! **Histoire** 1983;(52):50-9
**Panov IE** see **Gromov AP**
**Pansera MT:** Per un'antropologia filosofica freudiana: il valore della negazione. **Physis** 1982;24(1):76-108
**Pantaleoni M:** Perfezionamenti tecnici e metodologici ed apparecchiature per anestesia generale. **Minerva Anestesiol** 1982 Dec;48(12):879-86
**Pantó E:** Wachstum und Reifung der Stadtkinder in Abhängigkeit von soziodemographischen Faktoren. **Anthropol Anz** 1982 Mar;40(1):33-44
**Panzac D:** La population de l'empire Ottoman et de ses marges du XVe au XIX siècle: bibliographie (1941-1980) et bilan provisoire. **Rev Occident Musulman Mediterr** 1981;31(1):119-37
**Panzer D:** Zur historischen Entwicklung des Objektverständnisses der Sozialhygiene während der Entstehung der sozialistischen Gesellschaft am Beispiel der UdSSR. **Z Gesamte Hyg** 1983 Oct;29(10):581-4
**Pao-Min C:** Health and crime among Chinese-Americans: recent trends. **Phylon** 1981;42(4):356-68
**Pao-Min C:** The age and sex composition of Chinese-Americans: recent trends. **Asian Profile** 1980;8(5):409-20
**Paolinelli L:** Acciones de rehabilitación médica en Chile, 1952-1977. **Rev Med Chil** 1977 Oct;105(10):707-13
**Papaevangelou G** see **Halstead SB**
**Papalas AJ:** Medicinal bathing in mineral springs in fifth century B. C. Greece. **Clio Med** 1981 Dec;16(2/3):81-2
**Papàsogli G:** Giuseppe Moscati, 1880-1927: Leben eines heiligen Arztes. Stein am Rhein [Schweiz], Christiana-Verlag, 1982. 109 p.
**Papaxenopoulos A:** Zypriotische Medizin in der Antike. Diss., Bayerische Julius-Maximilians-Universität. Würzburg, 1981. iii, 104 p.
**Papers and exhibits on Paleopathology:** presented at the Annual Meeting of the Paleopathology Association. Niagara Falls, New York, 16. April, 1980.
**[Papers on Chinese medicine and on the study of medical history in China.] (Chi): Chung Hua I Shih Tsa Chih** 1980;10(1):1-64
**Papers on paleopathology:** presented at the Annual Meeting of the Paleopathology Association, 22 April, 1981. [Supplement to Paleopathology Newsletter, No. 34, June 1981] **Paleopathol Newsl** 1981 Jun;34:D1-D6
**Papers on Paleopathology presented at the Third European Members Meeting of the Paleopathology Association. 1980, Sept. 26-28. Caen, France.: Paleopathol Newsl** 1980 Dec;32 Suppl:C1-C18
**Papo I:** Izvještaj o četveromjesečnom radu ekipe SOVS-a. **Lijec Vjesn** 1979 Nov;101(11):707-8
**Papp J** see **Grynaeus T**
**Pappagianis D:** Dangerous dust. **Nat Hist** 1983;92(3):36-40
**Pappas CN:** The life and times of G. V. Black. Chicago, Quintessence Pub. Co., 1983. 128 p.
**Pappas DG:** Alexander Graham Bell: teacher of the deaf. **Am J Otol** 1983 Jan;4(3):263-5
**Pappas DG:** Barany's History of Vestibular Physiology. Translation and commentary. **Ann Otol Rhinol Laryngol [Suppl]** 1984 Mar-Apr;110:1-16
**Pappas DG, Galanos AN:** Prosper Ménière: beyond the controversial autopsy report. **South Med J** 1982 Apr;75(4):470-2
**Pappas DG:** Sir William Wilde: a historical review. **Ear Nose Throat J** 1983 Jun;62(6):58, 60-2
**Pappas DG:** The origin of aural instruments. **Am J Otol** 1979 Oct;1(2):121-4
**Pappenheim E:** More on the case of Anna O. **Am J Psychiatry** 1980 Dec;137(12):1625-6
**Pappenheimer JR:** Pavlov's contributions to physiology before 1900. **J Hist Behav Sci** 1981;17:239-41
**Papper EM, Mark LC, Ngai SH:** Anesthesiology: progress since 1940. Coral Gables, Fla., Univ. of Miami Press, [1973]. 192 p.
**Papper EM:** The fiftieth anniversary of the use of thiopentone in man. **Anaesthesia** 1984 Jun;39(6):517-9
**Paquet JB:** The gloving of a nurse (Caroline Hampton). **Nurs Success Today** 1984 Summer;1(2):44
**Paquin M:** Louise Soumande. In Dictionary of Canadian biography, 1701 to 1740. Volume 2, 1969. p. 613.
**Paracelsus-Forschung heute:** Bericht über den Jubiläumskongress 1976 und die 25 jährige Geschichte der Gesellschaft, mit Beiträgen von K. Goldammer, A. Dyk, S. Domandl. Wien, 1977. 51 p. (Salzburger Beiträge zur Paracelsusforschung, 15).
**Paracelsus in der Tradition:** Vorträge, Paracelsustag 1978. Wien, Verband der Wissenschaftlichen Gesellschaften Oesterreichs, 1980. 146p. (Salzburger Beiträge zur Paracelsusforschung, Folge 21). Contributions by W. Pagel, F. Baron, H. Rudolph, R. Dilg-Frank, A. Dyk, W. Schneider, A. Miller-Guinsburg, S. Domandl, L. Braun, H. M. Decker-Hauff.
**Paradis J, Postlewait T, ed:** Victorian science and Victorian values: literary perspectives. New York, New York Academy of Sciences, 1981. xiii, 362 p. (Annals of the New York Academy of Sciences, 360).
**Paradis JG:** T. H. Huxley, Man's place in nature. Lincoln, University of Nebraska Press, 1978. xi, 226 p.
**Parascandola J:** Chemistry and pharmacology in Britain 1840 1916. **Pharm Hist (London)** 1976 May;6(1):2
**Parascandola J, Swann J:** Development of Pharmacology in American Schools of Pharmacy. **Pharm Hist** 1983;25(3):95-115
**Parascandola J:** Gerty Theresa Radnitz Cori. In: Notable American women. The modern period. Cambridge, Mass., Belknap-Harvard Univ. Press, 1980. 4:165-7.
**Parascandola J:** John J. Abel and the early development of pharmacology at the Johns Hopkins University. **Bull Hist Med** 1982;56(4):512-27
**Parascandola J:** John J. Abel and the founding of ASPET. **Pharmacologist** 1984;26(1):37-40
**Parascandola J:** Maud Caroline Slye. In: Notable American women. The modern period. Cambridge, Mass., Belknap-Harvard Univ. Press, 1980. 4:651-2.
**Parascandola J:** Pharmaceutical history for the pharmacy student. With a commentary by J. K. Crellin. In J. J. Bylebyl, ed: Teaching the history of medicine at a medical center. Baltimore, London, Johns Hopkins University Press, 1982. (The Henry E. Sigerist supplements to the Bulletin of the History of Medicine; new ser., no. 7). p. 78-90.
**Parascandola J:** Reflections on the history of pharmacology. **Pharm Hist** 1980;22(4):131-40
**Parascandola J, Keeney E:** Sources in the history of American pharmacology. Madision, American Institute of the History of Pharmacy, 1983. 59 p.
**Parascandola J:** The search for the active oxytocic principle of ergot: laboratory science and clinical medicine in conflict. In Hickel E, Schröder G, ed: Neue Beiträge zur Arzneimittelgeschichte. Festschrift für Wolfgang Schneider zum 70. Geburtstag. Stuttgart, Wissenschaftliche Verlagsgesellschaft, 1982. p. 205-27.
**Parascandola J:** The theoretical basis of Paul Ehrlich's chemotherapy. **J Hist Med Allied Sci** 1981 Jan;36(1)19-43
**Parascandola J** see **McCormick JP**
**Parascandola JL, Bender GA:** Historical hobbies for the pharmacist. Symposium on historical hobbies for the pharmacist. Madison, Wis., 1974. iv, 57 p. (Publication/American Institute of the History of Pharmacy. no. 2)
**Parascandola J, ed:** The history of antibiotics. Madison, Wis., 1980. vi, 136 p. (Publication/American Institute of the History of Pharmacy. new series, no. 5)
**Paravicini Bagliani A:** A proposito dell'insegnamento di medicina allo Studium Curiae. In A. Maieru, A. Paravicini Bagliani, ed: Studi sul XIV secolo in memoria di Anneliese Maier. Rome, Storia e Letteratura, 1981. p. 395-413.
**Paravy P** see **Guillemain B**
**Pare A:** On monsters and marvels. Translated with an introduction and notes by J.L. Pallister. Chicago, London, University of Chicago Press, 1982. xxxii, 224 p.
**Paré A:** The classic. Compound fracture of leg, Paré's personal care (MII, 328). **Clin Orthop** 1983 Sep;178:3-6
**Paredes Salido F:** La cartilla de las compañias sanitarias de la armada en el siglo XIX. **Rev Gen Mar** 1981 Aug;201:137-9
**Parellada Feliu J:** Cinc manuscrits catalans escrits entre els anys 1749 i 1835. In Congrés International d'Història de la Medicina Catalana, 2nd, Barcelona, 1975. Llibre d'Actes. Barcelona, Socitra, 1977. p. 235-48.
**Parellada Feliu J:** Un text i vuit dibuixos teratològics d'un manuscrit català de l'any 1399. In Congrés International d'Història de la Medicina Catalana, 2nd, Barcelona, 1975. Llibre d'Actes. Barcelona, Socitra, 1977. p. 197-221.
**Parellada i Feliu D:** Comentaris al llibre 'Higiene del alma' del doctor Josep Call i Morros (editat a Barcelona l'any 1888). In Congrés International d'Història de la Medicina Catalana, 2nd, Barcelona, 1975. Llibre d'Actes. Barcelona, Socitra, 1977. p. 263-71.
**Parfit J:** The Oxford Board of Health 1831-1833. **Public Health** 1982 Jan;96(1):25-30
**Pargas K:** Bishop Charles Henry Brent (1862-1929)—a retrospective. 'That damned opium mess has started again'. **J Addict Res Found** 1979;8(9):7
**Pariente L:** De la synanche à l'angine. Paris, Pariente, 1982. 250 p.
**Pariente L:** Le De venarum ostiolis de Jerome Fabrice d'Acquapendente: sa place dans l'histoire de la découverte de la circulation du sang. Paris, Louis Pariente, 1981. 2 volumes.
**Pariente L, ed:** Les appareils de mesure du pouls et de la pression artérielle. Paris, L. Pariente, 1979. 113 p.
**Pariĭskaia TV** see **Orlova NV**
**Parin P:** Psychoanalyse als Gesellschaftskritik im Werk von Alexander Mitscherlich. **Psyche (Stuttg)** 1983 Apr;37(4):364-73
**Paris R** see **Vial F**
**Paris RR** see **Delaveau P**

Parisel F see Jurion F
Parish LC: Amerikanische dermatologische Zeitschriften und die New Yorker Dermatologische Gesellschaft. Hautarzt 1981 Mar;32(3):136-8
Parish LC, Crissey JT: Bibliography of secondary sources on the history of dermatology. Int J Dermatol 1981 Oct;20(8):555-61
Parish LC, Crissey JT: Bibliography of secondary sources on the history of dermatology: II. obituaries and biographies in English journals supplemented through 1980. Int J Dermatol 1981 Sep;20(7U):497-503
Parish LC, Crissey JT: Bibliography of secondary sources on the history of dermatology. III. Books, monographs, and chapters in English supplemented through 1980. Int J Dermatol 1981 Jun;20(5):390-2
Parish LC: The history of tropical dermatology and the 1907 International Congress of Dermatology. Int J Dermatol 1980 Oct;19(8):474-7
Parish LC see Crissey JT
Park CB: Preference for sons, family size, and sex ratio: an empirical study in Korea. Demography 1983 Aug;20(3):333-52
Park K: Albert's influence on late medieval psychology. In Weisheipl JA, ed: Albertus Magnus and the sciences. Toronto, Pontifical Institute of Mediaeval Studies, 1980. p. 501-35.
Park K, Daston LJ: Unnatural conceptions: the study of monsters in sixteenth- and seventeenth-century France and England. Past Present 1981;(92):20-54
Park RJ: The 'Enlightenment' in Spain: expressed concern for physical education in Spanish educational thought, 1765-1810. Can J Hist Sport Phys Educ 1978;9(2):1-19
Park RJ: The research quarterly and its antecedents. Res Q 1980 Mar;51(1):1-22
Park WM, Mourad K: Ossification and calcification of the posterior longitudinal ligament of the spine. Br J Radiol 1980 Apr;53(628):375-6
Parker EF: Eventful events in the history of cardiovascular surgery. J SC Med Assoc 1982 Aug;78(8):441-5
Parker GT: How to win friends and influence people: Dale Carnegie and the problem of sincerity. Am Q 1977;29(5):506-18
Parker HM: Invited paper delivered at the 25th Annual Meeting of the Health Physics Society. Protection programs of the Plutonium Project. Health Phys 1981 Oct;41(4):571-6
Parker JH see Whittaker DK
Parker JK, Carpenter EM: Julia Lathrop and the Children's Bureau: the emergence of an institution. Soc Serv Rev 1981;55(1):60-77
Parker RG: Academy of fine arts; print from a copper engraving, 1578, by Cornelis Cort after a drawing by Jan Van Der Straet, 1573. J Hist Med Allied Sci 1983 Jan;38(1):76-7
Parker W: Homosexuality in history; an annotated bibliography. J Homosex 1980-81 Fall-Winter;6(1-2):191-210
Parker WA see Baur FJ
Parkes AS: Sydney John Folley. In Dictionary of national biography, 1961-1970. Suppl. 8, 1981. p. 375-6.
Parkes D: History of narcolepsy. In Rose FC, Bynum WF, ed: Historical aspects of the neurosciences. New York, Raven, 1982. p. 151-63.
Parkes D, Schachter M: Meige, Brueghel or Blake? Aust Nurses J 1981 Feb;10(7):32-5
Parkhurst E see Breul FR
Parkinson JP: The Castle Hill lunatic asylum (1811-1826) and the origins of eclectic pragmatism in Australian psychiatry. Aust NZ J Psychiatry 1981 Dec;15(4):319-22
Parmeggiani L: L'opera di Bernadino Ramazzini nel campo della medicina del lavoro. Med Lav 1983 Nov-Dec;74(6):426-32
Parnas J: Thorvald Madsen 1870-1957. Leader in international public health. Dan Med Bull 1981;28(2):82-6
Parnitzke C, Schaeper M: Bedeutende Magdeburger antifaschistische Aerzte und die Entwicklung der Orthopädie in Magdeburg. Z Arztl Fortbild (Jena) 1980 Aug 15;74(16):781-6
Parr LJ: Early libraries for nurses in England, 1860-1914. J Librariansh 1980;12(2):102-14
Parra Hidalgo P, Marset Campos P, Ramos García E, et al: Cincuenta años de la Revista de Sanidad e Higiene Pública (1926-1975). Análisis bibliométrico de su producción científica. Rev Sanid Hig Publica (Madr) 1983 Sep-Oct;57(9-10):969-1038
Parra Hidalgo P: 'Marco téorico y conceptual de la atención médica primaria en Cuba'. Rev Sanid Hig Publica (Madr) 1980 Sep-Oct;54(9-10):959-1008
Parrés R: Las corrientes psiquiátricas contemporáneas. In Academia Nacional de Medicina. Libro conmemorativo del primer centenario. México, Comité Editorial de la Comisión Organizadora del Congreso del Centenario, 1964. Tome 2. p. 486-9.
Parrilla Hermida M: Apuntes historicos sobre la subdelegacion del promedicato en Cataluña. Asclepio 1981;33:391-405
Parrilla Hermida M: Biografia del doctor Jose Salvany Lleopart. Asclepio 1980;32:303-10
Parrilla Hermida M: Biografia del doctor Timoto O'Scalan---1726-1800. Asclepio 1980;32:287-93
Parrilla Hermida M: El doctor Cristobal Perez de Herrera. Presentacion de documentos ineditos. Asclepio 1978-79;30-31:371-6
Parrilla Hermida M: La direccion de Sanidad Militar---su primer director. Asclepio 1980;32:295-302
Parrilla Hermida M: Un hospital de la Armada en El Ferrol siglo XVI. Asclepio 1981;33:407-10
Parrish JA: Festschrift: Thomas B. Fitzpatrick--a powerful difference. J Invest Dermatol 1983 Jun;80 Suppl:3s-5s
Parrott JR, Harrison DB: Surgically dividing pianists' hands. J Hand Surg 1980 Nov;5(6):619
Parry NA: Pioneers of physical education in the 19th century: Alexander Alexander. [1849-1928]. Bull Hist Educ Soc 1978;22:21-38
Parry-Jones B see The preservation of medical and public health records
Parry-Jones WL: The development of the psychotherapies: a brief historical overview. In M. Weller, ed: The scientific basis of psychiatry. London, Baillière Tindall, 1983. p. 391-401.
Parry-Jones WL see Scull A, ed
Parson DO: The male labour force participation decision: health, reported health and economic incentives. Economica 1982;49(193):81-91
Parson T: The articulation of the personality and the social-action system: Sigmund Freud and Max Weber. In M. Albin, R. J. Devlin, G. Heeger, ed: New directions in psychohistory. The Adelphi papers in honor of Erik H. Erikson. Lexington, Toronto, D. C. Heath, 1980. p. 27-35.
Parsons ME: Mothers and matrons. Nurs Outlook 1983 Sep-Oct;31(5):274-8
Parsons ME see Duncan WA
Parsons W: Uninformed consent in 1942. N Engl J Med 1984 May 24;310(21):1397
Parsons-Smith BG: Sir Gordon Holmes. In Rose FC, Bynum WF, ed: Historical aspects of the neurosciences. New York, Raven, 1982. p. 357-70.
Parssinen TM, Kerner K: Development of the disease model of drug addiction in Britain, 1870-1926. Med Hist 1980 Jul;24(3):275-96
Parssinen TM: Professional deviants and the history of medicine: medical mesmerists in Victorian Britain. Sociol Rev [Monogr] 1979;27:103-20
Partanen J: Potreblenie alkogol'nykh napitkov i ego gosudarstvennoe regulirovanie. Sotsiol Issled 1981;1:178-86
Partsch KJ: Die zoologische Station in Neapel: Modell internationaler Wissenschaftszusammenarbeit. Göttingen, Vandenhoeck & Ruprecht, 1980. 369 p.
Partsch KJ: Die Zoologische Station in Neapel. Modell internationaler Wissenschaftszusammenarbeit. Gottingen, Vandenhoeck & Ruprecht, 1980. 369 p. (Studien zu Naturwissenschaft, Technik und Wirtschaft im Neunzehnten Jahrhundert, Bd. 11).
Pârvu E, Russo G: Une approche psychosociologique de lat tentative de suicide. Sante Publique (Bucur) 1981;24(1):61-5
Pascal JN: Bordeu, Bouvart et Rostain: trois médecins face à la tuberculose in 1772 (documents inédits). In J. Proust, ed: Recherches nouvelles sur quelques érivains des lumières (II). Montpellier, Univ. Paul Valéry, 1979. p. 63-71.
Pascarella F: Il colore degli occhi: 'teorie' del passato e 'conoscenze' attuali. Med Secoli 1979 Jan-Apr;16(1):105-12
Pascarella F: On 'The physician-writers from the 15th to the 20th century' by Arnaldo Cherubini. Rome, Arti Grafiche E. Cossidente, 1979.
Pascher F: George Miller MacKee (1878-1955): a memoir. J Am Acad Dermatol 1983 Jul;9(1):168-72
Pasiukov FV see Selivanov EF
Paskaukas RA: Sigmund Freud and Arthur Schopenhauer reexamined. In International Congress of the History of Medicine, 27th, Barcelona, 1980. Actas. Barcelona, Académia de Ciències Mèdiques de Catalunya i Balears, 1981. p. 125-9.
Paskauskas RA: Paracelsus and mental disorders. In International Congress of the History of Medicine, 27th, Barcelona, 1980. Actas. Barcelona, Académia de Ciències Mèdiques de Catalunya i Balears, 1981. p. 121-4.
Pasqualini RQ: Houssay y el serendipismo. Medicina (B Aires) 1981;41(6):827-30
Pasqualini RQ: La vigencia de los remedios. Medicina (B Aires) 1983;43(4):463-5
Passi S, Rothschild-Boros MC, Fasella P, et al: An application of high performance liquid chromatography to analysis of lipids in archaelogical samples. J Lipid Res 1981 Jul;22(5):778-84
Passmore R: Obituary Notice. Wallace Ruddell Aykroyd, CBE, MD, ScD (30 July 1899-7 February 1979). Br J Nutr 1980 Mar;43(2):245-50
Passmore R: Reflexions on energy balance. Proc Nutr Soc 1982 Jun;41(2):161-5
Passmore R, ed: Proceedings of the Royal College of Physicians of Edinburgh Tercentenary Congress, 1981. Edinburgh, Royal College of Physicians of Edinburgh, 1982. xvi, 416 p. (Publication No. 56)
Passouant P: Doctor Gelineau (1828-1906): narcolepsy centennial. Sleep 1981 Sep;4(3):241-6
Passouant P: La narcolepsie au temps de Gélineau. Hist Sci Med 1981;15(2):129-36
Passouant P: Le docteur Gélineau (1828-1906). Hist Sci Med 1981;15(2):137-43
Pasteels JJ: Albert Dalcq, 1893-1973. In Florilège des Sciences en Belgique - II. Bruxelles, Académie Royale de Belgique, 1980. p. 625-39.
Pasternak JL: An analysis of social perceptions of epilepsy: increasing rationalization as seen through the theories of Comte and Weber. Soc Sci Med [Med Psychol Med Sociol] 1981;15(3):223-9
Pastinszky I: A dermatovenerológia Hebrától napjainkig. Orv Hetil 1982 Apr 18;123(16):987-90
Pastinszky I: A száj müködése: harapás, evés, nevetés, beszéd, ízlelés a klasszikus közmondásokban és idézetekben. Fogorv Sz 1984 Jul;77(7):217-8
Pastinszky I: Stomatologia a klasszikus kózmondásokban és idézetekben. Fogorv Sz 1984 May;77(5):139-41
Pastore A: Peste e società. Studi Stor 1979;4:857-73
Pastore N: Dr. High on history. J Hist Behav Sci 1981 Oct;17(4):486-9
Pastushnyi SA see Frolov IT
Patai R: An unknown Hebrew medicl alchemist: a medieval treatise on the quinta essentia. Med Hist 1984 Jul;28(3):308-23

**Patai R:** Maria the Jewess--founding mother of alchemy. **Ambix** 1982 Nov;29(3):177-92

**Pataky L:** Az orthopantomográfia kialakulása Paatero munkásságának tükrében. **Fogory Sz** 1979 Sep;72(9):279-80

**Patel MR** see **Stricevic MV**

**Paterson GR, Neilson JB, Roland CG:** History of medicine. **Can Med Assoc J** 1982 Nov 15;127(10):948

**Paterson GR:** The Hannah Institute: promoting Canadian history of medicine. **Can Med Assoc J** 1983 Jun 1;128(11):1325-8

**Paterson H** see **Masters J**

**Paterson PY:** LT/EAE and the MS quest. Going to the dogs and rats to study the patient. **Cell Immunol** 1983 Nov;82(1):55-74

**The Paterson Laboratories, Manchester, England.: Oncology** 1981;38(1):59-61

**Patev E:** Peritonealna dializa--minalo, nastoiashte i budeshte. **Vutr Boles** 1980;19(1):7-11

**Pathak SK** see **Singh AN**

**Patočka F:** Počátky české mikrobiologie. **Cesk Epidemiol Mikrobiol Imunol** 1983 May;32(3):121-5

**Paton A:** Mission to Belsen 1945. **Br Med J [Clin Res]** 1981 Dec 19;283(6307):1656-9

**Paton D:** The surgery of A. Edward Maumenee. **Am J Ophthalmol** 1979 Sep;88(3 Pt 1):297-302

**Paton W:** Chemical transmission: exploitation and follow up. **Bull Mem Acad R Med Belg** 1982;137 Suppl:31-44

**Patrick JW:** Personal faith and the fear of death among divergent religious populations. **J Sci Stud Relig** 1979;18(3):298-305

**Patrick LL** see **Cotter JV**

**Patrick RC** see **Ibrahim MA**

**Patrimoine hospitalier de la Bourgogne:** [Dijon], Ministère de la Culture et de la Communication; Direction Régionale des Affaires Culturelles de Bourgogne, 1980. 163 p. Contributions by E. Pommier, J. Gaillard, S. Deyts, J. Richard, M. Guillaume, C. Lamarre-Tainturier.

**Patterson JA:** The tale of the psorosperm. **Am J Dermatopathol** 1979 Fall;1(3):229-35

**Patterson JN, Moore MJ:** Laboratory medicine and pathologists in Florida prior to 1950. **J Fla Med Assoc** 1980 Feb;67(2):97-102

**Patterson KD:** Health in colonial Ghana: disease, medicine, and socio-economic change, 1900-1955. Waltham, Mass., Crossroads Press, 1981. xiii, 187 p.

**Patterson KD:** Health in urban Ghana: the case of Accra 1900-1940 [1]. **Soc Sci Med [Med Anthropol]** 1979 Dec;13B(4):251-68

**Patterson KD:** Infectious diseases in twentieth-century Africa: a bibliography of their distribution and consequences. Waltham, Crossroads Press, 1979. xiii, 251 p.

**Patterson KD:** The veterinary department and the animal industry in the Gold Coast, 1909-1955. **Int J Afr Hist Stud** 1980;13(3):457-91

**Patterson T:** La fabbrica dei nasi. **Kos** 1984 Apr;1(3):75-90

**Patterson TJ:** Some Indian sources for the study of the history of medicine. **Indian Arch** 1980;29(1):27-30

**Patterson TJ:** The medical practice of the East India Company. **Soc Soc Hist Med Bull (Lond)** 1980 Jun;26:40-3

**Patterson KD, ed:** Infectious diseases in twentieth-century Africa: a bibliography of their distribution and consequences. Waltham, Mass., Crossroads Press of African Studies Association, 1979. xiii, 251 p.

**Patterson TJ, ed** see **Zeis E**

**Pattie FA:** A Mesmer-Paradis myth dispelled. **Am J Clin Hypn** 1979 Jul;22(1):29-31

**Pattison FL:** The Pattison-Miller quarrel. **Scott Med J** 1980 Jul;25(3):234-40

**Pattison I:** The Veterinary Surgeons Act, 1881. **Vet Rec** 1981 Feb 21;108(8):157-60

**Patton MA:** An early case of battle hysteria. **Br J Psychiatry** 1981 Feb 1;138:182-3

**Patton WK:** Deficit spending (Dr. William P.C. Barton). **US Navy Med** 1982 Feb;73(2):16-7

**Pattullo EL:** Reconciling risk and regulation. **Society** 1980;18(1):34-8

**Patureau N:** L'assistance à Tours au XVIIe siècle; la fondation de l'Hôpital Général de la Charité. In: Congrès National des Sociétés Savantes, 97e, Nantes, 1972. Actes. Paris, 1977. Histoire Moderne et Contemporaine, Tome 1. p. 431-43.

**Patz A:** Contributions of A. Edward Maumenee in the field of retinal and choroidal diseases. **Am J Ophthalmol** 1979 Sep;88(3 Pt 1):295-6

**Patz A:** Jonas S. Friedenwald, man of science. **Invest Ophthalmol Vis Sci** 1980 Oct;19(10):1139-49

**Patz A:** Retinal neovascularisation: early contributions of Professor Michaelson and recent observations. **Br J Ophthalmol** 1984 Jan;68(1):42-6

**Patzwald GA:** Discovering and recording chiropractic history: for a systematic program in the profession. **Chiropr Hist** 1981;1(1):5-9

**Pauchard D:** Neurasthénie, psychasthénie: evolution des concepts. **Rev Med Suisse Romande** 1982 Jun;102(6):621-7

**Paukov VS** see **Strukov AI**

**Paul CB:** Science and immortality. The eloges of the Paris Academy of Sciences (1699-1791). Berkeley, University of California Press, 1980. x, 202 p.

**Paul D:** Eugenics and the Left. **J Hist Ideas** 1984 Oct-Dec;45(4):567-90

**Paul DB:** A war on two fronts: J. B. S. Haldane and the response to lysenkoism in Britain. **J Hist Biol** 1983 Spring;16(1):1-37

**Paul JR, Bunnell WW:** Classics in infectious diseases. The presence of heterophile antibodies in infectious mononucleosis by John R. Paul and W. W. Bunnell. American Journal of the Medical Sciences, 1932.

**Paul U:** Das chirurgische Erbe. Albert Hoffa. **Zentralbl Chir** 1981;106(13):901-3

**Paul U:** Das chirurgische Erbe. Anton von Eiselsberg. **Zentralbl Chir** 1982;107(7):418-21

**Paul U:** Das chirurgische Erbe. Eduard Albert. **Zentralbl Chir** 1982;107(23):1535-7

**Paul U:** Das chirurgische Erbe. Franz König (1832-1910)--Weg und Wandel der Chirurgie seiner Zeit. **Zentralbl Chir** 1983;108(22):1451-6

**Paul U:** Das chirurgische Erbe: Johann von Mikulicz-Radecki. **Zentralbl Chir** 1981;106(7):469-72

**Paul U:** Das chirurgische Erbe. René Leriche. **Zentralbl Chir** 1983;108(18):1177-80

**Paul U:** Paul Friedrich Scheel zum 100. Geburtstag. **Beitr Orthop Traumatol** 1983 Oct;30(10):505-7

**Paul Revere, goldsmith: Dent Lab Rev** 1981 Feb;56(2):40

**Pauleikhoff B:** Das Menschenbild im Wandel der Zeit: Ideengeschichte der Psychiatrie und der klinischen Psychologie. Hürtgenwald, Pressler, 1983. 2 vol. 416 p., 439 p.

**Pauleikhoff B** see **Kraus A, ed**

**Paulenz H** see **Dittmann S**

**Pauling L** see **Dodson G**

**Paulseth JE** see **Rodger NW**

**Paulshock BZ:** Dr. Theodore de Mayerne. **JAMA** 1981;245:1732

**Paulshock BZ:** Tutankhamun and his brothers. Familial gynecomastia in the Eighteenth Dynasty. **JAMA** 1980 Jul 11;244(2):160-4

**Paulshock BZ:** When should a physician retire? - William Heberden's view. **Del Med J** 1983;55(6):359-60

**Paulshock BZ:** William Heberden and opium--some relief to all. **N Engl J Med** 1983 Jan 6;308(1):53-6

**Paulshock BZ:** William Heberden, M.D., and the end of theriac. **NY State J Med** 1982 Oct;82(11):1612-4

**Pauly PJ:** Jacques Loeb and the control of life: an experimental biologist in Germany and America, 1859-1924. Ph.D. Diss., The Johns Hopkins University. Baltimore, 1981. viii, 311 p.

**Pauly PJ:** The appearance of academic biology in late nineteenth-century America. **J Hist Biol** 1984 Fall;17(3):369-97

**Pauly PJ:** The Loeb-Jennings debate and the science of animal behavior. **J Hist Behav Sci** 1981 Oct;17(4):504-15

**Pauly PJ:** The political structure of the brain: cerebral localization in Bismarckian Germany. **Int J Neurosci** 1983 Oct;21(1-2):145-9

**Paung PP:** [The memoirs of Judy Chu] (Chi). **Hu Li Tsa Chih** 1980 Jul;27(3):63-71

**Pavan E:** Police des moeurs, sociètè et politique à Venise à la fin du Moyen Age. **Rev Hist (Paris)** 1980;264(2):241-88

**Pavel I:** Aperçu historique de l'existence du rôle du shunt disse-canalicule biliaire dans la sécrétion biliaire et dans la pathogénie de certains ictères. **Med Interne** 1981 Oct-Dec;19(4):389-96

**Pavel I:** The priority of N. C. Paulescu in the discovery of insulin. București, Editura Academiei Republicii Socialiste Romania, 1976. 251 p.

**Pavisic Z, Dugački V:** Značenje znanstvenog, stručnog i nastavnog rada prof. dr. Alberta Botterija za razvoj oftalmologije u Jugoslaviji. **Lijec Vjesn** 1980 Jan;102(1):43-7

**Pavlov AS:** Epidemiia travmatizma na fabrikakh i zavodakh Peterburga perioda kapitalizma. **Ortop Travmatol Protez** 1979 Jul;(7):64-5

**Pavlov AS:** Fabrichno-zavodskaia meditsina v Peterburge. **Feldsher Akush** 1981;46(2):41-3

**Pavlov AV:** Dostizheniia v bor'be infektsionnymi bolezniami v Ukrainskoĭ SSR za gody desiatoĭ piatiletki i dal'neĭshie zadachi po ikh profilaktike. **Zh Mikrobiol Epidemiol Immunobiol** 1982 Apr;(4):3-7

**Pavlov AV:** Istoricheskie preimushchestva sotsialisticheskogo zdravookhraneniia v oblasti profilaktiki infektsionnykh zabolevaniĭ. **Zh Mikrobiol Epidemiol Immunobiol** 1980 Aug;(8):3-8

**Pavlova V:** Istoriografiia meditsinskoĭ nauki v Bolgarii. **Sov Zdravookhr** 1980;(9):41-5

**Pavlovic BB:** Pismo Rista Jeremića povodom osnivanja sekcije za istoriju medicine i farmacije Srpskog lekarskog društva u Beogradu 12. II 1950 godine. **Srp Arh Celok Lek** 1981 Jul;109(7):955-8

**Pavlovičová L** see **Bunčáková V**

**Pavlovsky S, Dosne Pasqualini C:** XXV Aniversario 1956-1981: Instituto de Investigaciones Hematológicas Mariano R. Castex, Academia Nacional de Medicina, Buenos Aires. **Medicina (B Aires)** 1981;41 Suppl:1-4

**Pavluchkova AV:** Pervye sovetskie dispansery po bor'be s tuberkulezom u deteĭ (k Mezhdunarodnomu godu rebenka). **Probl Tuberk** 1979 Dec;(12):11-5

**Pawela T, Przepiórkowska E:** Przypadki schorzeń stomatologicznych leczonych w klinice chirurgicznej UJ w latach 1924-1939. **Czas Stomatol** 1983 Nov-Dec;36(11-12):869-74

**Pawlicka L** see **Olakowski T**

**Pawluch D:** Transitions in pediatrics: a segmental analysis. **Soc Probl** 1983;30(4):449-65

**Pawson BA:** History of retinoids. **J Am Acad Dermatol** 1982 Apr;6(4 Pt 2 Suppl):577-82

**Payne H, Luthe R:** Isaac Ray and forensic psychiatry in the United States. **Forensic Sci Int** 1980 Mar-Apr;15(2):115-27

**Payne JP:** Anaesthetic deaths. **Br J Hosp Med** 1983 Dec;30(6):411-4

**Payne LM:** A trap for the unwary. **J R Coll Physicians Lond** 1981;15:168

**Payne LM, Newman CE:** History of the College Library 9: Dr. Munk as Harveian Librarian 2 (1862-1870). **J R Coll Physicians Lond** 1978 Jan;12(2):189-95

**Payne LM, Newman CE:** The history of the College library: the eighteen-seventies. **J R Coll Physicians Lond** 1984 Jul;18(3):198-202

**Payton BW:** An historical survey of illustrations of the medicinal leech. **J Audiov Media Med** 1984 Jul;7(3):105-12

**Paz Torres M** see **Carrillo JL**

**Pazur JH:** Dexter French 1918-1981. **Adv Carbohydr Chem Biochem** 1984;42:1-13

**Peacher WG** see **Hsu HY**

**Peacock A:** The relationship between the soul and the brain. In Rose FC, Bynum WF, ed: Historical aspects of the neurosciences. New York, Raven, 1982. p. 83-98.

**Peacock EG:** Early Idaho panhandle doctor reached patients on horseback, boats and rails. **Pac Northwest** 1979;23(1):1-15

**Pearce JM:** The first attempts at removal of brain tumors. In Rose FC, Bynum WF, ed: Historical aspects of the neurosciences. New York, Raven, 1982. p. 239-42.

**Pearce TO:** Political and economic changes in Nigeria and the organization of medical care. **Soc Sci Med [Med Anthropol]** 1980 May;14(2):91-8

**Pearcy LT:** Galen and Stoic rhetoric. **Greek Roman Byz Stud** 1983;24:259-72

**Pearcy LT:** Melancholy rhetoricians and melancholy rhetoric: 'black bile' as a rhetorical and medical term in the second century A.D. **J Hist Med Allied Sci** 1984 Oct;39(4):446-56

**Pearl JL:** Witchcraft in New France in the seventeenth century: the social aspect. **Hist Reflect** 1977;4(2):191-205

**Pearle KM:** Arzteemigration nach 1933 in die USA: der Fall New York. **Medizinhist J** 1984;19(1-2):112-37

**Pearlman M:** Emotional factors in America's Western Pacific policy: Wood and Stimson in the Philippines. **J Psychohist** 1983 Fall;11(2):243-69

**Pearlman M:** Leonard Wood, William Muldoon and the medical profession: public health and universal military training. **N Engl Q** 1979;52(3):326-44

**Pearn J, O'Carrigan C, ed:** Australia's quest for colonial health: some influences on early health and medicine in Australia. Herston, Brisbane, Royal Children's Hospital, 1983. xii, 304 p.

**Pearn J:** Medical philately of Australia. Sydney, [s.n.], 1978. 32 p.

**Pearn J:** The discovery of neuronopathy and neuropathy as a cause of progressive paralysis in childhood. The historical origins of modern differential diagnosis in neuromuscular disease. **J Neurol Sci** 1984 Apr;64(1):99-107

**Pearson AA:** John and William Hunter: patrons of the arts. In: Congrès international d'histoire de la médecine, XXVe, Québec, 1976. Actes. Québec, 1977. p. 1053-62.

**Pearson CL:** 'Nine children were born': a historical problem from the Sugar Creek episode. **Brigham Young Univ Stud** 1981;21(4):441-4

**Pearson EF, Miles W:** Disinfection of mail in the United States. **Bull Hist Med** 1980 Spring;54(1):111-24

**Pearson EF:** First hospitals in Southern Illinois. **Proc Inst Med Chic** 1982 Apr-Jun;35(2):43-4

**Pearson EF:** Health care of the French in the Illinois country during the seventeenth and eighteenth centuries. In: Congrès international d'histoire de la médecine, XXVe, Québec, 1976. Actes. Québec, 1977. p. 1063-72.

**Pearson G:** Yorkshire dentists in the formative years of the B.D.A. **Br Dent J** 1981 Apr 21;150(8):231-2

**Pearson RW:** The Archives of Dermatology: the first hundred years. **Arch Dermatol** 1982 Oct;118(10):699-709

**Pearson ES, ed:** The history of statistics in the 17th and 18th centuries against the changing background of intellectual, scientific and religious thought. Lectures by Karl Pearson given at University College London during the academic sessions 1921-1933. New York, Macmillan, 1978. xix, 744 p.

**Peart WS:** Humors and hormones. **Harvey Lect** 1979;73:259-90

**Pease DC, Porter KR:** Electron microscopy and ultramicrotomy. **J Cell Biol** 1981 Dec;91(3 pt 2):287s-92s

**Pebley AR, Westoff CF:** Women's sex preferences in the United States: 1970 to 1975. **Demography** 1982 May;19(2):177-89

**Pechter EA, Sherman RA:** Maggot therapy: the surgical metamorphosis. **Plast Reconstr Surg** 1983 Oct;72(4):567-70

**Pecinjački S:** Podaci o kugi 1738. Godine u Bečkereku, Deski i Djali. **Naucni Sastanak Zb Rad Naucno Drus Istor Zdrav Kult Jugosl** 1975;(11):111-17

**Peck DL, Bharadwaj LK:** Personal stress and fatalism as factors in college suicide. **Soc Sci** 1980;55(1):19-24

**Peck H** see **Peck S**

**Peck S, Peck H:** Prosperity and decay: a portrait of the Dutch golden age. **Dent Abstr** 1980 Mar;25(3):116-8

**Peck S** see **Buchin ID**

**Peck W, Diethelm O:** Review of the Freud library. In International Congress of the History of Medicine, 27th, Barcelona, 1980. Actas. Barcelona, Acadèmia de Ciències Mèdiques de Catalunya i Balears, 1981. p. 130-3.

**Peck WH:** Mummies of ancient Egypt. In A. Cockburn, E. Cockburn, ed: Mummies, disease, and ancient cultures. Cambridge, Cambridge University Press, 1980. p. 11-28.

**Peck WH** see **Cockburn A**

**Peck WH** see **Reyman TA**

**Pecker A:** André Finot (24 mars 1884 - 3 janvier 1980). **Hist Sci Med** 1980;14(1):23-7

**Pecker A:** Gynäkologie und Geburtshilfe vom Altertum bis zum Anfang des 18. Jahrhunderts. In Sournia JC, Martiny M, Poulet J, ed: Illustrierte Geschichte der Medizin. Salzburg, Andreas, 1980. Vol. 3. p. 1023-73.

**Pecker A:** Nicolas Venette (1633?-1698) est-il le fils de Guy Patin. **Hist Sci Med** 1982;16(3):167-74

**Pecker J:** Thierry de Martel, 1875-1940. **Surg Neurol** 1980;13:401-3

**Pecorella Vergnano L** see **Libri e manoscritti di Haller, 1777-1977**

**Pediatric nurse pioneers (Helen Hogan): Am J Nurs** 1980;80:2084

**Pedicino V** see **Morricone A**

**Pedley CE:** A personal record of dentistry. **Tydskr Tandheelkd Ver S Afr** 1984 Jan;39(1):11-20

**Pedlow GW:** Marriage, family size, and inheritance among Hessian nobles, 1650-1900. **J Fam Hist** 1982 Winter;7(4):333-52

**Pedretti C, Keele K, ed al., ed:** Leonardo da Vinci: disegni anatomici dalla Biblioteca Reale di Windsor. Firenze, Barbèra, 1979. 159 p.

**Pédron F:** Histoire d'Ambroise, chirurgien du roi. Paris, Orban, 1980. 468 p.

**Peduzzi R, Piffaretti JC:** Ancylostoma duodenale and the Saint Gothard anaemia. **Br Med J [Clin Res]** 1983 Dec 24-31;287(6409):1942-5

**Peel J:** Changing patterns of contraception. **Proc Annu Symp Eugen Soc** 1981;16:41-8

**Peel J:** Sir Eardley Lancelot Holland. In Dictionary of national biography, 1961-1970. Suppl. 8, 1981. p. 525-7.

**Peel J:** The lives of the fellows of the Royal College of Obstetricians and Gynaecologists, 1929-1969. London, Heinemann, 1976. xviii, 390 p.

**Peel J, Robinson J:** The Oxford and Cambridge graduates' medical clubs. **Br Med J [Clin Res]** 1983 Dec 24-31;287(6409):1979-81

**Peeters A:** Pharmacopées et médecines traditionnelles: un exemple d'abus de langage. **J Agric Tradit Bot Appl** 1982;29(1):97-100

**Pegeron JP** see **Feinberg M**

**Peiró Rando E:** Notícies històriques sobre la medicina homeopàtica a Catalunya. In Congrés Internacional d'Història de la Medicina Catalana, 1st, Barcelona-Montpellier, 1970. Llibr d'Actes. Barcelona, Editorial Scientia, 1971. v 2, p 43-63

**Peitzman SJ:** Bright's disease and Bright's generation--toward exact medicine at Guy's Hospital. **Bull Hist Med** 1981;55(3):307-21

**Peitzman SJ:** Forgotten reformers: the American Academy of Medicine. **Bull Hist Med** 1984 Winter;58(4):516-28

**Peitzman SJ:** Lecturing in American medical schools. Tenacious tradition. **Arch Intern Med** 1983 Aug;143(8):1593-6

**Peitzman SJ:** The quiet life of a Philadelphia medical woman: Mary Willits (1855--1902). **J Am Med Wom Assoc** 1979 Dec;34(12):443-6, 448, 450, passim

**Peitzman SJ:** 'Thoroughly practical': America's polyclinic medical schools. **Bull Hist Med** 1980 Summer;54(2):166-87

**Peitzman SJ** see **Kaiser RM**

**Peiu N:** Din istoricul alimentării cu apă a orașului Iași în secolele XVIII și XIX. **Rev Med Chir Soc Med Nat Iasi** 1983 Oct-Dec;87(4):657-9

**Pejčic M:** Hadži Nešina buna, i kuga u Pirotu 1836-1837. godine. **Srp Arh Celok Lek** 1981 Sep;109(9):1223-31

**Pejčic M:** Lekari i narodna medicina u Pirotu pre oslobodjenja od Turaka. **Srp Arh Celok Lek** 1981 Dec;108(12):1349-55

**Pejčic M:** O nekim lekarima, apotekarima, i narodonoj medicini u Nišu za vreme Turaka (XIX vek). **Srp Arh Celok Lek** 1981 Oct;109(10):1405-12

**Pel JZ:** Uit de geschiedenis van het Middleburgse Gasthuis; het ziekenhuisperssoneel tijdens de overgangsfase van een 19e-eeuws gasthuis naar een 20e-eeuws ziekenhuis. **Ned Tijdschr Geneeskd** 1982 Sep 18;126(38):1741-5

**Peldán K:** Huvuddragen i farmaciens historia i Finland. **Sven Farm Tidskr** 1979;83:657-65

**Peleshchuk AP, Koliadenko VG, Zhukovskiĭ LI:** Ucheniki S. P. Botkina na Ukraine. **Klin Med (Mosk)** 1982 Sep;60(9):110-3

**Pélicier Y:** Beständigheit im Sinngehalt des lateinischen Vokabulars für 'La folie' (Verrücktheit). **Z Klin Psychol Psychother** 1982;30(1):68-76

**Pelicier Y:** Edouard Seguin et l'éducation spéciale. **Bull Acad Natl Med (Paris)** 1981 May;165(5):627-30

**Pelicier Y, Thuillier G:** Edouard Séguin (1812-1880). Nouveaux documents. Nevers, Centre Departemental de Documentation Pedagogique de Nevers, 1981. 211 p.

**Pélicier Y, Thuillier G:** Le fondateur de l'éducation des idiots: Edouard Séguin (1812-1880). **Paedagog Hist** 1980;20:129-52

**Pelicier Y, Thuillier G:** Pour une histoire de l'education des enfants idiots en France (1830-1914). **Rev Hist (Paris)** 1979;261(1):99-130

**Pélicier Y** see **Margolin JC**

**Pélicier Y** see **Vacola G**

**Pelikan J** see **Hamrum CL, ed**

**Pellegrino ED:** The sociocultural impact of twentieth-century therapeutics. In Vogel MJ, Rosenberg CE, ed: The therapeutic revolution. Philadelphia, 1979. p. 245-266.

**Peller S:** Cancer research since 1900. New York, Philosophical Library, 1979. xv, 394 p.

**Pelletier PA, ed:** Prominent scientists. An index to collective biographies. New York, Neal-Schuman, 1980. xxviii, 311 p.

**Pellicori SF** see **Miller VD**

**Pelling M:** A survey of East Anglian medical practitioners 1500-1640. **Local Popul Stud (Matlock)** 1980;:(25):54-5

**Pelling M:** Apothecaries and other medical practitioners in Norwich around 1600. **Pharm Hist (London)** 1983 Jun;13(2):5-8

**Pelling M:** Barbers and barber-surgeons: an occupational group in an English provincial town, 1550-1640. **Soc Soc Hist Med Bull (Lond)** 1981 Jun;28:14-6

**Pelling M:** Medical practice in the early modern period: trade or profession? **Soc Soc Hist Med Bull (Lond)** 1983 Jun;32:27-30

**Pelling M:** Occupational diversity: barbersurgeons and the trades of

Norwich, 1550–1640. **Bull Hist Med** 1982;56(4):484–511
**Pelling M:** Old people and poverty in early modern towns. **Soc Soc Hist Med Bull (Lond)** 1984 Jun;34:42–7
**Pelling M:** Social history of medicine and the geographers--a bibliography. **Soc Soc Hist Med Bull (Lond)** 1984 Dec;35:55–8
**Pelling M** see **Webster C, ed**
**Pelling M, ed:** Handlist of records of the Society of Medical Officers of Health deposited at the Wellcome Unit for the History of Medicine, Oxford, 4 May 1976, with later deposits and other locations. Oxford, Wellcome Unit for the History of Medicine, 1980 23 p. (Research Publications of the Wellcome Unit for the History of Medicine. Oxford, No. III).
**Pelner L:** The distinguished doctors Friedenwald. **Koroth** 1981;8(1–2):45–50
**Pelt JM** see **Fleurentin J**
**Peltier LF:** A brief historical note on the use of electricity in the treatment of fractures. **Clin Orthop** 1981 Nov–Dec;161:4–7
**Peltier LF:** A capite ad calcem--a parable for our time. **J Trauma** 1981 Feb;21(2):96–8
**Peltier LF:** Fractures of the distal end of the radius. An historical account. **Clin Orthop** 1984 Jul–Aug;(187):18–22
**Peltier LF:** Guerin versus Malgaigne: a precedent for the free criticism of scientific papers. **J Orthop Res** 1983;1(1):115–8
**Peltier LF:** Joseph François Malgaigne and Malgaigne's fracture. **Clin Orthop** 1980 Sep;(151):4–7
**Peltier LF:** Joseph Guichard Duverney (1648–1730). Champion of applied comparative anatomy. **Clin Orthop** 1984 Jul–Aug;(187):308–11
**Peltier LF:** The 'back school' of Delpech in Montpellier. **Clin Orthop** 1983 Oct;179:4–9
**Peltier LF:** The classic. Concerning traumatic malacia of the lunate and its consequences: degeneration and compression fractures. **Clin Orthop** 1980 Jun;149:4–8
**Peltier LF:** The classic: congenital osteomalacia. Olaus Jacob Ekman. **Clin Orthop** 1981 Sep;159:3–5
**Peltier LF:** The classic: qualities of intellectual order which the investigator should possess. Santiago Ramón y Cajal. **Clin Orthop** 1981;(160):2–13
**Peltier LF:** The classic. Separations of the epiphyses. By Jean Timothée Emile Foucher. 1867. **Clin Orthop** 1984 Sep;(188):3–9
**Peltier LF:** The classic. The growth of bone. Chapter III. Osteogenic power of bone bereft of periosteum. William Macewen, F.R.S. **Clin Orthop** 1983 Apr;(174):5–14
**Peltier LF:** Ununited fractures in children. James Paget, 1891. **Clin Orthop** 1982 Jun;(166):2–4
**Peluso A:** Patologia orale in una antica popolazione egiziana. **Dent Cadmos** 1980 Dec;48(12):9–28
**Pemmer H:** Schaustellungen von Abnormalitäten in Wien von der Mitte des 18. Jahrhunderts an. **Wien Geschichtsbl** 1968;23(1):265–70
**Pena Munoz C, Girón Irueste F:** Aspectos ineditos de la obra medica de Avenzoar: el prologo del 'Kitab al-Taysir'. Edicion, traduccion y comentarios. **Misc Estud Arabes Hebraicos** 1977;26(1):103–16
**Peña Muñoz C** see **Valverde JL**
**Peña Muñus C, ed:** Indice de sustancias medicinales citadas en el Kitab al-Kulliyyat de Averroes. Granada, Universidad de Granada, 1980. 18 [20] p. (Estudios del Departamento de Historia de la Farmacia y Legislacion Farmaceutica, 5).
**Peña Páez I de la, Viesca Treviño C, Casales Ortiz G:** Presencia de la cirugía española en México en el siglo XVIII. (Real Colegio de Cirugía). In International Congress of the History of Medicine, 27th, Barcelona, 1980. Actas. Barcelona, Académia de Ciències Mèdiques de Catalunya i Balears, 1981. p. 195–8.
**Peňáz J:** K úmrtí prof. MUDr. Vladislava Kruty, DrSc. **Cesk Fysiol** 1980 Mar;29(2):159–70
**Penco MA** see **Fenaroli G**
**Pendler MB:** Muzeĭ-usad'ba N. I. Pirogova (k 100-letiiu so dnia smerti N. I. Pirogova). **Feldsher Akush** 1981;46(12):40–2
**Pene P:** De Laveran aux conséquences médicales, sociales et économiques de sa découverte. **Bull Acad Natl Med (Paris)** 1980 Apr;164(4):382–92
**Penfield W:** Sir Gordon Morgan Holmes. In Dictionary of national biography, 1961–1970. Suppl. 8, 1981. p. 534–6.
**Penfold JB:** East Anglian bladder stone. **J R Soc Med** 1979 Sep;72(9):710–1
**Peng KL:** A Malay cultural explanation for epilepsy. **Aust NZ J Psychiatry** 1983 Dec;17(4):397–9
**Penington AH:** The Fiji School of Medicine--a brief history. **Hawaii Med J** 1984 Sep;43(9):314, 316, 318
**Penishkevich IF, Svitun VD:** Razvitie zdravookhraneniia za gody Sovetskoĭ vlasti na Bukovine. **Vrach Delo** 1983 Mar;(3):1–4
**Penkala D:** 'Hot' and 'cold' in the traditional medicine of Afghanistan. **Ethnomedizin** 1980;6(1–4):201–28
**Penland L:** A decade of dental health education: review of the 1970s. **Dent Hyg (Chic)** 1982 Sep;56(9):16–8, 20–2
**Penland LR:** Sex education in 1900, 1940 and 1980: an historical sketch. **J Sch Health** 1981 Apr;51(4):305–9
**Penman WR** see **Lansing DI**
**Penn RG:** The state control of medicines: the first 3000 years. **Br J Clin Pharmacol** 1979 Oct;8(4):293–305
**Penn RG:** Veterinary drugs: the beginnings of legislative control in the U.K. **Vet Res Commun** 1983 Dec;7(1–4):377–81
**Penneau D, Loriot J, Proteau J, et al:** La femme médecin à travers les âges et les pays. **Hist Sci Med** 1981;15(4):335–43
**Pennefather JP:** A surgeon with the Alberta Field Force. **Alberta Hist** 1978;26(4):1–14
**Pennelli N** see **Thiene G**
**Pennington C:** Tuberculosis. In Checkland O, Lamb M, ed: Health care as social history; the Glasgow case. Aberdeen, Aberdeen University Press, 1982. p. 86–99.
**Pennington G:** Frederick Rand Rogers: educational provocateur (1894–1972). **Can J Hist Sport Phys Educ** 1981;12(1):24–50
**Pennington TG:** The history of medical education in Nashville. **J Tenn Med Assoc** 1983 Jul;76(7):445–9
**Pennini de Vega E, Landáburu AJ, Kohn Loncarica AG, et al:** La inmigración médica española en la Argentina. In International Congress of the History of Medicine, 27th, Barcelona, 1980. Actas. Barcelona, Académia de Ciències Mèdiques de Catalunya i Balears, 1981. p. 188–94.
**Pensak ML, Yanagisawa E:** Tympanic membrane photography: historical perspective. **Am J Otol** 1984 Apr;5(4):324–32
**Pentogalos GE, Lascaratos JG:** A surgical operation performed on Siamese twins during the tenth century in Byzantium. **Bull Hist Med** 1984 Spring;58(1):99–102
**Penzholz H:** Development and present state of cerebellopontine angle surgery from the neuro- and otosurgical point of view. **Arch Otorhinolaryngol** 1984;240(2):167–74
**Peper W:** Der Chiropraktische Report. Heidelberg, Haug, 1978. 208 p.
**Peplau HE:** Some reflections on earlier days in psychiatric nursing. **J Psychosoc Nurs Ment Health Serv** 1982 Aug;20(8):17–24
**Pepłowska E** see **Felchner A**
**Péquignot H:** Société Médicale des Hôpitaux de Paris. **Ann Med Interne (Paris)** 1980;131(2):125–8
**Perakis CR** see **Reed K**
**Perälä M** see **Nieminewa K**
**Perazo N** see **Sociedad Venezolana de Historia de la medicina**
**Percebois G:** Il y un siècle, Laveran découvrit l'hématozoaire du paludisme. **Ann Med Nancy** 1981;20:549–58
**Percebois G:** Jean-Antoine Villemin, Vosgien de Prey, et la notion de contagiosité de la tuberculose. **Ann Med Nancy** 1979;18:685–98
**Perçebois G:** Jean-Antoine Villemin (1827–1892). In: Congrès National des Sociétés Savantes, 103e, Nancy, 1978. Comptes Rendus. Paris, 1978. Section des Sciences, Fasc. V. p. 31–41.
**Percebois G:** Laveran et le pays messin. **J Med Strasb** 1980;11:311–6
**Percebois G:** Le feu Saint-Antoine et les Antonins dans nos provinces de l'Est. **Acad Soc Lorraines Sci** 1978;17(1):19–36
**Percebois G:** Les Bulgares et la Faculté de Médecine de Nancy à la fin du XIXe siècle et au début du XXe siècle. In International Congress of the History of Medicine. 26th, Plovdiv, 1978. Actes du Congress. Sofia, 1981. Volume II. p. 179–82.
**Percy EC:** Sports medicine: its past, present and future. **Ariz Med** 1983 Nov;40(11):789–92
**Percze E:** A fogszabályozási ellátás megszervezése és kiépítése során szerzett 10 éves tapasztalatok, eredmények értékelése Bács-Kiskun megyében. **Fogorv Sz** 1982 Nov;75(11):338–41
**Perdriel G:** La médecine aéronautique dans l'armée de l'air. **Med Armees** 1980;8(10)spec:813–6
**Pereira CB, Galvao CA, Evans WG, et al:** A cephalometric evaluation of a Brazilian pre-historic man. **Tydskr Tandheelkd Ver S Afr** 1983 Oct;38(10):627–31
**Pereira I da R:** Processos de feitiçaria e de bruxaria na Inquisiçao de Portugal. **An Acad Port Hist** 1977;24(2):83–178
**Pereira M:** Alchimia medievale: alcuni studi recenti. **Ann Ist Mus Stor Sci Fir** 1984;9(2):89–98
**Pereira M:** Maternità e sessualità femminile nell' opera di Ildegarda di Bingen. Una proposta di lettura. **Quad Stor** 1980;2
**Pereira-Roque J** see **André R**
**Perekhrestenko PM** see **Piatak OA**
**Pérel L:** Conception pathogénique et traitement du cancer du sein au 18ème siècle. In: Congrès international d'histoire de la médecine, XXVe, Québec, 1976. Actes. Québec, 1977. p. 1073–80.
**Perelló J:** Historia de la otorrinolaringología en España. **An Otorrinolaringol Ibero Am** 1979;6(6):405–81
**Perelló J:** Los cantantes castrados. **An Otorrinolaringol Ibero Am** 1980;7(1):57–76
**Perello J:** The Bordeaux School of ENT in the nineteenth century as seen by a Spanish practitioner, Ricardo Botey. **Rev Laryngol Otol Rhinol (Bord)** 1980 Jan–Feb;101(1–2):15–30
**Perelló J:** The history of the International Association of Logopedics and Phoniatrics. Barcelona, Augusta, 1976. 73 p.
**Perelló J:** Un trauma acústico en el siglo XI. **An Otorrinolaringol Ibero Am** 1980;7(1):53–6
**Perepelkin VS** see **Agafonov VI**
**Perevodchikova NI, Garin AM:** Osnovnye étapy razvitiia klinicheskoĭ khimioterapii opukholeĭ v SSSR. **Vopr Onkol** 1982;28(5):31–8
**Pérez G:** Evolución de los recursos humanos y físicos de salud 1952–1977. **Rev Med Chil** 1977 Oct;105(10):732–8
**Pérez JL** see **Berciano J**
**Pérez L** see **Díaz-Briquets S**
**Pérez PJ, Arsuaga JL, Bermudez de Castro JM:** Atypical toothwear in fossil man. **Paleopathol Newsl** 1982 Sep;39:11–3
**Pérez PJ, Arsuaga JL de:** Estudio paleoepidemiológico y paleodemográfico de la necrópolis de Mirmad (Argin-Sur, Nubia sudanesa). In International Congress of the History of Medicine, 27th, Barcelona, 1980. Actas. Barcelona, Académia de Ciències Mèdiques de Catalunya i Balears, 1981. p. 596–602.
**Pérez Castro E:** Antologia urologica: Profesor Alexander von Lichtenberg (1880–1980). **Arch Esp Urol** 1980 Nov–Dec;33(6):529–38
**Pérez Gallardo R:** El monumento del Dr. Manuel Carmona y Valle.

**Bol Soc Mex Hist Filos Med** 1981 Mar;5(34):147–58
**Pérez García JM:** Los origenes de la Escuela de Veterinaria de Zaragoza. **Asclepio** 1982;34:101–80
**Pérez García JM** see **García Alfonso C**
**Pérez Loredo Díaz L:** Relato de acontecimientos sobresalientes en la enfermería sanitaria y asistencial 1943 a 1983. **Salud Publica Mex** 1983 Sep–Oct;25(5):509–12
**Perez Moreda V:** El paludismo en España a fines del siglo XVIII: la epidemia de 1786. **Asclepio** 1982;34:295–316
**Pérez Moreda V:** Las crisis de mortalidad en la España interior (siglos XVI–XIX). Madrid, Siglo XXI de España Editores, 1980. 526 p.
**Pérez Moreda V:** Un estudio evolutivo de la mortalidad: el ejemplo de otero de herreros a traves de sus registros parroquiales. **Estud Segov** 1973–74;25(73):37–52
**Pérez Moreda V** see **García Sanz A**
**Pérez-Olea J:** Don Augusto Orrego Luco. **Rev Med Chil** 1984 Feb;112(2):193–200
**Pérez Olea J:** Influencia de la biología en la medicina chilena. **Rev Med Chil** 1982 May;110(5):487–90
**Pérez Pabón MJ** see **Ramírez Ronda Ch**
**Perez Romero JA** see **Valverde JL**
**Pérez-Tamayo R** see **Jinich H**
**Perfil'ev GN:** Zemskaia meditsina v Krymu. **Sov Zdravookhr** 1981;(1):63–6
**Perfil'ev GN** see **Starchevskiĭ VS**
**Perich P:** Les foyers de trypanosomiase humaine africaine à Trypanosoma rhodesiense (vecteur Glossina morsitans) au Burundi. Aspects historiques et actuels. **Med Trop (Mars)** 1982 Jan–Feb;42(1):33–41
**Peričic S:** Oskudica i glad u dalmaciji u XIX i početkom XX stoljeća. **Rad Inst Hrvat Povij** 1980;13(1):1–31
**Pericle di Pietro:** Le fonti bibliografiche nella 'De morbis artificum diatriba' di Bernardino Ramazzini. **Hist Philos Life Sci** 1981;3(1):95–114
**Perin J:** Depedikulacija u uslovima partizanskog rata. **Lijec Vjesn** 1979 Nov;101(11):716–7
**Perin J:** Medicinsko–preventivni aspekti zdravstvene službe u narodnooslobodilačkom ratu. **Lijec Vjesn** 1979 Nov;101(11):663–8
**Perkin GD:** Arnold Bennett and medicine: with particular reference to his description of dressing apraxia. **Br Med J [Clin Res]** 1981 Dec 19;283(6307):1666–8
**Perkin GD:** Leber's optic atrophy. In Rose FC, Bynum WF, ed: Historical aspects of the neurosciences. New York, Raven, 1982. p. 463–72.
**Perkin GD, Handler CE:** Wernicke–Korsakoff syndrome. **Br J Hosp Med** 1983 Nov;30(5):331, 333–4
**Perkins JH:** Insects, food, and hunger: the paradox of plenty for U. S. entomology, 1920–1970. **Environ Rev** 1983;7(1):71–96
**Perkins JH:** Reshaping technology in wartime: the effect of military goals on entomological research and insect-control practices. **Technol Cult** 1978 Apr;19(2):169–86
**Perkins WJ:** Biomedical engineering--a reappraisal. **J Biomed Eng** 1984 Apr;6(2):157–9
**Perkovskiy AL:** Krizis demograficheskogo vosproizvodstva krepostnogo krest'yanstva rossii v pervoy polovine XIX stoletiya. Brachnost', Rozhdayemost', Smertnost' v Rossii i v sssr, Moskva, Statistika, 1977, p. 167–190.
**Perl G:** I was a doctor in Auschwitz. New York, Arno Press, 1979. 189 p.
**Perlmutter G:** History of the Achievement Medal. **Alpha Omegan** 1982 Sep;75(3):24–9
**Permiakov NK:** B. A. Petrov. Moskva, Meditsina, 1982. 170 p.
**Pernick MS:** A calculus of suffering: pain, anesthesia, and utilitarian professionalism in nineteenth-century American medicine. Ph.D. Diss. Columbia University. New York, 1979.
**Pernick MS:** Childhood death and medical ethics: an historical perspective on truth–telling in pediatrics. **Prog Clin Biol Res** 1983;139:173–88
**Pernick MS:** [History of] medical professionalism [in the United States]. In Reich WT, et al, ed: Encyclopedia of bioethics, v.3. New York, Free Press, 1978. p. 1028–34.
**Pernick MS:** The calculus of suffering in nineteenth–century surgery. **Hastings Cent Rep** 1983 Apr;13(2):26–36
**Pernin A, Vega DE:** Historia de la anestesia en el Uruguay. Montevideo, Roche, 1981. n. p.
**Pernow B:** Problem inom dagens medicinska högskola. **Sven Tidskr** 1981;68(7):338–44
**Peroff K, Podolak–Warren M:** Does spending on defence cut spending on health? A time–series analysis of the U. S. economy 1929–74. **Br J Polit Sci** 1979;9(1):21–39
**Péron Y** see **Dufour D**
**Perova M:** V poiskakh resheniia demograficheskikh problem. **Aziia Afr Segodnia** 1981;5:31–3
**Perrault JL** see **Audet–Lapointe P**
**Perrenoud A, Zumkeller D:** Caractères originaux de la démographie genevoise du XVIe siècle: structure ou conjoncture. **Ann Demogr Hist (Paris)** 1980;:125–41
**Perrenoud A:** Contribution à l'histoire cyclique des maladies. Deux cents ans de variole à Genève (1580–1810). In Imhof AE, ed: Mensch und Gesundheit in der Geschichte. Husum, Matthiesen, 1980. p. 175–98.
**Perrenoud A:** Les mécanismes de récupération d'une population frappée par la peste: L'épidémie de 1636–1640 à Genève. **Schweiz Z Gesch** 1978;28(3):265–88
**Perrenoud A:** Surmortalité féminine et condition de la femme (XVIIe–XIXe siècles). Une vérification empirique. **Ann Demogr Hist (Paris)** 1981;:89–104
**Perret GE:** Doctor Loyal Davis--the neurosurgeon. **Surg Gynecol Obstet** 1983 Aug;157(2):140–3
**Perret JJ** see **Tomlinson WK**
**Perret L:** Benedictus Olai: een nyttigh Läkere–Book 1578. Ett 400–årsminne. Några synpunkter på 1500–talets läkekonst. **Nord Medicinhist Arsb** 1980;Suppl 6:118–21
**Perret L:** Kropp, själ och ande i historisk belysning. **Nord Medicinhist Arsb** 1980;:53–8
**Perret L:** Medicin och medicinare vid Abo akademi under 1600–och 1700–talen. **Nord Medicinhist Arsbok** 1983;:71–81
**Perret L:** René Descartes--drottning Kristinas Cartesius--filosof, matematiker och medicinsk läromästare. **Nord Medicinhist Arsb** 1981;:52–8
**Perrin CE:** A reluctant catalyst: Joseph Black and the Edinburgh reception of Lavoisier's chemistry. **Ambix** 1982 Nov;29(3):141–76
**Perrin CE:** J. B. Van Mons' essai sur les principes de la chimie antiphlogistique: a mystery solved. **Ambix** 1984;31(1):1–5
**Perrin M** see **Lactance**
**Perritt RA:** Intraocular lens implantation from Ridley to the present: my 25 years' experience. **Int Ophthalmol Clin** 1979 Fall;19(3):11–31
**Perrot M:** De la nourrice à l'employée. Travaux de femmes dans la France du XIXe siècle. **Mouvement Soc** 1978 Oct–Dec;3–10
**Perrot M:** Sur la ségrégation de l'enfance au XIX siècle. **Psychiatr Enfant** 1982;25(1):179–206
**Perrot M** see **Dupâquier J**
**Perrot R** see **Hart GD, ed**
**Perry BD, Hedger RS:** History and epidemiology of foot–and–mouth disease in Zambia: a review. **Trop Anim Health Prod** 1984 May;16(2):107–14
**Perry C** see **Laurence JR**
**Perry CB:** Edward Jenner. **Ear Nose Throat J** 1984 Dec;63(12):605–17
**Perry CB:** The Bristol Royal Infirmary, 1904–1974. Bristol [Avon], Portishead Press, 1981. 130 p.
**Perry CW** see **Sheehan PW**
**Perry DS:** The early midwives of Missouri. **J Nurse Midwife** 1983 Nov–Dec;28(6):15–23
**Perry HO:** Department of Dermatology, Mayo Clinic. **Cutis** 1984 Sep;34(3):237–8
**Perry HO, Powell FC, Cooper AJ:** Paul A. O'Leary--dermatologist and teacher. **J Am Acad Dermatol** 1982 Nov;7(5):705–8
**Perry HO** see **Muller SA**
**Perry HS:** Clara Mabel Thompson. In: Notable American women. The modern period. Cambridge, Mass., Belknap–Harvard Univ. Press, 1980. 4:680–3.
**Perry HS:** Psychiatrist of America. The life of Harry Stack Sullivan. Cambridge, Belknap Press, 1982. 462 p.
**Perry PE** see **Aterman K**
**Perry PE** see **Cho LJ**
**Perry S:** Special report. The brief life of the National Center for Health Care Technology. **N Engl J Med** 1982 Oct 21;307(17):1095–100
**Perry T:** The 48th evacuation hospital. **RI Med J** 1982 Dec;65(12):493
**Persaud TV:** A brief history of anatomy at the University of Manitoba. **Anat Anz** 1983;153(1):3–31
**Perskiĭ EE** see **Nikitin VN**
**Person RS** see **Alekseev MA**
**Perspectivas de desarrollo del Instituto de Medicina Tropical 'Pedro Kourí': Rev Cubana Med Trop** 1979 Sep–Dec;31(3):161–3
**Perspectives in biorheology:** Festschrift for A. L. Copley. **Biorheology** 1981;18(3–6):305–729
**Persson LA** see **Brändström A**
**Persson O** see **Ahlström CG**
**Pertl E:** Pregled razvoja zdravstva v Laškem in njegovem okolišu. **Cas Zgodovino Narodop** 1976;12(2):358–91
**Pertl E:** Prvi slovenski zdravniki v Mariboru. **Zb Zgodovino Naravoslovja Teh** 1981;5–6:95–191
**Perugachi C** see **Barba J**
**Perutz MF** see **Dodson G**
**Peruzzi E:** Un trattato inedito di farmacologia di Gerolamo Fracastoro. **Rinascimento** 1978;18:183–228
**Pervomaĭskiĭ GS, Podolian VIa, Chagin KP, et al:** Rol' akademika Evgeniia Nikanorovicha Pavlovskogo v stanovlenii i razvitii parazitologii v SSSR (k 100–letiiu so dnia rozhdeniia). **Parazitologiia** 1984 Mar–Apr;18(2):89–98
**Perzigian AJ:** Allometric analysis of dental variation in a human population. **Am J Phys Anthropol** 1981 Mar;54(3):341–5
**Pescarini L** see **Lenarduzzi G**
**Pesce L:** Due inventari di libri del medico umanista trevigiano Nicolò Cesi. **Quad Stor Univ Padova** 1978;11:125–7
**Peschel ER:** 'Alchemy of the word'--language and 'the knife' a commentary on Richard Selzer's work. **Pharos** 1979 Winter;42(1):25–32
**Peschel ER** see **Peschel RE**
**Peschel RE, Peschel ER:** 'But what if she should die?'--case histories, literary histories: a discussion of maternal death in childbirth. **Pharos** 1981 Winter;44(1):11–8
**Peschel RE, Peschel ER:** Ritual and the death certificate: case histories, literary histories. **Pharos** 1983 Spring;46(2):11–6
**Pesenti Marañgon T:** 'Professores chirurgie', 'medici ciroici' e 'barbitonsores' a Padova nell' età di Leonardo Buffi da Bertipaglia (dopo il 1448). Quad. Stor Univ. Padova, 1978;11:1–38.
**Peset JL:** Cesare Lombroso y la psiquiatría de su tiempo: el caso U.S.A. In International Congress of the History of Medicine, 27th, Barcelona,

1980. Actas. Barcelona, Académia de Ciències Médiques de Catalunya i Balears, 1981. p. 134–9.
**Peset JL:** Epidemias y sociedad en la España del fin del antiguo regimen. In: Sociedad Española de Historia de la Medicina. V Congreso Nacional. Madrid, 1977. **Asclepio** 1977;29:37–65
**Peset JL, Nuñex D:** Filosofia, ciencia y alquimia en la ilustacion española. **Cuad Hispanoam** 1980;120(359):371–93
**Peset JL:** La sociedad enferma: algunas reflexiones sobre la muerte del presidente Carnot (1894). **Asclepio** 1983;35:177–88
**Peset JL, Arquiola E, Peset M, et al:** Los medicos y la peste de Valencia de 1647–1648. In: Sociedad Española de Historia de la Medicina. V Congreso Nacional. Madrid, 1977. **Asclepio** 1977;29:217–41
**Peset JL** see **Albarracín Teulón A**
**Peset JL** see **Peset M**
**Peset M, Mancebo MF, Peset JL:** Estudiantes medicos en Valencia durante la primera mitad del XVIII. **Asclepio** 1980;32:311–25
**Peset M, La Parra S, Mancebo MF, et al:** Gobierno y poder politico en la peste de Valencia de 1647–1648. In: Sociedad Española de Historia de la Medicina. V Congreso Nacional. Madrid, 1977. **Asclepio** 1977;29:243–63
**Peset M, La Parra S, Mancebo MF, et al:** Los bandoleros y la peste de Valencia de mediados del siglo XVII. In: Sociedad Española de Historia de la Medicina. V Congreso Nacional. Madrid, 1977. **Asclepio** 1977;29:265–82
**Peset M** see **Peset JL**
**Pesonen N:** Rovasti Wegelius ja hänen lääkärikirjansa. **Duodecim** 1984;100(2):72–9
**Pesquiès-Courbier S:** Le renouveau de la médecine aéronautique en France de 1945 à 1950. **Rev Hist Armees** 1982;3:102–9
**Peszke MA:** The historic antecedents to the current polemics on involuntary psychiatric hospitalization. **Compr Psychiatry** 1984 Mar–Apr;25(2):238–46
**Pětasedesátiny doc. MUDr. Z. Mařatky, DrSc.: Cesk Gastroenterol Vyz** 1979 Jun;33(4):236–47
**Petolski M:** Dr Józef Bednarz. **Przegl Lek** 1981;38(1):173–5
**Peter CH:** Der Briefwechsel zwischen Paulus Usteri und Melchior Aepli. Zürich, Juris Druck, 1983. 161 p. (Zürcher Medizingeschichtliche Abhandlungen, Neue Reihe, Nr. 155).
**Peter JP:** Les médecins français face au problème de l'inoculation variolique et de sa diffusion (1750–1790). **Ann Bretagne** 1979;86(3):251–64
**Peter JP:** Reparar el desorden del mundo: la medicina ilustrada ante la enfermedad epidemica (Bas-Poitou, 1784–1785). **Asclepio** 1983;35:3–26
**Péter L:** Juhász Gyula betegségtudata. **Orv Hetil** 1983 May 15;124(20):1205–7
**Péter L:** Móra Ferenc betegségei. Halálának 50. évfordulójára. **Orv Hetil** 1984 Feb 5;125(6):341–4
**Peter Brian Medawar: Cell Immunol** 1981 Aug;62(2):235–42
**Péterffy I:** Híradás két felvilágosodás kori jeles orvosról. **Orv Hetil** 1983 Jul 31;124(31):1895–6
**Peterman M** see **Ballstadt C**
**Peters BH** see **Levin HS**
**Peters D:** The British medical response to opiate addiction in the nineteenth century. **J Hist Med Allied Sci** 1981 Oct;36(4):455–88
**Peters D:** The pregnant Pamela: characterizations and popular medical attitudes in the 18th century. **Eighteenth Cent Stud** 1980–81;14:432–51
**Peters DS:** Das Biogenetische Grundgesetz--Vorgeschichte und Folgerungen. **Medizinhist J** 1980;15(1/2):57–69
**Peters L** see **Spor E, ed**
**Peters UH:** Anna Freud. Ein Leben für das Kind. München, Kindler, 1979. 309 p.
**Peters UH:** Hölderlin: Dichter, Kranker--Simulant? **Nervenarzt** 1981 May;52(5):261–8
**Peters UH, ed:** Psychiatrie. Weinheim, Beltz, 1983. 2 v. 588, 581 p. (Kindlers 'Psychologie des 20. Jahrhunderts'). Historical contributions by R. Tölle, H. Kindler, W. Schmitt, D. von Zerssen, Y. Fried, P. Berner.
**Petersdorf RG:** Landmark perspective: sulfadiazine. **JAMA** 1984 Mar 16;251(11):1475–6
**Petersdorf RG:** Managing the revolution in medical care. **J Med Educ** 1984 Feb;59(2):79–90
**Petersdorf RG:** The evolution of departments of medicine. **N Engl J Med** 1980 Aug 28;303(9):489–96
**Petersen ES:** Galen: the most maligned physician. **Proc Inst Med Chic** 1981;34:12
**Petersen JC, Markle GE:** Politics and science in the laetrile controversy. **Soc Stud Sci** 1979;9(2):139–66
**Petersen W:** Malthus. Cambridge, Mass. Harvard University Press, 1979. vi, 302 p.
**Petersen JC, ed** see **Markle GE**
**Peterson CD** see **Saddique A**
**Peterson CM:** Symposium on optimal insulin delivery. Introduction: History and goals of insulin treatment. **Diabetes Care** 1982 May–Jun;5 Suppl 1:1–5
**Peterson JA:** The impact of sanitary reform upon American urban planning, 1840–1890. **J Soc Hist** 1979;13(1):83–103
**Peterson M, Rose Cl:** Historical antecedents of normative vs pathologic perspectives in aging. **J Am Geriatr Soc** 1982 Apr;30(4):289–94
**Peterson MJ:** Gentlemen and medical men: the problem of professional recruitment. **Bull Hist Med** 1984 Winter;58(4):457–73
**Peterson MJ:** Specialist journals and professional rivalries in Victorian medicine. **Victorian Period Rev** 1979;12(1):25–32
**Peterson MJ** see **McCullough LB**
**Peterson RP ed** see **Licata SJ**
**Peterson W:** History of population theories. In Reich WT, et al, ed: Encyclopedia of bioethics, v.3. New York, Free Press, 1978. p. 1225–32.
**Pethö B:** A psychiatria mint történeti rendszer. **Orvostort Kozl** 1982;92(4):23–52
**Petit A:** L'esprit de la science anglaise et les Français au XIXème siècle. **Br J Hist Sci** 1984 Nov;17(57 pt 3):273–93
**Petit C:** Problèmes actuels de la génétique des populations. In Actes du Colloque R.A. Fisher.... Paris, 5–6 déc. 1979. p. 351–79. **Rev Synth (Paris)** 1981;102(103–104)
**Petit JG:** Folie, langage, pouvoirs en Maine-et-Loire, 1800–1841. **Rev Hist Mod Contemp** 1980 Oct–Dec;27:529–64
**Petitjean F, Bonnefoy JP, Caroli F, et al:** Le secteur et la loi du 30 juin 1838. **Ann Med Psychol (Paris)** 1982;140(3):301–19
**Petitjean F** see **Massé G**
**Petkova M:** Naukometrichna kharakteristika na publikanoto nauchno tvorchestvo na akad. Aleksi Pukhlev. **Vutr Boles** 1982;21(3):92–100
**Petkova M:** Naukometrichna kharakteristika na publikuvanoto nauchno tvorchestvo na professor Konstantin Chilov. **Vutr Boles** 1984;23(4):102–8
**Petkova M:** Seriĭni izdaniia na svetovnata zdravna organizatsiia naukometrichno prouchvane. **Vutr Boles** 1982;21(6):86–91
**Petlenko VP, Klishov AA:** Kletochnaia teoriia i teoriia kletok (k 100-letiiu so dnia smerti T. Shvanna). **Arkh Anat Gistol Embriol** 1982 Nov;83(11):17–27
**Peto M:** A népességnövekedés szabályozása az ókorban. **Orvostort Kozl** 1982;28(1–3):131–9
**Petot JM:** Mélanie Klein: le moi et le bon objet, 1932–1960. [Paris], Dunod, 1982. xvi, 303 p.
**Petr Andreevich Sokolov (k 80-letiiu so dnia rozhdeniia): Arkh Anat Gistol Embriol** 1980 Jul;79(7):118–20
**Petraccone C:** La difesa contro la peste: prevenzione e controllo dell'epidemia nelle pestilenze di Terra di Bari (1690–1692) e Noja (1815–1816). **Arch Stor Prov Napol** 1977;95:253–80
**Petrakis NL:** Diagonal earlobe creases, type A behavior and the death of Emperor Hadrian. **West J Med** 1980 Jan;132(1):87–91
**Petrányi L:** Markusovszky szellemének idézése a 3. évezred küszöbén. **Orv Hetil** 1984 Jun 17;125(25):1487–92
**Petrásek J, Adamec J:** Prof. MUDr. Emerich Maixner 1847--1920, významná osobnost počátku českého vnitřního lékařství. **Cas Lek Cesk** 1980 Jun 13;119(23–24):684–6
**Petrásek J:** Třicet let Slovenské akademie věd. **Cas Lek Cesk** 1983 Dec 16;122(50):1568
**Petrásek J:** 100 leté výročí odhalení desky J. E. Purkyněmu. **Cas Lek Cesk** 1983 Oct 14;122(41):1269–70
**Petrásek J** see **Adamec J**
**Petrenko VS:** Rozvytok fizychnoi kul'tury na seli USSR v 1951–1968. **Ukr Istor Zh** 1969;9:66–75
**Petrequin J:** Un manuel pour le service des malades. **Rev Infirm** 1982 Oct;32(16):17–9
**Petresco A** see **Marinesco M**
**Petrescu A:** Lumini în marele întuneric din istoria neurochirurgiei. **Rev Med Interna [Neurol Psihiatr]** 1981 Oct–Dec;26(4):311–4
**Petrescu A:** Simptoame neuropsihice consemnate în cronici şi vechi însemnări Româneşti. **Rev Med Interna [Neurol Psihiatr]** 1983 Apr–Jun;28(2):149–52
**Petrescu A** see **Marinescu M**
**Petrescu AD:** D. în secolul XVI, un clujean: medic de faimă europeană. **Mag Istor** 1976;10(12):27
**Petrescu G:** 125 de ani de la nasterea lui Sir Robert Philip (1856–1939). **Rev Ig [Pneumoftiziol]** 1982 Oct–Dec;31(4):383–4
**Petri G:** Sebészet és tudomány. **Orv Hetil** 1982 Jan 3;123(1):5–11
**Petrisko TW:** Schism and suppression: the elimination of medical protest schools, 1846–1939. **Chiropr Hist** 1982;2(1):35–9
**Petrocchi M:** Cassiodore, son temps et la Formula Comitis Archiatrorum. In International Congress of the History of Medicine. 26th, Plovdiv, 1978. Actes du Congress. Sofia, 1981. Volume II. p. 183–7.
**Petrociová O** see **Bartunek A**
**Petrov BD:** Akademii meditsinskikh nauk SSSR - 40 let. **Vestn Akad Med Nauk SSSR** 1984;(6):3–13
**Petrov BD:** Bor'ba s tuberkulezom v SSR, provodimaia v sootvetstvii s ideiami V. I. Lenina. **Probl Tuberk** 1980 Apr;(4):3–6
**Petrov BD:** Diagnostika v sisteme meditsinskikh vzgliadov Ibn Siny. **Klin Med (Mosk)** 1979 Dec;57(12):91–6
**Petrov BD:** I. A. Pribil' (k 200-letiiu so dnia rozhdeniia). **Zh Mikrobiol Epidemiol Immunobiol** 1983 Oct;(10):108–9
**Petrov BD:** Ibn-Sina--Avitsenna (K 1000-letiiu so dnia rozhdeniia). **Med Sestra** 1980 Aug;39(8):45–51
**Petrov BD:** Itogi i zadachi istoriko-meditsinskikh issledovaniĭ. **Sov Zdravookhr** 1982;(12):64–7
**Petrov BD:** Izuchenie nauchnogo naslediia S. P. Botkina. **Sov Zdravookhr** 1983;(2):57–9
**Petrov BD:** Meditsinskoe nasledie Ibn-Siny. **Sov Zdravookhr** 1980;(9):53–6
**Petrov BD:** O sozdanii polnoĭ istorii gigieny truda v Rossii i SSR. **Gig Tr Prof Zabol** 1980 Jun;(6):1–5
**Petrov BD:** 'Sposob sokhraneniia zdorov'ia morskikh sluzhiteleĭ'. **Gig Sanit** 1981 Feb;(2):42–3
**Petrov BD:** Study of Ibn Sina's medical heritage. In International Congress of the History of Medicine, 27th, Barcelona, 1980. Actas. Barcelona, Académia de Ciències Médiques de Catalunya i Balears, 1981. p. 746–9.
**Petrov BD:** Study on the medical heritage of Avicenna (Ibn Sina). In E. Schultheisz, ed: History of physiology. Oxford, Elmsford, New York,

Pergamon, 1981. xvi, 208 p. (Advances in Physiological Sciences. Proceedings of the 28th International Congress of Physiological Sciences, Budapest, 1980. Volume 21). p. 49–51.

**Petrov BD:** Trekhsotletie ukaza ob ospe (stranitsa istorii épidemiologii). **Zh Mikrobiol Epidemiol Immunobiol** 1981 Jun;(6):117–8

**Petrov BD:** Voprosy okhrany zdorov'ia v 'Kanone' Ibn-Siny (k 1000-letiiu so dnia rozhdeniia). **Gig Sanit** 1980 May;(5):22–5

**Petrov BD:** Zadachi istoriko-meditsinskikh issledovaniĭ v SSSR. **Sov Zdravookhr** 1980;(8):44–7

**Petrov IN:** P.G. Kornev i ego shkola. **Probl Tuberk** 1984 Jul;(7):73–5

**Petrov ME** see **Kamalov MKh**

**Petrov NS:** Idei S. P. Botkina v funktsional'noĭ gematologii i ikh dal'neishee razvitie. **Vestn Akad Med Nauk SSSR** 1983;(3):47–51

**Petrov NS, Georgievskiĭ AS, Antonov VB:** Sergeĭ Petrovich Botkin i voennaia meditsina (k 150-letiiu so dnia rozhdeniia). **Voen Med Zh** 1982;(9):64–6

**Petrov NS:** Sergeĭ Petrovich Botkin (k 150-letiius so dnia rozhdeniia). **Probl Gematol Pereliv Krovi** 1982 Dec;27(12):49–51

**Petrov P, Bussarsky VA:** Perspectives in international neurosurgery: neurosurgery in Bulgaria. **Neurosurgery** 1981 Dec;9(6):758

**Petrov RV:** Immunologiia ot Pastera do nashikh dnei. Moskva, Nauka, 1968. 101 p.

**Petrov VA** see **Gvozdev MP**

**Petrov VP, Shamko VI:** Oni zashchishchali Odessu. **Med Sestra** 1984 Apr;43(4):55–7

**Petrova L:** Die Bedeutung des Wassers in den volkstümlichen Bräuchen und in der Volksmedizin. In International Congress of the History of Medicine, 27th, Barcelona, 1980. Actas. Barcelona, Académia de Ciències Mèdiques de Catalunya i Balears, 1981. p. 603–9.

**Petrova LF** see **Kogan VI**

**Petrova LF** see **Kogan VIa**

**Petrova TA:** Razvitie khirurgii v dorevoliutsionnoĭ Karelii. **Sov Zdravookhr** 1981;(12):58–60

**Petrovic M** see **Stojan D**

**Petrovskaia EG** see **Sheĭman IB**

**Petrovskiĭ BV:** Petr Aleksandrovich Gertsen (k 80-letiiu Moskovskogo nauchno-issledovatel'skogo onkologicheskogo instituta im P. A. Gertsena). **Khirurgiia (Mosk)** 1983 Nov;(11):3–7

**Petrovskiĭ BV:** Ranenie na duéli i smert' A. S. Pushkina. **Klin Med (Mosk)** 1983 Apr;61(4):109–17

**Petrovskiĭ BV:** Sovetskaia khirurgiia za 60 let. **Klin Med (Mosk)** 1982 Dec;60(12):15–22

**Petrovskiĭ BV:** 60 let sovetskogo zdravookshraneiia. Moskva, Meditsina, 1977. 414 p.

**Petrovskiĭ KS:** Razvitie nauki o pitanii v SSSR. **Gig Sanit** 1982 Dec;(12):16–9

**Petrovskiĭ KS:** Razvitie sanitarnogo nadzora po gigiene pitaniia v SSSR za 60 let. **Gig Sanit** 1982 Sep;(9):21–3

**Petrovskiĭ KS, Novikov IV:** Zhurnalu 'Gigiena i sanitariia' 60 let. **Gig Sanit** 1982 Aug;(8):4–7

**Petrowa L:** Volksheilverfahren für Nervenkrankheiten im Bezirk Warna. In International Congress of the History of Medicine. 26th, Plovdiv, 1978. Actes du Congress. Sofia, 1981. Volume II. p. 71–2.

**Petrowskij KS, Novikov JV:** 60 Jahre 'Gigiena i sanitarija'. **Z Gesamte Hyg** 1983 Sep;29(9):564–5

**Petrun' AS** see **Maĭatruk PN**

**Petrun' AS** see **Maĭstruk PN**

**Petryszak NG:** Tabula rasa--its origins and implications. **J Hist Behav Sci** 1981 Jan;17(1):15–27

**Petsch K, Krekeler G, Otten JE:** Pathologische Veränderungen im alveolären Bereich an Funden einer historischen Grablege. **Dtsch Zahnarztl Z** 1982 Apr;37(4):358–60

**Petschauer P:** Growing up female in eighteenth-century Germany. **J Psychohist** 1983 Fall;11(2):167–207

**Pettener D:** Inbreeding secular changes in the Riomaggiore and Silla Valleys, Italy, from 1565 to 1980. **Acta Anthropogenet** 1981;5(4):271–8

**Pettus BE:** Osha inspection costs, compliance costs, and other outcomes: the first decade. **Policy Stud Rev** 1982;1(3):596–614

**Petty CS:** The medical examiner and medical education (Russell S. Fisher). **Hum Pathol** 1980 Mar;11(2):101–3

**Petty TL:** 25 years of Aspen Lung Conferences. **Chest** 1984 Jun;85(6 Suppl):1S

**Peumery JJ:** La prodigieuse carrière de Jean-François Coste (1741–1819) médicin-chef des armées. **Hist Sci Med** 1980;14(2):177–86

**Peumery JJ:** Une grande figure de la médecine et de la chirurgie française: Pierre-Jean Mauricheau-Beaupré (1778-1857). **Hist Sci Med** 1983;17(1):95–104

**Peutillot A:** Petite histoire de la vulgarisation en puériculture. **Soins Gynecol Obstet Pueric** 1982 Feb;(9):47–50

**Peyresblanques J:** Histoire de l'Hôpital de Dax au XIIIe siècle. **Bull Soc Borda** 1980;104(377):75–105

**Peyresblanques J:** Monsieur Vincent, ses maladies, ses médecins. **Hist Sci Med** 1982;16(4):253–61

**Peyton R:** A Webster parish country doctor's record. **North La Hist Assoc J** 1979;10(3):103–10

**Peyton W:** Tender loving care: a study of the doctors, their medicines and medical treatment during the American Civil War era. **Lincoln Her** 1982;84(2):106–13

**Pezin M** see **Devauchelle D**

**Pezzia A** see **Sawyer DR**

**Pezzuoli G** see **Montorsi W**

**Pfäfflin F, Gross J:** Involuntary sterilization in Germany from 1933 to 1945 and some consequences for today. **Int J Law Psychiatry** 1983;5(3-4):419–23

**Pfafrod GO** see **Derums VIa**

**Pfannkuche K, Schadewaldt H:** Die Bedeutung der Blutgefässe im Laufe der Entwicklung der Medizin. In Müller-Wiefel H, et. al., ed: Mikrozirkulation und Blutrheologie. Therapie der peripheren arteriellen Verschlusskrankheit. Baden-Baden, New York, Witzstrock, 1980. p. 4–9.

**Pfarrwaller-Stieve A:** Friedrich von Müller (1858–1941) und seine Stoffwechseluntersuchungen. Zürich, Juris Druck, 1983. 58 p. (Zürcher Medizingeschichtliche Abhandlungen, Neue Reihe, 156).

**Pfeffer R:** Professor Franz von Rinecker, 1811–1883. Diss., Bayerische Julius-Maximilians-Universität, Würzburg, 1981. 180 p.

**Pfeiffer S:** Paleopathology in an Iroquoian ossuary, with special reference to tuberculosis. **Am J Phys Anthropol** 1984 Oct;65(2):181–9

**Pfeiffer W** see **Poulet W**

**Pfister G:** The influence of women doctors on the origins of women's sports in Germany. In Borms J, Hebbelinck M, Venerando A, ed: Women and sport. Basel, Karger, 1981. p. 58–65.

**Pfister R:** 100 Jahre Dermatologie. **Fortschr Med** 1982 Dec 16;100(47-48):2214–21

**Pflug G:** Descartes und das mechanistische Menschenbild. **Medizinhist J** 1982;17(1/2):3–19

**Pfohl G:** Das philosophisch-philologische Element in der medizinischen Fakultät. **Med Welt** 1980 May 16;31(20):775–8

**Pfohl G:** Das philosophisch-philologische Element in der medizinischen Fakultät. Ein Beitrag der Medizingeschichte, mehr zu formen als zu informieren. I, II. **Med Welt** 1980 Apr 25, May 9;(17,19):644–6,730–3

**Pfohl G:** Humanitas Hippocratica. **ZFA (Stuttgart)** 1983 Dec 20;59(35-36):1943–54

**Pfohl G:** Medizin und Philologie--Allgemeine humanistische Bildung als Anliegen des Schweizer Medizinhistorikers Charles Lichtenthaeler. **Med Welt** 1980 Nov 7;31(45):1651

**Pfund N, Hofstadter L:** Biomedical innovation and the press. **J Commun** 1981;31(2):138–54

**Phaneuf MM:** Sanitation and cholera: Springfield and the 1866 epidemic. **Hist J West Mass** 1980;8(1):26–36

**A pharmaceutical museum: Pharm Hist (London)** 1977 Jul;7(2):4–5

**Pharmacist -cum-printer: Pharm Hist (London)** 1971 Dec;2(3):5–6

**Pharmacology of leadership: Practitioner** 1980 Feb;224(1340):119

**Pharoah PO, Alberman ED:** Mortality of low birthweight infants in England and Wales 1953 to 1979. **Arch Dis Child** 1981 Feb;56(2):86–9

**Phelps PD, Lloyd GA, Windle-Taylor PC, et al:** Mondini dysplasia. **Ann Otol Rhinol Laryngol** 1982 Mar–Apr;91(2 Pt 1):254

**Phelps WH:** John Gerard, the herbalist. **Library (Lond)** 1980 Mar;2(1):76–85

**Phil M** see **Jay M**

**Phillilps S:** Psychoanalysis and childhood education: a historical review. **Paedagog Hist** 1977;17(2):378–85

**Phillips CJ:** Rosetta Sherwood Hall. In: Notable American women. The modern period. Cambridge, Mass., Belknap-Harvard Univ. Press, 1980. 4:299–301.

**Phillips D** see **Dodson G**

**Phillips DP:** The influence of suggestion on suicide: substantive and theoretical implications of the Werther effect. **Am Sociol Rev** 1974;39(3):340–54

**Phillips DP** see **Bollen KA**

**Phillips GO:** Barbados' Battle Creek doctor Charles J. B. Cave 1879–1939. **Advent Herit** 1978;5(2):22–33

**Phillips JH:** Early Greek medicine and the poetry of Solon. **Clio Med** 1980;15(1/2):1–4

**Phillips JH:** Juxtaposed medical traditions: Pliny HN 27, 131. **Classical Philol** 1981;76(2):130–2

**Phillips JH:** Lucretius on the inefficiency of the medical arts: 6.1179 and 6.1226–38. **Classical Philol** 1982;77:233–5

**Phillips JH:** The emergence of the Greek medical profession in the Roman republic. **Trans Stud Coll Physicians Phila** 1980 Dec;5(2 no 4):267–75

**Phillips JH:** The etiology of disease: a Late Republican view. In International Congress of the History of Medicine, 27th, Barcelona, 1980. Actas. Barcelona, Académia de Ciències Mèdiques de Catalunya i Balears, 1981. p. 327–30.

**Phillips M:** Yorkshire, cradle of medical friends. **Pharm Hist (London)** 1984 Jun;14(2):6–9

**Phillips MJ** see **Burrow GN**

**Phillips PJ:** Kill or cure? Lotions, potions, characters & quacks of early Australia. Adelaide, Rigby, 1978. 157 p.

**Phillips R:** Family breakdown in late eighteenth-century France. Divorces in Rouen 1792–1803. Oxford and New York, clarendon Press, 1980. x, 244 p.

**Phillips TJ:** The intellectual roots of family practice. **Pharos** 1981 Winter;44(1):26–31

**Phillips VC** see **Bridson GD**

**Phillips WR:** Patients, pills, and professionals: the ethics of placebo therapy. **Pharos** 1981 Winter;44(1):21–5

**Phillips WR:** Sir James Mackenzie and family medicine. **Am Fam Physician** 1981 Jul;23(7):46, 50

**Phillips WR, Rosenberg J, ed:** The origins of modern treatment and education of physically handicapped children. Reprint of articles. New York, Arno, 1980. Various pagings. (The physically handicapped in society).

**Phipps A:** The runaway patient: a legend in oral circulation and the media. **Indiana Folkl** 1980;13(1-2):102–11

**Physician murderers and criminals: Forensic Sci Int** 1982 Jul–Aug;20(1):101–6

**Pi–Figueras J:** Els serveis de cirurgia moderna a l'Hospital de la Santa Creu i Sant Pau. In Congrés International d'Història de la Medicina Catalana, 2nd, Barcelona, 1975. Llibre d'Actes. Barcelona, Socitra, 1977. p. 157–61.

**Pi–Figueras J:** La cirugía moderna a Catalunya: de Cardenal al 1936. In Congrés Internacional d'Història de la Medicina Catalana, 1st, Barcelona–Montpellier, 1970. Llibr d'actes. Barcelona, Editorial Scientia, 1971. v 2, p. 193–212.

**Piaĭ LT, Kalnin VV:** Razvitie terapii v Tartuskom universitete. **Ter Arkh** 1984;56(3):44–6

**Pialoux P, Soudant J:** Geschichte der Hals–, Nasen– und Ohrenheilkunde. In Sournia JC, Martiny M, Poulet J, ed. Illustrierte Geschichte der Medizin. Salzburg, Andreas, 1980. Vol. 7. p. 2711–47.

**Piasecki E:** Umieralność niemowląt w parafii bejskiej. **Przeszlosc Demograf Pol** 1979;11:23–67

**Piatak OA, Perekhrestenko PM, Sadovskaia AG:** Programma issledonvaniĭ po istorii meditsiny i ee znachenie dlia dal'neĭshego razvitiia zdravookhraneniia, meditsinskogo obrazovaniia i meditsinskoĭ nauki v USSR. **Vrach Delo** 1981;(4):7–10

**Piatak OA, Perekhrestenko PM, Semenova NA:** 120 let meditsinskoĭ periodicheskoĭ pechati na Ukraine. **Vrach Delo** 1980 Oct;(10):1–5

**Piątkiewicz W** see **Brzozowski R**

**Piazza M** see **Disertori B**

**Picard C, Olivier A, Bertrand G:** The first human stereotaxic apparatus. The contribution of Aubrey Mussen to the field of stereotaxis. **J Neurosurg** 1983 Oct;59(4):673–6

**Picard C** see **Olivier A**

**Picard CW:** Vitamin B12: an area of darkness. **Br Med J** 1979 Oct 6;2(6194):867

**Picard JJ** see **Weets J**

**Picard JM, Aussedat M:** Historique de l'anesthésie par hypnose à Nancy. In: Congrès National des Sociétés Savantes, 103e, Nancy, 1978. Comptes Rendus. Paris, 1978. Section des Sciences, Fasc. V. p. 95–8.

**Picatoste y Patiño J, Martín García B:** La cistoscopia (1879–1979) (centenario de un invento trascendental). **Arch Esp Urol** 1980 Jul–Feb;33(1):1–18

**Picco C:** Das Biochemische Institut der Universität Zürich 1931–1981. Aarau, Verlag Sauerländer, 1981. 62 p. (Veröffentlichungen der Schweizerischen Gesellschaft für Geschichte der Medizin und der Naturwissenschaften, 37).

**Piccolo E:** L'elettrocardiografia a una svolta semeiologica. **G Ital Cardiol** 1981;11(1):1–3

**Piché V** see **Gregory JW**

**Picheau P:** Diagnostika i klassifikatsiia psikhicheskikh rasstroĭstv vo Frantsii (istoriia, sovremennye vzgliady i terminologicheskie sopostavleniia). **Zh Nevropatol Psikhiatr** 1982;82(8):103–10

**Pichot P:** Historical introduction to psychiatry. In M. Weller, ed: The scientific basis of psychiatry. London, Baillière Tindall, 1983. p. 34–46.

**Pichot P:** La recherche psychiatrique en France. **Ann Med Psychol (Paris)** 1981 Jun;139(6):640–3

**Pichot P:** Un siècle de psychiatrie. Neuilly–sur–Seine [France], Roche, [1983] 189 p.

**Pichot PJ:** The French approach to psychiatric classification. **Br J Psychiatry** 1984 Feb;144:113–8

**Pichulowa K** see **Janowiec M**

**Pickard HM:** Conservative dentistry in the past century. **Br Dent J** 1980 Jul 1;149(1):5–8

**Pickens DR:** Medical practice in early Nashville. **J Tenn Med Assoc** 1981 Sep;74(9):637–42

**Pickering G:** Walter Russell Brain. In Dictionary of national biography, 1961–1970. Suppl. 8, 1981. p. 127–9.

**Pickering G:** William Norman Pickles. In Dictionary of national biography, 1961–1970. Suppl. 8, 1981. p. 843–4.

**Pickering MJ:** A history of elderly exercises. **J Fla Med Assoc** 1980 Apr;67(4):398–400

**Pickett BH:** Remarks at the 20th anniversary celebration of the General Clinical Research Center. **Ala J Med Sci** 1984 Apr;21(2 Suppl 2):5–8

**Pickett J** see **Child abuse: historical perspective**

**Pickford M:** Ernest Basil Verney. In Dictionary of national biography, 1961–1970. Suppl. 8, 1981. p. 1035.

**Pickles M** see **Charlton C**

**Pickstone JV:** Bureaucracy, liberalism and the body in post–revolutionary France: Bichat's physiology and the Paris school of medicine. **Hist Sci** 1981 Jun;19(44 pt 2):115–42

**Pickstone JV:** Establishment and dissent in nineteenth–century medicine: an exploration of some correspondence and connections between religious and medical belief–systems in early industrial England. In Sheils WJ, ed: The Church and healing. Papers read at the twentieth summer meeting and the twenty–first winter meeting of the Ecclesiastical History Society. Oxford, Basil Blackwell for the Society, 1982. p. 165–89.

**Pickstone JV:** Ferriar's fever and Kay's cholera: disease and social structure in Cottonopolis. **Soc Soc Hist Med Bull (Lond)** 1980;27:19–22

**Pickstone JV:** Ferriar's fever to Kay's cholera: disease and social structure in cottonopolis. **Hist Sci** 1984 Dec;22(58 pt 4):401–19

**Pickstone JV:** Medical botany (self–help medicine in Victorian England). **Mem Proc Manch Lit Philos Soc** 1976–77;119:85–95

**Pickstone JV, Butler SV:** The politics of medicine in Manchester, 1788–1792: hospital reform and public health services in the early industrial city. **Med Hist** 1984 Jul;28(3):227–49

**Pictorius G:** Badenfahrtbüchlein. Wie und wo man richtig badet. Nachruck des Werkes aus dem Jahre 1560. U. Becker, ed., Basel and Wien; Herder, Freiburg, 1980. 111 p

**Pidrman V:** Hlavní směry činnosti katedry válečného vnitřního lékřství. K 25. výročí VLVDU JEvP. **Vnitr Lek** 1984 Jan;30(1):86–7

**Piechocki W:** Die Gesundheitsverhältnisse in der Stadt Halle im ausgehenden 19. Jahrhundert. **Wiss Beitr Martin Luther Univ Halle Wittenberg** 1983;5–R80:211–23

**Piechocki W:** Robert Kochs Aufenthalt in Halle zur Cholerabekämpfung im Spiegel der Presse (1893). **Wiss Beitr Martin Luther Univ Halle Wittenberg** 1983;5–R80:41–9

**Piechocki W** see **Kaiser W**

**Piel G** see **Tobach E**

**Pielat B:** Dur plamisty w poglądach Sebastiana Petrycego i Sebastiana Sleszkowskiego w i Połowie XVII wieku. **Arch Hist Med (Warsz)** 1980;43(4):393–406

**Pielmeyer K:** Statuten der deutschen medizinischen Fakultäten im Mittelalter. Ein Beitrag zur Geschichte des medizinischen Unterrichts an deutschen Universitäten anhand der Statuten der ersten 16 deutschen medizinischen Fakultäten von ihrer Gründung bis zum Ende des 16. Jahrhunderts. Diss. Bonn, 1981. 101 p.

**Pierard GE, Lapière CM:** Les corticostéroïdes à usage externe. Trente années d'utilisation et perspectives d'avenir. **Rev Med Liege** 1984 Feb 15;39(4):156–9

**Pierard GE, Lapiere CM:** Liège. The 'Ardent City' of Theodor Schwann and Tchantches. **Am J Dermatopathol** 1984 Feb;6(1):95–7

**Pierce EC:** Analysis of anesthetic mishaps. Historical perspectives. **Int Anesthesiol Clin** 1984 Summer;22(2):1–16

**Pierce J:** A dreaded disease. **Nurs Times** 1983 Jan 26–Feb 1;79(4):57–61

**Pierhal J:** Albert Schweitzer: biographie. München, Fischer, 1979 (1982 printing). 263 p.

**Pierhal J:** Albert Schweitzer. München, Kindler, 1979. 363 p.

**Pierre–Deschênes C:** Santé publique et organisation de la profession médicale au Quebec, 1870–1918. **Rev Hist Am Fr** 1981;35(3):355–75

**Pierson M** see **Neimann N**

**Pierson RR:** The double bind of the double standard: VD control and CWAC in World War II. **Can Hist Rev** 1981;62(1):31–58

**Pies E:** Ich bin der Doktor Eisenbarth. Arzt der Landstrasse. Eine Bildbiographie über das Leben und Wirken des volkstümlichen und berümten Chirurgen Johann Andreas Eisenbarth (1663–1727). Genf, Ariston, 1977. 306 p.

**Pies E:** Willem Piso (1611–1678): Begründer der kolonialen Medizin und Leibarzt des Grafen Johann Moritz von Nassau–Siegen in Brasilien: eine Biographie. Düsseldorf, Interma–Orb Verlagsgruppe, 1981. 227 p.

**Pietruschka WD** see **Hambsch K**

**Piffaretti JC** see **Peduzzi R**

**Piga Sánchez–Morate B:** Aspectos médico–legales del aborto. **An R Acad Nac Med (Madr)** 1982;99(1):51–70

**[Pigalle's bust of Dr. Maloët acquired by Fitzwilliam Museum, Cambridge, 1979.]: Burlington Mag** 1980 Jan;122:83

**Pigeaud J:** Cabanis et les rapports du physique et du moral. **Sci Tech Persp** 1981–82;1:8.1–.13

**Pigeaud J:** La maladie de l'ame: étude sur la relation de l'âme et du corps dans la tradition médico–philosophique antique.

**Pigeaud JM:** Du rhythme dans le corps. Quelques notes sur l'interprétation du pouls par le médecin Hérophile. **Bull Assoc Guillaume Bude** 1978;3:258–67

**Pigeaud JM:** Le rôle des passions dans la pensée médicale de Pinel à Moreau de Tours. **Hist Philos Life Sci** 1980;2(1):123–40

**Pigeaud JM** see **Grmek MD, ed**

**Pigem Serra JM:** Emilio Mira y López y su entorno. **Arch Neurobiol (Madr)** 1982 Mar–Apr;45(2):135–56

**Pighetti C:** L'antievoluzionismo nel Canada ottocentesco. **Physis** 1983;25(3):433–79

**Pihet C:** Les enfants abandonnés à Poitiers dans la seconde moitié du XVIIIe siècle (1755–1789). Maîtrise, Univ. de Poitiers, 1976, XII, 222 p.

**Pike JS, Ireland RL:** Pioneers in pedodontics. Kenneth Alexander Easlick, 1893–1979. **Pediatr Dent** 1982 Sep;4(3):268–9

**Pilarska–Machowicz A:** Rozwój diagnostyki bronchoskopowej. **Wiad Lek** 1982 Nov 1;35(19–20):1265–70

**Pilarska–Machowik A:** Rozwój diagnostyki bronchoskopowej. **Pieleg Polozna** 1983;(5):16–7

**Pilbeam D:** New hominoid skull material from the Miocene of Pakistan. **Nature** 1982 Jan 21–27;295(5846):232–4

**Pilbeam D:** The descent of hominoids and hominids. **Sci Am** 1984 Mar;250(3):84–96

**Pilcher GJ** see **Torrington M**

**Pilgrim I:** The too–good–to–be–true paradox and Gregor Mendel. **J Hered** 1984 Nov–Dec;75(6):501–2

**Pilipchuk NS, Pilipchuk VN:** K stoletiiu otkrytiia Robertom Kokhom vozbuditelia tuberkuleza. **Vrach Delo** 1982 Nov;(11):119–21

**Pilipchuk VN** see **Pilipchuk NS**

**Pilja M** see **Protic M**

**Pillai A** see **Vetschera T**

**Pillard E:** Nevada's treatment of the mentally ill, 1882–1961. **Nev Hist Soc Q** 1979;22(2):83–99

**Pillard RC:** Psychotherapeutic treatment for the invisible minority. **Am Behav Sci** 1982;25(4):407–22

**Pilleri G:** Josef Breuer, 1842–1925. Waldau-Bern (Schweiz), Verlag des Hiranatomischen Institutes, 1983. 81 p.

**Pilling R:** A horse on the street is a rare sight. **Am Hist Illus** 1982;17(6):42–4
**Pillsbury DM:** General Eisenhower's 'melanoma'. **J Am Acad Dermatol** 1981 May;4(5):631–2
**Pina L de, Meneses MO de:** Camilo e a historia da medicina. **Arch Hist Med Port** 1968–70;3(1–4):91–116
**Pina L de:** Farmacia ornamental uma historia portuense. **Arch Hist Med Port** 1968–70;3(1–4):117–36
**Pinchevskaia VI** see **Sheĭman IB**
**Pinchuk VG:** Razvitie ideĭ A. A. Bogomolets v oblasti izucheniia reaktivnosti organizma pri opukholevom protsesse. **Fiziol Zh** 1981 May–Jun;27(3):327–31
**Pinchuk VK** see **Lobzin VS**
**Pinckers AJ:** Leber's congenital amaurosis as conceived by Leber. **Ophthalmologica** 1979;179(1):48–51
**Pincu P:** Din istoricul unei farmacii bicentenare 'spiţeria mănăstirii neamţ'. **Rev Med Chir Soc Med Nat Iasi** 1980 Jan–Mar;84(1):137–9
**Pindborg JJ:** Nyt om Peking–manden og hans forgaengere. **Tandlaegebladet** 1981 Feb;85(3):82–5
**Pindborg JJ:** Victor Haderup. **Tandlaegebladet** 1984 Jun;88(11):411–6
**Pine C** see **Cash P**
**Pine Mountain--a clinic with a history: Front Nurs Serv Q Bull** 1984 Spring;59(4):19–28, 30
**Pineas R:** William Turner's Spirituall physik. **Sixteenth Cent J** 1983;14:387–98
**Pineau H:** Paul Broca et l'anthropologie. **Bull Acad Natl Med (Paris)** 1980;164(6):557–62
**Pineau H:** Paul Broca. L'anthropologiste et le biologiste. **Cah Anthropol** 1980;1–2:47–93
**Pineau H:** Remarque sur la bibliographie des oeuvres de Paul Broca. **Cah Anthropol** 1980;3–4:245–83
**Pineda L** see **Pinto–Cisternas J**
**Pinel P:** The clinical training of doctors. An essay of 1793. Ed. D. B. Weiner. Baltimore, Johns Hopkins University Press, 1980. 102 p. (Henry E. Sigerist suppl. to the Bull. Hist. Med. N.S. no. 3).
**Pinell P, Zafiropoulos M:** Un siècle d'échecs scolaires (1882–1982). Paris, Les Editions Ouvrières, 1983. (Collection Politique Sociale).
**Pines M:** Modern bioengineers reinvent human anatomy with spare parts. **Smithsonian** 1978;9(8):50–7
**Pines M:** The Foundations' Fund for Research in Psychiatry and the growth of research in psychiatry. **Am J Psychiatry** 1983 Jan;140(1):1–10
**Pines S:** The oath of Asaph the Physician and Yohanan Ben Zabda: Its relation to the Hippocratic Oath and the Doctrina duarum viarium of the Didaché. **Proc Isr Acad Sci Humanit** 1971–76;5:223–64
**Pingree D** see **Zimmermann F**
**Pinguet M:** 'Harakiri': L'art de l'éventrement au Japon. **Histoire** 1981;(31):10–8
**Pini UA:** Cristoforo Matteo Lusardi oculista giramondo. **Arch Stor Prov Parmensi** 1979;31:271–4
**Pini UA:** I medici parmigiani nelle poesie del Frugoni. Il medico dormiglione. **Minerva Med** 1980 Sep 22;71(35):2515
**Pini UA:** I medici parmigiani nelle poesie del Frugoni. L'Ippocrate dei mori, Medico freddoloso. **Minerva Med** 1980 Sep 19;71(34):2438–9
**Pini UA:** I medici parmigiani nelle poesie di Carlo Innocenzo Frugoni. **Minerva Med** 1980 Apr 7;71(14):1059–61
**Pini UA:** Medici e chirurghi parmigiani dell'ottocento. Notizie sulla vita e sulle opere. **Minerva Med** 1980 May 12;71(19–20):1393–8, 1461–6
**Pini UA:** Medici e chirurghi parmigiani dell'ottocento. Notizie sulla vita e sulle opere. III. **Minerva Med** 1980 Sep 1;71(31):2245–7 (continued periodically)
**Pinigin VV:** Pervyĭ vrach–iakut P.N. Sokol'nikov. **Sov Zdravookhr** 1979;(8):61–3
**Pinkerton JH:** Evory Kennedy: a master controversial. **Ir Med J** 1984 Mar;77(3):77–81
**Pinkerton JH:** John Creery Ferguson. Friend of William Stokes and pioneer of auscultation of the fetal heart in the British Isles. **Br J Obstet Gynaecol** 1980 Apr;87(4):257–60
**Pinkerton JH:** John Creery Ferguson 1802–1865: Physician and fetologist. **Ulster Med J** 1981;50(1):10–20
**Pinkerton JH:** Sir James Young Simpson: Irish influences. **Ir Med J** 1982 Jun;75(6):183–7
**Pinkham JR:** The dentist and child–patient encounter: an Adlerian analysis. **ASDC J Dent Child** 1982 Jul–Aug;49(4):266–72
**Pinkhas J** see **Weinberger A**
**Pinkus H:** Etiology of an anatomist's discoveries in dermatology. **Am J Dermatopathol** 1982 Apr;4(2):127–35
**Pinkus RL:** Innovation in neurosurgery: Walter Dandy in his day. **Neurosurgery** 1984 May;14(5):623–31
**Pinotti O:** Giulio Stella 1899–1978. **Arch Sci Biol (Bologna)** 1978 Jan–Dec;62(1–4):i–xiv
**Pinsent R:** The birth of an NHS practice. **Soc Soc Hist Med Bull (Lond)** 1983 Dec;33:11–2
**Pinsent RJ** see **Fry J**
**Pinsker H, Novick DM, Richman BL:** Hospital care at Second Avenue and East 17th Street, New York City, 1894–1984. **Bull NY Acad Med** 1984 Nov;60(9):905–24
**Pintaudi R:** Frammento di un trattato di materia medica in un Papiro Laurenziano (PL 68). **Z Papyrologie Epigraphik** 1976;23:203–7
**Pintér J:** Az urológia fejlődéséről 25 éves tapasztalat alapján. **Orv Hetil** 1980 Nov 2;121(44):2685–9
**Pinto LB:** The folk practice of gynecology and obstetrics in the Middle Ages. **Bull Hist Med** 1973 Sep–Oct;47(5):513–23
**Pinto–Cisternas J, Castelli MC, Pineda L:** La consanguinidad en la parroquia de Los Teques, Venezuela desde 1790 a 1869. **Acta Cient Venez** 1981;32(3):262–8
**Pinto–Cisternas J** see **Villarroel H**
**Pioneers in pedodontics: influential leaders of the past (John C. Brauer): Pediatr Dent** 1982 Jun;4(2):143–4
**Piontek J, Henneberg M:** Mortality changes in a Polish rural community (1350–1972) and estimation of their evolutionary significance. **Am J Phys Anthropol** 1981 Jan;54(1):129–38
**Piotrovskiĭ SM** see **Asimova MZ**
**Piotrowski A** see **Wardaszko–Lyskowska H**
**Piotrowski E:** Chirurgia starożytnego rzymu z okresu zagłady Pompei. **Wiad Lek** 1980 Jul 15;33(14):1175–8
**Piotrowski E:** Jan Mikulicz Radecki we Wrocławiu. **Arch Hist Med (Warsz)** 1979;42(3):351–7
**Piquer y Jover JJ:** Panorama històric de la radiologia a Catalunya. Barcelona, Asociación de Radiología y Electrología, 1971. 160 p.
**Pirchner F:** Wilhelm Weinberg's contribution to quantitative genetics. **Folia Mendeliana** 1978;13(63):261–6
**Pirmann F:** Fachkunde der Zahntechnik. **Zahntechnik (Geneve)** 1983;41(5):431–4, 436–8, 440–6 contd
**Piroli AT** see **Orsini M**
**Pirotte F:** Note sur l'évolution de la ladrerie de la Hesse à Tohogne. Du moyen âge à la fin de l'ancien régime. **Ann Inst Archeol Luxemb** 1975–76:106–7:163–81
**Pirozynski T** see **Bădărău GH**
**Pirsig W:** Hals–Nasen–Ohrenheilkunde im Werk des Ulmer Stadtarztes Johannes Scultetus (1595–1645). **HNO** 1984 Apr;32(4):149–54
**Pirsig W:** Historical notes and actual observations on the nasal septal abscess especially in children. **Int J Pediatr Otorhinolaryngol** 1984 Oct;8(1):43–54
**Pirsig W:** Septumdeviation 1882: Beginn der systematischen submukösen Septumchirurgie. **Laryngol Rhinol Otol (Stuttg)** 1982 Oct;61(10):547–51
**Pirsig W** see **Rodegra H**
**Pîrvulescu A** see **Pîrvulescu M**
**Pîrvulescu M, Pîrvulescu A:** Slănic Moldova, în documente ale trecutului. **Rev Med Chir Soc Med Nat Iasi** 1983 Oct–Dec;87(4):659–60
**Pisanó A:** El determinante germinal en la dinámica embriológica. **Acta Physiol Lat Am** 1979;29(1):7–13
**Piščevic S** see **Rich NM**
**Pisciotta AV:** Concepts of haemostasis and thrombosis: a study of the coagulation defect in hemophilia and in jaundice (Quick, Stanley–Brown and Bancroft 1935). Armand J. Quick (1894–1978)--a short biography. **Thromb Haemost** 1980 Aug 29;44(1):1–5
**Pisent RJ, ed** see **Fry J**
**Pisztora F:** A bel–, az elme és az ideggyógyászat viszonya hazánkban a századforduló körül. **Orv Hetil** 1982 Jun 27;123(26):1621–9
**Pisztora F, Ungvári G:** A gyógyítással és az orvostudomány haladásával kapcsolatos inventorius téveseszmék a XX. század elsö fel'eben. **Orv Hetil** 1980 Mar 23;121(12):716–7
**Pisztora F:** A kábítószer--fogyasztás a régi Vietnámban. Az ellene folytatott harc mai formái. **Orv Hetil** 1984 Oct 14;125(42):2569–72, 2575
**Pisztora F:** A schizophrenia és a paranoid kórformák gyógyítási kísérletei a Monarchia korabeli Magyarország különféle psychiátriai intézményeiben. **Orvostort Kozl** 1982;92(4):53–87
**Pisztora F:** A születési arisztokrácia súlya és a származási téveszmék gyakorisága a Monarchia társadalmában. **Orv Hetil** 1981 Jun 28;122(26):1593–5
**Pisztora F:** Evezredes–évszázados vallások és a religiózus megélés szélsőséges, valamint elmekóros formái a mai Indiában. **Orv Hetil** 1983 Mar 6;124(10):591–7
**Pisżtora F:** Tipikus társadalmi konfliktusok és reaktív neurosisok–psychosisok a Monarchia időszakában hazánkban. **Orv Hetil** 1980 Aug 10;121(32):1956–9
**Pisztora F** see **Farkas J**
**Pisztora F** see **Hörcsik E**
**Pisztora F** see **Martos G**
**Piternick LK:** Richard Goldschmidt, controversial geneticist and creative biologist: a critical review of his contribution. Basal, Boston, Birkhäuser, 1980. 153 p.
**Pitkänen K:** The changing features of mortality in Finland in the 18th and 19th centuries. The Fifth Scandinavian Demographic Symposium, 13–16 June 1979 at Hurdalssjen, Norway. **Scand Popul Stud** 1979;5:74–82
**Pitkänen K** see **Turpeinen O**
**Piton J** see **Delaunay A, ed**
**Pitot HC:** Landmark article (JAMA 1911;56:198). Transmission of a malignant new growth by means of a cell–free filtrate. By Peyton Rous. **JAMA** 1983 Sep 16;250(11):1445–9
**Pitronová B:** Hlavní rysy vývoje obyvatelstva severočeské hnědouhelné oblasti v období kapitalismu (do roku 1939). **Slezsky Sb** 1176–77;4:251–78
**Pitskhelauri GZ:** Aristotle's knowledge in the field of natural and medical sciences (on celebrating 2300 years since his death). **Sante Publique (Bucur)** 1980;23(4):375–9
**Pitskhelauri GZ:** Meditsina i vydaiushchiesia mediki srednevekovogo Vostoka. Tbilisi, Izd–vo Sabchota Sakartvelo, 1982. 234 p.
**Pitt B:** Insulin. **Br Herit** 1981;2(3):28–38
**Pittenger JC, Kuriloff P:** Educating the handicapped: reforming a radical law. **Public Interest** 1982;66:72–96
**Pittet–Faessler E:** Krankenpflege--Soins infirmiers à 75 ans. **Krankenpflege (Bern)** 1983 Jan;(1):17
**Pittman JA:** General Clinical Research Center. **Ala J Med Sci** 1984

de l'Institut de recherche universitaire d'histoire de la connaissance, des idées et des mentalités; no. 2).
**Poirier JL:** La réorganisation des études médicales selon Auguste Comte. In Poirier J, Poirier JL, ed: Médecine et philosophie à la fin du XIXe siècle. Paris, Université de Paris XII - Val de Marne, [1980?]. p. 47-59.
**Poirier S:** The physician and authority: portraits by four physician-writers. In Jones AH, ed: Images of healers. Albany, State University of New York Press, 1983. p. 21-40.
**Poirier S:** The Weir Mitchell rest cure: doctor and patients. **Womens Stud** 1983;10(1):15-40
**Poirier S:** Tobias Smollett, M.D.--expert on the body--and the bawdy. **Pharos** 1984 Winter;47(1):17-22
**Poirier JL, ed** see **Poirier J**
**Poitras JM:** Trotula of Salerno. **Md State Med J** 1980 Apr;29(4):62-4
**Pokar H** see **Brandt L**
**Pokorny L** see **Lounsbury JW**
**Pokrovskiĭ GA:** Razvitie nauchnykh issledovaniĭ vNII Proktologii za poslednie 10 let. **Khirurgiia (Mosk)** 1983 Mar;(3):40-5
**Pokrovskii AV, et al:** Sosudistyi zamenitel'iz veny pupochnogo kanatika novorozhdennogo. **Latv PSR Zinat Acad Vestis** 1981;12:80-7
**Pol LG** see **Eberstein IW**
**Poland UH:** Reflections on the Medical Library Association's international activities. **Bull Med Libr Assoc** 1982 Oct;70(4):359-68
**Polanyi TG** see **Simpson GT**
**Polenberg R:** The second victory of Anthony Comstock? **Society** 1982;19(4):32-8
**Polenova IV:** N. A. Iaroshenko i ucheniki S. P. Botkina. **Klin Med (Mosk)** 1982 Sep;60(9):117-9
**Poletaev SD, Sumbatov GA, Chausovskaia MM, et al:** Deiatel'nost' kafedry tuberkuleza Tsentral'nogo instituta usovershenstvovaniia vracheĭ v period 1931-1980 gg. **Probl Tuberk** 1980 Dec;(12):3-6
**Poletti R:** Il y a 75 ans naissait Le Bon Secours... 1905-1980. **Krankenpflege (Bern)** 1980 Nov;(11):567-9
**Polglase AL:** Rectal excision for cancer 1880 to 1980. **Med J Aust** 1981 Jan 10;1(1):3-4
**Poliak VE:** Voprosy okhrany zdorov'ia naroda v trudakh V. I. Lenina. **Feldsher Akush** 1980;45(4):5-7
**Poliakov AA** see **Shishkov VP**
**Poliakov IA, Kiselev IN:** Chislennost' i natsional'-nyi sostav naseleniia Rossii v 1917 godu. **Vopr Istor** 1980;6:39-49
**Poliakov VA:** K stoletiiu otkrytiia mestnoĭ anestezii. **Ortop Travmatol Protez** 1981 Sep;(9):65-8
**Polianskiĭ AA** see **Grando AA**
**Polikoff A:** The Interlake affair. **Wash Mon** 1971;3(1):7-17
**Politzer A:** History of otology. Volume I. From earliest times to the middle of the nineteenth century. An English translation by S. Milstein, C. Portnoff, A. Coleman from the original German edition (Stuttgart, 1907). Phoenix, Columella Press, 1981. xv, 324 p.
**Polk HC** see **Ray JW**
**Poll M:** Die Entwicklung der Gastroskopie. In M. Poll, ed: Gastro-Duodenoskopie. Grundlagen und Hinweise für die Praxis. Weinheim, Edition Medizin, 1982. p. 13-20.
**Poll M, Herlant-Meewis H:** Esquisse de l'histoire de la zoologie et de la biologie animale en Belgique depuis 1920. In Florilège des Sciences en Belgique - II. Bruxelles, Académie Royale de Belgique, 1980. p. 249-69.
**Pollack CV:** Electronic therapeutics of Albert Abrams, M.D. **Pharm Hist** 1984;26(2):109-13
**Pollack NS:** Medicine nineteenth-century style. **Echoes** 1981 Mar;20:4-5
**Pollak O:** The shadow of death over aging. **Ann Am Acad Polit Soc Sci** 1980; 447:71-7
**Pollak-Eltz A:** Folk-medicine in Venezuela. **Acta Ethnol Linguist** 1982;53:1-231
**Pollard C** see **Trautmann J**
**Pollard LJ:** Aging and slavery: gerontological perspective. **J Negro Hist** 1981 Fall;66:228-34
**Pollard MR:** Fostering competition in health care. **Proc Acad Polit Sci** 1980;33(4):158-67
**Pollay RW:** Pills, potions and palliatives: some of the social history of drug usage. **Hist Med (Lond)** 1975 Autumn-Winter;6(3-4):58-63
**Pollet M:** Naissances illégitimes, filles-mères et enfants trouvés à Grasse au XVIIIe siècle, 1751-1789. **Bull Inf Soc Demogr Hist** 1979;:5-21
**Pollitt R:** The wounding and treatment of William of Orange in 1582. **J Hist Med Allied Sci** 1982 Apr;37(2):135-58
**Pollitzer WS:** The development of genetics and population studies. **Am J Phys Antropol** 1981 Dec;56(4):483-9
**Pollock ML** see **Maud PJ**
**Pololian VIa:** Vazhneĭshie étapy sozdaniia ucheniia akademika E.N. Pavlovskogo o prirodnoĭ ochagovosti boleznei. **Vestn Akad Med Nauk SSSR** 1980;(10):10-4
**Polska bibliografia biezaca historii medycyny: Arch Hist Med (Warsz)** 1980;43(2):209-14
**Pol'ski MP:** K istorii organizatsii prodovol'stvennogo snabzhenia naseleniia v pervye gody sovetskoi vlasti. **Istor SSSR** 1974;6:149-62
**Pomata G:** Madri illegittime tra Ottocento e Novecento: storie cliniche e storie di vita. **Quad Stor** 1980;2
**Pombo MV** see **Franco Grande A**
**Pomel ML:** La médecine d'autrefois d'après des documents inédits. Le docteur Missoux (1800-1863). Rodez, Editions Subervie, 1979. 162 p.
**Pomerantz MB, Marr JS, Goldman WD:** Amebiasis in New York City 1958--1978: identification of the male homosexual high risk population. **Bull NY Acad Med** 1980 Mar;56(2):232-44
**Pomerleau CS** see **Morantz RM**
**Pomeroy SB:** Plato and the female physician ('Republic', 454d 2). **Am J Philol** 1978;99:496-500
**Pomianskaia NIu** see **Sheĭman IB**
**Pommerin R:** The fate of mixed blood children. **Ger Stud Rev** 1982;5(3):315-23
**Pommier E** see **Patrimoine hospitalier de la Bourgogne**
**Pomper P:** Nečaev, Lenin and Stalin: the psychology of leadership. **Jahrb Gesch Osteur** 1978;26(1):11-30
**Pompey H:** Pastoralmedizin--der Beitrag der Seelsorge zur psycho-physischen Gesundheit. Eine bibliographisch-historische Analyse. In Imhof AE, ed: Mensch und Gesundheit in der Geschichte. Husum, Matthiesen, 1980. p. 115-34.
**Pomponi F:** En amont de la mort: médecine et morbidité en Corse au XIXe siécle. **Etud Corses** 1979;7(12-13):251-73
**Ponak AM:** Unionized professionals and the scope of bargaining: a study of nurses. **Ind Labor Relat Rev** 1981;34(3):396-407
**Ponci R** see **Montanari L**
**Pond MA:** Block grants for health: a brief history of presidential initiatives. **Health Policy Q** 1982 Fall-Winter;2(3-4):180-98
**Pond MA:** Presidential initiatives in organizing health affairs: from Harding to Roosevelt. **Pres Stud Q** 1983;13(3):417-29
**Pond N:** Tennesse's Tyree Springs: the most celebrated watering place in the State. **Ky Folkl Rec** 1978;24(3-4):64-73
**Ponec DJ, Resnick D:** On the etiology and pathogenesis of porotic hyperostosis of the skull. **Invest Radiol** 1984 Jul-Aug;19(4):313-7
**Pongratz LJ** see **Brozek J**
**Pongratz LJ, ed** see **Baeyer WR von**
**Pongratz LJ, ed** see **Brozek J**
**Ponitz PV** see **Harris JE**
**Ponomarenko II** see **Shitskova AP**
**Ponomareva PA, Kuznetsova AI:** K 50-letiiu klinicheskikh pediatricheskikh kafedr II Moskovskogo meditsinskogo instituta im. N. I. Pirogova. **Pediatriia** 1981 Dec;(12):61-3
**Pons J, Davoust B, Pons ML:** Qui êtes-vous Monsieur Camille Bernard? **Ann Chir Plast Esthet** 1983;28(2):199-200
**Pons ML** see **Pons J**
**Pontalis JB:** Regards sur la psychanalyse en France. Paris, Gallimard, 1979. 301 p.
**Pontén J:** Gudar, präster och läkekonst. Södertälje, Axlings, 1980. 79 p. (Nordisk Medicinhistorisk Arsbok, Supplementum, VII).
**Pontius AA:** Face representation linked with literacy level in colonial American tombstone engravings and Third World preliterates' drawings. Toward a cultural-evolutional neurology. **Experientia** 1982 May 15;38(5):577-81
**Pontius AA:** Icono-diagnosis, a medical-humanistic approach, detecting Crouzon's malformation in Cook Islands' prehistoric art. **Perspect Biol Med** 1983 Autumn;27(1):107-20
**Pontuale L:** L'urbanistica 'risanatrice' a Napoli: meglio il colera? **Comunita** 1975;29(174):128-65
**Pontuch A:** Pokrokové tradície slovenského pôrodníctva. **Cesk Gynekol** 1981 Jul;46(6):423-6
**Poole JC, Holladay AJ:** Thucydides and the plague: a footnote. **Classical Q** 1982;32:235-6
**Poole JC, Holladay AJ:** Thucydides and the plague of Athens. **Classical Q** 1979;29:282-300
**Pooley FD** see **Hart GD, ed**
**Poorter DA de:** David Lipsius Iscanius, 17e-eeuws doctor medicus afkomstig uit Overijse. **Periodiek** 1980;35:16-22
**Poos LR:** Plague mortality and demographic depression in later medieval England. **Yale J Biol Med** 1981 May-Jun;54(3):227-34
**Popa LM, Repanovici R, Iliescu R:** Investigations in the field of recombinant DNA technology performed in the 'Stefan S. Nicoiau' Institute of Virology. **Virologie** 1984 Oct-Dec;35(4):315-22
**Pope BH** see **Boehm EH**
**Pope BH, ed:** Historical periodicals directory. Volume 2: Europe, West, North, Central and South. Santa Barbara, Oxford, ABC-Clio, 1983. xv, 597 p. (Clio Periodicals Directories).
**Popescu A** see **Milin M**
**Popescu V:** Centenar Robert Debré. **Rev Pediatr Obstet Ginecol [Pediatr]** 1983 Apr-Jun;32(2):97-100
**Popik SIa** see **Maĭatruk PN**
**Popik SIa** see **Maĭstruk PN**
**Popkowska N:** Przeglad problemów diagnostycznych i rehabilitacyjnych dzieci i młodzieży leczonej w Klinice Psychiatrii Akademii Medycznej w Lublinie w latach 1951-1971. **Psychiatr Pol** 1980 May-Jun;14(3):259-64
**Popov K** see **Davic P**
**Popov K** see **Sarac S**
**Popov M:** Novi materiali za istoriiata na veterinarnata meditsina u nas. **Vet Med Nauki** 1979;16(2):93-7
**Popov-Dragin O** see **Davic P**
**Popov MIa:** Ranenie i smert' bagrationa. **Vopr Istor** 1975;(3):211-4
**Popovic M:** Razvoj Instituta za pomorsku medicinu Ratne mornarice. **Vojnosanit Pregl** 1980 Sep-Oct;37(5):319-26
**Popp L:** Die Fleckfieber-Epidemie in Kulmbach im Jahre 1793. **Medizinhist J** 1981;16(3):257-69
**Popper H:** History of the American Association for the Study of Liver Diseases. **Hepatology** 1982 Nov-Dec;2(6):874-8
**Popper H:** Vienna and the liver. **Gastroenterology** 1984 May;86(5 Pt

1):982-6

**Popper L:** Die Entwicklung der Arbeitsmedizin in Osterreich und die sozialhygienische Tradition. **Arbeitsmed praventive Gesundheitspolitik** 1982;5:41-5

**Poppleston JA, McPherson MW:** The development of the archives of the history of American psychology. **Manuscripts** 1969;21(3):183-8

**Popplestone J** see **Robert I. Watson and the development of the history of psychology: a symposium**

**Popplestone JA, McPherson MW:** Pioneer psychology laboratories in clinical settings. In J. Brozěk, ed: Explorations in the history of psychology in the United States. Lewisburg, Bucknell University Press, 1984. p. 196-272.

**Popugaĭlo VM** see **Vaksman IA**

**Popushoĭ EP, Spineĭ LV:** A D. Kotsovskiĭ--vidnyĭ predstavitel' obshchestvennoĭ meditsiny Moldavii. **Sov Zdravookhr** 1980;(9):58-61

**Popushoĭ EP, Andrievskiĭ VA:** Iz istorii sozdaniia Kostiuzhenskoĭ psikhiatricheskoĭ lechebnitsy. **Sov Zdravookhr** 1984;(9):65-6

**Popushoĭ EP, Ioksa VA:** Mediko-geograficheskie opisaniia--vazhnyĭ istochnik izucheniia istorii metitsiny Moldavii. **Sov Zdravookhr** 1983;8:58-61

**Popushoĭ EP, Ioksa VA:** N. A. Doroshevskiĭ - peredovoĭ vrach, uchastnik revoliutsionne-demokraticheskogo dvizheniia. **Sov Zdravookhr** 1982;(11):55-7

**Popushoĭ EP, Ioksa VA:** N. P. Zubku-Kodrianu--progressivnyĭ vrach, vidnyĭ uchastnik revoliutsionno-demokraticheskogo dvizheniia. **Sov Zdravookhr** 1979;(3):59-63

**Popushoĭ EP, Ioksa VA:** Progressivnaia rol' vracha-revoliutsionera P. P. Tutyshkina v razvitii nauchnoĭ mysli v Moldavii. **Sov Zdravookhr** 1984;(4):69-71

**Popushoi EP:** Rol' meditsinskikh obvshchestv Moldavii v razvitii meditsinskoĭ mysli vo vtoroi polovine XIX--nachale XX veka. **Sov Zdravookhr** 1982;(1):65-8

**Popushoĭ EP, Ioksa VA:** Vklad A. V. Korchaka-Chepurkovskogo v razvitie zdravookhraneniia i bor'bu s épidemiiami v Moldavii. **Zh Mikrobiol Epidemiol Immunobiol** 1983 Oct;(10):109-11

**Popushoĭ EP, Ioksa VA:** Vklad nauchnykh meditsinskikh obshchestv Moldavskoĭ SSR v razvitie narodnogo zdravookhraneniia. **Sov Zdravookhr** 1984;(8):54-7

**Popushoĭ VP, Spineĭ LV:** Viktor Krésesku--vrach, revoliutsioner, pisatel'. **Sov Zdravookhr** 1981;(5):62-4

**Popv A:** Razvitie i segashno sŭstoianie na Katedrata po vŭtreshni bolesti. **Vutr Boles** 1981;20(6):6-11

**Porfilio RL** see **Ptalis P**

**Porkert M, Ullmann C:** Die chinesische Medizin. Düsseldorf, Wien, Econ Verlag, 1982. 416 p.

**Porkert M:** Sens et non-sens des recherches modernes sur la pharmacopée traditionnelle de la Chine. In Mazars G, ed: Les médecines traditionnelles de l'Asie. Strasbourg, Université Louis Pasteur, 1981. p. 49-56.

**Porksheian OKh** see **Mazurenko MD**

**Porst S:** Gynäkologie und Geburtshilfe bei Shakespeare. **Zentralbl Gynakol** 1984;106(12):863-75

**Porst S:** Gynäkologische, geburtshilfliche, embryologische und teratologische Beschreibungen im Werke Shakespeares. Würzburg, Horst Wellm, 1981. 178 p. (Dissertation, Julius-Maximilians-Universität Würzburg).

**Portal C, Rideau M, Viel C:** Quelques aspects de l'oeuvre de Duhamel de Monceau dans le domaine des sciences naturelles et des sciences physiques. In: Congrès National des Sociétés Savantes, 107e. Brest, 1982. Comptes Rendus, Paris, 1982. Section des Sciences, Fasc. IV. p. 341-50.

**Portele KA:** Die Henning-Moulagen des Pathologisch-anatomischen Bundesmuseums in Wien. **Med Lab (Stuttg)** 1979 Feb;32(2):41-3

**Portele KA:** Die Moulagensammlung des Pathologisch-Anatomischen Bundesmuseums in Wien. [Wien, Pathologisch-Anatomisches Bundesmuseum in Wien], 1977. 84 p.

**Porter GA:** Gouty nephropathy: fact or fiction? **Am J Kidney Dis** 1983 Mar;2(5):553-4

**Porter J:** Nursing in Imperial Russia. Nurses under siege. **Nurs Mirror** 1980 Oct 16;151(16):24-6

**Porter JR:** L'Hôpital-Général de Québec et le soin des aliénés (1717-1845). **Can Cathol Hist Assoc Study Sess** 1979;:23-55

**Porter KA** see **Starzl TE**

**Porter KR:** An informal tribute to George E. Palade. **J Cell Biol** 1983 Jul;97(1):D3-7

**Porter KR, Bennett HS:** Introduction; recollections on the beginnings of the Journal of Cell Biology. **J Cell Biol** 1981 Dec;91(3 pt 2):IX-XI

**Porter KR:** The cytomatrix: a short history of its study. **J Cell Biol** 1984 Jul;99(1 Pt 2):3s-12s

**Porter KR** see **Pease DC**

**Porter R:** Being mad in Georgian England. **Hist Today** 1981 Dec;31:42-8

**Porter R:** Cleaning up the Great Wen: public health and eighteenth-century London. **Soc Soc Hist Med Bull (Lond)** 1984 Dec;35:24-5

**Porter R:** Death and the doctors. **Med Hist** 1982 Jul;26(3):335-41

**Porter R:** Dictionaries and the history of science. **Hist Sci** 1980;18(2):148-50

**Porter R:** Le prospettive della 'follia': scienza, medicina, e letteratura nell'Inghilterra dell '700. **Intersezioni** 1982;2:55-76

**Porter R:** Medicina e illuminismo nell' Inghilterra del settecento. **Quad Stor** 1979;14(1):155-80

**Porter R:** Medicine and the Enlightenment in Eighteenth century England. **Soc Soc Hist Med Bull (Lond)** 1979 Dec;25:27-40

**Porter R:** Shutting people up. **Soc Stud Sci** 1982 Aug 3;12(3):467-76

**Porter R:** The descent of genius: Charles Darwin's brilliant career. **Hist Today** 1982 Jul;32:16-22

**Porter R:** The rage of party: a glorious revolution in English psychiatry? **Med Hist** 1983 Jan;27(1):35-50

**Porter R:** Was there a medical Enlightenment in 18th-century England? **Br J 18th-Cent Stud** 1982;5:49-63

**Porter R:** Was there a moral therapy in eighteenth century psychiatry? **Lychnos** 1981-82;:12-26

**Porter RW:** Variations in shape and size of the lumbar spinal canal. **Paleopathol Newsl** 1980 Dec;32:9-11

**Porter S** see **Roy I**

**Porter TM:** The calculus of liberalism: the development of statistical thinking in the social and natural sciences of the nineteenth century. Ph.D. Diss., Princeton University. Princeton, 1981. iv, 365 leaves.

**Porter R, ed:** Liber amicorum. Repertorio biografico di storia della medicina e delle scienze naturali. **Kos Liber Amicorum** 1984;1- (continued regularly)

**Porter R, ed** see **Bynum WF**

**Porter R, ed** see **Rousseau GS**

**Portmann G:** The old and new in Meniere's disease -- over 60 years in retrospect and a look to the future. **Otolaryngol Clin North Am** 1980 Nov;13(4):567-75

**Portmann G:** The 'Revue de Laryngologie' and the E. N. T. School of Bordeaux are a hundred years old. **Rev Laryngol Otol Rhinol (Bord)** 1980 Jan-Feb;101(1-2):1-14

**Portmann M, Bebear JP, Bagot D'Arc M:** L'histoire de l'otosclérose du XIXe siècle à 1952. **Acta Otorhinolaryngol Belg** 1982;36(2):297-305

**Portmann ML:** Der Basler Medizinprofessor Johann Jacob Harder (1656-1711) als Geburtshelfer. **Gesnerus** 1983;40(1-2):139-47

**Portmann ML:** Der Basler Stadtarzt Johannes Huber (1507-1571). **Gesnerus** 1981;38:81-91

**Portmann ML:** Relations d'Auguste Tissot (1728-1797), médecin à Lausanne, avec le patriciat bernois. **Gesnerus** 1980;37(1/2):21-7

**Portmann ML** see **Buess H**

**Portugal FH, Cohen JS:** A century of DNA: a history of the discovery of the structure and function of the genetic substance. Cambridge, MIT Press, 1977. xiii, 384 p.

**Portulov BM:** Torzhestvo ideĭ V. I. Lenina v meditsine. **Sov Med** 1980;(4):3-9

**Portwood D, Fielding A:** Privilege and the professions. **Sociol Rev** 1981 Nov;29(4):749-73

**Porubčinová Z:** Pokrokové tradice katedry sociálního lékařstvílékařské faculty UJEP v Brně. **Cesk Zdrav** 1983 Feb;31(2):71-6

**Porubský V** see **Kokavec M**

**Porus VN:** Ludwick Flecks's epistemological conception and contemporary discussion on the nature and dynamics of scientific knowledge. **Kwart Hist Nauki Tech** 1983;28(3-4):545-60

**Poser H** see **Hasler L, ed**

**Poses RM** see **Maulitz RC**

**Posinovec J:** Histologija i embriologija u djelu dra Ante Schwarza (u povodu 100. obljetnice njegove smrti). **Lijec Vjesn** 1980 Apr;102(4):208-10

**Posinovec J:** O hrvatskom stomatološkom nazivlju u drugoj polovici XIX. stoljeća. **Lijec Vjesn** 1980 May;102(5):282-3

**Posner E:** Josiah Wedgwood's doctors. **Pharm Hist (London)** 1973 Sep;3(2):2-5

**Posner E:** Milestones in the history of mineral dust pneumoconioses. In J. Cule, ed: Wales and medicine. London, British Society for the History of Medicine, 1975. p. 42-53.

**Posner MI** see **Hearst E, ed**

**Posner NA** see **Grossman E**

**Posner NA** see **Grossman EA**

**Posner RM:** Thomas Starr King and the mercy million. **Calif Hist Soc Q** 1964;43(4);291-308

**Pospísil L:** K prioritě objevu specifické imobilizace treponém. **Cesk Dermatol** 1981 Oct;56(5):346-8

**Possehl I:** Die Arzneitaxe--auch im 19. Jahrhundert ein Problem. **Beitr Gesch Pharm** 1980;8:61-3

**Possehl I:** Impfstoffe, Sera, Diagnostika - Resultate bakteriologischer und immunologischer Forschung. In Hickel E, Schröder G, ed: Neue Beiträge zur Arzneimittelgeschichte. Festschrift für Wolfgang Schneider zum 70. Geburtstag. Stuttgart, Wissenschaftliche Verlagsgesellschaft, 1982. p. 185-203.

**Possehl T:** Probleme der Arzneipreisgestaltung im 19. Jahrhundert. **Medizinhist J** 1981;16(4):358-90

**Post DL:** Floyd H. Allport and the launching of modern social psychology. **J Hist Behav Sci** 1980 Oct;16(4):369-76

**Post RJ** see **Crosskey RW**

**Postel J:** Les névroses. Evolution historique du concept de 1769 à nos jours. **Soins Psychiatr** 1982 Feb;(16):13-9

**Postel J:** Les premières expériences psychiatriques de Philippe Pinel à la Maison de santé Belhomme. **Can J Psychiatry** 1983 Nov;28(7):571-6

**Postel J, Quétel C, ed:** Nouvelle histoire de la psychiatrie. Toulouse, Privat, 1983. 774 p. Contributions by J. Bancaud, P. Berner, F. Bing.

**Postel J:** Un manuscrit inédit de Philippe Pinel sur 'Les guérisons opérées dans le 7ème emploi' de Bicêtre, en 1794. **Rev Int Hist Psychiatr** 1983;1(1):79-82

**Postel J** see **Gineste T**

**Postlewait T:** Bernard Shaw and science: the aesthetics of causality. In Paradis J, Postlewait T, ed: Victorian science and Victorian values: literary perspectives. New York, New York Academy of Sciences, 1981. p. 319-58.

**Prebluda HJ** see **Bing FC**

**Prebluda HJ** see **Day HG**

**Predy GN:** A brief history of public health in Alberta. **Can J Public Health** 1984 Sep–Oct;75(5):366–7

**Preiser G:** Wein im Urteil der griechischen Antike. In Völger G, ed: Rausch und Realität. Drogen im Kulturvergleich. Teil 1. Köln, Raufenstrauch-Joest-Museum für Völkerkunde der Stadt Köln, 1981. p. 296–303 (Materialienband zu einer Ausstellung 7. Aug. bis 11. Okt. 1981).

**Preiser G:** Wein im Urteil der Römer. In Völger G, ed: Rausch und Realität. Drogen im Kulturvergleich. Teil 1. Köln, Raufenstrauch-Joest-Museum für Völkerkunde der Stadt Köln, 1981. p. 304–8 (Materialienband zu einer Ausstellung 7. Aug. bis 11. Okt. 1981).

**Preiser G** see **Habrich C**

**Preisig R** see **Kotwas J**

**Preĭsman BS** see **Il'in II**

**Prem HJ:** Seuchengeschichte von Zentralmexiko im 16. Jahrhundert. Ein Modell für die heutige weltweite Seuchensituation? **Fortschr Med** 1981 Sep 24;99(36):1421–2

**Premio Abraham Horwitz. Dr. Martin M. Cummings: Bol Of Sanit Panam** 1984 Jan;96(1):73–8

**Premuda L:** Arthur Menzel (1844–1878), einer der liebsten und tüchtigsten Schüler und der treuesten Freunde Billroths, Primarchirung in Triest. **Gesnerus** 1981;38:191–205

**Premuda L:** Claude Bernard e gli indirizzi della fisiologia e della medicina nel secolo XIX. **Minerva Med** 1982 Feb 25;73(7):329–35

**Premuda L:** Considerazioni sull'illustrazione anatomica dall'antichità all'Ottocento. **Acta Med Hist Patav** 1980–81;27:31–40

**Premuda L:** Die Medizin in der Sicht eines italienischen Denkers der Aufklärung. **Gesnerus** 1983;40(3/4):249–56

**Premuda L:** G. B. Morgagni und seine Vorstellungen über die Methodik der Medizin. **Sudhoffs Arch** 1984;68(2):173–81

**Premuda L:** I fondamenti storici dell'ortognatodonzia. **Mondo Ortod** 1980 Mar–Apr;5(2):35–42

**Premuda L, Gasparini F:** La protesi dentaria: breve excursus storico. **G Stomatol Ortognatodonzia** 1982 Dec;1(4):7–10

**Premuda L:** La storia della medicina nelle facoltà mediche: ruolo e prospettive dell'insegnamento e della ricerca. **Acta Med Hist Patav** 1978–79;25:15–40

**Premuda L:** L'istanza sociale in Ramazzini pre-illuminista. **Med Lav** 1983 Nov–Dec;74(6):433–41

**Premuda L, Bonuzzi L:** Morgagni e la neuropatologia. **Acta Med Hist Patav** 1982–83;29:75–81

**Premuda L:** Schweizer Medizinstudenten und Arzte im Gebiet zwischen Padua und Triest. **Gesnerus** 1984;41(3–4):299–321

**Premuda L:** Significativi ritorni: Pierre Fauchard (1690–1761). **G Stomatol Ortognatodonzia** 1982 Apr–Jun;1(1):5–9

**Premuda L:** Storia della quarantena nei porti italiani. In Radovi sa Medunarodnog simpozija u povodu sestote obljetnice Dubrovacke karantene. Dubrovnik, 29 i 30. rujna 1977. Zagreb, 1980. p. 107–18.

**Premuda L:** The influence of the nineteenth-century Vienna School on Italian medicine: the roles of Padua and Trieste. In Stevenson LG, ed: A celebration of medical history. Baltimore, Johns Hopkins University Press, 1982. (The Henry E. Sigerist supplements to the Bulletin of the History of Medicine; new ser., no. 6). p. 180–99. With commentary by J. J. Bylebyl, p. 200–11.

**Premuda L:** The revival of the anatomico-clinical method in Padua: the fundamental contribution of F. S. Verson (1805–1849) from Trieste, a disciple of the Vienna School of Medicine. **Janus** 1980;67(1–2–3):31–9

**Premuda L** see **Albrecht von Haller, 1708–1777**

**Premuda L** see **Habrich C**

**Premuda L, et al:** L'illustrazione scientifica: ieri e oggi. **Acta Med Hist Patav** 1980–81;27:9–120

**Prentner H:** Geschichte der Urologie in Würzburg. Diss. Würzburg, 1981. 68 p.

**Preobrazhenskiĭ NA, Konstantinova NP:** Vsesoiuznoe nauchnoe obshchestvo otorinolaringologov k 60-letiiu obrazovaniia SSSR. **Vestn Otorinolaringol** 1982 Nov–Dec;(6):8–13

**Přerovsky J** see **Reinis Z**

**Prescott GW:** American Microscopical Society: the first one-hundred years. Part II. **Trans Am Microsc Soc** 1979 Apr;98(2):165–94

**Prescott JF:** The extensive medical writings of soldier-poet John McCrae. **Can Med Assoc J** 1980 Jan 12;122(1):110,113–4

**Prescott LF:** The Regional Poisoning Treatment Centre, Edinburgh. In Passmore R, ed: Proceedings of the Royal College of Physicians of Edinburgh Tercentenary Congress, 1981. Edinburgh, Royal College of Physicians of Edinburgh, 1982. p. 211–20.

**Presentación de José Vicente Bustillos. Una paradoja?: Rev Med Chil** 1983 Oct;111(10):1075–84

**Présentation des grands syndromes cliniques par atteinte focale des hémisphères cérébraux et par lésion du corps calleux. Données historiques: Rev Med Suisse Romande** 1984 Jul;104(7):477–91

**Presentation of the Gold Headed Cane to Arthur T. Hertig: Am J Pathol** 1979 Aug;96(2):365–8

**The preservation of medical and public health records:** (Research Publications of the Wellcome Unit for the History of Medicine, Oxford, No. I). Oxford, Wellcome Unit for the History of Medicine, 1979. 52 p. Contributions by C. Webster, P. Barnes, E. Freeman, H. Francis, B. Parry-Jones.

**The presidents: J Am Dent Assoc** 1979 Oct;99(4):601 (continued periodically)

**The presidents: J Am Dent Assoc** 1983 Oct;107(4):690 (continued periodically)

**The presidents. George Hoppin Çushing, 1871–1872: J Am Dent Assoc** 1979 Dec;99(6):956

**Presl J:** K stoletému výročí narození prof. MUDr. Jiřího Trapla--zakladatele československé perinatologie. **Cesk Gynekol** 1980 Sep;45(8):611–3

**Presly AS:** From madhouses to mental hospitals: does history repeat itself? **Scott Med J** 1983 Jan;28(1):71–4

**Pressat R:** Evolution des naissances en Chine. **Population** 1980;35(4–5):968–72

**Pressat R:** Mesures natalistes et relèvement de la fécondité en Europe de l'est. **Population** 1979;34(3):533–48

**Pressat R:** Pertes subies par la population de l'U.R.S.S. 1918–1958. **Population** 1979;34(6):1147–52

**Pressat R:** Situation démographique de l'U.R.S.S. à la veille de son cinquième recensement. **Population** 1979;34(4–5):845–68

**Pressley LC, ed** see **Wallace ER**

**Pressly JA** see **McBryde AM**

**Pressman D:** The development and use of radiolabeled antitumor antibodies. **Cancer Res** 1980 Aug;40(8 Pt 2):2960–4

**Pressman IaM:** E. A. Asratian i nauchnoe sodruzhestvo neĭrofiziologiov sotsialisticheskikh stran. **Zh Vyssh Nerv Deiat** 1983 Mar–Apr;33(2):211–5

**Preston B:** Further statistics of inequality. **Sociol Rev** 1979;27(2):343–50

**Preston CB** see **Pereira CB**

**Preston RD:** William Thomas Astbury. In Dictionary of national biography, 1961–1970. Suppl. 8, 1981. p. 41–2.

**Preston SH:** A halandóság és a gazdásagi fejlettség szintje közötti változó kapcsolat. **Demografia** 1976;19(2–3):228–55

**Preston SH** see **Johansson SR**

**Preston W:** Fear and loathing in addicted America. **Rev Am Hist** 1975;3(1):123–8

**Prestwich PE:** French workers and the temperance movement. **Int Rev Soc Hist** 1980;25(1):35–52

**Prestwich PE:** Temperance in France: the curious case of absinth. **Hist Reflect** 1979;6(2):301–19

**Preto P:** Peste e società a Venezia nel 1576. Vicenza, Neri Pozza Editore, 1978. 230 p.

**Pretresco A:** Dos conmemoraciones. **Rev Neuropsiquiatr** 1980 Jun;43(2):115–23

**Pretty GL, Calder A:** Mummification in Australia and Melanesia. In A. Cockburn, E. Cockburn, ed: Mummies, disease, and ancient cultures. Cambridge, Cambridge University Press, 1980. p. 194–210.

**Pretty GL** see **Pounder DJ**

**Preus A:** Biomedical techniques for influencing human reproduction in the fourth century B.C. **Arethusa** 1975;8:237–63

**Prevost A:** La selección natural en la evolución biológica. **Arbor** 1982;113(441–2):21–40

**Pribram KH** see **Kasschau RA**

**Price DB** see **Hand WD, ed**

**Price DE:** John Friend Mahoney. In Dictionary of American Biography, Suppl. 6, 1956–1960. p; 423–4, 1980.

**Price HH:** The Falklands: rate of British psychiatric combat casualties compared to recent American wars. **J R Army Med Corps** 1984 Jun;130(2):109–13

**Price JE:** Tuberculosis in west Texas, 1870–1940. Ph.D. Diss., University of Texas Grad Sch. of Biomed Sci. Galveston, 1982. x, 418 p.

**Price L:** Sydney Eye Hospital. **Br J Ophthalmol** 1982 Oct;66(10):617–21

**Price R:** Estado, iglesia, caridad y viruela: una crisis epidémica en la Ciudad de México 1797–98. **Bol Soc Mex Hist Filos Med** 1984 Mar;7(46):269–87

**Price R:** Hydropathy in England 1840–70. **Med Hist** 1981 Jul;25(3):269–80

**Price R:** Spanish medicine in the Golden Age. **J R Soc Med** 1979 Nov;72(11):864–74

**Price R:** St. Albans Medical Club. **J Int Wine Food Soc** 1979;6(1):7–12

**Price R:** State church charity and smallpox: an epidemic crisis in the City of Mexico 1797–98. **J R Soc Med** 1982 May;75(5):356–7

**Price R:** Wellcome Institute for the History of Medicine: American Collections. **Newsl Am Stud Libr Group** 1979;3:13

**Price R** see **Somolinos-Palencia J**

**Price R, ed:** An annotated catalogue of medical Americana in the Library of the Wellcome Institute for the History of Medicine. Books and printed documents 1557–1821 from Latin America and the Caribbean Islands and manuscripts from the Americas 1575–1927. London, Wellcome Institute for the History of Medicine, 1983. xix, 319 p.

**Prickler H:** Die Pestepidemie des Jahres 1600. **Burgenl Heimatbl** 1971;33(3):109–16

**Pridmore S:** The history of disease in Tasmania. **Mater Med Pol** 1980;12(4):302–3

**Priebe PM, Kauffman GB:** Making governmental policy under conditions of scientific uncertainty: a century of controversy about saccharin in Congress and the laboratory. **Minerva** 1980 Winter;18(4):556–74

**Prieto Cantero A** see **Garcia Gonzalez R**

**Prijs B:** Chymia Basiliensis: Episoden aus der Basler Chemiegeschichte. Basel; New York, Karger, 1983. x, 125 p.

**Prince AM:** Detection of the relation between the Australia antigen and hepatitis B virus. **Vox Sang** 1984;47(3):257–60

**Prince J:** Education for a profession: some lessons from history (Florence Nightingale). **Int J Nurs Stud** 1984;21(3):153–63

**Prindle RF:** Disinfection--yesterday and today. **Resid Staff Physician** 1977 Dec;23(12):suppl 1s–5s, 10s–11s

**Pringle JK, Saba SJ:** Langage médical et politique locale: l'urbanisme et la santé à Marseille à la fin de l'Ancien Régime. **Ann Midi** 1981;93(154):397-417

**Pringle KC:** Neonatal surgery: historical perspectives and a glimpse of the future. In Smith GF, Smith PN, Vidyasagar D, ed: Historical review and recent advances in neonatal and perinatal medicine. [Chicago?], Mead Johnson Nutritional Division, 1983. Vol. II. p. 85-105.

**Pringle KC** see **Smith GF**

**Prins G:** Disease at the crossroads: towards a history of therapeutics in Bulozi since 1876 [1]. **Soc Sci Med [Med Anthropol]** 1979 Dec;13B(4):285-315

**Prioleau E:** Leprosy. Reality and metaphor in literature. **Am J Dermatopathol** 1983 Aug;5(4):377-80

**Prioleau E:** The literary epidermists. **Am J Dermatopathol** 1981 Winter;3(4):359-60

**Pritchard A:** Alchemy: a bibliography of English-language writings. London, Routledge & Kegan Paul jointly with The Library Association, 1980. 439 p.

**Pritchet CD, ed:** Iohannis Alexandrini Commentaria in sextum librum Hippocratis Epidemiarum. Leiden, Brill, 1975. xi, 470 p.

**Pritikin RI:** History of the development of physical modalities in ophthalmology. In: Congrès international d'histoire de la médecine, XXVe, Québec, 1976. Actes. Québec, 1977. p. 1095-111.

**Probst C** see **Schweppe KW**

**Probst J:** Lorenz Heister, 1683-1758 Praeceptor Chirurgiae. **Unfallchirurgie** 1984 Feb;10(1):1-8

**Probst J:** Unfallmedizin und Lebensversicherungsmedizin. **Lebensversicherungsmedizin** 1982 Nov 25;34(9):193-4

**Proceedings of a symposium held to commemorate the bicentenary of Charles Waterton (1782-1865): Br J Anaesth** 1983 Mar;55(3):221-33

**Proceedings of the State Medical Convention, held in Raleigh, April, 1849, and Constitution and Medical Ethics of the Medical Society of the State of North Carolina, then adopted: NC Med J** 1982 Mar;43(3):212-21

**Procès-verbaux des délibérations du Collège de Pharmacie de Paris: Rev Hist Pharm (Paris)** 1981;28(248):45-8 (continued regularly)

**Procès-Verbaux des délibérations du Collège de Pharmacie, puis Société libre des Pharmaciens de Paris: Rev Hist Pharm (Paris)** 1982 Jun;29(253):109-14

**Procès-verbaux des délibérations du Collège de Pharmacie, puis Société libre des Pharmaciens de Paris: Rev Hist Pharm (Paris)** 1984 Mar;31(260):73-6

**Procès-verbaux des délibérations du Collège de Pharmacie, puis Société libre des Pharmaciens de Paris: Rev Hist Pharm (Paris)** 1984 Jun;31(261):171-6

**The process of child therapy: Publ Group Adv Psychiatry** 1982;11(111):3-220

**Procházka J:** Poznámky k rozvoji československé plicní chirurgie. **Cas Lek Cesk** 1984 Jan 27;123(4):85-8

**Proctor RC:** History of drinking in America. **South Med J** 1984 Jul;77(7):886-92

**Prof. Dr S. Halter (1916-1981): Arch Belg** 1984;42(7-8):349-89

**Profesor dr med. Stanisław Konopka (1896-1982). Wspomnienie: Pol Tyg Lek** 1983 Sep 5;38(36):1125-6

**Proffitt E:** Science and Romanticism. **Ga Rev** 1980;34(1):55-80

**Profile:** four academic pioneers who stayed to help the Health Center grow. **J Fla Med Assoc** 1980 Mar;67(3):298-301

**Prokhorov AA:** Dostizheniia gigieny na zheleznodorozhnom transporte. **Gig Sanit** 1982 Dec;(12):49-52

**Prokhorova G:** Prodovol'stvennaia problema kapitalizma. **Mirovaia Ekon Mezhdunar Otnosheniia** 1981;(9):81-91

**Prokhorova MI:** E. S. London i funktsional'naia neĭrokhimiia. **Nerv Sist** 1982;23:137-42

**Proklina TL** see **Borisenko NF**

**Prokof'eva-Bel'govskaia AA:** [G. A. Levitskiĭ and Soviet research on chromosome morphology.] (Rus). **Istor Biol Issled** 1978;7:46-64

**Prokop M:** Pro vorkutu, holod ta problemy samooborony narodu. **Sucasnist** 1980;(3):48-56

**Prokopec J:** Die Entwicklung des Gesundheitswesens in der CSSR. **Med Ges** 1979;(6):110-22

**Prokopec M** see **Pounder DJ**

**Prokupek J:** Dvacet roku výzkumného ústavu psychiatrického. **Cesk Psychiatr** 1981 Dec;77(6):361-3

**Prokupek J:** Pražská psychiatrická klinika před 50 lety. **Cesk Psychiatr** 1982 Apr;78(2):127-36

**Prölss E** see **Kössling FK**

**Prone A** see **Puech PF**

**Propach G:** Johann Heinrich Jung-Stilling (1740-1817) als Arzt. Köln, 1983. 410 p. (Arbeiten der Forschungsstelle des Instituts für Geschichte der Medizin der Universität zu Köln, Band 27).

**A propos du syndrome de Turner: LARC Med** 1981 Oct;1(1):63

**Propping P:** Genetic disorders presenting as 'schizophrenia'. Karl Bonhoeffer's early view of the psychoses in the light of medical genetics. **Hum Genet** 1983;65(1):1-10

**Propst A:** Bernd Lederer. **Verh Dtsch Ges Pathol** 1982;66:652-7

**Pros JR:** Padesát let gynekologické poradny pro sportovkyně. **Cesk Gynekol** 1983 Feb;48(1):55-6

**Proshansky HM, ed** see **Tobach E**

**Proskauer C:** A pictorial history of dentistry. **Tic** 1979 May;38(5):13-4 (continued periodically

**Proskauer C:** A pictorial history of dentistry. Part 1 -- prehistoric, Egyptian, Assyrian. **Tic** 1979 Feb;38(2):8-10 (continued periodically)

**Prosper Baumès, dermatologist of Lyon 1791-1871 and the Willan-Alibert controversy: Br J Dermatol** 1981 Dec;105(6):727-31

**Proteau J** see **Penneau D**

**Protic M, Sarac V, Pilja M, et al:** Stomatologija Vojvodine: razvojni put, stanje i perspektiva. **Med Pregl** 1982;35(11-12):499-502

**Protic M** see **Straser P**

**Protiva M:** Wývoj chemie psychofarmak za posledních 20 let. **Cesk Psychiatr** 1978 Dec;74(6):337-49

**Proudfit WL:** Origin of concept of ischaemic heart disease. **Br Heart J** 1983 Sep;50(3):209-12

**Proudfit WL:** The Fleece Medical Society. **Br Heart J** 1981 Dec;46(6):589-94

**Proudfoot AT:** The development of clinical toxicology in Edinburgh. In Passmore R, ed: Proceedings of the Royal College of Physicians of Edinburgh Tercentenary Congress, 1981. Edinburgh, Royal College of Physicians of Edinburgh, 1982. p. 204-10.

**Proust J:** Francis Anthonie, charlatan elisabéthain. In: Devins et charlatans au temps de la Renaissance. ed. M.T. Jones-Davies. Paris, Université, Centre de Recherches sur la Renaissance, 1979. p. 101-11.

**Proux C:** Geschichte der Radiotherapie. In Sournia JC, Martiny M, Poulet J, ed: Illustrierte Geschichte der Medizin. Salzburg, Andreas, 1980. Vol. 6. p. 2223-41.

**Prouzet J:** Le Service de Santé au cours des guerre de religion dans les pays d'Aude. **Bull Soc Etud Sci Aude** 1979, 1980;79:85-7

**Provine WB:** Francis B. Sumner and the evolutionary synthesis. **Stud Hist Biol** 1979;3:211-40

**Provine WB** see **Lewontin RC**

**Provine WB, ed** see **Mayr E**

**Pruett CE:** Naval medicine and modern sea power. **Nav Rev** 1965;10:238-59

**Pruett RC** see **Nussbaum JJ**

**Pruitt RD:** Symptoms, signs, signals, and shadows. The pathophysiology of angina pectoris--a historical perspective. **Mayo Clin Proc** 1983 Jun;58(6):394-8

**Pruitt RD:** William Osler and his Gulstonian lectures on malignant endocarditis. **Mayo Clin Proc** 1982 Jan;57(1):4-9

**Pruitt VD:** Yeats, the Mask, and the poetry of old age. **J Geriatr Psychiatry** 1982;15(1):99-112

**Prunet P:** Nouvelles technologies et vaccination antirabique. **Arch Inst Pasteur Tunis** 1982 March;59(1):115-20

**Prusiński A:** Professor dr hab. nauk med. Eufemiusz Herman - nestor polskiej neurologii (w 90 urodziny). **Neurol Neurochir Pol** 1982;(5-6):306-28

**Pruyser PW:** Religio medici: Karl A. Menninger, Calvinism and the Presbyterian Church. **J Presbyt Hist** 1981;59(1):59-72

**Prvi kongres liljećnika Narodnooslobodilačke Fronte Hrvatske:** Glina--Topusko--Slunj, 24--27. Veljače 1944. **Lijec Vjesn** 1979 Nov;101(11):686-90

**První české přednásky na Pražské lékařské fakultě - Kuřákovy přednásky z fysiologie: Cesk Fysiol** 1983;32(5):467-8

**Prydsö U** see **Helm S**

**Prygova NM:** Metody i vidy lecheniia u atstekov. **Klin Med (Mosk)** 1982 Feb;60(2):110-2

**Prygova NM:** O roli gosudarstva v meditsinskom dele atstekov (k voprosu ob izuchenii metsiny rabovladel'cheskikh obshchestv). **Sov Zdravookhr** 1981;(8):68-71

**Prygova NM:** Sanitariia i gigiena v atsteksom obshchestve (k istorii sanitarii i gigieny v Meksike). **Gig Sanit** 1981 Aug;(8):54-6

**Pryor EG:** The great plague of Hong Kong. **J Hong Kong Branch R Asiat Soc** 1975;15:61-70

**Pryor RJ:** Morbidity and minerals: health and mortality in Victoria in the 1850s. Canberra, Department of Demography, Australian National University, 1977. 26 leaves. (Working paper in demography, 5).

**Przepiórkowska E** see **Pawela T**

**Przyboś A:** Smierć wieźnia Stefana Przybosia w Mauthausen. **Przegl Lek** 1984;41(1):97-9

**Przychodzki M:** Dr Stanislaw Janiszewski. **Przegl Lek** 1981;38(1):180-2, 187-9

**Przychodzki M:** Lekarze Poznanscy w latach hitlerowskiej okupacji 1939-1945. **Przegl Zachod** 1977;33(1):106-39

**Przychodzki M:** Płk dr Eugeniusz Parczewski. **Przegl Lek** 1981;38(1):177-9

**Psatta DM:** Thirty years of research (II). **Neurol Psychiatr (Bucur)** 1982 Jan-Mar;20(1):3-28

**Pszczółkowska-Simiczyjew J:** Kształcenie pielegniarek ogólnych na dolnym śląsku w pierwszym xx-leciu Polski Ludowej. **Slaski Kwart Hist Sabotka** 1979;34(4):529-40

**Ptalis P, Porfilio RL:** The evolution of a State Department of Health: an example of the shift of the responsibility of health care from the private to the public sector. **Long Term Care Health Serv Adm Q** 1977 Summer;1(2):124-36

**Ptashekas RS:** K 25-letiiu patomorfologicheskoĭ laboratorii Litovskogo instituta ėksperimental'noĭ i klinicheskoĭ meditsiny. **Arkh Patol** 1983;45(12):76-8

**Ptashka EM** see **Kovaleva EP**

**Publications by John R. Lindsay: Ann Otol Rhinol Laryngol [Suppl]** 1983 Jan-Feb;102:33-6

**Puche J, Folch i Pi A:** El Doctor August Pi Sunyer. **Xaloc** 1980;16(105):10-2

**Püchel J:** Die Geschichte des German Hospital in London (1845 bis 1948). Münster, Murken-Altrogge, 1980. 207 p. (Studien zur Geschichte des Krankenhauswesens, 14).

**Puchkov IuG, Buslaeva MM, Volodina MN:** Georg Papanikolau (k 100-letiiu so dnia rozhdeniia). **Vopr Onkol** 1983;29(12):87-9

**Puchtler H, Meloan SN:** On Schiff's bases and aldehyde-fuchsin: a review from H. Schiff to R. D. Lillie. **Histochemistry** 1981;72(3):321-32

**Puciłowski O** see **Płaźnik A**

**Puckrein G:** Climate, health and black labor in the English Americas. **J Am Stud** 1979;13(2):179-93
**Puckrein GA:** Humoralism and social development in Colonial America. **JAMA** 1981 May 1;245(17):1755-7
**Puech PF, Prone A, Albertini H:** Reproduction expérimentale des processus d'altération de la surface dentaire par friction non abrasive et non adhésive: application à l'étude de l'alimentation de l'homme fossile. **C R Seances Acad Sci [III]** 1981 Nov 9;293(9):497-502
**Puech PF, Prone A:** Reproduction expérimentale des processus d'usure dentaire par abrasion: implications paléoécologiques chez l'homme fossile. **C R Acad Sci [D] (Paris)** 1979 Nov 19;289(13):895-8
**Puente Veloso S:** Aportación de la botánica a la medicina en el reinado de Carlos III. **An R Acad Nac Med (Madr)** 1982;99(3):437-501
**Puerto Sarmiento FJ:** Andrés Alcón (1782-1850), farmacéutico, político y profesor de Química. **Bol Soc Esp Hist Farm** 1984 Sep;35(139):143-64
**Puerto Sarmiento FJ, Cobo Cobo J:** La evolucion de la quimica farmaceutica durante el siglo XVIII. **Bol Soc Esp Hist Farm** 1983 Mar-Jun;34(133-134):25-33
**Puerto Sarmiento FJ:** Las luchas en torno al monopolio farmacéutico, vistas desde el Colegio de Farmacéuticos de Madrid, durante el periodo de la Junta Superior Gubernativa de Farmacia (1800-1839). **Bol Soc Esp Hist Farm** 1980 Mar-Jun;3(121-2):69-96
**Puerto Sarmiento FJ:** Las luchas en torno al monopolio farmacéutico vistas desde el Colegio de Farmacéuticos de Madrid (1839-1855). **Bol Soc Esp Hist Farm** 1980/81 Dec-Mar;31-32(124-5):9-33
**Puerto Sarmiento FJ** see **Folch Jou G**
**Pugh LG, Sutton JR:** Everest then and now. **Prog Clin Biol Res** 1983;136:415-30
**Pugin P** see **Hahnloser P**
**Pugliese P:** The scientific achievement of Robert Hooke: method and mechanics. Ph.D. Diss., Harvard University. Cambridge, 1982. xv, 353 leaves. (Pt. 1).
**Puhvel J** see **Hand WD, ed**
**Puig-Samper Mulero MA:** El Doctor Pedro Gonzalez de Velasco y la antropologia española en el siglo XIX. **Asclepio** 1982;34:327-37
**Puigvert A, Mallo N:** El sindrome próstato-hemorroidal. **Rev Clin Esp** 1983 Feb 15;168(3):217-9
**Puigvert A:** The young Albarrán in Spain. **Eur Urol** 1981;7(1):57-9
**Puissant A** see **Tsankov N**
**Pujadas Muñoz JJ** see **Comelles JM**
**Pujol F:** L'odontologie à la fin de l'empire romain: Caelius Aurelianus. **Chir Dent Fr** 1984 May 31;54(252):21-5
**Pulaski MS:** Understanding Piaget. Revised and expanded ed. New York, Harper & Row, 1980. xvii, 248 p.
**Pulatov AM:** Abuali Ibn-Sina (Avitsenna) i ego nauchno-meditsinskoe nasledie. **Vrach Delo** 1980 Sep;(9):1-6
**Pulatov RP** see **Shukurov AK**
**Pulewka P:** Neunzehn Jahre als Pharmakologe in der Türkei. **Ther Ggw** 1980 Feb;119(2):199-211
**Pulewka P:** Seit 56 Jahren Arzt und Forscher. **Ther Ggw** 1980;119:216-28
**Pullat R:** Istoricheskaia demografiia v SSR (znachenie, mesto, itogi i perspektivy razvitiia). **Probl Istor Demogr SSSR** 1977;8-17
**Pullat R** see **Mereste U**
**Pullen JJ:** Gentleman, this is no humbug. **Am Heritage** 1979;30(5):80-96
**Pulos L:** Mesmerism revisited: the effectiveness of Esdaile's techniques in the production of deep hypnosis and total body hypnoanaesthesia. **Am J Clin Hypn** 1980 Apr;22(4):206-11
**Puma A:** La Escuela de Alejandría y nuestro Occidente. **Med Secoli** 1981;17:237-44
**Puma A:** La escuela de Alejandría y nuestro occidente. In International Congress of the History of Medicine, 27th, Barcelona, 1980. Actas. Barcelona, Académia de Ciències Médiques de Catalunya i Balears, 1981. p. 610-5.
**Puma A:** Medicinas pretécnicas? In International Congress of the History of Medicine, 27th, Barcelona, 1980. Actas. Barcelona, Académia de Ciències Médiques de Catalunya i Balears, 1981. p. 616-20.
**Puma FA:** Cientificismo (enfermedad de nuestros días). **Rev Soc Venez Hist Med** 1981;30(45-46):57-83
**Puma FA:** Edad media y medicina. **Rev Soc Venez Hist Med** 1975-76;23(37):37-59
**Puma FA:** El significado historico de la anatomia. **Rev Soc Venez Hist Med** 1969-71;17-19(31-33):91-108
**Puma Fabricatore A:** Sobre la medicina romana autoctona. **Rev Soc Venez Hist Med** 1972-73;20-21(34-35):155-60
**Pumphrey RE** see **Breul FR**
**Punch TM:** Jonathan Prescott, M.D.: vincit qui patitur. **NS Hist Q** 1979;9(1):59-80
**Pünder T** see **Heinemeyer W**
**Punnett L:** Marie Elizabeth Zakrzewska 1829-1902. **Women Health** 1976 Jul-Aug;1(4):1-2
**Punnett L:** Women-controlled medicine--theory and practice in 19th century Boston. **Women Health** 1976 Jul-Aug;1(4)3-11
**Purcell EF, ed** see **Bowers JZ**
**Purévzhav T:** Razvitie rentgenoradiologicheskoĭ sluzhby v Mongol'skoĭ Narodnoĭ Respublike. **Vestn Rentgenol Radiol** 1981;(3):74-6
**Puric J, Obradovic M:** Radovi Stevana Koturovića i Bogoljuba Jovanovića o samoubistvima u Srbiji od 1845. do 1884. i od 1898. do 1907 godine. **Srp Arh Celok Lek** 1983 Apr;111(4):513-9
**Purkov J:** Razvoj neonatološke službe u Zrenjaninu. **Med Pregl** 1983 Jan;36(1-2):61-4
**Pursell CW** see **Durbin PT, ed**
**Purushothamacharyulu G:** Pandit D. Gopalacharyulu, regenerator of ayurveda. **Sachitra Ayurved** 1981 Mar;:194-200
**Purves SJ** see **Low MD**
**Pŭrvi Natsionalen kongres po istoriia na meditsinata:** Shumen, 9-11 oktomvri 1981 god: reziumeta. Bulgaria], Nauch. druzhestvo po istoriia na meditsinata v Bŭlgariia, [1981?]. 146 p.
**Püschel E:** 'Dictata' zu den Werken von Johannes de Gorter (1689-1762), professor in Harderwijk: medicinae compendium, praxis medicae systema und chirurgia repurgata. **Janus** 1980;67(1-2-3):41-57
**Püschel E:** Die Quarantäne auf Malta. Geschichte--Lazarettos und Hospital--Vorschriften. In Göpfert W, Otten HH, ed: Metavoeite: wandelt euch durch neues Denken. Düsseldorf, Triltsch, 1983. p. 95-105.
**Püschel E:** Die Seenotverbände der Deutschen Luftwaffe und ihr Sanitätsdienst 1939 1945. Düsseldorf, Droste, 1978. 180 p. ((Schriftenreihe Erfahrungen des deutschen Sanitätsdienst im zweiten Weltkrieg, 1).
**Püschel E:** Ein hundertjähriger Medizinstudenten-Stock. **Medizinhist J** 1983;18(3):260-5
**Püschel E** see **Habrich C**
**Putney DT:** Fighting the scourge: American Indian morbidity and federal policy, 1897-1928. Ph.D. Diss., Marquette University. Milwaukee, 1980. 355 leaves.
**Putnoky J:** The development of psychology in Hungary between 1945 and 1970. **Ann Univ Sci Budap Rolando Eotvos Nominatae** 1972;(3):95-102
**Putschar WG, Ortner DJ:** Zur Paläopathologie der Skelett-Missbildungen und -Dysplasien. **Verh Dtsch Ges Pathol** 1982;66:147-50
**Putschar WG** see **Ortner DJ**
**Putscher M:** Climbing Jacob's Ladder: on dreams. In: Congrèss international d'histoire de la médecine, XXVe, Québec, 1976. Actes. Québec, 1977. p. 1112-9.
**Putscher M:** Die Geschichte der Medizin zwischen normativem und historischem Denken. In International Congress of the History of Medicine. 26th, Plovdiv, 1978. Actes du Congress. Sofia, 1981. Volume II. p. 190 1.
**Putscher M:** Ein Totentanz von Tizian. Die 17 grossen Holzschnitte zur Fabrica Vesals (1538-1542). In Göpfert W, Otten HH, ed: Metavoeite: wandelt euch durch neues Denken. Düsseldorf, Triltsch, 1983. p. 23-40.
**Putscher M:** Jaspers und Van Gogh--oder über Krankheit und Kunst. **Janus** 1980;67(1-2-3):157-69
**Putscher M:** Le malattie nell'iconografia scientifica. **Acta Med Hist Patav** 1980-81:27:43-53
**Putscher M** see **Baur O**
**Putscher M, ed:** Rheinische Splitter und Augenblicke. Köln, Institut für Geschichte der Medizin der Universität zu Köln, 1976. 75 p.
**Puwalsi W** see **Stefański K**
**Puymèges D:** Les anatomies mouvantes. **Milieux** 1981-82;7-8:62-9
**Puzik VI** see **Strukov AI**
**Puzin D** see **La Salpêtrière**
**Pyke DA:** Claude Bernard et l'étiologie du diabète. **Journ Annu Diabetol Hotel Dieu** 1981;:153-61
**Pyke M:** Alfred Louis Bacharach. In Dictionary of national biography, 1961-1970. Suppl. 8, 1981, p. 59-60.
**Pyle GF, Rees PH:** Modeling patterns of death and disease in Chicago. **Econ Geogr** 1971;47(4):475-88
**Pyle GF:** The diffusion of cholera in the United States in the nineteenth century. **Geogr Anal** 1969;1:59-75
**Pyne RH** see **Allan P**
**Pyo YS** see **Kim JS**
**Pyrig LA, Mel'man NIa, Nemirovich LI:** K istorii nauchnykh issledovaniĭ po nefrologii v nefrologii v Ukrainskoĭ SSR. **Vrach Delo** 1983 Dec;(12):1-5
**Pytel' AIa:** Bol', prishedshaia iz glubiny vekov (k 375-letiiu so dnia rozhdeniia Rembrandta). **Sov Med** 1980;(12):98-9
**Pytel' AIa:** I. F. Zemmel'weis: ego bolezn' i prichina smerti. **Sov Med** 1979 Oct;(10):119-21
**Pytel' AIa:** Ioakhim Al'barran i ego rol' v razvitii urologii. **Urol Nefrol (Mosk)** 1981 Nov-Dec;(6):56-61
**Pytel' AIa:** Nicolaus Van Tul'p - vydaiushchiĭsia anatom i khirurg (k 340-letiiu opublikovania ego znamenitoĭ knigi 'Meditsinskie nabliudeniia'). **Khirurgiia (Mosk)** 1980 Aug;(8):117-9
**Pytel' AIa:** O pervykh kholetsistektomiiakh v Rossii. **Khirurgiia (Mosk)** 1981 Jan;(1):116-8
**Pytel' AIa:** Ob otkrytii Bil'gartsem vozbuditelia urinarnogo shistosomoza. **Urol Nefrol (Mosk)** 1980 May-Jun;(3):67-70
**Pytel' AIa:** Velikiĭ russkiĭ khirurg Nikolaĭ Ivanovich Pirogov (k 100-letiiu so dnia smerti). **Urol Nefrol (Mosk)** 1981 Jan-Feb;(1):3-8

# Q

**Qiu Renzong:** [On the origin of medicine ... from sorcery] (Chi). **Chin J Med Hist** 1981;11(1):6-10
**Quadagno JS:** Aging in early industrial society. Work, family, and social policy in nineteenth-century England. New York, Academic Press, 1982. xvi, 231 p. (Studies in Social Discontinuity).
**Quadagno JS:** From poor laws to pensions: the evolution of economic support for the aged in England and America. **Milbank Mem Fund Q** 1984 Summer;62(3):417-46
**Quaini M:** Il modello panoptico nel primo manicomio di Genova. **Mov Operaio Soc** 1980;3(4):395-404
**Quart L, Auster A:** The wounded vet in postwar film. **Soc Policy** 1982;13(2):24-31

**Quattlebaum JK:** Medicine in early Georgia (Savannah). **J Med Assoc Ga** 1983 Dec;72(12):829–32
**Qué es la Federación Odontológica Colombiana: Rev Fed Odontol Colomb** 1982 Jul–Sep;31(142):97–113
**Quen JM:** Forensic psychiatry. **JAMA** 1980 Jan 4;243(1):30
**Quen JM:** Isaac Ray and the development of American psychiatry and the law. **Psychiatr Clin North Am** 1983 Dec;6(4):527–37
**Quen JM:** Remarks on Doctor Isaac Ray (1807–1881). **RI Med J** 1980 Jun;63(6):217–9
**Quen JM** see **Carlson ET**
**Querner H:** 'Ein Wort über den Einfluss naturwissenschaftlicher Institute auf humane Bildung' (G. A. Goldfuss 1821). In Seidler E, Schott H, ed: Bausteine zur Medizingeschichte. Stuttgart, Steiner, 1984. p. 86–93.
**Querner H:** La cuestion metodologica en la biologia del siglo XIX. **Folia Hum (Barc)** 1981;19(225):595–611
**Querner H** see **Hasler L, ed**
**Questionnaire aux hôpitaux: Krankenpflege (Bern)** 1983 May;(5):32–4
**Quetel C:** L'asile d'aliénés en 1900. **Histoire** 1978;7:25–34
**Quétel C, ed** see **Postel J**
**Quevauviller A:** L'hygiène au XVIIIe siècle d'après l'abbé Jacquin. **Rev Hist Pharm (Paris)** 1980 Mar;27(244):24–38
**Queyrie G:** L'hôpital général de Tulle sous l'Ancien régime: etude économique et sociale (à suivre). **Bull Soc Lett Sci Arts Correze** 1982;85:72–91
**Qui BS** see **Yang KL**
**Quijano Narezo M:** México en las relaciones internacionales de salud. **Salud Publica Mex** 1983 Sep–Oct;25(5):519–23
**Quijano-Pitman F:** Desarrollo y estado actual de la cirugía del corazón. **Arch Inst Cardiol Mex** 1979 Sep–Oct;49(5):984–1002
**Quijano-Pitman F** see **Pacheco CR**
**Quilali air strip: Marine Corps Gaz** 1970;54(11):41–3
**Quin NE:** The impact of diseases on military operations in the Persian Gulf. **Milit Med** 1982 Sep;147(9):728–34
**Quindós LS** see **Fernández PL**
**Quinn FB** see **Clark WD**
**Quinn J:** Medical education in Mississippi. **J Miss State Med Assoc** 1981 Dec;22(12):325–9
**Quinn KF:** Banting and his biographers: maker of miracles, makers of myth. **Queens Q** 1982;89(2):243–59
**Quinn S:** [Development in nursing practice in the United Kingdom since 1948] (Jpn). **Kango** 1984 Jul;36(8):31–6
**Quinn S:** [Nursing in the European Community; nursing in Belgium]. **Kango** 1982 Mar;34(3):67–79
**Quinn S** see **Allan P**
**Quinn S, ed:** Nursing in the European community. London, Croom Helm, 1980. 192 p. With contributions by S. Russell, J. Delaide, K. Stallknecht, C. Allaire, R. Elster, I. Leydon, P. Breccia, D. Schol, M. Van Driel Krol, R. I. Emblin.
**Quiñones-Soto RA** see **Ramírez Ronda Ch**
**Quinta de Salud la Alianza, Barcelona:** 75 aniversari (1904–1979), editat per la 'Quinta de Salud la Alianza; dirigit y realitzat pel Servei Tecnic de Relacions Publiques de la Comission de Foment. Barcelona, Printer Industria Grafica S. A., 1979. 93 p.
**Quintana C:** Cincuentenario de la Facultad de Medicina de la Pontificia Universidad Católica de Chile. **Rev Med Chil** 1980 Jul;108(7):645–8
**Quintero García P:** Janusz Korczac. **Rev Soc Venez Hist Med** 1979;28(42):31–5
**Quintiliani R** see **Kotwas J**
**Quintyn JB:** Jozef Frans Kluyskens (1771–1843), eerste voorman van het Vlaams-Belgisch doktersgild. **Sartonia** 1980 Dec;49:1–37
**Quiroga M:** Juan Angel Farini, medico. **Bol Acad Nac Hist (Argentina)** 1967;40:348–53
**Quiroga MI:** La lepra, pasado y presente. Buenos Aires, Lopez, 1974. 195 p.
**Quiroga MI:** Un centro medico en Paris formado por colegas argentinos en 1901. **Bol Acad Nac Med B Aires** 1980;58:611–2
**Quisi Q** see **Armocida G**
**Quitt MH, ed** see **Fox VC**
**Qureshi IH** see **Said HM, ed**
**Qvist G:** John Hunter, 1728–1793. London, Heinemann, 1981. xvi, 216 p.

# R

**Raacke ID:** Agnes Fay Morgan. In: Notable American women. The modern period. Cambridge, Mass., Belknap-Harvard Univ. Press, 1980. 4:495–7.
**Raacke ID:** Herbert Mclean Evans (1882–1971). A biographical sketch. **J Nutr** 1983 May;113(5):929–43
**Raacke ID:** Jane Anne Russell. In: Notable American women. The modern period. Cambridge, Mass., Belknap-Harvard Univ. Press, 1980. 4:610–1.
**Raacke ID:** Marjorie Maxine Nelson. In Dictionary of American biography, 1961–1965. Suppl. 7, 1981. p. 568–9.
**Raalte M van** see **Horstmanhoff HF, ed**
**Raalte M van** see **Horstmanhoff HF, et al**
**Raalte M van, et al:** Epidemieën in Oudheid en Middeleeuwen. **Hermeneus Tijdschr Antieke Cult** 1979;51(2):57–169
**Rabasa SL:** Dificultades del neo-darwinismo a los 100 años de la muerte de Darwin (19–IV–1882). **Medicina (B Aires)** 1982;42(2):213–6
**Rabe V:** Ida Sophia Scudder. In: Notable American women. The modern period. Cambridge, Mass., Belknap-Harvard Univ. Press, 1980. 4:634–6.
**Rabel RJ:** Diseases of soul in Stoic psychology. **Greek Roman Byz Stud (Cambridge, Mass.)** 1981;22:385–93
**Rabgay L:** The origin and growth of medicine in Tibet. **Tibetan Med** 1981;3:3–31
**Rabin D** see **Rabin PL**
**Rabin PL, Rabin D:** Landmark perspective: The care of the patient. Francis Peabody revisited. **JAMA** 1984 Aug 10;252(6):819–20
**Rabinovich RS, Serdiuk GV, Egorysheva IV, et al:** Znamenatel'nye i iubileĭnye daty istorii kardiologii 1984. **Kardiologiia** 1984 Feb;24(2):124–5
**Rabinovich RS** see **Egorysheva IV**
**Rabinovich RS** see **Vengrova IV**
**Rabinovich MIa** see **Volokhov AA**
**Rabo M, Kullberg G:** [Swedish Nurses' Association's historical collection: witness to harsh conditions. Nursing departments.] (Swe) **Vardfacket** 1979;3(7):79–82
**Raboch J:** Historický vývoj lékařské sexuologie. **Cesk Psychiatr** 1982 Oct;78(5):353–7
**Race RR, Sanger R:** Fisher's contribution to Rh. **Vox Sang** 1982;43(6):354–6
**Race RR, Sanger R:** Some early and surprising blood group findings. **Vox Sang** 1983;44(2):126–8
**Rachal RE** see **Young RC Jr**
**Rachels J:** Can ethics provide answers? **Hastings Cent Rep** 1980 Jun;10(3):32–40
**Rachev RI:** Nachalo i razvitie na izkustvenoto osemeniavane na zhivoti v Shumenski okrŭg. **Vet Med Nauki** 1980;17(5):96–8
**Rachkov BM, Potanina MN:** Razvitie neĭrokhirurgii v Rossiĭskoĭ Federatsii. **Zh Vopr Neirokhir** 1982 Nov–Dec;(6):3–7
**Rachman AW, Raubolt RR:** The pioneers of adolescent group psychotherapy. **Int J Group Psychother** 1984 Jul;34(3):387–413
**Rachmanovna DO** see **Victorovich YV**
**Rachootin S** see **Bateson W**
**Rack HD:** Doctors, demons and early Methodist healing. In Sheils WJ, ed: The Church and healing. Papers read at the twentieth summer meeting and the twenty-first winter meeting of the Ecclesiastical History Society. Oxford, Basil Blackwell for the Society, 1982. p. 137–52.
**Racker E:** Resolution and reconstitution of biological pathways from 1919 to 1984. **Fed Proc** 1983 Sep;42(12):2899–909
**Rackham J:** Rattus rattus: the introduction of the black rat into Britain. **Antiquity** 1979;53:112–20
**Racz S:** Selected paragraphs from the 1789 edition of Samuel Rácz's textbook of physiology. With corresponding English translation by E. Kovács and C. Szabó. In E. Schultheisz, ed: History of physiology. Oxford, Elmsford, New York, Pergamon, 1981. xvi, 208 p. (Advances in Physiological Sciences. Proceedings of the 28th International Congress of Physiological Sciences, Budapest, 1980. Volume 21). p. 89–203.
**Radbill SX:** Arnold Lucius Gesell. In Dictionary of American biography, 1961–1965. Suppl. 7, 1981. p. 283–5.
**Radbill SX:** Infant feeding through the ages. **Clin Pediatr (Phila)** 1981 Oct;20(10):613–21
**Radbill SX:** Josef Hyrtl's Philadelphia connection. **J Hist Med Allied Sci** 1984 Apr;39(2):222–4
**Radbill SX:** Joseph Ioor Waring, 1897–1977. **J Hist Med Allied Sci** 1978 Jul;33(3):427–8
**Radbill SX:** Remarks on the Kate Hurd Mead lectures. **Trans Stud Coll Physicians Phila** 1977 Apr;44(4):179–81
**Radbill SX:** The cock as a symbol of medicine. **Adler Mus Bull** 1981;7(1):7–9
**Radbill SX** see **Cone TE**
**Radbill SX** see **Hand WD, ed**
**Radchenko VV:** Osoboe vnimanie podrastaiushchemu pokoleniiu (1917–1926 gg). **Sov Arkh** 1979(2):43–6
**Radcliff-Umstead D, ed:** Human sexuality in the Middle Ages and Renaissance. Pittsburgh, University of Pittsburgh Center for Medieval and Renaissance Studies, 1978. viii, 193 p. (University of Pittsburgh publications on the Middle Ages and the Renaissance, 4). Contributions by B. D. Palmer, J. Spisak, D. S. McCoy, T. G. Benedek, J. Schwartz, M. J. Thorssen, M. Novy, H. E. Faletti.
**Raddatz FJ:** Der Zahn, behandelt durch den Künstler. **Zahnarztl Mitt** 1983 Dec 1;73(23):2603–32
**Radford P:** Gilbert White: medical and social aspects of his letters. **Bristol Med Chir J** 1984 Apr;99(370):46–7
**Radhakrishna S** see **Sutherland I**
**Radice A** see **D'Amore C**
**Raditsa L:** Some sense about Wilhelm Reich. New York, Philosophical Library, 1978. 126 p.
**Radiukiewicz S:** Opieka nad matką i dzieckiem. **Pieleg Polozna** 1981;(6):1–3
**Radlitzki T:** Reshimot mimei hakibush hagermani Be-lvov (Lemberg), 1941–1943. **Yalkut Moreshet Period** 1976;21:7–34
**Radnabazar Zh:** Razvitie zdravookhraneniia v Mongol'skoĭ Narodnoi Respublike. **Sov Zdravookhr** 1983;(4):50–2
**Radner S:** Den selektiva angiografins bakgrund och begynnelse. **Sydsven Medicinhist Sallsk Arsskr** 1982;19:109–18
**Radnót M:** Ifj. Imre József (1884–1945). **Orv Hetil** 1984 Jun 10;125(24):1453–4
**Rado L:** Death redefined: social and cultural influences on legislation. **J Commun** 1971;31(1):41–7
**Radochoński M:** Ewolucja idei terapii rodszinnej w USA. **Psychiatr Pol** 1982;16(3):187–94
**Rádóczy G:** A Magyarországon Hivatalos gyógyszernormatívumok. **Orvostort Kozl** 1981;93–96(27 No 1–4):123–53
**Rádóczy G:** Norma Pauperum: Amtliche Standardrezeptsammlungen neben dem Arzneibuch in Ungarn. In Hickel E, Schröder G, ed: Neue Beiträge zur Arzneimittelgeschichte. Festschrift für Wolfgang Schneider zum 70.

Geburtstag. Stuttgart, Wissenschaftliche Verlagsgesellschaft, 1982. p. 71–80.
**Rádóczy G:** Régi gyógyszerészi mértékegységek és kialakulásuk története. **Orvostort Kozl** 1979;87–88(25 no 1–2):229–41
**Radosh M** see **Marcum JP**
**Radovi sa Medunarodnog simpozija u povodu sestote obljetnice Dubrovacke karantene:** Dubrovnik, 29. i 30. rujna 1977. Zagreb, Jugoslavenska Akademija Znanosti i Umjetnosti, 1980. 173 p.
**Radovic M, Taseski J:** Služba za transfuziju krvi i ratovi. **Vojnosanit Pregl** 1979 Sep–Oct;36(5):359–64
**Radt SL:** Zu Thukydides' Pestbeschreibung. **Mnemosyne** 1978;31:233–45; 1979;32:163
**Radziwiłł M** see **Kuźnicki L**
**Raf L:** Skandinaviska kirurger forst med beskrivning av tecken på appendicit. **Lakartidningen** 1984 Aug 8;81(32–33):2829–30
**Räf L** see **Husberg K**
**Räf PO** see **Thunberg CP**
**Rafaelsen OJ:** Thudichum: the founder of neurochemistry. In Rose FC, Bynum WF, ed: Historical aspects of the neurosciences. New York, Raven, 1982. p. 293–305.
**Rafail PA** see **Sokal MM**
**Rafajdusová I** see **Krahulec I**
**Raffel MW:** The U. S. health system. New York, Wiley, 1980. ix, 639 p.
**Raffel S:** Fifty years of immunology. **Annu Rev Microbiol** 1982;36:1–26
**Rafferty AM** see **Hardy L**
**Rafter GW:** Banting and Best and the sources of useful knowledge. **Perspect Biol Med** 1983 Winter;26(2):281–6
**Raghunathan K** see **Pandey AN**
**Ragsdale BD:** Gunshot wounds: a historical perspective. **Milit Med** 1984 Jun;149(6):301–15
**Ragsdale JS:** What did Thomas Jefferson mean by 'I have not yet lost a tooth by age'? **J Am Dent Assoc** 1984 Apr;108(4):643–4
**Ragumov RN, Aleskerov DSh:** Razvitie i dostizheniia rentgenologii i radiologii v Azerbaĭdzhane. **Vestn Rentgenol Radiol** 1982 Nov–Dec;(6):81–3
**Raheem Rafeeq MA** see **Ismail M**
**Rahim MA:** The contribution of Muslim medical scientists during the British period in India: a bibliography. **JPMA** 1980 Jan;30(1):17–21
**Rahimtoola SH:** The twenty-fifth anniversary of valve replacement: a time for reflection. **Circulation** 1985 Jan;71(1):1–3
**Rahman A, Alvi MA, Khan Ghori SA, et al:** Science and technology in Medieval India. A bibliography of source materials in Sanskrit, Arabic and Persian. New Delhi, Indian National Science Academy, 1982. xxxi, 719 p.
**Rahman F:** Essence and existence in Ibn Sina: the myth and the reality. **Hamdard** 1981;4(1):3–14
**Rahman F:** Islam and medicine: a general overview. **Perspect Biol Med** 1984 Summer;27(4):585–97
**Rahman SA:** Avicenna on digestion of food. **Bull Indian Inst Hist Med (Hyderabad)** 1981;1–4:59–63
**Rahman Baig MA:** Avicenna's principles of dietetics. **Bull Indian Inst Hist Med (Hyderabad)** 1981;1–4:95–8
**Rahn H** see **Robin ED, ed**
**Rai NP, Tiwari SK, Upadhya SD, et al:** The origin and development of pulse examination in Medieval India. **Indian J Hist Sci** 1981, reçu 1982;16(1):77–88
**Rai NP** see **Chaturvedi GN**
**Raics J:** Tauffer Vilmos mint szülészeti miniszteri biztos. **Orvostort Kozl** 1980;89–91(26 no 1–3):137–55
**Raimer SS** see **Smith EB**
**Rainer JK:** Cervical disc surgery––a historical review. **J Tenn Med Assoc** 1984 Jan;77(1):12–6
**Raines JR:** Dr. John McLoughlin. **JAMA** 1982 Mar 19;247(11):1566–7
**Rainger R:** The Henry Fairfield Osborn Papers at the American Museum of Natural History. **Mendel Newsl** 1980 Jun;(18):8–13
**Rains AJ:** A thought for Carl Langenbuch (1846–1901): a centenary. **Ann R Coll Surg Engl** 1982 Jul;64(4):268–9
**Rains AJ:** The continuing message. **Ann R Coll Surg Engl** 1984 May;66(3):151–8
**Rains AJ:** 'The Nightingale touch'. **J R Army Med Corps** 1982 Feb;128(1):4–17
**Raison A** see **Filliozat J**
**Raison A, ed:** La Haritasamhita: texte médical sanskrit; avec un index de nomenclature ayurvédique. Pondichéry, Institut français d'indologie, 1974. xlvi, 396 p. (Publications de l'Institut français d'indologie; no. 52).
**Raisz LG** see **Kahn AJ**
**Raiter AW:** Wspomnienia z piotrkowskiej partyanckiej słuzby sanitarnej. **Przegl Lek** 1981;38(1):155–9
**Raith L:** Johann Ernst Wichmann––ein zu Unrecht wenig bekannter Dermatologe des 18. Jahrhunderts. **Dermatol Monatsschr** 1983;169(11):725–7
**Raivio K:** Satavuotias duodecim-seura ja kehittyyä lääketiede. **Duodecim** 1981;97(20):1661–3
**Raj N:** The homoeopathic treatment of cholera; a historical study. **Bull Indian Inst Hist Med (Hyderabad)** 1978;8(1–4):39–43
**Rajkov M:** Jedan popis zdravstvenih radnika u velikokikindskom dištriktu 1875. Godine. **Naucni Sastanak Zb Rad Naucno Drus Istor Zdrav Kult Jugosl** 1976;(13):157–62
**Rajkovic D** see **Beric B**
**Raju TN:** Some famous 'high risk' newborn babies. In Smith GF, Smith PN, Vidyasagar D, ed: Historical review and recent advances in neonatal and perinatal medicine. [Chicago?], Mead Johnson Nutritional Division, 1983. Vol. II. p. 187–9.
**Raju TN:** Soranus of Ephesus: who was he and what did he do? In Smith GF, Smith PN, Vidyasagar D, ed: Historical review and recent advances in neonatal and perinatal medicine. [Chicago?], Mead Johnson Nutritional Division, 1983. Vol. II. p. 179–86.
**Raju TN** see **Smith GF**
**Rák K:** Korunk orvosi szakirodalma és a klinikai medicina. **Orv Hetil** 1980 Sep 14;121(37):2243–8
**Rak Y** see **Cronin JE**
**Rakic L:** Prilog proučuvanju zdravstvenih prilika u Bačkoj posle revolucije 1848–1849. **Naucni Sastanak Zb Rad Naucno Drus Istor Zdrav Kult Jugosl** 1980;21:149–52
**Rakitskaia TV** see **Borisenko NF**
**Rákóczi T:** Adatok az 1831. évi kolerajárvány Moson megyei történetéhez. Tanulmányok Györ és vidéke történetéböl (Gecsényi L., ed.), Györ, Györ-Sopron megyei l.sz. Levéltár, 1978, p. 71–8.
**Rakotonirina-Randriambeloma PJ** see **Coulanges P**
**Rakov PP:** Razvitie zdravookhraneniia Ul'ianovskoĭ oblasti za gody Sovetskoĭ vlasti. **Sov Med** 1980;(4):94–8
**Rakovec P** see **Musič D**
**Rakovskaia GG, Khokholia VP:** Kievskomu nauchno-issledovatel'skomu institutu klinicheskoĭ i éksperimental'noĭ khirurgii 10 let. **Klin Khir** 1982 May;(5):70–3
**Ralchs A, Rozman C:** Veintidós años después. Anotaciones para la historia de la Asociación Española de Hematología y Hemoterapia (AEHH). **Sangre (Barc)** 1982;27(3):377–85
**Rall JE:** Mones Berman––the man and his legacy to quantitative biology. **Am J Physiol** 1983 Nov;245(5 Pt 1):R618–9
**Rall P, Kirchhoff KT, Roberts J:** Professional attire at delivery, part I: an historical review. **J Nurse Midwife** 1984 Jul–Aug;29(4):251–6
**Rallu JL:** Evolution du nombre et de la composition des familles françaises entre 1975 et 1979. **Population** 1981;36(3):629–34
**Rallu JL:** La dépopulation des archipels du Pacifique: l'exemple de quatre villages de l'île Malekula. **Population** 1981;36(3):519–40
**Rallu JL:** Permanence des disparités régionales de la fécondité en Italie? **Population** 1983;38(1):29–59
**Rallu JL:** Situation démographique de la Polynésie Française. **Population** 1980;35(2):385–416
**Rallu JL** see **Festy P**
**Ram B:** Regional-sub-cultural explanations of black fertility in the United States. **Popul Stud** 1976;30(3):553ff
**Ram PC, Fordham EW:** An historical survey of bone scanning. **Semin Nucl Med** 1979 Jul;9(3):190–6
**Ram R, Schultz TW:** Life span, health, savings, and productivity. **Econ Dev Cult Change** 1979;27(3):399–421
**Rama Rao B, Reddy MV:** A note on Goraksanātha and his work Yogadipikā. **Bull Indian Inst Hist Med Hyderabad** 1982;12(1–4):34–44
**Rama Rao B:** Abhidhanaratnamala; a work with a new classification of Dravyas. **Bull Inst Hist Med (Hyderabad)** 1973 Oct;3(4):165–8
**Rama Rao B:** Bath in Ayurveda, Yoga and Dharmashastra. **Bull Indian Inst Hist Med Hyderabad** 1982;12(1–4):13–21
**Rama Rao B:** Bhishagratna Achanta Lakshmipathi, his dedicated service to Ayurveda. **Bull Indian Inst Hist Med (Hyderabad)** 1980;10(1–4):76–83
**Rama Rao B:** Contribution of Andhra to ayurveda in Sanskrit. **Bull Indian Inst Hist Med (Hyderabad)** 1978;8(1–4):8–13
**Rama Rao B:** Development of dravyaguna in India. **Bull Indian Inst Hist Med (Hyderabad)** 1978;8(1–4):1–7
**Rama Rao B:** Medical allusions in some inscriptions of Andhra Pradesh. **Bull Indian Inst Hist Med (Hyderabad)** 1975 Oct, 5(4):198–206
**Rama Rao B:** Rasapradipika; a Sanskrit medical work attributed to Bharadvaja. **Bull Indian Inst Hist Med (Hyderabad)** 1975 Jul;5(3):123–8
**Rama Rao B:** References to Ayurveda in the commentaries of Mallinatha. **Bull Indian Inst Hist Med (Hyderabad)** 1979;9:13–20
**Rama Rao B:** Water and usahpana in ayurvedic literature. **Bull Indian Inst Hist Med (Hyderabad)** 1980;10(1–4):1–6
**Rama Rao B** see **Pandey AN**
**Rama Rao B** see **Sarma CR**
**Rama Rao B** see **Venkata Reddy M**
**Rama Rao GS:** Contribution of Avicenna in therapeutics reflecting on modern medicine. **Bull Indian Inst Hist Med (Hyderabad)** 1981;1–4:118–22
**Ramadier JO:** La revue de chirurgie orthopédique et réparatrice de l'appareil moteur––90e anniversaire. **Rev Chir Orthop** 1981;67(3):161–3
**Ramage JA:** Thomas Hunt Morgan: family influences in the making of a great scientist. **Filson Club Hist Q** 1979;53(1):5–25
**Ramalingaswami V, Satyavati GV:** Sir Ram Nath Chopra. **Indian J Med Res** 1982 Dec;76 Suppl:V–VI
**Ramas M:** Freud's Dora, Dora's hysteria: the negation of a woman's rebellion. **Feminist Stud** 1980;6(3):472–510
**Ramaswamy S, Pace JL:** The medieval skeletal remains from St. Gregory's Church at Zejtun (Malta) Part I. Paleopathological studies. **Arch Ital Anat Embriol** 1979 Jan–Mar;84(1):43–53
**Ramaswamy S, Pace JL:** The medieval skeletal remains from St. Gregory's Church at Zejtun (Malta) Part II. Anthropological studies. **Arch Ital Anat Embriol** 1980;85(1):55–69
**Rambar AC:** Julius Hess, M.D. In Smith GF, Smith PN, Vidyasagar D, ed: Historical review and recent advances in neonatal and perinatal

medicine. [Chicago?], Mead Johnson Nutritional Division, 1983. Vol. II. p. 161-4.
**Rambar AC** see **Smith GF**
**Rambo LR:** Ethics, evolution, and the psychology of William James. **J Hist Behav Sci** 1980 Jan;16(1):50-7
**Ramer SC:** Childbirth and culture: midwifery in the nineteenth-century Russian countryside. In Ransel, David L., ed. The family in Imperial Russia. New lines of historical research. Urbana, U. of Illinois Press, 1978. p. 218-35.
**Ramírez EA:** Comentarios sobre la contribución del Dr. Ramón M. Suárez al estudio de la hipertensión arterial. **Bol Asoc Med PR** 1983 Nov;75(11):498-9
**Ramírez Almanza MA:** La formación de los médicos y su utilización en el área rural. **Salud Publica Mex** 1983 Sep-Oct;25(5):533-9
**Ramírez de Arellano AB:** Colonialism, Catholicism, and contraception: a history of birth control in Puerto Rico. Chapel Hill, University of North Carolina Press, 1983. xii, 219 p.
**Ramírez Oviedo A** see **Cueva J**
**Ramírez Ronda Ch, Bermúdez RH, Pérez Pabón MJ, et al:** Vacunación: principios y práctica 1980. Revisón y conceptos.--Parte I. Desarrollo histórico, efectos secundarios difteria, tétanos y tos ferina, poliomielitis y sarampión. **Bol Asoc Med PR** 1980 Jul;72(7):339-52
**Ramón Baltar Domínguez: Rev Esp Enferm Apar Dig** 1981 Oct;60(4):413-5
**Ramos J** see **Pacheco CR**
**Ramos MD** see **Carrillo JL**
**Ramos MR** see **Musto DF**
**Ramos P:** Crónica. La Asociación Mexicana de Gastroenterología. **Rev Gastroenterol Mex** 1981 Apr-Jun;46(2):71-3 contd.
**Ramos P:** El aprendizaje de la gastroenterología. **Rev Gastroenterol Mex** 1982 Jan-Mar;47(1):35-7
**Ramos P:** Etica médica en la era pretecnológica. **Gac Med Mex** 1980 Mar;116(3):102-8
**Ramos García E** see **Marset Campos P**
**Ramos García E** see **Parra Hidalgo P**
**Ramsey EM:** The story of spiral arteries. **J Reprod Med** 1981 Aug;26(8):393-9
**Ramsey FB:** January 1982: 75th birthday of the ISMA Journal; history and highlights, Indiana State Medical Association and its journal. **J Indiana State Med Assoc** 1982 Jan;75(1):14-9
**Ramsey LJ:** Bullet wounds and X-Rays in Britain's little wars. **J Soc Army Hist Res** 1982 Summer;:91-102
**Ramsey LJ:** Some notable early contributors to radiography--Thompson, Jackson and Campbell Swinton. **Radiography** 1980 Dec;46(552):289-97
**Ramsey M:** Medicina e politica di monopolio professionale nel XIX secolo. **Quad Stor** 1981;16(3):959-1011
**Ramsey M:** Popular medicine and medical power in France, 1707-1830. Ph.D. Diss. Harvard University. Cambridge, Mass., 1979.
**Ramsey M:** Sous le régime de la législation de 1803: trois enquêtes sur les charlatans au XIVe siècle. **Rev Hist Mod Contemp** 1980 Jul-Sept;27:485-500
**Ramsey M:** The repression of unauthorized medical practice in eighteenth-century France. **Eighteenth Cent Life** 1982;7(2):118-35
**Ramsey M:** Traditional medicine and medical enlightenment: the regulation of secret remedies in the ancien regime. **Hist Reflect** 1982;9(1-2):215-32
**Ramsey WO:** Hermetic sealing of root canals--the Greeks had a name for it. **J Endod** 1982 Mar;8(3):100
**Ramsøy NR:** Den norske folketellingsdatabanken: forskningspotensial belyst med eksempler. **Tidsskr Samfunnsforskning** 1981;22(4):287-308
**Ramzin MS:** Teratogene Wirkung von Medikamenten. **Gynakologe** 1982 Sep;15(3):136-42
**Ranade HG:** A note on 'Pata in Atharvaveda 2.27'. **Stud Hist Med** 1981 Sep;5(3):225-7
**Ranasinghe L:** Koch and Koch's bacillus: 100 years ago and today. **Ceylon Med J** 1982 Mar;27(1):1-5
**Ranasinghe L:** The medical writings of Dr. E. M. Wijerama. **Ceylon Med J** 1981 Mar;26(1):1-4
**Ranasinghe L** see **Aloysius DJ**
**Randall M:** La penetración imperialista y sus consecuencias para la mujer Latinoamericana. **Santiago (Cuba)** 1974;(15):227-47
**Randall S** see **Gelbier S**
**Randall SB** see **Gelbier S**
**Randolph ME:** A. Edward Maumenee--an appreciation. **Am J Ophthalmol** 1979 Sep;88(3 Pt 1):289-92
**Rangell L:** The Anna Freud experience. **Psychoanal Study Child** 1984;39:29-43
**Ranger T:** Medical science and pentecost: the dilemma of anglicanism in Africa. In Sheils WJ, ed: The Church and healing. Papers read at the twentieth summer meeting and the twenty-first winter meeting of the Ecclesiastical History Society. Oxford, Basil Blackwell for the Society, 1982. p. 333-65.
**Ranger T:** The Church and healing: introduction. In Sheils WJ, ed: The Church and healing. Papers read at the twentieth summer meeting and the twenty-first winter meeting of the Ecclesiastical History Society. Oxford, Basil Blackwell for the Society, 1982. p. xi-xxiv.
**Ranger TO:** Godly medicine: the ambiguities of medical mission in southeast Tanzania, 1900-1945. **Soc Sci Med [B]** 1981 Jul;15(3):261-77
**Rank BK:** George Grey Turner, F.R.A.C.S. (Hon). **Aust NZ J Surg** 1981 Dec;51(6):627-30
**Ranlett J:** The Smoke Abatement Exhibition of 1881. **Hist Today** 1981 Nov;31:10-3
**Ranney B:** Geschichte, Organisation und Praxis der amerikanischen Gynäkologie und Geburtshilfe. Eine Ubersicht. **Zentralbl Gynakol** 1984;106(9):626-32
**Ransel DL:** Recent Soviet studies in demographic history. **Russ Rev** 1981;40(2):143-57
**Ransford O:** 'Bid the sickness cease': disease in the history of black Africa. London, John Murray, 1983. x, 235 p.
**Ransom JF:** The origins of chiropractic physiological therapeutics: Howard, Forester and Schulze. **Chiropr Hist** 1984;4(1):47-52
**Ranum O, ed** see **Forster R**
**Rapaport FT:** Perspectives in transplantation. **Transplant Proc** 1981 Mar;13(1 pt 1):6-9
**Raphaël F:** La médecine populaire juive en Alsace. In Livet G, Schaff G, ed: Médecine et assistance en Alsace, XVIe-XXe siècle. Strasbourg, Istra, 1976. p. 287-302.
**Raphelson AC:** Psychology at Michigan: the Pillsbury years, 1897-1947. **J Hist Behav Sci** 1980 Oct;16(4):301-12
**Raphelson AC:** The history course as the capstone of the psychology curriculum. **J Hist Behav Sci** 1982 Jul;18(3):279-85
**Rapic S:** O zivotu i radu Ferde Kerna. In: I simpozij o historiji mikrobiologije i imunologije u Hrvatskoj do 1923. godine. Zagreb, Jugoslavenskoj akademiji, 1973. p. 85-93.
**Rapin M, Lemaire F:** La ventilation artificielle prolongée. 1954-1979. **Nouv Presse Med** 1979 Jan 13;8(2):89-92
**Rapp BA** see **Doszkoos TE**
**Rapp F** see **Guillemain B**
**Rapp G** see **Aufderheide AC**
**Rappard P:** La folie et l'Etat: aliénation mentale et aliénation sociale. Toulouse, Privat, 1981. 261 p.
**Rapson H:** The circulation of blood: a history. London, F. Muller, 1982. 132 p.
**Rascol A, Clanet M:** La sclérose en plaques. De Charcot et Vulpian à nos jours. **Rev Neurol (Paris)** 1982;138(12):921-30
**Rasheed BM:** Avicenna's influence on European medicine. **Bull Indian Inst Hist Med (Hyderabad)** 1981;1-4:99-102
**Rashevskaia AM** see **Zorina LA**
**Rashkind WJ:** Historical aspects of surgery for congenital heart disease. **J Thorac Cardiovasc Surg** 1982 Oct;84(4):619-25
**Rashkind WJ:** Tricuspid atresia: a historical review. **Pediatr Cardiol** 1982;2(1):85-8
**Rashkind WJ, ed:** Congenital heart disease. Stroudsburg, Pennsylvania, Hutchinson Ross, 1982. xv, 390 p. (Benchmark papers in human physiology, 16).
**Raska K:** How the smallpox programme began. **World Health Forum** 1981;2:290-1
**Raskin BV:** Razrabotka V. I. Leninym programmnykh zadach partii v oblasti zdravookhraneniia. **Zdravookhr Ross Fed** 1980;(4):9-13
**Raskin SP:** The pulmonary acinus: historical notes. **Radiology** 1982 Jul;144(1):31-4
**Rasmuson M** see **Hed HM**
**Rasmussen EG** see **Marvitz L**
**Rasmussen GL:** The history of hospital social work. **Tex Hosp** 1981 Feb;36(9):10-2
**Rasmussen L:** En forstander og hans assistent. **Dan Medicinhist Arbog** 1981;:130-40
**Rasmussen L, Wheatley DN:** The Biological Institute of the Carlsberg foundation: international centre for cell biology for 50 years. **Cell Biol Int Rep** 1983 Dec;7(12):1071-9
**Rasmussen P** see **Halaburt H**
**Rasmussen PG:** The history of veterinary roentgenology in Denmark 1895 - 1975. **Hist Med Vet** 1977;2(3):65-8
**Raso Rodríguez EJ:** Hitos cumbres en la historia de la cirugia. **Asclepio** 1980;32:333-9
**Raso Rodríguez EJ:** La evolucion historica de la profesion de instrumentista. **Asclepio** 1980;32:327-32
**Raspail S:** Raspail, savant et militant. **Histoire** 1978 Dec;7:89-91
**Rasporich AW, Getty IA:** George Verey. In Dictionary of Canadian biography, 1881-1890. 1982;11:900-1.
**Rasporich AW:** John Jeremiah Bigsby. In Dictionary of Canadian biography, 1881-1890. 1982;11:72-3.
**Rassengeschichte der Menscheit:** 7 vols. Vol. 1 ed. by K. Saller; Vols. 2-7 ed. by I. Schwidetzky. München und Wien, R. Oldenbourg Verlag, 1968-1979. Continuing.
**Rassengeschichte der Menschheit:** 8. Lieferung. Asien I: Japan, Indonesien, Ozeanien. München and Wien, Oldenbourg, 1981. 166 p. Contributions by H. Suzuki, S. Watanabe, J. Glinka, W. W. Howells, I. Schwidetzky.
**Rasuhin J:** Epidemiologija i profilaksa zaraznih bolesti u partizanskim prilikama. **Lijec Vjesn** 1979 Nov;101(11):714-6
**Rasuhin-Vekic N** see **Kraljevic M**
**Raszeja S:** Fifty years of the scientific work of Professor Boleslaw Popielski. **Forensic Sci Int** 1981 Mar-Apr;17(2):97-100
**Ratcliffe DS:** The evolution of medical societies in Britain---have they a future? **Bristol Med Chir J** 1979 Jan-Apr;94(349-350):3-10, 13-4
**Rathbun TA:** Morphological affinities and demography of metal-age Southwest Asian populations. **Am J Phys Anthropol** 1982 Sep;59(1):47-60
**Rather LJ:** On the source and development of metaphorical language in the history of Western medicine. In Stevenson LG, ed: A celebration of medical history. Baltimore, Johns Hopkins University Press, 1982. (The Henry E. Sigerist supplements to the Bulletin of the History of Medicine; new ser., no. 6). p. 135-53. With commentary by P. H. Niebyl, p. 154-6.
**Rather LJ:** The dream of self-destruction. Wagner's Ring and the modern

world. Baton Rouge, Louisiana State Univ. Press, 1979. xx, 215 p.
**Ratliff AH:** Ernest William Hey Groves and his contributions to orthopaedic surgery. **Ann R Coll Surg Engl** 1983 May;65(3):203-6
**Ratliff AH:** Ernest William Hey Groves and his contributions to orthopaedic surgery. **Bristol Med Chir J** 1983 Jul;98(367):98-103
**Ratnam SS, Karim SM, Ng CS, et al:** Research and development in obstetrics and gynaecology in the Department of Obstetrics and Gynaecology at the National University of Singapore. **Ann Acad Med Singapore** 1982 Jul;11(3):313-21
**Ratnoff WD:** A war with the molecules: Louis Pillemer and the history of properdin. **Perspect Biol Med** 1980;23(4):638-57
**Rattansi PM:** Medicine and the Puritan Revolution. **Soc Soc Hist Med Bull (Lond)** 1984 Jun;34:4-5
**Ratti A:** Antoinette Béclère e il Centro per le Relazioni internazionali in Radiologia. **Radiol Med (Torino)** 1982 Nov;68(11):785-7
**Ratti A:** I 75 anni della Deutsche Röntgengesellschaft. **Radiol Med (Torino)** 1980 Jul-Aug;66(7-8):481-4
**Rattner J:** Alexander Mitscherlich. In J. Rattner, ed: Wandlungen der Psychoanalyse. Wien, Europaverlag, 1980. p. 211-32.
**Rattner J:** Alfred Adler. New York, Frederick Ungar, 1983. 226 p.
**Rattner J:** Fritz Künkel. In J. Rattner, ed: Wandlungen der Psychoanalyse. Wien, Europaverlag, 1980. p. 141-63.
**Rattner J:** Karl Abraham. In J. Rattner, ed: Wandlungen der Psychoanalyse. Wien, Europaverlag, 1980. p. 9-29.
**Rattner J:** Medard Boss. In J. Rattner, ed: Wandlungen der Psychoanalyse. Wien, Europaverlag, 1980. p. 281-308.
**Rattner J:** Rollo May. In J. Rattner, ed: Wandlungen der Psychoanalyse. Wien, Europaverlag, 1980. p. 309-32.
**Rattner J:** Victor Emil von Gebsattel. In J. Rattner, ed: Wandlungen der Psychoanalyse. Wien, Europaverlag, 1980. p. 257-79.
**Rattner J, ed:** Wandlungen der Psychoanalyse. Wien, Europaverlag, 1980. 373 p.
**Ratzan RM:** 'No wreaths please': for William Carlos Williams. **Ann Intern Med** 1982 Dec;97(6):933-7
**Ratzmann GW, Jährig K:** Karl Stolte in seiner Zeit und für unsere Zeit. **Kinderarztl Prax** 1981 Dec;49(12):617-27
**Raubolt RR:** The history and development of adolescent group psychotherapy. Ph.D. Diss., The Fielding Institute, 1979. 172 leaves.
**Raubolt RR** see **Rachman AW**
**Rauch A:** Le souci du corps chez Condillac. **Stadion** 1977;3(1):60-89
**Rauchfuss A:** Zur korrekten Schreibweise des Namens von Prosper Menière und einige Anmerkungen zu Leben und Werk. **Laryngol Rhinol Otol (Stuttg)** 1984 Aug;63(8):381-5
**Rauhut K, ed** see **Klaschka F**
**Rausch U:** Das Medizinal- und Apothekenwesen der Landgrafschaft Hessen-Darmstadt und des Grossherzogtums Hessen unter besonderer Berücksichtigung der Provinz Starkenburg. Darmstadt, Marburg, Selbstverlag der Hessischen Historischen Kommission Darmstadt und der Historischen Kommission für Hessen 1978 (Quellen und Forschungen zur Hessischen Geschichte, Bd. 33). 588 p.
**Rausch VL, Freier EF:** Liver function tests. **Am J Med Technol** 1983 May;49(5):367-8
**Rausch DA, ed:** Civil War medicine: a patient's account. **Pa Folklife** 1977;26(5):46-8
**Rausky F:** Le discours freudien sur l'antisémitisme.
**Rausky F** see **Dupâquier J**
**Raven RW:** The surgeon and oncology. **Clin Oncol** 1984 Dec;10(4):311-8
**Ravenholt RT, Foege WH:** 1918 influenza, encephalitis lethargica, parkinsonism. **Lancet** 1982 Oct 16:2(8303):860-4
**Ravin AW:** Genetics in America: a historical overview. **Perspect Biol Med** 1978 Winter;21(2):214-31
**Ravin JG:** El Greco of Toledo. **Ohio State Med J** 1982 Nov;78(11):745-53
**Ravin JG:** Lethal ocular injuries. **J Pediatr Ophthalmol Strabismus** 1980 Jan-Feb;17(1):53-4
**Ravin JG:** Sir Arthur Conan Doyle and his mystical Ohio tour. **Ohio State Med J** 1983 Jun;79(6):425-7, 431-2
**Ravin JG:** Van Gogh's illness. **Ohio State Med J** 1981 Dec;77(12):699-702
**Ravines R:** Reconocimiento arqueologico en el rio corientes, nororiente del Peru. **Rev Mus Nac** 1978-80;44:111-38
**Ravitch MM:** A century of surgery. The history of the American Surgical Association. 2 vols. Philadelphia and Toronto, Lippincott, 1981.
**Ravitch MM, McAuley CE:** Airborne contamination of the operative wound. **Surg Gynecol Obstet** 1984 Aug;159(2):177-88
**Ravitch MM:** Development of intestinal anastomotic devices. **South Med J** 1982 Dec;75(12):1520-4
**Ravitch MM:** Progress in resection of the chest wall for tumor with reminiscences of Dr. Blalock. **Johns Hopkins Med J** 1982 Aug;151(2):43-53
**Ravitch MM:** Sir Astley Paston Cooper. **Bull Am Coll Surg** 1977 Feb;62(2):17-20
**Ravitch MM, Steichen FM:** Staples and staplers. **Adv Surg** 1984;17:241-79
**Ravitch MM:** The American Surgical Association. The peaks of excitement. **Ann Surg** 1980 Sep;192(3):282-7
**Ravitch MM:** The danger of stating an opinion or the hazards of going on record. **Surg Gynecol Obstet** 1980 Dec;151(6):810-6
**Ravitch MM:** The reception of new operations. **Ann Surg** 1984 Sep;200(3):231-46
**Ravitch MM:** The uses of medical history. **Pharos** 1983 Fall;46(4):2-6
**Ravitch MM** see **Steichen FM**
**Rawcliffe C:** Medicine and medical practice in later medieval London. **Guildhall Stud Lond Hist** 1981;5(1):13-25
**Rawcliffe C:** The hospitals of later medieval London. **Soc Soc Hist Med Bull (Lond)** 1983 Jun;32:24-6
**Rawcliffe C:** The hospitals of later medieval London. **Med Hist** 1984 Jan;28(1):1-21
**Rawlings DM:** The history of Hamot Medical Center. **J Erie Stud** 1981 Spring;10:1-16
**Rawlings FH:** Two 17th century women apothecaries. **Pharm Hist (London)** 1984 Sep;14(3):7
**Rawlings FH:** 18th century Bristol Poll Books; source list of apothecaries and chemists and druggists. **Pharm Hist (London)** 1973 May;3(1):5
**Rawlinson MC:** Psychiatric discourse and the feminine voice. **J Med Philos** 1982 May;7(2):153-77
**Rawn ML:** Some reflections on the work of Theodor Reik. **Psychoanal Rev** 1981-82 Winter;68(4):477-8
**Rawson E:** The life and death of Asclepiades of Bithynia. **Classical Q** 1982;32(2):358-70
**Ray BS:** The development of neurosurgery in New York City. **Bull NY Acad Med** 1979 Nov;55(10):916-38
**Ray DJ:** Mortuary art of the Alaskan Eskimos. **Am Indian Art Mag** 1982;7(2):50-7
**Ray JM:** The fractured hip: the historical development of fracture management. **Friends P. I. Nixon Med Hist Libr** 1980 Oct;9:1-9
**Ray JW, Polk HC:** The history of smallpox: an old story of current significance. **J Ky Med Assoc** 1980 Apr;78(4):206-12
**Ray LJ:** Models of madness in Victorian asylum practice. **Eur J Sociol** 1981;22(2):229-64
**Raymond JF de:** Querelle de l'inoculation, ou, Préhistoire de la vaccinaton. Paris, Vrin, 1982. 124 p.
**Raynaud P:** L'education specialisée en France, 1882-1982. **Esprit** 1982;5:79-99
**Raynier JP de:** L'Hôpital de l'Enfance de 1861 à 1979. **Rev Med Suisse Romande** 1980 Jun;100(6):557-65
**Razi Z:** Life, marriage and death in a medieval parish: economy, society and demography in Healesowen, 1270-1400. Cambridge, Cambridge University Press, 1980. xi, 162 p.
**Razumov VI** see **Kirsanov NA**
**Razumov VI** see **Stegunin SI**
**Razvitic A.I. Strukovym ucheniza o tuberculoza: Probl Tuberk** 1981 Apr;(4):3-6
**Razvitie nevrologicheskoĭ pomoshchi v Glavnom voennom klinicheskom gospitale imeni N. N. Burdenko (k 275-letiiu osnovaniia gospitalia): Voen Med Zh** 1982 Jul;(7):71-2
**Razvitie otorinolaringologii v Glavnom voennom klinicheskom gospitale imeni N. N. Burdenko (k 275-letiiu osnovaniia gospitalia): Voen Med Zh** 1982;(9):67-8
**Razzell P:** The conquest of smallpox: the impact of inoculation on smallpox mortality in eighteenth century England. Firle, Sussex, Caliban Books, 1977. x, 190 p.
**Reaching 'target zero':** The story of smallpox eradication in India. **WHO Chron** 1979 Oct;33(10):359-63
**Read H:** 'A hand to hold while dying': Dr. Charles A. Leale at Lincoln's side. **Lincoln Her** 1977;79:21-6
**Read MB:** A 19th-century weatherman, Dr. George Henry [sic] Fielding of Grove House, Tonbridge. **Cantium** 1972;3,4(4):99-100
**Read RC:** The development of inguinal herniorrhaphy. **Surg Clin North Am** 1984 Apr;64(2):185-96
**Read RD:** Marcy's priority in the development of inguinal herniorrphaphy. **Surgery** 1980 Nov;88(5):682-5
**Reale E:** Wissenschaftliche Arbeiten von H. von Mayersbach. **Mikroskopie** 1981;38(3-4):67-77
**Rebaudo D:** Le mouvement annuel de la population française rurale de 1670 à 1740. **Population** 1979;34(3):589-606
**Rebentisch E:** 100 Jahre Wehrmedizin. Arztliche Erfahrungen zwischen Krieg und Frieden. **Fortschr Med** 1984 Mar 8;102(9):225-31
**Rebérioux M** see **Dupâquier J**
**Rebollo M** see **Berciano J**
**Reboul G** see **Loustaud JP**
**Rebrikova NL, Mul'diiarov PIa:** Elektronno-mikroskopicheskoe izuchenie pergamenta. **Biull Eksp Biol Med** 1982 Dec;94(12):104-7
**Recensement des pharmacies hospitalières: Bull Soc Fr Hist Hop** 1979;(39):10-18
**Recent acquisitions of the manuscript division:** Carl R. Rogers papers. **Q J Libr Congr** 1978;35-258-9
**Rèche A:** Mille ans de médecine et de pharmacie à Bordeaux. Bordeaux, Mollat, 1980. 190 p.
**Rechenberg G** see **Erxleben DC**
**Rechsteiner J, Lockyer WJ, Friedman LI:** Overview, history, evaluation and future developments of the AutoGrouper 16-C. **Vox Sang** 1981;40(3):192-200
**Recht P:** La mesure de la santé. **Arch Belg** 1984;42(7-8):418-34
**Rechtman J:** De la brosse à dents à la brosse à bouche. **Soc Fr Hist Art Dent** 1979 Mar-Jun;(3-4):23-8
**Rechtman J:** De la brosse à dents à la brosse à bouche: deux siècles d'histoire (1780-1977). **Pedod Fr** 1978;12:299-311
**Rechtman J:** De l'asepsie... ou un siècle avant Semmelweis. **Hist Sci Med** 1980;14(2):165-70
**Rechtman J:** Jean-Paul Marat, ses origines, ses apports à la médecine. Agent secret? **Hist Sci Med** 1980;14:261-70
**Rechtman J:** La brosse à dents et son histoire (1780-1980). **Hist Sci Med** 1980;14(2):221-5
**Rechtman J:** L'asepsie et son histoire; le Dr Buchan précède le Dr

Semmelweis de plus d'un siècle (1769–1847). **Soc Fr Hist Art Dent** 1979 Sep–Dec;(5–6):15–17
**Rechtman J:** Le Dr. J.P. Marat et le secret professionnel. **Soc Fr Hist Art Dent** 1979 Sep–Dec;(5–6):22–5
**Rechtman J:** Un précurseur génial de la prévention et de la diététique, du bouche à bouche et du massage cardiaque externe de l'asepsie et parrain de J. P. Marat: Le docteur William Buchan (1729–1805). Diss. Paris VII, 1979. 115 p.
**Reckert H:** Das unbekannte Werk des Pathologen, Robert Carswell (1793–1857). Köln, 1982. 283 p. (Kölner medizinhistorische Beiträge, Band 22)
**Recollections & reflections:** Lawrence J. Henderson and George Sarton. **Isis** 1984 Mar;75(276):11–32
**Red Cross in philately: Scalpel Tongs** 1981;25:39–43
**The Red Cross: the first hundred years: MD** 1981 May;25(5):43–7
**Redden RB** see **Buus S**
**Redding JS:** A historical vignette: intensive care. **Respir Ther** 1979 Jan–Feb;9(1):74–6, 78
**Reddy CP, Surawicz B:** Terminology of tachycardias: historical background and evolution. **PACE** 1983 Sep;6(5 Pt 2):1123–42
**Reddy MV** see **Rama Rao B**
**Reddy PH** see **Caldwell JC**
**Reding MM:** History of the South Dakota State Medical Association Auxiliary 1910–1981. **SD J Med** 1981 May;34(5):72–3
**Redlich FC:** Medical ethics under National Socialism. In Reich WT, et al, ed: Encyclopedia of bioethics, v.3. New York, Free Press, 1978. p. 1015–20.
**Redman JF:** Partial nephretomy. **Urol Clin North Am** 1983 Nov;10(4):677–84
**Redondo A** see **Wertheimer P**
**Reece RD** see **Rodin AE**
**Reed A** see **Gregg JB**
**Reed ES:** Descartes' corporeal ideas hypothesis and the origin of scientific psychology. **Rev Metaphys** 1982;35:731–52
**Reed FA:** The fingermark. The prime piece of scientific evidence. **J Forensic Sci Soc** 1981 Jan;21(1):9–13
**Reed J:** Doctors, birth control, and social values, 1830–1970. In Vogel MJ, Rosenberg CE, ed: The therapeutic revolution. Philadelphia, 1979. p. 109–133.
**Reed J:** Katharine Dexter McCormick. In: Notable American women. The modern period. Cambridge, Mass., Belknap-Harvard Univ. Press, 1980. 4:440–2.
**Reed J:** Louise Frances Stevens Bryant. In Dictionary of American Biography, Suppl. 6, 1956–1960. p. 80–2, 1980.
**Reed J:** Margaret Sanger. In: Notable American women. The modern period. Cambridge, Mass., Belknap-Harvard Univ. Press, 1980. 4:623–7.
**Reed J:** Who invented the modern hospital and who should tell the story? **Rev Am Hist** 1981;9(1):29–33
**Reed J** see **Fee E**
**Reed J** see **Green D**
**Reed JF:** Samuel Clemens and family: the Hartfold connection and Hartford physicians. **Am J Surg** 1981 Apr;141(4):401–10
**Reed JH:** Brass butterflies or the thoughts of Mao Tse Tung: the sociology of schistosomiasis control in China. Ithaca, N.Y., Cornell U. Press. 1979. 280 p.
**Reed K, Perakis CR:** Medical historiography: its place in osteopathic medicine. Parts I and II. **J Am Osteopath Assoc** 1984 Jun;83(10):738–44
**Reed K, Grage TB:** Our surgical heritage. The Paget tradition revisited. **Am J Surg** 1982 Nov;144(5):498–503
**Reed LA:** Doctor Swan's restorative waters. **Wis Mag Hist** 1980–81;64(2):124–6
**Reed SC:** A short history of genetic counseling. Minneapolis, Dight Institute for Human Genetics of the Univ. of Minnesota, 1974. p. 1–10. (Bull. 14).
**Reed WG** see **Anderson RJ**
**Rees PH** see **Pyle GF**
**Rees RJ:** An appraisal of medical research in the treatment and control of leprosy. **Lepr India** 1982 Oct;54(4):783–800
**Rees WH:** The State Veterinary Service. **Vet Rec** 1982 Jun 26;110(26):606–10
**Reese WG:** Academic psychiatry in Arkansas. **J Arkansas Med Soc** 1981 Nov;78(6):220–33
**Reese WG:** 'Don't count the bricks'. Scientific contributions of W. H. Gantt. **Pavlov J Biol Sci** 1982 Jul–Sep;17(3):111–4
**Reese WG:** Early history of the Pavlovian Society. Twentyfive plus twentyfive. (W. Horsley Gantt). **Pavlov J Biol Sci** 1982 Oct–Dec;17(4):171–7
**Reese WJ:** After bread, education: nutrition and urban school children, 1890–1920. **Teach Coll Rec** 1980;81(4):496–525
**Reeves B** see **Low MD**
**Reeves C:** Illustrations of medicine in ancient Egypt. **J Audiov Media Med** 1980 Jan;3(1):4–13
**Reeves C** see **Thornton JL**
**Reeves WC, Emmons RW, Hardy JL:** Historical perspectives on California encephalitis virus in California. **Prog Clin Biol Res** 1983;123:19–29
**Reexamination of accoustic evidence in the Kennedy assassination: Science** 1982 Oct 8;218(4568):127–33
**Referent Robert Koch:** Der Entdecker des Tuberkulose-Erregers als sachverständiger Referent in der ersten Ausgabe der 'Fortschritte der Medicin'. **Fortschr Med** 1982 Jun 3;100(21):1012–3
**Reflections of the past: J Md State Dent Assoc** 1983 Aug;26(2):62–73
**Réflexions sur les soins infirmiers en psychiatrie:** L'equipe soignante de Castelluccio. **Soins Psychiatr** 1980 Mar 1;(1):3–8
**Refshauge WF, Walsh RJ:** Pitcairn Island: fertility and population growth, 1790–1856. **Ann Hum Biol** 1981 Jul;8(4):303–12
**Refsum S:** Some aspects of the history of neurology in Norway. In Rose FC, Bynum WF, ed: Historical aspects of the neurosciences. New York, Raven, 1982. p. 415–33.
**Regan LJ:** Malpractice: 25 years hasn't changed much. **Mich Med** 1981 Oct;80(29):550
**Regards sur la condition enfantine - XVIe–XXe siècles: Bull Soc Fr Hist Hop** 1980;(41):29–31
**Regato JA del:** Albert Soiland and the early development of therapeutic radiology in the United States. **Int J Radiat Oncol Biol Phys** 1983 Feb;9(2):243–53
**Regato JA del:** Enrico Fermi. **Int J Radiat Oncol Biol Phys** 1982 Aug;8(8):1393–416
**Regato JA del:** Francis Henry Williams. **Int J Radiat Oncol Biol Phys** 1983 May;9(5):739–49
**Regato JA del:** Max Planck. **Int J Radiat Oncol Bill Phys** 1979 Nov–Dec;5(11–12):2097–111
**Regaud J:** Claudius Regaud, (1870–1940): pionnier de la cancérologie, créateur de la Fondation Curie: chronique de sa vie et son oeuvre. Paris, Maloine, 1982. 233 p.
**Regelmann JP:** Die Geschichte des Lyssenkoismus. Frankfurt/Main, G. Fischer, 1980. 353 p.
**Regelmann JP:** Struktur des Arguments als Struktur der Geschichte?--oder: Paradigm lost! **Medizinhist J** 1982;17(1/2):37–53
**Reguero MA** see **Castellanos J**
**Rehder K, Shampo MA, Kyle RA:** Physician's personal in-flight medical kit. **JAMA** 1982 Feb 19;247(7):1011
**Rehfeldt FC:** George Goodfellow: practicing paradoxologist. **Tex Med** 1981;77(3):44–7
**Rehm WS:** In tribute to a living pioneer: Dr. Lyndon Edmund Lee. **Chiropr Hist** 1981;1(1):47–50
**Reich CV** see **Binford CH**
**Reich MR, Goldman RH:** Italian occupational health: concepts, conflicts, implications. **Am J Public Health** 1984 Sep;74(9):1031–41
**Reich MR** see **Lifton RJ**
**Reich W:** Psychiatry's second coming: the way we analyse now. **Encounter (Lond)** 1981;57(2):66–72
**Reich W:** The case of General Grigorenko: a psychiatric reexamination of a Soviet dissident. **Psychiatry** 1980 Nov;43(4):303–23
**Reich W:** The case of General Grigorenko: a second opinion. **Encounter (Lond)** 1980;54(4):9–24
**Reichard H** see **Olsson JE**
**Reichart B** see **Zenker R**
**Reichart PA:** Toothpastes containing betel nut (Areca catechu L.) from England of the nineteenth century. **J Hist Med Allied Sci** 1984 Jan;39(1):65–79
**Reichelt D:** Zur Entwicklung des Informationswesens im Fachgebiet und in der Gesellschaft. **Z Med Lab Diagn** 1983;24(7):408–14
**Reichert P:** A history of the development of cardiology as a medical specialty. **Clin Cardiol** 1978 Apr;1(1):5–15
**Reichsman F:** Life experiences and creativity of great composers: a psychosomaticist's view. **Psychosom Med** 1981 Aug;43(4):291–300
**Reid D:** De la médecine traditionnelle à la médecine préventive: analyse des réformes de santé au Québec. **Union Med Can** 1980 May;109(5):774–7
**Reid DD:** The historical background to wartime research in psychology and psychiatry in the Royal Air Force. In Dearnaley EJ, Warr PB, ed: Aircrew stress in wartime operations. London, New York, Academic Press, 1979. p. 1–8.
**Reid JA:** Was Anopheles Donaldi a vector of malaria in Kuala Lumpur, Malaysia, in the past? **Trans R Soc Trop Med Hyg** 1980;74(3):337–9
**Reid JD, Jedlicka D, Lee ES, et al:** Trends in black health. **Phylon** 1977;38(2):105–16
**Reid L:** Pollution: not a new problem for Missourians. **Gateway Herit** 1980;1(2):18–22
**Reid RA, Bartlett EE, Kozoll R:** The checkerboard area health system: delivering comprehensive care in a remote region of New Mexico. **Hum Organ** 1982;41(2):147–55
**Reid WA** see **Hamilton DN**
**Reier H:** Gesundheit, Krankheiten und Arzte bei den Goten. Kiel, 1981. 87 p.
**Reif AE:** Hippocrates and the biomedical scientist: the problems of controlling the dangers of science. **Minerva** 1980 Spring;18(1):29–50
**Reilly P:** The Virginia Racial Integrity Act revisited: the Plecker–Laughlin correspondence: 1928–1930. **Am J Med Genet** 1983 Dec;16(4):483–92
**Reimann R:** Das Bildungszentrum Essen des DBfK besteht zehn Jahre. **Krankenpflege (Frankfurt)** 1984 Jul–Aug;38(7–8):222–4
**Reimensnyder B:** Annotated bibliography of Pennsylvania folk medicine. **Pa Folklife** 1977;27(1):40–8
**Reimer H:** Robert Koch und die Rindertuberkulose. **Z Gesamte Hyg** 1982 Mar;28(3):156–60
**Reimer LW** see **Engelbrecht H**
**Reimer T:** Die Entwicklung der Flugmedizin in Deutschland. Köln, 1979. 282 p. (Kölner medizinhistorische Beiträge, Band 13)
**Reimers D:** Die interne Behandlung der Tuberkulose. **Prax Klin Pneumol** 1982 Nov;36(11):475–8
**Reimers D:** Tuberkulose und Kunst. **Med Welt** 1982 Mar 26;33(12):435–41
**Rein DB:** En République Démocratique d'Allemagne: population et politique. **Documents** 1979;34(4):131–7

**Rein DB:** Une attitude allemande face à l'évolution démographique. **Population** 1982;37(1):113–30
**Rein W** see **Mormont C**
**Reinders RC:** Toynbee Hall and the American settlement movement. **Soc Serv Rev** 1982;56(1):39–54
**Reingold N, Reingold IH, ed:** Science in America. A documentary history, 1900–1939. Chicago, London, Univ. of Chicago Press, 1981. xii, 490 p. (The Chicago history of science and medicine).
**Reingold N:** The scientist as troubled American. **Am Ind Hyg Assoc J** 1979 Dec;40(12):1107–13
**Reingold N** see **Whitaker MA**
**Reingold IH, ed** see **Reingold N**
**Reingold N, ed:** The papers of Joseph Henry. Volume 1. December 1797–October 1832. The Albany years. Washington, Smithsonian Institution Press, 1972. xxxix, 496 p.
**Reingold N, ed:** The papers of Joseph Henry. Volume 2. November 1832–December 1835. The Princeton Years. Washington, Smithsonian Institution Press, 1975. 524 p.
**Reinhardt UE:** Health insurance and cost-containment policies: the experience abroad. **Am Econ Rev** 1980;70(2):149–56
**Reinhold JG:** Adventures of a clinical chemist. **Clin Chem** 1982 Nov;28(11):2314–23
**Reinis Z:** Padesát let Ceskoslovenské kardiologické společnosti. **Cas Lek Cesk** 1979 Nov 9;118(45):1404–7
**Reinis Z:** Přehled 50 leté činnosti Cs. kardiologické spolčnosti. **Vnitr Lek** 1980 Apr;26(4):306–9
**Reinis Z, Gvozdják J, Widimský J, et al:** The fiftieth anniversary of the Czechoslovak Society of Cardiology. **Cor Vasa** 1979;21(6):445–9
**Reinstein H:** Laboratory medicine--then and now. **Am J Med Technol** 1982 Jun;48(6):427–9
**Reis CS:** A 'Doença crua e feia' em 'os lusíadas'. **An Inst Hig Med Trop (Lisb)** 1977–1978;5(1–4):127–69
**Reis CS, Jans GJ:** Sessão comemorativa do 7.o centenário de Pedro Hispano -- 20 de Maio de 1977. **An Inst Hig Med Trop (Lisb)** 1977–1978;5(1–4):3–19
**Reis DJ:** The brain and hypertension: reflections on 35 years of inquiry into the neurobiology of the circulation. **Circulation** 1984 Nov;70(5 Pt 2):III31–45
**Reis H** see **Fechner PU**
**Reis K:** Gesundheitserziehung in der DDR - Versuch einer historischen Betrachtung. **Z Gesamte Hyg** 1982 Apr;28(4):253–5
**Reis e Almeida FS:** Estomatologia sofrologia. **Rev Port Estomatol Cir Maxilofac** 1983 Apr–Jun;24(2):183–97
**Reiser S** see **Benison S**
**Reiser SJ:** Observer variance and error in clinical medicine. In: Congrès international d'histoire de la médecine, XXVe, Québec, 1976. Actes. Québec, 1977. p. 1120–7
**Reiser SJ:** Technology and the eclipse of individualism in medicine. **Pharos** 1982 Winter;45(1):10–5
**Reiser SJ:** Technology, specialization, and the allied health professions. **J Allied Health** 1983 Aug;12(3):177–82
**Reiser SJ:** Words as scalpels: transmitting evidence in the clinical dialogue. **Ann Intern Med** 1980 Jun;92(6):837–42
**Reiter A:** Ernst L. Kirchner--Psychoanalytische Perspektiven der Psychoökonomie seines künstlerischen Schaffens. **Confin Psychiatr** 1980;23(2):118–28
**Reiter PJ** see **Becke U**
**Reitman N:** The history of medicine and medical care in New Brunswick. **J Med Soc NJ** 1984 Sep;81(9):737–9
**Rejchrt B:** K počátkum Ceskoslovensko-sovětské spolupráce v oftalmologii. **Cesk Oftalmol** 1981 Sep;37(5):381–2
**Rejmanowski T:** Dzieje sióstr miłosierdzia w Szpitalu Powiatowym Sw. Antoniego we Włocławku (1877–1966). **Arch Hist Med (Warsz)** 1984;47(3):433–8
**Rektor I, Svejdová M, Hrazdira CL:** Epilepsie a sociální problematika epileptiku v minulosti. **Cas Lek Cesk** 1983 Feb 4;122(5):153–4
**Relethford JH:** Genetic structure and population history of Ireland: a comparison of blood group and anthropometric analyses. **Ann Hum Biol** 1983 Jul–Aug;10(4):321–33
**Relethford JH:** Isonymy and population structure of Irish isolates during the 1890s. **J Biosoc Sci** 1982 Apr;14(2):241–7
**Relethford JH, Lees FC:** The effects of aging and secular trend on adult stature in rural western Ireland. **Am J Phys Anthropol** 1981;55(1):81–8
**Religion et médecine populaires: Lemouzi** 1979;71:235–367
**Relman AS:** The Harvard Medical School Bicentennial. **N Engl J Med** 1982 Oct 7;307(15):943–4
**Relman AS:** Two hundred years young. **N Engl J Med** 1981 Oct 29;305(18):1088–9
**Remembering Maud Mellish Wilson: Mayo Alumnus** 1982 Apr;:18–20
**Remes NR:** The rural cemetery. **Nineteenth Century Fict** 1979;5(4):52–5
**Remini RV:** The final days and hours in the life of General Andrew Jackson. **Tenn Hist Q** 1980;39(2):167–77
**Remisová M, Janec M, Bruchâč D, et al:** Medici v Slovenskom národnom povstaní. **Bratisl Lek Listy** 1984 Sep;82(3):1142–52
**Remisová M:** Národnostná otázka v stavovskom živote lekárov na Slovensku v prvej CSR. **Cesk Zdrav** 1983 Jul;31(6):260–5
**Remisová M:** Slovenské národné povstanie a nový prístup k organizovaniu odborného spolkového života lekárov. **Bratisl Lek Listy** 1979 Aug;72(2):141–6
**Remley ML:** Jessie Hubbell Bancroft. In: Notable American women. The modern period. Cambridge, Mass., Belknap-Harvard Univ. Press, 1980. 4:46–7.
**Remmer H** see **Kotwas J**
**Remond R** see **Dupâquier J**
**Rémy B:** Répertoire épigraphique des médecins gaulois. **Rev Archeol Centre France** 1983;22(Dec):282
**Remy C, Aracil P:** Histoire de la chirurgie du strabisme. **J Fr Ophtalmol** 1984;7(6–7):493–8
**Ren M:** [The therapeutic custom handed down from the Meng He School] (Chi). **Chung Hua I Shih Tsa Chih** 1984;14(2):72–4
**Renaldo JJ:** A note on the history of medicine and a debate on Parnassus. **Bull Hist Med** 1979 Winter;53(4):606–13
**Renaudie M:** Etre généraliste il y a quatre siècles. Réalisme et fiction. **Hist Sci Med** 1984;18(2):173–9
**Rendell-Baker L:** Nineteenth-century resuscitation apparatus. **Anaesthesia** 1981 Nov;36(11):1058–9
**Rendell-Baker L:** Principles in design and function of mechanical ventilators. **Respir Ther** 1979 Jan–Feb;9(1):63–4, 66–9
**Rendinger C de:** Un apothicaire du 'Grand Siècle', Claude Bourdelin (1621–1699), de l'Académie des Sciences, sa vie et les événements de son temps. **Bull Ordre Natl Pharm** 1980 Sep;236:1415–24
**Rendulic M:** Demografska kretanja u hrvatskoj. **Ekon Pregl** 1971;22(7–8):340–51
**Rengei B** see **Földes V**
**Renger F:** Razvitie na khepatologiiata v GDR. **Vutr Boles** 1980;19(6):2–6
**Renger FG:** Zur Geschichte der Hepatologie von Galen bis Frerichs. **Dtsch Z Verdau Stoffwechselkr** 1982;42(5):193–202
**Renggli R:** Die Anfänge der Spirometrie im 19. Jahrhundert. **Gesnerus** 1981;38:247–58
**Renker K:** Zu einigen Prinzipien der medizinischen Betreuung der Bevölkerung. **Wiss Z Martin Luther Univ (Math)** 1976;25(2):79–89
**Renker K:** 25 Jahre Zeitschrift für die gesamte Hygiene. **Z Gesamte Hyg** 1979 Oct;25(10):792
**Renker K:** 30 Jahre Sozialhygiene an der Universität Halle. **Z Gesamte Hyg** 1980;26(2):116–21
**Renker U:** Zur Entwicklung des Betriebsgesundheitswesens in der DDR. **Wiss Z Martin Luther Univ (Math)** 1976;25(2):95–8
**Renkonen KO:** Old Chinese observation correlated to ABO groups. **Hum Genet** 1980;55(2):279
**Renner I:** Zur Entwicklungsgeschichte der Pharmakognosie als selbständiges Hochschulfach an der Ludwig-Maximilians-Universität Ingolstadt - Landshut - München. Stuttgart, Deutscher Apotheker Verlag, 1982. 377 p. (Quellen und Studien zur Geschichte der Pharmazie, Bd. 17).
**Renner M:** 'Krankenpflege' stellt sich vor. **Krankenpflege (Bern)** 1981 Dec;(12):58–9
**Renner M:** 75 Jahre Zeitschrift Krankenpflege. **Krankenpflege (Bern)** 1983 Jan;(1):57–65
**Rennison RW:** The supply of water to Newcastle upon Tyne and Gateshead, 1680–1837. **Archaeol Aeliana** 1977;5:5
**Rensch B** see **Mayr E**
**Renshon SA:** Life history and character development: some reflections on political leadership. In M. Albin, R. J. Devlin, G. Heeger, ed: New directions in psychohistory. The Adelphi papers in honor of Erik H. Erikson. Lexington, Toronto, D. C. Heath, 1980. p. 57–68.
**Rentchnick P:** Iode et goitre. A propos du 150e anniversaire de la mort du Dr Jean-François Coindet (12 juillet 1774–11 février 1834). **Med Hyg (Geneve)** 1984 Feb 15;42(1551):465–6, 469–70, 472–4, 477–8
**Repanovici R** see **Popa LM**
**Repetto R** see **Cook MS**
**A report on the quality of ambulance service as observed in 1862 by S. L. Abbot, Francis Minot. Transactions of the New York State Medical Society, 1863: NY State J Med** 1982 Mar;82(3):393–4
**Reproductive immunology. A festschrift in honor of Dr. Saul B. Gusberg.: Mt Sinai J Med (NY)** 1980 Sep–Oct;47(5):i–vii, 427–560
**The residents: MD** 1978 Jul;22(7):89–99
**Resnick D, Greenway G:** Distal femoral cortical defects, irregularities, and excavations. **Radiology** 1982 May;143(2):345–54
**Resnick D** see **Cone RO**
**Resnick D** see **Ponec DJ**
**Resnik SS:** The making of dermatologic surgeons. The first decade of the American Society for Dermatologic Surgery. **J Dermatol Surg Oncol** 1980 Dec;6(12):993–5
**Restak RM:** Psychiatry in America. **Wilson Q** 1983;7(4):94–125
**Restivo S** see **Collins R**
**Retamal P:** Consideraciones psicopatológicas sobre el diagnóstico de la enfermedad de Fedor Dostoyevski. **Actas Luso Esp Neurol Psiquiatr** 1983 May–Jun;11(3):231–4
**Retel-Laurentin A** see **Armagnac C**
**Retherford RD, Mirza GM:** Evidence of age exaggeration in demographic estimates for Pakistan. **Popul Stud** 1982 Jul;36(2):257–70
**Réthy L:** Medico-historical background of the possibility of introducing the compulsory and nation-wide immunization with combined vaccines in Hungary. **Ann Immunol hung** 1984;24:13–38
**Réti E:** A hazai orvosföldrajz története. **Foldr Kozl** 1979;103(1–3):177–80
**Réti E:** Early days of medicine in Hungary. **Ther Hung** 1981;29(4):194–6
**Réti E:** Idées d'avant-garde dans les thèses hongroises séculaires. **Orvostort Kozl** 1979;86(24 no 4):73–9
**Réti E:** Lenin, a modern egészségpolitika úttörője. **Orvostort Kozl** 85(24 No 3):77–84, 1978
**Reti E:** L'évolution des vues en démographie et en planification familiale. In: Congrès international d'histoire de la médecine, XXVe, Québec, 1976.

Actes. Québec, 1977. p. 229-35.
**Retief FP:** President J. H. Brand en sy siekte-geskiedenis. **S Afr Med J** 1981 Mar 14;59(11):384-6
**Retief FP:** The Medical University of Southern Africa after 5 years. **S Afr Med J** 1982 Nov 27;62(23)841-5
**Retnev VM:** 60 let kafedre gigieny truda i professional'nykh bolezneĭ. **Gig Tr Prof Zabol** 1984 May;(5):34-7
**Retsas S:** Medicine and the Olympic games of antiquity. **Hist Med (Lond)** 1981;9(1):4-7
**Retsinas J:** Smallpox vaccination: a leap of faith. **RI Hist** 1979;38(4):113-24
**Retterstøl N:** Gaustad sykehus 125 år (1855-1980). **Tidsskr Nor Laegeforen** 1980 Dec 10;100(34-36):2026-9
**Rettig A:** 35 Jahre Osterr. Krankenpflegeverband--Permanenz eines Auftrages oder einer Entwicklung. **Osterr Krankenpflegez** 1982;35(3):69-70
**Rettig RA:** Health care technology. Lessons learned from the end-stage renal disease experience. Santa Monica, Rand Corp., 1976. 36 p.
**Retzius AJ:** Fragmentum historiae pharmaceutices veterum. Med dansk oversaettelse, biografiske noter og kommentarer, ved N. W. Bruun, K. Baerentsen, V. G. Jensen. København, Dansk Farmacihistorisk Selskab, 1981. 152 p. (Theriaca, 20).
**Retzius' stilling i den svenske patologiske anatomi: Tandlaegebladet** 1979 Oct;83(18):659
**Reuben D** see **Blum L**
**Reulos M** see **Margolin JC**
**Reusch C:** Die medizinische Versorgung auf den französischen Westindischen Inseln im 18. Jhd. im Spiegel des Werkes von J.B. Dazille 'Les Maladies des Nègres, leurs causes, leur traitement, et les moyens de les prévenir.' Diss., Universität Düsseldorf. Düsseldorf, 1982. 117 p.
**Revel J** see **Forster R**
**Revenko TA, Matiashina OM, Sokolenko OM, et al:** Travmatologo-ortopedicheskaia nauka v Donbasse za gody sotsialisticheskogo stroitel'stva. **Ortop Travmatol Protez** 1983 March;(3):47-51
**Revenko TA, Matiashina OM, Tsimidanova NB, et al:** Travmatologo-ortopedicheskaia sluzhba v Donbasse za 60 let Soiuza SSR. **Vestn Khir** 1983;130(4):10-3
**Reverby S, Rosner D:** Beyond 'the great doctors.' In their: Health care in America. Philadelphia, Temple University Press, 1979. p. 3-16.
**Reverby S, Rosner D, ed:** Health care in America: essays in social history. Philadelphia, Temple University Press, 1979. 275 p.
**Reverby S:** Stealing the golden eggs: Ernest Amory Codman and the science and management of medicine. **Bull Hist Med** 1981 Summer;55(2):156-71
**Reverby S:** The search for the hospital yardstick: nursing and the rationalization of hospital work. In Reverby S, Rosner D, ed: Health care in America. Philadelphia, Temple University Press, 1979. p. 206-35.
**Reverend AP:** La enfermedad y los ultimos momentos de Simon Bolivar, libertador de Colombia y del Peru. **Rev Soc Bolivar Venez** 1980;37(128):57-94
**Reverte Coma JM:** El chamanismo en Panama. **Asclepio** 1980;32:341-52
**Reverte Coma JM:** El trabajo de campo en antropología médica. **Asclepio** 1983;35:69-115
**Reverte Coma JM:** La lepra en la historia. **Fontilles** 1980;12:565-92
**Reverzy JF:** Introduction au secteur psychiatrique, définitions et historique. **Soins Psychiatr** 1980 Oct;(5):3-8
**Reverzy JF:** La biocratie. Esquisse d'une histoire de la notion de prévention en médecine et en psychiatrie en Occident. **Soins Psychiatr** 1982 Feb;(16):27-35
**Reverzy JF:** Petite histoire de la psychiatrie de secteur. **Soins Psychiatr** 1982 Feb;(16):41
**Reverzy JF:** Pour une compréhension historique de la psychiatrie. **Soins Psychiatr** 1982 Feb;(16):3
**A review of dental radiography: J Am Dent Assoc** 1984 Apr;108(4):552-3
**Revolutionary doctors of Anne Arundel County: Md Geneal Soc Bull** 1978 Fall;19:303-7
**Revutskiĭ EL:** 50 let Respublikanskogo nauchnogo obshchestva terapevtov USSR. **Vrach Delo** 1981 Oct;(10):120-1
**Rex-Kiss B:** A vérátömlesztés története hazánkban - történeti elozmények és visszaemlékezés. **Orvostort Kozl** 1982;28(1-3):87-105
**Rex-Kiss B:** A vércsoportkutatás rövid története. **Orv Hetil** 1980 Sep 21;121(38):2335-9
**Rex-Kiss B:** A vitás származás vércsoport-vizsgálatokkal való tisztázásának története hazánkban. **Orvostort Kozl** 1979;86(24 no 4):39-54
**Rex-Kiss B:** Short history of blood group research. **Ther Hung** 1982;30(3):144-9
**Rey AO** see **Agüero I**
**Reyaz Ali Parvaz S** see **Hameed HA**
**Reyes H:** Cincuentenario de la revista chilena de pediatria. **Rev Med Chil** 1980 Jul;108(7):597-8
**Reyes RM** see **Aguirre Zozaya F**
**Reyman TA, Peck WH:** Egyptian mummification with evisceration per ano. In A. Cockburn, E. Cockburn, ed: Mummies, disease, and ancient cultures. Cambridge, Cambridge University Press, 1980. p. 85-100.
**Reyman TA, Dowd AM:** Processing of mummified tissue for histological examination. In A. Cockburn, E. Cockburn, ed: Mummies, disease, and ancient cultures. Cambridge, Cambridge University Press, 1980. p. 258-73.
**Reyman TA, Goodman M:** The histology of ancient mammoth tissue. **Paleopathol Newsl** 1981 Jan;33:13-5
**Reyman TA** see **Chapel A**
**Reyman TA** see **Cockburn A**
**Reyman TA** see **Cockburn E**
**Reyman TA** see **Kristen KT**
**Reyman TA** see **Millet NB**
**Reyman TA** see **El-Najjar MY**
**Reyment RA:** Moors and Christians: an example of multivariate analysis applied to human blood-groups. **Ann Hum Biol** 1983 Nov-Dec;10(6):505-21
**Reynaud G:** Un grand naturaliste méconnu: Constantin Samuel Rafinesque (1783-1840). **Marseille** 1978;112:61-70
**Reynolds D** see **Taylor W**
**Reynolds E:** A treatise of the passions and faculties of the soule of man (1640). Facsimile, with introduction by M. L. Wiley. Gainesville, Florida, Scholars' Facsimiles & Reprints, 1971. 585 p. in various pagings.
**Reynolds F:** [Grave robbing]. **Indiana Med Hist Q** 1978;4(1):5-13
**Reynolds G:** Infant mortality and sex ratios at baptism ... Willingham ... Cambridgeshire [1559-1812]. **Local Popul Stud (Matlock)** 1979;22:31-7
**Reynolds KJ:** Early days of Loma Linda.....and even before. **Advent Herit** 1975;2(1):42-50
**Reynolds MD:** The development of the concept of fibrositis. **J Hist Med Allied Sci** 1983 Jan;38(1):5-35
**Reynolds WA:** Late report of the first case of plasmapheresis for Waldenström's macroglobulinemia [1956] **JAMA** 1981;245:606-7
**Rezai RF:** Tribute to dental pioneer Friedrich Otto Walkhoff. **Quintessence Int** 1984 Jun;15(6):655-7
**Rezanov II:** Raboty sanitarnykh vracheĭ v trudakh V. I. Lenina. **Gig Tr Prof Zabol** 1983 Feb;(2):41-3
**Rezende de Castro Monteiro A:** 'Hypnotisme'. Analyse de la thèse présentée à la Faculté de Médecine de Rio de Janeiro par Francisco de Paula Fajardo Junior, en vue d'obtenir le grade de docteur en médecine - Rio de Janeiro, 1888. In: Congrès international d'histoire de la médecine, XXVe, Québec, 1976. Actes. Québec, 1977. p. 980-91.
**Rezhabi Y:** The disease of Rabbi Solomon ibn Gabirol. **Sinai** 1979;84:1-8
**Rheinberger HJ, McLaughlin P:** Darwin's experimental natural history. **J Hist Biol** 1984 Fall;17(3):345-68
**Rheinberger HJ:** Naudin, Darwin, Nägeli: Bemerkungen zu den Vererbungsvorstellungen des 19. Jahrhunderts. **Medizinhist J** 1983;18(3):198-212
**Rheinberger R:** Zum 200. Geburtstag von Landesphysikus Gebhard Schaedler. ein Liechtensteinischer Artzt als Pionier der Pockenschutzimpfung. **Jahrb Hist Ver Fuerst Liechtenstein** 1976;76:337-43
**Rhoades ER:** A seminar on antibiotics. **J Okla State Med Assoc** 1980 Jun;73(6):176-9
**Rhoades ER:** Medicine at Fort Sill, Indian Territory 1975-1880. **J Okla State Med Assoc** 1982 Feb;75(2):36-41
**Rhoads JE:** Development of surgical nutrition at the University of Pennsylvania. **JPEN** 1980 Sep-Oct;4(5):464-6
**Rhoads JE, Vars HM, Dudrick SJ:** The development of intravenous hyperalimentation. **Surg Clin North Am** 1981 Jun;61(3):429-35
**Rhoads JE:** The evolution of intravenous hyperalimentation. **World J Surg** 1982 Jan;6(1):144-8
**Rhoads PS:** James B. Herrick, M.D. Born August 11, 1861--Died March 7, 1954. **Proc Inst Med Chic** 1982 Jan-Mar;35(1):3-6
**Rhode BM** see **MacLean LD**
**Rhodes FH:** Gradualism, punctuated equilibrium and the Origin of Species. **Nature** 1983 Sep 22-28;305(5932):269-72
**Rhodes JS:** The Raleigh Academy of Medicine. **NC Med J** 1981 Apr;42(4):263-4
**Rhodes LC** see **Webb H**
**Rhodes M:** A pair of late medieval spectacles from the Trig Lane site. **Lond Archaeol** 1980;4:23-5
**Rhodes SL:** Trends in child development research important to day-care policy. **Soc Serv Rev** 1979;53(2):285-94
**Rhys Evans PH:** Prominent ears and their surgical correction. **J Laryngol Otol** 1981 Sep;95(9):9881-92
**Riabinina MA:** K istorii otkrytiia ritmiki élektricheskikh protsessov golovnogo mozga. **Zh Vyssh Nerv Deiat** 1981 Jan-Feb;31(1):192-5
**Riabov SI, Stavskaia VV:** Idei S. P. Botkina v nefrologii. **Klin Med (Mosk)** 1982 Sep;60(9):27-32
**Riabykh LD** see **Borisov EN**
**Riad N:** L'influence de la médecine pharaonique et arabe sur la médecine européenne et mondiale. In: Congrès international d'histoire de la médecine, XXVe, Québec, 1976. Actes. Québec, 1977. p. 1128-56.
**Rial Roade J:** Sources for studies of historical demography in Uruguay (1728-1860). **Lat Am Res Rev** 1980;15(2):180-200
**Riall CT:** Surgical and medical devices and their origins. Chapter XIV. Beginnings of modern surgery (Andreas Vesalius). **J Oper Room Res Inst** 1982 Sep;2(9):30-3
**Riall CT:** Surgical and medical devices and their origins. Chapter XIX. Surgical instrument manufacturers. **J Oper Room Res Inst** 1983 Apr;3(4):36-9
**Riall CT:** Surgical and medical devices and their origins. Chapter XVII. Surgical instrument manufacturers. **J Oper Room Res Inst** 1983 Jan;3(1):33-5, 38-9, 42
**Riall CT, Hilzinger F:** Surgical and medical devices and their origins. Chapter XVIII. Surgical instrument manufacturers. **J Oper Room Res Inst** 1983 Feb;3(2):34-9
**Riall CT:** Surgical and medical devices and their origins. Chapter XX. The Swedish influence. **J Oper Room Res Inst** 1983 Jun;3(6):18-9, 22, 24

**Riall CT:** Surgical and medical devices and their origins. William Harvey and circulation of the blood. Chapter XVI. **J Oper Room Res Inst** 1982 Nov;2(11):32-6
**Riall CT** see **Hughes WL**
**Riatsen VI:** Uspekhi zdravookhraneniia Estonii. **Sov Zdravookhr** 1982;(11):12-5
**Ribeiro LD** see **Veras RP**
**Ribeiro da Silva L:** Os Jesuitas e a assistencia medica no Brasil colonial. **Rev Inst Hist Geogr Bras** 1978 Jan-Mar;318:212-32
**Ribeiro de Araujo A:** O ensaio sobre as fracturas do cirurgiao Manuel Alves da Costa Barreto. **Rev Inst Hist Geogr Bras** 1977;317:100-31
**Ribeiro Filho BM** see **Ferreira LF**
**Ribnick R:** A short history of primate field studies: old world monkeys and apes. In F. Spencer, ed: A history of American physical anthropology, 1930-1980. New York, Academic Press, 1982. p. 49-73.
**Rice AL, Burstyn HL, Jones AG:** G. C. Wallich M.D.---megalomaniac or mis-used oceanographic genius? **J Soc Bibliogr Nat Hist** 1976;7(4):423-50
**Rice CN:** The history of the Society of State Directors of Health, physical education, and recreation, 1953-1976. Ed.D. Diss., University of Alabama. University, 1977. v, 199 p.
**Rice DP:** Health statistics: past and present. **N Engl J Med** 1981 Jul 23;305(4):219-20
**Rice EF:** Paulus Aegineta. In Cranz FE, Kristeller PO, ed: Catalogus translationum et commentariorum: Mediaeval and Renaissance Latin translations and commentaries. Annotated lists and guides. Vol. IV. Washington, D.C., Catholic University of America Press, 1980. p. 145-91.
**Rice EW:** Joseh H. Roe (1892-1967): American man of science, pioneer clinical chemist. **Clin Chem** 1984 Sep;30(9):1575-8
**Rice F:** Care and treatment of the mentally ill. In Checkland O, Lamb M, ed: Health care as social history; the Glasgow case. Aberdeen, Aberdeen University Press, 1982. p. 59-73.
**Rice JL:** Dostoevsky's medical history: diagnosis and dialectic. **Russ Rev** 1983;42(2):131-61
**Rice JL:** Russian stereotypes in the Freud-Jung correspondence. **Slavic Rev** 1982 Spring;41(1):19-34
**Rice RW:** Computers in dentistry. Part 1. **Chronicle** 1982 Sep;45(7):130-2
**Rice TB:** One hundred years medicine: Indianapolis, 1820-1920. **Indiana Med Hist Q** 1976;2(3):40-4
**Rich NM, Clagett GP, Salander JM, et al:** Surgical treatment of arterial and venous injuries. **Acta Chir Belg** 1982 Sep-Oct;(5):473-84
**Rich NM, Clagett GP, Salander JM, et al:** The Matas/Soubbotitch connection. **Surgery** 1983 Jan;93(1 Pt 1):17-9
**Rich NM** see **Wind GG**
**Rich RF** see **Markle GE**
**Richard A:** L'évolution de la condition militaire des chirurgiens-dentistes. **Bull Acad Chir Dent (Paris)** 1979-1980;25(25):59-69
**Richard J:** Psychohistory: an Australian perspective. **Hist Today** 1981 May;31:10-3
**Richard J** see **Patrimoine hospitalier de la Bourgogne**
**Richard M, Roy R:** La folie à travers les temps. **Infirm Can** 1983 Jun;25(6):17-20
**Richard Neuhold (17. 10. 1917 bis 14. 8. 1982): Verh Dtsch Ges Pathol** 1983;67:774-7
**Richards DW** see **Fishman AP**
**Richards E:** The German romantic concept of embryonic repetition and its role in evolutionary theory in England up to 1859. Ph. D. Diss. University of New South Wales, 1976.
**Richards E** see **Dorjee P**
**Richards EL:** 50 years ago--blazing the trail. **Alumni Mag** 1984;84(2):9-12
**Richards ND:** Morals and molars. Physical deterioration and the beginnings of the School Dental Service 1878 to 1921. **Br Dent J** 1982 Jul 6;153(1):35-6
**Richards P, Tucker WD, Srivastava SC:** Technetium-99m: an historical perspective. **Int J Appl Radiat Isot** 1982 Oct;33(10):793-9
**Richards RJ:** Christian Wolff's prolegomena to empirical and rational psychology: translation and commentary. **Proc Am Philos Soc** 1980 Jun;124(3):227-39
**Richards RJ:** Instinct and intelligence in British natural theology: some contributions to Darwin's theory of the evolution of behavior. **J Hist Biol** 1981 Fall;14(2):193-230
**Richards RJ:** The emergence of evolutionary biology of behaviour in the early nineteenth century. **Br J Hist Sci** 1982 Nov;15(51 pt 3):241-80
**Richards RJ:** The personal equation in science: William James's psychological and moral uses of Darwinian theory. **Harv Libr Bull** 1982 Oct;30(4):387-425
**Richards RJ:** Why Darwin delayed, or interesting problems and models in the history of science. **J Hist Behav Sci** 1983 Jan;19(1):45-53
**Richards T:** Farr sighted. **Br Med J [Clin Res]** 1983 May 28;286(6379):1736-7
**Richards T:** Weather, nutrition, and the economy: short-run fluctuations in births, deaths, and marriages, France 1740-1909. **Demography** 1983 May;20(2):197-212
**Richardson BD:** The historical background of research on diet and dental caries in South Africa. **Tydskr Tandheelkd Ver S Afr** 1982 May;37(5):327-33
**Richardson BD** see **Walker AR**
**Richardson C** see **Barlow J**
**Richardson FM:** Amateur Palestinian guerrilla. **J R Army Med Corps** 1980 Feb;126(1):48-54
**Richardson G:** Letitia Munson. In Dictionary of Canadian biography, 1881-1890. 1982;11:629-30.
**Richardson JP:** Surgeons, physicians, and cardiology. **Aust NZ J Surg** 1980 Dec;50(6):668-71
**Richardson JP:** The surgeon as medical practitioner: an historical appreciation of the role of surgery in the corpus medicum. **Aust NZ J Surg** 1980 Oct;50(5):550-5
**Richardson L:** Breakthrough to nursing: the black nurse's story. **Imprint** 1981 Dec;28(5):27, 60, 73
**Richardson P** see **Burke G**
**Richardson R:** A dissection of the Anatomy Act. **Soc Soc Hist Med Bull (Lond)** 1980 Jun;26:38-9
**Richardson R:** Old people's attitudes to death in the twentieth century. **Soc Soc Hist Med Bull (Lond)** 1984 Jun;34:48-51
**Richardson RG:** Dr. John Hall, Shakespeare's son-in-law. A vignette of Elizabethan medicine. **Practitioner** 1981 Apr;225(1354):593-5
**Richardson RG:** How sick was Napoleon? **Practitioner** 1981 Jan;225(1351):109-10
**Richardson WF:** Medicine: the art of guessing? **NZ Med J** 1984 Jul 11;97(759):453-5
**Richardson WJ:** Lacan's view of language and being. **Psychoanal Rev** 1982 Summer;69(2):229-33
**Richardson WJ:** Religion and mental health. In Reich WT, et al, ed: Encyclopedia of bioethics, v.3. New York, Free Press, 1978. p. 1064-71.
**Riché P:** Les 'Gouvernants' et les problèmes de population dans le Haut Moyen-Age (Ve-IXe siècles). **Ann Demogr Hist (Paris)** 1979;:301-9
**Richerson HB:** Hypersensitivity pneumonitis--pathology and pathogenesis. **Clin Rev Allergy** 1983 Dec;1(4):469-86
**Richler B:** Manuscripts of Avicenna's Kanon in Hebrew translation: a revised and up-to-date list. **Koroth** 1982 Aug;8(3/4):145-68
**Richler B:** Manuscripts of Moses ben Nahman's 'Torat ha-Adam'. **Koroth** 1983 Aug;8(7-8):265-7
**Richman BL** see **Pinsker H**
**Richman EA, Ortner DJ, Schulter-Ellis FP:** Differences in intracortical bone remodeling in three aboriginal American populations: possible dietary factors. **Calcif Tissue Int** 1979 Nov 6;28(3):209-14
**Richmond JB:** A conversation with Fidel Castro about health services. **N Engl J Med** 1984 Apr 12;310(15):994-5
**Richmond PA:** The germ theory of disease. In Lilienfeld AM, ed: Times, places, and persons. Baltimore, London, Johns Hopkins Univ. Press, 1980. (Sigerist suppl. to the Bull Hist Med, n.s., no 4) p. 84-93.
**Richou H, Chanoit PF:** Une expérience française: la loi sur les alcooliques présumés dangereux. **Drug Alcohol Depend** 1983 Aug;12(1):61-8
**Richter HR:** Perspectives in international neurosurgery: neurosurgery in Switzerland. **Neurosurgery** 1980 Dec;7(6):632-5
**Richter J** see **Gerecke K**
**Richter J** see **Miura T**
**Richter K:** Die II. Frauenklinik der Universität München und Richard Fikentscher. **MMW** 1983 Sep 23;125(38):827-30
**Richter T:** Das Sargassokraut in Vicente de Lardizábals Werk 'Consuelo de Navegantes' (Madrid 1772). Diss., Universität Düsseldorf. Düsseldorf, 1982. 111 p.
**Richter W:** Der Anteil des Griechischen an den vorklinischen Nomenklaturen und die didaktischen Konsequenzen für die fachsprachliche Ausbildung von Medizinstudenten. **Wiss Z Univ Rostock** 1979;28(3):145-50
**Richter W:** Janus Cornarius, ein 'philologischer Mediziner' des 16. Jahrhunderts, und seine Beziehungen zur Rostocker Universität. **Wiss Z Univ Rostock** 1978;27(3):181-9
**Richter W:** Palladius und sein Columella - Text im Buch über die Tiermedizin. **Wien Stud Z Klass Philol** 1978;12:249-71
**Richter-Bernburg L** see **Haddad FS**
**Richterová L:** Přispěvek k historii psychiatrie z doby před 'velkou přeměnou'. **Cesk Psychiatr** 1980 Apr;76(2):134-8
**Rick AM:** Analysis of animal remains from the Old Fort Point site, northern Alberta. **Can Hist Sites** 1981;(26):269-89
**Rickenbacher B:** Die Zahntechnik, von der Vergangenheit zur Gegenwart. **Zahntechnik (Geneve)** 1983;41(2):124-6
**Ricketts RM:** Perspectives in the clinical application of cephalometrics. The first fifty years. **Angle Orthod** 1981 Apr;51(2):115-50
**Rickham PP, Stauffer UG:** Exstrophy of the bladder progress of management during the last 25 years. **Prog Pediatr Surg** 1984;17:169-88
**Rickham PP:** Johannes Fatio: Sein Leben, sein Werk und sein schreckliches Ende. **Z Kinderchir** 1984 Oct;39(5):289-95
**Rico-Avello C:** La enigmatica sexualidad de La Monja-Alferez. **Asclepio** 1980;32:353-60
**Rico-Avello C:** Patologia en la conquista de Mejico. **Asclepio** 1978-79;30-31:377-87
**Ricoeur P** see **Smith JH, ed**
**Ricoy JR:** In memoriam: J. F. Tello. **Arch Neurobiol (Madr)** 1980 Nov-Dec;43(6):347-52
**Riddington Young J:** Medicus Magus. **J Hist Med Allied Sci** 1980 Jan;35(1):40-57
**Riddle JM:** A survey of ancient specimens by electron microscopy. In A. Cockburn, E. Cockburn, ed: Mummies, disease, and ancient cultures. Cambridge, Cambridge University Press, 1980. p. 274-86.
**Riddle JM, Mulholland JA:** Albert on stones and minerals. In Weisheipl JA, ed: Albertus Magnus and the sciences. Toronto, Pontifical Institute of Mediaeval Studies. 1980. p. 203-34.
**Riddle JM:** Dioscorides. In Cranz FE, Kristeller PO, ed: Catalogus translationum et commentariorum: mediaeval and Renaissance Latin translations and commentaries. Annotated lists and guides. Vol. IV.

Washington, D.C., Catholic University of America Press, 1980. p. 1-143.
**Riddle JM:** Gargilius Martialis as a medical writer. **J Hist Med Allied Sci** 1984 Oct;39(4):408-29
**Riddle JM, Vreeland JM:** Identification of insects associated with Peruvian mummy bundles by using scanning electron microscopy. **Paleopathol Newsl** 1982 Sep;39:5-9
**Riddle JM:** Marbode of Rennes' (1035-1123) De lapidibus, considered as a medical treatise with text, commentary and C. W. King's translation, together with text and translation of Marbode's minor works on stones. Wiesbaden, Steiner, 1977. 144 p. (Sudhoffs Archiv, Beihefte, Heft 20).
**Riddle JM:** Pseudo-Dioscorides' Ex herbis femininis and early medieval medical botany. **J Hist Biol** 1981 Spring;14(1):43-81
**Rideau M** see **Portal C**
**Rideout DF** see **Hart GD, ed**
**Ridlen SS:** Funerary art in the 1890's: a reflection of culture. **Pioneer Am Soc Trans** 1983;6:27-35
**Ridley JC** see **Dawson DA**
**Ridley M:** Coadaptation and the inadequacy of natural selection. **Br J Hist Sci** 1982 Mar;15((1 no 1):45-68
**Ridolphi N:** Création des pharmacies en Alsace (1870-1938). Mémoire de diplôme d'Etat de docteur en pharmacie, Université Louis-Pasteur, Strasbourg, 1983. 91 leaves.
**Rieber RW, Green M, ed:** Milestones in the history of forensic psychology and psychiatry; a book of readings. New York, Da Capo, 1981. xi, 271 p.
**Rieber RW, Salzinger K, ed:** Psychology; theoretical-historical perspectives. New York, Academic Press, 1980. xiv, 364 p.
**Rieber RW:** The Americanization of psychology before William James. In R. W. Rieber, K. Salzinger, ed: Psychology: theoretical-historical perspectives. New York, Academic Press, 1980. p. 103-23.
**Rieber RW, Salzinger K, ed:** The roots of American psychology: historical influences and implications for the future. (Conference on the roots of American psychology). New York, New York Academy of Sciences, 1977. 394 p.
**Rieber RW** see **Green M**
**Rieber RW, ed:** Wilhelm Wundt and the making of a scientific psychology. New York, Plenum, 1980. xii, 252 p. Includes contributions by S. Diamond, K. Danziger, A. L. Blumenthal, W. James, S. Feldman, H. K. Haebertin.
**Riecken WE** see **Cobb AB**
**Riedel K** see **Stefani FH**
**Riedl R** see **Lorenz K, ed**
**Riehm K:** Die Schädelstruktur des Frühmenschen als Ausdruck seines Waldlebens und seiner weiteren Entwicklung. **Gegenbaurs Morphol Jahrb** 1980;126(6):884-99
**Riera J:** Antonio Cibat y la catedra de fisica experimental de Barcelona (un proyecto de 1807). **Asclepio** 1980;32:383-8
**Riera J:** Cirurgía española ilustrada y su comunicación con Europa (Estudio y documentos de un influjo cultural). Valladolid, Universidad de Vallodolid, 1976. 332 p. (Acta Historico-Medica Vallisoletana, Monografias, VII)
**Riera J, Jiménez Muñoz JM:** Dos 'ordenanzas' sanitarias de Fernando VI. **Asclepio** 1980;32:389-99
**Riera J:** [Dr. Matias Nieto y Serrano and Romantic medicine in Spain.] (Spa) **Cuad Invest Hist** 1979;:3
**Riera J, Jiménez Muñoz JM:** El doctor Rossell y los temores en España por la peste de Milan (1629-1631). In: Sociedad Española de Historia de la Medicina. V Congreso Nacional. Madrid, 1977. **Asclepio** 1977;29:283-307
**Riera J:** El libro de la peste (1600) del doctor Antonio Ponce de Santa Cruz. In: Sociedad Española de Historia de la Medicina. V Congreso Nacional. Madrid, 1977. **Asclepio** 1977;29:319-29
**Riera J:** José Masdevall y la medicina española ilustrada (Enseñanza, epidemias y guerra a finales del siglo XVIII). Valladolid, Universidad de Valladolid, 1980. 257 p. (Acta Historico-Medica Vallisoletana, Monografias, X)
**Riera J:** Los viajes de estudios de Andres del Rio (un documento de 1794). **Asclepio** 1980;32:361-5
**Riera J:** Matias Nieto y Serrano (1813-1902) y la medicina romantica. **Asclepio** 1980;32:367-81
**Riera J:** Matías Nieto y Serrano (1813-1902) y la medicina romántica. **Cuad Invest Hist** 1979;3:275-306
**Riera J:** Medicinas y ciencia en la España ilustrada, epistolario y documentos, I. Valladolid, Universidad de Valladolid, 1981. 159 p. (Acta Historico-Medica Vallisoletana, Monografias, XII)
**Riera J:** Medicinas y ciencia en la España ilustrada, epistolario y documentos, I. Valladolid, Universidad de Valladolid, 1981. 159 p. (Acta Historico-Medica Vallisoletana, Monografias, XII)
**Riera J:** Noticia de una epidemia segoviana de viruela (1740-1741). In: Sociedad Española de Historia de la Medicina. V Congreso Nacional. Madrid, 1977. **Asclepio** 1977;29:309-17
**Riera J:** Planos de hospitales españoles del siglo XVIII existentes en el Archivo General de Simancas (inventario primero). Valladolid, Ediciones del Seminario de Historia de la Medicine, Universidad de Valladolid, 1975. 18 p., numerous plates. (Acta Historico-Medica Vallisoletana, Monografias, V)
**Riera J:** Valverde y la anatomía del Renacimiento. Valladolid, Ediciones de la Universidad de Valladolid, 1981. 63 p.
**Riera J** see **Albarracín Teulón A**
**Riera J** see **Jimenez Muñoz JM**
**Riera J** see **Mendez Alvaro F**
**Riera i Montserrat F:** Remeis amatoris, pactes amb el dimoni, encanteris, per a saber de persones absents, cercadors de tresors, remeis per a la salut: bruixes i bruixots davant la inquisició de Mallorca en el segle XVII. Barcelona, Pequña Biblioteca Calamus Scriptorius, 1979. 61 p.
**Riese W:** Selected papers on the history of aphasia. With an introduction by W. Gooddy. Edited with prefatory notes by R. Hoops, Y. Lebrun, E. Buyssens. Amsterdam, Swets and Zeitlinger, 1977. 144 p. (Neurolinguistics, 7).
**Riesenfeld SA:** [The development of] health insurance. In Reich WT, et al, ed: Encyclopedia of bioethics, v. 2. New York, Free Press, 1978. p. 637-42.
**Riet AV:** August Bier en de homoeopathie. Eindhoven, Gema, 1978. 320 p. (Diss. Amsterdam).
**Riet D:** Les déclarations de grossesses dans la région de Dinan à la fin de l'Ancien Régime. **Ann Bretagne** 1981;88(2):181-7
**Riethe P, Czarnetzki A:** Amalgam- und Goldfolienfüllung Anno Domini 1601. **Dtsch Zahnarztl Z** 1983 Jun;38(6):610-6
**Riethe P:** Geschichtliche Entwicklung der Amalgame. **Dtsch Zahnarztl Z** 1980;35(4):443-9
**Rife DC, et al:** Dr. Harold Cummins and dermatoglyphics. **Birth Defects** 1979;15(6):1-797, passim
**Rigau Pérez JG:** El Dr. Francisco Oller y el inicio de la salud pública moderna en Puerto Rico, 1790-1831. In International Congress of the History of Medicine, 27th, Barcelona, 1980. Actas. Barcelona, Académia de Ciències Médiques de Catalunya i Balears, 1981. p. 199-202.
**Rigau-Pérez JG:** Smallpox epidemics in Puerto Rico during the prevaccine era (1518-1803). **J Hist Med Allied Sci** 1982 Oct;37(4):423-38
**Rigault J:** Les membres de l'Académie des Sciences Arts et Belles-lettres de Dijon de 1798 à 1914. In: Congrès National des Sociétés Savantes, 100e, Paris, 1975. Actes. Paris, 1976. Histoire Moderne et Contemporaine et Histoire des Sciences. p. 145-50.
**Riggi G** see **Martinetto P**
**Rightmire GP:** Middle Pleistocene hominids from Olduvai Gorge, northern Tanzania. **Am J Phys Anthropol** 1980 Aug;53(2):225-41
**The rights of the child: Aust Paediatr J** 1982 Mar;18(1):6-12
**Rigler LG** see **Wangensteen OW, ed**
**Rihm A, Montag M, Mock HK:** A transition in nursing education. Santa Fe, Research Coordinating Unit, State Dept. of Education, 1967. viii, 114 p.
**Rihner F:** Alfred Hegar--Zum 150. Geburtstag. **Med Welt** 1980 Oct 17;31(42):1522-3
**Rihner F:** André Levert zum 200. Todestag. **MMW** 1980;122:1163-4
**Rihner F:** Jean Riolan der Jüngere. **Med Welt** 1981;32:476-8
**Rihner F:** Jean Riolan der Jüngere, 1580-1657. **MMW** 1980;122:1341-3
**Rihner F:** Professor Dr. Manfred Bleuler zum 80. Geburtstag. Zürich, Woodtli, 1982. 43 p.
**Rihner F:** Sir Alexander Fleming - zum 25. Todestag. **Med Welt** 1980;31:1564-5
**Říhová M:** Zamyšlení nad nejstarším lékařským prvotiskem pražské provenience. **Cas Lek Cesk** 1983 Aug 19;122(32-33):1020-2
**Rijlant P:** Results and perspectives in electrocardiology. **Adv Cardiol** 1981;28:1-8
**Rijlant P:** The coming of age of electrophysiology and electrocardiography. **NTM** 1980;17(1):108-23
**Riker DM:** Surgeon Hans Kierstede of New Amsterdam. **Halve Maen** 1983;57(3):11-3, 24
**Riley D:** 'The free mothers': pronatalism and working women in industry at the end of the last war in Britain. **Hist Workshop J** 1981;11:59-118
**Riley DP** see **Dodson G**
**Riley HD:** George Nicholas Papanicolaou. In Dictionary of American biography, 1961-1965. Suppl. 7, 1981. p. 598-9.
**Riley HD:** Homer William Smith. In Dictionary of American biography, 1961-1965. Suppl. 7, 1981. p. 699-700.
**Riley HD:** The history of histoplasmosis. **J Okla State Med Assoc** 1983 Feb;76(2):31-40
**Riley J:** The elephant man: 'Treat me as an equal' (John Merrick, Sir Frederick Treves). **Nurs Mirror** 1979 Nov 8;149(19):24-5
**Riley JC:** Mortality on long-distance voyages in the eighteenth century. **J Econ Hist** 1981;41(3):651-6
**Riley RH:** Historical data, Maryland State Department of Health, 1899-1932. **Md State Med J** 1980 Nov;29(11):92-7
**Riley RL:** Airborne contagion. Historical background. **Ann NY Acad Sci** 1980;353:3-9
**Riley RL:** The contagiosity of tuberculosis. **Schweiz Med Wochenschr** 1983 Jan 22;1113(3):75-9
**Riley RW:** A century of editors. **JAMA** 1983 Jul 8;250(2):230-5
**Riley TL** see **Massey EW**
**Rim HJ:** Therapy of fluke infections in the past. A review. **Arzneimittelforsch** 1984;34(9B):1127-9
**Ríman J:** From Mendel to molecular genetics and biotechnologies. **Folia Biol (Praha)** 1983;29(1):1-8
**Rimpela M** see **Vuori H**
**Rimpler M** see **Giebel G**
**Rinard RG:** The problem of the organic individual: Ernst Haeckel and the development of the biogenetic law. **J Hist Biol** 1981 Fall;14(2):249-76
**Rínchindorzh TS, Tuméngur Z:** Pomoshch' Sovetskogo Soiuza v razvitii zdravookhraneniia Mongol'skoĭ Narodnoĭ Respubliki. **Sov Zdravookhr** 1981;(8):59-62
**Rindfuss RR:** Changing patterns of fertility in the South: a social-demographic examination. **Soc Forces** 1978;57(2):621-35
**Rindfuss RR, Bumpass LL, Palmore JA, et al:** The transformation of Korean

child-spacing practices. **Popul Stud** 1982 Mar;36(1):87–104

**Ring J:** Zur Problematik der Dextran-Unverträglichkeit und ihrer spezifischen Prophylaxe durch Hapten-Hemmung. Ein Stück Geschichte angewandter Immunologie. **Fortschr Med** 1982 Nov 4;100(41):1917–21

**Ring M:** Dentures: the restoration of choice in the 1920s. **Dent Lab Rev** 1982 Aug;57(8):27, 34

**Ring M:** The age of cosmetic dentistry. **Dent Lab Rev** 1982 Nov;57(11):36

**Ring ME:** Fagan implant. **NY J Dent** 1984 Jun–Aug;54(5):194

**Ring ME:** Nothing new under the sun: an examination of newly discovered inventions and techniques. **J Am Dent Assoc** 1980 Jan;100(1):22–5

**Ring ME:** Oddments in dental history. **Bull Hist Dent** 1980 Apr;28(1):19–20 (continued periodically)

**Ring ME:** Oddments in dental history: a case of tooth implantation by the patient. **Bull Hist Dent** 1983 Apr;31(1):29

**Ring ME:** Oddments in dental history: down with toothbrushes – up with tobacco! **Bull Hist Dent** 1984;32(1):31–2

**Ring ME:** Oddments in dental history: the advertising, cut-rate dentist: a prophesy of a century ago. **Bull Hist Dent** 1982 Oct;30(2):115–6

**Ring ME:** Oddments in dental history: what every sea surgeon of around 1600 ought to know concerning treating teeth. **Bull Hist Dent** 1984 Oct;32(2):109–11

**Ring ME:** The rubber denture murder case: the true story of the vulcanite litigations. **Bull Hist Dent** 1984;32(1):3–18

**Ringertz NR:** Upptäckt av 'hoppande gener' hos majs gav 81-årig kvinna hela medicinpriset Barbara McClintock--en unik medicinsk nobelpristagare. **Lakartidningen** 1983 Oct 19;80(42):3908–10

**Rink E:** Technical Americana: a checklist of technical publications printed before 1831. Millwood, N. Y., Kraus International, 1981. 'Medical technology', p. 245–49.

**Rinn WA:** A medical anniversary. **Md State Med J** 1981 Dec;30(12):38

**Rinsler MG:** Spectroscopy, colorimetry, and biological chemistry in the nineteenth century. **J Clin Pathol** 1981 Mar;34(3):287–91

**Rintelen F:** Der Basler Chirurg und Rebell Johannes Fatio 1649–1691. **Gesnerus** 1983;40(1–2):149–58

**Rintelen F:** Geschichte der Medizinischen Fakultät in Basel 1900–1945. Basel/Stuttgart, Schwabe, 1980. 454 p.

**Rintelen F:** Von der Augenheilanstalt zur Universitätsaugenklinik in Basel. **Gesnerus** 1982;39(1):79–83

**Rintelen F:** Zum 100. Geburtstag von Alfred Vogt -- Versuch einer Würdigung seines wissenschaftlichen Werkes. **Klin Monatsbl Augenheilkd** 1979 Oct;175(4):439–41

**Rintelen F:** Zur Persönlichkeit Karl Gustav Jungs. **Gesnerus** 1982;39(2):237–42

**Rintelen F:** 75. Jahresversammlung der Schweizerischen ophthalmologischen Gesellschaft; zu ihrer Gründung und ihren Gründen. **Klin Monatsbl Augenheilkd** 1983 May;182(5):348–51

**Río Samper S del** see **Torres Ramírez C**

**Rioch MJ:** In memoriam: Abe Fortas. **Psychiatry** 1983;46(1):83–6

**Riopelle JL:** A la mémoire du Professeur Pierre Masson, Vingt ans après. **Union Med Can** 1979 May;108(5):473–6

**Riordan CE** see **Kleber HD**

**Riordan J, Countryman BA:** Basics of breastfeeding. Part I: Infant feeding patterns past and present. **JOGN Nurs** 1980 Jul–Aug;9(4):207–10

**Riou R** see **Martinon JF**

**Riou YF:** Un fragment d'un manuscrit disparu d'Oribase, C. L. A. 116 (Vatican, Urb. lat. 293, ff. 95–96, VIIIe siècle). **Scriptorium** 1979;33:235–7

**Rípodas Ardanaz D:** Fuentes inusuales en historia de la medicina hispanoamericana colonial. **Rev Indias** 1980;40(159–62):399–414

**Ripp GKh, Salamatov EI:** Uchastie medikov Zapadnoĭ Sibiri v lechenii ranenykh i bil'nykh voinov. **Voen Med Zh** 1980 Jun;(6):24–6

**Riquer JS** see **Flores y Troncoso FA**

**Rische H:** Moderne epidemiologische und pathogenetische Erkenntnisse, dargestellt am Beispiel der Cholera. **Z Erkr Atmungsorgane** 1983;161(1):65–73

**Rising JD:** Rambling recollections about the 'Postgraduate Department' -- now the Division of Continuing Education of the College of Health Sciences. **J Kans Med Soc** 1980 Mar;81(3):102, 156–8

**Risquez-Iribarren R:** Some aspects of social medicine in Venezuela. In: Congrès international d'histoire de la médecine, XXVe, Québec, 1976. Actes. Quebec, 1977. p. 237–45.

**Risse GB:** A letter to Benjamin Rush. **J Hist Med Allied Sci** 1980 Oct;35(4):461

**Risse GB:** Epidemics and medicine: the influence of disease on medical thought and practice. **Bull Hist Med** 1979 Winter;53(4):505–19

**Risse GB:** Erna Lesky and the history of medicine. **Bull Hist Med** 1981 Winter;55(4):575–80

**Risse GB:** From horse and buggy to automobile and telephone: medical practice in Wisconsin, 1848–1930. In Numbers RL, Leavitt JW, ed: Wisconsin medicine. Historical perspectives. Madison, University of Wisconsin Press, 1981. p. 25–45.

**Risse GB:** Historia de la medicina en los EE.UU.: nuevos enfoques de investigacion y enseñanza. **Bol Soc Mex Hist Filos Med** 1979 Sep;4(28):113–27

**Risse GB:** History of the concepts [of health and disease]. In Reich WT, et al, ed: Encyclopedia of bioethics, v. 2. New York, Free Press, 1978. p. 579–85.

**Risse GB:** La ecología de la enfermedad: tema de estudio médico-histórico. **Bol Soc Mex Hist Filos Med** 1984 Mar;7(46):289–304

**Risse GB:** Medical history in Latin America. **Clio Med** 1981 Apr;15(3–4):231–45

**Risse GB:** Medicine in New Spain: Institutions and practice 1570–1621. In International Congress of the History of Medicine, 27th, Barcelona, 1980. Actas. Barcelona, Acadèmia de Ciències Mèdiques de Catalunya i Balears, 1981. p. 207–11.

**Risse GB** see **Brieger GH**

**Risse GB** see **McCullough LB**

**Risse GB** see **Somolinos-Palencia J**

**Rissmann W:** Ernst Freiherr von Feuchtersleben (1806–1849). Sein Beitrag zur medizinischen Anthropologie und Psychopathologie. Freiburg im Breisgau, Schulz, 1980. 243 p. (Freiburger Forschungen zur Medizingeschichte, Neue Folge, Band 12).

**Risso M:** Institution psychiatrique, idéologie médicale et chronification. **Schweiz Arch Neurol Neurochir Psychiatr** 1980;126(2):327–35

**Rissom R:** Fritz Lenz und die Rassenhygiene. Husum, Matthiesen, 1983. 143 p. (Abhandlungen zur Geschichte der Medizin und der Naturwissenschaften, 47).

**Ritchey D:** The Baltimore theater and the yellow fever epidemic. **Md Hist Mag** 1972;67(3):298–301

**Ritchey FJ:** Medical rationalization, cultural lag, and the malpractice crisis. **Hum Organ** 1981;40(2):97–112

**Rits IA:** O razvitii rentgenologii v Sibiri. **Vestn Rentgenol Radiol** 1982 May–Jun;(3):90–2

**Ritt L** see **Bauer C**

**Ritter L:** Die Spezialgebiete der Medizin und ihre Geschichte. Darmstadt, Bläschke, 1978. 262 p.

**Ritter L** see **Back F**

**Riunione straordinaria dei Consigli Comunale e Provinciale in occasione del 1 centenario della morte di Francesco Rizzoli (24–5–1880) e della nascita di Vittorio Putti (1–3–1880): Chir Organi Mov** 1979 Jul–Aug;65(4):367–98

**Riva G:** Zum 50jährigen Bestehen der Schweizerischen Gesellschaft für Innere Medizin. **Schweiz Med Wochenschr [Suppl]** 1982;13:5–22

**Rival N:** Tabac, miroir du temps. Paris, Librairie Academique Perrin, 1981. 282 p.

**Rivera Nieves M** see **Colón Rourc C**

**Rivera Villanueva ZE:** The collection of the Boletín de la Asociación Médica de Puerto Rico and its preservation (1903–20). **Bol Asoc Med PR** 1984 Sep;76(9):394–6

**Rivero de la Calle M, Collado Lopez O:** Reporte sobre las primeras mediciones craneometricas de tipo comparativo realizadas en Cuba. [H. J. Dumont.]. **Cienc Habana Ser 9** 1976;6:3–27

**Rivero-Serrano O:** Restauración de la antigua Escuela de Medicina. **Gac Med Mex** 1980;116:429–30

**Rivero-Serrano O** see **Somolinos-Palencia J**

**Rivers JE** see **Stambolian G**

**Riverso E** see **Epistemologia, metodologia clinica e storia della scienza medica, 2**

**Rivet R:** A propos de l'oeuvre médicale du Baron Marchant (1767–1833). In: Congrès National des Sociétés Savantes, 103e, Nancy, 1978. Comptes Rendus. Paris, 1978. Section des Sciences, Fasc. V. p. 125–30.

**Rivet R:** Quelques aspects sanitaires de la Bretagne vus à travers les thèses des Facultés de médecine de Paris et de Strasbourg de l'an VII (1798) à 1870. In: Congrès National des Sociétés Savantes, 107e. Brest, 1982. Comptes Rendus, Paris, 1983. Section des Sciences, Fasc. IV. p. 241–52.

**Rivet R:** Un essai de journalisme médical en l'an VII (1799). In: Congrès National des Sociétés Savantes, 105e, Caen, 1980. Comptes Rendus, Paris, 1980. Section des Sciences, Fasc. V. p. 41–7.

**Rivet R:** Un médecin de Perpignan, professeur à l'Université de Montpellier: Joseph Anglada (1775–1833). In: Congrès National des Sociétés Savantes, 106e, Perpignan, 1981. Comptes Rendus. Paris, Bibliothèque Nationale, 1982. Fasc. IV. p. 111–7.

**Rivet R:** Usage médical du vin de Bordeaux au XVIIIe siècle. In: Congrès National des Sociétés Savantes, 104e, Bordeaux, 1979. Comptes Rendus. Paris, 1979. Section des Sciences, Fasc. IV. p. 121–31.

**Rivet R** see **Arvy L**

**Rivet R** see **Schiller J**

**Rix A:** Oklahoma's neurosurgical heritage. **J Okla State Med Assoc** 1980 Apr;73(4):112–8

**Rix KJ:** Boswell and his doctors. **Hist Med** 1981;9(1):9–12, 17

**Rixer A:** A magyar gyógyszerészi szaksajtó kialakulása és fejlődése a xix. században. **Acta Pharm Hung** 1983 Jul;53(4):183–90

**Rixer A:** A magyar nyelvü gyógyszerészeti szaksajtó kialakulása és jelenentősége 1831–1872 között. Diss., Budapest, 1976. 193 p.

**Riz R:** Geburtenrückgang in Südtirol. **Eur Ethn** 1980;37(1):14–9

**Rizzuti A:** Il dolore dei denti. **Dent Cadmos** 1981 May;49(5):75–6

**Rizzuti A:** Instituzione ed evoluzione dell'insegnamento dell'odontoiatria e genesi del dentista moderno. **Dent Cadmos** 1981 Jul;49(7):25–30

**Rizzuti A:** Odontoiatria del passato. Chirurgia e Medicina nel '700: nascita della Università moderna. **Dent Cadmos** 1982 Dec;50(12):59–61

**Rizzuti A:** Odontoiatria del passato. 'Matricole' di Dentista rilasciate nello Stato Pontificio. **Dent Cadmos** 1982 Nov;50(11):75–7

**Rizzuti A:** Odontoiatria del passato. Storia dell'amalgama dentale (I). **Dent Cadmos** 1983 Aug;51(8):69–73

**Roazen P:** A note on the Vienna Psychoanalytic Society: Felix Deutsch's letters, 1923 and 1935. **J Hist Behav Sci** 1984 Oct;20(4):359–62

**Roazen P:** Anorexia nervosa: Helene Deutsch, M.D. **Bull Menninger Clin** 1981 Nov;45(6):499–501

**Roazen P:** Erik H. Erikson's America: the political implications of ego psychology. **J Hist Behav Sci** 1980 Oct;16(4):333–41

**Roazen P:** Freud and America. **Soc Res (NY)** 1972;39(4):720–32

**Roazen P:** Paul Roazen on errors regarding Freud. **Int J Psychoanal** 1982;63(pt 2):260–1

**Roazen P:** The menopause. By Helene Deutsch. **Int J Psychoanal** 1984;65(Pt 1):55–62
**Roazen P:** Two cases of induced insanity. Helene Deutsch, Cambridge, Mass. **Int J Psychoanal** 1981;62(pt 2):139–50
**The Robb House: home of the Alachua County Medical Society and Auxiliary: J Fla Med Assoc** 1982 Aug;69(8):681–2
**Robb-Smith AH:** Egerton Y. Davis, M.D., and placentophagy. **Bull NY Acad Med** 1980 Mar;56(2):258–60
**Robb-Smith AH:** Osler's influence on haematology. **Blood Cells** 1981;7(3):513–36
**Robb-Smith AH:** The quatercentenary of the Lumleian Lecture. **J R Coll Physicians Lond** 1983 Jan;17(1):74–8
**Robbins C:** The collector's legacy. **MD** 1982 May;26(6):193–6, 201
**Robbins P:** Alas, Memphis! **Am Hist Illus** 1982;16(9):38–46
**Robbins P:** General Grant's calico colonel. **Am Hist Illus** 1979;14(1):4–7, 43–8
**Robbins T, Anthony D:** Deprogramming, brainwashing and the medicalization of diviant religious groups. **Soc Probl** 1982;29(3):283–97
**Robboy S** see **Côté RA**
**Roberson JW:** A view from Oklahoma, 1866–1868: the diary and letters of Dr. James Reagles, Jr., Assistant Surgeon, U. S. Army. **Red River Val Hist Rev** 1978;3(4):19–46
**Robert BP:** Origines du surréalisme. **Univ Ottawa Q** 1982;52(2):190–205
**Robert BP:** Profiles de 'La fruite des idées' et surréalisme. **Rev Univ Ottawa** 1977;47(3):345–64
**Robert E:** Les adresses de malades dans les Epidémies II, IV et VI. In La collection hippocratique et son rôle dans l'histoire de la médecine. Colloque de Strasbourg (23–27 octobre 1972) organisé par le Centre de Recherches sur la Grèce Antique, avec le concours des Facultés de Philosophie et des Langues Classiques. Leiden, E. J. Brill, 1975. p. 173–94.
**Robert F:** Hippocrate, Platon, Aristote et les notions de genre et d'espèce. **Hist Philos Life Sci** 1982;4(2):173–201
**Robert G:** La révocation de l'édit de Nantes et les professions de Santé. **Hist Sci Med** 1983;17(2):181–7
**Robert JC** see **Dechêne L**
**Robert JS:** Drink and industrial work discipline in 19th century Germany. **J Soc Hist** 1981;15(1):25–38
**Robert L:** Décret pour un médecin de Cos. **Rev Philol (Paris)** 1978;52(2):242–51
**Robert I. Watson and the development of the history of psychology: a symposium:** With contributions by E. S. Mills, E. R. Hilgard, B. Ross, J. Popplestone, M. W. McPherson, R. B. Evans, E. S. Goodman, J. Brožek. **J Hist Behav Sci** 1982 Oct;18(4):307–31
**Robert Koch: Probl Tuberk** 1982 Mar;(3):8–9
**Robert Koch: father of bacteriology and infectious diseases: Ceylon Med J** 1982 Mar;27(1):6–7
**Roberts A:** A history of the plague in England. **Nurs Times** 1979;75:777–9
**Roberts A:** Down the drain: cholera in Britain. **Nurs Times** 1984 Oct 10–16;80(41):40–3
**Roberts A:** The fifth little horseman. **Nurs Times** 1983 Nov 2–8;79(44):49–53
**Roberts A:** The plague in England. **Hist Today** 1980 Apr 30;:29–34
**Roberts A:** The pox and the people: a history of venereal diseases and sexual attitudes. **Nurs Times** 1982 Jul 14–20;78(28):1177–85
**Roberts CA:** Perspectives on 25 years of Canadian psychiatric research. **Psychiatr J Univ Ottawa** 1984 Sep;9(3):95–101
**Roberts DF:** Dermatoglyphics and human genetics. **Birth Defects** 1979;15(6):475–94
**Roberts GK:** The establishment of the Royal College of Chemistry: an investigation of the social context of early-Victorian chemistry. **Hist Stud Phys Sci** 1976;7:437–85
**Roberts GK:** The liberally-educated chemist: chemistry in the Cambridge Natural Science Tripos, 1851–1914. **Hist Stud Phys Sci** 1980;11(1):157–83
**Roberts J, Mendez-Bauer C:** A perspective of maternal position during labor. **J Perinat Med** 1980;8(6):255–64
**Roberts J** see **Rall P**
**Roberts JA:** Reginald Ruggles Gates. In Dictionary of national biography, 1961–1970. Suppl. 8, 1981. p. 424–5.
**Roberts KB:** Eustachius and his anatomical plates. **Newsl Can Soc Hist** 1979 Apr;:9–13
**Roberts KB:** Plague in 18th century Syria: the work of Alexander and Patrick Russell. In: Congrès international d'histoire de la médecine, XXVe, Québec, 1976. Actes. Québec, 1977. p. 1157.
**Roberts NJ:** Presidents's remarks. **Bull NY Acad Med** 1981 Oct;57(8):659–63
**Roberts R:** Pioneering, medicine and mind. **Australas Nurses J** 1982 Jun;11(5):16–23
**Roberts RE** see **Lee ES**
**Roberts RS:** A socio-historical view of the struggle for health in Zimbabwe. **Cent Afr J Med** 1979 Oct;25(10):235–6
**Roberts RS:** The first description of idiopathic thrombocytopaenic purpura and onyalai in Southern Africa? **Cent Afr J Med** 1980 Dec;26(12):257–8
**Roberts WC, Silver MA:** Norman Jefferis Holter and ambulatory ECG monitoring. **Am J Cardiol** 1983 Oct 1;52(7):903–6
**Roberts WC, Warnes CA:** The AJC in December 1958. **Am J Cardiol** 1983 Dec 1;52(10):1355
**Robertson D:** Magical medicine in Viking Scandinavia. **Med Hist** 1976 Jul;20(3):317–22
**Robertson D** see **Smith B**
**Robertson JH** see **Dodson G**
**Robertson RM** see **Smith B**
**Robetti I, Iorio M:** Università degli Studi di Torino, Istituto di Medicina Legale e delle Assicurazioni. **Minerva Stomatol** 1981 Jul–Aug;30(4):321–30
**Robicsek F:** An epitaph for cavopulmonary anastomosis. **Ann Thorac Surg** 1982 Aug;34(2):208–20
**Robicsek F:** The birth of the surgical stapler. **Surg Gynecol Obstet** 1980 Apr;150(4):579–83
**Robicsek F, Littmann L:** The first reported case of external heart massage (János Balassa). **Clin Cardiol** 1983 Nov;6(11):569, 571
**Robicsek F:** The smoking gods; tobacco in Maya art, history, and religion. Norman, Oklahoma, Univ. of Oklahoma Press, 1978. xxv, 233 p.
**Robillard D:** L'hôpital Notre-Dame de Montréal célèbre avec dynamisme 100 ans de progrès. **Can Med Assoc J** 1980 Apr 5;122(7):837–9
**Robin G** see **Hildesheimer F**
**Robin M:** Sheltering arms: the roots of child protection. In E. H. Newberger, ed: Child abuse. Boston, Little, Brown and Company, 1982. p. 1–21.
**Robin ED, ed:** Claude Bernard and the internal environment: a memorial symposium. New York, Dekker, 1979. xvi, 299 p. Historical contributions by J. Bernard, M. Bertrand, J. S. Fruton, R. H. Unger, J. P. Changeux, A. Cournand, F. Morel, R. Guillemin, H. Rahn, S. S. Cohen.
**Robins AH:** Did imprisonment ruin Oscar Wilde? **Practitioner** 1981 May;225(1355):773–5
**Robins L:** A short history of the modern struggle for national health insurance. **J Health Hum Resour Adm** 1983 Winter;5(3):252–65
**Robins R:** An old Cornish hand. **J Hand Surg [Br]** 1984 Jun;9(2):199–200
**Robins RS:** Disease, political events, and populations. In Rothschild H, ed: Biocultural aspects of disease. New York, Academic Press, 1981. p. 153–75.
**Robins RS, Rothschild H:** Hidden health disabilities and the presidency: medical management and political consideration. **Perspect Biol Med** 1981 Winter;24(2):240–53
**Robinson C** see **Wallace CE**
**Robinson DN:** System of modern psychology. New York, Columbia Univ. Press, 1979. xii, 333 p.
**Robinson DN:** The mind unfolded. Essays on psychology's historic texts. Washington, D. C., University Publications of America, 1978. xi, 539 p.
**Robinson DN** see **Hearst E, ed**
**Robinson DW:** The care of burns. Early history to present. **J Arkansas Med Soc** 1984 Apr;80(11):517–25
**Robinson G** see **Ebbert A, et al**
**Robinson G** see **Wilson LG, ed**
**Robinson GA:** The National Hospitals for Nervous Diseases, 1948–1982. London, The Board of Governors of the National Hospitals for Nervous Diseases, 1982. xvii, 133 p.
**Robinson HS:** Anderson Ruffin Abbott, MD, 1837–1913. **J Natl Med Assoc** 1980 Jul;72(7):713–6
**Robinson HS:** Furman Jeremiah Shadd, MD 1852–1908. **J Natl Med Assoc** 1980 Feb;72(2):151–3
**Robinson HS:** Robert and Roderick Badger, pioneer Georgia dentists. **Negro Hist Bull** 1961;24(4):77–80
**Robinson J** see **Peel J**
**Robinson JO:** The barber-surgeons of London. **Arch Surg** 1984 Oct;119(10):1171–5
**Robinson JO:** The failing health of Napoleon. **J R Soc Med** 1979 Aug;72(8):621–3
**Robinson JS:** Sciatica and the lumbar disk syndrome: a historic perspective. **South Med J** 1983 Feb;76(2):232–8
**Robinson K:** The crisis in general practice--1965. **Soc Soc Hist Med Bull (Lond)** 1983 Dec;33:15–6
**Robinson MC** see **Detre KC**
**Robinson PA:** The conception of death in Judaism in the Hellenistic and early Roman period. Ph.D. Diss., University of Wisconsin. Madison, 1978. ix, 176 leaves.
**Robinson PN:** The ANZAC link in the history of Harefield Hospital, Middlesex, England. **NZ Med J** 1983 Oct 26;96(742):807
**Robinson R** see **Dobbs R**
**Robinson RG:** JAMA at 100. **NZ Med J** 1983 Aug 24;96(738):654
**Robinson SA:** A historical development of midwifery in the black community: 1600–1940. **J Nurse Midwife** 1984 Jul–Aug;29(4):247–50
**Robinson T:** Baroque medicine: how a cup of Aunt Ida's hot air rescued a sailor. **Nurs Mirror** 1982 Jul 21;155(3):25
**Robinson WJ:** Physick in Bolton in 1779. **Pharm Hist (London)** 1981 Apr;11(1):6–7
**Robinson DN, ed:** Significant contributions to the history of psychology 1750–1920. Series A. Orientations. Volume I: E. Condillac, T. Brown. Washington, D. C., University Publications of America, 1977. Various pagings.
**Robinson MC, ed** see **Hoy SM**
**Robinton ED:** Anna Wessels Williams. In: Notable American women. The modern period. Cambridge, Mass., Belknap-Harvard Univ. Press, 1980. 4:737–9.
**Robinton ED:** Dorothy Reed Mendenhall. In: Notable American women. The modern period. Cambridge, Mass., Belknap-Harvard Univ. Press, 1980. 4:468–70.
**Robison DW:** Wisconsin and the mentally ill. A history of the 'Wisconsin Plan' of state and county care 1860–1915. New York, Arno Press, 1980. ix, 322 p. (Historical Issues in Mental Health).
**Robles C:** Los hospitales como microsociedades. **Gac Med Mex** 1980 Jan;116(1):1–8

**Robson A:** The significance of 'The maiden tribute of modern Babylon'. **Victorian Period Newsl** 1978;11(2):50–7
**Robson EB:** Gene mapping and chromosome 21: history and methodology. **Hum Gent [Supp]** 1981;2:147–53
**Rocchietta S:** Alchimia e medicina nel romanzo 'La rosticceria della regina Pedoca' di Anatole France. **Minerva Med** 1980 Oct 31;71(42):3091–2
**Rocchietta S:** Alcuni valzer viennesi di interesse medico. **Minerva Med** 1982 Oct 6;73(38):2603–4
**Rocchietta S:** Canzoni italiane correlate con la medicina e la farmacia. **Minerva Med** 1980 Oct 13;71(39):2861–70
**Rocchietta S:** Caricature di Daumier correlate alla medicina in una mostra commemorativa. **Minerva Med** 1981 May 7;72(18):1157–8
**Rocchietta S:** Due raffigurazioni di santa Apollonia. (sec. XVI e sec. XVIII). **Minerva Med** 1983 Oct 6;74(38):2215 6
**Rocchietta S:** Due secoli di canzoni inglesi con spunti medico-=farmaceutici. **Minerva Med** 1979 Sep 26;70(41):2839–43
**Rocchietta S:** Iconografia statuaria e pittorica di Santa Apollonia nel Duomo di Milano. **Minerva Med** 1981 Jan 14;72(1):45–9
**Rocchietta S:** Le edizioni italiane del ricettario di Madame Fouquet. **Minerva Med** 1981 Jan 21;72(2):111–2
**Rocchietta S:** Le pubblicazioni di storia della farmacia portoghese negli anni '70. **Minerva Med** 1980 Dec 15;71(50):3679–84
**Rocchietta S:** Libri di interesse medico stampati da Giambattista Bodoni (1740–1813). **Minerva Med** 1983 Oct 13;74(39):2327–8
**Rocchietta S:** Medici e speziali in tre romanzi de Voltaire. **Minerva Med** 1982 Feb 11;73(5):219–20
**Rocchietta S:** Musica e litotomia in una composizione di Marin Marais (1656–1728). **Minerva Med** 1983 Nov 16;74(44):2713
**Rocchietta S:** Musica e medicina negli scritti di Felice La Torre (1846–1923). **Minerva Med** 1980 Jul;71(27):1949–53
**Rocchietta S:** Musica e medicina negli scritti di Felice La Torre (1846–1923). **Minerva Ginecol** 1980 Oct;32(10):949–53
**Rocchietta S:** Sulle edizioni degli 'Antidotari' e di altre opere di J.-J. Wecker. **Minerva Med** 1981 Sep 19;72(34):2297
**Rocchietta S:** Un 'Christ à la pharmacie' ou 'Les Saints Côme et Damien'? **Rev Hist Pharm (Paris)** 1984 Jun;31(261):131–3
**Rocchietta S:** Una ricetta contro la gotta trascritta da Stendhal in italiano. **Minerva Med** 1981 Feb 25;72(6):305
**Rocchietta S:** Vita avventurosa di Johann Andreas Eisenbarth (1663–1727), chirurgo e medico girovago. **Minerva Med** 1981 Jan 28;72(3):173–4
**Rocchietta S:** Von der Apothekergilde während des 15. Jahrhunderts gestiftete Glasfenster im Dom von Mailand. **Beitr Gesch Pharm** 1981;31(13):97–100
**Roche D:** L'amour paternel à Paris au XVIIIe siècle. **Ann Demogr Hist (Paris)** 1983;:73–80
**Roche D** see **Forster R**
**Roche R:** L'apoplexie de Voltaire. **Hist Sci Med** 1981;15(2):145–9
**Rochefort DA:** Three centuries of care of the mentally disabled in Rhode Island and the nation, 1650–1950. **RI Hist** 1981;40(4):110–32
**Rochefort R, Devevey J:** Les jeunes médecins libéraux. Evolution de 1979 à 1982. **Cah Sociol Demogr Med** 1984 Apr–Jun;24(2):97–123
**Rochefrette J** see **Dumont M**
**Rocher GD de, ed** see **Joubert L**
**Rochford EB:** Stutterers' practices: folk remedies and therapeutic intervention. **J Commun Disord** 1983 Sep;16(5):373–84
**Rochford EB** see **Emerson RM**
**Rockett I** see **Yusuf F**
**Rockey D:** Speech disorder in nineteenth century Britain: the history of stuttering. London, Cromm Helm, 1980. 280 p.
**Rocko JM, Di Gioia JM:** Calot's triangle revisited. **Surg Gynecol Obstet** 1981 Sep;153(3):410–4
**Rocko JM** see **DiGioia JM**
**Roda JJ:** Histoire de la fondation du premier sanatorium populaire français. Ses origines et ses vingt-cinq premières années d'existence (Sanatorium Mangini Hauteville). Thèse. Lyon I, 1976. 85 p.
**Rodegra H:** Arztlicher Kunstfehler und Arzthaftung aus medizinhistorischer Sicht. **Med Welt** 1982 Sep 17;33(37):1256–61
**Rodegra H:** Das Gesundheitswesen der Stadt Hamburg im 19. Jahrhundert, unter Berücksichtigung der Medizinalgesetzgebung (1586–1818–1900). Wiesbaden, Steiner, 1979. 217 p. (Sudhoffs Archiv, Beihefte, Heft 21)
**Rodegra H:** Die Anfänge der Endoskopie. **Laryngol Rhinol Otol (Stuttg)** 1979 Sep;58(9):723–30
**Rodegra H:** Johann Carl Georg Fricke (1790–1841): Wegbereiter einer klinischen Chirurgie in Deutschland. Herzogenrath, Murken-Altrogge, 1983. 203 p. (Studien zur Geschichte des Krankenhauswesens, 20)
**Rodegra H:** Kindestötung und Verheimlichung der Schwangerschaft: eine sozialgeschichtliche und medizinsoziologische Untersuchung mit Einzelfallanalysen. Herzogenrath [Germany], Murken-Altrogge, 1981. 68 p.
**Rodegra H:** Philippe Pinels Ideen von der Befreiung der Irren und ihre Verwirklichung im norddeutschen Raum zu Beginn des 19. Jahrhunderts. **Med Welt** 1981 Feb 6;32(6):199–201
**Rodegra H:** Philippe Pinels Ideen von der Befreiung der Irren und ihre Verwirklichung im norddeutschen Raum zu Beginn des 19. Jahrhunderts. In International Congress of the History of Medicine, 27th, Barcelona, 1980. Actas. Barcelona, Académia de Ciències Mèdiques de Catalunya i Balears, 1981. p. 140–4.
**Rodegra H:** Qualitätssicherung in der Medizin unter medizinhistorischen Aspekten. **Med Welt** 1982 Nov 12;33(45):1607–10
**Rodegra H:** Zur Geschichte der Gesundheitserziehung in deutschen Schulen. **Med Welt** 1979 Oct 26;30(43):1615–20
**Rodegra H, Pirsig W:** Zur Geschichte der Versorgung von Mittelgesichtsverletzungen. **Laryngol Rhinol Otol (Stuttg)** 1980 Jul;59(7):412–7
**Rodegra H:** Zur Problematik des ärztlichen Kunstfehlers im 19. Jahrhundert. Arzthaftung im Beziehungsgeflecht von Recht und Medizin. **Med Welt** 1981 Mar 13;32(11):370–4
**Rodegra H** see **Goethe H**
**Rodegra H** see **Murken AH**
**Rödel V:** Gedanken zur Archivierung medizinischen Schriftguts. **Medizinhist J** 1984;19(3):167–72
**Rödel V:** Johann Christoph Gatterers 'Linnaeismus graphicus'. Klassifikation und Universalismus im 18. Jahrhundert. **Medizinhist J** 1982;17(3):215–38
**Rödel W:** Die wichtigsten Forderungen der revolutionären deutschen Sozialdemokratie zum Apothekenwesen ausgangs des 19. Jahrhunderts. **Pharmazie** 1983 Nov;38(11):772–4
**Rödel WG:** Mensch und Gesundheit in der Geschichte der Neuzeit. **Medizinhist J** 1984;19(1–2):138–47
**Rodero Vicente B:** Psiquiatría comunitaria: reforma psiquiátrica. **Rev Sanid Hig Publica (Madr)** 1982 Sep–Oct;56(9–10):941–51
**Rodero Vicente B** see **Fernández Felgueroso E**
**Rodger NW, Paulseth JE:** Hazards in managing diabetic acidosis. **Can Med Assoc J** 1981 Aug 15;125(4):335
**Rodgers BL:** The great depression, 1929–1940: an era of reform. **Va Nurse** 1984 Spring;52(1):12–3
**Rodgers GF:** A question of policy: is provision of special schools for defectives to be undertaken by this department? **Anzhes J** 1980;9(2):42–54
**Rodgers J:** Workhouse into hospital: not grim enough for Russia. **Health Soc Serv J** 1982 Feb 11;92(4783):180–1
**Rodgers JS:** 'Life' in the novel: Tristram Shandy and some aspects of eighteenth-century physiology. **Eighteenth Cent Life** 1980;6(1):1–20
**Rodin AE, Key JD:** Arthur Conan Doyle's thesis on tabes dorsalis. **JAMA** 1982 Feb 5;247(5):646–50
**Rodin AE, Key JD:** Assessment and significance of Arthur Conan Doyle's medical writings. **South Med J** 1982 Nov;75(11):1392–9
**Rodin AE:** Autoexperimentation with a drug by Arthur Conan Doyle. **J Hist Med Allied Sci** 1980 Oct;35(4):426–30
**Rodin AE:** Infants and gin mania in 18th-century London. **JAMA** 1981 Mar 27;245(12):1237–9
**Rodin AE:** Oslerian pathology: an assessment and annotated atlas of museum specimens. Lawrence, Kansas, Coronado, 1981. xviii, 250 p.
**Rodin AE, Reece RD:** The teaching of medical history by instructors from a variety of disciplines. With a commentary by L.G. Stevenson. In J. J. Bylebyl, ed: Teaching the history of medicine at a medical center. Baltimore, London, Johns Hopkins University Press, 1982. (The Henry E. Sigerist supplements to the Bulletin of the History of Medicine; new ser., no. 7). p. 152–60.
**Rodin AE** see **Key JD**
**Rodin MB** see **Fennel ML**
**Rodionov AV:** O partiïno-politicheskoï rabote sredi ranenykh i meditsinskogo personala vo vremia Kurskoï bitvy. **Voen Med Zh** 1984 Aug;(8):11–5
**Rodnan GP, Benedek TG:** Synovial fluid in antiquity. **Ann Rheum Dis** 1981 Feb;40(1):103
**Rodnan GP** see **Benedek TG**
**Rodowód przyszłości. 10:** Sekcja Pielęgniarek i Położnych ZZPSZ **Pieleg Polozna** 1982;(12):27–9
**Rodowód przyszłości. 4. Doskonalenie nauczycieli szkół medycznych: Pieleg Polozna** 1982;(6):22–3
**Rodowskas CA Jr:** A matter of degrees. **Drug Intell Clin Pharm** 1982 Jul–Aug;16(7–8):607–12
**Rodrigo A:** Doctor Trueta: héroe anónimo de dos guerras. Barcelona, Plaza & Janes, 1978. 294 p.
**Rodrigo Lizondo M:** La protesta de Valencia de 1318 y otros documentos inéditos referentes a Arnau de Vilanova. **Dynamis** 1981;1:241–73
**Rodrigues W** see **Goldberg HI**
**Rodríguez A:** Samuel Ramos: influencia de Adler y Jung en su estudio sobre el carácter del Mexicano. **Cuad Hispanoam** 1977;109(326–327):420–30
**Rodríguez E:** Las enfermedades mentales en la América precolombina. **Rev Enferm** 1984 Mar;7(67):73–5
**Rodríguez JF** see **Grinberg L**
**Rodríguez K** see **Gray L**
**Rodríguez Arroyo JL, Ivich Treviño MP:** Historia de la porcelana. **ADM** 1980 Jan–Feb;37(1):26–7
**Rodriguez-Castellon JA:** Selected items from the history of pathology – Girolamo Fracastoro (1478–1553). **Am J Pathol** 1980;101(1):62
**Rodríguez Domínguez J:** La Escuela de Salud Pública de México. **Salud Publica Mex** 1983 Sep–Oct;25(5):505–8
**Rodriguez Exposito C** see **Beauperthuy de Benedetti R**
**Rodríguez Galdo MX:** Hambre, epidemia y crisis demográfica en la Galicia litoral a mediados del siglo XIX. **Asclepio** 1983;35:53–68
**Rodríguez Galdo MX:** Hambre y enfermedad en Galicia a mediados del siglo XIX. In: Sociedad Española de Historia de la Medicina. V Congreso Nacional. Madrid, 1977. **Asclepio** 1977;29:331–41
**Rodríguez García JR:** Circulacion mundial de la obstetricia y ginecologia española a traves de Excerpta Medica (1951–71). **Asclepio** 1980;32:401–14
**Rodriguez Maffiotte C:** Consideraciones acerca de la obra 'Libro de anathomia del hombre', de Bernardino Montana de Monserrate. **Acta Med Tenerife** 1978;39:87–92
**Rodríguez Navarro M** see **Sociedad Venezolana de Historia de la medicina**

**Rodríguez Ocaña E:** Aproximacion al concepto y practica de la medicina social en Ludwig Teleky (1872–1957). **Dynamis (Spain)** 1982;2:299–323

**Rodríguez Ocaña E:** El cólera de 1834 en Granada. Enfermedad catastrófica y crisis social. Granada, Universidad de Granada, 1983. 170 p. (Colección Monográfica Universidad de Granada, 81).

**Rodriguez Ocaña E:** Higiene y terapeutica anticolericas en la primera epidemia de colera en España, 1833–1835. **Asclepio** 1982;34:71–100

**Rodriguez Ocaña E:** La dependencia social de un comportamiento científico: los médicos españoles y el cólera de 1833–35. **Dynamis** 1981;1:101–30

**Rodríguez Pazos M, Martí Lloret JB:** La aportacion de pedromata al derecho medico de su tiempo. **Asclepio** 1980;32:415–20

**Rodríguez Rebollo T** see **Zuluaga Gómez A**

**Rodríguez Sánchez A:** La natalidad ilegítima en Cáceres en el siglo XVI. **Rev Estud Extremenos** 1979;35(1):123–64

**Rodríguez Tejerina JM:** El doctorado en medicina en la Universidad de Mallorca. In Congrés International d'Història de la Medicina Catalana, 2nd, Barcelona, 1975. Llibre d'Actes. Barcelona, Socitra, 1977. p. 147–56.

**Rodríguez-Tejerina JM:** El pensamiento medico de Ramon Llull en la epoca de Miramar. **Asclepio** 1978–79,30–31:277–82

**Rodríguez Tejerina JM:** Historia de la medicina en Mallorca: desde sus orígenes hasta el siglo XVI. Palma de Mallorca, A. Rodríquez Tejerina, 1981. 249 p.

**Rodzik I** see **Labuda G**

**Roe DA:** Attempts at the eradication of pellagra: a historical review. In Lilienfeld AM, ed: Times, places, and persons. Baltimore, London, Johns Hopkins Univ. Press, 1980. (Sigerist suppl. to the Bull Hist Med, n.s., no 4) p. 62–78.

**Roe DA:** The insect theory of pellagra. **Fed Proc** 1981 Apr;40(5):1523–6

**Roe SA:** Matter, life, and generation. Eighteenth-century embryology and the Haller-Wolff debate. Cambridge, Cambridge University Press, 1981. 214 p.

**Roe W:** 'Science' in the practice of medicine: its limitations and dangers as exemplified by a study of the natural history of acute bronchial asthma in children. **Perspect Biol Med** 1984 Spring;27(3):386–400

**Roe SA, ed:** The natural philosophy of Albrecht von Haller. New York, Arno, 1981. Various pagings. Reprint of works published 1750–1936.

**Roed-Petersen K, Madsen CM:** Harald Hirschsprung (1830–1916). **Dan Medicinhist Arbog** 1980;:182–99

**Roeder BA:** Health care beliefs and practices among Mexican Americans: a review of the literature. **Aztlan** 1982;13(1–2):223–56

**Roeder PW** see **Sigelman L**

**Roemer F:** Plinius der Aeltere. (Annotated bibliog. 1964–77.) **Anz Altertumswiss** 1978;31:129–206

**Roentgenology 1902.: AJR** 1981 Mar;136(3):630–1

**Roesch P:** Médecins publics dans les cités grecques. **Hist Sci Med** 1984;18(3):279–93

**Roeske W:** Antonina Leśniewska, 1866–1937. [Warszawa], Zarzad Główny Polskiego Towarzystwa Farmaceutycznego, 1970. 26 p.

**Roeske W:** Ceramika apteczna z Proszkowa w Muzeum Farmacji Am w Krakowie. Krakow, 1978. 20 p.

**Roeske W:** Freski z dawnych polskich aptek. **Arch Hist Med (Warsz)** 1980;43(2):191–7

**Roeske W:** Geschichte der Pharmaziehistorik in Polen. In: Vorträge des Internationalen Pharmaziehistorischen Kongresses Innsbruck 1977. Stuttgart, Wissenschaftliche Verlagsgesellschaft, 1979. p. 155–61.

**Roeske W:** Lexicon Synonymorum Mineralo-Chymico-Pharmaceuticorum Trilingue Latino-Germano-Polonicum Collectum et Conscriptum a Johanne Stanko anno MCDLXXII (1472). In Hickel E, Schröder G, ed: Neue Beiträge zur Arzneimittelgeschichte. Festschrift für Wolfgang Schneider zum 70. Geburtstag. Stuttgart, Wissenschaftliche Verlagsgesellschaft, 1982. p. 29–39.

**Roeske W:** Muzeum Farmacji Akademii medycznej w Krakowie. Krakow, 1977. 22 p.

**Roesler HP:** Soemmerring--Denkmäler in Frankfurt am Main. **Nat Mus** 1978;108:345–53

**Rof Carballo MC:** Biografía y labor docente de Francisco Carbonell y Bravo. Diss. Barcelona, Facultad de Farmacia, Universidad de Barcelona, 1975. 189 p. (Publicaciones del Seminario de Historia de la Farmacia).

**Rof Carballo MC:** Le Dr. Jesús Isamat Vila, premier professeur d'histoire de la pharmacie de l'Université de Barcelone. In: Vorträge des Internationalen Pharmaziehistorischen Kongresses Innsbruck 1977. Stuttgart, Wissenschaftliche Verlagsgesellschaft, 1979. p. 189–94.

**Rof Carballo MC** see **Gomez Caamaño JL**

**Rofail FF:** Why Europe responded to the Muslims' medical achievements in the Middle Ages. **Arabica** 1978;25:292–309

**Rofail Farag F:** Why Europe responded to the Muslims' medical achievements in the Middle Ages. **Arabica** 1978;25:292–309

**Roger FH** see **Servais P**

**Roger J:** The living world. In G. S. Rousseau, R. Porter, ed. The ferment of knowledge. Studies in the historiography of eighteenth-century science. Cambridge, Cambridge University Press, 1980. p. 255–83.

**Roger J:** Two scientific discoveries: their genesis and destiny. In M. D. Grmek, R. S. Cohen, G. Cimino, ed: On scientific discovery. The Erice Lectures 1977. Dordrecht, D. Reidel, 1981. p. 229–37. (Boston Studies in the Philosophy of Science, v. 34).

**Rogers BO:** Hans Erni: humanistic and aesthetic artist. **Aesthetic Plast Surg** 1983;7(1):51–67

**Rogers BO:** Hippolyte Morestin (1869–1919). Part I: A brief biography. **Aesthetic Plast Surg** 1982;6(3):141–7

**Rogers BO:** History of cosmetic blepharoplasty. In S. J. Aston, et al., ed: Third international symposium of plastic and reconstructive surgery of the eye and adnexa. Baltimore, London, Williams & Wilkins, 1982. p. 276–81.

**Rogers BO:** Julius von Szymanowski (1829--1868). His life and contributions to plastic surgery. **Plast Reconstr Surg** 1979 Oct;64(4):465–78

**Rogers CC** see **O'Connell M**

**Rogers DE** see **McDermott W**

**Rogers FA:** The American Medical Association: yesterday, today and tomorrow. **J La State Med Soc** 1981 Sep;133(9):129–35

**Rogers FB:** Analytical psychology: Carl Jung and his circle. **Trans Stud Coll Physicians Phila** 1980 Dec;5(2 no 4):284–8

**Rogers FB:** Carl Jung and self-realization. **Penn Med** 1983 Oct;86(10):30, 32

**Rogers FB:** Charles E. Harris (1868–1947) of Hyannis, Massachusetts: family doctor and friend of mankind. **J Hist Med Allied Sci** 1983 Jul;38(3):339–42

**Rogers FB:** Dr. Edward F. Gleason (1869–1944) of Hyannis, Massachusetts, and the Cape Cod Hospital and Windmill. **J Hist Med Allied Sci** 1980 Oct;35(4):459–60

**Rogers FB:** Dr. Edward P. Crowell (1856–1934), Cape Codder, and the Black Slipper. **J Hist Med Allied Sci** 1981 Oct;36(4):493–4

**Rogers FB:** Dr. Samuel Pitcher (1824–1907): Cape Cod and Castoria. **J Hist Med Allied Sci** 1982 Jul;37(3):323–5

**Rogers FB:** Psychology in practice: a jungian perspective. **Del Med J** 1982 Mar;54(3):179–81

**Rogers FB:** The legacy of Carl Jung. **Trans Stud Coll Physicians Phila** 1979 Sep;5(1 No 3):211–14

**Rogers FB:** The origins of MEDLARS. In Stevenson LG, ed: A celebration of medical history. Baltimore, Johns Hopkins University Press, 1982. p. 77–84.

**Rogers FB** see **Blake JB, ed**

**Rogers IL:** John Mackieson. In Dictionary of Canadian biography, 1881–1890. 1982;11:565–6.

**Rogers J, Watt I, Dieppe P:** Arthritis in Saxon and mediaeval skeletons. **Br Med J [Clin Res]** 1981 Dec 19;283(6307)1668–70

**Rogers J, Dieppe P:** Lessons from paleopathology. **Practitioner** 1983 Jul;227(1381):1191–9

**Rogers JC:** Carle: concept and growth. A personal history. Urbana, Carle Foundation, 1978. xix, 228 p.

**Rogers JS:** 'Life' in the novel: Tristram Shandy and some aspects of 18th-century physiology. **Eighteenth Cent Life** 1980;6(1):1–20

**Rogers L:** Odabrana poglavlja iz ratne kirurgije 8. Britanske armije. **Lijec Vjesn** 1979 Nov;101(11):699–701

**Rogers P:** Florence Nightingale: the myth and the reality. **Nurs Focus** 1982 Jul;3(11):10

**Rogers R:** Metaphor: a psychoanalytic view. Berkeley, University of California Press, 1979. xi, 148 p.

**Rogers SL:** The shaman's healing way. Ramona, California, Acoma Books, 1976. 40 p.

**Rogers SL** see **Tyson RA**

**Rogers WW** see **Ward RD**

**Rogler LH** see **Cooney RS**

**Rogoll H, Späte HF:** Zur gesellschaftlichen Stellung des psychisch Kranken im Spiegel der Geschichte gesetzlicher Regelungen zur Einweisung in stationäre Einrichtungen. **Z Gesamte Hyg** 1983 Jan;29(1):37–9

**Rogowski J** see **Olakowski T**

**Rohde JR** see **Low AA**

**Rohland I, Keil G:** Randnotizen zum 'Schüpfheimer Kodex'. Teil I: Allgemeines und Textbestimmung der Traktate. **Gesnerus** 1983;40(3/4):257–74

**Rohr A von:** Die Medizinische Poliklinik der Universität Zürich 1835 bis 1983. Stuttgart; New York, Thieme, 1983. ix, 418 p.

**Röhrer H:** Friedrich Loeffler. Begründer der medizinischen Virusforschung vor 80 Jahren. **Hist Med Vet** 1979;4(2):46–8

**Röhrer-Ertl O:** Bemerkungen zur Identifikation des Hl. Emmeram aus St. Emmeram in Regensburg. Ein methodenkritischer Vergleich. **Anthropol Anz** 1981 Sep;39(3):173–88

**Röhrer-Ertl O:** Ein Beitrag zur historischen Vertiefung der Akzelerationsforschung: Längenwachstumsänderungen in einer Population vom Tell es Sultan/Jericho aus dem Präkeramischen Neolithikum (ca. 9000–6000 v. Chr.). **Arztl Jugendkd** 1984 Oct;75(5):292–302

**Röhrich H** see **Habrich C**

**Roĭ VP** see **Kovalev MM**

**Roisum KG** see **Lounsbury JW**

**Roitbak AI:** The importance of I. M. Sechenov's electrophysiological research. **Acta Neurobiol Exp (Warsz)** 1980;40(2):451–61

**Roĭtel'man AG:** Iz istorii razvitiia nezemskoĭ psikhiatricheskoĭ pomoshchi v Rossii vo vtoroĭ polovine XIX veka. **Zh Nevropatol Psikhiatr** 1981;81(9):1390–3

**Rojo Moreno J** see **Livianos Aldana L**

**Rojo Moreno L** see **Livianos Aldana L**

**Rojo Moreno M** see **Livianos Aldana L**

**Rojo Sierra M:** La vida de hoy y los trastornos psíquicos. **Actas Luso Esp Neurol Psiquiatr** 1983 Nov–Dec;11(6):433–41

**Rokhlin LL, Shereshevskiĭ AM:** Znamenatel'nye daty istorii psikhiatrii 1981 g. **Zh Nevropatol Psikhiatr** 1981;81(1):122–7

**Rokhlin LL, Shereshevskiĭ AM, Tom A:** Znamenatel'nye daty 1982 g. **Zh Nevropatol Psikhiatr** 1982;82(1):130–40

**Rokhlin LL, Shereshevskiĭ AM, Tom A:** Znamenatel'nye i iubileĭnye daty

nevropatologii i psikhiatrii 1983 g. **Zh Nevropatol Psikhiatr** 1983;83(1):122–33
**Rokhlin LL, Shereshevskiĭ AM, Tom A:** Znamenatel'nye i iubileĭnye daty nevropatologii i psikhiatrii 1984 g. **Zh Nevropatol Psikhiatr** 1984;84(2):271–80
**Rokkan S:** National primary socio-economic data structures: Norway. **Int Soc Sci J** 1978;30(3):621–52
**Rol' nauchnykh meditsinskikh obshchestv stomatologov v razvitii sovetskoĭ stomatologii: Stomatologiia (Mosk)** 1982;(6):4–6
**Roland CG:** Canadian medical journalism in the 19th century. **Can Med Assoc J** 1983 Feb 15;128(4):449–51, 454–9, 458–9
**Roland CG:** Dr. Earl Scarlett: melding tradition and beauty in historical writing. **Can Med Assoc J** 1980 Apr 5;122(7):822–6
**Roland CG:** Dr. James Bowman vs Canada: a struggle to obtain payment for government service. In: Congrès international d'histoire de la médecine, XXVe, Québec, 1976. Actes. Québec, 1977. p. 1158–69.
**Roland CG:** George William Campbell. In Dictionary of Canadian biography, 1881–1890. 1982;11:148–9.
**Roland CG:** Health and disease among the early Loyalists in Upper Canada. **Can Med Assoc J** 1983 Mar 1;128(5):587–95
**Roland CG:** John Fulton, In Dictionary of Canadian biography, 1881–1890. 1982;11:328–9.
**Roland CG:** Ontario medical periodicals as mirrors of change. **Ont Hist** 1980;72:3–15
**Roland CG:** Russell Morse Wilder. In Dictionary of American Biography, Suppl. 6, 1956–1960. p. 697–8, 1980.
**Roland CG:** Sir William Osler's dreams and nightmares. **Bull Hist Med** 1980 Fall;54(3):418–46
**Roland CG:** 'Sunk under the taxation of nature': malaria in Upper Canada. In Roland CG, ed: Health, disease and medicine. Toronto, Hannah Institute for the History of Medicine, 1984. p. 154–70.
**Roland CG:** The palpable Osler: a study in survival. **Perspect Biol Med** 1984;27(2):299–313
**Roland CG:** War amputations in Upper Canada. **Archivaria** 1980 Summer;10:73–84
**Roland CG** see **Paterson GR**
**Roland CG** see **Teigen PM, ed**
**Roland JL** see **Marchal P**
**Roland CG, ed:** Health, disease and medicine: essays in Canadian history. Proceedings of the First Hannah Conference on the History of Medicine, McMaster University, June 3–5, 1982. [Toronto?], Hannah Institute for the History of Medicine, 1984. 464 p.
**Role A:** La vie étrange d'un grand savant: le professeur Brown-Sequard, 1817–1894. Paris, Plon, 1977. 219 p.
**Roll-Hansen N:** E. S. Russell and J. H. Woodger: the failure of two twentieth-century opponents of mechanistic biology. **J Hist Biol** 1984 Fall;17(3):399–428
**Roll-Hansen N:** Eugenics before World War II; the case of Norway. **Hist Philos Life Sci** 1980;2(2):269–98
**Rollet C:** L'allaitement artificiel des nourrissons avant Pasteur. **Ann Demogr Hist (Paris)** 1983;:81–92
**Rollet C:** Nourrices et nourrissons dans le département de la Seine et en France de 1880 à 1940. **Population** 1982;37(3):573–604
**Rollet C:** Variole et mortalité des enfants au XVIIIe siècle. **Cah Hist** 1978;23(4):417–36
**Rollin BE** see **Rowan AN**
**Rollin HR:** Changing face of administration of mental hospitals. **J R Soc Med** 1981 Sep;74(9):641–4
**Rollin HR:** Crime and mental disorder. Daniel McNaughton, a case in point. **Med Leg J** 1982;50(Pt 3):102–13
**Rolls R:** Bark, blisters and the bathe: some problems of pain relief in former times. **J R Soc Med** 1982 Oct;75(10):812–9
**Rolls R:** The rise and fall of the Bath waters. **Soc Soc Hist Med Bull (Lond)** 1984 Dec;35:17–20
**Roloff JA, ed** see **Castaing L**
**Romanchuk KG:** Fluorescein. Physiochemical factors affecting its fluorescence. **Surv Ophthalmol** 1982 Mar–Apr;26(5):269–83
**Romanell P:** Medical history in the religious psychology of William James. In: Congrès international d'histoire de la médecine, XXVe, Québec, 1976. Actes. Québec, 1977. p. 1171–83.
**Romanell P:** The scientific and medical genealogy of Locke's 'historical, plain method'. **Trans Stud Coll Physicians Phila** 1983 Dec;5(5 no 4):339–52
**Romanenko AE:** Okhrana zdorov'ia materi i rebenka v Ukrainskoĭ SSR. **Pediatriia** 1982 Dec;(12):11–4
**Romanenko AE:** V.I. Lenin i zdravookhranenie Sovetskoĭ Ukrainy. **Vrach Delo** 1980 Mar;(3):1–7
**Romaniuk A:** Increase in natural fertility during the early stages of modernization: Canadian Indians case study. **Demography** 1981 May;18(2):157–72
**Romaniuk A:** Increase in natural fertility during the early stages of modernization: evidence from an African case study, Zaire. **Popul Stud** 1980;34(2):293–310
**Romano J:** Temples, asylums, hospitals --? **J Natl Assoc Priv Psychiatr Hosp** 1978 Summer;9(4):5–12
**Romano R:** Cocamania e cocainomania. **Belfagor** 1982;37(6):661–74
**Romanofsky P:** Ellen Culver Potter. In Dictionary of American Biography, Suppl. 6, 1956–1960. p. 515–16, 1980.
**Romanofsky P, ed** see **Chambers CA**
**Romanov NA** see **Stepanov PF**
**Romanova NN:** E. S. London's contribution to the problem of DNA structure. **Istor Biol Issled** 1983;9:166–75
**Romanyshyn RD:** Psychological life, from science to metaphor. Austin, University of Texas Press, 1982. xvii, 209 p.
**Romay Garcia Arias L:** La medicina en la obra literaria de Gustave Flaubert. **Galicia Clin** 1978;50:604, 671, 759
**Rome HP:** The troubled world of the psychiatric hospital: the deinstitutionalization problem. **J Natl Assoc Priv Psychiatr Hosp** 1977;9(2):4–13
**Romenskiĭ OIu** see **Kul'chitskiĭ KI**
**Romeo G:** X come cromosoma. **Kos** 1984 May;1(4):115–21
**Römer F:** Plinius der Aeltere. III. Bericht. **Anz Altertumswiss** 1978;31:129–206
**Romero H:** La planificación de familia en Chile, 1952–1977. **Rev Med Chil** 1977 Oct;105(10):724–30
**Romero H:** Población y planificación de familia. **Rev Med Chil** 1977 Dec;105(12):946–50
**Romero-Herrera AE** see **Barnhart MI**
**Romilly J de:** Théorie politique et théorie médicale dans la Grèce antique. **Actual Odontostomatol (Paris)** 1982;138:157–70
**Romm S, Zacher J:** Anna Coleman Ladd: maker of masks for the facially mutilated. **Plast Reconstr Surg** 1982 Jul;70(1):104–11
**Romm S:** Fritz Steinmann and the pin that bears his name. **Plast Reconstr Surg** 1984 Aug;74(2):306–10
**Romm S, Luce EA:** Hans Pichler: oral surgeon to Sigmund Freud. **Oral Surg** 1984 Jan;57(1):31–2
**Romm S:** Johann Friedrich August von Esmarch. **Plast Reconstr Surg** 1983 Feb;71(2):271–3
**Romm S:** Maurice Howe Richardson. **Plast Reconstr Surg** 1983 Mar;71(3):432–4
**Romm S:** Morris Joseph Asch. **Plast Reconstr Surg** 1983 May;71(5):724–8
**Romm S:** On the beauty of lips. **Clin Plast Surg** 1984 Oct;11(4):571–81
**Romm S:** Rejuvenation revisited. **Aesthetic Plast Surg** 1983;7(4):241–8
**Romm S:** The oral cancer of Sigmund Freud. In Romm S, ed: Symposium on historical perspectives of plastic surgery. Philadelphia, Saunders, 1983. p. 709–14.
**Romm S:** The person behind the name: Martin Kirschner. **Plast Reconstr Surg** 1983 Jul;72(1):104–7
**Romm S:** The persons behind the name: Charles Bingham Penrose. **Plast Reconstr Surg** 1982 Sep;70(3):397–9
**Romm S, ed:** Symposium on historical perspectives of plastic surgery. Philadelphia, Saunders, 1983. p. 593–716. (Clinics in plastic surgery, Oct. 1983, vol. 10, no. 4) Contributions by E. H. Christianson, D. Clark, B. F. Conroy, W. B. Davis, H. C. Greisman, E. A. Luce, M. H. McGrath, J. F. McMurry, W. O. Morain, A. D. Morani, R. F. Morgan, L. S. Nichter, M. A. Nichter, R. L. Ruberg, L. A. Sargent, J. Scarborough, R. R. Shah, C. N. Verheyden, A. F. Wallace, J. B. Zacher.
**Rommel J** see **Leonnard P**
**Romodanov AP:** Neirokhirurgiia Sovetskoĭ Ukrainy. **Zh Vopr Neirokhir** 1982 Sep–Oct;(5):9–11
**Ron M:** Catalog of the Sidney M. Edelstein Collection of the history of chemistry, dyeing and technology. Jerusalem, The Jewish National and University Library, 1981. 182 p.
**Rona E:** Laboratory contamination in the early period of radiation research. **Health Phys** 1979 Dec;37(6):723–7
**Ronchi L, Fronsini R:** Sviluppo e applicazioni cliniche dell'elettro-oculografia. Firenze, Baccini and Chiappi, 1975. 84 p.
**Roncière J de la, Fiessinger JN:** Maurice Raynaud, 1835–1881. **Rev Prat** 1981 Dec 1;31(55):3967–9
**Roney JL** see **Dubin JL**
**Ronkin ME** see **Alloway WJ**
**Rønnike F:** Arstidsfordeling for menneskets undfangelse i landene omkring Norskehavet--med specielt henblik på Nord-Norge. **Tidsskr Nor Laegeforen** 1981 Jan 20;101(2):151–5
**Ronsin F:** La classe ouvrière et le néo-Malthusianisme: l'exemple français avant 1914. **Mouvement Soc** 1979;106:85–117
**Ronsin F** see **Dupâquier J**
**Rook A, Newbold M:** David Edwardes: his activities at Cambridge. **Med Hist** 1975 Oct;19(4):389–92
**Rook A, Martin L:** John Addenbrooke M.D. (1680–1719). **Med Hist** 1982 Apr;26(2):169–78
**Rook A:** William Tilbury Fox (1836–1879): his contribution to tropical dermatology. **Int J Dermatol** 1981 Mar;20(2):140–2
**Rook A** see **Hart GD, ed**
**Rooke PT, Schnell RL:** Charlotte Whitton and the 'babies for export' controversy, 1947–48. **Alberta Hist** 1982;30(1):11–6
**Rooke PT, Schnell RL:** Child welfare in English Canada. **Soc Serv Rev** 1981;55(3):484–506
**Rooker C** see **Castaing L**
**Rooks JB, Fishman SH:** American nurse-midwifery practice in 1976–1977: reflections of 50 years of growth and development. **Am J Public Health** 1980 Sep;70(9):990–6
**Roos A, Boron WF:** The buffer value of weak acids and bases: origin of the concept, and first mathematical derivation and application to physico-chemical systems. The work of M. Koppel and K. Spiro (1914). **Respir Physiol** 1980 Apr;40(1):1–32
**Roos DA:** The 'aims and intentions' of Nature. In Paradis J, Postlewait T, ed. Victorian science and Vicorian values: literary perspectives. New York, New York Academy of Sciences, 1981. p. 159–80.
**Root-Bernstein RS:** Mendel and methodology. **Hist Sci** 1983 Sep;21(53 pt 3):275–95
**Roque MC:** As pestes medievais europeias e o 'regimento proueytoso contra

ha pestencça': Lisboa, Valentim Fernandes, 1495–1496: tentativa de interpretação à luz dos conhecimentos pestológicos actuais. Paris, Fundação Calouste Gulbenkian, Centro Cultural Português, 1979.
**Rosa E:** Medicina e salute pubblica a Bologna nel sei e settecento. **Quad Cult Bolognese** 1978 Dec;(2 no 8): 3–60
**Rosa JE, Madeira AA:** A fundação da faculdade de farmácia e odontologia de Santa Catarina antecedentes e funcionamento. **Rev Catarinense Odontol** 1979 Jan–Jun;6(1):7–20
**Rosa JE, Madeira AA:** Instituto Polytechnico--primeira instituição de ensino superior no Estado de Santa Catarina. **Rev Catarinense Odontol** 1978;5(1 Spec No):30–40
**Rosa JE** see **Madeira AA**
**Rosado A** see **Gómez P**
**Rosales VJ:** The medicotrophic syndrome: an acute modern phenomenon. **Unitas** 1970;43(4):30–59
**Rosborough JP** see **Criley JM**
**Roşca T:** Legioneloza (pneumonia veteranilor). **Rev Med Interna [Med Interna]** 1980 Jul–Aug;32(4):301–6
**Roscam Abbing HD:** International organizations in Europe and the right to health care. Antwerp, Boston, Kluwer–Deventer, 1979. xii, 278 p.
**Rose CH, Nansen P, Jørgensen RJ, et al:** Sheep farming in Greenland. Its history, managemental practices and disease problems. **Nord Vet Med** 1984 Mar–Apr;36(3–4):65–76
**Rose FC, Bynum WF, ed:** Historical aspects of the neurosciences. A festschrift for Macdonald Critchley. New York, Raven Press, 1982. xix, 537 p.
**Rose FC** see **Steiner TJ**
**Rose FL** see **Johnson AW**
**Rose G:** Professor D.D. Reid, MD Aberdeen, PHD DSc London, FRCP London. **J Epidemiol Community Health** 1978 Dec;32(4):229–34
**Rose H:** The social determinants of reproduction science and technology. In Knorr KD, et al, ed: Determinants and controls of scientific development. Dordrecht, Boston, D. Reidel, 1975. (Theory and decision library, v. 10). p. 407–30.
**Rose JC, Corn M:** Dr. E. and other patients: new lessons from old case reports. **J Hist Med Allied Sci** 1984 Jan;39(1):3–32
**Rose JC** see **Goodman AH**
**Rose M:** Curator of the dead: Thomas Hodgkin (1798–1866). London, Owen, 1981 148 p.
**Rose S** see **Lewontin R**
**Rose Cl** see **Peterson M**
**Rosegay H:** Cushing's legacy to transsphenoidal surgery. **J Neurosurg** 1981 Apr;54(4):448–54
**Roselli A:** Aristotele e il sistema della sensazione. **Physis** 1980;22(2):157–73
**Roselli A:** Problemi relativi ai trattati chirurgici De Fracturis e De Articulis. In La collection hippocratique et son rôle dans l'histoire de la médecine. Colloque de Strasbourg (23–27 octobre 1972) organisé par le Centre de Recherches sur la Grèce Antique, avec le concours des Facultés de Philosophie et des Langues Classiques. Leiden, E. J. Brill, 1975. p. 229–34.
**Rosen G:** Social medicine in the United States: The role of non-medical individuals and movements in its developments. In: Congrès international d'histoire de la médecine, XXVe, Québec, 1976. Actes. Québec, 1977. p. 247–74.
**Rosen G:** Urbanization, occupation and disease in the United States 1870–1920. The case of New York City. In Forbes EG, ed: Human implications of scientific advance. Edinburg, Edinburgh University Press, 1978. p. 224–50.
**Rosen G** see **Cohen IB, ed**
**Rosen H** see **Mikhail M**
**Rosen IL:** Aphrodisiacs in the kitchen. **J La State Med Soc** 1980 Oct;132(10):155–9
**Rosen J:** Of serpents and symbols. **J Am Dent Assoc** 1984 Apr;108(4):534
**Rosen PP:** Specimen radiography and the diagnosis of clinically occult mammary carcinoma. A brief historical review. **Pathol Annu** 1980;15(pt 1):225–37
**Rosen S:** The psychotherapeutic and hypnotherapeutic approaches of Milton H. Erickson, M.D. **Am J Psychoanal** 1984 Summer;44(2):133–45
**Rosenbaum MB:** Sir Thomas Lewis: a view from the south. **Br Heart J** 1981 Oct;46(4):349–50
**Rosenbaum M, ed:** Ethics and values in psychotherapy: a guidebook. New York, Free Press; London, Collier Macmillan; 1982. xvi, 464 p. Historical chapter by J. F. Drane.
**Rosenberg B:** Cultures complémentaires et nourritures de substitution au Maroc (XVe–XVIIIe siècle). **Ann Econ Soc Civilis** 1980;35:477–503
**Rosenberg C:** Science in American society; a generation of historical debate. **Isis** 1983 Sep;74(273):356–67
**Rosenberg CE:** From almshouse to hospital: the shaping of Philadelphia General Hospital. **Milbank Mem Fund Q** 1982 Winter;60(1):108–54
**Rosenberg CE:** Inward vision and outward glance: the shaping of the American hospital, 1880–1914. **Bull Hist Med** 1979 Fall;53(3):346–91
**Rosenberg CE:** Medical text and social context: explaining William Buchans's Domestic Medicine. **Bull Hist Med** 1983;57(1):22–42
**Rosenberg CE:** The therapeutic revolution: medicine, meaning, and social change in nineteenth-century America. **Perspect Biol Med** 1977 Summer;20(4):485–509
**Rosenberg CE:** The therapeutic revolution: medicine, meaning, and social change in nineteenth-century America. In Vogel MJ, Rosenberg CE, ed: The therapeutic revolution. Philadelphia, 1979. p. 3–25.
**Rosenberg CE** see **Ackerknecht EH**
**Rosenberg CE** see **Blake JB, ed**
**Rosenberg D:** Evolução do tratamento cirúrgico da úlcera duodenal. **Rev Hosp Clin Fac Med Sao Paulo** 1980 Oct;35(5):247–54
**Rosenberg MB:** Reforma social y conflicto político: La huelga médica como preludio a la guerra civil costarricense de 1948. **Rev Hist (Costa Rica)** 1977 Jul–Dec;3:149–70
**Rosenberg CE, ed** see **Vogel MJ**
**Rosenberg J, ed** see **Phillips WR**
**Rosenberger B:** Cultures complémentaires et nourritures de substitution au Maroc (XVe–XVIIIe siècle). **Ann Econ Soc Civilis** 1980;35(3–4):477–503
**Rosenberger B, Triki H:** Famines et épidémies au Maroc aux XVIe et XVIIe siècles. **Hesperis Tamuda** 1973;14:109–75
**Rosenberger HT:** Harriet Lane Johnston: pioneer advocate of special care for children with chronic diseases. **J Lanc Cty Hist Soc** 1972;76(1):1–28
**Rosenblatt A:** Concepts of the asylum in the care of the mentally ill. **Hosp Community Psychiatry** 1984 Mar;35(3):244–50
**Rosenfeld CP:** The medical history of Menilek II, Emperor of Ethiopia (1844–1913): a case of medical diplomacy. **Munger Afr Libr Notes** 1978(45–46):3–43
**Rosenfeld L:** Origins of clinical chemistry: the evolution of protein analysis. New York, Academic Press, 1982. xviii, 366 p.
**Rosenfeld LM:** Physiology at Jefferson Medical College (1842–1982). **Physiologist** 1984 Jun;27(3):113–27
**Rosenfield RE:** Immunobiology of the erythrocyte: perspectives since 1945. **Prog Clin Biol Res** 1980;43:13–7
**Rosengarten F:** A neglected Mayan galactagogue, Ixbut (Euphorbia lancifolia). **Bot Mus Leafl Harv Univ** 1978;26:277–309
**Rosengarten F:** A neglected Mayan galactagogue--ixbut (Euphorbia lancifolia). **J Ethnopharmacol** 1982 Jan;5(1):91–112
**Rosenheck S:** Money in the streets. **Work Pap Mag** 1982;9(2):19–23
**Rosenkötter L:** Alexander Mitscherlich als Chef und Lehrer. **Psyche (Stuttg)** 1983 Apr;37(4):346–51
**Rosenkötter L:** Die Idealbildung in der Generationenfolge. **Psyche (Stuttg)** 1981 Jul;35(7):593–9
**Rosenkötter L** see **Dahmer H**
**Rosenkötter L** see **Lohmann HM**
**Rosenkrantz BG:** Booby-hatch of booby-trap: a new look at nineteenth-century reform. **Soc Res (NY)** 1972;39(4):733–43
**Rosenkrantz BG:** Mad and bad in California. **Rev Am Hist** 1980;8(2):258–63
**Rosenkrantz BG:** Sara Claudia Murray Jordan. In: Notable American women. The modern period. Cambridge, Mass., Belknap-Harvard Univ. Press, 1980. 4:387–8.
**Rosenkrantz BG, Vinovskis MA:** Sustaining 'the flickering flame of life': accountability and culpability for death in ante-bellum Massachusetts asylums. In Reverby S, Rosner D, ed: Health care in America. Philadelphia, Temple University Press, p. 155–82.
**Rosenkrantz BG** see **Lomax EM**
**Rosenkrantz BG** see **Spicker SF**
**Rosenkrantz BG** see **Viseltear AJ**
**Rosenman S:** The late conceptualization of the self in psychoanalysis: the German language and Jewish identity. **J Psychohist** 1983 Summer;11(1):9–42
**Rosenow EC:** Osler--continuing education advocate. **Bull Am Coll Physicians** 1975 Aug;16(8):6–8
**Rosenthal F:** Cannabis and alcohol: the green and the red. **Adv Biosci** 1978 Jul 22–23;22–23:739–45
**Rosenthal MJ:** The structural approach to chiropractic: from Willard Carver to present practice. **Chiropr Hist** 1981;1(1):25–8
**Rosenthal MM:** Perspectivenes on women physicians in the USA through cross-cultural comparison: England, Sweden, USSR. **Int J Womens Stud** 1979;2(6):528–40
**Rosenthal MM, Greiner JR:** The barefoot doctors of China: from political creation to professionalization. **Hum Organ** 1982;41(4):330–41
**Rosenthal N:** The psychology of women. **Psychohist Rev** 1980;8(4):32–6
**Rosenthal PA, Eaton J:** Women MDs in America: 100 years of progress and backlash. **J Am Med Wom Assoc** 1982 May;37(5):129–33
**Rosenthal R:** Dr. Christopher Carli, pioneer physician of Minnesota. **Minn Med** 1982 Dec;65(12):765–8
**Rosenwaike I:** A note on new estimates of the mortality of the extreme aged. **Demography** 1981 May;18(2):257–66
**Rosenzweig E:** Porodništvo u starom Zagrebu (18. stoljeće). **Lijec Vjesn** 1981 Aug;103(8):363–6
**Rosenzweig KA:** Dental health service in the Cyprus detention camps, 1946–1948. **Bull Hist Dent** 1982 Oct;30(2):92–5
**Rosenzweig W:** Disease in art: a case for carcinoma of the breast in Michelangelo's La notte. **Paleopathol Newsl** 1983 Mar;41:8–11
**Roshchin AV, Kozik IV, Arkhangel'skaia LN, et al:** Piatidesiatiletie kafedry promyshlennoĭ gigeny Tsentral'nogo ordena Lenina instituta usovershenstvovaniia vracheĭ. **Gig Tr Prof Zabol** 1981 Aug;(8):37–41
**Roshchin AV:** 100-letie Ustava Moskovskogo gigienicheskogo obshchestva. **Gig Sanit** 1982;(5):48–9
**Rosický B:** Professor Evgenii Nikonorovich Pavlovsky--100 years since his birth. **J Hyg Epidemiol Microbiol Immunol** 1984;28(2):115–8
**Rosický B:** Razvitie ideĭ akademika E. N. Pavlovskogo v stranakh Tsentral'noĭ Evropy. **Med Parazitol (Mosk)** 1984 Mar–Apr;(2):21–8
**Rosin A:** Date de istoria medicinii privitoare la glaucom. **Viata Med [Medii Sanit]** 1980 Oct;28(10):233–5
**Rosinga WM:** Clinical trial under trial. **Pharm Weekbl [Sci]** 1983 Feb 25;5(1):1–8
**Rösler HP:** Samuel Thomas von Soemmerring (1755–1830), Aquarell, gemalt 1794 von seiner Frau Margarethe Elisabeth, geb. Grunelius

(1768-1802), Grösse des Bildovals 12,8 cm (Höhe): 11,5 cm (Breite) (Privatbesitz). **Medizinhist J** 1980;15(4):422-5

**Rosliakov AG, Konstantinov AA:** Pervyĭ meditsinskiĭ vuz na Sovetskom Dal'nem Vostoke. **Sov Zdravookhr** 1980;(4):67-70

**Rosliakova NA:** Contribution of academician P. K. Anokhin to physiology. **Agressologie** 1982;23(5):165-6

**Rosner D:** A once charitable enterprise: hospitals and health care in Brooklyn and New York, 1885-1915. Cambridge; New York, Cambridge University Press, 1982. ix, 234 p.

**Rosner D:** Business at the bedside: health care in Brooklyn, 1890-1915. **Health PAC Bull** 1980 Mar-Apr;11(4):23-31

**Rosner D:** Business at the bedside: health care in Brooklyn, 1890-1915. In Reverby S, Rosner D, ed: Health care in America. Philadelphia, Temple University Press, 1979. p. 117-31.

**Rosner D:** Gaining control: reform, reimbursement and politics in New York's community hospitals, 1890--1915. **Am J Public Health** 1980 May;70(5):533-42

**Rosner D:** Health care for the 'truly needy': nineteenth-century origins of the concept. **Milbank Mem Fund Q** 1982 Summer;60(3):355-85

**Rosner D:** Social control and social service: the changing use of space in charity hospitals. **Radic Hist Rev** 1979;21:183-97

**Rosner D** see **Markowitz GE**

**Rosner D** see **Reverby S**

**Rosner E:** 'Gewöhnung' an die Malaria in chinesischen Quellen des 18. Jhdts. **Sudhoffs Arch** 1984;68(1):43-60

**Rosner E:** Hohenheims Bergsuchtmonographie. **Medizinhist J** 1981;16(1-2):20-52

**Rosner E:** Hohenheims Weg von St. Gallen nach Augsburg (1531-1536). Wien, 1977. 91 p. (Salzburger Beiträge zur Paracelsusforschung, 16).

**Rosner E:** Zur Geschichte der Pocken in Innerasien. **Asiat Forsch** 1980;71:72-6

**Rosner E** see **Habrich C**

**Rosner F:** Ancient descriptions of hemophilia and preconception gender selection. **JAMA** 1984 Aug 17;252(7):900

**Rosner F:** Earliest description of gout. **Arthritis Rheum** 1983 Feb;26(2):236

**Rosner F, Bleich JD, ed:** Jewish bioethics. New York, Sanhedrin Press, 1979. xix, 424 p.

**Rosner F:** Julius Preuss. **Med Hist** 1975 Oct;19(4):376-88

**Rosner F:** Maimonides the physician: a bibliography. **Clio Med** 1980;15(1/2):75-9

**Rosner F:** Mandrakes and other aphrodisiacs in the Bible & Talmud. **Koroth** 1980 Jun;7(11-12):CCLXXVII-CCLXXXIV

**Rosner F:** Medicine in the Bible and the Talmud. Selections from classical Jewish sources. New York, KTAV Publishing House, Yeshiva University Press, 1977. xiii, 247 p. Includes Muntner S: Medicine in ancient Israel, p. 3-21.

**Rosner F:** Moses Maimonides' treatise on asthma. **Thorax** 1981 Apr;36(4):245-51

**Rosner F:** Moses Maimonides' Treatise on Asthma. **J Asthma** 1984;21(2):119-29

**Rosner F:** Moses Maimonides' treatise on poisons. **NY State J Med** 1980 Sep;80(10):1627-30

**Rosner F:** The medical writings of Moses Maimonides. **Clio Med** 1981 Sep;16(1):1-11

**Rosner F:** Therapeutic efficacy of chicken soup. **Chest** 1980;78:672-4

**Rosner LM:** Andrew Duncan M.D., F.R.S.E. (1744-1828). Edinburgh, History of Medicine and Science Unit, University of Edinburgh, [1981?]. [12] p.

**Rosner D, ed** see **Reverby S**

**Rosoff L:** Roger Bacon, William of Occam and Lord Houghton: guides for the perplexed physician. **Am J Surg** 1981 Jan;141(1):2-9

**Rosol Z:** Známý anglický kardiolog Thomas Lewis se narodil před 100 lety. **Vnitr Lek** 1982 Mar;28(3):297-9

**Ross B:** Edwin Ray Guthrie, Jr. In Dictionary of American Biography, Suppl. 6, 1956-1960. p. 261-3, 1980.

**Ross B:** In memoriam: Robert I. Watson, Sr. 1909-1980. **J Hist Behav Sci** 1981 Jan;17(1):1-2

**Ross B** see **Brozek J**

**Ross B** see **Robert I. Watson and the development of the history of psychology: a symposium**

**Ross D:** The development of the social sciences. In Oleson A, Voss J, ed: The organization of knowledge in modern America, 1860-1920. Baltimore and London, Johns Hopkins University Press, 1979. p. 107-38.

**Ross D:** Vision and the artist. **Occup Health (Lond)** 1980 Feb;32(2):68-73

**Ross D:** Woodrow Wilson and the case for psychohistory. **J Am Hist** 1982;69(3):659-68

**Ross DA:** Neglected bibliographical aspects of the works of Thomas Henry Huxley. **J Soc Bibliogr Nat Hist** 1978;8(4):401-20

**Ross E:** Rethinking 'the family'. **Radic Hist Rev** 1979 Spring/Summer;Spec:76-84

**Ross E:** 'The love crisis': couples advice books of the late 1970s. **Signs** 1980;6(1):109-22

**Ross HE, Bischof K:** Wundt's views on sensations of innervation: a reevaluation. **Perception** 1981;10(3):319-29

**Ross IK** see **Maddern GJ**

**Ross JA:** Men in battle. The factors affecting their lives and well-being. **J R Army Med Corps** 1980 Feb;126(1):4-17

**Ross JM, Slap JW, Gehrie MJ, et al:** George Klein's 'Psychoanalytic theory' in perspective. **Psychoanal Rev** 1980 Summer;67(2):161-216

**Ross JP, LeFanu WR, ed:** Lives of the Fellows of the Royal College of Surgeons of England 1965-1973. London, Pitman Medical, 1981. 405 p.

**Ross M:** The evolution of hospital care in Alberta. **Dimens Health Serv** 1980 Apr;57(4):A4

**Ross PJ:** The history of hypnosis in dentistry. **Bull Hist Dent** 1981;29(1):24-8

**Ross R:** Oppression, sexuality and slavery at the Cape of Good Hope. **Hist Reflect** 1979;6(2):421-33

**Ross RS:** A parlous state of storm and stress. The life and times of James B. Herrick. **Circulation** 1983 May;67(5):955-9

**Ross RT:** Statute and legislative history of the Federal Insecticide, Fungicide, and Rodenticide Act and its impact on agriculture. **J Environ Sci Health [B]** 1980;B15(6):665-76

**Ross WM:** Carcinoma of the breast in the section of radiology. **J R Soc Med** 1980 Oct;73(10):734-8

**Ross WM, Day MJ:** Mullard 4 MV linear accelerator at Newcastle upon Tyne. **Br J Radiol** 1981 Sep;54(645):819

**Ross WM:** The Institute: yesterday and tomorrow. **Br J Radiol** 1980 Feb;53(626):55-62

**Ross JC, et al** see **Harris P**

**Rosselli J:** The self-image of effeteness: physical education and nationalism in nineteenth-century Bengal. **Past Present** 1980;86:121-48

**Rosselli J:** The self-image of effeteness: physical education and nationalism in nineteenth-century Bengal. **Past Present** 1980;(86):221-48

**Rosser A:** Midsummer magic. **Nurs Times** 1983 Jun 22-9;79(25):50-1

**Rosser EM:** Campbell De Morgan and his spots. **Ann R Coll Surg Engl** 1983 Jul;65(4):266-8

**Rosset E:** Demographic factors concerning the re-polonization of western and northern territories. **Pol West Aff** 1970;11(1):67-88

**Rossi F:** Crisi di mortalità ad Adria nel contesto socio-ambientale dei secoli XVII-XIX. **Genus** 1977;33(3-4):83-118

**Rossi GF:** Perspectives in international neurosurgery: neurosurgery in Italy. **Neurosurgery** 1981 Jan;8(1):132-3

**Rossi L:** Il concetto di adattamento nella psicologia evoluzionistica di K. Lorenz e nell'epistemologia genetica di J. Piaget. **Stor Crit Psicol** 1984;5(2):301-17

**Rossi WA:** High heels. The agony and the ecstasy. **J Am Podiatry Assoc** 1981 Dec;71(12):698-9

**Rossier A:** L'enfant maudit. **Ann Pediatr (Paris)** 1980 Mar;27(3):195-6

**Rossier A:** Une jalousie mortelle (Honoré de Balzac). **Ann Pediatr (Paris)** 1981 Apr;28(4):298-300

**Rossiter MW:** The history and philosophy of science program at the National Science Foundation. **Isis** 1984 Mar;75(276):95-104

**Rossiter MW:** Women scientists in America. Struggles and strategies to 1940. Baltimore, London, Johns Hopkins University Press, 1982. xviii, 439 p.

**Rossiter MW:** 'Women's work' in science, 1880-1910. **Isis** 1980 Sep;71(258):381-98

**Rossiter MW** see **Wilson LG, ed**

**Rossiwall B** see **Scholz F**

**Rösslin E:** Der Swangern Frauwen und hebammen Rosengarten. Facsimile of Strasbourg edition of 1513. Einführung von H. M. Koelbing. Dietikon/Zürich, Stocker, 1976. 137 p.

**Rośu A:** Les conceptions psychologiques dans les textes médicaux indiens. Paris, Institut de civilisation indienne, 1978. xv, 287 p. (Publications de l'Institut de civilisation indienne. Série in-8; fasc. 43).

**Rosul S** see **Walewski W**

**Rotblat J** see **Lindop PJ**

**Roth G:** Ad salutem et prosperitatem hominum. Zur Entwicklung der ärztlichen Gelöbnisse in mittel- und osteuropäischen Staaten. In Ganzinger K, Skopec M, Wyklicky H, ed: Festschrift für Erna Lesky zum 70. Geburtstag. Wien, Brüder Hollinek, 1981. p. 67-73.

**Roth JK:** Verleihung des Ehrendoktors der Johann-Wolfgang-Goethe-Universität an Anna Freud. **Psyche (Stuttg)** 1982 Oct;36(10):951-3

**Roth MA:** With mercy toward all. Mercy Hospital, Cedar Rapids, Iowa, 1900-1978. Cedar Rapids, Stamats, 1979. vii, 104 p.

**Roth N:** Animal electricity. **Med Instrum** 1980 Jul-Aug;14(4):228

**Roth N:** Bugs and blasphemy: Andrew Crosse and the Acarus electricus. **Med Instrum** 1979 Nov-Dec;13(6):357

**Roth N:** Capturing the heart, 1880: Marey's cardiac tongs. **Med Instrum** 1980 Sep-Oct;14(5):285

**Roth N:** Electroresuscitation and the occult. **Med Instrum** 1980 Mar-Apr;14(2):120-1

**Roth N:** Electrotherapy, 19th-century neurasthenia, and the case of Alice James. **Med Instrum** 1981 Mar-Apr;15(2):116

**Roth N:** Hales's hydraulics: measuring blood pressure, 1706. **Med Instrum** 1981 Jan-Feb;15(1):66-7

**Roth N:** Life-and-death decisions: electrodiagnosis and premature burial. **Med Instrum** 1980 Nov-Dec;14(6):332

**Roth N:** Reviving resuscitation: 1900 -- present. **Med Instrum** 1980 May-Jun;14(3):160

**Roth N:** Tracking by telephone: locating the bullet in President Garfield, 1881. **Med Instrum** 1981 May-Jun;15(3):190

**Roth RR:** The foundation of bionics. **Perspect Biol Med** 1983 Winter;26(2):229-42

**Roth W:** Atherom auf einem Olgemälde Pinakothek in Brescia. **Hautarzt** 1983 Aug;34(8):407-8

**Roth W:** Differentialdiagnostische Erwägungen zu den Hauteffloreszenzen, dargestellt auf dem Sebastiansaltar Hans Holbeins d. A. **Hautarzt** 1980 Dec;31(12):662-4

**Roth W:** Lentigo maligna und Sclerodermia circumscripta auf Olgemälden

der Uffizien. **Hautarzt** 1982 Apr;33(4):229-30
**Roth Ulm HW** see **Poulet W**
**Roth-Woelfle L:** Jan Stephen van Kalkar als Illustrator der Anatomie des Andreas Vesal. **Imprimatur** 1980;8:11
**Roth-Wölfle L:** Jan Stephan von Kalkar als Illustrator der Anatomie des Andreas Vesal. **Imprimatur** 1980;9:86-100
**Rothe J, Ewert G:** Od pracovního společenství sociálních hygienikuke společnosti sociální hygieny NDR. **Cesk Zdrav** 1981 Jan;29(1):5-9
**Rothe J, Werner K, Kaiser W:** Sozialhygienische Konsequenzen aus der Klärung der Tuberkulose-Ätiologie durch Robert Koch. **Z Gesamte Hyg** 1982 Mar;28(3):176-9
**Rothe J** see **Ewert G**
**Rothe J** see **Kaiser W**
**Rothe R** see **Kolta KS**
**Rother P** see **Wendler D**
**Rothkopf A:** 'Das Narrenhaus' von W. Kaulbach und die Deutung des Bildes durch J. A. Schilling 1863. **Confin Psychiatr** 1980;23(1):51-64
**Rothlin M:** Koronarchirurgie vor 25 Jahren und heute. **Praxis** 1980 Dec 9;69(49):1839-43
**Röthlisberger P:** Charles Greene Cumston (1868-1928): Medizinhistoriker in zwei Kontinenten. **Gesnerus** 1984;41(1/2):137-51
**Rothman BK:** In labor. Women and power in the birthplace. New York, London, W.W. Norton, 1982. 320 p.
**Rothman BK:** Midwives in transition: the structure of a clinical revolution. **Soc Probl** 1983;30(3):262-71
**Rothman CM:** The varicocele--1800. **Urology** 1980 Jan;15(1):99-100
**Rothman D** see **Rosenkrantz BG**
**Rothman DJ:** Conscience and convenience. The asylum and its alternatives in progressive America. Boston, Toronto, Little, Brown and Company, 1980. xii, 464 p.
**Rothman DJ:** The limits of benevolence. **Soc Policy** 1981;12(1):24-8, 37-8
**Rothman KJ:** The rise and fall of epidemiology, 1950-2000 A.D. **N Engl J Med** 1981 Mar 5;304(10):600-2
**Rothman MA:** Unfinished business. **NY J Dent** 1980 Apr;50(4):134-5
**Rothman WA:** The hospital in literature. **Hosp Health Serv Adm** 1983 Jul-Aug;28(4):85-94
**Rothrock JC:** Nursing diagnosis: in the days of Florence Nightingale. **AORN J** 1984 Aug;40(2):189-90
**Rothschild H:** Diseases of the Jews. In his: Biocultural aspects of disease. New York, Academic Press, 1981. p. 531-55.
**Rothschild H** see **Robins RS**
**Rothschild L:** FDA's changing role in food safety. **FDA Consum** 1981 Jun;15(5):28-31
**Rothschild-Boros MC** see **Passi S**
**Rothschuh KE:** Aus der Geschichte der Naturheilbewegung (I). Ueber den 'Naturismus' als die weltanschauliche Grundlage der Naturheilbewegung. **ZFA (Stuttgart)** 1981 May 10;57(13):1011-8
**Rothschuh KE:** Aus der Geschichte der Naturheilbewegung (II). Die Entwicklung allgemeiner theoretischer Grundsätze in der Naturheilkunde des 19. Jahrhunderts. **ZFA (Stuttgart)** 1981 May 20;57(14):1091-100
**Rothschuh KE:** Aus der Geschichte der Naturheilbewegung (III). 'Vorläufer' des Rousseauschen Naturismus in der römischen Kaiserzeit. Die Philosophie der Stoa und die Methodische Medizin. **ZFA (Stuttgart)** 1981 May 31;57(15):1172-9
**Rothschuh KE:** Aus der Geschichte der Naturheilbewegung (IV). Hatte die Naturheilbewegung Vorläufer in der Renaissance? Montaigne, Paracelsus, Beobachtungsmedizin, Wasserheilkunde. **ZFA (Stuttgart)** 1981 Jun 10;57(16):1251-9
**Rothschuh KE:** Aus der Geschichte der Naturheilbewegung (IX). Körperkultur (Kleiderreform, Nacktkultur) aus dem Geiste der Lebensreform. **ZFA (Stuttgart)** 1983 Oct 10;59(28):1570-8
**Rothschuh KE:** Aus der Geschichte der Naturheilbewegung (V). Welche Umstände begünstigten die Entstehung der deutschen Naturheilbewegung im 19. Jahrhundert? **ZFA (Stuttgart)** 1981 Jun 20;57(17):1310-20
**Rothschuh KE:** Aus der Geschichte der Naturheilbewegung (VI). Zur Fortentwicklung und Pflege der Naturheilverfahren in der zweiten Hälfte des 19. Jahrhunderts. **ZFA (Stuttgart)** 1983 Apr 10;59(10):585-91
**Rothschuh KE:** Aus der Geschichte der Naturheilbewegung (VII). Die Heilkräfte von Licht, Luft und Erde. Arnold Rikli, Adolf Just und Pastor Felke. **ZFA (Stuttgart)** 1983 Jun 10;59(16):933-40
**Rothschuh KE:** Aus der Geschichte der Naturheilbewegung (VIII). Von der Naturheilbewegung zur Lebensreform. **ZFA (Stuttgart)** 1983 Sep 20;59(26):1446-53
**Rothschuh KE:** Das Buch 'Der Arzt' (1906) stammt nicht von Ernst Schweninger! **Medizinhist J** 1983;18(1-2):137-44
**Rothschuh KE:** Das Relevanzproblem in der Geschichte der theoretischen Medizin. Zugleich ein Beitrag zur Interpretation der Entwicklungsdynamik in den Wissenschaften von T. S. Kuhn und L. Fleck. In Ganzinger K, Skopec M, Wyklicky H, ed: Festschrift für Erna Lesky zum 70. Geburtstag. Wien, Brüder Hollinek, 1981. p. 75-86.
**Rothschuh KE:** Der Ausklang der wissenschaftlichen Iatromagie. **Ber Wissenschaftsgesch** 1981;4(1/2):51-60
**Rothschuh KE:** Die Konzeptualisierung der Medizin in Geschichte und Gegenwart. **Acta Hist Leopoldina** 1980;13:27-38
**Rothschuh KE:** Die Konzeptualisierung der Naturheilkunde im 19. Jahrhundert. **Gesnerus** 1981;38:175-90
**Rothschuh KE:** Ernst Schweninger (1850-1924). Zu seinem Leben und Wirken. Ergänzungen, Korrekturen. **Medizinhist J** 1984;19(3):250-8
**Rothschuh KE, Krafft F:** Forschungsberichte und Spezial-Bibliographien. **Ber Wissenschaftsgesch** 1978;1(3-4):201-15
**Rothschuh KE:** Iatromagie, Begriff, Merkmale, Motive, Systematik. Opladen, Westdeutscher Verlag, 1978. 60 p. (Vorträge. Geisteswissenschaften. Rheinisch-Westfälische Akademie der Wissenschaften, G 225).
**Rothschuh KE:** Medicina Historica. Zum Selbstverständnis der historischen Medizin. **Janus** 1980;67(1-2-3):7-19
**Rothschuh KE:** Medizinische Kulturgeschichte des Wassers. **ZFA (Stuttgart)** 1983 Mar 31;59(9):485-90
**Rothschuh KE:** Naturheilbewegung, Reformbewegung, Alternativbewegung. Stuttgart, Hippokrates, 1983. 148 p.
**Rothschuh KE:** Naturphilosophische Konzepte der Medizin aus der Zeit der deutschen Romantik. **Dtsch Vierteljahresschr Lit Wiss Geistesgesch** 1978;:243-66
**Rothschuh KE:** Richard Hermann Koch (1882-1949). **Medizinhist J** 1980;15(3):223-43
**Rothschuh KE:** Richard Hermann Koch (1882-1949): Arzt, Medizinhistoriker, Medizinphilosoph (Biographisches, Ergographisches). 1. Teil. Zur Biographie. **Medizinhist J** 1980;15(1/2):16-43
**Rothschuh KE:** Therapia rationalis systematica bei Friedrich Hoffmann (1660-1742). In Dilg P, et al., ed: Perspektiven der Pharmaziegeschichte. Graz, Austria, Akademische Druck- u. Verlagsanstalt, 1983. p. 269-80.
**Rothschuh KE:** Ursprünge und Wandlungen der physiologischen Denkweisen im 19. Jahrhundert. **Forschungsunternehm Fritz Thyssen Stift Stud Naturwiss Tech Wirtsch Neunzehn Jahrhundert** 1976;2:135-60
**Rothschuh KE** see **Hasler L, ed**
**Rothschuh KE** see **Mann G, ed**
**Rothstein WG:** Pathology: the evolution of a specialty in American medicine. **Med Care** 1979 Oct;17(10):975-88
**Roubert J:** L'adoption des enfants par des particuliers à Lyon sous l'ancien régime. **Bull Soc Fr Hist Hop** 1978;(36-37):41-67
**Roubert J:** Les archives médicales en France. **Archivaria** 1980;10:253-8
**Roubert J:** L'Hôtel-Dieu de Lyon au XVIIIe siècle. **Cah Rech Archit** 1980;6-7:134-41
**Roucoules L:** Paul Valery et l'art de guérir. **Bull Acad Chir Dent (Paris)** 1981-82;27(27):53-64
**Roudinesco E:** La bataille de cent ans. Histoire de la psychanalyse en France. Volume I. 1885-1939. Paris, Ramsay, 1982. 498 p.
**Rouillon A:** The International Union against Tuberculosis. **Tubercle** 1982 Dec;63(4):247-53
**Roulet JF, Ulrich-Bochsler S:** Zahnärztliche Untersuchung frühmittelalterlicher Schädel aus Biel-Mett. **SSO Schweiz Monatsschr Zahnheilkd** 1979 Jun;89(6):526-40
**Roulet JF** see **Wiederkehr M**
**Rouot J:** Die Zahnheilkunde in der Antike. In Sournia JC, Martiny M, Poulet J, ed: Illustrierte Geschichte der Medizin. Salzburg, Andreas, 1980. Vol. 2. p. 523-37.
**Rouslin S, ed** see **Smoyak SA**
**Rousseau A:** Laennec Celtisant. In: Congrès National des Sociétés Savantes, 97e, Nantes, 1972. Comptes Rendus. Paris, 1976. Section des Sciences, Tome 1. p. 9-19.
**Rousseau A** see **Huard P**
**Rousseau F:** Marie-Geneviève Parent. In Dictionary of Canadian biography, 1801 to 1820. Volume 5, 1983. p. 658-9.
**Rousseau F:** Marie-Vénérande Melançon. In Dictionary of Canadian biography, 1801 to 1820. Volume 5, 1983. p. 587-8.
**Rousseau GG** see **De Meyts P**
**Rousseau GS:** Ephebi, Epigoni, and Fornacalia: some meditations on the contemporary historiography of the eighteenth century. **Eighteenth Cent Stud** 1979;20:203-26
**Rousseau GS:** Literature and medicine: the state of the field. **Isis** 1981 Sep;72(263):406-24
**Rousseau GS:** Psychology. In G. S. Rousseau, R. Porter, ed: The ferment of knowledge. Studies in the historiography of eighteenth-century science. Cambridge, Cambridge University Press, 1980. p. 143-210.
**Rousseau GS:** Six new Hill letters. **Med Hist** 1984 Jul;28(3):293-302
**Rousseau GS, Porter R, ed:** The ferment of knowledge. Studies in the historiography of eighteenth-century science. Cambridge, Cambridge University Press, 1980. xiii, 500 p. including contributions by R. Harre, S. Schaffer, S. Shapin, H. J. Bos, J. L. Heilbron, E. G. Forbes, D. S. Cardwell.
**Rousseau GS** see **Lemay JA**
**Rousseau J:** Dièreville. In Dictionary of Canadian biography, 1701 to 1740. Volume 2, 1969. p. 188-9.
**Rousseau J:** Michel Sarrazin. In Dictionary of Canadian biography, 1701 to 1740. Volume 2, 1969. p. 593-600.
**Rousseau GS, ed:** The letters and papers of Sir John Hill 1714-1775. New York, AMS Press, 1982. li, 208 p.
**Roussel CI** see **Vial F**
**Roussel L** see **Girard A**
**Roussel M:** Ether et chaleur dans l'embryologie aristotélienne: influences archaïques. In: Mélanges d'études anciennes offerts à Maurice Lebel. St-Jean-Chrysostôme, Québec, 1980. p. 157-60.
**Roussel M:** Physique et biologie dans la 'Génération des animaux' d'Aristote. **Rev Etud Grec** 1980, reçu 1981:93(440-441):42-71
**Roussel Ch** see **Vial F**
**Rousselle A:** La sage-femme et le thaumaturge dans la Gaule tardive. Les sages-femmes ne font pas de miracles. **Rev Archeol Centre France** 1983;22(Dec):261-71
**Rousselle A:** Observation féminine et idéologie masculine: le corps de la

femme d'après les médecins grecs. **Ann Econ Soc Civilis** 1980;35:1089-115
**Rousselle A:** Porneia. De la maitrise du corps à la privation sensorielle. IIe-IVe siècles de l'ère chrétienne. Paris, Presses Universitaires de France, 1983. 254 p. (Les chemins de l'Histoire).
**Rousselle R:** Comparative psychohistory: snake-handling in Hellenistic Greece and the American South. **J Psychohist** 1984 Spring;11(4):477-89
**Rousselot Y:** De quelques influences qui se sont exercées sur R. Théophile Laennec et ce qui en résulta. In: Congrès National des Sociétés Savantes, 97e, Nantes, 1972. Comptes Rendus. Paris, 1976. Section des Sciences, Tome 1. p 37-45.
**Rousselot Y:** La conception de la schizophrénie chez Langfeldt. **Ann Med Psychol (Paris)** 1981;139(8):879-92
**Rousset JJ** see **Théodoridès J**
**Roustang F:** Dire mastery. Discipleship from Freud to Lacan. Translated by Ned Lukacher. Baltimore, London, Johns Hopkins University Press, 1982. (Translation of: Un destin si funeste).
**Roux L:** 'La sage-femme'. **Ann Demogr Hist (Paris)** 1984;:269-78
**Roux M:** Eloge de Charles Debray, 1907-1979. **Bull Acad Natl Med (Paris)** 1979 Dec;163(9):897-906
**Rouzeau L** see **Kernéis JP**
**Rovelli F:** Il 'giornale italiano di cardiologia': 10 anni di storia della cardiologia in Italia. **G Ital Cardiol** 1981;11 Suppl 1:1-7
**Rowan AN, Rollin BE:** Animal research - for and against: a philosophical, social, and historical perspective. **Perspect Biol Med** 1983 Autumn;27(1):1-17
**Rowbottom ME:** Dr. E. Ashworth Underwood (1899-1980). **Med Hist** 1980 Jul;24(3):349-52
**Rowe C:** Jean-Jacques Rousseau: ce qu'il pensait des médecins. **Bull Soc Hist Protestantisme Fr** 1978;124(4):501-17
**Rowe WF:** Discussion of 'George Armstrong Custer and the Battle of the Little Bighorn: homicide or mass suicide'. **J Forensic Sci** 1984 Jul;29(3):696-9
**Rowell M:** Russian medical botany before the time of Peter the Great. **Sudhoffs Arch** 1978;62(4):339-58
**Roweth B** see **Gould F**
**Rowland B:** Bishop Bradwardine on the artificial memory. **J Warburg Courtauld Inst** 1978;41:307-12
**Rowland B:** Chaucer's idea of the pardoner. **Chaucer Rev** 1979-80;14(2):138-54
**Rowland B:** Exhuming Trotula, sapiens matrona of Salerno. **Florilegium** 1979;1:42-57
**Rowland B, Jennings M:** Medieval multiple birth. **Neuphilol Mitt** 1980;81:169-73
**Rowland B** see **Medieval woman's guide to health**
**Rowland LP:** Changing approaches to the management of seizures: pharmacologic considerations. Introduction. **Epilepsia** 1982;23 Suppl 1:S1-4
**Rowland LP:** Thirty years of progress and problems in clinical neurology. **Ann Neurol** 1982 Apr;11(4):327-34
**Rowthorn AW:** A history of the evolution and development of therapeutic recreation services for special populations in the United States from 1918 to 1977. Ph.D. Diss. New York University. New York, 1978. 351 leaves.
**Roy B** see **Sutto C, ed**
**Roy I, Porter S:** The social and economic structure of an early modern suburb: the Tything at Worcester. **Bull Inst Hist Res** 1980;53:203-17
**Roy M** see **Barbeau A**
**Roy R** see **Richard M**
**Royal Alexandra's century of caring: Aust Nurses J** 1980 Nov;10(5):20-1
**Royal Australian College of General Practitioners:** The Royal Australian College of General Practioners, 1958-1978. [Sydney?] The College, [1979?] 130 p.
**Royer J, Haut J, Amalric P:** L'opération de la cataracte de Claude Monet, correspondence inédite du peintre et de G.-Clemenceau au docteur Coutela. **Hist Sci Med** 1984;18(2):109-27
**Royer J** see **Bailliart JP**
**Royle SA:** Clergymen's return to the 1831 census. **Local Hist** 1980;14(2):79-90
**Rozear MP, ed** see **Cebe B**
**Rozenshtraukh LS** see **Sokolov IuN**
**Róziewicz J:** Zwiazki Marii Skłodowskiej-Curie z nauka rosyjska i radziecka. **Kwart Hist Nauki Tech** 1984;29(3-4):535-55
**Rozman C** see **Ralchs A**
**Rozos B:** Pathological syndromes as mentioned by Xenophon in the march of the ten thousand. In International Congress of the History of Medicine. 26th, Plovdiv, 1978. Actes du Congress. Sofia, 1981. Volume II. p. 163-6.
**Rozos B:** The social care during the Eastern Middle Ages according to the sources. In: Congrès international d'histoire de la médecine, XXVe, Québec, 1976. Actes. Québec, 1977. p. 1184-95.
**Rozos B** see **Degleris N**
**Rozos BP** see **Degleris NE**
**Rózsa G:** 70 éve halt meg John Shaw Billings. **Orv Hetil** 1983 Sep 4;124(36):2191-2
**Rozsívalová E, Adamec J:** Podmínky vzniku I. ortopedické kliniky v Praze. **Cas Lek Cesk** 1979 Nov 16;118(46):1429-31
**Rozsívalová E:** Příspěvek k vývoji institucionální základny I. interní kliniky v Praze 1881-1938. **Cas Lek Cesk** 1981;120(50):1539-41
**Rozsívalová E, Fuchsová V:** Zájem lékařu o zdravotní stav dělnictva v druhých dvacetipěti ročnících Casopisu lékařu českých. **Cas Lek Cesk** 1981;120(52):1594-8
**Rozwadowska-Dowzenko M, Afek-Kamińska M:** Rys historyczny Towarzystawa Lekarskiego Warszawskiego w 160-lecie jego powstania. **Pol Tyg Lek** 1982 Apr 19;37(7):211-4
**Rubain TJ** see **Gordon EW**
**The rubber industry:** Historical overview. In IARC monographs on the evaluation of the carcinogenic risk of chemicals to humans. (Volume 28: The rubber industry). [Geneva], International Agency for Research on Cancer, 1982. p. 31-46.
**Rubenstein RL** see **Ostow M**
**Rubenstein S** see **Plaut EA**
**Ruberg RL, Shah RR:** Max Thorek: a surgeon for all seasons. In Romm S, ed: Symposium on historical perspectives of plastic surgery. Philadelphia, Saunders, 1983. p. 611-8.
**Ruberg RL** see **Romm S, ed**
**Rubin JA** see **Detre KC**
**Rubin JP:** Celsus' decircumcision operation: medical and historical implications. **Urology** 1980 Jul;16(1):121-4
**Rubin LP:** A young woman taken to the doctor by her family. Mezzotint by Johann Andreas Pfeffel after an original painting by Jan Josef Horemans. **J Hist Med Allied Sci** 1981 Oct;36(4):489
**Rubin LP:** Elizabeth Lee Hazen. In: Notable American women. The modern period. Cambridge, Mass., Belknap-Harvard Univ. Press, 1980. 4:326-8.
**Rubin LP:** Gladys Rowena Henry Dick. In: Notable American women. The modern period. Cambridge, Mass., Belknap-Harvard Univ. Press, 1980. 4:191-2.
**Rubin LP:** Styles in scientific explanations: Paul Ehrlich and Svante Arrhenius on immunochemistry. **J Hist Med Allied Sci** 1980 Oct;35(4):397-425
**Rubin S:** St Cuthbert of Lindisfarne: a medical reconstruction. **Trans Archit Archaeol Soc Durham Northumberl** 1978 Sep;4:101-3
**Rubin W:** Galdos y la medicina. **Atlantida** 1970;8(43):68-80
**Rubin W:** Pollock as Jungian illustrator: the limits of psychological criticism. **Art Am** 1979;67(7):104-23, (8):72-91
**Rubins JL:** Karen Danielson Horney. In: Notable American women. The modern period. Cambridge, Mass., Belknap-Harvard Univ. Press, 1980 4:351-4.
**Rubinstein BB:** Freud's early theories of hysteria. In R.S. Cohen, L. Laudan, ed: Physics, philosophy and psychoanalysis. Dordrecht, D. Reidel, 1983. p. 169-90.
**Rubio Vela A:** Una fundación burguesa en la Valencia medieval: El Hospital de En Clapers (1311). **Dynamis** 1981;1:18-49
**Ruck CA:** Mushrooms and philosophers. **J Ethnopharmacol** 1981 Sep;4(2):179-205
**Ruck CA:** The wild and the cultivated: wine in Euripides' Bacchae. **J Ethnopharmacol** 1982 May;5(3):231-70
**Ruckebusch Y:** An historical profile of veterinary pharmacology and therapeutics. **J Vet Pharmacol Ther** 1982 Mar;5(1):1-20
**Rucker CW:** A history of the ophthalmoscope. Rochester, Minn., Whiting Printers and Stationers, [1971]. 127 p.
**Rucker RD** see **Buchwald H**
**Rückleben H:** Deportation und Tötung von Geisteskranken aus den badischen Anstalten der Inneren Mission Kork und Mosbach. Karlsruhe, Evangelischer Presseverband für Baden, 1981. 104 p. (Veröffentlichungen des Vereins für Kirchengeschichte in der evangelischen Landeskirche in Baden, Band 33).
**Rudakova AIa:** Permskaia oblastnaia klinicheskaia bol'nitsa (k 150-letiiu bol'nitsy). **Sov Zdravookhr** 1984;(2):57-8
**Rudelic I:** Glagolijski grafiti kao svjedočanstva socijalnih i zdravstvenih prilka u Istri. **Lijec Vjesn** 1984 Jun;106(6):261-4
**Rüden AD von:** Medicina Graecensis. Das medizinisch-chirurgische Studium in Graz (1782-1862). Diss. Technischen Universität München, 1978. 195 p.
**Rudenko AK:** Muzeĭ istorii Donetskogo meditsinskogo instituta. **Sov Zdravookhr** 1980;(9):61-4
**Rudenko AK** see **Maĭatruk PN**
**Rudenko AK** see **Maĭstruk PN**
**Rudenko AT:** Kafedre cheliustno-litsevoĭ khirurgii so stomatologieĭ VMA imeni S. M. Kirova--50 let. **Voen Med Zh** 1980 Mar;(3):77
**Ruderman FA:** A placebo for the doctor. **Commentary** 1980;69(5):54-60
**Rudert H:** Von der sujbmukösen Septumresektion Killians über Cottles Septumplastik zur modernen plastischen Septumkorrektur und funktionellen Septo-Rhinoplastik. **HNO** 1984 Jun;32(6):230-3
**Rudichenko VF** see **Siniak KM**
**Rudney JD, Katz RV, Brand JW:** Interobserver reliability of methods for paleopathological diagnosis of dental caries. **Am J Phys Anthropol** 1983 Nov;62(3):243-8
**Rudnicki J:** Słuzba zdrowia l Polskiej Samodzielnej Brygady Spadochronowej w operacji 'Market-Garden'--relacje uczestników. **Arch Hist Med (Warsz)** 1984;47(1):127-31
**Rudnicky AI** see **Cole RA**
**Rudnyĭ NM:** Opyt meditsinskogo obespecheniia Voenno-Vozdushnykh Sil v Velikuiu Otechestvennuiu voĭnu. **Voen Med Zh** 1980 May;(5):34-7
**Rudolph ED:** The introduction of the Natural System of classification of plants to nineteenth century American students. **Arch Nat Hist** 1982 Apr;10(3):461-8
**Rudolph G:** Das Mechanismusproblem in der Physiologie des 19. Jahrhunderts. **Ber Wissenschaftsgesch** 1983;6(1-4):7-28
**Rudolph G:** Herkunft und Schicksal des Humor aqueus. Physiologische Untersuchungen im Vorfeld der Ätiologie des Glaukoms während des ersten Viertels des 20. Jahrhunderts. **Gesnerus** 1983;40(3/4):241-8
**Rudolph G:** Histoire mémorable d'une fille d'Anjou laquelle a été quatre ans sans user d'aucune nourriture que de peu d'eau commune; anorexie

mentale (?) au XVIe siècle. In: Congrès National des Sociétés Savantes, 93e, Tours, 1968. Comptes Rendus. Paris, 1971. Section des Sciences, Tome II. p. 17-29.
**Rudolph G:** Iconographie de La Mettrie (1709-1751) à propos de la découverte d'un portrait inconnu du médecin et philosophe breton. In: Congrès National des Sociétés Savantes, 91e, Rennes, 1966. Comptes Rendus. Paris, 1967. Section des Sciences. Tome 1, p. 171-9.
**Rudolph G:** Les relations entre Denis Papin (1647-1714) et Leibniz (1646-1716). In: Congrès National des Sociétés Savantes, 93e, Tours, 1968. Comptes Rendus. Paris, 1971. Sections des Sciences, Tome II. p. 55-68.
**Rudolph G:** Zwei Beiträge zur Geschichte der Balneologie. Die kulturgeschichtlichen und medizinischen Wurzeln des Bäderwesens. 100 Jahre wissenschaftliche Balneologie. Kassel, Meister, 1982. 132 p. (Schriftenreihe des Deutschen Bäderverbandes e.V., Heft 45).
**Rudolph G** see **Habrich C**
**Rudolph H:** Schriftauslegung und Schriftverständnis bei Paracelsus. **Medizinhist J** 1981;16(1-2):101-24
**Rudolph H** see **Paracelsus in der Tradition**
**Rudolph LI** see **Albin M**
**Rudolph SH** see **Albin M**
**Rudowska I, Rudzki E:** Dermatologiczna analiza ziołowych surowców kosmetycznych zalecanych w zielniku Falimirza z roku 1534. **Przegl Dermatol** 1983 Jul-Aug;70(4):429-37
**Rudowska I:** Kosmetyka zębów w starożytności. **Czas Stomatol** 1980 Aug;33(8):476-50
**Rudowska I:** Zródła kosmetyki leczniczej i upiększającej w starozytnym Egipcie. **Przegl Dermatol** 1981 Jan-Feb;68(1):123-8
**Rudowski W:** Ostatnia choroba Generała Stefana Grota-Roweckiego (1895-1944). **Arch Hist Med (Warsz)** 1983;46(4):487-502
**Rudowski W:** Polish contribution to the development of biomedical science. **Rev Pol Acad Sci (Warsz)** 1977;22:27-34
**Rudowski W:** Przemówienie z okazji jubileuszu xxx-lecia działalności Instytutu Hematologii. **Acta Haematol Pol** 1982 Jan-Jun;13(1-2):1-4
**Rudowski W, Kostrzewski J, Mossakowski M:** The twenty-fifth anniversary of the Polish Academy of Sciences and the twentieth anniversary of its medical science section. **Rev Pol Acad Sci (Warsz)** 1978;23(2):23-48
**Rudowski WJ:** Instytut Hematologii w Warszawie. Warszawa, Państwowy Zakład Wydawn. Lekarskich, 1976. 90 p.
**Rudzińska H** see **Olakowski T**
**Rudzki E** see **Rudowska I**
**Rueff J:** Ein schön lustig Trostbüchle von den Empfengknussen und Geburten der Menschen. 2 v. Facsimile of 1554 ed., with Einführung von H. M. Koelbing. Dietikon-Zürich, Verlag Bibliophile Drucke, 1981. 29, cxliii p.
**Ruel-Kellermann M:** Repères historiques de l'évolution du recours de l'odonto-stomatologie à la psychologie. **Inf Dent** 1981 Oct 1;63(33):3071-83
**Ruesch H:** Die Demographie der Alpen zwischen 1650 und 1850: Bericht über den heutigen Wissensstand und Fragen an die künftige Forschung. **Schweiz Z Gesch** 1979;29(1):159-80
**Ruestow EG:** Images and ideas: Leeuwenhoek's perception of the spermatozoa. **J Hist Biol** 1983 Summer;16(2):185-224
**Ruestow EG:** The rise of the doctrine of vascular secretion in the Netherlands. **J Hist Med Allied Sci** 1980 Jul;35(3):265-87
**Ruf E, ed** see **Jung-Merker L**
**Ruff CB:** Age differences in craniofacial dimensions among adults from Indian Knoll, Kentucky. **Am J Phys Anthropol** 1980 Jul;53(1):101-8
**Ruff PW:** Zum Wandel der gesellschaftlichen Stellung des medizinischen Wissenschaftlers im Deutschland des 19. Jahrhunderts. **Rostocker Wiss Hist Manuskripte** 1981;6:61-7
**Ruff PW** see **Löther R, ed**
**Ruffié J:** Darwin, cent ans après. **Biomed Pharmacother** 1982;36(3):170-3
**Ruffié J:** La signification du polymorphisme humain. **Rev Palais Decouv** 1983;11(107):46-51
**Ruffin CB:** Records of the Sellers Funeral Home, Chambersburg, Pennsylvania, relating to the black families of Franklin County, 1866-1933. **J Afro-Am Hist Geneal Soc** 1982;3(4):165-82; 1983;4(1):32-4
**Rufli T:** Lues-Serologie--gestern, heute und morgen. **Dermatologica** 1982 Oct;165(4):221-31
**Ruggiero G:** The status of physicians and surgeons in Renaissance Venice. **J Hist Med Allied Sci** 1981 Apr;36(2):168-84
**Ruggiero Pastura MG:** Una 'visita' del 1592 all'ospedale dei 'pazzarelli' di Roma. **Rass Arch Stato** 1972;32(1):47-67
**Ruhdorfer UE:** Die klinische Blutdruckmessung - rund 100 Jahre alt. **Osterr Arzteztg** 1982;37(4):193
**Ruhe CH:** Seventy-five years of American medical education: perceptions and reflections. **Conn Med** 1980 Feb;44(2):95-9
**Ruiloba J:** Listeriosis, toxoplasmosis y leptospirosis. In Academia Nacional de Medicina. Libro conmemorativo del primer centenario. México, Comité Editorial de la Comisión Organizadora del Congreso del Centenario, 1964. Tome 2. p. 532-5.
**Ruiz E** see **Bárcena A**
**Ruíz de Loyzaga S:** La epidemia de cólera de 1855 en Valdegovía. **Bol Inst Sancho Sabio** 1977;21:441-50
**Ruiz-Falcó López F:** Escuela Nacional de Sanidad. Problemática pasada, actual y futura. **Rev Sanid Hig Publica (Madr)** 1983 Mar-Apr;57(3-4):359-72
**Ruiz Naufal VM** see **Flores y Troncoso FA**
**Rujeola în judeţul Iaşi: 1951-1979: Rev Med Chir Soc Med Nat Iasi** 1980 Jul-Sep;84(3):406, 420, 436
**Rukavishnikova VM** see **Studnitsin AA**
**Rullière R, Heymans G, Chevalier P:** Abrégé d'histoire de la médecine. Paris, Masson, 1981. 376 p.
**Rullière R:** Die Kardiologie bis zum Ende des 18. Jahrhunderts. In Sournia JC, Martiny M, Poulet J, ed: Illustrierte Geschichte der Medizin. Salzburg, Andreas, 1980. Vol. 3. p. 1075-123.
**Rullière R:** Geschichte der Kardiologie im 19. und 20. Jahrhundert. In Sournia JC, Martiny M, Poulet J, ed: Illustrierte Geschichte der Medizin. Salzburg, Andreas, 1980. Vol. 4. p. 1251-309.
**Rulliere R, Heymans G, Vial F:** La version en langue française (1679) du Tractatus de Corde (1669) de Richard Lower. In International Congress of the History of Medicine, 27th, Barcelona, 1980. Actas. Barcelona, Acadèmia de Ciències Mèdiques de Catalunya i Balears, 1981. p. 331-5.
**Rullière R:** Les morts subites à la Cour de Louis XIV de 1690 à 1709, d'après Pierre Dionis. **Hist Sci Med** 1984;18(1):19-24
**Rulliere R** see **Berti Bock G**
**Rulliere R** see **Heymans G**
**Rullière R** see **Lellouch A**
**Rulliere R** see **Merlette B**
**Rulliere R** see **Vial F**
**Rumble W:** Homeopathy in the Lehigh Valley, 1881-1920. **Pa Mag Hist Biogr** 1980;104(4):474-90
**Rumer LZ** see **Krasil'shchikov MI**
**Rumiantsev GI, Korostelev NB:** Osnovanie kafedry gigieny v Moskovskom universitete (K 100-letiiu kafedry). **Gig Sanit** 1984 Aug;(8):41-4
**Rumiantsev GI** see **Kuz'min MK**
**Rumiantsev PP** see **Vorob'ev VI**
**Rumpf-Lehmann B:** Seltene Drogen von 'Dr. Dittrich aus Prag' in der Wigandschen Drogensammlung der Universität Marburg. **Beitr Gesch Pharm** 1982;31(16):123-6
**Rumpler K** see **Heilmittel aus Pflanzen und Tieren**
**Rumsey TJ:** 'The General' -- a history of Hennepin County Medical Center. Part II. **Minn Med** 1980 Feb;63(2):101-6
**Rundall TG:** Environmental selection and physician supply. **AJS** 1982 Mar;87(5):1090-1112
**Runyan WM:** Life histories and psychobiography. Explorations in theory and method. New York, Oxford, Oxford University Press, 1982. xiii, 288 p.
**Runyan WM:** Why did Van Gogh cut off his ear? The problem of alternative explanations in psychobiography. **J Pers Soc Psychol** 1981 Jun;40(6):1070-7
**Rupke NA:** The study of fossils in the Romantic philosophy of history and nature. **Hist Sci** 1983 Dec;21(54 Pt 4):389-413
**Rupp JP:** Gelbfieberabwehr in Mitteleuropa. Düsseldorf, Triltsch, 1981. 49 p. **Dusseld Arb Gesch Med Beihefte** 1981;6:1-49
**Ruppanner R** see **Goodger WJ**
**Rusakov AB:** Zhiznennyĭ i tvorcheskiĭ put' V. V. Gorinevskoĭ (K 100-letiiu so dnia rozhdeniia). **Ortop Travmatol Protez** 1983 Mar;(3):63-5
**Rusanov AA:** K stoletiiu rezektsii zheludka. **Vestn Khir** 1981 Sep;127(9):13-42
**Rusanov GA, Simbirtsev SA, Balanski R:** Sto godini ot publikuvaneto na truda na N. I. Pirogov vurkhu opita v meditsinata, pridobit vuv voĭnata za osvobozhdenieto na Bulgariia prez 1877-1878 g. **Khirurgiia (Sofiia)** 1979;32(3):247-53
**Rusch T:** Detmar Wilhelm Soemmerring, Leben und Werk. Diss. Mainz, 1981. 126 p.
**Ruscio KP:** A new regime in the republic of science. **Policy Stud Rev** 1983;2(4):790-4
**Ruse M:** Charles Darwin and group selection. **Ann Sci** 1980;37(6):615-30
**Ruse M:** Charles Darwin and the Beagle. **Wilson Q** 1982;6(1):164-75
**Ruse M:** Darwin's theory: an exercise in science. **New Sci** 1981;90:828-30
**Ruse M:** Medicine as social science: the case of Freud on homosexuality. **J Med Philos** 1981 Nov;6(4):361-86
**Ruse M:** Ought philosophers consider scientific discovery? A Darwinian case-study. In T. Nickles, ed: Scientific discovery: case studies. Dordrecht, D. Reidel, 1980. (Boston Studies in the Philosophy of Science, v. 60). p. 131-49.
**Ruse M:** The new dualism: 'Res Philosophica' and 'Res Historica.' In M. Ruse, ed: Nature animated. Historical and philosophical case studies in Greek medicine, nineteenth-century and recent biology, psychiatry, and psychoanalysis. Volume II. Dordrecht, D. Reidel, 1983. p. 3-25.
**Ruse M, ed:** Nature animated. Historical and philosophical case studies in Greek medicine, nineteenth-century and recent biology, psychiatry, and psychoanalysis. Papers deriving from the Third International Conference on the History and Philosophy of Science, Montreal, Canada, 1980. Volume II. Dordrecht, D. Reidel, 1983. xiii, 274 p.
**Rusek V:** Historie farmacie na farmaceutické fakultě University Karlovy. **Cas Lek Cesk** 1981 Jan 30;120(3-4):100-3
**Rusek V, Müller D:** Příspěvky k dějinám lékáren v Těšíně. **Cesk Farm** 1981 Jun;30(5):171-6
**Rusek V, Solich J:** Vědeckotechnická revoluce ve farmaceutických vědách a výzkumu. **Cesk Farm** 1982 Jun;31(5):145-8
**Rusek V** see **Melichar B**
**Rusiaev AP:** Znachenie dekreta o sanitarnykh organakh respubliki dlia razvitiia sanitarno-épidemiologicheskoĭ sluzhby v Belorusskoĭ SSR. **Gig Sanit** 1982 Sep;(9):12-4
**Rusiński M** see **Budnikowski A**
**Ruska E:** Die frühe Entwicklung der Elektronenlinsen und der Elektronenmikroskopie. **Acta Hist Leopoldina** 1979;12:7-136
**Ruska E:** The early development of electron lenses and electron microscopy. **Microsc Acta** 1980;(Suppl 5):1-140

**Russ, J:** Histoire de la folie [de] Michel Foucault: analyse critique. Paris, Hatier, 1979. 79 p.
**Russel ES:** A century of mammalian genetics and cancer, 1929–2029, a view at midpassage. **Prog Clin Biol Res** 1981;45:xi–xiv
**Russel G:** Writing and dyslexia--an historical analysis. **J Child Psychol Psychiatry** 1982 Oct;23(4):383–400
**Russell A:** Late effects--influence on the children of the concentration camp survivor. In Dimsdale, Joel E., ed: Survivors, victims, and perpetrators: Essays on the Nazi holocaust. Washington, Hemisphere Publ., 1980. p. 175–204.
**Russell AJ** see **Kean BH**
**Russell CA:** Science and social change in Britain and Europe, 1700–1900. New York, St. Martin's Press, 1983. xvii, 307 p.
**Russell GF:** History of writing and its relevance for the linguistic disorder in dyslexia: discussion paper. **J R Soc Med** 1982 Aug;75(8):631–40
**Russell HM, Weinberg J, ed:** The book of knowledge from the Mishnah Torah of Maimonides. Translated from the Hebrew. Edinburgh, Royal College of Physicians of Edinburgh, 1981. xi, 135 p. (Publication No. 55).
**Russell JC:** Werrett Wallace Charters, Sr. (1875–1952): his life, career and influence upon pharmaceutical education. Ph.D. Diss., Loyola University. Chicago, 1981. vii, 259 leaves.
**Russell JG:** The rationale of primitive delivery positions. **Br J Obstet Gynaecol** 1982 Sep;89(9):712–5
**Russell JR:** The three royal doctors of Betchworth. **Practitioner** 1981 Jul;225(1357):1070–1
**Russell MD** see **Wolpoff MH**
**Russell RL:** We worked hard, but we enjoyed it! General nurse training in NSW--the first 50 years. **Lamp** 1981 May;38(5 Suppl):57–63
**Russell S** see **Quinn S, ed**
**Russell WM** see **Hart GD, ed**
**Russell AW, ed:** The town and state physician in Europe from the Middle Ages to the Enlightenment. Wolfenbüttel, Herzog August Bibliothek, 1981. 156 p. (Wolfenbütteler Forschungen, 17).
**Russell KF, ed:** Catalogue of the historical books in the library of the Royal Australasian College of Surgeons. Melbourne, Queensberry Hill Press, 1979. vii, 152 p.
**Russet B:** Defense expenditures and national well-being. **Am Pol Sci Rev** 1982;76(4):767–77
**Russett CE:** Declaring the glory of God. **Hist Educ Q** 1980;20(2):217–21
**Russo A:** I 'semplici' nella Scuola Salernitana (Nota preliminare). **Rend Atti Accad Sci Med Chir** 128:55–75
**Russo A:** Il 'Petitorium' del 1614: prima farmacopea a stampa nel Regno di Napoli. In Hickel E, Schröder G, ed: Neue Beiträge zur Arzneimittelgeschichte. Festschrift für Wolfgang Schneider zum 70. Geburtstag. Stuttgart, Wissenschaftliche Verlagsgesellschaft, 1982. p. 107–10.
**Russo G** see **Pârvu E**
**Russo NF, ed** see **O'Connell AN**
**Rüster D:** Alte Chirurgie: Legende und Wirklichkeit. Berlin, VEB Verlag Volk und Gesundheit, 1984. 255 p.
**Rutkow BG** see **Rutkow IM**
**Rutkow IM, Rutkow BG, Ernst CB:** Letters of William Halsted and René Leriche: 'Our friendship seems so deep'. **Surgery** 1980 Dec;88(6):806–25
**Rutkow IM:** The letters of William Halsted and Alexis Carrel. **Surg Gynecol Obstet** 1980 Nov;151(5):676–88
**Rutkow IM:** The letters of William Halsted and Anton von Eiselsberg: a very special friendship. **Arch Surg** 1980 Aug;115(8):993–1001
**Rutkow IM:** William Halsted and Rudolph Matas: their unique alliance. **Surgery** 1980 May;87(5):524–38
**Rutkowska I:** Ludność świata i jej wyżywienie-kierunki zmian po kryzysie żywnościowym lat siedemdziesiątych. **Ekonomista** 1979;(2):445–63
**Rutkowska-Płachcińslak A:** Dżuma w Europie Zachodniej w XIV w. straty demograficzne i stutki psychiczne. **Przegl Hist** 1978;69(1):75–102
**Rutman AH** see **Rutman DB**
**Rutman DB, Rutman AH:** More true and perfect lists: the reconstruction of censuses for Middlesex County, Virginia, 1668–1704. **Va Mag Hist Biogr** 1980;88(1):37–74
**Rutman DB, Wetherell C, Rutman AH:** Rhythms of life: black and white seasonality in the early Chesapeake. **J Interdiscip Hist** 1980;11(1):29–53
**Rüttimann B:** Hippokratische 'Wirbelverrenkung'. **Gesnerus** 1983;40(1–2):159–66
**Rüttimann B:** Nelsons Oberarm-Amputation. **Z Orthop** 1982 Feb;120(1):86–8
**Rüttimann B:** Wilhelm Schulthess (1855–1917) und die Schweizer Orthopädie seiner Zeit. Zürich, Schulthess Polygraphischer Verlag, 1983. xv, 272 p.
**Rüttimann B:** Zur Geschichte der Krüppelfürsorge. **Gesnerus** 1980;37(3/4):199–214
**Rüttimann B** see **Boschung U**
**Rüttner JR:** Staublungenforschung in der Schweiz einst und jetzt. **Schweiz Med Wochenschr [Suppl]** 1983;15:51–61
**Ruzicka LT, Hansluwka H:** Mortality transition in South and East Asia: technology confronts poverty. **Popul Dev Rev** 1982;8(3):567–88
**Ryall RL, Marshall VR:** Measurement of urinary flow rate. **Urology** 1983 Nov;22(5):556–64
**Ryalls J:** Where does the term 'aphasia' come from? **Brain Lang** 1984 Mar;21(2):358–63
**Ryan MP:** Reproduction in American history. **J Interdiscip Hist** 1979;10(2):319–32
**Ryan MT, Fair MF:** The radiation warning symbol. **Health Phys** 1981 Aug;41(2):416–7
**Ryan S:** Reflections on the psychohistory of France, 1919–1940. **J Psychohist** 1983 Fall;11(2):225–41
**Ryan SJ, Mittl RN, Maumenee AE:** The disciform response: an historical perspective. **Albrecht Von Graefes Arch Klin Exp Ophthalmol** 1980;215(1):1–20
**Ryan TA:** Psychology at Cornell after Titchener: Madison Bentley to Robert Macleod, 1928–1948. **J Hist Behav Sci** 1982 Oct;18(4):347–69
**Ryant C:** Comment: oral history and gerontology. **Gerontologist** 1981 Feb;21(1):104–5
**Ryant C:** Oral history and psychohistory. **J Psychohist** 1981 Winter;8(3):307–18
**Rybak J:** Tradycje Krakowskiej Szkoły Położnych. **Pieleg Polozna** 1980;(3):25–7
**Rybicka E** see **Stefański K**
**Rybina AA** see **Khalmuradov AG**
**Rybová J:** Vývoj ideově výchovné práce Institutu pro další vzdělávání lékařu a farmaceutu. **Cas Lek Cesk** 1983 Oct 21;122(42):1291–4
**Rybus B** see **Sobień-Kopczyńska S**
**Rychlak JF:** Freud's confrontation with the telic mind. **J Hist Behav Sci** 1981;17:176–83
**Rychlak JF** see **Kasschau RA**
**Rychlak JF** see **Sharkey PW, ed**
**Ryckewaert A, Naveau B:** Les affections ostéo-articulaires de J.M. Charcot à nos jours. **Rev Neurol (Paris)** 1982;138(12):997–1008
**Ryckewaert A, Naveau B:** Principaux apports de Charcot et de Pierre Marie à la pathologie ostéo-articulaire. **Rev Rhum Mal Osteoartic** 1984 Jul–Sep;51(7–8):405–13
**Ryder NB:** The future of American fertility. **Soc Probl** 1979;26(3):359–70
**Ryder R:** [Nursing reformation in postwar Japan: a reflection on the period of occupation] (Jpn). **Kango Kyoiku** 1981 Oct;22(10):601–11
**Rye DH** see **Allan P**
**Rykushin IuP, Smorodintsev AA, Shliakhtenko LI, et al:** Professor V. A. Bashenin--odin iz osnovopolozhnikov otechestvennoĭ épidemiologii. **Zh Mikrobiol Epidemiol Immunobiol** 1983 Apr;(4):112–6
**Ryleeva RN** see **Studenikin MI**
**Ryn L:** Los Andes y la medicina. **Actas Luso Esp Neurol Psiquiatr** 1981 May–Jun;9(3):213–30, Jul–Aug;9(4):315–24
**Ryn L:** Medicina popular andina. **Actas Luso Esp Neurol Psiquiatr** 1982 Jan–Feb;10(1):33–42
**Ryn Z:** Antoni Kępiński we wspomnieniach. **Przegl Lek** 1983;40(12):881–4
**Ryn Z, Kłodziński S:** Głód w obozie koncentracyjnym. **Przegl Lek** 1984;41(1):21–37
**Ryn Z:** Zakopiańskie placówki słyzby zdrowia podczas okupacji hitlerowskiej. **Przegl Lek** 1981;38(1):114–21
**Ryn Z** see **Leśniak E**
**Ryslavy K:** Materialien zur Geschichte der Apotheken und Apotheker im Burgenland. Eisenstadt, Amt der Burgenländischen Landesregierung, Landesarchiv, 1979. 285 p. (Burgenländische Forschungen, Heft/68).
**Ryssing E:** Historien om Børnehospitalet i Rigensgade og Dronning Louises Børnehospital. **Dan Medicinhist Arbog** 1981;:58–92
**Rytand DA:** Sutton's or Dock's law? **N Engl J Med** 1980 Apr 24;302(17):972
**Rytter M** see **Gast W**
**Rywlin AM:** Non-Hodgkin's malignant lymphomas. Brief historical review and simple unifying classification. **Am J Dermatopathol** 1980 Spring;2(1):17–25
**Ryzhakova GI:** Itogi vypolneniia direktiv Dal'kraĭkoma VKP(b) po stroitel'stvu ob'ektov zdravookhraneniia v gody pervykh piatiletok (1928–1937). **Sov Zdravookhr** 1982;(8):55–7
**Ryzhikov KM, Sonin MD:** Biologicheskie problemy gel'mintologii. Kratkaia istoriia razvitiia issledovaniĭ v SSSR i vazhneĭshie dostizheniia. **Parazitologiia** 1982 Nov–Dec;16(6):433–40
**Ryzhkov SV** see **Samotokin BA**

## S

**Saarma IuM:** 100-letie kafedry i kliniki psikhiatrii v Tartu. **Zh Nevropatol Psikhiatr** 1981;81(11):1716–20
**Saavedra A:** Honorio Delgado y la psiquiatría Peruana. **Rev Neuropsiquiatr** 1980 Jun;43(2):67–86
**Saba SJ** see **Pringle JK**
**Sabagh G, Lopez D:** Religiosity and fertility: the case of Chicanas. **Soc Forces** 1980;59(2):431–9
**Sabagh G, Kim SB:** The relationship between migration and fertility in an historical context: the case of Morocco in the 1960s. **Int Migr Rev** 1980;14(4):525–38
**Saban R:** Le système veineux méningé de l'homme fossile de Biache-Saint-Vaast (Pas-de-Calais), d'après le moulage endocranien. **C R Acad Sci [D] (Paris)** 1979 Dec 10;289(15):1129–32
**Saban R:** Les sinus veineux méningés à travers les traités d'anatomie du XVe au XIXe siècle. In: Congrès National des Sociétés Savantes, 106e, Perpignan, 1981. Comptes Rendus. Paris, Bibliothèque Nationale, 1982. Fasc. IV. p. 119–31.
**Sabben-Clare EE, Bradley DJ, Kirkwood K, ed:** Health in tropical Africa during the colonial period: based on the proceedings of a symposium held at New College, Oxford, 21–23 March 1977. Oxford, Clarendon, 1980. ix, 276 p.
**Sabin AB:** Judaism and medicine. **Perspect Biol Med** 1983 Winter;26(2):188–97
**Sabin JA, Sanmartín Urchaga P:** Estudio comparado de las aportaciones iconográficas, en el sistema muscular, en las obras de Leonardo y Vesalio.

In International Congress of the History of Medicine, 27th, Barcelona, 1980. Actas. Barcelona, Académia de Ciències Médiques de Catalunya i Balears, 1981. p. 446–53.

**Sabin LE:** The French Revolution: the forgotten era in nursing history. **Nurs Forum** 1981;20(3):225–43

**Sabin TD:** The Penikese Hospital: a Massachusetts hospital for the treatment of Hansen's disease. **N Engl J Med** 1981 Jun 25;304(26):1610–2

**Sabiston DC:** Deryl Hart: leader in the development of the Duke University Medical Center. **NC Med J** 1983 Jul;44(7):441–2

**Sabiston DC:** Trendelenburg's classic work on the operative treatment of pulmonary embolism. **Ann Thorac Surg** 1983 May;35(5):570–4

**Sablik K:** Die Finanzierung des Wiener Allgemeinen Krankenhauses (gegründet 1784) durch Kaiser Joseph II. In Schmidtchen V, Jäger E, ed: Wirtschaft, Technik und Geschichte. Beiträge zur Erforschung der Kulturbeziehungen in Deutschland und Osteuropa. Festschrift für Albrecht Timm. Berlin, Verlag Ulrich Camen, 1980. p. 241–50.

**Sablik K:** Julius Tandler: Mediziner und Sozialreformer: eine Biographie. Wien, A. Schendl, 1983. 389 p.

**Sablosky AH:** The power of the forceps: a comparative analysis of the midwife--historically and today. **Women Health** 1976 Jan–Feb;1(1):10–13

**Sabo MO:** National health insurance and the states. **Publius** 1978;891):55–62

**Sabogal F** see **Sanz de Santamaría MC de**

**Sachs H** see **Jefferys M**

**Sacino G:** Singolari figure della tradizione medica popolare remota e recente nell'appennino centro–meridionale d'Italia: 'le janare', 'le masciare'. In: Congrès international d'histoire de la médecine, XXVe, Québec, 1976. Actes. Québec, 1977. p. 1196–207.

**Sackmann W:** Der Arzt und Biochemiker Emil Abderhalden (1877–1950) und seine Beziehungen zur Tiermedizin. **Schweiz Arch Tierheilkd** 1982 Jan;124(1):1–10

**Sackmann W:** Fleckfieber und Fleckfieberforschung zur Zeit des ersten Weltkrieges;zum Gedenken an Henrique da Rocha Lima (1879–1956). **Gesnerus** 1980;37(1/2):113–32

**Sackmann W:** Vor hundert Jahren: Robert Koch entdeckt den Erreger der Tuberkulose. **Schweiz Arch Tierheilkd** 1982 May;124(5):217–25

**Sadahiro U** see **Kato M**

**Saddique A, Peterson CD:** Thallium poisoning: a review. **Vet Hum Toxicol** 1983 Feb;25(1):16–22

**Sadegh–Zadeh K:** World 5 and medical knowledge. **J Med Philos** 1981 Aug;6(3):263–70

**Sadibelouiz M** see **Barbeau A**

**Sadler C:** Edith Cavell: from Blakeney Point to Brussels. **Nurs Mirror** 1982 Sep 15;155(11):52–4

**Sadler C:** Hospital report: a tradition for innovation. **Nurs Times** 1983 Sep 7;157(10):26–8

**Sadler C:** Hospital report: mixing the old with the new. **Nurs Mirror** 1984 Mar 21;158(12):23–6

**Sadovskaia AG** see **Piatak OA**

**Sadowska J:** Działalność Inspekcji Pracy w zakresie bezpieczeństwa i higieny w przemyśle łódzkim II Rzeczypospolitej. **Arch Hist Med (Warsz)** 1984;47(3):439–42

**Sadowska J:** Postulaty zdrowotne klasy robotniczej w rewolucji 1905–1907 roku. **Arch Hist Med (Warsz)** 1980;43(4):377–81

**Saegesser F:** César Roux (1857–1934) et son époque. **Rev Med Suisse Romande** 1984 Jun;104(6):403–64

**Saenz A, Boisvert H:** Correspondance inédite d'Albert Calmette (1863–1933). **Hist Sci Med** 1983;17(4):419–27

**Saenz A, Boisvert H:** Trois lettres de Louis Pasteur. **Hist Sci Med** 1981;15(4):327–33

**Saez A:** La fécondité en Espagne depuis le début du siècle. **Population** 1979;34(6):1007–21

**Safarov RN, Shtern MI, Fel'berg MB:** K istorii tuberkuleznoĭ bol'nitsy 'Zakhar'ino'. **Probl Tuberk** 1983 Feb;(2):70–3

**Saffirio L:** Razioni e salari in natura nell'antico Egitto. Considerazioni dietetiche e socio economiche. **Aegyptus (Milano)** 1977;57:14–78

**Saffron MH:** A sketch of medicine in New Jersey to 1825. **J Med Soc NJ** 1984 Sep;81(9):709–14

**Saffron MH:** Isidor Clinton Rubin. In Dictionary of American Biography, Suppl. 6, 1956–1960. p. 554–6, 1980.

**Saffron MH:** James Peter Warbasse. In Dictionary of American Biography, Suppl. 6, 1956–1960. p. 663–5, 1980.

**Saffron MH:** New Jersey or Massachusetts? **JAMA** 1981 May 22–29;245(20):2031–2

**Saffron MH:** Russell Story Fowler. In Dictionary of American Biography, Suppl. 6, 1956–1960. p. 214–15, 1980.

**Saffron MH:** The Academy of Medicine of New Jersey: a brief history. **J Med Soc NJ** 1984 Sep;81(9):785–8

**Safin MS** see **Lotsmanov IuA**

**Sagaert LLC:** Un grand chirurgien français: le docteur Achille–Cléophas Flaubert. **Hist Sci Med** 1980;14:449–52

**Sagan L** see **Jonsen AR**

**Saget H:** L'essor de la biologie moléculaire (1950–1965). Paris, Centre de Documentation Sciences Humaines, CNRS, xi, 1978. 43 p.

**Sági E:** A kinai gyógyszerészet a századfordulón. Diss., Budapest, 1979. 130 p.

**Sagne S:** The use of the scanning electron microscope with X–ray equipment for the analysis of elements in medieval bones. **Ossa** 1978;5:85–91

**Sagrera JE de** see **Cornet AM**

**Sagrera JE de** see **Escudero Mendo A**

**Sagrera JE de** see **Mendo AE**

**Saha MS:** The Carl Correns papers. **Mendel Newsl** 1981 Nov;21:1–6

**Sahakian WS:** Systematic social psychology. New York, Chandler, 1974. xiii, 589 p.

**Sahakian WS, ed:** History of psychology. A source book in systematic psychology. Revised edition. Itasca, Illinois, F. E. Peacock, 1981. xvi, 497 p.

**Sahli N:** Sexuality in 19th and 20th century America: the sources and their problems. **Radic Hist Rev** 1979;20:89–96

**Sai FT:** [Medical ethics in modern] sub–Saharan Africa. In Reich WT, et al, ed: Encyclopedia of bioethics, v. 2. New York, Free Press, 1978. p. 897–900.

**Said HM:** al–Tibb al–Islami. Dacca, Islamic Foundation Bangladesh, 1981. 202 p.

**Said HM:** Diseases of the liver: Greco–Arab concepts. Karachi, Hamdard Foundation Press, 1982. 131 p.

**Said HM:** Early hospitals in Turkey. **Med Times** 1981 Nov–Dec;16(11–12):8–14

**Said HM:** Greco–Arab concepts on cardiovascular diseases. Karachi, Pakistan, Hamdard Foundation Press, 1983. 201 p.

**Said HM:** Medicine in Turkey. **Med Times** 1981 Nov–Dec;16(11–12):4–8

**Said HM:** Medieval Chinese, Japanese and Arab medicine: reciprocal impact. In: Congrès international d'histoire de la médecine, XXVe, Québec, 1976. Actes. Québec, 1977. p. 1208–24.

**Said HM:** Zuviel Erfolg für Avicenna? **Med Welt** 1981 Sep 25;32(39):62–3

**Said M:** Greco–Arabic and modern Western Medicine: conflict or symbiosis? **Stud Philos Med** 1977 Mar;1(1):50–7

**Said HM, ed:** Pharmacy and medicine thru' the ages. Karachi, Hamdard Foundation, 1980. 264 p. Contributions by S. K. Hamarneh, Y. Ahmad, I. H. Qureshi, S. S. Ali, K. M. Habib, M. S. Akhtar, V. M. Tirmizi, M. Amin, M. Ashraf, M. K. Bhatty, S. F. Hussain, S. Mahdihassan, U. Schaffer, I. Haq.

**Saidi MH, Zainie CM:** Contraception and sterilization, a brief history. In their: Female sterilization, a handbook for women. New York, Garland, 1980. p. 1–14.

**Saĭfutdinov VA** see **Kamalov MKh**

**Saint André P:** The Marchoux Institute. **Lepr Rev** 1980 Mar;51(1):35–42

**Saint–Blanquat H de:** Tableaux de la médecine médiévale. **Sci Avenir** 1984;(445):58–63

**St. Clair RE:** Medical practitioners in early Auckland: part I. **Hist J (NZ)** 1982;40:9–11

**Saint–Denis A:** Institution hospitalière et société à Laon aux XIIe et XIIIe siècles. **Inf Hist** 1983;45(4):171–9

**St. Hoyme LE** see **Koritzer RT**

**St. John C:** Race differences in age at first birth and the pace of subsequent fertility: implications for the minority group status hypothesis. **Demography** 1982 Aug;19(3):301–14

**Saint–Maur PP:** Que pensait Laennec de l'anatomie pathologique? **Ann Pathol** 1981;1(4):249–50

**Saint–Pierre B** see **Sutto C, ed**

**Sainte–Fare–Garnot PN** see **Fourest HP**

**St–Pierre J** see **Mathieu J**

**St Vincent's Hospital, Sydney: 1857–1982: Med J Aust** 1982 Nov 27;2(11):532–3

**Saiz Moreno L:** Antiguas vías de circulación del ganado. La trashumancia del ganado merino en España y las epizootias. **Rev Sanid Hig Publica (Madr)** 1983 Nov–Dec;57(11–12):1229–53

**Saiz Moreno L:** La Sociedad Española de Higiene (un siglo al servicio de la Salud Pública). **Rev Sanid Hig Publica (Madr)** 1981 Sep–Oct;55(9–10):1073–100

**Sajner J:** Goethuv vztah k přírodním vědám, zvláště k lékařství. **Vnitr Lek** 1982 Jun;28(6):615–6

**Sajner J:** Patografická studie o Leoši Janáckovi. **Vnitr Lek** 1982 Aug;28(8):823–7

**Sajner J, Geus A:** Ueber eine Buchbesprechung von Jan Evangelista Purkyně. **J Soc Bibliogr Nat Hist** 1978 Nov;9(1):53–5

**Sájner J** see **Habrich C**

**Sajter V** see **Kukurová E**

**Sajter V** see **Kutarňa A**

**Sajter V** see **Tichý M**

**Sakai T:** [Morphology of premolar in primitive anthropoidea] (Jpn). **Shikai Tenbo** 1983 Jan;61(1):81–90

**Sakai–shi Ishikai, Kaishi Hensan Iinkai:** Nijugoshunen kinen Sakai–shi Ishikai shi. Sakai, Do Ishikai, Showa 52 nen, 1977. 822 p.

**Sakamoto T** see **Okamura H**

**Sakharchuk IM** see **Danilevskiĭ NF**

**Sakharchuk IM** see **Shalimov AA**

**Sakharov MI, Sorokin EIu:** Sverdlovskoe oblastnoe nauchnoe obshchestvo khirurgov (k 50–letiiu so dnia obrazovaniia). **Vestn Khir** 1982 May;128(5):136–7

**Saklad M:** Revolutionary ideas versus progress--in respiratory care. **Respir Care** 1977 Nov;22(11):1212–9

**Saklad SM:** Psychiatry in Rhode Island: 1725–1980. **RI Med J** 1980 Jun;63(6):207–16

**Sakowski RA** see **Miller JM**

**Saks FF** see **Zadorozhnyĭ AA**

**Sakula A:** Acceuil du livre 'De l'auscultation médiate' et du stéthoscope par les médecins de Grande–Bretagne. **Rev Palais Decouv** 1981 Aug;22:280–90

**Sakula A:** 'Amadeus' was Mozart poisoned? **Hist Med (Lond)** 1980 Jan–Feb;8(1):6–9

**Sakula A:** Augustus Bozzi Granville (1783–1872): London

physician-accoucheur and Italian patriot. **J R Soc Med** 1983 Oct;76(10):876–82
**Sakula A:** Baroness Burdett-Coutts' garden party: the International Medical Congress, London, 1881. **Med Hist** 1982 Apr;26(2):183–90
**Sakula A:** BCG: who were Calmette and Guérin? **Thorax** 1983 Nov;38(11):806–12
**Sakula A:** Bicentenary of Laennec's birth celebrated in Paris. **Med Hist** 1981;25:320–1
**Sakula A:** Blue plaques: London house of medicohistorical interest. **Br Med J [Clin Res]** 1982 Dec 18–25;285(6357):1799–800
**Sakula A:** Carlo Forlanini, inventor of artificial pneumothorax for treatment of pulmonary tuberculosis. **Thorax** 1983 May;38(5):326–32
**Sakula A:** Centenary of the discovery of the tubercle bacillus. **Lancet** 1982 Mar 27;1(8274):730
**Sakula A:** Dr. Thomas Hodgkin and Sir Moses Montefiore Bart--the friendship of two remarkable men. **J R Soc Med** 1979 May;72(5):382–7
**Sakula A:** Founding of the Athenaeum and Fellows of the Royal College of Physicians. **J R Coll Physicians Lond** 1983 Jul;17(3):206–7
**Sakula A:** In search of Hippocrates: a visit to Kos. **J R Soc Med** 1984 Aug;77(8):682–8
**Sakula A:** In search of Laënnec. **J R Coll Physicians Lond** 1981 Jan;15(1):55–7
**Sakula A:** Joseph Skoda 1805–81: a centenary tribute to a pioneer of thoracic medicine. **Thorax** 1981 Jun;36(6):404–11
**Sakula A:** Laennec's influence on some British physicians in the nineteenth century. **J R Soc Med** 1981 Oct;74(10):759–67
**Sakula A:** L'histoire du bacille tuberculeux telle qu'il nous la raconte dans 'La Ballade de la Seringue'. **Bull Int Union Tuberc** 1982 Sep–Dec;57(3–4):192–3
**Sakula A:** Moses Maimonides' treatise on asthma. **Thorax** 1981 Jul;36(7):560
**Sakula A:** Pierre Adolphe Piorry (1794–1879): pioneer of percussion and pleximetry. **Thorax** 1979 Oct;34(5):575–81
**Sakula A:** R.T.H. Laënnec 1781–1826, his life and work: a bicentenary appreciation. **Thorax** 1981 Feb;36(2):81–90
**Sakula A:** Ramazzini's De Morbis Artificum and occupational lung disease. **Br J Dis Chest** 1983 Oct;77(4):349–61
**Sakula A:** Robert Koch: centenary of the discovery of the tubercle bacillus, 1882. **Thorax** 1982 Apr;37(4):246–51
**Sakula A:** Robert Koch (1843–1910): founder of the science of bacteriology and discoverer of the tubercle bacillus. A study of his life and work. **Br J Dis Chest** 1979 Oct;73(4):389–94
**Sakula A:** Sir John Floyer's A Treatise of the Asthma (1698). **Thorax** 1984 Apr;39(4):248–54
**Sakula A:** The Betchworth Portraits: members of the family of William Harvey. **Med Hist** 1980 Jul;24(3):333–41
**Sakula A:** The story of the stethoscope. **Trans Med Soc Lond** 1981–82;98:27–31
**Sakula A:** The waters of Epsom Spa. **J R Coll Physicians Lond** 1982 Apr;16(2):124–8
**Sakurai K, Ogata T:** Japanese mummies. In A. Cockburn, E. Cockburn, ed: Mummies, disease, and ancient cultures. Cambridge, Cambridge University Press, 1980. p. 211–23.
**Sala Catalá J:** Cambio de paradigma y polemica cientifica entre los biologos expañoles (1860–1922). **Asclepio** 1982;34:239–63
**Sala Catalá J:** El evolucionismo en la practica cientifica de los biologos españoles del siglo XIX (1860–1907). **Asclepio** 1981;33:81–125
**Salaçin S:** Forensic medicine in Turkey. **Am J Forensic Med Pathol** 1982 Jun;3(2):179–80
**Salaeva ZM:** K istorii kliniki nervnykh bolezně Azerbaĭdzhanskogo orden Trudovogo Krasnogo Znameni gosudarstvennogo meditsinskogo instituta im. N, Narimanova. **Zh Nevropatol Psikhiatr** 1981;81(11):1720–1
**Salamatov EI** see **Ripp GKh**
**Salamon J:** The basic concept of psychical development in Soviet psychology and several of its variants. **Ann Univ Sci Budap Rolando Eotvos Nominatae** 1979;6:89–101
**Salander JM** see **Rich NM**
**Salas Sánchez M** see **Sanz de Santamaría MC de**
**Salazar JG, Espinosa JM:** A sociodemographic profile of Hispanic physicians in three United States metropolitan areas. **Aztlan** 1979;10:111–22
**Salden MJ:** Van doodstraft to straffeloosheid. **Spiegel Hist** 1982;17(11):559–65
**Salem J:** Coon dog graveyard. **South Exposure** 1979;7(3):27–9
**Salemme MA, Colani AM:** La valeur de la logique dans l'ancienne et la moderne science. In International Congress of the History of Medicine. 26th, Plovdiv, 1978. Actes du Congress. Sofia, 1981. Volume II. p. 94–6.
**Salemme MA** see **Stroppina L**
**Sales BD** see **Massad PM**
**Salfelder K, Novoa Montero D:** Patologos alemanes en Venezuela 1936–1981. Merida, Universidad de los Andes, 1982. 131 p.
**Salimbeni F:** Psicanalisi e storiografia: un problema pluridisciplinare. **Studium** 1981;77(5):565–80
**Salinas Cantú H:** Biografia del Dr. Jesus Ma. González Flores. **Humanitas** 1981;22:201–12
**Salinas Quiroga G:** Psicologia de los pueblos y del mexicano. **Humanitas** 1981;22:213–8
**Salk J:** The virus of poliomyelitis. From discovery to extinction. **JAMA** 1983 Aug 12;250(6):808–10
**Salkever DS:** Effects of children's health on maternal hours of work: a preliminary analysis. **South Econ J** 1980;47(1):156–66
**Saller K** see **Rassengeschichte der Menscheit**
**Salles-Cunha SX** see **Battocletti JH**
**Salmon JW** see **Garfield R**
**Salmon P:** Psychosociologie du collectionneur. **Rev Inst Sociol** 1977;2:271–87
**Salnikova GP:** Zhizn' i deiatel' nost' A.N. Rubakina. **Sov Med** 1981;(2):114–6
**Salokangas RK:** Hospital and outpatient care for psychotic patients during the last three decades. Subsequent hospital and outpatient treatment of psychotic patients hospitalized for the first time in 1949–50, 1959–60 or 1969–70. **Acta Psychiatr Scand** 1980 Jul;62(1):47–62
**Salomone G, Lambiase M:** Appunti storici sulla teoria del neurone. **Acta Neurol (Napoli)** 1983 Feb;5(1):62–76
**Salov VI:** Vtorzhenie psikhoanaliza v burzhuaznuiu istoriografiiu. (Rus). **Nov Noveishaia Istor** 1972;(4):89–105
**Salsburg D, Heath A:** When science progresses and bureaucracies lag: the case of cancer research. **Public Interest** 1981;65:30–9
**Salsbury D:** Step into the twenties with Jen-Sal's veterinary display. [An early 20th cent. veterinarian's office.] **Found News** 1979 Nov;:12–13
**Salter AL:** Veterinary life in the Boer War 1899–1902. Correspondence of James William Hall Masheter M.R.C.V.S. **Vet Hist** 1984;3(3):87–92
**Salter RB:** Scientific contributions to orthopaedic surgery by the staff of The Hospital for Sick Children, Toronto, 1875 to 1975. In: Congrès international d'histoire de la médecine, XXVe, Québec, 1976. Actes. Québec, 1977. p. 1225–43.
**Salter SS:** Toward community mental hygiene. A history of state policy in California, 1939–1969. Doctor of Social Welfare Diss. University of California. Berkeley, 1978. iv, 382 leaves.
**Saltzman BB:** Saga of America's first woman dental graduate. **Dent Stud** 1983 Oct;62(1):24–5
**Salukvadze SS:** Starodavnia apteka Vardziï. **Farm Zh** 1979;(6):66–9
**Salvat M:** L'accouchement dans la littérature scientifique médiévale. **Senefiance** 1980;9:87–106
**Salvetti ME:** Gefässpsychopathologie bei Richard von Krafft-Ebing (1840–1902). Bern, Huber, 1984. 125 p. (Berner Beiträge zur Geschichte der Medizin und der Naturwissenschaften, Neue Folge, Band 10)
**Salvini S:** La mortalità dei gesuiti in Italia nei secoli XVI e XVII. **Quad Depart Stat Univ Studi Fir** 1979;3:1–25
**Salzinger K, ed** see **Rieber RW**
**Samba Murthy KV** see **Rahman A**
**Sambin P:** Il dottorato padovano in medicina di Paolo da Middelburgo (1480). **Quad Stor Univ Padova** 1976–7;9–10:252–6
**Samborschi E, Baicu G, Suliman M, et al:** Die Tradition der Spezialitätenherstellung in Apotheken Rumäniens. In Hickel E, Schröder G, ed: Neue Beiträge zur Arzneimittelgeschichte. Festschrift für Wolfgang Schneider zum 70. Geburtstag. Stuttgart, Wissenschaftliche Verlagsgesellschaft, 1982. p. 81–5.
**Sambursky S:** Einheit und Einfachheit der Natur als Leitmotiv der Forschung. **Biomed Tech (Berlin)** 1979 Oct;24(10):230–6
**Samelson F:** A note on an unpublished article by John B. Watson. **J Hist Behav Sci** 1982 Jan;18(1):20–1
**Samion-Contet J, ed** see **Boulle L**
**Sammis S, Dummett E:** On display: the science and art of healing. **J Med Soc NJ** 1984 Sep;81(9):747–57
**Sammons JH, Miller JD, Hannon TF:** The Journal and publication in the other languages and countries. From hesitant beginnings to firm commitment. **JAMA** 1983 Jul 8;250(2):236–41
**Samoggia A** see **Bellettini A**
**Samotokin BA, Nechaĭ AI, Sitenko VM, et al:** Vladimir Nikolaevich Shamov (k 100-letiiu so dnia rozhdeniia). **Voen Med Zh** 1982 Jun;(6):73–4
**Samsonov MA:** Dostizheniia sovetskoĭ dietologii za piat'desiat let. **Vopr Pitan** 1980 Sep–Oct;(5):15–21
**Samuel R:** Henry Howard. In Dictionary of Canadian biography, 1881–1890. 1982;11:425–6.
**Samueloff S** see **Taylor W**
**Sananés R:** Homéopathie et langage du corps. Paris, Robert Laffont, 1982. 361 p.
**Sanazaro PJ:** Quality assurance in medicine: a brief historical perspective. **World Hosp** 1984 Apr;20(2):16–20
**Sanborn A:** The seed for a dream: M. Adelaide Nutting. **Alumni Mag** 1984 Jul;84(1):3–5
**Sances A** see **Battocletti JH**
**Sánchez F** see **Valverde JL**
**Sanchez F** see **Valverde Lopez JL**
**Sanchez Gozalbo A:** Boticarios, medicos y cirujanos en el Castellón del cuatrocientos. **Bol Soc Castell Cult** 1979;55(1):47–80
**Sanchez Granjel Santander L, Sanchez Granjel Santander M:** El libro medico español renacentista. Salamanca, Universidad de Salamanca, 1980. 41 p. (Trabajos de la Catedra de Historia de la Medicina, 5).
**Sanchez Granjel Santander M** see **Sanchez Granjel Santander L**
**Sanchez L. De Vinuesa F** see **Valverde JL**
**Sanchez-Moscoso A:** José Rodríguez Carracido. **Bol Soc Esp Hist Farm** 1971 Jun;22(86):54–84
**Sanchez-Moscoso Hermida A:** Distinción entre alimento y medicamento en un texto médico del siglo XVI. **Bol Soc Esp Hist Farm** 1980 Oct;31(123):151–90
**Sánchez-Moscoso Hermida A, Alfonso Galán MT:** Estudio histórico de una tesis de farmacia juzgada hace 100 años: 'Las divisiones de la naturaleza y de la ciencia', de Francisco Fernández Iparraguirre. **Bol Soc Esp Hist Farm** 1983;34(136):167–84
**Sánchez-Moscoso Hermida A:** La peligrosidad del medicamento a través del 'Discurso Farmacéutico sobre los Cánones de Mesué', de Miguel

Martínez de Leache (1652). **Bol Soc Esp Hist Farm** 1984 Jun;35(138):103-23
**Sánchez Reséndiz J, et al:** Investigaciones mexicans recientés sobre las propriedades medicinalesd del yumel (guatteria gaumeri). **Med Tradic** 1980;3(9):19-27
**Sanchez Tellez MC, Guerra F, Valverde JL:** La doctrina farmacéutica del Renacimiento en la obra de Francisco Hernández, c. 1515-1587. Granada, Universidad de Granada, Hospital Real, 1979. 140 p. (Estudios del Departamento de Historia de la Farmacia y Legislación Farmacéutica, Universidad de Granada, 6).
**Sánchez Téllez MC:** Remedios filipinos descritos por Fr. Antonio Mozo (1763). **Bol Soc Esp Hist Farm** 1983 Sep;135:95-100
**Sánchez Tellez MC** see **Valverde JL**
**Sanchez-Villacañas CM** see **Folch Jou G**
**Sancho Trabulo AA:** Perspectives in international neurosurgery: neurosurgery in Portugal. **Neurosurgery** 1982 Mar;10(3):409-10
**Sandbach FR:** The history of schistosomiasis research and policy for its control. **Med Hist** 1976 Jul;20(3):259-75
**Sandberg LG, Steckel RH:** Soldier, soldier, what made you grow so tall? A study of height, health and nutrition in Sweden, 1720-1881. **Econ Hist (Sweden)** 1980;23(2):91-105
**Sandblom P:** Skapande och Sjukdom. Hur lidande påverkar litteratur, konst och musik. Södertälje, Fingraf Tryckeri, 1983. 142 p. (Nordisk Medicinhistorisk Arsbok, Supplementum IX).
**Sandblom P:** The tragic development of socialized medicine in Sweden. **Bull Am Coll Surg** 1976 Feb;61(2):13-5
**Sande MA** see **Täuber MG**
**Sandelowski M:** Pain, pleasure, and American childbirth: from the twilight sleep to the Read Method, 1914-1960. Westport, Conn., Greenwood Press, 1984. xix, 152 p. (Contributions in Medical History, No. 13).
**Sanden B:** Gesundheitsfürsorge einst und jetzt. **ZFA (Stuttgart)** 1980 Mar;56(8):567-72
**Sander FM:** Individual and family therapy: toward an integration. New York Aronson, 1979. Historical chapters, p. 1-42, 89-109.
**Sanders ED** see **Davies NE**
**Sanders JH** see **Ward JO**
**Sanders RE:** History of the Illinois Association of School Nurses: the formative years. Ph.D. Diss., Southern Illinois University, Carbondale, 1979. viii, 175 leaves.
**Sanders V:** 'No ordinary case of a village apothecary': the doctor as hero in Harriet Martineaus's Deerbrook. **Notes Queries** 1983 Aug;30(4):293-4
**Sanderson CJ, Cote RJ, Levett JM, et al:** Acute aortic dissection. An historical review. **J R Coll Surg Edinb** 1982 Jul;27(4):195-9
**Sanderson ER:** Henri Hartmann and the Hartmann operation. **Arch Surg** 1980 Jun;115(6):792-3
**Sanderson WC:** Quantitative aspects of marriage, fertility and family limitation in nineteenth century America: another application of the Coale specifications. **Demography** 1979 Aug;16(3):339-58
**Sandführ K:** Das Verständnis vom Leben und vom Organismus im Werk von Johannes Müller (1801-1858). Die Eigenart des Lebendigen und die Methode seiner Erforschung. Diss, Bonn, 1979. 153 p.
**Sandifer SH:** Pellagra in South Carolina. **J SC Med Assoc** 1981 Dec;77(12):602-4
**Sandison AT:** Diseases in ancient Egypt. In A. Cockburn, E. Cockburn, ed: Mummies, disease, and ancient cultures. Cambridge, Cambridge University Press, 1980. p. 29-44.
**Sandison AT:** Glasgow and world medicine. **Pharm Hist (London)** 1971 Dec;2(3):1-2
**Sandler AM** see **Sandler J**
**Sandler B:** An unpalatable but popular gargle. **MIMS Mag** 1981 Jun 15;:59
**Sandler EM:** C. Louis Leipoldt--medical student extraordinary. **Adler Mus Bull** 1981 Oct;7(3):8-14
**Sandler I:** Pierre Louis Moreau de Maupertuis - a precursor of Mendel? **J Hist Biol** 1983 Spring;16(1):101-36
**Sandler IL:** Pierre Louis Moreau de Maupertuis--a precursor of Mendelian genetics?: an inquiry into the biological ideas of Maupertuis, the Mendelian principles of heredity and the nature of the precursor. Ph.D. diss. University of Washington. Seattle, 1979. 265 leaves.
**Sandler J:** Discussions with Anna Freud on The Ego and the Mechanisms of Defence: The Ego and the Id at Puberty. **Int J Psychoanal** 1983;64 (Pt 4):401-6
**Sandler J:** On the psychoanalytic theory of affects. A historical and developmental review. **Isr J Psychiatry Relat Sci** 1983;20(1-2):81-94
**Sandler J, Sandler AM:** The 'second censorship', the 'three box model' and some technical implications. **Int J Psychoanal** 1983;64 (Pt 4):413-25
**Sandmaier M:** Bacchantic maidens and temperance daughters: a historical perspective on female alcohol use. **Alcohol Health Res World** 1980 Summer;4(4):41-51
**Sandor RS, ed:** Bernheim's New studies in hypnotism. New York, International Universities Press, 1980. xix, 407 p. Translation of Hypnotisme, suggestion, psychothérapie: Etudes nouvelles, 1891.
**Sandos JA:** Prostitution and drugs: the United States Army on the Mexican-American border, 1916-1917. **Pac Hist Rev** 1980;49(4):621-45
**Sandoz Y:** Le droit d'initiative du Comité International de la Croix-Rouge. **Ger Yearb Int Law** 1979;22:352-73
**Sands D:** Using oral history to chart the course of illegal abortions in Montana. **Frontiers** 1983;7(1):32-7
**Sandson JI:** Medical education: past, present, and future. **RI Med J** 1984 Dec;67(12):537-42
**Sandu L** see **Curelaru I**
**Sandulesco C** see **Grmek MD, ed**
**Sandulescu C:** Primum non nocere: philological commentaries on a medical aphorism. **Acta Antiq Hung** 1965;13:359-368
**Sandusky WR:** Frank L. Meleney: pioneer surgeon-bacteriologist. **Arch Surg** 1983 Feb;118(2):151-5
**Sandyk R:** Brain development and the phylogenesis of writing and drawing direction. **S Afr Med J** 1982 Jul 10;62(2):43-4
**Sanfilippo J:** Bibliografía histórico-odontológica del Dr. Samuel Fastlicht. **Bol Soc Mex Hist Filos Med** 1984 Jun;7(47):317-24
**Sanfilippo J:** Homenaje a los fundadores de la odontologia en México. **ADM** 1980 Mar-Apr;37(2):82-4
**Sanfilippo J:** Semblanza del doctor Samuel Fastlicht. **Bol Soc Mex Hist Filos Med** 1984 Jun;7(47):309-15
**Sanfilippo J:** The life and accomplishments of Dr. Samuel Fastlicht. **Bull Hist Dent** 1983 Oct;31(2):87-92
**Sanfilippo B. J:** Bibliografia historia de la odontologia en Mexico. [Mexico City, Sociedad de la Historia y Filosofia de la Medicina], 1984. 23 p.
**Sanford JP:** Landmark perspective: Tularemia. **JAMA** 1983 Dec 16;250(23):3225-6
**Sanford WL:** The influenza epidemic of 1918 and its effects on the military. **Indiana Med Hist Q** 1983 Dec;9(4):16-22
**Sanger R** see **Race RR**
**Sanger G, ed:** The Charaka Club, 1898-1978. A history. New York, Charles C. Morchand, 1978. 260 p.
**Sangirardi J:** O índio e as plantas alucinógenas: tribos das 3 Américas e civilizações pré-colombianas. [S.l.], Alhambra, 1983. 207 p.
**Sanguinetti FA:** Reflexiones en torno a la historia de la medicina. **Rev Fac Cien Med Univ Nac Cordoba** 1981 Jan-Dec;39(1-4):81-6
**Sanitetskollegierne i Slesvig Holsten 1804-1864: Dan Medicinhist Arbog** 1980;:79-90
**Sanjeeva Rao I:** Surgical treatment of Fistula-in-Ano. Historical evolution of a technique. **Bull Inst Hist Med (Hyderabad)** 1973 Oct;3(4):169-72
**Sankaran JR:** Avicenna's thoughts and concepts of the pulse (sphygmology). **Bull Indian Inst Hist Med (Hyderabad)** 1981;1-4:64-74
**Sanmartín Urchaga P** see **Sabin JA**
**Sano K:** [Harvey Williams Cushing] (Jpn). **No Shinkei Geka** 1981 Jan;9(1):32-5
**Sano K:** Perspectives in international neurosurgery: neurosurgery in Japan. **Neurosurgery** 1980 Mar;6(3):337-9
**Sansoni J:** Considerazioni e riflessioni sul libro 'Lungo Viaggio nel Tunnel della Mallattia' di Gigi Ghirotti. **Prof Inferm** 1980 Jan-March;33(1):3-6
**Santamaría J** see **Edwards A**
**Santambrogio M:** Minima methodica: una rubrica che affronta problemi di metodo e di concetto, e intende stimolare nella cultura medica una riflessione 'di fondo'. (continued regularly). **Kos** 1984 Feb;1(1):16-8
**Santambrogio M** see **Camerino G**
**Santander FM:** Marco histórico para el análisis de las causas del descenso en la práctica de la lactancia materna. **Rev Chil Pediatr** 1982 Nov-Dec;53(6):607-14
**Santangelo MV:** The history and development of United States dental education. **J Dent Educ** 1981 Oct;45(10):619-27
**Santavý F:** Prof. Dr. chem. PhMr. Martin Ehrmann a jeho pusobení na medicínskochirurgickém učilišti v Olomouci v letech 1836--1866. **Cesk Farm** 1979 Jun;28(5):221-2
**Santoni-Rugiu P** see **Marsili A**
**Santonja R** see **Alegre Perez ME**
**Santopolo JL:** Norman W. Kingsley. 'He helped the dumb to speak'. **NY State Dent J** 1980;46:606, 608, 610
**Santoro C** see **Allison MJ**
**Santos GW:** History of bone marrow transplantation. **Clin Haematol** 1983 Oct;12(3):611-39
**Santos Filho LC** see **Bowers JZ**
**Santow G** see **Bracher MD**
**Santra SC** see **Lama S**
**Santurri EN:** Theodicy and social policy in Malthus' thought. **J Hist Ideas** 1982 Apr-Jun;43(2):315-30
**Sanz de Santamaría MC de, Salas Sánchez M, Sabogal F:** Aspectos psicosociales del aborto (mesa redonda). **Cuad Filos Let** 1980;3(2):85-105
**Sanz Diaz L** see **Folch Jou G**
**Sanz Diaz L** see **Javier Puerto F**
**Sanz Sanjosé MG, Merino Navarro JP:** Saneamiento y limpieza en Madrid, siglo XVIII. **An Inst Estud Madrilenos** 1976;(12):119-32
**Sanzharov BN:** Deiatel'nost' glavnykh épidemiologov frontov v 1941-1945 gg. **Voen Med Zh** 1980;(12):13-4
**Sapegina AV** see **Khromchenko OM**
**Sapińska I:** Rozwój refleksoterapii (akupunktury) w Zwiazku Radzieckim. **Wiad Lek** 1984 Aug 1;37(15):1233-7
**Sapira JD:** Quincke, de Musset, Duroziez, and Hill: some aortic regurgitations. **South Med J** 1981 Apr;74(4):459-67
**Sapov IA, Tiurin VI:** K 100-letiiu Kronshtadtskoĭ shkoly vodolazov. **Voen Med Zh** 1982 Aug;(8):70-2
**Sapp J:** The struggle for authority in the field of heredity, 1900-1932: new perspectives on the rise of genetics. **J Hist Biol** 1983 Fall;16(3):311-42
**Sapporo Ika Daigaku Soki 30-nenshi Henshu Iinkai:** Sapporo Ika Daigaku soki 30-nenshi (Showa 20 nen-Showa 50 nen). Sapporo, Japan, Sapporo Ika Daigaku Soki Sanjunenshi Kankokai, Showa 50 nen, 1975. 488 p.
**Sarac S, Lalic R, Jovanovic L, et al:** Stogodišnjica stomatologije u Somboru (1881-1981). **Med Pregl** 1982;35(11-12):497-8
**Sarac V** see **Protic M**
**Saraceno C:** Trent' anni di storia della famiglia Italiana. **Studi Stor** 1979;20(4):833-56

**Saraf PG, Cockett AT:** Marcello Malpighi--a tribute. **Urology** 1984 Jun;23(6):619-23

**Saragba M:** Histoire de la trypanosomiase ou maladie du sommeil en Oubangui-Chari (R. C. A.) de 1910 à 1950. 2 tomes. Thèse de doct., 3e cycle. Université de Provence, 1983. 630, 85 p.

**Sarason SB:** Psychology misdirected. New York, Free Press, 1981. xiii, 193 p.

**Sarazin M:** Le docteur Fournier de Lempdes (1783-1861). **Bull Hist Sci Auvergne** 1984;92(680):37-47

**Sarbaugh TJ:** A moral spectacle: American relief and the famine, 1845-1849. **Eire Irel** 1980;15(4):6-14

**Sardell A:** Neighborhood health centers and community-based care: federal policy from 1965 to 1982. **J Public Health Policy** 1983 Dec;4(4):484-503

**Sardi M:** Modelos de ejercicio de la odontologia en Venezuela desde Los años cuarenta. **Acta Odontol Venez** 1980 Jan-Apr;18(1):37-66

**Sardi PA:** Epidemiologia della tossicodipendenza e cicli storici di altri disturbi psichici. **Minerva Med** 1981 Sep 26;72(36):2447-52

**Sargent F:** Hippocratic heritage. A history of ideas about weather and human health. New York, Pergamon, 1982. xlii, 581 p. (Pergamon International Library of Science, Technology, Engineering and Social Studies).

**Sargent LA, Morgan RF, Davis WB:** John Staige Davis: pioneer American plastic surgeon. In Romm S, ed: Symposium on historical perspectives of plastic surgery. Philadelphia, Saunders, 1983. p. 653-6.

**Sargent LA** see **Romm S, ed**

**Saric M:** Institute for Medical Research and Occupational Health in Yugoslavia. Introduction. **Arh Hig Rada Toksikol** 1979;30 Suppl:5-9

**Sarich VM** see **Prager EM**

**Sariic P:** Je li Zabrebački kirurg Dragutin Schwarz uradio prvu nefrektomiju u Hrvatskoj? **Lijec Vjesn** 1980 Apr;102(4):205-7

**Sarkisov DS:** Dzh. B. Morgan'i (k 300-letiiu so dnia rozhdeniia). **Klin Med (Mosk)** 1983 Jan;61(1):110-4

**Sarkisov DS** see **Smol'iannikov AV**

**Sarkisov DS** see **Strukov AI**

**Sarma CR, Rama Rao B:** A note on the New Edition of Bhela Samhita. **Bull Indian Inst Hist Med (Hyderabad)** 1980;10(1-4):7-14

**Sarma CR, Rama Rao B:** Additional material in Astanga Sangraha. **Bull Indian Inst Hist Med (Hyderabad)** 1979;9:1-12

**Sarma CR, Rama Rao B:** Additional material in Astanga sangraha. **Bull Indian Inst Hist Med (Hyderabad)** 1980;10(1-4):23-33

**Sarma CR, Rama Rao B:** Urine in ancient ayurvedic literature. **Bull Indian Inst Hist Med (Hyderabad)** 1980;10(1-4):48-52

**Sărmąsanu-Cortez ML, Cortez P:** A great forerunner of the modern sanitary organization, Prof. Dr. Alexandru Obregia (1860-1937). **Sante Publique (Bucar)** 1979;22(4):387-93

**Sărmăşanu-Cortez ML, Cortez P:** Bernhard von Gudden şi drama de la lacul Starnberg (1824-1886). **Rev Med Interna [Neurol Psihiatr]** 1983 Jul-Sep;28(3):233-8

**Sărmăşanu-Cortez ML, Cortez P:** Dr. Hermann Simon, sitemul Gütersloh şi tratamentul activ al bolilor psihice. **Rev Med Interna [Neurol Psihiatr]** 1980 Oct-Dec;25(4):295-302

**Sărmăşanu-Cortez ML, Cortez P:** Dr. Ioan I. Popescu-Sibiu, promotor al psihanalizei şi neobosit animator al vieţii culturale din Romąnia (1901-1974). **Rev Med Interna [Neurol Psihiatr]** 1982 Oct-Dec;27(4):313-8

**Sărmăşanu-Cortez ML, Cortez PP:** Un distins psihiatru la confluenta dintre muzică şi medicină: dr. Stefan S. Braşcu (1895-1965). **Rev Med Interna [Neurol Psihiatr]** 1980 Apr-Jun;24(2):143-8

**Sărmăşanu-Cortez ML, Cortez P:** Un luptător neobosit pentru progresul psihiatriei româneşti: dr. Mircea Bruteanu (1882--1957). **Rev Med Interna [Neurol Psihiatr]** 1979 Apr-Jun;24(2):137-42

**Sărmăşeanu-Cortez ML** see **Cortez P**

**Sarnat HB:** The discovery, proof and reproof of neurosecretion (Speidel, 1917; Scharrer and Scharrer, 1934). **Can J Neurol Sci** 1983 Aug;10(3):208-12

**Sarnecka-Keller M:** Biochemia na Uniwersytecie Jagiellońskim: Przesylość i terazniejszość. **Stud Mater Dziejow Nauk Pol** 1981;25:87-105

**Sarre HJ:** Glomerulonephritis im Wandel der Zeit. Gedanken zu 40 Jahren Nephrologie. **Fortschr Med** 1982 Mar 4;100(9):364-73

**Sarre HJ, ed** see **Bock HE, ed**

**Sarro R:** Razon y sinrazon de las heterodoxias psicoanaliticas. **Asclepio** 1980;32:421-32

**Sartorius N:** La classification: une optique internationale. **Acta Psychiatr Belg** 1983 Mar-Apr;83(2):88-103

**Sáry G:** A megértés müvészete. **Orv Hetil** 1984 May 13;125(20):1210-1

**Sas M:** A hormonalis anticonceptio 25 éve. **Orv Hetil** 1982 Jan 24;123(4):195-200

**Sasaki C:** Scientific studies at Oxford and Cambridge in the seventeenth century - a research review. **Hist Sci** 1981;(20):57-75

**Sass H** see **Koehler K**

**Sass HM:** Reichsrundschreiben 1931: Pre-Nuremberg German regulations concerning new therapy and human experimentation. **J Med Philos** 1983 May;8(2):99-111

**Sass LJ:** Religion, medicine, politics and spices. **Appetite** 1981 Mar;2(1):7-13

**Sassão solene comemorativa do 75.o aniversário do Instituto de Higiene e Medicina Tropical--14 de Novembro de 1977: An Inst Hig Med Trop (Lisb)** 1977-1978;5(1-4):21-35

**Sastri R:** Bharata ke pranacarya: Aśivanikumara, Dhanvantari, Susruta, Atreya Punarvasu, Kaśyapa, Kumara Bhartr Jivaka, Caraka, Nagarjuna, Vagbhata sambandhi ayurvedika, aitihasika sahitya evam puratatva ke gambhira adhyayana, Bharatiya sabhyata, aura Samskrti ka gaveshana-purna paricaya. Dilli [Delhi, India], Atmarama, 1976. xvii, 895 p.

**Sastry VV:** Health habits of South Indians as recorded by Abbe J. A. Dubois. **Bull Indian Inst Hist Med (Hyderabad)** 1980;10(1-4):84-9

**Sastry VV:** Hortus Indicus Malabaricus (Garden of Malabar of India). **Bull Indian Inst Hist Med (Hyderabad)** 1975 Jul;5(3):143-9

**Sastry VV, Pandey AN:** Jajjata. **Bull Indian Inst Hist Med (Hyderabad)** 1975 Jul;5(3):115-22

**Sasvári L:** Emlékek és adatok az ingyenorvosok tiszteletére a magyarországi ortodoxok és görög katolikusok köréböl. **Orvostort Kozl** 1979;87-88(25 no 1-2):65-78

**Sasvári L:** Kiegészítö adatok a nöi beteg-ápolórendekröl. **Orv Hetil** 1982 Sep 12;123(37)2321-2

**Sasvári L:** Magyarországi egyházi betegellátó intézetek és testületek a XIX. század második felében. **Orvostort Kozl** 1982;28(1-3):209-18

**Sasvári L:** Nöi betegápoló rendek szerepe a hazai kórházak munkájában (1867-1918). **Orv Hetil** 1982 Apr 18;123(16):990-2

**Satin DG:** Erich Lindemann as humanist, scientist, and change agent. **Am J Community Psychol** 1984 Oct;12(5):519-27

**Satin DG:** Erich Lindemann: the humanist and the era of community mental health. **Proc Am Philos Soc** 1982 Aug;126(4):327-46

**Sato M:** Concept of shame and the mental health of Pacific Asian Americans. **Explor Ethnic Stud** 1980;3(1):3-12

**Satoh O:** [Transsphenoidal surgery for pituitary tumors: historical review and present trends] (Jpn). **No Shinkei Geka** 1984 Jan;12(1):7-26

**Satran R:** Les débuts de la Société française de neurologie. **Hist Sci Med** 1981;15(2):188-95

**Sattamini Duarte O:** Dr. José Maurício Nunes Garcia. **Rev Inst Hist Geogr Bras** 1971;291:92-103

**Saturno Canelón J:** Dos articulos odontologicos en la Gaceta Cientifica de Venezuela de 1877. **Acta Odontol Venez** 1980 Jan-Apr;18(1):87-95

**Saturno Hernández PJ:** Los medicos de la comarca de la huerta de Murcia. Numero, distribucion espacial, movilidad, grado de especializacion, tipo de ejercicio, edad y años de colegiacion. Evolucion de 1960 a 1974. **Asclepio** 1981;33:23-80

**Saturno Hernández PJ:** Los veterinarios de la comarca de la huerta de Murcia. Numero, distribucion espacial, movilidad, tipo de ejercicio, edad y años de colegiacion. Evolucion de 1960 a 1975. **Asclepio** 1980;32:433-52

**Saturno Hernández PJ** see **Marset Campos P**

**Satyavati GV** see **Ramalingaswami V**

**Sauer JE** see **Burnham JC**

**Sauerbrey B** see **Klessen D**

**Saueressig H:** Die Tuberkulose als Paradigma des Lebensgefühls. **Med Welt** 1982 Mar 26;33(12):428-34

**Saúl A, Latapí F:** La lepra en México. In Academia Nacional de Medicina. Libro conmemorativo del primer centenario. México, Comité Editorial de la Comisión Organizadora del Congreso del Centenario, 1964. Tome 2. p. 89-99.

**Saulsbury FT** see **Hayden GF**

**Saumande P:** La vie d'un pharmacien limousin à la fin du XIXe siècle d'après les documents d'archives de son officine. **Rev Hist Pharm (Paris)** 1982 Jun;29(253):91-4

**Saumande P:** Une collection d'instruments scientifiques anciens au Laboratoire de Physique pharmaceutique de la Faculté de Médecine et de Pharmacie de Limoges. **Bull Soc Archeol Hist Limousin** 1981;108:157-8

**Saunders AB** see **Halberstein RA**

**Saunders C:** A pioneering approach to the dying [interview by Laurence Dopson] **Nurs Times** 1984 Mar 28-Apr 3;80(13):16-8

**Saunders C:** Hospice care. **Indian J Cancer** 1979 Sep-Dec;16(3-4):1-4

**Saunders DM** see **Allan P**

**Saunders JB, Lee FR, ed:** The Manchu anatomy and its historical origin. Taipei, Li Ming Cultural Enterprise Co., 1981. 8, 180 p. English and Chinese.

**Saunders LZ:** Veterinary pathology in Russia, 1860-1930. Ithaca, Cornell University Press, 1980. xxi, 327 p.

**Saunders P:** Edward Jenner. The Cheltenham years 1795-1823. Being a chronicle of the vaccination campaign. Hanover, London, University Press of New England, 1982. xviii, 469 p.

**Sauri JJ:** Nacimiento del concepto de perversión. **Rev Neuropsiquiatr** 1979 Jun;42(2):71-85

**Saussure H** see **Gmelin OF**

**Sauvé R:** Legislative developments in Québec. **J Occup Med** 1982 Dec;24(12):981-4

**Sauvy A:** Science médicale et science économique. **Ann Med Interne (Paris)** 1982;133(3):216-21

**Sauzet R, ed** see **Margolin JC**

**Savage GH:** Psychiatry in the 1880s. **Psychol Med** 1984 Aug;14(3):723-4

**Savage R:** Croydon's local Board of Health in the early 1850s. **Proc Croydon Nat Hist Sci Soc** 1974;14(13)

**Savara BS** see **Boyd E**

**Savchenko NE:** Druzhba narodov i zdravookhranenie Belorussii. **Sov Zdravookhr** 1982;(12):19-22

**Savchenko NE, Shitikov BD:** Ob uspekhakh i tendentsiiakh razvitiia onkologicheskoĭ sluzhby v Belorusskoĭ SSR. **Vopr Onkol** 1982;28(12):13-20

**Savchenko NE:** Okhrana zdorov'ia deteĭ v Belorusskoĭ SSR. **Pediatriia** 1982 Dec;(12):15-8

**Säveland H** see **Ljunggren B**

**Savel'ev SA** see **Lur'e GO**

**Savel'ev VN:** Zdravookhranenie Udmurtii za 60 let Sovetskoĭ vlasti. **Med Sestra** 1982 Dec;41(12):23-30
**Savel'ev VN:** 60 let zdravookhraneniia avtonomii Udmurtii. **Sov Zdravookhr** 1981;(4):53-9
**Savel'ev VS:** N. I. Pirogov -- veljkiĭ russkiĭ khirurg i uchenyĭ. **Sov Med** 1981;(11):116-8
**Savic K** see **Borisev V**
**Savich VI, Maksimov SS, Gusakov IuA:** 50 let sudebno-meditsinskoĭ sluzhby Belorussii. **Sud Med Ekspert** 1980;23(3):57-8
**Savinov VA** see **Agababov SV**
**Savit TL:** The use of blacks for medical experimentation and demonstration in the old South. **J South Hist** 1982;48(3):331-48
**Savitskiĭ IV** see **Borisenko NF**
**Savitt TL:** Lincoln University Medical Department--a forgotten 19th century black medical school. **J Hist Med Allied Sci** 1985 Jan;40(1):42-65
**Savitt TL:** Medicine and slavery: the diseases and health care of blacks in antebellum Virginia. Urbana, University of Illinois Press, 1978. 332 p.
**Savitt TL:** Patient letters to an early nineteenth century Virginia physician. **J Fla Med Assoc** 1982 Aug;69(8):688-94
**Savitt TL:** Politics in medicine: the Georgia Freedmen's Bureau and the organization of health care, 1865-1866. **Civ War Hist** 1982;28(1):45-64
**Savitt TL:** Slave life insurance in Virginia and North Carolina. **J South Hist** 1977 Nov;43(4):583-600; 1978 Feb;44(1):163
**Savitt TL:** The invisible malady: sickle cell anemia in America, 1910-1970. **J Natl Med Assoc** 1981 Aug;73(8):739-46
**Savitt TL:** The social and medical history of crib death. **J Fla Med Assoc** 1979 Aug;66(8):853-9
**Savitt TL:** The use of Blacks for medical experimentation and demonstration in the Old South. **J South Hist** 1982 Aug;48(3):331-48
**Savitt TL:** Understanding the medical past through literature: bloodletting and the Louisiana swamp doctor. **J Okla State Med Assoc** 1982 Jul;75(7):174-7
**Savitt TL** see **Burns CR**
**Savitt TL** see **Kaufman M**
**Savitz HA:** Dreams in the Talmud: the prophets of yore had the noblest dream. **RI Med J** 1981 Sep;64(9):427-30
**Savodnik I, ed:** Concept and explanation in biology. Oceanside, Dabor, 1977. xvii, 240 p.
**Savodnik I, ed:** The origins of structure in biology. Oceanside, Dabor, 1977. xvi, 154 p.
**Savopoulos NM, ed:** The Baltimore College of Dental Surgery: heritage and history. Baltimore, Baltimore College of Dental Surgery, 1980?. 22 p.
**Sawada K:** [History of breast feeding in Japan]. (Jpn) **Josanpu Zasshi** 1979 Sep;33(9):596-604
**Sawday J:** The Leiden Anatomy Theatre as a source for Davenant's 'Cabinet of death' in Gondibert. **Notes Queries** 1983 Oct;30(5):437-9
**Sawicki B, Brońka E:** Karol Goebel - pierwszy docent stomatologii w Polsce. **Czas Stomatol** 1979 Aug;32(8):807-9
**Sawyer DJ:** The lady with the snake in her. **NY Folkl Q** 1969;25(4):299-305
**Sawyer DR, Allison MJ, Pezzia A, et al:** Crown dimensions of deciduous teeth from pre-Columbian Peru. **Am J Phys Anthropol** 1982 Dec;59(4):373-6
**Sawyer DR, Allison MJ, Pezzia A:** Elongated styloid process in a pre-Columbian Peruvian. **J Dent Res** 1980 Jan;59(1):79
**Sawyer DR, Logan WW, Oleru UG, et al:** The effect of attrition on the pre-Columbian Indian arch length. **J Dent** 1983 Jun;11(2):154-8
**Sawyer DR, Nwoku AL, Elzay RP, et al:** Two probable cases of a depression in the mandible caused by the submandibular salivary gland in Pre-Columbian Peruvians. **J Maxillofac Surg** 1981 Aug;9(3):194-6
**Sawyer RC:** Ordinary medicine for ordinary people: illness and its treatment in the East Midlands, 1600-1630. **Soc Soc Hist Med Bull (Lond)** 1983 Dec;33:20-3
**Sawyers JL** see **Herrington JL**
**Saxby MS:** Juvenile periodontitis: an historical review. **J Oral Rehabil** 1982 Sep;9(5):451-68
**Sayad EG:** Alexian Brothers' hospital: unique heritage. **Bull Mo Hist Soc** 1980;36(4):264-7
**Sayans Castaños M:** Importante impulso en el conocimiento cientifico dado por un medico placentino del siglo XVI. In: Sociedad Española de Historia de la Medicina. V Congreso Nacional. Madrid, 1977. **Asclepio** 1977;29:343-50
**Sayer K:** The ESRC Data Archive. **Soc Soc Hist Med Bull (Lond)** 1984 Dec;35:59-61
**Sayers BM** see **Bound JP**
**Sayili A:** Bizde tip ögretimi üzerine. **Belleten (Turk)** 1971;35(138):229-34
**Sayili A:** The emergence of the prototype of the modern hospital in medieval Islam. **Belleten (Turk)** 1980;44:279-86
**Sayre D, ed** see **Dodson G**
**Sbrana C:** Per una ricostruzione dell'antica biblioteca del Giardiono dei Semplici di Pisa. Nuovi Elementi. **Physis** 1982;24(3):423-34
**Scadding JG:** Maurice Davidson 1883-1967--progress in respiratory medicine since his time. **Postgrad Med J** 1984 Mar;60(701):178-82
**Scadding JG:** The eponymy of sarcoidosis. **J R Soc Med** 1981 Feb;74(2):147-57
**Scadding JG:** The Thoracic Society: a retrospect. **Thorax** 1983 Feb;38(2):88-92
**Scalabrin HR:** Heinrich Ludwig Attenhofer, 1783-1856. Arzt und Politiker. Zürich, Juris Druck, 1983. 67 p. (Zürcher Medizingeschichtliche Abhhandlungen, Neue Reihe, Nr. 158).
**Scalera V** see **Epistemologia, metodologia clinica e storia della scienza medica, 1**
**Scalettar R:** Presidential candidate disability. **JAMA** 1984 Jun 1;251(21):2811
**Scammon RE** see **Boyd E**
**Scandellari C** see **Epistemologia, metodologia clinica e storia della scienza medica, 2**
**Scandellari C** see **Federspil G**
**Scanlan TM:** La fonction de la mort dans la pensée sociale de Rousseau. **Univ Ottawa Q** 1981;51(1):91-7
**Scannell JG:** A sidelight of cholecystography. **Pharos** 1983 Summer;46(3):42
**Scannell JG:** Some thoracic surgeons of Boston--before the cardiac balloon went up. **Pharos** 1984 Fall;47(4):26-30
**Scarano GB:** Considerazioni storiche sull'uso dei sali d'oro nell'artrite reumatoide. **Med Secoli** 1982 May-Aug;19(2):175-91
**Scarano GB:** Le malattie della bocca e dei denti nell'opera di Girolamo Fabrizio d'Acquapendente. **Med Secoli** 1982 Jan-Apr;19(1):101-23
**Scarano JM** see **Berrance de Castro J**
**Scarborough J:** Classical antiquity: medicine and allied sciences. **Trends Hist** 1979 Fall-Winter;1(2):3-14
**Scarborough J:** Nicander: Theriaca 811. **Classical Philol** 1980;75:138-40
**Scarborough J:** On medications for burns in classical antiquity. In Romm S, ed: Symposium on historical perspectives of plastic surgery. Philadelphia, Saunders, 1983. p. 603-610.
**Scarborough J:** Roman medicine and public health. In Ogawa T, ed: Public health. Tokyo, Saikon, 1981. p. 33-74.
**Scarborough J:** Roman pharmacy and the eastern drug trade. **Pharm Hist** 1982;24(4):135-43
**Scarborough J:** The Galenic question. **Sudhoffs Arch** 1981;65(1):1-31
**Scarborough J:** The myth of lead poisoning among the Romans: an essay review. **J Hist Med Allied Sci** 1984 Oct;39(4):469-75
**Scarborough RR** see **Romm S, ed**
**Scarborough J, ed:** Society for Ancient Medicine newsletter. No. 1-10 (Apr. 1976-Sept. 1982). Continued periodically.
**Scarchuk JM, ed:** The first pharmacopoeia published in the Federated States of America, by William Brown, entitled Pharmacopoeia Simpliciorum et Efficiorum in Usum Nosocomii Militaris, published by Styner Cist. 1778. Coventry, Conn., the Author, 1976. xii, 32 p.
**Scardaville MC:** Alcohol abuse and tavern reform in late colonial Mexico City. **Hisp Am Hist Rev** 1980;60(4):643-71
**Scarlett C:** A tale of ratiocination: the death and burial of Edgar Allan Poe. **Md Hist Mag** 1978;73(4):360-74
**Scarpa A:** Pre-scientific medicines: their extent and value. **Soc Sci Med** 1981 May;15A(3):317-26
**Schachter M:** Alfred Adler (1870-1937), et sa psycho-pédagogie clinique. **Rev Hist Med Heb** 1981 Dec;139(34 no 4):53-6
**Schachter M:** Kallikreins and kinins, an overview: some thoughts old and new. **Adv Exp Med Biol** 1983;156:13-27
**Schachter M:** La personnalité de Frédéric II Le Grand, Roi de Prusse (1712-1786). Essai de psychologie adlérienne. **Hist Sci Med** 1984;18(2):181-7
**Schachter M:** Le malade Johann Wolfgang Goethe (1749-1832) et ses maladies (A l'occasion du 150e anniversaire de sa mort). **Hist Sci Med** 1982;16(2):81-8
**Schachter M:** Le professeur Erich Stern (1889-1959) psychiatre et psychologue. **Rev Hist Med Heb** 1980 Oct;134(33 no 3):53-4)
**Schachter M:** L'écrivain-médecin Arthur Schnitzler (1862-1931). **Prov Med** 1979;6/7:347-53
**Schachter M:** Marcel Proust (1871-1922), une étude psychopathographique. **Prov Med** 1980;:(3):61-75
**Schachter M** see **Parkes D**
**Schadewaldt H:** A propos de l'histoire de l'hygiène navale. In: Congrès National des Sociétés Savantes, 91e, Rennes, 1966. Comptes Rendus. Paris, 1967. Section des Sciences, Tome 1. p. 47-53.
**Schadewaldt H:** Albert Clemens Mooren als geschichtliche Persönlichkeit. **Jahrb Univ Dusseld** 1977-78;:259-68
**Schadewaldt H:** Anfänge der Medizinischen Mykologie in Deutschland. **Mykosen** 1981 Nov;24(11):654-67
**Schadewaldt H:** Anfänge der Röntgentherapie. **Schriftenr Dtsch Rontgenmus** 1983 Aug;5
**Schadewaldt H:** Arzt und Gesellschaft im Spannungsfeld der Geschichte. **Therapiewoche** 1983;33:6485-91
**Schadewaldt H:** Betrachtungen zur Entwicklung des medizinischen Buch- und Zeitschriftenwesens. In:Die Zeitung als Persönlichkeit. Festschrift Bringmann. Düsseldorf, 1982. p. 125-34.
**Schadewaldt H:** Das Badewesen in der Goethezeit. **Therapiewoche** 1982;32:4123-33
**Schadewaldt H:** Das Sargassokraut als Antiskorbutikum. In Dilg P, et al., ed: Perspektiven der Pharmaziegeschichte. Graz, Austria, Akademische Druck- u. Verlagsanstalt, 1983. p. 281-94.
**Schadewaldt H:** Das Verhältnis zur Krankheit im Wandel der Zeit. **Wien Med Wochenschr** 1980 Nov 15;130(21):673-82
**Schadewaldt H:** Der Rheumatismus und seine Behandlung im Wandel der Zeiten. **Z Rheumatol** 1983 Jul-Aug;42(4):139-44
**Schadewaldt H:** Der Schiffbruch der Méduse im Jahre 1816. In W. Treue, ed: Geschichte der französischen Marine. Herford, Mittler, 1982. p. 107-25.
**Schadewaldt H:** Der Zahnarzt in der Kunst. **Zahnarztl Mitt** 1983 Dec 16;73(24):2760, 2762-4, 2768-70
**Schadewaldt H:** Die Entdeckung des Tuberkuloseerregers durch Robert

**Schein CJ, Koch E:** Jenny Lind's concert in Göttingen. Billroth's letter to his mother. **NY State J Med** 1979 Oct;79(11):1786–1891
**Schein CJ:** The death of Ivan Ilych; an axiomatic hypothesis. **NY State J Med** 1981 Mar;81(3):416
**Scheinman MM:** The AJC in September 1959. **Am J Cardiol** 1984 Sep 1;54(6):702–3
**Scheiper R:** Zahnerkrankungen unserer Vorfahren, der Alamannen. **Zahnarztl Mitt** 1984 Feb 16;74(4):363–4, 367–8
**Scheips PJ:** Albert James Myer, an army doctor in Texas, 1854–1857. **Southwest Hist Q** 1978;82(1):1–24
**Scheithauer BW** see **Shenoy BV**
**Scheld HH, Mulch J, Schaper J, et al:** Myokardprotektion im Wandel der letzten 20 Jahre. **Med Welt** 1982 May 21;33(20):746–9
**Scheld HH, Mulch J, Walter P, et al:** 20 Jahre Herzklappenchirurgie. (2) Klinische Ergebnisse. **ZFA (Stuttgart)** 1981 Mar 31;57(9):645–51
**Scheld HH** see **Mulch J**
**Scheld WM, Mandell GL:** Landmark perspective. Sulfonamides and meningitis. **JAMA** 1984 Feb 10;251(6):791–4
**Scheller, EF:** Langlebigkeit mit Paracelsus-Arzneien: Versuch einer Geriatrie nach Paracelsus. Heidelberg, Haug, 1977. 150 p.
**Schellmann B:** Kunst und Pathologie: Joseph Beuys--'zeige deine Wunde'. **Pathologe** 1983 Nov;4(6):325–7
**Schenk J:** Homoseksualiteit in de Nederlandse beeldende kunst voor 1800. **Spiegel Hist** 1982;17(11):576–83
**Schenk J, ed** see **Hildesheimer F**
**Schepisi MA:** Il bilancio e le prospettive della psicoanalisi francese nella riflessione critica di alcuni protagonisti (1970–1980). **Stor Crit Psicol** 1984;5(2):345–71
**Scherg C:** Literatur als Lebenshilfe. Am Beispiel Thomas Manns. **Psyche (Stuttg)** 1982 Jul;36(7):630–61
**Scherlag BJ:** The development of the His bundle recording technique. **PACE** 1979 Mar;2(2):230–3
**Scherlis L:** Poetical version of the Rules of the Humane Society for recovering drowned persons. **Crit Care Med** 1981 May;9(5):430–1
**Scherrer P:** La débâcle de 1940: recueil des malades mentaux à l'Hôpital Psychiatrique d'Auxerre. **Ann Med Psychol (Paris)** 1984 Feb;142(2):266–70
**Scherrer RM:** Friedrich Hoffmanns Anweisung zu gesundem langen Leben, verglichen mit Hufelands Makrobiotik. Zürich, Juris, 1984. 47 p. (Zürcher Medizingeschichtliche Abhandlungen, Neue Reihe, Nr. 170)
**Schettler G:** Atherosclerosis during periods of food deprivation following World Wars I and II. **Prev Med** 1983 Jan;12(1):75–83
**Scheuch DW, Hoffmann H:** 20 Jahre Gesellschaft für Klinische Chemie und Laboratoriumsdiagnostik der DDR. **Z Med Lab Diagn** 1983;24(7):371–80
**Scheuermann A:** Die wissenschaftliche Gesellschaft als Medium des Fortschritts. **Tierarztl Prax** 1981:9(2):161–6
**Schiaffino A:** Fecondita e vita conjugale a Bologna nell'ultimo secolo: analisi longitudinale delle discendenze. **Inst Stat Q** 1979;3:199–275
**Schiaffino A:** Il declino della fecondità in ambiente urbano: Reggio Emilia fra otto e novecento. **Inst Stat Q** 1979;3:7–275
**Schiano Di Zenise M** see **D'Amore C**
**Schicke RK:** Sozialpharmakologie, makrosystemische Aspekte. **Fortschr Med** 1982 May 13;100(18):823–4, 845
**Schienbein G, Schienbein H:** 'Der Zähn stincken verbessern'--Zahnheilkunde in einem Kräuterbuch von 1602 (I, II). **Quintessenz** 1980 Jun-Jul;31(6,7):133–40, 165–70
**Schienbein H:** Die 'Neu-Vermehrte Heylsame Dreck-Apotheke' (1696/1734) des Hof- und Stadtarztes Christian Frantz Paulini. **Quintessenz** 1981 Sep;32(9):1699–1702
**Schienbein H** see **Geppert W**
**Schienbein H** see **Schienbein G**
**Schierhorn H:** Die Hirnanatomie im Spiegel der ersten 50 Bände des Anatomischen Anzeigers. **Anat Anz** 1981;150(1–2):77–118
**Schierhorn H:** Die Multinationalität der Anatomischen Gesellschaft und die Mehrsprachigkeit ihrer Versammlungen. **Anat Anz** 1980;148(2):168–206
**Schierhorn H:** Die Terata auf der Weltkarte des Richard de Haldingham (um 1280). **Gegenbaurs Morphol Jahrb** 1982;128(2):137–67
**Schierhorn H:** Egas Moniz, Wilhelm Löhr und die cerebrale Angiographie. Ein Streifzug durch die Entdeckungsgeschichte der Hirngefässe. **J Hirnforsch** 1981;22(5):491–515
**Schierhorn H:** Johann Friedrich Meckel d. J. als Begründer der wissenschaftlichen Teratologie. **Gegenbaurs Morphol Jahrb** 1984;130(3):399–439
**Schierhorn H:** Samuel Thomas Soemmerring (1755–1830) als Neuroanatom. **Z Mikrosk Anat Forsch** 1980;94(6):1051–76
**Schierhorn H:** Zur Säkularfeier von Robert Kochs Entdeckung des Tuberkulose-Bakteriums. **Z Mikrosk Anat Forsch** 1982;96(3):377–99
**Schiffczyk D:** Vom Therapiekonzept zur Architekturform. Betrachtungen über das Terrassenkrankenhaus. **Hist Hosp** 1979–80;13:177–96
**Schiffeler JW:** An essay on some of the fundamental philosophical tenets found in traditional Chinese medicine. **Chin Cult** 1976;17(4):141–7
**Schiffeler JW:** Chinese folk medicine: a study of the Shan-hai Ching. **Asian Folkl Stud** 1980;39(2):41–83
**Schilke JF** see **Boyd E**
**Schiller F:** A Möbius strip. Fin-de-siècle neuropsychiatry and Paul Möbius. Berkeley, University of California Press, 1982. 134 p.
**Schiller F:** A note on the Pickwickian syndrome and Felix Platter (1536–1614). **J Hist Med Allied Sci** 1985 Jan;40(1):66–7
**Schiller F:** Coenesthesis. **Bull Hist Med** 1984 Winter;58(4):496–515
**Schiller F:** Historical note on sleep and eye movements. **Sleep** 1984;7(3):199–201
**Schiller F:** Neurology: the electrical root. In Rose FC, Bynum WF, ed: Historical aspects of the neurosciences. New York, Raven, 1982. p. 1–11.
**Schiller F:** Paul Broca and the history of aphasia. **Neurosci Behav Physiol** 1983 May;33(5):667
**Schiller F:** Paul Broca, founder of French anthropology, explorer of the brain. Berkeley, University of California Press, 1979. ix, 350 p.
**Schiller F:** Reverend Wesley, Doctor Marat and their electric fire. **Clio Med** 1981 Apr;15(3–4):159–76
**Schiller F:** Semantics of sleep. **Bull Hist Med** 1982 Fall;56(3):378–97
**Schiller F:** Stepmother nature: a medico-historical scan. **Clio Med** 1979 May;13(3–4):201–18
**Schiller F:** Thomas de Quincey's lifelong addiction. **Perspect Biol Med** 1976 Autumn;20(1):131–41
**Schiller F:** When is posterior not dorsal but medial? **Neurology** 1984 Apr;34(4):511–4
**Schiller J:** Henri Dutrochet et la terminologie scientifique. In: Congrès National des Sociétés Savantes, 97e, Nantes, 1972. Comptes Rendus. Paris, 1976. Section des Sciences, Tome 1. p. 83–9.
**Schiller J, Rivet R:** La bibliographie à la Faculté de Médecine de Paris avant et pendant la Révolution. In: Congrès National des Sociétés Savantes, 91e, Rennes, 1966. Comptes Rendus. Paris, 1967. Section des Sciences, Tome 1. p. 247–54.
**Schiller J:** La notion d'organisation dans l'histoire de la biologie. Paris, Maloine, 1978. 133 p.
**Schiller J:** Les traductions en français des ouvrages scientifiques de Haller. In: Congrès National des Sociétés Savantes, 91e, Rennes, 1966. Comptes Rendus. Paris, 1967. Section des Sciences, Tome 1. p. 241–5.
**Schiller J:** Physiology and classification: historical relations. Paris, Maloine, 1980. xiii, 194 p.
**Schiller J** see **[The history of physiology:] essay review**
**Schiller N:** Henri Dutrochet contributions biographiques et iconographiques. In: Congrès National des Sociétés Savantes, 97e, Nantes, 1972. Comptes Rendus. Paris, 1976. Section des Sciences, Tome 1. p. 71–82.
**Schiller N:** L'iconographie de Claude Perrault (1613–1688). In: Congrès National des Sociétés Savantes, 91e, Rennes, 1966. Comptes Rendus. Paris, 1967. Section des Sciences, Tome 1. p. 217–34.
**Schilling R:** Bradford Hill's contribution to occupational health. **Stat Med** 1982 Oct-Dec;1(4):317–24
**Schilling RS:** Donald Hunter--the first editor of the British Journal of Industrial Medicine. **J Cell Biol** 1979 Aug;36(3):243
**Schimel JL:** Ralph M. Crowley: psychoanalytic pioneer. **J Am Acad Psychoanal** 1981 Oct;9(4):489–91
**Schimming I, Mann H:** Zur historischen Bedingtheit der Qualität ärztlicher Bewahrungspflicht für das menschliche Leben sowie der Betreuung Sterbender. **Z Arztl Fortbild (Jena)** 1984;78(16):693–4
**Schings HJ:** Melancholie und Aufklärung. Melancholiker und ihre Kritiker in Erfahrungsseelenkunde und Literatur des 18. Jahrhunderts. Stuttgart, Metzler, 1977. x, 476 p.
**Schinke SP** see **Gilchrist LD**
**Schipperges H:** Barmherzigkeit als Heilmittel bei Hildegard von Bingen. In Ganzinger K, Skopec M, Wyklicky H, ed: Festschrift für Erna Lesky zum 70. Geburtstag. Wien, Brüder Hollinek, 1981. p. 97–103.
**Schipperges H:** Bildung zu gesunder Vernunft. Zu einer wiederentdeckten Magazin der Aufklärung. **Arztebl Baden Wurttemberg** 1981;6
**Schipperges H:** Das medizinische Denken bei Albertus Magnus. In: Albertus Magnus, Doctor universalis, 1280/1980; hrsg. von G. Meyer, A. Zimmermann. Mainz, Matthias-Grünewald, 1980. p. 279–94.
**Schipperges H:** Der Arzt als Zeuge des Lebens. **Gesnerus** 1981;38:105–18
**Schipperges H:** Der Mensch und seine Welt bei Hildegard von Bingen. **Arzt Christ** 1978–79;1:2–7
**Schipperges H:** 'Der Mensch wird geringer'. Verliert die Medizin ihr Humanum? **Scheidewege** 1980;10(1):1–21
**Schipperges H:** Der Patient als Mensch. **Schleswig Holsteinisches Arztebl** 1979;11:609–14
**Schipperges H:** Diätetische Lebensführung nach der 'Regula Benedicti' bei Hildegard von Bingen. **Arzt Christ** 1980;2:87–97
**Schipperges H:** Die Kardinaltugenden im Weltbild der Hildegard von Bingen. **Grenzgeb Wiss** 1980;29(1):19–34
**Schipperges H:** Die Zähne und das Schöne im Wandel der Zeiten. **Dtsch Zahnarztl Z** 1981;36(7):406–13
**Schipperges H:** Eine 'summa medicinae' bei Albertus Magnus. **Jahrb Gorres Ges** 1981;:5–24
**Schipperges H:** Einheitsbestrebungen und Normbegriff auf der Naturforscherversammlung im 19. Jahrhundert. **Sudhoffs Arch** 1977;61(4):313–30
**Schipperges H:** Grundmuster und Richtlinien arabischer Diätetik. In Dilg P, et al., ed: Perspektiven der Pharmaziegeschichte. Graz, Austria, Akademische Druck- u. Verlagsanstalt, 1983. p. 295–309.
**Schipperges H:** Handschriftliche Funde zu den 'verdrängten Wissenschaften' in der Frühen Neuzeit. **Ber Wissenschaftsgesch** 1981;4(1/2):31–40
**Schipperges H:** Kranksein und Heilung bei Paracelsus. Wien, Verband der wissenschaftlichen Gesellschaften Oesterreichs, 1978. 32 p. (Salzburger Beiträge zur Paracelsusforschung, 18).
**Schipperges H:** Krankwerden und Gesundsein bei Novalis. **Dtsch Vierteljahresschr Lit Wiss Geistesgesch** 1978;226–42
**Schipperges H:** Paracelsus. Das Abenteuer einer sokratischen Existenz. Freiburg im Breisgau, Aurum Verlag, 1983. 108 p. (Reihe: Sokratische

Weisheit, Bd. 3).
**Schipperges H:** Sorge um den Kranken und Dienste am Kranken: ein Beitrag der Benediktiner zur Medizin des Abendlandes. **Arzt Christ** 1980;3:125–34
**Schipperges H:** Struktur und Funktion eines Instituts für Gesundheitsbildung. In R. Wittern, ed: Jahrbuch des Instituts für Geschichte der Medizin der Robert Bosch Stiftung. Stuttgart, Hippokrates Verlag, 1984. Bd. 1. p. 42–69.
**Schipperges H:** Vindication of the doctor's decisions. **Hexagon Roche** 1981;9(3):1–8
**Schipperges H:** Vom Physikus zum Arzt für Gesundheit. Verwurzelung, Entwicklung und Chancen des öffentlichen Gesundheitsdienstes. **Off Gesundheitswes** 1983 Jun;45(6):290–8
**Schipperges H:** Walther Schönfeld (1888–1977) und seine Verdienste als Medizinhistoriker. **Hautarzt** 1980 Aug;31(8):441–3
**Schipperges H** see **Engelhardt D von**
**Schipperges H** see **Habrich C**
**Schipperges H** see **Janzarik W ed**
**Schipperges H** see **Kraus A, ed**
**Schipperges H** see **Tellenbach H, ed**
**Schirmer F** see **Avellano E**
**Schirren C:** Niels Stensen – ein Pionier der Wissenschaft. **MMW** 1981;123:267–70
**Schlegel KF:** Der Körperbehinderte in Mythologie und Kunst. Stuttgart; New York, Thieme, 1983. 125 p.
**Schlegel KF:** Luzifer – ein orthopädischer Patient. In KF Schlegel, ed: Der Körperbehinderte in Mythologie und Kunst. Stuttgart, New York, Thieme, 1983. p. 19–27.
**Schlegel KF, ed:** Der Körperbehinderte in Mythologie und Kunst. Stuttgart, New York, Georg Thieme Verlag, 1983. 125 p.
**Schleiffer R:** Zur Methodologie von Psychopathologie und Historik. **Nervenarzt** 1980 Jan;51(1):17–21
**Schleppi JR:** 'It pays': John H. Patterson and industrial recreation at the National Cash Register Company. **J Sport Hist** 1979;6(3):20–8
**Schlesinger MC:** Snatched from oblivion: a Cambridge memoir. Boston, Little Brown, 1979. 243 p.
**Schlicke CP:** The Robinson affair. **Pac Northwest** 1983;27(2):81–93
**Schlicke CP:** West Coast medicine in 1776. **Pac Northwest** 1976 Winter;20:58–68
**Schlicke CP:** Working together. A history of a medical group practice, the Rockwood Clinic, Spokane, Washington. Fairfield, Wash. Ye Galleon Press, 1980. 187 p.
**Schliesser T:** Die Rindertuberkulose im Wandel der letzten 100 Jahre (1882–1982). **Prax Klin Pneumol** 1982 Mar;36(3):151–6
**Schliesser T:** Zur Geschichte und Entwicklung der Rindertuberkulose-Bekämpfung. **Zentralbl Bakteriol Mikrobiol Hyg [A]** 1982 Mar;251(3):326–40
**Schlissel CH:** A short history of dentistry in China from earliest times through 1900. **Bull Hist Dent** 1984;32(1):52–6
**Schlögel A:** Neuaufbau des Deutschen Roten Kreuzes nach dem II. Weltkrieg: Geschichte des DRK 1945–1950. Bonn, Das Deutsche Rote Kreuz, 1983. 120 p.
**Schlosser GA, Hrynyschyn K, Zornig C, et al:** Die Geschichte der Bauchdeckenschnitte. Historisches und Entwicklungstendenzen (I). **Med Welt** 1981 Oct 30;32(44):1672–6
**Schmacke N** see **Güse HG**
**Schmale AH** see **Ader R**
**Schmalhofer J:** Das Werk von Johann Florian Heller mit besonderer Berücksichtigung der Entstehung des ersten pathologisch-chemischen Laboratoriums am Allgemeinen Wiener Krankenhaus und der Ernennung Hellers zum Vorstand des Laboratoriums. Diss. Bonn, 1980. 201 p.
**Schmauss AK:** Das chirurgische Erbe. Johann Friedrich August von Esmarch--Leben und Werk (9. 1. 1823–23. 2. 1908). **Zentralbl Chir** 1983;108(24):1577–83
**Schmauss AK:** Die Geschichte der Gastrotomie zur Entfernung von Fremdkörpern. **Zentralbl Chir** 1982;107(22):1481–5
**Schmauss AK:** Zur Geschichte der chirurgischen Eingriffe am Magen. **Z Arztl Fortbild (Jena)** 1983;77(10):445–8
**Schmelz UO:** [Demography of Moslems and Christians in Jerusalem] (Heb). **Hamizrah Hehadash** 1979;28(1–2):40–73
**Schmelz UO:** Hamivneh hademografi shel ha'Aravim v'Hadruzim b'Yisrael. **Hamizrah Hehadash** 1979;28(3–4):244–54
**Schmid PC:** Zur Epidemiologie und Atiologie der Tuberkulose seit Robert Koch. Komplexes Ursachengefüge erfordert komplexe Strategien der Tuberkulose-Bekämpfung. **Fortschr Med** 1982 Mar 25;100(12):499–503
**Schmid R, Barbakow F, Mühlemann H, et al:** Amine fluoride and monofluorophosphate: I. Historical review of fluoride dentifrices. **ASDC J Dent Child** 1984 Mar–Apr;51(2):99–103
**Schmid R** see **Krebs H**
**Schmid-Kitsikis E:** Un certain regard sur l'oeuvre de N. Galifret-Granjon. **Psychiatr Enfant** 1984;27(1):35–48
**Schmid-Schönbein H:** Die Ursprünge der medizinischen Hämorheologie im 18. Jahrhundert: H. Boerhaave, A. v. Haller und G. van Swieten. **Vasa** 1984;Suppl 12:10–31
**Schmidhofer M** see **Dätwyler B**
**Schmidt A:** Die Geschichte der Methakrylate in der Stomatologie. **Zahntechnik (Berl)** 1978 Oct;19(10):436–44
**Schmidt C:** Alchemists, critics and psychohistorians. **J Psychohist** 1981 Winter;8(3):337–67
**Schmidt CG:** The group-fantasy origins of AIDS. **J Psychohist** 1984 Summer;12(1):37–78
**Schmidt DH** see **Maud PJ**
**Schmidt F:** Apothekerbildnisse auf Medaillen und Plaketten. **Beitr Gesch Pharm** 1981;31(13):100–1
**Schmidt G:** O znachenii otkrytiĭ Roberta Kokha dlia razvitiia bakteriologii i épidemiologii. **Zh Mikrobiol Epidemiol Immunobiol** 1983 Mar;(3):106–9
**Schmidt G:** Zur Bedeutung der Entdeckung Robert Kochs für die Entwicklungen der Bakteriologie. **Z Erkr Atmungsorgane** 1983;161(1):15–20
**Schmidt H:** Dr. med Marie-Elise Kayser in ihren Beziehungen zur Sowjetunion. **Beitr Gesch Univ Erfurt** 1979–83;19:299–303
**Schmidt H:** Zur Geschichte der Erfurter Kolonne des Arbeiter-Samariter-Bundes. **Beitr Gesch Univ Erfurt** 1979–83;19:283–91
**Schmidt H:** Zur Kostenfreiheit ärztlicher Hilfeleistung; eine Betrachtung aus Anlass des 90. Jahrestages des Erfurter Programms der SPD. **Beitr Gesch Univ Erfurt** 1979–83;19:265–70
**Schmidt H** see **Abe HR**
**Schmidt HD** see **Becker KH**
**Schmidt J:** Individuelle Rettungsmittel für Seenotfälle. In Göpfert W, Otten HH, ed: Metavoeite: wandelt euch durch neues Denken. Düsseldorf, Triltsch, 1983. p. 79–87.
**Schmidt M:** Zur Geschichte der tibetischen Ubersetzungen altindischer medizinischer Werke. In International Congress of the History of Medicine, 27th, Barcelona, 1980. Actas. Barcelona, Académia de Ciències Mèdiques de Catalunya i Balears, 1981. p. 336–9.
**Schmidt MS:** Why a separate organization for state boards? **Am J Nurs** 1980 Apr;80(4):724–6
**Schmidt P** see **Stambolian G**
**Schmidt PG:** Materielle und spirituelle Diät. Ein mittellateinischer Verstraktat des frühen 13. Jahrhunderts aus St. Albans. In Dilg P, et al., ed: Perspektiven der Pharmaziegeschichte. Graz, Austria, Akademische Druck- u. Verlagsanstalt, 1983. p. 311–23.
**Schmidt PJ:** Blood transfusion in the South before the war between the states. **South Med J** 1979 Dec;72(12):1587–9
**Schmidt PJ, Changus JE:** The bloodletters of Florida. **J Fla Med Assoc** 1980 Aug;67(8):743–7
**Schmidt PO:** Asylierung oder psychiatrische Familienpflege? Die Diskussionen in den Irrenärzteverbänden um die psychiatrische Versorgungsstruktur im 19. Jahrhundert. **Psychiatr Prax** 1983 Mar;10(2):56–9
**Schmidt R, Kludas A:** Die deutschen Lazarettschiffe im Zweiten Weltkrieg. Stuttgart, Motorbuch, 1978. 174 p.
**Schmidt R** see **Heilmittel aus Pflanzen und Tieren**
**Schmidt V:** Camille Pissarro, hans danske relationer og hans sygdom. **Dan Medicinhist Arbog** 1983;12:144–61
**Schmidt V:** Emil Abderhalden. Laege, professor, Geheimrat, kolonihavemand, afholdsmand -- og glemt! **Dan Medicinhist Arbog** 1979;116–29
**Schmidt V:** Hvad fejlede Florence Nightingale? **Sygeplejersken** 1980 Aug 6;80(31):4–10; Oct 5;67(17):16–21
**Schmidt V:** Klinisk kemi--medicinsk eller kemisk subspeciale? **Nord Med** 1983;98(1):26–7
**Schmidt V:** Zu dem medizinischen Traktat Pap. Laur. 68. **Z Papyrologie Epigraphik** 1977;24:151–4
**Schmidt WM:** Ethel Collins Dunham. In: Notable American women. The modern period. Cambridge, Mass., Belknap-Harvard Univ. Press, 1980. 4:212–3.
**Schmidt WM** see **Children's Bureau studies**
**Schmidt-Degenhard M:** Melancholie und Depression: zur Problemgeschichte der depressiven Erkrankungen seit Beginn des 19. Jahrhunderts. Stuttgart, Kohlhammer, 1983. 169 p.
**Schmidt-Glassner H** see **Kallinich G**
**Schmidt-Nielsen B:** A history of renal physiology at the Mount Desert Island Biological Laboratory. **Physiologist** 1983 Oct;26(5):260–6
**Schmidt-Nielsen B:** August and Marie Krogh and respiratory physiology. **J Appl Physiol** 1984 Aug;57(2):293–303
**Schmidt-Pospula M** see **Szymańska R**
**Schmidt-Tintemann U:** Plastische Chirurgie. Entwicklung in Deutschland. **MMW** 1983 Jul 1;125(26):566–8
**Schmidt-Voigt J:** Russische Ikonmalerei und Medizin. München, Thiemig. 1980. 168 p.
**Schmidtgall H:** Zur Rezeption von Harveys Blutkreislaufmodell in der englischen Wirtschaftstheorie des 17. Jahrhunderts. **Sudhoffs Arch** 1973;57(4):416–30
**Schmiking W, ed** see **Balde JH**
**Schmitt CB** see **Bono JJ**
**Schmitt JC:** The holy greyhound: Guinefort, healer of children since the thirteenth century. Cambridge, Cambridge University Press; Paris, Editions de la Maison des Sciences de l'Homme, 1983. 215 p. Translation of Le saint lévrier: Guinefort, guérisseur d'enfants depuis le XIIIe siècle, Paris, 1979.
**Schmitt JC** see **Guillemain B**
**Schmitt R:** Henri Loewel, chimiste alsacien, élève, collaborateur et ami du savant Angevin Michel-Eugène Chevreul. In: Congrès National des Sociétés Savantes, 93e, Tours, 1968. Comptes Rendus. Paris, 1971. Section des Sciences, Tome II. p. 175–88.
**Schmitt RC:** Health and medical firsts in Hawaii. **Hawaii Med J** 1981 Oct;40(10):284–9
**Schmitt W:** Das chirurgische Erbe. Alexis Carrel (1873–1944). **Zentralbl Chir** 1983;108(8):495–503
**Schmitt W:** Das chirurgische Erbe. Zur Geschichte der modernen Chirurgie; ein Abriss. Teil I. **Zentralbl Chir** 1982;107(12):727–36

**Schmitt W:** Das chirurgische Erbe. Zur Geschichte der modernen Chirurgie: ein Abriss. Teil II. **Zentralbl Chir** 1982;107(13):798–808
**Schmitt W:** Das Modell der Naturwissenschaft in der Psychiatrie im Ubergang vom 19. zum 20. Jahrhundert. **Ber Wissenschaftsgesch** 1983;6(1–4):89–101
**Schmitt W:** Grundlinien psychiatrischer Praxis bei Karl Jaspers. In Seidler E, Schott H, ed: Bausteine zur Medizingeschichte. Stuttgart, Steiner, 1984. p. 99–104.
**Schmitt W:** Magie und Mantik bei Hans Hartlieb. Wien, 1966. 25 p. (Salzburger Beiträge zur Paracelsusforschung, 6).
**Schmitt W:** Robert Koch, Mensch und Werk. **Zentralbl Chir** 1982;107(5–6):251–9
**Schmitt W** see **Janzarik W ed**
**Schmitt W** see **Peters UH, ed**
**Schmitt W** see **Tellenbach H, ed**
**Schmitt WM:** Die Sozialversicherung von 1883 bis 1962. **Zahnarzt** 1980 Jan;24(1):7–11
**Schmitz HH** see **Ocklitz HW**
**Schmitz R, Kuhlen FJ:** Anästhesie und Arzneimittelmissbrauch in peinlichen Gerichtsverfahren des 16. und 17. Jahrhunderts. In Göpfert W, Otten HH, ed: Metavoeite: wandelt euch durch neues Denken. Düsselfort, Triltsch, 1983. p. 189–99.
**Schmitz R:** 'Arzneimittelklassiker'. **Med Welt** 1983 Jul 15;34(28):799–803
**Schmitz R:** Der Anteil des Renaissance-Humanismus an der Entwicklung von Arzneibüchern und Pharmakopöen. In F. Krafft, D. Wuttke, ed: Das Verhältnis der Humanisten zum Buch. (Deutsche Forschungsgemeinschaft, Kommission für Humanismusforschung, Mitteilung 4.) Boppard: Boldt, 1977.
**Schmitz R:** Der Beginn der organischen Chemie und der Neo-Vitalismus von heute. In Seidler E, Schott H, ed: Bausteine zur Medizingeschichte. Stuttgart, Steiner, 1984. p. 105–11.
**Schmitz R:** Pharmazie und angewandte Naturwissenschaften in ihrer Beziehung zum Renaissance-Humanismus. In: Humanismusforschung seit 1945: Ein Bericht aus interdisziplinärer Sicht. (Deutsche Forschungsgemeinschaft, Kommission für Humanismusforschung, Mitteilung 2.) Boppard, Boldt, 1975. p. 185–91, 215–6.
**Schmuth GP:** Milestones in the development and practical application of functional appliances. **Am J Orthod** 1983 Jul;84(1):48–53
**Schmutz HK:** Die Gründung des Zürcher Lehrstuhles für Anthropologie. **Gesnerus** 1983;40(1–2):167–73
**Schmutz HK:** Rüdingers 'Atlas des peripherischen Nervensystems des menschlichen Körpers' mit Photographien von Joseph Albert; zur Frühgeschichte der medizinischen Photographie. **Gesnerus** 1980;37(1/2):83–90
**Schneck JM:** Brain injury, psychiatric sequelae, and surgical intervention in S. Weir Mitchell's Westways. **JAMA** 1983 Dec 9;250(22):3048
**Schneck JM:** Elisha Dick, Benjamin Rush, and George Washington. **JAMA** 1983 Jul 8;250(2):164
**Schneck JM:** S. Weir Mitchell and Oliver Wendell Holmes. A friendship and poetic tribute. **JAMA** 1981 Aug 28;246(9):974–8
**Schneck JM:** S. Weir Mitchell, M.D. (1829 to 1914) and D. Hayes Agnew, M.D. (1818 to 1892). Neuropsychiatrist's poetic tribute to a surgeon. **NY State J Med** 1982 Jul;82(8):1264–8
**Schneck JM:** S. Weir Mitchell, psychopathology, and 'The Waters of Oblivion'. **Am J Psychiatry** 1984 Jan;141(1):150–1
**Schneck JM:** Sigmund Freud, Josef Breuer, and Freud's self-observations on meralgia paresthetica. **NY State J Med** 1983 Jun;83(7):968–9
**Schneck JM:** William Pitcairn (1711–1791) and the Gold-Headed Cane. **JAMA** 1984 Apr 20;251(15):1952
**Schneck P:** Die Briefe Paul Ehrlichs an den Moskauer Mikrobiologen Georgij Norbertovič Gabričevskij. **NTM** 1982;19(2):81–7
**Schneck P:** Die medizinische Fakultät an der Universität Krakau zur Zeit des Herzogtums Warschau (1809–1815). **Arch Hist Med (Warsz)** 1979;42(2):251–5
**Schneck P:** Ernst Bumm (1858–1925) und die Gynäkologie seiner Zeit. Eine bioergographische Skizze anlässlich seines 125. Geburtstages. **Zentralbl Gynakol** 1983;105(10):662–5
**Schneck P:** Frauenheilkunde und Geburtshilfe in der Zeit des deutschen Faschismus 1933 bis 1945--Zum Schicksal der sozialen Gynäkologie im 'Dritten Reich'. **Z Gesamte Hyg** 1983 Oct;29(10):645–7
**Schneck P:** Iz istorii russko-nemetskikh meditsinskikh sviazeĭ. **Sov Zdravookhr** 1982;(4):61–3
**Schneck P:** Max Hirsch (1877–1948)--der Mitbegründer der sozialgynäkologischen Forschungrichtung. **Zentralbl Gynakol** 1983;105(24):1600–4
**Schneck P:** Standpunkte russischer und deutscher Geburtshelfer zur Problematik der Eklampsietherapie um die Wende vom 19. zum 20. Jahrhundert. **Z Gesamte Hyg** 1980;26(5):374–6
**Schneck P, Tutzke D:** Ueberblick über die Aktenbestände des Staatsarchivs Dresden zur Geschichte der deutsch-polnischen medizinischen Beziehungen im 18. Jahrhundert. **Arch Hist Med (Warsz)** 1979;42(2):205–9
**Schneck P:** Wilhelm Liepmann (1878–1939)--ein Gynäkologenschicksal zwischen Kaiserreich und faschistischer Diktatur. **Zentralbl Gynakol** 1984;106(17):1223–8
**Schneck P:** Wilhelm Liepmann (1878–1939) und die soziale Gynäkologie im Spiegel der Aktenbestände des Archivs der Humboldt-Universität zu Berlin. **NTM** 1980;17(2):102–20
**Schneck P:** Zum Wandel ärztlich-ethischer und deontologischer Auffassungen auf dem Gebiete der Frauenheilkunde während des ersten Drittels des 20. Jahrhunderts. **Z Gesamte Hyg** 1984 Apr;30(4):246–8
**Schneck P** see **Bazanov VA**
**Schneck P** see **Danilischina EI**
**Schneegans HJ:** Die Müttersterblichkeit im 17. bis 19. Jahrhundert. **Zentralbl Gynakol** 1982;104(22):1416–20
**Schneeloch NH:** 'Praecautien tegens de pest'. Pestgefahr in den Vereinigten Niederlanden 1720–1722. **Econ Soc Hist Jaarb** 1977;40:26–47
**Schneeweiss U:** Die Bedeutung der Entdeckung der Tuberkelbakterien für die Immunitäts- und Krankheitslehre. **Padiatr Grenzgeb** 1982;21(2):127–40
**Schneeweiss U:** Die Immunitätslehre im Lichte der Vorstellungen von Robert Koch. **Z Erkr Atmungsorgane** 1983;161(1):46–50
**Schneeweiss U:** Die Spezifitätslehre Robert Kochs; 100 Jahre Entdeckung der Tuberkelbakterien. **Medizinhist J** 1983;18(1–2):21–32
**Schneider DM** see **Breul FR**
**Schneider EC:** Mental retardation, state policy, and the Ladd School, 1908–1970. **RI Hist** 1981;40(4):133–43
**Schneider EC** see **Golden J**
**Schneider H:** Dr. August Heisler. Erinnerungen an einen grossen Arzt. **ZFA (Stuttgart)** 1983 May 10;59(13):774–6
**Schneider HG, Witte B:** Die Zeitschrift 'Deutsche Stomatologie/Stomatologie der DDR' in den Jahren 1961–1980. Eine Analyse ihrer Beiträge hinsichtlich Inhalt, Form und thematischer Trends. **Stomatol DDR** 1982 Jan;32(1):2–9
**Schneider HJ, Seiyfarth HH:** Die mikroskopische Harnsteinanalyse von den Anfängen 1879 bis zur Gegenwart. Jena, Friedrich-Schiller-Universität, 1980. 81 p.
**Schneider HJ, Doberentz D:** Zur Geschichte der Jenaer Harnsteinforschung. Mit einem vollständigen Abdruck der Dissertationsschrift Arno Krüches 'Ueber Struktur und Entstehung der Uratsteine' aus dem Jahre 1879. Jena, Friedrich-Schiller-Universität, 1979. 84, 42 p. (Jenaer Reden und Schriften).
**Schneider I:** Christiaan Huygens's contribution to the development of a calculus of probabilities. **Janus** 1980;67(4):269–79
**Schneider J:** Beiträge zur Geschichte der Wehrpharmazie von 1935–1945. Düsseldorf, Triltsch Druck, 1982. vi, 160 p. (Düsseldorfer Arbeiten zur Geschichte der Medizin, Beiheft VIII).
**Schneider LA:** The Rockefeller Foundation, the China Foundation, and the development of modern science in China. **Soc Sci Med** 1982;16(12):1217–21
**Schneider R:** Gibt es eine 'Problemkinderkurve' im HAWIK? Zur Geschichte von Intelligenztestergebnissen. **Prax Kinderpsychol Kinderpsychiatr** 1982 Nov–Dec;31(8):286–90
**Schneider S:** Commentaires sur l'article de Jacques-Louis Reverdin: 'des opérations modernes de cure radicale des hernies'. **Rev Med Suisse Romande** 1980 Dec;100(12):1097–101
**Schneider W:** Anleitung zum Gebrauch des Systema Pharmaceuticum. (Zur statistischen Auswertung von Quellen zur Arzneimittelgeschichte). Braunschweig, 1978. 67 p. (Veröffentlichungen aus dem Pharmaziegeschichtlichen Seminar der Technischen Universität Braunschweig, 18).
**Schneider W:** Arzneirezepte von Paracelsus. **Medizinhist J** 1981;16(1–2):151–66
**Schneider W:** Das Lot-Gewicht bei Paracelsus. In Dilg P, et al., ed: Perspektiven der Pharmaziegeschichte. Graz, Austria, Akademische Druck- u. Verlagsanstalt, 1983. p. 325–30.
**Schneider W:** Ein neuer Textbeleg vom Liber praeparationum. Wien, 1978. 51 p. (Salzburger Beiträge zur Paracelsusforschung, 19).
**Schneider W:** Entwicklung der pharmazeutischen Museologie in Deutschland. **Pharm Ztg** 1980 Jan 10;125(2):68–71
**Schneider W:** Pharmaziegeschichte und ihre Repräsentanten im 20. Jahrhundert. Zum 80. Geburtstag von Prof. Dr. Georg Edmund Dann. **Pharm Ztg** 1978;123:1265–71
**Schneider W:** Toward the improvement of the human race: the history of eugenics in France. **J Mod Hist** 1982;54(2):268–91
**Schneider W:** Ueber den Liber praeparationum des Paracelsus. **Sudhoffs Arch** 1980;64(1):69–78
**Schneider W** see **Domandl S, ed**
**Schneider W** see **Paracelsus in der Tradition**
**Schneider WH:** Chance and social setting in the application of the discovery of blood groups. **Bull Hist Med** 1983 Winter;57(4):545–62
**Schneider-Hiltbrunner V:** Wilhelm Fabry von Hilden 1560–1634. Verzeichnis der Werke und des Briefwechsels. Bern, Hans Huber, 1976. 172 p. (Berner Beiträge zur Geschichte der Medizin und der Naturwissenschaften, 8).
**Schneiderman L:** Henri Saint-Simon: his ideology and personality. **Am J Psychoanal** 1980 Winter;40(4):349–64
**Schneiderman MA:** Trends in cancer mortality and incidence in the United States: is the future clear or clouded? In V. Miké, K. E. Stanley, ed: Statistics in medical research. Methods and issues, with applications in cancer research. New York, John Wiley & Sons, 1982. p. 71–107.
**Schneiderman S:** Jacques Lacan, the death of an intellectual hero. Cambridge, Harvard University Press, 1983. vii, 182 p.
**Schnelbögl F:** Auerbacher Lebensbilder. Zum 500. Geburtsjahr Heinrich Stromers, genannt Auerbach. **Altnurnb Landsch** 1976;25(Sonderh. 1):1–26
**Schnell RL:** Contributions to psychohistory: IV. Individual experience in historiography and psychoanalysis: significance of Erik Erikson and Robert Coles. **Psychol Rep** 1980 Apr;46(2):591–612
**Schnell RL** see **Rooke PT**
**Schnelle T:** Ludwik Fleck – a classical scholar of the sociology of science and of epistemology. **Kwart Hist Nauki Tech** 1983;28(3–4):525–43
**Schnitzler H, Lieth H:** 25 year activities of the International Society of

Biometeorology and 25 year publication index. **Int J Biometeorol** 1983 Dec;27(4):287–434

**Schnorrenberg BB:** Is childbirth any place for a woman? The decline of midwifery in eighteenth-century England. **Stud Eighteenth Cent Cult** 1981;10:393–408

**Schnorrenberg BB:** Medical men of Bath. **Stud Eighteenth Cent Cult** 1984;13:189–203

**Schober K:** Das chirurgische Erbe: Vor etwa 100 Jahren (9). **Zentralbl Chir** 1979;104(12):798–9

**Schober KL:** Das chirurgische Erbe. Richard von Volkmann zum 150. Geburtstag am 17. 8. 1980. **Zentralbl Chir** 1980;105(24):1635–43

**Schober KL:** Das chirurgische Erbe. Theodor Billroth und die Karzinomchirurgie des Intestinaltraktes. **Zentralbl Chir** 1981;106(10):693–9

**Schober KL:** Das chirurgische Erbe. Theodor Billroth und seine norddeutsche Heimat. **Zentralbl Chir** 1982;107(20):1317–23

**Schober KL:** Das chirurgische Erbe: Tragische Chirurgenschicksale. 1882: Die Tragödie des Dr. Block. **Zentralbl Chir** 1984;109(5):366–73

**Schober KL:** Das chirurgische Erbe. Vor etwa hundert Jahren (27). **Zentralbl Chir** 1981;106(4):255–8 (continued periodically)

**Schober KL:** Gedächtnisvorlesung zum 150. Geburtstag von Richard von Volkmann, dem Mit-Gründer der Deutschen Gesellschaft für Chirurgie. **Langenbecks Arch Chir** 1981;355:597–606

**Schober KL:** Teodor Bil'rot i sovremennaia khirurgiia. **Khirurgiia (Mosk)** 1981 Feb;(2):116–7

**Schober KL:** The quotation about the heart. Comments on Theodor Billroth's attitude towards cardiac surgery. **Thorac Cardiovasc Surg** 1981 Jun;29(3):131–7

**Schober KL:** Vor etwa hundert Jahren. **Zentralbl Chir** 1980;105(6):401–3 (continued regularly)

**Schober KL, Simon G:** Vor etwa hundert Jahren (26). Exstirpation einer Niere bei Steinkranheit. **Zentralbl Chir** 1981;106(3):183–6

**Schober KL:** Vor etwa hundert Jahren (31). **Zentralbl Chir** 1981;106(11):733–6 (continued periodically)

**Schober KL:** Vor etwa hundert Jahren (41). **Zentralbl Chir** 1982;107(23):1538–40

**Schober KL:** Vor etwa 100 Jahren (8). Amputatio talo-calcanea von Dr. E. Blasius Geh. Medicinalrath und Professor in Halle. **Zentralbl Chir** 1979;104(11):739–41

**Schobloch R** see **Gürtler LG**

**Schoefer G:** Die chirurgische Behandlung der Lungentuberkulose. **Zentralbl Chir** 1982;107(5–6):285–94

**Schoen R, Nelson VE:** Mortality by cause among Spanish surnamed Californians, 1969–71. **Soc Sci Q** 1981;62(2):259–74

**Schoen WP:** The modern history of Loyola University Dental School. **CDS Rev** 1983 Jun;76(5):18–24

**Schoenberg B** see **Massey EW**

**Schoenberg BS:** Plague of pellagra. **South Med J** 1983 Mar;76(3):281–3

**Schoenberg BS** see **Schoenberg DG**

**Schoenberg BS** see **Steinfeld JL**

**Schoenberg DG, Schoenberg BS:** [Eponyms in medical history] **South Med J** 1979 Dec;72(12):1590–1 (continued periodically)

**Schoeneman TJ:** Criticisms of the psychopathological interpretation of witch hunts: a review. **Am J Psychiatry** 1982 Aug;139(8):1028–32

**Schoenfeld MR:** Nicolo Paganini--musical magician and Marfan mutant? **Med Times** 1980 Nov, 108(11):117–8, 120, 125

**Schoeninger MJ, DeNiro MJ, Tauber H:** Stable nitrogen isotope ratios of bone collagen reflect marine and terrestrial components of prehistoric human diet. **Science** 1983 Jun 24;220(4604):1381–3

**Schoental R:** A corner of history. Moses and mycotoxins. **Prev Med** 1980 Jan;9(1):159–61

**Schoental R:** Mozart's illnesses and death. **J R Soc Med** 1983 Dec;76(12):1079–80

**Schoental R:** Mycotoxins and the Bible. **Perspect Biol Med** 1984 Autumn;28(1):117–20

**Schoenwald RL:** The psychological study of history. In Iggers, GG, Parker HT, ed: International handbook of historical studies: contemporary research and theory. Westport, Conn., Greenwood, 1979. p. 71–85.

**Schoffeniels E:** In memoriam Marcel Florkin (Liège, 15 août 1900–3 mai 1979). Les chênes qu'on abat. **Rev Med Liege** 1979 Jun 1;34(11):481–7

**Schoffeniels E:** Marcel Florkin et les aspects moleculaires de la biologie. **Bull Mem Acad R Med Belg** 1979 Nov 24;134(10):604–16

**Schoffeniels E:** Marcel Florkin: founding father of comparative biochemistry. **Comp Biochem Physiol** 1980;67B:353–8

**Schoffeniels E** see **Lecomte J**

**Schöffler HH:** Die Akademie von Gondischapur. Aristoteles auf dem Wege in den Orient. Stuttgart, Freies Geistesleben, 1979. 154 p.

**Schofield R:** Microdemography and epidemic mortality: two case studies. In: Time, space and man, essays on microdemography. Uppsala, Almquist & Wiksell, 1979, p. 53–67.

**Schofield R** see **Charlton C**

**Schofield R** see **Webster C, ed**

**Schofield RE** see **Kieft L**

**Schofield RS** see **Wrigley EA**

**Schol D** see **Quinn S, ed**

**Scholle RH:** The best of American dentistry. **J Am Dent Assoc** 1982 Jun;104(6):962

**Scholle S:** Lanfranks 'Chirurgia Parva' in mittelniederfränkischer Ubertragung. Diss. Würzburg, 1978. Pattensen, Horst Wellm Verlag, 1978. 147 p. (Altdeutsche Lanfrank-Ubersetzungen, II, 1).

**Schöllgen G:** Das Problem einer Hitler-Biographie. **Neue Polit Lit** 1978;23(4):421–34

**Scholliers-van den Eeckhout P:** De geschiedenis van de 'Vondelingenbak' te Brussel. Conflicten tussen moraliteit en administratieve zuinigheid. **Ann Soc Belg Hist Hop** 1978;16:57–85

**Schollmayer E:** Skelettfunde aus fränkischen Reihengräberfriedhöfen in Eltville und Langenlonsheim. Vergleiche mit anderen merowingerzeitlichen Serien. **Z Morphol Anthropol** 1983;74(2):173–89

**Schölmerich P:** Historische Anmerkungen zum Begriff Myokarditis – Kardiomypathie. **Med Welt** 1984 Jan 13;35(1–2):109–13

**Scholz A:** Geburtshilfe vor 150 Jahren. **Z Arztl Fortbild (Jena)** 1980 Oct 1;74(19):930–3

**Scholz A:** Rudolph Leopold Mayer, Werk und Persönlichkeit. **Dermatol Monatsschr** 1981 Sep;167(9):582–6

**Scholz A:** Von kleinen und grossen Tumoren in der Kunst. **Hautarzt** 1982 Nov;33(11):598–604

**Scholz A:** Zur Geschichte der polnischen und deutschen Arzte-Exlibris. **Arch Hist Med (Warsz)** 1979;42(3):365–9

**Scholz F, Rossiwall B:** Taurodontismus: Eine anthropologische Streitfrage und ein Mikrosymptom für genetische Störungen. **Osterr Z Stomatol** 1981 Oct;78(10):373–8

**Scholz G:** Vom Hufbeschlag zur Huforthopädie. **DTW** 1981 Nov 5;88(11):475–9

**Schomburg E:** Sebastian Kneipp, 1821–1897. Bad Wörishofen, Kneipp-Verlag, 1976. 154 p.

**Schönbauer D, Dibold H:** Die Diätassistentin. Wien, Göschl, 1978. 223 p.

**Schönfeld J:** Zum Ursprung der Krankheitsbezeichnung 'Syphylis'. **Off Gesundheitswes** 1984 Feb;46(2):104–5

**Schönfeld J:** Zur Geschichte der Geschlechtskrankheiten. **Off Gesundheitswes** 1982 Oct;44(10):660–3

**Schönwetter HP:** Zur Geschichte der Akromegalie; mit besonderer Berücksichtigung der Frühgeschichte im Kanton Glarus. **Gesnerus** 1982;39(3–4):369–93

**Schoolman HM:** The clinician and the statistician. **Stat Med** 1982 Oct–Dec;1(4):311–6

**Schoolman HM** see **Doszkoos TE**

**Schöpf A:** Sigmund Freud. München, Beck, 1982. 244 p.

**Schopler E, Chess S, Eisenberg L:** Our memorial to Leo Kanner. **J Autism Dev Disord** 1981 Sep;11(3):257–69

**Schor I:** The continuing nursing education and adult education movements in the United States. **Nurs Forum** 1981;20(1):87–101

**Schorr A:** Die Verhaltens-Therapie: ihre Geschichte von den Anfängen bis zur Gegenwart. Weinheim, Beltz, 1984. 364 p.

**Schorr R** see **Dahm I**

**Schorske CF:** Freud: the psycho-archeology of civilizations. **Mass Hist Soc Proc** 1980;92:52–67

**Schoten EJ** see **Horstmanhoff HF, ed**

**Schoten EJ** see **Horstmanhoff HF, et al**

**Schott A:** Historical notes on the mechanism of closure of the atrioventricular valves. **Med Hist** 1980 Apr;24(2):163–84

**Schott B:** Histoire du syndrome de Guillain et Barré. **Rev Neurol (Paris)** 1982;138(12):931–8

**Schott GD:** Some neurological observations on Leonardo da Vinci's handwriting. **J Neurol Sci** 1979 Aug;42(3):321–9

**Schott H:** Der versteckte Poet in uns; zur Sprachtheorie in der naturphilosophischen Seelenlehre von Gotthilf Heinrich von Schubert (1780–1860). **Sudhoffs Arch** 1981;65(3):226–50

**Schott H:** Die Mitteilung des Lebensfeuers. Zum therapeutischen Konzept von Franz Anton Mesmer (1734–1815). **Medizinhist J** 1982;17(3):195–214

**Schott H:** Die 'Suggestion' und ihre medizinhistorische Bedeutung. In Seidler E, Schott H, ed: Bausteine zur Medizingeschichte. Stuttgart, Steiner, 1984. p. 111–21.

**Schott H:** Freuds Selbstanalyse (Freud und Fliess). In International Congress of the History of Medicine, 27th, Barcelona, 1980. Actas. Barcelona, Académia de Ciències Mèdiques de Catalunya i Balears, 1981. p. 145–8.

**Schott H:** Mesmer, Braid und Bernheim: zur Entstehungsgeschichte des Hypnotismus. **Gesnerus** 1984;41(1/2):33–48

**Schott H:** Traum und Geschichte. Zur Freudschen Geschichtsauffassung im Kontext der Traumdeutung. **Sudhoffs Arch** 1980;64(3):298–312

**Schott HG:** Elemente der Selbstanalyse in den 'Studien über Hysterie'. **Gesnerus** 1980;37(3/4):235–56

**Schott TE:** Paul Ramsey Hawley. In Dictionary of American biography, 1961–1965. Suppl. 7, 1981. p. 328–9.

**Schott H, ed** see **Seidler E**

**Schou M:** Lithium perspectives. **Neuropsychobiology** 1983;10(1):7–12

**Schouten J, Goltz D:** James Primrose und sein Kampf gegen die Theorie vom Blutkreislauf. **Sudhoffs Arch** 1977;61(4):331–52

**Schram R:** Britain's contribution to health and medicine in tropical countries through medical missions. **Trans R Soc Trop Med Hyg** 1981;75 Suppl:56–8

**Schramm A, Sperling M:** Ergotamin-Schäden einst und heute. Vom Antoniusfeuer zum Medikamentenschaden. **MMW** 1983 Jun 10;125(23):492–4

**Schramm E:** Linné, Gedner und die biologische Kontrolle. **Medizinhist J** 1984;19(3):244–9

**Schreiber HW:** Chirurgie im Wandel der Zeit 1945–1983. Berlin, New York, Springer-Verlag, 1983. xviii, 419 p.

**Schreiber HW:** Wo steht die Carcinom-Chirurgie des Magens 100 Jahre nach der ersten erfolgreichen Magenresektion durch Theodor Billroth? **Langenbecks Arch Chir** 1982;358:53–5

**Schreiber HW** see **Schlosser GA**

University of Minnesota Press, 1978. xiii, 277 p.

**Schwaber E** see **Goldberg A, ed**

**Schwaber J:** Hybridoma technology. **Science** 1982 May 21;216(4548):798

**Schwaber P:** Freud and the twenties. **Mass Rev** 1981;22(1):133–51

**Schwaber P:** Scientific art: the interpretation of dreams. **Colby Libr Q** 1977;13(1):5–18

**Schwaiberger R:** Zu einigen Aspekten der Entwicklung der Pharmazie im Rahmen der Aufklärung, beeinflusst durch hallesche Systematiker. **Rostocker Wiss Hist Manuskripte** 1981;6:35–44

**Schwan HP:** Biomedical engineering and basic research: historical perspectives. **Med Prog Technol** 1980 Jun;7(2–3):63–7

**Schwan HP:** Physical properties of biological matter: some history, principles, and applications. **Bioelectromagnetics** 1982;3(1):3–8

**Schwan HP:** Ultrasound and electromagnetic radiation in hyperthermia--a historical perspective. **Br J Cancer** 1982 Mar;45(5)Suppl:84–92

**Schwanitz HJ:** Homöopathie und Brownianismus 1795–1844. Zwei wissenschaftstheoretische Fallstudien aus der praktischen Medizin. Stuttgart Fischer, 1983. 202 p. (Medizin in Geschichte und Kultur, 15).

**Schwanitz HJ:** Vom Ausgestossenen zum Gesichtsversehrten - Ein Beispiel sozialer Diskriminierung aus der Geschichte der Medizin. **Hautarzt** 1984 Jan;35(1):45–9

**Schwann H:** Anton Jurasz's Bedeutung für die Rhinolaryngologie aus heutiger Sicht. **Arch Hist Med (Warsz)** 1979;42(3):317–21

**Schwann H, Wilke J:** 'Erbliche Taubheit' im Faschismus. **Z Gesamte Hyg** 1984 Apr;30(4):232–4

**Schwann H:** Richard Kochs Beziehungen zum Karl-Sudhoff-Institut. Archivstudie anlässlich seines 100. Geburtstages. **NTM** 1982;19(1):94–103

**Schwann H:** Zur Gestaltung spezieller Vorlesungen 'Geschichte der Zahnheilkunde' für Stomatologie-Studenten. **Stomatol DDR** 1982 Mar;32(3):229–33

**Schwann S:** Lekarze polscy w świetle historyczno-medycznego dzieła Grzegorza Matthiasa z XVIII wieku. **Arch Hist Med (Warsz)** 1979;42(2):217–22

**Schwartz B** see **Newell FW**

**Schwartz D:** Reminiscence: those fabulous forties. **Am J Nurs** 1981 Jul;81(7):1414

**Schwartz J** see **Radcliff-Umstead D, ed**

**Schwartz JH:** Dentofacial growth and development in Homo sapiens: evidence from perinatal individuals from Punic Carthage. **Anat Anz** 1982;152(1):1–26

**Schwartz JH** see **Tattersall I**

**Schwartz JI:** Public health: case studies on the origins of government responsibility for health services in the United States. Ithaca, N.Y., Environmental Health Planning Training Program, Dept. of City and Regional Planning, and the Program in Urban and Regional Studies, Cornell University, 1977, 1980 printing. vi, 208 p.

**Schwartz LL, Isser N:** Some involuntary conversion techniques. **Jew Soc Stud** 1981;43(1):1–10

**Schwartz RH:** The pneumatic otoscope, a new instrument for the examination of the tympanic membrane--E. Siegle. 1984. **Int J Pediatr Otorhinolaryngol** 1980 Sep;2(3):261–3

**Schwartz RJ, Weiss KM, Buchanan AV:** Looking into the black box: practical approaches to record linkage. **Ann Demogr Hist (Paris)** 1984;:119–28

**Schwartz RJ** see **Buchanan AV**

**Schwartz RM** see **Emerson RS**

**Schwarz H:** Darwinism between Kant and Haeckel. **J Am Acad Relig** 1980;48(4):581–602

**Schwarz HD:** Christian Theodor Lappe (1802–1877). **Pharm Ztg** 1977;122:338

**Schwarz J:** Yellow clover: Katharine Lee Bates and Katharine Coman. **Frontiers** 1979;4(1):59–67

**Schwarz M:** Psychohygienische Verhaltensgebote für schwangere Frauen in medizinischen Ratgebergüchern. Frankfurt am Main, Haag Herchen, 1983. iv, 382 p.

**Schwarz R** see **Klausch B**

**Schwarz R** see **Kyank H**

**Schwarz R** see **Pothoff PC**

**Schwarz S:** Asklepios a Temida. **Ginekol Pol** 1983 Oct;54(10):585–98

**Schwarz HD, ed** see **Hein WH**

**Schweber SS:** Darwin and the political economists: divergence of character. **J Hist Biol** 1980 Fall;13(2):195–289

**Schweber SS:** Essay review; early Victorian science: science in culture. **J Hist Biol** 1980 Spring;13(1):121–40

**Schwehn MR:** Making the world: William James and the life of the mind. **Harv Libr Bull** 1982 Oct;30(4):426–54

**Schwehn MR, ed:** A William James renaissance: four essays by young scholars. **Harv Libr Bull** 1982 Oct;30(4):367–480

**Schweier P:** Lebendige Pädiatrie. München, Marseille, 1983. 302 p.

**Schweiger K:** Medizinisches im Werk des Kirchenvaters Origenes. Diss., Universität Düsseldorf. Düsseldorf, 1983. 96 p.

**Schweiger O:** A tbc-elleni küzdelem eredményei Magyarországon 100 évvel a mycobacterium felfedezése után. **Orv Hetil** 1983 Jul 10;124(28):1667–70

**Schweighofer F:** Der Fall Schreber. **Psychother Psychosom Med Psychol** 1982 Jan;32(1):4–8

**Schweitzer J:** Sixty-two years of practice. **NY J Dent** 1980 Apr;50(4):135–7

**Schweitzer JM:** An evaluation of 50 years of reconstructive dentistry. Part I: Jaw relations and occlusion. **J Prosthet Dent** 1981 Apr;45(4):383–8

**Schweitzer JM:** An evaluation of 50 years of reconstructive dentistry. Part II: Effectiveness. **J Prosthet Dent** 1981 May;45(5):492–8

**Schwendinger K:** Krankheiten und Seuchen bei Mensch und Tier. **Montfort** 1965;17(3):308–12

**Schweppe KW, Probst C:** Die Versuche zur medikamentösen Karzinomtherapie des Anton Störck (1731 bis 1803). Ein Beitrag zur Geschichte der experimentellen Arzneimittelforschung in der älteren Wiener medizinischen Schule. In Ganzinger K, Skopec M, Wyklicky H, ed: Festschrift für Erna Lesky zum 70. Geburtstag. Wien, Brüder Hollinek, 1981. p. 105–22.

**Schweppe KW, Probst C:** Die Versuche zur medikamentösen Karzinomtherapie des Anton Störck (1731-1803). Ein Beitrag zur Geschichte der experimentellen Arzneimittelforschung in der älteren Wiener medizinischen Schule. **Wien Med Wochenschr** 1982 Mar 15;132(5):107–17

**Schwidetzky I** see **Rassengeschichte der Menscheit**

**Schwidetzky I** see **Rassengeschichte der Menschheit**

**Schyns C, Fossa A, Colaert J:** L'épidémie de choléra dans le Sud-Kivu. **Bull Seance Acad R Sci Outre Mer** 1979;(3):451–65

**Sciagura C** see **Ober WB**

**Science serving human needs: a history of Battelle Memorial Institute:** Columbus, Battelle, 1979. 16 p.

**Scientific essays on infectious diseases in honor of Dorothy M. Horstmann, M.D.: Yale J Biol Med** 1982 May–Aug;55(3–4):161–389

**Scigliano JA:** THC therapeutic research by independent and state-sponsored investigators: a historical review. **J Clin Pharmacol** 1981 Aug–Sept;21(8–9 Suppl):113S–121S

**Sclare AB:** John Carswell: a pioneer in Scottish psychiatry. **Scott Med J** 1981 Jul;26(3):265–70

**Scobey M** see **Kalisch PA**

**Scopa JP:** Boerhaave on alchemy. **Synthesis** 1979;4(4):24–37

**Scott CE** see **Sharkey PW, ed**

**Scott EL:** The origins of 'pneumatic medicine' and its practice in Manchester. **Mem Proc Manch Lit Philos Soc** 1974–75;117:75–92

**Scott HW:** A tribute to Barney Brooks, Alfred Blalock, and the Vanderbilt Surgical Staff (1925 to 1982). **South Med J** 1982 Dec;75(12):1439–52

**Scott J:** Taming a revolution the real achievements of early factory reformers. **Occup Health (Lond)** 1983 Oct;35(10):439–44

**Scott J** see **Hart GD**

**Scott JS** see **Walker JD**

**Scott JW:** Osler and the science of medicine. In: Congrès international de la médecine XXVe, Quebec, 1976. Actes. Québec, 1977. p. 1244–52.

**Scott LD** see **Hughes RE**

**Scott M:** 32,000 years of sutures. **NATNEWS** 1983 May;20(5):15–7

**Scott MH:** Say, 'Ah,' the story of a hundred years of medicine in Richland County, Wisconsin, 1840–1940. Richland Center, Wis., Richland County Pub., 1981. 262 p.

**Scott RB:** Historical review of legislative and national initiatives for sickle cell disease. **Am J Pediatr Hematol Oncol** 1983 Winter;5(4):346–51

**Scott WW:** Historical overview of the treatment of prostatic cancer. **Prostate** 1983;4(5):435–40

**Scott Adams: A continuing force in the age of discontinuity: Bull Am Soc Inf Sci** 1982 Dec;9(2):16–8

**Scott-Moncrieff R:** The classical period in chemical genetics; recollections of Muriel Wheldale Onslow, Robert and Gertrude Robinson and J. B. S. Haldane. **Notes Rec R Soc Lond** 1981;36(1):125–54

**The Scottish society of the history of medicine:** report of proceedings, session 1978–79. **Med Hist** 1980 Apr;24(2):209–13

**Scoville AB:** Insulin. **South Med J** 1983 Sep;76(9):1085–7

**Screbrny jubileusz: Pieleg Polozna** 1983;(5):28–9

**Screech MA:** A new look at 'Melencolia I'. **J Warburg Courtauld Inst** 1980;43:257–62

**Scriban R** see **Delaunay A, ed**

**Scribner Cl** see **Johnson KM**

**Scrimgeour EM:** Possible introduction of Huntington's chorea into Pacific Islands by New England whalemen. **Am J Med Genet** 1983 Aug;15(4):607–13

**Scrinivasan B** see **Huff DS**

**Scripcaru:** A century of forensic teachings research and medicolegal assistance in Iasi-Romania. **Am J Forensic Med Pathol** 1983 Dec;4(4):371–2

**Scripcaru G:** Traditia si actualitatea relatiei dintre învătămîntul medical si Societatea de Medici si Naturalisti. **Rev Med Chir Soc Med Nat Iasi** 1980 Oct–Dec;84(4):629–35

**Scripcaru G:** Un secol de învătămînt medical universitar la Iaşi. **Rev Med Chir Soc Med Nat Iasi** 1979 Oct–Dec;83(4):557–63

**Scrymgeour JM** see **Stubbe JH**

**Sct Apollonia og dansk odontologi: Tandlaegebladet** 1984 Jan;88(1):5–8

**Scull A:** A brilliant career? John Conolly and Victorian psychiatry. **Victorian Stud** 1984;27:203–35

**Scull A:** A convenient place to get rid of inconvenient people: the Victorian lunatic asylum. In King, Anthony D., ed.: Buildings and society: essays on the social development of the built environment. London, Routledge and Kegan Paul, 1980. p. 37–60.

**Scull A:** A new trade in lunacy: the recommodification of the mental patient. **Am Behav Sci** 1981;24(6):741–54

**Scull A:** Deinstitutionalization and the rights of the deviant. **J Soc Issues** 1981;37(3):6–20

**Scull A:** Humanitarianism or control? Some observations on the historiography of Anglo-American psychiatry. **Rice Univ Stud** 1981;67(1):21–41

**Scull A:** The domestication of madness. **Med Hist** 1983 Jul;27(3):233–48

**Scull A:** Was insanity increasing? A response to Edward Hare. **Br J Psychiatry** 1984 Apr;144:432–6

**Scull A, ed:** Madhouses, mad-doctors, and madmen. The social history of psychiatry in the Victorian era. Philadelphia, University of Pennsylvania Press, 1981. xv, 384 p. Contributions by W. F. Bynum, R. Cooter, N. J. Tomes, J. Walton, W. L. Parry-Jones, B. Sicherman, B. E. Blustein, M. J. Clark, E. Showalter, P. McCandless, R. Smith.
**Scully AL:** How the West was won ... by women doctors. **J Am Med Wom Assoc** 1982 Feb;37(2):36-7
**Scully D, Bart P:** A funny thing happened on the way to the orifice: women in gynecology textbooks. **Am J Sociol** 1973 Jan;78(4):1045-50
**Scully D:** [A history of] 'Baby catchers and uterus snatchers'. In her: Men who control women's health; the miseducation of obstetrician-gynecologists. Boston, Houghton Mifflin, 1980. p. 25-67.
**Seah CS:** Medical progress in Singapore--a review of the last three decades, 1951-1980. **Ann Acad Med Singapore** 1982 Jul;11(3):309-12
**Seal A:** Appendicitis: a historical review. **Can J Surg** 1981 Jul;24(4):427-33
**Seal SC:** Centenary of discovery of cholera vibrio. **Indian J Public Health** 1983 Jan-Mar;27(1):1-5
**Seal SC:** Centenary of discovery of cholera vibrio. **J Indian Med Assoc** 1983 Dec;81(11-12):210-2
**Seal SC:** Hundred years of malarial research. **J Indian Med Assoc** 1980 Apr 16;74(8):156-7
**Sealy WC:** The case of the fisherman with the fast pulse and the beginning of arrhythmia surgery. **NC Med J** 1983 Aug;44(8):489-90
**Seaman J** see **Condran GA**
**Seaman JD:** On phi-phenomena. **J Hist Behav Sci** 1984 Jan;20(1):3-8
**Séance du 11 octobre 1978:** Séance solennelle à la mémoire du Professeur Robert Deschiens (Professeur et Chef de Service honoraire à l'Institut Pasteur, Membre de l'Académie Nationale de Médecine, Secrétaire Général de la Société de Pathologie Exotique). **Bull Soc Pathol Exot Filiales** 1978;71 Spec No:499-511
**Searle CG:** A soldier pharmacist. **Pharm Hist (London)** 1974 Jan;4(1):2-3
**Searle GR:** Eugenics and class. In C. Webster, ed: Biology, medicine and society 1840-1940. Cambridge, Cambridge University Press, 1981. p. 217-42.
**Searle GR** see **Dupâquier J**
**Sears HF:** Soft tissue sarcoma: a historical overview. **Semin Oncol** 1981 Jun;8(2):129-32
**Sears RR:** Lewis Madison Terman. In Dictionary of American Biography, Suppl. 6, 1956-1960. p. 626-7, 1980.
**Sebald H:** Freud: instinctivist or behaviorist? The mirages of American sociology. **J Hist Sociol** 1982;4(2):64-89
**Sebastiani F:** Jean-Paul Marat, l'ami de la nature. **Physis** 1984;26(3):325-59
**Sebban:** Esquisse historique de la pratique dentaire populaire sous la Renaissance. **Soc Fr Hist Art Dent** 1979 Mar-Jun;(3-4):9-22
**Sebek V:** Josef Jerie--jeho život, doba, činnost, zásluhy. **Cesk Gynekol** 1980 Feb;45(1):55-68
**Sebrell WH:** History of pellagra. **Fed Proc** 1981 Apr;40(5):1520-2
**Sebrell WH:** Reflections on Nutrition Reviews from a clinical investigator. **Nutr Rev** 1982 Nov;40(11):326-8
**Secher O:** Fra Boston til Amaliegade; anaesthesiens vej til Danmark. **Dan Medicinhist Arbog** 1981;:25-56
**Sechzer JA:** Historical issues concerning animal experimentation in the United States. **Soc Sci Med [F]** 1981 Mar;15F(1):13-7
**Sechzer JA:** The ethical dilemma of some classical animal experiments. **Ann NY Acad Sci** 1983;406:5-12
**Sechzer JA:** The use of animals for experimentation in the United States. **Psychopharmacol Bull** 1981 Apr;17(2):88-91
**Secord JA:** Nature's fancy: Charles Darwin and the breeding of pigeons. **Isis** 1981;72:163-86
**Secret F:** Palingenesis, alchemy and metempsychosis in Renaissance medicine. **Ambix** 1979 Jul;26(2):81-92
**Secret F:** Réforme et alchimie. **Bull Soc Hist Protestantisme Fr** 1978;124:173-86
**Secret F:** Situation de la littérature alchimique en Europe, a la fin du XVIe et au début du XVIIe siècle. **Dix-Sept Siecle** 1978;30(3):135-44
**Secret F:** Un document oublié sur François Hotman et l'alchimie. **Bibl Hum Renaissance** 1980 May;42(2):435-46
**Seddon RP:** A cephalometric study of the Romano-British. **Eur J Orthod** 1984 Nov;6(4):303-12
**Sedgwick CE** see **Cady B**
**Sedgwick P:** Michel Foucault: the anti-history of psychiatry. **Psychol Med** 1981 May;11(2):235-48
**Sedgwick P:** Psycho politics: Laing, Foucault, Goffman, Szasz, and the future of mass psychiatry. New York, Harper & Row, 1982. 292 p.
**Sedláček K:** Sedesáté výrocí založení československé foniatrie prof. MUDr. Miloslavem Seemanem, DrSc. **Cesk Otolaryngol** 1982 Apr;31(2):65-8
**Sedler MJ:** Amendments to the Presidential papers. **Am J Psychiatry** 1982 Jan;139(1):136-7
**Sedler MJ:** Falret's discovery: the origin of the concept of bipolar affective illness. Translated by M. J. Sedler and Eric C. Dessain. **Am J Psychiatry** 1983 Sep;140(9):1127-33
**Sędzielowski Z** see **Kurzbauer R**
**Seed P:** The expansion of social work in Britain. London and Boston, Routledge and Kegan Paul, 1973. xi, 116 p.
**Seegers WH:** A personal perspective on hemostasis and thrombosis (1937-1981). **Semin Thromb Hemostas** 1981 Dec;7(3-4):177-307
**Seeman K, Lauren K:** Psychotherapy in Sweden: historical background, current status, and future projections. **Am J Psychother** 1984 Jan;38(1):97-110
**Seeman TE** see **Marcus AC**
**Seemayer TA:** The life and legacy of Professor Pierre Masson. **Am J Surg Pathol** 1983 Mar;7(2):179-83
**Seethalakshmi:** Nursing education through the ages. **Nurs J India** 1983 Oct;74(10):279-81
**Sefer M, Sefer M:** Evocare: Dumitru Combiescu (6 ianuarie 1887 - 25 noiembrie 1961)] (Rom). **Rev Ig [Bacteriol]** 1981 Jul-Sep;26(3):199-204
**Sefer M, Sefer M:** [10 years after the death of Professor Mihai Ciucă (18 July 1883 - 20 Feb. 1969). Mihai Ciucă and the study of bacteriophage, recorded in his working notebooks.] (Rum) **Rev Ig [Bacteriol]** 1979;24:123-6
**Sefer M** see **Sefer M**
**Sefrin P:** Notfall-Medizin heute. **Fortschr Med** 1982 Jul 22;100(27-28):1273-5
**Ségal A:** Le médecin principal de 1re classe Jean-Pierre Bonnafont (1805-1891); sa place prépondérante dans l'histoire de l'endoscopie aus XIXe siècle. **Hist Sci Med** 1983;17(1):63-70
**Segal A:** Les progrès de l'exploration visuelle des organes aux XVIIe et XVIIIe siècles. **Hist Sci Med** 1979;13(4):395-406
**Segal A** see **Hillemand P**
**Segal H:** Klein. Brighton, England, Harvester Press with Fontana Books, 1979. 189 p.
**Segal H:** Melanie Klein. New York, Viking, 1980. vii, 194 p.
**Segal H** see **Abrams RA**
**Segal N:** 150 de ani de existenţă a Secţiei de oftalmologie Oradea. **Rev Chir [Oftalmol]** 1981 Jan-Mar;25(1):75-9
**Segalen M:** Quelques réflexions pour l'étude de la condition féminine. **Ann Demogr Hist (Paris)** 1981;:11-22
**Segall H:** Dr. Harold Segall: a pioneer cardiologist reminisces. **Can Med Assoc J** 1982 May 1;126(9):1109-13-7
**Segall H:** N. C. Korotkoff and how he, a surgeon, discovered the sounds for measuring arterial pressure. In: Cóngrès international d'histoire de la médecine, XXVe, Québec, 1976. Actes. Québec, 1977. p. 1253-8.
**Segall HN** see **Korotkoff NS**
**Segebrecht W:** Krankheit und Gesellschaft. Zu E.T.A. Hoffmanns Rezeption der Bamberger Medizin. **Dtsch Vierteljahresschr Lit Wiss Geistesgesch** 1978;:267-90
**Segebrecht W:** Krankheit und Gesellschaft: zu E. T. A. Hoffmanns Rezeption der Bamberger Medizin. In Richard Brinkmann ed: Romantik in Deutschland: ein interdisziplinäres Symposion. Stuttgart, Metzler, 1978.
**Segelman AB, ed** see **Cowen DL**
**Séguin G:** Marie-Angélique Dussaus. In Dictionary of Canadian biography, 1801 to 1820. Volume 5, 1983. p. 293.
**Sehsuvaroglu BN:** Science and experimentation in Anatolian Turkey. In: Congrès international d'histoire de la médecine, XXVe, Québec, 1976. Actes. Québec, 1977. p. 1259-61.
**Seibel SD, Coura SH, Alho Filho JL:** Evolution de la politique brésilienne d'assistance psychiatrique et de santé mentale. **Ann Med Psychol (Paris)** 1979 Dec;137(10):1001-7
**Seibert S** see **Johnson LL**
**Seidel K:** Vergleichende Untersuchungen über die Häufigkeit des Auftretens degenerativer Wirbelsäulen-veränderungen bei Menschen des Neolitikums, des Mittelalters und der Jetztzeit. **Z Gesamte Inn Med** 1981 Mar;36(5):159-62
**Seidel T:** Medizinische Beobachtungen während der Weltumsegelung des Adam Johann von Krusenstern. Diss. Düsseldorf, 1979. 89 p.
**Seidel-Aprin H:** Zum Selbstmordgeschehen in der Bundesrepublik und den sozialistischen Staaten Osteuropas. Diss. Bonn, 1980. 94 p.
**Seidenschnur G:** Hans Hermann Schmid--Zum 100. Geburtstag. **Zentralbl Gynakol** 1984;106(18):1288-91
**Seidlein HJ** see **Friedrich C**
**Seidler E, Schott H, ed:** Bausteine zur Medizingeschichte. Heinrich Schipperges zum 65. Geburtstag. Stuttgart, Steiner, 1984. 154 p. (Sudhoffs Archiv, Beihefte, Heft 24)
**Seidler E:** Carl Gerhardt und seine Rede: 'Die Aufgaben und Ziele der Kinderheilkunde' (1879). **Monatsschr Kinderheilkd** 1983 Sep;131(9):545-8
**Seidler E:** Der 'kleine Patient'- traditionelle Probleme der Kindertherapie. **Monatsschr Kinderheilkd** 1982 Jun;130(6):332-6
**Seidler E:** Die Behinderten in Herten. **Gesnerus** 1982;39(1):133-40
**Seidler E:** Die Entwicklung des Rehabilitations-Verständnisses. **Krankenpflege (Frankfurt)** 1980 Oct;34(10):338-41
**Seidler E:** Die Freiburger Gobineau-Vereinigung und die Verbreitung des Arier-Gedankens in Deutschland. In Seidler E, Schott H, ed: Bausteine zur Medizingeschichte. Stuttgart, Steiner, 1984. p. 121-9.
**Seidler E:** Die Naturheilkundebewegung, ihre Systeme und Motive. In Dilg P, et al., ed: Perspektiven der Pharmaziegeschichte. Graz, Austria, Akademische Druck- u. Verlagsanstalt, 1983. p. 331-41.
**Seidler E, Kindt H, Schaub N:** Jaspers und Freud. **Sudhoffs Arch** 1978;62(1):37-63
**Seidler E:** Johann Friedrich Meckel the Younger (1781-1833). **Am J Med Genet** 1984 Aug;18(4):571-86
**Seidler E:** Le rôle de la méthode historique dans la médecine actuelle. In Poirier J, Poirier JL, ed: Médecine et philosohie à la fin du XIXe siècle. Paris, Université de Paris XII - Val de Marne, [1980?]. p. 149-55.
**Seidler E:** Wie wird man Arzt? Historische Grundformen der medizinischen Ausbildung. In R. Wittern, ed: Jahrbuch des Instituts für Geschichte der Medizin der Robert Bosch Stiftung. Stuttgart, Hippokrates Verlag, 1984. Bd. 1. p. 28-41.
**Seidler E** see **Eich W**
**Seidler FW:** Prostitution, Homosexualität, Selbstverstümmelung. Probleme der deutschen Sanitätsführung 1939-1945. Neckargemünd, Vowinkel, 1977. 323 p.

**Seidler MJ:** Kant and the stoics on suicide. **J Hist Ideas** 1983 Jul–Sep;44(3):429–53
**Seidler MJ:** The medical paradigm in Aristotelian ethics. **Thomist** 1978;42:400–33
**Seifert E** see **Simon P**
**Seifter E** see **Levenson SM**
**Seigworth GR:** Bloodletting over the centuries. **NY State J Med** 1980 Dec;80(13):2022–8
**Seiler FR** see **Gronski P**
**Seipel L, Breithardt G, Borggrefe M:** Die Entwicklung der klinischen Elektrophysiologie. Indikation, Komplikationen und Ergebnisse von 1296 invasiven elektrophysiologischen Untersuchungen 1971 bis 1981 in Düsseldorf. **Z Kardiol** 1984 Apr;73(4):194–8
**Seitelberger F:** The role of neuropathology in the neurosciences. In Rose FC, Bynum WF, ed: Historical aspects of the neurosciences. New York, Raven, 1982. p. 265–72.
**Seitelberger F** see **Hofecker G**
**Seitelberger F** see **Lorenz K, ed**
**Seivwright M:** The Florence Nightingale of Jamaica: Mary Seacole. **Jamaican Nurse** 1981 Dec;21(2):16
**Seiwa H:** An outline of the history of women and western sport in Japan. In Borms J, Hebbelinck M, Venerando A, ed: Women and sport. Basel, Karger, 1981. p. 52–7.
**Seiyfarth HH** see **Schneider HJ**
**Sejas García R** see **Wendorf de Sejas M**
**Seki M, Nonaka R:** [55 years of midwifery activities--oral history by Ms. Shin Tanaka]. (Jpn) **Josanpu Zasshi** 1981 Aug;35(8):600–9
**Seki T:** [Posthumous manuscripts: medicine and people in Britain] (Jpn). **Igakushi Kenkyu** 1978;51:1–25
**Sekscenski ES:** The health services industry: a decade of expansion. **Mon Labor Rev** 1981;104(5):9–16
**Sekuless P:** The first fifty years: an historical review of the Pharmacy Guild of Australia 1928–78. Canberra, Pharmacy Guild of Australia, 1978. 45 p.
**Selavan IC:** Angel in hell-with-the-lid-off. **Am J Nurs** 1980;80:2064–5
**Selby H** see **Johnston FE**
**Seldon A** see **Lindsay CM**
**Selected bibliography of Dr. J. Macura: Folia Microbiol (Praha)** 1980;25(2):81–5
**[Selected gems in medicine.] (Jpn).: Igaku Sensui** 1974–81 Oct–Dec;1–28: various pagings, issued irregularly
**Selections from Public health: reports and papers presented at meetings of the American Public Health Association (1884–1907). New York, Arno, 1977. Various paginations.:**
**Selections from Public health: reports and papers presented at the meetings of the American Public Health Association (1873–1883). New York, Arno, 1977. Various paginations.:**
**Selections from The health-education series. New York, Arno, 1977. Various paginations. (Reprint of articles published in Boston between 1906 and 1910).:**
**Selections from the Journal of the Massachusetts Association of Boards of Health (1891–1904). New York, Arno, 1977. Various paginations.:**
**Selective bibliography of Selma Fraiberg (1945–1982): Psychoanal Q** 1982;51(4):636–41
**Seletskiĭ AI:** Gegel' o patologii psikhiki--psikhoze i slaboumii. **Zh Nevropatol Psikhiatr** 1982;82(6):102–5
**Selezneva VT:** N. A. Russkikh--organizator bor'by s detskoĭ smertnost'iu (k 125-letiiu so dnia rozhdeniia). **Sov Zdravookhr** 1982;(7):64–7
**Seligman H** see **Kottek SS**
**Seligman S:** The royal maternity charity: the first hundred years. **Med Hist** 1980;24(4):403–18
**Selikoff IJ, Churg J, Hammond EC:** Classics in oncology: asbestos exposure and neoplasia. **CA** 1984 Jan–Feb;34(1):48–56
**Selikoff IJ** see **Lee DH**
**Selisskiĭ GD** see **Stoianov BG**
**Selivanov AP** see **Vankhanen VD**
**Selivanov EA** see **Bogomolova LG**
**Selivanov EF:** Meditsinskie muzei i vospitanie sovetskogo vracha. **Sov Med** 1982;(7):82–5
**Selivanov EF, Pasiukov FV:** Pamiatnik medikam Velikoĭ Otechestvennoĭ voĭny (o Voenno-meditsinskom muzee Ministerstva oborony SSSR). **Feldsher Akush** 1983 Nov;48(11):48–52
**Selivanov EF, Kantorovich MM:** Relikvii N. I. Pirogova v Voenno-meditsinskom muzee. **Voen Med Zh** 1983 Nov;(11):71–3
**Selivanov EF, Pasiukov FV:** 40-let Voenno-meditsinskogo muzeia. **Sov Zdravookhr** 1983;(2):67–70
**Selivanov EF** see **Selivanov VI**
**Selivanov EF** see **Varlamov VM**
**Selivanov VI, Tkhostov DR, Selivanov EF:** Lechbno- evakuatsionnaia kharakteristika ranenykh i bol'nykh, lechivshikhsia v gospital'noi baze tyla strany. **Voen Med Zh** 1980 Jun;(6):20–3
**Selivanov VI:** [Organization of rehabilitation of the wounded and sick during World War II in military hospitals]. (Rus) **Voen Med Zh** 1979 Nov;(11):74–5
**Selkurt EE:** Physiology at Indiana University School of Medicine-Indianapolis. **Physiologist** 1984 Oct;27(5):325–9
**Sell A, Madsen CB:** Radiumstationen in Aarhus from 1962 to 1984. **Acta Radiol [Oncol]** 1984;23(2–3):85–90
**Selleck AD:** William Cookworthy, an 18th century polymath. **Pharm Hist (London)** 1979 Dec;9(3):8–12
**Seller H:** Physiology at Heidelberg. **J Auton Nerv Syst** 1981 Apr;3(2–4):121–2
**Seller H** see **Brooks CM**
**Sellevold BJ:** Mandibular torus morphology. **Am J Phys Anthropol** 1980 Nov;53(4):569–72
**Sellors TH:** Sir Henry Sessions Souttar. In Dictionary of national biography, 1961–1970. Suppl. 8, 1981. p. 969–70.
**Selmanowitz VJ:** Impressions of Sechnin. Anatomy by slaughter. **NY State J Med** 1980 Dec;80(13):2016–21
**Selwyn S:** Pencillin pioneers. **J Antimicrob Chemother** 1980 Jan;6(1):151
**Selwyn S:** The evolution of the broad-spectrum penicillins. **J Antimicrob Chemother** 1982 Feb;9 Suppl B:1–10
**Selwyn S:** The first studies on the antibacterial effect of penicillium moulds between 1870 and 1876. In International Congress of the History of Medicine. 26th, Plovdiv, 1978. Actes du Congress. Sofia, 1981. Volume II. p. 192–5.
**Selwyn S:** The transition from mythology to medical microbiology in 1589. In: Congrès international d'histoire de la médecine, XXVe, Québec, 1976. Actes. Québec, 1977. p. 1262–73.
**Selzer R** see **Trautmann J, ed**
**Sembol J:** Dr Wacław Olszak. **Przegl Lek** 1981;38(1):169–73
**Semczuk B:** XXXV-lecie Lubelskiej Kliniki Otolaryngologicznej. **Otolaryngol Pol** 1980;34(1):113–6
**Semeniuk SI** see **Ignatovich FI**
**Semeniuta AIa** see **Dusmuratov MD**
**Semenov BF:** Razvitie ideĭ I.I.Mechnikova v oblasti immunologii. **Zh Mikrobiol Epidemiol Immunobiol** 1984 Jul;(7):50–4
**Semenov LK** see **Komkov GD**
**Semenov SV:** K istorii organizatsii gosudarstvennogo sanitarnogo nadzora na vodnom transporte v RSFSR. **Gig Sanit** 1984 Jan;(1):36–8
**Semenova EI:** Pervaia detskaia lechebnaia koloniia v Rossii (K 150-letiiu so dnia rozhdeniia D.I. Mendeleeva). **Pediatriia** 1984 Sep;(9):78–9
**Semenova NA** see **Piatak OA**
**Semenova VN** see **Lebedev DD**
**Semm K, Giese KP:** Ernst Gräfenberg, das Leben und Werk des Kieler Facharztes. Zum 100. Geburtstag am 26. September 1981. **Geburtshilfe Frauenheilkd** 1981 Jun;41(6):444–8
**Semm K, Giese KP:** Ernst Gräfenberg: the life and work of the specialist of Kiel on the hundredth anniversary of his birth on 26 September 1881. **Int J Fertil** 1983;28(3):141–8
**Semmelmann E:** Sykepleier i de 'gode gamle dager'. **Sykepleien** 1984 Jul 6;71(12):14–7
**Semorile A:** Aspectos sanitarios del terremoto de Mendoza de 1861. In Congreso de Historia de la Medicina Argentina [Transactions], 5th, Mendoza, 1983. p. 19–32.
**Semorile A:** Quienes ejercieron la medicina hasta el año 1.800. In Congreso de Historia de la Medicina Argentina [Transactions], 5th, Mendoza, 1983. p. 141–4.
**Sen A:** Ingredients of famine analysis: availability and entitlements. **Q J Econ** 1981;96(3):433–64
**Senchenkova EM:** [The importance of M. S. Tswett's investigations of the carotinoids.] (Rus). **Istor Biol Issled** 1978;7:65–92
**Senczek D:** Zur frühgeschichtlichen Entwicklung der tierärztlichen Nahrungsmittelhygiene aus freiberuflicher Sicht. **Z Ernaehrungwiss** 1980 Mar;19(1):40–6
**Sendler P:** Von der Krüppelheilanstalt zum Universitätsklinikum: die 'Hüfferstiftung' in Münster in Westfalen. Herzogenrath, Murken-Altrogge, 1984. 188 p. (Studien zur Geschichte des Krankenhauswesens, 17)
**Sendrail M:** La foi coranique et l'héritage médical grec. **Bull Assoc Guillaume Bude** 1977;:278–99
**Sendrail M** see **Histoire culturelle de la maladie**
**Senenko AN:** Obukhovskaia bol'nitsa (k 200-letiiu so dnia osnovaniia). **Klin Med (Mosk)** 1980 Feb;58(2):111–6
**Senft AW:** Parasitic disease and exploration: a glimpse of Central Africa in the 1860s. **RI Med J** 1983 Jan;66(1):31–6
**Senger HG:** Thomas Hirschhorn: ein Magdeburger Gelehrter des 15. Jahrhunderts. **Hist Jahrb** 1980;100:217–39
**Senior JE:** Hauksbee's prototypical electrostatic generator. **Med Instrum** 1983 Mar–Apr;17(2):126–7
**Senior JE:** The elusive search for electroanesthesia. **Med Instrum** 1984 Jan–Feb;18(1):86–7
**Senior N:** Aspects of infant feeding in 18th-century France. **Eighteenth Cent Stud** 1983;16:367–88
**Senn C** see **Zerobin K**
**Senn HJ:** Die medizinische Onkologie--eine fachliche und menschliche Herausforderung. **Wien Med Wochenschr** 1981;131(22):541–50
**Senning A:** Cardiac pacing in retrospect. **Am J Surg** 1983 Jun;145(6):733–9
**Senut B:** Quelques remarques à propos d'un humérus d'homino ide pliocène provenant de Chemeron (bassin du lac Baringo, Kenya). **Folia Primatol (Basel)** 1983;41(3–4):267–76
**Sepúlveda B:** La medicina en la seguridad social. In Academia Nacional de Medicina. Libro conmemorativo del primer centenario. México, Comité Editorial de la Comisión Organizadora del Congreso del Centenario, 1964. Tome 2. p. 678–83.
**Sepúlveda B:** Nuevas orientaciones de la medicina: los receptores celulares en terapéutica. I. Introducción. **Gac Med Mex** 1981 Dec;117(12):463–5
**Sepúlveda B** see **Jinich H**
**Sepúlveda B** see **Soberón G**
**Sepúlveda B** see **Somolinos-Palencia J**
**Sepúlveda MT:** Practicas medicas entre los purepecha prehispanicos. **Bol Soc Mex Hist Filos Med** 1980 Sep–Dec;5(32–33):67–81

**Sequeira MM:** A medicina moderna e os curandeiros. **Acta Med Port** 1980 Sep–Dec;2(5–6):439–41
**Serafin D:** Microsurgery: past, present, and future. **Plast Reconstr Surg** 1980 Nov;66(5):781–5
**Serdiuk AM:** Leninskim putem k novym svershenilam. **Vrach Delo** 1980 Apr;(4):1–7
**Serdiuk GV** see **Egorysheva IV**
**Serdiuk GV** see **Rabinovich RS**
**Serdiuk GV** see **Vengrova IV**
**Serebrennikov AB:** Dnevniki, memuary, épistoliarnye materialy kak istochniki dlia izucheniia istorii otechestvennoĭ meditsiny. **Sov Zdravookhr** 1981;(7):63–6
**Serebrennikov AB:** Khirurg L. A. Bekkers - uchenik N. I. Pirogova. **Klin Med (Mosk)** 1983 Mar;61(3):113–5
**Serebrennikov AB** see **Smol'iannikov AV**
**Serebrovskaja KB:** The role of scientific school in the formation of the new field of natural science. **Istor Biol Issled** 1983;9:145–58
**Serenko AF, Ermakov VV:** S. V. Kurashov--vydaiushchiĭsia deiatel' sovetskogo zdravookhraneniia. **Sov Zdravookhr** 1980;(10):45–8
**Serg E:** Ethnomedizin und Opfergegenstände auf Wallfahrtsorten in Ungarn. In International Congress of the History of Medicine. 26th, Plovdiv, 1978. Actes du Congress. Sofia, 1981. Volume II. p. 67.
**Sergeev TS** see **Alekseev GA**
**Sergeev VM, Levin AB:** Sovetskoe zdravookhranenie v kanun 60–letiia obrazovaniia SSSR. **Grudn Khir** 1982 Nov–Dec;(6):5–8
**Sergeĭ Sergeevich Mikhailov (k 60–letiiu so dnia rozhdeniia): Arkh Anat Gistol Embriol** 1980 Mar;78(3):121–5
**Sergienko VI** see **Zuev AI**
**Sergiev VP, Nikonova VA:** Raschet tendentsiĭ zabolevaemosti briushnym tifom na raznykh territoriiakh strany. **Zh Mikrobiol Epidemiol Immunobiol** 1980 Oct;(10):14–7
**Sergo E:** Gyermekágyas asszony étkeztetése Magyarországon. **Orvostort Kozl** 1982;28(1–3):245–50
**Seriano Lleras A** see **Bowers JZ**
**Serkov FN:** Fiziologicheskaia nauka v USSR za 60 let. **Fiziol Zh** 1982 Nov–Dec;28(6):643–52
**Serkov FN, Zadorozhnyĭ AG:** Nauchnaia deiatel'nost' Instituta fiziologii im. A. A. Bogomol'tsa AN USSR. K 50–letiiu so dnia osnovaniia. **Fiziol Zh** 1984 May–Jun;30(3):257–66
**Serkov FN:** Problemy normal'noĭ fiziologii v issledovaniiakh A. A. Bogomolets. **Fiziol Zh** 1981 May–Jun;27(3):438–43
**Serlin R:** Contraceptives: back to the barriers. **New Sci** 1981;91:281–4
**Sermonti G:** Gregor Mendel (1822–1884). **Riv Biol** 1984 Spring;77(1):105–13
**Sermonti G:** L'evoluzione e il metodo delle scienze biologiche. **Med Secoli** 1981 May–Aug;18(2):193–208
**Sermonti G:** Orpheus in Perugia. **Riv Biol** 1981 Winter;74(4):453–8
**Serna Gómez J:** Hospitales y beneficencia medicina y métodos curativos en la colonia. **Rev Acad Colomb Hist Ecles** 1973;8(29–30):101–21
**Sernett MC:** The rights of personhood: the Dred Scott case and the question of abortion. **Relig Life** 1980;49(4):461–76
**Seron X, Feyereisen P:** Cent ans de psychologie scientifique. **Rev Nouv** 1981;73(3):283–93
**Seror P:** Le rhumatisme blennorragique ancêtre des arthrites réactionnelles? **Presse Med** 1984 May 26;13(22):1359–63
**Serov VV:** M. N. Nikiforov i Moskovskaia shkola patologoanatomov (k 125–letiiu so dnia rozhdeniia). **Arkh Patol** 1984;46(2):3–12
**Serpa–Flores R:** La enseñanza de la historia de la medicina en la formación del médico. **Educ Med Salud** 1983;17(4):423–32
**Serrano P:** Avances en endocrinología. **Gac Med Mex** 1980 Oct;116(10):459–62
**Serre JL:** Mendel's rejection of the concept of blending inheritance. **Fundam Sci** 1981;2(1):55–66
**Serruys H:** Smallpox in Mongolia during the Ming and Ching dynasties. **Zentralasiat Stud** 1980;14:41–63
**Sersiron G:** La croix à double barre, symbole de l'UICT. Quelques informations sur ses origines. **Bull Int Union Tuberc** 1982 Sep–Dec;57(3–4):196–9
**Servais P, Roger FH:** Les archives médicales hospitalières: organisation et possibilités d'utilisation. **Ann Soc Belg Hist Hop** 1980;18:71–96
**Servat A, Servat C:** Pierre–Alphonse Doué, médecin de marine, médecin major de 'l'Aigle' à l'inauguration du canal de Suez. **Med Armees** 1981;9:453–68
**Servat C** see **Servat A**
**Servatinskiĭ GL** see **Mazurenko MD**
**Servít Z:** Počátky české novověké medicíny a biologie. Jan Marek Marci z Kronlandu (Joannes Marcus Marci, 1595–1667). Stručná biografie. **Cesk Fysiol** 1984;33(5):394–413
**Serý Z** see **Duda M**
**Ses MO de:** As dissertações finais centenárias da Escola Médico–Cirurgica do Porto - 1967. **Arch Hist Med Port** 1968–70;3(1–4):35–50
**Seshagiri Rao KL** see **Bleich JD**
**Sessão solene de homenagem ao Prof. Dr. Francisco Cambournac, por ocasião da atribuição do prémio e medalha da Fundação Léon Bernard pela Organização Mundial de Saúde--22 de Junho de 1978: An Inst Hig Med Trop (Lisb)** 1977–1978;5(1–4):37–53
**Sesti E** see **Adacher S**
**Sétáló G:** Az immunszövettani módszerek fejlődése és jelene. **Morphol Igazsagugyi Orv Sz** 1983 Apr;23(2):85–92
**Seters WH van** see **Palm LC**
**Setoguchi T:** [Paleontological view points on the morphological characteristics of human molar teeth. I (author's transl)] (Jpn). **Shikai Tenbo** 1981;(7):31–8
**Setoguchi T:** [Paleontological view points on the morphological characteristics of human molar teeth. II, III (author's transl)] (Jpn). **Shikai Tenbo** 1981;(8,9):319–25,441–8
**Settle EC, Ayd FJ:** Haloperidol: a quarter century of experience. **J Clin Psychiatry** 1983 Dec;44(12):440–8
**Seufert W, Seufert WD:** The recognition of leukemia as a systemic disease. **J Hist Med Allied Sci** 1982 Jan;37(1):34–50
**Seufert WD:** The chain osteotome by Heine. **J Hist Med Allied Sci** 1980 Oct;35(4):454–9
**Seufert WD** see **Seufert W**
**Severin SE:** V. V. Parin. Zhizn' i deiatel'nost'. **Vestn Akad Med Nauk SSSR** 1984;(4):3–7
**Severova EIa:** O proiskhozhdenii i ispol'zovanii termina 'lekarstvennaia bolezn''. **Sov Med** 1982;(5):113–5
**Sewall RB** see **Wand M**
**Seward M:** More than a century of change. **Br Dent J** 1980 Jul 1;149(1):35–6
**Sewell E** see **Trautmann J, ed**
**Sewerin I:** Fra katoderør til computer–tomografi. **Tandlaegebladet** 1983 Jun;87(11):383–8
**Sewering the cities. New York, Arno, 1977. Various paginations. Five reprinted articles by various authors, 1881–1914.:**
**Sexton PC:** The life of the homeless. **Dissent** 1983;30(1):79–84
**Seyda B:** Dzieje medycyny w zarysie. Warszawa, Państwowy Zakład Wydawn. Lekarskich, 1977. 606 p.
**Seyda B:** O nauczaniu historii medycyny w RFN. **Arch Hist Med (Warsz)** 1982;45(1–4):107–10
**Seymour H** see **Mauskopf SH**
**Seymour MC, et al, ed:** On the properties of things. John Trevisa's translation of Bartholomaeus Anglicus De proprietatibus rerum. A critical text. 2 vols. Oxford, Oxford University Press, 1975. xix, 1397 p.
**Sèze S de:** Histoire de la sciatique. **Rev Neurol (Paris)** 1982;138(12):1019–25
**Sèze S de:** Un demi siècle de rhumatologie: 1930–1980. **Bull Acad Natl Med (Paris)** 1980 Dec;164(9):807–21
**Sgibova LI** see **Gribanov ED**
**Shabashova NIa** see **Napalkov NP**
**Shabunin AV:** Efirnyĭ narkoz v pervyĭ god ego primeneniia v Rossii. **Sov Zdravookhr** 1983;8:62–4
**Shabunin AV:** K 150–letiiu izdaniia truda R. S. Chetyrkina 'Opyt voenno–meditsinskoĭ politsii ili pravila k sokhraneniiu zdorov'ia russkikh soldat v sukhoputnoĭ sluzhbe'. **Gig Sanit** 1984 Jun;(6):35–6
**Shabunin AV:** K 150–letiiu pervogo v Rossii perelivaniia krovi. **Akush Ginekol (Mosk)** 1982;(8):59–60
**Shabunin AV:** Kalinkinskiĭ khirurgicheskiĭ institut (k 200–letiiu so dnia osnovaniia). **Sov Zdravookhr** 1983;(11):66–7
**Shabunin AV:** Novye svedeniia o pervom perelivanii krovi v Rossii. **Sov Zdravookhr** 1982;(5):69–70
**Shabunin AV:** P. F. Lesgaft i razvitie fel'dshersko–akusherskogo obrazovaniia v Rossii. **Feldsher Akush** 1981;46(4):57–8
**Shabunin AV:** P. F. Lesgaft, 1837–1909. Moskva, Meditsina, 1982. 75 p.
**Shabunin AV:** Pervomu v Rossii perelivaniiu krovi--150 let. **Probl Gematol Pereliv Krovi** 1982 Aug;27(8):56–8
**Shabunin AV:** Prokhor Charukovskiĭ i ego 'Opyt sistemy prakticheskoĭ meditsiny' (k 150–letiiu so dnia vykhoda pervoĭ chasti truda). **Klin Med (Mosk)** 1983 Nov;61(11):145–7
**Shabunin AV:** Sto let otechestvennomu zubovrachebnomu obucheniiu. **Sov Zdravookhr** 1981;(11):52–3
**Shabunin AV:** Uchastie N.I. Pirogova v Obshchestve S.–Peterburgskikh prakticheskikh vracheĭ. **Sov Zdravookhr** 1983;(4):63–5
**Shabunin AV:** Vasiliĭ Ivanovich Priselkov--vidnyĭ deiatel' otechestvennyĭ meditsiny. **Sov Zdravookhr** 1984;(2):62–4
**Shabunin AV:** Vklad zhurnala 'Khirurgicheskiĭ vestnik' v razvitie khirurgicheskoĭ mysli v Rossii. **Vestn Khir** 1984 Aug;133(8):146–7
**Shackelford PG** see **White PJ**
**Shadbolt Y:** Nursing education - a major shift. **NZ Nurs J** 1983 Jan;76(1):6–9
**Shafar J:** The Brahms–Billroth friendship. **Br Med J** 1981;282:1775
**Shafer II** see **Napalkov PN**
**Shaffer AH** see **Friedman LJ**
**Shaffer AH** see **Himelhoch MS**
**Shafik Farid** see **Iskander Z**
**Shafranov BV:** Iz istorii gigieny promyshlennogo osveshcheniia v SSSR. **Gig Tr Prof Zabol** 1980 Jul;(7):46–7
**Shagdar L:** Otorinolaringologiia v Mongol'skoĭ Narodnoĭ Respublike. **Vestn Otorinolaringol** 1982 Mar–Apr;(2):59–62
**Shah M:** Tribhuvan University Institute of Medicine, Nepal. **Public Health Pap** 1980;2(71):81–96
**Shah RR** see **Romm S, ed**
**Shah RR** see **Ruberg RL**
**Shahar S:** Infants, infant care, and attitudes toward infancy in the medieval Lives of Saints. **J Psychohist** 1983 Winter;10(3):281–309
**Shakarian GA** see **Panosian GA**
**Shakhgel'diants AE:** Okhrana zdorov'ia promyshlennykh rabochikh v SSSR. **Sov Zdravookhr** 1980;(3):8–13
**Shakhmet AV:** Deiatel'nost' zhenotdelov Leningrada po okhrane materinstva i detstva (1926--1929). **Sov Zdravookhr** 1980;(4):64–6
**Shalaev NF:** Organizatsiia terapevticheskoĭ pomoshchi v Krasnoĭ Armii v gody inostrannoĭ voennoĭ interventsii i grazhdanskoĭ voĭny. **Voen Med Zh** 1982 Jun;(6):68–9
**Shalaev NF:** Terapevt, uchenyĭ i pedagog V.I. Glinchikov.

**Klin Med (Mosk)** 1984 Oct;62(10):146–9

**Shalaev NF:** Uchastie studentov Voenno-meditsinskoĭ akademii v revoliutsii 1905–1907 gg. **Sov Zdravookhr** 1980;(8):53–6

**Shalaev NF:** Vrach-bol'shevik I. D. Orakhelashvili. **Sov Zdravookhr** 1984;(1):51–3

**Shalagina TL** see **Dogel' LV**

**Shalganova IV** see **Roshchin AV**

**Shalimov AA, Kovalev MM, Sakharchuk IM:** Leninskaia druzhba narodov SSSR-reshaiushchee uslovie vosstanovleniia khirurgicheskikh kadrov Ukrainy posle ee osvobozhdeniia ot nemetsko-fashistskikh zakhvatchikov. **Klin Khir** 1982 Dec;(12):7–11

**Shalimov AA, Khokholia VP:** Zhurnalu 'Klinicheskaia khirurgiia' 60 let. **Klin Khir** 1981 Jun;(6):1–6

**Shalimov AA** see **Ternovoĭ KS**

**Shalybkova OP:** Rol' gipotermii v razvitii khirurgii serdtsa i sosudov. **Med Sestra** 1981 Jan;40(1):6–9

**Shamansky SL, Hamilton WM:** Is the public health nurse's bag anachronism? **Nurs Outlook** 1980 Jun;28(6):379–81

**Shamansurov SS, Madzhidova AT:** Ibn-Sina i bolezni detskogo vozrasta. **Pediatriia** 1980 Jul;(7):70–1

**Shambaugh GE:** French Keller Hansel and the history of allergy. **Arch Otolaryngol** 1983 Feb;109(2):126–9

**Shambaugh GE:** Pre and post-antibiotic otology. **Rev Laryngol Otol Rhinol (Bord)** 1980 Nov–Dec;101(11–12):529–36

**Shamin AN:** Issledovaniia po istorii biologii. **Vopr Istor Estestvozn Tekh** 1981;2:38–45

**Shamin AN:** Studies on the history of biochemistry. **Istor Biol Issled** 1983;9:4–15

**Shamin AN** see **Tovarova II**

**Shamko VI** see **Petrov VP**

**Shampo MA, Kyle RA:** [Contributions to the history of medical philately]. **JAMA** 1981 Dec 4;246(22):2572 (continued periodically)

**Shampo MA, Kyle RA:** Jacques-Alexandre-César Charles. **JAMA** 1984 May 18;251(19):2547

**Shampo MA** see **Kyle RA**

**Shampo MA** see **Rehder K**

**Shampo MA, ed** see **Kyle RA**

**Shandala MG:** Aleksandr Nikitich Marzeev (k 100-letiiu so dnia rozhdeniia). **Vrach Delo** 1983 May;5:119–21

**Shandala MG, Vaĭnrub EM, Kliuzko AS:** Edinstvo gigienicheskoĭ nauki i praktiki--osnovnoĭ printsip deiatel'nosti instituta (k 50-letiiu Kievskogo NII obshcheĭ i kommunal'noĭ gigieny im. A. N. Marzeeva). **Gig Sanit** 1981 Oct;(10):45–7

**Shandala MG, Kogan VIa:** Ot zemskogo sanitarnogo vracha do akademika (k 100-letiiu so dnia rozhdeniia A. N. Marzeeva). **Gig Sanit** 1983 Oct;(10):43–5

**Shandala MG:** Ozdorovlenie okruzhaiushcheĭ sredy--put' k obshchestvennomu zdorov'iu (k 50-letiiu Kievskogo NII obshcheĭ i kommunal'noĭ gigieny im. A. N. Marzeeva). **Vrach Delo** 1981 Sep;(9):1–5

**Shandling B:** History of the Canadian Association of Paediatric Surgeons. **J Pediatr Surg** 1979 Oct;14(5):509–10

**Shane KD:** New Mexico: salubrious El Dorado. **NM Hist Rev** 1981;56(4):387–99

**Shang ZJ:** [Survey of medicin 'Prescription for 52 diseases' (an old medicinal book)] (Chi). **Chung Yao Tung Pao** 1982;7(6):17–20

**Shankara MR, Venkataram BS, Leelavathy S:** A 19th century manuscript on traditional medicine. **Bull Indian Inst Hist Med (Hyderabad)** 1979;9:33–7

**Shankarashastry V:** The eminence of Lakshmipathi. **Bull Indian Inst Hist Med (Hyderabad)** 1980;10(1–4):62–8

**Shanks NJ, Al-Kalai D:** Arabian medicine in the middle ages. **J R Soc Med** 1984 Jan;77(1):60–5

**Shanley E:** The medicalisation of dying - 1. **Nurs Times** 1982 Aug 11–17;78(32):1360–2

**Shanley E** see **Davis B**

**Shannon GW, Cromley RG:** Philadelphia and the yellow fever epidemic of 1798. **Urban Geogr** 1982 Oct–Dec;3:355–70

**Shannon R:** [Re-evaluation of Florence Nightingale: a review of 'Florence Nightingale: Reputation and Power' by F. B. Smith] (Jpn). **Kango Kyoiku** 1982 Nov;23(11):677–85

**Shanzer S** see **Bender MB**

**Shapere D** see **Mayr E**

**Shapiro A** see **Bogdan R**

**Shapiro AK, Shapiro E:** Tourette syndrome: history and present status. **Adv Neurol** 1982;35:17–23

**Shapiro AL:** Private rights, public interest, and professional jurisdiction: the French public health law of 1902. **Bull Hist Med** 1980 Spring;54(1):4–22

**Shapiro AL:** Working class housing and public health in Paris, 1850–1902. Ph.D. Diss., Brown University. Providence, 1980. 338 leaves.

**Shapiro B, Frank RG:** English scientific virtuosi in the 16th and 17th centuries. Los Angeles, Clark Memorial Library, University of California, 1979, vii, 123 p.

**Shapiro B:** History and natural history in sixteenth- and seventeenth-century England: an essay on the relationship between humanism and science. In Shapiro, Barbara and Frank, Robert G. Jr., ed: English scientific virtuosi in the 16th and 17th centuries: Los Angeles, William Andrews Clark Memorial Lib., U. of California, 1980. p. 1–55.

**Shapiro D** see **Crowley JE**

**Shapiro E:** Robert Koch and his tuberculin fallacy. **Pharos** 1983 Fall;46(4):19–22

**Shapiro E:** The first textbook of electrocardiography. Thomas Lewis: Clinical Electrocardiography. **J Am Coll Cardiol** 1983 Apr;1(4):1160–1

**Shapiro E** see **Shapiro AK**

**Shapiro HD:** Getting back---and down---to basics. **Rev Am Hist** 1977;5(2):242–48

**Shapiro HL:** Peking man. London, George Allen & Unwin, 1976. 190 p.

**Shapiro LJ, Angorn RA, McCormick WC:** Look-alike prescription drugs. A historical perspective of the legal issues. **Am Pharm** 1982 Aug;22(8):26–30

**Shapiro MF:** Medical aid provided by American, Canadian and British Nationals to the Spanish Republic during the Civil War, 1936–1939. **Int J Health Serv** 1983;13(3):443–58

**Shapiro MF:** Medical aid to the Spanish Republic during the Civil War (1936–1939). **Ann Intern Med** 1982 Jul;97(1):119–24

**Sharaf M:** Fury on Earth. A biography of Wilhelm Reich. New York, St. Martin's Press/Marek, 1983. xiii, 550 p.

**Sharafiddinov TA** see **Abdullaev AKh**

**Sharipov MK:** Opyt raboty i dostizheniia sanitarno-épidemiologicheskoĭ sluzhby Uzbekskoĭ SSR. **Gig Sanit** 1982 Dec;(12):31–3

**Sharkey PW, ed:** Philosophy, religion and psychotherapy. Essays in the philosophical foundations of psychotherapy. Washington, University Press of America, 1982. xiii, 227 p. Contributions by R. Macklin, J. E. Morris, R. N. Sollod, J. Needleman, C. E. Scott, M. Friedman, J. F. Rychlak, E. Weisskopf-Joelson, T. S. Szasz, R. J. Sullivan.

**Sharma OA:** Avicenna's description of tuberculosis. **Bull Indian Inst Hist Med (Hyderabad)** 1981;1–4:83–6

**Sharma OP, James DG:** Did Osler's patient, Hannah W, have sarcoidosis? An historical footnote. **Chest** 1984 Aug;86(2):263–4

**Sharma OP:** Robert Willan remembered. **J Am Acad Dermatol** 1983 Dec;9(6):971–6

**Sharma PV:** Contributions of Sarngadhara in the field of materia medica and pharmacy. **Indian J Hist Sci** 1981, reçu 1982;16(1):3–10

**Sharma PV:** Dalhana's version of the Suśruta Samhita. **Bull Indian Inst Hist Med (Hyderabad)** 1979;9:27–32

**Sharma PV:** Fruits and vegetables in ancient India. Varanasi and Delhi, Chaukhambha Orientalia, 1979. xxvl, 188 p. (Jaikrishnadas Ayurveda Series, No. 28).

**Sharma RK, Dash B, ed:** Agniveśa Caraka samhita: text with English translation and critical exposition based on Cakrapani Datta's Ayurveda dipika. Vol I, Sutra Sthana. Varanasi: Chowkhamba Sanskrit Series Office, 1976. xlv, 619 p. (Chowkhamba Sanskrit Studies; 94).

**Sharma S, et al:** Realms of Ayurveda. Scientific excursions by nineteen scholars. New Delhi, Arnold-Heinemann, 1979. 336 p.

**Sharman IM:** Symposium on 'Vitamin A in nutrition and disease.' Historical introduction. **Proc Nutr Soc** 1983 Jan;42(1):1–5

**Sharman IM:** Vitamins: essential dietary constituents discovered. **Endeavour** 1977;1(3–4):97–102

**Sharmanov TSh:** Dostizheniia okhrany materinstva i detstva v Kazakhskoĭ SSR. **Pediatriia** 1982 Dec;(12):18–22

**Sharp ES:** Nurse-midwifery education: Its successes, failures, and future. **J Nurse Midwife** 1983 Mar–Apr;28(2):17–23

**Sharp RG:** Tribute to a great teacher. **S Afr Med J** 1979 Dec 15;56(25):1059–64

**Sharp S** see **Sutherland G**

**Sharpe WD:** Autopsies at Newark City Hospital, 1908 to 1911. **J Med Soc NJ** 1984 Jan;81(1):53–62

**Sharpless J:** Population redistribution in the American past: empirical generalizations and theoretical perspectives. **Soc Sci Q** 1980;61(3–4):401–17

**Sharrard WJ:** 90th anniversary of the Revue de Chirurgie Orthopédique: an outsider's view. **Rev Chir Orthop** 1981;67(3):165–6

**Shaternikov VA, Konyshev VA:** 50-ia godovshchina pervogo piatiletnego plana razvitiia narodnogo khoziaĭstva SSSR i nauka o pitanii v nasheĭ strane. **Vopr Pitan** 1979 Sep–Oct;(5):3–7

**Shatzmiller J:** Livres médicaux et éducation médicale: à props d'un contrat de Marseille en 1316. **Mediaev Stud** 1980;42:463–70

**Shavianidze GO** see **Shavianidze ON**

**Shavianidze ON, Shavianidze GO:** Kurort Tskhaltubo. **Vopr Kurortol Fizioter Lech Fiz Kult** 1984 Jul–Aug;(4):53–5

**Shaw A, Davis PD:** The lung ventilator--an engineering appraisal. **Eng Med** 1977 Jul;6(3):85–9

**Shaw AB:** East Anglian bladder stone. **J R Soc Med** 1979 Mar;72(3):222–8

**Shaw AB:** Paget's diseases. **Practitioner** 1980 Dec;224(1350):1323–7

**Shaw AB:** Sir Thomas Browne: the man and the physician. **Br Med J [Clin Res]** 1982 Jul 3;285(6334):40–2

**Shaw JA:** The postadolescent crisis of John Stuart Mill. **Adolesc Psychiatry** 1982;10:85–98

**Shaw LL** see **Emerson RM**

**Shaw R, Stubenbord WT:** Alexis Carrel, M.D.; contribution to kidney transplantation and preservation. **NY State J Med** 1980 Aug;80(9):1438–42

**Shaw S:** Seasonal foundations: Santa-the saint who founded hospitals. **Nurs Mirror** 1981 Dec 23–30;153(26):30–1

**Shchabad AL** see **Lopatkin NA**

**Shchepetova GA** see **Aleksandrovskiĭ BN**

**Shcherbina VP, Liashenko NI:** Akademik Evgeniĭ Nikanorovich Pavlovskiĭ (k 100-letiiu so dnia rozhdeniia). **Voen Med Zh** 1984 Feb;(2):65–8

**Shcherbina VP, Liashenko NI:** Vsia zhizn'--vdokhnovennyĭ trud. **Voen Med Zh** 1983 Mar;3:70–1

**Shcherbina VP** see **Pervomaĭskiĭ GS**

**Shcherbina VP** see **Shusterov AK**

**Shchetova GA** see **Aleksandrovskiĭ BN**

**Shdanov VM:** Molekularbiologie und Okologie der Virusgrippe. **Z Erkr Atmungsorgane** 1983;161(1):74–9

**Shea JJ:** Management of the stapes footplate with special reference to otosclerosis. **J Laryngol Otol** 1982 May;96(5):383–403

**Sheail P:** Hampshire man [Wilfred Buckley] and the quest for clean milk. **Hampshire** 1981 Mar;:60–2

**Shearer AW:** A commitment to excellence: a history of the School of Nursing, College of Allied Health Sciences, Thomas Jefferson University, 1891–1982. Wynnewood, Pa., Heden–Livingston, 1982. x, 148 p.

**Shearer D:** History of the Canterbury Medical Library 1934–1972. **NZ Libr** 1972 Oct;35(5):266–9

**Shearer J:** History of the Department of Nursing Education at the North Dakota State Hospital. **Prairie Rose** 1984 Oct–Dec;53(4):20–1

**Shearing SP:** Evolution of the posterior chamber intraocular lens. **J Am Intraocul Implant Soc** 1984 Summer;10(3):343–6

**Shedlin MG, Hollerbach PE:** Modern and traditional fertility regulation in a Mexican community: the process of decision making. **Stud Fam Plann** 1981 Jun–Jul:12(6–7):278–96

**Sheehan DV, Sheehan KH:** The classification of anxiety and hysterical states. Part I. Historical review and empirical delineation. **J Clin Psychopharmacol** 1982 Aug;2(4):235–44

**Sheehan E:** Victorian clitoridectomy: Isaac Baker Brown and his harmless operative procedure. **Med Anthropol Newsl** 1981;12(4):9–15

**Sheehan JC:** The enchanted ring. The untold story of penicillin. Cambridge, Mass., London, MIT Press, 1982. xvi, 224 p.

**Sheehan KH** see **Sheehan DV**

**Sheehan PW, Perry CW:** Methodologies of hypnosis. Hillsdale, N. J., Erlbaum, New York, Halsted Press, 1976. xiii, 329 p.

**Sheerin DJ:** A Carolingian cure recovered: Erasmus' citation of Hucbald of St. Amand's Ecloga de caluis. **Bibl Hum Renaissance** 1980 Jan;42(1):167–71

**Sheets–Johnstone M:** Why Lamarck did not discover the principle of natural selection. **J Hist Biol** 1982 Fall;15(3):443–65

**Sheets–Pyenson S:** Darwin's data: his reading of natural history journals, 1837–1842. **J Hist Biol** 1981 Fall;14(2):231–48

**Sheets–Pyenson S:** From the north to Red Lion Court: the creation and early years of the Annals of Natural History. **Arch Nat Hist** 1981 Oct;10(2):221–49

**Shegina F:** Survey of mental health services of hospitals in the greater Manila area. **Unitas** 1972;45(2):89–113

**Shehadi WH:** The biliary system through the ages. **Int Surg** 1979 Nov–Dec;64(6):63–78

**Shehadi WH:** X-ray tubes and other historic memorabilia. **Med Radiogr Photogr** 1981;57(2):preceding p 21

**Shehata MA:** History of laryngeal intubation. **Middle East J Anaesthesiol** 1981 Feb;6(1):49–53

**Shehata MA:** The larynx in Islamic medicine. **Middle East J Anaesthesiol** 1981 Jun;6(2):113–9

**Sheiham A** see **Dussault G**

**Sheil AG** see **Hall BM**

**Sheils WJ, ed:** The Church and healing. Papers read at the twentieth summer meeting and the twenty–first winter meeting of the Ecclesiastical History Society. Oxford, Basil Blackwell for the Society, 1982. xxiv, 440 p. (Studies in Church History, v. 19).

**Sheiman I:** Kapitalizm i problemy zdravo–okhraneniia. **Mirovaia Ekon Mezhdunar Otnosheniia** 1979;12:116–23

**Sheĭman IB, Petrovskaia EG, Pomianskaia NIu, et al:** Stanovlenie tsitologicheskoĭ diagnostiki vo L'vovskoĭ oblasti. **Lab Delo** 1984;(1):52–4

**Sheldon PB:** Mortar and pestle. **J Med Soc NJ** 1983 Feb;80(2):134

**Sheldon PB:** Wooden medicine chest. **J Med Soc NJ** 1983 May;80(5):383

**Sheldrick P:** 'Skinny bones' from the Dakhleh Oasis. **Paleopathol Newsl** 1980 Jun;(30):7–10

**Shelestov DK:** U istokov istoricheskoi demografii. **Vestn Mosk Univ Ser 8 Istor** 1982;(3):21–33

**Sheliuzhenko A:** Ekonomicheskie posledstviia poteri rabochego vremeni v sviazi s netrudosposobnost'iu po bolezni. **Ekon Sov Ukr** 1972;14(3):63–6

**Shell DH, Sparkman RS:** John Allan Wyeth, MD. Surgeon, soldier, author and founder of postgraduate medical education in America. **Am J Surg** 1980 Sep;140(3):447–56

**Shell DH:** John Bingham Roberts: Philadelphia plastic surgeon. **Plast Reconstr Surg** 1982 Jan;69(1):145–54

**Shellard EJ:** Jaborandi: a note on the contribution of E. M. Holmes to the identification of commercially available Pilocarpus and species. **J Ethnopharmacol** 1979 Dec;1(4):407–10

**Shellard EJ:** Some early women research workers in British pharmacy 1886–1912. **Pharm Hist (London)** 1982 Aug;12(2):2–3

**Shelley HS:** The Moll Collection on hypnotism at Vanderbilt. **Bull Med Libr Assoc** 1977 Jan;65(1):65–6

**Shelley WB:** Commentary: antihistamines and the treatment of urticaria. **Arch Dermatol** 1983 May;119(5):442–4

**Shelley WB:** Experimental disease in the skin of man. A review. **Acta Derm Venereol [Suppl] (Stockh)** 1982;108:1–38

**Shelley WB, Beerman H:** Jay Frank Schamberg (1870–1934). **Am J Dermatopathol** 1984 Oct;6(5):441–4

**Shelp EE:** The experience of illness: integrating metaphors and the transcendence of illness. **J Med Philos** 1984 Aug;9(3):253–6

**Shemluck M:** Medicinal and other uses of the Compositae by Indians in the United States and Canada. **J Ethnopharmacol** 1982 May;5(3):303–58

**Shen WW, Soldo JJ:** Symbol hunting in James Joyce's 'syphilizations'. **Arch Intern Med** 1981 Apr;141(5):691–2

**Shengelia MS:** Feudal Georgia translational medical literature (IX–I half of XIX century). In International Congress of the History of Medicine, 27th, Barcelona, 1980. Actas. Barcelona, Académia de Ciències Médiques de Catalunya i Balears, 1981. p. 340–5.

**Shengeliia GM:** 'Lechebnaia kniga––Karabadini' Z. Panaskerteli–Tsitsishvili. **Klin Med (Mosk)** 1981 Jun;59(6):110–2

**Shengeliia MS:** Georgievskiĭ traktat i istoriia russko–gruzinskikh vzaimootnosheniĭ v oblasti meditsiny. **Sov Zdravookhr** 1984;(3):54–5

**Shengeliia MS:** Izuchenie istorii meditsiny v soiuznykh respublikakh. **Sov Zdravookhr** 1982;(7):53–5

**Shenoy BV, Scheithauer BW:** Sir James Paget, F.R.S. **Mayo Clin Proc** 1983 Jan;58(1):51–5

**Sheon RP:** Transcutaneous electrical nerve stimulation. From electric eels to electrodes. **Postgrad Med** 1984 Apr;75(5):71–4

**Shepard FE** see **Burke GW**

**Shepard L** see **Maurizi AR**

**Shepardson M:** Changes in Navajo mortuary practices and beliefs. **Am Indian Q** 1978;4(4):383–96

**Shephard DA, Lévesque A, ed:** Norman Bethune. His time and his legacy. Ottawa, Canadian Public Health Association, 1982. xii, 253 p.

**Shephard L, ed:** Encyclopedia of occultism and parapsychology. A compendium of information on the occult sciences, magic, demonology, superstitions, spiritism, mysticism, metaphysics, psychical science, and parapsychology, with biographical and bibliographical notes and comprehensive indexes. Detroit, Gale, 1978. Two volumes.

**Shepherd J, Dawber RP:** The historical and scientific basis of cryosurgery. **Clin Exp Dermatol** 1982 May;7(3):321–8

**Shepherd JA:** Lawson Tait - disciple of Charles Darwin. **Br Med J [Clin Res]** 1982 May;284(6326):1386–7

**Shepherd JA:** Lawson Tait, the rebellious surgeon (1845–1899). Lawrence, Kansas, Coronado Press, xv, 249 p.

**Shepherd JJ:** Nutrition in the history of Tasmania. **JPEN J Parenter Enteral Nutr** 1980 May–Jun;4(3):312–3

**Shepherd M:** From social medicine to social psychiatry: the achievement of Sir Aubrey Lewis. **Psychol Med** 1980 May;10(2):211–8

**Shepherd M:** La découverte de la nature de la pellagre. Leçons d'une recherche épidémiologique et psychiatrique remarquable. **Acta Psychiatr Belg** 1983 May–Jun;83(3):295–303

**Shepherd M:** Social psychiatry and epidemiology. **Practitioner** 1983 Jan;227(1375):148–50

**Shepherd M:** The psycho–historians: a psychiatrist's skepticism. **Encounter (Lond)** 1979;52(3):35–42

**Shepherd MA:** Lunacy and labour. **Soc Stud Labour Hist** 1977;(34):61–9

**Shepherd RG:** Science news of controversy: the case of marijuana. **Journalism Monogr** 1979;62:1–36

**Shepherd RG:** Selectivity of sources: reporting the marijuana controversy. **J Commun** 1981;31(2):129–37

**Sheppard J:** Illustrations from the Wellcome Institute Library: Sir Leonard Rogers, FRS (1868–1962) and his papers. **Med Hist** 1983 Apr;27(2):214–5

**Sheppard J:** Illustrations from the Wellcome Institute Library: the Chain papers. **Med Hist** 1983 Oct;27(4):434–5

**Sheppard J** see **Davies C, ed**

**Sheppard J** see **Foster J**

**Sheptunova ZI:** Dzh R. Partington - vydaiushchiisia istorik khimii. **Vopr Istor Estestvozn Tekh** 1981;3:107–10

**Shereshevskiĭ AM:** Organizatsiia usovershenstvovaniia vracheĭ–psikhiatrov v Rossii. **Zh Nevropatol Psikhiatr** 1980;80(8):1230–4

**Shereshevskiĭ AM** see **Panchenko PM**

**Shereshevskiĭ AM** see **Rokhlin LL**

**Shereshevskiĭ GM:** O stanovlenii i razvitii gospital'nogo dela. **Voen Med Zh** 1983 Oct;10:67–9

**Shereshkov GM, Leont'ev PA:** Velikiĭ podvig sovetskogo naroda. **Vopr Okhr Materin Det** 1980 May;25(5):3–6

**Shergold PR** see **Nicholas S**

**Sheridan RB:** The Guinea surgeons on the middle passage: the provision of medical services in the British slave trade. **Int J Afr Hist Stud** 1981;14(4):601–25

**Sherlock S:** Landmark perspective: Landmarks in viral hepatitis. **JAMA** 1984 Jul 20;252(3):402–6

**Sherman ED:** David Ben–Gurion (1886–1973). **J Am Geriatr Soc** 1983 Aug;31(8):501–5

**Sherman ED:** Geriatric profile of Eleanor Roosevelt (1884–1962). **J Am Geriatr Soc** 1983 Jan;31(1):28–33

**Sherman H** see **Zinner ID**

**Sherman MH:** Psychosensory images from Virginia Woolf's 'A Sketch of the Past'. **Psychoanal Rev** 1983 Spring;70(1):33–9

**Sherman MH:** The paradox of Theodor Reik. **Psychoanal Rev** 1981–82 Winter;68(4):467–72

**Sherman PD:** Colour vision in the nineteenth century: the Young–Helmholtz–Maxwell theory. Bristol, Adam Hilger, 1981. xiii, 233 p.

**Sherman R:** Perspectives in management of trauma to the spleen. **J Trauma** 1980 Jan;20(1):1–13

**Sherman RA** see **Pechter EA**

**Sherman MH, ed:** Psychoanalysis and old Vienna: Freud, Reik, Schnitzler, Kraus. New York, Human Sciences Press, 1978. 192 p.

**Sherrard ML:** History of the Baltimore County Medical Association. **Md State Med J** 1983 May;32(5):332

**Sherrington A:** Canadian medical periodicals on microfiche. **Can Med Assoc J** 1981 Feb 15;124(4):361–2

**Sherrington A:** Seventy years of editorial excellence. **Can Med Assoc J**

1981 Jul 1;125(1):85, 88, 91-3

**Sherry S:** A tribute to Kenneth M. Brinkhous, M.D. **Thromb Haemost** 1979 Feb 28;40(1):3-23

**Sherwin-White SM:** The Coan school of medicine. In her: Ancient Cos. An historical study from the Dorian settlement to the Imperial period. Göttingen, Vendenhoeck & Ruprecht, 1978. p. 256-289 (Hypomnemata, 51).

**Sherwood RH:** Discovery of kerosene. **NS Hist Q** 1979;9(2):157-64

**Shestdeset godini Vissh veterinarnomeditsinski institut: Vet Med Nauki** 1982;19(7):3-5

**Shestdeset godini Vissh veterinarnomeditsinski institut: Vet Med Nauki** 1984;21(1):3-5

**Shetty PS:** A critical analysis of Avicenna's contribution to physiology. **Bull Indian Inst Hist Med (Hyderabad)** 1981;1-4:152-60

**Shevchenko IT:** K istorii protivorakovoĭ bor'by na Ukraine. **Klin Khir** 1982 May;(5):67-70

**Shewsbury JD:** A history of bubonic plague in the British Isles. Cambridge, University Press, 1970. xi, 661 p.

**Sheynin OB:** On the history of medical statistics. **Arch Hist Exact Sci** 1982;26(3):241-86

**Sheynin OB:** On the history of the statistical method in biology. **Arch Hist Exact Sci** 1980;22(4):323-71

**Shi NC:** Forensic laboratory work in Burma (with special reference to the Office of the Chemical Examiner, Burma). **Am J Forensic Med Pathol** 1980 Jun;1(2):173-6

**Shi Changyong:** [Life and chronology of Xue Lizhai.] (Chi). **Chin J Med Hist** 1981;11:65-9

**Shi Yuanyi:** [Advanced medical education in north-east China before the Liberation] (Chi). **Chung Hua I Shih Tsa Chih** 1981;11:70-4

**Shibaike N, Ogawa S:** [A historical study on formation of policy for 'Nambyo' (intractable diseases)] (Jpn). **Igakushi Kenkyu** 1978;50:49-59

**Shick TW:** Race, class, and medicine: 'Bad Blood' in twentieth-century America. **J Ethn Stud** 1982;10(2):97-105

**Shields EA:** A history of the United States Army Nurse Corps (female): 1901-1937. Ed. D. Diss., Columbia University Teachers College. New York, 1980. 232 leaves.

**Shields J** see **Hoffman W**

**Shields P:** Leipoldt the physician. **S Afr Med J** 1980;58:932-3

**Shields RT:** He helped shape Virginia: Dr. Wiliam Fleming, 1728-1795. **Va Med** 1982 Jul;109(7):441-5

**Shields SA:** The variability hypothesis: the history of a biological model of sex differences in intelligence. **Signs** 1982;7:769-97

**Shigematsu I, ed, Kawasaki T, ed, Kusakawa S, ed:** Kawasakibyo (MCLS) kenkyu no ayumi. Tokyo, Kindai Shuppan, 1976. ix, 224 p.

**Shih CJ:** Perspectives in international neurosurgery: neurosurgery in Taiwan. **Neurosurgery** 1979 Nov;5(5):637-40

**Shik LL:** Akademik V. V. Parin kak fiziolog. **Vestn Akad Med Nauk SSSR** 1984;(4):12-5

**Shiliaev VG** see **Volkov VV**

**Shils ME:** Historical aspects of minerals and vitamins in parenteral nutrition. **Fed Proc** 1984 Apr;43(5):1412-6

**Shima K:** [Endless voyage. The life of Ms. Shin Tanaka. 5. Chapter 2.] (Jpn). **Josanpu Zasshi** 1982 Nov;36(11):946-53 (continued regularly)

**Shima K:** [Endless voyage. The life of Ms. Shin Tanaka. 7. Chapter 2] (Jpn). **Josanpu Zasshi** 1983 Jan;37(1):72-9

**Shimabukuro R:** [History of the white nursing uniform. A study on the origin of the white uniform as the symbol of nursing] (Jpn). **Kurinikaru Sutadi** 1984 Jun;5(6):688-94

**Shimamura K:** [Chronological review of TB research - from a clinical viewpoint.] (Jpn). **Kekkaku** 1980;55:383-8

**Shimanine T** see **Kageyama K**

**Shimazono N:** Eiyogakushi. Tokyo: Asakura Shoten, Showa 53 nen [1978]. viii, 202 p.

**Shimizu K:** [Blood transfusion--practice at Komagome Municipal Hospital. 12. Progress in blood transfusion]. (Jpn) **Kangogaku Zasshi** 1979 Dec;43(12):1313-6

**Shimkin MB:** Roads to Oz. II. A personal account of some U.S.-USSR medical exchanges and contacts. 1942--1962. **Perspect Biol Med** 1979 Autumn;23(1):118-44

**Shimkin MB, ed:** Some classics of experimental oncology. 50 selections, 1775-1965. Bethesda, National Institutes of Health, 1980. 739 p. (NIH Publication No. 80-2150).

**Shimmura T:** [Development and alteration of medical system in the Ritsuryo code regimen] (Jpn). **Igakushi Kenkyu** 1978;49:27-30

**Shimmura T:** [Formation of the medical system in the Ritsyryo code regimen] (Jpn). **Igakushi Kenkyu** 1977;48:25-9

**Shimoosa T:** [History of dental prothesis and dental engineering] (Jpn). **Shikai Tenbo** 1982 Oct;60(4):731-44

**Shimoyama K:** [Care and nursing given at Koishikawa Clinic] (Jpn). **Kurinikaru Sutadi** 1983 Jul;4(7):837-42

**Shin JS:** Leprosy in Korea. **Nippon Rai Gakkai Zasshi** 1982 Oct-Dec;51(4):211-6

**Shin Y** see **Reid JD**

**Shinebourne EA:** Ethics of innovative cardiac surgery. **Br Heart J** 1984 Dec;52(6):597-601

**Shingarov GKh:** Filosofskie voprosy ucheniia o vyssheĭ nervnoĭ deiatel'nosti v tvorchestve E. A. Asratiana. **Zh Vyssh Nerv Deiat** 1983 Mar-Apr;33(2):204-10

**Shingarov GKh:** Gordost' russkoĭ nauki (k 150-letiiu so dnia rozhdeniia I. M. Sechenova). **Patol Fiziol Eksp Ter** 1979 Nov-Dec;(6):3-8

**Shingarov Gkh:** Teoreticheskie nasledie V. I. Lenina i nekotorye metodologicheskie problemy sovremennoĭ meditsiny. **Vestn Akad Med Nauk SSSR** 1980;(4):9-16

**Shingarov GKh** see **Asratian EA**

**Shinn M** see **Felton BJ**

**Shipek FE:** A native American adaptation to drought: the Kumeyaay as seen in the San Diego Mission records, 1770-1798. **Ethnohistory** 1981;28(4):295-312

**Shipitsina NK:** Vliianie issledovaniĭ V. N. Beklemisheva v oblasti obshcheĭ biologii, parazitologii i épidemiologii transmissivnykh bolezneŭ na razvitie étikh otrasleĭ nauki (k 90-letiiu so dnia rozhdeniia). **Med Parazitol (Mosk)** 1982 Mar-Apr;60(2):86-8

**Shipley M, Agass M, Bell A, et al:** The Quebec Medicare Programme. **R Soc Health J** 1982 Feb;102(1):37-8, 43

**Shipman P:** Applications of scanning electron microscopy to taphonomic problems. **Ann NY Acad Sci** 1981;376:357-85

**Shipov VL** see **Khokhlov LK**

**Shipp JC:** To serve the people: medical education and care in the People's Republic of China. **Ann Intern Med** 1982 Aug;97(2):277-9

**Shires GT:** The fourth surgical renaissance? **Ann Surg** 1980 Sep;192(3):269-81

**Shirkey HC:** Clinical pharmacy--past, present & future. **Drug Intell Clin Pharm** 1977 Nov;(11):674-7

**Shirokov IuG, Lebedeva NV, Koliadich MN:** Uchastie L. K. Khotsianova v rabote s'ezdov gigienistov i sanitarnykh vracheĭ. **Gig Sanit** 1983 Feb;(2):31-5

**Shishkin AP:** Bor'ba s detskoĭ smertnost'iu v pervye gody Sovetskoĭ vlasti. **Sov Zdravookhr** 1981;(12):46-50

**Shishkin AP:** Gosudarstvennyĭ institut sotsial'noĭ gigieny Narkomzdrava RSFSR i ego rol' v razvitii teorii i organizatsii sovetskogo. **Sov Zdravookhr** 1982;(6):59-62

**Shishkin AP:** Organizatsiia Narodnykh komissariatov zdravookhraneniia RSFSR i drugikh soiuznykh respublik (1918-1922) (K 65-letiiu sozdaniia Narodnogo komissariata zdravookhraneniia RSFSR). **Sov Zdravookhr** 1983;(8):47-51

**Shishkin AP:** Pervyĭ piatiletniĭ plan razvitiia zdravookhraneniia strany Sovetov. **Sov Zdravookhr** 1980;(9):46-9

**Shishkin AP:** Sozdanie seti institutov zdravookhraneniia i sotsial'noĭ gigieny v SSSR v 20-x--nachale 30-x godov. **Sov Zdravookhr** 1982;(10):57-61

**Shishkin AP:** Vazhnyĭ étap v stanovlenii sovetskogo zdravookhraneniia. **Sov Zdravookhr** 1983;(1):57-61

**Shishkin AP:** Voprosy profilaktiki v deiatel'nosti Gosudarstvennogo Instituta Sotsial'noĭ Gigieny Narkomzdrava RSFSR (k 65-letiiu obrazovaniia N rodnogo Komissariata Zdravookhraneniia RSFSR). **Sov Zdravookhr** 1983;6:55-8

**Shishkin NA, Orlova RV:** Stanovlenie aptechnoĭ sistemy v Iaroslavskoi oblasti. **Farmatsiia** 1980 Mar-Apr;29(2):52-5

**Shishkov VP, Poliakov AA:** Vsesoiuznyĭ tsentr sel'skokhoziaĭstvennoĭ nauki (k 50-letiiu VASKhNIL). **Veterinariia** 1979 Dec;(12):5-8

**Shitikov BD** see **Savchenko NE**

**Shitl'man NL** see **Egorysheva IV**

**Shitskova AP:** Moskovskomu ordena Trudovogo Krasnogo Znameni nauchno-issledova-tel'smkou institutu gigieny im. F. F. Erismana--60 let. **Gig Sanit** 1981 Jun;(6):27-31

**Shitskova AP:** Osnovnye itogi raboty Moskovskogo NII gigieny im. F. F. Erismana v desiatoĭ piatiletke po probleme 'Nauchnye osnovy gigieny pitaniia' (k 60-letiiu so dnia osnovaniia instituta). **Vopr Pitan** 1982 Mar-Apr;(2):64-7

**Shitskova AP, Novikov IV, Borisenkova RV, et al:** Stanovlenie sanitarnoĭ sluzhby RSFSR. **Gig Sanit** 1982 Sep;(9):6-11

**Shiva V, Bandyopadhyay J:** The large and fragile community of scientists in India. **Minerva** 1980 Winter;18(4):575-94

**Shivers FR** see **Capper J**

**Shizuoka-ken I:** Shizuoka-ken Ishikai nijunenshi. Shizuoka, Japan Do Ishikai, Showa 50 nen 1975. 13, 999 p.

**Shizusawa K:** [Columbus as the 1st known patient with Reiter's disease?] (Jpn). **Kango** 1981 Apr;33(4):83

**Shlepnina TG** see **Akulov KI**

**Shliakhtenko LI, Kryga LN, Liamtseva GA, et al:** Evoliutsiia épidemicheskogo protsessa virusnogo gepatita v Leningrade za 30 let. **Tr Inst Pastera** 1982;57:43-5

**Shliakhtenko LI** see **Rykushin IuP**

**Shliapak AE:** Partiĭno-politicheskaia rabota v ěvakogospitaliakh Kavkazskikh Mineral'nykh Vod. **Voen Med Zh** 1981 Nov;(11):69-70

**Shlykov IP, Dedov II:** Anatoliĭ Anatol'evich Voĭtkevich. **Arkh Anat Gistol Embriol** 1979 Dec;77(12):81-4

**Shmeleva VV** see **Shul'pina NB**

**Shmidt AA:** Stranitsy vospominanii o blokade goroda Lenina. **Latv PSR Zinat Akad Vestis** 1975;(5):10-7

**Shneidman ES:** The suicidal logic of Cesare Pavese. **J Am Acad Psychoanal** 1982 Oct;10(4):547-63

**Shoemaker P, Jones MV:** From infirmaries to intensive care: hospitals in Wisconsin. In Numbers RL, Leavitt JW, ed: Wisconsin medicine. Historical perspectives. Madison, University of Wisconsin Press, 1981. p. 105-31.

**Sholtes V** see **Black J**

**Shonick W:** Early developments and recent trends in the evolution of the local public hospital. **Annu Rev Public Health** 1984;5:53-81

**Shor MB** see **Shor RE**

**Shor RE, Shor MB, Williams DC:** The distinction between the antismoking and nonsmokers' rights movements. **J Psychol** 1980 Sep;106(First Half):129-46

**Shore MF:** Cecil Rhodes and the ego ideal. **J Interdiscip Hist** 1979;10(2):249–65
**Shore MF:** The psychogenic theory of history. **J Interdiscip Hist** 1979;9(3):517–23
**Shore MF** see **Albin M**
**Shorey JJ** see **Henker FO**
**Short AL:** Portraits, paintings and caricatures. **Pharm Hist (London)** 1970 Jun;1(5):10–11
**Short GR:** Postal and pharmaceutical history. **Pharm Hist (London)** 1974 Dec;4(3):5–6
**Short GR** see **Lothian A**
**Short RV:** The scientific contributions of Professor Emmanuel Ciprian Amoroso, CBE, TC, FRS. **J Reprod Fertil [Suppl]** 1982 Nov;31:1–8
**A short history of the dental drill: J Am Dent Assoc** 1984 Apr;108(4):572–3
**Shorter E:** L'âge des premières règles en France, 1750–1950. **Ann Econ Soc Civilis** 1981;36(3):495–511
**Shorter E:** Women's diseases before 1900. In M. Albin, R. J. Devlin, G. Heeger, ed: New directions in psychohistory. The Adelphi papers in honor of Erik H. Erikson. Lexington, Toronto, D. C. Heath, 1980. p. 183–208.
**Shorter E** see **Cutright P**
**Shorter FC** see **Ozbay F**
**Shortt HE:** Robert Thomson Leiper. In Dictionary of national biography, 1961–1970. Suppl. 8, 1981. p. 647–8.
**Shortt SE:** Andrew Macphail: the ideal in nature. In his The search for an ideal: six Canadian intellectuals and their convictions in an age of transition, 1890–1930. Toronto, Buffalo, University of Toronto Press, 1976. p. 12–38.
**Shortt SE:** Approaches to the physician's life. **Bull Hist Med** 1981 Spring;55(1):124–7
**Shortt SE:** Banting, insulin and the question of simultaneous discovery. **Queens Q** 1982;89(2):260–73
**Shortt SE:** 'Before the age of miracles': the rise, fall, and rebirth of general practice in Canada, 1890–1940. In Roland CG, ed: Health, disease and medicine. Toronto, Hannah Institute for the History of Medicine, 1984. p. 123–52.
**Shortt SE:** Cholera: doctors' dilemma, historians' delight. **Queens Q** 1981;88(1):130–4
**Shortt SE:** Clinical practice and the social history of medicine: a theoretical accord. **Bull Hist Med** 1981 Winter;55(4):533–42
**Shortt SE:** History in the medical curriculum. A clinical perspective. **JAMA** 1982 Jul 2;248(1):79–81
**Shortt SE:** Medical professionalization: pitfalls and promise in the historiography. **HSTC** 1981 Sep;19(5 no 3):210–9
**Shortt SE:** Physicians, science, and status: issues in the professionalization of Anglo-American medicine in the nineteenth century. **Med Hist** 1983 Jan;27(1):51–68
**Shortt SE:** R. M. Bucke: vital force, evolution and somatic psychiatry, 1862–1902. In International Congress of the History of Medicine, 27th, Barcelona, 1980. Actas. Barcelona, Acadèmia de Ciències Mèdiques de Catalunya i Balears, 1981. p. 149–53.
**Shortt SE, ed:** Medicine in Canadian society: historical perspectives. Montreal, McGill-Queen's University Press, 1981. xiii, 506 p. Reprinted articles by various authors.
**Shoshan A:** Rift Valley Fever and its relation to the 4th plague. **Koroth** 1980 Jun;7(11–12):810–3
**Shoshan B:** Notes sur les épidemies de peste en Egypte. **Ann Demogr Hist (Paris)** 1981;:387–404
**Shostak NA, Gorelova LE:** Kafedra fakul'tetskoĭ terapii II Moskovskogo meditsinskogo instituta im. I. N. Pirogova (k 70–letiiu so dnia osnovaniia). **Vopr Revm** 1980 Jan–Mar;(1):66–9
**Showa Byoin Kumiai:** Koritsu Showa Byoin gojunen no ayumi. Kodaira, Japan, Showa Byoin Kumiai, Showa 52 nen, 1977. xvii, iii, 384 p.
**Showalter E:** Victorian women and insanity. **Victorian Stud** 1980;23(2):157–81
**Showalter E** see **Scull A, ed**
**Shtel'makh NI** see **Chernenko VD**
**Shtenberg AI:** Osnovnye itogi razvitiia gigieny pitaniia. **Vopr Pitan** 1980 Sep–Oct;(5):9–15
**Shtenberg AI** see **Efremov VV**
**Shterev I:** 35 let samootverzhennogo truda. **Veterinariia** 1979 Nov;(11):12–4
**Shtern MI, Karinskaia GS:** Zemskiĭ vrach A. V. Ivanov. **Sov Zdravookhr** 1983;(8):64–7
**Shtern MI** see **Safarov RN**
**Shtern RD:** O prioritete opredeleniia limfomatoza zheludka otechestvennymi issledovateliami. **Arkh Patol** 1983;45(5):66–8
**Shtil'man NL** see **Idel'chik KhI**
**Shtil'man NL** see **Korotkikh RV**
**Shtil'man NL** see **Rabinovich RS**
**Shtil'man NL** see **Vengrova IV**
**Shtrom RS:** Meditsinskoe obsluzhivanie shakhterov i metallurgov Donbassa v gody pervoĭ piatiletki (k 50–letiiu pervoĭ piatiletki). **Sov Zdravookhr** 1980;(3):57–9
**Shu-Yuen Yim:** Famine relief statistics as a guide to the population of sixteenth-century China: a case-study of Honan province. **Ch'ing-Shih Wen-t'i** 1978;3(9):1–30
**Shugg D** see **Braithwaite PA**
**Shui-Meng NG** see **Smith PC**
**Shukla KP** see **Singhal GD**
**Shukurov AK, Pulatov RP:** [Development of health resort science and physiotherapy in Uzbekistan]. (Rus) **Vopr Kurortol Fizioter Lech Fiz Kult** 1979 Nov–Dec;(6):7–11
**Shulim JI:** The birth of a revolutionary: Robespierre in Artois. **Consortium Revolut Eur 1750–1850 Proc** 1977;:22–33
**Shulimin VA:** Osobennosti meditsinskogo obespecheniia 193–ĭ strelkovoĭ divizii v boiakh za Stalingrad. **Voen Med Zh** 1982 Nov;(11):61–2
**Shulman GL** see **Hearst E, ed**
**Shul'pina NB, Krasnov ML, Shmeleva VV:** Postdiplomnoe usovershenstvovanie oftal'mologov (k 50–letiiu Tsentral'nogo instituta usovershenstvovaniia vracheĭ). **Vestn Oftalmol** 1980 Sep–Oct;(5):7–10
**Shul'tsev GP:** Aleksandr Porfir'evich Borodin (k 150–letiiu so dnia rozhdeniia). **Klin Med (Mosk)** 1984 Jul;62(7):144–7
**Shul'tsev GP:** Khronologiia zhizni i deiatel'nosti Sergeia Petrovicha Botkina (k 150–letiiu so dnia rozhdenia). **Klin Med (Mosk)** 1983 Oct;61(10):142–8
**Shul'tsev GP:** Perechityvaia 'Klinicheskie Lektsii' S. P. Botkina (k 100–letiu so dnia izdaniia). **Klin Med (Mosk)** 1983 Oct;61(10):132–6
**Shul'tsev GP:** Razvitie kardiologii v trudakh uchenykh Tsentral'nogo instituta usovershenstvovaniia vracheĭ (k 50–letiiu Tsentral'nogo instituta usovershentsvovaniia vracheĭ. **Sov Med** 1980;(11):120–1
**Shul'tsev GP:** Vklad uchenykh Tsentral'nogo ordena Lenina instituta usovershenstvovaniia vracheĭ v razvitie sovetskoĭ terapii (k 50–letiiu instituta). **Klin Med (Mosk)** 1980 Jun;58(6):8–11
**Shul'tsev GP:** Vnutrennie bolezni v 'Klinicheskoĭ meditsine' za 1970–1979 gg. (obzor materialov.). **Klin Med (Mosk)** 1980 Aug;58(8):112–6
**Shul'tsev GP:** Zhizn' i deiatel'nost' Sergeia Petrovicha Botkina. **Klin Med (Mosk)** 1982 Sep;60(9):12–21
**Shultz SM, Wood MS:** Medical journals of Pennsylvania before the Civil War. **Trans Stud Coll Physicians Phila** 1983 Sep;5(5 No 3):244–70
**Shumacker HB:** A history of modern treatment of aortic aneurysms. **World J Surg** 1980 Sep;4(5):503–9
**Shumacker HB:** An American surgeon's contribution to Chinese health care. **Am J Surg** 1981 Mar;141(3):311–6
**Shumacker HB:** Better early than late. **Am J Surg** 1982 Aug;144(2):170–9
**Shumacker HB:** Extraperitoneal approach for vascular operations: retrospective review. **South Med J** 1982 Dec;75(12):1499–507, 1516
**Shumacker HB:** Leo Eloesser, M.D.: eulogy for a free spirit. New York, Philosophical Library, 1982. 483 p.
**Shumada IV, Gorodniaia VN:** K istorii Kievskogo obshchestva travmatologov-ortopedov. **Ortop Travmatol Protez** 1984 Aug;(8):69–73
**Shumada IV, Gorodniaia VN:** Rol' Kievskoĭ shkoly ortopedov v razvitii protezirovaniia i protezostroeniia na Ukraine. **Ortop Travmatol Protez** 1984 Jan;(1):69–70
**Shumsky NL** see **Knox PL**
**Shumway NE:** Heart transplantation. **J Arkansas Med Soc** 1982 Dec;79(7):221–7
**Shurygin DIa:** Razvitie ideĭ S. P. Botkina v oblasti épidemiologii. **Klin Med (Mosk)** 1982 Apr;60(4):112–5
**Shusterov AK, Shcherbina VP:** Nikolaĭ Aleksandrovich Kholodkovskiĭ (K 125–letiiu so dnia rozhdeniia). **Parazitologiia** 1983 Jul–Aug;17(4):322–4
**Shutka BV** see **Mel'man EP**
**Shuttleworth SA:** The language of science and psychology in George Eliot's Daniel Deronda. In Paradis J, Postlewait T, ed: Victorian science and Victorian values: literary perspectives. New York, New York Academy of Sciences, 1981. p. 269–98.
**Shutts D:** Lobotomy, resort to the knife. New York, Van Nostrand Reinhold, 1982. xxi, 284 p.
**Shuvalova EP:** Razvitie ideĭ S. P. Botkina v klinike infektsionnykh bolezneĭ. **Vestn Akad Med Nauk SSSR** 1983;(3):35–40
**Shvabe IuIa:** Lechenie travmaticheskikh povrezhdeniĭ v trudakh Ibn-Siny (Avitsenny) (k 1000–letiiu so dnia rozhdeniia Abu Ali Ibn-Siny). **Feldsher Akush** 1980;45(8):47–8
**Shvabe IuIa:** Voprosy travmatologii v trudakh Ibn-Siny (Avitsenny). **Ortop Travmatol Protez** 1979 Sep;(9):68–70
**Shyp NA:** Z istorii rozvytku medychnoi osvity v Rosii i na Ukraini v druhii polovyni 18 st. **Ukr Istor Zb** 1975;(11):97–104
**Sia CG** see **Harper RG**
**Sibatani A:** Two faces of molecular biology: revolution and normal science. **Riv Biol** 1981 Autumn;74(3):279–96
**Sibechi G:** Un doctor ieşean de prestigiu: Evstatie Rola. **Rev Med Chir Soc Med Nat Iasi** 1982 Jul–Sep;86(3):436, 440, 504
**Sibechi G:** Unele ştiri despre epidemia de holeră din Moldova anului 1848. **Rev Med Chir Soc Med Nat Iasi** 1983 Jul–Sep;87(3):406, 458, 470
**Síbl O:** Katedra otolaryngologie v rámci třicetileté činnosti institutu pro další vzdělávání lékařu a farmaceutu. **Cesk Otolaryngol** 1983 Jun;32(3):171–5
**Sicard A:** Allocution de André Sicard Président de L'Académie nationale de médecine. **Bull Acad Natl Med (Paris)** 1982 Dec;166(9):1243–9
**Sicard A:** Historique de l'Académie de Chirurgie. **Chirurgie** 1981;107(9):713–8
**Sicard A:** Hommage rendu au cimetière Saint-Pierre de Montmartre par l'Académie nationale de médecine au baron Antoine Portal, son fondateur, à l'occasion du 150e anniversaire de sa mort. **Hist Sci Med** 1983;17(2):195–8
**Sicard A:** L'aide des médecins de la Salpêtrière à la première expédition polaire de Jean-Baptiste Charcot. **Hist Sci Med** 1983;17(2):129–33
**Sicard A:** Un doyen misogyne et un recteur féministe. **Hist Sci Med** 1982;16(1):15–20
**Sícha V, Velková A:** K 25. výročí vzniku stomatologické katedry ILF. **Cesk Stomatol** 1981 Mar;81(2):81–5
**Sichel G:** Considerazioni sulla origine storica della biologia generale. **Med Secoli** 1981;17:163–87
**Sicherman B:** Alice Hamilton. In: Notable American women. The modern

period. Cambridge, Mass., Belknap-Harvard Univ. Press, 1980. 4:303-6.

**Sicherman B** see **Scull A, ed**

**Siclari A:** L'antropologia di Nemesio di Emesa. Padova, La Garangola, 1974. 318 p. (Filosofia e religione; 9).

**Sicuteri F:** The Enrico Greppi International Headache Award. A tribute to the memory of one of medicine's pioneers. **Cephalalgia** 1983 Mar;3(1):11-3

**Siddall AC:** Bloodletting in American obstetric practice, 1800-1945. **Bull Hist Med** 1980 Spring;54(1):101-10

**Siddall AC:** Chlorosis--etiology reconsidered. **Bull Hist Med** 1982 Summer;56(2):254-60

**Siddall AC:** George Chauncey Jameson, M.D., 1865-1948. From bloodletting to antibiotics. **Northwest Ohio Q** 1980;52(1):168-78

**Siddiqi T:** Ghalib and Unani medicine. **Stud Hist Med** 1979 Sep;3(3):181-98

**Siddiqi T:** Hakim Muhammad Akbar Arzani. **Stud Hist Med** 1981 Sep;5(3):167-224

**Siddiqi T:** Two eminent physicians (of Unani medicine) during Shah Jahan's reign. **Indian J Hist Sci** 1981;16(1):26-30

**Siddiqi T:** Unani medicine in India during the Delhi Sultanate. **Indian J Hist Sci** 1980 May;15(1):18-24

**Siddiqi T:** Unani medicine in India 1524 to 1605 A.D. **Indian J Hist Sci** 1981;16(1):22-5

**Siddiqi T:** Zubdat al-Hukama Allama Hakim Kabiruddin. **Stud Hist Med** 1981 Jun;5(2):87-132

**Siddiqui T:** Two eminent physicians (of Unani medicine) during Shah Jahan's reign. **Indian J Hist Sci** 1981, reçu 1982;16(1):26-30

**Siddiqui T:** Unani medicine in India. **Indian J Hist Sci** 1981, reçu 1982;16(1):22-5

**Sidel M** see **Sidel VW**

**Sidel VW, Sidel M:** Biomedical science and war. In Reich WT, et al, ed: Encyclopedia of bioethics, v.4. New York, Free Press, 1978. p. 1699-1704.

**Sidel VW** see **Tobach E**

**Sidel'nikov AI:** O nekotorykh osobennostiakh raboty otdel'nogo meditsinskogo batal'ona divizii v usloviiakh gorno-pustynnoĭ mestnosti (soobshchenie pervoe). **Voen Med Zh** 1983 Aug;8:20-5

**Sideman L** see **Winsten S**

**Sider D, McVaugh M:** Galen On tremor, palpitation, spasm, and rigor; Galeni De tremore, palpitatione, convulsione, et rigore. **Trans Stud Coll Physicians Phila** 1979 Sep;5(1 No 3):183-210

**Sidkar JC:** Phirangíroga (syphillis) and its management as described in Vaidyaka Samgraka, an old Gujarati manuscript of an unknown author (18th century A.D.). **Indian J Hist Sci** 1982;17(1):132-53

**Sídlo R:** Příspěvek k významu a metodice výuky dějin lékařství a zdravotnictví na lékařské fakultě. **Sb Ved Pr Lek Fak Univ Karlovy** 1979;22(5 Suppl):579-82

**Sidorenko GI:** Dostizheniia i perspektivy razvitiia sovetskoĭ gigienicheskoĭ nauki. **Gig Sanit** 1982 Dec;(12):4-9

**Sidorenko GI:** K 50-letiiu Instituta obshcheĭ i kommunal'noĭ gigieny im. A. N. Sysina AMN SSSR. **Gig Sanit** 1981 Oct;(10):41-5

**Sidorenko GI:** Razvitie obshcheĭ i kommunal'noĭ gigieny v SSSR za 60 let. **Gig Sanit** 1982 Sep;(9):17-21

**Sieber CF:** Johann Georg Amstein 'der Jüngere' (1819-1892): ein gelehrter Bündner Arzt und Naturforscher des 19. Jahrhunderts. Zürich, Juris Druck, 1984. 72 p. (Zürcher Medizingeschichtliche Abhandlungen, Neue Rheihe, Nr. 168).

**Siefert G, Stöckl T:** Die Entdeckung der Mastzellen durch den Freiburger Medizinstudenten Paul Ehrlich. **Medizinhist J** 1983;18(3):227-37

**Siefert H:** Emil Kraepelin. **Neue Dtsch Biogr** 1980;12:639-40

**Siefert H:** Hermann Knaus. **Neue Dtsch Biogr** 1980;12:163-4

**Siefert H:** Inkubation, Imagination und Kommunikation im antiken Asklepioskult. In Leuner H, ed: Katathymes Bilderleben. Ergebnisse in Theorie und Praxis. Bern, Stuttgart, Wien, Huber, 1980. p. 324-45.

**Siefert H:** Sigmund Freud, Georg Groddeck und die psychosomatische Medizin. **Prax Psychother Psychosom** 1979;24:63-78

**Siefert K:** An exemplar of primary prevention in social work: the Sheppard-Towner Act of 1921. **Soc Work Health Care** 1983 Fall;9(1):87-103

**Siefert H, ed** see **Fichtner G**

**Siegel AW, White SH:** The child study movement: early growth and development of the symbolized child. **Adv Child Dev Behav** 1982;17:233-85

**Siegel IM:** History through artifact. **IMJ** 1982 Sep;162(3):202-3, 217

**Siegel IM:** John B. Murphy - early American orthopaedic surgeon. **Int Surg** 1979 Jan-Feb;64(1):83-5

**Siegel JS:** On the demography of aging. **Demography** 1980 Nov;17(4):345-64

**Siegel LS:** Child health and development in English Canada, 1790-1850. In Roland CG, ed: Health, disease and medicine. Toronto, Hannah Institute for the History of Medicine, 1984. p. 360-80.

**Siegel RK, Hirschman AE:** Charvet and the first psychopharmacological studies on opium: a historical note and translation. **J Psychoactive Drugs** 1983 Oct-Dec;15(4):323-9

**Siegel RK:** Cocaine smoking. **J Psychoactive Drugs** 1982 Oct-Dec;14(4):271-359

**Siegel RK, Hirschman A:** Moreno and the first study on cocaine: a historical note and translation. **J Psychoactive Drugs** 1983 Jul-Sep;15(3):219-20

**Siegel S:** [Medical ethics in] contemporary Israel. In Reich ET, et al, ed: Encyclopedia of bioethics, v. 2. New York, Free Press, 1978. p. 895-6.

**Siegel S:** Wilkie Collins: Victorian novelist as psychopharmacologist. **J Hist Med Allied Sci** 1983 Apr;38(2):161-75

**Siegfried R** see **Forgan S, ed**

**Siegler AM, Grunebaum A:** The 100th anniversary of tubal sterilization. **Fertil Steril** 1980 Dec;34(6):610-3

**Sieiński W, Dąbska M:** Mięsaki kościotwórcze w materiale Zakładu Patologii Nowotworów Instytutu Onkologii w Warszawie w latach 1948-1977. **Nowotwory** 1979;Suppl:47-52

**Sieluźycki C:** Choroby Fryderyka Chopina, ich patogeneza i leczenie. **Arch Hist Med (Warsz)** 1981;44(3/4):237-56

**Siemen HL:** Das Grauen ist vorprogrammiert: Psychiatrie zwischen Fashismus und Atomkrieg. Giessen, Focus, 1982. 248 p.

**Sienkiewicz H:** Wspomnienie pośmiertne o doc. dr. med. Romanie Karwowskim. **Otolaryngol Pol** 1980;34(4):417-9

**Sieńkowski E:** Dr med. Leon Stanisław Szuman (1852-1920), chirurg, społecznik, poeta. **Arch Hist Med (Warsz)** 1984;47(1):133-41

**Sieńkowski E:** Ekslibris lekarski prof. dr Stanisława Sokoła. **Arch Hist Med (Warsz)** 1978;41(4):473-8

**Siesser WG:** Christian Gottfried Ehrenberg: Founder of micropaleontology. **Centaurus** 1981;25(3):166-88

**Sifneos PE:** A historical account of preventive psychiatry in the greater Boston area, 1942-1979. **Bibl Psychiatr** 1981;(160):1-6

**Sifneos PE:** Short-term dynamic psychotherapy: its history, its impact and its future. **Psychother Psychosom** 1981;35(4):224-9

**Sifontes JE, Valcárcel M:** Historical sketch -University Pediatric Hospital-1983. **Bol Asoc Med PR** 1983 Oct;75(10):444-5

**Sigelman CK** see **Sigelman L**

**Sigelman L, Roeder PW, Sigelman CK:** Social service innovation in the American states: deinstitutionalization of the mentally retarded. **Soc Sci Q** 1982;62(3):503-15

**Sighart H:** Die Behandlung der Tuberkulose vor Einführung der Chemotherapie. Pulmologisches Zentrum Stadt Wien/Osterreich. **Z Erkr Atmungsorgane** 1983;161(1):56-60

**Signoret JL:** La création de la chaire de Charcot. **Rev Neurol (Paris)** 1982;138(12):887-92

**Signoret JL, Castaigne P, Lhermitte F, et al:** Rediscovery of Leborgne's brain: anatomical description with CT scan. **Brain Lang** 1984 Jul;22(2):303-19

**Signoret JL:** Une leçon clinique a la Salpêtrière (1887) par André Brouillet. **Rev Neurol (Paris)** 1983;139(12):687-701

**Signoret JL** see **Alajouanine T**

**Signoret JL** see **Castaigne P**

**Signoret JL** see **Lhermitte F**

**Signorini I:** Transvestism and institutionalized homosexuality in North America. In: Congresso Intern. degli Americanisti, 40th, Italy, 1972. Atti. Vol. 2. p. 153-63.

**Sigron G:** Die Geschichte der Zahnmedizin in Graubünden. Zürich, Juris, 1981. 138 p. (Zürcher medizingeschichtliche Abhandlungen, Neue Reihe, 148).

**Sigron G:** Zahnheilkunde und Kieferchirurgie in Salerno. **SSO Schweiz Monatsschr Zahnheilkd** 1983 Jun;93(6):449-53

**Sigron G:** Zahnmedizin im Frühmittelalter. **Schweiz Monatsschr Zahnmed** 1984 Jan;94(1):49-56

**Sigsworth EM, Swan P:** An eighteenth-century surgeon and apothecary: William Elmhirst (1721-1773). **Med Hist** 1982 Apr;26(2):191-8

**Sigsworth EM, Swan P:** Para-medical provision in the West Riding. **Soc Soc Hist Med Bull (Lond)** 1981 Dec;29:37-9

**Sigsworth EM:** William Elmhirst 1721-1773: surgeon-apothecary--and medical frontiersman. **Pharm Hist (London)** 1984 Sep;14(3):6-7

**Siguan M:** La psicologia a Catalunya. Barcelona, Edicions 62, 1981. 268 p.

**Sigurosson S:** Tuberkulosens forkomst i Island. **Nord Medicinhist Arsbok** 1983;:135-48

**Sigvard J:** Cent ans de vie syndicale dans l'industrie pharmaceutique en France, 1880-1980. **Rev Hist Pharm (Paris)** 1982 Jun;29(253):115-23

**Sigvard J:** L'industrie du médicament en France: quelques points d'histoire. **Bull Acad Natl Med (Paris)** 1982 Jun;166(6):829-34

**Sihelvik L:** Diamond jubilee of the Vincentian Sisters of Charity. **Jednota Annu Furdek (US)** 1978;17:197-200

**Sijpesteijn PJ, ed** see **Harrauer H**

**Sikdar JC:** Jaina alchemy. **Indian J Hist Sci** 1980 May;15(1):6-17

**Sikorski J, Kłodiński S:** Mjr dr Marian Gustek. **Przegl Lek** 1981;38(1):182-4

**Sikorski J:** Płk dr Jan Bularski. **Przegl Lek** 1981;38(1):175-7

**Silber J:** Some demographic characteristics of the Jewish population in Russia at the end of the nineteenth century. **Jew Soc Stud** 1980;42(3-4):269-80

**Silberger J:** On the psychology of the aging woman. Mourning and transformation: how Mary Baker Eddy found in middle age a way of making a new life for herself. **J Geriatr Psychiatry** 1979;12(1):9-25

**Silgo Gamero J:** El servicio de sanidad en las guerras Carlistas. **Rev Hist Mil** 1969;13(26):93-103

**Sillman LR** see **Ostow M**

**Silló-Seidl G:** Arzte ohne Nobelpreis deren Entdeckungen Millionen Menschen geholfen haben. Genf, Ariston, 1978. 256 p.

**Silló-Seidl G:** Die Wahrheit über Semmelweis. Genf, Ariston Verlag, 1978. 214 p.

**Silló-Seidl G:** Kolletschkas Tod. **Beitr Gerichtl Med** 1979;37:415-7

**Silló-Seidl G:** Korányi Frigyes bécsi ösztöndíja. **Orvostort Kozl** 1979;87-88(25 no 1-2):311-3

**Sills A** see **Lounsbury JW**

**Sills DL** see **Merton RK**

**Silmser CR** see **Eichwald EJ**

**Silva B:** Administração e medicina. Goiânia, Goiás Brasil, Editora da

Universidade Federal de Goiás, [1979]. 48 p.
**Silva LR da:** Os Jesuitas e a assistência médica no Brasil colonial. **Rev Inst Hist Georgr Bras** 1978;318:212–32
**Silva Alvarez A:** Ensayo patobiografico sobre el Dr. Juan Pablo Rojas Paúl. **Bol Acad Nac Hist (Caracas)** 1981;64(256):859–68
**Silva Alvarez A:** Juicio critico y discurso de contestacion. **Rev Soc Venez Hist Med** 1977;25(39):93–8
**Silva Alvarez A:** Que haria y que no haria hoy Antonio Maria Pineda? **Rev Soc Venez Hist Med** 1980;29(43–44):125–30
**Silva Alvarez A** see **Sociedad Venezolana de Historia de la medicina**
**Silvay G, Griffin R:** The history and development of cardiovascular monitoring during anesthesia. **Mt Sinai J Med (NY)** 1984 Sep;51(5):560–3
**Silveira C** see **Marques Leal A**
**Silver GA** see **George Rosen: In Memoriam**
**Silver IA** see **McCullagh KG**
**Silver MA** see **Roberts WC**
**Silver P:** Auxiliary history is record of service. **J Miss State Med Assoc** 1981 Dec;22(12):316–8
**Silver P:** From chloroform to CT scans--doctors recall early days of practice. **J Miss State Med Assoc** 1981 Dec;22(12):312–5
**Silver P:** MSMA leadership is family tradition. **J Miss State Med Assoc** 1981 Dec;22(12):306–9
**Silver anniversary of the Advisory Committee on Medical Research: WHO Chron** 1984;38(1):8–16
**Silverblatt I:** The evolution of witchcraft and the meaning of healing in colonial Andean society. **Cult Med Psychiatry** 1983 Dec;7(4):413–27
**Silverman FN:** De l'art du diagnostic des nanismes et du diagnostic des nanismes dans l'art. **J Radiol** 1982 Feb;63(2):133–40
**Silverman HA** see **Lave JR**
**Silverman JA:** Richard Morton, 1637–1698. Limner of anorexia nervosa: his life and times. A tercentenary essay. **JAMA** 1983 Nov 25;250(20):2830–2
**Silverman M, Lee PR, Lydecker M:** Pills and the public purse: the routes to national drug insurance. Berkeley, University of California Press, 1981. xviii, 232 p.
**Silverman WA:** Incubator-baby side shows (Dr. Martin A. Couney). **Pediatrics** 64(2):127–41, Aug 79
**Silverman WA:** Medical inflation. **Perspect Biol Med** 1980 Summer;23(4):617–37
**Silverman WA:** Medicine's millenarianism. **Perspect Biol Med** 1981;24:339–51
**Silvers DN, Gorham JD:** Observations on a melanoma by William Norris, M.D., a country practitioner of the early 19th century. **Am J Dermatopathol** 1982 Oct;4(5):421–4
**Silverstein AM:** Contributions of A. Edward Maumenee to ocular immunology. **Am J Ophthalmol** 1979 Sep;88(3 Pt 1):302–5
**Silverstein AM:** Development of the concept of immunologic specificity: III. **Cell Immunol** 1983 May;78(1):174–90
**Silverstein AM:** Development of the concept of immunologic specificity: IV. **Cell Immunol** 1983 Sep;80(2):416–25
**Silverstein AM, Bialasiewicz AA:** History of immunology. A history of theories of acquired immunity. **Cell Immunol** 1980 Apr;51(1):151–67
**Silverstein AM:** History of immunology. Cellular versus humoral immunity: determinants and consequences of an epic 19th century battle. **Cell Immunol** 1979 Nov;48(1):208–21
**Silverstein AM:** History of immunology. Development of the concept of immunologic specificity, I. **Cell Immunol** 1982 Mar 1;67(2):396–409
**Silverstein AM:** History of immunology: development of the concept of immunologic specificity: II. **Cell Immunol** 1982 Jul 15;71(1):183–95
**Silverstein AM, Miller G:** History of immunology. The royal experiment on immunity: 1721–1722. **Cell Immunol** 1981 Jul 1;61(2):437–47
**Simberloff D:** Entropy, information and life: biophysics in the novels of Thomas Pynchon. **Perspect Biol Med** 1978 Spring;21(3):617–25
**Simbirtsev SA** see **Rusanov GA**
**Simco EL:** The history of perfumery. **Pharm Hist (London)** 1981;11(1):2–3
**Simenach BI** see **Korzh AA**
**Simeone FA:** Andreas Vesalius: anatomist, surgeon, count palatine, and pilgrim. **Am J Surg** 1984 Apr;147(4):432–40
**Simeone FA:** Studies of trauma and shock in man: William S. Stone's role in the military effort. **J Trauma** 1984 Mar;24(3):181–7
**Simeoni CE, Mouren MC, Aulas JJ:** Psychose et créativité. Réflexions à propos d'un peintre autiste: Sykvain Fusco. **Confin Psychiatr** 1980;23(3):151–63
**Simic V:** About correct and incorrect terminology in veterinary medicine. **Hist Med Vet** 1979;4(1):1–7
**Simili A:** Spigolature medicine fra gli inediti aldrovandiani. **Archiginnasio (Italy)** 1968–70;63–65(1):361–488
**Simkin RJ:** The inadequacy of health care of women. **Atlantis** 1979;4(2 pt 2):63–70
**Simko S** see **Krahulec I**
**Simmer HH:** Bilaterale Oophorektomie der Frau im späten 19. Jahrhundert. Zum methodologischen Wert der Kastration für die Entdeckung ovarieller Hormone. **Geburtshilfe Frauenheilkd** 1983 Jun;43 Suppl 1:54–9
**Simmer HH:** Die Anfänge der hormonalen Kontrazeption und die Münchener Medizinische Wochenschrift. **MMW** 1982 May 21;124(20):499–503
**Simmer HH:** Experimentelle Prüfungen der pflügerschen Reflexhypothese der Menstruation im späten 19. Jahrhundert. **Clio Med** 1980 Jul;14(3–4):235–54
**Simmer HH:** Innere Sekretion der Ovarien als Ursache der Menstruation. Halbans Falsifikation der Pflügerschen Hypothese. In Ganzinger K, Skopec M, Wyklicky H, ed: Festschrift für Erna Lesky zum 70. Geburtstag. Wien, Brüder Hollinek, 1981. p. 123–48.
**Simmer HH:** Medizin und Chemie um die Mitte des 19. Jahrhunderts in Erlangen: Eugen Franz Freiherr von Gorup-Besanez (1817–1878). **J Clin Chem Clin Biochem** 1981 Jul;19(7):497–509
**Simmer HH:** Organotherapie mit Ovarialpräparaten in der Mitte der neunziger Jahre des 19. Jahrhunderts; Medizinische und pharmazeutische Probleme. In Hickel E, Schröder G, ed: Neue Beiträge zur Arzneimittelgeschichte. Festschrift für Wolfgang Schneider zum 70. Geburtstag. Stuttgart, Wissenschaftliche Verlagsgesellschaft, 1982. p. 229–64.
**Simmer HH:** Santiago Ramón y Cajal und die Typologie des Wissenschaftlers. **Medizinhist J** 1981;16(4):414–23
**Simmer HH:** Zur Geschichte der hormonalen Auslösung einer echten Menstruation. Versuche an menstruierenden Affen und an Frauen in den frühen dreissiger Jahren unseres Jahrhunderts. In Göpfert W, Otten HH, ed: Metavoeite: wandelt euch durch neues Denken. Düsseldorf, Triltsch, 1983. p. 161–71.
**Simmer HH** see **Büttner J, ed**
**Simmer HH** see **Habrich C**
**Simmons CP:** Housing, health and educational facilities in the Indian coalfields during the colonial era. **South Asia** 1978;1(1):52–62
**Simmons GB, Smucker C, Bernstein S, et al:** Post-neonatal mortality in rural India: implications of an economic model. **Demography** 1982 Aug;19(3):371–89
**Simmons HG:** Explaining social policy: the English Mental Deficiency Act of 1913. **J Soc Hist** 1978;11(3):387–403
**Simmons HG:** From asylum to welfare. Downsview, Ont., National Institute on Mental Retardation, 1982. xv, 355 p.
**Simmons M:** Witchcraft and black magic: an interpretive view. **Palacio** 1974;80(2):5–11
**Simon A** see **Kaiser W**
**Simon F:** Latinčinár ako historik medicíny. **Cas Lek Cesk** 1984 Oct 12;123(40–41):1250
**Simon G:** Kosmetische Präparate vom 16. bis 19. Jahrhundert. Braunschweig, Deutscher Apotheker Verlag, 1983. 396 p. (Braunschweiger Veröffentlichungen zur Geschichte der Pharmazie und der Naturwissenschaften, Bd. 27).
**Simon G** see **Schober KL**
**Simon HA:** The behavioral and social sciences. **Science** 1980 Jul 4;209(4452):72–8
**Simon HR:** Die Bibliographie der Biologie. Eine analytische Darstellung unter wissenschaftshistorischen und informationstheoretischen Gesichtspunkten. Stuttgart, Hiersemann, 1977. x, 315 p. (Bibliothek des Buchwesens, Bd. 4).
**Simon I:** Die hebräische Medizin bis zum Mittelalter. In Sournia JC, Martiny M, Poulet J, ed: Illustrierte Geschichte der Medizin. Salzburg, Andreas, 1980. Vol. 3. p. 811–69.
**Simon I:** La vie et l'oeuvre des médecins juifs d'origine espagnole et portugaise du Moyen Age à la fin du XVIIIe siècle. **Rev Hist Med Heb** 1980 Mar–Apr;33(1):17–20 (continued periodically)
**Simon I:** Les notions de cardiologie bibliques et talmudiques. **Rev Hist Med Heb** 1984;37(1):3–6
**Simon I:** Les notions de cardiologie bibliques et talmudiques. **Rev Hist Med Heb** 1984 Jul;37(2):26–30
**Simon I:** L'influence hippocratique sur la médecine hébraique, surtout chez Assaph, Isaac Israèli et Maimonide. In La collection hippocratique et son rôle dans l'histoire de la médecine. Colloque de Strasbourg (23–27 octobre 1972) organisé par le Centre de Recherches sur la Grèce Antique, avec le concours des Facultés de Philosophie et des Langues Classiques. Leiden, E. J. Brill, 1975. 275–89.
**Simon K:** Hypnose--Geschichte und Anwendung heute. **Med Monatsschr Pharm** 1979 Apr;2(4):117–8
**Simon K** see **Bach A**
**Simon N:** 1979, au musée de l'Assistance publique de Paris. **Bull Soc Fr Hist Hop** 1980;(41):26–8
**Simon N** see **Garnot NS**
**Simon P, Seifert E:** Rollende Hilfsmittel fur Körperbehinderte als Gegenstand in der bildenden Kunst. In KF Schlegel, ed: Der Körperbehinderte in Mythologie und Kunst. Stuttgart, New York, Thieme, 1983. p. 89–125.
**Simon de Vallambert on the treatment of diarrhea in infants (1565): Pediatrics** 1982 Feb;69(2):163
**Simón Palmer M del C:** Las neurosis femeninas y la educación española. **Asclepio** 1983;35:327–42
**Simonin M:** Michel de Nostredame, Pierre Boaistuau, Chavigny et la peste aixoise de 1546. **Bibl Hum Renaissance** 1983;45(1):127–30
**Simonnet J:** L'hospice Saint-Charles d'Amiens. De sa fondation à 1900. Memoire de fin d'assistanant. E.N.S.P. de Rennes, 1977. 155 p.
**Simonov PV:** Half a century of pursuing the truth. Dedicated to the 80th anniversary of E. A. Asratyan. **Pavlov J Biol Sci** 1983 Apr–Jun;18(2):63–8
**Simonov PV:** Podkrepliaiushchaia funktsiia émotsiĭ (k 80-letiiu so dnia rozhdeniia Ezrasa Asratovicha Asratiana). **Fiziol Zh SSSR** 1983 May;69(5):577–86
**Simonov PV:** Polveka neotstupnykh iskaniĭ istiny (k 80-letiiu so dnia rozhdeniia E. A. Asratiana). **Zh Vyssh Nerv Deiat** 1983 Mar–Apr;33(2):197–203
**Simonovits I:** Emlékek az 1930–1944. Evi egyetemi diákmozgalomról és orvosmozgalomról. **Parttorteneti Kozl** 1980;26(2):130–41
**Simoons F:** Effects of culture: geographical and historical approaches. **Int J Obes** 1980;4(4):387–94

**Simpson AD:** Sir Robert Sibbald--the founder of the College. In Passmore R, ed: Proceedings of the Royal College of Physicians of Edinburgh Tercentenary Congress, 1981. Edinburgh, Royal College of Physicians of Edinburgh, 1982. p. 59-91.
**Simpson D** see **Curtis JB**
**Simpson GM:** A brief history of depot neuroleptics. **J Clin Psychiatry** 1984 May;45(5 pt 2):3-4
**Simpson GT, Polanyi TG:** History of the carbon dioxide laser in otolaryngologic surgery. **Otolaryngol Clin North Am** 1983 Nov;16(4):739-52
**Simpson HN:** Doctors afield: David Cobb, M.D. **N Engl J Med** 1980 Dec 25;303(26):1517-9
**Simpson HN:** Invisible armies. The impact of disease on American history. Indianapolis, Bobbs Merrill, 1980. xi, 239 p.
**Simpson J** see **Zellweger H**
**Simpson JA:** Electrophysiology of neuromuscular junction disease: an appreciation of the contributions of Edward H. Lambert. **Muscle Nerve** 1982;5(9S):S6-11
**Simri U:** Development of women's sport in the 20th century. In Borms J, Hebbelinck M, Venerando A, ed: Women and sport. Basel, Karger, 1981. p. 31-44.
**Simson JV:** Die Flussverunreinigungsfrage im 19. Jahrhundert. **Vierteljahrsschr Soz Wirtschgesch** 1978;65(3):370-90
**Simunovic V** see **Konjhodžic F**
**Sinclair HM:** Sherrington and industrial fatigue. **Notes Rec R Soc Lond** 1984 Sep;39(1):91-104
**Sinclair KB:** Britain's role in tropical veterinary medicine: past, present and future. **Trans R Soc Trop Med Hyg** 1981;75 Suppl:32-4
**Sindelář B:** Carodějnictví a jeho pronásledování u nás do r. 1526. **Sb Pr Filos Fak Brnenske Univ Rada Hist** 1981;30(28):177-206
**Sindelar JL:** Differential use of medical care by sex. **J Polit Econ** 1982;90(5):1003-19
**Sinding C:** Le concept de gène. Une approche épistémologique. **Arch Fr Pediatr** 1984 Jan;41(1):1-3
**Sindou M** see **Wertheimer P**
**Singapore General Hospital:** Singapore General Hospital 50th anniversary publication, 1926-1976. Singapore, [s. n., 1976?]. 128 p.
**Singer R, Wolff RG, Gladfelter BG, et al:** Pleistocene Macaca from Hoxne, Suffolk, England. **Folia Primatol (Basel)** 1982;37(3-4):141-52
**Singerman B:** DSM-III: historical antecedents and present significance. **J Clin Psychiatry** 1981 Nov;42(11):409-10
**Singh AN, Pathak SK, Singh RS:** Non-plant Vedic epithets in the Sanskrit nomenclature of Indian economic plants. **Stud Hist Med** 1982 Sep;6(3):225-30
**Singh AN, Singh RS:** On the identity of and Indo-Greek relation reflected in the plant-names and uses evinced in the Kautıliya Arthaśastra with particular reference to 'Kiratatikta' of 'Katuvarga' (group of spices). **Indian J Hist Sci** 1983 Nov;18(2):172-5
**Singh AN** see **Singh R**
**Singh AN** see **Singh RS**
**Singh BN:** Contribution of Madanapala Nighantu to the knowledge of Indian materia medica with particular reference to fig [Anjira] **Indian J Hist Sci** 1981, reçu 1982;16(1):89-94
**Singh LB** see **Singh RS**
**Singh M** see **Brahma B**
**Singh P:** The evolution of anxiety. In: Congrès international d'histoire de la médecine, XXVe, Québec, 1976. Actes. Québec, 1977. p. 1274-88.
**Singh R, Singh AN:** Socio-economic and trade relations of ancient India with the western world as reflected in plant names with particular reference to saffron (Kunkum/Kesara). **Stud Hist Med** 1981 Sep;5(3):228-32
**Singh RB:** Historical development of the laboratory services in Malaysia. **Malays J Pathol** 1982 Aug;5:23-32
**Singh RH** see **Singhal GD**
**Singh RN** see **Chauhan DK**
**Singh RS, Singh LB:** Aconites (Visas) in the Ayurvedic therapy (origin, sources, classification and historical antecedents). **Stud Hist Med** 1982 Jun;6(2):147-59
**Singh RS:** Contribution of Unani materia medicas to the identification of Vedic plants with special reference to Usana. **Indian J Hist Sci** 1981, reçu 1982;16(1):41-6
**Singh RS, Singh AN:** On the identity and economico-medicinal uses of hastikarnapalasa (Leea macrophylla Roxb., family: Ampelidaceae) as evinced in the ancient (Sanskrit) texts and traditions. **Indian J Hist Sci** 1981;16(2):219-22
**Singh RS, Vyas VD:** The identity and critical appraisal of the basis of nomenclature and ancient socio-cultural and geographico-historical reflections evinced with the Paninian perfume-plant/plant-part 'Kisara' (Panini IV. IV. 53). **Indian J Hist Sci** 1983 Nov;18(2):166-71
**Singh RS** see **Singh AN**
**Singh SB** see **Thakur RS**
**Singhal GD, Guru LV:** Anatomical and obstetric considerations in ancient Indian surgery: based on Sarirasthana of Susruta Samhita. Varanasi, India, Institute of Medical Sciences, Banaras Hindu University, 1973. L, 241 p.
**Singhal GD, Singh RH, Shukla KP:** Non-operative considerations in ancient Indian surgery: (based on Susruta Samhita, Cikitsa-Sthana, chapters 24-40). Varanasi, India, Institute of Medical Sciences, Banaras Hindu University, 1971. xlii, 396 p.
**Singleton WB:** The decade preceding the B.S.A.V.A. **Vet Hist** 1982/83;NS2(4):161-4
**Sinha A:** Physiological concepts in ancient and medieval India. In E. Schultheisz, ed: History of physiology. Oxford, Elmsford, New York, Pergamon, 1981. xvi, 208 p. (Advances in Physiological Sciences. Proceedings of the 28th International Congress of Physiological Sciences, Budapest, 1980. Volume 21). p. 61-75.
**Sinha DN:** Status of anatomy in the University of Bologna (13th to 18th century). **Stud Hist Med** 1982 Jun;6(3):141-6
**Siniak KM, Rudichenko VF:** Avksentiĭ Vasil'evich Korchak-Chepurkovskiĭ (k 125-letiiu so dnia rozhdeniia). **Vrach Delo** 1983 Apr;(4):118-21
**Siniak KM:** Epidemicheskie posledstviia vremennoĭ fashistskoĭ okkupatsii Ukrainskoĭ SSR i mery po ikh preodoleniiu. **Zh Mikrobiol Epidemiol Immunobiol** 1982 May;(5):11-4
**Siniak KM, Davidenko OS:** Materialisticheskoe ponimanie razvitiia épidemiologii. **Zh Mikrobiol Epidemiol Immunobiol** 1980 Sep;(9):12-7
**Sinigaglia G** see **Lanzavecchia P**
**Sinitsyn AM:** Zabota o ranenykh frontovikakh i invalidakh v gody otechestvennoi voiny. **Istor SSSR** 1973;(1):130-8
**Sinkovics JG:** Early history of specific antibody-producing lymphocyte hybridomas. **Cancer Res** 1981 Mar;41(3):1246-7
**Sinohara H:** [Archibald Edward Garrod (1857-1936): a biographical assay (author's transl)] (Jpn). **Seikagaku** 1980 Nov;52(11):1155-72
**Sinohara H:** [Eduard Buchner (1860-1917): a biographical essay] (Jpn). **Seikagaku** 1981;53(10):1139-60
**Sinohara H:** [James Batcheller Sumner (1887-1955): a biographical essay] **Seikagaku** 1979 Dec;51(12):1301-21
**Sinopeus DP** see **Krymkevich NI**
**Sinzinger H** see **Thakur ML**
**Sípek Z:** Na co umírali lidé v Morašicích na okrese znojemském v letech 1904-1949. **Cas Lek Cesk** 1984 Mar 16;123(11):331
**Sípek Z:** Norbert Mrštík. (1867-1905) Ze života venkovského lékaře na začátku 20. století. **Cas Lek Cesk** 1982 Jul 30;121(30):955-6
**Sipos G:** Egy 1495-re szóló érvágó kalendárium a fővárosi Szabó Ervin könyvtárban. **Magy Konyvsz** 1977;93(1):43-6
**Sipsma DH** see **Van Proosdij C**
**Sipukhin IaM:** Razvitie rentgenologii na Dal'nem Vostoke. **Vestn Rentgenol Radiol** 1982 Jan-Feb;(1):89-91
**Sipukhin IaM:** Vladimir Semenovich Kravchenko. K istorii otechestvennoi rentgenologii. **Vestn Rentgenol Radiol** 1983 May-Jun;(3):91-2
**Siqueira LF, de Almeida RG, Belda W:** Métodos tintoriais utilizados na identificação do Mycobacterium leprae. Revisão histórica. **Rev Saude Publica** 1984 Jun;18(3):246-58
**Sir Thomas Lewis centenary stamp: Lancet** 1981;ii:378
**Siraisi NG:** Some recent work on western European medical learning, ca. 1200-ca. 1500. In History of Universities, II, 1982. p. 225-38.
**Siraisi NG:** Taddeo Alderotti and his pupils. Two generations of Italian medical learning. Princeton, Princeton University Press, 1981. xxiii, 461 p.
**Siraisi NG:** The medical learning of Albertus Magnus. In Weisheipl JA, ed: Albertus Magnus and the sciences. Toronto, Pontifical Institute of Mediaeval Studies, 1980. p. 379-404.
**Sircus W:** Medical-surgical collaboration in the practice of gastroenterology. **Postgrad Med J** 1984 Nov;60(709):725-32
**Sîrghie E** see **Năstasă V**
**Sirkin M, Fleming M:** Freud's 'Project' and its relationship to psychoanalytic theory. **J Hist Behav Sci** 1982 Jul;18(3):230-41
**Sirota M:** On the Freud-Jung correspondence. **Mod Stud** 1977;2(3):45-8
**Sisaye S** see **Stommes E**
**Sisk TD:** External fixation. Historic review, advantages, disadvantages, complications, and indications. **Clin Orthop** 1983 Nov;(180):15-22
**Sitenko VM** see **Nechaĭ AI**
**Sitenko VM** see **Samotokin BA**
**Sitharamiah A:** Outline of history of Yoga. **Bull Indian Inst Hist Med (Hyderabad)** 1980;10(1-4):15-22
**Situación actual de la población indigena.: Am Indig** 1979;39:211-418
**Siudikas VP, Kutorga VV, Stalioraĭtite EI, et al:** Patologiia i ee prepodavanie v Vil'niusskom universitete (k 400-letiiu Vil'niusskogo universiteta i 200-letiiu meditsinskogo fakul'teta étogo universiteta). **Arkh Patol** 1980;42(9):70-5
**Siur HA** see **Bastenchuk AZ**
**Sivachenko TP** see **Kindzel'skiĭ LP**
**Sivolob NI:** Rol' A. N. Marzeeva v razvitii otechestvennoĭ gigieny (k 100-letiiu so dnia rozhdeniia). **Sov Zdravookhr** 1983;(8):54-6
**Sivolob NI:** Vklad I.V. Beliaeva v organizatsiiu sanitarnogo dela v Donbasse. **Sov Zdravookhr** 1984;(5):65-7
**Sizer SS:** New spirit, new flesh: the poetics of nineteenth-century mind-cures. **Soundings** 1980;63(4):407-22
**Sizov IE** see **Buranchiev AB**
**Sjöberg SG:** Magister Salomon Rummels libri medici. **Sydsven Medicinhist Sallsk Arsskr** 1982;19:119-36
**Sjöstrand T:** Magin i medicinen. **Lakartidningen** 1982 May 26;79(21):2137-40
**Sjöstrand T:** Medicinen i vetenskapshistorien. **Sydsven Medicinhist Sallsk Arsskr** 1980;:149-58
**Sjöstrand T:** Medicinsk vetenskap: Historik, teori och tillämpning. Stockholm, Natur och Kultur, 1979. 183 p.
**Sjövall H:** Vem skulle få vårda vad? Fackliga strider i 1600-talets Sverige. **Nord Medicinhist Arsb** 1980;:59-80
**Skachilov VA:** S. Ia. Elpat'evskiĭ v Ufimskoĭ ssylke. **Sov Zdravookhr** 1980;(8):56-9
**Skala E:** Kdo objevil krevní skupiny? **Cas Lek Cesk** 1984 Oct

19;123(42):1292-4
**Skalak R, Chien S:** Capillary flow: history, experiments and theory. **Biorheology** 1981;18(3-6):307-30
**Skalley M, Skalley R:** A medal for Marigold: Seattle's marine medic. Seattle, Superior Pub. Co., 1982. 150 p.
**Skalley R** see **Skalley M**
**Skaric J:** O osnutku i razvoju bakteriološke stanice u Splitu do 1923. god., s biografijom osnivača dr Josipa Skarića. In: I simpozij o historiji mikrobiologije i imunologije u Hrvatskoj do 1923. godine. Zagreb, Jugoslavenskoj akademiji, 1973. p. 95-105.
**Skarulis RI** see **Telichenas AI**
**Skarżyński Z:** Z problematyki przerywania clazy. **Panstwo Prawo** 1981;36(9-12):96-106
**Skerritt PW:** Anxiety and the heart--a historical review. **Psychol Med** 1983 Feb;13(1):17-25
**Skillman K:** The struggle to save a dental shrine. **Ohio Dent J** 1983 May;57(3):44-6
**Skinner BF:** Notebooks. Edited with an introduction by R. Epstein. Englewood Cliffs, Prentice-Hall, 1980. xiii, 386 p.
**Skinner BF:** Pavlov's influence on psychology in America. **J Hist Behav Sci** 1981;17:242-5
**Skinner BF:** The experimental analysis of operant behavior: a history. In R. W. Rieber, K. Salzinger, ed: Psychology: theoretical-historical perspectives. New York, Academic Press, 1980. p. 191-202.
**Skinner BF:** The shaping of a behaviorist. New York, Knopf, 1979. 373 p.
**Skinner G:** The history of surgical instruments. **Nurs Times** 1984 Jul 18-24;80(29):28-30
**Skinner GM:** The Wellcome Museum. **Sydsven Medicinhist Sallsk Arsskr** 1983;:13-22
**Skinner J:** 'Crisis mortality' in Buckinghamshire 1600-1750. **Local Popul Stud (Matlock)** 1982 Spring;28:67-72
**Skinner J:** Plague mortality in Buckinghamshire in the seventeenth century. **Rec Bucks** 1979;20(3):
**Skinner RE, Marcotte JM:** Bibliographic instruction in the health sciences: an historical review. **Med Ref Serv Q** 1982 Summer;1(2):53-76
**Skinner RE:** Narcotics, barred windows, and murder: the medical practitioner in the writings of Raymond Chandler. **Perspect Biol Med** 1983 Autumn;27(1):127-34
**Skinner RE:** Photography, advertising, and the history of medicine: notes on the medico-historical art of Lejaren a Hiller. **Watermark** 1983 Jan;6(2-3):11-2
**Skinner RE:** The historical work of William Dosité Postell, Sr. **Watermark** 1983 Fall;7(2):8-10
**Skinner RE:** The making of the air surgeon: the early life and career of David N. W. Grant. **Aviat Space Environ Med** 1983 Jan;54(1):75-82
**Skinner RE:** The roots of flight nursing: Lauretta M. Schimmoler and the Aerial Nurse Corps of America. **Aviat Space Environ Med** 1984 Jan;55(1):72-7
**Skinner RE:** The U. S. flight nurse: a supplementary bibliography. **Aviat Space Environ Med** 1983 Aug;54(8):735-7
**Skinner RE:** The U. S. flight nurse: an annotated historical bibliography. **Aviat Space Environ Med** 1981 Nov;52(11 pt 1):707-12
**Skinner RE, ed** see **Paddison RM**
**Skinsnes AV, Binford CH:** Leprosy research and the Public Health Service -- a brief chronological résumé. **Public Health Rep** 1980 May-Jun;95(3):210-2
**Skinsnes OK:** Leprosy in archeologically recovered bamboo book in China. **Int J Lepr** 1980 Sept;48(3):333
**Skipper JK, Hughes JE:** Podiatry: a medical care specialty in quest of full professional status and recognition. **Soc Sci Med** 1983;17(20):1541-8
**Skishkin AP:** Vazhnyĭ étap v razvitii planirovaniia sovetskoge zdravookhranenia. **Sov Zdravookhr** 1982;(3):61-4
**Skład osobowy władz Polskiego Towarzystwa Historii Medycyny i Farmacji: Arch Hist Med (Warsz)** 1984;47(2):269-85
**Skobulovich GV:** Itogi deiatel'nosti Amursjkogo otdeleniia Nauchnogo obshchestva épidemiologov, mikrobiologov i parazitologov za 25 let (1957-1982). **Zh Mikrobiol Epidemiol Immunobiol** 1984 Feb;(2):117-9
**Skodáček P:** Prof. MUDr Eduard Cmunt, prvý slovanský balneológ v Piešt'anoch. **Fysiatr Reumatol Vestn** 1984 Feb;62(1):44-6
**Skolnick M** see **Bardet JP**
**Skolnick M** see **Bean LL**
**Skolnick MH, Bean LL, Mineau GP, et al:** Etudes génétiques et démographiques et base de données généalogiques de l'Utah. **Ann Demogr Hist (Paris)** 1984;:103-13
**Skolnik H:** Historical deveopment of abstracting. **J Chem Inf Comput Sci** 1979 Nov;19(4):215-8
**Skopakov Kh:** N. I. Pirogov--genialen khirug i osnovopolozhnik na topografskata anatomiia. **Khirurgiia (Sofiia)** 1982;35(1):99-100
**Skopec M:** Anton Elfinger (1821-1864)--a forgotten medical illustrator. **Int J Dermatol** 1983 May;22(4):256-9
**Skopec M, Wyklicky H:** Die Heilpädagogische Abteilung der Universitäts-Kinderklink Wien--die älteste kinderpsychiatrische Forschungs- und Behandlungsstätte. **Erzieh Unterr** 1981 Oct;24:98-105
**Skopec M:** The development of hygiene in Austria. In Ogawa T, ed: Public health. Tokyo, Saikon, 1981. p. 129-44.
**Skopec M:** The Vienna Medical School. Vienna, Institute of the History of Medicine at the University of Vienna, [1983?]. 20 p.
**Skopec M:** Uber den 'Ring des Paracelsus'. **Osterr Arzteztg** 1981;36(24):4 pages (Sonderdruck)
**Skopec M** see **Ganzinger K**
**Skopec M** see **Wyklicky H**
**Skorecki J:** What have we learned about walking in twenty four centuries? **Manch Lit Phil Soc Mem Proc** 1977-80;120:56-71
**Skorogliadov AV:** K 50-letiiu so dnia organizatsii kafedry travmatologii, ortopedii i voenno- polevoĭ khirurgii II MOLGMI im. N.I. Pirogova. **Ortop Travmatol Protez** 1983 Dec;(12):60-1
**Skov H, Bastholm E, ed:** Petrus Severinus og hans Idea medicinae philosophicae. En dansk paracelsist. Copenhagen, Odense Universitetsforlag, 1979. 299 p. (Acta Historica Scientiarum et Medicinalium, 32).
**Skovránek V:** From the beginnings of infectious diseases control in USSR (a few notes on important jubilees). **J Hyg Epidemiol Microbiol Immunol** 1982;26(3):225-6
**Skovránek V:** Naše epidemiologie a mikrobiologie v posledních třiceti letech. **Cesk Epidemiol Mikrobiol Imunol** 1982 May;31(3):132-4
**Skovránek V:** Thirty years of the Czechoslovak sanitary and epidemiological service--1952-1982. **J Hyg Epidemiol Microbiol Immunol** 1982;26(4):329-33
**Skreb N, McKenzie J:** The early days of European Developmental Biology Organisation (E.D.B.O.). **Anat Anz** 1981;150(4):443-8
**Skripkin IuK, Turanov NM, Mordovtsev VN, et al:** Tsentral'nomu nauchno-issledovatel'skomu kozhno-venerologicheskomu institut--60 let. **Vestn Dermatol Venerol** 1981 Dec;(12):4-10
**Skrobacki A, Völker A:** Lekarz olsztyński, Joachim Kornalewskiijego rozprawa o koltunie z 1897 roku. **Komun Mazursko Warm** 1980;(2):155-67
**Skrobacki A:** Najstarszy na Warmii Polski regulamin szpitalny. **Komun Mazursko Warm** 1977;(3-4):447-54
**Skrobacki A:** Robert Koch in Wolsztyn. **Wiss Beitr Martin Luther Univ Halle Wittenberg** 1983;5-R80:51-61
**Skrobacki A, Völker A:** Ze starań Profesora Ludwika Bierkowskiego o pozyskanie katedry w berlinie w 1847 r. **Arch Hist Med (Warsz)** 1979;42(3):303-8
**Skrobacki A** see **Kaiser W**
**Skrupskelis IK** see **James W**
**Skrzypczak I** see **Słupczyński S**
**Skrzypek W:** Przypadek wyleczenia nosacizny u człowieka w 1828 r. **Arch Hist Med (Warsz)** 1983;46(3):325-32
**Skudarnova ZA:** Stanovlenie, razvitie i zadachi nevrologicheskoĭ sluzhby Smolenskoĭ oblasti. **Zh Nevropatol Psikhiatr** 1983;83(11):1732-4
**Skudder S, Barber LH:** The New Zealand nursing team at the Spanish Civil War. **NZ Med J** 1983 May 25;96(732):397-9
**Skulimowski M, Sliwinski S:** Joseph Dietl's contributions to European medicine development. In International Congress of the History of Medicine. 26th, Plovdiv, 1978. Actes du Congress. Sofia, 1981. Volume II. p. 96-7.
**Skulimowski M:** Mikołaj Kopernik, wybitny predstawiciel medycyny XVI wieku w Polsce. Kraków, Akademia Medyczna, 1978. 84 p.
**Skulimowski M, Sliwiński S:** Z przeszłości uzdrowiskowej Krzeszowic. **Wiad Lek** 1979 Nov 15;32(22):1651-4
**Skulimowski M, Sliwiński S:** Zwiazki Jana Nepomucena Rusta (1775--1840) z Krakowskim Fakultetem Medycznym. **Arch Hist Med (Warsz)** 1979;42(2):245-9
**Skulimowski MM:** Jan Baptysta van Helmont (1577-1644) odkrywca dwutlenku węgla (CO2). **Wiad Lek** 1980 Mar 15;33(6):495-7
**Skultans V:** English madness. Ideas on insanity, 1580-1890. London, Routledge & Kegan Paul, 1979. ix, 158 p.
**Skura MA:** The literary use of the psychoanalytic process. New Haven, London, Yale University, 1981. 280 p.
**Skvortsov VI, Skvortsova AI:** F. M. Dostoevskiĭ i meditsina. **Klin Med (Mosk)** 1982 Feb;60(2):112-6
**Skvortsov VIa:** O nekotorykh aspektakh istoricheskoĭ vzaimosviazi meditsiny i iskusstva. **Vestn Akad Med Nauk SSSR** 1982;(4):57-65
**Skvortsov VIa, Skvortsova AI:** Obrazy vracheĭ v proizvedeniiakh literatury i iskusstva. **Sov Zdravookhr** 1984;(9):59-62
**Skvortsova AI** see **Skvortsov VI**
**Skvortsova AI** see **Skvortsov VIa**
**Slack P:** The disappearance of plague: an alternative view. **Econ Hist Rev** 1981;34(3):469-76
**Slack P** see **Hart GD, ed**
**Slack P** see **Webster C, ed**
**Sladen A:** Landmark perspective: Closed-chest massage, Kouwenhoven, Jude, Knickerbocker. **JAMA** 1984 Jun 15;251(23):3137-40
**Slaff B:** The history of adolescent psychiatry. **Adolesc Psychiatry** 1981;9:7-21
**Slaney B:** The development of occupational health nursing. **Nursing (Oxford)** 1984 May;2(25):suppl 1-3
**Slaney BM** see **Allan P**
**Slap JW** see **Ross JM**
**Slater E:** Psychiatry in the thirties. **Contemp Rev** 1975;226(1309):70-5
**Slater S** see **Blum L**
**Slatter EM:** Illustrations from the Wellcome Institute Library: the new lazaretto at Siros (Syra), Greece, in 1840. **Med Hist** 1984 Jan;28(1):73-80
**Slaughter MM:** Universal languages and scientific taxonomy in the seventeenth century. Cambridge, Cambridge University Press, 1982. x, 277 p.
**Slavětinský M:** Jak se kdysi v Olomouci vzdělávali zdravotničtí pracovníci. **Cesk Gynekol** 1981 May;46(4):321-2
**Slavětinský M:** K dvoustému výročí vzniku lékařsko-chirurgického studia v Olomouci (1782-1875). **Cesk Zdrav** 1981 Oct;29(10):426-31
**Slavětinský M:** List z historie severomoravského zdravotnictví.

Vnitr Lek 1979 Dec;25(12):1219–21

**Slavětínský M:** Naši lékaři-archeologové. **Vnitr Lek** 1980 Mar;26(3):415–6

**Slavětínský M:** Poznámky k minulosti boje s TBC na Moravě. **Vnitr Lek** 1980;26(5):515–6

**Slavětínský M:** Předchudci československo-sovětských lékařských styku. **Cesk Zdrav** 1982 Sep;30(8–9):381–5

**Slavětínský M:** Připomínka prukopníka zestátněnú veřejného zdravotnictví z Moravy na sklonku minulého století. **Cesk Zdrav** 1980 May;28(5):219–20

**Slavětínský M:** Z historie poslední epidemie neštovic našich zemích. **Cesk Zdrav** 1980 Apr;28(4):172–4

**Slavinsky AT, Krauss JB:** Mutual withdrawal... or Gwen Tudor revisited. **Perspect Psychiatr Care** 1980 Sep–Oct;18(5):194–203

**Slenders J:** De Anatomische les van Dr. Zacheus de Jager (1640). **Tijdschr Geschied Geneeskd** 1981;4(4):159–67

**Slepushkin AN** see **Zhdanov VM**

**Slepushkina II** see **Borisenko NF**

**Slezák K:** Vývoj oboru 'Organizace a řízení vojenského zdravotnictví' za 25 let existence Vojenského lékařského výzkumného a doškolovacího ústavu J. E. Purkyně v Hradci Králové. **Cesk Zdrav** 1984 Jan;32(1):1–5

**Sligmann H:** [Some aspects of the physician's law in Jewish traditional sources] (Heb). **Harefuah** 1983 Apr 15;104(8):358–61

**Sliosberg R:** De la médecine à Saint-Germain en-Laye à travers les siècles. **Bull Soc Amis Vieux St.-Germain** 1978;30:17–33

**Sliwiński S:** Edward Korczyński (1844–1905) autor pierwszego opisu klinicznego zawału serca w medycynie polskiej. **Wiad Lek** 1979 Nov 15;32(22):1647–50

**Sliwiński S:** Miquel Serveto (1511–1553) -- odkrywca płucnego krążenia krwi. **Wiad Lek** 1980 Apr 1;33(7):589–91

**Sliwiński S:** Teoria Ibn an-Nafisa (1210–1288) krążenia płucnego krwi. **Wiad Lek** 1981 Mar 15;34(6):531–3

**Sliwiński S** see **Skulimowski M**

**Sloan AW:** Claude Bernard's philosophy of medical science. **S Afr Med J** 1984 May 19;65(20):817–9

**Sloan AW:** Highlights of physiological research at the University of Cape Town, 1912–1978. **S Afr Med J** 1979 Nov 24;56(22):974–6

**Sloan AW:** The Black Death in England. **S Afr Med J** 1981 Apr 25;59(18):646–50

**Sloan D:** Science in New York City, 1867 - 1907. **Isis** 1980 Mar;71(256):35–76

**Sloan DG:** The extent of contraceptive use and the social paradigm of modern demography. **Sociology** 1983;17(3):380–7

**Sloan FA, Steinwald B:** Effects of regulation on hospital costs and input use. **J Law Econ** 1980;23(1):81–109

**Sloan H:** Let us now praise famous men. **J Thorac Cardiovasc Surg** 1980 Aug;80(2):159–70

**Sloan JB:** The founding of the Naples Table Association for promoting scientific research by women, 1897. **Signs** 1978;4(1):208–16

**Sloan JW** see **Martin WR**

**Sloan PR:** Ontogeny and phylogeny. **Br J Hist Sci** 1980;13(1):50–5

**Sloan W, Stevens HA:** A century of concern: a history of the American Association on Mental Deficiency 1876–1976. Washington, American Association on Mental Deficiency, 1976, viii, 310p.

**Sloane DM:** Sex of privious children and intentions for further birth in the United States, 1965–1976. **Demography** 1983 Aug;20(3):353–67

**Slochower H:** The permanence of our Freudian heritage. **Mod Stud** 1977;2(3):13–18

**Slocum A:** Cornelius Packard Rhoads. In Dictionary of American Biography, Suppl. 6, 1956–1960. p. 537–8. 1980.

**Sloman JG** see **Mond HG**

**Slome C** see **Ibrahim MA**

**Slopek S:** Rozwój immunologii w Polsce w latach 1971–1975. **Nauka Pol** 1976;24(5):41–59

**Slosarová V, Tomanová M:** 100 let školího lékařství v Praze. **Cesk Pediatr** 1984 Jul;39(7):420–4

**Slotow M:** Medical Africana. **S Afr Med J** 1983 Jun 29;Spec No:43–6

**Slotow M:** The opening up of Africa. **S Afr Med J** 1981 Oct 3;60(14):557–8

**Sloyan PJ:** The day they shut down Birmingham. **Wash Mon** 1972;4(3):41–50

**Sluchanko BP:** Kerchenskoe meditsinskoe uchilishche im. Geroia Sovetskogo Soiuza glavstarshiny meditsinskoĭ sluzhby G. K. Petrovoĭ. **Med Sestra** 1983 Oct;42(10):56–8

**Słupczyński S, Skrzypczak I:** Cięia cesarskie wykonane w szpitalu miejskim w Lukowie w latach 1971–1978. **Ginekol Pol** 1979 Oct;50(10):855–8

**Slusarski W:** W pięćdziesiątą rocznicę śmierci Konstantego S. Janickiego (1876–1932). **Wiad Parazytol** 1983;28(5–6):507–15

**Small PA** see **El-Najjar MY**

**Small WE:** FDA: today's strengths built on turbulent past. **Am Pharm** 1980 Jan;20(1):25–7

**Small WE:** Pneumococcal pneumonia vaccine--strange success story. **Am Pharm** 1979 Dec;19(13):39

**Smallpox exhibit: Bull Hist Med** 1981 Spring;55(1):108–10

**Smandych R, Verdun-Jones SN:** Catch–22 in the nineteenth century: the evolution of the therapeutic confinement for the criminally insane in Canada, 1840–1900. **Crim Justice Hist** 1981;2:85–108

**Smeaton WA:** James Riddick Partington. In Dictionary of national biography, 1961–1970. Suppl. 8, 1981. p. 822–3.

**Smeaton WA:** Pharmacy in Revolutionary and Napoleonic Paris, 1789–1815. **Pharm Hist (London)** 1979 Apr;9(1):4–5

**Smeaton WA** see **Neville RG**

**Smekal FG** see **Speiser P**

**Smellie RM** see **Campbell N**

**Smereka J:** Rozprawy doktorskie obronione przez lekarzy polskich we Wrocławskiej Klinice Okulistycznej przed r. 1918. **Klin Oczna** 1979 Nov;81(11):635–6

**Smereka J** see **Heimrath T**

**Smereka J** see **Pacyńska M**

**Smeur EW, Smeur FA:** 'Krijg de pokken' -- een overwonnen verwensing. **Tijdschr Ziekenverpl** 1980 May 20;33(11):515–7

**Smeur FA** see **Smeur EW**

**Smíd F** see **Miřejovský P**

**Smil V:** Communist China's food: still a long way to go. **Issues Stud** 1980;16(4):37–44

**Smilor RW** see **Melosi MV, ed**

**Smirnov AN:** Razvitie terapii v SSSR. **Feldsher Akush** 1982;47(12):14–9

**Smirnov EI, Garin NS:** Agressivnaia sushchnost' amerikanskogo imperializma i vozmozhnye posledstviia primeneniia iadernogo oruzhiia. **Zh Mikrobiol Epidemiol Immunobiol** 1982 May;(5):3–11

**Smirnov EI, Garin NS:** S. P. Botkin o variabel'nosti klinicheskogo techeniia infektsionnykh bolezneĭ i épidemiologicheskikh aspektakh étoĭ problemy (K 150–letiiu so dnia rozhdeniia). **Vestn Akad Med Nauk SSSR** 1982;(10):3–9

**Smirnov EI, Garin NS:** Vklad S. P. Botkina v razvitie épidemiologii (k 150–letiiu so dnia rozhdeniia). **Zh Mikrobiol Epidemiol Immunobiol** 1982 May;(5):109–15

**Smirnov EI, Garin NS:** Voĭna i protivoépidemicheskaia zashchita. **Zh Mikrobiol Epidemiol Immunobiol** 1980 May;(5):6–10

**Smirnov EI:** Voĭna i voennaia meditsina, 1939–1945. Moskva, Meditsina, 1979. 524 p.

**Smirnov EI, Garin NS:** Znachenie nauchnogo nalslediia i deiatel'nosti Ia. L. Okunevskogo dlia sozdaniia dezinfektsionnogo i banno–prachechnogo dela v armii. **Voen Med Zh** 1979 Apr;(4):73–5

**Smirnov IN:** Problema integratsii znaniia v sovremennoi biologii. **Vopr Filos** 1981;11:38–50

**Smirnov VS** see **Nguyen TK**

**Smirnov VV, Bilaĭ VI:** Zhizn' i deiatel'nost' D. K. Zabolotnogo v Kieve. **Mikrobiol Zh** 1982 May–Jun;44(3):86–90

**Smirnov-Kamenskiĭ EA:** K 60–letiiu kardiologicheskoĭ kliniki im. V.I. Lenina v Kislovodske. **Vopr Kurortol Fizioter Lech Fiz Kult** 1983 Jan–Feb;(1):66–8

**Smirnova KV:** O razvitii ékologicheskoĭ parazitologii v Kazakhstane. **Parazitologiia** 1982 Jan–Feb;16(1):85–7

**Smirnova LI:** Girudoterapiia. **Feldsher Akush** 1983;48(1):58–60

**Smit P:** Jan Ingen-Housz (1730–1799): some new evidence about his life and work. **Janus** 1980;67(1–2–3):125–39

**Smit P** see **Palm LC**

**Smith AA** see **Kaltenbach RF**

**Smith AJ** see **Stubbe JH**

**Smith AM:** Getting the big picture in perspectivist optics. **Isis** 1981 Dec;72(264):568–89

**Smith AM:** Mercury poisoning and birth defects in Japan. **Women Health** 1978 Mar–Apr;3(2):9–12

**Smith AN:** Pringle's maneuver. **Curr Surg** 1982 Jan–Feb;39(1):12–7

**Smith B, Robertson RM, Robertson D:** An early Southern description of Curschmann's spirals. **Clin Notes Respir Dis** 1982 Summer;21(1):10–2

**Smith BA:** Irish prison doctors--men in the middle, 1865–90. **Med Hist** 1982 Oct;26(4):371–94

**Smith BE:** Black lung: the social production of disease. **Int J Health Serv** 1981;11(3):343–59

**Smith BL:** The brain drain re-emergent: foreign medical graduates in American medical schools. **Minerva** 1979 Winter;17(4):483–503

**Smith BT:** Marcia Crocker Noyes, medical librarian: the shaping of a career. **Bull Med Libr Assoc** 1974 Jul;62(3):314–24

**Smith C:** Medical radiology: its practical application 1895–1914. In Checkland O, Lamb M, ed: Health care as social history; the Glasgow case. Aberdeen, Aberdeen University Press, 1982. p. 100–116.

**Smith CA:** The Children's Hospital of Boston: 'built better than they knew'. Boston, Little, Brown, 1983. ix, 284 p.

**Smith CE:** The Broad Street pump revisited. **Int J Epidemiol** 1982 Jun;11(2):99–100

**Smith CM:** Control of tuberculosis in Delaware: an historical perspective on joint public and private involvement. **Del Med J** 1983 Oct;55(10):593–7

**Smith CU:** Don Juan and the vision of Vision. **Perception** 1981;10(4):435–53

**Smith CU:** Evolution and the problem of mind: part I. Herbert Spencer. **J Hist Biol** 1982 Spring;15(1):55–88

**Smith CU:** Evolution and the problem of mind: part II. John Hughlings Jackson. **J Hist Biol** 1982 Summer;15(2):241–62

**Smith CW** see **Woods R**

**Smith D:** A persistent rebel. **Am Hist Illus** 1981;15(9):28–35

**Smith DB, Delgado Escueta AV, Cramer JA, et al:** Historical perspective on the choice of antiepileptic drugs for the treatment of seizures in adults. **Neurology** 1983 Mar;33(3 Suppl 1):2–7

**Smith DB:** The science of medicine and the art of hypnosis. **Pharos** 1980 Winter;43(1):6–9

**Smith DC:** A renaissance for medical history. **J Hist Med Allied Sci** 1984 Oct;39(4):405–7

**Smith DC:** Dental materials today. Part 1: perspectives - past and present. **Ont Dent** 1980 Dec;57(12):16–9

**Smith DC:** Gerhard's distinction between typhoid and typhus and its reception in America, 1833–1860. **Bull Hist Med** 1980 Fall; 54(3):368–85

**Smith DC:** The emergence of organized clinical instruction in the nineteenth century American cities of Boston, New York and

Philadelphia. Ph.D. Diss. University of Minnesota. Minneapolis, 1979. 357 leaves.
**Smith DC:** The rise and fall of typhomalarial fever: I. origins. **J Hist Med Allied Sci** 1982 Apr;37(2):182–220
**Smith DC:** The rise and fall of typhomalarial fever: II. decline and fall. **J Hist Med Allied Sci** 1982 Jul;37(3):287–321
**Smith DC:** The triumph of scientific medicine in America: an essay review. **J Hist Med Allied Sci** 1982 Apr;37(2):231–5
**Smith DC:** William Budd manuscript at the National Library of Medicine. **J Hist Med Allied Sci** 1980 Jul;35(3):318–19
**Smith DC** see **Wangensteen OW, ed**
**Smith DG:** Federal health grants and regional health politics. **Publius** 1982;12(2):63–77
**Smith DG:** The voyage of the challenger. **Bookman** 1983 Apr;10(2):3–9
**Smith DP:** A reconsideration of Easterlin cycles. **Popul Stud** 1981 Jul;35(2):247–64
**Smith DS:** A community-based sample of the older population from the 1880 and 1900 United States manuscript census. **Hist Methods Newsl** 1978;11(2):67–74
**Smith DS:** The demographic history of colonial New England. **J Econ Hist** 1972;32(1):165–83
**Smith DS:** The estimates of early American historical demographers: two steps forward, one step back, what steps in the future? **Hist Methods Newsl** 1979;12(1):24–38
**Smith DS** see **Laslett P**
**Smith DS** see **Spicker SF**
**Smith DW:** Koch's postulates and the Koch phenomenon, an update. **Indian J Chest Dis Allied Sci** 1982 Apr–Sep;24(2–3):95–100
**Smith E:** The life of Sir Joseph Banks. New York, Arno Press, 1975. xvi, 348 p.
**Smith EB, Head ES, Raimer SS:** Dermatology on Galveston Island at the turn of the century. **Int J Dermatol** 1981 Jul–Aug;20(6):449–54
**Smith EB** see **Forgan S, ed**
**Smith EK:** History of the Pacific Northwest Section, AACC 1961–1981. **Clin Chem** 1981 May;27(5):762–4
**Smith EM** see **Cottam C**
**Smith FB:** Ethics and disease in the later nineteenth century: the Contagious Diseases Acts. **Hist Stud** 1971;15(57):118–35
**Smith FB:** Florence Nightingale. Reputation and power. London, Canberra, Croom Helm, 1982. xii, 216 p.
**Smith FH** see **Hinton RJ**
**Smith FN:** Swift and cannabis. **Am Notes Queries** 1983 Nov–Dec;22(3–4):37–9
**Smith FT:** Florence Nightingale: early feminist. **Am J Nurs** 1981 May;81(5):1021–4
**Smith FT:** [Florence Nightingale: early feminist] (Jpn). **Kango Kyoiku** 1982 Nov;23(11):671–6
**Smith G:** Ogston's Coccus: 102 years and still going strong. **South Med J** 1982 Dec;75(12):1559–62
**Smith G:** The physiology of air: eighteenth-century fever therapy in the advice literature. **Soc Soc Hist Med Bull (Lond)** 1984 Dec;35:21–3
**Smith GF:** Congenital abnormalities and genetic concepts in neonatology. In Smith GF, Smith PN, Vidyasagar D, ed: Historical review and recent advances in neonatal and perinatal medicine. [Chicago?], Mead Johnson Nutritional Division, 1983. Vol. II. p. 73–83.
**Smith GF, Smith PN, Vidyasagar D, ed:** Historical review and recent advances in neonatal and perinatal medicine. 2 vols. [Chicago?], Mead Johnson Nutritional Division, 1983. xxii, 212 p.; viii, 189 p. Historical contributions by B. F. Andrews, L. Ballowitz, L. J. Butterfield, V. Chernick, T. E. Cone, R. L. Day, M. L. Duxbury, D. Dye, L. M. Gartner, P. J. Goldstein, M. H. Greenberg, L. Johnson, A. Kaul, J. O. Klein, J. Lind, L. O. Lubchenco, N. M. Nelson, K. C. Pringle, T. N. Raju, A. C. Rambar, R. Sosa, M. T. Stahlman, L. Stern, K. Tarpey, A. Zipursky.
**Smith GF** see **Kaul A**
**Smith GH:** The excavation of the hospital of St. Mary of Ospringe, commonly called Maison Dieu. **Archaeol Cantiana** 1979,(1980);95:81–184
**Smith GJ:** Averill Abraham Liebow: contributions to pulmonary pathology. **Yale J Biol Med** 1981 Mar–Apr;54(2):139–46
**Smith H:** John Keats: poet, patient, physician. **Rev Infect Dis** 1984 May–Jun;6(3):390–404
**Smith HC:** Arthur Sinton Otis. In Dictionary of American biography, 1961–1965. Suppl. 7, 1981. p. 594–5.
**Smith HC:** Douglas Henry Fryer. In Dictionary of American Biography, Suppl. 6, 1956–1960. p. 222, 1980.
**Smith HE:** Doctors and society: a Northern Thailand study. **Soc Sci Med** 1982,16(5):515–26
**Smith HG:** Architecture, form and conservation in a spa town. **R Soc Health J** 1982 Oct;102(5):196–200
**Smith HH:** Life's a pleasant institution: the peregrinations of a Rockefeller doctor. Tucson, The Author, 1978. x, 254 p.
**Smith HL:** [Development of] heart transplantation. In Reich WT, et al, ed: Encyclopedia of bioethics, v. 2. New York, Free Press, 1978. p. 654–60.
**Smith J** see **Fischer JL**
**Smith JC, Weisstub DN:** The evolution of Western legal consciousness. **Int J Law Psychiatry** 1979;2(2):215–34
**Smith JD:** Kentucky Civil War recruits: a medical profile. **Med Hist** 1980 Apr;24(2):185–96
**Smith JL:** Sir Arbuthnot Lane, chronic intestinal stasis, and autointoxication. **Ann Intern Med** 1982 Mar;96(3):365–9
**Smith JM:** John Burdon Sanderson Haldane. In Dictionary of national biography, 1961–1970. Suppl. 8, 1981. p. 473–5.
**Smith JM:** The recent history of the treatment of asthma: a personal view. **Thorax** 1983 Apr;38(4):244–53
**Smith JM:** Thomas Huxley in Nashville. **Tenn Hist Q** 1974;33(2):191–203;(3):322–41
**Smith JP:** Mary Jane Seacole 1805–1881: a black British nurse. **J Adv Nurs** 1984 Sep;9(5):427–8
**Smith K:** Dr. Augusta Stowe-Gullen: a pioneer of social conscience. **Can Med Assoc J** 1982 Jun 15;126(12):1465–7
**Smith K:** Maude Abbott: pathologist and historian. **Can Med Assoc J** 1982 Oct 15;127(8):774–6
**Smith KC:** History of American Society for Photobiology (ASP). The first 10 years, and before. **Photochem Photobiol** 1982 May;35(5):597–614
**Smith KM:** Dr. James Barry: military man--or woman? **Can Med Assoc J** 1982 Apr 1;126(7):854–7
**Smith L:** The influence of tradition in nursing. **Nurs Times** 1982 Apr 28–May 4;78(17):suppl 12:45–8
**Smith LD:** Psychology and philosophy: towards a realignment, 1905–1935. **J Hist Behav Sci** 1981 Jan;17(1):28–37
**Smith MB:** Else Frenkel-Brunswik. In: Notable American women. The modern period. Cambridge, Mass., Belknap-Harvard Univ. Press, 1980. 4:250–2.
**Smith MG:** Resources for nursing history. **NZ Nurs J** 1983 Jan;76(1):26–7
**Smith MO** see **Hinton RJ**
**Smith MT, Hudson BL:** Isonymic relationships in the parish of Fylingdales, North Yorkshire, in 1851. **Ann Hum Biol** 1984 Mar–Apr;11(2):141–8
**Smith MW** see **Tokuhata GK**
**Smith NB:** The women who went to the war: the Union Army nurse in the Civil War. Ph.D. Diss., Northwestern Univ. Evanston, 1981. 183 p.
**Smith NW:** Illusions and counter-illusions or aesthetic effects in Greek temples? **Stor Crit Psicol** 1983 Dec;4(2):157–70
**Smith P, Tau S:** Dental pathology in the period of the Roman Empire: a comparison of two populations. **Ossa** 1978;5:35–41
**Smith P** see **Meir E**
**Smith PB:** Chemical glimpses of paradise. Springfield, Illinois, Charles C. Thomas, 1972. ix, 92 p.
**Smith PC:** Crisis mortality in the nineteenth century Philippines: data from parish records. **J Asian Stud** 1978;38(1):51–76
**Smith PC, Shui-Meng NG:** The components of population change in nineteenth-century South-east Asia: village data from the Philippines. **Popul Stud** 1982 Jul;36(2):237–55
**Smith PN** see **Smith GF**
**Smith R:** Criminal insanity: from a historical point of view. **Bull Am Acad Psychiatry Law** 1983;11(1):27–34
**Smith R:** History of the prison medical services. **Br Med J [Clin Res]** 1983 Dec 10;287(6407):1786–8
**Smith R:** Scientific thought and the boundary of insanity and criminal responsibility. **Psychol Med** 1980 Feb;10(1):15–23
**Smith R:** The first American officer wounded in World War I. **JAMA** 1982 Mar 26;247(12):1743
**Smith R:** Trial by medicine. Insanity and responsibility in Victorian trials. Edinburgh, Edinburgh University Press, 1981. ix, 238 p.
**Smith R:** Wilhelm Wundt resurrected. **Br J Hist Sci** 1982 Nov;15(51 pt 3):285–91
**Smith R** see **Scull A, ed**
**Smith RA:** Development of lung surgery in the United Kingdom. **Thorax** 1982 Mar;37(3):161–8
**Smith RD:** Avicenna and the Canon of Medicine: a millennial tribute. **West J Med** 1980 Oct;133(4):367–70
**Smith RD:** Paganini's hand. **Arthritis Rheum** 1982 Nov;25(11):1385–6
**Smith RD:** The cricket and the marionette. **South Med J** 1982 Jan;75(1):59–60
**Smith RD:** Tribute to Avicenna: one thousand years of the art of preserving health. **J Kans Med Soc** 1981;82:359–60, 372
**Smith RD** see **Markle GE**
**Smith RE:** Contributions of histochemistry to the development of the proteolytic enzyme detection system in diagnostic medicine. **J Histochem Cytochem** 1983 Jan;31(1A Suppl):199–209
**Smith RL** see **Neuberger A**
**Smith RM:** Fertility, economy, and household formation in England over three centuries. **Popul Dev Rev** 1981;7(4):595–622
**Smith RM:** The people of Tuscany and their families in the fifteenth century: Medieval or Mediterranean? **J Fam Hist** 1981 Spring;6(1):107–28
**Smith RM:** The structured dependency of the elderly: a twentieth-century creation? **Soc Soc Hist Med Bull (Lond)** 1984 Jun;34:35–41
**Smith RN:** D. J. A. McBride, MRCVS, 1843?–1889, itinerant professor extraordinary. **Vet Hist** 1981 N.Ser;2(1):3–25
**Smith S** see **Kohn D**
**Smith S** see **Stambolian G**
**Smith SB:** The great mental calculators: the psychology, methods, and lives of calculating prodigies, past and present. New York, Columbia University Press, 1983. xviii, 374 p.
**Smith SM:** Competency. **Psychiatr Clin North Am** 1983 Dec;6(4):635–50
**Smith SR:** Age in old England. **Hist Today** 1979;29(3):172–8
**Smith SR** see **Spicker SF**
**Smith T:** Document: [letter to Dr. Edward B. Krumbhaar]. **Trans Stud Coll Physicians Phila** 1981 Sep;5(3 no 3):214–5
**Smith T:** Prince of Wales's Hospital: prince and pauper. **Health Soc Serv J** 1981 Dec 17;91(4777):1552–4

**Smith T:** Royal Army Medical Corps. Into battle to save the casualties of war. **Health Soc Serv J** 1983 Aug 18;93(4860):994–5
**Smith T:** Victorian who sent a hospital to war. **Health Soc Serv J** 1983 May 5;93(4845):533–5
**Smith TF, Morowitz HJ:** Between history and physics. **J Mol Evol** 1982;18(4):265–82
**Smith TG:** Detaining the insane: detention hospitals, mental health, and frontier politics in Alaska, 1910–1915. **Pac Northwest Q** 1982;73(3):124–33
**Smith TW** see **Lamas GA**
**Smith WC:** Brief history of the treatment of disabled citizens--since the beginning of written history. **Am Correct Ther J** 1980 Nov–Dec;34(6):182–3
**Smith WD:** Erasistratus's dietetic medicine. **Bull Hist Med** 1982 Fall;56(3):398–409
**Smith WD:** Galen on Coans versus Cnidians. **Bull Hist Med** 1973 Nov–Dec;47(6):569–85
**Smith WD:** Under the influence. A history of nitrous oxide and oxygen anaesthesia. London, Macmillan, 1982. xxviii, 188 p.
**Smith WD** see **Grmek MD, ed**
**Smith WD** see **Lloyd GE**
**Smith WE:** Mormon sex standards on college campuses: or deal us out of the sexual revolution! **Dialogue** 1976;10(2):76–81
**Smith WS:** History of the control of some diseases of sheep and cattle in South Australia. **Aust Vet J** 1983 Apr;60(4):122–3
**Smith C, ed** see **Novotny A**
**Smith DC, ed:** 'On the causes of fevers' (1839) by William Budd. Baltimore and London, Johns Hopkins University Press, 1984. xi, 164 p. (Henry E. Sigerist Supplements to the Bulletin of the History of Medicine, n.s., no. 9)
**Smith ET, ed** see **Spears B**
**Smith JH, ed:** Kierkegaard's truth: the disclosure of the self. New Haven, London, Yale University, 1981. xvii, 438 p. (Psychiatry and the Humanities. Volume 5.) With contributions by P. L. Holmer, P. B. Armstrong, J. Collins, H. A. Durfee, W. Kerrigan, B. H. Kirmmse, L. H. Mackey, V. A. McCarthy, W. W. Meissner, P. Ricoeur, M. C. Taylor, M Theunissen.
**Smith (Lord of Marlow):** Annual oration on some lessons from the history of medicine. **Trans Med Soc Lond** 1977–78;94:86–94
**Smith RM, ed** see **Laslett P**
**Smith-Rosenberg C:** Sex as symbol in Victorian purity: an ethnohistorical analysis of Jacksonian America. In Demos, John and Boocock, Sarane Spence, ed: Turning points: historical and sociological essays on the family. Chicago, U. of Chicago Press, 1978. p. 212–47.
**Smith-Rosenberg C:** The new woman and the psycho-historian: a modest proposal. **Group Psychol Hist Newsl** 1975;4(3):4–11
**Smith WD, et al:** Reflections on black psychology. Washington, University Press of America, 1979. ix, 528 p.
**Smithcors JF:** Discovery of the arthropod vector of disease. **Mod Vet Pract** 1981 May;62(5):371–4
**Smithers DW:** Dicken's doctors. Oxford, New York, Pergamon, 1979. xiii, 111 p.
**Smithers DW:** The Barsetshire doctors. **Br Med J [Clin Res]** 1982 Dec 18–25;285(6357):1806–8
**Smits WH:** Prof. W.J. Roepke: Forty year link between science and practice. **Vet Q** 1984 Jul;6(3):105–6
**Smoje D** see **Sutto C, ed**
**Smola BK:** A study of the development of diploma and baccalaureate degree nursing education programs in Iowa from 1907–1978. Ph.D. Diss., Iowa State University. Ames, 1980. iv, 319 p.
**Smolenskiĭ VS, Tarasov KE:** Znachenie leninskogo ucheniia o dialekticheskoĭ vzaimosviazi ob'ektivnogo i sub'ektivnogo v oschchushcheniiakh dlia diagnostiki. **Klin Med (Mosk)** 1980 Sep;58(9):3–6
**Smol'iannikov AV:** Kafedre patologicheskoĭ anatomii Tsentral'nogo ordena Lenina instituta usovershenstvovannia vracheĭ 50 let. **Arkh Patol** 1980;42(12):59–61
**Smol'iannikov AV, Sarkisov DS, Serebrennikov AB:** N. I. Pirogov--velikiĭ uchenyĭ, vrach, grazhdanin. **Arkh Patol** 1982;44(9):3–13
**Smol'iannikov AV** see **Strukov AI**
**Smollich R:** Der Bisamapfel in Kunst und Wissenschaft. Stuttgart, Deutscher Apotheken Verlag, 1983. 342 p. (Quellen und Studien zur Geschichte der Pharmazie, Bd. 21).
**Smollich R:** Der Bisamapfel in Kunst und Wissenschaft. Stuttgart, Deutscher Apotheker Verlag, 1983. 342 p. (Quellen und Studien zur Geschichte der Pharmazie, Bd. 21)
**Smollon JF:** A review and history of endosseous implant dentistry. **Georgetown Dent J** 1979 Jan;63(1):33–45
**Smorodintsev AA:** K istorii izucheniia étiologii i vaktsinoprofilaktiki grippa (nauchnyĭ vklad v étu problemu kliniki M. D. Tushinshinskogo). **Klin Med (Mosk)** 1982 Jan;60(1):108–12
**Smorodintsev AA** see **Rykushin IuP**
**Smout C** see **Laslett P**
**Smoyak SA, Rouslin S, ed:** A collection of classics in psychiatric nursing literature. Thorofare, N. J., Slack, 1982. xi, 295 p.
**Smucker C** see **Simmons GB**
**Smyrniw W:** Tolstoy's depiction of death in the context of recent studies of the 'experience of dying.' **Can Slavonic Pap** 1979;21(3):367–79
**Smyth DH:** Sir Charles Arthur Lovatt Evans. In Dictionary of national biography, 1961–1970. Suppl. 8, 1981. p. 334–6.
**Smythies JR:** A visit to Dr. Jung. **Ala J Med Sci** 1981 Jan;18(1):93–4
**Snaedal G** see **Alfredsson JH**
**Snajder D:** Pola veka rada na eradikaciji difterije u našoj zemlji. **Srp Arh Celok Lek** 1983 Feb;111(2):239–48
**Snajdr J, Thiel L:** 30 let obvodního systému v CSSR--vývoj a perspektivy. **Cesk Zdrav** 1984 May;32(5):193–205
**Snape WJ, Wolfe EL:** Courage, compassion, and providence: Woodbury 1793. **Bull Gloucester Cty Hist Soc** 1984 Dec;19(6):41–4
**Snape WJ, Wolfe EL:** Preliminary report of yellow fever during the 18th century. **J Med Soc NJ** 1984 Sep;81(9):731–3
**Snape WJ, Wolfe EL:** The studies of yellow-fever by Noah Webster and John Conrad Otto at Red Bank, New Jersey. **Bull Gloucester Cty Hist Soc** 1984 Jun;19(4):25–32
**Snelders HA:** De chemische voordrachten van Wille de Loos (circa 1770). **Tijdschr Geschied Geneeskd** 1979;2(4):168–75
**Snelders HA:** De natuur- en scheikundige wetenschappen in de medische tijdschriften. **Ned Tijdschr Geneeskd** 1981 Apr 25;125(17):668–73
**Snelders HA:** Het chemisch laboratorium 'de Leeuwenbergh' te Utrecht (1845–1903). **Tijdschr Geschied Geneeskd** 1984;7(3):129–56
**Snelders HA:** Het fysisch-chemisch werk van de Rotterdamse arts Hendrik Willem Rouppe (1765–1816). **Tijdschr Geschied Geneeskd** 1981;4(1):25–44
**Snelders HA:** Het Gezelschap der Hollandsche Scheikundigen. Amsterdamse chemici uit het einde van de achttiende eeuw. Amsterdam, Rodopi, 1980. 111 p. (Nieuwe Nederlandse Bijdragen tot de Geschiedenis der Geneeskunde en der Natuurwetenschappen, no. 4).
**Snelders HA:** Hoofdstukken uit de geschiedenis van de scheikunde. 2e vermmerderde druk. Amsterdam, Rodopi, 1979. 175 p.
**Snelders HA:** Lambertus Bicker (1732–1801). An early adherent of Lavoisier in the Netherlands. **Janus** 1980;67(1–2–3):101–23
**Snelders HA:** Nederlandse apothekers en het acceptatieproces van Lavoisiers nieuwe scheikunde. **Pharm Weekbl** 1981 Nov 6;116(45):1401–6
**Snelders HA:** Science in the Low Countries during the sixteenth century. A survey. **Janus** 1983;70(3–4):213–27
**Snelders HA:** The Amsterdam pharmacist Willem van Barneveld (1747–1826) and the discovery of photosynthesis (1778). **Janus** 1981;68:1–14
**Snelders HA** see **Van der Leun C, ed:**
**Snelders HA, ed** see **Palm LC**
**Snell EE:** Lactic acid bacteria and identification of B-vitamins: some historical notes, 1937–1940. **Fed Proc** 1979 Dec;38(13):2690–3
**Snellen HA:** Birth and growth of the European Society of Cardiology. **Eur Heart J** 1980 Feb;1(1):5–7
**Snellen HA:** E. J. Marey and cardiology: physiologist and pioneer of technology, 1830–1904: selected writings in facsimile with comments and summaries, a brief history of life and work, and a bibliography. 264 p.
**Snellen HA, Dunning AJ, Arntzenius AC, ed:** History and perspectives of cardiology. Catheterization, angiography, surgery and concepts of circular control. The Hague, Leiden University Press, 1981. 204 p. Major historical contributions by L. Dexter, H. L. Abrams, H. Swan, A. C. Guyton, J. Sonolet.
**Snellen HA:** Thomas Lewis (1881–1945) and cardiology in Europe. **Br Heart J** 1981 Aug;46(2):121–5
**Snider GL:** Thirty years of mechanical ventilation. Changing implications. **Arch Intern Med** 1983 Apr;143(4):745–9
**Snively WD:** Daniel Drake: the Ohio Valley's man for all season. **Indiana Med Hist Q** 1976;2(4):61–4
**Snively WD:** 'We war perplext by a disease cald milksick'; the story of the pioneers' most dreaded plague. **Indiana Med Hist Q** 1974;1(2):31–5
**Snodgrass J:** William Healy (1869–1963): pioneer child psychiatrist and criminologist. **J Hist Behav Sci** 1984 Oct;20(4):332–9
**Snodgrass N:** BVA centenary. One Hundred years of Congress. **Vet Rec** 1982 Sep 18;111(12):251–4
**Snodgrass N:** BVA Centenary. The British Veterinary Association: an historical note. **Vet Rec** 1982 Mar 20;110(12):279–88
**Snoedal G:** Jordenmödrenes arbejde for 100 år siden. **Nord Medicinhist Arsb** 1982;:171–8
**Snook GA:** A short history of the anterior cruciate ligament and the treatment of tears. **Clin Orthop** 1983 Jan–Feb;(172):11–3
**Snook GA:** The history of sports medicine. **Am J Sports Med** 1984 Jul–Aug;12(4):252–4
**Snorrason E:** Den Habsburgske underkaebe. **Tandlaegebladet** 1982 May;86(8):277–80
**Snow D:** The progress of public health in Western Australia, 1829–1977. Perth, Public Health Department; Beaverton, Or., International Scholarly Book Services, 1981. xvi, 185 p.
**Snow LF:** Con men and conjure men: a ghetto image. In Jones AH, ed: Images of healers. Albany, State University of New York Press, 1983, p. 45–78.
**Snyder C:** A look at George Frick's Treatise on diseases of the eye. In: Congrès international d'histoire de la médecine, XXVe, Québec, 1976. Actes. Québec, 1977. p. 1289–1300.
**Snyder C:** Julius Hirschberg, the neglected historian of ophthalmology. **Am J Ophthalmol** 1981 May;91(5):664–76
**Snyder C** see **Lamping KA**
**Snyder CC:** The beginnings. **Clin Plast Surg** 1980 Apr;7(2):137–9
**Snyderman GS:** Witches, witchcraft, and Allegany Seneca medicine. **Proc Am Philos Soc** 1983;127(4):263–77
**Sobalski F:** Uwagi o pracownikach służby zdrowia w Czestochowie w XIX wieku. **Arch Hist Med (Warsz)** 1984;47(3):375–82
**Sobchuk GS, Klantsa PA:** N. I. Pirogov o nagrazhdenii zarubezhnykh uchenykh Russkimi orderami (Po neopublikovannym materialam). **Sov Zdravookhr** 1983;(4):65–8
**Sobchuk GS** see **Bilyk VD**
**Sobchuk GS** see **Klantsa PA**

**Sobchuk GS** see **Kul'chitskiĭ KI**

**Sobczak T:** Rozmiary spozycia mięsa i przetworów zbożowych w większych miastach Poznańskiego Pomorza i śląska w latach 1831-1861. **Kwart Hist Kultury Mater** 1979;27(1):17-30

**Soberón G, Sepúlveda B:** El Consejo de Salubridad General. **Salud Pubica Mex** 1983 Sep-Oct;25(5):483-7

**Sobień-Kopczyńska S, Gęsicka T, Rybus B, et al:** Epidemiologia choroby Wrzodowej u dzieci w latach 1968-1978 w dzielnicy Lódź-Bałuty. **Pediatr Pol** 1980 Apr;55(4):487-93

**Sobocki S, Maciałek E:** Rys historyczny towarzystw lekarskich w Jarosławiu. **Ann Univ Mariae Curie Sklodowska [Med]** 1978;33:353-9

**Sobocki S** see **Maciałek E**

**Sobolev VR:** K 50-letiiu kafedry mikrobiologii Tsentral'nogo ordena Lenina instituta usovershenstvovaniia vracheĭ. **Zh Mikrobiol Epidemiol Immunobiol** 1983 Mar;(3):113-5

**Sobolewicz T:** Wieźniowie w oświecimskiej kuchni obozowej. **Przegl Lek** 1984;41(1):111-5

**Sobolewicz T:** Z przeżyć w rewirze oświecimskim. **Przegl Lek** 1984;41(1):108-10

**Socarides CW:** Homosexuality. New York, Aronson, 1978. Historical chapters, p. 7-61.

**Sociedad Española de Historia de la Medicina:** V Congreso Nacional. Homenaje al Profesor Pedro Lain Entralgo. Madrid, 29-30 septiembre-1 octubre 1977. **Asclepio** 1977;29:1-358

**Sociedad Venezolana de Historia de la medicina:** En homenaje al Dr. Placido Daniel Rodriguez Rivero en el 100e aniversario de su nacimiento. Revista de la Sociedad Venezolana de Historia de la Medicina, 1977; 26(40), p. 11-85. Contributions by M. Rodríguez Navarro, G. Briceño Romero, D. W. Fernández Pérez, A. Osuna, C. R. Travieso, A. Silva Alvarez, N. Perazo, R. Beauperthuy de Benedetti, M. Granier-Doyaux, R. Caldera.

**Société française d'histoire des hôpitaux: [1978-79 prizes in hospital history]: Bull Soc Fr Hist Hop** 1980;(40):4-22

**Socknat TP:** The Canadian contribution to the China convoy. **Quaker Hist** 1980;69(2):69-90

**Södergård O:** La chirurgie de l'Abbé Poutrel. Texte picard de 1300 environ. **Acta Univ Lund** 1980;34:1-94

**Soderstrom L:** The Canadian experience. **Proc Acad Polit Sci** 1980;33(4):224-38

**Söderström N:** Infusum amarum alkalinum militare; en arabesk kring ett gammalt amarum. **Sydsven Medicinhist Sallsk Arsskr** 1982;19:137-43

**Sodini JP** see **Guillemain B**

**Soeur R:** Evocation du passé: le professeur Baron Seutin et sa réaction au bandage plâtré. **Rev Med Brux** 1983 Jun;4(6):447-9

**Soffer RN:** Ethics and society in England: the revolution in the social sciences, 1870-1914. Berkeley, University of California Press, 1978. ix, 325 p.

**Sogner S:** Om barnebegrensning i Norge ved sluten av 1800-tallet. **Heimen** 1981;18(9):577-85

**Sogner S** see **Charbonneau H**

**Sognnaes RF:** Hitler and Bormann identifications compared by postmortem craniofacial and dental characteristics. **Am J Forensic Med Pathol** 1980 Jun;1(2):105-15

**Sognnaes RF:** Preface to professional progress from Washington's old ivory relics to the modern Maryland bridge. **J Md State Dent Assoc** 1983 Aug;26(2):79-86

**Sognnaes RF:** President Washington's most famous dentures stolen from the Smithsonian. **J Am Dent Assoc** 1983 Feb;106(2):216-8

**Sohni H:** Die Medizin der Frühromantik. Novalis' Bedeutung für den versuch einer Umwertung der 'Romantischen Medizin.' Freiburg, Schulz, 1973. 270 p. (Freiburger Forschungen zur Medizingeschichte, Neue Folge, 2).

**Soiva K:** Juhlahaastattelu. **Katilolehti** 1980 Dec;85(12):408-11

**Sokal M** see **Brozek J**

**Sokal MM, Rafail PA:** A guide to manuscript collections in the history of psychology and related areas. Millwood, N.Y., Kraus International, 1982. xi, 212 p.

**Sokal MM:** James McKeen Cattell and American psychology in the 1920s. In J. Brozĕk, ed: Explorations in the history of psychology in the United States. Lewisburg, Bucknell University Press, 1984. p. 273-323.

**Sokal MM:** Science and James McKeen Cattell, 1894 to 1945. **Science** 1980 Jul 4;209(4452):43-52

**Sokal MM:** The origins of the psychological corporation. **J Hist Behav Sci** 1981 Jan;17(1):54-67

**Sokal MM, ed:** A guide to manuscript collections in the history of psychology and related areas. [Wellesley, Mass.], Wellesley College Colloquium on the History of Psychology, 1977. iii, 64 leaves.

**Sokal MM, ed:** An education in psychology: James McKeen Cattell's journal and letters from Germany and England. 1880-1888. Cambridge, Mass., MIT Press, 1981, xxvii, 372 p.

**Sokhin AA** see **Vankhanen VD**

**Sokolenko OM** see **Revenko TA**

**Sokoloff KL, Villaflor GC:** The early achievement of modern stature in America. **Soc Sci Hist** 1982;6(4):453-82

**Sokolov EI, Suvorova RV, Krechmer MI:** M. P. Mul'tanovskiĭ - vidnyĭ sovetskiĭ istorik meditsiny. **Sov Zdravookhr** 1983;(12):46-8

**Sokolov VE, Vorob'eva EI:** I. I. Shmal'gauzen i évoliutsionnaia morfologiia. **Arkh Anat Gistol Embriol** 1984 Jul;87(7):5-17

**Sokolov IuN, Rozenshtraukh LS:** Kafedre rentgenologii Tsentral'nogo instituta usovershenstvovaniia vrachei 50 let (kratkiĭ istoricheskiĭ ocherk). **Vestn Rentgenol Radiol** 1980 May-Jun;(3):75-8

**Sokolova LV:** Obzor: Problema vzaimodeĭstviia vozbuzhdeniia i tormozheniia pri formirovanii ucheniia A. A. Ukhtomskogo o printsipe dominanty. **Fiziol Zh SSSR** 1981 Jun;67(6):781-6

**Sokolova LV:** Uchenie A. A. Ukhtomskogo o dominante ka vektore povedeniia. **Nerv Sist** 1982;23:5-13

**Sokolova NF** see **Bogoliubov VM**

**Sokołowska-Pituchowa J:** Two monographs on the spinal cord vascularization. **Folia Morphol (Warsz)** 1980;39(1):1-8

**Sokołowski T:** Badanie ostrości wxroku przed 50 latami i dzfiś. **Klin Oczna** 1981;83(9):451

**Sol A del:** Ensayo histórico sobre las quemaduras en Cuba. La Habana, Editorial Científico-Técnica, 1979. 92 p.

**Solana RM:** Communication, language and family: a communicational analysis of Kafka's letter to his father. **Psychiatry** 1983 Nov;46(4):387-92

**Solar MA:** La atención médica en Chile, 1952-1977: una contribución a su estudio. **Rev Med Chil** 1977 Oct;105(10):701-6

**Solberg WU:** Cotton Mather's indebtedness to Marcello Malpighi. **J Hist Med Allied Sci** 1981 Jul;36(3):326-31

**Soldi A:** Agitare prima dell'uso. L'avventurosa storia dei medicamenti. Milano, Ferro, 1979. 176 p.

**Soldo JJ** see **Shen WW**

**Solé A** see **Darnés C**

**Solente G:** Le Musée de l'Hôpital Saint-Louis. **Am J Dermatopathol** 1983 Oct;5(5):483-9

**Soler J** see **Forster R**

**Solich J:** Prvních deset let farmaceutické fakulty University Karlovy. **Cesk Farm** 1980 Sep;29(7):217-25

**Solich J** see **Rusek V**

**Solimonov SL:** Mediko-sotsial'nye issledovaniia problemy narodonaseleniia Latviskoi SSR. **Latv PSR Zinat Acad Vestis** 1981;8:75-84

**Solís J** see **Germain J**

**Sollmann AH, Blaurock-Busch E:** Manipulative therapy of the spine: the development of 'manual medicine' in Germany and Europe. **Chiropr Hist** 1981;1(1):37-41

**Sollod RN:** Goodwin Watson's 1940 conference. **Am Psychol** 1981 Dec;36(12):1546-7

**Sollod RN** see **Sharkey PW, ed**

**Solnit AJ:** Anna Freud. December 3, 1895-October 9, 1982. **J Am Acad Child Psychiatry** 1984 Mar;23(2):233-6

**Solnit AJ, Newman LM:** Anna Freud: the child expert. **Psychoanal Study Child** 1984;39:45-63

**Solnit AJ:** Anna Freud 1895-1982. **Am J Psychiatry** 1983 Dec;140(12):1632-3

**Solnit AJ:** Anna Freud's contributions to child and applied analysis. **Int J Psychoanal** 1983;64 (Pt 4):379-90

**Solokhin AA:** K istorii poslediplomnogo obazovaniia sudebno-meditsinskikh ékspertov v SSSR (istoki, razvitie, stanovlenie). **Sud Med Ekspert** 1983 Apr-Jun;26(2):55-8

**Solomon N** see **Nyman GW**

**Solomon N** see **Wasserman H**

**Solomon NA** see **Demain Al**

**Solomon R, Barlow T, Kostal R:** The opiate trade of Taiwan and Japan: an historical note. **J Psychoactive Drugs** 1981 Jan-Mar;13(1):35-8

**Solomon R:** The rise and fall of the Laotian and Vietnamese opiate trades. **J Psychedelic Drugs** 1979 Jul-Sep;11(3):159-71

**Solomon-Bayet C:** L'interprétation historique des archives du Comité Nobel de Médecine, 1901-1920. **Soc Sci Inf** 1983;22:487-510

**Soloveĭ MG, Gribanov ED:** M. I. Pevzner--krupnyĭ sovetskiĭ terapevt-dietolog. **Feldsher Akush** 1983;48(2):52-3

**Solov'ev GS** see **Dunaev PV**

**Solov'eva IP** see **Mazurenko MD**

**Solov'eva VA:** K 100-letiiu otkrytiia Robertom Kokhom vozbuditelia tuberkuleza (1882-1982). **Sov Med** 1982;(3):120-2

**Solov'eva VA, ed:** Zhizn' deiatel'nost' Z. P. Solov'eva. Moskva, Meditsina, 1980. 205 p.

**Soloway RA:** Birth control, and the population question in England, 1877-1930. Chapel Hill, University of North Carolina Press, 1982. xix, 418 p.

**Sol'skiĭ IP:** Razvitie i dostizheniia akushersko-ginekologicheskoĭ sluzhby v USSR. **Akush Ginekol (Mosk)** 1982 Sep;(9):3-5

**Soltakhanov RM:** Iz istorii otkrytiia insulina. **Klin Med (Mosk)** 1982 Jul;60(7):118-20

**Soltani A:** Ancient Jundi-Shahpour and its role in medicine and pharmaceutical progress. In International Congress of the History of Medicine. 26th, Plovdiv, 1978. Actes du Congress. Sofia, 1981. Volume II. p. 196-202.

**Soltani A** see **Namigohar F**

**Soltani A** see **Yazdany S**

**Soma K** see **Miura F**

**Soman A:** La sorcellerie vue du Parlement de Paris au début du XVIIe siècle. In: Congrès National des Sociétés Savantes, 104e, Bordeaux, 1979. Actes. Paris, 1981. Histoire Moderne et Contemporaine, Tome 2. p. 393-405.

**Somenzi V** see **Epistemologia, metodologia clinica e storia della scienza medica, 2**

**Somló G:** Megemlékezés Diószsilágyi Sámuelröl Makón. **Orv Hetil** 1983 Jul 10;124(28):1705-6

**Sommer J:** Dusledky filozofické orientace pro farmacii. **Cesk Farm** 1982 Oct;31(8):297-302

**Sommer P:** Die ersten Jahrzehnte des Jenner-Kinderspitals in Bern. **Gesnerus** 1982;39(1):85-8

**Sommer R, Osmond H:** A bibliography of mental patients' autobiographies, 1960–1982. **Am J Psychiatry** 1983 Aug;140(8):1051–4

**Sommer R, Fjeld C:** Consumer protection programs in food cooperatives. **Policy Stud Rev** 1983;2(3):455–64

**Sommer R:** Zur Geschichte des Medizinal- und Apothekenwesens in einem kleinen souveränen Staat (Schaumburg-Lippe). Diss. Braunschweig, 1979. vi, 295 p. (Veröffentlichungen aus dem Pharmaziegeschichtlichen Seminar der Technischen Universität Braunschweig, 19).

**Somogyi E:** A tiszaeszlári vérvád a 100. évfordulóra. **Orv Hetil** 1982 Sep 5;123(36):2243–5

**Somogyi E:** A tiszaeszlári vérvád tanulságai (a budapesti egyetemi tanárok szerepe). **Orv Hetil** 1983 Jan 9;124(2):98–103

**Somogyi E:** Az orvosszakértöi felülvéleményezés történetéből. 25 éves az ETT Igazságügyi Bizottsága. **Orv Hetil** 1981 Nov 15;122(46):2851–3

**Somogyi E:** Korányi Frigyes közéleti munkássága. **Orv Hetil** 1984 Apr 29;125(18):1079–82

**Somogyi E:** Rupp N. János. **Orv Hetil** 1983 Nov 13;124(46):2821–2

**Somolinas Palencia J, Campillo Sainz C, Kumate J:** Conmemoración del sesquicentenario de la fundación del Establecimiento de Ciencias Médicas. **Gac Med Mex** 1983 Nov;119(11):471–4

**Somolinos d'Ardois G:** El fenomeno de fusion cultural y su trascendencica medica. México, Juan Somolinos Palencia, 1979. (Capitulos de Historia Medica Mexicana, II), p. 99–173.

**Somolinos d'Ardois G:** Francisco Bravo y su opera medicinalia. **Bol Inst Invest Bibliogr** 1970;4:337–88

**Somolinos D'Ardois G, Fernández del Castillo F:** Historia de la Academia Nacional de Medicina de México. In Academia Nacional de Medicina. Libro conmemorativo del primer centenario. México, Comité Editorial de la Comisión Organizadora del Congreso del Centenario, 1964. Tome 2. p. 513–21.

**Somolinos D'Ardois G:** Historia de la fundación de la Academia Nacional de Medicina y su tiempo. In Academia Nacional de Medicina. Libro conmemorativo del primer centenario. México, Comité Editorial de la Comisión Organizadora del Congreso del Centenario, 1964. Tome 2. p. 593–621.

**Somolinos d'Ardois G:** Medicina en las culturas mesoamericanas anteriores a la conquista. México, Rendón, for Sociedad Mexicana de Historia y Filosofía de la Medicina, 1978. Capitulos de historia medica Mexicana. I. 97 p.

**Somolinos d'Ardois G:** Relacion alfabetica de los profesionistas medicos, o en conexion con la medicina, que practicaron en territorio mexicano (1521–1618). México, Sociedad Mexicana de Historia y Filosofía de la Medicina, [1979?]. (Capitulos de historia medica mexicana, III). p. 175–312.

**Somolinos Palencia J:** Cristobal Mendez medico y cientifico del siglo XVI. **Bol Soc Mex Hist Filos Med** 1982 Jun;6(39):43–7

**Somolinos-Palencia J:** El doctor Rafael Lucio y las artes. **Gac Med Mex** 1980;116(9):422–8

**Somolinos Palencia J:** El expediente clínico y su importancia en la asistencia y educación médicas. I. El expediente clínico al través de la historia. **Gac Med Mex** 1980 Nov;116(11):477–81

**Somolinos Palencia J:** El tiempo medico de Don Vasco de Quiroga. **Bol Soc Mex Hist Filos Med** 1980 Sep-Dec;5(32–33):123–35

**Somolinos-Palencia J, Martínez-Cortés F, Sepúlveda B, et al:** Etapas de la educación médica en México. **Gac Med Mex** 1984 Jun;120(6):213–28

**Somolinos-Palencia J:** Gabino Barreda, el educador. **Gac Med Mex** 1981 Sep;117(9):377–81

**Somolinos-Palencia J, Risse GB, Price R, et al:** Homenaje a la Sociedad Mexicana de Historia y Filosofía de la Medicina. **Gac Med Mex** 1982 Dec;118(12):471–84

**Somolinos-Palencia J, Corvera-Bernardelli J:** Las casas de la Academia. **Gac Med Mex** 1982 Oct;118(10):403–17

**Somolinos-Palencia J:** René Teófilo Jacinto Laennec, a los 200 años de su nacimiento. **Gac Med Mex** 1981 Mar;117(3):122–6

**Somolinos Palencia J:** Roberto Koch. El descubrimiento del bacilo de la tuberculosis y su primera noticia en México. **Salud Publica Mex** 1982 May–Jun;24(3):237–40

**Somolinos Palencia J:** The Mexican Society of History and Philosophy of Medicine - past, present and future. **Clio Med** 1981;15:245–7

**Somolinas Palencia J:** Un hospital a raiz de la Conquista. **Bol Soc Mex Hist Filos Med** 1979 Jun;4(27):93–104

**Somolinos Palencia J:** Vision general de la medicina en la Nueva España durante el siglo XVI. **Bol Soc Mex Hist Filos Med** 1982 Sep;6(40):61–70

**Somolinos-Palencia J** see **Guarner V**

**Somweber E:** Der Zauberer und Hexenmeister Dr. Georg Iserin von Mazo. **Montfort** 1968;20(3):295–325

**Sonbol A:** The creation of a medical profession in Egypt during the nineteenth century: a study in modernization. Ph.D. Diss., Georgetown University. Washington, D. C., 1981. iv, 296 p.

**Sonbol A:** The creation of a medical profession in Egypt during the nineteenth century: a study in modernization. Washington, D.C., [s.n.], 1981. iv, 296 p.

**Sonderkamp JA** see **Fischer KD**

**Sondervorst FA:** Histoire de la medecine belge. Zaventem, Sequoia, 1981. xii, 326 p.

**Sondervost FA, Wery Ph:** Quelques aspects de l'histoire des organisations d'entraide et la médecine sociale en Belgique. In: Congrès international d'histoire de la médecine XXVe, Québec, 1976. Actes. Québec, 1977. p. 371–99.

**Sonenscher M** see **Jones C**

**Song GF** see **Yang WY**

**Sonin MD** see **Ryzhikov KM**

**Sonino M** see **Legrenzi P**

**Sonnedecker G:** Drug standards become official. In Young JH, ed: The early years of federal food and drug control. Madison, American Institute of the History of Pharmacy, 1982. p. 28–39.

**Sonnedecker G:** The American correspondence between George Urdang and Henry E. Sigerist 1941–1948. In Perspektiven der Pharmaziegeschichte. Festschrift für Rudolf Schmitz zum 65. Geburtstag. Graz, Akademische Druck- u. Verlagsanstalt. p. 343–63.

**Sonnedecker G:** The records of the American Association of Colleges of Pharmacy. **Pharm Hist** 1980;22(3):113–14

**Sonnedecker GS:** The Richtmann Archive at Auburn University. **Pharm Hist** 1984;26(4):179–81

**Sonneveld GJ** see **Hauben DJ**

**Sönnichsen N:** Zum 100. Jahrestag der Entdeckung des Erregers der Tuberkulose durch Robert Koch. **Dermatol Monatsschr** 1982 Mar;168(3):145–6

**Sonntag CD:** Zur Geschichte der Apothekenprivilegien im Gebiet des Herzogtums Kleve vom Vertrag zu Xanten (1614) bis zur Errichtung der Rheinprovinz (1822). Stuttgart, Deutscher Apotheker Verlag, 1982. v, 268, xviii p. (Quellen und Studien zur Geschichte der Pharmazie, Bd. 18).

**Sonolet J** see **Snellen HA**

**Sons HU:** Geschlechtskrankheiten während der Nachkriegszeit. Eine Untersuchung zur Epidemiologie der Gonorrhö und Lues und zur Reorganisation der Fürsorgeeinrichtungen in Nordrhein-Westfalen in den Jahren 1945–1949. **Med Welt** 1983 Oct 7;34(40):1124–6

**Sons HU:** Gesundheitspolitik während der Besatzungszeit: das öffentliche Gesundheitswesen in Nordrhein-Westfalen 1945–1949. Wuppertal, Hammer, 1983. 207 p.

**Sons HU:** Lebensbedingungen in Nordrhein-Westfalen nach dem Zweiten Weltkrieg. Teil 1: Die Situation. **Fortschr Med** 1984 Apr 5;102(13):93–5 (cont)

**Sons HU:** Öffentliches Gesundheitswesen und kommunale Selbstverwaltung in Nordrhein-Westfalen (britisches Besatzungsgebiet) 1945–1949. -- Die Kommunalisierung der Gesundheitsämter. **Off Gesundheitswes** 1983 Jul;45(7):343–8

**Sontag S:** Illness as metaphor. New York, Farrar, Straus and Giroux, 1978. 87 p.

**Sood RK:** Vital aspects of nursing: development of education and services. **Nurs J India** 1982 May;73(5):128–32

**Soong YL** see **Cho LJ**

**Sopronï L:** Nógrád megye gyógyszerészetének kialakualása és története 1701–1918-ig. Diss., Budapest, 1979. 133 p.

**Soprunov FF:** K 90-letiiu so dnia rozhdeniia Petra Grigor'evicha Sergieva (1893–1983). **Med Parazitol (Mosk)** 1983 Nov–Dec;(6):3–6

**Sorcinelli P:** Miseria e malattie nel XIX secolo. I ceti popolari nell'Italia centrale fra tifo petecchiale e pellagra. Milano, Franco Angeli, 1979. 285 p.

**Sorcinelli P** see **Anselmi S**

**Sordet D:** Un homme, une famille. Le médecin principal Pierre Spillmann, professeur agrégé du Val-de-Grâce, professeur à l'Ecole préparatoire de Médecine et de Pharmacie d'Alger (1833–1883). Lyon, Association corporative des Etudiants en Médecine de Lyon, 1978. 40 p. (Thèse, Lyon).

**Soren A, Waugh TR:** The historical evolution of arthrodesis of the foot. **Int Orthop** 1980;4(1):3–11

**Sorensen AA, Kunitz SJ:** The changing distribution of physicians in Regionville. **Rural Sociol** 1978;43(4):711–25

**Sørensen P:** Hospitaler og sygehuse i Kolding: er udgivet af Vejle amtsråds sygehusudvalg i anledning af hundredårsdagen for indvielsen af sygehuset i Sct. Jørgensgade i 1880. Kolding, Konrad Jørgensens bogtrykkeri, 1980. 167 p.

**Sørensen T:** James Blundell 27.XII.1790–15.I.1878. Professor i fysiologi og obstetrik ved Guy's Hospital 1823–1834. **Ugeskr Laeger** 1983 Jun 27;145 Spec No:5–49

**Sorenson AA:** Black Americans and the medical profession, 1930–1970. **J Negro Educ** 1972;41(4):337–42

**Soriano V:** Neurotransmitters. **Int J Neurol** 1979;13(1–4):9–23

**Sormani E:** Il fondo sulla stregoneria della Biblioteca Angelica di Roma. **Mem Riv Stor Donne** 1981;(1):114–5

**Sorní J, Suñé JM:** Barcelona. Baja edad media. Especieros o Boticarios? **Bol Soc Esp Hist Farm** 1983;34(136):139–50

**Sorní J, Suñé JM:** La farmacia en Barcelona desde Jaume I a Jaume II (1213–1327). **Bol Soc Esp Hist Farm** 1983 Sep;135:59–68

**Sorní J, Suñé JM:** Marcofilia farmacéutica española. III. **Bol Soc Esp Hist Farm** 1984 Sep;35(139):211–6

**Soroka AN** see **Kunovskiĭ BV**

**Soroka M:** Fifty years of progress in respiratory care. **Respir Ther** 1979 Jan–Feb;9(1):21, 24–9, 92–3

**Sorokin EIu** see **Sakharov MI**

**Sorokina TS:** Gippokrat i 'Gippokratov sbornik'. **Feldsher Akush** 1984 Mar;49(3):51–5

**Sorokina TS:** Grecheskaia mifologiia o vrachevanii i vrachevateliakh. **Feldsher Akush** 1983;48(6)::47–54

**Sorokina TS:** Meditsina doklassovogo obshchestva. **Feldsher Akush** 1983;48(1):49–52

**Sorokina TS:** Meditsina Drevnego Vostoka. **Feldsher Akush** 1983;48(3):50–3

**Sorokina TS:** Meditsina v Drevnem Rime. **Feldsher Akush** 1983 Dec;48(12):38–43

**Sorokina TS:** Meditsina v Vizantiĭskoĭ imperii. **Feldsher Akush** 1984

May;49(5):49-54
**Sorokina TS:** O drevneĭshikh sanitarno-tekhnicheskikh sooruzheniiakh. **Gig Sanit** 1980 Jul;(7):41-4
**Sorrel-Dejerine Y, Fardeau M:** Naissance et métamorphoses de la myopathie atrophique progressive de Landouzy et Déjerine. **Rev Neurol (Paris)** 1982;138(12):1041-51
**Sorsby A, Benjamin B, Bennett AG:** Steiger on refraction: a reappraisal. **Br J Ophthalmol** 1981 Dec;65(12):805-11
**Sosa R:** Maternal bonding: an overview. In Smith GF, Smith PN, Vidyasagar D, ed: Historical review and recent advances in neonatal and perinatal medicine. [Chicago?], Mead Johnson Nutritional Division, 1983. Vol. I. p. 123-38.
**Sosa R** see **Smith GF**
**Sosińska-Trawińska M, Sródka A:** O utworzeniu Wydziałów Lekarskich W polskich instytucjach naukowych. I. Polska Akademia Umiejętności (PAU). **Arch Hist Med (Warsz)** 1981;44(3/4):363-7
**Sosińska-Trawińska M:** Zalecenia lecznicze w chorobach dzieci zawarte w wybranych czasopismach nielekarskich XVIII w w Polsce. **Arch Hist Med (Warsz)** 1983;46(3):285-94
**Sosińska-Trawińska M** see **Kamińska-Axer M**
**Sosińska-Trawińska M** see **Sródka A**
**Sosnin VV:** Iaroslavskomu meditsinskomu uchilishchu--110 let. **Med Sestra** 1983 Sep;42(9):52-3
**Sosnovskiĭ AT, Eremenko SA, Korsun VF:** K 60-letiiu kafedry kozhnykh i venericheskikh bolezneĭ Minskogo meditsinskogo instituta. **Vestn Dermatol Venerol** 1984 Jan;(1):66-9
**Sospedra Ferrer R** see **Vázquez Albaladejo G**
**Soteras Elía B:** Centenario de la batalla de Oroquieta: primera actuacion de los camilleros de la Cruz Roja. **Pregon** 1972;(111):n p
**Soth DG:** The central processing department: a brief history. **HPN Hosp Purch News** 1983 Mar;7(3):10, 12-3
**Soto J** see **Fernández PL**
**Sotskov VG:** Ot kolonii dlia dushevnobol'nykh k oblastnoĭ psikhiatricheskoĭ bol'nitse (k 100-letiiu Psikhiatricheskoĭ bol'nitsy im. M. P. Litvinova). **Zh Nevropatol Psikhiatr** 1984;84(5):771-3
**Soubiran A, Théodoridès J:** Guillotin et la rage: un mémoire inédit. **Hist Sci Med** 1982;16(4):227-36
**Soudant J** see **Pialoux P**
**Soudek D:** Gregor Mendel and the people around him (commemorative of the centennial of Mendel's death). **Am J Hum Genet** 1984 May;36(3):495-8
**Soulié R:** Brucellosis: a case report dating from 650-700 A.D. **Paleopathol Newsl** 1982 Jun;38:7-10
**Soulié R** see **Wackenheim A**
**Soulie de Morant G:** Acuponcture. (Communications 1929-1951). Avant-propos par N. Soulié de Morant. Paris, Guy Trédaniel, 1979. 234 p.
**Soulier JP:** The history of PPSB. **Vox Sang** 1984;46(1):58-61
**Sourander P:** Drottning Christina och Giovanni Alfonso Borelli till 300-årsminnet av kinesiologins födelse. **Nord Medicinhist Arsb** 1982;:56-65
**Sourander P:** Edelfelts berömda pasteurporträtt - originalet och repliken. **Nord Medicinhist Arsbok** 1983;:149-54
**Sourander P:** Linnaeus and Neurology. **Sven Linnesallskap Arsskr** 1978; Commemorative Volume:88-117
**Sourander P** see **Breimer L**
**Sourkes TL** see **Jasper HH**
**Sournia JC:** Die arabische Medizin. In Sournia JC, Martiny M, Poulet J, ed: Illustrierte Geschichte der Medizin. Salzburg, Andreas, 1980. Vol. 2. p. 589-629.
**Sournia JC:** Die Sozialmedizin. In Sournia JC, Martiny M, Poulet J, ed: Illustrierte Geschichte der Medizin. Salzburg, Andreas, 1980. Vol. 6. p. 2149-93.
**Sournia JC, Manuila A:** Geschichte der medizinischen Fachsprache. In Sournia JC, Martiny M, Poulet J, ed: Illustrierte Geschichte der Medizin. Salzburg, Andreas, 1980. Vol. 8. p. 3093-107.
**Sournia JC:** Histoire et médecine. Paris, Fayard, 1982. 338 p.
**Sournia JC, Martiny M, Poulet J, et al., ed:** Illustrierte Geschichte der Medizin. Salzburg, Andreas, 1980. 9 vols. (Transl. of Histoire de la médecine de la pharmacie, de l'art dentaire, et de l'art vétérinaire, Paris, 1978).
**Sournia JC:** Le dossier médical du maréchal Blaise de Monluc (1500-1577). **Hist Sci Med**
**Sournia JC:** L'histoire de la médecine en France. **Clio Med** 1980;15(1/2):83-9
**Sournia JC:** Littré l'Académie de Médecine. **Bull Acad Natl Med (Paris)** 1981 Oct;165(7):941-7
**Sournia JC:** Remarques sur l'évolution de la protection sociale et sanitaire dans les pays en voie de développement. In: Congrès international d'histoire de la médecine, XXVe, Québec, 1976. Actes. Québec, 1977. p. 297-317.
**Sousa L de C:** Miguel Pereira: um cidadão exemplar. **Rev Inst Hist Geogr Bras** 1973;298:306-14
**Sousa Dias JP:** Problemas e perspectivas na historia das origens de farmacia em Portugal. **Farm Port** 1983 Jan-Feb;1::23-8
**Soutas-Little RW:** Louisa Burns memorial lecture: biomechanics and osteopathic manipulative treatment. **J Am Osteopath Assoc** 1983 Sep;83(1):63-5
**South A:** What Camp Custer brought to Battle Creek. **Chronicle** 1982;18(4):28-30
**Southgate MT:** A summer's reading: Virginia Woolf and her granddaughters. **Conn Med** 1981 Aug;45(8):483-6
**Southgate MT:** Vincent van Gogh, portrait of Dr. Gachet. **JAMA** 1981 Feb 20;245(7):657, 688
**Southgate VR:** Obituary. Dr. Christopher A. Wright. **Int J Parasitol** 1984 Jun;14(3):223-7
**Southwick HW:** The medical center. **Proc Inst Med Chic** 1980 Jul-Sep;33(3):85-7
**Soutter L, Surgeonor DM:** Reflections on blood transfusion (Carl W. Walter). **Am J Surg** 1984 Nov;148(5):562-4
**Souza L de C:** A medicina na guerra do Paraguai (Mato-Grosso) V. **Rev Hist (Brazil)** 1971;42(85):129-46
**Souza LC:** João Moniz Barreto de Aragão-médico militar e pioneiro da veterinária brasileira. **Rev Inst Hist Georgr Bras** 1974;305:51-68
**Souza LC:** Medicina militar brasileira: nomes marcantes et fatos notáveis. **Rev Inst Hist Geogr Bras** 1975;306:150-63
**Sovák M** see **Becker KP**
**Sovetskaia khirurgiia k 62-ĭ:** godovshchine Velikoĭ Oktiabr'skoĭ sotsialisticheskoĭ revoliutsii. **Vestn Khir** 1979 Nov;123(11):3-8
**Sovetskaia voenno-polevaia khirurgiia v Velikuiu Otechestvennuiu voinu 1941-1945 gg. i osnovnye napravleniia ee dal'neĭshego razvitiia: Khirurgiia (Mosk)** 1980 May;(5):3-8
**Sow I:** Psychiatrie dynamique africaine. Paris, Payot, 1977. 280 p.
**Sow M:** Des couleurs dans quelques traités de la collection hippocratique. Univ. de Strasbourg, Thèse de 3e cycle, 1979. lxiv, 402 p.
**Sowers JR:** Hypothalamic hormones. Stroudsburg, Pennsylvania, Dowden, Hutchinson & Ross, 1980. xviii, 342 p. (Benchmark Papers in Human Physiology, 14).
**Soyfer V:** Andrei Sakharov and the fate of biological science in the USSR. **J Craniofac Genet Dev Biol** 1984;4(3):173-8
**Spaar H:** Die Begründung der Vorzüge des Gesundheitsschutzes im Sozialismus und seiner gesetzmässigen Schranken im Kapitalismus im Lichte der Lehre von Karl Marx. **Z Gesamte Hyg** 1983 Oct;29(10):573-6
**Spady JG:** Dr. W. Montague Cobb: anatomist, physician, physical anthropologist, editor emeritus of the Journal of the National Medical Association, and first black president of NAACP. **J Natl Med Assoc** 1984 Jul;76(7):739-44
**Spaet TH** see **Nossel HL**
**Spagnoli PG:** High fertility in mid-nineteenth century France: a multivariate analysis of fertility patterns in the arrondissement of Lille. **Res Econ Hist** 1977;2:281-336
**Spagnoli PG:** Industrialization, proletarianization, and marriage: a reconsideration. **J Fam Hist** 1983 Fall;8(3):230-47
**Spagnoli PG:** Philippe Ariès, historian of the family. **J Fam Hist** 1981 Winter;6(4):434-41
**Spalding P:** Women in the Medical College of Georgia. **South Med J** 1981 Feb;74(2):221-4
**Spallanzani M:** Nuovi studi su Spallanzani e la biologia del '700. **Quad Stor** 1981;16(3):1080-90
**Spangler GM:** Suicide and social criticism: Durkheim, Dreiser, Wharton, and London. **Am Q** 1979;31(4):496-516
**Spängler H, Galle P:** 70 Jahre Unfallchirurgie an den Wiener Kliniken. **Wien Klin Wochenschr** 1981 Jun 26;93(13):423-8
**Spanhove J:** De Sieckenhuysen. **Ascania** 1977;20:33-61
**Spanier GB, Glick PC:** The life cycle of American families: an expanded analysis. **J Fam Hist** 1980 Spring;5(1):97-111
**Spann W:** Die Leichenschau bei Feuerbestattung. **Dtsch Med Wochenschr** 1980 Oct 3;105(40):1376-7
**Spann W:** Prof. Dr. med. Theo Morell, Hitlers Leibarzt. **MMW** 1983 Jun 17;125(24):534-6
**Spanos NP, Gottlieb J:** Demonic possession, mesmerism, and hysteria: a social psychological perspective on their historical interrelations. **J Abnorm Psychol** 88(5):527-46, Oct 79
**Spanos NP:** Ergotism and the Salem witch panic: a critical analysis and an alternative conceptualization. **J Hist Behav Sci** 1983 Oct;19(4):358-69
**Spanos NP** see **Stam HJ**
**Sparacia A:** Dal cerusico all'intensivoterapeuta (rassegna storica dell'emostasi). **Minerva Anestesiol** 1980 Jul;46(7):759-71
**Sparkman RS:** 100th anniversary of the first cholecystectomy. **Arch Surg** 1982 Dec;117(12):1525
**Sparkman RS** see **Shell DH**
**Sparre A:** Dagboksanteckningar från 1858. **Sydsven Medicinhist Sallsk Arsskr** 1981;:132-50
**Sparvieri F:** Teorie freudiane e psicologia aeronautica. **Riv Med Aeronaut Spaz** 1980 Jan-Jun;43(1-2):81-103
**Spasic B, Spasic S:** Razvoj službe za brigu o obolelim od dijabetesa u Surdulici. **Srp Arh Celok Lek** 1982 Nov;109(11):1519-26
**Spasic S** see **Spasic B**
**Spasokukotskiĭ IuA** see **Il'chevich NV**
**Späte HF, Thom A:** Psychiatrie im Faschismus--Bilanz der historischen Analyse. **Z Gesamte Hyg** 1980;26(8):553-60
**Späte HF** see **Rogoll H**
**Späth HU:** Der Hämatologe Albert Alder, 1888-1980. Zürich, Juris Druck, 1983. 81 p. (Zürcher Medizingeschichtliche Abhandlungen, Neue Reihe, 164).
**Spaulding J, Balch P:** A brief history of primary prevention in the twentieth century: 1908 to 1980. **Am J Community Psychol** 1983 Feb;11(1):59-80
**Spaulding WB:** Osler's roots in Dundas. **Ann R Coll Physicians Surg Can** 1982 May;15(3):219-22
**Spaulding WB:** Smallpox control in the Ontario wilderness, 1880-1910. In Roland CG, ed: Health, disease and medicine. Toronto, Hannah Institute for the History of Medicine, 1984. p. 194-214.

**Spavold J:** The sanitary pottery industries of South Debbyshire, 1840–1914. **Ind Archaeol Rev** 1981;5(2):143–54
**Spear DP:** California besieged: the foot-and-mouth epidemic of 1924. **Agric Hist** 1982;56(3):528–41
**Spear JL:** Filaments, females, families and social fabric: Carlyle's extension of a biological analogy. In Paradis J, Postlewait T, ed: Victorian science and Victorian values: literary perspectives. New York, New York Academy of Sciences, 1981. p. 69–84.
**Spears B, Swanson RA:** History of sport and physical activity in the United States. Ed. E. T. Smith. Dubuque, Iowa, Wm. C. Brown, 1978. xii, 402 p.
**Spears J:** Folk medicine and popular attitudes toward disease in the High Alps, 1780–1870. **Bull Hist Med** 1980 Fall;54(3):303–36
**Spears J, Sydenham D:** The evolution of medical practice in two marginal areas of the Western World, 1750–1830. **Hist Reflect** 1982;9(1–2):195–212
**Spears JV:** An epidemic among the Kgatla: the influenza of 1918. **Botsw Notes Rec** 1979;11:69–76
**Spears M** see **Moss C**
**Speck FL, Wheeland RG:** Cutaneous histopathology of southwestern American Indian mummies. **Int J Dermatol** 1984 Sep;23(7):487–92
**Specker H** see **Weiss C**
**Speckner W:** Carl Friedrich von Heusinger. Sein Leben und sein Wirken in Würzburg (1824–1829). Diss., Bayerische Julius-Maximilians-Universität, Würzburg, 1981. 154 p.
**Spector B:** The great Salk vaccine mess. **Antioch Rev** 1980;38(3):291–303
**Speer JB:** Pestilence and progress: health reform in Galveston and Houston during the nineteenth century. **Houston Rev** 1980 Fall;2:120–32
**Speiser P, Smekal FG:** Karl Landsteiner, Entdecker der Blutgruppen und Pionier der Immunologie. Biographie eines Nobelpreisträgers aus der Wiener Medizinischen Schule. 2., vollständig überarb. Aufl. Vienna, Hollinek, 1975. 207 p.
**Speiser P:** Rhesus-Prophylaxe. Zum 40. Todestag von Karl Landsteiner. **Wien Med Wochenschr** 1983 Dec 31;133(23–24):592–4
**Speiser P:** Vogts Lehrbuch und Atlas der Spaltlampenmikroskopie des lebenden Auges. **Gesnerus** 1981:38(3/4):339–45
**Speiser P** see **Bischoff P**
**Spelkoman D** see **Bogdan R**
**Spence DP:** Narrative truth and historical truth: meaning and interpretation in psychoanalysis. New York, W. W. Norton, 1982. 320 p.
**Spencer DG, Sturrock RD, Buchanan WW:** Ankylosing spondylitis: yesterday and today. **Med Hist** 1980 Jan;24(1):60–9
**Spencer EM:** Notes on the history of dental dispensaries. **Med Hist** 1982 Jan;26(1):47–66
**Spencer ER:** A society of physicians. An account of the activities of the members of the Massachusetts Medical Society 1923–1981. Boston, Massachusetts Medical Society, 1981. 410 p.
**Spencer ER:** The Massachusetts Medical Society bicentennial celebration. **N Engl J Med** 1981 Oct 15;305(16):953–4
**Spencer F, Erickson GE:** Charter members of the American Association of Physical Anthropologists. **Am J Phys Antropol** 1981 Dec;56(4):531–5
**Spencer F:** Samuel George Morton's doctoral thesis on bodily pain: the probable source of Morton's polygenism. **Trans Stud Coll Physicians Phila** 1983 Dec;5(5 no 4):321–38
**Spencer FC:** Intellectual creativity in thoracic surgeons. **J Thorac Cardiovasc Surg** 1983 Aug;86(2):163–79
**Spencer FJ:** The Gay Nineties: Oscar Wilde reconsidered. **MCVQ** 1981;16(3):67–70
**Spencer JD:** George Armstrong Custer and the Battle of the Little Bighorn: homicide or mass suicide? **J Forensic Sci** 1983 Jul;28(3):756–61
**Spencer S:** Delivering the woman artist from the silence of the womb: Otto Rank's influence on Anais Nin. **Psychoanal Rev** 1982 Spring;69(1):111–29
**Spencer F, ed:** A history of American physical anthropology, 1930–1980. New York, Academic Press, 1982. xvi, 495 p.
**Spengler JJ:** History of population policies. In Reich WT, et al, ed: Encyclopedia of bioethics, v.3. New York, Free Press, 1978. p. 1232–6.
**Speranskiĭ VS, Burdeĭ GD, Iudin KA:** Muzeĭ i biblioteka kafedry anatomii cheloveka Saratovskogo. **Arkh Anat Gistol Embriol** 1980 Jun;78(6):115–9
**Speransky LS, Bocharov VJ, Goncharov NI:** The personages of Jan Stephan van Calcar's frontispiece to Andreas Vesalius' book 'On the Structure of the Human Body'. **Anat Anz** 1983;153(5):465–79
**Sperduto K** see **Behn RD**
**Sperling M** see **Schramm A**
**Speroni Verner J:** Vida y obra de José Verocay. Montevideo, Universidad de la Republica, Division Publicaciones y Ediciones, 1980. 51 p.
**Speta F** see **Heilmittel aus Pflanzen und Tieren**
**Speta R** see **Heilmittel aus Pflanzen und Tieren**
**Sphon JA** see **Brumley WC**
**Spicer RD:** Infantile hypertrophic pyloric stenosis: a review. **Br J Surg** 1982 Mar;69(3):128–35
**Spicker SF, Van Tassel DD, Woodward KM, ed:** Aging and the elderly; humanistic perspectives in gerontology. Atlantic Highlands, New Jersey, Humanities Press, 1978. viii, 406 p. Historical contributions by D. E. Stannard, H. M. Stahmer, E. E. Whitehead, R. Freedman, S. S. Tamke, G. Berg, S. Gadow, B. G. Rosenkrantz, M. A. Vinovskis, S. R. Smith, D. Luke, W. G. Moss, D. Bronsen, D. S. Smith, T. W. Ganschow, D. Marquis, G. J. Gruman.
**Spicker SF, ed:** Organism, medicine, and metaphysics. Essays in honor of Hans Jonas on his 75th birthday May 10, 1978. Dordrecht and Boston, Reidel, 1978. xxvii, 330 p. Contributions by A. Lowe, M. Landmann, P. O. Kristeller, O. E. Guttentag, E. J. Cassell, L. R. Kass, M. Grene, C. Hartshorne, S. Donnelley, B. S. Currie, R. Kennington, W. Magnus, M. Greene, R. M. Zaner, J. N. Mohanty, H. Arendt.
**Spieckermann ML:** Deutsche Uebersetzungen englischer humanmedizinischer Werke 1680–1810. **Medizinhist J** 1984;19(3):280–4
**Spieckermann ML** see **Fabian B**
**Spiegel AD, Domanowski GF:** Beginnings of home health care: a brief history. **Pride Inst J Long Term Home Health Care** 1983 Summer;2(3):28–33
**Spiel W** see **Zur Geschichte der Psychiatrie in Wien**
**Spielmann J:** Az erdélyi néptáplálkozás kérdései Mátyus István müvében. **Nor Tannlaegeforen Tid** 1982 Jun 13;123(24):1495–8
**Spielmann J:** Egy XVII. századi magyar nyelvü orvosi kéziratról. **Orv Hetil** 1982 Jul 11;123(28):1748–51
**Spielmann J:** Ein siebenbürgischer Pionier der Nephrektomie: Josef Brandt (1838–1912). **Sudhoffs Arch** 1980;64(2):151–62
**Spielmann J, Spielmann M:** L'herbier de Joanus Kájoni. In: Congrès international d'histoire de la médecine, XXVe, Québec, 1976. Actes. Québec, 1977. p. 1301–15.
**Spielmann J:** Nyulas Ferenc emlékezete. **Orv Hetil** 1984 Jun 24;125(26):1578–81
**Spielmann J** see **Habrich C**
**Spielmann M** see **Spielmann J**
**Spielmeyer R:** The epic of Gilgamesh; resolution of concepts of evil and death in ancient Babylonia. **NY State J Med** 1979 Sep;79(10):1618–21
**Spiers CH:** The drug suppliers of George Washington and other Virginians. **Pharm Hist (London)** 1977 Mar;7(1):2–3
**Spiers FW:** 40 years of development in radiation protection. **Phys Med Biol** 1984 Feb;29(2):145–51
**Spiess EB:** Ching Chun Li, courageous scholar of population on genetics, human genetics, and biostatistics: a living history essay. **Am J Med Genet** 1983 Dec;16(4):603–30
**Spillane JD:** The evolution of the concepts of peripheral paralysis and of sensory ataxia in the 19th century. In Rose FC, Bynum WF, ed: Historical aspects of the neurosciences. New York, Raven, 1982. p. 23–36.
**Spina MB:** '... Nothing beats stamp collecting ...' **Tic** 1979;38(8):12–5
**Spineĭ LV** see **Popushoĭ EP**
**Spineĭ LV** see **Popushoĭ VP**
**Spink WW** see **Wangensteen OW, ed**
**Spira M, Hardy SB:** The history of Baylor College of Medicine affiliated residency in plastic surgery. **Ann Plast Surg** 1983 Oct;11(4):268–72
**Spirito A:** Breve istoria della 'rivista di biologia' con particolare riguardo all'ultimo trentennio. **Riv Biol** 1979 Jan–Jun;72(1–2):3–10
**Spiro HM:** Eppinger of Vienna: scientist and villain? **J Clin Gastroenterol** 1984 Dec;6(6):493–7
**Spisak J** see **Radcliff-Umstead D, ed**
**Spitzbart H:** Hugo Sellheim (1871 – 1936). **Zentralbl Gynakol** 1984;106(10):693–5
**Spitzer RL** see **Bayer R**
**Spitzy KH** see **Brandl E**
**Spitzy KH, ed, Lau I, ed:** Van Swietens Erbe: die Wiener Medizinische Schule heute in Selbstdarstellungen. Wien, Maudrich, 1982. 400 p.
**Spivak M:** Pour une approche renouvelée de l'histoire de l'éducation physique et du sport. **Hist Educ (France)** 1981;10:21–32
**Spivak M:** Quelques aperçus de la recherche en histoire de l'éducation physique et des sports en France. **Hist Educ (France)** 1981;10:1–19
**Spohr OH:** Dr. Med. Friedrich Ludwig Liesching. **Q Bull S Afr Libr** 1968;23(2):45–55
**Spor E, ed:** Das Theresienhospital. Ein Stück Düsseldorfer Stadtgeschichte 1288–1980. Düsseldorf, Triltsch, 1980. 128 p. Contributions by F. L. Greb, M. Antonina, L. Peters.
**Sporn MB:** Edward Charles Dodds: diethylstilbestrol. **Cancer Res** 1983 Sep;43(9):preceding 3981
**Sprague NF:** Operative arthroscopy. **Clin Orthop** 1982 Jul;(167):4–5
**Spranger H:** Daten und Fakten zur Entwicklung der Parodontologie in der Bundesrepublik Deutschland. **Dtsch Zahnarztl Z** 1981;36(7):445–8
**Spratt DM:** Dr Ian Murray Mackerras. **Int J Parasitol** 1980 Nov–Dec;10(5–6):329–36
**Spray W:** Down memory lane: obituary at Nottingham. **Nurs Mirror** 1980 Mar 27;150(13):27–8
**Spree R:** Die Entwicklung der differentiellen Säuglingssterblichkeit in Deutschland seit der Mitte des 19. Jahrhunderts. (Ein Versuch zur Mentalitäts-Geschichte). In Imhof AE, ed: Mensch und Gesundheit in der Geschichte. Husum, Matthiesen, 1980. p. 251–78.
**Spree R:** The German petite bourgeoisie and the decline of fertility. some statistical evidence from the late 19th and early 20th centuries. **Hist Soc Res** 1982;22:15–49
**Spree R:** The impact of the professionalization of physicians on social change in Germany during the late 19th and early 20th century. **Hist Soc Res** 1980;15:24–39
**Spree R** see **Labisch A**
**Spreitzer H:** Pestjahre in Mistelbach. **Unsere Heimat** 1970;41(3):132–6
**Spriggs AI** see **Grunze H**
**Spriggs EA:** Hector Gavin, MD, FRCSE (1815–1855) – his life, his work for the sanitary movement, and his accidental death in the Crimea. **Med Hist** 1984 Jul;28(3):283–92
**Spriggs EA:** The illnesses and death of Robert Walpole. **Med Hist** 1982 Oct;26(4):421–8
**Spring JH:** Psychologists and the war: the meaning of intelligene in the alpha and beta tests. **Hist Educ Q** 1972;12(1):3–16
**Sproul EE:** Acid phosphatase and prostate cancer: historical overview. **Prostate** 1980;1(4):411–3

**Stapiński A:** Powojenny wyż demograficzny a zapadalność na kiłę i rzeżączkę w Polsce. **Przegl Dermatol** 1979 Nov–Dec;66(6):667–72
**Stapleton B** see **Dupâquier J**
**Stapleton DH, Carter EC:** 'I have the itch of botany, of chemistry, of mathematics ... strong upon me': the science of Benjamin Henry Latrobe. **Proc Am Philos Soc** 1984 Sep;128(3):173–92
**Stapley EO** see **Woodruff HB**
**Stara JF** see **Dourson ML**
**Starchevskiĭ VS, Perfil'ev GN:** Ispol'zovanie kraevedcheskikh materialov v prepodavanii istorii meditsiny. **Sov Zdravookhr** 1982;(11):65–6
**Stare FJ:** Forty years of Nutrition Reviews. **Nutr Rev** 1982 Nov;40(11):321–5
**Starikov NM:** K 60-letiiu Tomskogo nauchno-issledovatel'skogo instituta kurortologii Minzdrava RSFSR. **Vopr Kurortol Fizioter Lech Fiz Kult** 1982 Jul–Aug;(4):66–7
**Starinskiĭ VV** see **Chissov Vi**
**Stark RB** see **Fisher GT**
**Starkey VL:** The way we were--Ohio State Dental Society, 1866. **Ohio Dent J** 1980 May;54(5):17–9
**Starna WA** see **Elting JJ**
**Starobinski J:** Breve storia della coscienza del corpo. **Intersezioni** 1981;1(1):27–43
**Starobinski J:** Chlorosis--the 'green sickness'. **Psychol Med** 1981 Aug;11(3):459–68
**Starobinski J:** D'Agrippa de Nettesheim à Montaigne: l'embarras de médecins devant l'origine de la semence. **Gesnerus** 1983;40(1–2):175–83
**Starobinski J:** Panorama succinct des sciences psychologiques entre 1575 et 1625. **Gesnerus** 1980;37(1/2):3–16
**Starobinski J:** Sur la chlorose. **Romantisme** 1981;31:113–30
**Starobinski J, ed** see **Cramer M**
**Starostin BA** see **Mikulinskij SR**
**Starr A** see **Freimanis I**
**Starr I:** Concerning Dr. Grayson Prevost McCouch with recollections of the earlier days of physiology in Philadelphia. **Neurol Res** 1983;5(1):1–17
**Starr P, Esping-Anderson G:** Passive intervention. **Work Pap New Soc** 1979;7(2):15–25
**Starr P:** The social transformation of American medicine. New York, Basic Books, 1982. xiv, 514 p.
**Starr P:** Transformation of defeat: the changing objectives of national health insurance, 1915–1980. **Am J Public Health** 1982 Jan;72(1):78–88
**Starr P** see **Hollingsworth R**
**Starr P** see **Navarro V**
**Starr P** see **Numbers RL, ed**
**Starzl TE:** Loyal Davis, surgery of the liver and transplantation of the kidney. **Surg Gynecol Obstet** 1983 Aug;157(2):160–3
**Starzl TE, Porter KA, Francavilla A:** The Eck fistula in animals and humans. **Curr Probl Surg** 1983 Nov;20(11):687–752
**Starzl TE:** The landmark identical twin case. **JAMA** 1984 May 18;251(19):2572–3
**Starzl TE:** The succession from kidney to liver transplantation. **Transplant Proc** 1981 Mar;13(1):50–4
**Starzycka M** see **Zygulska-Machowa H**
**Starzycki Z:** W 40 rocznice wprowadzenia penicyliny do leczenia kiły i rzeżaczki. **Przegl Lek** 1984;41(6):453–7
**Stasienko J** see **Jonecko A**
**Staszyc J:** Doktór Janusz Korczak -- lekarz, literat i twórca pedagogicznej koncepcji wychowania. **Ann Univ Mariae Curie Sklodowska [Med]** 1978;33:333–9
**The state and public welfare in nineteenth-century America:** Five investigations, 1833–1877. New York, Arno, 1976. Various pagings. Reprint of state documents. (Social Problems and Social Policy: The American Experience).
**Stäuble-Lipman Wulf, M:** De Quincey, Baudelaire, e i 'Paradisi artificiali'. **Nuova Antologia** 1972;514(2054):245–54
**Staude JR:** The adult development of C. G. Jung. Boston, Routledge & Kegan Paul, 1981. xxiv, 134 p.
**Stauffer RC** see **Kohn D**
**Stauffer UG** see **Rickham PP**
**Staum MS:** Cabanis. Enlightenment and medical philosophy in the French Revolution. Princeton, Princeton University Press, 1980. xi, 430 p.
**Staum MS** see **Greenbaum LS**
**Stavros T:** Erokles basiades o teleytaios iatrophilosophos. **Epeirotike Hestia** 1975;24(279 280):419–32
**Stavskaia VV** see **Riabov SI**
**Stawiarska B** see **Kucharz E**
**Stead EA:** Kempner revisited. **NC Med J** 1983 Apr;44(4):237–40
**Stearn WT:** From Theophrastus and Dioscorides to Sibthorp and Smith: the background and origin of the 'Flora Graeca'. **Biol J Linn Soc Lond** 1976;8:285–98
**Stearn WT:** Mediterranean and Indian species of Drimia (Liliaceae): a nomenclatural survey with special reference to the medicinal squill, D. maritima (syn. Urginea maritima). **Ann Mus Goulandris** 1978;4:199–210
**Stearns PN:** Old women: some historical observations. **J Fam Hist** 1980 Spring;5(1):44–57
**Stearns PN:** The modernization of old age in France: approaches through history. **Int J Aging Hum Dev** 1981;13(4):297–315
**Stebbins GL:** Darwin to DNA, molecules to humanity. San Francisco, Freeman, 1982. xiv, 491 p.
**Stebbins GL** see **Mayr E**
**Stebliak AG** see **Khokholia VP**
**Stechel RH:** Height and per capita income. **Hist Methods** 1983;16(1):1–7
**Steckel RH:** Antebellum southern white fertility: a demographic and economic analysis. **J Econ Hist** 1980;40(2):331–50
**Steckel RH:** Slave height profiles from coastwise manifests. **Explor Econ Hist** 1979;16(4):363–80
**Steckel RH:** Slave marriage and the family. **J Fam Hist** 1980 Winter;5(4):406–21
**Steckel RH:** The fertility of American slaves. **Res Econ Hist** 1982;7:239–86
**Steckel RH** see **Margo RA**
**Steckel RH** see **Sandberg LG**
**Steckelberg JM, et al:** Werner Forssmann (1904–1979) and his unusual success story. **Conn Med** 1981;45(2):110–2
**Stecko P:** O dalsza poprawe ochrony zdrowia. **Nowe Drogi** 1976;(6):51–62
**Steege MM:** Creating the pneumococcal pneumonia vaccine: a hundred-year story. **Conn Med** 1979 Nov;43(11):717–20
**Steel D:** Plague writing: from Boccaccio to Camus. **J Eur Stud** 1981;11(2):88–110
**Steele H:** The fortunes of economic reform legislation: the case of the Drug Amendments Act of 1962. **Am J Econ Sociol** 1966;25(1):39–52
**Steele JH:** International and world developments in veterinary public health with a comment on historical developments. **Int J Zoonoses** 1979 Jun;6(1):1–32
**Steele JP** see **Gregg JB**
**Steele RS, Swinney SV:** Freud and Jung: conflicts of interpretation. London, Boston, Routledge and Kegan Paul, 1982. x, 390 p.
**Steele TJ:** The death cart: it's place among the Santos of New Mexico. **Colo Mag** 1978;55(1):1–14
**Steen P:** Spas: pleasure of penance? **Hist Today** 1981 Sep;31:21–6
**Steendijk-Kuypers J:** De geneeskundige school te Hoorn (1825–1865). **Tijdschr Geschied Geneeskd** 1980;3(2):49–73
**Steendijk-Kuypers J:** De Hoornse Geneeskundige Genootschappen en hun ijver ten aanzien van de vaccinatie in de 19de EEUW. **Tijdschr Geschied Geneeskd** 1982;5(3):105–14
**Steenkamp WF:** The pharmaceutical industry in South Africa. **S Afr J Econ** 1979;47:75–89
**The 'Stefan S. Nicolau':** Institute of Virology on its 30th anniversary. **Virologie** 1979 Oct–Dec;30(4):253–5
**Stefánek B:** Zur Psychologie des slowakischen Politischen Realismus. **Bohemia Jahrb Coll Caroninum (Ger)** 1979;20:82–96
**Stefănescu P:** Drama otrăvirilor: dosare celebre. Bucuresti, Editura Medicală, 1980. 292 p.
**Stefani FH, Riedel K:** 400 Jahre Augendienst von George Bartisch (1535–1606). **Klin Monatsbl Augenheilkd** 1984 Jan;184(1):64–5
**Stefani WH:** The psycho-physiological effects of volume, pitch, harmony and rhythm in the development of Western art music: implications for a philosophy of music history. M. A. Thesis, Andrews University. Berrien Springs, 1981. 293 leaves.
**Stefanov I:** A népesedéspolitika jelenlegi problémái Bulgáriában. **Demografia** 1972;15(2):227–34
**Stefanovskaia NV** see **Kozliuk VM**
**Stefański K, Chudańska T, Jakubiak J, et al:** Przekrój działalności leczniczej Kliniki Chirurgii Szczękowej SS CMKP w Toruniu w latach 1972–1977. **Czas Stomatol** 1981 Mar;34(3):303–8
**Steffen C:** Eugène Apert (1868–1940). **Am J Dermatopathol** 1984 Jun;6(3):223–4
**Steffen C:** Jean-Nicolas Marjolin. **Am J Dermatopathol** 1984 Apr;6(2):163–5
**Steffen C:** Marjolin's ulcer. Report of two cases and evidence that Marjolin did not describe cancer arising in scars of burns. **Am J Dermatopathol** 1984 Apr;6(2):187–93
**Steffens G** see **Jackle P**
**Steffensen J:** Fra hedenskab til katolicisme, de medicinsk-historiske konsekvenser i Norden. **Nord Medicinhist Arsb** 1982;:149–56
**Steffensen J:** Islandske medicinhistoriske kilder, der ikke har påviselige forbilleder i samtidens Europa. **Nord Medicinhist Arsb** 1980;Suppl 6:94–105
**Stegunin SI, Palagin DA, Veselova AM:** Bor'ba Samarskikh bol'shevikov za okhranu zdorov'ia trudiashchikhsia v 1921–1922 gg. **Sov Zdravookhr** 1984;(5):61–4
**Stegunin SI, Razumov VI:** Pomoshch' narodov SSSR ranenym i bol'nym voinam Krasnoĭ Armii (1941–1945). **Sov Zdravookhr** 1982;(8):59–62
**Stegunin SI, Razumov VI:** Voprosy organizatsii pomoshchi ranenym voinam Krasnoĭ Armii v gody Velikoĭ Otechestvennoĭ voĭny na stranitsakh gazety 'Pravda'. **Sov Zdravookhr** 1984;(6):65–7
**Stehr S:** Zur Geschichte der Münchner Kinderheilkunde (1818 bis 1980, insbesondere die Zeit nach dem Zweiten Weltkrieg). Diss., Technischen Universität München, 1982. 178 p.
**Steichen FM, Ravitch MM:** History of mechanical devices and instruments for suturing. **Curr Probl Surg** 1982 Jan;19(1):1–52
**Steichen FM** see **Ravitch MM**
**Steifl A:** Die Braunkohle und das Egerer Becken. **Bohemia Jahrb Coll Caronium (Ger)** 1978;19:309–20
**Steiger K:** A hippokratészi orvostudomány természetfilozófiai elözményei. **Orvostort Kozl** 1981;93–96(27 No 1–4):17–23
**Steiger O** see **Dupâquier J**
**Steigleder GK:** Ixodes-ricinus-Spirochäten: wahrscheinlich Ursache der Acrodermatitis chronica atrophicans Herxheimer. **Dtsch Med Wochenschr** 1984 Jan 6;109(1):3–5
**Steimle R:** Albert Ehrmann (1821–1871). **Hist Sci Med** 1984;18(3):208–14
**Stein E** see **Bienia RA**
**Stein HF:** Historical understanding as sense of history: a psychoanalytic inquiry. **Psychoanal Rev** 1983 Winter;70(4):595–619

**Stein HF:** Implicit ideology in the psychoanalytic study of culture. **Psychohist Rev** 1981;10(2):91-108

**Stein HF:** Sittin' tight and bustin' loose: contradiction and conflict in midwestern masculinity and the psychohistory of America. **J Psychohist** 1984 Spring;11(4):501-12

**Stein J:** The bioethicists: facing matters of life and death. **Smithsonian** 1979;9(10):107-15

**Stein K** see **Kotek V**

**Stein K** see **Niklíček L**

**Stein R:** Mortality in the eighteenth-century French slave trade. **J Afr Hist** 1980, 21(1):35-41

**Steinberg A:** [Scientific pathology in the books of Talmud.] (Heb). **Harefuah** 1983 Mar 1;104(5):201-2

**Steinberg L:** Michelangelo and the doctors. **Bull Hist Med** 1982;56(4):543-53

**Steinberg ME:** Evolution and development of surface replacement arthroplasty. **Orthop Clin North Am** 1982 Oct;13(4):661-6

**Steinbock RT, ed:** Annotated bibliography [of paleopathology] **Paleopathol Newsl** 1984 Sep;(47):15-20

**Steinbrück P:** Der Erkenntnisprozess in Robert Koch auf seinem Wege zum Begründer der Tuberkulosebekämpfung. **Z Erkr Atmungsorgane** 1983;161(1):6-14

**Steinbruck P:** Hommage à Robert Koch, Sa vie et son oeuvre contre la tuberculose. **Bull Int Union Tuberc** 1981 Sep-Dec;56(3-4):115-9

**Steinbrück P:** Robert Koch und sein Werk. Seine Auswirkungen auf die Tuberkulosebekämpfung. **Z Erkr Atmungsorgane** 1982;158(1-2):5-23

**Steinbrück P:** 30 Jahre DDR -- 30 Jahre erfolgreicher Kampf um die Gesundheit unserer Bürger. **Z Erkr Atmungsorgane** 1979 Apr;153(11):3-4

**Steinebrunner WF:** Spitalarchitektur und Medizin im Zürich des 19. Jahrhunderts: die Planung des alten Kantonsspitals (1842) und des Burghölzlis (1870), ihre Vorbilder und medizinischen Experten. Zürich, Berichthaus, 1971. 104 p.

**Steiner BW:** From Sappho to Stand: historical perspective on crossdressing and cross gender. **Can J Psychiatry** 1981 Nov;26(7):502-6

**Steiner DF** see **Dodson G**

**Steiner H:** Freud against himself. **Perspect Biol Med** 1977 Summer;20(4):510-27

**Steiner I:** První popis 'senilního' amyloidu srdce--I. Soyka, 1876, Praha. **Cesk Patol** 1984 Feb;20(1):11-3

**Steiner ID** see **Hearst E, ed**

**Steiner M** see **Feinberg M**

**Steiner PE:** Medical history of a Civil War regiment: disease in the sixty-fifth United States colored infantry. Clayton, Mo., Institute of Civil War Studies, 1977. xxii, 137 p.

**Steiner TJ:** Development of the concept of supraspinal control. In Rose FC, Bynum WF, ed: Historical aspects of the neurosciences. New York, Raven, 1982. p. 37-43.

**Steiner TJ, Capildeo R, Rose FC:** The neurological tradition of Charing Cross Hospital. In Rose FC, Bynum WF, ed: Historical aspects of the neurosciences. New York, Raven, 1982. p. 347-56.

**Steiner W:** Fortschritte in der endoskopischen Larynxdiagnostik. **Ther Umsch** 1980 Dec;37(12):1021-8

**Steiner ER, et al** see **Gestewitz HR**

**Steinfeld AD, McDuff HC:** An ancient report of a dermoid cyst of the vagina. **Surg Gynecol Obstet** 1980 Jan;150(1):95-6

**Steinfeld JL, Summers N, Schoenberg BS:** Southern medicine in the Civil War. **South Med J** 1980 Apr;73(4):497-8

**Steinfeld JL:** Women and children last? Attitudes toward cigarette smoking and nonsmokers' rights, 1971. **NY State J Med** 1983 Dec;83(13):1257-8

**Steinhauer PD:** The Canadian Academy of Child Psychiatry. The development of child psychiatry in Canada. **J Am Acad Child Psychiatry** 1982 May;21(3):217-8

**Steinkamp U:** Zur Geschichte des Apothekenwesens in den Grafschaften und dem späteren Fürstentum Waldeck und Pyrmont von den Anfängen bis zur Gegenwart. Diss. rer. nat. Marburg, 1980. 278 p.

**Steinkrüger F** see **Kimmel K**

**Steinwald B** see **Sloan FA**

**Steinwendtner R** see **Heilmittel aus Pflanzen und Tieren**

**Stelle CC:** Americans and the China opium trade in the nineteenth century. New York, Arno Press, 1981. 154 p. (Also Diss, Chicago, 1938).

**Stembrowicz W:** Lekarze berlińscy pierwszej Połowy XIX wieku w relacjach lekarzy polskich. **Arch Hist Med (Warsz)** 1979;42(3):273-9

**Stembrowicz W:** Miscellanea prasy warszawskiej o służbie zdrowia w okresie Powstania Listopadowego. **Arch Hist Med (Warsz)** 1980;43(4):415-21

**Stembrowicz W:** Pruski kordon sanitarny w okresie wojny Polsko-Rosyjskiej (1830-1831). **Arch Hist Med (Warsz)** 1982;45(1-4):39-44

**Stembrowicz W:** Rys historyczny wojskowej służby zdrowia w okresie Powstania Listopadowego. **Arch Hist Med (Warsz)** 1981;44(2):129-41

**Stembrowicz W:** Tłumaczenie z jezyka łacińskiego pracy na stopień doktora medycyny z 1829 roku Józefa Lewickiego o osłuchiwaniu i opukiwaniu. **Arch Hist Med (Warsz)** 1984;47(1):49-74

**Stempel A** see **Wojtkowiak S**

**Stemvers FA:** Geslachtsziektenbestrijding 1850-1880. **Tijdschr Geschied Geneeskd** 1981;4(1):1-24

**Steneck NH:** Albert on the psychology of sense perception. In Weisheipl JA, ed: Albertus Magnus and the sciences. Toronto, Pontifical Institute of Mediaeval Studies, 1980. p. 263-90.

**Steneck NH:** Greatrakes the stroker: the interpretations of historians. **ISIS** 1982 Jun;73(267):161-77

**Steneck NH, Cook HJ, Vander AJ, et al:** The origins of U.S. safety standards for microwave radiation. **Science** 1980 Jun 13;208(4449):1230-7

**Steneck NH** see **Cook HJ**

**Stenfors LE** see **Hellström S**

**Stenn F:** The contributions of paleopathology to modern medicine. An update. **Arch Pathol Lab Med** 1981 Dec;105(12):633-7

**Stensman R:** The paraplegic Viking and the one-armed pianist--some well known persons with locomotor disability. **Scand J Rehabil Med [Suppl]** 1983;9:82-7

**Stent GS:** Max Delbrück, 1906-1981. **Genetics** 1982 May;101(1):1-16

**Stent GS:** To the Stockholm station: makers of the molecular-biological revolution. **Encounter (London)** 1980;54(3):79-85

**Stepak S:** Z dziejów Zakładu Wychowawczego dla Niewidomych we Lwowie w latach 1851-1918. **Klin Oczna** 1984 Apr;86(4):181-3

**Stepanov AA** see **Borisov EN**

**Stepanov PF, Romanov NA:** Istoriko-leksikologicheskiĭ aspekt russkoĭ anatomicheskoĭ terminologii. **Arkh Anat Gistol Embriol** 1980 Jun;78(6):111-5

**Stepanov PF, Romanov NA:** O russkoĭ osteologicheskoĭ terminologii XVIII v. **Arkh Anat Gistol Embriol** 1983 May;84(5):93-6

**Stepanskiĭ GA, Fomenko VN:** Sovetskaia toksikologicheskaia nauka i deiatel'nost' moskovskikh toksikologov (k 15-letiiu toksikologicheskoĭ sektsii Moskovskogo nauchnogo obshchestva farmakologov). **Farmakol Toksikol** 1980 Nov-Dec;43(6):747-50

**Stepansky P** see **Wallace ER**

**Stephan GE, McMullin DR, Stephan KH:** Statistical and historical analyses of nations which deviate from the size-density law. **Demography** 1982 Nov;19(4):567-76

**Stephan JC** see **Majnoni d'Intignano B**

**Stephan KH** see **Stephan GE**

**Stephan P:** Geburtlichkeit und Kindersterblichkeit in einem Dorf im 17. und 18. Jahrhundert. **Arztl Jugendkd** 1984 Jun;75(3):178-89

**Stephanos S:** Zur Problematik des omnipotenten Objekts - eine psychoanalytische Studie über Psoriasis. Ein Fall aus dem Jahre 802. **Krankenpfl J** 1984 Mar 1;22(3):20-3

**Stephen K:** Andrew Bell F.R.S.E. (1753-1832). Edinburgh, University of Edinburgh, 1982. [10 p.] (Scottish Men of Letters).

**Stephen K:** Robert Knox, M.D., F.R.S.E. (1791-1862). Edinburgh, University of Edinburgh, [1981]. 11 p. (Scottish men of medicine).

**Stephen RC** see **Dworkin AG**

**Stephen RL:** Artificial kidneys: past, present and future. **Ann Biomed Eng** 1980;8(4-6):487-502

**Stephens LD:** Joseph LeConte and the development of the physiology and psychology of vision in the United States. **Ann Sci** 1980 May;37(3):303-21

**Stephens LD:** Joseph LeConte. Gentle prophet of evolution. Baton Rouge, London, Louisiana State University Press, 1982. xix, 340 p.

**Stephens SD:** Centenary of British audiometry. London, Royal National Institute for the Deaf in collaboration with the British Society of Audiology, 1979. 40 p.

**Stephens SD:** David Edward Hughes and his audiometer. **J Laryngol Otol** 1979 Jan;93(1):1-6

**Stephens SD, Goodwin JC:** Non-electric aids to hearing: a short history. **Audiology** 1984;23(2):215-40

**Stephens SD:** Some historical aspects of ototoxicity. **Br J Audiol** 1982 May;16(2):76-80

**Stephens SD:** The British medical profession and the first audimeters. **J Laryngol Otol** 1981 Dec;95(12):1223-35

**Stephens SD:** The role of the state in hearing health care. **Br J Audiol** 1982 Nov;16(4):255-63

**Stephens SD:** The treatment of tinnitus--a historical perspective. **J Laryngol Otol** 1984 Oct;98(10):963-72

**Stephens SD** see **Mester AF**

**Stephens TD:** The Wolffian ridge: history of a misconception. **ISIS** 1982 Jun;73(267):254-9

**Stephenson GW:** A history of the Committee on Pre- and Postoperative Care. **Bull Am Coll Surg** 1981 Nov;66(11):21-2, 24, 26

**Stephenson GW:** Loyal Davis, M.D., Fellow of the American College of Surgeons. **Surg Gynecol Obstet** 1983 Aug;157(2):118-22

**Stephenson GW:** Martin and Mayo plant the seeds: a history of the international program. **Bull Am Coll Surg** 1980 Jul;65(7):22-8

**Stephenson GW:** The College's role in hospital standardization. **Bull Am Coll Surg** 1981 Feb;66(2):17-29

**Stephenson GW:** The Commission on Cancer: an historical review. **Bull Am Coll Surg** 1979 Sep;64(9):7-13

**Stephenson GW:** The Committee on Trauma: its men and its mission. **Bull Am Coll Surg** 1979 Oct;64(10):17-8, 22-6

**Stephenson HE:** Charles Claude Guthrie's contribution to cardiac resuscitation. **Crit Care Med** 1981 May;9(5):428-9

**Stephenson LW:** Reflections on the military involvement of a medical school. **Surg Gynecol Obstet** 1982 Jun;154(6):888-96

**Stephenson W:** Micheal Polanyi, science and belief. **Ethics Sci Med** 1980;7(2):97-110

**Stepney R:** The Indians' revenge or drunk without drinking. **Practitioner** 1980 Jan;224(1339):109-11

**Sterijev K, Utvic V:** Najsariji carski rez u Slavoniji (1694. godine). **Jugosl Ginekol Opstet** 1978 May-Aug;18(3-4):343-7

**Sterling Bunnell; 1882-1957: J Hand Surg** 1982 May;7(3):217-20

**Stern AC:** History of air pollution legislation in the United States. **J Air Pollut Control Assoc** 1982 Jan;32(1):44-61

**Stern D** see **Harper RG**

**Stern J:** The relationship between unemployment, morbidity and mortality

in Britain. **Popul Stud** 1983 Mar;37(1):61–74
**Stern L** see **Smith GF**
**Stern MB:** Margaret Fuller and the phrenologist-publishers. **Stud Am Renaiss** 1980;229:37
**Stern MJ** see **Katz MB**
**Stern WZ** see **Jacobson HG**
**Stern MB, comp:** A phrenological dictionary of nineteenth-century Americans. Westport, Conn., Greenwood Press, 1982. xx, 430 p.
**Sternbach G:** C.S. Campbell: Gamekeeper's thumb. **J Emerg Med** 1984;1(4):345–7
**Sternbach G:** Joseph Babinski: the phenomenon of the toes. **J Emerg Med** 1984;1(3):263–6
**Sternbach G:** William Osler: narcotic-induced pulmonary edema. **J Emerg Med** 1983;1(2):165–7
**Sternbach H:** Puerperal psychosis in America--1847. **Arch Gen Psychiatry** 1982 Feb;39(2):235–6
**Sternbach LH:** The benzodiazepine story. **J Psychoactive Drugs** 1983 Jan–Jun;15(1–2):15–7
**Sterns I:** Care of the sick brothers by the Crusader Orders in the Holy Land. **Bull Hist Med** 1983;57(1):43–69
**Steslicke WE:** Development of health insurance policy in Japan. **J Health Polit Policy Law** 1982 Spring;7(1):197–26
**Stetson CA** see **Barrow MV**
**Stetsula TI** see **Tret'iak TP**
**Stetten D:** High-powered research and the microscopic viewpoint. **J Med Educ** 1981 Jan;56(1):3–7
**Stettler A:** Lepra und Pest in der Antike. **Antike Welt** 1977;8(4):42–4
**Stettler A:** Vorläufige medizinhistorische und pathographische Bemerkungen zu Ulrich Bräker. **Gesnerus** 1983;40(1–2):185–92
**Stettler M** see **Albrecht von Haller, 1708–1777**
**Stetz MD:** Charles Dickens and 'The Sanatorium': an unpublished letter and manuscript. **Dickensian** 1980;76(390)22–30
**Steudel K:** New estimates of early hominid body size. **Am J Phys Anthropol** 1980 Jan;52(1):52–63
**Stevens EB:** The history of the Medical Group Management Association, 1926–1976. Denver, Medical Group Management Assn, 1976? ix, 135 p.
**Stevens HA** see **Sloan W**
**Stevens KM:** The pathophysiology of influenzal pneumonia in 1918. **Perspect Biol Med** 1981 Autumn;25(1):115–25
**Stevens P:** The health of Hampshire towns in an age of revolutions. **Pharm Hist (London)** 1981;11(2):4–5
**Stevens R:** 'A poor sort of memory': voluntary hospitals and government before the depression. **Milbank Mem Fund Q** 1982 Fall;60(4):551–84
**Stevens R:** Opening a hospital is easy--isn't it? an account of the commissioning of The William Harvey Hospital. Croydon, South East Thames Regional Health Authority, 1982. 52 p.
**Stevens R:** Sweet charity: state aid to hospitals in Pennsylvania, 1870–1910. **Bull Hist Med** 1984 Winter;58(4):474–95
**Stevens R:** Sweet charity: state aid to hospitals in Pennsylvania, 1870–1910. **Bull Hist Med** 1984 Fall;58(3):287–314
**Stevens R:** The changing idea of a medical specialty. **Trans Stud Coll Physicians Phila** 1980 Sep;5(2 no 3):159–77
**Stevens SM:** Alcohol and world view. A study of Passamaquoddy alcohol use. **J Stud Alcohol [Suppl]** 1981 Jan;9:122–42
**Stevenson AL:** The Canadian Medic-Alert Foundation. **Can Anaesth Soc J** 1983 Nov;30(6):573–4
**Stevenson D:** Sir Harry Guy Dain. In Dictionary of national biography, 1961–1970. Suppl. 8, 1981. p. 262.
**Stevenson G** see **Jacobs M**
**Stevenson JM:** Medicine in a nutshell. **J Indiana State Med Assoc** 1981 Oct;74(10):654–5
**Stevenson LG:** Cushion into launching pad; the fiftieth anniversary of the Institute of the History of Medicine. **Bull Hist Med** 1979 Winter;53(4):487–88
**Stevenson LG:** Exemplary disease: the typhoid pattern. **J Hist Med Allied Sci** 1982 Apr;37(2):159–81
**Stevenson LG:** Joseph Dietl, William Osler and the definition of therapeutic nihilism. In Ganzinger K, Skopec M, Wyklicky H, ed: Festschrift für Erna Lesky zum 70. Geburtstag. Wien, Brüder Hollinek, 1981. p. 149–52.
**Stevenson LG:** The Blake era at HMD. **Bull Hist Med** 1982;56(4):455–9
**Stevenson LG:** The emergence of American medicine in the nineteenth century. **Cah Hist Mond** 1968;11(3):455–66
**Stevenson LG:** The newest of old journals. **Bull Hist Med** 1980 Spring;54(1):1–3
**Stevenson LG** see **Bates DG**
**Stevenson LG** see **Ebbert A, et al**
**Stevenson LG** see **Joy RJ**
**Stevenson LG** see **Numbers RL, ed**
**Stevenson LG** see **Rodin AE**
**Stevenson LG** see **Teigen PM, ed**
**Stevenson LG, ed:** A celebration of medical history. The fiftieth anniversary of The Johns Hopkins Institute of the History of Medicine and The Welch Medical Library. Baltimore and London, Johns Hopkins University Press, 1982. vi, 228 p. (Henry E. Sigerist Supplements to the Bulletin of the History of medicine, new ser., no. 6)
**Stewart AB:** Sir William Allen Daley. In Dictionary of national biography, 1961–1970. Suppl. 8, 1981. p. 265–6.
**Stewart B:** CMA's Dr. T. Clarence Routley: 34 years of devoted service. **Can Med Assoc J** 1983 Sep 15;129(6):642–3, 645
**Stewart D:** Unapproved generics. A generation of confusion. **Am Pharm** 1980 Nov;20(11):12–7
**Stewart F:** Life and death in an Oxfordshire churchyard. **Local Hist** 1978;13(3):149–62
**Stewart FH:** The doctor who practiced in Miami. **J Fla Med Assoc** 1982 Aug;69(8):702–5
**Stewart HL:** Reflections on Colonel James Earle Ash on the occasion of his 100th birthday September 8, 1984. **Lab Invest** 1984 Jan;50(1):1–2
**Stewart J:** Women pioneers of medicine. **Midwife Health Visit Community Nurse** 1983 Jun;20(6):240, 242
**Stewart J** see **Ebers GC**
**Stewart JB:** The political economy of black male suicides. **J Black Stud** 1980;11(2):249–61
**Stewart KM:** Mortuary practices of the Mojave Indians. **Palacio** 1973;79(4):2–12
**Stewart L:** The edge of utility: slaves and smallpox in the early eighteenth century. **Med Hist** 1985 Jan;29(1):54–70
**Stewart MA:** The authenticity of Robert Boyle's anonymous writings on reason. **Bodleian Libr Rec** 1981 Aug;10(5):280–9
**Stewart MJ:** Moving the wounded. Litters, cacolets and ambulance wagons, U. S. Army, 1776–1876. Ft. Collins, Colorado, Old Army Press, 1979. 134 p.
**Stewart R:** Bethune. 2nd ed. Hamden, Connecticut, Archon, 1979. 210 p.
**Stewart R:** The mind of Norman Bethune. Toronto, Fitzhenry and Whiteside, 1977. ix, 150 p.
**Stewart RD:** Prehospital emergency care: historical foundations. **Top Emerg Med** 1979 Jul;1(2):11–5
**Stewart RF:** Nursing education in Texas 1890–1982. Part I. **Tex Nurs** 1982 Jun–Jul;56(6):19–22
**Stewart S:** Rational powwowing: an examination of choice among medical alternatives in rural York County, Pennsylvania. **Pa Folklife** 1976;26(1):12–7
**Stewart S:** Sharing more than marble palaces. **DAR Mag** 1981;115(3):188–91
**Stewart S** see **Laslett P**
**Stewart TD:** A tribute to the French forensic anthropologist Georges Fully (1926–1973). **J Forensic Sci** 1979 Oct;24(4):916–24
**Stewart TD:** Essentials of forensic anthropology, especially as developed in the United States. Springfield, Ill, Thomas, 1979. xvii, 300 p.
**Stewart TD:** J. Lawrence Angel. **Am J Phys Anthropol** 1979 Nov;51(4):509–16
**Stewart TD:** Pioneer contributions of Harris Hawthorne Wilder, Ph.D., to forensic sciences. **J Forensic Sci** 1982 Oct;27(4):754–62
**Stewart TD:** Responses of the human skeleton to changes in the quality of life. **J Forensic Sci** 1980 Oct;25(4):912–21
**Stewart TJ** see **Brod RL**
**Stewart WB:** Indian medicine in New Brunswick. In: Congrès international d'histoire de la médecine, XXVe, Québec, 1976. Actes. Québec, 1977. p. 1320–6.
**Stewart WH:** A warning against complacency. **NY State J Med** 1983 Dec;83(13):1256
**Stewart WJ:** Ross McIntire. In Dictionary of American Biography, Suppl. 6, 1956–1960. p. 413–14, 1980.
**Stewart-Robertson JC:** The well-principled savage, or the child of the Scottish enlightenment. **J Hist Ideas** 1981;42:503–25
**Steyer GE:** Joseph Hyrtl als komparativer Anatomiker. **Anat Anz** 1980;148(5):462–73
**Steyn RW:** Retrospections: a sketch of nautical psychiatry through World War II. **Milit Med** 1980 Jun;145(6):407–12
**Stiazhkov AV** see **Katsnel'bogen AG**
**Sticker A:** Agnes Karll, die Reformerin der deutschen Krankenpflege. Ein Wegweiser für heute zu ihrem 50. Todestag am 12. Februar 1927. Wuppertal, Aussat, 1977. 240 p.
**Sticker DA:** [Theodor Fliedner and nursing] (Jpn). **Sogo Kango** 1980;15(4):146–55
**Stickl H** see **Weber HG**
**Stickle DF:** Death and class in Baltimore: the yellow fever epidemic of 1800. **Md Hist Mag** 1979;74(3):282–99
**Stieb EW:** A century of formal pharmaceutical education in Ontario. **Can Pharm J** 1983;116(3):104–7; 116(4):153–7
**Stieb EW:** Some branches of Canadian pharmacy's family tree--how they sprouted and grew. **Can Pharm J** 1982 Oct;115(10):374–9
**Stieb EW:** Three centennials: a retrospective view of Canada's pure food and drug legislation. In: Congrès international d'histoire de la médecine, XXVe, Québec, 1976. Actes. Québec, 1977. p. 1327–40.
**Stieb EW** see **Hamarneh SK**
**Stieber MT, Karg AL, Connelly DM, et al:** Guide to the botanical records and papers in the archives of the Hunt Institute. **Huntia** 1981;4(1):3–89
**Stiebitz R, Teschler-Nicola M:** Pathologische Befunde am Kauapparat eines Schädels aus dem 6. Jh. n. Chr., Fundort: Schwechat, Niederösterreich. **Wien Klin Wochenschr** 1981 Nov 27;93(22):703–7
**Stiebitz R** see **Nicola M**
**Stiefvater EW, Stiefvater IR:** Chinesische Atemlehre und Gymnastik. 2. Auflage. Heidelberg, Haug, 1980. 121 p.
**Stiefvater IR** see **Stiefvater EW**
**Stielow F:** Health and pleasure seekers at the springs of Indiana: pamphlet literature in the Library of Congress. **Indiana Med Hist Q** 1982;8(1):4–7
**Stigler SM** see **Merton RK**
**Stiker HJ:** Corps infirmes et sociétés. Paris, Aubier Montaigne, 1982. 250 p.
**Stiller D** see **Marchette NJ**
**Stillwell GK:** Whence our academy? **Arch Phys Med Rehabil** 1983

Mar;64(3):97–100
**Stinaff R, Hollander L:** Origins of the American Academy of Dental Practice Administration. **J Dent Pract Adm** 1984 Jan–Mar;1(1):4–5
**Stine JK:** Eugene Jules Houdry. In Dictionary of American biography, 1961–1965. Suppl. 7, 1981. p. 367–9.
**Stinson JM:** Department of Physiology, Meharry Medical College, Nashville, Tennessee. **Physiologist** 1983 Jun;26(3):119–20
**Stirland A:** The burials from King Henry VIII's ship, the Mary Rose: an interim statement. **Paleopathol Newsl** 1984 Sep;(47):7–10
**Stirrat RL:** Shrines, pilgrimage and miraculous powers in Roman Catholic Sri Lanka. In Sheils WJ, ed: The Church and healing. Papers read at the twentieth summer meeting and the twenty-first winter meeting of the Ecclesiastical History Society. Oxford, Basil Blackwell for the Society, 1982. p. 385–413.
**Stitt RS** see **Young JH**
**Stobbe H:** Viktor Schilling 1883–1983. Sein hämatologisches Lebenswerk unter Bevorzugung der Tätigkeiten in Berlin. **Folia Haematol (Leipz)** 1983;110(5):630–3
**Stöber O:** Drudenfuss-Monographie. Linz, Stadt-Verlag Neydharting, 1981. 460 p.
**Stock CR:** Laryngoscopy. **Ear Nose Throat J** 1984 Oct;63(10):528–30
**Stocker IP** see **Cawson RA**
**Stocking GW:** Contradicting the doctor: Billy Hancock and the problem of baloma. **Hist Anthropol Newsl** 1977;4(1):4–7
**Stocking GW:** Innovation in the Malinowskian mode: an essay review of long-term field research in social anthropology. **J Hist Behav Sci** 1980 Jul;16(3):281–6
**Stockinger J** see **Stambolian G**
**Stöckl T** see **Siefert G**
**Stöcklin WH:** Sakpata, ein Beitrag Afrikanischer Medizinmänner zur Pockeneradikation. **Gesnerus** 1982;39(3–4):405–15
**Stockton JJ, ed:** A century of service. Veterinary medicine in Indiana, 1884–1984. Indianapolis, Indiana Veterinary Medical Association, 1984. 199 p.
**Stockwell RF:** Personalities of importance in the early days of New Zealand dentistry. **NZ Dent J** 1981 Jul;77(349):102–5
**Stockwell S:** Classics in oncology. George Thomas Beatson, M.D. (1848–1933). **CA** 1983 Mar–Apr;33(2):105–21
**Stoddard S:** The hospice movement. Briarcliff Manor, N. Y., Stein and Day, 1978. xviii, 266 p.
**Stoeckle DB, Carter RD:** Cupping in New York State--1978; historic review. **NY State J Med** 1980 Jan;80(1):117–20
**Stoeckle JD, Oliver LC, Hardy HL:** Women with asbestosis in a medical clinic: under reported women workers, delayed diagnosis and smoking. **Women Health** 1982 Spring;7(1):31–6
**Stoecklin WH:** Die Erfindung der Magensonde. Ein ethnomedizinischer Beitrag zur Prioritätsfrage. **Gesnerus** 1981;38:237–46
**Stoehr T:** Hawthorne's mad scientists: Pseudoscience and social science in nineteenth-century life and letters. Hamden, Conn., Shoestring Press, 1978. 313 p.
**Stoessel I:** Scheintod und Todesangst. Aeusserungsformen der Angst in ihren geschichtlichen Wandlungen (17.–20. Jahrhundert). Köln, 1983. 247 p. (Kölner medizinhistorische Beiträge, Band 30)
**Stoffel G:** Christian Friedrich Fritzsche, 1851–1938. Erster Glarner Spitalarzt und Beschreiber der Akromealie. Zürich, Juris Druck, 1983. 66 p. (Zürcher Medizingeschichtliche Abhandlungen, Neue Reihe, Nr. 161).
**Stoffregen M:** Nebennieren Anmerkungen zur vorendokrinologischen Ara. **Med Welt** 1980 Feb;31(8):295–301
**Stoffregen M:** Zur historischen Entwicklung der experimentellen Physiologie der Nebennierenrindensuffizienz. **Sudhoffs Arch** 1981;65(3):266–98
**Stoffregen M:** Zur Rolle histochemischer Phänomene bei der Erforschung und Systematisierung des chromaffinen Gewebes. **Medizinhist J** 1984;19(3):191–209
**Stoffregen MH:** Thomas Addison (1793–1860), zum 120. Todestag. **Med Welt** 1981;21:3–4
**Stofft H:** Bouestard, médecin des épidémies à Morlaix. **Hist Sci Med** 1984;18(3):223–45
**Stofft H:** Kergaradec à l'écoute du foetus. **J Gynecol Obstet Biol Reprod (Paris)** 1981;10(6):611–22
**Stofft H:** L'école des sages-femmes de Morlaix à fin du règne de Louis XV et sous le règne de Louis XVI. **Hist Sci Med** 1983;17(1):41–61
**Stoianov BG, Selisskiĭ GD:** Sostoianie dermatologicheskoĭ pomoshchi v gorodakh dorevoliutsionnoĭ Rossii. **Vestn Dermatol Venerol** 1981 May;(5):22–5
**Stoimenov G:** Istoriia na bŭlgarskoto akusherstvo i ginekologiia. **Akush Ginekol (Sofiia)** 1980;19(5–6):395–401
**Stojan D, Petrovic M:** Razvoj sanitetske opreme u Ratnom vazduhoplovstvu. **Vojnosanit Pregl** 1981 Jan–Feb;38(1):37–40
**Stokes GA:** Helen Flanders Dunbar. In: Notable American women. The modern period. Cambridge, Mass., Belknap-Harvard Univ. Press, 1980. 4:210–2.
**Stokstad EL:** Early work with folic acid. **Fed Proc** 1979 Dec;38(13):2696–8
**Stolinsky DC:** Trousseau's phenomenon. **Blood** 1983 Dec;62(6):1304
**Stoll C:** Nikolaus von Kues (1401–1464) und seine Bedeutung für die Naturwissenschaft. **Pharm Acta Helv** 1979;54(9–10):311–6
**Stollenwerk A:** Die Cholera im Regierungsbezirk Koblenz [1832]. **Jahrb Westdtsch Landesgesch** 1979;5:241–72
**Stollenwerk M:** Der Fakultätsneubau der Medizin in Aachen-Melaten. Versuch einer Deutung. In Göpfert W, Otten HH, ed: Metavoeite: wandelt euch durch neues Denken. Düsseldorf, Triltsch, 1983. p. 125–34.
**Stollenwerk M:** Die bauliche Entwicklung der Krankenversorgung der Industriestadt Stolberg im Rheinland vor dem Hintergrund der Ursprünge der Messingindustrie. **Hist Hosp** 1979–80;13:164–76
**Stollerman GH:** Landmark perspective: The historical role of the Dick test. **JAMA** 1983 Dec 9;250(22):3097–9
**Stolorow RD, Atwood GE:** Faces in a cloud: subjectivity in personality theory. New York, Aronson, 1979. 217 p.
**Stolorow RD** see **Goldberg A, ed**
**Stolt CM, Oberg L:** En ovariotomi i Borås 1814. **Sydsven Medicinhist Sallsk Arsskr** 1984;21:109–21
**Stoltz CR, Stoltz V:** Watertown District Medical Society (No. 2). **SD J Med** 1981 May;34(5):10–11
**Stoltz V** see **Stoltz CR**
**Stommes E, Sisaye S:** The development and distribution of health care services in Ethiopia: a preliminary review. **Can J Afr Stud** 1980;13(3):487–95
**Stone AA** see **Kuper A**
**Stone C, Lunde P:** Early Islamic hospitals: in the hospital bazaar. **Health Soc Serv J** 1981 Dec 17;91(4777):1548–51
**Stone GC** see **Dalitz RH**
**Stone I:** Eight decades of scurvy. **Australas Nurses J** 1979 Sep;8(11):28–30
**Stone I** see **Hamrum CL, ed**
**Stone J:** A lifetime of careful listening. A centennial retrospective on the work of William Carlos Williams (1883–1963). **JAMA** 1983 Sep 16;250(11):1421–5
**Stone JF** see **Fox DM**
**Stone LG:** Medical society of the county of Monroe; sesquicentennial–1971. **NY State J Med** 1980 Jun;80(7 Pt 1):1155–7
**Stone MH:** Modern concepts of emotion as prefigured in Descartes' 'Passions of the Soul'. **J Am Acad Psychoanal** 1980;8:473–95
**Stone MN:** The plumbing paradox: American attitudes toward late nineteenth-century domestic sanitary arrangements. **Winterthur Portf** 1979;14(3):283–309
**Stool SE:** A historical vignette: memoirs of an otologist's European study in 1883. **Am J Otol** 1983 Apr;4(4):346–9
**Stool SE, Brown SL:** Ellen James Patterns, MD. **Arch Otolaryngol** 1983 Jan;109(1):60–1
**Stool SE, Kemper M, Kemper B:** The compleat otolaryngologist: Burton Alexander Randall. **Laryngoscope** 1984 Jan;94(1):16–9
**Storch J, ed** see **Meilicke CA, ed**
**Storck H:** De genio loci dermatologiae Turicensis. **Hautarzt** 1980 Sep;31(9):505–9
**Storey JK:** Ultrasound in ophthalmic optics. **Ophthalmic Physiol Opt** 1981;1(3):133–57
**Stork A:** Sto deset let rozvoje I. interní kliniky v Praze. **Cas Lek Cesk** 1981 Oct 1;120(39):1169–73
**Stork G:** Samuel Marion McElvain: December 9, 1897–April 11, 1973. **Biogr Mem Natl Acad Sci** 1983;54:221–48
**Stork H:** La détermination du sexe dans la pédiatrie traditionnelle de l'Inde. In Mazars G, ed: Les médecines traditionnelles de l'Asie. Strasbourg, Université Louis Pasteur, 1981, p. 150–62.
**Stork H:** Principes de base des traitements psychiatriques dans l'Ayurveda. **Sci Orient** 1979;16:21–9
**Storm FK, Morton DL:** Localized hyperthermia in the treatment of cancer. **CA** 1983 Jan–Feb;33(1):44–56
**Storr A** see **Jung CG**
**Story DK:** A study of practical and associate degree nursing education in Iowa from 1918 to 1978. Ph. D. Diss., Iowa State University. Ames, 1980. iii, 308 leaves.
**Story of the Hosn Hospital: founded by American Hosn Welfare Association, New Kensington, Pennsylvania:** New Kensington, Pa., The Assn., [1971?]. 188 [152] p.
**Storzer GH** see **Stambolian G**
**Stossel JP:** Wie entsteht Arteriosklerose? **Med Klin** 1980 May 9;75(10):349–57
**Stott R:** The Scottish dimension of Enlightenment medicine; the political economy of health. **Soc Soc Hist Med Bull (Lond)** 1979 Dec;25:41–4
**Stout G:** A ledger stamped 'G.P'. **J R Coll Gen Pract** 1984 Apr;34(261):223–5
**Stout G:** Adult hypertrophic pyloric stenosis--a description in 1834? **J R Coll Gen Pract** 1983 Apr;33(249):239–41
**Stout G:** Any old iron. **MIMS Mag** 1981 Sept 1;:48–9
**Stout G:** The 1888 pneumonia in Middlesbrough. **J R Soc Med** 1980 Sep;73(9):664–8
**Stout SD:** Histological structure and its preservation in ancient bone. **Curr Anthropol** 1978;19:601–4
**Stowell RE:** Esmond R. Long, MD, 1890–1979. **Am J Pathol** 1980 Aug;100(2):321–5
**Straass G** see **Löther R, ed**
**Straight WM:** Florida and the Spanish flu. **J Fla Med Assoc** 1981 Aug;68(8):644–54
**Straight WM:** Florida medicine and the war between the states. **J Fla Med Assoc** 1980 Aug;67(8):748–60
**Straight WM:** Florida's medical historian--J. Webster Merritt. **J Fla Med Assoc** 1979 Aug;66(8):860–5
**Straight WM:** Fort Dallas, a most salubrious post. **J Fla Med Assoc** 1982 Aug;69(8):706–12
**Straight WM:** Throw downs, fixin, rooting and hexing. **J Fla Med Assoc** 1983 Aug;70(8):635–41
**Strandberg H:** Cupping, an old popular method of healing - a Finnish

20th century survival of ancient humoral pathology. In International Congress of the History of Medicine. 26th, Plovdov, 1978. Actes du Congress. Sofia, 1981. Volume II. p. 206–7.

**Strandberg H:** Nordiskt seminarium om folkmedicin på Kilen i Sideby, Kristinestad, Finland. **Nord Medicinhist Arsb** 1980;Suppl 6:139–42

**Strandberg H:** Sanitary regulations in calendars in public use to indicate the attitude to the preventive health care in Finland in the 17th and 18th centuries. In International Congress of the History of Medicine, 27th, Barcelona, 1980. Actas. Barcelona, Acadèmia de Ciències Mèdiques de Catalunya i Balears, 1981. p. 621–5.

**Strandberg H, ed:** Folk medicine in Finland. A bibliography. (In Finnish, English and German). Helsingin, Nordiskt Folkmedicinmuseum, 1977. 15 p. (Meddelanden Nr. 1).

**Strandell B:** Hur David Schulz von Schulzenheim fick sitt namn. **Nord Medicinhist Arsbok** 1983;:83–7

**Strandell B:** Linné och Stockholm. **Sven Farm Tidskr** 1979;83:677–84

**Strandell B:** Svenska medicinska medaljer. **Nord Medicinhist Arsb** 1980;Supp 6:52–6

**Strane S:** Childbirth - yesterday and today. **J Nurs Care** 1982 Apr;15(4):22–4

**Straser P, Protic M:** Pečat karlovačkog hirurško-berberskog esnafa iz XVIII veka. **Med Pregl** 1982;35(11–12):493

**Strassburg MA:** The global eradication of smallpox. **Am J Infect Control** 1982 May;10(2):53–9

**Stratone A** see **Stratone N**

**Stratone M:** Metoda analizei la E.B. Condillac. **Rev Med Chir Soc Med Nat Iasi** 1979 Jan–Mar;83(1):163–6

**Stratone M** see **Marinescu CG**

**Stratone N:** Filosofia în secolul 'luminilor'. **Rev Med Chir Soc Med Nat Iasi** 1983 Jul–Sep;87(3):509–11

**Stratone N, Stratone A:** Probleme de gnoseologie în lucrările doctorului Grigore T. Popa. **Rev Med Chir Soc Med Nat Iasi** 1979 Oct–Dec;83(4):713–6

**Stratone N:** Spaţiul si timpul in concepţia lui Vasile Conta (1845–1882). **Rev Med Chir Soc Med Nat Iasi** 1982 Jul–Sep;86(3):513–5

**Stratone N** see **Marinescu CG**

**Stratton R:** The Cherokee National Insane Asylum. **Bull Menninger Clin** 1983 May;47(3):266–8

**Stratton RJ** see **Johnson DL**

**Strauss JS:** The evolution of psychotherapeutic approaches for affective and schizophrenic disorders. In M. R. Zales, ed: Affective and schizophrenic disorders: new approaches to diagnosis and treatment. New York, Brunner/Mazel, 1983. p. 163–77.

**Strauss MJ:** The political history of the artificial heart. **N Engl J Med** 1984 Feb 2;310(5):332–6

**Strbánová S:** Biochemical journals and their profile in 1840–1930. **Acta Hist Rerum Nat Tech** 1981;16:149–95

**Strean HS** see **Freeman L**

**Streiff B:** Ernst Fuchs (1851–1930)--Gedächtnisvorlesung Wien 31. 5. 1984. **Klin Monatsbl Augenheilkd** 1984 Nov;185(5):316–20

**Streitmatter R:** John Blair Radford of Arnheim: New River Valley doctor and businessman. **Va Cavalcade** 1979;28(4):180–5

**Streitz JM, Aufderheide AC, El Najjar M, et al:** A 1,500-year-old bladder stone. **J Urol** 1981 Oct;126(4):452–3

**Strelka J** see **Kuniak B**

**Stremel RW:** Historical development of the anaerobic threshold concept. **Physiologist** 1984 Aug;27(4):295–8

**Stretton TB** see **Williams G**

**Streuli RA, Ultmann JE:** Non-Hodgkin's lymphomas: historical perspective and future prospects. **Semin Oncol** 1980 Sep;7(3):223–33

**Stricevic MV, Patel MR, Okazaki T, et al:** Karate: historical perspective and injuries sustained in national and international tournament competitions. **Am J Sports Med** 1983 Sep–Oct;11(5):320–4

**Strichartz GR** see **Wildsmith JA**

**Strickland WA:** Quinine pills, manufactured on the Missouri frontier (1832–1862). **Pharm Hist** 1983;25(2):61–8

**Strickland WA:** Requiem for a frontier physician: James W. Parker, M.D., doctor to the wagon trains and mountaineers of old Westport. **Mo Med** 1981 Oct;78(10):631–6

**Striežová V** see **Krahulec I**

**Strikovic J:** Analiza jednog samoubistva u delu Ive Andrića 'Na Drini Cuprija'. **Srp Arh Celok Lek** 1979 Sep;107(9):477–82

**Stringer CB** see **Cronin JE**

**Strizhkov IK, Suslov AI:** Noveishaia istoricheskaia literatura o bor'be na prodovol' stvennom fronte v gody grazhdanskoi voiny. **Vopr Istor** 1980;2:118–27

**Strmeň J:** Abraham Colles (1773–1843) a ním v roku 1814 popísaná zlomenina radia. **Rozhl Chir** 1984 Oct;63(10):701–4

**Strobusch AD, Jefferson JW:** The checkered history of lithium in medicine. **Pharm Hist** 1980;22(2):72–6

**Ströder J, Schuster J:** Estudio comparativo de la mortalidad infantil entre los niños Judios y no Judios en Europa Central y Oriental a finales del siglo diecinueve y principios del veinte. **Folia Hum (Barc)** 1983;21(240):1–10

**Stroh O:** Svenska röda korset i totalförsvaret. **K Krigsvetensk Akad Handl Tidskr** 1965;169:183–92

**Strohbach E** see **Khalatbari P**

**Strohmaier G:** Aerztliche Ausbildung im islamischen Mittelalter. **Klio** 1979;61:519–24

**Strohmaier G:** Der arabische Hippokrates. Bemerkungen zu einem Aufsatz von Dieter Irmer. **Sudhoffs Arch** 1980;64(3):234–49

**Strojnowski J:** Nowy obraz polskiej kultury w średniowieczu. **Arch Hist Med (Warsz)** 1983;46(1):21–8

**Strojnowski J:** Orientacja biologiczna a orientacja społeczna w medycynie w ujeciu historycznym. **Arch Hist Med (Warsz)** 1984;47(1):25–37

**Strojnowski J:** Stan zdrowotny i medycyna u Słowian według najdawniejszych kronik. **Arch Hist Med (Warsz)** 1979;42(1):93–105

**Strøm F** see **Keiser-Nielsen S**

**Ström J:** Männen bakom syndromet: Albert Stevens och Frank Johnson. Först att beskriva 'okänd infektionssjukdom'--allergi utlöst av läkemedel eller infektion. **Lakartidningen** 1983 Mar 16;80(11):1076–7

**Stromquist DL:** The true portraiture of a Roman youth; etching by Wenceslaus Hollar, 1641. New Haven, Yale Medical Library, Clements C. Fry Collection. **J Hist Med Allied Sci** 1983 Apr;38(2):176–7

**Strong B:** Ideas of the early sex education movement in America, 1890–1920. **Hist Educ Q** 1972;12(2):129–62

**Strong C:** Historical research: does it apply to health education? **Health Educ (Wash)** 1981 Jul–Aug;12(4):34–5

**Stroppiana L:** Correspondencia cientifica de 1858 entre el doctor Beauperthuy de Caracas y el doctor Socrate Cadet de Roma. **Rev Soc Venez Hist Med** 1979;28(42):37–44

**Stroppiana L:** Histoire et perspectives de la médecine sociale en Italie. In: Congrès international d'histoire de la médecine, XXVe, Québec, 1976. Actes. Québec, 1977. p. 321–31.

**Stroppiana L:** La moderne méthodologie scientifique dans le domaine de l'histoire de la medécine. In: International Congress of the History of Medicine, 26th, Plovdiv (Bulgaria), 1978. Actes du Congres, Vol. 1. Sofia, 1980. p. 80–1.

**Stroppina L, Salemme MA:** Le nouveau visage de la science et du savant au XXe siècle, après Einstein et Freud. In International Congress of the History of Medicine, 27th, Barcelona, 1980. Actas. Barcelona, Acadèmia de Ciències Mèdiques de Catalunya i Balears, 1981. p. 626–31.

**Strotzka H:** Laudatio auf Anna Freud. **Wien Klin Wochenschr** 1983 Jan 21;95(2):35–7

**Strotzka H** see **Zur Geschichte der Psychiatrie in Wien**

**Stroup A:** Christiaan Huygens & the development of the air pump. **Janus** 1981;68:129–58

**Strout C:** Henry James's dream of the Louvre, 'The Jolly Corner,' and psychological interpretation. **Psychohist Rev** 1979 Summer–Fall;8(1–2):47–52

**Strout C:** Psyche, Clio, and the artist. In M. Albin, R. J. Devlin, G. Heeger, ed: New directions in psychohistory. The Adelphi papers in honor of Erik H. Erikson. Lexington, Toronto, D. C. Heath, 1980. p. 97–115.

**Strozier CB:** A rationale for teaching psychohistory. **Group Psychol Hist Newsl** 1975;4(1):8–10

**Strozier CB:** Heinz Kohut and the historical imagination. **Psychohist Rev** 1978;7(2):36–9

**Strozier CB:** Springfield über alles: role playing and the teaching of psychohistory. **Group Psychol Hist Newsl** 1975;4(2):13–24

**Strozier CB** see **Goldberg A, ed**

**Strubel K:** Robert Koch und die Tuberkulose im Spiegel der halleschen Presse im ausgehenden 19. Jahrhundert. **Wiss Beitr Martin Luther Univ Halle Wittenberg** 1983;5–R80:225–42

**Strubell M, ed:** Trueta: surgeon in war and peace. The memoirs of Joep Trueta. London, Gollancz, 1980. 288 p.

**Struchkov VI:** Ivan Gur'evich Rufanov (k 100-letiiu so dnia rozhdeniia). **Sov Med** 1984;(7):114–5

**Struck HG, Fuchs C:** Zum Frühbild des Morbus Recklinghausen vorwiegend im Augenbereich in Verbindung mit Skelettveränderungen und einer Hypospadia glandis. **Wiss Z Martin Luther Univ (Math)** 1976;25(3):93–9

**Stručno-znanstveni sastanak u povodu tridesete obljetnice o snutka sekcije za hematologiju i transfuziologiju ZLH (1948–1978): Lijec Vjesn** 1981;103(3):105–30

**Struik DJ:** The land of Stevin and Huygens. A sketch of science and technology in the Dutch Republic during the Golden Century. Dordrecht, D. Reidel, 1981. xx, 162 p. (Studies in the History of Modern Science, v. 7).

**Strukov AI, Paukov VS, Kazantseva IA:** Druzhba i edinstvo narodov SSSR - zalog uspekhov narodnogo zdravookhraneniia. **Arkh Patol** 1982;44(11):3–16

**Strukov AI, Smol'iannikov AV, Sarkisov DS:** Razrabotka problem patologicheskoĭ anatomii v sisteme Akademii Meditsinskikh Nauk SSSR za 40 let ee sushchestvovaniia (1944–1984). **Arkh Patol** 1984;46(6):3–15

**Strukov AI, Puzik VI, Zemskova ZS, et al:** V. G. Shtefko i otechestvennaia shkola patologov-ftiziatrov. **Arkh Patol** 1984;46(2):81–5

**Struna NL:** Sport and colonial education: a cultural perspective. **Res Q Exerc Sport** 1981 Mar;52(1):117–35

**Strużak-Wysokińska M** see **Wysoki'nski A**

**Struzik T:** Metabolizm informacyjny Kępińskiego w świetle teorii informacji. **Przegl Lek** 1983;40(12):865–71

**Stryker S:** Social psychology: trends, assessment, and prognosis. **Am Behav Sci** 1981;24(3):386–406

**Strzałkowska W:** Rodowód przyszłości. 9. Klimat tamtych lat. **Pieleg Polozna** 1982;(11):31–2

**Strzelecka I:** Pierwszy szpital obozowy w Brzezince. **Przegl Lek** 1984;41(1):88–93

**Strzelecka I:** Rozwój szpitali obozowych w Oświecimiu-Brzezince. **Przegl Lek** 1984;41(1):84–8

**Strzelecki A:** O postawach wieźniów konspiratorów w Oświecimiu. **Przegl Lek** 1984;41(1):93–6

**Stuart D:** Urban Marks: 1880–1949. **Br Med J [Clin Res]** 1982 Jul

31;285(6338):345–7
**Stuart H:** A ninth century account of diets and Dies Aegyptiaci. **Scriptorium** 1979;33(2):237–44
**Stuart P** see **Orme JG**
**Stuart R, Stuart W:** John Marsh. **Pac Hist** 1980;24(3):369–75
**Stuart W** see **Stuart R**
**Stuart RB, ed:** Memoirs of a Council Bluffs druggist. **Palimpsest** 1980;61(3):66–79
**Stubbe JH, Scrymgeour JM, Smith AJ:** Medical background; History of Fremantle hospitals and doctors. [Nedlands], Published for the Fremantle Hospital Board by the Univ. of Western Australia Press, 1969. xxvi, 82 p.
**Stubberfield J** see **Maddern GJ**
**Stubbs HW** see **Wylie JA**
**Stubenbord WT** see **Shaw R**
**Stucke W:** Balintgruppen-Arbeit. **Med Monatsschr Pharm** 1982 Jun;5(6):176–82
**Stuckey RL:** Dr. William Darlington's botanical contacts on the western American frontier. **Trans Stud Coll Physicians Phila** 1983 Sep;5(5 No 3):213–43
**Stuckey RL:** Medical botany in the Ohio Valley (1800–1850). **Trans Stud Coll Physicians Phila** 1978 Jul;45(5):262–79
**Stucki JC** see **Cooper T**
**Studebaker GA:** Fifty years of hearing aid research: an evaluation of progress. **Ear Hear** 1980 Mar–Apr;1(2):57–62
**Studenikin MI, Ryleeva RN:** Pervyĭ nauchnyĭ tsentr okhrany materinstva idetstva v SSSR. **Pediatriia** 1982 Oct;(10):3–7
**Studer GC:** Powwowing: folk medicine or white magic? **Pa Mennon Heritage** 1980;3(3):17–23
**Studer KE, Chubin DE:** The cancer mission. Social contexts of biomedical research. Beverly Hills, London, Sage, 1980. 319 p. (Sage Library of Social Research, V. 103).
**Studnitsin AA, Rukavishnikova VM:** K 150-letiiu Zhana Al'freda Furn'e. **Vestn Dermatol Venerol** 1982 Apr;(4):75–7
**Studnitsin AA** see **Skripkin IuK**
**Stuhlhofer F:** Unser Wissen verdoppelt sich alle 100 Jahre. **Ber Wissenschaftsgesch** 1983;6(1–4):169–93
**Stukonis MK** see **Telichenas AI**
**Stukovský R** see **Andrik P**
**Stumpel AR:** Het Burgerziekenhuis te Amsterdam en de modernisering van de ziekenverpleging in de 19e eeuw. **Tijdschr Ziekenverpl** 1983 Jun 21;36(13):409–15
**Stumpf DA:** The founding of pediatric neurology in America. **Bull NY Acad Med** 1981 Nov;57(9):804–16
**Stupniker S:** Suspicious circumstances in Salem. **N Engl J Med** 1983 Nov 10;309(19):1194
**Stupp JA** see **Kahle E**
**Sturchio JL** see **Kevles DJ**
**Sturdza SA:** The activity of the Cantacuzino Institute in the field of tuberculosis. A review. **Arch Roum Pathol Exp Microbiol** 1982 Jul–Sep;41(3):195–204
**Sturgis KR:** The driftwood case: pioneering antipollution in Pennsylvania. **Trans Stud Coll Physicians Phila** 1982 Dec;5(4 no 4):259–71
**Sturm J:** Winds from the east - the cholera of '32. **Chronicle** 1982;4:24–7
**Sturrock J:** The Edinburgh Royal Maternity and Simpson Memorial Hospital. **J R Coll Surg Edinb** 1980 May;25(3):173–87
**Sturrock RD** see **Spencer DG**
**Sturrock RR:** William Ford Robertson (1867–1923): his study of neuroglia. **Med Hist** 1975 Oct;19(4):370–5
**Stürzbecher M:** Franz Schrakamp (1860–1920) Stadt- und Kreisarzt in Düsseldorf. **Clin Notes Respir Dis** 1980 May;42(5):289–92
**Stürzbecher M:** Quellen zur Geschichte der Medizin und des Gesundheitswesens in und über Berlin. **Baer Berl** 1977;26:113–8
**Stürzbecher M:** The physician in German-speaking countries from the Middle-Ages to the Enlightenment. In Russell AW, ed: The town and state physician in Europe from the Middle Ages to the Enlightenment. Wolfenbüttel, Herzog August Bibliothek, 1981. p. 123–29 (Wolfenbütteler Forschungen, 17).
**Stürzbecher M** see **Habrich C**
**Stutte H:** Ueber die Anfänge der 'Europäischen Kinderpsychiatrie'. **Acta Paedopsychiatr (Basel)** 1981 Jan;46(4):189–92
**Stutz GM:** Zur Geschichte der Zürcher Zahnärztegesellschaft. Zürich, Juris, 1984. 76 p. (Zürcher Medizingeschichtliche Abhandlungen, Neue Reihe, Nr. 172)
**Stutzman RH:** Harvey Washington Wiley; a famous Hoosier and 'The father of pure food'. **Indiana Med Hist Q** 1981;7(4):20–1
**Styblo K, Sutherland I:** Epidémiologie de la tuberculose chez l'enfant. **Bull Int Union Tuberc** 1982 Jun;57(2):134–41
**Stýblo K** see **Sutherland I**
**Stycos JM:** Recent trends in Latin American fertility. **Popul Stud** 1978;31(3):407–26
**Stycos JM:** The decline of fertility in Costa Rica: literacy, modernization and family planning. **Popul Stud** 1982 Mar;36(1):15–30
**Stypułkowska J:** 25 lat Kliniki Chirurgii Stomatologicznej AM w Krakowie. Historia i kierunki działalności. **Czas Stomatol** 1981 Jan;34(1):51–6
**Su TC** see **Wei DX**
**Suárez CV:** Ampulla of Vater---a misnomer. **Mt Sinai J Med (NY)** 1980 Jul–Aug;47(4):373–85
**Suassuna I** see **Milhomem AM**
**Subba Rao M:** Original observations of Filippo Pacini on vibrio cholera. **Bull Indian Inst Hist Med (Hyderabad)** 1978;8(1–4):32–8
**Subba Reddy BV** see **Gangadharam V**
**Subba Reddy DV:** Glimpses of health and medicine in Mauryan empire. Hyderabad, Upgraded Dept. of History of Medicine, Osmania Medical College, 1966. 97 p.
**Subba Reddy DV:** Glimpses of medicine in Rajatarangini; diseases, drugs, physicians and treatments in medieval Kashmir. **Bull Inst Hist Med (Hyderabad)** 1973 Oct;3(4):189–200
**Subba Reddy DV:** History of Siddha medicine; need for further detailed studies. **Bull Inst Hist Med (Hyderabad)** 1973 Oct;3(4):182–5
**Subba Reddy DV:** Major General S. L. Bhatia (1891–1982). **Bull Indian Inst Hist Med Hyderabad** 1982;12(1–4):88–91
**Subba Reddy DV:** Prelude to upgraded Department of History of Medicine, Hyderabad. **Bull Indian Inst Hist Med Hyderabad** 1982;12(1–4):92–9
**Subba Reddy DV:** Prof. Jean Filliozat (1906–1981). **Bull Indian Inst Hist Med Hyderabad** 1982;12(1–4):85–8
**Subba Reddy DV:** Wilhem Ten Rhyne (Rhijne) and his Treatise on Asiatic Leprosy; a medical classic by a Dutch physician in Java in the last quarter of 17th century. **Bull Indian Inst Hist Med (Hyderabad)** 1975 Jul;5(3):150–61
**Subba Reddy V:** History of Medicine in India. **Bull Indian Inst Hist Med (Hyderabad)** 1980;10(1–4):90–110
**Subrtová A, Cervený J:** About the history of caesarean section and its first performance in Prague in 1792. **Acta Univ Carol [Med] (Praha)** 1983;29(5–6):373–93
**Subrtová A:** Antonín Bohác--statistik a demograf: život a dílo. **Sb Nar Muzea Praze Rada A Hist** 1977;32(1–3):1–198
**Subrtová A:** Jean de Carro (1770–1857) - příspěvek k biografi. **Cas Nar Muz** 1980;149(1–2):45–61
**Subrtová A:** Johann Bapt. Michael Sagar (1732–1813). **Cas Nar Muz** 1981;150(3–4):153–90
**Suchi T:** The changing concept and classification of malignant lymphomas. **Jpn J Med** 1984 Feb;23(1):74–6
**Suchodolski B, Chmielewska-Szlajfer M:** Developmental tendencies of Polish 19th- and 20th century science against the background of world science. **Rev Pol Acad Sci (Warsz)** 1980;25(1–2):81–90
**Sucker U:** On the history of problems of scientific studies in the beginning of the XXth century in Germany. **Istor Biol Issled** 1983;9:191–200
**Suckling CW** see **Johnson AW**
**Sudhakara Reddy P** see **Gangadharam V**
**Suffolk horror story re-told: East Anglican Dly Times** 1980 Aug 27
**Sugar HS:** In appreciation of the contributions of Harry Searls Gradle. **Surv Ophthalmol** 1981 Nov–Dec;26(3):170–3
**Sugar HS, Foster CC:** Maximilian Salzmann. Ophthalmic pioneer and artist. **Surv Ophthalmol** 1981 Jul–Aug;26(1):28–30
**Sugar HS:** The filtering operations--past, present, and future. **Int Ophthalmol Clin** 1981 Spring;21(1):1–13
**Sugár I:** Az 'Egri Víz' története. **Orvostort Kozl** 1980;89–91(26 no 1–3):191–207
**Sugár L:** Morelli Gusztáv munkássága és szerepe a magyar parodontológiai oktatás kialakulásában. **Fogorv Sz** 1981 Feb;74(2):33–6
**Sugar O:** Doyle on tabes dorsalis. **JAMA** 1982 May 21;247(19):2659–60
**Sugden K:** Glimpses of medical history. **Br Dent J** 1981;150(3):75–6
**Sugden KC:** Dentists in the rare books. Joseph Audibran and incorruptible artificial teeth. **Br Dent J** 1983 Dec 24;155(12):420
**Sugden KC:** Dentists in the rare books. 2. Vittorio Cornelio. **Br Dent J** 1983 Oct 22;155(8):278
**Sugden KC:** Nicolas Dubois de Chemant and the disputed invention of mineral teeth. **Br Dent J** 1983 Sep 24;155(6):202
**Sugimoto S:** [An interpretation of a syndrome depicted in Buddhist cannon [sic] through Susruta Samhita] (Jpn). **Igakushi Kenkyu** 1980;54:12–7
**Sugimoto S:** [Makers of wooden denture bases] (Jpn). **Rinsho Shika** 1982;303:15–8
**Sugimoto S:** [Man-yo-shu and dentistry] (Jpn). **Rinsho Shika** 1982;(304):22–4
**Sugimoto S:** [Wooden denture bases] (Jpn). **Rinsho Shika** 1982;(304):19–21
**Sugita K:** Public health of ancient India. In Ogawa T, ed: Public health. Tokyo, Saikon, 1981. p. 75–81.
**Sugitachi G:** [Gen-etsu Kagawa and his obstetric practice] (Jpn). **Josanpu Zasshi** 1983 Jun;37(6):484–9
**Sugitani A:** [First successful case of intentional laparotomy (author's transl)]. (Jpn) **Nippon Geka Hokan** 1980 Jan 1;49(1):1–2
**Suitor JJ:** Husband's participation in childbirth: a nineteenth-century phenomenon. **J Fam Hist** 1981 Fall;6:278–93
**Sukhanov NV:** Meditsinakaia i trudovaia reabilitatsiia ranenykh v gospitaliakh Zapadnoĭ Sibiri v period Velikoĭ Otechestvennoĭ voiny. **Voen Med Zh** 1981;(7):72–4
**Sukharev AG, Fokina NS, Telenchi VI:** Kafedre Gigieny Deteĭ i Podrostkov Tsentral'nogo Ordena Lenina Instituta Usovershenstvovaniia Vracheĭ 50 let. **Gig Sanit** 1984 Aug;(8):38–40
**Sükösd L** see **Balogh J**
**Šůla L:** The 100th anniversary of the discovery of Koch's bacillus, the etiologic agent of tuberculosis. **J Hyg Epidemiol Microbiol Immunol** 1982;26(3):227–9
**Süle T:** Az Erzsébet Tudományegyetem Orvosi Kara, az önálló Pécsi Orvostudományi Egyetem rövid története és numizmatikai emlékei. **Orvostort Kozl** 1982;28(1–3):227–39
**Suleĭmenov AA, Balmukhanov SB, Abdrakhimov BE:** Onkologicheskaia sluzhba Kazakhstana za 60 let SSSR. **Vopr Onkol** 1982;28(9):3–7
**Sulestrowska H:** Zasługi prof. dr. Tadeusza Bilikiewicza dla rozwoju psychiatrii dziecięcej w Polsce. **Psychiatr Pol** 1982;16(4):321–8

**Suliman M** see **Samborschi E**
**Sullivan AM:** Nursing revisited: a tour of nursing history in Massachusetts. **Mass Nurse** 1983 Aug;52(8):9–10
**Sullivan CH, Krueger HW:** Carbon isotope analysis of separate chemical phases in modern and fossil bone. **Nature** 1981 Jul 23;292(5821):333–5
**Sullivan CH, Krueger HW:** Carbon isotope ratios of bone apatite and animal diet reconstruction. **Nature** 1983 Jan 13;301(5896):177–8
**Sullivan DJ:** Biological engineering. **Thought** 1981;56(221):199–211
**Sullivan E:** Ocular history of James Joyce. **Surv Ophthalmol** 1984 Mar–Apr;28(5):412–5
**Sullivan EJ:** Art in dermatopathology. Jusepe de Ribera. An interpreter of the skin through art. **Am J Dermatopathol** 1979 Summer;1(2):159–62
**Sullivan EJ:** Beauty marks or pigmented skin lesions? **Am J Dermatopathol** 1981 Fall;3(3):311–2
**Sullivan EJ:** Depictions of skin ailments in Western European and American art from the Middle Ages to the 20th century. **Am J Dermatopathol** 1982 Aug;4(4):343–52
**Sullivan EV:** The career and legacy of Jean Piaget. **Queens Q** 1981;88(2):341–52
**Sullivan LW:** The education of black health professionals. **Phylon** 1977;38(2):181–93
**Sullivan LW:** The Morehouse School of Medicine: a state of mind, of mission, and of commitment. **J Natl Med Assoc** 1983 Aug;75(8):837–9
**Sullivan LW:** The school of medicine at Morehouse College: status in 1979 and plans for the future. **J Med Assoc Ga** 1980 Aug;69(8):673–4
**Sullivan OR:** Who's testing black children and youth in the public schools? **Freedomways** 1981;21(2):114–8
**Sullivan RJ** see **Sharkey PW, ed**
**Sulloway FJ:** Darwin's conversion: the Beagle voyage and its aftermath. **J Hist Biol** 1982 Fall;15(3):325–96
**Sulloway FJ:** Freud as psychobiologist: a study in scientific revolution and revolutionary ideology. Ph.D. Diss. Harvard University. Cambridge, Mass., 1979.
**Sulloway FJ:** Freud, biologist of the mind: beyond the psychoanalytic legend. New York, Basic Books, 1979. xxvi, 612 p.
**Sulloway FJ:** Further remarks on Darwin's spelling habits and the dating of Beagle voyage manuscripts. **J Hist Biol** 1983 Fall;16(3):361–90
**Sulloway FJ:** Geographic isolation in Darwin's thinking: the vicissitudes of a crucial idea. **Stud Hist Biol** 1979;3:23–65
**Sulman AM:** Victor Vance Anderson. In Dictionary of American Biography, Suppl. 6, 1956–1960. p. 16–17, 1980.
**Sułowski Z:** Les mécanismes de l'expansion démographique des Juifs dans les villes de Pologne aux XVIe–XIXe siècles. **Zesz Nauk KUL** 1978;21:89–100
**Sulzberger MB:** My companions on the International Committee of Dermatology. **J Am Acad Dermatol** 1982 Feb;6(2):179–94
**Sulzberger MB:** Three lessons learned in Bloch's clinic. **Am J Dermatopathol** 1980 Winter;2(4):321–5
**Sulzberger! Biography, autobiography, iconography. A posthumous festschrift: Am J Dermatopathol** 1984 Aug;6(4):344–70
**Sumbatov GA** see **Poletaev SD**
**Sumii T:** [History of casting]. (Jpn) **Nippon Shika Ishikai Zasshi** 1979;32(4):367–73
**Summers GV:** Norman Bethune, Canadian surgeon: his Chinese connection. **Can J Surg** 1983 Jul;26(4):379–82
**Summers JL:** A century of health protection. **Can J Hosp Pharm** 1975 Sep–Oct;28(5):143
**Summers N** see **Steinfeld JL**
**Summerville J:** Educating black doctors: a history of Meharry Medical College. University, Ala., University of Alabama Press, 1983. xiii, 279 p.
**Summerville J:** Formation of a black medical profession in Tennessee, 1880–1920. **J Tenn Med Assoc** 1983 Oct;76(10):644–6
**Sumner E:** Psychiatry, 1. bordering on bedlam. **Nurs Mirror** 1980 Dec 4;151(23):16–8
**Sun RS:** Health services in the People's Republic of China: a blueprint for human and social development. Cambridge, Mass., Schenkman, 1980. xii, 123 p.
**Sun TH** see **Cho LJ**
**Sun TH** see **Freedman R**
**Sun Y:** [The historical materials of modern medical education in Nantong city: an early medical school solely established by Chinese] (Chi). **Chung Hua I Shih Tsa Chih** 1984;14(2):90–103
**Sunday ME:** Canada's Best. **Harv Med Alumni Bull** 1980 Dec;54(6):10–15
**Sunderland S:** Advances in diagnosis and treatment of root and peripheral nerve injury. **Adv Neurol** 1979;22:271–305
**Sunderman FW:** Trends in clinical science. **Ann Clin Lab Sci** 1980 Sep–Oct;10(5):361–7
**Sundin J, Tedebrand LG:** Dödlighet och sjuklighet i svenskjärnbruksmiljo, 1750–1875. **Scandia** 1981;47(1):67–108
**Suñe JM** see **Arques J**
**Suñé JM** see **Sorní J**
**Suñé JM** see **Valverde JL**
**Suñé JM, ed:** Pharmacopea cathalana sive antidotarium barcinonense. (Edición Facsímil). Barcelona, Catedra de Historia de la Farmacia y Legislacion Farmaceutica, Universidad de Barcelona, 1975. Various paginations.
**Sunseri AR:** The hazards of the trail. **Palacio** 1975;81(3):29–39
**Sunshine I:** Dr. Alexander O. Gettler's documentation of a radiation hazard. **Am J Forensic Med Pathol** 1983 Dec;4(4):307–9
**Supady J:** Ankieta statystyczna z 1931 r. na temat występowania nowotworów złośliwych w populacji II Rzeczypospolitej. **Wiad Lek** 1981 Feb 15;34(4):351–5
**Supady J:** Doświadczalne badania lekarzy polskich nad rakotwórczym działaniem smoły pogazowej i jej pochondnych (do 1939 r.). **Pol Tyg Lek** 1981 Mar 2;36(9):357–9
**Supady J:** Działalność Wileńskiego Komitetu do Zwalczania Raka w latach 1931--1936. **Nowotwory** 1979 May–Jun;29(2):151–6
**Supady J:** Powstanie i działalność stowarzyszenia 'Polski Instytut Przeciwrakowy' we Lwowie (1929–1939). **Wiad Lek** 1982 Nov 1;35(19–20):1301–3
**Supady J:** Serologia nowotworów w badaniach Ludwika Hirszfelda i jego współpracowników w okresie II Rzeczypospolitej. **Wiad Lek** 1981 Feb 1;34(3):257–62
**Supady J:** Udział lekarzy polskich w krajowych i międzynarodowych zjazdach onkologicznych w latach 1918–1938. **Nowotwory** 1979 Oct–Dec;29(4):315–20
**Supady J:** Wpływ wychowania i nauczania domowego oraz szkolnego na psychofizyczny rozwój młodzieży szlacheckiej w Polsce w XVIII w. **Wiad Lek** 1981 May 1;34(9):789–98
**Super JC:** Pan, alimentación y política en Querétaro a fines del siglo XVIII. **Hist Mex** 1980;30(2):247–72
**Super JC:** Sources and methods for the study of historical nutrition in Latin America. **Hist Methods** 1981;14(1):22–30
**Suppan W:** Biologische und kulturelle Bedingungen des Musikgebrauches. **Universitas (Stuttg)** 1982;37(12):1279–84
**Supply of manpower in selected health occupations: 1950–1990. Hyattsville, U. S. Bureau of Health Professions, 1980. xiii, 62 p:**
**Supuk A:** Sibenski onomastikon nakon kuge od 1649 godine. **Arh Vjesn** 1978–79;21–22:123–79
**Sur N:** The Bihar famine of 1770. **Indian Econ Soc Hist Rev** 1976;13(4):525–31
**Suransky VP:** A tyranny of experts. **Wilson Q** 1982;6(4):53–60
**Suratteau JR:** Contribution à l'étude des mouvements de population dans le canton et la ville de Berne à la fin du XVIIIe siècle. In: Congrès National des Sociétés Savantes, 92e, Strasbourg et Colmar, 1967. Actes. Paris, 1970. Section d'Histoire Moderne et Contemporaine, Tome 1. p. 177–272.
**Surawicz B** see **Reddy CP**
**Surgeonor DM** see **Soutter L**
**Susa E** see **Lontainé SZ**
**Suslov AI** see **Strizhkov IK**
**Suslov VS** see **Kovalev MM**
**Suslov VV, Gusakov NI:** K 200-letiiu ucheniia A. M. Shumlianskogo o pochke (1782–1982). **Urol Nefrol (Mosk)** 1983 Jan–Feb;(1):61–3
**Susser M:** The work of George Rosen: observations on a very small sample. **Int J Health Serv** 1980;10(2):323–8
**Susser M** see **Hansen H**
**Süsskind C:** The 'story' of nonionizing radiation research. **Bull NY Acad Med** 1979 Dec;55(11):1152–63
**Susskind JL:** Kathryn McHale. In Dictionary of American Biography, Suppl. 6, 1956–1960. p. 412–13, 1980.
**Sussman GD:** Selling mother's milk. The wet-nursing business in France, 1715–1914. Urbana, University of Illinois Press, 1982. xi, 210 p.
**Sussman GD:** The end of the wet-nursing business in France, 1874–1914. In R. Wheaton, T. K. Hareven, ed: Family and sexuality in French history. Philadelphia, University of Pennsylvania Press, 1980. p. 224–52.
**Sustic V:** Naša ratna zdravstvena služba i njezino značenje za zadatke u općenarodnoj obraini. (O nekim pitanjima iz kompenzacije sanitetskih kadrova i korištenja improvizacijama). **Lijec Vjesn** 1979 Nov;101(11):679–81
**Sutherland G:** Measuring intelligence: English local education authorities and mental testing 1919–1939. In C. Webster, ed: Biology, medicine and society 1840–1940. Cambridge, Cambridge University Press, 1981. p. 315–35.
**Sutherland G, Sharp S:** 'The fust official psychologist in the wurrld': aspects of the professionalization of psychology in early twentieth century Britain. **Hist Sci** 1980 Sep;18(41 pt 3):181–208
**Sutherland HD:** The metamorphosis of cardiac surgery in Australia. **J Thorac Cardiovasc Surg** 1980;80:808–23
**Sutherland I, Svandová E, Radhakrishna S:** The development of clinical tuberculosis following infection with tubercle bacilli. 1. A theoretical model for the development of clinical tuberculosis following infection, linking from data on the risk of tuberculous infection and the incidence of clinical tuberculosis in the Netherlands. **Tubercle** 1982 Dec;63(4):255–68
**Sutherland I, Bleiker MA, Meijer J, et al:** The risk of tuberculous infection in The Netherlands from 1967 to 1979. **Tubercle** 1983 Dec;64(4):241–53
**Sutherland I** see **Styblo K**
**Sutherland J** see **Franklin J**
**Sutherland JD:** The British object relations theorists: Balint, Winnicott, Fairbairn, Guntrip. **J Am Psychoanal Assoc** 1980;28(4):829–60
**Sutherland JM:** Multiple sclerosis: fifty years on. **Clin Exp Neurol** 1983;19:1–12
**Sutherland N:** 'To create a strong and healthy race': school children in the public health movement, 1880–1914. **Hist Educ Q** 1972;12(3):304–33
**Sutherland SK:** Useless X-rays. **Med J Aust** 1983 Aug 20;2(4):165
**Sutliff WD:** Histoplasmosis in Veterans Administration hospitals in middle America. **Mycopathologia** 1983;83(1):57–62
**Sutter J:** Aperçu historique de la psychopathologie française. **Acta Psychiatr Belg** 1983 Mar–Apr;83(2):104–14
**Sutto C, ed:** Le sentiment de la mort au Moyen Age. Etudes présentées

au Cinquième colloque de l'Institut d'études médiévales de l'Université de Montréal. Quebec, L'Aurore, 1979. Contributions by M. Hébert, R. Lavoie, B. Saint-Pierre, C. Dolan-Leclerc, B. Roy, R. M. Kully, A. Chené-Williams, P. Boglioni, G. H. Allard, E. Schulze-Busacker, D. Smoje.
**Sutton D:** Pilot surveys of Chinese shamans, 1875-1945: a spatial approach to social history. **J Soc Hist** 1981;15(1):39-50
**Sutton G:** Electric medicine and mesmerism. **Isis** 1981 Sep;72(263):375-92
**Sutton G:** The magnetic hands. **Med Instrum** 1984 Jul-Aug;18(4):247
**Sutton G:** The physical and chemical path to vitalism: Xavier Bichat's Physiological Researches on Life and Death. **Bull Hist Med** 1984 Spring;58(1):53-71
**Sutton GV:** A science for a polite society: Cartesian natural philosophy in Paris during the reigns of Louis XIII and XIV. Ph.D. Diss., Princeton University. Princeton, 1982. xi, 481 leaves.
**Sutton JR** see **Pugh LG**
**Sutton SB** see **Castleman B**
**Suvorov NF, Lange KA:** Sovětská fysiologie-hlavní etapy a tendence vývoje. **Cesk Fysiol** 1983;32(3):193-6
**Suvorov VIu, Bliumel' NF, Levtova KZ:** 50 Let Kafedre épidemiologii I Moskovskogo meditsinskogo instituta im. I. M. Sechenova. **Zh Mikrobiol Epidemiol Immunobiol** 1982 Jul;(7):102-6
**Suvorova KN** see **Anton'ev AA**
**Suvorova RV, Mikirtichan GL:** Metodicheskie voprosy prepodavaniia istorii meditsiny na pediatricheskikh fakul'tetakh. **Sov Zdravookhr** 1982;(1):58-61
**Suvorova RV** see **Sokolov EI**
**Suyehiro H, Asahino SN, Uesato G:** [The development of orthodontic treatment in America, the past, present, future] (Jpn). **Nippon Kyosei Shika Gakkai Zasshi** 1982 Mar;41(1):1-8
**Suzuki H** see **Rassengeschichte der Menschheit**
**Suzuki M:** [Past and present nursing in China] (Jpn) **Sogo Kango** 1982;17(4):59-74
**Suzuki S:** Kenko hoken kumiai hattatsu shi. Tokyo, Kitamura Shakai Hoken Shuppan, Showa 51 nen [1976]. 15, 362 p.
**Suzuki T, Hongo T, Yamamoto R:** Hair mercury levels of Japanese women during the period 1881 to 1968. **J Appl Toxicol** 1984 Apr;4(2):101-4
**Suzuki Y:** [Origin of cataract surgery (author's transl)] (Jpn). **Nippon Ganka Gakkai Zasshi** 1980;84(3):183-90
**Svaboe HM:** Sykepleiemuseet på Lovisenberg. **Sykepleien** 1983 Apr 21;70(7):12-3
**Svandová E** see **Sutherland I**
**Svarch Scharager N:** Obra y vida de Luis Pasteur. **Rev Cubana Med Trop** 1980 Jan-Apr;32(1):79-90
**Svebak S:** Helga Eng: a Norwegian precursor to Darrow and Lacey. **Psychophysiology** 1983 Sep;20(5):600-1
**Svejcar J:** Vznik a vývoj Ceskoslovenské spolupráce na poli doškolování pediatru. **Cesk Zdrav** 1983 Oct;31(10):401-7
**Svejdová M** see **Rektor I**
**Svetaĭlo EN:** Vydaiuschiĭsia uchenyĭ sovremennosti (k 100-letiiu so dnia rozhdeniia L. A. Orbeli). **Fiziol Zh SSSR** 1983 Feb;69(2):281-3
**Svinhufvud AC:** A Late Middle English treatise on horses edited from British Library Ms. Sloane 2584 ff 102-117b. **Acta Univ Stockh** 1978;47:1-281
**Svistunov RI:** Meditsinakaia deiatel'nost' Sof'i Perovskoĭ. **Feldsher Akush** 1984 Feb;49(2):47-50
**Svitun VD** see **Penishkevich IF**
**Swagerty WR** see **Dobyns HF**
**Swahn S:** Proust och läkarvetenskapen. **Sydsven Medicinhist Sallsk Arsskr** 1984;21:87-98
**Swain BK** see **Stricevic MV**
**Swain G:** Le sujet de la folie. Naissance de la psychiatrie. Toulouse, Edouard Privat, 1977. 174 p.
**Swain G:** Les métamorphoses de l'hystérie à la fin du XIX siècle. **Penelope** 1983;(8):13-4
**Swain HH:** G & G: the textbook which structured American pharmacology. **Pharmacologist** 1984;26(1):41-4
**Swain V:** No plaster saint! **Nurs Times** 1983 Mar 16-22;79(11):62-3
**Swain V:** Sir Jonathan Hutchinson 1828-1913: his role in the history of intussusception. **J Pediatr Surg** 1980 Apr;15(2):221-3
**Swain VA:** Some portraits of Sir Thomas Spencer Wells (1818-1897). **Ann R Coll Surg Engl** 1983 May;65(3):201-2
**Swain Gladys:** Une logique de l'inclusion: les infirmes du signe. **Esprit** 1982;5:61-75
**Swainson D:** William Henry Brouse. In Dictionary of Canadian biography, 1881-1890. 1982;11:114.
**Swales JK** see **McLachlan HV**
**Swales RJ:** Plague, population and ecology in early modern England. **Can J Hist** 1979;14(2):257-66
**Swan AV** see **Holland WW**
**Swan H** see **Snellen HA**
**Swan KG** see **DiGioia JM**
**Swan KG** see **Jain KM**
**Swan M:** Fitness to plead. **Br J Hosp Med** 1981 Nov;26(5):503, 505-9
**Swan P:** Cholera: a visitation on Victorian society. **Nurs Mirror** 1983 Oct 12;157(15):30-4
**Swan P** see **Sigsworth EM**
**Swan R:** Faith healing, Christian Science, and the medical care of children. **N Engl J Med** 1983 Dec 29;309(26):1639-41
**Swann J** see **Parascandola J**
**Swann JP:** The search for synthetic penicillin during World War II. **Br J Hist Sci** 1983 Jul;16(53 Pt 2):154-90
**Swanson BZ:** A dental Notgeld note. **Bull Hist Dent** 1982 Apr;30(1):27-30
**Swanson BZ:** Spain's private dental museum. **Bull Hist Dent** 1984;32(1):27-30
**Swanson BZ** see **Christen AG**
**Swanson RA** see **Spears B**
**Swantes HJ, Lamsfuss J:** Historische Beobachtungen über den Wetter- und Klimaeinfluss auf Krankheiten diskutiert aus heutiger Sicht. **Med Welt** 1981 Nov 20;32(47):1802-7
**Swartz T** see **Goldblum N**
**Swazey JP** see **Fox RC**
**Swedlund AC:** Historical demography as population ecology. **Annu Rev Anthropol** 1978;7:137-73
**Swedlund AC** see **Temkin-Greener H**
**Sweeney JK:** Earle Ensign Dickson. In Dictionary of American biography, 1961-1965. Suppl. 7, 1981. p. 182-3.
**Sweeney RE, Castleman B:** Asbestos disease and compensation. **Ann NY Acad Sci** 1979;330:273-80
**Swenson O:** Specialization: What it holds for the future of medicine. **Can J Surg** 1980 Mar;23(2):154-6
**Swenson RS:** Associate degree nursing: the gift of thirty years. **NLN Publ** 1983;23-1948:1-9
**Swensson RG** see **Weinberg MS**
**Swiątkowski S** see **Falkiewiczowa S**
**Swicegood G** see **Bean FD**
**Swiderski RM:** Chinese-American patent medicines. **Ethnomedizin** 1978-79;5(1-2):97-126
**Swierenga RP:** Dutch immigrant demography, 1820-1880. **J Fam Hist** 1980 Winter;5(4):390-405
**Swierenga RP:** Physicians and abortion reform in the nineteenth century: social control as the new orthodoxy. **Fides Et Hist** 1979;11(2):51-9
**Swift G:** Recollections and reflections: general practice since 1946. **J R Coll Gen Pract** 1982 Aug;32(241):471-9
**Swift G** see **Horder JP**
**Swift LL** see **McMartin DA**
**Swinney SV** see **Steele RS**
**Swinton WE:** Brains of dinosaurs. In Rose FC, Bynum WF, ed: Historical aspects of the neurosciences. New York, Raven, 1982. p. 473-9.
**Swinton WE:** Cadwallader Colden: physician, historian and government official. **Can Med Assoc J** 1981 Mar 15;124(6):805-9
**Swinton WE:** Charles Darwin as an 'invalid recluse'. **Can Med Assoc J** 1982 Nov 15;127(10):1042-5
**Swinton WE:** Dr. James Tytler: author, balloonist, encyclopedist. **Can Med Assoc J** 1981 Jan 15;124(2):216-23
**Swinton WE:** George Mellis Douglas: typhus and tragedy. **Can Med Assoc J** 1981 Dec 1;125(11):1284-6
**Swinton WE:** Rabelais' coarse humour was therapy for his patients. **Can Med Assoc J** 1981 Feb 15;124(4):500-4
**Swinton WE:** The hydrotherapy and infamy of Dr. James Gully. **Can Med Assoc J** 1980 Dec 20;123(12):1262-4
**Swinton WE:** The remarkable accomplishments of Dr. Peter Roget. **Can Med Assoc J** 1980 Nov 8;123(9):916-21
**Swinton WE** see **Hart GD, ed**
**Swintosky JV:** Maturing of pharmaceutical education. **Drug Intell Clin Pharm** 1976 Mar;10(3):153-60
**Swinyard EA:** History of the antiepileptic drugs. **Adv Neurol** 1980;27:1-9
**Swinyard EA:** Research and graduate education in pharmacy: looking back--looking forward. **Am J Pharm Educ** 1977 Nov;41(4):409-14
**Swoboda W:** 20 Jahre Osterreichische Gesellschaft für Kinderheilkunde. **Padiatr Padol** 1982;17(4):651-6
**Swoboda WW** see **Brücke EW von**
**Sydenham D** see **Spears J**
**Sydenham DM:** Practitioner and patient. The practice of medicine in eighteenth-century South Carolina. Ph.D. Diss. Johns Hopkins University. Baltimore, 1979. vii, 323 leaves.
**Sydney Hospital--a tribute: Lamp** 1983 Jan-Feb;40(1):14-6
**Sydow C von:** Notiser från Frans von Sydows utrikes studieresor 1861-1886. **Nord Medicinhist Arsb** 1984;:117-28
**Sykes WS:** Essays on the first hundred years of anaesthesia. 3 vols. Park Ridge, Illinois, Wood Library-Museum of Anesthesiology, 1982. 171, 187, 272 p. (Vols. 1 and 2 are reprints of 1960 ed; Vol. 3 is edited by R. H. Ellis)
**Syllaba J:** Rozvoj československé diabetologie v posledních 60 letech. **Vnitr Lek** 1984 Apr;30(4):401-5
**Sylvain P:** Jean-Etienne Landry. In Dictionary of Canadian biography, 1881-1890. 1982;11:483-6.
**Sylvestre PF:** Dossier historique: les religieuses infirmières en Ontario français. **Infirm Can** 1983 Nov;25(10):27-9
**Symons H, Nutton V, Schupbach W, et al:** [Manuscripts in the Wellcome Library] **Kos** 1984 Jun;1(5):5-26
**Symposium: adaptive grades in the evolution of primates: Z Morphol Anthropol** 1980;71(2):113-227
**Symposium on capillary permeability and mechanism of transport, American Physiological Society, New Orleans, 1979. A salute to Professor Hyman S. Mayerson.: Physiologist** 1980 Feb;23(1):34-93
**The symposium, part I:** Fifty years of change. **NY J Dent** 1980 Apr;50(4):127-37
**Synek VM:** Linnaeus--physician and king of flowers. **NZ Med J** 1984 Apr 25;97(754):267-9
**Synge RL:** Early work on Gramicidin S. In J. Parascandola, ed: The history of antibiotics. Madison, American Institute of the History of Pharmacy,

1980. p. 97–100.

**Syroka A:** Pojecie źródeł do historii medycyny i próba ich klasyfikacji. **Arch Hist Med (Warsz)** 1984;47(1):19–24

**Sytnik KM, Dyshlebyi PS:** Dialektika revoliutsii v estestvoznanii. **Vopr Filos** 1981;(3):42–56

**Szabadváry F:** Joseph Priestley születésének 250. évfordulójára. **Orv Hetil** 1983 Oct 16;124(42):2563–4

**Szabady E:** Crises of mortality in Hungary in the 19th century. In Charbonneau H, Larose A, ed: The great mortalities: methodological studies of demographic crises in the past. Liège, Belgium, Ordina Editions, 1980. p. 199–205.

**Szabó C** see **Racz S**

**Szabó G:** A gén fogalmának fejlödése. **Orv Hetil** 1982 Jan 31;123(5):259–65

**Szabó I:** A Koch bacilus 100 éve. **Orv Hetil** 1982 Jan 24,123(4).227–9

**Szabó I:** The influence of the discovery of Koch's bacterium on the Hungarians. **Indian J Chest Dis Allied Sci** 1982 Apr–Sep;24(2–3):175–8

**Szafrański P, Zagórski W, Filipowicz W:** Studies on protein biosynthesis at the Institute of Biochemistry and Biophysics, Polish Academy of Sciences, initiated by Professor J. Heller in 1956. **Acta Biochim Pol** 1984;31(1):9–16

**Szalay FS:** A critique of some recently proposed paleogene primate taxa and suggested relationships. **Folia Primatol (Basel)** 1982;37(3–4):153–62

**Szalay FS, Dagosto M:** Locomotor adaptations as reflected on the humerus of paleogene primates. **Folia Primatol (Basel)** 1980;34(1–2):1–45

**Szállá A:** Arthur Schnitzler és Georges Duhamel a Nyugatban. **Orv Hetil** 1982 Sep 5;123(36):2246–50

**Szállási A:** A fagyvilágmagyar orvosvándora. **Orv Hetil** 1984 Apr 1;125(14):835–7

**Szállási A:** A Nyugat, gyógyszerészei'. **Orv Hetil** 1982 Jan 24;123(4):229–32

**Szállási A:** A salvarsan felfedezésének visszhangja a Nyugat-ban. **Orv Hetil** 1980 Apr 20;121(16):966–7

**Szállási A:** Aki szerkesztönek született, az orvostudomány sem menti meg. **Orv Hetil** 1981 Apr 5;122(14):837–9

**Szállási A:** Arany János tanártársa Lengyel Dániel doktor. **Orv Hetil** 1983 Apr 3;124(14):833–4

**Szállási A:** Babits betegségei. **Orv Hetil** 1983 Nov 27;124(48):2940–2

**Szállási A:** Babits betegségei a tracheotomia elött. **Orv Hetil** 1981 Sep 6;122(36):2235–9

**Szállási A:** Csehov és Maugham a Nyugat kedvenc írói. **Orv Hetil** 1980 Jan 27;121(4):226–9

**Szállási A:** Diósszilágyi Sámuel, az írók orvosa és az orvosok írója. **Orv Hetil** 1981 Jun 14;122(24):1467–72

**Szállási A:** Donath Gyula és a Klinikai Füzetek. **Orv Hetil** 1984 Apr 15;125(16):960–3

**Szállási A:** Egy kolera-kiadvány 1831-böl. **Orvostort Kozl** 1979;87–88(25 no 1–2):307–9

**Szállási A:** Egy medikus müvészi metamorfózisa (100 éve születell Medgyessy Ferenc). **Orv Hetil** 1981 Mar 22;122(12):709–11

**Szállási A:** Fábián Dániel és József Attila. **Orv Hetil** 1983 Feb 20;124(8):464–6

**Szállási A:** Farkas Géza-akinek élete volt a fömüve. **Orv Hetil** 1984 Sep 16;125(38):2324–7

**Szállási A:** Fontos adalék a Tanácsköztársaság alkoholellenes küzdelméhez. **Orv Hetil** 1980 Aug 10;121(32):1955–6

**Szállási A:** Freud, Ferenczi és a Nyugat. **Orv Hetil** 1980 May 18;121(20):1207–8

**Szállási A:** [Gusztáv Rigler: prominent figure in Hungarian public health (1868–1930)] (Hun). **Orv Hetil** 1980;121:2209–11

**Szállási A:** Högyes Endre pesti kinevezésének centenáriuma. **Orv Hetil** 1983 Oct 30;124(44):2691–3

**Szállási A:** Id. Elischer Gyula élete––a mügyüjtés apológiája. **Orv Hetil** 1984 Oct 14;125(42):2567–9

**Szállási A:** Magyar orvosíró és az orosz forradalom. **Orv Hetil** 1984 Mar 18;125(12):712–5

**Szállási A:** Medgyessy Ferenc medikuskori rajzaiból. **Orvostort Kozl** 1979;87–88(25 no 1–2):315–9

**Szállási A:** Németh Lázzló és a Nyugat. **Orv Hetil** 1981 Jan 25;122(4):226–7

**Szállási A:** Nendtvich Károly orvosvegyész amerikai utazása 1855-ben. **Orv Hetil** 1984 Sep 2;125(36):2205–6, 2209–10

**Szállási A:** Orvosok a magyar irodalomban Földi Jánostól napjainkig. **Orv Hetil** 1982 Sep 19;123(38):2367–73

**Szállási A:** Orvosok és a Nyugat elsö évfolyamai. **Orv Hetil** 1979 Sep 23;120(38):2311–3

**Szállási A:** Ramón y Cajal und die ungarischen Arzte. In International Congress of the History of Medicine, 27th, Barcelona, 1980. Actas. Barcelona, Académia de Ciències Mèdiques de Catalunya i Balears, 1981. p. 632–5.

**Szállási A:** Rekviem a 'Gyógyászat'––ért Schachter Miksa szerkesztése ürügyén. **Orv Hetil** 1980 Dec 14;121(50):3073–6

**Szallasi A:** Reports by Hungarian physicians on North America in the nineteenth century. In: Congrès international d'histoire de la médecine, XXVe, Québec, 1976. Actes. Québec, 1977. p. 1341–6.

**Szállási A:** Székey Agoston––a szerkesztöi másodvonalból. **Orv Hetil** 1983 Jan 9;124(2):95–7

**Szállási A:** Szociálhigiéne, szociográfia, szépirodalom. **Orv Hetil** 1981 May 17;122(20)1199–202

**Szállási A:** 100 éve ismert a Pneumococcus pathogén természete. **Orv Hetil** 1984 Dec 9;125(50):3059–62

**Szállási A:** 100 éve szerzett oklevelet az elsö magyar orvosnö. **Orv Hetil** 1979 Aug 19;120(32):1950–2

**Szállási A:** 150 éve született Tóth N. János, az elsö dualista magyar szifidológus. **Orv Hetil** 1984 Jun 10;125(24):1457–8

**Szállási A:** 1925-ben alakult meg a Párizsi Magyar Egyesület. **Orv Hetil** 1980 Sept 21;121(38):2339–40

**Szaluta J:** Apotheosis to ignominy: the martyrdom of Marshal Pétain. **J Psychohist** 1980 Spring;7(4):415–53

**Szám I** see **Honti J**

**Szarek WA, Stacey M, Hay GW:** John Kenyon Netherton Jones (1912–1977). **Adv Carbohydr Chem Biochem** 1983;41:1–26

**Szarkowski JW, Wierzchowski KL:** Professor Józef Heller 1896–1982. **Acta Biochim Pol** 1984;31(1):5–8

**Szasz FM:** Francis Schlatter: the healer of the southwest. **NM Hist Rev** 1979;54(2):89–104

**Szasz T** see **Grenander ME**

**Szasz TS:** The lying truths of psychiatry. **J Libert Stud** 1979,3(2).121–39

**Szasz TS** see **Sharkey PW, ed**

**Szczepaniak AS:** Thomas Cromwell Corner, Baltimore Portrait artist. **Md State Med J** 1980 Apr;29(4):78–9

**Sze S:** The origins of the World Health Organization: a personal memoir, 1945–1948. Boca Raton, Fla. L.I.S.Z. Publications, [1982]. xiii, 31 p.

**Szegal B** see **McGuigan FJ**

**Székács I:** Freud és pszichoanalízis természettudományos alapjai. **Orv Hetil** 1982 Dec 12;123(50):3091–9

**Székács I:** Hári Pál emléke (1869–1933). **Orv Hetil** 1983 Jul 31;124(31):1889–94

**Szekér E:** Emléktábla-ayató ünnepség Balatonfüreden. **Orv Hetil** 1983 Feb 20;124(8):467–8

**Szekér E:** Hugonnaie Vilma balatonfüredi emlékezete. **Orv Hetil** 1982 Mar 7;123(10):611–2

**Szeleczky G:** Hüttl Tivadar centenáriumára. **Orv Hetil** 1984 Aug 19;125(34):2081–2

**Széll K:** A regionalis érzéstelenités helye a korszerü anaesthesiológiában. **Orv Hetil** 1982 Jul 4;123(27):1651–8

**Széll K:** Szemelvények a szombathelyi kórház történetéböl I. **Orv Hetil** 1979 Dec 16;120(50):3057–60

**Széll K:** Szemelvények a szombathelyi kórház történetéböl 1946-ig II. **Orv Hetil** 1980 Feb 10;121(6):346–9

**Szemkeö E:** A német orvostudomány szerepe a magyar –– orosz orvosi kapcsolatok XVIII –– XIX. századi történetében. **Orv Hetil** 1981 Jan 11;122(2):104, 107–8

**Szemkeö E:** Adalék Semmelweis életének utolsó heteihez. **Orv Hetil** 1980 Jul 27;121(30):1837–8

**Szemkeö E:** Die Teilnahme des ungarischen Landesrates für Gesundheitswesen an der Zusammenstellung eines internationalen Arzneibuches zur Zeit der Jahrhundertwende. In Hein WH, ed: Pharmaziehistorischer Kongress, Budapest, 1981. Stuttgart, Wissenschaftliche Verlagsgesellschaft, 1983. p. 129–33.

**Szemkeö E:** Ein Beitrag zu den letzten Wochen von Semmelweis. **Orvostort Kozl** 1979;87–88(25 no 1–2):291–7

**Szemkeö E** see **Kapronczay K**

**Szemraj-Lochynska A, Kempisty C:** Stan adaptacji do zycia na emeryturze nauczycieli akademickich represjonowanych przez hitleryzm. **Przegl Lek** 1981;38(1):33–6

**Szentágothai J:** Too 'much' and too 'soon'. A lifetime of inquiry into the functional organization of the nervous system. **Acta Biol Acad Sci Hung** 1982;33(2–3):107–26

**Szentgyörgyölgyi G:** 'Foltos' bürök. **Orv Hetil** 1981 Nov 1;122(44):2733–4

**Szentgyörgyvölgyi G:** Csáth Géza––Dr. Brenner József (1887–1919). **Orv Hetil** 1984 Sep 30;125(40):2446–8

**Szentgyörgyvölgyi G:** Egy régi hajdúszoboszlói gyógyszerész: Trocsányi Imre és köre. **Orv Hetil** 1982 Nov 28;123(48):2972–3

**Szentgyörgyvölgyi G:** Erdélyi történetírók egészségügyi közlései a török idökböl. **Orv Hetil** 1984 Apr 1;125(14):837–41

**Szentgyörgyvölgyi G:** Köleséri Sámuel pályája és jelleme. **Orvostort Kozl** 1981;93–96(27 No 1–4):183–7

**Szentgyörgyvölgyi G:** Szemelvények Debrecen gyógyítástörténeti múltiából. **Orv Hetil** 1982 May 2;123(18):1114–6

**Szepesi B:** Carp––a nutritional food: preliminary studies on the use of carp in the American diet. **J Nal Assoc** 1981;6(1–4):14–6

**Szerbák E:** Halál, temetés és búcsúztatás a XIX. század eleji Magyarországon. **Orvostort Kozl** 1980;89–91(26 no 1–3):175–90

**Szewko S** see **Markowski W**

**Szigetváry F:** Die Apotheke der Jesuiten von Köszeg. In Hein WH, ed: Pharmaziehistorischer Kongress, Budapest, 1981. Stuttgart, Wissenschaftliche Verlagsgesellschaft, 1983. p. 73–80.

**Szilagyi DE:** The elusive target: truth in scientific reporting. Comments on error, self-delusion, deceit, and fraud. **J Vasc Surg** 1984 Mar;1(2):243–53

**Szilágyi I:** Bethlen Gábor betegsége és halála. **Orv Hetil** 1984 May 13;125(20):1205–10

**Szilási A:** A magyar nyelvü belgyógyászati oktatás kezdete. **Orv Hetil** 1979 Oct 7;120(40):2435–7

**Szilvágyi I:** Fejér megye közegészségügyének története 1865–1903 között. **Orvostort Kozl** 1979;87–88(25 no 1–2):277–90

**Szlatky M:** Lippay János Posoni Kertjének orvos-botanikai vonatkozásai (1664–1667). **Orvostort Kozl** 1979;87(25 no 1–2):79–90

**Szlatky M:** Magyar nyelvü, kéziratos orvosló könyvek a 17. századból. **Magy Konyosz** 1980;96(2):131–48

**Szlatky M** see **Kádár Z**

**Szostak J:** Funkcja społeczna pierwszych zielników polskich. **Farm Pol** 1979;4:195–200

**Szostak J:** Scientia de simpliciis w pierwszych zielnikach polskich.

Arch Hist Med (Warsz) 1980;43(3):265-87
**Szpilczyński S:** A látás kérdése Witelon (Vitellio) Peri optices (1275) c. munkájában. **Orvostort Kozl** 1979;87-88(25 no 1-2)219-22
**Szpilczyński S:** Das traditionelle und progressive Gesicht der Medizin in der Renaissance-Epoche im Lichte der Polemik zwischen S. Simonius und N. Buccella nach dem Tode des Königs Stefan Batory. **Organon** 1979;15:229-37
**Szpilczyński S:** Jan Jonston z Szamotuł. Tytaniczny trud barokowego erudyty w świetle wielkiej dydaktyki. **Slaski Kwart Hist Sobotka** 1976;31(2):223-9
**Szpilczynski S:** La théorie de la vision chez Witelo 'Peri optikes', 1273. In: Congrès international d'histoire de la médecine, XXVe, Québec, 1976. Actes. Québec, 1977. p. 1347-53.
**Szpilczynski S** see **Barg L**
**Szpunar W:** Zgony z powodu gruźlicy w Lańcucie i okolicy w latach 1786-1970. Próba oceny epidemii. **Pneumonol Pol** 1981 Jul;49(7):527-35
**Sztanyik BL:** A sugárbiológia negyedszázada. **Orv Hetil** 1983 Sep 11;124(37):2223-32
**Sztanyik BL:** Curie és az orvostudomány. **Orv Hetil** 1981 Apr 19;;122(16):961-4
**Szüts T:** Ujabb adatok az 1831. Evi kolerajárvány történetéhez. **Orvostort Kozl** 1979;87-88(25 no 1-2):255-9
**Szwarc B:** Spis prac Prof. Tadeusza Krwawicza. **Klin Oczna** 1980 Jan;82(1):1-4
**Szwarczyński W:** Rozwój badań w dziedzinie oryginalnego polskiego leku syntetycznego. **Arch Hist Med (Warsz)** 1984;47(3):443-6
**Szwejcerowa A:** Marceli Nencki (1847-1901), pionnier de la biochimie. In International Congress of the History of Medicine. 26th, Plovdiv, 1978. Actes du Congress. Sofia, 1981. Volume II. p. 97-9.
**Szwejcerowa A:** O Towarzystwie Lekarzy Niemieckich w Paryzu. **Arch Hist Med (Warsz)** 1979;42(3):323-30
**Szwejcerowa A:** Siedziby Towarzystwa Lekarskiego Warszawskiego w latach 1820--1944. **Arch Hist Med (Warsz)** 1980;43(2):127-46
**Szyfman L:** Les prétendues falsifications d'Ernst Haeckel et son triomphe sur ses diffamateurs. **Bull Biol Fr Belg** 1980;113(4):375-406
**Szyfman L:** Remarques sur l'ouvrage d'Ernst Mayr: 'Lamarck Revisited'. **Bull Biol Fr Belg** 1977;111(3):209-29
**Szymańska R:** Karol Klecki (1866-1931) - wybitny patofizjolog i profesor Fakultetu Medycznego w Krakowie (w 50 rocznicę śmierci). **Pol Tyg Lek** 1981 Sep 21;36(38):1487-90
**Szymańska R, Schmidt-Pospuła M:** Z historii badań tadeusza Browicza (1847-1928) i Karola Kupffera (1829--1902) nad komórkami siateczkowo-śródbłonkowymi watroby. **Arch Hist Med (Warsz)** 1979;42(3):331-6
**Szymanski A:** On the uses of disinformation to legitimize the revival of the cold war: health in the U.S.S.R. **Sci Soc** 1981-82;45(4):453-74
**Szymanski B, Hieke M:** Zur Geschichte der Dentitionsforschung unter dem Gesichtspunkt der Entwicklungsdiagnostik. **Aerztl Jugendkd** 1981;72(5):304-26
**Szymczykiewicz K:** XXX lat działalności Instytutu Medycyny Pracy w Sosnowcu. **Med Pr** 1981;32(5):309-15
**Szymusik A** see **Fortuna D**

# T

**Tabanelli M:** Gli albori della chirurgia nelle Fiandre. Il libro del maestro Thomas Scellinck. Firenze, Leo S. Olschki, 1974. xxxviii, 284 p. (Biblioteca della 'Rivista di Storia delle Scienze Mediche e Naturali', v. 19).
**Tabeński Z:** Wkład polskich chirurgów w rozwój leczenia choroby Hirschsprunga u dzieci. **Pediatr Pol** 1981 Jun;56(6):695-7
**Tabolkina NM:** Okhrana materinstva i detstva v poslevoennom Leningrade (1945-1948). **Sov Zdravookhr** 1983;(7):67-9
**Tabor DC:** Ripe and unripe: concepts of health and sickness in Ayurvedic medicine. **Soc Sci Med** 1981;15B:439-55
**Taborko MM** see **Bakalkin GIa**
**Tabossi P** see **Job R**
**Tabutin D** see **Poulain M**
**Tachon J:** La revue 'Médecine Tropical'--retrospective. **Med Trop (Mars)** 1980 Nov-Dec;40(6):639-41
**Taddey G:** Pockenschutz in Hohenlohe. **Medizinhist J** 1983;18(4):313-23
**Tadeusz Bilikiewicz (1901-1980)---historyk medycyny i filozof: Kwart Hist Nauki Tech** 1981;26(2):435-48
**Tagger M:** Endodontic treatment in Israel. **Int Endod J** 1984 Jul;17(3):113-24
**Tagliavini A** see **Babini VP**
**Tagliavini R** see **Zanca A**
**Tagochi T:** [Nursing and nursing education in the past 35 years since the end of the Second World War. (1)] (Jpn) **Kango Kyoiku** 1981 Jan;22(1):34-40
**Tai E** see **Veatch RM**
**Taillefer J** see **Paiement B**
**Tainmont J:** La langue grecque classique et le vocabulaire ORL d'aujourd'hui. **Acta Otorhinolaryngol Belg** 1982;36(6):1039-60
**Tait HP:** The College and community health. In Passmore R, ed: Proceedings of the Royal College of Physicians of Edinburgh Tercentenary Congress, 1981. Edinburgh, Royal College of Physicians of Edinburgh, 1982. p. 162-78.
**Tait HP:** The McNeil Library and some of its notable volumes. **Univ Edinb J** 1980;29:313-7
**Tait HP:** Two tuberculosis anniversaries. **Practitioner** 1980 Oct;224(1348):1101-3
**Tait I:** History of our records. **Br Med J [Clin Res]** 1981 Feb 28;282(6265):702-4
**Tait JF, Tait SA:** Recent perspectives on the history of the adrenal cortex. **J Endocrinol** 1979 Oct;83(1):3P-24P
**Tait SA** see **Tait JF**
**Tajima Y:** [30 years of research using experimental animals--transition from bacteriology to the study of experimental animals] (Jpn). **Nippon Saikingaku Zasshi** 1984 Jul;39(4):739-43
**Takada M:** [Children who do not know Florence Nightingale: teaching of nursing history at a nursing school] (Jpn). **Kango Kyoiku** 1984 Dec;25(12):725-7
**Takagi K:** Arthroscope. Kenji Takagi. J. Jap. Orthop. Assoc., 1939. **Clin Orthop** 1982 Jul;(167):6-8
**Takahashi M:** [A tour of the areas related to Florence Nightingale. (1)] (Jpn). **Kango Kyoiku** 1981 Jan;22(1):54-60
**Takahashi M:** [Illustrated history of nursing - toward teaching of more attractive nursing history (3). The first nursing school in Japan and trained nurses] (Jpn). **Kango Kyoiku** 1983 Sep;24(9):560-3
**Takahashi M:** [Illustrated history of nursing--towards a more attractive study of nursing history] (Jpn). **Kango Kyoiku** 1984 Jan;25(1):46-9 contd
**Takahashi M:** [Illustrated nursing history--for teaching of more interesting nursing history (2). The image of midwives described in 'Fujin Juso' and 'Baba Hikken'] (Jpn). **Kango Kyoiku** 1983 Aug;24(8):496-9
**Takahashi M:** [Illustrated nursing history--teaching of more interesting nursing history (1). Focus on Japanese nursing history] (Jpn). **Kango Kyoiku** 1983 Jul;24(7):432-5
**Takahashi M:** [Mrs. Fuji Hirano, an early graduate of Jikei Hospital Nursing School] (Jpn). **Kango Kyoiku** 1983 Nov;24(11):686-91
**Takahashi M:** [Nurses in the history of nursing. (1) Masa Suzuki] (Jpn). **Kango Kyoiku** 1981 Jun;22(6):399-403
**Takâhashi M:** [Nurses in the history of nursing. (2). Kyo Takano] (Jpn). **Kango Kyoiku** 1981 Jul;22(7):451-6
**Takahashi M:** [Nurses in the history of nursing. (3). 'Infant Jesus' Mission and its nursing activities] (Jpn). **Kango Kyoiku** 1981 Aug;22(8):513-20
**Takahashi M:** [Nurses in the history of nursing (6). Mrs. Miki Sawada and a home nurse] (Jpn). **Kango Kyoiku** 1981 Nov;22(11):718-24
**Takahashi M:** [On participating in the tour of the 'Areas related to Nightingale' (2)] (Jpn). **Kango Kyoiku** 1981 Apr;22(4):262-7
**Takahashi M:** [Personalities in the history of nursing. (4). Ms. Chika Ozeki] (Jpn). **Kango Kyoiku** 1981 Sep;22(9)575-82
**Takahashi Y** see **Tsuboi Y**
**Takai S** see **Akiyoshi T**
**Takaki R:** Aesculapius was a white man: antebellum racism and male chauvinism at Harvard Medical School. **Phylon** 1978;39(2):128-34
**Takanishi R:** Childhood as a social issue: historical roots of contemporary child advocacy movements. **J Soc Issues** 1978;34(2):8-28
**Takáts L:** A magyarországi utolsó török háború egészségügyi ellátásának megszervezése 1788-89-ben. **Hadtortenelmi Kozl** 1966;13(1):40-63
**Takáts L, Fäller J, Leitner F:** Katonaegeszségügyi szolgálatunk megalakulása és müködése a felszabadulás évében (1945). **Hadtortenelmi Kozl** 1977;24(1):31-59
**Takazoe I** see **Moriyama N**
**Takeda Y, Zinnaka Y:** [Centenary of the discovery of Vibrio cholerae by Robert Koch] (Jpn) **Nippon Saikingaku Zasshi** 1984 Jul;39(4):709-12
**Takei Y:** [Administrative reform in 19th-century England, a result of the public health problem] (Jpn). **Shakai Keizai Shigaku** 1976;42(3):1-21
**Takei Y:** [The public health problem in Great Britain at the time of the Industrial Revolution] (Jpn). **Shakai Keizai Shigaku** 1974;40(4):1-24
**Takemi T** see **Unschuld PU**
**Takeshita YJ** see **Cho LJ**
**Takeuchi F** see **Okamura H**
**Takeyama M:** [Conclusion of the translation of the 'Life of Florence Nightingale'] (Jpn). **Sogo Kango** 1981 Aug;16(3):76-83
**Tal M:** Periodontal disease and oral hygiene. Described by Antoni van Leeuwenhoek. **J Periodontol** 1980 Nov;51(11):668-9
**Tal U:** On the study of the Holocaust and genocide. **Yad Vashem Stud Eur Jew Catastrophe Resist** 1979;13:7-52
**Talbot CH** see **Hand WD, ed**
**Talbot DM:** Federation of Specialty Nursing Organizations and the American Nurses' Association: a history. **Occup Health Nurs** 1981 Oct;29(10):27-33
**Talbott JH:** Gout therapy throughout the ages. **Med Times** 1981 Jan;109(1):2s-8s
**Talbott JH:** Medical maladies as seen by the artist. **JAMA** 1981 Feb 6;245(5):497-8
**Talbott MW:** Intraocular lenses and the Food and Drug Administration: regulation amid controversy. **Int Ophthalmol Clin** 1979 Fall;19(3):1-10
**Talenti M:** Cenni storici su la Farmacopea Ufficiale Italiana. **Nuovi Ann Ig Microbiol** 1982 Jul-Dec;33(4-6):889-99
**Talewski R:** Robert Koch 11.XII.1843--27.V.1910. **Pneumonol Pol** 1982 Nov;50(11):553-5
**Talewski R:** Zakopiański lekarz klimatyczny ministrem zdrowia (w czterdziestą rocznicę śmierci prof. Tomasza Janiszewskiego). **Arch Hist Med (Warsz)** 1980;43(3):331-41
**Tallberg M:** Sophie Mannerheim: en historisk beskrivning och analys av hennes verksamhet 1904-1928. **Vard Nord Utveckl Forsk** 1983 Spring;3(4):123-30
**Talmadge P** see **Evans RB**
**Talmage DW:** William Hay Taliaferro: February 10, 1895-December 21, 1973. **Biogr Mem Natl Acad Sci** 1983;54:375-407

**Talmor E, ed:** Malthus our contemporary. Contributions by K. W. Back, A. J. Field, L. Murard, P. Zylberman. **Hist Eur Ideas** 1983;4:121–214

**Talve I:** Piirilläkärit suomen kansan ravinnosta v. 1857–1870. **Kotiseutu** 1972;4–5:196–202

**Talyshinskiĭ AM:** K istorii éndotrakheal'nykh trukbok s manzhetkami i bronkhoblokatorov. **Anesteziol Reanimatol** 1980 Mar–Apr;(2):68–70

**Tamarina NA, Lange AB:** Razvitie ideĭ V. N. Beklemisheva v oblasti sravnitel'noĭ parazitologii. **Med Parazitol (Mosk)** 1982 Jan–Feb;51(1):3–9

**Tamáska P:** A boszorkányüldözések gazdasági és társadalmi háttere. **Orv Hetil** 1983 Sep 18;124(38):2322, 2325

**Tamáska P:** Az orvostörténet oktatásának és müvelésének története Csehországban. **Orv Hetil** 1984 Aug 5;125(32):1963–4

**Tambovtsev PD:** K istorii organizatsii i razvitiia sanatornoĭ pomoshchi detiam. **Pediatriia** 1983 Sep;:(9):71–3

**Tambovtsev PD:** K 25–letiiu detskogo pul'monologicheskogo sanatoriia im. M.S. Maslova. **Pediatriia** 1983 Jun;(6):74–5

**Tamburini C** see **Bernasconi M**

**TambyRaja RL** see **Ratnam SS**

**Tamke SS** see **Spicker SF**

**Tamminen S:** Varhainen väestökirjanpitokaava Maalahdella ja Sulvassa 1600–luvulla. **Hist Aikak** 1978;76(3):241–50

**Tammisto T:** Kipu muuttuvassa maailmassa. **Duodecim** 1981;97(14):1013–6

**Tamony P:** Tripping out from San Francisco. **Am Speech** 1981;56(2):98–103

**Tamura M:** [On research on Florence Nightingale -- a future overview] (Jpn). **Sogo Kango** 1980;15(4):18–21

**Tamura S:** [History of Czechoslovakia and its system for nursing education] (Jpn). **Kango Kyoiku** 1983 Oct;24(10):605–13

**Tan NC:** The Academy of Medicine of Singapore. **Ann Acad Med Singapore** 1982 Jul;11(3):307–8

**Tanabe K** see **Ueda M**

**Tanaka K, Uzawa Y, Hanashima T:** [Further and continuing education of nurses in Japan; historical overview by literature.] (Jpn). **Kango Tenbo** 1983 Nov;8(11):996–1005

**Tanaka M:** [Public health nurses of the Santama area (5). History of public health clinics in the past 40 years since their start: a visit with Ms. Miki Tanaka] (Jpn). **Hokenfu Zasshi** 1982 Aug;38(8):676–83

**Tanaka S** see **Seki M**

**Tang LC:** A personal and scientific biography of Dr. George C. Cotzias. **Neurotoxicology (Park Forest Il)** 1984 Spring;5(1):5–12

**Tang PS:** [An unfinished project--recollections of fifty years of physiological research] (Chi). **Sheng Li Ko Hsueh Chin Chan** 1984 Jul;15(3):193–7

**Tanitsu M:** [Medico-dental and pharmacological history--miscellaneous records (7)] (Jpn) **Dent Outlook** 1980;(7):114–5 (continued periodically)

**Tank MC:** Synopsis of the Brookings-Madison District medical community (No. 3). **SD J Med** 1981 May;34(5):12–3

**Tank RM:** Young children, families, and society in America since the 1820s: the evolution of health, education, and child care programs for preschool children. Ph.D. Diss., University of Michigan. Ann Arbor, 1980. v, 471 leaves.

**Tanneau Y:** L'ancienneté des bains de mer à Douarnenez. **Cah Iroise** 1979;26(2):78–81

**Tanner JM:** A history of the study of human growth. Cambridge, New York, Cambridge University Press, 1981. 499 p.

**Tanner-Weder C:** Alfred Brunner und die Entwicklung der Thoraxchirurgie. Zürich, Juris, 1980. 37p. (Zürcher Medizingeschichtliche Abhandlungen, Neue Reihe, Nr. 142).

**Tanselle GT** see **Teigen PM, ed**

**Tansey EM:** The life and works of Sir Alexander Crichton, F.R.S. (1763-1856): a Scottish physician to the Imperial Russian Court. **Notes Rec R Soc Lond** 1984;38(2):241–59

**Tansey V, Mekie DE:** Report of the Museum of the Royal College of Surgeons of Edinburgh. **J R Coll Surg Edinb** 1980 Mar;25(2):67–75 contd

**Tansey V, Mekie DE:** The museum of the Royal College of Surgeons of Edinburgh. **J R Coll Surg Edinb** 1980 Jul;25(4):248–56

**Tansey V, Mekie DE:** The Museum of the Royal College of Surgeons of Edinburgh. **J R Coll Surg Edinb** 1980 May;25(3):188–93 (continued periodically)

**Tansey V, Mekie DE:** The Museum of the Royal College of Surgeons of Edinburgh (Part 4). **J R Coll Surg Edinb** 1980 Nov;25(6):481–4

**Tanzer G:** Adolf Witzel (1847–1906) und die Zahnerhaltung. **Zahnarzt** 1984 Jan;28(1):49–52

**Tanzer G:** Aus der Geschichte der Zahnheilkunde. Giuseppangelo Fonzi, 13.7.1768–31.8.1840. **Zahnarzt** 1983 Dec;27(12):765–9

**Tanzer G:** Aus der Geschichte der Zahnheilkunde. Pierre Fauchard. **Zahnarzt** 1983 Nov;27(11):713–7

**Tanzer G:** Philipp Pfaff (1713–1766), seine Zeit und seine Vorgänger. **Zahnarzt** 1984 Feb;28(2):129–31

**Tanzer G:** Professor Dr. Alfred Gysi (1865–1957). **Zahnarzt** 1984 Jun;28(6):447–9

**Tanzer G:** Willoughby Dayton Miller (1853–1907). **Zahnarzt** 1984 May;28(5):375–6

**Taplin GV:** The history of lung imaging with radionuclides. **Semin Nucl Med** 1979 Jul;9(3):178–85

**Taplin GV, ed** see **Brucer M**

**Tappeiner J, Holubar K:** Ferdinand Ritter von Hebra: Person und Werk (1816 bis 1880). **Wien Klin Wochenschr** 1981 Sep 4;93(16):503–6

**Taquini AC:** XX aniversario de la Fundación de la Sociedad Argentina de Investigación Clínica. **Medicina (B Aires)** 1979 Nov–Dec;39(6):703–5

**Taramides G:** Ta dontia ton Kyprios tes neolithikos epoches (5800–3000 P.Ch.). **Odontostomatol Proodos** 1983 Jul–Aug;37(4):213–8

**Tarasenko IV** see **Kogan VI**

**Tarasenko NIu:** Gigiena truda i okhrana zdorov'ia trudiashchikhsia v rabotakh V. I. Lenina. **Gig Tr Prof Zabol** 1982 Apr;(4):1–3

**Tarasenko NIu, Moĭkin IuV, Anan'ev BV:** Razvitie ideĭ I. M. Sechenova v sovremennykh issledovaniiakh po gigiene i fiziologii truda. **Vestn Akad Med Nauk SSSR** 1981;(1):3–9

**Tarasenko NIu:** Rol' sanitarno-gigienicheskogo fakul'teta v podgotovke vracheĭ profilakticheskoĭ meditsiny i v razvitii gigieny truda (k 50–letiiu obrazovaniiu sanitarno-gigienicheskogo fakul'teta I Moskovskogo meditsinskogo instituta im I. M. Sechenova). **Gig Tr Prof Zabol** 1980 Oct;(10):29–32

**Tarasenko NIu** see **Moikin IuV**

**Tarasonov VM:** Vklad A.I. Tal'iantseva v éksperimental'noe issledovanie patologii serdechno sosudistoĭ sistemy. **Patol Fiziol Eksp Ter** 1980 Mar–Apr;(2):92–3

**Tarasov KE** see **Smolenskiĭ VS**

**Tarasov O:** Science in Soviet Moldavia. In Science and Technology: humanism and progress. Moscow, Social Science Today, 1981. Vol. 2, p. 53–66. (Problems of the Contemporary World, no. 96).

**Tarasov OF:** A. F. Tur: 1894–1974. Moskva, Meditsina, 1980. 125 p.

**Tarasov OI:** Iz istorii nauki v Moldavskoi SSR. **Vopr Istor Estestvozn Tekh** 1981;1:85–94

**Tareev EM:** Kollagenozy: évoliutsiia ucheniia i sovremennye kontseptsii. **Vopr Revm** 1982 Jul–Sep;(3):15–22

**Tareev EM:** P. E. Lukomskiĭ i stanovlenie sovetskoĭ kardiologii. **Kardiologiia** 1982 Feb;22(2):119–25

**Tareev EM:** Sergeĭ Petrovich Botkin i sovremennaia klinika. **Klin Med (Mosk)** 1982 Sep;60(9):4–11

**Tariq M** see **Khan AB**

**Tarmanowska B** see **Jaroszewski Z**

**Tarpey K** see **Dye D**

**Tarpey K** see **Smith GF**

**Tarr JA, Lamperes BC:** Changing fuel use behavior ... the Pittsburgh smoke control movement, 1940–1950. **J Soc Hist** 1981;14:561–88

**Tarr JA, Yosie T, McCurley J:** Disputes over water quality policy: professional cultures in conflict, 1900–1917. **Am J Public Health** 1980 Apr;70(4):427–35

**Tarr JA:** The separate vs. combined sewer problem: a case study in urban technology design choice. **J Urban Hist** 1979;5(3):308–39

**Tarr JA** see **Melosi MV, ed**

**Tarr JA, et al:** Water and wastes: a retrospective assessment of wastewater technology in the United States, 1800–1932. **Technol Cult** 1984 Apr;25(2):226–63

**Tarragó Valentines JF:** Un informe sobre el hospital de Santa Maria de Lerida, escrito en el siglo XIX por Marioano Olives. **Asclepio** 1980;32:453–6

**Tarsy D:** History and definition of tardive dyskinesia. **Clin Neuropharmacol** 1983 Jun;6(2):91–9

**Tartalja H:** [Doctors and biologists in Dubrovník.] (SCC) **Dubrovnik** 1975;18(3–4):5–51

**Tartalja H:** Geschichte der Pharmaziehistorik in Jugoslawien bis zum Jahre 1952. In: Vorträge des Internationalen Pharmaziehistorischen Kongresses Innsbruck 1977. Stuttgart, Wissenschaftliche Verlagsgesellschaft, 1979. p. 97–106.

**Tartalja H:** Mouvement social des pharmaciens en Croatie. **Orvostort Kozl** 1982;28(1–3):187–90

**Tartalja H:** Pharmacy in old Dubronik. In Veteris ragusae medicina et pharmacia. Zagreb, PLIVA, n.d. p. 49–77.

**Tartalja H:** Pomorska zdravstvena zaštita u narodnooslobodilackoj borbi. In Radovi sa Medunarodnog simpozija u povodu sestote obljetnice Dubrovacke karantene. Dubrovnik, 29 i 30. rujna 1977. Zagreb, 1980. p. 153–71.

**Taseski J** see **Radovic M**

**Tashima N:** Asian Americans in psychiatric systems. **Explor Ethnic Stud** 1979;2(1):11–21

**Tashjian LD:** Aspects of internalization and individuation: James Joyce's Portrait of the artist as a young man. **Adolesc Psychiatry** 1982;10:75–84

**Tashmukhamedov IR, Dzhuraev IN:** 60 let aptechnoĭ sistemy v Uzbekistane. **Farmatsiia** 1980 Mar–Apr;29(2):49–51

**Tasman W:** The history of Wills Eye Hospital. Hagerstown, Md., Harper & Row, 1980. ix, 135 p.

**Tatara K:** [Interim report on the future provision on medical and allied services, 1920 (I)] (Jpn). **Igakushi Kenkyu** 1978;51:42–51

**Tatarek K** see **Stefański K**

**Tatarinova SD** see **Ved'mina EA**

**Tate LG** see **Wright RK**

**Tateno Y** see **Yamaguchi C**

**Tateo F:** L'esperienza scientifica di A. de Ferrariis Galateo: Osservazioni sul De podagra. In S. Bertelli, G. Ramakus, ed: Essays presented to Myron P. Gilmore. Vol. 1. Florence, La Nuova Italia, 1978.

**Tatge RO:** A quarantine quandary; ship fever and yellow fever in Providence, Rhode Island, 1797. **Am Neptune** 1980;40(3):192–210

**Tatlock H:** Clarification of the cause of Fort Bragg fever (pretibial fever) - January 1982. **Rev Infect Dis** 1982 Jan–Feb;4(1):157–8

**Tatoń J:** Filozoficzna koncepcja człowieka a medycyna. **Pol Tyg Lek** 1983 Aug 15;38(33–34):1015–8

**Tattersall I, Schwartz JH:** A new genus and species of adapid primate from the middle Eocene of Alsace, and a new genus for 'Adapis' ruetimeyeri Stehlin, 1912. **Folia Primatol (Basel)** 1983;41(3–4):231–9

**Tattersall I** see **Eldredge N**

**Tattersall W** see **Hammarsten JF**

**Tatulian SA** see **Vorob'ev VI**
**Tatum HJ, Connell-Tatum EB:** Barrier contraception: a comprehensive overview. **Fertil Steril** 1981 Jul;36(1):1-12
**Tau S** see **Smith P**
**Tauber H:** 13C evidence for dietary habits of prehistoric man in Denmark. **Nature** 1981 Jul 23;292(5821):332-3
**Tauber H** see **Schoeninger MJ**
**Täuber MG, Sande MA:** Landmark perspective: the impact of penicillin on the treatment of meningitis. **JAMA** 1984 Apr 13;251(14):1877-80
**Taubert E:** Das chirurgische Erbe. Das Wirken Georg Axhausens an der Chirurgischen Klinik der Charité--Berlin. **Zentralbl Chir** 1983;108(14):913-7
**Taure Gómez C** see **Lentini J**
**Taureck R:** Die Bedeutung der Photographie für die medizinische Abbildung im 19. Jahrh, Köln, 1980, 258 p. (Kölner medizinhistorische Beiträge, 15).
**Taussig HB:** Little choice and a stimulating environment. **J Am Med Wom Assoc** 1981 Feb;36(2):43-4
**Tautz P, Hein G:** Frühformen orthopädischen Denkens und orthopädischer Methoden in den ersten 120 Jahren der Universität Halle (Saale) (III). Heinrich Bass (1690-1754), genannt, 'Bandagen-Bass'. **Beitr Orthop Traumatol** 1979;26(12):705-12
**Tavassoli M:** Selected items from the history of pathology - Giulio Bizzozero (1846-1901). **Am J Pathol** 1980;101(1):50
**Tavassoli M:** Selected items from the history of pathology - Robert Koch (1843-1910). **Am J Pathol** 1980;101(1):78
**Tavassoli M:** The cell theory: a foundation to the edifice of biology. **Am J Pathol** 1980 Jan;98(1):44
**Tayab M:** Clinical observations of Rāzi. **Stud Hist Med** 1982 Jun;6(2):79-121
**Taylor:** The natural history of preventive medicine, or breaking the chains of causation. **Br Med J** 1980 Sep 27;281(6244):849-53
**Taylor AE:** Dr. Mayerson, the scientist. **Physiologist** 1980 Feb;23(1):38-40
**Taylor AH:** American confrontation with opium traffic in the Philippines. **Pac Hist Rev** 1967;36(3):307-24
**Taylor B:** Free state physicians who served the confederacy: Medical doctors of Maryland in the CSA, by Daniel D. Hartzler. **Md State Med J** 1980 Apr;29(4):35-8
**Taylor B:** Health in history. Britain's Admiral Lord Horatio Nelson. **Md State Med J** 1979 Dec;28(12):35-50
**Taylor B** see **Wilson HB**
**Taylor CM:** W. E. B. Dubois's challenge to scientific racism. **J Black Stud** 1981;11(4):449-60
**Taylor DB:** Music in general hospital treatment from 1900 to 1950. **J Music Ther** 1981 Summer;18(2):62-73
**Taylor DC, March SM:** Hughlings Jackson's Dr Z: the paradigm of temporal lobe epilepsy revealed. **J Neurol Neurosurg Psychiatry** 1980 Sep;43(9):758-67
**Taylor DM:** Blutzellmarkierung: Rückblick und Ausblick. **Wien Klin Wochenschr** 1984 Feb 3;96(3):89-92
**Taylor DW:** Medical libraries and medical history. **NZ Libr** 1976 Apr;39(2):62-7
**Taylor DW:** Orthopaedics--a brief historical overview. **Australas Nurses J** 1981 Aug;10(8):24-5
**Taylor E:** Louville Eugene Emerson: psychotherapy, Harvard, and the early Boston scene. **Harv Med Alumni Bull** 1982 Spring;56(2):42-8
**Taylor E:** The electrified hand--psychotherapeutic implications. **Med Instrum** 1983 Jul-Aug;17(4):281-2
**Taylor E:** William James on psychopathology: the 1896 Lowell lectures on 'Exceptional mental states'. **Harv Libr Bull** 1982 Oct;30(4):455-79
**Taylor ES:** Commemorative issue: Georgeanna Seegar Jones, Howard W. Jones, Jr. Twenty-five years as editors-in-chief for Gynecology, Obstetrical & Gynecological Survey. **Obstet Gynecol Surv** 1982 Jun;37(6):355-84
**Taylor FK:** Disease concepts and the logic of classes. **Br J Med Psychol** 1981 Sep;54(pt 3):277-86
**Taylor FK:** On pseudo-hallucinations. **Psychol Med** 1981 May;11(2):265-71
**Taylor FK:** Sir Aubrey Lewis: Inquiries in Psychiatry; The State of Psychiatry; The Later Papers of Sir Aubrey Lewis. **Br J Psychiatry** 1983 Jul;143:89-93
**Taylor FK:** Sydenham's disease entities. **Psychol Med** 1982 May;12(2):243-50
**Taylor IG:** History and current practice in rehabilitation of deaf children. **Int Rehabil Med** 1983;5(2):82-5
**Taylor JH:** Disease, fire and water in the nineteenth century city: a bibliography. **Urban Hist Rev** 1979;8(1):113-5
**Taylor JH:** Fire, disease and water in Ottawa: an introduction. **Urban Hist Rev** 1979;8(1):7-37
**Taylor JL:** A backward glance; a forward view. **Med Leg J** 1981;49(pt 4):128-38
**Taylor JS:** The Cleveland Clinic Quarterly: the first fifty years. **Cleve Clin Q** 1982 Winter;49(4):149-58
**Taylor LS:** Organization for radiation protection: the operations of the ICRP and NCRP, 1928-1974. [Washington], U. S. Dept. of Energy. 1979. 2082 p. in various pagings.
**Taylor LS:** Technical accuracy in historical writing. **Health Phys** 1981 May;40(5):595-9
**Taylor LS:** The development of radiation protection standards (1925-1940). **Health Phys** 1981 Aug;41(2):227-32
**Taylor LS:** Who is the father of health physics? **Health Phys** 1982 Jan;42(1):92-2
**Taylor MC** see **Smith JH, ed**
**Taylor MR:** History of cosmetic color additive regulation: creative maneuvering by FDA bodes well for the future. **Food Drug Cosmet Law J** 1982 Apr;37(2):152-62
**Taylor PJ, Burridge J:** Trends in death, disablement, and sickness absence in the British Post Office since 1981. **Br J Ind Med** 1982 Feb;39(1):1-10
**Taylor R:** Doctors, paupers, and landowners. The evolution of primary medical care in Orkney. **North Scotl** 1981;4(1-2):113-20
**Taylor RC:** The politics of prevention. **Soc Policy** 1982;13(1):32-41
**Taylor RC:** Thomas Lewis and clinical research. **Br Med J** 1981;282:1976
**Taylor RG:** G. R. Girdlestone, M.D., F.R.C.S. **Clin Orthop** 1983 Mar;(173):125-9
**Taylor RW** see **Fergusson IL**
**Taylor S:** Surgical Research Society, 1954--79. **Lancet** 1979 Dec 8;2(8154):1234
**Taylor S:** Thomas Richardson Colledge FRCS, 1796-1879. **Ann R Coll Surg Engl** 1982 Jul;64(4):266-7
**Taylor SJ, Bogdan R:** Defending illusions: the institution's struggle for survival. **Hum Organ** 1980;39(3):209-18
**Taylor W, Wasserman D, Behrens V, et al:** Effect of the air hammer on the hands of stonecutters. The limestone quarries of Bedford, Indiana, revisited. **Br J Ind Med** 1984 Aug;41(3):289-95
**Teaford MF, Walker A:** Quantitative differences in dental microwear between primate species with different diets and a comment on the presumed diet of Sivapithecus. **Am J Phys Anthropol** 1984 Jun;64(2):191-200
**Teahan JF:** Warren Felt Evans and mental healing: romantic idealism and practical mysticism in nineteenth-century America. **Church Hist** 1979 Mar;48(1):63-80
**Tedebrand LG** see **Sundin J**
**Tedeschi CG, Merriam JC, et al:** Framingham medical reflections. Framingham, Mass., Tedeschi Library, Framingham Union Hospital, 1975. 120 p.
**Tedeschi G:** Jung-Freud: un dilemma inattuale. Roma, Astrolabio, 1979. 88 p.
**Tedeschi J** see **DelChicca S**
**Tedeschi LG:** George Burgess Magrath. Tribute to a resting lion. **Am J Forensic Med Pathol** 1980 Jun;1(2):169-72
**Tedeschi LG:** Shields Warren: the legend and the man. **Am J Forensic Med Pathol** 1980 Dec;1(4):297-301
**Tedeschi LG:** The Massachusetts Medico-Legal Society. The early years. **Am J Forensic Med Pathol** 1981 Sep;2(3):257-60
**Tedrow LM, Mahoney ER:** Trends in attitudes toward abortion: 1972-76. **Public Opin Q** 1979;43(2):181-9
**Teece WK:** John Ash. In Dictionary of Canadian biography, 1881-1890. 1982;11:32-3.
**Teeters NK** see **Breul FR**
**Teething troubles, 1921--1971. Part twelve: Dent Tech** 1980 Jan;33(1):11-2 (continued periodically)
**Teich M:** A history of biochemistry. **Hist Sci** 1980;18(1):46-67
**Teich M:** Ferment or enzyme: what's in a name? **Hist Philos Life Sci** 1981;3(2):193-215
**Teichman SL, Aldea PA:** Pioneers in pituitary physiology: Harvey Cushing and Nicolas Paulescu. **J Hist Med Allied Sci** 1985 Jan;40(1):68-72
**Teichman SL, Aldea PA:** The other side of the insulin story: Paulescu's contribution. **NY State J Med** 1984 Jun;84(6):312-6
**Teichmann E:** Glimpses into the North Dakota story. **Prairie Rose** 1980 Apr-Jun;59(2):10
**Teigen KH:** A note on the origin of the term 'nature and nurture': not Shakespeare and Galton, but Mulcaster. **J Hist Behav Sci** 1984 Oct;20(4):363-4
**Teigen PM:** Medical libraries and history of medicine libraries. **Newsl Libr Hist Health Sci** 1982 Jul;6(1):1-6
**Teigen PM:** This sea of simples; the materia medica in three early English receipt books. **Pharm Hist** 1980;22(3):104-8
**Teigen PM:** William Osler and comparative medicine. **Can Vet J** 1984;25:400-5
**Teigen PM, ed:** Books, manuscripts, and the history of medicine. Essays on the fiftieth anniversary of the Osler Library. New York, Science History Publications, 1982. 112 p. Contributions by L. G. Stevenson, C. G. Roland, R. J. Durling, E. Brodman, G. T. Tanselle, E. J. Freeman.
**Teimourian B, Adham MN:** Louis Ombredanne and the origin of muscle flap use for immediate breast mound reconstruction. **Plast Reconstr Surg** 1983 Dec;72(6):905-10
**Teir H:** Das Sanitätswesen der finnischen Truppen in Bulgarien sowie die Tätigkeit des finnischen Roten Kreuzes im Kriege von 1877-78 und die positiven Auswirkungen dieser Ereignisse auf die Entwicklung der finnischen Medizin und Krankenpflege. In International Congress of the History of Medicine. 26th, Plovdiv, 1978. Actes du Congress. Sofia, 1981. Volume II. p. 208.
**Teir H:** Medicinens historia som akademiskt undervisningsämne--erfarenheter från Finland. **Nord Medicinhist Arsb** 1980;Suppl 6:30-4
**Teitelbaum MS:** The population problem in demographic perspective. In Reich WT, et al, ed: Encyclopedia of bioethics, v.3. New York, Free Press, 1978. p. 1218-25.
**Tejada C** see **Bowers JZ**
**Telenchi VI** see **Sukharev AG**
**Tel'iatev IV** see **Georgievskiĭ AS**
**Telichenas AI, Gritsiute LA, Skarulis RI, et al:** Istoriia razvitiia onkologicheskoĭ sluzhby v Litovskoĭ SSR. **Vopr Onkol** 1982;28(11):8-11

**Tella A:** The practice of traditional medicine in Africa. **Niger Med J** 1979 May–Jun;9(5–6):607–12

**Telle J:** Die Schreibart des Paracelsus im Urteil deutscher Fachschriftsteller des 16. und 17. Jarhunderts. **Medizinhist J** 1981;16(1–2):78–100

**Telle J:** Manuscripta alchemica der Sammlung Mellon. Bemerkungen zum Katalog. **Suddtsch Opt Ztg** 1981;65(1):79–96

**Telle J:** Paracelsistische Sinnbildkunst. Bemerkungen zu einer Pseudo-'Tabula smaragdina' des 16. Jahrhunderts. In Seidler E, Schott H, ed: Bausteine zur Medizingeschichte. Stuttgart, Steiner, 1984. p. 129–39.

**Telle J:** Pharmazie und der gemeine Mann: Hausarznei und Apotheke in deutschen Schriften der frühen Neuzeit: Ausstellung der Herzog August Bibliothek Wolfenbüttel in der Halle des Zeughauses vom 23. August 1982 bis März 1983. Wolfenbüttel, Herzog August Bibliothek, 1982. 144 p.

**Tellenbach H:** Martin Bubers Einfluss auf die anthropologische Wende in der Medizin. **Nervenarzt** 1980 May;51(5):302–6

**Tellenbach H:** Zwang–Wahn–Schwermut–Melancholie: Dekompositionen normativer Seinsweisen. In Seidler E, Schott H, ed: Bausteine zur Medizingeschichte. Stuttgart, Steiner, 1984. p. 139–46.

**Tellenbach H** see **Janzarik W ed**

**Tellenbach H, ed:** Psychiatrische Therapie heute. Antike Diaita und moderne Therapeutik. Ein Symposium in Salzburg 1979. Stuttgart, Ferdinand Enke, 1982. 135 p. Contributions by P. L. Entralgo, D. Gracia-Guillen, H. Schipperges, W. Schmitt, K. P. Kisker, D. Wyss, W. Blankenburg.

**Telson H:** An explanation of the charm against measles. **J Hist Med Allied Sci** 1978 Jul;33(3):408

**Telson HW:** Une leçon du Docteur Charcot à la Salpêtrière. Lithograph by Eugene Pirodon after a painting (1887) by André Brouillet. **J Hist Med Allied Sci** 1980 Jan;35(1):58

**Temby KL:** Tracheobronchial hygieng circa 1900. **Respir Care** 1977 Aug;22(8):876

**Temin P:** Regulation and the choice of prescription drugs. **Am Econ Rev** 1980;70(2):301–5

**Temin P:** Taking your medicine. Drug regulation in the United States. Cambridge, Massachusetts, and London, Harvard Univ. Press, 1980. 274 p.

**Temin P:** The origin of compulsory drug prescriptions. **J Law Econ** 1979;22(1):91–106

**Temkin O, Frankena WK, Kadish SH:** Respect for life in medicine, philosophy, and the law. (Thalheimer lectures, 1975). Baltimore: Johns Hopkins Univ. Press, 1977. ix, 107 p.

**Temkin O:** Some moral implications of the concept of disease. In Ganzinger K, Skopec M, Wyklicky H, ed: Festschrift für Erna Lesky zum 70. Geburtstag. Wien, Brüder Hollinek, 1981. p. 153–60.

**Temkin O** see **Hilts VL**

**Temkin-Greener H, Swedlund AC:** A test of the child replacement hypothesis: nineteenth century Massachusetts. **Soc Biol** 1983 Summer;30(2):218–27

**Templado J:** Darwin: ayer y hoy. **Arbor** 1982;113(441–2):7–20

**Templar M:** Historical perspectives. **Nurs Mirror** 1984 Oct 24;159(15):vii–viii

**Templeton WL:** Artificial radionuclides in the oceans. In Sears M, Merriman D, ed: Oceanography, the past. New York, Springer, 1980. p. 420–37.

**Templin DW:** Some historical aspects of the treatment of hypothermia. **Alaska Med** 1984 Jan–Mar;26(1):13

**Ten Have HA:** Geneeskunde en filosofie, aspecten van een wisselvallige relatie. **Ned Tijdschr Geneeskd** 1982 Apr 10,126(15):668–73

**Ten year progress report of the Center for Population Research:** [Bethesda], The Center, 1978. 73 p.

**Tenenbaum L** see **Fraga M**

**Teng RS** see **Yang WY**

**Tengwall R:** A note on the influence of F. M. Alexander on the development of Gestalt therapy. **J Hist Behav Sci** 1981 Jan;17(1):126–30

**Tennant M:** Mrs. Grace Neill in the Department of Asylums, Hospitals and Charitable Institutions. **NZ J Hist** 1978 Apr 12;:3–16

**Tennstedt F** see **Labisch A**

**Teo SK, Chew CH:** Tuberculosis chemotherapy—developments in Singapore from 1957–1982. **Ann Acad Med Singapore** 1982 Jul;11(3):366–9

**Teodorovici G** see **Creteanu G**

**Teodorovici G** see **Marinescu CG**

**Teodorovici GF** see **Bădărău GH**

**Teplitsky PE, Grieman R:** History of formocresol pulpotomy. **Can Dent Assoc J** 1984 Aug;50(8):629–34

**Teppa S** see **Falkiewiczowa S**

**Tepun PD:** Deiatel'nost' partiĭnykh organizatsiĭ i naseleniia Severnogo Kavkaza po okazaniiu pomoshchi ranenym v gody Velikoĭ Otechestvennoĭ voĭny. **Sov Zdravookhr** 1980;(5):61–3

**Ter herinnering aan professor dr. jan hellemans:** **Tijdschr Gerontol Geriatr** 1982 Oct;13(5):171–8

**Teramo K:** Savusaunasta monitoroituun synnytyssaliin. **Duodecim** 1981;97(20):1682–9

**Teramoto M:** [Me and the Florence Nightingale letter collection] (Jpn). **Sogo Kango** 1982;17(4):35–8

**Terekhov NT:** Razvitie idei akademika A. A. Bogomol'tsa v sovremennoĭ transfuziologii. **Fiziol Zh** 1981 May–Jun;27(3):384–7

**Terencio de las Aguas J:** La lepra en el libro 'Doctrina de morbis cutaneis' de José Jacoba Plenck. **Fontilles** 1980;12:409–14

**Terencio de las Aguas J:** La lepra en el Reino de Valencia. **Fontilles** 1979;12(1):5–10

**Terencio de las Aguas J:** La lepra en el reino de Valencia. **Fontilles** 1977;11:237–40

**Terencio de las Aguas J:** La lepra en el Reino de Valencia (sigo XX). **Fontilles** 1978;11:465–6

**Terent'ev GV** see **Kul'chitskiĭ KI**

**Terent'eva LA** see **Makovskiĭ ChN**

**Tergolina U:** Le medaglie fatte coniare dal Nobile Collegio Chimico Farmaceutico di Roma. Nobile Collegio Chimico-Farmaceutico Roma, (Atti e Memorie) 1975 Jan–Mar; 5(1):13–6.

**Terlecki O:** Służba zdrowia Drugiego Korpusu Polskiego w bitwie o Monte Cassino. **Przegl Lek** 1980;37(1):92–100

**Ternberg JL:** Surgical treatment of idiopathic hyperinsulinemic hypoglycemia in children. First successful subtotal pancreatectomy with preservation of spleen reported by Evarts A. Graham (1934). **J Thorac Cardiovasc Surg** 1984 Nov;88(5 Pt 2):898–901

**Ternovoĭ KS:** Dostizheniia sovetskoĭ khirurgii (k 60–letiiu obrazovaniia SSSR). **Klin Khir** 1982 Dec;(12):1–7

**Ternovoĭ KS:** V. I. Lenin i okhrana zdorov'ia naroda. **Klin Khir** 1980 Apr;(4):1–7

**Ternovoĭ KS, Shalimov AA:** Vydaiushchiĭsia sovetskiĭ khirurg I. I. Dzhanelidze (k 100–letiiu so dnia rozhdeniia). **Klin Khir** 1983 Jul;(8):76–9

**Terrada ML** see **Lopez Piñero JM**

**Terrada ML, ed** see **López Piñero JM**

**Terreros DA, Grantham JJ:** Marshall Barber and the origins of micropipette methods. **Am J Physiol** 1982 Mar;242(3):F293–6

**Terrier G:** Louis Secrétan et les débuts de l'enseignement de l'ORL en Suisse Romande. **Acta Otorhinolaryngol Belg** 1982;36(2):306–10

**Terris M:** The complex tasks of the second epidemiologic revolution. **J Public Health Policy** 1983 Mar;4(1):8–24

**Terris M:** The epidemiologic tradition. **Public Health Rep** 1979 Jun;94(3):203–9

**Terris M:** The primacy of prevention. **Prev Med** 1981 Nov;10(6):689–99

**Terry JS, Herskovitz A, Fox DM:** Photographs tell more than meets the eye. **J Biol Photogr** 1980 Jul;48(3):111–5

**Terry LL:** The Surgeon General's first report on smoking and health. A challenge to the medical profession. **NY State J Med** 1983 Dec;83(13):1254–5

**Tertsionas PV** see **Chepulis SP**

**Terwiel BJ:** Tattooing in Thailand's history. **J R Asiat Soc GB Irel** 1979;156–66

**Terzioglu A:** Die Hofspitäler und andere Gesundheitseinrichtungen der osmanischen Palastbauten unter Berücksichtigung der Ursprungsfrage sowie ihre Beziehungen zu den Abendländischen Hofspitälern. München, Rudolf Trofenik, 1979. 303 p. (Beiträge zur Kenntnis Südosteuropas und des Nahen Orients, XXX).

**Terzioglu A, Krebs LM:** The development of surgery and of surgical clinics at the turn of the 20th century. Munich, (the authors), 1979. 69 p.

**Terzioglu A:** Zur Avicenna (Ibn Sina) – Forschung in der Türkei. In International Congress of the History of Medicine, 27th, Barcelona, 1980. Actas. Barcelona, Acadèmia de Ciències Mèdiques de Catalunya i Balears, 1981. p. 750–5.

**Terzioglu A** see **Habrich C**

**Tesař J:** Sto let českeho ústavu pro soudní lékařství v Praze. **Soud Lek** 1984 Aug;29(3):33–9

**Tesař J:** Sto let od vydání první učebnice soudního lékařství Josafem Reinsbergrem. **Cesk Patol** 1983 Aug;19(3):45–6

**Teschler-Nicola M** see **Stiebitz R**

**Tesh S:** Political ideology and public health in the nineteenth century. **Int J Health Serv** 1982;12(2):321–42

**Teske RH** see **Willett LB**

**Tesler DB:** Dostizheniia sanitarnoĭ sluzhby Turkmenistana. **Gig Sanit** 1982 Nov;(11):45–7

**Tesler DB:** Razvitie i dal'neĭshee sovershenstvovanie sanitarno–épidemiologicheskoĭ sluzhby Turkmenskoĭ SSR. **Gig Sanit** 1982 Dec;(12):40–3

**Tessar J:** Rozvoj soudniho lékařatví na Karlově Univerzitě. **Soud Lek** 1979;24(4):49–50

**Tessier JF:** L'hôpital de Ste-Marguerite de Cadillac et la littérature consacrée à Saint Jean de Dieu et ses disciples en France au XVIIe siècle. **Rev Fr Hist Livre** 1979;23:317–28

**Testoni G:** Una lettera di Cestoni a Vallisneri (1710). **Riv Biol** 1983 Spring;76(1):125–31

**Teteruck L** see **Teteruck WR**

**Teteruck WR, Boyd MA, Teteruck L:** The history of the dental aptitude test program in Canada. **Can Dent Assoc J** 1979 Aug;45(8):400–2

**Tétreault M:** Les maladies de la misère: aspects de la santé publique à Montréal, 1880–1914. **Rev Hist Am Fr** 1983;36(4):507–26

**Tetzner W:** Die Prognose und Behandlung der Tuberkulose in der vorchemotherapeutischen Ara. **Z Erkr Atmungsorgane** 1982;158(1–2):149–54

**Tetzner W:** Erfolgreiche Tuberkulosebekämpfung in der DDR. **Wiss Z Martin Luther Univ (Math)** 1976;25(2):99–103

**Teubel S:** Schulhygiene in der Zeit von 1870 bis 1900. Diss. Bonn, 1981. 149 p.

**Teulón AA:** La constitucion de la histologia celular: Schwann, Henle y Kölliker. **Asclepio** 1978–79;30–31:7–18

**Teuteberg HJ:** Der Verzehr von Nahrungsmitteln in Deutschland pro Kopf und Jahr seit Beginn der Industrialisierung (1850–1975). Versuch einer quantitativen Lang-Zeitanalyse. **Arch Sozialgesch** 1979;19:331–88

**Texter JH:** The President's dilemma, 1919 (Woodrow Wilson). **Va Med** 1980 Nov;107(11):756–62

**Teysseire D:** Pédiatrie des lumières: maladies et soins des enfants dans l'Encyclopédie et le Dictionnaire de Trévoux. Paris, Vrin, 1982. 255 p.
**Teysseire D** see **Bernier JJ**
**Thacker SB, Banta HD:** Benefits and risks of episiotomy: an interpretative review of the English language literature, 1860–1980. **Obstet Gynecol Surv** 1983 Jun;38(6):322–38
**Thackray A:** The pre-history of an academic discipline: the study of the history of science in the United States, 1891–1941. **Minerva** 1980 Autumn;18(3):448–73
**Thackray A** see **Durbin PT, ed**
**Thackray JC:** James Parkinson's Organic remains of a former world (1804–1811). **J Soc Bibliogr Nat Hist** 1976;7(4):45–66
**Thakral KK:** Techniques for extraction of foreign bodies from war wounds in medieval India. **Indian J Hist Sci** 1981, reçu 1982;16(1):11–6
**Thakur ML, Sinzinger H, Höfer R:** Radioisotopenmarkierung menschlicher Blutzellen--ein historischer Uberblick. **Wien Klin Wochenschr** 1984 Feb 3;96(3):87–8
**Thakur RS, Singh SB:** Artemisia: the sagebrush plant - a review. **Curr Res Med Aromat Plant** 1979;1:90–108
**Thaler L:** La génétique des populations dans la théorie moderne de l'évolution. In Actes du Colloque R.A. Fisher.... Paris, 5-6 déc. 1979. p. 351-79. **Rev Synth (Paris)** 1981;102(103–104)
**Thalidomide: 20 years on: Lancet** 1981 Sep 5;2(8245):510–1
**Thane P:** The perception and experience of old age 1945–1965. **Soc Soc Hist Med Bull (Lond)** 1984 Jun;34:52–4
**Thatte DG, Tiwari SP, Tiwari GP:** Techniques of venupuncture (śiravedha) in India in 18th century. **Indian J Hist Sci** 1981;16(2):181–8
**[The caricature of the teacher]: Indiana Med Hist Q** 1977;3(2):23–37
**'The Coast' Hospital: remember when?: Lamp** 1981 May;38(5 Suppl):17–9
**[The history of physiology:] essay review: Ann Sci** 1981;38(3):343–52
**[The need to preserve medical history records]: Evidence presented to the Public Records Committee.: Soc Soc Hist Med Bull (Lond)** 1979 Dec;25:68–76
**[The 1st quadrennial convention in commemoration of the diamond jubilee of the KNA] (Kor): Taehan Kanho** 1983 Sep 20;22(3):15–29
**Thébaud F:** Etre sage-femme entre les deux guerres: une profession en crise. **Penelope** 1981;(5):76–9
**Theil P:** Brève histoire de l'Ordre des Médecins. **Bull Acad Natl Med (Paris)** 1981 Jun;165(6):739–45
**Theil P:** Les premières radiographies faites en France, retrouvées à l'Académie Nationale de Médecine. **Bull Acad Natl Med (Paris)** 1980 Nov;164(8):752–6
**Theil P** see **Histoire culturelle de la maladie**
**Theilmann JM:** The miracles of King Henri VI of England. **Historian** 1980;42(3):456–71
**Theis HE** see **Winfree LT**
**Theisen WR:** 'Liber de visu': the Greco-Latin translation of Euclid's 'Optics'. **Mediaev Stud** 1979;41:44–105
**Theodor H** see **Dittmann S**
**Théodoridès J, Rousset JJ:** A propos de la découverte de Trichomonas tenax, Protozaire parasite de l'homme, par O. F. Müller. **Rev Hist Sci (Paris)** 1980 Apr;33(2):163–4
**Théodoridès J:** Antoine Portal et la rage (avec des documents inédits). In Ganzinger K, Skopec M, Wyklicky H, ed: Festschrift für Erna Lesky zum 70. Geburtstag. Wien, Brüder Hollinek, 1981. p. 161–5.
**Theodorides J:** Célébration du centenaire de la découverte par A. Laveran de l'Hématozoaire du paludisme. Strasbourg, 2–3 mai 1980. **Rev Hist Sci (Paris)** 1980;33(4):351–2
**Théodoridès J:** Claude Bernard et la microbiologie médicale. In: Congrès international d'histoire de la médecine, XXVe, Québec, 1976. Actes. Québec, 1977. p. 1354–60.
**Théodoridès J:** Claude Bernard et les parasites. (Contribution au centenaire de la mort de Claude Bernard). **Hist Nat** 1979;(14):31–8
**Théodoridès J:** Considerations on the medical uses of marine invertebrates. In Sears M. Merriman D, ed: Oceanography, the past. New York, Springer, 1980. p. 734–49.
**Théodoridès J:** Ernst Jünger ou 'l'oeil vivant'. **Gesnerus** 1983;40(1–2):193–202
**Théodoridès J:** Geschichte der Parasitologie. In Sournia JC, Martiny M, Poulet J, ed: Illustrierte Geschichte der Medizin. Salzburg, Andreas, 1980. Vol. 8. p. 2933–59.
**Théodoridès J:** Hippolyte Bernheim et la pathologie infectieuse. In: Congrès National des Sociétés Savantes, 103e, Nancy, 1978. Comptes Rendus. Paris, 1978. Section des Sciences, Fasc. V. p. 87–94.
**Théodoridès J:** Ibn Sina et la rage. In International Congress of the History of Medicine, 27th, Barcelona, 1980. Actas. Barcelona, Académia de Ciències Mèdiques de Catalunya i Balears, 1981. p. 756–60.
**Théodoridès J:** La contribution d'A. Laveran à l'étude des Sporozoaires (Hémosporidies exceptées) et des Myxosporidies. **Hist Nat** 1980–81;17–18:77–84
**Théodoridès J:** La médecine et les sciences dans les 'Notes journalières du général Foy'. **Hist Sci Med** 1980;14:305–15
**Théodoridès J:** L'abbé de Bap, curé de Sommières, et son prétendu remède antirabique. **Rev Hist Pharm (Paris)** 1979 Dec;26(243):269–79
**Théodoridès J:** Le docteur Basile Scrini (1869–1931) et la thérapeutique oculaire. **Rev Hist Pharm (Paris)** 1982 Jun;29(253):101–6
**Théodoridès J:** Les études sur la rage de deux médecins Lorrains: Pierre-Christophe Gorcy (1807–1821) et J. Camille Gorcy (1812). In: Congrès National des Sociétés Savantes, 103e, Nancy, 1978. Comptes Rendus. Paris, 1978. Section des Sciences, Fasc. v. p. 55–69.
**Théodoridès J, Ming Wong:** Les médecins nantais et l'histoire de la rage. In: Congrès National de Sociétés Savantes, 97e Nantes, 1972. Comptes Rendus. Paris, 1976. Section des Sciences, Tome 1. p. 91–7.
**Théodoridès J:** Les recherches histologiques sur la rage au 19e siècle. **Clio Med** 1981 Dec;16(2/3):83–92
**Théodoridès J:** Magendie et la pathologie infectieuse. **Hist Sci Med** 1983;17(4):367–80
**Théodoridès J:** Marcel Florkin (1900–1979). **Rev Hist Sci (Paris)** 1980 Jan;33(1):75–6
**Théodoridès J:** Marcel Florkin (1900–1979). **Hist Sci Med** 1980;14(2):145–50
**Théodoridès J:** 'Paris enragé'. **Rev Hist Pharm (Paris)** 1982;29(252):193–8
**Théodoridès J:** Pierre Chabbert (1924–1981). **Hist Sci Med** 1981;15(4):287–92
**Théodoridès J:** Quelle était la maladie décrite par l'historien Agathias (VIe siècle A.D.)? **Hist Sci Med** 1981;15(2):153–8
**Théodoridès J:** Rabies in Arabian medicine. **Stud Hist Med** 1980 Mar;4(1):13–22
**Théodoridès J:** Saints in medical history (a complement). **Clio Med** 1980 Jul;14(3–4):269–70
**Théodoridès J:** Sebastiano Rivolta (1832–1893) parasitologiste et microbiologiste. **Hist Sci Med** 1980;14(2):227–32
**Théodoridès J:** Un centenaire oublié: Casimir-Joseph Davaine (1812–1882). **Hist Sci Med** 1982;16(4):263–6
**Théodoridès J:** Un correspondant breton de la Société Royale de Médecine: Claude-Marie Robin de Keriavalle (1743–1785). In: Congrès National des Sociétés Savantes, 107e. Brest, 1982. Comptes Rendus, Paris, 1983. Section des Sciences, Fasc. IV. p. 225–39.
**Théodoridès J:** Un précurseur girondin de la pathologie infectieuse: Jean Hameau (1779–1851). In: Congrès National des Sociétés Savantes, 104e, Bordeaux, 1979. Comptes Rendus. Paris, 1979. Section des Sciences, Fasc. IV. p. 81–95.
**Théodoridès J:** Utilisation du sel et de l'eau de mer dans le traitement ancien de la rage. In: Congrès National des Sociétés Savantes, 99e, Besançon, 1974. Comptes Rendus. Paris, 1976. Section des Sciences, Fasc. V. p. 117–22.
**Théodoridès J** see **Florkin M**
**Théodoridès J** see **Huard P**
**Théodoridès J** see **Imbault-Huart MJ, ed**
**Théodoridès J** see **Mars FL**
**Théodoridès J** see **Soubiran A**
**Theophano J:** Feast, fast, and time. **Pa Folklife** 1978;27(3):25–32
**Theopold W:** Das Kind in der Votivmalerei. Munich, Karl Thiemig, 1981.
**Theopold W:** Paul Julius Möbius (1853–1907). **Medizinhist J** 1983;18(1–2):100–17
**Thermoz P** see **Alliez J**
**Theunissen B:** Theorie en praktijk van Cuviers Recherches sur les ossemens fossiles. **Tijdschr Geschied Geneeskd** 1983;6(1):1–17
**Theunissen M** see **Smith JH, ed**
**Thibault J:** Un accouchement laborieux. **Esprit** 1975;(5):696–703
**Thibaut-Payen J:** Les morts, l'Eglise et l'Etat: recherches d'histoire administrative sur la sépulture et les cimetières dans le ressort du parlement de Paris aux XVIIe et XVIIIe siècles. Paris, Lanore, 1977. (Also Thèse, Paris, 1974). 465 p.
**Thibodeau D:** Indexing medical history: a guide to the literature: an essay review. **Bull Hist Med** 1982 Summer;56(2):276–9
**Thibodeau D, ed:** A bibliography of the writings of Lloyd G. Stevenson. **Bull Hist Med** 1983 Summer;57(2):267–79
**Thie-Mummenthey G:** Vom Säuglingsheim zur Universitätskinderklinik. Die Entwicklung der Kinderklinik der Westfälischen Wilhelms-Universität Münster. Münster, Murken-Altrogge, 1980. 262 p. (Studien zur Geschichte des Krankenhauswesens, 10).
**Thiébaud M:** Traitement de l'ulcère gastro-duodénal. Point de vue du chirurgien. **Rev Med Suisse Romande** 1984 May;104(5):373–7
**Thiederman SB, ed** see **Hand WD**
**Thieffry S:** Avec Parrot, il y a un siècle, à l'Hospice des Enfants Assistés. **Ann Pediatr (Paris)** 1981 Jan;28(1):63–71
**Thieffry S:** La découverte de la syphilis congénitale par Jules Parrot à l'Hospice des Enfants Assistés il y a un siècle. **Bull Acad Natl Med (Paris)** 1980 Nov;164(8):725–9
**Thieffry S:** La vie quotidienne avec Robert Debré, pionnier de la pédiatrie: le médecin d'enfants, le chef de service, le chef d'école. **Bull Acad Natl Med (Paris)** 1982 Dec;166(9):1265–77
**Thiel C:** Folgen der Emigration deutscher und österreichischer Wissenschaftstheoretiker und Logiker zwischen 1933 und 1945. **Ber Wissenschaftsgesch** 1984;7(4):227–56
**Thiel L** see **Snajdr J**
**Thiele F:** Zur Notwendigkeit von Kuren--Definition, Indikation, Erfolgsaussichten, Wiederholung. **Off Gesundheitswes** 1982 Mar;44(3):169–75
**Thielemans MR:** Les sociétés scientifiques. **Rev Univ Brux** 1981;1–2:217–31
**Thiemer-Sachse U:** Hygiene und Heilkunde bei den Azteca zur Zeit der spanischen Eroberung. **Abh Ber Staatl Mus Voelkerkd Dres** 1978;36:151–213
**Thiene G, Pennelli N:** Terzo centenario della nascita di Giovanni Battista Morgagni (1682–1982): c'è ancora bisogno dell'autopsia? **G Ital Cardiol** 1983 Oct;13(10):262–4
**Thiery M:** Classic illustration. **Eur J Obstet Gynecol Reprod Biol** 1982 Dec;14(3):205–6
**Thiery M:** Het epos van de keizersnede. **Verh K Acad Geneeskd Belg** 1984;46(3):221–30
**Thiery M:** Historische beschouwingen over obstetrische wanverhouding.

**Verh K Acad Geneeskd Belg** 1983;45(6):509–32

**Thies AC** see **Titche LL**

**Thiess AM** see **Vetter L**

**Thigpen JT** see **Arseneau JC**

**Thill G** see **Marchal P**

**Thiriet F** see **Guillemain B**

**Thirty years of DNA--and after: Nature** 1983 Apr 14;302(5909):557–8

**Thirty years of drugs for hypertension: a festschrift for Sir John McMichael: Br J Clin Pharmacol** 1982 Jan;13(1):5–142

**Thiry U:** Le professeur Joseph Guislain (1797–1860), apôtre des aliénés. **Cah Biloque** 1980;30:35–40

**This B:** La requête des enfants à naître. Paris, Seuil, 1982. 256 p.

**This is the National League for Nursing:** New York, League, [1977?] 13 p

**Thiveaud D, Benejeam M:** La pharmacopée traditionnelle dans le département du lot. **Quercy Rech** 1982;(49–50):30–9

**Thivel A:** Cnide et Cos? Essai sur les doctrines médicales dans la collection hippocratique. Paris, Les Belles Lettres, 1981. 435 p. (Publications de la Faculté des Lettres et des Sciences Humaines de Nice, 21).

**Thivel A:** Le 'divin' dans la Collection hippocratique. In La collection hippocratique et son rôle dans l'histoire de la médecine. Colloque de Strasbourg (23–27 octobre 1972) organisé par le Centre de Recherches sur la Grèce Antique, avec le concours des Facultés de Philosophie et des Langues Classiques. Leiden, E. J. Brill, 1975. p. 57–76.

**Thivel A** see **Grmek MD, ed**

**Thoburn R, ed:** One hundred years of dentistry in Florida. Tampa, Florida Dental Education Foundation, 1983. xxxix, 412 p.

**Thoire V de:** L'Ordre Souverain de Malte au secours des lépreux. Vingt-cinq ans d'activité du CIOMAL 1958–1983. **Acta Leprol (Geneve)** 1983 Oct–Dec;(93):191–203

**Thom A:** Die spezifische Funktion sozialer und ideologischer Bedingungen in der Erkenntnisentwicklung der Medizin - methodologische Vorbestimmungen und Resultate bisheriger Forschungen. In International Congress of the History of Medicine, 26th, Plovdiv, 1978. Actes du Congress. Sofia, 1981. Volume II. p. 74–6.

**Thom A:** Ethische Prinzipien und moralische Normen ärztlichen Handelns--ihre Quellen, Begründungen und praktischen Funktionen. **Stomatol DDR** 1983 Feb;33(2):124–9

**Thom A:** Theorie und Empirie in der Entstehungsgeschichte der Bakteriologie - der Beitrag von Edwin Klebs zur Begründung der bakteriologischen Ara. **Wiss Beitr Martin Luther Univ Halle Wittenberg** 1983;5–R80:71–8

**Thom A:** Zur disziplinären Genese der Neurologie im ausgehenden 19. Jahrhundert--aus den Briefen Wilhelm Erbs an Adolf Strümpell. **Z Gesamte Inn Med** 1982 Jun 1;37(11):340–6

**Thom A:** Zur Geschichte der Psychiatrie im 19. Jahrhundert. Berlin, Volk und Gesundheit, 1984. 168 p.

**Thom A** see **Katzenstein A**

**Thom A** see **Späte HF**

**Thom D, Ineson A:** TNT poisoning among women workers in the First World War. **Soc Soc Hist Med Bull (Lond)** 1983 Dec;33:40–2

**Thom R** see **Waddington CH**

**Thom T:** Medicine in China: the continuing revolution - Part II. **J Okla State Med Assoc** 1982 Sep;75(9):308–12

**Thom T:** Medicine in China: the continuing revolution--part 1. **J Okla State Med Assoc** 1982 Aug;75(8):272–7

**Thomä H:** Von der Psychosomatischen Medizin zur Psychoanalyse--Heidelberg 1949–1967. **Psyche (Stuttg)** 1983 Apr;37(4):322–35

**Thomä H** see **Fischle-Carl H, ed**

**Thomae H** see **Brozek J**

**Thomann KD:** Wissenschaftliche Sozialhygiene und gesellschaftliche Praxis im Deutschen Reich. **Sudhoffs Arch** 1984;68(1):61–76

**Thomas B:** Feeding England during the Industrial Revolution: a view from the Celtic fringe. **Agric Hist** 1982;56(1):328–42

**Thomas C:** First suicide note? **Br Med J** 1980 Jul 26;281(6235):284–5

**Thomas C:** Inde: le pays du suicide? **Histoire** 1981;(30):81–3

**Thomas CB:** Fulfilling the promise: Hopkins women before World War II. **J Am Med Wom Assoc** 1981 Feb;36(2):40–3

**Thomas DM:** Freud and the 'White Hotel'. **Br Med J [Clin Res]** 1983 Dec 24–31;287(6409):1957–60

**Thomas EG:** Chelmsford and the Board of Health Report of 1849. **Essex J** 1979;14(1):

**Thomas EG:** The old Poor Law and medicine. **Med Hist** 1980 Jan;24(1):2–19

**Thomas G, Morgan-Witts M:** Anatomy of an epidemic. Garden City, N. Y., Doubleday, 1982. xv, 366 p.

**Thomas HD:** Fifty years of cardiology in Alabama. **J Med Assoc State Ala** 1981 Jul;51(1):19–20

**Thomas KB:** Attitudes to psychological illness in general practice. A historical cycle complete. **Br Med J [Clin Res]** 1981 Oct 31;283(6300):1157–8

**Thomas KB:** Sir Ivan Whiteside Magill, KCVO, DSc, MB, BCh, BAO, FRCS, FFARCS, (Hon), FFARCSI (Hon), DA. A review of his publications and other references to his life and work. **Anaesthesia** 1978 Jul–Aug;33(7):628–34

**Thomas KB:** Some early Welsh contributors to American medicine: the family of Jones. In J. Cule, ed: Wales and medicine. London, British Society for the History of Medicine, 1975. p. 10–22.

**Thomas L:** Dying as failure. **Ann Am Acad Polit Soc Sci** 1980;447:1–4

**Thomas L:** The right track. **Wilson Q** 1980;4(2):87–98

**Thomas L:** The youngest science. Notes of medicine-watcher. New York, Viking Press, 1983. xvi, 270 p.

**Thomas L:** Un manuel d'oculistique chinoise attribué a Sun Si-Miao des tang: le Yin hai jing wei. In Mazars G, ed: Les médecines traditionnelles de l'Asie. Strasbourg, Université Louis Pasteur, 1981. p. 85–92.

**Thomas LG** see **Grabowski HG**

**Thomas MO** see **Hunter JM**

**Thomas PH:** Dr. Thomas Williams of Swansea, 1818–65. In J. Cule, ed: Wales and medicine. London, British Society for the History of Medicine, 1975. p. 196–202.

**Thomas PH:** Professor Theophilus Redwood (1806–92). **Pharm Hist (London)** 1983 Jun;13(2):9–12

**Thomas RK:** The history of North American Indian alcohol use as a community based phenomenon. **J Stud Alcohol [Suppl]** 1981 Jan;9:29–39

**Thomas RZ:** An historical perspective: hospital planning and regulation from 1948 to 1978. **Hosp Health Serv Adm** 1982 Jul–Aug;27(4):66–77

**Thomas SJ:** Nostrum advertising and the image of woman as invalid in late Victorian America. **J Am Cult** 1982 Fall;5(3):104–12

**Thomas M, ed:** Urban and rural social conditions in industrial Britain; series 2. The reports [of the medical officers of health] to the Local Government Board 1869–1908. A complete listing and guide to the Harvester microfiche collection. Brighton, England, Harvester Press Microform Publications, 1979. 251 p.

**Thomasen AL:** Fra Trinitatis kirkes Loft til Universitetsbibliotekets 2. afdeling i følgeskab med Niels Stensen. **Ugeskr Laeger** 1983 Jun 27;145 Spec No:78–96

**Thomasen AL:** 'Historia animalium' contra 'Gynaecia' in der Literatur des Mittelalters. **Clio Med** 1980;15(1/2):5–23

**Thomasset C:** Quelques principes de l'embryologie médiévale (de Salerne à la fin du 13e siècle). **Senefiance** 1980;9:107–21

**Thomasset C** see **Jacquart D**

**Thomasson J:** Arbetsmiljö, förhandlingar, MBL, behörighet och utbildning. En kort berättelse om SHSTFs första fem år. **Vardfacket** 1982 Jan 14;6(1):34–6

**Thomasson WA:** Deadly legacy: dioxin and the Vietnam veteran. **Bull At Sci** 1979;35(5):15–19

**Thome AM** see **Goldberg HI**

**Thometz AC** see **Lambert JB**

**Thomford NR** see **Busnardo AC**

**Thomison JB:** Disease in Nashville: a short history. **J Tenn Med Assoc** 1983 Mar;76(3):151–5

**Thompson AC** see **Castagnino HE**

**Thompson DD, Trinkaus E:** Age determination of the Shanidar 3 Neanderthal. **Science** 1981 May 1;212(4494):575–7

**Thompson DD:** Forensic anthropology. In F. Spencer, ed: A history of American physical anthropology, 1930–1980. New York, Academic Press, 1982. p. 357–69.

**Thompson DD** see **Laughlin WS**

**Thompson EP:** Happy families. **Radic Hist Rev** 1979 Spring/Summer;Spec:42–50

**Thompson FG:** Assistant surgeon William Bradshaw, V.C. **Ir Sword** 1981;14(56):237–9

**Thompson HC:** 20th-century US child health care. Past, present, future. **Am J Dis Child** 1984 Sep;138(9):804–9

**Thompson HE:** Early history of the Medical Society of the U. S. and Mexico. **Ariz Med** 1982 Jan;39(1):55–8

**Thompson JA, Kronenfeld MR:** Graefenberg Medical Institute. **Ala J Med Sci** 1979 Oct;16(4):350–2

**Thompson JA** see **Weaver BL**

**Thompson JD:** The passionate humanist: from Nightingale to the new nurse. **Nurs Outlook** 1980 May;28(5):290–5

**Thompson JD:** [The passionate humanist: from Nightingale to the new nurse] (Jpn). **Sogo Kango** 1981;16(1):60–73

**Thompson K:** The notion of air purity in early California. **South Calif Q** 1972;54(3):203–10

**Thompson M:** Sixty years of progress: nursing and the times in U.S.A.--and in Vermont 1919–1920. **Vt Regist Nurse** 1980 Mar;:9–12

**Thompson M:** Sixty years of progress. Nursing and the times--in Vermont 1919: past/prospective. **Vt Regist Nurse** 1979 Dec;6–8

**Thompson ME:** Public health nursing faces challenges in rural health. **Vt Regist Nurse** 1981 May;:7–8, Jul; 3–4

**Thompson ME:** Sixty years of progress: nursing and the times in U. S. A. - and Vermont, 1919. An overview of nursing's accomplishment in World War I - under its chief - Jane A. Delano. **Vt Regist Nurse** 1979 Jul;:6–8

**Thompson RF** see **Hearst E, ed**

**Thompson RL, Chico C:** The first 40 years of osteopathic medicine in New Jersey. **J Med Soc NJ** 1984 Sep;81(9):798–801

**Thompson U:** Liverpool--'the home of orthopaedics'. **Physiotherapy** 1983 Jul 10;69(7):241–2

**Thompson WT:** Don't just do something.... **Va Med** 1980 Feb;107(2):146–9

**Thomsen M:** The history of burns treatment in Denmark. **Scand J Plast Reconstr Surg** 1984;18(1):7–9

**Thomsen M:** The Opera fire in Copenhagen. **Scand J Plast Reconstr Surg** 1984;18(1):3–5

**Thomson DM:** General practice and the Edinburgh Medical School: 200 years of teaching, care and research. **J R Coll Gen Pract** 1984 Jan;34(258):9–12

**Thomson EH:** Esther Pohl Lovejoy. In: Notable American women. The modern period. Cambridge, Mass., Belknap-Harvard Univ. Press, 1980. 4:424–6.

**Thomson EH:** Harvey Cushing, surgeon, author, artist. New York, Neale Watson Academic Publications, 1981, xvii, 347 p.

**Thomson EH:** John Farquhar Fulton. In Dictionary of American Biography, Suppl. 6, 1956–1960. p. 222–4, 1980.

**Thomson EH:** Madeline Earle Stanton, disciple: the years 1920 to 1941. **J Hist Med Allied Sci** 1981 Apr,36(2):151–67

**Thomson EH** see **George Rosen: In Memoriam**

**Thomson I:** The origins of physical education in state schools. **Scott Educ Rev** 1978;10(2)

**Thomson LR:** Medical illustration: our early years--reminiscing in letters: Harriet Blackstock Thomson to Ranice Crosby. **J Biocommun** 1981 Jul;8(2):13–5

**Thomson WA:** Presidential address to the British Academy of Forensic Sciences: an Edinburgh quintet. **Med Sci Law** 1982 Jul;22(3):154–67

**Thomson WA:** Rider Haggard and smallpox. **J R Soc Med** 1984 Jun;77(6):506–12

**Thomson WA:** The hospice tradition. **J R Soc Med** 1981 Feb;74(2):90–1

**Thonnier C** see **Buffat JJ**

**Thorburn AL:** Paul Ehrlich: pioneer of chemotherapy and cure by arsenic (1854–1915). **Br J Vener Dis** 1983 Dec;59(6):404–5

**Thorén L:** K. G. Lennander och kirurgien i Uppsala kring sekelskiftet. **Nord Medicinhist Arsb** 1984;:153–64

**Thorn GW:** A 50th anniversary celebration. **Transplant Proc** 1981 Mar;13(1):24–8

**Thorn GW** see **Hufnagel CA**

**Thorne AG, Wolpoff MH:** Regional continuity in Australasian Pleistocene hominid evolution. **Am J Phys Anthropol** 1981 Jul;55(3):337–49

**Thorne CB:** The watering spas of middle Tennessee. **Tenn Hist Q** 1970–71;29(4):321–59

**Thornton AD** see **Freedman R**

**Thornton EM:** Freud and cocaine: the Freudian fallacy. London, Blond & Briggs, 1983. 340 p.

**Thornton EM:** Images of cocaine. **Lancet** 1984 Jan 7;1(8367):46

**Thornton JL, Want PC:** Antique books in the library of the Royal College of Obstetricians and Gynaecologists. **Br J Obstet Gynaecol** 1981 Apr;88(4):337–45

**Thornton JL:** Jan Van Rymsdyk: medical artist of the eighteenth century. Cambridge, New York, Oleander Press, 1982. ix, 111 p.

**Thornton JL, Reeves C:** Medical book illustration: a short history. Cambridge, New York, Oleander Press, 1983. 142 p.

**Thornton JL, Want PC:** William Hunter (1718–1783) and his contributions to obstetrics. **Br J Obstet Gynaecol** 1983 Sep;90(9):787–94

**Thornton NT:** The power of Paracelsus. **Hist Med (Lond)** 1980 Jan–Feb;8(1):10–15

**Thornton R:** Demographic antecedents of a revitalization movement: population change, population size, and the 1890 Ghost Dance. **Am Sociol Rev** 1981;46(1):88–96

**Thorseth K:** Idraetsmedicin. **Ugeskr Laeger** 1981;143(34):2189–90

**Thorssen MJ** see **Radcliff-Umstead D, ed**

**Thorup OA:** Thomas Jefferson: founder of two medical schools. **Trans Am Clin Climatol Assoc** 1980;92:16–22

**Thould AK, Thould BT:** Arthritis in Roman Britain. **Br Med J [Clin Res]** 1983 Dec 24–31;287(6409):1909–11

**Thould BT** see **Thould AK**

**Thucydides:** The plague in Athens. Thucydides. The history of the Peloponnesian War. Translated by Thomas Hobbes. **NC Med J** 1980 Apr;41(4):230–2

**Thucydides and the Athenian plague: a reconsideration of the evidence: Pharm Hist (London)** 1984 Dec;14(4):6–7

**Thuen H:** 'Ad denne rent mekaniske vej ...': da tanken om hospitalisering av de sinnssvake kom til Norge. **Hist Tidsskr** 1982;61(4):313–32

**Thuillier G:** Pour une histoire du médicament en Nivernais, au XIXe siècle. **Rev Hist Econ Soc** 1975;53:73–98

**Thuillier G** see **Forster R**

**Thuillier G** see **Pelicier Y**

**Thulin KE:** Infektionernas förändrade sjukdomspanorama under 40 år. **Sydsven Medicinhist Sallsk Arsskr** 1981;:151–69

**Thulin L:** 'Om koppors ympande'--ett vaccinationens förstadium i 1700-talets Sverige. **Nord Medicinhist Arsb** 1981;59–73

**Thunberg CP:** Ma visite à l'Ecole Vétérinaire d'Alfort en 1771. **Hist Med Vet** 1977;2(4):123–6

**Thurer S:** Disability and monstrosity: a look at literary distortions of handicapping conditions. **Rehabil Lit** 1980 Jan–Feb;41(1–2):12–5

**Thuréus S:** Historiska glimtar och synpunkter på stomato-odontologi. **Nord Medicinhist Arsb** 1981;:176–82

**Thurston HI:** An historical perspective of continuing education in Kansas. Part I. **Kans Nurse** 1983 Jan;58(1):5–8

**Thurston HI:** An historical perspective of continuing education in Kansas. The 70's--voluntary to mandatory. Part II. **Kans Nurse** 1983 Mar;58(3):5–7, 18–9

**Thüry G:** Zur Infektkette der Pest in hellenistisch-römischer Zeit. In: 75 Jahre Anthropologische Staatssammlung München. Munich: Anthropologische Staatssammlung, 1977. p. 275–83.

**Tiberini ES:** Note sull'aborto e la contraccezione tra gli Nzema del Ghana. **Africa (Italy)** 1980;35(2):159–70

**Tiburskaia NA, Dukhanina NN:** Pamiati P. G. Shute (issledovaniia P. G. Shute shtammov Plasmodium vivax). **Med Parazitol (Mosk)** 1980 Jan–Feb;49(1):87–90

**Tichý M, Volná A:** Bratislavské roky profesora Brdlíka. **Cesk Zdrav** 1983 Jul;31(6):250–5

**Tichý M, Kukurová E, Beniak M, et al:** Historické okolnosti vzniku Ustavu pre lekársku fyziku. **Bratisl Lek Listy** 1984 Feb;81(2):235–9

**Tichý M, Ozorovský V, Beniak M, et al:** Pôsobenie profesora Reinsberga v akademických funkciách na LFUK v Bratislave (1925–1927). **Cesk Zdrav** 1984 Feb;32(2):68–73

**Tichý M, Kántorová V:** Vznik lekárskej fakulty UK Bratislave. 3. Nová situácia. **Bratisl Lek Listy** 1980 Dec;74(6):686–91

**Tichý M, Kántorová V:** Vznik lekárskej fakulty UK v Bratislave. 1. Možnosti štúdia medicíny na území slovenského etnika pred rokom 1918. **Bratisl Lek Listy** 1980 Apr;73(4):515–21

**Tichý M, Kántorová V:** Vznik lekárskej fakulty UK v Bratislave. 2. Usilie o založenie národnej univerzity a nové prúdy medzi lekármi. **Bratisl Lek Listy** 1980 Aug;74(2):234–40

**Tichý M, Kántorová V:** Vznik lekárskej fakulty UK v Bratislave. 4. Iniciatíva Hynkovej skupiny. **Bratisl Lek Listy** 1981 Jan;75(1):92–7

**Tichý M, Kántorová V:** Vznik lekárskej fakulty UK v Bratislave. 5. Misia dobrej vôle z Prahy. **Bratisl Lek Listy** 1981 Mar;75(3):372–8

**Tichý M, Kántorová V:** Vznik lekárskej fakulty UK v Bratislave. 6. Rokovanie V parlamente. **Bratisl Lek Listy** 1981;75(4):496–502

**Tichý M, Dedek J, Ozorovský V:** Začiatky lekárskej fakulty UK v Bratislave. **Cesk Zdrav** 1983 Feb;31(2):49–54

**Tichý M:** Začiatky lekárskej fakulty UK v Bratislave. 1. Prvý profesorský zbor. **Bratisl Lek Listy** 1982 Feb;77(2):235–40

**Tichy M:** Začiatky lekárskej fakulty UK v Bratislave. 3. Lekári a začiatky Univerzity Komenského. **Bratisl Lek Listy** 1982 Apr;77(4):488–94

**Tichý M, Dedek J, Krekáň J, et al:** Začiatky lekárskej fakulty UK v Bratislave. 4. Co predchádzalo vzniku Bratislavských lekárskych listov. **Bratisl Lek Listy** 1983;79(4):500–4

**Tichý M:** Začiatky lekárskej fakulty UK v Bratslave. 2. Prípravy na začatie výučby. **Bratisl Lek Listy** 1982 Mar;77(3):359–65

**Tichý M** see **Bečer A**

**Tichý M** see **Kokavec M**

**Tichý M** see **Moravec R**

**Tickamyer AR:** Women's roles and fertility intentions. **Pac Sociol Rev** 1979;22(2):167–84

**Tidrick RT** see **Busnardo AC**

**Tiedt N** see **Abe HR**

**Tielman RA:** De emancipatie van homoseksuelen in Nederland. **Spiegel Hist** 1982;17(11):572–5

**Tierney GD:** Botany and witchcraft. **Palacio** 1974;80(2):44–50

**Tiffany R:** The development of oncology nursing in the United Kingdom. **Prog Clin Biol Res** 1983;132E:435–40

**Tigbe JA:** 'Be it ever so little': reforming the insanity defense in the Progressive Era. **Bull Hist Med** 1983 Fall;57(3):397–411

**Tigertt HB, Tigertt WD:** Clara Louise Maass: a nurse volunteer for yellow fever inoculations--1901. **Milit Med** 1983 Mar;148(3):252–3

**Tigertt WD:** An annotated life of Egerton Yorrick Davis, M.D., an intimate of Sir William Osler. **J Hist Med Allied Sci** 1983 Jul;38(3):259–97

**Tigertt WD:** Anthrax. William Smith Greenfield, M.D., F.R.C.P., Professor Superintendent, the Brown Animal Sanatory Institution (1878–81). Concerning the priority due to him for the production of the first vaccine against anthrax. **J Hyg (Lond)** 1980 Dec;85(3):415–20

**Tigertt WD:** Noah Biggs, author, fl. 1651. **J Hist Med Allied Sci** 1983 Oct;38(4):452–5

**Tigertt WD** see **Tigertt HB**

**Tiglao T, Cruz WL:** Seven decades of public health in the Philippines (1898–1972). Tokyo, SEAMIC, 1975. xv, 310 p.

**Tijm W:** L'évolution de la consommation du fromage dans les hôpitaux de Clermont-Ferrand (1818–1952). **Cah Hist** 1979;24(1):71–8

**Tikhonov AF** see **Kuznetsov DN**

**Tikotin MA:** Peterburgskiĭ zhenskiĭ meditsinskiĭ institut v revoliutsionnom dvizhenii. **Sov Zdravookhr** 1981;(7):51–4

**Tikotin MA:** Voprosy obshchestvennoĭ gigieny na s'ezdakh russkikh estestvoispytateleĭ i vracheĭ. **Gig Sanit** 1981 Oct;(10):55–8

**Tilghman RC:** Captain James Cook (1728–1779). **Trans Am Clin Climatol Assoc** 1980;92:1–15

**Till R** see **Poch-Kalous M**

**Tillhagen CH:** Ingjald Reichborn-Kjennerud (1865–1949). **Arv** 1969–70;25–26:353–74

**Tillhagen CH:** Vögel in der Volksmedizin. **Ethnomedizin** 1978–79;5(3–4):263–86

**Tillier AM:** Evolution de la région symphysaire chez les homo sapiens juvéniles du paléolithique moyen: pech de l'azé 1, roc de marsal et la chaise 13. **C R Seances Acad Sci [III]** 1981 Nov 9;293(9):493–5

**Tillier AM, Genet-Varcin E:** La plus ancienne mandibule d'enfant découverte en France dans le gisement de La Chaise de Vouthon (Abri Suard) en Charente. **Z Morphol Anthropol** 1980;71(2):196–214

**Tilly LA:** Structure de l'emploi, travail des femmes et changements démographiques dans deux villes industrielles, Anzin et Roubaix, 1872–1906.. In: Le mouvement social. Paris, Les éditions ouvrières, 1978; 105:33–58.

**Tilney NL:** Carl Walter and the evolution of the Surgical Research Laboratory: 1937 through 1949. **Am J Surg** 1984 Nov;148(5):584–9

**Tilney NL:** Cushing, Cutler and the mitral valve. **Surg Gynecol Obstet** 1981 Jan;152(1):91–6

**Tilney NL:** Harvey Cushing and the Oxford connection. **Surg Gynecol Obstet** 1982 Jul;155(1):89–94

**Tilney NL:** Harvey Cushing and the surgical research laboratory. **Surg Gynecol Obstet** 1980 Aug;151(2):263–70

**Tilney NL:** The marrow of the tragedy (Harvey Cushing). **Surg Gynecol Obstet** 1983 Oct;157(4):380–8

**Tilney NL:** The original Peter Bent Brigham Hospital surgical staff.

**Surg Gynecol Obstet** 1981 Nov;153(5):741-6
**Timbal PC** see **Guillemain B**
**Timchenko GF** see **Ovchinnikov NM**
**Timio M:** Il rene artificiale: la storia di uno strumento per una vita semiartificiale. **Med Secoli** 1982;19(3):273-301
**Timmons CF:** Genetics of the eighteenth dynasty. **JAMA** 1981 Apr 17;245(15):1525
**Timofeeva GA, Valenkevich LN:** O podgotovke pediatricheskikh kadrov v SSSR. **Pediatriia** 1980;(1):3-5
**Timofeyev IS:** Izmeneniia v ponimanii predmeta istoriko-nauchnykh issledovanii. **Vopr Istor Estestvozn Tekh** 1981;(2):97-102
**Tindale WB** see **Black MM**
**Tindall G:** Bombay: City of gold. **Hist Today** 1982 May;32:15-21
**Tinkelenberg J:** On the morphology of creative forms and art. **Acta Morphol Neerl Scand** 1983 Mar;21(1):83-95
**Tipton DA, Mohler SR:** The Wright brothers: a personality profile. **Aviat Space Environ Med** 1983 Jun;54(6):560-2
**Tipton R:** Continued controversy: the Rutgers Medical School and the Library of Science and Medicine. **J Rutgers Univ Libr** 1983;45(1):1-24
**Tirmizi SM:** Ibn Sina as a scientist. **Stud Hist Med** 1981 Sep;5(3):233-8
**Tirmizi VM** see **Said HM, ed**
**Tischner J:** Refleksje nad dziełem Antoniego Kępińskiego. **Przegl Lek** 1983;40(12):855-9
**Tiser H, Mastný A:** O narození Napoleonova syna Orlíka. **Cesk Gynekol** 1982 Jul;47(6):442-4
**Tisseron S:** Une préhistoire de la psychiatrie? Plutôt quelques économies différentes de la folie. **Soins Psychiatr** 1982 Feb;(16):5-8
**Tissot SA:** De la santé des gens de lettres; présentation de F. Azouvi. Genève and Paris, Slatkine, 1981. viii, 246 p. Reprint of Lausanne ed., 1768.
**Titche LL, Wachter RD, Coulthard SW, et al:** Mastoiditis in prehistoric Arizona Indians. **Ariz Med** 1981 Sep;38(9):712-4
**Titche LL, Coulthard SW, Wachter RD, et al:** Prevalence of mastoid infection in prehistoric Arizona Indians. **Am J Phys Anthropol** 1981 Nov;56(3):269-73
**Title list for the history of science collection from the Library of the Jewish Theological Seminary of America:** Microfilm. 17 reels. Ann Arbor, University Microfilms International, 1980. 46 p.
**Tiukina AP:** S. A. Nikonov--vrach-revoliutsioner. **Sov Zdravookhr** 1984;(10):64-7
**Tiuliandin A, Vlasova-Leshtaeva TF:** Muzhestvo i miloserdie meditsinskikh sester. **Med Sestra** 1980 May;39(5):55-60
**Tiuliandin AD:** Dasha Sevastopol'skaia--pervaia sestra miloserdiia. **Med Sestra** 1982 Dec;41(12):60-1
**Tiuliandin AD:** Muzeĭ Sovetskogo Krasnogo Kresta. **Zdravookhr Ross Fed** 1980;(5):22-6
**Tiuliandin AD:** Sotrudnichestvo obshchestv Krasnogo Kresta SSSR i Bolgarii. **Sov Zdravookhr** 1982;(6):53-5
**Tiurin EI, Kovachev VI:** Kafedre rentgenologii i radiologii voenno-meditsinskoĭ akademii im. S. M. Kirova. **Vestn Rentgenol Radiol** 1981 Mar-Apr;(2):87-9
**Tiurin VI** see **Sapov IA**
**Tiurkian RA** see **Matveev MP**
**Tiutin LA** see **Kishkovskiĭ AN**
**Tiwari GP** see **Thatte DG**
**Tiwari SK** see **Chaturvedi GN**
**Tiwari SK** see **Rai NP**
**Tiwari SP** see **Thatte DG**
**Tjarks G, Fernández FM, Espinosa JC, et al:** La epidemia del cólera de 1856 en el valle central: analysis y consecuencias demográficas. **Rev Hist (Costa Rica)** 1976;2(3):81-129
**Tjarks GO, Espinoza Guadamuz JC, Paniagua Vargas C:** Un procedimiento estadístico para resolver muescas de población: el caso de Heredia. **Rev Hist (Costa Rica)** 1978;3(6):111-27
**Tkachenko BI, Voronenkova IA, Anoshina AA:** 50 let Otdela fiziologii vistseral'nykh sistem imeni akad. K. M. Bykova Instituta éksperimental'nŏ meditsiny AMN SSSR. **Fiziol Zh SSSR** 1981 Aug;67(8):1283-9
**Tkachenko SS, Andrianov VL, Kapitanaki IA:** K 125-letiiu so dnia rozhdeniia G. I. Turnera--osnovopolozhnika otechestvennoĭ travmatologii i ortopedii. **Ortop Travmatol Protez** 1984 Jun;(6):68-70
**Tkachenko VF:** K istorii Smelianskoĭ gorodskoĭ bol'nitsy im. N. A. Semashko. **Med Sestra** 1981 Dec;40(12):5-8
**Tkachuk VN:** Znamenatel'nye i iubileĭnye daty v istorii urologii i pogranichnykh oblastei v 1984 godu. **Urol Nefrol (Mosk)** 1984 Jan-Feb;(1):72-4
**Tkaczewski W:** Dwudziestopi ęciolecie Wojskowej Akademii Medycznej im. gen. dyw. prof. Bolesława Szareckiego. **Pol Tyg Lek** 1983 Jul 11-18;38(28-29):857-9
**Tkhostov DR** see **Selivanov VI**
**Tkocz I** see **Jensen KR**
**TNA and nursing in Texas: a 75-year perspective: Tex Nurs** 1982 Jan;56(1):12-3; Feb;56(2):6-7
**TNAI in retrospect:** The Agra Conference: 1909. **Nurs J India** 1983 Nov;74(11):300-9
**To honor A. Edward Maumenee: Am J Ophthalmol** 1979 Sep;88(3 Pt 1):285, 288-316
**Tobach E:** A brief history of the Psychology Section of The New York Academy of Sciences. In K. Salzinger, ed: Psychology in progress: an interim report. (Annals of the New York Academy of Sciences, vol. 270). New York, New York Academy of Sciences, 1976. p. 6-13.
**Tobach E, Proshansky HM, ed:** Genetic destiny: race as a scientific and social controversy. New York, AMS Press, 1976. 163 p. Contributions by A. Edel, R. Cancro, D. Layzer, H. Padfield, A. Chase, E. Drucker, V. W. Sidel, G. Piel, J. C. King, E. A. Mauss.
**Tobach E:** The relationship between Preyer's concept of psychogenesis and his views of Darwin's theory of evolution. **Z Psychol** 1983;191(4):388-95
**Tobias PV:** The natural history of the helicoidal occlusal plane and its evolution in early Homo. **Am J Phys Anthropol** 1980 Aug;53(2):173-87
**Tobin CE** see **Benjamin JA**
**Tocus EC, Nelson RC, Vocci FJ:** Regulatory perspectives and the benzodiazepines. **J Psychoactive Drugs** 1983 Jan-Jun;15(1-2):151-7
**Todd DM, Trickett EJ:** The 1978 Division 27 award for distinguished contributions to community psychology and community mental health: James G. Kelly. **Am J Community Psychol** 1979 Jun;7(3):239-61
**Todd EM:** The neuroanatomy of Leonardo Da Vinci. Ph.D. Diss., University of California, Los Angeles, 1981 xviii, 267 leaves.
**Todd EM:** The neuroanatomy of Leonardo da Vinci. Santa Barbara, Capra Press, 1983. 189 p.
**Todd J:** The history of the syndrome of Capgras. In Rose FC, Bynum WF, ed: Historical aspects of the neurosciences. New York, Raven, 1982. p. 117-25.
**Todd RG:** Some drugs of the 17th century. **Pharm Hist (London)** 1980 Aug;10(2):10-12
**Tode I:** [Significance of the letter 'u' in ancient Chinese. Did it mean caries or tooth?] (Jpn). **Shikai Tenbo** 1983 Nov;62(5):975-81
**Todericiu D:** Balthasar-Georges Sage (1740-1824) chimiste et minéralogiste français, fondateur de la première Ecole des Mines (1783). **Rev Hist Sci (Paris)** 1984 Jan;37(1):29-46
**Todericiu D:** Jean Hellot (1685-1766), savant chimiste, fondateur de la technologie chimique en France au XVIIIe siècle. In: Congrès National des Sociétés Savantes, 105e, Caen. Comptes Rendu, Paris. 1980. Section des Sciences, Fasc. 5. p. 201-11.
**Todericiu D:** Prolongements méconnus de la philosophie chimique de Jean-Baptiste Van Helmont (1578-1644) en Europe centrale et orientale. L'éloge à Van Helmont du savant roumain Démètre Cantémir (1701). **Bull Cl Sci Acad R Belg** 1979;65:228-38
**Todes DP:** Biological psychology and the Tsarist censor: the dilemma of scientific development. **Bull Hist Med** 1984 Winter;58(4):529-44
**Todes DP:** From radicalism to scientific convention: biological psychology in Russia from Sechenov to Pavlov. Ph.D. Diss., University of Pennsylvania. Philadelphia, 1981. v, 557 leaves.
**Todhunter EN:** Reflections on nutrition history. **J Nutr** 1983 Aug;113(8):1681-5
**Todhunter EN:** Some aspects of the history of nutrition and dietetics. **Ala J Med Sci** 1983 Oct;20(4):460-3
**Todisco O** see **Epistemologia, metodologia clinica e storia della scienza medica, 1**
**Todorov D:** D-r Neno TSarvulvanov. Sofiia, Meditsina i fizkultura, 1981. 113 p.
**Todorow A:** Die Entwicklung des Gesundheitswesens in der Volksrepublik Bulgarien. **Med Ges** 1979;(6):35-46
**Toellner R:** Decora Merenti. Glory, merit and science. Haller spellbound by the Newtonian star. **Janus** 1980;67(1-2-3):171-85
**Toellner R:** Die Bedeutung des physico-theologischen Gottesbeweises für die nachcartesianische Physiologie im 18. Jahrhundert. **Ber Wissenschaftsgesch** 1982;5:75-82
**Toellner R:** 'Ein Unding vor der Vernunft': Die generatio spontanea im Weltbild der aufgeklärten Naturforschung. In Dilg P, et al., ed: Perspektiven der Pharmaziegeschichte. Graz, Austria, Akademische Druck- u. Verlagsanstalt, 1983. p. 377-88.
**Toellner R:** Logical and psychological aspects of the discovery of the circulation of the blood. In M. D. Grmek, R. S. Cohen, G. Cimino, ed: On scientific discovery. The Erice Lectures 1977. Dordrecht, D. Reidel, 1981. p. 239-59. (Boston Studies in the Philosophy of Science, v. 34).
**Toellner R:** The historical preconditions for the origin of medical ethics committees in West Germany. **Metamedicine** 1981;2:275-82
**Toellner R** see **Albrecht von Haller, 1708-1777**
**Toellner R** see **Hasler L, ed**
**Tofte R:** Haukeland Sykepleierhøgskole 75 år: fra 'våkekoner' til moderne sykepleie. **Sykepleien** 1983 Jun 20;70(11):13, 17
**Tokin BP:** O nekotorykh problemakh émbriologii i teoreticheskoĭ biologii. **Arkh Anat Gistol Embriol** 1980 Dec;79(12):5-18
**Tokin BP, Ivanovo-Kazas OM, Gabaeva NS:** Vklad A. G. Knorre v razvitie sovremennoĭ émbriologii. **Arkh Anat Gistol Embriol** 1984 Jul;87(7):92-4
**Tokugawa S:** [Encounter with history of nursing: on Linda Richards and others] (Jpn). **Kango Kyoiku** 1982 Sep;23(9):539-43
**Tokuhata GK, Smith MW:** History of health studies around nuclear facilities: a methodological consideration. **Environ Res** 1981 Jun;25(1):75-85
**Tokunaga S:** [Scenes with illness. 8. Tragic past of the leprosy patients] (Jpn). **Kango Kyoiku** 1980 Aug;21(8):519-24
**Tokyo Seishin Byoin Kyokai:** Tokyo no shiritsu seishin byoin shi. Tokyo, Makino Shuppan, Showa 53 nen, 1978. 378 p.
**Tolins SH:** Treatment of varicose veins. An update. **Am J Surg** 1983 Feb;145(2):248-52
**Tölle R** see **Peters UH, ed**
**Tolmachev EP:** Nachal'nyĭ period razvitiia kosmonavtiki v SSSR (1917-1945). **Kosm Biol Aviakosm Med** 1982 Nov-Dec;16(6):7-15
**Tolmachov VF:** Rozvytok aptechnoĭ spravy na Donechchyni za roky Radians'koĭ vlady. **Farm Zh** 1980;(1):9-12

**Tolnay SE, Guest AM:** American family building strategies in 1900: stopping or spacing. **Demography** 1984 Feb 1;21(1):9–18
**Tolnay SE:** Black fertility in decline: urban differentials in 1900. **Soc Biol** 1980 Winter;27(4):249–60
**Tolnay SE:** Fertility of southern black farmers in 1900: evidence and speculation. **J Fam Hist** 1983 Winter;8(4):314–32
**Tolnay SE, Graham SN, Guest AM:** Own-child estimates of U. S. white fertility, 1886–1899. **Hist Methods** 1982;15(3):127–38
**Tolnay SE:** Trends in total and marital fertility for black Americans, 1886–1899. **Demography** 1981 Nov;18(4):443–63
**Tolo VT:** Progression in scoliosis. A 360 degrees change in 75 years. **Spine** 1983 May–June;8(4):373–7
**Tolosa ES, Klawans HL:** Meiges disease: a clinical form of facial convulsion, bilateral and medical. **Arch Neurol** 1979 Oct;36(10):635–7
**Tolpin M** see **Goldberg A, ed**
**Tolpin P** see **Goldberg A, ed**
**Tom A** see **Rokhlin LL**
**Tom SA:** The evolution of nurse–midwifery: 1900–1960. **J Nurse Midwife** 1982 Jul–Aug;27(4):4–13
**Tomanová M** see **Slosarová V**
**Tomaselli S:** The first person: Descartes, Locke and mind–body dualism. **Hist Sci** 1984;22(pt 2):185–205
**Tomashevich GV, ed:** Some of the incidents in the life of Mark De Mortie. **Afro–Am NY Life Hist** 1979;3(1):61–71
**Tomashuk IP** see **Novikov FG**
**Tomasi LT:** L'isola dei semplici. **Kos** 1984 Jun;1(5):61–84
**Tomaszewski W:** The Polish School of Medicine at the University of Edinburgh: an album. Edinburgh, W. Tomaszewski, 1983. 164 p.
**Tomes N:** Annie Warburton Goodrich. In: Notable American women. The modern period. Cambridge., Mass., Belknap–Harvard Univ. Press, 1980. 4:286–8.
**Tomes N:** Mary May Roberts. In: Notable American women. The modern period. Cambridge, Mass., Belknap–Harvard Univ. Press, 1980. 4:581–3.
**Tomes N:** The domesticated madman: changing concepts of insanity at the Pennsylvania Hospital, 1780–1830. **Pa Mag Hist Biogr** 1982;106(2):271–86
**Tomes NJ** see **Scull A, ed**
**Tomič–Karovic K:** Ljudevit Gutschy. In: I simpozij o historiji mikrobiologije i imunologije u Hrvatskoj do 1923. godine. Zagreb, Jugoslavenskoj akademiji, 1973. p. 107–17.
**Tomiček F, Křepelka J, Beran M:** In memoriam Doc. Dr. Ing. M. Semonského, DrSc. **Cesk Farm** 1979 Dec;28(9–10):362–6
**Tomich PQ, Barnes AM, Devick WS, et al:** Evidence for the extinction of plague in Hawaii. **Am J Epidemiol** 1984 Feb;119(2):261–73
**Tomini V** see **Epistemologia, metodologia clinica e storia della scienza medica, 2**
**Tomita T:** [Development of neurophysiology following the decrement–nondecrement controversy] (Jpn). **Nippon Seirigaku Zasshi** 1984;46(1):1–4
**Tomlinson WK, Perret JJ:** Jean–Charles Faget and the yellow fever controversy in New Orleans. In: Congrès international d'histoire de la médecine, XXVe, Québec, 1976. Actes. Québec, 1977. p. 1361–73.
**Tomlinson WK, Perret JJ:** Rudolph Matas father of cardiovascular surgery. In International Congress of the History of Medicine, 27th, Barcelona, 1980. Actas. Barcelona, Acadèmia de Ciències Mèdiques de Catalunya i Balears, 1981. p. 212–6.
**Töndury G:** Anatomie in Zürich. **Gesnerus** 1980;37(3/4):271–87
**Tong BR:** The ghetto of the mind: notes on the historical psychology of Chinese America. **Amerasia J** 1971;1(3):1–31
**Tonge CH:** Oral anatomy––progress of a discipline. **Br Dent J** 1981 Jul 7;151(1):3–5
**Tonge V:** Arthur Randell Jackson: 1877–1944. **Br Med J [Clin Res]** 1983 Jul 9;287(6385):97–8
**Tongiorgi Tomasi L:** Inventari della galleria e attivita iconografica dell'orto dei semplici dello studio pisano tra Cinque e Seicento. **Ann Ist Mus Stor Sci Fir** 1979;4(2):21–7
**Tonkikh AV:** K mekhanizmu sechenovskogo tormozheniia. **Zh Vyssh Nerv Deiat** 1980 Sep–Oct;30(5):1037–43
**Tonkin RE:** Mother Patrick Cosgrave, O.S.D. 1863–1900. **Zimbabwe Rhod Nurse** 1979;:46–54
**Toole HI:** Historical studies. Athens, [s.n.], 1984. 608 p. (Greek with English summaries) Includes a collection of the author's previously published essays, mostly on Greek medicine, with a short autobiographical sketch and bibliography.
**Tooley JB:** London scientific libraries in the nineteenth century. I: The springs of action. **Libr Hist** 1971;2(4):139–51
**Topelius C:** Om tandvärk och löständer. **Tandlakartidningen** 1981 May 15;73(10):565–9
**Topolnik E:** Razvoj veterinarske bakteriologije i imunologije u Hrvatskoj do god. In: I simpozij o historiji mikrobiologije i imunologije u Hrvatskoj do 1923. godine. Zagreb, Jugoslavenskoj akademiji, 1973. p. 119–26.
**Toporov GN:** Khirurgiia krovenosnykh sosudov v trudakh N. I. Pirogova (K stoletiiu vykhoda v svet piatogo izdaniia knigi N. I. Pirogova 'Khirurgicheskaia anatomiia arterial'nykh stvolov i fastsiĭ'. CPB, 1881–1882). **Klin Khir** 1982 Nov;(11):71–3
**Toporov GN:** N. I. Pirogov ob usovershenstvovanii meditsinkikh kadrov v Rossii (k 100–letiiu so dnia smerti N. I. Pirogova, 1810–1881 gg). **Sov Zdravookhr** 1982;(2):66–8
**Toppin EA:** Alma Cecelia Haupt. In Dictionary of American Biography, Suppl. 6, 1956–1960. p. 283–5, 1980.
**Torack RM:** Historical aspects of normal and abnormal brain fluids. **Arch Neurol** 1982 Apr;39(4):197–201; May;39(5):276–9
**Torack RM:** Historical aspects of normal and abnormal brain fluids. III. Cerebral edema. **Arch Neurol** 1982 Jun;39(6):355–7
**Torcida Valiente I** see **Fernández Felgueroso E**
**Torgersen J:** Medisineren John Locke og demokratiets ideer. **Samtiden (Norway)** 1970;79(1):29–43
**Törmä T:** Perspectives in international neurosurgery: neurosurgery in Finland. **Neurosurgery** 1981 Oct;9(4):479–81
**Tornero N:** O emprego de auxiliares de saúde em áreas em desenvolvimento: breve histórico. **Rev Saude Publica** 1979 Sep;13(3):254–61
**Toro C:** Sesquicentenario de la enseñanza médica. **Rev Chil Pediatr** 1983 Mar–Apr;54(2):81–2
**Törö I:** Service in biological sciences.... **Acta Biol Acad Sci Hung** 1980;31(1–3):5–12
**Toro Ibáñez MA:** Altruismo y cooperación: una interpretación darwinista. **Arbor** 1982;113(441–2):101–9
**Török B:** Langenbuch és Halpert Béla. Az elsö cholecytektómia centenáriumára. **Orv Hetil** 1983 Jun 26;124(26):1577–81
**Torok N:** Robert Bárány. **JAMA** 1980 Dec 5;244(22):2520
**Torp H:** 75 Jahre Fachzeitschrift: Dokumentation von Kontinuität und Wandel in der Krankenpflege. **Krankenpflege (Frankfurt)** 1981 Jun;35(6):235–7
**Torrance GM** see **Coburn D**
**Torrance TF:** The place of Michael Polanyi in the modern philosophy of science. **Ethics Sci Med** 1980;7(2):57–95
**Torre E:** Las 'Conclusiones' del doctor Estrada de Madrid, contra los 'Avisos particulares' del doctor Hidalgo de Aguero, sevillano. **Asclepio** 1978–79;30–31:389–401
**Torre JM:** Historia de la medicina potosina. Cuatro fases de su trayectoria. **Bol Soc Mex Hist Filos Med** 1984 Sep;7(48):351–92
**Torre JM:** La cardiologia en Nueva España durante el siglo XVI. **Bol Soc Mex Hist Filos Med** 1982 Sep;6(40):57–9
**Torre JM:** La contribución de Nueva España a la cardiología. **Arch Inst Cardiol Mex** 1980 Sep–Oct;50(5):623–9
**Torre JM:** Los balbuceos de la cardiologia mexicana. **Bol Soc Mex Hist Filos Med** 1980 Sep–Dec;5(32–33):109–22
**Torre JM:** Los balbuceos de la cardiología mexicana. **Prensa Med Mex** 1979 May–Jun;44(5–6):105–11
**Torre JM:** Panorama actual de la enseñanza de la medicina en México. In Academia Nacional de Medicina. Libro conmemorativo del primer centenario. México, Comité Editorial de la Comisión Organizadora del Congreso del Centenario, 1964. Tome 2. p. 702–5.
**Torre JM:** Publicaciones periódicas sobre cardiología en la actualidad. **Arch Inst Cardiol Mex** 1980 Nov–Dec;50(6):725–32
**Torrens PR:** Health insurance in the United States: implications for the United Kingdom. **Lancet** 1980 Jan 5;1(8158):27–31
**Torres CM:** Evidence for snuffing in the prehispanic stone sculpture of San Agustín, Colombia. **J Psychoactive Drugs** 1981 Jan–Mar;13(1):53–60
**Torres M:** La nueva perspectiva psicologica de Bolivar. **Bol Hist Antiq (Bogota)** 1980;67(728):69–85
**Torres Fontes J:** De historia médica murciana. I. Los médicos. Murcia, Academia Alfonso X El Sabio, Biblioteca Murciana de Bolsillo, 1980. 308 p.
**Torres–Gómez JM, García–Palmieri MR:** Datos biográficos del Dr. Ramón M. Suárez Calderón. **Bol Asoc Med PR** 1983 Nov;75(11):490
**Torres–Gómez JM:** Suárez, Ramón M., 1895–19811700 to PresentPuerto Rico **Bol Asoc Med PR** 1983 Nov;75(11):501–2
**Torres Medina J:** Los barcos hospitales en la campaña de Cuba. **Rev Hist Mil** 1970;14(29):161–86
**Torres Oliver LJ:** Historia del Hospital de la Caridad de Nuestra Señora de la Concepción de San Germán, Puerto Rico. **Cuatricenten San German** 1971;:235–72
**Torres Ramírez C, Aguilar Ruíz J, Zuluaga Gómez A, et al:** La cristalografía aplicada al análisis de los cálculos urinarios en España. Revisión histórica de la aportacion española al tema. **Arch Esp Urol** 1980 May–Jun;33(3):241–50
**Torres Ramírez C** see **Zuluaga Gómez A**
**Torrey EF:** Schizophrenia and civilization. New York, Aronson, 1980. ix, 230 p.
**Torrington M, Botha JL, Pilcher GJ, et al:** Association between familial hypercholesterolaemia and church affiliation. Is this the result of sociocultural isolation of migrant farmers in 19th–century South Africa? **S Afr Med J** 1984 May 12;65(19):762–7
**Torroncelli A, et al:** I manoscritti medici della Biblioteca Casanatense di Roma. **Kos** 1984 May;1(4):9–16
**Tort P:** L'Ordre et le monstres. Le débat sur l'origine des déviations anatomiques au XVIIIe siècle. Paris, Sycomore, 1980. 264 p.
**Torzhestvo leninskikh ideĭ: Voen Med Zh** 1980 Apr;(4):3–12
**Toscano Moreno J:** Los hospitales y la 'hospitalidad' de los franciscanos en la Nueva Galicia. **Bol Inst Invest Bibliogr** 1970;4:389–404
**Tota B:** The importance of comparative cardiology. **Comp Biochem Physiol [A]** 1983;76(3):401–3
**Tóth A:** Avicenna–kötet a keszthelyi Helikon Könyvtárban. Velencei kiadás, 1564. **Orv Hetil** 1980 Dec 28;121(52):3212–3
**Tóth A:** Hévízi érmek. **Orv Hetil** 1982 Jul 11;123(28):1751–3
**Tóth A:** Orvosok Széchenyi naplójában. **Orv Hetil** 1981 May 31;122(22):1329–37
**Tóth P:** A gyermekfogászat oktatásának 25 éve. **Fogorv Sz** 1980 Dec;73(12):377–8
**Tóth Z:** Az orvosdoktori értekezések jelentösége a gyógyszerészeti tudomanyok hazai kialakulásában és fejlödésében 1770–1848. Diss.,

Budapest, 1976. 131 p.
**Toti A:** Augusto Righi precursore della xeroradiografia. **Radiol Med (Torino)** 1979 Sep;65(9):615–6
**Totter JR, Darby WJ:** Paul Louis Day (1899–1980). A biographical sketch. **J Nutr** 1984 Feb;114(2):241–6
**Touati B:** Ambroise paré. **Rev Odontostomatol (Paris)** 1983 Mar–Apr;12(2):85
**Touati FO:** François d'Assise et la diffusion d'un modèle thérapeutique a XIIIe siècle. **Hist Sci Med** 1982;16(3):175–84
**Touati FO:** Une approche de la maladie et du phénomène hospitalier aux XIIe et XIIIe siècles: la léproserie du Grand-Beaulieu à Chartres. **Hist Sci Med** 1980;14:419–24
**Touhami M** see **Moussaoui D**
**Toujas R:** La lutte contre la mendicité à la fin du XVIIe siècle: l'établissement d'hôpitaux généraux dans la province ecclśiastique de Toulouse. In: Congrès National des Sociétés Savantes, 97e, Nantes, 1972. Actes. Paris, 1977. Histoire Moderne et Contemporaine, Tome 1. p. 389–401.
**Toulmin S** see **Kasschau RA**
**Touloukian RJ:** The legacy of Connecticut surgery: case histories revisited. **Conn Med** 1981 Apr;45(4):241–4
**Touraine JL** see **Woehrle R**
**Tournier-Lasserve C:** La Peyronie et la présence des chirurgiens militaires au sein de l'Académie de Chirurgie. **Chirurgie** 1981;107(9):719–22
**Tournier-Lasserve C:** Le Service de santé des armées et la recherche au fil du temps. **Med Armees** 1980,8(10)spec:851–6
**Tournier-Lasserve C:** Les chirurgiens militaires et l'Académie de médecine. **Bull Acad Natl Med (Paris)** 1982 May;166(5):601–8
**Toussaint R:** Médicinaire du 17e siècle provenant d'Aywaille. **Enquetes Mus Vie Wallonne** [1980?];13:205–20
**Touw M:** The religious and medicinal uses of Cannabis in China, India and Tibet. **J Psychoactive Drugs** 1981 Jan–Mar;13(1):23–34
**Tovarova II, Shamin AN:** Istoriia penitsillinov (k 100-letiiu so dnia rozhdeniia Aleksandra Eleminga). **Vopr Istor Estestvozn Tekh** 1981;3:65–75
**Tovbin MM:** Obshchestvo krasnogo kresta v SSSR (pervoe desiatiletie). **Vopr Istor** 1978;(4):204–10
**Tovmasian DA:** 50 let--45 vypuskov. **Veterinariia** 1979 Nov;(11):14–8
**Tower DB:** Hensing, 1719. An account of the first chemical examination of the brain and the discovery of phosphorus therein, set against the background of Europe in the 17th and early 18th centuries. A source book in the history of neurochemistry. New York, Raven, 1983. xvi, 407 p.
**Towers BA:** Health education policy 1916–1926: venereal disease and the prophylaxis dilemma. **Med Hist** 1980 Jan;24(1):70–87
**Towers BA:** The management and politics of a public exposé: the Prestwich Inquiry 1922. **J Soc Policy** 1984 Jan;13(1):41–61
**Towpik E:** Benjaminowskie Towarzystwo Lekarskie (1917–1918). **Arch Hist Med (Warsz)** 1982;45(1–4):101–5
**Toy EV:** The conservative connection: the chairman of the board took LSD before Timothy Leary. **Am Stud** 1980;21(2):65–77
**Toyohashi-shi Shika Ishikai shi:** Toyohashi, Japan, Toyohashi-shi Shika Ishikai, Showa 52 nen. [1977]. 755 p.
**Trabucchi C:** Riforma psichiatrica. I vecchi 'manicomi' e la riforma sanitaria. **Minerva Med** 1980 May 7;71(18):1281–5
**Tracy B:** Explorations in industry No. V. The 'ministering angel'. **Lamp** 1981 Dec;38(12):30–4
**Tracy GD:** Evolution of responsibilities in the care of health. **Med J Aust** 1980 Nov 29;2(11):591–6
**The traditional birth attendant in seven countries:** Case studies in utilization and training. **Public Health Pap** 1981;75:1–211
**Traer JF:** Marriage and the family in eighteenth-century France. Ithaca, Cornell University Press, 1980. 208 p.
**Träger O** see **Kaiser W**
**Tran Huan N:** Quelques aspects de la médecine et de la pharmacie au Vietnam. **Sci Orient** 1978;13:1–11
**Trandel-Korenchuk D, Trandel-Korenchuk K:** Entry into nursing practice: does nursing history repeat itself? **Nurse Pract** 1984 Mar;9(3):15–6, 21, 24–5
**Trandel-Korenchuk K** see **Trandel-Korenchuk D**
**Transcript of the amorial bearings of the Royal Australasian College of Radiologists in the letters patent: Australas Radiol** 1982;Spec. No.:3–4
**Tranter NL:** The demographic impact of economic growth and decline: Portpatrick, 1820–1891. **Scott Hist Rev** 1978 Apr;57:87–105
**Trapeznikov NN** see **Blokhin NN**
**Trapeznikova MF** see **Abramian AIa**
**Trapp F** see **Gumpert M**
**Tratner E:** A new Talmudic source on the history of diabetes (late onset). **Koroth** 1982 Aug;8(3/4):205–12
**Tratner E:** 1. Tracheotomy in the Hebrew translation of Ibn-Sina. 2. Intubation mentioned in the Talmud and by Jacob Ben Asher (14th Century). **Koroth** 1983 Aug;8(7–8):333–8
**Trattner WI:** Homer Folks. In Dictionary of American biography, 1961–1965. Suppl. 7, 1981. p. 250–2.
**Trattner WI** see **Breul FR**
**Traunfellner Z:** Polska medycyna sadowa drugiej połowy XIX wieku. **Arch Hist Med (Warsz)** 1979;42(1):45–60
**Trautman JR:** A brief history of Hansen's disease. **Bull NY Acad Med** 1984 Sep;60(7):689–95
**Trautmann J, Pollard C:** Literature and medicine. An annotated bibliography. Revised edition. Pittsburgh, University of Pittsburgh Press, 1982. xxi, 228 p. (Contemporary Community Health Series).
**Trautmann J:** Medical ethics in literature. In Reich WT, et al, ed: Encyclopedia of bioethics, v.3. New York, Free Press, 1978. p. 1008–15.
**Trautmann JC** see **Trautmann M**
**Trautmann M, Trautmann JC:** R. T. H. Laennec 1781–1826. Zum 200. Geburtstag des Autors der Auscultation médiate. **MMW** 1981 Nov 6;123(45):1717–20
**Trautmann J, ed:** Healing arts in dialogue. Medicine and literature. Carbondale, Edwardsville, Southern Illinois University Press, 1981. Contribution by N. C. Andreasen, R. Selzer, J. C. Cowan, I. Lawson, D. Levertov, E. Sewell, H. G. Moss. (Medical Humanities Series).
**Travers R:** Florey and Cairns--early work on penicillin. **Med J Aust** 1982 Jul 10;2(1):10–1
**Travieso CR:** Historia de la cirugia en Venezuela. **Rev Soc Venez Hist Med** 1975–76;23(37):21–35
**Travieso CR** see **Sociedad Venezolana de Historia de la medicina**
**Travill AA** see **Demaitre L**
**Trávníčkova E** see **Trojan S**
**Treacher A, ed** see **Wright P**
**Trease GE:** Claude Bernard 1813–1878. **Br J Pharm Pract** 1981;3(2):21–2
**Trease GE:** Elie Metchnikoff, 1845–1916. **Br J Pharm Pract** 1981;3(3):26–7
**Trease GE:** Joseph Lister, 1827–1912. **Br J Pharm Pract** 1981;2(10):34, 36
**Trease GE:** Robert Wilhelm Eberhard Bunsen (1811–1899). **Br J Pharm Pract** 1981;3(5):38–9
**Trease GE:** Rudolf Virchow 1821–1902. **Br J Pharm Pract** 1981;3(1):34–5
**Trease GE:** William Allen 1770–1843. **Br J Pharm Pract** 1981;3(4):33–4
**Trebach AS:** The heroin solution. New Haven, London, Yale University Press, 1982.
**Trebbin H:** Frühe Pathologie. **MMW** 1980 Feb 8;122(6):209–11
**Treccani A** see **Baume LG**
**Trecker JL:** Katharine Blunt. In: Notable American women. The modern period. Cambridge, Mass., Belknap-Harvard Univ. Press, 1980. 4:87–8.
**Treher W:** Jean-Jacques Rousseau oder die Anatomie eines Pulverfasses mit Betrachtungen über Georg Wilhelm Friedrich Hegel und Adolf Hitler verbunden zu einer Vergleichenden Psychopathologie der Funktionsschizophrenie. Emmendigen, W. Treher, 1982. 208 p.
**Treĭman VV:** F. G. Mukhamed'iarov--organizator Sovetskogo zdravookhraneniia v Tatarii. **Sov Zdravookhr** 1983;(7):71–2
**Trejo Rayón S** see **Juan López M**
**Treleven DE:** One hundred years of health and healing in rural Wisconsin. In Numbers RL, Leavitt JW, ed: Wisconsin medicine. Historical perspectives. Madison, University of Wisconsin Press, 1981. p. 133–53.
**Trenckmann U:** Das mikrobiologische Modell im theoretischen Denken der Psychiatrie. **Wiss Beitr Martin Luther Univ Halle Wittenberg** 1983;5–R80:301–6
**Trenckmann U, Ortmann F:** Das psychodynamische Krankheitskonzept der Romantik--Testfall für die Anwendung des Kuhnschen Paradigmabegriffs in einer Humanwissenschaft. **Z Psychol** 1980;188(3):331–9
**Trenckmann U:** Der Wandel der Epidemiologie in der Psychiatrie in der mikrobiologisch-antibiotischen Ara und seine Konsequenzen für das psychiatrische Denken im 19. und 20. Jahrhundert. **Z Gesamte Hyg** 1982 Mar;28(3):211–3
**Trenckmann U:** Vergleich der psychiatrischen Versorgungssysteme in Polen und Sachsen im 18. und 19. Jahrhundert. **Arch Hist Med (Warsz)** 1979;42(2):241–4
**Trenckmann U** see **Kaiser W**
**Trencséni T:** A 125 éves Orvosi Hetilap és szerkesztése az újraindulás óta. **Orv Hetil** 1982 Dec 26;123(52):3179–85
**Trends in biomedical research, 1901–1976:** Proceedings of the Second Rockefeller Archive Center Conference, December 10, 1976. North Tarrytown, The Center, 1977. 70 p. Contributions by R. S. Morison, A. M. Harvey, P. H. Mazumdar, S. Benison, M. Heidelberger, M. McCarty, E. H. Ahrens, A. Kappas.
**Trenn TJ:** Ludwik Fleck's 'On the question of the foundations of medical knowledge'. **J Med Philos** 1981 Aug;6(3):237–56
**Trenn TJ** see **Fleck L**
**Trent B:** Grosse Ile: island of the dead. **Can Med Assoc J** 1984 Oct 15;131(8):960–8
**Trente années d'existence:** Alsemberg, La Fondation, [1977?]. 23 p.
**Treolo J:** Seeing fingers: the ministry of the Christian Record Braille Foundation. **Advent Herit** 1982;7(2):28–37
**Trépanier P:** Victor Barbeau et Albiny Paquette. **Action Natl** 1978;68(4):324–30
**Treśc poprzednich zeszytów 'Przegladu lekarskiego' poświeconych zagadnieniom lekarskim okupacji hitlerowskiej: Przegl Lek** 1984;41(1):178–202
**Trethowan WH:** Ivor Gurney's mental illness. **Music Lett** 1981;62(3–4):300–9
**Tret'iak TP, Stetsula TI:** Zaslugi N. I. Pirogova v oftal'mologii. **Oftalmol Zh** 1981;36(8):506–8
**Trettin H:** Der Weg der Manuellen Lymphdrainage nach Vodder zur Therapeutischen Lymphdrainage nach Kuhnke/Asdonk--ein halbes Jahrhundert geschichtlicher Entwicklung der Odemtherapie. **Z Lymphol** 1983 Jul;7(1):47–9
**Treudley MB** see **Breul FR**
**Treuille H:** L'état des hôpitaux de pèlerins dans le Sud-Ouest de la France dans la seconde moitié du XVIIe siècle. In: Congrès National des Sociétés Savantes, 104e, Bordeaux, 1979. Actes. Paris, 1981. Histoire Moderne et Contemporaine, Tome 2. p. 35–50.

**Treuille H** see **La Coste-Messelière R de**

**Treutler H** see **Hambsch K**

**Treviño-García Manzo N, Kumate J, Alarcón-Segovia D, et al:** La Academia Nacional de Medicina en las actividades de investigación y enseñanza del país. **Gac Med Mex** 1983 Jul;119(7):274-88

**Treviño-Zapata N:** Valentín Gómez Farías. Patricio, precursor, médico y político. **Gac Med Mex** 1982 Jan;118(1):39-43

**Trevisani F, Moscheo R:** Between ancients and moderns: Tommaso Cornelio's medical teaching and an unpublished comment by him on the Galenic Ars parva. **Nouv Repub Lett** 1983;(2):59-73

**Trevisani F:** 'Ratio' und 'Experimentum': Johannes Bohn (1640-1718) und die italienische Experimentalphysiologie. **Clio Med** 1983 Mar;17(4):199-206

**Trevisani F:** Un corrispondente di Cartesio: alcune note su Lazare Meyssonnier (1611/12-1673), medico e astrologo lionese e sulla sua Belle Magie (1669). **Hist Philos Life Sci** 1979;1(2):285-308

**Trevor-Roper H:** Medicine in politics. **Am Scholar** 1981-82;51(1):23-41

**Trevor-Roper P:** The Noysome cataract. **Trans Ophthalmol Soc UK** 1980 Jul:100 (pt 2):299-308

**Trevor-Roper P:** Then and now--therapy. **Trans Ophthalmol Soc UK** 1980 Apr;100(pt 1):30-3

**Trevor-Roper PD:** Sir Henry Tristram Holland. In Dictionary of national biography, 1961-1970. Suppl. 8, 1981. p. 528-9.

**Triadan H:** Picasso--Pionier der Mundhygiene? **SSO Schweiz Monatsschr Zahnheilkd** 1983 Apr;93(4):250-1

**Trías de Gómez L, Pagán Ramos IH:** Organización del Museo de la Enfermería en Puerto Rico. **Bol Col Prof Enferm PR** 1983 Jun;9(34):24-5

**A tribute:** Michael E. DeBakey, M.D. **Compr Ther** 1984 Feb;10(2):3-5

**A tribute to Louis I. Grossman: J Endod** 1982 Jan;8(Spec issue):S1-48

**Tricard J** see **Biget JL**

**Trice ER:** Hugh Mercer: physician-hero of the American Revolution. **Va Med** 1981 Feb;108(2):104-6

**Trice ER:** Philip Syng Physick, father of American surgery. **Va Med** 1981 Jul;108(7):456-9

**Trice ER:** Theodorick Bland, Jr: Virginia physician, cuirassier. **Va Med** 1980 Feb;107(2):88-9

**Trickett EJ** see **Todd DM**

**Tricks N:** Man and medicine on Mendip. **Bristol Med Chir J** 1984 Apr;99(370):40-4

**Triebel-Schubert C:** Die Anfänge der Bonner akademischen Medizin. Johann Christian Friedrich Harless (1773-1853). **MMW** 1983 Oct 21;125(42):950-2

**Trifonov DN** see **Bykov GV**

**Triki H** see **Rosenberger B**

**Trimble MR:** Functional diseases. **Br Med J [Clin Res]** 1982 Dec 18-25;285(6357):1768-70

**Trincker DE:** Wilhelm Steinhausen (1887-1954). **Rev Physiol Biochem Pharmacol** 1980;87:25-32

**Tring FC:** Thomas Holloway and his patent pills. **Pharm Hist (London)** 1977 Dec;7(3):4-5

**Trinkaus E:** A history of Homo erectus and Homo sapiens paleontology in America. In F. Spencer, ed: A history of American physical anthropology, 1930-1980. New York, Academic Press, 1982. p. 261-80.

**Trinkaus E, Zimmerman MR:** Trauma among the Shanidar Neandertals. **Am J Phys Anthropol** 1982 Jan;57(1):61-76

**Trinkaus E** see **Thompson DD**

**Tripathi RD, Verma KC:** Contribution of Kaviraj Gangadhar Ray in the development of ayurvedic education. **Sachitra Ayurved** 1981 Mar;:190-3

**Triplet RG:** The relationship of Clark L. Hull's hypnosis research to his later learning theory: the continuity of his life's work. **J Hist Behav Sci** 1982 Jan;18(1):22-31

**Trisoglio M** see **Bellagarda M**

**Trivedi RP:** Glimpses of Ayurvedic contribution to paediatrics & allied subjects. **Sachitra Ayurved** 1981 Aug;:113-7

**Trocmé C:** Eléments pour une histoire de l'oedème pulmonaire. **Hist Sci Med** 1983;17(1):71-84

**Trocme C:** Esquisse d'une histoire de la pléthore, de la volémie et du retour veineux. **Hist Sci Med** 1981;15(1):69-80

**Trocme C:** L'atélectasie découverte et délaissée: Claude-Auguste Reynaud et Nicolas Bailly. **Hist Sci Med** 1979;13(4):441-50

**Troetel WM** see **Bolton S**

**Trofast J:** Jöns Jacob Berzelius och djurkemien. **Sydsven Medicinhist Sallsk Arsskr** 1981;:170-84

**Tröhler U:** Britische Spitäler und Polikliniken als Heil- und Forschungsstätten 1720-1820. **Gesnerus** 1982;39(1):115-31

**Tröhler U:** Klinisch-numerische Forschung in der britischen Geburtshilfe 1750-1820. **Gesnerus** 1981;38:69-80

**Tröhler U:** Medizin mit oder ohne Geschichte? **Praxis** 1981 Dec 15;70(51):2295-7

**Tröhler U:** Quantification in British medicine and surgery 1750-1830. Ph.D. Diss., University of London, 1978.

**Tröhler U:** Theodor Kocher und die neurotopographische Diagnostik: angewandte Forschung mit grundlegendem Ergebnis um 1900. **Gesnerus** 1983;40(1-2):203-14

**Tröhler U:** Towards clinical investigation on a numerical basis: James Lind at Haslar Hospital 1758-1783. In International Congress of the History of Medicine, 27th, Barcelona, 1980. Actas. Barcelona, Acadèmia de Ciències Mèdiques de Catalunya i Balears, 1981. p. 414-9.

**Tröhler U** see **Allgöwer M**

**Troianskiĭ AN:** Vklad prof. V. Iu. Kurliandskogo v razvitie nauchnykh problem ortopedicheskoĭ stomatologii (k 75-letiiu so dnia rozhdeniia). **Stomatologiia (Mosk)** 1983 Nov-Dec;62(6):75-6

**Troianskiĭ GN, Krechmer MI:** A. I. Evdokimov--odin iz osnovopolozhnikov sovetskoĭ stomatologii. **Sov Zdravookhr** 1984;(10):60-4

**Trojan S, Trávníčkova E:** Přednášky Vladimíra Tomsy. **Cesk Fysiol** 1979;80(5):471-2

**Trojan S:** 100 let od obnovení činnosti Ceské Lékařské fakulty. **Cesk Fysiol** 1982;31(6):481-2

**Trolander JA:** Lavinia Lloyd Dock. In Dictionary of American Biography, Suppl. 6, 1956-1960. p. 166-8, 1980.

**Trolle D:** The history of Caesarean section. Copenhagen, University Library, 1982. 109 p. (Acta Historica Scientiarum Naturalium Et Medicinalium, v. 33).

**Trombley S:** All that summer she was mad: Virginia Woolf and her doctors. **Soc Soc Hist Med Bull (Lond)** 1981 Jun;28:21-5

**Trombley S:** All that summer she was mad: Virginia Woolf, female victim of male medicine. New York, Continuum, 1982. ix, 338 p.

**Trompiz G:** Dogmas que se derrumban. **Rev Soc Venez Hist Med** 1981;30(45-46):101-3

**Troncale JA:** Nineteenth century neurology/psychiatry. **J Med Assoc State Ala** 1982 Aug;52(2):29-30, 32-5

**Tronnberg G:** S:ta Apollonia av Alexandra--tandlakarnas skyddshelgon. **Odontol Foren Tidskr** 1980 Dec;44(5):22-8

**Troschke J von:** Möglichkeiten und Grenzen ärztlicher Gesundheitsberatung. Freiburg, Gesomed, 1981. 373 p.

**Troshin AS** see **Vorob'ev VI**

**Trott NG** see **Mallard J**

**Trotter WR:** John Brown, and the nonspecific component of human sickness. **Perspect Biol Med** 1978 Winter;21(2):258-64

**Troupeau G** see **Ibn Masawayh Y**

**Trout GM:** The American Dairy Science Association: the third twenty-five years, 1957-1981. **J Dairy Sci** 1981 Jun;64(6):876-99

**Trovato F, Grindstaff CF:** Decomposing the urban-rural fertility differential: Canada, 1971. **Rural Sociol** 1980;45(3):448-68

**Trowell HC:** Ants distinguish diabetes mellitus from diabetes insipidus. **Br Med J [Clin Res]** 1982 Jul 17;285(6336):217

**Trüb CL, Eberhard W:** Arztliche Berufs- und Standeskunde im 16. und 17. Jahrhundert. **Med Welt** 1982 Oct 2;32(40):1504-9

**Trüb CL:** Die Terminologie und Definition Sozialmedizin und Sozialhygiene in den literarischen Sekundärquellen der Jahre 1900 bis 1960. Opladen, Westdeutscher Verlag, 1978. 87 p.

**Trüb CL:** Heilige und Krankheit. Stuttgart, Klett-Cotta, 1978. 307 p.

**Trubina LM:** K 100-letiiu fagotsitarnoĭ teorii I. I. Mechnikova. **Zh Mikrobiol Epidemiol Immunobiol** 1983 Dec;(12):99-101

**Trubnikov VF:** K 60-letiiu osnovanii kafedry ortopedii, travmatologii i voenno-polevoi khirurgii Khar'kovskogo meditsinskogo instituta. **Ortop Travmatol Protez** 1981 Sep;(9):68-70

**Truck B:** Mengele, l'ange de la mort. La vie diabolique du docteur Josef Mengele, médecin-chef du camp d'extermination d'Auschwitz. Paris, Presses de la cité, 1976. 248 p.

**Trueta J:** Els orígens del 'Welfare State' i de les lleis socials: Lluí Vives. In Congrés International d'Història de la Medicina Catalana, 2nd, Barcelona, 1975. Llibre d'Actes. Barcelona, Socitra, 1977. p. 39-47.

**Truman GL** see **Fel' II**

**Trumpener U:** The road to Ypres: the beginnings of gas warfare in World War I. **J Mod Hist** 1975;47(3):460-8

**Trümpy H:** Volkskundliche Uberlegungen zum Rauchen. **Ther Umsch** 1983 Feb;40(2):165-8

**Trusova TM** see **Bunchuk NV**

**Trussell J, Olsen R:** Evaluation of the Olsen technique for estimating the fertility response to child mortality. **Demography** 1983 Aug;20(3):391-405

**Trussell J** see **Fogel RW**

**Truupyl'd AIu:** Patologicheskaia anatomiia v Tartuskom universitete. **Arkh Patol** 1983;45(9):66-72

**Trynková O:** Některé metody středověkého léčení podle mistra Rhazesa a mistra Salicettiho. I. Rhazesovo a Salicettiho ranná lékařství a jejich vydavatelé. **Sb Lek** 1981;83(11-12):363-7

**Trynková O:** Některé metody středověkého léčení podle Mistra Rhazesa a Mistra Salicettiho. II. Uspěchy a neúspěchy středověkých léčitelu. **Sb Lek** 1982 Jan;84(1):25-32

**Trynková O:** Některé metody středověkého léčení podle mistra rhazesa a mistra Salicettiho. III. Výběr z anatomických pojmu užívaných ve středověké medicíně. **Sb Lek** 1982 Feb;84(2):59-63

**Trzydziestolecie sluzby zdrowia Ministerstwa Spraw Wewnetrznych w Olsztyńskiem, 1945-1975: materiały sesji naukowej, Olsztyn, 7 pazdziernika 1975:** Olsztyn, Wydano na zlecenie Tarchomińskich Zakładów Farmaceutycznych 'Polfa,' 1976. 106 p.

**Tsai C:** [Retrospect of a physiologist engaged in scientific research and education for 60 years] (Chi). **Sheng Li Ko Hsueh Chin Chan** 1982 Jul;13(3):193-200

**Ts'ai HC:** [Demographic methodology and its application to studies of historical populations] (Chi). **Ssu yu Yen** 1982;20(4):49-56

**Tsakok FH** see **Ratnam SS**

**Tsankov N, Puissant A:** Les dermatologistes bulgares à l'hôpital Saint-Louis et leurs relations avec la dermatologie française. **Hist Sci Med** 1980;14:349-56

**Tsao TF:** Endodontic treatment in China. **Int Endod J** 1984 Jul;17(3):163-75

**Tsaregorodtsev GI, Anokhin AM:** V. I Lenin i problemy okhrany zdorov'ia cheloveka v razvitom sotsialisticheskom obshchestve. **Ter Arkh** 1980;52(4):3-7

**Tschassovnikarov D, Markov G:** Personologische Untersuchungen über einige Urbilder im Schaffen von Hieronymus Bosch. **Psychiatr Neurol Med Psychol (Leipz)** 1980 Oct;32(10):623–30

**Tschikin SJ:** Die Entwicklung des Gesundheitswesens in der UdSSR. **Med Ges** 1979;(6):11–34

**Tschill Y:** Le bureau de bienfaisance de Mulhouse (1798–1848). In Livet G, Schaff G, ed: Médecine et assistance en Alsace, XVIe–XXe siècle. Strasbourg, Istra, 1976. p. 241–64.

**Tschinkel A:** Unser Bild. – Das 'Licht der Natur' [A. Tschinkel, 1964]. **Medizinhist J** 1981;16(1/2):196–8

**Tschofen H:** Die Drogenszene in Vorarlberg. Entwicklung und Abwehrmassnahmen. **Montfort** 1981;33(2):151–8

**Tsentral'nomu institutu tuberkuleza Ministerstva zdravookhraneniia SSSR 60 let: Probl Tuberk** 1982 May;(5):3–7

**Tsiklik AM:** K istorii vozniknoveniia i stanovleniia poliklinicheskoĭ. **Feldsher Akush** 1980;45(10):51–3

**Tsiklik AM:** S. M. Vasil'ev i ego klinicheskoe nasledie (K 125-letiiu so dnia rozhdeniia). **Ter Arkh** 1980;52(7):143–6

**Tsimidanova NB** see **Revenko TA**

**Tsitlanadze VG, Tskhomelidze NF, Melikishvili MN, et al:** K istorii razvitiia revmatologii v Gruzii. **Vopr Revm** 1982 Jul–Sep;(3):13–5

**Tskhomelidze NF** see **Tsitlanadze VG**

**Tsouyopoulos N:** Andreas Röschlaub und die Romantische Medizin. Die philosophischen Grundlagen der modernen Medizin. **Med Gesch Kult** 1982;14:1–259

**Tsouyopoulos N:** Andreas Röschlaub und die Romantische Medizin. Stuttgart, Fischer, 1982. 258 p. (Medizin in Geschichte und Kultur, 14).

**Tsouyopoulos N:** Auf der Suche nach einer adäquaten Methode für die Geschichte und Theorie der Medizin. Auseinandersetzung mit Ludwik Flecks 'Entstehung und Entwicklung einer wissenschaftlichen Tatsache'. **Medizinhist J** 1982;17(1/2):20–36

**Tsouyopoulos N:** Die neue Auffassung der klinischen Medizin als Wissenschaft unter dem Einfluss der Philosophie im frühen 19. Jahrhundert. **Ber Wissenschaftsgesch** 1978;1(1–2):87–100

**Tsouyopoulos N** see **Hasler L, ed**

**Tsubaki T:** [History of the Japanese Society of Neurology for 20 years (author's transl)]. (Jpn) **Rinsho Shinkeigaku** 1979 Dec;19(12):804–8

**Tsuboi Y, Haga S, Matsuda M, et al:** [Relationship between the Nightingale Nursing School and Tokyo Hospital Nursing School] (Jpn). **Sogo Kango** 1981;16(1):36–46

**Tsubota S:** [Public health nurses in the frontier of Hokkaido--a historical background] (Jpn). **Hokenfu Zasshi** 1982 Jan;38(1):50–6

**Tsubouchi Y** see **Cho LJ**

**Tsudechkis LM** see **Grigorash FF**

**Tsunoda F:** Hekiso, Nihon penishirin monogatari. Tokyo, Shinchosha, Showa 53 nen. [1978]. 237 p.

**Tsvang RL:** Sovetskaia meditsina v gody Velikoĭ Otechestvennoĭ voĭny. **Feldsher Akush** 1984 May;49(5):3–7

**Tsvetkov VL:** Srednie meditsinskie rabotniki Orlovskoĭ gubernii v XIX veke. **Med Sestra** 1983 Oct;42(10):49–50

**Tsyb AF:** Nauchno-issledovatel'skomu institutu meditsinskoĭ radiologii AMN SSSR-20 let. **Med Radiol (Mosk)** 1982 Sep;27(9):3–12

**Tsybul'kin AG:** Vklad Konstantina Monakova v izuchenie anatomii mozga. **Arkh Anat Gistol Embriol** 1979 Nov;77(11):115–7

**Tuan C** see **Cho LJ**

**Tubesing DA:** Whole person health care: an idea in evolution. Hinsdale, Il., Wholistic Health Centers, Inc.: distributed by Society for Wholistic Medicine, 1977. 52 p.

**Tubiana M:** Effets à long terme observés chez les survivants des explosions d'Hiroshima et Nagasaki. Implications pour l'évaluation des risques d'un guerre atomique. **Bull Mem Acad R Med Belg** 1982;137(8–9):533–41

**Tucat D:** Les sages-femmes parisiennes à la fin du XIXe siècle. **Penelope** 1981;(5):58–61

**Tuchman LR:** The Mount Sinai Journal: past. **Mt Sinai J Med (NY)** 1984 Jan–Feb;51(1):i–iv

**Tucker EB:** James Jackson Putnam: an American perspective on the social uses of psychoanalysis, 1895–1918. **N Engl Q** 1978;51(4):527–46

**Tucker EL:** A new letter by Thomas Holley Chivers. **Ga Hist Q** 1971;55(4):582–8

**Tucker GS:** Ida Henrietta Hyde: the first woman member of the society. **Physiologist** 1981 Dec;24(6):1–9

**Tucker L:** Aspirin--more roles for America's most widely used drug. **Am Pharm** 1979 Dec;19(13):26–7

**Tucker RA:** History of sizing of genitourinary instruments. **Urology** 1982 Sep;20(3):346–9

**Tucker RC:** A case of mistaken identity: djugashvili-Stalin. **Biography** 1982;5(1):17–24

**Tucker WD** see **Richards P**

**Tucker WS:** Osler and sleep apnea. **Arch Intern Med** 1984 May;144(5):1085

**Tudor C:** Răscoala de la 1888. **Rev Arhiv** 1978;40(3):348–9

**Tuffanelli DL:** 'Clinical significance of autoantibodies in pemphigus' by Chorzelski, Von Weiss and Lever, May 1966. Commentary: Clinical importance of autoantibodies in pemphigus. **Arch Dermatol** 1982 Oct;118(10):837–45

**Tuft L:** Allergy Practice during the early years. **Ann Allergy** 1982 Oct;49(4):238–43

**Tulloch JL:** The last 50 years of smallpox in Africa. **WHO Chron** 1980 Nov;34(11):407–12

**Tumbling walls:** The evolution of a community institution over 150 years: 1833, Maryborough District Lunatic Asylum for King's and Queen's Counties, Westmeath and Longford: 1925, Portlaoghise District Mental Hospital: 1983, St. Fintan's Psychiatric Hospital, clinics and community service. Portlaoise, Laois: Midland Health Board at St. Fintan's Hospital, in association with Relay Publications, Tyone, Nenagh, Tipperary, Ireland, 1983. 105 p.

**Tumbridge JE:** Home-workplace separation in Kingston: the legal and medical professions – past, present and future. **Urban Hist Rev** 1982;11(1):11–6

**Tumbridge JE:** Separation of [the doctor's] residence from workplace: a Kingston example. **Urban Hist Rev** 1979;(3):23–32

**Tumendemberel T:** The present situation and the experiment of the primary medical assistance development in the Mongolian People's Republic. **Sante Publique (Bucar)** 1979;22(1):3–13

**Tuméngur Z** see **Rinchindorzh TS**

**Tunell DN:** A regional history of Southern Branch, American Public Health Association. Ed.D. Diss., University of Alabama. University, Alabama, 1977. xv, 694 leaves.

**Tunis B:** George Longmore. In Dictionary of Canadian biography, 1801 to 1820. Volume 5, 1983. p. 501–3.

**Tunis B:** Inoculation for smallpox in the Province of Quebec, a re-appraisal. In Roland CG, ed: Health, disease and medicine. Toronto, Hannah Institute for the History of Medicine, 1984. p. 171–93.

**Tunis B:** Medical education and medical licencing in Lower Canada. **Soc Hist (Canada)** 1981;14(27):67–91

**Tunis B:** Public vaccination in Lower Canada, 1815–1823: controversy and a dilemma. **Hist Reflect** 1982;9(1–2):264–78

**Turanov NM** see **Skripkin IuK**

**Turbón D** see **Campillo D**

**Turchetti Grossi ML** see **Libri e manoscritti di Haller, 1777–1977**

**Turchini J:** Die französischen Schulen im Mittelalter. In Sournia JC, Martiny M, Poulet J, ed: Illustrierte Geschichte der Medizin. Salzburg, Andreas, 1980. Vol. 2. p. 767–92.

**Turegano Lopez A** see **Muñoz Calvo S**

**Turek K:** Działalność weterynaryjna fizyków szczecińskich w XVIII i XIX wieku. **Arch Hist Med (Warsz)** 1980;43(4):407–13

**Turiaf J:** Laennec et la pathologie respiratoire. **Bull Acad Natl Med (Paris)** 1981 Feb 17;Spec No:31–6

**Turk JL, Allen E:** Bleeding and cupping. **Ann R Coll Surg Engl** 1983 Mar;65(2):128–31

**Turk JL** see **Allen E**

**Turkevich NM** see **Diadiusha GF**

**Turkle S:** 'Mon oncle de Marienbad: sociobiology comes to the land of the structuralists. **Contemp Fr Civiliz** 1981–82;6(1–2):67–87

**Turkle S:** Psychoanalytic politics: Freud's French Revolution. Cambridge, MIT Press, 1981, c1978. x, 278 p.

**Turner CG, Bird J:** Dentition of Chilean paleo-Indians and peopling of the Americas. **Science** 1981 May 29;212(4498):1053–5

**Turner D:** A lost seventeenth century demographic crisis? The evidence of two counties. **Local Popul Stud (Matlock)** 1978;(21):11–18

**Turner GL:** Antique scientific instruments. Poole, Dorset, Blandford, 1980. 168 p.

**Turner GL** see **Maison Nachet**

**Turner H:** Henry Wellcome: the man, his collection and his legacy. London, Heinemann for the Wellcome Trust, 1980. 96 p.

**Turner I, Turner TD:** Ymarfer Fferylliaeth Meddygon Myddfai (The pharmacy of the physicians of Myddfai. **Pharm Hist (London)** 1983 Jun;13(2):2–5

**Turner J:** Reckoning with the beast. Animals, pain, and humanity in the Victorian mind. Baltimore, London, Johns Hopkins University Press, 1980. xii, 190 p. (The Johns Hopkins University Studies in Historical and Political Science; 98th ser., no. 2).

**Turner JC:** Kindness to animals: The animal-protection movement in England and America during the 19th century. Ph.D. diss., Harvard University. Cambridge, 1976.

**Turner MA** see **Craig RB**

**Turner PJ, Holtom DB:** The use of a fabric softener in the reconstitution of mummified tissue prior to paraffin wax sectioning for light microscopical examination. **Stain Technol** 1981 Jan;56(1):35–8

**Turner T, Lane D:** One hundred years of small animal practice. **Vet Rec** 1982 Dec 4;111(23):519–23

**Turner TB:** Joseph Earle Moore. In Dictionary of American Biography, Suppl. 6, 1956–1960. p, 460–1, 1980.

**Turner TB:** Women in medicine--a historical perspective. **J Am Med Wom Assoc** 1981 Feb;36(2):33–7

**Turner TD** see **Turner I**

**Turner GL'E:** Essays on the history of the microscope. Oxford, Senecio, 1980. 245 p. (Reprint of the author's journal articles).

**Turner-Warwick M:** The British Thoracic Society. **Thorax** 1982 May;37(5):321–3

**Turpeinen O:** Die Sterblichkeit an Pocken, Masern und Keuchhusten in Finnland in den Jahren 1751 bis 1865. In Imhof AE, ed: Mensch und Gesundheit in der Geschichte. Husum, Matthiesen, 1980. p. 135–61.

**Turpeinen O:** Infant mortality in Finland 1749–1865. **Scand Econ Hist Rev** 1979;27(1):1–21,67

**Turpeinen O:** Les causes des fluctuations annuelles du taux de mortalité finlandais entre 1750 et 1806. **Ann Demogr Hist (Paris)** 1980;:287–96

**Turpeinen O:** Monthly mortality in Finland in 1751–1806. **Yearb Popul Res Finl** 1979;17:59–73

**Turpeinen O:** Mortalitetskrisen i Finland åren 1788--1791. **Hist Tidskr Finl** 1981;66(1):14–34

**Turtle A:** Collections of early psychological laboratory apparatus in North America. **Newsl Australas Assoc Hist Philos Sci** 1977–78;9:4–5

**Turunen S** see **Achté K**

**Turupanov NL:** K istorii organizatsii besplatnoĭ lechebnitsy v Vologde. **Sov Med** 1982;(9):120–2
**Tutzke D:** Das sächsische Medizinalwesen um die Wende vom 19. zum 20. Jahrhundert. **Z Gesamte Hyg** 1983 Sep;29(9):556–9
**Tutzke D:** Geschichte der Medizin. Berlin, VEB Verlag Volk und Gesundheit, 1983. 248 p.
**Tutzke D:** Möglichkeiten und Bedeutung quantifizierbarer Aussagen in der medizingeschichtlichen Forschung. In International Congress of the History of Medicine. 26th, Plovdiv, 1978. Actes du Congress. Sofia, 1981. Volume II. p. 209–10.
**Tutzke D** see **Schneck P**
**Tutzke D, ed:** Geschichte der Medizin. Berlin, VEB Verlag, 1980. 247 p. Beiträge Von G. Harig, I. Winter.
**Tutzke D, ed:** Zur Entwicklung der Sozialhygiene im 19. und 20. Jahrhundert. Ausgewählte Beiträge vom I. Medizinhistorischen Symposium DDR–UdSSR, Halle (Saale) 1975. Berlin, Akademie für Aerztliche Fortbildung der DDR; Gesellschaft für Geschichte der Medizin in der DDR, 1976, xi, 277 p.
**Tuzova RV** see **Goregliad KhS**
**Tweney RD:** Isaac Newton's two uses of hypothetical reasoning: dual influences on the history of psychology. **Stor Crit Psicol** 1980;1(2):235–59
**Twentyman LR:** The nature of homoeopathy. **R Soc Health J** 1982 Oct;102(5):221–5
**Twin SL:** Ethel Perrin. In: Notable American women. The modern period. Cambridge, Mass., Belknap–Harvard Univ. Press, 1980. 4:539–41.
**Two jubilees in psychotherapy: Br Med J** 1980 Jul 26;281(6235):256–7
**The two manias: Br J Psychiatry** 1981 Sep;139:258–61
**Twumasi PA:** A social history of the Ghanaian pluralistic medical system. **Soc Sci Med [Med Anthropol]** 1979 Dec;13B(4):349–56
**Twumasi PA:** Colonialism and international health: a study in social change in Ghana. **Soc Sci Med [Med Anthropol]** 1981 Apr;15B(2):147–51
**Twumasi PA:** History of pluralistic medical systems: a sociological analysis of the Ghanaian case. **Issue** 1979;9(3):29–34
**Tybout RA** see **Horstmanhoff HF, ed**
**Tybout RA** see **Horstmanhoff HF, et al**
**Tychý M** see **Ozorovský V**
**Tyklina IG, Vol'f MSh:** Iz istorii Moskovskoĭ gorodskoĭ klinicheskoĭ psikhiatricheskoĭ bol'nitsy im. P. B. Gannushkina. **Med Sestra** 1984 Jul;43(7):45–6
**Tyler FB** see **Gatz M**
**Tyler HR, Tyler KL:** Charles Edouard Brown-Séquard: professor of physiology and pathology of the nervous system at Harvard Medical School. **Neurology** 1984 Sep;34(9):1231–6
**Tyler KL:** Classics in neurology. Fragments of neurologic history: 'Tetanoid Chorea' and progressive lenticular degeneration. **Neurology** 1983 Apr;33(4):461–2
**Tyler KL, McHenry LC:** Fragments of neurological history: the knee jerk and other tendon reflexes. **Neurosci Behav Physiol** 1983 May;13(5):609–10
**Tyler KL:** Hughlings Jackson: the early development of his ideas on epilepsy. **J Hist Med Allied Sci** 1984 Jan;39(1):55–64
**Tyler KL** see **Tyler HR**
**Tyler L** see **Kokaska CJ**
**Tyler VE:** Damiana - history of a herbal hoax. **Pharm Hist** 1983;25(2):55–60
**Tyler VE:** The case of Victor A. Reko--an unrecognized pioneer writer on New World hallucinogens. **J Nat Prod** 1979 Sep–Oct;42(5):489–95
**Tyler VE:** Three proprietaries and their claim as American 'Indian' remedies. **Pharm Hist** 1984;26(3):146–9
**Tymorek S** see **Westerman MP**
**Tymowski M:** Famines et épidémies à Oualata et à Tichit au XIXe siècle. **Afr Bull** 1978;27:35–53
**Tyndall RM:** A history of the Bellevue School for midwives 1911–1936. Diss (Ed D), Columbia University. New York, 1978. xi, 260 p.
**Tyor PL, Bell LV:** Caring for the retarded in America: a history. Westport, Conn., Greenwood, 1984. 215 p. (Contributions in Medical History, no. 15)
**Tyor PL:** Henry Herbert Goddard. In Dictionary of American Biography, Suppl. 6, 1956–1960. p. 240–1, 1980.
**Tyor PL** see **Zainaldin JS**
**Tyroler HA** see **Ibrahim MA**
**Tyson RA, Alcauskas ES, ed:** Catalogue of the Hrdlička paleopathology collection. Foreword and glossary by S. L. Rogers. Descriptions by C. F. Merbs. San Diego, San Diego Museum of Man, 1980. xi, 359 p.
**Tyszkiewicz J, Widy-Tyszkiewicz E:** Czynniki kształtujace zdrowie Polsce XIII–XV w. **Kwart Hist Kultury Mater** 1976;24(2):205–15
**Tyszkiewicz J:** Uwagi o historii medycyny w Polsce. **Kwart Hist Kultury Mater** 1975;23(2):245–54
**Tyszkiewicz J, Widy-Tyszkiewicz E:** Zdrowie i choroby w Polsce XIII–XV w. **Kwart Hist Kultury Mater** 1976;24(1):55–73
**Tytell P:** La plume sur le divan. Psychanalyse et littérature en France. Paris, Aubier Montaigne, 1982. 326 p.
**Tzonis A:** Un 'Mémoire sur les hôpitaux' de Condorcet. **Dix-Huit Siecle** 1977;9:109–14

# U

**U istochnikov mirovoĭ i otechestvennoĭ istorii meditsiny: Sov Med** 1983;6:107–8
**U. S. Bureau of Radiological Health:** Legislative history of Radiation control for health and safety act of 1968. Bureau of Radiological Health; Washington: for sale by the Supt. of Docs., U. S. Govt. Print. Off., 1975. 2 v. (ix, 1494 p.).
**Ubelaker D** see **Morse D**
**Ubelaker DH, Jantz RL:** Plains Caddoan relationships: the view from craniometry and mortuary analysis. **Nebr Hist** 1979;60(2):249–59
**Ubelaker DH:** Skeletal evidence for kneeling in prehistoric Ecuador. **Am J Phys Anthropol** 1979 Nov;51(4):679–86
**Ubelaker DH:** The development of American paleopathology. In F. Spencer, ed: A history of American physical anthropology, 1930–1980. New York, Academic Press, 1982. p. 337–56.
**Ubrizsy in Savoia A:** I rapport fra Carolus Clusius ed i naturalisti italiani del suo tempo. **Physis** 1978;20(1–4):49–68
**Uche C:** The contexts of mortality in Nigeria. **Genus** 1981;37(1–2):123–35
**Uchibori C:** [History of national public health activities in the Gunma Prefecture. 2. Stimulating seminars] (Jpn). **Hokenfu Zasshi** 1982 Feb;38(2):148–50
**Uchibori C:** [Personal record of the government-operated public health nursing activities at Gunma Prefecture. 8. The era of post-war confusion] (Jpn). **Hokenfu Zasshi** 1983 Jan;39(1):38–9
**Uchibori C:** [Problems faced by public health nurses during World War II] (Jpn). **Hokenfu Zasshi** 1982 Aug;38(8):694–6
**Uchibori C:** [Public health nursing activities in Gunma Prefecture: a personal history. At the end of World War II] (Jpn). **Hokenfu Zasshi** 1982 Nov;38(11):924–6
**Uchibori C:** [Reflection on public health nursing retraining seminars immediately after the Second World War] (Jpn). **Hokenfu Zasshi** 1983 Apr;39(4):294–6
**Uchikawa K:** Dr. Shiro Oshima (1934–1981). **Acarologia** 1982 Jun;23(2):99–101
**Uddin Siddiqui T** see **Durrany KS**
**Uddinahmed R:** Single drugs mentioned by Avicenna for cardiac ailments in his canon and Kitab-Ul-Adwiyyah Qalbiyyah. **Bull Indian Inst Hist Med (Hyderabad)** 1979;9:46–66
**Udelhoven P:** Die klassischen Penizilline halten die Stellung. **Med Welt** 1983 Dec 9;34(49):3
**Ueda M, Usui K, Kawasaki S, et al:** [History of public health nurses associated with Osaka public health clinics: social health of the Meiji, Taisho, and Showa eras and the birth of public health nurses] (Jpn). **Hokenfu Zasshi** 1981 Apr;37(4):250–7
**Ueno T:** [In memory of Prof. Heizo Nakamura] (Jpn) **Dent Outlook** 1980;55(5):921–6
**Uerckwitz J:** Zur Geschichte der Hygiene an der Universität Rostock. **Z Gesamte Hyg** 1981 Jul 7;27(7):501–3
**Uesato G** see **Suyehiro H**
**Uglov FG, Afanas'eva AV:** Iustin Iulianovich Dzhanelidze (k 100–letiiu so dnia rozhdeniia). **Vestn Khir** 1983 Aug;131(8):131–4
**Uglov FG, Golovin GV, Dutkevich IG:** Sovetskaia khirurgiia za 60 let Soiuza Sovetskikh Sotsialisticheskikh Respublik. **Vestn Khir** 1982 Dec;129(12):3–10
**Ugulava SN** see **Lukavskiĭ MI**
**Uhlenberg P:** Death and the family. **J Fam Hist** 1980 Fall;5(3):313–20
**Uhrig J** see **Dawson P**
**Uiblein P:** Beziehungen der Wiener Medizin zur Universität Padua im Mittelalter. Mit einem Konsilium des Stadtarztes von Udine Jeremias de Simeonibus für Herzog Albrecht VI von Osterreich. **Rom Hist Mitt** 1981;23:271–301
**Ujhely GB:** Jungian approach to clinical practice. **ANA Publ** (NP-59):319–32, 1979
**Ulanova IP** see **Korbakova AI**
**Ulfelder H:** The stilbestrol disorders in historical perspective. **Cancer** 1980 Jun 15;45(12):3008–11
**Ulitskaia NIa:** Istoriia sovetskoiĭ ftiziatrii. **Med Sestra** 1979 Oct;38(10)):48–9
**Ullman AH:** Analytical chemists on postage stamps. **Anal Chem** 1982 Jun;54(7):780A–785A
**Ullmann C** see **Porkert M**
**Ullmann E:** Adolf Witzel--Leben und Werk. **Stomatol DDR** 1981 Jul;31(7):535–41
**Ullmann M:** Die arabische Ueberlieferung der Werke des Rufus von Ephesos. In: International Symposium for the History of Arabic Science, 1st, University of Aleppo, 1976. Proceedings. Aleppo, Syria, 1976. Papers in European Languages, Vol. II. p. 348–57
**Ullmann M:** Die Schrift des Rufus von Ephesos über die Gelbsucht in arabischer und lateinischer Ubersetzung. Göttingen, Vandenhoeck & Ruprecht, 1983. 87 p. (Abhandlungen der Akademie der Wissenschaften in Göttingen, Philologisch–Historische Klass; Folge 3, No. 138).
**Ullmann M:** Die Tadkira des ibn as-Suwaidi, eine wichtige Quelle zur Geschichte der griechisch-arabischen Medicin und Magie. **Islam** 1977;54:33–65
**Ullmann M** see **Kudlien F**
**Ullmann M, ed:** Rufus von Ephesos Krankenjournale. Wiesbaden, Harrassowitz, 1978. 128 p.
**Ulman E** see **Detre KC**
**Ulmer L:** Mental retardation: evolution of care. **J Miss State Med Assoc** 1984 Feb;25(2):31–5
**Ulrich J:** Revmatická horečka na Mostecku--kdysi a dnes. **Vnitr Lek** 1983 Dec;29(12):1176–82
**Ulrich-Bochsler L** see **Kloiber A**
**Ulrich-Bochsler S, Schäublin E, Zeltner TB, et al:** Invalidisierende Wirbelsäulenverkrümmung an einem Skelettfund aus dem Frühmittelalter (7./8. bis Anfang 9. Jh.). Ein Fall einer wahrscheinlichen Spondylitis tuberculosa. **Schweiz Med Wochenschr** 1982 Sep 18;112(38):1318–23
**Ulrich-Bochsler S, Glowatzki G:** Ossäre Folgezustände einer langzeitig

unbehandelten osteomyelitis. Fallbeschreibung an einem mittelalterlichen Skelett. **Anthropol Anz** 1982 Mar;40(1):1-18
**Ulrich-Bochsler S, Glowatzki G, Zeltner T:** Ossäre Folgezustände einer unbehandelten Osteomyelitis. **Praxis** 1981 Oct;70(43):1913-8
**Ulrich-Bochsler S** see **Kloiber A**
**Ulrich-Bochsler S** see **Roulet JF**
**Ulrich-Bochsler S** see **Wiederkehr M**
**Ulstein M** see **Bergsjø P**
**Ultmann JE** see **Streuli RA**
**Umanskaia VV** see **Komarov BD**
**Umoh JU, Belino ED:** Rabies in Nigeria. A historical review. **Int J Zoonoses** 1979 Jun;6(1):41-8
**Un secol de activitate de medicină preventivă la Institutul de Medicină şi Farmacie din Iaşi (1882-1982): Rev Med Chir Soc Med Nat Iasi** 1983 Oct-Dec;87(4):707-25
**Un siècle d'oto-rhino-laryngologie: J Fr Otorhinolaryngol** 1983 Feb;32(2):81-110 contd
**Unda F:** Acciones de saneamiento ambiental del Servicio Nacional de Salud, 1952-1957. **Rev Med Chil** 1977 Oct;105(10):714-23
**Underhill D:** Government health insurance: an analysis of division. **Mich J Polit Sci** 1981;1(1):26-38
**[Understanding of man in education:** (3). 'Dusk of a Hermit' by Pestalozzi] (Jpn).
**Underwood BJ:** Studies in learning and memory: selected papers. New York, Praeger, 1982. x, 331 p.
**Underwood EJ:** The contribution of H. W. Bennetts to the solution and control of animal disease problems in Western Australia. **Hist Rec Aust Sci** 1980;5(1):59-67
**Une lettre de Louis Jouvet à la veille d'entreprendre ses études de pharmacie: Rev Hist Pharm (Paris)** 1981 Jun;28(249):121-4
**Unger CW:** The old Goschenhoppen Lutheran burial register: 1752-1772. **Pa Folklife** 1967-68;17(2):32-5
**Unger RH** see **Robin ED, ed**
**Ungerer GA:** Wilhelm Wundt als Psychologe und Politiker: Anmerkungen zur Biographie. **Psychol Rundschau** 1980;31:99-110
**Ungerer GA** see **Bringmann WG**
**Ungerer GA** see **Brozek J**
**Ungethüm M, Kolb W:** Elektro-Osteo-Stimulation, Teil 1. Historische Entwicklung und 'Stimulations'-Hypothesen. **Biomed Tech (Berlin)** 1982 Jun;27(6):130-5
**Ungureanu EM:** Contribuţia Academicianului Mihai Ciucă pe plan naţional şi internaţional în domeniul combaterii malariei. **Rev Med Chir Soc Med Nat Iasi** 1983 Oct-Dec;87(4):729-30
**Ungvári G:** Ujabb adatok Gulácsy Lajos betegségéhez. **Orvostort Kozl** 1982;92(4):113-8
**Ungvári G** see **Pisztora F**
**The University of Iowa College of Dentistry.: Dent Radiogr Photogr** 1980;53(1):preceding 1, 19-20
**University of North Carolina at Chapel Hill School of Dentistry: Dent Radiogr Photogr** 1981;54(1):preceding 1, 19-20
**Unna PG:** An exemplary instance of faulty scholarship. **Am J Dermatopathol** 1983 Dec;5(6):569-75
**Unschuld PU:** Arzneimittelmissbrauch und heterodoxe Heiltätigkeit im kaiserlichen China; ausgewählte Materialien zu Gesetzgebung und Rechtsprechung. **Sudhoffs Arch** 1977;61(4):353-86
**Unschuld PU:** Concepts of illness in ancient China: the case of demonological medicine. **J Med Philos** 1980;5(2):117-32
**Unschuld PU:** Das Ch'uan-ya und die Praxis chinesischer Landärzte im 18. Jahrhundert. **Sudhoffs Arch** 1978;62(4):378-407
**Unschuld PU:** Die Bedeutung der Ma-wang-tui-Funde für die chinesische Medizin- und Pharmaziegeschichte. In Dilg P, et al., ed: Perspektiven der Pharmaziegeschichte. Graz, Austria, Akademische Druck- u. Verlagsanstalt, 1983. p. 389-416.
**Unschuld PU:** Ginseng und 'Kostendämpfung im Gesundheitswesen'. Beiträge zu einer Diskussion im China der Kaiserzeit. **Asiat Forsch** 1980;71:128-32
**Unschuld PU, Jaggi OP, Kao JJ, et al:** [History of medical ethics: South and East Asia]. In Reich WT, et al, ed: Encyclopedia of bioethics, v.3. New York, Free Press, 1978. p. 901-30.
**Unschuld PU:** Ma-wang-tui materia medica: a comparative analysis of early Chinese pharmaceutical knowledge. **Zinbun** 1982;:(18):11-63
**Unschuld PU:** Medical ethics in imperial China: a study in historical anthropology. Berkeley, University of California Press, 1979. viii, 141 p. (Comparative Studies of Health Systems and Medical Care, 2).
**Unschuld PU:** Medizin in China: eine Ideengeschichte. München, Beck, 1980. 335 p.
**Unschuld PU:** The Chinese reception of Indian medicine in the first millennium A.D. **Bull Hist Med** 1979 Fall;53(3):329-45
**Unschuld PU:** The issue of structured coexistence of scientific and alternative medical systems: a comparison of East and West German legislation. **Soc Sci Med [Med Anthropol]** 1980 Feb;14B(1):15-24
**Unseld S:** Versuch, die Welt besser zu bestehen. **Psyche (Stuttg)** 1983 Apr;37(4):311-21
**Unusual blood evidence in a homicide a century ago: Am J Forensic Med Pathol** 1982 Sep;3(3):231-9
**Unver AS:** Les épidémies de choléra dans les terres balkaniques aux XVIIIe et XIXe siècles. **Etud Balk** 1973:4:89-97
**Upadhya SD** see **Rai NP**
**Uphoff MJ, Uphoff WH, Lewis RK:** Group Health: an American success story in prepaid health care. Minneapolis, Dillon Press, 1980. xvii, 173 p.
**Uphoff WH** see **Uphoff MJ**
**Uragoda CG, Aloysius DJ, Lionel ND:** A history of the Sri Lanka Medical Library. **Ceylon Med J** 1982 Jun;27(2):49-65
**Uragoda CG:** History of opium in Sri Lanka. **Med Hist** 1983 Jan;27(1):69-76
**Uragoda CG:** Some historical aspects of dermatology in Sri Lanka. **Int J Dermatol** 1984 Jan-Feb;23(1):78-80
**Uragoda CG** see **De Silva A**
**Uranga E:** Un ilustre anatónomo y cirujano con ideas necrofílicas del siglo XIX en Zaragoza. **Bol Real Soc Vascongada Amigos Pais** 1973;29(1-3):375-91
**Urbain JD:** Les cimétières d'occident: des sociétés de conservation. **Etudes (Fr)** 1982;357(2-3):193-204
**Urban A:** Konspiracyjna działalnść dydaktyczna profesor Janiny Kowalczykowej w okresie okupacji 1939-1944. **Patol Pol** 1980 Apr-Jun;31(2):161-9
**Urban F:** Historie vzájemných styku českých a ruských lékařu. **Cas Lek Cesk** 1984 Aug 17;123(33):1037
**Urbanek B:** Godzina W na Ochocie. **Pieleg Polozna** 1979;(8):25-6
**Urbanek B:** Z konspiracyjnej działalności sanitariuszek i pielęgniarek w okupowanej Warszawie. **Przegl Lek** 1980;37(1):137-41
**Urbani E** see **Epistemologia, metodologia clinica e storia della scienza medica, 2**
**Urbanová O** see **Krahulec I**
**Urge L** see **Linkesch W**
**Urmson WJ** see **Geerts A**
**Urquijo y Goitia JR de:** Madrid ante la epidemia de cólera de 1854-56. **Asclepio** 1983;35:27-51
**Urschel HC:** 'Life is short and the art long, the occasion instant, the experiment perilous, the decision difficult'. **Ann Thorac Surg** 1984 Jul;38(1):1-14
**Urzais Jimenez C:** Reseña historica de la enseñanza medica en Yucatan. **Bol Soc Mex Hist Filos Med** 1984 Dec;7(49):417-30
**Urzúa Merion H:** Estructuración inicial del Servicio Nacional de Salud. **Rev Med Chil** 1977 Oct;105(10):659-62
**Usbeck W:** 25 Jahre Medizinische Akademie Erfurt -- ihre Traditionen und ihr Weg. Begrüssungsansprache anlässlich der 12. Erfurter Konferenz über Hämostase und Thrombose. **Folia Haematol (Leipz)** 1979;106(5-6):653-5
**Uschmann G:** Haeckel's biological materialism. **Hist Philos Life Sci** 1979;1(1):101-18
**Uselding P:** In dispraise of the muckrakers: United States occupational mortality, 1890-1910. **Res Econ Hist** 1976;1:334-71
**Ushida N:** Etude comparative de la psychologie d'Aristote, d'Avicenne et de St. Thomas d'Aquin. Tokyo, Keio Institute of Cultural and Linguistic Studies, 1968. vi, 231 p. (Studies in the humanities and social relations; v. 11.).
**Ushmarov AK** see **Garmash VIa**
**Uslar D v.** see **Hasler L, ed**
**Usmanova RA:** Fiziologiia pishchevareniia v trudakh Ibn Siny. **Fiziol Zh SSSR** 1980 Sep;66(9):1424-8
**Usmanova RA:** Ibn Sina o Kostnoĭ i myshechnoĭ sisteme. **Arkh Anat Gistol Embriol** 1980 Sep;79(9):112-4
**Usov IN:** Belorusskomu nauchnomu obschchestvu detskikh vracheĭ 50 let. **Pediatriia** 1983 Nov;(11):72-4
**Usovich AK** see **Ibragimova ZI**
**Uspenskaia EP:** Mikhail Vasil'evich Chernorutskiĭ (k 100-letiiu so dnia rozhdeniia). **Ter Arkh** 1984;56(7):151-3
**Ustav zdravotní výchovy:** 20 years of health education in the Czech Socialist Republic. Prague, Institute of Health Education, 1973. 31 p.
**Ustinovich AK:** 50-letie Belorusskogo nauchno-issledovatel'skogo instituta okhrany materinstva i detstva. **Pediatriia** 1982 Jul;(7):74-6
**Ustrell Torrent JM:** El balneario de Vallfogona de Riucorb. **Asclepio** 1980;32:467-84
**Usui H** see **Yumaki M**
**Usui K** see **Ueda M**
**Usui T, Kodama K:** [At completion of the translation of the 'Notes on Lying-in Institutions'. A discussion] (Jpn) **Sogo Kango** 1984 Aug 15;19(3):79-91
**Usui T:** [The influence of Nightingale on my nursing activities] (Jpn) **Sogo Kango** 1980;15(4):37-45
**Uszkiewiczowa L:** Działalność profesora Stanisława Batawii w dziedzinie psychiatrii sądowej. **Psychiatr Pol** 1979 Sep-Oct;13(5):441-3
**Utevskaia LA** see **Nikitin VN**
**Utevskiĭ LA** see **Nikitin VN**
**Utrilla PN:** Lactancia mercenaria: otra expresion de la doble moral burguesa. **Asclepio** 1982;34:33-70
**Utterback N** see **McDonald MO**
**Utvic V** see **Sterijev K**
**Uvnäs B:** From physiologist to pharmacologist--promotion or degradation? Fifty years in retrospect. **Annu Rev Pharmacol Toxicol** 1984;24:1-18
**Uyer G:** Nursing education in Turkey: past and present. **Int J Nurs Stud** 1984;21(3):209-19
**Uzawa Y, Hanajima T:** [Modern nursing education observed in nursing text books-from 'Kongo Kokoroe' dated 1877 to those published by the end of World War II] (Jpn). **Kango Kyoiku** 1982 Sep;23(9):544-54
**Uzawa Y** see **Ishigaki Y**
**Uzawa Y** see **Kishi Y**
**Uzawa Y** see **Tanaka K**
**Uzhanskiĭ IaG:** K mekhanizmu stimuliatsii funksiĭ i regeneratsii kletok i tkaneĭ po A. A. Bogomol'tsa. **Fiziol Zh** 1981 May-Jun;27(3):322-6
**Uzhanskiĭ IaG:** K nauchno-literaturnomu nasledstvu akademika Aleksandra

Aleksandrovicha Bogomol'tsa (ob osobennostiakh pis'ma akademika A. A. Bogomol'tsa v nauchnykh trudakh). **Patol Fiziol Eksp Ter** 1981 Mar–Apr;(2):16–20

## V

**V. I. Lenin or razvitii fizicheskoĭ kul'tury i sporta: Voen Med Zh** 1980 Mar;(3):8–10

**V. I. Lenin'i stanovlenie sanatorno-kurortnogo dela v nasheĭ strane: Voen Med Zh** 1980 Fev;(2):7–9

**Vaccarezza RF:** Devoción a la causa de la salud: Fred Lower Soper. **Medicina (B Aires)** 1981;41(1):101–6

**Vacek Z:** Fakulta všeobechného lékařství současnosti. **Cas Lek Cesk** 1983 Oct 14;122(41):1265–8

**Vachon A:** Marguerite Dizy. In Dictionary of Canadian biography, 1701 to 1740. Volume 2, 1969. p. 189–90.

**Vacola G, Gayda M, Pélicier Y:** Philocalie d'une prière orthodoxe, aspects psycho-physiologiques. **Ann Med Psychol (Paris)** 1984 Mar;142(3):416–22

**Vadász I** see **Németh T**

**Vader JP:** August Forel defends the persecuted Persian Baha'is, 1925–27. **Gesnerus** 1984;41(1/2):53–60

**Vaeth JM:** Historical aspects of tylectomy and radiation therapy in the treatment of cancer of the breast. **Front Radiat Ther Oncol** 1983;17:1–10

**Vaeth JM:** Role of the pharmacist in cancer care throughout history. **Front Radiat Ther Oncol** 1980;15:1–4

**Vager EV** see **Strukov AI**

**Vagniluca G:** Epistemologia e psichiatria (II). **Sapienza** 1981;34(3):310–27

**Vago C** see **Delaunay A, ed**

**Vague J:** Die Geschichte der Endokrinologie bis zum Zweiten Weltkrieg. In Sournia JC, Martiny M, Poulet J, ed: Illustrierte Geschichte der Medizin. Salzburg, Andreas, 1980. Vol. 7. p. 2749–70.

**Vague J:** Geschichte der Endokrinologie nach dem Zweiten Weltkrieg. In Sournia JC, Martiny M, Poulet J, ed: Illustrierte Geschichte der Medizin. Salzburg, Andreas, 1980. Vol. 8. p. 3141–79.

**Vahey T, Brown D:** Comely Wenuhotep: computed tomography of an Egyptian mummy. **J Comput Assist Tomogr** 1984 Oct;8(5):992–7

**Vahiduddin S:** Body and soul. **Stud Philos Med** 1977 Mar;1(1):22–30

**Vahlquist B** see **Nordbring F**

**Vaĭl' SS:** M.M.Rudnev--odin iz osnovopolozhnikov otechestvennoĭ patologicheskoĭ anatomii (k 100-letiiu so dnia smerti). **Klin Med (Mosk)** 1979 Jul;57(7):107–10

**Vaillant JM** see **Bonneau E**

**Vaillant P** see **Guillemain B**

**Vainio K:** History of surgery of rheumatoid arthritis in Europe. **Scand J Rheumatol** 1983;12(2):65–8

**Vaĭnrub EM** see **Shandala MG**

**Vajda G:** La structure du corps humain d'après le commentaire de Dunash ben Tamin sur le 'Livre de la Création'. **J Semit Stud** 1978;23(1):88–94

**Vakhidov VV:** K 1000-letiiu Avitsenny. **Khirurgiia (Mosk)** 1980 Jul;(7):110–4

**Vaksman IA, Popugaĭlo VM:** Istoriia anesteziologii i reanimatsii v filatelii. **Anesteziol Reanimatol** 1984 Mar–Apr;(2):75–7

**Vaksman IA, Popugaĭlo VM:** Zhenshchiny mediki na pochtovykh markakh mira. **Feldsher Akush** 1984 Jul;49(7):38–43

**Valatkene R:** Kaunasskoe meditsinskoe uchilishche im. P. Mazhilisa. **Med Sestra** 1981 Apr;40(4):55–6

**Valcárcel M** see **Sifontes JE**

**Valderas JM:** Vuelve el lamarckismo? **Folia Hum (Barc)** 1981;19(216):57–65

**Valdés LM:** Ensayo sobre política de población 1970–1980 (planificación familiar). **Demogr Econ** 1980;14(4):467–80

**Valdez FM:** [Perspectives on Philippine nursing] (Jpn). **Kango** 1984 Jul;36(8):50–7

**Valdiserri RO:** Menstruation and medical theory: an historical overview. **J Am Med Wom Assoc** 1983 May–Jun;38(3):66–70

**Valdivia Ponce O:** Bases dinámicas de la psicoterapia tradicional. **Rev Neuropsiquiatr** 1979 Mar;42(1):31–46

**Valdivieso R:** La ley de medicina curativa para empleados y el Formulario Nacional de Medicamentos. **Rev Med Chil** 1977 Oct;105(10):663–7

**Válek A:** Ceskoslovenské nefrologické společnosti je dvacet let. **Cas Lek Cesk** 1982 May 7;121(18):568–71

**Válek A, Wing AJ:** Development of dialysis and transplant activity in the world during the seventies of the 20th century. **Z Exp Chir Transplant Kunstliche Organe** 1984;17(2):69–78

**Valencia-Parparcen J:** Cirrosis hepática. **GEN** 1981 Jan–Jun;35(1–2):43–97

**Valencia-Villa H:** Derecho y aborto: una relación de poder. **Cuad Filos Let** 1980;3(2):79–84

**Valenciano Gayá L:** Cajal (recuerdos y reflexiones de uno de sus últimos alumnos). **Arch Neurobiol (Madr)** 1983 Jul–Aug;46(4):272–81

**Valenciano Gayá L:** El Doctor Lafora y su época. Madrid, Morata, 1977. 226 p.

**Valenčik J** see **Blaták F**

**Valenkevich LN** see **Timofeeva GA**

**Valenstein AF:** Insight as an embedded concept in the early historical phase of psychoanalysis. **Psychoanal Study Child** 1981;36:307–15

**Valente V** see **Guidetti B**

**Valenti R:** Ongyilkosságok Budapesten 1881–82-ben. Egykorú boncjegyzőkönyvek összehasonlító vizsgálata. **Morphol Igazsagugyi Orv Sz** 1982 Jan;22(1):67–70

**Valentin F:** Wandel und Strukturveränderungen im Bereich der Inneren Medizin. **Internist (Berlin)** 1980 Apr;21(4):21–4

**Valentin H** see **Hollmann W**

**Valentin M:** Geschichte der Arbeitsmedizin. In Sournia JC, Martiny M, Poulet J, ed: Illustrierte Geschichte der Medizin. Salzburg, Andreas, 1980. Vol. 7. p. 2431–57.

**Valentin M, Niaussat PM:** Le rôle fondamental d'Amédée Lefèvre, médecin de la Marine (1798–1869), en médecine du travail et en histoire de la médecine. **Hist Sci Med** 1979;13(4):407–17

**Valentin M:** Louis-René Villermé (1782–1863); aperçu biographique. **Hist Sci Med** 1982;16(4):289–304

**Valentin M:** Travail des hommes et savants oubliés: histoire de la médecine du travail, de la sécurité: et l'ergonomie. [Paris], DOCIS, 1978. xi, 329 p.

**Valentin M** see **Monod H**

**Valentin M** see **Penneau D**

**Valentin M** see **Plessis JL**

**Valentin P:** Mit Brevier und Skalpell. Legendäre Bauchoperation Kaiser Heinrichs II. **Med Welt** 1982 Feb 19;33(7):260–2

**Valentin R:** Die Krankenbataillone. Sonderformationen der deutschen Wehrmacht im zweiten Weltkrieg. Düsseldorf, Droste, 1981. 250 p. (Schriftenreihe Erfahrungen des deutschen Sanitätsdienstes im zweiten Weltkrieg, 2).

**Valentine Mott: Surgery** 1979 Dec;86(6):906–7

**Valera Candel M** see **Marset Campos P**

**Valette G:** Allocution du Président de l'Académie Nationale de Médecine. **Bull Acad Natl Med (Paris)** 1980 Dec;164(9):801–4

**Valette G:** Auto-expérimentation en pharmacologie. **Bull Ordre Natl Pharm** 1978 Dec;217;1609–30

**Valette G:** Die Pharmakologie bei den Griechen und Römern. In Sournia JC, Martiny M, Poulet J, ed: Illustrierte Geschichte der Medizin. Salzburg, Andreas, 1980. Vol. 2. p. 496–521.

**Valette G:** Die pharmazeutische Lehre bei den mesopotamischen Völkern. In Sournia JC, Martiny M, Poulet J, ed: Illustrierte Geschichte der Medizin. Salzburg, Andreas, 1980. Vol. 2. p. 473–8.

**Valette S:** Die Pharmakologie im alten Agypten. In Sournia JC, Martiny M, Poulet J, ed: Illustrierte Geschichte der Medizin. Salzburg, Andreas, 1980. Vol. 2. p. 479–95.

**Valette S:** L'histoire de la pharmacie en France au XIXe siécle. In: Vorträge des Internationalen Pharmaziehistorischen Kongresses Innsbruck 1977. Stuttgart, Wissenschaftliche Verlagsgesellschaft, 1979. p. 73–80.

**Valette G, et al:** Centenaire de la mort de Paul Broca (1824–1880). **Bull Acad Natl Med (Paris)** 1980;164:535–62

**Valishin ES:** Aleksandr Grigor'evich Korotkov (K 60-letiiu so dnia Rozhdeniia). **Arkh Anat Gistol Embriol** 1981 May;80(5):122–5

**Valishin ES** see **Korotkov AG**

**Valla JP:** L'oeuvre psychothérapeutique de Déjerine. **Inf Psychiatr** 1978 Feb;54(2):171–8

**Vallaszky D:** Adatok Wallaszkay János, Pest város föorvosa életéhez. **Orvostort Kozl** 1979;87–88(25 no 1–2):249–53

**Vallat F:** Histoire de l'illustration dans l'anatomie vétérinaire française. Bayeux, Bayeusaine, 1973. 157 p.

**Vallaud D:** Infanticide et folie au XIX siècle. **Penelope** 1983;(8):51–3

**Valle AR** see **Valle RK**

**Valle RK, Valle AR:** La disertacion fisico-médica en la qual se prescribe un método seguro para preservar a los pueblos de viruelas hasta lograr la completa extincion de ellas en todo el reyno, by Dr. Francisco Gil. In International Congress of the History of Medicine, 27th, Barcelona, 1980. Actas. Barcelona, Académia de Ciències Médiques de Catalunya i Balears, 1981. p. 217–22.

**Valle RK, Valle AR:** Medicine and health among the Alta California mission Indians (1769–1834). In: Congrès international d'histoire de la médecine, XXVe, Québec, 1976. Actes. Québec, 1977., p. 1374–81.

**Vallee BL:** Metallothionein: historical review and perspectives. **Experientia [Suppl]** 1979;34:19–39

**Vallin J:** Tendances récentes de la mortalité française. **Population** 1983;38(1):77–105

**Vallin J** see **Nizard A**

**Vallin P** see **Dupâquier J**

**Vally G:** Ludovic cel stăruitor si misterioasa sa moarte. **Mag Istor** 1976;10(10):52–4

**Valtchev A** see **Hadjioloff A**

**Valtz A** see **Martinetto P**

**Valverde JL, Sánchez F, Vinuesa L:** Algunas consideraciones sobre la creación del empleo de boticario inspector de medicinas de la Armada. In International Congress of the History of Medicine, 27th, Barcelona, 1980. Actas. Barcelona, Académia de Ciències Médiques de Catalunya i Balears, 1981. p. 426–31.

**Valverde JL, Arrebola Nacle P:** Ayuda sanitaria de Felipe II a Francia. **Bol Soc Esp Hist Farm** 1982 Mar;33(130):123–9

**Valverde JL, Sánchez F, Vinuesa L:** Controversias jurisdiccionales del Protomedicato castellano. **Asclepio** 1978–79;30–31:403–23

**Valverde JL, Hidalgo J:** Documentos medicofarmaceuticos conservados en archivos de Sevilla. Salamanca, 1971. 120 p. (Cuadernos de Historia de la Medicina Española, Monografias, 17).

**Valverde JL, Sánchez Tellez MC:** Dos boticarios reales de origen frances del siglo XVII. **Ars Pharm** 1979;20:309–27

**Valverde JL, Munoz CP, ed:** El Formulario de los hospitales De Ibn Abi L-bayan. Introduccion, traduccion espanola y commentarios, con glosarios. Granada, Universidad de Granada, 1981. 256 p. (Cuadernos de historia de la farmacia, 8).

**Valverde JL, Peña Muñoz C:** El formulario de los hospitales' de Ibn Abi l-Bayan (S. XIII). In International Congress of the History of Medicine, 27th, Barcelona, 1980. Actas. Barcelona, Académia de Ciències Médiques

de Catalunya i Balears, 1981. p. 346–51.
**Valverde JL, Alvarez C, Suñé JM:** El primer 'Libro de botica' escrito en la España musulmana. **Bol Soc Esp Hist Farm** 1971 Jun;22(86):49–53
**Valverde JL, Bautista Méndez JL:** Estudio del 'Formulario medicinal de embarco para uso de los cirujanos de la Armada durante la navegación' de 1789. In International Congress of the History of Medicine, 27th, Barcelona, 1980. Actas. Barcelona, Acadèmia de Ciències Mèdiques de Catalunya i Balears, 1981. p. 420–5.
**Valverde JL, Peña-Muñoz C:** Ibn al-Hassa: Glosario sobre el 'Mansuri' de Razi. **Ars Pharm** 1980;21:317–32
**Valverde JL, Pena Muñoz C:** Ibn Al-Hašša Glosario sobre el Mansuri de Razi. **Ars Pharm** 1980;21(4):495–506
**Valverde JL, Sanchez Tellez MC:** Inventario de todos los efectos de la Botica del Monasterio de la Cartuja del Paular (1811). **Bol Soc Esp Hist Farm** 1980 Mar–Jun;31(121–2):51–67
**Valverde JL, Bautista Mendez MT, De Vinuesa FS:** La biblioteca de la Real Botica en 1816. **Bol Soc Esp Hist Farm** 1981 Jun;32(126):65–89
**Valverde JL, Bautista Mendez T:** La evolucion de las formas farmaceuticos a traves de textos españoles. II. Ungüentos. **Ars Pharm** 1980;21:291–315
**Valverde JL, Pérez Romero JA:** La sanidad en Navarra contemplada a través del hospital general de Pamplona en los siglos XVI al XVII. In International Congress of the History of Medicine, 27th, Barcelona, 1980. Actas. Barcelona, Acadèmia de Ciències Mèdiques de Catalunya i Balears, 1981. p. 636–43.
**Valverde JL, Lopez Andujar G:** Las disposiciones legales sobre el certificado de 'Limpieza de sangre' en relación al ejercicio profesional farmacéutico. **Bol Soc Esp Hist Farm** 1980 Oct;31(123):259–71
**Valverde JL, Bautista T, Montaña MT:** Libros de interés histórico-médico-farmaceútico conservados en la Biblioteca de la Real Academia de Medicina de Sevilla. Granada, Universidad de Granada, 1980. 130 p. (Cuadernos de Historia de la Farmacia, 6).
**Valverde JL, Sanchez L. De Vinuesa F:** Los inspectores de medicinas de la Armada en el siglo XVIII. **Bol Soc Esp Hist Farm** 1980 Oct;31(123):191–203
**Valverde JL, Arrebola Nacle P:** Los servicios farmacéuticos des los presidios menores de Africa. In International Congress of the History of Medicine, 27th, Barcelona, 1980. Actas. Barcelona, Acadèmia de Ciències Mèdiques de Catalunya i Balears, 1981. p. 644–9.
**Valverde JL, Martín Martín C:** Nuevas aportaciones al estudio del Tribunal del Real Protomedicato en México. In International Congress of the History of Medicine, 27th, Barcelona, 1980. Actas. Barcelona, Acadèmia de Ciències Mèdiques de Catalunya i Balears, 1981. p. 223–9.
**Valverde JL, Vinuesa SL de:** Panoramica legal de la introduccion de remedios quimicos en Navarra. **Llull (Spain)** 1978;2:81–94
**Valverde JL, Perez Romero JA:** Remedios secretos: expedientes de autorización en España en el siglo XVIII. **Bol Soc Esp Hist Farm** 1980 Mar–Jun;31(121–2):7–20
**Valverde JL, Martin C:** Situacion de los boticarios cubanos en sus relaciones con el Tribunal del Protomedicato S. XVIII. **Bol Soc Esp Hist Farm** 1982 Mar;33(129):3–7
**Valverde JL** see **Sanchez Tellez MC**
**Valverde López JL:** Estudio sobre los fueros y privilegios del Antiguo Colegio de Apotecarios de Valencia. [Granada], Universidad de Granada, 1979. 90 p.
**Valverde Lopez JL, Sanchez F, Vinuesa L, et al:** La dotacion de medicamentos en los buques de la Armada durante los siglos XVII y XVIII. Granada, Universidad de Granada, 1979. 60 [47] p.
**Valverde Lopez JL:** La experimentacion farmacologica sobre drogas americanas. (Discurso de ingreso, Academico Correspondiente Electo, 17 de marzo 1981.) Barcelona, Real Academia De Farmacia, 1981. 42 p.
**Valverde López JL, Vidal Casero MC:** Notas sobre médicos y cirujanos que trabajaron para el Jardín Botánico de Madrid. In International Congress of the History of Medicine, 27th, Barcelona, 1980. Actas. Barcelona, Acadèmia de Ciències Mèdiques de Catalunya i Balears, 1981. p. 650–5.
**Valvo JR, Cos LR, Cockett AT:** Giovanni Battista Morgagni: his contributions to urology. **Urology** 1983 Oct;22(4):452–7
**Van Cittert-Eymers JG** see **Van der Leun C, ed:**
**Van de Walle E** see **Dupâquier J**
**Van Driel Krol M** see **Quinn S, ed**
**Van Herwaarden J** see **Arts en sameleving. Medical history contributions by H. W. Pleket, J. Van Herwaarden, W. Frijhoff, C. Offringa, M. J. Van Lieburg, C. Bakker-Van der Kooij**
**Van Kampen NG** see **Van der Leun C, ed:**
**Van Lieburg MJ** see **Arts en sameleving. Medical history contributions by H. W. Pleket, J. Van Herwaarden, W. Frijhoff, C. Offringa, M. J. Van Lieburg, C. Bakker-Van der Kooij**
**Van Allen MW:** Landmark perspective: introduction of sodium diphenyl hydantoinate. **JAMA** 1984 Feb 24;251(8):1068–9
**Van Bekkum JG:** 75 jaar C. D. I. Ter introduktie. **Tijdschr Diergeneeskd** 1980 Aug 15;105(16):631–5
**Van Buren J:** Louisa May Alcott: a study in persona and idealization. **Psychohist Rev** 1981;9(4):282–99
**Van Buskirk EL:** Fort Wayne College of Medicine. Includes The practice of medicine in the Fort Wayne area written in 1889 by B. S. Woodworth. **Indiana Med Hist Q** 1977;3(2):4–6
**Van Buskirk EL:** The Fort Wayne Medical Schools 1876–1905 and the Union with Purdue University. **Indiana Med Hist Q** 1976 Summer;3(1):55–66
**Van Buyten L:** Drie 'doopregisters' van de Leuvense vondelingen (1745–1797). **Ann Soc Belg Hist Hop** 1979;17:31–69
**Vance G:** Nursing administration. **Aust Nurses J** 1983 Mar;12(1):12–4
**Vance G:** Reflections of nurse training. **Australas Nurses J** 1983 Jan–Feb;11(12):26–30
**Van Cittert-Eymers JG:** Joseph Mozes Son (1818–1884), een illuster tandmeester te Utrecht. **Tijdschr Geschied Geneeskd** 1978;2(2):62–9
**Vandam L, Volpitto PP:** The Genesis of contemporary American anesthesiology. Springfield, Thomas, 1982. xvi, 246 p.
**Vandam LD:** Anesthesiologists as clinicians. **Anesthesiology** 1980 Jul;53(1):40–8
**Vandam LD, Abbott JA:** Edward Gilbert Abbott: enigmatic figure of the ether demonstration. **N Engl J Med** 1984 Oct 11;311(15):991–4
**Vandam LD:** Impressions of anesthetics past. **Transplant Proc** 1981 Mar;13(1):61–4
**Vandam LD:** Intravenous anesthesia--history, currency, prospects. **Mt Sinai J Med (NY)** 1983 Jul–Aug;50(4):316–22
**Vandam LD:** Robert Hinckley's 'The First operation with ether'. **Anesthesiology** 1980 Jan;52(1):62–70
**Vande Kemp H:** The dream in periodical literature: 1860–1910. **J Hist Behav Sci** 1981 Jan;17(1):88–113
**Van de Walle E:** Motivation and technology in the decline of French fertility. In R. Wheaton, T. K. Hareven, ed: Family and sexuality in French history. Philadelphia, University of Pennsylvania Press, 1980. p. 135–78.
**Van de Walle E** see **Knodel J**
**Van den Nieuwenhuizen J:** Oorkondenboek van het Sint-Elizabeth-ospitaal te Antwerpen (1226–1355). Brussel, Paleis der Academiën, 1976. 414 p. (Koninklijke Commissie voor Geschiedenis).
**Vandenbroeke C:** De medische konsumptie sinds de 16e eeuw. **Handel Maatsch Geschied Oudheidk Gent** 1980;34:143–65
**Vandenbroeke C, Van Poppel F, Van Der Woude AM:** Le développement séculaire de la mortalité aux jeunes âges dans le territoire du Bénélux. **Ann Demogr Hist (Paris)** 1983;:257–89
**Vandenbroeke C:** Seksualiteit en huwelijksbeleving in Vlaanderen. **Spiegel Hist** 1979;14(7–8):425–33
**Vandenbroeke C:** Zuigelingensterfte, bevallingsstoornissen en kraambedsterfte (17–19de eeuw). **Bijdr Geschied Geneeskd** 1977;60:133–63
**Vander AJ** see **Cook HJ**
**Vander AJ** see **Steneck NH**
**Vander Elst E:** Die Geschichte der Orthopädie und der Traumatologie. In Sournia JC, Martiny M, Poulet J, ed: Illustrierte Geschichte der Medizin. Salzburg, Andreas, 1980. Vol. 5. p. 1655–1721.
**Van der Esch P:** Geschiedenis van het Staatstoezicht op Krankzinningen. 's-Gravenhage, Ministerium van Volksgezondheit en Milieuhygiene, 1975–1980. 3 volumes in 1.
**Van der Haegen H, De Vos R:** De cholera-epidemie te Leuven in 1849. **Driemaand Tijdschr Gemeentekrediet Belg** 1980;:197–210
**Van der Hammen L:** Type-concept, higher classification and evolution. **Acta Biotheor (Leiden)** 1981;30(1):3–48
**Van der Horst K:** Inventaire de la correspondance de Caspar Barlaeus (1602–1648). Assen, Van Gorcum, 1978. 214 p.
**Van der Horst PW:** Aelius Aristides and the New Testament. Leiden, E. J. Brill, 1980. ix, 115 p. (Studia ad Corpus Hellenisticum Novi Testamenti. Volumen Sextum.)
**Van der Kloot W:** Otto Loewi. In Dictionary of American biography, 1961–1965. Suppl. 7, 1981. p. 475–7.
**Van der Korst JK:** Bataafse geneeskunde in periodiek perspectief; in- en uitwendige historische aspecten van het Geneeskundig Magazijn (1801–1815). **Ned Tijdschr Geneeskd** 1981 Nov 28;125(48):1975–9
**Van der Korst JK:** Geneeskunde in de eerste internationale geleerdentijdschriften van Nederlandse origine (1680–1709). **Ned Tijdschr Geneeskd** 1981 Feb 28;125(9):355–60
**Van der Leun C, ed::** NG 200 – Natuurkundig Gezelschap te Utrecht 1777–1977. Utrecht, Natuurkundig Gezelschap te Utrecht, 1977. 143 p. With contributions by R. Hooykaas, J.G. van Cittert-Eymers, H.A.M. Snelders, N.G. van Kampen, P.H. Kylstra.
**Van der May-de Leur AP:** Moderne pelgrimage: Sint Elisabeth-expositie Marburg 1981. **Tijdschr Ziekenverpl** 1982 Feb 2;35(3):83–6
**Van der Molen HR:** Hommage à Jan ven Limborgh (1900–1984). **Phlebologie** 1984 Jul–Sep;37(3):XXV–XXXI
**Van der Molen HR:** Le développement de la phlébologie au cours des 30 dernières années (1948–1978). **Phlebologie** 1981 Jul–Sep;34(3):313–32
**Van der Peet R:** Florence Nightingale en haar visie op verplegen in relatie tot het leven en werk van Charles Darwin. **Tijdschr Ziekenverpl** 1983 Aug 23;36(17):530–6
**Van der Post L:** Jung and the story of our time. New York, Vintage Books, 1977. 276 p.
**Van der Sluis I:** Het recht om grootmoeder te doden. Korte geschiedenis van de euthanasiebeweging sinds 1870. Amsterdam, Buijten & Schipperheijn, 1977. 90 p.
**Van der Star P, ed:** Fahrenheit's letters to Leibniz and Boerhaave. Amsterdam, Rodopi, 1983. 195 p. (Nieuwe Nederlandse bijdragen tot de geschiedenis der geneeskunde en der natuurwetenschappen, no. 10).
**van der Veer R** see **van Ijzendoorn MH**
**Van der Woude AM:** Population developments in the Northern Netherlands (1500–1800) and the validity of the 'urban graveyard' effect. **Ann Demogr Hist (Paris)** 1982;:55–75
**Van Der Woude AM** see **Vandenbroeke C**
**Vanderbilt's history of nutrition collection bookplate: Nutr Hist Notes** 1979;5:2–7

**Vanderbilt's influence on world nutrition: Nutr Hist Notes** 1980;8:2–5; 1980;9:3–8; 1981;10:4–6

**Vanderdonck R:** De ontwikkeling van de tandheelkunde aan de RUG sinds 1930. **Rev Belge Med Dent** 1981;36(3):115–9

**VanderKuijp LW:** An index to Tibeto-Mongolian Materia Medica. **Can-Mong Rev** 1975;1(2):15–46

**Vanderpool HY:** Dominant health concerns in Protestantism. In Reich WT, et al, ed: Encyclopedia of bioethics, v.3. New York, Free Press, 1978. p. 1373–8.

**Vanderpool HY:** Miracle and faith healing. In Reich WT, et al, ed: Encyclopedia of bioethics, v.3. New York, Free Press, 1978. p. 1120–5.

**VanDeventer AD** see **Collins WE**

**Vandewiele LJ:** De realisaties van de Belgische apotekers in de 19e eeuw. **Sartonia** 1979 Mar;42:16–44

**Vandewiele LJ:** De ruime bijdrage van de Nederlandstalige botanisten op het gebied van de geneeskundige kruidenleer voor 1600. **Farm Tijdschr Belg** 1980;57:441–7

**Vandewiele LJ:** Een recept met gezegende distel uit Sint-Truiden anno 1456. **Pharm Weekbl** 1981 Nov 6;116(45):1406–8

**Vandewiele LJ:** Een vergeten Belgische farmakopee. Het dispensatorium van Triller. **Farm Tijdschr Belg** 1979;56:375–82

**Vandewiele LJ:** Geschiedenis van de farmacie in België met een inleiding tot de algemene geschiedenis van de farmacie. Beveren, Orion, 1981. 379 p.

**Vandewiele LJ:** Herodikos, de eerste sportarts. **Farm Tijdschr Belg** 1978;55:13–4

**Vandewiele LJ:** Historiek van de pharmacieopleiding in België. **Sartonia** 1979 Mar;42:6–15

**Vandewiele LJ:** Stenen in de Farmacie in de Leer bij Jacob van Maerlant. In Dilg P, et al., ed: Perspektiven der Pharmaziegeschichte. Graz, Austria, Akademische Druck- u. Verlagsanstalt, 1983. p. 419–30.

**Vandewiele LJ:** Van chemiatrie tot iatrochemie--van Paracelsus (1493–1541) tot Van Helmont (1579?–1644). **Farm Tijdschr Belg** 1980;57:25–30

**Van Dijk C** see **Majoor CL**

**Van Dijk JP:** Doodsoorzakenclassificaties van 1750 tot 1900. **Tijdschr Geschied Geneeskd** 1982;5(4):145–57

**Vane JR:** The research heritage of Henry Wellcome. **Pharm Hist (London)** 1980 Aug;10(2):2–8

**Vane JR:** The Wellcome centenary. Henry S. Wellcome, his research philosophy and current excitements. **Trans Med Soc Lond** 1980–81;97:41–50

**Van Egmond W:** New light on Paolo dell'Abbaco. **Ann Ist Mus Stor Sci Fir** 1977;2(2):3–21

**Van Elst H:** Jan Baptist Van Mons: aanhanger en verdediger van de leer van Lavoisier. **Farm Tijdschr Belg** 1980;57:145–58

**Vanes JM:** The Indiana University School of Dentistry in times of war. **Bull Hist Dent** 1980 Oct;28(2):91–5

**Van Eys J:** Nutritional therapy in childhood malignancies--a historical perspective. In Van Eys J, Seelig MS, Nichols BL, ed: Nutrition and cancer. New York and London, SP, 1979. P. 91–110.

**Van Gelder JB** see **Wittop Koning DA**

**Van Gerven DP:** The contribution of time and local geography to craniofacial variation in Nubia's Batn el Hajar. **Am J Phys Anthropol** 1982 Nov;59(3):307–16

**Van Gerven DP** see **Armelagos GJ**

**Van Gerven DP** see **Hummert JR**

**Van Ginneken J:** Bacteriological warfare. **J Contemp Asia** 1977;7(2):130–52

**VanHartesveldt FR:** Disease in the Western world: a review essay. **Teach Hist J Methods** 1980;5(1):75–81

**van Hoorn W:** Psychoanalysis, romanticism and biology. **Stor Crit Psicol** 1982 Jun;3(1):5–25

**Van Horn SH:** Women's roles: work and fertility for American women between 1900 and 1980. Ph.D. Diss., Carnegie-Mellon University. Pittsburgh, 1980. 344 leaves.

**Van Ijzendoorn MH, Van der Veer R:** Holzkamp's critical psychology and the functional-historical method: a critical appraisal. **Stor Crit Psicol** 1983;4(1):5–26

**van Ijzendoorn MH, Goossens FA, van der Veer R:** Klaus F. Riegel and dialectical psychology: in search for the changing individual in a changing society. **Stor Crit Psicol** 1984 Jun;5(1):5–28

**Van Kampen EJ, Jijlstra WG:** Haemoglobinometry: from estimation to reference method. **J Clin Chem Clin Biochem** 1981 Aug;19(8):517–9

**Van Keuren DK:** Human science in Victorian Britain: anthropology in institutional and disciplinary formation, 1863–1908. Ph.D. Diss., University of Pennsylvania. Philadelphia, 1982. vi, 329 p.

**Vankhanen NV** see **Levit AZ**

**Vankhanen VD, Grin' NV, Lastkov OA, et al:** Aktual'nye problemy gigieny Donbassa (k 50-letiiu so dnia osnovaniia Donetskogo meditsinskogo instituta im. M. Gor'kogo). **Gig Sanit** 1981 Aug;(8):51–3

**Van Lieburg MJ:** De dichter-medicus Daniël Jonctys (1611–1654), zijn strijd tegen het bijgeloof en zijn relatie tot Johan van Beverwijck, William Harvey en Daniël Sennert. **Tijdschr Geschied Geneeskd** 1979;2(4):137–67

**Van Lieburg MJ:** De genees- en heelkunde in de Noordelijke Nederlanden, gezien vanuit de stedelijke en chirurgijnsgilde-ordonnanties van de 16e eeuw. **Tijdschr Geschied Geneeskd** 1983;6(4):169–84

**Van Lieburg MJ:** De 'Materia Chirurgica' in de ordonnanties en examens der Noord-Nederlandse chirurgijnsgilden vóór 1600. **Pharm Weekbl** 1981;116(45):1393–8

**Van Lieburg MJ:** De syfilitische patiënt in de geschiedenis van het Nederlandse ziekenhuiswezen vóór 1900. **Tijdschr Soc Geschied** 1982;8:156–79

**Van Lieburg MJ:** Het medisch onderwijs te Rotterdam (1467–1967): een kort historisch overzicht. Amsterdam, Rodopi, 1978. 111 p. (Nieuwe Nederlandse Bijdragen tot de Geschiedenis der Geneeskunde, 3).

**Van Lieburg MJ:** The instrument-collection of Peter Vink, a chapter in the development of the surgical profession in the Netherlands during the 18th century. **Janus** 1980:67(1–2–3):207–19

**Van Loghem JJ:** Classic illustration (Sir Ronald Fisher). **Eur J Obstet Gynecol Reprod Biol** 1983 Oct;16(2):147–8

**Van Loghem JJ:** Introduction to a historical paper. An unusual case of intra-group agglutination by Philip Levine and Rufus E. Stetson. **Vox Sang** 1980;38(5):297–300

**Van Logtestijn JG:** 60 jaren V.V.D.O.---10 jaren afdeling technologie. **Tijdschr Diergeneeskd** 1980 Nov 1;105(21):883–4

**Van Malenstein MM:** Het Sint-Petersgasthuis te Culemborg een archief-studie vanuit medisch-historisch oogpunt. **Tijdschr Geschied Geneeskd** 1982;5(2):65–77

**Vann RT:** The new demographic history. Iggers, Georg G. and Parker, Harold T., ed: International Handbook of Historical Studies: Contemporary Research and Theory. Westport, Conn., Greenwood Press, 1979. p. 29–42.

**Van Noordwijk J:** Farmacologie, een erkende wetenschap. **Ned Tijdschr Geneeskd** 1983 Jul 9;127(28):1230–2

**van Oye E:** Enkele mijlpalen in de geschiedenis van de pneumoconiosen. **Arch Belg** 1984;42(5–6):289–93

**Van Patten HG:** The Arkansas Venereal Disease Program historical sketch and current trends. **J Arkansas Med Soc** 1984 Jan;80(8):365–6

**Van Poppel F** see **Vandenbroeke C**

**Van Praagh R, Van Praagh S:** Aristotle's 'triventricular' heart and the relevant early history of the cardiovascular system. **Chest** 1983 Oct;84(4):462–8

**Van Praagh S** see **Van Praagh R**

**Van Proosdij C, Sipsma DH:** Dertig jaar vaderlandse geschiedenis. De lijdensweg van de klinische geriatrie in Nederland. **Tijdschr Gerontol Geriatr** 1984 Feb;15(1):3–5

**Van Ree JM:** Nederlandse Farmacologie. I. Bouwstenen van de geneesmiddelentherapie: verantwoording. **Ned Tijdschr Geneeskd** 1983 Jul 9;127(28):1229–30

**Van Reenen JF:** Doctor 'Ribbebene' - cobbler, lumberman, dentist, politician and researcher. **Adler Mus Bull** 1983 Nov;Spec issue:53–7

**Van Rensburg BG:** Odontalgia--'n oorsig van die literatuur 1971–1980. **Tydskr Tandheelkd Ver S Afr** 1981 Dec;36(12):847–51

**Van Riet S, ed:** Avicenna Latinus. Liber de philosophia prima sive scientia divina, I–IV. Louvain, Peeters; Leiden, Brill, 1977. 225 p.

**Van Riper C:** An early history of ASHA. **ASHA** 1981 Nov;23(11):855–8

**Van Riper C:** My father, Doctor Van. Marquette, Mich., John M. Longyear Research Library, 1982. ix, 74 p.

**van Rood JJ:** Discovery of 4a and 4b. **Vox Sang** 1984;46(4):238–42

**Van Scott EJ, Yu RJ:** 'Ichthyosiform dermatoses' by Frost and Van Scott, August 1966. **Arch Dermatol** 1982 Oct;118(10):846–61

**Van Steijnen C:** Van gasthuis tot ziekenhuis; vier eeuwen St. Elisabeth's of Groote Gasthuis te Haarlem. **Ned Tijdschr Geneeskd** 1981 May 9;125(19):761–5

**Van Tassel DD** see **Spicker SF**

**Van Voorhis Wendler M:** Doctors and diseases on the Ohio frontier. **Ohio Hist** 1980 Spring;89(2):222–40

**Van Winter JM:** Het gebruik van cannabis in twee 15e-eeuwse kookboeken. **Farm Tijdschr Belg** 1980;57:411–9

**Van Zuylen J:** The microscopes of Antoni van Leeuwenhoek. **J Microsc** 1981 Mar;121(pt 3):309–28

**Van Zwanenberg D:** Interesting GPs of the past: George Stebbing: 1749–1825. **Br Med J [Clin Res]** 1981 Dec 5;283(6305):1517–8

**Van Zwanenberg D:** The training and careers of those apprenticed to apothecaries in Suffolk. 1815–1858. **Med Hist** 1983 Apr;27(2):139–50

**Vara López R:** Teodoro Billroth (con motivo del centenario de la primera gastrectomía). **An R Acad Nac Med (Madr)** 1981;98(2):283–310

**Varannai G** see **Huszár L**

**Varavej P:** The history of otorhinolaryngology in Thailand. **Adv Otorhinolaryngol** 1983;29:1–5

**Vardanian SA:** Ancient Armenian translations of the works of Syrian physicians. In International Congress of the History of Medicine, 27th, Barcelona, 1980. Actas. Barcelona, Académia de Ciències Mèdiques de Catalunya i Balears, 1981. p. 352–7.

**Varela G:** El tifo exantemático en México. In Academia Nacional de Medicina. Libro conmemorativo del primer centenario. México, Comité Editorial de la Comisión Organizadora del Congreso del Centenario, 1964. Tome 2. p. 524–7.

**Varenne E:** Traitée de médecine vétérinaire et de chirurgie par Bardon Jean, Maréchal-ferran à Cours. Explications de ce qui m'arrive dans mes exercices de vétérinaire. - Année 1870. Première partie: un maréchal-ferrand vétérinaire de la fin du XIX siècle. **Quercy Rech** 1982;(45–6):36–47

**Varga A:** Eksperimental'noe issledovanie faktorov testa Sondi. **Ann Univ Sci Budap Rolando Eotvos Nominatae** 1979;6:171–83

**Varga E:** Megemlékezés Went Istvánról. **Orv Hetil** 1983 Sep 18;124(38):2319–20

**Varga P:** Bacsó Bálint debreceni orvos-gyógyszerész élete és munkássága. **Orvostort Kozl** 1982;28(1–3):155–67

**Varga T** see **Lontainé SZ**

**Vargas M** see **Yáñez A**

**Vargas Fernández L:** En torno al primer caso de enfermedad de Addison descrito en Chile (1878). **Rev Med Chil** 1979 Jul;107(7):675-8
**Várhidy I:** Adatok a Budapesti központi tejesarnok szövetkezet szerepéről a főváros tejellátásában (1883-1916). **Agrartort Sz** 1978;20(1-2):172-80
**Varlamov VM, Selivanov EF:** Voenno-meditsinskomu muzeiu Ministerstva oborony SSSR - 40 let. **Voen Med Zh** 1982 Nov;(11):77-80
**Varma VP, Williams P, ed:** Piaget, psychology and education; papers in honour of Jean Piaget. Itasca, Illinois, Peacock, 1976. xiv, 233 p. Biographical chapters by E. A. Lunzer, p. xi-xiv, 3-14.
**Varotti C** see **Fanti PA**
**Vars HM:** Early research in parenteral nutrition. **JPEN** 1980 Sep-Oct;4(5):467-8
**Vars HM** see **Rhoads JE**
**Vartanian A:** Le frère de Maupertuis et l'homme machine. **Dix-huit Siecle** 1982;14:305-23
**Vas G, Hidvégi J:** Balassa érsebészeti munkásságáról. **Orv Hetil** 1983 Mar 20;124(12):709-10
**Vasanth P:** The life and deeds of late Dr. Achanta Lakshmipathi. **Sachitra Ayurved** 1981 Mar;:174-8
**Vasco Núñez P:** El primer Congreso Médico Internacional efectuado en la República de Panamá. **Rev Med Panama** 1984 May;9(2):164-71
**Vasconcellos I de:** Francisco de Paula Candido et son 'Rapport sur des mesures d'assainissement réclamées par cité de Rio de Janeiro et sur la fièvre jaune en particulier' - Typographie Nationale - Rio de Janeiro, 1854. In: Congrès international d'histoire de la médecine, XXVe, Québec, 1976. Actes. Québec, 1977. p. 1382-4.
**Vasconcellos Pedrosa MX de:** O ensino da anatomia no Brasil: saudação a Samuel Duarte Sattamini. **Rev Inst Hist Geogr Bras** 1971;291:83-91
**Vasconcelos D:** La enfermedad sagrada. Aspectos históricos y situación actual. **Gac Med Mex** 1982 Jan;118(1):35-7
**Vasconcelos R:** La academia y la evolución de la medicina en México desde la Independencia. In Academia Nacional de Medicina. Libro conmemorativo del primer centenario. México, Comité Editorial de la Comisión Organizadora del Congreso del Centenario, 1964. Tome 2. p. 621-9.
**Vasile R:** L'évolution démographique en Roumanie au cours des trois dernières décennies du XIXe siècle (II). **Rev Roum Hist** 1981;20(1):65-89
**Vasilenko VKh:** Metod Gippokrata. **Klin Med (Mosk)** 1983 Oct;61(10):3-12
**Vasilenko VKh:** Na grane antichnoĭ i novoĭ meditsiny. **Ter Arkh** 1983;55(1):133-9
**Vasilev D:** Borbata na BKP v pomosht na gladuvashtite v Suvestska Rusiia. **Izv Inst Istor BKP** 1968;18:339-65
**Vasilev D:** Izmenenie na zakonodatelstvoto, koeto regulira pravniia rezhim na izkustveniia abort v sveta prez poslednite 10 godini. **Akush Ginekol (Sofiia)** 1981;20(4):269-75
**Vasil'ev KG:** A. N. Sysin: 1879-1956. Moskva, Meditsina, 1981. 54 p.
**Vasil'ev KG, Vasil'ev KK:** K istorii likvidatsii natural'noĭ ospy v SSSR. **Vopr Virusol** 1982 Jan-Feb;(1):113-6
**Vasil'ev KG:** Metodologischeskie voprosy izucheniia otechestvennoi epidemiologii. **Zh Mikrobiol Epidemiol Immunobiol** 1982 Feb;(2):114-6
**Vasil'ev KG, Vasil'ev KK:** Rol' I. P. Franka a razvitii vysshego meditsinskogo obrazovaniia v Rossii. **Sov Zdravookhr** 1980;(10):62-5
**Vasil'ev KG, Vasil'ev KK:** Vrach-revoliutsioner V. L. Elin. **Sov Zdravookhr** 1983;(8):57-8
**Vasil'ev KK:** K istorii meditsinskikh obshchestv v Rossii. **Sov Zdravookhr** 1983;(1):71-3
**Vasil'ev KK:** K istorii zhurnala 'Gigiena i sanitariia'. **Gig Sanit** 1982 Sep;(9):51-2
**Vasil'ev KK:** Rol' A. N. Sysina v organizatsii i provendenii vserossiĭskikh (vsesoiuznykh) s'ezdov bakteriologov, épidemiologov i sanitarynykh vracheĭ. **Gig Sanit** 1980 Apr;(4):31-3
**Vasil'ev KK:** Rol' nauchnykh s'ezdov v nauchnoĭ meditsinskoĭ informatsii (iz istorii vserossiĭskikh i vsesoiuznykh s'ezdov bakteriologov, épidemiologov i sanitarnykh vracheĭ, 1918-1928 gg.) **Sov Zdravookhr** 1980;(6):58-60
**Vasil'ev KK:** Rol' pervykh Vserossiĭskikh sezdov bakteriologov i épidemiologov v bor'be s épidemiiami parazitarnykh tifov (k 60-letiiu IV sezda). **Zh Mikrobiol Epidemiol Immunobiol** 1981 Apr;(4):106-9
**Vasil'ev KK:** S'ezd, zalozhivshiĭ osnovy sanitarno-épidemiologicheskoĭ sluzhby SSSR (k 60-letiiu VI Vserossiĭskogo c'ezda bakteriologov i épidemiologov). **Zh Mikrobiol Epidemiol Immunobiol** 1982 Dec;(12):102-3
**Vasil'ev KK:** U istokov sanitarno-épidemiologicheskoĭ sluzhby sovetskogo zdravookhraneniia. **Med Sestra** 1983 Mar;42(3):46-8
**Vasil'ev KK:** 60 let VII Vserossi iskogo s'ezda bakteriologov, épidemiologov i sanitarnykh vracheĭ. **Zh Mikrobiol Epidemiol Immunobiol** 1983 Oct;(10):111-3
**Vasil'ev KK** see **Vasil'ev KG**
**Vasil'ev VI** see **Bunchuk NV**
**Vasilevskiĭ NN:** D. A. Biriukov, 1904-1969. Moskva, Meditsina, 1981 95 p.
**Vaskilampi T, Hänninen O:** Cupping as an indigenous treatment of pain syndromes in the Finnish culture and social context. **Soc Sci Med** 1982;16(21):1893-901
**Vaskilampi T** see **Hänninen O**
**Vasoli C:** The contribution of humanism to the birth of modern science. **Renaiss Reformation** 1979;3(1):1-15
**Vassilev V** see **Nikolaeva I**
**Vastyan EA:** Medicine and war. In Reich WT, et al, ed: Encyclopedia of bioethics, v.4. New York, Free Press, 1978. p. 1695-9.
**Vătămanu N:** Contribution à l'étude de la vie et de l'oeuvre di Giovanni Mascellini, médecin et secrétaire princier. **Rev Etud Sud Est Eur** 1978;16(2):269-87
**Vater G** see **Hiepe T**
**Vaubel E** see **Winau R**
**Vaughan L** see **Vaughan VH**
**Vaughan VH, Vaughan L:** Fifty years of service: The S. A. National Council for the Blind, 1929-1979. The story of the South African National Council for the Blind. Pretoria. S. A. National Council for the Blind, 1979. xii, 468 p.
**Vavilin PA:** A. P. Dobroslavin--ego obshchestvennaia i prakticheskaia deiatel'nost' (k 140-letiiu so dnia rozdeniia). **Gig Sanit** 1982 Sep;(9):53-6
**Vavilin PA:** Gigienicheskie prognozy v trudakh A. P. Dobroslavina. **Gig Sanit** 1980 May;(5):25-9
**Vavilin PA:** Rol' A. P. Dobroslavina v stanovlenii otechestvennoĭ gigienicheskoĭ nauki (k 90-letiiu so dnia smerti). **Gig Sanit** 1980 Mar;(3):45-7
**Vazquez C:** Sobre la cosmetica (zina) del S. XIV en Al-Andalus. **Bol Soc Esp Hist Farm** 1982 Mar;33(129):9-48
**Vázquez Albaladejo G, Sospedra Ferrer R:** Evolución de las técnicas quirúrgicas en el cáncer de mama. **Rev Esp Oncol** 1981;28(1):83-94
**Vázquez de Benito C, Herrera MT:** Dos capitulos ginecologicos: arabe y castellano. **Asclepio** 1981;33:183-241
**Vazquez de Benito MC, ed:** El libro del 'Amal man tabba li-man habba de Muhammad B. 'Abdallah B. Al-Jatib. Salamanca, Universidad de Salamanca, 1972. liii, 86 p. (Acta Salmanticensia, 66).
**Vazquez Leiva R** see **Weaver DS**
**Vdovin AI, Drobizhev VZ:** Sotsial'naia psikhologiia i nekotorye voprosy istorii sovetskogo obshchesta. **Istor SSSR** 1971;5:23-43
**Veatch RM, Tai E:** Talking about death: patterns of lay and professional change. **Ann Am Acad Polit Soc Sci** 1980;447:29-45
**Vecht RJ, Besterman EM, Bromley LL, et al:** Acute aortic dissection: historical perspective and current management. **Am Heart J** 1981 Dec;102(6 pt 1):1087-9
**Vedder JS:** Pediatric respiratory therapy of the 1930s. **Respir Ther** 1979 Jan-Feb;9(1):42, 44
**Ved'mina EA, Tatarinova SD:** 50-Letie kafedry mikrobiologii Tsentral'nogo ordena Lenina instituta usovershenstvovaniia vracheĭ. **Antibiotiki** 1982;27(9):714-5
**Vedrenne C** see **Huard P**
**Vega DE** see **Pernin A**
**Vega H:** Así sufrieron. Barcelona, Argos Vergara, 1981. 204 p.
**Vega Diaz F:** El corazón en la simbología y en la iconografía profana y religiosa. In Academia Nacional de Medicina. Libro conmemorativo del primer centenario. México, Comité Editorial de la Comisión Organizadora del Congreso del Centenario, 1964. Tome 2. p. 78-82.
**Vegetti M** see **Grmek MD, ed**
**Vegetti M** see **Manuli P**
**Végh F:** Jókai Mór Szájmütétje 1891-ben. **Orvostort Kozl** 1979;86(24 no 4):129-30
**Veidenheimer MC:** Presidential address. Who dug your well? **Dis Colon Rectum** 1982 Mar;25(2):85-9
**Veiga-Pires JA, Grainger RG:** Pioneers in angiography: The Portuguese School of Angiography. Lancaster, Boston, MTP Press, 1982. 131 p.
**Veispak T:** Rakvere elanikkonna suurus ja sotsiaalnestruktuur 17. sajandi lõpust 1780. Aastateni. **Esti NSV Tead Akad Toim** 1981;30(2):169-78
**Veith I:** Changing concepts of health care: an historian's view. **West J Med** 1980 Dec;133(6):532-8
**Veith I:** On privileged communication: a comparative study of several medical cases. **West J Med** 1983 Mar;138(3):437-40
**Veith I:** Psychologische Dimensionen der fernöstlichen Persönlichkeit. **Jahrb Univ Dusseld** 1977-78;:317-25
**Veith I:** The history of medicine dolls and foot-binding in China. **Clio Med** 1980 Jul;14(3-4):255-67
**Véjar-Lacave C:** El maestro Ignacio Chávez, la medicina y los problemas educacionales. **Gac Med Mex** 1980 Jan;116(1):43-6
**Vejnoska J:** Voluntarism: rich heritage of the alcohol field. **Alcohol Health Res World** 1982 Spring;6(3):4-7, 36-40
**Vejsiu Y** see **Misja V**
**Velasco B:** El hospital de convalescientes de Cuéllar. **Estud Segov** 1973;24(71-72):153-70
**Velasco D:** La psychiatrie infantile dans les pays en voie de développement. **Ann Med Psychol (Paris)** 1981 Jun;139(6):626-8
**Velasco Suárez C:** The Santorini valves. **Mt Sinai J Med (NY)** 1981 Mar-Apr;48(2):149-57
**Velasco-Suárez M:** El cerebro humano. Su evolución conceptual. **Gac Med Mex** 1982 Oct;118(10):395-402
**Velázquez Díaz G** see **Carrada Bravo T**
**Vélez Boza F:** Discurso pronunciado con motivo de la colocacion del retrato del Dr. Jesus Sanabria Bruzual en el salon de sesiones de la Sociedad Venezolana de Historia de la Medicina, el 12 de julio de 1978. **Rev Soc Venez Hist Med** 1980;29(43-44):63-71
**Vélez Boza F:** Estudio epidemiologico de la mortalidad por malformaciones congenitas letales en Venezuela, de 1950 a 1974. **Rev Soc Venez Hist Med** 1980;29(43-44):73-80
**Vélez Boza F:** Historia de la microscopia en Venezuela. **Rev Soc Venez Hist Med** 1981;30(45-46):125-97
**Velez Boza F:** Homenaje a la memoria del Dr. Jesus A. Yerena. **Rev Soc Venez Hist Med** 1975-76;23(37):91-100
**Vélez Boza F:** Licenciado Jose Maria Benitez; maestro en artes, médico y botánico. **Rev Soc Venez Hist Med** 1977;25(39):71-92
**Velez-I CG:** Se me acabó la canción: an ethnography of non-consenting

sterilizations among Mexican women in Los Angeles. Mora, Magdalena and Del Castillo, Adelaida R., ed. Mexican Women in the United States: Struggles past and present. Los Angeles, U. of California Chicano Studies Res. Center, 1980 p. 71-91.

**Velgos S:** Rozvoj stomatologichej vetvy lekárskej fakulty Univerzity Komensk'ho v Bratislave. **Cas Lek Cesk** 1979 Dec 21;118(51):1586-8

**Velikoretskiĭ AN:** Vzgliady N. I. Pirogova na preduprezhdenie zarazheniia ran. **Feldsher Akush** 1979 Sep;44(9):44-6

**Velkov DL** see **Kardashev TD**

**Velková A** see **Sícha V**

**Vella EE:** Belsen: medical aspects of a World War II concentration camp. Paper 1. **J R Army Med Corps** 1984 Feb;130(1):34-59

**Vella EE:** Brucellosis (the Corps disease). **J R Army Med Corps** 1983 Jun;129(2):97-100

**Velle K:** Gezondheidsopvoeding in België in de 19de eeuw. **Spiegel Hist** 1982;17(12):619-25

**Velter A, Lamothe MJ:** Les outils du corps. [Paris],? Hier et demain, 1978. 303 p.

**Veltheer W:** Erasmus, in de grond niet so slecht. **Spiegel Hist** 1982;17(4):190-6

**Veltheer W:** Het chirurgijnsgilde van Amersfoort. **Tijdschr Geschied Geneeskd** 1979;2(3):101-9

**Veltheer W:** History: the dawn of gastric resection. **Neth J Surg** 1981 Aug;33(3):107-14

**Vel'tishchev IuE:** A. A. Koltypin--uchenyĭ, vrach, obshchestvennyĭ deiatel' (k 100-letiiu so dnia rozhdeniia). **Pediatriia** 1983 Sep;(9):73-4

**Vencovský E:** Ceskoslovenský psychiatr spolupracovníkem profesora dr. Alberta Schweitzera v Lambarène. **Cesk Psychiatr** 1984 Apr;80(2):125-8

**Vencovský E:** Jubileum 40 let od založení nemocniční lužkové psychiatrické péče v Plzni. **Cesk Psychiatr** 1982 Dec;78(6):407-8

**Vencovský E:** Mudr. Josef Cermák a jeho zásluhy o vybudování psychiatrické léčebny v Cernovicích. **Cesk Psychiatr** 1984 Jun;80(3):200-3

**Vencovský E:** První nemocniční psychiatrické oddělení v Cechách. **Cesk Psychiatr** 1981 Jun;77(3):204-8

**Vendl L:** Dvacet let Detské nefrologické léčebny Miramonte v Mariánských Láznich. **Cesk Pediatr** 1982 Jul;37(7):419

**Venerando A, ed** see **Borms J**

**Vengrova IV:** Izuchenie zdorov'ia rabochikh Sibiri. **Sov Zdravookhr** 1982;(11):51-5

**Vengrova IV:** K. Marks i razvitie sotsial'noĭ gigieny. **Sov Zdravookhr** 1983;6:3-8

**Vengrova IV:** O deiatel'nosti pervykh Otechestvennykh fabrichnykh inspektorov (k 100-letiiu sozdaniia fabrichnoĭ inspektsii v Rossii). **Sov Zdravookhr** 1983;(3):61-5

**Vengrova IV, Danilishina EI:** Sotsial'no-gigienicheskie issledovaniia organizovannogo detskogo naseleniia v 20-e gody v Sibiri i Dal'nem Vostoke. **Sov Zdravookhr** 1981;(4):63-6

**Vengrova IV:** Sotsial'no-gigienicheskie issledovaniia 20-kh godov, posviashchennye sel'skomu pereselencheskomu naseleniiu Sibiri. **Sov Zdravookhr** 1981;(7):45-8

**Vengrova IV:** Translations of the classics of medicine in the USSR. In International Congress of the History of Medicine, 27th, Barcelona, 1980. Actas. Barcelona, Académia de Ciències Mèdiques de Catalunya i Balears, 1981. p. 358-62.

**Vengrova IV, Egorysheva IV, Rabinovich RS, et al:** Znamenatel'nye i iubileĭnye daty istorii fiziologii 1980 g. **Fiziol Zh SSSR** 65(9):1396-9, Sep 79

**Vengrova IV** see **Lotova EI**

**Venkat Rao B:** Development of naturopathy in Andhra Pradesh. **Bull Indian Inst Hist Med (Hyderabad)** 1979;9:41-5

**Venkata Reddy M, Rama Rao B:** A note on Kriya Yoga. **Bull Indian Inst Hist Med (Hyderabad)** 1980;10(1-4):69-75

**Venkata Reddy M:** Hatharatnavali of Srinivasabhatta, a late medieval treatise on yoga and tantra. **Bull Indian Inst Hist Med (Hyderabad)** 1979;9:74-81

**Venkataram BS** see **Shankara MR**

**Ventura P:** Freud e la giuridicità della coesistenza. Per un ritorno filosofico alla psicologia del profondo. Vol. I. La psicoanalisi individuale. Milano, Giuffrè, 1979. xvi, 420 p.

**Venturi D** see **Dreznik A**

**Venzlaff H:** Der marokkanische Drogenhändler und seine Ware. Wiesbaden, Steiner, 1977. 242 p.

**Veras RP, Ribeiro LD, Lima JC:** Notas sobre a evolução da escola médica no Brasil. **Educ Med Salud** 1983;17(4):398-413

**Veray FX:** Betances, el médico. **Bol Asoc Med PR** 1983 Mar;75(3):110-3

**Verbitskiĭ VM** see **Mirskiĭ MB**

**Verbov JL:** Mummified skin--an exercise in preservation. **Int J Dermatol** 1983 Jan-Feb;22(1):46-60

**Verbrugge MH:** Healthy animals and civic life: Sylvester Graham's physiology of subsistence. **Rev Am Hist** 1981;9(3):359-64

**Verbrugge MH:** The social meaning of personal health: The Ladies' Physiological Institute of Boston and vicinity in the 1850s. In Reverby S, Rosner D, ed: Health care in America. Philadelphia, Temple University Press, 1979. p. 45-66.

**Vercelli D** see **Camerino G**

**Vercellone A:** Vent'anni di nefrologia italiana. **Minerva Nefrol** 1979 Oct-Dec;26(4):443-8

**Verchere L:** Henri Lentulo, inventeur du bourre-pâte, 1889-1981. **Rev Odontostomatol (Paris)** 1981 Mar-Apr;10(2):175-7

**Verdan C:** Evolution historique de la chirurgie des tendons fléchisseurs. **Rev Med Suisse Romande** 1980 Jul;100(7):639-52

**Verdan C:** Geschichte der plastischen und wiederherstellenden Chirurgie. In Sournia JC, Martiny M, Poulet J, ed: Illustrierte Geschichte der Medizin. Salzburg, Andreas, 1980. Vol. 8. p. 2911-31.

**Verdan C:** Histoire de la chirurgie de la main. **Ann Chir** 1980 Nov;34(9):647-54

**Verdan C:** Historische Entwicklung der Beugesehnen-Chirurgie. **Handchirurgie** 1981;13(3-4):181-5

**Verdiglione A:** Fondations de la psychanalyse: la peste. Paris, Galilée/Spirali, 1981. 282 p.

**Verdoorn JA:** Arts en oorlog. Medische en sociale zorg voor oorlogsslachtoffers in de geschiedenis von Europa: inleiding in de medische polemologie. Amsterdam, Lynx, 1972. 2 v.

**Verdun-Jones SN** see **Smandych R**

**Verduzco Guerrero E:** La mortalidad por tuberbulosis en la República Mexicana durante el periodo 1963-1974. **SPM** 1980 Mar-Apr;22(2):191-28

**Verellen T:** Cosmas and Damian in the New Sacristy [Medici Chapel of San Lorenzo, Florence]. **J Warburg Courtauld Inst** 1979;42:274-7

**Vereninov AA** see **Braun AD**

**Verenkina TN, Markina LZ, Bashtanova LV:** Istoriia razvitiia bor'by s tuberkulezom v Sevastopole. **Probl Tuberk** 1984 Jan;(1):70-2

**Verenkina TN:** Vrachebnye obshchestva v dorevoliutsionnom Sevastopole. **Sov Zdravookhr** 1982;(6):68-71

**Verenkina TN, Davidiuk VG:** Zdravookhranenie Sebastopolia v pervye gody Sovetskoĭ vlasti (1920-1923). **Sov Zdravookhr** 1983;(11):54-7

**Veress O** see **Orosz L**

**Veretennikova VP** see **Vorob'ev IuI**

**Vergara de Campos A** see **Otero Chulian E**

**Verheyden CN:** The history of Dupuytren's contracture. In Romm S, ed: Symposium on historical perspectives of plastic surgery. Philadelphia, Saunders, 1983. p. 619-25.

**Verheyden CN** see **Romm S, ed**

**Verheyen H:** De zorg voor het gevonden kind te Antwerpen (1830-1870). **Ann Soc Belg Hist Hop** 1978;16:87-109

**Verkroost CM:** A. W. van Renterghem und Frederik van Eeden, zwei holländische Aerzte als Bahnbrecher auf dem Gebiete der psychischen Therapie. **Janus** 1980;67(1-2-3):191-9

**Verkuyl J:** Bezinning op family-planning in India. **Wereld Zending** 1973;2(5):328-36

**Verlinden C:** Ist mittelalterliche Sklaverei ein bedeutsamer demographischer Faktor gewesen? **Vierteljahrsschr Soz Wirtschgesch** 1979;66:153-73

**Verma A:** Birth control and planned parenthood in China. **China Rep (India)** 1971;7(2):41-8

**Verma KC** see **Tripathi RD**

**Verma RL:** Medical trends in Kashmir during Zain-ul-Abidin's reign. **Indian J Hist Sci** 1980 May;15(1):71-8

**Vermeersch AG:** L'enseignement de la médecine dentaire à l'Universitè Catholique de Louvain. **Rev Belge Med Dent** 1981;36(3):128-9

**Vermeulen CW:** For the greatest good to the largest number. A history of the Medical Center, the University of Chicago. Chicago, Univ. of Chicago, 1977. x, 129 p.

**Vermorel H:** Un trouble de mémoire sur l'Acropole, 1936-1904. **Rev Fr Psychanal** 1982;46(3):513-26

**Vernet Gines J:** Historia de la ciencia española. Madrid, Instituto de España, Cátedra Alfonso X el Sabio, 1975. 312 p.

**Vernia P:** La farmacopea Valenciana. Villarreal, Seriols-Sichet-Herrero, 1981. 168 p.

**Vernon C:** The early beginnings of the Association of Nurses. **Jamaican Nurse** 1981;21(1):9-10

**Vernon HA:** Medical crisis at Fort Niagara, 1779-80. **Niagara Frontier** 1977;24:89-94

**Vernon J:** The history of masking as applied to tinnitus. **J Laryngol Otol** 1981;4 Suppl:76-9

**Vernon JM** see **Grabowski HG**

**Veron C** see **Lanchou G**

**Véron J:** La mortalité en Asie Méridionale et Orientale. **Population** 1980;35(1):137-65

**Veron J** see **Curet M**

**Veronelli JC:** Medicina, gobierno y sociedad: evolución de las instituciones de atención de la salud en Argentina. Buenos Aires, El Coloquio, [1975]. 227 p.

**Veronese Ceseracciu E:** Ebrei laureati a Padova nel cinquecento. **Quad Stor Univ Padova** 1980;13:151-68

**Verseghi G:** A honvédorvosi kar vázlatos története 1968-1914 között. **Orv Hetil** 1980 Jul 13;121(28):1709-12

**Verslag van de bijzondere wetenschappelijke vergadering ter viering van het honderdvijfentwintigjarig bestaan der Vereniging Nederlands Tijdschrift voor Geneeskunde.: Ned Tijdschr Geneeskd** 1982 Jan 2;126(1):33-8

**Versluysen MC:** A forgotten chapter. **Nurs Times** 1981 Jul 15-21;77(29):1239

**Versluysen MC** see **Davies C, ed**

**Verso ML:** Airs, waters and places. **Victorian Hist J** 1977 Feb;48(1):6-21

**Verso ML:** Doctors and daguerrotypes. Contributions of medical men to the history of photography. **Victorian Hist Mag** 1969 Feb-May;40(155/6 No 1/2):3-24

**Verso ML:** Fifty years of the Red Cross Blood Transfusion Service in Victoria. **Victorian Hist J** 1980;51(4):218-36

**Verso ML:** The evolution of haemoglobinometry: and other essays on the history of haematology. Melbourne, Trefusis Publications, 1981. 105 p.

**Verso ML:** The history of medical history; with special reference to Australia. **Victorian Hist J** 1979 May;50(2):58–76

**Verstraete BC:** Homosexuality in ancient Greek and Roman civilization: a critical bibliography with supplement. Toronto, Canadian Gay Archives, 1982. 14 p.

**Verstraete BC:** Slavery and the social dynamics of male homosexual relations in ancient Rome. **J Homosex** 1980 Spring;5(3):227–36

**Vértes L:** Dr. Ivanchich Viktor. **Orv Hetil** 1984 Sep 16;125(38):2321–4

**Vértes L:** Elsö gerontológusunk: Rózsay József akadémikus. **Orv Hetil** 1983 Oct 16;124(42):2564–8

**Vértes L:** Georg Händel (Händel apja, a 'hallei chirurgus'). **Orv Hetil** 1980 Apr 6;121(14):851–3

**Vertinsky P:** Sexual equality and the legacy of Catharine Beecher. **J Sport Hist** 1979;6(1):38–49

**Vérut DD:** PreColombian dermatology and cosmetology in Mexico. [S.1]: Schering Corp. USA, 1973. [107 p].

**Verveen G:** Chirurgia: the handicraft of medicine. Philatelically illustrated historic survey of surgery. **Am J Surg** 1982 May;143(5):640–8

**Verveen G:** Venerologie auf Briefmarken; Philatelistisch illustrierte Geschichte der Venerologie. **Z Hautkr** 1981 Feb 15;56(4):227–33

**Verwer MA:** Diergeneeskunde--diergeneeskunst. **Tijdschr Diergeneeskd** 1983 Dec 15;108(24):964–9

**Verzeichnis der wissenschaftlichen Arbeiten von Erna Lesky:** In Ganzinger K, Skopec M, Wyklicky H, ed: Festschrift für Erna Lesky zum 70. Geburtstag. Wien, Brüder Hollinek, 1981. p. 193–203.

**Veselkin PN:** K 100–letiiu kafedry patologicheskoĭ fiziologii ordena Lenina Krasnoznamennoĭ voenno–meditsinskoĭ akademii im. S. M. Kirova. **Patol Fiziol Eksp Ter** 1980;(4):3–11

**Veselov EI, Belevitin AB:** A. V. Eliseev--vrach, puteshestvennik, uchenyĭ (k 125–letiiu so dnia rozhdeniia). **Voen Med Zh** 1984 Sep;(9):68–9

**Veselov NG** see **Andrianov VL**

**Veselova AM** see **Stegunin SI**

**Vester JW:** The valiant physicians. **Milit Med** 1982 Dec;147(12):1041–7

**Vet AC de:** Perspectives in international neurosurgery: neurosurgery in the Netherlands. **Neurosurgery** 1981 Jul;9(1):92–4

**Veterany Velikoĭ Otechestvennoĭ voĭny za 'kruglym stolom' redaktsii 'Voenno–medistinskogo zhurnala': Voen Med Zh** 1980 May;(5):14–20

**Veterinär–Medizinische Fakultät der Universität Zürich, 1902–1977: Jubiläumsschrift zum 75–jährigen Bestehen:** [Zürich, Veterinär–Medizinische Fakultät, Universität Zürich, 1977?].

**Vetro C:** Il colera del 1837 in provincia di Agrigento. **Arch Stor Sicil** 1975;4(1):57–90

**Vetschera T, Pillai A:** The use of hemp and opium in India. **Ethnomedizin** 1978–79;5(1–2):11–23

**Vetter L, Thiess AM:** 100 Jahre Frauenarbeit. Teil 1: Historische Entwicklung, Arbeitsschutz–Gesetzgebung. **Fortschr Med** 1983 Feb 10;101(6):206–10

**Vetter T:** Essai sur la littérature hippocratique au dix–huitième siècle. In La collection hippocratique et son rôle dans l'histoire de la médecine. Colloque de Strasbourg (23–27 octobre 1972) organisé par le Centre de Recherches sur la Grèce Antique, avec le concours des Facultés de Philosophie et des Langues Classiques. Leiden, E. J. Brill, 1975. p. 347–67.

**Vetter T:** Louis de la Forge (1632–1667?) angevin et fidèle adepte de la physiologie cartésienne. In: Congrès National des Sociétés Savantes, 93e, Tours, 1968. Comptes Rendus. Paris, 1971. Section des Sciences, Tome II. p. 31–50.

**Vetter T:** Témoignages du Strasbourgeois Victor Stoeber sur la médecine parisienne (1824–1825). **Gesnerus** 1983;40(1–2):215–22

**Vetter T:** Un siècle d'histoire de la circulation du sang, 1564–1664. [Bâle, Geigy, 1965]. 6 pts. in 1 v.

**Veylon R:** La photographie. Petit essai de 'psychopathologie'. **Nouv Presse Med** 1980 Jul 12–26;9(30):2073–5

**Veyne P:** La vie sexuelle dans l'Empire Romain. **Sci Avenir** 1977;365:698–703

**Vial F, Rullière R:** François Magendie. **Hist Sci Med** 1983;17(4):323–32

**Vial F, Merlette B, Roussel CI, et al:** Les livres médicaux de la Bibliothèque municipale de Laon. **Hist Sci Med** 1979;13(4):383–93

**Vial F, Merlette B, Paris R, et al:** Les recettes retenues par les Laonnois: observations médicales. **Hist Sci Med** 1980;14(1):61–9

**Vial F** see **Berti Bock G**

**Vial F** see **Heymans G**

**Vial F** see **Merlette B**

**Vial F** see **Rulliere R**

**Vial G:** Studien zum ersten altdeutschen Pferdearzneibuch des dänischen Lehnsmannes Mogens Sehestedt (1598–1657). Diss. Hannover, 1978. 272 p.

**Viana S:** El diario de una parroquia: Legrán. **Bol Inst Sancho Sabio** 1971;15:269–76

**Viaña Olaya R** see **Ordosgoitia Yarzagaray E**

**Vicente R de:** La investigación genética, entre la confusión y la esperanza. **Arbor** 1977;98(383):7–23

**Vickers DW:** The naive empiricism of an ancient medicine. **Apeiron** 1979;13(1):1–8

**Vickers ED:** F. Elisabeth Cromwell: Pensacola's pioneer nurse. **J Fla Med Assoc** 1983 Aug;70(8):642–6

**Vickers ED:** Pensacola's early hospitals. **J Fla Med Assoc** 1981 Aug;68(8):635–43

**Vickers HR:** Royal Naval Hospital Haslar 1940–44. **J R Nav Med Serv** 1984 Summer;70(2):103–9

**Victoria Ortiz M:** Vida y obra del doctor Areilza. Bilbao, La Gran Enciclopedia Vasca, 1975. 329 p.

**Victorovich YV, Rachmanovna DO:** Perspectives in international neurosurgery: neurosurgery in the Union of Soviet Socialist Republics. **Neurosurgery** 1981 Feb;8(2):283–4

**Vicziany M:** Coercion in a soft state: the family planning program of India. **Pac Aff** 1982;55(3):373–402;(4):557–92

**Vida M:** A Kozma- és Damján–tisztelet írásos és tárgyi emlékei Magyarországon. **Orvostort Kozl** 1980;89–91(26 no 1–3):257–65

**Vida M:** Az orvosi gyakorlat és a gyógyítószentek ikonográfiája a XIII–XIV. századi magyarországi falfestészetben. **Orvostort Kozl** 1979;87–88(25 no 1–2):13–63

**Vida M:** Tivadar Duka (1825–1908). **Orvostort Kozl** 1979;86(24 no 4):9–23

**Vida M:** Ursprung und Deutung der Verehrung der Heiligen Kosmas und Damian in Ungarn (11–14. Jahrhundert). **Orvostort Kozl** 1980;89–91(26 no 1–3):45–95

**Vida M:** Ursprung und Deutung des Kosmas–Damian–Kultes in Ungarn (11.–14. Jahrhundert). In Hein WH, ed: Pharmaziehistorischer Kongress, Budapest, 1981. Stuttgart, Wissenschaftliche Verlagsgesellschaft, 1983. p. 23–33.

**Vidal F:** [Bloodletting and dentistry in the 17th and 18th centuries.] (Fre). **Inf Dent** 1980;62:4059–64

**Vidal F:** Caelius Aurelianus et la douleur dentaire: 'de dolore dentium'. **Inf Dent** 1984 Jul 12–19;66(28–29):2875–88

**Vidal F, Buscaglia M, Vonèche JJ:** Darwinism and developmental psychology. **J Hist Behav Sci** 1983 Jan;19(1):81–94

**Vidal F:** La discontinuité de la douleur chez les physiologistes du XVIIIe siècle. **Inf Dent** 1983 Dec 8;65(43):4243–8

**Vidal F:** La pharmacologie bucco–dentaire au temps d'Auguste. **Chir Dent Fr** 1983 Mar 10;53(194):21–30

**Vidal F:** La thériaque--panacée des XVIe, XVIIe, et XVIIIe siècles. **Chir Dent Fr** 1984 Apr 26;54(247):27–32 contd

**Vidal F:** La thériaque--panacée des XVIe, XVIIe et XVIIIe siècles. **Chir Dent Fr** 1984 May 3;54(248):33–9 contd

**Vidal F:** Le Gayac, panacée du XVIe siècle. **Chir Dent Fr** 1983 Nov 24;53(226):37–42

**Vidal F:** L'Edit Royal de mai 1699--une date capitale pour l'odontologie. **Chir Dent Fr** 1981 Sep 3;51(123):25–37

**Vidal F:** Les anodins dans le traitement des douleurs dentaires aux XVIIe et XVIIIe siècles. **Inf Dent** 1982 Feb 25;64(8):695–703

**Vidal F:** Les drogues tirées du corps de l'homme dans la matière médicale du XVIIIe siècle. **Chir Dent Fr** 1983 Dec 15–22;53(229–230):49–52

**Vidal F:** Les drogues tirées du corps des animaux dans la matière médicale du XVIIIe siècle. **Chir Dent Fr** 1984 Feb 2;54(235):21–9

**Vidal F:** Les maîtrises en chirurgie au XVIIIe siècle. **Inf Dent** 1980 Jul 10;62(27):2345–54

**Vidal F:** Les saignées dan la médecine des XVIIe et XVIIIe siècles. **Chir Dent Fr** 1982 Dec 2;52(181):25–35

**Vidal F:** L'inflammation chez les physiologistes du XVIIIe siècle. **Chir Dent Fr** 1983 Oct 27;53(222):43–6

**Vidal F:** Medecine sacerdotale dans le monde antique. **Chir Dent Fr** 1983 Jun 2;53(206):37–5

**Vidal F:** Michel Servet (1511–1553). La découverte de la circulation du sang. **Chir Dent Fr** 1981 Apr;51(110):39–43

**Vidal F:** Odontoiatria del passato. Gli 'anodini' nel trattamento del mal di denti nel XVII e nel XVIII secolo. **Dent Cadmos** 1982 Jan;50(1):57–61

**Vidal F:** Odontoiatria del passato. L''Edit Royal' del maggio 1699. L''Editto' del 1699 y quello del 1768. **Dent Cadmos** 1982 Jan, Feb;50(1,2):57–63, 67–74

**Vidal F:** Odontoiatria del passato. Salasso e mal di denti nel XVII e nel XVIII sécolo. **Dent Cadmos** 1981 Mar;49(3):59–63

**Vidal F:** Un anesthésique vieux de 19 siècles: la mandragore. **Chir Dent Fr** 1982 Oct 7;52(173):21–6

**Vidal F:** Vers et carie dentaire chez les dentistes du XVIIIe siècle. **Chir Dent Fr** 1983 Jul 14–21;53(212–213):15–8

**Vidal F** see **Gauval VB**

**Vidal J:** External fixation. Yesterday, today, and tomorrow. **Clin Orthop** 1983 Nov;(180):7–14

**Vidal JL** see **Gracia D**

**Vidal Casero MC:** Aportacion a la historia del Jardin de Aclimatacion de San Lucard de Barrameda. **Bol Soc Esp Hist Farm** 1981 Dec;32(128):235–49

**Vidal Casero MC:** Plantas medicinales cultivadas en el Jardín Botánico con destino a las reales boticas de los hospitales militares del Campo de San Roque establecido en Algeciras. In International Congress of the History of Medicine, 27th, Barcelona, 1980. Actas. Barcelona, Acadèmia de Ciències Mèdiques de Catalunya i Balears, 1981. p. 656–62.

**Vidal Casero MC, Aguilera Guirao A:** Plantas medicinales cultivadas en el Jardín Botánico del Monasterio de Nuestra Señora de Carracido. In International Congress of the History of Medicine, 27th, Barcelona, 1980. Actas. Barcelona, Acadèmia de Ciències Mèdiques de Catalunya i Balears, 1981. p. 663–8.

**Vidal Casero MC** see **Valverde López JL**

**Vidon DJ:** Actualité des streptocoques un siècle après leur découverte. **Lyon Pharm** 1981 Apr;32(3):151–4

**Viduta VK:** Studenty–mediki v Tartuskom (Iur'evskom) Marksistskom kruzhke. **Sov Zdravookhr** 1983;(10):55–7

**Viduta VK:** Tobol'skaia fel'dsherskaia shkola i ee rol' v formirovanii revoliutsionerov. **Sov Zdravookhr** 1984;(8):57–9

**Viduta VK:** Vrach, revoliutsioner, uchenyĭ M. M. Chemodanov. **Sov Zdravookhr** 1983;(4):58–60

**Vidyasagar D, ed** see **Smith GF**

**Vié J:** Die grossen klassischen Traditionen von Hippokrates bis Pinel. In Sournia JC, Martiny M, Poulet J, ed: Illustrierte Geschichte der Medizin. Salzburg, Andreas, 1980. Vol. 6. p. 2008–33.
**Vié J, Baruk H:** Geschichte der Psychiatrie. In Sournia JC, Martiny M, Poulet J, ed: Illustrierte Geschichte der Medizin. Salzburg, Andreas, 1980. Vol. 6. p. 2003–7.
**Vieira e Silva D** see **Chapman AH**
**Viel B:** Fertility policies in the Latin American continent. **Proc Annu Symp Eugen Soc** 1981;16:15–22
**Viel C:** Quelques vers et écrits de jeunesse d'Henri Moissan. **Rev Hist Pharm (Paris)** 1984 Mar;31(260):5–12
**Viel C** see **Portal C**
**Viesca C** see **Flores y Troncoso FA**
**Viesca Treviño C:** El avicenismo. **Med Tradic** 1980;3(10):33–6
**Viesca Trevino C:** La medicina de Avicena. **Med Tradic** 1980;3(9):45–52
**Viesca Treviño C** see **Peña Páez I de la**
**Vieten B:** Medizinstudenten in Münster. Universität, Studentenschaft und Medizin 1905 bis 1945. Köln, Pahl-Rugenstein, 1982. 367 p.
**Vieuville P:** Duhamel et la médecine. **Hist Sci Med** 1980;14(1):71–6
**Vigani P:** Per una storia dell'assistenza in Lombardia: la pia casa degli incurabili di Abbiategrasso. **Risorgimento** 1982;34(1):48–64
**Vigarello G:** L'eau: Un imaginaire pédagogique dans la médecine des enfants aux XVIe–XVIIe et XVIIIe siècles. **Hist Philos Life Sci** 1981;3(2):171–91
**Vigarello G** see **Bernard M**
**Vigdorchuk IV** see **Napalkov PN**
**Vigliani F, Vigliani MC:** La strefopodia nella fantasia e nell'arte di Gustave Flaubert. **Chir Organi Mov** 1980 Jul–Aug;66(4):533–43
**Vigliani MC** see **Vigliani F**
**Vignati J:** Návrh na zřizení farmakologických oddělení u větších nemocnic. **Cas Lek Cesk** 1982 Dec 23;121(51):1590–1
**Vigue CL, Stanziale WG:** Recombinant DNA: history of the controversy. **Am Biol Teach** 1979;41:480–3, 491
**Vigue CL, Vigue LC:** The eugenics movement in America. **Essays Arts Sci** 1982;11:1–12
**Vigue LC** see **Vigue CL**
**Vikár G:** Emlékezés Anna Freudra. **Orv Hetil** 1983 Nov 13;124(46):2819–20
**Viksna D:** Kurortpilsetas Jurmala galvenas attistibas linijas socialisma celtniecibas posma (1940–1959). **Latv PSR Zinat Akad Vestis** 1979;6:9–20
**Viktor Petrovich Babmindra (k 60–letiiu so dnia rozhdeniia): Arkh Anat Gistol Embriol** 1983 Oct;85(10):102–4
**Vilain M:** Inventaire du fonds d'archives 'Service de santé et Croix–Rouge, 1831–1914'. Bruxelles, Musée royal de l'Armée, 1981. 25 p.
**Vilanilam JV:** A historical and socioeconomic analysis of occupational safety and health in India. **Int J Health Serv** 1980;10(2):233–49
**Vilaro de Descartes M:** Esbozo de una historía... educación de enfermería en la Universidad Católica de Puerto Rico. **Bol Col Prof Enferm PR** 1979 Sep;5(19):14
**Vilček E:** O prvom röntgenológovi z Moravy. **Cesk Radiol** 1980 Mar;34(2):138–43
**Vilček E:** O prvopočiatkoch rádiodiagnostiky a rádioterapie na Slovensku. **Bratisl Lek Listy** 1981;76(1):107–21
**Vilček E:** O zdravotnom stave P. O. Hviezdoslava. **Bratisl Lek Listy** 1983;79(1):117–22
**Vilenskiĭ IuG** see **Panchenko DI**
**Vilks IuK** see **Derums VIa**
**Villa R:** Le famiglie di Gheel: utopia, tradizione e storia nel trattamento della follia. **Studi Stor** 1980;21(3):503–26
**Villa R:** 'Pazzi e criminali': strutture istituzionali e pratica psichiatrica nei manicomi criminali italiani (1876–1915). **Mov Operaio Soc** 1980;3(4):369–93
**Villacorta Cifuentes JL:** Historia de la medicina, cirugia y obstetricia prehispanicas. Guatemala, [s. n.] 1976. 166 p.
**Villaflor GC** see **Sokoloff KL**
**Villanueva AR** see **Bassett EJ**
**Villar E** see **Fernández PL**
**Villard M:** Des hôpitaux de Marseille. **Marseille** 1980;122:93–104
**Villard M:** Des hôpitaux de Marseille. In: Marseille au XVIIème siècle. (Actes du 10ème Colloque de Marseille.) Marseilles Centre Méridional de Rencontres sur le XVIIe siècle. 1980.
**Villard P:** Pathologie et thérapeutique de l'ivresse dans l'Antiquité classique. **Hist Sci Med** 1982;16(3):193–8
**Villarroel H, Lazo B, Campusano C, et al:** Consanguinidad y migración en Viña del Mar durante 1888 a 1967. **Rev Med Chil** 1980 May;108(5):407–12
**Villaseñor RA:** Introduction to and historical overview of surgical procedures for the correction of refractive errors. **Int Ophthalmol Clin** 1983 Fall;23(3):1–9
**Villemin M:** Les vétérinaires français au XIXe siècle. Maisons–Alfort, Editions du point vétérinaire, [1982]. 319 p.
**Villeval G:** La Pharmacie de N.–D.–de-Lorette, à Alan. **Rev Comminges** 1975;88:307–13
**Villey R:** Die Medizin in Rom: Galen. In Sournia JC, Martiny M, Poulet J, ed: Illustrierte Geschichte der Medizin. Salzburg, Andreas, 1980. Vol. 2. p. 411–39.
**Villiers JC de:** Leipoldt as geneesheer. **S Afr Med J** 1980 Dec 6;58(23):921–5
**Villiers JC de, Keyser AL:** Lost hospitals of the Cape. **S Afr Med J** 1983 Jun 29;Spec No:33–9
**Vilmon G:** Orvosi közm'úvel'ódésünk – és könyvtáraink – h'óskora. **Orv Hetil** 1983 Feb 6;124(6):341–4
**Vilter RW:** The evolution of medical ethics. **Forum Med** 1980 Sep;3(9):576–80
**Viñas R** see **Campillo D**
**Vincelet L:** Asklépios, dieu grec de la médecine ou simple praticien grec mortel? **Arch Med Normandie** 1978 Oct, Dec;9(8,10):427–9, 543–4
**Vincent B:** Las epidemias en Andalucia durante el siglo XVI. In: Sociedad Española de Historia de la Medicina. V Congreso Nacional. Madrid, 1977. **Asclepio** 1977;29:351–8
**Viney W, Michaels T, Ganong A:** A note on the history of psychology in magazines. **J Hist Behav Sci** 1981;17:270–2
**Vingrys AJ** see **Cole BL**
**Viniaker H:** L'asthme et son environnement selon Sir John Floyer (1649–1734). **Hist Sci Med** 1984;18(1):77–82
**Vining JW:** Slater Burgesser and his famous spring. **West Ill Reg Stud** 1982;5(2):184–95
**Vining JW:** Versailles Mineral Springs: an historical geography. **Pioneer Am Soc Trans** 1982;5:37–43
**Vinogradova TI** see **Poletaev SD**
**Vinovskis MA:** Fertility in Massachusetts from the Revolution to the Civil War. New York, Academic Press, 1981. xii, 253 p.
**Vinovskis MA:** Mortality rates and trends in Massachusetts before 1860. **J Econ Hist** 1972;32(1):184–213
**Vinovskis MA:** The Jacobson life table of 1850: a critical reexamination from a Massachusetts perspective. **J Interdiscip Hist** 1978;8(4):703–24
**Vinovskis MA:** The 1789 life table of Edward Wigglesworth. **J Econ Hist** 1971;31(3):570–90
**Vinovskis MA** see **Hareven TK**
**Vinovskis MA** see **Rosenkrantz BG**
**Vinovskis MA** see **Spicker SF**
**Vinovskis MA, ed:** Studies in American historical demography. New York, Academic Press, 1979. 530 p. Reprinted articles by various authors.
**Vinuesa L** see **Valverde JL**
**Vinuesa L** see **Valverde Lopez JL**
**Vinuesa SL de** see **Valverde JL**
**Vipmanis VE, Magil'nitskiĭ SG:** Pamiatnye oftal'mologicheskie daty na 1984 g. **Vestn Oftalmol** 1984 Jan–Feb;(1):65–6
**Vipond M:** A Canadian hero of the 1920s: Dr. Frederick G. Banting. **Can Hist Rev** 1982;63(4):461–86
**Viqueira C:** Los hospitales para locos e 'inocentes' en hispanoamerica y sus antecedentes españoles. **Rev Esp Antropol Am** 1970;5:341–83
**Virágos-Kis E** see **Földes V**
**Virchow R:** A painting of lepers by Hans Holbein the Elder. **Am J Dermatopathol** 1984 Aug;6(4):377–8
**Viroulet JJ** see **Loustaud JP**
**Viseltear AJ:** Antecedents to contemporary health issues: history, politics, and the policy of health. With a commentary by B.G. Rosenkrantz. In J. J. Bylebyl, ed: Teaching the history of medicine at a medical center. Baltimore, London, Johns Hopkins University Press, 1982. (The Henry E. Sigerist supplements to the Bulletin of the History of Medicine; new ser., no. 7). p. 62–77.
**Viseltear AJ:** 'C.–E.A. Winslow and the early years of public health at Yale, 1915–1925'. **Yale J Biol Med** 1982 Mar–Apr;55(2):137–51
**Viseltear AJ:** Charles–Edward Amory Winslow. In Dictionary of American Biography, Suppl. 6, 1956–1960. p. 701–3, 1980.
**Viseltear AJ:** John R. Paul and the definition of preventive medicine. **Yale J Biol Med** 1982 May–Aug;55(3–4):167–72
**Viseltear AJ:** Looking back at tomorrow. Commencement address delivered at the Yale University School of Medicine, New Haven, Connecticut, May 24, 1981. **Yale J Biol Med** 1981 May–Jun;54(3):219–25
**Viseltear AJ:** The last illnesses of Robert and Horace Walpole. **Yale J Biol Med** 1983 Mar–Apr;56(2):131–52
**Viseltear AJ** see **George Rosen: In Memoriam**
**Viseltear AJ** see **Numbers RL, ed**
**Visita de Acarí (1593): Hist Cult (Peru)** 1973;7:129–209
**Visiting Nurse Service of Toledo––eighty–three years of caring: Caring** 1984 Apr;3(4):57–61
**The Visiting Nurses Association of Dayton and Montgomery County:** Celebrating 85 years of service. **Caring** 1983 Sep;2(9):18–22
**Visscher MB** see **Wangensteen OW, ed**
**Visser RP:** Arts en geneeskunde in de I83–eeuwse algemene tijdschriften. **Ned Tijdschr Geneeskd** 1981 May 16;125(20):792–4
**Visser RP:** Theorie en praktijk van Swammerdams wetenschappelijke methode in zijn entomologie. **Tijdschr Geschied Geneeskd** 1981;4(2):63–72
**Viswanathan R:** Robert Koch's contribution to medical science. **Indian J Chest Dis Allied Sci** 1982 Apr–Sep;24(2–3):65–7
**Vita a Laennec megemlékezés körül: Orv Hetil** 1981 Dec 13;122(50):3115–6
**Vitkov M** see **Dzhankov I**
**Vitoria M:** Universidad Padre Vitoria. Facultad de Medicina de Bilbao 1936–1937. **Gac Med Bilbao** 1981;78:1–54
**Vitoria Ortiz M:** Ollier et sa contribution à l'étude de l'appareil locomotor. In International Congress of the History of Medicine, 27th, Barcelona, 1980. Actas. Barcelona, Académia de Ciències Médiques de Catalunya i Balears, 1981. p. 680–9.
**Vittetoe MC:** Development of administrative roles for medical technologists. **Am J Med Technol** 1982 Sept;48(9):727–31
**Vivas JG:** Antecedentes históricos de la medicina en San Luis. In Congreso de Historia de la Medicina Argentina [Transactions], 5th, Mendoza, 1983. p. 197–200.
**Vives E, Campillo D:** Hipertrofia de un cornete nasal en una mujer procedente del cementerio medieval de Sant Marçal en Avinyó (Barcelona). In International Congress of the History of Medicine, 27th,

Barcelona, 1980. Actas. Barcelona, Acadèmia de Ciències Mèdiques de Catalunya i Balears, 1981. p. 669–70.

**Vives E, Campillo D:** Otoantritis en un individuo del dolmen del Torrent (Girona). In International Congress of the History of Medicine, 27th, Barcelona, 1980. Actas. Barcelona, Acadèmia de Ciències Mèdiques de Catalunya i Balears, 1981. p. 671–4.

**Vizioli R, De Rosa A:** Medical education and epilepsy. **Prog Clin Biol Res** 1983;124:361–70

**Vizkelety A** see **Kadár Z**

**Vklad farmakologov soiuznykh respublik v razvitie otechestvennoĭ farmakologii: Farmakol Toksikol** 1982 Nov–Dec;45(6):5–13

**Vklad sovetskikh voennykh medikov v pobedu nad militaristskoĭ Iaponieĭ.: Voen Med Zh** 1980 Sep;(9):17–21

**Vladár I:** Thököly Imre fejedelem megrokkanása. **Orv Hetil** 1979 Sep 23;120(38):2317–8

**Vladeck BC, Firman JP:** The aging of the population and health services. **Ann Am Acad Polit Soc Sci** 1983;(468):132–48

**Vladimirova LB, Gribanov ED:** A nagy magyar zeneszerzo, Liszt Ferenc és az ogyesszai gyermekkórház épületének története (orosz nyelven). **Orvostort Kozl** 1982;28(1–3):169–76

**Vladimirova LB, Gribanov ED:** Emblema meditsiny. **Feldsher Akush** 1981;46(4):58–60

**Vladimirova LB:** Sotsial'nye problemy meditsiny i gigieny na VII s'ezde russkikh estestvoispytateleĭ i vracheĭ. **Sov Zdravookhr** 1984;(1):54–7

**Vladimirova LB:** Voprosy bor'by s infektsionnymi zabolevaniiami na VII s'ezde russkikh estestvoispytateleĭ i vracheĭ (k 100–letiiu teorii fagotsitoza). **Zh Mikrobiol Epidemiol Immunobiol** 1984 Aug;(8):115–8

**Vladova MI** see **Bastenchuk AZ**

**Vlasak SM** see **Lambert JB**

**Vlasov AA:** Ikh trudom slaven kollektiv. **Voen Med Zh** 1982 Mar;(3):7–10

**Vlasova NA, Mokrovskaia AA:** 50 let dnevnomu logopedicheskomu polustatsionaru pri detskoĭ psikhiatricheskoĭ bol'nitse No. 6. **Zh Nevropatol Psikhiatr** 1980;80(10):1552–3

**Vlasova–Leshtaeva TF** see **Tiuliandin A**

**Vlček J, Klánova JV:** Akologický kabinet, jeho vznik a osudy. **Rozhl Chir** 1984 Feb;63(2):140–4

**Vlček J:** K historii stoletého trvání I. české chirurgické kliniky v Praze. **Cas Lek Cesk** 1983 Jul 15;122(28):865–70

**Vlietstra RE** see **Espinosa RE**

**Vocci FJ** see **Tocus EC**

**Vocht AM de:** Het gentse antwoord op de armoede: de sociale instellingen van wevers en volders te Gent in de late middeleeuwen. **Ann Soc Belg Hist Hop** 1981;:3–32

**Vodolagin MA:** Partiia––organizator pomoshchi ranenym boitsam i komandiram krasnoi armii v gody volikoi otechestvennoi voiny. **Vopr Istor KPSS** 1978;2:64–75

**Vodop'ianova ZK:** 'Nedelia rebenka' v Respublike Sovetov. **Vopr Istor** 1979;11:175–9

**Voelckel J:** L'école du Pharo. Tradition–permanence–avenir. **Med Trop (Mars)** 1980 Nov–Dec;40(6):635–8

**Voelckel J:** Les traditions du service outre–mer. **Med Armees** 1980;8(10)spec:807–12

**Voelker A** see **Kaiser W**

**Vogel C:** From firing to phenylbutazone in equine practice. **Vet Rec** 1982 Dec 4;111(23):523–5

**Vogel H:** Fraunhofer–Wappen auf einem Apothekenmörser aus dem 17. Jahrhundert. **Dtsch Apoth Ztg** 1980;120:2065–7

**Vogel MJ:** Ida Maud Canon. In Dictionary of American Biography, Suppl. 6, 1956–1960. p. 97–8, 1980.

**Vogel MJ:** Machine politics and medical care: the city hospital at the turn of the century. In Vogel MJ, Rosenberg CE, ed: The therapeutic revolution. Philadelphia, 1979. p. 159–175.

**Vogel MJ:** The invention of the modern hospital: Boston 1870–1930. Chicago, University of Chicago Press, 1980. 171 p.

**Vogel MJ, Rosenberg CE, ed:** The therapeutic revolution. Essays in the social history of American medicine. Philadelphia, University of Pennsylvania Press, 1979. xiii, 270 p.

**Vogel MJ:** The transformation of the American hospital, 1850–1920. In Reverby S, Rosner D, ed: Health care in America. Philadelphia, Temple University Press, 1979. p. 105–16.

**Vogel RJ** see **Blair RD**

**Vogel VJ** see **Hand WD, ed**

**Vogt DD, Montagne M:** Absinthe: behind the emerald mask. **Int J Addict** 1982 Aug;17(6):1015–29

**Vogt DD:** Absinthium: a nineteenth–century drug of abuse. **J Ethnopharmacol** 1981 Nov;4(3):337–42

**Vogt H:** Das Bild des Kranken. Die Darstellung äusserer Veränderungen durch innere Leiden und ihrer Heilmassnahmen von der Renaissance bis in unsere Zeit. 2d. ed. München, Bergmann, 1980. 384 p.

**Vogt H:** Medizinische Karikaturen von 1800 bis zur Gegenwart. 5th ed. München, Bergmann, 1980. 184 p.

**Vogt HH:** 100 Jahre Gram–Färbung. Ein Forschungsbeitrag aus den Anfängen dieser Zeitschrift. **Fortschr Med** 1984 Apr;102(16):94–5

**Vohora SB** see **Aslam M**

**Voigts LE:** British Library, Cotton Vitellius C. III, f. 82. **Old Engl Newsl** 1978 Fall;12(1):12–3

**Voigts LE:** British Library, Royal 12 D. XVII, f. 30v. **Old Engl Newsl** 1979 Fall;13(1):12–3

**Voigts LE** see **Levere TH, ed**

**Voisine N:** Marguerite Bourdon. In Dictionary of Canadian biography, 1701 to 1740. Volume 2, 1969. p. 92–3.

**Voitcu M** see **Năstasă V**

**Voĭtenko MF:** Organizatsiia meditsinskogo obespecheniia 64–ĭ armii pri vydvizhenii ee iz raĭona Stalingrada v novyĭ raĭon voennykh deĭstviĭ. **Voen Med Zh** 1984 Feb;(2):69–71

**Voĭtenko MF:** Organizatsiia meditsinskogo obespecheniia 7–ĭ gvardeĭskoĭ armii v Belgorodsko–Kharkovskoĭ nastupatel'noĭ operatsii (K 40–letiiu bitvy pod Kurskom). **Voen Med Zh** 1983 Aug;8:16–20

**Voĭtenko MF, Zil'berberg LB:** Organizatsiia raboty DMP pri massovom postuplenii ranenykh v period Velikoĭ Otechestvennoĭ voiny. **Voen Med Zh** 1983 Nov;(11):15–8

**Vojáček M:** Cíle a úkoly psychoterapie v díle Ernsta Kretschmera. **Cesk Psychiatr** 1979 Feb;75(1):69–72

**Vojtísek V:** Historie chirurgické kliniky lékařské fakulty hygienické Univerzity Karlovy v Praze. **Rozhl Chir** 1983 Jul;62(7):533–8

**Volbehr K:** Gesundheit an Bord. Kleine Geschichte der Hygiene und Arzneimittelversorgung auf Schiffen. Bremerhaven, Ditzen, 1979. 72 p. (Führer des Deutschen Schiffahrtsmuseums, Nr. 11).

**Voldman D:** Guérir du cancer et mourir de vieillesse: histoire de l'hospice Paul–Brousse de 1905 à 1975. **Asclepio** 1983;35:317–26

**Vol'f MSh** see **Tyklina IG**

**Volk L:** Episkopat und Kirchenkampf im Zweiten Weltkrieg. Lebensvernichtung und Klostersturm 1939–1941. **Stimmen Zeit** 1980;198(9):597–611

**Volk R:** Gesundheitswesen und Wohltätigkeit im Spiegel der byzantinischen Klostertypika. München, Institut für Byzantinistik und neugriechische Philologie der Universität München, 1983. lxxx, 326 p. (Miscellanea Byzantina monacensia, Heft 28)

**Volkan VD:** Cyprus––war and adaptation: a psychoanalytic history of two ethnic groups in conflict. Charlottesville, University Press of Virginia, 1979. xxviii, 192 p.

**Völker A:** Die Schwindsucht im halleschen Schrifttum des 18. Jahrhunderts. **Wiss Beitr Martin Luther Univ Halle Wittenberg** 1983;5–R80:203–10

**Völker A:** Markierungspunkte in der Geschichte der Parathyreoideaforschung. **Z Gesamte Inn Med** 1983 Aug 1;38(15):386–7

**Völker A:** Martin Luther und seine Arzte. Ein Beitrag zum Lutherjahr 1983. **Z Gesamte Inn Med** 1983 Oct 15;38(20):533–9

**Völker A** see **Kaiser W**

**Völker A** see **Skrobacki A**

**Volkert G:** Die Entwicklung der Körperbehindertenfürsorge. **ZFA (Stuttgart)** 1980 Apr 10;56(10):725–30

**Volkov MV, Mattis ER:** Osnovnye itogi napravleniia razvitiia Sovetskoĭ travmatologii i ortopedii. **Vestn Khir** 1982 Nov;129(11):3–9

**Volkov MV:** Tsentral'nomu institutu travmatologii i ortopedii im. N. N. Priorova––60 let. **Ortop Travmatol Protez** 1981;(4):1–5

**Volkov VV, Danilichev VF:** Professor A.V. Khodin – osnovatel' i pervyĭ redaktor–izdatel' 'Vestnika oftal'mologii' (k 100–letiiu zhurnala). **Vestn Oftalmol** 1984 Nov–Dec;(6):3–4

**Volkov VV, Shiliaev VG:** Voennaia Oftal'mologiia v period Velikoĭ Otechestvennoĭ Voĭny. **Voen Med Zh** 1980 May;(5):50–3

**Völksen W:** Die Stuckbilder der Berg–Apotheke in Clausthal–Zellerfeld. **Beitr Gesch Pharm** 1984;31(23):197–203

**Vollman RF:** Pathfinders 2: Wilhelm Hillebrand, first teacher of the sympto–thermic method. **Int Rev Nat Fam Plann** 1979;3:316–21

**Vollmer G** see **Lorenz K, ed**

**Volná A** see **Tichý M**

**Volodina MN** see **Buslaeva MM**

**Volodina MN** see **Puchkov IuG**

**Volokhov AA, Kolt'tsova MM, Kostandov EA, et al:** Institutu vyssheĭ nervnoĭ deiatel'nosti i neĭrofiziologii Adademii nauk 30 let. **Zh Vyssh Nerv Deiat** 1981 Jan–Feb;31(1):202–16

**Voloshin PV:** Razvitie nevrologicheskoĭ nauki na Ukraine za gody Sovetskoĭ vlasti. **Vrach Delo** 1983 Feb;(2):116–20

**Voloshin PV:** 60 let Khar'kovskomu nauchno–issledovatel'skomu institutu nevrologii i psikhiatrii im. V. P. Protopopova. **Zh Nevropatol Psikhiatr** 1983;83(5):780–3

**Volpitto PP** see **Vandam L**

**Vom Germanin zum Acylureidopenicillin.:** Forschung die Geschichte machte. Dokumentation einer wissenschaftlichen Revolution. Leverkusen, Bayer AG, 1980. 77 p.

**Von der Magie zur Medizin. In Becker U: Herders Gesundheitslexikon: Medizin von A biz Z. Freiburg, Herder, 1973. p. 13–36.:**

**Vondráček V:** Lékař dále vzpromíná (1920–1938). Praha, Avicenum, 1977. 481 p.

**Vonèche JJ** see **Vidal F**

**Von Endt DW, Ortner DJ:** Amino acid analysis of bone from a possible case of prehistoric iron deficiency anemia from the American Southwest. **Am J Phys Anthropol** 1982 Dec;59(4):377–85

**Von Paracelsus zu Goethe und Wilhelm von Humboldt:** Wien, Verband der Wissenschaftlichen Gesellschaften Osterreichs, 1981. 203 p.

**Voogd J:** Morphology and clinical neurology. The history and evolution of Wallenberg's syndrome. **Acta Morphol Neerl Scand** 1983 Mar;21(1):27–47

**Voorhees JJ:** 'Psoriasis as a possible defect of the adenyl cyclase–cyclic AMP Cascade' by Voorhees and Duell, October 1971. Commentary: Cyclic adenosine monophosphate regulation of normal and psoriatic epidermis. **Arch Dermatol** 1982 Oct;118(10):862–74

**Voorthuisen AE van** see **Falke TH**

**Vora E:** Evolution of race: a synthesis of social and biological concepts. **J Black Stud** 1981;12(2):182–91

**Vorob'ev AA:** O tendentsiiakh razvitiia sovremennoĭ immunologii.

**Zh Mikrobiol Epidemiol Immunobiol** 1979 Dec;(12):3–9
**Vorob'ev AI:** Ivan Mikhaĭlovich Sechenov. **Klin Med (Mosk)** 1980;58(11):105–8
**Vorob'ev AS** see **Orlova NV**
**Vorob'ev RI:** Istoriko-meditsinskie raboty I. A. Kassirskogo. **Feldsher Akush** 1984 Jul;49(7):44–6
**Vorob'ev RI** see **Zhuravleva TV**
**Vorob'ev VI, Krolenko SA, Rumiantsev PP, et al:** Adol'f Aronovich Lev (k 60–letiiu so dnia rozhdeniia). **Tsitologiia** 1983 Jul;25(7):852–9
**Vorob'ev IuI, Veretennikova VP:** 25 let kafedry rentgenologii i radiologii Moskovskogo meditsinskogo stomatologicheskogo instituta im. N. A. Semashko. **Vestn Rentgenol Radiol** 1980 Sep–Oct;(5):88–9
**Vorob'eva EI** see **Sokolov VE**
**Voronenkova IA** see **Tkachenko BI**
**Voronin LG:** Vysshaia nervnaia deiatel'nost' i psikhologiia. **Zh Vyssh Nerv Deiat** 1983 Jul–Aug;33(4):611–8
**Voronkov OV:** Iz istorii sozdaniia sapasov meditsinskogo imushchestva dlia obespecheniiavoĭsk na sluchaĭ voĭny (soobshchenie pervoe). **Voen Med Zh** 1984 Feb;(2):72–3
**Voronkov OV:** Iz istorii sozdaniia zapasov meditsinskogo imushchestva dlia obespecheniia voĭsk vo vremia voĭny (soobshchenie vtoroe). **Voen Med Zh** 1984 Oct;(10):66–8
**Voronkov OV:** Obespechenie meditsinskim imushchestvom voĭsk voennogo okruga vo vremia Velikoĭ Otechestvennoĭ voĭny. **Voen Med Zh** 1980 Oct;(10):19–22
**Voronkov OV:** Remont meditsinskogo imushchestva vo vremia Velikoĭ Otechestvennoĭ voĭny. **Voen Med Zh** 1982 May;(5):73–5
**Voronkov OV** see **Borisov EN**
**Voronov IB, Zeimal EV:** Obituary: Professor M. J. Michelson (died 16 August 1978). The contribution of Professor M. J. Michelson to comparative and evolutionary pharmacology. **Comp Biochem Physiol** 1979;62C(1):1–4
**Vorontsova EI, Moĭkin IuV:** V. I Lenin o profilakticheskom napravlenii sovetskogo zdravookhraneniia (k 110–ĭ godovshchine so dnia rozhdeniia Vladimira Il'icha Lenina). **Gig Tr Prof Zabol** 1980 Apr;(4):1–4
**Voskuil PH:** The epilepsy of Fyodor Mikhailovitch Dostoevsky (1821–1881). **Epilepsia** 1983 Dec;24(6):658–67
**Vosniuc R** see **Marinescu CG**
**Voss H:** Goethes Selbstzeugnisse über seine Beschäftigung mit 'organischen Naturen'. **Gegenbaurs Morphol Jahrb** 1979;125(5):687–736
**Voss H:** Goethes Selbstzeugnisse über seine Beschäftigung mit 'organischen Naturen'. II. Briefe (1776 bis 1817). **Gegenbaurs Morphol Jahrb** 1979;125(4):466–518
**Voss HJ:** Beitrag zur Seuchenlage in den Pferdebeständen einer Armee 1940/41 und zur Erfahrung als Leiter eines Seuchenlazarettes für Pferde. **DTW** 1981 Nov 5;88(11):483–6
**Voss J, ed** see **Oleson A**
**Voswinckel P:** Arzt und Auto: das Auto und seine Welt im Spiegel des Deutschen Arztblattes von 1907 bis 1975. Münster, Murken–Altrogge, 1981. iii, 194 p.
**Votavová J:** Prof. PhDr. PhMr. O. Tomíček a jeho analytická škola. **Cesk Farm** 1984 Jun;33(5):213–4
**Voth DE** see **Miller MK**
**Votočková J:** 130 let Helmholtzova oftalmoskopu. **Cesk Oftalmol** 1982 Jan;38(1):51–3
**Vovelle M:** A century and one–half of American epitaphs (1660–1813): toward the study of collective attitudes about death. **Comp Stud Soc Hist** 1980;22(4):534–47
**Vovelle M:** Rediscovery of death since 1960. **Ann Am Acad Polit Soc Sci** 1980;447:89–99
**Vovelle M:** The history of mankind in the mirror of death. **Proc Annu Meet West Soc Fr Hist** 1978;6:91–109
**Vovk IG:** Meropriiatiia KPSS po razvitiiu nardonogo zdravookhraneniia v predvoennye gody. **Voen Med Zh** 1980 Jun;(6):18–20
**Vovk IG:** Sovetskoe zdravookhranenie v gody pervykh piatiletok. **Voen Med Zh** 1981 Oct;(10):10–2
**Voyat G:** In tribute to Piaget: a look at his scientific impact in the United States. In R. W. Rieber, K. Salzinger, ed: Psychology: theoretical–historical perspectives. New York, Academic Press, 1980. p. 305–14.
**Voyatzakis E, et al:** [The research work of Sir Alexander Fleming] (Gre). **Mater Med Greca** 1981;9:367–76
**Voynovich P** see **Lewin PK**
**Vozchikov-Chernov SP:** V polevom podvizhnom gospitale. **Voen Med Zh** 1981 Nov;(11):70
**Vrbic V** see **Farcnik F**
**Vrebos J:** Jehan Yperman, medieval cleft lip surgeon. **Plast Reconstr Surg** 1982 Dec;70(6):762–5
**Vreeland JM, Cockburn A:** Mummies of Peru. In A. Cockburn, E. Cockburn, ed: Mummies, disease, and ancient cultures. Cambridge, Cambridge University Press, 1980. p. 135–74.
**Vreeland JM** see **Riddle JM**
**Vries A de:** The essence of medical ethics. **Biomed Pharmacother** 1982 Jan;36(1):59–65
**Vries PA de** see **Hendriks IH**
**Vukadinovic S:** Razvoj i zadaci pedijatrijske kardiologije. **Lijec Vjesn** 1979 Dec;101(12):733–6
**Vukas A:** Organizacija borbe protiv kožnih i spolnih bolesti i dosadašnji nedostaci u tom pogledu. **Lijec Vjesn** 1979 Nov;101(11):718–9
**Vuksanovic P** see **Goethe H**
**Vulcanescu R:** Les chevaux fantastiques et la psychothérapie populaire. In International Congress of the History of Medicine. 26th, Plovdiv, 1978. Actes du Congress. Sofia, 1981. Volume II. p. 83–5.
**Vuori H:** Lääketieteen historian tutkimuksesta. **Duodecim** 1980;96(1):9–17
**Vuori H, Rimpela M:** The development and impact of the medical model. **Perspect Biol Med** 1981 Winter;24(2):217–28
**Vuori H:** The World Health Organization and traditional medicine. **Community Med** 1982 May;4(2):129–37
**Vurgaft MB:** The 90th anniversary of Maklakov's applanation tomometer. **Am J Optom Physiol Opt** 1981 Feb;58(2):183–5
**Vutov M, Krumova E:** Razvitie na stomatologicnata pomost i obrazovanie v bulgariia. **Stomatologiia (Sofiia)** 1979 Mar–Apr;61(2):133–6
**Vutov M, Ivanova K:** Stomatologichnata pomost na podrastvastoto pokolenie u nas do September 9, 1944 godina. **Stomatologiia (Sofiia)** 1979 Nov–Dec;61(6):400–5
**Vutreshnata meditsina u nas prez poslednoto stoletie: Vutr Boles** 1979;18(5):1–9
**Vyas VD** see **Singh RS**
**Vyhnanek L:** 'Muggles,' 'Inchy,' and 'Mud': illegal drugs in New Orleans during the 1920's. **La Hist** 1981;22(3):253–79
**Vytrishchak VIa:** Vklad N. I. Pirogova v razvitie cheliustno–litsevoĭ khirurgii. **Voen Med Zh** 1982 Nov;(11):64–5
**Významné životné jubileum prof. MUDr. Adolfa Zácka: Cesk Zdrav** 1982 Dec;30(12):530–6
**Vzaimootnosheniia A.I. Gertsena i S. P. Botkina: Klin Med (Mosk)** 1983 Jun;61(6):108–10

## W

**Waas G:** Die Berufung von August Bier (1861–1949) an die Berliner Universität im Jahre 1907. **Z Arztl Fortbild (Jena)** 1980 Oct 15;74(20):982–7
**Wacek S:** Sytuacja zdrowotna Podola w świetle pism dr med Józefa Apolinarego Rollego. **Arch Hist Med (Warsz)** 1981;44(1):99–110
**Wachinger L:** Buber und Freud. **Stimmen Zeit** 1978;196(11):754–62
**Wachs GN:** The French school of dermatology. **Int J Dermatol** 1982 Jun;21(5):277–9
**Wachter MA de:** Is death and dying dying merely an ethical issue? **Ann Am Acad Polit Soc Sci** 1980;447:78–88
**Wachter RD** see **Titche LL**
**Wacke A:** Unfälle bei Sport und Spiel nach römischem und geltendem Recht. **Stadion** 1977;3(1):4–43
**Wackenheim A:** Die Entwicklung der menschlichen Hand in der Kunst. **Radiologe** 1982 May;22(5):195–8
**Wackenheim A, Dietemann J, Babin E, et al:** Hémi–occipitalisation de l'atlas chez un Mérovingien du bas Moyen Age. **J Radiol** 1981 Oct;62(10):545–7
**Wada J** see **al-Naaman YD**
**Waddington CH, Thom R:** On cell differentiation. **Riv Biol** 1981;74(1–2):213–27
**Waddington JL:** Ventricular enlargement in schizophrenia and the historical studies of John Haslam. **Am J Psychiatry** 1984 Dec;141(12):1640
**Waddy JL** see **Maddern GJ**
**Wade A:** 'Martindale'. The International Use of 'Martindale: the Extra Pharmacopoeia'. **Farm Tid** 1979 Dec 1;89(48):1001–4
**Wade N:** Hybridomas: the making of a revolution [news]. **Science** 1982 Feb 26;215(4536):1073–5
**Wade N:** The Nobel duel. Two scientists' 21–year race to win the world's most coveted research prize. Garden City, Anchor Press/Doubleday, 1981. 321 p.
**Wade NJ:** A note on the history of binocular microscopes. **Perception** 1981;10(5):591–2
**Wade-Jardetzky NG** see **Jardetzky O**
**Wadecki Z:** Nadgraniczny jubileusz. **Pieleg Polozna** 1984;(2):27
**Wagner BM:** Connective tissue disease––historical perspective. **Monogr Pathol** 1983;24:1–3
**Wagner D:** August Ferdynand Wolff und die Bedeutung der Semiotik. **Arch Hist Med (Warsz)** 1979;42(2):263–8
**Wagner D:** Die Epidemiologie in der Berliner medizinhistorischen Forschung des 19. Jahrhunderts. **Z Gesamte Hyg** 1980;26(12):920–3
**Wagner D:** Einige Aspekte von den Anfängen der experimentellen Desinfektionslehre. **Z Gesamte Hyg** 1982 Mar;28(3):172–6
**Wagner D:** The proletarianization of nursing in the United States. **Int J Health Serv** 1980;10(2):271–90
**Wagner D:** Zu August Hirschs epidemiologischer Reise an die Wolga im Jahre 1879 (ein Beispiel russisch–deutscher Zusammenarbeit auf medizinischem Gebiet. **Z Gesamte Hyg** 1980;26(5):377–8
**Wagner FB:** Revisit of Samuel D. Gross, M.D. **Surg Gynecol Obstet** 1981 May;152(5):663–74
**Wagner FB:** The founding fathers and centennial history of the Philadelphia Academy of Surgery. **Ann Surg** 1980 Jul;192(1):1–8
**Wagner G:** Robert Koch––Leistungen für die Menschheit. **Z Arztl Fortbild (Jena)** 1982 Jul 15;75(14):653–5
**Wagner GP** see **Lorenz K, ed**
**Wagner HJ:** Zur historischen Entwicklung des Begriffs 'Aerztlicher Kunstfehler'. **Z Rechtsmed** 1981;86(4):303–6
**Wagner JG:** History of pharmacokinetics. **Pharmacol Ther** 1981;12(3):537–62
**Wagner O** see **Oesterreich K**
**Wagner S** see **Jackle P**
**Wahab Zuhuri MA:** Influence on Ibn Sina on Unani medicine in subsequent ages. **Bull Indian Inst Hist Med (Hyderabad)** 1981;1–4:103–9
**Wahl RW:** Eponym: the loop of Henle. **South Med J** 1984 Apr;77(4):494–5

**Wahlberg P:** Tyreoidologi i Finland under 150 år. **Nord Medicinhist Arsb** 1984;:105–16

**Wahlquist WL:** Population growth in the Mormon core area: 1847–1890. Jackson, Richard H., ed. The Mormon role in the settlement of the West. 1978. Reprint ed., Provo, Utah, Brigham Young U. Pr., 1980. p. 107–34.

**Wahrman A:** The Philadelphia physician-factory. **J Hist Med Allied Sci** 1983 Jul;38(3):334–5

**Wain SL:** The controversy of unmodified versus citrated blood transfusion in the early 20th century. **Transfusion** 1984 Sep–Oct;24(5):404–7

**Wainapel SF:** Frederick Delius; medical assessment. **NY State J Med** 1980 Nov;80(12):1886–7

**Wainwright D** see **Cowell B**

**Waisman M:** Concepts of acne of the British school of dermatology prior to 1860. **Int J Dermatol** 1983 Mar;22(2):126–9

**Waisman M:** Historical note: Koebner on the isomorphic phenomenon. **Arch Dermatol** 1981 Jul;117(7):415

**Waite GM:** The indigenous medical system in East-Central African history. Ph.D. Diss., University of California, Los Angeles, 1981. xvi, 277 p.

**Waite RG:** The psychopathic god - Adolf Hitler. New York, Basic Books, 1977. xx, 482 p.

**Waites B** see **Evans B**

**Waites L:** American pioneers in the topic of word blindness. In Rose FC, Bynum WF, ed: Historical aspects of the neurosciences. New York, Raven, 1982. p. 115–6.

**Waitzkin H:** The social origins of illness: a neglected history. **Int J Health Serv** 1981;11(1):77–103

**Wajeman G:** Le Maître et l'hystérique. Paris, Navarin Editeur, 1982. 286 p. (Bibliothèque des Analytica).

**Wajs S:** O pierwszym zabiegu uranoplastyki w Polsce. **Czas Stomatol** 1980 Nov;33(11):1043–6

**Wajs S:** Obturatory stosowane w leczeniu protetycznym rozszczepów wrodzonych lub nabytych podniebienia twardego i miękkiego. Czesc III. **Nov Med Tekh** 1979 May–Jun;29(3):211–8

**Wajs S:** Sposoby znieczulenia stosowane przy usuwaniu zebow przed stu laty. **Czas Stomatol** 1979 Dec;32(12):1211–3

**Wajs S:** Sześćdziesifciolecie Państwowego Instytutu Dentystycznego. **Czas Stomatol** 1981 Aug;34(8):823–35

**Wajs S** see **Sródka A**

**Wakefield WL:** Heretics as physicians in the thirteenth century. **Speculum** 1982 Apr;57(2):328–31

**Wald FS** see **Foster Z**

**Wald HJ** see **Foster Z**

**Wald I** see **Mazurczak T**

**Waldeck-Semadeni EK:** Paul Julius Moebius, 1853–1907, Leben und Werk. Diss. Bern, 1980. 222 p.

**Walden DM:** Rebels among dissenters: a local history of chiropractic in Provo, Utah. **Chiropr Hist** 1984;4(1):55–61

**Waldenlind E** see **Ekbom K**

**Waldhauser H:** Zur Kur in Oesterreich, 'wo heilsam Wasser durch die Klüfte schleicht.' St. Pölten, Verlag Niederösterreichisches Pressehaus, 1980. 160 p.

**Waldinger RJ:** Virginia Apgar. In: Notable American women. The modern period. Cambridge, Mass., Belknap-Harvard Univ. Press, 1980. 4:27-8.

**Waldis V:** Der 'Stich' von 1564 - eine primäre Lungenpest. **Gesnerus** 1983;40(1–2):223–8

**Waldis V:** Hospitalisation und Absonderung in Pestzeiten--die Schweiz im Vergleich zu Oberitalien. **Gesnerus** 1982;39(1):71–8

**Waldis V:** Obrigkeitliche Massnahmen gegen die Pest in Stadt und Herrschaft Rheinfelden im 16. und 17. Jahrhundert. **Gesnerus** 1979;36(3–4):206–27

**Waldron G:** Sir Frederick Treves and the elephant man. **Lancet** 1980 Jul 5;2(8184):42

**Waldron HA:** A brief history of scrotal cancer. **Br J Ind Med** 1983 Nov;40(4):390–401

**Waldron HA:** Did the Mad Hatter have mercury poisoning? **Br Med J [Clin Res]** 1983 Dec 24–31;287(6409):1961

**Waldron HA:** Lead in bones: a cautionary tale. **Ecol Dis** 1982;1(2–3):191–6

**Waldron HA:** On the history of scrotal cancer. **Ann R Coll Surg Engl** 1983 Nov;65(6):420–2

**Waldron HA:** Richard Pulteney (1730–1801): Linnean botanist and cardiologist. **Trans Stud Coll Physicians Phila** 1980 Mar;5(2 no 1):31–40

**Waldron HA** see **Hart GD, ed**

**Waldron M** see **Levenson SM**

**Walewski W, Markowski W, Mosejczuk L, et al:** [35 years of service in medical supply to the Polish People's Forces]. (Rus) **Voen Med Zh** 1979 Nov;(11):67–8

**Walker A, Zimmerman MR, Leakey RE:** A possible case of hypervitaminosis A in Homo erectus. **Nature** 1982 Mar 18;296(5854):248–50

**Walker A:** Diet and teeth. Dietary hypotheses and human evolution. **Philos Trans R Soc Lond [Biol]** 1981 May 8;292(1057):57–64

**Walker A** see **Teaford MF**

**Walker AE:** The past four decades--experimental epilepsy. **Res Publ Assoc Res Nerv Ment Dis** 1983;61:1–17

**Walker AR, Richardson BD:** What did our forefathers eat? **S Afr Med J** 1981 Jan 3;59(1):3–4

**Walker B:** Meat preservation in Scotland. **R Soc Health J** 1981 Feb;101(1):19–28

**Walker FA:** Americanism versus Sovietism: a study of the reaction to the committee on the costs of medical care. **Bull Hist Med** 1979 Winter;53(4):489–504

**Walker J:** The British Red Cross in the Bromley area 1910–1919. **Bromley Local Hist** 1979;4:17–23

**Walker JB:** Charles John Bond of Leicester (1856–1939). **J R Soc Med** 1984 Apr;77(4):316–24

**Walker JD:** Family Medicine Education. A Kansas historical review, 1967–1982. **J Kans Med Soc** 1983 Mar;84(3):138–42

**Walker JD, Scott JS:** Location of mortality schedules of the United States decennial censuses, 1850–1900. **J Afro-Am Hist Geneal Soc** 1981;2(1):1–7

**Walker JM** see **Bülbring E**

**Walker LG:** L. L. Staton, M.D., and the first successful gastrostomy in America. **Surg Gynecol Obstet** 1984 Apr;158(4):387–8

**Walker LG** see **Chambers RW**

**Walker R:** The struggle against pulmonary tuberculosis in Australia, 1788–1950. **Hist Stud** 1983;20:439–61

**Walker RB:** Medical aspects of tobacco smoking and the anti-tobacco movement in Britain in the nineteenth Century. **Med Hist** 1980;24(4):391–402

**Walker RE:** Malleus and podagra: lead poisoning in horse and man. **Vet Hist** 1980/81, n.s.;1:118–36

**Walker RG:** Public death in the eighteenth century. **Res Stud** 1980;48(1):11–24

**Walker RM** see **Dobson J**

**Walker RT:** Joseph Whittlesey Noble: an American in Hong Kong. **J Am Dent Assoc** 1984 Nov;109(5):757

**Walker SS:** Witchcraft and healing in an African church. **J Relig Afr** 1979;10(2):127–138

**Walker W:** Harvey's contemporaries--science and society. **Scott Med J** 1981 Oct;26(4):356–63

**Walker WO:** Drug control in the Americas. Albuquerque, University of New Mexico Press, 1981. xvi, 287 p.

**Walkowitz JR:** Prostitution and Victorian society. Women, class, and the state. Cambridge, New York, Cambridge University Press, 1980. ix, 347 p.

**Wall HM:** Feminism and the New England Hospital, 1949–1961. **Am Q** 1980;32(4):435–52

**Wall JH:** Westchester County Medical Society and Westchester Division, New York Hospital-Cornell Medical Center; milestones in history. **NY State J Med** 1980 Nov;80(12):1884–5

**Wall R:** Inferring differential neglect of females from mortality data. **Ann Demogr Hist (Paris)** 1981;:119–40

**Wall R** see **Benson B**

**Wall WD:** Jean Piaget - 1896–1979. **J Child Psychol Psychiatry** 1982 Apr;23(2):97–104

**Wall R, ed** see **Charlton C**

**Wallace AF:** The influence of the Battle of Jutland on plastic surgery. In Romm S, ed: Symposium on historical perspectives of plastic surgery. Philadelphia, Saunders, 1983. p. 657–63.

**Wallace AF:** The progress of plastic surgery: an introductory history. Oxford, W. A. Meeuws, 1982. xii, 184 p.

**Wallace AF:** The surgery of beauty. **Trans Med Soc Lond** 1981–82;98:17–23

**Wallace AF** see **Romm S, ed**

**Wallace AR** see **McKinney HL, ed**

**Wallace B:** Changes in the genetic mentality. **Perspect Biol Med** 1984 Summer;27(4):598–610

**Wallace CE, Marshall FN, Robinson C:** A retrospective review of maternal and child health services at the Albert Schweitzer Hospital in rural Haiti. **Bull Pan Am Health Organ** 1982;16(1):7–16

**Wallace DJ:** Fibromyalgia: unusual historical aspects and new pathogenic insights. **Mt Sinai J Med (NY)** 1984 Apr;51(2):124–31

**Wallace DJ:** Thomsonians: the people's doctors. **Clio Med** 1980 Jul;14(3–4):169–86

**Wallace EM:** The first vaccinator. Benjamin Jesty of Yetminster and Worth Matravers and his family. Wareham and Swanage (England), Anglebury-Bartlett, 1981. 20 p.

**Wallace ER:** A commentary on the Freud-Jung letters. **Psychoanal Rev** 1980 Spring;67(1):112–37

**Wallace ER, Pressley LC, ed:** Essays in the history of psychiatry: a tenth anniversary supplementary volume to the Psychiatric Forum. Columbia, Wm. S. Hall Psychiatric Institute, 1980. xviii, 205 p. Contributions by E. Ackerknecht, R. Bosnak, E. T. Carlson, H. Decker, C. Fox, J. Gach, G. Gifford, M. Gildea, S. Jackson, O. Marx, W. McGuire, G. Mora, R. C. Powell, P. Stepansky.

**Wallace ER:** Freud and anthropology. A history and reappraisal. New York, International Universities Press, 1983. xi, 306 p. (Psychological Issues, Monograph 55).

**Wallace ER:** Historiography in history and psychoanalysis. **Bull Hist Med** 1983 Summer;57(2):247–66

**Wallace ER:** The primal parricide. **Bull Hist Med** 1980 Summer;54(2):153–65

**Wallace IR** see **Goodman WS**

**Wallace M** see **Fee E**

**Wallace M** see **Knightley P**

**Wallace WA:** Prelude to Galileo. Essays on medieval and sixteenth-century sources of Galileo's thought. Dordrecht, D. Reidel, 1981. xvi, 369 p. (Boston Studies in the Philosophy of Science, v. 62).

**Wallace B, ed** see **Lewontin RC**

**Walle E van de** see **Gutmann MP**

**Walle E van de** see **Laslett P**

**Waller T, Killion G:** Georgia folk medicine. **South Folkl Q** 1972;36(1):71–92

**Wallerstein RO:** ABIM certification revisited-what a difference 30 years make. **Trans Am Clin Climatol Assoc** 1982;94:182–9

**Wallerstein RS:** Anna Freud: radical innovator and staunch conservative. **Psychoanal Study Child** 1984;39:65–80
**Wallerstein RS** see **Goldberg A, ed**
**Wallerström A:** Johann Friedrich Struensee--en psykologisk gåta. **Nord Medicinhist Arsb** 1981;:74–87
**Wallerström A:** Levande tärd av maskar--terapeutisk användning av fluglarver. **Nord Medicinhist Arsb** 1980;:136–46
**Wallis R, et al** see **Morley P**
**Wallman LJ:** Shunting for hydrocephalus: an oral history. **Neurosurgery** 1982 Aug;11(2):308–13
**Wallner B:** The Middle English translation of Guy de Chauliac's Treatise on ulcers. Part II. Notes, glossary, marginalia. Book IV of the Great surgery. Edited from Ms. New York Academy of Medicine 12 and related mss. Stockholm, Almqvist & Wiksell International, 1983. 48 p. (Acta Universitatis Lundensis, Sectio I Theologica Juridica Humaniora 44).
**Wallot H:** A view on the socio-political history of psychiatric care in French-Canada with particular reference to Quebec asylums. **Soc Sci Med [Med Psychol Med Sociol]** 1980 Dec;14A(6):485–94
**Walls AF:** 'The heavy artillery of the missionary army': the domestic importance of the nineteenth-century medical missionary. In Sheils WJ, ed: The Church and healing. Papers read at the twentieth summer meeting and the twenty-first winter meeting of the Ecclesiastical History Society. Oxford, Basil Blackwell for the Society, 1982. p. 287–97.
**Walls E:** Observations on the New Orleans yellow-fever epidemic, 1878. **La Hist** 1982 Winter;23:60–7
**Walls E:** The introduction of prepayment medicine to Arkansas: the Trinity Hospital experience. **Arkansas Hist Q** 1983;42(1):3–26
**Walls HJ:** Henry Smith Holden. In Dictionary of national biography, 1961–1970. Suppl. 8, 1981. p. 524–5.
**Walls WK** see **Anning ST**
**Walravens H:** Alexander Tatarinov (1817–1886)--russischer Arzt und Sinologe, eine biobibliographische Skizze. **Sudhoffs Arch** 1980;64(4):392–6
**Walser HH:** Adolf Meyer--student of the Zurich psychiatric school. **Gesnerus** 1984;41(1/2):49–52
**Walser HH:** Der Weg der Schweizer Psychiatrie ins zwanzigste Jahrhundert. **Gesnerus** 1982;39(1):97–108
**Walser HH:** Geschichtliche Anmerkungen zum Problem der Aggressivität in der klinischen Psychiatrie. **Schweiz Arch Neurol Neurochir Psychiatr** 1981;129(1):83–91
**Walser HH:** Ist das Wohl des Landesherrn in Wein zu trinken? Carl und Gerhart Hauptmann bei August Forel in Zürich. **Gesnerus** 1981;38:207–14
**Walsh BM:** Health education and the demand for tobacco in Ireland, 1953–76: a note. **Econ Soc Rev (Irel)** 1980;11(2):147–51
**Walsh J:** New niche for science on reference shelf. **Science** 1981 Jan 16;211(4479):263–4
**Walsh J:** Science in transition, 1946 to 1962. **Science** 1980 Jul 4;209(4452):52–7
**Walsh J:** Who was William Doolin? **Ir Med J** 1983 Oct;76(10):436–7
**Walsh JP, Adelson R:** Health care: no time for placebos. **NY Aff** 1978;5(2):151–61
**Walsh LS:** 'Till death us do part': marriage and family in seventeenth-century Maryland. In Tate, TW, Ammerman, DL., ed. The Chesapeake in the seventeenth century: essays on Anglo-American society (Chapel Hill, U. of North Carolina Press for the Institute of Early American Hist. and Culture, 1979): 126–52.
**Walsh MR:** The rediscovery of the need for a feminist medical education. **Harv Educ Rev** 1979;49(4):447–66
**Walsh MR** see **Mandelbaum DR**
**Walsh RJ:** Adverse reactions to blood transfusion: introduction -- historical overview. **Anaesth Intensive Care** 1980 May;8(2):112–4
**Walsh RJ** see **Refshauge WF**
**Walsh W:** The Keatsian paradox: the hectic and the healthy. **Ann R Coll Surg Engl** 1984 Mar;66(2):139–44
**Walt AJ:** The world's best-known surgeon. **Surgery** 1983 Oct;94(4):582–90
**Walter CW:** Use of surgical rubber gloves. **Surgery** 1983 May;93(5):728–9
**Walter H:** Sándor Ferenczi. In J. Rattner, ed: Wandlungen der Psychoanalyse. Wien, Europaverlag, 1980. p. 53–86.
**Walter JD:** Charles W. Stearns and Norman W. Kingsley and the development of the artificial velum. **Bull Hist Dent** 1981 Oct;29(2):74–81
**Walter JD:** More on 'hare-lip'. **Cleft Palate J** 1984 Jan;21(1):44
**Walter P** see **Scheld HH**
**Walter-Janke Z:** Z dziejów służby zdrowia okupowanego Śląska. **Przegl Lek** 1980;37(1):104–12
**Walter Sandritter (7. 7. 1920 bis 12. 11. 1980): Verh Dtsch Ges Pathol** 1981;65:533–48
**Walters E** see **Wasserman H**
**Walters EM:** Infection control and the Renaissance. **Nurs Times** 1982 Feb 17–23;78(7):suppl 8
**Walters EM:** Infection control up to the Renaissance. **Nurs Times** 1981 Sep 2;77 Supp(36):JICN16–8
**Walters KA:** Mclean County and the influenza epidemic of 1918–1919. **J Ill State Hist Soc** 1981;74(2):130–44
**Walters V:** Class inequality and health care. London, Croom Helm, 1980. 175 p.
**Walters V:** State, capital, and labour: the introduction of Federal-Provincial insurance for physician care in Canada. **Can Rev Sociol Anthropol** 1982;19(2):157–72
**Walther H:** Ein Magister Ortolf de Bavaria in Paris. **Sudhoffs Arch** 1978;62(3):294–5
**Waltke R:** Moses Harris--inventor of the color wheel. **Dent Lab Rev** 1980 Apr;:24–5
**Walton E:** Royal Infirmary of Edinburgh: preserving a hospital's history. **Nurs Times** 1979 Jul 19;75(29):1239–40
**Walton J** see **Scull A, ed**
**Walton JC:** The state of medicine in 1912. **NC Med J** 1984 Feb;45(2):123–4
**Walton JK:** Lunacy in the Industrial Revolution: a study of asylum admissions in Lancashire, 1848–50. **J Soc Hist** 1979;13(1):1–22
**Walton JK:** Mad dogs and Englishmen: the conflict over rabies in late Victorian England. **J Soc Hist** 1979;13:219–39
**Walton MT:** Fifteenth century London medical men in their social context. Ph.D. Diss. The University of Chicago. Chicago, 1979.
**Walton MT:** Stinking air, corrupt water, and the English Sweat: a footnote to the quality of life in fifteenth-century London. **J Hist Med Allied Sci** 1981 Jan;36(1):67–8
**Walton MT:** Thomas Forestier and the 'False Lechys' of London. **J Hist Med Allied Sci** 1982 Jan;37(1):71–3
**Walton RG:** Women in social work. London, Boston, Routledge and Kegan Paul, 1975. xvi, 308 p.
**Wan Fang:** [Textual research on some ancient medical figures.] (Chi). **Chin J Med Hist** 1981;11:78–81
**Wan Fang:** Two questions about the Tian Sheng bronze statue for acupuncture of the Sung dynasty. (Chi). **Chin J Med Hist** 1981;11(1):62–4
**Wand M, Sewall RB:** 'Eyes be blind, heart be still': a new perspective on Emily Dickinson's eye problem. **N Engl Q** 1979;52(3):400–6
**Wand S:** After the first world war. **Br Med J [Clin Res]** 1983 Oct 1;287(6397):952–3
**Wang AG:** Establishment of a local psychiatric service. **Acta Psychiatr Scand** 1981 Aug;64(2):150–7
**Wang CL** see **Hilaski HJ**
**Wang GS** see **Yang KL**
**Wang JH** see **Wu BM**
**Wang Shu-huai:** Ya p'ien tu hai-kuang hsü erh shih san nien wen chüan tiao ch'a fen hsi. **Bull Inst Mod Hist Acad Sin** 1980;9:183–200
**Wang Xuetai:** [Research on the origin and development of acupuncture and moxibustion in China] (Chi). **Chung I Tsa Chih** 1979;20(8):59–64
**Wang Zhipu:** [Brief history of consumption-thirst syndrome (diabetes mellitus)] (Chi). **Chin J Med Hist** 1980;10:79–82
**Wangensteen OH:** A few renowned European military surgeons. In Ganzinger K, Skopec M, Wyklicky H, ed: Festschrift für Erna Lesky zum 70. Geburtstag. Wien, Brüder Hollinek, 1981. p. 167–84.
**Wangensteen OH:** Great opportunity: a binding summons to achieve. Musings upon surgical history. **Am J Surg** 1981 Nov;142(5):605–14
**Wangensteen OH:** Mandated celibacy in the academic arena. **Surg Gynecol Obstet** 1980 May;150(5):739–45
**Wangensteen OH:** Reflections on life's odyssey for medical school graduates. **Minn Med** 1980 May;63(5):341–5
**Wangensteen OH:** Surgery's reawakening. **Minn Med** 1979 Dec;62(12):879–82
**Wangensteen OH:** Teaching and learning: retrospect and prospect. **Proc Inst Med Chic** 1980 Apr–Jun;33(2):46–53
**Wangensteen OH:** The University of Glasgow and the Johns Hopkins schools of surgery. **Am J Surg** 1980 Jun;139(6):870–5
**Wangensteen OH** see **George Rosen: In Memoriam**
**Wangensteen OW, ed:** Elias Potter Lyon: Minnesota's leader in medical education. St. Louis, Green, 1981. 292 p. Contributions by J. A. Anderson, E. S. Benson, R. A. Good, J. C. Hinsey, C. H. Hodgson, L. P. Leone, R. J. McCollister, J. A. Myers, L. G. Rigler, H. G. Scheie, D. C. Smith, W. W. Spink, M. B. Visscher, J. H. Westerman, L. G. Wilson.
**Wankiewicz R:** Próba oceny działalności służby zdrowia w wojnie obronnej 1939 r. **Arch Hist Med (Warsz)** 1984;47(2):183–90
**Wankiewicz R:** Służba zdrowia Wojska Polskiego w bitwie nad Bzura. **Przegl Lek** 1984;41(1):68–79
**Wankmüller A, Cowen D, ed:** A visitor's view of American pharmacy, 1851. **Pharm Hist** 1981;23(2):101–3
**Wankmüller A:** Anfänge des Chemie- und Pharmaziestudiums in Stuttgart unter Professor Hermann Fehling. **Dtsch Apoth Ztg** 1982 Sep 9;122(36):1805–6
**Wankmüller A:** Deutschsprachige Lehrbücher der pharmazeutischen Technologie von 1845 bis 1945. **Dtsch Apoth Ztg** 1982 Oct 6;122(23):1236–9
**Wankmüller A:** Die Anfänge der Pharmazeutischen Gesellschaft Tübingen. **Dtsch Apoth Ztg** 1980 Jul 31;120(31):1460–2
**Wankmüller A:** Die Apotheker von Lenzburg im Kanton Aargau. Zum 25 jährigen Bestehen der Schweizerischen Gesellschaft für Geschichte der Pharmazie im Juni 1982. **Pharm Ztg** 1982 Jun 3;127(22):1207–8
**Wankmüller A:** Die Bibliothek der Internationalen Gesellschaft für Geschichte der Pharmazie. **Ber Wissenschaftsgesch** 1979;2(3–4):226–8
**Wankmüller A:** Die deutschen Lehrbücher von Ira Remsen. **Dtsch Apoth Ztg** 1979 Aug 30;119(35):1381–2
**Wankmüller A:** Die Pharmaziegeschichtsschreibung in Württemberg. In: Vorträge des Internationalen Pharmaziehistorischen Kongresses Innsbruck 1977. Stuttgart, Wissenschaftliche Verlagsgesellschaft, 1979. p. 63–9.
**Wankmüller A:** Die Schweizer Apotheker-Examen von 1874 bis 1880. **Pharm Ztg** 1979 Jun 14;124(24):1161–4
**Wankmüller A:** Die Tätigkeit deutscher Apotheker-Gehilfen in der Schweiz im 19. Jahrhundert. **Beitr Gesch Pharm** 1983;31(21):41–3
**Wankmüller A:** Entstehung des 'Grundriss der Geschichte der deutschen Pharmazie' von Adlung und Urdang. **Pharm Ztg** 1980;125:403–6
**Wankmüller A:** Hinweise zur Literatur für die Pharmaziegeschichte.

**Beitr Gesch Pharm** 1982;31(14):110-1
**Wankmüller A:** Hinweise zur Literatur für die Pharmaziegeschichte. 2. Deutschsprachige periodische Veröffentlichungen. **Beitr Gesch Pharm** 1981;31:86
**Wankmüller A:** Pharmaziestudenten in den Universitäts-Matrikeln. **Dtsch Apoth Ztg** 1979 Jun 14;119(24):945-7
**Wankmüller A:** Schlickums Lehrbuch für den Apothekerlehrling. **Dtsch Apoth Ztg** 1981 Sep 3;121(36):1921-3
**Wankmüller A:** [Studies in German pharmaceutical history] (Ger). **Beitr Wuerttemb Apothekengesch** 1978;12(2):33-64
**Wankmüller A** see **Hermann A**
**Wankmüllert A:** Studierende der Pharmazie an der Universität Strassburg vom Jahre 1872 an. **Pharm Ztg** 1982 Sep 9;127(36):1905-8
**Wannamaker LW:** The pathogenesis of rheumatic fever: Lewis Thomas and the Minnesota years. **Cell Immunol** 1983 Nov;82(1):82-7
**Want PC** see **Thornton JL**
**Waquet J** see **Antoine ME**
**Ward AR:** The passing of the Midwives' Act, 1902. **Midwives Chron** 1981 Jun;94(1121):190-4
**Ward JF:** Arthur F. Bentley and the foundations of behavioral science. **J Hist Behav Sci** 1981;17:222-31
**Ward JO, Sanders JH:** Nutritional determinants and migration in the Brazilian northeast: a case study of rural and urban Ceará. **Econ Dev Cult Change** 1980;29(1):141-63
**Ward PC** see **Ward WP**
**Ward PS:** An experiment in medical education: or How the College of Physicians and Surgeons of Chicago became The University of Illinois College of Medicine. In Cohen EP, ed: Medicine in transition. [Chicago], University of Illinois College of Medicine, 1981. p. 27-51.
**Ward PS:** Antibiotics and international relations at the close of World War II. In J. Parascandola, ed: The history of antibiotics. Madison, American Institute of the History of Pharmacy, 1980. p. 101-12.
**Ward PS:** The American reception of Salvarsan. **J Hist Med Allied Sci** 1981 Jan;36(1)44-62
**Ward PS:** 'Who will bell the cat?' Andrew C. Ivy and krebiozen. **Bull Hist Med** 1984 Spring;58(1):28-52
**Ward PS:** 100 years: a history [of the University of Illinois College of Medicine.] **Scope** 1981-82 centennial special;8(3):4-42
**Ward RD, Rogers WW:** Racial inferiority, convict labor, and modern medicine: a note on the Coalburg affair. **Ala Hist Q** 1982;44(3-4):203-10
**Ward T:** A century of achievement in oral surgery. **Br Dent J** 1980 Jul 1;149(1):25-7
**Ward WP, Ward PC:** Infant birth weight and nutrition in industrializing Montreal. **Am Hist Rev** 1984;89(2):324-45
**Wardaszko-Lyskowska H, Piotrowski A, Włosińska I:** Ewolucja celów, treści i form w programie dydaktycznym Kliniki Psychiatrycznej Akademii Medycznej w Warszawie. **Psychiatr Pol** 1982 Jan-Apr;16(1-2):73-6
**Wardell D:** Margaret Sanger: birth control's successful revolutionary. **Am J Public Health** 1980 Jul;70(7):736-42
**Warden GB** see **Cash P**
**Wards M** see **Loaring K**
**Ward's Island--a hospital of yesterday: Psychiatr News** 1979 Mar 16;14(6):4-5
**Wardwell WI:** The cutting edge of chiropractic recognition: prosecution and legislation in Massachusetts. **Chiropr Hist** 1982;2(1):55-65
**Ware F** see **West GP**
**Ware J, Hunt H:** The several lives of a Victorian vet. London, Bachman and Turner, 1979. 213 p.
**Warfe C:** The search for pure water in Ottawa: 1910-1915. **Urban Hist Rev** 1979;8(1):90-112
**Warick ER** see **Warick LH**
**Warick LH, Warick ER:** Transitional process and creativity in the life and art of Edvard Munch. **J Am Acad Psychoanal** 1984 Jul;12(3):413-24
**Warin RP:** Medicine and Bristol Zoo. **Bristol Med Chir J** 1982 Jul-Oct;97(363-364):4-11
**Waring JI:** A community fee bill for physicians, 1844. **J Hist Med Allied Sci** 1978 Jul;33(3):416-21
**Warkany J:** Friedrich Daniel von Recklinghausen and his times. **Adv Neurol** 1981;29:251-7
**Warkany J:** Laissez-faire in research. **J Am Coll Nutr** 1984;3(2):177-81
**Warkany J:** Prevention of congenital malformations. **Curr Probl Pediatr** 1983 May;13(7):1-26
**Warkany J:** The medical profession and congenital malformations (1900-1979). **Teratology** 1979 Oct;20(2):201-4
**Warner E:** The role of belief in healing. **Can Med Assoc J** 1983 May 1;128(9):1107-9
**Warner F:** Control of pollution. **Proc R Inst GB** 1979;51:95-119
**Warner HA** see **Aterman K**
**Warner JH:** A Southern medical reform: the meaning of the Antebellum argument for Southern medical education. **Bull Hist Med** 1983 Fall;57(3):364-81
**Warner JH:** 'Exploring the inner labyrinths of creation': popular microscopy in nineteenth-century America. **J Hist Med Allied Sci** 1982 Jan;37(1):7-33
**Warner JH:** Physiological theory and therapeutic explanation in the 1860s: the British debate on the medical use of alcohol. **Bull Hist Med** 1980 Summer;54(2):235-57
**Warner JH:** Therapeutic explanation and the Edinburgh bloodletting controversy: two perspectives on the medical meaning of science in the mid-nineteenth century. **Med Hist** 1980 Jul;24(3):241-58
**Warner JH** see **Numbers RL, ed**
**Warner MH:** Vindicating the minister's medical role: Cotton Mather's concept of the nishmath-chajim and the spiritualization of medicine. **J Hist Med Allied Sci** 1981 Jul;36(3):278-95
**Warnes CA** see **Roberts WC**
**Waroquy L** see **Desjeux P**
**Warren CA:** New forms of social control: the myth of deinstitutionalization. **Am Behav Sci** 1981;24(6):724-40
**Warren GB** see **Winslow JE**
**Warren JV:** Hippocrates--man and legend. **Forum Med** 1978 May;1(2):18-9
**Warren JV:** The evolution of the clinical investigator. **J Lab Clin Med** 1983 Mar;101(3):335-50
**Warren KS:** The bench and the bush in tropical medicine. **Am J Trop Med Hyg** 1981 Nov;30(6):1149 58
**Warren R:** Behavior of venous thrombi: historical observations. **Arch Surg** 1980 Oct;115(10):1151-4
**Warren R:** Landmark perspective: patent ductus arteriosus. **JAMA** 1984 Mar 2;251(9):1203-7
**Warren R:** Oliver Wendell Holmes, H.M.S. '36. **Harv Med Alumni Bull** 1982 Spring;56(2):20-6
**Warren S:** Shields Warren, M.D.: Excerpts from 'Medical aspects of the atomic bombings'. 1946. **Am J Forensic Med Pathol** 1980 Dec;1(4):303-7
**Warren WD:** Not for the profession ... for the people. **Ann Surg** 1983 Sep;198(3):241-50
**Warren WD:** Reflections on the early development of portacaval shunts. **Ann Surg** 1980 May;191(5):519-27
**Warren-Farrow D:** A perilous night. **Nurs Times** 1982 Jul 14-20;78(28):1203-4
**Warren JV, ed:** Cardiovascular physiology. Stroudsburg, Pennsylvania, Dowden, Hutchinson & Ross, 1975. xvi, 441 p. (Benchmark Papers in Human Physiology, 4).
**Warriner CK** see **Miller G**
**Warring FC:** A brief history of tuberculosis. **Conn Med** 1981 Mar;45(3):177-85
**Warrington-Türcke K:** 75th anniversary. The evolution of accountability in nursing in Canada. **Can Nurse** 1983 Oct;79(9):34-7
**Warzok R:** 125 Jahre Lehrstuhl für pathologische Anatomie an der Universität Greifswald. **Zentralbl Allg Pathol** 1982;126(5-6):405-15
**Waser PG:** Walter Rudolf Hess. Aus seinem Leben und seiner Tätigkeit an der Medizinischen Fakultät der Universität Zürich. **Gesnerus** 1982;39(2):279-86
**Waserman M:** An important John Shaw Billings find. **Bull Med Libr Assoc** 1984 Jan;72(1):23-5
**Waserman M, Clausen C, ed:** Bulletin of the History of Medicine. Index to volumes and supplements, 1933-1982. Baltimore, Johns Hopkins University Press, 1983. 195 p.
**Waserman M:** Sir James Y. Simpson and London's 'conservative and so curiously prejudiced' Dr. Ramsbotham. **Br Med J** 1980 Jan 19;280(6208):158-61
**Waserman MJ:** The emergence of modern child health care: pediatrics, public health, and the federal government. Ph.D. Diss., The Catholic University of America, Washington, D. C., 1982. v, 232 p.
**Washburn SL:** Fifty years of studies of human evolution. **Bull At Sci** 1982;38(5):37-43
**Waspomnienie pósmiertne o prof. dr med. Tadeuszu Bardadinie.: Otolaryngol Pol** 1980;34(1):I-VI
**Wassberg C:** The Swedish Hospital Medical Center, Seattle, Washington. **Swed-Am Hist Q** 1983;34(4):312-22
**Wassén SH:** On concepts of disease among Amerindian tribal groups. **J Ethnopharmacol** 1979 Oct;1(3):285-93
**Wassén SH** see **Holmstedt B**
**Wasserman D** see **Taylor W**
**Wasserman H, Solomon N, Alvarez R, et al:** Killing our own: the disaster of America's experience with atomic radiation. New York, Dell, 1982. xiii, 368 p.
**Wasserman M:** Alcohol, no! Gambling, yes: a matter of survival in Aztec society. **Br J Addict** 1982 Sep;77(3):283-6
**Wasserman M:** Aztec psychotherapy: a study of help-giving in ancient Mexico. **Int J Soc Psychiatry** 1982 Spring;28(1):54-9
**Wassermann GD:** On the nature of the theory of evolution. **Philos Sci** 1981;48(3):416-37
**Wasserstrom R** see **Chapin G**
**Wassilev W** see **Kühnel W**
**Wassilew W:** Die Medizin im alten Thrazien. In: International Congress of the History of Medicine, 26th, Plovdiv (Bulgaria), 1978. Actes du Congres, Vol. 1. Sofia, 1980. p. 79-80.
**Wasson RG:** The wondrous mushroom. Mycolatry in Mesoamerica. New York, McGraw-Hill, 1980. xxvi, 248 p.
**Wasson RG:** Traditional use in North America of Amanita muscaria for divinatory purposes. **J Psychedelic Drugs** 1979 Jan-Jun;11(1-2):25-8
**Wasti N:** A history of Iran-Pakistan medical relations. (Per) Rawalpindi, Iran Pakistan Institute of Persian Studies, 1974. 199 p.
**Waswo R:** The reaction of Juan Luis Vives to Valla's philosophy of language. **Bibl Hum Renaissance** 1980 Sep;42(3):595-609
**Waszyński E:** O mechanizmie żucia w 'Primitiae Physico-Medicae...' (1750-1753), pierwszym w Polsce czasopiśmie medycznym. **Czas Stomatol** 1984 Mar;37(3):227-32
**Waszyński E:** 'Primitiae physico-medicae ...' (1750-1753). Problematyka położniczo-ginekologiczna. **Arch Hist Med (Warsz)** 1984;47(3):447-61
**Waszyński E:** W dwusetną rocznicę urodzin Franciszka Izaaka Mayora (1779-1855), odkrywcy tonów serca płodu. **Ginekol Pol** 1980

Aug;51(8):765–6
**Watanabe K:** [History of nursing in the Taisho era.] (Jpn). **Kango Kyoiku** 1982 Jan 25;23(1):60–6 (continued regularly)
**Watanabe M:** The caloric theory of S. L. Metcalfe. **Br J Hist Sci** 1984 Jul;17(56 pt 2):210–3
**Watanabe N:** [On Siegemundine and her 'The most needed training in difficult and abnormal delivery'] (Jpn). **Josanpu Zasshi** 1980 Dec;34(12):812–7
**Watanabe S:** [Studies on the history of the anthropology of the Ainu skulls.] (Jpn). **Nihon I-Shigaku Zasshi** 1981;27:203–5
**Watanabe S** see **Rassengeschichte der Menschheit**
**Waterbolk TW** see **Alting MP**
**Waterman A** see **Dupâquier J**
**Waterman BB:** Memories of Malta 1940–42. **J R Nav Med Serv** 1984 Winter;70(3):182–5
**Watermann R:** Schwanns mikroskopische Forschungen und die Zellentheorie. Ein Beitrag zu seinem 100. Todestag. **Z Mikrosk Anat Forsch** 1982;96(6):1032–43
**Watermann RA:** Figures for bone-amputations, introduced by Zur Verth and regarding artificial limbs. In: Congrès international d'histoire de la médecine, XXVe, Québec, 1976. Actes. Québec, 1977. p. 1386–95.
**Watermann RA:** Mensch und Medizin zwischen Macht und Militär der römischen Kaiserzeit. Frankfurt am Main, Gerhard Michler, 1980. 204 p.
**Waters SC:** A country doctor of yesteryear: Samuel C. Waters (1861–1932) of Middletown, Indiana. **J Indiana State Med Assoc** 1983 Feb;76(2):144–5
**Watkin B:** Cottage hospitals: a study in technology and organisation. **Nurs Times** 1979 Jul 5;75(26):suppl 18:73–6
**Watkin B:** Ivory tower of strength: Hammersmith Hospital. **Health Soc Serv J** 1982 Apr 1;92(4790):394–7
**Watkin B:** St. Bernard's Hospital: pioneering a humane approach. **Health Soc Serv J** 1981 Dec 3;91(4775):1480–1
**Watkin B:** The National Health Service: the first phase, 1948–1974 and after. London, Boston, Allen and Unwin, 1978. 170 p.
**Watkin B:** Workhouse into hospital: a house of industry. **Health Soc Serv J** 1982 Mar 4;92(4786):273–5
**Watkin B** see **Allan P**
**Watkins AH:** James Scott, the famous surgeon of Bromley, 1770–1848. **Bromley Local Hist** 1979;4:41–7
**Watkins D:** The man who reformed hospital kitchens (Alexis Benoit Soyer). **Nurs Times** 1981 Nov 18–24;77(47):2029
**Watkins RN:** The Renaissance pater familias – 'Be ye perfect'. **Psychohist Rev** 1980;9:91–110
**Watkins SC, McCarthy J:** The female life cycle in a Belgian commune: La Hulpe, 1847–1866. **J Fam Hist** 1980 Summer;5(2):167–79
**Watne Al, Bartholomew S:** Giants in the hills: a brief history of the West Virginia Chapter, American College of Surgeons. **W Va Med J** 1982 Jul;78(7):168–71
**Watschinger B:** Klinische Nephrologie (Entwicklung und Aufgaben). **Wien Med Wochenschr** 1984 Jun 30;134(12):275–9
**Watson JA:** The residency program in otolaryngology at the Washington University School of Medicine. **Am J Otol** 1980;1:247–9
**Watson MH:** The early days of insulin in New Zealand. **NZ Med J** 1981 May 27;93(684):347–50
**Watson RI:** A methodological note on the research use of the Syntopicon. **J Hist Behav Sci** 1980 Jul;16(3):275–9
**Watson RI:** Basic writings in the history of psychology. New York, Oxford Univ. Press, 1979. xviii, 420 p.
**Watson RI** see **Brozek J**
**Watson RM, Harty FJ:** A coming of age. The British Endodontic Society. **Br Dent J** 1984 Jan 21;156(2):66–7
**Watson S:** Blue Cross idea began in Texas. **Tex Hosp** 1979 Jun;35(1):22–3
**Watson WF:** Development of the PVC endotracheal tube. **Biomaterials** 1980 Jan;1(1):41–6
**Watson WG:** Dentofacial orthopedics: fifty years of concern. **Am J Orthod** 1981 Nov;80(5):561–3
**Watson WG:** The journal––a record of professional transition and progress. **Am J Orthod** 1981 Feb;79(2):219–22
**Watson JM, ed** see **Fergusson IL**
**Watson-Jones R, Coltart WD:** The classic. Slow union of fractures with a study of 804 fractures of the shafts of the tibia and femur. **Clin Orthop** 1982 Aug;(168):2–16
**Watt DC:** Social psychiatry. **J R Soc Med** 1981 Feb;74(2):88–90
**Watt I** see **Rogers J**
**Watt J:** Doctors in the wars. **J R Soc Med** 1984 Apr;77(4):265–7
**Watt J:** Lettsomian lectures. Medical perspectives of some voyages of discovery. **Trans Med Soc Lond** 1979;95:61–91
**Watt J:** Nutrition in adverse environments, 1. Forgotten lessons of maritime nutrition. **Hum Nutr Appl Nutr** 1982 Feb;36(1):35–45
**Watt J:** Surgeons of the Mary Rose: the practice of surgery in Tudor England. **Mar Mirror** 1983;69:3–18
**Watt J:** The burns of seafarers under oars, sail and steam. **Injury** 1980 Jul;12(1):69–81
**Watt J:** The surgery of sea warfare from the galley to the nuclear age. **Trans Med Soc Lond** 1980–81;97:1–15
**Watt JA:** Sheep medicine: a century of progress. **Vet Rec** 1982 Jun 26;110(26):602–3
**Watt FB, ed** see **Hansen GA**
**Watters DR:** A Turlington balsam phial from Montserrat, West Indies: genuine or counterfeit? **Hist Archaeol** 1981;15(1):105–8
**Watterson P:** Environmental factors in infant and early childhood mortality decline in England and Wales, 1895 to 1910. **Soc Soc Hist Med Bull (Lond)** 1984 Dec;35:37–40
**Watterson J, ed:** Poetic justice; or, an illfated epic by Thomas Burke. **NC Hist Rev** 1978;55(3):339–46
**Wattley LA:** Male physicians and female health and sexuality in 19th century English and American society. **J Adv Nurs** 1983 Sep;8(5):423–8
**Watts CA:** General practice. **Br Med J** 1979 Oct 27;2(6197):1055–6
**Watts DC:** The Wellcome Museum of the History of Medicine. **Biochem Soc Trans** 1982 Jun;10(3):187–8
**Watts EA:** Down Memory Lane – a pioneer remembers. **Nurs J India** 1983 Nov;74(11):298–9
**Watts ES:** The biological race concept and diseases of modern man. In Rothschild H, ed: Biocultural aspects of disease. New York, Academic Press, 1981. p. 3–23.
**Watts RK:** Jewish fertility trends and differentials: an examination of the evidence from the census of 1970. **Jew Soc Stud** 1980;42(3–4):293–312
**Watts S:** Demographic facts as experienced by a group of families in eighteenth-century Shifnal, Shropshire. **Local Popul Stud (Matlock)** 1984;32:34–43
**Waugh ES, McGoldrick KE:** On the history of JAMWA. **J Am Med Wom Assoc** 1980 Jun;35(6):137–9
**Waugh MA:** Role played by Italy in the history of syphilis. **Br J Vener Dis** 1982 Apr;58(2):92–5
**Waugh TR** see **Soren A**
**Waugh W:** Breve storia dell'ortopedia. **Kos** 1984 Jun;1(5):33–44
**Waung WS:** Introduction of opium cultivation to China. **J Chin Univ Hong Kong** 1979;5(1):207–21
**Wawersik J:** Die Geschichte des Narkoseapparates in Grundzügen. **Anaesthesist** 1982 Oct;31(10):541–8
**Way EL:** History of opiate use in the Orient and the United States **Ann NY Acad Sci** 1982;398:12–23
**Way EL:** Hooked for thirty years: tales of an investigation. **Natl Inst Drug Abuse Res Monogr Ser** 1979;27:1–10
**Wayland JR** see **Higgins PG**
**Wayman A:** The human body as microcosm in India, Greek cosmology, and sixteenth-century Europe. **Hist Relig** 1982;22(2):172–90
**We walk the line: the struggle at preterm.: Radic Am** 1979;13(2):8–24
**Wear A:** Perceptions of health and environment in the settlement of North America in the early seventeenth century. **Soc Soc Hist Med Bull (Lond)** 1984 Dec;35:11–3
**Wear A:** William Harvey and the 'Way of the Anatomists'. **Hist Sci** 1983 Sep;21(53 pt 3):223–49
**Weaver B, Britt MC:** Dr. Lawrence Reynolds and his medical history collection. **Ala J Med Sci** 1984 Jul;21(3):311–7 contd
**Weaver B, Britt MC:** Dr. Lawrence Reynolds and his medical history collection. **Ala J Med Sci** 1984 Oct;21(4):441–7
**Weaver B:** Should women be admitted to medical school? The issue in the late 19th century. **South Med J** 1984 May;77(5):623–5
**Weaver BL, Thompson JA:** Women in medicine and the issue in late nineteenth-century Alabama. **Ala Hist Q** 1981;43(4):292–314
**Weaver CN** see **Glenn ND**
**Weaver DS, Vazquez Leiva R:** A survey of the paleopathology of the Vidor site, Guanacaste Province, Costa Rica. **Paleopathol Newsl** 1980 Jun;(30):6–7
**Weaver JA:** A hospital for all seasons. **Ulster Med J** 1984;53(1):18–32
**Weaver JL:** The politics of Latin American family-planning policy. **J Dev Areas** 1978;12(4):415–37
**Webb A:** A definitive history of the Raleigh Academy of Medicine. **NC Med J** 1981 Apr;42(4):260–2
**Webb AY** see **Bulgaro PJ**
**Webb CH:** An exciting half century in medicine. **Pharos** 1980 Winter;43(1):14–9
**Webb H, Rhodes LC:** The book of presidents: leaders of organized dentistry. [s.l., s.n.] 1977. [63] p.
**Webb ME:** A reexamination of the inception, development, and 'Newtonianism' of David Hartley's 'Observations on man.' Ph.D. Diss., University of Oklahoma, 1981. ix, 310 p.
**Webb WM:** There's a doctor in the library. The story of John Shaw Billings, M.D. (1838–1913). **J Indiana State Med Assoc** 1981 Jun;74(6):360–6
**Weber HG, Stickl H:** Auswirkungen der Urbanisation auf das Kind. **Off Gesundheitswes** 1982 Sep;44(9):560–5
**Weber M:** Kerners 'Kleksographien' und Rorschachs 'Psychodiagnostik'. **Gesnerus** 1984;41(1/2):101–9
**Weber S:** Zur Entstehung der Kieler Universitätskliniken im 19. Jahrhundert. **Hist Hosp** 1979–80;13:46–68
**Weber W:** Gerichtsärztlicher Beitrag zur Rekonstruktion eines Tötungs-deliktes zu Aachen 1734. **Beitr Gerichtl Med** 1984;42:373–8
**Weber W** see **Maurer HJ**
**Weber-Pieluszyńska H:** PTP w Katowicach. **Pieleg Polozna** 1983;(8–9):32
**Weber-Unger S:** Wahnsinn und Politik: zur neuen Psychiatrie in Italien. Frankfurt; New York, Campus Verlag, 1984. 181 p.
**Webster A:** Threefold cord of religion, science, and literature in the character of Sir Thomas Browne. **Br Med J [Clin Res]** 1982 Dec 18–25;285(6357):1801–2
**Webster C:** From Paracelsus to Newton. Magic and the making of modern science. The Eddington Memorial Lectures delivered at Cambridge University, November 1980. Cambridge, Cambridge University Press, 1982. 107 p.
**Webster C:** General practice under the panel – the last phase. **Soc Soc Hist Med Bull (Lond)** 1983 Jun;32:20–3
**Webster C:** Healthy or hungry thirties? **Hist Workshop J** 1982;13:110–29

endokrinen Verursachung der Menstruation. Diss. Erlangen-Nürnberg, 1980. 59 p.
**Weir DR:** Fertility transition in rural France, 1740–1829. Ph.D. Diss., Stanford University. Palo Alto, 1983. xiv, 366 p.
**Weir DR:** Rather never than late: celibacy and age at marriage in English cohort fertility, 1541–1871. **J Fam Hist** 1984 Winter;9(4):340–54
**Weir JA:** The army doctor looks at Indian medicine. **Denver West Roundup** 1977 Sep–Oct;33:12–28
**Weir JA:** The history of Fitzsimons Army Medical Center. **Denver West Roundup** 1980 Jan–Feb;36:3–14
**Weir JG:** The way they lived then. **Br Med J [Clin Res]** 1982 Dec 18–25;285(6357):1809–10
**Weir NF:** Theodor Billroth and Johannes Brahms--a thirty year friendship. **Hist Med (Lond)** 1975 Autumn–Winter;6(3–4):8–14
**Weir RB:** Obsessed with moderation: the drink trades and the drink question (1870–1930). **Br J Addict** 1984 Mar;79(1):93–107
**Weir RF:** Remarks on the gunshot wounds of the Civil War by Robert F. Weir. New York State Journal of Medicine, April, 1904. **NY State J Med** 1982 Mar;82(3):391–3
**Weisburger EK:** History of the Bioassay Program of the National Cancer Institute. **Prog Exp Tumor Res** 1983;26:187–201
**Weise M:** Experimental and clinical aspects of proteinuria. Introduction. **Contrib Nephrol** 1981;24:VI–IX
**Weise W:** Die Entdeckung des Erregers der Tuberkulose durch Robert Koch vor 100 Jahren. **MMW** 1982 Mar 26;124(12):299–300
**Weisert JJ:** Dr. Anthony Hunn: from storm and stress to tempest and sunshine. **Filson Club Hist Q** 1982;56(2):211–24
**Weishaar ME** see **Harbison SF**
**Weisheipl JA, ed:** Albertus Magnus and the sciences: commenmorative essays 1980. Toronto, Pontifical Institute of Mediaeval Studies, 1980. xiv, 657 p.
**Weisheit-Smith I** see **Jensen JE**
**Weismann G:** A fashion in metals. **Hosp Pract** 1982 Apr;17(4):33–4, 38, 42
**Weisner ME:** Early modern midwifery: a case study. **Int J Womens Stud** 1983;6(1):26–43
**Weispfenning I:** Pettenkofers Gesundheitswirtschaftslehre. Ein meilenstein in der Entwicklung des öffentlichen Gesundheitswesens. In Seidler E, Schott H, ed: Bausteine zur Medizingeschichte. Stuttgart, Steiner, 1984. p. 146–54.
**Weiss B:** Wissenschaftliche Bibliotheken in Madrid. **Biblos (Vienna)** 1980,29(1):18–26
**Weiss C, Specker H, Winckelmann HJ:** Die Medizinalgesetzgebung in Württemberg im 19. Jahrhundert. **MMW** 1983 Nov 4;125(44):1005–10
**Weiss EB** see **Weiss GN**
**Weiss GN, Weiss EB:** The health care profession on the threshold of the eighties: physician and nurse. **J La State Med Soc** 1980 Oct;132(10):151–4
**Weiss J:** Die Universitätshautklinik Hamburg-Eppendorf im Wandel der Zeit. **Hautarzt** 1981 Jan;32(1):28–32
**Weiss JB** see **Mawas LJ**
**Weiss KM, Chakraborty R:** Genes, populations, and disease, 1930–1980: a problem-oriented review. In F. Spencer, ed: A history of American physical anthropology, 1930–1980. New York, Academic Press, 1982. p. 371–404.
**Weiss KM** see **Buchanan AV**
**Weiss KM** see **Schwartz RJ**
**Weiss L:** The resurgence of biological psychiatry: new promise or false hope for a troubled profession. **Perspect Biol Med** 1977 Summer;20(4):573–85
**Weiss MG:** Critical study of Unmada in the early sanskrit medical literature. An analysis of ayurvedic psychiatry with reference to present-day diagnostic concepts. Ph.D. Diss., University of Pennsylvania. Philadelphia, 1977. 353 leaves.
**Weiss MM:** Fumigated mail. **J Ky Med Assoc** 1981 Jan;79(1):19–22
**Weiss P:** La Trepanacion ritual suprainiana--rasgo de culturas peruanas, encontrado también en México y Guatemala. **Bol Soc Mex Hist Filos Med** 1981 Sep;5(36):193–211
**Weiss RE:** Mother Joseph: the legendary nun who broke ground for women and men health administrators in the West. **Hosp Forum** 1981 Jan–Feb;24(1):17–8
**Weiss S** see **Bernische Liga gegen die Tuberkulose 1930–1980**
**Weiss Z** see **Kohn D**
**Weissauer W** see **Kotwas J**
**Weisse AB:** Conversations in medicine. **J Med Soc NJ** 1984 Jul;81(7):576–9
**Weisse AB** see **Mangel C**
**Weisser C:** Das Krankheitslunar aus medizinhistorischer Sicht. Ein Beitrag zur iatromathematisch-astrologischen Fachliteratur des Mittelalters. **Sudhoffs Arch** 1981;65(4):390–400
**Weisser C:** Der Braunsche Apparat zur Ather-Chloroform-Mischnarkose. Ein Beitrag zur Frühgeschichte der Kombinationsnarkose. **Anaesthesist** 1983 Aug;32(8):369–73
**Weisser C:** Der Ombrédannesche Ather-Inhalator. Ein Beitrag zur Geschichte der Ather-Apparatnarkose. **Anaesthesist** 1983 Feb;32(2):51–4
**Weisser C:** Studien zum mittelalterlichen Krankheitslunar. Ein Beitrag zur Geschichte laienastrologischer Fachprosa. Pattensen/Hannover, Horst Wellm, 1982. 468 p. (Würzburger medizinhistorische Forschungen, 21).
**Weisser U:** Beiträge Ibn Sina's zur Kenntnis der weiblichen Genitalien und zur Embryologie. Eine kritische Betrachtung. In International Congress of the History of Medicine, 27th, Barcelona, 1980. Actas. Barcelona, Académia de Ciències Médiques de Catalunya i Balears, 1981. p. 761–5.
**Weisser U:** Die hippokratische Lehre von den Siebenmonatskindern bei Galen und Tabit ibn Qurra. **Sudhoffs Arch** 1979;63(3):209–38
**Weisser U:** Ibn Qaiyim al-Gauziya über die Methoden der Embryologie. **Medizinhist J** 1981;16(3):227–39
**Weisser U:** Ibn Sina und die Medizin des arabisch-islamischen Mittelalters - Alte und neue Urteile und Vorurteile. **Medizinhist J** 1983;18(4):283–305
**Weisser U:** Künstliches Adrenalin. Der mühevolle Weg zur ersten Hormonsynthese. **Med Welt** 1980 Jan 4;31(1):40–4
**Weisser U:** The embryology of Yuhanna ibn Masawaith. **J Hist Arabic Sci** 1980;4(1):9–22
**Weisser U, ed:** Buch über das Geheimnis der Schöpfung und die Darstellung der Natur (Buch der Ursachen), von Pseudo-Apollonios von Tyana. Aleppo, Institute for the History of Arabic Science, University of Aleppo, 1979. 66 p. (Sources and Studies in the History of Arabic-Islamic Science, Natural Sciences Series 1).
**Weisskopf-Joelson E** see **Sharkey PW, ed**
**Weissman A:** The English romantics and modern psychology. **Centerpoint** 1975/76;1(4):9–15
**Weissman MB:** Elizabeth Burchenal. In: Notable American women. The modern period. Cambridge, Mass., Belknap-Harvard Univ. Press, 1980. 4:121–2.
**Weissmann A, Camisa C:** Friedrich Sigmund Merkel. **Am J Dermatopathol** 1982 Dec;4(6):521–35
**Weissmann G:** Against Aequanimitas. **Hosp Pract [Off]** 1984 Jun;19(6):159–69
**Weissmann G:** Bellevue: form follows function. **Hosp Pract** 1981 Aug;16(8):18, 21, 24–5
**Weissmann G:** Cholera at the Harvey. **Hosp Pract** 1982 Feb;17(2):129–31, 135–6
**Weissmann G:** Foucault and the bag lady. **Hosp Pract** 1982 Aug;17(8):28–9, 33–4, 39
**Weissmann G:** From Auden to arachidonate: a tribute and a hypothesis. **Cell Immunol** 1983 Nov;82(1):117–26
**Weissmann G:** In quest of Fleck: science from the holocaust. **Hosp Pract** 1980 Oct;15(10):48–9, 52, 54–5 passim
**Weissmann G:** Loeb and a Gloria. **Hosp Pract [Off]** 1984 Oct;19(10):65–74
**Weissmann G:** Proust in khaki. **Hosp Pract** 1983 Apr;18(4):56, 58, 62 passim
**Weissmann G:** The introduction is over. **Arthritis Rheum** 1983 Nov;26(11):1297–302
**Weisstub DN** see **Smith JC**
**Weisstub DN, ed:** Law and psychiatry in the Canadian context. New York, Pergamon Press, 1980. xlvi, 911 p.
**Weisz G:** Reform and conflict in French medical education, 1870–1914. In R. Fox, G. Weisz, ed: The organization of science and technology in France 1808–1914. Cambridge, Cambridge University Press, 1980. p. 61–94.
**Weisz G** see **Fox R**
**Weisz R:** Stress and mental health in a boom town. **Univ Wyo Publ** 1979;43:31–47
**Weisz-Maleček R** see **Kraljevic M**
**Weitzenhoffer AM:** What did he (Bernheim) say? A postscript and an addendum. **Int J Clin Exp Hypn** 1980 July;28(3):252–60
**Welch AD:** Folic acid: discovery and the exciting first decade. **Perspect Biol Med** 1983 Autumn;27(1):64–75
**Welch F** see **Dodson G**
**Welch JE:** Pioneering in health education and services at Amherst College. **J Am Coll Health** 1982 Jun;30(6):289–95
**Welch S** see **Combs MW**
**Wellborn MB:** Edwin Walker, M.D., Evansville, Indiana. **Indiana Med Hist Q** 1975;2(2):29–34
**Wellcome Institute for the History of Medicine and related Sciences, London:** Subject catalogue of the history of medicine and related sciences. 18 vols. München, Kraus-Thomson, 1980.
**Weller B:** The spy who nursed me (Edith Cavell). **Nurs Times** 1984 Oct 17–23;80(42):18–9
**Weller GR:** The delivery of health services in the Canadian north. **J Can Stud** 1981;16(2):69–80
**Weller RM:** Nitrous oxide in Bristol in 1836. A series of lectures by William Herepath (1796–1868). **Anaesthesia** 1983 Jul;38(7):678–82
**Wellmann J:** Culture and character: some perspectives from psychological anthropology for psychohistorians. **Group Psychol Hist Newsl** 1975;4(3):12–30
**Wells C, Woodhouse N:** Paget's disease in an Anglo-Saxon. **Med Hist** 1975 Oct;19(4):396–400
**Wells EB:** Scientists' libraries: a handlist of printed sources. **Ann Sci** 1983 Jul;40(4):317–89
**Wells EB:** The disease horse. **Factotum** 1981;12:14
**Wells LA:** Rural psychiatry on the nineteenth-century frontier: the career of Jacob Bowers. **Perspect Biol Med** 1981 Winter;24(2):270–81
**Wells RV:** Birth control: different conceptions. **J Interdiscip Hist** 1979;10(3):511–6
**Wells RV:** Women's lives transformed: demographic and family patterns in America, 1600–1970. In Berkin, CR, Norton MB, ed: Women of America: a history. Boston, Houghton Miffin, 1979. p. 16–33.
**Wells RV** see **Laslett P**
**Wells WC** see **McKinney HL, ed**
**Welsch M:** André Gratia, 1893–1950. In Florilège des Sciences en Belgique - II. Bruxelles, Académie Royale de Belgique, 1980. p. 663–72.
**Welsh JS:** The trial pharmacist. **Am Pharm** 19(5):16–7, 33, May 79
**Welsh ME:** A selected bibliography [on witchcraft]. **Palacio** 1974;80(2):51–4

**Welsh SO, Marston RM:** Review of trends in food use in the United States, 1909 to 1980. **J Am Diet Assoc** 1982 Aug;81(2):120-8
**Wendler D, Rother P:** Wilhelm His sen.--Leben und Wirken des bedeutenden Leipziger Morphologen. **Z Gesamte Inn Med** 1982 Dec;37(23):810-3
**Wendler M van Voorhis:** Doctors and diseases on the Ohio frontier. **Ohio Hist** 1980;89(2):222-42
**Wendler J, ed:** 75 Jahre Phoniatrie. Festschrift zu Ehren von Hermann Gutzmann sen. Berlin. Humboldt Universität, 1980. 240 p.
**Wendorf R:** 'Poor Collins' reconsidered. **Huntington Libr Q** 1979;42(2):91-116
**Wendorf de Sejas M, Sejas García R:** Medicina y psicologia tradicional de la region andina: bibliografía comentada. **Nuevos Libros** 1980;23-24:1-23
**Wendt V:** Heinrich A. Gottron: Leben und Werk. Lübeck, Hansisches Verlagskonto H. Scheffler, 1980. 99 p.
**Wendt V** see **Leyh F**
**Wengenmayer M** see **Bertram E**
**Wenneker M:** Huxley's ethical system: an alternative to evolutionary ethics. **Synthesis** 1980;5(1):13-44
**Wennig R:** Histoire de la toxicologie au Luxembourg. **Bull Soc Sci Med Grand Duche Luxemb** 1984;121(2):39-52
**Wens HM:** Johann Adam Kerstings Neujahrs-Kolleg an der Thierarzney-Schule (TAS), Hannover vom 3. Januar 1784. **DTW** 1981 Jan 5;88(1):35-8
**Wens HM:** Zur Geschichte der Tierkörperbeseitigung in Ober- und Nieder-österreich. **Zentralbl Bakteriol [B]** 1980 Mar;170(3-4):211-6
**Wente EF** see **Harris JE**
**Wentges RT:** Wilhelm Fliess en de nasale reflexneurose. **Ned Tijdschr Geneeskd** 1981 Feb 14;125(7):278-84
**Wenz W** see **Anger P**
**Wenzel M:** Goethes Morphologie in ihrer Beziehung zum darwinistischen Evolutionsdenken. **Medizinhist J** 1983;18(1-2):52-68
**Werdinger J:** Embryology at Woods Hole: the emergence of a new American biology. Ph.D. Diss., Indiana University. Bloomington, 1980. xii, 640 leaves.
**Wermut W:** Rodowody literackie niektórych zespołów klinicznych. **Psychiatr Pol** 1980 Jan-Feb;14(1):69-76
**Werner K:** Sozialhygienische Aspekte in der frühen Ara der Tuberkulose-Therapie. **Wiss Beitr Martin Luther Univ Halle Wittenberg** 1983;5-R80:273-7
**Werner K** see **Kaiser W**
**Werner K** see **Rothe J**
**Werner P:** Zur experimentellen Methode des Biochemikers Otto Heinrich Warburg. **Z Arztl Fortbild (Jena)** 1983;77(22):947-9
**Werner R:** Medicine men (traditional medical practitioners) in primary health care and the role of traditional medicine towards modern medicine. **Off Gesundheitswes** 1980;42(9):637-56
**Werner R:** Offentliches Gesundheitswesen, traditionelle chinesische Medizin, westliche Medizin, Barfussärzte und Heilmittelkunde in der Volksrepublik China. 1. Teil. **Off Gesundheitswes** 1981 Oct;43(10):480-99
**Werner-Brzezińska H:** Pierwotne mi ęsaki kościopochodne leczone w Instytucie Onkologii w latach 1947-1970. **Nowotwory** 1979;Suppl;117-21
**Werskey G:** The visible college. London, Allen Lane, 1978. 376 p.
**Wertelecki W** see **Plato CC**
**Wertenbaker L:** To mend the heart. New York, Viking Press, 1980. xiv, 344 p.
**Wertheim T:** Peripheral visual acuity: Th. Wertheim. **Am J Optom Physiol Opt** 1980 Dec;57(12):915-24
**Wertheimer M** see **Brozek J**
**Wertheimer P, David M, Sindou M, et al:** Naissance et croissance de la neurochirurgie. **Neurochirurgie** 1979;25(5-6):247-63
**Wertheimer R** see **Abbott P**
**Werthmann-Haas G:** Altdeutsche Ubersetzungen des Prager 'Sendbriefs' ('Missum imperatori') (= Untersuchungen zur mittelalterlichen Pestliteratur, I). Pattensen (Han.), Wellm, 1983. 317 p. (Würzburger medizinhistorische Forschungen, Bd. 27).
**Wertsch JV:** Trends in Soviet cognitive psychology. **Stor Crit Psicol** 1981;2(2):219-95
**Wertz DC:** What birth has done for doctors: a historical view. **Women Health** 1983 Spring;8(1):7-24
**Wery Ph** see **Sondervost FA**
**Wesley GR:** A history of hysteria. Washington, D. C., University Press of America, 1979. 172 p.
**Wespi HJ:** Die Salzjodierung als Vorläufer der Salzfluoridierung. **SSO Schweiz Monatsschr Zahnheilkd** 1982 Apr;92(4):273-89
**West CG:** A short history of the management of penetrating missile injuries of the head. **Surg Neurol** 1981 Aug;16(2):145-9
**West GP, Ware F:** A history of the overseas veterinary services. London, British Veterinary Assn., 1961-1973. 2 v.
**West JB:** Man at extreme altitude. **J Appl Physiol** 1982 Jun;52(6):1393-9
**West JB:** Stephen Hales: neglected respiratory physiologist. **J Appl Physiol** 1984 Sep;57(3):635-9
**West R:** An excursion into pharmacology: curare in medicine. **Med Hist** 1984 Oct;28(4):391-405
**West JB, ed:** Translations in respiratory physiology. Stroudsburg, Pennsylvania, Dowden, Hutchinson & Ross, 1975. 772 p. (Translations of 19th-20th century articles by various authors).
**Westaby D, Williams R:** The history injection sclerotherapy for esophageal varices. **Gastrointest Endosc** 1983 Nov;29(4):303-7
**Westbrooks B:** The troubled legacy of Harvey Lillard: the black experience in chiropractic. **Chiropr Hist** 1982;2(1):47-53
**Westendorf W** see **Deines H von**
**Westerman JH:** The joint commission on accreditation of hospitals: relations with the practicing physician--past, present and future. JCAH and the practicing physician: historical relationships and current issues. (First of two parts). **Conn Med** 1982 Jan;46(1):23-6
**Westerman JH:** The Joint Commission on Accreditation of Hospitals: relations with the practicing physician--past, present and future. JCAH and the practicing physician: present issues, current solutions and future considerations 2. **Conn Med** 1982 Feb;46(2):89-92
**Westerman JH** see **Wangensteen OW, ed**
**Westerman MP, Tymorek S:** A history of medical research at Mount Sinai Hospital Medical Center of Chicago. **Mt Sinai J Med (NY)** 1984 Apr;51(2):150-6
**Western JS** see **Najman JM**
**Western Countries Branch centenary celebrations: Br Dent J** 1979 Dec 4;147(11):315-6
**Westfall LG:** Immigrants in society. **Americas (Engl)** 1982;34(4):41-5
**Westfall RS:** Alchemy in Newton's library. **Ambix** 1984 Nov;31(3):97-101
**Westheimer G:** Helmholtz on eye movements. **Hum Neurobiol** 1984;3(3):149-52
**Westin M:** Så var det då. **Sjukskoterskan** 1984 Apr;:17-20
**Westing AH:** Research communication: war as a human endeavor: the high-fatality wars of the twentieth century. **J Peace Res** 1982;19(3):261-70
**Westoff CF** see **Pebley AR**
**Westphal J:** Das Hospital in Nordkirchen. Ein westfälisches Hospital der Barockzeit von Johann Conrad Schlaun. **Hist Hosp** 1979-80;13:119-34
**Wetherell C** see **Rutman DB**
**Wetzel N:** Loyal Davis; Allen Kanavel; surgery, gynecology and obstetrics, and the development of neurosurgery. **Surg Gynecol Obstet** 1983 Aug;157(2):135-9
**Weuffen W:** Der Beitrag Robert Koch zur Begründung der Desinfektionslehre und heutige Schwerpunkte der Desinfektionsforschung und -praxis. **Z Gesamte Hyg** 1982 Mar;28(3):167-71
**Weuffen W:** Der Beitrag Robert Kochs zur Begründung der Desinfektionslehre und heutige Schwerpunkte der Desinfektionsforschung und -praxis. **Z Erkr Atmungsorgane** 1983;161(1):28-35
**Weyrauch E:** Mahl-Zeiten. Beobachtungen zur sozialen Kultur des Essens in der Ständegesellschaft. In Imhof AE, ed: Leib und Leben in der Geschichte der Neuzeit. Berlin, Duncker & Humblot, 1983. p. 103-18.
**Whalen JM:** Edwin Arnold Vail. In Dictionary of Canadian biography, 1881-1890. 1982;11:896-7.
**Whaley J:** Mirrors of mortality: studies in the social history of death. New York, St. Martin's Press, 1982. viii, 252 p.
**Wharton M:** Sir Benjamin Brodie, Bt. (1783-1862). **Ann R Coll Surg Engl** 1983 Nov;65(6):418-9
**Wharton M:** Sir Gilbert Blane Bt (1749-1834). **Ann R Coll Surg Engl** 1984 Sep;66(5):375-6
**Wheatcroft SG:** Doctors and the Revolution in Russia. **Soc Soc Hist Med Bull (Lond)** 1984 Jun;34:19-24
**Wheatcroft SG:** Famine and epidemic crises in Russia, 1918-1922: the case of Saratov. **Ann Demogr Hist (Paris)** 1983;:329-52
**Wheatley DN** see **Rasmussen L**
**Wheaton R:** Family and sexuality in French history. Philadelphia, University of Pennsylvania Press, 1980. ix, 274 p.
**Wheeland RG** see **Speck FL**
**Wheeler CE:** Viewpoint: essay in response to republication of a biography (Florence Nightingale). **ANS** 1984 Jul;6(4):74-9
**Wheeler R:** Health and human resources. **New South** 1971;26(4):2-16
**Whelan WJ:** Use of liposomes in medicine. **Biochem Soc Trans** 1984 Apr;12(2):331-2
**Whelton MJ:** Perspective in liver disease: an Irish experience. **Ir J Med Sci** 1979 May-Jun;148(5-6):161-7
**When Harrogate was a spa: Nurs Times** 1982 Apr 21-27;78(16):suppl 11-3
**When 'more doctors smoked Camels':** Cigarette advertising in the Journal. **NY State J Med** 1983 Dec;83(13):1347-52
**Whitaker AH:** Pesticide use in early twentieth century animal disease control. **Agric Hist** 1980;54(1):71-81
**Whitaker MA:** Science, scientists and history of science. **Hist Sci** 1984 Dec;22(58 pt 4):421-4
**Whitby JD:** Alcohol in anaesthesia and surgical resuscitation. **Anaesthesia** 1980 May;35(5):502-5
**White B:** Public health and civic administration in nineteenth-century Glasgow. **Soc Soc Hist Med Bull (Lond)** 1983 Jun;32:37-9
**White BM:** Medical police. Politics and police: the fate of John Roberton. **Med Hist** 1983 Oct;27(4):407-22
**White BN, Holden JJ:** From genetic engineering to biotechnology. **Queens Q** 1982;89(3):538-49
**White D** see **Clark G**
**White E:** The inverted type: homosexuality as a theme in James Merrill's prophetic books. **J Homosex** 1983 Spring-Summer;8(3-4):47-52
**White E** see **Clark G**
**White FM:** Nosocomial infection control: scope and implications for health care--historical view. **Am J Infect Control** 1981 Aug;9(3):61-9
**White GC** see **Breul FR**
**White IR, MacDonald DM:** Thomas Addison, M.D. First dermatologist at Guy's Hospital. **J Am Acad Dermatol** 1982 Mar;6(3):426-30
**White JG** see **Dodson G**

**White JJ:** 'Classics' and total pneumonectomy. **Ann Thorac Surg** 1981 Aug;32(2):216
**White JM** see **Krantz JC**
**White JS:** The Hedden's Store handbook of proprietary medicines. Portland, Durham & Downey, 1974. 94 p.
**White LW:** Adapting commercial oxygen for medical use. **Respir Ther** 1979 Jan-Feb;9(1):30-2
**White LW:** Education of oxygen-treatment personnel, 1928-1948. **Respir Ther** 1979 Jan-Feb;9(1):35, 38-9
**White PJ, Shackelford PG:** Edward Jenner, MD, and the scourge that was. **Am J Dis Child** 1983 Sep;137(9):864-9
**White PJ:** Medical Leonardo of Boston, Oliver Wendell Holmes, M.D. (1809-1894): an evaluation of versatility. **Perspect Biol Med** 1981 Spring;24(3):411-21
**White PM** see **Whittet TD**
**White SH** see **Lerner RM, ed**
**White SH** see **Siegel AW**
**White TD** see **Kimbel WH**
**White WD:** The American hospital industry since 1900: a short history. **Adv Health Econ Health Serv Res** 1982;3:143-70
**White WE:** Monofluorophosphate--its beginning. **Caries Res** 1983;17 Suppl 1:2-8
**Whitefield M** see **Ashton RE**
**Whitehead CC:** Technical implications of the post-metapsychological era: toward a developmental psychoanalysis. **Int J Psychoanal Psychother** 1984-85;10:437-56
**Whitehead EE** see **Spicker SF**
**Whitehouse D** see **Passi S**
**Whitehouse FW:** Classification and pathogenesis of the diabetes syndrome: a historical perspective. **J Am Diet Assoc** 1982 Sep;81(3):243-6
**Whitehouse WL:** The British National Health Service. **Zentralbl Gynakol** 1984;106(14):1028-32
**Whiteley JM, ed:** The history of counseling psychology. Monterey, California, Brooks/Cole, 1980. xiii, 209 p. [Mostly reprinted articles by various authors]
**Whiteside HO:** The drug habit in nineteenth-century Colorado. **Colo Mag** 1978;55(1):46-68
**Whiteside N:** Central control and the approved societies: access to social support under the interwar health insurance scheme. **Soc Soc Hist Med Bull (Lond)** 1983 Jun;32:14-8
**Whiteside T:** The pendulum and the toxic cloud. The course of dioxin contamination. New Haven, London, Yale University Press, 1979. 205 p.
**Whitfield AG:** Disraeli's doctors. **J R Coll Physicians Lond** 1980 Jul;14(3):202-4
**Whitfield AG:** Physician to the Prince of Wales. **J R Coll Physicians Lond** 1983 Oct;17(4):231-4
**Whitfield AG:** Roger Marbeck--first Registrar. **J R Coll Physicians Lond** 1981 Jan;15(1):59-60
**Whitfield AG:** The kiss of death (Princess Alice). **Ann R Coll Surg Engl** 1979 Sep;61(5):390-2
**Whitfield AG:** The scholar prince. **J R Coll Physicians Lond** 1984 Jul;18(3):195-7
**Whitfield JB** see **Oppenheimer JM**
**Whitman M:** Toward a new psychology for nurses. **Nurs Outlook** 1982 Jan;30(1):48-52
**Whitney HA:** Let us now praise famous men... **Drug Intell Clin Pharm** 1983 Jan;17(1):45-7
**Whitney HA** see **McLeod DC**
**Whitrow M:** A classification scheme for the history of science, medicine and technology. In Forbes EG, ed: Human implications of scientific advance. Edinburgh, Edinburgh University Press, 1978. p. 518-30.
**Whittaker AP:** Source-material in the Winchester City Archives 1550-1981. **Pharm Hist (London)** 1981;11(1):5-6
**Whittaker DK, Molleson T, Bennett RB, et al:** The prevalence and distribution of dental caries in a Romano-British population. **Arch Oral Biol** 1981;26(3):237-45
**Whittaker DK, Parker JH, Jenkins C:** Tooth attrition and continuing eruption in a Romano-British population. **Arch Oral Biol** 1982;27(5):405-9
**Whittaker JA:** Distinguishing nurses 'from other types of frauds'. **RNABC News** 1984 Jul-Aug;16(4):20-3
**Whitten DO:** Medical care of slaves: Louisiana sugar region and South Carolina rice district. **South Stud** 1977;16:153-80
**Whitteridge D, Merton PA:** Charles Skinner Hallpike: 19 July 1900-26 September 1979. **Biogr Mem Fellows R Soc** 1984;30:283-95
**Whitteridge G:** Harvey and sensory neuropathy. **J R Coll Physicians Lond** 1981 Jan;15(1):61-2
**Whitteridge G:** Of the local movement of animals. **Proc R Soc Lond [Biol]** 1979 Nov 30;206(1162):1-13
**Whitteridge G:** The Piltdown Hippocrates. **Hist Sci** 1980 Sep;18(41 pt 3):226-30
**Whittet TD:** A survey of apothecaries' tokens including some previously unrecognised specimens. **Pharm J** 1982;228:719-24; 1983;230:133-40; 1983;231:42-5, 641-9; 1984;232:583-5, 790-2
**Whittet TD:** Botanic garden of the trustees of the Georgia colony at Savannah. **Pharm J** 1983;231:770-1
**Whittet TD:** John Badger, apothecaryite. **Pharm Hist (London)** 1973 May;3(1):2-4
**Whittet TD:** Project for a directory of provincial apothecaries. **Pharm Hist (London)** 1970 Mar;1(4):2-3
**Whittet TD:** Seen in west country. **Pharm Hist (London)** 1975 Aug;5(2):5-6
**Whittet TD, White PM:** Some midland apothecaries. **Pharm Hist (London)** 1978 Jul;8(2):6-8
**Whittet TD:** Some Oxford apothecaries. **J R Soc Med** 1979 Dec;72(12):940-5
**Whittet TD:** The Crown & Anchor and the arts and sciences. **Pharm Hist (London)** 1983 Sept;13(3-4):2-6, 5-8
**Whittet TD:** The octocentenary of the Pepperers' Gild. **Pharm Hist** 1980;22(3):111-13
**Whittet TD:** Two restored historical pharmacies. **Pharm Hist (London)** 1974 Jan;4(1):6
**Who was who in American history - science and technology:** (A component of Who's who in American history). Chicago, Marquis, 1976. xiii, 688 p.
**Whorton J:** 'Thialion!!!' Anatomy of a pseudo-ethical proprietary. **Pharm Hist** 1981;23(3):114-25
**Whorton J** see **Numbers RL, ed**
**Whorton JC:** 'Antibiotic abandon': the resurgence of therapeutic rationalism. In Parascandola J, ed: The history of antibiotics. Madison, American Institute of the History of Pharmacy, 1980. p. 125-136.
**Whorton JC:** 'Athlete's heart': the medical debate over athleticism, 1870-1920. **J Sport Hist** 1982;9(1):30-52
**Whorton JC:** Muscular vegetarianism: the debate over diet and athletic performance in the progressive era. **J Sport Hist** 1981;8(2):58-75
**Whorton JC:** 'Physiologic optimism': Horace Fletcher and hygienic ideology in progressive America. **Bull Hist Med** 1981 Spring;55(1):59-87
**Whyler FJ:** A history of Orpington Hospital. **Bromley Local Hist** 1979;4:24-31
**Whymant R:** The Butchers of Harbin. Experimentation on POWs--Japan, World War II. **Conn Med** 1983 Mar;47(3):163-5
**Whyte D:** A trying Chindit. **Br Med J [Clin Res]** 1982 Dec 18-25;285(6357):1776-9
**Wick DL:** Psychomythology: A phenomenological critique of psychohistory. **Dalhousie Rev** 1980;6(2):290-99
**Wickersheimer E** see **Keil G**
**Wickes HL:** History of nursing in the Army: behind the lines. **Nurs Mirror** 1981 Jul 8;153(2):23-4
**Wickes HL:** The Royal Army Dental Corps. **Br Dent J** 1980 Jun 3-17;148(11-12):269-70
**Wickramasinghe MB:** Malaria and its control in Sri Lanka. **Ceylon Med J** 1981 Sep;26(3):107-15
**Wickremesinghe C** see **Wijesinha S**
**Wickwar H, Bryan CS:** Broussais in Columbia, South Carolina - 1831. **J SC Med Assoc** 1981 Dec;77(12):615-22
**Widdess JD:** The Royal College of Surgeons in Ireland and its medical school, 1784-1984. Third edition. Dublin, Royal College of Surgeons in Ireland, 1984. x, 194 p.
**Widdowson EM:** Adventures in nutrition over half a century. **Proc Nutr Soc** 1980 Sep;39(3):293-306
**Widdowson EM:** The first fifty years. **Curr Concepts Nutr** 1984;13:1-20
**Widimský J** see **Reinis Z**
**Widlocher D:** L'hystérie, cent ans après. **Rev Neurol (Paris)** 1982;138(12):1053-60
**Widowski K** see **Lukázs J**
**Widy-Tyszkiewicz E** see **Tyszkiewicz J**
**Wieckowska E:** Formy opieki zdrowotnej na ziemiach polskich w końcu XIX wieku do lat 30 wieku XX. **Wiad Lek** 1984 Jul 1;37(13):1049-55
**Wieckowska E** see **Płonka-Syroka B**
**Wiederhold Rotter A:** La pediatría en la Provincia de Cautín en la década del 20 al 30. **Rev Chil Pediatr** 1981 Jan-Feb;52(1):75-81
**Wiederkehr M, Roulet JF, Ulrich-Bochsler S:** Zahnärztliche Untersuchung mittelalterlicher Schädel aus drei Regionen des Kantons Bern. **SSO Schweiz Monatsschr Zahnheilkd** 1982 Feb;92(2):127-36
**Wiegand R:** Thomas S. Szasz. In J. Rattner, ed: Wandlungen der Psychoanalyse. Wien, Europaverlag, 1980. p. 333-68.
**Wiegand W:** Die Antipyretikatherapie bei Carl Liebermeister. Diss. Bonn, 1981. 96 p.
**Wiegenstein JG:** Emergency medicine. **JAMA** 1980 Jun 6;243(21):2182-3
**Wiegert J:** Anfangsprobleme der Nahrungsmittelchemie in Deutschland unter besonderer Berücksichtigung pharmazeutischer Verhältnisse. Braunschweig, 1975. 180 p. (Veröffentlichungen aus dem Pharmaziegeschichtlichen Seminar der Technischen Universität Braunschweig, Band 15).
**Wielopolska H** see **Horbowska-Marzec H**
**Wiench P, ed:** Die grossen Arzte. Geschichte der Medizin in Lebensbildern. München, Kindler, 1982. 335 p.
**Wiener JD:** Ueber Kropf, Hypertyreose und Jodbehandlung. **Schweiz Med Wochenschr** 1980 Nov 22;110(47):1784-7
**Wier JA:** 19th century army doctors on the frontier and in Nebraska. **Nebr Hist** 1980;61(2):192-214
**Wier RA:** Federalism, interest groups, and parliamentary government: the Canadian Medical Association. **J Commonw Polit Stud** 1973;11(2):159-75
**Wierzchowski KL** see **Szarkowski JW**
**Wieth JO** see **Behnke O**
**Wietschoreck H:** Aethiops---eine neue Arzneimittelgruppe der Nachchemiatrie---und ihre Bedeutung in Verbindung mit anderen Antimon-Präparaten. (Ein Beispiel für den Einsatz chemischer Untersuchungen bei der Bearbeitung arzneimittelgeschichtlicher Fragen). In: Vorträge des Internationalen Pharmaziehistorischen Kongresses Innsbruck 1977. Stuttgart, Wissenschaftliche Verlagsgesellschaft, 1979. p. 49-55.

**Wietschoreck H:** Die historische Entwicklung von Tartarusverbindungen in Arzneimitteln unter besonderer Berücksichtigung von Tartarus Chalybeatus und Terra Foliata Tartari in der Nachchemiatrie. In International Congress of the History of Medicine, 27th, Barcelona, 1980. Actas. Barcelona, Académia de Ciències Mèdiques de Catalunya i Balears, 1981. p. 675–9.
**Wiewiórkowski M:** Chemia a biologia. **Nauka Pol** 1979;27(11):64–74
**Wiewiórowska M:** Koncepcja piel egniarstwa Florencji Nightingale. **Pieleg Polozna** 1981;(8):7–8
**Wiewiórowska M:** Koncepcja pielegniarstwa Florencji Nightingale. **Pieleg Polozna** 1981;(5):8
**Wiewiórowska M:** Koncepcja pielęgniarstwa Florencji Nightingale. **Pieleg Polozna** 1981;(6):10–2 contd
**Wiewiórowska M:** Koncepcja pielęgniarstwa Florencji Nightingale. **Pieleg Polozna** 1981;(7):9–10, 15
**Wiezorek WD** see **Niemann H**
**Wiggins SN:** The impact of regulation on pharmaceutical research expenditures: a dynamic approach. **Econ Inq** 1983;21(1):115–28
**Wigglesworth WC** see **Cash P**
**Wiglesworth FW:** Maude E. Abbott. **Perspect Pediatr Pathol** 1984 Winter;8(4):291–4
**Wigley SC:** The first hundred years of tuberculosis in New Guinea. In Winslow JH, ed: The Melanesian environment, Canberra, Anu Press, 1977, p. 471–84.
**Wijbenga A, Hutzinger O:** Chemicals, man and the environment: a historic perspective of pollution and related topics. **Naturwissenschaften** 1984 May;71(5):239–46
**Wijesinha CY** see **Wijesinha SS**
**Wijesinha S, Wickremesinghe C:** Surgery and hospitals in ancient Sri Lanka and India. **J R Coll Surg Edinb** 1981 Jul;26(4):245–9
**Wijesinha SS:** El Zahrawi (936–1013 AD), the father of operative surgery. **Ann R Coll Surg Engl** 1983 Nov;65(6):423
**Wijesinha SS, Wijesinha CY:** Surgery and hospitals: the Sri Lanka tradition. **Ceylon Med J** 1983 Mar;28(1):48–52
**Wikinski JA:** Apuntes para una historia de la anestesiologia venezolana. **Rev Soc Venez Hist Med** 1981;30(45–46):25–55
**Wikström-Haugen I:** Patienten im Sahlgren'schen Krankenhaus Göteborg 1782–1822. In Imhof AE, ed: Mensch und Gesundheit in der Geschichte. Husum, Matthiesen, 1980. p. 323–37.
**Wikström-Haugen I:** Syphilis in Sweden about 1800. In International Congress of the History of Medicine, 27th, Barcelona, 1980. Actas. Barcelona, Académia de Ciències Mèdiques de Catalunya i Balears, 1981. p. 690–9.
**Wilber JA:** The founding of Georgia and the discovery of blood pressure. **J Med Assoc Ga** 1981 May;70(5):333
**Wilberger JE:** Transplantation of central nervous tissue. **Neurosurgery** 1983 Jul;13(1):90–4
**Wilbur CK:** Revolutionary medicine 1700–1800. Chester, Connecticut, Glove Pequot Press, 1980. 80 p.
**Wilbur DA:** The inimitable surgeon Pleadwell. **US Navy Med** 1983 May–Jun;74(3):5–10
**Wilbush J:** Climacteric symptom formation: Donovan's contribution. **Maturitas** 1981 Aug;3(2):99–105
**Wilbush J:** Historical perspective: Tilt, E. J. and the change of life (1857)––the only work on the subject in the English language. **Maturitas** 1980 Dec;2(4):259–67
**Wilbush J:** La menespausie–––the birth of a syndrome. **Maturitas** 1979;1(3):145–51
**Wilcox HG:** A difficult pregnancy: embryologic development of American medical education. **Ala J Med Sci** 1981 Jan;18(1):86–92
**Wilcox HG:** The president ails: American medicine in retrospect (George Washington). **Eval Program Plann** 1981 Apr;53(4):201–10
**Wilcox J:** Problems in the Latin manuscript tradition of De differentia spiritus et animae by the physician Costa ben Luca (9/10 cent.). In International Congress of the History of Medicine, 27th, Barcelona, 1980. Actas. Barcelona, Académia de Ciències Mèdiques de Catalunya i Balears, 1981. p. 363–5.
**Wilcox J, Golden HH:** Prolific immigrants and dwindling natives?: fertility patterns in western Massachusetts, 1850 and 1880. **J Fam Hist** 1982 Fall;7(3):265–88
**Wilczyńska M:** Działalność Warszawskiej Podsekcji Ortodontycznej w latach 1956–78. **Czas Stomatol** 1980 May;33(5):475–8
**Wilde J:** Historische Aspekte zum Schneeberger Lungenkrebs. **Z Arztl Fortbild (Jena)** 1982 Feb;76(3):118–20
**Wilde SA** see **Kostychev SP**
**Wilder F:** The remarkable world of John Wesley, pioneer in mental health. Hicksville, Exposition Press, 1978. 192 p.
**Wildfuehr G:** Robert Koch, Begründer der modernen Mikrobiologie. **Z Gesamte Hyg** 1982 Mar;28(3):145–8
**Wildfuehr G:** 100 Jahre Hygiene in Leipzig. **Wiss Z Karl Marx Univ Math Natur Wiss Reihe** 1979;28:9–23
**Wildgoose M, Hadingham E, Hooper A:** The prehistoric hand pictures at Gargas: attempts at simulation. **Med Hist** 1982 Apr;26(2):205–7
**Wildhirt E:** Dreissig Jahre Hepatologie in Kassel. In Balde JH, Schmiking, W, ed: Festschrift zum 86. Deutschen Arztetag in Kassel. Kassel, Arztevereins, 1983. p. 99–104.
**Wildsmith JA, Strichartz GR:** Local anaesthetic drugs––an historical perspective. **Br J Anaesth** 1984 Sep;56(9):937–9
**Wilens S:** Ross Granville Harrison. In Dictionary of American Biography, Suppl. 6, 1956–1960. p. 281–3, 1980.
**Wiley ML** see **Reynolds E**
**Wilhelm Ebel, ed:** Göttinger Universitätsreden aus zwei Jahrhunderten (1737–1934). Göttingen, Vandenhoeck & Ruprecht, 1978. 650 p. (Reprinted lectures by various individuals).
**Wilk D:** David Israel Macht (1882–1961). **Koroth** 1983 Aug;8(7–8):305–17
**Wilk D:** In memoriam Dr. Leo Kanner, 1894–1981. **Koroth** 1982 Aug;8(3/4):213–20
**Wilk D** see **Kottek S**
**Wilke J** see **Schwann H**
**Wilken H:** Intrauterine und neonatale Infektionen. Geschichtlicher Rückblick. **Zentralbl Gynakol** 1983;105(16):1035–40
**Wilken U:** Zur Geschichte von Einstellungsdeterminanten gegen über Körperbehinderten. **Rehabilitation (Stuttg)** 1984 May;23(2):81–3
**Wilken U:** Zur geschichtlichen Entwicklung der Körperbehinderten-Selbsthilfe-Vereinigungen. **Rehabilitation (Stuttg)** 1983 May;22(2):65–8
**Wilkenson F:** Spotsylvania: reflections. How men die in battle. **Civ War Times Illus** 1983;22(2):16–8
**Wilkerson SY:** Mind over body. James Jackson Putnam and the impact of neurology on psychotherapy in late nineteenth-century America. Ph.D. Diss. Duke University. Durham, 1978. v, 377 leaves.
**Wilkie JS:** The history of health and medicine: a social history curriculum for secondary schools. D.A. Diss., Carnegie-Mellon University. Pittsburgh, 1982. 261 p.
**Wilkins EW:** Designation or dedication: seven men in the evolution of a trauma center. **Am J Surg** 1982 Apr;143(4):399–403
**Wilkins KS:** Attitudes to witchcraft and demonic possession in France during the 18th century. **J Eur Stud** 1973;3(4):348–62
**Wilkins RH:** Birth of a journal: the origin and early years of Neurosurgery. **Neurosurgery** 1982 Jun;10(6 Pt 2):820–6
**Wilkinson A:** Disease in the 19th century urban economy: the medical officer of health and the community. **Soc Soc Hist Med Bull (Lond)** 1980;27:24–6
**Wilkinson AW:** Development of modern neonatal surgery. **Trans Hunter Soc** 1978–80;37–38:65–83
**Wilkinson L:** 'The other' John Hunter, M.D., F.R.S. (1754–1809): his contributions to the medical literature, and to the introduction of animal experiments into infectious disease research. **Notes Rec R Soc Lond** 1982 Feb;36(2):227–41
**Wilkinson L:** Veterinary cross-currents in ideas on infectious diseases since Aristotle. **Vet Hist** 1980/81;1(n.s.):149–52
**Wilkinson L:** Veterinary cross-currents in the history of ideas on infectious disease. **J R Soc Med** 1980 Nov;73(11):818–27
**Wilkinson M:** Elizabeth Garrett Anderson and migraine. In Rose FC, Bynum WF, ed: Historical aspects of the neurosciences. New York, Raven, 1982. p. 165–9.
**Wilkoszewski E:** Z dziejów polskich czasopism pediatrycznych (lata 1908–1983). **Pediatr Pol** 1983 Aug–Sep;58(8–9):673–84
**Will H:** Die Geburt der Psychosomatik: Georg Groddeck, der Mensch und Wissenschaftler. München, Baltimore, Urban & Schwarzenberg, 1984. vi, 231 p.
**Will PE:** Chine: la terre des grandes famines. **Histoire** 1982;44:26–37
**Will the real 'father of dental education' please stand up? (John Harris): Ohio Dent J** 1980 May;54(5):19–20
**Willbanks OL, Willbanks SE:** Femoral neuropathy due to retroperitoneal bleeding. A red herring in medicine complicates anticoagulant therapy and influences the Russian Communist Revolution (Crown Prince Alexis, Rasputin). **Am J Surg** 1983 Feb;145(2):193–8
**Willbanks SE** see **Willbanks OL**
**Willcox RR:** The international venereological scene as viewed by Harrison and St Mary's. **Br J Vener Dis** 1982 Apr;58(2):72–85
**Willeford BR, ed** see **Kieft L**
**Willemot J:** Anatomie et traumatismes du nez. Septorhinoplastie. Nez et esthétique. **Acta Otorhinolaryngol Belg** 1981;35(2):201–350
**Willemot J:** Le nez et la gorge dans le poème de la médecine et le premier livre du Canon d'Avicenne. In International Congress of the History of Medicine, 27th, Barcelona, 1980. Actas. Barcelona, Académia de Ciències Mèdiques de Catalunya i Balears, 1981. p. 766–70.
**Willemot J:** L'endoscopie en oto-rhino-laryngologie de 1850 à 1950. **J Fr Otorhinolaryngol** 1983 Apr;32(4):233–6
**Willemot J:** Naissance et développement de l'oto-rhino-laryngologie dans l'histoire de la médecine. **Acta Otorhinolaryngol Belg** 1981;35(Suppl 3):393–1044
**Willemot J:** Rhinologie, Pharyngologie. **Acta Otorhinolaryngol Belg** 1981;35(2):11 200
**Willenegger H, Bandi W:** Werdegang und Aufgabe der AO-International. Teil 2. **Unfallchirurgie** 1984 Jun;10(3):107–9
**Willens SH:** Dr. Nathaniel Peabody and his book: The art of preserving teeth. **Bull Hist Dent** 1980 Oct;28(2):83–6
**Willett LB, Schanbacher FL, Teske RH:** Toxicology and the dairy industry: will problems outrun solutions? **J Dairy Sci** 1981 Jun;64(6):1483–93
**Willetts J** see **Shipley M**
**Willi Busanny-Caspari (8. 4. 1922 bis 7. 7. 1982): Verh Dtsch Ges Pathol** 1983;67:772–3
**Williams AR:** Victorian clinical photography. **J Audiov Media Med** 1982 Jul;5(3):100–3
**Williams CD:** Fifty years ago. Archives of Diseases in Childhood 1933. A nutritional disease of childhood associated with a maize diet. **Arch Dis Child** 1983 Jul;58(7):550–60
**Williams CM** see **Wilson CL**
**Williams CP:** Healing and evangelism: the place of medicine in later Victorian Protestant missionary thinking. In Sheils WJ, ed: The Church

and healing. Papers read at the twentieth summer meeting and the twenty-first winter meeting of the Ecclesiastical History Society. Oxford, Basil Blackwell for the Society, 1982. p. 271-85.
**Williams D, Young R:** Canadian food aid: surplus and hunger. **Int J** 1981;36(2):335-52
**Williams D, Williams G:** Every child a wanted child. Clarence James Gamble, M.D., and his work in the birth control movement. Ed. E. P. Flint. Boston, Harvard University Press for Countway Library of Medicine, 1978. xvii, 445 p.
**Williams DC** see **Shor RE**
**Williams DE:** Wendell Andrew Leroy Johnson. In Dictionary of American biography, 1961-1965. Suppl. 7, 1981. p. 395-6.
**Williams DF:** In search of perfect dental materials. **Br Dent J** 1981 Jul 7;151(1):24-7
**Williams DR:** Horses, pigeons, and the therapy of conversion: a psychological reading of Jonathan Edwards's theology. **Harv Theol Rev** 1981;74(4):337-52
**Williams E:** Diary of a VAD 1940-49. **Nurs Mirror** 1981 Jul 8;153(2):25-7 (continued regularly)
**Williams E:** Diary of a VAD 1940-9: cry havoc... **Nurs Mirror** 1981 Jul 1;153(1):25-8
**Williams E:** The history of brucellosis in Wales. In J. Cule, ed: Wales and medicine. London, British Society for the History of Medicine, 1975. p. 75-85.
**Williams G, Stretton TB, Leonard JC:** AIDS in 1959? **Lancet** 1983 Nov 12;2(8359):1136
**Williams G:** The age of miracles. Medicine and surgery in the nineteenth century. London, Constable, 1981. 234 p.
**Williams G** see **Williams D**
**Williams GR:** A history of appendicitis. With anecdotes illustrating its importance. **Ann Surg** 1983 May;197(5):495-506
**Williams H:** Public health and local history. **Local Hist** 1980;14(4):202-10
**Williams HB:** The McGill University plastic surgery program. **Ann Plast Surg** 1984 Nov;13(5):362-5
**Williams HE:** My four teachers. **Med J Aust** 1977 Dec 15;2(12):650-1
**Williams HH:** Icie Gertrude Macy Hoobler (1892-1984). A biographical sketch. **J Nutr** 1984 Aug;114(8):1351-62
**Williams JA:** Fourier analysis and homology of the first molars of the Palaeocene primate family Picrodontidae. **Arch Oral Biol** 1981;26(2):111-6
**Williams JE, Johns RB, Evans P:** The Gold-Headed Cane award of the Taylor-Jones County Medical Society. **Tex Med** 1981 Nov;77(11):50-1
**Williams K** see **Davies C, ed**
**Williams LE** see **Loken MK**
**Williams LP:** Album of science: the nineteenth century. New York, Scribner's, 1978. xiv, 413 p.
**Williams LP:** The history of science at Cornell University. **Hist Teacher** 1980;13(3):379-83
**Williams MR:** The scientific library of Charles Babbage. **Ann Hist Comput** 1981;3(3):235-40
**Williams MT:** New York's public baths: a case study in urban progressive reform. **J Urban Hist** 1981;7(1):49-81
**Williams PO** see **Bradburne P**
**Williams PV:** Primitive religion and healing. A study of folk medicine in North-East Brazil. Cambridge, England, and Totowa, New Jersey, D. S. Brewer and Rowman and Littlefield, 1979. xi, 212 p.
**Williams R** see **Westaby D**
**Williams S:** A 'Taylor made' practice. **Br Med J [Clin Res]** 1984 Jan 14;288(6411):116-8
**Williams S:** En tidlig dansk henrettelse: et kraniefund. **Tandlaegebladet** 1983 Oct;87(18):632-4
**Williams SE:** The use of beverage alcohol as medicine, 1790-1860. **J Stud Alcohol** 1980 May;41(5):543-66
**Williams TI, Withers S, ed:** A biographical dictionary of scientists. 3rd ed. London, A. & C. Black, 1982. xiv, 674 p.
**Williams WD:** Did Horace Wells stage a newspaper publicity scheme? Some unreported newspaper items. **Bull Hist Dent** 1983 Oct;31(2):93-8
**Williams WE:** The school physician's notebook: a cameo of William Carlos Williams. In Jones AH, ed: Images of healers. Albany, State University of New York Press, 1983. p. 3-8.
**Williams WH:** Norman Thomas Kirk. In Dictionary of American Biography, Suppl. 6, 1956-1960. p. 344-5, 1980.
**Williams P, ed** see **Varma VP**
**Williams TI, ed, Withers S, ed:** A biographical dictionary of scientists. New York, Wiley, [1974]. 641 p.
**Williamson DH** see **Kornberg H**
**Williamson GC** see **Moore PV**
**Williamson J:** Three views on geriatric medicine: 3. Notes on the historical development of geriatric medicine as a medical specialty. **Age Ageing** 1979 Aug;8(3):144-8
**Williamson JG:** British mortality and the value of life, 1781-1931. **Popul Stud** 1984 Mar;38(1):157-72
**Williamson R:** Sir Busick Harwood: a reappraisal. **Med Hist** 1983 Oct;27(4):423-33
**Willier BH, Oppenheimer JM, ed:** Foundations of experimental embryology. 2nd ed., enlarged and with a new introduction, by J. M. Oppenheimer. New York, Hafner, 1974. xx, 277 p. Selections from various authors.
**Willigan JD** see **Mineau GP**
**Williman JP, Kvarnes RG:** A medieval example of psychotherapy. **Psychiatry** 1984 Feb;47(1):93-5
**Willis E:** Sister Elizabeth Kenny and the evolution of the occupational division of labour in health care. **Aust NZ J Sociol** 1979;15(3):30-8
**Willis FN, Dean LM, Larsen L:** The first mental hospital for American Indians, 1900-1934. **Bull Menninger Clin** 1981 Mar;45(2):149-54
**[Willis Dew Gatch. Includes reprints of three of his articles.]: Indiana Med Hist Q** 1977;3(3):43-60
**Willison RG:** Dr. E. H. Lambert's contributions to electromyography. **Muscle Nerve** 1982;5(9S):S2-5
**Williston CL:** 1954-1984 with TMA: a look at 30 years of growth and change. **Tex Med** 1984 Jul;80(7):57-9
**Willmott S** see **Manson-Bahr PE**
**Willmott Dobbie BM:** An attempt to estimate the true rate of maternal mortality, sixteenth to eighteenth centuries. **Med Hist** 1982 Jan;26(1):79-90
**Willmuth LR:** Medical views of depression in the elderly: historical notes. **J Am Geriatr Soc** 27(11):495-9, Nov 79
**Willson PR:** Industrial health and rationalisation in an Italian light engineering firm: the Magneti Marelli in the Fascist period. **Soc Soc Hist Med Bull (Lond)** 1983 Dec;33:47-9
**Wilmanns JC:** Paroxysmal nocturnal hemoglobinuria first described in 1882 by Paul Strübing: an example of cooperation between clinical and basic research. **Blut** 1982 Dec;45(6):367-73
**Wilmer HA:** Defining and understanding the therapeutic community. **Hosp Community Psychiatry** 1981 Feb;32(2):95-9
**Wilson A:** Ignorant midwives - a rejoinder. **Soc Soc Hist Med Bull (Lond)** 1983 Jun;32:46-9
**Wilson A:** Oddity remembered: 1918 influenza epidemic. **Br Med J** 1981;282:1766
**Wilson A:** The way it used to be. In Aberdare. **Br Med J** 1981;282:1284-6
**Wilson AC** see **Prager EM**
**Wilson AF:** The Enlightenment and infant care. **Soc Soc Hist Med Bull (Lond)** 1979 Dec;25:44-7
**Wilson C:** Horace Evans. In Dictionary of national biography, 1961-1970. Suppl. 8, 1981. p. 336-7.
**Wilson C:** Lord of the underworld: Jung and the twentieth century. Wellingborough, Northamptonshire, Aquarian Press, 1984. 160 p.
**Wilson C:** Sensation and explanation: the problem of consciousness in Descartes. **Nat Syst** 1982;4:151-65
**Wilson C:** Sir Arthur William Mickle Ellis. In Dictionary of national biography, 1961-1970. Suppl. 8, 1981. p. 330-2.
**Wilson C:** The quest for Wilhelm Reich. Garden City, N.Y., Anchor, 1981. xv, 272 p.
**Wilson C** see **Knodel J**
**Wilson C** see **Lesthaeghe R**
**Wilson CB:** A decade of pituitary microsurgery. **J Neurosurg** 1984 Nov;61(5):814-33
**Wilson CE:** The Boston inoculation controversy: a revisionist interpretation. **Journalism Hist** 1980;7(1):16-9, 40
**Wilson CL, Williams CM:** Toward the biological control of insect pests: the rise of the International Center of Insect Physiology and Ecology. **Sci Public Aff Bull At Sci** 1973;29(3):10-16
**Wilson DC:** Ten fingers for God: [the complete biography of Dr. Paul Brand]. Nashville, Nelson Publ, 1983. vii, 275 p.
**Wilson E:** How pharmacy developed in the shadow of Parliament Hill. **Can Pharm J** 1982 Oct;115(10):369-73
**Wilson EO** see **Hamrum CL, ed**
**Wilson G:** Swallow it or rub it on: more mammoth cave remedies. **South Folkl Q** 1967;31(4):296-303
**Wilson G:** The first anaesthetic in Australia. **Anaesth Intensive Care** 1980 Aug;8(3):378-9
**Wilson G:** The pioneering anaesthetists of Australia. **Anaesth Intensive Care** 1979 Nov;7(4):311-21
**Wilson HB:** The Medical Annals Committee [interview by B. Taylor]. **Md State Med J** 1981 May;30(5):79-83
**Wilson HD:** A hundred years of the Ettles scholarship at the University of Edinburgh or 'Whatever happened to the likely lads (and lasses)?' **Med Educ** 1981 Nov;15(6):359-62
**Wilson HH:** The art of war and medical & surgical sciences of Hindus. Delhi, Nag Publishers, 1979. 44 p.
**Wilson HS:** Research in nursing has a history. **J Nurs Adm** 1984 Dec;14(12):4-5
**Wilson JG:** The evolution of teratological testing. **Teratology** 1979 Oct;20(2):205-11
**Wilson JL:** American Thoracic Society--five great teachers in the field of tuberculosis. **Am Rev Respir Dis** 1981 May;123(5):571-5
**Wilson JL:** 'The daily sanatorium routine was the treatment.' **Am Lung Assoc Bull** 1982 Mar;68(2):7-10
**Wilson JW:** Some aspects of medical services in the Trans-Mississippi Department of the Confederate States of America, 1863-1865. **J North LA Hist Assoc** 1981 Fall;12(4):123-46
**Wilson KS:** Mandibular reconstruction: introduction. **Otolaryngol Head Neck Surg** 1982 Sep-Oct;90(5):576
**Wilson L:** Schizophrenia in learned societies: professionalism vs. scholarship. **J Hist Med Allied Sci** 1981 Jan;36(1):5-8
**Wilson LB:** A women pioneer in a new profession, medical editing. **Mayo Alumnus** 1982 Apr;:20-3
**Wilson LB:** Les maladies des femmes: women, charlatanry, and professional medicine in eighteenth-century France. Ph.D. Diss., Stanford University. Palo Alto, 1982. vi, 449 p.
**Wilson LG:** Dorothy Schullian retires from the Journal. **J Hist Med Allied Sci** 1984 Oct;39(4):457-61

**Wilson LG:** Fevers and science in early nineteenth century medicine. **J Hist Med Allied Sci** 1978 Jul;33(3):386–407

**Wilson LG:** Madeline Earle Stanton 1898–1980. **Bull Med Libr Assoc** 1981 Jul;69(3):357–8

**Wilson LG:** Measure in everything: a decade of the journal. **J Hist Med Allied Sci** 1982 Oct;37(4):393–8

**Wilson LG** see **Ebbert A, et al**

**Wilson LG** see **Wangensteen OW, ed**

**Wilson RK:** Charles Henderson–a man stands tall. **J Med Assoc State Ala** 1982 Jun;51(12):41–3

**Wilson RN** see **Ibrahim MA**

**Wilson RT:** The incidence and control of livestock diseases in Darfur, Anglo-Egyptian Sudan, during the period of the condominium, 1916–1956. **Int J Afr Hist Stud** 1979,12(1).62–82

**Wilson S:** Death and the social historians: some recent books in French and English. **Soc Hist (Lond)** 1980;5(3):435–51

**Wilson TA** see **Gorman BM**

**Wilson TG:** Historical vignette. Sir Astley Cooper. **Am J Otol** 1984 Jul;5(5):411–4

**Wilson TH** see **Criado FJ**

**Wilson TS:** The National Health Service 1948–1980. In Checkland O, Lamb M, ed: Health care as social history; the Glasgow case. Aberdeen, Aberdeen University Press, 1982. p. 149–57.

**Wilson W:** Old ethics: new dilemmas. **Ulster Med J** 1982;51(1):23–34

**[Wilson L]:** The education of historians of medicine. **J Hist Med Allied Sci** 1982 Jul;37(3):265–8

**Wilson LG, ed:** Benjamin Silliman and his circle: Studies on the influence of Benjamin Silliman on science in America. Prepared in honor of Elizabeth H. Thomson. New York, Science History Publications, 1979. x, 227 p. Contributions by S. D Beckham, J. C. Greene, L. I. Kuslan, G. Robinson, M. W. Rossiter.

**Wilson, strokes, and zebras: N Engl J Med** 1983 Jan 20;308(3):163–4

**Wimberley T:** Toward national health insurance in the United States: an historical outline, 1910–1979. **Soc Sci Med [Med Econ]** 1980 Mar;14(1):13–25

**Wimmel B, Geus A, ed:** Die tiermedizinischen Zeitschriften des 18. Jahrhunderts. Stuttgart, Hiersemann, 1981. 200 p. (Indices naturwissenschaftlich-medizinischer Periodica bis 1850, 3).

**Wimmer J:** Die medizinisch-technische Assistentin in Osterreich: eine entwicklungsgeschichtliche Berufskunde oder eine berufskundliche Entwicklungsgeschichte. Wien, Maudrich, 1983. xii, 79 p.

**Winau R:** Bemerkungen zur 'Sprache' der Medizin. **Ber Wissenschaftsgesch** 1980;3(1–2):95–102

**Winau R, Vaubel E:** Chirurgen in Berlin. 100 Porträts. Berlin, New York, Walter de Gruyter, 1983. 106 p.

**Winau R:** Deutsche Gesellschaft für Geschichte der Medizin, Naturwissenschaft und Tecknik 1901–1976. Wiesbaden, Steiner, 1978. 164 p. (Beiträge zur Geschichte der Wissenschaft und der Technik, 15).

**Winau R:** Ernst Haeckels Vorstellungen von Wert und Werden menschlicher Rassen und Kulturen. **Medizinhist J** 1981;16(3):270–79

**Winau R:** James Israel, 1848–1926. Wiesbaden, F. Steiner, 1983. 256 p.

**Winau R** see **Berghaus A**

**Winau R** see **Habrich C**

**Winau R** see **Kotwas J**

**Winckelmann HJ** see **Weiss C**

**Wind GG, Rich NM:** Historical notes on surgical technique. In their Principles of surgical technique. The art of surgery. Baltimore, Munich, Urban & Schwarzenberg, 1983. p. 9–19.

**Winder M:** Il Buddha della medicina. **Kos** 1984 Apr;1(3):55–74

**Winder M:** Modern and traditional medicine: rivals or friends? Some solutions attempted by India, China, Japan and Tibetans in exile. **Bull Br Assoc Orient** 1979–80,N.Ser;11:35–9

**Winder M:** The buddhist antecedents of Tibetan medicine. **Tibet News Rev** 1981;2(1/2):29–34

**Windholz G:** Pavlov vs. Köhler. Pavlov's little-known primate research. **Pavlov J Biol Sci** 1984 Jan–Mar;19(1):23–31

**Windholz G:** Pavlov's position toward American behaviorism. **J Hist Behav Sci** 1983 Oct;19(4):394–407

**Windle WF:** Recollections of research in spinal cord regeneration. **Exp Neurol** 1981 Jan;71(1):1–5

**Windle-Taylor PC** see **Phelps PD**

**Windsor HM:** Direct blood transfusion. **Med J Aust** 1980 Feb 9;1(3):136

**Windstrup G:** Locke on suicide. **Polit Theory** 1980;8(2):169–82

**Winer JL** see **Moore C**

**Winfree LT, Theis HE, Griffiths CT:** Drug use in rural America: a cross-cultural examination of complementary social deviance theories. **Youth Soc** 1981;12(4):465–89

**Wing AJ** see **Válek A**

**Wing ES:** First American description of calcific aortic stenosis. **RI Med J** 1983 Jun;66(6):243–5

**Winge M:** James Lind Grundlaeggeren af den maritime medicin. **Dan Medicinhist Arbog** 1983;12:9–20

**Winge M:** Urban Bruun Aaskow. **Dan Medicinhist Arbog** 1981;:94–127

**Winkelman M** see **Krippner S**

**Winkelmann H:** Entbindungswissenschaft und Entbindungskunst bei Friedrich Benjamin Osiander. **Medizinhist J** 1983;18(4):306–12

**Winkelmann H, Mildner S:** Schriftenverzeichnis Hans-Heinz Eulner (19. 4. 1925 - 17. 10. 1980). **Medizinhist J** 1982;17(1/2):148–55

**Winkelmann O:** Werner Körte. **Neue Dtsch Biogr** 1980;12:395–6

**Winkelmann O:** Zur Erinnerung an Ernst von Düring-Pascha (1858–1944). In: First International Congress on the History of Turkish-Islamic Science and Technology, ITU 14–18 September 1981. Proceedings Vol. IV, p. 32–44.

**Winkelstein W:** A tribute to Abe Lilienfeld. **Am J Epidemiol** 1980 Aug;112(2):178–84

**Winkle S:** Johann Friedrich Struensee: Arzt, Aufklärer und Staatsmann: Beitrag zur Kultur-, Medizin- und Seuchengeschichte der Aufklärungszeit. Stuttgart, Fischer, 1983. 654 p.

**Winkleman M:** Institutional retreat. **NY Aff** 1980;6(3):80–3

**Winkler EA:** Ernst Unger: a pioneer in modern surgery. **J Hist Med Allied Sci** 1982 Jul;37(3):269–86

**Winkler H** see **Horn H**

**Winkler L:** Galens Schrift 'De Antidotis'. Ein Beitrag zur Geschichte von Antidot und Theriak. Diss. rer. nat. Marburg, 1980. 390 p.

**Winkler-Trachsel E:** Arnold Ott (1840–1910). Arzt und Dichter. Sein ärztliches Wirken. Zürich, Juris Druck, 1983. 83 p. (Zürcher Medizingeschichtliche Abhandlungen, Neue Reihe, Nr. 163).

**Winslow CE:** Health in the twentieth century. New York, Arno, 1977. Reprint of Winslow's The evolution and significance of the modern public health campaign (New Haven, 1923); and Winslow's A city set on a hill: The significance of the health demonstration at Syracuse, New York (Garden City, N. Y., 1934). Various paginations.

**Winslow CE:** The conquest of epidemic disease: a chapter in the history of ideas. Madison, University of Wisconsin Press, 1980 printing, c1971. viii, 411 p.

**Winslow JE, Warren GB:** Dental school capitation--an historical perspective. **J Dent Educ** 1981 Nov;45(11):759–62

**The Winslow tradition: J Public Health Policy** 1984 Sep;5(3):320–6

**Winsor MP:** Louis Agassiz and the species question. **Stud Hist Biol** 1979;3:89–138

**Winstanley J:** St Thomas Hospital a cradle of British ophthalmology. **Trans Ophthalmol Soc UK** 1982;102 (Pt 4):454–60

**Winsten S, Sideman L:** History of the Philadelphia Section, American Association for Clinical Chemistry. **Clin Chem** 1981 Jan;27(1):192–4

**Winter E:** Das Dekanatsbuch der Tübinger Medizinischen Fakultät 1808–1858 (Teil 1: 1808–1816). Text und Kommentar. Tübingen, Universitätsarchiv, 1979. 221 p.

**Winter G:** Zur Wirkungsgeschichte des frühmittelalterlichen 'Harnregelnkatalogs.' Diss., Universität Würzburg. Würzburg, 1981. 95 p.

**Winter I:** Die Zeitschrift 'Russische Medicinische Rundschau' als Mittlerin zwischen deutscher und russischer Medizin. **Z Gesamte Hyg** 1980;26(5):379–80

**Winter I** see **Tutzke D, ed**

**Winter JM:** Aspects of the impact of the first world war on infant mortality in Britain. **J Eur Econ Hist** 1982;11(3):713–38

**Winter JM:** Infant mortality, maternal mortality and public health in Britain in the 1930's. **J Eur Econ Hist** 1979;13(2):439–62

**Winter JM:** Military fitness and civilian health in Britain during the first World War. **J Contemp Hist** 1980;15(2):211–44

**Winter K:** Das Gesundheitswesen in der Deutschen Demokratischen Republik. Bilanz nach 30 Jahren. Berlin, Volk und Gesundheit, 1980. 223 p.

**Winter K:** Ein historischer Wendepunkt in der Geschichte von Naturwissenschaft und Medizin. Zum 100. Jahrestag der Entdeckung des Mycobacterium tuberculosis durch Robert Koch. **Z Arztl Fortbild (Jena)** 1982 Mar 15;76(6):229–30

**Winter ST, Ginott N:** Two pioneer paediatricians in Palestine under the Turks. **Adler Mus Bull** 1983 Nov;Spec issue:58–61

**Winter K, ed:** Das Gesundheitswesen in der Deutschen Demokratischen Republik. Berlin, Verlag Volk und Gesundheit, 1974. 209 p.

**Winters RW:** An historical review of the development of criteria for intravenous amino acid requirements. **Acta Chir Scand [Suppl]** 1983;517:7–15

**Winters RW, Heird WC, Dell RB:** History of parenteral nutrition in pediatrics with emphasis on amino acids. **Fed Proc** 1984 Apr;43(5):1407–11

**Winters SB:** The health of Edvard Beneš: an unpublished letter from 1948. **East Cent Eur** 1977;4:60–6

**Winton R:** Food and fitness at sea. **Med J Aust** 1980 Oct 18;2(8):411–2

**Winton R:** The nature of things: a history of the Royal College of Pathologists of Australasia. Sydney, The College, 1982. x, 120 p.

**Wintrobe B:** Mrs. Wintrobe writes about her husband. **Med Times** 1979 Nov;107(11):59–64

**Wintrobe M** see **Bernard J**

**Wintrobe MM:** Medical education in Utah. **West J Med** 1982 Apr;136(4):357–66

**Wintrobe MM:** Perspective in hematology. **Pharos** 1983 Winter;46(1):7–12

**Wirth J:** La jeune fille et la mort: recherches sur les themes macabres dans l'art germanique de la Renaissance. Genève, Droz, 1979. 194 p., 64 p. of plates. (Centre de recherches d'histoire et de philologie de la IVe section de l'Ecole pratique des hautes études. V, Hautes études médiévales et modernes; 36).

**Wirth M:** Das Leben und Wirken des Chirurgen Cajetan von Textor. Diss. Würzburg, 1980. 107 p.

**Wirthlin LS:** Joseph Smith's boyhood operation: an 1813 surgical success. **Brigham Young Univ Stud** 1981;21(2):131–54

**Wirz A:** Malaria-Prophylaxe und kolonialer Städtebau: Fortschritt als Rückschritt? **Gesnerus** 1980;37(3/4):215–34

**Wischermann H:** Mors meditans: Ein Beitrag zu drei Medaillen auf den Augsburger Arzt Occo III. **Arch Kulturgesch** 1978;58(2):432–3

**Wise RI:** Brucellosis in the United States. Past, present, and future.

**JAMA** 1980 Nov 21;244(20):2318-22
**Wiseman H:** Graduate medical education in Mobile. **J Med Assoc State Ala** 1983 Feb;52(8):43-9
**Wiser V:** Mary Engle Pennington. In: Notable American women. The modern period. Cambridge, Mass., Belknap-Harvard Univ. Press, 1980. 4:532-4.
**Wisner E** see **Breul FR**
**Wiśniewski L** see **Mazurczak T**
**Wisswaesser C:** Roots and ramifications of medicinal herbs in eighteenth-century North America. **Trans Stud Coll Physicians Phila** 1977 Apr;44(4):194-9
**Wit JG:** Institute of Veterinary Pharmacology, Pharmacy, and Toxicology: its research (1961-1980). **Tijdschr Diergeneeskd** 1981 Oct;106(20):suppl 3:169-75
**Witczak W:** Towarzystwo Paryskie Lekarzy Polskich (w 125 rocznice powstania). **Przegl Lek** 1984;41(4):325-7
**With TK:** A short history of porphyrins and the porphyrias. **Int J Biochem** 1980;11(3-4):189-200
**With TK:** Thirty years with biochemistry and clinic of porphyrias in man and animals. **Int J Biochem** 1980;12(5-6):985-8
**Withers S, ed** see **Williams TI**
**Withers S, ed** see **Williams TI, ed**
**Witkam HJ:** Catalogues of all the chiefest rarities in the Publick Anatomie Hall of the University of Leyden. Leiden, Witkam, 1980. xv, 86 leaves.
**Witkiewicz H:** Jubileusz Warszawskiej Szkoły Pielęgniarstwa. **Pieleg Polozna** 1982;(3):20-1
**Witkop CJ:** History of genetics in dentistry. **Birth Defects** 1980;16(5):13-26
**Witkowski JA:** Dr. Carrel's immortal cells. **Med Hist** 1980 Apr;24(2):129-42
**Witkowski JA:** Experimental pathology and the origins of tissue culture: Leo Loeb's contribution. **Med Hist** 1983 Jul;27(3):269-88
**Witkowski JA:** W. T. Astbury and Ross G. Harrison: the search for the molecular determination of form in the developing embryo. **Notes Rec R Soc Lond** 1980 Dec;35(2):195-219
**Witschel H:** Die Physiologie zu Erlangen von der Gründung der Universität bis zum Ausklang der Romantik. Erlangen, 1964. 141 p.
**Witt M, Early S:** The worker as safety inspector. **Work Pap New Soc** 1980;7(5):20-9
**Witte B** see **Schneider HG**
**Witten LC, Pachella R, ed:** Alchemy and the occult: a catalogue of books and manuscripts from the collection of Paul and Mary Mellon given to Yale University Library. Vols. 3 and 4: Manuscripts 1225-1922. With an introduction by P. Kibre and additional notes by W. McGuire. New Haven, Yale University Library, 1977. 853 p.
**Witten LC** see **Manuscripta alchemica der Sammlung Mellon: Bemerkungen zum Katalog**
**Wittenberg S:** Brock's research in stereopsis. **Am J Optom Physiol Opt** 1981 Aug;58(8):663-6, 667-70
**Wittenstein K** see **Kantrov I**
**Witter DA:** Witchcraft along the Rio Grande. **Palacio** 1974;80(2):21-37
**Wittern R:** Das Gift der frommen Denkart - Zur Pharmakologie des Schierlings in der Antike. In Hickel E, Schröder G, ed: Neue Beiträge zur Arzneimittelgeschichte. Festschrift für Wolfgang Schneider zum 70. Geburtstag. Stuttgart, Wissenschaftliche Verlagsgesellschaft, 1982. p. 15-28.
**Wittern R:** The Robert Bosch Foundation and the establishment of the Institute for the History of Medicine. **Clio Med** 1980;15(1/2):89-91
**Wittern R, ed:** Jahrbuch des Instituts für Geschichte der Medizin der Robert Bosch Stiftung. Band 1. Stuttgart, Hippokrates Verlag, 1984. 77 p.
**Wittern R, ed** see **Habrich C**
**Wittman E** see **Kiefer JH**
**Wittmann L** see **Pohlen M**
**Wittmers LE** see **Aufderheide AC**
**Wittop Koning AW** see **Hein WH**
**Wittop Koning DA:** De farmacie en de medische tijdschriften. **Ned Tijdschr Geneeskd** 1981 Dec 5;125(49):2021-4
**Wittop Koning DA, Van Gelder JB:** Die Offizin aus der Meteorologia philosophica-politica des Fr. Reinzer. **Beitr Gesch Pharm** 1984;31(24):210
**Wittop Koning DA:** Drei holländische Pharmaziehistoriker. In: Vorträge des Internationalen Pharmaziehistorischen Kongresses Innsbruck 1977. Stuttgart, Wissenschaftliche Verlagsgesellschaft, 1979. p. 129-39.
**Wittop Koning DA:** Ein Niederlassungszettel des Chymisten Mattheus Rabs. In Hickel E, Schröder G, ed: Neue Beiträge zur Arzneimittelgeschichte. Festschrift für Wolfgang Schneider zum 70. Geburtstag. Stuttgart, Wissenschaftliche Verlagsgesellschaft, 1982. p. 47-58.
**Wittop Koning DA** see **Blankaart S**
**Witzig JS:** Theodore Flournoy-a friend indeed. **J Anal Psychol** 1982 Apr;27(2):131-48
**Wladimirova LJ** see **Schtschepin OP**
**Włosińska I** see **Wardaszko-Lyskowska H**
**Woeber K:** Uber die historische Bedeutung der Bad Aachener Heilquellen für die Dermato-Venerologie. **Rehabilitation (Bonn)** 1981;34(3-4):17-25
**Woehrle R, Touraine JL, Garin JP, et al:** Comité de lecture d'une revue régionale. Fonctionnement et résultats. **Bull Soc Sci Med Grand Duche Luxemb** 1979;116(1):137-41
**Woerdeman MW:** The pre-constitutional years of the Dutch anatomical society. **Acta Morphol Neerl Scand** 1983 Mar;21(1):7-8
**Wójciak L, Mackowiak K:** Problemy stomatologii wieku rozwojowego w aspekcie rozwoju historycznego. **Czas Stomatol** 1979 Nov;32(11):1063-8
**Wójcik Z:** O Stasziou i nowych taszicianach. **Kwart Hist Nauki Tech** 1981;26:177-86
**Wojtkowiak S, Stempel A:** Z badań nad dziejami szkoleniowych bibliotek medycznych w Polskich Siłach Zbrojnych na Zachodzie w latach II wojny swiatowej. **Arch Hist Med (Warsz)** 1983;46(1):59-65
**Wolf E** see **Blake JB, ed**
**Wolf ES:** Tomorrow's self: Heinz Kohut's contribution to adolescent psychiatry. **Adolesc Psychiatry** 1980;8:41-50
**Wolf ES** see **Albin M**
**Wolf ES** see **Goldberg A, ed**
**Wolf F:** Universitätsprofessor Dr. Josef Hyrtl. **Osterr Gesch Kult** 1965;9(10):531-41
**Wolf JH** see **Habrich C**
**Wolf R:** Das Leben und Wirken von Carl Friedrich von Marcus (1802-1862). Diss. Würzburg, 1980. 141 p.
**Wolf S:** The psyche and the stomach. A historical vignette. **Gastroenterology** 1981 Mar;80(3):605-14
**Wolf SG:** Psychosocial and neural mechanisms in health and disease; historical perspectives. **J Okla State Med Assoc** 1982 Mar;75(3):53-61
**Wolf TH:** Florence Laura Goodenough. In: Notable American women. The modern period. Cambridge, Mass., Belknap-Harvard Univ. Press, 1980. 4:284-6.
**Wolfe C** see **Jenner CL, ed**
**Wolfe EL:** Calvin Ellis, the forgotten dean. **Harv Med Alumni Bull** 1982 Spring;56(2):27-31
**Wolfe EL** see **Benison S**
**Wolfe EL** see **Snape WJ**
**Wolfe MR:** Lucius Polk Brown and progressive food and drug control. Tennessee and New York City 1908-1920. Lawrence, Regents Press of Kansas, 1978. 194 p.
**Wolfe RJ:** Alaska's great sickness, 1900: an epidemic of measles and influenza in a virgin soil population. **Proc Am Philos Soc** 1982;126(1):91-121
**Wolfe RJ:** Jacob Bigelow's American medical botany 1817-1821. An examination of the origin, printing, binding and distribution of America's first color plate book. With special emphasis on the manner of making and printing its colored plates. North Hills, Pennsylvania, and Boston, Bird & Bull Press and Boston Medical Library, 1979. 121 p.
**Wölfel A:** Pflanzen in der Volksmedizin. Die volksmedizinischen Studien von Heinrich Marzell. Diss. Erlangen-Nürnberg, 1983. 117 p.
**Wolfensberger W:** Eulogy for a mentally retarded jester. **Ment Retard** 1982 Dec;20(6):269-70
**Wolfensberger W:** The extermination of handicapped people in World War II Germany. **Ment Retard** 1981 Feb;19(1):1-7
**Wolff E:** Le développement de la biologie du développement. **Bull Assoc Anat (Nancy)** 1980 Jun;64(185):135-42
**Wolff E:** The history and development of surgical tables for large animals. **VM SAC** 1981 Jul;76(7):1033-5
**Wolff H:** Billroth in Berlin. **Zentralbl Chir** 1982;107(20):1324-6
**Wolff HP** see **Wolff J**
**Wolff J, Wolff HP:** Die Förderung der Krankenpflege im vollentwickelten Kapitalismus durch Arzte an der Charité. Eine biographische Studies aus Anlass des 150 jährigen Bestehens der Ausbildung von Pflegekräften in Berlin. **Z Arztl Fortbild (Jena)** 1982 Sep 1;76(17):803-7
**Wolff J** see **Dupâquier J**
**Wolff JD:** Over chloroform-narcose en een Nederlandse pionier (S.N. Dentz Jr.). **Ned Tijdschr Geneeskd** 1981 Oct 17;125(42):1719-22
**Wolff M, Osborne JW, Hanson AL:** Mercury toxicity and dental amalgam. **Neurotoxicology (Park Forest Il)** 1983 Fall;4(3):201-4
**Wolff RG** see **Singer R**
**Wolfle D:** Science: a memoir of the 1960's and 1970's. **Science** 1980 Jul 4;209(4452):57-60
**Wolkinson BW, Barton D:** Arbitration and the rights of mentally handicapped workers. **Mon Labor Rev** 1980;103(4):41-7
**Wollman L:** Herbs and drugs. **J Am Soc Psychosom Dent Med** 1982;29(4):110
**Wollock JL** see **Carlson ET**
**Wolner E:** Die Chirurgie als Handwerk, Kunst und Wissenschaft. **Wien Klin Wochenschr** 1982 Mar 19;94(6):140-5
**Wolpoff MH, Russell MD:** Anterior dental cutting at Laetolil. **Am J Phys Anthropol** 1981 Jun;55(2):223-4
**Wolpoff MH** see **Thorne AG**
**Wolstenholme G:** Genetic engineering and public concern. **Clin Radiol** 1979 Nov;30(6):601-5
**Wolstenholme G** see **McCullough LB**
**Women in medicine: South Med J** 1981 Jun;74(6):775
**Women in psychiatry--a quiet revolution: Psychiatr News** 1980 Jul 18;15(14):7, 20-1
**Wondrák E:** Aerztliches und Arzttum im Werk von Ernst Weiss. In: Bilaterale Germanistenkommission CSSR-DDR. IV. Fachtagung ... 1977. Olomouc, Univerzita Palackého, 1979. pp. 142-54.
**Wondrák E:** Cesky anatom a patolog V. A. Bochdalek--100 let od smrti. **Cas Lek Cesk** 1983 Oct 28;122(43):1334-7
**Wondrák E:** Der Arzt und Dichter Laurentius Span (1530-1575). **Medizinhist J** 1983;18(3):238-49
**Wondrák E:** Die Anfänge der chirurgischen und geburtshilflichen Ausbildung in Mähren. In Ganzinger K, Skopec M, Wyklicky H, ed: Festschrift für Erna Lesky zum 70. Geburtstag. Wien, Brüder Hollinek, 1981. p. 185-92.
**Wondrák E:** Drei Bilder eines Arztes des 16. Jahrhunderts. **Medizinhist J** 1983;18(3):250-55
**Wondrák E:** Jaromír Mundy (1822-1894). Jeho podíl na vývoji záchranných služeb. **Cas Lek Cesk** 1982 Jan 29;121(4):116-9

**Wondrak E:** Johann Nepomuk Rust (1775–1840): der Lebensweg des Chirurgen und Förderers des jungen J.E. Purkyne. **Acta Univ Palacki Olomuc Fac Med** 1977;83:169–76
**Wondrák E:** Ke 100. výročí velkého výkonu v chirurgii žaludku. **Cas Lek Cesk** 1981 May 28;120(21):646–50
**Wondrák E:** Lékaři hanby. **Cas Lek Cesk** 1984 Aug 3;123(31):969–72
**Wondrák E:** Medicína na scestí. **Cas Lek Cesk** 1982 Jul;121(28):882–5
**Wondrák E:** Olomoucký Mistr Fridrich--zapomenutý lékař králuv a císařuv. **Cas Lek Cesk** 1984 May 4;123(18):551–2
**Wong A** see **Cimini TA**
**Wong EF:** Learned helplessness: the need for self-determination among the Chinese American elderly. **J Ethn Stud** 1980;8(2):45–62
**Wong HB:** Postgraduate medical education in Singapore. **Ann Acad Med Singapore** 1982 Jul;11(3):473–7
**Wong M:** Contribution à l'histoire des carences en Extrême-Orient: le béribéri. In: Congrès National des Sociétés Savantes, 93e, Tours, 1968. Comptes Rendus. Paris, 1971. Section des Sciences, Tome II. p. 9–15.
**Wong M:** Contributions récentes à l'histoire de la médecine chinoise. **Clio Med** 1981;15:260–2
**Wong M:** Die altchinesische Medizin. In Sournia JC, Martiny M, Poulet J, ed: Illustrierte Geschichte der Medizin. Salzburg, Andreas, 1980. Vol. 1. p. 49–89.
**Wong M:** Histoire du massage en Chine. In M. Wong: Les massages en médecine traditionnelle chinoise. Paris, Masson, 1984. p. 7–29.
**Wong M** see **Huard P**
**Wong PA:** Computed tomography in paleopathology: technique and case study. **Am J Phys Anthropol** 1981 May;55(1):101–10
**Wood BA, Abbott SA:** Analysis of the dental morphology of Plio-pleistocene hominids. I. Mandibular molars: crown area measurements and morphological traits. **J Anat** 1983 Jan;136 (Pt 1):197–219
**Wood BA, Abbott SA, Graham SH:** Analysis of the dental morphology of Plio-Pleistocene hominids. II. Mandibular molars--study of cusp areas, fissure pattern and cross sectional shape of the crown. **J Anat** 1983 Sep;137(Pt 2):287–314
**Wood BA:** Tooth size and shape and their relevance to studies of hominid evolution. **Philos Trans R Soc Lond [Biol]** 1981 May 8;292(1057):65–76
**Wood C:** Science and politics in the war on cattle diseases: the Kansas experience, 1900–1940. **Agric Hist** 1980;54(1):82–92
**Wood CH:** Infant mortality trends and capitalist development in Brazil: the case of Sao Paulo and Belo Horizonte. **Lat Am Perspect** 1977:4(4):56–65
**Wood CT:** The doctors' dilemma: sin, salvation, and the menstrual cycle in medieval thought. **Speculum** 1981;56(4):710–27
**Wood EH:** Four decades of physiology, musing, and what now. **Physiologist** 1982 Feb;25(1):19–32
**Wood G** see **Autian J**
**Wood M** see **Guha M**
**Wood MS** see **Shultz SM**
**Wood PB, Golinski JV:** Library and archive resources in the history of science and medicine at the University of Leeds. **Br J Hist Sci** 1981 Nov;14(3 no 48):263–81
**Wood RF:** Ophthalmology in colonial Queensland. **Aust J Ophthalmol** 1982 May;10(2):141–5
**Wood V:** Nursing education: the move from hospital schools of nursing--an historical perspective. **Int J Nurs Stud** 1984;21(3):183–92
**Woodall J:** The surgions mate. Facsimile of 1617 ed. Ed. J. Kirkup Bath, England, Kingsmead, 1978. xxxiv, 348 p.
**Woodall ME:** Ruolo e identita' dell'infermiere: riscoprire il pensiero di Florence Nightingale. **Prof Inferm** 1980 Oct-Dec;33(4):166–9
**Wooden AC:** Medical care in Islamic armies. In International Congress of the History of Medicine, 27th, Barcelona, 1980. Actas. Barcelona, Acadèmia de Ciències Mèdiques de Catalunya i Balears, 1981. p. 694–8.
**Wooden AC:** Medical services of the Roman army. In International Congress of the History of Medicine. 26th, Plovdiv, 1978. Actes du Congress. Sofia, 1981. Volume II. p. 211–3.
**Wooden WW:** Childhood and death: a reading of John Skelton's Phillip Sparrow. **J Psychohist** 1980 Spring;7(4):403–14
**Woodhall B:** Walter Dandy, M.D.: personal reminiscences. **Neurosurgery** 1979 Jan;4(1):3–6
**Woodham-Smith CB:** The great hunger, Ireland 1845-9. London, New England Library, 1979. 429 p.
**Woodhouse J:** Eugenics and the feeble-minded: the Parliamentary debates of 1912–14. **Hist Educ** 1982;11:127–37
**Woodhouse N** see **Wells C**
**Woodman RG:** Freud and Jung: the parting of the ways. **Queens Q** 1978;85(1):93–108
**Woodruff AW:** J M W Turner and some of his predecessors and successors, from the viewpoint of medical history. **J R Soc Med** 1980 May;73(5):381–92
**Woodruff HB:** A soil microbiologist's odyssey. **Annu Rev Microbiol** 1981;35:1–28
**Woodruff HB, Hernandez S, Stapley EO:** Evolution of an antibiotic screening programme. A tribute to Justo Martinez Mata. **Hindustan Antibiot Bull** 1979 Feb;21(3):71–84
**Woodruff HB** see **Helfand WH**
**Woodruff M:** The master surgeon. **J R Coll Surg Edinb** 1981 Sep;26(5):257–63
**Woodruff M** see **Nisbet NW**
**Woodruff NE:** The failure of relief during the Arkansas drought of 1930–1931. **Arkansas Hist Q** 1980;39(4):301–13
**Woods D:** Roche: blending independent and commercial research. **Can Med Assoc J** 1983 Oct 1;129(7):743–52
**Woods JO:** The history of medicine in Ireland. **Ulster Med J** 1982;51(1):35–45
**Woods R, Smith CW:** The decline of marital fertility in the late nineteenth century: the case of England and Wales. **Popul Stud** 1983 Jul;37(2):207–25
**Woodward AM:** The problematic science: psychology in nineteenth-century thought. New York, Praeger, 1982. xvii, 384 p.
**Woodward ER:** Dr. Dragstedt's first vagotomy. **World J Surg** 1983 Jul;7(4):554
**Woodward J:** The school medical officer 1880–1914. **Soc Soc Hist Med Bull (Lond)** 1980;27:30–1
**Woodward S** see **Kokaska CJ**
**Woodward TE:** The public's debt to military medicine. **Milit Med** 1981 Mar;146(3):168–73
**Woodward TE:** Yellow fever: from colonial Philadelphia and Baltimore to the mid-twentieth century. In Lilienfeld AM, ed: Times, places, and persons. Baltimore, London, Johns Hopkins Univ. Press, 1980. (Sigerist suppl. to the Bull Hist Med, n.s., no 4) p. 115–31.
**Woodward W** see **Brozek J**
**Woodward WR:** 'Visible colleges' and archives in Europe: first impressions. **J Hist Behav Sci** 1981;17:387–98
**Woodward WR:** William James's psychology of will: its revolutionary impact on American psychology. In J. Brozĕk, ed: Explorations in the history of psychology in the United States. Lewisburg, Bucknell University Press, 1984. p. 148–95.
**Woodward WR** see **High RP**
**Woodward KM, ed** see **Spicker SF**
**Wooley CF:** From irritable heart to mitral valve prolapse: the Osler connection. **Am J Cardiol** 1984 Mar 1;53(6):870–4
**Wooley CF:** From the 'irritable heart' of DaCosta to mitral valve prolapse: the development of medical thought about a constitutional, neuroendocrine cardiovascular process. **J Cardiogr** 1984 Oct;14 Suppl 5:9–10
**Wooley CF:** Jacob Mendez DaCosta: medical teacher, clinician, and clinical investigator. **Am J Cardiol** 1982 Nov;50(5):1145–8
**Woolfson RC:** Historical perspective on mental retardation. **Am J Ment Defic** 1984 Nov;89(3):231–5
**Woolrich J** see **Treviño-García Manzo N**
**Woolverton DK:** Taking stock: Med-Chi and its women members. **Md State Med J** 1983 Oct;32(10):787–91
**Woomert A** see **DeFriese GH**
**Woosley AI:** Fort Burgwin's hospital. **Palacio** 86(1):3–7, 36–9
**Wooten CW:** Unnoticed medical language in Demosthenes. **Hermes** 1979;107:157–60
**Wootton ID:** Earl Judson King. In Dictionary of national biography, 1961–1970. Suppl. 8, 1981. p. 612–3.
**Worboys M:** The development of the sanatorium treatment for consumption in Britain, 1880–1914. **Soc Soc Hist Med Bull (Lond)** 1984 Dec;35:41–3
**Work WP:** The American Board of Otolaryngology: 1950–1979. **Ann Otol Rhinol Laryngol [Suppl]** 1982 Mar-Apr;90:1–8
**Workman M:** Medical practice in Philadelphia at the time of the yellow fever epidemic, 1793. **Pa Folklife** 1978;27(4):33–9
**Works of the man:** extracts from research papers written or co-authored by Sir Gordon Arthur Ransome. **Ann Acad Med Singapore** 1979 Jan;8(1):13–26
**Worth D, Beck AM:** Multiple ownership of animals in New York City. **Trans Stud Coll Physicians Phila** 1981 Dec;5(3 no 4):280–300
**Worthington P** see **Moloney F**
**Wortis J:** How shock treatment came to America: what history teaches. **Biol Psychiatry** 1982 Nov;17(11):1203–5
**Wortis J:** Johannes Maargaard Nielsen, pioneer. **Biol Psychiatry** 1983 Feb;18(2):135–7
**Wortman R:** Power and responsibility in the upbringing of the nineteenth-century tsars. **Group Psychol Hist Newsl** 1976;4(4):18–27
**Woschick E:** Die kontrollierte Hypotension--Vergangenheit und Gegenwart. Eine Ubersicht. **Zentrabl Neurochir** 1984;45(1):1–10
**Wosh PJ:** Sound minds and unsound bodies: Massachusetts schools and mandatory physical training. **N Engl Q** 1982;55(1):39–60
**Wozniak KD:** Zur Bekämpfung der Geschlechtskrankheiten und der Berufsdermatosen in der DDR. **Wiss Z Martin Luther Univ (Math)** 1976;25(2):105–8
**Wren GR:** An historical view of health administration education. **Hosp Health Serv Adm** 1980 Summer;25(3):31–42
**Wren GR:** The first trained U. S. hospital administrator and his textbook. **Hosp Health Serv Adm** 1981 Winter;26(1):56–9
**Wren GR:** The history of osteopathic medicine in Georgia. Atlanta, Georgia State University, 1978. iii, 39 p. (Occasional publications of the Institute of Health Administration, Georgia State University, no. 18).
**Wright A:** An ethnography of the Navajo reproductive cycle. **Am Indian Q** 1982;6(1–2):52–70
**Wright A:** Scanning electron microscopy of the human organ of Corti. **J R Soc Med** 1983 Apr;76(4):269–78
**Wright A:** Some Yorkshire proprietaries. **Pharm Hist (London)** 1980 Dec;10(3):6–8
**Wright AJ** see **Aldrete JA**
**Wright D:** Moving the Wellcome Collection to the Science Museum. **Vet Hist** 1982 Summer;2(3):100–11
**Wright DJ:** John Hunter and venereal disease. **Ann R Coll Surg Engl** 1981 May;63(3):198–202
**Wright DJ** see **Mulhallen J**

Wright DS: Man-madè mineral fibres: a historical note. J Soc Occup Med 1980 Oct;30(4):138-40
Wright JC: Cancer chemotherapy: past, present, and future--Part I. J Natl Med Assoc 1984 Aug;76(8):773-84
Wright KW: From poorhouse to medical facility: genesis of Onondaga County Infirmary. NY State J Med 1979 Sep;79(10):1612-5
Wright MJ: History of academic psychology in Canada. Toronto, Hogrefe, 1982. x, 260 p.
Wright P, Treacher A, ed: The problem of medical knowledge. Examining the social construction of medicine. Edinburgh, Edinburgh University Press, 1982. 232 p.
Wright PW: A study in the legitimisation of knowledge: the 'success' of medicine and the 'failure' of astrology. Sociol Rev [Monogr] 1979;27:85-101
Wright PW: The radical sociology of medicine. Soc Stud Sci 1980;10(1):103-20
Wright RA see McDonald MO
Wright RC, Goldman L: Contact dermatitis: a historical perspective. Int J Dermatol 1979 Oct;18(8):665-8
Wright RJ see Graham FE
Wright RK, Tate LG: Forensic pathology. Last stronghold of the autopsy. Am J Forensic Med Pathol 1980 Mar;1(1):57-60
Wright RP: A Roman veterinary physician from the Thames Valley. Britannia 1977;8:279-82
Wright-St Clair RE: Early medical practitioners. NZ Med J 1980 Mar 12;91(655):190-1
Wright-St Clair RE: Influenza in New Zealand and the doctors who died from it. NZ Med J 1983 Oct 12;96(741):765-8
Wright-St Clair RE: Robert Hall Bakewell, letter writer. NZ Med J 1982 Nov 24;95(720):820-2
Wright-St Clair RE: The development of abdominal surgery in New Zealand. NZ Med J 1981 Apr;93(682):270-3
Wright-St Clair RE: The medical qualifications of Sir John Logan Campbell. NZ Med J 1983 Mar 23;96(728):212-3
Wrightson K see Laslett P
Wrigley EA: English mortality in the Industrial Revolution period. In Forbes EG, ed: Human implications of scientific advance. Edinburgh, Edinburgh University Press, 1978. p. 203-13.
Wrigley EA, Schofield RS: English population history from family reconsfitution: summary results 1600-1799. Popul Stud 1983 Jul;37(2):157-84
Wrigley EA: Marital fertility in seventeenth century Colyton. Econ Hist Rev 1978;31(3):429-36
Wrigley EA, Schofield RS: The population history of England, 1541-1871; a reconstruction. Cambridge, Mass., Harvard University Press, 1981. xv, 779 p.
Wrigley EA see Dupâquier J
Wrigley EA see Webster C, ed
Wrotnowska D: Jules Raulin, professeur au Lycée de Caen correspondance avec Pasteur. In: Congrès National des Sociétés Savantes, 105e, Caen, 1980. Comptes Rendus, Paris, 1980. Section des Sciences, Fasc. V. p. 109-120.
Wrotnowska D: La fièvre jaune. Séjour de Pasteur à Bordeaux, en septembre 1881. In: Congrès National des Sociétés Savantes, 104e, Bordeaux, 1979. Comptes Rendus. Paris, 1979. Section des Sciences, Fasc. IV. p. 109-20.
Wrotnowska D: Lettres de Le Dantec, disciple de Pasteur. In: Congrès National des Sociétés Savantes, 107e. Brest, 1982. Comptes Rendus, Paris, 1983. Section des Sciences, Fasc. IV. p. 253-64.
Wrotnowska D: Lettres inédites de Gilbert Déclat à Louis Pasteur. Hist Sci Med 1982;16(2):115-23
Wrotnowska D: Maladie des vers à soie: Pasteur s'intéresse à la race perpignanaise. In: Congrès National des Sociétés Savantes, 106e, Perpignan, 1981. Comptes Rendus. Paris, Bibliothèque Nationale, 1982. Fasc. IV. p. 197-208.
Wrotnowska D: Médecins polonais émigrés en Languedoc et dans les Pyrénées au XIXe siècle. In: Congrès National des Sociétés Savantes, 96e, Toulouse, 1971. Comptes Rendus. Paris, 1974. Histoires des Sciences, Tome 1. p. 175-92.
Wrotnowska D: Pasteur et Ferran y Clua, correspondance inédite. In International Congress of the History of Medicine, 27th, Barcelona, 1980. Actas. Barcelona, Académia de Ciències Mèdiques de Catalunya i Balears, 1981. p. 699-707.
Wrotnowska D: Pasteur et Victor Feltz de Nancy. Correspondance inédite. In: Congrès National des Sociétés Savantes, 103e, Nancy, 1978. Comptes Rendus. Paris, 1978. Section des Sciences, Fasc. V. p. 131-44.
Wrotnowska D: Pasteur, membre du Comice agricole de l'arrondissement de Lille. In: Congrès National des Sociétés Savantes, 101e, Lille, 1976. Comptes Rendus. Paris, 1976. Section des Sciences, Fasc. III. p. 133-44.
Wrotnowska D: Pasteur. Premières recherches sur les fermentations (1855-1857). Clio Med 1981 Apr;15(3-4):191-9
Wrotnowska D: Un ami de Pasteur: Charles Chappuis. In: Congrès National des Sociétés Savantes, 99e, Besançon, 1974. Comptes Rendus. Paris, 1976. Section des Sciences, Fasc. V. p. 171-84.
Wspomnienie o Profesorze Józefie Hellerze: Postepy Biochem 1982;28(4):387-90
Wu BM, Wang JH: Female cadaver in the Han Tomb No. 1. X-ray diffraction studies on two kinds of fibrous protein. Sci Sin 1980 Jul;23(7):915-22
Wu C see Brading DA
Wu K: [Ancient medical classic - the Papyrus Ebers] (Chi). Chung Hua I Shih Tsa Chih 1984;14(2):107-11
Wu M see Lo WH
Wu R: [Xue Shengbai's life and his scholarly method] (Chi). Chung Hua I Shih Tsa Chih 1984 Jan;14(1):7-9
Wu WQ: Neurosurgery in Tibet. Surg Neurol 1981 Jun;15(6):419-21
Wu Y: [An appraisal on Zhang Xichun's thought of amalgamating traditional Chinese medicine with western medicine] (Chi). Chung Hua I Shih Tsa Chih 1984 Jan;14(1):16-8
Wu YK: Reminiscence of personal association with American thoracic and cardiovascular surgery. Am J Surg 1980 Jun;139(6):765-70
Wu ZB see Yang WY
Wu Liangzuo: [On the medicine of the Tai Ping Heavenly Kingdom.] (Chi). Chin J Med Hist 1981;11:97-100
Wüger HJ: Die Darstellung des Schmerzes in der bildenden Kunst. Ther Umsch 1983 Aug;40(8):679-82
Wujastyk D: An alchemical ghost: the Rasaratnâkara by Nâgârjuna. Ambix 1984 Jul;31(2):70-83
Wujastyk D see Symons H
Wuketits FM: Das Kausalitätsproblem in der Evolutionslehre. Ein Beitrag zur Strukturgeschichte der Biologie. Medizinhist J 1980;15(4):392-402
Wuketits FM: Evolutionsmodelle in der Erklärung menschlicher Denkstrukturen im 19. Jahrhundert. Ber Wissenschaftsgesch 1983;6(1-4):115-22
Wuketits FM: Wissenschaftsgeschichte und gegenwärtige Theoriendiskussion in der Biologie. Nat Mus 1980;110:175-81
Wuketits FM, ed see Lorenz K, ed
Wülker G: Das grösste Volk der Erde: Bevölkerungsprobleme und Bevölkerungspolitik der Volksrepublik China. Eur Arch 1972;27(8):285-94
Wullstein HL: Das Schicksal unserer HNO-Zeitschrift bei der Neugründung nach dem Kriege. HNO 1980 Jan;28(1):33-4
Wunder JF see Breit DH
Wunderlich CA: Wien und Paris. Ein Beitrag zur Geschichte und Beurteilung der gegenwärtigen Heilkunde in Deutschland und Frankreich, 1841. Herausgegeben und eingeleitet von H. M. Koelbing. Bern, Huber, 1974. 159 p. (Hubers Klassiker der Medizin und der Naturwissenschaften, Bd. 13).
Wunderlich G: Die psychodynamische Theorie von Ideler (1835). Z Psychosom Med Psychoanal 1983;29(3):286-92
Wunderlich G: Kranheits- und Therapiekonzepte am Anfang der deutschen Psychiatrie (Haindorf, Heinroth, Ideler). Husum, Matthiesen, 1981. 132 p. (Abhandlungen zur Geschichte der Medizin und der Naturwissenschaften, 41).
Wunderlich P: Arthur Schlossmann (1867-1932) als Vorbild für unsere Zeit. Kinderarztl Prax 1982 Dec;50(12):589-95
Wunderlich P: Die Anfänge der Staatlichen Waisen-Fürsorge in Sachsen unter August dem Starken (Waldheim 1716). Kinderarztl Prax 1984 Nov;52(11):510-20
Wunderlich P: Ein Bericht aus dem Jahre 1838 über die Kliniken in Moskau und St. Petersburg. Z Gesamte Hyg 1980;26(5):381-2
Wunderlich P: Zur Geschichte der Universitäts-Kinderklinik in Breslau unter Adalbert Czerny (1863--1941) von 1894--1910. Arch Hist Med (Warsz) 1979;42(3):337-43
Wunderlich P: Zur Vorgeschichte und Geschichte der 'Kinderärztlichen Praxis' 4.: Weitere deutschsprachige Zeitschriften für Kinderheilkunde, die bis 1930 gegründet wurden. Kinderarztl Prax 1980 Jun;48(6):312-6
Wurbs W: Zur Klinik der Tuberkulose Erwachsener in der Gegenwart. Wiss Beitr Martin Luther Univ Halle Wittenberg 1983;5-R80:145-59
Wurgaft LD: Another look at Prospero and Caliban: magic and magical thinking in British India. Psychohist Rev 6(1):2-26, Summer 77
Wurmser L: Idealization and aggression in Beethoven's creativity. Am Imago 1979 Winter;36(4):328-44
Wussing H: 75 Jahre Karl-Sudhoff-Institut für Geschichte der Medizin und der Naturwissenschaften am Bereich Medizin der Karl-Marx-Universität. NTM 1981;18(1):2-3
Wuttke-Groneberg W: 'Parasitäre Glücksgefrässigkeit'. Irrationalismus in der Medizin. Bl Dtsch Int Polit 1980;25:572-83
Wyatt BW see Nadig P
Wyatt F: Erinnerungen vom ersten psychoanalytischen Kongress in Wiesbaden 1932. Psyche (Stuttg) 1984 Apr;38(4):360-7
Wyatt HV: Did thalidomide promote poliomyelitis following oral poliovirus vaccination in West Berlin in 1960? Perspect Biol Med 1983 Autumn;27(1):93-106
Wyatt HV: Provocation poliomyelitis: neglected clinical observations from 1914 to 1950. Bull Hist Med 1981 Winter;55(4):543-57
Wyczanski A: The social structure of nutrition: a case. Acta Pol Hist 1968;18:63-74
Wygant A: Shelley, Hawthorne, and Wells: images of medicine in early science fiction. Bookman 1981 Oct;8(8):3-8
Wygant LJ: Archives and manuscripts in the Moody Medical Library. Bookman 1983 Sep-Oct;10(5):3-8
Wygant LJ, ed: The Galveston smallpox quarantine camp in 1899. Bookman 1982;9(3):3-8
Wyk AJ: Medisyne uit Suid-Afrika vir die Keiser. Historia (S Afr) 1979;24(1):63-5
Wyklicky H: Arzt und Umwelt im 19. Jahrhundert. Prakt Arzt 1982 Feb;36:6-10
Wyklicky H: Economo als Psychiater. Osterr Arzteztg 1982;37(8):533
Wyklicky H: Förderer der Heilkunde. Medizin und Gesundheitswesen Josephs II. In: Was blieb von Joseph II.? Eine Dokumentation; Internationales Symposion Melk, 1980. [Vienna?], Edition Morgen, 1980.

p. 66–76.
**Wyklicky H:** Gedanken zur Geschichte der Allergie. In memoriam Clemens von Pirquet. **Wien Med Wochenschr** 1980 Feb 15;130(3):123–5
**Wyklicky H, Skopec M:** Ignaz Philipp Semmelweis, the prophet of bacteriology. **Infect Control** 1983 Sep–Oct;4(5):367–70
**Wyklicky H:** Maria Theresia und Joseph II. als Reformatoren des Gesundheitswesens in Oesterreich. **Wien Tierarztl Monatsschr** 1981;68(1):3–7
**Wyklicky H:** 'Prima inter pares' – Uber die Wiener interne Medizin am Beginn des 20. Jahrhunderts. **Wien Klin Wochenschr** 1983 Sep 16;95(17):601–6
**Wyklicky H:** The role of the Vienna Medical School in the investigation and treatment of infectious diseases. In [The Vienna Medical School]. Produced under a grant from the Squibb Institute for Medical Research, [1983]. p. 6–20.
**Wyklicky H:** Uber die Fürsorge Josephs II. für elternlose und kranke Kinder. **Padiatr Padol** 1982;17(2):437–40
**Wyklicky H:** Uber einige Aufgaben des medizinhistorischen Unterrichtes. **Wien Klin Wochenschr** 1981 Nov 13;93(21):660–5
**Wyklicky H:** Vor hundert Jahren. Billroths erste Pylorusresektion, seine diesbezüglichen Publikationen in der 'Wiener Medizinischen Wochenschrift' und ein Rückblick auf seine Zeit. **Wien Med Wochenschr** 1981 Jan 15;131(1):1–13
**Wyklicky H:** Warum sich ein Arzt mit Volkskunde beschäftigte. **Osterr Arzteztg** 1982 Jan 25;2
**Wyklicky H:** Zur Geschichte der Strahlentherapie in Oesterreich. **Wien Klin Wochenschr** 1980 Feb 29;92(5 Suppl 110):165–71
**Wyklicky H:** Zur hundertsten Wiederkehr der ersten Demonstration des Tuberkelbazillus durch Robert Koch (1843–1910). **Osterr Apoth Ztg** 1982 Apr 3;36(14):266–7
**Wyklicky H:** 100 Jahre Magenresektion. In H. Brunner, ed: Pathophysiologie und Pharmakotherapie des peptischen Geschwürs. München, Urban & Schwarzenberg, 1982. p. 123–32.
**Wyklicky H:** 175 Jahre Hygiene an Oesterreichs Universitäten. **Zentralbl Bakteriol [B]** 1981;172(6):441–53
**Wyklicky H** see **Skopec M**
**Wyklicky H** see **Zur Geschichte der Psychiatrie in Wien**
**Wyklicky H, ed** see **Ganzinger K**
**Wyler DJ:** Landmark perspective: The ascent and decline of chloroquine. **JAMA** 1984 May 11;251(18):2420–2
**Wylie EJ:** Vascular surgery—reflections of the past three decades. **Surgery** 1980 Dec;88(6):743–7
**Wylie HW:** Edvard Munch. **Am Imago** 1980 Winter;37(4):413–43
**Wylie JA, Linn IJ:** Observations upon the distribution and spread of the English sweating sickness (sudar anglicus) in Devon in 1551. **Devon Assoc Adv Sci** 1980;112:97–111
**Wylie JA, Collier LH:** The English sweating sickness (Sudor Anglicus): a reappraisal. **J Hist Med Allied Sci** 1981 Oct;36(4):425–45
**Wylie JA, Stubbs HW:** The plague of Athens, 430–428 B.C.: epidemic and epizoötic. **Classical Q** 1983;33:6–11
**Wylie MS:** Images of sickness and health in American medical thought: 1776–1800 and 1835–1865. Ph.D. Diss. American University. Washington, 1981. 541 p.
**Wyller I:** Et nytt år med 'gammel–nytt'? **Sykepleien** 1982 Jan 5;69(1):4–7
**Wyller I:** Sykepleiens historie og kvinnesynet. **Sykepleien** 1982 Nov 19;69(20):20–1
**Wyman AL:** John Nowell, an Elizabethan Fellow of the College of Physicians. **J R Coll Physicians Lond** 1984 Jul;18(3):166–9
**Wyman AL:** The surgeoness: the female practitioner of surgery 1400–1800. **Med Hist** 1984 Jan;28(1):22–41
**Wyman M:** Medicine and surgery in 1881. **N Engl J Med** 1981 Oct 29;305(18):1059–62
**Wymer JJ** see **Singer R**
**Wynder EL:** Some reflections on smoking and lung cancer. **J Thorac Cardiovasc Surg** 1984 Nov;88(5 Pt 2):854–7
**Wynes CE:** Dr. James Durham, mysterious eighteenth–century black physician: man or myth? **Pa Mag Hist Biogr** 1979;103(3):325–33
**Wyngaarden JB:** Nurturing the scientific enterprise. **J Med Educ** 1984 Mar;59(3):155–61
**Wynne–Edwards V** see **Dupâquier J**
**Wyrick R** see **Gutmann MR**
**Wyrost P:** A hundred years of Lvov Wrocxaw veterinary anatomy (1881–1981). **Folia Morphol (Warsz)** 1982;41(1):5–16
**Wyschogrod E:** Empathy and sympathy as tactile encounter. **J Med Philos** 1981 Feb;6(1):25–43
**Wysocka F, ed:** Głosy i teksty polskie w XV–wiecznym rekopisie lekarskim ze zbiorów Biblioteki Jagiellońskiej nr 132/60 akc. Komitet Jezykoznawstwa Pan. Wydawnictwa Zródłowe. Wrocław, Zakład Narodowy imienia Ossolińskich, 1971. 99 p.
**Wysokiński A:** Analiza rozwoju kadry lekarskiej w Europie w latach 1961–1975. **Wiad Lek** 1979 Nov 1;32(21):1573–7
**Wysoki'nski A, Strużak–Wysokińska M:** Ocena rozwoju stanu osobowego kadry farmaceutów w Europie w latach 1961–1975. **Wiad Lek** 1980 Mar 1;33(5):409–14
**Wysokiński A:** Rola Swiatowej Organizacji Zdrowia w życiu panstw i narodow. **Wiad Lek** 1979 Jul 15;32(14):1031–7
**Wyss D:** Die tiefenpsychologischen Schulen von den Anfängen bis zur Gegenwart. Entwicklung, Probleme, Krisen. Göttingen, Vandenhoeck & Ruprecht, 1977. xxxii, 562 p.
**Wyss D, Zacher A:** W. J. Revers' Bedeutung für die moderne Psychologie. Ein Uberblick. **Z Klin Psychol Psychother** 1983;31(2):137–48
**Wyss D** see **Tellenbach H, ed**
**Wyss E:** Erinnerungen an die Grippeepidemie im Aktivdienst 1918. **Berner Z Gesch Heimatkd** 1977;39:118–30
**Wyziembło M:** Losy polaków ... **Zesz Hist** 1974;(30):16–23

# X

**Xia ZY, Zhang MY:** History and present status of modern psychiatry in China. **Chin Med J [Engl]** 1981 May;94(5):277–82
**Xie Z:** [On the characteristics and contents of Dian Nan Ben Tsao: an extant work of materia medica featuring traditional medicine of both Chinese (Han) nationality and local minority nationalities] (Chi). **Chung Hua I Shih Tsa Chih** 1984 Jan;14(1):40–5
**Xie Zongwan:** [Present state and prospect of the study and systematization of works on Chinese materia medica written in past dynasties] (Chi). **J Tradit Chin Med** 1981;22(3):64–7
**Xiong T:** [Preliminary exploration on the materia medica from the localities inhabited by ancient China's minority nationalities] (Chi). **Chung Hua I Shih Tsa Chih** 1984;14(2):112–6
**Xirau R** see **Campillo–Sainz C**
**Xu X:** [An introduction to the pharmaceutical administration of ancient Chinese feudal dynasties] (Chi). **Chung Hua I Shih Tsa Chih** 1984;14(2):117–20
**Xue JN** see **Zheng GZ**
**XXXVI aniversario de la fundación del Instituto nacional de la nutrición Salvador Zubirán. Homenaje al Dr. Salvador Zubirán: Rev Invest Clin** 1983 Jan–Mar;35(1):85–103

# Y

**Yaffe G:** Wigan Dispensary. **Pharm Hist (London)** 1981;11(2):6
**Yagi K:** [Improvement of teaching/learning method of nursing history.] (Jpn). **Kango Tenbo** 1983 Nov;8(11):1041–50
**Yagisawa Y:** Early history of antibiotics in Japan. In J. Parascandola, ed: The history of antibiotics. Madison, American Institute of the History of Pharmacy, 1980. p. 69–90.
**Yakovlev PI** see **Livingston KE**
**Yaksh TL:** Obituary for Dr. Frederick W. L. Kerr. **Pain** 1984 Mar;18(3):217–20
**Yakushi Kenkyukai** see **Nagasaki–ken Yakuzaishikai**
**Yalow R:** Science and technology: problems and perceptions. In Cohen EP, ed: Medicine in transition. [Chicago], University of Illinois College of Medicine, 1981. p. 53–63.
**Yamada M, Horibe H, Fujimori K, et al:** Paleobiophysical studies on tooth tisues by microfluorometry and Raman–spectrometry. **Cell Mol Biol** 1979;25(3):167–72
**Yamada M** see **Fujimori K**
**Yamada S** see **Ono K**
**Yamagami K** see **Kato M**
**Yamagata S:** [Josen Morii and his medicine.] (Jpn). **Nihon I–Shigaku Zasshi** 1981;27(1):35–46
**Yamagata S:** [Studies of the pancreas –– historical survey]. (Jpn) **Nippon Rinsho** 1980;38(1):4–8
**Yamaguchi C:** [Betrachtungen über die frühesten physiologischen Arbeiten Hermann von Helmholtz, die zu seiner Entdeckung des Gesetzes von der Erhaltung der Energie führen] (Jpn). **Kagakushi Kenkyu** 1984;23(151):169–76
**Yamaguchi C, Yamanaka Y, Tateno Y:** Kakuigaku : kanri to hokisei. Institutional requirements and history of nuclear medicine. Tokyo, Jitsugyo Kohosha, Showa 53 nen. [1978]. 269 p.
**Yamaguchi Y:** [Life science. 5. Progress in medical research] (Jpn) **Kango Tenbo** 1980 Aug;5(8):722–9
**Yamakawa T:** Wonders in glycolipids––a historical view. **Adv Exp Med Biol** 1984;174:3–13
**Yamamoto R** see **Suzuki T**
**Yamamoto SI:** Cholera in Japan. In Ogawa T, ed: Public health. Tokyo, Saikon, 1981. p. 169–89.
**Yamamura K** see **Hanley SB**
**Yamanaka Y** see **Yamaguchi C**
**Yamashita S** see **Yamada M**
**Yamashita T** see **Yamada M**
**Yan YB, Chang NJ:** [Panel discussion: historical review of the nurses' status – educational perspective] (Kor). **Taehan Kanho** 1983 Sep 20;22(3):56–65
**Yanagisawa E** see **Pensak ML**
**Yanai Ishikai shi:** [Yanai, Japan], Yanai Ishikai, [1977]. 301 p.
**Yancey AG:** US postage stamp issued in honor of Charles R. Drew, MD, MDSc. **J Natl Med Assoc** 1982 Jun;74(6):561–5
**Yandle B:** A social regulation controversy: the cotton dust standard. **Soc Sci Q** 1982;63(1):58–69
**Yanes–Hoffman N:** Howard Rusk, MD: an equal chance. **JAMA** 1981 Oct 2;246(14):1503–5, 1509–10
**Yáñez A, Vargas M:** La tuberculosis en el mundo, historia antigua, problema actual. **Salud Publica Mex** 1982 May–Jun;24(3):261–7
**Yáñez Cortés RJ:** La intervención de conceptos psicoanalíticos en el pensamiento epistemológico de Gastón Bachelard. **Acta Psiquiatr Psicol Am Lat** 1979 Jun;25(2):135–41
**Yang D:** [10 kinds of symptom and sign of the pharynx and throat in ancient Chinese historical materials] (Chi). **Chung Hua I Shih Tsa Chih** 1984 Jan;14(1):4–6
**Yang KL, Qui BS, Zhang YE, et al:** Skin changes of 2,100 year old

Changsha female corpse. **Chin Med J [Engl]** 1982 Oct;95(10):765–76
**Yang WY, Wei DX, Song GF, et al:** Parasitologische Untersuchung einer alten Leiche aus der Chu–Dynastie der Streitenden Reiche aus dem Mazhuan–Grab Nr. 1, Kreis Jiangling, Provinz Hubei. **Acta Acad Med Wuhan** 1984;4(1):23–7
**Yang WY** see **Wei DX**
**Yankauer A:** Deregulation and the right to life. **Am J Public Health** 1981 Aug;71(8):797–8
**Yankauer A:** Refugees, immigrants, and the public health. **Am J Public Health** 1982 Jan;72(1):12–4
**Yaremovich AJ:** Collectivization through famine. **Ukr Q** 1978;34(4):349–62
**Yarington CT:** The evolution of reconstructive facial surgery. **Otolaryngol Clin North Am** 1983 May;16(2):305–8
**Yasuda T** see **Fukuyama K**
**Yasue M:** [On the ancient manuscript named 'A Togoku–ohayashi–ninjin'] (Jpn). **Yakushigaku Zasshi** 1983;18(2):87–94
**Yates D:** A fourteenth–century Latin poem on the art of the physician. **Bull Hist Med** 1980 Fall;54(3):447–50
**Yates F:** Sir Ronald Aylmer Fisher. In Dictionary of national biography, 1961–1970. Suppl. 8, 1981. p. 361–2.
**Yates FA:** The occult philosophy in the Elizabethan age. London, Boston, Routledge & Kegan Paul, 1979. x, 217 p.
**Yates W** see **Bleich JD**
**Yatsu M:** [Miscellaneous records of medico–dental and pharmacological history] (Jpn). **Shikai Tenbo** 1981;57(5):944–5 (continued regularly)
**Yatsu M:** [Miscellaneous records of medico–dental and pharmacological history (49). 'Jinrinkinmozui', a publication dated 1690 (3)] (Jpn). **Shikai Tenbo** 1984 Jan;63(1):194–5
**Yavenditti MJ:** The Hiroshima maidens and American benevolence in the 1950's. **Mid–Am** 1982;64(2):21–39
**Yazdany S, Soltani A:** The relationship between ancient Persia and Greece from medical point of view. In International Congress of the History of Medicine. 26th, Plovdiv, 1978. Actes du Congress. Sofia, 1981. Volume II. p. 114–5.
**Yazu M:** [Medico–dental and pharmacological history––miscellaneous records (1)] **Dent Outlook** 1980 Jan;(1):130–1 (contd. regularly)
**Yazu M:** [Teeth and toothache in the history of dentistry] (Jpn) **Dent Outlook** 1978;51(5):993–5
**Ybert G** see **Jolidon C**
**Yeazell RB, Maliszewski B, Constantikes A:** An exchange of letters between William and Alice James. **Psychohist Rev** 1979;8(1–2):53–9
**Yechezkel M, Deviri E, Levy MJ:** [Prosthetic heart valves––historical review] (Heb). **Harefuah** 1984 May 15;106(10):475–6
**Yellow fever studies. New York, Arno, 1977. Various paginations. Four reprinted articles by various authors, 1814–1915.:**
**Yellowlees WW:** Ill fares the land. **J R Coll Gen Pract** 1979 Jan;29(198):7–21
**Yépez Tamayo G:** Ensayo sobre la historia de las ciencias en Venezuela. **Bol Acad Nac Hist (Caracas)** 1975;58(231):573–95
**Yerkovic L** see **Edwards A**
**Yew E:** Medical inspection of immigrants at Ellis Island, 1891–1924. **Bull NY Acad Med** 1980 Jun;56(5):488–510
**Yim SY:** Famine relief statistics as a guide to the population of sixteenth century China: a case study of Honan Province. **Ch'ing–Shih Wen–t'i** 1978 Nov;3:1–30
**Ying YS** see **Zheng GZ**
**Yinyun Z:** Variability and evolutionary trends in tooth size of Gigantopithecus blacki. **Am J Phys Anthropol** 1982 Sep;59(1):21–32
**Yip KC:** Health and society in China: public health education for the community, 1912–1937. **Soc Sci Med** 1982;16(12):1197–205
**Yisai Y:** Abortion in Israel: social demand and political responses. **Policy Stud J** 1978;7(2):270–90
**Ylikahri R** see **Mäntylä I**
**Ylppö A:** Ensimmäinen Gunnar Soininen -luento. **Katilolehti** 1983 Mar;88(3):112–4
**Ylppö A:** Lapsen arvostuksesta vuosisatojen aikana. **Duodecim** 1981;97(6):300–5
**Yocum WS:** The cholesterol debates: some reminiscences on Dr. Irvine H. Page. **J Indiana State Med Assoc** 1980;73:567–8
**Yoder D** see **Hand WD, ed**
**Yoder D, ed:** Advertisements of urban healers. **Pa Folklife** 1978;27(3):44–8
**Yolton JW:** Perceptual cognition with Descartes. **Stud Cartesiana** 1981;2:63–83
**Yonace AH:** Morgagni's letters. **J R Soc Med** 1980 Feb;73(2):145–9
**Yonemoto S:** [Progress in life science and humanity––historical changes in the ideological background and the present status of life science] (Jpn). **Kango Gijutsu** 1981 Apr;27(6):739–44
**Yonkers AJ:** My specialty: otorhinolaryngology and maxillofacial surgery. **Nebr Med J** 1981 Jan;66(1):4–5
**York R:** The history of induction. **Midwife Health Visit Community Nurse** 1984 Apr;20(4):109–16
**Yorke C:** Anna Freud and the psychoanalytic study and treatment of adults. **Int J Psychoanal** 1983;64 (Pt 4):391–400
**Yorke C:** Anna Freud, CBE (1895–1982). **J Child Psychol Psychiatry** 1983 Jul;24(3):333–8
**Yoshida T:** [History of Dutch learning in Tokugawa Japan] (Jpn). **Kagakushi Kenkyu** 1984;23(150):73–80
**Yoshikawa R:** [Biography of Nightingale published in the early Meiji era – on 'Self–Help for Women'] (Jpn). **Sogo Kango** 1982;17(1):91–102
**Yoshpe RB** see **Ellencweig AY**
**Yosie T** see **Tarr JA**
**Yosie TF** see **Melosi MV, ed**
**You–chi T** see **Dodson G**
**Young CM:** Epidemics of infectious diseases in Australia prior to 1914. In Charbonneau H, Larose A, ed: The great mortalities: methodological studies of demographic crises in the past. Liège, Belgium, Ordina Editions, 1980. p. 207–27.
**Young DG** see **Christensen HA**
**Young DM:** Eugene H. Conner, M.D., KMA historian. **J Ky Med Assoc** 1982 Apr;80(4):224–6
**Young FG:** Alastair Campbell Frazer. In Dictionary of national biography, 1961–1970. Suppl. 8, 1981. p. 397–8.
**Young JH:** Adelle Davis. In: Notable American women. The modern period. Cambridge, Mass., Belknap–Harvard Univ. Press, 1980. 4:179–80.
**Young JH:** American health quackery: an historical view. **Ga J Sci** [1979?];38:33–40
**Young JH:** George Wilhelm Merck. In Dictionary of American Biography, Suppl. 6, 1956–1960. p. 447–8, 1980.
**Young JH:** Laetrile in historical perspective. **Conn Med** 1979 Aug;43(8):497–500
**Young JH:** Laetrile in historical perspective. In Markle GE, Petersen JC, ed: Politics, science and cancer: the laetrile phenomenon. Boulder, CO. Westview Press, for American Association for the Advancement of Science, Washington, D. C., 1980. p. 11–60.
**Young JH, Stitt RS:** Nutrition quackery. Upholding the right to criticize. **Food Technol** 1981 Dec;:42–7
**Young JH:** Nutritional eccentricities. In Neuberger A, Jukes TH, ed: Human nutrition: current issues and controversies. Lancaster, England, MTP Press, 1982. p. 217–32.
**Young JH:** Nutritional quackery. **Assoc Food Drug Off Q Bull** 1983 Jan;47:3–11
**Young JH:** Public policy and drug innovation. **Pharm Hist** 1982;24(1):3–31
**Young JH:** Self–dosage medicine in America, 1906 and 1981. **South Atl Q** 1981 Autumn;80(4):379–90
**Young JH:** The early years of federal food and drug control. Madison, Wis., 1982. 60 p. (Publication/American Institute of the History of Pharmacy. new series, no. 7)
**Young JH:** 'The foolmaster who fooled them'. **Yale J Biol Med** 1980 Nov–Dec;53(6):555–66
**Young JH:** The long struggle for the 1906 law. **FDA Consum** 1981 Jun;15(5):12–7
**Young JH:** The regulation of health quackery. **Pharm Hist** 1984;26(1):3–12
**Young JH:** 'This greasy counterfeit': butter versus oleomargarine in the United States Congress, 1886 (the Fielding H. Garrison Lecture). **Bull Hist Med** 1979 Fall;53(3):392–414
**Young JH:** Three southern food and drug cases. **J South Hist** 1983:49(1):3–36
**Young JH** see **Jenner CL, ed**
**Young LE** see **Napodano RJ**
**Young MJ** see **Maulitz RC**
**Young R** see **Williams D**
**Young RC Jr, Rachal RE, Cowan CL Jr:** Sarcoidosis––the beginning: historical highlights of personalities and their accomplishments during the early years. **J Natl Med Assoc** 1984 Sep;76(9):887–96
**Young TK:** Indian health services in Canada: a sociohistorical perspective. **Soc Sci Med** 1984;18(3):257–64
**Youtie LC:** A medical text (P. Corn. Inv. 47). **Z Papyrologie Epigraphik** 1978;29:279–86
**Youtie LC:** [Eye–salves.] **Bull Am Soc Papyrologists** 1979;16:149–51
**Youtie LC:** Two Michigan medical papyri [1. P. Mich. Inv. 1455; 2. P. Mich. Inv. 488 = P. Coll. Youtie II 87]. **Z Papyrologie Epigraphik** 1977;27:140–46
**Yoxen EJ:** Constructing genetic diseases. In P. Wright, A. Treacher, ed: The problem of medical knowledge. Examining the social construction of medicine. Edinburgh, Edinburgh University Press, 1982. p. 144–61.
**Yoxen EJ:** Scepticism about the centrality of technology transfer in the Rockefeller Foundation programme in molecular biology. **Soc Stud Sci** 1984 May;14(2):248–52
**Yturriaga Barberán JA de:** La Comunidad Económica Europea y la protección del medio acuático contra la contaminación. **Rev Inst Eur** 1976;3(3):691–99
**Yu RJ** see **Van Scott EJ**
**Yu S:** [Talks on the historical materials of medicine in Fujian Province] (Chi). **Chung Hua I Shih Tsa Chih** 1984;14(2):75–7
**Yu–chuan S:** Perspectives in neurosurgery: neurosurgery in the People's Republic of China. **Neurosurgery** 1981 Apr;8(4):497–500
**Yü Ming:** Barefoot doctors in mainland China: a unique medical corps. **Issues Stud** 1978;14(2):53–64
**Yuan Tien H:** Induced fertility transition: impact of population planning and socio–economic change in the People's Republic of China. **Popul Stud** 1984 Nov;38(3):385–400
**Yue J:** [Ancient Sino–Iraian medical exchanges as seen in Tanksuq–nameh] (Chi). **Chung Hua I Shih Tsa Chih** 1984 Jan;14(1):28–34
**Yumai M:** [Growing pain – a personal history (9)] (Jpn). **Sogo Kango** 1980;15(1):74–81
**Yumaki M, Kodama K:** [Changes in nursing during the 30 years after the war] (Jpn). **Kango** 1981 Jan;33(1):114–21 (continued periodically)
**Yumaki M, Kodama K, Usui H:** [Discussion: at the conclusion of 'Growing Pain'] (Jpn) **Sogo Kango** 1980;15(3):90–109
**Yumaki M:** [Nightingale's concept of God] (Jpn). **Sogo Kango** 1982;16(4):23–8
**Yumaki M, Kodama K:** [Transition in nursing in the 30 years since the end of World War II] (Jpn) **Kango** 1980 Nov;32(11):98–106

**Yumaki M:** [50 years of the studies on Florence Nightingale] (Jpn). **Sogo Kango** 1980;15(4):7-11

**Yusuf F, Rockett I:** Immigrant family patterns and differentials in Australia, 1971-76. **Popul Stud** 1981;35(3):413-24

# Z

**Zaar EI** see **Lozina-Lozinsky LK**

**Zabalogoitia GB:** Perspectives in international neurosurgery: neurosurgery in Spain. **Neurosurgery** 1984 Jan;14(1):111-2

**Zabarskas J:** Psychometric intelligence pattern of the native-born children of Lithuanian immigrants. **Lituanus** 1980;26(1):39-54

**Zabłotniak R:** Polacy studiujący medycynę i farmację w Kownie (1940 1944). **Przegl Lek** 1980;37(1):101-4

**Zablotniak R:** Polscy studenci medycyny i farmcji w uniwersytetach bejruckich (1941-1945). **Przegl Lek** 1981;38(1):124-5

**Zabłotniak R:** Polskie Towarzystwo Pomocy Ofiarom Wojny w Rosji (1914-1919). **Arch Hist Med (Warsz)** 1981;44(3/4):345-54

**Zabłotniak R:** Towarzystwo opieki nad nerwowo i umysłowo chorymi żydami w Warszawie (1906-1939). **Biul Zydowskiego Inst Hist Pol** 1981;1:37-44

**Zabludovskiĭ PE:** Istoriia meditsiny. Moskva, Meditsnina, 1981. 350 p.

**Zabludovskiĭ PE:** Izistorii professional'noĭ patologii i gigieny truda. **Gig Tr Prof Zabol** 1983 Dec;(12):40-2

**Zabludovskiĭ PE:** K 200-letiiu knigi 'Nastavlenie narodu v rassuzhdenii ego zdorov'ia'. **Feldsher Akush** 1982;47(4):52-3

**Zabludovskiĭ PE:** N. I. Pirogov i meditsinskiĭ trud zhenshchin. **Feldsher Akush** 1981;46(11):53-4

**Zabludovskiĭ PE:** Trudy nauchnykh uchrezhdeniĭ Ukrainskoĭ SSR k Pirogovskoĭ godovshchine. **Vrach Delo** 1983 Feb;(2):121-2

**Zabudlá K** see **Kokavec M**

**Zachariae H:** Changes in disease pattern in a skin clinic 1947 to 1977. **Acta Derm Venereol [Suppl] (Stockh)** 1979;59(85):199-205

**Zacharias KL:** The construction of a primate order: taxonomy and comparative anatomy in establishing the human place in nature, 1735-1916. Ph.D. diss. The Johns Hopkins University. Baltimore, 1980. 464 leaves.

**Zacher A:** Anthropologische Medizin im Wandel. Von Viktor von Weizsäcker zu Dieter Wyss. **Nervenarzt** 1983 Nov;54(11):598-603

**Zacher A** see **Wyss D**

**Zacher J** see **Romm S**

**Zacher JB** see **Romm S, ed**

**Zachert U, Zeidler U, ed:** Herzog August Bibliothek Wolfenbüttel. Verzeichnis medizinischer und naturwissenschaftlicher Drucke, 1472-1830. Band 1-4, Alphabetischer Index. Millwood, New York, Kraus International, 1982. 1857 p.

**Zachmann M** see **Landolt AM**

**Zack M** see **Caldwell GG**

**Zadecki J:** O Kępińskiego 'Schizofrenii'. **Przegl Lek** 1983;40(12):873-6

**Zadina R:** Casopis lékařu českých před sto lety. **Cas Lek Cesk** 1980 Jan 5;119(1):32

**Zadina R:** Casopis lékařučeských před sto lety. **Cas Lek Cesk** 1984 Jan 6;123(1):32

**Zadina R:** První sjezd českých lékařu a přírodozpytcu v Praze roku 1880. **Cas Lek Cesk** 1980 Jan 11;119(2):64

**Zadneprovski IA, Podol'ski AG:** Borisz Cezarevics Urlanisz (1906-1981). **Demografia** 1981;24(4):553-5

**Zadorozhnyĭ AA, Saks FF, Dolgikh VP, et al:** Erast Gavrilovich Salishchev (k 130-letiiu so dnia rozhdeniia). **Vestn Khir** 1982 Jul;129(7):140-3

**Zadorozhnyĭ AG** see **Serkov FN**

**Zafiropoulos M** see **Pinell P**

**Zagarra MJ:** Ludwig van Beethoven: hipótesis sobre su sordera. **CERON** 1979 Dec;4(3):7-9

**Zagórski W** see **Szafrański P**

**Zagrebin AM:** Kafedre anatomii cheloveka Izhevskogo meditsinskogo instituta 50 let. **Arkh Anat Gistol Embriol** 1984 Apr;86(4):91-5

**Zahlhaas G:** Die Fresken des römischen Thermengebäudes von Schwangau. **Antike Welt** 1978;9(4):13-23

**Zahn FW** see **Hahnloser P**

**Zahn WM:** Erik H. Erikson. In J. Rattner, ed: Wandlungen der Psychoanalyse. Wien, Europaverlag, 1980. p. 187-210.

**Zahradnický J:** 100 let od objevu puvodce tuberkulózy Robertem Kochem. **Cesk Epidemiol Mikrobiol Imunol** 1983 Jan;32(1):4-7

**Zaĭchenko LA** see **Klishov AA**

**Zaĭchik ASh:** Teoreticheskoe i prakticheskoe znachenie ucheniia o tsitotoksinakh. **Patol Fiziol Eksp Ter** 1981 Mar-Apr;(2):46-55

**Zaĭko NN:** A. A. Bogomolets kak pedagog. **Patol Fiziol Eksp Ter** 1981 Mar-Apr;(2):9-16

**Zaiko NN:** A. A. Bogomolets, zhizn i deiatel nost. K 100-letiiu so dnia rozhdeniia. **Fiziol Zh** 1981 May-Jun;27(3):291-301

**Zainaldin JS, Tyor PL:** Asylum and society: an approach to institutional change. **J Soc Hist** 1979;13(1):23-48

**Zainie CM** see **Saidi MH**

**Zajusz K, Ornowski J:** Rudolf Virchow a problemy niepodległościowe i społeczne narodu polskiego. **Arch Hist Med (Warsz)** 1979;42(3):285-9

**Zajusz K:** Z dziejów spółek Brackich. **Arch Hist Med (Warsz)** 1979;42(1):33-43

**Zakharov BI, Zakharov NP:** Priznaki ankiloziruiushchego spondiloartrita na iskopaemykh kostiakh liudeĭ, zhivshikh na territorii Sibiri. **Ortop Travmatol Protez** 1980 Apr;(4):46-7

**Zakharov BI, Zakharova NP, Beliaskiĭ EA:** Proiavleniia mielomnoĭ bolezni v kostiakh drevnikh liudeĭ. **Vopr Onkol** 1983;29(2):86-8

**Zakharov FG, Medik VA:** Razvitie zdravookhraneniia v Novgorodskoĭ gubernii v 1864-1917 gg. **Sov Zdravookhr** 1982;(7):59-61

**Zakharov FG, Medik VA, Bazylev AE:** Stanovlenie zdravookhraneniia Novgorodskoĭ gubernii (1917-1927). **Sov Zdravookhr** 1983;(1):68-71

**Zakharov FG, Medik VA, Bazylev AE:** Zdravookhranenie Novgorodskoĭ oblasti v poslevoennyĭ period. **Sov Zdravookhr** 1983;(4):53-5

**Zakharov NP** see **Zakharov BI**

**Zakharova LV:** Osobennosti klinicheskogo techeniia briushnogo tifa za 20 let (1959-1978). **Klin Med (Mosk)** 1981;59(7):98-103

**Zakharova NP** see **Zakharov BI**

**Zákonyi F:** Dr. Huray István, Balatonfüred föorvosa. **Orv Hetil** 1983 Sep 4;124(36):2192-4

**Zakusov VV:** Farmakologiia v Akademii meditsinskikh nauk SSSR. **Farmakol Toksikol** 1984 Jan-Feb;47(1):5-13

**Zalai K:** A gyógyszerészi szemlélet és gondolkodás változása századunkban Magyarországon. **Acta Pharm Hung** 1983 Jul;53(4):145-9

**Zalai K:** A gyógyszerügyi szervezéstudomány, a társadalmogyógyszerészet hazai és külföldi fejlödése. **Acta Pharm Hung** 1984 Jan;54(1):1-14

**Zalai K:** A Magyar Gyógyszerészeti Társaság ötven éve (1924-1974). Budapest, Magyar Gyógyszerészeti Társaság, 1974. 75 p.

**Zalai K:** Die Entwicklungsperioden der wissenschaftlichen Pharmazie in Ungarn. In Hein WH, ed: Pharmaziehistorischer Kongress, Budapest, 1981. Stuttgart, Wissenschaftliche Verlagsgesellschaft, 1983. p. 17-22.

**Zalai K:** Die Geschichte des Universitätsunterrichts der Pharmaziegeschichte in Ungarn. In: Vorträge des Internationalen Pharmaziehistorischen Kongresses Innsbruck 1977. Stuttgart, Wissenschaftliche Verlagsgesellschaft, 1979. p. 197-202.

**Zalai K:** Medizin-pharmazeutische Erwähnungen in einem ungarischen Codex des XII. Jahrhunderts. **Acta Pharm Hung** 1980 Mar;50(2):87-95

**Zalai K:** 'Systema Artis Pharmaceuticae'. La première dissertation à la Faculté Hongroise de médecine, présentée par Maritius Fabi. **Beitr Gesch Pharm** 1983;31(20):25-7

**Zalai K:** Vinum Tokajense passum. In Hickel E, Schröder G, ed: Neue Beiträge zur Arzneimittelgeschichte. Festschrift für Wolfgang Schneider zum 70. Geburtstag. Stuttgart, Wissenschaftliche Verlagsgesellschaft, 1982. p. 41-6.

**Zalai K** see **Bano-Fleischmann M**

**Zalai K** see **Fleishmann-Bánó M**

**Zalesova ZG:** The history of the establishment of the genetic role of DNA. **Istor Biol Issled** 1983;9:66-84

**Zallár A:** Huszonöt éve hunyt el jáki Gyula professzor. **Orv Hetil** 1983 Sep 18;124(38):2321-2

**Zambito RF:** A history of hospital dental practice. Part I and II. **New Dent** 1979 Oct-Nov;10(2-3):31-3, 35-8

**Zambon JV:** Brugmans, voorloper van Semmelweis. **Ned Tijdschr Geneeskd** 1983 Jun 11;127(24):1060-4

**Zambrano L, Jorge H:** Fecundidad y escolaridad en la ciudad de Mexico. **Demogr Econ** 1979;13(4):405-48

**Zanca A, Tagliavini R:** Iconografia dermatologica e venereologica: ieri e oggi. **Acta Med Hist Patav** 1980-81;27:81-97

**Zanca A:** Il Mal Francese. **Kos** 1984 Feb;1(1):77-92

**Zanca A, Zanca A:** Istituti Ospedalieri di Mantova, Mantova, Italy. **Int J Dermatol** 1980 Jan-Feb;19(1):55-8

**Zanca A** see **Zanca A**

**Zander E:** Was hat Schultz-Hencke uns heute noch zu sagen? **Z Psychosom Med Psychoanal** 1982;28(2):231-8

**Zander W:** Grusswort zum 25 jährigen Jubiläum der Zeitschrift für Psychosomatische Medizin und Psychoanalyse. **Z Psychosom Med Psychoanal** 1979 Oct-Dec;25(4):301-2

**Zaner RM** see **Spicker SF, ed**

**Zani A:** Le origini storiche dell'elettroencefalografia. **Stor Crit Psicol** 1981;2(1):119-84

**Zanjani SS:** George Springmeyer and the quarantine rebellion of 1902: student revolt reaches the University of Nevada. **Nev Hist Soc Q** 1980;23(4):283-9

**Zanobio B:** Contributi di Scuola Pavese allo sviluppo della chirurgia plastica. **Minerva Chir** 1983 Mar 31;38(6):297-302

**Zanobio B:** Je le pansai, Dieu le guérit. Gli aforismi di chirurgia militare di Louis Appia (1818-1898) sulla cura delle ferite d'armi da fuoco. **G Accad Med Torino** 1980;143(Spec No):7-95

**Zanobio B:** Le osservazioni clinico-anatomiche di Luigi Porta (1800-1875) sulle 'cotilitidi'. **Rend Ist Lomb Accad Sci Lett B** 1978;112:82-98

**Zapaśnik-Kobierska MH:** Działalność naukowo-dydaktyczna i społeczna zespołu klinik Państwowego Szpitala Klinicznego Nr 3. **Pediatr Pol** 1984 Sep;59(9):705-12

**Zapfe H:** Ein Schädel von Mesopithecus mit Biss-Spuren. **Folia Primatol (Basel)** 1981;35(4):248-58

**Zaprianov N, Nikolov I:** The share of the foreign 'Red Cross' societies in rendering help to the victims of the earthquake in Bulgaria, in the year of 1928. In International Congress of the History of Medicine. 26th, Plovdiv, 1978. Actes du Congress. Sofia, 1981. Volume II. p. 214.

**Zaprianov NI, Kazandzhiev NK:** D-r Stoian Chomakov. Sofiia, Meditsina i fizkultura, 1979.

**Zapryanov N:** Centennial anniversary of the Plovdiv State Hospital. **Folia Med (Plovdiv)** 1980;22(1):37-9

**Zaragoza JR:** Die Medizin in Mesopotamien. In Sournia JC, Martiny M, Poulet J, ed: Illustrierte Geschichte der Medizin. Salzburg, Andreas, 1980. Vol. 1. p. 91-107.

**Zaremba J** see **Mazurczak T**

**Zaretsky E:** A note on Marxism and psychoanalysis. **Marx Perspect**

**Zhurnalu 'Grudnaia khirurgiia' 20 let.: Grudn Khir** 1980 Jan–Feb;(1):5–6

**Zhurnalu 'Patologicheskaia fiziologiia i éksperimental'naia terapiia' 25 let: Patol Fiziol Eksp Ter** 1982 Jul–Aug;(4):3–10

**Zhurnalu 'Uspekhi sovremennoĭ biologii'--50 let:**

**Zhurnalu 40 let: Sov Zdravookhr** 1982;(6):3–7

**Ziedses des Plantes BG** see **Falke TH**

**Ziegelmayer G** see **Gürtler LG**

**Zieger W:** Zur 100. Wiederkehr des Geburtstages von Generaloberstabsveterinär Professor Dr. Curt Schulze. **DTW** 1981 Nov 5;88(11):449–52

**Ziegler CR:** The image of the physically handicapped in children's literature. New York, Arno, 1980. 156 p. (Also Ed. D. Diss. Philadelphia, Temple University, 1971).

**Zieliński K:** Ezras A. Asratyan. **Acta Neurobiol Exp (Warsz)** 1981;41(6):521–42

**Zieliński K:** Sixty years of the Nencki Institute of Experimental Biology. **Rev Pol Acad Sci (Warsz)** 1978;23(4):47–74

**Zieliński K** see **Brennan JF**

**Ziem G:** Medical education since Flexner. **Health PAC Bull** 1977;(76):8–14, 23

**Ziembicki W:** Zakład historii Medycyny we Lwowie. Kronika lat 1942–1944. **Arch Hist Med (Warsz)** 1981;44(2):189–215

**Ziemer PL, Kathren RL, ed:** Health physics: a backward glance. New York, Pergamon Press, 1980. 237 p.

**Zigiotti GL, Messerotti GF, Cavaliere F:** La chirurgia della palatoschisi dalle origini ai giorni nostri. **Minerva Med** 1983 Jan 14;74(1–2):59–68

**Zigmond D:** A psychosomatic approach. **Practitioner** 1982 Apr;226(1366):699, 701–2, 704 passim

**Zikakis JP:** Agricultural and food chemistry: accomplishments and perspectives. **J Agric Food Chem** 1983 Jul–Aug;31(4):672–5

**Zikeev PD:** Aleksandr Fleming (k 100–letiiu so dnia rozhdeniia). **Klin Med (Mosk)** 1983 Feb;61(2):110–2

**Zikeev PD:** Chrezvychaĭnyĭ kholernyĭ s'ezd Obshchestva russkikh vracheĭ v pamiat' N. I. Pirogova. **Sov Zdravookhr** 1981;(11):56–9

**Zil'berberg LB** see **Voĭtenko MF**

**Ziller R:** Zur Geschichte des künstlichen Gelenkersatzes. **Beitr Orthop Traumatol** 1984 Oct;31(10):526–32

**Zimbalist SE:** Historic themes and landmarks in social welfare research. New York, Harper & Row, 1977. xii, 432 p. (Harper Series in Social Work).

**Zimkin NV:** 60 let kafedre fiziologii Leningradskogo instituta fizicheskoĭ kul'tury imeni P. F. Lesgafta. **Fiziol Zh SSSR** 1979 Dec;65(12):1854–6

**Zimmerli W** see **Albrecht von Haller, 1708–1777**

**Zimmerman AN, Hülsmann WC:** The calcium paradox: historical remarks. **Eur Heart J** 1983 Dec;4 Suppl H:3–4

**Zimmerman BH** see **Zimmerman MR**

**Zimmerman BK:** An overview of regulatory responsibilities. **Basic Life Sci** 1982;21:439–60

**Zimmerman J:** Transcendent psychology: Erik H. Erikson, Erich Fromm, Karen Horney, Abraham H. Maslow, and Harry Stack Sullivan and the quest for a healthy humanity. Ph.D. Diss., Northwestern University. Evanston, 1982. vi, 498 p.

**Zimmerman L** see **Gregg JB**

**Zimmerman LJ, Gregg JB, Gregg PS:** Para–mortem osteopathology in the Crow Creek masacre victims. **SD J Med** 1981 Feb;34(2):7–12

**Zimmerman LJ** see **Gregg JB**

**Zimmerman MR:** Aleutian and Alaskan mummies. In A. Cockburn, E. Cockburn, ed: Mummies, disease, and ancient cultures. Cambridge, Cambridge University Press, 1980. p. 118–34.

**Zimmerman MR:** Annotated bibilography of paleopathology: 1970–1979. Part IV, T–Z and Index. **Trans Stud Coll Physicians Phila** 1980 Dec;5(2 no 4):289–314

**Zimmerman MR:** Annotated bibliography of paleopathology: 1970–1979. Part I, A–C. **Trans Stud Coll Physicians Phila** 1980 Mar;5(2 no 1):41–66

**Zimmerman MR:** Annotated bibliography of paleopathology: 1970–1979. Part II, D–J. **Trans Stud Coll Physicians Phila** 1980 Jun;5(2 no 2):112–43

**Zimmerman MR:** Annotated bibliography of paleopathology: 1970–1979; Part III, K–S. **Trans Stud Coll Physicians Phila** 1980 Sep;5(2 no 3):187–222

**Zimmerman MR:** Enterobiasis in precolumbian America. **Paleopathol Newsl** 1983 Jun;42:8

**Zimmerman MR:** The mummies of the tomb of Nebwenenef: paleopathology and archaeology. **J Am Res Cent Egypt** 1977;14:33–6

**Zimmerman MR:** The paleopathology of the human remains from Nebwenenef's tomb. Part II: The histologic findings. **Paleopathol Newsl** 1983 Jun;42:6–7

**Zimmerman MR, Zimmerman BH:** The paleopathology of the human remains from Nebwenenef's tomb--the 1979 season. **Paleopathol Newsl** 1980 Sep;(31):15–16

**Zimmerman MR** see **Millet NB**

**Zimmerman MR** see **Trinkaus E**

**Zimmerman MR** see **Walker A**

**Zimmerman M, et al:** Annotated bibliography [of Paleopathology]. **Paleopathol Newsl** 1980 Sep;(31):17–20. Continued regularly

**Zimmerman MR, et al:** The paleopathology of an Aleutian mummy. **Arch Pathol Lab Med** 1981 Dec;105(12):638–41

**Zimmermann A:** Pharmazeutisches aus dem Nachlassinventar des Octavianus Secundus Fugger (1549–1600). **Beitr Gesch Pharm** 1981;31(12):89–91

**Zimmermann F:** Les aspects médicaux du Yavanajataka (traité sankrit d'astrologie). **Sudhoffs Arch** 1981;65(3):299–305

**Zimmermann G, Liljeblad S, Frank A, et al:** The Indians have many terms for it: stuttering among the Bannock–Shoshoni. **J Speech Hear Res** 1983 Jun;26(2):315–8

**Zimmermann K** see **Zimmermann R**

**Zimmermann M:** Electrical stimulation of the human brain. **Hum Neurobiol** 1982;1(4):227–9

**Zimmermann MR:** A possible histiocytoma in an Egyptian mummy. **Arch Dermatol** 1981 Jun;117(6):364–5

**Zimmermann R, Zimmermann K:** Antike Tätowierungen aus heutiger Sicht. **Hautarzt** 1981 Jun;32(6):324–30

**Zimmermann RE:** The structure of mythos: on the cultural stability of alchemy. **Ambix** 1984 Nov;31(3):125–37

**Zimmermann V:** Der Rosmarin als Heilpflanze und Wunderdroge; ein Beitrag zu den mittelalterlichen Drogenmonographien. **Sudhoffs Arch** 1980;64(4):351–70

**Zimmermann V:** Ein besonderer Eid für die jüdischen Arzte und Wundärzte in Preussen. Ein Beitrag zur Geschichte der jüdischen Arzte in Deutschland. **Medizinhist J** 1982;17(1/2):78–88

**Zimolo A:** Kongelacije s naročitim osvrtom na preventivne mjere. **Lijec Vjesn** 1979 Nov;101(11):710–3

**Zimolo A:** Rad i značenje prvog kongresa liječnika Narodnooslobodilačke Fronte Hrvatske 24–27. 2. 1944. **Lijec Vjesn** 1979 Nov;101(11):674–8

**Zinevich VP:** Razvitie ideĭ A. N. Filatova po probleme parenteral'nogo pitaniia v khirurgii. **Vestn Khir** 1982 Oct;129(10):16–20

**Zingg W:** Historical use of hypothermia for cancer. **Can J Surg** 1983 Mar;26(2):97–8

**Zinnaka Y** see **Takeda Y**

**Zinner ID, Sherman H:** An analysis of the development of complete denture impression techniques. **J Prosthet Dent** 1981 Sep;46(3):242–9

**Zinsstag:** Memories of what mother told about her cousin Carl Gustav Jung. **J Am Soc Psychosom Dent Med** 1980;27(2):42–6

**Zipursky A:** The rise and fall of Rh disease. In Smith GF, Smith PN, Vidyasagar D, ed: Historical review and recent advances in neonatal and perinatal medicine. [Chicago?], Mead Johnson Nutritional Division, 1983. Vol. I. p. 99–106.

**Zipursky A** see **Smith GF**

**Zirinsky L:** The Leprosy Museum of Bergen. **St Mary Hosp Gaz** 1979 Autumn;85:23

**Zirnstein G:** Die Erforschung und Bewertung der Lebenserscheinung 'Variabilität' in der Biologie vor 1859. **NTM** 1981;18(2):58–78

**Zirnstein G:** Zur gesellschaftlichen Stellung der Wissenschaftler in der Geschichte von Evolutionstheorie und Vererbungsforschung. **Rostocker Wiss Hist Manuskripte** 1981;6:57–60

**Zivanovic S:** Povrede i prelomi kostiju u Srpskog srednjovekovnog stanoviništva iz nekropole Vajuga na Dunavu kod Kladova. **Srp Arh Celok Lek** 1982 Mar;110(3):273–89

**Zivanovic S** see **Burleigh R**

**Zivkovic K:** Dr Nikolaj S. Korotkov (13. II. 1874–1920). **Srp Arh Celok Lek** 1983 Jan;111(1):97–9

**Zivkovic K:** Sečanje na prof. Dr. Luisa A. Djuringa (23. XII 1854 – 8. V 1913). **Srp Arh Celok Lek** 1982 Apr;110(4):523–4

**Zivotní jubileum prof. MUDr. Frantiska Gazárka, CSc: Cesk Gynekol** 1983 Feb;48(1):75–80

**Zlotnik EN:** Razvitie neĭrokhirurgii v Belorusskoĭ SSR. **Zh Vopr Neirokhir** 1982 Nov–Dec;(6):7–9

**Zmirou–Lajuzan D:** L'hôpital Saint–Jacques de Bordeaux, du XIIe au XVIe siècle. Maîtrise, Univ. de Bordeaux, III, 1977. 309 p.

**Zmudzki A, Morawski J:** 25 lat przymusowego leczenia alkoholików w Polsce. **Psychiatr Pol** 1983 Mar–Apr;17(2):147–57

**Znachenie otkrytiia Roberta Kokha dlia razvitiia bakteriologii tuberkuleza: Probl Tuberk** 1982 Mar;(3):3–7

**Znamenatel'nye i iubileĭnye daty istorii meditsiny 1982 g: Sov Zdravookhr** 1981;(6):68–75

**Znamenatel'nye i jubileĭnye daty istorii morfologii v 1983 godu: Arkh Anat Gistol Embriol** 1982 Oct;83(10):109–10

**Znamenatel'nye i jubileĭnye daty istorii terapii 1980 g: Ter Arkh** 1979;51(11):131–3

**Znosko K** see **Kretowski J**

**Zoller H** see **Albrecht von Haller, 1708–1777**

**Zollinger RM:** Overview biography--Doctor Loyal Davis. **Surg Gynecol Obstet** 1983 Aug;157(2):111–3

**Zollinger RM:** The legacies of William Beaumont, pioneer investigator. **Pharos** 1983 Winter;46(1):20–3

**Zollinger RM** see **Murray JE**

**Zolotarev V:** Zapiska starshego vracha kreisera avrora. **Voen Istor Zh** 1976;(1):51–60

**Zolotnitskiĭ IaI:** O knige O. Kalinskogo 'Retseptura ili nastavlenie sochiniat' pravil'nye retsepty dlia studentov imperatorskoĭ mediko–khirurgicheskoĭ akademii'. **Klin Med (Mosk)** 1984 Apr;62(4):151

**Zolyomi ND:** Die Kochsche Entdeckung in der Pressburger Tagespresse. **Wiss Beitr Martin Luther Univ Halle Wittenberg** 1983;5–R80:79–84

**Zolyomi ND:** Ein Beitrag zur Entwicklung der Apothekenvisitationen in Ungarn des 17. und 18. Jahrhunderts. Von den Theriakvorführungen zur wissenschaftlich fundierten Apothekenvisitation. **Pharm Acta Helv** 1979;54(4):114–6

**Zolyomi ND:** L'acceptation des remèdes populaires par les médecins érudits. In: Congrès international d'histoire de la médecine, XXVe, Québec, 1976. Actes. Québec, 1977. p. 1396–1402.

**Zólyomi ND:** The development of the district medical officer in Hungary from the Middle–Ages to the 18th century. In Russell AW, ed: The town and state physician in Europe from the Middle Ages to the

Enlightenment. Wolfenbüttel, Herzog August Bibliothek, 1981. p. 131–40 (Wolfenbütteler Forschungen, 17).
**Zondek T:** Dr. Med. David Viet (1771–1814), eine Gestalt aus der Emanzipationszeit. **Bull Leo Beck Inst** 1976;15(52):49–7
**Zook CJ, Moore FD, Zeckhauser RJ:** 'Catastrophic' health insurance: a misguided prescription? **Public Interest** 1981;(62):66–81
**Zopf LC:** Iowa pharmacy, a century of service: a chronology of the Iowa Pharmacists Association, 1880–1980. West Des Moines, Rob Lee Hill Pub. Co., 1980. xv, 408 p.
**Zopff G:** Erinnerungen an die Anfänge des Berufsverbandes. **Chirurg** 1980 Aug;51(8):128–9
**Zorgniotti AW:** Bladder cancer in the pre-cystoscopic era. **Prog Clin Biol Res** 1984;162A:1–9
**Zorgniotti AW:** Suprapubic prostatectomy: an Anglo-American success story. In Hinman F., Boyarsky S, ed: Benign prostatic hypertrophy. New York, Springer-Verlag, 1983. p. 45–58.
**Zorgniotti AW:** The Civiale Remedial Agency. Urologic quackery in the gay nineties. **Urology** 1981 Jan;17(1):109–12
**Zorina LA, Rashevskaia AM:** Postdiplomnoe obuchenie vracheĭ na kafedre profpatologii (k 50-letiiu iubileiu Tsentral'nogo instituta usovershenstvovaniia vracheĭ). **Gig Tr Prof Zabol** 1980 Oct;(10):32–4
**Zorn E:** Geschichte und Bedeutung des Marinehospitals von Pola/Jugoslawien. **Hist Hosp** 1979–80;13:135–46
**Zorn W:** Medizinische Volkskunde als sozial-geschichtliche Quelle. Die bayerische Bezirksärzte-Landesbeschreibung von 1860/62. **Vierteljahrsschr Soz Wirtschgesch** 1982;69(2):219–31
**Zornig C** see **Schlosser GA**
**Zotter H, ed:** Antike Medizin. Die medizinische Sammelhandschrift Cod. Vindobonensis 93 in lateinischer und deutscher Sprache. Graz, Akademische Druck- und Verlagsanstalt, xxxii, 380 p.
**Zottl A:** Otto Rank: das Lebenswerk eines Dissidenten der Psychoanalyse. München, Kindler, 1982. 316 p.
**Zrubek H:** 35 lat w służbie macierzyństwa na Lubelszczyźnie. **Ginekol Pol** 1980 Dec;51(12):1057–61
**Zschoche S** see **Morantz RM**
**Zschock DK:** Health care financing in Central America and the Andean Region: a workshop report. **Lat Am Res Rev** 1980;15(3):149–68
**Zsebök Z:** Famous Hungarian doctors. **New Hung Q** 1982;23(85):131–4
**Zubirán S:** Informe de labores con motivo del XXXIII aniversario del Instituto Nacional de la Nutrición. **Rev Invest Clin** 1980 Jan–Mar;32(1):101–9
**Zubiri de Salinas R** see **Zubiri Vidal F**
**Zubiri García MD** see **Francès Causapè MC**
**Zubiri Vidal F, Zubiri de Salinas R:** Las epidemias de peste y cólera morbo-asiático en Aragón (Zaragoza, 1652 y 1885; Caspe, 1834; Alcañiz y Jaca, 1885). Zaragoza, Diputacion Provincial, Institucion 'Fernando el Catolico', [1980]. 195 p. (Temas Aragoneses, 32).
**Zubiri Vidal F:** Médicos aragoneses ilustres. Zaragoza, Diputación Provincial, Institución 'Fernando El Católico', [1983]. 395 p.
**Zubiri Vidal F, Zubiri de Salinas R:** Refranes médicos oidos en Aragón. **Cuad Aragon Hist Med Cienc (A)** 1978, 1980;2:1–99
**Zubrod CG:** Origins and development of chemotherapy research at the National Cancer Institute. **Cancer Treat Rep** 1984 Jan;68(1):9–19
**Zubrod CG:** The cure of cancer by chemotherapy – reflections on how it happened. (The fifth Myron Karon Memorial Lecture). **Med Pediatr Oncol** 1980;8:107–14
**Zuchowicz T** see **Drozdowski P**
**Zuck D:** Early opposition to obstetric anasthesia [letter] **Anaesthesia** 1981 May;36(5):538–42
**Zuck D:** John Hunter's treatment of gunshot wounds. **Ann R Coll Surg Engl** 1980 Jan;62(1):74–5
**Zucker GM, Clayman CB:** Landmark perspective: Bertram W. Sippy and ulcer disease therapy. **JAMA** 1983 Oct 28;250(16):2198–202
**Zuckerman A:** Scurvy and the ventilation of ships in the Royal Navy: Samuel Sutton's contribution. **Eighteenth Cent Stud** 1976/77;10:222–34
**Zuckerman AJ:** Palaeontology of smallpox. **Lancet** 1984 Dec 22;2(8417–18):1454
**Zuckerman L:** The launching of the Journal of Endocrinology and the founding of the Society for Endocrinology. **J Endocrinol** 1984 Jan;100(1):1–5
**Zuckermann C:** Realizaciónes en medicina asistencial. In Academia Nacional de Medicina. Libro conmemorativo del primer centenario. México, Comité Editorial de la Comisión Organizadora del Congreso del Centenario, 1964. Tome 2. p. 642–6.
**Zuev AI, Sergienko VI:** V. I. Lenin--organizator sovetskogo zdravookhraneniia. **Zh Ushn Nos Gorl Bolezn** 1980 Jan–Feb;1:1–6
**Zülch KJ:** Historical development of the classification of brain tumours and the new proposal of the World Health Organization (WHO). **Neurosurg Rev** 1981;4(3):123–7
**Zülch KJ:** Reflections on the surgery of the pineal gland (a glimpse into the past). Gleanings from medical history. **Neurosurg Rev** 1981;4(3):159–63
**Zuluaga Gómez A, Torres Ramírez C, Rodríguez Rebollo T, et al:** Análisis cristalográfico de lithiasis vesicales del siglo XIX. **Arch Esp Urol** 1982 Jul–Aug;35(4):234–45
**Zuluaga Gómez A** see **Torres Ramírez C**
**Zulueta J de** see **Bruce-Chwatt LJ**
**Zumkeller D** see **Perrenoud A**
**Zur Geschichte der Psychiatrie in Wien:** Psychiatry in Vienna. Eine Bilddokumentation. An illustrated documentation. With contributions by P. Berner, W. Spiel, H. Strotzka, H. Wyklicky. Wien, Brandstätter, 1983. 144 p.
**Zureck A:** 30 Jahre BCG-Impfung in der DDR – 20 Jahre BCG-Impfstoff aus Jena. **Z Erkr Atmungsorgane** 1982;158(1–2)168–84
**Zurfluh A:** A propos de la peste dans les Alpes: le canton d'Uri en 1629. **Ann Demogr Hist (Paris)** 1983;:353–68
**Zuring J:** Saint Côme et Saint Damien dans la philatélie. **Rev Hist Pharm (Paris)** 1984 Mar;31(260):69–72
**Zuylen J van:** On the microscopes of Antoni van Leeuwenhoek. **Janus** 1981;68:159–98
**Zuylen J van** see **Palm LC**
**Zvara V:** O vývoji a dalších perspektívach rozvoja chirurgických disciplín na lekárskej fakulte Univerzity Komenského v Bratislave. **Cas Lek Cesk** 1979 Dec 21;118(51):1583–5
**Zwanowetz G:** Herzog Sigismund von Osterreich in Gastein. **Mitt Ges Salzburger Landeskd** 1972–73;112–113(2):325–9
**Zwelling S:** Spiritualist perspectives on antebellum experience. **J Psychohist** 1982 Summer;10(1):3–25
**Zychowicz G** see **Markowski W**
**Zygulska-Machowa H, Starzycka M:** Professor Bolesław Wicherkiewicz jako współtwórca krakowskiej szkoły okulistycznej. **Klin Oczna** 1982 Sep;84(9):245–9
**Zykin LF, Metlin VN:** Nauchnaia deiatel'nost' professora V. V. Akimovicha. **Zh Mikrobiol Epidemiol Immunobiol** 1984 Apr;(4):113–4
**Zylberman P** see **Talmor E, ed**
**Zysk KG:** A note on ancient Indian medicine. **Bull Indian Inst Hist Med (Hyderabad)** 1978;8(1–4):14–23
**Zysset T** see **Kotwas J**

## 1

**100 anniversaire de la fondation de l'Ecole de Médecine dentaire de l'Université de Genève (1881–1981): SSO Schweiz Monatsschr Zahnheilkd** 1981 Oct;91(10):755–63
**100 de ani de la descoperirea de către Robert Koch a bacilului tuberculozei: Rev Ig [Pneumoftiziol]** 1982 Oct–Dec;31(4):289–90
**100 years ago: household medicine and treatment: the gospel according to Dr. Chase: One One** 1981 May–Jun;3(3):4–5
**14L 1000-letiiu so dnia rozhdenii a Abu Ali Ibn-Siny (980–1037): Zh Nevropatol Psikhiatr** 1980;80(8):1221–8
**150 years of factory inspectorate: J R Soc Health** 1983 Dec;103(6):244–5
**150e année:** La variole et son éradication. Contributions by L. Justin-Besançon, R. Fasquelle, J. Fasquelle, L. Jacques. **J Med Chir Prat** 1979 Sep;17–18:629–708
**(1816) Rum Hospital ... (1844) Infirmary-Dispensary ... (1881) Sydney Hospital ... (1982) ?: Med J Aust** 1982 Aug 21;2(4):198–200
**[1857–1982 – the National Danish Medical Society: 125th anniversary]: Ugeskr Laeger** 1982 Aug 30;144(35):2549–616
**1879–1979 – centenaire de la bibliothèque de l'Ecole Dentaire de Paris, Centre Français de Documentation Odonto-stomatologique.: Rev Odontostomatol (Paris)** 1980 Mar–Apr;9(2):13–5
**1947–1977: po povod zo godini na medidžinskiot fakultet Skopje: God Zb Med Fak Skopje** 1979 Jan;25:5–126
**1952–1982, 30e anniversaire de la Société suisse d'anesthésiologie et de réanimation:** [Switzerland: s.n., 1982?]. 72 p.

## 2

**22.500 thèses françaises de médecine publiées de 1796 à 1896:** Un monument de l'histoire de la médecine. Genève, Librairie Slatkine, 1982. Various paginations.
**25th anniversary issue of Australasian Radiology: Australas Radiol** 1982;Spec. No.:1–162

## 4

**40 aniversario del Institute Nacional de Cardiología de México: Arch Inst Cardiol Mex** 1984 Jul–Aug;54(4):411–26
**40 let nashemu zhunalu: Med Sestra** 1982 Aug;41(8):9–12

## 5

**50-lecie Zakładu Radiodiagnostyki Instytutu Onkologii im. Marii Skłodowskiej-Curie w Warszawie: Pol Przegl Radiol (Warszawa)** 1983 Jul–Aug;47(4):261–2

## 6

**60 ans déjà ...: Nurs Que** 1980 Nov–Dec;1(1):12–26
**60 Let deiatel'nosti zhurnala 'Akusherstvio i ginekologiia': Akush Ginekol (Mosk)** 1982;(12):16–7

## 7

**75 Jahre Zeitschrift Krankenpflege:** Krankenschwestern erinnern sich. **Krankenpflege (Bern)** 1983 Jan;(1):66–9
**75 years of caring: US Navy Med** 1983 May–Jun;74(3):14–7
**75 years of dedication and progress: American Dairy Science Association: J Dairy Sci** 1981 Jun;64(6):875–1526
**75 years of dental hygiene education.: Dent Hyg (Chic)** 1980 Mar;54(3):115–7

**75ème anniversaire de l'Institut de Médecine Tropicale du Service de Santé des Armées (le Pharo Marseille).: Med Trop (Mars)** 1980 Nov-Dec;40(6):591-604

**75th anniversary. CNA's twelve member association:** Without them where would we be? **Can Nurse** 1983 Oct;79(9):22-34

## 8

**[80th anniversary of the 'Zhurnal Nevropatologii i Psikhiatrii im. S. S. Korsakov'] (Rus): Zh Nevropatol Psikhiatr** 1981;81(1):3-5

# PART IV. INDEX TO JOURNAL ABBREVIATIONS

—A—

AAF Bijdr
A.A.G. BIJDRAGEN (Netherlands)
Aberdeen Univ Rev
ABERDEEN UNIVERSITY REVIEW (Gt Brit)
Abh Ber Staatl Mus Volkerkd Dres
ABHANDLUNGEN UND BERICHTE DES STAATLICHEN MUSEUMS FUR VOLKERKUNDE DRESDEN
Acad Bookman
ACADEMY BOOKMAN
Acad Soc Lorraines Sci
ACADEMIE ET SOCIETE LORRAINES DES SCIENCES (France)
Acadiensis
ACADIENSIS: JOURNAL OF THE HISTORY OF THE ATLANTIC REGION (Canada)
Acarologia
ACAROLOGIA (Paris)
Accad Naz Lincei Rome
ACCADEMIA NAZIONALE DEI LINCEI, ROME
Acquis Med Recent
ACQUISITIONS MEDICALES RECENTES (Paris)
Acta Acad Med Wuhan
ACTA ACADEMIAE MEDICINAE WUHAN (Wuhan)
Acta Anaesthesiol Belg
ACTA ANAESTHESIOLOGICA BELGICA (Bruxelles)
Acta Anaesthesiol Scand
ACTA ANAESTHESIOLOGICA SCANDINAVICA (Aarhus)
Acta Anthropogenet
ACTA ANTHROPOGENETICA (New Delhi)
Acta Antiq Hung
ACTA ANTIQUA HUNGARICA (Hungary)
Acta Belg Med Phys
ACTA BELGICA. MEDICA PHYSICA (Bruxelles)
Acta Biochim Pol
ACTA BIOCHIMICA POLONICA (Warszawa)
Acta Biol Acad Sci Hung
ACTA BIOLOGICA ACADEMIAE SCIENTIARUM HUNGARICAE (Budapest)
Acta Biotheor (Leiden)
ACTA BIOTHEORETICA (Leiden)
Acta Chir Belg
ACTA CHIRURGICA BELGICA (Bruxelles)
Acta Chir Iugosl
ACTA CHIRURGICA IUGOSLAVICA (Zagreb)
Acta Chir Orthop Traumatol Cech
ACTA CHIRURGIAE ORTHOPAEDICAE ET TRAUMATOLOGIAE CECHOSLOVACA (Praha)
Acta Chir Plast (Prague)
ACTA CHIRURGIAE PLASTICAE (Prague)
Acta Chir Scand [Suppl]
ACTA CHIRURGICA SCANDINAVICA. SUPPLEMENTUM (Stockholm)
Acta Cient Venez
ACTA CIENTIFICA VENEZOLANA (Caracas)
Acta Clin Belg
ACTA CLINICA BELGICA (Bruxelles)
Acta Cytol (Baltimore)
ACTA CYTOLOGICA (Baltimore)
Acta Derm Venereol [Suppl] (Stockh)
ACTA DERMATO-VENEREOLOGICA. SUPPLEMENTUM (Stockholm)
Acta Ethnol Linguist
ACTA ETHNOLOGICA ET LINGUISTICA (Austria)
Acta Gastroenterol Latinoam
ACTA GASTROENTEROLOGICA LATINOAMERICANA (Buenos Aires)
Acta Genet Med Gemellol (Roma)
ACTA GENETICAE MEDICAE ET GEMELLOLOGIAE (Roma)
Acta Haematol (Basel)
ACTA HAEMATOLOGICA (Basel)
Acta Haematol Pol
ACTA HAEMATOLOGICA POLONICA (Warszawa)
Acta Hist Leopoldina
ACTA HISTORICA LEOPOLDINA; ABHANDLUNGEN AUS DEM ARCHIV FUR GESCHICHTE DER NATURFORSCHUNG UND MEDIZIN DER DEUTSCHEN AKADEMIE DER NATURFORSCHER LEOPOLDINA (Leipzig)
Acta Hist Rerum Nat Tech
ACTA HISTORIAE RERUM NATURALIUM NEC NON TECHNICARUM (Praha)
Acta Leprol (Geneve)
ACTA LEPROLOGICA (Geneve)
Acta Med Hist Patav
ACTA MEDICAE HISTORIAE PATAVINA (Padua)
Acta Med Leg Soc (Liege)
ACTA MEDICINAE LEGALIS ET SOCIALIS (Liege)
Acta Med Pol
ACTA MEDICA POLONA (Warszawa)
Acta Med Port
ACTA MEDICA PORTUGUESA (Lisboa)
Acta Med Scand
ACTA MEDICA SCANDINAVICA (Stockholm)

Acta Med Tenerife
ACTA MEDICA DE TENERIFE (Santa Cruz de Tenerife)
Acta Med Venez
ACTA MEDICA VENEZOLANA (Caracas)
Acta Morphol Neerl Scand
ACTA MORPHOLOGICA NEERLANDO-SCANDINAVICA (LISSE)
Acta Mus Napocensis (Cluj)
ACTA MUSEI NAPOCENSIS. CLUJ, TRANSLVANIA, MUZEUL DE ISTORIE (Cluj)
Acta Neurobiol Exp (Warsz)
ACTA NEUROBIOLOGIAE EXPERIMENTALIS (Warszawa)
Acta Neurochir (Wien)
ACTA NEUROCHIRURGICA (Wien)
Acta Neurol (Napoli)
ACTA NEUROLOGICA (Napoli)
Acta Neurol [Quad]
ACTA NEUROLOGICA. QUADERNI (Napoli)
Acta Neurol Latinoam
ACTA NEUROLOGICA LATINOAMERICANA (Montevideo)
Acta Neurol Scand
ACTA NEUROLOGICA SCANDINAVICA (Copenhagen)
Acta Obstet Gynecol Scand
ACTA OBSTETRICA ET GYNECOLOGIA SCANDINAVICA (UMEA)
Acta Obstet Gynecol Scand [Suppl]
ACTA OBSTETRICIA ET GYNECOLOGICA SCANDINAVICA. SUPPLEMENT (UMEA)
Acta Odontol Venez
ACTA ODONTOLOGICA VENEZOLANA
Acta Otolaryngol [Suppl] (Stockh)
ACTA OTO-LARYNGOLOGICA. SUPPLEMENT (Stockholm)
Acta Otorhinolaryngol Belg
ACTA OTO-RHINO-LARYNGOLOGICA BELGICA (Bruxelles)
Acta Paediatr Hung
ACTA PAEDIATRICA HUNGARICA (Budapest)
Acta Paedopsychiatr (Basel)
ACTA PAEDPOSYCHIATRICA (Basel)
Acta Pathol Jpn
ACTA PATHOLOGICA JAPONICA (Tokyo)
Acta Pharm Hung
ACTA PHARMACEUTICA HUNGARICA (Budapest)
Acta Physiol Lat Am
ACTA PHYSIOLOGICA LATINO-AMERICANA (Buenos Aires)
Acta Physiol Pol
ACTA PHYSIOLOGICA POLONICA (Warszawa)
Acta Pol Hist
ACTA POLONIAE HISTORICA (Warszawa)
Acta Psiquiatr Psicol Am Lat
ACTA PSIQUIATRICA Y PSICOLOGICA DE AMERICA LATINA (Buenos Aires)
Acta Psychiatr Belg
ACTA PSYCHIATRICA BELGICA (Bruxelles)
Acta Psychiatr Scand
ACTA PSYCHIATRICA SCANDINAVICA (Copenhagen)
Acta Radiol [Oncol]
ACTA RADIOLOGICA. ONCOLOGY (Stockholm)
Acta Stomatol Croat
ACTA STOMATOLOGICA CROATICA (Zagreb)
Acta Trop (Basel)
ACTA TROPICA (Basel)
Acta Univ Carol [Hist] (Praha)
ACTA UNIVERSITATIS CAROLINAE-HISTORIA UNIVERSITATIS PRAGENSIS
Acta Univ Carol [Med] (Praha)
ACTA UNIVERSITATIS CAROLINAE; MEDICA (Praha)
Acta Univ Carol Philos Hist
ACTA UNIVERSITATIS CAROLINAE PHILOSOPHICA ET HISTORICA (Praha)
Acta Univ Lund
ACTA UNIVERSITATIS LUNDENSIS (Sweden)
Acta Univ Palacki Olomuc Fac Med
ACTA UNIVERSITATIS PALACKIANAE OLOMUCENSIS FACULTATIS MEDICAL (Praha)
Acta Univ Stockh
ACTA UNIVERSITATIS STOCKHOLMIENSIS (Sweden) STOCKHOLM STUDIES IN ENGLISH
Acta Urol Belg
ACTA UROLOGICA BELGICA (Bruxelles)
Acta Virol (Praha)
ACTA VIROLOGICA (Praha)
Acta Vitaminol Enzymol
ACTA VITAMINOLOGICA ET ENZYMOLOGICA (Milano)
Actas Dermosifiliogr
ACTAS DERMO-SIFILOGRAFICAS (Madrid)
Actas Luso Esp Neurol Psiquiatr
ACTAS LUSO-ESPANOLAS DE NEUROLOGIA, PSIQUIATRIA Y CIENCIAS DE AFINES (Madrid)
Action Natl
ACTION NATIONALE (Canada)
Actual Odontostomatol (Paris)
ACTUALITES ODONTO-STOMATOLOGIQUES (Paris)
Acupunct Electrother Res
ACUPUNCTURE AND ELECTRO-THERAPEUTICS RESEARCH (Oxford)
Adler
ADLER (Austria)
Adler Mus Bull
ADLER MUSEUM BULLETIN OF THE ADLER MUSEUM OF THE HISTORY OF MEDICINE (Johannesburg)
ADM
ADM: REVISTA DE LA ASOCIACION DENTAL MEXICANA (Mexico)
Adm Sci Q

ADMINISTRATIVE SCIENCE QUARTERLY (Ithaca NY)
Adolesc Psychiatry
ADOLESCENT PSYCHIATRY (New York)
Adv Biol Med Phys
ADVANCES IN BIOLOGICAL AND MEDICAL PHYSICS (New York)
Adv Biosci
ADVANCES IN THE BIOSCIENCES (Elmsford, NY)
Adv Carbohydr Chem Biochem
ADVANCES IN CARBOHYDRATE CHEMISTRY AND BIOCHEMISTRY (New York)
Adv Cardiol
ADVANCES IN CARDIOLOGY (Basel)
Adv Child Dev Behav
ADVANCES IN CHILD DEVELOPMENT AND BEHAVIOR (New York)
Adv Exp Med Biol
ADVANCES IN EXPERIMENTAL MEDICINE AND BIOLOGY (New York)
Adv Food Res
ADVANCES IN FOOD RESEARCH (New York)
Adv Health Econ Health Serv Res
ADVANCES IN HEALTH ECONOMICS AND HEALTH SERVICES RESEARCH (Greenwich Ct)
Adv Neurol
ADVANCES IN NEUROLOGY (New York)
Adv Otorhinolaryngol
ADVANCES IN OTO-RHINO-LARYNGOLOGY (Basel)
Adv Pediatr
ADVANCES IN PEDIATRICS (Chicago)
Adv Shock
ADVANCES IN SHOCK RESEARCH (New York)
Adv Surg
ADVANCES IN SURGERY (Chicago)
Adv Thanatol
ADVANCES IN THANATOLOGY (Edison NJ)
Advent Herit
ADVENTIST HERITAGE (Loma Linda CA)
Aegyptus (Milano)
AEGYPTUS; RIVISTA ITALIANA DI EGITTOLOGIA E DI PAPIROLOGIA (Milano)
Aesthetic Plast Surg
AESTHETIC PLASTIC SURGERY (New York)
Aevum
AEVUM (Italy)
Afr Bull
AFRICANA BULLETIN (Warsaw)
Afr Econ Hist
AFRICAN ECONOMIC HISTORY (US)
Afr Notes
AFRICAN NOTES (Nigeria)
Afr Soc Res
AFRICAN SOCIAL RESEARCH (Gt Brit)
Afr Stud Rev
AFRICAN STUDIES REVIEW (US)
Africa (Gt Brit)
AFRICA (Gt Brit)
Africa (Italy)
AFRICA (Italy)
Afro-Am NY Life Hist
AFRO-AMERICANS IN NEW YORK LIFE AND HISTORY (Buffalo NY)
Age Ageing
AGE AND AGEING (London)
Aged Care Serv Rev
AGED CARE AND SERVICES REVIEW (New York)
Agrartort Sz
AGRARTORT SZEMLE (Hungary)
Agressologie
AGRESSOLOGIE (Paris)
Agric Hist
AGRICULTURAL HISTORY (Berkeley CA)
AJR
AJR AMERICAN JOURNAL OF ROENTGENOLOGY (Baltimore)
AJS
AJS. AMERICAN JOURNAL OF SOCIOLOGY (Chicago)
Aktuel Gerontol
AKTUELLE GERONTOLOGIE (Stuttgart)
Aktuel Traumatol
AKTUELLE TRAUMATOLOGIE (Stuttgart)
Akush Ginekol (Mosk)
AKUSHERSTVO I GINEKOLOGIIA (Moskva)
Akush Ginekol (Sofiia)
AKUSHERSTVO I GINEKOLOGIIA; Supplement to SUVREMENNA MEDITSINA (Sofia)
Al-Arabi
AL-ARABI (Kuwait)
Ala Hist Q
ALABAMA HISTORICAL QUARTERLY (Montgomery AL)
Ala J Med Sci
ALABAMA JOURNAL OF MEDICAL SCIENCES (Birmingham AL)
Ala Med
ALABAMA MEDICINE (Montgomery AL)
Ala Rev
ALABAMA REVIEW (University AL)
Alaska J
ALASKA JOURNAL (Edmonds WA)
Alaska Med
ALASKA MEDICINE (Anchorage AK)
Alberta Hist
ALBERTA HISTORY (Canada)
Albion
ALBION (London)
Albrecht von Graefes Arch Klin Exp Opthalmol
ALBRECHT VON GRAEFES ARCHIV FUR KLINISCHE UND EXPERIMENTELLE OPHTHALMOLOGIE (Berlin)
Alcohol Alcohol
ALCOHOL AND ALCOHOLISM (Oxford)
Alcohol Health Res World

ALCOHOL HEALTH AND RESEARCH WORLD (Rockville MD)
Allerg Immunol (Leipz)
ALLERGIE UND IMMUNOLOGIE (Leipzig)
Alma Mater Philipp
ALMA MATER PHILIPPINA (Marburg)
Alpha Omegan
ALPHA OMEGAN (Beverly Hills)
Alt-Thuringen
ALT-THURINGEN (E Germany)
Altertum
DAS ALTERTUM (E Germany)
Altnurnb Landsch
ALTNURNBERGER LANDSCHAFT (Germany)
Alumni Bull Sch Dent Indiana Univ
ALUMNI BULLETIN—SCHOOL OF DENTISTRY, INDIANA UNIVERSITY (Indianapolis)
Alumni Mag
ALUMNI MAGAZINE (Baltimore)
Am Ann Deaf
AMERICAN ANNALS OF THE DEAF (Silver Spring MD)
Am Anthropol
AMERICAN ANTHROPOLOGIST (Washington)
Am Arch Rehabil Ther
AMERICAN ARCHIVES OF REHABILITATION THERAPY (Paramus NJ)
Am Behav Sci
AMERICAN BEHAVIORAL SCIENTIST (Beverly Hills CA)
Am Benedictine Rev
AMERICAN BENEDICTINE REVIEW (Atchison KS)
Am Biol Teach
AMERICAN BIOLOGY TEACHER (Washington)
Am Coll Physicians Obs
AMERICAN COLLEGE OF PHYSICIANS OBSERVER (Philadelphia)
Am Correct Ther J
AMERICAN CORRECTIVE THERAPY JOURNAL (Rehoboth Beach)
Am Econ Rev
AMERICAN ECONOMIC REVIEW (US)
Am Fam Physician
AMERICAN FAMILY PHYSICIAN (Kansas City MO)
Am Heart J
AMERICAN HEART JOURNAL (St Louis)
Am Heritage
AMERICAN HERITAGE (US)
Am Hist Illus
AMERICAN HISTORY ILLUSTRATED (Marion OH)
Am Hist Rev
AMERICAN HISTORICAL REVIEW (Washington)
Am Imago
AMERICAN IMAGO (New York)
Am Ind Hy Assoc J
AMERICAN INDUSTRIAL HYGIENE ASSOCIATION JOURNAL (Akron OH)
Am Indian Art Mag
AMERICAN INDIAN ART MAGAZINE (Scottsdale AZ)
Am Indian Q
AMERICAN INDIAN QUARTERLY (Hurst TX)
Am Indig
AMERICA INDIGENA (Mexico)
Am J Anat
AMERICAN JOURNAL OF ANATOMY (New York)
Am J Art Ther
AMERICAN JOURNAL OF ART THERAPY (Washington)
Am J Cardiol
AMERICAN JOURNAL OF CARDIOLOGY (New York)
Am J Chin Med
AMERICAN JOURNAL OF CHINESE MEDICINE (New York)
Am J Clin Hypn
AMERICAN JOURNAL OF CLINICAL HYPNOSIS (Minneapolis MN)
Am J Clin Oncol
AMERICAN JOURNAL OF CLINICAL ONCOLOGY (New York)
Am J Clin Pathol
AMERICAN JOURNAL OF CLINICAL PATHOLOGY (Philadelphia)
Am J Community Psychol
AMERICAN JOURNAL OF COMMUNITY PSYCHOLOGY (New York)
Am J Dermatopathol
AMERICAN JOURNAL OF DERMATOPATHOLOGY (New York)
Am J Dis Child
AMERICAN JOURNAL OF DISEASES OF CHILDREN (Chicago)
Am J Econ Sociol
AMERICAN JOURNAL OF ECONOMICS AND SOCIOLOGY (New York)
Am J Epidemiol
AMERICAN JOURNAL OF EPIDEMIOLOGY (Baltimore)
Am J Forensic Med Pathol
AMERICAN JOURNAL OF FORENSIC MEDICINE AND PATHOLOGY (New York)
Am J Gastroenterol
AMERICAN JOURNAL OF GASTROENTEROLOGY (New York)
Am J Hosp Pharm
AMERICAN JOURNAL OF HOSPITAL PHARMACY (Washington)
Am J Hum Genet
AMERICAN JOURNAL OF HUMAN GENETICS (Chicago)
Am J Ind Med
AMERICAN JOURNAL OF INDUSTRIAL MEDICINE (New York)
Am J Infect Control
AMERICAN JOURNAL OF INFECTION CONTROL

(St Louis)
Am J Kidney Dis
AMERICAN JOURNAL OF KIDNEY DISEASES (New York)
Am J Med
AMERICAN JOURNAL OF MEDICINE (New York)
Am J Genet
AMERICAN JOURNAL OF MEDICAL GENETICS (New York)
Am J Med Sci
AMERICAN JOURNAL OF THE MEDICAL SCIENCES (Thorofare NJ)
Am J Med Technol
AMERICAN JOURNAL OF MEDICAL TECHNOLOGY (Houston)
Am J Ment Defic
AMERICAL JOURNAL OF MENTAL DEFICIENCY (Washington)
Am J Nurs
AMERICAN JOURNAL OF NURSING (New York)
Am J Obstet Gynecol
AMERICAN JOURNAL OF OBSTETRICS AND GYNECOLOGY (Los Angeles)
Am J Occup Ther
AMERICAN JOURNAL OF OCCUPATIONAL THERAPY (Boston)
Am J Ophthalmol
AMERICAN JOURNAL OF OPTHALMOLOGY (Chicago)
Am J Optom Physicl Opt
AMERICAN JOURNAL OF OPTOMETRY AND PHYSIOLOGICAL OPTICS (Baltimore)
Am J Orthod
AMERICAN JOURNAL OF ORTHODONTICS (St. Louis)
Am J Orthop
AMERICAN JOURNAL OF ORTHOPEDICS (Houston)
Am J Otolaryngol
AMERICAN JOURNAL OF OTOLARYNGOLOGY (Cherry Hill NJ)
Am J Pathol
AMERICAN JOURNAL OF PATHOLOGY (Philadelphia)
Am J Pediatr Hematol Oncol
AMERICAN JOURNAL OF PEDIATRIC HEMATOLOGY/ONCOLOGY (New York)
Am J Pharm Educ
AMERICAN JOURNAL OF PHARMACEUTICAL EDUCATION (Des Moines IA)
Am J Philol
AMERICAN JOURNAL OF PHILOLOGY (Baltimore MD)
Am J Phys Anthropol
AMERICAN JOURNAL OF PHYSICAL ANTHROPOLOGY (New York)
Am J Physical
AMERICAN JOURNAL OF PHYSIOLOGY (Bethesda MD)
Am J Proctol Gastroenterol Colon Rectal Surg
AMERICAN JOURNAL OF PROCTOLOGY, GASTROENTEROLOGY AND COLON AND RECTAL SURGERY (Georgetown CT)
Am J Psychiatry
AMERICAN JOURNAL OF PSYCHIATRY (Washington)
Am J Psychoanal
AMERICAN JOURNAL OF PSYCHOANALYSIS (New York)
Am J Psychol
AMERICAN JOURNAL OF PSYCHOLOGY (Urban IL)
Am J Psychother
AMERICAN JOURNAL OF PSYCHOTHERAPY (Jamaica NY)
Am J Public Health
AMERICAN JOURNAL OF PUBLIC HEALTH (New York)
Am J Sociol
AMERICAN JOURNAL OF SOCIOLOGY (Chicago)
See AJS
Am J Sports Med
AMERICAN JOURNAL OF SPORTS MEDICINE (Baltimore)
Am J Surg
AMERICAN JOURNAL OF SURGERY (New York)
Am J Surg Pathol
AMERICAN JOURNAL OF SURGICAL PATHOLOGY (New York)
Am J Trop Med Hyg
AMERICAN JOURNAL OF TROPICAL MEDICINE AND HYGIENE (Lawrence KS)
Am J Hist
AMERICAN JEWISH HISTORY (US)
Am Lit
AMERICAN LITERATURE (Durham NC)
Am Lung Assoc Bull
AMERICAN LUNG ASSOCIATION BULLETIN (New York)
Am Med News
AMERICAN MEDICAL NEWS (Chicago)
Am Neptune
AMERICAN NEPTUNE; A QUARTERLY JOURNAL OF MARITIME HISTORY
Am Notes Queries
AMERICAN NOTES AND QUERIES (US)
Am Nurse
AMERICAN NURSE (Kansas City MO)
Am Pharm
AMERICAN PHARMACY (Washington)
Am Pol Sci Rev
AMERICAN POLITICAL SCIENCE REVIEW (Washington)
Am Psychol
AMERICAN PSYCHOLOGIST (Washington)
Am Q

AMERICAN QUARTERLY (Philadelphia)
Am Rev Can Stud
AMERICAN REVIEW OF CANADIAN STUDIES (Washington)
Am Rev Respir Dis
AMERICAN REVIEW OF RESPIRATORY DISEASE (New York)
Am Scholar
AMERICAN SCHOLAR (Washington)
Am Sci
AMERICAN SCIENTIST (New Haven)
Am Sociol Rev
AMERICAN SOCIOLOGICAL REVIEW (New York)
Am Speech
AMERICAN SPEECH (New York)
Am Stud
AMERICAN STUDIES (Lawrence KS)
Am Surg
AMERICAN SURGEON (Philadelphia)
Am Zool
AMERICAN ZOOLOGIST (Utica)
AMB
AMB; REVISTA DA ASSOCIACAO MEDICA BRASILEIRA (Sao Paulo)
Ambix
AMBIX; THE JOURNAL OF THE SOCIETY FOR THE STUDY OF ALCHEMY AND EARLY CHEMISTRY (London)
Amerasia J
AMERASIA JOURNAL (Los Angeles)
Americas
AMERICAS (Washington)
Amerikastudien
AMERIKASTUDIEN/AMERICAN STUDIES (W Germany)
An Acad Port Hist
ANAIS DA ACADEMIA PORTUGUESA DA HISTORIA (Portugal)
An Antropol
ANALES DE ANTROPOLOGIA (Mexico)
An Hist
ANAIS DE HISTORIA (Brazil)
An Hist Antigua Mediev
ANALES DE HISTORIA ANTIGUA Y MEDIEVAL (Argentina)
An Inst Estud Madrilenos
ANALES DEL INSTITUTO DE ESTUDIOS MADRILENOS (Spain)
An Inst Hig Med Trop (Lisb)
ANAIS DO INSTITUTO DE HIGIENE E MEDICINA TROPICAL (Lisboa)
An Med Cir
ANALES DE MEDICINA Y CIRUGIA (Barcelona)
An Otorrinolaringol Ibero Am
ANALES OTORRINOLARINGOLOGICOS IBERO-AMERICANOS (Barcelona)
An R Acad Farm (Madr)
ANALES DE LA REAL ACADEMIA DE FARMACIA (Madrid)
An R Acad Med Cir Cadiz
ANALES DE LA REAL ACADEMIA DE MEDICINA Y CIRUGIA DE CADIZ (Spain)
An R Acad Nac Med (Madr)
ANALES DE LA REAL ACADEMIA NACIONAL DE MEDICINA (Madrid)
An Soc Mex Hist Cienc Tec
ANALES DE LA SOCIEDAD MEXICANA DE HISTORIA DE CIENCIA Y TECHNOLOGIA
An Univ Bucur Istor
ANALELE UNIVERSITATII BUCURESTI; ISTORIE (Romania)
ANA Publ
AMERICAN NURSES ASSOCIATION PUBLICATIONS (Kansas City, MO)
Anaesth Intensive Care
ANAESTHESIA AND INTENSIVE CARE (Paddington NSW)
Anaesthesia
ANAESTHESIA (London)
Anal Chem
ANALYTICAL CHEMISTRY (Washington)
Anal Quant Cytol
ANALYTICAL AND QUANTITATIVE CYTOLOGY (St Louis)
Anat Anz
ANATOMISCHER ANZEIGER (Jena)
Anat Clin
ANATOMIA CLINICA (Berlin)
Anat Histol Embryol
ANATOMIA, HISTOLOGIA, EMBRYOLOGIA (Berlin)
Anat Rec
ANATOMICAL Record (New York)
Andrologia
ANDROLOGIA (Berlin)
Anesteziol Reanimatol
ANESTEZIOLOGIIA I REANIMATOLOGIIA (Moskva)
Aneath Analg
ANESTHESIA AND ANALGESIA (New York)
Aneath Prog
ANESTHESIA PROGRESS (Wellesley MA)
Anesthesiology
ANESTHESIOLOGY (Philadelphia)
Angew Parasitol
ANGEWANDTE PARASITOLOGIE (Jena)
Angiology
ANGIOLOGY (Great Neck NY)
Angle Orthod
ANGLE ORTHODONTIST (Appleton WI)
Anglican Theol Rev
ANGLICAN THEOLOGICAL REVIEW (Gt Brit)
Ann Acad Med Singapore
ANNALS OF THE ACADEMY OF MEDICINE, SINGAPORE (Singapore)
Ann Acad Med Stetin

ANNALES ACADEMIAE MEDICAE STETINENSIS (Warszawa)
Ann Allergy
ANNALS OF ALLERGY (Bloomington MN)
Ann Am Acad Polit Soc Sci
ANNALS OF THE AMERICAN ACADEMY OF POLITICAL AND SOCIAL SCIENCE (US)
Ann Anesthesiol Fr
ANNALES DE L'ANESTHESIOLOGIE FRANCAISE (Paris)
Ann Assoc Am Geogr
ANNALS OF THE ASSOCIATION OF AMERICAN GEOGRAPHERS (US)
Ann Biomed Eng
ANNALS OF BIOMEDICAL ENGINEERING (New York)
Ann Bretagne
ANNALES DE BRETAGNE ET DES PAYS DE L'OUEST (France)
Ann Cardiol Angeiol (Paris)
ANNALES DE CARDIOLOGIE ET D'ANGEIOLOGIE (Paris)
Ann Cerc Archeol Enghien
ANNALES DU CERCLE ARCHEOLOGIQUE D'ENGHIEN
Ann Cerc Archeol Mons
ANNALES DU CERCLE ARCHEOLOGIQUE DE MONS
Ann Chir
ANNALES DE CHIRURGIE (Paris)
Ann Chir Gynaecol
ANNALES CHIRURGIAE ET GYNAECOLOGIAE (Helsinki)
Ann Chir Plast
ANNALES DE CHIRURGIE PLASTIQUE (Paris)
Ann Chir Plast Esthet
ANNALES DE CHIRURGIE PLASTIQUE ET ESTHETIQUE (Paris)
Ann Clin Lab Sci
ANNALS OF CLINICAL AND LABORATORY SCIENCE (Philadelphia)
Ann Demogr Hist (Paris)
ANNALES DE DEMOGRAPHIE HISTORIQUE (Paris)
Ann Dermatol Venereol
ANNALES DE DERMATOLOGIE ET DE VENEREOLOGIE (Paris)
Ann Econ Soc Civilis
ANNALES ECONOMIE SOCIETE CIVILISATION (Paris)
Ann Emerg Med
ANNALS OF EMERGENCY MEDICINE (Dallas TX)
Ann Est
ANNALES DE L'EST (France)
Ann Frond Luigi Einaudi
ANNALI DELLA FONDAZIONE LUIGI EINAUDI (Italy)
Ann Fr Anesth Reanim
ANNALES FRANCAISES D'ANESTHESIE ET DE REANIMATION (Paris)
Ann Georg
ANNALES DE GEOGRAPHIE (France)
Ann Hist Comput
ANNALS OF THE HISTORY OF COMPUTING (Arlington VA)
Ann Hist Mantois
ANNALES HISTORIQUES DU MANTOIS (Mantes-la-Jolie, France)
Ann Hist Revolut Fr
ANNALES HISTORIQUES DE LA REVOLUTION FRANCAISE (France)
Ann Hum Biol
ANNALS OF HUMAN BIOLOGY (London)
Ann Immunol Hung
ANNALES IMMUNOLOGIAE HUNGARICAE (Budapest)
Ann Inst Archeol Luxemb
ANNALES DE L'INSTITUT ARCHEOLOGIQUE DU LUXEMBOURG (Luxembourg)
Ann Intern Med
ANNALS OF INTERNAL MEDICINE (Philadelphia)
Ann Iowa
ANNALS OF IOWA (Des Moines)
Ann Inst Giangiacomo Feltrinelli
ANNALI DELL'ISTITUTO GIANGIACOMO FELTRINELLI (Italy)
Ann Ist Mus Stor Sci Fir
ANNALI DELL'ISTITUTO E MUSEO DI STORIA DELLA SCIENZA DI FIRENZE (Italy)
Ann Ist Stor Italo-Ger
ANNALI ISTITUTO STORICO ITALO-GERMANICO (Trento)
Ann Ist Super Sanita
ANNALI DELL'ISTITUTO SUPERIORE DI SANITA (Roma)
Ann Med Interne (Paris)
ANNALES DE MEDECINE INTERNE (Paris)
Ann Med Nancy
ANNALES MEDICALES DE NANCY (Paris)
Ann Med Psychol (Paris)
ANNALES MEDICO-PSYCHOLOGIQUES (Paris)
Ann Midi
ANNALES DU MIDI (France)
Ann Mus Goulandris
ANNALES—MUSEI GOULANDRIS
Ann Neurol
ANNALS OF NEUROLOGY (Boston)
Ann Normandie
ANNALES DE NORMANDIE (France)
Ann NY Acad Sci
ANNALS OF THE NEW YORK ACADEMY OF SCIENCES (New York)
Ann Occup Hyg
ANNALS OF OCCUPATIONAL HYGIENE (Oxford)
Ann Ophthalmol

ANNALS OF OPHTHALMOLOGY (Harvard MA)
Ann Osp Maria Vittoria Torino
ANNALI DELL'OSPEDALE MARIA VITTORIA DI TORINO (Torino)
Ann Otol Rhinol Laryngol
ANNALS OF OTOLOGY, RHINOLOGY AND LARYNGOLOGY (St Louis)
Ann Otol Rhinol Laryngol [Suppl]
ANNALS OF OTOLOGY, RHINOLOGY AND LARYNGOLOGY, SUPPLEMENT (St. Louis)
Ann Pathol
ANNALES DE PATHOLOGIE (Paris)
Ann Pediatr (Paris)
ANNALES DE PEDIATRIE (Paris)
Ann Plast Surg
ANNALS OF PLASTIC SURGERY (Boston)
Ann R Australas Coll Dent Surg
ANNALS OF THE ROYAL AUSTRALASIAN COLLEGE OF DENTAL SURGEONS (Sydney)
Ann R Coll Physicians Surg Can
ANNALS OF THE ROYAL COLLEGE OF PHYSICIANS AND SURGEONS OF CANADA (Ottawa)
Ann R Coll Surg Engl
ANNALS OF THE ROYAL COLLEGE OF SURGEONS OF ENGLAND (London)
Ann Rheum Dis
ANNALS OF THE RHEUMATIC DISEASES (London)
Ann Sc Norm Super Pisa
ANNALI DELLA SCUOLA NORMALE SUPERIORE DI PISA (Pisa)
Ann Sci
ANNALS OF SCIENCE (London)
Ann Serv Antiq Egypte
ANNALES DU SERVICE DES ANTIQUITES DE L'EGYPTE (Egypt)
Ann Soc Belg Hist Hop
ANNALES DE LA SOCIETE BELGE D'HISTORIE DES HOPITAUX; ANNALEN VAN DE BELGISCHE VERENIGING VOOR HOSPITAAL-GESCHIEDENIS (Bruxelles)
Ann Soc Belg Med Trop
ANNALES DE LA SOCIETE BELGE DE MEDECINE TROPICALE (Antwerpen)
Ann Soc Emulation Bruges
ANNALES DE LA SOCIETE D'EMULATION DE BRUGES
Ann Surg
ANNALS OF SURGERY (Philadelphia)
Ann Trop Med Parasitol
ANNALS OF TROPICAL MEDICINE AND PARASITOLOGY (London)
Ann Univ Mariae Curie Sklodowska [Med]
ANNALES UNIVERSITATIS MARIAE CURIE-SKLODOWSKA. SECTIO D. MEDICINA (Lublin)
Ann Univ Sci Budap Rolando Eotvos Nominatae [Paedagog Psychol]
ANNALES UNIVERSITATIS SCIENTIARUM BUDAPESTINENSIS DE ROLANDO EOTVOS NOMINATAE. SECTIO PAEDAGOGICA ET PSYCHOLOGICA (Budapest)
Ann Wyo
ANNALS OF WYOMING (Cheyenne WY)
Annu Rev Anthropol
ANNUAL REVIEW OF ANTHROPOLOGY (Palo Alto CA)
Annu Rev Biochem
ANNUAL REVIEW OF BIOCHEMISTRY (Palo Alto CA)
Annu Rev Entomol
ANNUAL REVIEW OF ENTOMOLOGY (Palo Alto CA)
Annu Rev Genet
ANNUAL REVIEW OF GENETICS (Palo Alto CA)
Annu Rev Med
ANNUAL REVIEW OF MEDICINE (Palo Alto CA)
Annu Rev Microbiol
ANNUAL REVIEW OF MICROBIOLOGY (Palo Alto CA)
Annu Rev Neurosci
ANNUAL REVIEW OF NEUROSCIENCE (Palo Alto CA)
Annu Rev Nutr
ANNUAL REVIEW OF NUTRITION (Palo Alto CA)
Annu Rev Pharmacol Toxicol
ANNUAL REVIEW OF PHARMACOLOGY AND TOXICOLOGY (Palo Alto CA)
Annu Rev Physiol
ANNUAL REVIEW OF PHYSIOLOGY (Palo Alto CA)
Annu Rev Public Health
ANNUAL REVIEW OF PUBLIC HEALTH (Palo Alto CA)
Annu Soc Amis Vieux Strasb
ANNUAIRE DE SOCIETE DES AMIS DE VIEUX STRASBOURG (Strasbourg)
ANS
ANS. ADVANCES IN NURSING SCIENCE (Germantown MD)
Anthropol Anz
ANTHROPOLOGISCHER ANZEIGER (Stuttgart)
Anthropologica
ANTHROPOLOGICA (Canada)
Antibiotiki
ANTIBIOTIKI (Moskva)
Antike Welt
ANTIKE WELT; ZEITSCHRIFT FUR ARCHAEOLOGIE UND KULTURGESCHICHTE (Switzerland)
Antioch Rev
ANTIOCH REVIEW (US)
Antiq Class
L'ANTIQUITE CLASSIQUE (Belgium)
Antiquity
ANTIQUITY. A QUARTERLY REVIEW OF ARCHEOLOGY (Gt Brit)
ANU Hist J

A.N.U. HISTORY JOURNAL (Australia)
Anz Altertumswiss
ANZEIGER FUR DIE ALTERTUMSWISSENSCHAFT (Austria)
Anz Philol Hist Kl Osterr Akad Wiss
ANZEIGER DER PHILOLOGISCHEN-HISTORISCHEN KLASSE DER OSTERREICHISCHEN AKADEMIE DER WISSENSCHAFTEN (Austria)
Anzhes J
ANZHES JOURNAL; JOURNAL OF THE AUSTRALIAN AND NEW ZEALAND HISTORY OF EDUCATION SOCIETY (Australia)
AORN J
AORN JOURNAL (Denver CO)
Apeiron
APEIRON (Australia)
Apex
APEX (London)
Apoth J
APOTHEKER JOURNAL (MONATSMAGAZIN AUS WISSENSCHAFT UND PRAXIS)
Appetite
APPETITE (London)
Appl Neurophysiol
APPLIED NEUROPHYSIOLOGY (Basel)
Appl Res Ment Retard
APPLIED RESEARCH IN MENTAL RETARDATION (New York)
Apuntes Med Deportiva
APUNTES DE MEDICINA DEPORTIVA (Spain)
Arab Stud Q
ARAB STUDIES QUARTERLY (US)
Arabica
ARABICA (Netherlands)
Aramco World Mag
ARAMCO WORLD MAGAZINE (New York)
Arbeitsmed Praventive Gesundheitspolitik
ARBEITSMEDIZIN UND PRAVENTIVE GESUNDHEITSPOLITIK
Arbetarrorel Arsb
ARBETARRORELSENS ARSBOK (Sweden)
Arbor
ARBOR (Spain)
Arch Belg
ARCHIVES BELGES (Bruxelles)
Arch Belg Med Soc
ARCHIVES BELGES DE MEDICINE SOCIALE HYGIENE MEDECINE DU TRAVAIL ET MEDECINE LEGAL (Bruxelles)
Arch Biol (Liege)
ARCHIVES DE BIOLOGIE (Liege)
Arch Cas
ARCHIVNI CASOPIS (Czechoslovakia)
Arch Chir Neerl
ARCHIVUM CHIRURGICUM NEERLANDICUM (Wageningen)
Arch Dermatol
ARCHIVES OF DERMATOLOGY (Chicago)
Arch Dermatol Res
ARCHIVES OF DERMATOLOGICAL RESEARCH (Berlin)
Arch Dis Child
ARCHIVES OF DISEASE IN CHILDHOOD (London)
Arch Environ Health
ARCHIVES OF ENVIRONMENTAL HEALTH (Washington)
Arch Esp Urol
ARCHIVOS ESPANOLES DE UROLOGIA (Madrid)
Arch Fisiol
ARCHIVO DI FISIOLOGIA (Firenze)
Arch Fr Pediatr
ARCHIVES FRANCAISES DE PEDIATRIE (Paris)
Arch Franciscanum Hist
ARCHIVUM FRANCISCANUM HISTORICUM (Italy)
Arch Gen Psychiatry
ARCHIVES OF GENERAL PSYCHIATRY (Chicago)
Arch Gesch Buchwes
ARCHIV FUR GESCHICHTE DES BUCHWESENS
Arch Gesch Oberfranken
ARCHIV FUR DIE GESCHICHTE VON OBERFRANKEN
Arch Gynecol
ARCHIVES OF GYNECOLOGY (Munchen)
Arch Hist Doctrinale Litt Moyen Age
ARCHIVES D'HISTOIRE DOCTRINALE ET LITTERAIRE DU MOYEN AGE (Paris)
Arch Hist Exact Sci
ARCHIVE FOR HISTORY OF EXACT SCIENCES (Berlin)
Arch Hist Med (Warsz)
ARCHIWUM HISTORII MEDYCYNY (Warszawa)
Arch Hist Med Port
ARCHIVOS DE HISTORIA DA MEDICINA PORTUGUEZA (Oporto)
Arch Hyg
ARCHEIA HYGIENES (Athens)
Arch Iberoam
ARCHIVO IBERO-AMERICANO (Spain)
Arch Inst Cardiol Mex
ARCHIVOS DEL INSTITUTO DE CARDIOLOGIA DE MEXICO (Mexico)
Arch Inst Pasteur Madagascar
ARCHIVES DE L'INSTITUT PASTEUR DE MADAGASCAR (Tananarive)
Arch Inst Pasteur Tunis
ARCHIVES DE L'INSTITUT PASTEUR DE TUNIS (Tunis)
Arch Int Hist Idees
ARCHIVES INTERNATIONALES D'HISTOIRE DES IDEES (Netherlands)
Arch Int Hist Sci (Paris)
ARCHIVES INTERNATIONALES D'HISTOIRE DES SCIENCES (Paris)
Arch Int Physiol Biochim
ARCHIVES INTERNATIONALES DE PHYSIOL-

OGIE ET DE BIOCHIMIE (Liege)
Arch Intern Med
ARCHIVES OF INTERNAL MEDICINE (Chicago)
Arch Invest Med (Mex)
ARCHIVOS DE INVESTIGACION MEDICA (Mexico)
Arch Ital Anat Embriol
ARCHIVIO ITALIANO DI ANATOMIA E DI EMBRIOLOGIA (Firenze)
Arch Kriminol
ARCHIV FUR KRIMINOLOGIE (Lubeck)
Arch Kulturgesch
ARCHIV FUR KULTURGESCHICHTE (Cologne)
Arch Mal Coeur
ARCHIVES DES MALADIES DU COEUR ET DES VAISSEAUX (Paris)
Arch Med Normandie
ARCHIVES MEDICALES DE NORMANDIE (Le Havre)
Arch Mittelrheinischen Kirchengesch
ARCHIV DER MITTELRHEINISCHEN KIRCHENGESCHICHTE (W Germany)
Arch Monaldi
ARCHIVO MONDALDI PER LA TISIOLOGIA E LE MALATTIE DELL'APPARATO RESPIRATORIO (Napoli)
Arch Nat Hist
ARCHIVES OF NATURAL HISTORY (London)
Arch Neurobiol (Madr)
ARCHIVOS DE NEUROBIOLOGIA (Madrid)
Arch Neurol
ARCHIVES OF NEUROLOGY (Chicago)
Arch Ophthalmol
ARCHIVES OF OPHTHALMOLOGY (New York)
Arch Oral Biol
ARCHIVES OF ORAL BIOLOGY (Oxford)
Arch Otolaryngol
ARCHIVES OF OTOLARYNGOLOGY (Chicago)
Arch Otorhinolaryngol
ARCHIVES OF OTO-RHINO-LARYNGOLOGY (Berlin)
Arch Papyrusforsch
ARCHIV FUR PAPYRUSFORSCHUNG
Arch Pathol Lab Med
ARCHIVES OF PATHOLOGY AND LABORATORY MEDICINE (Chicago)
Arch Phys Med Rehabil
ARCHIVES OF PHYSICAL MEDICINE AND REHABILITATION (Chicago)
Arch Psychiatr Nervenkr
ARCHIV FUR PSYCHIATRIE UND NERVENKRANKHEITEN VEREINIGT MIT ZEITSCHRIFT FUR DIE GESAMTE NEUROLOGIE UND PSYCHIATRIE (Berlin)
Arch Psychol (Frankf)
ARCHIV FUR PSYCHOLOGIE (Frankfurt am Main)
Arch Roum Pathol Exp Microbiol
ARCHIVES ROUMAINES DE PATHOLOGIE EXPERIMENTALE ET DE MICROBIOLOGIE (Bucuresti)
Arch Sci
ARCHIVES DES SCIENCES (Geneva)
Arch Sci Biol (Bologna)
ARCHIVIO DI SCIENZE BIOLOGICHE (Bologna)
Arch Sozialgesch
ARCHIV FUR SOZIALGESCHICHTE (Bonn)
Arch Stor Ital
ARCHIVIO STORICO ITALIANO (Italy)
Arch Stor Prov Napol
ARCHIVIO STORICO PER LE PROVINCIA NAPOLETANE (Italy)
Arch Stor Prov Parmensi
ARCHIVIO STORICO PER LE PROVINCIA PARMENSI (Italy)
Arch Stor Pugliese
ARCHIVO STORICO PUBLIESE (Italy)
Arch Stor Sicil
ARCHIVIO STORICO SICILIANO (Italy)
Arch Surg
ARCHIVES OF SURGERY (Chicago)
Archaeol Aeliana
ARCHAEOLOGIA AELIANA (Northumberland Eng)
Archaeol Cantiana
ARCHAEOLOGIA CANTIANA (Kent)
Archaeol Korrespbl
ARCHAEOLOGISCHES KORRESPONDENZBLATT (Mainz)
Archaeology
ARCHAEOLOGY (Marrinsville NJ)
Archeologia
ARCHEOLOGIA: L'ARCHEOLOGIE DANS LE MONDE LE TOUT CE QUI CONCERNE LES RECHERCHES HISTORIQUES, ARTISTIQUES ET SCIENTIFIQUES SUR TERRE ET DANS LES MERS
Archiginnasio (Italy)
ARCHIGINNASIO (Italy)
Archivaria
ARCHIVARIA (Ottawa)
Arethusa
ARETHUSA (Buffalo NY)
Arh Hig Rada Toksikol
ARHIV ZA HIGIJENU RADA I TOKSIKOLOGIJU (Zagreb)
Arh Vjesn
ARHIVISKI VJESNIK (Yugoslavia)
Ariz Med
ARIZONA MEDICINE (Phoenix AZ)
Ariz West
ARIZONA AND THE WEST; A QUARTERLY JOURNAL OF HISTORY (Tucson)
Arkansas Archeol
ARKANSAS ARCHEOLOGIST (Fayetteville AR)
Arkansas Hist Q
ARKANSAS HISTORICAL QUARTERLY (Fayetteville AR)
Arkh Anat Gistol Embriol

ARKHIV ANATOMII, GISTOLOGII I EMBRIOLOGII (Leningrad)
Arkh Patol
ARKHIV PATOLOGII (Moskva)
Armed Forces Soc
ARMED FORCES AND SOCIETY (Chicago)
Army Q Def J
ARMY QUARTERLY AND DEFENSE JOURNAL (Gt Brit)
Arq Anat Antropol
ARQUIVO D'ANATOMICA ANTROPOLOGIA (Brasil)
Arq Neuropsiquiatr
ARQUIVOS DE NEURO-PSIQUIATRIA (Sao Paulo)
Ars Pharm
ARS PHARMACEUTICA (Granada)
Art Am
ART IN AMERICA (New York)
Arthritis Rheum
ARTHRITIS AND RHEUMATISM (Atlanta GA)
Artif Organs
ARTIFICIAL ORGANS (Cleveland OH)
Arts Auto
ARTS EN AUTO (Netherlands)
Arv
ARV (Sweden)
Arzneimittelforsch
ARZNEIMITTEL-FORSCHUNG (Aulendorf)
Arzt Christ
ARZT UND CHRIST (Salzburg)
Arztebl Baden Wurttemberg
ARZTEBLATT BADEN-WURTTEMBERG (Stuttgart)
Arztl Fortbild
ARZTLICHE FORTBILDUNG (Stuttgart)
Arztl Jugendkd
ARZTLICHE JUGENDKUNDE (Lepipzig)
Ascania
ASCANIA
Asclepio
ASCLEPIO; ARCHIVO IBEROAMERICANO DE HISTORIA DE LA MEDICINA Y ANTROPOLOGIA MEDICA (Madrid)
ASDC J Dent Child
ASDC JOURNAL OF DENTISTRY FOR CHILDREN (Chicago)
ASHA
ASHA (Washington)
Asian Folkl Stud
ASIAN FOLKLORE STUDIES
Asian Profile
ASIAN PROFILE (Hong Kong)
Asiat Forsch
ASIATISCHE FORSCHUNGEN (Wiesbaden)
Assoc Food Drug Off Q Bull
ASSOCIATION OF FOOD AND DRUG OFFICIALS QUARTERLY BULLETIN (Littleton CO)
Atenea (Puerto Rico)
ATENEA (Puerto Rico)
Atlantida
ATLANTIDA (Spain)
Atlantis
ATLANTIS (Canada)
Atti Accad Sci 1st Bologna
ATTI ACCADEMIA DE SCIENZE DELL'ISTITUTO DI BOLOGNA (Italy)
AUAA J
AUAA JOURNAL (Portland OR)
Audiology
AUDIOLOGY (Basel)
Ausgrab Funde
AUSGRABUNGEN UND FUNDE. NACHRICHTENBLATT FUR VOR-UND FRUHGESCHICHTE (Berlin)
Aust Agder Arv
AUST-AGDER ARV; ARBOK FOR A-AGDER MUSEET (Arendal)
Aust Dent J
AUSTRALIAN DENTAL JOURNAL (Sydney)
Aust Fam Physician
AUSTRALIAN FAMILY PHYSICIAN (Sydney)
Aust J Fr Stud
AUSTRALIAN JOURNAL OF FRENCH STUDIES (Melbourne)
Aust J Ophthalmol
AUSTRALIAN JOURNAL OF OPHTHALMOLOGY (Sydney)
Aust J Polit Hist
AUSTRALIAN JOURNAL OF POLITICS AND HISTORY (Australia)
Aust Libr J
AUSTRALIAN LIBRARY JOURNAL (Australia)
Aust Nurses J
AUSTRALIAN NURSES JOURNAL (West Perth)
Aust NZ J Med
AUSTRALIAN AND NEW ZEALAND JOURNAL OF MEDICINE (Sydney)
Aust NZ J Obstet Gynaecol
AUSTRALIAN AND NEW ZEALAND JOURNAL AND OBSTETRICS AND GYNAECOLOGY (Melbourne)
Aust NZ J Psychiatry
AUSTRALIAN AND NEW ZEALAND JOURNAL OF PSYCHIATRY (New South Wales)
Aust NZ J Sociol
AUSTRALIAN AND NEW ZEALAND JOURNAL OF SOCIOLOGY (Australia)
Aust NZ J Surg
AUSTRALIAN AND NEW ZEALAND JOURNAL OF SURGERY (Melbourne)
Aust Paediatr J
AUSTRALIAN PAEDIATRIC JOURNAL (Melbourne)
Aust Vet J
AUSTRALIAN VETERINARY JOURNAL (New South Wales)
Australas J Dermatol

AUSTRALASIAN JOURNAL OF DERMATOLOGY (New South Wales)
Australas Nurses J
AUSTRALASIAN NURSES JOURNAL (Port Adelaide)
Australas Radiol
AUSTRALASIAN RADIOLOGY (Sydney)
Auxiliaire
AUXILIAIRE (Montreal)
Avian Dis
AVIAN DISEASES (Kennett Square PA)
Aviat Space Environ Med
AVIATION, SPACE AND ENVIRONMENTAL MEDICINE (St Paul)
Aziia Afr Segodnia
AZIIA I AFRKA SEGODNIA (USSR)
Aztlan
AZTLAN (US)

—B—

Bar Berl
DER BAR VON BERLIN (Berlin)
Baptist Hist Heritage
BAPTIST HISTORY AND HERITAGE (Nashville TN)
Basic Life Sci
BASIC LIFE SCIENCES (New York)
Basler Z Gesch Altertumskd
BASLER ZEITSCHRIFT FUR GESCHICHTE UND ALTERTUMSKUNDE (Basel)
BC Stud
BRITISH COLUMBIA STUDIES (Canada)
Beaver
BEAVER MAGAZINE OF THE NORTH (Canada)
Behav Genet
BEHAVIOR GENETICS (New York)
Behav Res Ther
BEHAVIOR RESEARCH AND THERAPY (Oxford)
Behav Sci
BEHAVIORAL SCIENCE (Ann Arbor MI)
Behaviorism
BEHAVIORISM (Reno NV)
Beitr Gerichtl Med
BEITRAGE ZUR GERICHTLICHEN MEDIZIN (Vienna)
Beitr Gesch Pharm
BEITRAGE ZUR GESCHICHTE DER PHARMAZIE
Beitr Gesch Univ Erfurt
BEITRAGE ZUR GESCHICHTE DER UNIVERSITAT ERFURT (1392-1816) (Erfurt)
Beitr Heimatkd Stadt Kreis Nordhausen
BEITRAGE DER HEIMATKUNDE STADT KREIS NORDHAUSEN
Beitr Orthop Traumatol
BEITRAGE ZUR ORTHOPADIE UND TRAUMATOLOGIE (Berlin)
Beitr Wurttemb Apothekengesch
BEITRAGE ZUR WURTTEMBERGISCHEN APOTHEKENGESCHICHTE (Stuttgart)
Belfagor
BELFAGOR (Italy)
Belg Tijdschr Tandheelkd
BELGISCH TIJDSCHRIFT VOOR TANDHEELKUNDE
Belizean Stud
BELIZEAN STUDIES (Belize)
Bell Turk Tarih Kurumu
BELLETEN TURK TARIH KURUMU (Ankara)
Belleten (Turk)
BELLETEN (Turkey)
Bengal Past Present
BENGAL PAST AND PRESENT (India)
Ber Wissenschaftsgesch
BERICHTE ZUR WISSENSCHAFTSGESCHICHTE (Wiesbaden)
Ber Zusammenkunft Dtsch Ophthalmol Ges
BERICHT UBER DIE ZUSAMMENKUNFT DER DEUTSCHEN OPHTHALMOLOGISCHEN GESSELSCHAFT (Munchen)
Berl Munch Tierarztl Wochenschr
BERLINER UND MUNCHENER TIERARZTLICHE WOCHENSCHRIFT (Berlin)
Berner Z Gesch Heimatkd
BERNER ZEITSCHRIFT FUR GESCHICHTE DER HEIMATKUNDE (Bern)
Bibl Ec Chartres
BIBLIOTHEQUE DE L'ECOLE DES CHARTRES (Geneva)
Bibl Hum Renaissance
BIBLIOTHEQUE D'HUMANISME ET RENAISSANCE (Geneva)
Bibl Nutr Dieta
BIBLIOTHECA NUTRITIO ET DIETA (Basel)
Bibl Psychiatr
BIBLIOTHECA PSYCHIATRICA (Basel)
Bibliofilia
BIBLIOFILIA; RIVISTA DI STORIA DEL LIBRO E DI BIBLIOGRAFIA (Firenze)
Bibliotheck
BIBLIOTHECK; A SCOTTISH JOURNAL OF BIBLIOGRAPHICAL AND APPLIED TOPICS (Aberdeen)
Biblos (Vienna)
BIBLOS; OSTERREICHISCHE ZEITSCHRIFT FUR BUCH- UND BIBLIOTHEKSWESEN, DOCUMENTATION, BIBLIOGRAPHIE UND BIBLIOPHILIE
Biekorf
BIEKORF
Bijdr Geschied Geneeskd
BIJDRAGEN TOT DE GESCHIEDENIS DER GENEESKUNDE (Belgium)
Biochem Pharmacol
BIOCHEMICAL PHARMACOLOGY (Oxford)
Biochem Soc Trans
BIOCHEMICAL SOCIETY TRANSACTIONS (London)

Bioelectromagnetics
BIOELECTROMAGNETICS (New York)
Biofeedback Self Regul
BIOFEEDBACK AND SELF REGULATION (New York)
Biogr Mem Fellows R Soc
BIOGRAPHICAL MEMOIRS OF FELLOWS OF THE ROYAL SOCIETY (London)
Biogr Mem Natl Acad Sci
BIOGRAPHICAL MEMOIRS; NATIONAL ACADEMY OF SCIENCES OF THE UNITED STATES OF AMERICA (New York)
Biography
BIOGRAPHY (Honolulu HI)
Biol Bull Acad Sci USSR
BIOLOGY BULLETIN OF THE ACADEMY OF SCIENCES OF THE USSR (New York)
Biol J Linn Soc Lond
BIOLOGICAL JOURNAL OF THE LINNEAN SOCIETY OF LONDON (London)
Biol Nauki
BIOLOGICHESKIE NAUKI (Minsk)
Biol Psychiatry
BIOLOGICAL PSYCHIATRY (New York)
Biomaterials
BIOMATERIALS (Guilford)
Biomed Mass Spectrom
BIOMEDICAL MASS SPECTROMETRY (London)
Biomed Pharmacother
BIOMEDICINE AND PHARMACOTHERAPY (Paris)
Biomed Tech (Berlin)
BIOMEDIZINISCHE TECHNIK (Berlin)
Biometrics
BIOMETRICS (Washington)
Biorheology
BIORHEOLOGY (Oxford)
Biosci Rep
BIOSCIENCE REPORTS (London)
Biosystems
BIO SYSTEMS (Amsterdam)
Birth Defects
BIRTH DEFECTS ORIGINAL ARTICLE SERIES (New York)
Birth Fam J
BIRTH AND THE FAMILY JOURNAL (Berkeley)
Biul Bibl Jagiellon
BIULETYN-BIBLIOTEKI JAGIELLONSKIEJ (Cracow)
Biu Zydowskiego Inst Hist Pol
BIULETYN ZYDOWSKIEGO INSTYTUTU HISTROYCZNEGO (Warszawa)
Biull Espk Biol Med
BIULLETEN EKSPERIMENTALNOI BIOLOGI I MEDITSINY (Moskva)
Bl Dtsch Int Polit
BLATTER FUR DEUTSCHE INTERNATIONALE POLITIK (Cologne)
Black Scholar
BLACK SCHOLAR (Sausalito CA)
Blake Stud
BLAKE STUDIES (Normal IL)
Blood
BLOOD (New York)
Blood Cells
BLOOD CELLS (Berlin)
Blut
BLUT (Berlin)
Bodleian Libr Rec
BODLEIAN LIBRARY RECORD (Gt Brit)
Bogens Verden
BOGENS VERDEN (Copenhagen)
Bohemia Jahrb Coll Caroninum
BOHEMIA; JAHRBUCH DES COLLEGIUM CARONINUM (Munchen)
Bol Acad Nac Hist (Argentina)
BOLETIN DE LA ACADEMIIA NACIONAL DE LA HISTORIA (Argentina)
Bol Acad Nac Hist (Caracas)
BOLETIN DE LA ACADEMIA NACIONAL DE LA HISTORIA, CARACAS (Caracas)
Bol Acad Nac Med B Aires
BOLETIN DE LA ACADEMIA NACIONAL DE MEDICINA DE BUENOS AIRES (Buenos Aires)
Bol Asoc Med PR
BOLETIN DE LA ASOCIACION MEDICA DE PUERTO RICO (San Juan)
Bol Cent Estud Siglo XVIII
BOLETIN DEL CENTRO DE ESTUDIOS DEL SIGLO XVIII (Ovido Spain)
Bol Col Prof Enferm PR
BOLETIN — COLEGIO DE PROFESIONALES DE LA ENFERMERIA DE PUERTO RICO (San Juan)
Bol Cult Bibliogr (Bogota)
BOLETIN CULTURAL Y BIBLIOGRAFICO (Bogota)
Bol Estud Latinoam Caribe
BOLETIN DE ESTUDIOS LATINOAMERIKANOS Y DEL CARIBE (Amsterdam)
Bol Estud Med Biol
BOLETIN DE ESTUDIOS MEDICOS Y BIOLOGICOS (Mexico)
Bol Hist Antig (Bogota)
BOLETIN DE HISTORIA Y ANTIGUIDADES (Bogota)
Bol Inf Dent (Madr)
BOLETIN DE INFORMACION DENTAL (Madrid)
Bol Inst Estud Asturianos
BOLETIN DEL INSTITUTO DE ESTUDIOS ASTURIANOS (Spain)
Bol Inst Invest Bibliogr
BOLETIN DEL INSTITUTO DE INVESTIGA-CIONES BIBLIOGRAFICAS (Mexico)
Bol Inst Sancho Sabio
BOLETIN DE LA INSTITUCION SANCHO EL SABIO (Spain)
Bol Med Hosp Infant Mex
BOLETIN MEDICO DEL HOSPITAL INFANTIL DE

MEXICO (Mexico City)
Bol of Sanit Panam
BOLETIN DE LA OFICINA SANITARIA PANAMERICANA (Washington)
Bol Real Soc Vascongada Amigos Pais
BOLETIN-REAL SOCIEDAD VASCONGADA DE LOS AMIGOS DEL PAIS (Spain)
Bol Serv Odontol Sanit (Porto Alegre)
BOLETIN DO SERVICO DE ODONTOLOGIA SANITARIA DA SECRETARIA DA SAUDE DO RIO GRANDE DO SUL
Bol Soc Castell Cult
BOLETIN DE LA SOCIEDAD CASTELLONENSE DE CULTURA (Madrid)
Bol Soc Esp Hist Farm
BOLETIN DE LA SOCIEDAD ESPANOLA DE HISTORIA DE LA FARMACIA (Madrid)
Bol Soc Mex Hist Filos Med
BOLETIN DE LA SOCIEDAD MEXICANA DE HISTORIA Y FILOSOFIA DE LA MEDICINA (Mexico)
Boll Soc Ital Biol Sper
BOLLETTINO — SOCIETA ITALIANA BIOLOGIA SPERIMENTALE (Napoli)
Boll Stor Bibliogr Subalpino
BOLLETIN STORICO-BIBLIOGRAFICO SUBALPINO (Torino)
Boll Stor Pistoiese
BOLLETTINO STORICO PISTOIESE (Italy)
Book Collect
BOOK COLLECTOR (London)
Bookman
BOOKMAN (Galveston TX)
Bot Mus Leafl Harv Univ
BOTANICAL MUSEUM LEAFLETS-HARVARD UNIVERSITY (Cambridge MA)
Botsw Notes Rec
BOTSWANA NOTES AND RECORDS (Botswana)
Br Army Rev
BRITISH ARMY REVIEW
Br Book News
BRITISH BOOK NEWS (London)
Br Dent J
BRITISH DENTAL JOURNAL (London)
Br Dent Surg Assist
BRITISH DENTAL SURGERY ASSISTANT (Blackpool)
Br Heart J
BRITISH HEART JOURNAL (London)
Br Hist Illus
BRITISH HISTORY ILLUSTRATED (Gr Brit)
Br J Addict
BRITISH JOURNAL OF ADDICTION (Edinburgh)
Br J Anaesth
BRITISH JOURNAL OF ANAESTHESIA (London)
Br J Audiol
BRITISH JOURNAL OF AUDIOLOGY (London)
Br J Cancer
BRITISH JOURNAL OF CANCER (London)
Br J Clin Pharmacol
BRITISH JOURNAL OF CLINICAL PHARMACOLOGY (London)
Br J Clin Pract
BRITISH JOURNAL OF CLINICAL PRACTICE (London)
Br J Dermatol
BRITISH JOURNAL OF DERMATOLOGY (Oxford)
Br J Dis Chest
BRITISH JOURNAL OF DISEASE OF THE CHEST (London)
Br J Disord Commun
BRITISH JOURNAL OF DISORDERS OF COMMUNICATION (London)
Br J Educ Psychol
BRITISH JOURNAL OF EDUCATIONAL PSYCHOLOGY (London)
Br J Educ Stud
BRITISH JOURNAL OF EDUCATIONAL STUDIES (Oxfordshire Eng)
Br J 18th-Cent Stud
BRITISH JOURNAL FOR EIGHTEENTH-CENTURY STUDIES (Hampshire Eng)
Br J Hist Sci
BRITISH JOURNAL FOR THE HISTORY OF SCIENCE (Buckinghamshire Eng)
Br J Hosp Med
BRITISH JOURNAL OF HOSPITAL MEDICINE (London)
Br J Ind Med
BRITISH JOURNAL OF INDUSTRIAL MEDICINE (London)
Br J Law Soc
BRITISH JOURNAL OF LAW AND SOCIETY (Gt Brit)
Br J Med Psychol
BRITISH JOURNAL OF MEDICAL PSYCHOLOGY (Letchworth Eng)
Br J Nutr
BRITISH JOURNAL OF NUTRITION (London)
Br J Obstet Gynaecol
BRITISH JOURNAL OF OBSTETRICS AND GYNAECOLOGY (Oxford)
Br J Ophthalmol
BRITISH JOURNAL OF OPHTHALMOLOGY (London)
Br J Pharm Pract
BRITISH JOURNAL OF PHARMACEUTICAL PRACTICE (London)
Br J Philos Sci
BRITISH JOURNAL FOR THE PHILOSOPHY OF SCIENCE (London/New York)
Br J Plast Surg
BRITISH JOURNAL OF PLASTIC SURGERY (Edinburg)
Br J Polit Sci
BRITISH JOURNAL OF POLITICAL SCIENCE (Gr

Brit)
Br J Psychiatry
BRITISH JOURNAL OF PSYCHIATRY (London)
Br J Radiol
BRITISH JOURNAL OF RADIOLOGY (London)
Br J Rheumatol
BRITISH JOURNAL OF RHEUMATOLOGY (London)
Br J Sociol
BRITISH JOURNAL OF SOCIOLOGY (London)
Br J Surg
BRITISH JOURNAL OF SURGERY (London)
Br J Urol
BRITISH JOURNAL OF UROLOGY (Edinburgh)
Br J Vener Dis
BRITISH JOURNAL OF VENEREAL DISEASES (London)
Br Libr J
BRITISH LIBRARY JOURNAL (London)
Br Med Bull
BRITISH MEDICAL BULLETIN (London)
Br Med J
BRITISH MEDICAL JOURNAL (London)
Br Med J [Clin Res]
BRITISH MEDICAL JOURNAL [CLINICAL RESEARCH ED.] (London)
Br Vet J
BRITISH VETERINARY JOURNAL (London)
Brabantse Folkl
DE DRABANTSE FOLKLORE (Bruxelles)
Brain Dev
BRAIN AND DEVELOPMENT (Tokyo)
Brain Lang
BRAIN AND LANGUAGE (New York)
Bratisl Lek Listy
BRATISLAVSKE LEKARSKE LISTY (Bratislava)
Brigham Young Univ Stud
BRIGHAM YOUNG UNIVERSITY STUDIES (Provo UT)
Bristol Med Chir J
BRISTOL MEDICO-CHIRURGICAL JOURNAL (Bristol)
BRITANNIA (London)
Bromley Local Hist
BROMLEY LOCAL HISTORY (Kent)
Buch Augenarzt
BUCHEREI DES AUGENARZTES (Stuttgart)
Bull Acad Chir Dent (Paris)
BULLETIN DE L'ACADEMIE DE CHIRURGIE DENTAIRE (Paris)
Bull Am Acad Psychiatry Law
BULLETIN OF THE AMERICAN COLLEGE OF PHYSICIANS (Philadelphia)
Bull Am Coll Surg
BULLETIN OF THE AMERICAN COLLEGE OF SURGEONS (Chicago)
Bull Am Soc Inf Sci
BULLETIN OF THE AMERICAN SOCIETY FOR INFORMATION SCIENCE (Washington)
Bull Am Soc Anat (Nancy)
BULLETIN DE L'ASSOCIATION DES ANATOMISTES (Nancy)
Bull Assoc Guillaume Bude
BULLETIN DE L'ASSOCIATION GUILLAUME BUDE (Paris)
Bull At Sci
THE BULLETIN OF THE ATOMIC SCIENTISTS (Chicago)
Bull Audiophonol
BULLETIN D'AUDIOPHONOLOGIE (Paris)
Bull Biol Fr Belg
BULLETIN BIOLOGIQUE DE LA FRANCE ET DE LA BELGIQUE (Paris)
Bull Br Assoc Orient
BULLETIN OF THE BRITISH ASSOCIATION OF ORIENTALISTS
Bull Cl Sci Acad R Belg
BULLETIN DE LA CLASSE DES SCIENCES; ACADEMIE ROYALE DE BELGIQUE (Bruxelles)
Bull Coll Lib Arts (Taiwan)
BULLETIN OF THE COLLEGE OF LIBERAL ARTS, NATIONAL TAIWAN UNIVERSITY (Taiwan)
Bull Etud Port Bres
BULLETIN DES ETUDES PORTUGAISES ET BRESILIENNES (Portugal)
Bull Etud Valeryennes
BULLETIN DES ETUDES VALERYENNES (Montpellier)
Bull Gloucester Cty Hist Soc
BULLETIN OF THE GLOUCESTER COUNTY HISTORICAL SOCIETY (Woodbury NJ)
Bull Group Int Rech Sci Stomatol Odontol
BULLETIN DU GROUPEMENT INTERNATIONAL POUR LA RECHERCHE SCIENTIFIQUE EN STOMATOLOGIE ET ODONTOLOGIE (Bruxelles)
Bull Hist Dent
BULLETIN-HISTORY OF EDUCATION SOCIETY (Gloucestershire Eng)
Bull Hist Med
BULLETIN OF THE HISTORY OF MEDICINE (Baltimore)
Bull Hist Sci Auvergne
BULLETIN HISTORIQUE ET SCIENTIFIQUE DE L'AUVERGNE (France)
Bull Indian Inst Hist Med (Hyderabad)
BULLETIN OF THE INDIAN INSTITUTE OF THE HISTORY OF MEDICINE (Hyderabad)
Bull Inf Soc Demogr Hist
BULLETIN D'INFORMATION DE LA SOCIETE DE DEMOGRAPHE HISTORIQUE (Paris)
Bull Inst Archeol Liegeois
BULLETIN DE L'INSTITUT ARCHEOLOGIQUE LIEGEOIS (Liege)
Bull Inst Egypte (Cairo)
BULLETIN DE L'INSTITUT D'EGYPTE (Cairo)
Bull Inst Ethnol Acad Sin

BULLETIN. INSTITUTE OF ETHNOLOGY. ACADEMIA SINICA (Taipei)
Bull Inst Hist Res
BULLETIN OF THE INSTITUTE OF HISTORICAL RESEARCH (London)
Bull Inst Marit Trop Medi Gdynia
BULLETIN OF THE INSTITUTE OF MARITIME AND TROPICAL MEDICINE IN GDYNIA (Warszawa)
Bull Inst Mod Hist Acad Sin
BULLETIN OF THE INSTITUTE OF MODERN HISTORY. ACADEMIA SINICA (Taiwan)
Bull Int Union Tuberc
BULLETIN OF THE INTERNATIONAL UNION AGAINST TUBERCULOSIS (Paris)
Bull Leo Beck Inst
BULLETIN DES LEO BECK INSTITUTS (Israel)
Bull Liaison Assoc Amis Mus Pharm Montp
BULLETIN DE LIAISON-ASSOCIATION DES AMIS DE LA MUSEE DE LA PHARMACIE MONTPELLIER (France)
Bull Med Libr Assoc
BULLETIN OF THE MEDICAL LIBRARY ASSOCIATION (Chicago)
Bull Mem Acad R Med Belg
BULLETIN ET MEMOIRES DE L'ACADEMIE ROYALE DE MEDECINE DE BELGIQUE (Bruxelles)
Bull Mem Soc Fr Ophtalmol
BULLETINS ET MEMOIRES DE LA SOCIETE FRANCAISE D'OPHTALMOLOGIE (Paris)
Bull Menniger Clin
BULLETIN OF THE MENNINGER CLINIC (Topeka KS)
Bull Mich Dent Hyg Assoc
BULLETIN OF THE MICHIGAN DENTAL HYGIENISTS ASSOCIATION (Ypsilanti MI)
Bull NY Acad Med
BULLETIN OF THE NEW YORK ACADEMY OF MEDICINE (New York)
Bull Ninth Dist Dent Soc
BULLETIN OF THE NINTH DISTRICT DENTAL SOCIETY (White Plains NY)
Bull Ordre Natl Pharm
BULLETIN DE L'ORDRE NATIONAL DES PHARMACIENS (Paris)
Bull Pan Am Health Organ
BULLETIN OF THE PAN AMERICAN HEALTH ORGANIZATION (Washington)
Bull Pharm
BULLETIN DE PHARMACIE (Bruxelles)
Bull Phila Cty Dent Soc
BULLETIN OF THE PHILADELPHIA COUNTY DENTAL SOCIETY (Philadelphia)
Bull Physiopathol Respir (Nancy)
BULLETIN DE PHYSIO-PATHOLOGIE RESPIRATOIRE (Nancy)
Bull Prosthet Res
BULLETIN OF PROSTHETICS RESEARCH (Washington)
Bull Res Humanit
BULLETIN OF RESEARCH IN THE HUMANITIES (US)
Bull Rheum Dis
BULLETIN ON RHEUMATIC DISEASES (New York)
Bull Sch Orient Afr Stud
BULLETIN OF THE SCHOOL OF ORIENTAL AND AFRICAN STUDIES, UNIVERSITY OF LONDON (London)
Bull Schweiz Akad Med Wiss
BULLETIN DER SCHWEIZERISCHEN AKADEMIE DER MEDIZINISCHEN WISSENSCHAFTEN (Basel)
Bull Seances Acad R Sci Outre Mer
BULLETIN DES SEANCES DE L'ACADEMIE ROYALE DES SCIENCES D'OUTRE-MER (Bruxelles)
Bull Sect Geogr Com Trav Hist Sci
BULLETIN-SECTION DE GEOGRAPHIE COMITE DES TRAVAUX HISTORIQUES ET SCIENTIFIQUES (France)
Bull Soc Amis Vieux St Germain
BULLETIN DE LA SOCIETE DES AMIS DU VIEUX ST-GERMAIN (France)
Bull Soc Antiq Ouest Mus Poitiers
BULLETIN DE LA SOCIETE ANTIQUAIRES DE L'OUEST ET DES MUSEES DE POITIERS (France)
Bull Soc Archeol Hist Limousin
BULLETIN-SOCIETE ARCHEOLOGIQUE, ET HISTORIQUE DU LIMOUSIN (France)
Bull Soc Belge Ophtalmol
BULLETIN DE LA SOCIETE DE BORDA (France)
Bull Soc Etud Oceaniennes
BULLETIN-SOCIETE DES ETUDES OCEANIENNES (Tahiti)
Bull Soc Etud Sci Aude
BULLETIN DE LA SOCIETE D'ETUDES SCIENTIFIQUES DE L'AUDE (France)
Bull Soc Fr Hist Hop
BULLETIN DE LA SOCIETE FRANCAISE D'HISTOIRE DES HOPITAUX (Paris)
Bull Soc Hist Mod
BULLETIN DE LA SOCIETE D'HISTOIRE MODERNE (Paris)
Bull Soc Hist Portestantisme Fr
BULLETIN DE LA SOCIETE DE L'HISTOIRE DU PROTESTANTISME FRANCAIS (Paris)
Bull Soc Hist Sci Deux Sevres
BULLETIN-SOCIETE HISTORIQUE ET SCIENTIFIQUE DES DEUX SEVRES (Niort)
Bull Soc Lett Sci Arts Correze
BULLETIN DE LA SOCIETE DES LETTRES, SCIENCE ET ARTS DE LA CORREZE
Bull Soc Ophtalmol Fr
BULLETIN DES SOCIETES D'OPHTALMOLOGIES DE FRANCE (Paris)
Bull Soc Pathol Exot Filiales

BULLETIN DE LA SOCIETE DE PATHOLOGIE EXOTIQUE ET DE SES FILIALES (Paris)
Bull Soc R Vieux Liege
BULLETIN DE LA SOCIETE ROYALE DE VIEUX LIEGE (Belgium)
Bull Soc Sci Med Grand Duche Luxemb
BULLETIN DE LA SOCIETE DES SCIENCES MEDICALES DU GRAND-DUCHE DE LUXEMBORG (Luxemborg)
Burgenl Heimatbl
BURGENLANDISCHE HEIMATBLATTER (Austria)
Burlington Mag
BURLINGTON MAGAZINE (US)
Bus Hist Rev
BUSINESS HISTORY REVIEW (Cambridge MA)
Butil Informatiu Circ Farm
BUTILETI INFORMATIU DE CIRCULAR FARMACEUTICA (Barcelona)
Bygone Kent
BYGONE KENT (Kent)
Byzantinische Forsch
BYZANTINISCHE FORSCHUNG
Byzantion
BYZANTION (Bruxelles)

—C—

C R Acad Sci [D] (Paris)
COMPTES RENDUS HEBDOMADAIRES DES SEANCES DE L'ACADEMIE DES SCIENCES D: SCIENCE NATURELLES (Paris)
C R Seances Acad Sci [III]
COMPTES RENDUS DES SEANCES DE L'ACADEMIE DES SCIENCES. SERIE III, SCIENCES DE LA VIE (Paris)
CA
CA; A CANCER JOURNAL FOR CLINICIANS (New York)
Cah Am Lat
CAHIERS DES AMERIQUES LATINES (Paris)
Cah Anthropol
CAHIERS D'ANTHROPOLOGIE (Paris)
Cah Biloque
LES CAHIERS DE LA BILOQUE (GHENT)
Cah Clio
CAHIERS DE CLIO (Liege)
Cah Dix
CAHIERS DES DIX
Cah Etud Afr
CAHIERS D'ETUDES AFRICAINES (France)
Cah Haut Marnais
LES CAHIERS HAUT-MARNAIS (France)
Cah Hist
CAHIERS D'HISTORIE (France)
Cah Hist Mond
CAHIERS D'HISTOIRE MONDIALE. JOURNAL OF WORLD HISTORY. CUADERNOS DE HISTORIA MUNDIAL (France)
Cah Hist Seconde Guerre Mond
CAHIER D'HISTOIRE DE LA SECONDE GUERRE MONDIALE (Belgium)
Cah Int Hist Econ Soc
CAHIERS INTERNATIONAUX D'HISTOIRE ECONOMIQUE ET SOCIALE (Napoli)
Cah Iroise
CAHIERS DE L'IROISE (France)
Cah Monde Russe Sovietique
CAHIERS DU MONDE RUSSE ET SOVIETIQUE (France)
Cah Rech Archit
CAHIERS DE LA RECHERCHE ARCHITECTURAL
Cah Relig Afr
CAHIERS DES RELIGIONS AFRICAINES (Congo)
Cah Sociol Demogr Med
CAHIERS DE SOCIOLOGIE ET DE DEMOGRAPHIE MEDICALES (Paris)
Cah Tunis
CAHIERS TUNISIE (Tunisia)
CAL
CAL; CERTIFIED AKERS LABORATORIES (Chicago)
Calcif Tissue Int
CALCIFIED TISSUE INTERNATIONAL (Berlin)
Calif Hist Soc Q
CALIFORNIA HISTORICAL SOCIETY QUARTERLY (San Francisco)
Calif Nurse
CALIFORNIA NURSE (San Francisco)
Can Am Slav Stud
CANADIAN ANAESTHETISTS SOCIETY JOURNAL (Toronto)
Can Cathol Hist Assoc Study Ses
CANADIAN CATHOLIC HISTORIC ASSOCIATION. STUDY SESSION/SOCIETE CANADIENNE D'HISTOIRE DE L'EGLISE CATHOLIQUE. SESSIONS D'ETUDE (Ottawa)
Can Dent Assoc J
CANADIAN DENTAL ASSOCIATION JOURNAL. JOURNAL DE L'ASSOCIATION DENTAIRE CANADIENNE (Ottawa)
Can Geogr
CANADIAN GEOGRAPHIC (Canada)
Can Hist Assoc Hist Pap
CANADIAN HISTORICAL ASSOCIATION. HISTORICAL PAPERS (Ottawa)
Can Hist Rev
CANADIAN HISTORIAL REVIEW (Toronto)
Can Hist Sites
CANADIAN HISTORIC SITES (Canada)
Can J Afr Stud
CANADIAN JOURNAL OF AFRICAN STUDIES (Ottawa)
Can J Biochem
CANADIAN JOURNAL OF BIOCHEMISTRY (Ottawa)
Can J Biochem Cell Biol

CANADIAN JOURNAL OF BIOCHEMISTRY AND CELL BIOLOGY (Ottawa)
Can J Econ Polit Sci
CANADIAN JOURNAL OF ECONOMICS AND POLITICAL SCIENCE
Can J Hist
CANADIAN JOURNAL OF HISTORY (Saskatoon)
Can J Hist Sport Phys Educ
CANADIAN JOURNAL OF HISTORY OF SPORT AND PHYSICAL EDUCATION (Windsor Ont)
Can J Hosp Pharm
CANADIAN JOURNAL OF HOSPITAL PHARMACY (Weston)
Can J Nuerol Sci
CANADIAN JOURNAL OF NEUROLOGICAL SCIENCES (Winnipeg)
Can J Physiol Pharmacol
CANADIAN JOURNAL OF PHYSIOLOGY AND PHARMACOLOGY (Ottawa)
Can J Psychiatr Nurs
CANADIAN JOURNAL OF PSYCHIATRIC NURSING (New Westminister BC)
Can J Psychiatry
CANADIAN JOURNAL OF PSYCHIATRY. REVUE CANADIENNE DE PSYCHIATRIE (Ottawa)
Can J Psychol
CANADIAN JOURNAL OF PSYCHOLOGY (Toronto)
Can J Public Health
CANADIAN JOURNAL OF PUBLIC HEALTH (Ottawa)
Can J Surg
CANADIAN JOURNAL OF SURGERY (Ottawa)
Can Labour
CANADIAN LABOUR (Canada)
Can Med Assoc J
CANADIAN MEDICAL ASSOCIATION JOURNAL (Ottawa)
Can Ment Health
CANADA MENTAL HEALTH (Ottawa)
Can Mong Rev
CANADA-MONGOLIA REVIEW (Canada)
Can Nurse
CANADIAN NURSE (Montreal)
Can Pharm J
CANADIAN PHARMACEUTICAL JOURNAL (Ottawa)
Can Public Adm
CANADIAN PUBLIC ADMINISTRATION (Canada)
Can Rev Am Stud
CANADIAN REVIEW OF AMERICAN STUDIES (Winnipeg)
Can Rev Sociol Anthropol
CANADIAN REVIEW OF SOCIOLOGY AND ANTHROPOLOGY (Canada)
Can Slavonic Pap
CANADIAN SLAVONIC PAPERS
Can Vet J
CANADIAN VETERINARY JOURNAL (Ottawa)
Cancer
CANCER (Philadelphia)
Cancer Nurs
CANCER NURSING (New York)
Cancer Res
CANCER RESEARCH (Baltimore)
Cancer Treat Rep
CANCER TREATMENT REPORTS (Bethesda MD)
Cancer Treatment Review
CANCER TREATMENT REVIEWS (London)
Cantium
CANTIUM (Kent Eng)
Cardiovasc Clin
CARDIOVASCULAR CLINICS (Philadelphia)
Cardiovascular Res Cent Bull
CARDIOVASCULAR RESEARCH CENTER BULLETIN (Houston)
Caries Res
CARIES RESEARCH (Basel)
Caring
CARING (Washington)
Carinthia
CARINTHIA MITTEILUNGEN DES GESCHICHTSVEREINES FUR KARNTEN (Austria)
Caritas
CARITAS (Dublin)
Carmarthensh Hist
CARMARTHENSHIRE HISTORIAN (Gt Brit)
Carol J Pharm
CAROLINA JOURNAL OF PHARMACY (Chapel Hill NC)
Cas Lek Cesk
CASOPIS LEKARU CESKYCH (Praha)
Cas Nar Muz
CASOPIS NARODNIHO MUZEA (Czechoslovakia)
Cas Zgodovino Narodop
CASOPIS ZA ZGODOVINO IN NARODOPISJE (Yugoslavia)
Cathol Hist Rev
CATHOLIC HISTORICAL REVIEW (Washington)
CDS Rev
CDS REVIEW; CHICAGO DENTAL SOCIETY (Chicago)
Cell Biol Int Rep
CELL BIOLOGY INTERNATIONAL REPORTS (London)
Cell Immunol
CELLULAR IMMUNOLOGY (New York)
Cell Mol Biol
CELLULAR AND MOLECULAR BIOLOGY (Elmsford NY)
Cent Afr J Med
CENTRAL AFRICAN JOURNAL OF MEDICINE (Rhodesia)

Cent Eur Hist
CENTER EUROPEAN HISTORY (Atlanta GA)
Cent Mag
CENTER MAGAZINE (Santa Barbara CA)
Centaurus
CENTAURUS (Copenhagen)
Centen Rev
CENTENNIAL REVIEW (E Lansing MI)
Centerpoint
CENTERPOINT (US)
Cephalalgia
CEPHALALGIA (Oslo)
CERON
CERON; CENTRO DE ESTUDIOS DE RECURSOS ODONTOLOGICOS PARA EL NINO (Caracas)
Cesk Dermatol
CESKOSLOVENSKA DERMATOLOGIE (Praha)
Cesk Epidemiol Mikrobiol Imunol
CESKOSLOVENSKA EPIDEMIOLOGIE, MIKROBIOLOGIE, IMMUNOLOGIE (Praha)
Cesk Farm
CESKOSLOVENSKA FARMACIE (Praha)
Cesk Fysiol
CESKOSLOVENSKA FYSIOLOGIE (Praha)
Cesk Gastroenterol Vyz
CESKOSLOVENSKA GASTROENTEROLOGIE A VYZIVA (Praha)
Cesk Gynekol
CESKOSLOVENSKA GYNEKOLOGIE (Praha)
Cesk Oftalmol
CESKOSLOVENSKA OFTALMOLOGIE (Praha)
Cesk Otolaryngol
CESKOSLOVENSKA OTOLARYNGOLOGIE (Praha)
Cesk Patol
CESKOSLOVENSKA PATOLOGIE (Praha)
Cesk Pediatr
CESKOSLOVENSKA PEDIATRIE (Praha)
Cesk Psychiatr
CESKOSLOVENSKA PSYCHIATRIE (Praha)
Cesk Radiol
CESKOSLOVENSKA RADIOLOGIE (Praha)
Cesk Stomatol
CESKOSLOVENSKA STOMATOLOGIE (Praha)
Cesk Zdrav
CESKOSLOVENSKE ZDRAVOTNICTVI (Praha)
Ceylon Med J
CEYLON MEDICAL JOURNAL (Colombo)
Ch'ing-Shih Wen-t'i
CH'ING-SHIH WEN-T'I (Washington)
Chaucer Rev
CHAUCER REVIEW (University Park PA)
Chesopiean
CHESOPIEAN (Norfolk VA)
Chest
CHEST (Park Ridge IL)
Chi Sheng Chung Hsueh Yu Chi Sheng Chung Ping Tsa Chih
CHI SHENG CHUNG HSUEH YU CHI SHENG CHUNG PING TSA CHIH (Shanghai)
Chic Hist
CHICAGO HISTORY (Chicago)
Chin Cult
CHINESE CULTURE (Taiwan)
Chin J Med Hist
CHINESE JOURNAL OF MEDICAL HISTORY See Chung Hua I Shih Tsa Chih
Chin Med J [Engl]
CHINESE MEDICAL JOURNAL (Peking)
China Q
CHINA QUARTERLY (London)
China Rep (India)
CHINA REPORT (India)
Chir Dent Fr
CHIRURGIEN-DENTISTE DE FRANCE (Paris)
Chir Narzadow Ruchu Ortop Pol
CHIRURGIA NARZADOW RUCHU I ORTOPEDIA POLSKA (Warszawa)
Chir Organi Mov
CHIRURGIA DEGLI ORGANI DI MOVIMENTO (Bologna)
Chir Plast
CHIRURGICA PLASTICA (Berlin)
Chiropr Hist
CHIROPRACTIC HISTORY (Baltimore)
Chirurg
CHIRURG (Berlin)
Chirurgie
CHIRURGIE (Paris)
Chron Egypte
CHRONIQUE D'EGYPTE (Bruxelles)
Chron Okla
CHRONICLES OF OKLAHOMA (Oklahoma City OK)
Chronicle
CHRONICLE; OMAHA DISTRICT DENTAL SOCIETY (Omaha)
Chung Hsi I Chieh Ho Tsa Chih
CHUNG HSI I CHIEH HO TSA CHIH, CHINESE JOURNAL OF INTEGRATED TRADITIONAL AND WESTERN MEDICINE (Beijing)
Chung Hua I Shih Tsa Chih
CHUNG-HUA I SHIH TSA CHIH. CHINESE JOURNAL OF MEDICAL HISTORY (Peking)
Chung Hua Liu Hsing Ping Hsueh Tsa Chih
CHUNG-HUA LIU HSING PING HSUEH TSA CHIH (Peking)
Chung I Tsa Chih
CHUNG I TSA CHIH (Peking)
Chung Kuo I Hsueh Ko Hsueh Yuan Hsueh Pao
CHUNG-KUO I HSUEH KO HSUEH YUAN HSUEH PAO (Peking)
Chung Yao Tung Pao
CHUNG YAO TUNG PAO (Peking)
Church Hist
CHURCH HISTORY (Wallingford PA)
Ciba Found Symp
CIBA FOUNDATION SYMPOSIUM (Amsterdam)

Cienc Habana Ser 9
CIENCIAS — HABANA-SERIE 9 ANTROPOLOGIA Y PREHISTORIA, CUBA
Cinci Hist Soc Bull
CINCINNATI HISTORICAL SOCIETY BULLETIN (Cincinnati OH)
Circ Farm
CIRCULAR FARMACEUTICA (Barcelona)
Circ Res
CIRCULATION RESEARCH (Dallas TX)
Circulation
CIRCULATION (Dallas TX)
Civ War Hist
CIVIL WAR HISTORY (Kent OH)
Civ War Times Illus
CIVIL WAR TIMES ILLUSTRATED (Marion OH)
CLAO J
CLAO JOURNAL (New Orleans LA)
Classical Antiq
CLASSICAL ANTIQUITY (US)
Classical Philol
CLASSICAL PHILOLOGY (Chicago)
CLASSICAL Q
CLASSICAL QUARTERLY (London)
Classical Rev
CLASSICAL REVIEW (London)
Cleft Palate J
CLEFT PALATE JOURNAL (Pittsburgh)
Cleve Clin Q
CLEVELAND CLINIC QUARTERLY (Cleveland OH)
Clin Allergy
CLINICAL ALLERGY (Oxford)
Clin Biochem
CLINICAL BIOCHEMISTRY (Toronto)
Clin Cardiol
CLINICAL CARDIOLOGY (New York)
Clin Chem
CLINICAL CHEMISTRY (Winston-Salem NC)
Clin Exp Dermatol
CLINICAL AND EXPERIMENTAL DERMATOLOGY (Oxford)
Clin Exp Dial Apheresis
CLINICAL AND EXPERIMENTAL DIALYSIS AND APHERESIS (New York)
Clin Exp Neurol
CLINICAL AND EXPERIMENTAL NEUROLOGY (New York)
Clin Haematol
CLINICS IN HAEMATOLOGY (London)
Clin Immunol Immunopathol
CLINICAL IMMUNOLOGY AND IMMUNOPATHOLOGY (New York)
Clin Invest Med
CLINICAL AND INVESTIGATIVE MEDICINE. MEDECINE CLINIQUE ET EXPERIMENTALE (Oxford)
Clin Neuropharmacol
CLINICAL NEUROPHARMACOLOGY (New York)
Clin Neurosurg
CLINICAL NEUROSURGERY (Baltimorc)
Clin Notes Respir Dis
CLINICAL NOTES ON RESPIRATORY DISEASES (New York)
Clin Oncol
CLINICAL ONCOLOGY (London)
Clin Orthop
CLINICAL ORTHOPAEDICS AND RELATED RESEARCH (Philadelphia)
Clin Otolaryngol
CLINICAL OTOLARYNGOLOGY (Oxford)
Clin Pediatr (Phila)
CLINICAL PEDIATRICS (Philadelphia)
Clin Pharmacol Ther
CLINICAL PHARMACOLOGY AND THERAPEUTICS (St Louis)
Clin Physiol
CLINICAL PHYSIOLOGY (Oxford)
Clin Plast Surg
CLINICS IN PLASTIC SURGERY (Philadelphia)
Clin Radiol
CLINICAL RADIOLOGY (Edinburgh)
Clin Rev Allergy
CLINICAL REVIEWS IN ALLERGY (New York)
Clin Sci
CLINICAL SCIENCE (London)
Clin Ter
CLINICA TERAPEUTICA (Roma)
Clio
CLIO (US)
Clio Med
CLIO MEDICA (Amsterdam)
Coeur Med Interne
COEUR ET MEDECINE INTERNE (Paris)
Colby Libr Q
COLBY LIBRARY QUARTERLY (Waterville ME)
Cold Spring Harbor Symp Quant Biol
COLD SPRING HARBOR SYMPOSIA ON QUANTITATIVE BIOLOGY
Colo Mag
COLORADO MAGAZINE (Denver CO)
Colo Med
COLORADO MEDICINE (Denver CO)
Colo Q
COLORADO QUARTERLY (Boulder CO)
Com J Mediev Renaiss Stud
COMITATUS. JOURNAL OF MEDIEVAL AND RENAISSANCE STUDIES (Los Angeles)
Commentary
COMMENTARY (New York)
Community Dent Oral Epidemiol
COMMUNITY DENTISTRY AND ORAL EPIDEMIOLOGY (Copenhagen)
Community Health Stud
COMMUNITY HEALTH STUDIES (Adelaide)
Community Med
COMMUNITY MEDICINE (Bristol)

Community Ment Health J
COMMUNITY MENTAL HEALTH JOURNAL (New York)
Comp Biochem Physiol
COMPARATIVE BIOCHEMISTRY AND PHYSIOLOGY (Oxford)
Comp Biochem Physiol [A]
COMPARATIVE BIOCHEMISTRY AND PHYSIOLOGY A: COMPARATIVE PHYSIOLOGY (Oxford)
Comp Biochem Physiol [B]
COMPARATIVE BIOCHEMISTRY AND PHYSIOLOGY B: COMPARATIVE BIOCHEMISTRY (Oxford)
Comp Biochem Physiol [C]
COMPARATIVE BIOCHEMISTRY AND PHYSIOLOGY C: COMPARATIVE PHARMACOLOGY AND TOXICOLOGY (Oxford)
Comp Immunol Microbiol Infect Dis
COMPARATIVE IMMUNOLOGY, MICROBIOLOGY AND INFECTIOUS DISEASES (Oxford)
Comp Pol
COMPARATIVE POLITICS (Chicago)
Comp Stud Soc Hist
COMPARATIVE STUDIES IN SOCIETY AND HISTORY (Gt Brit)
Compend Contin Educ Dent
COMPENDIUM OF CONTINUING EDUCATION IN DENTISTRY (Lawrenceville NJ)
Compr Psychiatry
COMPREHENSIVE PSYCHIATRY (New York)
Compr Ther
COMPREHENSIVE THERAPY (Harvard MA)
Comput Biomed Res
COMPUTERS IN BIOMEDICAL RESEARCH (New York)
Comput Hum
COMPUTERS AND THE HUMANITIES (Amsterdam)
Computertomographie
COMPUTERTOMOGRAPHIE (Stuttgart)
Comunita
COMUNITA (Italy)
Conf Estud Hist Organ Cienc
CONFERENCIAS Y ESTUDIOS DE HISTORIA Y ORGANIZACION DE LA CIENCIA (Cuba)
Confin Psychiatr
CONFINIA PSYCHIATRICA (Basel)
Congr Pres J Cap Stud
CONGRESS AND THE PRESIDENCY; A JOURNAL OF CAPITAL STUDIES (US)
Conn Med
CONNECTICUT MEDICINE (New Haven CT)
Connaiss Pays Occident
CONNAISSANCE DU PAYS D'OCCIDENT (Montpellier)
Consortium Revolut Eur 1750–1850 Proc
CONSORTIUM ON REVOLUTIONARY EUROPE 1750–1850;PROCEEDINGS (US)
Consum Health Perspect
CONSUMER HEALTH PERSPECTIVES (New York)
Consum Rep
CONSUMER REPORTS (Mount Vernon NY)
Contact Dermatitis
CONTACT DERMATITIS (COPENHAGEN)
Contact Intraocular Lens Med J
CONTACT AND INTRAOCULAR LENS MEDICAL JOURNAL (St Louis)
Contemp Anesth Pract
CONTEMPORARY ANESTHESIA PRACTICE (Philadelphia)
Contemp Fr Civiliz
CONTEMPORARY FRENCH CIVILIZATION (US)
Contemp Rev
CONTEMPORARY REVIEW (Gt Brit)
Contemp Surg
CONTEMPORARY SURGERY (New York)
Contin Pract
ON CONTINUING PRACTICE (Canada)
Continuum
CONTINUUM (New York)
Contraception
CONTRACEPTION (Los Altos CA)
Contrat Soc
CONTRAT SOCIAL (Paris)
Contrib Nephrol
CONTRIBUTIONS TO NEPHROLOGY (Basel)
Controlled Clin Trials
CONTROLLED CLINICAL TRIALS (New York)
Cor Vasa
COR ET VASA (Prague)
Cortex
CORTEX (Milan)
CRC Crit Rev Diagn Imaging
CRC CRITICAL REVIEWS IN DIAGNOSTIC IMAGING (Cleveland OH)
Crim Justice Hist
CRIMINAL JUSTICE HISTORY (New York)
Crisis
CRISIS (New York)
Crit Care Med
CRITICAL CARE MEDICINE (New York)
Crit Rev Biomed Eng
CRITICAL REVIEWS IN BIOMEDICAL ENGINEERING (Boca Raton FL)
Crit Stor
CRITICA STORICA (Firenze)
Cron Pompeiane
CRONACHE POMPEIANE (Napoli)
Cuad Am
CUADERNOS AMERICANOS (Mexico)
Cuad Aragon Hist Med Cienc [A]
CUADERNOS ARAGONESES DE HISTORIA DE LA MEDICINA Y DE LA CIENCIA. Ser. A (Monografias) (Spain)

Cuad Aragon Hist Med Cienc [B]
CUADERNOS ARAGONESES DE HISTORIA DE LA MEDICINA Y DE LA CIENCIA. Ser. B (Spain)
Cuad Estud Gallegos
CUADERNOS DE ESTUDIOS GALLEGOS (Spain)
Cuad Filos Let
CUADERNOS DE FILOSOFIA Y LETRAS (Colombia)
Cuad Hispanoam
CUADERNOS HISPANOAMERICANOS (Spain)
Cuad Invest Hist
CUADERNOS DE INVESTIGACION HISTORICA (Spain)
Cuatricenten San German
EL CUATRICENTENARIO DE SAN GERMAN (San German Puerto Rico)
Cuban Stud
CUBAN STUDIES (Pittsburgh PA)
Cult Dev
CULTURES ET DEVELOPPEMENT (Belgium)
Cult Med Psychiatry
CULTURE, MEDICINE AND PSYCHIATRY (Dordrecht)
Cult Sc
CULTURA E SCUOLA (Roma)
Curationis
CURATIONIS (Pretoria)
Curr Alcohol
CURRENTS IN ALCOHOLISM (New York)
Curr Anthropol
CURRENT ANTHROPOLOGY. A WORLD JOURNAL OF THE SCIENCES OF MAN
Curr Concepts Nutr
CURRENT CONCEPTS IN NUTRITION (New York)
Curr Hist
CURRENT HISTORY (Philadelphia)
Curr Probl Clin Biochem
CURRENT PROBLEMS IN CLINICAL BIOCHEMISTRY (Zurich)
Curr Probl Pediatr
CURRENT PROBLEMS IN PEDIATRICS (Chicago)
Curr Probl Surg
CURRENT PROBLEMS IN SURGERY (Chicago)
Curr Res Med Aromat Plant
CURRENT RESEARCH ON MEDICINAL AND AROMATIC PLANTS (Lucknow)
Curr Surg
CURRENT SURGERY (Philadelphia)
Curr Top Microbiol Immunol
CURRENT TOPICS IN MICROBIOLOGY AND IMMUNOLOGY (Berlin)
Cutis
CUTIS (New York)
Cylchgrawn Llyfrgell Genedlaethol Cymru
CYLCHGRAWN LLYFRGELL GENEDLAETHOL CYMRU (Wales)
Cytometry
CYTOMETRY (New York)
Czas Stomatol
CZASOPISMO STOMATOLOGICZNE (Warszawa)
Czech Med
CZECHOSLOVAK MEDICINE (Prague)

—D—

Dacca Univ Stud [A]
DACCA UNIVERSITA STUDIES PART A (Bangladesh)
Daedalus
DAEDALUS; JOURNAL OF THE AMERICAN ACADEMY OF ARTS AND SCIENCES (Boston)
Dalhousie Rev
DALHOUSIE REVIEW (Canada)
Dan Med Bull
DANISH MEDICAL BULLETIN (Copenhagen)
Dansk Medicinhist Arbog
DANSK MEDICINHISTORISK ARBOG. KOEBENHAVNS UNIV. (Copenhagen)
DAR Mag
DAUGHTERS OF THE AMERICAN REVOLUTION MAGAZINE (US)
Deans List
DEANS LIST (Pittman NJ)
Deans Notes
DEANS NOTES (Pittman NJ)
Decouv Civilis
DECOUVERTE DES CIVILISATIONS (France)
Def Natl
DEFENSE NATIONALE (France)
Del Med J
DELAWARE MEDICAL JOURNAL (Wilmington DE)
Demogr Econ
DEMOGRAFIA Y ECONOMIA (Hungary)
Demografia
DEMOGRAFIA (Hungary)
Demography
DEMOGRAPHY (Ann Arbor MI)
Dent Abstr
DENTAL ABSTRACTS (Chicago)
Dent Assist
DENTAL ASSISTANT (Chicago)
Dent Cadmos
DENT CADMOS (Milano)
Dent Delin
DENTAL DELINEATOR (London)
Dent Echo (Heidelb)
DENTAL ECHO (Heidelberg)
Dent Health (London)
DENTAL HEALTH (London)
Dent Hyg (Chic)
DENTAL HYGIENE (Thorofare NJ)
Dent Lab Rev
DENTAL LABORATORY REVIEW (New York)
Dent Labor (Munch)
DENTAL LABOR (Munchen)
Dent Outlook

DENTAL OUTLOOK (Sydney)
Dent Radiogr Photogr
DENTAL RADIOGRAPHY AND PHOTOGRAPHY (Rochester NY)
Dent Stud
DENTAL STUDENT (Northfield IL)
Dent Tech
DENTAL TECHNICIAN (London)
Dentomaxillofac Radiol
DENTOMAXILLOFACIAL RADIOLOGY (Tokyo)
Denver West Roundup
DENVER WESTERN ROUNDUP (Boulder CO)
Dermatol Monatsschr
DERMATOLOGISCHE MONATSSCHRIFT (Leipzig)
Dermatologica
DERMATOLOGICA (Basel)
Desarro Econ
DESARROLLO ECONOM (Argentina)
Detroit Perspect
DETROIT IN PERSPECTIVE; A JOURNAL OF REGIONAL HISTORY (Detroit)
Dev Comp Immunol
DEVELOPMENTAL AND COMPARATIVE IMMUNOLOGY (Elmsford NY)
Dev Psychobiol
DEVELOPMENTAL PSYCHOBIOLOGY (New York)
Dev Toxicol Environ Sci
DEVELOPMENTS IN TOXICOLOGY AND ENVIRONMENTAL SCIENCE (Amsterdam)
Devon Assoc Adv Sci
DEVONSHIRE ASSOCIATION FOR THE ADVANCEMENT OF SCIENCE, LITERATURE AND ART. REPORT AND TRANSACTIONS (Devon)
Diabetes Care
DIABETES CARE (New York)
Diabetologia
DIABETOLOGIA (Berlin)
Diagn Imag Clin Med
DIAGNOSTIC IMAGING IN CLINICAL MEDICINE (Basel)
Diagn Imaging
DIAGNOSTIC IMAGING (Basel)
Dialogue (Canada)
DIALOGUE; CANADIAN PHILOSOPHICAL REVIEW (Canada)
Dialogue J Mormon Thought
DIALOGUE: A JOURNAL OF MORMON THOUGHT (Arlington VA)
Dickensian
THE DICKENSIAN (London)
Dig Dis Sci
DIGESTIVE DISEASES AND SCIENCES (New York)
Dimens Health Serv
DIMENSIONS IN HEALTH SERVICE (Toronto)
Diogenes
DIOGENES (Italy)
Dis Colon Rectum
DISEASES OF THE COLON AND RECTUM (Philadelphia)
Dissent
DISSENT (New York)
Dix-Huit Siecle
DIX-HUITIEME SIECLE (Paris)
Doc Hist Vocab Sci
DOCUMENTS POUR L'HISTOIRE DU VOCABULAIRE SCIENTIFIQUE (Paris)
Doc Ophthalmol
DOCUMENTA OPHTHALMOLOGICA (The Hague)
Documents
DOCUMENTS (Paris)
Donauraum
DONAURAUM (Vienna)
Draco Med
DRACO PRO MEDICO (Lund)
Drei Z Wiss Kunst Soz Leben
DIE DREI ZEITSCHRIFT FUR WISSENSCHAFT, KUNST UND SOZIALES LEBEN (Stuttgart)
Driemaand Tijdschr Gemeentekrediet Belg
DRIEMAANDELIJKS TIJDSCHRIFT GEMEENTEKREDIET VAN BELGIE
Drug Alcohol Depend
DRUG AND ALCOHOL DEPENDENCE (Lausanne)
Drug Intell Clin Pharm
DRUG INTELLIGENCE AND CLINICAL PHARMACY (Cincinnati OH)
Dtsch Aussenpolit
DEUTSCH AUSSENPOLITIK (E Germany)
Dtsch Arztebl
DEUTSCHES ARZTEBLATT; ARZTLICHE MITTEILUNGEN (Kohn)
Dtsch Apoth Ztg
DEUTSCHE APOTHEKER ZEITUNG (Stuttgart)
Dtsch Jahrb Volkskd
DEUTSCHES JAHRBUCH FUR VOLKSKUNDE (E GERMANY)
Dtsch Med Wochenschr
DEUTSCHE MEDIZINISCHE WOCHENSCHRIFT (Stuttgart)
Dtsch Vierteljahresschr Lit Wiss Geistesgesch
DEUTSCHE VIERTELJAHRESSCHRIFT FUR LITERATURWISSENSCHAFT UND GEISTESGESCHICHTE (Stuttgart)
Dtsch Z Philos
DEUTSCHE ZEITSCHRIFT FUR PHILOSOPHIE (Berlin)
Dtsch Z Verdau Stoffwechselkr
DEUTSCHE ZEITSCHRIFT FUR VERDAUUNGS- UND STOFFWECHSELKRANKHEITEN (Leipzig)
Dtsch Zahnarztl Z
DEUTSCHE ZAHNARZTLICHE ZEITSCHRIFT (Munchen)
DTW
DTW. DEUTSCHE TIERARZTLICHE WOCHENSCHRIFT (Hannover)
Dublin Hist Rec
DUBLIN HISTORICAL RECORD (Ireland)

Dubrovnik
DUBROVNIK (Yugoslavia)
Dusseld Arb Gesch Med
DUSSELDORFER ARBEITEN ZUR GESCHICHTE DER MEDIZIN (Dusseldorf)
Dusseld Arb Gesch Med (Beih)
DUSSELDORFER ARBEITEN ZUR GESCHICHTE DER MEDIZIN; BEIHEFT (Dusseldorf)
Duodecim
DUODECIM (Helsinki)
Durham Univ J
DURHAM UNIVERSITY JOURNAL (Gt Brit)
Dynamis
DYNAMIS, ACTA HISPANICA AD MEDICINAE SCIENTIARUMQUE HISTORIAM ILLUSTRANDAM (Granada)

—E—

Ear Hear
EAR AND HEARING (Baltimore)
Ear Nose Throat J
EAR, NOSE, AND THROAT JOURNAL (New York)
Early Am Lit
EARLY AMERICAN LITERTURE (Amherst MA)
East Afr Med J
EAST AFRICAN MEDICAL JOURNAL (Nairobi)
East Anglican Dly Times
EAST ANGLICAN DAILY TIMES
East Cent Eur
EAST CENTRAL EUROPE (US)
East Horiz
EASTERN HORIZON (Hong Kong)
East Tenn Hist Soc Publ
EAST TENNESSEE HISTORICAL SOCIETY'S PUBLICATIONS (Knoxville TN)
Echoes
ECHOES (Columbus OH)
Ecol Dis
ECOLOGY OF DISEASE (Oxford)
Econ Bot
ECONOMIC BOTANY (Bronx NY)
Econ Dev Cult Change
ECONOMIC DEVELOPMENT AND CULTURAL CHANGE (Chicago)
Econ Geogr
ECONOMIC GEOGRAPHY (Worcester MA)
Econ Hist (Sweden)
ECONOMY AND HISTORY (Sweden)
Econ Hist Rev
ECONOMIC HISTORY REVIEW (Gt Brit)
Econ Inq
ECONOMIC INQUIRY (US)
Econ Soc Hist Jaarb
ECONOMISCH- EN SOCIAAL-HISTORISCH JAARBOEK (The Hague)
Econ Soc Rev (Irel)
ECONOMIC AND SOCIAL REVIEW (Ireland)
Econ Stor
ECONOMIA E STORIA (Italy)
Economica
ECONOMICA (Gt Brit)
Educ Med Salud
EDUCATION MEDICA Y SALUD (Washington)
EEG EMG
EEG/EMG (Stuttgart)
Eesti NSV Tead Akad Toim
EESTI NSV TEADUSTE AKADEEMIA TOIMETISED USSR
Egeszsegneveles
EGESZSEGNEVELES
Egypt J Psychiatry
EGYPTIAN JOURNAL OF PSYCHIATRY (Cairo)
Eigen Schoon Brabander
EIGEN SCHOON EN DE BRABANDER (Bruxelles)
Eighteenth Cent Life
EIGHTEENTH CENTURY LIFE (Pittsburgh PA)
Eightenth Cent Stud
EIGHTEENTH CENTURY STUDIES (Columbus OH)
Eighteenth Cent Theory Interpret
EIGHTEENTH CENTURY; THEORY AND INTERPRETATION (Lubbock TX)
Eire Irel
EIRE-IRELAND (St Paul MN)
EITV
E-ITV (US)
Ekon Pregl
EKONOMSKI PREGLED (Yugoslavia)
Ekon Sov Ukr
EKOMONIKA SOVETSKOI UKRAINY (USSR)
Ekonomista
EKONOMISTA (Poland)
Electroencephalogr Clin Neurophysiol
ELECTROENCEPHALOGRAPHY AND CLINICAL NEUROPHYSIOLOGY (Limerick)
Ellenika
ELLENIKA (Greece)
Emerg Med Serv
EMERGENCY MEDICAL SERVICES (Sherman Oaks CA)
Empedocle
EMPEDOCLE (Palermo)
Employee Benefit Plan Rev
EMPLOYEE BENEFIT PLAN REVIEW (Chicago)
Encounter (Lond)
ENCOUNTER (London)
Endeavour
ENDEAVOUR (Oxford)
Endocrinol Exp (Bratisl)
ENDOCRINOLOGIA EXPERIMENTALIS (Bratislava)
Endokrinologie
ENDOKRINOLOGIE (Leipzig)
Enfoque
ENFOQUE (Sao Paulo)
Eng Med

ENGINEERING IN MEDICINE (London)
Engl Lang Notes
ENGLISH LANGUAGE NOTES (Boulder CO)
Enquetes Mus Vie Wallonne
ENQUETES DE LA MUSEE DE LA VIE WALLONNE (Belgium)
Environ Health Perspect
ENVIRONMENTAL HEALTH PERSPECTIVES (Research Triangle Park, NC)
Environ Res
ENVIRONMENTAL RESEARCH (New York)
Epeirotike Hestia
EPEIROTIKE HESTIA (Greece)
Epet Etaireias Stereoelladikon Meleton
EPETIRIS ETAIREIAS STEREOELLADIKON MELETON (Greece)
Epilepsia
EPILEPSIA (New York)
Episteme
EPISTEME (Roma)
Equine Vet J
EQUINE VETERINARY JOURNAL (London)
Ergonomics
ERGONOMICS (London)
Erzieh Unterr
ERZIEHUNG UND UNTERRICHT (Vienna)
Esprit
ESPRIT (France)
Essays Arts Sci
ESSAYS IN ARTS AND SCIENCES
Essex Inst Hist Collect
ESSEX INSTITUTE HISTORICAL COLLECTIONS (Salem MA)
Essex J
ESSEX JOURNAL (Gt Brit)
Estodont Press
ESTODONT PRESS (Madrid)
Estud Cent Am
ESTUDIOS CENTRO AMERICANOS (El Salvador)
Estud Cult Nahuatl
ESTUDIOS DE CULTURA NAHUATL (Mexico)
Estud Duesto
ESTUDIOS DE DUESTO (Bilboa)
Estud Hist Novohisp
ESTUDIOS DE HISTORIA NOVOHISPANA (Mexico)
Estud Segov
ESTUDIOS SEGOVIANOS (Spain)
Estudis
ESTUDIS (Spain)
Ethics Sci Med
ETHICS IN SCIENCE AND MEDICINE (Oxford)
Ethiop Med J
ETHIOPIAN MEDICAL JOURNAL (Addis Ababa)
Ethnicity
ETHNICITY (US)
Ethnohistory
ETHNOHISTORY (Tucson AZ)
Ethnol Fr
ETHNOLOGIE FRANCAISE (Paris)
Ethnomed
ETHNOMEDIZIN; ETHNOMEDICINE. ZEITSCHRIFT FUR INTERDISCIPLINARE FORSCHUNG. JOURNAL FOR INTERDISCIPLINARY RESEARCH (Hamburg)
Etud Anglaises
ETUDES ANGLAISES (Philadelphia)
Etud Balk
ETUDES BALKANIQUES (Bulgaria)
Etud Corses
ETUDES CORSES (Ajaccio)
Etud Int
ETUDES INTERNATIONALES (Canada)
Etud Philos
ETUDES PHILOSOPHIQUES (Paris)
Etudes (Fr)
ETUDES (Paris)
Eur Arch
EUROPA ARCHIV (West Germany)
Eur Ethn
EUROPA ETHNICA (Austria)
Eur Heart J
EUROPEAN HEART JOURNAL (London)
Eur J Obstet Gynecol Reprod Biol
EUROPEAN JOURNAL OF OBSTETRICS, GYNECOLOGY AND REPRODUCTIVE BIOLOGY (Amsterdam)
Eur J Orthod
EUROPEAN JOURNAL OF ORTHODONTICS (London)
Eur J Pediatr
EUROPEAN JOURNAL OF PEDIATRICS (Berlin)
Eur J Sociol
EUROPEAN JOURNAL OF SOCIOLOGY (Gt Brit)
Eur Stud Rev
EUROPEAN STUDIES REVIEW (London)
Eur Urol
EUROPEAN UROLOGY (Basel)
Eval Program Plann
EVALUATION AND PROGRAM PLANNING (Elmsford NY)
Evol Psychiatr (Paris)
EVOLUTION PSYCHIATRIQUE (Paris)
Except Child
EXCEPTIONAL CHILDREN (Reston VA)
Exp Hematol
EXPERIMENTAL HEMATOLOGY (New York)
Exp Neurol
EXPERIMENTAL NEUROLOGY (New York)
Experientia
EXPERIENTIA (Basel)
Experientia [Suppl]
EXPERIENTIA. SUPPLEMENTUM (Basel)
Explor Econ Hist
EXPLORATIONS IN ECONOMIC HISTORY (New York)
Explor Ethnic Stud

EXPLORATIONS IN ETHNIC STUDIES (US)

—F—

Factotum
FACTOTUM
Fam Plann Perspect
FAMILY PLANNING PERSPECTIVES (New York)
Fam Process
FAMILY PROCESS (New York)
Farm Pol
FARMACJA POLSKA (Warsaw)
Farm Port
FARMACIA PORTUGUESA
Farm Tijdschr Belg
FARMACEUTISCH TIJDSCHRIFT VOOR BELGIE (Bruxelles)
Farm Tid
FARMACEUTISK TIDENDE (Copehhagen)
Farm Univers
FARMACIA UNIVERSAL (Spain)
Farm Zh
FARMATSEVTYCHNYI ZHURNAL (Kiev)
Farmaco [Prat]
FARMACO, EDIZIONE PRATICA (Pavia)
Farmakol Toksikol
FARMAKOLOGIIA I TOKSIKOLOGIIA (Moskva)
Farmatsiia
FARMATSIIA (Moskva)
FDA Consum
FDA Consumer (Washington)
FEBS Lett
FEBS LETTERS (Amsterdam)
Fed Proc
FEDERATION PROCEEDINGS (Bethesda MD)
Feldsher Akush
FEL'DSHER I AKUSHERKA (Moskva)
Femina
FEMINA (Sao Paulo)
Feminist Stud
FEMINIST STUDIES (College Park MD)
Fertil Steril
FERTILITY AND STERILITY (Birmingham AL)
Fides Et Hist
FIDES ET HISTORIA (Terre Haute IN)
Figueres
FIGUERES (Spain)
Filson Club Hist Q
FILSON CLUB HISTORY QUARTERLY (Louisville KY)
Fiziol Zh
FIZIOLOGICHESKII ZHURNAL (Moskva)
Fiziol Zh SSSR
FIZIOLOGICHESKII ZHURNAL SSSR IMENI I.M. SECHENOVA (Moskva)
Fla Dent J
FLORIDA DENTAL JOURNAL (Tampa)
Fla Hist Q
FLORIDA HISTORICAL QUARTERLY (Tampa)
Fla Nurse
FLORIDA NURSE (Orlando)
Flammes Fumee
FLAMMES FUMEES
Flash Inf
FLASH-INFORMATIONS (Bruxelles)
Flintknappers Exch
FLINTKNAPPERS EXCHANGE (US)
Florilegium
FLORILEGIUM
FNIB
FNIB; FEDERATION NATIONALE DES INFIRMIER(E)S BELGES (Bruxelles)
Fogorv Sz
FOGORVOSI SZEMLE (Budapest)
Foldr Kozl
FOLDRAJZI KOZLEMNYEK (Hungary)
Folia Biol (Praha)
FOLIA BIOLOGICA (Praha)
Folia Haematol (Leipz)
FOLIA HAEMATOLOGICA. INTERNATIONALES MAGAZIN FUR KLINISCHE UND MORPHOLOGISCHE BLUTFORSCHUNG (Leipzig)
Folia Hum (Barc)
FOLIA HUMANISTICA; CIENCIAS, ARTES, LETRAS (Barcelona)
Folia Med Cracov
FOLIA MEDICA CRACOVIENSIA (Warszawa)
Folia Mendeliana
FOLIA MENDELIANA (Brno)
Folia Morphol (Praha)
FOLIA MORPHOLOGICA (Praha)
Folia Morphol (Warsz)
FOLIA MORPHOLOGICA (Warszawa)
Folia Phoniatr (Basel)
FOLIA PHONIATRICA (Basel)
Folia Primatol (Basel)
FOLIA PRIMATOLOGICA (Basel)
Folkl Brabancon
FOLKLORE BRABANCON (Belgium)
Folklore
FOLKLORE (London)
Fontilles
FONTILLES. REVISTA DE LEPROLOGIA (Valencia)
Food Drug Cosmet Law J
FOOD, DRUG, COSMETIC LAW JOURNAL (New York)
Food Res Inst Stud
FOOD RESEARCH INSTITUTE STUDIES IN AGRICULTURAL ECONOMICS TRADE AND DEVELOPMENT (Stanford CA)
Food Technol
FOOD TECHNOLOGY (Chicago)
Foreign Aff
FOREIGN AFFAIRS (New York)
Foreign Policy

FOREIGN POLICY (New York)
Fogorv Sz
FOGORVOSI SZEMLE (Budapest)
Forschungsunternehm Fritz Thyssen Stift Stud Naturwiss Tech Wirtsch Neunzehn Jahrhundert
FORSCHUNGSUNTERNEHMEN DER FRITZ THYSSEN STIFTUNG STUDIEN ZUR NATURWISSENSCHAFT, TECHNIK UND WIRTSCHAFT IM NEUNZEHNTEN JAHRHUNDERT (Gottingen)
Fortschr Kieferorthop
FORTSCHRITTE DER KIEFERORTHOPADIE (Munchen)
Fortschr Med
FORTSCHRITTE DER MEDIZIN (Leipzig)
Fortschr Neurol Psychiatr
FORTSCHRITTE DER NEUROLOGIE-PSYCHIATRIE (Stuttgart)
Forum Med
FORUM ON MEDICINE (Philadelphia)
Found News
FOUNDATION NEWS (Wellcome) (Gt Brit)
Fr Am Rev
FRENCH-AMERICAN REVIEW (Fort Worth TX)
Fr Hist Stud
FRENCH HISTORICAL STUDIES (Baton Rouge LA)
Francia
FRANCIA: FORSCHUNGEN ZUR WESTEUROPAISCHEN GESCHICHTE (Munchen)
Freedomways
FREEDOMWAYS (New York)
Friends P.I. Nixon Med Hist Libr
FRIENDS OF THE P.I. NIXON MEDICAL HISTORICAL LIBRARY
Front Nurs Serv Q Bull
FRONTIER NURSING SERVICE QUARTERLY BULLETIN (Lexington Ky)
Front Radiat Ther Oncol
FRONTIERS OF RADIATION THERAPY AND ONCOLOGY (Basel)
Frontiers
FRONTIERS (Boulder CO)
Fruhmittelalt Stud
FRUHMITTELALTERLICHE STUDIEN (Berlin)
Fukuoka Igaku Zasshi
FUKUOKA IGAKU ZASSHI. FUKUOKA ACTA MEDICA (Fukuoka)
Fundam Sci
FUNDAMENTA SCIENTIAE (Oxford)
Fysiatr Reumatol Vestn
FYSIATRICKY A REUMATOLOGICKY VESTNIK (Praha)

—G—

G Accad Med Torino
GIORNALE DELLA ACCADEMIA DI MEDICINA DI TORINO (Torino)
G Batteriol Virol Immunol
GIORNALE DI BATTERIOLOGIA, VIROLOGIA ED IMMUNOLOGIA (Torino)
G Clin Med
GIORNALE DI CLINICA MEDICA (Bologna)
G Crit Filos Ital
GIORNALE CRITICO DELLA FILOSOFIA ITALIANA (Firenze)
G Ital Cardiol
GIORNALE ITALIANO DI CARDIOLOGIA (Roma)
G Ital Med Lav
GIORNALE ITALIANO DI MEDICINA DEL LAVORO (Pavia)
G Stomatol Ortognatodonzia
GIORNALE DI STOMATOLOGIA E DI ORTOGNATODONZIA (Orderzo)
Ga Histo Q
GEORGIA HISTORICAL QUARTERLY (Savannah GA)
Ga J Sci
GEORGIA JOURNAL OF SCIENCE (US)
Ga Nurse
GEORGIA NURSING (Atlanta GA)
Ga Pharm Q
GEORGIA PHARMACIST QUARTERLY (US)
Ga Rev
GEORGIA REVIEW (Athens GA)
Gac Med Bilbao
GACETA MEDICA DE BILBAO (Bilbao)
Gac Med Mex
GACETA MEDICA DE MEXICO (Mexico)
Galicia Clin
GALICIA-CLINICA (La Coruna)
Gard Hist
GARDEN HISTORY (Surrey)
Gastroenterology
GASTROENTEROLOGY (Baltimore)
Gastrointest Endosc
GASTROINTESTINAL ENDOSCOPY (Baltimore)
Gastrointest Radiol
GASTROINTESTINAL RADIOLOGY (Berlin)
Gateway Herit
GATEWAY HERITAGE (St Louis Mo)
Gaz Inst Med Lab Sci
GAZETTE OF THE INSTITUTE OF MEDICAL LABORATORY SCIENCES (London)
Gaz Med Fr
GAZETTE MEDICALE DE FRANCE (Paris)
Geburtshilfe Frauenheilkd
GEBURTSHILFE UND FRAUENHEILKUNDE (Stuttgart)
Gegenbaurs Morphol Jahrb
GEGENBAURS MORPHOLOGISCHES JAHRBUCH (Leipzig)
Gematol Transfuziol
GEMATOLOGIIA I TRANSFUZIOLOGIIA (Moskva)
GEN
GEN (Caracas)
Gen Dent

GENERAL DENTISTRY (Chicago)
Gen Hosp Psychiatry
GENERAL HOSPITAL PSYCHIATRY (New York)
Gen Pharmacol
GENERAL PHARMACOLOGY (Oxford)
Geneeskd Gids
GENEESKUNDIGE GIDS (The Hague)
Genetics
GENETICS (Austin TX)
Genetika
GENETIKA (Moskva)
Geneva Afr
GENEVA AFRICA (Geneva)
Genus
GENUS (Roma)
Geogr Anal
GEOGRAPHICAL ANALYSIS (Columbus OH)
Geogr Med
GEOGRAPHIA MEDICA (Budapest)
Geography
GEOGRAPHY (London)
Georgetown Dent J
GEORGETOWN DENTAL JOURNAL (Washington)
Ger Stud Rev
GERMAN STUDIES REVIEW (Tempe AZ)
Ger Yearb Int Law
GERMAN YEARBOOK OF INTERNATIONAL LAW (W Germany)
Gerontologist
GERONTOLOGIST (Washington)
Gesammelte Aufs Kulturgesch Spaniens
GESAMMELTE AUFSATZE DER KULTURGESCHICHTE SPANIENS
Gesch Wiss Unterr
GESCHICHTE IN WISSENSCHAFT UND UNTERRICHT (W Germany)
Gesnerus
GESNERUS (Aarau)
Gig Sanit
GIGIENA I SANITARIIA (Moskva)
Gig Tr Prof Zabol
GIGIENA TRUDA I PROFESSIONALNYE ZABOLEVANIIA (Moskva)
Ginecol Obstet Mex
GINECOLOGIA Y OBSTETRICIA DE MEXICO (Mexico)
Ginekol Pol
GINEKOLOGIA POLSKA (Warszawa)
Glas Srp Akad Nauka [MED]
GLAS. SRPSKA AKADEMIJA NAUKA I UMETNOSTI, ODELJENUE MEDICINSKIH NAUKA (Belgrade)
Glotta
GLOTTA, ZEITSCHRIFT FUR GRIECHISCHE UND LATEINISCHE SPRACHE (Gottingen)
God Drus Istor Bosne Herceg
GODISNJAK DRUSTVA ISTORICARA BOSNE I HERCEGOVINE (Yugoslavia)
God Zb Med Fak Skopje
GODISEN ZBORNIK NA MEDICINSKIOT FAKULTET VO SKOPJE (Yugoslavia)
Gold Bull
GOLD BULLETIN-CHAMBER OF MINES OF SOUTH AFRICA RESEARCH ORGANIZATION (South Africa)
Goriski Letnik
GORISKI LETNIK (Yugoslavia)
Goteb Etnogr Mus
GOTEBORGS ETHNOGRAFISKA MUSEUM ARSTRYCK (Sweden)
Grants Mag
GRANTS MAGAZINE (New York)
Greek Roman Byz Stud
GREEK, ROMAN AND BYZANTINE STUDIES (Cambridge MA)
Grenzgeb Wiss
GRENZGEBIETE DER WISSENSCHAFT
Groniek
GRONIEK; ONAFHANKELIJK GRONINGS HISTORISCH TIJDSCHRIFT (Netherlands)
Group Psychol Hist Newsl
GROUP FOR THE USE OF PSYCHOLOGY IN HISTORY NEWSLETTER (Springfield IL)
Growth
GROWTH (Philadelphia)
Grudn Khir
GRUDNAIA KHIRURGIIA (Moskva)
Guam Rec
GUAM RECORDER (US)
Guatem Indig
GAUTEMALA INDIGENA (Guatemala)
Guildhall Stud Lond Hist
GUILDHALL STUDIES IN LONDON HISTORY (Gt Brit)
Gutenberg Jahrb
GUTENBERG JAHRBUCH (Mainz)
Gynakologe
GYNAKOLOGE (Berlin)
Gynecol Oncol
GYNECOLOGIC ONCOLOGY (New York)

—H—

Hacettepe Sosyal Bilimler Derg
HACETTEPE SOSYAL VE BESERI BILIMLER DERGISI (Turkey)
Hades
HADES (Antwerp)
Hadtortenelmi Kozl
HADTORTENELMI KOZLEMENYEK (Hungary)
Haematologia (Budap)
HAEMATOLOGIA (Budapest)
Haematologica (Pavia)
HAEMATOLOGICA (Pavia)
Haemostasis
HAEMOSTASIS (Basel)

Halve Maen
HALVE MAEN (New York)
Hamdard
HAMDARD. THE ORGAN OF THE INSTITUTE OF HEALTH AND TIBBI RESEARCH (Karachi)
Hamizrah Hehadash
HAMIZRAH HEHADASH (Israel)
Hampshire
HAMPSHIRE (Gt Brit)
Hand
HAND; JOURNAL OF THE BRITISH SOCIETY FOR SURGERY OF THE HAND (Brentwood)
Handchirurgie
HANDCHIRURGIE (Erlangen)
Handel Maasch Geschied Oudheidk Gent
HANDELINGEN DER MAATSCHAPPIJ VOOR GESCHIEDENIS EN OUDHEIDKUNDE TE GENT (Belgium)
Hansenol Int
HANSENOLOGIA INTERNATIONALIS (Sao Paulo)
Harefuah
HAREFUAH (Tel Aviv)
Harv Educ Rev
HARVARD EDUCATIONAL REVIEW (Cambridge MA)
Harv Libr Bull
HARVARD LIBRARY BULLETIN (Cambridge MA)
Harv Mag
HARVARD MAGAZINE (Cambridge MA)
Harv Med Alumni Bull
HARVARD MEDICAL ALUMNI BULLETIN (Boston)
Harv Theol Rev
HARVARD THEOLOGICAL REVIEW (Cambridge MA)
Harvey Lect
HARVEY LECTURES (New York)
Hasifrut
HASIFRUT (Tel Aviv)
Hastings Cent Rep
HASTINGS CENTER REPORT (New York)
Hautarzt
HAUTARZT (Berlin)
Hawaii J Hist
HAWAIIAN JOURNAL OF HISTORY (Honolulu)
Hawaii Med J
HAWAII MEDICAL JOURNAL (Honolulu HI)
Health Bull (Edinb)
HEALTH BULLETIN (Edinburgh)
Health Educ (Wash)
HEALTH EDUCATION (Washington)
Health PAC Bull
HEALTH-PAC BULLETIN (New York)
Health Phys
HEALTH PHYSICS (Elmsford NY)
Health Policy Educ
HEALTH POLICY AND EDUCATION (Amsterdam)
Health Policy Q
HEALTH POLICY QUARTERLY (New York)
Health Popul Perspect Issues
HEALTH AND POPULATION; PERSPECTIVES AND ISSUES (New Delhi)
Health Serv Rep
HEALTH SERVICES REPORTS (Rockville MD)
Health Soc Serv J
HEALTH AND SOCIAL SERVICE JOURNAL (London)
Health Soc Work
HEALTH AND SOCIAL WORK (Washington)
Health Values
HEALTH VALUES (Thorofare NJ)
Health Visit
HEALTH VISITOR (London)
Hefte Unfallheilkd
HEFTE ZUR UNFALLHEILKUNDE (Berlin)
Heimen
HEIMEN (Norway)
Helmantica
HELMANTICA; REVISTA DE HUMANIDADES CLASICAS (Spain)
Helv Archaeol
HELVETICA CHIRURGICA ACTA (Basel)
Henry Ford Hosp Med J
HENRY FORD HOSPITAL MEDICAL JOURNAL (Detroit)
Hepatology
HEPATOLOGY (Baltimore)
Herbal Rev
HERBAL REVIEW (US)
Hereditas
HEREDITAS (Lund)
Hermathena
HERMATHENA (Ireland)
Hermeneus Tijdschr Antieke Cult
HERMENEUS; TIJDSCHRIFT VOOR DE ANTIEKE CULTUUR (Netherlands)
Hermes
HERMES; ZEITSCHRIFT FUR KLASSISCHE PHILOLOGIE (Wiesbaden)
Hesperis Tamuda
HESPERIS—TAMUDA (Morocco)
Hess Familienkd
HESSISCHE FAMILIENKUNDE (W Germany)
Hexagon Roche [Engl]
HEXAGON ROCHE (ENGLISH EDITION) (Basel)
Hillside J Clin Psychiatry
HILLSIDE JOURNAL OF CLINICAL PSYCHIATRY (New York)
Hindustan Antibiot Bull
HINDUSTAN ANTIBIOTICS BULLETIN (Primpri)
Hisp Am Hist Rev
HISPANIC AMERICAN HISTORICAL REVIEW (Durham NC)
Hisp Antiq
HISPANIA ANTIGUA (Spain)
Hispania

HISPANIA (Madrid)
Hist Aikak
HISTORIALLINEN AIKAKAUSKIRJA (Helsinki)
Hist Anthropol Newsl
HISTORY OF ANTHROPOLOGY NEWSLETTER (Chicago)
Hist Archaeol
HISTORICAL ARCHAEOLOGY (Washington)
Hist Arkisto (Finl)
HISTORIALLINEN ARKISTO (Finland)
Hist Cult (Peru)
HISTORIA Y CULTURA (Peru)
Hist Educ
HISTORY OF EDUCATION (Gt Brit)
Hist Educ (France)
HISTOIRE DE L'EDUCATION (Paris)
Hist Educ Q
HISTORY OF EDUCATION QUARTERLY (New York)
Hist Eur Ideas
HISTORY OF EUROPEAN IDEAS (Gt Brit)
Hist Foren Arsskr
HISTORIELARARNAS FORENINGS ARSSKRIFT (Sweden)
Hist Hosp
HISTORIA HOSPITALIUM; MITTEILUNGEN DER DEUTSCHEN GESELLSCHAFT FUR KRANKENHAUSGESCHICHTE (Dusseldorf)
Hist J (Gt Brit)
HISTORICAL JOURNAL (Gt Brit)
Hist J (NZ)
HISTORICAL JOURNAL (New Zealand)
Hist J West Mass
HISTORICAL JOURNAL OF WESTERN MASSACHUSETTS (US)
Hist Jahrb
HISTORISCHES JAHRBUCH (Freiburg)
Hist Jahrb Stadt Linz
HISTORISCHES JAHRBUCH DER STADT LINZ (Austria)
Hist Litteraturhist Studier (Finl)
HISTORISKA OCH LITTERATURHISTORISKA STUDIER (Finland)
Hist Mag Protest Episc Church
HISTORICAL MAGAZINE OF THE PROTESTANT EPISCOPAL CHURCH (Austin TX)
Hist Med
HISTORY OF MEDICINE (London)
Hist Med Vet
HISTORIA MEDICINAE VETERINARIAE (Copenhagen)
Hist Methods
HISTORICAL METHODS (US)
Hist Methods Newsl
HISTORICAL METHODS NEWSLETTER (US)
Hist Mex
HISTORIA MEXICANA (Mexico)
Hist Nat
HISTOIRE ET NATURE; CAHIERS DE L'ASSOCIATION POUR L'HISTOIRE DES SCIENCES DE LA NATURE (Paris)
Hist Pap Can Hist Assoc
HISTORICAL PAPERS CANADIAN HISTORICAL ASSOCIATION (Canada)
Hist Philos Life Sci
HISTORY AND PHILOSOPHY OF THE LIFE SCIENCES. SECTION II OF PUBBLICAZIONI DELLA STAZIONE ZOOLOGICA DI NAPOLI (Firenze)
Hist Rec Aust Sci
HISTORICAL RECORD OF AUSTRALIAN SCIENCE (Australia)
Hist Reflect
HISTORICAL REFLECTIONS (Canada)
Hist Relig
HISTORY OF RELIGIONS (Chicago)
Hist Sci
HISTORIA SCIENTIARUM (Tokyo)
Hist Sci
HISTORY OF SCIENCE (Gr Brit)
Hist Sci Med
HISTOIRE DES SCIENCES MEDICALES (Asnieres)
Hist Soc Res
HISTORICAL SOCIAL RESEARCH (W Germany)
Hist Stud
HISTORICAL STUDIES (Melbourne)
Hist Stud Phys Sci
HISTORICAL STUDIES IN THE PHYSICAL SCIENCES (Berkeley CA)
Hist Teach
HISTORY TEACHER (Long Beach CA)
Hist Tidskr
HISTORISK TIDSKRIFT (Stockholm)
Hist Tidskr Finl
HISTORISK TIDSKRIFT FOR FINLAND (Helsinki)
Hist Tidsskr
HISTORISK TIDSSKRIFT (Oslo)
Hist Today
HISTORY TODAY (Gr Brit)
Hist Workshop J
HISTORY WORKSHOP; A JOURNAL OF SOCIALIST HISTORIANS (Oxford)
Hist Z
HISTORISCHE ZEITSCHRIFT (Munchen)
Histochem J
HISTOCHEMICAL JOURNAL (London)
Histochemistry
HISTOCHEMISTRY (Berlin)
Histoire
HISTOIRE (France)
Historia (Argentina)
HISTORIA (Argentina)
Historia (S Afr)
HISTORIA (S Africa)
Historian
HISTORIAN (US)

Historie
HISTORIE (Denmark)
History
HISTORY (London)
HNO
HNO (Berlin)
Hokenfu Zasshi
HOKENFU ZASSHI. JAPANESE JOURNAL FOR PUBLIC HEALTH NURSE (Tokyo)
Horizon
HORIZON. A MAGAZINE OF THE ARTS (New York)
Horm Behav
HORMONES AND BEHAVIOR (New York)
Hosp Adm Can
HOSPITAL ADMINISTRATION IN CANADA (Don Mills)
Hosp Community Psychiatry
HOSPITAL AND COMMUNITY PSYCHIATRY (Washington)
Hosp Eng
HOSPITAL ENGINEERING (London)
Hosp Financ Manage
HOSPITAL FINANCIAL MANAGEMENT (Oak Brook IL)
Hosp Forum
HOSPITAL FORUM (San Francisco)
Hosp Health Serv Adm
HOSPITAL AND HEALTH SERVICES ADMINISTRATION (Chicago)
Hosp Libr
HOSPITAL LIBRARIES (Oak Park IL)
Hosp Pract
HOSPITAL PRACTICE (New York)
Hosp Pract [Off]
HOSPITAL PRACTICE (OFFICE EDITION) (New York)
Hosp Prog
HOSPITAL PROGRESS (St Louis)
Hospitals
HOSPITALS (Chicago)
Houston Rev
HOUSTON REVIEW; HISTORY AND CULTURE OF THE GULF COAST (Houston TX)
HPN Hosp Purch News
HPN. HOSPITAL PURCHASING NEWS (Northfield, IL)
HSTC Bull
HSTC BULLETIN (Canada)
Hu Li Tsa Chih
HU LI TSA CHIH; JOURNAL OF NURSING (Taipei)
Hum Biol
HUMAN BIOLOGY (Detroit)
Hum Dev
HUMAN DEVELOPMENT (Basel)
Hum Ecol
HUMAN ECOLOGY (New York)
Hum Genet
HUMAN GENETICS (Berlin)
Hum Genet [Suppl]
HUMAN GENETICS, SUPPLEMENT (Berlin)
Hum Hered
HUMAN HEREDITY (Basel)
Hum Neurobiol
HUMAN NEUROBIOLOGY (New York)
Hum Nutr Appl Nutr
HUMAN NUTRITION. APPLIED NUTRITION (London)
Hum Organ
HUMAN ORGANIZATION (Washington)
Hum Pathol
HUMAN PATHOLOGY (Philadelphia)
Hum Physiol
HUMAN PHYSIOLOGY (New York)
Hum Toxicol
HUMAN TOXICOLOGY (Basingstoke Hampshire)
Humanitas
HUMANITAS; JOURNAL OF THE INSTITUTE OF MAN (Mexico)
Huntia
HUNTIA (Pittsburgh)
Huntington Libr Q
HUNTINGTON LIBRARY QUARTERLY; A JOURNAL FOR THE HISTORY AND INTERPRETATION OF ENGLISH AND AMERICAN CIVILIZATION (San Marino CA)
Hypertension
HYPERTENSION (Dallas TX)

—I—

IARC Sci Publ
IARC SCIENTIFIC PUBLICATIONS (Lyon)
Igaku Kenkyu
IGAKU KENKYU. ACTA MEDICA (Fukuoka)
Igaku Sensui
IGAKU SENSUI (Tokyo)
Igakushi Kenkyu
IGAKUSHI KENKYU. STADIUM HISTORIAE MEDICAE (Osaka)
Ill Dent J
ILLINOIS DENTAL JOURNAL (Chicago)
Illimani
ILLIMANI (Bolivia)
Image (IN)
IMAGE (Indianapolis IN)
Image J Nurs Sch
IMAGE—THE JOURNAL OF NURSING SCHOLARSHIP (Indianapolis IN)
Imago Mundi
IMAGO MUNDI; A REVIEW OF EARLY CARTOGRAPHY
IMJ
IMJ ILLINOIS MEDICAL JOURNAL (Chicago)
Immun Infekt
IMMUNITAT UND INFEKTION (Munchen)

Immunogenetics
IMMUNOGENETICS (New York)
Imprimatur
IMPRIMATUR
Imprint
IMPRINT (New York)
Ind Archaeol
INDUSTRIAL ARCHAEOLOGY (Gt Brit)
Ind Archaeol Rev
INDUSTRIAL ARCHAEOLOGY REVIEW (London)
Ind Labor Relat Rev
INDUSTRIAL AND LABOR RELATIONS REVIEW (US)
Indian Arch
INDIAN ARCHIVES (India)
Indian Econ Soc Hist Rev
INDIAN ECONOMIC AND SOCIAL HISTORY REVIEW (India)
Indian Heart J
INDIAN HEART JOURNAL (Bombay)
Indian J Am Stud
INDIAN JOURNAL OF AMERICAN STUDIES (India)
Indian J Cancer
INDIAN JOURNAL OF CANCER (Bombay)
Indian J Chest Dis Allied Sci
INDIAN JOURNAL OF CHEST DISEASES AND ALLIED SCIENCES (New Delhi)
Indian J Hist Sci
INDIAN JOURNAL OF THE HISTORY OF SCIENCE (Calcutta)
Indian J Med Res
INDIAN JOURNAL OF MEDICAL RESEARCH (New Delhi)
Indian J Med Sci
INDIAN JOURNAL OF MEDICAL SCIENCES (Bombay)
Indian J Pathol Microbiol
INDIAN JOURNAL OF PATHOLOGY AND MICROBIOLOGY (Chandigarh)
Indian J Pediatr
INDIAN JOURNAL OF PEDIATRICS (Calcutta)
Indian J Public Health
INDIAN JOURNAL OF PUBLIC HEALTH (Calcutta)
Indian Pol Sci Rev
INDIAN POLITICAL SCIENCE REVIEW (India)
Indian Pract
INDIAN PRACTITIONER (Bombay)
Indiana Folkl
INDIANA FOLKLORE (Bloomington)
Indiana Med
INDIANA MEDICINE (Indianapolis IN)
Indiana Med Hist Q
INDIANA MEDICAL HISTORY QUARTERLY (Indianapolis)
Indiana Soc Stud Q
INDIANA SOCIAL STUDIES QUARTERLY (Muncie)
Inf Dent
INFORMATION DENTAIRE (Paris)
Inf Hist
INFORMATION HISTORIQUE (Paris)
Inf Pharm
INFORMATIONS PHARMACEUTIQUES (Paris)
Inf Psychiatr
INFORMATION PSYCHIATRIQUE (Paris)
Infect Control
INFECTION CONTROL (Thorofare NJ)
Infection
INFECTION (Munchen)
Infirm Can
INFIRMIERE CANADIENNE
Infirm Fr
INFIRMIERE FRANCAISE (Paris)
Injury
INJURY; BRITISH JOURNAL OF ACCIDENT SURGERY (Bristol)
INS Rep
INS REPORTER (US)
Inst Stat Q
INSTITUTO DI STATISTICA-QUADERNO
Int Anesthesiol Clin
INTERNATIONAL ANESTHESIOLOGY CLINICS (Boston)
Int Arch Occup Environ Health
INTERNATIONAL ARCHIVES OF OCCUPATIONAL AND ENVIRONMENTAL HEALTH (Berlin)
Int Endod J
INTERNATIONAL ENDODONTIC JOURNAL (Oxford)
Int J
INTERNATIONAL JOURNAL (Canada)
Int J Addict
INTERNATIONAL JOURNAL OF THE ADDICTIONS (New York)
Int J Afr Hist Stud
INTERNATIONAL JOURNAL OF AFRICAN HISTORICAL STUDIES (New York)
Int J Aging Hum Dev
INTERNATIONAL JOURNAL OF AGING AND HUMAN DEVELOPMENT (Farmingdale NY)
Int J Appl Radiat Isot
INTERNATIONAL JOURNAL OF APPLIED RADIATION AND ISOTOPES (Elmsford NY)
Int J Artif Organs
INTERNATIONAL JOURNAL OF ARTIFICIAL ORGANS (Milano)
Int J Biochem
INTERNATIONAL JOURNAL OF BIOCHEMISTRY (Oxford)
Int J Biometeorol
INTERNATIONAL JOURNAL OF BIOMETEOROLOGY (Amsterdam)
Int J Cardiol
INTERNATIONAL JOURNAL OF CARDIOLOGY

(Amsterdam)
Int J Chronobiol
INTERNATIONAL JOURNAL OF CHRONOBIOLOGY (London)
Int J Clin Exp Hypn
INTERNATIONAL JOURNAL OF CLINICAL AND EXPERIMENTAL HYPNOSIS (New York)
Int J Clin Pharmacol Ther Toxicol
INTERNATIONAL JOURNAL OF CLINICAL PHARMACOLOGY, THERAPY, AND TOXICOLOGY (Munchen)
Int J Comp Sociol
INTERNATIONAL JOURNAL OF COMPARATIVE SOCIOLOGY (Toronto)
Int J Contemp Sociol
INTERNATIONAL JOURNAL OF CONTEMPORARY SOCIOLOGY (Raleigh NC)
Int J Dermatol
INTERNATIONAL JOURNAL OF DERMATOLOGY (Philadelphia)
Int J Epidemiol
INTERNATIONAL JOURNAL OF EPIDEMIOLOGY (London)
Int J Fertil
INTERNATIONAL JOURNAL OF FERTILITY (Stockholm)
Int J Group Psychother
INTERNATIONAL JOURNAL OF GROUP PSYCHOTHERAPY (New York)
Int J Gynaecol Obstet
INTERNATIONAL JOURNAL OF GYNAECOLOGY AND OBSTETRICS (Stockholm)
Int J Gynecol Pathol
INTERNATIONAL JOURNAL OF GYNECOLOGICAL PATHOLOGY (New York)
Int J Health Serv
INTERNATIONAL JOURNAL OF HEALTH SERVICES (Westport CT)
Int J Law Psychiatry
INTERNATIONAL JOURNAL OF LAW AND PSYCHIATRY (Elmsford NY)
Int J Lepr
INTERNATIONAL JOURNAL OF LEPROSY (Washington)
Int J Middle East Stud
INTERNATIONAL JOURNAL OF MIDDLE EAST STUDIES (Gt Brit)
Int J Neurol
INTERNATIONAL JOURNAL OF NEUROLOGY (Montevideo)
Int J Neurosci
INTERNATIONAL JOURNAL OF NEUROSCIENCE (London)
Int J Nurs Stud
INTERNATIONAL JOURNAL OF NURSING STUDIES (Oxford)
Int J Obes
INTERNATIONAL JOURNAL OF OBESITY (London)
Int J Oral Myol
INTERNATIONAL JOURNAL OF ORAL MYOLOGY (Nacogdoches TX)
Int J Parasitol
INTERNATIONAL JOURNAL FOR PARASITOLOGY (Oxford)
Int J Pediatr Otorhinolaryngol
INTERNATIONAL JOURNAL OF PEDIATRIC OTORHINOLARYNGOLOGY (Amsterdam)
Int J Periodontics Restorative Dent
INTERNATIONAL JOURNAL OF PERIODONTICS AND RESTORATIVE DENTISTRY (Chicago)
Int J Polit
INTERNATIONAL JOURNAL OF POLITICS (White Plains NY)
Int J Psychoanal
INTERNATIONAL JOURNAL OF PSYCHOANALYSIS (London)
Int J Psychoanal Psychother
INTERNATIONAL JOURNAL OF PSYCHOANALYTIC PSYCHOTHERAPY (New York)
Int J Psychosom
INTERNATIONAL JOURNAL OF PSYCHOSOMATICS (Philadelphia)
Int J Radiat Oncol Biol Phys
INTERNATIONAL JOURNAL OF RADIATION ONCOLOGY, BIOLOGY, PHYSICS (Elmsford NY)
Int J Soc Psychiatry
INTERNATIONAL JOURNAL OF SOCIAL PSYCHIATRY (London)
Int J Womens Studd
INTERNATIONAL JOURNAL OF WOMENS STUDIES (Canada)
Int J Zoonoses
INTERNATIONAL JOURNAL OF ZOONOSES (Taipei)
Int Migr Rev
INTERNATIONAL MIGRATION REVIEW (Staten Island NY)
Int Opthalmol Clin
INTERNATIONAL OPHTHALMOLOGY CLINICS (Boston)
Int Organ
INTERNATIONAL ORGANIZATION (Boston)
Int Orthop
INTERNATIONAL ORTHOPAEDICS (Berlin)
Int Pharmacopsychiatry
INTERNATIONAL PHARMACOPSYCHIATRY (Basel)
Int Rehabil Med
INTERNATIONAL REHABILITATION MEDICINE (Basel)
Int Rev Nat Fam Plann
INTERNATIONAL REVIEW OF NATURAL FAMILY PLANING (Collegeville MN)
Int Rev Soc Hist
INTERNATIONAL REVIEW OF SOCIAL HISTORY

(Netherlands)
Int Soc Sci J
INTERNATIONAL SOCIAL SCIENCE JOURNAL (France)
Int Surg
INTERNATIONAL SURGERY (Chicago)
Int Wiss Korresp Gesch Dtsch Arb-bew
INTERNAZIONALE WISSENSCHAFTLICHE KORRESPONDENZ ZUR GESCHICHTE DER DEUTSCHEN ARBEITERBEWEGUNG (W Germany)
Interam Rev Bibliogr
INTER-AMERICAN REVIEW OF BIBLIOGRAPHY (Washington)
Interdiscip Sci Rev
INTERDISCIPLINARY SCIENCE REVIEWS
Internist (Berlin)
INTERNIST (Berlin)
Intersezioni
INTERSEZIONI; RIVISTA DI STORIA DELLE IDEE
Intervirology
INTERVIROLOGY (Basel)
Invest Econ
INVESTIGACION ECONOMICA (Mexico)
Invest Hist
INVESTIGACIONES HISTORICAS (Valladolid)
Invest Ophthalmol Vis Sci
INVESTIGATIVE OPHTHALMOLOGY AND VISUAL SCIENCE (St Louis)
Invest Radiol
INVESTIGATIVE RADIOLOGY (Philadelphia)
Invest Urol
INVESTIGATIVE UROLOGY (Baltimore)
Investor Owned Hosp Rev
INVESTOR-OWNED HOSPITAL REVIEW (Little Rock AR)
Iowa Dent J
IOWA DENTAL JOURNAL (Des Moines IA)
Iowa Med
IOWA MEDICINE (Des Moines IA)
Ir Econ Soc Hist
IRISH ECONOMIC AND SOCIAL HISTORY (Gt Brit)
Ir J Med Sci
IRISH JOURNAL OF MEDICAL SCIENCE (Dublin)
Ir Med J
IRISH MEDICAL JOURNAL (Dublin)
Ir Sword
IRISH SWORD (Ireland)
Iraq
IRAQ (Gt Brit)
Isis
ISIS (Philadelphia)
Islam
ISLAM: ZEITSCHRIFT FUR GESCHICHTE UND KULTUR DES ISLAMISCHEN ORIENTS (Berlin)
Islam Stud
ISLAMIC STUDIES (Islamabad)
Isr Ann Psychiatry
ISRAEL ANNALS OF PSYCHIATRY AND RELATED DISCIPLINES (Jerusalem)
Isr J Med Sci
ISRAEL JOURNAL OF MEDICAL SCIENCES (Tel Aviv)
Isr J Psychiatr Relat Sci
ISRAEL JOURNAL OF PSYCHIATRY AND RELATED SCIENCES (Jerusalem)
Issue
ISSUE; A QUARTERLY JOURNAL OF OPINION (US)
Issues Health Care Women
ISSUES IN HEALTH CARE OF WOMEN (New York)
Issues Stud
ISSUES AND STUDIES (Taiwan)
Istor Biol Issled
ISTORIKO-BIOLOGICHESKIE ISSLEDOVANIIA (Moskva)
Istor Filol Zh
ISTORIKO-FILOLOGICHESKII ZHURNAL
Istor Pregl
ISTORICHESKI PREGLED (Bulgaria)
Istor SSSR
ISTORIIA SSSR (USSR)
Isotr Zap Acad Nauk SSSR
ISTORICHESKIE ZAPISKI AKADEMII NAUK SSSR (USSR)
Istor Zapisi
ISTORIJSKI ZAPISI (Yugoslavia)
Iyodenshi To Seitai Kogaku
IYODENSHI TO SEITAI KOGAKU. JAPANESE JOURNAL OF MEDICAL ELECTRONICS AND BIOLOGICAL ENGINEERING (Tokyo)
Izv Inst Istor
IZVESTIIA NA INSTITUTA ZA ISTORIIA (Bulgaria)
Izv Inst Istor BKP
IZVESTIIA NA INSTITUTA PO ISTORIIA NA BKP (Bulgaria)

## —J—

J Abnorm Psychol
JOURNAL OF ABNORMAL PSYCHOLOGY (Washington)
J Addict Res Found
JOURNAL-ADDICTION RESEARCH FOUNDATION (Toronto)
J Adolesc
JOURNAL OF ADOLESCENCE (London)
J Adolesc Health Care
JOURNAL OF ADOLESCENT HEALTH CARE (New York)
J Adv Nurs
JOURNAL OF ADVANCED NURSING (Oxford)
J Afr Hist
JOURNAL OF AFRICAN HISTORY (Gt Brit)
J Afro-Am Hist Geneal Soc
JOURNAL OF THE AFRO-AMERICAN

HISTORICAL AND GENEALOGICAL SOCIETY
J Agric Food Chem
JOURNAL OF AGRICULTURAL AND FOOD CHEMISTRY (Washington)
J Agric Tradit Bot Appl
JOURNAL D'AGRICULTURE TRADITIONNELLE ET DE BOTANIQUE APPLIQUEE (JATBA) (France)
J Agric Trop Bot Appl
JOURNAL D'AGRICULTURE TROPICALE ET DE BOTANIQUE APPLIQUEE
J Air Pollut Control Assoc
JOURNAL OF THE AIR POLLUTION CONTROL ASSOCIATION (Pittsburgh PA)
J Ala Dent Assoc
JOURNAL—ALABAMA DENTAL ASSOCIATION (Birmingham AL)
J Allergy Clin Immunol
JOURNAL OF ALLERGY AND CLINICAL IMMUNOLOGY (St Louis)
J Allied Health
JOURNAL OF ALLIED HEALTH (Thorofare NJ)
J Am Acad Child Psychiatry
JOURNAL OF THE AMERICAN ACADEMY OF CHILD PSYCHIATRY (New Haven CT)
J Am Acad Dermatol
JOURNAL OF THE AMERICAN ACADEMY OF DERMATOLOGY (St Louis)
J Am Acad Psychoanal
JOURNAL OF THE AMERICAN ACADEMY OF PSYCHOANALYSIS (New York)
J Am Acad Relig
JOURNAL—AMERICAN ACADEMY OF RELIGION
J Am Coll Cardiol
JOURNAL OF THE AMERICAN COLLEGE OF CARDIOLOGY (New York)
J Am Acad Dermatol
JOURNAL OF THE AMERICAN ACADEMY OF DERMATOLOGY (St Louis)
J Am Coll Health
JOURNAL OF AMERICAN COLLEGE HEALTH (Washington)
J Am Coll Nutr
JOURNAL OF THE AMERICAN COLLEGE OF NUTRITION (New York)
J Am Cult
JOURNAL OF AMERICAN CULTURE (Bowling Green OH)
J Am Dent Assoc
JOURNAL OF THE AMERICAN DENTAL ASSOCIATION (Chicago)
J Am Folkl
JOURNAL OF AMERICAN FOLKLORE
J Am Geriatr Soc
JOURNAL OF THE AMERICAN GERIATRICS SOCIETY (Philadelphia)
J Am Hist
JOURNAL OF AMERICAN HISTORY (Bloomington IN)
J Am Inst Soc Ger Russ
JOURNAL OF THE AMERICAN HISTORICAL SOCIETY OF GERMANS FROM RUSSIA (US)
J Am Inst Homeopath
JOURNAL OF THE AMERICAN INSTITUTE OF HOMEOPATHY (Washington)
J Am Intraocul Implant Soc
JOURNAL — AMERICAN INTRA-OCULAR IMPLANT SOCIETY (Santa Monica CA)
J Am Med Rec Assoc
JOURNAL OF THE AMERICAN MEDICAL RECORD ASSOCIATION (Chicago)
J Am Med Wom Assoc
JOURNAL OF THE AMERICAN MEDICAL WOMEN'S ASSOCIATION (New York)
J Am Oil Chem Soc
JOURNAL OF THE AMERICAN OIL CHEMISTS' SOCIETY (Chicago)
J Am Optom Assoc
JOURNAL OF THE AMERICAN OPTOMETRIC ASSOCIATION (St Louis)
J Am Orient Soc
JOURNAL: AMERICAN ORIENTAL SOCIETY (US)
J Am Osteopath Assoc
JOURNAL OF THE AMERICAN OSTEOPATHIC ASSOCIATION (Chicago)
J Am Podiatry Assoc
JOURNAL OF THE AMERICAN PODIATRY ASSOCIATION (Washington)
J Am Psychoanal Assoc
JOURNAL OF THE AMERICAN PSYCHOANALYTIC ASSOCIATION (New York)
J Am Res Cent Egypt
JOURNAL-AMERICAN RESEARCH CENTER IN EGYPT (US)
J Am Soc Psychosom Dent Med
JOURNAL OF THE AMERICAN SOCIETY OF PSYCHOSOMATIC DENTISTRY AND MEDICINE (Buffalo NY)
J Am Stud
JOURNAL OF AMERICAN STUDIES (Gt Brit)
J Am Vet Med Assoc
JOURNAL OF THE AMERICAN VETERINARY MEDICAL ASSOCIATION (Chicago)
J Anal Psychol
JOURNAL OF ANALYTICAL PSYCHOLOGY (London)
J Anat
JOURNAL OF ANATOMY (London)
J Androl
JOURNAL OF ANDROLOGY (Philadelphia)
J Antimicrob Chemother
JOURNAL OF ANTIMICROBIAL CHEMOTHERAPY (London)
J Appl Bacteriol
JOURNAL OF APPLIED BACTERIOLOGY (London)
J Appl Biochem

JOURNAL OF APPLIED BIOCHEMISTRY (New York)

J Appl Physiol
JOURNAL OF APPLIED PHYSIOLOGY: RESPIRATORY, ENVIRONMENTAL AND EXERCISE PHYSIOLOGY (Bethesda, MD)

J Appl Toxicol
JOURNAL OF APPLIED TOXICOLOGY (New York)

J Ariz Hist
JOURNAL OF ARIZONA HISTORY (Tucson AZ)

J Arkansas Med Soc
JOURNAL OF THE ARKANSAS MEDICAL SOCIETY (Fort Smith AR)

J Asian Stud
JOURNAL OF ASIAN STUDIES (Ann Arbor MI)

J Asiat Soc
JOURNAL OF THE ASIATIC SOCIETY (India)

J Assoc Off Anal Chem
JOURNAL — ASSOCIATION OF OFFICIAL ANALYTICAL CHEMISTS (Washington)

J Assoc Physicians India
JOURNAL OF THE ASSOCIATION OF PHYSICIANS OF INDIA (Bombay)

J Asthma
JOURNAL OF ASTHMA (New York)

J Asthma Res
JOURNAL OF ASTHMA RESEARCH (Baltimore)

J Auckl-Waikato Hist Soc
JOURNAL OF THE AUCKLAND-WAIKATO HISTORICAL SOCIETY (New Zealand)

J Audiov Media Med
JOURNAL OF AUDIOVISUAL MEDIA IN MEDICINE (London)

J Autism Dev Disord
JOURNAL OF AUTISM AND DEVELOPMENTAL DISORDERS (New York)

J Auton Nerv Syst
JOURNAL OF THE AUTONOMIC NERVOUS SYSTEM (Amsterdam)

J Auton Pharmacol
JOURNAL OF AUTONOMIC PHARMACOLOGY (North Ferriby, Yorkshire)

J Behav Med
JOURNAL OF BEHAVIORIAL MEDICINE (New York)

J Behav Ther Exp Psychiatry
JOURNAL OF BEHAVIOR THERAPY AND EXPERIMENTAL PSYCHIATRY (Elmsford NY)

J Belge Med Phys Rehabil
JOURNAL BELGE DE MEDECINE, PHYSIQUE ET DE REHABILITATION. BELGISCH TIJDSCHRIFT VOOR FYSISCHE GENEESKUNDE EN REHABILITATIE (Bruxelles)

J Bicommun
JOURNAL OF BIOCOMMUNICATIONS (San Francisco)

J Biol Chem
JOURNAL OF BIOLOGICAL PHOTOGRAPHY (Durham NC)

J Biomech Eng
JOURNAL OF BIOMECHANICAL ENGINEERING (New York)

J Biosoc Sci
JOURNAL OF BIOSOCIAL SCIENCE (Colchester)

J Black Stud
JOURNAL OF BLACK STUDIES (Beverly Hills CA)

J Br Stud
JOURNAL OF BRITISH STUDIES (Chicago)

J Bus
JOURNAL OF BUSINESS (Chicago)

J Calif Great Basin Anthropol
JOURNAL OF CALIFORNIA AND GREAT BASIN ANTHROPOLOGY (US)

J Can Church Hist Soc
JOURNAL OF THE CANADIAN CHURCH HISTORICAL SOCIETY (Canada)

J Can Stud
JOURNAL OF CANADIAN STUDIES (Canada)

J Cardiogr
JOURNAL OF CARDIOGRAPHY (Tokyo)

J Cardiovasc Surg (Torino)
JOURNAL OF CARDIOVASCULAR SURGERY (Torino)

J Cell Biol
JOURNAL OF CELL BIOLOGY (New York)

J Cell Physiol [Supp]
JOURNAL OF CELLULAR PHYSIOLOGY. SUPPLEMENT (New York)

J Chem Inf Comput Sci
JOURNAL OF CHEMICAL INFORMATION AND COMPUTER SCIENCES (Washington)

J Cherokee Stud
JOURNAL OF CHEROKEE STUDIES (Cherokee NC)

J Child Psychol Psychiatry
JOURNAL OF CHILD PSYCHOLOGY AND PSYCHIATRY AND ALLIED DISCIPLINES (Oxford)

J Chin Univ Hong Kong
JOURNAL OF THE CHINESE UNIVERISTY OF HONG KONG (Hong Kong)

J Chronic Dis
JOURNAL OF CHRONIC DISEASES (St Louis)

J Church State
JOURNAL OF CHURCH AND STATE (Waco TX)

J Clin Chem Clin Biochem
JOURNAL OF CLINICAL CHEMISTRY AND CLINICAL BIOCHEMISTRY (Berlin)

J Clin Endocrinol Metab
JOURNAL OF CLINICAL ENDOCRINOLOGY AND METABOLISM (Philadelphia)

J Clin Eng
JOURNAL OF CLINICAL ENGINEERING (City of Industry CA)

J Clin Gastroenterol
JOURNAL OF CLINICAL GASTROENTEROLOGY (New York)

J Clin Invest

JOURNAL OF CLINICAL INVESTIGATION (New York)
J Clin Oncol
JOURNAL OF CLINICAL ONCOLOGY (New York)
J Clin Pathol
JOURNAL OF CLINICAL PATHOLOGY (London)
J Clin Pharmacol
JOURNAL OF CLINICAL PHARMACOLOGY (New York)
J Clin Psychiatry
JOURNAL OF CLINICAL PSYCHIATRY (Memphis TN)
J Clin Psychopharmacol
JOURNAL OF CLINICAL PSYCHOPHARMACOLOGY (Baltimore)
J Colo Dent Assoc
JOURNAL OF THE COLORADO DENTAL ASSOCIATION (Denver CO)
J Commonw Comp Polit
JOURNAL OF COMMONWEALTH AND COMPARATIVE POLITICS (Gt Brit)
J Commonw Polit Stud
JOURNAL OF COMMONWEALTH POLITICAL STUDIES (Gt Brit)
J Commun
JOURNAL OF COMMUNICATION (Philadelphia)
J Commun Disord
JOURNAL OF COMMUNICATION DISORDERS (Amsterdam)
J Comp Neurol
JOURNAL OF COMPARATIVE NEUROLOGY (New York)
J Comput Assist Tomogr
JOURNAL OF COMPUTER ASSISTED TOMOGRAPHY (New York)
J Contemp Asia
JOURNAL OF CONTEMPORARY ASIA (Sweden)
J Contemp Hist
JOURNAL OF CONTEMPORARY HISTORY (Gt Brit)
J Craniofac Genet Dev Biol
JOURNAL OF CRANIOFACIAL GENETICS AND DEVELOPMENTAL BIOLOGY (New York)
J Cutan Pathol
JOURNAL OF CUTANEOUS PATHOLOGY (Copenhagen)
J Cyclic Nucleotide Res
JOURNAL OF CYCLIC NUCLEOTIDE RESEARCH (New York)
J Dairy Sc
JOURNAL OF DAIRY SCIENCE (Champaign IL)
J DC Dent Soc
JOURNAL — DISTRICT OF COLUMBIA DENTAL SOCIETY (Washington)
J Dent
JOURNAL OF DENTISTRY (Bristol)
J Dent Assoc S Afr
JOURNAL OF THE DENTAL ASSOCIATION OF SOUTH AFRICA (Cape Town)
J Dent Assoc Thai
JOURNAL OF THE DENTAL ASSOCIATION OF THAILAND (Bangkok)
J Dent Educ
JOURNAL OF DENTAL EDUCATION (Washington)
J Dent Pract Adm
JOURNAL OF DENTAL PRACTICE ADMINISTRATION (Philadelphia)
J Dent Res
JOURNAL OF DENTAL RESEARCH (Houston TX)
J Dermatol Surg Oncol
JOURNAL OF DERMATOLOGIC SURGERY AND ONCOLOGY
J Dev Areas
JOURNAL OF THE DEVELOPING AREAS (Macomb IL)
J Dev Stud
JOURNAL OF DEVELOPMENT STUDIES (Gt Brit)
J Early Repub
JOURNAL OF THE EARLY REPUBLIC (Indianapolis IN)
J Econ Hist
JOURNAL OF ECONOMIC HISTORY (Wilmington DE)
J Econ Soc Hist Orient (Netherl)
JOURNAL OF THE ECONOMIC AND SOCIAL HISTORY OF THE ORIENT (Netherlands)
J Ecumenical Stud
JOURNAL OF ECUMENICAL STUDIES (Philadelphia)
J Educ Adm Hist
JOURNAL OF EDUCATIONAL ADMINISTRATION AND HISTORY (Yorkshire Eng)
J Egypt Archeol
JOURNAL OF EGYPTIAN ARCHEOLOGY
J Egypt Med Assoc
JOURNAL OF THE EGYPTIAN MEDICAL ASSOCIATION (Cairo)
J Egypt Soc Parasitol
JOURNAL OF THE EGYPTIAN SOCIETY OF PARASITOLOGY (Cairo)
J Electrocardiol
JOURNAL OF ELECTROCARDIOLOGY (South Burlington VT)
J Emerg Med
JOURNAL OF EMERGENCY MEDICINE (New York)
J Emerg Med Serv JEMS
JOURNAL OF EMERGENCY MEDICAL SERVICES: JEMS (Morristown NJ)
J Endocrinol
JOURNAL OF ENDOCRINOLOGY (London)
J Endocrinol Invest
JOURNAL OF ENDOCRINOLOGICAL INVESTIGATION (Milano)
J Endod
JOURNAL OF ENDODONTICS (Chicago)

J Environ Sci Health [B]
JOURNAL OF ENVIRONMENTAL SCIENCE AND HEALTH. PART B: PESTICIDES, FOOD CONTAMINANTS, AND AGRICULTURAL WASTES (New York)
J Epidemiol Community Health
JOURNAL OF EPIDEMIOLOGY AND COMMUNITY HEALTH (London)
J Erie Stud
JOURNAL OF ERIE STUDIES (Erie PA)
J Ethn Stud
JOURNAL OF ETHNIC STUDIES (Bellingham WA)
J Ethnopharmacol
JOURNAL OF ETHNOPHARMACOLOGY (Lausanne)
J Eur Econ Hist
JOURNAL OF EUROPEAN ECONOMIC HISTORY (Italy)
J Eur Stud
JOURNAL OF EUROPEAN STUDIES (Gt Brit)
J Exp Anal Behav
JOURNAL OF THE EXPERIMENTAL ANALYSIS OF BEHAVIOR (Bloomington IN)
J Exp Med
JOURNAL OF EXPERIMENTAL MEDICINE (New York)
J Fac Med Baghdad
JOURNAL OF THE FACULTY OF MEDICINE, BAGHDAD (Iraq)
J Fam Hist
JOURNAL OF FAMILY HISTORY (Minneapolis MN)
J Fam Pract
JOURNAL OF FAMILY PRACTICE (New York)
J Fla Med Assoc
JOURNAL OF THE FLORIDA MEDICAL ASSOCIATION (Jacksonville FL)
J Forensic Sci
JOURNAL OF FORENSIC SCIENCES (Philadelphia)
J Forensic Sci Soc
JOURNAL — FORENSIC SCIENCE SOCIETY (London)
J Fr Ophtalmol
JOURNAL FRANCAIS D'OPHTALMOLOGIE (Paris)
J Fr Otorhinolaryngol
JOURNAL FRANCAIS D'OTO-RHINO-LARYNGOLOGIE, AUDIOPHONOLOGIE, CHIRURGIE MAXILLO-FACIALE (Villeurbanne)
J Genet Hum
JOURNAL DE GENETIQUE HUMAINE (Geneva)
J Geriatr Psychiatr
JOURNAL OF GERIATRIC PSYCHIATRY (New York)
J Gerontol Nurs
JOURNAL OF GERONTOLOGICAL NURSING (Thorofare NJ)
J Gynecol Obstet Biol Reprod (Paris)
JOURNAL DE GYNECOLOGIE, OBSTETRIQUE ET BIOLOGIE DE LA REPRODUCTION (Paris)
J Hand Surg [Am]
JOURNAL OF HAND SURGERY (St Louis)
J Hand Surg [Br]
JOURNAL OF HAND SURGERY (Endinburgh)
J Health Hum Resour Adm
JOURNAL OF HEALTH AND HUMAN RESOURCES ADMINISTRATION (Montgomery AL)
J Health Polit Policy Law
JOURNAL OF HEALTH POLITICS, POLICY AND LAW (Durham NC)
J Health Soc Behav
JOURNAL OF HEALTH AND SOCIAL BEHAVIOR (Washington)
J Hered
JOURNAL OF HEREDITY (Washington)
J Hirnforsch
JOURNAL FUR HIRNFORSCHUNG (Berlin)
J Hist Arabic Sci
JOURNAL FOR THE HISTORY OF ARABIC SCIENCE (Aleppo)
J Hist Behav Sci
JOURNAL OF THE HISTORY OF THE BEHAVIORAL SCIENCES (Brandon VT)
J Hist Biol
JOURNAL OF THE HISTORY OF BIOLOGY (Dordrecht)
J Hist Geogr
JOURNAL OF HISTORICAL GEOGRAPHY (New York)
J Hist Ideas
JOURNAL OF THE HISTORY OF IDEAS (Philadelphia)
J Hist Med Allied Sci
JOURNAL OF THE HISTORY OF MEDICINE AND ALLIED SCIENCES (New Haven CT)
J Hist Philos
JOURNAL OF THE HISTORY OF PHILOSOPHY (San Diego CA)
J Hist Sociol
JOURNAL OF THE HISTORY OF SOCIOLOGY (Brookline MA)
J Histochem Cytochem
JOURNAL OF HISTOCHEMISTRY AND CYTOCHEMISTRY (Baltimore)
J Homosex
JOURNAL OF HOMOSEXUALITY (New York)
J Hong Kong Branch R Asiat Soc
JOURNAL OF THE HONG KONG BRANCH OF THE ROYAL ASIATIC SOCIETY (Hong Kong)
J Hyg (Lond)
JOURNAL OF HYGIENE (London)
J Hyg Epidemiol Microbiol Immunol
JOURNAL OF HYGIENE, EPIDEMIOLOGY, MICROBIOLOGY AND IMMUNOLOGY (Praha)
J Ill State Hist Soc
JOURNAL OF THE ILLINOIS STATE HISTORICAL SOCIETY (Springfield IL)
J Immunol

JOURNAL OF IMMUNOLOGY (Baltimore)
J Immunol Methods
JOURNAL OF IMMUNOLOGICAL METHODS (Amsterdam)
J Ind Econ
JOURNAL OF INDUSTRIAL ECONOMICS (Oxford)
J Indian Hist
JOURNAL OF INDIAN HISTORY (India)
J Indian Med Assoc
JOURNAL OF THE INDIAN MEDICAL ASSOCIATION (Calcutta)
J Indiana State Med Assoc
JOURNAL OF THE INDIANA STATE MEDICAL ASSOCIATION (Indianapolis IN)
J Individ Psychol
JOURNAL OF INDIVIDUAL PSYCHOLOGY (Chicago)
J Infect
JOURNAL OF INFECTION (Chicago)
J Infect Dis
JOURNAL OF INFECTIOUS DISEASES (Chicago)
J Int Wine Food Soc
JOURNAL OF THE INTERNATIONAL WINE AND FOOD SOCIETY
J Interam Stud World Aff
JOURNAL OF INTERAMERICAN STUDIES AND WORLD AFFAIRS (Beverly Hills CA)
J Interdiscip Hist
JOURNAL OF INTERDISCIPLINARY HISTORY (Cambridge MA)
J Invest Dermatol
JOURNAL OF INVESTIGATIVE DERMATOLOGY (Baltimore)
J Iowa Med Soc
JOURNAL OF THE IOWA MEDICAL SOCIETY (Des Moines IA)
J Ir Coll Physicians Surg
JOURNAL OF THE IRISH COLLEGE OF PHYSICIANS AND SURGEONS (Dublin)
J Ir Dent Assoc
JOURNAL OF THE IRISH DENTAL ASSOCIATION (Dublin)
J Kans Med Soc
JOURNAL OF THE KANSAS MEDICAL SOCIETY (Topeka KS)
J Ky Med Assoc
JOURNAL OF THE KENTUCKY MEDICAL ASSOCIATION (Louisville KY)
J La State Med Soc
JOURNAL OF THE LOUISIANA STATE MEDICAL SOCIETY (New Orleans LA)
J Lab Clin Med
JOURNAL OF LABORATORY AND CLINICAL MEDICINE (St Louis)
J Lanc Cty Hist Soc
JOURNAL OF THE LANCASTER COUNTY HISTORICAL SOCIETY (Lancaster PA)
J Laryngol Otol
JOURNAL OF LARYNGOLOGY AND OTOLOGY (Asford)
J Lat Am Stud
JOURNAL OF LATIN AMERICAN STUDIES (Gt Brit)
J Law Econ
JOURNAL OF LAW AND ECONOMICS (Chicago)
J Learn Disabil
JOURNAL OF LEARNING DISABILITIES (Chicago)
J Leo Med (Chicago)
JOURNAL OF LEGAL MEDICINE (Long Island City NY)
J Libert Stud
JOURNAL OF LIBERTARIAN STUDIES (New York)
J Libr Hist
JOURNAL OF LIBRARY HISTORY, PHILOSOPHY, AND COMPARATIVE LIBRARIANSHIP (Austin TX)
J Librariansh
JOURNAL OF LIBRARIANSHIP (London)
J Lipid Res
JOURNAL OF LIPID RESEARCH (Bethesda MD)
J Long Term Care Adm
JOURNAL OF LONG TERM CARE ADMINISTRATION (Silver Spring MD)
J Mal Vasc
JOURNAL DES MALADIES VASCULAIRES (Paris)
J Malays Branch R Asiat Soc
JOURNAL — MALAYSIAN BRANCH — ROYAL ASIATIC SOCIETY (Singapore)
J Maxillofac Surg
JOURNAL OF MAXILLOFACIAL SURGERY (Stuttgart)
J Md State Dent Assoc
JOURNAL OF THE MARYLAND STATE DENTAL ASSOCIATION (Baltimore)
J Med Assoc Ga
JOURNAL OF THE MEDICAL ASSOCIATION OF GEORGIA (Atlanta GA)
J Med Assoc State Ala
JOURNAL OF THE MEDICAL ASSOCIATION OF THE STATE OF ALABAMA (Montgomery AL)
J Med Chir Prat
JOURNAL DE MEDECINE ET DE CHIRURGIE PRATIQUES (Paris)
J Med Educ
JOURNAL OF MEDICAL EDUCATION (Washington)
J Med Eng Technol
JOURNAL OF MEDICAL ENGINEERING AND TECHNOLOGY (London)
J Med Entomol
JOURNAL OF MEDICAL ENTOMOLOGY (Honolulu HI)
J Med Ethics
JOURNAL OF MEDICAL ETHICS (London)
J Med Lyon
JOURNAL DE MEDECINE DE LYON (Lyon)
J Med Philos

JOURNAL OF MEDICINE AND PHILOSOPHY (Chicago)
J Med Primatol
JOURNAL OF MEDICAL PRIMATOLOGY (New York)
J Med Soc NJ
JOURNAL OF THE MEDICAL SOCIETY OF NEW JERSEY (Trenton NJ)
J Med Strasb
JOURNAL DE MEDECINE DE STRASBOURG (Paris)
J Med Syst
JOURNAL OF MEDICAL SYSTEMS (New York)
J Mediev Renaiss Stud
JOURNAL OF MEDIEVAL AND RENAISSANCE STUDIES (Durham NC)
J Microsc
JOURNAL OF MICROSCOPY (Oxford)
J Microsurg
JOURNAL OF MICROSURGERY (New York)
J Miss Dent Assoc
JOURNAL — MISSISSIPPI DENTAL ASSOCIATION (McComb MS)
J Miss Hist
JOURNAL OF MISSISSIPPI HISTORY (Jackson MS)
J Miss State Med Assoc
JOURNAL OF THE MISSISSIPPI STATE MEDICAL ASSOCIATION (Jackson MS)
J Mod Afr Stud
JOURNAL OF MODERN AFRICAN STUDIES (New York)
J Mod Hist
JOURNAL OF MODERN HISTORY (Chicago)
J Mol Cell Cardiol
JOURNAL OF MOLECULAR AND CELLULAR CARDIOLOGY (London)
J Mol Evol
JOURNAL OF MOLECULAR EVOLUTION (Berlin)
J Music Ther
JOURNAL OF MUSIC THERAPY (Lawrence KS)
J NAL Assoc
JOURNAL OF NAL ASSOCIATION (US)
J Nat Prod
JOURNAL OF NATURAL PRODUCTS (Columbus OH)
J Natl Assoc Priv Psychiatr Hosp
JOURNAL — NATIONAL ASSOCIATION OF PSYCHIATRIC HOSPITALS (Leonia NJ)
J Natl Med Assoc
JOURNAL OF THE NATIONAL MEDICAL ASSOCIATION (New York)
J Negro Educ
JOURNAL OF NEGRO EDUCATION (Washington)
J Negro Hist
JOURNAL OF NEGRO HISTORY (Washington)
J Nerv Ment Dis
JOURNAL OF NERVOUS AND MENTAL DISEASE (Baltimore)
J Neurol Neurosurg Psychiatry
JOURNAL OF NEUROLOGY, NEUROSURGERY AND PSYCHIATRY (London)
J Neurol Sci
JOURNAL OF THE NEUROLOGICAL SCIENCES (Amsterdam)
J Neurosurg
JOURNAL OF NEUROSURGERY (Baltimore)
J North LA Hist Assoc
JOURNAL NORTH LOUISIANA HISTORICAL ASSOCIATION (Ruston LA)
J Nucl Med
JOURNAL OF NUCLEAR MEDICINE (New York)
J Nucl Med Allied Sci
JOURNAL OF NUCLEAR MEDICINE AND ALLIED SCIENCES (Torino)
J Nurs Adm
JOURNAL OF NURSING ADMINISTRATION (Wakefield)
J Nurs Care
JOURNAL OF NURSING CARE (New York)
J Nurse Midwife
JOURNAL OF NURSE MIDWIFERY (New York NY)
J Nutr
JOURNAL OF NUTRITION (Bethesda MD)
J Occup Med
JOURNAL OF OCCUPATIONAL MEDICINE (Chicago)
J Okla State Med Assoc
JOURNAL — OKLAHOMA STATE MEDICAL ASSOCIATION (Oklahoma City OK)
J Oper Room Res Inst
JOURNAL OF THE OPERATING ROOM RESEARCH INSTITUTE (Totowa NJ)
J Oral Implantol
JOURNAL OF ORAL IMPLANTOLOGY (Abington MA)
J Oral Rehabil
JOURNAL OF ORAL REHABILITATION (Oxford)
J Oral Surg
JOURNAL OF ORAL SURGERY (Chicago)
J Orthop Res
JOURNAL OF ORTHOPAEDIC RESEARCH (New York)
J Otolaryngol
JOURNAL OF OTOLARYNGOLOGY (Toronto)
J Pac Hist
JOURNAL OF PACIFIC HISTORY (Australia)
J Parasitol
JOURNAL OF PARASITOLOGY (Lawrence KS)
J Pastoral Care
JOURNAL OF PASTORAL CARE (Kutztown PA)
J Peace Res
JOURNAL OF PEACE RESEARCH (Oslo)
J Pediatr
JOURNAL OF PEDIATRICS (St Louis)
J Pediatr Ophthalmol Strabismus
JOURNAL OF PEDIATRIC OPHTHALMOLOGY

AND STRABISMUS (Thorofare NJ)
J Pediatr Orthop
JOURNAL OF PEDIATRIC ORTHOPEDICS (New York)
J Pediatr Surg
JOURNAL OF PEDIATRIC SURGERY (New York)
J Perinat Med
JOURNAL OF PERINATAL MEDICINE (Berlin)
J Periodontol
JOURNAL OF PERIODONTOLOGY (Chicago)
J Pers Soc Psychol
JOURNAL OF PERSONALITY AND SOCIAL PSYCHOLOGY (Washington)
J Physiol (Lond)
JOURNAL OF PHYSIOLOGY (Cambridge)
J Polit
JOURNAL OF POLITICS (Gainesville FL)
J Polit Econ
JOURNAL OF POLITICAL ECONOMY (Chicago)
J Polynesian Soc
JOURNAL OF THE POLYNESIAN SOCIETY (New Zealand)
J Pop Cult
JOURNAL OF POPULAR CULTURE (Bowling Green OH)
J Postgrad Med
JOURNAL OF POSTGRADUATE MEDICINE (Bombay)
J Presbyt Hist
JOURNAL OF PRESBYTERIAN HISTORY (Philadelphia)
J Prosthet Dent
JOURNAL OF PROSTHETIC DENTISTRY (St Louis)
J Protozool
JOURNAL OF PROTOZOOLOGY (New York)
J Psychedelic Drugs
JOURNAL OF PSYCHEDELIC DRUGS (Madison WI)
J Psychiatr Nurs
JOURNAL OF PSYCHIATRIC NURSING AND MENTAL HEALTH SERVICES (Thorofare NJ)
J Psychiatr Res
JOURNAL OF PSYCHIATRIC RESEARCH (Oxford)
J Psychoactive Drugs
JOURNAL OF PSYCHOACTIVE DRUGS (San Francisco)
J Psychohist
JOURNAL OF PSYCHOHISTORY (New York)
J Psychol
JOURNAL OF PSYCHOLOGY (Provincetown MA)
J Psychosoc Nurs Ment Health Serv
JOURNAL OF PSYCHOSOCIAL NURSING AND MENTAL HEALTH SERVICES (Thorofare NJ)
J Public Health Dent
JOURNAL OF PUBLIC HEALTH DENTISTRY (Raleigh NC)
J Public Health Policy
JOURNAL OF PUBLIC HEALTH POLICY (Burlington VT)
J R Army Med Corps
JOURNAL OF THE ROYAL ARMY MEDICAL CORPS (London)
J R Asiat Soc GB Irel
JOURNAL — ROYAL ASIATIC SOCIETY OF GREAT BRITAIN AND IRELAND (London)
J R Aust His Soc
JOURNAL OF THE ROYAL AUSTRALIAN HISTORICAL SOCIETY (Australia)
J R Coll Gen Pract
JOURNAL OF THE ROYAL COLLEGE OF GENERAL PRACTITIONERS (London)
J R Coll Physicians Lond
JOURNAL OF THE ROYAL COLLEGE OF PHYSICIANS OF LONDON (London)
J R Coll Surg Edinb
JOURNAL OF THE ROYAL COLLEGE OF SURGEONS OF EDINBURGH (Edinburgh)
J R Nav Med Serv
JOURNAL OF THE ROYAL NAVAL MEDICAL SCIENCE (Alverstoke)
J R Soc Health
JOURNAL OF THE ROYAL SOCIETY OF HEALTH (London)
J R Soc Med
JOURNAL OF THE ROYAL SOCIETY OF MEDICINE (London)
J R Stat Soc
JOURNAL OF THE ROYAL STATISTICAL SOCIETY (London)
J Radiol
JOURNAL DE RADIOLOGIE (Paris)
J Rehabil
JOURNAL OF REHABILITATION (Washington)
J Relig
JOURNAL OF RELIGION (Chicago)
J Relig Afr
JOURNAL OF RELIGION IN AFRICA (Leiden)
J Reprod Fertil
JOURNAL OF REPRODUCTION AND FERTILITY (Oxford)
J Reprod Fertil [Suppl]
JOURNAL OF REPRODUCTION AND FERTILITY, SUPPLEMENT (Oxford)
J Reprod Med
JOURNAL OF REPRODUCTIVE MEDICINE (Chicago)
J Reticuloendothel Soc
JOURNAL OF THE RETICULOENDOTHELIAL SOCIETY (Winston-Salem NC)
J Rheumatol
JOURNAL OF RHEUMATOLOGY (Toronto)
J Rutgers Univ Libr.
JOURNAL OF RUTGERS UNIVERSITY LIBRARY (New Burnswick NJ)
J S Afr Vet Assoc
JOURNAL OF THE SOUTH AFRICAN VETERINARY ASSOCIATION (Pretoria)

J San Diego Hist
JOURNAL OF SAN DIEGO HISTORY (San Diego CA)

J Sc Med Assoc
JOURNAL OF THE SOUTH CAROLINA MEDICAL ASSOCIATION (Columbia SC)

J Sch Health
JOURNAL OF SCHOOL HEALTH (Kent OH)

J Sci Stud Relig
JOURNAL FOR THE SCIENTIFIC STUDY OF RELIGION (Notre Dame IN)

J Semit Stud
JOURNAL OF SEMITIC STUDIES (Gt Brit)

J Siam Soc
JOURNAL OF THE SIAM SOCIETY (Thailand)

J Small Anim Pract
JOURNAL OF SMALL ANIMAL PRACTICE (Oxford)

J Soc Army Hist Res
JOURNAL OF THE SOCIETY FOR ARMY HISTORICAL RESEARCH (London)

J Soc Bibliogr Nat Hist
JOURNAL OF THE SOCIETY FOR THE BIBLIOGRAPHY OF NATURAL HISTORY (London)

J Soc Hist
JOURNAL OF SOCIAL HISTORY (Pittsburgh PA)

J Soc Issues
JOURNAL OF SOCIAL ISSUES (US)

J Soc Occup Med
JOURNAL OF THE SOCIETY OF OCCUPATIONAL MEDICINE (Edinburgh)

J Soc Policy
JOURNAL OF SOCIAL POLICY (London)

J South Afr Stud
JOURNAL OF SOUTHERN AFRICAN STUDIES (Gt Brit)

J South Hist
JOURNAL OF SOUTHERN HISTORY (Athens GA)

J Speech Hear Disord
JOURNAL OF SPEECH AND HEARING DISORDERS (Rockville MD)

J Speech Hear Res
JOURNAL OF SPEECH AND HEARING RESEARCH (Rockville MD)

J Sport Hist
JOURNAL OF SPORT HISTORY (University Park PA)

J Sports Med Phys Fitness
JOURNAL OF SPORTS MEDICINE AND PHYSICAL FITNESS (Torino)

J Sri Lanka Branch R Asiat Soc
JOURNAL OF THE SRI LANKA BRANCH OF THE ROYAL ASIATIC SOCIETY (Sri Lanka)

J Steroid Biochem
JOURNAL OF STEROID BIOCHEMISTRY (Oxford)

J Stud Alcohol
JOURNAL OF STUDIES ON ALCOHOL (New Brunswick NJ)

J Stud Alcohol [Suppl]
JOURNAL OF STUDIES ON ALCOHOL. SUPPLEMENT (New Brunswich NJ)

J Submicrosc Cytol
JOURNAL OF SUBMICROSCOPIC CYTOLOGY (Bologna)

J Surg Oncol
JOURNAL OF SURGICAL ONCOLOGY (New York)

J Tenn Dent Assoc
JOURNAL OF THE TENNESSEE DENTAL ASSOCIATION (Nashville TN)

J Tenn Med Assoc
JOURNAL OF THE TENNESSEE MEDICAL ASSOCIATION (Nashville TN)

J Thorac Cardiovascular Surg
JOURNAL OF THORACIC AND CARDIOVASCULAR SURGERY (St Louis)

J Toxicol Clin Toxicol
JOURNAL OF TOXICOLOGY. CLINICAL TOXICOLOGY (New York)

J Toxiocl Environ Health
JOURNAL OF TOXICOLOGY AND ENVIRONMENTAL HEALTH (Washington)

J Tradit Chin Med
JOURNAL OF TRADITIONAL CHINESE MEDICINE (Beijing)

J Trauma
JOURNAL OF TRAUMA (Baltimore)

J Trop Med Hyg
JOURNAL OF TROPICAL MEDICINE AND HYGIENE (London)

J Trop Pediatr
JOURNAL OF TROPICAL PEDIATRICS (London)

J Urban Hist
JOURNAL OF URBAN HISTORY (Beverly Hills CA)

J Urol
JOURNAL OF UROLOGY (Baltimore)

J Urol (Paris)
JOURNAL D'UROLOGIE (Paris)

J Vasc Surg
JOURNAL OF VASCULAR SURGERY (St Louis)

J Vet Med Educ
JOURNAL OF VETERINARY MEDICAL EDUCATION (Knoxville TN)

J Vet Pharmacol Ther
JOURNAL OF VETERINARY PHARMACOLOGY AND THERAPEUTICS (Oxford)

J W Va Hist Assoc
JOURNAL OF THE WEST VIRGINIA HISTORICAL ASSOCIATION (Huntington WV)

J Warburg Courtauld Inst
JOURNAL OF THE WARBURG AND COURTAULD INSTITUTE (London)

Jaarb Kunst Oudheidk Kring Deinze
JAARBOEK VAN DE KUNST-OUDHEIDKUNDIGE KRING DEINZE

Jabega (Malaga)
JABEGA (Malaga)

Jahrb Coburg Landesstift
JAHRBUCH DER COBURGER LANDESSTIFTUNG
Jahrb Gesch
JAHRBUCH FUR GESCHICHTE (Berlin)
Jahrb Gesch Osteur
JAHRBUCHER FUR GESCHICHTE OSTEUROPAS (Wiesbaden)
Jahrb Gesch Staat Wirtsch Ges Lateinam
JAHRBUCH FUR GESCHICHTE VON STAAT WIRTSCHAFT UND GESELLSCHAFT LATEINAMERIKAS (Cologne)
Jahrb Gorres Ges
JAHRBUCH DER GORRES GESELLSCHAFT
Jahrb Hist Ver Furst Liechtenstein
JAHRBUCH DES HISTORISCHEN VEREINS FUR DAS FURSTENTUM LIECHTENSTEIN (Liechtenstein)
Jahrb Inst Dtsch Gesch
JAHRBUCH DES INSTITUTS FUR DEUTSCHE GESCHICHTE (Israel)
Jahrb Krit Med
JAHRBUCH FUR KRITISCHE MEDIZIN (Berlin)
Jahrb Landeskd Niederosterr
JAHRBUCH FUR LANDESKUNDE VON NIEDEROSTERREICH (Vienna)
Jahrb Univ Dusseld
JAHRBUCH DER UNIVERSITAT DUSSELDORF (Dusseldorf)
Jahrb Westdtsch Landesgesch
JAHRBUCH WESTDEUTSCHE LANDESGESCHICHTE
JAMA
JOURNAL OF THE AMERICAN MEDICAL ASSOCIATION (Chicago)
Jamaican Nurse
JAMAICAN NURSE (Jamaica)
Janus
JANUS; REVUE INTERNATIONALE DE L'HISTOIRE DES SCIENCES, DE LA MEDECINE, DE LA PHARMACIE ET DE LA TECHNIQUE (Netherlands)
JAOA
JAOA. JOURNAL OF THE AMERICAN OSTEOPATHIC ASSOCIATION (Chicago)
JCU
JCU; JOURNAL OF CLINICAL ULTRASOUND (Denver CO)
JDBP
JDPP. JOURNAL OF DEVELOPMENTAL AND BEHAVIORAL PEDIATRICS (Baltimore)
Jednota Annu Furdek (US)
JEDNOTA ANNUAL FURDEK (US)
Jerus Stud Arabic Islam
JERUSALEM STUDIES OF ARABIC ISLAM
Jew Q Rev
JEWISH QUARTERLY REVIEW (Philadelphia)
Jew Soc Stud
JEWISH SOCIAL STUDIES (New York)
Jimbun Chiri
JIMBUN CHIRI (Tokyo)
JNCI
JNCI. JOURNAL OF THE NATIONAL CANCER INSTITUTE (Bethesda MD)
JNE
JNE; JOURNAL OF NURSING EDUCATION (Thorofare NJ)
JNM
JNM; JOURNAL OF NUCLEAR MEDICINE (New York)
JOGN Nurs
JOGN NURSING (Hagerstown MD)
Johns Hopkins Med J
JOHNS HOPKINS MEDICAL JOURNAL (Baltimore)
JOM
JOM. JOURNAL OF OCCUPATIONAL MEDICINE (Chicago)
Jordemodern
JORDEMODERN (Stockholm)
Josanpu Zasshi
JOSANPU ZASSHI. JAPANESE JOURNAL FOR MIDWIVES (Tokyo)
Journ Annu Diabetol Hotel Dieu
JOURNEES ANNUELLES DE DIABETOLOGIE DE L'HOTEL-DIEU (Paris)
Journalism Hist
JOURNALISM HISTORY (Northridge CA)
Journalism Monogr
JOURNALISM MONOGRAPHS (Minneapolis MN)
JPEN
JPEN. JOURNAL OF PARENTERAL AND ENTERAL NUTRITION (Baltimore)
JPMA
JPMA. JOURNAL OF THE PAKISTAN MEDICAL ASSOCIATION (Karachi)
Jpn Heart J
JAPANESE HEART JOURNAL (Tokyo)
Jpn J Med
JAPANESE JOURNAL OF MEDICINE (Tokyo)
Jpn J Ophthalmol
JAPANESE JOURNAL OF OPHTHALMOLOGY (Tokyo)
Jpn Stud Hist Sci
JAPANESE STUDIES IN THE HISTORY OF SCIENCE (Okayama)
Jugosl Ginekol Opstet
JUGOSLAVENSKA GINEKOLOGIJA I OPSTETRICIJA (Zagreb)
Jyske Saml
JYSKE SAMLINGER (Denmark)

—K—

K Krigsvetensk Akad Handl Tidskr
KUNGLIGA KRIGSVETENSKAPS AKADEMIENS HANDLINGAR OCH TIDSKRIFT (Sweden)
Kagakushi Kenkyu

KAGAKUSHI KENKYU (Tokyo) JOURNAL OF HISTORY OF SCIENCE, JAPAN
Kampo No Rinsho
KAMPO NO RINSHO (Tokyo)
Kango
KANGO (Tokyo)
Kango Gijutsu
KANGO GIJUTSU. JAPANESE JOURNAL OF NURSING ART (Tokyo)
Kango Kenkyu
KANGO KENKYU. JAPANESE JOURNAL OF NURSING RESEARCH (Tokyo)
Kango Kyoiku
KANGO KYOIKU. JAPANESE JOURNAL OF NURSES EDUCATION (Tokyo)
Kango Tenbo
KANGO TENBO. JAPANESE JOURNAL OF NURSING SCIENCE (Tokyo)
Kangogaku Zasshi
KANGOGAKU ZASSHI. JAPANESE JOURNAL OF NURSING (Tokyo)
Kans Hist
KANSAS HISTORY (Topeka KS)
Kans Nurse
KANSAS NURSE (Topeka KS)
Kardiol Pol
KARDIOLOGIA POLSKA (Warszawa)
Kardiologiia
KARDIOLOGIIA (Moskva)
Karolinska Forb Arsb
KAROLINSKA FORBUNDETS ARSBOK (Sweden)
Katilolehti
KATILOLEHTI; TIDSKRIFT FOR BARNMORSKOR (Helsinki)
Kekkaku
KEKKAKU (Tokyo)
Khirurgiia (Mosk)
KHIRURGIIA (Moskva)
Khirurgiia (Sofiia)
KHIRURGIIA (Sofiia)
Kidney Int [Suppl]
KIDNEY INTERNATIONAL. SUPPLEMENT (New York)
Kinderarztl Prax
KINDERARZTLICHE PRAXIS (Leipzig)
King Faisal Spec Hosp Med J
KING FAISAL SPECIALIST HOSPITAL MEDICAL JOURNAL (Riyadh)
Kiva
KIVA (Tucson AZ)
Kleio
KLEIO (Netherlands)
Kleio (S Afr)
KLEIO (South Africa)
Klin Anasthesiol Intensivther
KLINSCHE ANASTHESIOLOGIE UND INTENSIVTHERAPIE (Berlin)
Klin Khir
KLINICHESKAIA KHIRURGIIA (Kiev)
Klin Med (Mosk)
KLINICHESKAIA MEDITSINA (Moskva)
Klin Monatsbl Augenheilkd
KLINISCHE MONATSBLATTER FUR AUGENHEILKUNDE (Stuttgart)
Klin Oczna
KLINIKA OCZNA (Warszawa)
Klin Padiatr
KLINISCHE PADIATRIE (Stuttgart)
Klio
KLIO: BEITRAGE ZUR GESCHICHTE DER HISTORISCHEN KUNST (Berlin)
Koinonia
KOINONIA (Nashville TN)
Koku Eisei Gakkai Zasshi
KOKU EISEI GAKKAI ZASSHI (Tokyo)
Kokubyo Gakkai Zasshi
KOKUBYO GAKKAI ZASSHI. THE JOURNAL OF THE STOMATOLOGICAL SOCIETY, JAPAN (Tokyo)
Komun Mazursko Warm
KOMUNIKATY MAZURSKO WARMINSKIE (Poland)
Koroth
KOROTH (Jerusalem)
Kos
KOS (Milano)
Kos Liber Amicorum
KOS LIBER AMICORUM (Milano)
Kosm Biol Aviakosm Med
KOSMICHESKAIA BIOLOGIIA I AVIAKOSMICHESKAIA MEDITSINA (Moskva)
Kotiseutu
KOTISEUTU (Helsinki)
Krankenhausazt
KRANKENHAUSARZT (Leipzig)
Krankenpfl J
KRANKENPFLEGE JOURNAL (Wurzburg)
Krankenpflege (Bern)
KRANKENPFLEGE (Bern)
Krankenpflege (Frankfurt)
KRANKENPFLEGE (Frankfurt)
Krankenpflege Soins Infirm
KRANKENPFLEGE. SOINS INFIRMIERS (Bern)
Krober Antropol Soc Pap
KROBER ANTHROPOLOGICAL SOCIETY PAPERS (Berkeley CA)
Kronika (Yugosl)
KRONIKA (Yugoslavia)
Kult Spoleczenstwo
KULTURA I SPOLECZENSTWO (Poland)
Kurinikaru Sutadi
KURINIKARU SUTADI. CLINICAL STUDY (Tokyo)
Kurtrier Jahrb
KURTRIER JAHRBUCH
Kvartalsskr Sven Nationalforen Hjart Lungsjukd
KVARTALSSKRIFT, SVENSKA NA-

TIONALFORENINGEN MOT HJART-OCH LUNGS-JUKDOMAR (Stockholm)
Kwart Hist
KWARTALNIK HISTORYCZNY (Poland)
Kwart Hist Kultury Mater
KWARTALNIK HISTORII KULTURY MATERIALNEJ (Poland)
Kwart Hist Nauki Tech
KWARTALNIK HISTORII NAUKI I TECHNIKI (Poland)
Kwartaal Teken
KWARTAAL EN TEKEN
Ky Dent J
KENTUCKY DENTAL JOURNAL (Louisville KY)
Ky Folkl Rec
KENTUCKY FOLKLORE RECORD (Bowling Green KY)

—L—

La Hist
LOUISIANA HISTORY (Baton Rouge LA)
La Pharm
LOUISIANA PHARMACIST (New Orleans LA)
Lab Anim Sci
LABORATORY ANIMAL SCIENCE (Joliet IL)
Lab Delo
LABORATORNOE DELO (Moskva)
Lab Invest
LABORATORY INVESTIGATION (Baltimore)
Lab World
LAB WORLD (Philadelphia)
Labour
LABOUR (Canada)
Labour Hist
LABOUR HISTORY (Australia)
Lakartidningen
LAKARTIDNINGEN (Stockholm)
Lamp
LAMP (Sydney)
Lancet
LANCET (London)
Landscape
LANDSCAPE (Berkeley CA)
Langenbecks Arch Chir
LANGENBECKS ARCHIV FUR CHIRURGIE (Berlin)
LARC Med
LARC MEDICAL (Lille)
Laryngol Rhinol Otol (Stuttg)
LARYNGOLOGIE, RHINOLOGIE, OTOLOGIE (Stuttgart)
Laryngoscope
LARYNGOSCOPE (St Louis)
Lat Am Perspect
LATIN AMERICAN PERSPECTIVES (US)
Lat Am Res Rev
LATIN AMERICAN RESEARCH REVIEW (Chapel Hill NC)
Latomus
LATOMUS: REVUE D'ETUDES LATINES (Belgium)
Latv PSR Zinat Acad Vestis
LATVIJAS PSR ZINATNU AKADEMIJAS VESTIS (USSR)
Law Soc Rev
LAW AND SOCIETY REVIEW (Denver CO)
League Exch
LEAGUE EXCHANGE (New York)
Lebensversicherungsmedizin
LEBENSVERSICHERUNGSMEDIZIN (Karlsruhe)
Leber Magen Darm
LEBER, MAGEN, DARM (Baden-Baden)
Leg Med
LEGAL MEDICINE (Philadelphia)
Leg Med Q
LEGAL MEDICAL QUARTERLY (Toronto)
Lemouzi
LEMOUZI (Tulle)
Lepr India
LEPROSY IN INDIA (New Delhi)
Lepr Rev
LEPROSY REVIEW (London)
Leveltari Sz
LEVELTARI SZEMLE (Hungary)
Leyte-Samar Stud
LEYTE-SAMAR STUDIES (Philippines)
Liberian Stud J
LIBERIAN STUDIES JOURNAL (Newark DE)
Libr Hist
LIBRARY HISTORY (London)
Libr Q
LIBRARY QUARTERLY (Chicago)
Libr Trends
LIBRARY TRENDS (Urbana IL)
Library (Lond)
LIBRARY; TRANSACTIONS OF THE BIBLIOGRAPHICAL SOCIETY (London)
Liet Istor Metrast
LIETUVOS ISTORIJOS METRASTIS (USSR)
Life Sci
LIFE SCIENCES (Oxford)
Ligament (Montp)
LIGAMENT (MONTPELLIER)
Lijec Vjesn
LIJECNICKI VJESNIK (Zagreb)
Lille Med
LILLE MEDICAL (Lille)
Lincoln Her
LINCOLN HERALD (Harrogate TN)
Lipp Mitt Gesch Landeskd
LIPPISCHE MITTEILUNGEN AUS GESCHICHTE UND LANDESKUNDE (W Germany)
Lituanus
LITUANUS (Chicago)
Liverp Classical Mon
LIVERPOOL CLASSICAL MONTHLY
Livrustkammaren

LIVRUSTKAMMAREN (Sweden)
Llafur J Soc Stud Welsh Labour Hist
LLAFUR: JOURNAL OF THE SOCIETY FOR THE STUDY OF WELSH LABOUR HISTORY (Gt Brit)
Llull (Spain)
LLULL. BOLETIN DE LA SOCIEDAD ESPANOLA DE HISTORIA DE LAS CIENCIAS (Madrid)
Local Hist
LOCAL HISTORIAN (London)
Local Popu Stud (Matlock)
LOCAL POPULATION STUDIES MAGAZINE AND NEWSLETTER (Matlock)
Lond Archaeol
LONDON ARCHAEOLOGIST (London)
Long Term Care Health Serv Adm Q
LONG TERM CARE AND HEALTH SERVICES ADMINISTRATION QUARTERLY (Greenvale NY)
Luso-Braz Rev
LUSO-BRAZILIAN REVIEW (Madison WI)
Lychnos
LYCHNOS; LARDOMSHISTORISKA SAMFUNDETS ARSBOK. ANNUAL OF THE SWEDISH HISTORY OF SCIENCE SOCIETY (Stockholm)
Lymphology
LYMPHOLOGY (Stuttgart)
Lyon Pharm
LYON PHARMACEUTIQUE (Lyon)

—M—

Mag Istor
MAGAZIN ISTORIC (Romania)
Magy Traumatol Orthop Helyreallito Sebesz
MAGYAR TRAUMATOLOGIA, ORTHOPAEDIA ES HELYREALLITO SEBESZET (Budapest)
Magy Tud
MAGYAR TUDOMANY (Hungary)
Magy Konyvxa
MAGYAR KNOYVSZEMLE (Hungary)
Mainfrank Jahrb
MAINFRANKISCHES JAHRBUCH FUR GESCHICHTE UND KUNST (Wurzburg)
Majallat al-Puhuth al-Tarikhiya (Lybia)
MAJALLAT AL-PUHUTH AL-TARIKHIYA (Lybia)
Major Probl Clin Surg
MAJOR PROBLEMS IN CLINICAL SURGERY (Philadelphia)
Malays J Pathol
MALAYSIAN JOURNAL OF PATHOLOGY (Kuala Lumpur)
Man
MAN; JOURNAL OF THE ROYAL ANTHROPOLOGICAL INSTITUTE (Gt Brit)
Man Med
MAN AND MEDICINE (New York)
Manch Lit Phil Soc Mem Proc
MANCHESTER LITERARY AND PHILOSOPHICAL SOCIETY MEMOIRS AND PROCEEDINGS (Lancashire)
Mankind
MANKIND (Los Angeles)
Mankind Q
MANKIND QUARTERLY (Gt Brit)
Manuscripts
MANUSCRIPTS (Burbank CA)
Mar Mirror
MARINER'S MIRROR (London)
Marine Corps Gaz
MARINE CORPS GAZETTE (Quantico VA)
Marseille
MARSEILLE. REVUE MUNICIPALE (France)
Marx Perspect
MARXIST PERSPECTIVES (New York)
Mass Hist Soc Proc
MASSACHUSETTS HISTORICAL SOCIETY. PROCEEDINGS (Boston)
Mass Nurse
MASSACHUSETTS NURSE (Boston)
Mass Rev
MASSACHUSSETS REVIEW (US)
Masterkey Ind Lore Hist
MASTERKEY FOR INDIAN LORE AND HISTORY (Los Angeles)
Masui
MASUI. JAPANESE JOURNAL OF ANESTHESIOLOGY (Tokyo)
Mater Med Greca
MATERIA MEDICA GRECA
Mater Med Pol
MATERIA MEDICA POLONA (Warszawa)
Maturitas
MATURITAS (Amsterdam)
Max Planck Ges Ber Mitt
MAX-PLANCK GESELLSCHAFT: BERICHTE UND MITTEILUNGEN (W Germany)
Mayo Alumnus
MAYO ALUMNUS
Mayo Clin Proc
MAYO CLINIC PROCEEDINGS (Rochester MN)
McGill J Educ
MCGILL JOURNAL OF EDUCATION (Montreal)
MCN
MCN; AMERICAN JOURNAL OF MATERNAL CHILD NURSING (New York)
MCVQ
MCVQ; MEDICAL COLLEGE OF VIRGINIA QUARTERLY (Richmond VA)
MD
MD (New York)
Md Geneal Soc Bull
MARYLAND GENEALOGICAL SOCIETY BULLETIN (US)
Md Hist
MARYLAND HISTORIAN (College Park MD)
Md Hist Mag
MARYLAND HISTORICAL MAGAZINE (Baltimore)

Md Pharm
MARYLAND PHARMACIST (Baltimore)
Md State Med J
MARYLAND STATE MEDICAL JOURNAL (Baltimore)
Med Anthropol Newsl
MEDICAL ANTHROPOLOGY NEWSLETTER (Washington)
Med Arh
MEDICINSKI ARHIV (Sarajevo)
Med Armees
MEDECINE ET ARMEES (Paris)
Med Bull Instanbul Med Fac
MEDICAL BULLETIN OF ISTANBUL MEDICAL FACULTY (Istanbul)
Med Care
MEDICAL CARE (Philadelphia)
Med Clin (Barc)
MEDICINA CLINICA (Barcelona)
Med Educ
MEDICAL EDUCATION (Oxford)
Med Esp
MEDICINA ESPANOLA (Valencia)
Med Ges
MEDIZIN UND GESELLSCHAFT (Jena)
Med Gesch Kult
MEDIZIN IN GESCHICHTE UND KULTUR (Stuttgart)
Med Group Manage
MEDICAL GROUP MANAGEMENT (Denver CO)
Med Hist
MEDICAL HISTORY (London)
Med Hist (Barc)
MEDICINA E HISTORIA (Barcelona)
Med Hyg (Geneve)
MEDICINE ET HYGIENE (Geneve)
Med Hypotheses
MEDICAL HYPOTHESES (Montreal)
Med Inf (Lond)
MEDECINE ET INFORMATIQUE. MEDICAL INFORMATICS (London)
Med Instrum
MEDICAL INSTRUMENTATION (Arlington VA)
Med Interne
MEDECINE INTERNE (Bucuresti)
Med J Aust
MEDICAL JOURNAL OF AUSTRALIA (Sydney)
Med Lab (Stuttg)
MEDIZINISCHE LABORATORIUM (Stuttgart)
Med Lab Sci
MEDICAL LABORATORY SCIENCES (London)
Med Lav
MEDICINA DEL LAVORO (Milano)
Med Law
MEDICINE AND LAW (Berlin)
Med Leg J
MEDICO-LEGAL JOURNAL (Cambridge Eng)
Med Mark Media
MEDICAL MARKETING AND MEDIA (Stamford CT)
Med Monatsschr Pharm
MEDIZINISCHE MONATSSCHRIFT FUR PHARMAZEUTEN (Stuttgart)
Med News
MEDICAL NEWS (New York)
Med Parazitol (Mosk)
MEDITSINSKAIA PARAZITOLOGIIA I PARAZITARNYE BOLEZNI
Med Pediatr Oncol
MEDICAL AND PEDIATRIC ONCOLOGY (New York)
Med Pharm (Tokyo)
MEDICAL PHARMACY (Tokyo)
Med Phys
MEDICAL PHYSICS (Lancaster PA)
Med Pr
MEDYCYNA PRACY (Warszawa)
Med Pregl
MEDICINSKI PREGLED (Novi Sad)
Med Prog Technol
MEDICAL PROGRESS THROUGH TECHNOLOGY (Berlin)
Med Radiogr Photogr
MEDICAL RADIOGRAPHY AND PHOTOGRAPHY (Rochester NY)
Med Radio (Mosk)
MEDISINSKAIA RADIOLOGIIA (Moskva)
Med Ref Serv Q
MEDICAL REFERENCE SERVICES QUARTERLY (New York)
Med Sci Law
MEDICINE, SCIENCE AND THE LAW (Brentford Middlesex)
Med Secoli
MEDICINA NEI SECOLI (Roma)
Med Sestra
MEDITSINSKAIA SESTRA (Moskva)
Med Soziol
MEDIZINISCHE SOZIOLOGIE (Frankfurt)
Med Tekh
MEDITSINSKAIA TEKHNIKA (Moskva)
Med Times
MEDICAL TIMES (Manhasset NY)
Med Tradic
MEDICINA TRADICIONALE (Mexico)
Med Trop (Mars)
MEDECINE TROPICALE; REVUE DU SERVICE DE SANTE DES TROUPES DE MARINE (Marseille)
Med Unserer Zeit
MEDIZIN IN UNSERE ZEIT (Weinheim)
Med Weit
MEDIZINISCHE WELT (Stuttgart)
Mediaev Stud
MEDIAEVAL STUDIES (Toronto)
Medicamentum
MEDICAMENTUM

Medicina (B Aires)
MEDICINA (Buenos Aires)
Medita
MEDITA (Solothurn)
Medizinhist J
MEDIZINHISTORISCHES JOURNAL (Hildesheim)
Melanges Archeol Hist Ec Fr Rome
MELANGES D'ARCHEOLOGIE ET HISTORIE DE L'ECOLE FRANCAISE DE ROME
Melanges Casa Velasquez
MELANGES DE LA CASA VELASQUEZ (Paris)
Mem Acad Sci Arts B-Lett Dijon
MEMOIRES DE L'ACADEMIE DES SCIENCES, ARTS ET BELLES-LETTRES DE DIJON
Mem Acad Sci Inscr B-Lett Toulouse
MEMOIRES DE L'ACADEMIE DES SCIENCES, INSCRIPTIONS ET BELLES-LETTRES DE TOULOUSE
Mem Col Nac (Mex)
MEMORIA DEL COLEGIO NACIONAL (Mexico)
Mem Inst Oswaldo Cruz
MEMORIAS DO INSTITUTO OSWALDO CRUZ (Rio de Janeiro)
Mem Proc Manch Lit Philos Soc
MEMOIRS AND PROCEEDINGS OF THE MANCHESTER LITERARY AND PHILOSOPHICAL SOCIETY (Gt Brit)
Mem Publ Soc Sci Arts Lett Hainaut
MEMOIRES ET PUBLICATIONS DE LA SOCIETE DES SCIENCES DES ARTS ET DES LETTRES DU HAINAUT (Belgium)
Mem Riv Stor Donne
MEMORIA; RIVISTA STORIA DELLE DONNE (Italy)
Mem Soc Agric Commer Sci Arts Marne
MEMOIRES DE LA SOCIETE D'AGRICULTURE COMMERCE SCIENCES ET ARTS DU DEPARTEMENT DE LA MARNE, CHALONS SUR MARNE
Mendel Newsl
MENDEL NEWSLETTER; ARCHIVAL RESOURCES FOR THE HISTORY OF GENETICS AND ALLIED SCIENCES ISSUED BY THE LIBRARY OF THE AMERICAN PHILOSOPHICAL SOCIETY (Philadelphia)
Mennon Q Rev
MENNONITE QUARTERLY REVIEW (Goshen IN)
Ment Retard
MENTAL RETARDATION (Washington)
Mesopotamia Q
MESOPOTAMIA QUARTERLY (Iraq)
Metab Bone Dis Relat Res
METABOLIC BONE DISEASE AND RELATED RESEARCH (Paris)
Metab Pediatr Syst Ophthalmol
METABOLIC, PEDIATRIC AND SYSTEMIC OPHTHALMOLOGY (Elmsford NY)
Metamedicine
METAMEDICINE (Dordrecht)
Methodist Hist
METHODIST HISTORY (Lake Junaluska NC)
Methods Biochem Anal
METHODS OF BIOCHEMICAL ANALYSIS (New York)
Methods Cell Biol
METHODS IN CELL BIOLOGY (New York)
Methods Find Exp Clin Pharmacol
METHODS AND FINDINGS IN EXPERIMENTAL AND CLINICAL PHARMACOLOGY (Barcelona)
Methods Inf Med
METHODS OF INFORMATION IN MEDICINE (Stuttgart)
Mich Acad
MICHIGAN ACADEMICIAN (Ann Arbor MI)
Mich Hist
MICHIGAN HISTORY (Lansing MI)
Mich Hosp
MICHIGAN HOSPITALS (Lansing MI)
Mich J Polit Sci
MICHIGAN JOURNAL OF POLITICAL SCIENCE (US)
Mich Jew Hist
MICHIGAN JEWISH HISTORY (Detroit)
Mich Med
MICHIGAN MEDICINE (East Lansing MI)
Mich Q Rev
MICHIGAN QUARTERLY REVIEW (Ann Arbor MI)
Michael Hist Jews Diaspora
MICHAEL: ON THE HISTORY OF THE JEWS IN THE DIASPORA (Israel)
Microbiol Rev
MICROBIOLOGICAL REVIEWS (Washington)
Microbios
MICROBIOS (Cambridge Eng)
Microsc Acta
MICROSCOPICA ACTA (Stuttgart)
Microscope
MICROSCOPE (London)
Mid-Am
MID-AMERICA (Chicago)
Midcont J. Archaeol
MIDCONTINENTAL JOURNAL OF ARCHAEOLOGY (Kent OH)
Middle East J. Anaesthesiol
MIDDLE EAST JOURNAL OF ANAESTHESIOLOGY (Beirut)
Middle East Stud
MIDDLE EASTERN STUDIES (London)
Midl Hist
MIDLAND HISTORY (Gt Brit)
Midstream
MIDSTREAM (New York)
Midwest Q
MIDWEST QUARTERLY (Pittsburg KS)
Midwife Health Visit Community Nurse
MIDWIFE HEALTH VISITOR AND COMMUNITY NURSE

Midwives Chron
MIDWIVES CHRONICLE (London)
Migr Today
MIGRATION TODAY (US)
Mikrobiol Zh
MIKROBIOLOGICHESKII ZHURNL (Kiev)
Mikroskopie
MIKROSKOPIE (Wein)
Milbank Mem Fund Q
MILBANK MEMORIAL FUND QUARTERLY; HEALTH AND SOCIETY (New York)
Milieux
MILIEUX (France)
Milit Aff
MILITARY AFFAIRS (Manhattan KS)
Milit Med
MILITARY MEDICINE (Washington)
Milit Rev
MILITARY REVIEW (Fort Leavenworth KS)
Militargesch
MILITARGESCHICHTE (E Germany)
Milw Hist
MILWAUKEE HISTORY (Milwaukee WI)
MIMS Mag
MIMS MAGAZINE: MONTHLY INDEX OF MEDICAL SPECIALTIES (London)
Mind
MIND (Oxford)
Minerva
MINERVA (New York)
Minerva Anestesiol
MINERVA ANESTESIOLOGICA (Torino)
Minerva Chir
MINERVA CHIRURGICA (Torino)
Minerva Ginecol
MINERVA GINECOLOGICA (Torino)
Minerva Med
MINERVA MEDICA (Torino)
Minerva Nefrol
MINERVA NEFROLOGICA (Torino)
Minerva Pediatr
MINERVA PEDIATRICA (Torino)
Minerva Psichiatr
MINERVA PSICHIATRICA (Torino)
Minerva Stomatol
MINERVA STOMATOLOGICA (Torino)
Minn Hist
MINNESOTA HISTORY (St Paul MN)
Minn Med
MINNESOTA MEDICINE (St Paul MN)
Mirovaia Ekon Mezhdunar Otnoscheniia
MIROVAIA EKONOMIKA I MEZHDUNARODNYE OTNOSHENIIA (USSR)
Misc Am Philos Soc
MISCELLANEA OF THE AMERICAN PHILOSOPHICAL SOCIETY (Philadelphia)
Misc Estud Arabes Hebraicos
MISCELANEA DE ESTUDIOS ARABES Y HEBRAICOS (Spain)
Miss Q
MISSISSIPPI QUARTERLY (US)
Mitt Forschungsbeitr Cusanusges
MITTEILUNGEN UND FORSCHUNGSBEITRAGE DER CUSANUS-GESELLSCHAFT
Mitt Ges Salzburger Landeskd
MITTEILUNGEN DER GESELLSCHAFT FUR SALZBURGER LANDESKUNDE (Austria)
Mitt Krems Stadtarch
MITTEILUNGEN DES KREMSER STADTARCHIVS (Austria)
MMG
MMG; MEDIZIN MENSCH GESELLSCHAFT (Stuttgart)
MMW
MMW. MUNCHENER MEDIZINISCHE WOCHENSCHRIFT (Munchen)
MMWR
MMWR. MORBIDITY AND MORTALITY WEEKLY REPORT (Atlanta GA)
Mnemosyne
MNEMOSYNE; BIBLIOTHECA CLASSICA BATAVIA (Leiden)
Mo Hist Rev
MISSOURI HISTORICAL REVIEW (Columbia MO)
Mo Med
MISSOURI MEDICINE (St Louis)
Mobius
MOBIUS (San Francisco)
Mod Asian Stud
MODERN ASIAN STUDIES (Gt Brit)
Mod China
MODERN CHINA (US)
Mod Jud
MODERN JUDAISM (US)
Mod Med (Stuttg)
MODERNE MEDIZIN (Stuttgart)
Mod Probl Pharmacopsychiatry
MODERN PROBLEMS OF PHARMACOPSYCHIATRY (Basel)
Mod Schoolman
MODERN SCHOOLMAN
Mod Stud
MODERNIST STUDIES (Canada)
Mod Vet Pract
MODERN VETERINARY PRACTICE (Wheaton IL)
Mol Biol Biochem Biophys
MOLECULAR BIOLOGY, BIOCHEMISTRY AND BIOPHYSICS (Berlin)
Mol Cell Biochem
MOLECULAR AND CELLULAR BIOCHEMISTRY (The Hague)
Mon Labor Rev
MONTHLY LABOR REVIEW (US)
Mon Rev
MONTHLY REVIEW (US)
Monatsschr Kinderheilkd

MONATSSCHRIFT KINDERHEILKUNDE (Berlin)
Mondo Cinese
MONDO CINESE (Italy)
Mondo Ortod
MONDO ORTODONTICO (Milano)
Mondae Credito
MONDAE Y CREDITO (Spain)
Monit Farm Ter
MONITOR DE LA FARMACIA Y DE LA TERAPEUTICA (Madrid)
Monit Pharm Lab
MONITEUR DES PHARMACIES ET DES LABORATOIRES (Paris)
Monogr Pathol
MONOGRAPHS IN PATHOLOGY (Baltimore)
Montana
MONTANA: MAGAZINE OF WESTERN HISTORY (Helena MT)
Montfort
MONTFORT (Austria)
Montreal Gen Hosp News
MONTREAL GENERAL HOSPITAL NEWS (Montreal)
Morfol Norm Patol
MORFOLOGIA NORMAL Y PATOLOGIA (Granada)
Morphol Embryol (Bucur)
MORPHOLOGIE ET EMBRYOLOGIE (Bucuresti)
Morphol Igazsagugyi Orv Sz
MORPHOLOGIAI ES IGAZSAGUGYI ORVOSI SZEMLE (Budapest)
Mouvement Soc
MOUVEMENT SOCIAL (France)
Mov Operaio Soc
MOVIMENTO OPERAIO E SOCIALISTA (Italy)
Moyen Age
LE MOYEN AGE (Bruxelles)
Mt Sinai J Med (NY)
MOUNT SINAI JOURNAL OF MEDICINE (New York)
Munger Afr Libr Notes
MUNGER AFRICANA LIBRARY NOTES (US)
Mus Geneve
MUSEE DE GENEVE (Switzerland)
Muscle Nerve
MUSCLE AND NERVE (New York)
Music Lett
MUSIC AND LETTERS (London)
Muslim World
MUSLIM WORLD (Hartford CT)
Mycopathologia
MYCOPATHOLOGIA (The Hague)
Mykosen
MYKOSEN (Berlin)

—N—

N Engl Galaxy
NEW ENGLAND GALAXY (Sturbridge MA)
N Engl Hist Geneal Regist
NEW ENGLAND HISTORICAL AND GENEALOGICAL REGISTER (Boston)
N Engl J Med
NEW ENGLAND JOURNAL OF MEDICINE (Boston)
N Engl Q
NEW ENGLAND QUARTERLY (Brunswick ME)
Nachrichtenbl Dtsch Ges Gesch Med Naturwiss Tech
NACHRICHTENBLATT DER DEUTSCHEN GESELLSCHAFT FUR GESCHICHTE DER MEDIZIN, NATURWISSENSCHAFT UND TECHNIK (Frankfurt)
Nada
NADA (Zimbabwe)
Nagarjun
NAGARJUN (Calcutta)
Nahrung
NAHRUNG (Berlin)
Nar Azii Afriki
NARODY AZII AFRIKI (USSR)
Nasza Przeslosc
NASZA PRZESLOSC (Poland)
Nat Hist
NATURAL HISTORY (New York)
Nat Immun Cell Growth Regul
NATURAL IMMUNITY AND CELL GROWTH REGULATION (Basel)
Nat Mus
NATUR AND MUSEUM (Frankfurt am Main)
Nat Syst
NATURE AND SYSTEM (Tucson AZ)
Nationalocon Tidsskr
NATIONALOCONOMISK TIDSSKRIFT (Copenhagen)
Natl Civ Rev
NATIONAL CIVIC REVIEW (New York)
Natl Forum Hosp Health Aff
NATIONAL FORUM ON HOSPITAL AND HEALTH AFFAIRS (Durham NC)
Natl Inst Drug Abuse Res Monogr Ser
NATIONAL INSTITUTE ON DRUG ABUSE RESEARCH MONOGRAPH SERIES (Rockville MD)
NATNEWS (Matlock Eng)
NATNEWS
Nature
NATURE (London)
Naturwiss Rundsch
NATURWISSENSCHAFTLICHE RUNDSCHAU (Stuttgart)
Naturwissenschaften
NATURWISSENSCHAFTEN (Berlin)
Naucni Sastanak Zb Rad Naucno Drus Istor Zdrav Kult Jugosl
NAUCNI SASTANAK ZBORNIK RADOVA — NAUCNO DRUSTVO AZ ISTORIJU ZDRAVSTVENE KULTURE JUGOSLAVIJE (Yugoslavia)
Nauka Pol

THE HISTORY OF MEDICINE (France)
Newsl Libr Hist Health Sci
NEWSLETTER OF THE ASSOCIATION OF LIBRARIANS IN THE HISTORY OF THE HEALTH SCIENCES (Baltimore)
Newsl Optom Hist Soc
NEWSLETTER OF THE OPTOMETRIC HISTORICAL SOCIETY (St Louis)
Newsl Soc 17th Centry Fr Stud
NEWSLETTER-SOCIETY OF 17TH CENTURY FRENCH STUDIES
Niagara Frontier
NIAGARA FRONTIER (Buffalo NY)
Niedersachs Zahnarztebl
NIEDERSACHSISCHES ZAHNARZTEBLATT (Hannover)
Niger Med J
NIGERIAN MEDICAL JOURNAL (Lagos)
Nihon I-Shigaku Zasshi
NIHON I-SHIGAKU ZASSHI (Tokyo) JOURNAL OF THE JAPANASE SOCIETY OF THE MEDICAL HISTORY
Nihonshi Kenkyu
NIHONSHI KENKYU (Japan)
Nineteenth Century Fict
NINETEENTH CENTURY FICTION (US)
NIPH Ann
NIPH ANNALS (Oslo)
Nippon Gan Chiryo Gakkai Shi
NIPPON GAN CHIRYO GAKKAI SHI. JOURNAL OF JAPAN SOCIETY FOR CANCER THERAPY (Kyoto)
Nippon Ganka Gakkai Zasshi
NIPPON GANKA GAKKAI ZASSHI. ACTA SOCIETATIS OPHTHALMOLOGICAE JAPONICAE (Tokyo)
Nippon Geka Hokan
NIPPON GEKA HOKAN. ARCHIV FUR JAPANISCHE CHIRURGIE (Kyoto)
Nippon Ika Daigaku Zasshi
NIPPON IKA DAIGAKU ZASSHI. JOURNAL OF THE NIPPON MEDICAL SCHOOL (Tokyo)
Nippon Kyosei Shika Gakkai Zasshi
NIPPON KYOSEI SHIKA GAKKAI ZASSHI. JOURNAL OF JAPAN ORTHODONTIC SOCIETY (Tokyo)
Nippon Naika Gakkai Zasshi
NIPPON NAIKA GAKKAI ZASSHI. JOURNAL OF JAPANESE SOCIETY OF INTERNAL MEDICINE (Tokyo)
Nippon Rai Gakkai Zasshi
NIPPON RAI GAKKAI ZASSHI. JAPANESE JOURNAL OF LEPROSY (Japan)
Nippon Rinsho
NIPPON RINSHO. JAPANESE JOURNAL OF CLINICAL MEDICINE (Osaka)
Nippon Saikingaku Zasshi
NIPPON SAIKINGAKU ZASSHI. JAPANESE JOURNAL OF BACTERIOLOGY (Tokyo)
Nippon Sanka Fujinka Gakkai Zasshi
NIPPON SANKA FUJINKA GAKKAI ZASSHI. ACTA OBSTETRICA ET GYNAECOLOGICA JAPONICA (Tokyo)
Nippon Seirigaku Zasshi
NIPPON SEIRIGAKU ZASSHI. JOURNAL OF THE PHYSIOLOGICAL SOCIETY OF JAPAN (Tokyo)
Nippon Shika Hyoron
NIPPON SHIK HYORON. NIPPON DENTAL REVIEW (Tokyo)
Nippon Shika Ishikai Zasshi
NIPPON SHIKA ISHIKAI ZASSHI. JOURNAL OF THE JAPAN DENTAL ASSOCIATION (Tokyo)
Nippon Shokakibyo Gakkia Zasshi
NIPPON SHOKAKIBYO GAKKAI ZASSHI. JAPANESE JOURNAL OF GASTROENTEROLOGY (Tokyo)
NJ Hist
NEW JERSEY HISTORY (Newark NJ)
NJ J Pharm
NEW JERSEY JOURNAL OF PHARMACY (Trenton NJ)
NJ Nurse
NEW JERSEY NURSE (Trenton NJ)
NLN Publ
NLN PUBLICATIONS; NATIONAL LEAGUE FOR NURSING (New York)
NM Hist Rev
NEW MEXICO HISTORICAL REVIEW (Albuquerque NM)
No Shinkei Geka
NO SHINKEI GEKA. NEUROLOGICAL SURGERY (Tokyo)
No To Hattatsu
NO TO HATTATSU (Tokyo)
No To Shinkei
NO TO SHINKEI. BRAIN AND NERVE (Tokyo)
Noesis
NOESIS (Bucharest)
Nor Tannlaegeforen Tid
NORSKE TANNLAEGEFORENINGS TIDENDE (Oslo)
Nor Teol Tidsskr
NORSK TEOLOGISK TIDSSKRFT (Norway)
Nord Med
NORDISK MEDICIN (Stockholm)
Nord Medicinhist Arsb
NORDISK MEDICINHISTORISK ARSBOK (Stockholm)
Nord Vet Med
NORDISK VETERINAERMEDICIN (Copenhagen)
North La Hist Assoc J
NORTH LOUISIANA HISTORICAL ASSOCIATION JOURNAL (Ruston LA)
North Scotl
NORTHERN SCOTLAND (Gt Brit)
Northeast Folkl
NORTHEAST FORKLORE (Orono ME)

Northeast Nev Hist Soc Q
NORTHEASTERN NEVADA HISTORICAL SOCIETY QUARTERLY (Elko NV)
Northwest Dent
NORTHWEST DENTISTRY (St Paul MN)
Northwest Ohio Q
NORTHWEST OHIO QUARTERLY (Maumee)
Notes Queries
NOTES AND QUERIES (London)
Notes Rec R Soc Lond
NOTES AND RECORDS OF THE ROYAL SOCIETY OF LONDON (London)
Nouv Com Int Cathol Infirm Assist Med Soc
NOUVELLES — COMITE INTERNATIONAL CATHOLIQUE DES INFIRMIERES ET ASSISTANTES MEDICO-SOCIALES (Bruxelles)
Nouv Presse Med
NOUVELLE PRESSE MEDICALE (Paris)
Nouv Repub Lett
NOUVELLES DE LA REPUBLIQUE DES LETTRES (Napoli)
Nouv Rev Deux Mondes
NOUVELLE REVUE DES DEUX MONDES (France)
Nouv Rev Fr Hematol
NOUVELLE REVUE FRANCAISE D'HEMATOLOGIE (Heidelberg)
Nov Med Tekh
NOVOSTI MEDITSINSKOI TEKHNIKI (Moskva)
Nov Noveishaia Istor
NOVAIA I NOVEISHAIA ISTORIIA (USSR)
Nowe Drogi
NOWE DROGI (Poland)
Nowotwory
NOWOTWORY (Warszawa)
NS Hist Q
NOVA SCOTIA HISTORICAL QUARTERLY (Canada)
NS Hist Rev
NOVA SCOTIA HISTORICAL REVIEW (Canada)
NS Hist Soc Collect
NOVA SCOTIA HISTORICAL SOCIETY COLLECTIONS (Canada)
NTM
NTM; SCHRIFTENREIHE FUR GESCHICHTE DER NATURWISSENSCHAFTEN TECHNIK UND MEDIZINE (Leipzig)
Nueva Enferm
NUEVA ENFERMERIA (Madrid)
Nuevos Libros
NUEVOS LIBROS (Centro Portales Cochabamba)
Nuova Antologia
NUOVA ANTOLOGIA (Italy)
Nuova Riv Stor
NUOVA RIVISTA STORICA (Italy)
Nuovi Ann Ig Microbiol
NUOVI ANNAL D'IGIENE E MICROBIOLOGIA (Roma)
Nurs Care see J Nurs Care
JOURNAL OF NURSING CARE (New York)
Nurs Careers
NURSING CAREERS (Encino CA)
Nurs Clin North Am
NURSING CLINICS OF NORTH AMERICA (Philadelphia)
Nurs Focus
NURSING FOCUS (London)
Nurs Forum
NURSING FORUM (Hillsdale NJ)
Nurs Health Care
NURSING AND HEALTH CARE (Westport CT)
Nurs J India
NURSING JOURNAL OF INDIA
Nurs Leadersh
NURSING LEADERSHIP (Thorofare NJ)
Nurs Mirror
NURSING MIRROR (Sussex)
Nurs Montreal
NURSING MONTREAL (Canada)
Nurs Outlook
NURSING OUTLOOK (New York)
Nurs Que
NURSING QUEBEC (Montreal)
Nurs Res
NURSING RESEARCH (New York)
Nurs Success Today
NURSING SUCCESS TODAY (Thorofare NJ)
Nurs Times
NURSING TIMES (London)
Nurse Pract
NURSE PRACTITIONER (Trenton NJ)
Nursing (Oxford)
NURSING (OXFORD)
Nutr Hist Notes
NUTRITION HISTORY NOTES
Nutr Rev
NUTRITION REVIEWS (New York)
NY Aff
NEW YORK AFFAIRS (US)
NY Folkl
NEW YORK FOLKLORE (US)
NY Folkl Q
NEW YORK FOLKLORE QUARTERLY (Cooperstown NY)
NY Hist
NEW YORK HISTORY (Cooperstown NY)
NY J Dent
NEW YORK JOURNAL OF DENTISTRY (New York)
NY State Dent J
NEW YORK STATE DENTAL JOURNAL (New York)
NY State J Med
NEW YORK STATE JOURNAL OF MEDICINE (Lake Success NY)
NZ Dent J
NEW ZEALAND DENTAL JOURNAL (Dunedin)
NZ J Hist

NEW ZEALAND JOURNAL OF HISTORY (New Zealand)
NZ Libr
NEW ZEALAND LIBRARIES (New Zealand)
NZ Med J
NEW ZEALAND MEDICAL JOURNAL (Dunedin)
NZ Nurs J
NEW ZEALAND NURSING JOURNAL (Wellington)

—O—

OAZ Osterr Apoth Ztg
OAZ. OSTERREICHISCHE APOTHEKER ZEITUNG (Vienna)
Obstet Gynecol
OBSTETRICS AND GYNECOLOGY (New York)
Obstet Gynecol Annu
OBSTETRICS AND GYNECOLOGY ANNUAL (New York)
Obstet Gynecol Surv
OBSTETRICAL AND GYNECOLOGICAL SURVEY (Baltimore)
Occas Pap Farlow Herb Cryptogam Bot Harv Univ
OCCASIONAL PAPERS-FARLOW HERBARIUM OF CRYPTOGAMIC BOTANY HARVARD UNIVERSITY (US)
Occup Health (Lond)
OCCUPATIONAL HEALTH (London)
Occup Health Saf
OCCUPATIONAL HEALTH NURSING (Thorofare NJ)
Occup Health Saf
OCCUPATION HEALTH AND SAFETY (Waco TX)
Oceania
OCEANIA (Sydney)
Odontol Foren Tidskr
ODONTOLOGISKA FORENINGENS TIDSKRIFT (Stockholm)
Odontostomatol Proodos
ODONTOSTOMATOLOGIKE PROODOS (Athens)
Off Gesundheitswes
OFFENTLICHE GESUNDHEITSWESEN (Stuttgart)
Offarm
OFFARM
Oftalmol Zh
OFTAL'MOLOGISCHESKII ZHURNAL (Odessa)
OH
OH. OSTEOPATHIC HOSPITALS (Park Ridge IL)
Ohio Dent J
OHIO DENTAL JOURNAL (Columbus OH)
Ohio Hist
OHIO HISTORY (Columbus OH)
Ohio State Med J
OHIO STATE MEDICAL JOURNAL (Columbus OH)
Okla Nurse
OKLAHOMA NURSE; OKLAHOMA STATE NURSES ASSOCIATION (Oklahoma City OK)
Old Engl Newsl
OLD ENGLISH NEWSLETTER (Columbus OH)
Old Northwest
OLD NORTHWEST (Oxford OH)
Omvardaren
OMVARDAREN (Sweden)
Oncol Nurs Forum
ONCOLOGY NURSING FORUM (New York)
Oncology
ONCOLOGY (Basel)
One One
ONE ON ONE (Salt Lake City UT)
Ons Heem
ONS HEEM
Ont Dent
ONTARIO DENTIST (Toronto)
Ont Hist
ONTARIO HISTORY (Toronto)
Oostvlaam Zanten
OOSTVLAAMSE ZANTEN
Oper Dent
OPERATIVE DENTISTRY (Seattle WA)
Ophthalmic Physiol Opt
OPHTHALMIC AND PHYSIOLOGICAL OPTICS (Oxford)
Ophthalmic Surg
OPHTHALMIC SURGERY (Thorofare NJ)
Ophthalmologica
OPHTHALMOLOGICA (Basel)
Ophthalmology
OPHTHALMOLOGY (Philadelphia)
Oral Hist
ORAL HISTORY (Essex Eng)
Oral Hist Rev
ORAL HISTORY REVIEW (Denton TX)
Oral Surg Oral Med Oral Path
ORAL SURGERY, ORAL MEDICINE AND ORAL PATHOLOGY (St Louis)
Orchester
ORCHESTER (W Germany)
Oreg Hist Q
OREGON HISTORICAL QUARTERLY (Portland OR)
Organon
ORGANON (Warsaw)
Oriente Mod
ORIENTE MODERNO (Roma)
Orthod Fr
ORTHODONTIE FRANCAISE (Lyon)
Orthop Clin North Am
ORTHOPEDIC CLINICS OF NORTH AMERICA (Philadelphia)
Orthop Nurs
ORTHOPEDIC NURSING (Pitman NJ)
Orthop Prax
ORTHOPAEDISCHE PRAXIS (Ulzen)
Ortop Travmatol Protez
ORTOPEDIIA, TRAVMATOLOGIIA I PROTEZIROVANIE (Moskva)
Orv Hetil

ORVOSI HETILAP (Budapest)
Orvostort Kozl
ORVOSTORTENETI KOZLEMENYEK (Budapest)
OSSA
OSSA (Solna)
Osterr Arch Kirchenr
OSTERREICHISCHES ARCHIV FUR KIRCHENRECHT (Austria)
Osterr Arzteztg
OSTERREICHISCHE ARZTEZEITUNG (Austria)
Osterr Gesch Kult
OSTERREICH IN GESCHICHTE UND KULTUR (Austria)
Osterr Gesch Lit
OSTERREICH IN GESCHICHTE UND LITERATUR (Austria)
Osterr Krankkkenplfegez
OSTERREICHISCHE KRANKENPFLEGEZEITSCHRIFT (Vienna)
Osterr Monatsh
OSTERREICHISCHE MONATSHEFTE (Austria)
Osterr Osthefte
OSTERREICHISCHE OSTHEFTE (Vienna)
Osterr Z Stomatol
OSTERREICHISCHE ZEITSCHRIFT FUR STOMATOLOGIE (Vienna)
Osteuropa
OSTEUROPA (Stuttgart)
Otolaryngol Clin North Am
OTOLARYNGOLOGIC CLINICS OF NORTH AMERICA (Philadelphia)
Otolaryngol Head Neck Surg
OTOLARYNGOLOGY AND HEAD AND NECK SURGERY (Rochester MN)
Otolaryngol Pol
OTOLARYNGOLOGIA POLSKA (Warszawa)
Outlook Mag
OUTLOOK MAGAZINE
Oxf Slav Pap
OXFORD SLAVONIC PAPERS (London)

—P—

Pa Folklife
PENNSYLVANIA FOLKLIFE (Lancaster PA)
Pa Herit
PENNSYLVANIA HERITAGE (Harrisburg PA)
Pa Hist
PENNSYLVANIA HISTORY (University Park PA)
Pa Mag Hist Biogr
PENNSYLVANIA MAGAZINE OF HISTORY AND BIOGRAPHY (Philadelphia)
Pa Mennon Heritage
PENNSYLVANIA MENNONITE HERITAGE (Lancaster PA)
Pac Aff
PACIFIC AFFAIRS (Canada)
Pac Hist
PACIFIC HISTORIAN (Stockton CA)
Pac Hist Rev
PACIFIC HISTORICAL REVIEW (Berkeley CA)
Pac Northwest
PACIFIC NORTHWESTERNER (Spokane WA)
Pac Northwest Q
PACIFIC NORTHWEST QUARTERLY (Seattle WA)
Pac Sociol Rev
PACIFIC SOCIOLOGICAL REVIEW (US)
Pace
PACE. PACING AND CLINICAL ELECTROPHYSIOLOGY (Mount Kisco NY)
Padiatrie Grenzgeb
PADIATRIE UND GRENZGEBIETE (Berlin)
Padiatr Padol
PADIATRIE UND PADOLOGIE (Wien)
Paedagog Hist
PAEDAGOGICA HISTORICA (Belgium)
Pain
PAIN (Amsterdam)
Palacio
EL PALACIO (Santa Fe NM)
Paleopathol Newsl
PALEOPATHOLOGICAL NEWSLETTER (Detroit)
Palimpsest
PALIMPSEST (Iowa City IA)
Pandore
PANDORE (France)
Panstwo Prawo
PANSTWO I PRAWO (Poland)
Pap Far East Hist
PAPERS ON FAR EASTERN HISTORY (Australia)
Pap Slov Stud
PAPERS IN SLOVENE STUDIES (US)
Papua New Guinea Med J
PAPUA NEW GUINEA MEDICAL JOURNAL (Port Moresby)
Parameters
PARAMETERS (US)
Paraplegia
PARAPLEGIA (Edinburgh)
Parassitologia
PARASSITOLOGIA (Roma)
Parol Passato
LA PAROLA DEL PASSATO; RIVISTA DI STUDI ANTICHI (Napoli)
Partisan Rev
PARTISAN REVIEW (New Brunswick NJ)
Parttorteneti Kozl
PARTTORTENETI KOZLEMENYEK (Hungary)
Past Present
PAST AND PRESENT (Gt Brit)
Pathol Annu
PATHOLOGY ANNUAL (New York)
Pathol Res Pract
PATHOLOGY, RESEARCH AND PRACTICE (Stuttgart)
Pathologe

PATHOLOGE (Berlin)
Pathologica
PATHOLOGICA (Genoa)
Pathologist
PATHOLOGIST (Skokie IL)
Patma-Banasirakam Handes. Ist-Filol Zh
PATMA-BANASIRAKAM HANDES. ISTORKO-FILOLOGICHESKII TERAPIIA (Moskva)
Patol Fiziol Eskp Ter
PATOLOGICHESKAIA FIZIOLOGIIA I EKSPERIMENTALNAIA
Patol Pol
PATOLOGIA POLSKA (Warszawa)
Patterns Prejudice
PATTERNS OF PREJUDICE (Gt Brit)
Pavlov J Biol Sci
PAVLOVIAN JOURNAL OF BIOLOGICAL SCIENCE (Philadelphia)
Pearson Mus Monogr Ser
PEARSON MUSEUM MONOGRAPH SERIES (Springfield IL)
Peasant Stud
PEASANT STUDIES (Pittsburgh)
Pediatr Akush Ginekol
PEDIATRIIA AKUSHERSTVO I GINEKOLOGIIA (Kiev)
Pediatr Ann
PEDIATRIC ANNALS (New York)
Pediatr Cardiol
PEDIATRIC CARDIOLOGY (New York)
Pediatr Dent
PEDIATRIC DENTISTRY (Chicago)
Pediatr Nurs
PEDIATRIC NURSING (Pitman NJ)
Pediatr Pathol
PEDIATRIC PATHOLOGY (Washington)
Pediatr Pol
PEDIATRIA POLSKA (Warszawa)
Pediatr Res
PEDIATRIC RESEARCH (Baltimore)
Pediatrics
PEDIATRICS (Evanston IL)
Pediatriia
PEDIATRIIA (Moskva)
Pedod Fr
PEDODONTIE FRANCAISE (Paris)
Penelope
PENELOPE, POUR L'HISTOIRE DES FEMMES
Penn Med
PENNSYLVANIA MEDICINE (Harrisburg PA)
Peptides (Fayetteville)
PEPTIDES (Fayetteville)
Percept Mot Skills
PERCEPTUAL AND MOTOR SKILLS (Missoula MT)
Percept Psychophys
PERCEPTION AND PSYCHOPHYSICS (Austin TX)
Perception
PERCEPTION (London)
Periodico
EL PERIODICO (Spain)
Periodiek
PERIODIEK
Perspect Biol Med
PERSPECTIVES IN BIOLOGY AND MEDICINE (Chicago)
Perspect Pedagog (Barc)
PERSPECTIVAS PEDAGOGICAS (Barcelona)
Perspect Pediatr Pathol
PERSPECTIVES IN PEDIATRIC PATHOLOGY (Chicago)
Perspect Psychiatr Care
PERSPECTIVES IN PSYCHIATRIC CARE (Hillsdale NJ)
Pharm Acta Helv
PHARMACEUTICA ACTA HELVETIAE (Zurich)
Pharm Hist
PHARMACY IN HISTORY (Madison WI)
Pharm Hist (London)
PHARMACEUTICAL HISTORIAN (London)
Pharm Ind
DIE PHARMAZEUTISCHE INDUSTRIE (W Germany)
Pharm Int
PHARMACY INTERNATIONAL (Amsterdam)
Pharm J
PHARMACEUTICAL JOURNAL (London)
Pharm Times
PHARMACY TIMES (Port Washington NY)
Pharm Unserer Zeit
PHARMAZIE IN UNSERER ZEIT (Weinheim)
Pharm Weekbl
PHARMACEUTISCH WEEKBLAD (The Hague)
Pharm Ztg
PHARMAZEUTISCHE ZEITUNG (Frankfurt)
Pharmacol Ther
PHARMACOLOGY AND THERAPEUTICS (Oxford)
Pharmacologist
PHARMACOLOGIST (Washington)
Pharmacopsychiatria
PHARMACOPSYCHIATRIA (Stuttgart)
Pharmazie
PHARMAZIE (Berlin)
Pharos
PHAROS OF ALPHA OMEGA ALPHA HONOR MEDICAL SOCIETY (Menlo Park CA)
Philologus
PHILOLOGUS. ZEITSCHRIFT FUR KLASSISCHE PHILOLOGIE (Berlin)
Philos Sci
PHILOSOPHY OF SCIENCE (Baltimore)
Philos Trans R Soc Lond [Biol]
PHILOSOPHICAL TRANSACTIONS OF THE ROYAL SOCIETY OF LONDON. SERIES B: BIOLOGICAL SCIENCES (London)
Phlebologie
PHLEBOLOGIE (Paris)

York)
Presence Afr
PRESENCE AFRICAINE (Paris)
Presse Med
PRESSE MEDICALE (Paris)
Prev Med
PREVENTIVE MEDICINE (New York)
Pride Inst J Long Term Home Health Care
PRIDE INSTITUTE JOURNAL OF LONG TERM HOME HEALTH CARE (New York)
Probe (Lond)
PROBE (London)
Probl Gematol Pereliv Krovi
PROBLEMY GEMATOLOGII I PERELIVANIA KROVI (Moskva)
Probl Istor Demogr SSSR
PROBLEMY ISTORICHESKOI DEMOGRAFII SSSR
Probl Khig
PROBLEMI NA KHIGIENATA (Sofia)
Probl Tuberk
PROBLEMY TUBERKULEZA (Moskva)
Proc Acad Polit Sci
PROCEEDINGS OF THE ACADEMY OF POLITICAL SCIENCE (New York)
Proc Am Antiq Soc
PROCEEDINGS OF THE AMERICAN ANTIQUARIAN SOCIETY (Worcester MA)
Proc Am Philos Soc
PROCEEDINGS OF THE AMERICAN PHILOSOPHICAL SOCIETY (Philadelphia)
Proc Annu Meet West Soc Fr Hist
PROCEEDINGS OF THE ANNUAL MEETING OF THE WESTERN SOCIETY FOR FRENCH HISTORY (Santa Barbara CA)
Proc Annu Symp Eugen Soc
PROCEEDINGS OF THE ANNUAL SYMPOSIUM OF THE EUGENICS SOCIETY (New York)
Proc Aust Assoc Neurol
PROCEEDINGS OF THE AUSTRALIAN ASSOCIATION OF NEUROLOGISTS (Melbourne)
Proc Camb Mass Hist Soc 1973-5
PROCEEDINGS OF THE CAMBRIDGE MASSACHUSETTS HISTORICAL SOCIETY 1973-1975
Proc Clin Dial Transplant Forum
PROCEEDINGS OF THE CLINICAL DIALYSIS AND TRANSPLANT FORUM (Washington)
Proc Consort Revolutionary Eur
PROCEEDINGS OF THE CONSORTIUM ON REVOLUTIONARY EUROPE 1750-1850 (US)
Proc Croydon Nat Hist Sci Soc
PROCEEDINGS OF THE CROYDON NATURAL HISTORY AND SCIENTIFIC SOCIETY (Surrey Eng)
Proc Finn Dent Soc
PROCEEDINGS OF THE FINNISH DENTAL SOCIETY (Helsinki)
Proc Huguenot Soc Lond
PROCEEDINGS OF THE HUGUENOT SOCIETY OF LONDON (London)
Proc Inst Med Chic
PROCEEDINGS OF THE INSTITUTE OF MEDICINE OF CHICAGO (Chicago)
Proc Isr Acad Sci Humanit
PROCEEDINGS ISRAEL ACADEMY OF SCIENCES AND HUMANITIES (Israel)
Proc Leeds Philos Lit Soc [Lit Hist Sect]
PROCEEDINGS - LEEDS PHILOSOPHICAL AND LITERARY SOCIETY (LITERARY AND HISTORICAL SECTION) (Gt Brit)
Proc Nutr Soc
PROCEEDINGS OF THE NUTRITION SOCIETY (London)
Proc R Inst GB
PROCEEDINGS OF THE ROYAL INSTITUTE OF GREAT BRITAIN
Proc R Soc Lond [Biol]
PROCEEDINGS OF THE ROYAL SOCIETY OF LONDON. SERIES B: BIOLOGICAL SCIENCES (London)
Proc SC Hist Assoc
PROCEEDINGS OF THE SOUTH CAROLINA HISTORICAL ASSOCIATION (Greenville SC)
Proc Soc Exp Biol Med
PROCEEDINGS OF THE SOCIETY FOR EXPERIMENTAL BIOLOGY AND MEDICINE (New York)
Proc Somerset Archaeol Nat Hist Soc
PROCEEDINGS OF THE SOMERSET ARCHAEOLOGICAL AND NATURAL HISTORY SOCIETY (Gt Brit)
Prof Inferm
PROFESSIONI INFERMIERISTICHE (Roma)
Profiles Hosp Mark
PROFILES IN HOSPITAL MARKETING (Lancaster (PA)
Prog Allergy
PROGRESS IN ALLERGY (Basel)
Prog Biochem Pharmacol
PROGRESS IN BIOCHEMICAL PHARMACOLOGY (Basel)
Prog Brain Res
PROGRESS IN BRAIN RESEARCH (Amsterdam)
Prog Cardiovasc Dis
PROGRESS IN CARDIOVASCULAR DISEASES (New York)
Prog Clin Biol Res
PROGRESS IN CLINICAL AND BIOLOGICAL RESEARCH (New York)
Prog Exp Tumor Res
PROGRESS IN EXPERIMENTAL TUMOR RESEARCH (Basel)
Prog Food Nutr Sci
PROGRESS IN FOOD AND NUTRITION SCIENCE (Oxford)
Prog Lipid Res
PROGRESS IN LIPID RESEARCH (Oxford)
Prog Med Virol
PROGRESS IN MEDICAL VIROLOGY (Basel)

Prog Neurobiol
PROGRESS IN NEUROBIOLOGY (Oxford)
Prog Pediatr Surg
PROGRESS IN PEDIATRIC SURGERY (Munchen)
Prologue J Nat Arch
PROLOGUE; JOURNAL OF THE NATIONAL ARCHIVES (Washington)
Prostate
PROSTATE (New York)
Prosthet Orthot Int
PROSTHETICS AND ORTHOTICS INTERNATIONAL (Hellerup)
Protet Stomatol
PROTETYKA STOMATOLOGICZNA (Warszawa)
Prov Med
PROVENCE MEDICALE (Marseille)
Provence Hist
PROVENCE HISTORIQUE (Marseille)
Przegl Dermatol
PRZEGLAD DERMATOLOGICZNY (Warszawa)
Przegl Epidemiol
PRZEGLAD EPIDEMIOLOGICZNY (Warszawa)
Przegl Hist
PRZEGLAD HISTORYCZNY (Warszawa)
Przegl Lek
PRZEGLAD LEKARSKI (Krakow)
Przegl Zachod
PRZEGLAD ZACHODNI (Poland)
Przeszlosc Demograf Pol
PRZESZLOSC DEMOGRAFICZNA POLSKI (Warszawa)
Psyche (Stuttg)
PSYCHE (Stuttgart)
Psychiatr Clin North Am
PSYCHIATRIC CLINICS OF NORTH AMERICA (Philadelphia)
Psychiatr Enfant
PSYCHIATRIE DE L'ENFANT (Paris)
Psychiatr Hosp
PSYCHIATRIC HOSPITAL (Washington)
Psychiatr J Univ Ottawa
PSYCHIATRIC JOURNAL OF THE UNIVERSITY OF OTTAWA. REVUE DE PSYCHIATRIE DE L'UNIVERSITE D'OTTAWA (Ottawa)
Psychiatr Neurol Med Psychol (Leipz)
PSYCHIATRIE, NEUROLOGIE UND MEDIZINISCHE PSYCHOLOGIE (Leipzig)
Psychiatr News
PSYCHIATRIC NEWS (Washington)
Psychiatr Pol
PSYCHIATRIA POLSKA (Warszawa)
Psychiatr Q
PSYCHIATRIC QUARTERLY (New York)
Psychiatry
PSYCHIATRY (Washington)
Psychoanal Q
PSYCHOANALYTIC QUARTERLY (New York)
Psychoanal Rev
PSYCHOANALYTIC REVIEW (London)
Psychoanal Study Child
PSYCHOANALYTIC STUDY OF THE CHILD (New York)
Psychohist Rev
PSYCHOHISTORY REVIEW (Springfield IL)
Psychol Issues
PSYCHOLOGICAL ISSUES (New York)
Psychol Med
PSYCHOLOGICAL MEDICINE (London)
Psychol Rep
PSYCHOLOGICAL REPORTS (Missoula MT)
Psychol Rev
PSYCHOLOGICAL REVIEW (Washington)
Psychol Rundschau
PSYCHOLOGISCHE RUNDSCHAU (Gottingen)
Psychoneuroendocrinology
PSYCHONEUROENDOCRINOLOGY (Oxford)
Psychopharmacol Bull
PSYCHOPHARAMACOLOGY BULLETIN (Rockville MD)
Psychophysiology
PSYCHOPHYSIOLOGY (Madison WI)
Psychosom Med
PSYCHOSOMATIC MEDICINE (New York)
Psychother Psychosom
PSYCHOTHERAPY AND PSYCHOSOMATICS (Basel)
Psychother Psychosom Med Psychol
PSYCHOTHERAPIE, PSYCHOSOMATIK, MEDIZINISCHE PSYCHOLOGIE (Stuttgart)
Publ Group Adv Psychiar
PUBLICATION - GROUP FOR THE ADVANCEMENT OF PSYCHIATRY (New York)
Publ Inst Fr Indologie
PUBLICATIONS DE L'INSTITUT FRANCAIS D'INDOLOGIE (Pondicherie India)
Publ Mus Farm
PUBLICACIONES DEL MUSEO DE LA FARMACIA (Buenos Aires)
Public Adm
PUBLIC ADMINISTRATION (London)
Public Health
PUBLIC HEALTH (London)
Public Health Pap
PUBLIC HEALTH PAPERS (Geneva)
Public Health Rep
PUBLIC HEALTH REPORTS (Hyattsville MD)
Public Health Rev
PUBLIC HEALTH REVIEW (Tel Aviv)
Public Hist
PUBLIC HISTORIAN (Santa Barbara CA)
Public Interest
PUBLIC INTEREST (New York)
Public Opin Q
PUBLIC OPINION QUARTERLY (US)
Public Welf
PUBLIC WELFARE (Chicago)

Publius
PUBLIUS (US)
Pulse
PULSE OF THE MONTANA STATE NURSES ASSOCIATION (Helena MT)

—Q—

Q Bull S Afr Libr
QUARTERLY BULLETIN - SOUTH AFRICAN LIBRARY (South Africa)
Q J Econ
QUARTERLY JOURNAL OF ECONOMICS (Cambridge MA)
Q J Libr Congr
QUARTERLY JOURNAL OF THE LIBRARY OF CONGRESS (Washington)
Q J Med
QUARTERLY JOURNAL OF MEDICINE (Oxford)
Q Rev Biol
QUARTERLY REVIEW OF BIOLOGY (Stony Brook NY)
Q Rev Econ Bus
QUARTERLY REVIEW OF ECONOMICS AND BUSINESS (Urbana IL)
Qadmoniot
QADMONIOT (Israel)
QRB
QRB. QUALITY REVIEW BULLETIN (Chicago)
Quad Cult Bolognese
QUADERNI CULTURALI BOLOGNESE (Italy)
Quad Depart Stat Univ Studi Fir
QUADERNI DEL DEPARTIMENTO STATISTICO UNIVERSITA DEGLI STUDI DI FIRENZE (Italy)
Quad Stor
QUADERNI DI STORIA (Italy)
Quad Stor Univ Padova
QUADERNI PER LA STORIA DELL UNIVERSITA DI PADOVA (Italy)
Quaker Hist
QUAKER HISTORY (Haverford PA)
Queens Q
QUEENS QUARTERLY (Canada)
Quercy Rech
QUERCY RECHERCHE (Cahors)
Quintessence Int
QUINTESSENCE INTERNATIONAL (Berlin)
Quintessenz
QUINTESSENZ (Berlin)
Quintessenz J
QUINTESSENZ JOURNAL (Berlin)
Quintessenz Zahntech
QUINTESSENZ DER ZAHNTECHNIK (Berlin)

—R—

R Soc Health J
ROYAL SOCIETY OF HEALTH JOURNAL (London)
Race Cl
RACE AND CLASS (London)
Rad Inst Hrvat Povij
RADOVI; INSTITUT ZA HRVATSKU POVIJEST (Yugoslavia)
Radiat Med
RADIATION MEDICINE (Tokyo)
Radic Am
RADICAL AMERICA (Somerville MA)
Radic Hist Rev
RADICAL HISTORY REVIEW (New York)
Radiobiol Radiother (Berl)
RADIOBIOLOGIA, RADIOTHERAPIA (Berlin)
Radiography
RADIOGRAPHY (London)
Radiol Manage
RADIOLOGY MANAGEMENT (Boston)
Radiol Med (Torino)
RADIOLOGIA MEDICA (Torino)
Radiol Technol
RADIOLOGIC TECHNOLOGY (Baltimore)
Radiologe
RADIOLOGE (Berlin)
Radiology
RADIOLOGY (Easton PA)
Rass Arch Stato
RASSEGNA DEGLI ARCHIVI DI STATO (Roma)
Rass Lett Ital
RASSEGNA DELLA LETTERATURA ITALIANA (Roma)
Real Acad Med Zaragoza
REAL ACADEMIA DE MEDICINA DE ZARAGOZA (Spain)
Reason
REASON (US)
Rec Bucks
RECORDS OF BUCKINGHAMSHIRE (Gt Brit)
Rec Columb Hist Soc
RECORDS OF THE COLUMBIA HISTORICAL SOCIETY (Washington)
Recenti Prog Med
RECENTI PROGRESSI IN MEDICINA (Roma)
Rech Amerindiennes Que Bull Inf
RECHERCHES AMERINDIENNES AU QUEBEC BULLETIN D'INFORMATION (Montreal)
Rech Sociogr
RECHERCHES SOCIOGRAPHIQUES (Quebec)
Recherche
LA RECHERCHE (Paris)
Record
RECORD
Red River Val Hist Rev
RED RIVER VALLEY HISTORICAL REVIEW (Durant OK)
Regist Ky Hist Soc
REGISTER OF THE KENTUCKY HISTORICAL SOCIETY (Frankfort KY)
Regul Toxicol Pharmacol

REGULATORY TOXICOLOGY AND PHARMACOLOGY (New York)
Rehabil Lit
REHABILITATION LITERATURE (Chicago)
Rehabilitation (Bonn)
REHABILITATION; SOZIALMEDIZIN PHYSIKALISCHEMEDIZIN PRAVENTIVMEDIZIN (Bonn)
Rehabilitation (Stuttg)
REHABILITATION (Stuttgart)
Relig Life
RELIGION IN LIFE (Nashville, TN)
Renaiss Q
RENAISSANCE QUARTERLY (New York)
Renaiss Reformation
RENAISSANCE & REFORMATION (Canada)
Rend Atti Accad Sci Med Chir
RENDICONTI ED ATTI DELLA ACCADEMIA DI SCIENZE MEDICHE E CHIRURGICHE (Naples)
Rend Ist Lomb Accad Sci Lett B
RENDICONTI-ISTITUTO LOMBARDO ACCADEMIA DI SCIENZE E LETTERE B SCIENCE BIOLOGICHE E MEDICHE (Italy)
Reproduccion
REPRODUCCION (Madrid)
Res Econ Hist
RESEARCH IN ECONOMIC HISTORY (US)
Res Nurs Health
RESEARCH IN NURSING AND HEALTH (New York)
Res Publ Assoc Res Nerv Ment Dis
RESEARCH PUBLICATIONS—ASSOCIATION FOR RESEARCH IN NERVOUS AND MENTAL DISEASE (Baltimore)
Res Q
RESEARCH QUARTERLY (Washington)
Res Q Exerc Sport
RESEARCH QUARTERLY FOR EXERCISE AND SPORT (Washington)
Res Stud
RESEARCH STUDIES. A QUARTERLY PUBLICATION OF WASHINGTON STATE UNIVERSITY (US)
Resid Staff Physician
RESIDENT AND STAFF PHYSICIAN (Port Washington NY)
Respir Care
RESPIRATORY CARE (Philadelphia)
Respir Physiol
RESPIRATION PHYSIOLOGY (Amsterdam)
Respir Ther
RESPIRATORY THERAPY (Los Angeles)
Retina
RETINA (Philadelphia)
Reumatizam
REUMATIZAM (Zagreb)
Reumatologia
REUMATOLOGIA (Warszawa)
Rev Acad Colomb Hist Ecles
REVISTA DE LA ACADEMIA COLOMBIANA DE HISTORIA ECLESIASTICA (Colombia)
Rev Alsace
REVUE D'ALSACE (France)
Rev Am Hist
REVIEWS IN AMERICAN HISTORY (Baltimore MD)
Rev Arch Bibl Mus
REVISTA DE ARCHIVOS, BIBLIOTECAS Y MUSEOS (Madrid)
Rev Archeol Centre France
REVUE ARCHEOLOGIQUE DU CENTRE DE LA FRANCE
Rev Arhiv
REVISTA ARHIVELOR (Bucuresti)
Rev Asoc Odontol Argent
REVISTA DE LA ASOCIACION ODONTOLOGICA ARGENTINA (Buenos Aires)
Rev Assoc Paul Cir Dent
REVISTA DA ASSOCIACAO PAULISTA DE CIRURGIOES DENTISTAS (Sao Paulo)
Rev Auvergne
REVUE D'AUVERGNE (France)
Rev Belge Hist Milit
REVUE BELGE D' HISTOIRE MILITAIRE (Belgium)
Rev Belge Med Dent
REVUE BELGE DE MEDECINE DENTAIRE (Bruxelles)
Rev Bibl Nac Jose Marti
REVISTA DE LA BIBLIOTECA NACIONAL "JOSE MARTI" (Cuba)
Rev Bras Malariol Doencas Trop
REVISTA BRASILEIRA DE MALARIOLOGIA E DOENCAS TROPICAIS (Rio de Janeiro)
Rev Catarinense Odontol
REVISTA CATARINENSE DE ODONTOLOGIA (Brasil)
Rev Chil Pediatr
REVISTA CHILENA DE PEDIATRIA (Santiago)
Rev Chir [Oftalmol]
REVISTA DE CHIRURGIE, ONCOLOGIE, RADIOLOGIE, ORL, OFTALMOLOGIE, STOMATOLOGIE. SERIA: OFTAMLOLOGIE (Bucuresti)
Rev Chir [Otorinolaringol]
REVISTA DE CHIRURGIE, OTORINOLARINGOLOGIE (Bucharest)
Rev Chir Orthop
REVUE DE CHIRURGIE ORTHOPEDIQUE ET REPARATRICE DE L'APPAREIL MOTEUR (Paris)
Rev Clin Esp
REVISTA CLINICAL ESPANOLA (Madrid)
Rev Col Nac Enferm
REVISTA DEL COLEGIO NACIONAL DE ENFERMERAS (Mexico)
Rev Comminges
REVUE DE COMMINGES (France)
Rev Cubana Med Trop
REVISTA CUBANA DE MEDICINA TROPICAL (Havana)

Rev Dent (St Domingo)
REVISTA DENTAL (Santo Domingo)
Rev Deux Mondes
REVUE DES DEUX MONDES (France)
Rev Econ Stat
REVIEW OF ECONOMICS AND STATISTICS (Cambridge MA)
Rev Enferm
REVISTA DE ENFERMERIA (Barcelona)
Rev Environ Health
REVIEWS ON ENVIRONMENTAL HEALTH (Tel Aviv)
Rev Esc Enferm USP
REVISTA DA ESCOLA DE ENFERMAGEN DA UNIVERSIDADE DE SAO PAULO (Brazil)
Rev Esp Anestesiol Reanim
REVISTA ESPANOLA DE ANESTESIOLOGIA Y REANIMACION (Barcelona)
Rev Esp Antropol Am
REVISTA ESPANOLA DE ANTROPOLOGIA AMERICANA
Rev. Esp Endodoncia
REVISTA ESPANOLA DE ENDODONCIA (Madrid)
Rev Esp Enferm Apar Dig
REVISTA ESPANOLA DE LAS ENFERMEDADES DEL APARATO DIGESTIVO (Madrid)
Rev Esp Estomatol
REVISTA ESPANOLA DE ESTOMATOLOGIE (Barcelona)
Rev Esp Invest Sociol
REVISTA ESPANOLA DE INVESTIGACIONES SOCIOLOGICAS (Spain)
Rev Esp Oncol
REVISTA ESPANOLA DE ONCOLOGIA (Madrid)
Rev Estud Extremenos
REVISTA DE ESTUDIOS EXTREMENOS (Spain)
Rev Estud Hisp
REVISTA DE ESTUDIOS HISPANOLA
Rev Ethnol Que
REVUE D'ETHNOLOGIE QUEBEC
Rev Etud Comp Est Quest
REVUE D'ETUDES COMPARATIVES EST-QUEST (France)
Rev Etud Grec
REVUE DES ETUDES GRECQUES (Paris)
Rev Etud Ital
REVUE DES ETUDES ITALIENNES (Paris)
Rev Estud Juives
REVUE DES ETUDES JUIVES. HISTORIA JUDAICA (France)
Rev Etud Sud Est Eur
REVUE DES ETUDES SUD-EST EUROPEENNES (Romania)
Rev Fac Cienc Med Univ Nac Cordoba
REVISTA DE LA FACULTAD DE CIENCIAS MEDICAS/UNIVERSIDAD NACIONAL DE CORDOBA (Cordoba)
Rev Fac Odontol Univ Nac Colomb
REVISTA DE LA FACULTAD DE ODONTOLOGIA DE LA UNIVERSIDAD NACIONAL DE COLOMBIA (Colombia)
Rev Fed Odontol Colomb
REVISTA DE LA FEDERACION ODONTOLOGICA COLOMBIANA (Colombia)
Rev Fom Soc
REVISTA DE FOMENTO SOCIAL (Madrid)
Rev Fr Hist Livre
REVUE FRANCAISE D'HISTOIRE DU LIVRE (Bordeaux)
Rev Fr Hist Outre Mer
REVUE FRANCAISE D'HISTOIRE D'OUTRE-MER (Paris)
Rev Fr Mal Respir
REVUE FRANCAISE DES MALADIES RESPIRATOIRES (Paris)
Rev Fr Psychanal
REVUE FRANCAISE DE PSYCHANALYSE (Paris)
Rev Gastroenterol Mex
REVISTA DE GASTROENTEROLOGIA DE MEXICO (Mexico)
Rev Gen Mar
REVISTA GENERAL DE MARINA (Madrid)
Rev Hist (Brazil)
REVISTA DE HISTORIA (Brazil)
Rev Hist (Costa Rica)
REVISTA DE HISTORIA (Costa Rica)
Rev Hist (Paris)
REVUE HISTORIQUE (Paris)
Rev Hist Am Argent
REVISTA DE HISTORIA AMERICANA Y ARGENTINA (Mendoza)
Rev Hist Am Fr
REVUE D'HISTOIRE DE L'AMERIQUE FRANCAISE (Canada)
Rev Hist Armees
REVUE HISTORIQUE DES ARMEES (France)
Rev Hist Bordeaux Dep Gironde
REVUE HISTORIQUE DE BORDEAUX ET DU DEPARTMENT DE LA GIRONDE (Bordeaux)
Rev Hist Deuxieme Guerre Mond
REVUE D'HISTOIRE DE LA DEUXIEME GUERRE MONDIALE (France)
Rev Hist Eccles
REVUE D'HISTOIRE ECCLESIASTIQUE (Belgium)
Rev Hist Econ Soc
REVUE D'HISTOIRE ECONOMIQUE ET SOCIALE (Paris)
Rev Hist Med Heb
REVUE D'HISTOIRE DE LA MEDECINE HEBRAIQUE (Paris)
Rev Hist Mil
REVISTA DE HISTORIA MILITAR (Madrid)
Rev Hist Mod Contemp
REVUE D'HISTOIRE MODERNE ET CONTEMPORAINE (Paris)
Rev Hist Pharm (Paris)

REVUE D'HISTOIRE DE LA PHARMACIE (Paris)
Rev Hist Philos Relig
REVUE D'HISTOIRE ET DE PHILOSOPHIE RELIGIEUSES (Paris)
Rev Hist Sci (Paris)
REVUE D'HISTOIRE DES SCIENCES (Paris)
Rev Hosp Clin Fac Med Sao Paulo
REVISTA DO HOSPITAL DAS CLINICAS: FACULDADE DE MEDICINA DA UNIVERSIDADE DE SAO PAULO (Sao Paulo)
Rev Ig [Bacteriol]
REVISTA DE IGIENA, BACTERIOLOGIE, VIRUSOLOGIE, PARAZITOLOGIE, EPIDEMIOLOGIE, PNEUMOFTIZIOLOGIE. BACTERIOLOGIA, VIRUSOLOGIA, PARAZITOLOGIA, EPIDEMIOLOGIA (Bucuresti)
Rev Indias
REVISTA DE INDIAS (Madrid)
Rev Infect Dis
REVIEWS OF INFECTIOUS DISEASES (Chicago)
Rev Infirm
REVUE DE L'INFIRMIERE (Paris)
Rev Inst Eur
REVISTA DE INSTITUCIONES EUROPEAS (Madrid)
Rev Inst Hist Geogr Bras
REVISTA DO INSTITUTO HISTORICO E GEOGRAFICO BRASILEIRO (Brazil)
Rev Inst Hyg Mines (Hasselt)
REVUE DE L'INSTITUT D'HYGIENE DES MINES (Hasselt)
Rev Inst Napoleon (Paris)
REVUE DE L'INSTITUT NAPOLEON (Paris)
Rev Inst Sociol
RVUE DE L'INSTITUT DE SOCIOLOGIE (Belgium)
Rev Int Hist Psychiatr
REVUE INTERNATIONALE D'HISTOIRE DE LA PSYCHIATRIE
Rev Int Trach Pathol Ocul Trop Subtrop
REVUE INTERNATIONALE DU TRACHOME ET DE PATHOLOGIE OCULAIRE TROPICALE ET SUBTROPICALE (France)
Rev Int Trach Pathol Ocul Trop Subtrop Sante Publique
REVUE INTERNATIONALE DU TRACHOME ET DE PATHOLOGIE OCULAIRE TROPICALE ET SUBTROPICALE ET DE SANTE PUBLIQUE (Annonay)
Rev Invest Clin
REVISTA DE INVESTIGACION CLINICA (Caracas)
Rev Istor
REVISTA DE ISTORIE (Romania)
Rev Laryngol Otol Rhinol (Bord)
REVUE DE LARYNGOLOGIE OTOLOGIE-RHINOLOGIE (Bordeaux)
Rev Louisiane-La Rev
REVUE DE LOUISIANE-LOUISIANA REVIEW (US)
Rev Louvre Mus Fr
REVUE—LOUVRE ET DES MUSEES DE FRANCE
Rev Mar
REVISTA DE MARINA (Chile)
Rev Med Brux
REVUE MEDICALE DE BRUXELLES (Bruxelles)
Rev Med Chil
REVISTA MEDICA DE CHILE (Santiago)
Rev Med Chir Soc Med Nat Iasi
REVISTA MEDICO-CHIRURGICALA A SOCIETATII DE MEDICI SI NATURALISTI DIN IASI (IASI)
Rev Med Interna [Med Interna]
REVISTA DE MEDICINA INTERNA, NEUROLOGIE, PSIHIATRIE, NEUROCHIRURGIE, DERMATO VENEROLOGIE. SERIA: MEDICINA INTERNA (Bucuresti)
Rev Med Interna [Neurol Psihiatr]
REVISTA DE MEDICINA-INTERNA, NEUROLOGIE, PSIHIATRIE, NEUROCHIRURGIE, DERMATO VENEROLOGIE. NEUROLOGIE, PSIHIATRIE, NEUROCHIRURGIE (Bucuresti)
Rev Med Liege
REVUE MEDICALE DE LIEGE (Liege)
Rev Med Panama
REVISTA MEDICA DE PANAMA (Panama)
Rev Med Suisse Romande
REVUE MEDICALE DE LA SUISSE ROMANDE (Lausanne)
Rev Med Univ Navarra
REVISTA DE MEDICINA DE LA UNIVERSIDAD DE NAVARRA (Pamplona)
Rev Metaphys
REVIEW OF METAPHYSICS (Washington)
Rev Mex Cienc Polit Soc
REVISTA MEXICANA DE CIENCIAS POLITICAS Y SOCIALES (Mexico)
Rev Mus Nac
REVISTA DEL MUSEO NACIONAL (Peru)
Rev Neurol (Paris)
REVUE NEUROLOGIQUE (Paris)
Rev Neuropsiquiatr
REVISTA DE NEURO-PSIQUIATRIA (Lima)
Rev Nord
REVUE DU NORD (France)
Rev Nouv
REVUE NOUVELLE (Belgium)
Rev Occident Musulman Mediterr
REVUE DE L'OCCIDENT MUSULMAN ET DE LA MEDITERRANEE (France)
Rev Odontol P R
REVISTA ODONTOLOGICA DE PUERTO RICO (Santurce)
Rev Sci Hum
REVUE DES SCIENCES HUMAINES (France)
Rev Odontostomatol (Paris)
REVUE D'ODONTO-STOMATOLOGIE (Paris)
Rev Otoneuroopthalmol
REVUE D'OTO-NEURO-OPTHALMOLOGIE (Paris)
Rev Palais Decour

REVUE DU PALAIS DE LA DECOUVERTE (Paris)
Rev Paul Med
REVISTA PAULISTA DE MEDICINA (Sao Paulo)
Rev Pediatr Obstet Ginecol [Pediatr]
REVISTA DE PEDIATRIE, OBSTETRICA SI GINECOLOGIE. PEDIATRIA (Bucuresti)
Rev Philol (Paris)
REVUE DE PHILOLOGIE DE LITTERATURE ET D'HISTOIRE ANCIENNE (Paris)
Rev Physiol Biochem Pharmacol
REVIEWS OF PHYSIOLOGY BIOCHEMISTRY AND PHARMACOLOGY (Berlin)
Rev Pol Acad Sci (Warsz)
REVIEW OF THE POLISH ACADEMY OF SCIENCES (Warszawa)
Rev Port Estomatol Cir Maxilofac
REVISTA PORTUGUESA DE ESTOMATOLIGIA E CIRURGIA MAXILOFACIALE (Lisbon)
Rev Port Farm
REVISTA PORTUGUESA DE FARMACIA (Lisbon)
Rev Prat
LA REVUE DU PRATICIEN (Paris)
Rev Radic Polit Econ
REVIEW OF RADICAL POLITICAL ECONOMICS (US)
Rev Rhum Mal Osteoartic
REVUE DU RHUMATISME ET DES MALADIES OSTEO-ARTICULAIRES (Paris)
Rev Roum Hist
REVUE ROUMAINE D'HISTOIRE (Romania)
Rev Sanid Hig Publica (Madr)
REVISTA DE SANIDAD E HIGIENE PUBLICA (Madrid)
Rev Saude Publica
REVISTA DE SAUDE PUBLICA (Sao Paulo)
Rev Sci Hum
REVUE DES SCIENCES HUMAINES (France)
Rev Soc Bolivar Venez
REVISTA DE LA SOCIEDAD BOLIVARIANA DE VENEZUELA (Venezuela)
Rev Soc Econ
REVIEW OF SOCIAL ECONOMY (US)
Rev Soc Venez Hist Med
REVISTA DE LA SOCIEDAD VENEZOLANA DE HISTORIA DE LA MEDICINA (Caracas)
Rev Stomatol Chir Maxillofac
REVUE DE STOMATOLOGIE ET DE CHIRURGIE MAXILLO-FACIALE (Paris)
Rev Synth (Paris)
REVUE DE SYNTHESE (Paris)
Rev Trav Acad Sci Morales Polit
REVUE DES TRAVAUX DE L'ACADEMIE DES SCIENCES MORALES ET POLITIQUES ET COMTES RENDUS DE SES SEANCES (France)
Rev Univ Brux
REVUE DE L'UNIVERSITE DE BRUXELLES (Bruxelles)
Rev Univ Complut Madr
REVISTA DE LA UNIVERSIDAD COMPLUTENSE DE MADRID (Spain)
Rev Univ Ottawa
REVUE DE L'UNIVERSITE D'OTTAWA (Canada)
Rheinische Vierteljahrsbl
RHEINISCHE VIERTELJAHRSBLATTER (Bonn)
Rheinisches Arztebl
RHEINISCHES ARZTEBLATT (Cologne)
Rheinisches Mus Philol
RHEINISCHES MUSEUM FUR PHILOLOGIE (Frankfurt am Main)
Rheinl Mus Bonn
RHEINLAND MUSEUM IN BONN
Rheumatol Rehabil
RHEUMATOLOGY AND REHABILITATION (London)
Rhodesiana
RHODESIANA
RI Hist
RHODE ISLAND HISTORY (Providence)
RI Med J
RHODE ISLAND MEDICAL JOURNAL (Providence RI)
Rice Univ Stud
RICE UNIVERSITY STUDIES (Houston)
Rinascimento
RINASCIMENTO (Florence)
Rinsho Byori
RINSHO BYORI. JAPANESE JOURNAL OF CLINICAL PATHOLOGY (Tokyo)
Rinsho Ketsueki
RINSHO KETSUIKI. JAPANESE JOURNAL OF CLINICAL HEMATOLOGY (Tokyo)
Rinsho Kyobu Geka
RISHO KYOBU GEKA (Tokyo)
Rinsho Shika
RINSHO SHIKA (Kyoto)
Rinsho Shinkeigaku
RINSHO SHINKEIGAKU. CLINICAL NEUROLOGY (Tokyo)
Risorgimento
RISORGIMENTO (Milan)
Riv Biol
RIVISTA DI BIOLOGIA (Perugia)
Riv Filol Istruz Classica
RIVISTA DI FILOLOGIA E DI ISTRUZIONE CLASSICA (Torino)
Riv Filos
RIVISTA DI FILOSOFIA (Turin)
Riv Int Sci Sociali
RIVISTA INTERNAZIONALE DI SCIENZE SOCIALI (Milano)
Riv Ital Stomatol
RIVISTA ITALIANA DI STOMATOLOGIA (Venezia)
Riv Med Aeronaut Spaz
RIVISTA DI MEDICINA AERONAUTICA E SPAZIALE (Roma)
Riv Mil

RIVISTA MILITAIRE (Roma)
Riv Odontoiatr Amici Brugg
RIVISTA DI ODONTOIATRIA DEGLI AMICI DI BRUGG (Asti)
RN Id
RN IDAHO (Boise ID)
RNABC News
RNABC NEWS; REGISTERED NURSES ASSOCIATION OF BRITISH COLOMBIA (Vancouver BC)
ROFO
ROFO, FORTSCHRITTE AUF DEM GEBIETE DER RONTGENSTRAHLEN UND DER NUKLEARMEDIZIN (Stuttgart)
Rom Hist Mitt
ROMISCHE HISTORISCHE MITTEILUNGEN (Vienna)
Romantisme
ROMANTISME; REVUE DU DIX-NEUVIEME SIECLE (France)
Rontgenblatter
RONTGEN-BLATTER (Wuppertal)
Rostocker Wiss Hist Manuskripte
ROSTOCKER WISSENSCHAFTLICH-HISTORISCHE MANUSKRIPTE
Rostrum
ROSTRUM
Rozhl Chir
ROZHLEDY V CHIRURGII (Praha)
Ruperto Carola
RUPERTO CAROLA (HEIDELBERG)
Rural Sociol
RURAL SOCIOLOGY (Madison WI)
Russ Rev
RUSSIAN REVIEW (Stanford)

—S—

S Afr J Econ
SOUTH AFRICAN JOURNAL OF ECONOMICS (South Africa)
S Afr J Surg
SOUTH AFRICAN JOURNAL OF SURGERY (Johannesburg)
S Afr Med J
SOUTH AFRICAN MEDICAL JOURNAL (Cape Town)
SAAD Dig
SAAD DIGEST. SOCIETY FOR THE ADVANCEMENT OF ANAESTHESIA IN DENTISTRY (London)
Saalburg Jahrb
SAALBURG JAHRBUCH (Berlin)
Sachitra Ayurved
SACHITRA AYURVED
Saeculum (Freiburg)
SAECULUM; JAHRBUCH FUR UNIVERSALGESCHICHTE (Freiburg)
Salud Bucal
SALUD BUCAL (Buenos Aires)
Salud Publica Mex
SALUD PUBLICA DE MEXICO
Salzburger Beitr Paracelsusforsch
SALZBURGER BEITRAGE ZUR PARACELSUS-FORSCHUNG (Salzburg)
Samtiden (Norway)
SAMTIDEN (Norway)
San Jose Stud
SAN JOSE STUDIES (US)
Sangre (Barc)
SANGRE (Barcelona)
Sante Publique (Bucur)
SANTE PUBLIQUE (Bucuresti)
Santiago (Cuba)
SANTIAGO (Cuba)
Saopcenja
SAOPCENJA (Yugoslavia)
Sapienza
SAPIENZA (Italy)
Sartonia
SARTONIA (Gent Belgium)
Sask Hist
SASKATCHEWAN HISTORY (Canada)
Sb Arch Pr
SBORNIK ARCHIVNICH PRACI (Czechoslovakia)
Sb Lek
SBORNIK LEKARSKY (Praha)
Sb Nar Muzea Praze Rada A Hist
SBORNIK NARODNIHO MUZEA V PRAZE RADA A: HISTORIE (Czechoslovakia)
Sb Nar Muzea Praze Rada C Lit Hist
SBORNIK NARODNIHO MUZEA V PRAZE RADA C: LITERARNI HISTORIE (Czechoslovakia)
Sb Pr Filos Fak Brnenske Univ Rada Hist
SBORNIK PRACI FILOSOFICKE FAKULTY BRNENSKE UNIVERSITY: RADA HISTORICKA (Czechoslovakia)
Sb Ved Pr Lek Fak Univ Karlovy
SBORNIK VEDECKYCH PRACI LEKARSKE FAKULTY KARLOVY UNIVERZITY V HRADCI KRALOVE (Praha)
SC Hist Illus
SOUTH CAROLINA HISTORY ILLUSTRATED (US)
SC Hist Mag
SOUTH CAROLINA HISTORICAL MAGAZINE (US)
Scalpel Tongs
SCALPEL AND TONGS (Salem VA)
Scan Electron Microsc
SCANNING ELECTRON MICROSCOPY (Chicago)
Scand Econ Hist Rev
SCANDINAVIAN ECONOMIC HISTORY REVIEW (Finland)
Scand J Dent Res
SCANDINAVIAN JOURNAL OF DENTAL RESEARCH (Copenhagen)
Scand J Gastroenterol
SCANDINAVIAN JOURNAL OF GASTROENTEROLOGY (Oslo)

Scand J Hist
SCANDINAVIAN JOURNAL OF HISTORY (Stockholm)
Scand J Immunol
SCANDINAVIAN JOURNAL OF IMMUNOLOGY (Oxford)
Scand J Plast Reconstr Surg
SCANDINAVIAN JOURNAL OF PLASTIC AND RECONSTRUCTIVE SURGERY (Stockholm)
Scand J Psychol
SCANDINAVIAN JOURNAL OF PSYCHOLOGY (Stockholm)
Scand J Rehabil Med [Suppl]
SCANDINAVIAN JOURNAL OF REHABILITATION MEDICINE. SUPPLEMENT (Stockholm)
Scand J Rheumatol
SCANDINAVIAN JOURNAL OF RHEUMATOLOGY (Stockholm)
Scand J Soc Med
SCANDINAVIAN JOURNAL OF SOCIAL MEDICINE (Stockholm)
Scand J Soc Med [Suppl]
SCANDINAVIAN JOURNAL OF SOCIAL MEDICINE. SUPPLEMENT (Stockholm)
Scand J Urol Nephrol
SCANDINAVIAN JOURNAL OF UROLOGY AND NEPHROLOGY (Stockholm)
Scand Popul Stud
SCANDINAVIAN POPULATION STUDIES (Oslo)
Scandia
SCANDIA (Lund)
Schaffhauser Beitr Vaterl Gesch
SCHAFFHAUSER BEITRAGE ZUR VATERLANDISCHEN GESCHICHTE (Switzerland)
Scheidewege
SCHEIDEWEGE
Schizophr Bull
SCHIZOPHRENIA BULLETIN (Rockville MD)
Schleswig Holsteinisches Arztebl
SCHLESWIG-HOLSTEINISCHES ARZTEBLATT (W Germany)
Schr Gesch Kult Alten Orients
SCHRIFTEN ZUR GESCHICHTE UND KULTUR DES ALTEN ORIENTS (E Germany)
Schriftenr Dtsch Rontgenmus
SCHRIFTENREIHE DEUTSCHES RONTGENMUSEUM
Schweiz Apoth Ztg
SCHWEIZERISCHE APOTHEKER-ZEITUNG (Lausanne)
Schweiz Arch Neurol Neurochir Psychiatr
SCHWEIZER ARCHIV FUR NEUROLOGIE, NEUROCHIRURGIE UND PSYCHIATRIE (Zurich)
Schweiz Arch Tierheilkd
SCHWEIZER ARCHIV FUR TIERHEILKUNDE (Zurich)
Schweiz Arzteztg
SCHWEIZERISCHE ARZTEZEITUNG; BULLETIN DES MEDECINS SUISSES; BOLLETTINO DEI MEDICI SVIZZERI (Bern)
Schweiz Med Wochenschr
SCHWEIZERISCHE MEDIZINISCHE WOCHENSCHRIFT. JOURNAL SUISSE DE MEDECINE (Basel)
Schweiz Med Wochenschr [Suppl]
SCHWEIZERISCHE MEDIZINISCHE WOCHENSCHRIFT. SUPPLEMENTUM (Basel)
Schweiz Monatsschr Zahnmed
SCHWEIZERISCHE MONATSSCHRIFT FUR ZAHNMEDIZIN (Zurich)
Schweiz Rundsch Med Prax
SCHWEIZERISCHE RUNDSCHAU FUR MEDIZIN PRAXIS (Bern)
Schweiz Spital
SCHWEIZER SPITAL (Switzerland)
Schweiz Z Gesch
SCHWEIZERISCHE ZEITSCHRIFT FUR GESCHICHTE (Switzerland)
Sci Am
SCIENTIFIC AMERICAN (New York)
Sci Avenir
SCIENCES ET AVENIR (Paris)
Sci Cult
SCIENCE AND CULTURE (India)
Sci Orient
SCIENTIA ORIENTALIS (France)
Sci Public Aff Bull At Sci
SCIENCE AND PUBLIC AFFAIRS; BULLETIN OF THE ATOMIC SCIENTISTS (US)
Sci Sin
SCIENTIA SINICA (Peking)
Sci Soc
SCIENCE AND SOCIETY (New York)
Sci Tech Perspect
SCIENCES ET TECHNIQUES EN PERSPECTIVE
Sci Total Environ
SCIENCE OF THE TOTAL ENVIRONMENT (Amsterdam)
Science
SCIENCE (Washington)
Scientia
SCIENTIA (Milano)
Scope
SCOPE. OFFICE OF PUBLIC AFFAIRS, UNIVERSITY OF ILLINOIS AT THE MEDICAL CENTER (Chicago IL)
Scott Educ Rev
SCOTTISH EDUCATIONAL REVIEW (Gt Brit)
Scott Hist Rev
SCOTTISH HISTORICAL REVIEW (Gt Brit)
Scott Med J
SCOTTISH MEDICAL JOURNAL (Glasgow)
Scriptorium
SCRIPTORIUM; REVUE INTERNATIONALE DES ETUDES RELATIVES AUX MANUSCRITS (Belgium)

SD J Med
SOUTH DAKOTA JOURNAL OF MEDICINE (Sioux Falls)
Sefarad
SEFARAD (Madrid)
Seikagaku
SEIKAGAKU. JOURNAL OF JAPANESE BIOCHEMICAL SOCIETY (Tokyo)
Seishin Shinkeigaku Zasshi
SEISHIN SHINKEIGAKU ZASSHI. PSYCHIATRIA ET NEUROLOGIA JAPONICA (Tokyo)
Sem Hop Paris
SEMAINE DES HOPITAUX DE PARIS (Paris)
Sem Med
LA SEMANA MEDICA (Buenos Aires)
Semin Arthritis Rheum
SEMINARS IN ARTHRITIS AND RHEUMATISM (New York)
Semin Nucl Med
SEMINARS IN NUCLEAR MEDICINE (New York)
Semin Oncol
SEMINARS IN ONCOLOGY (New York)
Semin Perinatol
SEMINARS IN PERINATOLOGY (New York)
Semin Roentgenol
SEMINARS IN ROENTGENOLOGY (New York)
Semin Thromb Hemost
SEMINARS IN THROMBOSIS AND HEMOSTASIS (New York)
Semin Urol
SEMINARS IN UROLOGY (New York)
Senefiance
SENEFIANCE (France)
Ser Libr
SERIALS LIBRARIAN (US)
Sex Transm Dis
SEXUALLY TRANSMITTED DISEASES (Philadelphia)
Shakai Keizai Shigaku
SHAKAI-KEIZAI-SHIGAKU (Japan)
Shakespeare Stud
SHAKESPEARE STUDIES
She Hui K'ohsueh Lun Ts'ung
SHE HUI K'OHSUEH LUN T'SUNG (Journal of Social Science) (Taiwan)
Sheng Li Ko Hsueh Chin Chan
SHENG LI KO HSUEH CHIN CHAN (Peking)
Shigaku
SHIGAKU. ONDONTOLOGY (Tokyo)
Shigaku Zasshi
SHIGAKU ZASSHI (Japan)
Shi-ta Hsueh-pao
SHIH-TA HSUEH-PAO (Taiwan)
Shikai Tenbo
SHIKAI TENBO. DENTAL OUTLOOK (Tokyo)
Shikwa Gakuho
SHIKWA GAKUHO (Tokyo)
Shvut (Israel)
SHVUT (Israel)
Signs
SIGNS; JOURNAL OF WOMEN IN CULTURE AND SOCIETY (US)
Sinai
SINAI
Singapore Libr
SINGAPORE LIBRARIES
Singapore Med J
SINGAPORE MEDICAL JOURNAL (Singapore)
Sitzungsber Osterr Akad Wiss Philos Hist Kl
SITZUNGSBERICHTE DER OSTERREICHISCHEN AKADEMIE DER WISSENSCHAFTEN, PHILOSOPHISCH-HISTORISCH KLASSE (Vienna)
Sixteenth Century J
SIXTEENTH CENTURY JOURNAL (US)
Sjukskoterskan
SJUKSKOTERSKAN (Stockholm)
Slaski Kwart Hist Sobotka
SLASKI KWARTALNIK HISTORYCZNY SOBOTKA (Poland)
Slav East Eur Rev
SLAVONIC AND EAST EUROPEAN REVIEW (London)
Slavic Rev
SLAVIC REVIEW (Chicago)
Sleep
SLEEP (New York)
Slezsky Sb
SLEZSKY SBORNIK (Czechoslovakia)
Smithsonian
SMITHSONIAN (Washington)
Snakeroot Extr
SNAKEROOT EXTRACT. A NEWSLETTER OF INDIANA MEDICAL HISTORY (US)
Soc Amis Arts Sci Tournus
SOCIETE DES AMIS DES ARTS ET DES SCIENCES DE TOURNUS (France)
Soc Biol
SOCIAL BIOLOGY (Chicago)
Soc Casework
SOCIAL CASEWORK (New York)
Soc Hist Archeol Molsheim Environs Annu
SOCIETE D'HISTOIRE ET D'ARCHEOLOGIE DE MOLSHEIM ET ENVIRONS. ANNUAIRE (France)
Soc Econ Stud
SOCIAL AND ECONOMIC STUDIES (Jamaica)
Soc Forces
SOCIAL FORCES (US)
Soc Fr Hist Art Dent
SOCIETE FRANCAISE D'HISTOIRE DE L'ART DENTAIRE (Paris)
Soc Gen Physiol Ser
SOCIETY OF GENERAL PHYSIOLOGISTS SERIES (New York)
Soc Hist (Canada)
SOCIAL HISTORY (Canada)
Soc Hist (Lond)

SOCIAL HISTORY (London)
Soc Policy
SOCIAL POLICY (US)
Soc Probl
SOCIAL PROBLEMS (Buffalo NY)
Soc Psychiatry
SOCIAL PSYCHIATRY (Berlin)
Soc Res (NY)
SOCIAL RESEARCH (New York)
Soc Sci
SOCIAL SCIENCE (Winfield KS)
Soc Sci Hist
SOCIAL SCIENCE HISTORY (Beverly Hills CA)
Soc Sci Inf
SOCIAL SCIENCE INFORMATION (Gt Brit)
Soc Sci J
SOCIAL SCIENCE JOURNAL (Fort Collins CO)
Soc Sci Med
SOCIAL SCIENCE AND MEDICINE (Oxford)
Soc Sci Med [A]
SOCIAL SCIENCE AND MEDICINE. PART A, MEDICAL SOCIOLOGY (Oxford)
Soc Sci Med [B]
SOCIAL SCIENCE AND MEDICINE. PART B, MEDICAL ANTHROPOLOGY (Oxford)
Soc Sci Med [D]
SOCIAL SCIENCE AND MEDICINE. PART D, MEDICAL GEOGRAPHY (Oxford)
Soc Sci Med [F]
SOCIAL SCIENCE AND MEDICINE. PART F, MEDICAL AND SOCIAL ETHICS (Oxford)
Soc Sci Med [Med Anthropol]
SOCIAL SCIENCE AND MEDICINE. MEDICAL ANTHROPOLOGY (Oxford)
Soc Sci Med [Med Econ]
SOCIAL SCIENCE AND MEDICINE. MEDICAL ECONOMICS (Oxford)
Soc Sci Med [Med Geogr]
SOCIAL SCIENCE AND MEDICINE. MEDICAL GEOGRAPHY (Oxford)
Soc Sci Med [Med Psychol Med Sociol]
SOCIAL SCIENCE AND MEDICINE. MEDICAL PSYCHOLOGY AND MEDICAL SOCIOLOGY (Oxford)
Soc Sci Q
SOCIAL SCIENCE QUARTERLY (Austin TX)
Soc Sci Res Counc Items
SOCIAL SCIENCE RESEARCH COUNCIL ITEMS (US)
Soc Secur Bull
SOCIAL SECURITY BULLETIN (Washington)
Soc Serv Rev
SOCIAL SERVICE REVIEW; DEVOTED TO THE SCIENTIFIC AND PROFESSIONAL INTERESTS OF SOCIAL WORK (Chicago)
Soc Soc Hist Med Bull (Lond)
SOCIETY FOR THE SOCIAL HISTORY OF MEDICINE-BULLETIN (London)
Soc Stor
SOCIETA E STORIA
Soc Stud Labour Hist
SOCIETY FOR THE STUDY OF LABOUR HISTORY (Gt Brit)
Soc Stud Sci
SOCIAL STUDIES OF SCIENCE (London)
Soc Work Health Care
SOCIAL WORK IN HEALTH CARE (New York)
Socialmed Tidsskr
SOCIALMEDICINSK TIDSSKRIFT (Stockholm)
Societas
SOCIETAS; A REVIEW OF SOCIAL HISTORY (US)
Society
SOCIETY (US)
Social Anal
SOCIOLOGICAL ANALYSIS (US)
Sociol Health Illn
SOCIOLOGY OF HEALTH AND ILLNESS (Henley-on-Thames)
Sociol Inq
SOCIOLOGICAL INQUIRY (US)
Sociol Q
SOCIOLOGICAL QUARTERLY (US)
Sociol Rev
SOCIOLOGICAL REVIEW (Keele)
Sociol Rev [Monogr]
SOCIOLOGICAL REVIEW MONOGRAPH (Keele)
Sociol Soc Res
SOCIOLOGY AND SOCIAL RESEARCH (US)
Sociology
SOCIOLOGY (Gt Brit)
Sogo Kango
SOGO KANGO. COMPREHENSIVE NURSING, QUARTERLY (Tokyo)
Soins
SOINS (Paris)
Soins Gynecol Obstet Pueric
SOINS. GYNECOLOGIE, OBSTETRIQUE, PUERICULTURE (Paris)
Soins Gynecol Obstet Pueric Pediatr
SOINS. GYNECOLOGIE, OBSTETRIQUE, PUERICULTURE, PEDIATRIE (Paris)
Soins Psychiatr
SOINS PSYCHIATRIE (Paris)
Sotsiol Issled
SOTSIOLOGICHESKIE ISSLEDOVANIA (USSR)
Soud Lek
SOUDNI LEKARSTVI (Praha)
Soundings
SOUNDINGS (Nashville TN)
South Asia
SOUTH ASIA (Australia)
South Atl Q
SOUTH ATLANTIC QUARTERLY (Durham NC)
South Calif Q
SOUTHERN CALIFORNIA QUARTERLY (Los Angeles)

South Econ J
SOUTHERN ECONOMIC JOURNAL (US)
South Exposure
SOUTHERN EXPOSURE (Durham NC)
South Folkl Q
SOUTHERN FOLKLORE QUARTERLY (US)
South Hist
SOUTHERN HISTORY (Gt Brit)
South Hosp
SOUTHERN HOSPITALS (Charlotte NC)
South Indian Stud (NC)
SOUTHERN INDIAN STUDIES (Chapel Hill NC)
South Med J
SOUTHERN MEDICAL JOURNAL (Birmingham AL)
South Q
SOUTHERN QUARTERLY (US)
South Stud
SOUTHERN STUDIES; AN INTERDISCIPLINARY JOURNAL OF THE SOUTH (US)
Southeast Asia Libr Group Newsl
SOUTHEAST ASIA LIBRARY GROUP NEWSLETTER
Southeast Eur
SOUTHEASTERN EUROPE (US)
Southwest Hist Q
SOUTHWESTERN HISTORICAL QUARTERLY (Austin TX)
Sov Arkh
SOVETSKIE ARKHIVY (USSR)
Sov Etnogr
SOVETSKAIA ETNOGRAFIIA (USSR)
Sov Med
SOVETSKAIA MEDITSINA (Moskva)
Sov Stud Hist
SOVIET STUDIES IN HISTORY (White Plains NY)
Sov Union
SOVIET UNION (Pittsburgh PA)
Sov Zdravookhr
SOVETSKOE ZDRAVOOKHRANENIE (Moskva)
Soz Praventivmed
SOZIAL- UND PRAVENTIVMEDIZIN (Solothurn)
Spec Collect
SPECIAL COLLECTIONS (New York)
Spec Educ Forward Trends
SPECIAL EDUCATION; FORWARD TRENDS (London)
Spec Law Dig Health Care (Mon)
SPECIALTY LAW DIGEST. HEALTH CARE (MONTHLY) (Washington)
Speculum
SPECULUM; A JOURNAL OF MEDIAEVAL STUDIES (Cambridge MA)
Spiegel Hist
SPIEGEL HISTORIAEL (Netherlands)
Spine
SPINE (Hagerstown MD)
SPM
SPM. SALUD PUBLICA DE MEXICO (Mexico)
Srp Arh Celok Lek
SRPSKI ARHIV ZA CEOPKUPNO LEKARSTVO (Beograd)
SSO Schweiz Monatsschr Zahnheilkd
SSO; SCHWEIZERISCHE MONATSSCHRIFT FUR ZAHNHEILKUNDE (Zurich)
Ssu yu Yen
SSU YU YEN (Taiwan)
St Mary Hosp Gaz
ST MARY'S HOSPITAL GAZETTE (London)
St Thomas Hosp Gaz
ST THOMAS'S HOSPITAL GAZETTE (London)
Stadion
STADION (Cologne)
Stain Technol
STAIN TECHNOLOGY (Baltimore)
Stanford Fr Rev
STANFORD FRENCH REVIEW (US)
Stat Med
STATISTICS IN MEDICINE (Chichester)
State Gov
STATE GOVERNMENT (Lexington KY)
Stimmen Zeit
STIMMEN DER ZEIT (Freiburg)
Stomatol DDR
STOMATOLOGIE DER DDR (Berlin)
Stomatol Vjesn
STOMATOLOSKI VJESNIK. STOMATOLOGICAL REVIEW (Sarajevo)
Stomatologia (Athenai)
STOMATOLOGIA (Athenai)
Stomatologiia (Mosk)
STOMATOLOGIIA (Moskva)
Stomatologiia (Sofiia)
STOMATOLOGIIA (Sofiia)
Stor Crit Psicol
STORIA E CRITICA DELLA PSICOLOGIA (Bologna)
Strategy Tactics
STRATEGY AND TACTICS (US)
Strenna Stor Bolognese
STRENNA STORICA BOLOGNESE
Stud Am Renaiss
STUDIES IN THE AMERICAN RENAISSANCE (US)
Stud Burke Time
STUDIES IN BURKE AND HIS TIME (US)
Stud Cartesiana
STUDIA CARTESIANA (Amsterdam)
Stud Comp Int Dev
STUDIES IN COMPARATIVE INTERNATIONAL DEVELOPMENT (US)
Stud Eighteenth Cent Cult
STUDIES IN EIGHTEENTH-CENTURY CULTURE (US)
Stud Fam Plann
STUDIES IN FAMILY PLANNING (New York)
Stud Filoz
STUDIA FILOZOFICZNE (Poland)
Stud Hist Biol

STUDIES IN HISTORY OF BIOLOGY (Baltimore MD)
Stud Hist Med
STUDIES IN HISTORY OF MEDICINE (New Delhi)
Stud Hist Philos Sci
STUDIES IN HISTORY AND PHILOSOPHY OF SCIENCE (Oxford)
Stud Mater Dziejow Nauk Pol
STUDIA I MATERIALY Z DZIEJOW NAUKI POLSKIEJ (Warszawa)
Stud Mediev
STUDI MEDIEVALI (Italy)
Stud Mediev Cult
STUDIES IN MEDIEVAL CULTURE (Kalamazoo MI)
Stud Philol
STUDIES IN PHILOLOGY (Chapel Hill NC)
Stud Philos Med
STUDIES IN PHILOSOPHY OF MEDICINE (New Delhi)
Stud Sov Thought
STUDIES IN SOVIET THOUGHT (Netherlands)
Studi Francesi
STUDI FRANCESI (Italy)
Studi Romani
STUDI ROMANI (Roma)
Studi Stor
STUDI STORICI ISTITUTO GRAMISCI EDITORE (Italy)
Studies
STUDIES; AN IRISH QUARTERLY REVIEW OF LETTERS, PHILOSOPHY AND SCIENCES (Ireland)
Studium Hist
STUDIUM HISTORIKE (Albania)
Studium
STUDIUM (Roma)
Sucasnist
SUCASNIST (W Germany)
Sud Med Ekspert
SUDEBNO-MEDITSINSKAIA EKSPERTIZA (Moskva)
Suddtsch Optikerztg
SUDDEUTSCHE OPTIKERZEITUNG (Stuttgart)
Sudhoffs Arch
SUDHOFFS ARCHIV; ZEITSCHRIFT FUR WISSENSCHAFTSGESCHICHTE (Wiesbaden)
Suicide Life Threat Behav
SUICIDE AND LIFE-THREATENING BEHAVIOR (New York)
Surg Annu
SURGERY ANNUAL (New York)
Surg Clin North Am
SURGICAL CLINICS OF NORTH AMERICA (Philadelphia)
Surg Gynecol Obstet
SURGERY, GYNECOLOGY AND OBSTETRICS (Chicago)
Surg Neurol
SURGICAL NEUROLOGY (New York)
Surgery
SURGERY (St Louis)
Surv Ophthalmol
SURVEY OF OPHTHALMOLOGY (Boston)
Surv Sources Newsl
SURVEY OF SOURCES NEWSLETTER (US)
Survey
SURVEY (London)
Sven Farm Tidskr
SVENSK FARMACEUTISK TIDSKRIFT (Stockholm)
Sven Linnesallskap Arsskr
SVENSKA LINNESALLSKAPETS ARSSKRIFT (Uppsala)
Sven Tidskr
SVENSK TIDSKRIFT (Sweden)
Swed Am Hist Q
SWEDISH-AMERICAN HISTORICAL QUARTERLY (US)
Swed Dent J
SWEDISH DENTAL JOURNAL (Jonkoping)
Swed Pioneer Hist Q
SWEDISH PIONEER HISTORICAL QUARTERLY (Chicago)
Swiss Dent
SWISS DENT (Zurich)
Sydsven Medicinhist Sallsk Arsskr
SYDSVENSKA MEDICINHISTORISKA SALLSKAPETS ARSSKRIFT (Lund)
Sygeplejersken
SYGEPLEJERSKEN (Copenhagen)
Sykepleien
SYKEPLEIEN (Oslo)
Synthese
SYNTHESE (Finland)
Synthesis (Mass)
SYNTHESIS (Cambridge MA)
Szazadok
SZAZADOK (Hungary)

—T—

Taehan Kanho
TAEHAN KANHO. KOREAN NURSE (Seoul)
Tandlaegebladet
TANDLAEGEBLADET (Copenhagen)
Tandlakartidningen
TANDLAKARTIDNINGEN (Stockholm)
Tandteknikern
TANDTEKNIKERN (Uppsala)
Tanpakushitsu Kakusan Koso
TANPAKUSHITSU KAKUSAN KOSO. PROTEIN, NUCLEIC ACID, ENZYME (Tokyo)
Tanzan Notes Rec
TANZANIA NOTES AND RECORDS (Tanzania)
Tarih Dergesi (Turkey)
TARIH DERGESI (Turkey)
Teach Coll Rec
TEACHERS COLLEGE RECORD (New York)

Teach Hist J Methods
TEACHING HISTORY: A JOURNAL OF METHODS (US)
Tech Hosp
TECHNICA HOSPITALARIA (Caracas)
Technikgeschichte
TECHNIKGESCHICTE (W Germany)
Technol Cult
TECHNOLOGY AND CULTURE (US)
Technologia
TECHNOLOGIA (Belgium)
Tenn Folkl Soc Bull
TENNESSEE FOLKLORE SOCIETY BULLETIN (US)
Tenn Hist Q
TENNESSEE HISTORICAL QUARTERLY (Nashville TN)
Ter Arkh
TERAPEVTICHESKII ARKHIV (Moskva)
Teratology
TERATOLOGY (New York)
Tex Hosp
TEXAS HOSPITALS (Dallas TX)
Tex Med
TEXAS MEDICINE (Austin TX)
Tex Nurs
TEXAS NURSING (Austin TX)
Tex Rep Biol Med
TEXAS REPORTS ON BIOLOGY AND MEDICINE (Galveston TX)
Tex Stud Lit Land
TEXAS STUDIES IN LITERATURE AND LANGUAGE (Austin TX)
Thalassia Salentina
THALASSIA SALENTINA (Italy)
Ther Ggw
THERAPIE DER GEGENWART (Munchen)
Ther Hung
THERAPIA HUNGARICA (Budapest)
Ther Recreation J
THERAPEUTIC RECREATION JOURNAL (Arlington VA)
Ther Umsch
THERAPEUTISCHE UMSCHAU (Bern)
Therapie
THERAPIE (Paris)
Therapiewoche
THERAPIEWOCHE (W Germany)
Theriaca
THERIACA (Copenhagen)
Third Repub
THIRD REPUBLIC (US)
Thomist
THOMIST (Washington)
Thorac Cardiovasc Surg
THORACIC AND CARDIOVASCULAR SURGEON (Stuttgart)
Thorax
THORAX (London)
Thought
THOUGHT (US)
Thromb Haemost
THROMBOSIS AND HAEMOSTASIS (Stuttgart)
Thromb Res
THROMBOSIS RESEARCH (Elmsford NY)
Thromb Res [Suppl]
THROMBOSIS RESEARCH. SUPPLEMENT (Elmsford NY)
Tibet News Rev
TIBET NEWS REVIEW
Tibetan Med
TIBETAN MEDICINE (India)
TIC
TIC; TICONIUM (Albany)
Tidsskr Nor Laegeforen
TIDSSKRIFT FOR DEN NORSKE LAEGEFORENING (Oslo)
Tidsskr Rettsvitenskap
TIDSSKRIFT FOR RETTSVITENSKAP (Oslo)
Tidsskr Samfunnsforskning
TIDSSKRIFT FOR SAMFUNNSFORSKNING (Norway)
Tidsskr Tandlaeger
TIDSSKRIFT FOR TANDLAEGER (Copenhagen)
Tierarztl Prax
TIERARZTLICHE PRAXIS (Munchen)
Tijdschr Diergeneeskd
TIJDSCHRIFT VOOR DIERGENEESKUNDE (Amsterdam)
Tijdschr Gerontol Geriatr
TIJDSCHRIFT VOOR GERONTOLOGIE EN GERIATRIE (Deventer)
Tijdschr Geschied Geneeskd Natuurwet Wiskd Tech
TIJDSCHRIFT VOOR DE GESCHIEDENIS DER GENEESKUNDE, NATUURWETENSCHAPPEN, WISKUNDE EN TECHNIEK (Amsterdam)
Tijdschr Kindergeneeskd
TIJDSCHRIFT VOOR KINDERGENEESKUNDE (Amsterdam)
Tijdschr Soc Geschied
TIJDSCHRIFT VOOR SOCIALE GESCHIEDENIS (Assen)
Tijdschr Ziekenverpl
TIJDSCHRIFT VOOR ZIEKENVERPLEGING (Amsterdam)
Tirol Heimat
TIROLER HEIMAT (Austria)
Tirol Heimatbl
TIROLER HEIMATBLATTER (Austria)
Tissue Ccell
TISSUE AND CELL (Edinburgh)
Todays OR Nurse
TODAYS OR NURSE (Throfare NJ)
Tohogaku
TOHOGAKU (Japan)
Tokushima J Exp Med

TOKUSHIMA JOURNAL OF EXPERIMENTAL MEDICINE (Tokushima)
Top Clin Nurs
TOPICS IN CLINICAL NURSING (Germantown MD)
Top Emerg Med
TOPICS IN EMERGENCY MEDICINE (Germantown MD)
Top Health Care Financ
TOPICS IN HEALTH CARE FINANCING (Rockville MD)
Torax
TORAX (Uruguay)
Tort Stat Tanulin
TORTENETI STATISZTIKAI TANULMANYOK (Hungary)
Tortenelmi Sz
TORTENELMI SZEMLE (Hungary
Toxicol Eur Res
TOXICOLOGICAL EUROPEAN RESEARCH, RECHERCHE EUROPEENNE EN TOXICOLOGIE (Puteaux)
Toyoschi Kenkyu
TOYOSCHI KENKYU (Japan)
Tr Inst Pastera
TRUDY INSTITUTA IMENI PASTERA (Leningrad)
Trap Inst Cajal Invest Biol
TRABAJOS DEL INSTITUTO CAJAL DE INVESTIGACIONES BIOLOGICAS (Madrid)
Traditio
TRADITIO; STUDIES IN ANCIENT AND MEDIEVAL HISTORY, THOUGHT AND RELIGION (New York)
Trans Action
TRANS-ACTION (US)
Trans Am Clin Climatol Assoc
TRANSACTIONS OF THE AMERICAN CLINICAL AND CLIMATOLOGICAL ASSOCIATION (Baltimore MD)
Trans Am Microsc Soc
TRANSACTIONS OF THE AMERICAN MICROSCOPICAL SOCIETY (Lawrence KS)
Trans Am Soc Artif Intern Organs
TRANSACTIONS-AMERICAN SOCIETY FOR ARTIFICIAL INTERNAL ORGANS (Washington)
Trans Archit Archaeol Soc Durham Northumberl
TRANSACTIONS-ARCHITECTURAL AND ARCHAEOLOGICAL SOCIETY OF DURHAM AND NORTHUMBERLAND (Gt Brit)
Trans Camb Bibliogr Soc
TRANSACTIONS OF THE CAMBRIDGE BIBLIOGRAPHICAL SOCIETY (Gt Brit)
Trans Hunter Archaeol Soc
TRANSACTIONS - HUNTER ARCHAEOLOGICAL SOCIETY (Sheffield)
Trans Hunter Soc
TRANSACTIONS OF THE HUNTERIAN SOCIETY (London)
Trans Jew Hist Soc Engl
TRANSACTIONS OF THE JEWISH HISTORICAL SOCIETY OF ENGLAND (London)
Trans Kans Acad Sci
TRANSACTIONS OF THE KANSAS ACADEMY OF SCIENCE (Lawrence KS)
Trans Med Soc Land
TRANSACTIONS OF THE MEDICAL SOCIETY OF LONDON (London)
Trans Ophthalmol Soc UK
TRANSACTIONS OF THE OPHTHALMOLOGICAL SOCIETIES OF THE UNITED KINGDOM (London)
Trans R Hist Soc
TRANSACTIONS OF THE ROYAL HISTORICAL SOCIETY (London)
Trans R Soc Can
TRANSACTIONS OF THE ROYAL SOCIETY (London)
Trans R Soc Trop Med Hyg
TRANSACTIONS OF THE ROYAL SOCIETY OF TROPICAL MEDICINE AND HYGIENE (London)
Trans Stud Coll Physicians Phila
TRANSACTIONS AND STUDIES OF THE COLLEGE OF PHYSICIANS OF PHILADELPHIA (Baltimore MD)
Trans Thoroton Soc
TRANSACTIONS OF THE THOROTON SOCIETY (Gt Brit)
Transfusion
TRANSFUSION (Philadelphia)
Transplant Proc
TRANSPLANTATION PROCEEDINGS (New York)
Trav Soc Pharm Montp
TRAVAUX DE LA SOCIETE DE PHARMACIE DE MONTPELLIER (France)
Trends Hist
TRENDS IN HISTORY (New York)
Trop Anim Health Prod
TROPICAL ANIMAL HEALTH AND PRODUCTION (Edinburgh)
Trop Doct
TROPICAL DOCTOR (London)
Tsitol Genet
TSITOLOGIIA I GENETIKA (Kiev)
Tsitologiia
TSITOLOGIIA (Moskva)
Tubercle
TUBERCLE (Edinburgh)
Tunis Med
TUNISIE MEDICALE (Tunis)
Turk Hemsire Derg
TURK HEMSIRELER DERGISI
Turk J Pediatr
TURKISH JOURNAL OF PEDIATRICS (Ankara)
Turun Hist Ark (Finl)
TURUN HISTORIALLINEN ARKISTO (Finland)
Tydskr Tandheelkd Ver S Afr
TYDSKRIF VAN DIE TANDHEELKUNDIGE VERENIGING VAN SUID AFRICA (Cape Town)

—U—

Udim
UDIM (Germany)
Ugeskr Laeger
UGESKRIFT FOR LAEGER (Copenhagen)
Uirusu
UIRUSU (Kyoto)
Ukr Biokhim Zh
UKRAINSKII BIOKHIMICHESKII ZHURNAL (Moscow)
Ukr Istor Zh
UKRAINSKYI ISTORYCHNYI ZHURNAL (USSR)
Ukr Q
UKRAINIAN QUARTERLY (New York)
Ukr Rev (Lond)
UKRAINIAN REVIEW (London)
Ulster Folklife
ULSTER FOLKLIFE (Gt Brit)
Ulster Med J
ULSTER MEDICAL JOURNAL (Belfast)
Ultrasound Med Biol
ULTRASOUND IN MEDICINE AND BIOLOGY (Oxford)
Ultrastruct Pathol
ULTRASTRUCTURAL PATHOLOGY (New York)
Unesco Cour
UNESCO COURIER (Paris)
Unfallchirurgie
UNFALLCHIRURGIE (Munchen)
Unifarma
UNIFARMA
Union Med Can
UNION MEDICALE DU CANADA (Montreal)
Unitas
UNITAS (Philippines)
Univ Edinb J
UNIVERSITY OF EDINBURGH JOURNAL (Edinburgh)
Univ Ottawa Q
UNIVERSITY OF OTTAWA QUARTERLY (Ottawa)
Univ Wyo Publ
UNIVERSITY OF WYOMING PUBLICATIONS (US)
Universitas (Stuttg)
UNIVERSITAS (Stuttgart)
Unsere Heimat
UNSERE HEIMAT (Vienna)
Ups J Med Sci
UPPSALA JOURNAL OF MEDICAL SCIENCES (Uppsala)
Urban Geogr
URBAN GEOGRAPHY
Urban Hist Rev
URBAN HISTORY REVIEW (Canada)
Urban Hist Yearb
URBAN HISTORY YEARBOOK (Gt Brit(
Urban Soc Change Rev
URBAN AND SOCIAL CHANGE REVIEW (US)
Urol Clin North Am
UROLOGIC CLINICS OF NORTH AMERICA (Philadelphia)
Urol Nefrol (Mosk)
UROLOGIIA I NEFROLOGIIA (Moskva)
Urol Surv
UROLOGICAL SURVEY (Baltimore)
Urology
UROLOGY (Ridgewood NJ)
US Navy Med
US NAVY MEDICINE (Washington)
Usp Fiziol Nauk
USPEKHI FIZIOLOGICHESKIKH NAUK (Moskva)
Usp Sovrem Biol
USPEKHI SOVREMENNOI BIOLOGII (Moskva)
Utah Hist Q
UTAH HISTORICAL QUARTERLY (Salt Lake City UT)

—V—

Va Cavalcade
VIRGINIA CAVALCADE (Richmond)
Va Dent J
VIRGINIA DENTAL JOURNAL (Richmond)
Va Law Rev
VIRGINIA LAW REVIEW (Charlottesville VA)
Va Mag Hist Biogr
VIRGINIA MAGAZINE OF HISTORY AND BIOGRAPHY (Richmond)
Va Med
VIRGINIA MEDICAL (Richmond VA)
Va Nurse
VIRGINIA NURSE (Richmond)
Va Q Rev
VIRGINIA QUARTERLY REVIEW (US)
Vard Nord Utveckl Forsk
VARD I NORDEN. UTVECKLING OCH FORSKNING (Copenhagen)
Vardfacket
VARDFACKET (Stockholm)
Vasa
VASA; ZEITSCHRIFT FUR GEFASSKRANKEITEN (Bern)
Veltro
IL VELTRO; RIVISTA DELLA CIVILTA ITALIANA (Roma)
Verh Anat Ges
VERHANDLUNGEN DER ANATOMISCHEN GESELLSCHAFT; ERGANZUNGSHEFT ZUM ANATOMISCHEN ANZEIGER (Jena)
Verh Dtsch Ges Herz Kreislaufforsch
VERHANDLUNGEN DER DEUTSCHEN GESELLSCHAFT FUR HERZ- UND KREISLAUF-FORSCHUNG (Darmstadt)
Verh Dtsch Ges Pathol
VERHANDLUNGEN DER DEUTSCHEN GESELLSCHAFT FUR PATHOLOGIE (Stuttgart)

Verh K Acad Geneeskd Belg
VERHANDELINGEN - KONINKLIJKE ACADEMIE VOOR GENEESKUNDE VAN BELGIE (Bruxelles)
Vestn Akad Med Nauk SSSR
VESTNIK AKADEMII MEDITSINSKIKH NAUK SSSR (Moskva)
Vestn Dermatol Venerol
VESTNIK DERMATOLOGII I VENEROLOGII (Moskva)
Vestn Khir
VESTNIK KHIRURGII IMENI I.I. GREKOVA (Leningrad)
Vestn Mosk Univ Ser 8 Istor
VESTNIK MOSKOVSKOGO UNIVERSITETA, SERIA 8: ISOTRIIA (USSR)
Vestn Oftalmol
VESTNIK OFTALMOLOGII (Moskva)
Vestn Otorinolaringol
VESTNIK OTO-RINO-LARINGOLOGII (Moskva)
Vestn Rentgenol Radiol
VESTNIK RENTGENOLOGII I RADIOLOGII (Moskva)
Vet Clin North Am [Small Anim Pract]
VETERINARY CLINICS OF NORTH AMERICA. SMALL ANIMAL PRACTICE (Philadelphia)
Vet Hist
VETERINARY HISTORY (London)
Vet Hum Toxicol
VETERINARY AND HUMAN TOXICOLOGY (Manhattan KS)
Vet Med (Praha)
VETERINARNI MEDICINA (Praha)
Vet Med Nauki
VETERINARNOMEDITSINSKI NAUKI (Sofia)
Vet Q
VETERINARY QUARTERLY (The Hague)
Vet Rec
VETERINARY RECORD (London)
Vet Res Commun
VETERINARY RESEARCH COMMUNICATIONS (Amsterdam)
Veterinariia
VETERINARIIA (Moskva)
Viata Med [Medii Sanit]
VIATA MEDICALA; REVISTA DE INFORMARE PROFESIONALA SI STIINTIFICA A CADRELOR MEDII SANITARE (Bucuresti)
Victorian Hist J
VICTORIAN HISTORICAL JOURNAL (Australia)
Victorian Hist Mag
VICTORIAN HISTORICAL MAGAZINE (Melbourne)
Victorian Period Newsl
VICTORIAN PERIODICALS NEWSLETTER (Bloomington IN)
Victorian Period Rev
VICTORIAN PERIODICAL REVIEW (Canada)
Victorian Stud
VICTORIAN STUDIES; A QUARTERLY JOURNAL OF THE HUMANITIES, ARTS AND SCIENCES (Bloomington IN)
Vierteljahrsh Zeitgesch
VIERTELJAHRSHEFTE FUR ZEITGESCHICHTE (W Germany)
Vierteljahrsschr Soz Wirtschgesch
VIERTELJAHRSSCHRIFT FUR SOZIAL - UND WIRTSCHAFTSGESCHICHTE (W Germany)
Virchows Arch [A]
VIRCHOWS ARCHIV. A. PATHOLOGICAL ANATOMY AND HISTOPATHOLOGY (Berlin)
Virchows Arch [Pathol Anat]
VIRCHOWS ARCHIV. A. PATHOLOGICAL ANATOMY AND HISTOLOGY (Berlin)
Virologie
VIROLOGIE (Bucuresti)
Vision Res
VISION RESEARCH (Oxford)
Vlaam Stam
VLAAMSE STAM (Belgium)
VM SAC
VM/SAC (Bonner Springs KS)
Vnitr Lek
VNITRNI LEKARSTVI (Praha)
Voen Istor Zh
VOENNO-ISTORICHESKII ZHURNAL (USSR)
Voen Med Zh
VOENNO-MEDITSINSKII ZHURNAL (Moskva)
Vojnois Glas
VOJNOISTORIJSKI GLASNIK (Yugoslavia)
Vojnosanit Pregl
VOJNOSANITETSKI PREGLED (Belgrade)
Volkskunde
VOLKSKUNDE (Belgium)
Volunt Action Leadersh
VOLUNTARY ACTION LEADERSHIP (Washington)
Vopr Filos
VOPROSY FILOSOFII (USSR)
Vopr Istor
VOPROSY ISTORII (USSR)
Vopr Istor Estestvozn Tekh
VOPROSY ISTORII ESTESTVOZNANITA I TEKHNIKI (USSR)
Vopr Istor KPSS
VOPROSY ISTORII KPSS (USSR)
Vopr Kurortol Fizioter Lech Fiz Kult
VOPROSY KURORTOLOGII, FIZIOTERAPII I LECHEBNOI FIZICHESKOI KULTURY (Moskva)
Vopr Okhr Materin Det
VOPROSY OKHRANY MATERINSTVA I DETSTVA (Moskva)
Vopr Onkol
VOPROSY ONKOLOGII (Leningrad)
Vopr Pitan
VOPROSY PITANIIA (Moskva)
Vopr Psikhol
VOPROSY PSIKHOLOGII (Moskva)
Vopr Revm

VOPROSY REVMATIZMA (Moskva)
Vopr Virusol
VOPROSY VIRUSOLOGII (Moskva)
Vox Sang
VOX SANGUINIS (Basel)
Vrach Delo
VRACHEBNOE DELO (Kiev)
Vt Hist
VERMONT HISTORY (Montpelier VT)
Vt Regist Nurse
VERMONT REGISTERED NURSE (Burlington VT)
Vutr Boles
VUTRESHNI BOLESTI (Sofia)

—W—

W Va Hist
WEST VIRGINIA HISTORY (Charleston WV)
Wa Va Med J
WEST VIRGINIA MEDICAL JOURNAL (Charleston WV)
Waage
DIE WAAGE; ZEITSCHRIFT DER CHEMIE GRUNENTHAL
Warwickshire Hist
WARWICKSHIRE HISTORY (Warwick Eng)
Wash Mon
WASHINGTON MONTHLY (Washington)
Watermark
WATERMARK. NEWSLETTER OF THE ASSOCIATION OF LIBRARIANS IN THE HISTORY OF THE HEALTH SCIENCES
Welsh Hist Rev
WELSH HISTORY REVIEW. CYLCHGRAWN HANES CYMRU (Gt Brit)
Wereld Zending
WERELD EN ZENDING (Netherlands)
West Eur Polit
WEST EUROPEAN POLITICS (London)
West Folkl
WESTERN FOLKLORE (US)
West Hum Rev
WESTERN HUMANITIES REVIEW (US)
West Ill Reg Stud
WESTERN ILLINOIS REGIONAL STUDIES (Macomb IL)
West Indian Med J
WEST INDIAN MEDICAL JOURNAL (Kingston)
West J Med
WESTERN JOURNAL OF MEDICINE (San Francisco)
West J Nurs Res
WESTERN JOURNAL OF NURSING RESEARCH (Anaheim CA)
West Polit Q
WESTERN POLITICAL QUARTERLY (US)
West States Jew Hist Q
WESTERN STATES JEWISH HISTORICAL QUARTERLY (US)
West Tenn Hist Soc Pap
WEST TENNESSEE HISTORICAL SOCIETY PAPERS (Memphis TN)
West Tex Hist Assoc Yearb
WEST TEXAS HISTORICAL ASSOCIATION YEARBOOK (US)
WHO Chron
WHO CHRONICLE (Geneva)
Wiad Lek
WIADOMOSCI LEKARSKIE (Warszawa)
Wiad Parazytol
WIADOMISCI PARAZYTOLOGICZNE (Warszawa)
Wien Geschichtsbl
WIENER GESCHICHTSBLATTER (Austria)
Wien Klin Wochenschr
WIENER KLINISCHE WOCHENSCHRIFT (Wien)
Wien Stud Z Klass Philol
WIENER STUDIEN. ZEITSCHRIFT FUR KLASSISCHE PHILOLOGIE (Austria)
Wien Tierarztl Monatsschr
WIENER TIERARZTLICHE MONATSSCHRIFT (Austria)
William Mary Q
WILLIAM AND MARY QUARTERLY (Williamsburg VA)
Wilson Libr Bull
WILSON LIBRARY BULLETIN (New York)
Wilson Q
WILSON QUARTERLY (US)
Winterthur Portf
WINTERTHUR PORTFOLIO (US)
Wis Mag Hist
WISCONSIN MAGAZINE HISTORY (Madison WI)
Wis Med J
WISCONSIN MEDICAL JOURNAL (Madison WI)
Wiss Beitr Martin Luther Univ Halle Wittenberg
WISSENSCHAFTLICHE BEITRAGE DER MARTIN-LUTHER-UNIVERSITAT HALLE-WITTENBERG (Halle)
Wiss Z Friedrich Schiller Univ (Gesellsch)
WISSENSCHAFTLICHE ZEITSCHRIFT DER FRIEDRICH-SCHILLER-UNIVERISTAT, JENA. GESELLSCHAFTS- UND SPRACHWISSENSCHAFTLICHE REIHE (Jena)
Wiss Z Humboldt Univ Berl [Ges Sprachwiss]
WISSENSCHAFTLICHE ZEITSCHRIFT DER HUMBOLDT-UNIVERSITAT ZU BERLIN. GESELLSCHAFTS- UND SPRACHWISSENSCHAFTLICHE REIHE (Berlin))
Wiss Z Karl Marx Univ [Math Naturwiss Wiss]
WISSENSCHAFTLICHE ZEITSCHRIFT DER KARL-MARX-UNIVERSITAT: MATHEMATISCH-NATURWISSENSCHAFTLICHE REIHE (Leipzig)
Wiss Z Martin Luther Univ (Math)
WISSENSCHAFTLICHE ZEITSCHRIFT; MARTIN-LUTHER-UNIVERSITAT, HALLE-WITTENBERG. MATHEMATISCH-NATURWISSENSCHAFTLICHE

REIHE (Halle-Witenberg)
Wiss Z Martin Luther Univ (Ges Sprachwiss)
WISSENSCHAFTLICHE ZEITSCHRIFT; MARTIN-LUTHER-UNIVERSITAT, HALLE-WITTENBERG. GESELLSCHAFTS-UND SPRACHWISSENSCHAFTLICHE REIHE (Germany)
Wolfenbutteler Renaiss Mitt
WOLFENBUTTELER RENAISSANCE MITTEILUNGEN (Hamburg)
Women Health
WOMEN AND HEALTH (New York)
Womens Stud
WOMEN'S STUDIES (US)
Work Pap Mag
WORKING PAPERS MAGAZINE (US)
Work Pap New Soc
WORKING PAPERS FOR A NEW SOCIETY (US)
World Archaeol
WORLD ARCHAEOLOGY (Gt Brit)
World Health Forum
WORLD HEALTH FORUM (Geneva)
World Hosp
WORLD HOSPITALS (Oxford)
World J Surg
WORLD JOURNAL OF SURGERY (New York)
World Polit
WORLD POLITICS (US)
World Rev Nutr Diet
WORLD REVIEW OF NUTRITION AND DIETETICS (Basel)

—X—

Xaloc
XALOC (Mexico)

—Y—

Yad Vashem Stud Eur Jew Catastrophe Resist
YAD VASHEM STUDIES ON THE EUROPEAN JEWISH CATASTROPHE AND RESISTANCE (Israel)
Yakushigaku Zasshi
YAKUSHIGAKU ZASSHI. JOURNAL OF JAPANESE HISTORY OF PHARMACY (Tokyo)
Yale J Biol Med
YALE JOURNAL OF BIOLOGY AND MEDICINE (New Haven CT)
Yalkut Moreshet Period
YALKUT MORESHET PERIODICAL (Israel)
Yearb Popul Res Finl
YEARBOOK OF POPULATION RESEARCH IN FINLAND
York State Tradit
YORK STATE TRADITION (New York)
Youth Soc
YOUTH AND SOCIETY (Beverly Hills CA)

—Z—

Z Allg Wissenschaftstheorie
ZEITSCHRIFT FUR ALLGEMEINE WISSENSCHAFTSTHEORIE (Wiesbaden)
Z Alternsforsch
ZEITSCHRIFT FUR ALTERNSFORSCHUNG (Dresden)
Z Angew Bader Klimaheilkd
ZEITSCHRIFT FUR ANGEWANDTE BADER- UND KLIMAHEILKUND (Stuttgart)
Z Arztl Fortbild (Jena)
ZEITSCHRIFT FUR ARZTLICHE FORTBILDUNG (Jena)
Z Bayer Landesgesch
ZEITSCHRIFT FUR BAYERISCHE LANDESGESCHICHTE (Muchen)
Z Bevolkerungswiss
ZEITSCHRIFT FUR BEVOLKERUNGSWISSENSCHAFT
Z Dtsch Altert Dtsch Lit
ZEITSCHRIFT FUR DEUTSCHES ALTERTUM UND DEUTSCHE LITERATUR
Z Entwicklungspsychol Padagog Psychol
ZEITSCHRIFT FUR ENTWICKLUNGSPSYCHOLOGIE UND PADAGOGISCHE PSYCHOLOGIE (Hamburg)
Z Erkr Atmungsorgane
ZEITSCHRIFT FUR ERKRANKUNGEN DER ATMUNGSORGANE (Leipzig)
Z Ernahrungswiss
ZEITSCHRIFT FUR ERNAHRUNGSWISSENSCAFT. JOURNAL OF NUTRITIONAL SCIENCES (Darmstadt)
Z Exp Chir
ZEITSCHRIFT FUR EXPERIMENTELLE CHIRURGIE (Berlin)
Z Exp Chir Transplant Kunstliche Organe
ZEITSCHRIFT FUR EXPERIMENTELLE CHIRURGIE, TRANSPLANTATION, UND KUNSTLICHE ORGANE (Berlin)
Z Gastroenterol
ZEITSCHRIFT FUR GASTROENTEROLGIE (Munchen)
Z Geburtshilfe Perinatol
ZEITSCHRIFT FUR GEBURTSHILFE UND PERINATOLOGIE (Stuttgart)
Z Gerontol
ZEITSCHRIFT FUR GERONTOLOGIE (Darmstadt)
Z Ges Schleswig Holstein Gesch
ZEITSCHRIFT DER GESELLSCHAFT FUR SCHLESWIG-HOLSTEINISCHE GESCHICHTE (W Germany)
Z Ges Z Gesamte Hyg
ZEITSCHRIFT FUR DIE GESAMTE HYGIENE UND IHRE GRENZGEBIETE (Berlin)
Z Gesamte Inn Med
ZEITSCHRIFT FUR DIE GESAMTE INNERE

MEDIZIN UND IHRE GRENZGEBIETE (Leipzig)

Z Geschichtswiss
ZEITSCHRIFT FUR GESCHICHTSWISSENSCHAFT (E Germany)

Z Hautkr
ZEITSHRIFT FUR HAUTKRANKHEITEN (Berlin)

Z Hist Ver Steiermark
ZEITSCHRIFT DES HISTORISCHEN VEREINS FUR STEIERMARK (Austria)

Z Kardiol
ZEITSCHRIFT FUR KARDIOLOGIE (Darmstadt)

Z Kinderchir
ZEITSCHRIFT FUR KINDERCHIRURGIE (Stuttgart)

Z Kirchengesch
ZEITSCHRIFT FUR KIRCHENGESCHICHTE (Stuttgart)

Z Klin Psychol Psychother
ZEITSCHRIFT FUR KLINISCHE PSYCHOLOGIE UND PSYCHOTHERAPIE (Munchen)

Z Lymphol
ZEITSCHRIFT FUR LYMPHOLOGIE. JOURNAL OF LYMPHOLOGY (Stuttgart)

Z Med Lab Diagn
ZEITSCHRIFT FUR MEDIZINISCHE LABORATORIUMSDIAGNOSTIK (Berlin)

Z Mikrosk Anat Forsch
ZEITSCHRIFT FUR MIKROSKOPISCH-ANATOMISCHE FORSCHUNG (Leipzig)

Z Morphol Anthropol
ZEITSCHRIFT FUR MORPHOLOGIE UND ANTHROPOLOGIE (Stuttgart)

Z Orthop
ZEITSCHRIFT FUR ORTHOPADIE UND IHRE GRENZGEBIETE (Stuttgart)

Z Ostforsch
ZEITSCHRIFT FUR OSTFORSCHUNG (Marburg)

Z Papyrologie Epigraphik
ZEITSCHRIFT FUR PAPYROLOGIE UND EPIGRAPHIK (Bonn)

Z Plast Chir
ZEITSCHRIFT FUR PLASTISCHE CHIRURGIE (Stuttgart)

Z Psychol
ZEITSCHRIFT FUR PSYCHOLOGIE MIT ZEITSCHRIFT FUR ANGEWANDTE PSYCHOLOGIE (Leipzig)

Z Psychosom Med Psychoanal
ZEITSCHRIFT FUR PSYCHOSOMATISCHE MEDIZIN UND PSYCHOANALYSE (Gottingen)

Z Rechtsmed
ZEITSCHRIFT FUR RECHTSMEDIZIN. JOURNAL OF LEGAL MEDICINE (Berlin)

Z Rheumatol
ZEITSCHRIFT FUR RHEUMATOLOGIE (Darmstadt)

Z Urol Nephrol
ZEITSCHRIFT FUR UROLOGIE UND NEPHROLOGIE (Leipzig)

Z Versuchstierkd
ZEITSCHRIFT FUR VERSUCHSTIERKUNDE (Jena)

Zahn Mund Kieferheilkd
ZAHN-, MUND- UND KIEFERHEILKUNDE MIT ZENTRALBLATT (Leipzig)

Zahnarzt
ZAHNARZT (Munich)

Zahnarztebl Baden Wurttemb
ZAHNARZTEBLATT BADEN-WURTTEMBERG (Stuttgart)

Zahnarztl Mitt
ZAHNARZTLICHE MITTEILUNGEN (Cologne)

Zahnarztl Prax
ZAHNARZTLICHE PRAXIS (Berlin)

Zahntechnik (Berl)
ZAHNTECHNIK (Berlin)

Zahntechnik (Geneve)
ZAHNTECHNIK (Geneve)

Zb Drus Nauke
ZBORNIK ZA DRUSTVENE NAUKE (Yugoslavia)

Zb Istor (Yugoslavia)
SEE: Naucni Sastanak Zb Rad Naucno Drus Istor Zdrav Kult Jugosl

Zb Zgodovino Naravoslovja Teh
ZBORNIK ZA ZGODOVINO NARAVOSLOVJA IN TEHNIKE (Yugoslavia)

Zdravookhr Kirg
ZDRAVOOKHRANENIE KIRGIZII (Frunze)

Zdravookhr Ross Fed
ZDRAVOOKHRANENIE ROSSIISKOI FEDERATSII (Moskva)

Zeitgesch
ZEITGESCHICHTE (Austria)

Zentralasiat Stud
ZENTRALASIATISCHE STUDIEN (W Germany)

Zentralbl Allg Pathol
ZENTRALBLATT FUR ALLGEMEINE PATHOLOGIE UND PATHOLOGISCHE ANATOMIE (Jena)

Zentralbl Arbeitsmed Arbeitsschutz Prophyl
ZENTRALBLATT FUR ARBEITSMEDIZIN ARBEITSSCHUTZ UND PROPHYLAXE (Heidelberg))

Zentralbl Bakteriol [B]
ZENTRALBLATT FUR BAKTERIOLOGIE. I. ABT. ORIGINALE REIHE B: HYGIENE, KRANKENHAUSHYGIENE, BETRIEBSHYGIENE, PRAVENTIVE MEDIZIN (Stuttgart)

Zentralbl Bakeriol [Orig B]
ZENTRALBLATT FUR BAKTERIOLOGIE, PARASITENKUNDE, INFEKTIONSKRANKHEITEN UND HYGIENE. I. ABT. ORIGINALE. REIHE B: HYGIENE, PRAVENTIVE MEDIZIN (Stuttgart)

Zentralbl Bakteriol Mikrobiol Hyg [A]
ZENTRALBLATT FUR BAKTERIOLOGIE, MIKROBIOLOGIE UND HYGIENE. I. ABT. ORIGINALE. A: MEDIZINISCHE MIKROBIOLOGIE, INFEKTIONSKRANKHEITEN

UND PARASITOLOGIE (Stuttgart)
Zentralbl Bakteriol Mikrobiol Hyg [B]
ZENTRALBLATT FUR BAKTERIOLOGIE MIKROBIOLOGIE UND HYGIENE. I. ABT. ORIGINALE. B: UMWELTHYGIENE, KRANKENHAUSHYGIENE, ARBEITSHYGIENE, PRAVENTIVE MEDIZIN (Stuttgart)
Zentralbl Chir
ZENTRALBLATT FUR CHIRURGIE (Leipzig)
Zentralbl Gynakol
ZENTRALBLATT FUR GYNAKOLOGIE (Leipzig)
Zentralbl Neurochir
ZENTRALBLATT FUR NEUROCHIRURGIE (Leipzig)
Zentralbl Veterinarmed [A]
ZENTRALBLATT FUR VETERINARMEDIZIN REIHE A (Berlin)
Zentralbl Veterinarmed [B]
ZENTRALBLATT FUR VETERINARMEDIZIN. REIHE B (Berlin)
Zesz Hist
ZESZYTY HISTORYCZNE (France)
Zesz Nauk KUL
ZESZYTY NAUKOWE KUL (Poland)
ZFA
ZFA. ZEITSCHRIFT FUR ALTERNSFORSCHUNG (Berlin)
ZFA (Dresden)
ZFA; ZEITSCHRIFT FUR ALTERNSFORSCHUNG (Dresden)
ZFA (Stuttgart)
ZFA; ZEITSCHRIFT FUR ALLGEMEINMEDIZIN (Stuttgart)
Zh Evol Biokhim Fiziol
ZHURNAL EVOLIUTSIONNOI BIOKHIMII I FIZIOLOGII (Moskva)
Zh Mikrobiol Epidemiol Immunobiol
ZHURNAL MIKROBIOLOGII, EPIDEMIOLOGII I IMMUNOBIOLOGII (Moskva)
Zh Nevropatol Psikhiatr
ZHURNAL NEVROPATOLOGII I PSIKHIATRII IMENI S.S. KORSAKOVA (Moskva)
Zh Ushn Nos Gorl Bolezn
ZHURNAL USHNYKH, NOSOVYKH I GORLOVYKH BOLEZNEI (Kiev)
Zh Vopr Neirokhir
ZHURNAL VOPROSY NEIROKHIRURGII IMENI N.N. BURDENKO (Moskva)
Zh Vyssh Nerv Deiat
ZHURNAL VYSSHEI NERVNOI DEIATELNOSTI IMENI I.P. PAVLOVA (Moskva)
Zimbabwe Rhod Nurse
ZIMBABWE RHODESIA NURSE (Salisbury)
Zinbun
ZINBUN (Japan)
Zion
ZION (Israel)
Zobozdrav Vestn
ZOBOZDRAVSTVENI VESTNIK (Ljubljana)
Zwingliana
ZWINGLIANA (Switzerland)
ZWR
ZWR (Heidelberg)
Zygon
ZYGON (US)

[redacted]